Hematology

Hematology

3rd Edition

WILLIAM J. WILLIAMS, M.D.

Edward C. Reifenstein Professor of Medicine and Chairman of the Department of Medicine, Upstate Medical Center, State University of New York

ERNEST BEUTLER, M.D.

Chairman, Division of Basic and Clinical Research; Head, Department of Hematology and Oncology, Scripps Clinic and Research Foundation, La Jolla, CA.; Clinical Professor of Medicine, University of California at San Diego, La Jolla, CA.

ALLAN J. ERSLEV, M.D.

Cardeza Research Professor of Medicine, Jefferson Medical College of Thomas Jefferson University; Director, Cardeza Foundation for Hematologic Research

MARSHALL A. LICHTMAN, M.D.

Professor of Medicine and Radiation Biology and Biophysics; Co-Chief, Hematology Unit; and Senior Associate Dean for Academic Affairs and Research, University of Rochester School of Medicine and Dentistry

McGRAW-HILL BOOK COMPANY

New York St. Louis San Francisco Auckland Bogotá Guatemala Hamburg Johannesburg Lisbon London Madrid Mexico Montreal New Delhi Panama Paris San Juan São Paulo Singapore Sydney Tokyo Toronto

NOTICE

Medicine is an ever-changing science. As new research and clinical experience broaden our knowledge, changes in treatment and drug therapy are required. The editors and the publisher of this work have made every effort to ensure that the drug dosage schedules herein are accurate and in accord with the standards accepted at the time of publication. Readers are advised, however, to check the product information sheet included in the package of each drug they plan to administer to be certain that changes have not been made in the recommended dose or in the contraindications for administration. This recommendation is of particular importance in regard to new or infrequently used drugs.

HEMATOLOGY

234567890 D O W D O W 89876543

This book was set in Palatino by Ruttle, Shaw & Wetherill, Inc. The editors were Robert P. McGraw and Moira Lerner; the production supervisors were Jeanne Skahan and Avé McCracken. R. R. Donnelley & Sons was printer and binder.

Library of Congress Cataloging in Publication Data
Main entry under title:

Hematology.

Includes bibliographical references and index.
1. Blood–Diseases. 2. Hematology.
I. Williams, William J. (William Joseph), date. [DNLM: 1. Hematologic diseases. WH100 H487]
RC633.H43   1983   616.1′5   83-5388
ISBN 0-07-070377-9

Contents

List of Contributors

SAMUEL K. ACKERMAN, M.D.
Division of Biochemistry and Biophysics, National Center for Drugs and Biologics, Bethesda, Maryland.

CHESTER A. ALPER, M.D.
Professor of Pediatrics, Harvard Medical School. Scientific Director, Center for Blood Research, Senior Associate in Hematology and Oncology, Children's Hospital Medical Center, Boston, Massachusetts.

DAVID L. ARONSON, M.D.
Chief, Coagulation Branch, National Center for Drugs and Biologics, Bethesda, Maryland.

RICHARD H. ASTER, M.D.
Clinical Professor of Medicine, Medical College of Wisconsin. President, Blood Center of Southeastern Wisconsin, Milwaukee, Wisconsin.

JEAN ATWATER, B.S., MT (ASCP)
Late Research Associate Professor of Medicine, Jefferson Medical College of Thomas Jefferson University; Late Senior Member, Cardeza Foundation for Hematologic Research, Philadelphia, Pennsylvania.

ARTHUR BANK, M.D.
Professor of Medicine and Professor of Human Genetics, Columbia University, New York, New York.

PETER M. BANKS, M.D.
Consultant in Surgical Pathology and Director of Lymphoma Laboratory, Mayo Clinic and Mayo Foundation, Rochester, Minnesota.

WILLIAM S. BECK, M.D.
Professor of Medicine and Tutor in Biochemical Sciences, Harvard University; Director of the Hematology Research Laboratory, Massachusetts General Hospital, Boston, Massachusetts.

DANIEL E. BERGSAGEL, M.D., D. PHIL.
Professor of Medicine, University of Toronto; Chief of Medicine, Princess Margaret Hospital, Toronto, Ontario, Canada.

NATHANIEL I. BERLIN, M.D.
Teuton Professor of Medicine and Director, Cancer Center, Northwestern University, Chicago, Illinois.

MARCEL BESSIS, M.D.
Professor of Medicine (Hematology), School of Medicine, University of Paris; Director, Institut de Pathologie Cellulaire, Hôpital de Bicêtre, Paris, France.

ROBERT F. BETTS, M.D.
Associate Professor of Medicine and Member, Infectious Diseases Unit, University of Rochester School of Medicine and Dentistry, Rochester, New York.

ERNEST BEUTLER, M.D.
Chairman, Division of Basic and Clinical Research; Head, Department of Hematology and Oncology, Scripps Clinic and Research Foundation, La Jolla, CA.; Clinical Professor of Medicine, University of California at San Diego, La Jolla, CA.

KARL G. BLUME, M.D.
Director, Department of Hematology and Bone Marrow Transplantation, City of Hope National Medical Center, Duarte, California. Professor, University of Freiburg, Germany.

JOHN M. BOWMAN, M.D.
Professor of Pediatrics, Faculty of Medicine, University of Manitoba; Medical Director, Rh Laboratory, Health Sciences Center, Winnipeg, Manitoba, Canada.

LAURENCE A. BOXER, M.D.
Professor of Pediatrics, University of Michigan School of Medicine; Director of Pediatric Hematology/Oncology, C.S. Mott Children's Hospital, Ann Arbor, Michigan.

JAMES K. BRENNAN, M.D.
Associate Professor of Medicine, University of Rochester School of Medicine and Dentistry, Rochester, New York.

PAUL A. BUNN, JR., M.D.
Associate Professor of Medicine, Uniformed Services University of the Health Sciences; Head, Cellular Kinetic Section, National Cancer Institute-Navy Medical Oncology Branch, National Naval Medical Center, Bethesda, Maryland.

RICHARD A. BURNINGHAM, M.D.
Portland Clinic, Portland, Oregon.

DENNIS A. CARSON, M.D.
Associate Member, Department of Basic and Clinical Research, Research Institute of Scripps Clinic, Scripps Clinic and Research Foundation, La Jolla, California.

PETER A. CASSILETH, M.D.
Professor of Medicine and Associate Chief, Hematology-Oncology Section, School of Medicine, University of Pennsylvania, Philadelphia, Pennsylvania.

FRANCIS V. CHISARI, M.D.
Associate Member, Department of Basic and Clinical Research, Research Institute of Scripps Clinic, Scripps Clinic and Research Foundation, La Jolla, California; Adjunct Professor, University of California, San Diego, California.

CHARLES G. COCHRANE, M.D.
Member, Department of Immunology, Research Institute of Scripps Clinic, Scripps Clinic and Research Foundation, La Jolla, California; Adjunct Professor of Pathology, University of California, San Diego, California.

NEIL R. COOPER, M.D.
Member, Department of Immunology, Research Institute of Scripps Clinic, Scripps Clinic and Research Foundation, La Jolla, California.

RICHARD A. COOPER, M.D.
Professor of Medicine and Chief, Hematology-Oncology Section, University of Pennsylvania School of Medicine, Philadelphia, Pennsylvania.

WILLIAM H. CROSBY, M.D.
Colonel, Medical Corps, Walter Reed Army Institute of Research, Washington, D.C.

FREDERICK R. DAVEY, M.D.
Professor of Pathology, Associate Professor of Medicine, and Director of Blood Bank, State University of New York Upstate Medical Center, Syracuse, New York.

STEVEN D. DOUGLAS, M.D.
Professor of Pediatrics and Microbiology, University of Pennsylvania School of Medicine; Director, Division of Allergy-Immunology-Pulmonology, The Children's Hospital of Philadelphia, Philadelphia, Pennsylvania.

ANN DVORAK, M.D.
Associate Professor of Pathology, Harvard Medical School; Pathologist, Beth Israel Hospital, Boston, Massachusetts.

HAROLD F. DVORAK, M.D.
Mallinckrodt Professor of Pathology, Harvard Medical School; Chief, Department of Pathology, Beth Israel Hospital, Boston, Massachusetts.

ALLAN J. ERSLEV, M.D.
Cardeza Research Professor of Medicine, Jefferson Medical College of Thomas Jefferson University; Director, Cardeza Foundation for Hematologic Research, Philadelphia, Pennsylvania.

VIRGIL F. FAIRBANKS, M.D.
Professor of Medicine and Laboratory Medicine, and Consultant, Mayo Clinic, Rochester, Minnesota.

CLEMENT A. FINCH, M.D.
Professor of Medicine, School of Medicine, University of Washington, Seattle, Washington.

STUART C. FINCH, M.D.
Professor of Medicine, College of Medicine and Dentistry of New Jersey-Rutgers Medical School; Chief of Medicine, Cooper Hospital, University Medical Center, Camden, New Jersey.

CHARLES W. FRANCIS, M.D.
Assistant Professor of Medicine, University of Rochester School of Medicine and Dentistry, Rochester, New York.

EDWARD C. FRANKLIN, M.D.
Late Professor of Medicine, Chairman, Rheumatic Diseases Study Group, and Director, Irvington House Institute, New York University Medical Center, New York, New York.

BRUCE FURIE, M.D.
Associate Professor of Medicine, Tufts University School of Medicine; Chief, Coagulation Unit, New England Medical Center, Boston, Massachusetts.

STEPHEN J. GALLI, M.D.
Assistant Professor of Pathology, Harvard Medical School; Director, Autopsy Service, Beth Israel Hospital, Boston, Massachusetts.

FRANK H. GARDNER, M.D.
Professor of Medicine and Director, Division of Hematology-Oncology, Department of Medicine, University of Texas Medical Branch, Galveston, Texas.

ELOISE R. GIBLETT, M.D.
Research Professor of Medicine, University of Washington School of Medicine; Executive Director, Puget Sound Blood Center, Seattle, Washington.

FRANCES McNIELL GILL, M.D., M.P.H.
Associate Professor of Pediatrics, Children's Hospital of Philadelphia, University of Pennsylvania School of Medicine, Philadelphia, Pennsylvania.

DAVID W. GOLDE, M.D.
Professor of Medicine and Chief, Division of Hematology and Oncology, School of Medicine, University of California at Los Angeles, Los Angeles, California.

HARVEY M. GOLOMB, M.D.
Associate Professor of Medicine and Chief, Hematology and Oncology, University of Chicago School of Medicine, Chicago, Illinois.

ARLAN J. GOTTLIEB, M.D.
Professor of Medicine and Chief, Section of Hematology, Department of Medicine, State University of New York, Upstate Medical Center, Syracuse, New York.

HARVEY R. GRALNICK, M.D.
Chief, Hematology Service, Clinical Pathology Department, National Institutes of Health, Bethesda, Maryland.

JEROME E. GROOPMAN, M.D.
Assistant Professor of Medicine, Division of Hematology-Oncology, Department of Medicine, University of California at Los Angeles Medical Center, Los Angeles, California.

EDWARD S. HENDERSON, M.D.
Professor of Medicine, State University of New York at Buffalo, New York; Chief, Medical Oncology, Roswell Park Memorial Institute, Buffalo, New York.

ROBERT S. HILLMAN, M.D.
Professor of Medicine, University of Vermont School of Medicine; Chief of Medicine, Maine Medical Center, Portland, Maine.

HOLM HOLMSEN, Ph.D.
Professor of Biochemistry, Department of Biochemistry, University of Bergen, Bergen, Norway.

CECIL HOUGIE, M.D.
Professor of Pathology, School of Medicine, University of California, San Diego; Director of Coagulation Laboratory, University Hospital Medical Center, La Jolla, California.

JOHN R. HUDDLESTONE, M.D.
Assistant Member, Department of Immunology, Research Institute of Scripps Clinic, Scripps Clinic and Research Foundation, La Jolla, California.

ERIC A. JAFFE, M.D.
Professor of Medicine, Cornell University Medical College, New York, New York.

JAMES H. JANDL, M.D.
George Richards Minot Professor of Medicine, Harvard Medical School, Boston, Massachusetts.

ALAN J. JOHNSON, M.D.
Professor of Medicine, New York University Medical Center, New York, New York.

BARRY H. KAPLAN, M.D., Ph.D.
Associate Professor of Medicine, Albert Einstein College of Medicine, Bronx, New York.

SIMON KARPATKIN, M.D.
Professor of Medicine, New York University Medical Center, New York, New York.

HAEWON CHANG KIM, M.D.
Assistant Professor of Pediatrics, University of Pennsylvania School of Medicine; Attending Hematologist, Director of Blood Bank, Donor Center, and Transfusion Center, The Children's Hospital of Philadelphia, Philadelphia, Pennsylvania.

DONNA D. KOSTYU, Ph.D.
Medical Research Associate, Duke Medical Center, Durham, North Carolina.

WANDA KUHL, B.A., B.S.
Scientific Associate, Department of Basic and Clinical Research, Research Institute of Scripps Clinic, Scripps Clinic and Research Foundation, La Jolla, California.

STEPHEN A. LANDAW, M.D., Ph.D.
Professor of Medicine, State University of New York Upstate Medical Center; Associate Chief of Staff, Research and Development, Veterans Administration Medical Center, Syracuse, New York.

JOHN LASZLO, M.D.
Professor of Medicine and Director, Clinical Programs, Duke Comprehensive Cancer Center, Duke Medical Center, Durham, North Carolina.

JOHN P. LEDDY, M.D.
Professor of Medicine and Microbiology and Chief, Clinical Immunology Unit, University of Rochester School of Medicine and Dentistry, Rochester, New York.

LAWRENCE S. LESSIN, M.D.
Professor of Medicine and Pathology and Director, Division of Hematology and Oncology, George Washington University School of Medicine, Washington, District of Columbia.

ERIC P. LESTER, M.D.
Assistant Professor of Medicine, Section of Hematology-Oncology, The University of Chicago School of Medicine, Chicago, Illinois.

MARSHALL A. LICHTMAN, M.D.
Professor of Medicine and of Radiation Biology and Biophysics, Co-Chief, Hematology Unit, Senior Associate Dean for Academic Affairs and Research, University of Rochester School of Medicine and Dentistry, Rochester, New York.

VICTOR J. MARDER, M.D.
Professor of Medicine, Co-Chief, Hematology Unit, University of Rochester School of Medicine and Dentistry, Rochester, New York.

S. P. MASOUREDIS, M.D., Ph.D.
Professor of Pathology, School of Medicine, and Director, University Hospital Blood Bank, University of California, San Diego, La Jolla, California.

CHARLES F. MOLDOW, M.D.
Associate Professor of Medicine, University of Minnesota School of Medicine; Chief, Medical Service, Veterans Administration Medical Center, Minneapolis, Minnesota.

TIMOTHY W. MORGAN, M.D.
Associate Pathologist and Director of Hematology Laboratory, Saint Joseph Hospital, Denver, Colorado.

SCOTT MURPHY, M.D.
Professor of Medicine, Jefferson Medical College of Thomas Jefferson University; Member, Cardeza Foundation for Hematologic Research, Philadelphia, Pennsylvania.

DOUGLAS A. NELSON, M.D.
Professor of Pathology and Director, Hematology Section, Division of Clinical Pathology, Department of Pathology, State University of New York Upstate Medical Center, Syracuse, New York.

W. STEPHEN NICHOLS, JR., M.D.
Associate Clinical Member, Department of Pathology and Head, Immunopathology Section, Scripps Clinic and Research Foundation; Assistant Clinical Professor, Department of Pathology, University of California, San Diego, School of Medicine, La Jolla, California.

JACOB NUSBACHER, M.D.
Professor of Medicine, University of Pittsburgh School of Medicine; Executive Vice President and Medical Director, Central Blood Bank of Pittsburgh, Pittsburgh, Pennsylvania.

FRANK A. OSKI, M.D.
Professor and Chairman, Department of Pediatrics, State University of New York Upstate Medical Center, Syracuse, New York.

CHARLES H. PACKMAN, M.D.
Associate Professor of Medicine, University of Rochester School of Medicine and Dentistry, Rochester, New York.

D. ELLIOT PARKS, Ph.D.
Assistant Member, Department of Immunology, Research Institute of Scripps Clinic, Scripps Clinic and Research Foundation, La Jolla, California.

JEAN-MICHEL PAULUS, M.D., Ph.D.
Chargé de cours associé at the Belgian Fund for Scientific Research, University of Liège, Liège, Belgium; and Professor associé at the University of Paris-Sud, Institute de Pathologie Cellulaire, Inserm U 48, Hôpital de Bicêtre, Paris, France.

BERNARD J. POIESZ, M.D.
Assistant Professor of Medicine, State University of New York Upstate Medical Center, Syracuse, New York; Chief, Oncology Section, Syracuse Veterans Administration Medical Center; Research Investigator, Barbara Kopp Research Center, Auburn, New York.

F. STANLEY PORTER, M.D.
Professor and Chairman, Department of Pediatrics, Eastern Virginia Medical School; Physician-in-Chief, Children's Hospital of the King's Daughters, Norfolk, Virginia.

PETER J. QUESENBERRY, M.D.
Byrd S. Leavell Professor of Medicine and Chief, Division of Hematology-Oncology, University of Virginia School of Medicine, Charlottesville, Virginia.

HELEN M. RANNEY, M.D.
Professor and Chairperson, Department of Medicine, University of California, San Diego, California.

EMILY G. REISNER, Ph.D.
Medical Research Assistant Professor of Microbiology-Immunology, and Director of Transfusion Service, HLA Laboratory, Duke University, Durham, North Carolina.

STEPHEN H. ROBINSON, M.D.
Professor of Medicine, Harvard Medical School; Chief, Hematology Division, and Clinical Director, Department of Medicine, Beth Israel Hospital, Boston, Massachusetts.

FRED S. ROSEN, M.D.
James L. Gamble Professor of Pediatrics, Harvard Medical School; Chief, Division of Immunology, Children's Hospital Medical Center, Boston, Massachusetts.

WENDELL F. ROSSE, M.D.
Florence McAlister Professor of Medicine and Chief, Division of Hematology-Oncology, Duke University Medical Center, Durham, North Carolina.

R. WAYNE RUNDLES, M.D., Ph.D.
Professor Emeritus, Duke University Medical Center, Durham, North Carolina.

ELIAS SCHWARTZ, M.D.
Professor of Pediatrics and Human Genetics, University of Pennsylvania School of Medicine; Director, Division of Hematology, Children's Hospital of Philadelphia, Philadelphia, Pennsylvania.

JEAN A. SHAFER, B.A., M.S.
Assistant Professor of Medicine and Pathology, University of Rochester School of Medicine and Dentistry, Rochester, New York.

VIJAY S. SHARMA, Ph.D.
Associate Professor of Medicine in Residence, University of California at San Diego, La Jolla, California.

STEPHEN B. SHOHET, M.D.
Professor of Medicine and Chief of Hematology, Cancer Research Institute, University of California at San Francisco, San Francisco, California.

ROBERT SILBER, M.D.
Professor of Medicine and Director, Division of Hematology, New York University School of Medicine, New York, New York.

MURRAY N. SILVERSTEIN, M.D., Ph.D.
Professor of Medicine, Mayo Graduate School, and Chairman, Division of Hematology, Mayo Clinic, Rochester, Minnesota.

JOSEPH E. SMITH, D.V.M., Ph.D.
Professor of Pathology, Kansas State University School of Veterinary Medicine, Manhattan, Kansas.

THOMAS P. STOSSEL, M.D.
Professor of Medicine, Harvard Medical School, Chief, Hematology-Oncology Unit, Massachusetts General Hospital, Boston, Massachusetts.

DONALD P. TSCHUDY, M.D.
Senior Investigator, Metabolism Branch, National Cancer Institute, National Institutes of Health, Bethesda, Maryland.

JOHN E. ULTMANN, M.D.
Professor of Medicine and Director, Cancer Research Center, University of Chicago School of Medicine, Chicago, Illinois.

WILLIAM N. VALENTINE, M.D.
Professor of Medicine, School of Medicine, University of California at Los Angeles, Los Angeles, California.

DAVID J. WEATHERALL, M.A., M.D., F.R.S.
Nuffield Professor of Clinical Medicine and Honorary Director of the MRC Molecular Haematology Unit, University of Oxford, Oxford, England.

IRWIN M. WEINSTEIN, M.D.
Clinical Professor of Medicine, School of Medicine, University of California at Los Angeles School of Medicine, Los Angeles, California.

HARVEY J. WEISS, M.D.
Professor of Medicine, Columbia University College of Physicians and Surgeons; Director, Division of Hematology-Oncology, St. Luke's-Roosevelt Center, New York, New York.

LEON WEISS, M.D.
Grace Lansing Lambert Professor of Cell Biology and Chairman, Department of Animal Biology, School of Veterinary Medicine, University of Pennsylvania; Professor of Medicine (Division of Hematology), School of Medicine, University of Pennsylvania, Philadelphia, Pennsylvania.

JAMES G. WHITE, M.D.
Professor, Departments of Pediatrics, Laboratory Medicine, and Pathology, University of Minnesota School of Medicine, Minneapolis, Minnesota.

WILLIAM J. WILLIAMS, M.D.
Edward C. Reifenstein Professor of Medicine, and Chairman of the Department of Medicine, Upstate Medical Center, State University of New York, Syracuse, New York.

MARJORIE B. ZUCKER, Ph.D.
Professor of Pathology, New York University School of Medicine, New York, New York.

DOROTHEA ZUCKER-FRANKLIN, M.D.
Professor of Medicine, New York University School of Medicine, New York, New York.

Preface

The purpose of this book remains the same as that stated in the preface to the first edition: to provide clinicians—in practice or in training—investigators, and students with a ready source of detailed information regarding the whole of hematology as it applies to the human being, with emphasis on the biochemical and physiological approach to the field. The organization of the book continues to evolve. We have retained the concept of presentation of general information followed by discussions of specific topics, and to further that end, the broad discussions of clinical manifestations of hematologic disorders have been moved to the front of the book. A new chapter on "Comparative Hematology" has been added under "General Hematology," and under "Replacement Therapy" we have added chapters on marrow transplantation and on hemapheresis procedures. The concept of the hemopoietic stem cell is emphasized by organization of the relevant information in a new part entitled "The Hemopoietic Stem Cell." In this part, the concept of the hemopoietic stem cell is reviewed, followed by a classification of stem cell disorders and then discussions of the specific diseases.

Extensive new material has been added throughout the book, and in several places the presentation has been reorganized for greater clarity. Thus the discussion of the metabolic aspects of vitamin B_{12} and folic acid have been included in a separate chapter under "Biochemistry and Function of the Erythrocyte," and the megaloblastic anemias and the hereditary nonspherocytic hemolytic anemias are consolidated into single chapters. The hemoglobinopathies have been separated according to their clinical manifestations rather than grouped on the basis of the presence of abnormal hemoglobin.

With the completion of the second edition, Dr. R. Wayne Rundles reached the retirement age established by the editorial board, and in this edition his place has been taken by Dr. Marshall A. Lichtman. Dr. Rundles' keen editorial skills, profound wisdom, and gentle humor contributed enormously to the development of the first two editions of the book. Fortunately, he has remained as a contributor, and we are grateful for his continuing interest.

The multiauthor approach has been retained in order to present authoritative, up-to-date information on all topics. In the initial planning of this project it was agreed that there should be rotation of authors, and that has now been instituted. As a consequence, a number of new authors appear in this edition, and we here formally express our deep appreciation for the contributions of our retiring authors, and for the extensive efforts made by all contributors to this book.

In this edition, we have revised and expanded the color plates to contain much new material. We have retained a number of the excellent photographs prepared by Mr. Carl Bishop, of the Duke University Medical Center (Plates 1 and 11, Plates 4-1 to 4-4, and Plates 6-1 and 6-2) and added others prepared by Ms. Jean A. Shafer, of the University of Rochester Medical Center (Plates 2, 3, 4-5 to 4-12, 5, 6-3 to 6-10, 7, and 8). Dr. Peter M. Banks contributed the photomicrographs of the lymphomas (Plates 9 and 10).

Our staff associates deserve far more recognition than can possibly be communicated by simple acknowledgment of their attention to seemingly endless detail: Sophia Antczak, Sally Burke, Terri Gelbart, Marjorie Jordahl, Marianne Moss, Beth Bush, Doris Riso, Ilene Roberts, Rosemarie Silvano, Margaret Snyder, and Carol West.

William J. Williams
Ernest Beutler
Allan J. Erslev
Marshall A. Lichtman

Hematology

PART ONE

The patient with hematologic disease

Clinical evaluation of the patient

CHAPTER 1

Approach to the patient

WILLIAM J. WILLIAMS

The care of a patient begins with a systematic attempt to determine the nature of the illness by eliciting and recording an adequate medical history and performing a physical examination. The physician should identify the important symptoms and obtain as much relevant information as possible about their origin and evolution and about the general health of the patient by appropriate questions designed to explore the patient's recent and remote experience. Hereditary and environmental factors should be carefully sought and evaluated. The physician follows the medical history with a physical examination, again to provide a general survey of the patient's health status and to permit a careful search for signs of the illnesses suggested by the history. The process of history taking is nearly always extended during the physical examination, so that these two activities should be considered as a unit and as providing the basic information for further diagnostic probes.

Primary hematologic diseases are uncommon, while hematologic manifestations secondary to other diseases occur frequently. For example, the signs and symptoms of anemia and the presence of enlarged lymph nodes are common clinical findings that may be related to hematologic disease, but they occur even more frequently as secondary manifestations of disorders not considered primarily hematologic. A wide variety of diseases may produce signs or symptoms of hematologic illness. Thus, in patients with metastatic carcinoma, all the signs and symptoms of anemia may be elicited and lymphadenopathy may be pronounced, but additional findings are usually present that indicate primary involvement of some system besides the blood and lymph nodes. In this discussion, therefore, emphasis is placed on the clinical findings resulting from either primary hematologic disease or the complications of hematologic disorders in order to avoid presenting an extensive catalog of signs and symptoms encountered in general clinical medicine.

In each discussion of specific diseases in subsequent chapters, the signs and symptoms that accompany the particular disorder are presented and the clinical find-

ings are covered in detail. In this chapter the signs and symptoms that may result from hematologic diseases or their complications are presented in the format of the standard review of systems and the physical examination, essentially along anatomic lines. This general presentation may provide suggestions as to possible diagnoses based on the data derived from the history and the physical examination.

History

DRUGS AND CHEMICALS

Drugs Drug therapy, either self-prescribed or ordered by a physician, is extremely common in our medicated society. Drugs often induce or aggravate hematologic disease, and it is therefore essential that a careful history of drug ingestion, including beneficial and adverse reactions, be obtained from all patients. It must be remembered that drugs taken regularly become a part of the patient's way of life and are often forgotten or are not recognized as "drugs." Agents such as mild analgesics, laxatives, tranquilizers, and sedatives are often in this category. Further, drugs may be ingested in unrecognized form, such as antibiotics in food or quinine in "gin and tonic." Specific, persistent questioning, often on several occasions, may be necessary before a complete history of drug use is obtained.

Chemicals In addition to drugs, most people are exposed regularly to a variety of chemicals in the environment, some of which may be potentially harmful agents in hematologic disease. Similarly, occupational exposure to chemicals must be considered. When a toxin is suspected, the patient's daily activities and environment must be carefully reviewed, since significant exposure to toxic chemicals may occur incidentally.

GENERAL SYMPTOMS

Performance status (PS) is a useful concept in establishing the seriousness of the patient's disability at the outset and in evaluating the effects of therapy. A widely used set of criteria for evaluating performance status is presented in Table 1-1.

Weight loss is a frequent accompaniment of many serious diseases, including primary hematologic entities, but it is often not present or, at most, is mild. Weight loss may occur early in a patient with a lymphoma, but usually this is a relatively late finding. Some patients with leukemia will lose weight rapidly, but many do not and may appear to be in good health for much of the course of their disease. Patients with pernicious anemia may lose weight, but this is unusual. Many "wasting" diseases, such as disseminated carcinoma or tuberculosis, cause anemia, and pronounced emaciation should suggest one of these diseases rather than anemia as the primary disorder.

Fever is a common manifestation of the lymphomas or leukemias, either as a result of the disease itself or

TABLE 1-1 Criteria of performance status (PS)

Able to carry on normal activity; no special care is needed.	100%	Normal; no complaints; no evidence of disease.
	90%	Able to carry on normal activity; minor signs or symptoms of disease.
	80%	• Normal activity with effort; some signs or symptoms of disease.
Unable to work; able to live at home; care for most personal needs; a varying amount of assistance is needed.	70%	Cares for self; unable to carry on normal activity or to do active work.
	60%	Requires occasional assistance but is able to care for most personal needs.
	50%	Requires considerable assistance and frequent medical care.
Unable to care for self; requires equivalent of institutional or hospital care; disease may be progressing rapidly.	40%	Disabled; requires special care and assistance.
	30%	Severely disabled; hospitalization is indicated though death not imminent.
	20%	Very sick; hospitalization necessary; active supportive treatment necessary.
	10%	Moribund; fatal processes progressing rapidly.
	0%	Dead.

SOURCE: Karnofsky [1].

because of occult secondary infection. In patients with "fever of unknown origin," these diseases, and particularly Hodgkin's disease, should be considered. Myelofibrosis may also cause fever. In some patients with severe pernicious anemia or hemolytic anemia, fever may be pronounced. *Chills* accompany severe hemolytic processes. *Night sweats* suggest the presence of low-grade fever and may occur in patients with lymphoma or leukemia.

Fatigue, malaise, and *lassitude* are such common accompaniments of both physical and emotional disorders that their evaluation is difficult and often impossible. In patients with serious disease, these symptoms may be readily explained by fever, muscle wasting, or other associated findings. Patients with anemia frequently complain of fatigue, malaise, or lassitude, and these symptoms may accompany the hematologic malignancies. Fatigue or lassitude may occur with iron deficiency in the absence of sufficient anemia to account for the symptom. In slowly developing chronic anemias, the patient may not recognize reduced exercise tolerance, etc., except in retrospect, after a remission has been induced by appropriate therapy.

Weakness may accompany anemia or the wasting of malignant processes, in which cases it is manifest as a *general* loss of strength or reduced capacity for exercise. The weakness may be *localized* as a result of neurologic complications of hematologic disease. In pernicious anemia there may be weakness of the lower extremities, accompanied by numbness, tingling, and unsteadiness of gait. Weakness of one or more extremities in patients with leukemia, myeloma, or lymphoma may signify central or peripheral nervous system invasion or compression. Myopathy secondary to malignancy occurs

with the hematologic malignancies and is usually manifest as weakness of proximal muscle groups. Foot drop or wrist drop may occur in lead poisoning, amyloidosis, or the "collagen" diseases—disorders that may have hematologic manifestations as well. Paralysis may occur in acute intermittent porphyria.

SPECIFIC SYMPTOMS

NERVOUS SYSTEM
Headache may be due to a number of causes related to hematologic diseases. Anemia or polycythemia may cause mild to severe headache. Invasion or compression of the brain by leukemia or lymphoma or infection of the central nervous system by *Cryptococcus* or tuberculosis may also cause headache in patients with hematologic malignancies. Hemorrhage into the brain or subarachnoid space in patients with thrombocytopenia or other bleeding disorders may cause sudden, severe headache.

Paresthesias may occur because of peripheral neuropathy in pernicious anemia or secondary to hematologic malignancy or amyloidosis. Probably the most common cause of paresthesias in patients with hematologic diseases is therapy with vincristine.

Confusion may accompany malignant or infectious processes involving the brain, sometimes as a result of the accompanying fever; it may also occur with severe anemia. Glucocorticoid therapy may cause confusion. It is extremely important to recognize confusion or apparent senility as a manifestation of pernicious anemia. Frank psychosis may develop in acute intermittent porphyria or with glucocorticoid therapy.

Impairment of consciousness may be due to increased

intracranial pressure secondary to hemorrhage or tumor in the central nervous system. It may also accompany severe anemia or polycythemia, or it may be due to hyperviscosity secondary to a paraprotein in the plasma.

EYES

Visual disturbances may be manifestations of anemia or polycythemia. Occasionally blindness may result from retinal hemorrhages secondary to anemia and thrombocytopenia. Diplopia or disturbances of ocular movement may occur with orbital tumors or paralysis of the third, fourth, or sixth cranial nerves because of compression by tumor.

EARS

Vertigo, tinnitus, and "roaring" in the ears may occur with marked anemia.

NASOPHARYNX AND MOUTH

Epistaxis may occur with any bleeding disorder. *Anosmia* or *olfactory hallucinations* occur in pernicious anemia. The nasopharynx may be invaded by a malignant tumor, with the symptoms dependent on the structures invaded. *Sore tongue* occurs in pernicious anemia and may accompany iron deficiency or vitamin deficiencies. *Macroglossia* occurs in amyloidosis. *Bleeding gums* may occur with bleeding disorders. *Ulceration* of the tongue or oral mucosa may be severe in the leukemias or in patients with neutropenia. *Dryness of the mouth* may be due to hypercalcemia, secondary, for example, to plasma cell myeloma. *Dysphagia* may be seen in patients with severe mucous membrane atrophy associated with chronic iron-deficiency anemia.

NECK

Painless swelling in the neck is characteristic of lymphoma but may be due to a number of other diseases as well. Occasionally, the enlarged nodes of lymphomas may be tender or painful because of secondary infection or rapid growth. *Diffuse swelling* of the neck and face may occur with obstruction of the superior vena cava due to lymphoma.

CHEST AND HEART

Both *dyspnea* and *palpitation*, usually on effort but occasionally at rest, may occur because of anemia. *Congestive cardiac failure* may supervene, and *angina pectoris* may become manifest in anemic patients. The impact of anemia on the circulatory system depends in part on the rapidity with which it develops, and chronic anemia may become severe without producing major symptoms; with acute blood loss, the patient may be in shock with a nearly normal hemoglobin level. *Cough* may result from enlarged mediastinal nodes. *Chest pain* may arise from involvement of the ribs or sternum with lymphoma or multiple myeloma, nerve-root invasion or compression, or herpes zoster; the pain of herpes zoster may precede the skin lesions by several days. *Tenderness*

of the sternum may be quite pronounced in chronic myelogenous or acute leukemia or if the sternal marrow is invaded by lymphoma or myeloma.

GASTROINTESTINAL SYSTEM

Dysphagia has already been mentioned under "Nasopharynx." *Anorexia* frequently occurs but usually has no specific diagnostic significance. Hypercalcemia and azotemia cause anorexia, nausea, and vomiting. A variety of ill-defined gastrointestinal complaints grouped under the heading "indigestion" may occur with hematologic diseases. *Abdominal fullness, belching,* or *discomfort* may occur because of a greatly enlarged spleen, but such splenomegaly may also be entirely asymptomatic. *Abdominal pain* may arise from intestinal obstruction by lymphoma, retroperitoneal bleeding, lead poisoning, ileus secondary to therapy with the *Vinca* alkaloids, acute hemolysis, allergic purpura, the abdominal crises of sickle cell disease, or acute intermittent porphyria. *Diarrhea* is now infrequent in pernicious anemia. It may be prominent in the various forms of intestinal malabsorption, although significant malabsorption may occur without diarrhea. Malabsorption may be a manifestation of small bowel lymphoma. *Gastrointestinal bleeding* related to thrombocytopenia or other bleeding disorder may be entirely occult but often is manifest as *hematemesis* or *melena*. *Constipation* may occur in the patient with hypercalcemia or in one receiving treatment with the *Vinca* alkaloids.

GENITOURINARY SYSTEM

Impotence or *bladder dysfunction* may occur with spinal cord or peripheral nerve damage due to one of the hematologic malignancies or with pernicious anemia. Priapism may occur in leukemia or sickle cell disease. *Hematuria* may be a manifestation of any of the bleeding disorders. *Red urine* may also occur with intravascular hemolysis (hemoglobinuria), myoglobinuria, or porphyrinuria. Injection of anthracycline drugs or ingestion of drugs such as Pyridium regularly causes the urine to turn red, and ingestion of beets may cause red urine in iron-deficient patients. Beeturia also occurs as a benign genetic disorder. *Amenorrhea* may accompany any serious disease. It may also be induced by certain drugs, such as antimetabolites or alkylating agents. *Menorrhagia* is of great significance in the etiology of iron deficiency, and care must be taken to obtain an accurate history of the extent of menstrual blood loss. Menorrhagia may occur in patients with bleeding disorders.

BACK AND EXTREMITIES

Back pain may accompany acute hemolytic reactions or be due to involvement of bone or the nervous system in malignant disease.

Arthritis or *arthralgia* may occur with gout secondary to increased uric acid production in patients with hematologic malignancies, myelofibrosis, or hemolytic anemia. They also occur in the plasma cell dyscrasias, acute leukemias, and sickle cell disease without evidence of gout, and in allergic purpura. Arthritis may accompany hemochromatosis. Hemarthroses in patients with severe bleeding disorders cause marked joint pain. Rheumatoid arthritis or systemic lupus erythematosus may present as anemia or thrombocytopenia, respectively, and arthritis may occur as a later manifestation. *Shoulder pain* on the left may be due to infarction of the spleen. *Bone pain* may occur with bone involvement by the hematologic malignancies or metastatic tumor; it is common in the congenital hemolytic anemias, such as sickle cell anemia, and may occur in myelofibrosis. In patients with Hodgkin's disease, ingestion of alcohol may induce pain at the site of any lesion, including those in bone. *Edema* of the lower extremities, sometimes unilateral, may occur because of obstruction to veins or lymphatics by enlarged lymph nodes. *Leg ulcers* are a common complaint in sickle cell anemia and occur rarely in other hereditary anemias.

SKIN

Skin manifestations of hematologic disease are of great importance and include changes in texture or color, itching, and the presence of specific or nonspecific lesions. The *texture* of the skin in iron-deficient patients may become dry, the hair dry and fine, and the nails brittle. In myxedema, which may present with anemia, the skin is dry, coarse, and scaly. *Jaundice* may be apparent with pernicious anemia or congenital or acquired hemolytic anemia. The skin of patients with pernicious anemia is said to be "lemon yellow" because of the simultaneous appearance of jaundice and pallor. Jaundice may also occur in patients with hematologic diseases as a result of liver involvement or biliary tract obstruction. *Pallor* is a common accompaniment of anemia, although some severely anemic patients may have a ruddy complexion. Widespread *erythroderma* occurs in some cases of chronic lymphocytic leukemia or lymphocytic lymphoma, and in mycosis fungoides (Sézary syndrome). Patients with hemachromatosis may have *bronze* or *grayish* pigmentation of the skin. *Cyanosis* occurs with methemoglobinemia, either hereditary or acquired, sulfhemoglobinemia, abnormal hemoglobins with low oxygen affinity, and primary and secondary polycythemia. Cyanosis of the ears or the fingertips may occur after exposure to cold in individuals with cryoglobulins or cold agglutinins.

Itching may occur in the absence of any visible skin lesions in Hodgkin's disease and may be extreme. Mycosis fungoides or other lymphomas with skin involvement may also present as itching. A significant number of patients with polycythemia vera will complain of itching after bathing.

Petechiae and *ecchymoses* are most often seen in the extremities in patients with thrombocytopenia, nonthrombocytopenic purpura, or other bleeding disorders. Unless secondary to trauma, these lesions usually are painless, although the lesions of autoerythrocyte sensitivity and erythema nodosum are painful. *Easy bruising* is a common complaint, especially among women, and usually no abnormalities are found after detailed study. This symptom may indicate a mild congenital bleeding disorder, such as von Willebrand's disease or one of the thrombocytopathies.

Infiltrative lesions may occur in the leukemias and lymphomas and are sometimes the presenting complaint. *Necrotic lesions* may occur with intravascular coagulation, as in purpura fulminans, or rarely with exposure to cold in patients with circulating cryoproteins or cold agglutinins.

FAMILY HISTORY

A carefully obtained family history may be of great importance in the study of patients with hematologic disease. In the case of hemolytic disorders, questions should be asked regarding jaundice, anemia, and gallstones in relatives. In patients with disorders of hemostasis, particular attention must be given to bleeding manifestations in family members. In the case of autosomal recessive disorders such as pyruvate kinase deficiency the parents are usually not affected, but a similar clinical syndrome may have occurred in siblings. It is particularly important to inquire about siblings who may have died in infancy, since these may be forgotten, especially by older patients. When sex-linked inheritance is suspected, it is necessary to inquire about symptoms in the maternal grandfather, maternal uncles, male siblings, and nephews. In patients with disorders with dominant inheritance, such as hereditary spherocytosis, one may expect to find that one of the parents and possibly siblings and children of the patient have stigmata of the disease.

Physical examination

A detailed physical examination should be performed on every patient, with sufficient attention paid to all systems to obtain a full evaluation of the general health of the individual. Certain body areas are especially pertinent to hematologic disease and therefore deserve special attention. These are the skin, eyes, tongue, lymph nodes, skeleton, spleen and liver, and nervous system.

SKIN

Pallor and flushing   The color of the skin is due to the pigment contained therein and to the blood flowing through the skin capillaries. The component of skin color related to the blood may be a useful guide to anemia or polycythemia, since pallor may result when the hemoglobin level is reduced and redness when the hemoglobin level is increased. The amount of pigment in the skin will modify skin color and may mislead the clinician, as in individuals with pallor due to decreased pigment, or make skin color useless as a guide because of the intense pigmentation present.

Alterations in blood flow and in hemoglobin content

may change skin color; this too may mislead the clinician. Thus emotion may cause either pallor or blushing. Exposure of the skin to cold or heat may similarly cause pallor or blushing. Chronic exposure to wind or sun may lead to permanent redness of the skin, and chronic ingestion of alcohol to a flushed face. The degree of erythema of the skin can be evaluated by pressing the thumb firmly against the skin, as on the forehead, so that the capillaries are emptied, and then comparing the color of the compressed spot with the surrounding skin immediately after the thumb is removed.

The mucous membranes and nail beds are usually more reliable guides to anemia or polycythemia than the skin. The conjunctivae and gums may be inflamed, however, and therefore not reflect the hemoglobin level, or the gums may appear pale because of pressure from the lips. The gums and the nail beds may also be pigmented and the capillaries correspondingly obscured. In some individuals, the color of the capillaries does not become fully visible through the nails unless pressure is applied to the fingertip, either laterally or on the end of the nail.

The palmar creases are useful guides to the hemoglobin level and appear pink in the fully opened hand unless the hemoglobin is 7 g/dl or less. Liver disease may induce flushing of the thenar and hypothenar eminences of the palm, even in patients with anemia.

Cyanosis The detection of cyanosis, like the detection of pallor, may be made difficult by skin pigmentation. Cyanosis is a function of the total amount of reduced hemoglobin, methemoglobin, or sulfhemoglobin present. The minimum amount of these pigments causing detectable cyanosis is about 5 g of reduced hemoglobin, 1.5 to 2 g of methemoglobin, and 0.5 g of sulfhemoglobin per deciliter of blood.

Jaundice Jaundice may be observed in the skin of individuals who are not otherwise deeply pigmented or in the conjunctivae or the mucous membranes. The patient should be examined in daylight rather than under incandescent light, because the yellow color of the latter masks the yellow color of the patient. The jaundice is due to actual staining of the skin by bile pigment, and bilirubin glucuronide (direct-reacting or conjugated bilirubin) stains the skin more readily than the unconjugated form. Jaundice of the skin may not be visible if the bilirubin level is below 2 to 3 mg/dl. Yellow pigmentation of the skin may also occur with carotenemia, especially in young children.

Petechiae and ecchymoses Petechiae are small (1 to 3 mm), round, red or brown lesions resulting from hemorrhage into the skin and are present primarily in areas with high venous pressure, such as the lower legs. These lesions do not blanch on pressure, and this can be demonstrated most readily by compressing the skin with a glass microscope slide. Petechiae may occasionally be elevated slightly, but this finding suggests a vasculitis as well as the hemorrhage. Ecchymoses may be of various sizes and shapes and may be red, purple, blue, or yellowish green, depending on the intensity of the skin hemorrhage and its age. They may be flat or elevated; some are painful and tender. The lesions of hereditary hemorrhagic telangiectasia are small, flat, nonpulsatile, and violaceous. They blanch with pressure.

Excoriation Itching may be intense in some hematologic disorders such as Hodgkin's disease, even in the absence of skin lesions. Excoriation of the skin from scratching is the only physical manifestation of this severe symptom.

Leg ulcers Open ulcers or scars from healed ulcers are often found in the region of the internal or external malleoli in patients with sickle cell anemia and, rarely, in other hereditary anemias.

Nails Detection of pallor and rubor by examining the nails was discussed earlier. The fingernails in chronic, severe iron-deficiency anemia may be ridged longitudinally and flattened or concave rather than convex. The latter change is referred to as *koilonychia* and is uncommon in present practice.

EYES
Jaundice, pallor, or *plethora* may be detected from examination of the eyes. Jaundice is more readily detected in the sclerae than in the skin. Ophthalmoscopic examination is also essential in patients with hematologic disease. *Retinal hemorrhages* and *exudates* occur in patients with severe anemia and thrombocytopenia. These hemorrhages are usually the typical "flame-shaped" hemorrhages, but they may be quite large and elevate the retina so that they may appear as a darkly colored tumor. Round hemorrhages with white centers are also often seen. *Dilatation of the veins* may be seen in polycythemia; in patients with macroglobulinemia, the veins are engorged and segmented, resembling link sausages.

MOUTH
Pallor of the mucosa has already been discussed. *Ulceration* of the oral mucosa occurs commonly in neutropenic patients. In leukemia there may also be infiltration of the gums with swelling, redness, and bleeding. *Bleeding* from the mucosa may occur with the hemorrhagic disease. A dark line of lead sulfide may be deposited in the gums at the base of the teeth in lead poisoning. The *tongue* may be completely smooth in pernicious anemia and iron-deficiency anemia. Patients with an upper dental prosthesis may also have papillary atrophy, presumably on a mechanical basis. The tongue may be smooth and red in patients with nutritional deficiencies. This may be accompanied by fissuring at the corners of the mouth, but fissuring may also be due to ill-fitting dentures.

LYMPH NODES

Lymph nodes are widely distributed in the body, and in disease any node or group of nodes may be involved. The major concern on physical examination is the detection of enlarged or tender nodes in the cervical, axillary, epitrochlear, inguinal, or femoral regions. Under normal conditions in adults, the only readily palpable lymph nodes are in the inguinal region, where several firm nodes 0.5 to 2 cm long are normally attached to the dense fascia below the inguinal ligament and in the femoral triangle. In children, multiple small (0.5 to 1 cm) nodes may be palpated in the cervical region as well. Supraclavicular nodes may sometimes be palpable only when the patient performs the Valsalva maneuver.

Enlarged lymph nodes are ordinarily detected in the superficial areas by palpation, although they are sometimes large enough to be seen. Palpation should be gentle and is best performed with a circular motion of the fingertips, using slowly increasing pressure.

Nodes too deep to palpate may be detected by radiologic examination, including computerized tomography, or by ultrasound. Enlarged nodes deep in the axillae may be visualized by mammographic or xerographic techniques. Enlargement of mediastinal lymph nodes can be demonstrated by standard x-ray examination or by tomography. Lymphangiography involving the injection of iodinated contrast media into the lymphatics of the dorsum of the feet has become a standard procedure for the diagnosis and management of diseases which involve lymph channels and lymph nodes (see Chaps. 118 and 119). Nodes of abnormal size or configuration may be identified by this means in the femoral, iliac, and paraaortic areas and occasionally in the mediastinal or left supraclavicular areas. The radiopaque oil is retained in the nodes for at least 3 to 6 months, and during this time, changes due to disease or to therapy may be followed by serial x-ray films. Inferior vena cavograms or pyelograms are occasionally useful to show gross displacement of organs or urinary tract obstruction by enlarged lymph nodes.

CHEST

Increased rib or sternal tenderness is an important physical sign often ignored. Increased bone pain may be generalized, as in leukemia, or spotty, as in plasma cell myeloma or in metastatic tumors. The superficial surfaces of all bones should be examined thoroughly by applying intermittent firm pressure with the fingertips to locate potential areas of disease.

SPLEEN

The normal adult spleen is usually not palpable on physical examination but occasionally may be felt. Palpability of the normal spleen may be related to body habitus [2], but there is disagreement on this point [3]. Enlarged spleens may be detected by percussion, although palpation is a far more reliable method. Some enlarged spleens may be visible through the abdominal wall.

The normal spleen weighs about 150 g and lies in the peritoneal cavity against the diaphragm and the posterolateral abdominal wall at the level of the lower three ribs. As it enlarges it remains close to the abdominal wall, while the lower pole moves downward, anteriorly, and to the right. Spleens enlarged only 40 percent above normal may be palpable [4], but significant splenic enlargement may occur and the organ still not be felt on physical examination [5–11]. A good but imperfect correlation has been reported between spleen size estimated from radioisotope scanning and spleen weight determined after splenectomy or at autopsy [7–9]. Although it is common to fail to palpate an enlarged spleen on physical examination, palpation of a normal-sized spleen is quite unusual [11], and therefore a palpable spleen is nearly always a significant physical finding.

In examining for an enlarged spleen, it should be remembered that the organ lies just beneath the abdominal wall and that it is identified by its movement during respiration. The splenic notch may be evident if the organ is moderately enlarged. During the examination the patient lies in a relaxed, supine position. The examiner, standing on the patient's right, gently palpates the left upper abdomen with the left hand while exerting pressure forward with the palm of the right hand placed over the lower ribs posterolaterally. If nothing is felt, the palpation should be performed repeatedly, moving the examining hand about 2 cm toward the inguinal ligament each time. It is often advantageous to carry out the examination initially with the patient lying on the right side with knees flexed and to repeat it with the patient supine.

It is not always possible to be sure that a left upper-quadrant mass is spleen; masses in the stomach, colon, kidney, or pancreas may mimic splenomegaly on physical examination. When there is uncertainty regarding the nature of a mass in the left upper quadrant, radiologic examinations will usually permit accurate diagnosis (see Chap. 4 for radioisotope scanning of the spleen).

LIVER

Palpation of the edge of the liver in the right upper quadrant of the abdomen is commonly used to detect hepatic enlargement, although the inaccuracies of this method have been demonstrated [6,11,12]. It is necessary to determine both the upper and lower borders of the liver by percussion in order properly to assess liver size [12–14]. The normal liver may be palpable as much as 4 to 5 cm below the right costal margin but is usually not palpable in the epigastrium. The height of liver dullness is best measured in a specific line 8, 10, or 12 cm to the right of the midline. Techniques should be standardized so that serial measurements can be made. The vertical span of the normal liver determined in this manner will range about 10 cm in an average-size man and about 2 cm smaller in women. Because of variations introduced by technique, each physician should determine the normal values for liver dullness by his or her own procedure. Correlation of radioisotope imaging data with results from routine physical examinations indicates that often a liver of normal size is considered enlarged on physical examination and an enlarged liver is considered normal [11]. Radioisotope imaging may be useful in demonstrating localized infiltrative lesions.

NERVOUS SYSTEM

A thorough evaluation of neurologic function is necessary in many patients with hematologic disease. Vitamin B_{12} deficiency impairs cerebral, olfactory, spinal cord, and peripheral nerve function, and severe chronic deficiency may lead to irreversible neurologic degeneration. Leukemic meningitis, often manifested by headache, visual impairment, or cranial nerve dysfunction, is becoming increasingly common. Tumor growth in the brain or spinal cord compression may be due to malignant lymphoma or plasma cell myeloma. A variety of neurologic abnormalities may develop in patients with various leukemias and lymphomas as a consequence of infiltration, bleeding, or infection.

References

1. Karnofsky, D. A., Abelmann, W. H., Craver, L. F., and Burchenal, J. H.: The use of the nitrogen mustards in the palliative treatment of carcinoma. *Cancer* 1:634, 1948.
2. Dell, J. M., Jr., and Klinefelter, H. F., Jr.: Roentgen studies of the spleen. *Am. J. Med. Sci.* 24:437, 1946.
3. McIntyre, O. R., and Ebaugh, F. G., Jr.: Palpable spleens in college freshmen. *Ann. Intern. Med.* 66:301, 1967.
4. Blackburn, C. R. B.: On the clinical detection of enlargement of the spleen. *Aust. Ann. Med.* 2:78, 1953.
5. Holzbach, R. T., Clark, R. E., Shipley, R. A., Kent, W. B., III, and Lindsay, G. E.: Evaluation of spleen size by radioactive scanning. *J. Lab. Clin. Med.* 60:902, 1962.
6. Riemenschneder, P. A., and Whalen, J. P.: The relative accuracy of estimation of enlargement of the liver and spleen by radiologic and clinical methods. *Am. J. Roentgenol.* 94:462, 1965.
7. Rollo, F. D., and DeLand, F. H.: The determination of spleen mass from radionuclide images. *Radiology* 97:583, 1970.
8. Larson, S. M.: Dimensions of the normal adult spleen scan and prediction of spleen weight. *J. Nucl. Med.* 12:123, 1971.
9. Silverman, S., DeNardo, G. L., Glatstein, E., and Lipton, M. J.: Evaluation of the liver and spleen in Hodgkin's disease. II. The value of splenic scintigraphy. *Am. J. Med.* 52:362, 1972.
10. Brubaker, L. H., and Johnson, C. A.: Correlation of splenomegaly and abnormal neutrophil pooling (margination). *J. Lab. Clin. Med.* 92:508, 1978.
11. Halpern, S., et al.: Correlation of liver and spleen size: Determinations by nuclear medicine studies and physical examination. *Arch. Intern. Med.* 134:123, 1974.
12. Naftalis, J., and Leevy, C. M.: Clinical estimation of liver size. *Am. J. Dig. Dis.* 8:236, 1963.
13. Peternel, W. W., Schaefer, J. W., and Schiff, L.: Clinical evaluation of liver size and hepatic scintiscan. *Am. J. Dig. Dis.* 11:346, 1966.
14. Castell, D. O., O'Brien, K. D., Muench, H., and Chalmers, T. C.: Estimation of liver size by percussion in normal individuals. *Ann. Intern. Med.* 70:1183, 1969.

CHAPTER 2

Examination of the blood

WILLIAM J. WILLIAMS

Examination of the blood is performed in almost all patients with major illnesses because of the importance of determining the presence of anemia and leukocytosis. Other abnormalities may also be detected in the blood, by either quantitative or qualitative studies. The so-called routine procedures are covered in this chapter, while special procedures are discussed in the appropriate sections of the book; some methods are presented in detail in the Appendix. This discussion is concerned only with the formed elements. The basic aspects of the study of coagulation and hemostasis are discussed in Chaps. 129 and 137. Other studies on the blood which do not bear on primary hematologic disease are not reviewed in this book.

Measurement of hemoglobin

Hemoglobin is intensely colored, and this property has been utilized in methods to estimate this component of blood. Hemoglobin in blood is a mixture of hemoglobin, oxyhemoglobin, carboxyhemoglobin, methemoglobin, and minor amounts of other forms of this pigment. It is necessary to prepare a stable derivative involving all the forms of hemoglobin in the blood in order to measure this compound accurately. The cyanmethemoglobin (hemiglobincyanide, cyanferrihemoglobin) derivative [1] can be conveniently and reproducibly prepared and is now widely used for hemoglobin estimations [2]. All forms of hemoglobin are readily converted to cyanmethemoglobin except for sulfhemoglobin, which is rarely present in significant amounts. Cyanmethemoglobin can be measured accurately by its absorbance at 540 nm in a photometer. Errors in hemoglobin determinations are those of dilution and estimation of the color. Turbidity from improperly lysed cells or from high concentrations of paraprotein may also lead to erroneous results. The normal values for adults are presented in Table 2-1. The mean hemoglobin level in blacks of both sexes and all ages has been found to be about 0.5 to 1 g/dl below the mean for comparable whites [3–6].

The reproducibility of hemoglobin measurement using the cyanmethemoglobin method in an automated system is presented in Table 2-2. Estimation of hemoglobin levels manually by the same method gives comparable reproducibility [7].

TABLE 2-1 Blood cell values in a normal population

	Men	*Women*
White cell count,†		
× 10³/μl blood	7.25 (3.9–10.6)*	7.28 (3.5–11.0)
Red cell count,		
× 10⁶/μl blood	5.11 (4.4–5.9)	4.51 (3.8–5.2)
Hemoglobin,		
g/dl blood	15.5 (13.3–17.7)§	13.7 (11.7–15.7)§
Hematocrit,		
percent	46.0 (39.8–52.2)	40.9 (34.9–46.9)
Mean corpuscular volume,		
μm³/red cell	90.1 (80.5–99.7)	90.4 (80.8–100.0)
Mean corpuscular hemoglobin,		
pg/red cell	30.2 (26.6–33.8)	30.2 (26.4–34.0)
Mean corpuscular hemoglobin		
concentration, g/dl RBC	33.9 (31.5–36.3)	33.6 (31.4–35.8)
Platelet count,		
× 10³/μl blood	295 (150–440)	295 (150–440)

*The range given is the mean ± 2 standard deviations.
†The International Committee for Standardization in Hematology has recommended that the following units be used (SI units): white cell count, "number × 10⁹/l," red cell count, "number × 10¹²/l," and hemoglobin, "g/dl" (dl = deciliter). The hematocrit (packed cell volume) is given as a number, e.g., 0.41, without designated units. Units of liter per liter are implied. Mean corpuscular volume is given as "fl" (femtoliters), mean corpuscular hemoglobin as "pg" (picograms), and mean corpuscular hemoglobin concentration as "g/dl." Platelets are reported as "number × 10⁹/l."
§The mean hemoglobin level of blacks of both sexes and all ages has been reported to be 0.5 to 1.0 g/dl below the mean for comparable whites [3–6].
NOTE: The studies were performed on 186 normal adult men and 270 normal adult women, with the Coulter Counter Model S, except for the platelet counts, which were done on 50 normal adult men and 50 normal adult women using a Coulter Counter Model S-plus. The platelet count data were provided by Dr. Frederick R. Davey and the remainder of the data by Dr. Arthur S. Schneider.

Measurement of the hematocrit[1]

The portion of the blood occupied by erythrocytes—the *hematocrit*—may be determined by subjecting the blood to sufficient centrifugal force to pack the cells in as small a volume as possible [8]. In electronic instruments the hematocrit is calculated from the erythrocyte count and the mean corpuscular volume (see below). Determination of the hematocrit requires an anticoagulant which does not change the volume of the erythrocytes, such as heparin [8], a mixture of potassium and ammonium oxalate [9], or dipotassium or tripotassium EDTA [10,11].

The hematocrit is expressed as a percentage, or as a ratio in the SI system (Table 2-1). The errors in estimating hematocrit by centrifugation arise from changes in cell volume induced by preparing the blood for the determination, from inadequate mixing of the sample, and from inadequate centrifugation. The hematocrit may be determined on a "macro" scale, using relatively low-speed centrifugation in tubes 3 mm in diameter, or on a "micro" scale, using capillary tubes and high-speed centrifugation. The amount of plasma remaining in the packed cells varies somewhat with the method used,

but it is on the order of 1 to 4 percent [12–15]. The hematocrit determined on a macro scale [12–15] is subject to error from increased plasma trapping with high packed cell volumes [13,16] and may be disproportionately low with low packed cell volumes [13,16]. This error is due, at least in part, to the greater centrifugal force exerted near the bottom of the tube in the centrifuge, which causes relatively greater packing at the tip of the tube and relatively less near the meniscus [13]. This problem appears not to occur to the same extent with the micro technique [14,15], probably because much greater centrifugal forces are used.

The hematocrit of blood containing abnormal red cells is relatively increased, apparently due to increased plasma trapping caused by the abnormal cells. Thus plasma trapping as high as 6 percent has been observed in iron deficiency anemia and as high as 30 percent after anaerobic incubation of blood from patients with sickle cell anemia [16]. High values for plasma trapping have also been found in thalassemia [17] and spherocytosis [18]. This artifactual increase in the hematocrit leads to errors in calculation of red cell indices and has introduced some confusion when values obtained by manual methods are compared with those determined with automated cell counters. Present-day electronic cell counters determine the hematocrit by summation of individual red cell volumes measured directly [19]. Since the electronic instruments require calibration for estimation of the hematocrit, it is possible to adjust the

[1] Although the term *hematocrit* was originally defined as the tube in which blood is centrifuged to determine the volume of packed cells or the centrifuge used for this purpose, it has come to mean the packed cell volume itself and will be used in that sense here.

TABLE 2-2   Reproducibility of automated hemotologic values

	1	2	3	4
Number of samples	23	14	21	19
White cell count, $\times 10^3/\mu l$ blood:*				
Mean	5.07	12.31	12.74	11.76
Standard deviation	0.19	0.39	0.40	0.31
Coefficient of variation	3.72	3.16	3.18	2.64
Red cell count, $\times 10^6/\mu l$ blood:*				
Mean	3.32	5.13	5.19	5.10
Standard deviation	0.04	0.06	0.12	0.08
Coefficient of variation	1.16	1.19	2.22	1.51
Hemoglobin, g/dl blood:*				
Mean	10.3	15.91	15.48	15.17
Standard deviation	0.1	0.19	0.17	0.23
Coefficient of variation	1.11	1.22	1.08	1.54
Volume-packed RBC, ml/dl blood:*				
Mean	30.0	45.75	43.80	43.54
Standard deviation	0.3	0.81	1.16	0.55
Coefficient of variation	1.03	1.78	2.64	1.26
Mean corpuscular volume, μm^3/red cell:*				
Mean	89.6	88.76	83.33	84.53
Standard deviation	1.5	1.40	1.59	1.08
Coefficient of variation	1.64	1.58	1.91	1.27
Mean corpuscular hemoglobin, pg/red cell:*				
Mean	30.6	30.83	29.41	29.34
Standard deviation	0.5	0.37	0.86	0.58
Coefficient of variation	1.60	1.19	2.92	1.99
Mean corpuscular hemoglobin concentration, percent:*				
Mean	33.8	34.90	35.45	34.78
Standard deviation	0.5	0.63	1.07	0.50
Coefficient of variation	1.44	1.80	3.03	1.44

*See second footnote to Table 2-1 for SI units.
NOTE: The data represent the results of repetitive determinations by a Coulter Counter Model S.

Column 1: A pool of whole blood, anticoagulated with ACD, was repetitively sampled as every fifth sample during a routine series of laboratory determinations and represents a measure of in-run variability.

Columns 2 to 4: Repetitive sampling once daily of aliquots from a preserved whole blood reference material. This represents day-to-day variability.

instrument to give a hematocrit value equal to that obtained by centrifugation when studying normal blood. The coefficient of variation in the hematocrit determined by centrifugation is 1 to 2 percent [20] and is somewhat less than 1 percent with electronic methods [19]. Normal values are presented in Table 2-1. The hematocrit, like hemoglobin concentration [3–6], is lower in blacks than in whites [21].

Cell counts

Determination of the number of leukocytes, erythrocytes, and platelets in the blood has long been a fundamental procedure in hematology. Manual methods provide satisfactory measurement of the leukocyte and platelet counts [22,23], but the erythrocyte count is quite inaccurate when performed manually [19]. Electronic cell counting methods are now widely used and permit accurate enumeration of all three formed elements, including the erythrocyte. In this section the general principles of cell counting are discussed.

PRINCIPLES OF CELL COUNTING
In order to obtain useful quantitative data, the number of cells in an accurately diluted, precisely measured sample of blood must be reproducibly counted.

Dilution   The dilution must be performed as accurately as possible, and since the number of cells in blood is enormous, the dilution must be great (up to 1:50,000). Therefore, the volume of blood used is small and the errors of measurement are potentially large. The blood may be diluted manually or mechanically [24].

The extent of dilution is dictated by the numbers of the particular formed element usually found in the blood. For example, dilution will be greater for the erythrocyte count than for the leukocyte count.

The diluting fluid is chosen to permit the formed element under study to be counted selectively. Thus for erythrocyte counts the diluting fluid merely dilutes the blood while preserving erythrocyte morphology. In the methods for counting leukocytes, the fluid lyses the erythrocytes while preserving the leukocytes. Some methods for platelet counting employ this same principle.

Sampling A precisely measured sample of the diluted blood must be obtained, and the cells must be evenly distributed in the sample. For manual counting, a "counting chamber" is used which permits examination of a precise volume of the diluted blood determined by a grid inscribed in the base of a chamber of exact depth. In automated counting methods the number of cells in an exact volume of cell suspension is determined.

Counting Counting may be performed visually or by automated means. Visual counting may be done under the bright-field or phase-contrast microscope. The cells to be counted are identified and enumerated by the operator. Care must be exercised to count *all* the appropriate cells in the area defined by the grid. Automated counting may be done utilizing either impedance (conductivity) [25–27] or optical systems [28–31].

ERRORS OF COUNTING
The errors inherent in cell counts are those of diluting the blood, distribution of cells in the diluting fluid, precision of sampling of the diluted blood, and enumeration of the cells. This last source of error arises because of superimposition of cells or abnormalities in the size or shape of the cells so that they are misinterpreted visually or by the detection device in automated methods.

STATISTICAL CONSIDERATIONS
When randomly distributed blood cells are counted by either manual or automated techniques, the variation among repetitive observations theoretically follows a Poisson distribution. A characteristic of such distributions is that the standard deviation of the repeated observations is equal to the square root of the mean number of cells counted for each observation. Ideally, then, it is desirable to count very large numbers of cells in order to achieve the highest degree of precision. To achieve, for example, a coefficient of variation of 2 percent, one would have to count no less than 2500 blood cells. It is obvious that automated techniques permit the enumer-

ation of vastly greater numbers of cells than is possible by manual methods. A second consideration is that as the number of cells counted increases, there is a greater chance that two or more cells will be sensed as one by the detecting device, producing a progressive negative error due to coincidence. Techniques for minimizing or correcting for coincidence error have thus been a requirement for automated cell-counting devices.

AUTOMATED METHODS FOR ROUTINE HEMATOLOGIC DETERMINATIONS
Before the advent of automated instruments, the most numerous determinations performed in the hematology laboratory were hemoglobin concentration, hematocrit, white cell count, and qualitative and quantitative microscopic evaluation of the stained blood film. Less frequent measurements included enumeration of red blood cells, reticulocytes, and platelets and the derivation of red cell indices. Of these measurements, only the hemoglobin and hematocrit determinations can be performed by simple, rapid, and highly reproducible manual techniques. In contrast, manual methods of cell counting have been time-consuming and tedious and have been associated with a low degree of precision. In one study [19], reproducibility for carefully performed manual red cell counts as expressed by the coefficient of variation was 8.2 percent. It is likely that more casually performed day-to-day enumerations in busy laboratories have a coefficient of variation as high as 15 to 20 percent. The variability in manual platelet counting is at least this great [23] and may be greater when platelets are reduced in number. The lack of precision of red cell counting can have a secondary effect on two of the erythrocyte indices, the mean corpuscular hemoglobin and the mean corpuscular volume (see below), both of which are calculated from the red cell count.

The practical problems associated with the satisfactory performance of these studies have been a major impetus for the development of automated techniques, and an ever-increasing availability and utilization of automated instrumentation has resulted. Most such equipment is very expensive; however, the improved efficiency has tended to lower the overall costs of laboratory tests. In addition, automated analysis can minimize random technical errors, thus adding to the reliability of laboratory data.

AUTOMATED CELL COUNTERS
Erythrocytes, leukocytes, and platelets may all be counted automatically by electrical impedance [19,25–27] or optical [28–31] methods.

Erythrocyte counts

ELECTRICAL IMPEDANCE METHODS
The electrical impedance method is utilized in the Coulter [19,25–27], Celloscope [32], and Ultra-Flo 100 [33–35] instruments. In these systems a suspension of

blood cells in a metered volume of an electrolyte medium flows through a small orifice. An electric current is applied between platinum electrodes on either side of the orifice. Since each cell is a relative nonconductor, there is a momentary decrease in conductance that corresponds to the passage of each cell through the orifice. This results in a series of pulses which can be counted electronically. With appropriate standardization and correction for coincidence and dilution factor, the number of pulses can be expressed as a blood cell count. In addition, the magnitude of each pulse is proportional to the volume of displaced electrolyte. Electronic averaging of the pulse heights has been employed as a direct measurement of the mean corpuscular volume of erythrocytes [19].

The pulses generated by passage of the cells through the orifice are distorted unless the particle passes through the center of the opening. Such distorted pulses may be misinterpreted by the detection system with resulting inaccuracies in the estimated cell volumes [36]. The accuracy of the analysis may be improved by electronic editing of the data to reject distorted peaks, analysis of the distorted peaks to provide correction of the aberrance, or modification of the flow system to ensure a central position for the particle in the aperture (hydrodynamic focusing) [35,37,38]. Instruments incorporating each of these modifications have improved precision and accuracy and provide reliable estimates of the mean corpuscular volume. Such instruments may be used to count platelets as well as erythrocytes in diluted whole blood [33–35].

Red cells are counted in diluted blood that contains leukocytes and platelets as well as red cells. In the less-sophisticated instruments, leukocytes are counted along with the red cells, but since the number of red cells usually exceeds that of the white cells by a factor of 500 or more, the error in the red cell count due to the presence of white cells is usually negligible. The error progressively increases, however, as the white count rises, and red cell volume measurements are significantly altered when the white cell count exceeds 50,000 per microliter. Platlets are so small that they do not introduce errors in the red cell count. Leukocyte counting usually is performed after lysis of the red cells by surface-active agents [27]. Platelet counting can be performed on platelet-rich plasma after removal of red cells by sedimentation or centrifugation [23,39] or on diluted blood [33–35].

OPTICAL METHODS
The Hemalog [28–30] and ELT-8 [31] instruments utilize optical detection systems. Cells may be counted optically utilizing a system in which a photoelectric cell detects light which is refracted, diffracted, or scattered by cells passing through a small illuminated area in the optical system. The photoelectric cell generates electrical pulses of magnitude proportional to the size of the particle. As with the electrical impedance systems, the pulses can be counted and also used to determine par-

ticle size. Optical systems have been developed which will count erythrocytes, leukocytes, and platelets with precision equivalent to or better than that of the electrical impedance methods [28–31].

Determination of size and hemoglobin content of erythrocytes

In characterizing the blood of patients with anemia, it is useful to know the size of the erythrocytes, the amount of hemoglobin in each erythrocyte, and the concentration of hemoglobin in the erythrocytes. Indeed, these quantities have been the basis for the classifications of anemia or morphologic grounds, e.g., hypochromic microcytic anemia, macrocytic anemia, etc. [40]. Erythrocyte size and hemoglobinization can be estimated visually on stained films of the blood or can be calculated quantitatively from the hemoglobin, erythrocyte count, and packed cell volume [41]. Obviously, calculation of these quantities involves the errors of the individual determinations, and they must be interpreted with this in mind. With the advent of the more accurate methods of erythrocyte counting, however, the reliability of these indices has increased greatly, and as discussed above, they may be calculated automatically by some of the more elaborate electronic instruments now available. The average volume of the erythrocytes is determined directly with electronic cell counters [19].

Mean corpuscular volume (MCV) [41]   The volume of the erythrocytes can be calculated from the erythrocyte count, which measures the number of cells per microliter of blood, and the packed cell volume, which measures the proportion of the blood occupied by the erythrocytes expressed as volume rather than percent. This is most conveniently calculated as follows:

$$MCV = \frac{\text{volume of packed erythrocytes/1000 ml blood}}{\text{erythrocyte count, millions/microliter}}$$

The MCV is measured in cubic micrometers of femtoliters (fl). The normal values are presented in Table 2-1.

The MCV is also measured by electronic cell counters, usually by dividing the summation of the cell volumes by the erythrocyte count [19,31,36]. This value is thus quite independent of the hematocrit and can be measured with excellent precision in the newer instruments [19,31,36]. However, a number of sources of error are inherent in the electronic methods [36–38]. Thus an improper lower threshold may obviate detection of the smallest microcytes and lead to an overestimation of the MCV. Inclusion of leukocytes because of ineffective upper-threshold settings will have the opposite effect, as will cells passing eccentrically through the aperture of an impedance instrument with consequent generation of an artifactually large pulse [36–38]. The MCV determined with electronic instruments tends to be smaller than that determined by manual methods because the hematocrit contains a small amount of trapped plasma, which leads to overestimation of the packed-cell volume and therefore of the MCV [12–15,19,31,36]. All electronic counters require calibration for the MCV determination, and the output of the instrument can easily by adjusted to correspond to the values obtained by the traditional methods. Although discrepancies occur between results produced by manual methods and by electronic methods, the agreement is usually close, and data obtained by properly standardized methods of either type are useful clinically [19,31,32].

Mean corpuscular hemoglobin [41]   The amount of hemoglobin per cell can be evaluated from the mean corpuscular hemoglobin (MCH), which is calculated by dividing the amount of hemoglobin in 1 liter of blood by the number of erythrocytes per microliter of blood, in millions, as follows:

$$MCH = \frac{\text{hemoglobin, in grams/1000 ml blood}}{\text{erythrocyte count, millions/microliter}}$$

The MCH is determined as micromicrograms, or picograms (pg), of hemoglobin per cell. The normal values are presented in Table 2-1. The MCH is calculated automatically in the multichannel instruments currently on the market.

Mean corpuscular hemoglobin concentration (MCHC) [41]   The concentration of hemoglobin in the erythrocytes is determined by dividing the amount of hemoglobin per deciliter of blood by the packed cell volume expressed as a percentage. This quotient is multiplied by 100 to permit the MCHC to be expressed as a percentage quantity. The calculation is

$$MCHC = \frac{\text{hemoglobin, in g/dl} \times 100}{\text{packed cell volume, percent}}$$

The MCHC thus measures the concentration of hemoglobin in grams per deciliter of erythrocytes or as a percentage. The normal values are presented in Table 2-1. Using data obtained by manual methods, the MCHC is the most accurate of the quantities used to characterize erythrocytes, because it does not involve the erythrocyte count, the least accurate of the three parameters used to evaluate these cells. However, the MCHC, as originally derived, is susceptible to the variations in hematocrit resulting from increased retention of plasma in the column of packed cells when abnormal cells are present [15,17,18]. The most frequent problem encountered is iron deficiency anemia, where classically the MCHC is low [40,41] but has been reported to be normal when determined by electronic methods [42]. It has been suggested that the hypochromia observed on blood films from patients with iron deficiency anemia [43] is due to small, thin cells containing a normal concentration of hemoglobin [42].

Although the MCV, and therefore the MCHC, determined electronically may be lower than that obtained manually, there is generally good agreement between the values obtained by the two methods [19,31]. However, systematic comparisons have not been made in disease states [16]. When determined by manual methods, abnormal indices are found in only 50 to 70 percent of patients with hypochromic or macrocytic anemias. The concern that hypochromic microcytic anemias will be detected less readily by electronic instruments than by manual methods has not been substantiated [16].

It must be emphasized that the MCV, MCH, and MCHC are average quantities and therefore may not detect abnormalities in blood with mixed-cell populations. For example, patients with sideroblastic anemia have a dimorphic blood picture, with both hypochromic and normochromic cells. The indices may be in the normal range, and the important finding of the mixed-cell population would not be detected if one relied on the indices alone. Examination of the blood film is therefore an essential part of the study of the blood, since it may lead to detection of abnormalities which would otherwise be missed.

Leukocyte counts

Leukocyte counts are performed on blood samples appropriately diluted with a solution which causes lysis of the erythrocytes (e.g., urea or a detergent) [19,27,31]. The cells are counted using one of the electronic cell counters discussed above or by manual methods [see, for example, Ref. 44]. The values obtained in a study of a normal population are presented in Table 2-1, and the reproducibility of the values obtained with an automated method are presented in Table 2-2. Manual counting has a coefficient of variation of 6.5 percent with normal or elevated leukocyte counts and 15 percent with low leukocyte counts [22]. Changes in the leukocyte count in children are discussed later in this chapter.

Platelet counts

Platelet counts may also be performed by automated methods [23,29,30]. With electrical impedance methods, platelet-rich plasma obtained either by sedimentation [23] or by low-speed centrifugation [39] may be used, or diluted whole blood may be employed in instruments incorporating hydrodynamic focusing or electronic editing to ensure accurate sizing of the particles being counted [33–35]. In the electrical impedance methods utilizing whole blood, the red cell count must be determined independently and subtracted from the total particle count (red cells plus platelets) to obtain the platelet count [33]. The optical methods utilize either platelet-rich plasma [29] or diluted blood in which red cells are lysed with urea or similar solutions [30]. In methods using platelet-rich plasma, the plasma platelet count must be converted to a blood platelet count by a correction factor based on the hematocrit [23]. Large platelets will not be counted by automated methods, and nucleated red cells, fragments of leukocytes, and red cell ghosts may be counted as platelets [23,29,30,33–35]. These problems are identified by some instruments [33–35], and manual counts can then be performed. Falsely low platelet counts may also be obtained by automated methods if platelet agglutinins or adsorption of platelets to leukocytes (platelet satellitism) are present [45] (see Chap. 141).

Manual methods, such as that of Brecher and Cronkite [46], are also used. That method utilizes phase-contrast microscopy and 10 percent ammonium oxalate as the diluting fluid. The means of platelet counts performed by this method on venous and on capillary blood were 248,000 and 242,000, respectively, but the coefficient of variation using venous blood was 11 percent, while that with capillary blood was 24 percent [47]. The mean platelet count by another direct method was 246,000, with a coefficient of variation of 23 percent [20]. In another study the coefficient of variation for the manual method using venous blood was found to be 16.6 percent, while that for the automated method was about 4 percent [23]. The range of normal for platelet counts is probably from about 150,000 to 440,000. All platelet counts, electronic or manual, should be verified by examination of a properly prepared, stained blood film.

Platelet volume may be measured by electronic counting devices [48] (see Chaps. 130 and 131). Platelet volume varies with the interval between specimen collection and counting and the anticoagulant [49] and must be determined under carefully controlled conditions [48,49].

Normal hematologic values as determined by automated equipment

The results of a survey of a normal adult population utilizing the Coulter Counter Model S are shown in Table 2-1. These data are strikingly similar to studies performed by classical manual methods. The changes that occur in these values in childhood are discussed below.

Examination of blood films

Microscopic examination of the blood spread on a glass slide or cover slip yields useful information regarding all the formed elements of the blood. The technique of preparing a blood film and staining with Wright's stain is described in Chap. A1. Blood films may also be prepared mechanically (see pp. 20–21). The information which can be derived from study of the film is discussed here. It must be remembered that the process of preparing a thin blood film involves mechanical trauma to the cells during the spreading process.

Further, the cells flatten on the glass during drying, and the fixation and staining involve exposure to methanol and water. Artifacts obviously are induced, and films must be evaluated with this in mind. Blood films must be examined under oil-immersion magnification in order to appreciate the necessary details of the cells.

EXAMINATION OF WET PREPARATIONS
It is sometimes advantageous to examine fresh blood under the microscope to avoid artifacts of fixation or staining. This is readily accomplished by sealing a small drop of blood diluted with isotonic sodium chloride beneath a coverslip on a glass slide. Buffered glutaraldehyde will preserve the cells for reexamination at a later time. Petroleum jelly or Aquaphor may be used to seal the coverslip to the slide. Wet preparations are employed to detect sickling (Chap. A10), and spherocytes may be readily detected in this manner. Wet preparations should be examined to be sure that erythrocyte abnormalities seen on fixed smears are not artifacts of drying or staining. Phase-contrast microscopy permits study of cellular detail in unstained, wet preparations [50].

SUPRAVITAL STAINING
Supravital staining [51–53] may offer advantages in studying leukocyte morphology, since the cells are not subjected to mechanical trauma and fragile cells remain intact. Further, mitochondria may be demonstrated in this manner, and other characteristics of the cells may permit identification of cell type, which is not possible in fixed smears. Supravital staining is essential for the demonstration of certain inclusions in erythrocytes. These are *Heinz bodies,* the reticulum in *reticulocytes,* and *hemoglobin H inclusions.* The techniques for demonstrating these are presented in the Appendix, Chaps. A2, A4, and A6.

ERYTHROCYTE MORPHOLOGY
The stained film should be sufficiently thin that the erythrocytes do not touch and therefore do not distort one another. Erythrocytes should be examined for size, shape, hemoglobin concentration and distribution, staining properties, distribution on the film, and inclusions. The abnormalities of erythrocyte morphology that occur in disease are presented briefly here and are discussed in more detail in Chap. 29 and in the description of specific diseases.

SIZE (see Plate 3)
Normal erythrocytes studied on dried films are nearly uniform in size, with a normal distribution about a mean of 7.2 to 7.9 μm. Erythrocyte size can be evaluated by use of a micrometer disc inserted into the microscope, although experienced morphologists usually evaluate erythrocyte size without this aid. Macrocytes may be seen in a number of disease states. Cells are considered to be macrocytes if their diameters exceed 9 μm. Macrocytes may have a normal appearance, except for

their size, or may have decreased hemoglobin concentration, abnormal hemoglobin distribution (targeting), or abnormal shape. Reticulocytes appear in stained films as large, bluish cells, often referred to as *polychromatophilic macrocytes. Microcyte* is the term used to describe a small cell, i.e., one less than 6 μm in diameter. Microcytes usually have normal or diminished hemoglobin concentration, but if the cells look small because they are spherocytic, the hemoglobin concentration may appear to be increased (see below).

SHAPE
The normal erythrocyte is round. The term *poikilocytosis* is used to describe variations in the shape of erythrocytes. Various-shaped abnormalities are found in small numbers of cells in blood from anemic patients. Accurate interpretation of shape changes requires recognition of the predominant shape abnormality. The following variations may be observed (see also Chap. 29).

Elliptocytes Elliptical or oval cells are seen in normal blood and in increased numbers in anemia. In hereditary elliptocytosis (Chap. 56), these and other elongated forms may account for 25 to 90 percent of the erythrocytes.

Spherocytes Spherocytes appear as small, densely staining cells and are seen in hereditary spherocytosis (Chap. 55) and in acquired hemolytic anemias (see Plate 3).

Dacryocytes These cells have assumed the shape of a teardrop or pear. They occur in increased numbers in myelofibrosis.

Sickled cells These cells occur in patients with sickle cell disease, but are usually seen only in small numbers on dried films because the hemoglobin becomes oxygenated during the drying process and only the irreversibly sickled cells remain. The cells assume a wide variety of shapes, most often appearing as elongated crescents. Cells resembling sickled cells may occasionally be seen in normal blood, but these can usually be differentiated by the lack of any sharp projections.

Schizocytes These are fragmented cells which appear in a variety of sizes and shapes from small triangular forms to normal-sized cells with grossly irregular outlines.

Echinocytes These cells are characterized by multiple spiny projections regularly distributed over the cell surface. The cells are morphologically identical with crenated normal erythrocytes.

Acanthocytes Acanthocytes are cells whose surfaces present several irregular projections of relatively large size. They are characteristic of the syndrome of acanthocytosis (Chap. 57).

HEMOGLOBIN CONCENTRATION AND DISTRIBUTION
(see Plate 3)
The normal erythrocyte appears as a disc with a rim of hemoglobin and a clear central area. The central pallor normally occupies less than one-half the diameter of the cells, but there is often variation within the film in that in some areas the central pallor may not be detected at all. Variations in hemoglobin concentration may be observed, usually in the direction of reductions in hemoglobin in those conditions characterized by diminished hemoglobin synthesis. Spherocytes, however, appear to be more densely stained because of their increased thickness, and large cells may not show central pallor for the same reason. *Hypochromia,* or decreased hemoglobin in the erythrocytes, may range from a slight, barely detectable increase in the central pallor of the cells to such extreme reduction that only a thin rim of hemoglobin is visible. The difficulties in evaluating hemoglobin concentration from examination of the blood film are discussed in Chap. 48.

The hemoglobin may be abnormally distributed in the erythrocytes, particularly in a form of cell in which there is a spot or disc of hemoglobin in the center surrounded by a clear area which is in turn surrounded by a rim of hemoglobin at the outer edge of the cell, giving the appearance of a target—a *target cell.* The central disc of hemoglobin may be small and lightly stained or may be densely stained and occupy more than one-third the diameter of the cell. Target cells are often hypochromic as well as showing the abnormal distribution of hemoglobin. Hemoglobin C disease is characterized by many target cells, and in some cases rod-shaped crystals of hemoglobin C are observed in the erythrocytes.

STAINING PROPERTIES (see Plate 3)
The hemoglobin in the erythrocyte stains pink to red, but some cells have a grayish or bluish hue. This is called *polychromatophilia* and when seen in macrocytes suggests that the cell is a reticulocyte. Generalized gray or blue staining of the red cells is an artifact (see Chap. A1).

DISTRIBUTION OF ERYTHROCYTES
Erythrocytes are usually distributed evenly throughout the film. In some films the cells become aligned in aggregates (*rouleau*) resembling stacks of coins. Such rouleau formation may be an artifact but often is due to the presence of a paraprotein and suggests the diagnosis of plasma cell myeloma or macroglobulinemia.

INCLUSIONS
Inclusions may be observed in erythrocytes on films stained with Wright's stain. Other inclusions are visible only in supravitally stained films and are discussed under that heading. The following are seen in fixed, stained erythrocytes:

Nuclei In disease, nucleated red cells appear in the peripheral blood. These are usually orthochromatic erythroblasts, with fully hemoglobinized cytoplasm and small, pyknotic nuclei, but in patients with severe anemia they may be grossly immature promegaloblasts. Nucleated red cells may appear in the peripheral blood when the marrow is subjected to intense stimulation, as in response to acute hemorrhage, acute anoxemia with congestive heart failure, or severe hemolytic anemia, as well as in pernicious anemia, leukemia, and marrow metastases. The presence of these cells in the peripheral blood should be considered an important indication of serious disease, except in asplenic individuals.

Howell-Jolly bodies   These are small, well-defined, round, densely staining basophilic inclusion bodies about 1 μm in diameter, which usually occur singly but sometimes in multiples. They appear after splenectomy and are also seen in cases of severe anemia from a variety of causes. They contain DNA and may be chromosomal remnants or nuclear fragments [54].

Cabot rings   These are blue-staining, threadlike inclusions in the red cells in severe anemia. They may appear as rings, figures-of-eight, or twisted and convoluted in a variety of shapes. They may occupy the entire periphery of the cell but frequently are much smaller. They are not often seen. It has been postulated that they are remnants of the mitotic spindle [55], but others have found that they contain histone and iron [56].

Basophilic stippling   This term refers to the presence in erythrocytes of coarse or fine, punctate basophilic inclusions which may vary in size, shape, and distribution. This *diffuse basophilic stippling* may be seen in a variety of anemias. Coarse basophilic stippling occurs to an extreme degree in lead poisoning, with involvement of up to 1 to 2 percent of the cells. A special form of basophilic stippling occurs in conditions in which iron granules are present in the red cells. These granules stain blue with Wright's stain but are also stained by the Prussian blue reaction (see Chap. A3). The iron granules are called *Pappenheimer bodies* when observed in Wright-stained films. Basophilic stippling is prominent in pyrimidine-5'-nucleotidase deficiency, possibly because of failure to degrade ribosomes [57,58]. The basophilic stippling of lead poisoning may be due to the inhibition of the nucleotidase by lead [58].

Parasites   Malaria and *Babesia* parasites are seen in the red cells of patients suffering from these diseases (see Chap. A5). Malaria parasites are associated with Schüffner's dots in vivax malaria. These are red-staining inclusions within the red cells but discrete from the parasites.

ERYTHROCYTE ARTIFACTS
Artifacts may appear in some part of nearly every blood film. It is essential to have a well-prepared blood film and to examine a number of different areas of the smear to be sure that one is observing a real abnormality. Artifacts may involve erythrocytes, leukocytes, or platelets. Improper staining may cause all the cells to be excessively blue, red, dark, or pale. The polychrome stains are relatively insoluble in water and may precipitate on the surface of the film during the staining procedure. The stain may precipitate as fine granules on or around erythrocytes or leukocytes or may be deposited at random over large areas of the slide.

Vacuolation of the erythrocyte   In some blood films a variable number of erythrocytes will appear to contain one or several vacuoles of variable size distributed irregularly through the cytoplasm, but usually near the center of the cell. These vacuoles appear to expand as the focus is moved from the plane of the cell, and this phenomenon is the basis for their recognition.

Target cells   In a few areas of a film there may be a number of erythrocytes with the configuration of target cells. In such instances these target cells must be considered artifacts, since in those pathologic conditions characterized by target cells, they are evenly distributed over the slide.

Loss of central pallor   Again, in some parts of a blood film there may be cells which appear as solid red discs without the usual central pallor. Such cells are readily differentiated from spherocytes because of their nearly normal size and uneven distribution in the smear.

Distortion of shape   Distortion of shape may occur in some films as a result of the cells pressing upon one another. Such cells may assume a variety of forms, including teardrop, oblong, etc. This artifact can be recognized readily because the abnormal shapes of adjacent cells are complementary, reminiscent of a jigsaw puzzle.

Crescent cells   These are large, pale cells which have assumed a crescent shape during preparation of the blood film.

Crenated cells (echinocytes)   Crenated cells are covered with small projections which may have sharp or rounded ends. The formation of echinocytes is discussed in Chap. 29.

PLATELET MORPHOLOGY AND NUMBERS
Platelets appear in normal blood as small blue bodies with red or purple granules. Normal platelets average about 1 to 2 μm in diameter but show wide variation in shape from round to elongated, cigar-shaped forms. A rough estimate of the platelet count can be made by observation of the stained blood film. If the platelet count is normal, several platelets (individually or in small clumps) should be visible in each oil-immersion field. There should be one platelet present for every 10 to 20 erythrocytes. This study should be made on all films of peripheral blood. In improperly prepared films the platelets may form large aggregates in some areas and

TABLE 2-3   Normal leukocyte count, differential count, and hemoglobin concentration at various ages

Age	Leukocytes, total	Neutrophils Total	Band	Segmented	Eosinophils	Basophils	Lymphocytes	Monocytes	Hemoglobin, g/dl blood
12 mo	11.4(6.0–17.5)	3.5(1.5–8.5)	0.35	3.2	0.30(0.05–0.70)	0.05(0–0.20)	7.0(4.0–10.5)	0.55(0.05–1.1)	11.6(9.0–14.6)
		31	*3.1*	*28*	*2.6*	*0.4*	*61*	*4.8*	
4 yr	9.1(5.5–15.5)	3.8(1.5–8.5)	0.27(0–1.0)	3.5(1.5–7.5)	0.25(0.02–0.65)	0.05(0–0.20)	4.5(2.0–8.0)	0.45(0–0.8)	12.6(9.6–15.5)
		42	*3.0*	*39*	*2.8*	*0.6*	*50*	*5.0*	
6 yr	8.5(5.0–14.5)	4.3(1.5–8.0)	0.25(0–1.0)	4.0(1.5–7.0)	0.23(0–0.65)	0.05(0–0.20)	3.5(1.5–7.0)	0.40(0–0.8)	12.7(10.0–15.5)
		51	*3.0*	*48*	*2.7*	*0.6*	*42*	*4.7*	
10 yr	8.1(4.5–13.5)	4.4(1.8–8.0)	0.24(0–1.0)	4.2(1.8–7.0)	0.20(0–0.60)	0.04(0–0.20)	3.1(1.5–6.5)	0.35(0–0.8)	13.0(10.7–15.5)
		54	*3.0*	*51*	*2.4*	*0.5*	*38*	*4.3*	
21 yr	7.4(4.5–11.0)	4.4(1.8–7.7)	0.22(0–0.7)	4.2(1.8–7.0)	0.20(0–0.45)	0.04(0–0.20)	2.5(1.0–4.8)	0.30(0–0.8)	♂15.8(14.0–18.0)
		59	*3.0*	*56*	*2.7*	*0.5*	*34*	*4.0*	♀13.9(11.5–16.0)

NOTE: Values are expressed as "cells $\times 10^3/\mu l$." The numbers in italic type are percentages.
SOURCE: P. L. Altman and D. S. Dittmer (eds.), *Blood and Other Body Fluids*. Federation of American Societies for Experimental Biology, Washington, 1961. By permission.

appear to be diminished or absent in others. The occurrence of giant platelets or platelet masses may indicate a myeloproliferative disorder (Chaps. 23 through 26) or absence of the spleen.

PLATELET ARTIFACTS

Superimposition   A platelet will occasionally overlie an erythrocyte, where it may be mistaken for an inclusion body or a parasite. The differentiation depends on the observation of a halo around the platelet, determination that it lies above the plane of the erythrocyte, and observation of the characteristics of a normal platelet in the "inclusion."

Aggregation   As noted above platelets may form masses in some films. These are readily recognized, but this maldistribution may create a mistaken impression of thrombocytopenia if the aggregates are not detected. Platelet clumping may be due to platelet agglutinins in the blood [45] (see Chap. 141).

Platelet satellitism   On some blood films, for unknown reasons, platelets adhere to neutrophils and can be observed surrounding these cells in large numbers [45].

LEUKOCYTE MORPHOLOGY

In examining films made on a glass slide, it must be remembered that the distribution of leukocytes is not uniform and the larger cells, such as monocytes and polymorphonuclear leukocytes, will tend to be concentrated on the edges and at the end of the film [59]. With cover-slip preparations this uneven distribution is less likely to occur. In patients with leukopenia it may be necessary to concentrate the leukocytes by centrifuging blood anticoagulated with EDTA or heparin and preparing films from the top layer of the packed cells. This "buffy coat" contains primarily leukocytes and platelets. The cells which normally are found in peripheral blood are polymorphonuclear leukocytes of the neutrophilic, eosinophilic, and basophilic types; lymphocytes; and monocytes. These cell types are described below, and normal values for the differential count are presented in Table 2-3. More detailed discussions of the morphology of these cells are found in Chaps. 80, 90, 91, 94, and 101.

POLYMORPHONUCLEAR LEUKOCYTES

Neutrophils are round cells ranging from 10 to 14 μm in diameter (see Plate 1). The nucleus is lobulated, with from two to five lobes connected by a thin thread of chromatin. The chromatin stains purple and is coarse and arranged in clumps. The nucleus of from 1 to 16 percent of the neutrophils from female patients may have an appendage shaped like a drumstick and attached to one lobe by a thin strand of chromatin (Plate 1). A similar appendage attached by a broad base also occurs. The cytoplasm is pink and contains many small purple granules distributed evenly throughout the cell, although they may not be apparent when they lie over the nucleus.

Bands or *stabs* are identical to mature polymorphonuclear leukocytes except that the nucleus is U-shaped or has rudimentary lobes connected by a thick band rather than a thread (see Plate 1).

Eosinophils are round cells of approximately the same size as neutrophils. The nucleus usually has only two lobes. The chromatin pattern is the same as that in the neutrophil, but the nucleus tends to be more lightly stained. The differentiating characteristic of these cells is the presence of many refractile, orange-red granules which are distributed evenly through the cell and may be visible overlying the nucleus (see Plate 1). These granules are larger than those in the neutrophil and are more uniform in size. Occasionally some of the granules in eosinophils stain light blue rather than orange-red.

Basophils are similar to the other polymorphonuclear cells, but the nucleus may stain more faintly than in the other forms, and the large deeply basophilic granules are fewer in number and less regular in size and shape than in the eosinophil. The granules are visible overlying the nucleus and, in some cells, almost completely obscure the lightly stained nuclear chromatin (see Plate 1).

LYMPHOCYTES

Lymphocytes in peripheral blood are usually small, about 10 μm in diameter, but larger forms up to 20 μm are seen. The small lymphocyte is round and contains a relatively large, round, densely stained nucleus in which the chromatin is distributed in coarse masses (see Plate 1). The nuclear membrane is dense. The cytoplasm is scanty and stains pale blue. It may contain a few large red granules (azurophilic granules). There is often a perinuclear clear zone. In the large lymphocytes the nucleus is relatively small and the chromatin distribution is less coarse than that in the small lymphocyte. The nucleus is usually round but may be oval or indented. The cytoplasm is abundant and may contain a few red (azurophilic) granules. The outline of the cytoplasm is often distorted by adjacent erythrocytes.

MONOCYTES

These are the largest cells in the peripheral blood, usually measuring from 15 to 22 μm in diameter. The nucleus is of various shapes—round, kidney-shaped, oval, or lobulated—and frequently appears to be folded (see Plate 1). The chromatin is arranged in fine strands with sharply defined margins. The cytoplasm is light blue or gray and contains numerous, fine lilac or purple granules.

LEUKOCYTE INCLUSIONS

In addition to the granules normally present in leukocytes, there may be inclusions indicative of disease.

Increased size of granules   In some patients the granules of the neutrophils are larger than normal and stain more darkly, often assuming a dark blue-black color. This has been called *toxic granulation*. These granules should not be confused with large basophilic granules. In *Alder's anomaly*, coarse, dark granules are found in the polymorphonuclear leukocytes and large azurophilic granules are found in the polymorphonuclear leukocytes and in some lymphocytes and monocytes. In *gargoylism*, the leukocytes contain similar abnormal granules, which are sometimes called *Reilly bodies*. Huge misshapen granules are found in the polymorphonuclear leukocytes and giant azurophilic granules are present in the lymphocytes in patients exhibiting the *Chédiak-Higashi anomaly* (see Fig. 89-1).

Light-blue cytoplasmic inclusions   Light-blue, round or oval bodies about 1 to 2 μm in diameter may be seen in the cytoplasm of neutrophils of patients with infections or burns and with the Chédiak-Higashi anomaly. These have been named *Döhle bodies*. Similar inclusions are seen in patients with the May-Heggelin anomaly.

Auer rods   These are sharply outlined, red-staining rods found in the cytoplasm in immature cells in the blood of patients with acute myelogenous or monocytic leukemia (see Plate 7).

LEUKOCYTE ARTIFACTS

Size   Granulocytes and monocytes will appear to be small in the thick parts of a film because they retained a more spherical shape while the film dried.

Compression of cells   Leukocytes may be compressed by surrounding erythrocytes with consequent distortion of the outline of the cytoplasm or nucleus.

Crushed cells   During the process of preparing the film, leukocytes may be damaged, with consequent alteration in their appearance and staining. In some damaged leukocytes the cytoplasm may appear intact but the nucleus appears enlarged, with alteration of the chromatin so that the strands appear more homogeneous, stain with a distinct reddish hue, and are more widely separated. Such cells may appear to have a large blue nucleolus and may resemble reticulum cells. These cells have been called *basket cells*. More extensively damaged cells are also seen in which the cytoplasmic membrane has been stripped from the nucleus, leaving the distorted nucleus lying free or surrounded by granules which have spilled from the cytoplasm.

Radial segmentation of the nuclei (Reider cells)   Use of oxalated blood to prepare films results in the appearance of abnormal segmentation of the nuclei of leukocytes. This segmentation differs from that of the granulocytes in that the lobes appear to radiate from a single point, giving a clover-leaf or cartwheel picture. Extensive changes can occur within an hour or two in oxalated blood. Less extensive changes occur with other anticoagulants, including EDTA.

Vacuolation   Vacuoles may develop in the nucleus and cytoplasm of leukocytes from blood anticoagulated with EDTA. Vacuoles may be associated with swelling of the nuclei and loss of granules from the cytoplasm [11].

"Pseudophagocytosis"   Occasionally a small lymphocyte or, more often, an erythrocyte will lie atop a granulocyte and monocyte and thus appear to have been ingested. The true position of such cells can be suspected because they will be surrounded by a halo and will come into sharp focus in a plane above that of the larger cell.

Endothelial cells   If the blood film is prepared from the first drop of blood issuing from the fingertip wound, endothelial cells may be present singly or in clumps.

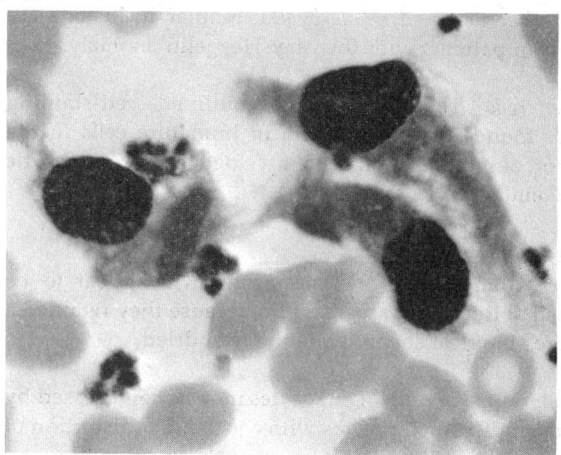

FIGURE 2-1 Endothelial cells in blood film. (Courtesy of Dr. H. A. Wurzel.)

Such cells are illustrated in Fig. 2-1. These cells appear quite immature and may be misinterpreted as blasts or metastatic tumor cells.

AUTOMATED DIFFERENTIAL LEUKOCYTE COUNTING

Automated differential leukocyte-counting devices have been developed using either flow systems [60–62], with analysis of cell size and biochemical parameters, or pattern recognition of cells on fixed and stained blood films [63–67]. The flow systems permit rapid analysis of large numbers of cells, thus increasing the precision of the count and detecting cells which are present in small numbers. Measurements of light scattering [60–62] are utilized to distinguish cell size. Methods have been developed for obtaining differential leukocyte counts based on volume alone [68–74]. In other systems the cells are further characterized by measuring light absorption, either of unstained cells or after staining, or fluorescence of cell constituents after staining with fluorescent dyes [60,62,75]. In some systems, two or more parameters, such as light scattering and light absorption at one or more wavelengths, can be measured simultaneously [61,62]. Some cell properties can be measured without fixation, minimizing the introduction of artifacts and permitting subsequent cell sorting for further study [76]. Using a slit-scan system with a band of light only a few micrometers in width, it is possible to determine the ratio of nuclear diameter to cell diameter for individual cells [60]. Interference by red cells is minimized by treating the samples with lytic reagents, and cell ghosts are eliminated from consideration by utilizing a suspending medium of refractive index such that they are not detected [61]. Platelets are sufficiently small that they do not interfere. Single cells must be presented to the analytical component of the system, and this is accomplished by utilizing a flow cell with a narrow sample stream (e.g., 60 μm). To avoid occlusion of the small capillary tube in the flow cell by cell clumps or debris, the cell suspension is sheathed by a layer of inert liquid of refractive index identical to that of the sample fluid [61,62,77].

The Hemalog D white cell differential system is a flow device which classifies cells by size and staining properties [61]. Basophils are identified in one channel, monocytes in a second channel, and a combination of lymphocytes, neutrophils, eosinophils, "large unclassified cells," and "high peroxidase cells" in a third channel. Basophils are detected after staining with Alcian blue dye, using a technique (low pH, quaternary ammonium salts, and lanthanum ions) which minimizes nuclear staining with that dye. Monocytes are identified as large cells which stain intensely for nonspecific esterase activity measured with α-naphthylbutyrate substrate and coupling of the α-naphthol product with diazotized basic fuchsin. Inhibitors of neutrophil and plasma esterases are added to the reaction mixture. Neutrophils and eosinophils are identified after peroxidase staining, utilizing a mixture of 4-chloro-1-naphthol and H_2O_2 at pH 3.2. Cells are fixed with formaldehyde prior to staining in order to ensure localization of the enzyme. Eosinophils are differentiated from neutrophils by their more intense peroxidase stain. A small proportion of neutrophils stain more intensely than the remainder ("high peroxidase cells") but are differentiated from eosinophils by light scattering. Monocytes, atypical lymphocytes, and immature granulocytes do not stain with the peroxidase reagents and are detected as "large unstained cells." Lymphocytes are identified as small unstained cells.

This system permits classification of 10,000 cells per minute in each channel. The results agree with manual differential counts of 200 or more cells [78,79]. This system has also been used for analysis of variations in the basophil count in disease [80,81], and it and similar systems have been utilized for study of leukemia [82–84] and monocyte esterase activity [85]. It has proved useful in detecting abnormalities in peroxidase levels in leukocytes [81,86]. Platelet satellitism may cause an artifactual increase in the number of high-peroxidase-activity cells detected by the Hemalog D [87]. A modified version of this instrument (Technicon H 6000) utilizes only the peroxidase and basophil channels and provides an automatically prepared and stained blood film for examination if necessary [88].

The theory and equipment design of flow systems for single-cell analysis are well developed and will certainly continue to be improved. Significant limitations are the availability of specific stains and markers [89–92] and the establishment of the clinical and biological significance of the data. Interpretation of discrepancies between the data generated by the automatic systems and that resulting from traditional methods of differential counting is a problem at present. Extensive research will be required to establish the role of these new instruments in clinical practice.

Pattern-recognition systems employ blood films prepared on glass slides by the traditional smear ("wedge") technique [67,93] or by a "spinner" method [66,94]. The spinner technique produces even distribution of cells on the slide by centrifugal force applied by rapid rotation of the slide after a blood sample has been placed on its surface. The stained cells are examined by digital image processing, utilizing a television microscope system interfaced with a computer [63–67]. The slide is automatically moved on a mechanical stage and cells are centered in the image field. Color differences are measured by consecutive scans of the cell using color filters selected as appropriate for the stain used [64,65]. Cytologic features such as cell size, nuclear density, cytoplasmic color, and cytoplasmic texture are evaluated, and normal patterns are established for cells of known classes [64]. The characteristics of the unknown cells are compared with the known patterns in the computer memory, and the cell is identified as a particular type if a sufficient number of matching features are present. Lymphocytes, monocytes, neutrophils, eosinophils, and basophils can be classified accurately by such methods [64].

Commercial machines using these principles have been developed. One of the earliest instruments of the type was the LARC (Leukocyte Automatic Recognition Computer) [66], which incorporated a computerized stage that recorded the coordinates of each cell counted so that unclassified cells could be reviewed visually by the operator. The LARC gave results comparable to standard procedures, except that band neutrophil counts were higher and segmented neutrophil counts lower than those obtained with manual methods [95]. Abnormal cells were reliably detected by the automatic system [95,96]. The LARC is no longer commericially available.

The Hematrak system also utilizes a computerized pattern-recognition method to identify nucleated cells on Wright's-stained blood films prepared by the wedge or spinner technique [67,96–99]. The technician reviews the slide for quality of preparation and staining, evaluates red cell morphology and platelet count, selects an area of the slide suitable for differential leukocyte counting, and activates the electronic system. The machine can be instructed to stop for any unidentified cells so that the technician can provide visual identification. The system recognizes segmented neutrophils, bands, lymphocytes, monocytes, eosinophils, and basophils. Counts obtained with the instrument agree satisfactorily with those obtained manually or with other machines [96,99].

Another instrument, the "diff 3 System," utilizes a stained blood film to perform a differential leukocyte count, evaluate red cell morphology, and estimate number of platelets (high, normal, low). It has been reported to function satisfactorily in a clinical setting, except for inaccuracies in estimating hypochromia [100].

The ADC500 instrument classifies 500 nucleated cells on stained spun blood films [101,102]. Eleven categories are identified automatically, and the operator has the option to review any category. Classification of 500 cells improves the precision of the method over those using 100 cell counts [101,102]. Artifacts on the spun smears occur occasionally and reduce the accuracy of the method [101]. The number of monocytes detected by the ADC500 appears to be greater than that obtained by manual methods [102], possibly because of the use of spun blood films rather than wedge smears in the ADC500 [102].

The Honeywell ACS 1000 locates nucleated cells on stained wedge blood films [103]. The cells may be viewed through a microscope, or the images may be projected on a television screen for interpretation by the operator [103]. The blood film is scanned automatically at a rate which is adjustable by the operator. The speed of operation may not be greater than that achieved by a skilled technician using manual methods, although the instrument does provide for rapid scanning of blood films [103].

Other systems which permit identification of additional leukocyte types [104] and evaluation of unstained erythrocytes on blood films using Soret absorption [100] have been proposed. As with the flow systems, detailed evaluations of the pattern-recognition methods under field conditions will be required to define their role in clinical hematology.

The development of automated leukocyte differential counting systems has led to increased interest in the statistical significance of the leukocyte differential count. In the classical manual methods, counts of 100 cells are generally accepted, although large errors are inherent in such small numbers [106]. The automated instruments provide ready access to classification of several thousand cells in the flow systems and several hundred in the pattern-recognition systems. The computer systems which are integral parts of these instruments can be adapted to calculate and report the reliability of the data [101,102]. Implementation of these concepts and further control of variables such as time of specimen collection [107] and method of specimen preparation [93] to improve precision of the determinations will enhance the clinical utility of the differential leukocyte count of the future.

The need for examination of the blood film

The quantitative determinations discussed earlier in this chapter—hemoglobin, hematocrit, and erythrocyte, platelet, and leukocyte counts—permit description of the blood in sufficient detail that the physician will often recognize the need for further study if there is such a need. The probability of detecting early abnormalities, such as incipient pernicious anemia, is further increased if the MCH, MCV, and MCHC are provided by the automatic counting device, or calculated, assuming that the erythrocyte counts have been performed

TABLE 2-4   Diseases in which the blood count may be normal but examination of the blood film will suggest the disorder

Disease	Findings on blood film
Compensated acquired hemolytic anemia	Spherocytosis, polychromatophilia, erythrocyte agglutination
Hereditary spherocytosis	Spherocytosis, polychromatophilia
Hemoglobin C disease	Target cells
Thalassemia trait	Hypochromia, target cells
Elliptocytosis	Elliptocytes
Lead poisoning	Basophilic stippling
Incipient pernicious anemia or folic acid deficiency	Macrocytosis, hypersegmented neutrophils
Multiple myeloma, macroglobulinemia	Rouleau formation
Malaria, babesiosis	Parasites in the erythrocytes
Consumptive coagulopathy	Schizocytes
Mechanical hemolysis	Schizocytes
Severe infection	Relative increase in neutrophils; increased band forms
Infectious mononucleosis	Atypical lymphocytes
Agranulocytosis	Decreased neutrophils, relative increase in lymphocytes
Allergic reactions	Eosinophilia
Chronic lymphocytic leukemia (early)	Relative lymphocytosis
Acute leukemia (early)	Blast forms

with sufficient accuracy. A significant number of diseases involving both erythrocytes and leukocytes may not be detected by these studies but are suggested from examination of a stained blood film. The best person to examine the blood film is the physician who is experienced in interpreting blood cell morphology and has sufficient knowledge of the patient to direct his or her attention along specific lines. While some technicians are very skillful in evaluating blood films, routine examination by such personnel may fail to discover abnormalities which are readily appreciated when the blood film is viewed with complete understanding of the clinical circumstances.

A number of diseases in which the blood counts may be normal but in which examination of the blood film will suggest the disorder are listed in Table 2-4.

Changes in the leukocyte count and hemoglobin level with age

The normal differential leukocyte count varies with age (Table 2-3). As described in Chap. 5, in the first few days polymorphonuclear neutrophils are predominant, but thereafter lymphocytes account for the majority of leukocytes. This persists up to about 4 to 5 years of age, when the polymorphonuclear leukocyte again becomes the predominant cell and remains so throughout the rest of childhood and adult life. Changes in the leukocyte count in old age are discussed in Chap. 6. The leukocyte count may decrease slightly in old age, due to a fall in the lymphocyte count. Leukopenia, due primarily to neutropenia, has been reported to occur frequently in

blacks in the United States [108–112]. Leukopenia has also been reported in African blacks [113,114].

Another parameter which varies with age is hemoglobin level (Table 2-3). Changes in hemoglobin in the neonatal period are discussed in Chap. 5. After the first week or two of extrauterine life, the hemoglobin and hematocrit fall from levels of about 17 g/dl and 54 percent, respectively, to levels of about 12 g/dl and 35 percent by 2 months of age. Thereafter the levels remain relatively constant throughout the first year of life. Although the lower limit of normal values throughout childhood is presented as 9 g/dl in many studies, it is likely that this level of hemoglobin is found only in children with nutritional deficiency, and any child with a hemoglobin level below 11 g/dl or hematocrit of less than 33 percent should be considered to be anemic [5,115–118]. Changes in hemoglobin levels in the elderly are discussed in Chap. 6.

Storage of anticoagulated blood prior to examination

Anticoagulated venous blood is often used for laboratory study, and occasionally it is desirable to repeat tests on blood which has been stored for several hours. It is therefore important to have some idea of the storage properties of the formed elements in anticoagulated blood. Some data on storage stability are presented in Table 2-5.

Blood films should be prepared promptly in order to avoid artifacts in the leukocytes, such as radial segmentation of the nuclei (see above).

TABLE 2-5   Effects of anticoagulants on stability of blood formed elements on storage

Anticoagulant	Storage temperature	Hours of storage without change in the parameter measured				
		Hemoglobin	Hematocrit	Platelet count	White cell count	Reticulocyte count
EDTA*	4°	48	48	24	48	48
	23°	48	24	5	24	48
EDTA†	8°	—	—	—	24	—
	25°	—	—	—	24	—
Double oxalate†	8°	—	—	—	24	—
	25°	—	—	—	6	—
ACD†	8°	—	—	—	24	—
	25°	—	—	—	24	—

*Data of Lampasso [119]
†Data of Gagon et al. [22].

References

1. Crosby, W. M., Munn, J. J., and Furth, F. W.: Standardizing a method for clinical hemoglobinometry. *U.S. Armed Forces Med. J.* 5:693, 1954.

2. International Committee for Standardization in Haematology: Recommendations for haemoglobinometry in human blood. *Br. J. Haematol. [Suppl.]* 13:71, 1967.

3. Garn, S. M., Smith, N. J., and Clark, D. C.: Lifelong differences in hemoglobin levels between blacks and whites. *J. Natl. Med. Assn.* 67:91, 1975.

4. Kraemer, M. J., McFarland, R. M., Dillon, T. L., and Smith, N. J.: Letter to the editor. *Am. J. Clin. Nutr.* 28:566, 1975.

5. Dallman, P. R., Barr, G. D., Allen, C. M., and Shinefield, H. R.: Hemoglobin concentration in white, black and Oriental children: Is there a need for separate criteria in screening for anemia? *Am. J. Clin. Nutr.* 31:377, 1978.

6. Garn, S. M., Ryan, A. S., Owen, G. M., and Abraham, S.: Income matched black-white hemoglobin differences after correction for low transferrin saturations. *Am. J. Clin. Nutr.* 34:1645, 1981.

7. Henry, J. B.: *Todd-Sanford-Davidsohn: Clinical Diagnosis and Management by Laboratory Methods*, 16th ed. Saunders, Philadelphia, 1979, p. 869.

8. Wintrobe, M. M.: Macroscopic examination of the blood. *Am. J. Med. Sci* 185:58, 1933.

9. Heller, V. G., and Paul, H.: Changes in cell volume produced by varying concentrations of different anticoagulants. *J. Lab. Clin. Med.* 19:777, 1934.

10. Hadley, G. G., and Weiss, S. P.: Further notes on use of salts of ethylenediamine tetraacetic acid (EDTA) as anticoagulants. *Am. J. Clin. Pathol.* 25:1090, 1955.

11. Sacker, L. S.: Specimen Collection, in *Quality Control in Haematology*, edited by S. M. Lewis and J. F. Coster. Academic, London, 1975, p. 211.

12. Chaplin, H., Jr., and Mollison, P. L.: Correction for plasma trapped in the red cell column of the hematocrit. *Blood* 7:127, 1952.

13. Owen, C. A., Jr., and Power, M. H.: Intercellular plasma of centrifuged human erythrocytes as measured by means of iodo¹³¹ albumin. *J. Appl. Physiol.* 5:323, 1953.

14. Garby, L., and Vuille, J. C.: The amount of trapped plasma in a high speed microcapillary hematocrit centrifuge. *Scand. J. Lab. Clin. Invest.* 13:642, 1961.

15. England, J. M., Walford, D. M., and Waters, D. A. W.: Reassessment of the reliability of the hematocrit. *Br. J. Haematol.* 23:247, 1972.

16. Fairbanks, V. A.: Nonequivalence of automated and manual hematocrit and erythrocyte indices. *Am. J. Clin. Pathol.* 73:55, 1980.

17. Enconomou-Marrou, C., and Tsenghi, C.: Plasma trapping in the centrifuged red cells of children with severe thalassemia. *J. Clin. Pathol.* 18:203, 1965.

18. Furth, F. W.: Effect of spherocytosis on volume of trapped plasma in a high speed micro-capillary hematocrit centrifuge. *J. Lab. Clin. Med.* 48:421, 1956.

19. Pinkerton, P. H., Spence, I., Ogilvie, J. C., Ronald, W. A., Marchant, P., and Ray, P. K.: An assessment of the Coulter Counter Model S. *J. Clin. Pathol.* 23:68, 1970.

20. Biggs, R., and MacMillan, R. L.: The errors of some haematological methods as they are used in a routing laboratory. *J. Clin. Pathol.* 1:269, 1948.

21. McDonough, J. R., et al.: The relationship of hematocrit to cardiovascular states of health in the Negro and white population of Evans County, Georgia. *J. Chron. Dis.* 18:243, 1965.

22. Gagon, T. E., Athens, J. W., Boggs, D. R., and Cartwright, G. E.: An evaluation of the variance of leukocyte counts as performed with the hemocytometer, Coulter and Fisher instruments. *Am. J. Clin. Pathol.* 46:684, 1966.

23. Bull, B. S., Schneiderman, M. A., and Brecher, G.: Platelet counts with the Coulter Counter. *Am. J. Clin. Pathol.* 44:678, 1965.

24. Bull, B. S.: Aids to electronic platelet counting. *Am. J. Clin. Pathol.* 54:707, 1970.

25. Brecher, G., Schneiderman, M., and Williams, G. Z.: Evaluation of an electronic blood cell counter. *Am. J. Clin. Pathol.* 26:1439, 1956.

26. Mattern, C. F., Brackett, F. S., and Olson, B. J.: Determination of number and size of particles by electronic gating. I. Blood cells. *J. Appl. Physiol.* 10:56, 1957.

27. Richar, W. J., and Breakell, E. S.: Evaluation of an electronic particle counter for the counting of white blood cells. *Am. J. Clin. Pathol.* 31:384, 1959.

28. Saunders, A. M., and Scott, F.: Hematologic automation by use of continuous flow systems. *J. Histochem. Cytochem.* 22:707, 1974.

29. Simmons, A., Schwebbauer, M. L., and Earhart, C. A.: Automated platelet counting with the AutoAnalyzer. *J. Lab. Clin. Med.* 77:656, 1971.

30. Brittin, G. M., Dew, S. A., and Fewell, E. K.: Automated optical counting of blood platelets. *Blood* 38:422, 1971.

31. Lewis, S. M., and Bentley, S. A.: Haemocytometry by laser-beam optics: Evaluation of the Hemac 630L. *J. Clin. Pathol.* 30:54, 1977.

32. Lappin, T. R. J., Lamont, A., and Nelson, M. G.: An evaluation of the Celloscope 401 electronic blood cell counter. *J. Clin. Pathol.* 25:539, 1972.

33. Shulman, G., and Yapit, M. K.: Whole-blood platelet counts with an impedance-type particle counter. *Am. J. Clin. Pathol.* 73:104, 1980.

34. Day, H. J., Young, E., and Helfrich, M.: An evaluation of a whole-blood platelet counter. *Am. J. Clin. Pathol.* 73:588, 1980.

35. Bacus, J. W., Watt, S., and Trobaugh, F. E., Jr.: Clinical evaluation of a new electrical impedance instrument for counting platelets in whole blood. *Am. J. Clin. Pathol.* 73:655, 1980.

36. England, J. M., and Down, M. C.: Measurement of the mean cell volume using electronic particle counters. *Br. J. Haematol.* 32:403, 1976.

37. Spielman, L., and Goren, S. L.: Improving resolution in Coulter counting by hydrodynamic focusing. *J. Coll. Interface Sci.* 26:175, 1968.

38. Schulz, J., and Thom, R.: Electrical sizing and counting of platelets in whole blood. *Med. Biol. Eng.* 11:447, 1973.

39. Fry, G. L., and Hoak, J. C.: Improved method for electronic counting of platelets. *J. Lab. Clin. Med.* 74:536, 1969.

40. Wintrobe, M. M.: Anemia: Classification and treatment on the basis of differences in the average volume and hemoglobin content of the red corpuscles. *Arch. Intern. Med.* 54:256, 1934.

41. Wintrobe, M. M.: The size and hemoglobin content of the erythrocyte. *J. Lab. Clin. Med.* 17:899, 1932.

42. Rose, M. S.: Epitaph for the M.C.H.C. *Br. Med. J.* 4:169, 1971.

43. Beutler, E.: The red cell indices in the diagnosis of iron deficiency anemia. *Ann. Intern. Med.* 50:313, 1959.

44. Henry, J. B.: *Todd-Sanford-Davidsohn: Clinical Diagnosis and Management by Laboratory Methods*, 16th ed. Saunders, Philadelphia, 1979, p. 881.

45. Kjeldsberg, C. R., and Hershgold, E. J.: Spurious thrombocytopenia. *JAMA* 227:628, 1974.

46. Brecher, G., and Cronkite, E. P.: Morphology and enumeration of human blood platelets. *J. Appl. Physiol.* 3:365, 1958.

47. Brecher, G., Schneiderman, M., and Cronkite, E. P.: The reproducibility and constancy of the platelet count. *Am. J. Clin. Pathol.* 23:15, 1953.

48. Paulus, J.-M.: Platelet size in man. *Blood* 46:321, 1975.

49. Bull, B. S., and Zucker, M. B.: Changes in platelet volume produced by temperature, metabolic inhibitors, and aggregating agents. *Proc. Soc. Exp. Biol. Med.* 120:296, 1965.

50. Bessis, M.: Phase contrast microscopy and electron microscopy applied to the blood cells. *Blood* 10:272, 1955.

51. Sabin, F. R.: Studies of living human blood-cells. *Bull. Johns Hopkins Hosp.* 34:277, 1923.

52. Doan, C. A., Cunningham, R. S., and Sabin, F. R.: Experimental studies on the origin and maturation of avian and mammalian red blood cells. *Contrib. Embryol.* 16:163, 1925.

53. Schwind, J. L.: The supravital method in the study of the cytology of blood and marrow cells. *Blood* 5:597, 1950.

54. Discombe, G.: L'Origine des corps de Howell-Jolly et des anneaux de Cabot. *Sang* 29:262, 1948.

55. Picard, D.: Nature et signification des auneaux de Cabot des hématies. *Comptes Rendu Soc. Biol. (Paris)* 147:1451, 1953.

56. Kass, L.: Origin and composition of Cabot rings in pernicious anemia. *Am. J. Clin. Pathol.* 64:53, 1975.

57. Valentine, W. N., Fink, K., Paglia, D. E., Harris, S. R., and Adams, W. S.: Hereditary hemolytic anemia with human erythrocyte pyrimidine-5'-nucleotidase deficiency. *J. Clin. Invest.* 54:866, 1974.

58. Valentine, W. N.: The Stratton lecture: Hemolytic anemias and inborn errors of metabolism. *Blood* 54:549, 1979.

59. Davidson, E.: The distribution of cells in peripheral blood smears. *J. Clin. Pathol.* 11:410, 1958.

60. Fulwyler, M. J.: Status quo in flow-through cytometry. *J. Histochem. Cytochem.* 22:605, 1975.

61. Mansberg, H. P., Saunders, A. M., and Groner, W.: The Hemalog D white cell differential system. *J. Histochem. Cytochem.* 22:711, 1974.

62. Curbelo, R., Schildkraut, E. R., Hirchfeld, T., Webb, R. H., Block, M. J., and Shapiro, H. M.: A generalized machine for automated flow cytology system design. *J. Histochem. Cytochem.* 24:388, 1976.

63. Ingram, M., and Preston, K., Jr.: Automatic analysis of blood cells. *Sci. Am.* 223(5):73, 1970.

64. Bacus, J. W., and Gose, E. E.: Leukocyte pattern recognition. *IEEE Trans. Systems, Man, and Cybernetics* SMC-2:513, 1972.

65. Brenner, J. T., Gelsema, E. S., Necheles, T. F., Neurath, P. W., Selles, W. D., and Vastola, E.: Automated classification of normal and abnormal leukocytes. *J. Histochem. Cytochem.* 22:697, 1974.

66. Megla, G. K.: The LARC automatic white blood cell analyzer. *Acta Cytol.* 17:3, 1973.

67. Dutcher, T. F., Benzel, J. E., Egan, J. J., Hart, D. J., and Christopher, E. A.: Evaluation of an automated differential leukocyte counting system. I. Instrument description and reproducibility studies. *Am. J. Clin. Pathol.* 62:525, 1974.

68. Gauthier, J., and Harel, P.: Human leukocytes: Their size distribution and mean corpuscular volume. *Can. Med. Assoc. J.* 97:793, 1967.

69. Oberjat, T. E., Zucher, R. M., and Cassen, B.: Rapid and reliable differential counts on dilute leukocyte suspensions. *J. Lab. Clin. Med.* 76:518, 1970.

70. Humphries, R. K., and Miller, R. G.: Volume analysis of human peripheral blood leukocytes. *Ser. Haematol.* 4:142, 1972.

71. Hughes-Jones, N. C., Norley, I., Young, J. M. S., and England, J. M.: Differential white cell counts by frequency distribution analysis of cell volumes. *J. Clin. Pathol.* 27:673, 1974.

72. England, J. M., Hewer, M. G., Bashfor, C. C., Hughes-Jones, N. C., and Down, M. C.: Simple method for automating the differential leucocyte-count. *Lancet* 1:492, 1975.

73. England, J. M., Down, M. C., Bashfor, C. C., and Sabry-Grant, R.: Differential leucocyte-counts on Coulter counter Model S. *Lancet* 1:1134, 1976.

74. Wycherly, P. A., and O'Shea, M. J.: Abridged differential leucocyte counts provided by a Coulter Channelyzer in a routine haematology laboratory. *J. Clin. Pathol.* 31:271, 1978.

75. Van Dilla, M. A., Trujillo, T. T., Mullaney, P. F., and Coulter, J. R.: Cell microfluorometry: A method for rapid fluorescence measurement. *Science* 163:1213, 1969.

76. Steinhamp, J. A., Fulwyler, M. J., Coulter, J. R., Hieber, R. D., Horney, J. L., and Mullaney, P. F.: A new multiparameter separator for microscopic particles and biological cells. *Rev. Sci. Instrum.* 44:1301, 1973.

77. Crossland-Taylor, P. J.: A device for counting small particles suspended in a fluid through a tube. *Nature* 171:37, 1953.

78. Pierre, R. V., and O'Sullivan, M. B.: Evaluation of the Hemalog D automated differential leukocyte counter. *Mayo Clin. Proc.* 49:870, 1974.

79. Simmons, A., and Elbert, G.: Hemalog-D and manual differential leukocyte counts: A laboratory comparison of results obtained with blood of hospitalized patients. *Am. J. Clin. Pathol.* 64:512, 1975.

80. Gilbert, H. S., and Ornstein, L.: Basophil counting with a new staining method using Alcian blue. *Blood* 46:279, 1965.

81. Gilbert, H. S.: The clinical application of automated cytochemical techniques in patient management. *Adv. Automated Anal.* 3:51, 1973.

82. Buchner, T., Hiddemann, W., Schneider, R., and Kamanabroo, D.: Zur Praparation von Blut- und Knochenmarkzellen fur die Impulszytophotometrie. *Blut* 28:191, 1974.

83. Ross, D. W., and Bardwell, A.: Automated cytochemistry and the white cell differential in leukemia. *Blood Cells* 6:455, 1980.

84. Arlin, Z. A., Fried, J., and Clarkson, B. O.: Human acute leukemia, in *Flow Cytometry and Sorting*, edited by M. R. Melamud, R. F. Mullaney, and M. L. Mendelsohn. Wiley, New York, 1979, p. 531.

85. Kaplow, L. S., Dauber, H., and Lerner, E.: Assessment of monocytic esterase activity by flow cytophotometry. *J. Histochem. Cytochem.* 24:363, 1976.

86. Bozdech, M. J., Bainton, D. F., and Mustacchi, P.: Partial peroxidase deficiency in neutrophils and eosinophils associated with neurologic disease. Histochemical, cytochemical and biochemical studies. *Am. J. Clin. Pathol.* 73:409, 1980.

87. Larson, J. H., and Pierre, R. V.: Platelet satellitism as a cause of abnormal Hemalog D differential results. *Am. J. Clin. Pathol.* 68:758, 1977.

88. Pierre, R. V.: Automation of blood film preparation and staining utilizing the Technicon autoslide. *Blood Cells* 6:471, 1980.

89. Ornstein, L., and Ansley, H. R.: Spectral matching of classical cytochemistry to automated cytology. *J. Histochem. Cytochem.* 22:453, 1974.

90. Kaplow, L. W.: The application of cytochemistry to automation. *J. Histochem. Cytochem.* 25:990, 1977.

91. Saunders, A. M.: The automation of cytochemical methods for automated cytophotometers. *J. Histochem. Cytochem.* 25:1001, 1977.

92. Adams, L. R., Bourgeois, D., and Kamentsky, L. A.: Cytofluorographic differential leukocyte count, in *Flow Cytometry and Sorting*, edited by M. R. Melamud, P. F. Mullaney, and M. L. Mendelsohn. Wiley, New York, 1979, p. 547.

93. Wenk, R. E.: Comparison of five methods for preparing blood smears. *Am. J. Med. Technol.* 42:71, 1976.

94. Ingram, M., and Minter, P. M.: Semi-automatic preparation of cover glass blood smears using a centrifugal device. *Am. J. Clin. Pathol.* 51:214, 1969.

95. Cotter, D. A., and Sage, B. H. L.: Performance of the LARC™ classifier in clinical laboratories. *J. Histochem. Cytochem.* 24:202, 1976.

96. Rosvoll, R. V., Mengason, A. P., Smith, L., Patel, H. J., Maynard, J., and Connor, F.: Visual and automated differential leukocyte counts. A comparison of three instruments. *Am. J. Clin. Pathol.* 71:695, 1979.

97. Benzel, J. E., Egan, J. J., Hart, D. J., and Christopher, E. A.: Evaluation of an automated differential leukocyte counting system. II. Normal cell identification. *Am. J. Clin. Pathol.* 62:530, 1974.

98. Egan, J. J., Benzel, J. E., Hart, D. J., and Christopher, E. A.: Evaluation of an automated differential leukocyte counting system. III. Detection of abnormal cells. *Am. J. Clin. Pathol.* 62:537, 1974.

99. Basterfield, P. J., and Slade D. B.: Evaluation of the Hematrak white cell differential counting machine. *Med. Lab. Sci.* 35:283, 1978.

100. Schoentag, R. A., and Pedersen, J. T.: Evaluation of an automated blood smear analyzer. *Am. J. Clin. Pathol.* 71:685, 1979.

101. Kingsley, T. C.: The automated differential: Pattern recognition systems, precision, and the spun smear. *Blood Cells* 6:493, 1980.

102. Daoust, P. R.: The clinical detection of variations in the concentrations of leukocyte types: A laboratory comparison of 100-cell manual differential counts on wedge smears and 500-cell counts by the ADC500. *Blood Cells* 6:489, 1980.

103. Clowes, M., Giles, C., Ibbotson, R. M., and Johnson, P. H.: Evaluation of the Honeywell ACS 1000 leucocyte differential counter. *J. Clin. Pathol.* 33:145, 1980.

104. Tycko, D. H., Anbalagan, S., Liu, H. C., and Ornstein, L.: Automatic leukocyte classification using cytochemically stained smears. *J. Histochem. Cytochem.* 24:178, 1976.

105. Bacus, J. W., Belanger, M. G., Aggarwal, R. K., and Trobaugh, F. E., Jr.: Image processing for automated erythrocyte classification. *J. Histochem. Cytochem.* 24:195, 1976.

106. Rumke, C. L., Bezemer, P. D., and Kuik, D. J.: Normal values and least significant differences for differential leukocyte counts. *J. Chronic Dis.* 28:661, 1975.

107. Statland, B. E., Winkel, P., Harris, S. C., Burdsall, M. J., and Saunders, A. M.: Evaluation of biologic sources of variation of leukocyte counts and other hematological quantities using very precise automated analyzers. *Am. J. Clin. Pathol.* 69:48, 1977.

108. Brown, G. O., Jr., Hertig, F. K., and Hamilton, J. R.: Leukopenia in negroes. *N. Engl. J. Med.* 275:1410, 1966.

109. Orfanakis, N. G., Ostlund, R. E., Bishop, C. R., and Athens, J. W.: Normal blood leukocyte concentration values. *Am. J. Clin. Pathol.* 53:647, 1970.

110. Karayalcin, G., Rosher, F., and Sawitsky, A.: Pseudoneutropenia in Negroes. A normal phenomenon. *N.Y. State J. Med.* 72:1815, 1972.

111. Caramihai, E., Karayalcin, G., Aballi, A. J., and Lanzkowsky, P.: Leukocyte count differences in healthy white and black children 1 to 5 years of age. *J. Pediatr.* 86:252, 1975.

112. Mason, B., Lessin, L., and Schechter, G. P.: Marrow granulocyte reserves in black Americans. Hydrocortisone-induced granulocytosis in the "benign" neutropenia of the black. *Am. J. Med.* 67:201, 1979.

113. Shaper, A. G., and Lewis, P.: Genetic neutropenia in people of African origin. *Lancet* 2:1021, 1971.

114. Ezeilo, G. C.: Non-genetic neutropenia in Africans. *Lancet* 2:1003, 1972.

115. Mauer, A. M.: *Pediatric Hematology.* McGraw-Hill, New York, 1969, chap. 1, p. 5.

116. Brigety, R. E., and Pearson, H. A.: Effects of dietary and iron supplementation on hematocrit levels of preschool children. *J. Pediatr.* 76:757, 1970.

117. Owen, G. M., Nelson, C. E., and Garry, P. J.: Nutritional status of preschool children: Hemoglobin, hematocrit, and plasma iron values. *J. Pediatr.* 76:761, 1970.

118. Dallman, P. R., and Siimes, M. A.: Percentile curves for hemoglobin and red cell volume in infancy and childhood. *J. Pediatr.* 94:26, 1979.

119. Lampasso, J. A.: Changes in hematologic values induced by storage of ethylenediaminetetraacetate human blood for varying periods of time. *Am. J. Clin. Pathol.* 49:443, 1968.

CHAPTER 3

Examination of the marrow

WILLIAM J. WILLIAMS

Examination of the marrow is critically important in the study and management of a wide variety of hematologic disorders. Marrow may be obtained for examination without significant risk or discomfort and is quickly and easily processed for examination.

At birth all bones contain hemopoietic marrow. Fat cells begin to replace hemopoietic marrow in the extremities in the fifth to seventh year, and by adulthood the hemopoietic marrow is limited to the axial skeleton and the proximal portions of the extremities [1,2].

Fatty marrow appears yellow, while hemopoietic marrow looks red. Red marrow does contain fat, however, and fat droplets are visible grossly in aspirated marrow specimens. Histologically, yellow marrow consists almost entirely of fat cells and supporting connective tissue, while red marrow contains an abundance of hemopoietic cells along with fat cells and connective tissue.

The marrow fills the spaces between the trabeculae of bone in the marrow cavity. It is soft and friable and can be readily aspirated or biopsied with a needle. The structure and function of the marrow are discussed in Chap. 12 and the distribution of marrow in the skeleton in Chaps. 5 and 12.

Methods of sampling marrow

Marrow for clinical examination may be obtained by aspiration through a needle, by biopsy utilizing a special needle, or by open surgical biopsy with a trephine.

MARROW ASPIRATION

The site chosen for the aspiration depends on the age of the patient and the skill and experience of the operator. Most marrow aspirates from both children and adults are now obtained through the iliac crest at the posterior superior iliac spine (Fig. 3-1) in association with biopsy of the marrow using a Jamshidi needle [3] (Fig. 3-1). In adults, the sternum and the anterior iliac crest are also utilized (Fig. 3-2). The spinous processes of the vertebrae, the ribs, or other marrow-containing bones may be used occasionally. In children less than 1 year old, the anteromedial surface of the tibia is sometimes employed, while in older children, the iliac crests or the spines of the most prominent vertebral segments (L1 or L2) may be employed. The hazards of marrow aspiration are very small indeed when the procedure is carefully performed. Penetration of the bone with damage to the underlying structures is possible with all marrow

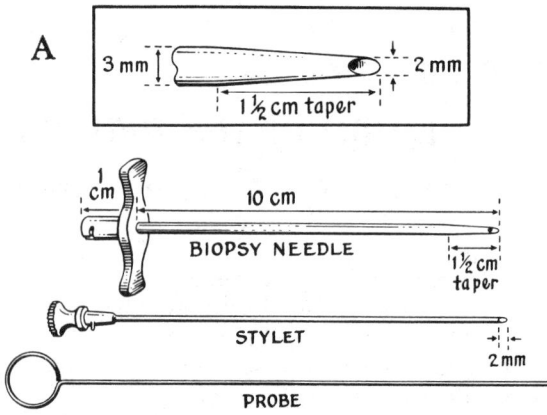

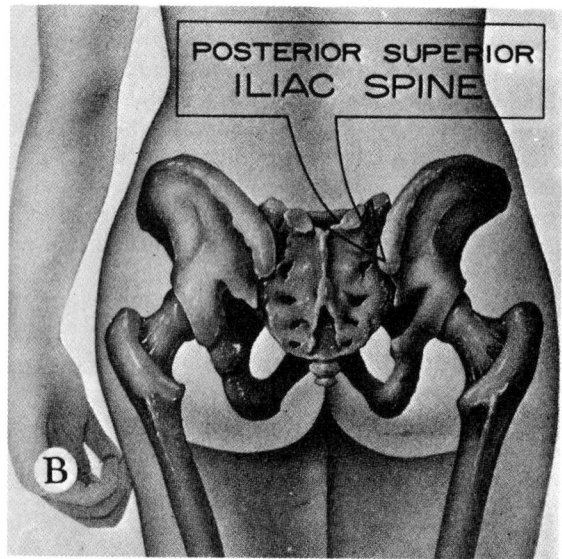

FIGURE 3-1 (*A*) Jamshidi biopsy instrument. (*B*) Site of marrow biopsy. [(*A*) From Jamshidi and Swaim [3] by permission; (*B*) from Ellis, Jensen, and Westerman [5] by permission.]

by a slight, rapid forward movement accompanied by a sudden increase in the ease of advancing the needle. The stylet of the needle is removed promptly, the hub is attached to a 10- or 20-ml syringe, and about 0.2 to 0.5 ml of fluid is aspirated. This is accompanied by suction pain, which may be quite uncomfortable to the patient but lasts only a few seconds at most. The needle is removed from the bone immediately after the marrow has been aspirated. Pressure is applied by the patient or the operator's assistant for a brief period to ensure hemostasis. In the thrombocytopenic patient, firm pressure should be applied for at least 10 to 15 min.

The fluid aspirated is blood that contains light-colored particles of marrow from 0.5 to 1 mm in diameter. They are often readily visible in the syringe but may not be detected until the syringe contents are discharged on a glass slide to prepare films.

Occasionally nothing enters the syringe when aspiration is performed. This may mean the needle is not properly placed in the marrow cavity. It may be cautiously advanced 1 to 2 mm after reinserting the obturator and aspiration attempted again, or it may be more desirable to remove the needle from the bone and reinsert it in a nearby site in the anesthetized area. The thickness of the bone must be kept in mind when attempting to adjust the needle in the bone. Occasionally the needle must be rotated on its longitudinal axis, or in a larger orbit, in order to loosen the marrow mechanically before it can be aspirated. If a small amount of blood was aspirated, it is wise to use a new needle because of the probability of clotting of the aspirate when it is finally obtained. Aspiration with a 50-ml syringe may succeed when failure has been encountered with a smaller syringe. Leukemic marrow may be so densely packed in the bone as to resist all attempts at aspiration, in which case biopsy is necessary. The marrow in myelofibrosis also may be impossible to aspirate. The commonest cause of failure to obtain marrow is faulty

aspirations, but the hazard is greatest in sternal aspirations. It must be remembered that the sternum at the second interspace in only about 1 cm thick in the adult [4].

Several different types of needles are available for marrow aspiration, most of which are satisfactory. An 18-gauge needle is sufficiently large to permit aspiration of adequate specimens; larger needles are unnecessary. Sterile precautions must be observed. The skin over the puncture site is shaved if necessary and cleansed with a disinfectant solution, and the skin, subcutaneous tissues, and periosteum are infiltrated with a local anesthetic solution such as 1% procaine or 1% lidocaine. The patient may experience discomfort during infiltration of the periosteum. After the anesthesia has taken effect, the marrow needle is inserted through the skin, subcutaneous tissue, and cortex of the bone with a slight twisting motion. Penetration of the cortex can be sensed

FIGURE 3-2 Sites used for marrow aspiration. (Modified from S. O. Schwartz, W. H. Hartz, Jr., and J. H. Robbins, *Hematology in Practice.* McGraw-Hill, New York, 1961, part 1, p. 36.)

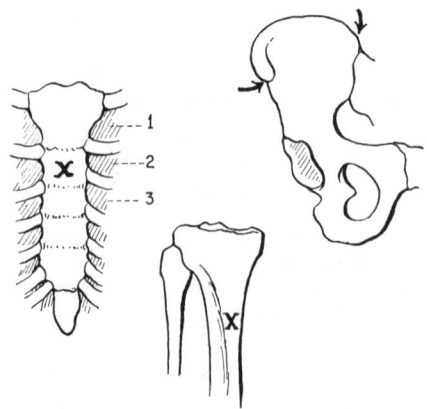

positioning of the needle, and a second attempt at aspiration will usually succeed.

NEEDLE BIOPSY

Needle biopsy is usually performed with the Jamshidi needle [3]. The Westerman-Jensen modification of the Vim-Silverman needle [5] may also be used. With these needles the ileum is biopsied at the posterior superior iliac spine (Fig. 3-1) with the patient prone or in the left or right lateral decubitus position. Sterile precautions must be followed and adequate local anesthetic administered. It may be advisable to give the apprehensive patient meperidine and atropine prior to the procedure. The Jamshidi instrument, which yields excellent biopsy material, is illustrated in Fig. 3-1. This device consists of a cylindrical needle of constant bore except for a concentrically tapered distal portion ending in a sharp, beveled cutting tip. The stylet fits precisely inside the opening at the tapered tip, interlocks at the hub of the needle, and extends 1 to 2 mm beyond the end of the needle. After anesthetizing the skin and periosteum of the biopsy site, a 3-mm incision is made in the skin, and the needle, with obturator in place, is inserted into the skin incision and through the subcutaneous tissue to the cortex of the bone. The needle is directed toward the anterior superior iliac spine and advanced with a twisting motion. Penetration of the cortex is sensed by a decreased resistance to forward movement of the needle. The obturator is then removed and the needle slowly advanced with reciprocal clockwise-counterclockwise twisting motions around the long axis. After sufficient penetration of the bone (up to about 3 cm), the needle is rotated several times on its axis and withdrawn about 2 to 3 mm. The needle is then reinserted to the original depth at a slightly different angle, with care not to bend the needle, and rotated several times in order to free the specimen from attachments in the marrow cavity. Next the needle is slowly withdrawn, using the same twisting motion employed during insertion. The core of marrow inside the needle is removed by inserting the probe through the cutting tip and extruding the specimen through the hub of the needle. Touch preparations or films may be made before fixation of the specimen in 95% Zenker's solution—5% glacial acetic acid [3]. The smaller size of the cutting aperture relative to the bore of the shaft of the Jamshidi instrument yields a specimen which fits loosely inside the needle and is therefore less subject to compression, distortion, or fragmentation. This technique reliably produces biopsy specimens of good quality [3,6] and is now widely used.

OPEN SURGICAL BIOPSY

Discussion of the technique involved in open biopsy is beyond the scope of this book. With the advent of the biopsy needles described above open biopsies are rarely necessary but may be performed during "staging" procedures for malignant lymphomas (see Chaps.

118 and 119) or for the diagnosis of deeply situated bone lesions.

Preparation of marrow for study

FILMS

Aspirated marrow is discharged onto a glass slide for preparation of a film. Thin films may be prepared in the same manner as blood films, using slides or cover slips. The objective is to make a thin film of a cellular particle of marrow, and usually the results are best if the films are prepared rapidly and with a minimum of manipulation of the specimen. If cover slips are used, it is best to discharge the aspirate on a slide so that the particles may be identified. Excess blood may be aspirated back into the syringe or allowed to drain off by tilting the slide. One or more particles may then be transferred to a clean cover slip, using the corner of a slide or cover slip, and a film prepared. Alternatively, particles may be drawn into the tip of a white cell diluting pipette, placed on a cover slip, and the film prepared. Some hematologists recommend that the marrow be aspirated into a syringe rinsed with sterile heparin solution to avoid clotting of the specimen. Heparinization of the aspirate is not necessary if the operator works rapidly, and it may introduce artifacts.

It is useful to prepare a thick smear of marrow by discharging a drop or two of the aspirate on a slide, covering the aspirate with a second slide, pressing these gently together to express most of the blood into a gauze sponge, and then pulling the slides apart longitudinally. Such preparations may contain an increased number of broken cells if too much pressure is applied, but they provide a large number of particles from which cellularity of the marrow may be estimated and which are essential for estimation of the amount of hemosiderin present.

TOUCH PREPARATIONS

Although biopsy or autopsy specimens will be examined histologically, touch preparations should be made from all biopsy or autopsy material. The surface of the biopsy with exposed marrow may be touched to a glass slide in several places and lifted directly up without smearing. Such preparations are allowed to dry and are stained in the same manner as films. Touch preparations are essential to determine cytologic details not visible in the unusual histologic preparations. Touch preparations from spleen specimens obtained surgically or at autopsy may also be helpful in some cases.

PREPARATION OF HISTOLOGIC SECTIONS

A variety of techniques have been advocated for preparing aspirated material for histologic study. All are designed to collect a sufficient number of particles in a small volume so that adequate sections may be prepared. This may be accomplished by discharging the marrow aspirate onto a glass slide, allowing the particles to settle for a few seconds, and then gently tilting the slide so that the excess blood runs off. The particles are then pushed together with an applicator stick and the remaining blood allowed to clot. The clot is then promptly fixed in Zenker's formol solution. The clot may be folded inside a small piece of lens paper to ensure that it will not disintegrate when placed in the fixative.

Examination of marrow films

Marrow films or touch preparations are stained by one of the polychrome techniques, usually Wright's stain or Wright's stain followed by Giemsa stain. The techniques are described in Chap. A1. The stained slides are first examined grossly to detect the presence of marrow particles. These appear as darkly stained blue or purple irregularly shaped areas on the film, contrasting with the even violet or pink areas representing stained erythrocytes.

Unless marrow particles are present, one cannot evaluate cellularity or hemosiderin content or even be certain that any abnormal cells present were derived from the marrow in patients who have such abnormal cells in the blood. The marrow film should be examined under low-power magnification to assess the relative amounts of fat and hemopoietic cells and the number of megakaryocytes, plasma, and mast cells present. Low-power examination will also permit detection of normal giant cells, such as osteoclasts or osteoblasts, groups of malignant cells, Gaucher cells, lymph follicles, and granulomas. The entire film should be examined, including the particles, and higher magnification employed to study any abnormalities discovered.

Megakaryocytes are described in detail in Chap. 130 and illustrated in Plate 2. They are large cells (30 to 150 μm) with darkly stained, irregularly lobed nuclei. The cytoplasm is blue "cotton candy"–textured and usually contains many red granules. About half of the megakaryocytes should have platelets adjacent to their periphery.

Mast cells are readily recognized by their content of dark-blue granules, which usually completely fill the cytoplasm and may obscure the nucleus. The cells are round or spindle-shaped and are often located deep in the particles, frequently lying along blood vessels. The nucleus is often not visible, but when seen, it is round or oval with a vesicular chromatin pattern.

Osteoclasts and *osteoblasts* are uncommon and are seen more frequently in marrow obtained from children and from adults with osteoblastic tumors or hyperparathyroidism. Osteoclasts are large cells and may be more than 100 μm in diameter (see Plate 11). They contain multiple nuclei, which have a moderately fine chromatin pattern and contain nucleoli. The cytoplasm varies from slightly basophilic to intensely acidophilic.

It contains acidophilic granules. Osteoclasts may contain coarse debris.

Osteoblasts are usually oval cells up to 30 μm in diameter (see Plate 11). They often occur in groups. The nucleus is usually eccentric and is relatively small. The chromatin pattern is coarse, and there are one to three nucleoli. The cytoplasm is light blue and may contain a few red granules. Osteoblasts may be mistaken for plasma cells.

Gaucher cells and other lipid-laden macrophages are described in Chap. 99.

MARROW NECROSIS
Necrosis of the marrow may occur in a variety of disorders, particularly sickle cell disease and neoplastic processes involving the marrow [7–10]. Aspirates of necrotic marrow stained with polychrome stains contain cells with indistinct margins and intensely basophilic nuclei surrounded by acidophilic material [7–10]. Sections of marrow stained with hematoxylin and eosin or with polychrome stains show loss of normal marrow architecture, indistinct cellular margins, and a background of amorphous eosinophilic material [8–10]. Nucleated red cells are seen in the blood in nearly all cases of significant marrow necrosis, and immature white cells are frequently present. Nearly all patients are anemic, and thrombocytopenia occurs frequently [8–10].

Patients with severe weight loss may develop gelatinous transformation of the marrow, characterized by amorphous extracellular material, fat atrophy, and marrow hypoplasia [11–13]. The findings of gelatinous transformation are reversible [11,12]. The extracellular material is mucopolysaccharide [12,13].

MARROW DIFFERENTIAL COUNT
After the low-power survey, the films should be examined under oil-immersion magnification to determine the various hemopoietic cell types present. Because a large number of cell types are normally present and their distribution is irregular, it is necessary to identify and tabulate a large number of cells. A total of 300 to 500 nucleated cells is necessary to obtain a significant differential count and estimate the myeloid/erythroid ratio, (M/E ratio, sometimes called the granulocyte/erythroid ratio), both useful parameters in evaluating the state of the marrow. Normal values for these determinations are presented in Table 3-1, including data for infants from birth to 18 months of age [14]. Between birth and 1 month there is an increase in lymphocytes and a decrease in erythroid and granulocytic precursors. After 1 month the marrow differential count varies little to age 18 months, the duration of the study [14]. The range of normal for all cell types is broad, and differential counts and M/E ratios are to be considered rough guides to the character of the marrow as a whole.

The cellular composition of the marrow specimen depends in part on the volume aspirated [15,18]. The

TABLE 3-1   Normal values for bone marrow differential cell count according to several authors

Type of cell	Rosse et al. [14] Infants tibial marrow 0 month (n = 57)	1 month (n = 7)	18 mo (n = 19)	Glaser et al. [4] Subjects aged 1–20 sternal marrow, 1 ml aspirated	Osgood and Seaman [15] Adult sternal marrow, 0.5–10 ml aspirated	Vaughan and Brockmyre [16] Adult sternal marrow, 3 ml aspirated	Wintrobe [17] Adults
Myeloblast	–	–	–	1.2 (0–3)	0.4 (0–1)	1.3 (0–3)	2 (0.3–5)
Promyelocyte	0.79 ± 0.91	0.76 ± 0.65	0.64 ± 0.59	1.8 (0–4)	1.4 (0–3)	–	5 (1–8)
Myelocyte	3.95 ± 2.93	2.50 ± 1.48	2.49 ± 1.39	16.5 (8–25)	4.2 (0–12)	8.9 (3–15)	–
Neutrophilic							12 (5–19)
Eosinophilic							1.5 (0.5–3)
Basophilic							0.3 (0–0.5)
Metamyelocyte	19.37 ± 4.84	11.34 ± 3.59	12.42 ± 4.15	23 (14–34)	6.5 (3–10)	8.8 (4–15)	22 (13–22)
Band form	28.89 ± 7.56	14.10 ± 4.63	14.20 ± 5.63	–	24 (17–33)	23.9 (12–34)	
Segmented							
Neutrophil	7.37 ± 4.64	3.64 ± 2.97	6.31 ± 3.91	12.9 (4.5–29)	15 (5–25)	18.5 (0–32)	20 (7–30)
Eosinophil	2.70 ± 1.27	2.61 ± 1.40	2.70 ± 2.16	–	2 (0–4)	1.9 (0–6)	2 (0.5–4)
Basophil	0.12 ± 0.20	0.07 ± 0.16	0.10 ± 0.12	–	0.2 (0–5)	0.2 (0–1)	0.2 (0–0.7)
Lymphocyte	14.42 ± 5.54	47.05 ± 9.24	43.55 ± 8.56	16 (5–36)	14 (3–25)	16.2 (8–26)	10 (3–17)
Monocyte	0.88 ± 0.85	1.01 ± 0.89	2.12 ± 1.59	–	2 (0–4)	2.4 (0–6)	–
Plasma cell	0.00 ± 0.02	0.02 ± 0.06	0.06 ± 0.08	–	–	0.3 (0–1.5)	0.4 (0–2)
Reticular cell	–	–	–	–	–	0.3 (0–1)	0.2 (0.1–0.2)
Proerythroblast	0.02 ± 0.06	0.10 ± 0.14	0.08 ± 0.13	0.5 (0–1.5)	0.2 (0–1)		4 (1–8)
Erythroblast						9.5 (2–18)	18 (7–32)
Basophilic	0.24 ± 0.25	0.34 ± 0.33	0.50 ± 0.34	1.7 (0–5)	2 (0–4)		
Polychromatophilic	13.06 ± 6.78	6.90 ± 4.45	6.97 ± 3.56	18 (5–34)	6 (4–8)		
Orthochromatic	0.09 ± 0.73	0.54 ± 1.88	0.44 ± 0.49	2.7 (0–8)	3 (1–5)		
Megakaryocyte	0.06 ± 0.15	0.05 ± 0.09	0.07 ± 0.12	–	–	1–38/50 low-power fields	–
Transitional cells*	1.18 ± 1.13	1.95 ± 0.94	1.99 ± 1.00	–	–	–	–
Broken cell	5.79 ± 2.78	5.50 ± 2.46	5.05 ± 2.15	–	19 (10–30)	7.9 (2–16)	–
M/E ratio	4.4:1	4.4:1	4.8:1	2.9:1 (1:1–5:1)	3.6:1 (2:1–8:1)	3.5:1–30:1	3:1–4:1

*Transitional cells are intermediate in size between lymphocytes and blast cells. They have fine chromatin and a small amount of basophilic cytoplasm. They are morphologically similar to blast cells.

proportion of polymorphonuclear neutrophils is increased with large volumes of aspirate, probably because of dilution of marrow cells by mature granulocytes in the blood. Intravenously administered ^{51}Cr-labeled erythrocytes and ^{125}I-labeled serum albumin have been used to estimate the admixture of nucleated cells from blood with those from marrow in sternal marrow aspirates [19]. In patients with hematologic disease, from 6 to 93 percent of the nucleated cells were derived from the blood. In 65 percent of the specimens, less than one-third of the cells were from the blood. The greatest admixture occurred in patients with leukemia. In healthy volunteers, from $14 ± 8$ percent (standard deviation) (range 3 to 37 percent) of the cells in the marrow aspirate were derived from the blood.

The nucleated cells found in normal marrow are mature granulocytes and their precursors, erythroid precursors, lymphocytes in varying stages of development, plasma cells, monocytes, macrophages (histiocytes), reticular cells, and megakaryocytes. In addition, a number of unusual cells may be encountered, such as phagocytic cells and "grape" cells.

The characteristics of each cell type are briefly described and the nomenclature is discussed. Further details of the morphology of these cells are found in

chapters in the special hematology parts of the book (see discussion of erythrocyte precursors, Chap. 29; granulocyte series, Chaps. 80, 90, and 91; monocyte series, Chap. 94; lymphocytes and plasma cells, Chaps. 101 and 102).

GRANULOCYTES

The term *granulocytes* is used to refer to the precursors and mature forms of those leukocytes characterized by neutrophilic, eosinophilic, or basophilic granules in their cytoplasm in the more mature stages of development. This series is sometimes referred to as the *myeloid series*. The recognized developmental forms are described in the following paragraphs.

Myeloblast (see Plate 2)   This cell is large, about 14 to 18 μm in diameter on a dried film, and is usually round. The nucleus occupies most of the cell. The chromatin is fine and the nuclear membrane is thin. There are from two to five nucleoli. The cytoplasm is basophilic but less so than is that of the erythroid series. There are no granules.

Promyelocyte (see Plate 6)   This cell is larger than the myeloblast. The chromatin pattern is coarser than that of the myeloblast. Nucleoli are often present. The cytoplasm is basophilic and is characterized by the presence of a variable number of large red granules. These are the so-called nonspecific or azurophilic granules and in the marrow usually mark the cell as a granulocyte precursor, although they occur in lymphocytes and reticular cells as well.

Myelocyte (see Plate 2) This cell is smaller than the myeloblast or promyelocyte. The nucleus is round or oval and is often located eccentrically. The chromatin pattern is coarser than that of the promyelocyte. Nucleoli are not present. There are a variable number of specific granules in the cytoplasm. These may be neutrophilic (fine, lilac color), eosinophilic (larger, round, regular in size, orange-red in color), or basophilic (larger still, few in number, irregular in size, deep blue in color). The cytoplasm is only slightly basophilic.

Metamyelocyte (see Plate 2) This cell is about the same size as the myelocyte and resembles it closely, except that the nucleus is indented, the chromatin is more coarse, and the cytoplasm is less basophilic.

Band form or stab cell (see Plate 2) This type of cell is characterized by a nucleus which is horseshoe-shaped or lobulated but not segmented in that the rudimentary lobes are connected by a thick band of chromatin rather than the thin thread which characterizes the mature polymorphonuclear leukocyte. The cytoplasm is yellowish pink or nearly colorless. Fine neutrophilic granules are abundant in the cytoplasm.

Polymorphonuclear leukocytes (see Plate 1) These are described in Chap. 2. They differ from the band cell only in the multilobed character of the nucleus.

ERYTHROID CELLS
The nomenclature suggested by different authors for erythroid cells is more varied than that for the myeloid series. Some commonly used systems are presented in Table 3-2.

The term *megaloblast* has been used to denote the earliest precursor of the normal erythrocyte, as in the system proposed by Sabin [20], or as a specific term to indicate the abnormal cells in pernicious anemia and related disorders, as in the systems used by Wintrobe [17], Custer [21], and others. These different usages have generated considerable controversy in the past, and some confusion still remains regarding the precise definitions of the terms *megaloblast* and *megaloblastic*, as is discussed in Chap. 47.

In this book we have chosen a nomenclature system which recognizes the marked morphologic differences among all stages in red cell development in normal persons and in patients with vitamin B_{12} or folic acid deficiency and related disorders (Table 3-2).

The erythroid cells which may be seen in normal marrow are described briefly here. More detailed descriptions of normal red cell precursors are presented in Chap. 29. The megaloblastic series is described in Chaps. 29 and 47.

Proerythroblast (see Plate 3) This is a large round cell, measuring from 15 to 20 μm in diameter. The nucleus occupies most of the cell and is densely stained. The chromatin is present in a fine reticular or stippled pattern. Nucleoli are present and are often bluish. The cytoplasm is deeply basophilic.

Basophilic erythroblast (see Plate 3) This cell is smaller than the proerythroblast, and the nucleus occupies less of the cell. The chromatin pattern is stippled, and the small, condensed masses of chromatin are sharply defined and separated by colorless parachromatin. The cytoplasm is deeply basophilic.

Polychromatophilic erythroblast (see Plate 3) This cell is smaller than the basophilic erythroblast. The nucleus occupies even less of the cell, and the chromatin pattern is more condensed, with larger masses of chromatin sharply defined by clear parachromatin. The nuclear membrane is dense. The cytoplasm is gray or grayish-pink because of the presence of hemoglobin.

TABLE 3-2 Systems classifying red blood cells

This book		Wintrobe [17]		Sabin [20]
Normal	Abnormal (pernicious anemia)	Normal	Abnormal (pernicious anemia)	
Proerythroblast	Promegaloblast	Pronormoblast	Promegaloblast	Megaloblast
Basophilic erythroblast	Basophilic megaloblast	Basophilic normoblast	Basophilic megaloblast	Early erythroblast
Polychromatophilic erythroblast	Polychromatophilic megaloblast	Polychromatophilic normoblast	Polychromatophilic megaloblast	Late erythroblast
Orthochromatic erythroblast	Orthochromatic megaloblast	Orthochromatic normoblast	Orthochromatic megaloblast	Normoblast
Reticulocyte*	Reticulocyte	Reticulocyte*	Reticulocyte	Reticulocyte
Erythrocyte	Macrocyte	Erythrocyte	Macrocyte	Erythrocyte

*Reticulocytes are identified by supravital staining. On blood films stained with polychrome stains reticulocytes appear as polychromatophilic macrocytes.

Orthochromatic erythroblast (see Plate 3) This cell is only slighly larger than the mature erythrocyte. The nucleus is small and pyknotic. The cytoplasm is red, like that of the mature erythrocyte.

Polychromatophilic macrocyte (reticulocyte) and erythrocyte (see Plate 3) Polychromatophilic macrocytes are large, anucleate cells with bluish or gray cytoplasm. Reticulocytes appear as polychromatophilic macrocytes on blood films stained with polychrome stains. The blue or gray color of the cytoplasm is due to cytoplasmic RNA. Erythrocyte morphology is the same as that seen in the blood (see Chaps. 2 and 29).

MONOCYTES

Monocytes in normal marrow are identical morphologically to those in the peripheral blood (see Plate 1) (Chaps. 2 and 94). *Monoblasts* are described but cannot be distinguished from myeloblasts except perhaps if the nucleus is indented or appears to be folded.

LYMPHOCYTES

In normal marrow lymphocytes occur in the mature form, although immature forms may be seen occasionally. The *lymphoblast* is usually indistinguishable from the myeloblast, although it is said to have fewer nucleoli (one to two), a dense nuclear membrane, and a perinuclear clear zone. The *prolymphocyte* is a smaller round cell, with a round nucleus occupying most of the cell. The chromatin is condensed, and nucleoli may be present. The nuclear membrane is dense and there is a perinuclear clear zone. The *lymphocyte* is a smaller cell, often only slightly larger than the erythrocyte (see Plate 1). These are described in Chaps. 2 and 101. They may be confused with erythroid precursors, but the chromatin is quite distinctive in the two types of cells. *Large lymphocytes* may also be seen.

PLASMA CELLS

Normal plasma cells vary somewhat in size but are usually 12 to 16 μm in diameter (see Chap. 102). They are round or oval. The nucleus is small, round, eccentrically placed, and stained densely purple. The chromatin is coarse and clumped. There are no nucleoli. The cytoplasm is deep blue, often with a paranuclear clear zone. Small vacuoles are commonly seen in normal plasma cells. Binucleate forms are often present in normal marrow.

RETICULUM CELLS

The term *reticulum cell* has been used for a wide variety of cells. It usually describes a large cell, 20 to 30 μm in diameter, which is round or oval and may have an irregular outline. The nucleus occupies about one-half of the cell. The chromatin often stains with a reddish hue and is present in coarse strands. There may be one or more blue-staining nucleoli. The cytoplasm is lightly stained and contains a variable number of large red granules (azurophilic granules) (see Plate 2). Some reticulum cells may contain phagocytosed material and may in fact be macrophages. Occasionally a large (30 to 80 μm) cell with a small round nucleus with condensed chromatin may be seen. The cytoplasm may be blue and homogeneous, or it may give a foamy appearance, with clear areas in the cytoplasm separated by blue strands of cytoplasm. The latter cells may be lipoid-containing macrophages similar to those seen in the lipoidoses but are normal variants in some cases. Cells in which the clear areas are round and regular may remind one of a bunch of grapes and are called "grape cells." The significance of these unusual cells is unknown.

Examination of thin sections of marrow

After fixation, marrow biopsy specimens may be sectioned and stained by standard procedures. Plastic embedding of marrow biopsies permits preparation of sections approximately 2 μm thick [22–27]. Such sections may be stained or subjected to histochemical procedures, with improved identification of cells and accuracy of diagnosis [24,26,27] (see Plate 8). Both hematoxylin-eosin and Giesma stains are employed [6,28]. Sections are particularly valuable in estimating marrow cellularity and detecting myelofibrosis and infiltrative diseases of the marrow, such as granulomas, lipid storage diseases, or lymphomatous or carcinomatous invasion [5,6,15]. These disorders are discussed in detail in the appropriate chapters of this book.

Examination of iron stores

Every marrow examination should include evaluation of the iron stores. This is accomplished by staining a marrow film or section by the Prussian blue technique (see Chap. A3). Marrow macrophages are evaluated for storage iron and erythroblasts are examined for the presence of iron granules in the cytoplasm (sideroblasts). Erythroblasts are readily identified by their small size and the size, shape, and chromatin pattern of the nucleus. Normally 20 to 50 percent of erythroblasts contain a few such granules. Interpretation of marrow films stained for iron is presented in Chap. A3 and in the discussion of specific diseases.

References

1. Piney, A.: Anatomy of bone marrow. *Br. Med. J.* 2:792, 1922.
2. Custer, R. P., and Ahlfeldt, F. E.: Studies on the structure and function of bone marrow. II. Variations in cellularity in various bones with advancing years of life and their relative response to stimuli. *J. Lab. Clin. Med.* 17:960, 1932.
3. Jamshidi, K., and Swaim, W. R.: Bone marrow biopsy with unaltered architecture: A new biopsy device. *J. Lab. Clin. Med.* 77:335, 1971.
4. Glaser, K., Limarzi, L. R., and Poncher, H. G.: Cellular composition of the bone marrow in normal infants and children. *Pediatrics* 6:789, 1950.

5. Ellis, L. D., Jensen, W. N., and Westerman, M. P.: Needle biopsy of bone and marrow. An experience with 1 445 biopsies. *Arch. Intern. Med.* 114:213, 1964.

6. Bearden, J. D., Ratkin, G. A., and Coltman, C. A.: Comparison of the diagnostic value of bone marrow biopsy and bone marrow aspiration in neoplastic disease. *J. Clin. Pathol.* 27:738, 1974.

7. Brittin, G. M., and Brecher, G.: Appearance of bone marrow smears with necrotic tumor cells. *Blood* 38:229, 1971.

8. Brown, C. H., III: Bone marrow necrosis. A study of seventy cases. *Johns Hopkins Med. J.* 131:189, 1972.

9. Kiraly, J. F., III, and Wheby, M. S.: Bone marrow necrosis. *Am. J. Med.* 60:361, 1976.

10. Norgard, M. J., Carpenter, J. T., Jr., and Conrad, M. E.: Bone marrow necrosis and degeneration. *Arch. Intern. Med.* 139:905, 1979.

11. Mant, M. J., and Faragher, B. S.: The haematology of anorexia nervosa. *Br. J. Haematol.* 23:737, 1972.

12. Tavassoli, M., Eastlund, D. T., Yam, L. T., Neiman, R. S., and Finkel, H.: Gelatinous transformation of bone marrow in prolonged self-induced starvation. *Scand. J. Haematol.* 16:311, 1976.

13. Seaman, J. P., Kjeldsberg, C. R., and Linker, A.: Gelatinous transformation of the bone marrow. *Hum. Pathol.* 9:685, 1978.

14. Rosse, C., Krauner, M. J., Dillon, T. L., McFarland, R., and Smith, N. J.: Bone marrow cell populations of normal infants: the predominance of lymphocytes. *J. Lab. Clin. Med.* 89:1225, 1977.

15. Osgood, E. E., and Seaman, A. J.: The cellular composition of normal bone marrow as obtained by sternal puncture. *Physiol. Rev.* 24:46, 1944.

16. Vaughan, S. L., and Brockmyre, F.: Normal bone marrow as obtained by sternal puncture. *Blood* (special issue) 1:54, 1947.

17. Wintrobe, M. M.: *Clinical Hematology*, 6th ed. Lea & Febiger, Philadelphia, 1968, chap. 1.

18. Dresch, C., Faille, A., Poirier, O., and Kadouche, J.: The cellular composition of the granulocyte series in the normal human bone marrow according to the volume of the sample. *J. Clin. Pathol.* 27:106, 1974.

19. Holdrinet, R. S. G., v. Egmond, J., Wessels, J. M. C., and Haanen, C.: A method for quantification of peripheral blood admixture in bone marrow aspirates. *Exp. Hematol.* 8:103, 1980.

20. Sabin, F. R.: Bone marrow. *Physiol. Rev.* 8:191, 1928.

21. Custer, R. P.: *An Atlas of the Blood and Bone Marrow*, 2d ed. Saunders, Philadelphia, 1974, chap. 1, p. 7.

22. Rosenberg, M., Bartl, P., and Leško, J.: Water-soluble methacrylate as an embedding medium for the preparation of ultrathin sections. *J. Ultrastruct. Res.* 4:298, 1960.

23. Ashford, A. E., Allaway, W. G., and McCully, M. E.: Low temperature embedding in glycol methacrylate for enzyme histochemistry in plant and animal tissues. *J. Histochem. Cytochem.* 20:986, 1972.

24. Block, M.: Bone marrow examination. Aspiration of core biopsy, smear or section, hematoxylin-eosin or Romanowsky stain—Which combination? *Arch. Pathol. Lab. Med.* 100:454, 1976.

25. Bennett, H. S., Wyrick, A. D., Lee, S. W., and McNeil, J. H., Jr.: Science and art in preparing tissues embedded in plastic for light microscopy, with special reference to glycol methacrylate, glass knives and simple stains. *Stain Tech.* 51:71, 1976.

26. Moosavi, H., Lichtman, M. A., Donnelly, J. A., and Churukian, M. T.: Plastic-embedded human marrow biopsy specimens. Improved histochemical methods. *Arch. Pathol. Lab. Med.* 105:269, 1981.

27. Beckstead, J. H., Halverson, P. S., Ries, C. A., and Bainton, D. F.: Enzyme histochemistry and immunohistochemistry on biopsy specimens of pathologic human bone marrow. *Blood* 57:1088, 1981.

28. Cramer, A. D., Rogers, E. R., Parker, J. W., and Lukes, R. J.: The Giemsa stain for tissue sections: An improved method. *Am. J. Clin. Pathol.* 59:148, 1973.

CHAPTER 4

Radioisotope imaging procedures in evaluating patients with hematologic disorders

STEPHEN A. LANDAW

Many isotopically labeled compounds are available for evaluation of patients with hematologic disease [1,2]. The most versatile of the isotopes used in labeling is ^{99m}Tc, which by virtue of differences in its chemical formulation, can be used to image the extracellular space (as pertechnetate), the monocyte-macrophage system (as sulfur colloid), blood pools (albumin or erythrocytes), the spleen (heat-damaged erythrocytes), or cortical bone (various phosphate complexes). This chapter will briefly outline the various areas in hematology in which isotopic scanning may be of value and some of the limitations of these techniques. In view of recent progress in the general field of imaging, the position of isotopic scanning relative to other techniques (x-ray, lymphangiography, ultrasound, and computed tomography) is summarized in Table 4-1.

Erythroid marrow

Isotopes of iron (^{52}Fe and ^{59}Fe) can be used to generate images of active erythropoiesis and sites of iron storage. In the normal adult, erythropoietic marrow is invariably found throughout the central portion of the skeleton (ribs, spine, pelvis, scapula, and clavicle), with the exception of the caudal half of the sacrum. Despite individual variation, erythropoietic marrow is usually confined to the proximal quarter of the humerus and femur, and extension beyond the proximal one-third of these bones is considered abnormal (Fig. 4-1). Initial uptake of radioactive iron in the spleen indicates the presence of extramedullary erythropoiesis in that organ, although care should be taken to ensure that there is no colloidal iron in the preparation used. Serial imaging studies, possible only with ^{59}Fe because of the short half-life of ^{52}Fe, can be used to delineate effective and ineffective erythropoiesis, as well as splenic sequestration of red cells. Abnormal marrow patterns due to myelofibrosis, radiation treatment [14,15], or malignant disease, can also be detected, although special equipment and long imaging times are required for adequate resolution of the high-energy gamma emissions of ^{59}Fe.

Because ^{52}Fe is not generally available and ^{59}Fe is difficult to image, attempts have been made to follow the

TABLE 4-1   Comparison of various scanning techniques in hematology

Disorder/organ system	Techniques	References
Mass lesions, liver	Ultrasound, computed tomography, ^{99m}Tc colloid	[3–5]
Multiple myeloma	X-ray, gallium, ^{99m}Tc phosphate complexes	[6,7]
Spleen, size	X-ray, ultrasound, ^{99m}Tc colloid	[8]
Spleen, lymphomatous involvement	Ultrasound, ^{99m}Tc colloid	[9]
Iliac and paraaortic nodes, lymphomatous involvement	Lymphangiography, gallium 67	[10–12]

distribution of marrow elements using agents other than radioactive iron. Since carrier-free ^{111}indium chloride can bind to transferrin and small amounts may be incorporated into the erythron, it has been suggested that this agent is a satisfactory substitute. However, overall kinetics of indium and iron are not generally comparable [2]. Since ^{111}In distribution partially mimics that of the monocyte-macrophage system, and since ^{111}In can be taken up by certain tumors, it is not correct to equate its uptake with erythropoiesis in all instances [16]. However, in selected cases, distribution of ^{111}In in the marrow, but not in the liver or spleen, has been shown to correlate with ^{59}Fe kinetics and marrow biopsy in patients with myelofibrosis [17]. In conjunction with marrow biopsy, indium scanning may be useful in the evaluation of cytopenias in lymphoma [18]. In aplastic anemia, indium scanning with [19] or without [20] simultaneous ^{99m}Tc colloid scanning correlated well with clinical severity and prognosis. However, in view of partial comparability of indium and iron, plus the high radiation dose delivered with ^{111}In, indium scanning is not recommended as a clinical routine [2].

Monocyte-macrophage marrow

Any radioactive colloid of the proper size, labeled with ^{99m}Tc, ^{113m}In, or ^{198}Au, can be used to visualize the monocyte-macrophage system within the marrow. In the normal subject, the various components of hemopoietic marrow (megakaryocytic, granulopoietic,

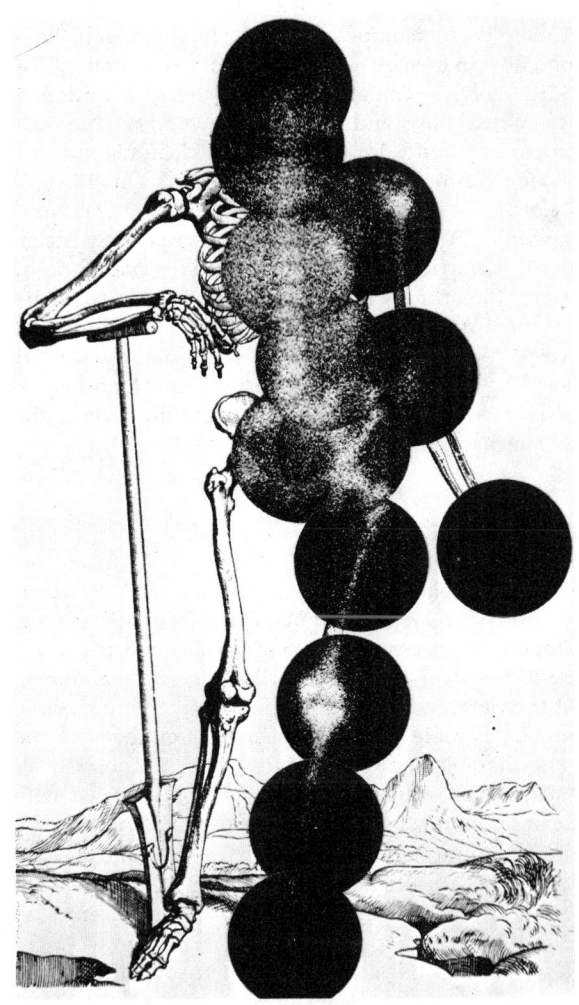

FIGURE 4-1   Extension of marrow into knee, ankle, and elbow in patient with severe hemolytic anemia of 3 years' duration. (Van Dyke and Anger [13]. **Reproduced by permission of** *Journal of Nuclear Medicine.*)

TABLE 4-2   Indications for use of marrow scanning in clinical hematology

1. When marrow biopsies disagree with clinical findings
2. Demonstration of sites of extramedullary hemopoiesis [27]
3. To determine whether significant medullary erythropoiesis exists before removing the spleen in myelofibrosis
4. To determine whether marrow failure is due to tumor infiltration (patchy encroachments), radiation (failure restricted to radiation fields [15]), or suppression by chemotherapy
5. Demonstration of onset of "spent" phase of polycythemia vera [26]
6. Evaluation of procedures designed to alter marrow function [28]
7. Suspected marrow infarction [29]
8. To determine appropriate site(s) for marrow aspiration or biopsy

erythropoietic, and the monocyte-macrophage system) are invariably linked together [21,22] and therefore have the same distribution. However, in the presence of disease or radiation treatment, erythropoietic function can cease within the marrow or spleen, with [23] or without [24] intact function of the monocyte-macrophage system, so that radioactive colloid and radioactive iron studies may give differing information [14,25,26]. Indications for marrow scanning are given in Table 4-2.

Bone imaging

Distribution of the positron emitter ^{18}F and of various phosphate complexes of [99m]Tc (polyphosphate, pyrophosphate, diphosphonate, etc.) is primarily the result of variations in cortical bone blood flow. Because of ease of labeling and availability, the latter agents are now routinely used for cortical bone scanning and have wide applicability in the demonstration of bone infarcts, aseptic necrosis, metastatic disease, foci of tumor or infection, fractures, and the like [29–32].

Using these isotopes, a markedly increased bone blood flow in myelofibrosis has been demonstrated [33]. Additionally, a similarity between the distribution of bone blood flow and hemopoietic marrow has also become apparent [34], suggesting a close relationship between perfusion and marrow growth. In multiple myeloma it is generally agreed that isotopic bone imaging with ^{99m}Tc phosphate complexes is relatively insensitive in detecting areas of disease and that radiography remains the primary method of evaluation of skeletal involvement with this disease (Table 4-1). It is important always to remember the nonspecific nature of ^{99m}Tc phosphate complex uptake by cortical bone (or other tissues), as well as the need for correlation with radiographic changes.

Spleen and liver

Radioactive colloids are routinely employed for determination of organ size and parenchymal distribution of isotope [35]. In certain cases, especially when the left lobe of the liver extends into the left upper abdomen and interferes with interpretation of splenic images, it may be desirable to obtain special oblique views or to image the spleen alone. For this latter purpose, heat-damaged or chemically damaged red cells labeled with ^{51}Cr or ^{99m}Tc may be used. Such cells will localize in the spleen without significant hepatic uptake and are the agents of choice when searching for an accessory spleen [2]. Indications for splenic scanning are outlined in Table 4-3.

Use of radioactive colloids for staging of patients with lymphoma can often lead to erroneous results. Thus organomegaly, patchy isotope uptake, and even focal

TABLE 4-3   Indications for spleen scintigraphy

1. Objective determination of spleen position and size
2. Quantitative determination of spleen size
3. Differential diagnosis of left upper quadrant masses
4. Demonstration of accessory spleens
5. Demonstration of parenchymal lesions: infarcts, cysts, necrosis, abscesses, tumors, lacerations
6. Demonstration of splenic aplasia or functional asplenia [39]
7. Follow-up of spleen size and function, especially during therapy
8. Measurement of splenic red blood cell mass [40]

SOURCE: Modified from Fischer and Wolfe [38].

defects have occasionally proved on laparotomy to be due to causes other than malignancy (false-positive reaction) [36,37]. Similarly, small areas of involvement less than 2 to 3 cm in diameter may be missed with current imaging equipment (false-negative reaction). Thus liver-spleen imaging cannot take the place of definitive biopsy techniques for the determination of the presence or absence of lymphomatous involvement.

Tumor scanning agents

Carrier-free ^{67}Ga citrate and ^{111}In-Bleomycin are the main agents used to determine the extent of metastatic spread of malignancies as lymphoma [41]. These agents have often indicated areas of involvement when the results with other techniques (radiography, lymphangiography, closed biopsy) were negative, although the reverse is often also the case. Localized gallium uptake may also be observed in nonmalignant processes such as abscess, active granulomatous disease, and Bleomycin lung toxicity; in marrow biopsy sites and surgical incisions, active epiphyses, the nasopharynx (interfering with evaluation of Waldeyer's ring), and the salivary glands (interfering with evaluation of cervical adenopathy); and in *Pneumocystis carinii* infection, radiation pneumonitis, and the normal lung after lymphangiography [42]. Gallium localization was present in about two-thirds of biopsy-proven sites of Hodgkin's disease [11] and in about one-half of biopsy-proven sites in non-Hodgkin's lymphomas [12]. Overall accuracy was best in cervical and thoracic regions and worst in abdominal and inguinal areas. The histologic variant seems to be of importance in overall accuracy in lymphoma, with large cell lymphomas (and perhaps also Burkitt's) showing better overall uptake [12,42]. In Hodgkin's disease, all variants showed similar uptake except for lower uptake in the lymphocyte-predominant type [11].

Although gallium accuracy does not achieve that of staging laparotomy, it can be a useful adjunct, especially when used for follow-up studies or in patients who cannot undergo laparotomy or lymphangiography [43]. The nonspecificity of gallium uptake can on occasion be a helpful property. For example, it can localize in abscesses, even in leukopenic subjects [44]. It appears that a tumor-specific agent is not yet available, although investigative approaches using labeled antibodies directed against tumor antigens may be fruitful [45,46].

Scanning with labeled platelets and leukocytes

The lipid-soluble agent 8-hydroxyquinoline (oxine) is capable of chelating ^{111}In and labeling platelets and leukocytes, which allows study of cellular kinetics and permits scanning procedures to detect sites of cellular localization [47]. Thus ^{111}In-labeled autologous [48] or homologous ABO-matched [49] granulocytes have accurately and rapidly (30 min to 4 h) identified known sites of infection in human subjects. Similarly, ^{111}In-labeled platelets have been shown to localize in experimental venous thrombi [50], coronary artery bypass grafts [51], and accessory spleens [52].

References

1. Freeman, L. M., and Blaufox, M. D.: Hematological studies with radionuclides. *Semin. Nucl. Med.* 5:1, 1975.

2. McIntyre, P. A.: Newer developments in nuclear medicine applicable to hematology, in *Progress in Hematology*, edited by E. B. Brown. Grune & Stratton, New York, 1977, vol. 10, pp. 361–409.

3. Grossman, Z. D., Wistow, B. W., Bryan, P. J., Dinn, W. M., McAfee, J. G., and Kieffer, S. A.: Radionuclide imaging, computed tomography, and gray-scale ultrasonography of the liver: A comparative study. *J. Nucl. Med.* 18:327, 1977.

4. Petasnick, J. P., Ram, P., Turner, D. A., and Fordham, E. W.: The relationship of computed tomography, gray-scale ultrasonography and radionuclide imaging in the evaluation of hepatic masses. *Semin. Nucl. Med.* 9:8, 1979.

5. Snow, J. H., Goldstein, H. M., and Wallace, S.: Comparison of scintigraphy, sonography, and computed tomography in the evaluation of hepatic neoplasms. *Am. J. Roentgenol.* 132:915, 1979.

6. Woolfended, J. M., Pitt, M. J., Durie, B. G. M., and Moon, T. E.: Comparison of bone scintigraphy and radiography in multiple myeloma. *Radiology* 134:723, 1980.

7. Waxman, A. D., et al.: Radiographic and radionuclide imaging in multiple myeloma: The role of gallium scintigraphy: Concise communication. *J. Nucl. Med.* 22:232, 1981.

8. Aito, H.: The estimation of the size of the spleen by radiological methods. A comparative radiographic, gamma imaging and ultrasonic study. *Ann. Clin. Res. 6 (Suppl. 15): 1*, 1974.

9. Glees, J. P., Taylor, K. J. W., Gazet, J. C., Peckham, M. J., and McCready, V. R.: Accuracy of gray scale ultrasonography of liver and spleen in Hodgkin's disease and the other lymphomas compared with isotope scans. *Clin. Radiol.* 28:233, 1977.

10. Rudders, R. A., McCaffrey, J. A., and Kahn, P. C.: The relative roles of gallium-67-citrate scanning and lymphangiography in the current management of malignant lymphoma. *Cancer* 40:1439, 1977.

11. Johnston, G. S., Go, M. F., Benua, R. S., Larson, S. M., Andrews, G. A., and Hubner, K. F.: Gallium-67 citrate imaging in Hodgkin's disease: Final report of cooperative group. *J. Nucl. Med.* 18:692, 1977.

12. Andrews, G. A., Hubner, K. F., and Greenlaw, R. H.: Gallium-67 citrate imaging in malignant lymphoma: Final report of cooperative group. *J. Nucl. Med.* 19:1013, 1978.

13. Van Dyke, D., and Anger, H. O.: Patterns of marrow hypertrophy and atrophy in man. *J. Nucl. Med.* 6:109, 1965.

14. DeGowin, R. L., Chaudhuri, T. K., Christie, J. H., Callis, M. N., and Mueller, A. L.: Marrow scanning in evaluation of hemopoiesis after radiotherapy. *Arch Intern. Med.* 134:297, 1974.

15. Knospe, W. H., Rayudu, V. M. S., Cardello, M., Friedman, A. M., and Fordham, E. W.: Bone marrow scanning with [52]iron ([52]Fe). *Cancer* 37:1432, 1976.

16. Merrick, M. V., Gordon-Smith, E. C., Lavender, J. P., and Szur, L.: A comparison of ^{111}In with [52]Fe and ^{99m}Tc-sulfur colloid for bone marrow scanning. *J. Nucl. Med.* 16:66, 1975.

17. McNeil, B. J., Holman, B. L., Button, L. N., and Rosenthal, D. S.: Use of indium chloride scintigraphy in patients with myelofibrosis. *J. Nucl. Med.* 15:647, 1974.

18. Gilbert, E. H., Glatstein, E., Goris, M. L., and Earle, J. D.: Value of [111]indium chloride bone marrow scanning in the differential diagnosis of blood count depression in lymphoma. *Cancer* 41:143, 1978.

19. Najean, Y., LeDanvic, M., LeMercier, N., Pecking, A., Colonna, P., and Rain, J. D.: Significance of bone-marrow scintigraphy in aplastic anemia: Concise communication. *J. Nucl. Med.* 21:213, 1980.

20. McNeil, B. J., Rappeport, J. M., and Nathan, D. G.: Indium chloride scintigraphy: An index of severity in patients with aplastic anaemia. *Br. J. Haematol.* 34:599, 1976.

21. Greenberg, M. L., Atkins, H. L., and Schiffer, L. M.: Erythropoietic and reticuloendothelial function in bone marrow in dogs. *Science* 152:526, 1966.

22. Nelp, W. B., Larson, S. M., and Lewis, R. J.: Distribution of the erythron and the RES in the bone marrow organ. *J. Nucl. Med.* 8:430, 1967.

23. Szur, L., Pettit, J. E., Lewis, S. M., Bruce-Tagoe, A. A., and Short, M. D.: The effect of radiation on splenic function in myelosclerosis: Studies with [52]Fe and [99]Tc[m]. *Br. J. Radiol.* 46:295, 1973.

24. Rubin, P., Landman, S., Mayer, E., Keller, B., and Ciccio, S.: Bone marrow regeneration and extension after extended field irradiation in Hodgkin's disease. *Cancer* 32:699, 1973.

25. Van Dyke, D., Shkurkin, C., Price, D., Yano, Y., and Anger, H. O.: Differences in distribution of erythropoietic and reticuloendothelial marrow in hematologic disease. *Blood* 30:364, 1967.

26. Van Dyke, D., Lawrence, J. H., and Anger, H. O.: Whole-body marrow distribution studies in polycythemia vera, in *Symposium on Myeloproliferative Disorders of Animals and Man*. United States Atomic Energy Commission, Division of Technical Information CONF-680529, 1970, p. 721.

27. Robinson, A. E., Rosse, W. F., and Goodrich, J. K.: Intrathoracic extramedullary hematopoiesis: A scan diagnosis. *J. Nucl. Med.* 9:416, 1968.

28. Van Dyke, D., and Harris, N.: Bone marrow reactions to trauma. *Blood* 34:257, 1969.

29. Alavi, A., Schumacher, R., Dorwart, B., and Kuhl, D. E.: Bone marrow scan evaluation of arthropathy in sickle cell disorders. *Arch. Intern. Med.* 136:436, 1976.

30. Hammel, C. F., DeNardo, S. J., DeNardo, G. L., and Lewis, J. P.: Bone marrow and bone mineral scintigraphic studies in sickle cell disease. *Br. J. Haemat.* 25:593, 1973.

31. Bell, E. G., Subramanian, G., Blair, R. J., and McAfee, J. G.: Bone scanning in pediatrics, in *Pediatric Nuclear Medicine*, edited by A. E. James, Jr., H. N. Wagner. Jr., and R. E. Cooke. Saunders, Philadelphia, 1974, p. 335.

32. Silberstein, E. B., Saenger, E. L., Tofe, A. J., Alexander, G. W., and Park, H-M.: Imaging of bone metastases with ^{99m}Tc-Sn-EHDP (diphosphonate), ^{18}F, and skeletal radiography. *Radiology* 107:551, 1973.

33. Van Dyke, D., et al.: Markedly increased bone blood flow in myelofibrosis. *J. Nucl. Med.* 12:506, 1971.

34. Van Dyke, D.: Similarity in distribution of skeletal blood flow and erythropoietic marrow. *Clin. Orthop.* 52:37, 1967.

35. De Land, F. H., and Wagner, H. N.: *Atlas of Nuclear Medicine*, vol. 3: *Reticuloendothelial System, Liver, Spleen, and Thyroid*. Saunders, Philadelphia, 1972.

36. Lipton, M. J., DeNardo, G. L., Silverman, S., and Glatstein, E.: Evaluation of the liver and spleen in Hodgkin's disease. I. The value of hepatic scintigraphy. *Am. J. Med.* 52:356, 1972.

37. Silverman, S., DeNardo, G. L., Glatstein, E., and Lipton, M. J.: Evaluation of the liver and spleen in Hodgkin's disease. II. The value of splenic scintigraphy. *Am. J. Med.* 52:362, 1972.

38. Fischer, J., and Wolf, R.: *Nuclear Medicine in Hematology*. Farbewerke Hoechst, 1968.

39. Pearson, H. A., Cornelius, E. A., Schwartz, A. D., Zelson, J. H., Wolfson, S. L., and Spencer, R. P.: Transfusion-reversible functional asplenia in young children with sickle-cell anemia. *N. Engl. J. Med.* 283:334, 1970.

40. Glass, H. I., deGarreta, A. C., Lewis, S. M., Grammaticos, P., and Szur, L.: Measurement of splenic red-blood-cell mass with radioactive carbon monoxide. *Lancet* 1:669, 1968.

41. Jones, S. E., and Salmon, S. E.: The role of radionuclides in clinical oncology. *Semin. Nucl. Med.* 6:331, 1976.

42. Richman, S. D., Levenson, S. M., Jones, A. E., and Johnston, G. S.: Radionuclide studies in Hodgkin's disease and lymphomas. *Semin. Nucl. Med.* 5:103, 1975.

43. Turner, D. A., Fordham, E. W., Ali, A., and Slayton, R. E.: Gallium-67 imaging in the management of Hodgkin's disease and other malignant lymphomas. *Semin. Nucl. Med.* 8:205, 1978.

44. Milder, M. S., Glick, J. H., Henderson, E. S., and Johnston, G. S.: [67]Ga scintigraphy in acute leukemia. *Cancer* 32:803, 1973.

45. Order, S. E., et al.: Radionuclide immunoglobulin lymphangiography: A case report. *Cancer 35*:1487, 1975.

46. Ettinger, D. S., Dragon, L. H., Klein, J., Sgagias, M., and Order, S. E.: Isotopic immunoglobulin in an integrated multimodal treatment program for primary liver cancer: A case report. *Cancer Treat. Rep. 63*:131, 1979.

47. McAfee, J. G., and Thakur, M. L.: Survey of radioactive agents for in vitro labeling of phagocytic leukocytes. I. Soluble agents. *J. Nucl. Med. 17*:480, 1976.

48. Thakur, M. L., Lavender, J. P., Arnot, R. N., Silvester, D. J., and Segal, A. W.: Indium-lll-labeled autologous leukocytes in man. *J. Nucl. Med. 18*:1012, 1977.

49. Dutcher, J. P., Schiffer, C. A., and Johnston, G. S.: Rapid migration of ^{111}indum-labeled granulocytes to sites of infection. *N. Engl. J. Med. 304*:586, 1981.

50. Wistow, B. W., Grossman, Z. D., Subramanian, G., and McAfee, J. G.: Localization of fresh experimental venous thrombi in rabbits using ^{99m}Tc-oxine-labeled autologous platelets. *Radiology 123*:787, 1977.

51. Dewanjee, M. K., Fuster, V., Kaye, M. P., and Josa, M.: Imaging platelet deposition with ^{111}In-labeled platelets in coronary artery bypass grafts in dogs. *Mayo Clin. Proc. 53*:327, 1978.

52. Davis, H. H., Varki, A., Heaton, W. A., and Siegel, B. A.: Detection of accessory spleens with indium-lll-labeled autologous platelets. *Am. J. Hematol. 8*:81, 1980.

Epochal hematology

CHAPTER 5

Hematology of the newborn

ELIAS SCHWARTZ
FRANCES M. GILL

There are important hematologic differences between the newborn infant and the older child and adult. These are related to the embryologic development of the fetus, the interaction between the fetus and the mother, and the changes necessary to adapt to extrauterine life. Even among newborns there are differences between those infants born after a term gestation and those born prematurely. This chapter discusses only the normal findings in the newborn infant.

Fetal hemopoiesis

PRODUCTION OF FETAL HEMOPOIETIC CELLS

The three major sites of fetal hemopoiesis are the yolk sac, the liver, and the marrow. Erythropoiesis begins in the 19-day embryo [1,2]. The earliest hemopoietic cells, called *hemocytoblasts* or *stem cells*, are derived from the vessels of the yolk sac. Erythropoiesis is primarily intravascular and megaloblastic. Erythropoiesis stops in the yolk sac by the eleventh week of gestation.

Erythropoietic activity is present in the liver of the 6-week embryo [1]. This organ is the primary source of red blood cells from the ninth to the twenty-fourth week of gestation. Hepatic erythropoiesis is extravascular, with late cells entering the vascular space. Erythropoiesis also occurs to a lesser extent in connective tissue, kidney, spleen, thymus, and lymph nodes.

Erythropoiesis is first seen in the marrow of the 10- to 11-week embryo [1,2]. Erythropoietic activity increases rapidly in the ensuing weeks, and the marrow is the major site of hemopoiesis after the twenty-fourth week of gestation. Fetal erythropoiesis is almost entirely megaloblastic through the first 11 weeks of gestation and remains partially so until the fifth day of postnatal life. The number of circulating nucleated red cells is greatest in the early embryo, comprising 50 percent of the red cells in the 8-week embryo, 10 percent in the 11-week stage, and only 0.6 percent in the 19-week embryo

[2]. After the fifteenth postnatal day, hemopoiesis is normally confined to the marrow.

Granulopoiesis is present in the liver parenchyma and in some areas of connective tissue in the 7-week embryo, but the amount in these tissues is small. Granulopoiesis begins in the marrow in the tenth to eleventh week of gestation and increases rapidly. Circulating leukocytes in small numbers are present at the eleventh week of gestation [2]. Lymphopoiesis has not been observed in the yolk sac but is present in the lymph plexuses at 9 weeks and in the lymph glands at 11 weeks of gestation. Circulating lymphocytes are seen in the 9-week embryo [2]. Lymphocyte subpopulations may be detected as early as 13 weeks of gestation in fetal livers [3]. Megakaryocytes are present in the yolk sac and liver by 6 weeks of gestation, the spleen by 10 weeks, and the marrow by 13 weeks of gestation. They are constantly present in the marrow thereafter [2].

PRODUCTION OF FETAL HEMOGLOBINS

The earliest globin chains in the embryo are the zeta (ζ), which is an alpha-type chain (α), and the epsilon (ϵ), which is similar to the later gamma (γ) chain [4,5]. Hemoglobin Gower 1 ($\zeta_2\epsilon_2$) is the major hemoglobin of embryos of less than 5 to 6 weeks of gestation [6]. Hemoglobin Gower 2 ($\alpha_2\epsilon_2$) has been found in embryos with a gestational age as low as 4 weeks and is absent in embryos older than 13 weeks [7]. Hemoglobin Portland ($\zeta_2\gamma_2$) is found in young embryos but persists in infants with homozygous α thalassemia [5]. Synthesis of the ζ and ϵ chains decreases as that of α and γ chains increases. This progression occurs about the time that the liver replaces the yolk sac as the main site of erythropoiesis [4].

Hemoglobin F ($\alpha_2\gamma_2$) is also present in very young embryos and is the major hemoglobin of fetal life [8]. It constitutes 90 to 95 percent of the total hemoglobin in the fetus until about 34 to 36 weeks of gestation. Synthesis of hemoglobin A (Hb A) can be demonstrated in fetuses as young as 9 weeks of gestation [9,10]. In fetuses of 9 to 21 weeks of gestation, the amount of Hb A rises from 4 to 13 percent of the total hemoglobin [10]. After 34 to 36 weeks of gestation, the percentage of Hb A rises further, while that of Hb F decreases. The amount of Hb F in blood varies in term infants from 53 to 95 percent of total hemoglobin [11,12]. The mean synthesis of Hb F in term infants was found to be 59.0 ± 10 percent (1 standard deviation) [13].

The fetal hemoglobin concentration in blood decreases after birth by approximately 3 percent per week and is generally less than 2 to 3 percent of the total hemoglobin by 6 months of age. This rate of decrease in Hb F production is closely related to the gestational age of the infant and does not appear to be affected by the changes in environment and oxygen tension that occur at the time of birth [14].

Increased proportions of Hb F at birth have been reported in infants who are small for gestational age,

TABLE 5-1   Red cell values for term infants during the first 12 weeks of life*

Age	Hb, g/100 ml ±SD	RBC × 10⁶ ±SD	Hematocrit, % ±SD	MCV, μm³ ±SD	MCHC, % ±SD	Reticulocytes, % ±SD
Days:						
1	19.3±2.2	5.14±0.7	61±7.4	119±9.4	31.6±1.9	3.2±1.4
2	19.0±1.9	5.15±0.8	60±6.4	115±7.0	31.6±1.4	3.2±1.3
3	18.8±2.0	5.11±0.7	62±9.3	116±5.3	31.1±2.8	2.8±1.7
4	18.6±2.1	5.00±0.6	57±8.1	114±7.5	32.6±1.5	1.8±1.1
5	17.6±1.1	4.97±0.4	57±7.3	114±8.9	30.9±2.2	1.2±0.2
6	17.4±2.2	5.00±0.7	54±7.2	113±10.0	32.2±1.6	0.6±0.2
7	17.9±2.5	4.86±0.6	56±9.4	118±11.2	32.0±1.6	0.5±0.4
Weeks:						
1–2	17.3±2.3	4.80±0.8	54±8.3	112±19.0	32.1±2.9	0.5±0.3
2–3	15.6±2.6	4.20±0.6	46±7.3	111±8.2	33.9±1.9	0.8±0.6
3–4	14.2±2.1	4.00±0.6	43±5.7	105±7.5	33.5±1.6	0.6±0.3
4–5	12.7±1.6	3.60±0.4	36±4.8	101±8.1	34.9±1.6	0.9±0.8
5–6	11.9±1.5	3.55±0.2	36±6.2	102±10.2	34.1±2.9	1.0±0.7
6–7	12.0±1.5	3.40±0.4	36±4.8	105±12.0	33.8±2.3	1.2±0.7
7–8	11.1±1.1	3.40±0.4	33±3.7	100±13.0	33.7±2.6	1.5±0.7
8–9	10.7±0.9	3.40±0.5	31±2.5	93±12.0	34.1±2.2	1.8±1.0
9–10	11.2±0.9	3.60±0.3	32±2.7	91±9.3	34.3±2.9	1.2±0.6
10–11	11.4±0.9	3.70±0.4	34±2.1	91±7.7	33.2±2.4	1.2±0.7
11–12	11.3±0.9	3.70±0.3	33±3.3	88±7.9	34.8±2.2	0.7±0.3

*Capillary blood samples. The RBC count and MCV measurements were made on an electronic counter.
SOURCE: Adapted from Matoth et al. [24].

who have experienced chronic intrauterine anoxia, or who have trisomy 13 [15–18]. Decreased levels of Hb F at birth are found in trisomy 21 [19]. Persistence of the embryonic hemoglobins Gower 1, 2, and Portland has been described in some infants with developmental abnormalities.

Neonatal hemopoiesis

NORMAL VALUES

The mean hemoglobin level in cord blood is 16.8 g/dl, with 95 percent of the values falling between 13.7 and 20.1 [20]. This variation reflects perinatal events, particularly asphyxia [21], and also the amount of blood transferred from the placenta to the infant after delivery. Delay of cord clamping may increase the blood volume of the infant by as much as 55 percent [22]. Normally, the hemoglobin and hematocrit values rise in the first several hours of life because of the movement of plasma from the intravascular to the extravascular space [23]. A venous hemoglobin concentration of less than 14 g/dl in a term infant and/or a fall in hemoglobin or hematocrit level in the first day of life are abnormal. Normal red cell values from capillary blood samples are given in Table 5-1 for term infants in the first 12 weeks of life [24]. The hemoglobin level at birth has been reported to be lower in the premature than in the term infant [25,26], and the reticulocyte and nucleated red cell counts are higher. In another study of premature infants, the mean hemoglobin level of capillary blood on the first postnatal day was constant at about 19 g/dl despite gestational ages ranging from 24 to 37 weeks [27]. The mean hematocrit level was also constant, but the red cell count rose and the mean corpuscular volume decreased as gestational age increased. Infants who are small for their gestational ages have higher red cell counts, hematocrit levels, and hemoglobin concentrations [26,28], but the reticulocyte counts are compatible with their gestational age [29]. Capillary hemoglobin and hematocrit values in newborns are higher than those in simultaneous venous samples, probably because of circulatory factors [30]. Venous blood determinations should be used in sick newborns to ensure that accurate values are obtained.

The reticulocyte count is high at birth but falls to less than 1 percent by the sixth day of life [31]. The red cell, hemoglobin, and hematocrit values decrease only slightly during the first week but decline more rapidly in the following 5 to 8 weeks [24]. Physiologic anemia of the newborn develops at this time [32]. When the hemoglobin concentration falls to a level of about 11 g/dl, erythropoietic activity begins to increase. The lowest hemoglobin values in the term infant occur at about 2 months of age [33]. In the premature infant the fall in hemoglobin level is more pronounced, and the nadir may be reached by the fifth week. The mean hemoglobin level at 2 months in one study of premature infants was 9.4 g/dl with a 95 percent range of 7.2 to 11.7 g/dl [34]. The mean values for iron-sufficient premature infants attained those of term infants by 4 months for red cell count, 5 months for hemoglobin level, and 6 months for mean corpuscular volume and mean corpuscular hemoglobin [34].

The red cells of the newborn are markedly macrocytic

at birth, but the mean cell volume and diameter begin to fall after the first week, reaching adult values by the ninth week [24,33]. The mean corpuscular hemoglobin concentration averages 31.6 percent at birth and rises thereafter. A blood film from a newborn infant shows macrocytic, normochromic cells, polychromasia, and a few nucleated red blood cells. Even in healthy infants there may be mild anisocytosis and poikilocytosis. From 3 to 5 percent of the red cells may show fragmentation, target formation, and distortion of shape. Nucleated red blood cells are not normally found in the blood after 3 to 5 days of life, even in premature infants, but may be present in markedly elevated numbers in the presence of hemolysis or hypoxia.

The values for the white cell count and differential count during the first 2 weeks of life are given in Table 5-2. The absolute number of polymorphonuclear neutrophils rises in both term and premature infants in the first 24 h of life [35]. In term infants in this study the mean value rose from 8000 per microliter to a peak of 13,000 and then fell to 4000 per microliter by 72 h of age, remaining at this level through the following 7 days. In the premature infant the mean values for neutrophils were 5000 per microliter at birth, 8000 at 12 h, and 4000 at 72 h. The mean count then fell gradually to 2500 per microliter by the twenty-eighth day of life. The level after the first 72 h was very stable for an individual infant, whether term or premature. Earlier forms, including an occasional promyelocyte and blast cell, may be seen in the blood of healthy infants in the first few days of life and are more frequent in premature than in term infants [35]. Polymorphonuclear leukocytes are the predominant cells in the first few days of life. As their number decreases, the lymphocyte becomes the most numerous cell and remains so during the first 4 years of life. An absolute eosinophil count of greater than 700 per microliter was found in 76 percent of premature infants at 2 to 3 weeks of age. The onset of the eosinophilia coincided with the establishment of steady weight gain in the infants [36].

There is active hemopoiesis in the marrow at birth [37,38]. The amount of erythropoiesis decreases markedly during the first week. The average number of nucleated red cells falls from 41,000 per microliter on day 1 to 7000 by day 9 [38]. The myeloid to erythroid ratio rises from a value of 1.9:1 on day 1 to 6.7:1 on day 8 [37]. Lymphocytes comprise about 14 percent of the marrow cells at birth, but after the first month of life constitute about 50 percent of the marrow cells. The average cell counts of marrows of healthy children over the first 18 months of life have been determined [39] (see Chap. 3).

The serum iron level in cord blood of the normal infant is elevated, the mean value in one series of 320 infants being 154 μg/dl with a standard deviation of 41 [40]. In a study of infants on an iron-supplemented diet, the median serum iron level fell from 125 μg/dl at 1 month of age to 77 μg/dl at 6 months of age. The total iron-binding capacity rose throughout the first year of life. The median transferrin saturation fell from 67 percent at 0.5 months to 23 percent at 1 year, with saturations as low as 10 percent observed in the absence of iron deficiency [41]. Serum ferritin levels in these iron-sufficient infants were high at birth, the mean being 160 μg/liter, rose further during the first month, and then fell to a mean of 31 μg/liter by 12 months of age [42]. The amount of stainable iron present in the marrow at birth is small but increases in both the term and premature infant during the first weeks of life. Stainable marrow iron begins to decrease after 2 months and is gone by 4 to 6 months in term infants and even earlier in premature infants [43].

The mean value for total blood volume in the first 3 days of life is 86.3 ml/kg for the term infant and 89.4 ml/kg for the premature infant [44]. The blood volume per kilogram decreases over the ensuing weeks, reaching a mean value of about 65 ml/kg by 3 to 4 months of age. The mean red cell mass during the first 3 days of life for full-term or premature infants is about 45 ml/kg, falling to 18.8 ml/kg at 60 to 130 days of age [44].

TABLE 5-2 The white cell count and the differential count during the first 2 weeks of life

Age	Leukocytes	Neutrophils			Eosinophils	Basophils	Lymphocytes	Monocytes
		Total	Seg.	Band				
Birth:								
Mean	18,000	11,000	9400	1600	400	100	5500	1050
Range	9.0–30.0	6.0–26	–	–	20–850	0–640	2.0–11.0	0.4–3.1
Mean %	–	61	52	9	2.2	0.6	31	5.8
7 days:								
Mean	12,200	5500	4700	830	500	50	5000	1100
Range	5.0–21.0	1.5–10.0	–	–	70–1100	0–250	2.0–17.0	0.3–2.7
Mean %	–	45	39	6	4.1	0.4	41	9.1
14 days:								
Mean	11,400	4500	3900	630	350	50	5500	1000
Range	5.0–20.0	1.0–9.5	–	–	70–1000	0–230	2.0–17.0	0.2–2.4
Mean %	–	40	34	5.5	3.1	0.4	48	8.8

SOURCE: P. L. Altman and D. S. Dittmer, *Blood and Other Body Fluids.* Federation of American Societies for Experimental Biology, Washington, 1961.

The life-span of the red cells in the newborn infant is shorter than that of adult red cells. The average of several studies of mean half-life of newborn red cells labeled with chromium was 23.3 days in term infants and 16.6 days in premature infants. When corrected for the elution rate of chromium from newborn cells, the estimate of mean red cell survival in the newborn is 60 to 80 days [45]. The reasons for this shortened survival are unclear, but the known differences between newborn and adult red cells may be contributing factors.

Erythroid functions

Erythropoietin seems to be involved in red cell production in the marrow phase of fetal erythropoiesis during the third trimester [46]. The level of erythropoietin rises with gestational age and reaches significant levels after 34 weeks of gestation [26]. In healthy infants, erythropoietin falls to an undetectable level after birth [26,47], but is again measurable after the sixtieth day of life [48]. However, if there is sufficient stimulus, such as hemolytic anemia or cyanotic congenital heart disease, the newborn infant is able to produce erythropoietin [47]. In healthy premature infants, erythropoietin, as measured by a radioimmunoassay, was again detectable when the hemoglobin level fell to 11 to 13 g/dl. In infants with a lower percentage of Hb F (as from transfusion) and consequently better oxygen delivery, erythropoietin did not rise until the hemoglobin fell 2 to 3 g lower [49].

OXYGEN DELIVERY

The oxygen affinity of cord blood is greater than that of maternal blood, since the affinity of Hb F for 2,3-DPG and ATP is less than that of Hb A [50]. The red cell oxygen equilibrium curve of the newborn is shifted to the left of that of the adult. The mean P_{50} at 1 day of age in one study of term infants was 19.4 ± 1.8 mmHg, as compared with the normal adult value of 27.0 ± 1.1 mmHg [51]. After birth, the oxygen equilibrium curve shifts gradually to the right, reaching the position of the adult curve by 4 to 6 months of age. The shift to the left is even more pronounced in the premature infant, and the shift to the adult position is more gradual. The position of the curve in the premature infant correlates with gestational age rather than with postnatal age [51].

Levels of 2,3-DPG have been reported to be lower in newborn red cells than in adult cells and even more decreased in the red cells of premature infants [52]. The levels of ATP and ADP were found to be higher in the red cells of term and premature infants than in adult cells [53]. A recent study suggests that 2,3-DPG and ATP levels are normal in the red cells of term infants if corrected for the red cell age [54].

NEONATAL RED CELLS

The viscosity of blood from the newborn increases in relation to hematocrit [55–57]. Newborn infants with hematocrit values of greater than 65 to 70 percent may become symptomatic because of increased viscosity. Hyperviscosity has been found in 5 percent of infants in one series [58] and in 18 percent of infants who were small for gestational age in another [59].

The deformability of the newborn erythrocyte is less than that of adult cells [60]. The decrease in filterability of cord cells cannot be explained by the observed differences in mean corpuscular volume or in the numbers of white cells or reticulocytes.

Many differences have been found between the metabolism of the red cells of newborn infants and adults [61,62]. Some of the differences may be explained by the younger mean cell age in the newborn, but others seem to be unique properties of the fetal cell. If cells of a similar young age are compared, the glucose consumption in newborn cells is lower than that in adult cells, suggesting a difference in red cell glycolysis [63]. Elevated levels of glucose phosphate isomerase, glyceraldehyde-3-phosphate dehydrogenase, phosphoglycerate kinase, and enolase beyond those explainable by the young cell age have been found in neonatal cells [52,64]. The level of phosphofructokinase is low in red cells from term and premature infants [52,53,64]. The pentose phosphate shunt is active in red cells of term and premature infants [68]. Lower-than-adult activities have been found for several other red cell enzymes, including NADP-dependent methemoglobin reductase [66], glutathione peroxidase [67], and catalase [68].

The membrane of the fetal red cell also shows differences from that of the adult red cell. Stromal ouabain-sensitive ATPase is decreased in neonatal cells [69]. Flux studies show that the active potassium influx is significantly less in neonatal red cells, but sodium influx is the same [70]. Newborn cells are more sensitive to osmotic hemolysis and to oxidant injury than are adult cells. Newborn red cells have higher total lipid, phospholipid, and cholesterol per cell than adult red cells [71,72]. The patterns of phospholipid and phospholipid fatty acid composition also differ from those in adult red cells. Red cells of newborns have the same pattern of membrane proteins on polyacrilamide gel electrophoresis [73] and the same electrophoretic mobility [74] as do red cells from adults. After trypsin treatment of newborn and adult cells, however, there is a difference in electrophoretic mobility, suggesting that the fetal membrane protein may be different [74]. The relationship of the metabolic and membrane alterations in neonatal red cells to their shorter life-span is not clear.

Phagocyte functions

Bacterial infections are a major cause of morbidity and mortality in the newborn period [75]. The infections are frequently due to organisms of low virulence in normal children and adults, including *Staphylococcus*, Lancefield group B β-hemolytic streptococci, *Pseudomonas*, and other gram-negative bacilli. Several features of the cellular defense mechanisms and humoral immunity of the newborn differ from those found later in life, and any or all of these may be in part responsible for the unusual susceptibility to infection noted in the neonatal period.

The absolute number of neutrophils and monocytes in the blood of term and premature infants is usually greater than that found in older children (Table 5-2), but the neutrophil count tends to be lower in the premature than in the term infant, with a more striking shift to the left [76]. Serum and urinary colony-stimulating activity are elevated during the period of neutrophilia [77]. Eosinophilia is common in premature infants, with 76 percent developing absolute eosinophilia (>700 per microliter), the infants in the lower gestational age having the highest incidence and counts [78,79]. It appears to be aggravated by the use of total parenteral nutrition, endotracheal intubation, and blood transfusions.

Engulfment and destruction of bacteria by neutrophils depend on opsonin activity of the plasma, chemotaxis, phagocytosis, and the bacteriocidal capacity of the leukocyte. The serum factors necessary for optimal phagocytosis (opsonins) include the immunoglobulins and complement components. In term infants, opsonin activity for *Staphylococcus aureus* and group B strepococcus is normal [80,81], but it is low for yeast [82] and *Escherichia coli* [81]. In premature infants, opsonin activity for *Pseudomonas aeruginosa* is normal [83], but it is low for *S. aureus* and *Serratia marcescens* [80]. The decreased opsonin activity for some organisms in premature infants has been attributed to diminished IgG levels, since additional IgG will correct the opsonic defect both in vivo and in vitro [80]. The classical and alternative complement pathways are decreased in activity and in levels of individual components in many newborns. The mean level of C3, the first common component of the two pathways of complement activation, is about 60 to 74 percent of that in normal adults [84–86]. There is no transplacental transfer of this protein, and levels in infants are lower than those in their mothers [84]. Since heterozygotes for C3 deficiency have levels comparable with those seen in the normal newborn and are entirely healthy [87], the decreased C3 levels alone probably do not result in increased susceptibility to infection in the newborn. Total hemolytic complement (CH_{50}) and alternative pathway activity (PH_{50}) in newborns are lower than in adults, as are mean levels of C1q, C2 to C9, factor B, properdin, C3bINA, and β1H [85,86,88]. In general, the mean levels in full-term infants are greater than 50 percent of those in normal controls and may be somewhat less in premature babies. There is considerable overlap between levels in infants and in controls. Using mother-infant paired sera to study opsonic activity, uptake of *E. coli* strains which are opsonized by the alternative complement pathway was decreased in infants, while uptake of strains requiring the classical pathway was normal, indicating a functional deficiency in the alternative pathway [89].

Chemotactic function of leukocytes is low in neonates, while random mobility is normal [90–92]. Neonatal serum does not generate as much chemotactic factor as does adult serum, even after the addition of purified C3.

Phagocytosis of bacteria and latex granules by neutrophils from premature and full-term infants is normal [80–83,93,94]. Bactericidal activity varies according to the conditions of testing and the clinical status of the neonates. The intracellular killing of *S. aureus* and *Serratia marcescens* in cells from most term and low-birth-weight infants is normal [80,95], as is that of *E. coli* in full-term infants [81]. Similar studies have shown defective bactericidal activity against *S. aureus* in some infants in the first 12 h of life [93], *P. aeruginosa* in cells from premature infants [83], and *C. albicans* in granulocytes from term and premature infants [96]. With bacteria/neutrophil ratios of 1:1, newborn cells kill *S. aureus* and *E. coli* as effectively as controls do; however, at the higher ratio of 100:1, killing and oxidative response as measured by chemoluminescence are markedly depressed, although phagocytosis is normal [94]. Depressed activity has also been found in cells from newborns who have had clinical stress, either from infection or other disorders, shown both as decreased chemoluminescence and impaired bactericidal activity against *S. aureus*, *E. coli*, and group B streptococci [97–99]. The decreased granulocyte function shown in these studies is also found in liquid culture, where neutrophils from newborns do not survive as long as those from controls, perhaps because of decreased resistance to autooxidation [100]. Although superoxide dismutase levels are normal in neutrophils from newborns, glutathione peroxidase and catalase levels are decreased [101]. The relationship of these in vitro cellular defects to bacterial infections in the newborn is still not clear.

Monocytes from newborn infants have normal Nitro Blue Tetrazolium (NBT) reduction [102], antibody-dependent cellular cytotoxicity [103], and in vitro killing of *S. aureus* and *E. coli* [104]. They are slower than monocytes from adults in phagocytosis of polystyrene spheres [105], and they also do not appear to generate ATP [106].

Thymus functions

CELLULAR IMMUNITY

The absolute number of lymphocytes in the newborn is equivalent to that in older children (Table 5-2), with lower values in premature infants at birth [96]. Large lymphocytes comprise 90 percent of the total at birth, with a decrease in absolute number to 3 days of age, followed by an increase [107]. The rise after 3 days may reflect antigenic stimulation in the extrauterine environment. Small lymphocytes are few at birth but increase during the first 2 weeks to approximately 35 percent of the total lymphocytes. Thymus-derived cells (T cells) develop early in gestation [108], and the absolute number of T cells in blood of newborns is similar to that of adults [109], as are percentages of T-helper and T-suppressor cells [110]. Most responses of the cellular-immunity system are present in the newborn, although some are decreased in comparison with adults [111]. The in vitro response to phytohemagglutinin of cord blood lymphocytes is increased [112,113]. Inoculation with bacillus Calmette-Guérin (BCG) at birth elicits delayed hypersensitivity to tuberculin in the same time interval as is observed in adults [114]. The response of the newborn to 2,4-dinitrofluorobenzene, a potent inducer of delayed hypersensitivity, is not as regular as that seen in older children [115]. Cord blood T cells from term or preterm newborns have a potent suppressive effect on cell-mediated immunity responses of lymphoid cells from adults, even without stimulation of the cord blood cells by mitogens [116,117].

HUMORAL IMMUNITY

The humoral immunity system (B cells) also develops early in gestation [108], but it is not fully active until after birth. In the newborn, 10 to 20 percent of lymphocytes have surface-membrane–bound immunoglobulin, with all classes represented [118]. As in adults, the percentages of specific immunoglobin markers are not related to relative serum immunoglobulin levels. Variation in antibody response to specific antigens relates to the interaction of macrophages, T cells, and B cells; B lymphocytes appear to be well represented in newborns [119].

The fetus has a low synthesis of immunoglobulins, presumably because of the sheltered environment in utero. Animals kept germ-free after birth similarly have a scarcity of plasma cells and markedly decreased production of immunoglobulins [120]. IgG levels of full-term infants are similar to maternal levels because of transplacental transfer [121]. IgM, IgD, and IgE do not cross the placenta [121,122], and the levels of these immunoglobulins and IgA are low or not detectable at birth. Breast feeding provides some transfer of T and B antibodies, lysozyme, lactoferrin, monocytes, and lymphocytes to the infant, particularly in colostrum, perhaps aiding in protection against infection [123,124]. Although the newborn infant can produce specific IgG antibody [125], only small amounts of IgG are usually produced by the fetus. IgG levels in premature infants are reduced in relation to gestational age because of the low placental transport early in pregnancy [126–128]. The ability of the fetus to produce IgM and IgA with appropriate stimuli is indicated by the presence of these antibodies in many newborn infants who have had prenatal infections [129] and by the presence of IgM isohemagglutinins in more than one-half of full-term newborn infants [130]. In human newborn and in fetal animals, the IgM response is predominant, and the appearance of IgG after exposure to specific antigens is delayed. These differences from the adult may relate to functional immaturity of B and T lymphocytes [110,131–133], to increased activity of suppressor T cells [131], and perhaps to altered macraphage function as well [134].

The neonate may have severe infections from viruses such as herpes simplex that are usually not major pathogens later in life. The interferon response of leukocytes from newborns and the induction of natural killer cytotoxicity are normal [135,136].

Splenic hypofunction or asplenia is accompanied by an unusual susceptibility to severe infection in children with sickle cell disease [137], congenital asplenia [138], thalassemia [139], and other chronic systemic disorders [140]. The large number of "pocked" erythrocytes seen in neonates (especially prominent in premature infants) indicates monocyte-macrophage hypofunction in these infants [141,142]. Howell-Jolly bodies are not seen as commonly and were present only transiently in 1 of 76 term and 4 of 82 healthy premature infants [143].

Hemostatic functions

PLATELETS

The mean platelet count in infants at term is slightly lower than that found in older children and adults. In 193 healthy infants in two studies, the mean count was 223,000 per microliter in the first 2 days of life, with a range from 84,000 to 478,000 per microliter [144,145]. Most values were between 100,000 and 350,000 per microliter. At birth the platelet counts of premature infants have the same mean value and range observed in full-term newborn infants [145–147]. Platelet counts of less than 100,000 per microliter are common in infants admitted to a high-risk nursery for other reasons [148], in small-for-date infants [149], and in newborns with trisomy syndromes [150]. In high-risk infants without major clinical complications, the incidence of thrombocytopenia was much lower than in sick infants, with 22 percent of "healthy" term babies and 35 percent of "healthy" preterm infants having low platelet counts at some point during their stay in the hospital compared with greater than 72 percent of sick infants [148].

Although healthy newborn infants have a normal bleeding time [151], laboratory studies show impairment of platelet function, including clot retraction, release of platelet factors 3 and 4 and ADP, and aggregation with epinephrine, collagen, thrombin, and ADP [152–154]. Increased bilirubin levels do not cause further impairment of platelet aggregation [155]. In infants of mothers ingesting aspirin, there is markedly decreased aggregation in response to collagen [153,156], indicating further impairment of ADP release. Increased clinical bleeding may occur in newborns whose mothers have taken aspirin during the week before delivery [154,156,157].

Newborn infants commonly have petechiae [158], particularly on the head, neck, and shoulders, after vertex deliveries. Petechiae are usually not present in infants delivered by cesarean section. They are presumably due to trauma associated with passage through the birth canal and disappear within a few days.

CLOTTING FACTORS

The concentration of specific coagulation factors in the fetus depends on the balance of rates of placental transfer from the mother, endogenous synthesis in the fetus, and catabolism or consumption of the factors. The transfer of plasma proteins from mother to fetus is only partially dependent on molecular weight. IgG molecules are readily transported across the placenta, while the much larger IgM molecules are not. Haptoglobin, ceruloplasmin, IgA, and C3 are relatively excluded by the placenta, however, even though their molecular weights approximate that of IgG. Fibrinogen [159] and factor VIII [160] do not readily cross the placenta. These two proteins are synthesized by the fetus, and the levels are lower than those found in the mother [161–163]. The relative catabolic rates of these and other coagulation factors in mother and neonate have not been determined.

Levels of prothrombin [164], of factors V [161], VII [165], IX, X [161], XI [165], and XII [166], and of plasminogen [167] are reduced in the newborn infant in comparison with the mother [163], indicating reduced placental transfer, increased catabolism, or both. There are conflicting data about factor XIII levels in the newborn, with both decreased [168,169] and elevated [163] values in relation to the mother being reported. In comparison with older children or adults, rather than with pregnant women at term, values of fibrinogen, prothrombin, factors VII, IX, X, XI, and XII, Fletcher and Fitzgerald factors, plasminogen, and antithrombin III in the full-term newborn infant are decreased, while factors V and XIII and fibrinogen split products are usually normal [147,163,170–173]. Factor VIII coagulant activity, related antigen, and ristocetin cofactor activity are elevated in healthy term infants [174].

Although marked variations in prothrombin times in newborns have been reported in several studies, more recent results indicate that the values do not differ much from those in normal adults, with the range in term and premature infants extending to values about 2 to 3 s longer than in controls [175]. The partial thromboplastin time has a very wide range in healthy term and preterm infants.

The factors dependent on vitamin K synthesis, II (prothrombin), VII, IX, and X, decrease during the first 3 to 4 days, a fall which may be lessened in some infants by administration of vitamin K [176]. Inactive prothrombin molecules have been found in the plasma of newborns, but in contrast to earlier observations [177] they disappear after administration of vitamin K [178]. The low levels of factor IX at birth are not improved with oral administration of vitamin K, and there is no evidence of inactive factor IX molecules [179].

Fibrinogen, factors II, VII, and X [180], factor VIII (coagulent activity and antigen levels), and factor IX are all lower in fetuses of gestational ages of 12 to 24 weeks than in full-term infants [181]. Factor V is at the same level as in full-term infants. In a group of healthy infants born at 27 to 42 weeks of gestation, determinations of fibinogen, prothrombin, factors II, VII, and X, and factor VIII in the newborn period showed higher levels with increasing gestational age, while factors V and IX levels did not vary with gestational age [147]. In a study of thriving infants of 26 to 29 weeks of gestational age compared with normal-term infants, decreases in levels of factors II, V, VII, XI, and XII, Fitzgerald and Fletcher factors, and antithrombin III were present in the younger groups, while levels of factor VIII, fibrinogen, fibrin degradation products, and factor VII-X complex were comparable in the groups [182]. Factor XIII levels are normal in premature infants [183]. There are no significant differences in mean prothrombin time determinations between premature and full-term infants who have not received vitamin K [184]. Premature infants given vitamin K have a longer mean prothrombin time than term infants similarly treated. In some small infants there is no improvement in prothrombin time or levels of prothrombin and of factors VII and X after the intramuscular administration of vitamin K [176,185]. These results suggest a greater degree of "immaturity" of the liver in the small infants.

Low-birth-weight infants have significant bleeding more often than do full-term newborn infants. Increased capillary fragility is frequently found in premature infants in the first 2 days after birth and is not associated with thrombocytopenia [176]. Bleeding under the scalp or in other superficial areas may be due to trauma coupled with increased capillary fragility. The more serious disorders of periventricular-intraventricular hemorrhage and pulmonary hemorrhage are probably not due primarily to coagulation disorders, although such disorders may increase the bleeding [186]. Hypoxia seems to affect the clotting status of low-birth-weight infants [187]. Many infants with markedly abnormal prothrombin times have had hypoxia during delivery or shortly thereafter [184]. Cardiovascular collapse seen with episodes of cardiac arrest or with profound shock may cause disseminated intravascular coagulation and generalized bleeding [175]. In many sick premature infants, a combination of shock, sepsis, liver immaturity, hypoxia, and other factors may make a careful analysis of the pathogenesis of coagulation abnormalities very difficult.

References

1. Bloom, W., and Bartelmez, G. W.: Hematopoiesis in young human embryos. *Am. J. Anat.* 67:21, 1940.
2. Gilmour, J. R.: Normal hemopoiesis in intrauterine and neonatal life. *J. Pathol.* 52:25, 1942.
3. Gupta, S., Pahwa, R., O'Reilly, R., Good, R. A., and Siegal, F. P.: Ontogeny of lymphocyte subpopulation in human fetal liver. *Proc. Natl. Acad. Sci. U.S.A.* 73:919, 1976.
4. Gale, R. E., Clegg, J. B., and Huehns, E. R.: Human embryonic haemoglobins Gower 1 and Gower 2. *Nature* 280:162, 1979.
5. Kamuzora, H., and Lehmann, H.: Human embryonic haemoglobins including a comparison by homology of the human ζ and α chains. *Nature* 256:511, 1975.
6. Hecht, F., Motulsky, A. G., Lemire, R. J., and Shepard, T. E.: Predominance of hemoglobin Gower 1 in early human embryonic development. *Science* 152:91, 1966.

7. Huehns, E. R., Dance, N., Beaven, G. H., Hecht, F., and Motulsky, A. G.: Human embryonic hemoglobins. *Cold Spring Harbor Symp. Quant. Biol.* 29:327, 1964.

8. Pataryas, H. A., and Stomatoyannopoulos, G.: Hemoglobins in human fetuses: Evidence of adult hemoglobin production after the 11th gestational week. *Blood* 39:688, 1972.

9. Thomas, E. D., Lochte, H. L., Jr., Greenough, W. B., III, and Walls, M.: In vitro synthesis of foetal and adult haemoglobin by foetal haematopoietic tissues. *Nature* 185:396, 1960.

10. Kazazian, H. H., and Woodhead, A. P.: Hemoglobin A synthesis in the developing fetus. *N. Engl. J. Med.* 289:58, 1973.

11. Kirschbaum, T.: Fetal hemoglobin content of cord blood determined by column chromatography. *Am. J. Obstet. Gynecol.* 84:1375, 1962.

12. Armstrong, D., Schroeder, W. A., and Fenninger, W.: A comparison of the percentage of fetal hemoglobin in human umbilical cord blood as determined by chromatography and by alkali denaturation. *Blood* 22:554, 1963.

13. Bard, H.: The effect of placental insufficiency on fetal and adult hemoglobin synthesis. *Am. J. Obstet. Gynecol.* 120:67, 1974.

14. Bard, H.: Postnatal fetal and adult hemoglobin synthesis in early preterm newborn infants. *J. Clin. Invest.* 52:1789, 1973.

15. Bard, H., Makowski, E. L., Meschia, G., and Battaglia, C. F.: The relative rates of synthesis of hemoglobins A and F in red cells of newborn infants. *Pediatrics* 45:766, 1970.

16. Bromberg, Y. N., Abrahamov, A., and Salzberger, M.: The effect of maternal anoxemia on the foetal haemoglobin of the newborn. *J. Obstet. Gynecol. Br. Commonw.* 63:875, 1956.

17. Huehns, E. R., Hecht, F., Keil, J. V., and Motulsky, A. G.: Developmental hemoglobin anomalies in a chromosomal triplication. *Proc. Natl. Acad. Sci. U.S.A.* 51:89, 1964.

18. Lee, C. S. N., et al.: The D_1 trisomy syndrome: Three subjects with unequally advancing development. *Johns Hopkins Med. J.* 118:374, 1966.

19. Wilson, M. G., Schroeder, W. A., and Graves, D. A.: Postnatal change of hemoglobins F and A_2 in infants with Down's syndrome (G trisomy). *Pediatrics* 42:349, 1968.

20. Marks, J., Gairdner, D., and Roscoe, J. D.: Blood formation in infancy. III. Cord blood. *Arch. Dis. Child.* 30:117, 1955.

21. Linderkamp, O., Versmold, H. T., Messow-Zahn, K., Müller-Holve, W., Riegel, K. P., and Betke, K.: The effect of intra-partum and intra-uterine asphyxia on placental transfusion in premature and full-term infants. *Eur. J. Pediatr.* 127:91, 1978.

22. Yao, A. C., Hirvensalo, M., and Lind, J.: Placental transfusion rate and uterine contraction. *Lancet* 1:380, 1968.

23. McCue, C. M., Garner, F. B., Hurt, W. G., Schelin, E. C., and Sharpe, A. R., Jr.: Placental transfusion. *J. Pediatr.* 72:15, 1968.

24. Matoth, Y., Zaizor, R., and Varsano, I.: Postnatal changes in some red cell parameters. *Acta Paediatr. Scand.* 60:317, 1971.

25. Burman, D., and Morris, A. F.: Cord hemoglobin in low birth weight infants. *Arch. Dis. Child.* 49:382, 1974.

26. Meberg, A.: Haemoglobin concentrations and erythropoietin levels in appropriate and small for gestational age infants. *Scand. J. Haematol.* 24:162, 1980.

27. Zaizov, R., and Matoth, Y.: Red cell values on the first postnatal day during the last 16 weeks of gestation. *Am. J. Hematol.* 1:275, 1976.

28. Humbert, J. R., Abelson, H., Hathaway, W. E., and Battaglia, F. C.: Polycythemia in small for gestational age infants. *J. Pediatr.* 75:1812, 1969.

29. Lockridge, S., Pass, R., and Cassady, G.: Reticulocyte counts in intrauterine growth retardation. *Pediatrics* 47:919, 1971.

30. Linderkamp, O., Versmold, H. T., Strohhacker, I., Messow-Zahn, K., Riegel, K. P., and Betke, K.: Capillary-venous hematocrit differences in newborn infants. *Eur. J. Pediatr.* 127:9, 1977.

31. Seip, M.: The reticulocyte level and the erythrocyte production judged from reticulocyte studies in newborn infants during the first week of life. *Acta Paediatr. Scand.* 44:355, 1955.

32. Stockman, J. A., III, and Oski, F. A.: Physiological anaemia of infancy and the anaemia of prematurity. *Clin. Haematol.* 7:3, 1978.

33. Saarinen, U. M., and Siimes, M. A.: Developmental changes in red blood cell counts and indices of infants after exclusion of iron deficiency by laboratory criteria and continuous iron supplementation. *J. Pediatr.* 92:412, 1978.

34. Lundström, U., Siimes, M. A.: Red blood cell values in low-birth-weight infants: Ages at which values become equivalent to those of term infants. *J. Pediatr.* 96:1040, 1980.

35. Xanthou, M.: Leucocyte blood picture in healthy full-term and premature babies during neonatal period. *Arch. Dis. Child.* 45:242, 1970.

36. Gibson, E. L., Vaucher, Y., and Corrigan, J. J., Jr.: Eosinophilia in premature infants: Relationship to weight gain. *J. Pediatr.* 95:99, 1979.

37. Shapiro, L. M., and Bassen, F. A.: Sternal marrow changes during the first week of life. *Am. J. Med. Sci.* 202:341, 1941.

38. Gairdner, D., Marks, J., and Roscoe, J. D.: Blood formation in infancy: The normal bone marrow. *Arch. Dis. Child.* 27:128, 1952.

39. Rosse, C., Kraemer, M. J., Dillon, T. L., McFarland, R., and Smith, N. J.: Bone marrow cell populations of normal infants: The predominance of lymphocytes. *J. Lab. Clin. Med.* 89:1225, 1977.

40. Weipple, G., Pantlitschko, M., Bauer, P., and Lund, S.: Normal values and distribution of serum iron in cord blood. *Clin. Chim. Acta* 44:147, 1973.

41. Saarinen, U. M., and Siimes, M. A.: Developmental changes in serum iron, total iron-binding capacity, and transferrin saturation in infancy. *J. Pediatr.* 91:875, 1977.

42. Saarinen, U. M., and Siimes, M. A.: Serum ferritin in assessment of iron nutrition in healthy infants. *Acta Paediatr. Scand.* 67:745, 1978.

43. Seip, M., and Halvorsen, S.: Erythrocyte production and iron stores in premature infants during the first months of life: The anemia of prematurity—Etiology, pathogenesis, iron requirement. *Acta Paediatr. Scand.* 45:600, 1956.

44. Bratteby, L. E.: Studies on erythro-kinetics in infancy. XI. The change in circulating red cell volume during the first five months of life. *Acta Paediatr. Scand.* 57:215, 1968.

45. Pearson, H. A.: Life-span of the fetal red blood cell. *J. Pediatr.* 70:166, 1967.

46. Finne, P. H., and Halvorsen, S.: Regulation of erythropoiesis in the fetus and newborn. *Arch. Dis. Child.* 47:683, 1972.

47. Halvorsen, S.: Plasma erythropoietin levels in cord blood and in blood during the first week of life. *Acta Paediatr. Scand.* 52:425, 1963.

48. Mann, D. L., Sites, M. L., Donati, R. M., and Gallagher, N. I.: Erythropoietic stimulating activity during the first ninety days of life. *Proc. Soc. Exp. Biol. Med.* 118:212, 1965.

49. Stockman, J. A., III, Garcia, J. F., and Oski, F. A.: The anemia of prematurity: Factors governing the erythropoietin response. *N. Engl. J. Med.* 296:647, 1977.

50. Bauer, C., Ludwig, I., and Ludwig, M.: Different effects of 2,3-diphosphoglycerate and adenosine triphosphate on oxygen affinity of adult and fetal hemoglobin. *Life Sci.* 7:1339, 1968.

51. Oski, F. A., and Delivoria-Papadopoulos, M.: The red cell, 2,3-diphosphoglycerate, and tissue oxygen release. *J. Pediatr.* 77:941, 1970.

52. Oski, F. A.: Red cell metabolism in the newborn infant. V. Glycolytic intermediates and glycolytic enzymes. *Pediatrics* 44:84, 1969.

53. Gross, R. T., Schroeder, E. A. R., and Brounstein, S. A.: Energy metabolism in the erythrocytes of premature infants compared to full term newborn infants and adults. *Blood* 21:755, 1963.

54. Travis, A. F., Kumar, S. P., Delivoria-Papadopoulos, M.: Red cell metabolic alterations in postnatal life in term infants: Glycolytic intermediates and adenosine triphosphate. *Pediatr. Res.* 15:34, 1981.

55. MacIntosh, T. F., and Walker, C. H. M.: Blood viscosity in the newborn. *Arch. Dis. Child.* 48:547, 1973.

56. Bergqvist, G.: Viscosity of the blood in the newborn infant. *Acta Paediatr. Scand.* 63:858, 1974.

57. Bergqvist, G., and Zetterstrom, R.: Blood viscosity and peripheral circulation in newborn infants. *Acta Paediatr. Scand.* 63:865, 1974.

58. Wirth, F. H., Goldberg, K. E., and Lubchenco, L.: Neonatal hyperviscosity. I. Incidence. *Pediatrics* 63:833, 1979.

59. Hakanson, D. O., and Oh. W.: Hyperviscosity in the small-for-gestational age infant. *Biol. Neonate* 37:190, 1980.

60. Gross, G. P., and Hathaway, W. E.: Fetal erythrocyte deformability. *Pediatr. Res.* 6:593, 1972.

61. Zipursky, A.: The erythrocytes of the newborn infant. *Semin. Hematol.* 2:167, 1965.
62. Oski, F. A., and Komazawa, M.: Metabolism of the erythrocytes of the newborn infant. *Semin. Hematol.* 12:209, 1975.
63. Oski, F. A., and Smith, C. A.: Red cell metabolism in the premature infant. III. Apparent inappropriate glucose consumption for cell age. *Pediatrics* 41:473, 1968.
64. Konrad, P. N., Valentine, W. N., and Paglia, D. E.: Enzymatic activities and glutathione content of erythrocytes in the newborn: Comparison with red cells of older normal subjects and those with comparable reticulocytosis. *Acta Haematol.* 48:193, 1972.
65. Oski, F. A.: Red cell metabolism in the premature infant. II. The pentose phosphate pathway. *Pediatrics* 39:689, 1967.
66. Ross, J. D.: Deficient activity of DPNH-dependent methemoglobin diaphorase in cord blood erythrocytes. *Blood* 21:51, 1963.
67. Gross, R. T., Bracci, R., Rudolph, N., Schroeder, E., and Kochen, J. A.: Hydrogen peroxide toxicity and detoxification in erythrocytes of newborn infants. *Blood* 29:481, 1967.
68. Jones, P. E. H., and McCance, R. A.: Enzyme activities in the blood of infants and adults. *Biochem. J.* 45:464, 1949.
69. Whaun, J. M., and Oski, F. A.: Red cell stromal adenosine triphosphatase (ATPase) of newborn infants. *Pediatr. Res.* 3:105, 1969.
70. Blum, S. F., and Oski, F. A.: Red cell metabolism in the newborn infant. IV. Transmembrane potassium flux. *Pediatrics* 43:396, 1969.
71. Crowley, J., Ways, P., and Jones, J. W.: Human fetal erythrocyte and plasma lipids. *J. Clin. Invest.* 44:989, 1965.
72. Neerhout, R. C.: Erythrocyte lipids in the neonate. *Pediatr. Res.* 2:172, 1968.
73. Shapiro, D. L., and Pasqualini, P.: Erythrocyte membrane proteins of premature and full-term newborn infants. *Pediatr. Res.* 12:176, 1978.
74. Kosztolányi, G., and Jobst, K.: Electrokinetic analysis of the fetal erythrocyte membrane after trypsin digestion. *Pediatr. Res.* 14:138, 1980.
75. Siegel, J. D., and McCracken, G. H., Jr.: Sepsis neonatorum. *N. Engl. J. Med.* 304:642, 1981.
76. Coulombel, L., Dehan, M., Tchernia, G., Hill, C., and Vial, M.: The number of polymorphonuclear leukocytes in relation to gestational age in the newborn. *Acta Paediatr. Scand.* 68:709, 1979.
77. Barak, Y., Blachar, Y., and Levin, S.: Neonatal neutrophilia: Possible role of a humoral granulopoietic factor. *Pediatr. Res.* 14:1026, 1980.
78. Gibson, E. L., Vaucher, Y., and Corrigan, J. J., Jr.: Eosinophilia in premature infants: Relationship to weight gain. *J. Pediatr.* 95:99, 1979.
79. Bhat, A. M., and Scanlon, J. W.: The pattern of eosinophilia in premature infants. *J. Pediatr.* 98:612, 1981.
80. Forman, M. L., and Stiehm, E. R.: Impaired opsonic activity but normal phagocytosis in low-birth-weight infants. *N. Engl. J. Med.* 281:926, 1969.
81. Dossett, J. H., Williams, R. C., Jr., and Quie, P. G.: Studies on interaction of bacteria, serum factors and polymorphonuclear leukocytes in mothers and newborns. *Pediatrics* 44:49, 1969.
82. Miller, M. E.: Phagocytosis in the newborn infant: Humoral and cellular factors. *J. Pediatr.* 74:255, 1969.
83. Cocchi, P., and Marianelli, L.: Phagocytosis and intracellular killing of *Pseudomonas aeruginosa* in premature infants. *Helv. Pediatr. Acta* 22:110, 1967.
84. Propp, R. P., and Alper, C. A.: C'3 synthesis in the human fetus and lack of transplacental passage. *Science* 162:672, 1968.
85. Johnston, R. B., Jr., Altenburger, K. M., Atkinson, A. W., Jr., and Curry, R. H.: Complement in the newborn infant. *Pediatrics* 64:781, 1979.
86. Strunk, R. C., Fenton, L. J., and Gaines, J. A.: Alternative pathway of complement activation in full term and premature infants. *Pediatr. Res.* 13:641, 1979.
87. Alper, C. A., Propp, R. P., Klemperer, M. R., and Rosen, F. S.: Inherited deficiency of the third component of human complement. *J. Clin. Invest.* 48:553, 1969.
88. Davis, C. A., Vallota, E. H., and Forristal, J.: Serum complement levels in infancy: Age-related changes. *Pediatr. Res.* 13:1043, 1979.
89. Mills, E. L., Björksten, B., and Quie, P. G.: Deficient alternative complement pathway activity in newborn sera. *Pediatr. Res.* 13:1341, 1979.
90. Miller, M. E.: Chemotactic function in the neonate. Humoral and cellular aspects. *Pediatr. Res.* 5:487, 1971.
91. Klein, R. B., Fischer, T. J., Gard, S. E., Biberstein, M., Rich, K. C., and Stiehm, E. R.: Decreased mononuclear and polymorphonuclear chemotaxis in human newborns, infants, and young children. *Pediatrics* 60:467, 1977.
92. Tono-oka, T., Nakayama, M., Uehara, H., and Matsumoto, S.: Characteristics of impaired chemotactic function in cord blood leukocytes. *Pediatr. Res.* 13:148, 1979.
93. Coen, R., Grush, O., and Kander, E.: Studies of bactericidal activity and metabolism of the leukocyte in full-term neonates. *J. Pediatr.* 78:400, 1969.
94. Mills, E. L., Thompson, T., Björksten, B., Fillipovich, D., and Quie, P. G.: The chemiluminescence response and bactericidal activity of polymorphonuclear neutrophils from newborns and their mothers. *Pediatrics* 63:429, 1979.
95. Park, B. H., Holmes, B., and Good, R. A.: Metabolic studies on newborn leukocytes. *Pediatr. Res.* 3:376, 1969 (abstract).
96. Xanthou, M., Valassi-Adam, E., Kintronidou, E., and Matsaniotis, N.: Phagocytosis and killing ability of *Candida albicans* by blood leucocytes of healthy term and preterm babies. *Arch. Dis. Child.* 50:72, 1975.
97. Wright, W. C., Jr., Ank, B. J., Herbert, J., and Stiehm, E. R.: Decreased bactericidal activity of leukocytes of stressed newborn infants. *Pediatrics* 56:569, 1975.
98. Shigeoka, A. O., Santos, J. I., and Hill, H. R.: Functional analysis of neutrophil granulocytes from healthy, infected, and stressed neonates. *J. Pediatr.* 95:454, 1979.
99. Shigeoka, A. O., Charette, R. P., Wyman, M. L., and Hill, H. R.: Defective oxidative metabolic responses of neutrophils from stressed neonates. *J. Pediatr.* 98:392, 1981.
100. Strauss, R. G., and Synder, E. L.: Neutrophils from human infants exhibit decreased viability. *Pediatr. Res.* 15:794, 1981.
101. Strauss, R. G., Synder, E. L., Wallace, P. O., and Rosenberger, T. G.: Oxygen-detoxifying enzymes in neutrophils of infants and their mothers. *J. Lab. Clin. Med.* 95:897, 1980.
102. Kretschmer, R. R., Papierniak, C. K., Stewardson-Krieger, P., Bamzai, A. K., and Gotoff, S. P.: Quantitative nitrobluetetrazolium reduction by normal newborn monocytes. *J. Pediatr.* 91:306, 1977.
103. Milgrom, H., and Shore, S. L.: Assessment of monocyte function in the normal newborn infant by antibody-dependent cellular cytoxicity. *J. Pediatr.* 91:612, 1977.
104. Orlowski, J. P., Sieger, L., and Anthony, B. F.: Bactericidal capacity of monocytes of newborn infants. *J. Pediatr.* 89:797, 1976.
105. Schuit, K. E., and Powell, D. A.: Phagocytic dysfunction in monocytes of normal newborn infants. *Pediatrics* 65:501, 1980.
106. Das, M., Henderson, T., and Feig, S. A.: Neonatal mononuclear cell metabolism: Further evidence for diminished monocyte function in the neonate. *Pediatr. Res.* 13:632, 1979.
107. Andersen, V., and Andersen, E.: Changes in blood lymphocytes during the neonatal period. *Acta Paediatr. Scand.* 63:266, 1974.
108. Pabst, H. F.: Ontogeny of the immune response as a basis of childhood diseases. *J. Pediatr.* 97:519, 1980.
109. Wara, D. W., and Barrett, D. J.: Cell-mediated immunity in the newborn: Clinical aspects. *Pediatrics* 64:822, 1979.
110. Hayward, A. R., and Lydard, P. M.: B cell function in the newborn. *Pediatrics* 64:758, 1979.
111. Stiehm, E. R., Winter, H. S., and Bryson, Y. F.: Cellular (T cell) immunity in the human newborn. *Pediatrics* 64:814, 1979.
112. Carr, M. C., Stites, D. P., and Fudenberg, H. H.: Cellular immune aspects of the human fetal-maternal relationship. I. In vitro response of cord blood lymphocytes to phytohemagglutinen. *Cell. Immunol.* 5:21, 1972.
113. Papiernick, M.: Comparison of human foetal with child blood lymphocytic kinetics. *Biol. Neonate* 19:163, 1971.
114. Gaisford, W.: The protection of infants against tuberculosis. *Br. Med. J.* 2:1164, 1955.
115. Uhr, J. W., Dancis, J., and Neumann, C. G.: Delayed-type hypersensitivity in premature neonatal humans. *Nature* 187:1130, 1960.

116. Olstone, M. B. A., Tishon, A., and Moretta, L.: Active thymus-derived suppressor lymphocytes in human cord blood. *Nature* 269:333, 1977.
117. Abedin, M., and Kirkpatrick, C. H.: Immunosuppressive activity of cord blood leukocytes. *Pediatrics* 66:405, 1980.
118. Stern, C. M. M.: Changes in lymphocytes subpopulations in the blood of healthy and sick newborn infants. *Pediatr. Res.* 13:792, 1979.
119. Lawton, A. R., and Cooper, M. D.: B cell ontogeny: Immunoglobulin genes and their expression. *Pediatrics* 64:750, 1979.
120. Gustafsson, B. E., and Laurell, C. B.: Gamma globulin production in germ free rats after bacterial contamination. *J. Exp. Med.* 110:675, 1959.
121. Gitlin, D.: The differentiation and maturation of specific immune mechanisms. *Acta Pediatr. Scand.* [Suppl.] 172:60, 1967.
122. Stiehm, E. R.: Fetal defense mechanisms. *Am. J. Dis. Child.* 129:438, 1975.
123. Pitt, J.: Breast milk and the high-risk baby: Potential benefits and hazards. *Hosp. Prac.* 14:81, 1979.
124. Narayaran, I., Prakash, K., Balax, S., Verma, R. K., and Gujral, V. V.: Partial supplementation with expressed breast-milk for prevention of infection in low-birth-weight infants. *Lancet* 2:561, 1980.
125. Rothberg, R. M.: Immunoglobin and specific antibody synthesis during the first weeks of life of premature infants. *J. Pediatr.* 75:391, 1969.
126. Harworth, J. C.: Norris, M., and Dilling, L.: A study of the immunoglobulins in premature infants. *Arch. Dis. Child.* 40:243, 1965.
127. Thom, H., McKay, E., and Gray, D. W. G.: Protein concentrations in the umbilical cord plasma of premature and mature infants. *Clin. Sci.* 33:433, 1967.
128. Yeung, C. Y., and Hoffs, J. R.: Serum-γ-G-globulin levels in normal, premature, postmature, and "small-for-dates" newborn babies. *Lancet* 1:1167, 1968.
129. Sever, J. H. (ed.): Immunological responses to perinatal responses to perinatal infections. *J. Pediatr.* 75:1111, 1969.
130. Thomaidis, T., Agathopoulos, A., and Matsaniotis, N.: Natural isohemagglutinin production by the fetus. *J. Pediatr.* 74:39, 1969.
131. Morito, T., Bankhurst, A. D., and Williams, R. C., Jr.: Studies of human cord blood and adult lymphocyte interactions with in vitro immunoglobulin production. *J. Clin. Invest.* 64:990, 1979.
132. Miyagawa, Y., Sugita, K., Komiyama, A., and Akabane, T.: Delayed in vitro immunoglobulin production by cord lymphocytes. *Pediatrics* 65:497, 1980.
133. Ferguson, A. C., and Cheung, S. C.: Modulation of immunoglobulin M and G synthesis by monocytes and T lymphocytes in the newborn infant. *J. Pediatr.* 98:385, 1981.
134. Blaese, R. M., Poplack, D. G., and Muchmore, A. V.: The mononuclear phagocyte system: Role in expression of immunocompetence in neonatal and adult life. *Pediatrics* 64:829, 1977.
135. Ray, C. G.: The ontogeny of interferon production by human leukocytes. *J. Pediatr.* 76:94, 1970.
136. Kohl, S., Frazier, J. J., Greenberg, S. B., Pickering, L. K., and Loo, L.: Interferon induction of natural killer cytoxicity in human neonates. *J. Pediatr.* 98:379, 1981.
137. Pearson, H. A., Spencer, R. T., and Cornelius, E. A.: Functional asplenia in sickle-cell anemia. *N. Engl. J. Med.* 281:923, 1969.
138. Kevy, S. V., Tefft, M., Vawter, G. F., and Rosen, F. S.: Hereditary splenic hypoplasia. *Pediatrics* 42:752, 1968.
139. Smith, S. C., Erlandson, M. E., Stern, G., and Hilgartner, M. W.: Postsplenectomy infection in Cooley's anemia. *N. Engl. J. Med.* 266:737, 1962.
140. Erkalis, A. J., Kevy, S. V., Diamond, L. K., and Gross, R. E.: Hazard of overwhelming infection after splenectomy in childhood. *N. Engl. J. Med.* 276:1225, 1967.
141. Holroyde, C. P., Oski, F. A., and Gardner, F. H.: The "pocked" erythrocyte. *N. Engl. J. Med.* 281:516, 1969.
142. Freedman, R. M., Johnston, D., Mahoney, M. J., and Pearson, H. A.: Development of splenic reticuloendothelial function in neonates. *J. Pediatr.* 96:466, 1980.
143. Padmanabhan, J., Risenberg, H. M., and Rowe, R. D.: Howell-Jolly bodies in the peripheral blood of full-term and premature neonates. *Johns Hopkins Med. J.* 132:146, 1973.

144. Ablin, A. R., Kushner, J. H., Murphy, A., and Zippin, C.: Platelet enumeration in the neonatal period. *Pediatrics* 28:822, 1961.
145. Aballi, A. J., Puapondh, Y., and Desposito, F.: Platelet counts in thriving premature infants, *Pediatrics* 42:685, 1968.
146. Fogel, B. J., Arais, D., and Kung, F.: Platelet counts in healthy premature infants. *J. Pediatr.* 73:108, 1968.
147. Sell, E. J., and Corrigan, J. J.: Platelet counts, fibrinogen concentrations, and factor V and factor VII levels in healthy infants according to gestational age. *J. Pediatr.* 82:1028, 1973.
148. Mehta, P., Vasa, R., Neumann, L., and Karpatkin, M.: Thrombocytopenia in the high-risk infant. *J. Pediatr.* 97:791, 1980.
149. Meberg, A., Halvorsen, S., and Ørstavik, I.: Transitory thrombocytopenia in small-for-dates infants, possibly related to maternal smoking. *Lancet* 2:303, 1977.
150. Thüring, W., and Tönz, O.: Neonatale Thrombozytenwerte be: Kindern mit Down-Syndrom und anderen autosomalen Trisomien. *Helv. Paediat. Acta* 34:545, 1979.
151. Feusner, J. H.: Normal and abnormal bleeding times in neonates and young children utilizing a fully standardized template technic. *Am. J. Clin. Pathol.* 74:73, 1980.
152. Mull, M. M., and Hathaway, W. E.: Altered platelet function in newborns. *Pediatr. Res.* 4:229, 1970.
153. Corby, D. G., and Schulman, I.: The effects of antenatal drug administration on aggregation of platelets of newborn infants. *J. Pediatr.* 79:307, 1971.
154. Stuart, M. J.: Platelet function in the neonate. *Am. J. Pediatr. Hematol./Oncol.* 1:227, 1979.
155. Higsönmez, G., and Prozorova-Zamani, V.: Platelet aggregation in neonates by hyperbilirubinemia. *Scand. J. Haematol.* 24:67, 1980.
156. Blieyer, W. A., and Breckenridge, R. T.: Studies on the detection of adverse drug reactions in the newborn. II. The effects of prenatal aspirin on newborn hemostasis. *JAMA* 213:2049, 1970.
157. Haslam, R. R., Eckert, H., and Gillam, G. L.: Hemorrhage in a neonate possibly due to a maternal ingestion of salicylate. *J. Pediatr.* 84:556, 1974.
158. Poley, J. R., and Stickler, G. B.: Petechiae in the newborn infant. *Am. J. Dis. Child.* 102:365, 1961.
159. Gitlin, D., Kumate, J., Urrusti, J., and Morales, C.: The selectivity of the human placenta in the transfer of plasma proteins from mother to fetus. *J. Clin. Invest.* 43:1938, 1964.
160. Baehner, R. L., and Strauss, H. S.: Hemophilia in the first year of life. *N. Engl. J. Med.* 275:524, 1966.
161. Nossel, H. L., Lanzkowsky, P., Levy, S., Mibashan, R. S., and Hensen, J. D. L.: A study of coagulation factor levels in women during labor and in their newborn infants. *Throm. Diath. Haemorrh.* 16:185, 1966.
162. Preston, A. E.: The plasma concentrations of factor VIII in the normal population. I. Mothers and babies at birth. *Br. J. Haematol.* 10:110, 1964.
163. Biland, L., and Duckert, F.: Coagulation factors of the newborn and his mother. *Thromb. Diath. Haemorrh.* 29:644, 1973.
164. Dyggve, H.: Prothrombin and proconvertin in the newborn and during the first year of life. *Acta Paediatr.* 47:251, 1958.
165. Hilgartner, M. W., and Smith, C. H.: Plasma thromboplastin antecedant (factor XI) in the neonate. *J. Pediatr.* 66:747, 1965.
166. Kurkcuoglu, M., and McElfresh, A. E.: The Hageman factor: Determination of its concentration during the neonatal period and presentation of a case of Hageman factor deficiency. *J. Pediatr.* 57:61, 1960.
167. Beller, F. K., Douglas, G. W., and Epstein, M. D.: The fibrinolytic enzyme system in the newborn. *Am. J. Obstet. Gynecol.* 96:977, 1966.
168. Stroder, J.: Uber den fibrinstabilisierenden Faktor (FSf) in den verschiedenen Lebensabschnitten und bei bestimmten Krankheiten des Kindes. *Ann. Paediatr.* 203:393, 1964.
169. Rosti, D.: Il Fattore XIII nel periodo neonatale. *Boll. Soc. Ital. Biol. Sper.* 45:1220, 1969.
170. Bleyer, W. A., Hakami, N., and Shepard, T. H.: The development of hemostatis in the human fetus and newborn infant. *J. Pediatr.* 79:838, 1971.
171. Teger-Nilsson, A.: Antithrombin in infancy and childhood. *Acta Pediatr. Scand.* 64:624, 1975.

172. Hathaway, W. E.: The bleeding newborn. *Semin. Hematol.* 12:175, 1975.

173. Gordon, E. M., Ratnoff, O. D., Saito, H., Gross, S., and Jones, P. K.: Studies on some coagulation factors (Hageman factor, plasmas prekallikrein, and high molecular weight kininogen) in the normal newborn. *Am. J. Pediatr. Hematol./Oncol.* 2:213, 1980.

174. Johnson, S. S., Montgomery, R. R., and Hathaway, W. E.: Newborn factor VIII complex: Elevated activities in term infants and alterations in electrophoretic mobility related to illness and activated coagulation. *Br. J. Haematol.* 47:597, 1981.

175. Zipursky, A., deSa, D., Hsu, E., Johnston, M., and Milner, R.: Clinical and laboratory diagnosis of hemostatic disorders in newborn infants. *Am. J. Pediatr. Hematol./Oncol.* 1:217, 1979.

176. Aballi, A. J., and deLamerens, S.: Coagulation changes in the neonatal period and in early infancy. *Pediatr. Clin. North Am.* 9:785, 1962.

177. Muller, A. D., van Doorm, J. M., and Hemker, H. C.: Heparin-like inhibitor of blood coagulation in normal newborns. *Nature* 267:616, 1977.

178. Muntean, W., Petek, W., Rosanelli, K., and Mutz, I. D.: Immunologic studies of prothrombin in newborns. *Pediatr. Res.* 13:1262, 1979.

179. Schettini, F., DeMattia, O., Altomare, M., and Montagna, O.: Postnatal development of factor IX. *Acta Paediatr. Scand.* 69:53, 1980.

180. Owren, P. A., and Aas, K.: The control of dicumarol therapy and the quantitative determination of prothrombin and proconvertin. *Scand. J. Clin. Invest.* 3:201, 1951.

181. Holmberg, L., Henriksson, P., Ekelund, H., and Astedt, B.: Coagulation in the human fetus. Comparison with term newborn infants. *J. Pediatr.* 85:860, 1974.

182. Barnard, D. R., Simmons, M. A., and Hathaway, W. E.: Coagulation studies in extremely premature infants. *Pediatr. Res.* 13:1330, 1979.

183. Schettini, F., Lattanzi, E., Violante, N., and Rana, N.: Il Factore XIII (FSF) nel neonata immaturo. *Boll. Soc. Ital. Biol. Sper.* 42:924, 1966.

184. Aballi, A. J.: The action of vitamin K in the neonatal period. *South. Med. J.* 58:48, 1965.

185. Gray, O. P., Ackerman, A., and Fraser, A. J.: Intracranial haemorrhage and clotting in low-birth-weight infants. *Lancet* 1:543, 1968.

186. Volpe, J. J.: Neonatal intraventricular hemorrhage. *N. Engl. J. Med.* 304:886, 1981.

187. Appleyard, W. J., and Cottom, D. G.: Effect of asphyxia on thrombotest values in low birthweight infants. *Arch. Dis. Child.* 45:705, 1970.

CHAPTER 6

Hematology in the aged

WILLIAM J. WILLIAMS

Life expectancy has increased in recent decades. For example, in the United States in 1978, life expectancy at birth was 73.3 years, whereas in 1900 it was 49.2 years [1]. Of 100,000 white female babies born in 1978, over 36,000 are expected to live to age 85 [1]. As a result, physicians are increasingly concerned with the care of elderly patients and are frequently called upon to interpret hematologic data in the context to the age of the patient. In this chapter some theoretical considerations of the effects of aging on hemopoiesis and the presently recognized age-dependent hematologic changes are discussed.

Theoretical considerations of aging

Throughout embryogenesis and early infancy, nearly all cells of the body have mitotic capacity. Subsequently certain cells of the body lose their ability to divide (e.g., nervous tissue, muscles [2,3]). Others continue to divide until full growth has been achieved. Thereafter they usually do not divide at a significant rate, except under conditions of stress, when they become capable of rapid cell division. These cells are said to be "intermittently mitotic" or "dicontinuous replicators" and are exemplified by hepatic cells or renal tubular cells [2,3]. Finally, cells of certain organs, such as the marrow or gastrointestinal mucosa, are continuously mitotic throughout life [2,3]. Studies of diploid human cells maintained in continuous culture have led to the assertion that there is a finite limit to the number of divisions a cell may undergo [4]. This concept has major implications for hemopoiesis in the aged, since it raises the possibility of exhaustion of marrow stem cells with extreme aging. There is evidence from studies of mouse marrow that the stem cell reserve has limited proliferative capacity [5-9], which decreases with aging of the donor animal [8,10,11]. Cells from organs other than marrow have been shown to have limited proliferative capacity both in vitro [12,13] and in vivo [14], which in some cases decreases with aging of the donor animal [4]. The period of time required for cells to grow out from an explant also increases as the donor animal ages [15]. However, some evidence indicates that the in vitro lifespan of diploid cells may be related to factors other than chronologic age [16].

Senescent mice have lower packed red cell volumes than mature mice [17]. However, marrow cells from old donor mice functioned as well as those from young donors when transplanted into old recipient mice [18]. Further, the impaired response of the marrow to hemorrhage in old mice was not improved by transplantation of marrow from young mice, suggesting that the hemopoietic defect was not intrinsic to the marrow cells [19]. Theoretical and experimental considerations suggest that the effects of aging on marrow proliferative capacity may not have clinical significance within existing animal life-spans [8,9,18,20].

Total and differential leukocyte count

In childhood the normal total and differential leukocyte counts vary with age, as discussed in Chap. 2 (Table 2-3) and Chap. 5 (Table 5-2). There is no variation in the total or differential leukocyte count through middle age. No gross changes occur in old age. Normal leukocyte and neutrophil counts were found in a nonagenarian population [21]. Some investigators have found that above age 65 the total leukocyte count tends to be lower in both sexes, due primarily to a decrease in the lymphocyte count [22–27] (e.g., total WBC 3100–8500; neutrophils, mean 65 ± 10 percent [standard deviation]; lymphocytes 30 ± 9 percent [standard deviation] [22]). Others have reported a decrease in the leukocyte count due to a fall in both the lymphocyte and the neutrophil counts in women, but not in men, over the age of 50 [28,29]. The absolute lymphocyte count has also been reported to be unchanged in the aged [30–33].

Lymphocyte function

There is some disagreement with regard to the relative proportions of thymus-derived lymphocytes (T cells) and marrow-derived lymphocytes (B cells) in the blood of elderly people compared with young adults. Thus, in some studies the percentage of T and B cells was unchanged in older subjects [26,31,33–36], while in others the percentage of T cells was decreased [24,37–39] and that of B cells increased [24,40] in the elderly. In one study [24] B cells accounted for 35 ± 12 percent (standard deviation) of the lymphocytes in the blood of individuals 60 to 95 years old and 22 ± 6 percent in adults from 18 to 51 years old. Lymphopenia occurs in the aged (see above), with the result that the absolute number of B cells may be the same as in younger adults (mean of approximately 600 cells per microliter in each group), while the absolute number of T cells is decreased (mean of approximately 1100 per microliter in the aged and 1700 in the younger adults) [24]. Decreases in null cells [26] and B cells [41] have also been reported with increasing age. T-cell subsets may also vary with age [41,42]. In lymph nodes the number of germinal centers and the proportion of the node occupied by the paracortical and medullary areas vary with the age of the individual and the site of the node [43].

Lymphocytes from aged subjects may show significantly less mitogenic response to plant mitogens and in mixed lymphocyte cultures [23,34,35,40,44,45], although not all investigators have obtained this result [26,36]. The impaired response of lymphocytes from older patients to mitogens has been reported to be due to a decreased number of mitogen-responsive cells and their failure to undergo clonal expansion [35]. Lymphocytes obtained from aged subjects were less likely to effect antibody-mediated cytolysis than lymphocytes from younger subjects [46]. Cell-mediated cytotoxicity is also depressed in older individuals [36]. Deficient lymphocyte function in vivo in elderly individuals is implied from studies of induction of dinitrochlorobenzene sensitivity [47], of cutaneous delayed hypersensitivity reactions [45,48,49], and of the lymphocyte transfer reaction [50]. The IgG antibody response to *Salmonella* flagellin, presumably a T cell–dependent response, is reduced in subjects over age 60 compared with that seen in younger individuals [45].

Immunoglobulin levels vary with age, sex, race, prior infection, etc., and therefore present a wide range of normal, which makes interpretation difficult [51–56]. Immunoglobulin levels in the newborn are discussed in Chap. 5. IgG levels fall in the first few months of life and then slowly rise to reach adult levels at ages 5 to 16 [51–54]. IgA levels increase slowly throughout childhood and appear to reach adult levels in parallel with IgG levels [51–53], but a slower rise has been observed [54]. IgM concentrations show an initial rapid rise and possibly achieve adult levels at the age of 1 year [52], although other studies show a further increase with age throughout childhood [51].

In apparently normal people, IgG and IgM levels reach a peak in early adult life and then fall slowly, so that by the sixth decade the levels are significantly lower than those in young adults [55–57]. Most studies have shown a subsequent increase in γ-globulin levels in the elderly [23,56–58]. Increases in IgG and IgA levels are found in about two-thirds of those above the age of 50 [57].

Antibody responses to pneumococcal polysaccharide immunization and to influenza vaccination are reduced in older individuals [59,60]. The ineffective response to influenza vaccine is associated with a deficiency of Ig-bearing blood lymphocytes [60]. An increased prevalence of autoantibodies has also been reported in older people [24,45,47,58,61,62]. This may be due to deficient suppressor T-cell activity in older patients [63,64]. Monoclonal plasma immunoglobulins (benign monoclonal gammopathy) are found with increasing frequency with age [65], reaching 3 percent in people over 70 [66] and nearly 6 percent in those from 80 to 89 [65] (see Chap. 113).

Leukocyte response to infection

It is generally held that the leukocyte count does not rise as high in response to infection in elderly individuals as in young people and that often the principal manifestation of a leukocyte response is an increase in the number of band forms in an otherwise normal leukocyte count [67,68]. However, in two series of cases of acute appendicitis, the leukocytosis of patients over 60 was the same as that found in younger patients [69,70]. The disease was more advanced in the older patients, but the authors concluded that the leukocytosis generally reflected the severity of the process. In a study of the leukocyte response to bacteria pyrogen, it was found that the total leukocyte count and the proportion of neutrophils rise much less in individuals over the age of 70 than in young adults [71]. Similarly, the neutrophilic leukocytosis which occurs at 5 h after the oral administration of 40 mg prednisolone is diminished in patients over 55 years of age [72]. These studies suggest a diminished marrow granulocyte reserve (Chap. 84) in the elderly. Leukocyte function and serum opsonic capacity have been reported to be well preserved in elderly individuals [33].

Hemoglobin level

Another parameter which varies with age is hemoglobin level. Changes in hemoglobin levels in the neonatal period are discussed in Chap. 5 (Table 5-1), and those in childhood and adolescence in Chap. 2 (Table 2-3). Nearly all studies have shown that the hemoglobin level falls in men after middle age. Thus the mean hemoglobin level ranged between 15.3 and 12.4 g/dl in studies of men over 60 years of age [21,30,73–83]. In a group of men aged 96 to 106 years, the mean hemoglobin level was 12.4 g/dl [21]. The lowest levels are generally found in the oldest patients (Fig. 6-1). The hemoglobin levels in women also decrease with age, with the mean level ranging from 13.8 to 11.7 [21,30,73–77,79–83]. The decrease in hemoglobin level in women was relatively less than that in men, and in some studies the hemoglobin level was nearly the same in the aged of both sexes [30,73,83]. In some studies the hemoglobin level has not been found to decrease with age [84].

In one group of 229 elderly patients living at home, 37 were found to have hemoglobin levels below 12.0 g/dl. Nineteen of these had iron deficiency, associated in one case with folate deficiency and in three others with vitamin B_{12} deficiency. In 11 other subjects, 10 of whom were female, no cause could be determined for the decreased hemoglobin level [79]. In other studies, iron deficiency has also been responsible for the low hemoglobin levels in the majority of asymptomatic elderly people [81]. Unexplained anemia has been frequently observed in other studies of elderly people [83]. Iron absorption is not impaired in elderly people, but utilization of orally administered iron for hemoglobin production is reduced [85]. Great caution must be exercised in concluding that anemia in an older person is due solely to the patient's age and not to some specific disease, such as an occult neoplasm.

Erythrocyte 2,3-diphosphoglycerate (2,3-DPG)

The erythrocyte 2,3-DPG level has been reported to fall with age from a mean value of 14.9 μmol/g hemoglobin at age 18 to 24 to 13.9 μmol/g hemoglobin at age 75 to 84 [84]. This decrease is statistically significant, although it could account for only a slight change in oxygen affinity and therefore is of doubtful physiologic significance.

Osmotic fragility

The osmotic fragility is increased in older individuals in comparison with younger subjects [86,87]. This phe-

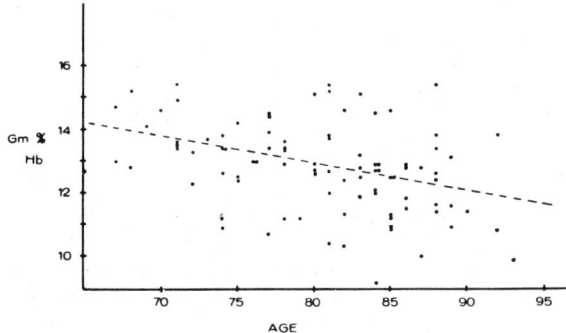

FIGURE 6-1 Hemoglobin level as a function of age. Hemoglobin was estimated on arterial blood drawn from apparently physically well individuals who had been recumbent overnight. The actual values may therefore be lower than would be obtained using venous blood from ambulatory patients (see Table 2-1). The relative values demonstrate a decrease in hemoglobin level with age. (From Smith and Whitelaw [78], by permission.)

nomenon may be related to the increased MCV and decreased MCHC of the red cells of older people [87]. The rate of hemolysis, in contrast, is more rapid in older individuals, perhaps due to changes in the erythrocyte membrane [87].

Serum iron and iron-binding capacity

In individuals of both sexes with normal hemoglobin levels, and presumably with normal iron stores, the serum iron level falls after the age of 30 from a mean of about 130 μg/dl in males and 116 μg/dl for females to a mean at age 71 to 80 of about 75 μg/dl in men and 66 μg/dl in women [88]. Levels of 50 μg/dl were found in 40 percent of men and women above the age of 50 [89]. The iron-binding capacity also falls in the elderly [90,91].

Serum ferritin

Serum ferritin levels rise from a median of 25 μg/liter to 94 μg/liter in males in the third decade and then increase slowly thereafter to a median of 124 μg/liter above age 45 [92]. Ferritin levels in females remain low to middle age and then increase from a median of 25 μg/liter to 89 μg/liter in women at menopause [92]. Serum ferritin levels appear to reflect iron stores in elderly people [83].

Serum vitamin B_{12} and folate levels

Individuals with reduced intrinsic-factor secretion and persistent low serum vitamin B_{12} levels but without anemia or central nervous system disorder have been described as having "latent pernicious anemia" [93]. Low serum vitamin B$_{12}$ levels without anemia occur in a significant proportion of elderly people [77,94–96]. Thus in one study the serum vitamin B$_{12}$ level was below the lower limit of "normal" (150 pg/ml) in 80 of 533 nonanemic individuals over the age of 65 [77]. In some patients, the mean serum vitamin B$_{12}$ levels ranged from 109 to 122 ng/liter over a 4-year period without development of anemia or other signs of vitamin B$_{12}$ deficiency [97]. Vitamin B$_{12}$ absorption was normal in many of the patients in which it was measured [94,95]. A group of subjects with low vitamin B$_{12}$ levels was studied further to evaluate the effects of vitamin B$_{12}$ therapy. Since macrocytic anemia and neuropathy were absent, psychiatric state and "well-being" were evaluated. It was found in a controlled trial that vitamin B$_{12}$ injections had no greater beneficial effect than placebo (phenol red) [98]. The significance of low serum vitamin B$_{12}$ level without anemia and with normal vitamin B$_{12}$ absorption remains uncertain.

Both serum [77,96] and red cell [77] folate levels were below the usual lower limit of normal (3 μg/liter) in a small proportion (3–7 percent) of both males and females over the age of 65. Similar low levels were also found in the same proportion of young people who were clinically well and apparently on a normal diet [96], creating uncertainty regarding the "normal" level of serum folate and making the interpretation of these results difficult. None of the patients with low serum folate levels were anemic, and the significance of these findings is uncertain.

The mean corpuscular volume (MCV) increases slightly but significantly with age [80–82,87,99–101]. Cigarette smoking may also cause an increase in the MCV [100,101], and it has been reported that older persons who smoke may have MCVs of 100 μm^3 or more in the absence of any demonstable cause of macrocytosis [101].

Platelets

No age-related changes in the platelet count have been reported [30].

Increased plasma levels of two platelet α-granule constituents, β-thromboglobulin and platelet factor IV have been found in individuals over 65 years of age in comparison with younger individuals [102,103]. Statistically significantly higher levels were found in elderly women compared with elderly men, but in the younger age groups no sex differences were found [102]. The significance of these findings is uncertain.

Marrow

The cellularity of the marrow decreases in old age, as estimated from the studies of histologic sections [104,105]. Studies of marrow from the anterior iliac crest [93] have demonstrated a progressive decrease in cellularity from 80 to 100 percent to about 50 percent over the first 30 years of life. Cellularity of about 40 percent has been found in sternal marrow from normal adults [106]. In iliac crest marrow there is a plateau of about 50 percent cellularity to age 65, when a decrease in cellularity to about 30 percent occurs over the succeeding decade [105]. This latter decline may be due to an increase in fat related to osteoporosis with reduction of the volume of cancellous bone rather than to a decrease in hemopoietic cells. The distribution of hemopoietic cells in marrow is uneven, and estimation of cellularity from observation of a few fields of a single slide may be misleading.

Chromosome studies

Several studies have demonstrated that aneuploidy due to an XO (45,X) chromosome pattern occurs frequently in karyotypes derived from direct marrow preparations from elderly men [107–111]. The Y chromosome is not missing in cultured peripheral blood leukocytes [107,108,110]. The number of individuals with loss of the Y chromosome in some karyotypes increases with age, but the degree of Y chromosome loss does not [110]. From 12 to 35 percent of men over the age of 60 were missing the Y chromosome from some karyotypes, whereas 0 to 5 percent of males under age 60 had missing Y chromosomes [108,110,111]. In one study, marrow preparations from 75 percent of 23 men over the age of 80 contained the 45,X chromosome pattern in some karyotypes [110].

Erythrocyte sedimentation rate

The erythrocyte sedimentation rate increases significantly with age [112–115]. Mean values of 14 mm/h (Westergren) and individual values as high as 69 mm/h were found in apparently well women aged 70 to 89 years who were followed for 3 to 11 years [115]. The erythrocyte sedimentation rate is of limited value in detecting disease in elderly patients.

Plasma coagulation factors

Factor VIII coagulant activity increased with age in two studies but was not influenced by age in a third [116–118]. In one study the plasma factor VIII coagulant activity increased from 101 percent at 17 to 29 years to 132 percent at 60 to 79 years in males and from 89 percent at 17 to 29 years to 105 percent at 60 to 79 years in females [116]. Plasma levels of fibrinogen [118,119] and factors V [118], VII [117,118], and IX [117] have also been reported to increase with age. Fibrinogen levels were uninfluenced by age up to 65 years in one study [117]. The increase in fibrinogen concentration may be related to the increase in sedimentation rate [114] (see above). The partial thromboplastin time has been reported to shorten with increasing age, beginning in childhood [120].

References

1. Life Tables, 1978: *Vital Statistics of the United States*, vol. II, sec. 5. U.S. Department of Health and Human Services, National Center for Health Statistics, Hyattsville, Md., 1980.
2. Post, J., and Hoffman, J.: Cell renewal patterns, *N. Engl. J. Med.* 279:248, 1968.
3. Goldstein, S.: The biology of aging. *N. Engl. J. Med.* 285:1120, 1971.
4. Hayflick, L.: The limited *in vitro* lifetime of human diploid cell strains. *Exp. Cell Res.* 37:614, 1965.
5. Cudkowicz, G., Upton, A. C., Shearer, G. M., and Hughes, W. L.: Lymphocyte content and proliferative capacity of serially transplanted mouse bone marrow. *Nature* 201:165, 1964.
6. Siminovitch, L., Till, J. E., and McCulloch, E. A.: Decline in colony-forming ability of marrow cells subjected to serial transplantation into irradiated mice. *J. Cell. Comp. Physiol.* 64:23, 1964.
7. Vos, O., and Dolans, M. J. A. S.: Self-renewal of colony forming units (CFU) in serial bone marrow transplantation experiments. *Cell Tissue Kinet.* 5:371, 1972.
8. Harrison, D. E.: Normal production of erythrocytes by mouse marrow continuous for 13 months. *Proc. Natl. Acad. Sci. U.S.A.* 70:3184, 1973.
9. Relucke, U., Burlington, H., Cronkite, E. P., and Laissue, J.: Hayflick's hypothesis: An approach to in vivo testing. *Fed. Proc.* 34:71, 1975.
10. Yuhas, J. M., and Storer, J. B.: The effect of age on two modes of radiation death and on hematopoietic cell survival in the mouse. *Radiat. Res.* 32:596, 1967.
11. Davis, M. L., Upton, A. C., and Satterfield, L. C.: Growth and senescence of the bone marrow stem cell pool in RFM/Un mice. *Proc. Soc. Exp. Biol. Med.* 137:1452, 1971.
12. Swim, H. E., and Parker, R. F.: Culture characteristics of human fibroblasts propagated serially. *Am. J. Hyg.* 66:235, 1957.
13. Hayflick, L., and Moorhead, P. S.: The serial cultivation of human diploid cell strains. *Exp. Cell Res.* 25:585, 1961.
14. Daniel, C. W., and Young, L. J. T.: Influence of cell division of aging process: Life span of mouse mammary epithelium during serial propagation in vivo. *Exp. Cell Res.* 65:27, 1971.
15. Soukupová, M., Holečková, E., and Hnevkovsky, P.: Changes of the latent period of explanted tissues during ontogenesis, in *Aging in Cell and Tissue Culture*, edited by E. Holečková and V. J. Cristofalo. Plenum, New York, 1970, p. 41.
16. Goldstein, S., Moerman, E. J., Soelder, J. S., Gleason, R. E., and Barnett, D. M.: Chronologic and physiologic age affect replicative lifespan of fibroblasts from diabetic, prediabetic, and normal donors. *Science* 199:781, 1978.
17. Finch, C. E., and Foster, J. R.: Hematologic and serum electrolyte values of the C57BL/6J male mouse in maturity and senescence. *Lab. Anim. Sci.* 23:339, 1973.
18. Harrison, D. E.: Normal function of transplanted marrow cell lines from aged mice. *J. Gerontol.* 30:279, 1975.
19. Harrison, D. E.: Defective erythropoietin responses of aged mice not improved by young marrow. *J. Gerontol.* 30:286, 1975.
20. Lajtha, L. B., and Schofield, R.: Regulation of stem cell renewal and differentiation of possible significance in aging. *Adv. Gerontol. Res.* 3:131, 1971.
21. Zaino, E. C.: Blood counts in the nonagenarian. *N.Y. State J. Med.* 81:1199, 1981.
22. Caird, F. I., Andrews, G. R., and Gallie, T. B.: The leukocyte count in old age. *Age Aging* 1:239, 1972.
23. Conrad, R. A., Demoise, C. F., Scott, W. A., and Makar, M.: Immunohematological studies of Marshall Islanders sixteen years after fallout radiation exposure. *J. Gerontol.* 26:28, 1971.
24. Díaz-Jouanen, E., Strickland, R. G., and Williams, R. C., Jr.: Studies of human lymphocytes in the newborn and the aged. *Am. J. Med.* 58:620, 1975.
25. MacKinney, A. A., Jr.: Effect of aging on the peripheral blood lymphocyte count. *J. Gerontol.* 33:213, 1978.
26. Jamil, N. A. K., and Millard, R. E.: Studies of T, B, and "null" blood lymphocytes in normal persons of different age groups. *Gerontol.* 27:79, 1981.
27. Polednak, A. P.: Age changes in differential leukocyte count among female adults. *Hum. Biol.* 50:30, 1978.
28. Allan, R. N., and Alexander, M. K.: A sex difference in the leukocyte count. *J. Clin. Pathol.* 21:691, 1968.
29. Cruickshank, J. M., and Alexander, M. K.: The effect of age, sex, parity, haemoglobin level, and oral contraceptive preparations on the normal leukocyte count. *Br. J. Haematol.* 18:541, 1970.
30. Shapleigh, J. B., Mayes, S., and Moore, C. V.: Hematologic values in the aged. *J. Gerontol.* 7:207, 1952.
31. Davey, F. R., and Huntington, S.: Age-related variation in lymphocyte subpopulations. *Gerontol.* 23:381, 1977.
32. Sparrow, D., Silbert, J. E., and Rowe, J. W.: The influence of age on peripheral lymphocyte count in men: A cross-sectional and longitudinal study. *J. Gerontol.* 35:163, 1980.
33. Phair, J. P., Kauffman, C. A., Bjornson, A., Gallagher, J., Adams, L., and Hess, E. V.: Host defenses in the aged: Evaluation of components of the inflammatory and immune responses. *J. Infect. Dis.* 138:67, 1978.
34. Weksler, M. E., and Hütteroth, T. H.: Impaired lymphocyte function in aged humans. *J. Clin. Invest.* 53:99, 1972.
35. Inkeles, B., Innes, J. B., Kuntz, M. M., Kadish, A. S., and Weksler, M. E.: Immunological studies of aging. III. Cytokinetic basis for the impaired responses of lymphocytes from aged humans to plant lectins. *J. Exp. Med.* 145:1176, 1977.
36. Becker, M. J., Farkas, R., Schneider, M., Drucker, I., and Klajman, A.: Cell-mediated cytotoxity in humans: Age-related decline as measured by a xenogeneic assay. *Clin. Immunol. Immunopathol.* 14:204, 1979.
37. Augener, W., Cohnen, E., Reuter, A., and Brittinger, E.: Decrease of T lymphocytes during aging. *Lancet* 1:1164, 1974.
38. Carosella, E. D., Mochanko, K., and Braum, M.: Rosette-forming T cells in human peripheral blood at different ages. *Cell. Immunol.* 12:323, 1974.
39. Smith, M. A., Evans, J., and Steel, C. M.: Age-related variation in proportion of circulating T cells. *Lancet* 2:922, 1974.
40. Del PozoPerez, M. A., Prieto Valtuena, J., Gonzales Builabert, M. I., and Velasso Alonso, R.: Effect of age and sex on T and B lymphocytic populations in man. *Biomedicine* 19:340, 1973.
41. Cobleigh, M. A., Braun, D. P., and Harris, J. E.: Age-dependent changes in human peripheral blood B cells and T-cell subsets: Correlation with mitogen responsiveness. *Clin. Immunol. Immunopathol.* 15:162, 1980.
42. Birnbaum, G., and Swick, L.: Human suppressor lymphocytes. II. Changes in concanavalin A inducible suppressor cells with age. *J. Gerontol.* 36:410, 1981.
43. Luscieti, P., Hubschmid, T., Cottier, H., Hess, M. W., and Sobin, L. H.: Human lymph node morphology as a function of age and site. *J. Clin. Pathol.* 33:454, 1980.
44. Pisciotta, A. V., Westring, D. W., DePrey, C., and Walsh, B.: Mitogenic effect of phytohemagglutinin at different ages. *Nature* 215:193, 1967.
45. Roberts-Thomson, I. C., Whittingham, S., Youngchaiyud, U., and Mackay, I. R.: Ageing, immune response, and mortality. *Lancet* 2:368, 1974.
46. McConnachie, P. R., Rachelefsky, G., Stiehm, E. R., and Terasaki, P. I.: Antibody-dependent lymphocyte killer function and age. *Pediatrics* 52:795, 1973.
47. Waldorf, D. S., Willkens, R. F., and Decker, J. L.: Impaired delayed hypersensitivity in an aging population: Association with antinuclear antibody and rheumatoid factor. *JAMA* 203:111, 1968.
48. Giannini, D., and Sloan, R. S.: Tuberculin survey of 1285 adults, with special reference to the elderly. *Lancet* 1:525, 1957.
49. Toh, B. H., Roberts-Thompson, I. C., Mathews, J. D., Whittingham, S., and Mackay, I. R.: Depression of cell mediated immunity in old age and immunopathic diseases, lupus erythematosus, chronic

hepatitis and rheumatoid arthritis. *Clin. Exp. Immunol.* 14:193, 1973.

50. Andersen, E.: The influence of age on transplantation immunity: Reactivity to normal lymphocyte transfer at different ages. *Scand. J. Haematol.* 9:621, 1972.

51. Stiehm, E. R., and Fudenberg, H. H.: Serum levels of immunoglobulins in health and disease: A survey. *Pediatrics* 37:715, 1966.

52. Buckley, R. H., Dees, S. C., and O'Fallon, W. M.: Serum immunoglobulins. I. Levels in normal children and in uncomplicated childhood allergy. *Pediatrics* 41:600, 1968.

53. Rowe, D. S., McGregor, I. A., Smith, S. J., Hall, P., and Williams, K.: Plasma immunoglobulin concentrations in a West African (Gambian) community and in a group of healthy British adults. *Clin. Exp. Immunol.* 3:63, 1968.

54. Stoop, J. W., Zegers, B. J. M., Sander, P. C., and Ballieux, R. E.: Serum immunoglobulin levels in healthy children and adults. *Clin. Exp. Immunol.* 4:101, 1969.

55. Buckley, C. E., III, and Dorsey, F. C.: The effect of aging on human serum immunoglobulin concentrations. *J. Immunol.* 105:964, 1970.

56. Buckley, C. E., III, and Dorsey, F. C.: Serum immunoglobulin levels throughout the life-span of healthy man. *Ann. Intern. Med.* 75:673, 1971.

57. Buckley, C. E., III, Buckley, E. G., and Dorsey, F. C.: Longitudinal changes in serum immunoglobulin levels in older humans. *Fed. Proc.* 33:2036, 1974.

58. Walford, R. L.: *The Immunological Theory of Aging*, Munksgaard, Copenhagen, 1969, p. 40.

59. Ammann, A. J., Schiffman, G., and Austrian, R.: The antibody responses to pneumococcal capsular polysaccharides in aged individuals. *Proc. Soc. Exp. Biol. Med.* 164:312, 1980.

60. Phair, J., Kauffman, C. A., Bjornson, A., Adams, L., and Linnemann, C., Jr.: Failure to respond to influenza vaccine in the aged: Correlation with B-cell number and function. *J. Lab. Clin. Med.* 92:822, 1978.

61. Whittingham, S., Irwin, J., Mackay, I., Marsh, S., and Cowling, D. C.: Autoantibodies in healthy subjects. *Australas. Ann. Med.* 18:130, 1969.

62. Hooper, B., Whittingham, S., Mathews, J. P., Mackay, I. R., and Curhow, D. H.: Autoimmunity in a rural community. *Clin. Exp. Immunol.* 12:79, 1972.

63. Hallgren, H. M., and Yunis, E. J.: Suppressor lymphocytes in young and aged humans. *J. Immunol.* 118:2004, 1977.

64. Kishimoto, S., Tomino, S., Mitsuya, H., and Fujiwara, H.: Age-related changes in suppressor functions of human T cells. *J. Immunol.* 123:1586, 1979.

65. Axelsson, U., Bachmann, R., and Hällén, J.: Frequency of pathological proteins (M-components) in 6,995 sera from an adult population. *Acta Med. Scand.* 179:235, 1966.

66. Hällén, J.: Frequency of "abnormal" serum globulins (M-components) in the aged. *Acta Med. Scand.* 173:737, 1963.

67. Thomas, J. H., and Powell, D. E. B.: *Blood Disorders in the Elderly.* John Wright and Sons, Bristol, 1971, p. 18.

68. Thorbjarharson, B., and Loehr, W. J.: Acute appendicitis in patients over the age of sixty. *Surg. Gynecol. Obstet.* 125:1277, 1967.

69. Peltokallio, P., and Jauhiainen, K.: Acute appendicitis in the aged patient: Study of 300 cases after the age of 60. *Arch. Surg.* 100:140, 1970.

70. Sasso, R. D., Hanna, E. A., and Moore, D. L.: Leukocyte and neutrophil counts in acute appendicitis. *Am. J. Surg.* 120:563, 1970.

71. Timaffy, M.: A comparative study of bone marrow function in young and old individuals. *Gerontol. Clin. (Basel)* 4:13, 1962.

72. Cream, J. J.: Prednisolone-induced granulocytosis. *Br. J. Haematol.* 15:259, 1968.

73. Freiman, H. D., Tauber, S. A., Tulsky, E. G.: Iron absorption in the healthy aged. *Geriatrics* 18:716, 1963.

74. Parsons, P. L., Withey, J. L., and Kilpatrick, G. S.: The prevalence of anaemia in the elderly. *Practitioner* 195:656, 1965.

75. Myers, A. M., Saunders, C. R. G., and Chalmers, D. G.: The haemoglobin level of fit elderly people. *Lancet* 2:261, 1968.

76. Cruickshank, J. M.: Some variations in the normal haemoglobin concentration. *Br. J. Haematol.* 18:523, 1970.

77. Elwood, P. C., Shinton, N. K., Wilson, C. I. D., Sweetnam, P., and Frazer, A. C.: Haemoglobin, vitamin B_{12} and folate levels in the elderly. *Br. J. Haematol.* 21:557, 1971.

78. Smith, J. S., and Whitelaw, D. M.: Hemoglobin values in the elderly. *Can. Med. Assoc. J.* 105:816, 1971.

79. McLennan, W. J., Andrews, G. R., Macleod, C., and Caird, F. I.: Anaemia in the elderly. *Q. J. Med.* 42:1, 1973.

80. Kelly, A., and Munan, L.: Haematologic profile of natural populations: Red cell parameters. *Br. J. Haemat.* 35:153, 1977.

81. Htoo, M. S., Kofkoff, R. L., and Freedman, M. L.: Erythrocyte parameters in the elderly: An argument against new geriatric normal values. *J. Am. Geriatr. Soc.* 27:547, 1979.

82. Jernigan, J. A., Gudat, J. C., Blake, J. L., Bowen, L., and Lezotte, D. C.: Reference values for blood findings in relatively fit elderly persons. *J. Am. Geriatr. Soc.* 28:308, 1980.

83. Lipschitz, D. A., Mitchell, C. O., and Thompson, C.: The anemia of senescence. *Am. J. Hematol.* 11:47, 1981.

84. Purcell, Y., and Borzović, B.: Red cell 2,3-diphosphoglycerate concentration in man decreases with age. *Nature* 251:511, 1974.

85. Marx, J. J. M.: Normal iron absorption and decreased red cell iron uptake in the aged. *Blood* 53:;204, 1979.

86. Detraglia, M., Cook, F. B., Stasiw, D. M., and Cerny, L. C.: Erythrocyte fragility in aging. *Biochim. Biophys. Acta.* 345:213, 1974.

87. Araki, K., and Rifkind, J. M.: Age dependent changes in osmotic hemolysis of human erythrocyte. *J. Gerontol.* 35:499, 1980.

88. Pirrie, R.: The influence of age upon serum iron in normal subjects. *J. Clin. Pathol.* 5:10, 1952.

89. Powell, D. E. B., Thomas, J. H., and Mills, P.: Serum iron in elderly hospital patients. *Gerontol. Clin. (Basel)* 10:21, 1968.

90. Rechenberger, J.: Über die Eisenbildungskapazität des Blutserums in den verscheidenen Lebensaltern. *Z. Alternsforsch.* 9:98, 1955.

91. Powell, D. E. B., and Thomas, J. H.: The iron-binding capacity of serum in elderly hospital patients. *Gerontol. Clin. (Basel)* 11:36, 1969.

92. Cook, J. D., Finch, C. A., and Smith, N. J.: Evaluation of the iron status of a population. *Blood* 48:449, 1976.

93. Callander, S. T., and Spray, G. H.: Latent pernicious anemia. *Br. J. Haematol.* 8:230, 1962.

94. Henderson, J. G., Strachen, R. W., Swanson Beck, J., Dawson, A. A., and Daniel, M.: The antigastrin-antibody test as a screening procedure for vitamin B_{12} deficiency in psychiatric practice. *Lancet* 2:809, 1966.

95. Hansen, T., Rafaelsen, O. J., and Rodbro, P.: Vitamin B_{12} deficiency in psychiatry. *Lancet* 2:965, 1966.

96. Girdwood, R. H., Thompson, A. D., and Williamson, J.: Folate status in the elderly. *Br. Med. J.* 2:670, 1967.

97. Pathy, M. S., and Newcombe, R. G.: Temporal variation of serum levels of vitamin B_{12}, folate, iron, and total iron-binding capacity. *Gerontology* 26:34, 1980.

98. Hughes, D., Elwood, P. C., Shinton, N. K., and Wrighton, R. J.: Clinical trial of the effect of vitamin B_{12} in elderly subjects with low serum B_{12} levels. *Br. Med. J.* 2:458, 1970.

99. Okuno, T.: Red cell size as measured by the Coulter model S. *J. Clin. Pathol.* 25:599, 1972.

100. Okuno, T.: Smoking and blood changes. *JAMA* 225:1387, 1973.

101. Helman, N., and Rubenstein, L. S.: The effects of age, sex, and smoking on erythrocytes and leukocytes. *Am. J. Clin. Pathol.* 63:35, 1975.

102. Ludlam, C. A.: Evidence for the platelet specificity of β-thromboglobulin and studies on its plasma concentration in healthy individuals. *Br. J. Haematol.* 41:271, 1979.

103. Zahavi, J., Jones, N. R. G., Leyton, J., Dubiel, M., and Kakkar, V. V.: Enhanced in vivo platelet "release reaction" in old healthy individuals. *Thrombosis Res.* 17:329, 1980.

104. Custer, R. P., and Ahlfeldt, F. E.: Studies on the structure and function of the bone marrow. *J. Lab. Clin. Med.* 17:960, 1932.

105. Hartsock, R. J., Smith, E. B., and Petty, C. S.: Normal variations with aging on the amount of hematopoietic tissue in bone marrow from the anterior iliac crest. *Am. J. Clin. Pathol.* 43:326, 1965.

106. Beutler, E., Drennan, W., and Block, M.: The bone marrow and liver in iron-deficiency anemia: A histopathologic study of sections with special reference to the stainable iron content. *J. Lab. Clin. Med.* 43:427, 1954.

107. O'Riordan, M. L., Berry, E. W., and Tough, I. M.: Chromosome studies on bone marrow from a male control population. *Br. J. Haematol. 19*:83, 1970.
108. Pierre, R. V., Hoagland, H. C.: 45 X cell lines in adult men: Loss of Y chromosome, a normal aging phenomenon? *Mayo Clin. Proc. 46*:52, 1971.
109. Walker, L. M. S.: The chromosomes of bone-marrow cells of haematologically normal men and women. *Br. J. Haematol. 21*:455, 1971.
110. Pierre, R. V., and Hoagland, H. C.: Age-associated aneuploidy: Loss of Y chromosome from human bone marrow cells with aging. *Cancer 30*:889, 1972.
111. Sandberg, A. A., and Sakural, M.: The missing Y chromsome and human leukaemia. *Lancet 1*:375, 1973.
112. Boyd, R. V., and Hoffbrand, B. I.: Erythrocyte sedimentation rate in elderly hospital in-patients. *Br. Med. J. 1*:901, 1966.
113. Böttiger, L. E., and Svedberg, C. A.: Normal erythrocyte sedimentation rate and age. *Br. Med. J. 2*:85, 1967.
114. Sharland, D. E.: Erythrocyte sedimentation rate: The normal range in the elderly. *J. Am. Geriatr. Soc. 28*:346, 1980.
115. Sparrow, D., Rowe, J. W., and Silbert, J. E.: Cross-sectional and longitudinal changes in the erythrocyte sedimentation rate in man. *J. Gerontol. 36*:180, 1981.
116. Cooperberg, A. A., and Teitelbaum, J.: The concentration of antihaemophilic globulin (AHG) related to age. *Br. J. Haematol. 6*:281, 1960.
117. Dodds, W. J., Moynihan, A. C., Benson, R. E., and Hall, C. A.: The value of age- and sex-matched controls for coagulation studies. *Br. J. Haematol. 29*:305, 1975.
118. Meade, W. W., and North, W. R. S.: Population-based distributions of haemostatic variables. *Br. Med. Bull. 33*:283, 1977.
119. Steinmann, B.: Über Beziehungen zwischen Cholesterin und Fibrinogenkeit, Thromboembolien und Atherosklerose. *Gerontologia 10*:100, 1964.
120. Cawkwell, R. C.: Patient's age and the activated partial thromboplastin time test. *Thromb. Haemost. 39*:780, 1978.

Clinical manifestations of hematologic disorders

CHAPTER 7

Clinical manifestations of hemopoietic stem cell disorders

MARSHALL A. LICHTMAN

The classification of hemopoietic stem cell diseases is outlined in Chap. 19. The principal clinical manifestations of these disorders reflect their pathogenesis and result from a lack of adequate concentrations of normal blood cells and from the physical and metabolic effects of abnormal blood cells. In the myeloaplastic disorder aplastic anemia, failure of stem cells to proliferate and differentiate leads to severe pancytopenia. In the chronic myeloproliferative syndromes, overproduction of blood cell precursors in marrow results in an excessive number and turnover of erythrocytes (polycythemia vera), granulocytes (chronic myelogenous leukemia), or platelets (primary thrombocythemia). In the acute myeloproliferative disease acute myelogenous leukemia, proliferation and accumulation of leukemia blast cells result in suppressed normal hemopoiesis and anemia, thrombocytopenia, and often neutropenia, as well as in the deleterious effects of leukemic blast cells in tissues and in the circulation. In the myelodysplastic syndromes or preleukemias, ineffective hemopoiesis leads to cytopenias and the production of dysfunctional cells. The clinical manifestations are principally the result of lack of adequate concentrations of normal blood cells, which leads to signs of anemia, infection, and sometimes abnormal bleeding.

Deficiency, excess, or dysfunction of blood cells

Alterations in blood cell concentrations are the primary manifestations of hemopoietic stem cell disorders. The clinical manifestations of deficiencies or excesses of individual blood cell types are described in the chapters on clinical manifestations of disorders of erythrocytes (Chap. 8), granulocytes and monocytes (Chap. 9), and platelets (Chap. 11).

Several hemopoietic stem cell diseases have as frequent manifestations qualitative abnormalities of blood cells. Abnormal red cell shapes, red cell or granulocyte enzyme deficiencies, abnormal neutrophil granules, bizarre nuclear configurations, disorders of neutrophil chemotaxis, phagocytosis or microbial killing, giant platelets, abnormal platelet granules, and disturbed platelet function can occur in some patients with preleukemia, acute myelogenous leukemia (AML), and agnogenic myeloid metaplasia. In preleukemia and AML, the effects of severe cytopenia usually dominate and the disturbances of cell function are less important. In agnogenic myeloid metaplasia and primary thrombocythemia, functional platelet abnormalities may contribute to the hemorrhagic diathesis, especially if surgery or injury occurs. Paroxysmal nocturnal hemoglobinuria is a hemopoietic stem cell lesion in which a highly specific alteration in blood cell membranes renders the cells exquisitely sensitive to complement lysis. Patients with chronic myelogenous leukemia (CML) or polycythemia vera do not usually have functional abnormalities of cells, although in the latter disease neutrophils are often activated with heightened metabolic rates and enhanced phagocytosis.

Secondary clinical manifestations occur as a result of the proliferation and accumulation of the malignant (leukemic) cells themselves.

Effects of leukemic blast cells

GRANULOCYTIC SARCOMAS

Granulocytic sarcomas (also called chloromas or myeloblastomas) are discrete tumors of leukemic myeloblasts and partially matured granulocytes that form in soft tissues, periosteum, bone, skin, lymph nodes, gastrointestinal tract, pleura, testes, and other sites [1–9]. They can develop in patients with AML or the accelerated phase of CML or may be the first manifestation of a myelogenous leukemia, preceding the onset in marrow and blood by months or years [4,6,7,9]. Granulocytic sarcomas are frequently mistaken for large cell (histiocytic) lymphomas because of the similarity of their histopathology in biopsy specimens from soft tissues. The presence of eosinophils or other granulocytes may arouse suspicion of a granulocytic sarcoma; however, chloracetate esterase or antilysozyme immunoperoxidase stains will establish the granulocytic nature of the process, and these should be performed on biopsies of such lesions [9].

Monocytomas are more diffuse tumorous collections of leukemic promonocytes or monoblasts that invade skin, gingiva, anal canal, lymph nodes, or central nervous system of patients with AML and a predominance of leukemic monocytes [10–16]. Leukemic monocytes tend to mature to the point at which they develop many of the cytoplasmic and membrane features required for motility and tissue entry [12,13]. Moreover, monocytes proliferate and survive in tissues for long periods. Consequently, this AML phenotype has a higher frequency of overt infiltrative tissue lesions than other forms of AML.

RELEASE OF PROCOAGULANTS

Microvascular thrombosis is a feature of the hypergranular progranulocytic type of AML [17–20], although it can occur rarely in other forms of acute leukemia as well [16,21,22]. The leukemic progranulocytes are thought to liberate procoagulants, probably from their granules, which can initiate disseminated intravascular coagulation.

HYPERLEUKOCYTIC SYNDROMES

A small proportion of cases of acute and chronic myelogenous leukemia manifest extraordinarily high blood leukocyte counts [23–25]. These patients present special problems because of the effects of blast cells in the microcirculation of the lung, brain, and other organs [26–33] and the metabolic effects that result when massive numbers of leukemic cells in blood, marrow, and tissues are killed by cytotoxic drugs. Leukemic blast cell concentrations over 50,000 per microliter are usually required to produce such problems. The hyperleukocytic syndrome occurs much more frequently in myelogenous leukemias than in lymphocytic leukemias [23,24]. This difference is explained in part by the smaller cell volume of leukemic lymphocytes (200 μm^3) than that of lymphoblasts (300 μm^3) or myeloblasts (400 μm^3).

The viscosity of blood is usually not increased in hyperleukocytic leukemias because of the concomitant reduction in hematocrit [23]. Occasional patients with CML or hyperleukocytic patients transfused excessively with red cells may have an increase in blood viscosity above normal [25].

Leukoocclusion and vascular invasion in small vessels of the lung, brain, or other sites have been identified in pathologic studies [24]. Since viscosity in the microcirculation is thought to be a function of the plasma viscosity and the deformability of individual cells in capillaries, leukocytes should transiently raise the viscosity in such small channels. Flow in microchannels will fall if poorly deformable blast cells enter capillary channels. With high leukocyte counts, chronically reduced flow may reduce oxygen transport to tissues, since the probability of leukocytes being in microchannels should be increased as a function of white cell count. Moreover, trapped leukemic cells have an oxygen consumption rate that could contribute to deleterious effects in the microcirculation [34].

High leukemic blast cell counts in acute and chronic myelogenous leukemia may be associated with pulmonary signs, such as tachypnea, dyspnea, and hypoxia, or nervous system signs, such as delerium, ataxia, visual blurring, papilledema, retinal vein distention, or intracranial hemorrhage [24,26–33]. Sudden death may occur, usually as a result of intracranial hemorrhage [32,33]. Thus hyperleukocytosis should be treated promptly with leukapheresis with a centrifuge technique (blast cells are poorly adherent) and with cytotoxic therapy. Leukapheresis may reverse the hyperleukocytic syndrome, can be used immediately without having to wait for the effect of allopurinol to reduce the risk of uric acid nephropathy, and can reduce the extent of cytolysis-induced hyperuricemia, hyperkalemia, and hyperphosphatemia by reducing the tumor cell mass [26,35,36].

Thrombocythemic syndromes

Hemorrhagic and thrombotic episodes can be the presenting manifestation of thrombocythemia or can develop during the course of primary thrombocythemia. Arterial vascular insufficiency and venous thrombosis are the major vascular manifestations of thrombocythemia. Peripheral vascular insufficiency with gangrene and cerebral vascular thrombi can occur. Thrombosis of superficial or deep veins of the extremities occurs frequently. Mesenteric, hepatic, portal, splenic, or penile venous thrombosis can develop. Hemorrhage is a frequent manifestation of thrombocythemia and often occurs concomitantly with thrombotic episodes. Gastrointestinal hemorrhage and cutaneous hemorrhage, the latter especially after trauma, are most frequent, but bleeding from other sites also can occur (see Chap. 26).

Systemic symptoms

Fever, weight loss, and malaise occur as an early manifestation of AML. At the time of diagnosis, fever is present in nearly 50 percent of patients [37]. Systemic infection is relatively uncommon at the time of diagnosis in AML [37,38]. However, fever during cytotoxic therapy, when neutrophil counts are extremely low, is nearly always a sign of infection [39]. Fever also may be a manifestation of the acute leukemic transformation of CML [40] and can occur in some patients with preleukemia [41].

Weight loss occurs in nearly one-fifth of patients with AML [35]. Loss of well-being, reduction in tolerance to exertion, and similar feelings may be out of proportion to the extent of anemia and may not be corrected by red cell transfusions; their pathogenesis is still unknown.

Metabolic signs

Hyperuricemia and hyperuricosuria are very common manifestations of the acute and chronic myeloproliferative diseases [42]. Acute gouty arthritis and hyperuricosuric nephropathy are less common. If therapy is instituted without reduction in plasma uric acid and without adequate hydration, saturation of the urine with uric acid can lead to precipitation of urate (gravel) and obstructive uropathy. If the uropathy is severe, urine flow can be obliterated and renal failure can ensue. Hyponatremia can occur in AML and in some cases is a result of inappropriate antidiuretic hormone secretion [43]. It also can be the result of an osmotic diuresis of urea, creatinine, urate, and other substances released from blast cells and wasting muscles. Hypokalemia is commonly seen in AML, and it has been thought to be caused by injury to the kidney by increased plasma and urine lysozyme and subsequent kaliuresis [44]. The hypokalemia is related to excessive urinary potassium loss, but the correlation with lysozymuria is imperfect [45,46], and other mechanisms are probably responsible in most cases, including osmotic diuresis and tubular dysfunction. Kaliuretic antibiotics, often used in patients with AML, may accentuate the hypokalemia.

Hypercalcemia occurs in about 2 percent of patients with myelogenous leukemia [47]. Several causes have been proposed, including bone resorption as a result of leukemic infiltration. This explanation is in keeping with the normal serum inorganic phosphate in most patients. Occasional patients have had hypercalcemia and hypophosphatemia, and ectopic parathyroid hormone secretion by leukemic blast cells was strongly suggested in one carefully studied case [48]. Lactic acidosis has also been observed in association with myelogenous leukemia [49,50], although the mechanism is obscure. Hypoxia can result from hyperleukocytic syndrome as a consequence of pulmonary vascular leukostasis [29,30]. Hypophosphatemia can occur because of rapid utilization of plasma inorganic phosphate in some cases of myelogenous leukemia with a high blood blast cell count and a high fraction of proliferative cells [51].

Factitious laboratory results

Elevation of serum potassium has resulted from the release of potassium from platelets or, less often, leukocytes in patients with myeloproliferative diseases and extreme elevations in these blood cell concentrations [51–56]. If blood is collected in a tube that contains an anticoagulant and the plasma is removed after high-speed centrifugation, the potassium concentration is normal. Glucose can be falsely decreased, especially since autoanalyzer techniques call for the omission of glycolytic inhibitors such as sodium fluoride in collection tubes [56,57]. Blood with high leukocyte counts that stands prior to separation of the plasma may have a significant amount of plasma glucose utilized by leukocytes. Factitious hypoglycemia can also occur as a result of red cell utilization of glucose, especially in polycythemic patients. True hypoglycemia has been observed rarely in patients with leukemia [58]. Blood oxygen content also can be lowered spuriously as a result of utilization by large numbers of leukocytes [34,59,60].

Specific organ involvement

Myeloproliferative diseases lead to disturbances principally in marrow, blood, and spleen. Although clusters of cells may be found in all organs, major infiltrates and organ dysfunction are unusual. In AML and the acute phase of CML, clinically significant infiltration of the larynx [61], central nervous system [62], heart [63], lungs [64–66], bone [67], joints [68,69], gastrointestinal tract [70,71], kidney [72], skin [73], or virtually any other organ may occur.

Splenic enlargement is a feature of the acute and chronic myeloproliferative diseases. In AML, palpable splenomegaly is present in about one-third of cases and is usually slight in extent. In the chronic myeloproliferative diseases, palpable splenomegaly is present in a high proportion of cases (polycythemia vera, 80 percent; CML, 90 percent; and agnogenic myeloid metaplasia, 100 percent). In primary thrombocythemia, splenic enlargement is present in about 60 percent of patients. A predisposition to silent splenic vascular thrombi and splenic atrophy analogous to that which occurs in sickle cell anemia has been postulated for the lower frequency of splenic enlargement. Early satiety, left upper quadrant discomfort, bladder irritation, and splenic infarctions with painful perisplenitis, diaphragmatic pleuritis, and shoulder pain may occur in patients with splenomegaly, especially in the acute phase of CML and in myeloid metaplasia. In the latter disease, the spleen can become enormous, occupying the left hemiabdomen. Blood flow through the splenic vein can be so great as to lead to portal hypertension and gastroesophageal varices [74]. Usually, reduced hepatic venous compliance is also present. Bleeding and, occasionally, encephalopathy can result from the portosystemic venous shunts [75].

Transitions among stem cell diseases

Certain hemopoietic stem cell disorders undergo evolution into others, and their clinical manifestations can change accordingly. Polycythemia vera has a predisposition to evolve into agnogenic myeloid metaplasia, and paroxysmal nocturnal hemoglobinuria into aplastic anemia. CML has a very high probability of terminating in acute leukemia (~80 percent), preleukemia has an intermediate probability (~35 percent), and agnogenic myeloid metaplasia (~15 percent) and primary thrombocythemia (10 percent) have a lower probability of such a transformation. AML occurs in less than 1 to 2 percent of patients with paroxysmal nocturnal hemoglobinuria, aplastic anemia, or polycythemia vera not treated with cytotoxic drugs or ^{32}P. The latter agents increase the likelihood of acute leukemia to about 10 percent in patients with polycythemia vera.

References

1. Wiernik, P. H.: Granulocytic sarcoma (chloroma). *Blood* 35:361, 1970.
2. Muss, H. B., and Moloney, W. C.: Chloroma and other myeloblastic tumors. *Blood* 42:721, 1973.

3. Brugo, E. A., Larkin, E., Molina-Escobar, T., and Costanzi, J.: Primary granulocytic sarcoma of the small bowel. *Cancer 35:*1333, 1975.
4. Sears, H. F., and Reid, J.: Granulocytic sarcoma. *Cancer 37:*1808, 1976.
5. Krishnamurthy, M., Nusbacher, N., Elguezabal, A., and Seligman, B. R.: Granulocytic sarcoma of brain. *Cancer 39:*1542, 1977.
6. Long, J. C., and Mihm, M. C.: Multiple granulocytic tumors of the skin. *Cancer 39:*2004, 1977.
7. Krause, J. R.: Granulocytic sarcoma preceding acute leukemia. *Cancer 44:*1017, 1979.
8. Cheson, B. D., and Christiansen, R. M.: Cutis verticis gyrata. *Am. J. Hematol. 8:*415, 1980.
9. Neiman, R. S., et al.: Granulocytic sarcoma. *Cancer 48:*1426, 1981.
10. Marks, M. M.: Monocytic leukemia. Oral and anorectal involvement. *J. Int. Coll. Surg. 20:*750, 1953.
11. Flandrin, C., Daniel, M.-Th., Blanchet, Ph., Briere, J., and Bernard, J.: La Leucémie aiguë monocytaire. *Nouv. Rev. Fr. Hematol. 11:*241, 1971.
12. Lichtman, M. A., and Weed, R. I.: Peripheral cytoplasmic characteristics of leukemia cells in monocytic leukemia. Relationship to clinical manifestations. *Blood 40:*52, 1972.
13. Schiffer, C. A., Sanel, F. T., Stechmuller, B. K., and Wiernik, P.: Functional and morphologic characteristics of the leukemic cells of a patient with acute monocytic leukemia. Correlation with clinical features. *Blood 46:*17, 1975.
14. Shaw, M. T.: The distinctive features of acute monocytic leukemia. *Am. J.. Hematol. 4:*97, 1978.
15. Cuttner, J., et al.: Association of monocytic leukemia in patients with extreme leukocytosis. *Am. J. Med. 69:*555, 1980.
16. McKenna, R. N., Bloomfield, E. D., Dick, F., Nesbit, M. E., and Brunning, R. D.: Acute monoblastic leukemia. Diagnosis and treatment of ten cases. *Blood 46:*481, 1975.
17. Didisheim, P., Tranbold, J. S., Vanderwoort, L. E., and Mibashan, R. S.: Acute promyelocytic leukemia with fibrinogen and factor V deficiencies. *Blood 23:*717, 1964.
18. Gralnick, H. R., and Sultan, C.: Acute promyelocytic leukaemia: Haemorrhagic manifestations and morphologic criteria. *Br. J. Haematol. 29:*373, 1975.
19. Groopman, J., and Ellman, L.: Acute promyelocytic leukemia. *Am. J. Hematol. 7:*395, 1979.
20. Daly, P. A., Schiffer, C. A., and Wiernik, P. H.: Acute promyelocytic leukemia: Clinical management of 15 patients. *Am. J. Hematol. 8:*347, 1980.
21. Rosner, F., Dobbs, J. V., Ritz, N. D., and Lee, S. L.: Disturbances of hemostasis in acute myeloblastic leukemia. *Acta Haematol. 43:*65, 1970.
22. Gralnick, H., Marchesi, S., and Givelber, H.: Intravascular coagulation in acute leukemia: Clinical and subclinical abnormalities. *Blood 40:*709, 1972.
23. Lichtman, M. A.: Rheology of leukocytes, leukocyte suspensions and blood in leukemia: Possible relationship to clinical manifestations. *J. Clin. Invest. 52:*350, 1973.
24. McKee, L. C., and Collins, R. D.: Intravascular leukocyte thrombi and aggregates as a cause of morbidity and mortality in leukemias. *Medicine 53:*463, 1974.
25. Lichtman, M. A., and Rowe, J.: Hyperleukocytic leukaemias. *Blood 60:*279, 1982.
26. Stirling, M. L., Parker, A. C., Keller, A. J., and Urbaniak, S. J.: Leukapheresis for papillaedma in chronic granulocytic leukaemia. *Br. Med. J. 2:*676, 1977.
27. Dearth, J. C., Fountain, K. S., Smithson, W. A., Burgert, E. O., Jr., and Gilchrist, G. S.: Extreme leukemic leukocytosis (blast crisis) in childhood. *Mayo Clin. Proc. 53:*207, 1978.
28. Preston, F. E., Sokol, R. J., Lilleyman, J. S., Winfield, P. A., and Blackburn, E. K.: Cellular hyperviscosity as a cause of neurologic symptoms in leukemia. *Br. Med. J. 1:*476, 1978.
29. Vernant, J. P., Brun, B., Mannoni, P., and Dreyfus, B.: Respiratory distress of hyperleukocytic granulocytic leukemias. *Cancer 44:*264, 1979.
30. Karp, D. D., Beck, R., and Cornell, C. J., Jr.: Chronic granulocytic leukemia with respiratory distress. *Arch. Intern. Med. 141:*1353, 1981.
31. Suri, R., Goldman, J. M., Catovsky, D., Johnson, S. A., Wiltshaw, E., and Galton, D. A. G.: Priapism complicating chronic granulocytic leukemia. *Am. J. Hematol, 9:*295, 1980.

32. Fritz, R. D., Forkner, C. E., Freireich, E. J., Frei, E., and Thomas, L. B.: The association of fatal intracranial hemorrhage and "blastic crisis" in patients with acute leukemia. *N. Engl. J. Med. 261:*59, 1959.
33. Freireich, E. J., Thomas, L. B., Frei, E., III, Fritz, R. D., and Forkner, C. E., Jr.: A distinctive type of intracerebral hemorrhage associated with "blastic crisis" in patients with leukemia. *Cancer 13:*146, 1960.
34. Lichtman, M. A., and Kearney, E. A.: The filterability of normal and leukemic leukocytes. *Blood Cells 2:*491, 1976.
35. Eisenstaedt, R. S., and Berkman, E. M.: Rapid cytoreduction in acute leukemia. *Transfusion 18:*113, 1978.
36. Lane, T. A.: Continuous-flow leukapheresis for rapid cytoreduction in leukemia. *Transfusion 20:*455, 1980.
37. Burke, P. J., Braine, H. G., Rathbun, H. K., and Owens, A. H., Jr.: The clinical significance of fever in acute myelocytic leukemia. *Johns Hopkins Med. J. 139:*1, 1976.
38. Burns, C. P., et al.: Analysis of the presenting features of adult acute leukemia. *Cancer 47:*2460, 1981.
39. Goodall, P. T., and Vosti, K. L.: Fever in acute myelogenous leukemia. *Arch. Intern. Med. 135:*1197, 1975.
40. Theologides, A.: Unfavorable signs in patients with chronic myelogenous leukemia. *Ann. Intern. Med. 76:*95, 1972.
41. Zanger, B., Dorsey, H. N.: Fever—A manifestation of preleukemia. *JAMA 236:*1266, 1976.
42. Sandberg, A. A.: Studies in leukemia. I. Uric acid excretion. *Blood 11:*154, 1956.
43. Mir, M. A., and Delamore, I. W.: Hyponatremia syndrome in acute myeloid leukemia. *Br. Med. J. 1:*52, 1974.
44. Muggia, F. M., Heineman, H. O., Farhangi, M., and Oggerman, E. F.: Lysozymuria and renal tubular dysfunction in monocytic and myelomonocytic leukemia. *Am. J. Med. 47:*351, 1969.
45. Mir, M. A., and Delamore, I. W.: Metabolic disorders in acute myeloid leukaemia. *Br. J. Hematol. 40:*79, 1978.
46. Mir, M. A., Brabin, B., Tang, O. T., Leyland, M. J., and Delamore, I. W.: Hypokalemia in acute myeloid leukemia. *Ann. Intern. Med. 82:*54, 1975.
47. Jordan, G. W.: Serum calcium and phosphorous abnormalities in leukemia. *Am. J. Med. 41:*381, 1966.
48. Zidar, B. L., Shadduck, R. K., Winkelstein, A., Zeigler, Z., and Hawker, C. D.: Acute myeloblastic leukemia and hypercalcemia. *N. Engl. J. Med. 295:*692, 1976.
49. Roth, G. J., and Porte, D., Jr.: Chronic lactic acidiosis and acute leukemia. *Arch. Intern. Med. 125:*317, 1970.
50. Warner, R. A., Wiernik, P. H., and Thompson, W. L.: Metabolic and therapeutic studies of a patient with acute leukemia and severe lactic acidosis of prolonged duration. *Am. J. Med. 55:*255, 1973.
51. Zamkoff, K. W., and Kirshner, J. J.: Marked hypophosphatemia associated with acute myelomonocytic leukemia. *Arch. Intern. Med. 140:*1523, 1980.
52. Meyerson, R. M., and Frumin, A. M.: Hyperkalemia associated with myeloproliferative disorders. *Arch. Intern. Med. 106:*479, 1960.
53. Ingram, R. H., Jr., and Seki, M.: Pseudohyperkalemia with thrombocytosis. *N. Engl. J. Med. 267:*895, 1962.
54. Bellevue, R., Dosik, H., Spergel, G., and Gussoff, B. D.: Pseudohyperkalemia and extreme leukocytosis. *J. Lab. Clin. Med. 85:*660, 1975.
55. Chumbley, L. C.: Pseudohyperkalemia in acute myelocytic leukemia. *JAMA 211:*1007, 1970.
56. Salomon, J.: Spurious hypoglycemia and hyperkalemia in myelomonocytic leukemia. *Am. J. Med. Sci. 267:*359, 1974.
57. Messeloff, C. R., Stolz, C., and Schoenfeld, M. R.: Factitious hypoglycemia in chronic myelogenous leukemia. *NY State J. Med. 64:*551, 1964.
58. Tashima, C. K., Cala, R. G., and Thomas, W.: Symptomatic hypoglycemia in terminal leukemia. *JAMA 204:*399, 1968.
59. Hess, C. E., Nichols, A. B., Hunt, W. B., and Suratt, P. M.: Pseudohypoxemia secondary to leukemia and thrombocytosis. *N. Engl. J. Med. 301:*361, 1979.
60. Fox, M. J., Brody, J. S., Weintraub, L. R., Szymanski, J., and O'Donnell, C.: Leukocytic larceny: A cause of spurious hypoxemia. *Am. J. Med. 67:*742, 1979.
61. Ti, M., et al.: Acute leukemia presenting as laryngeal obstruction. *Cancer 34:*427, 1974.
62. Davies-Jones, G. A. B., Preston, F. E., and Timperley, W. R.: Neuro-

logic complications in clinical haemotology, in *Leukemia*. Blackwell Scientific, Oxford, 1980, p. 36.

63. Roberts, W. C., Bodey, G. P., and Wertlake, P. T.: The heart in leukemia. *Am. J. Cardiol. 21*:388, 1968.

64. Green, R. A., and Nichols, N. J.: Pulmonary involvement in leukemia. *Am. Rev. Respir. Dis. 80*:833, 1959.

65. Green, R. A., Nichols, N. J., and King, E. J.: Alveolar-capillary block due to leukemic infiltration of the lung. *Am. Rev. Respir. Dis. 80*:895, 1959.

66. Bodey, G. P., et al.: Pulmonary complications of acute leukemia. *Cancer 19*:781, 1966.

67. Thomas, L. B., et al.: The skeletal lesions of acute leukemia. *Cancer 14*:608, 1961.

68. Silverstein, M. N., and Kelley, P. J.: Leukemia with osteoarticular symptoms and signs. *Ann. Intern. Med. 59*:637, 1963.

69. Weinberger, A., et al.: Arthritis in acute leukemia. *Arch. Intern. Med. 141*:1183, 1981.

70. Prolla, J. C., and Kirsner, J. B.: The gastrointestinal lesions and complications of the leukemias. *Ann. Intern. Med. 61*:1084, 1964.

71. Steinberg, D., Gold, J., and Broden, A.: Necrotizing enterocolitis in leukemia. *JAMA 131*:538, 1973.

72. Uno, Y.: Histopathological study of leukemic cell infiltration in the kidney. *Med. J. Osaka U. 18*:185, 1967.

73. Gunz, F., and Baikie, A. G.: Pathology of leukemic tissue in *Leukemia*, 3d ed. Grune & Stratton, New York, 1974, p. 223.

74. Rosenbaum, D. L., Murphy, G. W., and Swishes, S. N.: Hemodynamic studies of the portal circulation in myeloid metaplasia. *Am. J. Med. 41*:360, 1966.

75. Schwartz, S. I.: Myeloproliferative disorders. *Ann. Surg. 182*:464, 1975.

CHAPTER *8*

Clinical manifestations of erythrocyte disorders

ALLAN J. ERSLEV

Anemia

The clinical manifestations of anemia are to some extent determined by their specific etiology and pathogenesis. Certain signs and symptoms, however, are general and can be attributed to a reduction in oxygen-carrying capacity. Although some of these are caused directly by tissue hypoxia, the majority are related to compensatory mechanisms called into action to prevent or ameliorate destructive tissue anoxia.

Tissue hypoxia occurs when the pressure head of oxygen in the capillaries is too low to provide distant cells with enough oxygen for their metabolic needs. This may happen despite the presence of several times the needed oxygen in the circulating blood. Using approximate figures for a normal adult, the red cell mass has to provide the tissues with about 250 ml/min of oxygen to support life. Since the oxygen-carrying capacity of normal blood is 1.34 ml per gram hemoglobin, or about 20 ml/dl of normal blood, and the cardiac output is about 5000 ml/min, 1000 ml/min of oxygen is made available at the tissue level. The extraction of one-fourth of this amount will reduce the oxygen tension of 100 mmHg in the arterial end of the capillary to 40 mmHg in the venous end. This partial extraction will maintain a diffusion pressure throughout the capillaries sufficient to provide all cells within a truncated cone segment with enough oxygen for their metabolism (Fig. 8-1). In anemia, the extraction of the same amount of oxygen would lead to greater hemoglobin desaturation and a lower oxygen tension at the venous end of the capillary. Since this would result in destructive cellular hypoxia or anoxia in the immediate vicinity, compensatory and frequently symptomatic adjustment in the supply of blood and oxygen must be mobilized in order to keep the oxygen gradient almost unchanged.

DECREASED OXYGEN CONSUMPTION

A decrease in the rate of aerobic metabolism would undoubtedly ameliorate the effect of anemia. However, within the tissues, cellular metabolism proceeds at a normal rate as long as molecular oxygen is available. The overall oxidative metabolism in anemia may actually be 10 to 15 percent higher than normal because of the metabolic cost of cardiac and pulmonary overactivity [1].

DECREASED OXYGEN AFFINITY

One of the earliest and least problem-causing adjustments of oxygen delivery is a decrease in the affinity of hemoglobin for oxygen. This will permit increased oxygen extraction without jeopardizing oxygen pressure [2–4]. Since there is no consistent decrease in the pH of blood or evidence of impaired CO_2 removal from the tissues, the observed change in oxygen affinity cannot be accounted for by a simple acid Bohr shift in the dissociation curve. However, the red cells of patients with anemia generate increased amounts of 2,3-diphosphoglycerate [4], and this phosphate compound has the capacity to combine with deoxygenated hemoglobin and decrease its affinity for oxygen [5,6]. The reason for increased synthesis of 2,3-diphosphoglycerate in anemia is not clear, but it probably is caused primarily by a change in the intracellular pH of red cells. Deoxygenated hemoglobin is more alkaline than oxyhemoglobin, and alkalosis is a potent stimulator of glycolysis and the production of 2,3-diphosphoglycerate. In addition, the binding of 2,3-diphosphoglycerate to deoxygenated hemoglobin may diminish the intracellular pool of free 2,3-diphosphoglycerate and thereby remove product inhibition of 2,3-diphosphoglycerate mutase, the enzyme responsible for its synthesis [6,7]. A similar accumulation of 2,3-diphosphoglycerate has been demonstrated in red cells of patients with altitude hypoxia [8] and with other types of acute or chronic hypoxemia [9,10]. However, in these conditions the rise in 2,3-diphosphoglycerate may merely compensate for

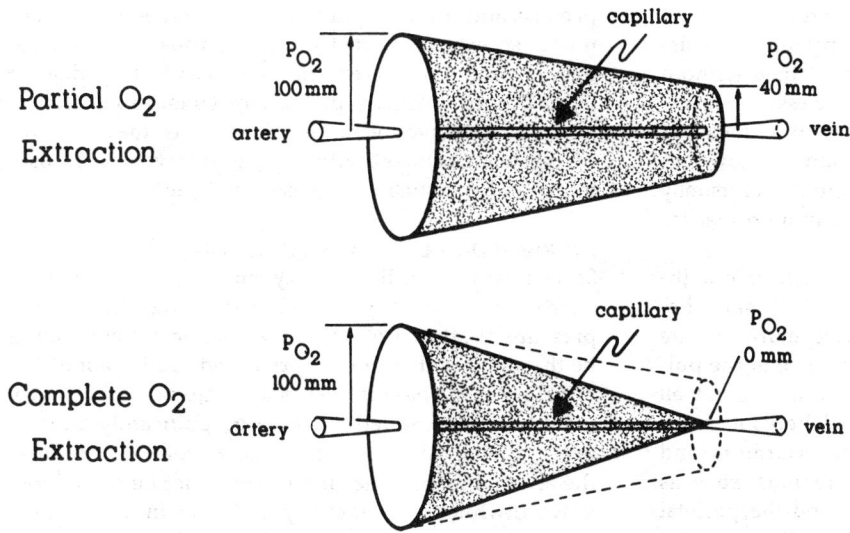

FIGURE 8-1 Theoretical tissue segment provided with oxygen from one capillary. With an arterial diffusion pressure of oxygen of 100 mmHg and partial oxygen extraction resulting in a venous oxygen pressure of 40 mmHg, one capillary can provide oxygen to cells within a truncated cone segment. With complete oxygen extraction, however, oxygen cannot be supplied to cells within a rim of tissue around the apex of the cone.

the left shift in the oxygen dissociation curve induced by hyperventilation alkalosis [11].

INCREASED TISSUE PERFUSION

The effect of a decreased oxygen-carrying capacity on the tissue tension of oxygen can be offset if, by using all potential capillary channels, the distance from tissue cells to oxygen supply is reduced.

Since the blood volume in anemia is not changed significantly (Fig. 8-2) [12], increased tissue perfusion has to be performed selectively with blood shunted from presumably nonvital donor areas to oxygen-sensitive recipient organs. The major donor areas for the redistribution of blood in moderate acute anemia in the experimental animal are the mesenteric and iliac beds [13]. However, in human chronic anemia the donor areas appear to be the cutaneous tissue [14] and the kidneys [15]. Vasoconstriction and oxygen deprivation in the subcutaneous tissue appear to be well tolerated, but will cause pallor far in excess of actual reduction in oxygen-carrying capacity. Although the kidney can hardly be thought of as a nonvital area, the oxygen supply under normal conditions is in excess of oxygen demands. The arteriovenous oxygen difference in the kidney is as low as 1.4 ml/dl [16] (as compared with the myocardium, where it may be as high as 20 ml/dl), indicating that even a severe reduction in the kidney perfusion will not limit oxidative cellular metabolism. The effect on renal excretory mechanisms is also slight, since the reduction in renal blood flow is offset by the high "plasma-crit" and, even in severe anemia with the renal blood flow reduced by almost 50 percent, the renal plasma flow is only moderately curtailed.

The benefits derived from a redistribution of blood

are obvious, and the organs with the most pressing need for oxygen, such as myocardium, brain, and muscles, will to a great extent be unhampered by a moderate reduction in oxygen-carrying capacity.

INCREASED CARDIAC OUTPUT

An increase in cardiac output is an excellent but metabolically expensive compensatory device [17–19]. It will decrease the fraction of oxygen which needs to be extracted during each circulation and thereby keep the oxygen pressure high. Since the viscosity of blood from

FIGURE 8-2 Relation between hematocrit and total blood volume in normal individuals and in patients with anemia and polycythemia. (Huber, Lewis, and Szur [12].)

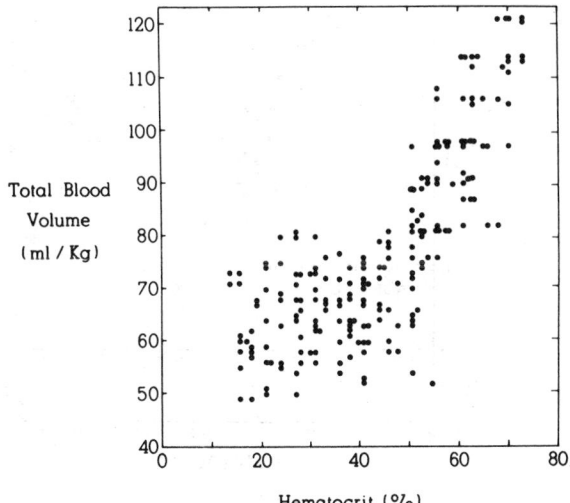

anemic patients is lower than normal, and since selective vascular dilatation will decrease peripheral resistance, a high cardiac output can be maintained without any increase in blood pressure. Nevertheless, a measurable increase in the resting cardiac output does not occur until the hemoglobin concentration is below 7 g/dl, and clinical signs of cardiac hyperactivity are usually not present until the hemoglobin concentration reaches even lower levels [20].

Signs of cardiac hyperactivity include tachycardia, increased arterial and capillary pulsation, and many hemodynamic murmurs [21]. The cardiac murmurs are usually systolic and heard best at the apex or at the pulmonary area. Diastolic murmurs are unusual, but all murmurs in an anemic patient should be considered hemodynamic until proved otherwise. Murmurs and bruits have been described in many regions, such as over the jugular vein, the closed eye, and the parietal region of the skull. Their characteristic feature is that they disappear promptly after the hemoglobin concentration has been restored to normal [22].

The normal myocardium will tolerate a prolonged period of sustained hyperactivity. However, angina

pectoris and high-output failure may supervene if anemia is so extreme that it impairs coronary oxygen demands or if the patient has coronary artery disease [23,24]. Cardiomegaly, pulmonary congestion, ascites, and edema have been observed, and they call for emergency treatment with oxygen, intravenous furosemide, and transfusion of packed red cells.

INCREASED PULMONARY FUNCTION
Since blood, regardless of oxygen-carrying capacity, is nearly completely oxygenated in the lungs, the oxygen pressure of arterial blood in the anemic patient should be the same as that in the normal individual, about 100 mmHg. An increase in respiratory rate or vital capacity would not be expected to decrease significantly the oxygen gradient from ambient air to alveolar air or across the alveolar membrane, and it would not be considered a worthwhile compensatory mechanism in anemia. Nevertheless, exertional dyspnea and orthopnea are characteristic clinical manifestations of anemia [25,26]. In some instances the pulmonary hyperactivity can be related to incipient congestive failure, but in most patients it almost appears to be an inappropriate response to hypoxia or hypercapnia in the respiratory center [17].

INCREASED ERYTHROPOIETIC ACTIVITY
The most appropriate of the compensatory adjustments is an increase in the rate of red cell production. The release of erythropoietin is inversely related to red cell mass and hemoglobin concentration [27], and with the exception of renal disease and various debilitating illnesses, erythropoietin is available in all kinds of anemia. Currently available assay techniques cannot always demonstrate increased concentrations of erythropoietin in serum of patients with moderate anemia. However, radioimmunoassays [28] and bioassays of plasma concentrates [29] (Fig. 8-3) have disclosed erythropoietin titers ranging from 10 mU/ml at normal hematocrit values to 10,000 units or more per milliliter in severe anemia.

The triggering mechanism for increased erythropoietin production is probably renal tissue hypoxia, although hypoxia in extrarenal sites may also play a role (see Chap. 38).

In patients with a marrow capable of response to erythropoietin, increased erythroid activity can occasionally be recognized clinically by sternal tenderness and by diffuse bone aches or pains. "Stress reticulocytes" with increased volume and reticulum appear, and nucleated red cells may be observed [30,31]. Even in patients with inadequate marrow mass, increased concentrations of erythropoietin may be inferred from the presence of abnormally large reticulocytes [30] and by a shortened transit time [32].

UNCORRECTED TISSUE HYPOXIA
Despite the mobilization of compensatory mechanisms, a certain residual degree of tissue hypoxia remains.

FIGURE 8-3   Erythropoietin titers in plasma of normal individuals and patients with anemia uncomplicated by renal disease or inflammatory disease. The lower limit of accuracy of the erythropoietin assay is 3 mU/ml and is indicated by a broken line.

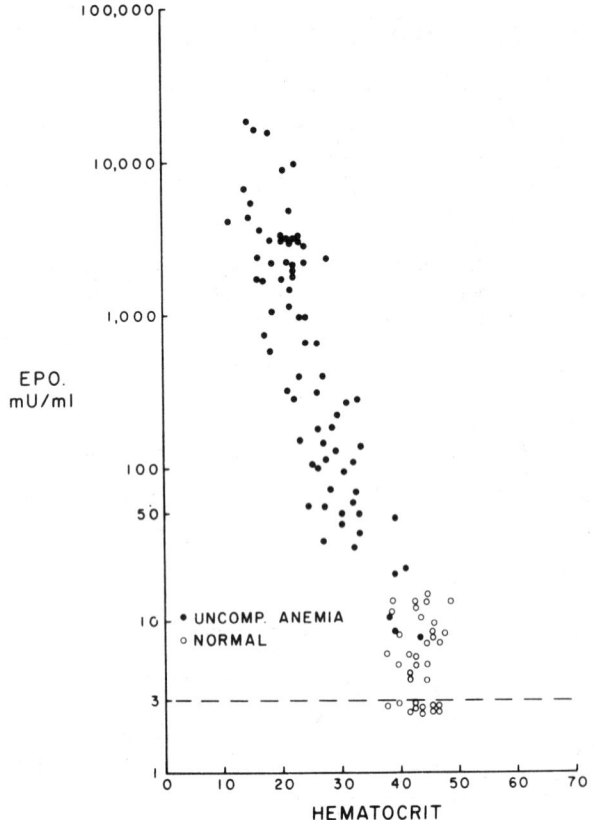

Some of this contributes the necessary driving force to sustain cardiovascular and renal adjustments, but tissue hypoxia per se may cause disturbing and even disabling symptoms. Angina pectoris, intermittent claudication, and night cramps are muscular signs of tissue hypoxia; headache, lightheadedness, tinnitus, roaring in the ears, and faintness are cerebral signs. A number of diffuse gastrointestinal and genitourinary symptoms have been associated with anemia, but it is uncertain whether they should be attributed to tissue hypoxia, to compensatory redistribution of blood, or to the underlying cause of anemia.

Erythrocytosis

The clinical and laboratory features of patients with erythrocytosis depend primarily on the etiology of the underlying disorder and are described in the appropriate chapters. However, the production and presence of an increased number of red cells are associated with certain general effects on marrow function, blood viscosity, and blood volume.

MARROW FUNCTION
Under normal conditions, the rate of red cell production is adjusted to maintain the red cell mass at about 30 ml per kilogram of body weight. Since the life-span of the red cells in polycythemia is normal, a mere doubling of the daily rate of red cell production would be adequate to maintain a red cell mass of 60 ml/kg or, in other words, to maintain a very substantial erythrocytosis. Consequently, the morphology and volume of the marrow are only moderately altered in polycythemia in comparison with the changes observed in some types of anemia, in which the rate of red cell production may be 6 to 10 times normal. The increased rate of red cell production and destruction is reflected by some increase in uric acid and bilirubin levels, but secondary gout and splenomegaly are usually signs of a myeloproliferative disorder rather than of erythrocytosis alone.

VISCOSITY AND BLOOD VOLUME
A sustained increase in red cell production will lead to an increase in both hematocrit and blood volume (see Fig. 8-2) [12]. The associated increase in viscosity and vascular volume are responsible for many of the signs and symptoms of polycythemia. The characteristic "ruddy cyanosis" in patients with polycythemia vera is caused by excessive deoxygenation of blood flowing sluggishly through dilated cutaneous vessels. Nonspecific symptoms such as headaches, dizziness, tinnitus, or a feeling of fullness of face and head are probably also caused by a combination of increased viscosity and vascular dilatation [33]. Hemorrhages from the nose or stomach in patients with normal platelets and coagulation proteins can be attributed to capillary distention, but circulatory stagnation causing ischemia and ne-

crosis is probably contributory. Thromboses are common in polycythemia vera, but they also occur in erythrocytosis when aggravated by plasma loss (dehydration) or by alveolar hypoventilation [34]. It has been claimed that the risk of angina pectoris and coronary thrombosis in patients with mild erythrocytosis is increased, but statistical analyses have yielded equivocal results [35–38]. It has also been stated that cerebral blood flow is materially reduced in patients with elevated hematocrit values [39]. Similar reductions, however, were found in individuals with high normal hematocrit values and may have little practical significance. Since judicious phlebotomies are quite harmless in the middle-aged, high-risk male population, it seems justifiable from a pragmatic, although not scientifically proved, point of view, to recommend phlebotomies in this group of patients when the hematocrit is above 53 percent.

At hematocrit readings higher than 50 percent, the viscosity of blood increases exponentially (Fig. 8-4). The resulting sluggishness of blood flow will decrease the transport of oxygen with optimal values found at hematocrit readings between 40 and 45 percent. In a study of the red cells from a number of animal species, it was found that the optimal value of oxygen transport corresponds closely to the normal hematocrit level of these animals [40] and may explain the evolutionary choice of certain hematocrit levels as "normal." The decrease in oxygen transport at high hematocrit readings was com-

FIGURE 8-4 Viscosity of heparinized normal human blood related to hematocrit (hct.). Viscosity is measured with an Ostwald viscosimeter at 37°C and expressed in relation to viscosity of saline solution. Oxygen transport is computed from hct. and O_2 flow (1/viscosity) and is recorded in arbitrary units.

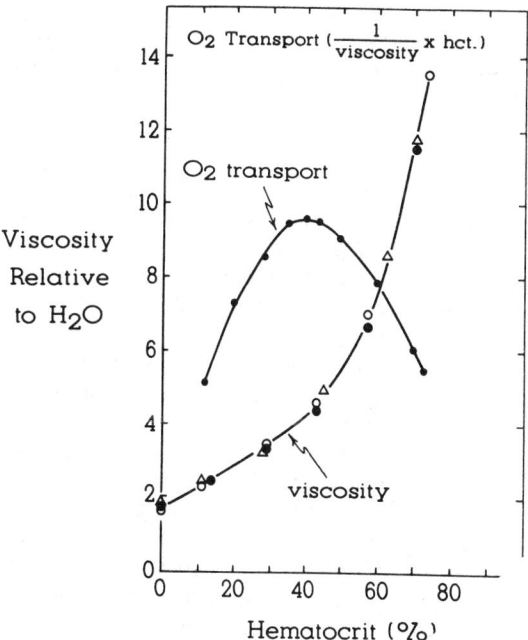

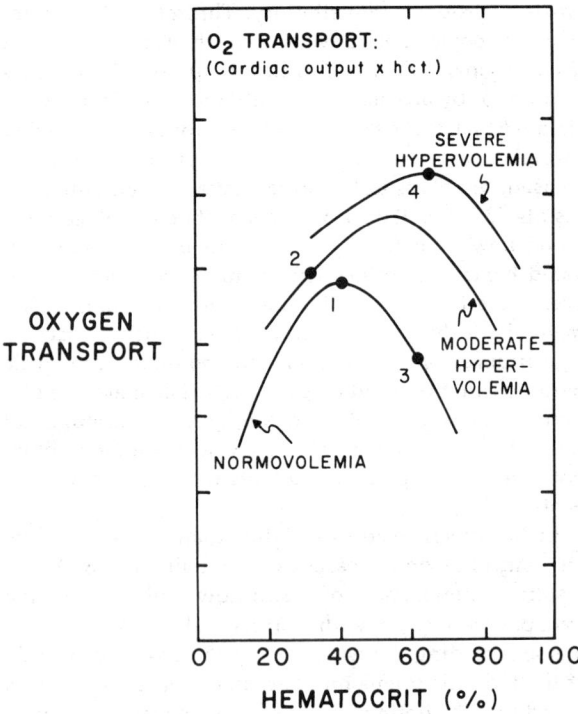

O₂ TRANSPORT: (Cardiac output x hct.)

SEVERE HYPERVOLEMIA

OXYGEN TRANSPORT

MODERATE HYPER-VOLEMIA

NORMOVOLEMIA

HEMATOCRIT (%)

FIGURE 8-5 Oxygen transport at various hematocrit levels in normovolemic, mildly hypervolemic, and severely hypervolemic individuals. The oxygen transport is estimated by multiplying hematocrit by cardiac output. As can be seen in 1, the optimal oxygen transport for the normovolemic subjects is at a hematocrit of about 45 percent with a progressive rise in the optimal hematocrit as the blood volume increases. A suboptimal hematocrit in a hypervolemic person (anemia of pregnancy), as in 2, may be associated with a higher oxygen transport than that of a normovolemic person with normal hematocrit. However, a high hematocrit without increase in blood volume (3) may be associated with an absolute reduction in oxygen transport and tissue hypoxia. Only high hematocrit coupled with high blood volume (4) enhances oxygen transport to the tissues. (Adapted from Murray et al. [41] and Thorling and Erslev [42].)

puted from viscosity data on blood in vitro and confirmed by direct measurements of cardiac output [41] or tissue tension of oxygen [42] in animals with normovolemic polycythemia. Such animals were also found to have decreased resistance to stress [42,43] and did not seem to have any of the adaptive advantages we associate with secondary polycythemia. However, absolute polycythemia is not normovolemic but accompanied by an increase in blood volume, which in turn enlarges the vascular bed and decreases the peripheral resistance. Since the blood pressure remains stable, these peripheral vascular changes must be associated with an increased cardiac output and an increased oxygen transport (cardiac output × hematocrit). Using measurements of cardiac output in dogs [41], and tissue oxygen tension in rats and mice [42], it is possible to construct curves

(Fig. 8-5) which relate oxygen transport to hematocrit in normovolemic and hypervolemic states. These curves show that hypervolemia per se will increase oxygen transport and that the optimum oxygen transport in these conditions is found at higher hematocrit values than in normovolemic states. Consequently, secondary compensatory polycythemia is indeed of benefit, but this benefit is derived both from the increase in oxygen-carrying capacity and from the associated increase in blood volume and tissue perfusion.

Increased viscosity has also been thought to play a role in the suppression of erythropoiesis observed in transfusion polycythemia [44,45]. This suggestion has been as difficult to test or substantiate [46] as the proposal that polycythemia causes the release of humoral inhibitors of erythropoietin or of erythropoiesis [47]. At present it seems more probable that a transfusion-induced increase in oxygen supply to the kidney is responsible for a decreased production of erythropoietin and in turn for the decrease in red cell production [27].

References

1. Brannon, E. S., Merrill, A. J., Warren, J. V., and Stead, E. A., Jr.: The cardiac output in patients with chronic anemia as measured by the technique of right arterial catheterization. *J. Clin. Invest.* 24:332, 1945.
2. Rodman, T., Close, H. P., and Purcell, M. K.: Oxyhemoglobin dissociation curve in anemia. *Ann. Intern. Med.* 52:295, 1960.
3. Edwards, M. J., Novy, M. J., Walters, C. L., and Metcalfe, J.: Improved oxygen release: An adaptation of mature red cells to hypoxia. *J. Clin. Invest.* 47:1851, 1968.
4. Pollock, A., and Cotter, K. P.: Oxygen transport in anemia. *Br. J. Haematol.* 25:631, 1973.
5. Torrance, J., Jacobs, P., Lenfant, C., and Finch, C. A.: Intraerythrocytic adaptation to anemia. *Blood* 34:843, 1969.
6. Bellingham, A. J., and Grimes, A. J.: Red cell, 2,3-diphosphoglycerate. *Br. J. Haematol.* 25:555, 1973.
7. Oski, F. A., Gottlieb, A. J., Miller, W. W., and Delivoria-Papadopoulos, M.: The effects of deoxygenation of adult and fetal hemoglobin on the synthesis of red cell 2,3-diphosphoglycerates and its in vivo consequences. *J. Clin. Invest.* 49:400, 1970.
8. Lenfant, C., et al.: Effect of altitude on oxygen binding by hemoglobin and on organic phosphate levels. *J. Clin. Invest.* 47:2652, 1968.
9. Metcalfe, J., Dhindsa, D. S., Edwards, M. J., and Mourdjinis, A.: Decreased oxygen affinity of blood for oxygen in patients with low-output heart failure. *Circ. Res.* 25:47, 1969.
10. Oski, F. A., Gottlieb, A. J., Delivoria-Papadopoulos, M., and Miller, W. W.: Red-cell 2,3 diphosphoglycerate levels in subjects with chronic hypoxemia. *N. Engl. J. Med.* 280:1165, 1969.
11. Finch, C. A., and Lenfant, C.: Oxygen transport in man. *N. Engl. J. Med.* 286:407, 1972.
12. Huber, H., Lewis, S. M., and Szur, L.: The influence of anaemia, polycythaemia and splenomegaly on the relationship between venous haemotocrit and red-cell volume. *Br. J. Haematol.* 10:567, 1964.
13. Vatner, S. F.: Effects of hemorrhage on regional blood flow distribution in dogs and primates. *J. Clin. Invest.* 54:225, 1974.
14. Abramson, D. J., Fierst, S. M., and Flachs, K.: Resting peripheral blood flow in the anemic state. *Am. Heart J.* 25:609, 1954.
15. Bradley, S. E., and Bradley, G. P., Renal function during chronic anemia in man. *Blood* 2:192, 1947.
16. Wesson, L. G.: *Physiology of the Kidney.* Grune & Stratton, New York, 1968, p. 28.
17. Sproule, B. J., Mitchell, J. H., and Miller, W. F.: Cardiopulmonary

physiological responses to heavy exercise in patients with anemia. *J. Clin. Invest.* 39:378, 1960.

18. Roy, S. B.: Hemodynamic effect of chronic severe anemia. *Circulation* 28:346, 1963.

19. Duke, M., and Abelman, W. H.: The hemodynamic response to chronic anemia. *Circulation* 39:503, 1969.

20. Sharpey-Schafer, E. P.: Cardiac output in severe anemia. *Clin. Sci.* 5:125, 1944.

21. Wintrobe, M. M.: The cardiovascular system in anemia. *Blood* 1:121, 1946.

22. Wales, R. T., and Martin, E. A.: Arterial bruits in anemia. *Br. Med. J.* 2:1444, 1963.

23. Zoll, P. M., Wessler, S., and Blumgart, H. L.: Angina pectoris: A clinical and pathologic correlation. *Am. J. Med.* 11:331, 1951.

24. Bartels, E. C.: Anemia as the cause of severe congestive heart failure. *Ann. Intern. Med.* 11:400, 1937.

25. Varat, M. A., Adolph, R. J., and Fowler, N. O.: Cardiovascular effects of anemia. *Am. Heart J.* 83:415, 1972.

26. Blumgart, H. L., and Altschule, M. D.: Clinical significance of cardiac and respiratory adjustments in chronic anemia. *Blood* 3:329, 1948.

27. Adamson, J. W.: The erythropoietin/hematocrit relationship in normal and polycythemic man: Implications of marrow regulation. *Blood* 32:597, 1968.

28. Sherwood, J. B., and Goldwasser, E.: A radioimmunoassay for erythropoietin. *Blood* 54:885, 1979.

29. Erslev, A. J., Caro, J., Miller, O., and Silver, R.: Plasma erythropoietin in health and disease. *Ann. Clin. Lab. Sci.* 10:250, 1980.

30. Hillman, R. S., and Finch, C. A.: Erythropoiesis: Normal and abnormal. *Semin. Hematol.* 4:327, 1967.

31. Ward, H. P., and Halman, J.: The association of nucleated red cells in the peripheral smear with hypoxemia. *Ann. Intern. Med.* 67:1190, 1967.

32. Finch, C. A., et al.: Ferrokinetics in man. *Medicine (Baltimore)* 49:17, 1970.

33. Dintenfass, L.: A preliminary outline of the blood high viscosity syndromes. *Arch. Intern. Med.* 118:427, 1966.

34. Monge, C. M., and Monge, C. C.: *High Altitude Diseases: Mechanism and Management.* Thomas, Springfield, Ill., 1966, p. 34.

35. Burch, G. E., and DePasquale, N. P.: Hematocrit, viscosity and coronary blood flow. *Dis. Chest* 48:225, 1965.

36. Mayer, G. A.: Hematocrit and coronary heart disease. *Can. Med. Assoc. J.* 93:1151, 1965.

37. Conley, C. L., Russell, R. P., Thomas, C. B., and Tumulty, P. A.: Hematocrit values in coronary artery disease. *Arch. Intern. Med.* 113:170, 1969.

38. Hershberg, P. J., Wells, R. E., and McGandy, R. B.: Hematocrit and prognosis in patients with acute myocardial infarction. *JAMA* 219:855, 1972.

39. Thomas, D. J., et al.: Cerebral blood flow in polycythemia. *Lancet* 2:161, 1977.

40. Stone, H. O., Thompson, H. K., Jr., and Schmidt-Nielsen, K.: Influence of erythrocytes on blood viscosity. *Am. J. Physiol.* 214:913, 1968.

41. Murray, J. F., Gold, P., and Johnson, B. L., Jr.: The circulatory effects of hematocrit variations in normovolemic and hypervolemic dogs. *J. Clin. Invest.* 42:1150, 1963.

42. Thorling, E. B., and Erslev, A. J.: The "tissue" tension of oxygen and its relation to hematocrit and erythropoiesis. *Blood* 31:332, 1968.

43. Smith, E. E., and Crowell, J. W.: Role of an increased hematocrit on altitude acclimatization. *Aerosp. Med.* 38:39, 1967.

44. Erslev, A. J.: The erythropoietic effect of hematocrit variations in normovolemic rabbits. *Blood* 27:629, 1966.

45. Kilbridge, T. M., Fried, W., and Heller, P.: The mechanism by which plethora suppresses erythropoieses. *Blood* 33:104, 1969.

46. Erslev, A. J., and Thorling, E. B.: Effect of polycythemic serum on the rate of red cell production. *Ann. N.Y. Acad. Sci.* 149:173, 1968.

47. Whitcomb, W. H., Moore, M. Z., and Rhodes, J. P.: Influence of polycythemia and anemic plasma on erythrocyte iron incorporation in the plethoric hypoxic mouse. *J. Lab. Clin. Med.* 73:584, 1969.

CHAPTER 9

Clinical manifestations of granulocyte and monocyte disorders

MARSHALL A. LICHTMAN

The clinical manifestations of granulocyte disorders may result from too many or too few cells or from the replacement of normal by dysfunctional cells. Clinical manifestations are also related to the severity and duration of the abnormality.

The ill effects of too few or dysfunctional neutrophils are principally the result of infection. An isolated deficiency of monocytes rarely occurs, and thus the effects of pure monocytopenia must be inferred. The combined deficit of neutrophils and monocytes characteristic of aplastic anemia, hairy cell leukemia, and cytotoxic therapy is likely to lead to a susceptibility to a broader spectrum of infectious agents. The functions of eosinophils and basophils are less well understood than those of neutrophils and monocytes, and isolated deficiencies of the former cells are extremely rare. Thus less is known of the effects of their absence from the blood and tissues. Eosinophilia and basophilia are more common events, and some information on the effect of excessive concentrations of eosinophils and basophils has been deduced from the manifestations of patients with chronic elevations of these two cell types. In these circumstances, chemical mediators contained in eosinophil or basophil granules may reach a high enough concentration in blood or tissues to lead to deleterious effects. Increased concentrations of normal neutrophils or monocytes per se have not been associated with clinical manifestations, although increased concentrations of leukemic neutrophil or monocyte precursors can produce clinical manifestations of hyperleukocytosis, such as stupor, visual impairment, and skin infiltrates.

Neutropenia

The lower limit of the normal neutrophil count is about 1800 neutrophils per microliter in white subjects [1–3] and 1400 neutrophils per microliter in black subjects [4–6]. The decrement in neutrophil concentration to a chronic, new steady state between 1800 and 1000 cells per microliter usually poses little threat in the otherwise healthy individual. As the neutrophil count drops further, the risk of infection increases, and chronically neutropenic subjects with counts less than 500 cells per microliter are likely to develop recurrent infections [7].

The relationship of frequency or type of infection to neutrophil concentration is an imperfect one. The cause of the neutropenia, the relationship to monocytopenia, lymphopenia, concurrent use of alcohol or glucocorticoids, and other factors can influence the likelihood of infection. Infections in neutropenic subjects not otherwise compromised are most likely to result from gram-positive cocci and usually are superficial, involving skin, oropharynx, bronchi, anal canal, or vagina. However, any site may become infected, and gram-negative organisms, viruses, or opportunistic organisms may be responsible.

A decrease in neutrophil count can occur abruptly or gradually. One type of drug-induced neutropenia is distinguished by the rapidity of onset. This abrupt-onset neutropenia is more likely to be severe and lead to symptoms. If the neutrophil count approaches zero (agranulocytosis), high fever, chills, necrotizing oral ulcers (agranulocytic angina), and prostration may occur, presumably as a result of sepsis [8–10]. As the disease progresses, headache, stupor, and rash may develop. In the preantibiotic era, chronic agranulocytosis had a fatality rate approaching 100 percent. Even with bactericidal, broad-spectrum antibiotics, severe neutropenia or agranulocytosis is a serious illness with a high fatality rate.

There is a decrease in the formation of pus in patients with severe neutropenia [11,12]. Exudate-poor infections occur in patients with *chronic hypoplastic neutropenias* of the congenital or acquired type. This failure to suppurate can be misleading to the clinician and delay the identification of the site of infection because minimal physical or radiographic findings develop. For example, lack of pneumonic consolidation is characteristic of pneumonia in granulocytopenic subjects. Exudate, swelling, heat, and regional adenopathy are much less prevalent in granulocytopenic patients. Fever is common, and local pain, tenderness, and erythema are nearly always present despite a marked reduction in neutrophils [13].

The mechanism of neutropenia, as well as the severity of the deficiency of cells, plays a role in clinical manifestations. *Chronic idiopathic (benign) neutropenia*, which is associated with normal granulopoiesis in the marrow, is asymptomatic for prolonged periods, sometimes in the face of neutrophil counts approaching zero [14,15]. Presumably the delivery of neutrophils from marrow to tissues is high enough to prevent infection despite the lower blood-pool size. Monocyte counts are normal, and this may also aid in host defenses, since these cells are effective phagocytes.

Chronic idiopathic (symptomatic) neutropenia is often associated with pyoderma and otitis media in children [16]. The former is usually caused by *Staphylococcus aureus, Escherichia coli,* and *Pseudomonas* spp., and the latter is usually the result of infection by pneumococci or *Pseudomonas aeruginosa.* Unexplained chronic gingi-

vitis may also be a manifestation of chronic neutropenia [17]. Pneumonia, lung abscesses, stomatitis, hepatic abscesses, or infections in other sites may occur [18,19].

Chronic cyclic neutropenia is characterized by periodic oscillations of neutrophils, with the nadir occurring at about 3-week intervals [20–22]. During neutropenia, patients develop malaise; fever; buccal, labial, or lingual ulcers; and cervical adenopathy. Furuncles, carbuncles, cellulitis, infected cuts with lymphangitis, chronic gingivitis, and abscesses of the axilla or groin also may occur. Although severe infections, such as pneumonia, peritonitis, necrotizing colitis, or septicemia, may occur and lead to fatality, life-threatening complications are uncommon.

Some individuals may have neutropenia because a larger proportion of their blood neutrophils is in the marginal rather than the circulating pool. The total blood neutrophil pool is normal, and infections do not result from this atypical distribution of neutrophils [23]. This type of alteration has been called *pseudoneutropenia.*

Qualitative neutrophil abnormalities

Neutrophil function depends on the ability of neutrophils to adhere to endothelium, move, respond to chemotactic gradients, ingest microorganisms, and kill ingested pathogens. Loss of any of these functions can predispose to infection. Defects in each step of the neutrophil's participation in the inflammatory response have been identified [24–26]. Defects in cytoplasmic contractile proteins, granule synthesis or contents, or intracellular enzymes may underly a movement, ingestion, or killing defect. These defects may be congenital or acquired. Chronic granulomatous disease [27,28] and Chédiak-Higashi disease [29] are two examples of the former. Among the acquired disorders are those extrinsic to the cell, such as in the movement, chemotactic, or phagocytic defects of diabetes mellitus [30–32], alcohol abuse [32,33], or glucocorticoid excess [34]. Acquired intrinsic disorders are usually manifestations of stem cell diseases like preleukemia [35].

Severe defects in bacterial killing, such as occurs in chronic granulomatous disease, results in *S. aureus, Klebsiella-Aerobacter, E. coli,* and other catalase-positive bacterial infections. Suppurative lymphadenitis, pneumonia, dermatitis, hepatic abscesses, osteomyelitis, and stomatitis occur, and chronic granulomatous reactions in these sites give the disease its name. Fatality rates have been high. Functional disorders may be severe, as in chronic granulomatous disease, or mild, predisposing to infection relatively infrequently and responding readily to antibiotics. Severe functional disorders like chronic granulomatous disease result in suppurative lesions because neutrophil influx into inflammatory foci is not impaired, whereas agranulocytosis is associated with nonsuppurative lesions.

Neutrophilia

An overabundance of neutrophils has not been shown to result in specific clinical manifestations. Neutrophils can transiently be seen to occlude capillaries, as determined by supravital microscopy, and investigators have postulated that such occlusions may reduce local blood flow and contribute to the development of ischemia. Recently, under special experimental conditions, coronary flow has been found to be impaired as a result of neutrophil occlusion.

In acute and chronic myelogenous leukemia, an excessive concentration of blast cells (>100,000 blast cells per microliter) has been associated with intracerebral hemorrhage, stupor, papilledema, priapism, or pulmonary insufficiency [36]. These manifestations, referred to as the "hyperleukocytic syndrome," are thought to result from the microvascular effects of poorly deformable leukemic blast cells [37] (see Chap. 7).

Monocytopenia

Isolated monocytopenia does not occur, and thus the manifestations of such a clinical state must be largely inferred [38]. Moreover, neutrophils, endothelial cells, and other cell types can substitute in part for some monocyte functions. Monocytes are effective phagocytes that seem to be involved in the ingestion of certain organisms such as mycobacteria, listeria, brucella, trypanosomes, and other granuloma-producing organisms. Thus their deficiency or functional abnormality might predispose to such infections. Since monocytes process some antigens, play a role in immune suppression, and secrete numerous monokines, such as plasminogen activator, complement components, prostaglandins, hemopoietic mediators, elastase, and others, their deficiency has the potential of influencing many functions and systems. A monocytopenia occurs after glucocorticoid administration and monocyte entry into inflammatory sites is reduced [39]. This may contribute to the predisposition of glucocorticoids to lead to infections in which monocytes may have a principal role as protective cells, such as infections resulting from fungi, mycobacteria, and other opportunistic organisms. Dysfunctional monocytes, incapable of killing ingested microoganisms, are present in chronic granulomatous disease [40], as well as in stem cell disease, such as AML [41].

Monocytosis

Benign monocytosis is not associated with specific clinical manifestations. Acute myelogenous leukemia with a predominance of monocytes is associated with a predisposition to troublesome tissue infiltrates, especially in the gingiva, lymph nodes, meninges, and anal canal [42,43]. Release of procoagulants leading to intravascular coagulation also occurs (see Chap. 7).

Eosinophilia

The association of myocardial endomyofibrosis, peripheral neuropathy, diffuse central nervous system involvement, bronchial asthma, and pulmonary fibrosis with hypereosinophilic syndromes has long suggested that eosinophil constituents released in tissues produce organ damage, especially of heart, lung, and nervous system [44,45]. An assocation of hypereosinophilia and thrombosis has also been implied [46]. Demonstration of the toxicity of a major basic protein, a key constituent of eosinophil granules, when applied to intestine, skin, and trachea suggests that it may be pathogenic in the tissue damage associated with eosinophilia [47,48].

Basophilia and mastocytosis

Marked increases in the numbers of blood basophils occur nearly exclusively as a feature of the myeloproliferative disease chronic myelogenous leukemia or, rarely, acute basophilic leukemia. Those features which may be specifically related to basophilia include a propensity to a shocklike state attributed to release of biogenic amines, since increased quantities of histamine and glycosaminoglycan are in plasma and are excreted in the urine [49,50].

Excessive circulating mast cells are associated with reddish-brown macules and papules that urticate on gentle abrasion, develop pruritis, and may form bullae [51]. Flushing, headache, palpitation, hypotension, and diarrhea have also been associated with chemical mediators, especially histamine released from mast cells [52,53]. Chronic bone resorption has been associated with mast cells, perhaps as a consequence of release of heparinoid substances [54].

References

1. Orfanakis, N. G., Ostlund, R. E., Bishop, C. R., and Athens, J. W.: Normal blood leukocyte concentration values. *Am. J. Clin. Pathol.* 53:649, 1970.
2. Rumke, C. L., Brezemer, P. D., and Kuik, D. J.: Normal values and least significant differences for differential leukocyte counts. *J. Chronic Dis.* 28:661, 1975.
3. England, J. M., and Bain, B. J.: Total and differential leukocyte count. *Br. J. Haematol.* 33:1, 1976.
4. Broun, G. O., Herbeg, F. K., and Hamilton, J. R.: Leukopenia in Negroes. *N. Engl. J. Med.* 275:1410, 1966.
5. Rippey, J. J.: Leukopenia in West Indians and Africans. *Lancet* 2:44, 1967.
6. Karayalcin, G., Rosner, F., and Saurtsky, A.: Pseudoneutropenia in Negroes. *N.Y. State J. Med.* 72:1815, 1972.
7. Bodey, G. P., Buckley, M., and Sathe, Y. S.: Quantitative relationships between circulating leukocytes and infection in patients with acute leukemia. *Ann. Intern. Med.* 64:328, 1966.
8. Kracke, R. R.: Recurrent agranulocytosis. *Am. J. Clin. Pathol.* 1:385, 1931.
9. Gorlin, R. J., and Chaudhry, A. P.: The oral manifestations of cyclic (periodic) neutropenia. *Arch. Dermatol.* 82:344, 1960.
10. Levine, S.: Neutropenia with marked periodontal lesions. *Oral Surg.* 12:310, 1959.

11. Boggs, D. R.: The cellular composition of inflammatory exudates in human leukemia. *Blood* 15:466, 1960.
12. Dale, D. C., and Wolff, S. M.: Skin window studies of the acute inflammatory responses of neutropenic patients. *Blood* 38:138, 1971.
13. Sickles, E. A., Green, W. H., and Wiernick, P. H.: Clinical presentation of infection in granulocytopenic patients. *Arch. Intern. Med.* 135:715, 1975.
14. Kyle, R. A., and Linman, J. W.: Chronic idiopathic neutropenia: Newly recognized entity? *N. Engl. J. Med.* 179:1015, 1968.
15. Kyle, R. A.: Natural history of chronic idopathic neutropenia. *N. Engl. J. Med.* 302:908, 1980.
16. Pincus, S. H., Boxer, L. A., and Stossel, T. P.: Chronic neutropenia in childhood. *Am. J. Med.* 61:849, 1976.
17. Kyle, R. A., and Linman, J. W.: Gingivitis and chronic idiopathic neutropenia. *Mayo Clin. Proc.* 45:494, 1970.
18. Doan, C. A.: The neutropenic state. *JAMA* 99:194, 1932.
19. Dale, D. C., Guerry, D. N., Wewerka, J. R., Bull, J. M., and Chusid, M. J.: Chronic neutropenia. *Medicine* 58:128, 1979.
20. Wright, D. G., Dale, D. C., Fauci, A. S., and Wolff, S. M.: Human cyclic neutropenia: Clinical review and long-term follow-up of patients. *Medicine* 60:1, 1981.
21. Joyce, R. A., Boggs, D. R., and Chervenick, P. A.: Neutrophil kinetics in hereditary and congenital neutropenias. *N. Engl. J. Med.* 295:1385, 1976.
22. Morley, A. A., Carew, J. P., and Backie, A. G.: Familial cyclic neutropenia. *Br. J. Haematol.* 13:719, 1967.
23. Joyce, R. A., Boggs, D. R., Hasiba, U., and Srodes, C. H.: Marginal neutrophil pool size in normal subjects and neutropenic patients as measured by epinephrine infusion. *J. Lab. Clin. Med.* 88:614, 1976.
24. Lehrer, R. I.: The role of phagocyte function in resistance to infection. *Calif. Med.* 114:17, 1971.
25. Baehner, R. L.: Disorders of leukocytes leading to recurrent infection. *Pediatr. Clin. North Am.* 19:935, 1972.
26. Gallin, J. I., et al.: Disorders of phagocyte chemotaxis. *Ann. Intern. Med.* 92:520, 1980.
27. Quie, P. G.: Chronic granulomatous disease of childhood. *Adv. Pediatr.* 16:287, 1969.
28. Babior, B. M.: Oxygen dependent microbial killing by phagocytes. *N. Engl. J. Med.* 298:721, 1978.
29. Padgett, G. A.: Comparative studies of susceptibility of infection in Chediak-Higaski syndrome. *J. Pathol. Bacteriol.* 95:509, 1968.
30. Mowat, A. G., and Baum, J.: Chemotaxis of polymorphonuclear leukocytes from patients with diabetes mellitus. *N. Engl. J. Med.* 284:621, 1971.
31. Tan, J. S., et al.: Neutrophil dysfunction in diabetes mellitus. *J. Lab. Clin. Med.* 85:26, 1975.
32. Brayton, R. G., Stokes, P. E., Schwartz, M. S., and Louria, D. B.: Effect of alcohol and various diseases on leukocyte mobilization, phagocytosis, and intracellular killing. *N. Engl. J. Med.* 282:123, 1970.
33. Liu, Y. K.: The effect of alcohol on granulocytes and lymphocytes. *Semin. Hematol.* 17:130, 1980.
34. Dale, D. C., Fauci, A. S., Dupont, G., IV, and Wolff, S. M.: Comparison of agents producing a neutrophilic leukocytosis in man: Hydrocortisone, prednisone, endotoxin and etiocholanoline. *J. Clin. Invest.* 56:808, 1975.
35. Breton-Gorius, J.: Abnormalities of granulocytes and megakaryocytes in preleukemic syndromes, in *Preleukemia*, edited by F. Schmalzl and K.-P. Helbriegel. Springer-Verlag, Berlin, 1979, p. 24.
36. Lichtman, M. A., and Rowe, J.: Hyperleucocytic leukaemias. *Blood* 60:279, 1982.
37. Lichtman, M. A.: Rheology of leukocytes, leukocyte suspensions and blood in leukemia: Possible relationship to clinical manifestations. *J. Clin. Invest.* 52:350, 1973.
38. Nathan, C. F., Murray, H. W., and Cohn, Z. A.: The macrophage as an effector cell. *N. Engl. J. Med.* 303:622, 1980.
39. Fauci, A. S., and Dale, D. C.: Alternate-day prednisone therapy and human lymphocyte subpopulations. *J. Clin. Invest.* 55:22, 1975.
40. Rodey, G. E., et al.: Defective bactericidal activity of monocytes in fatal granulomatous disease. *Blood* 23:813, 1969.
41. Cline, M. J.: Defective mononuclear phagocyte function in patients with myelomonocytic leukemia and in some patients with lymphoma. *J. Clin. Invest.* 52:2185, 1973.
42. Lichtman, M. A., and Weed, R. I.: Peripheral cytoplasmic characteristics of leukocytes in monocytic leukemia: Relationship to clinical manifestations. *Blood* 40:52, 1972.
43. Shaw, M. T.: The distinctive features of acute monocytic leukemia. *Am. J. Hematol.* 4:97, 1978.
44. Chusid, M. J., Dale, D. C., and West, B. C.: The hypereosinophilic syndrome. *Medicine* 54:1, 1975.
45. Solley, G. O., et al.: Endomyocardiopathy with eosinophilia. *Mayo Clin. Proc.* 51:697, 1976.
46. Ishii, T., Koide, O., Hosoda, Y., and Takahashi, R.: Hypereosinophilic multiple thrombosis. *Angiology* 28:361, 1977.
47. Frigas, E., Loegering, D. A., and Gleich, G. J.: Cytotoxic effects of the guinea pig eosinophil major basic protein on tracheal epithelium. *Lab. Invest.* 42:35, 1980.
48. Wassom, D. L., et al.: Elevated serum levels of the eosinophil granule major basic protein in patients with eosinophilia. *J. Clin. Invest.* 67:651, 1981.
49. Shibata, A., et al.: Cytological studies on basophilic leukocytes. *Acta Haematol. Jap.* 29:879, 1966.
50. Youman, J. D., Taddeini, L., and Cooper, T.: Histamine excess symptoms in basophilic chronic granulocytic leukemia. *Arch. Intern. Med.* 131:560, 1973.
51. Klaus, S. N., and Winkelmann, R. K.: The clinical spectrum of urticaria pigmentosa. *Mayo Clin. Proc.* 40:923, 1965.
52. Demis, D. J.: The mastocytosis syndrome. Clinical and biological studies. *Ann. Intern. Med.* 59:194, 1963.
53. Kaliner, M. A.: The mast cell: A fascinating riddle. *N. Engl. J. Med.* 301:498, 1979.
54. Frame, B., and Nixon, R. K.: Bone-marrow mast cells in osteoporosis of aging. *N. Engl. J. Med.* 279:626, 1968.

CHAPTER 10

Clinical manifestations of lymphocytic disorders

MARSHALL A. LICHTMAN

B-lymphocyte disorders

IMMUNOGLOBULIN DEFICIENCY AND MONOCLONAL PROTEINS

The clinical manifestations of B-lymphocyte disorders include the consequences of B-lymphocyte deficiency, dysfunction, or malignant transformation and may consist of a specific deficiency of one of the immunoglobulin (Ig) types or of several or all normal Ig molecules (panhypogammaglobulinemia) [1–3]. Inability to synthesize or secrete antibodies impairs phagocytosis because of the inability to opsonize microorganisms. Increased susceptibility to infection results [4,5].

B lymphocytes may undergo malignant transformation and clonal proliferation and may secrete monoclonal proteins inappropriately. In the case of monoclonal IgM, IgA, and some molecular species of IgG, hyperviscosity of blood may occur because of enhanced erythrocyte-erythrocyte aggregation (pathologic rouleaux) [6]. Headache, dizziness, diplopia, stupor, and retinal venous engorgement may result. Monoclonal proteins can also interact with cell surfaces and impair granulocyte [7] or platelet function [8] or interact with coagulation proteins to impair their function in hemostasis [9,10]. Excessive excretion of light chains of Ig can lead to several types of renal tubular dysfunction and renal insufiency [11]. IgM deposited in glomerular tufts can also lead to renal disease [12].

Formation of autoreactive antibodies spontaneously or in relationship to a B-lymphocyte tumor can lead to autoimmune hemolytic anemia, autoimmune thrombocytopenia, or rarely, autoimmune neutropenia [13]. Antibodies directed against tissues can lead to autoimmune thyroiditis, aspermia, adrenalitis, encephalitis, or other organ involvement [13].

MARROW AND OTHER TISSUE INFILTRATION

B lymphocytes in marrow or peripheral lymphatic structures may undergo malignant transformation [14]. Rather extensive marrow infiltrates with well-differentiated B lymphocytes can occur with minimal impairment of hemopoiesis. Early stages of chronic lymphocytic leukemia or macroglobulinemia are examples of tumors of this type. Eventually, proliferation of malignant B lymphocytes in marrow can lead to suppression of hemopoiesis and varying combinations of anemia, granulocytopenia, and thrombocytopenia [15]. Proliferation of B lymphocytes can lead to any combination of enlargement of superficial or deep lymph nodes or the spleen. B-cell lymphomas tend to involve isolated lymph node groups, whereas B-cell chronic lymphocytic leukemia tends to involve many superficial and deep lymph node–bearing areas and the spleen [16]. Prolymphocytic leukemia [17] and hairy cell leukemia [18], two uncommon B-lymphocyte tumors, have a propensity for marrow involvement and massive splenic infiltration and enlargement.

LYMPHOKINE-INDUCED DISORDERS

In addition to the consequences of monoclonal Ig and tumor proliferation noted above, certain malignant B-lymphocyte tumors, especially multiple myeloma, elaborate chemical mediators that contribute to the morbidity of the disease. Osteoclast activating factor (OAF), a lymphokine that stimulates osteoclast proliferation and activity leading to extensive osteolysis, severe bone pain, and pathologic fractures, is the best characterized of these chemical mediators [19].

T-lymphocyte disorders

IMPAIRED IMMUNOREGULATION

The clinical manifestations of deficiencies or excesses of T lymphocytes depend on the subset (i.e., function) of T lymphocytes involved. Delayed hypersensitivity is normally mediated by T cells. A deficit or functional dis-turbance in T cells can impair the inflammatory response important in the reaction to mycobacteria, listeria, brucella, fungi, and other organisms associated with immune granuloma formation, a tissue response that is a complex interaction between T lymphocytes, macrophages, B lymphocytes, neutrophils, and eosinophils [20].

After an allograft, donor T lymphocytes can be provoked to initiate the graft-versus-host reaction. The acute form of the reaction can lead to a profound dermatitis, hepatitis, and gastroenteritis mediated by alloaggressive T cells [21]. The chronic syndrome simulates collagen vascular diseases. Scleroderma, xerophthalmia, xerostomia, pulmonary insufficiency, and wasting occur. Eosinophilia, hypergammaglobulenemia, development of autoantibodies, and plasmacytosis also can occur [23]. The apparent dysregulation in B-lymphocyte behavior (excessive, purposeless Ig production) is thought to be the result of the inactivation of a T-lymphocyte subset, the cells that suppress B lymphocyte's antibody synthesis. Lymphocytic tumors of suppressor T-cell phenotypes may, on the other hand, cause hypogammaglobulinemia as a result of an inappropriate suppression of normal B-lymphocyte function [22]. Infection with classical or opportunistic pathogens is a common complication of both acute and chronic graft-versus-host disease. A similar qualitative reaction, albeit more limited, is seen in mononucleosis that results from Epstein-Barr virus infection. This disease is initiated by a viral infection of B lymphocytes that provokes a reaction by T lymphocytes, principally cytotoxic and suppressor T-cell subsets. It is largely T lymphocytes that proliferate and contribute to lymphocytosis, lymphadenopathy, splenomegaly, hepatitis, and occasionally, involvement of other organs [24].

ORGAN INFILTRATION

Malignancy of T lymphocytes can cause leukemias or lymphomas which, in addition to lymph node and spleen enlargement, often are associated with skin, mediastinal, and central nervous system involvement [25]. The predilection for skin involvement is particularly notable in cutaneous T-cell lymphomas, which may produce a severe desquamating erythroderma in Sézary cell syndrome and a variety of tumorous infiltrative lesions in mycosis fungoides [26]. Mediastinal lymph node enlargement is a frequent feature of T-cell acute lymphocytic leukemia and T-cell lymphocytic lymphoma [27,28]. In both diseases, a high frequency of involvement of the leptomeninges and structures that traverse the subarachnoid space, such as cranial and peripheral nerves, occurs.

Systemic symptoms

Large-cell lymphoma, poorly differentiated lymphoma, and Hodgkin's disease are frequently associated with fever, night sweats, weight loss, and anorexia [29–31].

Pruritis is common in Hodgkin's disease, and its severity parallels disease activity [32]. Localized or disseminated herpes zoster also has a heightened frequency in lymphomas and Hodgkin's disease, affecting about 10 percent of patients sometime during the course of their illness [33]. Systemic systems may be present in Hodgkin's disease in the absence of obvious, bulky lymph node or splenic tumors, whereas in well-differentiated small-cell lymphomas, such as chronic lymphocytic leukemia and Waldenström's macroglobulinemia, fever, night sweats, and significant weight loss are uncommon, despite generalized lymphadenopathy and splenomegaly. When fever is troublesome in chronic lymphocytic leukemia and macroglobulinemia, it is usually related to infection.

Metabolic signs

Lymphocytic malignancies are associated with the most dramatic metabolic disturbances associated with cancers [34]. These abnormalities, including hyperuricemia and hyperuricosuria of an extreme degree, can occur because of an extremely high proliferative rate, a high death fraction of cells, and therefore, an enormous turnover of nucleoproteins. Hyperuricemic renal failure can occur at the time of presentation prior to cytotoxic therapy, requiring urgent hemodialysis therapy. Burkitt's lymphoma or leukemia is particularly likely to result in an extreme degree of hyperuricemia prior to cytotoxic therapy [35]. Following treatment of lymphomas or lymphocytic leukemias, because of their sensitivity to cytotoxic drugs and glucocorticoids, massive hyperuricemia, hyperuricosuria, hyperkalemia, and hyperphosphatemia can result. Precipitation of uric acid in the renal tubules and collecting system can lead to acute obstructive nephropathy and renal failure if precautions, such as pretreatment with allopurinol and hydration, are not taken.

Hypercalcemia and calciuria are common complications of multiple myeloma because of osteolysis. Hypercalcemia may also occur during the course of lymphomas [36]. Metabolic studies suggest that several mechanisms may be causal, including ectopic parathormone elaboration, excessive bone resorption, and impaired bone formation.

Extranodal involvement

The salivary glands [37], endocrine glands [38], central nervous system [39], skin [40], joints [41], heart [42], lung [43], kidney [44], bowel [45], bone [46,47], and, less frequently, other sites may be involved by lymphoma or lymphocytic leukemia. The disease may begin with an extranodal tumor, or the tumor may develop during the course of the disease [48,49].

References

1. Rosen, F. S., and Janeway, C. A.: The gamma globulins. III. The antibody deficiency syndromes. *N. Engl. J. Med.* 275:709, 1966.
2. Horowitz, S. D., and Hong, R.: The pathogenesis and treatment of immunodeficiency. *Monogr. Allergy* 10:1, 1977.
3. Waldman, T. A.: Primary immunodeficiency diseases, in *Rheumatology and Immunology*, edited by A. S. Cohen. Grune & Stratten, New York, 1979, pp. 442–451.
4. Stossel, T. P.: Phagocytosis: Recognition and ingestion. *Semin. Hematol.* 12:83, 1975.
5. Meyers, B. R., Hirschman, S. Z., and Axelrod, J. A.: Current patterns of injection in multiple myeloma. *Am. J. Med.* 52:87, 1972.
6. McGrath, M. A., and Penny, R.: Paraproteinemia: Blood hyperviscosity and clinical manifestations. *J. Clin. Invest.* 58:1155, 1976.
7. Penny, R., and Galton, D. A. G.: Studies on neutrophil function. II. Pathologic aspects. *Br. J. Haematol.* 12:633, 1966.
8. Pachter, et al.: Bleeding, platelets and macroglobulinemia. *Am. J. Clin. Pathol.* 31:467, 1959.
9. Perkins, H. A., McKenzie, M. R., and Fudenberg, H. H.: Hemostatic defects in dysproteinemias. *Blood* 35:695, 1970.
10. Lackner, H.: Hemostatic abnormalities associated with dysproteinemias. *Semin. Hematol.* 10:125, 1978.
11. Martinez-Maldenado, M., Yium, J., Suki, W. N., and Eknoyan, G.: Renal complications in multiple myeloma. *J. Chronic Dis.* 24:221, 1971.
12. Morel-Maroger, L., et al.: Pathology of the kindey in Waldenström's macroglobulinemia. *N. Engl. J. Med.* 283:123, 1970.
13. Vaughan, J. H.: Autoimmune and histocompatibility (HLA)-associated diseases: General considerations, in *Immunological Diseases*, 3d ed., edited by M. Santer. Little, Brown, Boston, 1978.
14. Aisenberg, A. C.: Cell-surface markers in lymphoproliferative disease. *N. Engl. J. Med.* 304:331, 1981.
15. Bloomfield, C. D., McKenna, R. W., and Brunning, R. D.: Significance of haematologic parameters in the non-Hodgkin's lymphoma. *Br. J. Haematol.* 32:41, 1976.
16. Sweet, D. L., Jr., Golomb, H. M., and Ultmann, J. E.: The clinical features of chronic lympocytic leukemia. *Clin. Hematol.* 6:185, 1977.
17. Galton, D. A. G., et al.: Prolymphocytic leukemia. *Br. J. Haematol.* 27:7, 1974.
18. Golomb, H. M., Catovsky, D., and Golde, D. W.: Hairy cell leukemia. A clinical review based on 71 cases. *Ann. Intern. Med.* 89:684, 1978.
19. Mundy, G. R., et al.: Evidence for the secretion of an osteoclast stimulating factor in myeloma. *N. Engl. J. Med.* 291:1041, 1974.
20. Warren, K. S.: Granulomatous inflammation, in *Inflammation*, edited by I. H. Lepow. Academic, New York, 1972.
21. Thomas, E. D., et al.: Bone marrow transplantation. *N. Engl. J. Med.* 292:895, 1975.
22. Broder, S., Uchiyama, T., and Waldmann, T. A.: Current concepts in immunoregulatory T-cell neoplasms. *Cancer Treat. Rep.* 63:607, 1979.
23. Shulman, H. M., et al.: Chronic graft-versus-host syndrome in man. *Am. J. Med.* 69:204, 1980.
24. DeWaele, M., Thielemans, C., and VanCamp, B. K. G.: Characterization of immunoregulatory T-cells in EBV-induced infectious mononucleosis by monoclonal antibodies. *N. Engl. J. Med.* 304:460, 1981.
25. Safai, B., and Good, R. A.: Lymphoproliferative disorders of the T-cell series. *Medicine* 59:335, 1980.
26. Lutzer, M. A., et al.: Cutaneous T-cell lymphomas: The Sézary syndrome, mycosis fungoides and related disorders. *Ann. Intern. Med.* 83:534, 1975.
27. Nathwani, B. N., et al.: Malignant lymphoma, lymphoblastic. *Cancer* 38:964, 1976.
28. Lilleyman, J. S., and Sugden, P. J.: T-lymphoblastic leukemia and the central nervous system. *Br. J. Cancer* 43:320, 1981.
29. Rosenberg, S., Diamond, H. D., Jaslowitz, B., and Craver, L. F.: Lymphosarcoma. *Medicine* 40:31, 1961.
30. Lobel, M., Boggs, D. R., and Wintrobe, M. M.: The clinical significance of fever in Hodgkin's disease. *Arch. Intern. Med.* 117:335, 1960.
31. Gordon, H. W., Wilson, W. W., and Beutler, E.: Response of the fever

of Hodgkin's disease to nitrogen mustard. *Cancer Chemother. Rep.* 53:127, 1969.

32. Feiner, A. S., Mahmood, T., and Wallner, S. F.: Prognostic importance of pruritis in Hodgkin's disease. *JAMA* 240:2738, 1978.
33. Goffinet, D. R., Glatstein, E. J., and Mengan, T. C.: Herpes zoster–varicella infections and lymphoma. *Ann. Intern. Med.* 76:235, 1972.
34. Muggia, F. M., Ball, T. J., and Ultmann, J. E.: Allopurinol in the treatment of neoplastic disease complicated by hyperuricemia. *Arch. Intern. Med.* 120:12, 1967.
35. Cohen, L. F., Balow, J. E., MaGrath, I. T., Poplack, D. G., and Ziegler, J. L.: Acute tumor lysis syndrome. *Am. J. Med.* 68:4862, 1980.
36. Moses, A. M., and Spencer, H.: Hypercalcemia in patients with malignant lymphoma. *Ann. Intern. Med.* 59:531, 1963.
37. Hayman, G. A., and Wolff, M.: Malignant lymphoma of the salivary glands. *Am. J. Clin. Pathol.* 65:421, 1976.
38. Compagno, J., and Oertel, J. E.: Malignant lymphoma and other lymphoproliferative disorders of the thyroid gland. *Am. J. Clin. Pathol.* 74:1, 1980.
39. Bunn, P. A., Jr., Schein, P. S., Banks, P. M., and DeVita, V. T., Jr.: Central nervous system complications in patients with diffuse histiocytic and undifferentiated lymphoma: Leukemia revisited. *Blood* 47:3, 1976.
40. Fisher, E. R., Park, E. J., and Wechsler, H. L.: Histologic identification of malignant lymphoma cutis. *Am. J. Clin. Pathol.* 65:149, 1976.
41. Fink, C. W., Windmiller, J., and Sartain, P.: Arthritis as the presenting feature of childhood leukemia. *Arthritis Rheum.* 15:347, 1972.
42. Roberts, W. C., Glancy, D. L., and DeVita, V. T., Jr.: Heart in malignant lymphoma. *Am. J. Cardiol.* 22:85, 1968.
43. Hilbun, B. M., and Chavez, C. M.: Lymphoma of the lung. *J. Thorac. Cardiovasc. Surg.* 53:721, 1967.
44. Kuly, J. M., et al.: Renal complications of lymphoma. *Ann. Intern. Med.* 71:1159, 1969.
45. Hande, K. R., et al.: Diffuse histiocytic lymphoma involving the gastrointestinal tract. *Cancer* 41:1984, 1978.
46. Hustu, H. O., and Pinkel, D.: Lymphosarcoma, Hodgkin's disease, and leukemia in bone. *Clin. Orthop.* 52:83, 1967.
47. Reimer, R. R., et al.: Lymphoma presenting in bone. *Ann. Intern. Med.* 87:50, 1977.
48. Freeman, C., et al.: Occurrence and prognosis of extranodal lymphoma. *Cancer* 29:252, 1972.
49. Rudders, R. A., et al.: Primary extranodal lymphoma. *Cancer* 42:406, 1978.

CHAPTER *11*

Clinical manifestations of disorders of hemostasis

WILLIAM J. WILLIAMS

Internal or external bleeding is an extremely common accompaniment of trauma. The normal hemostatic mechanisms are sufficient to seal small vessels promptly, and even major trauma may not cause alarming hemorrhage. However, bleeding from larger vessels may require intervention, often in the form of externally applied pressure or by means of a suture or ligature.

Failure of the hemostatic mechanism

When the normal hemostatic mechanism fails, spectacular hemorrhage may follow minor trauma or may arise apparently spontaneously. This abnormal bleeding tendency may be manifested anywhere in the body in disorders of hemostasis resulting from abnormalities of either platelets or plasma coagulation factors. However, disorders of hemostasis may also be a result of vascular abnormalities which may cause localized bleeding, such as that which occurs at the site of the vascular malformations of hereditary hemorrhagic telangiectasia or in areas of vasculitis in some forms of nonthrombocytopenic purpura, such as allergic purpura. The vascular abnormalities may be widespread in the skin, for example, and be manifested with bleeding from multiple loci. In such cases, determination that the bleeding is caused by widespread local lesions rather than by some general disorder may be difficult.

Abnormal bleeding due to deficiencies or abnormalities of platelets presents a clinical picture distinct from that due to deficiencies or abnormalities of plasma coagulation factors. As discussed in Chap. 129, platelets are primarily responsible for the cessation of bleeding in small vessels, and a prolonged bleeding time and petechial hemorrhages are the hallmarks of abnormalities of these components of the hemostatic system. Petechiae are apparent on the skin and the visible mucous membranes, but they may be widespread throughout the body, including the retinae and internal organs. However extensive, bleeding associated with platelet abnormalities is still manifested primarily as bleeding from small vessels. Bleeding resulting from platelet abnormalities tends to stop promptly with local pressure and not to recur when the pressure is removed.

On the other hand, bleeding resulting from abnormalities of the plasma coagulation factors does not give rise to superficial hemorrhages of the type found with thrombocytopenia, for example, because in coagulation disorders the platelets function in a nearly normal fashion and the bleeding time is normal. Abnormalities of the plasma coagulation factors result in hemorrhages deeper in the body, such as subcutaneous or intramuscular hematomas, or bleeding into joint spaces. The latter form of bleeding, in the absence of major local trauma, is highly characteristic of severe plasma coagulation factor disorders. External bleeding associated with abnormalities of the plasma coagulation factors responds only slowly to local pressure, and it is likely to recur several hours after the local pressure is removed.

The occurrence of superficial bleeding with platelet disorders and deeper bleeding with coagulation disorders is a clinically useful point, but it must be remembered that platelets and plasma coagulation factors are interdependent in hemostasis. Thrombin formation is essential for hemostasis, not only because it leads to fibrin formation but also because of its additional catalytic effects on factors V and VIII, its activating effects on factor XIII, and its role in platelet aggregation. The importance of these latter functions is apparent from comparison of the relatively mild bleeding tendencies in patients with afibrinogenemia, where thrombin formation is normal, with the severe bleeding tendencies of patients with hemophilia, where thrombin formation is markedly impaired. A severe coagulation defect may so interfere with thrombin formation as to give rise to some abnormalities of platelet function and petechial bleeding. Further, defects in the platelet system and in the plasma coagulation factors may coexist, as in patients with von Willebrand's disease or the defibrination syndrome and in people who suffer severe hemorrhage with replacement by banked blood which is deficient in factors V and VIII and in platelets.

Both the superficial bleeding of platelet abnormalities and the deep bleeding of plasma coagulation factor abnormalities may appear "spontaneously" as well as after significant trauma. In any form of "spontaneous" bleeding, e.g., gastrointestinal or intrauterine bleeding, it is important to search for a local lesion, such as peptic ulcer or intrauterine polyp, which may be the site of the hemorrhage. In addition to abnormal bleeding, delayed wound healing occurs in factor XIII deficiency (Chap. 154) and in some forms of dysfibrinogenemia (Chap. 153). Although not obviously related to bleeding, this manifestation may be due to formation of abnormal fibrin which is an ineffective matrix for fibroblastic proliferation.

LEVELS OF PLATELETS ASSOCIATED WITH BLEEDING
One clinical enigma has been the lack of an obvious relationship between the platelet count and bleeding manifestations. Some patients with severe thrombocytopenia will have no hemorrhagic manifestations, while others with a less severe decrease in the number of platelets will have marked bleeding. This dissociation may be explained by variations in platelet function. In patients with normally functioning platelets, the bleeding time correlates well with the platelet count [1]. In idiopathic thrombocytopenic purpura, platelet function is enhanced because of the presence of young platelets, and the bleeding time is relatively short. Patients with qualitative platelet abnormalities or von Willebrand's disease may have prolonged bleeding times with normal platelet counts [1].

A careful study has shown that the tendency of patients with acute leukemia to bleed can be related inversely to the platelet count: the lower the platelet count, the greater the probability of serious hemorrhage [2–5]. Major hemorrhages were unusual with platelet counts greater than 20,000 per microliter [2–5]. In one study of patients with aplastic anemia, major bleeding occurred only with platelet counts below 5000 per microliter [4]. In that study, blood loss was greater in patients receiving therapy with antibiotics or prednisone [4]. It is generally stated that platelet counts of about 50,000 will prevent hemorrhage during surgical procedures, if the platelets are functioning normally. Vascular function is another determinant of petechial bleeding, and in some patients with thrombocytopenia, glucocorticoid therapy may cause the disappearance of petechiae without any change in the platelet count [6]. Anemia is also a factor, for retinal hemorrhages occur more often in patients with thrombocytopenia who are also anemic than in patients with thrombocytopenia alone [7]. The presence of local lesions may lead to bleeding in thrombocytopenia, with cessation of the bleeding problem when the local lesion is corrected. Finally, associated abnormalities in the coagulation factors may also play a role, as in the defibrination syndrome or following massive hemorrhage, as noted above.

Elevated platelet counts may also be accompanied by bleeding, particularly in patients with myeloproliferative disorders. In such cases, the correlation between platelet count and bleeding is quite imperfect, and the patient with a markedly elevated platelet count may either bleed or develop thrombosis.

LEVELS OF COAGULATION FACTORS ASSOCIATED WITH BLEEDING
Correlation between the level of a plasma coagulation factor and bleeding is much better than that between thrombocytopenia and bleeding, although in an individual case there may be exceptions to this from time to time. This correlation is established most clearly in classic hemophilia (Chap. 152). With each of the coagulation factors, the minimum hemostatic level has been determined from clinical studies on replacement therapy. There is wide variation, from less than 1 percent of mean normal for factor XIII to 15 to 20 percent of mean normal for factor VIII. These data are presented for all the coagulation factors in Table 167-2. As with platelet abnormalities, extraneous influences such as local lesions may cause bleeding in patients with coagulation factor levels at which one would not expect hemorrhage to occur.

HYPERCOAGULABILITY
The complex interactions of platelets, coagulation factors, plasma inhibitors, blood flow, and vessel wall that lead to thrombosis are presented in Chap. 160. The effects of the thrombosis are local and depend on restriction of blood flow because of the vascular occlusion.

More generalized intravascular clotting (Chap. 158) involves all reactants of the hemostatic system also and leads to consumption of platelets and plasma coagulation factors and to deposition of fibrin in small vessels. Thrombocytopenia and depletion of coagulation factors lead to a marked bleeding tendency, with blood both oozing from venipuncture sites and infiltrating deeper tissues. Occlusion of both small and large vessels may occur, with infarction of the tissues supplied by the vessels, or hemolytic anemia may be induced, probably from the mechanical trauma to erythrocytes passing through intravascular fibrin deposits (Chap. 64).

Clinical manifestations of disorders of hemostasis

HISTORY
The history is extremely important in evaluating patients with disorders of hemostasis. The duration of the bleeding disorder must be determined, since many of these disorders are inherited. Careful questioning may be necessary to reveal a lifelong history.

BRUISING
Bruising is a frequent complaint and occurs often in apparently normal people, especially in women. Small bruises have little significance, but bruises of more than 6 cm in diameter may be significant, particularly if they occur without trauma that the patient remembers. Petechiae and bruising occur most frequently on the lower extremities but may be seen on any part of the body.

SPONTANEOUS BLEEDING
Spontaneous bleeding, as from the gums or nose, suggests abnormalities of platelets but is more often caused by local trauma without an associated hemostatic disorder. Gastrointestinal and genitourinary bleeding may occur spontaneously with disorders either of platelets or of plasma factors. Spontaneous hemarthroses are indications of a severe coagulation factor disorder.

EXCESSIVE BLEEDING AFTER TRAUMA
It is often difficult to evaluate the significance of a history of heavy bleeding after a dental extraction, a surgical wound, or an accidental laceration unless the medical record is available. The extent of hemorrhage is likely to be exaggerated by the patient and his or her family, but it is wise to accept the patient's story at face value. Bleeding from a circumcision is suggestive of an inherited coagulation disorder. Dental extractions are a very common major stress of the hemostatic mechanism, and a prior history of bleeding following an extraction is important. In evaluating this history, one must consider the number of teeth extracted, the location of the teeth which were extracted, the time of onset and duration of the hemorrhage, and the extent of the blood loss.

FAMILY HISTORY
The family history of patients with factor VIII and factor IX deficiency usually shows the characteristic pattern of sex-linked inheritance (Chap. 16), although about one-third of all hemophilic patients have a negative family history. Careful questioning is necessary, since sex-linked disorders may skip generations (Fig. 152-5) or the patient may not be aware of bleeding disorders in maternal uncles or in relatives who died at an early age. Von Willebrand's disease is usually inherited as a dominant trait, but it may also appear as a recessive trait. The remainder of the disorders appear to be inherited as autosomal recessive traits (Chap. 152).

PHYSICAL EXAMINATION
The physical examination of patients with hemorrhagic disorders may permit evaulation of the type of skin bleeding (petechiae, bruising) or the presence of hemarthroses, hematomas, or local bleeding sites. Residual joint deformities from old hemarthroses may be present.

LABORATORY STUDIES
In the evaluation of a patient with a presumed coagulation disorder, it is customary to perform a series of tests to detect abnormalities which may involve certain groups of the coagulation factors ("screening tests") and then proceed to more specific studies if abnormalities are detected in these tests. One difficulty with this approach is the relative insensitivity of some of the screening tests, so that patients with mild disorders may not be detected. It is important to recognize this limitation of the screening tests when evaluating patients with a questionable history of a bleeding disorder.

The relationship of the level of a coagulation factor to the detection of abnormality in various coagulation tests has been studied in classic hemophilia. The whole-blood clotting time is prolonged only when the factor VIII level is about 1 percent [8]. This is clearly an insensitive test, but it has some use as a screening test, since if it is prolonged, it suggests a severe abnormality, and it also provides clotted blood, which can be incubated at 37°C to examine for the presence of fibrinolysis and clot retraction. The activated partial thromboplastin time is abnormal with factor VIII and factor IX levels of 30 to 40 percent [9,10] and is therefore a useful screening test.

The usual screening tests for platelet function are the bleeding time, clot retraction test, and platelet count. The usual screening tests for the coagulation factors are the activated partial thromboplastin time, prothrombin time, and thrombin time. Specific factor deficiencies can be diagnosed using modifications of the activated partial thromboplastin time. The results that one would expect in these tests in patients with platelet abnormalities or abnormalities of specific coagulation factors are presented in Table 137-1.

In patients who have a definite history of previous abnormal bleeding and give abnormal results in any of the screening tests, the diagnosis of a significant coagulation abnormality is assured. Similarly, in those with a questionable bleeding history and an abnormal screening test, the diagnosis of a coagulation disorder would be highly likely. In patients with a questionable bleeding history and negative screening tests, further studies should be performed if the patient is to be operated on or is likely to be at high risk of exposure to trauma, although this decision must be based on the history obtained. It is better to err in the direction of performing too many tests than to reassure a patient that she or he has no coagulation disorder when in fact there is a deficiency so mild as to escape detection by the usual screening procedures, or the patient has von Willebrand's disease and the laboratory tests are transiently normal (see Chap. 155). Massive bleeding may occur in patients with coagulation disorders which appear to be minor in terms of the laboratory data, and caution is the rule in evaluating these patients.

References

1. Harker, L. A., and Slichter, S. J.: The bleeding time as a screening test for evaluation of platelet function. *N. Engl. J. Med. 287*:155, 1972.

2. Freirich, E.: Effectiveness of platelet transfusions in leukemia and aplastic anemia. *Transfusion 6*:50, 1966.

3. Roy, A. J., Jaffe, N., and Djerassi, I.: Prophylactic platelet transfusions in children with acute leukemia: A dose response study. *Transfusion 13*:283,1973.

4. Slichter, S. J., and Harker, L. A.: Thrombocytopenia: Mechanisms and management of defects in platelet production. *Clin. Haematol. 7*:523, 1978.

5. Slichter, S. J.: Controversies in platelet transfusion therapy. *Ann. Rev. Med. 31*:509, 1980.

6. Robson, H. N., and Duthie, J. J. R.: Capillary resistance and adrenocortical activity. *Br. Med. J. 2*:971, 1950.

7. Rubenstein, R. A., Yanoff, M., and Albert, D. A.: Thrombocytopenia, anemia and retinal hemorrhages. *Am. J. Ophthalmol. 65*:435, 1968.

8. Langdell, R. H.: Transfusion therapy in hemophilia, in *Hemophilia and Hemophilioid Diseases,* edited by K. M. Brinkhous. University of North Carolina Press, Chapel Hill, 1957, p. 189.

9. Proctor, R. R., and Rapaport, S. I.: The partial thromboplastin time and kaolin. *Am. J. Clin. Pathol. 36*:212, 1961.

10. Goulian, M., and Beck, W. S.: The partial thromboplastin time test. *Am. J. Clin. Pathol. 44*:1, 1965.

PART TWO *General hematology*

Structure and function of hemopoietic organs

CHAPTER *12*

Structure and function of the marrow

ALLAN J. ERSLEV
LEON WEISS

The marrow, one of the largest organs in the body, is in human beings the principal site for blood cell formation. In the normal adult its daily production and export of blood cells amount to about 2.5 billion red cells, 2.5 billion platelets, and 1.0 billion granulocytes per kilogram of body weight. This rate of production is adjusted to actual needs and can be varied from nearly zero to many times normal. The marrow is also responsible for the production of monocytes and of virgin, uncommitted lymphocytes, and as part of the monocyte-macrophage system it is involved in antibody synthesis and in the recognition and removal of senescent and abnormal cells. Despite the relative ease with which it can be sampled and examined, the marrow has been a difficult organ to study because of its complex cellular composition. However, recent technical improvements in cell separation and in vivo and in vitro culture techniques have led to a better understanding of its role in cellular and humoral homeostasis.

Until the late nineteenth century, blood cell formation was thought to be the prerogative of the lymph nodes or the liver and spleen. In 1868, Neuman [1] and Bizzazero [2] independently observed nucleated blood cells in material squeezed from ribs of human cadavers and proposed that the marrow is the major source of blood cells. This concept was vigorously opposed by many contemporary hematologists, and it was first accepted after the prestigious physiologist Claude Bernard had presented and endorsed Neuman's findings at the Academy of Science in Paris [3]. During the next decade, postmortem examinations of the marrow yielded considerable information about the morphology of immature blood cells, but a dynamic understanding of their maturation, proliferation, and relation to disease had to await in vivo marrow sampling and better staining methods.

The first in vivo marrow biopsy was probably made in 1876 by Mosler [4], who used a regular wood drill to obtain marrow particles from a patient with leukemia. Despite the obvious diagnostic advantages of this approach, 50 years passed before Arinkin's studies in 1929 established marrow aspiration as a safe, easy, and useful technique [5]. With the help of the Romanovsky and supravital staining techniques and improved methods for sectioning, the morphology and interrelationships of blood and marrow cells were clarified and the existence of definite cell lines established.

During the last 25 years, kinetic studies of marrow cells have confirmed the existence of a cellular hierarchy dimly envisioned by the great morphologists at the turn of the century. These studies have shown that cell lines consist of differentiated end cells with a finite functional life-span, capable of proliferation when young but without the capacity for self-renewal. Sustained cellular production, on the other hand, depends on the presence of pools of stem cells capable both of differentiation into specific cell lines and of continuous self-replication [6]. The proliferative activity of these stem cell pools was found to involve humoral feedback from peripheral target tissues [7] as well as cell-to-cell interactions within the microenvironment of the marrow [8].

Structure

The emergence of cavities within bone occurs in the human being at about the fifth fetal month, and these cavities soon become the exclusive site for myeloid and megakaryocytic proliferation. Erythropoietic activity at that time is confined to the liver and spleen, and it is not until the end of the last trimester that the microenvironment in the marrow becomes attractive to erythroblasts (Fig. 12-1). At birth, the bone cavities are the only sites of hemopoietic activity and are completely engorged with hemopoietic cells [9]. Consequently, any increase in cellular production may lead to a spillover of marrow elements into blood, and the presence of immature cells in the blood of infants does not have the same serious implications as in an adult. Neither has the

FIGURE 12-1 Expansion and recession of hemopoietic activity in extramedullary and medullary sites.

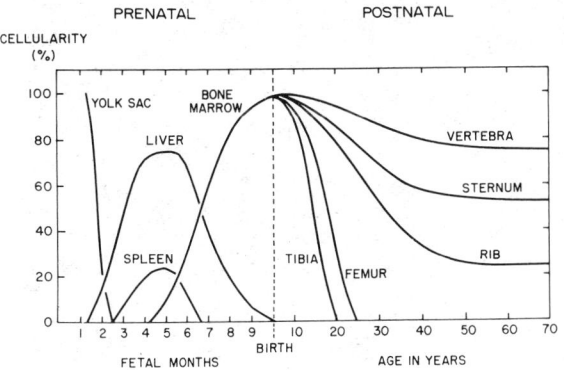

presence of many small mononuclear cells in the marrow of infants and children [10]. In the newborn, the relative number of these lymphocyte-like cells is very low, but within one month it rises to about 40 percent. Such percentage is maintained until late childhood, when it slowly decreases to adult values of about 20 percent.

By the fourth year, a significant number of fat cells have appeared in the diaphysis of the long bones [11]. These space-occupying cells slowly replace hemopoietic elements and expand centripetally until at about the age of 18, hemopoietic marrow is found only in the vertebrae, ribs, skull, pelvis, and proximal epiphyses of the femurs and humeri. Since the ratio between the number of precursor cells in the marrow and the number of mature cells in blood is the same at all ages, the available marrow space must have expanded faster than the blood volume. Direct measurements of the volume of bone cavities support this conclusion by revealing that the bone cavity volume increases from 1.4 percent of body weight at birth to 4.8 percent in the adult [9,12], while the blood volume decreases from 8 percent of body weight in the newborn to about 7 percent in the adult [13]. Owing to bone resorption and bone remodeling, the expansion of marrow space continues throughout life, resulting in a further gradual increase in the amount of fatty tissue in all bone cavities, especially in peripheral bones.

The preference of hemopoietic tissue for centrally located bones is still a puzzle. Higher central tissue temperature with greater vascularity has been invoked to explain this hemopoietic distribution [14]. However, complete reactivation of peripheral fatty marrow in the rat demands more than merely increased environmental temperature, suggesting that there is an inherent determinant of the cellularity of marrow in different sites [15,16].

Despite the unequal distribution of fat, a single

FIGURE 12-2   The venous vessels of the marrow appear here in an arborizing pattern: smaller venous sinuses converge into large venous sinuses. The central longitudinal vein lies in the lower right-hand corner. The orifices in its wall represent the entrance of its tributary venous sinuses [17].

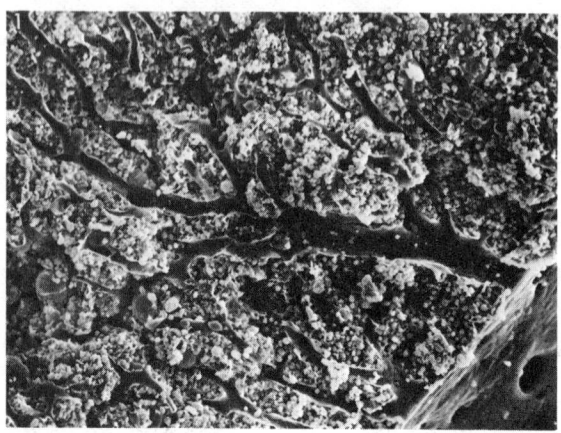

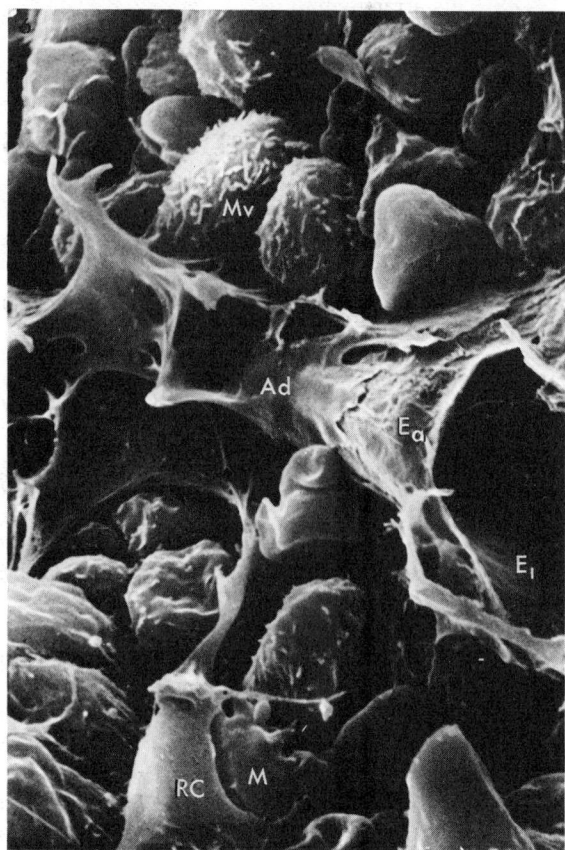

FIGURE 12-3   A vascular sinus crosses the field from left to right, coming out toward the surface, its lumen exposed at the right-hand margin of the field. Both the luminal (E_l) and the adventitial (E_a) surfaces of the endothelium can be seen. The broad cytoplasmic expanse of an adventitial reticular cell (Ad) covers much of the outside surface of the vascular sinus and branches richly, far out into the hemopoietic compartment. Its processes pass between hemopoietic cells and at one place reticular cell cytoplasm (RC) almost completely envelops a myelocyte (M). Several cells bearing microvilli (Mv) lie close against the adventitial surface of the sinus at its upper aspect. These microvilli may well have developed preparatory to transmural passage of these cells. Many hemopoietic cells have been removed in this preparation by the loosening effects of perfusion. Those which remain are somewhat separated from one another [17].

biopsy sample of marrow tissue from the posterior iliac crest or the sternum can usually be trusted to reflect total hemopoietic marrow activity. In some illnesses, however, multiple samplings, marrow imaging, or radioisotope turnover studies may be required in order to measure accurately the size and function of the marrow mass (see Chaps. 3 and 4).

Structurally, the marrow consists of hemopoietic cells lying in a meshwork of vessels and branched fibroblastic cells [17–19]. The blood supply is derived from the nutrient artery of the bone and the cortical capillaries, which communicate to form an endosteal network that in turn drains through marrow sinuses into a central sinus [20]. This arrangement may provide hemopoietic cells with a high concentration of chemicals from the cortical bone or may possibly expose hemopoietic cells to a low P_{O_2} claimed to facilitate blood cell formation [21]. The most distinctive elements in the vasculature are the venous sinuses, large thin-walled vessels which constitute the outflow system carrying blood cells into the circulation (Fig. 12-2). The walls of these vessels consist of endothelial cells which form a complete cover but with loose overlapping junctions and a basement membrane. The outside surface is clothed by large, broad cells which branch into the perivascular space and thereby provide a scaffolding for the hemopoietic cells and such associated cells as macrophages and mast cells. These branched cells are termed adventitial reticular cells and may be derived from fibroblasts (Fig. 12-3). Their branches in the perivascular hemopoietic space are closely associated with slender extracellular fibers (reticular fibers), which can be distinctively impregnated with silver and which support and compartmentalize the hemopoietic tissue. Reticular cells appear to play a major role in the creation of the hemopoietic-inductive microenvironment (HIM) [8,22], which makes the marrow the prime site for production, sorting, and homing of hemopoietic cells. Furthermore, they may provide a filler for unused space by becoming gelatinous or fatty [23] (Fig. 12-4). Such fat cells occupy about 50 percent of active red marrow and almost 100 percent of yellow inactive marrow. Their fat content has been shown not to undergo lipolysis in response to starva-

FIGURE 12-4 A venous sinus (S) runs vertically on the right. Its endothelium (En) shows well in its upper portion. At least five of its adventitial cells have become fatty and spherical. From the lumen of the sinus the spherical protruding shapes of these cells can be seen through the endothelium. They are directly visible on the adventitial surfaces which face upon hemopoietic cells. The adventitial surface of each fat cell is covered by cytoplasmic processes of reticular cells, as seen well on the two near fat cells. Such processes may spring from the fat cell and branch into the hemopoietic compartment *(arrows)*. Hemopoietic cells are found on the left-hand portion of the field. The processes of reticular cells (RC) can be seen lying between them [17].

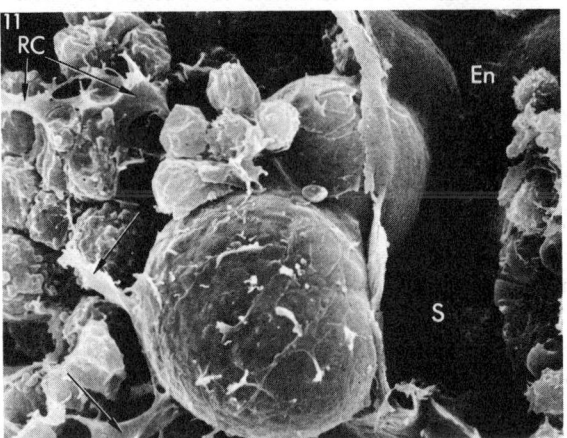

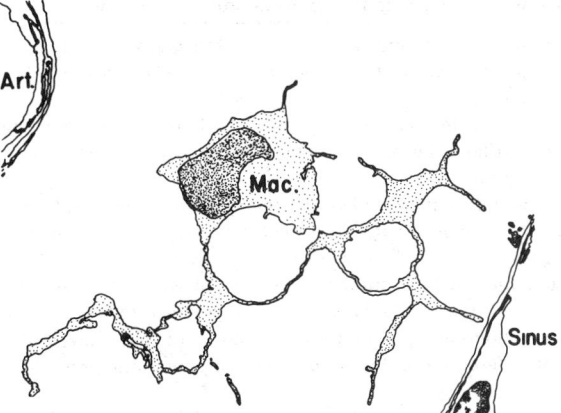

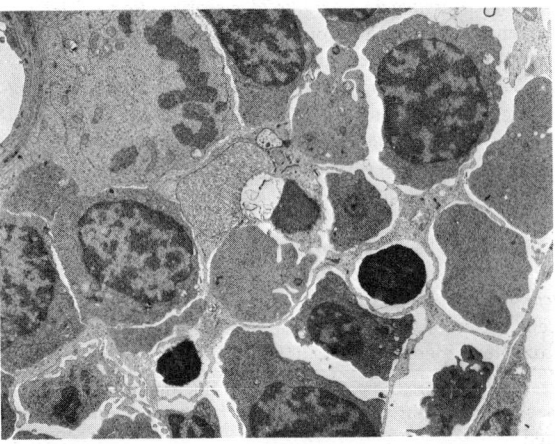

FIGURE 12-5 As seen from the tracing, a single macrophage (Mac.) extends long, slender, branching processes which enclose erythroblasts in different degrees of maturation. This is the central macrophage in an erythroblastic island. The island lies between an arterial vessel in the left upper corner (Art.) and a venous sinus (Sinus) in the right lower corner. Cell separation induced by preparatory perfusion is valuable in loosening hemopoietic cells so that they can fall out of the tissue and reveal the macrophages and reticular cells. Compare with Fig. 12-3 [17].

tion [24], an appropriate feature if their function is to occupy space rather than to store energy. Other claimed functions, such as phagocytosis and differentiation to hemic cells, have not been established.

In the reticular stroma, hemopoietic cells lie in cords or wedges between the vascular sinuses. Erythroblasts lie close against the outside surface of the vascular sinuses in distinctive clusters, erythroblastic islands [25]. These consist of one or more concentric circles of erythroblasts closely surrounding a macrophage. The inner erythroblastic shells are less mature than the peripheral ones. The central macrophage sends out extensive slender membranous processes which envelop each erythroblast and phagocytize defective erythroblasts and extruded nuclei (Fig. 12-5). Since macrophages produce a burst-promoting activity (BPA) capable of stimulating early erythroid stem cells, it is pos-

TABLE 12-1 Stem cell* definition and nomenclature

Pluripotential (totipotential) *(colony-forming unit — lymphoid, hemopoietic = CFU-LH; colony-forming unit — lymphoid, myeloid = CFU-LM):*
    Cells capable of extensive, possibly lifelong, self-renewal and of differentiation to hemopoietic and lymphopoietic progenitor cells.

Multipotential (pluripotential) *(colony-forming unit — spleen = CFU-S; colony-forming unit — neutrophil, erythroid, monocyte, megakaryocyte = CFU-NEMM):*
  Hemopoietic progenitor cells capable of self-renewal and of differentiation to unipotential hemopoietic progenitor cells.
  Lymphopoietic progenitor cells capable of self-renewal and of differentiation to unipotential lymphopoietic progenitor cells.

Bipotential *(colony-forming unit — neutrophil, monocyte = CFU-NM; colony-forming unit — erythroid, mekaryocytic = CFU-EM):*
  Progenitor cells capable of limited self-renewal and of differentiation to two cell lines.

Unipotential *(burst-forming unit — erythroid = BFU-E; colony-forming unit — erythroid = CFU-E; colony-forming unit — neutrophil = CFU-N; colony forming unit — monocyte = CFU-M; colony-forming unit — eosinophil = CFU-Eo; colony-forming unit — basophil = CFU-Baso; colony-forming unit — megakaryocyte = CFU-Meg):*
  Progenitor cells capable of limited self-renewal and of differentiation to one cell line.

Precursor cells
  Cells incapable of self-renewal and morphologically recognizable as members of a single, fully differentiated cell line.

---

*The cells listed are those for which convincing evidence exists. It seems likely that additional types of stem cells will be identified.

sible that these shells of maturing erythroblasts are the end result of a stem cell induced to proliferate by macrophage-released BPA. Megakaryocytes also lie directly outside the vascular wall and discharge platelets through small apertures in the endothelium. Scanning electron microscopic data indicate that cytoplasm peels off the megakaryocyte and enters the sinuses in ribbons, which separate into individual platelets in the vascular lumen [26]. Granulocytes differentiate deeper in the hemopoietic cords, away from the vascular sinuses. When they reach the metamyelocyte stage, they appear to move to the wall of the vascular sinus, cross the wall, and enter the circulation. Lymphocytes and monocytes seem to concentrate about arterial vessels, near the center of the hemopoietic cords.

The cellular interactions associated with the passage of maturing blood cells into the circulation begin with the displacement of the reticular cell cover of the outside surface of the vascular sinus. The blood cells then penetrate the basement membrane and the endothelial cells, and enter the lumen of the vascular sinus [27]. In the case of the red cells, the macrophage of the erythroblastic island promotes preparative extrusion of the right pycnotic nuclei and in addition may interact with the reticular cells and endothelium to facilitate passage. The extent of reticular cell cover appears to depend on

the degree of erythropoietic activity [28]. It has been reported that erythropoietin may act directly on this cover, since after erythropoietin administration the adventitial reticular cells are displaced from the wall before erythroblasts begin to proliferate [29]. The apertures through which the white and red cells pass develop in the endothelial cytoplasm rather than between cells. They probably develop in relation to cell passage and are absent otherwise [30].

The nerve supply to the marrow is extensive and seems to be responsive to intramedullary pressure. These nerves may transmit information to the vessel walls about changes in growth pressure within the hemopoietic compartments. If so, they could adjust the blood flow and cellular release to the rate of cellular proliferation [31].

Function

STEM CELLS

The principal adjustment of blood cell formation is exerted at the level of the stem cells. In the marrow, stem cells constitute a pool of morphologically similar but functionally dissimilar cells capable of both self-renewal and differentiation. They range from pluripotential with an extensive, possibly lifelong capacity for self-renewal to unipotential, committed to a single cell line and with very limited capacity for self-renewal. The latter cells are often called progenitor cells, intermediate between undifferentiated stem cells and differentiated marrow precursor cells. Table 12-1 and Fig. 12-6 outline nomenclature and current concepts of the position of stem cells in the kinetics of blood cell formation.

The earliest marrow stem cell is a pluripotential cell common to both marrow cells and lymphocytes. It has been identified by in vivo and in vitro studies of mice, and it appears to be involved in some leukemias [32]. Normally, however, it probably is dormant throughout life. The next step, the multipotential marrow stem cell, provides cellular backup for stem cell pools committed to either erythroid, granulocytic, or megakaryocytic cell lines. These pools provide offspring of increasing differentiation and responsiveness to specific "poietins" or stimulators until finally they transform into the appropriate blast cell [6] (see Chap. 18).

Morphologically, stem cells of different potentials probably all look alike [33]. Pluripotential stem cells isolated from human blood have been identified as small non-T and non-B lymphocytes [34]. Studies of erythropoietin-stimulated marrow [35] and of hemopoietic colony-forming cells [36] suggest that committed stem cells also resemble small- to medium-sized lymphocytes.

Functionally, stem cells are identified by their capacity to repopulate the marrow after hemopoietic injury and by their ability to grow and differentiate in in vitro cultures. It was known for many years that lethally irradiated mice could be salvaged by marrow transplanta-

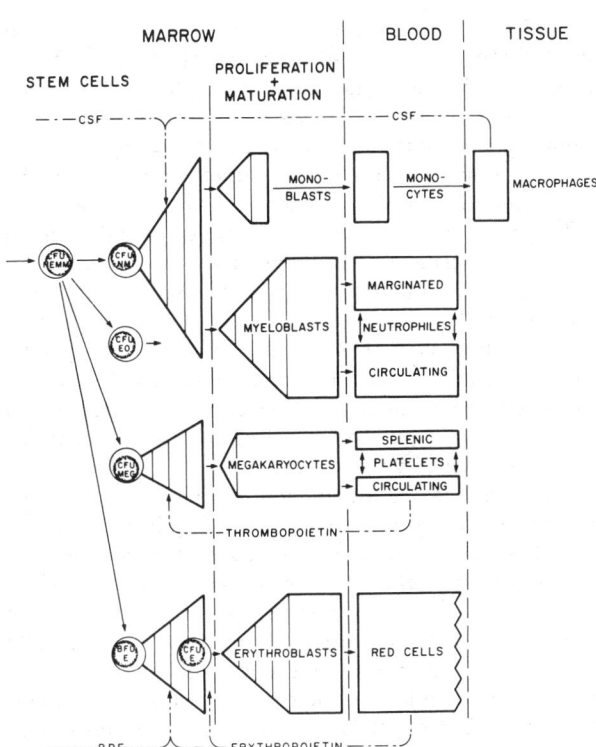

FIGURE 12-6 Schematic outline of marrow cell kinetics. CFU-NEMM = Colony-forming unit—neutrophil, erythroid, monocyte, megakaryocyte (also called CFU-S, or colony-forming unit—spleen); CFU-NM = colony-forming unit—neutrophil, monocyte (also called CFU-C, or colony-forming unit—culture); CFU-EO = colony-forming unit—eosinophil; CFU-MEG = colony-forming unit—megakaryocyte; CFU-E = colony-forming unit—erythroid; BFU-E = burst-forming unit—erythroid; CSF = colony-stimulating factor (also called CSA, or colony-stimulating activity); BPF = burst-promoting factor (also called BPA, or burst-promoting activity).

tion from normal isogenic donors. In 1961, Till and Mc-Cullough [37] discovered distinct colonies of marrow in and on the spleen 7 to 10 days after injecting small numbers of marrow cells into irradiated mice (Fig. 12-7). About half these colonies were composed of erythroid cells alone; the other half were granulocytic, megakaryocytic, or mixed [38,39]. Retransplantation of cells from colonies of a single cell type led to colonies with the same distribution of pure- and mixed-cell populations [40]. Chromosomal studies showed that the colonies were clonal, derived from single cells [36]. It was concluded that the responsible cells were true multipotential stem cells. In the mouse there are about 10 to 30 of these multipotential colony-forming units (CFU-S, S denoting spleen) per 10,000 nucleated marrow cells [41].

The observed kinetics of these cells have provided us with a model of normal cellular development. After the injection of marrow suspension into the irradiated mouse, single stem cells sequestered by the spleen will undergo a number of mitotic divisions and produce minute clonal colonies of undifferentiated stem cells

[42]. After the fifth day they become responsive to various effectors and begin to form pure or mixed marrow colonies. This final differentiation depends on short-range signals from the immediate environment and long-range signals from circulating poietins. Stem cell colonies on the surface of the spleen primarily become erythroid, while stem cell colonies inside the spleen or in the marrow cavity primarily become granulocytic and megakaryocytic. These observations suggest the effect of a hemopoietic-inductive microenvironment (HIM) with a modifying influence of stem cells and their path of differentiation [8,43]. The actual induction and subsequent rate of growth of the erythroid colonies depend on erythropoietin. Erythroid colonies emerge and become large and easy to recognize in the presence of erythropoietin but are hardly visible in its absence [44,45]. Similar dependence on poietins is probably true for granulocytic and megakaryocytic colonies, but so far the effect of their presumed poietins has been difficult to study in vivo.

In vitro studies of marrow cultured in a semisolid medium have confirmed and further elaborated on the differentiation steps observed in spleen colonies. They have disclosed the presence of erythropoietin-dependent differentiation and the growth of erythroid-committed stem cells and colony-stimulating-factor (CSF)–dependent differentiation and growth of granulocytic and monocytic committed stem cells [46]. The initial ac-

FIGURE 12-7 Each white, raised plaque on the surface of these murine spleens represents a splenic marrow colony. They were found 7 to 10 days after the infusion of a suspension of marrow cells into an irradiated isogeneic host, and each colony was derived from the growth and differentiation of a single multipotential stem cell.

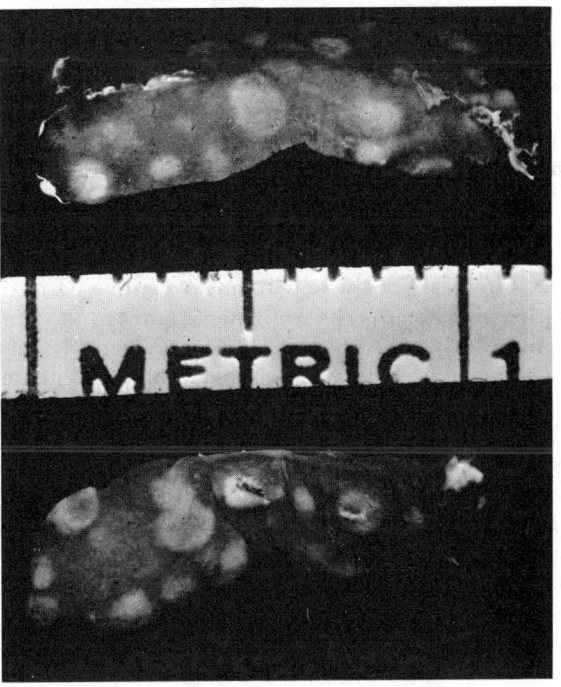

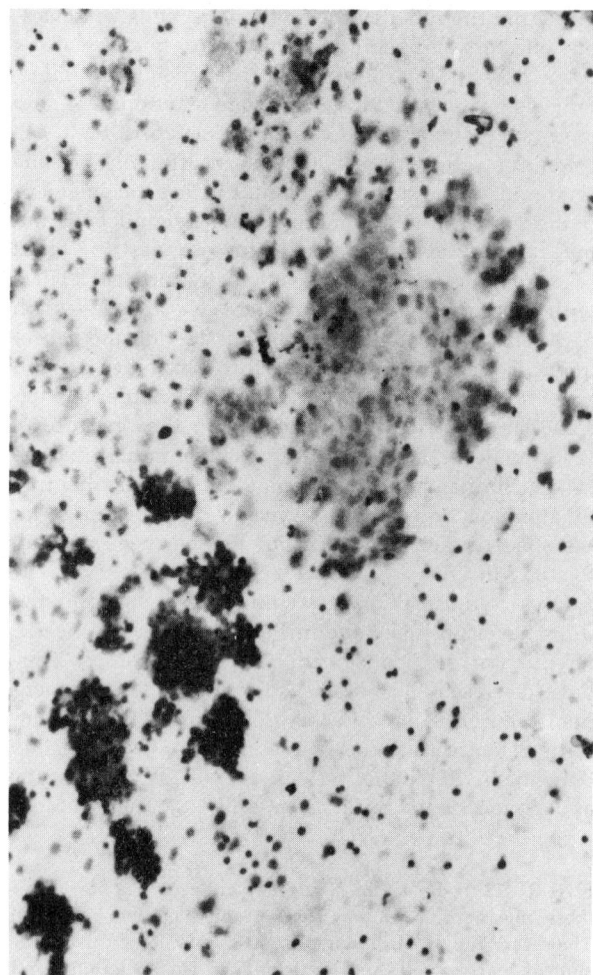

FIGURE 12-8   Growth of one erythroid burst (BFU-E, darkly strained group) and one neutrophil-monocyte colony (CFU-NM, lighter-stained group) on semisolid agar in the presence of both erythropoietin and colony-stimulating activity.

tivation and multiplication of multipotential stem cells can now be studied in a semisolid culture medium. The requirement for an adequate HIM is met by a "stroma" consisting of endothelial cells, macrophages, fat cells, and other tissue cells deposited on the surface of a plastic culture flask. In this environment marrow-derived multipotential stem cells will emerge, grow, and form colonies, and in the presence of erythropoietin or colony-stimulating factors (CSF), they will differentiate into normal marrow elements [47,48].

The turnover of multipotential stem cells must be slow, since injections in vivo or in vitro of tritiated thymidine in lethal concentrations cause only moderate reductions in the number of CFU-S [49]. Consequently, it appears that the committed stem cell pools need only occasional replenishment and that the CFU-S provide a backup triggered into action by signals from the committed stem cells [50,51]. Such signals could be generated by cellular depletion or injury and may be transmitted directly by cell-cell interactions [52]. Although multipotential stem cells have a remarkable capacity for self-renewal and replacement of depleted committed stem cells [53], there appears to be a limit, and after a number of serial transplantations or repeated exposures to destructive radiation or chemotherapeutic agents, the multipotential stem cells become exhausted [54]. This exhaustion may be permanent and suggests either a limit on the capacity for self-renewal or a loss of nonrenewable multipotential stem cells during each regenerative effort.

Committed stem cells and their response to specific poietins are described in detail in Chaps. 38 and 84. Here it will suffice to mention certain features which determine their place in the proliferation and maturation sequence of marrow cells.

The presence of a hierarchy of unipotential stem cells committed to granulocytopoiesis, erythropoiesis, or megakaryocytopoiesis was first suspected as a result of studies of transplanted spleen colonies and first established by studies of in vitro cultures of marrow. The granulocytic colonies which emerge in vitro are usually made up of both neutrophils and monocytes and originate from a single cell, the so-called CFU-C (C for culture) or CFU-NM (N for neutrophils and M for monocytes), which in about 5 to 10 days proliferate into thousands of descendants [55,56] (Fig. 12-8). Since recognizable granulopoietic precursor cells in the marrow divide about 4 to 6 times with an amplification factor of about 30, a number of preceding divisions (about 5 to 6) must have taken place in order for one CFU-C to have produced these thousands of descendants. The addition of radioactive thymidine of high specific activity will kill most of the CFU-C, indicating, not surprisingly, that they are in a very active cell cycle [57]. Initiation of proliferation and maturation is dependent on certain glycoproteins referred to as colony-stimulating factors (CSF). These proteins can functionally be divided into subclasses dependent on their cellular origin and their capacity to support differentiation of CFU-C into granulocytic, monocytic, or mixed colonies [58]. CSF is present in both plasma and urine and has been isolated from lymphocytes, macrophages, and endothelial cells, especially after stimulation by antigens or endotoxin. It actually seems possible that all tissues are capable of releasing such stimulators. It has been suggested that CSF may have two major in vitro actions. One is directed at the proliferation of early committed stem cells, not only those committed to the neutrophilic-monocytic line, but also those committed to the erythroid and megakaryocytic lines [59]. The second action, however, is specific and involves the final differentiation of CFU-C to myeloblasts or monoblasts.

The in vivo role, if any, of these CSF is still not resolved. It seems most unlikely that they would play no part in the complex positive- or negative-feedback systems which control granulocytopoiesis and monocytopoiesis. However, attempts to stimulate granulocytopoiesis in vivo by injecting crude or pure CSF have

TABLE 12-2 Normal differentiated marrow cell kinetics

| | Marrow | | |
Cell type	Number, cells/kg	Transit time, days	Production cells/kg/day
I. Red cells:			
Erythroblasts	5.3×10^9	$\simeq 5.0$	3.0×10^9
Reticulocytes	8.2×10^9	2.8	3.0×10^9
II. Megakaryocytes	15×10^6	$\simeq 7$	2.0×10^6
III. Granulocytes:			
Proliferation pool	2.1×10^9	$\simeq 5.0$	0.85×10^9
Postmitotic pool	5.6×10^9	6.6	0.85×10^9

SOURCE: Finch et al. [69].

not been uniformly successful [60], suggesting that short-range feedback from the microenvironment may be more important than long-range feedback via specific CSF.

Stem cells committed to the erythroid cell line will also grow in vitro but will only differentiate to hemoglobin-containing erythroblasts if erythropoietin is present [61,62]. Within 1 to 2 days of the plating of marrow in erythropoietin-containing semisolid media, small colonies emerge, grow into colonies containing up to 64 erythroblasts, and then disappear. They and their responsible stem cells are called CFU-E. In the presence of large amounts of erythropoietin, new colonies appear some days later and grow into huge macroscopic aggregates of thousands of erythroblasts. Because of their irregular outline with numerous CFU-E subcolonies, they are called bursts and the responsible stem cell is called burst-forming unit—erythroid, or BFU-E (Fig. 12-8).

Although large amounts of erythropoietin initiate the proliferation of BFU-E, this action may be caused by impurities in the preparation rather than by erythropoietin per se. Other substances derived from T lymphocytes or macrophages are effective as burst-promoting activities (BPA) or burst-promoting factors (BPF). They are currently believed to control the early proliferation of committed stem cells, while erythropoietin controls the final differentiation into proerythroblasts [63].

Stem cells committed to megakaryocytes have been identified and their proliferation and differentiation found to be influenced by various stimulating factors, including erythropoietin [64–67]. However, megakaryocytic colonies are rarely pure, and it has been difficult to study their kinetics, especially the effect of thrombopoietic substances isolated from plasma or urine.

PRECURSOR CELLS
After final blast transformation of committed stem cells, the erythroid and granulocytic blast cells undergo three to five mitotic divisions, while the megakaryocytic blast cells divide perhaps once and then undergo three to five endomitotic nuclear divisions (see Fig. 12-6). Concomitant with nuclear proliferation, the cytoplasm begins specific maturation, a process which continues several days beyond the last mitotic division. The erythroblastic nucleus is extruded spontaneously or by mechanical enucleation, and the maturing reticulocytes and granulocytes are ready for release. This release, however, is usually delayed for a number of days and appears to be controlled by releasing factors produced in response to the peripheral needs for blood cells [68]. Since the circulating neutrophil mass is much smaller than the postmitotic marrow pool of maturing neutrophils, this pool serves as an important reserve, and adjustments in its rate of release play a considerable role in the mobilization of neutrophils for defense. The circulating red cell mass, however, is too large to be affected materially by changes in the rate of release of reticulocytes, and adjustments in this release are of questionable functional significance. Adjustments, if any, in the release of platelets are also of unknown functional significance.

Data on the number of differentiated cells in the marrow of humans have been obtained primarily by the study of films and sections relating differential counts of marrow samples to their content of injected radioactive iron. A number of assumptions and approximations have to be made, but the summary data given in Table 12-2 agree well with many other observations on the cellular content and kinetics of normal and abnormal marrows.

References

1. Neuman, E.: Ueber die Bedeutung des Knochenmarks für die Blutbildung. *Cbl. Med. Wiss*, 6:689, 1868.
2. Bizzazero, G.: Sulla fungione ematopoietica del midollo delle ossa. *Gazz. Med. Ital-Lomb.*, vol. 46, 1868.
3. Neuman, E.: Du Role de la möelle des os dans la formation du sang. *C. R. Acad. Sci. (Paris)*, vol. 68, no. 19, 1869.
4. Mosler, F.: Klinische Symptome und Therapie der medullären Leukemi. *Berl. Klin. Woehenschr.* 13:233, 1876.
5. Arinkin, M. J.: Die intravitale Untersuchungsmetodik des Knochenmarks. *Folia Haematol. (Leipz.)* 38:233, 1929.
6. Lajtha, L. G.: The common ancestral cell, in *Blood Pure and Eloquent*, edited by M. M. Wintrobe. McGraw-Hill, New York, 1980, p. 81.
7. Erslev, A. J.: Feedback circuits in the control of stem cell differentiation. *Am. J. Pathol.* 65:629, 1971.
8. Trentin, J. J.: Determination of bone marrow stem cell differentiation by stroma hemopoietic inductive microenvironment (HIM). *Am. J. Pathol.* 65:621, 1971.

9. Hudson, G.: Bone marrow volume in the human foetus and newborn. *Br. J. Haematol. 11:*446, 1965.

10. Rosse, C., Kraemer, M. J., Dillon, T. L., McFarland, R., and Smith, N. J.: Bone marrow cell populations of normal infants: The predominance of lymphocytes. *J. Lab. Clin. Med. 89:*1225, 1977.

11. Custer, R. P., and Ahlfeldt, F. E.: Studies on the structure and function of the bone marrow. *J. Lab. Clin. Med. 17:*960, 1932.

12. Mechanik, N.: Untersuchunge über das Gewicht des Knochenmarks des Menschen. *Z. Ges. Anat. 79:*58, 1926 (summarized by R. E. Ellis, *Phys. Med. Biol. 5:*255, 1961).

13. Gregersen, M. I., and Rawson, R. A.: Blood volume. *Physiol. Rev. 39:*307, 1969.

14. Huggins, C., and Blocksom, B. H., Jr.: Changes in outlying bone marrow accompanying a local increase in temperature within physiologic limits. *J. Exp. Med. 64:*253, 1936.

15. Maniatis, A., Tavassoli, M., and Crosby, W. H.: Factors affecting the conversion of yellow to red marrow. *Blood 37:*581, 1971.

16. Crosby, W. H.: Experience with injured and implanted bone marrow: Relation of function to structure, in *Hemopoietic Cellular Proliferation,* edited by F. Stohlman, Jr. Grune & Stratton, New York, 1970, p. 87.

17. Weiss, L.: The hemopoietic microenvironment of the bone marrow: An ultrastructural study of the stroma in rats. *Anat. Rev. 186:*161, 1976.

18. Lichtman, M. A.: The ultrastructure of the hemopoietic environment of the marrow: A review. *Exp. Hematol. 9:*391, 1981.

19. DeBruyn, P. P. H.: Structural substrates of bone marrow function. *Semin. Hematol. 18:*179, 1981.

20. Brookes, M.: *The Blood Supply of Bone.* Butterworths, London, 1971.

21. Bradley, T. R., Hodgson, G. S., and Rosendaal, M.: The effect of oxygen tension on haemopoietic and fibroblast cell proliferation in vitro. *J. Cell. Physiol. 97:*517, 1978.

22. Bentley, S. A.: Bone marrow connective tissue and the haemopoietic microenvironment. *Br. J. Haematol. 50:*1, 1982.

23. Bathija, A., Davis, S., and Trubowitz, S.: Marrow adipose tissue: Response to erythropoiesis. *Am. J. Hematol. 5:*315, 1978.

24. Bathija, A., Davis, S., and Trubowitz, S.: Bone marrow adipose tissue: Response to acute starvation. *Am. J. Hematol. 6:*191, 1979.

25. Bessis, M.: L'Ilot érythroblastique, unité fonctionelle de la moelle osseuse. *Rev. Hématol. 13:*8, 1958.

26. Lichtman, M. A., et al.: Parasinusoidal location of megakaryocytes in marrow. A determinant of platelet release. *Am. J. Hematol. 4:*303, 1978.

27. Tavassoli, M.: The marrow-blood barrier. *Br. J. Haematol. 41:*297, 1979.

28. Aoki, M., and Tavassoli, M.: Dynamics of red cell egress from bone marrow after blood letting. *Br. J. Haematol. 49:*337, 1981.

29. LeBlond, P. F., Chamberlain, J. K., and Weed, R. I.: Scanning electron microscopy of erythropoietin-stimulated bone marrow. *Blood Cells 1:*639, 1975.

30. Chamberlain, J. K., and Lichtman, M. A.: Marrow cell egress: Specificity of the site of penetration into the sinus. *Blood 52:*959, 1978.

31. Fliedner, T. M., Calvo, W., Haas, R., Forteza, J., and Bohne, F.: Morphologic and cytogenetic aspects of bone marrow stroma, in *Hemopoietic Cellular Proliferation,* edited by F. Stohlman, Jr. Grune & Stratton, New York, 1970, p. 67.

32. Boggs, D. R.: Clonal origin of leukemia: Site of origin in the stem cell hierarchy and the significance of chromosomal changes. *Blood Cells 7:*205, 1981.

33. von Bekkum, D. W., van den Engh, G. J., Wagemaker, G., Bol, S. J. L., and Visser, J. W. M.: Structural identity of the pluripotential hemopoietic stem cell. *Blood Cells 5:*143, 1979.

34. Barr, R. D., and Whang-Peng, J.: Hemopoietic stem cells in human peripheral blood. *Science 190:*284, 1975.

35. Fliedner, T. M., Calvo, W., Haas, R., Forteza, J., and Bohne, F.: Morphologic and cytogentic aspects of bone marrow stroma, in *Hemopoietic Cellular Proliferation,* edited by F. Stohlman, Jr. Grune & Stratton, New York, 1970, p. 67.

36. Moore, M. A. S., Williams, N., and Metcalf, D.: Purification and characterization of the in vitro colony forming cells in monkey hemopoietic tissue. *J. Cell Physiol. 79:*283, 1972.

37. Till, J. E., and McCulloch, E. A.: A direct measurement of the radiation sensitivity of normal mouse bone marrow. *Radiat. Res. 14:*213, 1961.

38. Lewis, J. P., and Trobaugh, F. E., Jr.: Hematopoietic stem cells. *Nature 204:*589, 1964.

39. Curry, J. L., and Trentin, J. J.: Hemopoietic spleen colony studies. I. Growth and differentiation. *Dev. Biol. 15:*395, 1967.

40. Wu, A. M., Till, J. E., Siminovitch, L., and McCulloch, E. A.: A cytological study of the capacity for differentiation of normal hemopoietic colony-forming cells. *J. Cell. Physiol. 69:*177, 1967.

41. Lewis, J. P., Passovoy, M., Freeman, M., and Trobaugh, F. E., Jr.: The repopulation potential and differentiation capacity of hematopoietic stem cells from the blood and bone marrow of normal mice. *J. Cell. Physiol. 71:*121, 1968.

42. Hasthorpe, S., and Hodgson, G.: Proliferation of erythroid and granulocyte progenitors in the spleen as a function of stem cell dose. *Cell. Tissue Kinet. 10:*43, 1977.

43. Wolf, N. S.: Dissecting the hematopoietic microenvironment. Evidence for a positive short range stimulus for cellular proliferation. *Cell. Tissue Kinet. 11:*335, 1978.

44. Till, J. E., Siminovitch, L., and McCulloch, E. A.: The effect of plethora on growth and differentiation of normal hemopoietic colony forming cells transplanted in mice of genotype W/W^v. *Blood 29:*102, 1967.

45. O'Grady, L. F., Lewis, J. P., and Trobaugh, F. E., Jr.: The effect of erythropoietin on differentiated erythroid precursors. *J. Lab. Clin. Med. 71:*693, 1968.

46. Quesenberry, P., and Levitt, L.: Hematopoietic stem cells. *N. Engl. J. Med. 301:*755, 1979.

47. Dexter, T. M., Allen, T. D., and Lajtha, L. G.: Conditions controlling the proliferation of hematopoietic stem cells in vitro. *J. Cell. Physiol. 91:*335, 1977.

48. Hocking, W. G., and Golde, D. W.: Long-term human bone marrow cultures. *Blood 56:*118, 1980.

49. Becker, A. J., McCulloch, E. A., Siminovitch, L., and Till, J. E.: The effect of differing demands for blood cell production on DNA synthesis by hemopoietic colony-forming cells of mice. *Blood 26:*296, 1965.

50. Porteous, D. D., and Lajtha, L. G.: On stem cell recovery after irradiation. *Br. J. Haematol. 12:*177, 1966.

51. Stohlman, F., Jr.: Regulation of red cell production, in *Formation and Destruction of Blood Cells,* edited by T. J. Greenwalt and G. A. Jamieson. Lippincott, Philadelphia, 1970, p. 650.

52. McCulloch, E. A., and Till, J. E.: Cellular interactions in the control of hemopoiesis, in *Hemopoietic Cellular Proliferation,* edited by F. Stohlman, Jr. Grune & Stratton, New York, 1970, p. 15.

53. Harrison, D. E.: Normal function of transplanted marrow cell lines from aged mice. *J. Gerontol. 30:*279, 1975.

54. Hellman, S., Botnick, L. E., Hannon, E. C., and Vigneulle, R. M.: Proliferative capacity of murine hematopoietic stem cells. *Proc. Natl. Acad. Sci. U.S.A. 75:*490, 1978.

55. Bradley, T. R., and Metcalf, D.: The growth of mouse bone marrow cells in vitro. *Aust. J. Exp. Biol. Med. Sci. 44:*287, 1966.

56. Pluznik, D. H., and Sacks, L.: The induction of clones of normal mast cells by a substance from conditioned medium. *Exp. Cell. Res. 43:*553, 1966.

57. Lajtha, L. G., Pozzi, L. V., Schofield, R., and Fox, M.: Kinetic properties of haemopoietic stem cells. *Cell Tissue Kinet. 2:*39, 1969.

58. Burgess, A. W., and Metcalf, D.: The nature and action of granulocyte-macrophage colony stimulating factors. *Blood 56:*947, 1980.

59. Metcalf, D., Johnson, G. R., and Burgess, A. W.: Direct stimulation by purified GM-CSF of the proliferation of multipotential and erythroid precursor cells. *Blood 55:*138, 1980.

60. Metcalf, D., and Stanley, E. R.: Haematological effects in mice of partially purified colony stimulating factor (CSF) prepared from human urine. *Br. J. Haematol. 21:*481, 1971.

61. Stephenson, J. K., Axelrod, A. A., McLeod, D. L., and Shreeve, M. M.: Induction of colonies of hemoglobin-synthesizing cells by erythropoietin in vitro. *Proc. Natl. Acad. Sci. U.S.A. 68:*1542, 1971.

62. Gregory, C. J., and Eaves, A. C.: Human marrow cells capable of erythropoietic differentiation in vitro. Definition of three erythroid colony responses. *Blood 49:*855, 1977.

63. Iscove, N. N.: Erythropoietin-independent stimulation of early erythropoiesis in adult marrow cultures by conditioned media from

lectin-stimulated mouse spleen cells, in *Hematopoietic Cell Differentiation*, edited by D. W. Golde, M. J. Cline, D. Metcalf, and C. F. Fox. Academic, New York, 1978, p. 25.

64. Metcalf, D., MacDonald, H. R., Odartchenko, N., and Sordat, B.: Growth of mouse megakaryocytic colonies in vitro. *Proc. Natl. Acad. Sci. U.S.A.* 72:1744, 1975.

65. Nakoff, A., and Bryan, J. E.: Megakaryocyte proliferation and its regulation as revealed by CFU-M analysis, in *Hematopoietic Cell Differentiation*, edited by D. W. Golde, M. J. Cline, D. Metcalf, and C. F. Fox. Academic, New York, 1978, p. 241.

66. Freedman, M. H., McDonald, T. P., and Saunders, E. F.: Differentiation of murine marrow megakaryocyte progenitors (CFU-M): Humoral control in vitro. *Cell. Tissue Kinet.* 14:53, 1981.

67. Mazur, E. M., Hoffman, R., and Bruno, E.: Regulation of human megakaryocytopoiesis. An in vitro analysis. *J. Clin. Invest.* 68:733, 1981.

68. Lichtman, M. A., Chamberlain, J. K., and Santillo, P. A.: Factors thought to contribute to the regulation of egress of cells from marrow, in *The Year in Hematology*, Plenum, New York, 1978, p. 243.

69. Finch, C. A., Harker, L. A., and Cook, J. D.: Kinetics of the formed elements of human blood. *Blood* 50:699, 1977.

CHAPTER *13*

Structure and function of the lymphoid tissues

W. STEPHEN NICHOLS, Jr.
FRANCIS V. CHISARI

The immune system, which defends against foreign pathogens with cells of the lymphoid series, displays the following characteristics:

It discriminates between self and foreign antigens, which may be in soluble form or bound to microbial agents or cells. Foreign antigens may gain access to the body through contact, invasion, ingestion, or inhalation. Host cells may be targets of immune reactivity if they are altered by disease, trauma, or mutation to appear foreign (altered self). This alteration can lead to autoimmune destruction of the cells bearing altered self antigens.

It maintains responsiveness to foreign antigens throughout life by the generation of immunologic diversity. This diversity is maintained even in the absence of exposure to antigen.

It remembers previous antigenic exposure and mounts an accelerated and heightened (anamnestic) response to a second encounter with antigen.

It monitors antigens throughout the body and mobilizes an appropriate local or systemic response.

The lymphoid tissues are primarily concerned with host defense. At the cellular level they consist of a complex assortment of lymphocytes and phagocytic cells whose functional activities are orchestrated to produce a coordinated protective response to foreign pathogens.

The lymphocytes confer exquisite antigenic specificity to the response and also express several important effector functions in classical humoral and cell-mediated immunity. Lymphocyte subsets also display several nonspecific effector functions and regulate the immune system so that normal responses occur.

The phagocytic cells of the monocyte-macrophage series serve a primitive scavenger function and also cooperate with the lymphocytes in immune responsiveness, such as antigen presentation and lymphocyte activation and proliferation. Macrophages under the influence of immunoglobulins and other soluble products of lymphocytes (lymphokines) function as a major effector limb of the immune response.

The lymphoid tissues consist of fixed and circulating elements. The fixed lymphoid cells include the lymphocytes; the monocyte-macrophage system of the marrow, thymus, spleen, and lymph nodes; and the lymphoid and phagocytic cells found in the submucosa of the gastrointestinal tract (Peyer's patches), respiratory tract, and liver (Kupffer cells). The circulating lymphoid cells are the lymphocytes and cells of the monocyte-macrophage series present in the blood, and a dynamic equilibrium exists between the fixed and circulating compartments that facilitates the delivery of organ-specific maturational influences (e.g., thymosin) on the circulating cells, permits rapid and localized responsiveness to anatomically segregated antigens, and fosters communication and integration of functionally diverse responses to an antigenic stimulus.

Characteristics of lymphocytes and macrophages

The initiation and coordination of the immune response is mediated by surface-membrane receptors on the cells of the lymphoid system [1]. Receptors for nonself (i.e., antigen) are essential for recognition, activation, and cell-cell communication. Receptors for self (histocompatibility antigens) are also important in the immune response [2].

Other receptors important in the immune response can differentiate cellular subsets within the lymphoid system [3,4]. For example, B lymphocytes possess surface-membrane IgM and IgD, receptors for the Fc region of IgG and other immunoglobulin classes, and several complement components and activation products. B lymphocytes are the antibody-forming cells of the lymphoid system and develop in or under the influence of the bursa of Fabricius in birds and the bursa equivalent (e.g., marrow) in mammals [5].

T lymphocytes, the primary effectors of cell-mediated

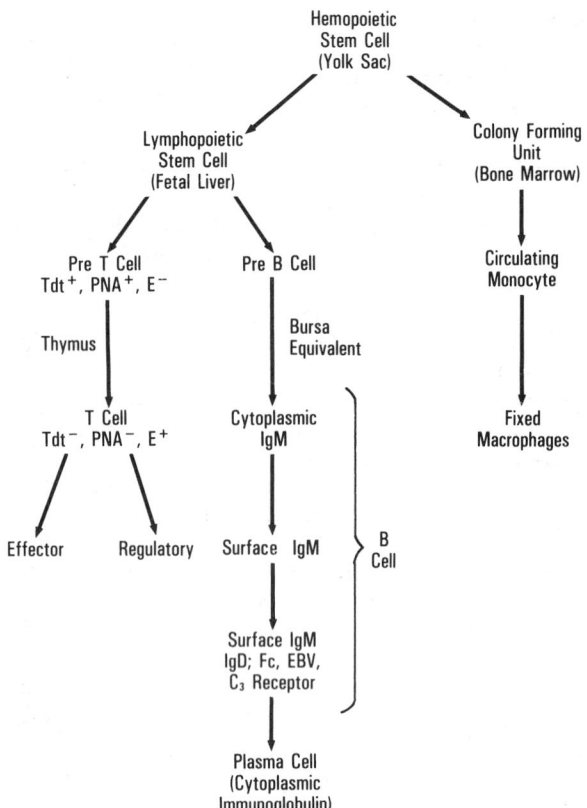

FIGURE 13-1 Ontogeny of mononuclear cells of the lymphoid system. Tdt = terminal deoxynucleotidyl transferase; PNA = peanut agglutinin; E = sheep red blood cell receptor; EBV = Epstein-Barr virus receptor.

immunity and immunoregulation, arise in all species under the influence of the thymus [5]. Individual T-cell subsets have surface-membrane receptors for the Fc region of IgG (Tγ cells) and IgM (Tµ cells) and function as suppressors and helpers of the immune response, respectively [6]. T cells also express surface-membrane receptors for sheep erythrocytes and are commonly identified by their ability to bind and form rosettes (E rosettes) with these cells. E-rosette formation can occur as a high-affinity process (at 37°C) and as a low-affinity process (at 4°C), and different lymphocyte subsets that are physically separable and morphologically distinct are responsible for these two phenomena. Although the precise role of this receptor is unclear, a number of reports describing T-cell activation as a consequence of E-rosette formation have been published. Monoclonal antibodies specific for many of the T-lymphocyte subsets have been developed [7]. A detailed discussion of these antibodies and the other T-cell markers is found in Chaps. 105 and 106.

A separate subset of cells that lacks the B-cell markers (membrane-bound immunoglobulin) and T-cell markers (high-affinity E-rosette formation), referred to as *null cells,* is thought to be responsible for two distinct forms of cell-mediated cytotoxicity, natural killer cell function (N-K cells) and antibody-dependent cellular cytotoxicity (K cells), which are discussed in Chap. 105. These cells are not strictly null, since they bear surface-membrane receptors for the Fc region of IgG [8] and form low-affinity rosettes with sheep erythrocytes [9]. Although they have a similar surface-membrane phenotype as Tγ cells, they do not function as T-suppressor cells, from which they are separable by their affinity for sheep erythrocytes. These cells also are larger and more granular (large granular lymphocytes) than classic Tγ cells [10]. For these reasons there is controversy over their classification. Nonetheless, they constitute a distinct subset on the basis of functional, morphologic, and surface-membrane characteristics.

Cells of the monocyte-macrophage series also display surface-membrane Fc and complement receptors [3]. Additionally, they have a high affinity for glass and plastic surfaces (adherence) and, by definition, are phagocytic.

Generally, multiple marker systems are employed for enumeration of lymphocyte subpopulations, and systems employing phagocytosis or adherence are used to separate monocytes from other mononuclear cells. About 75 percent of normal blood lymphocytes are T cells, about 10 percent are B cells, and 15 percent are null cells that lack classical T or B markers. The distinguishing characteristics of cell subsets are discussed in detail in Chap. 105.

Ontogeny of the mononuclear cells of the lymphoid system

Lymphocyte markers have permitted delineation of the development (ontogeny) of the mononuclear cells of the lymphoid system (see Chap. 106). The major lymphocyte classes and cells of the monocyte-macrophage series originate from stem cells [5] found in hemopoietic tissue, including the blood islands of the yolk sac, the fetal liver and spleen, and the marrow (Fig. 13-1). A common lymphopoietic stem cell gives rise to daughter cells which develop, subsequently, along B- or T-cell lines. T-lymphocyte progenitors migrate to the thymus, where they undergo a series of differentiation steps under the influence of hormone-like substances such as thymopoietin, a polypeptide that is produced by thymic epithelial cells [11]. Within the thymus, immature (pre-T) cells are found in the thymic cortex and contain terminal deoxynucleotidyl transferase (Tdt) and receptors for peanut agglutinin [13], but they lack receptors for sheep red blood cells. As they proliferate and differentiate, the pre-T cells move into the thymic medulla, where they lose Tdt and peanut agglutinin receptors and gain receptors for sheep red blood cells. Within the thymus, T lymphocytes develop the ability to recognize antigen through an interaction with self-antigens expressed on thymic epithelial cells or thymic macrophages. Following intrathymic development, thymocytes migrate to peripheral lymphoid tissues, where they undergo additional differentiation and are found in the white pulp of the spleen, paracortex of the lymph nodes, and the interfollicular areas of gastrointestinal lymphoid tissues, as well as in the lymph and blood.

The pre-B cell originates in the fetal liver and migrates to the bursa of Fabricius in birds and to a bursa equivalent in mammals. The bursa equivalent is thought to be the marrow in humans, although this is not yet established. Within the bursa or its equivalent, the B cell undergoes an orderly sequence of differentiation and development. The earliest stage is represented by cells containing cytoplasmic IgM but lacking membrane immunoglobulin. This cell differentiates within the bursa equivalent and loses cytoplasmic IgM while acquiring surface-membrane IgM. At this point the B cell lacks surface-membrane IgD, complement receptors, Fc receptors, or Ia antigens. This primitive lymphocyte with surface-membrane IgM is the precursor of the entire pool of B cells containing surface-membrane immunoglobulins of the other heavy-chain classes, indicating that a switch in the class of immunoglobulin expressed on an individual cell must occur during development [14]. With further development, surface-membrane IgD is acquired [15]. This immunoglobulin is found on a great majority of adult B cells and is thought to function as a membrane receptor. Following activation, adult B cells lose membrane IgD and differentiate into plasma cells containing cytoplasmic but lacking surface-membrane immunoglobulin. Prior to plasma cell differentiation, the adult B cell expresses surface-membrane Fc receptors, C3 receptors, and receptors for the Epstein-Barr virus (EBV) [16]. Throughout development, pre-B cells and B cells alike express Ia antigens, unlike the T cell, which acquires these antigens only when activated [17]. Ia antigens, products of the immune response (Ir) genes or closely related genes in the major histocompatibility complex, are two-chain glycoproteins which play a critical role in the regulation of the immune response. They are present as surface markers on B lymphocytes, macrophages, null cells, and activated T cells and are also structural components on antigen-specific helper and suppressor factors derived from T cells.

Cells of the monocyte-macrophage series derive from hemopoietic stem cells but differentiate along a different pathway from the lymphocytes. The monocyte-macrophage precursor develops in the marrow. Its progeny circulate as blood monocytes, where they acquire receptors for certain complement components and the Fc region of IgG [18]. The circulating monocyte is considered an immature precursor of the fixed-tissue macrophage, which also expresses Ia antigens on its membrane.

The structures and function of marrow and spleen are discussed in Chaps. 12 and 14. Here the distribution and organization of cells in their other lymphoid organs, viz., thymus, lymph nodes, and accessory tissues, will be considered [19].

The thymus

The thymus develops at about the eighth week of gestation. It arises from the third and fourth branchial pouches as an epithelial organ populated by lymphoid cells, the thymocytes. The thymus is a bilobed organ which increases in size through fetal and postnatal life until puberty, when it weighs about 40 g. In adulthood the thymus steadily involutes and becomes frankly atrophic in old age.

The thymus is divided into cortical and medullary structures with a lobular architecture formed by capsular septations (Fig. 13-2). The cortex of the thymus consists of small and medium-sized thymocytes, epithelial cells, and macrophages. The thymocytes are predominant in number, are densely packed, and appear as lymphocytes of slightly variable size with scattered, rare mitoses. The epithelial cells are stellate, reveal interepithelial desmosomal connections, and appear to adhere to thymocytes at times, while macrophages are primarily located near the corticomedullary junction. Thymic epithelium is thought to play a role in inducing maturation of thymocytes within the cortex, the site of thymic differentiation. Progressive differentiation of precursor cells to T cells takes place, the cells then moving to the medulla and finally migrating to other lymphoid organs through the blood.

The medulla of the thymus forms the central core of the organ, and it extends into each lobular cortical division. The medulla of the thymus contains loosely arranged mature thymocytes and epithelial cells and rather characteristic small corpuscular bodies composed of partially degenerated, concentric, squamous-appearing epithelial cells called *Hassall's corpuscles*, which are of no known functional significance.

FIGURE 13-2 **Structure of the thymus. Immature thymocytes populate the cortex, maturing toward the medullary region. Abbreviations are those used in Fig. 13-1. (Modified from L. Weiss,** *The Cells and Tissues of the Immune System: Structures, Functions, Interactions.* **Prentice-Hall, Englewood Cliffs, N.J., 1972.)**

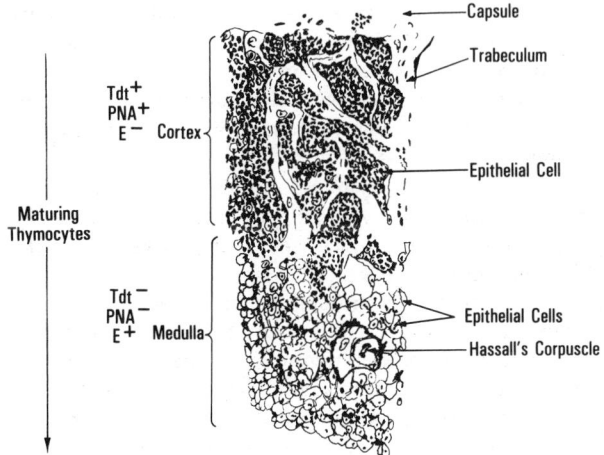

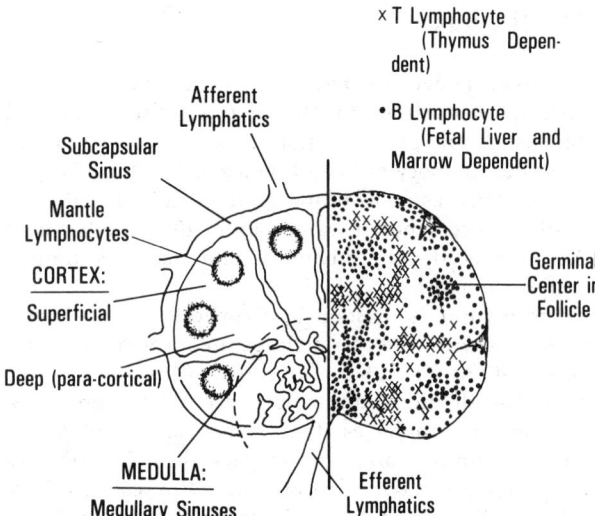

FIGURE 13-3 Structure of the lymph node. T and B indicate areas rich in T and B lymphocytes. (Modified from J. W. Alexander and R. Good, *Fundamentals of Clinical Immunology.* Saunders, Philadelphia, 1977.)

Capillary blood vessels are present in the thymic cortex and medulla. Vessels of the cortex appear relatively impermeable to plasma proteins when compared with medullary vessels, perhaps serving to isolate maturing thymocytes from influences exterior to the thymus.

Prothymocytes originate in the marrow and migrate to the thymus, where maturation occurs. Maturation can be followed because of the sequential acquisition by thymocytes of the various cell markers unique to the T-cell lineage. The so-called theta, or Thy-1, antigen appears on immature as well as mature mouse thymocytes [20]. Tdt adds nucleotides to single-stranded DNA without requiring a template. It is found in prothymocytes and immature thymocytes, but it is absent in mature T cells [12]. Tdt is found in certain neoplastic lymphoid cells, such as those of acute lymphoblastic leukemia, thus allowing classification of such diseases as thymic-derived.

Interestingly, thymic extracts are capable of inducing the appearance of thymic markers among marrow cells in culture. The differentiation of thymocytes, therefore, has been suggested to be under partial control of hormonal influences, such as thymopoietin and thymosin, as mentioned above.

With aging, the thymus becomes atrophic, with the disappearance of thymocytic populations and finally with fatty involution. However, it is likely that the thymus retains a degree of function throughout life.

The thymus in some species has already conferred maturation of the T component by birth, and subsequent removal of the thymus may have little effect. However, certain animals require the presence of an intact thymus for up to several days following birth for maturation of the T-lymphocyte system. Removal of the thymus at birth in these animals results in a profound

defect in cell-mediated immunity. Animals undergoing neonatal thymectomy may become chronically infected and either fail to thrive or undergo physical runting. Thymic hypoplasia or aplasia in humans results in DiGeorge's syndrome, with T-cell deficiency and often lethal infection early in life. Prolonged survival following thymic transplantation and subsequent T-cell reconstitution has been reported.

Lymph nodes

Lymph nodes (Fig. 13-3) are encapsulated, dense collections of lymphocytes, plasma cells, and macrophages organized along the course of large blood vessels throughout several regions of the body, including the abdomen, axilla, inguinal area, and neck. The capsule of the lymph node is perforated by afferent lymphatic channels that drain lymph from regional tissues. The lymph node, in turn, empties into efferent lymphatic vessels which eventually drain into larger lymphatic channels such as the thoracic duct.

Lymphocytes within the lymph node are partially organized by fibrous trabeculae that extend from the capsule. Numerous cortical follicles consist of dense numbers of lymphocytes situated between trabeculae. The capsule and trabeculae serve as a scaffolding for lymphatic spaces, the subcapsular and cortical sinuses, which are continuous with medullary sinuses and the efferent lymphatics. Arterial and venous structures, including a rich network of postcapillary venules, complete the chief architectural components of the lymph nodes.

Lymphoid follicles are nodules predominantly of small B lymphocytes. Each follicle contains a central zone of proliferating cells called a *germinal center*, a pale area when viewed histologically. Germinal centers contain large lymphocytes and macrophages with abundant cytoplasm. Surrounding the lymphoid follicles of the superficial cortex are sheets of lymphocytes that extend to the deep cortex, the so-called paracortex, and then blend into medullary cords of cells.

The paracortex is formed mostly of T lymphocytes, with a ratio of T cells to B cells of about 3:1. The medulla, however, contains mostly B cells and macrophages. Superficial cortex and medulla of the lymph nodes are thus rich in B cells, the thymic-independent areas, while the deep cortex is enriched with T cells, the thymic-dependent area. Thymic aplasia results in depletion of the deep cortex, while a nearly normal component of B cells remains within the superficial cortex. The major T-cell population found within the lymph node consists of helper T cells [21]. The location of the T cells in the paracortical area indicates that T cells in the lymph node play a primary role in the induction of B-cell responses.

During antigen stimulation of lymph nodes, the follicles enlarge and the germinal centers become prominent. Antigens entering the lymph node are first trapped by macrophages in the sinuses and in the deep cortex. Subsequently, lymphocytes recognize and interact with partially degraded macrophage-entrapped antigen. Antibody first forms among B cells by B-cell interaction with T cells and macrophages adjacent to follicles. When an immune response has previously occurred, antigen may also be entrapped within the superficial cortex, there to be bound within stimulated germinal centers by specialized dendritic, reticular macrophages in the form of antigen-antibody complexes. No definite role has been attributed to this latter process, although immunologic memory may arise or be enhanced by similar processes.

Lymphocytes present within the follicular B region display convoluted nuclei and may be identified by their surface-membrane IgM or IgD receptors, which are detectable by immunofluorescence microscopy. B lymphocytes outside the follicular areas generally contain nonconvoluted nuclei and may display only faint surface-membrane immunoglobulin.

Large numbers of T lymphocytes circulate between the blood and the lymph nodes [22]. Lymphocytes primarily enter the lymph nodes through the blood by means of the postcapillary venules near the follicles, eventually reentering the blood through the efferent lymphatics. Following the entrance of antigen into the lymph node, there is a decrease in numbers of lymphocytes in efferent lymphatics. Within days, the lymphocytes proliferate and increased numbers of cells exit the lymph node. The T lymphocytes are primed to recognize and destroy antigen and become dispersed throughout the blood and tissues. The B lymphocytes differentiate into plasma cells that produce antigen-specific antibody. The plasma cells are prominent in follicles but eventually reach the superficial and deep cortical areas of the nodes as well as the medullary cords.

Spleen

The role of the spleen is similar to that of the lymph node, which is to clear antigen from the blood. The splenic architecture is also parallel to that of the lymph node, consisting of a white pulp composed of lymphoid tissues that surrounds vessels called *penicilliary arterioles* and a red pulp that contains red blood cells and sinuses. The red and white pulps are rich in phagocytes. Thymic-dependent lymphocytes of the white pulp surround the blood vessels in a periarteriolar sheath. The thymic-independent areas comprised of B cells are the follicular areas with germinal activities located adjacent to the bifurcation of the penicilliary arterioles. Plasma cells are found surrounding the white pulp. The spleen is discussed in detail in Chap. 14.

Accessory lymphoid tissues

Solitary lymph nodules with follicular and germinal center structures occur in the mucosa and submucosa of the respiratory tract, the gastrointestinal tract (particularly within the ileum), the urinary tract, and the vagina.

During states of chronic inflammation, lymphoid nodules with marked follicular activity may form as a localized center of lymphoid function. Waldeyer's ring of pharyngeal lymphoid tissues and Peyer's patches in the ileum contain prominent aggregated nodular lymphoid tissue. These accessory lymphoid organs differ from the thymus, lymph nodes, and spleen by the lack of a capsule separating the lymphoid tissue from the surrounding tissues. No efferent or afferent lymphatic vessels are present in the accessory lymphoid tissues.

Peyer's patches found in the lamina propria of the small intestine (beneath the mucosa near the ileocolonic junction) consist of up to 50 or more lymphoid nodules, which may be covered by a single layer of columnar epithelium. They are well developed in youth and regress with age. Peyer's patches and the genitourinary and respiratory lymphoid nodules are involved in the immune response to local mucosal assault by antigen related to microorganisms and other foreign substances. In the lung, lymphoid tissue actually increases with age and is infiltrated with trapped, inspissated particulate matter such as anthracotic particles.

Respiratory and gastrointestinal mucosal tissues are rich in plasma cells and eosinophils [23]. The plasma cells are a source of secretory immunoglobulin which is transferred into the lumina of the bronchi and gastrointestinal tract. The majority of plasma cells in the mucosa of the bronchi and gut contain IgA. IgA is released from the plasma cell and then combined with a secretory piece most likely synthesized within the mucosal epithelium. IgA is secreted across the microvilli of mucosal epithelium and prevents pathogenic colonization of mucosal membranes. Lymphoid nodules along mucosa-lined tracts serve as precursors of IgA-producing cells, and the lymphoid nodules act to preserve integrity against many microorganisms and antigens. Microfolds overlying specialized epithelial cells in the gut transport antigenic material by pinocytosis with subsequent immunization and IgA secretion.

The function of accessory lymphoid tissue is exemplified by examination of the lung and liver. The lung is exposed to up to 10,000 liters of air every 24 h, and this air contains a large number of particles. Protective immunity through an active lymphoid system within the lung results in IgA secretion. However, the lung appears to be capable of localized immunologic reaction by cell- as well as antibody-mediated mechanisms. Lung damage occurs secondary to immunologic reaction *in situ*. Some cases of asthma and pneumonia, for instance, result in severe respiratory damage. One of the interesting findings in respiratory sarcoidosis, a chronic granulomatous inflammatory disease of unknown etiology, is the presence of numerous activated T lymphocytes within alveolar structures [24]. In contrast, normal lung tissue contains mostly large numbers of alveolar macrophages. The mechanisms for sensitization and activation of lymphoid cells in the lung have stimulated interest in the pathogenesis of hypersensitivity-type disease of the lung.

Alveolar macrophages reside within the lung and,

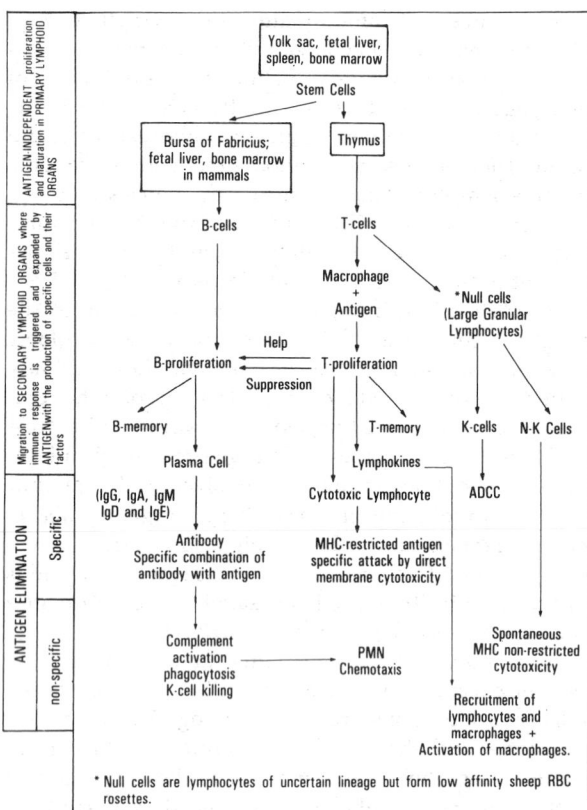

FIGURE 13-4 Components of the immune response. ADCC = antibody-dependent cell-mediated cytotoxicity; K = killer; NK = natural killer; MHC = major histocompatibility complex; PMN = polymorphonuclear leukocyte. (Modified from W. G. Reeves and E. J. Holborow, General introduction, in *Immunology in Medicine: A Comprehensive Guide to Clinical Immunology*, edited by W. G. Reeves and E. J. Holborow. Grune & Stratton, New York, 1977.)

like the Kupffer cells of the liver sinusoids, offer large reservoirs of macrophages for processing antigen. Most recently, macrophage binding and phagocytosis of antigen-antibody immune complexes have been found to be abnormal in the liver [25] and spleen [26] in mice and humans, respectively, in autoimmune diseases.

The tonsils are covered by variable epithelial surfaces, depending on the location of the tissue, with deep, branching depressions, the crypts. Fused lymphatic nodules lie adjacent to the crypts, and germinal centers are prominent. A pseudocapsule of condensed connective tissue surrounds the tonsils, and septae within the structures form lobulations. Lymphocytic and plasma-cell infiltration of overlying epithelium and crypts is present.

The immune response—a brief overview

The immune response to foreign antigens is a highly developed and coordinated series of cellular interactions among macrophages, lymphocytes, and, by their

soluble products, inflammatory cells that contain lysosomal enzymes and other phlogogenic molecules (Fig. 13-4). Control of the immune response is effected by a complex series of interactions between inducer, regulatory, and effector cells within the lymphoid system.

The immune response is initiated by a process involving nonspecific, nonsaturable binding of immunogens by macrophages and presentation of the macrophage-bound immunogen to antigen-reactive T cells. The cellular cooperation involved in antigen presentation requires that the T cell recognize and interact with macrophage surface-membrane proteins encoded by the major histocompatibility complex (MHC). The necessity for the presence of the MHC antigen in cell-cell interaction is known as *MHC restriction*.

The interaction of immunogen-presenting macrophages with antigen-reactive T cells stimulates the latter to differentiate into cells with either regulatory or effector capabilities [27,28]. Regulatory T cells interact with MHC determinants on B cells and effector T cells to produce a coordinated humoral and cellular immune response to the initiating antigen [29]. Such regulatory systems are also important for the development of immunologic tolerance [30]. Defective immunoregulation is thought to play an important role in the development of autoimmune diseases, immunodeficiency states, and perhaps lymphoproliferative disorders.

The expansion of specific immunologic responsiveness is antigen-dependent. The second exposure to antigen leads to augmented activation of immune effector systems by T- and B-cell memory, resulting in specific antigen elimination [7]. In the delayed-type response (T-cell mediated), cytotoxic killer lymphocytes direct a specific attack at the level of cell membranes. Lymphokines, the chemical mediators of cellular immunity, recruit lymphocytes and activate macrophages for augmentation of response. The antibody response [31] is carried out partly through complement activation [32], opsonization, and antibody-dependent cell-mediated cytotoxicity by K cells. Polymorphonuclear leukocytes (PMNs) may be attracted to the site of reaction through chemotactic phenomena that serve to heighten the local inflammatory response.

The integration of all these functions into a coherent, directed immune response results in protection of the host against pathogens (nonself) and preservation of somatic integrity in the form of immunologic tolerance to self-antigen.

References

1. Katz, D. H.: *Lymphocyte Differentiation, Recognition, and Regulation.* Academic, New York, 1977.
2. Zinkernagel, R. M., and Doherty, P. C.: MHC-restricted cytotoxic T cells: Studies on the biological role of polymorphic major transplantation antigens determining T cell restriction-specificity, function, and responsiveness. *Adv. Immunol.* 27:52, 1979.
3. Aisenberg, A. C.: Current concepts in immunology: Cell surface markers in lymphoproliferative disease. *N. Engl. J. Med.* 304:331, 1981.

4. McKenzie, I. F. C., and Potter, T.: Murine lymphocyte surface antigens. *Adv. Immunol.* 27:179, 1979.
5. Stites, D. P., Caldwell, J., Carr, M. C., and Fudenberg, H. H.: Ontogeny of immunity in humans. *Clin. Immunol. Immunopathol.* 4:519, 1975.
6. Moretta, L., Webb, S. R., Grossi, C. E., Lydyard, P. M., and Cooper, M. D.: Functional analyses of human T cell subpopulations: Help and suppression of B cell responses by T cells bearing receptors for IgM or IgG. *J. Exp. Med.* 146:184, 1977.
7. Reinherz, E. L., Kung, P. C., Goldstein, G., Levy, R. H., and Schlossman, S. F.: Discreet stages of human intrathymic differentiation analysis of normal thymocytes and leukemic lymphoblasts of T-cell lineage. *Proc. Natl. Acad. Sci. U.S.A.* 77:1588, 1980.
8. Lobo, P., Westervett, F. B., and Horwitz, D. A.: Identification of two populations of immunoglobulin bearing lymphocytes in man. *J. Immunol.* 114:116, 1975.
9. West, W. H., Boozer, R. B., and Heberman, R. B.: Low affinity E-rosette formation by the human K cell. *J. Immunol.* 120:90, 1978.
10. Timonen, T., Ortaldo, J. R., and Heberman, R. B.: Characteristics of human large granular lymphocytes and relationship to natural killer and K cells. *J. Exp. Med.* 153:569, 1981.
11. Goldstein, C. S.: Serologic and genetic aspects of murine Ia antigens. *Transplant. Rev.* 30:299, 1976.
12. Bollum, F. J.: Terminal deoxynucleotidyl transferase: A hematopoietic cell marker. *Blood* 54:1203, 1979.
13. Raisner, Y., Biniaminor, M., and Rosenthal, E.: Interaction of peanut agglutinin with normal human lymphocytes and leukemic cells. *Proc. Natl. Acad. Sci. U.S.A.* 76:447, 1979.
14. Lawton, A. R., and Cooper, M. D.: Modification of B lymphocyte differentiation by anti-immunoglobulins. *Contemp. Top. Immunobiol.* 3:193, 1974.
15. Vitetta, E. S., and Uhr, J. W.: IgD and B cell differentiation. *Immunol. Rev.* 37:50, 1978.
16. Greaves, M. F., Brown, G., and Rickinson, A: Receptors for Epstein-Barr virus on human B lymphocytes. *Clin. Immunol. Immunopathol.* 3:514, 1975.
17. David, C. S.: Serologic and genetic aspects of murine Ia antigens. *Transplant. Rev.* 30:299, 1976.
18. Zuckerman, S. H., and Douglas, S. D.: Dynamics of the macrophage plasma membrane. *Ann. Rev. Microbiol.* 33:267, 1979.
19. Douglas, S. D., and Ackerman, S. K.: Anatomy of the immune system. *Clin. Hematol.* 6:299, 1977.
20. Cantor, H., and Boyse, E. A.: Lymphocytes as models for the study of cellular differentiation. *Immunol. Rev.* 33:105, 1977.
21. Poppema, S., Bhan, A. K., Reinherz, E. C., McCluskey, R. T., and Schlossman, S. F.: Distribution of T cell subsets in human lymph nodes. *J. Exp. Med.* 153:30, 1981.
22. Ford, W. L.: Lymphocyte migration and immune responses. *Prog. Allergy* 19:1, 1975.
23. Tomasi, T. B., Larson, L., Challacombe, S., and McNabb, P.: Mucosal immunity: The origin and migration patterns of cells in the secretory system. *J. Allergy Clin. Immunol.* 65:12, 1980.
24. Crystal, R. G., et al.: Pulmonary sarcoidosis: A disease characterized and perpetuated by activated lung T lymphocytes. *Ann. Intern. Med.* 94:73, 1981.
25. Magilavy, D. B., Rifai, A., and Plotz, P. H.: An abnormality of immune complex kinetics in murine lupus. *J. Immunol.* 126:770, 1981.
26. Frank, M. M., Hamburger, M. I., Lawley, T. J., Kimberly, R. P., and Plotz, P. H.: Defective reticuloendothelial system Fc-receptor function in systemic lupus erythematosus. *N. Engl. J. Med.* 300:518, 1979.
27. Rosenthal, A. S.: Regulation of the immune response—Role of the macrophage. *N. Engl. J. Med.* 303:1153, 1980.
28. Rosenthal, A. S.: Determinant selection and macrophage function in genetic control of the immune response. *Immunol. Rev.* 40:136, 1978.
29. Cantor, H., and Boyse, E. A.: Regulation of the immune response by T-cell subclasses. *Contemp. Top. Immunobiol.* 7:47, 1977.
30. Talal, N.: Autoimmunity and the immunologic network. *Arthritis Rheum.* 21:853, 1978.
31. Spiegelberg, H. L.: Biological activities of immunoglobulins of different classes and subclasses. *Adv. Immunol.* 19:259, 1974.
32. Müller-Eberhard, H. J.: Complement. *Ann. Rev. Biochem.* 44:697, 1975.

CHAPTER 14

Structure and functions of the spleen

WILLIAM H. CROSBY

The spleen is a fascinating organ with a 2000-year history of being the source of the "black bile" and all its sinister implications for body and mind [1]. Although this mystic effect has made a mark on our linguistic legacy, the spleen itself has been found to be an expendable organ that functions primarily as a line filter in the portal circulation. It removes particulate material from the blood and gives to the blood some cells and proteins. It is an extremely vascular organ with several specialized vascular structures essential to its function. Blood flow through the normal spleen is about 300 ml/min, and the spleen, when drained of blood after splenectomy, weighs about 80 g [2]. Thus the spleen makes up about 0.1 percent of the total body weight (80/70,000) but receives about 6 percent of the cardiac output (300/5000). In 2000 persons who suffered violent deaths, the average postmortem splenic weight was about 135 g [3]. The weight of apparently normal spleens was as low as 100 and as high as 250 g. Obviously, the term *normal* may be subject to considerable latitude of interpretation in the case of the spleen. The adult human spleen contains about 140 billion cells, somewhat less than half of which are capable of phagocytosis. Increased requirement for phagocytosis, as in hereditary spherocytosis, results in enlargement of the spleen, with the cell content increasing about eightfold [4].

Structure of the spleen

THE VASCULATURE

The fibrous capsule of the spleen projects trabeculae into the parenchyma, providing a scaffolding along which the arteries and veins penetrate from the hilus. Smaller arteries emerge from the trabeculae surrounded by a lymphatic sheath. Branches from these "central arteries" take off at almost right angles, consistent with a plasma-skimming function. It is characteristic of the splenic circulation that the arteries emerging from the sheath do not terminate in capillaries connecting to veins. Anatomically, they are open-ended, indicating that blood is dumped into the splenic cords. The venous system collects the blood from these cords through splenic sinusoids into larger veins and thence to the hilus via the trabecular scaffold. "Skimmed" plasma returns to the circulation via lymphatics which also exit along the trabeculae [5] (Fig. 14-1).

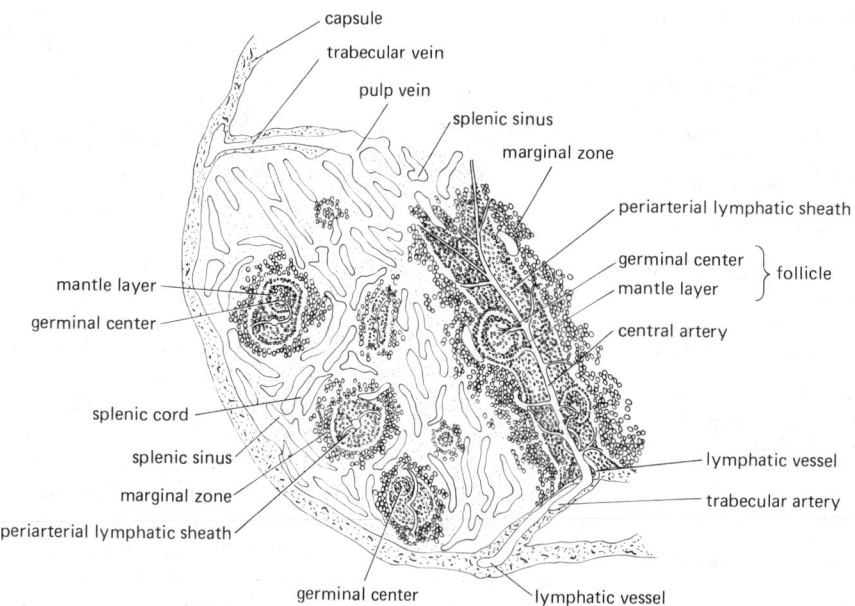

FIGURE 14-1   **The structure of the spleen. White pulp is composed of the periarterial lymphatic sheath (PLS) and the germinal centers. One PLS is shown sectioned longitudinally; several are sectioned radially. Red pulp is the area of splenic cords and sinuses. Marginal zone is indicated. In the human spleen the penicillar arteries loop back to supply the germinal follicles [70]. The short branch from the central artery to the follicle, shown above, is characteristic of other mammalian spleens. (Weiss and Tavassoli [16].)**

There has been controversy over whether the circulation through the red pulp is "open" or "closed" [6]. Does blood move from the arteries through *closed* channels into the sinuses or does it empty from the ends of arteries into the *open* meshwork of the cords and come into the venous system through interstices of the walls of the sinuses? Some studies indicate the former. Swift currents of blood stream rapidly across the cords, while a small amount moves sluggishly through the red pulp [7]. Other studies [6] as well as histologic observations [5], however, have demonstrated few direct connections from the arterial to the venous system. It seems reasonable to conclude that there are de facto courses through the cords which may have no endothelial walls. The cells that move *slowly* through the cords may take minutes to traverse these few millimeters; yet it is known that blood flows through the normal human spleen at a rate of 300 ml/min. At this rate, not every cell could go through the cordal filter every time. There must be rapid shunts across the spleen.

THE PARENCHYMA

The spleen is divided into three parts: the white pulp, the red pulp, and between red and white, the marginal zone. Each part has three components: vessels, reticular cells, and free cells within a reticular meshwork.

The *white pulp* [8] is seen grossly as points on the cut surfaces of the spleen and in histologic sections as small discs surrounded by the vaster matrix of red pulp. In three dimensions the white pulp is a cylindrical periar-

terial lymphatic sheath surrounding the central artery (Fig. 14-1). Eccentric within the sheath are germinal centers encased by a shell of small lymphocytes, the mantle layer.

The vessels are branches of the central artery which take off at right angles. Some terminate within the white pulp, some in the marginal zone, and others, often the larger ones, in the red pulp. Plasma skimming probably minimizes the number of red cells released into the white pulp, while larger terminal arterioles carry a concentrated mix of red cells into the red pulp.

The reticular meshwork of the white pulp forms the structural fabric. At the periphery of the sheath it forms a fine radial net, but the interior is an intricate, almost random interlacing. The fibers of the periarterial sheath have a particular affinity for the T lymphocytes that comprise the lymphocytic component of the sheath, entrapping and retaining them as they arrive via the circulating blood [8]. The reticular structure also supports the germinal centers with a shell of fibrils.

Free cells in the white pulp are predominantly small lymphocytes. There are few granulocytes and plasma cells and even fewer red cells. Macrophages abound, as in all parts of the spleen. In the germinal centers large and medium-size lymphocytes are present, together with many macrophages. The mantle of the germinal center consists almost entirely of small lymphocytes.

The *marginal zone* [9] is peripheral to the radial layers of reticulum that bound the periarterial sheath (Fig. 14-1). Vessels are end arterioles arising from the central artery. The reticulum of the marginal zone is dense. This network receives many if not most of the terminal arterioles. The free cells are blood cells emerging from the arterial endings, a fair number of macrophages, and many medium-size lymphocytes. The cells are not so tightly packed as in the white pulp. Although the marginal zone is clearly demarcated from the periarterial sheath, its outer margin blends imperceptibly with the red pulp, so that some sinusoids of the red pulp come quite close to the periphery of the sheath.

The *red pulp* [10] vessels are primarily arteries derived from the central artery and branching to penetrate the lymphatic sheath or extending beyond the termination of that periarterial cylinder. Some of these branches end in the marginal zone; others cross into the red pulp. The area between the marginal zone and the sinuses comprises the splenic cords (cords of Billroth). The splenic sinus has been compared to a loosely assembled barrel. The staves are long, slender endothelial cells lying side by side. The hoops are a net of fibers; they are, in fact, the vessel's discontinuous basement membrane (Fig. 14-3). Cells in transit across the pulp cords enter the sinus through slits between the endothelial cells (Figs. 14-4 and 14-5).

The reticulum of the red pulp (Fig. 14-2) intermingles with that of the marginal zone on the one hand, and on the other it forms the perisinusal mantle. The reticular cells of the mantle give off fibers that surround the sinus and other fibers that commingle with the meshwork of the cords.

The free cells of the cords are, of course, erythrocytes and granulocytes of the blood, lymphocytes from wherever, and numerous macrophages.

FIGURE 14-2 Scanning electron micrograph of sinus viewed from the outside suspended in a mesh of cordal reticulum. The surface of the sinus consists of folded flattened reticular cells which have processes continuous with branches of reticular cells in the splenic cords. This provides some indication of the denseness of the thicket through which blood cells are filtered as they move across the splenic cords. Tissue dried by freeze drying, causing maximal retraction and shrinkage. ×6750. (Weiss [5].)

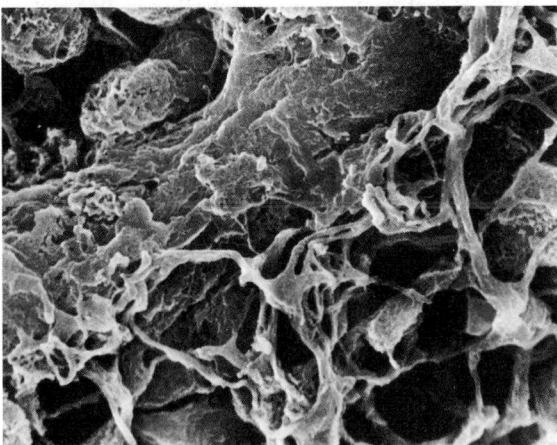

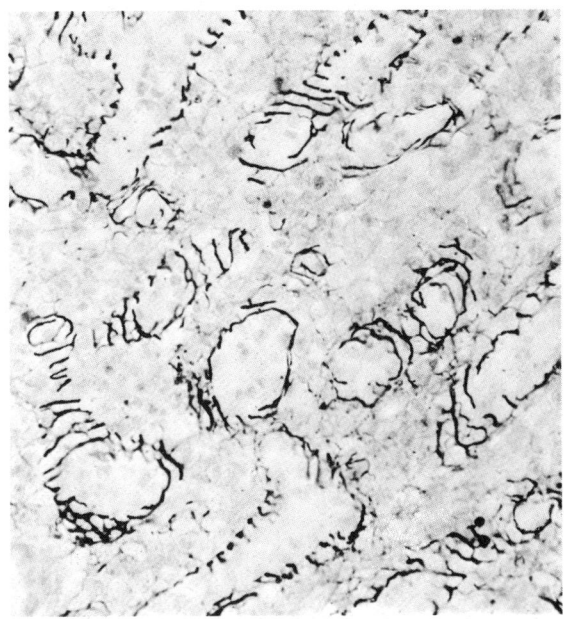

FIGURE 14-3 Red pulp of human spleen stained to show discontinuous basement membrane of the sinusoids. The straps and stippling represent hoops of reticulum that encircle the sinuses. In some of the cords between the sinuses are branches of reticulin that connect with processes from cordal reticulum cells (see Fig. 14-2). Thin section (3 μm); Gomori's reticulin stain. ×300. (Courtesy of L. T. Yam.)

Functions of the spleen

IMMUNE FUNCTION

The spleen performs in concert with other immunologically active organs. It contains a concentration of immunologically active cells, captures circulating antigens, provides an arena for their interaction, and is a major site of IgM production. For example, during primary antibody response to *Salmonella* flagella, tagged antigen is immediately concentrated in the red pulp, especially in macrophages [11]. At 1 h the concentration there has diminished, and the label is most heavily concentrated in the marginal zone. At 2 h the label is in the small lymphocytes surrounding the germinal centers, and at 4 h the germinal center itself has been penetrated. At 48 h the germinal center is the only place where antigen persists, having faded first from the red pulp and later from the marginal zone. In secondary antibody response the sequence is the same but the tempo is faster.

The first observable cellular response to antigenic stimulus is at 24 h, with the appearance of large plasmablasts in the white pulp, the periarterial lymphatic sheath [12]. These cells move toward the perimeter of the sheath, and at 2 days plasmablasts are present in the red pulp, clustered especially at the arterial terminals. At 4 days many plasma cells are present in the red pulp. There is also activity in germinal centers, which enlarge,

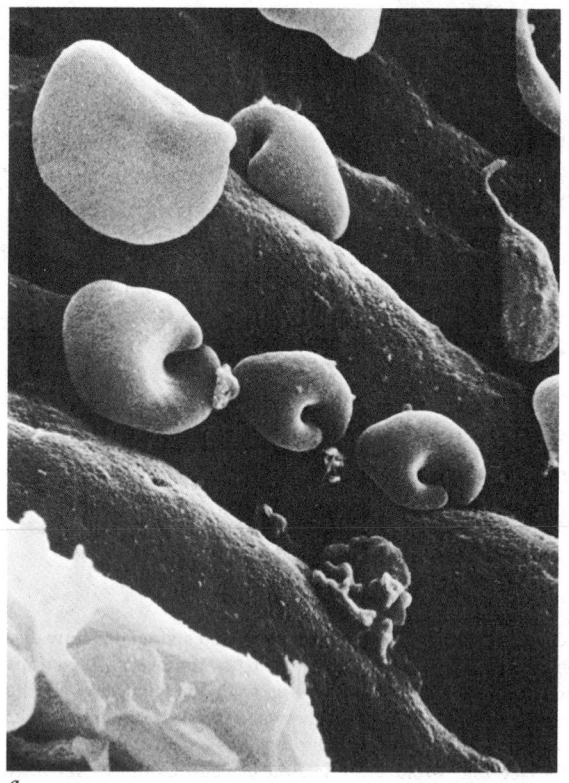

a

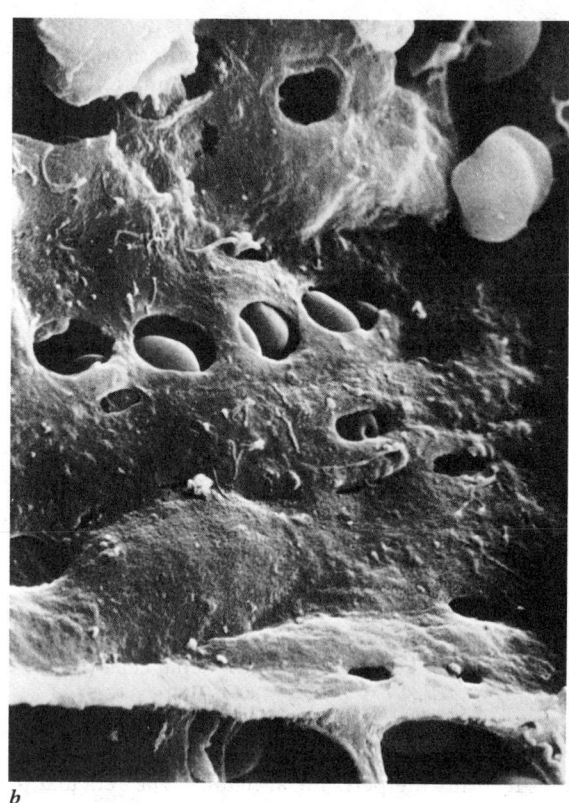

b

FIGURE 14-4   Scanning electron micrograph of inner surface of sinus of rat spleen. (*a*) Erythrocytes squeezing through intercellular interstices of the sinus wall. Normal animal. ×8500. (*b*) Erythrocytes have been converted to stomatocytes by injection of antiserum 24 h earlier. Because of rigidity and shape change the cells cannot pass through the sinus filter. Dilation of orifices is probably due to stretching by acute splenic enlargement and to intrasplenic pressure. ×5100. (Courtesy of A. de Boisfleury and N. Mohandas.)

with the presence of many mitoses. After 10 days the centers gradually diminish in size, becoming normal at about 4 weeks. During the immune response the spleen enlarges as a result of cellular proliferation and the entrapment of blood lymphocytes.

FILTER FUNCTION

The intricate meshwork of splenic reticulum, the concentration of free and sessile macrophages, and the pseudobarrier at the sinus wall all serve to slow the passage of blood and to bring its components into leisurely association with functional components of the spleen [13–16].

The absence of red cells in the white pulp indicates that the arteries that empty there carry almost pure plasma, bringing soluble antigens into the concentration of lymphocytes. The arteries that empty into the marginal zone and the red pulp carry a more concentrated slurry of blood cells and other particles, which crowd across the cords, running the gauntlet of free macrophages, phagocytic reticular cells, and littoral cells of the sinuses, which may also be phagocytic [9].

Phagocytosis, the primary immunologic event when particulate or cellular antigens are involved, is also the terminal event for damaged or otherwise defective red cells. Most granulocytes probably die in the body's tissue spaces, and platelets may be consumed in the line of hemostatic duty. But most red cells are destroyed by phagocytosis, many of them in the spleen.

Red cell destruction by the spleen requires preliminary changes that result, among other things, in a lack of deformability. This may result from stiffening of the cytoplasm, as in sickle cell anemia or Heinz body anemia, from loss of red cell surface membrane, or from rigidity of membrane protein [17] (Fig. 14-4).

CULLING

The ability of the spleen to recognize and remove from the blood the cells that are worn out or otherwise defective, such as sensitized platelets or spherocytic red cells, denatured red cells, and red cells infected with plasmodia or hemobartonella, has been designated *culling* [18–22]. Removal of bacteria, especially pneumococci, is also a splenic function, and splenectomy exposes both experimental animals [23] and patients [24] to the risk of developing bacteremia.

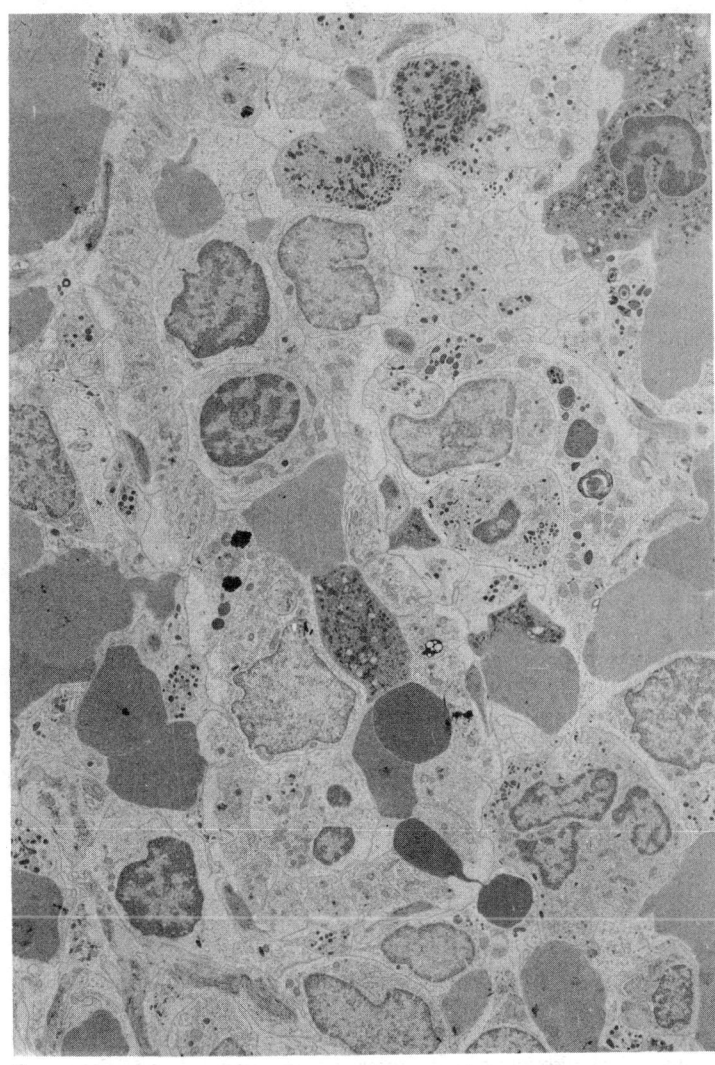

a

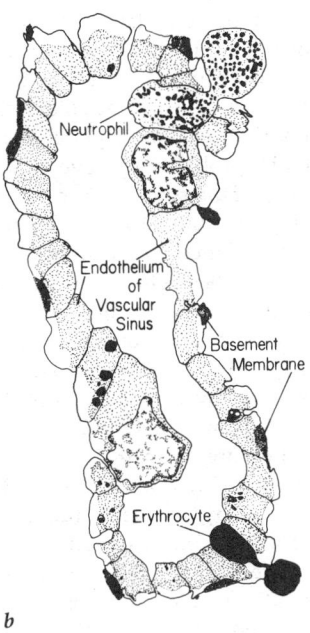

b

FIGURE 14-5 Transmission electron micrograph (×5000, reproduced at 63 percent of original print size) of a sinus of a human spleen showing the entrance, at opposite sides of an erythrocyte (bottom) and a neutrophil (top). Endothelial nuclei protrude into the sinus lumen. (Weiss [4].)

PITTING

Pitting is the ability of the spleen to remove particulate inclusions from red cells without destroying the cell itself [18,25]. Electron microscopic studies of rat spleen following a dose of phenylhydrazine demonstrate that pitting is accomplished at the wall of the sinus [13,20,21]. The drug causes formation of Heinz bodies, hard spheres of denatured hemoglobin. Red cells carried across the splenic cords return to the venous circulation by squeezing through the slits in the sinus wall. The deformable cytoplasm does this easily, but the rigid Heinz body is held up and ultimately is detached from the red cell along with a rim of membrane and a film of hemoglobin. The rejected inclusion is ingested by the perisinusoidal phagocytes. Other red cell inclusions, such as malarial parasites, bartonella, and piroplasma organisms, are also removed by the spleen [20]. Splenectomy results in greatly increased parasitization of red cells in infected hosts and greatly increased susceptibility to such infections [26,27].

IRON REUTILIZATION

Hemolytic anemias provide examples of the manner in which the structure of the spleen participates in iron metabolism. In hereditary spherocytosis (HS), most of the red cell destruction occurs in the spleen, in and around the sinuses where the reticular cells are phagocytic [14]. These cells are adept at removing iron from the ingested, degraded hemoglobin and transferring it into the plasma so that it can be returned to the marrow. In HS and in autoimmune hemolytic anemia, many red cells are destroyed by the wandering macrophages in the cords. They become engorged with iron and are stagnated, some even piling up together to form masses of hemosiderin. The spleen in this sort of disease is characteristically siderotic [28] even when the patient may otherwise be iron-deficient.

POOLING

Pooling by the spleen has come to mean that the concentration of one or another cell is greater in the splenic blood than in the circulating blood [29]. The spleen does, of course, accumulate lymphocytes from the blood in the white pulp [4]. Pooling has been demonstrated for platelets and also for reticulocytes. In the normal human about 30 percent of platelets are pooled in the spleen [30,31], probably by reversible adhesion to reticulum fibers of the splenic filter [5]. There is no significant pooling of granulocytes or mature red cells [29]. Reticulocytes retained by the spleen [32] may lose those metabolic organelles which remain from the erythroblastic phases of their career. Mitochondria, for example, cluster at the edge of the erythrocyte, where, surrounded by a thin rim of cytoplasm, they are extruded to be picked up by cordal macrophages [33]. Nuclear remnants (the Howell-Jolly bodies) and other large inclusion bodies are probably removed by the pitting function at the sinus wall [18]. Reticulocytes in the spleen also undergo some reduction of surface area. After a normal spleen has been removed, the average red cell surface is larger [34]; the difference in surface-to-volume ratio results in the postsplenectomy target cell. In the spherocytic hemolytic anemias, whether due to antibodies or to hereditary deformity, the red cells in the splenic pulp may have pieces of their own cytoplasm pinched off [19]. The change increases the spherocytic deformity of the red cells, making them more rigid and increasing the liability to capture by phagocytes.

Pooling by the spleen does not cause differences in cell concentration in splenic artery versus splenic vein. The concentration of platelets may be higher in the spleen than in the blood, but when a state of equilibrium exists, the number of platelets entering and leaving the spleen is the same.

RESERVOIR FUNCTION

During sleep, as much as one-third of a dog's red cells become sequestered in a greatly expanded spleen. This results in a corresponding decrease of the blood hematocrit. When the animal awakens, especially if alarmed, the spleen contracts and the sequestered cells are injected into the circulation. The hematocrit reading immediately rises [35]. The human spleen has little if any reservoir function under normal circumstances [36,37]. In the splenomegalic crisis of hemoglobin SC disease, the rapidly expanding spleen may capture many of the red cells, causing a shocklike state. Similar rapidly developing splenomegaly may occur in the blackwater crises of falciparum malaria (Chap. 70).

BLOOD VOLUME REGULATION

The spleen may exert some control over plasma volume and albumin synthesis. In most patients with chronic massive splenomegaly, the plasma volume and total albumin mass are expanded beyond normal [38,39]. The degree of expansion is greatly in excess of the amount of plasma present in the spleen itself [39,40]. Following removal of the spleen, the abnormality of the plasma volume and of albumin synthesis is only gradually corrected [39,40]. It may require 6 months before the

plasma and albumin mass finally level off at a lower, stabilized size. The feedback effect that the spleen exerts on plasma volume and albumin synthesis is not understood.

In animals with splenic reservoir function, such as the dog, removal of the spleen is followed by a gradual loss of about 30 percent of the red cell mass owing to reduction of erythropoiesis [41]. The nucleated red cell mass of the marrow is proportionately reduced [42]. The change evidently is not a result of loss of the splenic reservoir. Tightly wrapping the spleen *in situ,* for example, does not result in loss of red cell mass, although the reservoir cannot function [35].

HEMATOPOIETIC FUNCTION

Direct In utero the human spleen is a hematopoietic organ until the fifth month. After this time the spleen does not appear to provide an adequate microenvironment for hematopoiesis. Myeloid metaplasia in the adult spleen involves only abnormal marrow elements such as the neoplastic cells of myelogenous leukemia or polycythemia vera. The spleen may trap circulating marrow cells in syndromes of high marrow output [43], but the presence of these scattered cells in the splenic filter is quite different from the overgrowth that is characteristic of the myeloproliferative diseases.

The lymphocytic cell line does proliferate in the spleen: witness the mitoses in the germinal centers. It seems probable that some lymphocytes and plasma cells originate in the spleen. In older treatises it has been claimed that all or most of the monocytes are generated by the spleen, but there is no evidence for this claim.

Indirect Evidence in humans for inhibitory splenic humoral activity against human marrow is weak. After removal of a normal spleen, the platelet count and leukocyte count increase to a greater degree than after laparotomy without splenectomy, but the surge is temporary, and unless there are postsplenectomy complications, the counts usually return to nearly normal levels within 30 days [44,45].

In some animals, however, evidence of a splenic humoral effect upon the marrow is a bit more substantial. In the rat, for example, the platelet count remains elevated after splenectomy, and this is associated with a measurable increase of megakaryocytes in the marrow [46]. The increase, some 25 percent, seems to be more than enough to compensate for any loss of the megakaryocytes normally present in the spleen. Consequently, in the rat the spleen may normally exert some inhibitory effect on the megakaryocytes. The postsplenectomy granulocyte count also remains elevated [47].

Splenic size

The size of the spleen appears to be under some humoral control. Implantation of isologous splenic fragments into splenectomized rats results in the development of reconstituted splenunculi, the total weights of which equal the weights of the animals' own spleens [48]. Successful implants thus seem to be aware of one another and limit their total size accordingly. Also, successful grafts inhibit subsequent implantations. However, when splenunculi are challenged, for example, with a *Bartonella* infection, they do grow larger [27]. Embryologically, the multilobular splenic anlage may fail to fuse, so that instead of a single spleen there are two spleens on separate pedicles. The weight of the two equals the weight of a single normal spleen [49], suggesting some exchange of information concerning size between the pair.

Late in life the human spleen undergoes involution. The spleen of the octogenarian weighs, on average, considerably less than the spleen of younger people: 70 g versus 135 g [1]. The involution does not cause signs of asplenia in the blood.

In certain disorders the spleen becomes smaller than normal, sometimes nonexistent. This occurs regularly in sickle cell anemia [50] and frequently in primary thrombocythemia [51], where sequestration of firmly sickled red cells or massive clots of platelets cause infarctions and gradual destruction of the spleen. In other diseases, especially ulcerative colitis and celiac disease, the spleen becomes atrophic without infarction [52,53]. Evidence of atrophy is the presence of Howell-Jolly bodies in the blood, remnants of the erythroblast nucleus which are normally removed by the spleen's pitting function. Autoantibodies are sometimes found in patients with splenic atrophy associated with celiac disease or ulcerative colitis. The combination has been interpreted as evidence for a generalized dysfunction of the monocyte-macrophage system [52]. In splenic atrophy the numbers of Howell-Jolly bodies may be greater than after surgical removal of the spleen, signifying that a more than normal number of inclusion-bearing red cells escape from the marrow; the marrow's pitting function may also have a somewhat diminished efficiency.

In Fanconi's hypoplastic-marrow syndrome the spleen is often quite small [54]. This, together with the atrophic marrow, may represent a generalized failure of mesenchymal organs to develop properly or abnormal involution of these organs. Congenital asplenia, however, is not associated with marrow aplasia but often occurs together with situs inversus and other developmental anomalies of the heart [55]. In newborn infants with congenital heart disease, the spleen may be present but nonfunctional [56]. In this circumstance the splenic filter may be clogged with Heinz body–containing red cells. As the child matures, splenic function develops. In sickle cell anemia the spleen may be present but nonfunctional because its filters become clogged with sickled red cells. Splenic function, demonstrated by the absence of Howell-Jolly bodies, can be reestablished by washing out the sickled red cells by exchange transfusions [57].

Absence of the spleen, whether surgical or congenital, is associated with an increased risk of severe, abrupt infection from encapsulated bacteria, especially pneumococcus and *Hemophilus influenzae* [24]. This may be related to removal of these organisms by the splenic filter or to the formation by the spleen of opsonizing IgM [58] or other opsonizing agents [59]. The risk is especially high in younger children [60].

Postsplenectomy state

Hematologic changes which occur in normal persons following splenectomy provide information about the normal functions of the spleen [61]. Red cells become thinner, probably because the surface area remains somewhat greater than normal [62]. This results in the appearance of target cells on the blood smear [63]. Howell-Jolly bodies are always present [64]. They are found in about 1 percent of red cells [63], and there may be occasional siderocytes [65] and acanthocytes [66]. There are also "pocked" red cells in which the pocks on the surface represent inclusions retained within the cell after splenectomy [18,67]. Oxidative drugs such as phenacetin can provoke Heinz bodies in normal splenectomized persons but not in those with spleens. In the former, Heinz bodies once formed may persist in circulating erythrocytes for weeks after the patient stops taking the drug [68]. Nucleated red cells are not present in the blood of normal persons after splenectomy. The reticulocyte count remains normal. The life-span of the normal red cell is not extended or shortened. Whatever normal hemolytic function the spleen possesses is quickly and completely taken up by other organs [61]. Normal persons do not develop anemia or polycythemia after splenectomy [34,61].

The leukocyte count, after an immediate postsplenectomy surge, settles to a level usually within the normal range. In about 25 percent of patients it may be higher [64]. On average it is increased by about 40 percent: neutrophils are up by 35 percent, lymphocytes by 45 percent, and monocytes by almost 100 percent [44]. Eosinophilia with elevation up to 15 percent is not uncommon [64]. Epinephrine injection causes a brief leukocytosis after splenectomy, as it does before [69]: the splenic pool contains no sequestered leukocytes.

In hematologically normal people [45] the platelet count, after a postsplenectomy surge, becomes normal within a month [70]. Epinephrine injection after splenectomy does not provoke thrombocytosis, as it does when the spleen is present [30,69], probably because platelets are normally sequestered in the splenic pool [30].

When the spleen is present, normal fluctuations in white counts tend to be moderate. When the spleen is absent, the variations tend to be greater. Multiple examinations, rather than one, are necessary to evaluate "abnormal" findings in spleenless subjects. Abnormal counts, when conspicuous and persistent, should bring to mind something other than the postsplenectomy state [64].

In about 50 percent of splenectomized patients, there appears to be regrowth of splenic tissue [72]. These "born again" spleens may eliminate the hematologic postsplenectomy changes and reduce the threat of fatal pneumococcemia.

References

1. Crosby, W. H.: The spleen, in *Blood, Pure and Eloquent,* edited by M. M. Wintrobe. McGraw-Hill, New York, 1980, p. 96.
2. Koyama, K.: Hemodynamics of the spleen in Banti's syndrome. *Tohoku J. Exp. Med.* 93:199, 1967.
3. Krumbhaar, E. B., and Lippincott, S. W.: The postmortem weight of the "normal" human spleen at different ages. *Am. J. Med. Sci.* 197:344, 1939.
4. Jandl, J. H., Files, N. M., Barnett, S. B., and MacDonald, R. A.: Proliferative response of the spleen and liver to hemolysis. *J. Exp. Med.* 122:299, 1965.
5. Weiss, L.: The spleen, in *Histology,* 5th ed., edited by L. Weiss. McGraw-Hill, New York, 1981.
6. Chen, L.-T.: Microcirculation of the spleen: An open or closed circulation? *Science* 201:157, 1978.
7. McCuskey, R. S., Meineke, H. A., and Townsend, S. F.: Studies in hemopoietic microenvironment. I. Changes in microvascular system and stroma during erythropoietic regeneration and suppression in the spleens of CF 1 mice. *Blood* 39: 697, 1972.
8. Weiss, L.: The white pulp of the spleen. *Johns Hopkins Med. J.* 115:99, 1964.
9. Weiss, L.: The structure of intermediate vascular pathways in the spleen of rabbits. *Am. J. Anat.* 113:51, 1963.
10. Chen, L.-T., and Weiss, L.: Electron microscopy of the red pulp of human spleen. *Am. J. Anat.* 134:425, 1972.
11. Nossal, G. J. V., Austin, C. M., Pye, J., and Mitchell, J.: Antigens in immunity. XII. Antigen trapping in the spleen. *Int. Arch. Allergy* 29:368, 1966.
12. Langevoort, H. L.: The histophysiology of the antibody response. I. Histogenesis of the plasma cell reaction in rabbit spleen. *Lab. Invest.* 12:106, 1963.
13. Chen, L.-T., and Weiss, L.: The role of the sinus wall in the passage of erythrocytes through the spleen. *Blood* 41:529, 1973.
14. Rappaport, H., and Molnar, Z.: Fine structure of the red pulp of the spleen in hereditary spherocytosis. *Blood* 39:81, 1972.
15. Weed, R. I., and Weiss, L.: The relationship of red cell fragmentation occurring within the spleen to cell destruction. *Trans. Assoc. Am. Phycicians* 79:426, 1966.
16. Weiss, L., and Tavassoli, M.: Anatomical hazards to the passage of erythrocytes through the spleen. *Semin. Hemat.* 7:372, 1970.
17. Weed, R. I.: The importance of erythrocyte deformability. *Am. J. Med.* 49:147, 1970.
18. Koyama, S., Aoki, S., and Deguchi, K.: Electron microscopic observations of the splenic red pulp with special reference to the pitting function. *Mei Med. J.* 14:143, 1964.
19. Weed, R. I., and Weiss, L.: The relationship of red cell fragmentation occurring within the spleen to cell destruction. *Trans. Assoc. Am. Physicians* 79:426, 1966.
20. Schnitzer, B., Sodeman, T. M., Mead, M. L., and Contacos, P. G.: An ultrastructural study of the red pulp of the spleen in malaria. *Blood* 41:207, 1973.
21. Rifkind, R. A.: Heinz body anemia, and ultrastructural study. II. Red cell sequestration and destruction. *Blood* 26:433, 1965.
22. Tavassoli, M., and McMillan, R.: Structure of spleen in idiopathic thrombocytopenic purpura. *Am. J. Clin. Pathol.* 64:180, 1975.
23. Brown, E. J., Hosea, S. W., and Frank, M. M.: The role of the spleen in experimental pneumococcal bacteremia. *J. Clin. Invest.* 67:975, 1981.
24. Bisno, A. L.: Hyposplenism and overwhelming pneumococcal infection: A reappraisal. *Am. J. Med. Sci.* 262:101, 1971.
25. Crosby, W. H.: Siderocytes and the spleen. *Blood* 12:165, 1957.
26. Conrad, M. E., and Dennis, L. H.: Splenic function in experimental malaria. *Am. J. Trop. Med. Hyg.* 17:170, 1968.
27. Crosby, W. H., and Benjamin, N. R.: Frozen spleen reimplanted and challenged with *Bartonella. Am. J. Pathol.* 39:119, 1961.
28. Rappaport, H., and Crosby, W. H.: Autoimmune hemolytic anemia. II. Morphologic observations and clinico-pathologic correlations. *Am. J. Pathol.* 33:429, 1967.
29. Jandl, J. H., and Aster, R. H.: Increased splenic pooling and the pathogenesis of hypersplenism. *Am. J. Med. Sci.* 253:383, 1967.
30. Aster, R. H.: Pooling of platelets in the spleen: Role in the pathogenesis of "hypersplenic thrombocytopenia." *J. Clin. Invest.* 45:645, 1966.
31. Penny, R., Rozenberg, M. C., and Firkin, B. G.: The splenic platelet pool. *Blood* 27:1, 1966.
32. Berendes, M.: The proportion of reticulocytes in the erythrocytes of the spleen. *Blood* 14:558, 1959.
33. Matsumoto, N., Ishihara, T., Miwa, S., and Uchino, F.: The mechanism of mitochondrial extrusion from reticulocytes in the spleen from patients with erythrocyte pyruvate kinase (PK) deficiency. *Acta Haematol. Jpn.* 37:25, 1974.
34. Crosby, W. H.: Normal functions of the spleen relative to red blood cells: A review. *Blood* 14:399, 1959.
35. Areas Elenas, N., Ewald, R., and Crosby, W. H.: The reservoir function of the spleen and its relation to postsplenectomy anemia of the dog. *Blood* 24:299, 1964.
36. Ebert, R. V., and Stead, E. A.: Demonstration that in normal man no reserves of blood are mobilized by exercise, epinephrine, and hemorrhage. *Am. J. Med. Sci.* 202:655, 1941.
37. Fudenberg, H., Baldini, M., Mahoney, J. P., and Dameshek, W.: The body hematocrit/venous hematocrit and the "splenic reservoir." *Blood* 17:71, 1961.
38. Pryor, D. S.: The mechanism of anemia in tropical splenomegaly. *Q. J. Med.* 36:337, 1967.
39. Blendis, L. M., Ramboer, C., and Williams, R.: Studies on the hemodilutional anemia of splenomegaly. *Eur. J. Clin. Invest.* 1:54, 1970.
40. Hess, C. E., Ayers, C. R., Sandusky, W. R., Carpenter, M. A., Wetzel, R. A., and Mohler, D. N.: Mechanism of dilutional anemia in massive splenomegaly. *Blood* 47:629, 1976.
41. Waldmann, T. A., Weissman, S. M., and Berlin, N.: The effect of splenectomy on erythropoiesis in the dog. *Blood* 15:873, 1960.
42. Alexanian, R., McAlexander, R. A., and Donohue, D. M.: Effect of splenectomy on bone marrow cellularity in the dog. *Texas Rep. Biol. Med.* 23:562, 1965.
43. Yam, L. T., McMillan, R., Tavassoli, M., and Crosby, W. H.: Splenic hemopoiesis in idiopathic thrombocytopenic purpura. *Am. J. Clin. Pathol.* 62:830, 1974.
44. McBride, J. A., Dacie, J. V., and Shapley, R.: The effect of splenectomy on the leukocyte count. *Br. J. Haematol.* 14:225, 1968.
45. Hirsh, J., and Dacie, J. V.: Splenectomy, thrombocytosis and thromboembolism. *Br. J. Haematol.* 12:44, 1966.
46. Matter, M., Hartmann, J. R., Kautz, J., DeMarsh, Q. B., and Finch, C. A.: A study of thrombocytopoiesis in induced acute thrombocytopenia. *Blood* 15:174, 1960.
47. Palmer, J. G., Kemp, I., Cartwright, G. E., and Wintrobe, M. M.: Studies on the effect of splenectomy on the total leukocyte count in the albino rat. *Blood* 6:3, 1951.
48. Tavassoli, M.: Limitation of splenic growth as studied by heterotopic splenic implants. *Blood* 46:631, 1975.
49. Connor, L. A.: Double spleen. *Proc. N.Y. Pathol. Soc.* 1901:102, 1899–1900.
50. Blaustein, A. U., and Diggs, L. W.: Pathology of the spleen, in *The Spleen,* edited by A. U. Blaustein. McGraw-Hill, New York, 1963, pp. 45–178.
51. Hardesty, R. M., and Wolff, H. H.: Haemorrhagic thrombocythaemia: A clinical and laboratory study. *Br. J. Haematol.* 1:390, 1955.
52. Wardrop, C. A. J., Dagg, J. H., Lee, F. D., Singh, H., Dyet, J. F., and Moffat, A.: Immunologic abnormalities in splenic atrophy. *Lancet* 2:4, 1975.
53. Ryan, F. P., Smart, R. C., Holdsworth, C. D., et al.: Hyposplenism in inflammatory bowel disease. *Gut* 19:50, 1978.
54. Garriga, S., and Crosby, W. H.: The incidence of leukemia in families of patients with hypoplasia of the marrow. *Blood* 14:1008, 1959.

55. Putschar, W. G. J., and Manion, W. C.: Congenital absence of the spleen and associated anomalies. *Am. J. Clin. Pathol.* 26:429, 1956.

56. Pearson, H. A., Schiebler, G. L., and Spencer, R. P.: Functional hyposplenia in cyanotic congenital heart disease. *Pediatrics* 48:277, 1971.

57. Pearson, H. A., Cornelius, E. A., Schwartz, A. D., Zelson, J. H., Wolfson, S. L., and Spencer, R. P.: Transfusion-reversible functional asplenia in young children with sickle-cell anemia. *N. Engl. J. Med.* 283:334, 1970.

58. Schumacher, M. J.: Serum immunoglobulin and transferrin levels after childhood splenectomy. *Arch. Dis. Child.* 45:114, 1970.

59. Najjar, V. A., and Constantopoulos, A.: A new phagocytosis-stimulating tetrapeptide hormone, tuftsin, and its role in disease. *J. Reticuloend. Soc.* 12:197, 1972.

60. Walker, W.: Splenectomy during childhood in England and Wales. *Br. J. Haematol.* 28:145, 1974.

61. Crosby, W. H.: Hyposplenism: An inquiry into normal functions of the spleen. *Annu. Rev. Med.* 14:349, 1963.

62. Crosby, W. H.: The pathogenesis of spherocytes and leptocytes (target cells). *Blood* 7:261, 1952.

63. Singer, K., Miller, E. B., and Dameshek, W.: Hematologic changes following splenectomy in man with particular reference to target cells. *Am. J. Med. Sci.* 202:171, 1941.

64. Lipson, R. L., Bayrd, E. D., and Watkins, C. H.: The postsplenectomy blood picture. *Am. J. Clin. Pathol.* 32:526, 1959.

65. Douglas, A. S., and Dacie, J. V.: Incidence and significance of iron-containing granules in human erythrocytes and their precursors. *J. Clin. Pathol.* 6:307, 1953.

66. Dean, H. W.: Acanthocytes after splenectomy. *N. Engl. J. Med.* 279:947, 1968.

67. Holroyde, C. P., Oski, F. A., and Gardner, F. H.: The "pocked" erythrocytes. *N. Engl. J. Med.* 281:516, 1969.

68. Selwyn, J. G.: Heinz bodies in red cells after splenectomy and after phenacetin administration. *Br. J. Haematol.* 1:173, 1955.

69. Griffoni, V., Scaltrini, G. C., Confalonieri, C., and Conigliaro, S.: La Prova dell' adrenaline in ematologia. *Haematologica* 44:393, 1959.

70. Zuricker, M.: Beitrage zum Einfluss der Splenectomie auf Blutbild und Knochenmarksausstrich. *Folia Haematol. (Leipz)* 74:109, 1956.

71. Snook, T.: The origin of the follicular capillaries in the human spleen. *Am. J. Anat.* 144:13, 1975.

72. Pearson, H. A., Johnston, D., Smith, K. A., et al.: The born-again spleen. Return of splenic function after splenectomy for trauma. *N. Engl. J. Med.* 198:1389, 1978.

The inflammatory response

CHAPTER 15

The biochemistry and biologic activities of the complement and contact systems

NEIL R. COOPER
CHARLES G. COCHRANE

In plasma there are four principal systems of proteins in which the components undergo sequential proenzyme-enzyme reactions. These are the complement, contact (Hageman factor, factor XII), clotting, and fibrinolytic systems. These four systems have the capacity to act in concert and cross-activate one another. They generally participate in the defense of the host and in maintenance of homeostasis; however, they also play roles in the pathogenesis of inflammatory injury. Components of these systems are known to interact with cells, leading to stimulation of their function, and various cells are known to release activators of the plasma protein components of these systems.

The complement system

Complement is the term applied to a plasma effector system with diverse biological activities ranging from direct mediation of an acute inflammatory reaction to destruction of many different kinds of cells, bacteria, and viruses. Complement, through hormone-like properties of some of its factors, can also recruit other humoral and cellular effector systems, which in turn can induce directed migration of leukocytes, trigger histamine release from mast cells, stimulate the release of lysosomal constituents from phagocytes, and initiate the directed migration of leukocytes.

PROTEINS AND REACTION MECHANISMS

THE PROTEINS
Some complement components or factors are designated numerically, for example, C1, C2, C3, C4, while others are known by letters or names with historical signifi-

cance, such as factor B, factor D, properdin, or β1H. The terminology for a few of the proteins is based on their function within the complement system, that is, C3b inactivator, C1 inhibitor. A bar placed over the term for a complement protein denotes an active enzyme. Fragments of the complement proteins generated during the activation processes are denoted by a lower-case letter following the symbol for the component, that is, C3a, factor Bb.

The constituents of the complement system are 20 normal plasma proteins which range from 25,000 to more than 500,000 daltons in molecular weight and from α to slow γ in electrophoretic mobility (Table 15-1). They are immunologically non-cross-reactive and, except for a few which apparently arose by gene duplication, chemically distinct. Together their concentration represents approximately 15 percent of the plasma globulins. Except for three of the proteins, all circulate as individual noncomplexed molecules.

GENERAL FEATURES OF THE ACTIVATION PROCESSES
The complement proteins acquire the ability to interact with each other, with antibody and other proteins, and with biological membranes following a series of activation processes. Activation thus enables the separate complement components or factors to become members of a functionally integrated system. Activation is a dynamic process, since each component of the complement system must be activated sequentially under appropriate conditions for the reaction to progress.

There are two general features of the activation processes shared by a number of the individual steps in the complement sequence [1–4]. The first of these is activation by limited proteolytic cleavage, generally of a single bond. C1r, C1s, C2, C3, C4, C5, and factor B are activated by limited proteolytic cleavage. The second general feature of the activation processes is the formation of large multimolecular protein-protein complexes that contain up to five different complement proteins depending on the reaction step involved. The most important of these protein-protein complexes is the C5b–9 complex, which is able, in its nascent form, to disrupt lipid bilayer membranes. Components activated partly or completely by protein-protein complexing are C1, C2, C3, C4, C5, C6, C7, C8, C9, factor B, and properdin. Other complex plasma effector systems, such as the coagulation and kinin-forming systems, are also activated by combinations of limited proteolytic cleavage and protein-protein complexing reactions.

REACTION PATHWAYS
There are two parallel but independent mechanisms or pathways leading to activation of the terminal, biologically important portion of the complement sequence (Fig. 15-1). These activation pathways, termed the *classical* and *alternative* or *properdin pathways*, respectively, are triggered by different substances. Each involves the reaction steps of several complement components. The two activation pathways converge at the midpoint of the complement system at the C3 reaction

TABLE 15-1   Properties of the complement components and complement regulators

Name	Molecular weight	Electrophoretic mobility	Approximate plasma concentration, $\mu g/ml$
Classical pathway:			
C1q	410,000	γ_2	70
C1r	190,000	β	34
C1s	87,000	α	31
C2	117,000	β_1	25
C3	185,000	β_1	1600
C4	206,000	β_1	600
Properdin or alternative pathway:			
C3	185,000	β_1	1600
Factor B	95,000	β_2	200
Factor D	25,000	α	1
Factor I (C3b inactivator)	88,000	β	34
Factor H (βIH)	150,000	β_1	500
Properdin	224,000	γ_2	25
Membrane attack mechanism:			
C5	180,000	β_1	85
C6	128,000	β_2	75
C7	121,000	β_2	55
C8	153,000	γ_1	55
C9	72,000	α	60
Complement regulators:			
C1 inhibitor	105,000	α_2	137
C4 binding protein	>500,000	β	—
Factor I (C3b inactivator)	88,000	β	34
Factor H (βIH)	150,000	β_1	500
Properdin	185,000	γ_2	25
S protein	80,000	α	>300
Anaphylatoxin inactivator	300,000	α	
Abnormal proteins:			
C3 nephritic factor	180,000	γ	—

step, and the remainder of the reaction sequence, involving the reactions of C5 through C9, is common to both pathways. This later portion of the reaction sequence is termed the *membrane attack mechanism* because of its ability to lyse or otherwise damage cellular membranes. In addition, there are control proteins that act to modulate and inhibit various reaction steps.

THE CLASSICAL PATHWAY

The classical pathway comprises the reaction steps of C1, C2, C3, and C4. The pathway may be subdivided into two functional units: (1) activation of C1 and (2) generation of two related complex enzymes, $\overline{C42}$ and $\overline{C423}$ [5–7].

The first component of the classical pathway, C1, is

FIGURE 15-1   Activation pathways of the complement system. Details of the system are presented in the text.

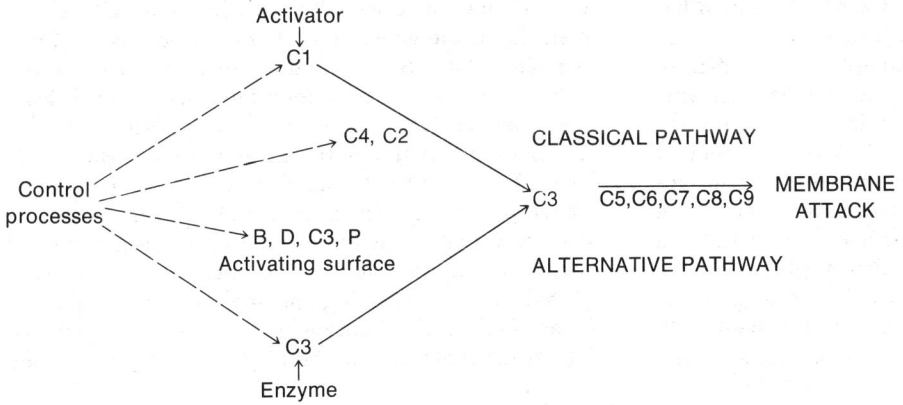

readily activated by immune complexes and aggregated immunoglobulins. Human immunoglobulins belonging to the IgM class and to the IgG1, IgG2, and IgG3 subclasses are capable of initiating the classical pathway. C1 may also be activated in the absence of antibody by a large number of different substances, including a polypeptide located on the external surface of retroviruses, C-reactive protein in complex with phosphorylcholine, its natural substrate, polyanions such as DNA or RNA, certain cellular membranes, and lipid A of lipopolysaccharides. The structural or chemical features responsible for C1 binding and activation are not yet known.

C1 in normal plasma is a trimolecular calcium-dependent complex of three different proteins, C1q, C1r, and C1s [8]. Activation of C1 is initiated by the binding of the entire molecule to the Fc portion of antibody molecules [9] or to structural features on the various non-immune activators [10]. C1q is an unusual molecule chemically in that it contains a large collagen-like sequence [11]. Ultrastructurally it is also striking because it resembles a bouquet of six tulips [12]. It is through the C1q subunit that C1 binds to immune complexes [13]. This ability of C1q to bind to immune complexes has led to its widespread use as a detector for immune complexes in clinical laboratories. The binding of C1 to an activator initiates a series of intramolecular changes which leads to limited proteolytic cleavage of each of the two polypeptide chains of C1r [14], a process which converts C1r from a zymogen into an enzyme of the serine esterase type [14,15]. The newly activated C1r enzyme cleaves C1s, thereby converting C1s from a zymogen into an active protease, also of the serine esterase type [16,17]. With the cleavage and thus activation of the C1s subcomponent, C1 activation is completed.

Activated C1s in $\overline{C1}$ mediates the formation of another complement enzyme, $\overline{C42}$, which is assembled from two precursor molecules, C4 and C2 [18]. C4 is first cleaved by $\overline{C1s}$ and $\overline{C1}$ into a small fragment, C4a, which has biological activity as considered below, and a larger fragment, C4b. The cleavage reaction engenders several sites in C4b. One of these, a labile binding site, enables C4b, for a brief period of time after formation, to bind to immune complexes and biological membranes [19], while another site in C4b serves as an acceptor for the larger fragment of C2, or C2a, which has been similarly cleaved and activated by $\overline{C1s}$ in $\overline{C1}$ [18,20]. The protein-protein complex thus formed, C4b2a or $\overline{C42}$, is an indigenous complement enzyme that assumes the function of continuing the ongoing complement reaction. Although $\overline{C42}$ may be generated in the fluid phase, only those complexes on the surface of a target cell efficiently mediate the next step in the reaction sequence. The $\overline{C42}$ enzyme cleaves C3, the component in highest concentration in plasma, into a small fragment, C3a, which has potent biological activity as discussed below, and a large fragment, C3b [18,21]. C3b, like C4b, has a short-lived binding site

[22], which permits the attachment of this molecule to the membrane of the activator in a cluster-type distribution around the $\overline{C42}$ enzyme. The labile binding sites in C3 and C4 contain the amino acid sequence -Cys-Gly-Glu-Glu- with the Cys and second Glu residues joined by a thiolester bond [23,24]. With cleavage of C3 into C3b by $\overline{C42}$, the thiolester apparently undergoes stress-mediated hydrolysis and the acyl group of the glutamyl residue forms a covalent bond with a reactive hydroxyl or amino group on the activator surface. As with C4, a major proportion of C3 molecules undergoing cleavage fail to achieve binding. In all probability these represent molecules in which the glutamyl residue has reacted with water. The binding of C3b molecules in close proximity to the bound $\overline{C42}$ complexes generates yet another enzyme, $\overline{C423}$, or more properly, $\overline{C4b2a3b}$, which has C5 as its substrate. The proteolytic cleavage of C5 by $\overline{C423}$ triggers the formation of the membrane attack complex, as described below.

The classical complement pathway therefore consists of a series of enzyme-substrate and protein-protein interactions leading to the sequential formation of several complement enzymes. The reactions involved are highly specific, and other molecules cannot substitute for the required complement components. In addition, since the reactions are enzymatically mediated, there is a considerable turnover of molecules of C2, C3, C4, and C5 at the respective steps in the reaction and an accumulation of reaction products free in the plasma. Since some of these reaction products have biologic activity, it is evident that a relatively small stimulus to complement activation may lead to considerable generation of these biologically active products.

THE ALTERNATIVE OR PROPERDIN PATHWAY

The alternative or properdin complement activation pathway consists of the reaction steps involving factor B, factor D, factor H, factor I, C3, and properdin (P). This pathway is parallel to, but distinct from, the classical activation pathway with which it converges at the C3 step. It may be divided into two functional units: initiation and amplification [25].

The alternative pathway is triggered in a different manner than the classical pathway. The initial requirement is for the generation of small amounts of C3b in the circulation. Since mixtures of purified native C3 and factors B and D were found to generate a C3-cleaving enzyme [26,27], the possibility existed that a minor subpopulation of the C3 molecules might behave like C3b, a form of C3 long known to generate a C3-cleaving enzyme with factors B and D. However, the discovery that C3 with its internal thiolester cleaved was C3b-like in functional properties strongly suggested that a C3-cleaving enzyme in the circulation, or in purified C3 preparations, represented C3 which had lost its internal thiolester bond [28]. The thiolester bond has been found to hydrolyze in aqueous buffers at a slow but finite rate consistent with this hypothesis [28]. Most likely, therefore, thiolester-hydrolyzed C3, that is, $C3(H_2O)$, interacts with factors B and D to form $C3(H_2O)B$ or, more properly, $\overline{C3(H_2O),Bb}$, which efficiently cleaves C3 into C3a and C3b. In addition to the preceding steady-state mechanism of generation of a C3b-like molecule, C3b may sporadically appear in the circulation as a consequence of classical pathway activation or as a result of direct C3 cleavage by tissue enzymes or enzymes of the fibrinolytic or coagulation system. Such C3b would interact with factors B and D to form the C3-cleaving enzyme $\overline{C3bBb}$. Although most of the C3b molecules generated by any of the mechanisms just described are rapidly inactivated by factors I and H, a certain minor proportion becomes covalently bound to cell and membrane surfaces via an ester or amide linkage with the glutamyl residue of the thiolester, as described earlier. On most surfaces, the bound C3b molecules are also rapidly cleaved and inactivated by the concerted action of factors H and I. On the surface of activators, including a number of polysaccharides, lipopolysaccharides, viruses, bacteria, fungi, and certain cells and parasites [25], a different series of events follows. On such surfaces, the bound C3b is "protected" from destruction by factors H and I [29]. This surface-bound protected C3b interacts with factors B and D to form $\overline{C3bBb}$, which cleaves large amounts of C3, some of which also arrives on the surface of the activator. This additional C3b, also protected from destruction by factors H and I, interacts with additional factors B and D and forms more $\overline{C3bBb}$. $\overline{C3bBb}$ is rendered more efficient in C3 cleavage by properdin (P), which binds to the complex forming $\overline{C3bPBb}$, a more stable form of the enzyme. Properdin attachment also slows the spontaneous dissociation of factor Bb. The cyclic amplifying system, in conjunction with the crucial protected surface, represents the key events in activation of the alternative pathway.

Many of the C3b molecules generated by surface-bound $\overline{C3bBb}$ or $\overline{C3bPBb}$ bind to the surface of the activator particle in close proximity to these enzymes. This results in the formation of modified enzymes, $\overline{C3b_nBb}$ or $\overline{C3b_nPBb}$ ($n > 1$), which have the ability to cleave C5 and initiate the membrane attack mechanism. The catalytic site of these enzymes resides in the factor B moiety.

A pathologic member of this pathway, C3 nephritic factor, is found in the circulation of some patients with hypocomplementemic mesangiocapillary nephritis. This protein is an autoantibody directed to the $\overline{C3bBb}$ complex of the alternative pathway [30].

THE REACTIONS OF C5–C9: THE MEMBRANE ATTACK MECHANISM

The membrane attack mechanism includes the reaction steps of C5, C6, C7, C8, and C9 [31,32]. This cytolytic pathway is initiated by C5 cleavage induced by the $\overline{C423}$, $\overline{C3b_nBb}$, or $\overline{C3b_nPBb}$ enzymes of the classical and alternative pathways. The products of C5 cleavage are C5a, a molecule with potent biological activities, as considered below, and C5b, the larger fragment which initiates the self-assembly of the C5b–9 membrane attack complex. C5b–9, a large multimolecular complex containing C5b, C6, C7, C8, and C9, is the fully assembled cytolytic principle of the complement system. C5b has the ability to bind to C6 and C7, thus forming the C5b67 complex to which C8 and several C9 molecules bind [33]. Progressive assembly of the C5b–9 complex is associated with increasing hydrophobicity and ability to bind phospholipids and membrane analogs [34]. Thus, as the complexes form, they acquire the ability to bind to membranes. This process, however, is modulated by a normal serum protein, S, which is able to bind to the forming C5b–9 complex [35]. C5b–9 complexes which have interacted with S or with SC5b–9 are unable to attach to membranes and thus are cytolytically inactive.

Membrane leakage, in the case of cell-bound attack complexes, begins at the C8 stage; however, the lytic process is greatly accelerated by C9. The precise mechanism by which the C5b–9 complex disrupts cellular membranes is not fully elucidated [31,32,36]. It is likely, however, that the attachment and insertion of the strongly lipid-binding C5b–9 complex into lipid bilayer membranes leads to a reorientation and reorganization of the bilayer structure. By this means it is likely that channels appear in the lipid bilayer which permit the passage of ions, water, and cellular constituents.

CONTROL MECHANISMS OF THE COMPLEMENT SYSTEM

This potent system is under precise control and regulation. The regulatory processes are complex and involve various kinds of labile sites and decay processes as well as the action of a group of regulatory proteins. All these proteins interact only with the activated forms of the molecule involved. They include a multispecific protease inhibitor, C1 inhibitor, which binds to and rapidly inactivates the activated forms of C1r and C1s [2]. This molecule thus regulates the first step of the classical pathway. The regulatory proteins include also C4-binding protein, which binds to C4b and serves as a cofactor for factor I, a proteolytic enzyme which degrades C4b into smaller inactive fragments [37]. Also included among the control proteins is factor H, a protein which binds to C3b and serves as a cofactor for C3b cleavage and degradation by factor I [38,39]. The S protein binds to the forming C5b–9 complex and modulates the cytolytic function of this complex on membranes [35]. Finally, the control proteins include the anaphylatoxin inactivator which removes the C-terminal arginine of C3a, C4a, C5a, respectively, and thereby abrogates some of the biological activities of these complement activation peptides [40].

Biological consequences of complement activation

The biological activities of the activated complement system can be grouped into three broad categories (Table 15-2). First, complement is able to produce a number of ultrastructural changes in lipid-containing biological membranes which may result in a number of effects ranging from functional impairment to cytotoxic and cytolytic damage. Second, effector cells which possess specific receptors for various bound complement compounds or fragments thereof may interact with the bound complement molecules and form rosettes or cellular aggregates with the target cells. The third category of complement biology relates to the hormone-like activities of the small cleavage products of C3, C4, and C5 — C3a, C4a, and C5a, respectively.

COMPLEMENT-MEDIATED DAMAGE TO BIOLOGICAL MEMBRANES

Complement is able to mediate the lytic destruction of many kinds of cells, including erythrocytes, lymphocytes, platelets, bacteria, and viruses, although with greatly varying degrees of efficiency in each instance [41]. Either complement pathway may trigger the membrane attack complex to produce cytolytic damage. Some cells are quite resistant to destruction by complement even in the presence of marked complement activation on the cell surface. There are several reasons why complement may fail to lyse cells, including *antigenic modulation,* a phenomenon whereby antibody alters the distribution of antigen on the cell surface, a spatial arrangement of antigenic sites which does not facilitate complement activation in a region of the membrane susceptible to lysis, or a lack of binding sites for the late-reacting complement components. Most commonly, however, complement fails to produce lysis because of the nature and structure of the cell wall or membrane or because the cell repairs the complement-mediated damage. Factors in addition to complement may also be required, as in the lysis of gram-negative bacteria.

As the complement components free in serum become attached to the surfaces of cells and other biologic membranes, there are changes in membrane electrical charge and environment due to the accumulation of complement proteins on the cell surface. Complement action produces circular lesions having a diameter of 8 to 12 nm in many types of membranes. These lesions, which are C5b–9 complexes inserted into the cellular membrane, are the sites of lytic membrane damage. The possible mechanisms by which the C5b–9 complex disrupts cellular lipid bilayer membranes leading to lysis were considered above under "The Membrane Attack Mechanism."

COMPLEMENT RECEPTOR INTERACTIONS

Human neutrophils, polymorphonuclear leukocytes, B lymphocytes, and erythrocytes have specific receptors on their surfaces for the larger cleavage fragment of C3 and C4 [42,43]. These cells are able to bind C3b and C4b regardless of whether the b fragments are free in solution or are themselves bound, via their labile binding sites, to an immune complex or target cell. Thus C3b and C4b molecules may serve as a bridge between a target cell or immune complex which bears these fragments and a responding or effector cell. Such interactions may trigger various cellular responses depending on the type of responding cell (Table 15-2). In the case of phagocytic cells, interaction mediates adherence with the target cell or complex. In this manner, the complement fragments may facilitate phagocytosis stimulated directly or through IgG Fc interaction. In some cases, the complement fragments alone suffice to trigger ingestion. Human B lymphocytes also have receptors for C3b and C4b. Although the biological significance of the presence of the receptor on these cells is unclear, this reaction brings antigens in direct surface contact with potential antibody-forming cells. Bound complement components may play a role in this manner in the induction of an immune response.

C3b receptors are also present on human erythrocytes and platelets from many nonprimate species. The biological significance of attachment of complexes or cells bearing C3b to human erythrocytes, a reaction termed *immune adherence,* is not clear, although it may be an immobilizing mechanism important in dealing with pathogenic agents.

Specific cellular receptors for other breakdown products of C3b, i.e., for C3b cleaved by factors H and I, for C3d, a further degradation product, and for other complement molecules have also been described. The biological roles played by interactions of effector cells with these complement components are under active investigation.

TABLE 15-2   Biological consequences of complement action

Complement-mediated damage to biological membranes:
  Ultrastructural changes and cytotoxic effects
  Disruption of lipid bilayer envelopes of cells, bacteria, viruses
Complement receptor interactions:
  Opsonization, phagocytosis
  Clearance from the circulation
  Role in induction of an immune response
Biological effects of complement cleavage fragments:

C3a, C4a, C5a	Release of vasoactive amines from cells
	Smooth muscle contraction
	Enhanced vascular permeability
	Induced release of lysosomal enzymes
C5a	Chemotaxis
	Granulocyte aggregation
	Stimulation of oxidative metabolism
	Stimulation of release of slow-reacting substance of anaphylaxis (SRS-A)

BIOLOGICAL EFFECTS OF COMPLEMENT CLEAVAGE FRAGMENTS

The smaller fragments of C3, C4, and C5—C3a, C4a, and C5a, respectively—are known as *anaphylatoxins* [44]. These hormonelike peptides induce smooth-muscle contraction, enhance vascular permeability, release mediators such as histamine from mast cells and basophils, and induce lysosomal enzyme release from granulocytes (Table 15-2). In addition to these properties of the C3a, C4a, and C5a peptides, C5a is chemotactic and thus able to induce the migration of leukocytes into an area of complement activation. C5a also has a number of other properties, including granulocyte aggregation and activation of intracellular processes in certain cells which leads to various effects such as release of oxygen metabolites and slow-reacting substance of anaphylaxis (SRS-A).

Most of the C3a and C4a effects are abrogated by antihistamines and thus are dependent on histamine released as a consequence of C3a and C4a interaction with mast cells and basophils. Some of the effects are also sensitive to the action of the anaphylatoxin inactivator, a serum enzyme that removes the C-terminal arginine residue from these peptides. Although antihistamines and the control enzyme inhibit some of the effects of C5a, C5a desarg, lacking the C-terminal arginine, retains significant chemotactic, granulocyte aggregating, and intracellular activating ability.

A comparison of the primary structures of C3a, C4a, and C5a [44] indicates that they are genetically related. They also share a number of the same biological actions, as noted above. Despite these facts, the C3a and C5a anaphylatoxins interact with distinct cell-surface receptors and thus are biologically distinct.

Biological importance of the complement system

The in vitro biological reactions considered above are individual aspects of an integrated system able to produce inflammation and thereby to facilitate the localization of an infective agent. Thus the anaphylatoxin activities lead to histamine release and consequent contraction of smooth muscle, increased vascular permeability, and edema. The chemotactic C5a peptide triggers an influx of leukocytes which remain fixed in the area of complement activation through attachment to specific sites on bound C3b and C4b molecules. Phagocytosis or release of lysosomal and other constituents facilitates the destruction of an infective agent. Released enzymes activate more complement and amplify the process.

Evidence for the biological importance of this system in vivo in host defense has come from studies of experimentally induced diseases in animals, from human immunologic disease processes, and from the markedly increased susceptibility to infection and predisposition to certain diseases which characterize some congenital or acquired deficiencies of complement components or complement regulators in humans.

In induced diseases in animals, the role of complement in producing the inflammatory aspects of the disease has been defined [45,46]. In several such examples, tissue damage does not occur if complement participation is prevented by in vivo destruction of complement or by use of antibodies rendered unable to fix complement.

A number of human diseases bear certain hallmarks which imply the participation of complement. These include reduced levels of the components in the circulation, deposition of complement components in sites of tissue injury, and leukocyte infiltration [4,6,31,47]. Metabolic studies with purified radiolabeled complement components in a number of infections and auto-immune-type diseases have documented in vivo complement activation [48].

The role of complement in the maintenance of a normal state of health is dramatically illustrated by the predisposition to disease or susceptibility to infection which characterizes congenital deficiency of certain of the complement components or their regulators [4,47,49] (Table 15-3). Congenital deficiency of C1 inhibitor permits uncontrolled activation of the classical pathway, as in hereditary angioedema. Over half of the more than 50 reported individuals with hereditary deficiencies of the classical pathway—C1r, C1s, C4, and C2—are clinically ill and suffer from several diseases, including systemic lupus erythematosus, glomerulonephritis, and repeated infections. Most of the relatively few individuals found with genetic deficiencies of C3 or its regulator, factor I, suffer from recurrent life-threatening infections. More than half of the approximately 30 individuals with inherited deficiencies of the terminal components—C5, C6, C7, and C8—have recurrent infections with *Neisseria* organisms (gonococcus or meningococcus).

The genes for C2, C4, and factor B (but not other complement components) are encoded within the major histocompatibility complex in humans [4,47,49]. It is not clear how the absence of a complement component or a regulator predisposes to diseases. Genes within

TABLE 15-3   Inherited complement deficiencies

Component lacking	Disease association
C1r, C1s, C2, C4	Systemic lupus erythematosus and systemic lupus erythematosus-like syndrome, dermatomyositis, glomerulonephritis
C3, C5, factor I	Recurrent pyogenic infections (pneumococcus, staphylococcus, streptococcus)
C6, C7, C8	*Neisseria* infections, healthy
C1 inhibitor	Hereditary angioedema

this region are of fundamental importance to immune recognition, regulation, and responses, and these unexplained relationships suggest major but as yet unknown physiologic roles for the complement system in vivo.

The contact (Hageman factor, factor XII) system

DESCRIPTION OF COMPONENTS AND SCHEME OF PATHWAYS

The components of the contact system and their physical characteristics are presented in Table 15-4. The central components of the contact system include Hageman factor (clotting factor XII), prekallikrein, high-molecular-weight kininogen, and clotting factor XI. These components, upon activation of the system, can activate the fibrinolytic, intrinsic clotting, and extrinsic clotting systems, as shown in Fig. 15-2. It is not clear how extensively the extrinsic clotting system or the fibrinolytic systems are activated by Hageman factor (factor XII), and kallikrein, respectively, because these reactions have been demonstrated only with isolated components. As noted in Fig. 15-2, Hageman factor (factor XII), prekallikrein, and high-molecular-weight kininogen interact on a negatively charged surface, leading to the activation of Hageman factor (factor XII) and prekallikrein, as will be discussed below. The activated Hageman factor (factor XIIa) on the surface, if in contact with factor XI, can activate factor XI, leading to stimulation of the intrinsic clotting system (Fig. 15-2). In addition, activated Hageman factor (factor XIIa), in the presence of tissue factor, can stimulate factor VII and thereby the extrinsic clotting system. The fact that these initial events take place on a negatively charged surface constitutes the reason for designating this the *contact system.*

MOLECULAR MECHANISM OF ACTIVATION OF THE CONTACT SYSTEM

When plasma contacts a negatively charged surface, Hageman factor (factor XII) binds rapidly to the surface and, in the presence of prekallikrein and high-molecular-weight kininogen, is rapidly cleaved into two disulfide-linked peptide chains with molecular weights of 52,000 and 28,000 daltons (site 1, Fig. 15-3). Cleavage then occurs on the N-terminal side of the disulfide

bridge (site 2), allowing the smaller chain which bears the enzymatic site of Hageman factor (factor XII) to dissociate into the fluid phase [51]. The larger fragment remains surface-bound, presumably by virtue of positively charged amino acid residues in the heavy chain. In a clear departure from the complement and coagulation systems, the proteins of the contact system do not require metal ions for activation.

The enzyme in plasma responsible for the rapid cleavage of Hageman factor (factor XII) is kallikrein. Its precursor, prekallikrein, is itself cleaved into heavy and light chains and activated by Hageman factor. Thus a reciprocal activation by these two molecules was proposed as a mechanism of activation of the contact system [52]. The reciprocal enzymatic cleavage and activation of Hageman factor (factor XII) and prekallikrein is augmented by the fact that when bound to the surface, Hageman factor (factor XII) is more than 100-fold more susceptible to enzymatic cleavage [53]. In the absence of prekallikrein, Hageman factor (factor XII) is cleaved and activated slowly, suggesting that other enzymes, such as factor XI and plasmin, may play a secondary role. However, in the absence of prekallikrein, the clotting and kinin-generating activities are markedly retarded [54].

Prekallikrein and factor XI exist in plasma as a complex with high-molecular-weight kininogen [55,56]. The high-molecular-weight kininogen acting stoichiometrically with Hageman factor (factor XII) [57] brings prekallikrein and factor XI to the surface, where they are able to interact with Hageman factor (factor XII) [58]. The light chain of high-molecular-weight kininogen bears a domain extremely rich in histidine residues which apparently is responsible for the adherence of the molecule to negatively charged surfaces [59]. A portion of the light chain is also responsible for the complexing of high-molecular-weight kininogen with prekallikrein and factor XI [60,61]. Thus high-molecular-weight kininogen acts as a cofactor in a stoichiometric relation with Hageman factor (factor XII) to promote the reciprocal activation of prekallikrein and Hageman factor (factor XII) [57,62] and the cleavage and activation of factor XI by Hageman factor (factor XII).

Kallikrein rapidly dissociates from high-molecular-weight kininogen on the surface and cleaves and activates other surface-bound Hageman factor (factor XII) molecules [63]. The dissociated kallikrein also rapidly cleaves high-molecular-weight kininogen both on the

TABLE 15-4 Physical properties of the central components of the contact activation system of human plasma

	Molecular weight, daltons	*Concentration in citrated plasma, µg/ml*	*pI*
Hageman factor (factor XII)	74,000 to 80,000	24–40	6.8
Prekallikrein	80,000 to 85,000	50	8.5–9.0
Factor XI	160,000 (dimer)	4	8.5–9.0
High-molecular-weight kininogen	110,000	70	4.5

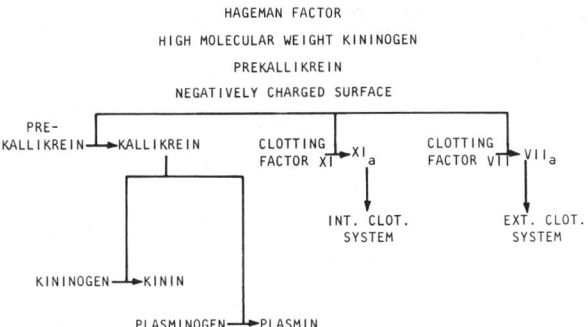

FIGURE 15-2 Activation sequences of the contact system. The sequences are initiated when the three proteins at the top of the diagram interact with a negatively charged surface. The activated Hageman factor (factor XIIa) may then convert prekallikrein to kallikrein, clotting factor XI to XIa, and clotting factor VII to VIIa as shown.

surface and in fluid phase. This fluid-phase action of kallikrein probably accounts for a great majority of the burst of activity of the contact system.

The initial event that triggers the activation of Hageman factor (factor XII) and prekallikrein is not precisely understood. The concept that Hageman factor (factor XII) is activated upon binding to a surface in the absence of other proteins has been questioned. [50]. In the absence of prekallikrein or high-molecular-weight kininogen, Hageman factor (factor XII) still becomes surface-bound, but it does not activate and does not undergo cleavage for several minutes (well after the burst of activity seen in normal plasma [64]. Single-chain zymogen Hageman factor (factor XII) binds [³H]DFP extremely slowly, and this is not influenced by contact with a surface [65,66]. By contrast, kallikrein-activated two-chain Hageman factor (factor XIIa) binds [³H]DFP rapidly. A plausible explanation for the initiating mechanism for the burst of activity is that Hageman factor (factor XII) and prekallikrein are "active zymogens." Like trypsinogen, these molecules expose the active site for a finite period. If brought into contact with a substrate molecule, cleavage during this moment could take place. Once one of the two becomes fully activated, reciprocal activation could ensue. The fluid-

phase movement of kallikrein could then rapidly disseminate the reaction.

A summary of the molecular assembly leading to the activation of Hageman factor (factor XII) is given in Fig. 15-4a. At the upper left portion of the figure, Hageman factor (factor XII) and the complex of prekallikrein and high-molecular-weight kininogen are depicted in the plasma. It should be noted that factor XI and high-molecular-weight kininogen also exist in plasma as a complex. When presented with a negatively charged surface (right side of the figure), Hageman factor (factor XII) and the complex of prekallikrein and high-molecular-weight kininogen become bound to the surface. This occurs by virtue of positively charged residues on the heavy chain of Hageman factor (factor XII) and a histidine-rich portion of the light chain of high-molecular-weight kininogen. The Hageman factor (factor XII) and prekallikrein are thus brought into apposition and activation of each takes place. This is aided by apparent conformational changes occurring in the Hageman factor (factor XII) upon surface contact in that the surface-bound molecule is approximately 100 times more sensitive to enzymatic cleavage than the unbound Hageman factor (factor XII). The molecular assembly presumed to lead to activation of factor XI is shown in Fig. 15-4b. The molecules are similar to those in Fig. 15-4a. Kallikrein (Kal) has come from a complex such as that in Fig. 15-4a since kallikrein, but not factor XI, rapidly dissociates from the surface and is more than tenfold more active in stimulating Hageman factor.

NEGATIVELY CHARGED SURFACES THAT ACTIVATE THE CONTACT SYSTEM

A variety of substances have been shown to activate the contact system. A list of nonorganic and organic agents that have been studied appears in Table 15-5.

The importance of negative charges on the surface has been shown by relating the capacity of surfaces to bind basic dyes with their ability to promote activation of Hageman factor (factor XII) and induce clotting [67]. In addition, pretreatment of surfaces with molecules bearing positive charges, such as silicone, hexadimethrine bromide, or cytochrome c, prevents activation of the contact system [68,69].

A discussion of the capacity of several biologically important agents to induce activation of the contact system is given in Ref. 50. The agents include components of connective tissues, e.g., collagen and vascular basement membranes, monosodium urate crystals, bacterial lipopolysaccharides and sulfatides which serve to activate, and antigen-antibody complexes which do not.

The most prominent effect of negatively charged surfaces is undoubtedly produced by the ability of the negative charges to bind Hageman factor (factor XII) and high-molecular-weight kininogen firmly and induce a conformational change in Hageman factor (factor XII) which renders it more susceptible to proteolytic cleavage and activation by kallikrein, as

FIGURE 15-3 Cleavage and activation of Hageman factor (factor XII) by kallikrein. The cleavage occurs initially at site 1, which is associated with activation of the Hageman factor. Cleavage at site 2 follows and results in the release of the active fragment (M_r 28,000 daltons) into fluid phase. The N-terminal end of the molecule is on the left.

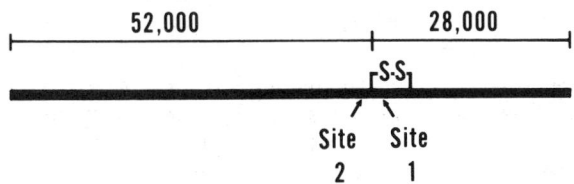

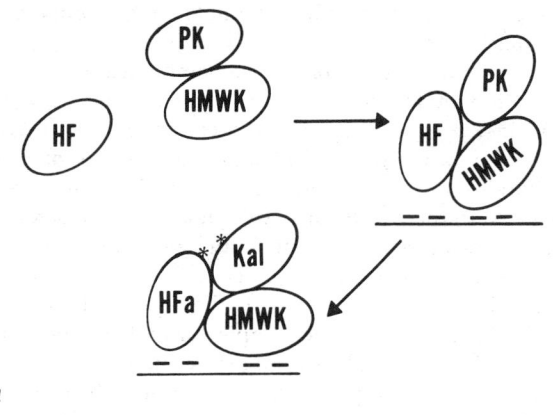

a

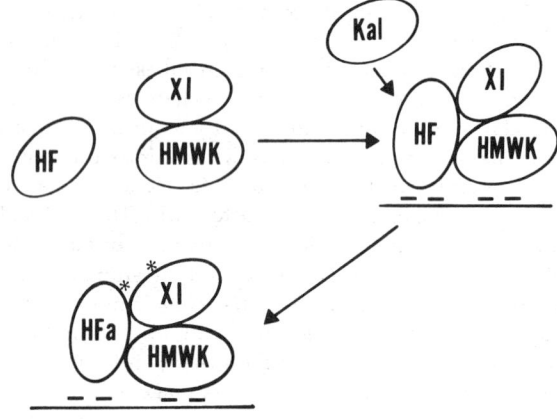

b

FIGURE 15-4 (*a*) **Presumptive assembly of molecules of the contact system on a negatively charged surface to induce activity (see text).** (*b*) **Presumptive assembly of molecules inducing activity of factor XI. Factor XI is dimeric. See text for explanation. HF = Hageman factor (factor XII); HFa = activated Hageman factor (factor XIIa); PK = prekallikrein; Kal = kallikrein; HMWK = high-molecular-weight kininogen; * = active site.**

noted above. The high-molecular-weight kininogen apparently brings its complexed prekallikrein into apposition with the Hageman factor (factor XII). Thus the surface assembles the key components of the system. The complex of factor XI and high-molecular-weight kininogen is also apparently assembled with Hageman factor (factor XII), although the data indicate that the Hageman factor (factor XII) in this latter complex is activated by kallikrein in fluid phase rather than by the factor XI.

REGULATION OF THE CONTACT SYSTEM

INHIBITION OF SURFACE ACTIVATION
Binding of Hageman factor (factor XII) to the surface is inhibited by proteins, including plasma proteins in general. This appears to be competitive in nature, although positively charged proteins are the best. Small, positively charged molecules also prevent activation of the system, even though Hageman factor (factor XII)

TABLE 15-5 Surface activators of the contact system

Inorganic substances	Organic substances
Silica dioxide	Microcrystalline sodium urate
Glass	Bacterial lipopolysaccharide
Kaolin	Ellagic acid
Diatomaceous earth	Carrageenan
Asbestos	Collagen (active, inactive)
Talc	Vascular basement membrane
	Articular cartilage, chrondroitin sulfate
Celite	Long-chain fatty acids
	Heparin
Calcium pyrophosphate	Dextran sulfate
	Glycolipids (sulfatides, ganglioside)
	Skin
	Barium carbonate
	Sulfated cellulose

can bind to the surface. Presumably the competition for negative charges on the surface prevents either conformational changes from occurring in the Hageman factor or prevents appropriate assembly of the trimolecular complex. Among the small, competing molecules that act in this capacity are silicone, hexadimethrine bromide, cytochrome c, lysozyme, polylysine, and protamine.

INHIBITION OF ACTIVATED COMPONENTS
Hageman factor (factor XII) The major inhibitor of enzymatically active Hageman factor (factor XIIa) is C1 inhibitor (C1-In). The reaction between C1 inhibitor and activated Hageman factor (factor XIIa) is stoichiometric and resists boiling in 1% sodium dodecylsulfate. Both forms of activated Hageman factor (M_r 80,000 and 28,000 daltons) bind and are inactivated by C1 inhibitor. A secondary inhibitor in plasma is antithrombin III. The capacity of both this inactivator and C1 inhibitor to inactivate Hageman factor (factor XIIa) is augmented by heparin.

Kallikrein α_2-Macroglobulin and C1 inhibitor are the principal inhibitors of kallikrein, with α_2-macroglobulin accounting for the majority of inhibitor activity.

Factor XI C1 inhibitor and antithrombin III, but not α_2-macroglobulin, account for the inhibition of factor XI in plasma.

THE RELATIONSHIP OF CELLS AND COMPONENTS OF THE CONTACT SYSTEM

ACTIVATION OF COMPONENTS OF THE CONTACT SYSTEM BY CELLULAR CONSTITUENTS
Endothelial cells contain membrane- or vesicle-bound enzymes capable of activating Hageman factor (factor XII). The Hageman factor (factor XII) is cleaved so as to generate the disulfide-linked fragment (M_r 28,000 daltons) which contains the active site [70] (Fig. 15-3).

The enzyme responsible could be distinguished from plasmin and kallikrein and may be related to the plasminogen activator associated with the same cell fractions.

Isolated *mast cells* from human lung tissue and washed fragments of human lung, when stimulated with anti-IgE or sensitized with IgE antibody followed by specific antigen, release several enzymes capable of cleaving Hageman factor (factor XII) and prekallikrein and of releasing bradykinin from high-molecular-weight kininogen [71–73]. In addition to proteolytic enzymes, mast cells contain negatively charged glycosaminoglycans. These substances can act as a surface to activate the contact system similar to kaolin, glass, etc. Thus the mast cells and the allergic reaction may relate closely to the contact system by providing both a negatively charged surface and enzymes capable of activating the system.

Proteolytic enzymes of *neutrophilic leukocytes* have been implicated in the activation of the contact system. Incubation of normal but not Hageman factor–deficient (factor XII–deficient) plasma with human peripheral leukocytes (principally neutrophils) releases kinin activity and depletes available kininogen [74–79]. However, a question as to whether neutrophil elastase is responsible for a direct action on high-molecular-weight kininogen has been in dispute [76–79].

REACTIONS OF COMPONENTS OF THE
CONTACT SYSTEM WITH CELLS
An initial observation that kallikrein induced chemotactic movement of human neutrophils [80] remained unconfirmed by others. The difficulty in repeating the observation may be explained by the finding that when C5 is present, chemotaxis of rabbit neutrophils is generated by kallikrein [81]. Presumably, small amounts of C5a are generated by the kallikrein.

The contact system proteins may activate on the surface of stimulated platelets. ADP-stimulated platelets exert a procoagulant activity in plasma that is partially dependent upon Hageman factor (factor XII) [82]. Stimulated platelets augment the activation of Hageman factor (factor XII) by kallikrein and the activation of factor XI by Hageman factor–dependent (factor XII–dependent) and –independent mechanisms.

PATHOPHYSIOLOGIC ACTIONS OF THE
COMPONENTS OF THE CONTACT SYSTEM

HAGEMAN FACTOR (FACTOR XII) AND THE
PERMEABILITY FACTOR OF DILUTION (PF/DIL)
Activation of the contact system has long been associated with the generation of a permeability activity [83]. Hageman factor, when activated, induces an increased vascular permeability [84] with as little as 1 ng (3×10^{-10} M), yielding increased vascular permeability [85]. This is about 10 to 100 times more active than bradykinin.

Dilution of plasma in the presence of a negatively charged surface induces a factor (PF/dil) that increases the permeability of blood vessels [86,87]. The PF/dil was later found to be identical to activated Hageman factor (factor XIIa) [88], since the activity and radiolabeled Hageman factor (factor XII) were simultaneously removed from diluted plasmas upon absorption with insolubilized antibodies to Hageman factor (factor XII).

Arterial hypotension is induced by protein preparations that have been shown to contain active Hageman factor (factor XIIa) [89], and purified activated Hageman factor (factor XIIa) has recently been shown in the authors' laboratory to induce profound hypotension and leukopenia.

Leukocyte accumulation in vascular beds in rabbit ear chambers results when human Hageman factor (factor XII) is applied. The reaction reaches a maximum in about 90 minutes [90].

High-molecular-weight kininogen High- and low-molecular-weight kininogens are the parent molecules of bradykinin. Kallikrein releases bradykinin by proteolytic cleavage only from high-molecular-weight kininogen. Thus during activation of the contact system, only high-molecular-weight kininogen is involved. Other arginine proteases release kinin from low-molecular-weight kininogen. Aside from the biologically potent bradykinin, high-molecular-weight kininogen also contains a histidine-rich fragment which lies at the immediate N-terminal side of bradykinin on the light chain of the parent molecule. In the case of bovine high-molecular-weight kininogen, this fragment is released by the action of kallikrein and has been shown to increase vascular permeability and contract smooth muscle [91,92]. While its potency is less than that of bradykinin when tested in soluble form, it must be remembered that the high concentration of histidine residues is responsible for anchoring the parent molecule to negatively charged structures. Since such structures could be vascular basement membranes, the biologic importance of this fragment could be great.

Bradykinin The physiologic and pathologic effects of bradykinin are of extreme diversity and have received intensive study over the past three to four decades. Increase in vascular permeability, smooth-muscle contraction, diminished arterial resistance and hypotension, vascular margination and infiltration of leukocytes into tissues, and pain are among the common responses to bradykinin. Bradykinin has been found in plasma and joint fluid in experimental and clinical inflammatory disease. The reader is referred to compilations of studies of kinins [93–95].

CONTACT ACTIVATION SYSTEM AND THE
PLASMA RENIN–ANGIOTENSIN SYSTEM
The plasma kallikrein–kinin system and the plasma renin–angiotensin system exhibit a number of interesting relationships. Bradykinin is hypotensive, whereas angiotensin II is hypertensive. The dipeptidase-converting enzyme, found principally in pul-

monary endothelium, generates angiotensin II from a less active peptide, angiotensin I, by cleaving off a dipeptide. The same proteolytic enzyme destroys bradykinin by eliminating its C-terminal dipeptide, Phe-Arg.

It has been shown that in vitro activation of plasma prorenin can be effected via factor XIIa and kallikrein. Experiments employing plasmas deficient in Hageman factor (factor XII) or prekallikrein indicated that these proteins are essential for these in vitro activations of prorenin [96,97]. Normal prorenin activation is restored by addition of kallikrein to plasma deficient in Hageman factor (factor XII), but not by addition of activated Hageman factor of M_r 28,000 daltons to prekallikrein-deficient plasma [98,99]. Prekallikrein apparently influences the physiologic percentage of renin versus prorenin, since the level of prorenin is abnormally high and the level of renin is abnormally low in plasma from patients with prekallikrein deficiency [98]. Thus a connection between the contact system and the prorenin-angiotensin system is apparent.

THE PARTICIPATION OF THE CONTACT SYSTEM IN DISEASE

It is clear from the preceding discussion that the components of the contact system can contribute to pathophysiologic changes. It has been difficult, as with the complement system, to define with consistency any essential participation of the components in a given disease, since several pathways can participate simultaneously, making it difficult to identify the essentiality of any one. This reasoning also applies to the phenomenon that with factor XI or Hageman factor (factor XII) deficiency (and prekallikrein and high-molecular-weight kininogen deficiency as well), there is little tendency for individuals to bleed. Only in occasional patients with a deficiency of factor XI is this seen, although the numbers of patients with deficiencies of the other contact system proteins are too few to draw firm conclusions. The extrinsic clotting system is functional in such individuals and probably provides adequate clotting when required in vivo.

There is growing evidence that components of the contact system participate in several human diseases. These include bacteremic shock, arthritis, allergic and anaphylactic reactions, hereditary angioedema, and others. Much of this information has been reviewed [50]. With purified components and sensitive means of detection, significant progress should be made in analyzing the role of these proteins in various diseases.

References

1. Reid, K. B. M., and Porter, R. R.: The proteolytic activation systems of complement. *Ann. Rev. Biochem. 50*:433, 1981.
2. Cooper, N. R., and Ziccardi, R. J.: The nature and reaction of complement enzymes, in *Proteolysis and Physiological Regulation*, edited by D. W. Ribbons and K. Brew. Academic, New York, 1976, Miami Winter Symposium, vol. 11, pp. 167–187.
3. Müller-Eberhard, H. J.: Complement. *Ann. Rev. Biochem. 44*:697, 1975.
4. Day, N. K., and Good, R. A. (eds.): *Comprehensive Immunology, Biological Amplification Systems in Immunology*. Plenum, New York, 1977, vol. 2.
5. Cooper, N. R.: Activation of the complement system. *Contemp. Top. Mol. Immunol. 2*:155, 1974.
6. Cooper, N. R.: Laboratory evaluation of complement activation, in *Future Perspectives in Clinical Laboratory Immunoassays*, edited by R. M. Nakamura. Liss, New York, 1980, pp. 393.
7. Porter, R. R., and Reid, K. B. M.: Activation of the complement system by antibody antigen complexes: The classical pathway. *Adv. Prot. Chem. 33*:1, 1979.
8. Lepow, H., Naff, G. B., Todd, E. W., Pensky, J., and Hinz, C. F.: Chromatographic resolution of the first component of complement into three activities. *J. Exp. Med. 117*:983, 1963.
9. Taranta, A., and Franklin, E. C.: Complement fixation by antibody fragments. *Science 134*:1981, 1961.
10. Cooper, N. R., Jensen, F. C., Welsh, R. M., Jr., and Oldstone, M. B. A: Lysis of RNA tumor viruses by human serum: Direct antibody independent triggering of the classical complement pathway. *J. Exp. Med. 144*:970, 1976.
11. Calcott, M. A., and Müller-Eberhard, H. J.: C1q protein of human complement. *Biochemistry 11*:3443, 1972.
12. Shelton, E., Yonemasu, K., and Stroud, R. M.: Ultrastructure of human complement component C1q. *Proc. Natl. Acad. Sci. U.S.A. 69*:65, 1972.
13. Müller-Eberhard, H. J.: Complement. *Ann. Rev. Biochem. 38*:389, 1969.
14. Ziccardi, R. J., and Cooper, N. R.: Activation of C1r by proteolytic cleavage. *J. Immunol. 116*:504, 1976.
15. Valet, G., and Cooper, N. R.: Isolation and characterization of the proenzyme form of the C1s subunit of the first complement component. *J. Immunol. 112*:339, 1974.
16. Becker, E. L.: Concerning the mechanism of complement action. II. The nature of the first component of guinea pig complement. *J. Immunol. 77*:469, 1956.
17. Lepow, I. H., Ratnoff, O. D. Rosen, F. S., and Pillemer, L.: Observations on a pro-esterase associated with partially purified first component of human complement. *Proc. Soc. Exp. Biol. Med. 92*:32, 1956.
18. Müller-Eberhard, H. J., Polley, M. J., and Calcott, M. A.: Formation and functional significance of a molecular complex derived from the second and fourth component of human complement. *J. Exp. Med. 125*:359, 1967.
19. Müller-Eberhard, H. J., and Lepow, I. H.: C1 esterase effect on activity and physicochemical properties of the fourth component of complement. *J. Exp. Med. 121*:819, 1965.
20. Polley, M. J., and Müller-Eberhard, H. J.: The second component of human complement. Its isolation, fragmentation by C1 esterase and incorporation into C3 convertase. *J. Exp. Med. 128*:533, 1968.
21. Bokisch, V. A., Müller-Eberhard, H. J., and Cochrane, C. G.: Isolation of a fragment (C3a) of the third component of human complement containing anaphylatoxin and chemotactic activity and a description of an anaphylatoxin inactivator of human serum. *J. Exp. Med. 129*:1109, 1969.
22. Müller-Eberhard, H. J., Dalmasso, A. P., and Calcott, M. A.: The reaction mechanism of βIC globulin in immune hemolysis. *J. Exp. Med. 123*:33, 1966.
23. Tack, B. F., Harrison, R. A., Janatova, J., Thomas, M. L., and Prahl, J. W.: Evidence for the presence of an internal thiolester bond in the third component of human complement. *Proc. Natl. Acad. Sci. U.S.A. 77*:5764, 1980.
24. Campbell, F. D., Gagnon, J., and Porter, R. R.: Amino acid sequence around the proposed thiolester bond of human complement component C4 and comparison with the corresponding sequences from C3 and α2 macroglobulin. *Biosci. Rep. 1*:423, 1981.
25. Müller-Eberhard, H. J., and Schreiber, R. D.: Molecular biology and chemistry of the alternative pathway of complement. *Adv. Immunol. 29*:1, 1980.
26. Fearon, D. T., and Austen, K. F.: Initiation of C3 cleavage in the alternative complement pathway. *J. Immunol. 115*:1357, 1975.
27. Pangburn, M. K., and Müller-Eberhard, H. J.: Relation of a putative

thiolester bond in C3 to activation of the alternative pathway and the binding of C3b to biological targets to complement. *J. Exp. Med.* 152:1102, 1980.

28. Pangburn, M. K., Schreiber, R. D., and Müller-Eberhard, H. J.: Formation of the initial C3 convertase of the alternative complement pathway: Acquisition of C3b like activities by spontaneous hydrolysis of the putative thiolester in native C3. *J. Exp. Med.* 154:856, 1981.

29. Fearon, D. T., and Austen, K. F.: Activation of the alternative complement pathway with rabbit erythrocytes by circumvention of the regulatory action of endogenous control proteins. *J. Exp. Med.* 146:22, 1977.

30. Daha, M. R., Fearon, D. T., and Austen, K. F.: C3 nephritic factor (C3NeF): Stabilization of fluid phase and cell bound alternative pathway convertase. *J. Immunol.* 116:1, 1976.

31. Müller-Eberhard, H. J.: Complement reaction pathways, in *Progress in Immunology.* Academic, 1980, vol. IV, pp. 1001–1024.

32. Mayer, M. M.: Mechanism of cytolysis by complement. *Proc. Natl. Acad. Sci. U.S.A.* 69:2954, 1972.

33. Podack, E. R., Biesecker, G., Kolb, W. P., and Müller-Eberhard, H. J.: The C5b–6 complex: Reaction with C7, C8, C9. *J. Immunol.* 121:484, 1978.

34. Podack, E. R., Biesecker, G., and Müller-Eberhard, H. J.: Membrane attack complex of complement: Generation of high affinity binding site, by fusion of five hydrophilic plasma proteins. *Proc. Natl. Acad. Sci. U.S.A.* 76:897, 1979.

35. Podack, E. F., and Müller-Eberhard, H. J.: Isolation of human S-protein, an inhibitor of the membrane attack complex of complement. *J. Biol. Chem.* 254:9908, 1979.

36. Esser, A. F., Kolb, W. P., Podack, E. R., and Müller-Eberhard, H. J.: Molecular reorganization of lipid bilayers by complement: A possible mechanism for membranolysis. *Proc. Natl. Acad. Sci. U.S.A.* 76:1410, 1979.

37. Fujita, T., Gigli, I., and Nussenzweig, V.: Human C4 binding protein. I. Role in proteolysis of C4b and C3b inactivator. *J. Exp. Med.* 148:1044, 1978.

38. Whaley, K., and Ruddy, S.: Modulation of C3b hemolytic activity by a plasma protein distinct from C3b inactivator. *Science* 193:1011, 1976.

39. Pangburn, M. K., Schreiber, R. D., and Müller-Eberhard, H. J.: Human complement C3b inactivator: Isolation, characterization and demonstration of an absolute requirement for the serum protein β1H for cleavage of C3b and C4b in solution. *J. Exp. Med.* 146:257, 1977.

40. Bokisch, V. A., and Müller-Eberhard, H. J.: Anaphylatoxin inactivator of human plasma: Its isolation and characterization as a carboxypeptidase. *J. Clin. Invest.* 49:2427, 1970.

41. Esser, A. E.: Interactions between complement proteins and biological and model membranes, in *Biological Membranes,* edited by D. Chapman. Academic, London, 1982, vol. 4, p. 277.

42. Ross, G. D.: Analysis of the different types of leukocyte complement receptors and their interaction with the complement system. *J. Immunol. Methods* 37:197, 1980.

43. Fearon, D. T.: Identification of the membrane glycoprotein that is the C3b receptor of the human erythrocyte, polymorphonuclear leukocyte, B lymphocyte and the monocyte. *J. Exp. Med.* 152:20, 1980.

44. Hugli, T. E.: The structural basis for anaphylatoxin and chemotactic functions of C3a, C4a and C5a. *CRC Crit. Rev. Immunol.* 1(4):321, 1981.

45. Dixon, F. J., and Wilson, C. B.: Immunologic renal injury produced by formation and deposition of immune complexes, in *Immunologic Mechanisms of Renal Disease; Contemporary Issues in Nephrology,* edited by C. B. Wilson, B. M. Brenner, and J. H. Stein. Churchill Livingstone, New York, 1979, vol. 3, p. 1.

46. Cochrane, C. G., and Dixon, F. J.: Antigen-antibody complex induced disease, in *Textbook of Immunopathology,* edited by P. A. Miescher and H. J. Müller-Eberhard. Grune & Stratton, New York, 1976, vol 1, p. 137.

47. Opferkuch, W., Rother, K., and Schultz, D. R. (eds.): *Clinical Aspects of the Complement System.* Thieme, Stuttgart, 1978.

48. Ruddy, S., et al.: Human complement metabolism: An analysis of 144 studies. *Medicine* 54:165, 1975.

49. Lachmann, P. J., and Rosen, F. S.: Genetic defects of complement in man. *Springer Seminar Immunopathol.* 1:339, 1978.

50. Cochrane, C. G., and Griffin, J. H.: The biochemistry and pathophysiology of the contact system of plasma, in *Advances in Immunology,* edited by F. J. Dixon and H. G. Kunkel. Academic, New York, 1982, vol. 33.

51. Revak, S. D., and Cochrane, C. G.: The relationship of structure and function in human Hageman factor. The association of enzymatic and binding activities with separate regions of the molecule. *J. Clin. Invest.* 57:852, 1976.

52. Cochrane, C. G., Revak, S. D., and Wuepper, K. D.: The activation of Hageman factor in solid and fluid phases. A critical role. *J. Exp. Med.* 138:1564, 1973.

53. Griffin, J. H.: The role of surface in the surface-dependent activation of Hageman factor (factor XII). *Proc. Natl. Acad. Sci. U.S.A.* 75:1998, 1978.

54. Wuepper, K. D.: Prekallikrein deficiency in man. *J. Exp. Med.* 138:1345, 1973.

55. Mandle, R., Colman, R. W., and Kaplan, A. P.: Identification of prekallikrein and high molecular weight kininogen as a complex in human plasma. *Proc. Natl. Acad. Sci. U.S.A.* 11:4179, 1976.

56. Thompson, E., Mandle, R., and Kaplan, A. P.: Association of factor XI and high molecular weight kininogen in human plasma. *J. Clin. Invest.* 60:1376, 1977.

57. Griffin, J. H., and Cochrane, C. G.: Mechanisms for the involvement of high molecular weight kininogen in surface-dependent reactions of Hageman factor. *Proc. Natl. Acad. Sci. U.S.A.* 73:2554, 1976.

58. Wiggins, R. C., Bouma, B. N., Cochrane, C. G., and Griffin, J. H.: Role of high molecular weight kininogen in surface-binding and activation of coagulation factor XI and prekallikrein (Hageman factor, contact activation, fibrinolysis). *Proc. Natl. Acad. Sci. U.S.A.* 74:4636, 1977.

59. Han, Y. N., Komiya, M., Iwanaga, S., and Suzuki, T.: Studies on the primary structure of bovine high molecular weight kininogen. *J. Biochem.* 77:55, 1975.

60. Waldman, R., et al.: Significant role of fragment 1-2 plus light chain of bovine high molecular weight kininogen in contact mediated coagulation. *Thromb. Haemost.* 38:14, 1977.

61. Thompson, R. E., Mandle, R., and Kaplan, A. P.: Characterization of human MWK kininogen: Procoagulant activity associated with the light chain of kinin-free HMW-kininogen. *J. Exp. Med.* 147:488, 1978.

62. Meier, H. K., Webster, M. E., Mandle, R., Colman, R. W., and Kaplan, A. P.: Enhancement of surface dependent Hageman factor activation by high molecular weight kininogen. *J. Clin. Invest.* 60:18, 1977.

63. Cochrane, C. G., and Revak, S. D.: Dissemination of contact activation in plasma by plasma kallikrein. *J. Exp. Med.* 152:608, 1980.

64. Revak, S. D., Cochrane, C. G., and Griffin, J. H.: The binding and cleaving characteristics of human Hageman factor during contact activation. A comparison of normal plasma with plasmas deficient in factor XI, prekallikrein, or high molecular weight kininogen. *J. Clin. Invest.* 59:1167, 1977.

65. Griffin, J. H.: Molecular mechanism of surface-dependent activation of Hageman factor (coagulation factor XII). *Fed. Proc.* 36:324, 1977.

66. Fujikawa, K., Walsh, K. A., and Davie, E. W.: Isolation and characterization of bovine factor XII (Hageman factor). *Biochemistry* 16:2270, 1977.

67. Margolis, J.: The interrelationship of coagulation of plasma and release of peptides. *Ann. N.Y. Acad. Sci.* 104:133, 1963.

68. Eisen, V.: Effect of hexadimethrine bromide on plasma kinin formation, hydrolysis of p-tosyl-L-arginine methylester and fibrinolysis. *Br. J. Pharmacol.* 22:87, 1964.

69. Nossel, H. L., Rubin, H., Drillings, H., and Haich, R.: Inhibition of Hageman factor activation. *J. Clin. Invest.* 47:1172, 1968.

70. Wiggins, R. C., Loskutoff, D. J., Cochrane, C. G., Griffin, J. H., and Edgington, T. S.: Activation of rabbit Hageman factor by homogenates of cultured rabbit endothelial cells. *J. Clin. Invest.* 65:197, 1980.

71. Newball, H. H., Talamo, R., and Lichtenstein, L.: Release of leukocyte kallikrein mediated by IgE. *Nature* 254:635, 1975.

72. Newball, H. H., Berninger, R. W., Talamo, R. C., and Lichtenstein, L. M.: Anaphylactic release of a basophil kallikrein-like activity. I.

Purification and characterization. *J. Clin. Invest. 64:*457, 1979.

73. Newball, H. H., Talamo, R., and Lichtenstein, L.: Anaphylactic release of a basophil kallikrein-like activity. II. A mediator of immediate hypersensitivity reactions. *J. Clin. Invest. 64:*466, 1979.

74. Melmon, K. L., and Cline, M. J.: Interaction of plasma kinins and granulocytes. *Nature 213:*90, 1967.

75. Melmon, K. L., and Cline, M. J.: The interaction of leukocytes and the kinin system. *Biochem. Pharmacol. 17 (Suppl.):*271, 1968.

76. Movat, H. Z., Habal, F. M., and MacMorine, D. R. L.: Neutral proteases of human PMN leukocytes with kininogenase activity. *Int. Arch. Allergy. Appl. Immunol. 50:*257, 1976.

77. Wasi, S., Movat, H. Z., Pass, E., and Chan, J. Y. C.: Production, conversion and destinations of kinins by human neutrophil leukocyte proteases, in *Neutral Proteases of Human Polymorphonuclear Leukocytes,* edited by K. Havermann and A. Janoff. Urban and Schwartzenback, Baltimore-Munich, 1978, p. 245.

78. Fritz, H.: Necessity for critical consideration of the homogeneity of polymorphonuclear leukocyte protease applied to biological systems: Failure to detect intrinsic kininogenase activity in PMN elastase, in *Neutral Proteases of Human Polymorphonuclear Leukocytes,* edited by K. Havermann and A. Janoff. Urban and Schwartzenback, Baltimore-Munich, 1978. p. 261.

79. Dittmann, B., Weimer, R., Mindermann, R., and Ohlsson, K.: The effect of human granulocyte proteinases on kininogens, in *Kinins— II; Systemic Proteases and Cellular Function,* edited by S. Fujii, H. Moriya, and T. Suzuki. Plenum, New York, 1979, p. 297.

80. Kaplan, A. P., and Austen, K. F.: The fibrinolytic pathway of human plasma. Isolation and characterization of the plasminogen proactivator. *J. Exp. Med. 136:*1378, 1972.

81. Wiggins, R. C., Giclas, P. C., Henson, P. M.: Chemotactic activity generated from the fifth component of complement by plasma kallikrein of the rabbit. *J. Exp. Med. 153:*1391, 1981.

82. Walsh, P. N.: The effects of collagen and kaolin on the intrinsic coagulant activity of platelets. Evidence for an alternative pathway in intrinsic coagulation not requiring factor XII. *Br. J. Haematol. 22:*393, 1972.

83. Armstrong, D., Keele, C. A., Jipson, J. B., and Stewart, J. W.: Development of pain-producing substance in human plasma. *Nature 174:*791, 1954.

84. Ratnoff, O. D., and Miles, A. A.: The induction of permeability increasing activity in human plasma by activated Hageman factor. *Br. J. Exp. Pathol. 45:*328, 1964.

85. Yamamoto, T., and Cochrane, C. G.: Guinea pig Hageman factor as a vascular permeability enhancement factor. *Am. J. Pathol. 105:*164, 1981.

86. Miles, A. A., and Wilhelm, D. L.: Enzyme-like globulins from serum reproducing the vascular phenomena of inflammation. I. An activatable permeability factor and its inhibitors in guinea-pig serum. *Br. J. Exp. Pathol. 36:*71, 1955.

87. Wilhelm, D. L., Mill, P. J., Sparrow, E. M., Mackey, M. E., and Miles, A. A.: Enzyme-like globulins from serum reproducing the vascular phenomena of inflammation. IV. Activatable permeability factor and its inhibitor in the serum of the rat and the rabbit. *Br. J. Exp. Pathol. 39:*228, 1958.

88. Johnston, A. R., Cochrane, C. G., and Revak, S. D.: The relationship between PF/dil and activated human Hageman factor. *J. Immunol. 113:*103, 1974.

89. Alving, B. M., et al.: Hypotension association with prekallikrein activator (Hageman-factor fragments) in plasma protein fraction. *N. Engl. J. Med. 299:*66, 1978.

90. Graham, R., Ebert, R. H., Ratnoff, O. D., and Moses, J. M.: Pathogenesis of inflammation. II. *In vivo* observations of the inflammatory effects of activated Hageman factor and bradykinin. *J. Exp. Med. 121:*807, 1965.

91. Matheson, R. T., et al.: Flaujeac factor deficiency. Reconstitution with highly purified bovine high molecular weight-kininogen and delineation of a new permeability-enhancing peptide released by plasma kallikrein from bovine high molecular weight-kininogen. *J. Clin. Invest. 58:*1395, 1976.

92. Oh-Ishi, S., Katori, M., Han, Y. N., Kanagawa, S., Kato, H., and Suzuki, T.: Possible physiological role of new peptide fragments released from bovine high molecular weight kininogen by plasma kallikrein. *Biochem. Pharmacol. 26:*115, 1977.

93. Pisano, J. J., and Austen, K. F. (eds.): *Chemistry and Biology of the Kallikrein-Kinin System in Health and Disease.* DHEW Publication No. (NIH) 76–791, 1976.

94. Fujii, S., Moriya, H., and Suzuki, T. (eds.): *Kinins II.* Plenum, New York, 1979.

95. Erdos, E. (ed.): Bradykinin, kallidin, and kallikrein (supplement), in *Handbook of Experimental Pharmacology.* Springer-Verlag, New York, 1979, vol. 25.

96. Osmond, D. H., Lo, E. K., Loh, A. Y., Zingg, E. A., and Hedlin, A. H.: Kallikrein and plasmin as activators of inactive renin. *Lancet 2:*1375, 1978.

97. Millar, J. A., Clappison, B. H., and Johnston, C. I.: Kallikrein and plasmin as activators of inactive renin. *Lancet 2:*1376, 1978.

98. Derkx, F. H. M., Bouma, B. N., Schalekamp, M. P. A., and Schalekamp, M. A. D. H.: An intrinsic factor XII-prekallikrein-dependent pathway activates the human plasma renin-angiotensin system. *Nature 280:*315, 1979.

99. Sealey, J., Atlas, S. A., Laragh, J. H., Silverberg, M. J., and Kaplan, A. P.: Initiation of plasma prorenin activation by Hageman factor-dependent conversion of plasma prekallikrein to kallikrein. *Proc. Natl. Acad. Sci. U.S.A. 76:*5914, 1979.

Genetics

CHAPTER 16

Genetic principles

ERNEST BEUTLER

All the information required for the development of a complete adult organism is contained in a single cell, the zygote. This includes the data needed for the synthesis of all the enzymes of energy metabolism; the plasma proteins, including the clotting factors and complement components; the transport proteins; proteins that form the membranes of cells, and those that participate in the synthesis of complex lipids, carbohydrates, lipoproteins, and glycoproteins. It contains all the information required for the formation of cells, the regulation of their proliferation, their assembly into tissues, and the development of these tissues into organs.

Understanding how this massive amount of information is coded has been one of the major advances of modern biology. The information is all contained in chromosomal polynucleotides, deoxyribonucleic acid (DNA). DNA contains only four different bases—adenine, guanine, thymine, and cytosine. It is in the form of a double helix in which adenine is always paired with thymine and guanine is always paired with cytosine. It is this pairing of bases which makes possible the accurate replication of the genetic code during cell division: when the two DNA strands separate, the bases of the separate strands pair with the complementary bases so that two double strands that are identical with the original double strand are formed.

The sequence of base pairs in the DNA strand specifies the sequence of amino acids in proteins. Each base cannot represent a single amino acid, since only four bases are found in DNA and there are 20 commonly occurring amino acids in proteins. Similarly, pairs of bases are not sufficient; they could code for only 16 amino acids. A triplet code is therefore the minimum number of bases which would be required to code for 20 amino acids. The genetic code has been found in fact to consist of triplets: each amino acid is specified by one or more sequences of three bases. Long stretches of the triplet code are colinear with the amino acid sequence of the protein the synthesis of which the gene specifies, but these stretches are separated by intervening se-quences or introns that do not code for the amino acid sequence of the protein. Moreover, DNA does not directly assemble amino acids into protein. This assembly is carried out through a mechanism which involves another polynucleotide, ribonucleic acid (RNA). Messenger ribonucleic acid (mRNA) polymerizes, using the nuclear DNA as a template, and moves into the cytoplasm. After the intervening sequences which have been transcribed into RNA are excised, the processed messenger forms a template for the linear assembly of amino acids in the order which was specified by the DNA.

Chromosomes

It has been known since the early part of this century that genetic information is carried on the chromosomes. Indistinct, tangled threads during most of the cell cycle, chromosomes condense into clearly visible rodlike structures in metaphase. The development of relatively simple techniques for short-term in vitro culture of cells, arrest of cell division at metaphase with colchicine, and the preparation of chromosome "spreads" have made it possible to count, sort, and classify human chromosomes in health and in disease. The development of special methods of staining, especially with Giemsa stain and quinacrine mustard, has disclosed characteristic banding patterns in chromosomes which allow differentiation of similar but distinct chromosome pairs to a degree not previously possible. Figure 16-1 illustrates the normal human karyotype as prepared from a dividing blood cell, presumably a lymphocyte. The chromosomes are arranged into groups which depend on their size and the position of the centromere (the last portion of the chromosome to divide during mitosis).

When chromosome preparations are made from the blood of persons without circulating blast cells, most of the dividing cells are lymphocytes. Such preparations are very useful in the detection of chromosomal abnormalities which affect all body cells. In Down's syndrome, for example, there are three chromosomes 21, designated *trisomy 21*; most patients with Turner's syndrome have an XO karyotype, indicating only one X chromosome and no Y chromosome; in Klinefelter's syndrome, there are two or more X chromosomes and one Y chromosome (XXY). To detect chromosomal abnormalities in the myeloid series it is necessary to examine a marrow aspirate, unless substantial numbers of early myeloid cells are present in the peripheral circulation. A high percentage of patients with chronic myelogenous leukemia manifest a characteristic translocation from the long arm of chromosome 22, usually to the long arm of chromosome 9 [2] (Fig. 16-2). The chromosome with the deletion, designated the *Philadelphia chromosome* after the city in which it was discovered by Nowell and Hungerford [3], is a hallmark of chronic

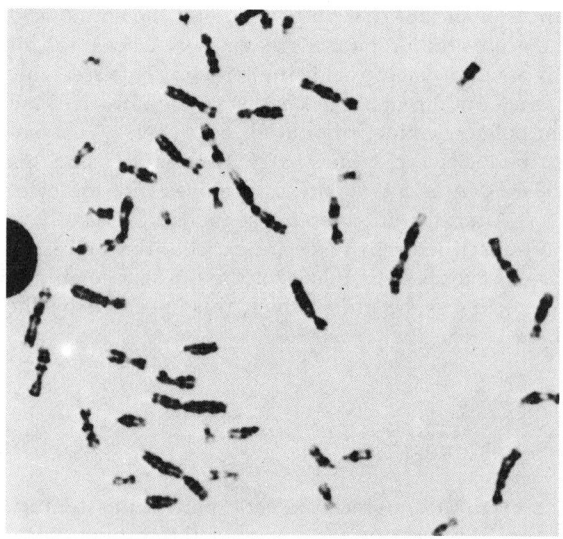

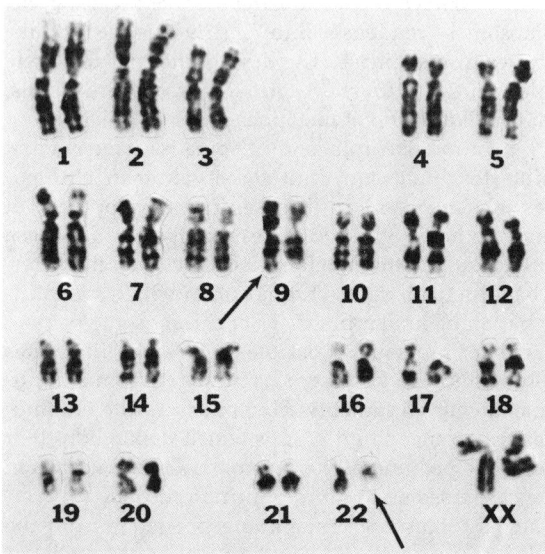

FIGURE 16-1   A normal male human marrow-cell karyotype stained with the acetic-saline-Giemsa method [1] to show the banding pattern of the chromosomes. (Courtesy of Dr. Raymond Teplitz.)

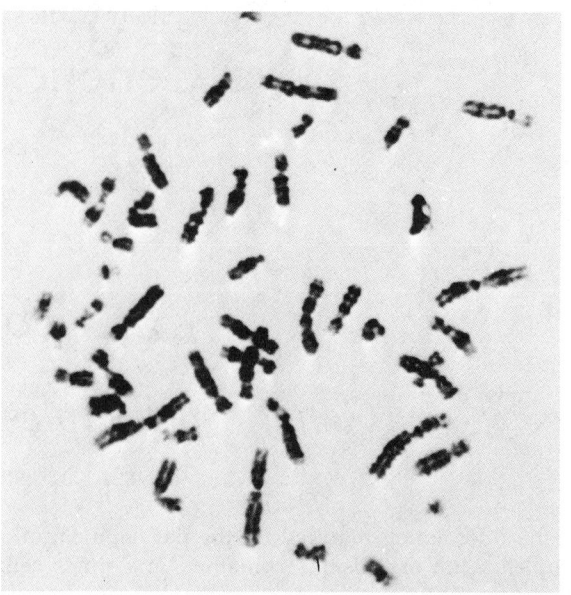

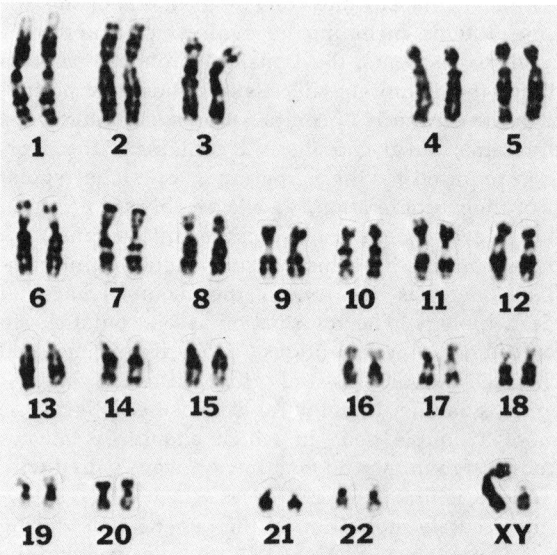

FIGURE 16-2   Karyotype of a marrow cell from a female patient with chronic granulocytic leukemia. A fragment has been lost from chromosome 22 and translocated to chromosome 9. The preparation is stained with the acetic-saline-Giemsa method [1] to show banding pattern. (Courtesy of Dr. Raymond Teplitz.)

myelogenous leukemia (see Chap. 24). Sporadic reports of chromosomal abnormalities in chronic lymphocytic leukemia presumably represent coincidental deviations of the karyotype from normal and bear no etiologic relationship to this disorder (Chap. 115).

In acute leukemia, striking abnormalities in chromosome number (aneuploidy) and type are often observed. Although there is not a characteristic pattern of abnormality, as is observed in chronic granulocytic leukemia, it has been shown that certain abnormal chromosome patterns are encountered repeatedly among such patients [4,5].

Linkage

In somatic cells chromosomes are present in pairs—one pair of sex chromosomes (two X chromosomes in females and an X and a Y in males) and, in humans, 22 pairs of autosomes. One chromosome of each pair is distributed into the gametes, so that eggs and sperm of humans each contain 23 chromosomes.

If two genes are located on different chromosomes or are far apart on the same chromosome, they are said to be *unlinked*: the offspring of a carrier of these two genes has one chance in two of inheriting each of the mutant genes, and the probability of inheriting each of the mutant genes, one or the other, both, or neither is governed purely by the laws of chance. For example, if a woman is a carrier of hereditary spherocytosis (HS) and of sickle cell trait, two genes which are presumably on different autosomes, the probabilities of inheritance of HS, on the one hand, and sickle cell trait, on the other, are entirely independent. One-fourth the offspring will inherit both HS and sickle cell trait, one-fourth the offspring will inherit neither, one-fourth will inherit only sickle cell trait, and one-fourth will inherit only HS.

If the two genes in question are close together on the same chromosome, however, the situation may be quite different. For example, the genes for hemophilia A and for glucose-6-phosphate dehydrogenase (G-6-PD) deficiency are both sex-linked. If a woman carried both these genes on one of her X chromosomes, the probability of her child's inheriting either both the abnormal genes or neither of the abnormal genes is much greater than the probability of its inheriting one or the other. Yet the inheritance of only one of these two genes is not an impossibility, because of the phenomenon of crossing-over during meiosis. In the course of the formation of germ cells, homologous pairs of chromosomes come into side-by-side apposition and exchange chromosomal material. Thus two genes which were originally on the same chromosome may find themselves on separate chromosomes after germ-cell formation (see Fig. 16-3). The probability of their being separated during meiosis is a function of their distance from one another on the chromosome, and this distance is expressed in terms of *map units*. It is not unusual for genes on the same chromosome to be so far apart that the probability of their finding themselves in separate germ cells is just as great as if they had been on separate chromosomes. For this reason, genes on the same chromosome may be linked but can also be unlinked; in the latter case they are referred to as *syntenic*. G-6-PD and hemophilia A are both on the X chromosome with a map distance estimated at approximately 4 units [6]. Therefore, if two mutant genes at this locus are on the same chromosome

in a female, there is a 4 percent chance of the genes being in separate gametes. The genes for both G-6-PD and the Xg blood group are also on the X chromosome, but are apparently unlinked [7].

Gene duplication

Crossing-over during meiosis usually occurs with great precision. Homologous genes pair with each other, and although genes which were together on one chromosome before meiosis may now be on opposite chromosomes of the pair, each chromosome still contains a complete set of genes (Fig. 16-3). Occasionally, however, an error occurs and pairing during meiosis is imperfect. Under these circumstances—unequal crossing-over (Fig. 16-4)—one of the daughter chromosomes contains a duplicated gene, while the other one exists with a deleted gene.

Once a duplication has occurred, further duplications occur more readily, because pairing of the first of the duplicate genes on one chromosome with the second gene of the duplicate on the other produces one chromosome with a triplicated gene and one with a single gene. Duplication has probably played a very important role in the course of evolution [8], because the presence of two genes with the same function allows experiments of nature, mutations, to occur on one of the genes without totally losing the original function, which is still carried out by the duplicate. Examples of the results of gene duplication abound in hematology, particularly with respect to the hemoglobin loci. The α-chain loci are duplicated, and there are also two nearly identical copies of the γ-chain locus (see Chap. 60). Furthermore, the close similarity of their amino acid sequence and the fact that they are tightly linked indicate that the β, γ, and δ loci represent the result of duplication of a single ancestral gene. The process of unequal crossing-over takes place not only between genes, but also within genes. When this occurs, one would anticipate that a portion of the amino acid sequence of a protein is represented twice on one chromosome and is missing on

FIGURE 16-3   Schematic representation of equal crossing-over during meiosis. There has been an exchange of chromosomal material between the maternally derived and paternally derived chromosome, but all genes are represented on the products of the crossover.

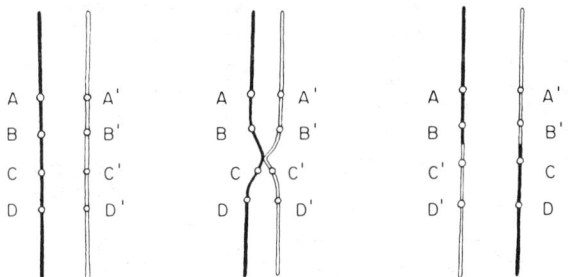

FIGURE 16-4   Schematic representation of unequal crossing-over during meiosis. Crossing-over has occurred between non-homologous sites of the paternally derived and maternally derived chromosome. As a result, one of the two chromosomes formed contains a duplicated C locus, while the other has had this locus deleted.

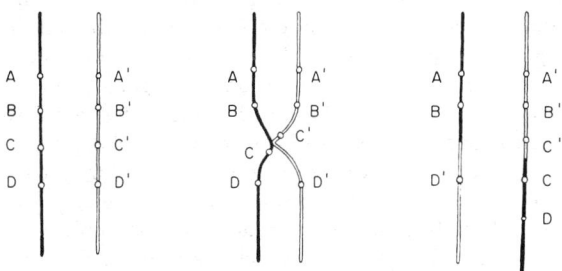

the other. The Lepore hemoglobins, leading to a thalassemic clinical state, are the best example of this type of unequal crossing-over (see Fig. 16-4). These abnormal hemoglobins have the amino acid sequence of the δ chain at the amino end and the sequence of the β chain at the carboxyl end (see Chap. 50). The complement to this kind of abnormality, the "anti-Lepore" hemoglobin, has also been found.

Dominance

The concept of dominant and recessive inheritance is one of the most deeply ingrained in our genetic thinking. It has long played a primary role in the introduction of every high school student of biology to genetics and is used extensively in the classification of genetic disease. It is often implied that genes are dominant or recessive. This is incorrect. It is disease states or phenotypes which are dominant or recessive. The gene for sickle cell hemoglobin is expressed in the heterozygous state, so that the carrier of this gene has sickle cell trait. Sickle cell trait is therefore dominant, but sickle cell disease, which occurs in the homozygote, is recessive. Virtually all genes are expressed in the heterozygous state, but it may require a considerable degree of biochemical sophistication to detect this expression.

X linkage and X inactivation

Although the X chromosome is involved, at least indirectly, in the sex-determination process, most of the genes on the X chromosome have nothing whatsoever to do with sex determination. Hematologically, the more important of these "sex-linked" genes include those which code for G-6-PD, phosphoglycerate kinase, factor VIII, factor IX, Bruton-type agammaglobulinemia, and chronic granulomatous disease.

The chromosomal complement of males differs from that of females in that males have one X chromosome and one Y chromosome, while females have two X chromosomes. However, early in embryonic development, one of the two X chromosomes of somatic cells of female mammals has become geneticaly inactive: in some cells, the paternally derived chromosome is inactivated; in others, the maternally derived chromosome is inactivated. Inactivation remains fixed, so that all the progeny of the cell in which the maternally derived X chromosome is inactive show only the gene products from the paternal X. Female heterozygotes for sex-linked genes such as G-6-PD deficiency, phosphoglycerate kinase deficiency, or factor VIII or factor IX deficiency are therefore the mosaic of cells, some of which manifest the full-blown deficiency, as it is found in affected males, and some of which are normal. The final proportion of cells with one or the other X chromosome

active depends upon random factors, i.e., the binomial probability distribution, and on selection between cell populations which may occur following the inactivation process [9,10]. The process of X inactivation is not only useful in understanding the expression of X-linked diseases in women, but it has also been valuable in studying the possible clonal origin of a variety of disorders. As shown in Fig. 16-5, the progeny of a single cell of a female heterozygous for an X-linked gene will manifest only the phenotype of the original cell. Examination of electrophoretically distinguishable variants of G-6-PD has made it possible to demonstrate in this way that the red cells are a clone in chronic myelogenous leukemia [11], probably in acute myelogenous leukemia [12,13], and in paroxysmal nocturnal hemoglobinuria [14]. This indicates that each of these disorders arises through transformation of a single cell and that in the case of the leukemias, erythroid cells as well as leukocytes are part of the malignant clone.

The pattern of genetic transmission of sex-linked genes is characteristic: a father cannot transmit a sex-linked gene to his son; the offspring is a boy by virtue of the fact that he inherited the father's Y chromosome, not his X chromosome. Conversely, it is a truism that males always inherit sex-linked genes from their mother and that the mother must therefore be either heterozygous or homozygous for the gene. Because of X inactivation, however, the degree of expression of X-linked genes in females is highly variable. This is why, even with the most sophisticated methodology, it is not always possible to detect the heterozygous state in the mother of an affected individual.

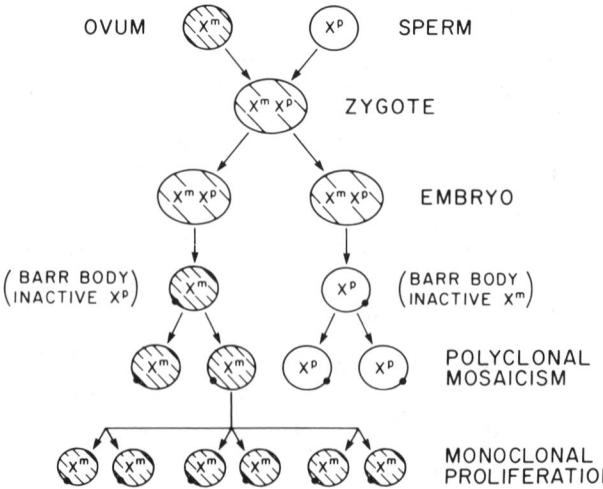

FIGURE 16-5 At fertilization, the female zygote inherits one maternal chromosome (X^m) and one paternal X chromosome (X^p). At some time early in embryogenesis, one X in each cell is inactivated at random and condenses to form the Barr body. The active X remains active not only for the lifetime of that cell, but also for the lifetime of all its progeny. A tumor with a clonal origin will consist entirely of cells in which either X^m or X^p is active, but not both. A tumor with a multicentric origin may contain both X^m and X^p cells.

Types of mutations

Mutations can occur either in structural genes (the part of the DNA which specifies the amino acid sequence of protein), in the poorly understood regulatory apparatus which determines whether or not a gene will be available for transcription (the process of being copied by RNA) and/or translation (the process of making a polypeptide on the mRNA template) or in portions of the DNA which have no known function.

Errors in the base sequence of the structural gene result in failure to form any of the protein, in the formation of a very unstable protein which may never appear in the fully assembled form, or in the formation of an abnormal protein. The latter circumstance appears to be the most common. The abnormal protein may maintain all, some, or none of the functional properties of the normal protein. Even when it has lost the functional properties of the original protein, it may retain the antigenic properties, and it is then designated *cross-reacting material* (CRM). Its stability may be normal or reduced. Mutations which result in the formation of stable proteins with normal functional properties are clinically not significant, but they may be very valuable from the point of view of population and family studies or as genetic markers for various types of biologic investigations. Some "deficiencies" of enzymes are also clinically harmless. For example, genetic absence of the glycosyl transferases, which convert the H antigen to the A or B antigen (see Chap. 161), results in the appearance of blood group O, surely a clinical state which cannot be considered a disease. Genetic variants which reach a frequency of more than 1 percent in a population are known as *polymorphisms*. Sometimes genetic variants such as the sickle cell gene or the G-6-PD deficiency gene reach polymorphic levels because the deleterious effect which they may have is counterbalanced by a beneficial effect on survival, such as increased resistance to malaria. They are known as *balanced polymorphisms*. Mapping DNA with the aid of restriction endonucleases has shown that a marked variability may exist in the nucleotide sequences outside of structural genes. Since probes for the globin chains were the first to become generally available for the study of human populations, it is in the areas flanking the structural genes for the globin chains that such variability was first appreciated [15]. Similar degrees of variability is being found outside the other structural genes. Such nontranscribed DNA sequences may be very permissive in that alterations in the sequence may not have any discernible effect. Thus considerable heterogeneity of the flanking nucleotide sequences probably exists and may prove to be very useful in linkage and population studies.

All cells receive the same complement of genes. Some enzymes are tissue-specific, and even some enzymes which appear to perform the same function are coded by different genes in different tissues. For example, the pyruvate kinase of leukocytes and that of erythrocytes are under separate genetic control (see Chap. 59). In most instances, however, a mutation which affects an enzyme in red cells will also affect the same enzyme in white cells, in liver, in brain, and in other tissues.

The types of enzyme deficiencies encountered clinically are limited by the ability of the affected individual to survive. Thus complete absence of a key glycolytic enzyme is incompatible with the basic process of energy metabolism and would almost surely be lethal long before birth. The inheritance of an enzyme with catalytic activity but with reduced stability, however, would not produce nearly as catastrophic a result. Most tissues would be able to replace the mutant enzyme by further synthesis, but not the long-lived anucleate erythrocyte. Thus many of the enzyme defects which are observed in humans are clinically apparent only in the red blood cell and represent mutations which affect primarily the stability of enzyme proteins.

Detailed study of gene regulation in *Escherichia coli* led to emergence of the elegant concept of an operon regulated by a repressor or activator substance synthesized by a regulator gene [16]. There are, no doubt, also complex systems which regulate the activity of genes in man, but little is known of these mechanisms. Regulatory mutations should result in the formation of an altered quantity of the normal gene product. Of all the diseases of man, the thalassemias seem best to fulfill these requirements. The study of this group of diseases is yielding much additional information about mechanisms of human gene regulation.

The family history

A carefully taken family history can give a physician considerable insight into the nature of a hematologic disorder. It is important, of course, to ascertain whether another member of the family has had a similar disease. In the case of patients with anemia, this is often difficult, since so many women have a history of anemia, usually due to iron deficiency. To estimate the severity of anemia it is particularly germane to inquire whether transfusion was required. A history of gallstones, particularly at an early age, may indicate that a hemolytic disorder was present. Similarly, episodes of jaundice in family members may be the only clue to the existence of familial hemolytic anemia.

Presence of the disease in one of the parents strongly suggests a dominant mode of transmission. If neither parent is affected but several sibs have the disease, an autosomal recessive transmission is more likely. Consanguinity of the parents of the patient makes it highly probable that a disease is an autosomal recessive disorder. Occurrence primarily in male sibs and maternal uncles, with mild or absent manifestations of the disease in the mother, suggests a sex-linked mode of inheritance. Father-to-son transmission rules out sex linkage.

Lack of any family history does not rule out the genetic basis of a disease. In some instances, the disease may be so mild in other family members that it is not recognized. Whenever possible, the family members should be examined, rather than relying solely on history. In some instances, of course, the gene mutation causing the disorder may have arisen in the generation in which the disease presents.

Once the mode of genetic transmission is clear, the diagnostic alternatives have been narrowed considerably. For example, methemoglobinemia transmitted as an autosomal dominant disorder is due to hemoglobin M, while methemoglobinemia transmitted as an autosomal recessive disorder is due to NADH diaphorase deficiency. Hemolytic anemia with autosomal dominant transmission is likely to be due to hereditary spherocytosis, but sex-linked transmission of the hemolytic state suggests a deficiency of glucose-6-phosphate dehydrogenase or, more rarely, phosphoglycerate kinase. A bleeding disorder which is transmitted in a sex-linked fashion may be due to a deficiency of factor VIII or factor IX, but autosomal recessive inheritance should suggest to the physician a deficiency of other clotting factors, such as factors X, XI, or V. Thus careful analysis of the family history not only will make possible more appropriate genetic counseling to the patient and family, but also will shorten the road to a correct diagnosis.

References

1. Sumner, A. T., Evans, H. J., and Buckland, R. A.: New technique for distinguishing between human chromosomes. *Nature [New Biol.]* 232:31, 1971.
2. Rowley, J. D.: A new consistent chromosomal abnormality in chronic myelogenous leukaemia identified by quinacrine fluorescence and Giemsa staining. *Nature (Lond.)*, 243:290, 1973.
3. Nowell, P. C., and Hungerford, D. A.: Chromosomes studies in human leukemia. II. Chronic granulocytic leukemia. *J. Natl. Cancer Inst.* 27:1013, 1961.
4. Rowley, J. D.: Nonrandom chromosomal abnormalities in hematologic disorders of man. *Proc. Natl. Acad. Sci. U.S.A.* 72:152, 1975.
5. Trujillo, J. M., Cork, A., Hart, J. S., George, S. L., and Freireich, E. J.: Clinical implication of aneuploid cyto-genetic profiles in adult acute leukemia. *Cancer* 33:824, 1974.
6. Boyer, S. H., and Graham, J. B.: Linkage between the X chromosome loci for glucose-6-phosphate dehydrogenase electrophoretic variation and hemophilia A. *Am. J. Hum. Genet.* 17:320, 1965.
7. Siniscalco, M., et al.: Failure to detect linkage between Xg and other X-borne loci in Sardinians. *Ann. Hum. Genet.* 29:231, 1966.
8. Ohno, S.: *Evolution by Gene Duplication.* Springer-Verlag, New York, 1970.
9. Gartler, S. M., and Linder, D.: Developmental and evolutionary implications of the mosaic nature of the G-6-PD system. *Cold Spring Harbor Symp. Quant. Biol.* 29:253, 1964.
10. Beutler, E.: The distribution of gene products among populations of cells in heterozygous humans. *Cold Spring Harbor Symp. Quant. Biol.* 29:261, 1964.
11. Fialkow, P. J., Gartler, S. M., and Yoshida, A.: Clonal origin of chronic myelocytic leukemia in man. *Proc. Natl. Acad. Sci. U.S.A.* 58:1468, 1967.
12. Beutler, E., West, C., and Johnson, C.: Involvement of the erythroid series in acute myeloid leukemia. *Blood* 53:1203, 1979.
13. Wiggans, R. G., Jacobson, R. J., Fialkow, P. J., Woolley, P. V., MacDonald, J. S., and Schein, P. S.: Probable clonal origin of acute myeloblastic leukemia following radiation and chemotherapy of colon cancer. *Blood* 52:659, 1978.
14. Oni, S. B., Osunkoya, B. O., and Luzzatto, L.: Paroxysmal nocturnal hemoglobinuria: Evidence for monoclonal origin of abnormal red cells. *Blood* 36:145, 1970.
15. Kan, Y. W., Lee, K. Y., and Furbetta, M.: Polymorphism of DNA sequence in the beta-globin gene region. *N. Engl. J. Med.* 302:185, 1980.
16. Changeux, J. P.: The control of biochemical reactions. *Sci. Am.* 212:36, 1965.

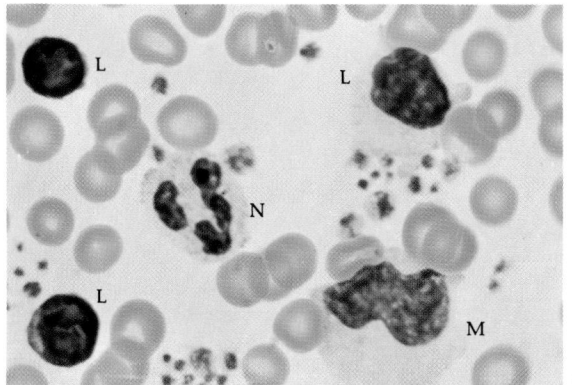

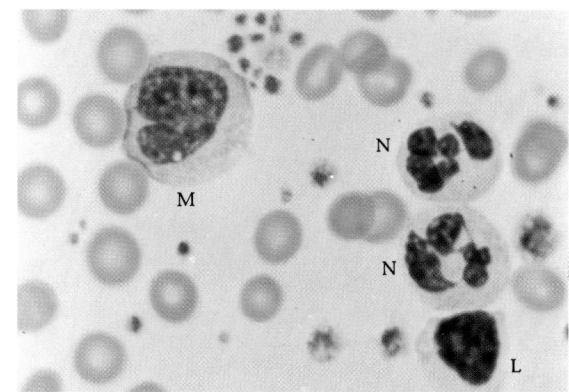

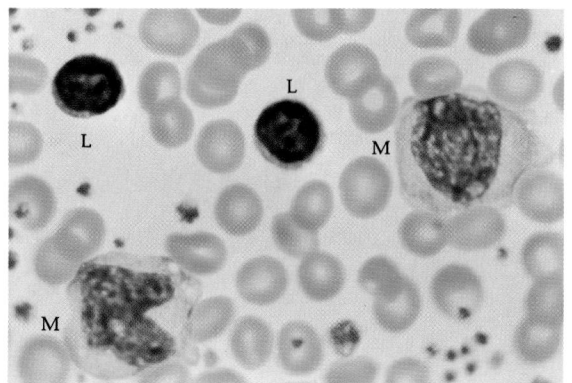

1-1,2,3 Normal blood. The film was prepared from the buffy coat of blood from a normal donor. The number of platelets and leukocytes is therefore increased above normal. L, lymphocytes; M, monocytes; N, polymorphonuclear neutrophils. Wright's stain, original magnification ×1000.

1-4 Hypersegmented polymorphonuclear neutrophils from the blood of a patient with pernicious anemia. The cells are large and the nuclei show increased lobulation. Wright's stain, original magnification ×1000.

1-5 Neutrophils from normal blood. Two mature polymorphonuclear neutrophils are on the left, while on the right is a non-segmented (band or stab) form, with a "drumstick" attached to the upper pole of the nucleus. Wright's stain, original magnification ×1000.

1-6 A mature eosinophil (left) and two mature basophils (right) from normal blood. Wright's stain, original magnification ×1000.

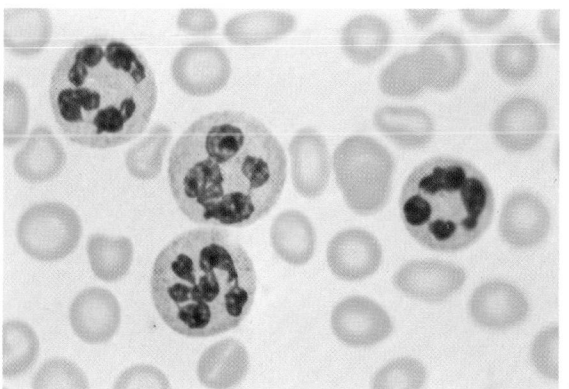

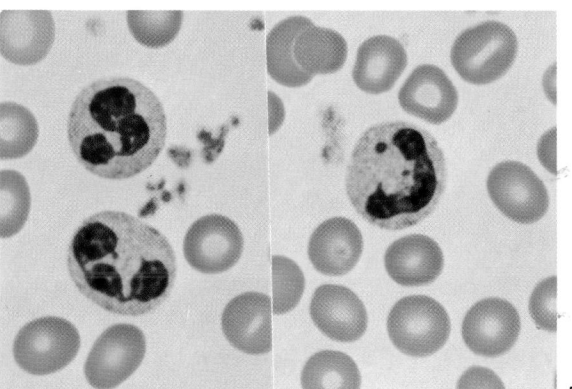

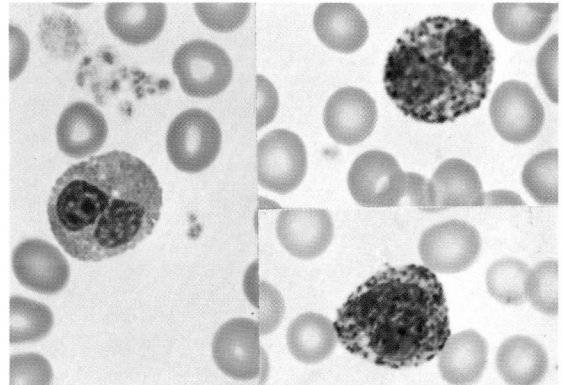

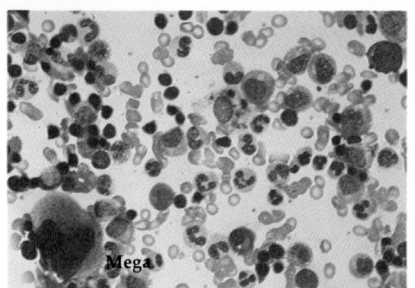

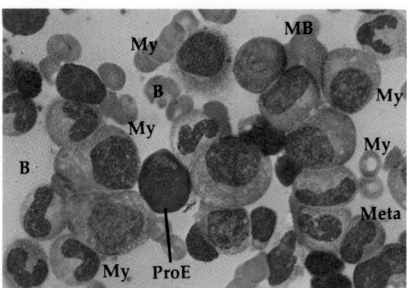

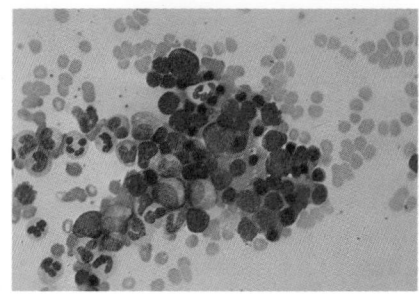

2-1 Normal marrow. Film of a normal marrow aspirate showing predominantly granulopoiesis. A megakaryocyte (Mega) is shown at the lower left. Wright's stain, original magnification ×500.

2-2 Normal marrow. Film of an aspirate of normal marrow showing predominantly granulopoiesis, including a myeloblast (MB), neutrophilic myelocytes (My), metamyelocytes (Meta), and bands (B), and a proerythroblast (ProE). Wright's stain, original magnification ×1000.

2-3 Normal marrow. A film of normal marrow showing predominantly erythropoiesis. All of the darkly staining cells are erythroid precursors in various stages of development. Wright's stain, original magnification ×500.

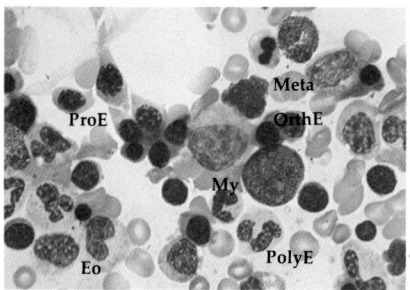

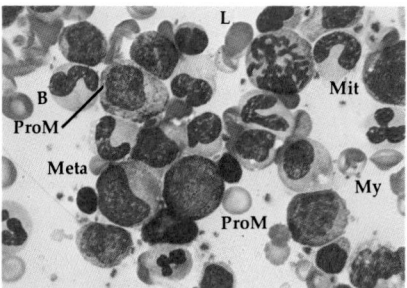

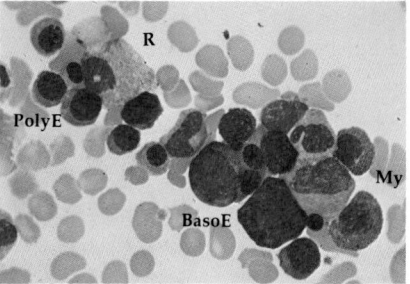

2-4 Normal marrow. A film of normal marrow showing eyrthropoiesis, including a proerythroblast (ProE), polychromatophilic erythroblasts (PolyE), and orthochromatic erythroblasts (OrthE). Also identified are a myelocyte (My) and a metamyelocyte (Meta).

2-5 Normal marrow. A film of normal marrow showing a promyelocyte (ProM), several myelocytes (My), a metamyelocyte (Meta), several band forms (B), and a lymphocyte (L). A mitotic figure is apparent as well (Mit). Wright's stain, original magnification ×1000.

2-6 Normal marrow. A film of normal marrow showing erythropoiesis, including basophilic erythroblasts (BasoE), and polychromatophilic erythroblasts (PolyE). A reticulum cell (R) and myelocyte (My) are also shown. Wright's stain, original magnification ×1000.

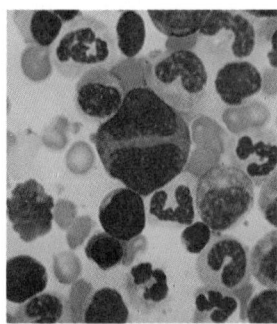

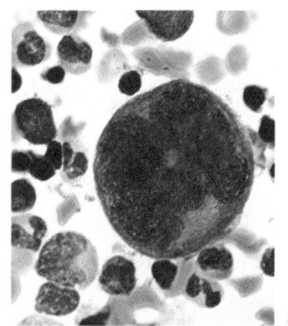

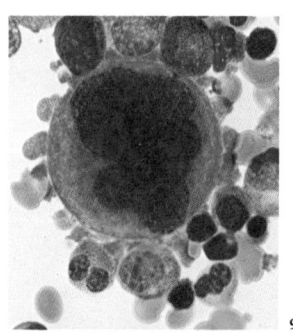

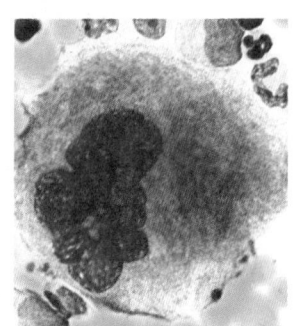

2-7 Normal marrow. A megakaryoblast, or stage I megakaryocyte. Wright's stain, original magnification ×500. **2-8** Normal marrow. Promegakaryocyte, also called a stage II or basophilic megakaryocyte. Wright's stain, original magnification ×500. **2-9** Normal marrow. Promegakaryocyte, also called a stage II or basophilic megakaryocyte. Wright's stain, original magnification ×500. **2-10** Normal marrow. A mature megakaryocyte, also called a state III, acidophilic, or granular megakaryocyte. Wright's stain, original magnification ×500.

PLATE 2 Normal marrow

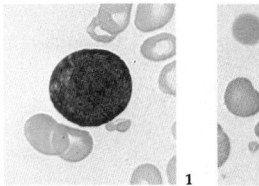 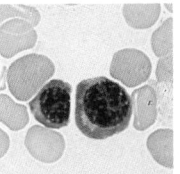 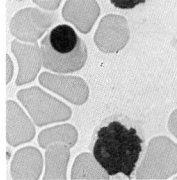 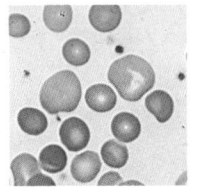

Series A
Normal erythropoiesis

1 Proerythroblast. **2** Basophilic erythroblast. **3.** Polychromatophilic erythroblast. **4.** Polychromatophilic erythroblast. **5** Orthochromatic erythroblast. **6** Polychromatophilic macrocytes (reticulocytes).

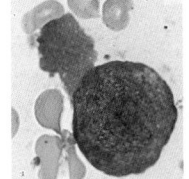 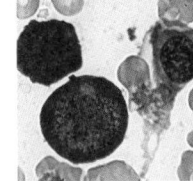 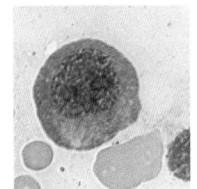 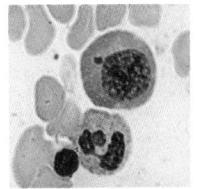 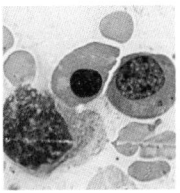 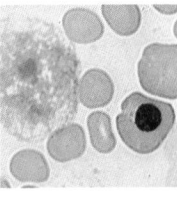

Series B
Megaloblastic erythropoiesis

1 Promegaloblast. **2** Basophilic megaloblast. **3** Polychromatophilic megaloblast. **4** Polychromatophilic megaloblast. **5** Orthochromatic megaloblast. **6** Orthochromatic megaloblast and macrocyte.

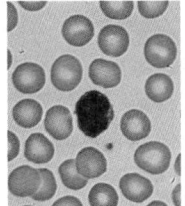 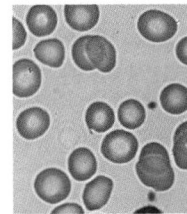 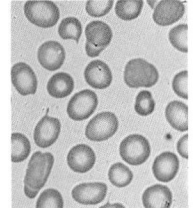 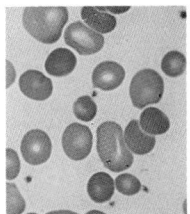 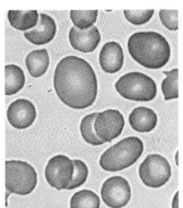 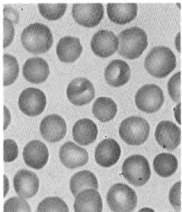

Series C
Erythrocyte morphology

1 Normal erythrocytes. **2** Slight hypochromia and microcytosis in early iron deficiency anemia. **3** Severe hypochromia and microcytosis in iron deficiency anemia. **4** Polychromatophilia. **5** Macrocytosis. **6** Spherocytosis.

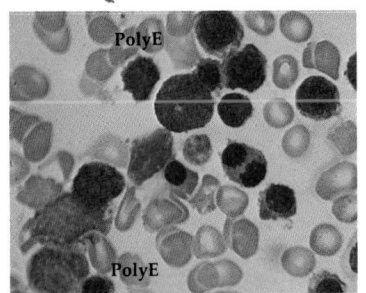 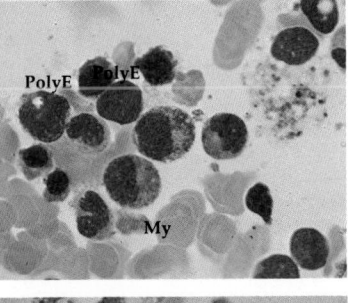 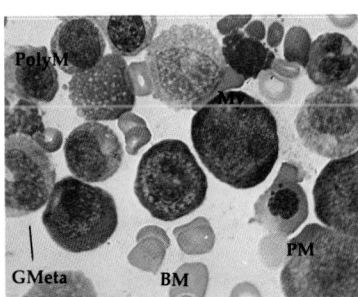

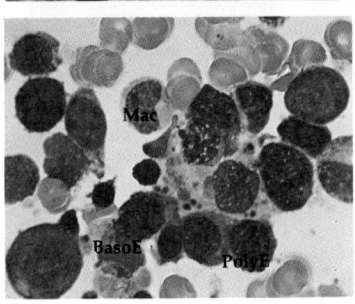 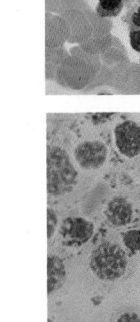 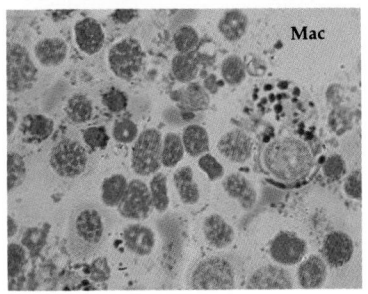 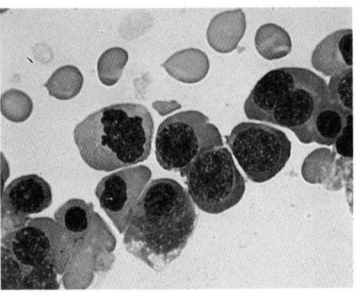

Series D
Abnormal erythropoiesis

1 Hypoferremic erythropoiesis in iron deficiency anemia. The predominant cell is a polychromatophilic erythroblast (PolyE). **2** Hypoferremic erythropoiesis in the anemia of chronic disease. Polychromatophilic erythroblasts (PolyE) and myelocytes (My) are the predominant cells. **3** Megaloblastic erythropoiesis. A promegaloblast (PM), basophilic megaloblast (BM), and polychromatophilic megaloblasts (PolyM) are seen. Other cells are a myelocyte (My) and a giant metamyelocyte (GMeta). **4** Sideroblastic erythropoiesis. An erythroid island consisting of an iron-laden macrophage (Mac) surrounded by polychromatophilic erythroblasts (PolyE) is shown, along with a basophilic erythroblast (BasoE). **5** Sideroblastic erythropoiesis. The marrow film was stained by the Prussian blue technique. Many sideroblasts are present along an iron-laden macrophage (Mac). **6** Dyserythropoiesis. Grossly abnormal erythroblasts in a patient with erythroleukemia.

Note: All films were stained with Wright's stain except as noted. Original magnification ×1000.

Erythrocyte morphology   **PLATE 3**

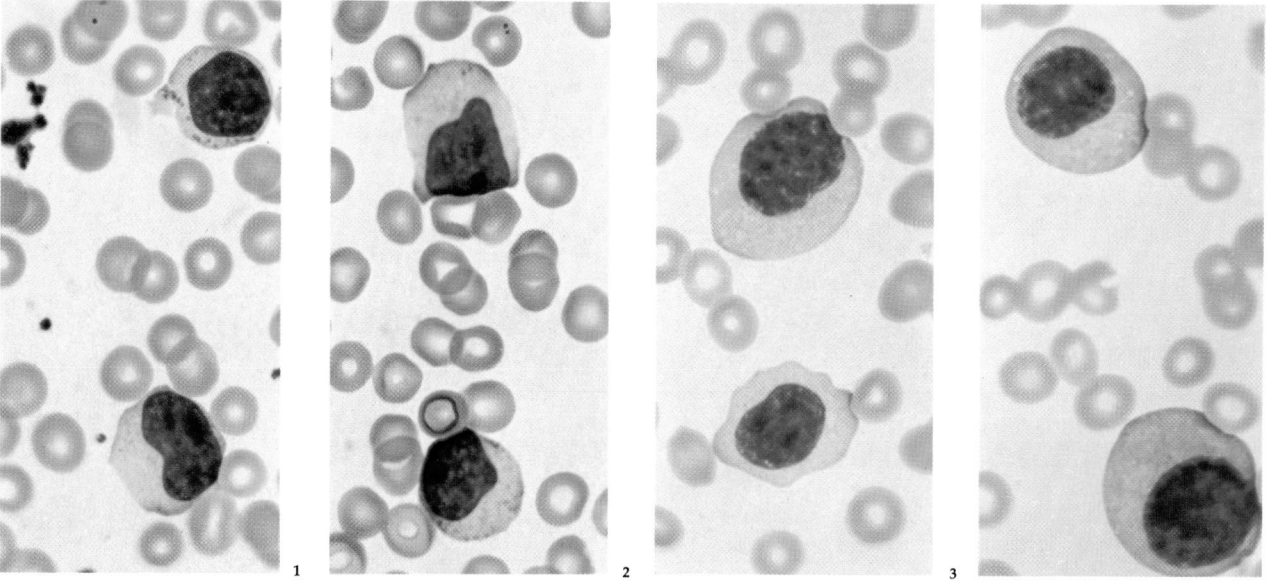

4-1,2,3,4 Atypical lymphocytes from the blood of a patient with infectious mononucleosis.

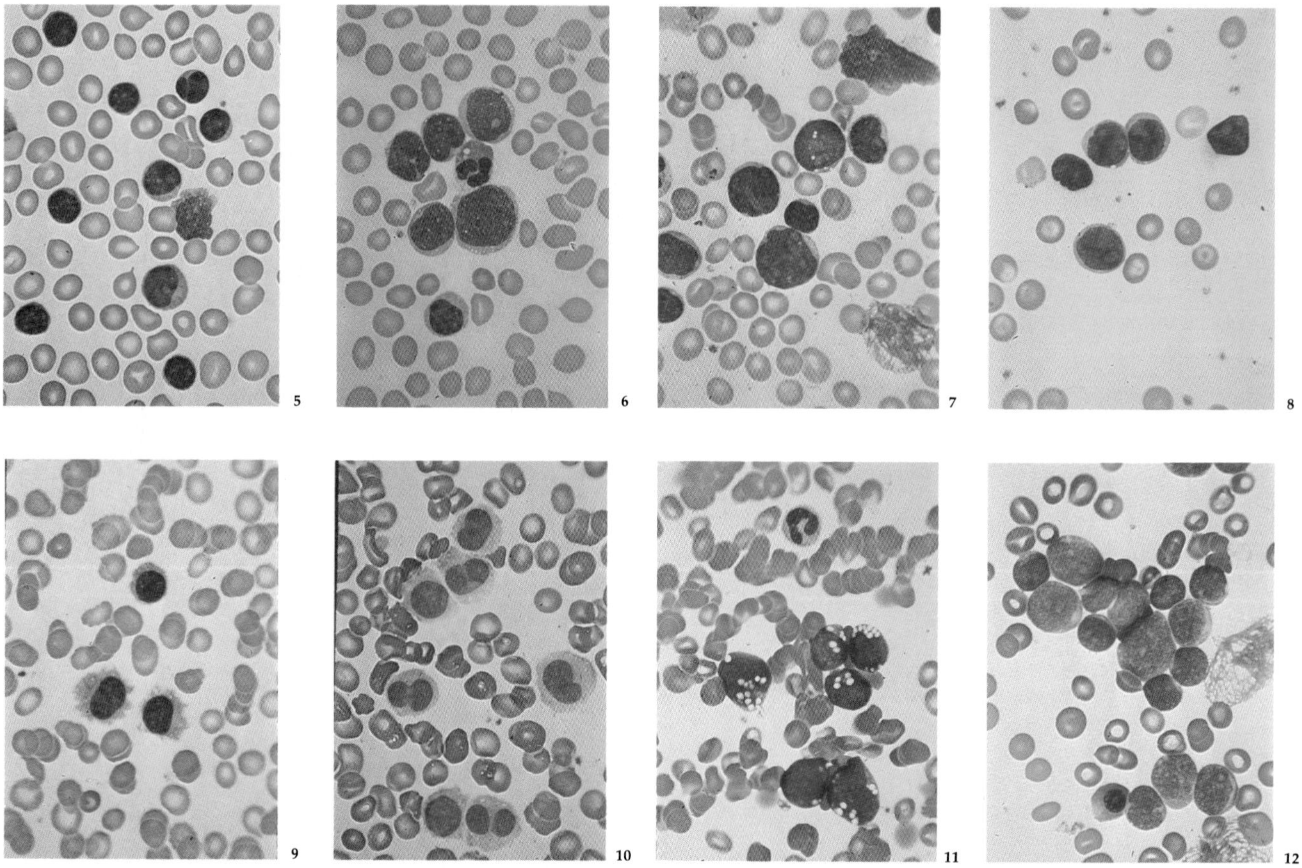

4-5 Chronic lymphocytic leukemia. **4-6** Lymphoma cell leukemia. **4-7** Prolymphocytic leukemia. **4-8** Sézary cells. **4-9** Hairy cells, lymphocytoid. **4-10** Hairy cells, monocytoid. **4-11** Burkitt's cell leukemia. **4-12** Acute lymphocytic leukemia.

Note: All cells on this plate, Wright's stain, original magnification ×1000.

PLATE 4   Abnormal lymphocytes

Comparative hematology

CHAPTER 17

Comparative hematology

JOSEPH E. SMITH

Hematologic data have been collected from relatively few of the several thousand species of animals in existence and even among these, normal values have been difficult to determine. Blood has often been collected from animals that were parasitized, anesthetized, or kept in abnormal environments [1], and furthermore the values for healthy individuals are influenced by age, sex, breed, training, sampling technique, diet, time of day, and time of season. Despite these difficulties, comparative hematology has yielded valuable information about blood and its function in both human beings and animals. The readers should refer to several excellent books which describe the hematology of various types of animals [1–8]. The data compiled in the tables in this chapter have been selected from the literature and include only determinations which are considered methodologically and statistically to be reliable.

Erythrocytes

Although the respiratory pigments of invertebrates are dissolved in blood, such pigments are confined to cells in the circulation of vertebrates. This change does not affect the viscosity of blood materially, but it does provide the respiratory pigments with an appropriate colloid environment and most importantly allows respiratory function to be regulated [9]. The oxygen affinity of hemoglobin of most species except Feloidea (cats) and some ruminants (such as sheep, cows, llamas, etc.) is regulated or influenced by the intracellular concentration of certain phosphates and their capacity to bind to hemoglobin. In mammals, embryos of birds, some turtles, and some amphibians the crucial phosphate is 2, 3-DPG, in fish it is ATP and/or GTP, and in birds, some turtles, and some fish it is inositol pentaphosphate [10].

Erythrocytes of birds, fish, amphibians, and reptiles are nucleated and ellipsoidal [11]. The volume of nucleated erythrocytes is generally large, with those of the *Amphiuma* (13,800 fl) being the largest described. Ellipsoidal but nonnucleated erythrocytes occur in Camelidae (camels, llamas, etc.) [11]. Sickling occurs commonly in several species of deer, sheep, goats, genets,

and mongooses, but is not associated with hematologic abnormalities [12].

The hemoglobin concentration and the packed cell volume of mammals are relatively uniform, but the number of erythrocytes varies considerably (Table 17-1). Consequently, the mean red cell volume ranges from 5 to 220 fl and the mean red cell diameter from 1.5 to 12.4 μm. Except for Camelidae, erythrocyte osmotic fragility decreases [13] and erythrocyte deformability increases [14] as cell volume increases. The erythrocyte life-span of mammals is finite and can be estimated by the equation $T = 68.9M^{0.132}$, where T is time in days and M is the body weight of adults in kilograms [15].

Generally, human erythrocytes and erythrocytes of most (but not all) mammals depend on similar metabolic pathways. Inherited disorders of animals provide valuable models for human erythrocyte disorders (Table 17-2) [16].

Leukocytes

Both the total number of white cells and the neutrophil/lymphocyte ratio vary among species (Table 17-1). In domestic animals the magnitude of the total leukocyte response to disease correlates directly with the neutrophil/lymphocyte ratio characteristic of the species when healthy [2].

Both lymphocytes and monocytes of vertebrates are similar, but the polymorphonuclear leukocytes vary in both morphology and staining characteristics. Granulocytes of some species contain both eosinophilic and neutrophilic granules and are called *heterophils*. Furthermore eosinophilic granules vary in size, shape, number, and staining characteristics [1]. The degree of nuclear lobulation varies. Nuclei with little lobulation are present in some rodents; hypersegmented nuclei are present in most nonhuman primates.

Disorders of leukocyte (Table 17-3) and immune function (Tables 17-4 and 17-5) in animals have provided valuable models for similar human disorders.

Hemostasis

The blood platelet count varies widely among mammals. The count may be as low as 100,000 per microliter in dolphins and some Equidae and greater than 1 million per microliter in elephants and rats. Platelets of some species (e.g., rabbit, rat, mouse, guinea pig, cow, sheep, and horse) are smaller than human platelets; some (dog and pig) are the same size; and some (cat) are larger. Platelet size does not correlate with animal size or erythrocyte size [17]. Animals with nearly all of the inherited and acquired thrombotic and hemostatic disorders are available (Tables 17-6 and 17-7) and have been successfully utilized in comparative hematology [18].

Stem cells

Inherited abnormalities in the proliferation of progenitor cells have been identified in several animal species (Table 17-8).

TABLE 17-1 Blood cell values in selected mammals (mean ± standard deviation)

Species	No.	RBC, ×10⁶/μl	Hb, g/dl	PCV, %	WBC, ×10³/μl	N, %	L, %	M, %	E, %	B, %	Platelets, ×10³/μl	Reference
Marsupialia:												
Hairy-nose wombat	22	4.68 ± 0.51	12.8 ± 1.5	39.7 ± 4.5	10.0 ± 4.0	54.3 ± 23.8	49.6 ± 26.5	0.1 ± 0.3	5.5 ± 6.8	0		[19]
Rat kangaroo	5	9.03 ± 0.55	14.5 ± 1.4	47.0 ± 3.4	8.06 ± 2.59	24.2 ± 6.5	68.5 ± 7.7	3.3 ± 2.5	4.0 ± 1.5	0.8 ± 0.6		[20]
Red kangaroo	10	5.3 ± 0.4	16.8 ± 1.1	48.7 ± 2.9	5.5 ± 1.7	61.8 ± 25.4	32.7 ± 11.8	5.4 ± 3.1	1.8 ± 0.6	0		[21]
Virginia opossum	14	4.27 ± 0.52	12.0 ± 2.1	35.2 ± 5.7	18.9 ± 4.5	34.4 ± 12.2	53.9 ± 19.1	0.6 ± 0.6	7.3 ± 4.0	0.4 ± 0.5	503 ± 287	[22]
Woolly opossum	57	4.7 ± 0.5	13.8 ± 1.8	37.0 ± 5.7	11.8 ± 5.3	33.6 ± 5.4	57.0 ± 5.7	1.2 ± 1.9	6.0 ± 8.4	0.8 ± 1.5	630 ± 225	[23]
Insectivora:												
Hedgehog	3	5.03 ± 0.35	11.2 ± 0.3	33.7 ± 2.1	3.27 ± 1.69	69.3 ± 4.5	24.0 ± 5.0	3.7 ± 0.6	3.0 ± 1.0	0	143 ± 99	[24]
Mole	3	4.72 ± 0.36	17.4 ± 0.9	48.7 ± 1.5	11.2 ± 6.63	78.3 ± 8.7	17.7 ± 8.5	2.7 ± 0.6	1.3 ± 0.6	0	244 ± 78	[24]
Primates:												
Black howler monkey	8	3.81 ± 0.86	11.4 ± 1.9	37.1 ± 6.0	14.1 ± 7.0	59.7 ± 6.1	37.9 ± 6.8	1.9 ± 1.0	0.6 ± 0.6	0		[25]
Bonnet monkey	45	5.61 ± 0.67	12.9 ± 1.2	47.8 ± 2.8	10.3 ± 2.43	55.1 ± 8.3	39.8 ± 6.7	2.5	3	0.5		[26]
Brown stump-tail macaque	10	4.70 ± 0.81	12.1 ± 1.5	37.2 ± 5.2	19.6 ± 5.97	39.6 ± 17.1	47.5 ± 15.1	2.5 ± 1.4	9.8 ± 8.3	0.4 ± 0.7		[3]
Celebes black ape	5	6.26 ± 0.50	12.0 ± 1.9	42.3 ± 1.9	15.5 ± 3.10	39.0 ± 11.0	54.0 ± 10.9	1.9 ± 1.2	4.9 ± 2.9	0.4 ± 0.5		[3]
Chimpanzee	175	4.57 ± 0.62	12.5 ± 1.5	39.7 ± 5.0	12.5 ± 5.14	63.1 ± 16.4	32.8 ± 15.3	1.1 ± 1.3	2.6 ± 3.2	0.2 ± 0.5	349 ± 133	[3]
Drill	5	4.82 ± 0.46	12.7 ± 0.6	41.2 ± 2.6	10.1 ± 3.27	53.6 ± 15.5	41.0 ± 13.4	3.6 ± 2.7	1.4 ± 1.3	0.4 ± 0.5		[3]
Gibbon	25	5.74 ± 0.60	13.9 ± 1.8	44.8 ± 4.4	7.82 ± 3.27	46.0 ± 19.1	48.5 ± 19.5	2.7 ± 3.0	2.1 ± 3.7	0.5 ± 0.9	210 ± 61	[3]
Gorilla	58	4.41 ± 0.40	11.7 ± 1.2	39.1 ± 3.8	10.7 ± 4.78	59.3 ± 17.3	36.0 ± 6.2	1.9 ± 2.0	2.4 ± 2.7	0.1 ± 0.4		[3]
Java macaque	21	5.98 ± 0.73	11.5 ± 1.1	39.9 ± 3.6	12.7 ± 4.21	51.7 ± 13.6	42.2 ± 12.8	2.9 ± 2.3	2.7 ± 3.6	0.5 ± 0.8	393 ± 61.6	[3]
Langur	16	4.72 ± 0.76	11.5 ± 1.8	44.0 ± 1.8	9.54 ± 1.81	65.1 ± 4.23	31.7 ± 4.46	2	0	0		[26]
Lesser bushbaby (female)	13	6.61 ± 0.34	15.8 ± 1.4	45.8 ± 2.9	9.04 ± 2.60	18.9 ± 10.6	72.7 ± 20.3	3.2 ± 1.8	2.4 ± 0.5	0	591 ± 200	[27]
Moor macaque	4	5.45 ± 0.36	12.2 ± 0.3	40.0 ± 2.9	12.2 ± 1.62	43.2 ± 18.7	44.8 ± 19.0	4.5 ± 2.5	7.0 ± 8.0	0.5 ± 0.6		[3]
Orangutan	149	4.21 ± 0.55	10.8 ± 1.4	36.7 ± 4.0	13.6 ± 5.48	55.5 ± 14.8	39.7 ± 13.8	1.8 ± 2.1	2.6 ± 2.8	0.1 ± 0.4	417 ± 129	[3]
Owl monkey	157	5.17 ± 0.84	14.3 ± 1.1	42.0 ± 5.4	12.7 ± 4.7	55.4 ± 7.6	35.5 ± 18.3	0	9.5 ± 9.2	0	397 ± 109	[28]
Pig-tailed macaque	9	5.95 ± 0.57	11.3 ± 1.3	41.8 ± 4.8	11.8 ± 2.65	50.1 ± 3.4	44.9 ± 3.9	2.3 ± 1.7	2.0 ± 1.5	0.7 ± 0.6		[3]
Rhesus macaque	750	5.61 ± 0.58	12.3 ± 1.1	42.1 ± 3.2	10.1 ± 3.64	39.7 ± 17.1	55.2 ± 16.6	1.1 ± 1.6	3.3 ± 3.1	0.3 ± 0.5	418 ± 115	[3]
Squirrel monkey (female)	31	6.87 ± 0.57	13.7 ± 1.2	41.1 ± 3.3	11.2 ± 5.2	52.9 ± 16.9	38.9 ± 11.3	2.0 ± 1.8	6.2 ± 6.1	0.1 ± 0.3	448 ± 64	[29]
Stump-tailed macaque	36	4.86 ± 0.41	12.7 ± 1.1	37.8 ± 3.1	9.28 ± 2.19	38.2 ± 18.3	54.1 ± 17.4	0.36 ± 0.68	7.5 ± 6.3	0.17 ± 0.38	353 ± 94	[30]
Treeshaw	45	6.42 ± 0.93	13.9 ± 1.2	43.4 ± 4.3	4.41 ± 1.92	14.4 ± 10.3	80.0 ± 13.6	0.4 ± 0.6	3.8 ± 3.5	0.8 ± 1.7		[31]
White-face monkey	14	4.92 ± 0.72	14.4 ± 1.8	47.0 ± 6.7	16.0 ± 8.4	55.6 ± 6.6	40.9 ± 6.7	1.8 ± 1.1	1.6 ± 2.2	0		[25]

TABLE 17-1 Blood cell values in selected mammals (mean ± standard deviation) (Continued)

Species	No.	RBC, ×10⁶/μl	Hb, g/dl	PCV, %	WBC, ×10³/μl	N, %	L, %	M, %	E, %	B, %	Platelets, ×10³/μl	Reference
Lagomorpha:												
Alaskan snowshoe hare	55	6.36 ± 1.23	12.3 ± 2.6	39 ± 7	3.02 ± 1.52	27 ± 19	68 ± 20	2.8 ± 3.5	1.9 ± 2.6	0.5 ± 0.8		[32]
Domestic rabbit	24	6.05 ± 0.61	12.9 ± 1.3	41.2 ± 3.2	9.79 ± 3.21	45.2 ± 13.1	45.3 ± 13.0	4.6 ± 3.1	1.9 ± 1.5	3.0 ± 2.3	343 ± 120	[2]
Jackrabbit	17	7.79 ± 0.51	16.0 ± 1.2	47.6 ± 2.9	7.46 ± 3.15	48.8 ± 34.6	44.2 ± 32.2	3.9 ± 3.0	2.6 ± 2.9	0.5 ± 0.7	449 ± 215	[2]
Rodentia:												
Alaskan brown lemming	19	10.7 ± 1.42	14.2 ± 1.3	44 ± 4	2.5 ± 0.97	49 ± 16	45 ± 16	4 ± 3	2 ± 2	0		[33]
Canadian beaver	13	3.86 ± 0.82	12.9 ± 1.2	38.1 ± 2.6	11.8 ± 4.27	69.1 ± 12.6	27.8 ± 12.7	1.2 ± 1.1	0.8 ± 1.2	0		[34]
Chinchilla (female)	52	6.6 ± 1.4	11.7 ± 1.4	38.3 ± 5.8	8.0 ± 6.5	53.6 ± 17.3	44.6 ± 15.8	1.2 ± 1.4	0.5 ± 1.4	0.4 ± 1.4	298 ± 149	[35]
Deer mouse	19	11.8 ± 2.06	15.0 ± 1.5	49 ± 4	3.68 ± 2.33	25 ± 15	67 ± 15	3 ± 2	5 ± 2	0.1 ± 0.3		[33]
Eastern meadow mouse		13.3 ± 2.6	14.9 ± 1.3	47 ± 5	4.3 ± 1.9	13 ± 10	78 ± 14	5 ± 5	3 ± 3	0.2 ± 0.4		[36]
Egyptian spiny rat	21	7.58 ± 1.35	13.9 ± 1.1	44 ± 3	16.8 ± 4.39	5 ± 4	92 ± 5	0.8 ± 1.1	3 ± 2	0.1 ± 0.4		[33]
Golden hamster		7.5 ± 2.4	16.8 ± 1.2	52.5 ± 2.3	5.24 ± 1.20	20 ± 6.0	61 ± 7.5	3.0 ± 0.5	1.8 ± 0.2	0		[37]
Greenland collared lemming		10.6 ± 1.7	15.2 ± 1.6	50 ± 4	2.7 ± 1.6	16 ± 13	79 ± 15	3 ± 3	0.6 ± 1.0	0.1 ± 0.2		[36]
Guinea pig	31	4.92 ± 0.54	12.4 ± 1.3	41.2 ± 3.6	11.2 ± 2.84	26.7 ± 12.9	67.8 ± 14.1	3.1 ± 3.1	2.2 ± 2.2	0.2 ± 0.2	530 ± 149	[2]
Mongolian gerbil (female)	10	8.85 ± 0.51	15.0 ± 0.4	46.8 ± 1.4	8.70 ± 0.42	23.4 ± 12.2	74.8 ± 12.4	0.3	1.2	0.1		[38]
Mouse	111	8.25 ± 0.90	13.1 ± 1.5	40.4 ± 3.8	6.33 ± 3.72	21.0 ± 11.5	74.3 ± 13.1	2.4 ± 2.0	1.5 ± 1.6	0.1 ± 0.4	1,163 ± 382	[2]
Multimammate mouse (female)	32	7.30 ± 0.58	12.9 ± 0.9	38.8 ± 3.0	7.53 ± 2.1	18.4 ± 7.24	78 ± 7.9	1.9 ± 1.2	1.7 ± 2.1	0	289 ± 56	[39]
Northern red-back vole		11.5 ± 3.1	15.5 ± 1.3	49 ± 4	3.1 ± 2.3	19 ± 12	73 ± 12	4 ± 5	3 ± 3	0.3 ± 0.7		[36]
Rat	134	7.83 ± 0.62	14.8 ± 0.8	46.1 ± 2.5	9.98 ± 2.68	25.0 ± 8.2	71.7 ± 8.7	2.5 ± 2.0	1.7 ± 1.3	0.1 ± 0.3	1,043 ± 200	[2]
Raton de campo	20	8.39 ± 1.1	15.1 ± 1.6	49 ± 6	7.38 ± 2.4	33 ± 20	58 ± 21	2 ± 2	6 ± 4	0.4 ± 1.1		[36]
Tundra vole		13.4 ± 1.5	16.0 ± 1.3	48 ± 4	3.8 ± 1.5	10 ± 9	86 ± 10	1 ± 2	1 ± 1	0.1 ± 0.3		[33]
Vesper mouse	19	11.6 ± 2.22	16.1 ± 1.3	45 ± 6	4.06 ± 1.27	7 ± 6	85 ± 8	2 ± 2	5 ± 4	0.1 ± 0.3		[36]
Vole		11.9 ± 1.3	14.7 ± 1.4	45 ± 4	4.4 ± 2.0	25 ± 17	65 ± 17	5 ± 4	4 ± 5	0.3 ± 0.5		[36]
Cetacea:												
Amazon dolphin	8	3.85 ± 0.4	13.8 ± 0.8	41.0 ± 3.5	13.4 ± 2.62	66.5 ± 15.0	20.5 ± 7.5	3.5 ± 3.0	4.5 ± 3.5	0		[40]
Beluga whale	27	3.47 ± 0.61	18.1 ± 1.1	44.6 ± 2.9	10.0 ± 1.72	50.0 ± 6.5	27.0 ± 8.0	3.0 ± 1.2	15.2 ± 4.6	0		[40]
Bottlenose dolphin	52	3.87 ± 2.27	14.6 ± 1.4	43.6 ± 3.6	11.3 ± 4.24	61.0 ± 12.0	18.0 ± 8.2	2.0 ± 1.8	17.0 ± 9.3	1		[60]
Killer whale	4	4.03 ± 0.3	16.2 ± 0.85	45.2 ± 4.7	8.62 ± 2.55	72.0 ± 9.1	19.0 ± 8.0	4.0 ± 1.7	2.0 ± 1.6	1		[40]
Pacific striped dolphin	8	5.60 ± 0.5	19.0 ± 3.5	52.4 ± 3.5	6.29 ± 1.54	42.0 ± 12.5	28.0 ± 9.3	4.3 ± 3.3	22.0 ± 12.0	1		[40]
Pilot whale	6	3.7 ± 0.38	15.8 ± 1.2	45.0 ± 3.5	11.5 ± 3.16	60.1 ± 11.9	18.8 ± 6.2	2.6 ± 1.5	7.0 ± 9.2	0		[40]
Pinnipedia:												
California sea lion	8	4.38 ± 0.7	15.0 ± 2.1	45 ± 5	9.23 ± 1.55	64 ± 13	28 ± 10	4 ± 2	4 ± 4		0	[41]
Gray seal	6	5.04 ± 0.41	19.1 ± 2.2	57.2 ± 5.8	10.6 ± 3.06	65 ± 8	19 ± 8	0	2.8 ± 2.7		0	[42]
Harbor seal	5	5.45 ± 0.7	19 ± 1.3	52.0 ± 6.0	8.01 ± 1.0	60 ± 21	33 ± 22	4 ± 2	1 ± 1		0	[41]
Sirenia:												
Florida manatee	2	3.62 ± 0.24	14.8 ± 0.7	46.6 ± 0.5	9.30 ± 1.28	56.2 ± 15.8	34.0 ± 16.5	3.1 ± 0.3	5.2 ± 0.2	0.5 ± 0.5		[43]

TABLE 17-1 Blood cell values in selected mammals (mean ± standard deviation) (Continued)

Species	No.	RBC $\times 10^6/\mu l$	Hb g/dl	PCV %	WBC $\times 10^3/\mu l$	N, %	L, %	M, %	E, %	B, %	Platelets, $\times 10^3/\mu l$	Reference
Carnivora:												
Cat (male)	32	7.40 ± 0.20	10.7 ± 0.4	41.4 ± 1.2	17.4 ± 1.20	58.3 ± 7.8	32.0 ± 5.8	2.8 ± 0.8	6.9 ± 1.75	0	235 ± 65	[4]
Coyote	42	7.7 ± 1.0	14.7 ± 1.9	49.0 ± 5.9	8.90 ± 2.90	69.7 ± 7.2	20.9 ± 6.7	3.3 ± 1.2	5.9 ± 3.1	0.1 ± 0.3		[44]
Dog (male)	18	6.98 ± 0.6	17.1 ± 0.9	53.9 ± 2.7	12.9 ± 2.4	61.2 ± 14.7	29.7 ± 6.2	2.3 ± 0.1	4.6 ± 2.7	0.1 ± 0.1		[4]
Raccoon	10	7.32 ± 1.18	13.1 ± 2.4	40.0 ± 7.1	10.9 ± 4.3	66.4 ± 16.8	29.1 ± 15.5	3.6 ± 2.2	0.9	0		[45]
Proboscidea:												
Indian elephant	6	2.88 ± 0.59	12.2 ± 2.4	36.7 ± 6.9	12.7 ± 1.7	10.3 ± 3.6	73.2 ± 3.1	3.2 ± 4.3	13.2 ± 2.8	0		[46]
Perissodactyla:												
Donkey	30	6.56 ± 0.82	11.6 ± 1.9	36.4 ± 4.1	14.5 ± 3.13	38.1 ± 10.1	47.2 ± 12.4	3.2 ± 2.8	6.9 ± 4.1	0	418 ± 110	[47]
Horse	147	9.0 ± 1.2	14.4 ± 1.7	41 ± 4.5	5.5	9.05 ± 1.80	52.6 ± 8.7	38.7 ± 8.7	4.3 ± 2.4	3.4 ± 2.6	0.5 ± 0.6	[2]
White rhinoceros	16	6.99 ± 0.56	16.3 ± 1.6	43.1 ± 3.2	11.0 ± 4.75	52.1 ± 32.4	36.5 ± 11.8	2.7 ± 1.3	7.1 ± 3.2	0		[48]
Zebra	5	8.3 ± 0.6	15.4 ± 1.1	44 ± 4.0	8.30 ± 1.20	67.0 ± 10.0	16.8 ± 10	3.0 ± 1.0	1.5 ± 1.0	0		[1]
Artiodactyla:												
American bison	163	10.1 ± 1.43	17.0 ± 1.4	47.1 ± 4.1	8.03 ± 1.41	63.8 ± 8.0	24.9 ± 6.4	6.3 ± 4.2	4.0 ± 3.3	0.8 ± 1		[49]
Bighorn sheep	16	9.0 ± 0.9	12.3 ± 1.6	35 ± 3.9	4.7 ± 1.1	62 ± 18.7	34 ± 17.8	1 ± 1.9	2 ± 2.9	0		[50]
Black buck	3	13.5 ± 0.76	17.5 ± 0.5	48.7 ± 0.6	4.43 ± 1.29	41.7 ± 32.2	55.3 ± 31.9	2.3 ± 0.6	0.3 ± 0.6	0.3 ± 0.6		[2]
Cattle	81	5.95 ± 0.76	11.3 ± 1.5	33.7 ± 4.1	7.03 ± 1.96	29.1 ± 9.2	51.4 ± 11.8	8.3 ± 2.7	9.9 ± 11.9	0		[51]
Dorcas gazelle	55	13.8 ± 2.2	16.3 ± 1.9	46.7 ± 5.1	6.2 ± 2.6	62.9 ± 38.7	33.9 ± 19.3	0	3.2 ± 4.8	0		[52]
Dromedary camel	10	7.24 ± 0.84	13.1 ± 1.6	27 ± 4.1	18.1 ± 2.51	50.6 ± 8.4	39.7 ± 5.8	3.0 ± 1.3	6.5 ± 3.8	0.1 ± 0.1		[53]
Fallow deer (female)	28	9.59 ± 1.40	15.9 ± 1.8	41.4 ± 4.4	4.69 ± 1.86	51.6 ± 16.2	30.5 ± 16.2	5.5 ± 5.2	5.0 ± 5.2	0		[54]
Giraffe	14	12.4 ± 3.4	13.5 ± 2.4	38.8 ± 5.8	13.5 ± 4.2	69.6 ± 27.4	22.2 ± 11.1	1.5 ± 2.2	2.2 ± 2.2	3.0 ± 4.4		[55]
Goat (female)	50	12.7 ± 2.63	11.1 ± 1.8	28.7 ± 4.5	8.08 ± 2.51	49.0 ± 10.7	42.3 ± 10.4	3.1 ± 2.5	1.9 ± 1.6	0.1 ± 0.3		[56]
Hog	34	6.88 ± 0.09	41.4 ± 4.6	13.4 ± 0.2	19.6 ± 0.84	32.1 ± 2.8	53.8 ± 2.0	4.8 ± 0.3	3.0 ± 0.2	0.1 ± 0.1	425 ± 12.8	[5]
Sheep (female)	26	11.6 ± 0.67	11.0 ± 0.62	34.1 ± 1.3	7.30 ± 1.20	28.0 ± 6.7	62.0 ± 6.6	2.0 ± 0.6	8.0 ± 2.2	0	320 ± 71.0	[4]
Water buffalo	50	6.54 ± 0.77	11.1 ± 1.0	31 ± 2	9.68 ± 1.79	32.9 ± 8.74	52.7 ± 12.0	5.9 ± 2.6	6.9 ± 4.6	1.4 ± 1.0		[57]

TABLE 17-2 Inherited erythrocyte defects of animals

Disease	Inheritance	Species	Reference
Acatalasemia	AR	Mouse, guinea pig	[58,59]
	N	Dog, duck	[60,61]
Congenital porphyria	AR	Cow	[62]
	N	Fox squirrel	[63]
	AD	Cat, hog	[64,65]
Cysteine transport deficiency	AR	Sheep	[66]
Glucose-6-phosphate dehydrogenase deficiency	U	Dog	[67]
Glutathione deficiency	AR	Sheep	[68]
Hereditary elliptocytosis	AR	Dog	[69]
Hereditary spherocytosis	AR	Deer mouse	[70]
Hereditary stomatocytosis	AR	Dog	[71]
Iron-utilization defects:			
Flexed-tail	AR	Mouse	[72]
Microcytic anemia	AR	Mouse	[72]
Sex-linked anemia	XR	Mouse	[72]
Methemoglobin reductase deficiency	U	Dog	[73,74]
Polycythemia	AR	Cow	[75]
Pyruvate kinase deficiency	AR	Dog	[76]
Spectrin deficiency:			
Hemolytic anemia	AR	Mouse	[77]
Jaundiced	AR	Mouse	[77]
Normoblastic anemia	AR	Mouse	[77]
Spherocytosis	AR	Mouse	[77,78]
Thalassemia		Mouse	[79]

NOTE: AD = autosomal dominant; AID = autosomal incomplete dominant; AR = autosomal recessive; N = normal for species; U = unknown; XR = X-linked.

TABLE 17-3 Inherited abnormalities of neutrophils and macrophages

Disease	Inheritance	Species	Reference
Canine granulocytopathy syndrome	AR	Dog	[81]
Chédiak-Higashi syndrome	AR	Mink, cow, cat, whale, beige mouse	[82–85]
Macrophage defect	AR	Mouse	[86]
Pelger-Huët syndrome	AD	Rabbit, dog	[87,88]

NOTE: AD = autosomal dominant; AR = autosomal recessive.
SOURCE: Perryman and Magnuson [80].

TABLE 17-4 Immunodeficiencies of animals

Disease	Inheritance	Species	Reference
T cell:			
Hairlessness and immunodeficiency	AR	Guinea pig, mouse, rat	[89–91]
Hereditary athymia, asplenia	AD	Mouse	[92]
Hypopituitary dwarf	AR	Mouse, dogs	[93,94]
Lethal trait A46	AR	Cattle	[95]
B cell:			
Agammaglobulinemia	U	Horse	[96,97]
Dysgammaglobulinemia	U	Chicken	[98]
Hereditary asplenia	AD	Mouse	[99]
IgA deficiency	U	Chicken	[100]
IgG$_2$ deficiency	U	Cow	[101]
IgM deficiency	U	Horse	[97]
Immune defective	XR	Mouse	[102]
Combined T and B cell:			
Monogenic	AR	Horse, mouse	[103,104]
Digenic	AR and XR	Mouse	[105]

NOTE: AD = autosomal dominant; AR = autosomal recessive; U = unknown; XR = X-linked.
SOURCE: Perryman and Magnuson [80].

TABLE 17-5   Inherited deficiencies of complement

Deficient component	Inheritance	Species	Reference
C1	AID	Chicken	[106]
C2	AID	Guinea pig	[107]
C3	AID	Dog	[108]
C4	AID	Guinea pig, rat	[109,110]
C5	AID	Mouse	[111]
C6	AID	Hamster, rabbit	[106,112]

NOTE: AID = autosomal incomplete dominant.

TABLE 17-6   Congenital disorders of coagulation in animals

Deficient factor	Trivial name of disease	Inheritance	Species	Reference
I	Afibrinogenemia	AID	Goat	[114]
	Hypofibrinogenemia	AID	Dog	[115]
	Dysfibrinogenemia	AR	Dog	[113]
II	Hypoprothrombinemia	AID	Dog	[116]
VII		AID	Dog	[113,117]
VIII	Hemophilia A	XR	Cat, dog, horse	[118,119]
VIII	Von Willebrand's disease	AR	Dog	[120]
		AID	Hog, dog, rabbit	[121,122]
IX	Hemophilia B	XR	Dog	[119]
X		AID	Dog	[123]
XI		AID	Cow, dog	[124,125]
XII	Hageman trait	AR	Cats	[126]
		N	Marine mammals, reptiles, birds	[127,128]

NOTE: AID = autosomal incomplete dominant; AR = autosomal recessive; N = normal for species; XR = X-linked.
SOURCE: Dodds [113].

TABLE 17-7   Inherited platelet function defects

Disease	Inheritance	Species	Reference
Arachidonate insensitivity	U	Dog	[129]
Familial thrombopathia	AR	Cow, dog	[113,130]
Storage pool disease	AR	Mouse, rat	[131,132]
Thrombasthenic thrombopathia	AR	Dog	[133]

NOTE: AR = autosomal recessive; U = unknown.
SOURCE: Dodds [113].

TABLE 17-8   Inherited disorders of hemopoietic cell proliferation

Disease	Inheritance	Species	Reference
Cyclic hemopoiesis	AR	Dog	[134]
Hertwig's anemia	AR	Mouse	[135]
Steel (sl) anemia (8 alleles)	AR	Mouse	[135]
White-spotting (W) anemia (37 alleles)	AR	Mouse	[136]

NOTE: AR = autosomal recessive.

References

1. Hawley, C. M.: *Comparative Mammalian Haematology,* Heinemann, London, 1975.
2. Schalm, O. W., Jain, N. C., and Carroll, E. J.: *Veterinary Hematology,* 3d ed., Lea & Febiger, Philadelphia, 1975.
3. Huser, H.-J.: *Atlas of Comparative Primate Hematology,* Academic, New York, 1970.
4. Mitruka, B. M., and Rawnsley, H. M.: *Clinical Biochemical and Hematological Reference Values in Normal Experiment Animals,* Masson Publishing USA, New York, 1977.
5. Archer, R. K., and Jeffcott, L. B.: *Comparative Clinical Haematology,* Blackwell Scientific, Oxford, 1977.
6. Duncan, J. R., and Prasse, K. W.: *Veterinary Laboratory Medicine,* The Iowa State University Press, Ames, 1977.
7. Schalm, O. W.: *Manual of Feline and Canine Hematology,* Veterinary Practice Publishing Company, Culver City, 1980.
8. Andrew, W.: *Comparative Hematology,* Grune & Stratton, New York, 1965.
9. Schmidt-Nielsen, K., and Taylor, C. R.: Red blood cells: Why or why not? *Science 162:*274, 1968.
10. Bunn, H. F.: Evolution of mammalian hemoglobin function. *Blood 58:*189, 1982.
11. Gulliver, G.: Observations on the sizes and shapes of the red corpuscles of the blood of vertebrates, with drawings of them to a uniform scale, and extended and revised tables of measurement. *Proc. Zool. Soc. Lond.* 1875, p. 474.
12. Butcher, P., and Hawkey, C.: Red blood cell sickling in mammals, in *The Comparative Pathology of Zoo Animals,* edited by R. J. Montali and G. Migaki. Smithsonian Institution Press, Washington, D.C., 1980, pp. 633–641.
13. Coldman, M. F., Gent, M., and Good, W.: Relationships between osmotic fragility and other species-specific variables of mammalian erythrocytes. *Comp. Biochem. Physiol. 34:*759, 1970.
14. Smith, J. E., Mohandas, N., and Shohet, S. B.: Marked variability in erythrocyte deformability among various mammals. *Am. J. Physiol. 236:*H725, 1979.
15. Vacha, J.: Critical comparative review of the life span of red blood cells in mammals. *Acta. Sc. Nat. Brno. 13:*1, 1979.
16. Smith, J. E.: Animal models of human erythrocyte metabolism, in *Animal Models of Inherited Metabolic Disease,* edited by R. J. Desnick, R. G. Scarpelli, and D. F. Patterson. Alan R. Liss, New York, 1982.
17. Prost-Dvojakovic, R. J., Le Tohic, F., and Boulard, C.: Study of platelet volumes and diameters in 11 mammals, in *Platelets: Recent Advances in Basic Research and Clinical Aspects,* edited by O. N. Ulutin and J. V. Jones. Elsevier, New York, 1975, pp. 30–36.
18. Dodds, W. J.: Introduction to hemorrhagic diseases, in *Spontaneous Animal Models of Human Disease,* edited by E. J. Andrews, B. C. Ward, and N. H. Altman. Academic, New York, 1979, vol. 1, p. 266.
19. Gaughwin, M. D., Judson, G. J.: Haematology and clinical chemistry of hair-nosed wombats (*Lasiorhinus latifrons*). *J. Wildl. Dis. 16:*275, 1980.
20. Moore, W., Jr., and Gillespie, L. J.: Hemogram of the rat kangaroo, *Potorous tridactylus. Am. J. Vet. Res. 29:*1073, 1968.
21. Wilson, G. R., and Hoskins, L.: Haematology and blood chemistry of the red kangaroo *Megaleia rufa* in captivity. *Aust. Vet. J. 51:*146, 1975.
22. Timmons, E. H., and Marques, P. A.: Blood chemical and hematological studies in the laboratory-confined, unanesthetized opossum, *Didelphis virginiana. Lab. Anim. Care 19:*342, 1969.
23. Rothstein, R., and Hunsaker, D., II: Baseline hematology and blood chemistry of the South American woolly opossum, *Caluromys derbianus. Lab. Anim. Care 22:*227, 1972.
24. Quilliam, T. A., Clarke, J. A., and Salsbury, A. J.: The ecological significance of certain new haematological findings in the mole and hedgehog. *Comp. Biochem. Physiol. 40A:*89, 1971.
25. Porter, J. A., Jr.: Hematologic values of the black spider monkey (*Ateles fusciceps*), red spider monkey (*Ateles geoffroyi*), white face monkey (*Cebus capucinus*), and black howler monkey (*Alouatta villosa*). *Lab. Anim. Sci. 21:*426, 1971.
26. Jayaraman, S., Hurkadli, K., and Rao, S. S.: Hematological data of the laboratory-maintained bonnet (*Macaca radiata*) and the langur (*Presbytis entellus entellus*) monkeys. *Folia Primatol. 29:*98, 1978.
27. Haines, D. E., Holmes, K. R., and Brett, I. J.: The hemogram of the colonized lesser bushbaby (*Galago senegalensis*). *Folia Primatol. 14:*95, 1971.
28. Wellde, B. T., Johnson, A. J., Williams, J. S., Langbehn, H. R., and Sadun, E. H.: Hematologic, biochemical, and parasitologic parameters of the night monkey (*Aotus trivirgatus*). *Lab. Anim. Care 21:*575, 1971.
29. Capel-Edwards, K., and Hall, D. E.: Haematological observations on the squirrel monkey. *Folia Primatol. 12:*142, 1970.
30. Vondruska, J. F.: Certain hematologic and blood chemical values in adult stumptailed macques (*Macaca arctoides*). *Lab. Anim. Care 20:*97, 1970.
31. Hunt, R. D., and Chalifoux, L.: The hemogram of the tree shrew (*Tulpaia glis*). *Folia Primatol. 7:*34, 1967.
32. Dieterich, R. A., and Feist, D. D.: Hematology of Alaskan snowshoe hares (*Lepus americanus macfarlani*) during years of population decline. *Comp. Biochem. Physiol. 66A:*545, 1980.
33. Dieterich, R. A.: Hematologic values for six standardized wild rodent species. *Am. J. Vet. Res. 34:*431, 1973.
34. Patenaude, R. P., and Genest, F. B.: The hematology and chromosomes of the Canadian beaver (*Castor canadensis*). *J. Zoo Anim. Med. 8(3):*6, 1977.
35. Strike, T. A.: Hemogram and bone marrow differential of the chinchilla. *Lab. Anim. Care 20:*33, 1970.
36. Clark, J. D., Loew, F. M., and Olfert, E. D.: Rodents, in *Zoo and Wild Animal Medicine,* edited by M. E. Fowler. Saunders, Philadelphia, 1978, pp. 457–478.
37. Desal, R. G.: Hematology and microcirculation, in *The Golden Hamster: Its Biology and Use in Medical Research,* edited by R. A. Hoffman, P. F. Robinson, and H. Magalhaes. Iowa State University Press, Ames, 1968, pp. 185–194.
38. Mays, A., Jr.: Baseline hematological and blood biochemical parameters of the mongolian gerbil (*Meriones unguiculatus*). *Lab. Anim. Care 19:*838, 1969.
39. Martin, K., and Rutty, D. A.: Haematological values of the multimammate mouse *Praomys (Mastomys) natalensis. Lab. Anim. 3:*27, 1969.
40. MacNeill, A. C.: Blood values for some cetaceans. *Can. Vet. J. 16:*187, 1975.
41. Sweeney, J. C.: Procedures for clinical management of pinnipeds. *J. Am. Vet. Med. Assoc. 165:*811, 1974.
42. Greenwood, A. G., Ridgway, S. H., and Harrison, R. J.: Blood values in young gray seals. *J. Am. Vet. Med. Assoc. 159:*571, 1971.
43. White, J. R., Harkness, D. R., Isaacks, R. E., and Duffield, D. A.: Some studies on blood of the Florida manatee, *Trichechus manatus latirostris. Comp. Biochem. Physiol. 55A:*413, 1976.
44. Gates, N. L., Goering, E. K.: Hematologic values of conditioned, captive wild coyotes. *J. Wildl. Dis. 12:*402, 1976.
45. Strolle, L. A., Nielsen, S. W., and Diters, R. W.: Bone marrow and hematologic values of wild raccoons. *J. Wildl. Dis. 14:*409, 1978.
46. Lewis, J. H.: Comparative hematology: Studies on elephants, *Elephas maximus. Comp. Biochem. Physiol. 49A:*175, 1974.
47. Brown, D. G., and Cross, F. H.: Hematologic values of burros from birth to maturity: Cellular elements of peripheral blood. *Am. J. Vet. Res. 30:*1921, 1969.
48. Seal, U. S., Barton, R., Mather, L., and Gray, C. W.: Baseline laboratory data for the white rhinoceros (*Ceratotherium simum simum*). *J. Zoo Anim. Med. 7(1):*11, 1976.
49. Mehrer, C. F.: Some hematologic values of bison from five areas of the United States. *J. Wildl. Dis. 12:*7, 1976.
50. McDonald, S. E., Paul, S. R., and Bunch, T. D.: Physiologic and hematologic values in Nelson desert bighorn sheep, *J. Wildl. Dis. 17:*131, 1981.
51. Holman, H. H.: The blood picture of the cow. *Br. Vet. J. 111:*440, 1955.
52. Bush, M., Smith, E. E., and Custer, R. S.: Hematology and serum chemistry values for captive Dorcas gazelles: Variations with sex, age and health status. *J. Wildl. Dis. 17:*135, 1981.
53. Banerjee, S., Bhattacharjee, R. C., and Singh, T. I.: Hematological

studies in the normal adult Indian camel *(Camelus dromedarius).* *Am. J. Physiol. 203:*1185, 1962.

54. English, A. W., and Lepherd, E. E.: The haematology and serum biochemistry of wild fallow deer *(Dama dama)* in New South Wales. *J. Wildl. Dis. 17:*289, 1981.

55. Bush, M., Custer, R. S., and Whitla, J. C.: Hematology and serum chemistry profiles of giraffes *(Giraffa camelopardalis):* Variations with sex, age, and restraint. *J. Zoo Anim. Med. 11:*122, 1980.

56. Holman, H. H., and Dew, S. M.: The blood picture of the goat. I. The two-year-old female goat. *Res. Vet. Sci. 4:*121, 1963.

57. Jain, N. C., Vegad, J. L., Jain, N. K., and Shrivastava, A. B.: Haematological studies on normal lactating Indian water buffaloes. *Res. Vet. Sci. 32:*52, 1982.

58. Feinstein, R. N., Howard, J. B., Braum, J. T., and Seaholm, J. E.: Acatalasemic and hypocatalasemic mouse mutants. *Genetics 53:*923, 1966.

59. Rader, T.: Inheritance of hypocatalasaemia in guinea pigs. *J. Genet. 57:*169, 1960.

60. Feinstein, R. N., Faulhaber, J. T., and Howard, J. B.: Acatalasemia and hypocatalasemia in the dog and the duck. *Proc. Soc. Exp. Biol. Med. 127:*1051, 1968.

61. Nakamura, H., Yoshiya, M., Kaziro, K., and Kikuchi, G.: Anenzymia catalasea, a type of constitutional abnormality. Physiological significance of catalase in the animal organism. *Proc. Jpn. Acad. 28:*59, 1952.

62. Levin, E. Y.: Uroporphyrinogen III cosynthetase in bovine erythropoietic porphyria. *Science 161:*907, 1968.

63. Levin, E. Y., and Flyger, V.: Erythropoietic porphyria of the fox squirrel *Sciurus niger. J. Clin. Invest. 52:*96, 1973.

64. Glenn, B., Gleen, H., Omtvedt: Congenital porphyria in the domestic cat. Preliminary investigations on inheritance pattern. *Am. J. Vet. Res. 29:*1653, 1968.

65. With, T. K.: Porphyrias in animals. *Clin. Haematol. 9:*345, 1980.

66. Young, J. D., Ellory, J. C., and Tucker, E. M.: Amino acid transport defect in glutathione-deficient sheep erythrocytes. *Nature 245:*156, 1975.

67. Smith, J. E., Ryer, K., and Wallace, L.: Glucose-6-phosphate dehydrogenase deficiency in a dog. *Enzyme 21:*379, 1976.

68. Smith, J. E.: Glutathione deficiency and partial γ-glutamylcysteine synthetase in sheep. *Am. J. Pathol. 82:*147, 1976.

69. Smith, J. E., Moore, K., Arens, M., Rinderknecht, G. A., and Ledet, A.: Unpublished observations, 1982.

70. Anderson, R. S., Huestis, R. R., and Motulsky, A. G.: Hereditary spherocytosis in the deer mouse. Its similarity to the human disease. *Blood 15:*491, 1960.

71. Pinkerton, P. H., Fletch, S. M., Brueckner, P. J., and Miller, D. R.: Hereditary stomatocytosis with hemolytic anemia in the dog. *Blood 44:*557, 1974.

72. Pinkerton, P. H., and Bannerman, R. M.: Nonimmune anemias, in *Introduction in Spontaneous Animal Models of Human Disease,* edited by E. J. Andrews, B. C. Ward, and N. H. Altman. Academic, New York, 1979, vol. 1, pp. 233–236.

73. Harvey, J. W., Ling, G. V., and Kaneko, J. J.: Methemoglobin reductase deficiency in a dog. *J. Am. Vet. Med. Assoc. 164:*1030, 1974.

74. Letchworth, G. J., Bentinck-Smith, J., Bolton, G. R., Wootton, J. F., and Family, L.: Cyanosis and methemoglobinemia in two dogs due to a NADH methemoglobin reductase deficiency. *J. Am. Anim. Hosp. Assoc. 13:*75, 1977.

75. Tennant, B., Asbury, A. C., Laben, R. C., Richards, W. P. C., Kaneko, J. J., and Cupps, P. T.: Familial polycythemia in cattle. *J. Am. Vet. Med. Assoc. 150:*1493, 1967.

76. Searcy, G. P., Tasker, J. B., and Miller, D. R.: Animal model of human disease: Pyruvate kinase deficiency in dogs. *Am. J. Pathol. 94:*689, 1979.

77. Lux, S. E., Pease, B., Tomaselli, M. B., John, K. M., and Bernstein, S. E.: Hemolytic anemias associated with deficient or dysfunctional spectrin, in *Normal and Abnormal Red Cell Membranes,* edited by S. E. Lux and V. T. Marchesi. Allan R. Liss, New York, 1979, pp. 463–469.

78. Greenquist, A. C., Shohet, S. B., and Bernstein, S. E.: Marked reduction of spectrin in hereditary spherocytosis in the common house mouse. *Blood 51:*1149, 1978.

79. Martinell, J., Whitney, J. B., III, Popp, R. A., Russell, L. B., and Anderson, W. F.: Three mouse models of human thalassemia. *Proc. Natl. Acad. Sci. 78:*5056, 1981.

80. Perryman, L. E., and Magnuson, N. S.: Immunodeficiency disease in animals, in *Animal Models of Inherited Metabolic Disease,* edited by R. J. Desnick, D. G. Scarpelli, and D. F. Patterson. Alan R. Liss, New York, 1982.

81. Renshaw, H. W., Davis, W. C., and Renshaw, S. J.: Canine granulocytopathy syndrome: Defective bactericidal capacity of neutrophils from a dog with recurrent infections. *Clin. Immunol. Immunopathol. 8:*385, 1979.

82. Padgett, G. A., Leader, R. W., Gorham, J. R., and O'Mary, C. C.: The familial occurrence of the Chediak-Higashi syndrome in mink and cattle. *Genetics 49:*505, 1964.

83. Kramer, J. W., Davis, W. C., and Prieur, D. J.: The Chediak-Higashi syndrome of cats. *Lab. Invest. 36:*554, 1977.

84. Taylor, R. F., and Farrell, R. K.: Light and electron microscopy of peripheral blood neutrophils in a killer whale affected with Chediak-Higashi syndrome. *Fed. Proc. 32:*822, 1973.

85. Lutzner, M. A., Lowrie, C. T., and Jordan, H. W.: Giant granules in leukocytes of the beige mouse. *J. Hered. 58:*299, 1967.

86. Vogel, S. N., Weinblatt, A. C., and Rosentreich, D. L.: Inherent macrophage defects in mice, in *Immune Defects of Laboratory Animals,* edited by M. E. Gershwin and B. Merchant. Plenum, New York, 1980, vol. 1, pp. 327–357.

87. Nachtsheim, H.: Pelger-anomaly in man and rabbit: Mendelian character of nuclei of leukocytes. *J. Hered. 41:*131, 1950.

88. Schalm, O. W.: Interesting features in canine leukocytes. *Calif. Vet. 19:*25, 1965.

89. O'Donoghue, J. L., and Reed, C.: The hairless immune-deficient guinea pig, in *Immune Defects of Laboratory Animals,* edited by M. E. Gershwin and B. Merchant. Plenum, New York, 1981, vol. 1, pp. 285–308.

90. Fogh, J., and Giovanella, B. C.: *The Nude Mouse in Experimental and Clinical Research,* Academic, New York, 1978.

91. Festing, M. F.: Athymic nude rats, in *Immune Defects of Laboratory Animals,* edited by M. E. Gershwin and B. Merchant. Plenum, New York, 1981, vol. 1, pp. 267–283.

92. Erickson, K. L., and Gershwin, M. E.: Hereditarily athymic-asplenic (Lasat) mice, in *Immune Defects of Laboratory Animals,* edited by M. E. Gershwin and B. Merchant. Plenum, New York, 1981, vol. 1, pp. 297–308.

93. Duquesnoy, R. J., and Pedersen, G. M.: Immunologic and hematologic deficiencies of the hypopituitary dwarf mouse, in *Immune Defects of Laboratory Animals,* edited by M. E. Gershwin and B. Merchant. Plenum, New York, 1981, vol. 1, pp. 309–324.

94. Roth, J. A., et al.: Thymic abnormalities and growth hormone deficiency in dogs. *Am. J. Vet. Res. 41:*1256, 1980.

95. Andresen, E., Flagstad, T., Basse, A., and Brummerstedt, E.: Evidence of a lethal trait, A46, in Black Pied Danish cattle of Friesian descent. *Nord. Vet. Med. 22:*319, 1970.

96. Banks, K. L., McGuire, T. C., and Jerrells, T. R.: Absence of B lymphocytes in a horse with primary agammaglobulinemia. *Clin. Immunol. Immunopathol. 5:*282, 1976.

97. Perryman, L. E., and McGuire, T. C.: Evaluation for immune system failures in horses and ponies. *J. Am. Vet. Med. Assoc. 176:*1374, 1980.

98. Bennedict, A. A., Gershwin, M. E., and Abplanalp, H.: Inherited dysgammaglobulinemia of chickens, in *Immune Defects of Laboratory Animals,* edited by M. E. Gershwin and B. Merchant. Plenum, New York, 1981, vol. 1, pp. 139–161.

99. Welles, W. L., and Battisto, J. R.: The significance of hereditary asplenia for immune competence, in *Immune Defects of Laboratory Animals,* edited by M. E. Gershwin and B. Merchant. Plenum, New York, 1981, vol. 1, pp. 191–212.

100. Luster, M. I., Bacon, L. D., Rose, N. R., and Leslie, G. A.: Immunogenetic and ontogenetic studies of chickens with selective IgA-deficiency and autoimmune thyroiditis. *Cell. Immunol. 32:*417, 1977.

101. Nansen, P.: Selective immunoglobulin deficiency in cattle and susceptibility to infection. *Acta Pathol. Microbiol. Scand. Sect. B 80:*49, 1972.

102. Scher, I.: B-lymphocyte development and heterogeneity: Analysis with the immune-defective CBA/N mouse strain, in *Immune De-*

fects of Laboratory Animals, edited by M. E. Gershwin and B. Merchant. Plenum, New York, 1981, vol. 1, pp. 163–190.

103. McGuire, T. C., and Perryman, L. E.: Combined immunodeficiency of Arabian foals, in *Immune Defects of Laboratory Animals*, edited by M. E. Gershwin and B. Merchant, Plenum, New York, 1981, vol. 2, pp. 185–203.

104. Kincade, P. W.: Hemopoietic abnormalities in New Zealand Black and motheaten mice, in *Immune Defects of Laboratory Animals*, edited by M. E. Gershwin and B. Merchant, Plenum, New York, 1981, vol. 2, pp. 125–142.

105. Azar, H. A., Hansen, C. T., and Costa, J.: N:NIH(S)ll-nu/nu mice with combined immunodeficiency: A new model for human tumor heterotransplantation. *J. Nat. Cancer Inst.* 65:421, 1980.

106. Hammer, C. H., Gaither, T., and Frank, M. M.: Complement deficiencies of laboratory animals, in *Immune Defects of Laboratory Animals*, edited by M. E. Gershwin and B. Merchant, Plenum, New York, 1981, vol. 2, pp. 207–240.

107. Bitter-Suerman, D., Hoffman, T., Burger, R., and Hadding, U.: Linkage of total deficiency of the second component (C2) of the complement system and of genetic C2-polymorphism to the major histocompatibility complex of the guinea pig. *J. Immunol.* 127:608, 1981.

108. Winkelstein, J. A., Cork, L. C., Griffin, D. E., Griffin, J. W., Adams, R. J., and Price, D. L. Genetically determined deficiency of the third component of complement in the dog. *Science* 212:1169, 1981.

109. Ellman, L., Green, I., and Frank, M. M.: Genetically controlled total deficiency of the fourth component of complement in the guinea pig. *Science* 170:74, 1970.

110. Arroyave, C. M., Levy, R. M., and Johnson, J. S.: Genetic deficiency of the fourth component of complement (C4) in Wistar rats. *Immunology* 33:453, 1970.

111. Nilsson, U. R., and Muller-Eberhard, H. J.: Deficiency of the fifth component of complement in mice with an inherited complement defect. *J. Exp. Med.* 125:1, 1967.

112. Rother, K., Rother, U., Muller-Eberhard, H. J., and Nilsson, U.: Deficiency of the sixth component of complement in rabbits with an inherited complement defect. *J. Exp. Med.* 124:773, 1966.

113. Dodds, W. J.: Second international registry of animal models of thrombosis and hemorrhagic diseases. *ILAR News* 24:R1, 1981.

114. Breukink, J. H., Hart, H. C., Arkel, C., Veldon, N. A., and Watering, C. C.: Congenital afibrinogenemia in goats. *Zentralbl. Veterinaermed. Reihe A* 19:661, 1972.

115. Kammerman, B., Gmur, J., and Stunzi, H.: Afibrinogenamie beim hund. *Zentralbl. Veterinaermed. Reihe A* 18:192, 1971.

116. Dodds, W. J.: Hemostasis and coagulation, in *Clinical Biochemistry of Domestic Animals*, 3d ed., edited by J. J. Kaneko. Academic, New York, 1980, pp. 671–718.

117. Mustard, J. E., Secord, D., Hoeksema, T. D., Downie, H. G., and Rowsell, H. C.: Canine factor VII deficiency. *Br. J. Haematol.* 8:43, 1962.

118. Cotter, S. M., Brenner, R. M., and Dodds, W. J.: Hemophilia A in three unrelated cats. *J. Am. Vet. Med. Assoc.* 172:166, 1978.

119. Graham, J. B., Brinkhous, K. M., and Dodds, W. J.: Canine and equine hemophilia, in *Handbook of Hemophilia*, edited by K. M. Brinkhous and H. C. Hemker. Excerpta Medica, Amsterdam, 1975, pp. 119–139.

120. Dodds, W. J.: Further studies of canine von Willebrand's disease. *Blood* 45:221, 1975.

121. Dodds, W. J., Webster, W. P., Brinkhous, K. M., Owen, C. A., and Bowie, E. J. W.: Porcine and canine Von Willebrand's disease, in *Handbook of Hemophilia*, edited by K. M. Brinkhous and H. C. Hemker, Excerpta Medica, Amsterdam, 1975, pp. 141–148.

122. Benson, R. E., and Dodds, W. J.: Autosomal factor VIII deficiency in rabbits: Size variations of rabbit factor VIII. *Thromb. Haemost.* 38:380, 1977.

123. Dodds, W. J.: Canine factor X (Stuart-Prower factor) deficiency. *J. Lab. Clin. Med.* 82:560, 1973.

124. Kociba, G. J., Ratnoff, O. D., Loeb, W. F., Wall, R. L., and Heider, L. E.: Bovine plasma thromboplastin antecedent (factor XI) deficiency. *J. Lab. Clin. Med.* 74:37, 1969.

125. Dodds, W. J., and Kull, J. E.: Canine factor XI (plasma thromboplastic antecedent) deficiency. *J. Lab. Clin. Med.* 78:746, 1971.

126. Green, R. A., and White, F.: Feline factor XII (Hageman) deficiency. *Am. J. Vet. Res.* 38:893, 1977.

127. Ratnoff, O. D.: The biology and pathology of the initial stages of blood coagulation. *Prog. Hematol.* 5:204, 1966.

128. Robinson, A. J., Kropatkin, M., and Aggeler, P. M.: Hageman factor (factor XII) deficiency in marine mammals. *Science* 166:1420, 1969.

129. Johnson, G. J., Rao, G. H. R., Leis, L. A., and White, J. G.: Effect of agents that alter cyclic AMP on arachidonate-induced platelet aggregation in the dog. *Blood* 55:722, 1980.

130. Johnstone, I. B., and Lotz, F.: An inherited platelet function defect in basset hounds. *Can. Vet. J.* 20:211, 1979.

131. Novak, E. K., Hui, S. W., and Swank, R. T.: The mouse pale ear pigment mutant as a possible animal model for human platelet storage pool deficiency. *Blood* 57:38, 1981.

132. Raymond, S. L., and Dodds, W. J.: Characterization of the fawn-hooded rat as a model for hemostatic studies. *Thromb. Diath. Haemorrh.* 33:361, 1975.

133. Raymond, S. L., and Dodds, W. J.: Platelet membrane glycoproteins in normal dogs and dogs with hemostatic defects. *J. Lab. Clin. Med.* 93:607, 1979.

134. Lund, J. E., Padgett, G. A., and Ott, R. L.: Cyclic neutrophilia in grey collie dogs. *Blood* 29:452, 1967.

135. Russell, E. S.: Hereditary anemias of the mouse: A review for geneticists. *Adv. Genets.* 20:357, 1979.

136. Geissler E. N., McFarland, E. C., and Russell, E. S.: Analysis of pleiotropism at the dominant white-spotting (W) locus of the house mouse: A description of ten new W alleles. *Genetics* 97:337, 1981.

PART THREE *The hemopoietic stem cell*

The concept of the hemopoietic stem cell

CHAPTER 18

Hemopoietic stem cells

PETER J. QUESENBERRY

Definition

A number of cellular systems are made up by a few undifferentiated progenitor cells with the capacity for self-renewal and proliferation and by many differentiated cells with specific functions. During embryogenesis, most systems depend on continuous renewal from primitive progenitor cells, but in adult life, only a few tissues retain this dependency. In the liver, progenitor cells are dormant and only become activated after major cellular depletion, such as after partial hepatectomy. However, progenitor cells for the cells of skin, gastrointestinal epithelium, lymphoid tissue, and marrow are active throughout life. These crucial progenitor cells are also called stem cells, and our working definition for a stem cell is a cell with a capacity for self-renewal, proliferation, and differentiation.

Hemopoietic stem cells

The existence of a common stem cell for erythrocytes, platelets, and leukocytes is a theoretically attractive tenet in hematology and has been supported experimentally by recent studies on the clonality of hemopoietic stem cells in chronic myelogenous leukemia [1] and polycythemia vera [2]. Early arguments centered on whether stem cells were unipotential or pluripotential [3,4], but studies on both mice and humans have provided convincing evidence for the existence of a complex concatenated system. According to this, the most primitive of stem cells are pluripotential and have an extensive capacity for self-renewal. Their more differentiated progenies are unipotential for either erythroid, granulocytic, or megakaryocytic lines and have only limited capacity for self-renewal [5–9]. In addition, other data have suggested the existence of stem cells bipotential for megakaryocytopoiesis and erythropoiesis [10] or tripotential for all three cell lines [11]. (See Table 12-1 for a summary of current nomenclature.) A number of humoral substances and local environmental influences act at various points on proliferation and differentiation in this system [12–15]. A model of hemopoiesis based on these features is presented in Fig. 18-1.

Colony-forming units — spleen (CFU-S)

The cellular basis for hemopoietic repopulation was established in the early 1950s in studies on lethally irradiated mice [16–19]. A possible assay for repopulating stem cells was introduced by Till and McCulloch [5], who showed that mouse marrow cells, when injected into lethally irradiated syngeneic mice, are capable of forming discrete nodules of marrow cells in the spleens 8 to 10 days after intravenous injection. These nodules are called spleen colonies and consist of erythroid, granulocytic, megakaryocytic, and undifferentiated cells, either as pure populations or in varying mixtures [20–22]. Erythroid colonies predominate, with varying proportions of granulocytic, megakaryocytic, and undifferentiated colonies. After extended growth, most colonies become mixed [21]. The cells that formed these colonies were termed colony-forming units — spleen (CFU-S). In general, with some very important exceptions (see below), the number of CFU-S in murine marrow populations correlates with the ability of that marrow to repopulate the hemopoietic system of a lethally irradiated mouse.

In order to establish the CFU-S as a hemopoietic pluripotential stem cell, it was first necessary to determine whether or not the erythroid, granulocyte, and megakaryocyte components of the colonies were derived from a single cell. Clonality, or single-cell origin, of these nodules was initially suggested by radiation survival curves and the linear relation between cells injected and colonies formed [5]. This concept was further supported by injection of marrow cells with radiation-induced chromosome markers into irradiated mice; some of the resulting spleen colonies showed abnormal karyotypes in 95 to 99 percent of the metaphases [23]. Studies using a similar model showed that unique karyotypic markers are present in both ^{55}Fe-labeled erythroid and peroxidase-positive granulocytic cells [24]. The single-cell origin of these spleen colonies was also confirmed by injecting a mixture of normal and syngeneic cells with translocation chromosomal markers [25] into irradiated animals. The resulting colonies contained metaphases which were either normal or showed a marker; no mixed karyotypes were observed.

These observations have demonstrated the capacity of a single progenitor cell for extensive proliferation and differentiation into the three major hemopoietic cell lines. In order to qualify as a true stem cell, however, demonstration of a capacity for self-renewal was necessary. This was achieved by dissecting out single-cell–derived splenic colonies 10 to 14 days after injection,

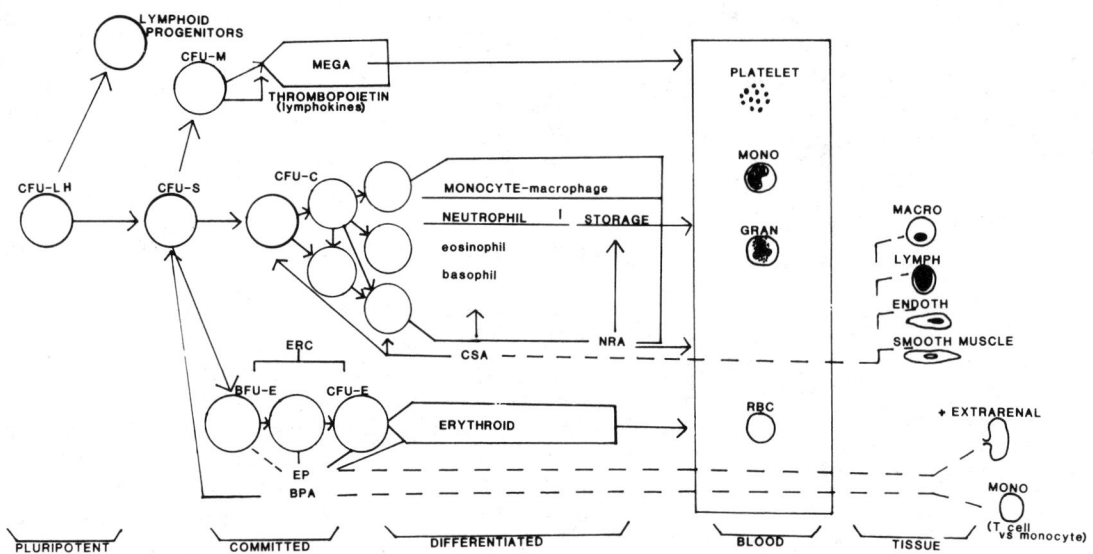

FIGURE 18-1   Model of Hemopoiesis. EP = erythropoietin; MACRO = macrophage; LYMPH = lymphocyte; ENDOTH = endothelial cell; MEGA = megakaryocyte; NRA = neutrophil-releasing activity; GRAN = granulocyte; MONO = monocyte; RBC = red blood cell; CFU-M = colony-forming unit−megakaryocyte; CFU-C = colony-forming unit−culture (granulocyte-monocyte stem cell); CFU-E = erythroid colony-forming unit; ERC = erythropoietin-responsive cell compartment; BFU-E = burst-forming unit−erythroid; CFU-LH = colony-forming unit−lymphoid-hemopoietic.

reinjecting a suspension of these cells into new irradiated recipients, and determining the number of new CFU-S generated per spleen colony [26]. The number of new colonies per dissected colony ranged from 0 to 1000. Pure colonies of any one type contained CFU-S that could form colonies of all three types after transplantation [20,27], clearly demonstrating the capacity of some CFU-S for extensive self-renewal.

The existence of a similar pluripotential stem cell in human marrow can be inferred from a number of observations. The success of marrow engraftment in patients with aplastic anemia who receive marrow from identical twins strongly suggests the existence of a cell in human marrow analogous to CFU-S [28]. The recently described in vitro assay of a cell (CFU-GEMM) giving rise to four hemopoietic lines (granulocytes, erythrocytes, monocytes, and megakaryocytes) also supports the presence of a CFU-S analog in human marrow [29], although the self-renewal capacity of the cell assayed is still in question. Perhaps the most impressive evidence for the existence of pluripotential stem cells in human marrow can be derived from analysis of several hematologic diseases which appear to represent neoplastic transformations of human stem cells. Chronic myelogenous leukemia (CML) is characterized in 90 percent of cases by a disease-specific marker chromosome, the Philadelphia chromosome (Chap. 24). It is present in erythroid, granulocytic, and megakaryocytic cells and suggests that a cell common to these lines is primarily affected in this disease [1]. However, a disease-specific marker chromosome could be caused by a single insult to a number of different cell lines and thus is not definite proof of

clonality. More convincing evidence of the clonal origin of cells can be derived from studies of cells with X-linked isoenzymes of glucose-phosphate dehydrogenases (G-6-PD). X chromosomes are randomly inactivated early in embryogenesis, and thus individuals heterozygous for an X-linked characteristic, such as G-6-PD isoenzymes A and B, will have a mixture of cells with either isoenzyme A or B [30]. However, if a cellular population originates from a single cell, then only one isoenzyme will be found (see Fig. 16-5). Studies in CML patients heterozygous for G-6-PD isoenzymes A and B demonstrated one isoenzyme type in platelets, red cells, and granulocytes and both types in fibroblasts and lymphocytes [31]. Studies in polycythemia vera using G-6-PD isoenzyme as cell markers have similarly shown that red cells, platelets, and granulocytes are clonally derived, whereas lymphocytes and fibroblasts are not [2]. These lines of evidence strongly suggest that a single hemopoietic pluripotential stem cell for all three hemopoietic lines exists in humans.

Colony-forming units−lymphoid, hemopoietic (CFU-LH)

The capacity of CFU-S to give rise to lymphocytes was questioned in early studies because lymphoid progenitors were not present in spleen colonies. However, a common marker chromosome could be observed in spleen-colony cells and lymphoid cells repopulating lymph nodes, thymus, and spleen [32–34], suggesting the existence of a primitive stem cell (CFU-LH) which gives rise to hemopoietic CFU-S and to lymphoid stem cells. Studies utilizing G-6-PD clonal markers indicated that non-T lymphocytes may also be clonal in CML and suggested that in some patients the neoplastic transformation may involve a stem cell common to the pluripotential hemopoietic stem cell and to the lymphoid system [35]. This is also suggested by observations that blast cells from some patients with CML in blast crisis contain terminal deoxynucleotidyl transferase, a DNA-synthetic enzyme whose expression is ordinarily restricted to primitive cells in the thymus and prothymocytes in the marrow [36,37]. However, the most definite demonstration of a stem cell for both hemopoietic and lymphoid lines has come from transplantation studies in stem cell-deficient W/W^v mice. These mice were repopulated with progressive dilutions of marrow that contained irradiation-induced chromosomal markers [38]. In some mice, CFU-S, marrow, spleen, and thymus cells, as well as phytohemagglutinin- and lipopolysaccharide-stimulated spleen cells, contained large proportions of cells bearing the same chromosome marker, indicating repopulation of hemopoietic and lymphopoietic cells by a single primitive stem cell (CFU-LH). Heterogeneity within the stem cell population was clearly shown by the observations that in some mice, only marrow cells and CFU-S had a common chromosomal marker, while in others, the chromosomal marker was restricted to thymus cells and phytohemagglutinin-stimulated spleen cells (i.e., T lymphocytes). Thus it appeared that in some animals the classical CFU-S with a restriction to myeloid trilineage differentiation repopulated the animal, while in others only a T-lymphocyte progenitor engrafted. These studies and others indicate that the stem cell compartments probably consist of cell populations with varying degrees of self-renewal and proliferative and differentiative potential and that there is a continuum of these cells rather than sharply defined cell compartments. However, it is helpful conceptually to regard general classes of stem cells as compartmentalized, keeping in mind that the transition from one stem cell compartment to another may be gradual and that there appears to be marked heterogeneity within a defined stem cell compartment. This general concept is presented in Fig. 18-2.

Humoral mediators of CFU-S

Humoral factors are important in determining spleen-colony growth and differentiation. Reduced erythropoietin levels induced either by plethora of host mice or antierythropoietin antibodies result in a decrease in erythroid colonies and an increase in undifferentiated colonies [15,39–40]. The undifferentiated colonies contain pluripotential stem cells and another population of stem cells apparently committed to erythropoiesis [14,15,41,42]. Administration of erythropoietin to plethoric mice as late as 7 to 9 days after injection of marrow

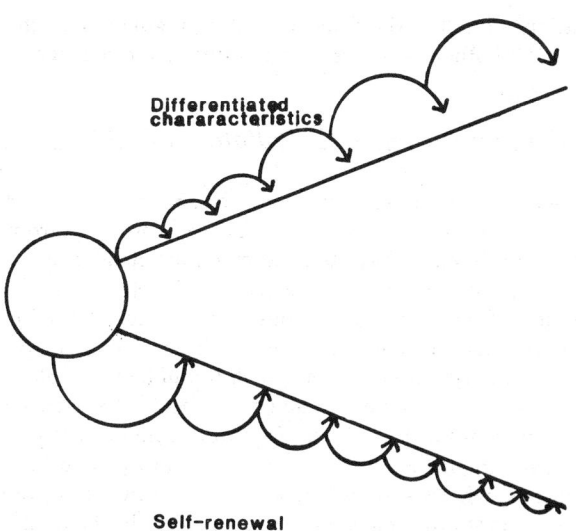

FIGURE 18-2 Stem cell model. Progressive loss of self-renewal with acquisition of differentiated characteristics.

converted the undifferentiated colonies of 100 to 200 cells to erythroid colonies containing 2 to 4×10^4 cells within 2 days. Other studies indicate that erythropoietin does not affect replication of CFU-S [15,43,44]. Studies utilizing in vitro clonal assays (see below) suggest that mitogen-stimulated spleen cells (or mononuclear cells) elaborate a substance termed burst-promoting activity (BPA) or factor (BPF), which may act at a primitive erythroid and possibly pluripotential stem cell level to induce both proliferation and acquisition of receptors for erythropoietin [45–49]. The production of BPA in vivo may explain the increase of erythropoietin-sensitive progenitors in spleen colonies from mice with depressed erythropoietin levels. Conditioned medium from mitogen-stimulated spleen cells contains an activity which induces CFU-S to synthesize DNA and to differentiate as well as to potentiate and stimulate granulocyte-macrophage colony formation [50,51]. These activities appear to be mediated by glycoproteins and are partially separable from each other and from BPA by polyacrylamide gel electrophoresis. Purified mouse lung granulocyte-macrophage colony-stimulating activity (CSA) or factor (CSF), previously considered to act specifically at the committed granulocyte-macrophage stem cell level, may also be capable of inducing four to five divisions of primitive cells which form erythroid or trilineage multipotential colonies in vitro [52,53]. These latter colonies are also directly stimulated by conditioned media from mitogen-stimulated spleen cells. Other activities which appear to act relatively early in the stem cell differentiation hierarchy include the erythroid-enhancing activity derived from a T-lymphoblast cell line [54] and the substances which induce giant macrophage colonies in vitro [55]. The relationship of these activities to marrow-derived stimulators and suppressors of CFU-S DNA synthesis is not yet clear [56,57]. It does seem apparent, however, that a variety of cell-derived factors act as regulators at the CFU-S or other closely related primitive stem cell levels.

Microenvironmental mediators of CFU-S

The local environment appears to be another important determinant of CFU-S differentiation. These environmental influences have been termed the hematopoietic-inductive microenvironment (HIM) [15,32]. The distribution of hemopoietic colonies in the spleen following administration of marrow CFU-S to irradiated recipients supports the concept of HIM. About half the spleen colonies are located on the spleen surface and 80 percent are erythroid or mixed [58]. Erythroid colonies are also present in the red pulp but not in empty lymphoid follicles, whereas granulocytic colonies grow along the trabeculae of the spleen or in subcapsular sheets. Megakaryocyte colonies usually grow beneath the capsule [32]. Further evidence of environmental influences is provided by the observations that colonies of hemopoietic cells in the spleen are usually erythroid, while in the marrow they are predominately granulocytic [12,32,59,60]. Furthermore, when irradiated marrow stroma is implanted into the spleens of lethally irradiated mice and a marrow cell suspension injected, colonies that form in the marrow stroma are mostly granulocytic, while those that form in the spleen are mostly erythroid. Colonies at the interface are mixed [12]. Studies of the genetically anemic *Sl/Sl^d* mutant mouse have provided additional support for the importance of HIM. These mice have a normal stem cell compartment, but their stroma cannot support normal hemopoiesis. Transplantation of their marrow cells can repopulate lethally irradiated mice, and their anemia can be cured by engraftment of normal stromal elements [61,62].

The effect of HIM is also seen when animals are exposed to granulopoietic stresses. The marrow shows increased granulopoiesis, while the spleen becomes predominantly an erythroid organ [63,64].

The introduction of a method for long-term mouse marrow culture has provided the opportunity to study stromal regulation of hemopoiesis [65,66]. This system permits long-term maintenance of in vitro hemopoiesis, including granulocytes, megakaryocytes, macrophages, CFU-S, granulocyte-macrophage stem cells, megakaryocytic stem cells, and late and early erythroid progenitors (BFU-E/CFU-E), along with an adherent stromal layer [66–70]. Lymphopoiesis is also supported in this system [71]. The stromal component of the murine system appears to consist of macrophages, hemopoietic cells, fibroblasts, endothelial cells, and "reticular cells" [72,73]. Initially, giant fat cells were thought to be essential for appropriate stromal function, but other data suggest that this represents an epiphenomenon and may signal eventual decline of the stromal cells [74]. Hemopoietic stem cells with increased proliferative potential appear to exist in intimate association with the stromal cells

[75]. This system opens the way for a detailed investigation of stromal regulation of hemopoiesis. The *Sl/Sl^d* stromal defect can be demonstrated in the in vitro system [76], and studies in the Golden Syrian hamster [77] have suggested that marrow-adherent cells in vitro not only support hemopoiesis with predominantly granulocytic differentiation, but may actually actively suppress erythroid differentiation. It appears that the stromal cells are radioresistant [78] and can produce colony-stimulating activity (CSA) in vitro [79]. Defective hemopoietic stroma has been observed in animals or patients after irradiation [80,81], and some patients with aplastic anemia or congenital hypoplastic anemia may also have a microenvironmental abnormality [82,83]. In mice, transplantation of cultured marrow under the kidney capsule has demonstrated that marrow stromal cells can be transplanted, form marrow architecture, and be repopulated by host stem cells [84]. Further evidence suggests that transplantation of marrow stromal cells may be important in hemopoietic marrow grafting [85]. A long-term culture system of human marrow [86] should allow for more detailed elucidation of the role of stroma in hemopoietic regulation.

Kinetics of CFU-S

A great deal of physiologic information is available on murine CFU-S. In the adult mouse they are present primarily in the marrow, with only about 2 percent in the spleen [5,32,87,88]. There are even fewer CFU-S in the blood, and the rare CFU-S detected in other tissues can probably be accounted for by contamination with blood [87,88]. The original source of CFU-S in adult animals is controversial; studies in avian species indicate that they derive mainly from the intraembryonic mesenchyme [89], while studies in murine species suggest that they originate in the yolk sac and migrate to the fetal liver and then to the marrow [90]. However, regardless of their origin, in adult mice, CFU-S are localized almost exclusively in the marrow, spleen, and blood. Hypoxia, anemia, or injection of antigens or endotoxin lead to decreased marrow and increased blood and spleen concentrations, suggesting migration of CFU-S from the marrow to the spleen [91–95]. Studies in mice subjected to lethal doses of irradiation except for one limb, protected with a lead shield, have proved that stem cell migration occurs and probably accounts for repopulation of irradiation-depleted marrow and spleen [96,97].

Most CFU-S appear to be out of cell cycle (G$_0$ phase) or have a relatively long generation time, as determined by "cell suicide" experiments with high-specific-activity tritiated thymidine or hydroxyurea [98–100]. Suicide experiments involve the killing of cells during the DNA synthesis (S) phase of the cell cycle, which lasts from 30 minutes to 2 hours; such experiments provide a "window" on the position of the stem cells within the generative cycle of the cell (Fig. 18-3). In most studies, these

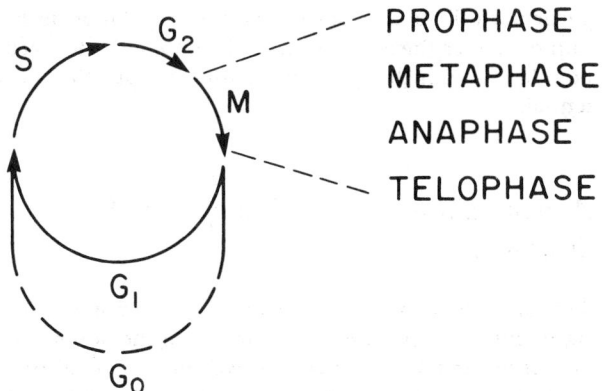

FIGURE 18-3 **The generative cycle of somatic cells consists of several distinct stages: G_1 is the period of cytoplasmic activity in preparation for cellular duplication; S is the synthetic period covering DNA replication; and G_2 is the premitotic resting period of a tetraploid cell. M is the mitotic period, which can be subdivided into a** *prophase,* **during which the nuclear membrane is dissolved and tetraploid chromosomes are found; a** *metaphase,* **during which spindle fibers connect centrioles with tetraploid chromosomes; an** *anaphase,* **during which the tetraploid chromosomes are separated into diploid chromosomes and pulled toward the centrioles; and a** *telophase,* **during which diploid nuclei are formed and the cell divides into two daughter cells. G_0 is a resting period, with cytoplasmic activity but no immediate preparation for cellular duplication.**

agents have had relatively little effect on CFU-S, indicating that CFU-S are not in cycle or that the generation time of the cell is relatively long. However, this is strain-dependent, with some strains showing substantial killing by S-phase-specific agents [101,102]. The CFU-S can be induced to proliferate rapidly by depopulation of the marrow. When moderate marrow depopulation is induced, CFU-S respond by increased differentiation and proliferation; however, when the CFU-S compartment has been reduced to less than 10 percent of normal by irradiation, there is no differentiation until self-replication partially restores the compartment [103]. This observation suggests that when marrow is severely depopulated, a mechanism exists that can induce CFU-S to enter the cell cycle and restore the number of these cells prior to differentiation. After restoration of CFU-S levels, differentiation then proceeds. As noted earlier, other studies suggest that marrow cells themselves can elaborate factors which either induce CFU-S into cycle or block cycle activation [104].

A number of mechanisms have been implicated in triggering CFU-S into S phase. Stimulation of both beta adrenergic and cholinergic receptors induces proliferation of CFU-S, and this effect appears to be mediated by the adenyl cyclase system [105–108]. In addition, calcium fluxes, androgens, and stimulation of histamine receptors also stimulate CFU-S proliferation [109–111]. Less well defined serum factors [112] or products of T lymphocytes or monocytes [45–49, 113] also appear to

act at the CFU-S level, inducing both increased proliferation and differentiation. The relationship of these entities to the CFU-S cell-cycle-active agents described above is unclear [56,57].

A number of studies have addressed the question of the total proliferative potential of CFU-S. As outlined above, the CFU-S has the ability to self-replicate extensively, but there is a limit, as suggested by the eventual decline of self-renewal and repopulating potential on serial transplantation [114]. A similar decline in self-renewal can be observed in long-term cultures [75]. Under ordinary circumstances, the renewal potential of the pluripotential stem cell appears to exceed the lifespan of the murine species under study; therefore mice do not show an exhaustion of stem cells with aging. However, therapy with alkylating agents decreases the capacity of murine CFU-S for self-renewal and limits the repopulating potential of stem cells [115–117]. In addition, in vitro studies suggest that stimulation of CFU-S by lithium in long-term cultures leads to an accelerated decline in self-renewal of these stem cells [79]. Such limitations on proliferative capacity of hemopoietic stem cells may have clinical relevance to the late sequelae of irradiation or chemotherapy.

Morphologically, the CFU-S resemble "transitional" lymphocytes [118]. Cell separation studies have indicated that most CFU-S are monuclear cells resembling lymphocytes but with distinct ultrastructural characteristics [119,120]. Furthermore, CFU-S appear to consist of extremely heterogenous cell population, as determined by analysis of self-replicative potential [26], adherence, cell size, density, lectin binding, and differentiation [5,121–124]. In addition, distinct differences in position within the cell cycle, repopulating potential, and possibly differentiation exist among marrow, blood, and splenic CFU-S [125,126]. Antigenic determinants on CFU-S are less well characterized. However, studies using mouse brain antisera with anti-CFU-S activity have shown that there are populations of antigen-negative and antigen-positive CFU-S [127,128]. Other antigen systems detected on murine CFU-S include H-2K, D, H-21-E, theta, and on rat CFU-S, Thy 1 [129,130].

CFU-S in murine species can be cryopreserved with retention of the capacity to form colonies and the potential for repopulation [131–133]. Stromal cells necessary for long-term culture can be cryopreserved in a similar manner [134]. These basic observations have been utilized in the development of programs using cryopreserved marrow for transplantation in humans.

Other assays exist for pluripotential stem cells in murine species. These involve sublethal whole-body irradiation or lethal irradiation of the whole body except for one leg that is protected by a lead shield [134–136]. The latter model appears to involve endogenous transplantation from a shielded leg to the spleen. In both techniques, splenic colonies grow from residual stem cells and have been referred to as *endogenous colony-formation assays.* These techniques investigate two variables: cell migration and stem cell numbers. The endogenous techniques avoid the use of transplantation. Some workers suggest that CFU-S in the S phase may not tolerate transplantation well [137]. If this is true, the exogenous transplantation technique may preferentially assay noncycling CFU-S and underestimate the number of CFU-S in cell cycle. The endogenous technique is not suitable for many studies of stem cell kinetics, but whether the transplantation technique adequately measures all CFU-S remains open to debate.

An important experimental consideration with regard to assaying CFU-S involves determination of the number that actually end up "seeding" the spleen. Neither the endogenous nor exogenous spleen-colony techniques measure all the stem cells, since only a few of the transplanted or endogenous cells actually seed the spleen. Since the percentage that do seed the spleen may change with various experimental manipulation, this could be a critical factor in interpreting data from various experiments. The transplantation fraction (f fraction) has been determined by several techniques [44,138,139], which have yielded estimates ranging from 3 to 24 percent. Previous exposure of donor cells to irradiation, endotoxin, or vinblastine decrease the f fraction [60,140,141].

Although a large volume of data has been generated on the CFU-S as a pluripotential repopulating stem cell, there may be other marrow stem cells which correlate more exactly with marrow repopulation and which have more self-renewing, proliferative, and differentiative potential. The stem cell identified in plasma-clot diffusion-chamber cultures, termed colony-forming unit—diffusion chamber (CFU-D), may be a cell at the same stage as the CFU-S or possibly more primitive [142,143]. This stem cell is assayed by culturing marrow in semisolid plasma clots in diffusion chambers which have been implanted into the peritoneal cavity of mice. After various periods of time, colonies with granulocytes, macrophages, or, less commonly, erythrocytes and megakaryocytes are found. The CFU-D appear to be similar to the CFU-S with regard to cell-cycle status, cell size, and density, but they appear to differ with regard to differential preservation after cryopreservation and sensitivity to hypotonic lysis [134,143–146]. This particular assay, while cumbersome, is applicable to both humans and mice and as such may provide a means of studying primitive pluripotential stem cells in humans. Marrow from 5-fluorouracil pretreated animals has been found to have an increased ability to repopulate lethally irradiated mice [56,147,148]. This ability correlates with the presence of a stem cell which could be grown in soft agar cultures and which produces huge macrophage colonies. This stem cell has been termed high proliferative potential–CFC (HPP-CFC), and the assay appears to correlate more closely with repopulation potential than does CFU-S. Others have suggested that the primitive erythroid colony-forming cell (see below) may also represent a stem cell at the CFU-S level or earlier [149]. Thus while the CFU-S gives us much insight into primitive stem cell compartments, it is not yet clear whether this

particular cell, as assayed by the transplantation technique, defines the most primitive hemopoietic stem cell population with the greatest marrow repopulating potential.

Animal and human models of CFU-S dysfunction

Several animal models have provided important insights into the regulatory mechanisms in hemopoiesis. The Sl/Sl^d and W/W^v mice are two important murine models of hemopoietic insufficiency. The Sl/Sl^d mouse appears to have a stromal defect resulting in macrocytic anemia and other more subtle defects of hemopoiesis [61,62,150], whereas the W/W^v mice have a defect in the CFU-S compartment. These latter mice also suffer from prominent macrocytic anemia and lesser defects in megakaryocytopoiesis and granulopoiesis [112,151,152]. The defect in the W/W^v mouse may be the absence of a regulatory T lymphocyte, which is critical in determining CFU-S differentiation and proliferation [153,154].

Clinical studies on some patients with aplastic anemia or congenital hypoplastic anemia have suggested the existence of stromal defects such as has been demonstrated in the Sl/Sl^d mouse [82,83]. Other studies have indicated possible T-cell or mononuclear-cell abnormalities in the genesis of aplastic anemia in humans and have suggested that regulatory cells such as have been demonstrated in the W/W^v mouse may be abnormal in certain cases of marrow insufficiency [155–159]. In general, however, data on the existence of these regulatory mechanisms in humans and their disorders in aplastic anemia are relatively unconvincing [160,161].

Another animal model of stem cell deficiency is cyclic neutropenia in the gray collie dog [162,163]. In this disorder, neutrophils, eosinophils, lymphocytes, reticulocytes, and platelets all cycle [162]. The cycle length is about 11 days for each cell type, but all cycles are out of phase with each other. This recessive disease results in severe infections and premature death. It can be cured or transferred to a normal litter mate by marrow transplantation, demonstrating that the defect lies either in the stem cells or in transplantable regulatory cells [164]. Additional studies suggest that the basic defect is at the stem cell level and that other changes are secondary [165–167]. Cycling in these animals can be eliminated by daily endotoxin treatment [165]. The administration of lithium carbonate eliminates the severe recurrent neutropenia, normalizes the monocyte, reticulocyte, and platelet counts, and ameliorates the anemia [168]. Further studies utilizing long-term culture systems suggests that lithium may be acting on the pluripotential stem cell in this setting [79]. Studies in outbred animals treated with cyclophosphamide suggest that moderate marrow hypoplasia leads to cyclical neutropenia, while more severe hypoplasia causes a severe steady-state neutropenia [169]. These data taken together suggest that cyclical hemopoiesis in the gray collie represents a moderate decrease in the number of CFU-S. A similar disorder exists in humans in which monocyte, lymphocyte, reticulocyte, and platelet populations also cycle at an interval of approximately 3 weeks [163]. Alternate-day steroid therapy stabilizes the cycling and prevents infections in humans with cyclic neutropenia [170]. Lithium administration to humans with this disorder has in general been ineffectual.

In summary, the experimentally defined pluripotential stem cell in the marrow appears to be a slowly cycling cell with a capacity for extensive self-renewal and differentiation. This stem cell gives rise to megakaryocyte, erythroid, and granulocyte-monocyte progenitors, but probably not lymphocytes. There is evidence that a more primitive stem cell exists that gives rise to CFU-S and lymphocytes, and this cell or other more primitive cells may correlate more closely than the CFU-S with repopulating potential in certain experimental situations. The CFU-S appears to be influenced by the microenvironment, factors from mitogen-stimulated mononuclear cells, factors derived from marrow cell populations, cell depopulation, and less well defined humoral factors. Figure 18-4 shows a model of CFU-S regulation.

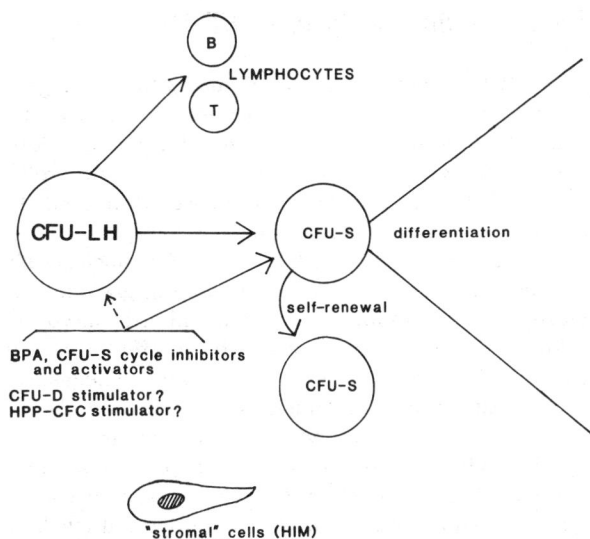

FIGURE 18-4 Model of pluripotential stem cell (CFU-S) regulation. CFU-LH = lymphoid-hemopoietic colony-forming unit common progenitor; CFU-S = colony-forming unit—spleen; HIM = hemopoietic inductive environment; BPA = burst-promoting activity; HPP-CFC = high proliferative potential colony-forming cell; CFU-D = colony-forming unit—diffusion chamber.

Erythroid-committed stem cells (CFU-E and BFU-E)

At the time of the introduction of the assay for the pluripotential stem cells, evidence accumulated for the existence of an intermediate compartment of stem cells committed to erythropoiesis. Previous studies had demonstrated a humoral agent, named erythropoietin, that controlled the rate of red cell production [171,172] (see Chap. 38). Erythropoietin is a glycoprotein with a molecular weight of 32,000 daltons [173] and is produced largely by the kidney in response to renal tissue hypoxia [174,175]. However, 10 to 15 percent appears to be of extrarenal, probably hepatic, origin [176–179]. Erythropoietin was the first humoral agent shown to affect hemopoietic differentiation [180–181]. It acts primarily on cells not morphologically recognizable as erythroblasts and transforms these cells to proerythroblasts [182]. The target cells are rapidly proliferating and behave kinetically both in vivo and in vitro as a more differential progeny of CFU-S [7,15,43,44,183–186]. They are termed erythropoietin-responsive cells and were the first intermediate class of stem cells demonstrated experimentally.

Studies utilizing in vitro clonal culture systems have more precisely defined this compartment of committed erythroid stem cells [7,184,185]. Two separate classes of erythroid stem cells were recognized using the plasma-clot culture technique [184]. A stem cell with extensive proliferative potential requiring high levels of erythro-

poietin and a relatively long culture period was termed a burst-forming unit—erythroid (BFU-E). This cell appeared to be analogous to the erythropoietin-committed stem cell studied with in vivo techniques. A more differentiated stem cell close to the proerythroblast in the differentiation pathway was termed colony-forming unit—erythroid (CFU-E); the CFU-E gave rise to small clusters of erythroid cells after several days of culture and required relatively small amounts of erythropoietin. Further studies in both humans and murine species have indicated that there may be classes of erythroid stem cells intermediate between the CFU-E and BFU-E [187,188]. There is also evidence for an erythroid stem cell more primitive than the conventional BFU-E with a high proliferative and differentiative capacity and first seen at 9 to 12 days of culture in murine species [149]. Further studies have also indicated that many of the erythroid stem cells may be bipotential and be capable of producing megakaryocytes [10]. Clonality of these bipotential erythroid-megakaryocyte stem cells was established with sex-chromosome markers [10]. CFU-E proliferate more rapidly than BFU-E [189,190]. Moreover, actinomycin administration or induction of plethora selectively ablates the CFU-E compartment but increases the number of marrow BFU-E [191–193]. These observations suggest that the CFU-E is a mature descendant of the more primitive BFU-E and depends upon erythropoietin in vivo for its existence. However, the BFU-E and other more primitive erythroid stem cells appear to respond to erythropoietin by differentiating into the CFU-E, but they are not maintained by erythropoietin.

Burst-promoting activity (BPA)

As described above, conditioned media from mitogen-stimulated mononuclear cells appear to reduce the amount of erythropoietin required for the development of bursts and to allow for the survival and proliferation of BFU-E, even if the addition of erythropoietin to the cultures is delayed for as long as 3 days [45–49]. The conditioned media derived from these mononuclear cells also appear to be capable of stimulating granulocyte, macrophage, eosinophil, erythroid, and megakaryocyte colonies [192,193]. The granulocyte, macrophage, and eosinophil stimulators are separable, but the megakaryocyte- and erythroid-stimulating activities are always associated with granulocyte, macrophage, and eosinophil activities. Thus it is not clear at present whether one molecule is capable of stimulating all four colony types, possibly acting at a very primitive cell level, or whether multiple, closely related factors are involved. Gel filtration indicates an apparent molecular weight of 37,000 daltons for each of the factors [52]. Pokeweed mitogen-stimulated spleen cells were also capable of stimulating erythroid colonies from fetal liver without the addition of exogenous erythropoietin [47]. It has been proposed that this burst-promoting activity (BPA) or factor (BPF) acts at the pluripotential stem cell level to allow proliferation and survival of early stem cells. Subsequent differentiation is then characterized by a progressive increase in pathway-specific receptors, either erythropoietin receptors or possibly granulocyte-macrophage colony-stimulating activity (CSA) receptors [48]. A number of hormones potentiate the effects of erythropoietin in vitro, including androgenic steroids, particularly those of an angular (5B) configuration [194,195], dexamethasone [196] (but not other glucocorticoids [194]), growth hormone [197], and thyroid hormone [198].

Granulocyte- and monocyte-committed stem cells (CFU-GM)

A precise definition of regulation of granulopoiesis has not been achieved. In contrast to the erythroid system, there is no practical method for reversibly suppressing granulocyte production, there are a large number of apparently unrelated stimuli affecting granulopoiesis, and there is no specific radioactive label for newly produced granulocytic-monocytic cells. However, in vitro clonal assays have provided the analytic tool for the elucidation of control mechanisms involved in granulocyte, monocyte, and eosinophil production and for the definition of the granulocyte, monocyte, and eosinophil stem cell compartment. In these culture systems, single cells proliferate in the presence of substances termed colony-stimulating activity (CSA) or factor (CSF) to form colonies consisting of up to several thousands of granulocyte- and monocyte-macrophages [6,199–201]. These clonal culture systems are applicable to most mamma-

lian species, including dogs, monkeys, cows, pigs, and humans. The single-cell origin of these colonies has been established by cell-transfer experiments. Further analysis of clonal growth has demonstrated subpopulations of progenitor cells which tend to differentiate into granulocytes or into macrophages. Each progenitor responds to a CSA specific for its type. However, there are other populations of cells which appear to respond to both factors with the production of colonies whose predominant cell type is related to the type of factor utilized [202,203]. In addition, some mixed granulocyte-macrophage colonies have been shown to be single-cell-derived [202]. Additional data have suggested that eosinophil colony-forming cells represent a separate population which responds to different factors [204–206]. Cells that give rise to all these colonies were termed colony-forming units in culture (CFU-C) and appear to be separate from populations of CFU-S, BFU-E, or CFU-Meg [7,9,99,100,121–123,207–212]. CFU-C have a relatively high proliferation rate [99,100,207], can be partially separated from CFU-S by velocity, density, and adherence separation techniques [122], and are kinetically different from CFU-S [208–211]. In rats, clear physical separations of CFU-S and CFU-C have been accomplished [213]. In general, the CFU-C have limited capacity for self-renewal compared with the CFU-S [214] and show a marked heterogeneity manifest by different colony size, cell density and size [121,122], and sensitivity to CSA [215,216].

Morphologically, CFU-C resembles either a primitive blast cell or, similar to the CFU-S, a transitional lymphocyte [118–120,202].

Colony-stimulating activity (CSA)

The growth of CFU-C in vitro has an absolute requirement for CSA [217,218]. As noted above different CSAs have different propensities for inducing differentiation along the granulocyte or macrophage pathway, and there probably exists a number of different CSAs acting at different levels of differentiation. It would appear that CSA is analogous to erythropoietin, representing a regulator of granulocyte-macrophage differentiation acting at the committed or relatively differentiated stem cell level. If CSA is not present, no colonies form. Moreover, CSA is required during the whole culture period or growth will cease [219,220]. CSA has been detected in biological fluids and is extractable from most tissues of all mammalian species studied. Thus far CSA has been derived from macrophages and monocytes [221–223], activated lymphocytes [224,225], endothelial cells [226,227], and vascular smooth muscle [228]. A number of cell lines, transformed cells, or malignant tissues also produce CSA in vitro, but the physiologic relevance of this is unknown [229,230]. Serum CSA levels in vivo appear to be determined at least in part by exposure to bacterial antigens or breakdown products [64,231,232]. In most situations in which an increased need for granulocytes or monocytes is present, serum or tissue levels of CSA have been found to be elevated.

Biochemical characterization of various CSA species has been carried out by a number of workers [229,234–241]. The CSA termed CSF-I [242–244], which induces largely macrophage differentiation, has been purified to homogeneity and appears to consist of two polypeptide chains, disulfide bonded, each chain with a molecular weight of 14,000 daltons. Molecular weight estimates for CSA have a range from 40,000 to 86,000 daltons, perhaps reflecting different degrees of glycosylation. However, removal of these carbohydrate groups has had no basic effect on CSA activity. Radioimmunoassays and receptor assays have been developed utilizing CSF-I purified from mouse cells [245,246]. Studies based on these techniques suggest that CSA is rapidly bound to macrophage progenitor cells and to their more differentiated progeny and then internalized and degraded. A granulocyte-differentiation CSA derived from murine lung–conditioned media has been extensively purified [236]. This CSA is a glycoprotein with a molecular weight of approximately 23,000 daltons. Further work with purified CSAs and their antibodies should provide major insights into the regulation of granulopoiesis.

The mechanisms controlling CSA levels in vivo have been the subject of intensive study. It has been reported that lactoferrin derived from mature granulocytes blocks the production or release of CSA by nonstimulated monocytes [247] but does not block endotoxin-stimulated production of CSA. This has led to the proposal that lactoferrin may be a physiologic regulator of granulopoiesis. As granulocyte levels begin to rise, granulocyte-derived lactoferrin inhibits granulocyte-monocyte production by blocking evolution of monocyte CSA unless there is a continuing stimulus, such as might be provided by unresolved infection. Others have proposed that prostaglandin E produced by monocytes and macrophages may function as a direct inhibitor of macrophage progenitors [248,249]. In addition, prostaglandins appear to be increased in response to elevated levels of CSA, providing the potential for a feedback regulatory system [250]. This area remains controversial, since some workers have failed to demonstrate inhibition by lactoferrin [251] and others have indicated that lactoferrin may act via a T lymphocyte [252]. Vascular endothelium may be a more potent source of CSA than monocytes because it responds to endotoxin, granulocytes, granulocyte lysates, and even lactoferrin by increased CSA production [227,228]. All in all, the mode of regulation of CSA levels in vivo remains at present unanswered.

A number of other possible regulators of granulocyte, monocyte, and macrophage production have been described. There are high- and low-molecular-weight inhibitors of in vitro CFU-C growth [253,254], granulocytic chalones [255], and substances which potentiate in vitro growth of CFU-C without intrinsic CSA activity [256–258], but their physiologic relevance is unclear. Modulation of granulocyte production by factors acting

at more primitive stem cells, such as burst-promoting activity, diffusion-chamber granulocytic-stimulating activity, or the activity necessary for induction of high proliferative potential CFU-C growth, remain to be defined.

Another potential regulator of granulocyte-monocyte levels in blood is the humoral factor termed *neutrophil-releasing activity*, which induces the release of mature granulocytes from the marrow granulocyte reserve pool [259,260]. This activity and CSA evolve in many of the same situations, but they are separate entities [64,261].

A model for the regulation of granulocyte, eosinophil, and monocyte production is presented in Fig. 18-5.

Megakaryocytic-committed stem cells (CFU-Meg)

Megakaryocytes are derived from CFU-S, and their differentiation is determined, at least in part, by microenvironmental location. Megakaryocytopoiesis and platelet production are stimulated by thrombocytopenia and suppressed by thrombocytosis [262,263]. A number of studies have indicated that regulation of platelet production depends on the humoral substance called *thrombopoietin* [264–266], and various assays for this entity have been proposed [267–269]. It has been suggested that small acetylcholinesterase-positive mononuclear cells in rats are megakarycote precursors [270], but their roles as stem cells remain problematic. Studies on the cloning of megakaryocytic colonies in vitro in the presence of conditioned media from murine

FIGURE 18-5 Model of granulopoiesis. MB = myeloblast or monoblast; MONO = monocyte; PMN = polymorphonuclear leukocyte; CSA = colony-stimulating activity; CFU-S = colony-forming unit–spleen; CFU-C = colony-forming unit–culture (granulocyte-monocyte stem cell); EOS = eosinophil; NEUT = neutrophil; BASO = basophil.

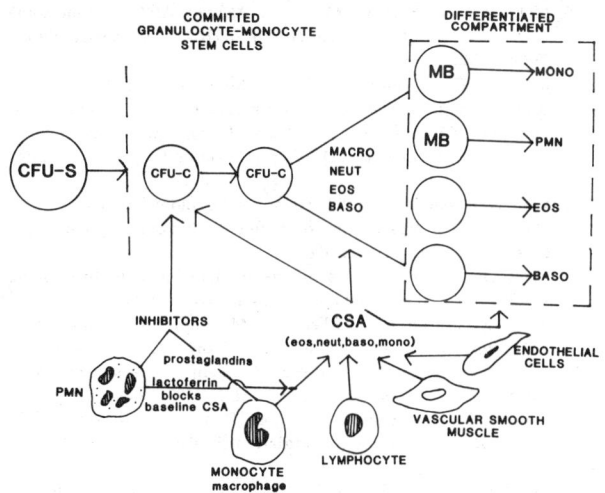

(Role of HPP-CFC/CFU-D stimulators not yet clear)

lymphocytes stimulated by pokeweed mitogen or 2-mercaptoethanol have indicated the existence of an intermediate compartment of stem cells committed to megakaryocytopoiesis [9,271,272]. Megakaryocyte colony-forming units have also been grown from human blood and have been identified with an antiplatelet glycoprotein antiserum probe. The growth of these colonies was enhanced by sera from patients with aplastic anemia, but not with erythropoietin- or thrombopoietin-containing material [273]. Data on the kinetics and control of these compartments, cell-cycle status, and differentiation potential remain areas of ongoing research. Clonal assay methods should allow for a clear definition of the megakaryocytic stem cell compartment and its regulation.

References

1. Whang, J., Frei, E., III, Tjio, J. H., Carbone, P. P., and Brecher, G.: The distribution of the Philadelphia chromosome in patients with chronic myelocytic leukemia. *Blood* 22:664, 1963.
2. Adamson, J. W., Fialkow, P. J., Murphy, S., Prchal J. F., and Steinmann, L.: Polycythemia vera: Stem cell and probable clonal origin of the disease. *N. Engl. J. Med.* 295:913, 1976.
3. Maximow, A. A.: Relation of blood cells to connective tissues and endothelium. *Physiol. Rev.* 4:533, 1924.
4. Sabin, F. R., Miller, F. R., Smithburn, K. C., Thomas, R. M., and Hummell, L. E.: Changes in the bone marrow and blood cells of developing rabbits. *J. Exp. Med.* 64:97, 1936.
5. Till, J. E., and McCulloch, E. A.: A direct measurement of the radiation sensitivity of normal mouse bone marrow cells. *Radiat. Res.* 14:213, 1961.
6. Bradley, T. R., and Metcalf, D.: The growth of mouse bone marrow cells in-vitro. *Aust. J. Exp. Biol. Med. Sci.* 44:287, 1966.
7. Axelrad, A. A., McLeod, D. L., Shreeve, M. M., and Health, D. S.: Properties of cells that produce erythrocytic colonies in-vitro, in *Hemopoiesis in Culture: Second International Workshop,* edited by W. A. Robinson. DHEW Publication No. NIH Government Printing Office, Washington, 1973, p. 226.
8. Pike, B. L., and Robinson, W. A.: Human bone marrow colony growth in agar-gel. *J. Cell. Physiol.* 76:77, 1970.
9. Nakeff, A., Dicke, K. A., and Van Noord, M. J.: Megakaryocytes in agar culture of mouse bone marrow. *Ser. Haematol* 8:4, 1975.
10. McLeod, D. L., Shreeve, M. L., and Axelrad, A. A.: Chromosome marker evidence for bipotentiality of BFU-E. *J. Supramolec. Struct.* (Suppl. 4):211, 1980.
11. Johnson, G. R., and Metcalf, D.: Multi-potential hemopoietic colony formation in agar cultures stimulated by spleen conditioned medium, in *Experimental Hematology Today, 1980,* edited by S. J. Baum, G. D. Ledney, and D. W. Van Bekkum. Karger, Basel, 1980, p. 29.
12. Wolf, N. S., and Trentin, J. J.: Hemopoietic colony studies. V. Effect of hemopoietic organ stroma on differentiation of pluripotent stem cells. *J. Exp. Med.* 127:205, 1968.
13. Reissmann, K. R.: Studies on the mechanism of erythropoietic stimulation in parabiotic rats during hypoxia. *Blood* 5:372, 1950.
14. Bleiberg, I., Liron, M., and Feldman, M.: Studies on the regulation of hemopoietic spleen colonies. *Blood* 29:469, 1967.
15. Curry, J. L., Trentin, J. J., and Wolf, N.: Hemopoietic spleen colony studies. II. Erythropoiesis. *J. Exp. Med.* 125:703, 1967.
16. Ford, C. E., Hamerton, J. L., Barnes, D. W. H., and Loutit, J. F.: Cytological identification of radiation-chimaeras. *Nature* 177:452, 1956.
17. Lindsley, D. L., Odell, T. T., Jr., and Tausche, F. G.: Implantation of functional erythropoietin elements following total-body irradiation. *Proc. Soc. Exp. Biol. Med.* 90:512, 1955.
18. Mitchison, N. A.: The colonisation of irradiated tissue by transplanted spleen cells. *Br. J. Exp. Pathol.* 37:239, 1956.
19. Nowell, P. C., Cole, L. J., Habermeyer, J. G., and Roan, P. L.: Growth and continued function of rat marrow cells in x-radiated mice. *Cancer Res.* 16:258, 1956.
20. Lewis, J. P., and Trobaugh, F. E., Jr.: Haematopoietic stem cells. *Nature* 204:589, 1964.
21. Curry, J. L., and Trentin, J. J.: Hemopoietic spleen colony studies. IV. Phytohemagglutinin and hemopoietic regeneration. *J. Exp. Med.* 126:819, 1967.
22. Fowler, J. H., Wu, A. M., Till, J. E., McCulloch, E. A., and Siminovitch, L.: The cellular composition of hemopoietic spleen colonies. *J. Cell. Physiol* 69:65, 1967.
23. Becker, A. J., McCulloch, E. A., and Till, J. E.: Cytological demonstration of the clonal nature of spleen colonies derived from transplanted mouse marrow cells. *Nature* 197:452, 1963.
24. Wu, A. M., Till, J. E., Siminovitch, L., and McCulloch, E. A.: A cytological study of the capacity for differentiation of normal hemopoietic colony-forming cells. *J. Cell. Physiol.* 69:177, 1967.
25. Welshons, W. J.: Detection and use of cytological anomalies in the mouse, in *Mammalian Cytogenetics and Related Problems in Radiobiology,* edited by C. Pavan et al. Pergamon, Oxford, 1964, p. 233.
26. Siminovitch, L., McCulloch, E. A., and Till, J. E.: The distribution of colony-forming cells among spleen colonies. *J. Cell Comp. Physiol.* 62:327, 1963.
27. Juraskova, V., and Tkadlecek, L.: Character of primary and secondary colonies of haematopoiesis in the spleen of irradiated mice. *Nature* 206:951, 1965.
28. Thomas, E. D., Rudolph, R. H., Fefer, A., Storb, R., Slichter, S., and Buckner, C. D.: Isogeneic marrow grafting in man. *Exp. Hematol.* 21:16, 1971.
29. Fauser, A. A., and Messner, H. A.: Identification of megakaryocytes, macrophages and eosinophils in colonies of human bone marrow containing neutrophilic granulocytes and erythroblasts. *Blood* 53:1023, 1979.
30. Fialkow, P. J.: Clonal origin of human tumors. *Biochim. Biophys. Acta* 458:283, 1976.
31. Fialkow, P. J., Jacobson, R. J., and Papayannopoulou, T.: Chronic myelocytic leukemia: Clonal origin in stem cell common to the granulocyte, erythrocyte, platelet and monocyte/macrophage. *Am. J. Med.* 63:125, 1977.
32. Curry, J. L., and Trentin, J. J.: Hemopoietic spleen colony studies. I. Growth and differentiation. *Dev. Biol.* 15:395, 1967.
33. Curry, J. L., Trentin, J. J., and Cheng, U.: Hemopoietic spleen colony studies. III. Hemopoietic nature of spleen colonies induced by lymph node or thymus cells, with or without phytohemagglutinin. *J. Immunol.* 99:907, 1967.
34. Trentin, J., Wolf, N., Cheng, U., Fahlberg, W., Weiss, D., and Bonhag, R.: Antibody production by mice repopulated with limited numbers of clones of lymphoid cell precursors. *J. Immunol.* 98:1326, 1967.
35. Fialkow, P. J., Denman, A. M., Jacobson, R. J., and Lowenthal, M. N.: Chronic myelocytic leukemia: Origin of some lymphocytes from leukemic stem cells. *J. Clin. Invest.* 62:815, 1978.
36. Baltimore, D., Silverstone, A. E., and Kung, P. C.: What cells contain terminal deoxynucleotidyl transferase? in *The Generation of Antibody Diversity: A New Look,* edited by A. J. Cunningham. Academic, New York, 1976, p. 21.
37. McCaffrey, R., Harrison, T. A., Parkman, R., and Baltimore, D.: Terminal deoxynucleotidyl transferase activity in human leukemic cells and in normal human thymocytes. *N. Engl. J. Med.* 292:775, 1975.
38. Abramson, S., Miller, R. G., and Phillips, R. A.: The identification in adult bone marrow of pluripotent and restricted stem cells of the myeloid and lymphoid systems. *J. Exp. Med.* 145:1567, 1977.
39. Schooley, J. C., and Garcia, J. F.: Some properties of serum obtained from rabbits immunized with human urinary erythropoietin. *Blood* 25:204, 1965.
40. Lange, R. D., McDonald, T. P., and Jordan, T.: Antisera to erythropoietin: Partial characterization of two different antibodies. *J. Lab. Clin. Med.* 73:78, 1969.
41. Feldman, M., Bleiberg, I., and Liron, M.: Regulation of intrasplenic

formation of erythroid clones. *Ann. N.Y. Acad. Sci. 129*:864, 1966.

42. Feldman, M., Yaffe, D., Liron, M., and Bleiberg, I.: Regulatory mechanisms controlling the stability of cell differentiation. *Cancer Res. 26*:2041, 1966.

43. O'Grady, L. F., Lewis, J. P., and Trobaugh, F. E., Jr.: The effect of erythropoietin on differentiated erythroid precursors. *J. Lab. Clin. Med. 71*:693, 1968.

44. Schooley, J. C.: The effect of erythropoietin on the growth and development of spleen colony-forming cells. *J. Cell. Physiol. 68*:249, 1966.

45. Nathan, D. G., et al.: Human erythroid burst-forming unit: T cell requirement for proliferation in-vitro. *J. Exp. Med. 147*:324, 1978.

46. Axelrad, A. A., McLeod, D. L., Suzuki, S., and Shreeve, M. M.: Regulation of the population size of erythropoietic progenitor cells, in *Differentiation of Normal and Neoplastic Hematopoietic Cells*, edited by B. Clarkson, P. A. Marks, and J. E. Till. Cold Spring Harbor Laboratory, Cold Spring Harbor, New York, 1978, p. 155.

47. Johnson, G. R., and Metcalf, D.: Pure and mixed erythroid colony formation in-vitro stimulated by spleen conditioned medium with no detectable erythropoietin. *Proc. Natl. Acad. Sci. U.S.A. 74*:3879, 1977.

48. Iscove, N. N.: Erythropoietin-independent stimulation of early erythropoiesis in adult marrow cultures by conditioned media from lectin-stimulated mouse spleen cells, in *Hematopoietic Cell Differentiation*, edited by D. W. Golde, et al. Academic, New York, 1978, p. 37.

49. Abboud, C. N., DiPersio, J. F., Brennan, J. K., and Lichtman, M. A.: Erythropoietic enhancing activity (EEA) secreted by the human cell line, GCT. *J. Supramolec. Struct. 13*:199, 1980.

50. Lö Wenberg, B., and Dicke, K. A.: Induction of proliferation of haemopoietic stem cells in culture. *Exp. Hematol. 5*:319, 1977.

51. Wagemaker, G.: Early erythropoietin-independent stage of in-vitro erythropoiesis: Relevance to stem cell differentiation, in *Experimentation Hematology Today, 1980*, edited by S. J. Baum, G. D. Ledney, and D. W. van Bekkum. Karger, Basel, 1980, p. 47.

52. Metcalf, D., and Johnson, G. R.: Interactions between purified GM-CSF, purified erythropoietin and spleen conditioned medium on hemopoietic colony formation in-vitro. *J. Cell. Physiol. 99*:159, 1979.

53. Metcalf, D., Johnson, G. R., and Burgess, A. W.: Direct stimulation by purified GM-CSF of the proliferation of multipotential and erythroid precursor cells. *Blood 55*:138, 1980.

54. Golde, D. W., Bersch, N., Quan, S. G., and Lusis, A. J.: Production of erythroid potentiating activity by a human T-lymphoblast cell line. *Proc. Natl. Acad. Sci. U.S.A. 77*:593, 1980.

55. Bradley, R. R., and Hodgson, G. S.: Detection of primitive macrophage progenitor cells in mouse bone marrow. *Blood 54*:1446, 1979.

56. Lord, B. I., Mori, K. J., Wright, E. G., and Lajtha, L. G.: An inhibitor of stem cell proliferation in normal bone marrow. *Br. J. Haematol. 34*:441, 1976.

57. Lord, B. I., Mori, K. J., and Wright, E. G.: A stimulator of stem cell proliferation in regenerating bone marrow. *Biomedicine 27*:223, 1977.

58. Lewis, J. P., O'Grady, L. F., and Trobaugh, F. E., Jr.: Studies of hematopoiesis: Significance of haematopoietic colonies formed on the surface of spleens. *Cell Tissue Kinet. 1*:101, 1968.

59. Brecher, G., and Smith, W. W.: Dissociation between spleen colony formation and bone marrow recovery in colchicine-treated irradiated mice. *Radiat. Res. 25*:176, 1965.

60. Savage, A. M.: Hematopoietic recovery in endotoxin-treated lethally x-irradiated BUB mice. *Radiat. Res. 23*:180, 1964.

61. McCulloch, E. A., Siminovitch, L., Till, J. E., Russell, E. S., and Bernstein, S. E.: The cellular basis of the genetically determined hemopoietic defect in anemic mice of genotype Sl/Sl^d. *Blood 26*:399, 1965.

62. Bernstein, S. E.: Tissue transplantation as an analytic and therapeutic tool in hereditary anemias. *Am. J. Surg. 119*:448, 1970.

63. Twentyman, P. R.: The effects of repeated doses of endotoxin on erythropoiesis in the normal and splenectomized mouse. *Br. J. Haematol. 22*:169, 1972.

64. Quesenberry, P., Halperin, J., Ryan, M., and Stohlman, F., Jr.: Tolerance to the granulocyte-releasing and colony-stimulating factor elevating effects of endotoxin. *Blood 45*:789, 1975.

65. Friedenstein, A. J., Chailakhjan, R. K., and Lalykina, K. S.: The development of fibroblast colonies in monolayer cultures of guinea-pig bone marrow and spleen cells. *Cell Tissue Kinet. 3*:393, 1970.

66. Dexter, T. M., Allen, T. D., and Lajtha, L. G.: Conditions controlling the proliferation of haemopoietic stem cells in-vitro. *J. Cell. Physiol. 91*:335, 1977.

67. Testa, N. G., and Dexter, T. M.: Long-term production of erythroid precursor cells (BFU) in bone marrow cultures. *Differentiation 9*:193, 1977.

68. Williams, N. H., Jackson, H., Sheridan, A. P. C., Murphy, M. J., Elste, A., and Moore, M. A. S.: Regulation of megakaryopoiesis in long-term murine bone marrow cultures. *Blood 51*:245, 1978.

69. Williams, N. H., Jackson, H., and Rabellino, E. M.: Proliferation and differentiation of normal granulopoietic cells in continuous bone marrow cultures. *J. Cell. Physiol. 93*:435, 1977.

70. Greenberger, J. S.: Sensitivity of corticosteroid dependent insulin-resistant lipogeneses in marrow preadipocytes of obese diabetic (db/db) mice. *Nature (London) 275*:752, 1978.

71. Schrader, J. W., and Schrader, S.: In-vitro studies on lymphocyte differentiation. I. Long-term in-vitro culture of cells giving rise to functional lymphocytes in irradiated mice. *J. Exp. Med. 148*:823, 1978.

72. Allen, T. D., and Dexter, T. M.: Cellular interrelationships during in-vitro granulopoiesis. *Differentiation 6*:191, 1976.

73. Bentley, S. A., and Foidart, J. M.: Some properties of marrow derived adherent cells in tissue culture. *Blood 56*:1006, 1980.

74. Greenberger, J. S., Davisson, P. B., and Gans, P. J.: Murine sarcoma viruses block corticosteroid-dependent differentiation of bone marrow preadipocytes associated with long-term in-vitro hemopoiesis. *Virology 95*:317, 1979.

75. Mauch, P., Greenberger, J. S., Botnick, L., Hannon, E., and Hellman, S.: Evidence for structural variation in self-renewal capacity within long-term bone marrow cultures. *Proc. Natl. Acad. Sci. U.S.A. 77*:2927, 1980.

76. Dexter, T. M., and Moore, M. A. S.: In-vitro duplication and "cure" of haemopoietic defects in genetically anaemic W/W^v and Sl/Sl^d mice. *Nature 269*:412, 1977.

77. Eastment, E., and Ruscetti, F. W.: Generation of erythropoiesis in long-term bone marrow suspension cultures. *J. Supramolec. Struct. Cell Biochem. (Suppl. 5)*:111, 1981 (abstract).

78. Quesenberry, P. J.: Personal observations, 1981.

79. Levitt, L., and Quesenberry, P.: The effect of lithium on murine hematopoiesis in a liquid culture system. *N. Engl. J. Med. 302*:713, 1979.

80. Chamberlain, W., Borone, J., Kedo, A., and Fried, W.: Lack of recovery of murine hematopoietic stromal cells after irradiation-induced damage. *Blood 44*:385, 1974.

81. Rubin, P., Landman, S., Mayer, E., Keller, B., and Ciccio, S.: Bone marrow regeneration and extension after extended field irradiation in Hodgkin's disease. *Cancer 32*:699, 1973.

82. Knospe, W. H., and Crosby, W. H.: Aplastic anemia: A disorder of the bone-marrow sinusoidal micro-circulation rather than stem-cell failure? *Lancet 20*:22, 1971.

83. Ershler, B. B., Ross, J., Finlay, J., and Shahidi, N. T.: Bone marrow microenvironment defect in congenital hypoplastic anemia. *New Engl. J. Med. 302*:1321, 1980.

84. Friedenstein, A. J., Chailakhjan, R. K., Latsinik, N. V., Panasyuk, A. F., and Keilis-Borok, I. V.: Stomal cells responsible for transferring the microenvironment of the hemopoietic tissues. *Transplantation 17*:331, 1974.

85. Werts, E. D., Gibson, D. P., Knapp, S. A., and Degowin, R. L.: Stromal cell migration precedes hemopoietic repopulation of bone marrow after irradiation. *Radiat. Res. 81*:20, 1980.

86. Gartner, S., and Kaplan, H. S.: Long-term culture of human bone marrow cells. *Proc. Natl. Acad. Sci. U.S.A. 77*:4756, 1980.

87. Siminovitch, L. J., Till, J. E., and McCulloch, E. A.: Radiation responses of hemopoietic colony-forming cells derived from different sources. *Radiat. Res. 24*:482, 1965.

88. Barnes, D. W. H., and Loutit, J. F.: Haemopoietic stem cells in the peripheral blood. *Lancet 2*:1138, 1967.

89. Le Douarin, N. M.: Ontogeny of hematopoietic organs studied in avian embryo interspecific chimeras, in *Differentiation of Normal*

and Neoplastic Hematopoietic Cells, edited by B. Clarkson, P. A. Marks, and J. E. Till. Cold Spring Harbor Laboratory, Cold Spring Harbor, New York, 1978, p. 5.

90. Moore, M. A. S., and Metcalf, D.: Ontogeny of haemopoietic system: Yolk sac origin on in-vivo and in-vitro colony forming cells in the developing mouse embryo. *Br. J. Haematol. 18:*279, 1970.

91. Quesenberry, P. J., Morley, A., Ryan, M., Howard, D., Stohlman, F., Jr.: The effect of endotoxin on murine stem cells. *J. Cell. Physiol 82:*239, 1973.

92. Hanks, G. E., and Ainsworth, E. J.: Endotoxin protection and colony-forming units. *Radiat. Res. 32:*367, 1964.

93. Rencricca, N. J., Rizzoli, V., Howard, D., and Stohlman, F., Jr.: Stem cell migration and proliferation during severe anemia. *Blood 36:*764, 1970.

94. Rickard, K. A., et al.: Myeloid stem cell kinetics during erythropoietin stress. *Br. J. Haematol 20:*537, 1971.

95. Quesenberry, P. J., Levin, J., Zuckerman, K., Rencricca, N., Sullivan, R., and Tyler, W.: Stem cell migration induced by erythropoietin or haemolytic anemia: The effects of actinomycin and endotoxin contamination of erythropoietin preparations. *Br. J. Haematol. 41:*253, 1979.

96. Hanks, G. E.: In-vitro migration of colony-forming units from shielded bone marrow in the irradiated mouse. *Nature 203:*1393, 1964.

97. Maloney, M. A., and Patt, H. M.: Migration of cells from shielded to irradiated marrow. *Blood 39:*804, 1972.

98. Becker, A. J., McCulloch, E. A., Siminovitch, L., and Till, J. E.: The effect of differing demands for blood cell production on DNA synthesis by hemopoietic colony-forming cells of mice. *Blood 26:*296, 1965.

99. Rickard, K. A., Shadduck, R. K., Howard, D. E., Stohlman, F., Jr.: A differential effect of hydroxyurea on hemopoietic stem cell colonies in-vitro and in-vivo. *Proc. Soc. Exp. Biol. Med. 134:*152, 1970.

100. Iscove, N. N., Till, J. E., and McCulloch, E. A.: The proliferative states of mouse granulopoietic progenitor cells. *Proc. Soc. Exp. Biol. Med. 134:*33, 1970.

101. Blackett, N. M., Millard, R. E., and Belcher, H. M.: Thymidine suicide in-vivo and in-vitro of spleen colony forming and agar colony forming cells of mouse bone marrow. *Cell Tissue Kinet. 7:*309, 1974.

102. Quesenberry, P., and Stanley, K.: A statistical analysis of murine stem cell suicide techniques. *Blood 56:*1000, 1980.

103. Chervenick, P. A., Boggs, D. R.: Patterns of proliferation and differentiation of hematopoietic stem cells after compartment depletion. *Blood 37:*568, 1971.

104. Toksöz, D., Dexter, T. M., Lord, B. I., Wright, E. G., and Lajtha, L. G.: The regulation of hemopoiesis in long-term bone marrow cultures. II. Stimulation and inhibition of stem cell proliferation. *Blood 55:*931, 1980.

105. Przala, F., Gross, D. M., Beckman, B., and Fisher, J. W.: Influence of albuterol on erythropoietin production and erythroid progenitor cell activation. *Am. J. Physiol. 236:*H422, 1979.

106. Byron, J. W.: Evidence for a β-adrenergic receptor initiating DNA synthesis in haemopoietic stem cells. *Exp. Cell. Res. 71:*228, 1972.

107. Byron, J. W.: Molecular basis for the triggering of hemopoietic stem cells into DNA synthesis, in *Hemopoiesis in Culture: Second International Workshop*, edited by W. A. Robinson. DHEW Publication No. NIH 74-205, Government Printing Office, Washington, 1974, p. 91.

108. Byron, J. W.: Manipulation of the cell cycle of the hemopoietic stem cell. *Exp. Hematol. 3:*44, 1975.

109. Byron, J. W.: Analysis of receptor mechanisms involved in the hemopoietic effects of androgens; use of the *Tfm* mutant. *Exp. Hematol. 5:*429, 1977.

110. Byron, J. W.: Mechanisms for histamine H_2-receptor induced cell-cycle changes in the bone marrow stem cell. *Agents Actions 7:*209, 1977.

111. Gallien-Lartigue, O.: Calcium and ionophore A-23187 as initiators of DNA replication in the pluripotent haemopoietic stem cell. *Cell Tissue Kinet. 9:*533, 1976.

112. Tyler, W. S., Stohlman, F., Jr., and Chovaniec, M.: Effect of a congenital defect in hemopoiesis on myeloid growth and the stem cell (CFU) in an in-vitro culture system. *Blood 47:*413, 1976.

113. Goodman, J. W.: Cellular interaction between thymocytes and transplanted marrow stem cells. *Transplant. Proc. 3:*430, 1971.

114. Siminovitch, L., Till, J. E., and McCulloch, E. A.: Decline in colony-forming ability of marrow cells subjected to serial transplantation into irradiated mice. *J. Cell. Comp. Physiol. 64:*23, 1964.

115. Botnick, L. E., Hannon, E. C., and Hellman, S.: Limited proliferation of stem cells surviving alkylating agents. *Nature 262:*68, 1976.

116. Hellman, S., Botnick, L. E., Hannon, E. C., and Vigneulle, R. M.: Proliferative capacity of murine hematopoietic stem cells. *Proc. Natl. Acad. Sci. U.S.A. 75:*490, 1978.

117. Botnick, L. E., Hannon, E. C., and Hellman, S.: Multisystem stem cell failure after apparent recovery from alkylating agents. *Cancer Res. 38:*1942, 1978.

118. Moffat, D. J., Rosse, C., and Yoffey, J. M., Jr.: Identity of the hematopoietic stem cell. *Lancet 2:*547, 1967.

119. Van Bekkum, D. W., Van Noord, M. J., Maat, B., and Dicke, K.: Attempt at identification of hematopoietic stem cells in mouse. *Blood 38:*547, 1971.

120. Rubinstein, A. S., and Trobaugh, F. E., Jr.: Ultrastructure of presumptive hematopoietic stem cells. *Blood 42:*61, 1973.

121. Worton, R. G., McCulloch, E. A., and Till, J. E.: Physical separation of hemopoietic stem cells forming colonies in culture. *J. Cell. Physiol. 74:*171, 1969.

122. Haskill, J. S., McNeil, T. A., and Moore, M. A. S.: Density distribution analysis of in-vivo and in-vitro colony forming cells in bone marrow. *J. Cell. Physiol. 75:*167, 1970.

123. Metcalf, D., Moore, M. A. S., and Shortman, K.: Adherence column and buoyant density separation of bone marrow stem cells and more differentiated cells. *J. Cell. Physiol. 78:*441, 1971.

124. Nicola, N. A., Metcalf, D., Von Melchner, H., and Burgess, A. W.: Isolation of murine fetal hemopoietic progenitor cells and selective fractionation of various erythroid precursors. *Blood 58:*376, 1981.

125. Schofield, R.: A comparative study of the repopulating potential of grafts from various haemopoietic sources: CFU repopulation. *Cell Tissue Kinet. 3:*119, 1970.

126. Vos, O., and Dolmans, J. A. S.: Self-renewal of colony forming units (CFU) in serial bone marrow transplantation experiments. *Cell Tissue Kinet. 5:*371, 1972.

127. Golub, E. S.: Brain-associated stem cell antigen shared by brain and hemopoietic stem cells. *J. Exp. Med. 136:*369, 1972.

128. Levitt, L., Quesenberry, P., Monette, F., Zuckerman, K., Sullivan, R., and Ryan, M.: Utilization of mouse stem cell depleted marrow in the study of diffusion chamber myelopoiesis. *Proc. Soc. Exp. Biol. Med. 167:*188, 1981.

129. Goldschneider, I., Gordon, L. K., and Morris, R. J.: Demonstration of Thy-1 antigen on pluripotent hemopoietic stem cells in the rat. *J. Exp. Med. 148:*1351, 1978.

130. Fitchern, J. H., Foon, K. A., and Cline, M. J.: The antigenic characteristics of hematopoietic stem cells. *N. Engl. J. Med. 305:*17, 1981.

131. Gray, J. L., Robinson, W. A.: In-vitro colony formation by human bone marrow cells after freezing. *J. Lab. Clin. Med. 81:*317, 1973.

132. Lewis, J. P., Trobaugh, F. E., Jr.: The assay of the transplantation potential of fresh and stored bone marrow by two in-vitro systems. *Ann. N.Y. Acad. Sci. 114:*677, 1964.

133. Schaefer, U. W., Dicke, K. A., and Van Bekkum, D. W.: Recovery of haemopoiesis in lethally irradiated monkeys by frozen allogeneic bone marrow grafts. *Eur. J. Clin. Biol. Res. 17:*483, 1972.

134. Boswell, S., Niskanen, E., and Quesenberry, P.: Personal observations, 1981.

135. Marsh, J. C., Boggs, D. R., Bishop, C. R., Chervenick, P. A., Cartwright, G. E., and Wintrobe, M. M.: Factors influencing hematopoietic spleen colony formation in irradiated mice. I. The normal pattern of endogenous colony formation. *J. Exp. Med. 126:*833, 1967.

136. Hanks, G. E.: In-vivo migration of colony-forming units from shielded bone marrow in the irradiated mouse. *Nature 203:*1393, 1964.

137. Lajtha, L. G.: Bone marrow stem cell kinetics. *Semin. Hematol. 4:*293, 1967.

138. Siminovitch, L., McCulloch, E. A., and Till, J. E.: The distribution of colony-forming cells among spleen colonies. *J. Cell. Comp. Physiol. 62:*327, 1963.

139. Matioli, G. T., Vogel, H., and Niewisch, H.: The dilution factor of

intravenously injected hemopoietic stem cells. *J. Cell. Physiol.* 72:229, 1968.

140. Smith, W. W., Wilson, S. M., and Fred, S. S.: Kinetics of stem cell depletion and proliferation: Effects of vinblastine and vincristine in normal and irradiated mice. *J. Natl. Cancer Inst.* 40:847, 1968.

141. Fred, S. S., and Smith, W. W.: Induced changes in transplantability of hemopoietic colony-forming cells. *Proc. Soc. Exp. Biol. Med.* 128:364, 1968.

142. Steinberg, H. N., Handler, E. S., and Handler, E. D.: Assessment of erythrocytic and granulocytic colony formation in an in-vivo plasma clot diffusion chamber culture system. *Blood* 47:1041, 1976.

143. Niskanen, E., and Cline, M. J.: Differentiation of subpopulations of human and murine hemopoietic stem cells by hypotonic lysis. *J. Clin. Invest.* 65:285, 1980.

144. Niskanen, E., and Cline, M. J.: Growth of mouse and human bone marrow in diffusion chambers in mice. Development of myeloid and erythroid colonies and proliferation of myeloid stem cells in cyclophosphamide and erythropoietin-treated mice. *Cell Tissue Kinet.* 12:59, 1979.

145. Jacobsen, N., Broxmeyer, H. E., Grossbard, E., and Moore, M. A. S.: Colony-forming units in diffusion chambers (CFU-D) and colony-forming units in agar culture (CFU-C) obtained from normal human bone marrow: A possible parent progeny relationship. *Cell Tissue Kinet.* 12:213, 1979.

146. Niskanen, E. O., Wells, J. R., Quesenberry, P. J., and Cline, M. J.: Effect of cryopreservation on recovery of cells forming colonies in diffusion chambers in mice (CFU-D). *Exp. Hematol.* 9:411, 1981.

147. Hodgson, G. S., and Bradley, T. R.: Properties of haematopoietic stem cells surviving 5-fluorouracil treatment: Evidence for a pre-CFU-S cell? *Nature* 281:381, 1979.

148. Bertoncello, I., Bradley, T. R., and Hodgson, G. S.: Characterization and enrichment of macrophage progenitor cells from normal and 5-fluorouracil treated mouse bone marrow by unit gravity sedimentation. *Exp. Hematol.* 9:604, 1981.

149. Humphries, R. F., Eaves, A. C., and Eaves, C. J.: Expression of stem cell behavior during macroscopic burst formation in-vitro, in *Experimental Hematology Today, 1980*, edited by S. J. Baum, G. D. Ledney, and D. W. Van Bekkum. Karger, Basel, 1980, p. 39.

150. Ebbe, S., Phalen, E., and Stohlman, F., Jr.: Abnormalities of megakaryocytes in Sl/Sl^d mice. *Blood* 42:865, 1973.

151. Ebbe, S., Phalen, E., and Stohlman, F., Jr.: Abnormalities of megakaryocytes in W/W^v mice. *Blood* 42:857, 1973.

152. Lewis, J. P., O'Grady, L. F., Bernstein, S. E., Russell, E. S., and Trobaugh, F. E., Jr.: Growth and differentiation of transplanted W/W^v marrow. *Blood* 30:601, 1967.

153. Sharkis, S. J., Spivak, J. L., Ahmed, A., and Sensenbrenner, L. L.: The regulation of hematopoiesis by anti-theta sensitive cells (TSRC), in *Proceedings of the Conference on Aplastic Anemia: A Stem Cell Disease, San Francisco, June 1979*. U.S. Dept. of Health and Human Services, PHS, NIH, June 1981.

154. Wiktor-Jedrzejczak, W., Sharkis, S., Ahmed, A., and Sell, K. W.: Theta-sensitive cell and erythropoiesis: Identification of a defect in W/W^v anemic mice. *Science* 196:313, 1977.

155. Jeannet, M., Rubinstein, A., Pelet, B., and Kummer, H.: Prolonged remission of severe aplastic anemia after ALG pretreatment and HLA semi-incompatible bone-marrow cell transfusion. *Transplant. Proc.* 6:359, 1974.

156. Thomas, E. D., et al.: Recovery from aplastic anemia following attempted marrow transplantation. *Exp. Hematol.* 4:97, 1976.

157. Baran, D. T., Griner, P. F., and Klemperer, M. R.: Recovery from aplastic anemia after treatment with cyclophosphamide. *N. Engl. J. Med.* 295:1522, 1976.

158. Kagan, W. A., et al.: Aplastic anemia: Presence in human bone marrow of cells that suppress myelopoiesis. *Proc. Natl. Acad. Sci. U.S.A.* 73:2890, 1976.

159. Hoffman, R., Zanjani, E. D., Lutton, J. D., Zalusky, R., and Wasserman, L. R.: Suppression of erythroid-colony formation by lymphocytes from patients with aplastic anemia. *N. Engl. J. Med.* 296:10, 1977.

160. Singer, J. W., et al.: Effect of peripheral blood lymphocytes from patients with aplastic anemia on granulocytic colony growth from HLA-matched and -mismatched marrows: Effect of transfusion sensitization. *Blood* 52:37, 1978.

161. Sullivan, R., Quesenberry, P., Parkman, R., Zuckerman, K., Rappeport, J., and Ryan, M.: Aplastic anemia. Lack of inhibitory effect of bone marrow lymphocytes on in-vitro granulopoiesis. *Blood* 56:625, 1980.

162. Dale, D. C., Alling, D. W., and Wolff, S. M.: Cyclic hematopoiesis: The mechanism of cyclic neutropenia in grey collie dogs. *J. Clin. Invest.* 51:2197, 1972.

163. Guerry, D., IV, Dale, D. C., Omine, M., Perry, S., and Wolff, S. M.: Periodic hematopoiesis in human cyclic neutropenia. *J. Clin. Invest.* 52:3220, 1973.

164. Dale, D. C., and Graw, R. G., Jr.: Transplantation of allogeneic bone marrow in canine cyclic neutropenia. *Science* 183:83, 1974.

165. Lange, R. D., Jones, J. B., Jones, E. S., Ichiki, A. T., and Yang, T. J.: Regulation of erythropoiesis in grey collies with cyclic hematopoiesis, in *Erythropoiesis*, edited by K. Nakao, J. W. Fisher, and F. Takaku. University Park Press, Baltimore, 1975, p. 255.

166. Guerry, D., Adamson, J. W., Dale, D. C., and Wolff, S. M.: Human cyclic neuthropenia: Urinary colony-stimulating factor and erythropoietin levels. *Blood* 44:257, 1974.

167. Greenberg, P. L., Bax, I., Levin, J., and Andrews, T. M.: Alteration of colony-stimulating factor output, endotoxemia and granulopoiesis in cyclic neutropenia. *Am. J. Hematol.* 1:375, 1976.

168. Hammond, W. P., and Dale, D. C.: Canine cyclic hematopoiesis (CH): Treatment with lithium. *Clin. Res.* 27:461A, 1979.

169. Morley, A., Stohlman, F., Jr.: Cyclophosphamide-induced cyclical neutropenia: An animal model of a human periodic disease. *N. Engl. J. Med.* 282:643, 1970.

170. Wright, D. G., Fauci, A. S., Dale, D. C., and Wolff, S. M.: Correction of human cyclic neutropenia with prednisolone. *N. Engl. J. Med.* 298:295, 1978.

171. Erslev, A. J.: Humoral regulation of red cell production. *Blood* 8:349, 1953.

172. Plzak, L. F., Fried, W., Jacobson, L. O., and Bethard, W. F.: Demonstration of stimulation of erythropoiesis by plasma from anemic rats using Fe^59. *J. Lab. Clin. Med.* 46:671, 1955.

173. Miyake, T., Kung, C. K.-H., and Goldwasser, E.: Purification of human erythropoietin. *J. Biol. Chem.* 252:5558, 1977.

174. Jacobson, L. O., Goldwasser, E., Fried, W., and Plzak, L.: Role of the kidney in erythropoiesis. *Nature.* 179:633, 1957.

175. Erslev, A. J.: The renal biogenesis of erythropoietin. *Am. J. Med.* 58:25, 1975.

176. Fried, W.: The liver as a source of extrarenal erythropoietin. *Blood* 40:671, 1973.

177. Peschle, C., et al.: Hepatic erythropoietin: Enhanced production in anephric rats with hyperplasia of Kupffer cells. *Br. J. Haematol.* 32:105, 1976.

178. Erslev, A. J., et al.: Renal and extrarenal erythropoietin production in anemic rats. *Br. J. Haematol.* 45:65, 1980.

179. Rich, I., Anselstelter, V., Heit, W., and Kubanek, B.: Release of erythropoietin (Ep) from macrophages by treatment with silica. *J. Supramolec. Struct. (Suppl. 4)*:141, 1980.

180. Erslev, A. J.: The effect of anemic anoxia on the cellular development of nucleated red cells. *Blood* 14:386, 1959.

181. Alpen, E. L., and Cranmore, D.: Cellular kinetics and iron utilization in bone marrow as observed by Fe^59 radioautography. *Ann. N.Y. Acad. Sci.* 77:753, 1959.

182. Filmanowicz, E., and Gurney, C. W.: Studies on erythropoiesis, XVI. Response to a single dose of erythropoietin in polycythemic mouse. *J. Lab. Clin. Med.* 57:65, 1961.

183. Bruce, W. R., and McCulloch, E. A.: The effect of erythropoietic stimulation on the hemopoietic colony-forming cells of mice. *Blood* 23:216, 1964.

184. McLeod, D. L., Shreeve, M. M., and Axelrad, A. A.: Improved plasma culture system for production of erythrocytic colonies in-vitro: Quantitative assay method for CFU-E. *Blood* 44:517, 1974.

185. Iscove, N. N., and Sieber, F.: Erythroid progenitors in mouse bone marrow detected by macroscopic colony formation in culture. *Exp. Hematol.* 3:32, 1975.

186. Porteous, D. D., and Lajtha, L. G.: Restoration of stem cell function after irradiation. IV. Kinetics of erythropoiesis and sites of action of erythropoietin. *Ann. N.Y. Acad. Sci.* 149:151, 1968.

187. Gregory, C. J.: Erythropoietin sensitivity as a differentiation marker in the hemopoietic system: Studies of three erythropoietic colony responses in culture. *J. Cell. Physiol.* 89:289, 1976.

188. Monette, F. C., et al.: Cell-cycle properties and proliferation kinetics of late erythroid progenitors in murine bone marrow. *Exp. Hematol.* 8:484, 1980.

189. Hara, H., and Ogawa, M.: Erythropoietic precursors in mice under erythropoietic stimulation and suppression. *Exp. Hematol.* 5:141, 1977.

190. Iscove, N. N.: The role of erythropoietin in regulation of population size and cell cycling of early and late erythroid precursors in mouse bone marrow. *Cell Tissue Kinet.* 10:323, 1977.

191. Zuckerman, K. S., Sullivan, R., and Quesenberry, P. J.: Effects of actinomycin D in-vivo on murine erythroid stem cells. *Blood* 51:957, 1978.

192. Johnson, G. R., and Metcalf, D.: Nature of cells forming erythroid colonies in agar after stimulation by spleen conditioned medium. *J. Cell. Physiol.* 94:243, 1978.

193. Aye, M. T.: Erythroid colony formation in cultures of human marrow. Effect of leukocyte conditioned medium. *J. Cell. Physiol.* 91:69, 1977.

194. Adamson, J. W., Popovic, W. J., and Brown, J. E.: Hormonal control of erythropoiesis, in *Hematopoietic Cell Differentiation*, edited by D. W. Golde, et al. Academic, New York, 1978, p. 53.

195. Moriyama, Y., and Fisher, J. W.: Effects of testosterone and erythropoietin on erythroid colony formation in rabbit bone marrow cultures. *Life Sci.* 15:1181, 1974.

196. Golde, D. W., Bersch, N., and Cline, M. J.: Potentiation of erythropoiesis in-vitro by dexamethasone. *J. Clin. Invest.* 57:57, 1976.

197. Golde, D. W., Bersch, N., and Li, C. H.: Growth hormone: Species-specific stimulation of erythropoiesis in-vitro. *Science* 196:1112, 1977.

198. Golde, D. W., Bersch, N., Chopra, I. J., and Cline, M. J.: Thyroid hormones stimulate erythropoiesis in-vitro. *Br. J. Haematol.* 37:173, 1977.

199. Pluznik, D. H., and Sachs, L.: The cloning of normal "mast" cells in tissue culture. *J. Cell. Comp. Physiol.* 66:319, 1965.

200. Bradley, T. R., Telfer, P. A., and Fry, P.: The effect of erythrocytes on mouse bone marrow colony development in-vitro. *Blood* 38:353, 1971.

201. Paran, M., and Sachs, L.: The single cell orgin of normal granulocyte colonies in-vitro. *J. Cell. Physiol.* 73:91, 1969.

202. Moore, M. A. S., Williams, N., and Metcalf, D.: Purification and characterization of the in-vitro colony forming cells in monkey hemopoietic tissue. *J. Cell. Physiol.* 79:283, 1972.

203. Metcalf, D.: Clonal analysis of proliferation and differentiation of paired daughter cells: Action of granulocyte-macrophage colony-stimulating factors on granulocyte-macrophage precursors. *Proc. Natl. Acad. Sci.* 77:5327, 1980.

204. Metcalf, D.: *Hemopoietic Colonies: In-Vitro Cloning of Normal and Leukemic Cells.* Springer-Verlag, Berlin, 1977, p. 140.

205. Metcalf, D., Parker, J., Chester, H. M., and Kincade, P. W.: Formation of eosinophilic-like granulocytic colonies by mouse bone marrow cells in-vitro. *J. Cell. Physiol.* 84:275, 1974.

206. Basten, A., and Beeson, P. B.: Mechanism of eosinophilia. II. Role of the lymphocyte. *J. Exp. Med.* 131:1288, 1970.

207. Lajtha, L. G., Pozzi, L. V., Schofield, R., and Fox, M.: Kinetic properties of haemopoietic stem cells. *Cell Tissue Kinet.* 2:39, 1969.

208. Rickard, K. A., Morley, A., Howard, D., and Stohlman, F., Jr.: The in-vitro colony-forming cell and the response to neutropenia. *Blood* 37:6, 1971.

209. Morley, A., Rickard, K. A., Howard, D., and Stohlman, F., Jr.: Studies on the regulation of granulopoiesis. IV. Possible humoral regulation. *Blood* 37:14, 1971.

210. Chen, M. G., and Schooley, J. C.: Recovery of proliferative capacity of agar colony-forming cells and spleen colony-forming cells following ionizing radiation or vinblastine. *J. Cell. Physiol.* 75:89, 1970.

211. Sumner, M. A., Bradley, T. R., Hodgson, G. S., Cline, M. J., Fry, P. A., and Sutherland, L.: The growth of bone marrow cells in liquid culture. *Br. J. Haematol.* 23:221, 1972.

212. Sutherland, D. J. A., Till, J. E., and McCulloch, E. A.: Short-term cultures of mouse marrow cells separated by velocity sedimentation. *Cell Tissue Kinet.* 4:479, 1971.

213. Goldschneider, I., Metcalf, D., Battye, F., and Mondel, T.: Analysis of rat hemopoietic cells on the fluorescence-activated cell sorter. *J. Exp. Med.* 152:419, 1980.

214. Moore, M. A. S., and Williams, N.: Functional morphologic, and kinetic analysis of the granulocyte-macrophage progenitor cell, in *Hemopoiesis in Culture: Second International Workshop*, edited by W. A. Robinson. DHEW Publication No. NIH 74-205, Government Printing Office, Washington, 1974, p. 17.

215. Metcalf, D., and MacDonald, H. R.: Heterogeneity of in-vitro colony- and cluster-forming cells in the mouse marrow: segregation by velocity sedimentation. *J. Cell. Physiol.* 85:643, 1975.

216. Metcalf, D.: Studies on colony formation in-vitro by mouse bone marrow cells. II. Action of colony-stimulating factor. *J. Cell Physiol.* 76:89, 1970.

217. Brennan, J. K., et al.: Chemical mediators of granulopoiesis: A review. *Exp. Hematol.* 8:441, 1980.

218. Burgess, A. W., and Metcalf, D.: The nature and action of granulocyte-macrophage colony stimulating factors. *Blood* 56:947, 1980.

219. Metcalf, D., and Foster, R.: Bone marrow colony-stimulating activity of serum from mice with viral-induced leukemia. *J. Natl. Cancer Inst.* 39:1235, 1967.

220. Paran, M., and Sachs, L.: The continued requirement for inducer for the development of macrophage and granulocyte colonies. *J. Cell. Physiol.* 72:247, 1968.

221. Golde, D. W., and Cline, M. J.: Identification of the colony-stimulating cell in human peripheral blood. *J. Clin. Invest.* 51:2981, 1972.

222. Chervenick, P. A., and LoBuglio, A. F.: Human blood monocytes: Stimulators of granulocyte and mononuclear colony formation in-vitro. *Science* 178:164, 1972.

223. Moore, M. A. S., and Williams, N.: Physical separation of colony-stimulating cells from in-vitro colony forming cells in hemopoietic tissues. *J. Cell. Physiol.* 80:195, 1972.

224. Parker, J. W., and Metcalf, D.: Production of colony-stimulating factor in mitogen-stimulated lymphocyte cultures. *J. Immunol.* 112:502, 1974.

225. Cline, M. J., and Golde, D. W.: Production of colony-stimulating activity by human lymphocytes. *Nature* 248:703, 1974.

226. Knudtzon, S., and Mortensen, B. I.: Growth stimulation of human bone marrow cells in agar culture by vascular cells. *Blood* 46:937, 1975.

227. Quesenberry, P., and Gimbrone, M.: Endothelium as a regulator of granulopoiesis: Studies on production of colony-stimulating activity by cultured endothelial cells. *Blood* 56:1060, 1980.

228. Quesenberry, P. J., Gimbrone, M. A., Doukas, M. A., and Goldwasser, E.: Vascular derived tissues as a source of colony-stimulating activity (CSA). *Clin. Res.* 29:830A, 1981.

229. Guez, M., and Sachs, L.: Purification of the protein that induces cell differentiation to macrophages and granulocytes. *FEBS Lett.* 37:149, 1973.

230. Austin, P. E., McCulloch, E. A., and Till, J. E.: Characterization of the factor in L-cell conditioned medium capable of stimulating colony formation by mouse marrow cells in culture. *J. Cell Physiol.* 77:121, 1971.

231. Metcalf, D.: Acute antigen-induced elevation of serum colony stimulating factor (CSF) levels. *Immunology* 21:427, 1971.

232. Quesenberry, P., Cohen, H., Levin, J., Sullivan, R., Bealmear, P., and Ryna, M.: Effects of bacterial infection and irradiation on serum colony-stimulating factor levels in tolerant and nontolerant, CF_1 mice. *Blood* 51:229, 1978.

233. Greenberg, P. L., Levin, J., and Andrews, T. M.: Alteration of colony-stimulating factor output, endotoxemia, and granulopoiesis in cyclic neutropenia. *Am. J. Hematol.* 1:375, 1976.

234. Stanley, E. R., and Metcalf, D.: Purification and properties of human urinary colony-stimulating factor (CSF), in *Cell Differentiation*, edited by R. Harris, P. Allin, and D. Viza. Munksgaard, Copenhagen, 1972, p. 272.

235. Lind, D. E., Bradley, M. L., Gunz, F. W., and Vincent, P. C.: The non-equivalence of mouse and human marrow culture in assay of granulopoietic stimulatory factors. *J. Cell. Physiol.* 83:35, 1974.

236. Burgess, A. W., Camakaris, J., and Metcalf, D.: Purification and properties of colony-stimulating factor from mouse lung-conditioned medium. *J. Biol. Chem.* 252:1998, 1977.

237. Stanley, E. R., Cifone, M., Heard, P. M., and Defendi, V.: Factors regulating macrophage production and growth: Identity of colony-stimulating factor and macrophage growth factor. *J. Exp. Med.* 143:631, 1976.

238. Landau, T., and Sachs, L.: Activation of a differentiation-inducing protein by adenine and adenine containing nucleotides. *FEBS Lett.* 17:339, 1971.

239. Price, G. B., Senn, J. S., McCulloch, E. A., and Till, J. E.: The isolation and properties of granulocyte colony-stimulating activities from medium conditioned by human peripheral leukocytes. *Biochem. J.* 148:209, 1975.

240. Price, G. B., McCulloch, E. A., and Till, J. E.: A new low molecular weight granulocyte colony-stimulating activity. *Blood* 42:341, 1973.

241. Burgess, A. W., Wilson, E. M. A., and Metcalf, D.: Stimulation by human placental conditioned medium of hemopoietic colony formation by human marrow cells. *Blood* 49:573, 1977.

242. Stanley, E. R., Guilbert, L. J., Das, S. K., and Forman, L.: Colony-stimulating factor and the regulation of macrophage production. *J. Supramolec. Struct. (Suppl. 4):*120, 1980.

243. Wu, M.-C., Miller, A. M., and Yunis, A. A.: Immunological and functional differences between human type I and II colony-stimulating factors. *J. Clin. Invest.* 67:1588, 1981.

244. Guilbert, L. J., and Stanley, E. R.: Specific interaction of murine colony-stimulating factor with mononuclear phagocytic cells. *J. Supramolec. Struct. (Suppl. 4):*176, 1980.

245. Shadduck, R. K., Pigoli, G., and Waheed, A.: The role of colony-stimulating factor in granulopoiesis. *J. Supramolec. Struct. (Suppl. 4):*116, 1980.

246. Waheed, A., and Shadduck, R. K.: Purification and properties of L-cell derived colony-stimulating factor. *J. Lab. Clin. Med.* 94:180, 1979.

247. Broxmeyer, H. E., Smithyman, A., Eger, R. R., Meyers, P. A., and deSousa, M.: Identification of lactoferrin as the granulocyte derived inhibitor of colony-stimulating activity (CSA) production. *J. Exp. Med.* 148:1052, 1978.

248. Kurland, J. I., Bockman, R. S., Broxmeyer, H. E., and Moore, M. A. S.: Limitation of excessive myelopoiesis by the intrinsic modulation of macrophage-derived prostaglandin E. *Science* 199:552, 1978.

249. Pelus, L. M., Broxmeyer, H. E., Kruland, J. I., and Moore, M. A. S.: Regulation of macrophage and granulocyte proliferation. Specificities of prostaglandin E and lactoferrin. *J. Exp. Med.* 150:277, 1979.

250. Kurland, J. I.: Dependence upon colony-stimulating factor for the synthesis of prostaglandin E by normal and neoplastic mononuclear phagocytes, in *Hematopoietic Cell Differentiation,* edited by D. W. Golde, Academic, New York, 1978, p. 479.

251. Winton, E. F., Kinkade, J. M., Vogler, W. R., Parker, M. B., and Barnes, K. C.: In-vitro studies of lactoferrin and murine granulopoiesis. *Blood* 57:574, 1981.

252. Rigas, V. D., Bagby, G. C., Bennett, R. M., and Gorewal, H. S.: Interaction of lactoferrin, monocytes and T-lymphocytes in the regulation of granulopoiesis in-vitro. *Clin. Res.* 29:346A, 1981.

253. Chan, S. H., Metcalf, D., and Stanley, E. R.: Stimulation and inhibition by normal human serum of colony formation in-vitro by bone marrow cells. *Br. J. Haematol.* 20:329, 1971.

254. Metcalf, D.: Inhibition of bone marrow colony formation in-vitro by dialysable products of normal and neoplastic haemopoietic cells. *Aust. J. Exp. Biol. Med. Sci.* 49:351, 1971.

255. Rytömma, T.: Granulocyte chalone and antichalone, in *Hemic Cells In-Vitro,* edited by P. Farnes. Williams & Wilkins, Baltimore, 1969, p. 47.

256. McNeill, T. A.: Antigenic stimulation of bone marrow colony forming cells. I. Effect of antigens on normal bone marrow cells in-vitro. *Immunology* 18:39, 1970.

257. Bradley, T. R., Telfer, P. A., and Fry, P.: The effect of erythrocytes on mouse bone marrow colony development in-vitro. *Blood* 38:353, 1971.

258. Metcalf, D., MacDonald, H. R., and Chester, H. M.: Serum potentiation of granulocyte and macrophage colony formation in-vitro. *Exp. Hematol.* 3:261, 1975.

259. Gordon, A. S., Handler, E. S., Siegel, C. D., Dornfest, B. S., and LoBue, J.: Plasma factors influencing leukocyte release in rats. *Ann. N.Y. Acad. Sci.* 113:766, 1964.

260. Boggs, D. R., Marsh, J. C., Chervenick, P. A., Cartwright, G. E., and Wintrobe, M. M.: Neutrophil releasing activity in plasma of normal human subjects injected with endotoxin. *Proc. Soc. Exp. Biol. Med.* 127:689, 1968.

261. Broxmeyer, H., Van Zant, G., Zucali, J. R., LoBue, J., and Gordon, A. S.: Mechanisms of leukocyte production and release. XII. A comparative assay of leukocytosis-inducing factor (LIF) and the colony-stimulating factor (CSF). *Proc. Soc. Exp. Biol. Med.* 145:1262, 1974.

262. Odell, T. T., Jr., Jackson, C. W., Friday, T. J., and Charsha, D. E.: Effect of thrombocytopenia on megakaryocytopoiesis. *Br. J. Haematol.* 17:91, 1969.

263. Shulman, N. R., Marder, V. J., and Weinrach, R. S.: Similarities between known antiplatelet antibodies and the factor responsible for thrombocytopenia in idiopathic purpura: Physiologic, serologic and isotopic studies. *Ann. N.Y. Acad. Sci.* 124:499, 1965.

264. Cooper, G. W.: The regulation of thrombopoiesis, in *Regulation of Hematopoiesis,* edited by A. S. Gordon, Appleton-Century-Crofts, New York, 1970, vol. 2, p. 161.

265. Abildgaard, C. F., and Simone, J. V.:Thrombopoiesis. *Semin Hematol.* 4:424, 1967.

266. Odell, T. T. Jr., McDonald, T. P., and Detwiler, T. C.: Stimulation of platelet production by serum of platelet-depleted rats. *Proc. Soc. Exp. Biol. Med.* 108:428, 1961.

267. Evatt, B. L., and Levin, J.: Measurement of thrombopoiesis in rabbits using 75selenomethionine. *J. Clin. Invest.* 48:1615, 1969.

268. Penington, D. G.: Isotope bioassay for "thrombopoietin." *Br. Med. J.* 1:606, 1970.

269. McDonald, T. P.: The hemagglutination-inhibition assay for thrombopoietin. *Blood* 41:219, 1973.

270. Jackson, C. W.: Cholinesterase as a possible marker for early cells of the megakaryocytic series. *Blood* 42:413, 1970.

271. Metcalf, D., MacDonald, H. R., Odartchenko, N., and Sordat, B.: Growth of mouse megakaryocyte colonies in-vitro. *Proc. Natl. Acad. Sci. U.S.A.* 72:1744, 1975.

272. McLeod, D. L., Shreeve, M. M., and Axelrad, A. A.: Induction of megakaryocyte colonies with platelet formation in-vitro. *Nature* 261:492, 1976.

273. Mazur, E. M., Hoffman, R., and Bruno, E.: Regulation of human megakaryocytopoiesis. An in vitro analysis. *J. Clin. Invest.* 68:733, 1981.

Hemopoietic stem cell disorders — classification

CHAPTER *19*

Classification of the hemopoietic stem cell disorders

MARSHALL A. LICHTMAN

The hemopoietic stem cell disorders are a group of diseases that are thought to result from an injury to a primitive blood progenitor cell pool, which may function under normal conditions as the stem cell pool for blood cell production. The wide variability in the morphologic expression (phenotype) of hemopoietic stem cell diseases is related to the intrinsic capabilities of stem cells to take various commitment pathways and to proceed through many levels of differentiation and maturation.

Stem cells and normal hemopoiesis

Hemopoiesis is the process of progenitor cell proliferation, differentiation, and maturation that provides terminally differentiated red cells, neutrophils, eosinophils, basophils, monocytes, and platelets [1–4]. Although it is a continuum, one can consider hemopoiesis as having five major levels (Fig. 19-1). The first and most primitive level is the pluripotential stem cell pool.

A *stem cell pool* is defined as one from which cells are recruited to differentiation pathways, but in which cell proliferation leads to a replacement of recruited cells such that the cell pool is sustained for very long periods without requiring influx of cells from a more primitive compartment. This capability is referred to as *self-renewal*. The pluripotential pool is the stem cell compartment for hemopoiesis and lymphopoiesis in the adult mouse and rat [5–7]. Although a pluripotential cell pool is probably present during ontogeny in human beings, it is uncertain if this is the functioning stem cell pool after birth.

In healthy individuals, lymphopoiesis and hemopoiesis appear to be sustained by separate stem cell compartments. These two distinct cell compartments compose the second level of hemopoiesis shown in Fig. 19-1. The common hemopoietic stem cell pool is capable of providing progenitors for the six types of blood cells, and the common lymphopoietic stem cell pool is capable of providing progenitors for the various T-lymphocyte subsets and B-lymphocyte idiotypic classes. Their stemness implies that they maintain their pool size by proliferation and not by influx of cells from the pluripotential stem cell pool, at least for extended periods.

PROGENITOR CELL POOLS

By a process of differentiation, the common stem cell pools provide cells that develop into several progenitor cells committed to a specific cell lineage. In the case of hemopoiesis, these cells ultimately become committed, unipotential progenitor cells for each of the six blood cell types, and they represent the third level of hemopoiesis shown in Fig. 19-1. These committed progenitor cells can proliferate into visible colonies of cells in a viscous culture medium and are referred to as *colony-form-*

FIGURE 19-1 The functioning stem cell pool in mice is thought to be at level 1, the pluripotential cells. In healthy human beings, two stem cell pools may be operative; these are the cell pools at level 2. Cells at level 3 have become sensitive to specific cytopoietic hormones, such as erythropoietin, thrombopoietin, or neutropoietin. The committed progenitor cells at this level of differentiation are referred to as colony-forming units (CFU) or colony-forming cells (CFC), since they form colonies of cells in semisolid medium in the presence of the appropriate stimulating hormone. These hormones are capable of inducing proliferation and maturation of these committed progenitor cells so that they achieve level 4, at which the first morphologically identifiable precursors are present, such as myeloblasts and proerythroblasts, and ultimately level 5, the level of fully matured blood cells. (Modified from *Hematology and Oncology,* edited by M. A. Lichtman. Grune & Stratton, New York, 1980. Used with permission.)

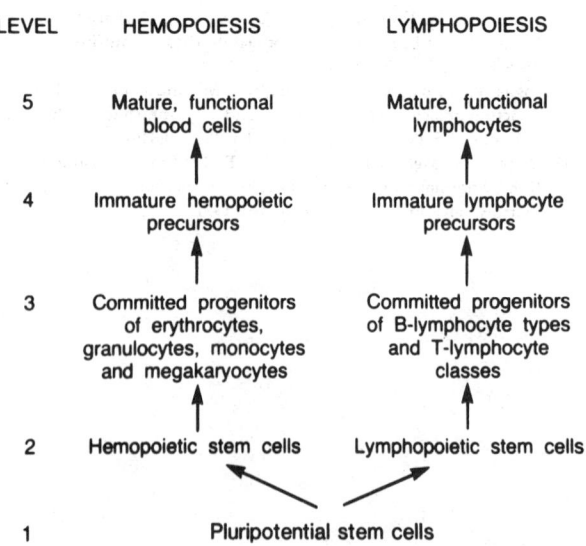

LEVEL	HEMOPOIESIS	LYMPHOPOIESIS
5	Mature, functional blood cells	Mature, functional lymphocytes
4	Immature hemopoietic precursors	Immature lymphocyte precursors
3	Committed progenitors of erythrocytes, granulocytes, monocytes and megakaryocytes	Committed progenitors of B-lymphocyte types and T-lymphocyte classes
2	Hemopoietic stem cells	Lymphopoietic stem cells
1	Pluripotential stem cells	

ing cells (CFC) or *colony-forming units* (CFU), with a suffix identifying the cell line, e.g., CFU-N for the cell that generates neutrophil colonies. Cells at this level of hemopoiesis are referred to as *committed stem cells* by many authors. Since they show very limited self-renewal capability, the term *progenitor cell* has been suggested as a better designation, limiting the term *stem cell* to one that demonstrates substantial self-renewal.

PRECURSOR CELLS

The committed progenitors develop into the precursors of blood cells, such as proerythroblasts, myeloblasts (granuloblasts), and megakaryoblasts. These cells are designated as level 4 in Fig. 19-1. The designation *precursor* has been suggested for those marrow cells that are morphologically identifiable as being part of a specific cell lineage, such as myeloblasts, progranulocytes, and myelocytes. The precursors develop sequentially until they become fully mature, functional blood cells, designated as level 5. The reader is referred to the preceding chapter for further details of hemopoiesis.

Categories of hemopoietic stem cell disorders

Injury to the hemopoietic stem cell pool can result in several of the most serious hematologic disorders. The hemopoietic stem cell diseases can be grouped into three categories by the principal pathogenetic process involved in their expression (Table 19-1).

MYELOAPLASIA

Aplastic pancytopenia, traditionally called *aplastic anemia*, is the result of aplasia of the hemopoietic stem cell compartment and leads to a deficiency of all derivatives of the hemopoietic stem cell pool. Usually lymphocytes are present in normal numbers and remain functionally intact [8,9]. Moderate decreases in lymphocytes occur in

TABLE 19-1 Pluripotential or hemopoietic stem cell disorders

MYELOAPLASIA
Aplastic pancytopenia (aplastic anemia)
MYELODYSPLASIA
Dyshemopoietic (preleukemic) syndromes (see Table 24-1 for further breakdown)
MYELOPROLIFERATION
Chronic:
Polycythemia vera
Chronic myelogenous leukemia
Idiopathic myelofibrosis
Primary thrombocythemia
Subacute:
Atypical myeloproliferative syndromes
Oligoblastic (smoldering) leukemia
Acute:
Acute myelogenous leukemia (see Table 19-2 for further breakdown)

occasional patients, and this is the result usually of a B-lymphocyte deficiency [10]. Careful evaluation of the lymphoid system in myeloaplasia has not been made. Thus it is possible that lymphocytic progenitors may be affected in aplastic anemia in occasional patients. This would place the site of injury closer to the pluripotential stem cell pool (level 1) in that subgroup of individuals.

MYELODYSPLASIA

The myelodysplasias are a subgroup of hemopoietic stem cell diseases in which dyshemopoiesis is the most characteristic feature [11]. *Dyshemopoiesis* refers to abnormalities in differentiation or maturation of blood cells that lead to morphologic and biochemical alterations in the cells. Chromosome abnormalities can occur. Ineffective erythropoiesis is a common feature, and ineffective granulopoiesis and thrombopoiesis also can occur. Myeloaplasia or myeloproliferation can occur in myelodysplastic conditions as well. There are often combinations of these pathogenetic mechanisms or switches from one mechanism to another during the course of the illness.

The preleukemia syndrome is a group of myelodysplastic conditions in which ineffective hemopoiesis, abnormal morphology, chromosome abnormalities, and biochemical abnormalities of hemopoietic and blood cells can occur. Several hemopoietic stem cell disorders, including idiopathic refractory sideroblastic anemia, idiopathic refractory nonsideroblastic anemia, pancytopenia with hyperplastic marrow, and paroxysmal nocturnal hemoglobinuria, are dysplasias with a heightened likelihood of evolution to acute myelogenous leukemia (AML) compared with that of healthy population (see Chap. 22).

MYELOPROLIFERATION

The chronic myeloproliferative diseases are polycythemia vera, chronic myelogenous leukemia (CML), and primary thrombocythemia. All are thought to be stem cell disorders characterized by a striking overaccumulation either of erythrocytes (polycythemia), granulocytes (leukemia), or platelets (thrombocythemia).

Idiopathic myelofibrosis is often associated with an overaccumulation of granulocytes and platelets and is traditionally grouped with the chronic myeloproliferative diseases. However, ineffective hemopoiesis, cytopenias, myeloaplasia, and myelodysplasia can also occur, highlighting the overlapping expression of pathogenetic mechanisms. Marked megakaryocytic hyperplasia and extensive fibrosis in marrow are very characteristic findings in nearly all cases. The fibroplasia is thought to be the result of the release of a growth factor for fibroblasts by the abnormal and numerous megakaryocytes and thus a secondary feature of the disease.

Splenic enlargement is very frequent in each of the chronic myeloproliferative syndromes, but it is uncommon in the myelodysplastic diseases and does not occur in the myeloaplastic disorder aplastic anemia. Each of the chronic myeloproliferative diseases may transform into acute myelogenous leukemia (AML). CML has the highest likelihood of this transformation.

The subacute myeloproliferative diseases include the oligoblastic (smoldering) leukemias and a variety of uncommon atypical myeloproliferative syndromes. They produce more morbidity than the chronic syndromes, and patients tend to have shorter life-spans [12–16]. These subacute myeloproliferative diseases often present evidence for a leukemic state, including the presence of low concentrations of leukemic blast cells in marrow and often blood, as well as anemia, thrombocytopenia, and sometimes prominent monocytic maturation of cells.

The acute myeloproliferative diseases include the phenotypic variants of AML listed in Table 19-2. Morphologic and histochemical characteristics of cells on stained films of blood and marrow provide the major basis for the classification of AML [17–19]. The prevailing attitude is to look on AML as a single disease with many forms of morphologic expression. This variation is consistent with the behavior of normal hemopoietic stem cells, which are capable of differentiation into several cell types. Hence partial differentiation of leukemic cells may allow one or another cell type to predominate. There is little evidence for a fundamental difference in the cause, pathogenesis, or behavior of these different morphologic variants of AML. There are important epiphenomena related to special features of certain morphologic types, such as tissue infiltration (monocytic leukemia), intravascular coagulation (progranulocytic leukemia), cardiac and lung disease (eosinophilic leukemia), myelofibrosis (megakaryocytic leukemia), and others (see Chap. 28).

TABLE 19-2   Phenotypic variants of myelogenous leukemia

TYPES OF ACUTE MYELOGENOUS LEUKEMIA
(POORLY DIFFERENTIATED CELLS PREDOMINATE)

Myeloblastic (granuloblastic)	Eosinophilic*
Monocytic	Basophilic†
Myelomonocytic (granulomonoblastic)	Erythroid
Progranulocytic	Megakaryocytic‡

TYPES OF CHRONIC MYELOGENOUS LEUKEMIA
(BETTER-DIFFERENTIATED CELLS PREDOMINATE)

Granulocytic: Classical, Ph¹-positive (90%) Atypical, Ph¹-negative (10%)	Basophilic, Ph¹-positive†
Granulomonocytic or monocytic, usually Ph¹-negative	Eosinophilic, Ph¹-positive*

*Most cases are Ph¹-negative AML-eosinophilic type; rarely they may be variants of CML and contain the Ph¹ chromosome.
†Rare cases of basophilic leukemia are Ph¹-negative and are variants of AML; most cases have the Ph¹ chromosome and evolve from CML.
‡Some cases are associated with intense myelofibrosis. The syndrome of acute myelofibrosis may be a type of megakaryocytic leukemia.

Pathogenesis of hemopoietic stem cell diseases

The pathogeneses of AML and CML have been intensively studied [20]. In AML, the disturbance in the stem cell pool results in a clone of cells that is unable to mature or is severely defective in maturation. Proliferation of primitive progenitors is also excessive when considered in absolute terms, i.e., the total number of blast cells proliferating. The abnormality of the stem cell pool in CML is reflected in a marked increase in proliferation of marrow granulocytic and often of megakaryocytic progenitor and precursor cells. Erythropoiesis is usually impaired. Maturation of cells is disordered, but not so severely as in AML; hence the predominant leukemic cells in the blood are amitotic, mature, or partially matured cells, such as segmented neutrophils and myelocytes, erythrocytes, and platelets.

Since a stem cell pool is a site of injury in AML and CML, erythropoiesis and thrombopoiesis as well as granulopoiesis are considered to be leukemic. The involvement of all blood cell lines, as a consequence of the leukemic lesion originating in a stem cell pool in AML and CML, has been strongly suggested by the qualitative abnormalities of structure and function of each cell lineage in many subjects with leukemia and by studies of chromosome composition of cells in leukemia [21]. In AML and CML, erythroblasts, megakaryocytes, and granulocyte precursors may contain an identical chromosomal abnormality. These findings have been taken as evidence for a stem cell lesion in AML and CML [21].

Studies of the X-chromosome-linked isoenzymes glucose-6-phosphate dehydrogenase types A and B in patients with myelogenous leukemia are consistent with a clonal origin of the disease [22–24], as are studies of a patient with a sex-chromosome mosaic [25].

The Ph¹ chromosome is usually present in all hemopoietic cell metaphases even after treatment. Thus a normal hemopoietic clone is not evident overtly, although Ph¹-negative cells have been observed occasionally after intensive and standard treatment [26]. In vitro studies also suggest that dual populations can exist [27].

The current basis for chemotherapy of AML is that two competing stem cell pools, a leukemic and a normal or nearly normal pool, are present in the hemopoietic stem cell compartment and that the extreme reduction of the leukemic cell pool by cytotoxic drugs permits emergence and regrowth of the normal clones and cells. Such a change is supported by the disappearance of cells with abnormal karyotypes during remission in patients with AML. Intensive cytotoxic therapy has resulted in a high frequency of remission in patients with AML. CML has not responded to intensive therapy frequently enough to justify such an approach. The reasons why a clone change does not occur as readily in CML is not clear. It appears to be related to a higher resistance of the leukemic stem cell pool to suppression by chemotherapy in CML. A schematic representation of the defective hemopoiesis in myelogenous leukemia is shown in Fig. 19-2.

Phenotype of hemopoietic stem cell diseases as a result of the matrix of commitment and maturation

The phenotype of the hemopoietic stem cell diseases represents the interaction of the commitment (vertical) ordinal and the maturation (horizontal) continuum. The vertical ordinal is the expression of the hemopoietic stem cell pool's ability to differentiate into erythroid, granulocytic (neutrophilic, basophilic, eosinophilic), monocytic, and megakaryocytic precursors (Fig. 19-3).

The horizontal continuum is the differentiation-maturation pathway. The differentiation pathway is invisible to morphologic examination and represents the changes in cells from the primitive stem cell to the committed unipotential progenitor. Maturation represents the sequence of changes from a unipotential progenitor through a sequence of precursors to the terminally differentiated blood cell, including progression from proerythroblast to erythrocyte or myeloblast to segmented granulocyte, monocyte, or megakaryocyte. This matrix, composed of the options of commitment to different lineages and the stages of differentiation and maturation at which partial or complete arrests occur, results in the wide array of morphologic syndromes induced by a disturbance of the stem cell pool (Fig. 19-3).

In the stem cell diseases in which chronic myeloproliferation dominates the clinical picture, one of the cell lines, for example, erythrocytes, granulocytes, or platelets, tends to accumulate in the blood to a more prominent extent and results in a phenotypic expression of the disease that determines the nosology. Moreover, differentiation and maturation are better preserved. In

FIGURE 19-2 The current understanding of hemopoiesis in myelogenous leukemia. The malignant process is believed to reside in a hemopoietic stem cell. This cell is represented at level 2 in Fig. 19-1. This pool of cells is capable of multivariate commitment to leukemic erythroid, granulocytic, and megakaryocytic precursors. In most cases, granulocytic commitment predominates, and myeloblasts and promonocytes or their immediate derivatives are the dominant cell types. Multiplication of these precursors leads to the accumulation of leukemic blast cells in the marrow. The multiplying blast cells can take one of three paths. The leukemic blast cells may become amitotic (sterile) and effete and die. Alternatively, the blast cells may stop dividing for prolonged periods (blasts in G_0), but have the potential to reenter the mitotic cycle. Third, the blast cells may divide and undergo varying degrees of maturation. The maturation may lead to terminally differentiated cells, such as red cells, segmented neutrophils, monocytes, or platelets. A severe block in maturation is characteristic of AML, whereas a high proportion of leukemic blast cells mature in CML. The disturbance in commitment and maturation in myelogenous leukemia is quantitative, and thus many patterns are possible.

At least four major steps in hematopoiesis are regulated: stem cell proliferation, commitment to one of the three major hemopoietic cell lines (red cells, granulocytes, platelets), multiplication and maturation of early committed cells, and release of mature cells into the blood. These control points are partially or totally defective in myelogenous leukemia. (Reprinted from *Hematology and Oncology*, edited by M. A. Lichtman. Grune & Stratton, New York, 1980. Used with permission.)

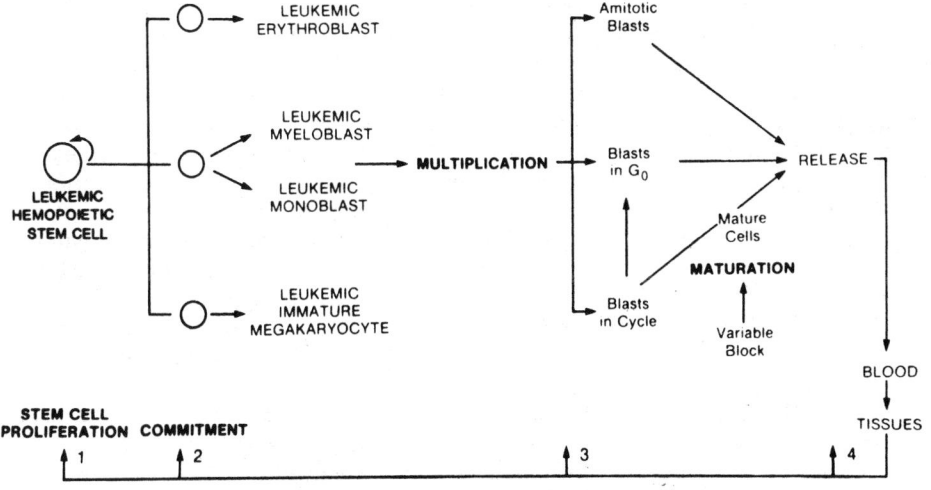

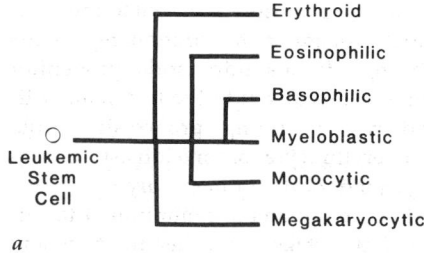

Erythroid
Eosinophilic
Basophilic
Myeloblastic
Monocytic
Megakaryocytic

Leukemic
Stem
Cell

a

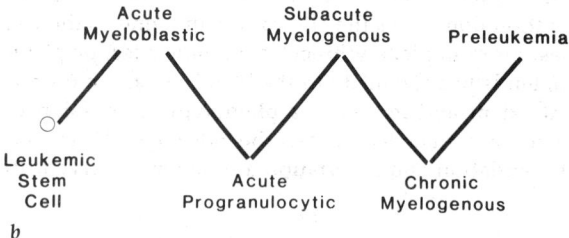

Acute
Myeloblastic

Subacute
Myelogenous

Preleukemia

Leukemic
Stem
Cell

Acute
Progranulocytic

Chronic
Myelogenous

b

FIGURE 19-3   **Myelogenous leukemia has a wide spectrum of morphologic expression as well as a wide spectrum in the maturation of leukemic cells into recognizable precursors. This phenotypic variation is a consequence of the fact that the leukemic lesion resides in a cell pool normally programmed to be capable of many different commitment decisions. (*a*) The morphologic variants of AML can be considered vertical (commitment) variants, in which the cells derived from one of the vertical options of commitment accumulate prominently (e.g., leukemic erythroblasts, leukemic monocytes, etc.) (*b*) Acute myeloblastic leukemia, progranulocytic leukemia, subacute leukemia, and chronic leukemia can be considered horizontal (maturation) variants, in which blocks at different levels of maturation are present.**

the poorly differentiated acute myeloproliferative disease (AML), the phenotypic expression may be predominantly myeloblastic (granuloblastic), erythroid, monocytic, megakaryocytic, or combinations thereof. Certain patterns are favored. Thus, in AML, myeloblastic leukemia and monocytic leukemia or combinations of the two are more common than erythroid, megakaryocytic, or eosinophilic leukemia. AML, however, usually has a disturbance in all cell lines. Thus in myeloblastic or myelomonocytic leukemia there are often overt, qualitative abnormalities of erythroblasts and megakaryocytes. The phenotypic abnormalities of the latter two lineages may not be great enough or evident enough for the observer to designate them as erythroid or megakaryocytic leukemia. The distinction, however, is a quantitative one and has not proved important from the standpoint of choice of primary therapy.

The horizontal continuum of maturation can be completely or partially blocked at various levels, leading to morphologic variants such as acute myeloblastic, progranulocytic, oligoblastic, subacute, or chronic myelogenous leukemia, or to preleukemia.

Hemopoietic versus pluripotential progenitor cell pool as site of the lesion

The site of the lesion of the disorders under consideration is not precisely defined. Most evidence in the past has suggested that the lesion is in the hemopoietic stem cell pool, since at their inception, the diseases rarely involve lymphocytes. Early studies in CML patients emphasized the absence of the Ph[1] chromosome in phytohemagglutinin-stimulated lymphocytes, now known to be principally T lymphocytes [21]. The absence of overt lymphoid aplasia in aplastic anemia or the involvement of lymphocytes in AML supported this thesis also. Similarly, in patients with lymphoid tumors, such as acute lymphocytic leukemia (ALL), in which lymphoblasts had abnormal chromosome markers, the hemopoietic precursors did not share the abnormality.

Recent observations of five types suggest that disturbances thought to be in a hemopoietic stem cell pool may reside in some cases in the pluripotential stem cell compartment or somewhere between the two compartments. First, there is the documentation of a lymphoid type of metamorphosis of CML, agnogenic myeloid metaplasia, and polycythemia vera [28–30]. This occurs in at least 10 percent of cases in CML. Cells appear that bear the Ph[1] chromosome, but they are indistinguishable from malignant lymphocytes, usually of B-cell or pre-B-cell type. Second, there is the high frequency of the Ph[1] chromosome in cases of de novo acute lymphoblastic leukemia, especially in adults [31], and in rare cases of multiple myeloma [32]. Third, X-chromosome-linked isoenzymes of glucose-6-phosphate dehydrogenase, used to establish the clonogenicity of CML, have permitted identification of monoclonal isoenzyme phenotypes in lymphocytic cells as well as hemopoietic cell derivatives in some cases of CML [33,34] and preleukemia [35]. Fourth, cells in CML that have been induced to proliferate in vitro by EB virus infection, which are presumptive B lymphocytes, have been shown to contain the Ph[1] chromosome [36], as have B lymphocytes isolated from the blood of some CML patients. Thus the leukemic hemopoietic stem cell in CML has a propensity to dedifferentiate into lymphoid cells as a result of the neoplastic process or the process can be initiated in some cases farther back in the differentiation scheme, closer to the level of the pluripotential stem cell. Fifth, there are increasing reports of myelogenous leukemia or preleukemic abnormalities of hemopoietic cells in untreated patients with lymphocyte malignancies, and less frequently the reverse [37–48]. In contrast, the B-lymphocyte malignancy chronic lymphocytic leukemia (CLL) has been observed in patients with CML, but CLL lymphocytes have not contained the Ph[1] chromosome, suggesting that an independent clone was involved in the lymphoid tumor in these cases [49,50]. The evidence for the level in hemopoiesis that is involved in these disorders is not definitive, and in CML and AML it may exist at level 1, between levels 1 and 2, or at level 2 in different subjects (see Fig. 19-1).

A recent analysis of cases of AML in young girls and elderly women who were double heterozygotes for isotypes A and B of the enzyme glucose-6-phosphate dehydrogenase has suggested that the AML clone in the girls was restricted to the granulocyte-monocyte pathway, but in the elderly patients monoclonality was expressed in all cell lines in keeping with all prior studies of CML and AML by enzyme or chromosome markers [51,52]. These findings raise the possibility that a leukemic transformation in the young can occur between levels 2 and 3 in Fig. 19-1 and result in a true acute "granulocytic" leukemia.

Quantitativeness of hemopoietic stem cell lesions

The lesions of the hemopoietic stem cell compartment are qualitative in the sense that there is a distinct alteration from normal in the function of the cell pool, and this is a reflection of a qualitative change in the genome of hemopoietic cells. This qualitative change, however, is such that a wide expression of the lesion can occur, and this expression can mimic the options of commitment and maturation expected of normal hemopoietic cells. Although most cases tend to conform to readily recognized patterns, the opportunity for a large number of variations on the more common themes is possible.

Thus many mixed and so-called in-between syndromes occur in which features of myelodysplasia and myeloproliferation of different cell lineages are present. For example, extreme thrombocytosis may accompany CML or agnogenic myeloid metaplasia. Erythrocytosis may accompany CML rarely. Preleukemic states may have mixtures of anemia, granulocytopenia, and thrombocytosis or anemia, granulocytosis, and thrombocytosis rather than pancytopenia. Qualitative abnormalities of erythroblast development may result in acquired α thalassemia (hemoglobin H disease) in patients with agnogenic myeloid metaplasia or other stem cell diseases. Qualitative abnormalities of either red cell, granulocyte, or platelet structure or functions may be more or less prominent in a given patient. In AML, unusual patterns of phenotypic expression occur. For example, one may see patients in whom leukemic erythroblast and monocyte or eosinophil and monocyte proliferation and maturation are prominent. Indeed there is so much opportunity for variation in disease expression among patients with AML that it is unusual to see patients whose phenotypes are identical to others. Choice of treatment is little affected by these variations. The decision to treat and which drugs to use are greatly influenced by whether a patient has a chronic, subacute, or acute myeloproliferative disease; by the rate of progression of the disease; and by the severity of cytopenias. The diagnostician and therapist usually can identify variants as diseases of the hemopoietic stem cell and can manage them as dictated by their manifestations regardless of precise subclassification.

References

1. McCulloch, E. A., Mak, T. W., Price, G. B., and Till, J. E.: Organization and communication in populations of normal and leukemic cells. *Biochim. Biophys. Acta 355:* 260, 1974.
2. Lajtha, L. G.: Hemopoietic stem cells. *Br. J. Haematol. 29:*529, 1975.
3. Cronkite, E. A.: Hemopoietic stem cells, in *An Analytical Review of Hemopoiesis,* edited by H. Ioachin. Pathobiology Annual, vol. 5, Appleton-Century-Crofts, New York, 1975, p. 35.
4. Quesenberry, P., and Levitt, L.: Hematopoietic stem cells. *N. Engl. J. Med. 301:*755, 819, 868, 1979.
5. Wu, A. M., Till, J. E., Siminovitch, L., and McCulloch, E. A.: Cytological evidence for a relationship between normal hematopoietic colony-forming cells and cells of the lymphoid system. *J. Exp. Med. 127:*455, 1967.
6. Nowell, P. C., Hirsch, B. E., Fox, D. H., and Wilson, D. B.: Evidence for the existence of multipotential lymphohemopoietic stem cells in adult rat. *J. Cell. Physiol. 75:*151, 1970.
7. Abramson, J., Miller, R. G., and Phillips, R. A.: The identification in adult bone marrow of pluripotent and restricted stem cells of the myeloid and lymphoid systems. *J. Exp. Med. 145:*1567, 1977.
8. Mohler, D. N., and Leavell, B. S.: Aplastic anemia: An analysis of 50 cases. *Ann. Intern. Med. 21:*379, 1958.
9. Najean, Y., and Pecking, A., for the Cooperative Group for the Study of Aplastic and Refractory Anemia: Prognostic factors in acquired aplastic anemia. *Am. J. Med. 67:*564, 1979.
10. Morley, A., Holmes, K., and Forbes, I.: Depletion of B lymphocytes in chronic hypoplastic marrow failure (aplastic anemia). *Aust. N.Z. J. Med. 4:*538, 1974.
11. Bessis, M.: Hemopoietic dysplasia. *Blood Cells 2:*11, 1976.
12. Knospe, W. H.: Smoldering acute leukemia. *Arch. Intern. Med. 127:*910, 1971.
13. Geary, C. G.: Chronic myelomonocytic leukemia. *Br. J. Haematol. 30:*289, 1975.
14. Zittouw, R.: Subacute and chronic myelomonocytic leukemia. A distinct haematologic entity. *Br. J. Haematol. 32:*1, 1976.
15. Cohen, J. R.: Subacute myeloid leukemia. *Am. J. Med. 66:*959, 1979.
16. Sexauer, J.: Subacute myelomonocytic leukemia. *Am. J. Med. 57:*853, 1974.
17. Flandrin, G.: Cytological classification of acute leukemia: A survey of 1,400 cases. *Blood Cells 1:*7, 1975.
18. Gralnick, H. R.: Classification of acute leukemia. *Ann. Intern. Med. 87:*740, 1977.
19. Hayhoe, F. G. J., and Cawley, J. C.: Acute leukemia. Cellular morphology, cytochemistry, and fine structure. *Clin. Hematol. 1:*49, 1972.
20. Killman, S.-A.: A hypothesis concerning the relationship between normal and leukemic hematopoiesis in acute myeloid leukemia, in *Hematopoietic Cellular Proliferation,* edited by F. Stohlman. Grune & Stratton, New York, 1970.
21. Sandberg, A. A.: The leukemias: Chronic granulocytic leukemia, in *The Chromosomes in Human Cancer and Leukemia.* Elsevier, North-Holland, New York, 1980, chap. 10.
22. Fialkow, P. J., Gartler, S. M., and Yoshida, A.: Clonal origin of chronic myelocytic leukemia in man. *Proc. Natl. Acad. Sci. U.S.A. 58:*1468, 1967.
23. Fialkow, P. J.: Chronic myelogenous leukemia: Clonal origin in a stem cell common to granulocyte, erythrocyte, platelet and monocyte and macrophage. *Am. J. Med. 63:*125, 1977.
24. Wiggans, R. G.: Probable clonal origin of acute myeloblastic leukemia following radiation and chemotherapy of colon cancer. *Blood 52:*659, 1978.
25. Moore, M. A. S., Ekert, H., Fitzgerald, M. G., and Camichael, A.: Evidence for the clonal origin of chronic myeloid leukemia from a sex chromosome mosaic. *Blood 43:*15, 1974.

26. Finney, R.: Chronic granulocytic leukemia with Ph[1] negative cells in bone marrow and a ten year remission after busulfan hypoplasia. *Br. J. Haematol. 23*:283, 1972.

27. Chervenik, P. A.: Human leukemic cells:*In vitro* growth of colonies containing the Philadelphia (Ph[1]) chromosome. *Science 174*:1134, 1971.

28. Joseph, R. R., Zarafonetis, C. J. D., and Durant, J. R.: Lymphoma in chronic granulocytic leukemia. *Am. J. Med. Sci. 257*:417, 1966.

29. Boggs, D. R.: Hematopoietic stem cell theory in relation to possible lymphoblastic conversion of chronic myeloid leukemia. *Blood 44*:449, 1974.

30. Sarin, R. B., Anderson, P. N., and Gallo, R. C.: Terminal deoxynucleotidyl transferase activities in human blood leukocytes and lymphoblast cell lines: High levels in lymphoblast cell lines and in blast cells of some patients with chronic myelogenous leukemia in acute phase. *Blood 47*:11, 1976.

31. Catovsky, D.: Ph1-positive acute leukemia and chronic granulocytic leukemia: One or two diseases. *Br. J. Haematol. 42*:493, 1979.

32. Van Den Berghe, H., et al.: Philadelphia chromosome in human multiple myeloma. *J. Natl. Cancer Inst. 63*:11, 1979.

33. Fialkow, P. J., Denman, A. M., Jacobson, R. J., and Lowenthal, M. N.: Chronic myelocytic leukemia: Origin of some lymphocytes from leukemic stem cells. *J. Clin. Invest. 62*:815, 1978.

34. LeBien, T. W., Hozier, J., Minowada, J., and Kersey, J. H.: Origin of chronic myelocytic leukemia in a precursor of pre-B-lymphocytes. *N. Engl. J. Med. 301*:144, 1979.

35. Prchal, J. T., Throckmorton, D. W., Caroll, A. J., Fuson, E. W., Gams, R. A., and Prchal, J. F.: A common progenitor for human myeloid and lymphoid cells. *Nature 274*:590, 1978.

36. Martin, P. J., Najfield, V., Hansen, J. A., Penfold, G. K., Jacobsen, R. J., and Fialkow, P. J.: Involvement of the B-lymphoid system in chronic myelogenous leukemia. *Nature 287*:49, 1980.

37. MacSween, J. M., and Langley, G. R.: Light-chain disease (hypogammaglobulinemia and Bence-Jones proteinuria) and sideroblastic anemia—Preleukemic chronic granulocytic leukemia. *Can. Med. Assoc. J. 106*:995, 1972.

38. Tursz, T., Flandun, G., Bronet, J.-C., Briere, J., and Seligmann, M.: Simultaneous occurrence of acute myeloblastic leukaemia and multiple myeloma without previous chemotherapy. *Br. Med. J. 2*:642, 1974.

39. Hamilton, P. J.: Concomitant myeloblastic and lymphoblastic leukaemia. *Lancet 1*:373, 1976.

40. Hoffman, R., Estren, S., Kopel, S., Marks, S. M., and McCaffrey, R. P.: Lymphoblastic-like leukemic transformation of polycythemia vera. *Ann. Intern. Med. 89*:71, 1978.

41. Cleary, B., Binder, R. A., Kales, A. N., and Veltri, B. J.: Simultaneous presentation of acute myelomonocytic leukemia and multiple myeloma. *Cancer 41*:1381, 1978.

42. Barr, R. D., and Watt, J.: Preliminary evidence for the common origin of a lympho-myeloid complex in man. *Acta Haematol. 60*:29, 1978.

43. Lawlor, E., McCann, S. R., Whelan, A., Greally, J., and Temperley, I. J.: Acute myeloid leukaemia occurring in untreated chronic lymphatic leukaemia. *Br. J. Haematol, 43*:369, 1979.

44. Barton, J. C., Conrad, M. E., and Parmley, R. T.: Acute lymphoblastic leukemia in idiopathic refractory sideroblastic anemia. *Am. J. Hematol. 9*:109, 1980.

45. Iland, H., Chan, W., and Vincent, P. C.: Myeloproliferative and lymphoproliferative disorders in the same patient. *Aust, N.Z. J. Med. 10*:650, 1980.

46. Polliack, A., Prokocimer, M., and Matzner, Y.: Lymphoblastic leukemic transformation (lymphoblastic crisis) in myelofibrosis and myeloid metaplasia. *Am. J. Hematol. 9*:211, 1980.

47. Berkowitz, L. R., Ross, D. W., and Orringer, E. P.: Hairy cell leukemia with acquired dyserythropoiesis. *Arch. Intern. Med. 140*:554, 1980.

48. Martelli, M. F., Falini, B., Rambotti, P., Tonato, M., and Davis, S.: Sideroblastic anemia associated with hairy cell leukemia. *Cancer 48*:762, 1981.

49. Wheng, J., Gralnick, H. R., Johnson, R. E., Lee, E. C., and Lear, A.: Chronic granulocytic leukemia (CGL) during the course of chronic lymphocytic leukemia (CLL): Correlation of blood, marrow, and spleen morphology and cytogenetics. *Blood 43*:333, 1974.

50. Vilpo, J. A., Klemi, P., Lassila, O., and de la Chappelle, A.: Concomitant presentation of two chronic leukemias. Evidence for independent clonal evolution. *Am. J. Hematol. 8*:205, 1980.

51. Fialkow, P. J., et al.: Acute nonlymphocytic leukemia: Heterogeneity of stem cell origin. *Blood 57*:1068, 1981.

52. Fialkow, P. J., et al.: Acute nonlymphocytic leukemia: Expression in cells restricted to granulocyte and monocytic differentiation. *N. Engl. J. Med. 301*:1, 1979.

Hemopoietic stem cell disorders — aplastic

CHAPTER *20*

Aplastic anemia

ALLAN J. ERSLEV

Aplastic anemia is a stem cell disorder characterized by fatty replacement of hemopoietic tissue and pancytopenia. The reduction in functional marrow mass is believed to be caused by toxic, radiant, or immunologic injury to marrow stem cells or their microenvironment, reducing their capacity for normal cellular renewal. The remaining active marrow is usually scattered uniformly throughout the marrow cavities but occasionally may be confined to small pockets surrounded by fatty tissue. These pockets can be extremely cellular, but the overall functional capacity of the marrow, as assessed by blood counts and iron clearance studies, is reduced.

In 1888, Paul Ehrlich reported the case of a 21-year-old woman who had died from severe anemia and neutropenia and on postmortem examination was found to have a yellow, hypocellular marrow [1]. This may have been the first description of an illness which subsequently was given the name aplastic anemia by Chauffard in 1904 [2]. During the next few decades, numerous cases of so-called aplastic anemia were reported, and there was a mounting realization of the possible relation between x-rays or certain chemicals and marrow failure. Since in vivo marrow examination did not become routine until the 1930s, the term aplastic anemia was used interchangeably with other terms for marrow failure, such as primary refractory anemia, aregenerative anemia, aleukemia hemorrhagica, panmyelophthisis, toxic paralytic anemia, Fanconi's anemia, Estren-Dameshek anemia, Diamond-Blackfan anemia, and, of course, hypoplastic anemia. In 1941, Bomford and Rhoads [3] made a major attempt to classify pancytopenia according to marrow morphology. Unfortunately, this attempt did not resolve the problem of terminology, and aplastic anemia continued to be used as a synonym for diseases as disparate as pure red cell aplasia, aplastic crisis, refractory normoblastic anemia, pancytopenia with hyperactive marrow, and pancytopenia with hypoactive marrow. Despite our still limited knowledge of the pathophysiology of marrow failure, it seems appropriate now to split rather than to lump, and in this chapter the term aplastic anemia will be restricted to pancytopenia caused by the decreased functional capacity of a hypoplastic, fatty marrow.

Etiology and pathogenesis

The development of a fatty, inactive marrow and pancytopenia has been associated with prior exposure to drugs and chemicals, to radiation, and to a variety of diseases (Table 20-1)) Unfortunately, establishment of a cause is in most cases merely an educated guess supported by statistical correlations or suggestive temporal relationships. When it is not possible to hazard even a guess, the aplastic anemia is designated as idiopathic, a confession of ignorance we have to make in about 50 percent of the cases. Obviously, even in these cases there must be some constitutional or environmental etiologic factor, and in industrial society the possibilities for unrecognized exposure to potentially toxic compounds seem almost limitless. Many of the chemicals used in the household and in the cosmetic industry contain complex benzene radicals, and the widespread use of insecticides, fertilizers, and food supplements makes even our "daily bread" suspect.

Despite difficulties in pinpointing a cause in patients with aplastic anemia, it is mandatory that a serious attempt be made in each case. The patients should particularly be queried about model building, painting, and other hobbies, daily activities, and medications, and a thorough history of occupational exposures to chemicals or to radiant energy should be obtained. A great deal of ingenuity and persistence may be demanded of the physician [4]. It is essential to remember that aspirin, sleeping tablets, laxatives, and antihistamines are frequently not considered medications by the patient and that the term drug today often is interpreted to mean an illegal mood-altering chemical rather than a therapeutic agent.

Regardless of exact etiology, aplastic anemia is proba-

TABLE 20-1 Etiologic classification of aplastic anemia

IDIOPATHIC
Constitutional (Fanconi's anemia)
Acquired

SECONDARY
Chemical and physical agents:
  Drugs
  Nonpharmacologic chemicals
  Radiation
Infectious:
  Viral: hepatitis
  Bacterial: miliary tuberculosis
Metabolic:
  Pancreatitis
  Pregnancy
Immunologic:
  Humoral
  Cellular
Paroxysmal nocturnal hemoglobinuria

bly caused by failure of pluripotential stem cells with secondary depletion of hemopoietic precursor cells and fatty marrow replacement [5–8]. The early committed stem cells, i.e., CFU-C, BFU-E, and CFU-M, are believed to be capable of limited self-renewal in addition to continuous proliferation and differentiation. However, if impaired or depleted, they must be replenished from a compartment of pluripotential stem cells (CFU-S). If this compartment fails to respond appropriately to emergency signals from the committed stem cells, marrow hypoplasia and sustained pancytopenia ensue.

Failure of the pluripotential stem cell compartment may be caused by either stem cell dysfunction or stem cell depletion. Stem cell dysfunction could occur if the microenvironment were damaged or if the stem cells themselves were altered. Although the success of marrow transplantation appears to rule out the presence of a detrimental microenvironment, the possible cotransplantation of a missing environmental helper cell keeps this option open [9]. A stem cell alteration which selectively would impede stem cell renewal could also lead to aplastic anemia. However, such an alteration would probably have to be clonal, and it is difficult to envision a clone capable of suppressing normal clones but permitting engraftment of stem cells from an identical twin.

Stem cell depletion, however, could explain sustained underproduction of normal cells as well as successful transplantation of compatible stem cells. Early studies involving retransplantation of CFU-S through generations of irradiated mice had suggested that the normal CFU-S compartment is nearly inexhaustible [10]. However, more recent studies have shown that regeneration after repeated depletions actually becomes less and less efficient until it fails altogether [11]. Furthermore, in humans, repeated exposure to non-cycle-active chemotherapeutic agents such as busulfan or nitrosourea leads to prolonged and often irreversible reductions in the number of stem cells [12]. Similarly, the number of CFU-S in mice exposed to busulfan can be shown to be permanently reduced even though pancytopenia is not present, so-called latent aplasia [13]. Consequently, it is possible that the capacity for stem cell regeneration is finite and that aplastic anemia develops when injury to pluripotential stem cells has reduced their number to a level inadequate for the sustained maintenance of committed stem cell compartments. Overactivity of the remaining stem cells with rapid cellular transit of their progeny could explain the appearance of small CFU-C colonies [14] and the production of macrocytic "stress erythrocytes" with increased amounts of fetal hemoglobin [15–18].

In order to explain that exposure to concentrations of drugs or chemicals generally considered innocuous in some individuals causes stem cell failure and aplastic anemia in others, it appears necessary to invoke an element of hypersensitivity. This vulnerability may be caused by a genetic or acquired defect in drug elimination or detoxification or by a genetic or acquired vulnerability of stem cells. Heterozygotes for the gene for Fanconi's constitutional aplastic anemia [19] or for the genes controlling cellular uptake and processing of folic acid [20] are hematologically normal but could represent an important subpopulation with vulnerable stem cells. Acquired "latent aplasia" with predisposition to the development of further stem cell damage may also be quite common but not easily demonstrable in humans. In mice it has been shown convincingly that animals with busulfan-induced "latent aplasia" are, for example, excessively vulnerable to chloramphenicol [21].

Immunologic rejection of stem cells can undoubtedly cause aplastic anemia in some patients, but the frequency of this mechanism is still hotly debated. Coculture of marrow or blood lymphocytes from patients with aplastic anemia and normal individuals have revealed the presence of suppressor or killer lymphocytes [22,23]. However, careful review of the cases and the techniques employed has led to the conclusion that in many instances the suppressor or killer lymphocytes were not primary but rather secondary to transfusions of HLA-incompatible blood [24,25]. Nevertheless, in the few patients with no preceding transfusions and in the patients in whom the lymphocytes suppress autologous marrow [26] the evidence for a pathogenic role of cellular immunity is very strong. Furthermore, immunosuppressive therapy has caused complete hemopoietic recovery in some patients [27], and even transplantation between identical twins has in a few instances required concurrent immunosuppression in order to be successful [28,29]. Although circulating anti-stem cell antibodies have been demonstrated [30,31], immunologic rejection, when it occurs, is generally believed to be due to cellular rejection.

A defect in the marrow microenvironment leading to inadequate stem cell function has been found to cause pancytopenia in strains of inbred mice [32] and has been postulated to be of pathogenetic significance in humans as well. The high initial take of transplanted marrow in patients with aplastic anemia suggests that an abnormal microenvironment is of only occasional pathogenetic significance.

DRUGS AND CHEMICALS

CHLORAMPHENICOL (CHLOROMYCETIN)
Among the many drugs and chemicals which have been associated with the development of aplastic anemia, chloramphenicol is undoubtedly the one regarded with the greatest suspicion. This drug was introduced in 1948, and because of its wide antibiotic spectrum and ease of administration, it rapidly became one of the most popular antibiotics. In 1952, after a few unheeded warnings, a number of reports suddenly appeared strongly associating chloramphenicol treatment with the onset of aplastic anemia [33]. Since then there have been hundreds of additional reports which, abetted by malpractice suits and senatorial interest, have led to the acceptance of chloramphenicol as a potentially danger-

ous antibiotic [34–36] whether administered by mouth or intravenously [320]. Data accumulated by the American Medical Association in 1967 [37] show that of 771 cases of pancytopenia suspected of being drug-related and reported to the AMA, 338 cases, or 44 percent, followed the use of chloramphenicol. Of even greater importance was the finding that of these 338 cases, 154 had received chloramphenicol as the only drug administered in the previous 6 months. In a tabulation of 787 cases of aplastic anemia reported between 1970 and 1977, 164, or 21 percent, followed the use of chloramphenicol [38]. However, a bad reputation leads to increased suspicion, and any patients with pancytopenia and the slightest previous exposure to chloramphenicol will be designated as suffering from chloramphenicol-induced aplastic anemia. Nevertheless, chloramphenicol has achieved its bad reputation with good reason, and it should be used with great caution and respect. The actual risk of developing fatal aplastic anemia after being treated with chloramphenicol is low, about 1 in 20,000 to 30,000 [39,40], but this is still 13 times the risk of developing fatal idiopathic aplastic anemia [41].

Concomitantly with the realization that chloramphenicol can induce prolonged, self-sustaining marrow hypoplasia, it was found that it also can cause a brief, reversible marrow suppression in many, if not all, exposed patients [42,43]. This drug-dependent marrow failure is associated with an increase in serum iron (Fig. 20-1) [44] and with vacuolization of marrow cells (Fig. 20-2) [45,46].

FIGURE 20-1 The effect of a chloramphenicol analog on serum iron and blood counts. Similar effects are seen with chloramphenicol itself. (Weisberger [41].)

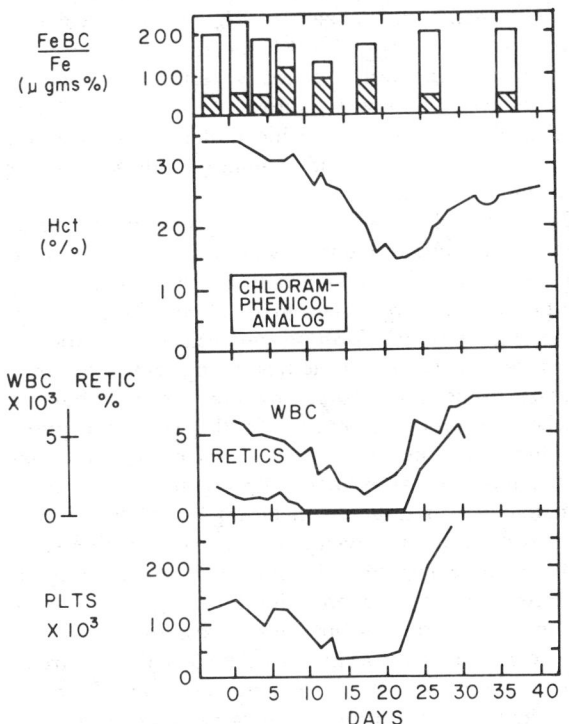

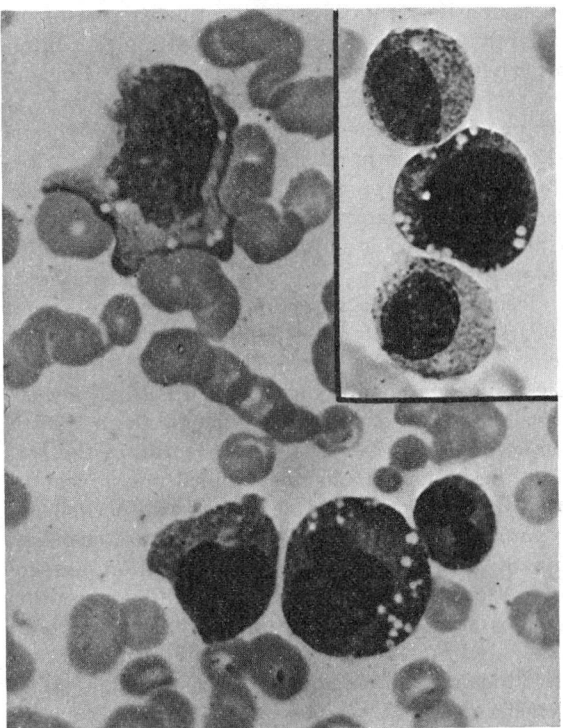

FIGURE 20-2 Vacuolization of marrow cells in a patient treated with chloramphenicol. (Courtesy of R. W. Rundles.)

It has been tempting to consider this marrow suppression as being an early, still reversible manifestation of impending chloramphenicol-induced aplastic anemia. Consequently, it has been recommended that marrow suppression heralded by an increase in serum iron, decrease in reticulocytes, and vacuolization of marrow cells should be an absolute indication for the discontinuation of the drug [47]. However, some physicians have continued to use chloramphenicol despite these early warnings and apparently have not encountered serious consequences [48,49]. Furthermore, an analysis of 94 cases of chloramphenicol-induced marrow failure led to the conclusion that the two conditions are independent [50]. One is described as a reversible marrow suppression occurring during drug administration and directly related to length of drug exposure and to amount of drug used. It is uncertain whether or not this suppression is of clinical consequence, but it presumably does not lead to marrow aplasia. The other is described as a frequently irreversible type of marrow aplasia occurring some time after the drug has been discontinued and not related to the amount or length of drug exposure. The basic difference between the pathogenesis of these two disorders is presumed to be that in one chloramphenicol affects the maturation and proliferation of differentiated cells, rendering them temporarily ineffective, and in the other chloramphenicol changes the genetic structure of the stem cells rendering them permanently incapable of differentiation. However, the similarities between the two disorders cannot be disregarded. An analysis of 408 cases reported to the American Medical

Association Registry did not permit separation of the cases into two distinct groups [34]. Until further information has been provided, it seems prudent to consider the early drug-induced suppression of the marrow a warning which, whenever clinically appropriate, should be heeded in order to reduce the possibility that a benign, reversible suppression might become a dangerous, irreversible marrow aplasia.

Chloramphenicol is a nitrobenzene compound with a dichloracetamide side chain. Such chemical compounds have been regarded with great suspicion since Kracke and Parker in the early 1930s pointed out that they were often responsible for agranulocytosis [51]. Although there is no experimental support for this suspicion, almost all hydrocarbons involved etiologically in aplastic anemia contain the benzene ring. In addition, the spatial configuration of chloramphenicol resembles the pyrimidine nucleotide uridine-5-phosphate, a challenging similarity [52] since it could explain a proposed competitive inhibition of chloramphenicol on messenger RNA formation. In the bacterial cell this competition appears to lead to impaired formation of peptide bonds and reduced protein synthesis [53], but the mode of action in the mammalian marrow cell is still unknown. In this cell, impaired protein synthesis appears to be restricted to the protein synthesis which takes place independently in the mitochondria [54,55]. The synthesis of mitochondrial ferrochelatase has been singled out as particularly vulnerable to chloramphenicol [56].

In suspension cultures of intact marrow cells, chloramphenicol has been found to decrease iron uptake, amino acid incorporation, heme synthesis, and synthesis of DNA and RNA [57–59]. This inhibitory action occurs only when marrow cells or reticulocytes are exposed to chloramphenicol in concentrations 5 to 10 times those observed in vivo. At more clinically important concentrations, however, chloramphenicol has been demonstrated to inhibit colony growth of CFU-C [60]. The physiologic relevance of the in vitro test is supported by the fact that glucuronidation of chloramphenicol renders the drug inert both in vivo and in vitro [58]. Nevertheless, it is probably unrealistic to equate drug-induced alterations of the metabolism of differentiated cells in vitro with the stem cell injury which must underlie the development of aplastic anemia. Possibly of more relevance is the observation [61] that chloramphenicol can cause vacuolization of chromosomes. Such chromosomal change could lead to irreversible and self-perpetuating changes in the stem cells [62], resulting in aplastic anemia, acute leukemia [63–65], or paroxysmal nocturnal hemoglobinuria [66].

Although it is possible that the toxic alteration of the genome is a chance phenomenon, it seems more likely that there is an underlying genetic or acquired stem cell hypersensitivity to chloramphenicol. Some, but not all, studies have suggested that marrow from patients who have recovered from chloramphenicol-induced marrow hypoplasia or marrow from relatives of chloramphenicol victims may be more sensitive in vitro to the inhibitory

action of chloramphenicol than normal marrow [31,67,68]. Furthermore, latent marrow damage induced in mice by busulfan renders the marrow excessively sensitive to the effect of chloramphenicol [21]. There is also some reason [44] for believing that individual differences in the rate or extent of chloramphenicol detoxification play a role [69,70]. An immunologic mechanism has been proposed with rejection of the marrow either by anti-stem cell antibodies or by sensitized lymphocytes. However, the only evidence for this idea is the fact that chloramphenicol can act as a haptene and cause the production of specific humoral antibodies [71] and that steroids or splenectomy occasionally can induce a remission. Unfortunately, a suitable animal model for the study of chloramphenicol toxicity has not been developed; so we have to accept its capricious toxic actions as another example of "pharmacogenetic polymorphism" [72].

BENZENE (BENZOL)

Since the turn of the century it has been recognized that benzene and benzene derivatives are of potential toxicity to the marrow [73]. The extensive use of benzene as a solvent in industry has led to numerous attempts to define its toxicity and to establish safe limits. The early regulations defined safe limits as less than 100 parts per million, but present federal regulations limit the safe industrial level to 10 parts per million [74]. A recent attempt by the Occupational Safety and Health Administration (OSHA) to reduce the acceptable limit to 1 part per million was, however, not accepted by the U.S. Supreme Court [75]. Unfortunately, the manufacture of many solvents used in the home is not carefully controlled, and these may contain significant amounts of benzene. Although benzene, C_6H_6, is highly volatile, with a boiling point of 80°C, the distillation process used in the preparation of many petroleum products, such as paint removers, kerosene, degreasers, Stoddard's solvent, etc., is often incomplete, and uncertain quantities of benzene may remain in these popular household solvents.

Benzene will cause marrow suppression and occasionally leukemia in laboratory animals [76,77]. In mice it appears that benzene acts both by suppressing DNA synthesis of differentiated marrow cells [78] and by damaging the colony-forming stem cells [79]. Studies in rats have suggested that the hematologically toxic compounds in benzene poisoning are various phenolic breakdown products, especially the diphenol pyrocatechin (pyrocatechol) [80]. In humans, benzene exposure has been associated with a confusing array of hematologic abnormalities including hemolytic anemia, marrow hyperplasia, myeloid metaplasia, lymphopenia, and acute myelogenous leukemia, but the most common toxic result is pancytopenia due to a hypoplastic marrow or to a hyperplastic but ineffective marrow [81–85].

Pancytopenia may occur years after actual exposure to benzene, but such delayed reactions should always be suspected of being coincidental rather than related. In most cases, the marrow depression appears shortly after exposure to the chemical, with a close relation between amounts and duration of exposure and degree of marrow suppression. The subsequent development of leukemia in patients with pancytopenia due to a hyperplastic but ineffective marrow has occurred frequently enough to consider benzene a potential leukemogenic agent [81–85].

OTHER CHEMICALS AND DRUGS

A great number of chemicals structurally related to benzene are used in industry, on the farm, and at home [86], but although they all should be suspect, only a few have convincingly been associated with the development of aplastic anemia. The insecticides pentachlorophenol, lindane, and DDT [87–89] have been shown to have potential marrow-toxic properties, and exposure to trinitrotoluene [90] in industry or toluene among glue sniffers [91] or glue users [92] is also hazardous.

Table 20-2 lists drugs and key references [93–177] to studies which have shown a suggestive cause-effect relation between drug administration and the development of aplastic anemia. Spurred on by the sudden realization of the potential toxicity of chloramphenicol, the American Medical Association Council on Drugs in 1955 established a Sub-Committee on Drug-Induced Blood Dyscrasias. This committee was charged with developing a reporting system which would give the medical profession early warning of possible hematologic side effects of new drugs. As such, the system seems to have failed, since almost all information about toxic side effects has been provided through other channels, such as from manufacturers, clinical trials, and case reports. However, thousands of reports sent in to the AMA from this country and abroad [37] have provided useful data in the assessment of the relative toxicity of drugs. In order to evaluate these data, it is of importance that they be correlated with a rough estimate of the total consumption of the individual drugs and that the appropriate adjustment be made. In the majority of patients, several drugs had been administered prior to the onset of aplastic anemia; so the cases in which only one drug had been administered take on an added significance. Similarly, drugs administered with other medication considered "innocent" should be regarded with more suspicion than drugs administered along with other drugs already suspected of causing marrow damage. An attempt has been made in Table 20-2 to separate these categories. However, it should be emphasized that a drug generally considered innocent, such as aspirin, has been reported by some to cause aplastic anemia [94,95], and that current conclusions about potential marrow toxicity still rest on judgment and experience—hallowed but very vulnerable criteria.

From the many reports of single cases, it is difficult to gain much information except that most drugs on occasion have been associated with the development of marrow hypoplasia and that some, such as the hydantoins, pyrazolones, sulfonamides, and gold preparations, ap-

pear to have an unusual affinity for this association. The only drug for which statistically significant toxicity data are available is quinacrine (Atabrine). During World War II [164], the incidence of fatal aplastic anemia was found to be 3 for 100,000 quinacrine-treated soldiers as compared with 0.2 for 100,000 untreated soldiers. This incidence of about 1 in 30,000 is not far from what has been suggested for the incidence of fatal chloramphenicol-induced aplastic anemia [35,178], although the pathogenesis may well be quite different. Quinacrine-induced aplastic anemia, for example, occurs while the drug is being administered and in about 50 percent of the cases is associated with skin lesions, suggesting a hypersensitivity reaction.

RADIATION

The biologic effect of radiation depends on the amount of radiant energy absorbed by the tissues (measured in rads) and the specific radiosensitivity of the tissue. The highly penetrating radiant energy delivered by x-rays, γ-rays, or neutrons is effective at a distance, but the pathway of α and β particles is so short that it is necessary to introduce the radiant source directly into the tissues. Here the radiant energy generates electrons and causes a wave of ionizations and further energy release. One rad is defined as the radiation dose which causes 10^{12} primary ionizations per gram of tissue or releases 100 ergs of energy per gram of tissue. The absorbed energy, when greater than the energy of chemical bonds, will cause random molecular changes with the formation of ions, peroxides, and other free radicals which in turn may transfer the absorbed energy to large, critical macromolecules [179–181]. As a guide to radiation exposure and its potential dangers, Table 20-3 lists some published figures [182–185] relating to whole-body radiation.

Extremely high radiant energies such as those released in laboratory or reactor accidents or by extracorporeal irradiation of blood can cause damage to mature, differentiated cells [186,187], but otherwise only organ systems with a rapid cellular turnover are vulnerable. The radiosensitivity of these systems can be ranked in the following order [188]: (1) germinal epithelium of the testes, (2) hemopoietic cells, (3) intestinal epithelium, and (4) basal layers of the skin.

Exposure to lethal or sublethal amounts of whole-body radiation results in extensive cell death in the two critical cellular systems, marrow and intestine, and the patients may succumb from the combined effect of acute marrow aplasia and intestinal ulcerations. If the patient lives through the first crucial 3- to 6-week period, surviving stem cells will effect slow marrow regeneration. This regeneration may completely restore marrow function to normal, but in some cases the stem cells have become permanently damaged and ineffective. Such damage can lead to chronic marrow hypoplasia with various degrees of pancytopenia, or it can cause the formation of a hyperplastic but ineffective marrow displaying multinucleated giant cells, asymmetric mitotic

TABLE 20-2   Drugs associated with the development of aplastic anemia

Generic name	No. of patients receiving drug alone or drug in combination with nontoxic drugs [37]	No. of patients receiving drug in combination with potentially toxic drug [37]	References
Acetazolamide	3	7	[93]
Acetophenetidin	3	31	
Acetylsalicylic acid	7	90	[94,95]
Amodiaquine hydrochloride	2		
Amphotericin B	1	1	[96]
Carbamazepine		2	[97–99]
Carbimazole			[100,101]
Chloramphenicol	182	156	See text
Chlordiazepoxide hydrochloride	2	7	[102]
Chlorothiazide	2	13	
Chloroquine			[103]
Chlorpheniramine	2	15	[104,105]
Chlorpromazine	3	18	[106,107]
Chlorpropamide	4	2	[108]
Cimetidine			[109,110]
Colbutamide			[111]
Colchicine	2	3	[112–115]
Diphenylhydantoin sodium	3	21	[116,117]
Epinephrine	2	4	
Ethosuximide	1	1	[118]
Flucytosine			[119]
Gamma benzene hexachloride			[120]
Gold salts	8	2	[121–123]
Ibuprofen			[124]
Indomethacin			[125–127]
Lithium			[128,129]
Mepazine	4	1	
Meprobamate		15	[130,131]
Mercurochrome			[132]
Methazolamide			[133]
Methicillin sodium			[134,135]
Methimazole	1	1	[136,137]
Methyldopa			[138,139]
Methylphenylhydantoin			[140,141]

divisions, and foci of arrested or short-lived blast cells [189]. In addition, it has been proposed that injury to hypothetical "vascular stem cells" will change the "vascular microenvironment" or "stroma" in the marrow and interfere with marrow regeneration after irradiation [190,191].

In the marrow the cellular elements most sensitive to acute radiation-induced change are the erythroid cells, followed by the myeloid cells and the megakaryocytes [192–195]. The reticulum cells, plasma cells, and fibroblasts are presumably quite radioresistant. Because of the long life-span of circulating red blood cells, the red cell count changes slowly, but careful enumeration of reticulocytes will disclose early impairment in erythroid function. There may be an initial rise in granulocyte count caused by a sudden release of granulocytes from the marrow depots, but leukopenia follows shortly [196]. The almost immediate reduction in lymphocytes cannot be explained by damage of lymphocytopoietic cells, since even short-lived lymphocytes have a long intermitotic phase [197]. It is more likely that radiant

energy directly or indirectly exerts a "lymphocytolytic" effect similar to that observed after steroid administration. In addition, radiant energy causes changes in the genetic structure of some lymphocytes, and it is possible to observe bilobed cells, cytoplasmic inclusions, and chromosomal changes in lymphocytes months to years after radiation exposure [198,199]. Thrombocytopenia usually occurs after the onset of reticulocytopenia and neutropenia and may also be the last to disappear in the recovery phase. This sequence of events is not invariable and is influenced by bleeding, infections, or other mechanisms. The blood picture of chronic postirradiation aplastic anemia is similar to that seen in idiopathic aplastic anemia.

Long-term continuous exposure to small amounts of external radiation (as by radiologists) [200] or to internally deposited radium [201] or thorium [202] has been followed by the development of aplastic anemia. There are also reports that aplastic anemia may occur months or years after a brief exposure to radiation, such as that of patients treated with x-rays for spondylitis [203,204],

TABLE 20-2   Drugs associated with the development of aplastic anemia *(Continued)*

Generic name	No. of patients receiving drug alone or drug in combination with nontoxic drugs [37]	No. of patients receiving drug in combination with potentially toxic drug [37]	References
Methylthiouracil			[142]
Methyprylon			[143]
Metolazone			[144]
Naproxen			[145]
Oxyphenbutazone			[146]
Penicillin	4	91	
Penicillamine			[147,148]
Phenacemide			[149]
Phenantoin	9	14	[150]
Phenylbutazone	18	22	[151–155]
Piperacetazine			[156]
Potassium perchlorate	6	4	[157,158]
Primidone	2	6	
Prochlorperazine	1	9	[159]
Propylthiouracil			[160,161]
Pyrilamine maleate		3	[162]
Pyrimethamine	2	3	[163]
Quinacrine hydrochloride	3	2	[164–166]
Quinidine	1	2	[167]
Salicylamide	2	3	
Streptomycin		31	[168]
Sulfadimethoxine	2	4	[169]
Sulfamethoxazole-trimethoprim			[170]
Sulfamethoxypyridazine	3	11	[171,172]
Sulfaphenazole	2		[173]
Sulfathiazole	2		
Sulfisoxazole	3	30	
Sulfonamides	4	17	
Sulindac			[174]
Thiacetazone	2	1	
Thiocyanate			[175]
Tolbutamide	7	5	[176,177]
Trimethadione	2	4	

SOURCE: AMA *Registry* and key case reports.

but these reports are difficult to evaluate. Among the survivors of the atomic bombing of Nagasaki, only a very few developed delayed aplastic anemia [205,206]. The problem here is the same as the problem that arises in cases of aplastic anemia diagnosed months after exposure to chloramphenicol or years after exposure to benzene. There is no way in which we experimentally can establish a cause-effect relation, and the etiologic designation becomes a question of judgment and possibly personal bias.

MISCELLANEOUS ACQUIRED CAUSES

Aplastic anemia has been reported as a sequel to several diseases. Hepatitis, in particular, has been associated with an especially malignant form of aplastic anemia [207–210]. It is tempting to assume that hepatic dysfunction may lead to impaired detoxification of a potentially myelotoxic compound, but there is no evidence to support such a sequence. An autoimmune mechanism may be responsible, but the most attractive explanation is that the virus involved in hepatitis in some way inter-

TABLE 20-3   Relative magnitudes of radiation exposure (whole-body exposure)

Observations	Rads
Few if any symptoms	0–125
Reversible symptoms and signs	125–250
Irreversible signs and occasional mortality	250–400
50% mortality	500
100% mortality	700
Doubling of spontaneous mutations	5–150
Maximum permissible occupational exposure in adults	5.0/year
Radiation from naturally occurring radionuclides and from cosmic radiation:	
Sea level	0.10/year
5000 feet	0.14/year
Radiation from fallout (atomic bomb debris)	0.002/year
Radiation from diagnostic radioisotope studies:	
Red blood cell life-span (50 μCi ^{51}Cr)	0.04
Ferrokinetic studies (10 μCi ^{59}Fe)	0.04
Shilling test (1 μCi ^{60}Co)	0.02
Blood volume (10 μCi ^{131}I)	0.01
Thyroid scan (75 μCi ^{131}I)	0.1

feres with the self-perpetuating function of marrow stem cells. Other viruses can cause hemodepression [211,212], and serum from patients with infectious hepatitis has been reported to produce chromosomal abnormalities in cultured leukocytes [213].

Miliary tuberculosis is reputed to have the potential for inducing pancytopenia and aplastic anemia [214, 215]. However, in the majority of cases, it causes a dysfunction of the marrow rather than aplasia, and the associated fever, weight loss, and splenomegaly usually set it apart from acquired idiopathic aplastic anemia. Paroxysmal nocturnal hemoglobinuria is regularly associated with a pancytopenia, and an increasing number of cases have been reported of aplastic anemia with complement-sensitive red cells [216] and of paroxysmal nocturnal hemoglobinuria merging into classic aplastic anemia [217–220]. The relation between these two acquired marrow disorders and their occasional association with acute myelogenous leukemia are challenging but still quite obscure [63]. Isolated cases have been reported of aplastic anemia occurring in association with pancreatic dysfunction [221], pregnancy [222–224], diffuse fasciitis [26], and disseminated lupus erythematosus [27,225], but the cause-effect relation has been tenuous. Of special interest is the type of aplastic anemia which has been observed after transfusion of whole blood or marrow to immunodeficient children [226–230]. This response resembles the graft-versus-host reaction observed after marrow transplantation in irradiated animals [231] and humans [232] and appears to represent an immunologic rejection of marrow stem cells [233] or structural cells [234]. The recent demonstration of suppressor or killer lymphocytes in marrow or blood from some patients with aplastic anemia [26, 27] as well as the occasional remissions observed after immunosuppressive therapy [23,235] have suggested that such a rejection may occur more often than previously thought.

CONSTITUTIONAL CAUSES

In 1927, Fanconi described the cases of three brothers with aplastic anemia and multiple congenital abnormalities [236]. Since then, many hundreds of similar cases have been reported, and it has become apparent that congenital marrow hypoplasia can occur with and without associated visceral or bony malformations and with and without definite family histories of this condition [237–239]. At the present time, the designation constitutional aplastic anemia is used to describe this confusing group of diseases or syndromes of suspected inherited origin [34]. It includes in addition to Fanconi's anemia, familial aplastic anemia without physical abnormalities, and congenital amegakaryocytic thrombocytopenia [34]. The term Fanconi's anemia is usually applied only to familial marrow hypoplasia which becomes manifest in the first decade of life and is associated with various malformations [240], such as brown skin pigmentations, hypoplasia of the kidney and spleen, absent or hypo-

plastic thumb or radius, microcephaly, and mental and sexual retardation.

The lack of consistent familial or genetic background has suggested that an induced change in fetal development is responsible for the congenital abnormalities [237]. However, an autosomal recessive inheritance could explain that only a few homozygotes exhibit both aplastic anemia and physical abnormalities. It has even been estimated that the frequency of heterozygotes in the population is between 1 in 300 and 1 in 600 [241,242]. These individuals may have excessively vulnerable marrow and could conceivably develop idiopathic aplastic anemia after exposure to unrecognized chemical toxins. Mapping the chromosomal pattern of marrow cells has been hampered by the scarcity of cells available for study, and most chromosomal studies have been carried out on fibroblasts and transformed lymphocytes. These cells display an unusually high incidence of chromosomal gaps and breaks, chromatid exchanges, and endoduplication [243–245]. The significance of such changes has been disputed, since they are also observed in many unrelated conditions, and in some cases they could have been induced by therapy [246]. Furthermore, they have been found primarily in lymphocytes which apparently are not involved in the basic marrow disorder. Nevertheless, it is tempting to speculate that inherited or induced chromosomal abnormalities may result in the emergence of cell lines with low fertility. The high incidence of leukemia found in patients with Fanconi's anemia [242,245,247] also suggests a correlation between the disease process and the observed chromosomal changes. Cultures of stem cells from marrow and blood have consistently revealed a scarcity of hemopoietic progenitors [248] similar to the findings in acquired aplastic anemia.

Clinical features

The onset of aplastic anemia is often insidious, and the patient is usually first brought to the physician's attention when the disease has progressed so far that one of the late consequences of pancytopenia has become manifest: weakness and fatigue because of anemia, fever or infections because of neutropenia, and bruises or nosebleeding because of thrombocytopenia. Because of the nonspecific nature of many of these symptoms and signs, they are frequently treated symptomatically until purpura, with its more serious connotations, forces a thorough hematologic evaluation. Physical examination may be quite unremarkable, revealing only slight pallor and a few petechiae in areas exposed to continuous or intermittent high venous pressure, such as ankles or supraclavicular regions. When purpuric spots are present, they can be observed anywhere and are usually related to trauma. Hemorrhages with or without central pallor are regularly found in the retinas, and these, along with traces of blood in the gum margins, are important signs. The general pallor has frequently gone unnoticed by the patient and his family unless there has been an abrupt change in hemoglobin concentration due to nasal or gastrointestinal blood loss. Overt inflammatory lesions in the mouth or around the rectum are later manifestations.

In the early phase of the disease a palpable spleen is very unusual and should always lead to a questioning of the diagnosis of aplastic anemia. However, splenomegaly does not rule out this disorder, and actually an enlarged spleen is found in some cases in the final stages of the disease or on postmortem examination. In one series, 3 of 39 patients with aplastic anemia developed splenomegaly [249], whereas in another series, splenomegaly was present in 17 of 50 patients [250]. Most of these patients had been followed and treated for a prolonged period of time before they died from infections or other complications, and the splenomegaly may in part have been caused by transfusion hemosiderosis or by reactive hyperplasia. It is most unusual, too, to find hepatomegaly or general enlargement of lymph nodes at the time of diagnosis.

Laboratory features

According to our diagnostic criteria, pancytopenia is an invariable finding in aplastic anemia. The degree of severity may vary, and the total white blood cell count may be less abnormal than the absolute number of granulocytes, but it is still a good rule to question the diagnosis unless red cell count, white cell count, and platelet count are all below normal values.

In aplastic anemia the red cells are usually normochromic and macrocytic, displaying slight changes in size and shape [216]. The reticulocyte percentage ranges from 0 to as high as 5 percent, but the absolute number of reticulocytes is usually subnormal. It has been pointed out that many of the reticulocytes are large and immature, possibly reflecting an increased concentration of erythropoietin, a short bone marrow transit time [251], and the production of stress erythrocytes [14]. The presence of nucleated red cells in the blood film is an unusual finding and suggests marrow dysfunction rather than marrow hypoplasia.

Absolute granulocytopenia is always present and is responsible for the leukopenic part of pancytopenia. The magnitude of absolute granulocytopenia is of considerable importance for the immediate prognosis. As a rough guide, an absolute granulocyte count of less than 200 per microliter suggests imminent danger of infectious complications. An assessment of granulocyte reserve might be more meaningful, but the present quantitation of this reserve by marrow examination or by the granulocytic response to endotoxin, glucocorticoids, or etiocholanolone [252] is still less dependable than the peripheral granulocyte count (Chap. 85). Monocytopenia is usually present [253], but lymphocyte pro-

duction is not considered to be impaired. The absolute lymphocyte count, however, is often decreased and is, of course, always decreased when the total white cell count is less than about 1500 cells per microliter (the lower limit of the normal absolute lymphocyte count). The kinetic and functional significance of this decrease is not known, since both immunoglobulin production and delayed hypersensitivity are usually unimpaired [254].

It is rare that a diagnosis of aplastic anemia is made without the presence of thrombocytopenia. Because of the insidious onset of aplastic anemia, it is not certain which of the marrow elements is affected first. However, during spontaneous or induced recovery, thrombopoiesis appears to be the last function to be restored to normal, and many patients continue to have decreased platelet counts for years after other abnormalities have disappeared.

Tests of hemostasis are generally normal except for those such as bleeding time, capillary fragility, or clot retraction, which reflect the low platelet count. Serum iron concentration is increased with an almost complete saturation of iron-binding capacity. This increase may be the first sign of erythroid suppression and is of considerable screening value in patients receiving potentially toxic drugs such as chloramphenicol [40]. Other ferrokinetic studies reveal a prolonged clearance time of injected iron and a subnormal incorporation of iron into circulating red cells [255] (Fig. 20-3). Such data indicate an overall reduction in erythroid iron-consuming activity and constitute one of the diagnostic criteria for aplastic anemia. Pancytopenia with hyperplastic marrow is associated with a rapid disappearance of iron into the marrow, but with an ineffective utilization of iron and a low iron incorporation into circulating red cells [256] (see Chap. A19).

The plasma iron turnover rate, as calculated from the concentration of serum iron, plasma volume, and iron clearance time and expressed in milligrams of iron per deciliter of blood per 24 h, is rarely much lower than the normal values of 0.6 to 0.8 mg/dl of blood per 24 h. The reason for the maintenance of a normal plasma turnover despite an aplastic marrow appears to be an increased incorporation of iron into other tissues owing to high serum iron concentrations. This incorporation, which normally constitutes only 0.1 to 0.2 mg/dl of blood per 24 h is corrected for in the "erythron turnover," rendering this value a better measure of erythroid hypoplasia than plasma turnover [257]. External organ scanning (Fig. 20-3) indicates that most of the extramedullary incorporation is contributed by the liver. In general, it should be emphasized that erythrokinetic tests having low base-line values such as plasma iron turnover or reticulocyte count are poorly designed for the measurement of subnormal marrow activities and should be used primarily for the measurement of increased rates of red cell production. Decreased red cell production is better gauged by the disappearance rate of iron as

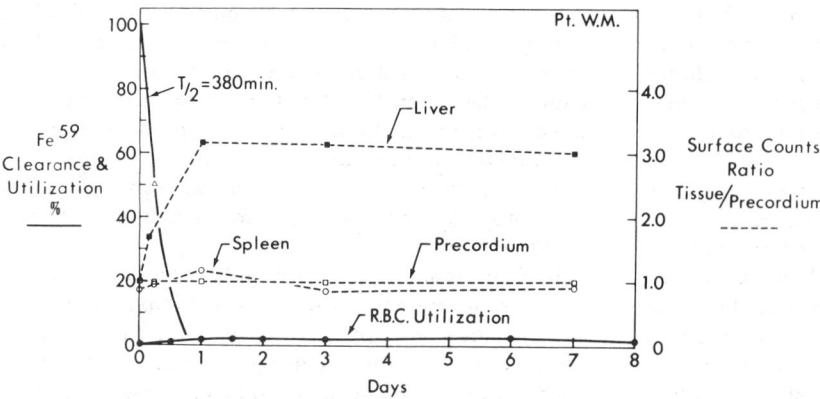

FIGURE 20-3 Ferrokinetics in a patient with severe aplastic anemia. The $T_{1/2}$ of clearance of injected radioactive iron is markedly prolonged, while the utilization of the iron for red blood cell formation is nearly absent. Most of the radioactive iron is found in the liver.

expressed by the half-life of injected radioactive iron (^{59}Fe) or by red cell iron utilization (Fig. 20-4).

The life-span of red cells in patients with aplastic anemia is difficult to assess because of transfusions, hemorrhages, and infections. In the early phases of the illness, measurements of the life-span of radioactive chromium (^{51}Cr)-labeled red cells, the haptoglobin levels, or the fecal urobilinogen excretion are usually normal [250]. Later on there may be evidence of premature red cell destruction [216], but it is not clear whether this is a result of intrinsic abnormalities of the red cells or of extrinsic complications.

Erythropoietin titers in plasma and the 24-h urinary excretion rates of erythropoietin usually exceed those found in most other types of anemia at the same hemoglobin concentration [258–260]. This curious finding has suggested that active marrow consumes erythropoietin and that the high levels in aplastic anemia reflect decreased consumption [261]. However, a more likely explanation is that the oxygen affinity of erythrocytes from patients with aplastic anemia is higher than that from patients with hemolytic anemia. Measurements of the 2,3-diphosphoglycerate (2,3-DPG) content of the relatively old erythrocytes in aplastic anemia have disclosed a much lower content than in the young erythrocytes in hemolytic anemia [262]. Consequently, the oxygen affinity must be higher in aplastic anemia, resulting in a more pronounced tissue hypoxia and erythropoietin release at a given hemoglobin concentration. Because of the high daily excretion of erythropoietin, urine from patients with aplastic anemia has been used profitably for the preparation of erythropoietin concentrates.

Of interest, but still inadequately explained, is the finding of an increase in fetal hemoglobin [18]. In adults, substantial increases are rare, but in children the concentration of fetal hemoglobin has been reported to be as high as 1.5 g/dl. It has been stated that a high level of fetal hemoglobin suggests a good prognosis [263], but more recent studies [264] do not support such a relationship.

Aspiration from marrow cavities can frequently be performed without the characteristic suction pain, and it yields thin bloody material with a few spicules. Smears made from these spicules reveal fatty material with diffuse, sparse accumulation of mononuclear lymphocytoid cells, phagocytizing reticulum cells, conspicuous mast cells, and plasma cells. There are a few myeloid cells, principally of the myelocytic and promyelocytic variety, and an often almost complete absence of megakaryoctes. Nucleated red cells are also decreased in number, but may be the most numerous cell type. In some instances, the immature erythroid cells appear abnormal, with megaloblastic features and incomplete terminal divisions [12].

Iron stain will disclose many siderotic granules inside or outside the macrophages, but only rarely is cytoplasmic iron found in the few remaining nucleated red cells [265].

In order to assess the total morphologic and functional capacity of the marrow, aspirations from several different sites should be performed. Although carefully prepared smears from marrow spicules may provide as good a sampling as marrow cores obtained with a Jamshidi needle, a marrow biopsy specimen is usually required for a definite diagnosis of aplastic anemia [266]. This is a requirement made necessary because a hypocellular "dry tap" caused by marrow replacement by lymphatic tissue or cancer metastases may be misinterpreted as suggesting hypoplastic marrow. It must be recognized that any spot sampling of an organ as large as the marrow may be misleading, and that the posterior iliac bone cavity may contain excessive amounts of fat. Nevertheless, several fatty, cell-poor marrow specimens constitute strong evidence for a general marrow hypoplasia.

Quite frequently, small foci of hypercellular marrow may be encountered. When they are lymphoid, they are compatible with a diagnosis of aplastic anemia, but if they are made up by erythroid or myeloid cells, they can be diagnostically confusing and suggest refractory erythroblastic anemia, Di Guglielmo syndrome, or aleu-

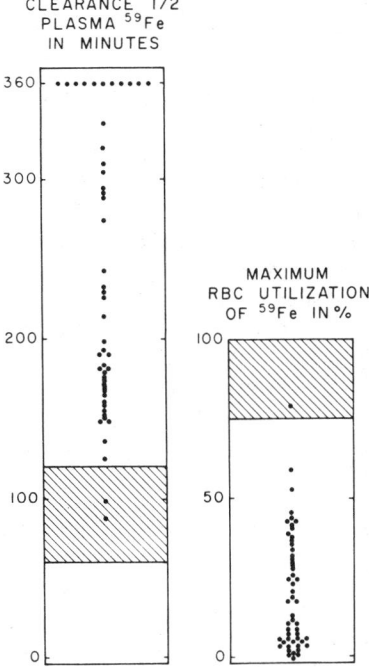

CLEARANCE T/2
PLASMA ^{59}Fe
IN MINUTES

MAXIMUM
RBC UTILIZATION
OF ^{59}Fe IN %

FIGURE 20-4 **Plasma clearance and red blood cell utilization of ^{59}Fe in 50 patients with aplastic or hypoplastic anemia.**

kemia leukemia. However, iron-turnover measurements and further marrow sampling should clarify the picture. The finding of such foci is of uncertain prognostic importance, since they may reflect the last surviving elements of an injured marrow or they may herald recuperation and marrow renewal [13]. Attempts to quantitate total hemopoietic marrow mass by body scanning with radioactive technetium sulfur colloid, which is picked up by phagocytic cells, or indium chloride [267], which binds to transferrin, have in some cases led to useful information as to the extent of aplasia (Chap. 4).

Differential diagnosis

Pancytopenia is a feature common to many diseases, and below are listed the disorders which should be considered in the diagnostic evaluation of patients with pancytopenia:

1. Aplastic anemia
2. Marrow replacement
    a. Myelofibrosis, myelosclerosis
    b. Osteopetrosis
    c. Metastatic carcinoma
    d. Acute leukemia
    e. Multiple myeloma
    f. Hodgkin's disease, lymphoma
    g. Gaucher's disease, Niemann-Pick disease, Letterer-Siwe disease
    h. Refractory erythroblastic anemia
    i. Di Guglielmo syndrome
3. Hypersplenism
    a. Congestive splenomegaly
    b. Hodgkin's disease, lymphoma, leukemia
    c. Gaucher's disease, Niemann-Pick disease, Letterer-Siwe disease
    d. Kala azar, sarcoidosis
    e. Primary splenic pancytopenia
4. Infection
    a. Miliary tuberculosis
    b. Disseminated fungus disease
    c. Fulminating septicemia
    d. Malaria
5. Deficiency disease
    a. Vitamin B_{12} and folic acid deficiency
    b. Pyridoxine deficiency
6. Consumptive coagulopathy
7. Paroxysmal nocturnal hemoglobinuria

In order to establish a diagnosis of aplastic anemia, the marrow has to be not only functionally, but also structurally hypoplastic, and the diagnosis rests on marrow aspirations or biopsies yielding fatty, hypocellular material.

Therapy

The major aims in the conservative management of a patient with aplastic anemia are to remove the patient from suspected causative agents and to "buy time," i.e., to keep the patient active and comfortable until he or she may experience a spontaneous remission. Attempts to induce a remission through the use of myelostimulatory drugs, such as steroids and androgens, have been moderately successful in children but generally discouraging in adults. Marrow replacement by means of transplantation is gaining in reputation and in severe cases may be the treatment of choice [5].

SUPPORTIVE THERAPY
As far as possible, the patient should be permitted to participate in normal work, play, or school activities. Restrictions or safeguards are best managed by the patient and his family after they have received frank and realistic information about the danger of the disease and the aims of therapy. The incidence of skin infections may be reduced by the use of antiseptic soaps, and the risks of hemorrhage decreased by the use of electric razors, soft toothbrushes, and stool softeners and by avoidance of intramuscular injections. Menstrual bleeding does not often cause problems unless the platelet count is severely depressed. Suppressive hormonal therapy with an anovulatory agent such as norethynodrel is an effective means of regulating or abolishing excessive menstrual flow, but it must be remembered that "breakthrough" bleeding will occur in patients maintained continuously on these drugs.

REPLACEMENT THERAPY

The use of blood and blood components is described in Chaps. 164 to 166 and will be merely outlined here. Transfusion with packed red cells is indicated when hemoglobin concentration approaches symptom-causing levels. An ambulatory, afebrile patient with a hemoglobin concentration of 8 g/dl is usually asymptomatic, and such a patient may tolerate 6 to 7 g/dl without any subjective discomfort. These levels can often be maintained without supplementary transfusions even by a severely impaired marrow. The need for blood occurs primarily when bleeding, fever, or inflammation causes a premature loss or destruction of red cells.

Multiple transfusions and the possible increase in iron absorption caused by anemic hypoxia may cause hemochromatosis with hepatic and pancreatic fibrosis and splenomegaly. Attempts to reduce this iron load by the administration of deferoxamine [268] or other chelating agents are rarely carried out, presumably because hemochromatosis is considered one of the minor problems among the host of life-threatening complications of aplastic anemia.

Platelet transfusion has been an increasingly important tool in the prevention and treatment of hemorrhages in patients with aplastic anemia. Platelets properly prepared at room temperature and administered within 10 h from the time of harvesting have a nearly normal life-span and, with carefully spaced transfusions, can maintain the platelet count at fairly safe levels (>20,000 per microliter) for considerable lengths of time. In the absence of adequate means for platelet typing, it can be anticipated that the beneficial effect of platelet transfusion will gradually diminish by the emergence of antibodies (Fig. 20-5) [269,270]. The effectiveness of platelet transfusions is also curtailed by fever and infections, and in the final phase of severe aplastic anemia, it may be almost impossible to elicit a platelet rise even after massive platelet transfusion. Nevertheless, when used sparingly and judiciously, and especially if HLA-compatible donors are available, platelet transfusions can check acute thrombocytopenic bleeding and prevent hemorrhagic complications for months and even for years.

Transfusion of granulocytes obtained by continuous-flow centrifugation [271] or filtration leukopheresis [272] of blood from family members or HLA-compatible donors is being used more and more. Except during preparations for marrow transplantation [273], prophylactic granulocyte transfusions in patients with aplastic anemia do not appear to be justified [274]. However, as part of the therapy for septicemias, especially gram-negative, a short course of granulocyte transfusions is appropriate if the WBC is low. The use of patients with chronic granulocytic leukemia as donors, despite their high number of potentially phagocytic granulocytes, is probably no longer defensible [275].

ANTIBIOTIC THERAPY

Infections in patients with aplastic anemia call for early and intense antibiotic therapy. As soon as fever or local signs suggest infection, cultures should be obtained of blood, throat, urine, and all suspected inflammatory lesions, and the patient should be started on bactericidal, broad-spectrum antibiotics. An aminoglycoside with a cephalosporin or penicillin are good initial drugs [276] unless bacteriologic smears or the character of the infection indicates the use of other antibiotics. When reports from the cultures and sensitivity studies are available, the therapy obviously will have to be changed appropriately. Unfortunately, informative results are not always forthcoming from the bacteriology laboratory, and the possibility of infections in unusual areas such as the meninges or by unusual organisms such as saprophytic bacteria or fungi have to be considered. As in patients treated with immunosuppressive drugs [277], infections induced by *Listeria, Nocardia, Histoplasma, Aspergillus*, and *Candida* have become of increasing importance, since they are virtually unopposed in the granulocytopenic and frequently steroid-treated patient. The use of preventive antibiotic therapy is usu-

FIGURE 20-5 Progressive decrease in effectiveness of platelet transfusions in a patient with aplastic anemia. (Faltwo and Freireich [269].)

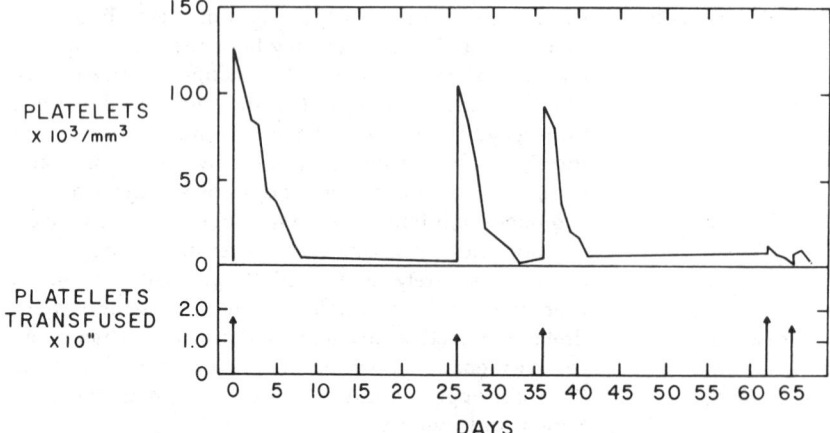

ally scorned by experts, although it must be conceded that adequate data for the evaluation of its beneficial or detrimental effects on patients with severe aplastic anemia are not available. Several investigators have recommended the use of preventive nonabsorbable antibiotics for severe agranulocytosis [226,227], but their extraordinary cost and frequent gastrointestinal side effects make them less than ideal. The use of oral trimethoprim/sulfamethoxazole is better tolerated and may reduce the incidence not only of enterobacterial infections but also of *Pneumocystis carinii* pneumonitis [278]. Despite intensive diagnostic and therapeutic efforts, not all fevers can be traced to infections, and some may respond dramatically to steroids. Such fevers may be caused by necrotic tissue or hematomas, but it seems prudent always to react to a fever as though it were caused by an external, treatable agent.

REVERSE OR COMPLETE ISOLATION

Although many, if not most, infectious complications originate on the skin or in the gastrointestinal tract, it is advisable to attempt to reduce environmental possibilities for transmission of pathogens. When the absolute granulocyte count is above 500 per microliter, only general instruction of the patient and family of the danger of infections appears to be necessary. In case of granulocyte counts below 200 per microliter, reverse isolation is in order. However, this reverse isolation should be kept at a reasonable level and should consist mainly of a reduction of exposure to crowds or visitors, thorough hand washing with an antiseptic soap before all personal contacts, and the use of face masks. The strict use of gowns and gloves in the hospital may be of benefit, but it undoubtedly reduces the effectiveness of day-to-day nursing care. This is even more true of the use of large protective devices such as the "life islands." In one study of patients with severe granulocytopenia, the combined use of preventive nonabsorbable antibiotics and a strict isolator system reduced the incidence of infections to about 30 percent of what might have been expected [279]. However, the logistics and expense of maintaining patients in life islands are almost forbidding [280]. It is possible that a system of laminar airflow away from the patient may provide needed protection with less interference with nursing care [281].

IMMUNOSUPPRESSION

The in vitro evidence for an autoimmune pathogenesis in at least some patients with aplastic anemia has stimulated interest in immunosuppression as treatment. In the past, the use of glucocorticoids in the supportive management of patients with aplastic anemia has been both recommended [282,283] and condemned [5,264,284]. Since sustained and transient remissions may occur after treatment with adrenal steroids, a therapeutic trial for 2 to 4 weeks can be justified [285]. However, if there is no effect on cellular production, therapy beyond that point should be restricted to amelioration of specific complications. In addition to immuno-

suppression, steroids appear to lessen vascular fragility and thrombocytopenic hemorrhage, reduce idiopathic fevers that are unresponsive to antibiotic therapy, and decrease febrile toxicity. Steroids may also reduce shortening of cellular life-span, one of the late but serious consequences of multiple transfusions and intermittent inflammatory episodes. These borderline beneficial effects should be balanced against the many potentially dangerous side effects of prolonged steroid therapy. If more than 20 mg per day of prednisone or prednisone equivalents is needed, a sober appraisal of the indications for steroid therapy should be made, since the increased potential for gastrointestinal hemorrhage and unchecked disseminated infections is of particular concern in patients with aplastic anemia.

The use of cyclophosphamide [286], 6-mercaptopurine (6-MP) [235], or antilymphocyte globulin [287–289] has been reported to result in complete remission in some cases. However, immunosuppression is usually associated with stem cell suppression, and the decision to use such drugs in patients with limited or absent marrow reserve should be taken most reluctantly.

SPLENECTOMY

Splenectomy as a means to improve marrow function has been recommended [290–292]. Impressive case reports have been listed, but it is generally conceded that splenectomy in the majority of patients with aplastic anemia has not been followed by a hemopoietic remission. At the present time there is no known theoretical reason why splenectomy should improve marrow function. Nevertheless, splenectomy can increase the effective life-span of the available circulating blood cells, particularly in patients in whom transfusion hemosiderosis or recurrent inflammatory complications have caused splenomegaly and hypersequestration. In such patients, splenectomy may be followed by a significant decrease in transfusion requirements and in an increase in the number of circulating platelets and granulocytes [269]. With the availability of platelet transfusion, the surgical risk has decreased considerably, and splenectomy should always be considered as a potentially valuable measure when pancytopenia becomes unmanageable [282].

MYELOSTIMULATORY THERAPY

Many compounds and procedures have been claimed to have myelostimulatory properties, and there are spectacular case reports to back up such claims. The long list of therapeutic remedies includes yellow marrow extract, iron, vitamin B_{12}, splenectomy, cobalt, irradiation, normal plasma, phytohemagglutinins, and more recently, bolus of methylprednisolone [293], ceruloplasmin [294], etiocholanolone [295], and lithium [296]. A critical appraisal of the effectiveness of these agents in aplastic anemia leads to the conclusion that in many cases the disease treated was pancytopenia rather than true aplastic anemia and, as a group, pancytopenia includes many potentially treatable diseases as well as diseases with a high incidence of spontaneous remission. However, there are impressive data relating to remissions induced by androgens [283,297–299]. In 1953, Kennedy and Gilbertson [300] showed that pharmacologic doses of testosterone would induce erythrocytosis in women with breast cancer, and subsequent studies [301] have established androgens as therapeutically useful stimulants of erythropoiesis in patients with myelofibrosis and refractory anemia. The mode of action is still controversial, but it appears to involve increased release of erythropoietin [302] and increased marrow responsiveness to erythropoietin [303]. Such mechanisms may explain the erythropoietic effect of androgens in some types of anemia, but the usefulness of androgens in aplastic anemia would have to demand the presence of a stimulating effect directly on the marrow stem cells. Some studies indicate that the 5β configuration of androgenic steroids has such an effect while the 5α configuration is responsible for increased erythropoietin production or release [299]. Despite many prospective and retrospective studies, no agreement as to the therapeutic effectiveness of androgens in aplastic anemia has been reached. It is accepted by all that impressive remissions, especially in less severe cases, may occur, but the rating of overall effectiveness ranges from very poor [304] to quite good [305,306].

In view of the occasional good response to androgens (Fig. 20-6), a therapeutic trial of a synthetic oral testosterone preparation such as oxymetholone (3 to 5 mg/kg per day) is probably indicated. Nandrolone decanoate, 3 to 5 mg/kg given intramuscularly once a week, has also been shown to be effective, but the intramuscular injections can cause problems in a thrombocytopenic patient. A definitive response may appear only slowly, and when first started, androgen treatment should be continued for at least 4 months. If not effective then, it should be discontinued in order not to add acne, fluid retention, hirsutism, and cholestatic jaundice to an already miserable disease. Because of often irreversible growth retardation and vocal cord changes, androgens should only be given to children with great reluctance.

MARROW REPLACEMENT

Transplantation of normal multipotential marrow stem cells to a patient with aplastic anemia has a great deal of appeal (see Chap. 168). The feasibility of this procedure was first established in patients with healthy identical twins. Transplantation of normal twin marrow resulted in immediate takes and cures and showed that aplastic anemia, at least in these cases, is caused by a failure of stem cells rather than a failure of the marrow microenvironment. A subsequent report [25] on transplantation between identical twins indicates that in some cases an element of autoimmunity exists and has to be overcome by immunosuppression. Immunosuppression is necessary in all other cases, even between perfectly matched siblings. However, the results, especially in the pediatric age group, have been remarkable, with a gradual improvement in technique and survival [308–311]. Of 73

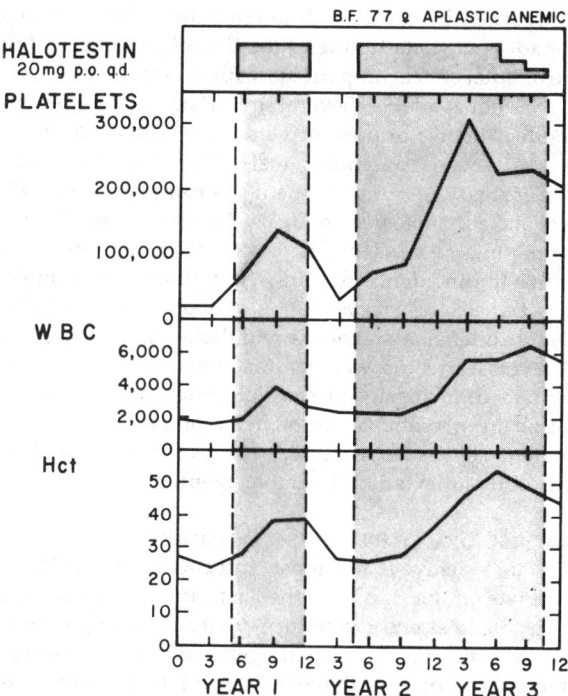

FIGURE 20-6 Blood cell response to the administration of fluoxymesterone (Halotestin) in a patient with severe aplastic anemia.

patients with severe aplastic anemia transplanted with marrow from HLA-identical siblings, 95 percent demonstrated engraftment and 40 percent were alive with complete hematologic restoration [310]. Similar results on 159 transplanted cases have been reported from Europe [311]. When untransfused and therefore unsensitized patients 30 years or younger were analyzed separately, 80 percent were found to be alive with functioning grafts [312]. These remarkable results, however, were not achieved easily. The recipients had to be conditioned for acceptance of the marrow graft by receiving cyclophosphamide or total-body irradiation 24 h after an infusion of buffy coat cells or platelet-rich plasma from the donor. This conditioning presumably will eliminate clones of cells capable of reacting against the graft. The infusion of marrow cells was followed by prolonged immunosuppressive therapy with methotrexate or antilymphocyte serum in order to prevent a graft-versus-host reaction.

Many clinicians feel that marrow transplantation has become the treatment of choice for the young patient with an HLA-compatible sibling. Nevertheless, the overall mortality from immunosuppression and graft-versus-host diseases in the adult is such that others feel that only patients with a particularly poor prognosis, i.e., total marrow aplasia or posthepatitic marrow failure, should be considered for transplantation. Unfortunately, the decision to recommend a marrow transplantation has to be made early, lest blood and platelet transfusions cause irreversible sensitization of the patient. At present, marrow transplantation must be considered a challenging and hopeful procedure, but not a procedure to be undertaken lightly.

Course and prognosis

Aplastic anemia may be a brief, overwhelming disease, with death occurring within a few months, or a protracted, smoldering disease lasting many years. The overall mortality in adults with aplastic anemia has been reported to be about 65 to 75 percent, and the median survival about 3 months [282,313,314].

There are only few prognostic leads when the patient is first seen. Clinically it appears that patients who develop aplastic anemia in conjunction with the exposure to a marrow toxin do better than patients with idiopathic aplastic anemia or aplastic anemia which first becomes manifest some time after exposure to the suspected toxic agent. In general, the more severe the pancytopenia and marrow aplasia, the worse the prognosis, but attempts have been made to refine predictions by the construction of prognostic indices [315–317]. When steady progression of the disease process has been established, or when the marrow aplasia follows an attack of infectious hepatitis, the mortality in adults is exceedingly high. Of patients experiencing a remission, it has been observed [282] that one-third were cured, one-third continued to have a low but tolerable platelet count, and one-third developed therapeutic dependence on steroids or androgens.

The prognosis in children with acquired aplastic anemia is slightly better than that in adults, with 50 percent of children surviving, whether treated with supportive care alone [318] or with myelostimulatory agents [264,319]. Constitutional aplastic anemia is reportedly uniformly fatal unless responsive to continuous testosterone therapy.

References

1. Ehrlich, P.: Uber einen Fall von Anamie mit Bemerkungen über regenerative Veranderungen des Knochenmarks. *Charite Ann.* 13:300, 1888.
2. Chauffard, M.: Un Cas d'anémie pernicieuse aplastique. *Bull. Soc. Med. Hop. Paris* 21:313, 1904.
3. Bomford, R. R., and Rhoads, C. P.: Refractory anemia. *Q. J. Med.* 10:175, 1941.
4. Williams, D. M., Lynch, R. E., and Cartwright, G. E.: Drug-induced aplastic anemia. *Semin. Hematol.* 10:195, 1973.
5. *Proceedings of the Conference on Aplastic Anemia: A Stem Cell Disease,* edited by A. S. Levine. N.I.H. publication no. 81-1008, Washington, 1981.
6. Boggs, D. R., and Boggs, S. S.: The pathogenesis of aplastic anemia: A defective pluripotent hematopoietic stem cell with inappropriate balance of differentiation and self-replication. *Blood* 48:71, 1976.
7. Appelbaum, F. R., and Fefer, A.: The pathogenesis of aplastic anemia. *Semin. Hematol.* 18:241, 1981.
8. Gale, R. P., et al.: Aplastic anemia: Biology and treatment. *Ann. Intern. Med.* 95:477, 1981.
9. Sharkis, S. J., et al.: Antitheta-sensitive regulatory cell (TSRC) and hematopoiesis: Regulation and differentiation of transplanted stem cells in W/W anemic and normal mice. *Blood* 52:802, 1978.
10. Harrison, D. E.: Normal function of transplanted marrow cell lines from aged mice. *J. Gerontol.* 30:279, 1975.
11. Hellman, S., Botnick, L. E., Hannon, E. C., and Vigneulle, R. M.: Proliferative capacity of murine hematopoietic stem cells. *Proc. Natl. Acad. Sci. U.S.A.* 75:490, 1978.
12. Lohrmann, H.-P.: Tolerance of hemopoiesis for repeated cytotoxic drug therapy. *Blut* 39:237, 1979.
13. Morley, A., and Blake, J.: An animal model of chronic aplastic marrow failure. I. Late marrow failure after busulfan. *Blood* 44:49, 1974.
14. Trainor, K. J., Morley, A. A., and Seshadri, R. S.: A proliferative defect of marrow cells in experimental chronic hypoplastic marrow failure (aplastic anemia). *Exp. Hematol.* 8:674, 1980.
15. Frisch, B., Lewis, S. M., and Sherman, D.: The ultrastructure of dyserythropoiesis in aplastic anemia. *Br. J. Haematol.* 29:545, 1975.
16. Kansu, E., and Erslev, A. J.: Aplastic anemia with "hot pockets." *Scand. J. Haematol.* 17:326, 1976.
17. Alter, B. P.: Fetal erythropoiesis in stress hematopoiesis. *Exp. Hematol.* 7:200, 1979.
18. Shahidi, N. T., Gerald, P. S., and Diamond, L. K.: Alkali-resistant hemoglobin in aplastic anemia of both acquired and congenital types. *N. Engl. J. Med.* 266:177, 1962.
19. Swift, M.: Fanconi's anaemia: Cellular abnormalities and clinical predisposition to malignant diseases, in *Congenital Disorders of Erythropoiesis, Ciba Foundation Symposium 37.* Elsevier, Amsterdam, 1976, p. 115.
20. Branda, R. F., Moldow, C. F., MacArthur, J. R., Wintrobe, M. M., Anthony, B. K., and Jacob, H. S.: Folate-induced remission in aplastic anemia with familial defect of cellular folate uptake. *N. Engl. J. Med.* 298:469, 1978.
21. Morley, A., Trainor, K., and Remes, J.: Residual marrow damage: Possible explanation for idiosyncrasy to chloramphenicol. *Br. J. Haematol.* 32:525, 1976.
22. Hoffman, R., Zanjani, E. D., Lutton, J. D., Zalusky, R., and Wasserman, L. R.: Suppression of erythroid-colony formation by lymphocytes from patients with aplastic anemia. *N. Engl. J. Med.* 296:10, 1977.
23. Kagan, W. A., Ascensao, J. L., Fialk, M. A., Coleman, M., Valera, E. B., and Good, R. A.: Studies on the pathogenesis of aplastic anemia. *Am. J. Med.* 66:444, 1979.
24. Singer, J. W., et al.: Effect of peripheral blood lymphocytes from patients with aplastic anemia on granulocytic colony growth from HLA-matched and -mismatched marrows: Effect of transfusion sensitization. *Blood* 52:37, 1978.
25. Sullivan, R., et al.: Aplastic anemia: Lack of inhibitory effect of bone marrow lymphocytes on in vitro granulopoiesis. *Blood* 56:625, 1980.
26. Nissen, C., Cornu, P., Gratwohl, A., and Speck, B.: Peripheral blood cells from patients with aplastic anaemia in partial remission suppress growth of their own bone marrow precursors in culture. *Br. J. Haematol.* 45:233, 1980.
27. Speck, B., et al.: Immunologic aspects of aplasia. *Transplant. Proc.* 10:131, 1978.
28. Royal Marsden Hospital Bone Marrow Transplantation Team: Failure of syngeneic bone marrow graft without preconditioning in post-hepatitis marrow aplasia. *Lancet* 2:742, 1977.
29. Appelbaum, F. R., Fefer, A., Cheever, M. A., et al.: Treatment of aplastic anemia by bone marrow transplantation in identical twins. *Blood* 55:1033, 1980.
30. Hoffman, R., Dainiak, N., Sibreck, L., Pober, J. S., and Waldron, J. A.: Antibody-mediated aplastic anemia and diffuse fasciitis. *N. Engl. J. Med.* 300:718, 1979.
31. Fitchen, J. J., Cline, M. J., Saxon, A., and Golde, D. W.: Serum inhibitors of hematopoiesis in a patient with aplastic anemia and systemic lupus erythematosus. *Am. J. Med.* 66:537, 1979.
32. Bernstein, S. E., Russell, E. S., and Keighley, G.: Two hereditary mouse anemias (se/se^d and w/w^v) deficient in response to erythropoietin. *Ann. N.Y. Acad. Sci.* 149:475, 1968.
33. Dameshek, W.: Chloramphenicol (Chloromycetin) and the bone marrow. *Blood* 7:755, 1952 (editorial).
34. Best, W.: Chloramphenicol-associated blood dyscrasias. *JAMA* 201:181, 1967.
35. Yunis, A. A.: Chloramphenicol-induced bone marrow suppres-

sion. *Semin. Hematol.* 10:225, 1973.

36. Polak, B. C. P., Wesseling, H., Schut, D., Herxheimer, A., and Meyler, L.: Blood dyscrasias attributed to chloramphenicol: A review of 576 published and unpublished cases. *Acta Med. Scand.* 192:409, 1972.
37. Tabulation of reports compiled by the panel on hematology of the registry on adverse reactions council on drugs. American Medical Association, May 1965 and June 1967.
38. Alter, B. P., Potter, N. V., and Li, F. P.: Classification and aetiology of the aplastic anaemias. *Clin. Haematol.* 7:431, 1978.
39. Smick, K., Condit, P. K., Proctor, R. L., and Sutcher, V.: Fatal aplastic anemia: An epidemiological study of its relationship to the drug chloramphenicol. *J. Chronic Dis.* 17:899, 1964.
40. Modan, B., Segal, S., Shani, M., and Sheba, C.: Aplastic anemia in Israel: Evaluation of the etiologic role of chloramphenicol on a community-wide basis. *Am. J. Med. Sci.* 270:441, 1975.
41. Wallerstein, R. O., Condit, P. K., Kasper, C. K., Brown, J. W., and Morrison, F. R.: Statewide study of chloramphenicol therapy of fatal aplastic anemia. *JAMA* 208:2045, 1969.
42. Erslev, A. J.: Hematopoietic depression induced by chloromycetin. *Blood* 8:170, 1953.
43. Krakoff, J. H., Karnofsky, D. A., and Burchenal, J. H.: Effect of large doses of chloramphenicol on human subjects. *N. Engl. J. Med.* 253:7, 1955.
44. Weisberger, A. S.: Mechanisms of action of chloramphenicol. *JAMA* 209:97, 1969.
45. Rosenbach, L. M., Caviles, A. P., and Mitus, W. J.: Chloramphenicol toxicity: Reversible vacuolization of erythroid cells. *N. Engl. J. Med.* 263:724, 1960.
46. McCurdy, P. R.: Chloramphenicol bone marrow toxicity. *JAMA* 176:588, 1961.
47. Erslev, A. J., and Wintrobe, M. M.: Detection and prevention of drug-induced blood dyscrasias. *JAMA* 181:114, 1962.
48. Waisbren, B. A., Simski, C., and Change, P. L.: Administration of maximum doses of chloramphenicol. *Am. J. Med. Sci.* 245:35, 1963.
49. Lloyd, A. V. C., Grimes, G., Khaw, K. T., and Schwachman, H.: Chloramphenicol for long-term therapy of cystic fibrosis. *JAMA* 184:1001, 1963.
50. Yunis, A. A., and Bloomberg, G. R.: Chloramphenicol toxicity: Clinical features and pathogenesis. *Prog. Hematol.* 4:138, 1964.
51. Kracke, R. R., and Parker, F. P.: The etiology of granulopenia (agranulocytosis) with particular reference to the drugs containing the benzene ring. *J. Lab. Clin. Med.* 19:799, 1934.
52. Jardetzky, O.: Studies on the mechanism of action of chloramphenicol. I. The conformation of chloramphenicol in solution. *J. Biol. Chem.* 238:2498, 1963.
53. Brock, T. D.: Chloramphenicol. *Bacteriol. Rev.* 25:32, 1961.
54. Yunis, A. A., Smith, U. S., and Restrepo, A.: Reversible bone marrow suppression from chloramphenicol: A consequence of mitochondrial injury. *Arch. Intern. Med.* 126:272, 1970.
55. Firkin, F. C.: Mitochondrial lesions in reversible erythropoietin depression due to chloramphenicol. *J. Clin. Invest.* 51:2085, 1972.
56. Manyan, D. R., Arimura, G. K., and Yunis, A. A.: Chloramphenicol-induced erythroid suppression and bone marrow ferrochelatase activity in dogs. *J. Lab. Clin. Med.* 79:137, 1972.
57. Yunis, A. A., and Harrington, W. J.: Patterns of inhibition by chloramphenicol of nucleic acid synthesis in human bone marrow and leukemia cells. *J. Lab. Clin. Med.* 56:831, 1960.
58. Erslev, A. J., and Iossifides, J. A.: In vitro action of chloramphenicol and chloramphenicol analogues on the metabolism of human immature red blood cells. *Acta Haematol. (Basel)* 28:1, 1962.
59. Ward, H. P.: The effect of chloramphenicol on RNA and heme synthesis in bone marrow cultures. *J. Lab. Clin. Med.* 68:400, 1966.
60. Ratzan, R. J., Moore, M. A. S., and Yunis, A. A.: Effect of chloramphenicol and thiamphenicol on the in vitro colony-forming cell. *Blood* 43:363, 1974.
61. Mitus, W. J., and Coleman, N.: In vitro effect of chloramphenicol on chromosomes. *Blood* 35:689, 1970.
62. Dameshek, W.: Riddle: What do aplastic anemia, paroxysmal nocturnal hemoglobinuria (PNH) and "hypoplastic" leukemia have in common? *Blood* 30:251, 1967 (editorial).
63. Mukerji, P. S.: Acute myeloblastic leukemia following chloramphenicol treatment. *Br. Med. J.* 1:1286, 1957.
64. Cohen, T., and Creger, W. P.: Acute myeloid leukemia following seven years of aplastic anemia induced by chloramphenicol. *Am. J. Med.* 43:762, 1967.
65. Brouer, M. J., and Dameshek, W.: Hypoplastic anemia and myeloblastic leukemia following chloramphenicol therapy. *N. Engl. J. Med.* 277:1003, 1967.
66. Quagliana, J. M., Cartwright, G. E., and Wintrobe, M. M.: Paroxysmal nocturnal hemoglobinuria following drug-induced aplastic anemia. *Ann. Intern. Med.* 61:1045, 1964.
67. Nagao, I., and Mauer, A. M.: Concordance for drug-induced aplastic anemia in identical twins. *N. Engl. J. Med.* 281:7, 1969.
68. Howell, A., Andrews, T. M., and Watts, R. W.: Bone marrow cells resistant to chloramphenicol in chloramphenicol-induced aplastic anemia. *Lancet* 1:65, 1975.
69. Kunin, C. M., Glazko, A. J., and Finland, M.: Persistence of antibiotics in blood of patients with acute renal failure. II. Chloramphenicol and its metabolic products in the blood of patients with severe renal disease or hepatic cirrhosis. *J. Clin. Invest.* 38:1498, 1959.
70. Yunis, A. A., Miller, A. M., Salem, Z., Corbett, M. D., and Arimura, G. K.: Nitroso-chloramphenicol: Possible mediator in chloramphenicol-induced aplastic anemia. *J. Lab. Clin. Med.* 96:36, 1980.
71. Hamburger, R. N.: Passive immune kill and pseudoautoimmune disease: A proposed model for chloramphenicol-induced aplastic anemia. *Int. Med. Digest* 3:21, 1968.
72. Price Evans, D. A.: Pharmacogenetics. *Am. J. Med.* 34:639, 1963.
73. Bowditch, M., Elkins, H. B., Hunter, F. T., Mallory, T. B., Gall, E. A., and Brickley, W. J.: Chronic exposure to benzene (Benzol). *J. Ind. Hyg. Toxicol.* 21:321, 1939.
74. Elkins, H. B., and Pagnatta, L. D.: Benzene content of petroleum solvents. *Arch. Ind.* 13:51, 1956.
75. Carter, L. J.: Dispute over cancer risk quantification. *Science* 203:1324, 1979.
76. Steinberg, B.: Bone marrow regeneration in experimental benzene intoxication. *Blood* 4:550, 1949.
77. Latta, J. S., and Davies, L. T.: Effects on the blood and hemopoietic organs of the albino rat of repeated administration of benzene. *Arch. Pathol.* 31:55, 1941.
78. Kissling, M., and Speck, B.: Further studies on experimental benzene induced aplastic anemia. *Blut* 25:97, 1972.
79. Uyeki, E. M., Ashkar, A. E., Shoeman, D. W., and Bisel, T. U.: Acute toxicity of benzene inhalation to hemopoietic precursor cells. *Toxicol. Appl. Pharmacol.* 40:49, 1977.
80. Snyder, R., Andrews, L. S., Lee, E. W., Witmer, C. M., Reilly, M., and Kocsis, J. J.: Benzene metabolism and toxicity, in *Biological Reactive Intermediates*, edited by Jallow et al. Plenum, New York, 1977, p. 286.
81. Erf, L. A., and Rhoads, C. P.: The hematological effects of benzene (benzol) poisoning. *J. Ind. Hyg. Toxicol.* 21:421, 1939.
82. DeGowin, R. L.: Benzene exposure and aplastic anemia followed by leukemia fifteen years later. *JAMA* 185:748, 1963.
83. Vigliani, E. C.: Leukemia associated with benzene exposure. *Ann. N.Y. Acad. Sci.* 271:143, 1976.
84. Aksoy, M., Dinçol, K., Erdein, S., and Dinçol, G.: Acute leukemia due to chronic exposure to benzene. *Am. J. Med.* 52:160, 1972.
85. Aksoy, M., Dinçol, K., Akgün, T., Erdein, S., and Dinçol, G.: Haematological effects of chronic benzene poisoning in 217 workers. *Br. J. Ind. Med.* 28:296, 1971.
86. Toughill, P. J., and Wilcox, R. G.: Aplastic anemia and hair dye. *Br. Med. J.* 1:502, 1976.
87. Loge, J. P.: Aplastic anemia following exposure to benzene hexachloride (Lindane). *JAMA* 193:110, 1965.
88. Sanchez-Medal, L., Castanedo, J. P., and Garcia-Rojas, F.: Insecticides and aplastic anemia. *N. Engl. J. Med.* 269:1365, 1963.
89. Roberts, H. J.: Aplastic anemia due to pentochlorophenol. *N. Engl. J. Med.* 305:1650, 1981.
90. Crawford, M. A. D.: Aplastic anemia due to trinitrotoluene intoxication. *Br. Med. J.* 2:430, 1954.
91. Powers, D.: Aplastic anemia secondary to glue sniffing. *N. Engl. J. Med.* 272:700, 1965.
92. Roodman, G. D., Reese, E. P., Jr., and Cardamone, J. M.: Aplastic anemia associated with rubber cement used by a marathon runner. *Arch. Intern. Med.* 140:703, 1980.
93. Wisch, N., Fishman, F. J., Siegel, R., Glass, J. L., and Leopold, J.:

Aplastic anemia resulting from the use of carbonic anhydrase inhibitors. *Am. J. Ophthalmol.* 75:132, 1973.

94. Wijnja, L., Snigder, J. A. M., and Neiweg, H. O.: Acetylsalicylic acid as a cause of pancytopenia from bone-marrow damage. *Lancet* 2:768, 1966.

95. Eldar, M., Aderka, D., Shoenfeld, Y., et al.: Aspirin-induced aplastic anemia. *S. Afr. Med. J.* 9:318, 1979.

96. Brandriss, M. W., Wolff, S. M., Moores, R., and Stohlman, F., Jr.: Anemia induced by amphotericin. *JAMA* 189:663, 1964.

97. Dyer, N. H., Hughes, D. T., and Jenkins, G. C.: Aplastic anaemia after carbamazepine. *Br. Med. J.* 1:108, 1966.

98. Arieff, A. J., and Mier, M.: Three deaths from aplastic anemia due to Tegretol. *Neurology (Minneap.)* 16:107, 1966.

99. Pisciotta, A. V.: Hematologic toxicity of carbamazepine. *Adv. Neurol.* 11:355, 1975.

100. Richardson, J. S., Sarkany, I., and Campbell, C. D.: Fatal case of marrow asplasia after treatment with carbimazole. *Br. Med. J.* 1:364, 1964.

101. Burrell, C. D.: Fatal aplastic anemia after treatment with carbimazole. *Br. Med. J.* 1:1456, 1956.

102. Menon, G. N.: Hypoplastic anemia: An unusual complication of chlordiazepoxide hydrochloride therapy. *Postgrad. Med. J.* 41:282, 1965.

103. Nagaratham, N., Chetiyawardana, A. D., and Rajiyah, S.: Aplasia and leukemia following chloroquine therapy. *Postgrad. Med. J.* 54:108, 1978.

104. Kanoh, T., Jingami, H., and Uchino, H.: Aplastic anemia after prolonged treatment with chlorpheniramine. *Lancet* 1:546, 1977.

105. Spry, C. J.: Chlorpheniramine-induced bone marrow suppression. *Lancet* 1:545, 1976.

106. Mansour, N., and Brown, G. O.: Depression of erythropoiesis associated with chlorpromazine therapy. *Arch. Intern. Med.* 119:113, 1967.

107. McKinney, W. T., Jr.: Pancytopenia due to chlorpromazine. *Am. J. Psychiatry* 123:879, 1967.

108. Recker, R. R., and Hynes, H. E.: Pure red blood cell aplasia associated with chlorpropamide therapy. *Arch. Intern. Med.* 123:445, 1969.

109. Chang, H. K., and Morrison, S. L.: Bone-marrow suppression associated with cimetidine. *Ann. Intern. Med.* 91:580, 1979.

110. Tonkonow, B., and Hoffman, R.: Aplastic anemia and cimetidine. *Arch. Intern. Med.* 140:1123, 1980.

111. Traumann, K. J., Grom, E., and Schwartzkopf, H.: Pancytopenia in diabetes mellitus treatment with colbutamide. *Dtsch. Med. Wochenschr.* 100:250, 1975.

112. Boruchow, I. B.: Bone marrow depression associated with acute colchicine toxicity in the presence of hepatic dysfunction. *Cancer* 19:541, 1966.

113. Malawista, E. E.: Marrow aplasia induced by colchicine. *Arthritis Rheum.* 21:735, 1978.

114. Liu, Y. K., Hymowitz, R., and Carroll, M. G.: Marrow aplasia induced by colchicine. *Arthritis Rheum.* 21:731, 1978.

115. Bismuth, C., Gaultier, M., and Conso, F.: Aplasie médullaire aprés intoxication aigué a la colchicine. *Nouv. Presse med.* 6:1625, 1977.

116. Robins, M. M.: Aplastic anemia secondary to anticonvulsants. *Am. J. Dis. Child.* 104:614, 1962.

117. Sperberg, M.: Diagnostically confusing complications of diphenylhydantoin therapy: A review. *Ann. Intern. Med.* 59:914, 1963.

118. Weinstein, A. J., and Allen, R. J.: Hypoplastic anemia with Zarontin. *Am. J. Dis. Child.* 111:63, 1966.

119. Meyer, R., and Axelrod, J. L.: Fatal aplastic anemia resulting from flucytosine. *JAMA* 228:1573, 1974.

120. Hans, R. J.: Aplastic anemia associated with gamma-benzene hexachloride. *JAMA* 236:1009, 1976.

121. Wohlenberg, H.: Aplastic anemia following gold therapy: Report on a late reaction and review of 32 case reports of world literature. *Med. Welt* 23:971, 1972.

122. Kay, A.: Depression of bone marrow and thrombocytopenia associated with chrysotherapy. *Ann. Rheum. Dis.* 32:277, 1973.

123. Shearer, C. A., and Parker, W. A.: Chrysotherapy-induced aplastic anemia. *Am. J. Hosp. Pharm.* 35:1095, 1978.

124. Gryfe, C. I.: Agranulocytosis and aplastic anemia possibly due to ibuprofen. *Can. Med. Assoc. J.* 114:877, 1976.

125. Fredrick, G. R., and Tanaka, K. R.: Fatal anemia due to in-

domethacin. *N. Engl. J. Med.* 279:1290, 1968.

126. Shearer, C. A.: Indomethacin and aplastic anemia. *Can. Med. Assoc. J.* 118:18, 1978.

127. Menkes, E., and Kutas, G. J.: Fatal aplastic anemia following indomethacin ingestion. *Can. Med. Assoc. J.* 117:118, 1977.

128. Hussain, M. Z., Khan, A. G., and Chaudhry, Z. A.: Aplastic anemia associated with lithium therapy. *Can. Med. Assoc. J.* 108:724, 1973.

129. Jefferson, J. W.: Aplastic anemia associated with lithium. *Lancet* 1:413, 1975.

130. Cromie, B. W.: Meprobamate and aplastic anemia. *Br. Med. J.* 1:562, 1964.

131. Anastassiades, C.: Pancytopenia and meprobamate. *Br. Med. J.* 1:349, 1971.

132. Slee, P. H., DenOllolander, G. F., and DeWolff, F. A.: A case of merbromin (Mercurochrome) intoxication possibly resulting in aplastic anemia. *Acta. Med. Scand.* 205:463, 1979.

133. Gangitano, J. L., Foster, S. H., and Contro, R. M.: Nonfatal methazolamide-induced aplastic anemia. *Am. J. Ophthalmol.* 86:138, 1978.

134. McElfresh, A. E., and Huand, N. N.: Bone-marrow depression resulting from the administration of methicillin: With a comment on the value of serum iron determination. *N. Engl. J. Med.* 266:246, 1962.

135. Levitt, B. H., Gottlieb, A. J., Rosenberg, I. R., and Klein, J. J.: Bone marrow depression due to methicillin, a semisynthetic penicillin. *Clin. Phamacol. Ther.* 5:301, 1964.

136. Edel, S. L., and Bartuska, D. G.: Aplastic anemia secondary to methimazole: Case report and review of hemetologic side effects. *J. Am. Med. Wom. Assoc.* 30(10):412, 1975.

137. Rosenberg, A. H.: Methimazole-induced aplastic anemia. *Conn. Med.* 34:32, 1970.

138. Devlin, J. C.: Depression of erythropoiesis with methyldopa. *Br. Med. J.* 2:1184, 1965.

139. Durge, N. G., Vyas, H. D., and Ward, R. L.: Marrow aplasia and Methyldopa. *Lancet* 1:695, 1968.

140. Pearson, D. H., Peck, J. L., and Livingston, S.: Fatal aplastic anemia following therapy with Nuvarone (3-methyl-5-phenylhydantoin): A case report. *Bull. Johns Hopkins Hosp.* 91:341, 1952.

141. Isaacson, S., Gold, J. A., and Ginsberg, V.: Fatal aplastic anemia after therapy with Nuvarone (3-methyl-5-phenylhydantoin). *JAMA* 160:1311, 1956.

142. Kurata, N., Murakami, T., Hojo, K., and Fujimura, T.: An autopsy case of panmyelophthisis after treatment with methylthiouracil. *Acta Haematol. Jap.* 27:580, 1964.

143. McLaren, G. D., Donkas, M. A., and Muir, W. A.: Methyprylon-induced bone marrow suppression in siblings. An inherited defect. *JAMA* 240:1744, 1978.

144. Suh, K., and Sood, R.: Hypoplastic anemia associated with metolazone. *JAMA* 242:139, 1979.

145. Arnold, A., and Heimpel, A. J.: Aplastic anemia after naproxen. *Lancet* 1:8163, 1980.

146. Pilewski, R. M., Ellis, L. D., Sapira, J. D., and Mark, R.: Oxyphenbutazone and aplastic anemia. *Am. J. Med.* 53:693, 1972.

147. Weiss, A. S., Markenson, J. A., Weiss, M. S., and Kammerer, W. H.: Toxicity of D-penicillamine in rheumatoid arthritis. A report of 63 patients including two with aplastic anemia and one with the nephrotic syndrome. *Am. J. Med.* 64:114, 1978.

148. Bourke, B., Maimi, R. N., Griffits, J. D., and Scott, J. T.: Fatal marrow aplasia in patients on penicillamine. *Lancet* 1:515, 1976.

149. Simpson, T. W., Wilson, E. B., Jr., and Zimmerman, S. G.: Fatal aplastic anemia occurring during anti-convulsant therapy: Probable idiosyncrasy to Phenurone. *Ann. Intern. Med.* 32:1224, 1950.

150. Witkind, E., and Waid, M. E.: Aplasia of the bone marrow during mesantoin therapy. *JAMA* 147:757, 1951.

151. Cameron, A., Eisen, A. A., and Niranjan, L. M.: Aplastic anemia due to phenylbutazone. *Postgrad. Med. J.* 42:49, 1966.

152. McCarthy, D. D., and Chalmers, T. M.: One case each of agranulocytosis and aplastic anemia reported after treatment with phenylbutazone. *Can. Med. Assoc. J.* 90:1061, 1964.

153. Cunningham, J. L., Leyland, M. J., Delamore, J. W., and Price Evans, D. A.: Acetanilide oxidation in phenylbutazone-associated hypoplastic anaemia. *Br. Med. J.* 3:313, 1974.

154. Bottiger, L. E.: Phenylbutazone, oxyphenbutazone and aplastic anemia. *Br. Med. J.* 2:265, 1977.

155. Inman, W. H.: Study of fatal bone marrow depression with special reference to phenylbutazone and oxyphenbutazone. *Br. Med. J.* 1:1500, 1977.

156. Yeung, K.-Y., and Corn, M.: Fatal aplastic anemia with piperacetazine therapy. *Ann. Intern. Med.* 31:411, 1974.

157. Krevans, J. R., Asper, S. P., and Reinhoff, W. F.: Fatal asplastic anemia following use of potassium perchlorate in thyrotoxicosis. *JAMA* 181:162, 1962.

158. Barzilai, D., and Sheinfeld, M.: Fatal complications following use of potassium perchlorate in thyrotoxicosis (aplastic anemia): Report of two cases and a review of the literature. *Isr. J. Med. Sci.* 2:453, 1966.

159. Bhaskaran, K., Subrahmanyan, P., and Nand, D. S.: Fatal bone marrow aplasia complicating prochlorperazine therapy. *Am. J. Psychiatry* 119:373, 1962.

160. Martelo, O. J., Katims, R. B., and Yunis, A. A.: Bone marrow aplasia following propylthiouracil therapy: Report of a case with complete recovery. *Arch. Intern. Med.* 120:587, 1967.

161. Aksoy, M., and Erdem, S.: Aplastic anemia due to propylthiouracil. *Lancet* 1:1379, 1968.

162. Glassmire, C. R.: Fatal pancytopenia following antihistamine administration (pyrilamine and tripelennamine). *J. Maine Med. Assoc.* 42:83, 1951.

163. TenPas, A., and Abraham, J. P.: Hematologic side-effects of pyrimethamine in the treatment of ocular toxoplasmosis. *Am. J. Med. Sci.* 249:448, 1966.

164. Custer, R. P.: Aplastic anemia in soldiers treated with Atabrine (quinacrine). *Am. J. Med. Sci.* 212:211, 1946.

165. Paton, M. D., Riddell, J. M., and Strong, J. A.: Aplastic anemia following Mepacrine (quinacrine) therapy of lupus erythematosus. *Lancet* 1:281, 1955.

166. Biro, R., and Leone, N.: Aplastic anemia induced by quinacrine. *Arch. Dermatol.* 92:574, 1965.

167. Barzel, U. S.: Quinidine sulfate-induced hypoplastic anemia and agranulocytosis. *JAMA* 201:325, 1967.

168. Womack, C. R., and Reiner, C. B.: Fatal aplastic anemia due to streptomycin: Case report and brief review of the literature. *Ann. Intern. Med.* 34:759, 1951.

169. Dunning, A. M.: Pathologic changes in blood and bone marrow following sulfadimethoxine (Madribon). *Ned. Tijdschr. Geneeskd.* 106:1729, 1962.

170. Tulloch, A. L.: Pancytopenia in an infant associated with sulfamethoxazole-trimethoprim therapy. *J. Pediatr.* 88:499, 1976.

171. Holsinger, D. R., Hanlon, D. G., and Welch, J. S.: Fatal aplastic anemia following sulfamethoxypyridazine therapy. *Mayo Clin. Proc.* 33:679, 1958.

172. Johnson, D. R., and Korst, D. R.: Pancytopenia associated with sulfamethoxypyridazine administration. *JAMA* 175:967, 1961.

173. Spracklen, F.: Fatal aplastic anemia following sulfaphenazole (Orisulf) therapy. *Postgrad. Med. J.* 39:488, 1963.

174. Miller, J. L.: Marrow aplasia and sulindac. *Ann. Intern. Med.* 92:129, 1980.

175. Frohman, L. A., and Klocke, F. J.: Recurrent thiocyanate intoxication with pancytopenia, hypothyroidism and psychosis. *N. Engl. J. Med.* 268:701, 1963.

176. Jost, F.: Blood dyscrasias associated with tolbutamide therapy. *JAMA* 169:1468, 1959.

177. Chapman, I., and Cheung, W. H.: Pancytopenia associated with tolbutamide therapy. *JAMA* 186:595, 1963.

178. Bottiger, L. E., and Westerholm, B.: Aplastic anemia. II. Drug-induced aplastic anaemia. *Acta Med. Scand.* 192:319, 1972.

179. Patt, H. M., and Quastler, H.: Radiation effects on cell renewal and related system. *Physiol. Rev.* 43:357, 1963.

180. Puck, T. T.: The action of radiation on mammalian cells. *Am. Naturalist* 94:95, 1960.

181. Borel, V. P., Fliedner, T. M., and Archambean, J. O.: *Mammalian Radiation Lethality.* Academic, New York, 1965.

182. Pollard, E. C.: The biological action of ionizing radiation. *Am. Sci.* 57:206, 1969.

183. Morgan, K. Z., and Turner, J. E.: *Principles of Radiation Protection.* Wiley, New York, 1967.

184. National Council on Radiation Protection and Measurements. N.C.R.P. Report 33, 1969.

185. Adelstein, S. J.: The risk benefit ratio in nuclear medicine. *Hosp. Prac.* 141:1973.

186. Lawrence, J. S., Dowdy, A. H., and Valentine, W. N.: Effects of radiation on hemopoiesis. *Radiology* 51:400, 1948.

187. Storb, R., Epstein, R. B., Buckner, C. D., and Thomas, E. D.: Treatment of chronic lymphocytic leukemia by extracorporeal irradiation. *Blood* 31:490, 1968.

188. Cronkite, E. P., and Bond, V. P.: *Radiation Injury in Man.* Charles C Thomas, Springfield, Ill., 1960.

189. Jacobson, L. O., Marks, E. K., and Lorenz, E.: The hematological effects of ionizing radiations. *Radiology* 52:371, 1949.

190. Knospe, W. H., Blom, J., and Crosby, W. H.: Regeneration of locally irradiated bone marrow. II. Induction of regeneration in permanently aplastic medullary cavities. *Blood* 31:400, 1968.

191. Chertkov, J. L., Novikova, M. N., Nemenova, N. M., and Malanina, V. N.: Hematopoiesis in long-term survival following supralethal irradiation and bone marrow transplantation in dogs. *Blood* 32:895, 1968.

192. Wald, W., Thoma, F. E., Jr., and Broun, G., Jr.: Hematologic manifestation of radiation exposure in man. *Prog. Hematol.* 3:1, 1962.

193. Mathé, G.: Total body irradiation injury: A review of the disorders of the blood and hematopoietic tissues and their therapy, in *Nuclear Hematology,* edited by E. Szirmai. Academic, New York, 1965, p. 275.

194. Adelstein, S. J., and Dealy, J. B., Jr.: Hematologic responses to human whole body irradiation. *Am. J. Roentgenol.* 93:927, 1965.

195. Cronkite, E. P.: Radiation induced aplastic anemia. *Semin. Hematol.* 4:273, 1967.

196. Brown, W. M. C., and Abbatt, J. D.: Effect of a single dose of x-rays on the peripheral blood count of man. *Br. J. Haematol.* 1:75, 1955.

197. Ford, W. L., and Gowans, J. L.: The traffic of lymphocytes. *Semin. Hematol.* 6:67, 1969.

198. Dickle, A., and Hempelman, L. H.: Morphologic changes in the lymphocytes of persons exposed to ionizing radiation. *J. Lab. Clin. Med.* 32:1045, 1947.

199. Roy-Taranger, M., Mayaud, G., and Davydoff-Alibert, S.: Lymphocytes binuclées dans le sang d'individus irradiés a faible dose. *Fr. Etudes Clin. Biol.* 10:958, 1965.

200. Warren, S.: Effects of radiation on normal tissues. *Arch. Pathol.* 34:443, 1942.

201. Martland, H. S.: The occurrence of malignancy in radioactive persons. *Am. J. Cancer* 15:2435, 1931.

202. Duane, G. W.: Aplastic anemia fourteen years following administration of Thorotrast. *Am. J. Med.* 23:499, 1957.

203. Von Swaay, H.: Spate Folgen von Rontgenbestrahlung beim rheumatischen Krankheiten. *Z. Rheumaforsch.* 17:129, 1958.

204. Court-Brown, W. M., and Doll, R.: *Leukemia and Aplastic Anemia in Patients Irradiated for Ankylosing Spondylitis.* Med. Res. Council Special Rep. 295, H.M. Stationery Office, London, 1957.

205. Lange, R. D., Wright, S. W., Tomonage, M., Kurasaki, H., Matsouke, S., and Matsunage, H.: Refractory anemia occurring in survivors of the atomic bombing in Nagasaki, Japan. *Blood* 10:312, 1955.

206. Kirshbaum, J. D., Matsno, T., Sato, K., Ischimarn, M., Tsucchmoto, T., and Ishimarn, T.: A study of aplastic anemia in an autopsy series with special reference to atomic bomb survivors in Hiroshima and Nagasaki. *Blood* 38:17, 1971.

207. Levy, R. N., Sawitsky, A., Florman, A. L., and Rubin, E.: Fatal aplastic anemia after hepatitis. *N. Engl. J. Med.* 273:1118, 1965.

208. Rubin, E., Gottlieb, C., and Vogel, P.: Syndrome of hepatitis and aplastic anemia. *Am. J. Med.* 45:88, 1968.

209. Camitta, B. M., Nathan, D. G., Forman, E. N., Parkman, R., Rappeport, J. J., and Orellana, T. D.: Posthepatitic severe aplastic anemia: An indication for early bone marrow transplantation. *Blood* 43:473, 1974.

210. Hagler, L., Pastore, R. A., and Bergin, J. J.: Aplastic anemia following viral hepatitis: Report of two fatal cases and literature review. *Medicine (Baltimore)* 54:139, 1975.

211. Raksen, A. R., Richter, P., Tallal, L., and Cooper, L. Z.: Hematologic effects of intrauterine rubella. *JAMA* 199:111, 1967.

212. Shadduck, R. K., et al.: Aplastic anemia following infectious mononucleosis: Possible immune etiology. *Exp. Hematol.* 7:264, 1979.

213. Mella, B., and Lang, D. J.: Leukocyte mitosis: Suppression in vitro

associated with acute infectious hepatitis. *Science* 155:80, 1967.

214. Fountain, J. R.: Blood changes associated with disseminated tuberculosis. *Br. Med. J.* 2:76, 1954.

215. Cooper, W.: Pancytopenia associated with disseminated tuberculosis. *Ann. Intern. Med.* 50:1497, 1959.

216. Lewis, S. M.: Red-cell abnormalities and haemolysis in aplastic anaemia. *Br. J. Haematol.* 8:322, 1962.

217. Dacie, J. V., and Lewis, S. M.: Paroxysmal nocturnal haemoglobinuria: Variation in clinical severity and association with bone marrow hypoplasia. *Br. J. Haematol.* 7:442, 1961.

218. Dacie, J. V.: Paroxysmal nocturnal haemoglobinuria. *Proc. R. Soc. Med.* 56:587, 1963.

219. Lewis, S. M., and Dacie, J. V.: The aplastic anemia: Paroxysmal nocturnal haemoglobinuria syndrome. *Br. J. Haematol.* 13:236, 1967.

220. Gardner, F. H., and Blum, S. F.: Aplastic anemia in paroxysmal nocturnal hemoglobinuria: Mechanisms and therapy. *Semin. Hematol.* 4:250, 1967.

221. Shwachman, H., Diamond, L. K., Oski, F. A., and Khaw, K. T.: The syndrome of pancreatic insufficiency and bone marrow dysfunction. *J. Pediatr.* 65:645, 1964.

222. Lachmann, A., Lund, E., and Vinther-Poulsen, N.: Severe refractory anemia in pregnancy. *Acta Obstet. Gynecol. Scand.* 33:395, 1954.

223. Evans, J. L.: Aplastic anemia in pregnancy remitting after abortion. *Br. Med. J.* 3:166, 1968.

224. Goldstein, J. M., and Coller, B. S.: Aplastic anemia in pregnancy: Recovery after normal spontaneous delivery. *Ann. Intern. Med.* 82:537, 1975.

225. Dubois, E. L., and Tuffanelli, D. L.: Clinical manifestations of systemic lupus erythematosus. *JAMA* 190:104, 1964.

226. Hathaway, W. E., Githens, J. H., Blackburn, W. R., Fulginiti, V. A., and Kempe, C. H.: Aplastic anemia, histiocytosis and erythrodermia in immunologically deficient children. *N. Engl. J. Med.* 273:953, 1965.

227. Miller, M. E.: Thymic dysplasia ("Swiss agammaglobulinemia"). I. Graft vs. host reaction following bone marrow transfusion. *J. Pediatr.* 70:730, 1967.

228. Hathaway, W. E., et al.: Graft vs. host reaction (human runt disease) following a single blood transfusion. *JAMA* 201:1015, 1967.

229. Naiman, J. L., Punnett, H. H., Lischner, H. W., Destine, M. L., and Arey, J. B.: Possible graft-versus-host reaction after intrauterine transformation for HR erythroblastosis foetalis. *N. Engl. J. Med.* 281:697, 1969.

230. Meuwissen, H. K., Gatti, R. A., Terasaki, P. J., Hong, R., and Good, R. A.: Treatment of lymphopenic hypogammaglobulinemia and bone marrow aplasia by transplantation of allogenic marrow: Crucial role of histocompatibility matching. *N. Engl. J. Med.* 281:691, 1969.

231. Barnes, D. W. H., and Mole, R. H.: Aplastic anemia in sublethally irradiated mice given allogeneic lymph node cells. *Br. J. Haematol.* 13:482, 1967.

232. Mathe, G., et al.: Immunogenetic and immunological problems of allogeneic haemopoietic radiochimaeres in man. *Scand. J. Haematol.* 4:193, 1967.

233. Meuwissen, H. J., Stutman, O., and Good, R. A.: Functions of the lymphocytes. *Semin. Hematol.* 6:28, 1969.

234. Knospe, W. H., and Crosby, W. H.: Aplastic anaemia: A disorder of the bone marrow sinusoidal microcirculation rather than stem cell failure. *Lancet* 2:20, 1971.

235. Bacigalupo, A., et al.: Severe aplastic anemia: Correlation of in vitro tests with clinical response to immunosuppression in 20 patients. *Br. J. Haematol.* 47:423, 1981.

236. Fanconi, G.: Familiare infantile perniziosartige Anamie (pernizioses Blutbild und Konstitution). *Jahrb. Kiherh.* 117:257, 1927.

237. Fanconi, G.: Familial constitutional panmyelopathy, Fanconi's anemia (F.A.) I. Clinical aspects. *Semin. Hematol.* 4:233, 1967.

238. Beard, M. E. J., et al.: Fanconi's anaemia. *Q. J. Med.* 166:403, 1973.

239. O'Gorman Hughes, D. W.: Aplastic anemia in childhood. III. Constitutional aplastic anemia and related cytopenias. *Med. J. Aust.* 1:519, 1974.

240. Juhl, J. H., Wesenberg, R. L., and Gwinn, J. L.: Roentgenographic findings in Fanconi's anemia. *Radiology* 89:646, 1967.

241. Schroeder, T. M., Tilgen, D., Krüger, J., and Vogel, F.: Formal genetics of Fanconi's anemia. *Hum. Genet.* 32:257, 1976.

242. Swift, M.: Fanconi anaemia: Cellular abnormalities and clinical predisposition to malignant disease, in *Congenital Disorders of Erythropoiesis, Ciba Foundation Symposium 37*. Elsevier, Amsterdam, 1976, p. 115.

243. Bloom, G. E., Warner, S., Gerald, P. S., and Diamond, L. K.: Chromosome abnormalities in constitutional aplastic anemia. *N. Engl. J. Med.* 274:8, 1966.

244. Schmid, W.: Familial constitutional panmyelopathy, Fanconi's anemia (F.A.). II. A discussion of the cytogenetic findings. *Semin. Hematol.* 4:241, 1967.

245. Schroeder, T. M., and Kurth, R.: Spontaneous chromosomal breakage and high incidence of leukemia in inherited disease. *Blood* 37:96, 1971.

246. Latt, S. A., Stetten, G., Juergens, L. A., Buchanan, G. R., and Gerald, P. S.: Induction by alkylating agents of sister chromatid exchanges and chromatid breaks in Fanconi's anemia. *Proc. Natl. Acad. Sci. U.S.A.* 72:4066, 1975.

247. Garriga, S., and Crosby, W. H.: Incidence of leukemia in families of patients with hypoplasia of marrow. *Blood* 14:1008, 1959.

248. Saunders, E. F., and Freedman, H. H.: Constitutional aplastic anemia: Defective haemotopoietic stem cell growth in vitro. *Br. J. Haematol.* 40:277, 1978.

249. Scott, J. L., Cartwright, G. E., and Wintrobe, M. M.: Acquired aplastic anemia: An analysis of thirty-nine cases and reviews of the pertinent literature. *Medicine (Baltimore)* 38:119, 1959.

250. Mohler, D. N., and Leavell, B. S.: Aplastic anemia: An analysis of 50 cases. *Ann. Intern. Med.* 49:326, 1958.

251. Hillman, R. S., and Finch, C. A.: Erythropoiesis: Normal and abnormal. *Semin. Hematol.* 4:327, 1967.

252. Dale, D. C., Fanci, A. S., Guerry, D., IV, and Wolff, S. M.: Comparison of agents producing a neutrophilic leukocytosis in man. Hydrocortisone, prednisone, endotoxin, and etiocholanolone. *J. Clin. Invest.* 56:808, 1975.

253. Twomey, J. J., Douglass, C. C., and Sharkey, O., Jr.: The monocytopenia of aplastic anemia. *Blood* 41:187, 1973.

254. Effenbein, G. J., et al.: The immune system in 40 aplastic anemia patients receiving conventional therapy. *Blood* 53:652, 1979.

255. Finch, C. A., et al.: Ferrokinetics in man. *Medicine (Baltimore)* 49:17, 1970.

256. Najean, Y., Meeks-Bith, L., Bernard, C., Boiron, M., Bousser, J., and Bernard, J.: Isotopic study of the erythrokinetics in 31 cases of chronic idiopathic pancytopenia with histologically normal or rich marrow. *Sang* 30:101, 1959.

257. Cook, J. D., Marsaglia, G., Eschbach, J. W., Funk, D. D., and Finch, C. A.: Ferrokinetics: A biologic model for plasma iron exchange in man. *J. Clin. Invest.* 49:197, 1970.

258. Lange, R. D., McCarthy, J. M., and Gallagher, N. J.: Plasma and urinary erythropoietin in bone marrow failure. *Arch. Intern. Med.* 108:850, 1961.

259. Hammond, G. D., Ishikawa, A., and Keighley, G.: Relationship between erythropoietin and severity of anemia in hypoplastic and hemolytic states, in *Erythropoiesis*, edited by L. O., Jacobson and M. Doyle. Grune & Stratton, New York, 1962, p. 351.

260. Alexanian, R.: Erythropoietin excretion in bone marrow failure and hemolytic anemia. *J. Lab. Clin. Med.* 82:438, 1973.

261. Stohlman, F., Jr.: Erythropoiesis. *N. Engl. J. Med.* 267:342, 1962.

262. Opalinski, A., and Beutler, E.: Creatine, 2-3-diphosphoglycerate and anemia. *N. Engl. J. Med.* 285:483, 1971.

263. Bloom, G. E., and Diamond, L. K.: Prognostic value of tetal hemoglobin levels in acquired aplastic anemia. *N. Engl. J. Med.* 278:304, 1968.

264. Li. F. P., Alter, B. P., and Nathan, D. G.: The mortality of acquired aplastic anemia in children. *Blood* 40:153, 1972.

265. Nixon, R. K., and Olson, J. P.: Diagnostic value of marrow hemosiderin patterns. *Ann. Intern. Med.* 69:1249, 1968.

266. Jamshidi, K., and Swain, W. R.: Bone marrow biopsy with unaltered architecture. *J. Lab. Clin. Med.* 77:335, 1971.

267. McNeil, B. J., Rappaport, J. M., and Nathan, D. G.: Indium chloride scintigraphy: An index of severity in patients with aplastic anemia. *Br. J. Haematol.* 34:599, 1976.

268. Cooper, B., Bunn, H. F., Propper, R. D., et al.: Treatment of iron overload in adults with continuous parenteral desferrioxamine. *Am. J. Med.* 63:958, 1977.

269. Faltwo, F. A., and Freireich, E. J.: Effect of splenectomy on the response to platelet transfusion in three patients with aplastic anemia. *N. Engl. J. Med.* 274:242, 1966.

270. Freireich, E. J., Klinman, A., Gaydas, L. A., Mantel, N., and Frei, E., III: Response to repeated platelet transfusions from the same donor. *Ann. Intern. Med.* 59:227, 1963.

271. McCredie, K. B., Freireich, E. J., and Hester, J. P.: Leukocyte transfusion therapy for patients with host-defense failure. *Transplant. Proc.* 5:1285, 1973.

272. Higby, D. J., Yates, J. W., Henderson, E. S., and Holland, J. F.: Filtration leukapheresis for granulocyte transfusion therapy. *N. Engl. J. Med.* 292:761, 1975.

273. Clift, R. A., Sanders, J. E., Thomas, E. D., Williams, B., and Backner, C. D.: Granulocyte transfusions for the prevention of infection in patients receiving bone marrow transplants. *N. Engl. J. Med.* 298:1052, 1978.

274. Rosenhein, H. S., Farewell, V. T., Price, T. H., Larson, E. B., and Dale, D. C.: The cost effectiveness of therapeutic and prophylactic leukocyte transfusion. *N. Engl. J. Med.* 302:1058, 1980.

275. Yankee, R. A., Freireich, E. J., Carbone, P. P., and Frei, E., III: Replacement therapy using normal and chronic myelogenous leukemia leukocytes. *Blood* 24:844, 1964.

276. Gurwith, M. J., Brunton, J. L., and Lank, B. A.: Granulocytopenia in hospitalized patients. II. A prospective comparison of two antibiotic regimens in the empiric therapy of fever. *Am. J. Med.* 64:127, 1978.

277. Young, L. S.: Infection in the compromised host. *Hosp. Pract.* 16:73, 1981.

278. Gurwith, M. J., Brunton, J. L., Lank, B. A., Hardin, G. K. M., and Ronald, A. R.: A prospective controlled investigation of prophylactic trimethoprim/sulfamethoxazole in hospitalized granulocytopenic patients. *Am. J. Med.* 66:248, 1979.

279. Levitan, A. A., and Perry, S.: The use of an isolator system in cancer chemotherapy. *Am. J. Med.* 44:234, 1968.

280. Pizzo, P. A.: The value of protective isolation in preventing nosocomial infections in high risk patients. *Am. J. Med.* 70:631, 1981.

281. Levine, A. S., et al.: Environments and prophylactic antibiotics. *N. Engl. J. Med.* 288:477, 1973.

282. Vincent, P. C., and DeGruchy, G. C.: Complications and treatment of acquired aplastic anemia. *Br. J. Med. Hematol.* 13:977, 1967.

283. Shahidi, N. T., and Diamond, L. K.: Testosterone-induced remission in aplastic anemia of both acquired and congenital types. *N. Engl. J. Med.* 264:953, 1961.

284. Huguley, C. M., Jr.: Drug-induced blood dyscrasias, in *Disease-a-Month,* edited by H. F. Dowling. Year Book, Chicago, October 1963.

285. Bagby, G. C., Goodnight, S. H., Mooney, W. M., and Richert-Bae, K.: Prednisone responsive aplastic anemia: A mechanism of glucocorticoid action. *Blood* 54:322, 1979.

286. Griner, P. F.: A survey of the effectiveness of cyclophosphamide in patients with severe aplastic anemia. *Am. J. Hematol.* 8:55, 1980.

287. Speck, B., Gluckman, E., Haak, H. L., and Van Rood, J. J.: Treatment of aplastic anemia by antilymphocyte globulin with and without allogenic bone marrow infusion. *Lancet* 2:1145, 1977.

288. Gluckman, E., et al.: Treatment of severe aplastic anemia with antilymphocyte globulin and androgens. *Exp. Hematol.* 6:679, 1978.

289. Pedersen-Bjerggaard, J., Ernst, P., and Nissen, N. J.: Severe aplastic anemia with complete autologous marrow reconstitution following treatment with antilymphocyte globulin. Report of a case and review of the literature. *Scand. J. Haematol.* 21:14, 1978.

290. Estren, S., and Dameshek, W.: Familial hypoplastic anemia of childhood: Report of eight cases in two families with beneficial splenectomy in one case. *Am. J. Dis. Child.* 73:671, 1947.

291. Heaton, L. D., Crosby, W. H., and Cohen, A.: Splenectomy in the treatment of hypoplasia of the bone marrow: With a report of twelve cases. *Ann. Surg.* 146:637, 1957.

292. Koch, J. L.: Aplastic anemia and splenectomy. *Arch. Intern. Med.* 119:305, 1967.

293. Bacigalupo, A., et al.: Bolus methylprednisolone in severe aplastic anemia. *N. Engl. J. Med.* 301:501, 1979.

294. Shimizu, M.: Clinical results on the use of human ceruloplasmin in aplastic anemia. *Transfusion* 19:742, 1979.

295. Besa, E. C., et al.: Aetiocholanolone and prednisone therapy in patients with severe bone marrow failure. *Lancet* 1:728, 1977.

296. Blum, S. F.: Lithium therapy of aplastic anemia. *N. Engl. J. Med.* 300:677, 1979.

297. Sanchez-Medal, L., Pizzuto, J., Torre-Lopez, E., and Derbez, R.: Effect of oxymetholone in refractory anemia. *Arch. Intern. Med.* 113:721, 1964.

298. Allen, D. M., Fine, M. H., Nechles, T. F., and Dameshek, W.: Oxymetholone therapy in aplastic anemia. *Blood* 32:83, 1968.

299. Hast, R., et al.: Oxymetholone treatment in agenerative anemia. II. Remission and survival—a prospective study. *Scand. J. Haematol.* 16:90, 1976.

300. Kennedy, B. J., and Gilbertson, A. S.: Increased erythropoiesis induced by androgenic-hormone therapy. *N. Engl. J. Med.* 256:719, 1953.

301. Shahidi, N. T.: Androgens and erythropoiesis. *N. Engl. J. Med.* 289:72, 1973.

302. Rishpon-Meyerstein, N., Kilbridge, T., Simone, J., and Fried, W.: The effect of testosterone on erythropoietin levels in anemic patients. *Blood* 31:453, 1968.

303. Naets, J. P., and Wittek, M.: The mechanism of action of androgens on erythropoiesis. *Ann. N.Y. Acad. Sci.* 149:366, 1968.

304. Camitta, B. C., and Thomas, E. D.: Severe aplastic anemia: A prospective study of the effect of androgens or transplantation on haematological recovery and survival. *Clin. Haematol.* 7:587, 1978.

305. Van Hengstum, M., Steenbergen, J., and Haanen, C.: Clinical course in 28 unselected patients with aplastic anemia treated with anabolic steroids. *Br. J. Haematol.* 41:323, 1979.

306. Najean, Y., Pecking, A., and Le Danvic, M.: Androgen therapy of aplastic anaemia—A prospective study of 352 cases. *Scand. J. Haematol.* 22:343, 1979.

307. Pillow, R. P., Epstein, R. B., Buckner, C. D., Giblett, E. R., and Thomas, E. D.: Treatment of bone-marrow failure by isogenic marrow infusion. *N. Engl. J. Med.* 275:94, 1966.

308. Storb, R., et al.: Allogeneic marrow grafting for treatment of aplastic anemia. *Blood* 43:157, 1974.

309. Camitta, B. M., et al.: Severe aplastic anemia: A prospective study of the effect of early marrow transplantation on acute mortality. *Blood* 48:63, 1976.

310. Storb, R., Prentice, R. L., and Thomas, E. D.: Treatment of aplastic anemia by marrow transplantation from HLA identical siblings. Prognostic factors associated with graft versus host disease and survival. *J. Clin. Invest.* 59:625, 1977.

311. Gluckman, E., et al.: Bone marrow transplantation in severe aplastic anaemia: A survey of the European Group for Bone Marrow Transplantation (E.G.B.M.T.). *Br. J. Haematol.* 49:165, 1981.

312. Storb, R., Thomas, E. D., Buckner, C. D., et al.: Marrow transplantation in thirty "untransfused" patients with severe aplastic anemia. *Ann. Intern. Med.* 92:30, 1980.

313. Lewis, S. M.: Course and prognosis in aplastic anemia. *Br. Med. J.* 1:1027, 1965.

314. Lynch, R. E., Williams, D. M., Reading, J. C., and Cartwright, G. E.: The prognosis in aplastic anemia. *Blood* 45:517, 1975.

315. Najean, Y., and Pecking, A.: Prognostic factors in acquired aplastic anemia. A study of 352 cases. *Am. J. Med.* 67:564, 1979.

316. Hellriegel, K. P., Zinger, M., and Gross, R.: Prognosis in acquired aplastic anemia. An approach in the selection of patients for allogenic bone marrow transplantation. *Blut* 34:11, 1977.

317. Sleijfer, D. Th., Mulder, N. H., and Nieweg, H. O.: The value of prognostic indicies in aplastic anemia. *Blut* 42:69, 1981.

318. Heyn, R. M., Ertel, I. J., and Tubergen, D. G.: Course of acquired aplastic anemia in children treated with supportive care. *JAMA* 208:1372, 1969.

319. Desposito, F., Akatsuka, J., Thatcher, L. G., and Smith, N. J.: Bone marrow failure in pediatric patients. *J. Pediatr.* 64:683, 1964.

320. Plaut, M. E., and Best, W. R.: Aplastic anemia after parenteral chloramphenicol: Warning renewed. *N. Engl. J. Med.* 306:1486, 1982.

Hemopoietic stem cell disorders — myelodysplastic

CHAPTER *21*

Paroxysmal nocturnal hemoglobinuria

ERNEST BEUTLER

Definition and history

Commonly regarded as a type of hemolytic anemia, paroxysmal nocturnal hemoglobinuria (PNH) is in reality a stem cell disorder characterized by the formation of defective platelets and granulocytes as well as abnormal erythrocytes. The name suggests that cyclic variation in hemoglobinuria is an important feature of this disease. However, in many patients, hemoglobinuria is quite irregular in its occurrence, and the central diagnostic feature of PNH is the increased sensitivity of the red blood cells to the hemolytic action of complement.

In a scholarly historical review of PNH, Crosby [1] attributed the first definitive account of this disease to Strübing [2], who in 1882 described a patient with hemoglobinuria after sleep. The patient's plasma was red, and Strübing suggested that the erythrocytes were being destroyed within the bloodstream. He also detected in the urine a fine-grained yellowish-brown material, which must have been hemosiderin. Hijmans Vandenbergh [3] demonstrated that erythrocytes from a similar patient were lysed in normal serum as well as in the patient's serum if the mixture was acidified with carbon dioxide. Marchiafava and Micheli also were early students of the disease, and for the time it was often designated as the Marchiafava-Micheli syndrome, an appellation which has gradually fallen into disuse.

Etiology and pathogenesis

THE CAUSE OF PNH

PNH is an acquired disorder; it has been reported in only one of a pair of identical twins [4]. This sets it apart from all the other intrinsic abnormalities of the erythrocyte. In heterozygotes for glucose-6-phosphate dehydrogenases (G-6-PD) A and B who have PNH, the ab-

normal cells manifest a single G-6-PD type [5]. This indicates that PNH cells are a clone, and that they presumably arise, like a neoplasm, from the transformation of a single cell. The abnormal clone appears to arise most commonly in a damaged marrow; many patients with PNH have a prior history of idiopathic aplastic anemia [6], but PNH has also been reported following drug-induced aplastic anemia [7]. The marrow karyotype in PNH is usually normal [8], but occasionally, aneuploidy has been observed [9]. Although in a clonal disorder only a single abnormal population is anticipated, more than one population of abnormal red cells with respect to complement sensitivity is often observed in PNH [10]. It may be that additional somatic mutations occur, producing subclones of the original abnormal clone, or that the development of additional populations is a function of red cell aging or other types of environmental conditioning.

THE NATURE OF THE MEMBRANE DEFECT

The characteristic abnormality of PNH erythrocytes is their increased sensitivity to complement-mediated lysis, whether the complement is activated by the classic or the alternative pathway (see Chap. 15). Activation of complement may be achieved by lowering of pH, as in the acid hemolysis test; by reducing ionic strength, as in the sucrose hemolysis test [11]; by cobra venom [12]; by increasing the magnesium concentration [13]; or by antibodies [14]. Using graded amounts of complement, it is possible to identify several populations of cells, which have been designated PNH I, PNH II, and PNH III, manifesting progressively increasing sensitivity to complement lysis [10], and increasing amounts of C3 are deposited on the PNH membranes.

The basic membrane defect in PNH red cells which leads to increased complement sensitivity has, in spite of extensive investigation, remained obscure. The lipid composition of PNH red cell membranes shows no characteristic abnormality [15]. Although an abnormality of the electrophoretic pattern of detergent-solubilized red cell membranes has been described [16], this finding has not been consistent [17]. The acetylcholinesterase activity of the red cell membrane is markedly diminished in PNH [18,19], and the severity of the enzyme deficiency tends to parallel the severity of the disease [20]. However, inhibition of acetylcholinesterase by drugs [21] or its hereditary absence [22] does not result in hemolysis or in complement sensitivity, and the acetylcholinesterase deficiency of PNH cells is clearly a secondary manifestation of the disorder. It has been possible to simulate the PNH defect in red cells by treating them with high concentrations of sulfhydryl compounds [23–25], but the resemblance of these cells to true PNH cells is probably more apparent than real, and the significance of this phenomenon with respect to the basic defect is obscure. Even less is known about the membrane defect of granulocytes and platelets, but in common with red cells, both show increased sensitivity to complement-mediated lysis [26]. Chemotactic responses of PNH granulocytes are also impaired [27].

Clinical features

HEMOGLOBINURIA

The nocturnal hemoglobinuria from which PNH derives its name, i.e., the passage of red or brownish urine in the morning on rising, occurs in only a minority of patients. When hemoglobinuria does follow the classical cyclic pattern, the hemoglobinuria occurs during sleep, regardless of the time of day [28]. It was originally believed that nocturnal hemoglobinuria was a function of a lowered blood pH during sleep, but this has proved not to be the case [29]. A factor which may be important and which seems not to have been considered is that hemoglobinuria may be the result of the production of increased numbers of abnormal cells rather than of an increase in hemolytic processes.

In most patients with PNH, hemoglobinuria is irregular in its occurrence. Bouts of hemolysis may be initiated by infections, surgery, and possibly even strenuous exercise [30]. Transfusion with whole blood often seems to exacerbate hemolysis, possibly by increasing the supply of some of the components of the complement system. It has been suggested that the injection of contrast dyes, as in intravenous pyelography or myelography, can precipitate hemolysis by activating complement [31].

CHRONIC HEMOLYSIS

Patients with PNH manifest all the clinical and laboratory signs of chronic hemolytic anemia.

IRON DEFICIENCY

Iron deficiency is often a manifestation of PNH because of iron loss in the urine both in the form of hemosiderin and hemoglobin. The administration of iron to iron-deficient patients sometimes results in overt signs of hemolysis manifested by the appearance of frank hemoglobinuria. Although this effect of iron has sometimes been attributed to its peroxidatic effect increasing damage to the red cell membrane [32], it seems more likely that it is due to increased production of both normal and abnormal red cells by the marrow, the newly formed abnormal cells undergoing hemolysis [33].

BLEEDING

Thrombocytopenia may be very severe in patients with PNH, and extensive hemorrhagic complications may be a prominent part of the clinical presentation of PNH.

THROMBOSES

Venous thromboses represent one of the most frequent clinical manifestations of PNH. The Budd-Chiari syndrome, resulting from hepatic vein thrombosis, is a particularly common development which has an ominous prognosis [34,35]. Pain in the abdomen or in the lower part of the back also appears to be more common in patients with PNH than in those with other types of hemolytic anemia. The abdominal pain is often colicky in nature and the abdomen is tender on palpation. Frank intestinal infarction or bleeding into the intestinal wall has sometimes been found [36,37].

RENAL MANIFESTATIONS

A variety of abnormalities of renal functions are observed. These include hyposthenuria, abnormal tubular function, and declining creatinine clearance. Hypertension was observed in 8 of a series of 21 patients who had been followed for a long period of time. Radiologic findings included enlarged kidneys and the presence of cortical infarcts, cortical thinning, and papillary necrosis. Most patients have some episodes of hematuria and proteinuria distinct from hemoglobinuria [31].

Acute diminution of renal functions has been observed during episodes of severe hemoglobinuria [38]. Renal failure that develops gradually during the course of the disease and terminates in uremia has also been reported [39].

NEUROLOGIC MANIFESTATIONS

Severe headaches or pains in the eyes occur in patients with PNH without the presence of any objectively demonstrable neurologic abnormalities. These complications may well be due to small venous occlusions. Frank cerebral venous thrombosis is a grave and fortunately uncommon complication of PNH [40].

Although thrombotic complications occur in other forms of hemolytic anemia as well, they are particularly prominent and severe in PNH. The reason for this is not entirely clear, but it may be related to activation of platelets by complement or to the intravascular release of ADP from red cells, leading to platelet aggregation.

Laboratory features

BLOOD

Anemia may be very severe, but in some cases the hemoglobin concentration of the blood is normal. A mild to moderate reticulocytosis is usually present; the reticulocyte count tends to be somewhat lower than in other patients with chronic hemolysis who manifest the same degree of anemia. A modest degree of macrocytosis commensurate with the increased reticulocyte count is usually present. However, if the patient has become iron-deficient, the red cells may be microcytic and hypochromic. Erythrocytes from patients with PNH manifest increased sensitivity to complement lysis and a decrease in membrane acetylcholinesterase activity. These characteristics of PNH red cells are discussed below under "Diagnosis."

The leukocyte count is characteristically low, principally because of a diminution of the number of granulocytes. The leukocyte alkaline phosphatase activity is diminished [41,42]. The platelet count is characteristically low but may occasionally be normal.

MARROW

The erythroid hyperplasia which is characteristic of other hemolytic disorders is usually present in the marrow of patients with PNH. However, the marrow cellularity is generally not greatly increased, and it may even be aplastic. Stainable iron is often absent.

URINE

Hemoglobin is sometimes but by no means always present in the urine. Hemoglobin casts may be present. Hemosiderinuria is one of the most constant features of the disease and is of considerable diagnostic importance.

Diagnosis

The diagnosis of PNH should be entertained in any patient with pancytopenia of unknown origin, particularly when accompanied by reticulocytosis. The most convenient screening tests for PNH are the sucrose hemolysis test [43] (see Chap. A14) and the examination of urine for hemosiderin (see Chap. A3). If the sucrose hemolysis test is positive, the diagnosis should be confirmed using the complete Ham acid hemolysis test [28] (see Chap. A14). The latter test establishes that (1) hemolysis is a property of the patient's erythrocytes, (2) hemolysis requires the presence of serum, (3) the hemolytic effect of the serum is increased by acidification, (4) the hemolytic properties of serum are destroyed by heating, and (5) the hemolytic properties of heated serum are not restored by guinea pig serum. Many other methods have been used in the past to demonstrate the abnormality of PNH cells. Such methods, including the thrombin activation test [44] and the increased sensitivity of PNH cells to isoimmune antibodies [45], are largely of historical interest. The quantitative measurement of lysis of red cells by graded amounts of complement is used to measure the proportion of PNH II and PNH III cells [46]. Other findings which aid in the diagnosis of PNH include the decrease in acetylcholinesterase activity of the red cells, particularly of the upper layer of erythrocytes after centrifugation, and the decrease in leukocyte alkaline phosphatase activity.

Occasionally, the characteristically complement-sensitive red cells cannot be demonstrated in patients with well-established PNH. This probably occurs when the production of PNH cells is relatively low and most of the PNH cells which have been delivered to the circulation have already been destroyed. Thus a single normal sucrose hemolysis test cannot be considered absolute evidence that a patient does not have PNH. Hemosiderinuria is a more constant feature of the disease and is helpful in identifying the occasional patient who may have PNH with a transiently normal sucrose hemolysis test.

Differential diagnosis

Thrombocytopenia and leukopenia are features of PNH which help to differentiate this disorder from other types of hemolytic anemia. Hemosiderinuria, a constant feature of PNH, does not usually occur in other forms of hemolytic anemia, except for those in which there is considerable intravascular destruction of erythrocytes, such as in the hemolytic anemia associated with prosthetic cardiac valves. Although the acronym *HEMPAS* (Hereditary Erythroblastic Multinuclearity with a Positive Acidified Serum lysis test) would imply that confusion might occur between this arcane disorder and PNH, there should be no difficulty in distinguishing HEMPAS from PNH (see Chap. 46). Lysis of HEMPAS cells is due to the presence in normal serum of antibodies to unusual antigens on the surface of HEMPAS cells, the serum of the patients lacking the required alloantibody. Thus HEMPAS cells will not lyse in their own serum. Moreover, HEMPAS is a hereditary disorder and is not associated with leukopenia or thrombocytopenia.

The possibility of the existence of PNH deserves consideration in any patient presenting with aplastic anemia. PNH arises within the context of such marrow failure states. When such patients manifest moderate numbers of reticulocytes in the blood, tests for PNH may demonstrate that a complement-sensitive clone has appeared. A search for PNH may also occasionally prove rewarding in the case of patients with repeated unexplained thrombotic episodes.

Therapy

Treatment of PNH consists chiefly of supportive measures such as transfusion, antibiotics, and anticoagulants as may be required. Suitable patients may be cured by marrow transplantation.

TRANSFUSIONS

Transfusions with red cells is often necessary in the management of patients with severe PNH. Pyrogenic transfusion reactions are common in patients with PNH, and an increase in hemolysis of the patient's own cells often follows transfusion. These adverse effects of transfusion may often be controlled by the administration of washed red cells.

IRON THERAPY

The iron deficiency which often occurs in patients with PNH because of the urinary loss of iron should be treated. The oral administration of iron is usually entirely satisfactory (see Chap. 48). Although an increase in hemoglobinuria may occur during iron therapy because of increased production of PNH cells by the marrow, administration of iron may lessen the requirements for blood transfusion.

STEROIDS

Both androgenic and glucocorticoids have been used in the treatment of PNH. Fluoxymestrone (Halotestin) in doses of 20 to 30 mg per day usually produces some increase in the hemoglobin concentration of the blood

[47]. The administration of glucocorticoids has also been reported to be useful [48,49]. Doses ranging from 20 to 60 mg of prednisone on alternate days may be tried. In view of the potential side effects, particularly when these drugs are administered chronically, steroid therapy should be limited to those patients whose transfusion requirement is significantly decreased at well-tolerated doses.

ANTICOAGULANTS

Although the prophylactic use of anticoagulants in PNH was advocated in the past [50], no clear-cut evidence that the long-term use of such agents alters the course of the disease has emerged. The principal role of anticoagulants in the management of PNH is in the treatment of thrombotic complications such as the Budd-Chiari syndrome [34]. Sometimes a trial of anticoagulation therapy is undertaken with patients who have repeated episodes of abdominal and back pain, but the usefulness of this approach cannot be considered to be established.

SPLENECTOMY

Splenectomy is not usually indicated in the treatment of PNH, although isolated patients with a favorable response have been reported [51]. Because of the considerable risk of thromboembolic complications in patients with PNH, elective surgery of any type, including splenectomy, is best avoided.

MARROW TRANSPLANTATION

As in other stem cell disorders, marrow transplantation is an effective, albeit high-risk, method for the treatment of PNH [52] (see Chap. 168).

OTHER TREATMENTS

Hemolysis may be diminished temporarily by the infusion of a dextran solution [53,54], but this measure does not seem to have a role in the clinical management of PNH. An effort to treat PNH utilizing the antimetabolite 6-mercaptopurine to suppress the PNH clone has been reported [55]. Although some selective suppression of PNH cells was documented, this did not prove to be of any clinical value.

Course and prognosis

The clinical course of PNH is enormously variable. In rare instances, the patient may succumb to this disease within a few months of the first onset of symptoms. Other patients experience a chronic course in which the severity of the disease may wax and wane as the normal cells and the PNH clone alternately appear to gain ascendancy. Sometimes the abnormal clone disappears altogether and the patient appears to be cured. As with so many other diseases, initial reports tended to emphasize the more severely affected patients, so the prognosis was generally deemed to be very grave. As physi-

cians developed a higher index of suspicion concerning this disorder, and as simplified methods for diagnosis became available, milder cases were diagnosed, and these tend to have the better long-term outlook. Nonetheless, even today the disease must be considered a very serious one, and most patients eventually succumb to its complications. The most commonly lethal of these are probably thrombotic episodes such as the Budd-Chiari syndrome, but the various complications of pancytopenia may also lead to death, and in a few patients the terminal episode has been the development of acute leukemia [56].

References

1. Crosby, W. H.: Paroxysmal nocturnal hemoglobinuria. A classic description by Paul Strübing in 1882, and a bibliography of the disease. Blood 6:270, 1951.
2. Strübing, P.: Paroxysmale Haemoglobinurie. Dtsch. Med. Wochenschr. 8:1, 1882.
3. Hijmans Van Den Bergh, A. A.: Ictère hemolytique avec crises hemoglobinuriques fragilité globulaire. Rev. Med. 31:63, 1911.
4. Freman, H., Hill, R., Edwards, A. M., and Wolowyk, M. W.: Paroxysmal nocturnal hemoglobinuria in an identical twin. Can. Med. Assoc. J. 109:1002, 1973.
5. Oni, S. B., Osunkoya, B. O., and Luzzatto, L.: Paroxysmal nocturnal hemoglobinuria: Evidence for monoclonal origin of abnormal red cells. Blood 36:145, 1970.
6. Dacie, J. V.: The Haemolytic Anaemias, part 4. Grune & Stratton, New York, 1967.
7. Quagliana, J. M., Cartwright, G. E., and Wintrobe, M. M.: Paroxysmal nocturnal hemoglobinuria following drug-induced aplastic anemia. Ann. Intern. Med. 61:1045, 1964.
8. Beutler, E., Ohno, S., Goldenburg, E. W., and Yettra, M.: Chromosome-21 and paroxysmal nocturnal hemoglobinuria. Blood 24:160, 1964.
9. Fleischman, T., and Bodor, F.: Aneuploidy in paroxysmal nocturnal hemoglobinuria. Acta Haematol. 44:251, 1970.
10. Rosse, W. F.: Variations in the red cells in paroxysmal nocturnal haemoglobinuria. Br. J. Haematol. 24:327, 1973.
11. Jenkins, D. E., Jr., Hartmann, R. C., and Kerns, A. L.: Serum-red cell interactions at low ionic strength: Erythrocyte complement coating and hemolysis of paroxysmal nocturnal hemoglobinuria. J. Clin. Invest. 46:453, 1967.
12. Kabakci, T., Rosse, W. F., and Logue, G. L.: The lysis of paroxysmal nocturnal hemoglobinuria red cells by serum and cobra venom factor. Br. J. Haematol. 23:693, 1972.
13. May, J. E., Rosse, W., and Frank, M. M.: Paroxysmal nocturnal hemoglobinuria. Alternate-complement-pathway-mediated lysis induced by magnesium. N. Engl. J. Med. 289:705, 1973.
14. Rosse, W. F., and Dacie, J. V.: Immune lysis of normal human and paroxysmal nocturnal hemoglobinuria (PNH) red blood cells. I. The sensitivity of PNH red cells to lysis by complement and specific antibody. J. Clin. Invest. 45:736, 1966.
15. De Gier, J., and Van Deenen, L. L. M.: Phospholipid and fatty acid characteristics of erythrocytes in some cases of anaemia. Br. J. Haematol. 10:246, 1964.
16. Righetti, P. G., Perrella, M., Zanella, A., and Sirchia, G.: The membrane abnormality of the red cell in paroxysmal nocturnal haemoglobinuria. Nature [New Biol.] 245:273, 1973.
17. Jackson, P., and Whittaker, M.: Evidence for an abnormality in the erythrocyte membranes of patients having paroxysmal nocturnal haemoglobinuria and aplastic anemia. Clin. Chim. Acta 41:299, 1972.
18. De Sandre, G., and Ghiotto, G.: An enzymic disorder in the erythrocytes of paroxysmal nocturnal haemoglobinuria; a deficiency in acetylcholinesterase activity. Br. J. Haematol. 6:39, 1960.

19. Auditore, J. V., and Hartmann, R. C.: Paroxysmal nocturnal hemoglobinuria. II. Erythrocyte acetylcholinesterase defect. *Am. J. Med.* 27:401, 1959.

20. Metz, J., Bradlow, B. A., Lewis, S. M., and Dacie, J. V.: The acetylcholinesterase activity of the erythrocytes in paroxysmal nocturnal haemoglobinuria in relation to the severity of the disease. *Br. J. Haematol.* 6:372, 1960.

21. Metz, J., Stevens, K., Van Rensburg, N. J., and Hart, D.: Failure of invivo inhibition of acetylcholinesterase to affect erythrocyte life-span: The significance of the enzyme defect in paroxysmal nocturnal haemoglobinuria. *Br. J. Haematol.* 7:458, 1961.

22. Johns, R. J.: Familial reduction in red-cell cholinesterase. *N. Engl. J. Med.* 267:1344, 1962.

23. Sirchia, G., Ferrone, S., and Mercuriali, F.: The action of two sulfhydryl compounds on normal human red cells: Relationship to red cells of paroxysmal nocturnal hemoglobinuria. *Blood* 25:502, 1965.

24. De Sandre, G., Vettore, L., Corrocher, R., Cortesi, S., and Perona, A.: Ham-positive red cells induced in vitro by N-acetylcysteine or D-penicillamine. *Br. J. Haematol.* 15:437, 1968.

25. Kann, H. E., Jr., Mengel, C. E., Meriwether, W. D., and Ebbert, L.: Production of in vitro lytic characteristics of paroxysmal nocturnal hemoglobinuria erythrocytes in normal erythrocytes. *Blood* 32:49, 1968.

26. Aster, R. V., and Enright, S. E.: A platelet and granulocyte defect in paroxysmal nocturnal hemoglobinuria: Usefulness for detecting platelet antibodies. *J. Clin. Invest.* 48:1199, 1969.

27. Craddock, P. R., Fehr, J., and Jacob, H. S.: Complement-mediated granulocyte dysfunction in paroxysmal nocturnal hemoglobinuria. *Blood* 47:931, 1976.

28. Ham, T. H.: Studies on destruction of red blood cells. I. Chronic hemolytic anemia with paroxysmal nocturnal hemoglobinuria: An investigation of the mechanism of hemolysis, with observations on five cases. *Arch. Intern. Med.* 64:1271, 1939.

29. Crosby, W. H.: Paroxysmal nocturnal hemoglobinuria. Relation of the clinical manifestations to underlying pathogenic mechanisms. *Blood* 8:769, 1953.

30. Blum, S. F., Sullivan, J. M., and Gardner, F. H.: The exacerbation of hemolysis in paroxysmal nocturnal hemoglobinuria by strenuous exercise. *Blood* 30:513, 1967.

31. Clark, D. A., Butler, S. A., Braren, V., Hartmann, R. C., and Jenkins, D. E., Jr.: The kidneys in paroxysmal nocturnal hemoglobinuria. *Blood* 57:83, 1981.

32. Mengel, C. E., Kann, H. E., Jr., and O'Malley, B. W.: Increased hemolysis after intramuscular iron administration in patients with paroxysmal nocturnal hemoglobinuria: Report of six occurrences in four patients, and speculations on a possible mechanism. *Blood* 26:74, 1965.

33. Rosse, W. F., and Gutterman, L. G.: The effect of iron therapy in paroxysmal nocturnal hemoglobinuria. *Blood* 36:559, 1970.

34. Hartmann, R. C., Luther, A. B., Jenkins, D. E., Jr., Tenorio, L. E., and Saba, H. I.: Fulminant hepatic venous thrombosis (Budd-Chiari syndrome) in paroxysmal nocturnal hemoglobinuria: Definition of a medical emergency. *Johns Hopkins Med. J.* 146:247, 1980.

35. Leibowitz, A. I., and Hartmann, R. C.: Annotation: The Budd-Chiari syndrome and paroxysmal nocturnal haemoglobinuria. *Br. J. Haematol.* 48:1, 1981.

36. Blum, S. F., and Gardner, F. H.: Intestinal infarction in paroxysmal nocturnal hemoglobinuria. *N. Engl. J. Med.* 274:1137, 1966.

37. Lee, B. C. P.: Paroxysmal nocturnal haemoglobinuria presenting as acute abdominal emergency. *Br. J. Radiol.* 46:467, 1963.

38. Rubin, H.: Paroxysmal nocturnal hemoglobinuria with renal failure. *JAMA* 215:433, 1971.

39. Blaisdell, R. K., Priest, R. E., and Beutler, E.: Paroxysmal nocturnal hemoglobinuria: A case report with a negative Ham presumptive test associated with serum properdin deficiency. *Blood* 13:1074, 1958.

40. Johnson, R. V., Kaplan, S. R., and Blailock, E. R.: Cerebral venous thrombosis in paroxysmal nocturnal hemoglobinuria (Marchiafava-Micheli syndrome). *Neurology* 20:681, 1970.

41. Beck, W. S., and Valentine, W. N.: Biochemical studies on leucocytes. II. Phosphatase activity in chronic lymphatic leukemia, acute leukemia, and miscellaneous hematologic conditions. *J. Lab. Clin. Med.* 38:245, 1951.

42. Lewis, S. M., and Dacie, J. V.: Neutrophil (leucocyte) alkaline phosphatase in paroxysmal nocturnal haemoglobinuria. *Br. J. Haematol.* 11:549, 1965.

43. Hartmann, R. C., and Jenkins, D. E., Jr.: The "sugar-water" test for paroxysmal nocturnal hemoglobinuria. *N. Engl. J. Med.* 275:155, 1965.

44. Crosby, W. H.: Paroxysmal nocturnal hemoglobinuria. A specific test for the disease based on the ability of thrombin to activate the hemoglobin factor. *Blood* 5:843, 1950.

45. Dacie, J. V.: Diagnosis and mechanism of hemolysis in chronic hemolytic anemia with nocturnal hemoglobinuria. *Blood* 4:1183, 1949.

46. Rosse, W. F.: Variations in the red cells in paroxysmal nocturnal haemoglobinuria. *Br. J. Haematol.* 24:327, 1973.

47. Hartmann, R. C., Jenkins, D. E., Jr., McKee, L. C., nad Heyssel, R. M.: Paroxysmal nocturnal hemoglobinuria: Clinical and laboratory studies relating to iron metabolism and therapy with androgen and iron. *Medicine (Baltimore)* 45:331, 1966.

48. Fudenberg, H., Palmer, W. L., and Kirsner, J. B.: Paroxysmal nocturnal hemoglobinuria: Report of a case with rare hemoglobinuria treated with corticotropin. *Am. J. Med. Sci.* 227:32, 1954.

49. Firkin, F., Goldberg, H., and Firkin, B. G.: Glococorticoid management of paroxysmal nocturnal hemoglobinuria. *Aust. Ann. Med.* 17:127, 1968.

50. Crosby, W. H.: Paroxysmal nocturnal hemoglobinuria: Plasma factors of the hemolytic system. *Blood* 8:444, 1953.

51. Melkild, A., and Morstad, K. S.: A case of paroxysmal nocturnal haemoglobinuria splenectomized twice. *Acta Med. Scand.* 164:299, 1959.

52. Storb, R., et al.: Paroxysmal nocturnal haemoglobinuria and refractory marrow failure treated by marrow transplantation. *Br. J. Haematol.* 24:743, 1973.

53. Stratton, F., Wilkinson, J. F., and Israels, M. C. G.: Clinical dextran for acute episodes in paroxysmal nocturnal hemoglobinuria. *Lancet* 1:831, 1958.

54. Gardner, F. H., and Laforet, M. T.: The use of clinical dextran in patients with paroxysmal nocturnal hemoglobinuria. *J. Lab. Clin. Med.* 55:946, 1960.

55. Beutler, E., and Collins, Z.: The effect of 6-mercaptopurine (6-MP) administration in paroxysmal nocturnal hemoglobinuria (PNH), in *Proceedings of the 10th International Congress of Hematology,* Stockholm, Sweden, Aug. 30–Sept. 4, 1964.

56. Zittoun, R., Bernadou, A., James, I. M., Soria, J., and Bousser, J.: Acute myelomonocytic leukaemia: A terminal complication of paroxysmal nocturnal haemoglobinuria. *Acta Haematol.* 53:241, 1975.

CHAPTER *22*

Dyshemopoietic (preleukemic) disorders

MARSHALL A. LICHTMAN
JAMES K. BRENNAN

Definition and history

There are two major types of preneoplastic state. One type is the predisposition of certain disorders or circumstances to eventuate in a higher incidence of cancer than in the population at large. An example of this circumstance is the heavily irradiated population, in whom leukemia occurs with a markedly heightened frequency. The two-hit theory of leukemogenesis (carcinogenesis) holds that cancer is a multistep event [1]. The first step, e.g., retrovirus insertion into the genome, "promotes" a predisposed state in which a tumor is "initiated" after a second insult, e.g., excessive irradiation. The second type of preneoplasia is a dysplasia of tissues, which is reflected in cytologic changes that experience has shown to be a harbinger of malignancy. In this type of preneoplasia, multiple hits have occurred, but in some individuals, the result is dysplasia rather than neoplasia. Neoplasia ultimately emerges because of genetic instability and clonal succession.

Preleukemia corresponds to the type of preneoplasia that is a dysplasia. It is an overt abnormality of the marrow associated with increased proliferation and inadequate maturation of marrow precursor cells that results in cytopenias in varying combinations and severity. Qualitative abnormalities of cell shape, organelle structure, and biochemical pathways and function can occur. The range of quantitative and qualitative alterations is broad, explaining the wide array of clinical patterns. Thus preleukemia can occur with isolated refractory anemia and a nearly normal appearing marrow or with severe pancytopenia, profoundly hypercellular marrow, and bizarre alterations in blood cell shape, size, and structure. The term *preleukemia* refers to disorders that antedate acute myelogenous leukemia (AML) or acute lymphocytic leukemia (ALL), but the latter are very rare (see below).

The boundary between preleukemia and leukemia is indistinct, leading to disagreement about classification. It is our view that if small proportions of leukemic blast cells are present in marrow, the diagnosis of oligoblastic leukemia should be made, maintaining the important principle that the presence of tumor cells should be the key determinant of the histopathologic diagnosis, as in other tissues. These oligoblastic leukemias are analogous to the minimal-deviation tumors that develop during experimental carcinogenesis studies (Table 22-1).

Since most patients with preleukemia do not develop overt leukemia, other terms such as *dyshemopoietic syndrome* or *myelodysplastic syndrome* have been suggested as more accurate alternatives. The term *preleukemia* is commonly used, however, to describe these syndromes. Even though patients with the clinical findings of preleukemia may not develop overt AML, their risk of doing so is about 1000 to 10,000 times that of the general population.

In the early twentieth century, physicians became aware that patients could experience extended periods of refractory anemia or other cytopenias prior to the appearance of morphologic evidence of AML [2–5]. Chevaliar, in 1942, discussed formally the "odo-leukemias." He chose the Greek word *odo*, meaning "threshold," to highlight disorders that were on the threshold of leukemia. Terms such as *herald state of leukemia, refractory anemia, sideroachrestic anemia, idiopathic refractory sideroblastic anemia, pancytopenia with hyperplastic marrow*, and others were coined to describe these various manifestations of the dyshemopoietic diseases.

Patients with dyshemopoietic states have had refractory cytopenias for months or years prior to their developing AML [6–20]. Cytogenetic analysis [21] and marrow cell culture studies [22–25], as well as more standard blood cell studies [26], have established the close association of dyshemopoietic states and AML, and these two disorders are considered to be part of a spectrum of marrow disease (see Chap. 19).

Etiology, pathogenesis, and inheritance

The etiology of preleukemia, like that of other stem cell disorders, is unknown. RNA viruses are likely to be involved, since they are known to cause leukemia in many animal species [27] in which a preleukemic phase occurs. Somatic mutation has also been considered as an etiologic factor, a mechanism that is not mutually exclusive with an RNA virus etiology [28,29]. Radiation [30,31] and chemical leukemogens [31–33] are initiating factors [34]. Aging is important, since preleukemia is unusual under the age of 40 years [18,19], and aging has been related to the multihit theory of carcinogenesis [35].

Preleukemia is thought to result from a lesion in the pluripotential or hemopoietic stem cell pool and evolves from the clonal expansion of a single stem cell or a very small number of such cells (see Chap. 19). The clonal origin of preleukemia is supported by studies of a woman who was a double heterozygote for glucose-6-phosphate dehydrogenase isoenzymes A and B and who had a preleukemic syndrome. Her hemopoietic

TABLE 22-1   Prodromal (preleukemias) and minimal deviation (oligoblastic leukemias) hemopoietic stem cell diseases

PRELEUKEMIC STATES
Ineffective hemopoiesis and dyshemopoiesis dominate:
Pancytopenia with hyperplastic marrow [9,12,15,17]
Bicytopenia with hyperplastic marrow [9,15,17]
Idiopathic refractory sideroblastic anemia [93–95,97,98]
Idiopathic refractory nonsideroblastic anemia [17,20,87]
Hypoplastic hemopoiesis dominates:
Amegakaryocytic thrombocytopenia [99]
Chronic hypoplastic neutropenia [100–102]
Erythroid aplasia [96]
Aplastic anemia [110–111]
Paroxysmal nocturnal hemoglobinuria–aplastic anemia syndrome [112–117]
OLIGOBLASTIC LEUKEMIAS
Refractory anemia with excessive myeloblasts [121–123]
Smoldering myelogenous leukemia [124–129]
ATYPICAL MYELOPROLIFERATIVE SYNDROMES
Chronic myelomonocytic leukemia [130–137]

NOTE: Acute and chronic myeloproliferative diseases are listed in Table 19-1. Syndromes in which hypoplastic hemopoiesis is the dominant abnormality are uncommon antecedants of AML.

progenitors and lymphocytes had only one isoenzyme present, supporting the concept of clonal expansion of a diseased multipotential stem cell [36].

The major specific pathophysiologic mechanism in the preleukemic syndrome is ineffective hemopoiesis, i.e., defective maturation of marrow precursor cells [24,37–39]. The proliferation of progenitor and early precursor cells is usually normal or enhanced, resulting in a hypercellular marrow despite the failure to accumulate adequate numbers of fully matured cells. Mild shortening of cell life-span contributes to the cytopenias [12].

One family in which myelodysplastic states were found in several members has been reported [40]. It is probable that, like familial leukemia, such relationships occur occasionally.

A protracted preleukemic disorder lasting for from 1 to 20 years occurs in about 5 to 10 percent of patients with AML prior to onset [41].

Clinical features

Preleukemic syndromes are more frequent in men than in women, and over 85 percent of patients are over 40 years of age at the time of diagnosis. The disorder does occur occasionally in children and young adults. Patients can be asymptomatic or have symptoms associated with anemia, such as weakness, loss of a sense of well-being, and exertional dyspnea [12,18,19]. A small proportion of patients have infections related to granulocytopenia or hemorrhage related to thrombocytopenia. Palpable hepatomegaly occurs in about 5 percent and palpable splenomegaly in about 10 percent of patients. Pallor associated with anemia is present in nearly 50 percent of patients. Rarely, patients have fever unrelated to infection [42]. Arthralgias are the principal initial complaint in many patients.

Laboratory features

BLOOD

Anemia is present in over 85 percent of patients [20,21]. The mean cell volume (MCV) is often increased. Red cell shape abnormalities are present in many patients, and red cell shape abnormalities often are patternless (anarchic) with a variety of shapes, including oval, elliptical, tear-drop, spherical, and fragmented, but there is a spectrum of findings, and some patients have only slight anisocytosis. Basophilic stippling of red cells occurs. Nucleated red cells can be found on the blood film. Other abnormalities of red cells also occur, such as increased proportions of hemoglobin F [43], abnormal red cell enzyme activities, especially acquired pyruvate kinase deficiency [44–48], enhanced sensitivity of membranes to complement [19], and modification of red cell antigens [49–52]. Acquired hemoglobin H disease, which reflects an acquired decrease in the rate of α chain synthesis in erythroblasts, can occur rarely [53].

Neutropenia occurs in about 50 percent of patients. The proportion of monocytes is often increased [54]. Morphologic abnormalities of neutrophils can occur, especially the acquired Pelger-Huet anomaly in which the nuclei of neutrophils are unilobed or bilobed, the latter with a pince-nez-shaped nucleus [6,18,19]. Neutrophil alkaline phosphatase activity is decreased in some patients [19]. Defective primary granules of abnormal size and shape and with decreased myeloperoxidase content may be present [55]. Specific neutrophil granules may be decreased in number, producing hypogranular cells [56]. Bactericidal and chemotactic capability may be impaired [57]. Muramidase (lysozyme) activity in blood and urine may be increased [58], a reflection of granulocytic hyperplasia and heightened monocytopoiesis and monocyte turnover.

Thrombocytopenia occurs in about 25 percent of patients, but it is often mild in extent. Abnormal platelet morphology consisting of large platelets and platelets with poor granulation or a large, fused central granule may be present [59,60]. Abnormal platelet function may contribute to easy bruising or excessive bleeding. Decreased platelet aggregation in response to collagen or epinephrine is a frequent functional abnormality [61].

Serum lactic dehydrogenase and uric acid may be increased, principally as a result of the ineffective hemopoiesis and high death fraction of maturing marrow precursors.

Marrow

MORPHOLOGY

Marrow cellularity is usually normal or increased. Rarely, it may be decreased and may simulate hypoplastic anemia, although islands of hemopoiesis are present. Erythroid hyperplasia is frequent, and very large or small erythroblasts, nuclear fragmentation, stippled erythroblasts, and poor hemoglobinization may be seen [18,19,62]. Erythroblasts may resemble megaloblasts with macroerythroblasts, nuclear-cytoplasmic maturation asynchrony, and nuclear fragmentation or nuclear remnants in erythroblasts. This pattern is referred to as *megaloblastoid erythropoiesis*, although *dyserythropoiesis* is a more accurate description.

Pathologic sideroblasts may be present. These include erythroblasts with an increased number and size of siderosomes (cytoplasmic ferritin-containing vacuoles) or erythroblasts with mitochondrial iron aggregates, which when very prominent take the form of a partial or complete circumnuclear ring of iron globules. Macrophage iron is often increased. Some observers believe that ringed sideroblasts are less often associated with progression to leukemia than are sideroblasts with increases in cytoplasmic ferritin [63,64]. Others dispute this conclusion [54].

Granulocytic hyperplasia is frequent [18,19]. Monocytes also can be increased in number. Abnormalities of granulocytes include hypogranulation and a monocytoid appearance of neutrophilic granulocytes and the Pelger-Huet nuclear abnormality of mature neutrophils. Progranulocytes and myelocytes may be increased. Blast cells are not increased in true preleukemia, although observers differ on what proportion of blast cells should be considered preleukemia as opposed to oligoblastic leukemia. Some series include patients with 10 to 40 percent blast cells and progranulocytes as preleukemic. The number of plasma cells may be slightly increased. Megakaryocytes are present in normal or increased numbers. Micromegakaryocytes (dwarf megakaryocytes) may occur [56]. The number of megakaryocytes with unilobed or bilobed nuclei may be increased [65,66]. All the morphologic aberrations of blood cells seen in preleukemia can be seen in AML as well, contributing to the argument that they represent different stages of a single disorder.

MARROW CULTURE

The clonal growth of marrow granulocytic progenitors in soft agar or analogous viscous culture systems may be abnormal in some patients with preleukemia [22,67–73]. Colony-forming units for neutrophils and monocytes (CFU-NM) are decreased. Very small colonies or clusters often dominate the cultures. Abnormally small and infrequent CFU-NMs may be found when blood neutrophil and monocyte counts are nearly normal. Maturation defects have been identified in culture. Occasionally, overabundant growth is present. Usually, cell culture results become more abnormal as the blood cell abnormalities in the patient worsen. In overt AML, CFU-NM growth is usually absent. Some studies indicate that very abnormal growth of small clusters is a poor prognostic sign and may be a harbinger of overt leukemia. Erythroid progenitors are responsive to erythropoietin and are identifiable in normal or excessive numbers [74]. Biochemical abnormalities of erythroid precursors in preleukemia have been found [75].

Cytogenic studies

Most patients with preleukemia have a normal karyotype; however, an altered number or form of chromosomes may occur in as many as one-third of patients with preleukemia [21,76–85]. The chromosome abnormalities are nonrandom and often involve chromosomes that are abnormal in patients with AML.

Common abnormalities include an extra chromosome 8 or 9; loss of the long arm of chromosome 5, 20, or 21; and monosomy for chromosome 7. A preleukemic syndrome manifested by refractory anemia and associated with deletion of the long arm of chromosome 5 (5q-) has received particular attention. The refractory anemia is associated with marked dyserythropoiesis, erythroid multinuclearity, and hypolobulated megakaryocytes [86–90]. In some of these cases, an associated deletion of the long arm of chromosome 21 (21q-) has occurred

along with thrombocytosis [91]. Isolated deletions of chromosome 21 also have been reported in patients with primary thrombocythemia [92]. The prognostic significance of chromosome abnormalities is uncertain. Some observers believe them to be associated with an earlier development of AML, but all studies do not confirm this impression. Indeed, loss of the long arm of chromosome 5 has been associated with a better prognosis than cases with other abnormal karyotypes.

The proportion of cases of preleukemia with chromosome abnormalities is difficult to assess because the definition of preleukemia is imprecise. Inclusion of cases with refractory anemia with excess myeloblasts may increase the proportion of cases with abnormalities. Some scientists consider the presence of chromosome abnormalities in themselves indicative of leukemia, or at least of a malignant clone in marrow, regardless of the histopathology present. This criterion is probably too sensitive to be clinically useful. In general, prevalence of chromosome abnormalities and the likelihood of progression to AML are both a function of the number of cell lines involved and the severity of the cytopenias.

Specific dyshemopoietic disorders

SYNDROMES WITH A PROPENSITY FOR LEUKEMIC TRANSFORMATION (PRELEUKEMIA)

ISOLATED ANEMIA

Preleukemia can present as idiopathic refractory sideroblastic anemia or refractory normocytic or macrocytic anemia with little overt involvement of granulocytes or megakaryocytes [93–98]. Most patients are over 40 years of age, but rare cases can occur in children or young adults. Idiopathic refractory sideroblastic anemia may be associated with a dimorphic red cell morphology: a population of hypochromic cells and one of normochromic cells. The percentage of reticulocytes is normal or slightly increased, but the absolute reticulocyte count is low for the degree of anemia. Falsely elevated reticulocyte counts may occur because of the failure to subtract stippled red cells, which take up the new methylene blue stain. Other features of this disorder are described in Chap. 54. In refractory macrocytic anemia, mean cell volume is often slightly or moderately increased, the absolute reticulocyte count is low for the blood hemoglobin concentration, plasma vitamin B_{12} and folic acid levels are normal, and other features of megaloblastic anemias are absent. The frequency of evolution of these syndromes to AML has not been quantified carefully, but it is probably in the range of 10 to 20 percent of patients [95,105]. Pure red cell aplasia has been reported to precede AML, but this is a very rare event [96].

ISOLATED THROMBOCYTOPENIA

Amegakaryocytic thrombocytopenia is a very rare preleukemic syndrome, although bona fide cases have transformed into AML months or years later [99].

ISOLATED NEUTROPENIA

Chronic neutropenic states are rare antecedents of AML. Congenital hypoplastic neutropenia (Kostmann's syndrome) has evolved into AML [100,101]. The evolution of Shwachman's syndrome (neutropenia and exocrine pancreatic insufficiency) into acute leukemia has been documented [102]. Six of eight children with this disorder developed AML and two developed ALL. A related disorder, Pearson's syndrome (sideroblastic anemia and exocrine pancreatic insufficiency), is a putative preleukemic disorder in children [103]. Acquired chronic hypoplastic neutropenia is a very rare antecedent of AML, and few documented cases have been reported.

PANCYTOPENIAS

Most patients with preleukemia present with anemia, neutropenia, and thrombocytopenia; anemia and neutropenia; or anemia and thrombocytopenia. In these patients, the clinical and laboratory features described previously usually lead to a diagnosis of a dyshemopoietic state, especially in the patient over 40 years of age [6,9,12,18,19,104–109].

APLASTIC ANEMIA, PAROXYSMAL NOCTURNAL HEMOGLOBINURIA, AND EOSINOPHILIC FASCIITIS

AML occurs in a small fraction of patients (~5 percent) with acquired aplastic anemia [110,111]. Since aplasia itself is a disease with a high early mortality rate, the propensity to leukemia may be greater than is apparent.

Paroxysmal nocturnal hemoglobinuria is a hemopoietic stem cell disease that has a propensity for development of marrow hypoplasia (see Chap. 21). AML may ensue in some patients [112–117]. It can be considered a preleukemic syndrome with a very low incidence of leukemic transformation. There is a propensity for all hemopoietic stem cell disorders to undergo transformation to myelogenous leukemia (see Chap. 19).

Eosinophilic fasciitis mimics the cutaneous manifestations of scleroderma. Symmetrical swelling and induration of arms and legs, sparing the hands and feet, are common [118]. Eosinophilia and hypergammaglobulinemia are frequent, and aplastic anemia has been associated with the disease [119]. An immune mechanism has been postulated for all the manifestations of the disease. In one series of 12 patients, 2 developed myeloproliferative disorders, one of which was AML [120].

OLIGOBLASTIC LEUKEMIA

REFRACTORY ANEMIA WITH EXCESS MYELOBLASTS (RAEM)

This disorder is grouped by some among the preleukemic states and is referred to by the acronym RAEM [121–123]. It consists of chronic refractory anemia, granulocytopenia, and/or thrombocytopenia. Myeloblasts and progranulocytes constitute from 5 to 40 percent of nucleated marrow cells. Most patients are males, and three-quarters of patients are over 50 years of age. Median survival of patients is about 10 months.

Refractory anemia with excess myeloblasts and pancytopenia with hyperplastic marrow with evident leukemic blast cells can be considered to be oligoblastic leukemias [124–129]. These disorders have protracted (smoldering) courses in comparison with classical AML.

CHRONIC MYELOMONOCYTIC LEUKEMIA

Chronic myelomonocytic leukemia is another syndrome that is included by some among the preleukemic disorders. Chronic myelomonocytic leukemia is characterized by anemia, monocytosis usually in excess of 1000 monocytoid cells per microliter, granulocytic hyperplasia of marrow, abnormal myelocytes, and increased myeloblasts, monoblasts, and progranulocytes in marrow [130–135]. The disease afflicts those over 50 years of age in most cases. The onset is usually insidious, and weakness, infection, or excessive bleeding may bring patients to medical attention. Blood hemoglobin concentration is slightly to moderately decreased, and white cell counts are normal or moderately elevated with a very high proportion of monocytes. Immature granulocytes may be present in the blood. Thrombocytopenia is present in most patients. Slight hepatomegaly and splenomegaly occur in about a third of patients. The marrow is hypercellular, with the dominant cells being early myelocytes. A high proportion of cells have obvious nucleoli, although the chromatin pattern is coarser than that of a typical myeloblast. Monocytoid cells are usually present in marrow. Despite thrombocytopenia, megakaryocytes are usually present in marrow. Plasma and urine lysozymes are nearly always elevated. The disease may evolve into a more florid blastic leukemia. The response to cytotoxic treatment is poor, and symptomatic therapy with component transfusion and antibiotics is the preferable management.

Chronic myelomonocytic leukemia is an atypical myeloproliferative disease closely related to subacute or chronic myelogenous and chronic monocytic leukemias. It is difficult to consider it a preleukemic syndrome except in the same sense that CML is an antecedent to a more acute form of leukemia. Chronic monocytic dyscrasia [136] and chronic monocytic leukemia [137] are closely related to chronic myelomonocytic leukemia and can terminate in acute myelogenous leukemia.

Prodromal syndromes antedating lymphocytic leukemia

The term *preleukemia* usually implies that the condition under consideration is an antecedent of myelogenous leukemia. AML often begins with a protracted period (weeks to months) of symptoms or signs preceding clinical diagnosis, and a proportion of cases, perhaps as many as 5 to 10 percent, are preceded by an overt dyshemopoietic syndrome. Acute lymphocytic leukemia (ALL) usually begins explosively, and it is rare for symptoms to be present for more than a few weeks prior to diagnosis. Intermediate syndromes, e.g., smoldering or oligoblastic lymphocytic leukemia, or preleukemic syndromes are exceedingly rare.

Apparent aplastic anemia [138–144] or erythroid hypoplasia [145] has been described as an antecedent to ALL in a few children. The aplasia is promptly improved by glucocorticoids, and ALL ensues quickly, usually within 1 to 8 months. The brief interval between remission of aplastic anemia and the onset of leukemia in most patients suggests that the foci of leukemia, inapparent on marrow biopsy, may in some way initiate the aplasia. Remission of aplasia followed shortly by ALL has occurred in the absence of glucocorticoid or other specific therapy in several cases. Rare cases of adult ALL have developed after sideroblastic anemia [146].

PRELEUKEMIA PRECEDING OR EMERGING IN LYMPHOID MALIGNANCIES – OTHER THAN ACUTE LYMPHOCYTIC LEUKEMIA

Sideroblastic anemia sometimes associated with qualitative disorders of other blood cell lines (such as thrombopathy) has developed in patients who have had, or later developed, a lymphoproliferative disease such as hairy cell leukemia, lymphocytic lymphoma, myeloma, chronic lymphocytic leukemia, and Hodgkin's disease [147–154]. The sideroblastic anemia in these cases was not preceded by cytotoxic therapy. Similar associations have been reported in patients who have received chemotherapy or radiotherapy for a lymphoproliferative disease or a solid tumor, and preleukemic syndromes in these patients have usually been presumed to be the result of treatment [155].

Differential diagnosis

Preleukemia should be considered in patients, especially if over 40 years of age, with unexplained cytopenias and cellular marrows. Suspicion should be heightened if the MCV is high normal or increased, if more than one cell line is involved, and if abnormalities of red cell shape or leukocyte and platelet morphology are present. Giant platelets and neutrophils with Pelger-Huet nuclear abnormalities in the blood are two prime examples of such changes.

Megaloblastic anemia as a result of vitamin B_{12} or folic acid deficiency is an important consideration in the differential diagnosis. Paroxysmal nocturnal hemoglobinuria (PNH) may also be confused with other preleukemic syndromes, especially in the state of PNH in which pancytopenia and marrow hypofunction are present. Congenital dyserythropoietic anemias are extremely rare, have an onset in early life, and often have a familial pattern. Moreover, abnormalities are confined to erythroid cells (see Chap. 46). Since many patients with dyshemopoietic disorders present with pancytopenia, the blood counts alone raise the possibility of acute leukemia, aplastic anemia, multiple myeloma, hairy cell leukemia, and other disorders associated with the failure of normal hemopoiesis. Careful scrutiny of the blood film and marrow as well as other features of the clinical picture will usually clarify the situation.

Management

Cytopenias that are not troublesome should not be treated. Transfusion of blood components when necessary is the mainstay of treatment. Regular transfusion of red cells may be used for those who do not adapt to moderate anemia or in whom medical conditions, such as angina pectoris, require a higher packed red cell volume. Thrombocytopenia is often not so severe as to require treatment. Asymptomatic neutropenia should not be treated, but fever should be evaluated promptly and proven or suspected infection treated vigorously with bactericidal antibiotics.

Androgens have not been useful in this or related disorders [156]. Rare cases may show minor improvement, but the likelihood of substantial improvement is low. Glucocorticoid use has no sound physiological basis, although occasional cases have shown improvement in blood cell counts [19]. Improvement of marrow cell growth in vitro in the presence of a glucocorticoid was shown to predict its efficacy in the 10 percent of patients who showed a response [157]. Protracted use of glucocorticoids may increase the risk of infection, especially with opportunistic organisms. Cytotoxic therapy with currently available drugs and dosage schedules is not useful in preleukemia syndromes and can worsen the cytopenias and shorten the life of patients so treated.

A retrospective analysis of the treatment of 235 putative cases of AML identified 20 who had oligoblastic leukemia, including 13 with refractory anemia with excess myeloblasts and 7 with chronic myelomonocytic leukemia. Three patients with refractory anemia and excess blast cells achieved complete remissions lasting 14 to more than 36 months [158]. These patients were young and had no prior exposure to chemotherapy. The median survival of the remaining 17 patients was 1 month with aggressive treatment. If sideroblastic anemia is present, a trial of pyridoxine, 200 mg per day for 6 to 8 weeks, may be administered. Significant responses are very infrequent. Patients with splenomegaly have occasionally responded to splenectomy, but the risk of surgery in elderly cytopenic subjects is high. Since cytopenias are the result principally of ineffective production of blood cells, splenectomy is not likely to produce dramatic results. The rare young patient with a preleukemic syndrome and a histocompatible sibling donor may be considered for marrow transplantation [159].

Course and prognosis

The type of preleukemic syndrome determines, in part, the morbidity of the disease and the likelihood of transformation into AML or a fatal outcome during the preleukemic period. Refractory sideroblastic or macrocytic anemia without other cytopenias may persist for years without morbidity [95,104]. Red cell transfusions may be required. AML develops in about 10 percent of such patients [95,105,106]. In patients with multicytopenias, morbidity is greater; severe infections, excessive bleeding, and severe anemia and lassitude may occur [107]. Mortality from infection or hemorrhage occurs in about 25 percent of patients. Acute myelogenous leukemia develops in about 50 percent of patients. Median survival of patients with multicytopenias is probably less than 1 year. Statistics on patients with preleukemia are difficult to interpret, because classification as preleukemia versus oligoblastic leukemia is difficult and most studies have been retrospective, using selected samples of patients.

In general, a greater likelihood of transformation to overt AML is implied by involvement of more cell lines, more severe cytopenias, more overt qualitative disorders of cells, chromosome abnormalities, and abnormalities of marrow cell growth in culture (excessive growth or suppressed growth).

References

1. Ashley, D. B.: The two "hit" and multiple "hit" theories of carcinogenesis. *Br. J. Cancer* 23:313, 1969.
2. Sinck, F., and Kohn, E.: Gleichzeitiges bestehen perniziöser Anämie und chronisher myeloisher Leukamie. *Folia Haematol.* 42:180, 1930.
3. Elman, C., and Marshall, S.: Anaemia of pernicious type. Complicated by diabetes mellitus and terminating in acute myeloid leukaemia. *Lancet* 2:1094, 1936.
4. Chevalier, P.: Sur la terminologie des leucoses et des affections frontières. Les odo-leucoses. *Sang.* 15:587, 1942–3.
5. Hamilton-Paterson, J. L.: Preleukaemic anaemia. *Acta Haematol.* 2:309, 1949.
6. Block, M., Jacobson, L. O., and Bethard, W. J.: Preleukemic acute human leukemia. *JAMA* 152:1018, 1953.
7. Meacham, C. G., and Weisberger, A. S.: Early atypical manifestations of leukemia. *Ann. Intern. Med.* 41:780, 1956.
8. Williams, M. J.: Myeloblastic leukemia preceded by prolonged hematological disorder. *Blood* 10:502, 1955.
9. Vilter, R. W., Jarrold, T., Will, J. J., Mueller, J. F., Friedman, B. I., and Hawkins, V. R. : Refractory anemia with hyperplastic bone marrow. *Blood* 15:1, 1960.
10. Blair, T. R., Bayrd, E. D., and Pease, G. I.: Atypical leukemia. *JAMA* 198:139, 1966.
11. Salomon, H., and Tatarsky, I.: Preleukemic leukemia. *Isr. J. Med. Sci.* 5:1178, 1969.
12. Schiller, M., Rachmilewitz, E. A., and Izak, G.: Pancytopenia with hypercellular hemopoietic tissue. *Isr. J. Med. Sci.* 5:69, 1969.
13. Saarni, M. I., and Linman, J. W.: Preleukemia. *Am. J. Med.* 55:38, 1973.
14. Fisher, W., et al.: "Preleukemia." A myelodysplastic syndrome often terminating in acute leukemia. *Arch. Intern. Med.* 132:226, 1973.
15. Linman, J. W., and Saarni, M.I.: The preleukemic syndrome. *Semin. Hematol.* 11:93, 1974.
16. Kamada, N., and Uchino, H.: Haematologic abnormalities in six cases with the preleukemic stage for 5–13 years. *Acta Haematol. Jpn,* 37:32, 1974.
17. Pierre, R. V.: Preleukemic states. *Semin. Hematol.* 11:73, 1974.
18. Dreyfus, B.: Preleukemic states. *Blood Cells* 2:33, 1976.
19. Linman, J. W., and Bagby, G. C., Jr.: The preleukemic syndrome: Clinical and laboratory features, natural course and management. *Blood Cells* 2:11, 1976.
20. Linman, J. W., and Bagby, G. C., Jr: The preleukemic syndrome (hemopoietic dysplasia). *Cancer* 42:854, 1978.
21. Pierre, R. V.: Cytogenetic studies in preleukemia: Studies before and after transition to acute leukemia in 17 subjects. *Blood Cells* 1:163, 1975.
22. Greenberg, P. L., Nichols, W. C., and Schrier, S. L.: Granulopoiesis in acute myeloid leukemia and preleukemia. *N. Engl. J. Med.* 284:1225, 1971.
23. Senn, J. S., and Pinkerton, P. H.: Defective in vitro colony formation by human bone marrow preceding overt leukemia. *Br. J. Haematol.* 23:277, 1972.
24. Golde, D. W., and Cline, M. J.: Human preleukemia—Identification of a maturation defect in vitro. *N. Engl. J. Med.* 288:1083, 1973.
25. Dormer, P.: Bone marrow cell kinetics in patients with pancytopenia, in *Preleukemia,* edited by F. Schmalzl and K.-P. Helbriegel. Springer-Verlag, Berlin, 1979, p. 91.
26. Koeffler, H. P., and Golde, D. W.: Human preleukemia. *Ann. Intern. Med.* 93:347, 1980.
27. Bishop, J. M.: The molecular biology of RNA tumor viruses. *N. Engl. J. Med.* 303:675, 1980.
28. Passarge, E., and Bartram, C. R.: Somatic recombination as possible prelude to malignant transformation. *Birth Defects* 12:177, 1976.
29. Knudson, A. G.: Mutation and human cancer. *Adv. Cancer Res.* 17:317, 1973.
30. Kamada, N., and Uchins, H.: Preleukemic states in atomic bomb survivors. *Blood Cells* 2:57, 1976.
31. Renoux, M., et al.: Erythrocyte abnormalities induced by chemotherapy and radiotherapy: Induction of preleukemic states? *Br. J. Haematol.* 21:323, 1978.
32. Tulliez, M., Ricard, M. F., Jan, F., and Sultan, C.: Preleukaemic abnormal myelopoiesis induced by chlorambucil. *Scand. J. Haematol.* 13:179, 1974.
33. Van den Berghe, H., Lovwagie, A., Broeckart-Van Orshoven, A., David, G., and Verwilghen, R.: Chromosome analyses in two unusual malignant blood disorders presumably induced by benzene. *Blood* 53:558, 1979.
34. Kitahara, M., Cosgriff, T. M., and Eyre, H. J.: Sideroblastic anemia as a preleukemic event in patients treated for Hodgkin's disease. *Ann. Intern. Med.* 92:625, 1980.
35. Armitage, P., and Doll, R.: The age-distribution of cancer and a multistage theory of carcinogenesis. *Br. J. Cancer* 8:1, 1954.
36. Prchal, J. T., Throckmorton, D. W., Caroll, A. J., Fuson, E. W., Gams, R. A., and Prchal, J. F.: A common progenitor for human myeloid and lymphoid cells. *Nature* 274:590, 1978.
37. Quiesser, U., Olischläger, A., Queisser, W., and Heimpel, H.: Cell proliferation in the "preleukemic" phase of acute leukemia. *Acta Haematol.* 47:21, 1972.
38. Fischer, M., Mitzou, P. S., and Hubner, K.: Myelopoietic cell proliferation in granulocytopenia of refractory anemia and preleukemia states with hyperplastic bone marrow. *Klin. Wochenschr.* 54:211, 1976.
39. Mitzou, P. S., Fischer, M., and Hubner, K.: Proliferation of ineffective erythropoiesis with nuclear abnormalities and megaloblastoid appearance in preleukemia. *Acta Haematol.* 54:271, 1975.
40. Li, F. P., Marchetto, D. J., and Vawter, G. F.: Acute leukemia and preleukemia in eight males in a family: An X-linked disorder? *Am. J. Hematol.* 6:61, 1979.
41. Boggs, D. R., Wintrobe, M. M., and Cartwright, G. E.: The acute leukemias. *Medicine* 41:163, 1962.

42. Zanger, B., and Dorsey, H. N.: Fever—A manifestation of preleukemia. *JAMA* 236:1266, 1976.

43. Rochant, H., Dreyfus, B., Gouguerra, M., and Hoi Tant-Hot: Hypothesis: Refractory anemias, preleukemic conditions, and fetal erythropoiesis. *Blood* 39:721, 1972.

44. Bovin, R., Galand, C., and Dreyfus, B.: Activités enzymatiques erythrocytaires au cours des anémies réfractaires. *Nouv. Rev. Fr. Hematol.* 9:105, 1969.

45. Valentine, W. N., Komad, P. N., and Paglia, D. E.: Dyserythropoiesis, refractory anemia and "preleukemia": Metabolic features of the erythrocytes. *Blood* 41:857, 1973.

46. Arnold, H., Blume, K. G., Lohr, G. W., Boulard, M., and Najean, Y.: "Acquired" red cell enzyme defects in hematologic diseases. *Clin. Chim. Acta* 57:187, 1974.

47. Bowin, P., Galand, C., Hakim, J., and Kahn, A.: Acquired erythroenzymopathies in blood disorders. *Br. J. Haematol.* 31:531, 1975.

48. Helmstadter, V., Arnold, H., Blume, K. G., Uhl, N., and Hunstein, W.: Acquired pyruvate kinase deficiency with hemolysis in preleukemia. *Acta Haematol.* 57:339, 1977.

49. Dreyfus, B., et al.: Anomalies of the blood group antigens and erythrocyte enzymes in two types of chronic refractory anemia. *Br. J. Haematol.* 16:303, 1969.

50. Salmon, C.: A tentative approach to variation in ABH and associated erythrocyte antigens. *Semin. Hematol.* 2:3, 1969.

51. Salmon, C., et al.: Étude des modifications des antigenes de groupes sanguins dans 11 cas "d'anémies réfractaires." *Nouv. Rev. Fr. Hematol.* 9:113, 1969.

52. Salmon, C.: Blood group changes in preleukemic states. *Blood Cells* 2:211, 1976.

53. Streichman, S., Tatarski, I., and Manaster, J.: Red cell inclusion bodies in a case of preleukemia. *Scand. J. Haematol.* 22:263, 1979.

54. Economopolus, T., et al.: Myelodysplastic syndrome. *Acta Haematol.* 65:97, 1981.

55. Breton-Gorius, J., Houssay, D., and Dreyfus, B.: Partial myeloperoxidase deficiency in a case of preleukaemia. I. Studies of fine structure and peroxidase synthesis of promyelocytes. *Br. J. Haematol.* 30:273, 1975.

56. Breton-Gorius, J.: Abnormalities of granulocytes and megakaryocytes in preleukemic syndromes, in *Preleukemia*, edited by F. Schmalzl and K.-P. Helbriegel. Springer-Verlag, Berlin, 1979, p. 24.

57. Breton-Gorius, J., Houssay, D., Vilde, J. L., and Dreyfus, B.: Partial myeloperoxidase deficiency in a case of preleukaemia. II. Defects of degranulation and abnormal bactericidal activity of blood neutrophils. *Br. J. Haematol.* 30:279, 1975.

58. Youman, J. D., III, Saarni, M. I., and Linman, J. W.: Diagnostic value of muramidase (lysozyme) in acute leukemia and preleukemia. *Mayo Clin. Proc.* 45:219, 1970.

59. Maldonado, J. E., and Pierre, R. V.: The platelet in preleukemia and myelomonocytic leukemia. *Mayo Clin. Proc.* 50:575, 1975.

60. Maldonado, J. E.: Platelet granulopathy. A new morphologic feature in preleukemia and myelomonocytic leukemia. *Mayo Clin. Proc.* 51:452, 1976.

61. Pintado, T., and Maldonado, J. E.: Ultrastructure of platelet aggregation in refractory anemia and myelomonocytic leukemia. *Mayo Clin. Proc.* 51:443, 1976.

62. Reizenstein, P., Lagerlof, B., Skarberg, K. O., Carlmark, B., Jores, S., and Kock, Y.: Alterations in erythropoiesis preceding leukemia. *Acta Haematol.* 54:152, 1975.

63. Hast, R.: Studies on preleukemia. II. Clinical and prognostic significance of sideroblasts in aregenerative anaemia with hypercellular bone marrow. *Scand. J. Haematol.* 21:396, 1978.

64. Hast, R., and Reizenstein, P.: Sideroblastic anemia and development of leukemia. *Blut* 42:203, 1981.

65. Smith, W., et al.: Atypical megakaryocytes in the preleukemic phase of AML. *Blood* 42:535, 1973.

66. Queisser, W., Queisser, U., Ansmann, M., Brunner, G., Hoelzer, D., and Heimpel, H.: Megakaryocyte polyploidization in acute leukemia and preleukemia. *Br. J. Haematol.* 28:261, 1974.

67. Faille, A., Najean, Y., Dresch, C., and Poirer, O.: Cell culture studies in 19 cases of refractory anaemia: Comparison of clinical data with in vivo erythrokinetic studies. *Scand. J. Haematol.* 19:39, 1977.

68. Beran, M., and Hast, R.: Studies in human preleukemia. II. In vitro colony forming capacity in a regenerative anaemia with hypercellular bone marrow. *Scand. J. Haematol.* 21:139, 1978.

69. Koeffler, H. P., and Golde, D. W.: Cellular maturation in human preleukemia. *Blood* 52:355, 1978.

70. Verma, D. S., Spitzer, G., Dicke, K. A., and McCredie, K. B.: In vitro agar culture patterns in preleukemia and their clinical significance. *Leukemia Res.* 3:41, 1979.

71. Lidbeck, J.: In vitro colony and cluster growth in haemopoietic dysplasia (the preleukaemic syndrome). I. Clinical correlations. *Scand. J. Haematol.* 24:412, 1980.

72. Senn, J. S., Curtro, J. E., Pinkerton, P. H., Till, J. E., and McCulloch, E. A.: The distribution of marrow granulopoietic progenitors among patients with preleukemia. *Leukemia Res.* 4:409, 1980.

73. Lidbeck, J.: In vitro colony and cluster growth in haemopoietic dysplasia (the preleukaemic syndrome). II. Identification of a maturation defect in agar cultures. *Scand. J. Haematol.* 25:113, 1980.

74. Koeffler, H. P., Cline, M. J., and Golde, D. W.: Erythropoiesis in preleukemia. *Blood* 51:1013, 1978.

75. Lourenco, G., Embury, S., Schrier, S. L., and Kedes, L. H.: Decreased ribosomal RNA content and in vitro RNA synthesis in purified bone marrow erythroblasts of patients with idiopathic ineffective erythropoiesis and DiGuglielmo disease. *Am. J. Hematol.* 5:169, 1978.

76. Rowley, J. D., Blaisdell, R. K., and Jacobson, L. O.: Chromosome studies in preleukemia. I. Aneuploidy of group C chromosomes in three patients. *Blood* 27:782, 1966.

77. Lisker, R., Cobo de Gutierrez, A., and Velazques-Ferrari, M.: Longitudinal bone marrow chromosome studies in potential leukemic myeloid disorders. *Cancer* 31:509, 1973.

78. Yamada, K., and Furusawa, S.: Preferential involvement of chromosomes no. 8 and no. 21 in acute leukemia and preleukemia. *Blood* 47:679, 1976.

79. Helbriegel, K.-P.: Chromosome findings in preleukemia, in *Preleukemia*, edited by F. Schmalzl and K.-P. Helbriegel. Springer-Verlag, Berlin, 1979, p. 68.

80. Nowell, P. C.: Marrow chromosome studies in "preleukemia." *Cancer* 28:513, 1971.

81. Nowell, P., and Finan, T.: Chromosome studies in preleukemia states. *Cancer* 42:2254, 1978.

82. Streuli, R. A., Tests, J. R., Vardiman, J. W., Golomb, H. M., and Rowley, J. D.: Dysmyelopoietic syndrome: Sequential clinical and cytogenetic studies. *Blood* 55:636, 1980.

83. Testa, J. R., Kinnealey, A., Rowley, J. D., Golde, D. W., and Potter, D.: Deletion of the long arm of chromosome 20 in myeloid disorders. *Blood* 52:868, 1978.

84. Second International Workshop on Chromosomes in Leukemia. Chromosomes in preleukemia. *Canc. Genet. Cytogenet.* 2:108, 1980.

85. Humbert, J. R., Hathaway, W. E., Robinson, A., Peakman, D. C., and Githens, J. H.: Preleukemia in children with a missing bone marrow C chromosome and a myeloproliferative disorder. *Br. J. Haematol.* 21:705, 1971.

86. Van den Berge, H., Cassiman, J. J., David, G., Fryns, J. P., Michaux, J. L., and Sokal, G.: Distinct haematological disorder with deletion of long arm of a number 5 chromosome. *Nature* 251:437, 1974.

87. Sokal, G., et al.: A new hematologic syndrome with a distinct karyotype. The 5q-chromosome. *Blood* 46:519, 1975.

88. Kaffe, S., Hsu, L. F. Y., Hoffman, R., and Hirschhorn, K.: Association of 5q- and refractory anemia. *Am. J. Hematol.* 4:269, 1978.

89. Mahmood, T., Robinson, W. A., Hamstia, R. D., and Wallner, S. F.: Macrocytic anemia, thrombocytosis and nonlobulated megakaryocytes: The 5q-syndrome, a distinct entity. *Am. J. Med.* 66:946, 1979.

90. Jume'an, H. G., and Libnoch, J. A.: 5q-myelodysplasia terminating in acute leukemia. *Ann. Intern. Med.* 91:748, 1979.

91. Van den Berghe, H., Petit, P., Broeckaert-Van Orshoven, A., Louwagie, A., DeBaere, H., and Verwilghen, R.: Simultaneous occurrence of 5q- and 21q- in refractory anemia with thrombocytosis. *Cancer Genet. Cytogenet.* 1:63, 1979.

92. Petit, P., and Van den Berge, H.: A chromosomal abnormality (21q-) in primary thrombocytosis. *Hum. Genet.* 50:105, 1979.

93. Kuschner, J. P., Lee, G. R., Wintrobe, M. M., and Cartwright, G. E.: Idiopathic refractory sideroblastic anemia. *Medicine* 50:139, 1971.

94. Dameshek, W.: Sideroblastic anaemia: Is this a malignancy? *Br. J. Haematol. 11:*52, 1965.

95. Cheng, D. S., Kuschner, J. P., and Wintrobe, M. M.: Idiopathic refractory sideroblastic anemia. *Cancer 44:*724, 1979.

96. Peschle, C.: Pure red cell aplasia type III progression to acute myeloid leukemia and absence of the IgG inhibitor to erythropoiesis, in *Preleukemia,* edited by F. Schmalzl and K.-P. Helbriegel. Springer-Verlag, Berlin, 1979, p. 12.

97. Hayhoe, F. G. J., and Quaglino, D.: Refractory sideroblastic anaemia and erythremic myelosis: Possible relationships and cytochemical observations. *Br. J. Haematol. 6:*381, 1960.

98. Abrahamson, J. R., and Edgington, S. T.: Sideroblastic anemia associated with cytogenetic aberration of bone marrow cells. *Am. J. Clin. Pathol. 57:*348, 1972.

99. Stoll, D. B., Blum, S., Pasquale, D., and Murphy, S.: Thrombocytopenia with decreased megakaryocytes. *Ann. Intern. Med. 94:*170, 1981.

100. Gilman, P. A., Jackson, D. P., and Guild, H. G.: Congenital agranulocytosis: Prolonged survival and terminal acute leukemia. *Blood 36:*576, 1970.

101. Rosen, R. B., and Kang, S.-J.: Congenital agranulocytosis terminating in acute myelomonocytic leukemia. *J. Pediatr. 94:*406, 1979.

102. Woods, W. G., Roloff, J. S., Lukens, J. N., and Krivit, W.: The occurrence of leukemia in patients with the Shwachman's syndrome. *J. Pediatr. 99:*425, 1981.

103. Pearson, H. A., et al.: A new syndrome of refractory sideroblastic anemia with vacuolization of marrow precursors and exocrine pancreatic dysfunction. *J. Pediatr. 95:*976, 1979.

104. Reizenstein, P., and Lagerlof, B.: Aregenerative anemia with hypercellular sideroblastic marrow. *Acta Haematol. 47:*1, 1972.

105. Lewy, R. I., Kansu, E., and Gabuizda, T.: Leukemia in patients with acquired idiopathic sideroblastic anemia. *Am. J. Hematol. 6:*323, 1979.

106. Ricci, P., Baccarani, M., Zaccaria, A., Santucci, M. A., and Tura, S.: Clinical contribution to the knowledge of hemopoietic dysplasias: Long-term follow-up of 13 patients with refractory anemia. *Acta Haematol. 60:*10, 1978.

107. Heimpel, H., Drings, P., Mitrou, P., and Queiber, W.: Verlauf und prognostische Kriteuen bei Patienten mit ''Praleukamie.'' *Klin. Wochenschr. 57:*21, 1979.

108. Vilter, R. W., Will, J. J., and Jarrold, T.: Refractory anemia with hyperplasic bone marrow (aregenerative anemia). *Semin. Hematol. 4:*175, 1967.

109. Dawdson, S. P., Davis, L. J., and Innes, J.: Studies in refractory anaemie. III. Refractory anaemies with cellular marrow. *Edinburgh Med. J. 50:*431, 1943.

110. Alter, B. P., Potter, N. U., and Li, F. P.: Classification and aetiology of the aplastic anemias. *Clin. Haematol. 7:*431, 1978.

111. Hellriegel, K. P., Fohlmeister, I., and Schaefer, H. E.: Aplastic anemia terminating in leukemias, in *Aplastic Anemia,* edited by H. Heimpel, E. C. Gordon-Smith, W. Heit, and B. Kubanek. Springer-Verlag, Berlin, 1979, p. 47.

112. Jenkins, D. S., and Hartmann, R. C.: Paroxysmal nocturnal hemoglobinuria terminating in acute myeloblastic leukemia. *Blood 33:*274, 1969.

113. Holden, D., and Lichtman, H.: Paroxysmal nocturnal hemoglobinuria with acute leukemia. *Blood 33:*283, 1969.

114. Kaufmann, R. W., Schecter, G. P., and McFarland, W.: Paroxysmal nocturnal hemoglobinuria terminating in acute granulocytic leukemia. *Blood 33:*287, 1969.

115. Carmel, R., Coltman, C. A., Jr., Yatteau, R. R., and Costanzi, J. J.: Association of paroxysmal nocturnal hemoglobinuria with erythroleukemia. *N. Engl. J. Med. 283:*1329, 1970.

116. Zittoun, R., Bernadore, A., James, J. M., Soria, J., and Bousser, J.: Acute myelomonocytic leukemia—Terminal complications of paroxysmal nocturnal hemoglobinuria. *Acta Haematol. 53:*241, 1975.

117. Cowell, D. E., Pasquale, D. N., and Dekker, P.: Paroxysmal nocturnal hemoglobinuria terminating as erythroleukemia. *Cancer 43:*1914, 1979.

118. Moore, T. L., and Zuckner, J.: Eosinophilic fasciitis. *Semin. Arthritis Rheum. 9:*228, 1980.

119. Hoffman, R., Dainiak, N., Sibrack, L., Pober, J. S., and Waldron, J. A., Jr.: Antibody-mediated aplastic anemia and diffuse fasciitis. *N. Engl. J. Med. 300:*718, 1979.

120. Michet, C. J., Jr., Doyle, J. A., and Ginsburg, W. W.: Eosinophilic fasciitis. *Mayo Clin. Proc. 56:*27, 1981.

121. Dreyfus, B., Rochant, H., Sultan, C., Clauvel, J. P., Yvart, J., and Chesneau, A. M.: Les anémies réfractaires avu excés des myeloblastes dans la moelle. Etude de 11 observations. *Nouv. Presse Med. 78:*359, 1970.

122. Najean, Y., and Pecking, A.: Refractory anemia with excess of myeloblasts in the bone marrow. A clinical trial of androgens in 90 cases. *Br. J. Haematol. 37:*23, 1977.

123. Najean, Y., and Pecking, A.: Androgen therapy in the refractory anemia with excess myeloblasts in the bone marrow, in *Preleukemia,* edited by F. Schmalzl and K.-P. Helbriegel. Springer-Verlag, Berlin, 1979, p. 154.

124. Rheingold, J. J., Kaufman, R., Adelson, E., and Lear, A.: Smoldering acute leukemia. *N. Engl. J. Med. 268:*812, 1963.

125. Khamsi, F., Carstairs, K. C., and Scott, J. G.: Smoldering acute leukemia, in *Proc. XIII Congr. Int. Soc. Hematol.* Lehmann Verlag, Munich, 1970, p. 192.

126. Knospe, W. H., and Gregory, S. A.: Smoldering acute leukemia. Clinical and cytogenic studies in six patients. *Arch. Intern. Med. 127:*910, 1971.

127. Bernard, J., Izrael, V., and Jacquillat, C.: Les Leucémies oligoblastiques. *Nouv. Presse Med. 4:*943, 1975.

128. Izrael, V., et al.: Donníes nouvelles sur les leucémies oligoblastiques. *Nouv. Presse Med. 4:*947, 1975.

129. Spitzer, G., Verma, D. S., Dicke, K. A., Smith, T., and McCredie, K. B.: Subgroups of oligoleukemia as identified by in vitro agar culture. *Leukemia Res. 3:*29, 1979.

130. Miescher, P. A., and Farquet, J. J.: Chronic myelomonocytic leukemia in adults. *Semin. Hematol. 11:*129, 1974.

131. Sexauer, J., Kass, L., and Schnitzer, B.: Subacute myelomonocytic leukemia. *Am. J. Med. 57:*853, 1974.

132. Geary, C. G., et al.: Chronic myelomonocytic leukemia. *Br. J. Haematol. 30:*289, 1975.

133. Zittoun, R.: Subacute and chronic myelomonocytic leukemia. *Br. J. Haematol. 32:*1, 1976.

134. Cohen, J. R., Creger, W. P., Greenberg, P. L., and Schrier, S. L.: Subacute myeloid leukemia. *Am. J. Med. 66:*959, 1979.

135. Skinnider, L. F., Card, R. T., and Padmanabh, S.: Chronic myelomonocytic leukemia. *Am. J. Clin. Pathol. 67:*339, 1977.

136. Pretlow, T. G.: Chronic monocytic dyscrasia culminating in acute leukemia. *Am. J. Med. 46:*130, 1969.

137. Sinn, C. M., and Dick, F. W.: Monocytic leukemia. *Am. J. Med. 20:*588, 1956.

138. Bernard, J.: Les Aplasies pre-leucémiques. *Nouv. Rev. Fr. Hematol. 9:*41, 1969.

139. Melhorn, D. K., Gross, S., and Neuman, A. J.: Acute childhood leukemia presenting as aplastic anemia. The response to corticosteroids. *J. Pediatr. 77:*647, 1970.

140. Shackelford, G. D., Bloomberg, G., and McAlister, W. H.: The value of roentgenography in differentiating aplastic anemia from leukemia masquerading as aplastic anemia. *Am. J. Roentgenol. Rad. Ther. 116:*651, 1972.

141. Rokica-Milewska, R., and Derulsak, D.: Aplastic anemia in the early period of acute leukemia in childhood. *Mater. Med. Pol. 6:*24, 1974.

142. Toledano, S. R.: Preleukemia phase in childhood acute lymphoblastic leukemia. *J. Pediatr. 91:*507, 1977.

143. Sills, R. H., and Stockman, J. A., III: Preleukemia states in children with acute lymphoblastic leukemia. *Cancer 48:*110, 1981.

144. Beatnach, F., Chessells, J. M., and Greaves, M. F.: The aplastic presentation of childhood leukemia: A feature of common ALL. *Br. J. Haematol. 49:*387, 1981.

145. DeAlarcon, P., Miller, M., and Stuart, M. J.: Erythroid hypoplasia: An unusual presentation of childhood leukemia. *Am. J. Dis. Child. 132:*763, 1978.

146. Barton, J. C., Conrad, M. E., and Parmley, R. T.: Acute lymphoblastic leukemia in idiopathic refractory sideroblastic anemia. *Am. J. Hematol. 9:*109, 1980.

147. MacSween, J. M., and Langley, G. R.: Light-chain disease and

sideroblastic anemia — Preleukemic chronic granulocytic leukemia. *Can. Med. Assoc. J. 106*:995, 1972.

148. Trachida, L., Palutke, M., Poylik, M. D., and Prasad, A. S.: Primary acquired sideroblastic anemia preceding monoclonal gammopathy and malignant lymphoma. *Am. J. Med. 55*:559, 1973.

149. Papayannis, A. G., Stathakis, N. E., Kyrkou, K., Panani, A., and Gardikos, C.: Primary acquired sideroblastic anemia associated with chronic lymphocytic leukemia. *Br. J. Haematol. 28*:125, 1974.

150. Berkowitz, L. R., Ross, D. W., and Orringe, E. P.: Hairy cell leukemia with acquired dyserythropoiesis. *JAMA 140*:554, 1980.

151. Martelli, M. F., Falini, B., Rambotti, P., Touato, M., and Davis, S.: Sideroblastic anemia associated with hairy cell leukemia. *Cancer 48*:762, 1981.

152. Catovsky, D., Shaw, M. T., Hoffbrand, A. V., and Dacie, J. V.: Sideroblastic anemia and its association with leukemia and myelomatosis. A report of five cases. *Br. J. Haematol. 20*:385, 1971.

153. Tranchida, L., Palutke, M., Poylik, M. D., and Prasad, A. S.: Primary acquired sideroblastic anemia preceding monoclonal gam-mopathy and malignant lymphoma. *Am. J. Med. 55*:559, 1973.

154. Dahlke, M. A., and Nowell, P. C.: Chromosomal abnormalities and dyserythropoiesis in the preleukaemic phase of multiple myeloma. *Br. J. Haematol. 31*:111, 1975.

155. Khaleeli, M., Keane, W. M., and Lee, G. R.: Sideroblastic anemia in multiple myeloma: A preleukemic change. *Blood 41*:17, 1973.

156. Najean, Y., and Pecking, A.: Refractory anemia with excess of blast cells, prognostic factors and effect of treatment with androgens or cytosine arabinoside. *Cancer 44*:1976, 1979.

157. Bagby, G. C., Jr., Gabourel, J. D., and Linman, J. W.: Glucocorticoid therapy in the preleukemic syndrome (hemopoietic dysplasia). *Ann. Intern. Med. 92*:55, 1980.

158. Armitage, J. O., Dick, F. R., Needleman, S. W., and Burns, C. P.: Effect of chemotherapy for the dysmyelopoietic syndrome. *Cancer Treat. Rep. 65*:601, 1981.

159. Bhaduri, S., et al.: A case of preleukemia — Reconstitution of normal marrow function after bone marrow transplantation (BMT) from identical twins. *Blut 38*:145, 1979.

Hemopoietic stem cell disorders— myeloproliferative disorders

CHAPTER 23

Polycythemia vera

SCOTT MURPHY

Definition and history

Polycythemia vera is a hemopoietic stem cell disorder characterized by sustained cellular proliferation. This proliferation is first of all expressed by an increase in the production of red cells, and an absolute increase in erythroid mass is the *sine qua non* for making the diagnosis. The other expressions of myeloid proliferation, leukocytosis and thrombocytosis, with their associated manifestations of splenomegaly, myeloid metaplasia, and myelofibrosis, are variably expressed at the onset and during the progression of the disease. Management depends on recognition of evolving pathophysiologic patterns and anticipation of possible complications.

In 1892, Vaquez [1] first described polycythemia vera as an autonomous erythrocytosis. However, neither he nor Osler, who further delineated the disease in 1903 [2], recognized the presence of generalized myeloproliferation. Increased granulocytic and megakaryocytic activity were first described by Türk in 1904 [3] and by Hutchinson and Miller in 1906 [4]. The evolution of the disease to an anemic phase was reported by Freund in 1919 [5] and by Minot and Buckman in 1923 [6]. In 1935, Hirsch [7] described the replacement of hemopoietic marrow by fibrous and sclerotic tissue, and the complete natural history and course of the disease were outlined by Rosenthal and Bassen in 1938 [8].

Etiology and pathogenesis

The cause of polycythemia vera is completely unknown, but several mechanisms have been proposed to explain the pathogenesis of the panmyelosis. These include unregulated neoplastic proliferation of marrow cells, increased proliferation of normal marrow cells in response to an abnormal myeloproliferative factor [9], and increased sensitivity of marrow cells to normal regulatory factors, such as erythropoietin [10]. Recent studies of these possible mechanisms have been aided by observations of female patients heterozygous for the X-linked glucose-6-phosphate dehydrogenase (G-6-PD) gene [11] (see Fig. 16-5). In a study of two such patients with polycythemia vera, skin fibroblasts representative of somatic cells contained both type A and B isoenzymes [12]. In otherwise normal women, an equivalent distribution of isoenzyme types would be found in blood cells. However, in these patients, only a single enzyme, type A, was found in erythrocytes, granulocytes, and platelets. These observations virtually exclude the possibility that polycythemia vera results from accelerated activity of normal marrow. They strongly suggest that the disease has a unicellular origin and that it is clonal, at least at the time of study. The involvement of erythrocytes, granulocytes, and platelets suggests that the cell of origin is an abnormal pluripotential hemopoietic stem cell. Lymphocytes contained both enzymes, which shows that either lymphocytes are not involved in this clonal expansion or large numbers of lymphocytes, present at the time of study, are the progeny of cells whose origin preceded the onset of the disease. Furthermore, similar to idiopathic myelofibrosis [13,14], the marrow fibrosis that develops during the course of some patients appears to be a reactive phenomenon and not the result of proliferation of fibroblasts derived from the polycythemia vera clone. Normal megakaryocytes and platelets contain growth factors that stimulate the proliferation of fibroblasts [15], and it has been proposed that intramedullary release of growth factors by abnormal megakaryocytes results in the characteristic hyperplasia of fibroblasts [16].

Information concerning the relationship between the polycythemia vera clone and residual normal stem cells has been obtained from studies of erythroid (CFU-E) and granulocytic (CFU-C) colony-forming units during culture of marrow cells in semisolid media. Formation of CFU-E from normal marrow requires the addition of exogenous erythropoietin [17]. However, marrow from patients with polycythemia vera will form CFU-E without exogenous erythropoietin, so-called endogenous CFU-E [18]. Studies in two G-6-PD heterozygotes in remission showed that all endogenous CFU-E arise from the polycythemia vera clone, but that the addition of erythropoietin stimulates the formation of CFU-E from both the polycythemia vera clone and from normal residual stem cells [19]. CFU-C of both enzyme types were also found in these cultures [20]. These studies imply that normal residual stem cells are present in the marrow, but that their proliferation is inhibited by an unknown mechanism that gives the polycythemia vera clone a growth advantage.

Since the addition of crude erythropoietin antibodies to the culture medium substantially reduces the number of endogenous CFU-E, it has been proposed that these colonies are not autonomous, but merely exessively sensitive to extremely low levels of erythropoietin present in the culture medium [10,17]. By inference, precursors of granulocytes and platelets would be excessively responsive to physiologic mediators as well. Unfortunately, the available assays for erythropoietin are not sufficiently sensitive to detect the extremely low levels that may be present in patients with polycythemia vera.

Epidemiologic aspects

Accurate information on the incidence of polycythemia vera is not available, but it would appear to be a relatively uncommon disorder. Thus the minimum annual incidence rate was found to be four to five new cases per million population in the Baltimore area [21].

Polycythemia vera is a disease of the middle and later years of life, the peak age of onset being in the 50- to 60-year-old group, with a wide range of distribution from adolescence to old age [22]. Males are affected slightly more frequently than females. A recent survey of the literature identified nine childhood cases [23]. No preponderance of any particular national, geographic, or religious group was noticed in one large series [25]. Only four well-substantiated familial occurrences of polycythemia vera have been reported [26].

Clinical features

The onset of polycythemia vera is usually insidious and often first suspected after a routine blood count discloses an elevated hemoglobin or hematocrit level. In some cases it may not be diagnosed until after the occurrence of a dramatic complication, such as a major thrombosis or hemorrhage.

The symptoms of this disease are characteristically varied and nonspecific and may be referrable to almost every organ system [22]. Most of the symptoms are related to circulatory disturbances resulting from the increase of red cell mass. The resultant hypervolemia and hyperviscosity cause vascular distention, impairment of blood flow, stasis, and ultimately, tissue hypoxia [27,28] (see Chap. 8). The high hematocrit may enhance thrombus formation by facilitating movement of platelets to the endothelial surface [29]. It has been suggested [30] that the coexistent thrombocytosis interacts with hypervolemia and hyperviscosity to increase the incidence of thrombosis, thromboembolism, and hemorrhage, which is already high in the advanced age group of these patients.

Symptoms related to circulatory disturbances in the central nervous system occur most frequently and are probably related to the decrease in cerebral blood flow observed in patients with even mild polycythemia [28,31]. Headache, dizziness, vertigo, and tinnitus are often present. Visual disturbances are common and include blurred vision, scotomata, and diplopia. Cardiovascular symptoms include angina pectoris or inter-mittent claudication. Gastrointestinal symptoms are frequent and include pain or hemorrhage related to peptic ulcer, which has four to five times the normal incidence in patients with polycythemia vera [32]. Early satiety and fullness as well as abdominal pain may be related to peptic ulcers or to splenomegaly.

A common complaint is pruritus, which occurs in about 40 percent of patients and is often most troublesome after a warm bath or shower. The pathogenesis of the itching and urticaria that occurs in 10 percent of the patients is not known, but it may be related to increased histamine release by granulocytes [33].

Thrombosis and hemorrhage occur in about 40 percent of patients and are a significant cause of morbidity and mortality [25,34–36]. The most frequent sites of arterial occlusion are the peripheral, cerebral, and coronary vascular systems. Thrombophlebitis with pulmonary embolism are found more commonly than mesenteric, splenic, hepatic, and portal venous occlusions. However, polycythemia vera is still a major cause for such intraabdominal emergencies [37,38].

Spontaneous minor hemorrhagic phenomena, such as epistaxis, gingival bleeding, and ecchymoses, are common [25,34,37,39]. More serious, often life-threatening hemorrhages may occur in patients with peptic ulcer and uncontrolled disease [32].

The same factors that contribute to thrombosis and hemorrhage often give rise to serious problems during and following surgery [40,41]. More than 75 percent of patients with uncontrolled polycythemia vera who undergo surgery develop hemorrhagic or thrombotic complications, and approximately one-third die as a result. A dramatic reduction in these complications occurs with adequate control of the disease.

The most common physical finding is plethora or ruddy cyanosis of the face, nose, ears, and lips. The conjunctiva and retina and the mucous membranes of the mouth also appear congested. Fundoscopic examination often reveals the retinas to be deeply colored with markedly engorged retinal veins. Arterial hypertension is common and may improve with reduction of the blood volume [22,25].

The only physical finding that is significant in the differential diagnosis of polycythemia vera is splenomegaly. It is present in about three-fourths of patients with polycythemia vera at the time of diagnosis [22]. The enlargement is usually moderate, and marked splenomegaly is rare in early disease. Roentgenograms of the abdomen or radioisotopic scanning of the spleen may sometimes demonstrate an enlarged spleen that cannot be detected on physical examination [42]. Splenic enlargement is not due to the expanded blood volume per se, since there is usually little or no diminution in spleen size when blood volume is reduced by phlebotomy, and splenomegaly is not seen in patients with secondary polycythemia vera. Extramedullary hemopoiesis and proliferation of splenic reticulum have been suggested as responsible for the enlargement, but the exact cause has still not been defined [43].

Modest enlargement of the liver is present in about one-third of patients at the time of diagnosis, and the enlargement tends to increase as the disease progresses.

Laboratory features

ERYTHROCYTES

The diagnosis of polycythemia vera requires the demonstration of an increased red cell mass at some time during the course of the disease. The red cell mass should be measured directly, since it cannot always be deduced from the hemoglobin or hematocrit determinations or the red cell count [22]. The plasma volume is within the normal range in the majority of patients, but it may be increased, particularly in patients with pronounced hepatosplenomegaly [44].

Different patterns of erythropoiesis have been demonstrated during the course of polycythemia vera [45]. Early in the disease, erythropoiesis is characterized by increased red cell production at intramedullary sites associated with a normal red cell life-span. Ferrokinetic studies at this time reveal accelerated plasma iron turnover, reflecting increased erythropoietic activity. There is initial rapid accumulation of radioactive iron in the marrow and subsequent complete incorporation in circulating erythrocytes [46]. As the disease progresses, extramedullary ineffective hemopoiesis occurs with progressive shortening of the red cell life-span secondary to increasing splenic sequestration [45,47].

Changes in red cell morphology accompany these changes in patterns of erythropoiesis. Early in the course of the disease, red cell morphology is usually normal unless iron deficiency is present. Mild anisocytosis, poikilocytosis, polychromatophilia, and a rare erythroblast may be present in the blood film. In some cases there is an increased percentage of cells containing hemoglobin F [48]. As the disease progresses, striking morphologic changes occur, reflecting the increasing degrees of extramedullary ineffective hemopoiesis. Thus marked anisocytosis and poikilocytosis are seen with ovalocytes, elliptocytes, and teardrop forms, and increasing numbers of nucleated red cells appear in the peripheral blood.

GRANULOCYTES

Leukocytosis with a relative and absolute granulocytosis occurs in about two-thirds of cases [22]. It is usually moderate in degree (12,000 to 25,000 per microliter), but extreme degrees (50,000 to 100,000 per microliter) are sometimes observed, particularly late in the course. A moderate shift to the left in the granulocyte series frequently accompanies the increase in granulocytes, and an occasional metamyelocyte, myelocyte, or even earlier form may be seen in the blood. An increase in the absolute basophil count (above 65 per microliter) is observed in about two-thirds of patients [33]. Utilizing DF^{32}P-labeled granulocytes, it has been demonstrated that there is an increase in the total blood granulocyte pool size in all polycythemia vera patients with peripheral blood granulocyte counts greater than 10,000 per microliter [49]. This granulocytosis reflects a significant increase in granulocyte production. The daily granulocyte turnover rate may range from normal to as much as 12 times normal. As far as is known, granulocyte function is normal [50].

PLATELETS AND COAGULATION

Thrombocytosis is present in about 50 percent of patients at the time of diagnosis [22]. The degree of thrombocytosis is usually modest, with platelet counts in the range of 450,000 to 800,000 per microliter, but occasionally counts of a million or more may be seen. The platelet life-span is minimally reduced, and there is a moderate increase in the size of the splenic platelet pool [51]. Thus the degree of elevation of the platelet count may underestimate the increased rate of platelet production so characteristic of this disorder. Estimates of volume of marrow megakaryocytes are increased in accord with the increase in rate of platelet production, suggesting that thrombopoiesis is effective. Reduction of red cell mass with phlebotomy is not associated with an increase in platelet count or rate of platelet production in contrast to the reactive thrombocytosis observed secondary to bleeding in normal individuals [52]. This presumably reflects the relative autonomy of cell production in this disorder.

Morphologic and functional abnormalities of platelets also occur. The blood film often reveals a small population of abnormally large platelets with deficient granulation [53]. Platelets from the majority of patients show some abnormality in studies of aggregation with ADP, epinephrine, and collagen [54]. However, these in vitro tests correlate very poorly with clinical episodes of thrombosis and hemorrhage, so their meaning is obscure. The bleeding time, which is the best measurement of platelet function in vivo, is almost always normal, even in patients with hemorrhagic manifestations [54,55].

The prothrombin time, partial thromboplastin time, and fibrinogen level are usually normal. The ratio of anticoagulant to plasma must be considered in blood collection in order to prevent excessive concentration of anticoagulant in plasma from blood with high hematocrit readings.

MARROW

Excessive hemopoiesis in polycythemia vera results in hyperplasia of erythroid, myeloid, and megakaryocytic elements within those areas of the skeleton which normally contain active marrow [56] and minimal extension of the active hemopoietic marrow peripherally into the proximal portions of the humerus and femur [47].

Marrow specimens obtained by needle aspiration or biopsy are hypercellular with decreased fat in nearly all cases. Because of granulocytic hyperplasia, the hypercellularity is much more pronounced than in the secondary polycythemias. Megakaryocytes are increased in size and, most strikingly, in number [57]. Stainable marrow iron is decreased or absent in the majority of cases [58]. This is presumably related to chronic occult blood loss or utilization of iron during expansion of the red cell mass. Sectioned biopsy specimens are superior to aspirates for determining cellularity and are essential for determining the presence and extent of myelofibrosis and osteosclerosis [59]. Fibrosis is rare at the time of diagnosis, but a significant increase in reticulin content can be demonstrated by silver stain in 10 to 20 percent of marrow specimens. Progression to the spent phase of postpolycythemic myeloid metaplasia is accompanied by an increased prominence of the normal reticulin network, the development of abnormally coarse reticulin fibers, and ultimately, frank myelofibrosis. The development of marrow fibrosis is accompanied by extension of hemopoietic marrow into the periphery of the extremities and the development of extramedullary hemopoiesis [47].

URIC ACID

The excessive cellular proliferation in this disease results in increased synthesis and degradation of nucleoprotein and the production of increased amounts of uric acid [60]. Thus hyperuricemia and hyperuricosuria are present in about 40 percent of patients at the time of diagnosis. Both tend to increase in frequency and severity as the disease progresses. Most patients remain asymptomatic, but approximately 5 to 10 percent develop symptoms and signs of gout [61].

ARTERIAL OXYGEN SATURATION

Nearly all patients with polycythemia vera have a near-normal arterial oxygen saturation [62]. Mild degrees of unsaturation may occur in some patients, and in one study, arterial oxygen saturation was found to be between 88 and 92 percent in 10 percent of well-documented cases [22]. The pathogenesis of this unsaturation is not clear, since pulmonary-function testing is generally normal. Pulmonary capillary blood volume and the size of the pulmonary vascular bed may be reduced in some patients with resultant abnormalities in the ventilation-perfusion relationship [63]. In addition, in vitro oxygen consumption in arterial blood samples will continue even at low temperatures if the leukocyte and platelet counts are high and the specimen is not analyzed promptly [64]. Thus the hypoxemia may be spurious. In any event, an arterial oxygen saturation greater than 92 percent is characteristic of polycythemia vera, and a normal value is helpful in excluding erythrocytosis secondary to pulmonary and cardiac conditions.

ERYTHROPOIETIN

Absent or reduced erythropoietin levels have been found in plasma and urine of patients with polycythemia vera in marked contrast to the increased levels found in most cases of secondary polycythemia [65] (Fig. 23-1). The routine biologic assay for erythropoietin is, unfortunately, crude and laborious, and measure-

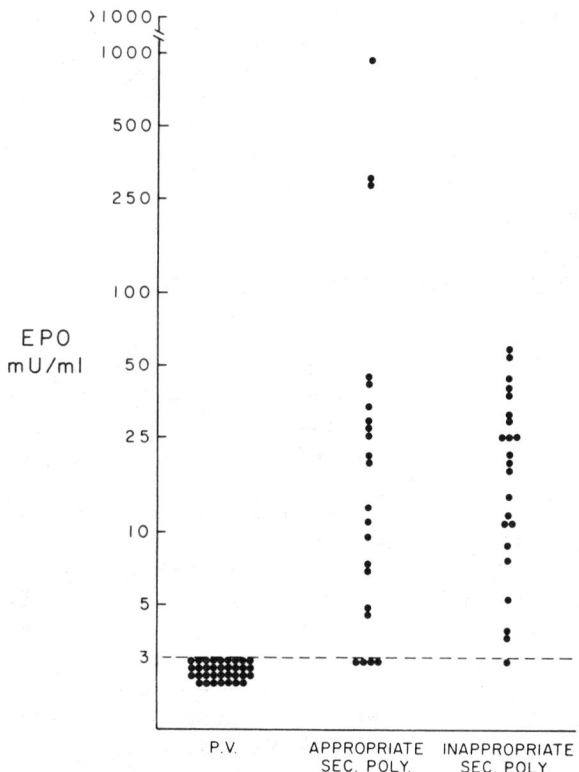

FIGURE 23-1 Plasma erythropoietin in the polycythemias. Erythropoietin titers as measured by bioassay of concentrates prepared from plasma of patients with hematocrits greater than 53 percent [65]. In uncontrolled polycythemia vera, plasma erythropoietin is below the limits of detection (3 mU/ml). Elevated levels are characteristic of most cases of secondary polycythemia. Similar findings have been reported for radioimmunoassay [66].

ments of erythropoietin levels have not been of much use clinically. Recently, however, a radioimmune assay for erythropoietin has been developed and holds the promise of becoming a useful test in the differential diagnosis of the polycythemias [66].

ERYTHROID STEM CELLS

Erythroid stem cells can be demonstrated and characterized by culturing mononuclear cells obtained from either marrow or blood. Normal erythroid stem cells will grow on semisolid media and form erythroblastic colonies, but only in the presence of erythropoietin [10]. Erythroid stem cells obtained from patients with polycythemia vera, on the other hand, will form colonies in the absence of added erythropoietin [10,17–19] (Fig. 23-2). The emergence of such so-called endogenous colonies is characteristic of autonomous erythroid stem cells and, consequently, could be of diagnostic importance in rare cases.

LEUKOCYTE ALKALINE PHOSPHATASE

The alkaline phosphatase activity of mature polymorphonuclear leukocytes is usually increased in polycythemia vera. Thus approximately 70 percent of patients

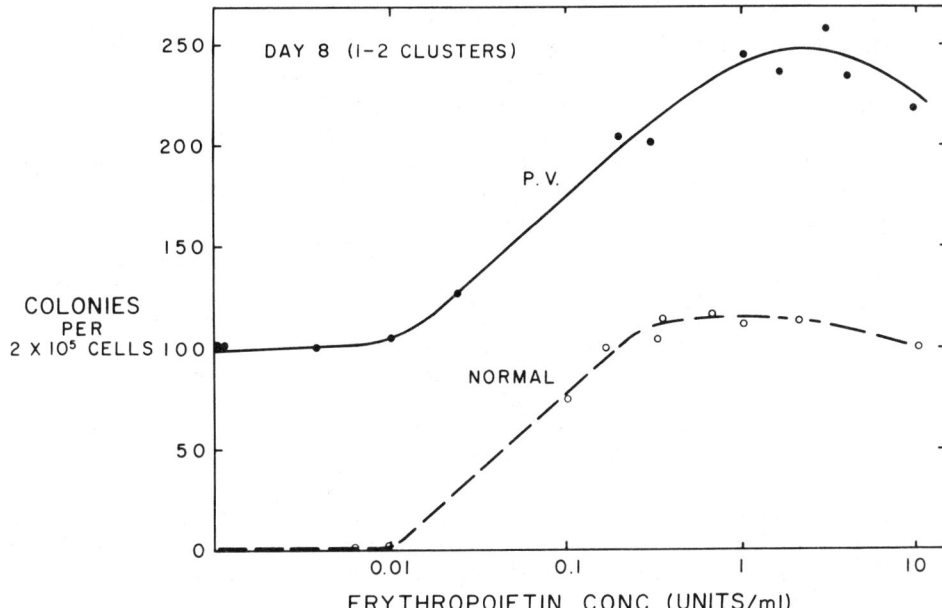

FIGURE 23-2 Early burst-forming colonies in marrow obtained from normals and from patients with polycythemia vera and plated on semisolid media in the presence of various amounts of erythropoietin. (Data from Eaves and Eaves [17].)

have leukocyte alkaline phosphatase (LAP) "scores" above the upper limits of normal, while the remainder have normal LAP values [22]. No clinical or hematologic differences are apparent in patients with normal LAP activity as compared with those with increased LAP activity [67,68]. The LAP activity of individual patients tends to remain within a fairly narrow range during the course of the disease, regardless of treatment or disease transition to "spent" polycythemia [67].

LAP determination is of limited value in helping to differentiate polycythemia vera from other forms of erythrocytosis in which normal activity is the rule. An elevated LAP activity is, at best, confirmatory, and a normal LAP score does not exclude the diagnosis. Furthermore, a variety of nonspecific stimuli (e.g., fever, infection, inflammation, corticosteroids) may elevate the LAP activity in a patient with secondary polycythemia.

VITAMIN B_{12} AND B_{12}-BINDING CAPACITY

Serum vitamin B_{12} content and the capacity of the serum to bind additional vitamin B_{12} added in vitro (expressed as unsaturated B_{12} binding capacity, or $UB_{12}BC$) are both increased in many patients with uncontrolled polycythemia vera. Vitamin B_{12} levels above 900 pg/ml are found in about one-third of patients before treatment or during relapse [22]. Similarly, the serum $UB_{12}BC$ level is increased to values above 2200 pg/ml in about three-fourths of these patients [69]. Thus serum vitamin B_{12} content is within the normal range in approximately two-thirds of all instances in which the $UB_{12}BC$ is elevated. This is unlike the situation in chronic myelogenous leukemia, in which a concomitant rise in serum vitamin B_{12} level accompanies the rise in $UB_{12}BC$.

The source of the increased amounts of vitamin B_{12} and B_{12}-binding protein in serum is complex. Plasma contains three vitamin B_{12}-binding proteins: transcobalamin I, II, and III [70]. Transcobalamin II is immunologically distinct from I and III, contains no carbohydrate, and is not commonly elevated in polycythemia vera. Transcobalamins I and III belong to a group of immunologically indistinguishable glycoproteins known as R-type vitamin B_{12}-binding proteins [71]. They differ in sialic acid content and, therefore, electrophoretic mobility. The increase in $UB_{12}BC$ in chronic myelogenous leukemia is predominantly due to an increase in transcobalamin I, while in polycythemia vera it is predominantly related to an increase in transcobalamin III [72]. However, there is considerable overlap. Both proteins are released by granulocytes and their precursors, and serum levels correlate with the rate of granulocyte turnover. When present, these abnormalities help to distinguish polycythemia vera from other types of erythrocytosis [73]. Furthermore, serum $UB_{12}BC$ levels correlate with disease activity and provide an index of therapeutic control [69,73].

CYTOGENETICS

Reports of abnormal cytogenetic findings of marrow cells in polycythemia vera must be interpreted with caution, since in many cases, the patients have been previously treated with myelosuppressive therapy, which may have been responsible for the changes seen. For example, chromosomal abnormalities (deletions, translocations, clones of abnormal cells) were found in marrow cells of 66 percent of 32 patients previously treated with ^{32}P [74]. However, in a large series of previously untreated patients, chromosomal abnormalities were found in only 26 percent [75]. Aneuploidy was the most common abnormality; an extra C-group chromosome and low mitotic index were also noted.

MISCELLANEOUS LABORATORY FINDINGS

Elevated blood and urine histamine levels are present in the majority of patients with uncontrolled polycythemia vera [33]. The source of the elevation is uncertain, but blood histamine is contained almost entirely within circulating leukocytes, and the activity of histidine decarboxylase, the enzyme responsible for the conversion of histidine to histamine, is increased in the leukocytes of patients with polycythemia vera [76]. Mean serum lysozyme (muramidase) levels are significantly elevated in patients with polycythemia vera, although most individual values are within the normal range [77]. This increase is thought to reflect granulocytic hyperplasia. Serum iron levels are frequently decreased, reflecting therapeutic or spontaneous blood loss. Hyperkalemia has been reported in polycythemia vera and other myeloproliferative disorders associated with thrombocytosis. Since plasma potassium concentration is usually normal, the increased serum concentration is probably spurious and related to potassium release from platelets during coagulation of the blood in vitro [78]. Similarly, glucose levels may fall significantly in vitro if the patient has high cell counts and the specimen is allowed to rest at room temperature for a significant period of time prior to analysis.

Diagnosis and differential diagnosis

Polycythemia vera is a rather well defined disease entity, and in the fully developed case, the diagnosis should present little difficulty. The following criteria, adopted in 1968 by the national Polycythemia Vera Study Group, serve to document the presence of the disease and differentiate it from other forms of polycythemia. The diagnostic criteria have been classified according to their relative significance in two categories:

Category A

   A1. Increased red cell mass (measured with ^{51}Cr-labeled red cells); males $\geq$ 36 ml/kg; females $\geq$ 32 ml/kg

   A2. Normal arterial oxygen saturation: $\geq$ 92 percent

   A3. Splenomegaly

Category B

   B1. Thrombocytosis: platelets $\geq$ 400,000 per microliter

   B2. Leukocytosis: white count $\geq$ 12,000 per microliter (in absence of fever or infection)

   B3. Elevated leukocyte alkaline phosphatase score: >100 in absence of fever or infection

   B4. Elevated serum vitamin B_{12} or unbound B_{12}-binding capacity: B_{12} > 900 pg/ml; $UB_{12}BC$ > 2200 pg/ml

The diagnosis of polycythemia vera is acceptable if (1) all three parameters from category A are present or (2) the combination of an elevated red cell mass and normal arterial oxygen saturation is present with any two parameters from caterogy B.

The most common type of "polycythemia" referred to a hematologist for evaluation is really no polycythemia at all, but an entity variously known as *relative polycythemia, stress erythrocytosis,* or *spurious erythrocytosis* [79]. This entity, discussed in Chap. 74, is characterized by an elevated venous hematocrit, a normal or near-normal red cell mass, and, especially in smokers, a decreased plasma volume. It is not a hematologic disorder, but it can be differentiated with certainty from the true erythrocytoses only by measurement of the red cell mass and plasma volume.

Once an absolute erythrocytosis has been documented, a distinction must be made between polycythemia vera and the secondary polycythemias (see Table 23-1). A normal chest x-ray and electrocardiogram, along with a normal arterial oxygen saturation, help to exclude cardiopulmonary disease. Search for an occult erythropoietin-producing neoplasm should be carried out with, at least, an intravenous pyelogram and a liver scan. Measurement of the P_{50} of the oxygen-hemoglobin dissociation curve excludes an abnormal hemoglobin. Carboxyhemoglobin should be measured if the patient is a smoker, since an elevated blood carbon monoxide level leads to reduction in the P_{50} and subsequent increase in red cell volume to the abnormal range [80]. In a difficult case, one may be helped by an erythropoietin assay (Fig. 23-1) and a marrow culture designed to identify endogenous erythroid colonies.

The criteria of the Polycythemia Vera Study Group have been useful, but they have been criticized as so restrictive as to exclude valid cases. Certainly some patients present with only a few features of the disease and then develop a more characteristic and complete clinical picture as time passes. In addition, there are examples of pure erythrocytosis with no primary cause and no accompanying leukocytosis, thrombocytosis, or splenomegaly. In one large series [81] of such cases, only 12 percent evolved into a classical picture or polycythemia vera. In two patients with pure erythrocytosis, undetectable plasma erythropoietin levels and endogenous CFU-E formation were documented, suggesting that the erythroid compartment in these patients behaves as in typical polycythemia vera [82]. At present, the relationship between this entity and typical polycythemia vera is uncertain.

Therapy

Management of the patient with polycythemia vera requires understanding of the underlying pathophysiology and an appreciation of the chronic, progressive nature of the disease and the complications that may occur as a result of both the disease and its treatment. There

TABLE 23-1   Findings of value in the differential diagnosis of polycythemia
vera from secondary polycythemia and spurious erythrocytosis

Findings	Polycythemia vera	Secondary polycythemia	Spurious erythrocytosis
Red blood cell mass	Increased	Increased	Normal
Splenomegaly	Present	Absent	Absent
Arterial oxygen saturation	Normal	Decreased or normal	Normal
Thrombocytosis	Present	Absent	Absent
Blood histamine	Increased	Normal	Normal
Serum $UB_{12}BC$	Increased	Normal	Normal
Serum vitamin B_{12}	Increased	Normal	Normal
Leukocyte alkaline phosphatase	Increased	Normal	Normal
Marrow	Panhyperplasia	Erythroid hyperplasia	Normal
Basophil count	Increased	Normal	Normal
Leukocytosis	Present	Absent	Absent
Erythropoietin	Decreased	Increased	Normal
Serum iron	Decreased	Normal	Normal

are two main approaches to the management of the erythrocytotic stage of the disease. The first is to remove the end product of red cell proliferation by the use of phlebotomy; the second is to attempt to control the proliferative process by the use of a myelosuppressive agent. In practice, one often resorts to both approaches sequentially or in combination, depending on the predominant disease manifestations at any particular time.

Phlebotomy can reduce the increased blood volume to normal within a relatively short period of time, thereby relieving the patient of many distressing symptoms and at the same time reducing the risk of thrombosis or hemorrhage. Phlebotomies of 350 to 500 ml may be performed every other day until the hematocrit is reduced to the normal range. This regimen is well tolerated by nearly all patients, although smaller phlebotomies of 200 to 300 ml may be desirable in elderly patients or those with cardiovascular disease, in whom rapid hemodynamic changes are undesirable. In emergencies, such as an impending vascular occlusion, or in preparation of the patient for urgent surgery, intensive phlebotomy accompanied by plasma infusion may be lifesaving. Certainly phlebotomy should be the initial therapy prescribed at the time of diagnosis.

Since each 500-ml phlebotomy removes approximately 200 mg of iron, patients managed in this manner for a period of time become iron-deficient. Development of a microcytic cell population may allow the maintenance of a normal hematocrit level with red cell counts of 6 to 8 million per microliter. This iron-deficient hypochromic microcytic polycythemia may be associated at times with such symptoms as glossitis, cheilosis, dysphagia, anorexia, weight loss, and asthenia. These symptoms are reversed by iron administration, but concurrent iron therapy will increase the frequency with which phlebotomy will be required. If phlebotomy is selected as the sole means of chronic therapy, one needs to choose an upper limit of hematocrit above which the patient will be bled. This level has generally been considered to be 50 percent. However, in recent studies, an increase in vascular complica-

tions and a decrease in cerebral blood flow and mental alertness were observed to begin at hematocrits above 46 percent [28,31,83]. Iron-deficient red cells have decreased deformability and may make a greater contribution to whole-blood viscosity than normal cells [84]. It is possible that more aggressive phlebotomy, reducing the hematocrit to levels in the low forties, would decrease the incidence of vascular complications seen in patients treated with phlebotomy alone [85].

Phlebotomy is useful only in removing the end product of red cell proliferation and has no suppressive effect on myeloproliferation. It does not relieve pruritus or symptoms related to hepatosplenomegaly. It does not control thrombocytosis, and both retrospective and prospective studies have suggested that its use as sole therapy is associated with an increased risk of thrombotic and hemorrhagic complications [85,86]. Control of these manifestations requires myelosuppressive therapy.

Radioactive phosphorus (^{32}P), first used in the treatment of polycythemia vera in 1940 [87], is still probably the simplest and most convenient form of myelosuppressive therapy. When administered orally or intravenously, ^{32}P enters the miscible body phosphate pool and is concentrated to some degree by mitotically active cells in the marrow, liver, and spleen. The intravenous route is preferred in order to circumvent variability in gastrointestinal absorption. Following an initial series of phlebotomies to decrease the expanded blood volume, thus reducing the immediate threat of thrombosis or hemorrhage, 3 to 5 mCi of ^{32}P (2.3 mCi/m²) is given intravenously. As with any form of myelosuppressive therapy, there is a latent period before the maximum effects of therapy are seen. One cannot expect suppression of marrow proliferation, reduction in spleen size, and normalization of the hematologic picture until 2 to 3 months after onset of therapy. Often a second small dose of 2 to 3 mCi of ^{32}P is required 12 to 16 weeks after the initial injection in order to bring the disease under complete control. ^{32}P affords satisfactory control of the disease in 75 to 85 percent of cases [25,36,39]. Remissions frequently last 6 to 24 months and sometimes longer. Once remission has occurred, follow-up visits need to be made only every 2 to 3 months. Marrow hypoplasia and dangerous degrees of leukopenia or thrombocytopenia are rarely produced.

Interest in other forms of myelosuppressive therapy in polycythemia vera stems primarily from concern regarding the leukemogenic role of ^{32}P and other forms of ionizing radiation. While a small background incidence of acute leukemia seems to be characteristic of the natural history of polycythemia vera, retrospective studies have suggested that its incidence is increased after radiation exposure. In one series [88], the incidence of acute leukemia in ^{32}P-treated patients was 14 percent. Calculations suggested that this incidence was 20 to 40 times greater than that expected for a population of normal human subjects exposed to similar radiation doses and times at risk. These considerations imply that the polycythemia vera clone may be more susceptible to radiation-induced leukemia than normal marrow cells.

As other modes of therapy were sought, impressive results were obtained using alkylating agents such as busulfan (Myleran), chlorambucil (Leukeran), cyclophosphamide (Cytoxan), and melphalan (Alkeran) [89–91]. Busulfan and melphalan have generally been used with a starting dose of 4 to 6 mg daily, chlorambucil with a dose of 6 to 10 mg daily, and cyclophosphamide with a dose of 100 to 150 mg daily. Therapy can be initiated while the hematocrit is being reduced to normal levels by phlebotomy. The blood count must be checked frequently (every 2 to 3 weeks) and necessary adjustments made in dosage. As with ^{32}P, a satisfactory response can be expected in about 85 percent of patients [91]. The maximum response to therapy with busulfan and chlorambucil occurs in approximately 2 to 4 months. The delay may be somewhat shorter with cyclophosphamide and melphalan. A decrease in the elevated white cell and platelet counts is generally observed first, the hematocrit level being the last parameter to be controlled. Most patients have some reduction in spleen size, commonly to an extent that it is no longer palpable. Undesirable thrombocytopenia (platelet counts less than 100,000 per microliter) occurs infrequently with chlorambucil and cyclophosphamide and is reversible with cessation of therapy. Busulfan and melphalan, however, may produce more severe thrombocytopenia in about 25 percent of patients. In many instances, this platelet depression may be long-lasting and difficult to manage [92]. Chronic busulfan administration has also been associated with other untoward effects, such as skin pigmentation and pulmonary fibrosis [93], and it should be used with caution. However, it may be particularly useful in patients whose hematocrit is easily controlled by phebotomy but who have significant thrombocytosis. The use of cyclophosphamide is associated with gastrointestinal distress, dysuria, hematuria, and alopecia. Chlorambucil and melphalan are generally better tolerated. If drug therapy is stopped soon after the hematologic picture returns to normal, relapse occurs relatively rapidly [91].

The mean duration of unmaintained response with chlorambucil, melphalan, and cyclophosphamide is about 5 to 6 months. Remissions induced by busulfan are longer-lived, the mean approaching 1 year. Remissions can be prolonged by maintenance therapy.

The benefits and risks of these therapeutic approaches were examined in a prospective randomized trial that compared treatment with phlebotomy alone, an alkylating agent (chlorambucil) supplemented by phlebotomy, and ^{32}P supplemented by phlebotomy [94]. After 14 years of study, there were no statistically significant differences in survival. However, the causes of death were markedly influenced by therapy [85]. The risk of acute leukemia among patients treated with chlorambucil was 13.5 times greater than that among patients treated with phlebotomy and 2.3 times greater than that among patients treated with ^{32}P (Fig. 23-3). Leukemia in this population of patients is characteristically refractory to therapy [95]. Although the leukemogenic potential of alkylating agents was not appreciated when the study was begun, the intervening years have documented the increased incidence of leukemia in patients treated with alkylating agents for management of multiple myeloma, Hodgkin's disease, and carcinoma of the breast and ovary [96–98]. It is important to recognize, however, that in a parallel study in Europe [99] busulfan given intermittently was found to be less leukemogenic, indicating that this potential may be dependent on both the alkylating agent employed and its schedule of administration. In addition, the prospective randomized trial showed an increased incidence of nonhematologic malignancies of rapidly proliferating tissue (gastrointestinal tract and skin) in patients treated with chlorambucil and ^{32}P as compared with phlebotomy alone [115].

In contrast, there was a significant excess of severe thrombotic episodes in patients treated with phlebotomy alone, particularly during the first 3 years of treatment. The risk was markedly increased in patients over 70 years of age and in those with a history of a thrombotic event prior to entry. Risk was not associated with hematocrit level or platelet count either at entry into the study or at the time of the thrombosis [100]. In a second study [101], phlebotomy was supplemented with aspirin, 300 mg three times daily, and dipyridamole, 75 mg three times daily, in an attempt to inhibit platelet function and reduce the incidence of thrombosis. The rate of thrombosis was not reduced, and there was a significant increase in the rate of gastrointestinal hemorrhage requiring hospitalization. Thus the use of these platelet-function inhibitors was deleterious.

In summary, older patients and patients with previous thrombotic events should not be treated with phlebotomy alone, but rather with some form of myelosuppression. In the younger patient, phlebotomy alone is acceptable if the patient is maintained free of complications of the disease. For the younger patient who requires myelosuppression, there is an urgent need for effective agents whose use will not be complicated by subsequent malignant transformation. In preliminary

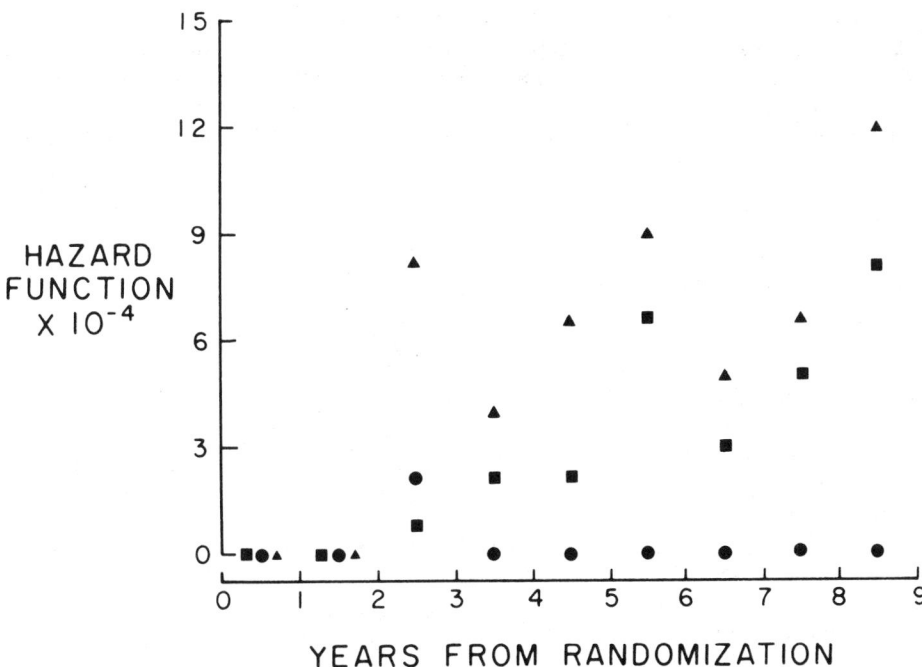

FIGURE 23-3   Hazard function for acute leukemia in polycythemia vera. Patients were randomized to be treated with phlebotomy alone (●), chlorambucil plus phlebotomy (▲), or ^{32}P plus phlebotomy (■). The hazard function is the incidence rate of leukemia in each study year, assuming survival without leukemia to the start of that year. The incidence of leukemia is significantly increased in patients treated with chlorambucil compared with patients treated with phlebotomy alone. (Redrawn from Berk et al. [94]. Used with permission.)

studies [116], hydroxyurea appears to be such an agent.

Acute gouty arthritis in polycythemia vera is treated in the same manner as in primary gout, with colchicine, phenylbutazone, or corticosteroids. Chronic gouty complications may be reduced if myelosuppressive therapy is used to control cellular proliferation, thereby reducing nucleoprotein turnover and the level of serum and urinary uric acid. For patients who do not receive myelosuppressive therapy, the introduction of the xanthine oxidase inhibitor allopurinol has been an important therapeutic advance [102]. This agent, given orally at a dose of 300 mg daily, blocks the formation of uric acid from its precursors, results in fall in serum uric acid levels and urinary uric acid excretion, and reduces the incidence of chronic gouty complications.

Pruritis may be severe and disabling in some patients. It is generally improved by myelosuppressive therapy, but it may persist even when the blood picture and physical examination are entirely normal. Antihistamines usually are not effective, although cyproheptadine may be of benefit. Recently, cholestyramine [103] and cimetidine [104] have been reported to be useful.

Course and prognosis

The course of a patient with polycythemia vera is dominated by the development of complications secondary to the natural history of the disease and its treatment.

SPENT PHASE OF POLYCYTHEMIA VERA

The duration of the erythrocytotic phase of polycythemia vera is quite variable, but in many cases the disease eventually enters a period during which the hematocrit remains at normal levels without treatment for many months or several years. This "spent" phase is characterized by increasing anemia, often associated with continued or increased proliferation of the other cell types in both intramedullary and extramedullary sites.

Approximately 5 to 15 percent of patients develop the complete picture of postpolycythemic myeloid metaplasia with myelofibrosis in the marrow. In one series [105], the interval from diagnosis of polycythemia to the development of this complication was from 5 to 13 years. This complication appears to be an integral part of the natural history of polycythemia vera. At the onset of the erythrocytotic phase, patients who will develop myeloid metaplasia cannot be distinguished from those who will not [105]. In contrast to acute leukemia, it has not been related to a particular mode of therapy. The major sites of myeloid metaplasia are the spleen and liver, although lymph nodes and kidneys may also be involved. As the disease progresses, enlargement of the liver and, particularly, of the spleen becomes more pronounced. Eventually these organs may fill a large part of the abdominal cavity, producing gastrointestinal symptoms and debilitation on a mechanical basis. The enlarging spleen causes another potentially serious problem by sequestering and destroying red cells, platelets, and white cells. Furthermore, splenomegaly is accompanied by an increased plasma volume, which results in a further reduction of the hemoglobin concentration [44]. Any combination of cytopenias may therefore result [107]. However, leukocytosis and thrombocytosis may persist despite progressive anemia. Thus the clinical picture is not fundamentally different from agnogenic myeloid metaplasia.

Treatment of this phase of the disease is usually difficult. It is primarily symptomatic and has relatively little impact on life expectancy. In several series, median survival has been approximately 2 years [106,108]. Myelosuppressive therapy may be indicated to control thrombocytosis, leukocytosis, or splenomegaly, but even small doses of cytotoxic drug or ^{32}P may upset an already delicate balance and produce severe anemia or pancytopenia. Treatment of the anemia requires recognition of the many causative factors involved. Deficiencies of iron, folic acid, and vitamin B_{12} may be present and should be corrected. If significant shortening of the red cell life-span is demonstrated, treatment with corticosteroids may be helpful [105]. If anemia is due largely to ineffective erythropoiesis or absolute failure of red cell production, the administration of testosterone or one of the related anabolic steroids should be tried [109]. Often, all regimens are ineffective, and periodic transfusions with packed red cells are required. Splenectomy is often considered, but there is a 5 to 15 percent incidence of significant surgical morbidity and mortality in this group of patients [110,111]. Extreme degrees of thrombocytosis with thrombotic or hemorrhagic complications may result, particularly in patients who have thrombocytosis preoperatively. Marked hepatic enlargement may ensue, but this may be part of the natural history of the disease. Nonetheless, splenectomy may be of benefit in carefully selected patients with marked shortening of red cell survival, severe thrombocytopenia, or abdominal symptoms on a mechanical basis. One can expect the best results with the fewest complications if there is adequate functional marrow and a low or normal platelet count preoperatively. If a patient with severe mechanical symptoms is too ill for surgery, irradiation may produce relief for several months [112]. However, the patient must be monitored with great care, since even a few hundred rads can result in severe pancytopenia.

PREGNANCY
Pregnancy in polycythemia vera, although uncommon, has little, if any, effect on the disease. However, polycythemia vera apparently has an adverse effect on pregnancy, as indicated by an increased incidence of infertility, preeclampsia, fetal wastage, and premature births [113]. Severe postpartum hemorrhage may also occur [114].

LIFE EXPECTANCY
Thrombosis and hemorrhage account for approximately 40 percent of deaths in most large series. Acute leukemia and myeloid metaplasia each account for another 15 percent. In a large prospective study [94], the 6-year

mortality in patients treated with chlorambucil or with phlebotomy alone was twice the expected mortality in the American population of comparable age and sex and slightly (1.3 times) greater in those treated with ^{32}P. The median survival times ranged from 8 years in patients receiving chlorambucil to 10 years in patients treated with ^{32}P.

References

1. Vaquez, H. M.: Sur une forme spéciale de cyanose s'accompagnant d'hyperglobulie excessive et persistante. C. R. Soc. Biol. (Paris) 44:384, 1892.
2. Osler, W.: Chronic cyanosis with polycythemia and enlarged spleen: A new clinical entity. Am. J. Med. Sci. 126:187, 1903.
3. Türk, W.: Beitrage zur Kenntnis des Symptomenbildes Polycythamie mit Milztumor und Zyanose. Wien. Klin. Wochenschr. 17:153, 1904.
4. Hutchinson, R., and Miller, C. H.: A case of splenomegalic polycythaemia, with report of post-mortem examination. Lancet 1:744, 1906.
5. Freund, H.: Polyzythamie mit Ausgang in pernisiose anamie. Munch. Med. Wochenschr. 66:84, 1919.
6. Minot, G. R., and Buckman, T. E.: Erythremia (polycythemia rubra vera), the development of anemia, the relation to leukemia, consideration of the basal metabolism in blood formation and destruction and fragility of the red cells. Am. J. Med. Sci. 166:469, 1923.
7. Hirsch, R.: Generalized osteosclerosis with chronic polycythemia vera. Arch. Pathol. 19:91, 1935.
8. Rosenthal, N., and Bassen, F. A.: Course of polycythemia. Arch. Intern. Med. 62:903, 1938.
9. Ward, H. P., Vautrin, R., and Kurnick, J.: Presence of a myeloproliferative factor in patients with polycythemia vera and agnogenic myeloid metaplasia. I. Expansion of the erythropoietin-responsive stem cell compartment. Proc. Soc. Exp. Biol. Med. 147:305, 1974.
10. Zanjani, E. D., Lutton, J. D., Hoffman, R., and Wasserman, L. R.: Erythroid colony formation by polycythemia vera bone marrow in vitro. Dependence on erythropoietin. J. Clin. Invest. 59:841, 1977.
11. Fialkow, P. J.: The origin and development of human tumors studied with cell markers. Physiol. Med. 291:26, 1974.
12. Adamson, J. W., Fialkow, P. J., Murphy, S., Prchal, J. F., and Steinmann, L.: Polycythemia vera: Stem-cell and probable clonal origin of the disease. N. Engl. J. Med. 295:913, 1976.
13. Van Slyck, E. J., Weiss, L., and Dully, M.: Chromosomal evidence for the secondary role of fibroblastic proliferation in acute myelofibrosis. Blood 35:729, 1970.
14. Jacobson, R. J., Salo, A., and Fialkow, P. J.: Agnogenic myeloid metaplasia: A clonal proliferation of hematopoietic stem cells with secondary myelofibrosis. Blood 51:189, 1978.
15. Castro-Malaspina, H., Rabellino, E. M., Yen, A., Nachman, R. L., and Moore, M. A. S.: Human megakaryocyte stimulation of proliferation of bone marrow fibroblasts. Blood 57:781, 1981.
16. Groopman, J. E.: The pathogenesis of myelofibrosis in myeloproliferative disorders. Ann. Intern. Med. 92:857, 1980.
17. Eaves, C. J., and Eaves, A. C.: Erythropoietin (Ep) dose-response curves for three classes of erythroid progenitors in normal human marrow and in patients with polycythemia vera. Blood 52:1196, 1978.
18. Prchal, J. F., and Axelrad, A. A.: Bone-marrow responses in polycythemia vera. N. Engl. J. Med. 290:1382, 1974.
19. Prchal, J. F., Adamson, J. W., Murphy, S., Steinmann, L., and Fialkow, P. J.: Polycythemia vera. The in vitro response of normal and abnormal stem cell lines to erythropoietin. J. Clin. Invest. 61:1044, 1978.
20. Singer, J. W., et al.: Polycythemia vera. Increased expression of normal committed granulocytic stem cells in vitro after exposure of marrow to tritiated thymidine. J. Clin. Invest. 64:1320, 1979.
21. Modan, B.: An epidemiological study of polycythemia vera. Blood 26:657, 1965.

22. Berlin, N. J.: Diagnosis and classification of the polycythemias. *Semin. Hematol.* 12:339, 1976.

23. Danish, E. H., Rasch, C. A., and Harris, J. W.: Polycythemia vera in childhood: Case report and review of the literature. *Am. J. Hematol.* 9:421, 1980.

24. Modan, B.: Polycythemia: A review of epidemiological and clinical aspects. *J. Chronic Dis.* 18:605, 1965.

25. Lawrence, J. H.: *Polycythemia: Physiology, Diagnosis and Treatment Based on 303 Cases.* Modern Medical Monographs, Grune & Stratton, New York, 1955.

26. Ratnoff, W. D., and Gress, R. E.: The familial occurrence of polycythemia vera: Report of a father and son, with consideration of the possible etiologic role of exposure to organic solvents, including tetrachloroethylene. *Blood* 56:233, 1980.

27. Castle, W. B., and Jandl, J. H.: Blood viscosity and blood volume: Opposing influences upon oxygen transport in polycythemia. *Semin. Hematol.* 3:193, 1966.

28. Humphrey, P. R. D., et al.: Cerebral blood-flow and viscosity in relative polycythaemia. *Lancet* 2:873, 1979.

29. Turitto, V. T., and Weiss, H. J.: Red blood cells: Their dual role in thrombus formation. *Science* 207:541, 1980.

30. Dawson, A. A., and Ogston, D.: The influence of the platelet count on the incidence of thrombotic and haemorrhagic complications in polycythaemia vera. *Postgrad. Med. J.* 46:76, 1970.

31. Willison, J. R., et al.: Effect of high haematocrit on alertness. *Lancet* 1:846, 1980.

32. Tinney, W. S., Hall, B. E., and Giffin, H. Z.: Polycythemia vera and peptic ulcer. *Mayo Clin. Proc.* 18:24, 1943.

33. Gilbert, H. S., Warner, R. R. P., and Wasserman, L. R.: A study of histamine in myeloproliferative disease. *Blood* 28:795, 1966.

34. Chievitz, E., and Thiede, T.: Complications and causes of death in polycythemia vera. *Acta Med. Scand.* 172:513, 1962.

35. Videbaek, A.: Polycythaemia vera. Course and prognosis. *Acta. Med. Scand.* 138:179, 1950.

36. Perkins, J., Israels, M. C. G., and Wilkinson, J. F.: Polycythaemia vera: Clinical studies on a series of 127 patients managed without radiation therapy. *Q. J. Med.* 33:499, 1964.

37. Parker, R. G. F.: Occlusion of the hepatic veins in man. *Medicine* 38:369, 1959.

38. Noble, J. A.: Hepatic vein thrombosis complicating polycythemia vera. *Arch. Intern. Med.* 120:105, 1967.

39. Wasserman, L. R.: Polycythemia vera—Its course and treatment: Relation to myeloid metaplasia and leukemia. *Bull. N.Y. Acad. Med.* 3:343, 1954.

40. Rigby, P. G., and Leavell, B. S.: Polycythemia vera: A review of fifty cases with emphasis on risk of surgery. *Arch. Intern. Med.* 106:622, 1960.

41. Wasserman, L. R., and Gilbert, H. S.: Surgical bleeding in polycythemia vera. *Ann. N.Y. Acad. Sci.* 115:122, 1964.

42. Westin, J., Lanner, L.-O., Larsson, A., and Weinfeld, A.: Spleen size in polycythemia. *Acta Med. Scand.* 191:263, 1972.

43. Berg, B., Stahl, E., and Soderstrom, N.: The cytology of spleen aspiration in uncomplicated polycythemia vera. *Scand. J. Haematol.* 10:59, 1973.

44. Blendis, L. M., Ramboer, C., and Williams, R.: Studies on the haemodilution anemia of splenomegaly. *Eur. J. Clin. Invest.* 1:54, 1970.

45. Pollycove, M., Winchell, H. S., Lawrence, J. H.: Classification and evolution of patterns of erythropoiesis in polycythemia vera as studied by iron kinetics. *Blood* 28:807, 1966.

46. Ellis, L. D., Westerman, M. P., and Balcerzak, S. P.: The effect of iron stores on ferrokinetics in polycythemia. *Br. J. Haematol.* 13:892, 1967.

47. VanDyke, D., Lawrence, J. H., and Anger, H. O.: *Whole-Body Marrow-Distribution Studies in Polycythemia Vera.* U.S. Atomic Energy Commission Symposium Series, no. 19, 1970.

48. Hoffman, R., et al.: Fetal hemoglobin in polycythemia vera: Cellular distribution in 50 unselected patients. *Blood* 53:1148, 1979.

49. Athens, J. W., et al.: Leukokinetic studies. XI. Blood granulocyte kinetics in polycythemia vera, infection and myelofibrosis. *J. Clin. Invest.* 44:778. 1965.

50. Ghosh, M. L., Hudson, G., and Blackburn, E. K.: Skin window studies in polycythaemia rubra vera. *Br. J. Haematol.* 29:461, 1975.

51. Kutti, J., Ridell, B., Weinfeld, A., and Westin, J.: The relation of thrombokinetics to bone marrow megakaryocytes and to the size of the spleen in polycythaemia vera. *Scand. J. Haematol.* 10:88, 1973.

52. Kutti, M., and Weinfeld, A.: Platelet survival in active polycythaemia vera with reference to the haematocrit level. An experimental study before and after phlebotomy. *Scand. J. Haematol.* 8:405, 1971.

53. Zeigler, A., Murphy, S., and Gardner, F. H.: Microscopic platelet size and morphology in various hematologic disorders. *Blood* 51:479, 1978.

54. Berger, S., Aledort, L. M., Gilbert, H. S., Hanson, J. P., and Wasserman, L. R.: Abnormalities of platelet function in patients with polycythemia vera. *Cancer Res.* 33:2683, 1973.

55. Murphy, S., Davis, J. L., Walsh, P. N., Gardner, F. H.: Template bleeding time and clinical hemorrhage in myeloproliferative disease. *Arch. Intern. Med.* 138:1251, 1978.

56. Ellis, J. T., and Peterson, P.: The bone marrow in polycythemia vera. *Pathol. Ann.* 14:383, 1979.

57. Lundin, P. M., Ridell, B., and Weinfeld, A.: The significance of bone marrow morphology for the diagnosis of polycythaemia vera. *Scand. J. Haematol.* 9:271, 1972.

58. Ellis, L. D., Jensen, W. N., and Westerman, M. P.: Marrow iron: An evaluation of depleted stores in a series of 1,332 needle biopsies. *Ann. Intern. Med.* 61:44, 1964.

59. Burston, J., and Pinniger, J. L.: The reticulin content of bone marrow in haematological disorders. *Br. J. Haematol.* 9:172, 1963.

60. Yu, T. F., Weissmann, B., Sharney, L., Jupfer, S., and Gutman, A. B.: On the biosynthesis of uric acid from glycine-N^{15} in primary and secondary polycythemia. *Am. J. Med.* 21:901, 1956.

61. Yu, T. F.: Secondary gout associated with myeloproliferative diseases. *Arthritis Rheum.* 8:765, 1965.

62. Murray, J. F.: Classification of polycythemic disorders with comments on the diagnostic value of arterial blood oxygen analysis. *Ann. Intern. Med.* 64:892, 1966.

63. Lertzman, M., Frome, B. M., Israels, L. G., and Cherniack, R. M.: Hypoxia in polycythemia vera. *Ann. Intern. Med.* 60:409, 1964.

64. Fox, M. J., Brody, J. S., Weintraub, L. R., Szymanski, J., and O'Donnell, C.: Leukocyte larceny: A cause of spurious hypoxemia. *Am. J. Med.* 67:742, 1979.

65. Ersley, A. J., Caro, J., Kansu, E., Miller, O., and Cobbs, E.: Plasma erythropoietin in polycythemia. *Am. J. Med.* 66:243, 1979.

66. Koeffler, H. P., and Goldwasser, E.: Erythropoietin radioimmunoassay in evaluating patients with polycythemia. *Ann. Intern Med.* 94:44, 1981.

67. Meislin, A. G., Lee, S. L., and Wasserman, L. R.: Leukocyte alkaline phosphatase activity in hematopoietic disorders. *Cancer* 12:760, 1959.

68. Anstey, L., Kemp, N. H., Stafford, J. L., and Tanner, R. K.: Leukocyte alkaline phosphatase activity in polycythaemia rubra vera. *Br. J. Haematol.* 9:91, 1963.

69. Gilbert, H. S., Krauss, S., Pasternack, B., Herbert, V., and Wasserman, L. R.: Serum vitamin B_{12} content and unsaturated vitamin B_{12}-binding capacity in myeloproliferative disease. *Ann. Intern. Med.* 71:719, 1969.

70. Burger, R. L., Schneider, R. J., Mehlman, C. S., and Allen, R. H.: Human plasma R-type vitamin B_{12}-binding proteins. *J. Biol. Chem.* 250:7707, 1975.

71. Jacob, E., Baker, S. J., and Herbert, V.: Vitamin B_{12}-binding proteins. *Physiol. Rev.* 60:918, 1980.

72. Zittoun, J., Zittoun, R., Marquet, J., and Sultan, C.: The three transcobalamins in myeloproliferative disorders and acute leukaemia. *Br. J. Haematol.* 31:287, 1975.

73. Rachmilewitz, B., Manny, N. and Rachmilewitz, M.: The transcobalamins in polycythaemia vera. *Br. J. Haematol.* 19:453, 1977.

74. Kay, H. E. M., Lawler, S. D., and Millard, R. E.: The chromosomes in polycythemia vera. *Br. J. Haematol.* 12:507, 1966.

75. Wurster-Hill, D., et al.: Cytogenetic studies in polycythemia vera. *Semin. Hematol.* 13:13, 1976.

76. Krauss, S., Gilbert, H. S., and Wasserman, L. R.: Leukocyte histidine decarboxylase: Properties and activity in myeloproliferative disorders. *Blood* 31:699, 1968.

77. Binder, R. A., and Gilbert, H. S.: Muramidase in polycythemia vera. *Blood* 36:228, 1970.

78. Hartmann, R. C.: Pseudokalemia, in *The Platelet*, edited by K. M.

Brinkhous, R. W. Shermer, and F. K. Mostofi. Williams & Wilkins, Baltimore, 1971, p. 344.

79. Weinreb, N. J., and Shih, C. F.: Spurious polycythemia. *Semin. Hematol.* 12:397, 1975.

80. Smith, J. R., and Landaw, S. A.: Smoker's polycythemia. *N. Engl. J. Med.* 298:5, 1978.

81. Najean, Y., Triebel, F., and Dresch, C.: Pure erythrocytosis: Reappraisal of a study of 51 cases. *Am. J. Hematol.* 10:129, 1981.

82. Greenberg, B. R., and Golde, D. W.: Erythropoiesis in familial erythrocytosis. *N. Engl. J. Med.* 296:1080, 1977.

83. Pearson, T. C., and Wetherley-Mein, G.: Vascular occlusive episodes and venous haematocrit in primary proliferative polycythaemia. *Lancet* 2:1219, 1978.

84. Hutton, R. D.: The effect of iron deficiency on whole blood viscosity in polycythaemic patients. *Br. J. Haematol.* 43:191, 1979.

85. Wasserman, J. D.: Influence of therapy on causes of death in polycythemia vera. *Clin. Res.* 29:573A, 1981.

86. Modan, B., and Lilienfeld, A. M.: Polycythemia vera and leukemia — The role of radiation treatment: A study of 1,222 patients. *Medicine* 44:305, 1965.

87. Lawrence, J. H.: Nuclear physics and therapy: Preliminary report on a new method for the treatment of leukemia and polycythemia. *Radiology* 35:51, 1940.

88. Lawrence, J. H., Winchell, H. S., and Donald, W. G.: Leukemia in polycythemia vera. Relationship to splenic myeloid metaplasia and therapeutic radiation dose. *Ann. Intern. Med.* 70:763, 1969.

89. Killman, S., and Cronkite, E. P.: Treatment of polycythemia vera with Myleran. *Am. J. Med. Sci.* 241:218, 1961.

90. Logue, G. L., Gutterman, J. V., McGinn, T. G., Laszlo, J., and Rundles, R. W.: Melphalan therapy of polycythemia vera. *Blood* 36:70, 1970.

91. Gilbert, H. S.: Problems relating to control of polycythemia vera: The use of alkylating agents. *Blood* 32:500, 1968.

92. Stuart, J. J., Crocker, D. L., and Roberts, H. R.: Treatment of busulfan-induced pancytopenia. *Arch. Intern. Med.* 136:1181, 1976.

93. Kyle, R. A., Schwartz, R. S., Oliner, H. L., and Dameshek, W.: A syndrome resembling adrenal cortical insufficiency associated with long term busulfan (Myleran) therapy. *Blood* 18:497, 1961.

94. Berk, P., et al.: Increased incidence of acute leukemia in polycythemia vera associated with chlorambucil therapy. *N. Engl. J. Med.* 304:441, 1981.

95. Weinfeld, A., Westin, J., Ridell, B., and Swolin, B.: Polycythaemia vera terminating in acute leukaemia. A clinical cytogenetic and morphologic study in 8 patients treated with alkylating agents. *Br. J. Haematol.* 19:255, 1977.

96. Rosner, F., and Grunwald, H.: Hodgkin's disease and acute leukemia: Report of 8 cases and review of the literature. *Am. J. Med.* 58:339, 1975.

97. Carey, R. W., Holland, J. F., Sheehe, P. R., Graham, S.: Association of cancer of the breast and acute myelocytic leukemia. *Cancer* 20:1080, 1967.

98. Rosner, F., and Grunwald, H.: Multiple myeloma terminating in acute leukemia: Report of 12 cases and review of the literature. *Am. J. Med.* 57:927, 1974.

99. Brodsky, I.: Busulphan treatment of polycythaemia vera. *Br. J. Haematol.* 52:1, 1982.

100. Wasserman, L. R., et al.: Influence of therapy on causes of death in polycythemia vera. *Clin. Res.* 29:573A, 1981.

101. Tartaglia, A. P., et al.: Aspirin and Persantine do not prevent thrombotic complications in patients with polycythemia vera treated with phlebotomy. *Blood* 58:240a, 1981.

102. Rundles, R. W., Metz, E. N., and Siberman, H. R.: Allopurinol the treatment of gout. *Ann. Intern. Med.* 64:299, 1966.

103. Chanarin, I., and Szur, L.: Relief of intractable pruritus in polycythemia rubra vera with cholestyramine. *Br. J. Haematol.* 29:669, 1975.

104. Harrison, A. R., Littenberg, G., Goldstein, L., and Kaplowitz, N.: Pruritus, cimetidine and polycythemia. *N. Engl. J. Med.* 300:433, 1979.

105. Bouroncle, B. A., and Doan, C. A.: Myelofibrosis clinical, hematologic and pathologic study of 110 patients. *Am. J. Med. Sci.* 243:697, 1962.

106. Silverstein, M. N.: Postpolycythemia myeloid metaplasia. *Arch. Intern. Med.* 134:113, 1974.

107. Rosenthal, D. S., and Moloney, W. C.: Myeloid metaplasia: A study of 98 cases. *Postgrad. Med.* 45:136, 1969.

108. Meytes, D., Katz, D. and Ramot, B.: Prognostic parameters in myeloid metaplasia: Agnogenic versus postpolycythemic. *Isr. J. Med. Sci.* 12:534, 1976.

109. Gardner, F. H., and Nathan, D. G.: Androgens and erythropoiesis: III. Further evaluation of testosterone treatment of myelofibrosis. *N. Engl. J. Med.* 274:420, 1966.

110. Benbassat, J., Penchas, S., and Ligumski, M.: Splenectomy in patients with agnogenic myeloid metaplasia: An analysis of 321 published cases. *Br. J. Haematol.* 42:207, 1979.

111. Silverstein, M. N., and ReMine, W. H.: Splenectomy in myeloid metaplasia. *Blood* 53:515, 1979.

112. Greenberger, J. S., Chaffey, J. T., Rosenthal, D. S., and Moloney, W. C.: Irradiation for control of hypersplenism and painful splenomegaly in myeloid metaplasia. *Int. J. Radiat. Oncol. Biol. Phys.* 2:1083, 1977.

113. Centrole, A. L., Freda, R. N., and McGowan, L.: Polycythemia rubra vera in pregnancy. *Obstet. Gynecol.* 30:657, 1967.

114. Harris, R. E., and Conrad, F. G.: Polycythemia vera in the childbearing age. *Arch. Intern. Med.* 120:697, 1967.

115. Berk, P. D., et al.: Non-hematologic malignancies in patients receiving myelosuppressive treatment for polycythemia vera. *Clin. Res.* 30:558A, 1982.

116. Donovan, P. B., et al.: Hydroxyurea, an effective agent for the treatment of polycythemia vera. *Clin. Res.* 30:315A, 1982.

CHAPTER *24*

Chronic myelogenous leukemia

R. WAYNE RUNDLES

Definition and history

Chronic myelogenous leukemia (CML) was the first type of leukemia to be discovered [1–3]. It is a neoplastic disease that results from the development of an abnormal hemopoietic stem cell which gives rise to progeny that have the Philadelphia (Ph[1]) chromosome. The clinical manifestations of the disease relate to excessive and unrestrained growth of blood cell progenitors in the marrow. Large numbers of immature and mature granulocytic cells accumulate in the blood, and extramedullary myelopoiesis produces gross enlargement of the spleen and liver. In most cases, the proliferation of hemopoietic cells can be suppressed by cytotoxic drug therapy for 1 to 4 years, but eventually, disease progression or transition to acute leukemia develops in most patients. During the terminal months of the disease, therapeutic agents, including those useful in the treatment of acute leukemia, are ineffective. Death results from inanition, organ infiltration with leukemic cells, infection, or hemorrhage.

Etiology and pathogenesis

Chronic myelogenous leukemia and related myeloproliferative entities are regarded as neoplastic diseases [4]. Many of the morphologic stigmata of neoplasia arising from other tissues occur in CML [4]: immature and abnormal cells varying in size and shape, with large nuclei, prominent nucleoli, an increased number of mitotic figures, and chromosomes anomalies. Abnormalities can be demonstrated that involve nucleoli, nucleosomes, Golgi bodies, endoplasmic reticulum, and mitochondria [5]. In CML, about 90 percent of patients have a unique abnormality, the Ph^1 (Philadelphia) chromosome in which part of the long arm of chromosome 22 has been translocated, usually to chromosome 9 (see below).

Clues to the etiology of CML are not evident in most patients, although antecedent causes have been identified [6]. These relate to the virtually pathognomonic Ph^1 chromosome, which may be produced by irradiation and possibly other agents which damage hemopoietic cells [4,7]. When multiple leukemogenic factors operate, each one may potentiate the risk of all the others [8]. Evidence indicates that CML develops with or following the appearance in the marrow of an abnormal stem cell from which a new clone proliferates. The latter has selective growth advantages and in the course of time, after many cell generations, suppresses or replaces normal marrow progenitors.

RADIATION LEUKEMOGENESIS

The acute inflammatory effect of irradiation on the conjunctiva and skin was recognized within a few months after W. K. von Röntgen discovered x-rays in November 1895, and the more chronic, destructive effect of x-rays and radium on blood cells and their precursors in humans was well documented during the first decade of this century [9,10]. Early hematologic changes appeared to be reversible, but after a certain amount of exposure, they became permanent.

Reports of leukemia developing in physicians and others who had been exposed to radiation for some period appeared, and then large-scale surveys showed that the overall incidence of leukemia in physicians was 1.7 times that of the general population [11]. This increase was the result of a high rate among radiologists, in whom the incidence of leukemia was 9 times that of other practitioners [12–14]. In physicians, the excessive mortality from leukemia occurred within the first 5 years of their exposure to radiation [15]. The incidence of leukemia among radiologists has fallen in recent years, coincident with the use of better-shielded radiation apparatus and the more systematic use of monitoring devices [4,14].

The exposure of Japanese in Hiroshima and Nagasaki to the atomic bomb explosions in 1945 provided a unique demonstration of the leukemogenic effects of a single dose of radiation [16–20]. After a latent period of about 3 years, the annual incidence of leukemia in the survivors gradually increased to a maximum some 7 years after the explosion and then began to fall. Fourteen years after the explosion, the rate still exceeded the national average. The risk for those nearest the hypocenter, who received the greatest irradiation, was about 50 times that of persons who were in the nonirradiated periphery [18,19]. For a high-level single-dose exposure, the increased incidence of leukemia was approximately linear with dose, but the effect of smaller amounts of irradiation was less predictable [20]. In almost all instances the leukemia was acute or chronic myelogenous or an atypical variant, such as myelofibrosis, the types prone to occur in the Japanese people. The incidence of leukemia in the offspring of persons exposed to atomic bomb irradiation was not increased [21], and there was no demonstrable increase in mutation rate [22].

The leukemogenic effects of therapeutic irradiation in humans have been documented most clearly by careful studies of a large group of patients with ankylosing spondylitis treated by radiotherapy in Great Britain [23–25]. After a latent period, which again averaged about 6 years, the incidence of leukemia increased to become nearly 13 times that of the general population. The leukemia was chronic myelogenous in almost every instance. While the incidence of leukemia may be slightly increased in ankylosing spondylitis itself, the exposure to radiation seemed to be the factor of major importance [26,27]. The risks of radiation therapy given for thymic enlargement in infancy [28–30], chronic infections [4,31], and carcinomas [4,32]; of ^{131}I administration for hyperthyroidism [33]; and of diagnostic x-ray procedures during pregnancy [34,35] are less but statistically significant [4].

An increased incidence of leukemia following irradiation has been observed in many animal species [36–39], including rodents, beagles, and miniature swine, but its pathogenesis has been studied in greatest detail in mice. In certain strains, leukemia is increased from 7 to as much as 30 percent by irradiation. Irradiation leukemogenesis in mice involves many modifying factors, such as direct and indirect cellular effects, the kinetics of cell division, organ specificity, hormone influences, and the activation of occult viral infection, all of which have been reviewed extensively [4,40–42].

CHEMICAL LEUKEMOGENS

Despite the scientific importance of ionizing radiation as an etiologic factor in CML, not more than 1 person in 15 or 20 who develop the disease has had unusual exposure to any form of radiation or to the solvents, drugs, and chemicals discussed below. Identification of chemical leukemogens has been difficult, since our society offers a plethora of candidates. Any chemical capable of damaging hemopoietic stem cells is potentially leukemogenic.

The only chemical that has been clearly identified as one that increases the incidence of myelogenous leukemia in humans is benzene in heavy occupational exposure [43–45]. The development of myelogenous leukemias [45] and persistent chromosome abnormalities in exposed persons known to have had neutropenia [46] is especially significant. The leukemogenic importance of other widely distributed chemicals, such as sedatives, solvents, antibiotics, analgesics, and insecticides, that may produce adverse hemopoietic reactions is still uncertain.

CYTOGENETICS

Improved methods for studying human metaphase cells [47] have led to remarkable advances in knowledge of chromosome abnormalities in the leukemias. Short-term culture of marrow cells with colchicine treatment showed that aneuploidy and morphologic abnormalities of chromosomes occurred in some patients with acute leukemia [47,48]. The application of this method to blood leukocytes led to the recognition of the minute abnormal Ph[1] chromsome, which had been overlooked earlier in preparations made from cultured marrow [49–53].

The description of the Ph[1] chromosome, a member of the G group (number 22) missing approximately half its longer arm, was a notable advance in the understanding of CML. It is present in about 90 percent of patients with typical disease manifestations and was usually absent in other myeloproliferative variants [53–56]. Studies of marrow using a direct method that required no culture confirmed its specificity for the hemopoietic cells in CML [52,53]. The granulocytic, megakaryocytic, and erythroid cells had the Ph[1] chromosome, but the lymphocytes and fibroblasts had normal chromosomes [52]. When one of a pair of identical twins developed CML, the abnormal chromosome was present in only the affected member [57–59]. The Ph[1] chromosome thus was an acquired or induced abnormality and was found to persist in precursors during remissions of the disease and in the abnormal myeloblasts when CML became acute [60,61].

Ionizing radiation was shown to produce a number of chromosome abnormalities, including the Ph[1] chromosome in occasional cells in normal persons [7,24,60]. Those who developed CML following irradiation usually had the Ph[1] chromosome [60].

In the early 1970s, DNA-binding fluorescent agents and Giemsa-stain banding were developed to study human chromosome structure [61,62]. The Ph[1] chromosome was confirmed as being derived from chromosome 22, which had lost the distal half of its long arm [63]. With the new techniques, the Ph[1] chromosome could be distinguished from the trisomy 21 chromosome anomaly involved in Down's syndrome [64]. Study of chromosome 22 showed that it was the chromosome uniquely involved in patients with CML, and that its distribution in cells supported the unicellular (clonal) nature of the disease [65]. The Ph[1] chromosome was shown to represent a translocation and not a deletion [66]. The displaced fragment of chromosome 22 most frequently became attached to chromosome 9, but occasionally to other chromosomes [66–72]. Using the chromosome nomenclature in which the short arm of a chromosome is designated p and the long arm q, the Ph[1] chromosome in CML is designated t(9+;22q−) [73–74]. In 5 percent of patients with Ph[1]-positive CML, unusual or complex translocations involve recipient chromosomes other than number 9 or rearrangements, including multiple chromosomes, chromosome breaks, or chromatin loss [70–76]. The clinical features of the disease in these patients and their response to treatment, course, and survival are about the same as in those with the standard Ph[1] translocation. The crucial event in the pathogenesis of CML appears to be the abbreviation of chromosome 22.

When CML undergoes exacerbation or becomes acute, the Ph[1] chromosome persists, but in about 80 percent of patients, additional chromosome rearrangements, additions, or deletions develop. The most common of these are (1) duplication of the Ph[1] chromosome, (2) an extra chromosome 8, or (3) isochromosomes for the long arm of number 17 (17q) [70–76].

While about 90 percent of patients with CML have the Ph[1] chromosome when the disease is first discovered, a few patients develop the anomaly later. Rarely, a mixture of abnormal and normal cell lines persists indefinitely. Patients who are Ph[1]-negative tend to have atypical disease. Their clinical course is usually more acute and their response to therapy less satisfactory, but some seem to have an unusually chronic form of the disease [77–78].

The cytogenetic findings suggested that CML is a monoclonal disease, i.e., that it arises from a single cell. Confirmatory evidence was obtained from studies of women with CML who also were heterozygotes for the X-linked glucose-6-phosphate dehydrogenase (G-6-PD) enzyme [79]. If the CML cells were unicellular in origin, they should contain only one of the two G-6-PD enzymes, while if their origin was multicellular, both isoenzymes should be present [80]. Three Negro women with typical CML, one untreated and one undergoing busulfan therapy, who were heterozygous for the common isoenzyme of G-6-PD were selected for study and enzyme assays of their granulocytes, red cells, and fibroblasts from skin biopsies carried out. Only one isoenzyme (type A) was demonstrable in erythrocyte and granulocyte preparations, while fibroblasts from cell cultures in each patient contained both A and B isoenzymes.

Leukemic granulocytes containing only one isoenzyme were found in additional patients [81–83], and a single isoenzyme was found also in platelets and monocyte-macrophage cells cultured from the blood of patients with CML [83]. Heterogeneity occurred in some patients with more acute disease variants [84].

PATHOGENESIS

In 1971, hematologic remissions lasting several months were reported to occur in about 30 percent of patients with CML in blast cell transformation following treatment with vincristine and prednisone, the drugs considered most effective in the treatment of acute lymphoblastic leukemia [85]. Further studies showed that the leukemic cells in the patients who responded appeared to be lymphoblastic rather than myeloid, and cytogenetically frequently hypodiploid [86]. Another characteristic of the blast cells in the responding CML subpopulation was the presence of the DNA polymerase, terminal deoxynucleotidyl transferase (TdT), generally regarded as a biochemical marker of early T lymphocytes or null cells of lymphoid origin [87–91]. TdT was not found in granulocytes during the chronic phase of CML. While not all patients with CML in the acute phase responded to the administration of vincristine and prednisone, there were no responses among those who lacked the enzyme [90]. There were no distinguishing morphologic features by which TdT-containing blast cells could be identified with certainty.

Renewed interest in the acute phase of CML has shown that this progression is heterogeneous [92,93]. Granulocytic abnormalities predominate in most patients, but the transformation can involve erythroblasts primarily and resemble erythroleukemia in some patients, or it can evolve as acute myelomonocytic, basophilic, or megakaryocytic leukemia, acute myelofibrosis, or lymphoblastic leukemia [83,84,94–98].

The first evidence of some link between myelogenous and lymphocytic leukemias came with the finding that the Ph[1] chromosome occurs in the blast cells of some patients who apparently have acute lymphocytic leukemia (ALL) [99–101]. It now appears that about one-quarter of adults with ALL, in whom the undifferentiated cells are indistinguishable from those of the childhood disease, have the Ph[1] chromosome. Myeloblasts in patients with CML in the acute phase contain "acute lymphoblastic leukemia–associated" and Ia-like antigens and have the phenotype of pre-B lymphocytes [97]. Antisera raised against cells from patients with myelogenous and lymphocytic leukemias show some evidence of overlapping cytotoxicity [102].

The finding of lymphoid cell phenotypes in CML has suggested that the malignant lesion does not involve the hemopoietic stem cell primarily but the preceding pluripotent stem cell (see Fig. 19-1). Thus the pluripotent stem cell may be the target for malignant transformation, and if damage by radiation or mutagenic chemicals occurs at slightly different stages of development, the result could be some variation in early disease manifestations and exaggerated heterogeneity during the acute phase of the disease. Mitotic abnormalities would ordinarily lead to cell death, but in some instances, leukemic stem cells seem to survive better, proliferate excessively, or grow independently of normal regulatory forces. Progeny of the abnormal stem cells transmit the new growth potential to their cellular descendants and, after a "preleukemic" growth period of 2 to 4 years, replace in part or completely normal hemopoietic elements. By the time CML is clinically or hematologically detectable, most, if not all, of the myeloid cells in the marrow are Ph[1]-positive. The production of too many or too few erythroid elements or platelets may be prominent features in individual patients [4,103–105].

Reasons for the growth advantage of leukemic cells which eventually produces a five- to tenfold increase in the mass of myeloid tissue have not been identified [106–109]. The intravascular life-span of granulocytes in CML is prolonged, in proportion to their degree of immaturity [106]. In the fully developed disease, an increase in the total amount of proliferative tissue in the marrow and extramedullary sites and the premature release of granulocytes from the marrow are the most prominent abnormalities.

Once the disease is established, the Ph[1] chromosome-containing cells are liable to additional chromosome aberrations, or possibly the etiologic factor continues to operate and induce further cytogenetic changes. The inherent tendency for CML to undergo slow or rapid exacerbation 1 to 4 years after its appearance is its most notorious feature. Once this occurs, fever, cytopenias, increasingly abnormal cellular morphology, and extramedullary hemopoiesis develop, all of which are progressive and increasingly refractory to therapy. The new cell species progressively lose their capacity to differentiate or to function normally. The development of new karyotypic abnormalities may precede the appearance of any other sign of acute transformation [111–112]. New leukemic clones may appear in the spleen [113–115] or the lymph nodes [76] late in the course of the disease.

INCIDENCE

Chronic myelogenous leukemia accounts for about 20 percent of all cases of leukemia in Western countries, and the death rate from it is about 1 per 100,000 population per year [4]. The incidence of CML in recent years does not seem to be increasing like that of acute leukemia in adults and chronic lymphocytic leukemia [116]. CML occurs rarely during the first few months of life, when its course is relatively acute. There is no well-defined hereditary liability to the development of CML, and children born of mothers who have the disease are not affected. The typical disease is occasionally seen in adolescents, but the great majority of patients are aged 25 to 60 years. The peak incidence of CML in the past has been in the fourth decade of life, but it is shifting to a later age [116].

Leukemias of all types tend to occur more commonly in men than in women. A comprehensive tabulation showed the male/female ratio for all leukemias to be 57 to 43 [116]. Forty or fifty years ago, 60 percent of patients with CML were men [4]. The appearance and course of the disease is identical in both sexes.

Clinical features

ONSET

The signs and symptoms of CML develop insidiously at first, but tend to become continuously worse if treatment is not given. The discovery of CML at an asymptomatic stage by finding splenomegaly or hematologic abnormalities during routine examinations is uncommon. If the granulocytic leukocytosis of CML is discovered by routine blood counts before there are symptoms or physical signs, overt disease usually becomes manifest within a few weeks or months. On rare occasions, leukocytosis with an abnormally high granulocyte percentage or with undue granulocyte immaturity may occur after acute hemorrhage or during the course of an infection. The leukocytosis may persist or recur and in retrospect prove to have been an early manifestation of CML. Once well-defined physical and hematologic abnormalities are present, spontaneous remissions rarely if ever occur.

SYMPTOMS

The earliest symptoms of CML are usually malaise, fatigue, lack of exercise tolerance, pallor, and weight loss. These symptoms are associated with the development of some degree of anemia and, frequently, elevation of the metabolic rate. Aching in the bones that contain red marrow or discomfort and fullness in the upper abdomen associated with enlargement of the spleen and liver are common symptoms that develop as the disease progresses. Rarely, bleeding manifestations—retinal hemorrhages, ecchymoses, or hematuria—may occur in patients who have too many, too few, or abnormal platelets. Individuals with latent gout may develop acute arthritis or have uric acid urinary stones as a consequence of the increased nucleic acid breakdown. Rare symptoms of CML include peripheral vascular insufficiency and priapism, usually associated with extraordinarily high leukocyte counts and/or thrombocytosis.

SIGNS

Pallor, warm moist skin, low-grade fever, and splenomegaly may be present. Increased tenderness in the lower half of the sternum is characteristic of CML in relapse. Bone tenderness develops whenever a considerable increase in marrow cellularity occurs within a short period of time.

Patients with CML who have a hypercellular marrow for a long time may develop diffuse demineralization of the "short bones," and occasionally multiple osteolytic lesions may be visible in roentgenograms. As the disease progresses, the bones may become exquisitely tender to pressure, and aching along the spine and about the pelvis may increase until it becomes a major complaint.

Punctuate retinal hemorrhages and exudates or bruises and ecchymoses over the extremities are frequent in CML. The lymph nodes are rarely enlarged in patients with typical CML, though node enlargement may be a feature of the acute transformation phase. Skin infiltration or exfoliation, destructive bone or joint lesions, or granulomatous sarcomas (chloromas, myeloblastomas) are usually indicative of an acute stage or form of myelogenous leukemia (see below).

In untreated disease, the spleen continues to enlarge until it becomes palpable and eventually may fill half the abdomen. The development of splenomegaly is usu-

ally accompanied by some degree of hepatomegaly. Anorexia is then a common symptom. Patients complain of having a reduced food capacity, and weight loss may be rapid. If the disease is allowed to progress without treatment or relapses between courses of therapy, the above signs become more pronounced, and when remission in the disease is induced by treatment, the signs gradually regress. The disease manifestations respond to therapy promptly at first, but after a period of 1 to 4 years, when the more acute phase develops, signs and symptoms of poorly controlled disease persist (see below under "Therapy").

Laboratory features

BLOOD FINDINGS

Examination of the blood film in CML usually shows a diagnostic profusion of granulocytic elements. When the granulocytic leukocytosis is pronounced, the blood resembles marrow in which granulocytes have largely displaced fat, early erythroid precursors, plasma cells, and megakaryocytes. The blood abnormalities seen in typical patients with moderately advanced disease are shown in Table 24-1.

Granulocytes in all stages of development are present in the blood and appear to be normal in morphology. The most mature cells are ordinarily present in greatest number and the less mature in diminishing frequency. Myeloblasts and promyelocytes should not exceed 10 percent [104]. In CML there is no "gap" or hiatus in the granulocytic series. If a patient with early disease is observed without treatment for a few weeks or months, the total number of granulocytes in the circulating blood ordinarily rises progressively. Some patients may have a conspicuous increase in the number of eosinophils or basophils in the blood, and this is often regarded as a poor prognostic sign. A third or more of patients with CML have pronounced thrombocytosis [103–105]. In these patients, fragments of megakaryocyte nuclei may be found occasionally in the blood. A small number of nucleated red blood cells, sometimes with immature and/or megaloblastoid features, are often present.

Anemia is almost always a feature of active CML, and it generally increases in severity as the disease advances. The anemia is usually normocytic and normochromic; ordinarily there is little evidence of iron deficiency, accelerated red cell hemolysis, or erythrocyte abnormality. As myeloid overgrowth progresses, the number of erythroid elements in the marrow is reduced and the red cells may show variation in size and shape. Reticulocytes are generally normal or slightly increased in number. Some shortening of red cell survival occurs in the presence of gross splenomegaly, but immune hemolysis does not occur. On rare occasions, anemia develops that responds to splenectomy, but the major cause of anemia in CML is a decrease in erythropoiesis.

On rare occasions, too, erythrocytosis and thrombocytosis may develop at early stages of the disease, even to a degree that suggests polycythemia vera, or they may appear after myeloid overgrowth has been controlled by

TABLE 24-1 Typical blood abnormalities in patients with moderately severe chronic myelogenous leukemia

Hemoglobin, g/dl	9–12
Red blood cells, $\times 10^{12}$ per liter	3–4.5
White blood cells, $\times 10^9$ per liter	50–250
Volume packed red cells, %	28–35
Packed white cell layer, mm	3–15
Packed platelet layer, mm	1–2
Platelets, $\times 10^9$ per liter	250–1000
Reticulocytes, %	1–3
Differential white cell count, %:	
PMN neutrophils	35–20
Nonsegmented bands	25–30
Metamyelocytes	12–18
Myelocytes	6–10
Promyelocytes	2–4
Myeloblasts	1–3
Eosinophils	4–4
Basophils	4–5
Lymphocytes	5–1
Monocytes	5–2
Nucleated RBC	1–3

therapy. These responses are consistent with the evidence that the stem cell clone that produces CML affects precursors of erythrocytes and platelets as well as granulocytes.

MARROW FINDINGS

Marrow is markedly hypercellular, and fat is practically absent. Granulocytic cells are greatly increased in number, and the granulocytic/erythroid ratio is 10 to 50:1 rather than the normal 2 to 5:1. Granulocytes in the marrow resemble those in the blood, but they are less mature. Mitotic figures are usually increased, often being four to five times that in normal marrow. The number of eosinophils and basophils in the marrow may be increased too, usually in proportion to their number in the blood. In patients with thrombocytosis, the number of megakaryocytes in the marrow is proportionately increased [117].

Different proliferative capabilities of individual cell lines have been observed in patients with CML who developed chronic blood loss anemia, or after they had had a series of phlebotomies [118]. Patients with iron-deficiency anemia developed pronounced erythroblastic hyperplasia in their marrow. The administration of iron increased the rate of red cell production to about twice normal, but not to the extent one would expect in normal persons or in those with hemolytic disease. Pronounced hyperplasia of red cell precursors was produced by normal erythropoietic stimuli in spite of the malignant proliferation of granulocytes. Control of the latter required busulfan or ^{32}P therapy, since it was not notably suppressed by the erythroid proliferation [118].

HYPERMETABOLISM

The increased metabolic rate in patients with CML associated with such symptoms as weight loss, increased sweating, and fever is roughly proportional to the sever-

ity of anemia, organomegaly, and the number and immaturity of the leukocytes [119,120].

Primary disturbances in thyroid function have not occurred, and antithyroid therapy has little effect on the hypermetabolism or on other manifestations of leukemia [121]. The metabolic rate becomes normal with effective antileukemic therapy.

CHEMICAL ABNORMALITIES

URIC ACID

An increased production of uric acid with hyperuricosuria and hyperuricemia occurs in untreated CML [122–126]. Uric acid excretion is often two to three times normal in patients with active CML, and if aggressive therapy leads to rapid cell lysis, excretion of the additional purine load may produce urinary tract blockage [127]. The formation of urinary urate stones is common in patients with CML, and some with latent gout may develop acute gouty arthritis or nephropathy [128]. The likelihood of complications from urate overproduction is greatly increased by starvation, acidosis, renal disease, and diuretic drug therapy [129].

Although the increased uric acid excretion in CML results from the breakdown of granulocytes, it is not a quantitative measure of cell turnover, since xanthine and hypoxanthine are salvaged and reutilized [130]. Search for abnormal purines in the urine of patients with leukemia has not been successful [126].

LEUKOCYTE ALKALINE PHOSPHATASE

A striking decrease in neutrophil alkaline phosphatase levels can be demonstrated by both histochemical and biochemical techniques [131–134]. About 20 percent of normal mature granulocytes give a positive alkaline phosphatase reaction. In infections, pregnancy, polycythemia vera, and in some patients with other myeloproliferative variants, the alkaline phosphatase content of neutrophils is strikingly increased [135]. The considerable reduction in the amount of alkaline phosphatase in the neutrophils of CML may be helpful in differential diagnosis. The enzyme activity also may be reduced in paroxysmal nocturnal hemoglobinuria, hypophosphatasia, in some patients with agnogenic myeloid metaplasia, and after androgen treatment.

The presence of the Ph¹ chromosome in granulocytes and the reduction in alkaline phosphatase levels are independent variables and have no obvious quantitative relationship. The enzyme activity has not been associated with any specific neutrophil granule, and in CML there is no evidence that an antigenically normal but enzymatically defective alkaline phosphatase is present [137–140].

SERUM VITAMIN B$_{12}$

The serum vitamin B$_{12}$ level in patients with CML is increased to approximately 15 times normal [141]. The increase is proportional to the height of the leukocyte count in untreated patients, but it is still four times normal in patients who have normal white cell counts during remissions. Patients with other chronic myeloproliferative diseases and some with acute leukemia have high serum vitamin B_{12} levels too, while those with acute and chronic lymphocytic leukemia, including those with extremely high white cell counts, have normal levels [142].

The concentration of vitamin B_{12} in normal and leukemic leukocytes is low in comparison with other body tissues, but both normal and leukemic granulocytes contain a vitamin B_{12}-binding protein similar to transcobalamin I (TC I) [143–149]. The TC I binding protein in CML is somewhat different from that in polycythemia vera. The abnormally high levels of vitamin B_{12} in the serum of patients with CML apparently come from the breakdown of granulocytes. With treatment of the disease, the high levels fall slowly toward normal [136]. The persistence of increased amounts of viatmin B_{12} in the plasma when the disease is in remission may be an indication of "ineffective myelopoiesis" in the marrow or extramedullary sites and in other situations may provide a measure of granulocyte turnover [148–151].

SERUM LACTIC DEHYDROGENASE AND K+
The level of serum lactic dehydrogenase (LDH) is considerably elevated in CML, as it is in acute leukemia [152]. Pseudohyperkalemia due to the release of potassium from white cells during clotting can occur [153].

GRANULOCYTE FUNCTION
The neutrophilic granulocyte is a highly differentiated cell, but evidence of defective function before or after antileukemic treatment in CML is meager [154–164]. The most important, if not the sole, function of granulocytes is to prevent bacterial invasion of the tissues by phagocytosis and destruction of microorganisms. Patients with CML, during relapse and in remission, are not especially vulnerable to infection. The absolute number of mature granulocytes in the blood is usually increased. The intravascular sojourn of granulocytes in CML seems to be prolonged, and while they disappear into the tissues, oral secretions [155], etc., they do not appear in inflammatory lesions [156–157]. Most studies have shown that the immature granulocytes of CML generally phagocytize poorly, but the cells present during remissions in the disease phagocytize normally [159–164]. In some patients, macrophages in the marrow show prominent phagocytic activity, becoming engorged with glycolipids, and resemble Gaucher's cells [165] (see Plate 5).

Differential diagnosis

The diagnosis of CML can be made accurately in patients by the study of a well-stained blood film and examination of the marrow. Scarcely any other disease can produce such an outpouring of myelocytes, metamyelocytes, and mature neutrophils with a variable number of eosinophils, basophils, and a few erythrocyte precur-

sors. The differentiation of CML from other chronic myeloproliferative diseases may be difficult on occasion. Teardrop red cells are suggestive of myelofibrosis, but some patients with typical CML have marrow fibrosis [166–169] (see chap. 25). Masses of platelets around megakaryocyte nuclei and a minor degree of granulocytic immaturity are typical of primary thrombocythemia. An undue number of erythrocyte precursors with bizarre nuclei or inclusions and malformed red cells are characteristic of erythroleukemia.

CML may be overlooked in persons who lack some typical features of the disease. An occasional patient with nascent CML may not have sternal tenderness, and in 1 patient out of 20, splenomegaly may not be demonstrable. The elevated granulocyte count may fluctuate somewhat in patients with early disease, or it may appear only during infection or glucocorticoid therapy or after hemorrhage. In rare instances of "neutrophilic leukemia," the granulocytes in the circulating blood and marrow may show virtually no immaturity [169,170]. A type of familial myeloproliferative disease that closely resembles myelogenous leukemia has been described in children [171].

Leukoerythroblastic reactions, referring to the presence of a few immature granulocytes and nucleated red cells in the circulating blood with a normal or modestly elevated total leukocyte count, occur in patients with shock, brisk hemolysis, hemorrhage, metastatic tumor in the marrow, plasma cell myeloma, varieties of hereditary anemia, and megaloblastic anemia [172,173]. Examination of the marrow usually clarifies the diagnosis in these instances.

A conspicuous nonleukemic granulocytic leukocytosis may be produced by extensive metastatic tumor (with or without hemorrhage or necrosis), some infections, rebound after drug or infectious depression of marrow function, Hodgkin's disease, and ACTH or glucocorticoid therapy. Standard diagnostic procedures, examination of the marrow, and a short period of observation are usually sufficient to clarify the diagnosis.

Leukemoid reactions in which blood abnormalities resemble those of myelogenous leukemia were reported frequently in the past, mostly in the preantibiotic era and before the day of frequent marrow examinations. The suspicion of leukemoid reaction arises now whenever active tuberculosis is discovered in a patient with leukemia who has not been under observation [174]. Patients with hematologic malignances seem to be especially vulnerable to the hematogenous spread of tuberculosis [175], and control of the infection rarely if ever changes the abnormal blood picture.

The most common leukemoid reaction, however, occurs in patients with infection or tumor who have a pronounced granulocytic leukocytosis and in whom monocytes are mistaken for myelocytes. In most of these patients, very few granulocytes even as immature as metamyelocytes are present in the blood; the alkaline phosphatase level in the granulocytes is increased and the Ph[1] chromosome is always absent.

VARIANTS OF CML

Eosinophilic leukemia is a rare entity, and its distinction from benign hypereosinophilic syndromes can be difficult [176–179]. An abnormal karyotype is indicative of a neoplastic process. Most patients with eosinophilic leukemia have been Ph[1]-negative.

Extreme basophilia may occur in patients with CML. This usually represents a progressive phase of the disease [180], but the marrow and blood basophilia may be so predominant as to be called basophilic leukemia. The Ph[1] chromosome may be present in primitive marrow cells and the disease represents a prognostically unfavorable variant of CML. It can be associated with unusual hemorrhagic manifestations, symptoms of histamine excess, or skin lesions resembling urticaria pigmentosa.

Subacute or chronic myelomonocytic leukemia is a CML variant in which there is a greater proportion of myelocytes and monocytes in the blood and marrow. The white cell count tends to be lower than in typical CML, and the response to treatment is more unpredictable. The Ph[1] chromosome is usually absent. When the abnormal cell population consists largely of well-differentiated monocytic cells, the entity may be referred to as chronic monocytic leukemia.

CML in childhood is a rare entity, and although the disease is somewhat heterogeneous, it tends to evolve in one of two patterns: in children usually 1 to 2 years of age, the course is almost always rapidly progressive, while in those 10 to 12 years of age or older, the disease may be more chronic and typical of the disease seen in adults [181–186]. Several children 2 to 3 years of age have been studied in whom the hemoglobin and red cell enzyme pattern reverted to a fetal type: the fetal hemoglobin increased to 40 to 70 percent, hemoglobin A_2 became very low, and carbonic anhydrase activity was negligible. In these instances, the abnormal leukemic stem cells apparently originate from a clone established in the prenatal period [187,188]. Leukemic involvement of the erythroid cells has been observed [189]. Patients with panmyelopathy have had evidence of prominent monocytic involvement on marrow culture [190].

Therapy

RADIATION

Irradiation was first used in the treatment of CML by Pusey in 1902 [191]. In 1924, Minot, Buckman, and Isaacs published their classic paper on CML documenting the age and sex incidence, clinical features, data relating to prognosis, and changes produced by irradiation therapy [192]. In 78 patients treated with intensive irradiation, the duration of life averaged 3.5 years compared with slightly over 3 years in 52 patients who were given no specific therapy. The major benefit from irradiation was the almost uniform and gratifying relief of symptoms, the alleviation of physical and hematologic abnormalities, and a significant increase in living

efficiency. The standard treatment for CML for the next 15 years was local x-ray or radium therapy given over the spleen, long bones, or areas of leukemic infiltration. Total-body, or "spray," irradiation then began to gain favor [193], and finally radioactive phosphorus (^{32}P) was introduced and evaluated [194,195].

In 1951, Shimkin and his collaborators published a comprehensive study of the incidence, distribution, and fatality of leukemia in the San Francisco area during the years 1910–1948 [196]. Despite advances in diagnostic methods, better medical care, improved radiologic equipment, the introduction of ^{32}P as a therapeutic agent, etc., the survival of patients with CML had not changed appreciably over the decades. Five to ten percent of patients died during the first year of their disease, the median survival was 3.1 years, and about 15 percent lived 5 years or longer.

CHEMOTHERAPY

The era of antitumor chemotherapy, having been on the threshold of discovery by Paul Ehrlich in the late 1890s [197], began in 1942 when Goodman and Gilman discovered during World War II that nitrogen mustard compounds could suppress the growth of lymphoid tissue and some rapidly dividing cells. A large series of nitrogen mustard derivatives were synthesized later and tested for antitumor activity [198,199].

The hoped-for broad spectrum of antitumor activity or agents with highly selective antitumor effects in the nonhematopoietic neoplasms was not found, but compounds with improved pharmacologic properties were developed which are now in wide use. Ethyl carbamate (urethan) was introduced as an antileukemic agent and found to produce unique biologic and antitumor effects, but side reactions reduced its clinical efficacy [200]. Busulfan (1,4-dimethanesulfonyoxybutane; Myleran) was developed as a sulfonic acid alkylating compound and found to produce granulocytopenia in experimental animals [201], and a selective antileukemic effect in CML [202].

A dozen or more chemotherapeutic agents with a variety of chemical structures have shown significant degrees of activity against CML (Table 24-2). None appears to be more effective than busulfan. One group reported a median survival of 42 months in a group of 30 patients treated with busulfan [209]. Three died in less than 1 year, but at least four patients lived more than 5 years. Patients treated with busulfan live longer and better than untreated patients and as long as those treated with ^{32}P or x-ray. Side reactions to the chemical were infrequent. The response to successive courses of therapy tended to become less and the periods of remission shorter, but control of the disease was satisfactory until the acute phase developed. This occurred unpredictably in over two-thirds of the patients, abruptly or gradually over a period of months, with the onset of anemia, thrombocytopenia, increasing immaturity of the granulocytes, fever, and hepatosplenomegaly.

The clear superiority of busulfan over radiotherapy in

TABLE 24-2 Chemotherapeutic agents with significant activity in chronic myelogenous leukemia

Agent	References
Sulfonic acid esters:	
Busulfan	[104,202–209, 212–217]
Dihydroxybusulfan	[218]
Dimethanesulfonate	[219]
Nitrogen mustards, HN_2:	[220]
Triethylene melamine, TEM	[208,220,221]
Chlorambucil	[104,222,223]
L-Phenylalanine mustards, melphalan, L-sarcolysin	[224,225]
Uracil mustard	[226–228]
Cyclophosphamide	[215,228]
Antipurines:	
6-Mercaptopurine and 6-substituted derivatives	[210,213,229,230]
Thioguanine, thioguanosine	[231–233]
Antipyrimidines, urethan:	[200]
6-Azauridine	[210,234]
Colchicine and derivatives	[210,213,235–240]
Vinca alkaloids, vinblastine	[210,241–243]
Hydroxyurea	[244–248]
Dibromannitol	[249–254]

the treatment of CML was demonstrated in a cooperative trial involving 102 patients [214]. The form of treatment was determined by a randomized procedure, and subsequent analysis showed that there was no major difference in disease characteristics in the two groups of patients. Busulfan and radiotherapy were compared with reference to the control of spleen size, efficacy in restoring and maintaining a satisfactory hemoglobin level, adverse side effects, the prevailing clinical status of patients, and their survival. Although splenomegaly could be controlled equally well with both modalities, every other manifestation of CML was controlled better with busulfan. The median survival of the busulfan-treated group was almost 1 year longer than for those given irradiation, and the period for which 20 percent survived was 18 months longer. Blast cell transformation was the cause of death in 70 percent of the patients. The incidence of acute exacerbation was the same in both groups.

Busulfan and the two nitrogen mustard derivatives that are most generally effective in the treatment of CML, uracil mustard and melphalan [224–225], are used in approximately the same manner. Six to eight milligrams of busulfan or melphalan, or half this amount of uracil mustard, is given by mouth daily, before breakfast in one dose, for 10 to 14 days. The white cell count is determined once or twice a week, and when it begins to fall, the dose of the chemical is reduced. The maintenance dose of busulfan or melphalan may be as little as 2 to 6 mg per week. A period of 2 to 3 months is ordinarily required to correct the major clinical and hematologic evidences of the disease, and it is usually advisable to continue therapy for several additional weeks to ensure a long remission [209–212]. While interrupted courses of

therapy are preferred to avoid undue depression of marrow function, close control of the disease may be important in prolonging survival [196]. If cytopenia, particularly thrombocytopenia, is produced by busulfan, it may persist for several months. With any type of active chemotherapy, the dose of the agent must be carefully monitored and adjusted with reference to blood counts.

The leukocyte alkaline phosphatase level returns to normal in perhaps 50 to 60 percent of patients with CML during therapy and is generally regarded as a favorable prognostic sign [4,210]. Splenomegaly, eosinophilia, and/or basophilia may persist in some or recur quickly between courses of therapy. The prognosis is poorer in these patients, but there is no assured way to change the therapeutic strategy and improve their prospects.

None of the standard therapeutic agents or regimens used in the treatment of CML, however, eliminates the Ph^1 chromosome from cells in the bone marrow more than temporarily (see below). Cytogenetic studies in patients who would ordinarily qualify as having a complete clinical and hematologic remission show that upward of 90 percent of the dividing cells in the marrow still contain the abnormal chromosome [60,210]. The accidental or intentional production of severe and lasting cytopenia by busulfan or other agents in CML produces somewhat longer remissions but does not eliminate the abnormal chromosome or materially alter the subsequent evolution of the disease [210].

The first objective in treating CML is to control the abnormal myeloid proliferation with optimal selectivity, but individual peculiarities of the disease and complications prohibit stereotyped management. Busulfan has a profound effect on the platelets, and its use in patients with thrombocytopenia is hazardous. Cyclophosphamide or a thiopurine is a far safer agent to use in these patients [215,228,231–233]. After some years of busulfan therapy, pulmonary fibrosis, skin pigmentation, hypogonadism, and/or a syndrome with some features of Addison's disease may develop [4,257]. This necessitates an immediate halt in the use of busulfan, but the toxicity is often irreversible. The syndrome does not occur with the use of melphalan. Extreme leukocytosis increases the risk of cerebrovascular complications and may require leukapheresis or aggressive therapy with hydroxyurea, 4 to 6 g daily for 3 to 6 days to reduce the white cell count. Hydroxyurea can be employed for primary treatment of CML also, but it is more difficult to use than busulfan. Although its effects are rapid, disease control is labile. Enlargement of the spleen may persist in some instances and be a source of discomfort when all other manifestations of the disease are well controlled. This complication often responds at least temporarily to local radiation therapy. Iron and/or folic acid deficiency occur in CML, but manifestations of vitamin B_{12} deficiency are rare, even though abnormal binding of the vitamin occurs [258].

The anemia associated with active CML regresses with suppression of excessive myeloid proliferation. In rare instances it persists, however, and may be associated with the virtual disappearance of erythroid precursors from the marrow. The administration of pharmacologic doses of androgens may be helpful in these instances. Rarely, evidence of "hypersplenism" develops, often with additional cytopenias. If the marrow is cellular and contains an adequate number of precursor cells, splenectomy may be worthwhile, despite the risk of uncontrolled platelet proliferation (see below).

When hyperuricemia is present before treatment of CML is initiated, hydration and pretreatment with allopurinol for 1 to 2 days are advisable. The xanthine oxidase inhibitor is also useful in controlling chronic hyperuricemia and hyperuricosuria when these persist despite optimal control of the underlying disease [122–130].

PREGNANCY

The treatment of leukemia during pregnancy poses a particular dilemma. Children born of leukemic mothers are not affected by the disease, but irradiation and all chemotherapeutic agents are potentially harmful to the growing fetus [259–260]. Antileukemia therapy should be delayed as long as practical in early pregnancy and then given as cautiously as possible.

Gestation has progressed to a normal termination in many women with CML who have been treated with either antipurines or alkylating agents [260–266]. Leukapheresis may become the optimal treatment (see below). Most standard antileukemic agents affect eosinophils and basophils less than neutrophilic granulocytes. Eosinophilic leukemia is a heterogeneous entity, and its course is usually more acute than chronic [267–269]. This type of leukemia has been refractory to common therapeutic agents, but good remissions have been reported recently with the use of vincristine and hydroxyurea [243]. Basophilia in excess of 15 to 20 percent is generally reported as a poor prognostic sign. Basophilic leukemia may not be recognized before the phase of acute exacerbation, and the results of therapy have usually been poor [270].

As each new agent effective in controlling the major signs, symptoms, and hematologic abnormalities in CML appeared, its long-term effect in eliminating Ph[1] chromosome-containing myeloid precursors, and possibly in delaying or preventing the development of acute transformation, was explored. No single agent is effective in this regard, even when severe pancytopenia is produced intentionally or accidentally [271–274]. Clinical trials have been carried out rotating different agents to forestall "resistance," and antimetabolites have been substituted for the alkylating agents to avoid the additional leukemogenic effects of the latter [275–276]. There is no evidence that more complete remissions were produced or that there is a significant prolongation of the chronic phase of CML. Newer agents, such as doxorubicin, rubidomycin (daunorubicin), bleomycin, cytosine arabinoside, and L-aspariginase, and newer procedures, such as splenectomy and leukapheresis, were used in increasingly complicated and aggressive regimens. In some instances, the Ph[1]-positive cells in the marrow could be eliminated temporarily, and in some patients, a mixture of normal and abnormal cell types was observed along with some improvement in overall survival [273–276]. Benefit from or a definite role for immunotherapy in standard therapy was not substantiated [277–279].

SPLENECTOMY

Splenectomies performed in patients with CML during periods of exacerbation have usually had very poor results. Splenectomy may be beneficial in some individuals who develop unusual complications, such as thrombocytopenia, neutropenia, or increased red cell destruction [280–283]. The discovery that myeloid elements obtained from the spleen sometimes have a different karyotype than those in the circulating blood and marrow was interpreted as evidence that abnormal cell clones might originate in the spleen before disseminating to other tissues [284,285]. The possible benefit of elective splenectomy during the chronic phase of the disease was then investigated in many clinics [286–288]. With suitable preoperative and perioperative management, the mortality and morbidity with the procedure were not excessive [287]. The hazards of extreme postsplenectomy thrombocytosis [289] were avoided by excluding those patients with evidence of myelosclerosis or by using chemotherapy to reduce the platelet count to low normal preoperatively. The basic evolution of CML does not appear to be greatly altered by splenectomy, but 10 percent of patients seem to be benefited [287]. In one study involving 26 patients, elective splenectomy appeared to produce a significant postponement of acute transformation [286]. Although early splenectomy in CML generally does not prolong survival, the procedure reduces myeloid cell sequestration and possibly the generation of abnormal myeloid clones. It may avert the development of painful splenomegaly in those with advancing disease, and in patients with cytopenias, the tolerance to chemotherapy may be increased and the requirement for blood and platelet transfusions reduced. At the present time, there is no really effective means of treating the acute phase of the disease, when splenomegaly is most troublesome. Subjecting patients to splenectomy at this juncture is rarely beneficial.

LEUKAPHERESIS

Techniques for the removal of leukocytes from the blood were developed as an outgrowth of blood fractionation research carried out in World War II. With the development of continuous-flow closed-system centrifugation, platelets and granulocytes could be obtained for the first time in great enough numbers to be effective in the transfusion of patients with acute leukemia. With the first available equipment, patients with untreated CML were obviously the most suitable donors. This provided a unique opportunity to study the biologic and antileukemic effects of the procedure [290–294]. With repeated and intensive leukapheresis, enormous numbers of leukocytes could be removed from the blood, and with improved methodology, there was evidence finally that clinical symptoms could be relieved promptly in a large percentage of patients with reduction in organomegaly and leukocytosis [292–294]. Cyclical fluctuation in disease activity [295–297] and other variables may have accounted for some differences in therapeutic effect. Hyperuricemia and thrombocytopenia were never a major problem. Anemia requiring transfusions, however, was produced frequently by the removal of the more buoyant reticulocytes from the blood by the centrifugation procedure [294]. The relative importance in disease control of removing young myeloid cells and of circulating hemopoietic stem cells from the blood is unclear.

An increased number of hemopoietic progenitor cells was found in the blood of patients after they have been given doxorubicin and cyclophosphamide chemotherapy for a variety of malignancies [298]. The granulocyte progenitor cells disappeared from the blood 1 week after treatment, but then they returned to reach a peak of 10 times the pretreatment level in 21 days. On some occasions, as much as a twentyfold increment was found. Thus leukapheresis appeared to be a feasible method to collect an adequate number of hemopoietic progenitor cells that could be frozen, stored, and serve as an autologous graft later for patients given intensive cytotoxic drug therapy for the acute phase of CML.

In patients with untreated CML, the number of granulocyte progenitors was about three times normal in marrow and greatly increased in the blood, somewhat in proportion to the degree of blood granulocytosis [299,300]. After repeated leukaphereses had been carried out, the total number of leukocytes and granulocyte progenitors collected appeared to greatly exceed the number lost from the circulation [301,302]. This was interpreted as indicating that leukocytes and progenitors must have been mobilized from the marrow and spleen storage sites during the procedure. Studies were then carried out to determine optimal conditions for freezing, storing, and reconstituting hemopoietic stem cells. Methods were developed by which buffy-coat cells obtained during the chronic phase of the leukemia could be stored to use as an autograft later in the course of the disease [301,302]. In the first five patients with advanced CML who were pretreated with cytotoxic drugs plus radiotherapy and then given autologous buffy-coat leukocyte transfusions, a rapid restoration of normal blood counts was produced in three. Moreover, it appeared that lymphoid, as well as myeloid, reconstitution was accomplished [302]. The use of cytotoxic drugs, irradiation, splenectomy, and buffy-coat marrow transplantations at earlier stages of disease evolution is now being investigated.

Considerable encouragement has been provided by the report of a possible cure in patients with CML in whom the Ph¹-positive clone was eradicated by aggressive chemotherapy and irradiation, following which the marrow was repopulated with marrow obtained from normal identical twins [303].

Acute transformation

The accelerated, transformation or acute "myeloblastic crisis" phase of CML is an intrinsic feature of the disease and does not represent resistance to any one agent or therapeutic modality. All agents and treatment procedures ordinarily effective during the earlier phase of the disease are relatively impotent at this juncture. With new treatment programs it may be more important to recognize the earliest evidence of acute transformation, the point at which more aggressive therapeutic measures may need to be considered. As the acute disease progresses, it becomes increasingly refractory to treatment.

The acute phase of CML is clinically and hematologically heterogeneous [92,93]. In most series of patients, a few die from marrow hypoplasia, sometimes attributable to chemotherapy or irradiation, and 15 percent die from intercurrent diseases. About 80 percent of individuals with CML die as a result of acute transformation. The so-called myeloblastic crisis occurs in about 5 to 10 percent of patients. These individuals may have what appears to be well-controlled disease when they abruptly develop severe pancytopenia and are found to have a large number of blast cells in the blood and marrow. In the majority of patients, the disease gradually becomes less responsive to therapy over a period of months, and more severe symptoms develop: fever, sweating, aching in the bones, increasing hepatosplenomegaly, and weight loss. Marrow cell morphology becomes more abnormal [304], with the development of eosinophilia, basophilia, deformed red cells, atypical neutrophils, and thrombocytopenia. All these manifestations become increasingly refractory to therapy as the new cell species lose their capacity to differentiate [110,305–308].

In a recent study of the morphologic features of the blast crisis in CML, about 70 percent of the patients had a myeloblastic tranformation, including nearly 10 percent with a predominance of erythroblasts in the bone marrow [309]. The remainder had a lymphoblastic transformation as described earlier. There was no great difference in the clinical features of the two groups. Anemia and marrow megakaryocytosis occurred more frequently in the myeloblastic group and thrombocytopenia in the lymphoblastic group. Varying degrees of myelofibrosis were present in 40 percent of patients. Extramedullary leukemia with tumors or diffuse infiltration involving the skin, mucous membranes, lymph nodes, orbit, pleurae, synovia, extradural tissues, peripheral nerves, and meninges occurred in nearly 40 percent [309]. Other patients have been reported who developed erythroleukemia [94,98], refractory or sideroblastic anemia, rarely with acquired hemoglobin H disease [310], or myelofibrosis with destructive bone lesions [310–312]. The pattern of blastic transformation may be discordant with variation in the time and severity of involvement of different cell lines [112].

Several indicators are potentially useful in predicting the imminence of acute transformation in CML as well as in monitoring responses to therapy. Two to four months before the acute phase appears, new chromosome abnormalities superimposed on the Ph[1] cell line may be present [75,76,101,313]. With effective therapy, the original Ph[1] chromosome status present during the chronic phase of the disease may be restored. Other indicators of acute transformation are impairment of granulocyte cell growth in marrow cultures [314,315] and increasing TdT in marrow cells [316].

Treatment of the blast phase of CML has been notoriously difficult and mostly unrewarding. Short remissions have been produced in a few patients, both in those who are Ph[1]-positive and in those who are Ph[1]-negative, by the use of multiagent regimens developed for the treatment of acute leukemia [317–322]. Splenectomy early in the course of chronic disease has been claimed to postpone transformation and avert complications that might otherwise interfere with subsequent therapy [280–283]. Leukapheresis apparently does not prevent or delay transformation [290–294]. The type of cellular transformation that has evolved in individual patients provides a guide to the choice of the most promising chemotherapeutic agents to use initially. A large portion of the 20 percent of patients who have lymphoblastic marrow morphology or who are TdT-positive [91] responds to treatment with prednisone and vincristine [85,86,94,273]. Hypodiploidy is a favorable cytogenetic finding [86]. Blast cells of patients with advanced disease are extraordinarily resistant to aggressive chemotherapy and radiotherapy [276,322]. The elimination of abnormal cell lines by aggressive measures in those with advanced disease followed by the transplantation of marrow from HLA-identical siblings was rarely successful [322], in contrast to the results in grafting marrow from identical twins during the chronic phase of the disease [303].

Course and prognosis

The clinical course of chronic myelogenous leukemia, which was referred to earlier in some detail, can be divided into three phases: (1) a phase during which abnormal granulocytes proliferate until symptoms and signs of CML are produced, which lead to its recognition; (2) the chronic "treatable" phase, which usually lasts from 1 to 5 years; and (3) the accelerated phase, which usually lasts from 2 to 6 months.

An accurate prognosis cannot be made when CML first appears, even when factors such as the rapidity of onset and severity of symptoms, size of the spleen, degree of anemia, level of the white cell count, immaturity of the granulocytes, the presence of severe thrombocytopenia or thrombocytosis, or unrelated diseases are considered. Ph[1]-positive patients generally have a longer survival than those who are Ph[1]-negative, and women with CML survive longer than men [323]. If myeloblasts represent more than 10 percent of the leukocytes, the disease may behave more like subacute than chronic leukemia.

The development of fever, enlarged superficial lymph nodes, destructive bone lesions, hypercalcemia [324, 325], more pronounced basophilia or eosinophilia, or extramedullary tissue infiltration are unfavorable signs and may signify the presence or the imminent development of acute transformation. An incomplete response to therapy or short remissions between courses of treatment are usually associated with more severe disease. Granulocytic sarcomas (chloroma) are usually indicative of more acute disease [326–332].

Attempts to avert disease progression and to forestall the eventual development of the acute phase of the disease, which causes the death of the great majority of the patients with CML, have been unsuccessful. Aggressive programs of combination chemotherapy have occasionally resulted in karyotype conversion in Ph[1]-positive patients [275,276,302,320–322]. Nonconversions, or the persistence of Ph[1]-positive cells, probably identifies the proportion of cells that has not been, and possibly cannot be, eliminated with a given therapeutic regimen [322]. The existence of a normal population of cells or chromosomal mosaicism may be associated with prolonged remissions in the disease [333].

The likelihood of progression in a given instance is always difficult to predict. In some patients, chronic disease evolves into acute within a few weeks time, while in others it remains chronic for many years. The onset of the accelerated or acute phase of CML is often subtle and difficult to pinpoint, but its recognition is becoming more important, since it marks the point at which conventional therapeutic strategy should be reviewed.

References

1. Craige, D.: Case of disease of the spleen in which death took place in consequence of the presence of purulent matter in the blood. *Edinburgh Med. Surg. J.* 64:400, 1845.
2. Bennett, J. H.: Case of hypertrophy of the spleen and liver, in which death took place from suppuration of the blood. *Edinburgh Med. Surg. J.* 64:413, 1845.
3. Virchow, R.: Weisses Blut. *Froiep's Notizen* 36:151, 1845.
4. Damesek, W., and Gunz, F.: *Leukemia*, 2d ed. Grune & Straton, New York, 1964.
5. Bessis, M.: *Living Blood Cells and Their Ultrastructure.* Springer-Verlag, New York, 1973.
6. Burnet, M.: Leukaemia as a problem in preventive medicine. *N. Engl. J. Med.* 259:423, 1958.
7. Goh, K.: Total-body irradiation and human chromosomes: Cytogenic studies of the peripheral blood and bone marrow leukocytes seven years after total-body irradiation. *Radiat. Res.* 35:155, 1968.
8. Gibson, R. W., et al.: Leukemia in children exposed to multiple risk factors. *N. Engl. J. Med.* 279:906, 1968.
9. Rolleston, H.: Critical review: The harmful effects of irradiation (x-rays and radium). *Q. J. Med.* 24:101, 1930.
10. Martland, H.S.: The occurrence of malignancy in radioactive persons: A general review of data gathered in the study of the radium dial painters, with special reference to the occurrence of osteogenic sarcoma and the inter-relationship of certain blood diseases. *Am. J. Cancer* 15:2435, 1931.
11. Henshaw, P. S., and Hawkins, J.W.: Incidence of leukemia in physicians. *J. Natl. Cancer Inst.* 4:339, 1944.
12. March, H. C.: Leukemia in radiologists, *Radiology* 43:275, 1944.
13. March, H. C.: Leukemia in radiologists in a 20 year period. *Am. J. Med. Sci.* 220:282, 1950.

14. March, H. C.: Leukemia in radiologists, ten years later. Am. J. Med. Sci. 242:137, 1961.

15. Peller, S., and Pick, P.: Leukemia and other malignant disease in physicians. JAMA 147:893, 1951.

16. Lange, R. D., Moloney, W. C. and Yamawaki, R.: Leukemia in atomic bomb survivors. I. General observations. Blood 9:574,1954.

17. Moloney, W. C., and Lange, R. D.: Cytologic and biochemical studies on the granulocytes in early leukemia among atomic bomb survivors. Texas Rep. Biol. Med. 12:887, 1954.

18. Moloney, W. C.: Leukemia in survivors of atomic bombing. N. Engl. J. Med. 253:88, 1955.

19. Heyssel, R., Brill, A. M., Woodbury, L. A., Nishimura, E. T., Ghose, T., Hoshino, T., and Yamasaki, M.: Leukemia in Hiroshima atomic bomb survivors. Blood 15:313, 1960.

20. Cronkite, E. P., Moloney, W. C., and Bond, V. P.: Radiation leukemogenesis: An analysis of the problem. Am. J. Med. 28:673, 1960.

21. Hoshino, R., Kato, H., Finch, S. C., and Hrubec, Z.: Leukemia in offspring of atomic bomb survivors. Blood 30:719, 1967.

22. Neel, J. V., et al.: Search for mutations affecting protein structure in children of atomic bomb survivors: Preliminary report. Proc. Natl. Acad. Sci. U.S.A. 77:4221, 1980.

23. Court Brown, W. M., and Abbatt, J. D.: The incidence of leukaemia in ankylosing spondylitis treated with x-rays: A preliminary report. Lancet 1:1283, 1955.

24. Buckton, K. E., Jacobs, P. A., Court Brown, W. M., and Doll, R.: A study of the chromosome damage persisting after x-ray therapy for ankylosing spondylitis. Lancet 2:676, 1962.

25. Court Brown, W. M., and Doll, R.: Adult leukaemia. Br. Med. J. 1:1063, 1959; and 1:1753, 1960.

26. Silberberg, D. H., Frohman, L. A., and Duff, I. F.: The incidence of leukemia and related diseases in patients with rheumatoid (ankylosing) spondylitis treated with x-ray therapy. Arthritis Rheum. 3:64, 1960.

27. Graham, D. C.: Leukemia following x-ray therapy for ankylosing spondylitis. Arch. Intern. Med. 105:51, 1960.

28. Simpson, C. L., Hempelmann, L. H., and Fuller, L. M.: Neoplasia in children treated with x-rays in infancy for thymic enlargement. Radiology 64:840, 1955.

29. Latourette, H. B., and Hodges, F. J.: Incidence of neoplasia after irradiation of thymic region. Am. J. Roentgenol. 82:667, 1959.

30. Murray, R. Heckel, P., and Hempelmann, L. H.: Leukemia in children exposed to ionizing irradiation. N. Engl. J. Med. 261:585, 1959.

31. Gavosto, F., Pileri, A., and Pegoraro, L: X-rays and Philadelphia chromosome. Lancet 1:1336, 1965.

32. Moloney, W. C.: Leukemia and exposure to x-ray. Blood 14:1137, 1959.

33. Saenger, E. L., Thomas, G. E., and Tompkins, E. A.: Incidence of leukemia following treatment of hyperthyroidism. JAMA 205:855, 1968.

34. Court Brown, W. M., Doll, R., and Hill, A. B.: Incidence of leukaemia after exposure to diagnostic radiation in utero. Br. Med.J. 2:1539, 1960.

35. Graham, S., et al.: Preconception, intrauterine, and postnatal irradiation as related to leukemia, in Epidemiological Approaches to the Study of Cancer and Other Chronic Diseases, edited by William Haenszel. National Cancer Institute, Monograph 19, 1966, p. 347.

36. Henshaw, P. S: Leukemia in mice following exposure to x-rays. Radiology 43:279, 1944.

37. Furth, J., and Furth, O. B.: Neoplastic diseases produced in mice by general irradiation with x-rays. Incidence and type of neoplasm. Am. J. Cancer 28:54, 1936.

38. Mole, R. H.: The development of leukaemia in irradiated animals. Br. Med. Bull. 14:174, 1958.

39. Dungworth, D. L., Goldman, M., Switzer, J. W., and McKelvie, D. H.: Development of a myeloproliferative disorder in beagles continuously exposed to 90Sr. Blood 34:610, 1969.

40. Kaplan, H. S.: On the etiology and pathogenesis of the leukemias: A review. Cancer Res. 14:535, 1954.

41. Upton, A. C., Wolff, F. F., Furth, J., and Kimball, A. W.: A comparison of the induction of myeloid and lymphoid leukemias in x-radiated RF mice. Cancer Res. 18:842, 1958.

42. Bowditch, M., Elkins, H. B., Hunter, F. T., Mallory, T. B., Gall, E. A., and Buckley, W. J.: Chronic exposure to benzene (benzol). J. Industr. Hyg. Toxicol. 21:321, 1939.

43. Rawson, R., Parker, F., Jr., and Jackson, H., Jr.: Industrial solvents as possible etiologic agents in myeloid metaplasia. Science 93:541, 1941.

44. Infante, P. F., Rinsky, R. A., Wagoner, J. K., and Young, R. J.: Leukemia in benzene workers. Lancet 2:76, 1977.

45. Vigliani, E. C., and Saita, G.: Benzene and leukemia, N. Engl. J. Med. 271:872, 1964.

46. Tough, I. M., and Court Brown, W. M.: Chromosome aberrations and exposure to ambient benzene. Lancet 1:684, 1965.

47. Ford, C. E., Jacobs, P. A., and Lajtha, L. G.: Human somatic chromosomes. Nature 181:1565, 1958.

48. Baikie, A. G., Court Brown, W. M., Jacobs, P. A., and Milne, J. S.: Chromosome studies in human leukaemia. Lancet 2:425, 1959.

49. Nowell, P. C., and Hungerford, D. A.: A minute chromosome in human chronic granulocytic leukemia. Science 132:1497, 1960.

50. Nowell, P. C., and Hungerford, D. A.: Chromosome studies on normal and leukemic human leukocytes. J. Natl. Cancer Inst. 25:85, 1960.

51. Nowell, P. C., and Hungerford, D. A.: Chromosome studies in human leukemia. II. Chronic granulocytic leukemia. J. Natl. Cancer Inst. 27:1013, 1961.

52. Baikie, A. G., Court Brown, W. M., Buckton, K. E., Harnden, D. G., Jacobs, P. A., and Tough, I. M.: A possible specific chromosome abnormality in human chronic myeloid leukaemia. Nature 188:1165, 1960.

53. Sandberg, A. A., Ishihara, T., Crosswhite, L. H., and Hauschka, T. S.: Comparison of chromosome constitution in chronic myelocytic leukemia and other myeloproliferative disorders. Blood 20: 393, 1962.

54. Whang, J., Frei, E., III, Tijo, J. H., Carbone, P. P., and Brecker, G.: The distribution of the Philadelphia chromosome in patients with chronic myelogenous leukemia. Blood 22:664, 1963.

55. Goh, K., and Swisher, S. N.: Specificity of the Philadelphia chromosome: Cytogenic studies in cases of chronic myelocytic leukemia and myeloid metaplasia. Ann. Intern. Med. 61:609, 1964.

56. Krauss, S., Sokal, J. E., and Sandberg, A. A.: Comparison of Philadelphia chromosome-positive and -negative patients with chronic myelocytic leukemia. Ann. Intern. Med. 61:625, 1964.

57. Jacobs, E. M., Luce, J. K., and Cailleau, R.: Chromosome abnormalities in human cancer: Report of patient with chronic myelocytic leukemia and his non-leukemic monozygotic twin. Cancer 19:869, 1966.

58. Goh, K. O., and Swisher, S. N.: Chronic myelocytic leukemia and identical twins. Arch. Intern. Med. 120:214, 1967.

59. Bauke, J.: Chronic myelocytic leukemia. Cancer 24:643, 1969.

60. Tough, I. M.: Cytogenetic studies in cases of chronic myeloid leukemia with a previous history of radiation, in Current Research in Leukemia, edited by F. G. J. Hayhoe. Cambridge University Press, London, 1965, p. 47.

61. Caspersson, T., Zech, L., Johansson, C., and Modest, E. J.: Identification of human chromosomes by DNA-binding fluorescent agents. Chromosoma 30:215, 1970.

62. Summer, A. T., Evans, H. J., and Buckland, R. A.: New technique for distinguishing between human chromosomes. Nature 232:31, 1971.

63. Capersson, T., Gahrton, G., Lindsten, J., and Zech, L.: Identification of the Philadelphia chromosome as a number 22 by quinacrine mustard fluorescence analysis. Exp. Cell Res. 63:238, 1970.

64. O'Riordan, M. L., Robinson, J. A., Buckton, K. E., and Evans, H. J.: Distinguishing between the chromosomes involved in Down's syndrome (trisomy 21) and chronic myeloid leukaemia (Ph1) by fluorescence. Nature 230:167, 1971.

65. Gahrton, G., Lindsten, Jr., and Zech, L.: Origin of the Philadelphia chromosome: Tracing of chromosome 22 to parents of patients with chronic myelocytic leukemia. Exp. Cell. Res. 79:246, 1973.

66. Rowley, J. D.: A new consistent chromosome abnormality in chronic myelogenous leukemia identified by quinacrine fluorescence and Giemsa staining. Nature 243:290, 1973.

67. Engel, E., McGee, B. J., Flexner, J. M., Russel, M. T., and Myers, B. J.:

Philadelphia chromosome (Ph¹) translocation in an apparently Ph¹ negative, minus 22, case of chronic myeloid leukemia. *N. Engl. J. Med. 291*:154, 1974.

68. Engel, E., McGee, B. J., Flexner, J. M., and Krantz, S. B.: Translocation of the Philadelphia chromosome onto the 17 short arm in chronic myeloid leukemia: A second example. *N. Engl. J. Med. 293*:666, 1975.

69. Whang-Peng, J., Lee, E. C., and Knutsen, T. A.: Genesis of the Ph¹ chromosome. *J. Natl. Cancer Inst. 52*:1035, 1974.

70. Gahrton, G., Lindsten, J., and Zech, L.: Involvement of chromosomes 8, 9, 19, and 22 in Ph¹ positive and Ph¹ negative chronic myelocytic leukemia in the chronic or blastic stage. *Acta Med. Scand. 196*:355, 1974.

71. Mammon, Z., Grinblat, J., and Joshua, H.: Philadelphia chromosome with t(6;22) (p25;q12). *N. Engl. J. Med. 294*:827, 1976.

72. Hayata, I., Sakurai, M., Kakati, S., and Sandberg, A. A.: Chromosomes and causation of human cancer and leukemia. XVI. Banding studies of chronic myelocytic leukemia, including five unusual Ph¹ translocations. *Cancer 36*:1177, 1975.

73. Rowley, J. D.: Chromosomes in leukemia and lymphoma. *Semin. Hematol. 15*:301, 1978.

74. van den Berghe, H., et al.: First international workshop on chromosomes in leukemia. *Cancer Res. 38*:867, 1978.

75. Sandberg, A. A.: Chromosomes and causation of human cancer and leukemia. XL. The Ph¹ and other translocations in CML. *Cancer 46*:2221, 1980.

76. Kohno, S., and Sandberg, A. A.: Chromosomes and causation of human cancer and leukemia: Usual and unusual findings in Ph¹-positive CML. *Cancer 46*:2227, 1980.

77. Ezdinli, E. Z., Sokal, J. E., Crosswhite, L., and Sandberg, A. A.: Philadelphia-chromosome-positive and -negative chronic myelocytic leukemia. *Ann. Intern. Med. 72*:175, 1970.

78. Sakurai, M., Hayata, I., and Sandberg, A. A.: Prognostic value of chromosomal findings in Ph¹-positive chronic myelocytic leukemia. *Cancer Res. 36*:313, 1976.

79. Linder, D., and Gartler, S. M.: Glucose-6-phosphate dehydrogenase mosaicism. *Science 150*:67, 1965.

80. Beutler, E., Collins, Z., and Irvin, L. E.: Value of genetic variants of glucose-6-phosphate. *N. Engl. J. Med. 276*:389, 1967.

81. Fialkow, P. J., Gartler, S. M., and Yoshida, A.: Clonal origin of chronic myelocytic leukemia in man. *Proc. Natl. Acad. Sci. U.S.A. 58*:1468, 1967.

82. Barr, R. D., and Fialkow, P. J.: Clonal origin of chronic myelocytic leukemia. *N. Engl. J. Med. 289*:307, 1973.

83. Fialkow, P. J., and Jacobson, R. J.: Papayannopoulou T: Chronic myelocytic leukemia: Clonal origin in a stem cell common to the granulocytic, erythrocyte, platelet and monocyte/macrophage. *Am. J. Med. 63*:125, 1977.

84. Fialkow, P. J., et al.: Acute nonlymphocytic leukemia: Expression in cells restricted to granylocytic and monocytic differentiation. *N. Engl. J. Med. 301*:1, 1979.

85. Canellos, G. P., DeVita, V. T., Whang-Peng, J., and Carbone, P. P.: Hematologic and cytogenetic remission of blastic transformation in chronic granulocytic leukemia. *Blood 38*:671, 1971.

86. Rosenthal, S., Canellos, G. P., Whang-Peng, J., and Gralnick, H. R.: Blast crisis of chronic granulocytic leukemia: Morphologic variants and therapeutic implications. *Am. J. Med. 63*:542, 1977.

87. McCaffey, R., Harrison, T. A., and Parkman, R.: Terminal deoxynucleotidyl transferase activity in human leukemic cells and in normal human thymocytes. *N. Engl. J. Med. 292*:775, 1975.

88. Coleman, M. S., Greenwood, M. F., Hutton, J. J., Bollum, F. J., Lampkin, B., and Holland, P.: Serial observations on terminal deoxynucleotidyl transferase activity and lymphoblast surface markers in acute lymphoblastic leukemia. *Cancer Res. 36*:120, 1976.

89. Srivastava, B. I., Sahai, K., Sohaib, A., Minowada, J., Gomez, G. A., and Rakowski, I.: Terminal deoxynucleotidyl transferase activity in blastic phase of chronic myelogenous leukemia. *Cancer Res. 37*:3612, 1977.

90. Marks, S. M., Baltimore, D., and McCaffey, R.: Terminal transferase as a predictor of initial responsiveness to vincristine and prednisone in blastic chronic myelogenous leukemia. *N. Engl. J. Med. 298*:812, 1978.

91. Beutler, E., and Blume, K. G.: Terminal deoxynucleotidyl transferase: Biochemical properties, cellular distribution, and hematologic significance, in *Progress in Hematology*, edited by F. B. Brown. Grune & Stratton, New York, 1979, vol. 11, pp. 47–63.

92. Boggs, D. R.: Hematopoietic stem cell theory in relation to possible lymphoblastic conversion of chronic myeloid leukemia. *Blood 44*:449, 1974.

93. Shaw, M. T., Bottomley, R. H., Grozea, P. N., and Nordquist, R. E.: Heterogeneity or morphological, cytochemical, and cytogenetic features in the blastic phase of chronic granulocytic leukemia. *Cancer 35*:199, 1975.

94. Rosenthal, S., Canellos, G. P., and Gralnick, H. R.: Erythroblastic transformation of chronic granulocytic leukemia. *Am. J. Med. 63*:116, 1977.

95. Udomratn, T., Steinberg, M. H., Dreiling, B. J., and Lockhard, V.: Circulating micromegakaryocytes signaling blast formation of chronic myeloid leukaemia. *Scand. J. Haematol. 16*:394, 1976.

96. Fialkow, P. J., Denman, A. M., Jacobson, R. J., and Lowenthal, M. N.: Chronic myelocytic leukemia: Origin of some lymphocytes from leukemic stem cells. *J. Clin. Invest. 62*:815, 1978.

97. LeBien, T. W., Hozier, J., Minowada, J., and Kersey, J. H.: Origin of chronic myelocytic leukemia in a precursor of pre-B lymphocytes. *N. Engl. J. Med. 301*:144, 1979.

98. Neiman, R. S.: Erythroblastic transformation in myeloproliferative disorders (confirmation by an immunohistologic technique). *Cancer 46*:1636, 1980.

99. Propp, S., and Lizzi, F. A.: Philadelphia chromosome in acute lymphocytic leukemia (brief report). *Blood 36*:353, 1970.

100. Philip, P., Muller-Berat, N., and Killmann, S.: Philadelphia chromosome in acute lymphocytic leukemia. *Hereditas 84*:231, 1976.

101. Alimena, G.: Meeting report: Second International Workshop on Chromosomes in Leukemia. *Cancer Res. 40*:4826, 1980.

102. Metzgar, R. S., and Mohanakumar, T.: Tumor-associated antigens of human leukemia cells. *Semin. Hematol. 15*:139, 1978.

103. Minot, G. R., and Buckman, T. E.: The blood platelets in the leukemias. *Am. J. Med. Sci. 169*:477, 1925.

104. Rundles, R. W., et al.: Comparison of chlorambucil and myleran in chronic lymphocytic and granulocytic leukemia. *Am. J. Med. 27*:424, 1959.

105. Mason, J. E., Jr., DeVita, V. T., and Canellos, G. P.: Thrombocytosis in chronic granulocytic leukemia: Incidence and clinical significance. *Blood 44*:483, 1974.

106. Athens, J. W., et al.: Leukokinetic studies. X. Blood granulocyte kinetics in chronic myelocytic leukemia. *J. Clin. Invest. 44*:765, 1965.

107. Chervenick, P. A., and Boggs, D. R.: Granulocyte kinetics in chronic myelocytic leukemia. *Ser. Haematol. 1*:24, 1968.

108. Ogawa, M., Fried, J., Sakai, Y., Strife, A., and Clarkson, B. D.: Studies of cellular proliferation in human leukemia. VI. The proliferative activity, generation time, and emergence time of neutrophilic granulocytes in chronic granulocytic leukemia. *Cancer 25*:1031, 1970.

109. Price, G. B., and McCulloch, E. A.: Cell surfaces and the regulation of hemopoiesis. *Semin. Hematol. 15*:283, 1978.

110. Peterson, L. C., Bloomfield, C., and Brunning, R. D.: Blast crisis as an initial or terminal manifestation of chronic myeloid leukemia. A study of 28 patients. *Am. J. Med. 60*:209, 1976.

111. Nigam, R., and Dosik.: Chronic myelogenous leukemia presenting in the blastic phase and its association with a 45 XO Ph¹ karyotype. *Blood 47*:223, 1976.

112. Gall, J. A., Boggs, D. R., Chervenick, P. A., Pan, S., and Fleming, R. B.: Discordant patterns of chromosome changes and myeloblast proliferation during the terminal phase of chronic myeloid leukemia. *Blood 47*:347, 1976.

113. Mitelman, F., Brandt, L., and Nilsson, P. G.: Cytogenetic evidence for splenic origin of blastic transformation in chronic myeloid leukemia. *Scand. J. Haematol. 13*:87, 1974.

114. Mitelman, F., Nilsson, P. G., and Brandt, L.: Brief communication: Abnormal clones resembling those seen in blast crisis arising in the spleen in chronic myelocytic leukemia. *J. Natl. Cancer Inst. 54*:1319, 1975.

115. Brandt, L., Mitelman, F., and Panani, A.: Cytogenetic differences between bone marrow and spleen in a case of agnogenic myeloid

metaplasia developing blast crisis. *Scand. J. Haematol. 15:*187, 1975.

116. Cutler, S. J., Axteel, L., and Heise, J.: Ten thousand cases of leukemia: 1940–62. *J. Natl. Cancer Inst. 39:*993, 1967.

117. Leitner, S. J.: *Bone Marrow Biopsy,* translated by C. J. C. Britton and E. Neumark. Grune & Stratton, New York, 1949.

118. Goodman, S. B., and Block, M. H.: Increased red blood cell production in chronic myelocytic leukemia. *JAMA 200:*141, 1967.

119. Lennox, W. G., and Means, J. H.: Study of basal and nitrogenous metabolism in case of acute leukemia during roentgen ray treatment. *Arch. Intern. Med. 32:*705, 1923.

120. Riddle, M. C., and Sturgis, C. C.: Basal metabolism in chronic myelogenous leukemia. *Arch. Intern. Med. 39:*255, 1927.

121. Albright, E. C., and Middleton, W. S.: The uptake of radioactive iodine by the thyroid gland of leukemic patients. *Blood 5:*764, 1950.

122. Sandberg, A. A., Cartwright, G. E., and Wintrobe, M. M.: Studies on leukemia. I. Uric acid excretion. *Blood 11:*154, 1956.

123. Krakoff, I. H., and Balis, M. E.: Abnormalities of purine metabolism in human leukemia. *Ann. N.Y. Acad. Sci. 113:*1043, 1964.

124. Krakoff, I. H.: Studies of uric acid biosynthesis in the chronic leukemias. *Arthritis Rheum. 8:*772, 1965.

125. Rundles, R. W.: Uric acid metabolism in leukemia and lymphoma, in *Proceedings of the International Conference of Leukemia-Lymphoma,* edited by C. J. D. Zarafonetis. Lea & Febiger, Philadelphia, 1968, p. 385.

126. Wyngaarden, J. B.: Gout, in *The Metabolic Basis of Inherited Disease,* 2d ed., edited by J. B. Stanbury, J. B. Wyngaarden, and D. S. Fredrickson. McGraw-Hill, New York, 1966, p. 667.

127. Kravitz, S. C., Diamond, H. D., and Craver, L. F.: Uremia complicating leukemia chemotherapy. *JAMA 146:*1595, 1951.

128. Yü, T.: Secondary gout associated with myeloproliferative diseases. *Arthritis Rheum. 8:*765, 1965.

129. Rundles, R. W., Metz, E. N., and Silberman, H. R.: Allopurinol in the treatment of gout. *Ann. Intern. Med. 64:*229, 1966.

130. Rundles, R. W., Wyngaarden, J. B., Hitchings, G. H., and Elion, G. B.: Drugs and uric acid. *Annu. Rev. Pharmacol. 9:*345, 1969.

131. Wachstein, M.: Alkaline phosphatase activity in normal and abnormal human blood and bone marrow cells. *J. Lab. Clin. Med. 31:*1, 1946.

132. Beck, W. S., and Valentine, W. N.: Biochemical studies on leukocytes. II. Phosphatase activity in chronic lymphatic leucemia, acute leucemia and miscellaneous hematologic conditions. *J. Lab. Clin. Med. 38:*245, 1951.

133. Beck, W. S., and Valentine, W. N.: The aerobic carbohydrate metabolism of leukocytes in health and leukemia. II. The effect of various substances and coenzymes on glycolysis and respiration. *Cancer Res. 12:*823, 1952.

134. Kaplow, L. W.: A histochemical method for localizing and evaluating leukocyte alkaline phosphatase activity in smears of blood and marrow. *Blood 10:*1023, 1955.

135. Mitus, W. J., Mednicoff, I. B., and Dameshek, W.: Alkaline phosphatase of mature neutrophils in various "polycythemias." *N. Eng. J. Med. 260:*1131, 1959.

136. Tanaka, K. R., Valentine, W. N., and Fredericks, R. E.: Diseases or clinical conditions associated with low leukocyte alkaline phosphatase. *N. Engl. J. Med. 262:*912, 1960.

137. Ullyat, J. L., and Bainton, D. F.: Azurophil and specific granules of blood neutrophils in chronic myelogenous leukemia: An ultrastructural and cytochemical analysis. *Blood 44:*469, 1974.

138. Teplitz, R. L., Rosen, R. B., and Teplitz, M. R.: Granulocytic leukemia, Philadelphia chromosome and leukocyte alkaline phosphatase. *Lancet 2:*418, 1964.

139. Rosenblum, D., and Petzold, S. J.: Neutrophil alkaline phosphatase: Comparison of enzymes from normal subjects and patients with polycythemia vera and chronic myelogenous leukemia. *Blood 45:*335, 1975.

140. Winkelstein, A., Goldberg, L. S., Tishkoff, G. H., and Sparkes R. S.: Leukocyte alkaline phosphatase and the Philadelphia chromosome. *Arch. Intern. Med 119:*291, 1967.

141. Beard, M. F., Pitney, R. W., and Sanneman, E. H.: Serum concentrations of vitamin B 12 in patients from leukemia. *Blood 9:*789, 1954.

142. Beard, M. F., Pitney, W. R., Sanneman, E. H. Kakol, M. J., and Moorhead, H. H.: Serum concentrations of vitamin B 12 in acute leukemia. *Ann. Intern. Med. 41:*323, 1954.

143. Pitney, W. R., Beard, M. F., and van Loon, E. J.: Observations on the bound form of vitamin B_{12} in human serum. *J. Biol. Chem. 207:*143, 1954.

144. Stevenson, T. D., and Beard, M. F.: Serum vitamin B_{12} content in liver disease. *N. Engl. J. Med. 260:*206, 1959.

145. Weinstein, I. B., and Watkin, D. M.: Co^{58} B_{12} absorption, plasma transport and excretion in patients with myeloproliferative disorders, solid tumors, and non-neoplastic diseases. *J. Clin. Invest. 39:*1667, 1960.

146. Hall. C. A.: The plasma disappearance of radioactive vitamin B_{12} in myeloproliferative diseases and other blood disorders. *Blood 18:*717, 1961.

147. Retief, F. P., Vandenplas, L., and Visser, H.: Vitamin B 12 binding proteins in liver disease. *Br. J. Haematol. 16:*231, 1969.

148. Zittoun, J., Zittoun, R., Marquet, J., Sultan, C.: The three transcobalamins in myeloproliferative disorders and acute leukaemia. *Br. J. Haematol. 31:*287, 1975.

149. Hall, C. A.: Transcobalamins I and II as natural transport proteins of vitamin B_{12}. *J. Clin. Invest. 56:*1125, 1975.

150. Gilbert, H. S., Krauss, S., Pasternack, B., Herbert, V., and Wasserman, L. R.: Serum vitamin B_{12} content and unsaturated vitamin B_{12} binding capacity in myeloproliferative disease. *Ann. Intern. Med. 71:*719, 1969.

151. Scott, J. M., Bloomfield, F. J., Stebbins, R., and Herbert, V.: Studies on derivation of transcobalamin III from granulocytes: Enhancement by lithium and elimination by fluoride of in vitro increments in vitamin B_{12}-binding capacity. *J. Clin. Invest. 53:*228, 1974.

152. Magill, G. B., Wroblewski, F., and LaDue, J. S.: Serum lactic dehydrogenase and serum transaminase in human leukemia. *Blood 14:*870, 1959.

153. Bronson, W. R.: Pseudohyperkalemia due to release of potassium from white blood cells during clotting. *N. Engl. J. Med. 274:*369, 1966.

154. Perry, S., Godwin, H. A., and Zimmerman, T. S.: Physiology of the granulocyte. *JAMA 203:*937, 1968.

155. Galbraith, P. R.: Studies on longevity, sequestration and release of leukocytes in chronic myelogenous leukemia. *Can. Med. Assoc. J. 95:*511, 1966.

156. Boggs, D. R.: The cellular composition of inflammatory exudates in human leukemias. *Blood 15:*466, 1960.

157. Hirschberg, N.: Phagocytic activity in leukemia. *Am. J. Med. Sci. 197:*706, 1939.

158. Braude, A. I., Feltes, J., and Brooke, M.: Differences between the activities of mature granulocytes in leukemic and normal blood. *J. Clin. Invest. 33:*1936, 1954.

159. Brandt, L.: Studies on the phagocytic activity on neutrophilic leukocytes: Phagocytic activity of neutrophilic leukocytes in chronic myeloid leukemia. *Scand. J. Haematol. ,Suppl. 2:*35, 1967.

160. Whang-Peng, J., Perry, S., and Knutsen, T.: Maturation and phagocytosis by chronic myelogenous leukemia cells *in vitro. J. Natl. Cancer Inst. 38:*969, 1967.

161. Sbarra, A. J., Shirley, W., Selvaraj, R. J., McRipley, R. J., and Rosenbaum, E.: The role of the phagocyte in host parasite interactions. III. The phagocytic capabilities of leukocytes from myeloproliferative and other neoplastic disorders. *Cancer Res. 25:*1199, 1965.

162. Kalinske, R. W., and Hoeprich, P. D.: Engulfment and bactericidal capabilities of peripheral blood leukocytes in chronic leukemias. *Cancer 23:*1094, 1969.

163. Whittaker, J. A., Khurshid, M., and Hughes, H. R.: Neutrophil function in chronic granulocytic leukaemia before and after Busulphan treatment. *Br. J. Haematol. 28:*541, 1974.

164. Odelberg, H., Olofsson, T., and Olsson, I.: Granulocyte function in chronic granulocytic leukaemia. I. Bactericidal and metabolic capabilities during phagocytosis in isolated granulocytes. *Br. J. Haematol. 29:*427, 1975.

165. Lee, R. E., and Ellis, L. D.: The storage cells of chronic myelogenous leukemia. *Lab. Invest. 24:*261, 1971.

166. Laszlo, J.: Myeloproliferative disorders (MPD): Myelofibrosis myelosclerosis, extramedullary haematopoiesis, undifferentiated MPD, and haemorrhagic thrombocythaemia. *Semin. Hematol. 12:*75, 1975.

167. Clough, V., Geary, C. G., Hashini, K., Davson, J., and Knowlson, T.: Myelofibrosis in chronic granulocytic leukaemia. *Br. J. Haematol. 42:*515, 1979.

168. Petit, J. E., Lewis, S. M., and Nicholas, A. W.: Transitional myelo-proliferative disorder. *Br. J. Haematol.* 43:167, 1979.

169. Jackson, I. M. D., and Clark, R. M.: A case of neutrophilic leukemia. *Am. J. Med. Sci.* 249:72, 1965.

170. Rubin, H.: Chronic neutrophilic leukemia. *Ann. Intern. Med. 66*:93, 1966.

171. Randall, D. L., Reiquam, C. W., Githens, J. H., and Robinson, A.: Familial myeloproliferative disease: New syndrome closely simulating myelogenous leukemia in childhood. *Am. J. Dis. Child.* 110:479, 1965.

172. Strauss, M. B., Brokow, R., and Chapman, C. B.: Leukemoid bone marrow in pernicious anemia. *Am. J. Med. Sci.* 223:54, 1952.

173. Levine, P. H., and Hamstra, R. D.: Megaloblastic anemia of pregnancy simulating acute leukemia. *Ann. Intern. Med.* 71: 1141, 1969.

174. Twomey, J. J., and Leavell, B. W.: Leukemoid reactions to tuberculosis. *Arch. Intern. Med.* 116:21, 1965.

175. Morrow, L. B., and Anderson, R. E.: Active tuberculosis in leukemia: Malignant lymphoma and myelofibrosis. *Arch. Pathol.* 79:484, 1965.

176. Kauer, G. L., and Engle, R. L., Jr.: Eosinophilic leukaemia with Ph¹-positive cells, *Lancet* 2:1340, 1964.

177. Benvenisti, D. S., and Ultmann, J. E.: Eosinophilic leukemia: Report of five cases and review of literature. *Ann. Intern. Med.* 71:731, 1969.

178. Flannery, E. P., Dillon, D. E., Freeman, M. V. R., Levy, J. D., D'Ambrosio, U., and Bedynek, J. L.: Eosinophilic leukemia with fibrosing endocarditis and short Y chromosome. *Cancer* 29:660, 1972.

179. Chusid, M. J., Dale, D. C., West, B. C., and Wolff, S. M.: The hypereosinophilic syndrome: Analysis of fourteen cases with review of the literature. *Medicine* 54:1, 1975.

180. Youman, J. D., Taddeini, L., and Cooper, T.: Histamine excess symptoms in basophilic chronic granulocytic leukemia. *Arch. Intern. Med.* 131:560, 1973.

181. Cooke. J. V.: Chronic myelogenous leukemia in children. *J. Pediatr.* 42:537, 1953.

182. Barrett, O'N., Jr., Conrad, M., and Crosby, W. H.: Chronic granulocytic leukemia in childhood. *Am. J. Med. Sci.* 240:587, 1960.

183. Reisman, L. E., and Trujillo, J. M.: Chronic granulocytic leukemia of childhood: Clinical and cytogenic studies. *J. Pediatr.* 62:710, 1963.

184. Hardisty, R. M., Speed, D. E., and Till, M.: Granulocytic leukemia in childhood. *Br. J. Hematol.* 10:551, 1964.

185. Pochedly, C.: Unusual manifestations of chronic granulocytic leukemia in a child. *Cancer* 24:1017, 1969.

186. Hays, T., Morse, H., Peakman, D., Rose, B., and Robinson, A.: Cytogenic studies of chronic myelocytic leukemia in children and adolescents. *Cancer* 44:210, 1979.

187. Weatherall, D. J., Edwards, J. A., and Donohoe, W. T. A.: Haemoglobin and red cell enzyme changes in juvenile myeloid leukaemia. *Br. Med. J.* 1:679, 1968.

188. Weatherall, D. J., and Brown, M. J.: Juvenile chronic myeloid leukemia. *Lancet* 1:526, 1970.

189. Sheridan, B. L., et al.: The patterns of fetal haemoglobin production in leukaemia. *Br. J. Haematol.* 32:487, 1976.

190. Altman, A. J., Palmer, C. G., and Baehner, R. L.: Juvenile "chronic granulocytic" leukemia: A panmyelopathy with prominent monocytic involvement and circulating monocyte colony-forming cells. *Blood* 43:341, 1974.

191. Pusey, W. A.: Report of cases treated with roentgen rays. *JAMA* 38:911, 1902.

192. Minot, G. R., Buckman, T. E., and Isaacs, R.: Chronic myelogenous leukemia: Age incidence, duration and benefit derived from irradiation. *JAMA* 82:1489, 1924.

193. Osgood, E. E.: Titrated, regularly spaced radioactive phosphorus or spray roentgen therapy of leukemias. *Arch. Intern. Med.* 87:329, 1951.

194. Lawrence, J. H., Dobson, R. L., Low-Beer, B. V. A., and Brown, B. R.: Chronic myelogenous leukemia. *JAMA* 136:672, 1948.

195. Reinhard, E. H., Neely, L., and Samples, D. M.: Radioactive phosphorus in the treatment of chronic leukemias: Long-term results over a period of 15 years. *Ann. Intern. Med.* 50:942, 1959.

196. Shimkin, M. B., Mettier, S. R., and Bierman, H. R.: Myelocytic leukemia: An analysis of incidence, distribution and fatality, 1910–1948. *Ann. Intern. Med.* 35:194, 1951.

197. Schmidt, L. H.: Introductory remarks, comparative clinical and biological effects of alkylating agents. *Ann. N.Y. Acad. Sci.* 68:661, 1958.

198. Gilman, A., and Phillips, F. S.: The biological actions and therapeutic applications of the B-chloroethyl amines and sulfides. *Science* 103:409, 1946.

199. Bergel, F.: Design of alkylating agents for selectivity of action. *Ann. N.Y. Acad. Sci.* 68:1238, 1958.

200. Paterson, E., Haddow, A., ApThomas, I., and Watkinson, J. M.: Leukemia treated with erethane compared with deep x-ray therapy. *Lancet* 1:677, 1946.

201. Haddow, A., and Timmis, G. M.: Myleran in chronic myeloid leukemia: Chemical constitution and biological action. *Lancet* 1:207, 1953.

202. Galton, D. A. G.: Myleran in chronic myeloid leukaemia. *Lancet* 1:208, 1953.

203. Galton, D. A. G., and Till, M.: Myleran in chronic myeloid leukaemia. *Lancet* 1:425, 1955.

204. Blackburn, E. K., King, G. M., and Swan, H. T.: Myleran in treatment of chronic myeloid leukemia. *Br. Med. J.* 1:835, 1956.

205. Human, G. A., and Gellhorn, A.: Myleran therapy in malignant neoplastic disease: Use of 1,4-dimethanesulfonyloxybutane with emphasis on chronic granulocytic leukemia. *JAMA* 161:844, 1956.

206. Schilling, R. F., and Meyer, O. O.: Treatment of chronic granulocytic leukemia with 1,4-dimethanesulfonoxybutane (Myleran). *N. Engl. J. Med.* 254:986, 1956.

207. Unugur, A., Schulman, E., and Dameshek, W.: Treatment of granulocytic leukemia with Myleran. *N. Engl. J. Med.* 256:727, 1957.

208. Bethell, F. H.: Myleran and triethylene melamine in the treatment of chronic granulocytic leukemia. *Ann. N.Y. Acad. Sci* 68:996, 1958.

209. Haut, A., Abbott, W. S., Wintrobe, M. M., and Cartwright, G. E.: Busulfan in the treatment of chronic myelocytic leukemia: The effect of long term intermittent therapy. *Blood* 17:1, 1961.

210. Carbone, P. P., Tijo, J. H., Whang, J., Block, J. B., Kremer, W. B., and Frei, E.: The effect of treatment in patients with chronic myelogenous leukemia: Hematologic and cytogenetic studies. *Ann. Intern. Med.* 59:622, 1963.

211. Huguley, C. M., Jr., et al.: Comparison of 6-mercaptopurine and busulfan in chronic myelocytic leukemia. *Blood* 21:89, 1963.

212. Galton, D. A. G.: Problems in the management of the myeloproliferative states. *Ser. Haematol.* 1:37, 1965.

213. Tijo, J. H., Carbone, P., Whang, J., and Frei, E.: The Philadelphia chromosome and chronic myelogenous leukemia. *J. Natl. Cancer Inst.* 36:567, 1966.

214. Report of the Medical Research Council's Working Party for Therapeutic Trials in Leukaemia: Chronic granulocytic leukaemia: Comparison of radiotherapy and busulphan therapy. *Br. Med. J.* 1:201, 1968.

215. Kaung, D. T., Close, H. P., Whittington, R. M., and Patno, M. E.: Comparison of busulfan and cyclophosphamide in the treatment of chronic myelocytic leukemia. *Cancer* 27:608, 1971.

216. Gollerkeri, M. P., and Shah, G. B.: Management of chronic myeloid leukemia: A five-year survey with a comparison of oral busulfan and plenic irradiation. *Cancer* 27:596, 1971.

217. Conrad, F. G.: Survival in chronic granulocytic leukemia: Splenic irradiation vs busulfan. *Arch. Intern. Med.* 131:684, 1973.

218. Loeb, V., Jr.: Dihydroxybusulfan (NSC-39069) in chronic myelocytic leukemia and miscellaneous malignant neoplasms. *Cancer Chemother. Rep.* 42:39, 1964.

219. Van Dyk, J. J., Falkson, G., and Falkson, H. C.: Clinical experience with 1,4-dihydtacryloylpiperazine, dimethanesulfonate (NSC-47774). *Cancer Chemother. Rep.* 52:275, 1968.

220. Karnofsky, D. A.: Summary of results obtained with nitrogen mustard in the treatment of neoplastic disease. *Ann. N.Y. Acad. Sci.* 68:899, 1958.

221. Rundles, R. W., Coonrad, E. V., and Willard, N. L.: Summary of results obtained with TEM. *Ann. N.Y. Acad. Sci.* 68:926, 1958.

222. Krakoff, I. H., Karnofsky, D. A., and Burchenal, J. H.: Remissions induced by chlorambucil in chronic granulocytic leukemia. *JAMA* 166:629, 1958.

223. Rundles, R. W., Grizzle, J., Bono, V. H., Jonsson, U., Huguley, C. M., and Corley, C. C., Jr.: Comparison of CB-1348 (chlorambucil, Leukeran) and CB-1364. *Cancer Chemother. Rep* 16:223, 1962.

224. Hauch, T., Logue, G., Laszlo, J., Cox, E., and Rundles, R. W.: Treat-

ment of chronic granulocytic leukemia with melphalan. *Blood* 51:571, 1978.

225. Seeler, R. A., and Hahn, K. O.: Chronic granulocytic leukemia responding to Melphalan. *Cancer* 27:284, 1971.

226. Shanbrom, E., Miller, S., Haar, H., and Opfell, R.: Therapeutic spectrum of uracil-mustard, a new antitumor drug. *JAMA* 174:1702, 1960.

227. Wilkinson, J. F., Bourne, M. S., and Israels, M. C. G.: Treatment of leukemias and reticuloses with uracil mustard. *Br. Med. J.* 1:1563, 1963.

228. Frommeyer, W. B., Jr.: Comparison of cyclophosphamide (Cytoxan) and uracil mustard (U-8344) in chronic granulocytic leukemia. *Cancer* 17:288, 1964.

229. Burchenal, J. H., et al.: Clinical evaluation of a new antimetabolite, 6-mercaptopurine, in the treatment of leukemia and allied diseases. *Blood* 8:965, 1953.

230. Rundles, R. W., Laszio, J., Itoga, T., Hobson, J. B., and Garrison, F. E.: Clinical and hematologic study of 6-[(1'-methyl-4'-nitro-5'-imidazolyl)thio] purine (B.W. 57-322) and related compounds. *Cancer Chemother. Rep.* 14:99, 1961.

231. Rundles, R. W., Fulmer, T. E., Doyle, R. T., and Gore, T. W.: Effect of 2-amino-6-[(1'-methyl-4'-nitro-5'-imidazolyl)thio] purine (B.W. 57-323) on neoplastic disease in man. *Cancer Chemother. Rep.* 8:66, 1960.

232. Krakoff, I. H., Ellison, R. R., and Tan, C. T. C.: Clinical evaluation of thioguanosine. *Cancer Res.* 21:1015, 1961.

233. Spiers, A. S. D., Galton, D. A. G., Kaur, J., and Goldman, J. M.: Thioguanine as primary treatment for chronic granulocytic leukemia. *Lancet* 1:829, 1975.

234. Fallon, H. J., Frei, E., III, and Freireich, E. J.: Correlation of the biochemical and clinical effects of 6-azauridine in patients with leukemia. *Am. J. Med.* 33:526, 1962.

235. Moeschlin, S., Meyer, H., and Lichtman, A.: Ein neues Colchicum-Nebenalkaloid (Demecolcin Ciba) als Cytostaticum Myeloischer Leukamien. *Schweiz. Med. Wochenschr.* 83:990, 1953.

236. Jaffe, I. A., and Hyman, G. A.: Hematologic toxicity after the use of desacetylmethylcolchicine in the treatment of gouty arthritis. *N. Engl. J. Med.* 257:157, 1957.

237. Dittman, W. A., and Ward, J. R.: Demecolcine toxicity. *Am. J. Med.* 27:519, 1959.

238. Lessman, E. M., and Sokal, J. E.: A colchicine derivative in therapy of chronic myelocytic leukemia. *JAMA* 175:741, 1961.

239. Lessner, H., Jonsson, U., Loeb, V., and Larsen, W.: Preliminary clinical experience with trimethylcolchicinic acid methyl ether *d*-tartrate (TMCA) in various malignancies. *Cancer Chemother. Rep.* 27:33, 1963.

240. Stolinsky, D. C., et al.: Clinical trial of trimethylcolchicinic acid methyl ether *d*-tartrate (TMCA: NSC036354) in advanced cancer. *Cancer Chemother. Rep.* 51:25, 1967.

241. Hill, J. M., and Loeb, E.: Treatment of leukemia, lymphoma, and other malignant neoplasms with vinblastine. *Cancer Chemother. Rep.* 15:41, 1961.

242. Johnson, I. S.: Historical background of vinca alkaloid research and areas of future interest. *Cancer Chemother. Rep.* 52:455, 1968.

243. Chusid, M. J., and Dale, D. C.: Eosinophilic leukemia: Remission with vincristine and hydroxyurea. *Am. J. Med.* 59:297, 1975.

244. Kennedy, B. J., and Yarbro, J. W.: Metabolic and therapeutic effects of hydroxyurea in chronic myelogenous leukemia. *Trans. Assoc. Am. Physicians* 78:391, 1965.

245. Kennedy, B. J.: Hydroxyurea therapy in chronic myelogenous leukemia. *Cancer* 29:1052, 1972.

246. Vogler, W. R., Horwitz, S., and Groth, D. P.: Studies in the effects of hydroxyurea and other anticancer drugs upon pyrimidine metabolism. *Cancer Res.* 29:1371, 1969.

247. Schwartz, J. H., and Canellos, G. P.: Hydroxyurea in the management of the hematologic complications of chronic granulocytic leukemia. *Blood* 46:11, 1975.

248. Yataganas, X., Strife, A., Perez, A., and Clarkson, B.: Cell kill kinetics with hydroxyurea. *Med. Pediatr. Oncol.* 2:39, 1976.

249. Eckhardt, S., Sellei, C., Horvath, I. P., and Institorisz, L.: Effects of 1,6-dibromo-1, 6-dideoxy-*d*-mannitol on chronic granulocytic leukemia. *Cancer Chemother. Rep.* 33:57, 1963.

250. Casazza, A. R., Cahn, E. L., and Carbone, P. P.: Preliminary studies with dibromomannitol (NSC-94100) in patients with chronic myelogenous leukemia. *Cancer Chemother. Rep.* 51:91, 1967.

251. Ramanan, C. V., and Israels, M. C. G.: Treatment of chronic myeloid leukaemia with dibromomannitol. *Lancet* 2:125, 1969.

252. Eckhardt, S.: Clinical pharmacology of dibromohexitols, in *Chronic Myeloid Leukaemia*, edited by S. Tura and M. Baccarani. St. Orsola University Hospital, Bologna, 1972, p. 125.

253. Tura, S., et al.: Dibromomannitol and chronic myeloid leukaemia: Results of a cooperative study, in *Chronic Myeloid Leukaemia*, edited by S. Tura and M. Baccarani. St. Orsola University Hospital, Bologna, 1972, p. 136.

254. Canellos, G. P., Young, R. C., Nieman, P. E., and DeVita, V. T. Jr.: Dibromomannitol in the treatment of chronic granulocytic leukemia: A prospective randomized comparison with busulfan. *Blood* 45:197, 1975.

255. Tough, I. M., et al.: Chronic myeloid leukemia: Cytogenic studies before and after splenic irradiation. *Lancet* 2:115, 1962.

256. Whang-Peng, J., Canellos, G. P., Carbone, P. P., and Tijo, J. H.: Clinical implications of cytogenic variants of chronic myelocytic leukemia (CML). *Blood* 32:755, 1968.

257. Kyle, R. A., Schwartz, R. W., Olner, H. B., and Dameshek, W.: Syndrome resembling adrenal cortical insufficiency associated with long term busulfan (Mylean) therapy. *Blood* 18:497, 1961.

258. Sage, R. E.: Polycythemia rubra vera with pernicious anemia: Some observations on vitamin B_{12} metabolism. *Blood* 5:920, 1950.

259. Ask-Upmark, E.: Another follow-up study of children born of mothers with leukemia. *Acta Med. Scand.* 175:391, 1964.

260. Sokal, J. E., and Lessmann, E. M.: Effects of cancer chemotherapeutic agents on the human fetus. *JAMA* 172:1765, 1960.

261. Reyes, G. R., and Perez, R. T.: Leukemia and pregnancy: Observation of a case treated with busulfan (Mylean). *Blood* 18:764, 1961.

262. White, L. V. G.: Busulfan in pregnancy. *JAMA* 179:973, 1962.

263. Dennis, L. H., and Stein, S.: Busulfan in pregnancy: Report of a case. *JAMA* 192:715, 1965.

264. Earll, J. M., and May, R. L.: Busulfan therapy of myelocytic leukemia during pregnancy. *Am. J. Obstet. Gynecol.* 92:580, 1965.

265. Dugdale, M., and Fort, T.: Busulfan treatment of leukemia during pregnancy: Case report and review of literature. *JAMA* 199:131, 1967.

266. Richard, H. G. H., and Spiers, A. S. D.: Chronic granulocytic leukaemia in pregnancy. *Br. J. Radiol.* 48:261, 1975.

267. Benvenisti, D. S., and Ultman, J. E.: Eosinophilic leukemia. *Ann. Intern. Med.* 71:731, 1969.

268. Goh, D., Swisher, S. N., and Rosenberg, C. A.: Cytogenic studies in eosinophilic leukemia. *Ann. Intern. Med.* 62:80, 1965.

269. Gruenwalk, H., Kiossoglou, K. A., Mitus, W. J., and Dameshek, W.: Philadelphia chromosome in eosinophilic leukemia. *Am. J. Med.* 39:1003, 1965.

270. Kyle, R. A., and Pease, G. L.: Basophilic leukemia. *Arch. Intern. Med.* 118:205, 1966.

271. Monfardini, S., Gee, T., Fried, J., and Clarkson, B.: Survival in chronic myelogenous leukemia: Influence of treatment and extent of disease at diagnosis. *Cancer* 31:492, 1973.

272. Hayes, D. M., Ellison, R. R., Glidewell, O., Holland, J. F., and Silver, R. T.: Chemotherapy, for the terminal phase of chronic myelocytic leukemia. *Cancer Chemother. Rep.* 58:233, 1974.

273. Spiers, A. S. D.: The treatment of chronic granulocytic leukemia (annotation). *Br. J. Haematol.* 32:291, 1976.

274. Allan, N. D., Duvall, E., and Stockdill, G.: Combination chemotherapy for chronic granulocytic leukaemia. *Lancet* 2:523, 1978.

275. Cunningham, I., et al.: Results of treatment of Ph+ chronic myelogenous leukemia with an intensive treatment regimen (L-5 protocol). *Blood* 53:375, 1979.

276. Sharp, J. D., et al.: Karyotypic conversion in Ph^1-positive chronic myeloid leukaemia with combination chemotherapy. *Lancet* 2:1370, 1979.

277. Fairley, G. H.: Immunotherapy in the management of myelogenous leukemia. *Arch. Intern. Med.* 136:1406, 1976.

278. Sokal, J. E.: Immunotherapy for chronic granulocytic leukaemia. *Clin. Haematol.* 6:129, 1977.

279. Murphy, S., and Hersh, E. Immunotherapy of leukemia and lymphoma. *Semin. Hematol.* 15:181, 1978.

280. Jonsson, U., Hansen-Pruss, O. C., and Rundles, R. W.: Hemolytic

anemia in myelogenous leukemia with splenectomy. *Blood* 5:920, 1950.

281. Green, T. W., Conley, C. L., Ashburn, L. I., and Peters, H. R.: Splenectomy for myeloid metaplasia of the spleen. *N. Engl. J. Med.* 248:211, 1953.

282. Canellos, G. P., Norkland, J., and Carbone, P. P.: Splenectomy for thrombocytopenia in chronic granulocytic leukemia. *Ann. Intern. Med.* 76:447, 1972.

283. Spiers, A. S. D., et al.: Splenectomy for complications of chronic granulocytic leukaemia. *Lancet* 2:7936, 1975.

284. Mitelman, F., Brandt, L., and Nilsson, P. G.: Cytogenetic evidence for splenic origin of blastic transformation in chronic myeloid leukaemia. *Scand. J. Haematol.* 13:87, 1974.

285. Gomez, G., Hossfeld, D. K., and Sokal, J. E.: Removal of abnormal clone of leukaemic cells by splenectomy. *Br. J. Haematol.* 2:421, 1975.

286. Spiers, A. S. D., et al.: Chronic granulocytic leukaemia: Effect of elective splenectomy on the course of disease. *Br. Med. J.* 1:175, 1975.

287. Gomez, G. A., Sokal, J. E., Mittelman, A., and Aungst, C. W.: Splenectomy for palliation of chronic myelocytic leukemia. *Am. J. Med.* 61:14, 1976.

288. Ihde, D. C., Canellos, G. P., Schwartz, J. H., and DeVita, V. T.: Splenectomy in the chronic phase of chronic granulocytic leukemia. Effects in 32 patients. *Ann. Intern. Med.* 84:17, 1976.

289. Bensinger, T. A., Logue, G. L., and Rundles, R. W.: Hemorrhagic thrombocythemia: Control of postsplenectomy thrombocytosis with melphalan. *Blood* 36:61, 1970.

290. Vallejos, C. S., McCredie, K. B., Britten, G. M., and Freireich, E. J.: Biological effects of repeated leukapheresis of patients with chronic myelogenous leukemia. *Blood* 42:925, 1973.

291. Fortuny, I. E., Crandall, L., McCullough, J., Theologides, A., Kennedy, B. J.: Leukapheresis in the management of chronic leukemia. *Minnesota Med.* 56:674, 1973.

292. Lowenthal, R. M., et al.: Intensive leukapheresis as initial therapy for chronic granulocytic leukaemia. *Blood* 46:835, 1975.

293. Hadlock, D. C., Fortuny, I. E., McCullough, J., and Kennedy, B. J.: Continuous flow centrifuge leucapheresis in the management of chronic myelogenous leukaemia. *Br. J. Haematol.* 29:443, 1975.

294. Lowenthal, A. M.: Chronic leukaemias: Treatment by leukapheresis. *Exp. Hematol.* 5:(Suppl.)73, 1977.

295. Vodopick, H., Rupp, E. M., Edwards, C. L., Goswitz, F. A., and Beauchamp, J. J.: Spontaneous cyclic leukocytosis and thrombocytosis in chronic graulocytic leukaemia. *N. Engl. J. Med.* 286:284, 1972.

296. Gatti, R., et al.: Cyclic leukocytosis in chronic myelogenous leukemia: New perspectives on pathogenesis and therapy. *Blood* 41:771, 1973.

297. Rodriguez, A. R., and Lutcher, C. L.: Marked cyclic leukocytosis-leukemia in chronic myelogenous leukemia. *Am. J. Med.* 60:1041, 1976.

298. Richman, C. M., Weiner, R. S., and Yankee, R. A.: Increase in circulating stem cells following chemotherapy in man. *Blood* 47:1301, 1976.

299. Goldman, J. M., Th'ng, K. H., and Lowenthal, R. M.: In vitro colony forming cells and colony stimulating factor in chronic granulocytic leukaemia. *Br. J. Cancer* 30:12, 1974.

300. Goldman, J. M., Th'ng, K. H. Gatovsky, D., and Galton, D. A. G.: Production of colony-stimulating factor by leukemic leukocytes. *Blood* 47:381, 1976.

301. Goldman, J. M.: Circulating stem cells: Effects of leukapheresis. *Exp. Hematol.* 5:85, 1976.

302. Goldman, J. M.: Modern approaches to the management of chronic granulocytic leukaemia. *Semin. Hematol.* 15:420, 1978.

303. Fefer, A., et al.: Disappearance of Ph¹-positive cells in four patients with chronic granulocytic leukemia after chemotherapy, irradiation and marrow transplantation from an identical twin. *N. Engl. J. Med.* 300:333, 1979.

304. Bainton, D. F., Lawrence, M. F., and Shohet, S. B.: Abnormalities in granule formation in acute myelogenous leukemia. *Blood* 49:693, 1977.

305. Canellos, G. P., DeVita, V. T., Wang-Peng, J., and Carbone, P. P.: Hematologic and cytogenetic remission of blast transformation in chronic granulocytic leukemia. *Blood* 38:671, 1971.

306. Bornstein, R. S., Nesbit, M., and Kennedy, B. J.: Chronic myelogenous leukemia presenting in blastic crisis. *Cancer* 30:939, 1972.

307. Beard, M. E. J., et al.: Blast crisis of chronic myeloid leukaemia (CML): Presentation stimulating acute lymphoid leukaemia (ALL). *Br. J. Haematol.* 34:167, 1976.

308. Gustavsson, A., Mitelman, F., and Olsson, I.: Acute myeloid leukaemia with the Philadelphia chromosome. *Scand. J. Haematol.* 19:449, 1977.

309. Rosenthal, S., Canellos, G. P., DeVita, V. T., and Gralnick, H. R.: Characteristics of blast crisis in chronic granulocytic leukemia. *Blood* 49:705, 1977.

310. Yoo, D., Schecter, G. P., Amigable, A. N., and Nienhuis, A. W.: Myeloproliferative syndrome with sideroblastic anemia and acquired hemoglobin H disease. *Cancer* 45:78, 1980.

311. Chabner, B. A., Haskell, Cm., and Canellos, G. P.: Destructive bone lesions in chronic granulocytic leukemia. *Medicine* 48:401, 1969.

312. Kosmidis, P. A., Palacas, C. G., and Axelrod, A. R.: Diffuse purely osteolytic lesions in myelofibrosis. *Cancer* 46:2263, 1980.

313. Rowley, J. D.: Ph¹-positive leukemia, including chronic myelogenous leukemia. *Clin. Haematol.* 9:55, 1980.

314. Moore, M. A. S.: Prediction of relapse and remission in AML by marrow culture criteria. *Blood Cells* 2:109, 1976.

315. Moore, M. A. S.: In vitro culture studies in chronic granulocytic leukemia. *Clin. Haematol.* 6:97, 1977.

316. Ross, D. D., Wiernik, M. D., Sarin, P. S., and Wang-Peng, J.: Loss of terminal deoxynucleotidyl transferase (TdT) activity as a predictor of emergence of resistance to chemotherapy in a case of chronic myelogenous leukemia in blast crisis. *Cancer* 44:1566, 1979.

317. Vallejos, C. S., Trujillo, J. M., Cork, A., Bodey, G. P., McCredie, D. B., and Freireich, E. J.: Blastic crisis in chronic granulocytic leukemia: Experience in 39 patients. *Cancer* 34:1806, 1974.

318. Spiers, A. S. D., Costello, C., Catovsky, D., Galton, D. A. G., and Goldman, J. M.: Chronic granulocytic leukaemia: Multiple-drug chemotherapy for acute transformation. *Br. Med. J.* 3:77, 1974.

319. Gomez, G. A., Sokal, J. E., and Aungst, C. W.: Chemotherapy of the terminal phase of chronic myelocytic leukemia with combinations of colchicine derivatives and purine analogs. *Leukemia Res.* 2:141, 1976.

320. Beard, M., Gauci, C., Sikora, E., Kirk, B., and Fairley, G.: Blast crisis of chronic myeloid leukaemia: The effect of intensive chemotherapy. *Scand. J. Haematol.* 16:258, 1976.

321. Mandelli, F., Amadori, S., Alimena, G., Annino, L., Nardelli, S., and Papa, G.: Experience on the treatment of chronic myelocytic leukaemia (CML) in blastic crisis. *Scand. J. Haematol.* 19:495, 1977.

322. Doney, K., Buckner, C. D., Sale, G. E., Ramberg, R., Boyd, C., and Thomas, E. D.: Treatment of chronic granulocytic leukemia by chemotherapy, total body irradiation and allogeneic bone marrow transplantation. *Exp. Hematol.* 6:738, 1978.

323. Kardinal, C. G., Bateman, J. R., and Weiner, J.: Chronic granulocytic leukemia: Review of 536 cases. *Arch. Intern. Med.* 136:305, 1976.

324. Haskell, C. M., DeVita, V. T., and Canellos, G. P.: Hypercalcemia in chronic granulocytic leukemia. *Cancer* 27:872, 1971.

325. Walter, R. M., and Greenberg, B. R.: Hypercalcemia in the accelerated phase of chronic myelogenous leukemia. *Cancer* 46:1174, 1980.

326. Wiercik, P. H., and Serpick, A. A.: Granulocytic sarcoma (chloroma). *Blood* 35:361, 1970.

327. Pascoe, H. R.: Tumors composed of immature granulocytes occurring in the breast in chronic granulocytic leukemia. *Cancer* 25:697, 1970.

328. Fayami, A. O., Gerber, M. A., Cohen, I., Davis, S., and Rubin, A. D.: Myeloid sarcoma. Review of the literature and report of a case. *Cancer* 32:253, 1973.

329. Rosenoff, S. H., Canellos, G. P., O'Connell, M., and Wiernik, P. H.: Mediastinal adenopathy in granulocytic leukemia. *Arch. Intern. Med.* 134:135, 1974.

330. Lieu, P. I., Ishimaru, T., McGregor, D. H., Okada, H., and Steer, A.: Autopsy study of granulocytic sarcoma (chloroma) in patients with myelogenous leukemia, Hiroshima-Nagasaki 1949–1969. *Cancer* 31:948, 1973.

331. Krause, J. R.: Granulocytic sarcoma preceding acute leukemia: A report on six cases. *Cancer* 44:1017, 1979.

332. McCarty, K. S., Wortman, J., Daly, J., Rundles, R. W., and Hanker,

J. S.: Chloroma (granulocytic sarcoma) without evidence of leukemia: Facilitated light microscopic diagnosis. *Blood* 56:104, 1980.

333. Golde, D. W., Bersch, N. L., and Sparkes, R. S.: Chromosomal mosaicism associated with prolonged remission in chronic myelogenous leukemia. *Cancer* 37:1849, 1976.

CHAPTER 25

Agnogenic myeloid metaplasia

MURRAY N. SILVERSTEIN

Definition and history

Agnogenic myeloid metaplasia is a chronic myeloproliferative disorder characterized by (1) splenomegaly, (2) immature granulocytes and erythroblasts in the blood, (3) distorted and teardrop-shaped red cells, and (4) some degree of marrow fibrosis. The disorder was originally described by Heuck [1] in 1879 under the title "Two Cases of Leukemia and Peculiar Blood and Bone Marrow Findings." He recognized that the findings in these two patients differed from those of chronic myelogenous leukemia by the prominence of marrow fibrosis and of extramedullary hemopoiesis in the liver and spleen.

Etiology and pathogenesis

Agnogenic myeloid metaplasia has a close pathogenetic relationship to the other chronic myeloproliferative diseases, such as polycythemia vera, chronic myelogenous leukemia, and primary thrombocythemia [2], each of which is thought to result from a hemopoietic stem cell lesion.

Studies in women heterozygous for isotypes A and B of the enzyme glucose-6-phosphate dehydrogenase (G-6-PD) support the hypothesis that the hemopoietic abnormalities in agnogenic myeloid metaplasia arise from a single multipotential stem cell, since blood cells have one enzyme isotype [3,4]. In contrast, the marrow fibroblasts contain G-6-PD A and G-6-PD B, the typical mosaicism expected in tissue. Chromosomal aberrations in the blood cells of patients with agnogenic myeloid metaplasia have not been present in the patient's fibroblasts [5]. Thus the marrow fibroblasts are not derived from the abnormal clone and their proliferation represents a secondary effect.

The etiology of agnogenic myeloid metaplasia is unknown. Lesions similar to the human disease have been produced in murine species by (1) chemical agents such as lead acetate and saponin, (2) viruses, (3) estrogenic hormones, (4) immunologic reactants, (5) industrial solvents such as benzene, and (6) ionizing radiation. In all experimental models, a common mechanism observed prior to the onset of myelofibrosis is the development of severe vascular injury to the marrow [6]. The disease in murine species, produced by whatever means, leads to a rapidly developing clinical picture of severe pancytopenia, extramedullary hemopoiesis, and marrow fibrosis with subsequent rapid demise of the animals.

In humans, exposure to benzene or its derivatives has been associated with an increased frequency of myelofibrosis. Ionizing radiation may be a factor in the development of some cases, since an increased incidence of myelofibrosis has been reported in survivors of the Hiroshima atomic bomb blast [7] and in patients with polycythemia vera treated with ^{32}P [8]. Immunologic mechanisms have also been associated with human agnogenic myeloid metaplasia, as noted by its development in patients with lupus erythematosus [9] and the high incidence of immune complexes in patients [10].

The pathogenesis of the fibrosis is controversial, but the G-6-PD and chromosomal data indicate that the fibrosis is provoked by the hemopoietic process. Platelets and megakaryocytes contain a potent growth factor which stimulates fibroblastic proliferation [11]. Thus the proliferation of megakaryocytes and the release of platelet growth factor for fibroblasts could be important in the occurrence of fibrosis. In agnogenic myeloid metaplasia there is a progressive insolubilization of collagen as the disease process continues [12].

Myelofibrosis develops in about 15 percent of patients with polycythemia vera (postpolycythemia myeloid metaplasia) and can be related to previous ^{32}P therapy [8]. About 10 percent of patients with classic agnogenic myeloid metaplasia eventually develop acute myelogenous leukemia [13].

Clinical features

Most patients are in the sixth and seventh decades of life when the disease is diagnosed [6,14]. Males are a little more frequently affected than females. Less than 30 cases of the disorder have been reported in patients below the age of 30 [15]. Approximately one-third of patients are asymptomatic at the time of their diagnosis. They are either discovered by the abnormalities observed in the blood or by the finding of a large spleen on physical examination.

Most of this group have symptoms or signs of anemia, such as weakness, fatigue, exertional dyspnea, palpitations, or pallor. Patients may complain of a dragging sensation in the left upper abdomen or of early satiety resulting from the pressure of the enlarged spleen on the gastric outlet. Splenic infarction with severe left upper quadrant pain may occur in occasional patients. Petechiae or ecchymoses secondary to thrombocytopenia, qualitative platelet defects, or disseminated intravascular coagulation are often present.

Splenomegaly is present in all patients. The spleen is

mildly enlarged in one-third of patients, is enlarged to greater than 5 cm below the left costal margin in one-third, and fills the entire left side of the abdomen in the remaining third [6]. Splenomegaly is due to extramedullary hemopoiesis in the spleen plus a markedly increased blood flow through the celiac axis to the spleen. Hepatomegaly is observed in the majority of patients and may be the result of a marked increase in blood flow to the liver from the spleen [6]. Although extramedullary hemopoiesis occurs frequently in the liver in the nonsplenectomized patient, it is unusual for it to account for excessive hepatomegaly. Jaundice or ascites has been observed in occasional patients.

Laboratory features

A normocytic-normochromic anemia develops in about two-thirds of patients [6]. A few patients may develop a hypochromic-microcytic anemia secondary to gastrointestinal bleeding from either varices or a peptic ulcer. In nearly all patients, ineffective erythropoiesis is present, and in half the anemic patients there is a shortened red cell survival time. Overt, severe hemolytic anemia may occur and is nearly always antiglobulin test negative. Red cell mass and plasma volume measurements may detect hypervolemia, which can explain in part the low hemoglobin concentration that results from the expanded plasma volume and the hemoconcentration in a massively enlarged spleen. Thrombocytopenia develops in about a third of patients. Thrombocytosis is present in a similar proportion, and platelet counts in excess of 600,000 per microliter occur in about 10 percent of patients. Fifteen percent of the patients develop leukopenia. Blood films reveal a leukoerythroblastic reaction, i.e., granulocyte immaturity and erythroblasts in the blood. Accompanying this reaction is significant tear-drop poikilocytosis (Fig. 25-1). Teardrop red cells are present in virtually every oil-immersion field on the blood film. Following removal of the spleen, the teardrop red cells either disappear or are reduced in frequency, suggesting that injury during splenic passage is important in their formation [16].

Marrow aspirates are usually hypocellular but can be hypercellular (10 percent of patients) or normocellular (5 percent of patients). Marrow biopsy sections contain varying degrees of reticulin or collagen fibrosis in all patients.

Defects in hemostasis are common [6]. In addition to thrombocytopenia, almost all patients have an abnormal second wave of platelet aggregation in response to collagen and epinephrine [17]. The prothrombin time is prolonged in most patients, often resulting from a deficiency of factor V. A few patients have the classic laboratory profile of disseminated intravascular coagulation (DIC), which is characterized by low levels of factors V and VIII, thrombocytopenia, and the presence of increased levels of fibrin split products. Most patients with this profile do not have bleeding manifestations and thus have "the syndrome of inapparent DIC" [6].

Other laboratory findings include an elevation of leukocyte alkaline phosphatase scores in some patients [18], elevation in serum uric acid concentrations, and a decrease in serum albumin and cholesterol levels [19]. Patients with agnogenic myeloid metaplasia and polycythemia vera have a high frequency of serum monoclonal immunoglobulins [6], although several population studies have shown similar frequencies in aged healthy individuals.

Chromosomal abnormalities occur frequently [20,21], but no specific abnormality that is predictive of either the clinical course or of transformation into acute leukemia has been observed. Trisomy and monosomy involving the C group of chromosomes are the most common

FIGURE 25-1 Blood films from two patients with agnogenic myeloid metaplasia. (*a*) Characteristic teardrop poikilocytes, a nucleated red cell, and a segmented neutrophil are evident. (*b*) Teardrop red cells, a nucleated red cell, and a promyelocyte are present.

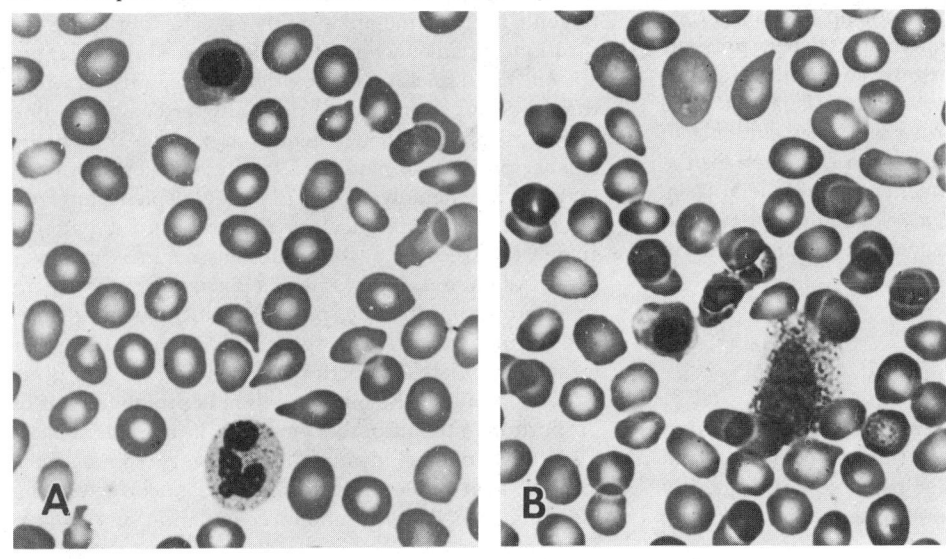

abnormality. Patients with classic agnogenic myeloid metaplasia, both clinically and at autopsy, have been described who have the Ph[1] chromosome in their marrow cells [6]. About one-half the patients will develop radiographic evidence of bone change, usually increased bone density due to osteosclerosis [22]. Osteolytic lesions are rare and should alert the clinician to the possibility of a leukemic transformation to granulocytic sarcoma (chloroma) [6,23].

Differential diagnosis

The most frequent lesion to be considered in the differential diagnosis of agnogenic myeloid metaplasia is chronic myelogeneous leukemia. In chronic myelogenous leukemia, the white cell count is over 30,000 per microliter in most patients and over 100,000 per microliter in half the patients. In myelofibrosis, the white count is usually less than 30,000 per microliter. In chronic myelogenous leukemia, red cell shape is normal or slightly perturbed, whereas in myelofibrosis, teardrop poikilocytes are present in every oil-immersion field. The marrow in chronic myelogenous leukemia shows intense granulocytic hyperplasia and very slight or absent fibrosis. In myelofibrosis, the marrow is normal or hypocellular with moderate to marked fibrosis. The presence of the Ph[1] chromosome also would point toward myelogenous leukemia. Most cases are readily separable on the basis of these laboratory studies. Metastatic carcinoma and tuberculous or fungal involvement of the marrow can cause myelofibrosis [24,25]. Rapid progression of disease and other clinical considerations may point to carcinoma or infection. The demonstration of metastatic carcinoma cells or organisms in the marrow indicates the etiology of the underlying myelofibrosis in these cases. Postpolycythemia myeloid metaplasia is defined by a foregoing history of polycythemia vera. Rarely, a patient with agnogenic myeloid metaplasia may be confused with one exhibiting a dyshemopoietic (preleukemic) state. Reticulin staining of the marrow and spleen size can help to differentiate these diseases. Hairy cell leukemia, when it presents with pancytopenia, splenomegaly, and a fibrotic marrow, can mimic myeloid metaplasia. Usually careful scrutiny of the blood and marrow will show evidence of the abnormal mononuclear cell which characterizes the disease. Also, features of agnogenic myeloid metaplasia, such as nucleated red cells, myeloid immaturity, and teardrop red cells, may be absent from the blood film in patients with hairy cell leukemia.

Acute myelofibrosis

Acute myelofibrosis (or acute myelosclerosis) is a syndrome characterized by anemia, thrombocytopenia, and intense myelofibrosis. Neither palpable splenomegaly nor teardrop poikilocytosis are present. The leukocyte count may be low or moderately elevated. Myeloblasts are usually present in the blood. The clinical course is accelerated from that in agnogenic myeloid metaplasia and survival beyond 1 year is unusual [26,27]. Acute myelofibrosis may be a variant of acute megakaryocytic leukemia [29,30]. The myelofibrosis is thought to be caused by the stimulatory effect of the primitive hemopoietic cells (megakaryoblasts) on marrow fibroblasts. Almost all patients with acute myelofibrosis have been found at autopsy to have acute leukemia. (See Chap. 28.) Several patients have had successful treatment with intensive chemoradiotherapy and marrow transplantation. Marrow fibrosis has disappeared with the eradication of the disease and successful transplant [28].

Treatment

Patients with agnogenic myeloid metaplasia who are asymptomatic when first seen are best left untreated. Approximately 80 percent of the asymptomatic patients with agnogenic myeloid metaplasia seen at diagnosis will remain stable for 5 years [6]. The major problem requiring therapy is anemia. In those patients with severe normocytic-normochronic anemia, androgen therapy may be helpful. Prospective studies of the role of androgens suggest that the anemia may improve in about 50 percent of treated patients [6]. Either oxymetholone in doses up to 200 mg per day orally or testosterone enanthate in doses of 200 to 400 mg intramuscularly every 3 to 4 weeks can be used. While patients are on oxymethalone therapy, careful monitoring of liver function tests is essential. Since one-half of patients with normocytic, normochromic anemia have shortened red cell survival, glucocorticoids can be considered. Thus one out of every two patients with normocytic, normochromic anemia may benefit from treatment with androgens and glucocorticoids. For patients with significant hemolytic anemia, a trial of prednisone in doses of 30 to 60 mg per day is recommended.

Splenectomy is important in the management of agnogenic myeloid metaplasia [31–34]. The four major indications for splenectomy include (1) painfully enlarged spleen, (2) refractory hemolytic anemia, (3) refractory thrombocytopenia, and (4) portal hypertension. In one series, 50 patients had splenectomy; 26 of 27 patients splenectomized for pain, 5 of 9 patients splenectomized for refractory hemolysis, 4 of 10 patients splenectomized for refractory thrombocytopenia, and 4 of 4 patients splenectomized for portal hypertension had improvement. All patients should have a partial thromboplastin time, prothrombin time, platelet count, bleeding time, and fibrinogen and fibrin split products measured prior to surgery. Platelet-function studies can be useful as well, especially if the bleeding time is prolonged out of proportion to the thrombocytopenia. If the patient has a qualitative platelet dysfunction, surgery can be performed after platelet transfusion has corrected the bleeding time. Patients who on coagulation survey have findings of disseminated intravascular coagulation are at serious risk of hemorrhage with surgery and should not have the procedure. Mean survival following splenectomy is 25 months. The procedure does not seem to alter the overall clinical course, and patients die of the same causes as patients who have not had splenectomy.

Patients with myeloid metaplasia can develop portal hypertension and varices because of an enormous splenic blood flow and increased resistance to blood flow in the liver [35]. Patients who are operated on for portal hypertension and bleeding varices should have circulatory dynamic studies performed at the time of surgery. In those patients in whom the hepatic wedge-pressure elevations are a result of the markedly increased blood flow from the spleen to the liver, the curative procedure for portal hypertension is splenectomy. In those patients who have portal hypertension as a result of intrahepatic block, a splenorenal shunt rather than a portacaval shunt is recommended [6].

Chemotherapy and radiation therapy have been employed in patients with myeloid metaplasia. Either modality will reduce the size of the spleen to half its pretreatment size. However, within 3 to 4 months, splenomegaly usually recurs, and few patients treated with either modality can be expected to maintain a reduced spleen size for 1 year [6]. Therapy with hydroxyurea, however, is indicated in the group of patients who develop compensatory hepatic myeloid metaplasia with marked hepatomegaly following splenectomy.

Radiotherapy is indicated for patients with myeloid metaplasia in three situations [6]: (1) acute splenic infarction (in which doses of 50 to 200 rads will produce a rapid amelioration of pain); (2) ascites when megakaryocytes are demonstrated in the ascitic fluid (this finding suggests that myeloid metaplasia of the peritoneum is the etiology of the ascites, and cautious low-dose total abdominal radiation may produce a disappearance of peritoneal lesions with disappearance of ascites); and (3) focal areas of severe bone pain, which usually represent either acute leukemia or a granulocytic sarcoma (in which focal radiation therapy can lead to marked amelioration of pain). Hematologic remission has been described in one case of myeloid metaplasia by bilateral iliac-crest marrow curettage [36]. Investigative approaches to the disease include the use of agents that prevent collagen formation, such as monoamineoxidase inhibitors and such lysylaldehyde chelators as dehydroproline.

Course and prognosis

Some patients with agnogenic myeloid metaplasia remain asymptomatic for at least 5 years. The 5-year survival is about 60 percent of that expected for age- and sex-matched controls [6]. The common causes of death include degenerative vascular disease (i.e., acute myocardial infarction or congestive heart failure) in 35 percent of cases, hemorrhage in 25 percent of cases, acute

leukemia in 25 percent of cases, and infection in 15 percent of cases [37]. Certain clinical measures are important prognostic indicators at the time of diagnosis. Those patients who are asymptomatic, not anemic, not thrombocytopenic, and do not have enlarged livers tend to do better than their symptomatic, anemic, thrombocytopenic, or hepatomegalic counterparts. Sex and the size of the spleen at diagnosis have no prognostic value. Patients with significant ineffective erythropoiesis, accelerated hemolysis, and diminution of total red cell mass may have a poorer survival than patients without these features [38]. Rare patients who develop acquired hemoglobin H disease [39] or acute lymphocytic leukemia [40] have been reported. Extremely rare spontaneous improvement in marrow function also has been reported [41,42].

References

1. Heuck, G.: Zwei Fälle von leukämie mit eigenthümlichem blut-resp knoch en marksbefund. *Virchows Arch.* [*Pathol. Anat.*] 78:475, 1879.
2. Silverstein, M. N.: Myeloproliferative disease: Their shifting spectrums. *Postgrad. Med.* 43:167, 1968.
3. Jacobson, R. S., Salo, A., and Fialkow, P. S.: Agnogenic myeloid metaplasia: A clonal proliferation of hematopoietic stem cells with secondary myelofibrosis. *Blood* 51:189, 1978.
4. Kahn, A., et al.: A deficient G-6-PD variant with hemizygous expression in blood cells of a woman with primary myelofibrosis. *Humangenetik* 30:41, 1975.
5. Van Slyck, E. J., Weiss, L., and Dully, M.: Chromsomal evidence for the secondary role of fibroblastic proliferation in acute myelofibrosis. *Blood* 36:729, 1970.
6. Silverstein, M. N.: *Agnogenic Myeloid Metaplasia.* Publishing Science Corp., Boston, 1975.
7. Anderson, R. E., Hoshino, T., and Yamamoto, T.: Myelofibrosis with myeloid metaplasia in survivors of the atomic bomb in Hiroshima. *Ann. Intern. Med.* 60:1, 1964.
8. Silverstein, M. N.: The evolution into and the treatment of late-stage polycythemia vera. *Semin. Hematol.* 3:79, 1976.
9. Rosen, P. S., et al.: Systemic lupus erythematosus (SLE) and myelofibrosis: A possible pathogenic relationship. *Clin. Res.* 21:565, 1973.
10. Lewis, C. M., and Pegrum, G. D.: Immune complexes in myelofibrosis: A possible guide to management. *Br. J. Haematol.* 39:233, 1978.
11. Ross, R., and Vogel, R.: The platelet-derived growth factor. *Cell* 14:203, 1980.
12. Charron, D., et al.: Biochemical and histological analysis of bone marrow collagen in myelofibrosis. *Br. J. Haematol.* 41:151, 1979.
13. Silverstein, M. N., Brown, A. L., Jr., and Linman, S. W.: Idiopathic myeloid metaplasia: Its evolution into acute leukemia. *Arch. Intern. Med.* 132:709, 1973.
14. Bouroncle, B., and Doan, C. A.: Myelofibrosis. *Am. J. Med. Sci.* 243:697, 1962.
15. Boxer, L. A., Camitta, B. M., Berenberg, W., and Fanning, J. P.: Myelofibrosis–myeloid metaplasia in childhood. *Pediatrics* 55:861, 1975.
16. DiBella, N. J., Silverstein, M. N., and Hoagland, H. C.: Effect of splenectomy on teardrop-shaped erythrocytes in agnogenic myeloid metaplasia. *Arch. Intern. Med.* 137:380, 1977.
17. Neemeh, J. A., Bowie, E. J. W., Thompson, J. H., Didisheim, P., and Owen, C. A., Jr.: Quantitation of platelet aggregation in myeloproliferative disorders. *Am. J. Clin. Pathol.* 57:336, 1972.
18. Silverstein, M. N., and Elveback, L. R): Leukocyte alkaline phosphatase in agnogenic myeloid metaplasia. *Am. J. Clin. Pathol.* 61:307, 1974.
19. Gilbert, H. S., et al.: Characterization of hypocholesterolemia in myeloproliferative diseases. *Am. J. Med.* 71:595, 1981.

20. Whang-Peng, J., et al.: Cytogenetic studies in patients with myelosclerosis and myeloid metaplasia. *Leukemia Res. 21*:41, 1977.
21. Nowell, P. C., and Finian, J. B.: Cytogenetics of acute and chronic myelofibrosis. *Virchows Archiv. [Cell Pathol.] 29*:45, 1978.
22. Killmann, S.-A.: Myelofibrosis. *Clin. Orthop. 52*:95, 1967.
23. Ward, H. P., and Block, M. H.: The natural history of agnogenic myeloid metaplasia (AMM) and a critical evaluation of its relationship with the myeloproliferative syndrome. *Medicine (Baltimore) 50*:357, 1971.
24. Kiely, J. M., and Silverstein, M. N.: Metastatic carcinoma simulating agnogenic myeloid metaplasia. *Cancer 24*:1041, 1969.
25. Silverstein, M. N., Martin, W. J., and Bahn, R. C.: Fever, polycythemia and lip ulcer. *Minn. Med. 47*:569, 1964.
26. Lewis, S. M., and Szur, L.: Malignant myelosclerosis. *Br. J. Med. 1*:472, 1963.
27. Bergsman, K. L., and Van Slyck, E. J.: Acute myelofibrosis. *Ann. Intern. Med. 74*:232, 1971.
28. Wolf, J. L., et al.: Reversal of acute malignant myelosclerosis by allogenic bone marrow transplantation. *Blood 59*:191, 1982.
29. Breton Gorius, S., Daniel, M., Flandrin, G., and Kinet-Dendel, C.: Fine structural and peroxidase activity of circulating micromegakaryoblasts and platelets in a case of acute myelofibrosis. *Br. J. Haematol. 25*:331, 1973.
30. den Ottolander, G. J., et al.: Megakaryoblastic leukaemia (acute myelofibrosis): A report of three cases. *Br. J. Haematol. 42*:9, 1979.
31. Silverstein, M. N., and ReMine, W. H.: Sex, splenectomy and myeloid metaplasia. *JAMA 227*:424, 1974.
32. Silverstein, M. N., and ReMine, W. H.: Splenectomy in agnogenic myeloid metaplasia. *Blood 53*:515, 1979.
33. Mulder, H., Steenbergen, J., and Haanen, C.: Clinical course and survival after elective splenectomy in 19 patients with primary myelofibrosis. *Br. J. Haematol. 35*:419, 1977.
34. Benbassat, J., Penchas, S., and Ligumski, M.: Splenectomy in patients with agnogenic myeloid metaplasia: An analysis of 321 published cases. *Br. J. Haematol. 42*:207, 1979.
35. Rosenbaum, D. L., Murphy, G. W., and Swisher, S. N.: Hemodynamic studies of the portal circulation in myeloid metaplasia. *Am. J. Med. 41*:360, 1966.
36. Matzner, Y., et al.: Sustained haematological remission after bone marrow curettage in a case of primary myelosclerosis. *Scand. J. Haematol. 20*:168, 1979.
37. Silverstein, M. N., and Linman, J. W.: Causes of death in agnogenic myeloid metaplasia. *Mayo Clin. Proc. 44*:36, 1969.
38. Najean, Y., et al.: Erythrokinetic studies in myelofibrosis. *Br. J. Haematol. 40*:205, 1978.
39. Veer, A., Kosciolek, B. A., Bauman, A. W., and Rowley, P. T.: Acquired hemoglobin H disease in idiopathic myelofibrosis. *Am. J. Hematol. 6*:199, 1979.
40. Polliack, A., Prokocimer, M., and Matzner, Y.: Lymphoblastic leukemic transformation (lymphoblastic crisis) in myelofibrosis and myeloid metaplasia. *Am. J. Hematol. 9*:211, 1980.
41. Shreiner, D. P.: Spontaneous hematologic remission in agnogenic myeloid metaplasia. *Am. J. Med. 60*:1014, 1976.
42. Kelemen, E., Kraszuai, G., Endes, P., and Szinay, G.: Chronic idiopathic myelofibrosis. A reversible disease? *Acta Haematol. 57*:171, 1977.

CHAPTER 26

Primary thrombocythemia

MURRAY N. SILVERSTEIN

Primary thrombocythemia, the least common of the chronic myeloproliferative diseases, is defined by (1) a platelet count in excess of 1 million per microliter, (2) profound megakaryocytic hyperplasia in the marrow with a background of myriad platelets, (3) the absence of the Philadelphia chromosome, (4) the absence of an increased red cell mass, and (5) the absence of a disorder associated with reactive thrombocytosis, such as severe iron deficiency, lung cancer, or a collagen disease (see Chap. 145) [1]. Ancillary features include a mild neutrophilic leukocytosis in most patients, palpable splenomegaly in about half the patients, and a microcytic-hypochromic anemia in some patients as a result of chronic blood loss.

Primary thrombocythemia was initially described by Epstein and Goedel in 1934 [2]. Synonyms for the syndrome include *idiopathic,* or *essential, thrombocythemia, primary hemorrhagic thrombocythemia,* and *primary thrombohemorrhagic thrombocythemia.* Several reviews of the syndrome have been published [3–10].

Etiology and pathogenesis

The etiology of thrombocythemia is unknown, although pathogenetically it is closely related to the other chronic myeloproliferative diseases, i.e., polycythemia vera, chronic myelogenous leukemia, and agnogenic myeloid metaplasia. Studies on three affected women who were heterozygous for glucose-6-phosphate dehydrogenase isoenzymes A and B have established primary thrombocythemia, like the other chronic myeloproliferative diseases, to be a clonal disorder originating in a multipotential stem cell [11]. Primary thrombocythemia is so closely related to the other chronic myeloproliferative diseases that in one series of 50 patients with thrombocythemia [1], two patients developed polycythemia vera, two developed acute myelogenous leukemia, two developed agnogenic myeloid metaplasia, and two evolved into a syndrome indistinguishable from chronic myelogenous leukemia within 1 to 5 years of the diagnosis of thrombocythemia.

Most patients are over 50 years of age, but the disease occurs occasionally in patients aged 20 to 40 years [12]. In older patients, the combination of increased platelets and degenerative vascular disease may lead to serious bleeding or thrombosis. Bleeding may occur as a result of three mechanisms: (1) an initial intravascular thrombosis with distal infarction, ulceration of the infarct, and bleeding; (2) platelet functional abnormalities; and (3) consumption of coagulation factors. The occurrence of thrombosis is related to platelet hyperaggregability [13,14]. Silent infarctions of the spleen secondary to splenic vascular thrombosis may occur in over 20 percent of patients. This is thought to induce splenic atrophy and lead to the high proportion of patients without splenomegaly when compared with the other chronic myeloproliferative diseases. Patients with this syndrome who have an enlarged spleen have a longer survival than those who do not, perhaps because sequestration of platelets in the spleen is beneficial to them. The markedly elevated platelet count is the result of a marked increase in platelet production, which averages about six times normal [15]. Survival of the platelets is usually normal or slightly decreased.

CLINICAL FEATURES

Essential thrombocythemia usually appears between the ages of 50 and 70 years. Males and females are equally affected [7–10]. Approximately 20 percent of patients are asymptomatic when first seen, especially younger patients. The diagnosis is discovered after the incidental finding of an elevated platelet count or of splenomegaly. Eighty percent of patients are symptomatic when diagnosed. Patients may be evaluated for unexplained anemia, hemorrhage, a thrombotic episode, or suspicion of leukemia. Sixty percent of the symptomatic patients have bleeding that is most frequently from the gastrointestinal tract, occasionally with massive hematemesis or melena. Skin or mucous membrane bleeding, epistaxis, spontaneous hematomas, or more rarely, bleeding in other sites may occur [3–10,13]. The diagnosis of thrombocythemia also may be made because of investigation of protracted bleeding following surgery.

Both venous and arterial thrombosis occur in about one-third of patients. Peripheral arterial lesions, including gangrene of the toes, livedo reticularis, and erythromelalgia, are most common [7,10,13], but thrombosis in the internal carotid artery or other visceral sites may occur [17]. Venous thrombi are most often in the lower extremities, but renal vein thrombosis leading to the nephrotic syndrome and mesenteric, hepatic, portal, and splenic thromboses also have occurred.

Splenomegaly is found in about 60 percent of patients and is usually of a slight degree. In most patients, the spleen extends less than 6 cm below the left costal margin. Slight hepatomegaly is present in 40 percent of patients.

LABORATORY FEATURES

In nearly all patients, the platelet count is persistently elevated to levels greater than 1 million per microliter. Occasional patients have counts between 750,000 and 1 million per microliter. Striking platelet aggregates, giant platelets, megakaryocyte cytoplasmic fragments, and unusually shaped platelets are present on the blood films [15]. Wide variation in platelet size is present [17].

Megakaryocytic hyperplasia and a markedly hypercellular marrow specimen are present in all patients. The marrow background invariably reveals myriads of platelet aggregates. Megakaryocytes are large with abundant cytoplasm and often with many nuclear lobes. In a small number of cases, the megakaryocytes may appear bizarre. Granulocytic and erythrocytic precursors are present in the marrow in increased numbers. The iron content is either normal or increased, in sharp contrast with the decreased content seen in polycythemia vera. Slight increases in marrow reticulin have been noted in some patients.

More than half the patients have microcytic-hypochromic anemia secondary to blood loss from the gastrointestinal tract during the course of the disease. A mild neutrophilic leukocytosis with white counts ranging from 12,000 to 20,000 per microliter is present in most patients. In some patients, the blood abnormalities of asplenia secondary to autosplenectomy occur, including nucleated red cells and red cells with Howell-Jolly bodies. The leukocyte alkaline phosphatase score is usually normal. Serum vitamin B_{12} and vitamin B_{12} binding capacity are elevated in one-third of patients.

The majority of patients with primary thrombocythemia have normal chromosomes, but a deletion of the long-arm of chromosome number 21 (21q-) has been reported in some patients [18,19]. There is no relationship between chromosomal aberrations and the evolution into other acute or chronic myeloproliferative diseases.

Abnormalities of platelet aggregation occur in about 50 percent of patients. These abnormalities result from a defective response of the platelets to epinephrine and collagen. Spontaneous aggregation has been reported in some patients with primary thrombocythemia [14]. Lesions that appear identical to duodenal ulcers in gastrointestinal x-rays occur in nearly half the patients with thrombocythemia [7].

DIFFERENTIAL DIAGNOSIS

Primary thrombocythemia should be differentiated from the other chronic myeloproliferative diseases that can occasionally be associated with extreme thrombocytosis, as well as from those diseases in which there is a secondary rise of the platelet count. The secondary causes of thrombocytosis include chronic iron deficiency, removal of the spleen, inflammatory diseases such as rheumatoid arthritis and inflammatory bowel disease, and malignancies, including lung and pancreatic carcinomas and Hodgkin's disease. Secondary thrombocytosis also may be seen following hemorrhage or severe hemolysis (see Chap. 145).

The finding of sustained and unexplained elevation of the platelet counts of greater than 1 million per microliter suggests the presence of a myeloproliferative disease. When there is associated splenomegaly, the absence of an increased red cell mass, the absence of the Philadelphia chromosome, and the characteristic marrow findings with the presence of stainable iron, a diagnosis of thrombocythemia can be established. In polycythemic patients who have massive gastrointestinal hemorrhage and thrombocytosis, the disease can be mistaken initially for primary thrombocythemia. Eventually, an increase in red cell mass, characteristic of polycythemic patients, permits one to differentiate the two disorders. Uncomplicated polycythemia vera may be differentiated from thrombocythemia by the presence of an increased red cell mass, a high leukocyte alkaline phosphatase score, and the virtual absence of marrow iron.

Chronic myelogenous leukemia may rarely be preceded by, or occasionally associated with, extreme thrombocytosis. It usually can be identified by the presence of neutrophilic leukocytosis (> 30,000 per microliter), profound myeloid hyperplasia with a myelocyte bulge in the marrow, the presence of the Philadelphia chromosome, and a low leukocyte alkaline phosphatase activity.

Agnogenic myeloid metaplasia also may occasionally be associated with thrombocytosis and can be differentiated from primary thrombocythemia by the massive splenomegaly, teardrop red cells, nucleated red cells, myeloid immaturity in the blood film and the fibrosis, and marked increase in reticulin fibers with silver stains of the marrow.

In conditions unrelated to intrinsic marrow disease that are characterized by thrombocytosis, the platelet count is usually less than 1 million per microliter, and the lesions producing secondary thrombocytosis are evident on clinical evaluation. If no secondary cause for a mildly elevated platelet count can be uncovered, it is possible that one is dealing with early primary thrombocythemia, since a proportion of cases may present with platelet counts between 700,000 and 1 million per microliter.

TREATMENT

Patients who are asymptomatic and older than 50 years when first seen should be treated so as to lower the elevated platelet count. A number of agents have been effective, including ^{32}P, L-phenylalanine mustard, busulfan, uracil mustard, and more recently, hydroxyurea. In a retrospective study, ^{32}P appeared more efficacious than busulfan [7]. In a subsequent prospective study, phenylalanine mustard was as effective as ^{32}P in controlling thrombocythemia. Doses of phenylalanine mustard can vary from 1 to 4 mg per day orally. Approximately 70 percent of patients so treated will have a normalization of the platelet count within 3 months, and 90 percent of the patients should be in complete remission within 6 months. Doses of ^{32}P of 2.3 mCi/m² intravenously are almost equally as effective as L-phenylalanine mustard. After ^{32}P, the platelet count begins to fall in a month and reaches its nadir in about 6 to 8 weeks. Hydroxyurea (15 to 30 mg/kg) is effective in lowering the platelet count. Toxicity with L-phenylalanine mustard, ^{32}P, and hydroxyurea is minimal. Retreatment within 3 to 6 months may be necessary following initial reduction of the

platelet count with any type of treatment. Iron therapy in iron-deficient patients may help correct anemia and reduce the contribution of hypoferremia to the thrombocytosis.

In older patients who present with acute bleeding, especially massive gastrointestinal hemorrhage, the platelet count should be decreased as rapidly as possible. Plateletpheresis in emergency situations associated with thrombocythemia is rapidly effective [20,21]. Nitrogen mustard in doses of 0.4 mg/kg intravenously also can bring about a rapid reduction in the platelet count [7], as can hydroxyurea therapy.

A close interrelationship may exist between platelet hyperaggregability and thrombosis [14]. The use of platelet antiaggregating agents, such as acetylsalicylic acid and dipyridamole, has been effective in normalizing platelet aggregability, although their ultimate role in treatment has not been established. Conceivably, those patients with mild elevation of platelet count, e.g., between 750,000 and 1.5 million per microliter, might be effectively treated with this approach.

Although primary thrombocythemia is typically a disease of older patients, the syndrome has been described in young individuals. In a study of 10 patients below the age of 30 years with classic thrombocythemia, no hemorrhagic or thrombotic problems existed prior to diagnosis and none developed during a follow-up interval of from 14 months to 10 years [12]. Platelet-function studies in 6 of these 10 patients revealed variable aggregation with ADP and absent aggregation with epinephrine. One patient demonstrated spontaneous platelet aggregation. Only one patient was given specific chemotherapy, and this was prior to 1973. Since none of these patients has had a serious bleeding or thrombotic accident, primary thrombocythemia occurring in young patients can be a benign disease, at least for an extended period. Aggressive or repeated chemotherapy to lower the platelet count in these patients seems unwarranted in view of the potential mutagenic consequences of these agents. Plateletpheresis should be done whenever elective surgery is considered or prior to childbirth. In at least five instances, the use of plateletpheresis has completely controlled the platelet count; two patients delivered healthy children with no maternal complications, and three patients had elective surgery with no difficulty.

PROGNOSIS

About 80 percent of patients will survive 1 year, and at least 50 percent of patients live 5 years [1,7]. Patients who have splenic atrophy from repeated infarctions tend to have more difficulty than those with splenomegaly. Bleeding and thrombosis are constant threats in older patients when the platelet count is elevated. In younger patients, the prognosis appears excellent; however, as these patients reach the fifth and sixth decades of life, it will be important to see whether there is increased morbidity or mortality or evolution into another myeloproliferative disease.

References

1. Silverstein, M. N.: Myeloproliferative diseases. *Postgrad. Med.* 61:206, 1977.
2. Epstein, E., and Goedel, A.: Hämorrhagische thrombocythämie bei vasculärer schrumpfmilz. *Virchows Arch.* [*Pathol. Anat.*] 293:233, 1934.
3. Hardisty, R. M., and Wolff, H. H.: Haemorrhagic thrombocythemia: A clinical and laboratory study. *Br. J. Haematol.* 1:390, 1955.
4. Spaet, T. H., Bauer, S., and Melamud, S.: Hemorrhagic thrombocythemia. *Arch. Intern. Med.* 98:377, 1956.
5. Fanger, H., Cella, L. J., Jr., and Lichtman, H.: Thrombocythemia. Report of 3 cases and review of the literature. *N. Engl. J. Med.* 250:456, 1958.
6. Kupfer, H. G., et al.: Essential thrombocythemia. *Ann. Intern. Med.* 48:685, 1958.
7. Silverstein, M. N.: Primary or hemorrhagic thrombocythemia. *Arch. Intern. Med.* 122:18, 1968.
8. Gunz, F. W.: Hemorrhagic thrombocythemia: A critical review. *Blood* 15:706, 1960.
9. Ozer, F. L., et al.: Primary hemorrhagic thrombocythemia. *Am. J. Med.* 28:807, 1960.
10. Lewis, S. M., Szur, L., and Hoffbrand, A. V.: Thrombocythemia. *Clin. Hematol.* 1:339, 1972.
11. Fialkow, P. J., Faguet, G. B., Jacobson, R. J., Vardya, K., and Murphy, S.: Evidence that essential thrombocythemia is a clonal disorder with origin in a multipotent stem cell. *Blood* 58:916, 1981.
12. Hoagland, H. C., and Silverstein, M. N.: Primary thrombocythemia in the young patients. *Mayo Clin. Proc.* 53:578, 1978.
13. Singh, A. K., and Wetherley-Mein, G.: Microvascular occlusive lesions in primary thrombocythemia. *Br. J. Haematol.* 36:553, 1977.
14. Wu, K. K.: Platelet hyperaggregability and thrombosis in patients with thrombocythemia. *Ann. Intern. Med.* 88:7, 1978.
15. Weinfeld, A., Branehög, I., and Kutti, J.: Platelets in the myeloproliferative syndrome. *Clin. Hematol.* 4:373, 1975.
16. Hussain, S., Schwartz, J. M., Friedman, S. A., and Chua, S. N.: Arterial thrombosis in essential thrombocythemia. *Am. Heart J.* 96:31, 1978.
17. Holme, S., Simmonds, M., Ballek, R., and Murphy, S.: Comparative measurements of platelet size by Coulter counter, microscopy of blood smears and light transmission studies. *J. Lab. Clin. Med.* 97:610, 1981.
18. Zaccarria, A., and Tura, S.: A chromosomal abnormality in primary thrombocythemia. *N. Engl. J. Med.* 298:1422, 1978.
19. Fuscaldo, K. E., et al.: Correlation of a specific chromosomal marker, 21q-, and retroviral indicators in patients with thrombocythemia. *Cancer Lett.* 6:51, 1979.
20. Pamlilio, A. L., and Reiss, R. F.: Therapeutic plateletpheresis in thrombocythemia. *Transfusion* 19:147, 1979.
21. Younger, J., and Umlas, J.: Rapid reduction of platelet count in essential thrombocythemia by discontinuous flow plateletpheresis. *Am. J. Med.* 64:659, 1978.

CHAPTER 27

Acute leukemia—general considerations

EDWARD S. HENDERSON

Definition and history

Acute leukemia (AL) is a malignant disease that is thought to originate either in the lymphopoietic stem cell (acute lymphocytic leukemia, ALL) or in the hemopoietic stem cells (acute myelogenous leukemia, AML). Either tumor is characterized by uncontrolled growth of these cells to poorly differentiating lymphoblasts in ALL or poorly differentiating myeloblasts in AML. The leukemic blast cells accumulate in the marrow and suppress the growth and differentiation of normal hemopoietic cells. Thus, both AML and ALL result in the diminished production of normal erythrocytes, granulocytes, and platelets. This deficiency of normal cells leads to the most important manifestations of this disease: weakness, fatigue, and pallor as a result of anemia, infection as a result of granulocytopenia, and hemorrhage as a result of thrombocytopenia.

Less frequent manifestations of the disease are produced by accumulations of leukemic cells in sites other than marrow. These myeloblastomas or lymphoblastomas can occur in skin, paranasal sinuses, bones, breasts, gonads, lymph nodes, and other sites.

Chronic "splenic" myelogenous leukemia was described almost simultaneously by Craige, Bennett, and Virchow in 1844. Neumann was the first to identify leukemia as a disease involving the marrow. Acute leukemia was defined as a separate clinical entity in 1889 by Epstein, and later, further morphologic characterizations were made when polychrome stains became available for the study of blood cells.

The term *acute leukemia* is not as descriptive of the disease now as it was in the nineteenth century. The term *acute* has become obsolescent for young patients because of advances in treatment. Many patients with ALL and some with AML have prolonged periods of good health because of successful treatment, and some have been considered cured of their disease. Thus many patients with ALL have a better prognosis than those with chronic myelogenous leukemia. (CML). The term *leukemia*, originally *weisses blut* or *white blood*, was introduced because of the enormous accumulation of white cells found in a patient with far-advanced chronic leukemia by Virchow. Although patients with chronic leukemia always have an elevation in white cell count, many patients with acute leukemia have low or normal total leukocyte counts. Thus the term *acute leukemia* is often a misnomer, but it is time-honored as a disease category.

Classification

Acute leukemia can be subclassified into three broad categories on the basis of light microscopy with polychrome stains, cytochemical reactions, and electron microscopy combined with cytochemistry (Table 27-1). These categories are acute lymphocytic leukemia (ALL), acute myelogenous leukemia (AML), and acute undifferentiated leukemia (AUL). ALL cells are agranular blast cells that do not stain for peroxidase but do stain with periodic acid Schiff reagents. AML blast cells may have granules and stain with peroxidase, chloracetate esterase, or non specific esterase. They also may contain Auer rods, cigar-shaped violaceous cytoplasmic inclusions, structures that do not develop in lymphoblasts. In rare cases, leukemic cells cannot be classified by current techniques into one of these two major categories and can be referred to as AUL.

Subclassification of AML into the types listed in Table 19-2 is made largely by morphology and by cytochemistry. Subclassification of ALL is made on the basis of morphology and immunologic tests for cytoplasmic immunoglobulin, surface immunoglobulin, receptors for sheep red cells, content of terminal deoxynucleotidyl transferase, and reactivity with anti-T-cell, anti-B-cell, and anti-non-T, non-B (null) leukemic cell-surface antibodies. The latter reagent has been used to define a type of ALL that is called *common-type ALL* because it has surface antigens in common with a pool of null cell ALL populations (see Chap. 114). Descriptions of the subcategories of AML are given in Chap. 28, "Acute Myelogenous Leukemia," and of ALL in Chap. 114, "Acute Lymphocytic Leukemia."

Occurrence

Acute leukemias, taken collectively, are relatively common diseases. The incidence in the United States and in most Western European countries is 3.5 cases per 100,000 inhabitants per year. This rate is comparable to that of cancer of the esophagus and malignant melanoma and makes acute leukemia the twentieth cause of death among cancers at all ages and the most common malignant disease in childhood. ALL and AML are about equal in overall incidence, but the former is much more common in childhood and the latter is the predominant type in adults. The incidence of acute leukemia, like most cancers, increases with age [1] (Fig. 27-1), except for ages 2 through 9, during which time there is a high frequency of common-type ALL. The overall incidence in males as compared with that in females is 1.3:1, the discrepancy being chiefly due to a greater incidence of acute leukemia in young boys and older men [1].

The reported incidence of acute leukemia is relatively low in non-Caucasian children, although similar in adults of different races (Fig. 27-2). Among Caucasians, it occurs frequently in Jews. Acute leukemia, especially in children, is apparently more frequent in industrialized countries and in urban areas. These differences have been variable, however, and may reflect standards of medical care and accuracy of diagnosis and reporting for different racial, ethnic, and economic groups. Some studies have suggested an increase in ALL among rural as compared with urban populations [2,3].

Etiology

The cause of human acute leukemia is unknown. It is probable that no single factor is responsible. Several influences may operate to produce the disease. High-dose irradiation, chronic benzene exposure, or Down's syndrome alone do not produce leukemia in the majority of the individuals affected, although they increase its incidence substantially. In inbred animal strains with high leukemic susceptibility, some individuals never become leukemic. However, if such animals are exposed to radiation or chemical carcinogens, there is an in-

TABLE 27-1   Classification of major types of acute leukemia

Cytologic features	Myelogenous (AML)	Lymphocytic (ALL)	Undifferentiated (AUL)
Auer rods	Present occasionally	Absent	Absent
Phi bodies	Often present	Absent	Absent
Peroxidase, Sudan black, Chloracetate esterase	Often positive	Negative	Negative
Periodic acid Schiff	Usually negative	Usually positive	Negative
Immunologic features of lymphocytes (cALLa, T- or B-cell features)	Absent	Present	Absent
Terminal deoxynucleotidyl transferase	Rare	Present	Absent

NOTE: See text for further details. cALLa is the acronym for common-type ALL antigen. Subclassification of AML is described in Chap. 19, "Classification of the Hemopoietic Stem Cell Disorders," and in Chap. 28, "Acute Myelogenous Leukemia," and of ALL in Chap. 114, "Acute Lymphocytic Leukemia."

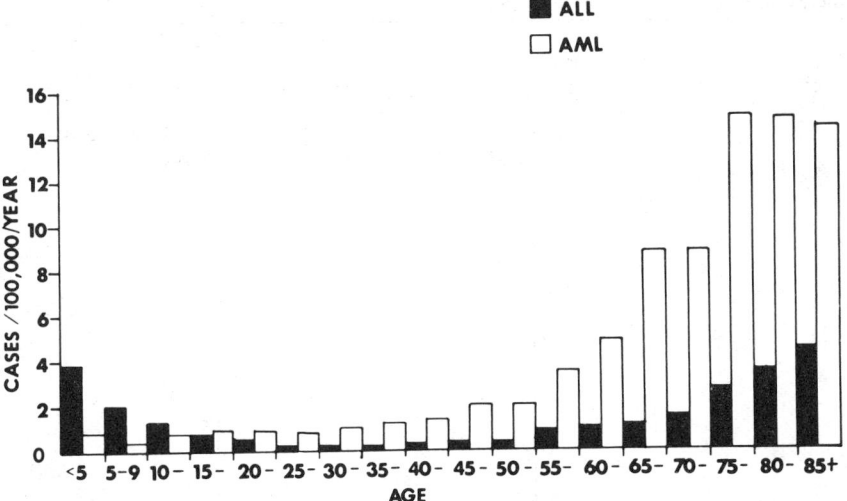

FIGURE 27-1 Incidence, by year of age, of acute lymphocytic leukemia (ALL, *black bars*), and of acute myelogenous leukemias (AML, *open bars*) in the United States. (Data derived from the *Third National Cancer Survey* of 1969–1971 [1].)

creased likelihood that the disease will develop. In most instances, leukemia results from the concatenation of host susceptibility factors, chemical or physical injury to chromosomes, and in animals and presumably in humans, the incorporation of genetic information of viral origin into susceptible stem cells.

HEREDITARY FACTORS

An inherited susceptibility to leukemia is suggested by the increased incidence of the disease observed in certain high-risk families and in association with specific hereditable syndromes and by the high frequency of concordant leukemia in monozygous twins [4]. Estimates of the incidence of acute leukemia in such in-

stances is presented in Table 27-2. The greatest risk is found in the identical twin of a child who has leukemia (usually ALL) before the age of 8 years. Approximately 20 percent of such individuals will manifest the disease within 1 year of their twin's diagnosis [3]. The risk subsequently declines to that of nonidentical siblings of leukemic individuals, which is about five times that of the general population. In such cases, however, factors other than heredity, e.g., intrauterine infection, radiation, or drug exposure, may play a role. In at least one case, leukemic cells from one twin have crossed the common placenta to involve the second twin, with karyotypically identical disease presenting in both infants at 15 months of age [6].

FIGURE 27-2 Incidence of acute leukemia by age and race in the United States annually. (Data compiled by the *Third National Cancer Survey* of 1969–1971 [1].)

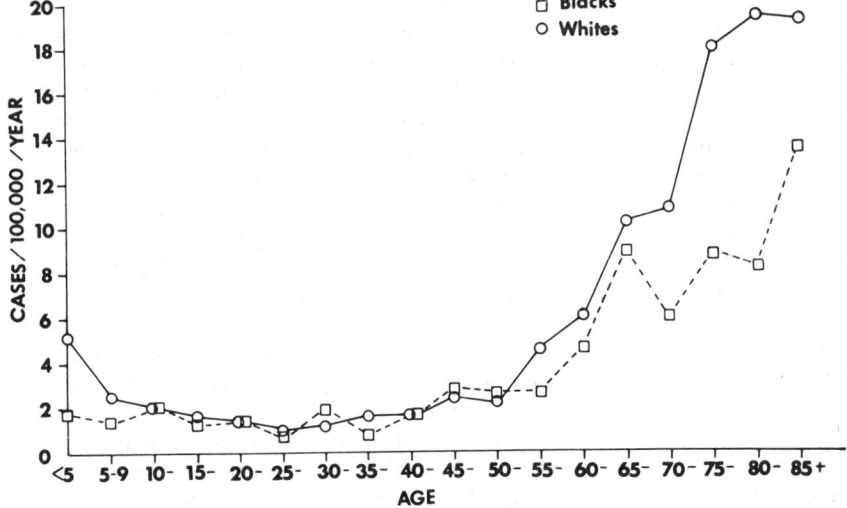

TABLE 27-2   Factors associated with an increased frequency of acute leukemia

	Type of AL	Approximate risk of AL (where known)
1. Genetic conditions:*		
Identical sibling with leukemia	AML, ALL	20% (below age 10)
Nonidentical sibling with leukemia	AML, ALL	10/100,000/year‡
Down's syndrome	AML, ALL	50/100,000/year
Bloom's syndrome	AML	50%
Fanconi's anemia	AML	
Ataxia telangiectasia	ALL	
Kleinfelter's syndrome	AML	
Osteogenesis imperfecta	ALL	
Wiskott-Aldrich syndrome	AML	
2. Acquired diseases:		
Chronic myelogenous leukemia	AML, ALL	75%
Myelofibrosis	AML	10%
Polycythemia vera†	AML	10%
Primary thrombocythemia	AML	
Paroxysmal nocturnal hemoglobinuria	AML	
Dyshemopoietic syndromes (preleukemia)	AML	50%
Sideroblastic anemia, idiopathic refractory	AML	10%
Multiple myeloma†	AML	≤ 1000/100,000/year
Hodgkin's disease†	AML	≤ 100/100,000/year
Carcinoma of ovary, breast†	AML	
3. Exposures:		
Radiation	AML, ALL	Up to 80/100,000 year
Benzene (chronic)	AML	13/100,000/year
Alkylating agents	AML	Up to 1000/100,000/year
Chloramphenicol	AML	

*Established factors in italics.
†Treatment related (in toto or in part).
‡May reflect the high incidence in certain cancer families.

The hereditary basis for leukemia in high-risk families is somewhat more convincing. In the families so affected, concordance, i.e., simultaneous diagnosis, is unusual, but an increased risk of leukemia continues throughout life. In apparently normal family members who have no evidence of disease at the time of study, definite abnormalities in immunologic function or cellular susceptibility to virus transformation may be demonstrated that is similar to that seen in the relatives who have developed leukemia [7,8].

Hereditary or congenital disorders, such as Down's syndrome, Bloom's syndrome, Fanconi's anemia, ataxia telangiectasia, and congenital agammaglobulinemia, are also prone to terminate in acute leukemia [4]. The first three entities are associated with chromosomal abnormalities—stable trisomy 21 in the case of Down's syndrome and multiple breaks and endoreduplication of cells in cultures in Bloom's and Fanconi's diseases. Furthermore, somatic cells in these conditions appear to be unusually susceptible to virus transformation in vitro [8]. In ataxia telangiectasia and congenital agammaglobulinemia, chromosomal abnormalities are not detectable by current methods, but deficiencies in humoral or cellular immunity exist. Although the similarity between these various abnormalities and the defects induced by irradiation or those observed in certain "leukemia families" may be more apparent than real,

they provide leads for biologic and epidemiologic investigation.

PREDISPOSING HEMATOLOGIC DISEASES
Some hematologic diseases acquired during life have a remarkable tendency to terminate as acute leukemia. This development sometimes appears to be a coincidence, or it may relate to treatment given for the underlying disease or reflect an intrinsic predetermination for the disease.

There is a strikingly high frequency of acute leukemia in the chronic myeloproliferative disease, CML. Over 70 percent of patients die of a transformation to acute leukemia. Agnogenic myeloid metaplasia, primary thrombocythemia, and polycythemia vera may also terminate in acute leukemia, although the frequency is much lower than in CML. ^{32}P or chlorambucil treatment of polycythemia vera increases the likelihood of development of leukemia several times. The dyshemopoietic syndromes terminate in acute leukemia in about one-half the cases, and these syndromes have been referred to as *preleukemias* for that reason. Paroxysmal nocturnal hemoglobinuria, a hemopoietic stem cell disease, also can terminate in acute leukemia.

Acute leukemia has been less commonly noted in patients with chronic lymphocytic leukemia, multiple myeloma, Hodgkin's disease, and non-Hodgkin's lymphoma. The leukemia in such cases usually has the morphologic and histochemical features of myeloblastic, erythroblastic, or myelomonocytic leukemia. In some cases of "blastic transformation" of CML, the cells resemble lymphoblasts morphologically, and the abnormal cells have high concentrations of terminal deoxynucleotidyl transferase, an enzyme characteristically present in thymic lymphocytes and some cases of acute lymphoblastic leukemias [9–14]. Antileukemic treatment is rarely effective [14].

IRRADIATION

The leukemogenic potential of ionizing radiation has been demonstrated in animals and in humans. Physicians and scientists exposed to excessive amounts of radiation during the early years of research on the medical application of x-rays, patients given chronic low-dose radiotherapy for rheumatoid spondylitis, and persons exposed acutely to radiation during the nuclear attacks on Hiroshima and Nagasaki have all been found to have an increased incidence of leukemia [15,16]. In the latter instances, the amount and quality of radiation exposure have been carefully investigated, and a linear relation has been demonstrated between cumulative doses of 100 to 900 rads and the subsequent incidence of leukemia [10]. Outside this range of exposure, data regarding the incidence of leukemia are incomplete, but of greatest practical interest is the lack of convincing evidence that radiation doses of less than 100 rads increase the incidence of leukemia. However, the danger of radiation in utero may be greater than that observed postnatally [17]. The leukemia associated with irradiation is usually acute, although the incidence of CML, myelofibrosis, and other myeloproliferative diseases is also somewhat increased. The increased incidence of leukemia following the atomic bomb explosions in Japan included both ALL and AML. The relative frequency of the two types of acute leukemia paralleled their usual age-related incidence, suggesting that host factors may determine the susceptibility to leukemogenesis in individuals exposed to irradiation.

Total-body and extended-field radiation produces both myelosuppression and immunosuppression. Chromosomal breaks and recombinations can be observed for many months after radiation therapy is given or diagnostic x-ray contrast studies are performed. Radiation causes reversible breaks in double-stranded DNA and at the same time induces oncogenic virus replication and shedding in vitro, and presumably in vivo, from cells containing viral genetic information. The relative importance of these several phenomena in leukemogenesis is unknown, but nevertheless, radiation remains the most conclusively identified leukemogenic factor in human beings.

CHEMICALS

The production of leukemia in animals by exposure to certain chemicals has been demonstrated, and several compounds have been associated with the genesis of human leukemia. Among them, however, only benzene, its congener toluene, and alkylating agents have been documented well enough to assign them causative roles. The occurrence of acute leukemia in workers exposed to benzene was reported in 1908 [18], and numerous other reports have appeared subsequently [19–22]. In many cases, marrow hypoplasia and/or pancytopenia occurred first, leading in some instances to the diagnosis of preleukemia. In some series, erythroleukemia was the predominant type of acute leukemia encountered, while in others, the leukemic subcategories were comparable to those expected to occur in the general adult population. Seventy to eighty percent overall were classified as one or another form of AML [22]. The duration of benzene exposure prior to the diagnosis of leukemia was usually 5 years or more, but an occasional patient was exposed for a little as 1 year. The incidence of acute leukemia in shoe workers exposed to benzene in Istanbul was 13 per 100,000, two to three times greater than the incidence of acute leukemia generally [22].

Similar but less convincing reports have implicated chloramphenicol and phenylbutazone as leukemogenic [23–25]. The number of cases reported has been too few in comparison with the total amount of these drugs used to establish a definite cause-and-effect relationship. In most but not all cases, a preleukemic phase of marrow hypoplasia had been suspected or documented, and as with benzene, the type of leukemia was usually AML. All three chemicals can produce marrow hypoplasia, as well as chromosome breakage and fragmentation both in vivo and in vitro.

Leukemia also may be produced by multiagent anticancer chemotherapy. A few suggestive reports appeared a decade or more ago, but since 1970, excluding those instances of blastic transformation in patients with CML and other myeloproliferative diseases, hundreds of individuals given cytotoxic drug chemotherapy have developed AML [26–29]. Virtually all were given one or another of the alkylating agents, either alone or in combination with other antineoplastic drugs. Most of them had been given radiotherapy as well. Patients given a nonalkylating cytotoxic agent as sole antitumor therapy have not been reported to develop acute leukemia as a second neoplasm. AML has been diagnosed in an individual given methotrexate for psoriasis.

These associations indicate that alkylating agents and possibly other anticancer drugs predispose the recipient to leukemia. Like the situation observed with radiation, benzene, chloramphenicol, phenylbutazone, and most hereditary disorders associated with acute leukemia, the use of antitumor agents is frequently associated with chromosomal breakage and some degree of marrow dysfunction. In addition, alkylating agents are markedly immunosuppressive and in mice can lead to the enhancement of tumor growth and reduction of immunologic resistance to neoplasms [26,30].

The majority of patients with post-alkylating-agent acute leukemia have been treated for neoplasms of lymphocytic origin or for tumors that produce immunologic deficiency, e.g., multiple myeloma, lymphocytic lymphoma, chronic lymphocytic leukemia, and Hodgkin's disease. In all these entities, acute leukemia can develop in the absence of either radiation or alkylating-agent therapy [31–33]. Given the success of modern chemotherapy and radiotherapy for these malignant disorders, the number of untreated patients will undoubtedly remain too small for a valid estimation to be made of the risk of leukemia. It is possible that the apparent increase in acute leukemia in part reflects the nature of the underlying tumor, coupled with the increased longevity owing to chemotherapy.

Acute leukemia has, however, occurred in patients with carcinoma of the ovary [34,35], lung, and breast after 16 to 91 months of alkylating-agent therapy [36,37]. About one-half of these patients were not given radiotherapy. The leukemia observed in these patients was AML. The erythroleukemic type was associated somewhat more often with ovarian cancer. Subtle impairment of immunologic function has been reported in patients with far-advanced solid tumors, but it is generally much less severe than that seen regularly in lymphomas and multiple myelomas.

VIRUSES

The viral cause of leukemia in mammals has been documented. Leukemia in mice, cats, cattle, sheep, and primates has, for example, been shown to be caused by ribonucleic acid (RNA) viruses potentially capable of horizontal infectivity through the formation and extrusion of type C virus particles. These viruses are capable of forming a deoxyribonucleic acid (DNA) copy (provirus) of their RNA sequences through the mediation of their endogenous enzyme RNA-directed DNA polymerase (reverse transcriptase). The reverse transcriptases of the several type C leukemogenic viruses are strikingly similar in their substrate and primer requirements. Furthermore, while base sequences of the viral genomes vary from species to species, the degree of molecular similarity (homology) that has been demonstrated has been greater than would be anticipated by chance. Thus these viruses are descendants of a common ancestor, and their individual variations have accumulated through millennia of passages through different endemic hosts.

Viruses as a cause of leukemia in the human have been discussed for decades. Following the initial demonstration by Gross that a virus causes murine leukemia and lymphoma [38], cellular particles morphologically indistinguishable from type C viruses were demonstrated in electron micrographs of human leukemia cells and plasma [39,40]. Later, a reverse transcriptase similar to that of oncogenic viruses in lower species was identified in spleen cells in a child with myelofibrosis [41] and in leukemic cells of human origin [42,43]. In 1970, identical type C viruses were isolated from lymphosarcoma arising in an Old World monkey (the gibbon) and a fibrosarcoma of a New World primate (the woolly monkey) [44,45]. Viral RNA, the homologous DNA (provirus), and viral-induced antigens were detectable in the neoplastic cells from both primates.

Studies of leukocytes from normal New World monkeys and gibbons did not reveal the same viral stigmata, thus suggesting that the leukemia-associated virus was acquired rather than inherited in the genetic material of the victim. Several investigators have detected reverse transcriptase and viral RNA that are strikingly similar to that of the gibbon and woolly monkey in leukemic cells derived from patients with AML [41,46–48]. Similarly, both the reverse transcriptase and major structural proteins of the primate viruses and viruses shown to bud from certain of the AML culture lines [49] appear to be immunologically identical [48,49]. To date, provirus has not been positively identified in humans, although DNA sequences other than those normally present in human tissues have been identified in leukemic tissue, most notably in leukemic patients whose healthy identical twins had no identifiable DNA abnormalities in their circulating leukocytes [50]. In summary, there is increasingly convincing evidence to show that at least some acute leukemias are *associated* with a transmissible (infectious) RNA virus closely related to the leukemogenic viruses of lower mammals [51]. How and when these viruses gain access to hemopoietic cells, what exact role they play, and what underlies the susceptibility of blood cells to lysogeny and transformation remain virtually unknown.

Acute leukemia can originate *de novo* in recipients of allogenic marrow from HLA identical siblings of the opposite sex [52–54]. Three recipients given marrow as grafts in the treatment of acute leukemia had acute leukemia recur that bore the karyotype of the donor. In these instances, the second leukemia was morphologically identical to the original disease. These patients were given radiation therapy, chemotherapy, and the immunosuppressive therapy related to allogenic marrow engraftment. The third received cyclophosphamide alone as preparation for grafting and for immunosuppression [53]. The donor marrow cells were not exposed to radiation or drugs at any time prior to engraftment. Posttransplantation leukemia has not been observed to date in patients with aplastic anemia who have undergone similar grafting procedures.

The schema of leukemogenesis presented in Fig. 27-3 is consistent with our knowledge. This hypothesis requires a multiplicity of factors, hereditary, environmental, and acquired, to be present in order for leukemia to develop as a clinical entity. Leukemogenesis is presented as a series of separate steps, each one increasing the likelihood of overt acute leukemia. Given a genetic predisposition and/or an acquired instability of nuclear DNA, exposure to a human leukemogenic virus leads to incorporation of viral sequences into the host genome. Therefore, any stress during which stem cell replication is stimulated carries a risk that a clone of

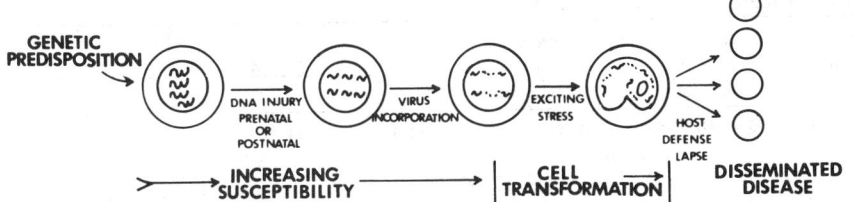

FIGURE 27-3 Hypothetical schema of the genesis of human acute leukemia. Its development as a clinical entity apparently requires a multiplicity of factors, hereditary, environmental, and acquired as outlined, in addition to some degree of immunologic deficiency. Some of the events indicated may overlap.

malignant cells will develop and expand. This clone may lie dormant or be capable, during lapses of homeostasis, of expanding sufficiently to cause detectable marrow infiltration and ineffective hemopoiesis. Although the schema suggest a sequence of events, it is likely that some steps coincide. However, it is improbable that an isolated exposure to an oncogenic virus or to radiation, for example, or a transient lapse in immunologic responsiveness per se would result in leukemia.

Pathophysiology

Acute leukemia is the result of the malignant transformation of primitive hemopoietic cells in the case of AML or of primitive lymphopoietic cells in the case of ALL. In either disease it is proposed that the malignant process evolves from a single cell (unicentric origin, clonal expansion) and that the proliferation eventually suppresses the growth of normal hemopoietic progenitors that cohabit the marrow spaces. Leukemic blast cells frequently have a slower rate of cell replication than do normal myeloblasts, promyelocytes, and myelocytes [54–57] (Table 27-3). These findings have been variable and are difficult to interpret because growth slows when tumor cell mass increases, cell populations under study are heterogeneous in growth characteristics, and the precise normal cell types with which to compare leukemia cell growth is arguable. Nonetheless, there is usually a slower cell mitotic cycle time for leukemic blast cells than for normal precursors.

The precise reasons for the growth advantage of leukemic cells and for the suppression of normal hemopoiesis are not known. Results of studies that have correlated blood cell production or numbers of hemopoietic progenitor cells that grow in culture in overt leukemia or in preleukemia have indicated that hemopoiesis may be severely impaired before there is a large blast cell content in marrow [63–66]. Studies of granulocyte-monocyte progenitors have shown that leukemic blast cells can suppress growth of colonies from these normal progenitors in viscous culture, but it is different reproducing the cellular densities and relationships that exist in vivo in culture dishes and thus it is difficult to draw strong inferences from such studies.

No single mechanism seems to be responsible for the ineffective hemopoiesis in leukemia. Decreased numbers of neutrophil-monocyte progenitors (CFU-NM) and deficient and/or abnormal amounts of humoral regulators of myelopoiesis have been obsered in patients with acute leukemia [67–69], but marked variability in these results has been reported. In patients who respond to therapy and in whom a complete remission is achieved, CFUc numbers and the production of colony-stimulating factors become normal, both qualitatively and quantitatively [63,64,67,68]. With recurrence of the overt disease hemopoiesis deteriorates and abnormalities in progenitors and regulators return.

At the present time, the pancytopenia associated with leukemia is considered to represent a deficiency in normal stem cell proliferation and differentiation, although a failure in the production of humoral stimulators or the release of humoral inhibitors of normal hemopoietic stem cells could also be present. The level of hemopoiesis at which leukemic involvement occurs and whether acute leukemia is a monoclonal disease have not been established. The basic lesion in CML resides in the hemopoietic multipotent marrow stem cells [70,71]. This has not been proved for preleukemia or for AML or ALL [72]. Although abnormalities of erythrocytic and megakaryocytic cell production, morphology, and function have been documented in AML and preleukemia, these dysplastic features have not been conclusively shown to be primary phenomena. For example, the dysplastic erythroblasts of erythroleukemia, a variant of AML in which such cells are predominant, have been shown to respond to erythropoietin in a qualitatively normal fashion [73,74], and they have not been clearly identified as having cytogenetic abnormalities. However, abnormalities in the appearance and function of mature granulocytes [75–80] and platelets [81] and in immunologic reactivity have been demonstrated in patients with overt acute leukemia [82], thus showing effects of the disease beyond simple reduction in the number of normal cells. In myelogenous leukemias, differentiated metamyelocytes, myelocytes, and granulocytes retain stigmata of leukemia; e.g., cytogenetic abnormalities and Auer rods have been identified in vivo and in vitro [77–79,83]. In AML, the largest pools of segmented neutrophils were observed in patients with the

TABLE 27-3   Cell cycle kinetics of normal and acute leukemia cells in the bone marrow

Type of cell	Approx. total number	Total number of stem cells	Growth fraction, % (labeling index)	T_g	S	G_2	M	G_1
					Median duration			
Acute leukemia	1×10^{12}	2×10^{11}	ALL: 2–8	60 h	20 h			
			AML:					
			Large blast 10–50	2–10 d	20 h	2–3 h	1 h	<1 h
			Small blast 5–10					>10 d
Normal marrow	8×10^{11}	5×10^{10}						
Erythroblasts	2.5×10^{11}	—			>13 h			
Myeloblasts	0.09×10^{11}	—	85	24 h	< 24 h			
Promyelocytes	0.34×10^{11}	—	65	60 h	≤24 h			
Myelocytes	1.3×10^{11}	—	30	54 h	≤24 h			
			Small, 10–20					
			Large, 70					
Metamyelocytes, bands, polys	4×10^{11}	—	0					

NOTE: T_g = generation time; S = DNA synthesis phase; G_1 = phase of cycle before DNA synthesis phase; G_2 = phase of cycle after DNA synthesis phase; M = mitosis; h = hour; d = day.
SOURCE: Combined estimates from Clarkson [57], Cronkite [58], Cronkite and Vincent [59], Stryckmanns et al. [60], Harrison [61], Lajtha and Oliver [62], and Bull et al. [63].

highest total leukocyte counts in relapse (thus the largest circulating blast counts), an unexpected finding more consistent with differentiation of leukemic cells than with leukemia-induced inhibition of normal stem cells [80]. Established leukemic cell lines of murine [85,87,88] and human origin [89,90] can be stimulated to mature in the presence of either physiologic or nonphysiologic stimuli. These studies suggest that the progression and regression of acute leukemia may depend at least in part on microenvironmental factors rather than solely on the presence or absence of transformed hemopoietic stem cells.

Finally, there is the question of whether leukemia represents the growth of a clone or clones of malignant cells existing in parallel with normal hemopoietic tissue or whether the disease is a pervasive defect involving all replicating elements. The answer to this question depends on the detection of specific markers of malignancy in individual blood and marrow cells. Of the various immunologic, morphologic, and biochemical approaches to the identification of leukemic cells, only cytogenetic evaluation provides reliable information. Abnormal karyotypes are seen in slightly less than half of all individuals with acute leukemia, and in such cases, estimates of normal and abnormal cell populations can be made [92]. Exhaustive cytogenetic analysis of acute leukemia in patients followed through multiple relapses and remissions have in almost all instances demonstrated the coexistence of normal and abnormal karyotypes. The latter predominate during overt phases of disease activity and become rare or undetectable during periods of complete remission [92–95]. At present it appears that acute leukemia is a disease in which normal and malignant cells coexist and compete for ascendance within blood-forming organs. In those patients in whom the number of cytogenetically normal cells is reduced or absent, suggesting a more pervasive malignancy, the response to treatment and later recovery of normal hemopoiesis are less common [92,95].

Clinical features

The signs and symptoms that may be produced by acute leukemia are outlined in Table 27-4 in parallel with major laboratory abnormalities and pathophysiologic considerations. Most of the common systemic manifestations, such as fatigue, weakness, bruising, fever, and weight loss, are nonspecific. Symptoms of more diagnostic importance, which may reflect the growth or infiltration of leukemic cells in the marrow, include persistent or recurrent skeletal pain or tenderness, especially of the lower sternum, and occasionally swelling of the large joints. Children with these symptoms may be thought to have rheumatic fever or adults some type of arthritis unless hematologic studies are carried out.

Enlargement of the superficial lymph nodes, liver, and spleen occur commonly in acute leukemia. The incidence and degree of organ infiltration vary somewhat with the different types of leukemia (see Table 27-5). Organomegaly is not always the result of leukemic cell infiltration. Splenomegaly and renal enlargement have been reported with normal architecture, presumably the result of increased metabolic activity secondary to the presence of leukemic tissue elsewhere in the body [96–98]. The most important tissue involvement, however, in all forms of leukemia is the infiltration of marrow by leukemic cells; this interferes with growth of normal hemopoietic progenitor cells and thus with the production of erythrocytes, granulocytes, and platelets. These cytopenias result in a high frequency of infection and bleeding.

Less-common manifestations of acute leukemia include retinal hemorrhages in patients with thrombocytopenia, gum hypertrophy in granulocytic or monocytic leukemia, and the development of extranodal masses in the subcutaneous tissues, bones, orbits, breasts, or testes. Leukemic myeloblasts in soft tissues are frequently mistaken for lymphoid cells when studied by

TABLE 27-4   Clinical features of acute leukemia related to pathophysiology

Symptoms	Signs	Laboratory abnormalities	Cause
Fatigue, weakness	Pallor, lethargy, weakness	Anemia, hypocalcemia, hypercalcemia, hypomagnesemia	Marrow failure, release of cellular ions and metabolites
Weight loss	Weight loss		Reduced food intake, anemia, hepatosplenomegaly, increased catabolism
Bleeding in skin, mucous membranes, gums, gastrointestinal, genitourinary tracts	Purpura, gum oozing or hypertrophy, hematuria, melena	Thrombocytopenia; hypofibrinogenemia; reduced factors V, VIII; increased fibrin split products	Marrow failure, DIC*
Infection of skin, throat, gums, respiratory or urinary tracts	Fever, chills, tissue infiltrates, pyodermia gangrenosum	Granulocytopenia, x-ray evidence of pneumonia, sinusitis, etc., positive cultures	Marrow failure, granulocytopenia, immunodeficiency
Headache, nausea, vomiting, blurred vision, cranial nerve dysfunction	Papilledema, cranial nerve palsy, meningeal irritation	Spinal fluid pleocytosis, reduced CSF sugar, increased CSF protein	Meningeal, CNS, or nerve infiltration and/or compression
Bone pain and tenderness	Increased bone tenderness	Periosteal elevation, bone destruction by x-ray, abnormal bone marrow pressure, fibrosis	Local leukemic infiltration
Abdominal fullness, anorexia	Hepatosplenomegaly, abdominal tenderness	Hyperfibrinogenemia; elevated SGOT, SGPT; alkaline phosphatase	Infiltration of abdominal viscera
Enlarged lymph nodes or tumor masses	Enlarged lymph nodes, masses in node areas, skin, breast, testes	Abnormal biopsy, liver, spleen, and bone scans	Local tumor growth or infiltration
Oliguria	Oliguria	Concentrated urine, elevated BUN, elevated uric acid	Dehydration, uric acid nephropathy, DIC
Obstipation	Abdominal fullness, tenderness	Abnormal scans or x-ray contrast studies	Local infiltration, obstruction; calcium/magnesium imbalance

* Disseminated intravascular coagulation.

hematoxylin and eosin staining. If masses are removed for histologic study, fresh imprints should be made and processed with polychrome peroxidase and chloracetate stains in addition to hematoxylin and eosin so that the hemopoietic origin of the malignant cells can be recognized. Failure to do this may lead to incorrect diagnoses, such as lymphoma or anaplastic carcinoma, as well as to inappropriate management.

Meningeal leukemia is present at the time of diagnosis in about 2 percent of patients and occurs in the absence of specific CNS treatment in up to 70 percent of patients with ALL and with much less frequency (~5 percent) in AML patients at some time during the course of the illness. Headache, blurred vision, nausea and vomiting, or cranial nerve palsies may provide the first diagnostic clue to the presence of leukemia.

Laboratory features

Patients with signs or symptoms should have an examination of the blood. If anemia, granulocytopenia, or thrombocytopenia is present, or if there are abnormal cells in the blood, a marrow examination should be per-

formed. Acute leukemia is widespread at the time of presentation, and marrow obtained from any of the usual sites of hemopoiesis will be satisfactory, excluding any area to which intensive radiation therapy has been administered. The site usually preferred for safety and simplicity is the posterior iliac crest.

Aspirates are ideal for morphologic studies using Wright's or Wright-Giemsa polychrome stains, immunological assessment, histochemical staining, and cultures for clonogenicity and for cytogenetic studies. Sections of needle core biopsy specimens are often required for the identification of granulomas, lymphomatous foci, or carcinoma metastases, as well as for the estimation of total marrow cellularity. Particles obtained by either aspiration or needle biopsy are suitable for most purposes, but biopsy is required whenever adequate marrow particles cannot be obtained by aspiration. Features that aid in the differentiation of ALL from AML, including morphologic, histochemical, and immunologic, are summarized in Table 27-1.

A requirement for the diagnosis of acute leukemia is that the disease, during its untreated phase, show evidence of progression. This is usually implicit in the striking marrow changes and in the aberrations of cell

TABLE 27-5 Approximate frequency of organ infiltration in acute leukemia

	Acute lymphocytic		Acute myelogenous	
Organ	Percent on initial exam	Percent at autopsy	Percent on initial exam	Percent at autopsy
Lymph nodes	80	90	10–60*	50
Liver	75	90	40	90
Spleen	70	90	35	90
Bone and joint†	11	15	2	5
Lungs	5	50	5	50
Heart	2	35	2	35
Kidneys	30	30	20	30
Gastrointestinal	5	10	—	10
Central nervous system	4	75	1	27
Skin	1	—	3	10
Mediastinum	2	—	1	—

* Higher values are for children.
† Extramedullary symptoms and signs.

production and function. In 15 percent of cases, however, the degree of infiltration or the degree of marrow dysfunction may be borderline, and malignancy can be suspected only on clinical and morphologic grounds. Preleukemia or smoldering or oligoblastic leukemias fall into this category. In most of these instances, blood cell production is severely limited, but the patient may be maintained in reasonably good health for months or years by the use of blood transfusions alone. The presence of Auer rods or cytogenetic abnormalities may confirm the presence of a malignant cell line, although such stigmata are often missing. Smoldering leukemia frequently runs a protracted course and is poorly responsive to antileukemic cytotoxic therapy. From a pragmatic point of view, it should not be considered as acute leukemia until there is evidence of progressive marrow infiltration and clinical deterioration.

Leukemia-associated antigens

The presence on human leukemic cells of antigenic determinants specific for this malignant disease has been predicted for years and supported by some immunologic studies applied to patients, relatives, and other contacts. Numerous reports of leukemia-associated antigens have been published using mixed tumor cell lymphocyte reactions, humoral immunofluorescence, cytotoxicity, and delayed skin hypersensitivity [99,100]. Several groups of investigators [101–104] studying identical twins have demonstrated immunologic recognition of leukemic blast cells in mixed cell cultures by the leukemic member of the twinship. Blast cell recognition by the clinically normal twin has been inconsistent, some reacting and some not reacting to isologous leukemic cells. Patients with leukemia have been able to mount immunologic reactions against leukemogenic animal viruses [105], and oncor-

navirus proteins have been detected on their leukemia cells [48,49]. However, whether the immunologic reactions are directed toward leukemia-specific antigens as opposed to leukemia-associated antigens derived from viruses or other agents causally unrelated to the origin and propagation of the malignancy remains unclear. A series of xenogenic antisera have been produced from leukemic tissues per se and/or membrane extracts of leukemic tissue. After exhaustive adsorption to remove known normal xenogenic and allogenic reactivities, it has been possible to demonstrate relatively specific in vitro reactions to cells from patients with leukemia or other myeloproliferative and lymphoproliferative disorders [100,102]. The specificities of these antisera vary, some being reactive to lymphoblasts only, some to specific subsets of normal lymphocytes, some to both ALL and CLL, some to AML and CML, and some to all forms of leukemia. In addition, highly purified antisera and monoclonal antibodies can identify leukemic cells that share surface features. The best studied of these antisera identify a subcategory of immunologically null (non-T, non-B) ALL cells [103,104] that carries a surface complex referred to as *common ALL antigen* (cALLa).

Differential diagnosis

Acute leukemia is rarely overlooked or misdiagnosed. Acute leukemia may simulate other diseases. Failure to recognize clues from the physical examination (e.g., minute petechial hemorrhages, minimal enlargement of superficial lymph nodes, hypertrophy of the gums, increased sternal tenderness) or omission of a study of the cells in the blood, as well as marrow examination when indicated, may subject patients to irrelevant diagnostic and therapeutic procedures (see Chaps. 28 and 114).

Therapy

See Chaps. 28 and 114.

Course and complications

CYTOPENIAS
Acute leukemia can be associated with many complications. Virtually all of them are aggravated by treatment, and many may be directly attributable to therapy. In Table 27-6, the common complications of acute leukemia are listed together with their estimated frequency as presenting clinical problems and as a cause of death.

Leukemic cell proliferation itself is rarely lethal. Rather, the disease terminates fatally because of secondary problems, the most important of which are infection, hemorrhage, and renal and hepatic insufficiency (Table 27-7).

TABLE 27-6   Complications of acute leukemia

Type of complication	Complication	Frequency as presenting feature, %	Frequency as cause of death, %
Hematologic	Granulocytopenia with infection	19	70
	Thrombocytopenia with bleeding	18	10
	Anemia, symptomatic	17	<1
Nutritional	Weight loss	12	—
Metabolic	Hyperuricemia	36	1
	Hypocalcemia	30	1
	Hypercalcemia	5	<1
	Disseminated intravascular coagulation	5	<5
	Hepatic insufficiency	<1	5
Infiltrative	Meningeal leukemia and sequelae	2	5
	Superior mediastinal obstruction	2	<1
	Leukostasis	5	2
	Solid hemopoietic tumors (myeloblastoma)	2	—
	Severe bone pain	7	—
	Gum hypertrophy	5	—

Leukemic cells tend to accumulate within the marrow and at some point begin to interfere with normal hemopoiesis. At least 90 percent of the morbidity of leukemia can be attributed to pancytopenia, which is worsened by therapy [105–107]. Anemia, thrombocytopenia, and granulocytopenia occur concomitantly. Red cell deficiencies are the most readily corrected. The most serious complications are infection and bleeding.

METABOLIC EFFECTS

The second major cause of morbidity in leukemia relates to the production or release by leukemic cells of nucleic acid metabolites, intracellular electrolytes, and biologically active enzymes. Of these products, the most important clinically is uric acid (see "Uric Acid Nephropathy," later in this chapter).

The release of phosphates, sulfates, and other organic anions from leukemic cells can lead to reductions in the serum concentrations of calcium and magnesium [108–110]. The release of procoagulants from leukemic blast cells may initiate intravascular coagulation and produce hemorrhage associated with depletion of fibrinogen, factors VIII, V, and X, and activation of plasminogen [111–113] (see "Bleeding," below). These metabolic abnormalities tend to be most severe in patients with very proliferative disease and parallel the amount of leukemic tissue present. They may be aggravated by successful therapy, which increases cytolysis and the release of cellular contents into fluid compartments.

INFILTRATES

The third most frequent cause of morbidity in acute leukemia is extramedullary leukemic cell infiltration. As outlined in Table 29-5, leukemic cells can be identified in virtually all tissues of the body during relapse. These infiltrates are usually diffuse, but they may grow as tumors. In contrast to lymphomas and other solid tumors, leukemic infiltration rarely leads to obstruction of hollow viscera, or of blood vessels, or to major aberrations in organ function other than that of the marrow. However, infiltrates occasionally accumulate in anatomically confined spaces, such as the mediastinum, where superior vena cava obstruction may be produced, or the central nervous system, with resultant cranial nerve palsy or communicating hydrocephaly (see "Meningeal Leukemia," below). Rarely, blast cells infiltrate subcutaneous tissues, the breasts, bones (especially the orbit and long bones), or the gonads before there is detectable involvement of the marrow. In such cases, the biopsy findings will be those of lymphoblastic lymphoma or myeloblastoma (chloroma). Extramedullary leukemic infiltrations usually do not develop, however, until late in the course of the disease.

INFECTION

INCIDENCE

Infection is currently the most serious complication of leukemia. The most significant infectious agents are listed in Table 27-7 together with the more important predisposing factors and recommendations for therapy. Most infections are caused by microbes indigenous to human beings and their environment, and in particular to the hospital wherein treatment is administered. With advances in antibiotic therapy, the spectrum of agents causing severe and fatal infections has changed both for leukemia and for other severe debilitating illnesses, reflecting for the most part the emergence of pathogens relatively resistant to available drugs.

PREDISPOSING FACTORS

The underlying cause of infection is the breakdown of normal defense mechanisms. Natural barriers to infection, the mucous membranes, an intact integument, adequate inflammatory responses, and cellular and humoral immunity are all to varying degrees disrupted by leukemia and its treatment. The clearest correlation between the incidence of infection and host defense capability involves the production and distribution of granulocytes and macrophages, which are required for an appropriate inflammatory response. Qualitative granulocyte abnormalities have been noted [75–79], but quantitative deficits are more important [114]. In the absence of local injury, the incidence of infection remains normal as long as the granulocyte count in the blood is 1000 per microliter or more. The incidence of both minor and severe uncontrolled infections rises progressively as the number of granulocytes falls below that level. The risk of infection at any level of blood granulocytes is proportional also to the duration of the granulocytopenia. Thus a short period of granulocytopenia, produced with chemotherapy, poses less danger than the more prolonged granulocytopenia related to leukemic infiltration itself.

Lymphocytopenia has also been advanced as a cause of increased infection [114], along with chronic immunosuppression produced by antileukemic medications [115,116]. During leukemic relapse, however, granulocytopenia and lymphocytopenia are most often concordant phenomena, so that it is difficult to separate the contribution each makes in the pathogenesis of infection. During remission, the number of granulocytes rarely falls to critical levels, while immunosuppression is often maintained. During this phase, virus and protozoal infections are most common [106,107,117].

Leukemia therapy injures the gastrointestinal mucosa, creating portals of entry for autochthonous bacteria from oral, nasopharyngeal, and intestinal reservoirs. Bacterial invasions are likely to occur at times of marrow suppression also, which enhances the possibility of local or systemic infection. These can be minimized by topical (and peroral) antisepsis and antibiotics, as discussed below, but these measures cannot resolve established infections, particularly when local necrosis has led to structural changes of the mucosa.

Thrombocytopenia probably increases the likelihood of infection by permitting local bleeding. Fever increases the risk of hemorrhage associated with thrombocytopenia, thus completing the vicious cycle of infection and hemorrhage [105,118,119].

Finally, venipunctures, finger sticks, marrow aspiration and biopsies, lumbar punctures, etc., which are so often required for the study and follow-up of patients with leukemia, provide potential routes for the entry of pathogens, as do intravenous injections and infusions. All these procedures should be prescribed judiciously and carried out with meticulous asepsis.

TREATMENT OF BACTERIAL INFECTIONS

The diagnosis of infection in patients with acute leukemia and the identification of the pathogenic organism are difficult. Controversy still exists as to the origin of fever in leukemia, but the weight of evidence suggests that, except for drug fever and reactions to blood products, most fevers are of infectious origin. In the absence of clear evidence to the contrary, the febrile patient should be assumed to have an infection rather than a re-

TABLE 27-7   Infection in acute leukemia—major etiologic agents

Type of infection	Organism	Predisposing cause	Treatment
Bacterial	Pseudomonas aeruginosa	Granulocytopenia	Appropriate antibiotics and granulocytes
	Escherichia coli	Granulocytopenia	
	Staphylococcus aureus	Granulocytopenia	
	Klebsiella aerobacter	Granulocytopenia	
	Proteus vulgaris	Granulocytopenia	
	Bacteroides spp.	Granulocytopenia	
	Clostridium spp.	Granulocytopenia	
Fungal	Candida spp.	Granulocytopenia, immunosuppression, antibiotics	Granulocytes, amphotericin, ketoconazole
	Aspergillus		
	Phycomycetes		
Protozoal	Pneumocystis carinii	Immunosuppression	Trimethaprim sulfa, pentamidine
	Toxoplasma gondii	Immunosuppression	Pyrimethamine and sulfonamide
Viral	Herpes zoster/varicella virus	Immunosuppression	Zoster immune antisera
	Cytomegalovirus	Immunosuppression	

action to the underlying disease. In practice, the patient should be examined for any localizing signs or symptoms of infection, blood cultures secured, and direct smears from the urine sediment and sputum or any other clinically apparent site of infection examined. Patients who develop a sustained or intermittent fever greater than 38.5°C or signs of major organ inflammation should be given antibiotic therapy promptly. Such treatment should be instituted before the organism or organisms are positively identified by culture or otherwise and should include broad-spectrum antibiotics bactericidal to *Staphylococcus aureus, Pseudomonas*, and gram-negative enteric bacilli. As soon as more definitive evidence as to the cause and extent of infection is available, the anti-infectious regimen should be suitably modified if necessary. If defervescence occurs quickly, antibiotic administration should be continued for at least 5 days, until cultures show no pathogens and the clinical signs of infection have resolved. Longer administration of antibiotics should be considered if granulocyte production remains subnormal, i.e., if the patient is not entering remission [120,121]. Patients fail to respond to antibacterial therapy for two major reasons: (1) use of the wrong antibiotics for the pathogenic microorganism, and (2) granulocytopenia. In the latter instance, the transfusion of 1×10^{10} or more granulocytes daily for 4 or more days may lead to resolution of the infection without change in antibiotics [118,119]. If the infection and/or fever persists, a complete reevaluation of the patient is necessary.

NONBACTERIAL MICROBES AND THEIR TREATMENT
In the latter circumstance, more consideration should be given to possible nonbacterial causes of infection, particularly pathogenic fungi (especially *Candida, Aspergillus*, and Phycomycetes), viruses, or protozoa such as *Toxoplasma gondii* and *Pneumocystis carinii*. Visceral candidiasis is usually accompanied by detectable lesions in the oropharynx or esophagus together with organisms demonstrable in the urine or stool. Rising titers of complement-fixing antibodies are occasionally observed [122]. Both *Candida* and *Aspergillus* can cause a variety of lung infiltrates visualized by x-ray examination. Lung or liver biopsy may on occasion be required for diagnosis. Cytomegalovirus infection is common in immunosuppressed patients, but since infectious exposure increases with age, even virus isolation and rising antibody titers may not be conclusively diagnostic. The histopathologic findings of typical giant nuclei when present are relatively definitive. Toxoplasmosis may present with fever, enlarged lymph nodes, splenomegaly, and atypical lymphocytes in the blood, and toxoplasma granulomas sometimes occur within the central nervous system. The Sabin dye exclusion test and complement fixation aid in the diagnosis.

Pneumocystis carinii lung involvement is of increasing clinical importance. Its absolute frequency is rising, particularly during remissions in the malignant condition. The paucity of early symptoms, even in patients with rapidly advancing disease, often leads to a fatal delay in diagnosis and treatment. Fever, malaise, and nonproductive cough are often the only symptoms of infection even when chest roentgenograms may show extensive pulmonary infiltration. The condition may remain stable for days or weeks, but frequently the patient deteriorates rapidly with progressive dyspnea, hypoxia, and respiratory failure. Individuals are rarely salvaged after respiratory insufficiency develops. *Pneumocystis carinii* cannot be diagnosed at the present time by culture or serologic means. As a general rule, diagnosis depends on the identification of organisms by lung biopsy. A high index of suspicion should be maintained for patients receiving immunosuppressive drugs who develop fever, pulmonary infiltrates, and a nonproductive cough without signs and symptoms of pleuritis.

The effectiveness of treatment for common bacterial infections in patients with leukemia varies from excellent to nil. Gram-positive organisms, including staphylococci, are generally effectively controlled with semisynthetic penicillins, cephalosporins, and aminoglycosides, such as gentamicin and tobramycin. Gram-negative coliforms and *Pseudomonas* are usually sensitive to aminoglycosides and semisynthetic penicillins, such as carbenicillin or tobramycin, especially when there are an adequate number of granulocytes. Toxoplasmosis and *Pneumocystis* can be controlled by pentamidine, pyrimethamine, or most effectively, trimethoprim-sulfa [123] when diagnosed early. On the other hand, there is no consistently effective treatment for virus infections and most visceral mycoses. Some strains of *Candida* and *Aspergillus* are marginally sensitive to amphotericin and 5-fluorocytosine in vivo, and such newer agents as myconizol and ketoconazole are promising [124]. Infections that originate and progress in the presence of severe cytopenia or immunologic deficiency are most difficult to control with drugs. In these circumstances, the induction of remission in the leukemia or recovery from drug-induced aplasia and immune depression is requisite for survival. If normal hematologic and immunologic functions, can be restored, many of these infections, despite their ominous extent and severity, rapidly resolve.

PROPHYLACTIC MEASURES
Because of the autochthonous origin of most pathogens and the importance of host factors in the pathogenesis of infections in leukemic patients, a variety of prophylactic measures have been and are being evaluated. Polyvalent vaccines against strains of *Pseudomonas* have failed to reduce the incidence of infection by these organisms [125]. Decontamination, air filtration, and patient isolation techniques have reduced the incidence of infections and their associated mortality [126], but this approach is costly and time-consuming and does not control infections existing at the time of diagnosis and at the start of antileukemic therapy.

The management of the infected patient with leukemia in relapse is perhaps the most challenging problem of therapy. Antileukemic therapy is becoming more effective, but the use of some of the most effective agents may be compromised by the presence of infection and antibiotic complication, especially the nephrotoxicity of aminoglycosides and amphotericin. All drugs used to treat leukemia are either myelotoxic or immunosuppressive, or both, but the effective control of major infections requires that remission in the leukemia be induced by the most efficient regimen. Although there are no infallible guidelines, the optimal treatment of infection generally should be given for 2 to 4 days before antileukemic drug administration is begun. Antileukemic therapy can then be initiated using the most effective regimen determined by prior drug trials. Initiating cytostatic chemotherapy before the best possible preparation is made courts disaster, while failing to provide the best known remission induction therapy simply perpetuates the basic hematologic defects that allowed the infection to originate and propagate in the first place.

Infections that develop during remissions in acute leukemia may be related to excessive chemotherapy. If marrow function is reasonably normal, the temporary suspension of cytostatic therapy may aid in controlling the infection without adding materially to the risk of relapse in the malignant disease.

BLEEDING

Hemorrhage and infection were about equally important in causing death in patients with acute leukemia until platelet transfusion was developed [105]. At the present time only about 15 percent of deaths in acute leukemia are the direct result of hemorrhage. Bleeding, usually minor, is a common early symptom or sign of the disease and is usually due to thrombocytopenia. There is an inverse relation between platelet level and the risk of hemorrhage [128]. Bleeding with platelet counts below 30,000 per microliter is rare unless local ulceration, infection, fever, or intravascular coagulation are present. Bleeding due to defective platelet function is very rare.

Thrombocytopenia leads in most instances to scattered hemorrhages, or petechiae, in the skin, mucous membranes, retina, and serosal surfaces. Microscopic hematuria is common, but gross hematuria is rare. Intracranial bleeding is generally subarachnoid when it occurs. Confluent ecchymoses, major gastrointestinal hemorrhage, or destructive intracerebral bleeding due to thrombocytopenia alone are uncommon. Platelet transfusions, e.g., 10 units per square meter of body surface area from random donors are usually adequate for the treatment or prophylaxis of thrombocytopenic bleeding. Later in the disease, if the recipient has been immunized against the histocompatibility antigens of the donor platelets, histocompatible platelets should be used. Sibling donors are an important source of such platelets. In patients who are infected, or febrile, or who show evidence of disseminated intravascular coagulation (DIC), the platelet requirement may be greatly increased.

DIC is being diagnosed with increasing frequency in acute leukemia. It occurs almost exclusively during relapse, when leukemic cells are abundant and intracellular procoagulants are released in large quantities [112]. The condition is most frequently associated with hypergranular acute promyelocytic leukemia, in which large primary cytoplasmic granules and multiple or branched Auer rods are prominent [129,130]. A rare microgranular variety has also been identified that has the same propensity for DIC [131]. DIC is also common in acute monocytic leukemia [132], but it may occur in any type of AML and possibly in atypical lymphocytic forms as well. Cytostatic therapy may temporarily increase the severity of DIC, and unless the coagulopathy is controlled before therapy, the mortality during remission induction may be high.

DIC should be considered in patients with severe bleeding, particularly in those with large confluent ecchymoses, or when brisk local bleeding follows venipuncture or marrow aspiration. Typically, DIC reduces multiple clotting factors: platelets, factor VIII, factor V, factor X, prothrombin, and fibrinogen. Secondarily, fibrinolysis is activated and leads to the appearance of circulating fibrin and fibrinogen degradation products (FDP). Since platelet counts are generally low in leukemia due to underproduction and fibrinogen is usually elevated above the normal range for unknown reasons [111], the diagnosis of DIC can be obscured. Increased levels of FDP, decreasing concentrations of fibronogen, and low plasma plasminogen are the most reliable laboratory indications of DIC in leukemic subjects [112].

Clinically significant DIC may require treatment with heparin and replacement of plasma factors and platelets before cytotoxic therapy is initiated [112,113]. It may be necessary to continue treatment until the bulk of the leukemic cell mass has been destroyed, generally 2 weeks. ϵ-Aminocaproic acid (EACA) and other fibrinolysis inhibitors never should be given without prior heparinization lest DIC be aggravated and irreversible thrombosis of organs (especially the renal cortex) occur. EACA may be useful therapy in rare instances of leukemia cell production of plasminogen activator [133].

Occasional patients with AML or ALL may present with disease-related isolated factor deficiencies in the apparent absence of DIC or liver failure. Fibrinogen is most often depressed, but specific deficiencies of factor V, factor VIII and factor X, and factor XIII have been identified [134,135]. Whether these result from specific inhibitors of synthesis or product or from antibodies directed against these factors is not known. The deficits correct themselves when remission is achieved and require appropriate replacement only if clotting factors become dangerously low.

Toxic effects of drugs on the liver and gastrointestinal tract commonly depress the levels of clotting factors. Low levels of fibrinogen and other coagulation proteins synthesized in the liver may result from hepatotoxicity from antimetabolites, steroids, and especially L-asparaginase. Fortunately, these deficits rarely cause overt bleeding and usually regress rapidly with cessation of therapy. In the case of asparaginase, it is usually possible to continue treatment without bleeding complications despite persistent fibrinogenopenia.

HYPERLEUKOCYTIC LEUKEMIAS

Patients with AML, CML, and occasionally ALL may develop leukocyte counts that result in symptoms or signs attributable to the effects of masses of immature cells on flow of blood. Stupor, coma, retinal engorgement, papilledema, and priapism have been ascribed to leukostasis. Another specific lesion of leukostasis, in which leukemic blast cells from intravascular aggregates infiltrate and injure the endothelium of small arteries and veins, also is seen in patients with large masses of circulating blast cells [136,137]. These lesions occur rarely if the blast cell count is less than 150,000 per microliter but become progressively more common above this level. The vascular injury commonly leads to extensive local hemorrhage and can occur in any organ. If leukostatic hemorrhage occurs within the central nervous system, it is almost always fatal, and the few individuals who survive have severe neurologic handicaps. Since prevention is the only practical solution to this problem, vulnerable patients should be treated early with cytoreductive therapy. Rapidly active cytolytic drugs, with or without cranial radiotherapy of 500 to 1000 rads, and leukapheresis are the most promising therapeutic approaches. Whenever possible, remission induction therapy should be instituted before the blast cells have reached a dangerous level.

URIC ACID NEPHROPATHY

Uric acid is the normal end product of human nucleic acid degradation. It is mainly excreted by the kidneys at a normal rate of 300 to 500 mg per day. While it is reasonably soluble in alkaline solutions, it precipitates readily at a low pH. In patients with untreated acute leukemia or with leukemia in relapse, the body pool of urate may expand manyfold. Renal clearance and urine concentration of urate may increase to the point at which it precipitates in the renal tubules, producing renal failure. This complication is potentially fatal and may contraindicate the administration of antileukemic drugs that are excreted by the kidney.

Uric acid nephropathy can be prevented in most cases by ensuring an adequate urine flow, combined with the inhibition of uric acid production by 5-hydroxypyrazolopyrimidine (allopurinol). Immediately after the diagnosis of acute leukemia is made, dehydration should be corrected and a urine flow of 100 ml/h maintained by oral and, if necessary, parenteral fluid administration. Allopurinol should be started in a dose of 100 to 200 mg/m² every 6 h. In cases of established nephropathy, sodium bicarbonate should be given to alkalinize the urine and solubilize the urate crystals. A trial of mannitol diuresis may be warranted, and ureteral lavage may be required to relieve acute renal pelvis and ureteral obstruction in some instances. If these measures fail, hemodialysis should be employed, with platelet and clotting factor replacement when necessary.

Unless restoration of renal function is accomplished, there is little prospect of successful antileukemic therapy. On occasion, however, even in the face of renal insufficiency, remission induction drugs are given despite the risk. The usual doses of vincristine and prednisone for ALL or cytosine arabinoside for AML may be given or, alternatively, a single dose of nitrogen mustard. The latter may temporarily arrest leukemic cell proliferation and buy time for the correction of the uric acid nephropathy.

MENINGEAL LEUKEMIA

Leukemic infiltration of the meninges is not strictly a complication of acute leukemia but a direct result of leukemic cell growth and spread. It may develop gradually or appear suddenly during periods of remission when other signs of disease are absent.

Meningeal leukemia occurs more frequently in children than in adults, and more often in acute lymphocytic than in other types of leukemia regardless of age. The risk of overt meningeal leukemia has been estimated at 3.8 percent per month for the first 24 months and 2.0 percent thereafter in children with acute leukemia [138]. In adults, the risk per month increases from 0.8 percent at the time of diagnosis to nearly 4 percent 3 years after the diagnosis [139]. The overall clinical and autopsy incidence of meningeal leukemia in the latter study was 74 percent for ALL and 27 percent for AML. Meningeal leukemia in AML is much more common in children than in adults. In all categories there is an inverse relation between patient age and the length of survival and a direct relation between the development of meningeal leukemia, other manifestations of leukemic activity, and the incidence of extramedullary leukemic infiltrations elsewhere in the body. Despite occasional reports to the contrary, there is no consistent correlation between sex, initial blast cell count or platelet counts in the peripheral blood, and the subsequent development of meningeal leukemia.

The arachnoid is the primary site of involvement in meningeal leukemia [140,141]. Leukemic cells may be blood-borne or derived from the marrow spaces of the calvarium. As they accumulate in the leptomeninges, they produce a barrier to cerebrospinal fluid flow that results in increased intraventricular pressure and hydrocephaly. Encroachment on and infiltration into subjacent neural tissue develops, and concomitantly leukemic cells migrate into perineural spaces in sufficient numbers to cause compression of the cranial nerves where they traverse osseous foramina. The combination of increased intracranial pressure and cranial nerve injury produces the papilledema and cranial nerve palsies that often accompany meningeal leukemia.

The signs and symptoms of meningeal leukemia are those of increased intracranial pressure (nausea, vomiting, headache, bradycardia, elevated blood pressure, blurred vision, and nerve palsies) particularly of the Vth, VIth, VIIth, VIIIth, and IXth cranial nerves. When any relevant sign or symptom develops, the spinal fluid should be examined promptly. Spinal fluid pleocytosis with the presence of abnormal cells usually makes the diagnosis a simple one, but even with cell concentration techniques, between 5 and 15 percent of patients with arachnoid infiltration will not have identifiable leukemic cells in the spinal fluid [142]. Moreover, CT scans are of little value in identifying this disorder [143].

Prognosis

The survival of patients with acute leukemia has lengthened during the last two decades with the development of increasingly more effective antileukemic regimens, coupled with the increased availability of blood component transfusion support, better antibiotics, and better understanding and treatment of the diverse complications of the disease. The length of survival for the vast majority of patients depends on the duration of the first complete remission. Survival is inextricably linked accordingly, to the response to remission induction and maintenance treatments. The survival of nonresponsive patients is little changed today from the approximately 2.5 months' median survival that prevailed in the 1950s for patients with acute leukemia.

As treatment has improved, a number of prognostic factors have been recognized (Table 27-8). A major factor is the age of the patient, independent of the leukemic subcategory. The best responses frequently are seen by patients with common-type ALL, frequently but not exclusively occurring between 2 and 10 years of age. Teenagers, young adults, and children less than 2 years of age have a higher frequency of ALL with mediastinal masses, undifferentiated leukemia, of AML and a less favorable response rate and survival. The response rate

and survival in all forms of AML are poorer at the extremes of age, in infancy and in the elderly.

Three additional prognostic characteristics are the morphologic, immunologic, and cytogenetic characteristics of the acute leukemia. At all ages, the reponse in ALL exceeds that in AML. In childhood, the median survival for ALL exceeds 5 years, while that for AML remains at best half as long. The proportion of children who survive 5 years free of disease is over 50 percent with ALL and only 15 percent with AML. Recent advances in the treatment of AML may reduce this disparity, but the morphologic type of the acute leukemia is likely to remain an important determinant of survival.

Among ALL types, B-cell and T-cell forms respond less often and less durably to current treatment than does null-cell ALL. In children and young adults, the presence of a large mediastinal mass, often but not always seen in T-cell ALL, is associated with early relapse and attenuated survival. In fact, this clinical feature may account entirely for the poor prognosis attributed to T-cell ALL, since patients with T-cell ALL and normal mediastinal configurations have been shown to have excellent survival [144]. Patients whose leukemic blasts exhibit abnormal karyotypes respond and survive less well than those with apparently normal chromosomes on cytogenetics examination [92,95].

Other prognostically important factors include infection, leukemic meningitis, severe metabolic or cardiovascular disturbances at the time of diagnosis, and marked elevation in the number of circulating blast cells to produce leukostasis. Of less prognostic effect are the initial platelet count, blast cell labeling indices, the number of normal marrow progenitor cells in viscous culture, the immunologic competence, and race [145–148]. Sex, the presence or absence of enlarged lymph nodes, and the initial hemoglobin level have no clear relation to response and survival.

With the exception of smoldering leukemia, in which the evolution of the disease may be protracted and for which cytostatic treatment is rarely effective, prognostic factors are related primarily to the susceptibility of the malignant cell line to cytotoxic drugs and to the ability of the patient to tolerate aggressive treatment.

TABLE 27-8 Prognostic factors in acute leukemia

Established factors indicative of a favorable prognosis:
  Response to therapy: Long duration of complete remission
  Age: 2 to 9 years
  Leukemic subtype:
    ALL better than AML or AUL
    Immunologic: Prognosis of common ALL cell type better than T- or B-cell ALL
  Cytogenetics: Normal karyotype; Ph¹-negative (ALL)
  Race: Caucasian
  Initial WBC or blast cell count below 50,000 per microliter
  Absence of mediastinal widening and infiltration
  Absence of CNS or testicular leukemia
  Absence of other major illnesses
  Acute onset, no preleukemia, no prior malignancy or cytotoxic therapy
Controversial in regard to prognostic significance:
  Infection at time of diagnosis
  Gross obesity
  Hepatosplenomegaly
  Certain leukemic subtypes, e.g., prolymphoblastic, promyelocytic
  Blast cell labeling index
  Number of progenitor cells in culture marrow
  Pre- or posttherapy immunocompetence

References

1. *Third National Cancer Survey: Incidence Data*, edited by S. J. Cutler and J. L. Young, Jr. National Cancer Institute Monograph, no. 41, Government Printing Office, Washington, 1975, p. 102.
2. Blair, A., and Thomas, T. L.: Leukemia among Nebraska farmers: A death certificate study. *Am. J. Epidemiol.* 110:264, 1979.
3. Burmeister, L. F.: Cancer mortality in Iowa farmers, 1971–78. *J. Natl. Cancer Inst.* 66:461, 1981.
4. Miller, R. W.: Relation between cancer and congenital defects: An epidemiological evaluation. *J. Natl. Cancer Inst.* 40:1079, 1968.
5. Miller, R. W.: Deaths from childhood cancer in sibs. *N. Engl. J. Med.* 279:122, 1968.
6. Chaganti, R. S. K., Miller, D. R., Meyers, P. A., and German, J.: Cytogenetic evidence of the intrauterine origin of acute leukemia in monozygotic twins. *N. Engl. J. Med.* 300:1032, 1979.
7. Snyder, A. L., Henderson, E. S., Li, F. P., and Todaro, G. J.: Possible

inherited leukemogenic factors in familial acute myelogenous leukemia. *Lancet* 1:586, 1970.

8. Miller, R. W., and Todaro, G. J.: Viral transformation of cells from persons at high risk of cancer. *Lancet* 1:81, 1969.

9. McCaffrey, R., Harrison, T. A., Parkman, R., and Baltimore, D.: Terminal deoxynucleotidyl transferase in human leukemic cells and in human thymocytes. *N. Engl. J. Med.* 292:775, 1975.

10. Sarin, P. S., Anderson, P. M., and Gallo, R. C.: Terminal deoxynucleotidyl transferase activities in human leukocytes and lymphoblast cell lines: High levels in lymphoblast cell lines and in blast cells of some patients with chronic myelogenous leukemia in acute phase. *Blood* 47:11, 1976.

11. Bollum, F. J.: Terminal deoxynucleotidyl transferase as a hematopoietic cell marker. *Blood* 54:1203, 1979.

12. Srivastava, B. I. S., Khan, S. A., Minowada, J., Rakowski, I., and Henderson, E. S.: Terminal deoxynucleotidyl transferase activity, blast cell characteristics, and response to chemotherapy in adult acute leukemia. *Leukemia Res.* 4:209, 1980.

13. Canellos, G. R., DeVita, V. T., Whang-Peng, J., and Carbone, P. P.: Hematologic cytogenetic remission of blastic transformation in chronic granulocytic leukemia. *Blood* 38:671, 1971.

14. Preisler, H. D., and Lyman, G. H.: Acute myelocytic leukemia subsequent to therapy for a different neoplasm. Clinical features and response to therapy. *Am. J. Hematol.* 3:209, 1977.

15. Court-Brown, W. M., and Abbott, J. D.: The incidence of leukemia in ankylosing spondylitis treated with x-rays. *Lancet* 1:1283, 1955.

16. Brill, A. B., Tomonoga, M., and Heyssel, R. M.: Leukemia in man following exposure to ionizing irradiation: Summary of findings in Hiroshima and Nagasaki and comparison to other human experience. *Ann. Intern. Med.* 56:590, 1962.

17. Bross, I. D., and Natarajan, N.: Leukemia from low-level irradiation: Identification of susceptible children. *N. Engl. J. Med.* 257:107, 1972.

18. LeNoir et Claude: Sur un cas de purpura attribué à l'intoxication per le benzine. *Bull. Mem. Soc. Med. Hop. Paris* 14:1251, 1897.

19. Browning, E.: *Toxicity and Metabolism of Industrial Solvents.* Elsevier, Amsterdam, 1966, p. 41.

20. Goguel, A., Cavigneaux, A., and Bernard, J.: Les Leucémies benzéniques. *Bull. Inst. Natl. Sante Rech. Med.* 22:421, 1967.

21. Vigliani, E. C., and Saita, G.: Benzene and leukemia. *N. Engl. J. Med.* 271:872, 1964.

22. Aksoy, M., Erdem, S., and Din Col, G.: Leukemia in shoeworkers exposed chronically to benzene. *Blood* 44:837, 1974.

23. Cohen, T., and Creger, W. P.: Acute myeloid leukemia following seven years of aplastic anemia induced by chloramphenicol. *Am. J. Med.* 43:762, 1967.

24. Brauer, M. J., and Dameshek, W.: Hypoplastic anemia and myeloblastic leukemia following chloramphenicol therapy. *N. Engl. J. Med.* 277:1003, 1967.

25. Dougan, L., and Woodliff, A. J.: Acute leukemia associated with phenylbutazone treatment: A review of the literature and report of a further case. *Med. J. Aust.* 1:217, 1965.

26. Sieber, S. M., and Adamson, R. H.: Toxicity of antineoplastic agents in man: Chromosomal aberrations, antifertility effects, congenital abnormalities, and carcinogenic potential, in *Advances in Cancer Research,* edited by G. Klein, S. Weinhouse, and A. Haddow. Academic, New York, 1975, vol. 22, pp. 57–144.

27. Rosner, F., and Grunwald, H.: Hodgkin's disease terminating in acute leukemia. Report of eight cases and review of the literature. *Am. J. Med.* 58:339, 1975.

28. Rosner, F., Carey, R. W., and Zarrabi, M. H.: Breast cancer and acute leukemia: Report of 24 cases and review of the literature. *Am. J. Hematol.* 4:151, 1978.

29. Landaw, S. A.: Acute leukemia in polycythemia vera. *Semin. Hematol.* 13:33, 1976.

30. Makinodan, T., Santos, J. W., and Quinn, R. P.: Immunosuppressive drugs. *Pharmacol. Rev.* 22:189, 1970.

31. Videbaek, A.: Unusual cases of myelomatosis. *Br. Med. J.* 2:326, 1971.

32. Turz, T., Flandrin, G., Brouet, J. C., Briere, J., and Seligman, M.: Simultaneous occurrence of acute myeloblastic leukemia and multiple myeloma without previous chemotherapy. *Br. Med. J.* 2:642, 1974.

33. Bloomfield, C. D., and Brunning, R. D.: Acute leukemia as a terminal event in non-leukemic hematopoietic disorders. *Semin. Oncol.* 3:297, 1976.

34. Greenspan, E. M., and Tung, B. G.: Acute meyloblastic leukemia after cure of ovarian cancer. *JAMA* 230:418, 1974.

35. Kaslow, R. A., Wisch, N., and Glass, J. L.: Acute leukemia following cytoxic chemotherapy. *JAMA* 219:75, 1972.

36. Garfield, D. H.: Acute erythromegakaryocytic leukemia after treatment with cytostatic agents. *Lancet* 2:1037, 1970.

37. Zarrabi, M. H., and Rosner, F.: Acute myeloblastic leukemia following treatment for non-hematopoietic cancers: Report of 19 cases and review of the literature. *Am. J. Hematol.* 7:357, 1979.

38. Gross, L.: "Spontaneous" leukemia developing in C3H mice following inoculation in infancy with AK leukemic extracts of AK embryos. *Proc. Soc. Exp. Biol. Med.* 76:27, 1951.

39. Dmolchowski, L., et al.: Electron microscopic studies of human leukemia and lymphoma. *Cancer* 20:760, 1967.

40. Dalton, A. J., Moloney, J. B., Porter, G. H., Frei, E., and Mitchell, E. Z.: Studies on murine and human leukemia. *Trans. Assoc. Am. Physicians* 77:52, 1964.

41. Chandra, P., Steel, L. K., Laube, H., and Kornhuber, B.: Expression of C-type viral information in tissues of patients with preleukemic disorders: Myelofibrosis and granulocytic sarcoma associated with acute myelomonocytic leukemia (A.M.M.L.) in children, in *Antiviral Mechanisms in the Control of Neoplasia,* edited by P. Chandra. Plenum, New York, 1979, p. 117.

42. Gallo, R. C., Yang, S. S., and Ting, R. C.: RNA dependent DNA polymerase of human acute leukemic cells. *Nature* 228:927, 1970.

43. Baxt, W., Hehlman, R., and Spiegelman, S.: Human leukemic cells contain reverse transcriptase associated with a high molecular weight virus-related RNA. *Nature* 244:72, 1972.

44. Kawakami, T. G., Huff, S. D., Buckely, P. M., Dungworth, D. L., Snyder, S. P., and Gilden, R. V.: C-type virus associated with Gibbon lymphosarcoma. *Nature* 235:170, 1972.

45. Theilin, G. H., Gould, D., Fowler, M., and Dungworth, D. L.: C-type virus in human tissues of a woolly monkey (*Lagothix* spp.) with fibrosarcoma. *J. Natl. Cancer Inst.* 47:881, 1971.

46. Gallagher, R. E., and Gallo, R. C.: Type C RNA tumor virus isolated from cultured human acute myelogenous leukemia cells. *Science* 187:350, 1975.

47. Mak, T. W., Kurtz, S., Manaster, J., and Houseman, D.: Viral-related information on oncornavirus-like particles isolated from cultures of marrow cells from leukemic patients in relapse and remission. *Proc. Natl. Acad. Sci. U.S.A.* 72:623, 1975.

48. Todaro, G. J., and Gallo, R. C.: Immunological relationship of DNA polymerase from human acute leukemia cells and primate and mouse leukemia virus reverse transcriptase. *Nature* 244:206, 1973.

49. Scherr, C. J., and Todaro, G. J.: Primate type-C virus p30 antigen in cells from humans with acute leukemia. *Science* 187:855, 1975.

50. Baxt, W. G., Yates, J. W., Wallace, H. J., Holland, J. F., and Spiegelman, S.: Leukemia-specific DNA sequences in leukocytes of the leukemic member of identical twins. *Proc. Natl. Acad. Sci. U.S.A.* 70:2629, 1973.

51. Bishop, J. M.: The molecular biology of RNA tumor viruses. *N. Engl. J. Med.* 303:675, 1980.

52. Fialkow, P. J., Thomas, E. D., Bryant, J. I., and Neiman, P. E.: Leukaemic transformation of engrafted human marrow cells *in vivo. Lancet* 1:251, 1971.

53. Thomas, A. D., Bryant, J. I., and Buckner, C. D.: Leukemic transformation of human marrow cells in vivo. *Lancet* 1:1310, 1972.

54. Elfenbein, G. J., et al.: Cytogenetic evidence for recurrence of acute myelogenous leukemia after allogeneic bone marrow transplantation in donor hematopoietic cells. *Blood* 52:627, 1978.

55. Gavosta, F., Pileri, A., and Peforaso, L.: Proliferation kinetics of acute leukemic cell in relation to the chemotherapy. *Acta Genet. Med. Gemellol. (Roma)* 17:30, 1968.

56. Mauer, A. M., Lampkin, B. C., Evert, C. F., and McWilliams, N. B.: Cell kinetic patterns in human acute leukemia: Evidence for control mechanisms. *Bibl. Haematol.* 39:1014, 1973.

57. Clarkson, B. D.: *Review of Recent Studies of Cellular Proliferation in Acute Leukemia.* National Cancer Institute Monograph, no. 30. Government Printing Office, Washington, 1969, p. 81.

58. Cronkite, E. P.: Granulocytic models: Effect on chemotherapy. *N.*

Engl. J. Med. 282:683, 1970.

59. Cronkite, E. P., and Vincent, P. C.: Granulocytopoiesis, in *Hemopoietic Cellular Proliferation,* edited by F. Stohlman, Jr. Grune & Stratton, New York, 1959, p. 1.

60. Stryckmanns, P., Cronkite, E. P., Fache, J., Fliedner, T. M., and Ramos, J.: Deoxyribonucleic acid synthesis time in human beings. *Nature* 211:717, 1966.

61. Harrison, W. J.: The total cellularity of the bone marrow in man. *J. Clin. Pathol.* 15:254, 1962.

62. Lajtha, L. A., and Oliver, R.: Studies on the kinetics of erythropoiesis: A model of the erythron, in *CIBA Foundation Symposium,* edited by G. E. W. Wolstenholme and W. O'Connor. Little, Brown, Boston 1960, p. 289.

63. Bull, J. M., Duttera, M. J., Stushick, E. D., Northrup, J., Henderson, E. S., and Carbone, P. P.: Serial in vitro marrow culture on acute myelocytic leukemia. *Blood* 42:679, 1973.

64. Duttera, M. J., Bull, J. M., Northrup, J. D., Henderson, E. S., and Carbone, P. O.: Serial in vitro marrow culture in acute lymphocytic leukemia. *Blood* 42:687, 1973.

65. Greenberg, P. L., Nichols, W. C., and Schrier, S. L.: Granulocytopoiesis in acute myeloid leukemia and preleukemia. *N. Engl. J. Med.* 284:1225, 1971.

66. Hoelzer, D., Harriss, E. B., Jäger, C., Haas, R. J., and Fliedner, T. M.: Effect of the acute rat leukemia L5222 on bone marrow stroma cells. *Cancer Res.* 34:1892, 1974.

67. Moore, M. A. S., Williams, N., and Metcalf, D.: In vitro colony formation by normal and leukemic human hematopoietic cells: Interaction between colony-forming and colony-stimulating cells. *J. Natl. Cancer Inst.* 50:591, 1973.

68. Messner, H. A., Till, J. E., and McCulloch, E. A.: Interacting cell populations affecting granulopoietic colony formation by normal and leukemic human marrow cells. *Blood* 44:671, 1974.

69. Robinson, W. A., and Pike, B. L.: Colony growth of human bone marrow cells *in vitro,* in *Hemopoietic Cellular Proliferation,* edited by F. Strohlman, Jr. Grune & Stratton, New York, 1970, p. 249.

70. Fialkow, P. J.: Use of glucose-6-phosphate dehydrogenose markers to study human myeloproliferative disorders, in *Modern Trends in Human Leukemia III,* edited by R. Neth, R. C. Gallo, P. H. Hofschneider, and K. Mannweiler. Springer, Berlin, 1979, p. 53.

71. Whang-Peng, J., Canellos, G. P., Carbone, P. P., and Tjio, J. H.: Clinical implications of cytogenetic variants in chronic myelocytic leukemia (CML). *Blood.* 33:824, 1968.

72. Fialkow, P. J., et al.: Acute non-lymphocytic leukemia: Expression in cells restricted to granulocytic/monocytic differentiation. *N. Engl. J. Med.* 301:1, 1979.

73. Gabuzda, T. G., Shute, H. E., Erslev, A. J.: Regulation of erythropoiesis in erythroleukemia. *Arch. Intern. Med.* 123:60, 1969.

74. Adamson, J. W., and Finch, C. A.: Erythropoietin and the regulation of erythropoiesis in DiGuglielmo's syndrome. *Blood* 36:590, 1970.

75. Bannerjee, T. K., Senn, H., and Holland, J. F.: Comparative studies on localized leukocyte mobilization in patients with chronic myelocytic leukemia. *Cancer* 29:637, 1972.

76. Skeel, R. T., Yankee, R. A., and Henderson, E. S.: Hexosemonophosphate shunt activity in circulating phagocytes in patients with acute lymphocytic leukemia. *J. Lab. Clin. Med.* 77:975, 1971.

77. Leder, L. D.: A case of acute leukemia with pseudo-Pelger cells containing Auer bodies. *Acta Haematol. (Basel)* 42:58, 1969.

78. Davies, A. R., and Schmitt, R. G.: Auer bodies in mature neutrophils. *JAMA* 203:895, 1968.

79. Catovsky, D., Galton, D. A. G., and Robinson, J.: Myeloperoxidase deficient neutrophils in acute myeloid leukemias. *Scand. J. Haematol.* 9:142, 1972.

80. Galbraith, P. R., Chikappa, G., and Abu-Zahra, H. T.: Patterns of granulocyte kinetics in acute myelogenous and myelomonocytic leukemia. *Blood* 36:371, 1970.

81. Henderson, E. S., and Goldstein, I. M.: Platelets in leukemia, in *The Platelet,* edited by K. Brinkhaus and F. K. Mostofi. Williams & Wilkins, Baltimore, 1971, p. 315.

82. Broder, S., Poplack, D., Whang-Peng, J., Durm, M., Goldman, C., Mull, L., and Waldman, T. A.: Characterization of a suppressor-cell leukemia. Evidence for the requirement of an interaction of two T-cells in the development of human suppressor effector cells. *N. Engl. J. Med.* 298:66, 1978.

83. Moore, M. A. S., and Metcalf, D.: Cytogenetic analysis of human acute and chronic myeloid leukemic cells cloned in agar culture. *Int. J. Cancer* 11:143, 1973.

84. Friend, C., Scher, W., Holland, J. G., and Sato, T.: Hemoglobin synthesis in murine virus-induced leukemic cells in vitro. *Proc. Natl. Acad. Sci. U.S.A.* 68:378, 1971.

85. Hayashi, M., Fibach, F., and Sachs, L.: Control of normal differentiation of myeloid leukemic cells: Normal differentiation in aneuploid leukemic cells and the chromosome binding pattern of D+ and D− clones. *Int. J. Cancer* 14:40, 1974.

86. Preisler, H. D., Christoff, G., and Taylor, E.: Cryoprotective agents as inducers of erythroleukemia cell differentiation in vitro. *Blood* 47:363, 1976.

87. Ichikawa, Y.: Differentiation of a cell line of myeloid leukemia. *J. Cell. Physiol.* 74:223, 1969.

88. Miller, A. M., Marmor, J. B., Page, P. L., Russell, J. L., and Robinson, S. H.: Unregulated growth of murine leukemia cells and suppression of normal granulocyte growth in diffusion chamber cultures. *Blood* 47:737, 1977.

89. Collins, S. J., Gallo, R. C., and Gallagher, R. E.: Continuous growth and differentiation of human myeloid leukemic cells in suspension culture. *Nature* 270:347, 1977.

90. Koeffler, H. P., and Golde, D. W.: Acute myelogenous leukemia: A human cell line responsive to colony stimulating activity. *Science* 200:1153, 1978.

91. Burke, P. S., Karp, J. F., Braine, H. G., and Vaughan, W. P.: Timed sequential therapy of human leukemia based upon the response of leukemic cells to humoral growth factors. *Cancer Res.* 37:2138, 1977.

92. Sandberg, A. A., and Horsfeld, D. K.: Chromosomal abnormalities in human neoplasia. *Ann. Rev. Med.* 21:379, 1970.

93. Whang-Peng, J., Freireich, E. J., Oppenheim, J. J., Frie, E., III, and Tjio, H. J.: Cytogenetic studies in 45 patients with acute lymphocytic leukemia. *J. Natl. Cancer Inst.* 42:881, 1969.

94. Whang-Peng, J., Henderson, E. S., Knutson, T., Freireich, E. J., and Gart, J. J.: Cytogenetic studies in acute myelocytic leukemia with special emphasis on the occurrence of the Ph¹ chromosome. *Blood* 36:448, 1970.

95. Rowley, J. D.: Chromosome abnormalities in human leukemia. *Ann. Rev. Genet.* 14:17, 1980.

96. Frei, E., Bentzel, C. J., Rieselbach, R., and Block, J. B.: Renal complications of neoplastic disease. *J. Chronic Dis.* 16:757, 1963.

97. LePrise, P. Y., Toujas, L., Grandhour, C., and Lessard, M.: Splenomegaly and ALL. *Lancet* 1:1035, 1980.

98. Monoharan, A., Goldman, J. M., Lampert, I. A., Catovsky, D., Lauria, F., and Galton, D. A. G.: Significance of splenomegaly in childhood acute lymphoblastic leukaemia in remission. *Lancet* 1:449, 1980.

99. Murphy, S., and Hersh, E.: Immunotherapy of leukemia and lymphoma. *Semin. Hematol.* 15:181, 1978.

100. Metzger, R. S., and Mohanakumar, R.: Tumor associated antigens of leukemia cells. *Semin. Hematol.* 15:138, 1978.

101. Greaves, M. F., Brown, G., Rapson, N. T., and Lister, T. A.: Antisera to acute lymphoblastic leukemia cells. *Clin. Immunol. Immunopathol.* 4:67, 1975.

102. Durantez, A., Zighelboim, J., Thieme, T., and Fahey, J. L.: Antigens shared by leukemic blast cell and lymphoblastoid cell lines detected by lymphocyte-dependent antibody. *Cancer Res.* 35:2693, 1975.

103. Pesando, J. M., Ritz, J., Lazarus, H., Costello, S. B., and Schlossman, S. F.: Leukemia associated antigens in ALL. *Blood* 54:1240, 1979.

104. Greaves, M. F., and Lister, T. A.: Prognostic importance of immunologic markers in adult acute lymphoblastic leukemia. *N. Engl. J. Med.* 304:119, 1981.

105. Hersh, E. M., Bodey, G. P., Nies, B. A., and Freireich, E. J.: Causes of death in acute leukemia. *JAMA* 193:105, 1965.

106. Levine, A. S., Graw, R. G., and Young, R. C.: Management of infections in patients with leukemia and lymphoma: Current concepts and experimental approaches. *Semin. Hematol.* 9:141, 1972.

107. Ketchel, S. J., and Rodriguez, V.: Acute infections in cancer patients *Semin. Oncol.* 5:167, 1978.

108. Zusman, J., Brown, B. M., and Nesbit, M. E.: Hyperphosphatemia,

hyperphosphaturia, and hypocalcemia in acute lymphoblastic leukemia. *N. Engl. J. Med. 289:*1335, 1973.

109. Clarkson, D. R., Blondin, J., and Cryer, P. E.: Phosphate depletion and glucocorticoid induced hyperphosphatemia in lymphoblastic leukemia. *Metabolism 22:*611, 1973.

110. Jaffe, N., Kim, B. S., and Vawter, G. F.: Hypocalcemia: A complication of childhood leukemia. *Cancer 29:*392, 1972.

111. Brakman, P., Snyder, J., Henderson, E. S., and Astrup, T.: Blood coagulation and fibrinolysis in acute leukemia. *Br. J. Haematol. 18:*135, 1970.

112. Gralnick, H. R.: Marchesi, S., and Givelber, H.: Intravascular coagulation in acute leukemia: Clinical subclinical abnormalities. *Blood 40:*709, 1972.

113. Drapkin, R. L., et al.: Prophylactic heparin therapy in acute promyelocytic leukemia. *Cancer 41:*2484, 1978.

114. Bodey, G. P., Buckley, M., Sathe, Y. S., and Freireich, E. J.: Quantitative relationships between circulating leukocytes and infections in patients with acute leukemia. *Ann. Intern. Med. 64:*328, 1966.

115. Borella, L., Green, A. A., and Webster, R. G.: Immunological rebound after cessation of long-term chemotherapy in acute leukemia. *Blood 40:*42, 1972.

116. Hersh, E. M., Whitecar, J. P., McCredie, K. B., Bodey, G. P., and Freireich, E. J.: Chemotherapy, immunocompetence, immunosuppression and prognosis in acute leukemia. *N. Engl. J. Med. 285:*1211, 1971.

117. Simone, J.: Acute lymphoblastic leukemia in childhood. *Semin. Hematol. 11:*25, 1974.

118. Higby, D. J., Yates, J. W., Henderson, E. S., and Holland, J. F.: Filtration leukapheresis for granulocyte transfusion therapy. *N. Engl. J. Med. 292:*761, 1975.

119. Higby, D. J., and Burnett, D.: Granulocyte transfusions: Current status (review). *Blood 55:*2, 1980.

120. Bjornsson, S., Preisler, H., and Henderson, E. S.: A study of antibiotic therapy in fever of unknown origin in neutropenic cancer patients. *Med. Pediatr. Oncol. 3:*379, 1977.

121. Pizzo, P. A., et al.: Duration of empivic antibiotic therapy in granulocytopenic patients with cancer. *Am. J. Med. 67:*194, 1979.

122. Preisler, H. D., Hasenclever, H. F., and Henderson, E. S.: Anticandida antibodies in patients with acute leukemia: A prospective study. *Am. J. Med. 51:*352, 1971.

123. Hughes, S. W. T., et al.: Successful chemoprophylaxis for pneumocystis *Carninii* pneumonitis. *N. Engl. J. Med. 297:*1419, 1977.

124. Restrepo, A., Stenens, D. A., and Utz, J. P. (eds.): First international symposium on ketoconazole. *Rev. Infect. Dis 2(4):*519, 1980.

125. Hagbin, M., Armstrong, D., and Murphy, M. L.: Controlled prospective trail of *Pseudomonas aeruginosa* vaccine in children with acute leukemia. *Cancer 32:*761, 1973.

126. Preisler, H. D., and Bjornsson, S.: Protected environment unit in the treatment of acute leukemia. *Semin. Oncol. 2:*369, 1975.

127. Chang, Y. Y., Rodriguez, V., Narboni, G., Bodey, G. P., Luna, M. A., and Freireich, E. J.: Causes of death in adults with acute leukemia. *Medicine 55:*259, 1976.

128. Gaydos, L. A., Freireich, E. J., and Mantel, N.: The quantitative relation between platelet count and hemorrhage in patients with acute leukemia. *N. Engl. J. Med. 266:*905, 1962.

129. Didisheim, P., Trombold, J. S., Vandervoot, R. L. E., and Songin-Mibashan, R.: Acute promyelocytic leukemia with fibrinogen and factor V deficiencies. *Blood 23:*717, 1964.

130. Dietrich, M., Rasche, H., and Kubanek, B.: Coagulation disorder in acute leukemia as a prognostic factor. *Adv. Biosci. 14:*175, 1975.

131. Golomb, H. M., Rowley, J. D., Vardiman, J. W., Testa, J. R., and Butler, A.: "Microgranular" acute promyelocytic leukemia: A distinct clinical, ultrastructural, and cytogenetic entity. *Blood 55:*253, 1980.

132. McKenna, R., Bloomfield, C. D., Nesbit, M., and Brunning, R. S.: Nonspecific esterase positive acute leukemia: A distinctive cytologic and clinical entity. *Proc. A.A.C.R./A.S.C.O. 16:*61, 1975.

133. Wuenschmann-Henderson, B., Goldstein, I., Henderson, E. S., and Astrup, T.: Variations in fibrinolytic activity of leukemic cell lines. *Fed. Proc. 30:*822, 1971.

134. Gralnick, H., and Henderson, E. S.: Acquired coagulation factor deficiencies in leukemia. *Cancer 26:*1097, 1970.

135. Rasche, H., Dietrich, M., Gaus, W., and Schleyer, M.: Factor XIII activity and fibrin subunit structure in acute leukemia. *Biomedicine 21:*61, 1974.

136. Moore, E. W., Thomas, L. B., Shaw, R. K., and Freireich, E. J.: The central nervous system in acute leukemia. *Arch. Intern. Med. 105:*451, 1960.

137. McKee, C., Jr., and Collins, R. D.: Intracellular leukocyte thrombi and aggregates as a cause of morbidity and mortality in leukemia. *Medicine (Baltimore) 53:*463, 1974.

138. Evans, A., Gilbert, E. J., Zandstra, R.: The increasing incidence of central nervous system leukemia in children. *Cancer 26:*404, 1970.

139. Wolk, R. N., Masse, S. R., Conklin, R., and Freireich, E. J.: Incidence of central nervous system leukemia in adults. *Cancer 33:*863, 1974.

140. Thomas, L. B.: Pathology of leukemia in the brain and meninges: Postmortem studies of patients with acute leukemia and of mice given inoculations of L1210 leukemia. *Cancer Res. 25:*1555, 1965.

141. Price, R. A., and Johnson, W. W.: The central nervous system in childhood leukemia. I. The arachnoid. *Cancer 31:*520, 1973.

142. Nies, B. A., Thomas, L. B., and Freireich, E.: Meningeal leukemia: A follow-up study. *Cancer 18:*546, 1965.

143. Enzmann, D. R., Krikorian, J., and Yorke, C.: Computed tomography in leptomeningeal spread of tumors. *J. Comput. Assist. Tomogr. 2:*448, 1978.

144. Hann, H. W. L., Lustbader, E. D., Evan, A. E., Toledano, S. R., Lillie, P. D., and Jasko, L. B.: Lack of influence of T-cell marker and importance of mediastinal mass on the prognosis of acute lymphocytic leukemia of childhood. *J. Natl. Cancer Inst. 66:*285, 1981.

145. Wiernik, P. H., and Serpick, A. A.: Factors affecting remission and survival in adult acute nonlymphocytic leukemia (ANLL). *Medicine (Baltimore) 49:*505, 1970.

146. Boggs, D., Wintrobe, M. M., and Cartwright, G. E.: The acute leukemias. *Medicine (Baltimore) 41:*163, 1962.

147. Simone, J.: Prognostic factors in childhood lymphocytic leukemia. *Adv. Biosci. 14:*27, 1975.

148. Pierce, M. I., Borges, N. H., Heyn, R., Wolff, J. A., and Gilbert, E. S.: Epidemiological factors and survival experience in 1770 children with acute leukemia treated by members of Children's Cancer Group A. *Cancer 23:*1296, 1969.

149. Keating, M. J., et al.: Factors related to length of complete remission in adult acute leukemia. *Cancer 45:*2017, 1980.

CHAPTER *28*

Acute myelogenous leukemia

EDWARD S. HENDERSON

Definition

Acute myelogenous leukemia (AML) is a malignant disease of the multipotential hemopoietic stem cells. The disease is thought to originate in marrow, although cells with proliferative capabilities escape, circulate, and can be found in most tissues after the disease is established. The cell pool that sustains the malignant process (leukemic multipotential stem cell pool) is capable of a spectrum of differentiation, and thus several morphologic variants of AML may occur. Qualitative abnormalities of cell structure and abnormal chromosomal patterns in developing leukemic erythroid, granulocytic, and megakaryocytic cells have supported the concept of an early multipotential stem cell lesion. The results of studies of X-linked enzyme isotypes and cytogenetics in two children with AML have been exceptions to this concept [1]; however, the weight of evidence in adults supports the involvement of all hemopoietic cell lineages in most patients with AML studied prior to treatment (see Chap. 19).

Incidence

Acute myelogenous leukemia is the predominant form of leukemia during the neonatal period, but it represents a small proportion of cases during childhood and in early adulthood. From middle age onward, the incidence increases progressively until it reaches about 15 per 100,000 persons in the eighth and ninth decades of life [2]. AML accounts for 20 percent of the acute leukemias in children and 80 percent of the acute leukemias in adults [2,3]. AML is slightly more common in males, but there is little difference in incidence between black and white races at any age. Unlike ALL, AML is probably increasing in incidence in the industrialized nations. [4]. Also in contrast to ALL, it is the type of leukemia that develops most frequently from an antecedent preleukemic disorder (see Chap. 22) or as a complication of chemotherapy or irradiation. For a further discussion of the pathogenesis of AML, see Chap. 19, and for discussion of the predisposing factors in AML, see Chap. 27.

Classification

Several variants of AML can be identified by morphologic features of blood films using polychrome stains and by the histochemical reaction of cells. These morphologic variants are considered to be manifestations of a leukemic lesion in the multipotential hemopoietic stem cell. Each morphologic variant is characterized by proliferation of leukemic cells in marrow and by the suppression of hemopoiesis leading to anemia, thrombocytopenia, and frequently granulocytopenia. The morphologic variants have special clinical features as a result of the effects of the different types of leukemic cells (Table 28-1).

Clinical features

The most important features of AML which occur in all variants are the result of suppression of normal hemopoiesis. Anemia leads to pallor, fatigue, weakness, palpitations, and exertional dyspnea. Weakness and fatigue on exertion can be out of proportion to the extent of the anemia. Thrombocytopenia can result in easy bruising, petechiae, epistaxis, gingival bleeding, or conjunctival hemorrhages. Less often, gastrointestinal, genitourinary, nervous system, or bronchopulmonary hemorrhage can occur. Granulocytopenia may predispose to a variety of infections. Pyogenic infections of the skin and infected cuts or minor wounds are most common; however, pneumonia, pyelonephritis, meningitis, or other specific infections can occur, but they are unusual at presentation of the disease. Major bacterial infections become a more serious problem after cytotoxic treatment is instituted. Infections with opportunistic organisms (protozoa, certain viruses, or fungi) are also more common later in the disease after treatment is instituted and severe marrow aplasia occurs.

Anorexia and weight loss are frequent findings. Fever is present in many patients at the time of diagnosis [5,6]. Palpable splenomegaly occurs in about one-third of patients. Hepatomegaly and lymphadenopathy are infrequent.

Bone tenderness or aching and joint pains can occur. Synovitis results most commonly from leukemic infiltration, although acute gouty arthritis as a result of hyperuricemia can occur. Infiltrates of leukemic cells in many organs are common, but functional impairment is rare. Collections of leukemic blast cells referred to as *granulocytic sarcomas* can occur in soft tissues, gonads, breasts, bones, lymph nodes, paranasal sinuses, and other sites. Rarely, granulocytic sarcomas may precede the involvement of marrow and blood by months or years (see Chap. 7).

Laboratory features

BLOOD AND MARROW FINDINGS

Anemia and thrombocytopenia are nearly constant features of the disease. Leukopenia or normal total leukocyte counts with neutropenia occur in at least half the patients. Patients with markedly elevated leukocyte counts may have normal or slightly elevated absolute neutrophil counts despite a very low proportion of neutrophils. Poikilocytosis and anisocytosis of red cells, nucleated red cells, giant platelets, platelets with abnormal granules, unilobed or bilobed neutrophils, hypogranular neutrophils, and other qualitative abnormalities of cells may be present in the blood film.

The diagnosis of AML depends on identification of leukemic (abnormal) blast cells in marrow and blood. In most cases, the blast cells can be identified in the blood and range from 15 to 95 percent of the blood cells. The marrow can contain anywhere from a few percent to nearly 100 percent leukemic blast cells. In rare patients with severe leukopenia, blast cells may be difficult to identify in blood but are present in the marrow. Aspiration of marrow occasionally may be difficult ("dry tap") and a biopsy will show extensive infiltration with leukemic blast cells. Varying degrees of dysplastic blood cell maturation may be present. Dysplastic erythroblasts, progranulocytes, myelocytes, monocytes, or megakaryocytes may be present in the marrow. Maturation abnormalities affect the more mature marrow cells

TABLE 28-1   Morphologic variants of acute myelogenous leukemia

Variant	Cytologic features	Special clinical features
1. Acute myeloblastic leukemia	1. Myeloblasts are usually large; nuclear cytoplasmic ratio 1:1. Cytoplasm usually contains granules and occasionally Auer bodies. Nucleus shows fine reticular pattern and distinct nucleoli. 2. Leukemic cells are sudanophilic. They are positive for myeloperoxidase and chloroacetate esterase, negative for nonspecific esterase, and negative or diffusely positive for PAS (no clumps or blocks). 3. Electron microscope (EM) shows primary cytoplasmic granules.	1. Most common in adults, and most frequent variety in infants.
2. Acute progranulocytic leukemia	1. Leukemic cells resemble progranulocytes. They have large atypical primary granules. Branched or adherent Auer rods are common. 2. Histochemical features similar to those in AML. Peroxidase intensely positive.	1. Usually in adults. 2. DIC* very common.
3. Acute myelomonocytic leukemia	1. Both myeloblastic and monoblastic leukemia cells in blood and marrow. 2. Peroxidase-, Sudan-, chloroacetate esterase–, and nonspecific esterase–positive cells.	1. Indistinguishable clinically from myeloblastic leukemia. 2. Slightly elevated serum and urine muramidase.
4. Acute monocytic leukemia	1. Leukemic cells are large and often bizarre; nuclear cytoplasmic ratio 1:1 or less. Cytoplasm contains fine granules. Auer rods are rare. Nucleus is often convoluted and contains 1 to 4 large nucleoli. 2. Histochemically, nonspecific esterase–positive, inhibited by NaF; Sudan-, peroxidase-, and chloroacetate esterase–negative. PAS occurs in granules and blocks. 3. Cytoplasmic microfibrils demonstrable by EM.	1. Usually in children or young adults. 2. Gum, CNS lymph node and extramedullary infiltrations are common. 3. DIC* occurs. 4. Plasma and urine muramidase moderately elevated.
5. Acute erythroleukemia	1. Abnormal erythroblasts are in abundance initially in marrow and often in blood. Later the morphologic findings are indistinguishable from those of AML. 2. Erythroblasts are usually strongly PAS-positive.	1. May have long prodromal period.
6. Acute megakaryocytic leukemia	1. Large and small megakaryoblasts with high nucleus/cytoplasmic ratio, pale agranular cytoplasm. 2. Peroxidase-negative, platelet peroxidase–positive, occasionally strongly PAS-positive.	1. High blood blast counts and organ infiltration are rare. 2. Markedly elevated LDH. 3. Myelofibrosis and "dry taps" common.
7. Eosinophilic leukemia	1. Many eosinophils and eosinophilic precursors in marrow and blood.	1. Pulmonary, cardiac, and CNS manifestations more frequent.
8. Basophilic leukemia	1. Many basophils and basophilic precursors in marrow and blood.	1. Skin lesions and elevated blood and urine histamine may be present.

* Disseminated intravascular coagulation.

as well. Myelocytes, metamyelocytes, and polymorphonuclear leukocytes may have poorly developed specific granulation. Acquired Pelger-Huet cells (monolobed or bilobed neutrophils) may also be noted. Normal erythropoiesis, granulopoiesis, and megakaryopoiesis are usually markedly decreased.

Morphologically there are two pathognomonic signs which distinguish myeloblasts from lymphoblasts: peroxidase activity by histochemical stains or the presence in blast cells of Auer rods. Either finding is considered pathognomonic of myeloblasts (AML). Auer rods are tubular or oval structures about 1 μm in length which may be found in an occasional leukemic blast cell in all varieties of AML. These rods are derived from the primary or azurophilic granule. Auer rods or atypical primary granules appear in about 10 percent of cases of AML. "Phi bodies," small, fusiform, peroxidase-positive structures thought to be Auer rod precursors, have been identified in the cells of a very high percentage of patients with AML [7,8]. Leukemic myeloblasts give positive reactions for either myeloperoxidase, Sudan black B, or naphthol AS-D-chloroacetate esterase staining and do not contain the large clumps of periodic acid–Schiff staining material that are typical of leukemic lymphoblasts.

BLOOD CHEMICAL FINDINGS

Metabolic abnormalities are frequently present in patients with AML [9]. Hyperuricemia is very frequent. Elevation in serum lactic dehydrogenase can occur. Occasionally, hypercalcemia, hypokalemia, hyperphosphatemia, lactic acidosis, or hypoxemia are present (see Chap. 7).

Morphologic variants

ERYTHROLEUKEMIA

Erythroleukemia is a variant of AML which was first described by DiGuglielmo [10]. It makes up about 3 percent of all cases of acute leukemia and is rare in childhood. It occurs with greater than expected frequency following radiation or cytotoxic drugs. It also may develop from a prexisting hemopoietic stem cell disease [11–13]. In its early stage, erythroleukemia has been referred to as *erythremic myelosis* because the dominant changes in the blood are anemia, bizarre red cell morphology with marked anisocytosis, poikilocytosis, anisochromia, nucleated red cells, and intense erythroid hyperplasia in the marrow [14–16]. The erythroblasts in the marrow are extremely abnormal with giant and multinucleated forms, nuclear budding, and nuclear fragmentation. There may be nearly normal granulopoiesis and thrombopoiesis in this phase of the disease. This severe dyserythropoietic phase may be protracted or may evolve rapidly into one in which myeloblasts are more prominent in the marrow, amegakaryocytic thrombocytopenia occurs, and impairment of granulopoiesis is present—a phase which more closely fits the

typical description of erythroleukemia. The disease may evolve into a more florid acute myelogenous leukemia with a replacement of marrow by leukemic blast cells. There are, however, many variations on the classical theme of a three-stage evolution: erythremic myelosis, erythroleukemia, and acute myelogenous leukemia. Thus there is a spectrum from idiopathic refractory anemia (preleukemia) through erythroleukemia in which dyserythropoiesis may be a prominent feature, although qualitative abnormalities of erythroblasts become more profound in erythroleukemia [17].

Studies of erythropoiesis in erythroleukemia have shown markedly ineffective erythropoiesis [18]. Although erythropoiesis is severely disordered, some of the normal regulatory system remains, since hypertransfusion decreases both erythropoietin levels and abnormal erythropoiesis [19,20]. The cell mitotic cycle of erythroblasts is prolonged as a result of slowing of DNA synthesis and arrest of cells during the premitotic stage of the cell cycle [18]. The red cell morphology may resemble that observed in megaloblastic anemias, although serum vitamin B_{12} and folic acid levels are normal or high, and treatment with these vitamins does not correct the abnormalities in erythropoiesis.

Cytogenetic abnormalities including chromosome fragmentation, marker chromosomes, and aneuploidy are present in about half the cases [21–24]. Immunologic abnormalities are more common than in any other myeloproliferative disease [16,25]. These features include hypergammaglobulinemia, positive Coombs' test, antinuclear antibody, and rheumatoid factor. Rarely, the positive Coombs' test is associated with severe hemolysis requiring glucocorticoid therapy. Anemia is present in virtually every case. Absolute reticulocytopenia is usually present. Leukocyte count varies from markedly reduced to markedly elevated. Thrombocytopenia is very common but not invariable, and thrombocytosis occurs occasionally [14–16]. The proportion of blast cells in the marrow varies from 1 to 50 percent at the time of diagnosis. Hepatomegaly and splenomegaly occur infrequently. Rheumatic complaints are prominent in patients with erythroleukemia. Synovitis, serositis, and effusions which respond to anti-inflammatory agents occur with unexpected frequency [16].

Erythroleukemia can have an indolent course during the erythremic myelosis phase. In patients with significant replacement of marrow with blast cells and severe cytopenias, treatment is warranted. Regimens used for acute myeloblastic leukemia are efficacious in erythroleukemia, and results correspond to those of myeloblastic leukemia.

PROGRANULOCYTIC LEUKEMIA

Progranulocytic leukemia is one of the most virulent variants of AML in part because it is often associated with intense disseminated intravascular coagulation and occasionally with very high blast cell counts [26–40]. It is characterized by the presence of progranulocytes that contain numerous prominent primary granules with wide variation in size and intense staining characteristics [37,39]. Auer rods can be present in some of the cells, and occasional cells contain multiple Auer rods ("faggots") [35,37]. The progranulocytes stain intensely for peroxidase activity. A distinctive cytogenetic abnormality, the translocation of a portion of chromosome 17 to 15 (t15q+:17q−) occurs in about half the cases [21,41–45]. In most cases, disseminated intravascular coagulation (DIC) is correlated with the presence of the abnormal granules rather than with the proportion of promyelocytes. In rare cases, referred to as *microgranular progranulocytic leukemia,* the granules are so minute that they can be seen only by electron microscopy [46]. The 15:17 translocation and the propensity to DIC is retained in such cases. Several studies have suggested that the granules in the leukemic progranulocytes contain procoagulants that initiate DIC in the patients [33]. Fibrin thrombi are present in many vascular beds in autopsied patients.

This variant of AML can occur at any age and comprises about 10 percent of cases of AML. Bleeding occurs in nearly all patients, and skin, mucosal, uterine, and gastrointestinal hemorrhages may be present. Pulmonary or intracranial hemorrhages can occur and lead to death. The hemorrhagic tendency is a result of intravascular thrombosis and consumption of coagulation factors and secondary activation of fibrinolysis. Hemorrhage is frequently out of proportion to the degree of thrombocytopenia. Thrombosis is largely microvascular and can lead to glomerular occlusion and renal failure; thrombi can also occur in larger arteries, leg veins, and visceral veins.

Other presenting symptoms and signs are similar to those of acute myeloblastic leukemia. The prothrombin time and partial thromboplastin time are prolonged in over two-thirds of patients. The plasma fibrinogen level is often decreased, and some believe that its concentration has prognostic implications in that patients with fibrinogen levels less than 100 mg/dl do not have as good results from therapy as those with higher concentrations.

The response of this variant of AML was poor prior to the availability of anthracycline antibiotics [32]. Daunorubicin or doxorubicin have greatly increased the frequency of remission and should be used in treatment. Heparin therapy should be used in patients with evidence of DIC [41,42,47]. Replacement of platelets and consumed coagulation factors after heparin is started is important. The hemorrhagic diathesis in progranulocytic leukemia may be mediated in different ways in some patients. Rarely, primary fibrinolysis may be present or degradation of coagulation factors may occur by granule enzymes released into plasma. Thus heparin therapy should be evaluated carefully to ensure that the therapist is getting the expected result. Heparin blocks the microvascular thrombosis, conserves coagulation factors, and may therefore lessen bleeding. If microvascular thrombosis is not present, heparin will worsen bleeding.

MONOCYTIC LEUKEMIA

Acute monocytic leukemia is characterized by blood and marrow cells that either appear to be monocytic or appear to be large blast cells [48–59]. These leukemic monoblasts have special ultrastructural features that include nuclear irregularity, nuclear blebs, abundant cytoplasm with numerous pinocytotic vesicles, and perinuclear fibrillar bands [48]. Both well-differentiated and poorly differentiated leukemic monocytes have granules which stain for α-naphthylbutyrate esterase [49,53,55,57,58], a reaction characteristically inhibited by sodium fluoride. Leukemic monocytes can perform erythrophagocytosis in vivo, can phagocytize particles or bacteria in vitro, and have membrane Fc receptors and specific surface antigens [50,54,56]. Marrow monoblasts tend to be less differentiated morphologically than blood promonocytes or monocytes, although the latter can be functionally impaired and unable to kill ingested microorganisms.

Acute monocytic leukemia is prone to high total leukocyte counts, as well as to infiltration of gingiva, lungs, meninges, colon, rectum, lymph nodes, bladder, and larynx [49–51,59]. Plasma and urinary muramidase levels are usually elevated [52,59]. Therapy for this variant of AML is similar to that for myeloblastic leukemia, and the results are about the same. There is a significantly increased propensity to meningeal leukemia [60], and some workers suggest that prophylactic intrathecal treatment should be given to younger patients who have a good remission, especially if initial total leukocyte count is very high.

MEGAKARYOBLASTIC LEUKEMIA AND ACUTE MYELOFIBROSIS

Megakaryoblastic leukemia [61–65] and acute myelofibrosis [66–68] have been described as separate entities. The diagnosis of megakaryoblastic leukemia has been facilitated by high-resolution histochemistry [63], and the frequent coincidence and possible identity of megakaryoblastic leukemia and acute myelofibrosis [64,68] have been suggested. The clinical course of both diseases rarely exceeds 1 year from earliest symptoms to death. A period of several months from initial symptoms to diagnosis is common. A megakaryoblastic variant of AML can be the terminal event of CML [69,70].

Patients usually present with pancytopenia. Pallor, weakness, and excessive bleeding are common. Elevated leukocyte counts, lymphadenopathy, or hepatosplenomegaly are rarely present at the time of diagnosis. Later in the course of the disease, high blood blast cell counts develop. Marrow aspiration is often not diagnostic ("dry tap"). The extensive marrow reticulin fibrosis impairs aspiration of cells. Marrow biopsy reveals infiltration with a mixture of small and large blast cells which may resemble abnormal megakaryoblasts. The small blast cells usually have a high nuclear cytoplasmic ratio, moderately fine chromatin with distinct nuclei, and pale blue agranular cytoplasm with cytoplasmic protrusions. In contrast to other myelogenous leukemias, the blast cells are peroxidase-negative. Confirmation of their megakaryoblastic nature may require electron microscopy coupled with a specific histochemical test for platelet peroxidase [63]. The more-differentiated megakaryocytes can stain with periodic acid–Schiff reagents and contain sodium fluoride-inhibitable nonspecific esterase. They are negative for α-naphthylbutyrate esterase, a pattern consistent with megakaryocyte origin [64]. Occasionally, the demarcation membrane system characteristic of normal megakaryocyte cytoplasm can be seen in the blast cells by electron microscopy.

Blood and marrow granulocytes have normal leukocyte alkaline phosphatase levels. The serum lactic acid dehydrogenase is frequently strikingly increased and has an isomorphic pattern unlike that seen with other myeloproliferative disorders. Treatment with cytotoxic drugs has not been successful in producing remissions.

EOSINOPHILIC LEUKEMIA
Eosinophilic leukemia is a variant of AML that is highlighted by a high proportion of cells with eosinophilic granules in blood and marrow [71–75]. In rare cases, the marrow cells contain the Philadelphia chromosome (Ph¹) and are presumably variants of CML [76]. More commonly, eosinophilic leukemia exhibits features of AML with increased blast cells in marrow, suppression of hemopoiesis, and a predisposition toward progressive congestive heart failure, respiratory distress, central nervous system disturbances, and fever associated with sustained blood hypereosinophilia [77–79]. Hepatosplenomegaly is common. Marrow examination reveals hypereosinophilia with marked degrees of immaturity and often cytogenetic abnormalities of eosinophils. The Ph¹ chromosome is characteristically absent [80]. Eosinophilic leukemia may be difficult to differentiate from hypereosinophilic syndromes [81, 82]. Rarely, episodes of reactive eosinophilia that occur with acute lymphocytic leukemia or T-cell lymphoblastic lymphoma can simulate eosinophilic leukemia [83]. Treatment of acute eosinophilic leukemia is the same as that used for other types of AML and includes cytosine arabinoside and an anthracycline antibiotic. Vincristine and hydroxyurea can produce salutory results [84], but clinical trials have not been conducted with these agents and their general usefulness has not been established.

BASOPHILIC LEUKEMIA
Acute basophilic leukemia is an extremely rare variant of AML. The blood leukocyte count is usually elevated, and a proportion of the cells are basophils [85–88]. The marrow is cellular with a high proportion of blasts and early and late basophilic myelocytes. Special staining with toluidine blue or astra blue may be necessary to distinguish basophilic from neutrophilic promyelocytes and myelocytes. Electron microscopy can be useful in identifying basophilic granules [89]. Intravascular coagulation and hemorrhage are uncommon presenting features in patients with basophilic leukemia, whereas they are very common in progranulocytic leukemia, with which basophilic leukemia can be confused if the basophilic early myelocytes are mistaken for progranulocytes. Urticaria and elevated blood histamine levels occur in patients with basophilic leukemia. Most cases of basophilic leukemia have a chronic course and evolve as a phase of Ph¹-positive CML. Immature basophils undergoing mitosis can be shown to contain the Ph¹ chromosome in such cases [90]. Treatment for acute (Ph¹-negative) basophilic leukemia is similar to that for other variants of AML.

OLIGOBLASTIC (SMOLDERING) LEUKEMIA
In a small proportion of cases (~ 10 percent), patients may have anemia, leukopenia and thrombocytopenia, and a small proportion of blast cells in marrow (5 to 20 percent). A plateau of disease activity may develop and last for several months or even years. Such cases have been termed *oligoblastic*, or *smoldering, leukemia* [91,92]. The clinical course of the untreated disease is protracted, but eventually the disease becomes more severe. The marrow cellularity in patients with oligoblastic leukemia may be increased, normal, or occasionally decreased in the early stages, and it contains less than 20 percent myeloblasts. Since the smoldering disease progresses very slowly during early stages and responds poorly to cytocidal therapy, these patients are best treated with transfusions of red cells and other symptomatic measures until evidence of more rapid progression and clinical deterioration occurs.

NEONATAL LEUKEMIA
Several varieties of acute leukemia occur in neonates, and their frequency in infants with Down's syndrome is about 12 times greater than that in other infants [93–95]. Purpura and enlargement of the liver and spleen are almost invariably present in patients with neonatal leukemia, and about one-half of the reported cases have had nodular skin infiltrates [96]. Fever, failure to gain weight, and diarrhea are characteristic of AML when it occurs at this age. Transient congenital myeloproliferative disorders that mimic myelogenous leukemia also occur in neonates with Down's syndrome [97–99]. These transient syndromes regress spontaneously. In the transient myeloproliferative syndromes in infants with Down's syndrome, there are no cytogenetic abnormalities other than trisomy 21. In infants who have Down's syndrome and abnormalities indicative of myelogenous leukemia, cytotoxic therapy should be withheld until disease progression is clearly demonstrated in order to distinguish neonatal leukemia from transient myeloproliferative disease. Permanent spontaneous remissions have also been reported in infants with "congenital leukemia" who do not have Down's syndrome. In most of these infants, blast cells disappear from the blood and marrow by 4 months of age. The pathogenesis of these unusual reactions is not understood.

Therapy

Almost all patients with AML should receive cytotoxic chemotherapy. However, patients who have smoldering leukemia are best treated with symptomatic, supportive measures until the phase of increasing myeloblastic proliferation is reached.

Marrow failure and pancytopenia are the major causes of morbidity and mortality in virtually all patients with AML, and thus rapid restoration of normal hemopoiesis is the therapeutic goal. Leukemic blast cell infiltration seems to impair marrow function to a disproportionate degree [100], so a pronounced reduction in leukemic blast cells is usually required before hemopoiesis improves. Agents capable of destroying leukemic blast cells are nonspecific, and every regimen in current use for the treatment of AML injures the stem cells and progenitors for normal hemopoiesis. Complete remissions are rarely achieved without the production of severe marrow hypoplasia and more severe pancytopenia. The treatment of AML requires facilities for the transfusion of red cells, platelets, and granulocytes, as well as facilities for the diagnosis and management of unusual infections. The increased ability of normal stem cells to recover their ability to proliferate and differentiate leads to remissions in acute leukemia.

In the initial appraisal of AML it is necessary to define the extent to which marrow, renal, and hepatic functions are compromised. The presence of disease-related complications such as DIC and hyperuricemia and the presence of cardiovascular disease, diabetes mellitus, or infections should be considered. Allopurinol administration (300 to 900 mg per day orally or intravenously) and hydration and high urine flow are important to minimize the renal injury that may occur from hyperuricemia and hyperuricosuria. Severe anemia should be corrected and platelet transfusions given to patients with thrombocytopenia and hemorrhagic manifestations. Some therapists prefer to give platelets prophylactically if the platelet count is less than 10,000 per microliter. The plasma fibrogen level, prothrombin time, partial thromboplastin time, and fibrin degradation products (FDP) should be determined before treatment is initiated in all patients with AML. Patients with evidence of DIC should be considered for heparin treatment before antileukemic therapy is started. This complication should be suspected in those patients with large numbers of leukemic progranulocytes and blast cells with Auer rods.

Patients with blast counts greater than 100,000 per microliter require prompt treatment to prevent serious and often fatal complications of leukostatic thrombosis and hemorrhage. Cytoreduction therapy can be initiated simultaneously with supportive measures. Leukapheresis and cytotoxic drug therapy can be given to reduce blast cell count rapidly. Leukapheresis therapy is especially useful in hyperleukocytic patients, since it can reduce blood leukemic cell concentration within several hours without contributing to the release of uric acid. Cytotoxic drug therapy with either hydroxyurea, 6 to 10 g per day orally for 3 to 6 days, or with cytosine arabinoside and an anthracycline antibiotic should be started also. During the first few days of therapy, the maintenance of adequate renal function is critical. Every effort should be made to maintain urine flow of 100 ml/$(m^2 \cdot h)$ through hydration and, if necessary, osmotic diuresis or furosemide administration. Allopurinol should be started promptly to decrease the formation of uric acid during cytotoxic therapy, even in individuals in whom the initial serum uric acid level is only slightly elevated.

REMISSION-INDUCTION TREATMENT

The cytotoxic therapy of AML rests on two key tenets: first, that two competing clones of cells are present in marrow — a normal and a leukemic clone — and second, that profound reduction in the leukemic cell populations is necessary to permit a clone change. The latter necessity leads to iatrogenic, severe, transient aplastic pancytopenia and the requirement for component blood cell transfusion and usually antimicrobial therapy as important adjuncts to cytotoxic treatment.

Most patients can be treated within 36 hours after admission to a hospital. The proportion of patients with AML who achieve a complete remission has increased to 70 percent of those treated. This improvement is the result of the discovery of cytosine arabinoside (ara-C) and the anthracycline antibiotics daunorubicin and doxorubicin, one or both of which have been included in successful current regimens. The chemical and pharmacologic features of these compounds and others with lesser degrees of activity against AML are listed in Table 28-2.

CYTOSINE ARABINOSIDE (ara-C, CYTOSAR)

Cytosine arabinoside is a synthetic pyrimidine antimetabolite which was found to have significant activity against mouse leukemia L1210 in 1965. Subsequently, numerous clinical trials have demonstrated that ara-C is a useful antileukemic agent, particularly in the treatment of AML. It is minimally toxic to tissues other than the marrow, gastrointestinal epithelium, rapidly dividing lymphocytes, and the germinal epithelium of hair follicles. The predominant effect of ara-C is the destruction of both normal and malignant blood progenitor cells. The drug inhibits DNA polymerase and thus is cytocidal only during the period of the DNA synthesis (S phase of the cell mitotic cycle) [101]. There is conflicting evidence as to whether or not it inhibits the progression of cells from the pre-S phase of cell growth (G_2) into the S phase [102]. However, ara-C has no effect on nondividing cells and no vesicant activity. It can thus be given with minimal local toxicity by the intravenous, subcutaneous, intramuscular, or intrathecal route. It is poorly absorbed from the gastrointestinal tract.

Following parenteral administration, ara-C is rapidly converted to uracil arabinoside, a virtually nontoxic metabolite. The enzyme catalyzing this conversion, cy-

TABLE 28-2   Characteristics of drugs effective in the treatment of acute myelogenous leukemia

Agent	Class	Mechanism of antitumor action	Usual dose, route, schedule	Pharmacology	Limiting toxicity
Daunorubicin (DNR)	Anthracycline antibiotic	Binds to DNA; inhibits DNA and RNA synthesis	40–60 mg/m² IV daily for 3–5 days	Plasma $T_{1/2}$ 45 min; metabolized in liver	Acute: Reversible myelosuppression Chronic: Cumulative myocardial fibrosis
Doxorubicin (DOX)	Anthracycline antibiotic	Same as DNR	30–45 mg/m² daily for 3–5 days	Plasma $T_{1/2}$ 5 h; metabolized in liver and elsewhere; excreted by kidney; excluded from CSF	Acute: Reversible myelosuppression Chronic: Cumulative cardiac fibrosis
Cytosine arabinoside (ara-C)	Pyrimide antimetabolite	Inhibits DNA synthesis (inhibits DNA polymerase and nucleotide reductase)	100 mg/m² IV or subcutaneously every 12 h for 7–10 days; 50 mg intrathecal every 4–7 days for CNS leukemia	Plasma $T_{1/2}$ 30 min; metabolized to ara-U in liver; excreted by kidney; slow entry into CSF	Acute: Reversible myelosuppression
6-Thioguanine (TG)	Purine antimetabolite	Inhibits de novo purine synthesis; incorporated into DNA	80–100 mg/m² PO or IV* every 12 h for 7–10 days	Plasma $T_{1/2}$ 80 min; metabolized in liver, blood cells, etc.; excreted by kidney; very slow entry into CSF	Reversible myelosuppression
6-Mercaptopurine (MP)	Purine antimetabolite	Inhibits de novo purine synthesis	80–100 mg/m² PO or IV* daily or every 12 h for 7–10 days	Plasma $T_{1/2}$ 90 min; metabolized in liver and elsewhere (by xanthine oxidase); excreted by kidney; enters CSF very slowly.	Reversible myelosuppression
5-Azacytidine*	Pyrimidine antimetabolite	Inhibits DNA, RNA, and protein synthesis; incorporated into DNA and RNA	100–250 mg/m² IV daily for 5–10 days	Plasma $T_{1/2}$ 90 min; excreted 80% in urine; slow entry into CSF	Reversible myelosuppression Reversible emesis, nausea, vomiting, orthostatic hypotension
Methylglyoxal-bis-guanylhydrazone* (methyl-GAG)	Unknown	Unknown; inhibits S-adenosylmethionine decarboxydase	150 mg/m² IV daily or 250–350 mg/m² IV twice a week	Not metabolized; excreted by kidney slowly; (?) accumulates in body; plasma $T_{1/2}$ 2 h; does not enter CSF	Myelosuppression, mucositis, polyserositis, vasculitis, related to cumulative dose
4'-(9-Acridynyl-amino)-methana-sulfon-M-anisidide (AMSA)	Unknown	Binds to DNA; inhibits DNA and RNA synthesis	90 mg/m² IV daily for 7 days	Unknown	Myelosuppression

* Investigational drug application.

tosine deaminase, is found to a varying degree in most tissues. Rapid deamination occurs in the plasma, and the half-life is less than 30 minutes. Thus the effect of single injections of even massive doses of ara-C is very short, being cytocidal to only the small proportion of cells that are in DNA synthesis during the few minutes that native drug is present in the tissues. Consequently, ara-C should be given either by frequent intermittent doses or by continuous infusion to be effective in reducing cell populations [103–105]. Other factors which condition the effect of ara-C are intracellular concentrations of cytidine kinase—necessary for phosphorylation of ara-C to its biologically active triphosphate form—and the level of deoxycytidine [106] and possibly other

nucleosides and nucleotides involved with DNA synthesis. The degree of retention of ara-CTP, a phosphorylated product of ara-C, in leukemic cells in vitro has proved to be a reliable indicator of the duration of ara-C induced and maintained remissions [107]. Both ara-C and uracil arabinoside are excreted through the kidneys, but since in vivo catabolism is the critical mechanism of detoxification, ara-C can be given in therapeutic amounts despite severe renal failure.

DAUNORUBICIN AND DOXORUBICIN

Daunorubicin, a naturally occurring antibiotic, was isolated from Streptomyces ceruleorubidus and S. peucetius early in the 1960s and was introduced into clinical trials in 1964 [108]. Daunorubicin is strikingly toxic to the marrow and effective against both AML and ALL. The drug intercalates in DNA, causing diminution of DNA and RNA synthesis and inhibition of DNA polymerase. It appears to be most toxic during the S phase and the G_2 growth phase. Daunorubicin is poorly absorbed when given orally. When given subcutaneously or intramuscularly, it binds rapidly to most macromolecules. If given carefully by intravenous infusion, its acute toxicity can be limited to myelosuppression, nausea, vomiting, and alopecia. The major limiting factor in the use of daunorubicin is neither its acute local nor systemic toxicity, but rather a late, usually irreversible, dose-related cardiomyopathy. This toxicity occurs most commonly in older individuals. It is uncommon unless the cumulative dose level exceeds 500 mg/m². There is no way to avoid or reverse cardiac toxicity, so the total dose used in maintenance or reinduction therapy should be limited. Daunorubicin is metabolized largely by the liver and excreted by the kidneys. A lower dose should be employed when the function of either of these organs is impaired. Hydroxydaunorubicin (doxorubicin, Adriamycin) exhibits antileukemic and toxic effects similar to those of daunorubicin but at slightly lower doses. Other anthracyclines, such as aclacinomycin, are under investigation in the hope of finding less cardiotoxic, but comparably antileukemic drugs.

5-AZACYTIDINE
5-Azacytidine is another synthetic antimetabolite of the pyrimidine family. Like ara-C, it is most active against dividing cells, particularly during their late G_1 and S phases. It must be given parenterally, and it is highly effective against AML [109,110]. In addition to being toxic to marrow, it regularly causes severe nausea and vomiting and occasionally orthostatic hypotension. Unlike ara-C, it has activity at high doses during all phases of the cell cycle and may indeed have some effect on nonreplicating cells [111]. 5-Azacytidine is still classified as an investigational drug.

6-THIOGUANINE
6-Thioguanine (TG), a purine antimetabolite, has only modest activity as a remission-induction agent in AML. Its major role in the treatment of acute leukemia is administration in combination with ara-C. The resultant combination is more effective and somewhat less toxic than ara-C alone. 6-Thioguanine is well absorbed when given orally. It is metabolized by the liver and excreted by the kidneys. Toxicity is relatively mild, but includes anorexia, nausea, suppression of granulocyte proliferation, and possibly adverse hepatic effects.

METHYLGLYOXAL-bis-GUANYLHYDRAZONE
Methylglyoxal-bis-guanylhydrazone (methyl-GAG) is a synthetic drug with an undetermined mode of action which has a profound toxicity on the marrow, mucosal surfaces, and connective tissues. It is of historical interest because it is the first compound discovered that was capable of producing remissions in a high proportion of patients with AML [112].

4'(9-ACRIDINYLAMINO)-METHANSULFON-M-ANISIDIDE (AMSA)
4'(9-Acridinylamino)-methansulfon-M-anisidide is a DNA intercalating agent which has shown consistent activity in initial clinical trials in AML and marginal activity in ALL [113]. It is being investigated further as a component of multidrug induction and maintenance protocols.

OTHER ANTILEUKEMIC AGENTS
Vincristine (V), glucocorticoids, 6-mercaptopurine (MP), methotrexate (MTX), and cyclophosphamide all have modest degrees of anti-AML effect when given as single agents [114–120] (Table 28-3). These agents have been incorporated into a large number of combination-drug regimens. Their pharmacology and toxicology are discussed in reference to acute lymphocytic leukemia (ALL), for which they are more applicable (see Chap. 114).

TABLE 28-3   Acute myelogenous leukemia treatment—remission-induction response to single drugs

Drugs	Dose and schedule*	Children No.	Children %CR*	Adults No.	Adults %CR*	References
Vincristine (V)	2 mg/m² each week	14	36	7	0	[114,115]
Prednisone (P)	40 mg/m² daily or bid	54	24	39	15	[116,117]
6-Mercaptopurine (MP)	90 mg/m² daily	11	9	31	10	[118]
Methotrexate (MTX)	5 mg daily	9	11	34	3	[118]
	1.25–2.5 mg every 6 h			29	3	[119]
Cyclophosphamide (Cyclo)	2 mg/kg daily or 10 mg/kg weekly			21	0	[120]
Cytosine arabinoside (ara-C)	10–30 mg/m² daily			98	16	[121]
	150–200 mg/m² daily for 5 days	12	25			[122]
	67 mg/m² every 8 h for 5 days			51	31	[123]
Daunorubicin (DNR)	30–60 mg/m² daily for 3–7 days	35	37	61	34	[124]
AMSA	90 mg/m² daily IV for 7 days				32	[113]
Methyl-GAG	150 mg/m² daily			31	45	[112]
5-Azacytidine	150–400 mg/m² daily for 5 days	11	27	18	16	[109,110]

* CR = complete remission.

DRUG COMBINATIONS

The current strategy for induction treatment in AML is to administer a potent multiple-drug regimen continuously or intermittently long enough to eliminate the leukemic blast cells in the marrow. The most successful regimens reported to date have used combinations of daunorubicin, or of its congener, doxorubicin, and ara-C [121-133], with or without 6-thioguanine. Other less effective combinations include ara-C plus 6-thioguanine [104], ara-C plus cyclophosphamide [123,126,134], and 6-mercaptopurine plus methotrexate [135-137]. Vincristine and prednisone have been added to these regimens by some therapists, although the role of these latter two agents in the treatment of AML is uncertain and regimens without them are as effective as those with them.

The reported remission rates from such combinations have varied from about 25 to 80 percent (Table 28-4). The most successful regimens, capable of producing 60 percent or more complete remissions in large series, cause severe marrow hypoplasia in virtually every pa-tient [104,105,129-133]. Less rigorous schedules and lower doses have not been as effective. For example, combinations of the daunorubicin and ara-C have resulted in higher rates of remission and shorter periods of granulocytopenia as the course of treatment was extended from 4 to 10 days [125,129-131,138-141] (Table 28-5). Thus the highest initial response rate, the lowest mortality, and the longest median survivals have been produced by the intensive use of the most rapidly acting myelotoxic chemicals (Table 28-6). Throughout the treatment, attention must be given to patient support, comparable to that given during the initial 24 h of management and continued for the 4 to 10 or more weeks, in order to avoid fatal infection, bleeding, or organ failure.

REMISSION MAINTENANCE

Remission maintenance has not been as successful in AML as it has been in ALL. Although a few studies have shown no advantage from the administration of drugs during periods of remission in AML [121,142], others

TABLE 28-4   Acute myelogenous leukemia treatment—remission induction with drug combinations

Regimen	Drugs*	Children		Adults		References
		No.	%CR	No.	%CR	
POMP (NCI)*	V, P, MP, MTX	12	75	39	44	[138]
POMP (MDA)	V, P, MP, MTX			51	26	[135]
POMP/PRVD (NCI)	V, P, MP, MTX, ara-C, DNR	24	71	24	38	[136,137]
COAP (SWOG)	V, P, ara-C, cyclo			57	46	[123]
L6 (SKI)	ara-C, TG			88	56	[104]
CALGB	ara-C, TG	47	43	66	36	[139]
Barts/Marsden	DNR 1 day, ara-C 5 days			72	54	[125]
CALGB 7122	DNR 2 days, ara-C 5 days	18	56	74	43	[136]
CALGB 7421	DNR 3 days, ara-C 7 days			44	77	[127]
A-OAP (MDA)	DOX, V, P, ara-C					[126]
University of Washington	V, P, TG, ara-C, DNR			46	70	[128]
7+3 (Pennsylvania)	DOX 3 days, ara-C 7 days			21	67	[130]
950501 (RPMI)	DOX 3 days, ara-C 7 days			21	67	[129]
970701 (RPMI)	DOX 3 days, ara-C 10 days	11	91	46	72	[134,140]
TAD (UCLA)	DNR, ara-C, TG			28	79	[132]
TAD (SKI)	DNR, ara-C, TG				78	[133]

* NCI = National Cancer Institute; MDA = M. D. Anderson Hospital and Tumor Clinic; SWOG = Southwestern Cooperative Group; SKI = Sloan Kettering Institute for Cancer Research; CALGB = Cancer Leukemia Group B; RPMI = Roswell Park Memorial Institute; and UCLA = University of California at Los Angeles.
NOTE: Refer to Tables 28-2 and 28-3 for meanings of abbreviations.

TABLE 28-5   Remission induction for acute myelogenous leukemia—combinations of daunorubicin (DNR) and cytosine arabinoside (ara-C)

Dose and schedule		No. of patients	%CR	Reference
ara-C	DNR			
80 mg/m² daily for 1-4 days	60 mg/m² (one dose)	45	40	[141]
2 mg/kg daily for 1-5 days	1.5 mg/kg (one dose)	72	54	[125]
100 mg/m² daily for 1-5 days	45 mg/m² daily for 2 days	74	43	[139]
100 mg/m² daily for 1-5 days	45 mg/m² daily for 2 days	43	53	[127]
100 mg/m² daily for 1-7 days	45 mg/m² daily for 1-3 days	43	77	[127]
100 mg/m² daily for 1-10 days	DRN 45 mg/m² daily or ADN 30/mg/m² daily for 1-3 days	46	72	[129]

NOTE: See Tables 28-2 and 28-3 for meanings of abbreviations.

have reported longer durations of remissions when maintenance treatment was given [121,123,129,131,142–146] (Table 28-7). It is still unclear, however, whether this represents the effect of patient selection, the form of maintenance therapy given, or the nature and effectiveness of the initial regimen used to induce remission.

The value of immunotherapy during remission is in doubt. Specific active immunotherapy with irradiated leukemic blast cells or nonspecific active immunotherapy with strains of bacillus Calmette-Guérin (BCG), or with methanol-extracted residues of BCG, have been reported to produce an increased duration of remission and survival [145–148]. Subsequent controlled studies have confirmed a slight increase in survival in some instances [149,150] and no improvement in others [131,151].

Many of the uncertainties regarding the value of maintenance chemotherapy in AML reflect a lack of sensitive markers of disease activity. Those which are useful during relapse, such as serum or urine muramidase levels, and morphologic, immunologic, biochemical, and cytogenic markers of leukemic cells disappear and become unusable during complete remission.

MARROW TRANSPLANTATION

Of all recent experimental approaches, marrow stem cell transplantation has proved the most successful, so much so in fact that it has become a treatment of choice in younger patients with closely matched donors. Two transplantation centers have shown convincingly that marrow ablation followed by transplantation of compatible marrow during remission allows excellent anti-

TABLE 28-6   Acute myelogenous leukemia—reported survivals

Treatment	No. of Patients	Median survival, months	At 1 year, %	At 2 years, %	Reference
POMP	39	6.5	40	20	[142]
POMP	51	7	30	18	[135]
DNR, V, P, ara-C, TG	31	8			[128]
P, ara-C, C, V, BCNU	29	8.5	45	28+	[144]
Methyl-GAG	31	9			[112]
7122A	31	10	48	26	[105]
L6	88	11	47	28	[104]
950501/970701	67	11	45	35	*
TAD					[132]

*Unpublished observations, H. D. Preisler et al., Roswell Park Memorial Institute, 1981.
NOTE: See Tables 28-1 through 28-3 for abbreviations.

TABLE 28-7   Acute myelogenous leukemia treatment—remission-maintenance regimens

Regimen Induction	Maintenance	No. of patients	Median months of complete remission	Reference
ara-C	ara-C	18	10.7	[125]
ara-C	ara-C	18	2.3–7.5	[121]
ara-C	No treatment	6	1.2	[121]
POMP	POMP	38	7	[142]
ara-C + TG	ara-C, TG, MTX, Cyclo, DNR, BCNU, hydroxyurea	49	10	[143]
ara-C, V, Cyclo	BCNU, Cyclo	13	22	[144]
COAP	COAP (Cyclo, V,	44	10	[123]
	P, ara-C)	32	20	[134]
OAP	OAP (V, P, ara-C)	33	11.5	[143]
OAP	OAP + BCG	20	21	[126]
DOX-OAP	OAP + BCG	44	13	[146]
ara-C + DNR	ara-C + DNR + TG	19	7	
ara-C + DNR	ara-C + DNR + TG + BCG + leukemic cells	23	11	
ara-C + TG ± DNR	MTX ± (Cyclo + V),	26	7.5	[151]
	MTX + BCG ± (Cyclo + V)	22	11	
ara-C + DNR	ara-C + TG, ara-C + DNR, ara-C + Cyclo	10	5	[147]
ara-C + DNR	ara-C + TG, ara-C + DNR, ara-C + Cyclo, + VCNase-treated leukemic cells	7	16+	*
ara-C + DOX	ara-C + DOX, ara-C + Cyclo, ara-C + TG, MeGAG ± VCNase-treated leukemic cells	63	15	*

*Unpublished observations, H. D. Preisler et al., Roswell Park Memorial Institute, 1981.
NOTE: BCNU = bis-β-chloroethyl nitrosourea; see Tables 20-2 and 20-3 for meanings of other abbreviations.

tumor effects and decreases graft-versus-host reactions and peritransplant infection [152,153]. Results of grafts achieved during the first remission are superior to those observed during a second remission, presumably because antileukemic effects of drugs and irradiation are superior during the initial period [152,154]. However, marrow grafting is difficult in older patients, and most long-term survivors have been under 40 years of age at the time of engraftment (Table 28-8).

All the methods of treating AML are based on the concept that leukemia requires the ablation of all pathologic cells for control or cure. The validity of this theory, proposed by Ehrlich early in the twentieth century [155], has been challenged by observations of human leukemic cell differentiation in vivo and in vitro [156–159], by the identification of endogenous stimuli to both normal and leukemia cell replication and maturation [160,161], and by the induction of differentiation and loss of cloning potential in animal cell lines using membrane-active agents [162–164]. Since the primary defect in leukemia is the lack of stem cell maturation, the use of such chemical agents to overcome the block could eliminate the need for cytolytic treatment.

Prognosis

Prior to the introduction of chemotherapy for acute leukemia 35 years ago, the median survival of patients with AML was about 3 months [165,166]. The 5-year survival of adults treated in the 1950s and 1960s was only 2 percent. Despite occasional successes, the overall outlook changed very little until the 1970s. Now, drug combinations are capable of inducing a complete remission in the majority of patients with AML. Median survival times have increased to over 1 year [105,126,129–131,142] (Table 28-6), and 20 percent of patients are living 5 years or longer after diagnosis. Morphologic and immunologic features of AML cells appear to have little effect on survival if proper treatment and support are available. As with other acute leukemias, patients without gross cytogenetic alterations respond better than those with karyotype abnormalities [45,167]. The outlook is least favorable for individuals less than 1 year or more than 60 years of age, for patients with serious concomitant hematologic or metabolic disorders [142,168–174], and for patients who have developed AML after receiving cytotoxic drug or radiation therapy for other neoplasms [174]. Thus, despite the impressive advances in therapy during the last few years, AML remains a fatal disease for most patients.

References

1. Fialkow, P. J., et al.: Acute non-lymphocytic leukemia: Heterogeneity of stem cell origin. Blood 57:1068, 1981.
2. Third Cancer Survey: Incidence Data, edited by S. J. Cutler and J. L. Young, Jr. National Cancer Institute Monograph 41, Washington, D.C., 1975.
3. Hayhoe, F. G. J.: Clinical and cytological recognition and differentiation of the leukemias, in Proceedings of the International Conference on Leukemia-Lymphoma, edited by C. J. D. Zarafonetis. Lea & Febiger, Philadelphia, 1968, p. 307.
4. Fraumeni, J. A., Jr., and Miller, R. W.: Epidemiology of human leukemia: Recent observations. J. Natl. Cancer Inst. 38:593, 1967.
5. Goodall, P. T., and Vosti, K. L.: Fever in acute myelogenous leukemia. Arch. Intern. Med. 135:1197, 1975.
6. Burke, P. J., Braine, H. G., Rathbun, H. K., and Owens, A. H.: The clinical significance and management of fever in acute myelocytic leukemia. Johns Hopkins Med. J. 139:1, 1976.
7. Hanker, J. S., et al.: The light microscopic demonstration of hydroxyperoxide-positive phi bodies and rods in leukocytes in acute myeloid leukemia. Histochem. J. 58:241, 1978.
8. Hanker, J. S., et al.: Facilitated light microscopic cytochemical diagnosis of acute myelogenous leukemia. Cancer Res. 39:1635, 1979.
9. O'Regan, S., et al.: Electrolytes and acid-base disturbances in the management of leukemia. Blood 49:345, 1977.
10. di Guglielmo, G.: Uno Caso di eritroleucemia. Folia Med. 13:386, 1917.
11. Eastman, P., Wallerstein, R. O., and Schrier, S. L.; Conversion of polycythemia vera to chronic di Guglielmo's syndrome. JAMA 204:1141, 1968.
12. Carmel, R., Coltman, C. A., Yatteau, R. F., and Costanzi, J. J.: Association of paroxysmal nocturnal hemoglobinuria with erythroleukemia. N. Engl. J. Med. 283:1329, 1970.
13. Shaw, M. T., Bottomley, S. S., Bottomley, R. H., and Hussein, K. K.: The relationship of erythromonocytic leukemia to other myeloproliferative disorders. Am. J. Med. 55:542, 1973.
14. Sheets, R. F., Drevets, C. C., and Hamilton, H. C.: Erythroleukemia (di Guglielmo's syndrome). Arch. Intern. Med. 111:77, 1963.
15. Scott, R. B., Ellison, R. R., and Ley, A. B.: A clinical study of twenty cases of erythroleukemia (di Guglielmo's syndrome). Am. J. Med. 37:162, 1964.
16. Hetzel, P., and Gee, T. S.: A new observation in the clinical spectrums of erythroleukemia. Am. J. Med. 64:765, 1978.
17. Eastman, P. M., Schwartz, R., and Schrier, S. L.: Distinction beteen ineffective erythropoiesis and di Guglielmo's disease: Clinical and biochemical differences. Blood 40:487, 1972.
18. Crossen, P. E., Fitzgerald, P. H., Menzies, R. C., and Brehaut, L. A.: Chromosomal abnormality, megaloblastosis, and arrested DNA syntheses in erythroleukemia. J. Med. Genet. 6:95, 1969.
19. Gabuzda, T. G., Shute, H. E., and Erslev, A. J.: Regulation of erythropoisis in erythroleukemia. Arch. Intern. Med. 123:60, 1969.
20. Adamson, J. W., and Finch, C. A.: Erythropoietin and the regula-

TABLE 28-8   Results of allogenic marrow transplantations

Institution	Time of transplant	Percent long-term unmaintained remission	References
Seattle	First remission	60	[152,154]
	First relapse	17	
	Second remission	14	
City of Hope	Remission	70	[153]
	Relapse	<10	
	Partial remission	55	

tion of erythropoiesis in di Guglielmo's syndrome. *Blood* 36:590, 1970.

21. Sandberg, A. A.: *The Chromosomes in Human Cancer and Leukemia.* Elsevier, New York, 1980.

22. Heath, C. W., Bennett, J. M., Whang-Peng, J., Berry, E. W., and Wiernick, P.: Cytogenic findings in erythroleukemia. *Blood* 33:453, 1969.

23. Williams, D. M., Scott, C. D., and Beck, T. M.: Premature chromosome condensation in human leukemia. *Blood* 47:687, 1976.

24. Sakurai, M., and Sandberg, A. A.: Chromosomes and causation of human cancer and leukemia. XIII. An evaluation of karyotypic findings in erythroleukemia. *Cancer* 37:790, 1976.

25. Finkel, H. E., Brauer, M. J., Taub, R. N., and Dameshek, W.: Immunologic aberrations in the Di Guglielmo syndrome. *Blood* 28:634, 1966.

26. Hillstad, L. K.: Acute promyelocytic leukemia. *Acta Med. Scand.* 159:189, 1957.

27. Didisheim, P., Trombold, J. S., Vandervoort, R. L. E., and Mibashan, R. S.: Acute promyelocytic leukemia with fibrinogen and factor V deficiencies. *Blood* 23:717, 1964.

28. Baker, W. G., et al.: Hypofibrinogenemic hemorrhage in acute myelogenous leukemia treated with heparin. *Ann. Intern. Med.* 61:116, 1964.

29. Pittman, G. R., Senshauser, D. A., and Lowney, J. F.: Acute promyelocytic leukemia. *Am. J. Clin. Pathol.* 46:214, 1966.

30. Cooperberg, A. A.: Acute promyelocytic leukemia. *Can. Med. Assoc. J.* 97:57, 1967.

31. Gralnick, H. R., and Abrell, E.: Studies of the procoagulant and fibrinolytic activity of promyelocytes in acute promyelocytic leukemia. *Br. J. Haematol.* 24:89, 1973.

32. Bernard, J., Weil, M., Boiron, M., Jacquillat, C., Flandria, G., and Gemon, M. F.: Acute promyelocytic leukemia: Results of treatment by daunorubicin. *Blood* 41:489, 1973.

33. Stavem, P.: Hypergranular acute promyelocytic leukemia with intravascular coagulation. *Scand. J. Haematol.* 11:249, 1973.

34. Sultan, C., Heilmann-Gouault, M., and Tulliez, M.: Relationship between blast-cell morphology and occurrence of a syndrome of disseminated intravascular coagulation. *Br. J. Haematol.* 24:255, 1973.

35. Breton-Gorius, J., and Houssay, D.: Auer bodies in acute promyelocytic leukemia: Demonstration of their fine structure and peroxidase localization. *Lab. Invest.* 28:135, 1973.

36. Gralnick, H. R., and Tan, H. K.: Acute promyelocytic leukemia. *Hum. Pathol.* 5:661, 1974.

37. Gralnick, H. R., and Sultan, C.: Acute promyelocytic leukaemia: Hemorrhagic manifestation and morphologic criteria. *Br. J. Haematol.* 29:373, 1975.

38. Collins, A. J., et al.: Acute promyelocytic leukemia. *Arch. Intern. Med.* 138:1677, 1978.

39. Groopman, J., and Ellman, L.: Acute promyelocytic leukemia. *Am. J. Hematol.* 7:395, 1979.

40. Daly, P. A., Schiffer, C. A., and Wiernik, P. H.: Acute promyelocytic leukemia. Clinical management of 15 patients. *Am. J. Hematol.* 8:347, 1980.

41. Rowley, J. D., Golomb, H. M., and Dougherty, C.: 15/17 translocation, a consistent chromosomal change in acute promyelocytic leukemia. *Lancet* 1:549, 1977.

42. Scheres, J. M. J. C., Hustinx, T. W. J., de Vaan, G. A. M., and Rutten, F. J.: 15/17 translocation in acute promyelocytic leukemia. *Hum. Genet.* 43:115, 1978.

43. Testa, J. R., et al.: Hypergranular promyelocytic leukemia (APL): Cytogenetic and ultrastructural specificity. *Blood* 52:272, 1978.

44. Teerenhovi, L., et al.: Uneven geographical distribution of 15:17 translocation in acute promyelocytic leukemia. *Lancet* 2:797, 1978.

45. Rowley, J. D.: Chromosome abnormalities in human leukemia. *Ann. Rev. Genet.* 14:17, 1980.

46. Golomb, H. M., Rowley, J. D., Vardiman, J. W., Testa, J. R., and Butler, A.: "Microgranular" acute promyelocytic leukemia: A distinct clinical, ultrastructural, and cytogenetic entity. *Blood* 55:253, 1980.

47. Drapkin, R. L., et al.: Prophylactic heparin therapy in acute promyelocytic leukemia. *Cancer* 41:2484, 1978.

48. Freeman, A. I., and Journey, L. J.: Ultrastructural studies on monocytic leukemia. *Br. J. Haematol.* 20:225, 1971.

49. Shaw, M. T.: The distinctive features of acute monocytic leukemia. *Am. J. Hematol.* 4:97, 1978.

50. Straus, D. J.: The acute monocytic leukemias. *Medicine (Baltimore)* 59:409, 1980.

51. Lichtman, M. A., and Weed, R. I.: Peripheral cytoplasmic characteristics of leukocytes in monocytic leukemia: Relationship to clinical manifestations. *Blood* 40:52, 1972.

52. Ohta, H., and Nagose, H.: Serial estimation of serum, urine and leukocyte muramidase (lysozyme) in monocytic leukemia. *Acta Haematol.* 46:257, 1971.

53. McKenna, R. W., Bloomfield, C. D., Dick, F., Nesbit, M. E., and Brunning, R. D.: Acute monoblastic leukemia: Diagnosis and treatment of ten cases. *Blood* 46:481, 1975.

54. Baker, M. A., Falk, R. E., and Greaves, M. R.: Detection of monocytic specific antigen on human acute leukaemia cells. *Br. J. Haematol.* 32:13, 1976.

55. Brynes, R. K., et al.: Acute monocytic leukemia. *Am. J. Clin. Pathol.* 65:471, 1976.

56. Koziner, B., et al.: Cell markers in acute monocytic leukemia. *Blood* 49:895, 1977.

57. Shaw, M. T., and Nordquist, R. E.: "Pure" monocytic or histiomonocytic leukemia: A revised concept. *Cancer* 35:208, 1975.

58. McKenna, R., Bloomfield, C. D., Nesbit, M., and Brunning, R. S.: Nonspecific esterase positive acute leukemia: A distinctive cytologic and clinical entity. *Proc. Amer. Assoc. Canc. Res./Amer. Soc. Clin. Oncol.* 11:61, 1975.

59. Cuttner, J., et al.: Association of monocytic leukemia in patients with extreme leukocytosis. *Am. J. Med.* 69:555, 1980.

60. Meyer, R. J., et al.: Central nervous system involvement at presentation in acute granulocytic leukemia: A prospective cytocentrifuge study. *Am. J. Med.* 68:691, 1980.

61. McDonald, J. B., and Hamrick, J. G.: Acute megakaryocytic leukemia. *Arch. Intern. Med.* 81:73, 1948.

62. Allegra, S. R., and Broderick, P. A.: Acute aleukemic megakaryocytic leukemia: Report of a case. *Am. J. Clin. Pathol.* 55:197, 1971.

63. Breton-Gorius, J., Reyes, F., Duhamel, G., Majman, A., and Gorin, N. C.: Megakaryoblastic acute leukemia: Identification by the ultrastructural demonstration of platelet peroxidase. *Blood* 51:45, 1978.

64. DenOttolander, G. J., et al.: Megakaryoblastic leukemia (acute myelofibrosis): A report of three cases. *Br. J. Haematol.* 42:9, 1979.

65. Habib, A., Lee, H., and Chan, M.: Acute myelogenous leukemia with megakaryocytic myelosis. *Am. J. Clin. Pathol.* 74:705, 1980.

66. Lewis, S. M., and Szur, L.: Malignant myelosclerosis. *Br. Med. J.* 2:472, 1963.

67. Bergsman, K. L., and Van Slyck, E. J.: Acute myelofibrosis. *Ann. Intern. Med.* 74:232, 1971.

68. Breton-Gorius, J., Daniel, M. T., Flandrin, G., Kinet-Deuoel, C.: Fine structure and peroxidase activity of circulating micromegakaryoblasts and platelets in a case of acute myelofibrosis. *Br. J. Haematol.* 25:331, 1973.

69. Hossfield, D. K., Tormey, D., and Ellison, R. R.: Ph¹-positive megakaryoblastic leukemia. *Cancer* 36:576, 1975.

70. Bain, B., et al.: Megakaryoblastic transformation of chronic granulocytic leukemia. *J. Clin. Pathol.* 30:235, 1977.

71. Evans, T. S., and Nesbit, R. R.: Eosinophilic leukemia. *Blood* 4:603, 1949.

72. Fadell, E. J., Crone, R. I., Leonard, M. E., and Altamarino, M. D.: Eosinophilic leukemia. *Arch. Intern. Med.* 99:819, 1957.

73. Chen, H. P., and Smith, H. S.: Eosinophilic leukemia. *Ann. Intern. Med.* 52:1343, 1960.

74. Bentley, H. P., Reandon, A. E., Knoedler, J. P., and Krivit, W.: Eosinophilic leukemia, report of a case, with review and classification. *Am. J. Med.* 30:310, 1961.

75. Benvenisti, D. S., and Ultmann, J. E.: Eosinophilic leukemia. *Ann. Intern. Med.* 71:731, 1969.

76. Gruenwald, H., Krossoglou, K. A., Mitus, W. J., and Damashek, W.: Philadelphia chromosome in eosinophilic leukemia. *Am. J. Med.* 39:1003, 1965.

77. Roberts, W. C., Liegler, D. G., and Carbone, P. P.: Endomyocardial disease and eosinophilia. *Am. J. Med.* 46:28, 1969.

78. Flannery, E. P., et al.: Eosinophilic leukemia with fibrosing endocarditis and short Y chromosome. *Ann. Intern. Med.* 77:223, 1972.

79. Yam, L. T., Li, C. Y., Necheles, T. F., and Katayama, I.: Pseudoeosinophilia, eosinophilic endocarditis, and eosinophilic leukemia. *Am. J. Med.* 53:193, 1972.

80. Goh, K., Swisher, S. N., and Rosenberg, C. A.: Cytogenic studies in eosinophilic leukemia. *Ann. Intern. Med.* 62:80, 1965.

81. Karle, H., and Videback, A.: Eosinophilic leukemia or a collagen disease with eosinophilia. *Dan. Med. Bull.* 13:41, 1966.

82. Chusid, M. J., Dale, D. C., Wolff, S. M., and West, B. C.: The hypereosinophilic syndrome: Analyses of fourteen cases with review of the literature. *Medicine (Baltimore)* 54:1, 1975.

83. Catovsky, D., et al.: The association of eosinophilia with lymphoblastic leukemia or lymphoma: A study of seven patients. *Br. J. Haematol.* 45:523, 1980.

84. Dale, D. C., and Chusid, M. J.: Eosinophilic leukemia. Remission with vincristine and hydroxyurea. *Am. J. Med.* 59:297, 1975.

85. Lennert, K., Köster, E., and Martin, H.: Über die mastzellenleukaemic. *Acta Haematol.* 16:255, 1956.

86. Kyle, R. A., and Pease, G. L.: Basophilic leukemia. *Arch. Intern. Med.* 118:205, 1966.

87. Schubert, J. F. C., and Martin, H.: Observations on 7 patients with "blood mast cell leukemia." *Klin. Wochenschr.* 46:929, 1968.

88. Quattrin, N.: Leucémies aiguës à basophiles. *Nouv. Rev. Fr. Hematol.* 13:745, 1973.

89. Cecio, A., Dini, E., and Quattrin, N.: Preliminary observations with the electron microscope of two cases of acute basophilic leukemia. *Boll. Soc. Ital. Biol. Sper.* 46:459, 1970.

90. Goh, K.-O., and Anderson, F. W.: Cytogenetic studies in basophilic chronic myelocytic leukemia. *Arch. Pathol. Lab. Med.* 103:288, 1979.

91. Reingold, J. J., Kaufman, R., Adelson, E., and Lear, A.: Smoldering acute leukemia. *N. Engl. J. Med.* 268:812, 1963.

92. Knospe, W. H., et al.: Smoldering acute leukemia. *Arch. Intern. Med.* 127:910, 1971.

93. Schunk, G. J., and Lehman, W. L.: Mongolism and congenital leukemia. *JAMA* 155:250, 1954.

94. Krivit, W., and Good, R. A.: Simultaneous occurrence of mongolism and leukemia: Report of a nationwide survey. *Am. J. Dis. Child.* 94:289, 1957.

95. Rosner, F., and Lee, S.: Down's syndrome and acute leukemia: Myeloblastic or lymphoblastic. *Am. J. Med.* 53:203, 1972.

96. Reimann, D. L., Clemens, R. L., and Pillsbury, W. A.: Congenital acute leukemia: Skin nodules, a first sign. *J. Pediatr.* 46:415, 1955.

97. Van Eys, J., and Flexner, J. M.: Transient spontaneous remission in a case of untreated congenital leukemia. *Am. J. Dis. Child.* 118:507, 1969.

98. Ross, J. D., Moloney, W. C., and Desforges, J. F.: Ineffective regulation of granulopoiesis masquerading as congenital leukemia in a mongoloid child. *J. Pediatr.* 63:1, 1963.

99. Weinstein, H. J.: Congenital leukemia and the neonatal myeloproliferative disorders associated with Down's syndrome. *Clin. Hematol.* 7:147, 1978.

100. Bull, J. M., Duttera, M. J., Northrup, J. D., Henderson, E. S., Stachick, E. D., and Carbone, P. P.: Serial in vitro bone marrow culture in acute myelocytic leukemia. *Blood* 42:679, 1973.

101. Graham, F. L., and Whitmore, G. F.: Studies in mouse L-cells on the incorporation of β-arabinofuranosylcytosine into DNA and on inhibition of DNA polymerase by β-arabinofuranosylcytosine-5'-triphosphate. *Cancer Res.* 30:2636, 1970.

102. Edelstein, M., Vietti, T., and Valoriote, F.: Schedule-dependent syngergism for the combination of β-arabinofuranosylcytosine and daunorubicin. *Cancer Res.* 34:293, 1974.

103. Skipper, H. E., Schabel, F. M., Jr., and Wilcox, W. S.: Experimental evaluation of potential anticancer agents. XXI. Scheduling of arabinosylcytosine to the advantage of its S-phase specificity against leukemia cells. *Cancer Treat. Rep.* 51:125, 1967.

104. Clarkson, B. D.: Acute myelocytic leukemia in adults. *Cancer* 30:1572, 1972.

105. Yates, J. W., Wallace, H. J., Ellison, R. R., and Holland, J. F.: Cytosine arabinoside and daunomycin therapy in nonlymphocytic leukemia. *Cancer Treat. Rep.* 57:485, 1973.

106. Tattersall, M. H., Ganeshaguru, K., and Hoffbrand, A. V.: Mechanisms of resistance of human acute leukemia cells to cytosine arabinoside. *Br. J. Haematol.* 27:39, 1974.

107. Rustum, Y. M., and Preisler, H. D.: Correlation between leukemic cell retention of β-arabinosylcytosine-5-triphosphate and response to therapy. *Cancer Res.* 39:42, 1979.

108. Bernard, J., Jacquillat, C., and Weil, M.: Treatment of the acute leukemias. *Semin. Hematol.* 9:181, 1972.

109. Karon, M., Sieger, L., Leimbroch, S., Finklestein, J. Z., Nesbit, M. E., and Swaney, J. J.: 5-Azacytidine: A new agent active for the treatment of acute leukemia. *Blood* 42:359, 1973.

110. McCredie, K. B., Bodey, G. P., and Burgess, M. A.: Treatment of acute leukemia with 5-azacytidine (NSC-102816). *Cancer Treat. Rep.* 57:319, 1973.

111. Presant, C. A., Vietti, T., and Valeriote, F.: Kinetics of both leukemic and normal cell population reduction following azacytidine. *Cancer Res.* 35:1926, 1975.

112. Levin, R. H., Henderson, E. S., Karon, M., and Freireich, E. J.: Treatment of acute leukemia with methylglyoxal-bis-guanylhydrazone (methyl-GAG). *Clin. Pharmacol. Ther.* 6:31, 1965.

113. Legha, S. S., Keatin, M. J., Zander, A. R.: 4'-(9-Aridinylamino)-methansulfon-M-aniside (AMSA): A new drug effective in the treatment of adult acute leukemia. *Ann. Intern. Med.* 93:17, 1980.

114. Karon, M., et al.: The role of vincristine in the treatment of childhood acute leukemia. *Clin. Pharmacol. Ther.* 7:332, 1966.

115. Cline, M. J., and Rosenbaum, E.: Prediction of in vivo cytotoxicity of chemotherapeutic agents by their in vitro effect on leukocytes from patients with acute leukemia. *Cancer Res.* 28:2516, 1968.

116. Wolff, J. A., Brubaker, C. A., and Murphy, M. L.: Prednisone therapy of acute childhood leukemia: Prognosis and response in 330 treated patients. *J. Pediatr.* 70:626, 1967.

117. Working Party on the Evaluation of Different Methods of Therapy in Leukaemia: Treatment of acute leukaemia in adults: Comparison of steroid and mercaptopurine therapy alone and in conjunction. *Br. Med. J.* 1:1383, 1966.

118. Frei, E., III, et al.: The effectiveness of anti-leukemic agents in inducing and maintaining remission in children with acute leukemia. *Blood* 26:642, 1965.

119. Vogler, W. R., Huguley, C. M., Jr., and Rundles, R. W.: Comparison of methotrexate with 6-mercaptopurine prednisone in treatment of acute leukemia in adults. *Cancer* 20:1221, 1967

120. Hoogstraten, B.: Cyclophosphamide (Cytoxan) in acute leukemia. *Cancer Treat. Rep.* 16:167, 1962.

121. Ellison, R. R., et al.: Arabinosyl cytosine: A useful agent in the treatment of acute leukemia in adults. *Blood* 32:507, 1968.

122. Wang, J. J., Selawry, O. S., Vietti, T. J., and Bodey, G. P.: Prolonged infusion of arabinosyl cytosine in childhood leukemia. *Cancer* 25:1, 1970.

123. Bodey, G. P., et al.: Chemotherapy of acute leukemia: Comparison of cytarabine alone and in combination with vincristine, prednisone, and cyclophosphamide. *Arch. Intern. Med.* 133:260, 1974.

124. Weil, M., Glidewell, O., and Jacquillat, C.: Daunorubicin in the therapy of acute granulocytic leukemia. *Cancer Res.* 33:921, 1973.

125. Crowther, D., et al.: Management of adult acute myelogenous leukemia. *Br. Med. J.* 1:131, 1973.

126. McCredie, K. B., Bodey, G. P., Freireich, E. J., Hester, J. P., Rodriguez, V., and Keating, M. J.: Chemoimmunotherapy of adult acute leukemia. *Cancer* 47:1256, 1981.

127. Rai, K. R., Holland, J. F., and Glidewell, O.: Improvement in remission induction therapy of acute myelocytic leukemia. *Proc. Amer. Assoc. Canc. Res./Amer. Soc. Clin. Oncol.* 16:265, 1975.

128. Glucksberg, H., et al.: Combination chemotherapy for acute nonlymphoblastic leukemia in adults. *Cancer Treat. Rep.* 59:1131, 1975.

129. Preisler, H. D., et al.: Treatment of acute nonlymphocytic leukemia: Use of anthracycline-cytosine arabinoside induction therapy and a comparison of two maintenance regimens. *Blood* 53:455, 1979.

130. Cassileth, P. A., and Katz, M. E.: Chemotherapy for adult acute nonlymphocytic leukemia with daunorubicin and cytosine arabinoside. *Cancer Treat. Rep.* 61:1441, 1977.

131. Preisler, H. D., Bjornsson, S., Henderson, E. S., Hryniak, W., and Higby, D. J.: Remission induction in acute nonlymphocytic leuke-

mia: Comparison of a 7-day and a 10-day infusion of cytosine arabinoside in combination with Adriamycin. *Med. Pediatr. Oncol. 7:269, 1979.*

132. Gale, R. R., and Cline, M. J.: High remission induction rate in acute myeloid leukemia. *Lancet 1:497, 1977.*

133. Arlin, Z., Gee, T., Fried, J., Koenigsberg, E., Wolmark, N., and Clarkson, B.: Rapid induction of remission in acute nonlymphocytic leukemia. *Proc. Amer. Assoc. Canc. Res./Amer. Soc. Clin. Oncol. 20:112, 1979 (abstract 239).*

134. Whitecar, J. R., Jr., Bodey, G. P., Freireich, E. J., McCredie, K. B., and Hart, J. S.: Cyclophosphamide, vincristine, arabinosyl cytosine and prednisone (COAP): Combination chemotherapy for adult acute leukemia. *Cancer Treat. Rep. 56:543, 1972.*

135. Rodriguez, V., Hart, J. S., Freireich, E. J.: POMP combination, chemotherapy of adult acute leukemia. *Cancer 32:69, 1973.*

136. Pizzo, P. A., Henderson, E. S., and Leventhal, B. G.: Acute myelogenous leukemia in children: A preliminary report of combination chemotherapy. *J. Pediatr. 88:125, 1976.*

137. Leventhal, B. G., and Henderson, E. S.: Therapy of acute leukemia with drug combinations which include asparaginase. *Cancer 28:825, 1971.*

138. Henderson, E. S.: Treatment of acute leukemia. *Ann. Intern. Med. 69:628, 1968.*

139. Wallace, H. J., et al.: Therapy of acute myelocytic leukemia, acute leukemia group B studies, in *Therapy of Acute Leukemias*, edited by F. Mandelli, S. Amadori, and G. Mariani. Centro Minerva Medica, Rome, 1975, p. 255.

140. Preisler, H. D., Browman, G., and Tebbi, C.: Acute myeloblastic leukemia remission and maintenance therapy in patients thirty years of age and less, in *Major Advances in Prediatric and Adolescent Oncology*. G. K. Hall, Boston, 1982.

141. Palva, I., et al.: Treatment of acute leukemia in adults using the combinations of cyclophosphamide, cytosine arabinoside and prednisone or daunorubicin, cytosine arabinoside and prednisone, in *Therapy of Acute Leukemias*, edited by F. Mandelli, S. Amadori, and G. Mariani. Centro Minerva Medica, Rome, 1975, p. 477.

142. Henderson, E. S.: Clinical course of treated and untreated adult acute leukemia. *Hematol-Bluttransfusion 8:89, 1969.*

143. Clarkson, B. D.: Considerations of cell kinetic principles to strategy of treating leukemia, in *Cancer Chemotherapy: Fundamental Concepts and Recent Advances.* Yearbook, Chicago, 1975, p. 19.

144. Manaster, J.: Remission maintenance of acute nonlymphoblastic leukemia with BCNU (NSC 409962) and cyclophosphamide (NSC-26271). *Cancer Treat. Rep. 59:537, 1975.*

145. Gutterman, J. V., et al.: Chemo-immunotherapy of adult acute leukemia: Prolongation of remission in myeloblastic leukaemia with BCG. *Lancet 2:1405, 1974.*

146. Powles, R. L., et al.: Immunotherapy for acute myelogenous leukemia. *Br. J. Cancer 28:365, 1973.*

147. Bekesi, J. G., Holland, J. F., Yates, J. W., Henderson, E. S., and Fleminger, R.: Chemotherapy of acute myelocytic leukemia with neuraminidase treated allogeneic leukemic cells. *Proc. Amer. Assoc. Canc. Res./Amer. Soc. Clin. Oncol. 16:121, 1975.*

148. Weiss, D. W., Stupp, Y., Many, N., and Izak, G.: Treatment of acute myelocytic leukemia (AML) patients with the MER tubercle bacillus fraction: A preliminary report. *Transplant. Proc. 7(Suppl. 1):545, 1975.*

149. Lindemalm, C. S. N., et al.: Adjuvant immunotherapy in acute nonlymphocytic leukaemia. *Cancer Immunol. Immunother. 4:179, 1978.*

150. Harris, R., et al.: Active immunotherapy and the induction of second and subsequent remissions. *Br. J. Cancer 37:282, 1978.*

151. Vogler, W. R., et al.: A randomized clinical trial of C. G. in myeloblastic leukemia, in *Immunotherapy of Cancer: Present Status*

of Trials in Man, edited by T. W. Windhorst. Raven Press, New York, 1978, p. 365.

152. Thomas, E. D., et al.: Marrow transplantation for acute nonlymphoblastic leukemia in first remission. *N. Engl. J. Med. 301:597, 1979.*

153. Blume, K. G., et al.: Bone marrow ablation and allogeneic marrow transplantation in acute leukemia. Clinical candidacy and outcome. *N. Engl. J. Med. 302:1041, 1980.*

154. Thomas, E. D., et al.: One hundred patients with acute leukemia treated by chemotherapy, total body irradiation, and allogeneic marrow transplantation. *Blood 49:511, 1977.*

155. Ehrlich, P.: Principles of cancer chemotherapy, in *The Collected Papers of Paul Ehrlich*, edited by F. Himmelweit. Pergamon, New York, 1980, vol. 3, p. 505.

156. Metcalf, D.: The nature of leukaemia: Neoplasm or disorder of haemopoietic regulation? *Med. J. Aust. 2:739, 1971.*

157. Leder, L. D.: A case of acute leukemia with pseudo-Pelger cells containing Auer bodies. *Acta Haematol. (Basel) 42:58, 1969.*

158. Davies, A. R., and Schmitt, R. G.: Auer bodies in mature neutrophils. *JAMA 203:895, 1968.*

159. Catovsky, D., Galton, D. A. G., and Robinson, J.: Myeloperoxidase deficient neutrophils in acute myeloid leukemias. *Scand. J. Haematol. 9:142, 1972.*

160. Messner, H. A., Till, J. E., and McCulloch, E. A.: Interacting cell populations affecting granulopoietic colony formation by normal and leukemic human marrow cells. *Blood 44:671, 1974.*

161. Moore, M. A. S., Williams, N., and Metcalf, D.: In vitro colony formation by normal and leukemic human hematopoietic cells: Interaction between colony forming and colony stimulating cells. *J. Natl. Cancer Inst. 50:591, 1973.*

162. Friend, C., Preisler, H. D., and Scher, W. S.: Studies on the control of differentiation of murine virus-induced erythroleukemic cells. *Curr. Top. Dev. Biol. 8:81, 1974.*

163. Preisler, H. D., and Lyman, G.: Differentiation of erythroleukemia cells in vitro: Properties of chemical inducers. *Cell Diff. 4:179, 1975.*

164. Lotem, J., and Sachs, L.: Control of normal differentiation of myeloid leukemic cells. VI. Inhibition of cell multiplication and the formation of macrophages. *J. Cell. Physiol. 85:587, 1975.*

165. Tivey, H.: The natural history of untreated acute leukemia. *Ann. N.Y. Acad. Sci. 60:322, 1954.*

166. Bierman, H. R., Cohen, P., McClelland, J. N., and Shimkin, M. B.: The effect of transfusion and antibiotics upon the duration of life in children with lymphogenous leukemia. *J. Pediatr. 37:455, 1950.*

167. Sakurai, M., and Sandberg, A. A.: Chromosomes and causation of human cancer and leukemia. II. Prognostic and therapeutic value of chromosomal findings in acute myeloblastic leukemia. *Cancer 33:1548, 1974.*

168. Boggs, D. R., Wintrobe, M. M., and Cartwright, G. E.: The acute leukemias: Analysis of 322 cases and review of the literature. *Medicine (Baltimore) 41:163, 1962.*

169. Wiernik, P. N., and Serpick, A. A.: Factors affecting remission and survival in adult acute nonlymphocytic leukemia (ANLL). *Medicine (Baltimore) 49:505, 1970.*

170. Beard, M. E. J., and Fairley, G. H.: Acute leukemias in adults. *Semin. Hematol. 11:5, 1974.*

171. Bernard, J., Weil, M., and Jacquillat, C.: Prognostic factors in human acute leukemias. *Adv. Biosci. 14:97, 1975.*

172. Henderson, E. S., et al.: Factors influencing prognosis in adult myelocytic leukemia. *Adv. Biosci. 14:72, 1975.*

173. Keating, M. J., et al.: Factors related to length of complete remission in adult acute leukemia. *Cancer 45:2017, 1980.*

174. Preisler, H. D., and Lyman, G. H.: Acute myelocytic leukemia subsequent to therapy for a different neoplasm. Clinical features and response to therapy. *Am. J. Hematol. 3:209, 1977.*

PART FOUR   *The erythrocyte*

Morphology of the erythron

CHAPTER 29

Morphology of the erythron

MARCEL BESSIS
LAWRENCE S. LESSIN
ERNEST BEUTLER

Morphology of erythropoiesis in adult man

The total mass of erythropoietic cells and circulating erythrocytes may be viewed as a functional, though dispersed, organ and has been termed the *erythron* (Fig. 29-1). The successive morphologic alterations observed through the developmental spectrum from proerythroblast to erythrocyte reflect the functional specialization of these cells and their maturation. The production of hemoglobin and enzymes requires (1) nuclear synthesis of coded messenger RNA, which passes through nuclear pores into the erythroblast cytoplasm; (2) the nucleolar production of ribosomes, which similarly pass to cytoplasm and organize along strands of messenger RNA into polyribosomes, the functional units of protein synthesis; and (3) the formation and later loss of mitochondria, which are required in immature forms to provide high-energy phosphates for amino acid activation and binding to transfer RNA and to serve as the site for the enzymatic synthesis of heme. The Golgi apparatus, where sugars are presumably added in the synthesis of glycoproteins, is progressively reduced with cellular maturation. Erythroblast maturation, which permits the potential development of 16 mature erythrocytes from a single proerythroblast via four mitotic divisions in a 72-h period, is reflected in its nuclear morphology (Fig. 29-1).

The maturing erythroblast rids itself in an extremely efficient manner of organelles not essential to specific tasks in the production of the erythrocyte. Any alteration in the synchronized sequence of maturation and amplification—as imposed by a deficiency or metabolic inhibition of the utilization of iron, folic acid, vitamin B_6 or B_{12}; by defective globin synthesis in thalassemia; or by defective heme synthesis in lead toxicity—gives rise to a defective erythrocyte with morphologic expression of its biochemical errors. It may also result in morphologic evidence of metabolic dyssynchronism in the developing erythroblast, such as defective hemoglobinization, megablastosis, maturation arrest, or iron-laden mitochondria.

THE ERYTHROBLASTIC ISLAND (Fig. 29-2)

The anatomic unit of erythropoiesis in the normal adult is the *erythroblastic island* [1]. It consists of one or two centrally located macrophages, surrounded by erythroblasts of all stages of maturation which remain in contact with the body of the macrophage or its long cytoplasmic extensions throughout development. Phase-contrast microscopic observations and microcinematography reveal that the macrophage is not passive or sessile but is in a dynamic state. Its pseudopodium-like cytoplasmic extensions move rapidly among the surrounding wreath of erythroblasts, producing intimate but fleeting intercellular contact [1] (Fig. 29-2). When viewed three-dimensionally with the scanning electron microscope, the erythroblastic island is a spongelike structure in which erythroblasts lie in surface invaginations of the macrophage. As the erythroblast matures, it moves away from the main body of the macrophage, leaving in its wake a developing series of red cell precursors, from proerythroblast to orthochromatic erythroblast, along the cytoplasmic extension [2]. When sufficiently mature for nuclear expulsion, the erythroblast detaches from the cytoplasmic extension of the macrophage, makes contact with the antisinusoidal aspect of the endothelial cell, and traverses this cell or passes between two cells, usually leaving its nucleus behind to be phagocytosed and destroyed by the macrophage. Thus, via diapedesis from erythroblastic island into the marrow sinus, the reticulocyte is born.

While retaining its close association with the macrophage for a mean period of 72 h, the erythroblast undergoes four mitotic divisions and synthesizes 80 percent of the total hemoglobin of the mature erythrocyte. It is probable that this relationship is a functional one: the macrophages play an active role in the microenvironment of the maturing erythroblast and supply it with undefined nutrient substances [1]. An activity which promotes growth of erythroid cells in culture has been isolated from media "conditioned" by macrophages. Electron microscopic studies reveal that small droplets of fluid are internalized by the developing erythroid cells, particularly when they are in contact with the macrophage. This process has been termed *rhopheocytosis*. Molecules of ferritin can be seen in these vacuoles, and they may well contain other substances which are of importance to the developing erythroblast. It has been suggested that such factors decrease the requirement for erythropoietin in culture [3].

The erythroblastic island is, however, a fragile structure which is usually disrupted by the negative pressure employed in obtaining a marrow specimen by needle aspiration (Fig. 29-2*a*). Remnant groups of erythroblasts

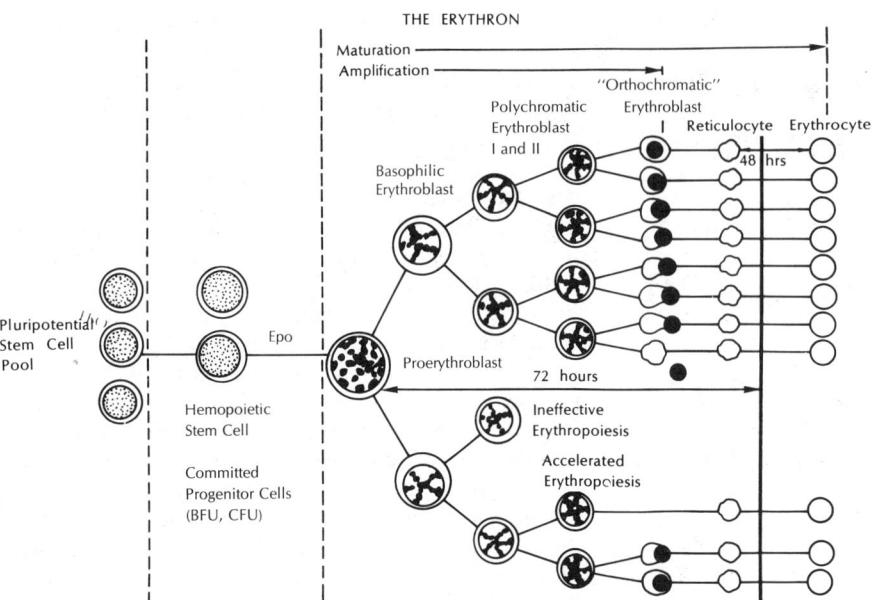

FIGURE 29-1   The erythron. The erythropoietic organ and circulating red cell mass constitute the erythron. Depicted here are the composition of the erythron and the maturation and amplification of the red cell series. Pluripotential stem cells are recruited into the pool of committed erythropoietin-responsive stem cells. Under the stimulus of erythropoietin (Epo), these committed cells differentiate into proerythroblasts. Normal maturation occurs by four mitotic divisions, during which the proerythroblast matures to the reticulocyte by a continual differentiation process, passing through three arbitrarily defined stages: the basophilic erythroblast, polychromatophilic erythroblasts I and II, and the orthochromatic erythroblast, which by ejection of its nucleus emerges as a reticulocyte. Amplification results from maturational divisions such that each proerythroblast results in a potential 16 reticulocytes. The maturation process requires a period of approximately 72 h. In the ensuing 48 h, the circulating reticulocyte matures into an erythrocyte. Ineffective erythropoiesis, with failure of erythroblast maturation and intramedullary cell destruction, and accelerated erythropoiesis, with skipped maturational divisions, are also illustrated.

in progressive stages of maturation, occasionally with one or several juxtaposed to a macrophage or cell fragment, are often encountered in stained films of marrow aspirates. Similarly, apparently extracellular iron may actually be a fragment of a disrupted macrophage. Biopsy techniques which preserve the histologic relationships of marrow cells permit demonstration in the living state of erythroblastic islands, particularly in careful teased specimens, with the phase-contrast microscope, or by electron microscopy of sections of marrow particles (Fig. 29-2b and c). In clinical situations with accelerated erythroblastic activity, such as acute hemolytic anemia and erythroleukemia, intact erythroblastic islands may be encountered in marrow films.

MARROW IRON METABOLISM

In normal man, the marrow macrophage plays a major role in iron conservation. Aged and damaged erythrocytes, recognized and entrapped within the microcirculation of the red marrow, are phagocytosed by the macrophage. The primary phagosome containing the engulfed red cell is approached by lysosomes which release their lytic enzymes into the phagosome. Within 60 min the digestion of the engulfed red cell is evidenced by degeneration of the membrane into a multilaminar myelin

figure and replacement of the hemoglobin portion of the digested red cell by particles identifiable as ferritin (Fig. 29-3a). The ferritin particles may be dispersed or may exist in aggregates either free within the cytoplasm of the macrophage or in membrane-bound vacuoles, occasionally with a hexagonal paracrystalline arrangement (Fig. 29-3b and c). These aggregates may be as large as 100 μm in diameter and represent the major part of *hemosiderin,* seen as brown masses in unstained marrow and giving the typical Prussian blue reaction with ferrocyanide. X-ray diffraction and high-resolution electron microscopy (Fig. 29-3d) of the ferritin molecule show that it consists of a protein shell and a central micelle of ferric hydroxide [1]. The molecule is 100 to 110 Å in diameter.

Hemosiderin arising from digestion of the aged erythrocyte in macrophages is the major form of storage iron in man. Although composed primarily of ferritin, it appears to exist in a variety of chemical forms, with the iron-protein complex mixed with lipids, saccharides, copper, and calcium [5]. Similarly, several morphologic types of hemosiderin can be identified in the macrophage by electron microscopy [1].

The incorporation of iron into protoporphyrin, catalyzed by heme synthase, occurs in the mitochondria.

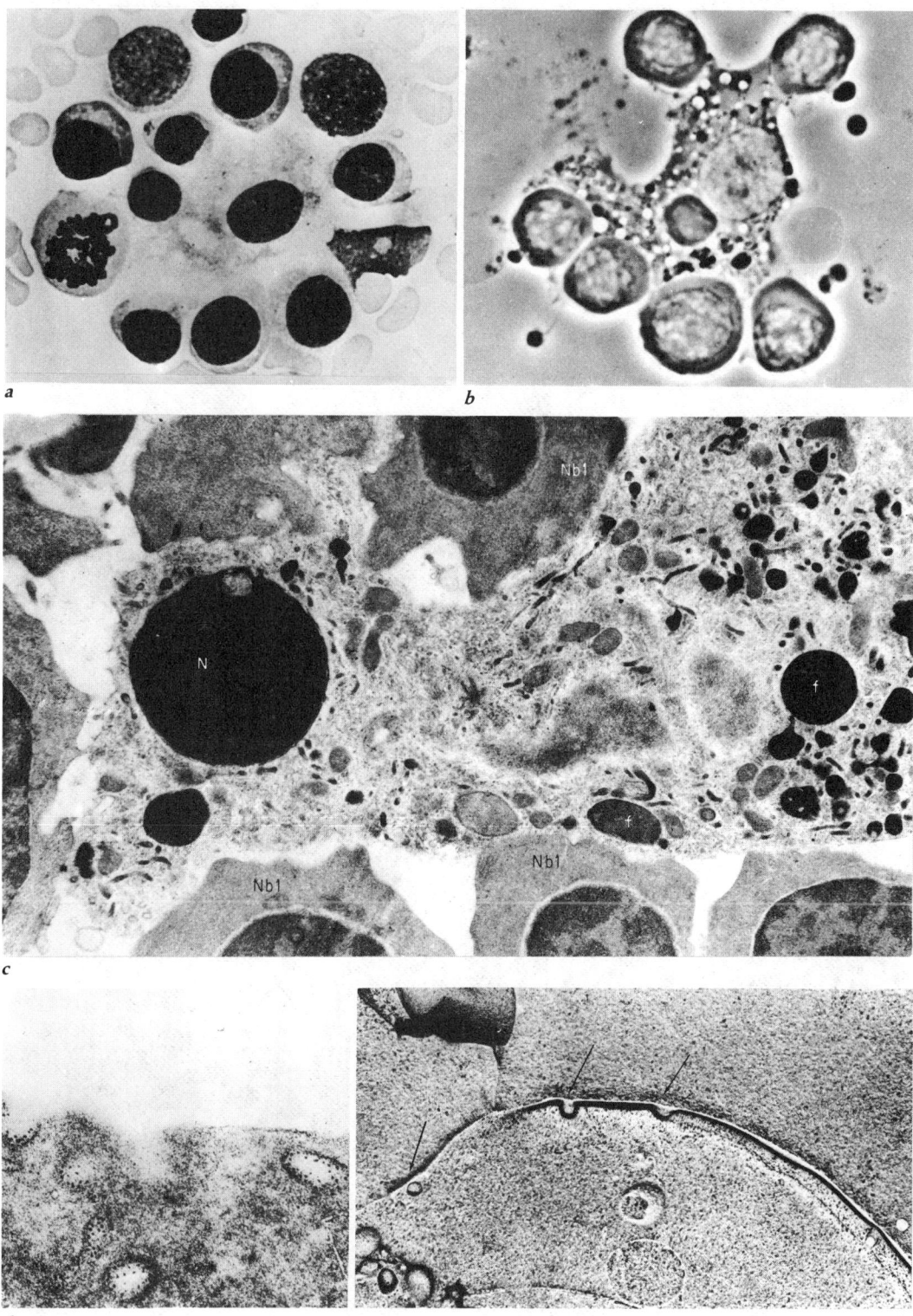

FIGURE 29-2 Erythroblastic island and rhopheocytosis. (*a*) Erythroblastic island as seen in a Giemsa-stained marrow. (*b*) Erythroblastic island in the living state seen in the phase-contrast microscope. The macrophage shows dynamic movement in relation to its surrounding erythroblasts. (*c*) Electron micrograph of a portion of an erythroblastic island shows dense ferritin (f) aggregates within the cytoplasm of the macrophage and an ingested pyknotic erythroblast nucleus (N). Close contact between the erythroblasts and the macrophage is seen. (*d*) Erythroblast margin showing the presence of ferritin on the cell surface and within micropinocytotic vesicles. Ferritin molecules appear to be membrane-fixed, and the membrane invaginates to incorporate the ferritin into the erythroblast cytoplasm. (*e*) Rhopheocytosis viewed by freeze etching with stages of invagination and micropinocytosis of the erythroblast membrane.

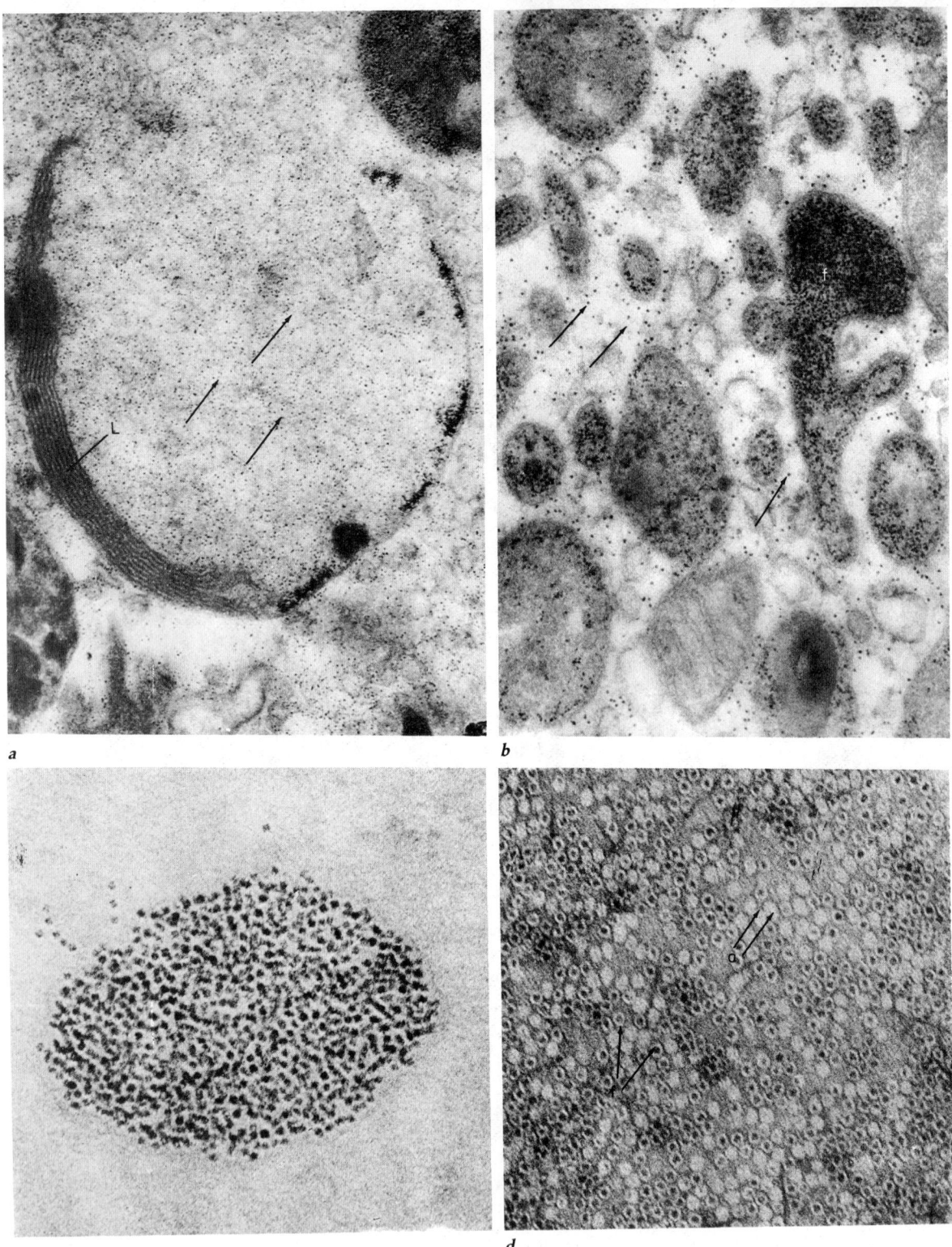

a

b

c

d

FIGURE 29-3 Ferritin and hemosiderin. (*a*) Electron micrograph of a portion of a macrophage showing the digestion of a phagocytized erythrocyte; the membrane is broken down to a multi-laminar lipid structure (L) and the hemoglobin iron into ferritin particles (*arrows*). (*b*) Ferritin is stored in the macrophage, free within the cytoplasm (*arrows*), and in membrane-bound vesicles. Large vesicles containing dense aggregations of ferritin (f) are seen on light microscopy as brown masses, staining blue with ferricyanide, identifying them as hemosiderin. (*c*) Membrane-bound erythroblast siderosome has an internal composition of individual ferritin molecules. (*d*) Electron micrograph of negatively stained ferritin and apoferritin mixture, showing the ferritin molecule (f) with its protein coat and central dense iron core; apoferritin molecules (a) lack the central iron cores [4].

In disorders in which an abnormality in heme or globin synthesis exists (sideroblastic anemia, lead intoxication) or with delayed turnover of iron, electron-dense, particulate iron accumulates between the cristae of the mitochondria [6]. These intramitochondrial masses of iron have been termed *ferruginous micelles* [6].

MATURATION OF THE ERYTHROBLASTIC SERIES

The morphology of the erythroblastic series closely corresponds to the biochemical events of the developing erythroblast. The 48 to 72 h during which the committed erythropoietic stem cell, under the stimulation of erythropoietin, differentiates from the proerythroblast to the reticulocyte are characterized by cell maturation and amplification. During this period, specialized organelles such as mitochondria, Golgi apparatus, polyribosomes, and siderosomes—the cellular machinery for the synthesis of hemoglobin, enzymes, and stromal proteins—are developed. After the expulsion of the nucleus, the activity of the protein-synthesizing apparatus is diminished, and these organelles lose their utility and gradually disappear. The disappearance of organelles continues during the 48 h of maturation of the reticulocyte and represents the morphologic equivalent of this diminution of protein synthesis. As measured on stained marrow films, the erythroblast diminishes in mean diameter from 25 μm to 9 μm as it develops from proerythroblast to orthochromatic erythroblast. This reduction in size is largely due to a reduction in absolute size of the nucleus, with a relative increase in the volume of cytoplasm.

The appearance of the nucleus correlates well with its functional state. From the proerythroblast to the first polychromatophilic erythroblast, three mitoses occur (Fig. 29-1). At the early stage of development, the nuclear chromatin is loosely arranged in fine strands and aggregates. The nucleus is marked by the presence of a nucleolus in which ribosomal and transfer RNA are produced. As the cell matures and the need for ribosome production diminishes, the nucleolus becomes inactive and gradually disappears. As the mitotic divisions occur and the cell matures, the nuclear chromatin becomes clumped and compressed, a process known as *pyknosis*. With the fourth maturational division the pyknotic process accelerates, and a completely pyknotic nucleus results. In stained films of marrow, immature cells are intensely basophilic because of the presence of large numbers of polyribosomes. The basophilia gradually diminishes as hemoglobin production increases and the polyribosomes are diluted with increasing amounts of hemoglobin. The intense basophilia due to the large numbers of ribosomes fades to polychromatophilia and finally to acidophilia, due to the increasing amount of hemoglobin prior to the ejection of the erythroblast nucleus.

Spectrophotometric studies confirm that during the course of maturation the quantity of RNA in the cytoplasm decreases in a linear fashion [7]. The synthesis of RNA appears to diminish at the stage of the basophilic erythroblast [7]. Although the total quantity of protein with the developing erythroblast decreases until the polychromatophil stage, probably because of the diminution of the cytoplasmic volume, there is a relative increase in the quantity of hemoglobin. Electron microscopic studies have permitted quantitative analyses of the distribution and growth of polyribosomes within the erythroblast [8]. They are generally composed of two to six ribosomes arranged along a messenger RNA filament specific for a globin chain (see Chap. 32). Polyribosomes form early in the development of the erythroblast, are relatively stable, and persist through the later stages of maturation.

THE ERYTHROBLAST SERIES (Plate 3)

THE HEMOPOIETIC STEM CELL
The recognizable cells in the erythron arise from a hemopoietic stem cell which is not morphologically recognizable. This cell is discussed in detail in Chap. 18.

PROERYTHROBLAST
The proerythroblast (Fig. 29-4) is a large cell, 20 to 25 μm in diameter, irregularly rounded or slightly oval, whose nucleus occupies approximately 80 percent of its area.

The nucleus contains fine chromatin delicately distributed in small clumps, with one or several well-defined nucleoli, which are often somewhat acidophilic when stained with Wright's stain. In sections of normal marrow examined by electron microscopy, the proerythroblast is difficult to find and relatively rarely noted. It is among the largest cells and has the characteristics of an immature cell. Numerous polyribosomes, arranged in groups of two or six, are dispersed throughout the cytoplasm, giving the proerythroblast intense basophilia when stained with the usual stains. At high magnification, ferritin molecules can be seen dispersed singly throughout the cytoplasm, and rhopheocytosis is easily observed at cell margins (Fig. 29-2*d*). Variable amounts of glycogen are present in the proerythroblast cytoplasm.

BASOPHILIC ERYTHROBLAST
In the stained film of the marrow the basophilic erythroblast is smaller in size than the proerythroblast, measuring 16 to 18 μm (Fig. 29-5). The nucleus occupies three-fourths of the cell area. At this stage it begins to show characteristic dark-violet heterochromatin interspersed with pink-staining euchromatin distributed into clumps linked by irregular linear strands, often with a wheel-spoke or clockface arrangement. The cytoplasm stains deep blue, leaving a perinuclear halo and the justanuclear clear zone which represents the Golgi apparatus. The basophilia in this cell also is due to the presence of polyribosomes. Small amounts of cytoplasmic glycogen can be demonstrated cytochemically, particularly in pathologic erythroblasts.

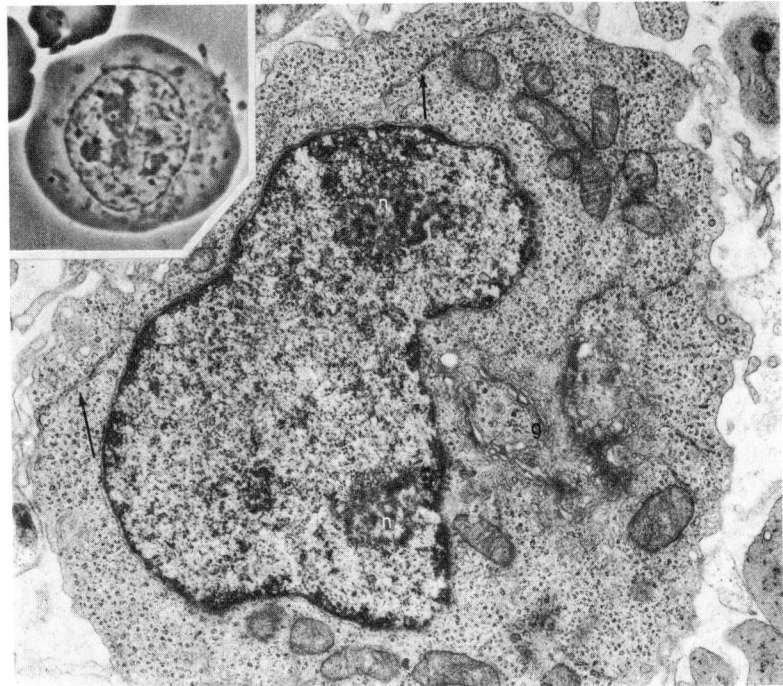

FIGURE 29-4 Proerythroblast. Phase-contrast micrograph (inset) of a proerythroblast showing the immature nucleus with nucleoli and finely dispersed nuclear chromatin. Centrosome (juxtanuclear clear zone) is apparent with its dense accumulation of mitochondria. Electron microscope section of the proerythroblast shows nucleoli (n) in contact with the nuclear membrane. Chromatin is finely dispersed and forms small aggregates in the fixed nuclear membrane. The perinuclear canal is narrow but well defined. Polyribosome groups, many in helical configurations, are dispersed throughout the cytoplasm. The Golgi apparatus (g) is well developed, and regions of endoplasmic reticulum (*arrows*) are seen.

FIGURE 29-5 Basophilic erythroblast. Phase-contrast photomicrograph (*inset*) shows increased clumping of the nuclear chromatin and further rounding of the cell, with aggregation of the mitochondria and centrosome into the regions of nuclear indentation. Electron microscopic section shows clumping of the nuclear chromatin, nuclear pores (p), organization of the nucleoli, increased density of polyribosomes (pr), well-developed Golgi apparatus (g), and a decrease in content of smooth endoplasmic reticulum.

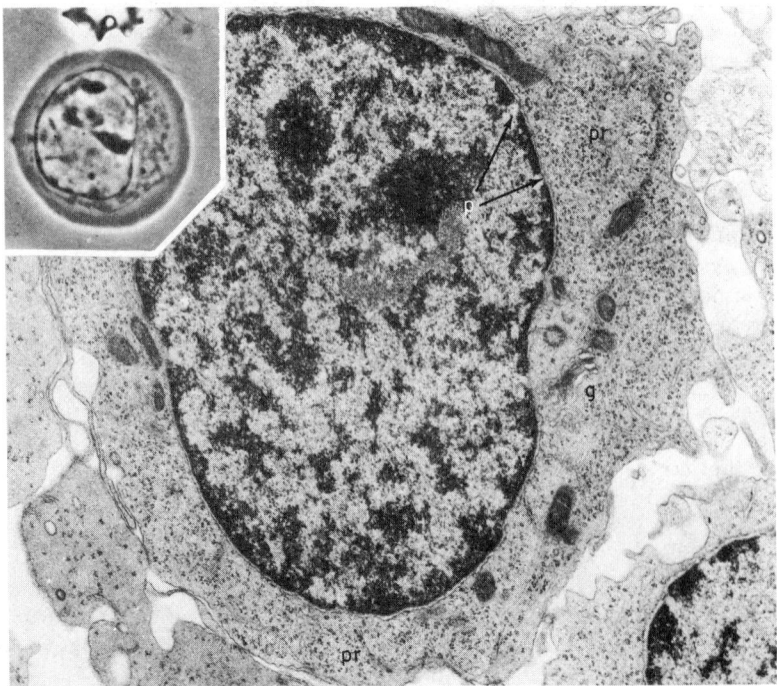

When examined with the electron microscope, the nucleolus appears less well defined, and heterochromatin aggregation is increased compared with earlier stages. As this cell approaches a mitotic division, chromatin becomes more dispersed and more linear in appearance. Polyribosomes are extremely numerous throughout the cytoplasm. Microtubules are evident in the basophilic erythroblast, often appearing in bundles within an excrescence of the cell margin or arranged in an arcuate band. Microfilaments can be seen close to the nuclear membrane. Siderosomes, membrane-bound or free masses of ferritin, are scattered in the cytoplasm. Individually dispersed ferritin molecules may also be identified. As the erythroblast matures, the ferritin tends to group into small masses. In many regions, ferritin molecules appear intimately related to the external aspect of the cell membrane. The basophilic erythroblast undergoes one mitotic division. It is often encountered in early telophase with the remnant of a bridge between two daughter cells.

POLYCHROMATOPHILIC ERYTHROBLAST

Following the second mitotic division of the erythropoietic series, the erythroblast develops increasing amounts of hemoglobin within the cytoplasm. Its polyribosome content is thus diluted, and it assumes a polychromatophilic appearance on the Wright's-stained marrow film (Fig. 29-6). The polychromatophilic erythroblast is smaller than the basophilic erythroblast, measuring approximately 12 to 15 μm in diameter. The nucleus occupies less than half of the cell area and is usually eccentric. The nuclear heterochromatin is dispersed into well-defined clumps spaced regularly about the nucleus, producing a checkerboard pattern. The nucleolus is lost, but the perinuclear halo is preserved. The cytoplasm shows a mixed basophilic and acidophilic coloration, giving the cell a variegate or greenish color on Wright's stain.

Electron microscopy of the polychromatophilic erythroblast reveals increased aggregation of nuclear heterochromatin. The polyribosome content of the cell has become significantly diluted by hemoglobin. Rhopheocytosis is still apparent at the cell margins, and this cell is commonly found in close contact with a macrophage. Siderosomes can be identified within the cytoplasm [9], and singly dispersed ferritin molecules are also encountered. This normal distribution of ferritin iron in the erythroblast characterizes the *normal sidero-*

FIGURE 29-6 Polychromatophilic erythroblast. Phase-contrast micrograph (*inset*) demonstrates a diminution in the size of this cell in comparison with its precursor, with further clumping of nuclear chromatin to give the nucleus a checkerboard appearance. The centrosome is condensed, and a perinuclear halo has developed. Electron microscopic section demonstrates relative reduction of the density of polyribosomes and dilution by the moderately osmophilic hemoglobin in the cytoplasm. Nuclear chromatin shows a marked increase in clumping, and nuclear pores (P) are enlarged.

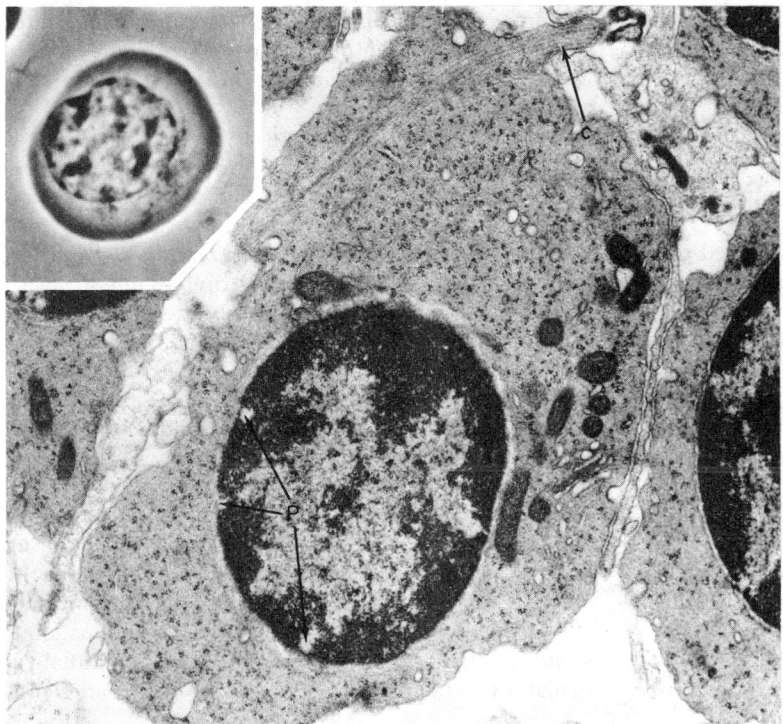

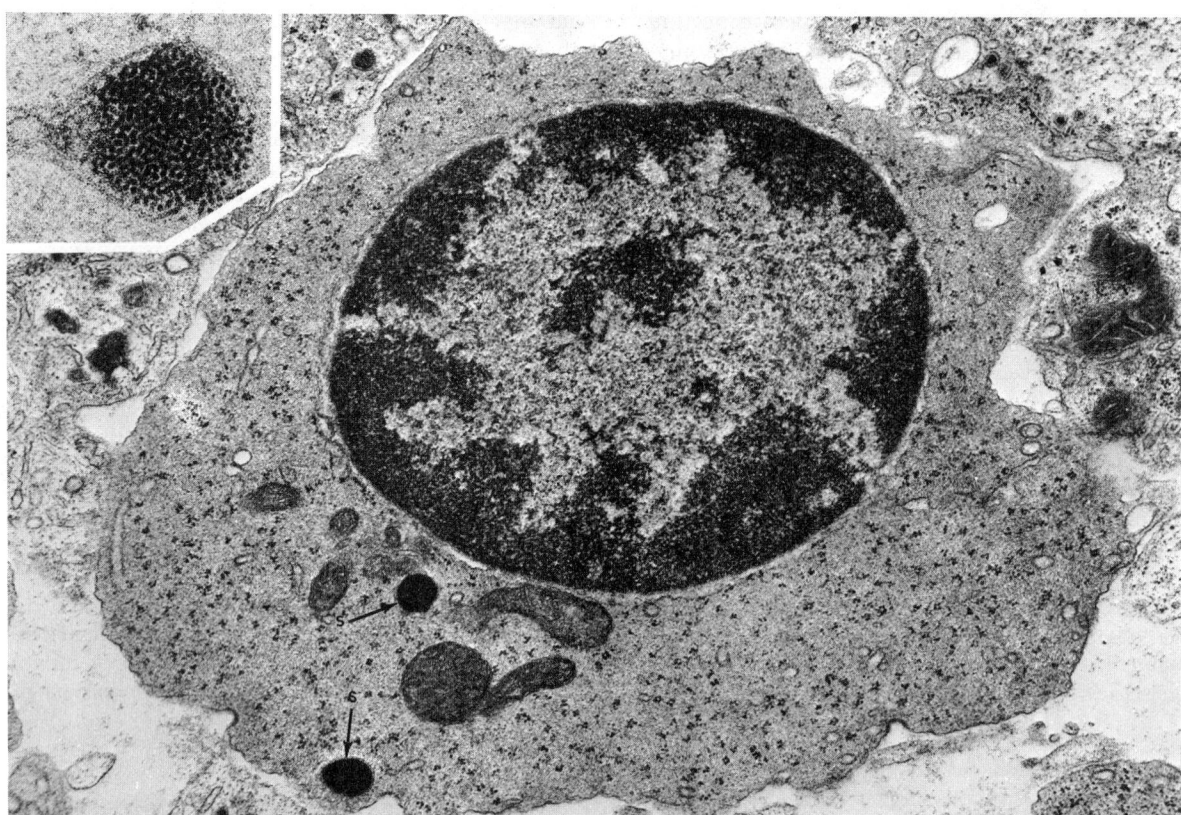

FIGURE 29-7 Depicted here is the normal sideroblast, a polychromatophilic erythroblast, containing several siderosomes (s) within its cytoplasm. At higher magnification (*inset*) these are seen to be membrane-bound vacuoles containing a tightly packed aggregate of ferritin molecules.

blast (Fig. 29-7). Under normal conditions mitochondrial iron is usually not apparent at electron microscopic resolution, although iron is known to be incorporated into protoporphyrin by mitochondrial heme synthase.

ORTHOCHROMATIC ERYTHROBLAST
After the final mitotic division of the erythropoietic series, the relative proportion of hemoglobin increases within the erythroblast to give it a relatively uniform, or orthochromatic, staining appearance (Fig. 29-8). This cell is, in fact, polychromatophilic, retaining mixed coloration on Wright's stain as a result of persistence of signficant numbers of mono- and polyribosomes. Nuclear pyknosis has increased to the point where the nucleus appears most completely dense and measurably decreased in size. This cell, the smallest of the erythroblast series, varies from 10 to 15 μm in diameter. Its nucleus occupies approximately one-fourth of the cell area and is eccentric. In the phase-contrast microscope, the erythroblast at this stage has taken on striking motility and manifests undulating movements, probably in preparation for ejection of its nucleus [1]. When examined with the electron microscope, the cell is characterized by irregular borders, reflecting its motile state. The nucleus is eccentric; the heterochromatin forms large masses. The cytoplasmic polyribosomes are fur-

ther diluted by the moderately osmophilic hemoglobin, and increasing numbers of di- and monoribosomes are present, reflecting dispersion of polyribosomes. Mitochondria are reduced in number and size, some of them already showing degeneration.

BIRTH OF THE RETICULOCYTE
Under in vitro conditions, expulsion of the nucleus requires a 10-min period [1]. The erythroblast displays increasing undulating movements, and the nucleus is lost, with several dynamic contractions around the midportions of the cell (Fig. 29-9). The cell divides unequally, so that a smaller portion contains only the nucleus and a thin rim of cytoplasm with its hemoglobin [1]; the larger portion becomes the reticulocyte. On stained films, partial expulsion is often seen; the nucleus then has an hourglass or dumbbell appearance. Under physiologic conditions the expelled nucleus is quickly ingested by a macrophage (Fig. 29-2a to c). Any increase in erythropoietic activity associated with the increased rate of removal of erythroblast nuclei with their surrounding "corona" of hemoglobin will lead to an increase in the "early peak" of stercobilin which occurs in normal man [10]. The release of reticulocytes into the venous sinusoids may be influenced by the marrow adventitial reticular cell, which retracts its covering cytoplasmic pro-

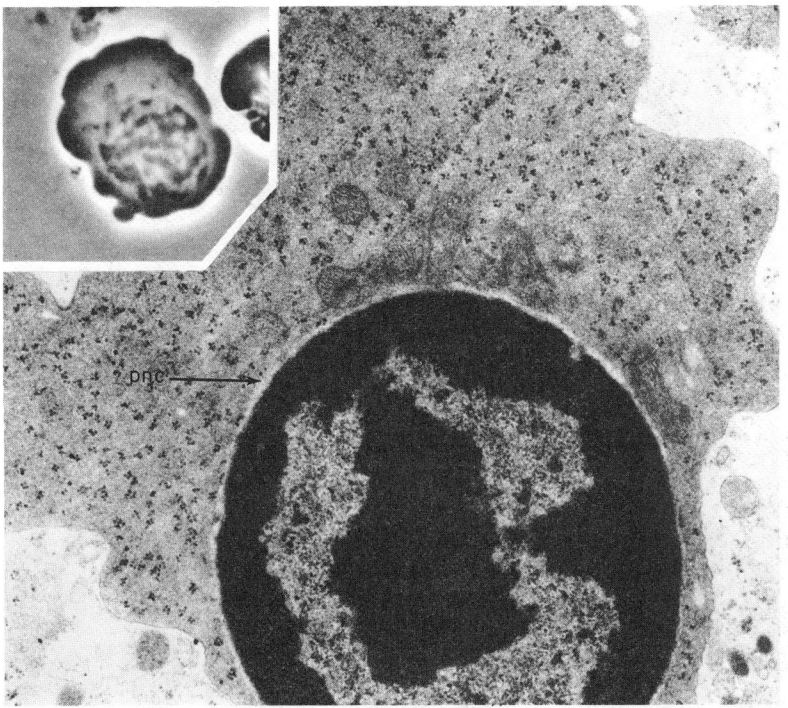

FIGURE 29-8 Orthochromatic erythroblast. Phase-contrast appearance of this cell in the living state (*inset*) shows the irregular borders indicative of the characteristic motility of this cell, the eccentric nucleus making contact with the plasmalemma, further pyknosis of the nuclear chromatin, and condensation of the centrosome. Electron microscopic section shows further dilution of polyribosomes, some of which appear to be disintegrating into monoribosomes, by the increasing hemoglobin. The number of mitochondria is decreased, and some exhibit degeneration. Nuclear chromatin is clumped into large masses and a perinuclear canal (pnc) is seen.

cesses, possibly in response to erythropoietin, to permit reticulocyte access to the circulation via fenestrations in sinus endothelial cells [1].

MATURATION OF THE RETICULOCYTE

After expulsion of the nucleus and diapedesis into the marrow capillary, the orthochromatic erythroblast has emerged as a reticulocyte, retaining mitochondria, small numbers of ribosomes, the centriole, and remnants of the Golgi bodies (Fig. 29-10). The reticulocyte contains no endoplasmic reticulum. Supravital staining of the reticulocyte with brilliant cresyl blue or new methylene blue produces aggregates of deep-blue-staining material arranged in reticular strands. This is the artifact which gives the reticulocyte its name; it is due to precipitation and aggregation of ribosomes, mitochondria, and other organelles by these dyes [11].

Maturation of the circulating reticulocyte requires from 24 to 48 h. During this period the reticulocyte synthesizes the remaining 20 percent of the red cell hemoglobin content and undertakes autophagy and ejection of unneeded organelles [12].

Observed in the living state in the phase-contrast microscope, the reticulocyte is a motile, irregularly shaped cell with its organelles corresponding to granulations grouped around an indentation or hilum (Fig. 29-10a to d). The cell displays nondirectional dynamic movement, with regional expansion and retraction of cytoplasm; the hilar portion remains relatively stable.

Reticulocytes vary from 10 to 15 μm in diameter, slightly larger than normal erythrocytes. With accelerated erythropoietic activity, erythrocyte diameter may approach twice that of normal erythrocytes following nuclear expulsion from a less mature, larger erythroblast.

So-called supravital stains employed for identification of reticulocytes actually kill the cells and lead to the production of an artifactual reticulofilamentous substance. The stains usually employed are brilliant cresyl blue or new methylene blue. In the usual blood film, dried in air and stained with Wright's or Giemsa stain, the reticulocytes can be identified by their slight diffuse basophilia, often referred to as *polychromatophilia*. They appear round in contour and are slightly larger than mature erythrocytes. Combined supravital (brilliant cresyl blue or new methylene blue) and postvital staining (Wright's or Giemsa) demonstrates that the reticulofilamentous structures and polychromatophilia exist in the same cell [13]. Scanning and transmission electron microscopic studies of the reticulocyte, employing the technique of moulage, as well as studies with the scanning electron microscope show the multilobular surface configuration of the reticulocyte and confirm in three dimensions that the reticulocyte is an irregular cell with a region of hilar indentation and points of retraction (Fig. 29-11) [11]. On electron microscopic section, reticulocytes are easy to recognize by their irregular shape and the presence of multiple remnant organelles.

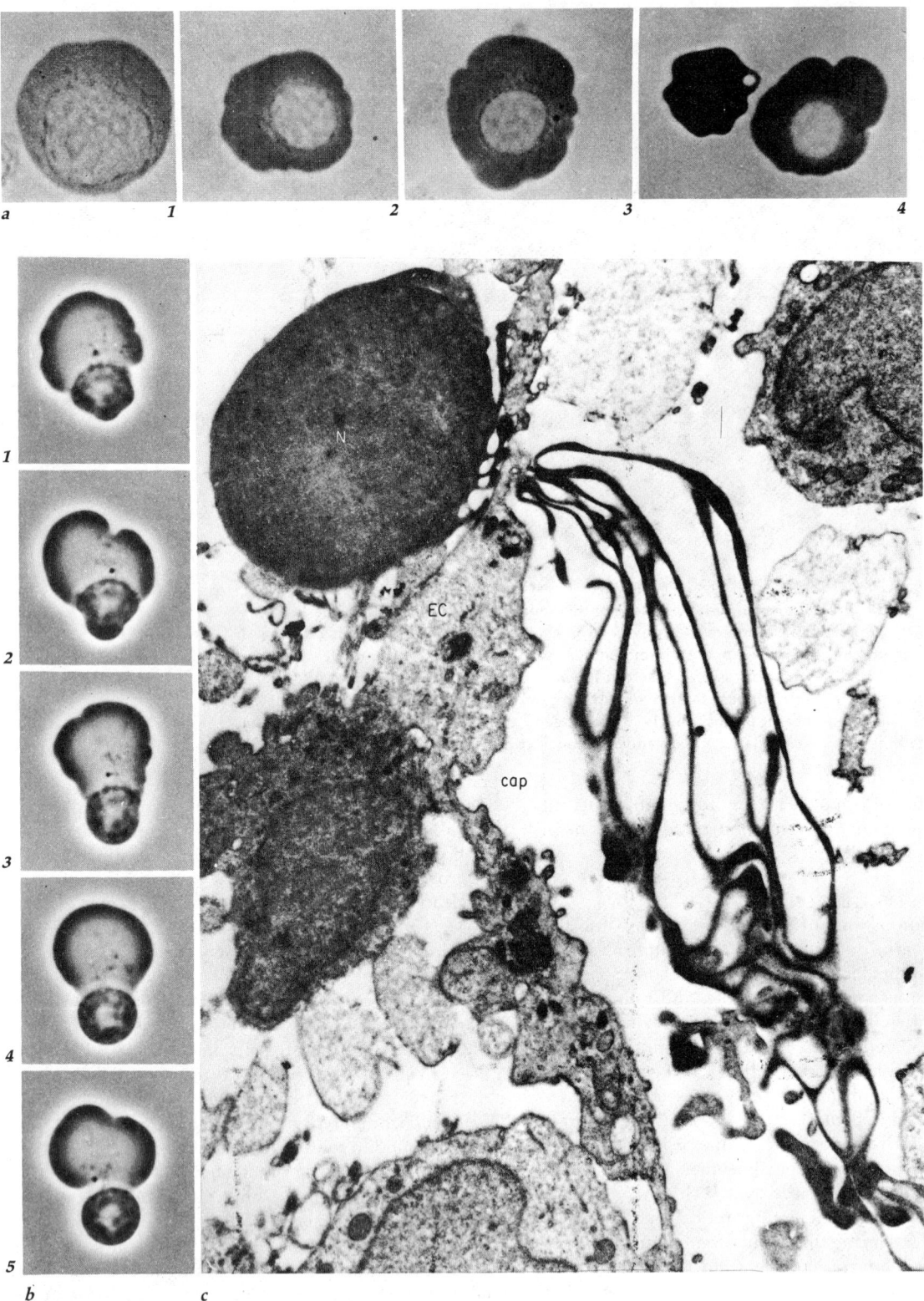

FIGURE 29-9 Soret absorption micrograph of developing erythroblasts and ejection of the erythroblast nucleus. (*a*) Erythroblast series from the basophilic erythroblast (1) through the orthochromatophilic erythroblast (3) and reticulocyte (4) are observed in the living state with Soret absorption (414 nm), showing the increase in Soret absorption (hemoglobin content) as the erythroblast develops from the basophilic erythroblast to the reticulocyte (left to right). (*b*) Portions of a phase-contrast microcinematography film of the ejection of the nucleus by an orthochromatic normoblast (1–5). Note the dynamic alterations in the shape of the cell, the undulating contractions and constrictions across the cell as nuclear ejection occurs. (*c*) Electron micrograph depicts ejection of the normoblast nucleus (N) and diapedesis of the resultant reticulocyte across the endothelial cell (EC) into the sinusoidal capillary space (cap). The reticulocyte is markedly deformed during this sieving process but quickly resumes its characteristic shape.

266

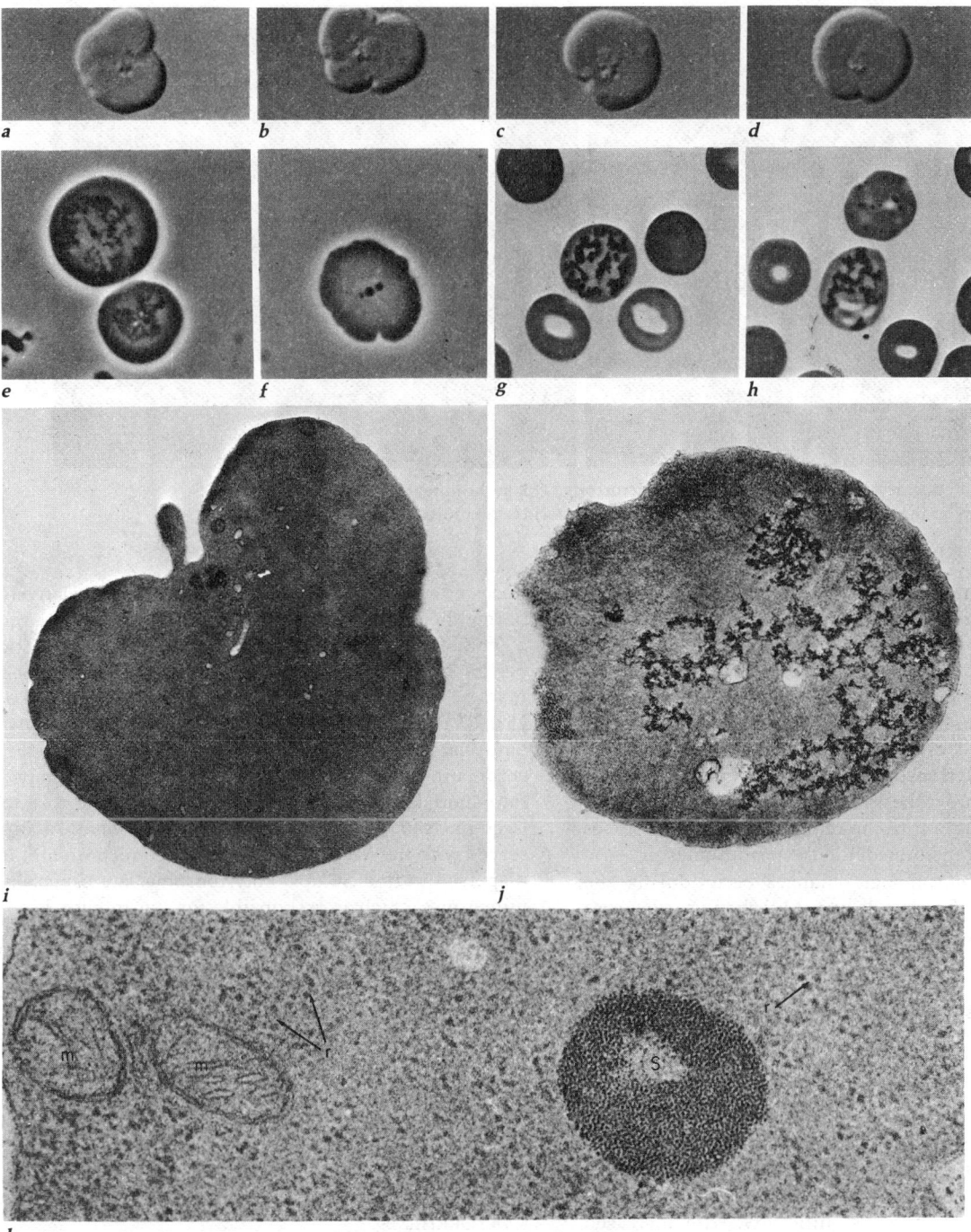

FIGURE 29-10   Reticulocytes. (*a–d*) Film clips from phase-contrast microcinematography of the same reticulocyte showing its irregularity and its motility. Note that the organelles appear as bumps on the surface and are grouped about the hilum of the cell. (*e*) Reticulocytes viewed by phase-contrast microscopy after staining with new methylene blue. The reticulofilamentous substance precipitated by the stain is apparent (*f*) Phase-contrast micrograph of a reticulocyte in the living state after vital staining with neutral red. (*g,h*) Reticulocytes on dried film after supravital staining with new methylene blue. The deep-blue-staining microfilamentous substance is the artifact which identifies these cells. (*i*) Electron microscopic section of a reticulocyte prior to supravital staining. Note the organelles grouped about the hilum of this irregular cell, with clear vacuoles distributed about the cytoplasm. (*j*) Reticulocyte sectioned after new methylene blue staining. Note the precipitate composed largely of ribosomes and stained with coprecipitation of mitochondria ferritin and other organelles. (*k*) Highly magnified portion of a reticulocyte showing mono- and polyribosomes (r) dispersed throughout the cytoplasm, mitochondria (m), and sidero-some (s) composed of ferritin molecules.

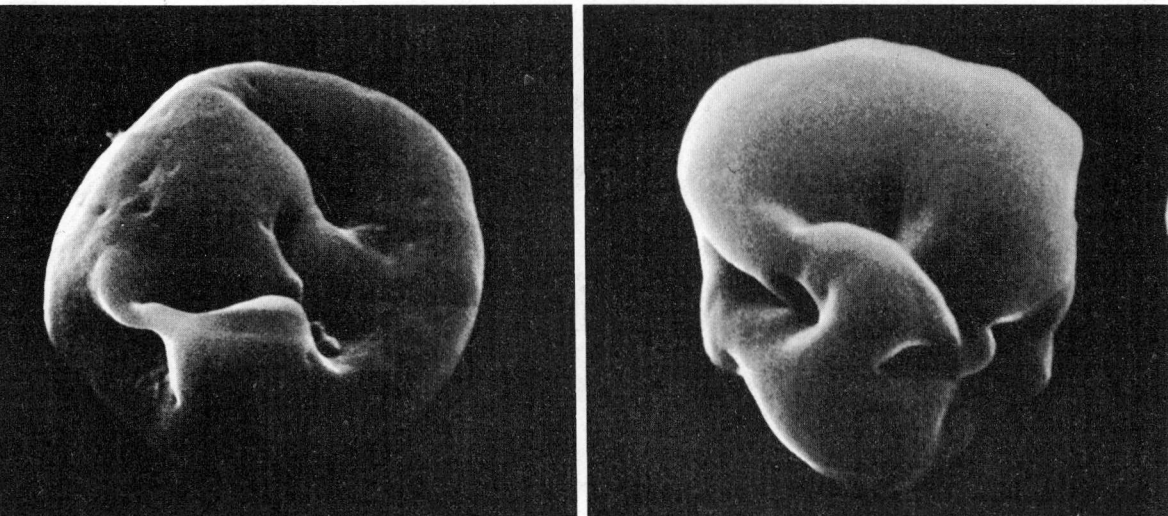

FIGURE 29-11   Reticulocytes on stereoscan electron microscopy. This technique provides a three-dimensional view of the surface configuration of the reticulocytes, invaginations, and projections.

Small mitochondria are generally grouped in the hilar region of the reticulocyte with small, smooth vesicles and an occasional centriole. It is from this region of the cell that the nucleus has separated. Ribosomes are dispersed throughout the cytoplasm as poly- or mono-ribosomes (Fig. 29-10k). It has been shown that in the "young" reticulocyte 88 percent of the ribosomes are in the form of polyribosomes, apparently in relation to the rate of protein synthesis. With its diminution during the 48-h maturation of the reticulocyte, polyribosomes are gradually transformed into monoribosomes.

Numerous morphologic changes occur during the maturation of the reticulocyte. Mitochondria decrease significantly in size and number and show degeneration, with loss of cristae and vacuolization, as their metabolic activity decreases. Reticulocytes eject degenerating organelles by autophagy during their maturation [12]. In this process, small vacuoles encircle organelles to be ejected and fuse into a single autophagosome, which then ejects its contents into the extracellular space.

Under normal conditions, reticulocytes may contain small quantities of iron in the form of clumps of hemosiderin or ferritin. These cells are often called *siderocytes*. Under pathologic conditions, the quantity and distribution of iron may change significantly, with increased siderosomes and intramitochondrial iron.

PATHOLOGIC ERYTHROBLASTS

MEGALOBLASTIC SERIES (Plate 3)

Megaloblastic maturation of the erythroid series occurs as a result of disturbances of DNA synthesis such as that due to a deficiency of vitamin B_{12} or folic acid (see Chap. 34). It is characterized by an asynchrony of nuclear and cytoplasmic development referred to as *cytonuclear dissociation,* which results from a decreased rate of DNA synthesis [14]. In the megaloblastic series, a lag in

nuclear development occurs in the presence of relatively normal hemoglobinization of the cytoplasm. The large megaloblasts resemble those from the mesoblastic period of embryonic erythropoiesis. On the stained marrow film, the *promegaloblast* is a slightly oval cell of 25 to 35 μm, with a large, eccentric nucleus. It has a juxtanuclear clear zone and a perinuclear halo. The nuclear chromatin is finely granular and occasionally clumped into short rods or masses. Nuclei contain one to four large nucleoli. The cytoplasm is intensely blue. As observed with the electron microscope, heterochromatin is dispersed in fine clumps. Polyribosomes are especially numerous, which is responsible for the intense basophilia. The *basophilic megaloblast* and *polychromatophilic megaloblast* are successive stages in the development of the megaloblastic series which bridge the gap between the promegaloblast and the orthochromatic megaloblast. Their development parallels that of the erythroblastic series, with a progressive decrease in cytoplasmic basophilia. The *orthochromatic megaloblast* is the smallest cell of the megaloblastic series, measuring 10 to 13 μm in diameter. Howell-Jolly bodies are frequent at this stage in the development of a megaloblast.

KARYORRHEXIS

Karyorrhexis is characteristic of certain dyserythropoietic anemias (Chap. 46) and of arsenic poisoning [15–17]. In these states, the erythroblast nucleus shows accelerated pyknosis, which begins prematurely at the polychromatophilic erythroblast stage and is marked by clumping of the basichromatin and reduction in nuclear size. The nuclei become polylobular or cloverleaf, and internuclear bridging, with thin strands of chromatin connecting two cells, is frequently seen. This suggests that the final mitotic division of the polychromatophil erythroblast is incomplete. Pyknotic nuclei with cloverleaf forms and multiple nuclear fragments characterize the orthochromatic erythroblast in this series.

DEFECTIVE HEMOGLOBINIZATION

Abnormalities in hemoglobin synthesis such as are found in iron deficiency [1], lead poisoning, anemia of chronic disease, and thalassemia manifest themselves as a second type of cytonuclear dissociation, the reverse of that seen in the megaloblastic anemias. Nuclear development parallels that of the normal cell, but the cytoplasm retains its basophilia throughout the polychromatophil erythroblast stage. Cells are smaller than those of the normal series and often display ragged, irregular cell borders, attributed to marked endovesiculation at the surface [1]. The persistent polychromatophilia is due to a decreased amount of hemoglobin and an excess of polyribosomes, attributed to defective hemoglobin synthesis. In iron-deficiency anemia, intracellular iron content is reduced or absent; in other defects of hemoglobin synthesis, excessive amounts of iron may be present in erythroid cells.

VACUOLIZATION OF ERYTHROBLASTS

Vacuolization of both cytoplasm and nucleus of the erythroblast occurs as a manifestation of chloramphenicol toxicity [18]. Clear nuclear cytoplasmic vacuoles are particularly prominent in basophilic and polychromatophilic erythroblasts. The vacuoles may number from 3 to 20 per cell and range up to 1 μm in diameter. They do not stain with Sudan (lipid) or periodic acid–Schiff (polysaccharide) stains. Similar vacuoles are also commonly seen in patients with erythroid suppression following acute alcoholism [19]. In this case, vacuolization is seen primarily in proerythroblasts and basophilic erythroblasts. Alcohol-induced vacuoles, produced in vitro in cultured human erythroblasts, appear to occur by surface invagination [20]. Electron microscopic studies of vacuolated erythroblasts from patients with acute alcoholism show marked surface irregularity and endovesiculation.

PATHOLOGIC SIDEROBLASTS

The pathologic sideroblast characterizes some of the refractory anemias, pyridoxine-responsive anemia, thalassemia, chloramphenicol toxicity, occasionally vitamin B_{12} or folic acid deficiency, and a large number of hypochromic, hypersideremic anemias [21,22]. Its presence suggests an abnormality of heme synthesis in the erythroblast. Marrow films stained for iron characteristically show small particles of iron up to 0.5 μm in diameter arranged in a ring about the nucleus. Hence they have been termed *ringed sideroblasts* [23] (see Chap. 54). Electron microscopic studies have revealed these iron granulations to be located between the cristae of mitochondria [24,25] (Fig. 29-12). In the living erythroblast, these mitochondria are dispersed in the cytoplasm and are more numerous in the region of the Golgi apparatus. On preparations of the dried film, they tend to form a perinuclear collar or ring. Phase-contrast microscopy of

FIGURE 29-12 The pathological sideroblast is an erythroblast characterized by the presence of intramitochondrial deposits of iron—ferruginous micelles (fm). Intramitochondrial iron may accumulate to the point of complete obliteration of the mitochondria. At higher magnification (*inset*), iron deposits can be seen in the intercristal spaces of the mitochondrion.

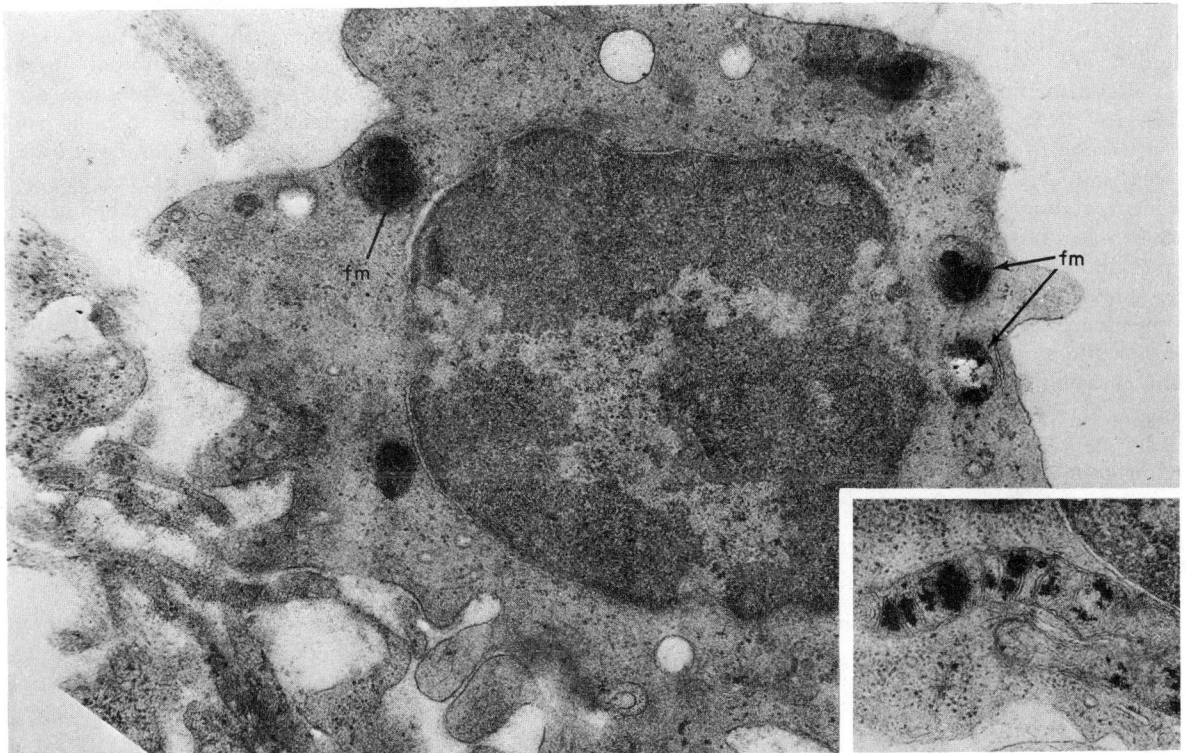

TABLE 29-1   Erythrocyte and reticulocyte inclusions

Inclusions	Composition	Cell type	Appearance on Wright's-stained film	Appearance in the living state
"Reticulo filamentous substance"	Artifactual aggregation of ribosomes	Reticulocyte	Invisible	Visible after postvital staining
Basophilic stippling	Pathologic precipitation of ribosomes	Reticulocyte	Dispersed blue granulations	Visible after concentration of the medium
Howell-Jolly bodies	Nuclear fragment containing aberrant chromosomes	Reticulocyte; rarely erythrocyte	Dense blue spherical granule	Visible
Azurophilic granulations	Nuclear rest, from karyorrhexis	Reticulocyte	Few small, dense blue granules	Visible only after hemolysis
Siderosomes	Iron-containing granule (+ Perl's reaction)	Reticulocyte	Invisible	Visible only after hemolysis
Pappenheimer bodies	Basophilic body which may contain iron	Reticulocyte	Small, dense blue granule	Visible only after hemolysis
Cabot rings	Spindle remnant (?)	Reticulocytes	Ring or figure-eight strand stained purple	Visible only after hemolysis
Heinz bodies	Denatured hemoglobin	Erythrocytes and occasionally reticulocytes	Rarely visible	Refractile inclusions (stained with methylene or Nile blue dyes)

the normal erythroblast shows the tendency of the mitochondria to be distributed about the nucleus. Most characteristic of the pathologic sideroblast is the dense, finely granular material—ferruginous micelles—morphologically different from cytoplasmic ferritin, found between the mitochondrial cristae [1]. Within a single cell, mitochondria may show varying degrees of iron incorporation; some may be markedly distended and nearly destroyed by iron, whereas others contain only small amounts of electron-dense material in spaces between cristae [1]. Other nuclear and cytoplasmic abnormalities may appear in association with the abnormal deposition of iron in the pathologic sideroblast. Cytonuclear asynchrony similar to that seen in the megaloblast may be present, cytoplasmic glycogen is often increased, and polyribosomes may be decreased and monoribosomes increased in number.

PATHOLOGY OF THE RETICULOCYTE

By light microscopy, the reticulocyte may show pathologic alterations of size or tinctorial properties or the presence of inclusion bodies. The majority of pathologic inclusions usually attributed to erythrocytes are actually found in reticulocytes (see Table 29-1). These consist of nuclear or cytoplasmic remnants derived from the late-stage normoblasts.

MACRORETICULOCYTES

In the presence of an intense erythropoietin response to an acute anemia or large injections of erythropoietin, reticulocytes may reach up to two times their normal size with a corresponding increase in their hemoglobin content. This is a normal response of the erythropoietic system to severe stress, and these large reticulocytes are referred to as "stress" reticulocytes [26]. Whether the doubling of the size is due to one less mitotic division than normal in the process of amplification or to some other phenomenon is not yet clear. In contrast, even under moderate erythropoietic stress, some of the reticulocytes in the marrow pool are shifted to the circulating pool to compensate the anemia, and these reticulocytes are referred to as "shift" reticulocytes [27]. Shift reticulocytes can be either of normal size or large depending on whether the cells being shifted from the marrow are of normal size or macro-stress reticulocytes [26,28].

HOWELL-JOLLY BODIES [29]

Howell-Jolly bodies are small nuclear remnants which have the color of a pyknotic nucleus on the Wright's-stained film and give a positive Feulgen reaction for DNA [30]. They are spherical in shape, usually no larger than 0.5 μm in diameter. Generally only one is present in each red cell, but they may be numerous. In pathologic situations, they appear to represent chromosomes which have been separated from the mitotic spindle during abnormal mitosis [31]. Under normal conditions, they seem to arise from nuclear fragmentation (karyorrhexis) or incomplete expulsion of the nucleus [32] and are pitted from reticulocytes in their passage through the interendothelial slits of the splenic sinus. They are characteristically seen in splenectomized persons and in those with hemolytic anemia, hyposplenism, or megaloblastic anemia.

CABOT RINGS

The ringlike figure seen in reticulocytes in megaloblastic anemias, sometimes twisted into a figure eight, is designated a *Cabot ring*. It is a thin strand, often concentric with the cell membrane, and stains red-violet on Wright's stain. As a rule, one is seen per cell, but rarely several may be encountered. Although it has been proposed that this circular strand represents a remnant of the nuclear membrane or a part of the mitotic spindle apparatus, cytochemical and electron microscopic studies have failed to reveal the origin of the Cabot ring [33].

BASOPHILIC STIPPLING

Basophilic stippling consists of granulations of variable size and number, staining deep blue with Wright's stain. This *punctate basophilia* represents an alteration of the normal polychromatophilia of the reticulocyte. Coarse stippling is characteristic of lead intoxication and thalassemia and has been associated with numerous pathologic states in which the biosynthesis of hemoglobin is altered [34]. Electron microscopic studies have shown that the granulations of basophilic stippling represent aggregated ribosomes [34]. These clumps do not preexist in the red cell but appear during the course of drying and staining of the cell. They may also include degenerating mitochondria and siderosomes. In conditions such as lead intoxication, the altered reticulocyte polyribosomes appear to have a greater propensity to form aggregates after postvital staining and dehydration. As a result, the basophilic granulation appears larger and is referred to as *coarse basophilic stippling* [34]. Collection of blood in ethylenediaminetetraacetic acid may result in disappearance of basophilic stippling [35].

SIDEROSOMES AND PAPPENHEIMER BODIES

Normal or pathologic cells containing siderosomes, or "iron bodies," are usually reticulocytes. In the pathologic state, the iron granulations are larger and more numerous, and electron microscopy has shown that many of these are mitochondria containing ferruginous micelles, rather than the ferritin aggregates which characterize the normal siderocyte [24]. Siderosomes are usually found in the cell periphery, whereas basophilic stippling tends to be distributed homogeneously throughout the cell. Siderosomes staining with Wright's stain have been called *Pappenheimer bodies* [36]. Electron microscopy of these bodies shows that the iron is often contained within a lysosome, as confirmed by the presence of acid phosphatase [37]. They often also contain degenerating mitochondria, ribosomes, and other cellular remnants.

STRUCTURE AND SHAPE OF THE ERYTHROCYTE

THE RESTING ERYTHROCYTE

The normal resting form of the erythrocyte is a biconcave disc. All of the factors necessary for the maintenance of this form are not understood, but variations in the shape and dimensions of the red cell can be useful in the differential diagnosis of anemias. Normal human red cells have a diameter of 7.5 to 8.3 μm, which decreases slightly with cell age. They are 1.7 μm thick and have an average volume of 83 μm^3 and a surface area of approximately 145 μm^2. Size variation of approximately 5 percent occurs among normal red cells. The normal erythrocyte stains reddish-brown in Wright's-stained blood films and stains pink with Giemsa stain. The center of the cell is relatively pale, with the stained portion distributed peripherally, reflecting its biconcave disc shape. Red cells on dried blood films are 0.6 μm thick, having lost about two-thirds of their normal thickness [1]. Many artifacts can be produced in the preparation of the blood film. They may result from contamination of the glass slide or cover slip with traces of fat, detergent, or other impurities [38]. Friction and surface tension involved in preparation of the blood film produce fragmentation, "doughnut cells" or annulocytes, crescent-shaped cells, etc. [38]. Examined in the living state with the phase-constrast microscope, normal red cells are seen as small biconcave discs, yellow or slightly red-brown in color, with a central clear area. Mature human red cells are easily deformable, with a tendency to reassume the biconcave disc shape. Observed in the phase contrast or interference microscope, the red cell shows a characteristic internal scintillation known as *red cell flicker* [39]. Anything which interferes with molecular motion, such as crystallization, sickling crenation, or fixation, will arrest red cell flicker. It is thought to represent molecular motion of the hemoglobin within the red cell.

Freeze-etching (freeze-fracture-replication) studies of red cells frozen after cryoprotection in the living state (such that postthawing viability is preserved) provides another technique for study of the ultrastructure of the red cell membrane [40].

VARIATION OF RED CELL SHAPE IN THE CIRCULATION

The shape of the red cell is the product of multiple forces and depends on the environment of the cell, its metabolic status, and its age. Within the circulation, the red cell traverses blood vessels of varying diameters and flow rates, exhibiting a variety of dynamic transitions of form. The red cell spends most of its circulatory life within the capillary channels of the microcirculation. During its 100- to 120-day life-span it travels a distance of approximately 175 miles. In the capillaries, deform-

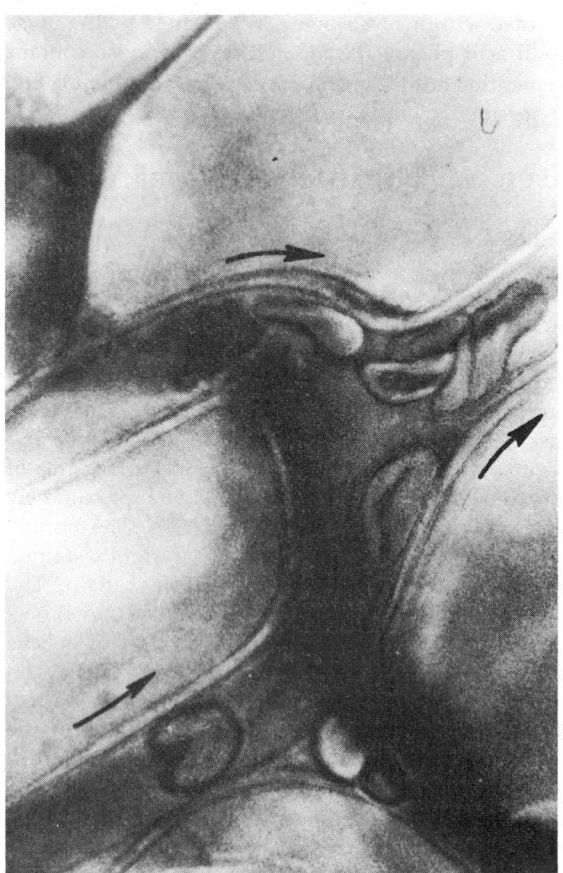

FIGURE 29-13 Dynamic alteration of red cell shape in the microcirculation. Reproduction of a single frame from microcinematographic study of blood flow in the capillary circulation. The direction of flow is indicated by arrows. ×1000. (Lessin, Klug, and Jensen [46], by permission.)

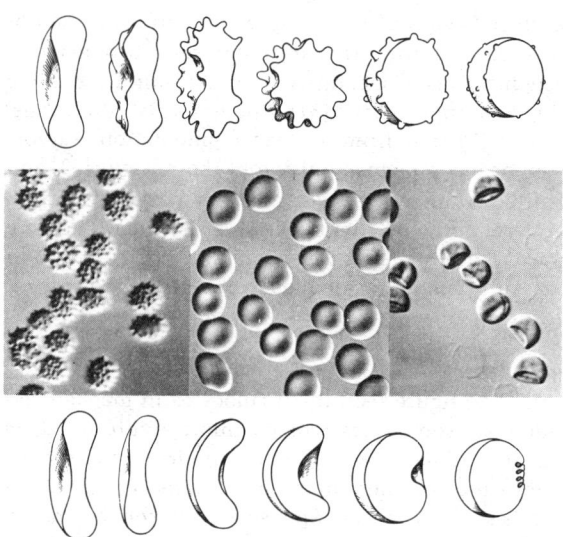

FIGURE 29-14 The discocyte-echinocyte and the discocyte-stomatocyte transformation. The upper panel schematically depicts the echinocytic transformation as induced by an anionic phenothiazine derivative. The lower panel schematically depicts stomatocyte formation as induced by a cationic phenothiazine derivative. The microscopic appearance in wet preparations, of stomatocytes (*left*), discocytes (*middle*), and echionocytes (*right*) is shown in the center panel.

ability of the red cell becomes the primary rheologic determinant of blood viscosity and flow [41]. At slow flow rates, red cell aggregation is seen in capillaries, where the cells assume a variety of irregular, ellipsoid, and hemispheric shapes (Fig. 29-13). They travel in aggregates of two to a dozen cells, forming rouleaux in regions of circulatory standstill or very slow flow [42]. Within large vessels, aggregation is disrupted by the increased shear forces. Pathologic conditions that alter the vascular channel may also influence the dynamics of red cell shape. In vessels narrowed or traversed by platelet clumps or fibrin strands, red cells will undergo cleavage and fragmentation as they are propelled across fibrin strands or platelet dendrites [43]. Red cells negotiating branching points of the microcirculation or bypassing a circulatory obstruction show striking deformation as they squeeze through openings as small as one-twentieth of the cell diameter.

NOMENCLATURE OF COMMON RED CELL SHAPES
Although in 1948 Ponder defined the red cell shape transitions identifiable with the light microscope [44],

the introduction of many new descriptive terms and attempts to associate specific cell alterations with disease states or mechanisms has led to much confusion. The advent of the scanning electron microscope, with its resolving power to 100 Å and great depth of resolution, provided an opportunity to define the shape transitions of the red cell in three-dimensional fashion. An international terminology using uniform Greek word stems has been introduced to describe cells on the basis of their three-dimensional morphology [45] (Table 29-2).

The *discocyte* is the red cell in its resting or steady state. It is a biconcave disc.

The most common transitional red cell form is the *echinocyte*, which passes through progressive stages from biconcave disc to crenated sphere. Intermediate spiculated stages (I to III) are shown in Fig. 29-14 [46]. Echinocyte III bears 10 to 30 short projections, equally spaced over the entire cell surface. It progresses from a spiculated disc to a sphere with a nearly complete loss of spicules. Under experimental conditions, the discocyte-echinocyte transformation can be produced and reversed very rapidly without loss of volume or membrane or hemolysis.

The *acanthocyte* is similar to the echinocyte when observed on a dried stained blood film. It is, however, easily distinguished from the echinocyte when viewed in the living state under the phase microscope or three-dimensionally with the scanning electron microscope. This cell has an irregular shape with 2 to 10 spicules of variable length, often appearing as clublike projections.

TABLE 29-2   Nomenclature of red cell shapes and associated disease states

Terminology (Greek meaning)	Old terms, synonyms	Description	Micrograph	Associated disease states
Discocyte (disc)	Biconcave disc	Biconcave disc form of RBC		
Echinocyte (I–III) (sea urchin)	"Burr cell," crenated cell, "berry cell"	Spiculated RBC with short, equally spaced projections over entire surface; progressing from the "crenated disc" (echinocyte I) to the crenated sphere (echinocyte IV—not shown) with nearly complete loss of spicules		Uremia Pyruvate kinase deficiency Low-potassium red cells Immediately posttransfusion with aged or metabolically depleted blood Carcinoma of stomach and bleeding peptic ulcers
Acanthocyte (spike)	"Spur cell," acanthoid cell	Irregularly spiculated RBC with projections of varying length and position		Abetalipoproteinemia Alcoholic liver disease Postsplenectomy state Malabsorptive states
Stomatocyte (I–III) (mouth)	Mouth cell, cup form, mushroom cap, uniconcave disc, microspherocyte	Bowl-shaped RBC with single concavity progressing from shallow bowl (I) to near sphere with small dimple (seen as mouth-shaped form in peripheral smear)		Hereditary spherocytosis Hereditary stomatocytosis Alcoholism, cirrhosis, obstructive liver disease Erythrocyte sodium-pump defect
Spherostomatocyte (sphere)	Spherocyte, prelytic sphere, microspherocyte	Spherical RBC with dense hemoglobin content; SEM shows a persistent minimal dimple		Hereditary spherocytosis (cells actually spherostomatocytes) Immune hemolytic anemia Posttransfusion Heinz body hemolytic anemia Water-dilution hemolysis Fragmentation hemolysis
Schizocyte (cut)	Schistocyte, helmet cell, fragmented cell	Split RBC, often showing half-disc shape with two or three pointed extremities; may be small, irregular fragment		Microangiopathic hemolytic anemia (TTP, DIC, vasculitis, glomerulonephritis, renal-graft rejection) Heart-valve hemolysis (prosthetic or pathologic valves) Severe burns March hemoglobinuria
Elliptocyte (oval)	Ovalocyte	Oval to elongated ellipsoid cell (with polarization of hemoglobin)		Hereditary elliptocytosis Thalassemia Iron deficiency Myelophthisic anemias Megaloblastic anemias
Drepanocyte (sickle)	Sickle cell	Cells containing polymerized hemoglobin S showing varying shapes from bipolar spiculated forms to holly-leaf and irregularly spiculated forms		Sickle cell disorders (SS, S-trait, SC, SD S-thalassemia, etc.) Hemoglobinopathy C-Harlem Hemoglobin Memphis/S

TABLE 29-2 Nomenclature of red cell shapes and associated disease states (*Continued*)

Terminology (Greek meaning)	Old terms, synonyms	Description	Micrograph	Associated disease states
Codocyte (bell)	Target cell	On SEM examination, these bell-shaped cells assume a target shape on dried films of blood		Obstructive liver disease Hemoglobinopathies (S, C) Thalassemia Iron deficiency Postsplenectomy state LCAT deficiency
Dacryocyte (tear)	Teardrop cell, tennis racket cell, poikilocyte	Cells with a single, elongated or pointed extremity		Myelofibrosis with myeloid metaplasia Myelophthisic anemias Thalassemias
Leptocyte (thin)	Thin cell, wafer cell	Thin, flat cell with hemoglobin at periphery		Thalassemia Obstructuve liver disease (± iron deficiency)
Keratocyte (horn)	Horn cell	Spicules result from ruptured vacuole; cell appears like half-moon or spindle		DIC or vascular prosthesis

The *stomatocyte*, the second most common transitional form of the red cell, is basically a bowl-shaped cell with a single concavity, or dimple. It derives its name from the fact that in stained smears the rim of the cell folds over to produce a "mouth-shaped" appearance, with a slot replacing the rounded central pallor of the biconcave disc. When seen in three dimensions, the stomatocyte has a stoma, or single concavity, on one surface. Under experimental conditions and in some human disease states, the cell is seen to progress from a shallow bowl to a near sphere with a small dimple, or stoma, through progressive stages referred to as stomatocyte I to III [1].

Notwithstanding the time-honored use of the word, *spherocytes* are not truly spherical cells. Their thickness is increased, so that the central concavity is greatly reduced and may be overlooked. On scanning electron microscopic examination, the spherocyte frequently bears a small dimple or irregular area, suggesting derivation from a stomatocyte. Experimentally, spherocytes may also be derived from echinocytes which, upon maximal crenation, lose their spicules and become spheres (spheroechinocytes), with small surface remnants of spicules.

Schizocyte refers to a red cell fragment which characteristically assumes a half-disc shape with two or three pointed extremities. Because it is produced by physical cleavage or fragmentation of the red cell, it is smaller than the normal discocyte and may display a variety of fragmented shapes.

The *elliptocyte* is basically an oval biconcave disc showing varying degrees of elliptical aberration from a slightly oval to an almost cylindrical, bipolar, elongated cell.

Drepanocyte is a term which describes the sickle cell and a variety of shapes induced by the polymerization of sickle hemoglobin. Such cells vary in shape from bipolar, spiculated forms to cells with long, irregular spicules and holly-leaf configurations.

The *codocyte*, the true circulating form of the target cell, is a bell-shaped cell which assumes a target configuration when dried on a slide in the preparation of a blood film [38]. On a flat surface, the codocyte tends to invert its concavity into a central projection into which hemoglobin redistributes to produce a central density (target) on the blood film, with a three-dimensional "Mexican hat" configuration.

Dacryocyte refers to cells characterized by a single elongated or pointed extremity. This cell shape has previously been referred to as a *teardrop cell* or *tail poikilocyte*.

The *leptocyte* is a wafer-thin cell which is generally large in diameter and displays a thin rim of hemoglobin at the periphery with a large area of central pallor. Such a cell reflects an increased surface/volume ratio.

Keratocytes are red cells with a relatively normal cell volume which have been deformed so that they present with two or more points.

Any shape variation of the red cell may be described precisely, if necessary, by the use of compound terms such as "spherostomatocyte." The addition of modifiers such as "micro-" to denote volume may add to descriptive precision, as in "microspherocyte" or "macroleptocyte."

PHYSIOLOGIC AND PATHOLOGIC TRANSITIONS OF RED CELL SHAPE

NORMAL RED CELL AGING

The shape of the reticulocyte changes continually because of internal movement. It has excess membrane and a convoluted region at the cell hilum from which nuclear ejection occurred. For a 2-day period, remodeling of cell shape results in shedding of membrane, water, and organelles unnecessary to the function of the mature red cell. This transition results in the generation of the discocyte, which during its 100- to 120-day course through the hazardous biophysical and biochemical circulatory environment loses its membrane by gradual, symmetric fragmentation [47]. It is eventually transformed to a dense cell with increased corpuscular hemoglobin concentration, metabolic depletion, and decreased deformability [48]. Changes in the shape and physical and chemical characteristics of the red cell mark its senescence and may play a role in its recognition as effete by the monocyte-macrophage system, particularly as it is sieved through the spleen [49] (Chap. 14).

THE DISCOCYTE-ECHINOCYTE-STOMATOCYTE EQUILIBRIUM

The discocyte-echinocyte-stomatocyte transformation is basic to red cell physiology and common to a variety of alterations of in vitro conditions and pathologic clinical states. Transformation of a discocyte to an echinocyte is the largely reversible development of spiculated red cells containing an average of 10 to 30 short, regularly spaced spicules of uniform height [1]. At early stages of transformation, echinocytes generated by extrinsic factors can usually be reversed by washing of the cells in fresh plasma. If the cells remain in the presence of the transforming agent, membrane and spicules are gradually lost until the cell becomes a spheroechinocyte that has lost the capacity to revert to the discocyte form. The discocyte-echinocyte transformation appears to occur without significant alteration of red cell volume. It may take place in milliseconds, with reversal occurring almost as rapidly. In contrast, the transformation of a discocyte to a stomatocyte consists of transition to a bowl-shaped, uniconcave cell, with progressive loss of the concavity until the cell becomes nearly spherical. The discocyte-echinocyte-stomatocyte transformations can be viewed as opposite phenomena and are produced by substances that act antagonistically [50,51]. Agents and conditions which can produce these changes are listed in Table 29-3. The formation of echinocytes may be due to an increase in the area of the outer leaflet of the lipid bilayer as compared with the inner leaflet. Conversely, the stomatocytic transformation may be due to an increase in the relative area of the inner leaflet [52], but the mechanism of such changes remains unknown [53]. The spherocytes of hereditary spherocytosis seem, in fact, to

TABLE 29-3   Agents and conditions which produce echinocytic and stomatocytic changes in erythrocytes

ECHINOCYTOGENIC AGENTS		
Fatty acids (oleate)	Dioxopyrazolidines:	Repetitive saline
Alkylsulfonates	Phenylbutazone	washing
Dihydroxybenzenes	Phenopyrazone	High (alkaline) pH
Substituted benzoates:	Indomethacin	"Alkaline glass effect"
Salicylate	Furosemide	ATP depletion
Gentisate	Barbiturates	
Ethacrynic acid	Phloretin	
2,4-Dinitrophenol	Phlorhizin	
Lysolecithin	Tannic acid	
(aged plasma)	Thiosemicarbazone	
Ethanol	Dipyridamole	
Butanol	Alkylpyridinium chlorides	
Bile acids	Uranyl salts	
STOMATOCYTOGENIC AGENTS		
Alkylammonium chlorides	Phenylamine	Low (acid) pH
Phenothiazines:	Verapamil	Cationic detergents
Chlorpromazine	Papaverine	
Local anesthetics:	Primaquine	
Cinchocaine	Chloroquine	
Tetracaine	Benzydamine	
Procaine	Colchicine	
Antihistamines:	Vincristine	
Pheniramine	Vinblastine	
Brompheniramine	LSD	
Bampine	Triton X	
Propranolol	Tween 80	
Hexobendine	Vitamin A or E	

SOURCE: Modified from Deuticke [50] and Weed and Chailley [51].

be stomatocytic forms displaying a progression of stomatocytic alterations from uniconcave discs to spherostomatocytes [54].

THE CODOCYTE

The codocyte, or target cell, is characterized by relative membrane excess due to either increased red cell surface area or decreased intracellular hemoglobin content. In patients with obstructive hepatic disease, an increased total membrane cholesterol content resulting from a decrease in lecithin cholesterol acetyl transferase (LCAT) activity with a significant increase in the cholesterol/phospholipid ratio [55] leads to an absolute increase in cell surface area. In iron-deficiency anemia and thalassemia, codocytes have relatively excess membrane because of the reduced quantity of intracellular hemoglobin.

THE ACANTHOCYTE [56]

Acanthocytes are generated from normal red blood cells under conditions that alter their membrane lipid content. The mechanism of acanthocyte formation is unknown. Once produced, the shape is irreversible. A markedly increased membrane cholesterol/lecithin ratio is common to acanthocytes from patients with hepatocellular liver disease and abetalipoproteinemia.

THE DISCOCYTE-DREPANOCYTE TRANSFORMATION

The sickle cell, or drepanocyte, displays a characteristic variation of form on stained blood films. Most commonly encountered is the fusiform cell in the shape of a crescent with two pointed extremities. Such cells persist in well-oxygenated preparations of sickle cell blood and have been referred to as *irreversibly sickled cells* [57]. In addition to these bipolar drepanocytes, examination of deoxygenated sickle cell preparations in the phase-contrast microscope reveals varied cell forms characterized by pointed extremities in various holly-leaf and poikilocytic configurations, many containing multiple spicules several microns in length. The spicules are quite fragile and easily evulse from the cell. As deoxygenation proceeds, the cell loses its flicker before shape change is evident [58]. This is followed by slight deformations at the border of the discocyte, with displacement of the hemoglobin to one region of the cell. After a few minutes of deoxygenation, characteristic spicules appear and the cell elongates and becomes rigid. Areas within the spicules and the cell center manifest varying degrees of birefringence, indicating an organization of hemoglobin molecules within the cell [59]. The hemoglobin S polymers are rods of 150 to 180 Å in diameter, which appear to be composed of monomolecular filaments of 60 to 70 Å in diameter intertwined into a six-stranded helix [60]. In partially sickled cells such polymers display random orientation, but as cells become more tightly sickled, polymeric rods of hemoglobin S undergo lateral alignment into paracrystals. The polymers of intracellular hemoglobin are long parallel rods aligned with the long axis of the cell or spicule. Upon reoxygenation, the sickled drepanocyte reverts to the dis-

cocyte form and in so doing loses membrane as the retraction of long spicules occurs, accompanied by the process of microspherulation and fragmentation [61]. The unsickling process also leads to the formation of micro-Heinz bodies that adhere to the internal surface of the red cell membrane and contribute to the increased membrane rigidity and cation leak [62]. With repetitive sickle-unsickle cycles, membrane damage accumulates until the cells become incapable of reversion to the biconcave disc shape even in the presence of high oxygen tension and in the absence of internal polymers. They thus become irreversibly sickled cells. The irreversibly sickled cell has a high hemoglobin concentration, increased cation permeability with decreased potassium and increased sodium content, and markedly decreased cellular deformability [57].

SHAPE ALTERATION IN HEINZ BODY–CONTAINING CELLS

Heinz bodies are particles of denatured proteins, primarily hemoglobin, which form as a consequence of chemical insult (Chap. 65), from hereditary defects of the hexosemonophosphate shunt (Chap. 58), or in the thalassemias (Chap. 50) or unstable hemoglobin syndromes (Chap. 61). The binding of denatured hemoglobin to the membrane leads to altered cation permeability with loss of water and potassium, sodium gain, and early ATP depletion [63]. Portions of the membrane damaged by Heinz body fixation may be lost from the cell by microspherulation or fragmentation, leading to spherocyte formation [64]. Heinz bodies appear as small rounded or angular inclusions measuring from 0.3 to 2 μm in diameter by light microscopy. They are easily seen in the phase-contrast or the interference microscope and strongly absorb Soret band (414 nm) light. Vital staining with crystal violet, new methylene blue, or brilliant cresyl blue easily demonstrates these inclusions. They persist after hemolysis and usually appear to be attached to the cell membrane. Heinz bodies are seen in films stained with May-Grunwald-Giemsa but are invisible in Wright's-stained films. In the electron microscope they appear as dense masses which begin to form in the center of the cell and then become attached to the red cell membrane [65]. Freeze-etch studies show Heinz bodies to occur as dense submembrane hemoglobin aggregates affixed to the internal membrane surface or as isolated large masses of denatured hemoglobin producing marked distortion of the overlying membrane [64]. The attachment of the Heinz body to the membrane causes a rearrangement of membrane-associated particles, with aggregation of these particles over the Heinz body regions, suggesting that denatured hemoglobin may be attached to membrane glycophorin and other proteins.

Electron microscopic studies have confirmed Heinz's original observations [66] of the inability of rigid Heinz bodies to traverse the interepithelial slits of the splenic sinus. These inclusion bodies are left behind in the perisinusoidal red pulp for phagocytosis by macrophages [67].

THE SCHIZOCYTE

Fibrin strands on the altered wall of blood vessels or damaged prostheses may arrest the progress of erythrocytes through the circulation. As the bloodstream pulls the red cell beyond its attachment, it is stretched and develops two portions connected by a thin band [43]. Often the red cell becomes free from its attachment, but sometimes it is fragmented into two pieces, often unequal in size. Alternatively, the inner surfaces of the membranes may become fused and the cell subsequently break into two pieces.

Another form of schizocyte has been designated a "bite" cell. It apparently arises when a substantial portion of the red cell is removed along with a Heinz body.

THE SPHEROCYTE

As described above, the normal red cell aging process results in progressive sphering of the red cell by symmetric membrane loss and decrease in surface/volume ratio. A variety of other conditions may accelerate this aging process or result in spherocyte formation by other mechanisms. Red cells sensitized with antibodies, complement, or immune complexes undergo loss of cholesterol and thus of surface area, displaying the increased osmotic fragility of the spherical cell [68]. Heinz body formation leads to membrane depletion by fragmentation, with spherocyte formation [67]. A spherogenic mechanism common to both Heinz body hemolytic anemias and immune hemolysis is partial phagocytosis of portions of the cell containing aggregates of denatured hemoglobin [67] and portions of the sensitized membrane [69], respectively. Another rare cause of intravascular spherocytosis is *water dilutional hemolysis*, occurring when distilled water is infused into the circulation or in drowning [70]. In patients with hereditary spherocytosis, a spectrum of abnormal cells varying from normal discocytes to stomatocytes, spherostomatocytes, and dense microspherocytes is seen [54]. The characteristic cell type is a spherocyte of low to normal corpuscular volume, high hemoglobin concentration, and significant reduction in surface/volume ratio (see Chap. 55).

CRYSTAL CELLS OF HEMOGLOBIN C DISEASE

In splenectomized patients with homozygous hemoglobin C disease, as many as 10 percent of the circulating cells may contain tetrahedral crystals [71]. In blood films of nonsplenectomized patients, crystal cells are rare. Crystal cells may be produced by dehydration of the red cells between slide and cover slip for a 24-h period [72]. Hypertonic dehydration of red cells in a 3% NaCl buffer for 4 to 12 h produces 50 to 75 percent crystal cells in the blood of patients with homozygous hemoglobin C disease; lower percentages occur in hemoglobin SC and other hemoglobin C variants. These crystals are birefringent and strongly absorb Soret light [73]. In cells not containing crystals the hemoglobin molecules appear to be partially aggregated in the cytoplasm. With dehydration, the first change is a central condensation of the hemoglobin, which on electron microscopy shows in-

creased molecular packing until a paracrystalline alignment can be seen at the cell periphery. As dehydration proceeds, the paracrystalline pattern can be seen to move into a more uniform crystalline arrangement within the cell. Molecular subunits in a tetragonal or hexagonal arrangement may be identified within the hemoglobin C crystals [73].

KERATOCYTES OR "HORN CELLS"

Keratocytes are erythrocytes with one or more notches. These cells differ from schizocytes in that their hemoglobin content is normal or only slightly lower than normal; they have not been formed by the bisection of a red cell. Rather they may arise when the opposing interior walls of a markedly deformed red cell become adherent. This forms a pseudovacuole, and the resulting cell has been referred to as a prekeratocyte. Within a short time the pseudovacuole ruptures, leaving a notch with bordering spicules or "horns."

ELLIPTOCYTES

In blood films of normal subjects, elliptical or oval cells usually constitute less than 1 percent of the erythrocytes. In most anemias the number can increase to as much as 10 percent. In hereditary elliptocytosis, up to 70 percent of the cells may be oval to elliptical (see Chap. 60). The form may vary from slight elliptical distortion to extreme pencil or cigar shapes in which hemoglobin appears concentrated at the extremities of the cell.

Hereditary ovalocytosis has been associated with a missing band 4.1 on SDS-gel electrophoresis [74,75].

OSMOTIC BEHAVIOR

The red cell behaves as an osmometer [44]. When placed in a hypertonic solution, it shrinks and becomes very flat; when placed in a hypotonic solution, it quickly swells, first becoming dome-shaped and then spherical. If the medium is sufficiently hypotonic, red cells swell to their critical hemolytic volume, holes greater than 100 Å in size appear [76], and the hemoglobin suddenly exits from the cell. Alternatively, a large tear may develop in the red cell membrane, allowing release of the contents. Following hemolysis (exit of the hemoglobin), the holes or tears close and the membrane resumes its original biconcave disc shape.

FRAGMENTATION

Heat can produce striking alterations of red cell form [77]. Temperatures in excess of 49°C cause sphering. Small spherical fragments bud from the cell surface, and the red cells become transformed into many small, round fragments. Such fragments are often seen after severe burns.

DEFORMABILITY

An important determinant of the survival of a red cell in the circulation is its deformability. The extent to which a red cell can be deformed can be estimated by measuring its ability to flow through a very narrow aperture such as the lumen of a micropipette or the holes in a nucleopore filter, or by observing its change of shape when exposed to a defined shear force. The latter measurements can be made either visually, using an instrument which has been designated a rheoscope [78], or by measuring the change in the defraction pattern produced when a laser beam traverses the erythrocytes, using an instrument which has been named an ektacytometer [79].

The deformability of red cells in such systems represents a complex of several different factors. Most important of these are the surface/volume ratio of the cell, the internal viscosity, and the deformability of the membrane itself. The membrane of the erythrocyte offers very little resistance to bending, but it cannot stretch. Thus, a perfectly spherical erythrocyte cannot be deformed without rupturing the membrane. The large amount of membrane redundancy present in the normal disc-shaped red cell permits extensive deformation of shape. However, the internal viscosity of the erythrocyte probably depends largely upon the interactions between closely packed hemoglobin molecules. To some extent, the contributions of these three factors to red cell deformability can be separated. Suspension of the red cells in a hypotonic medium hydrates the interior of the cell and markedly reduces cellular viscosity. In contrast, a decreased surface/volume ratio causes a marked decrease in deformability as cell volume is increased by suspension in hypotonic media [80]. Decreased membrane flexibility may be detected by measuring deformability at very low shear stresses [80].

By use of the shear force viscometer it has been calculated that the force necessary to deform a red cell is 3 to 60×10^{-8} dynes per square centimeter [81]. The normal red cell can easily traverse a $3\text{-}\mu m$ micropore filter at pressures encountered in capillaries and can enter a 2.5- to $3.0\text{-}\mu m$ capillary micropipette in characteristic form, trailing a small spherule of hemoglobin-filled membrane which eventually enters the pipette [81].

In man and other mammalian species, the splenic filter bed represents the primary microcirculatory test of red cell deformability (see Chap. 14). Red cells with decreased deformability, unable to negotiate the interendothelial slits of the splenic sinus, are phagocytized by nearby phagocytic cells [82]. Cells in passage through the interendothelial slits of the spleen, as well as those traversing micropore filters of $3\text{-}\mu m$ pipettes in vitro, may be transformed transiently or permanently into teardrop and other poikilocytic shapes [83].

References

1. Bessis, M.: *Living Blood Cells and Their Ultrastructure.* Springer-Verlag, Berlin, 1973.
2. Mohandas, N., and Prenant, M.: Three-dimensional model of bone marrow. *Blood* 51:633, 1978.
3. Kurland, J. I., Meyers, P. A., and Moore, M. A. S.: Synthesis and release of erythroid colony and burst-potentiating activities by purified populations of murine peritoneal macrophages. *J. Exp. Med.* 151:839, 1980.
4. Bessis, M., and Breton-Gorius, J.: Iron metabolism in the bone mar-
row as seen by electron microscopy: A critical review. *Blood* 19:635, 1962.
5. Richter, G. W., and Bessis, M.: Commentary on hemosiderin. *Blood* 25:370, 1965.
6. Bessis, M., and Breton-Gorius, J.: Ferritin and ferruginous micelles in normal erythroblasts and hypochromic hypersideremic anemias. *Blood* 14:423, 1959.
7. Grasso, J. A., Woodard, J. W., and Swift, H.: Cytochemical studies of nucleic acids and proteins in erythrocytic development. *Proc. Natl. Acad. Sci.* 50:134, 1963.
8. Rifkind, R. A., Danon, D., and Marks, P. A.: Alterations in polyribosomes during erythroid cell maturation. *J. Cell Biol.* 22:599, 1964.
9. Howell, H.: The life history of the formed elements of the blood, especially the red blood corpuscules. *J. Morphol.* 4:57 (pl. IV), 1891.
10. Bessis, M., Breton-Gorius, J., and Thiery, J. P.: Role possible de l'hemoglobine accompagnant le noyau des erythroblastes dans l'origine de la stercobiline éliminée précocement. *C. R. Acad. Sci. (Paris)* 252:2300, 1961.
11. Bessis, M., and Breton-Gorius, J.: Le reticulocyte: Coloration vitale et microscopic electronique. *Nouv. Rev. Fr. Hematol.* 4:77, 1964.
12. Simpson, C. F., and Kling, J. M.: The mechanism of mitochondrial extrusion from phenylhydrazine-induced reticulocytes in the circulating blood. *J. Cell Biol.* 36:103, 1968.
13. Isaacs, R.: The refractive granule red blood corpuscule: Its behavior and significance. *Anat. Rec.* 29:299, 1924–1925.
14. Yoshida, Y., Toda, A., Shirakawa, S., Wakisaka, G., and Uchino, H.: Proliferation of megaloblasts in pernicious anemia as observed from nucleic acid metabolism. *Blood* 31:292, 1968.
15. Limarzi, L. R.: The effect of arsenic (Fowler's solution) on erythropoiesis. *Am. J. Med. Sci.* 206:339, 1943.
16. Crookston, J. H., et al.: Hereditary erythroblastic multinuclearity associated with a positive acidified-serum test: A type of congenital dyserythropoietic anaemia. *Br. J. Haematol.* 17:11, 1969.
17. Wolff, J. A., and Von Hofe, F. H.: Familial erythroid multinuclearity. *Blood* 6:1274, 1951.
18. Saidi, P., Wallerstein, R. O., and Aggeler, P. M.: Effect of chloramphenicol on erythropoiesis. *J. Lab. Clin. Med.* 57:247, 1961.
19. McCurdy, P. R., Pierce, E., and Rath, C. E.: Abnormal bone marrow morphology in acute alcoholism. *N. Engl. J. Med.* 266:505, 1962.
20. Yeung, K. Y., Klug, P. P., Brown, M., and Lessin, L. S.: Mechanism of alcohol induced vacuolization in human bone marrow cells. *Blood* 42:998, 1973.
21. Mollin, D. L.: Sideroblasts and sideroblastic anaemia. *Br. J. Haematol.* 11:41, 1965.
22. Bessis, M., and Jensen, W. N.: Sideroblastic anaemia, mitochondria and erythroblastic iron. *Br. J. Haematol.* 11:49, 1965.
23. Bowman, W. D., Jr.: Abnormal (ringed) sideroblasts in various hematologic disorders. *Blood* 18:662, 1961.
24. Bessis, M., and Breton-Gorius, J.: Iron particles in normal erythroblasts and normal pathological erythrocytes. *J. Biophys. Biochem. Cytol.* 3:503, 1957.
25. Bessis, M., and Breton-Gorius, J.: Différences entre sideroblastes normaux et pathologiques: Étude au microscope électronique. *Nouv. Rev. Fr. Hematol.* 2:629, 1962.
26. Brecher, G., Haley, J. E., Prenant, M., and Bessis, M.: Macronormoblasts, macroreticulocytes and macrocytes. *Blood Cells* 1:547, 1975.
27. Reiff, R. H., Nutter, J. Y., Donohue, D. M., and Finch, C. A.: The relative number of marrow reticulocytes. *Am. J. Clin. Pathol.* 30:199, 1958.
28. Mel, H. C., Prenant, M., and Mohandas, N.: Reticulocyte motility and form: Studies on maturation and classification. *Blood* 49:1001, 1977.
29. Jolly, J.: Recherches sur la formation des globules rouges des mammiferes. *Arch. Anat. Microsc.* 9:133, 1907.
30. Discombe, G.: L'Origine des corps de Howell-Jolly et des anneaux de Cabot. *Sangre* 29:262, 1948.
31. Koyama, S.: Studies on Howell-Jolly body. *Acta Haematol. Jpn.* 23:20, 1960.
32. Rondanelli, E. G., Trenta, A., Magliulo, E., Vannini, V., and Gerna, G.: Morphogenese des micronoyauc supplementaires (pseudocorps de Jolly) dans le cellules erythropoietiques irradiées. *Acta Haematol.* 35:232, 1966.

33. Van Oye, E.: L'Origine des anneaux de Cabot. *Rev. Hematol. 9*:173, 1954.

34. Jensen, W. N., Moreno, G. D., and Bessis, M.: An electron microscopic description of basophilic stippling in red cells. *Blood 25*:933, 1965.

35. Ben-Bassat, I., Brok-Simoni, F., Kende, G., Holtzmann, F., and Ramot, B.: A family with red cell pyrimidine 5'-nucleotidase deficiency. *Blood 47*:919, 1976.

36. Pappenheimer, A. M., Thompson, W. P., Parker, D. D., and Smith, K. E.: Anaemia associated with unidentified erythrocytic inclusions. *Q. J. Med. Sci. 14*:75, 1945.

37. Kent, G., Minick, O. T., Volini, F. I., Orfei, E., and Madera-Orsini, F.: Autophagic vacuoles (lysosomes) in human erythrocytes: Their role in red cell maturation and the effect of the spleen on their disposal. *J. Cell Biol. 27*:51A, 1965.

38. Bessis, M.: *Blood Smears Reinterpreted,* translated by G. Brecher. Springer International, New York, 1977, p. 220.

39. Burton, A. L., Anderson, W. L., and Andrews, A. V.: Quantitative studies on the flicker phenomenon in the erythrocytes. *Blood, 32*:819, 1968.

40. Weinstein, R. S., Khodadad, J. K., and Steck, T. L.: Fine structure of the band 3 protein in human red cell membranes: Freeze-fracture studies. *J. Supramol. Struct. 8*:325, 1978.

41. Lessin, L. S., Kurantsin-Mills, J., and Weems, H. B.: Deformability of normal and sickle erythrocytes in a pressure-flow filtration system. *Blood Cells 3*:241, 1977.

42. Branemark, P.-I., and Bagge, U.: Intravascular rheology of erythrocytes in man. *Blood Cells 3*:11, 1977.

43. Bull, B. S., and Kuhn, I. N.: The production of schistocytes by fibrin strands (a scanning electron microscopy study). *Blood 35*:104, 1970.

44. Ponder, E.: *Hemolysis and Related Phenomena.* Grune & Stratton, New York, 1948.

45. Bessis, M., Weed, R., and LeBlond, P. (eds.): *Red Cell Shape: Physiology, Pathology, Ultrastructure.* Springer-Verlag, New York, 1973.

46. Lessin, L., Klug, P., and Jensen, W.: Clinical implications of red cell shape. *Adv. Intern. Med. 21*:451, 1976.

47. Weed, R. I., and Reed, C.: Membrane alterations and red cell destruction. *Am. J. Med. 41*:681, 1966.

48. Feo, C. J.: Influence de l'age et de la concentration en hemoglobine sur la deformabilite des erythrocytes. *Nouv. Rev. Fr. Hematol. 21 (Suppl.)*:60, 1979.

49. DeBoisfleury, A., and Mohandas, N.: Antibody-induced spherocytic anemia. II. Splenic passage and sequestration of red cells. *Blood Cells 3*:197, 1977.

50. Deuticke, B.: Transformation and restoration of biconcave shape of human erythrocytes by amphiphilic agents and changes of ionic environment. *Biochem. Biophys. Acta 163*:494, 1968.

51. Weed, R. I., and Chailley, B.: Calcium-pH interactions in the production of shape change in erythrocytes, in *Red Cell Shapes: Physiology, Pathology and Ultrastructure,* edited by M. C. Bessis, R. I. Weed, and P. F., LeBlond, Springer-Verlag, New York, 1973, p. 55.

52. Sheetz, M., and Singer, S. J.: Biological membranes as bilayer couples: A molecular mechanism of drug-erythrocyte interactions. *Proc. Natl. Acad. Sci. U.S.A. 71*:4457, 1974.

53. Conrad, M. J., and Singer, S. J.: Evidence for a large internal pressure in biological membranes. *Proc. Natl. Acad. Sci. U.S.A. 76*:5202, 1979.

54. LeBlond, P. F., DeBoisfleury, A., and Bessis, M.: La Forme des erythrocytes dan la spherocytose hereditaire. *Nouv. Rev. Fr. Hematol. 13*:873, 1973.

55. Cooper, R. A., and Jandl, J. H.: Bile salts and cholesterol in the pathogenesis of target cells in obstructive jaundice. *J. Clin. Invest. 47*:809, 1968.

56. Bessis, M.: *Blood Smears Reinterpreted,* translated by G. Brecher. Springer International, New York, 1977, p. 66.

57. Bertles, J. F., and Milner, P. F. A.: Irreversibly sickled erythrocytes: A consequence of the heterogeneous distribution of hemoglobin type in sickle cell anemia. *J. Clin. Invest. 47*:1731, 1968.

58. Padilla, F., Bromberg, P. A., and Jensen, W. N.: The sickle-unsickle cycle: A cause of cell fragmentation leading to permanently deformed cells. *Blood 41*:653, 1973.

59. Bessis, M., Normarski, G., Thiery, J. P., and Breton-Gorius, J.: Études sur la falciformation des globules rouges au microscope polarisant et au microscope electronique. *Rev. Hematol. 13*:249, 1958.

60. White, J. G.: The fine structure of sickled hemoglobin in situ. *Blood 31*:561, 1968.

61. Jensen, W. N., and Lessin, L. S.: Membrane alterations associated with hemoglobinopathies. *Semin. Hematol. 7*:409, 1970.

62. Lessin, L., and Wallas, C. P.: Biochemical basis for membrane alterations in the irreversibly sickled cell. *Blood 42*:978, 1973.

63. Jacob, H. S.: Mechanism of Heinz body formation and attachment to red cell membrane. *Semin. Hematol. 7*:341, 1970.

64. Lessin, L. S.: Membrane ultrastructure of normal sickled and Heinz body erythrocytes by freeze-etching, in *Red Cell Shape,* edited by M. Bessis, R. Weed, and P. LeBlond. Springer-Verlag, New York, 1973, p. 151.

65. Rifkind, R. A., and Danon, D.: Heinz body anemia: An ultrastructure study. I. Heinz body formation. *Blood 25*:885, 1965.

66. Heinz, R.: Über Blutdegeneration und Regeneration. *Beitr. Pathol. 29*:299, 1901.

67. Rifkind, R. A.: Heinz body anemia: An ultrastructural study. II. Red cell sequestration and destruction. *Blood 26*:433, 1965.

68. Cooper, R. A.: Loss of membrane components in pathogenesis of antibody induced spherocytosis. *J. Clin. Invest. 51*:16, 1972.

69. Rabinovitch, M.: Phagocytosis: The engulfment stage. *Semin. Hematol. 5*:134, 1968.

70. Landsteiner, E. K., and Finch, C. A.: Hemoglobinemia accompanying transurethral resection of the prostate. *N. Engl. J. Med. 237*:310, 1947.

71. Diggs, L. W., Kraus, A. P., et al.: Intraerythrocytic crystals in a white patient with hemoglobin C in absence of other types of hemoglobin. *Blood 9*:1172, 1954.

72. Charache, S., Conley, C. L., Waugh, D. F., Ugovetz, R. J., and Spurell, J. R.: Pathogenesis of hemolytic anemia in homozygous hemoglobin C disease. *J. Clin. Invest. 46*:1795, 1967.

73. Lessin, L. S., Jensen, W. N., and Ponder, E.: Molecular mechanism of hemolytic anemia in homozygous hemoglobin C disease. *J. Exp. Med. 130*:443, 1969.

74. Feo, C. J., Fischer, S., Piau, J. P., Grange, M. J., and Tchernia, G.: Premiere observation de l'absence d'une proteine de la membrane erythrocytaire (bande 4-1) dans un cas d'anémie elliptocytaire familiale. *Nouv. Rev. Fr. Hematol. 22*:315, 1980.

75. Alloisio, N., Dorleac, E., Girot, R., and Delaunay, J.: Analysis of the red cell membrane in a family with hereditary elliptocytosis—total or partial of protein 4.1. *Hum. Genet. 59*:68, 1981.

76. Seeman, P.: Transient holes in the erythrocyte membrane during hypotonic hemolysis and stable holes after hemolysis by saponin and lysolecithin. *J. Cell Biol. 32*:55, 1967.

77. Ham, T. H., Shen, S. C., Fleming, E. M., and Castle, W. B.: Studies on the destruction of red blood cells. *Blood 3*:373, 1948.

78. Schmid-Schönbein, H., v. Gosen, J., Heinich, L., Klose, H. J., and Volger, E.: A counter-rotating "rheoscope chamber" for the study of the microrheology of blood cell aggregation by microscopic observation and microphotometry. *Microvas. Res. 6*:366, 1973.

79. Bessis, M., Mohandas, N., and Feo, C.: Automated ektacytometry: A new method of measuring red cell deformability and red cell indices. *Blood Cells 6*:315, 1980.

80. Mohandas, N., Clark, M. R., Jacobs, M. S., and Shohet, S. B.: Analysis of factors regulating erythrocyte deformability. *J. Clin. Invest. 66*:563, 1980.

81. Holwill, M. E. J.: Deformation of erythrocytes by trypanosomes. *Exp. Cell Res. 37*:306, 1955.

82. Chien, S.: Principles and techniques for assessing erythrocyte deformability. *Blood Cells 3*:71, 1977.

83. Weiss, L., and Tavassoli, M.: Anatomical hazards to the passage of erythrocytes through the spleen. *Semin. Hematol. 7*:372, 1970.

Biochemistry and function of the erythrocyte

CHAPTER 30

Composition of the erythrocyte

ERNEST BEUTLER

The erythrocyte is a complex cell. The membrane is composed of lipids and proteins, and the interior of the cell contains metabolic machinery designed to maintain hemoglobin function. Each component of red blood cells may be expressed as a function of red cell volume, grams of hemoglobin, or square centimeters of cell surface. These expressions are usually interchangeable, but under certain circumstances each may have specific advantages. However, because disease may produce changes in the average red cell size, hemoglobin content, or surface area, the use of any of these measurements individually may, at times, be misleading. For convenience and uniformity, data in the accompanying tables (Tables 30-1 through 30-9) have been expressed in terms of cell constituent per milliliter of red cell and per gram of hemoglobin; in many instances this has required recalculation of published data. These recalculations assume a hematocrit value of 45 percent and 33 g Hb per deciliter red cells. The reference on which each value is based is the first number presented in the last column of each table. Where applicable, additional confirmatory references (second set of bracketed numbers) are shown. Additional data and references may be found elsewhere [91,92]. In some instances, only the percentage of the total of the type of constituent present is given. Data regarding activities of red cell enzymes are presented in Chap. 35.

TABLE 30-1   Human erythrocyte protein and water content

Component	RBC, mg/ml	Reference
Water	721 ± 17.3	[1,2]
Total protein	371	[2,3] [4,5]
Nonhemoglobin protein	9.2	[2,3]
Insoluble stroma protein	6.3	[3]
Protein from enzymes	2.9	[3]

TABLE 30-2   Human erythrocyte lipids

Lipid	mg/ml RBC	mg/g Hb	Reference
Total lipid	5.10 ± 0.51	15.45 ± 1.54	[6]
Phospholipid	2.98 ± 0.2	9.03 ± 0.61	[6]
Plasmalogen	0.56	1.69	[6]
Total cholesterol (unesterified)	1.20 ± 0.08	3.63 ± 0.21	[6,7]
Fatty acids	2.00	6.06	[6]
Other	0.92 ± 0.18	2.78 ± 0.54	[6]
FATTY ACIDS AS PERCENT OF TOTAL FATTY ACID			
Lauric (n-C_{12})		0.3	[8]
Myristic (n-C_{14})		0.8	[8]
Pentoenoic (n-C_{15})		0.3	[8]
Palmitoleic (16:1)		1.1	[8]
Palmitic (n-C_{16})		41.0	[8]

TABLE 30-2   Human erythrocyte lipids *(Continued)*

Lipid	mg/g Hb	Reference
FATTY ACIDS AS PERCENT OF TOTAL FATTY ACID		
(C_{17}) branched	0.3	[8]
(n-C_{17})	0.3	[8]
Linoleic	15.3	[8]
Oleic	18.9	[8]
Oleic isomer	Trace	[8]
Stearic (n-C_{18})	7.9	[8]
Arachidonic (20:4)	7.9	[8]
C_{22} unsaturated (a)	2.5	[8]
C_{22} unsaturated (b)	2.0	[8]
LONG-CHAIN ALDEHYDE AS PERCENT OF TOTAL ALDEHYDES		
n-C_{14}	Trace	[8]
Branched C_{15}	0.8	[8]
n-C_{15}	0.6	[8]
Highly branched C_{16}	Trace	[8]
C_{16} monoene	0.4	[8]
n-C_{16}	24.2	[8]
Highly branched C_{17}	1.7	[8]
Branched C_{17}	7.5	[8]
n-C_{17}	1.3	[8]
C_{18} monoene	6.0	[8]
Isomeric C_{18} monoene	2.8	[8]
n-C_{18}	42.5	[8]
Unknown C_{19}	2.9	[8]
Unknown C_{20}	3.1	[8]
Unknown C_{21}	5.6	[8]
FATTY ACIDS AS PERCENT OF TOTAL FATTY ACIDS OF NEUTRAL LIPIDS		
n-C_{10}	0–0.6	[9]
n-C_{12}	1.1–2.2	[9]
n-C_{14}	5.9–17.3	[9]
16:1	3.2–6.0	[9]
n-C_{16}	15.2–22.6	[9]
18.2 and 3	11.4–21.1	[9]
18:1	28.8–29.1	[9]
n-C_{18}	5.7–10.7	[9]
Unsaturated $C_{19}A$	Trace	[9]
Arachidonic	7.4–8.3	[9]
Polyunsaturated C_{20}	Trace	[9]

NOTE: The results are shown as mean ± standard deviation.

TABLE 30-3   Human erythrocyte phospholipids

Lipid	Amount	Reference
Total phospholipids	2.98 ± 0.20 mg/ml RBC	[6]
Cephalin	1.17 (0.38–1.91) mg/ml RBC	[6]
Ethanolamine phosphoglyceride	29% total phospholipid	[6]
Mean plasmalogen content	67% ethanolamine phosphoglyceride	[6]
Serine phosphoglyceride	10% total phospholipid	[6]
Mean plasmalogen content	8% of serine phosphoglyceride	[6]
Lecithin	0.32 (0.03–0.95) mg/ml	[10]
Sphingomyelin	0.12–1.13 mg/ml	[10]
Lysolecithin	1.8 ± 2% of total phospholipids	[11]

NOTE: The results are shown as mean ± standard deviation.

TABLE 30-4   Fatty acid compositions of erythrocyte phospholipids (mole percent)

Shorthand designation	Mixed phospholipids (methanol fraction)	Ethanolamine	Serine	Choline	Reference
12:0	0.1	...	...	0.1	[6]
14:0	0.5	0.2	Trace	0.5	[6]
15:0	0.3	0.2	Trace	0.3	[6]
16:0	28.8	18.9	7.1	33.0	[6]
cis $16:1^9$	0.7	0.6	0.4	0.1	[6]
17:0	0.4	Trace	0.3	0.5	[6]
18:0	15.1	8.0	41.6	11.7	[6]
cis $18:1^9$	18.3	21.6	7.9	17.9	[6]
trans $18:1^9$	2.9	3.6	5.1	2.7	[6]
cis, cis $18:2^{9,12}$	10.6	7.0	2.8	18.2	[6]
cis,cis,cis $18:3^{9,12,15}$	...	Trace	...	...	[6]
19:0 iso or ante-iso	Trace	0.2	...	...	[6]
20:0	0.1	...	Trace	0.2	[6]
$20:1^{11}$	0.2	0.3	Trace	0.2	[6]
$20:2^{8,11}$	...	Trace	...	...	[6]
$20:2^{11,14}$	0.1	0.1	...	0.2	[6]
$20:3^{5,8,11}$	1.6	1.0	2.1	1.6	[6]
$20:4^{5,8,11,14}$	10.8	21.9	19.7	5.0	[6]
$20:5^{5,8,11,14,17}$	0.8	1.4	0.3	0.5	[6]
Unknown (22:unsat.?)	1.7	4.7	2.2	0.3	[6]
22:5	0.7	0.8	0.9	1.7	[6]
22:5	2.3	2.3	2.0	2.7	[6]
$22:5^{7,10,13,16,19}$	1.0	...	...	1.0	[6]
$22:6^{4,7,10,13,16,19}$	2.1	3.9	4.2	1.1	[6]
14:0	Trace	...	...	0.8	[6]
Branched 15:0	2.8	2.6	5.5	...	[6]
15:0 iso or ante-iso	0.1	...	0.4	...	[6]
15:0	0.2	0.3	...	...	[6]
15:0	0.2	0.3	...	...	[6]
Unknown	0.1	...	1.6	1.0	[6]
cis $16:1^9$	Trace	...	...	0.2	[6]
16:0	18.2	15.9	17.1	49.8	[6]
Branched 17:0 unsat.?	0.9	1.5	...	...	[6]
Branched 17: unsat.?	2.4	3.0	...	...	[6]
Branched 17:0	5.8	5.5	11.3	6.9	[6]
17:0 iso or ante-iso	1.1	0.8	0.7	2.9	[6]
cis,cis $18:2^{9,12}$	Trace	...	1.4	...	[6]
cis $18:1^9$	6.8	7.0	5.4	5.3	[6]
18:1 isomer	13.2	18.8	10.5	7.7	[6]
18:0	37.1	40.4	32.3	19.2	[6]
Unknown	1.3	2.1	...	...	[6]

TABLE 30-5 Nucleotides

Compound	μmol/ml RBC	μmol/g Hb	Reference
Adenosine monophosphate	0.021 ± 0.003	0.062 ± 0.010	[12] [13–18]
Adenosine diphosphate	0.216 ± 0.036	0.635 ± 0.105	[12] [13–17]
Adenosine triphosphate	1.35 ± 0.035	4.05 ± 0.105	[19] [14–16,18,20–22]
Cyclic adenosine monophosphate	0.015 ± .0024	0.044 ± .007	[23]
Cyclic guanosine monophosphate	0.013 ± .0042	0.038 ± .012	[23]
Guanosine diphosphate	0.018 ± 0.005	0.054 ± 0.015	[14]
Guanosine triphosphate	0.052 ± 0.012	0.157 ± 0.036	[13] [14]
Inosine monophosphate	0.031 ± 0.005	0.0939 ± 0.015	[14] [18]
Nicotinamide adenine dinucleotide*	0.04	0.121	[20] [17,18]
Nicotinamide adenine dinucleotide phosphate*	0.031 ± 0.003	0.093 ± 0.009	[24] [14,17,18]
Total nucleotide	1.534 ± 0.033	4.648 ± 0.099	[25]
Uridine diphos- phoglucose	0.031 ± 0.005	0.094 ± 0.015	[14] [26]
Uridine diphosphate N-acetyl glucosamine	0.018	0.085	[26]

* Total (reduced + oxidized).
NOTE: The results are given as mean ± standard deviation.

TABLE 30-6 Amino acids and other nitrogen-containing compounds

Compound	μmol/ml RBC	μmol/g Hb	Reference
Alanine	0.275 ± 0.060	0.809 ± 0.176	[27] [28,29,30,31]
α-Amino butyrate	0.016 ± 0.009	0.047 ± 0.026	[27] [28,29]
Arginine	0.040 ± 0.013	0.118 ± 0.038	[27] [28,29,32,33]
Asparagine	0.121 ± 0.041	0.356 ± 0.121	[27] [28]
Aspartate	0.306 ± 0.081*	0.900 ± 0.238	[27]
Citrulline	0.036 ± 0.005*	0.106 ± 0.262	[27]
Glutamate	0.265 ± 0.089	0.779 ± 0.262	[27] [29]
Glutamine	0.624 ± 0.136	1.835 ± 0.400	[27] [29,34]
Glycine	0.347 ± 0.070	1.020 ± 0.206	[27] [28]
Histidine	0.086 ± 0.013	0.253 ± 0.038	[27] [29,33,35]
Isoleucine	0.058 ± 0.013	0.171 ± 0.038	[27] [28]
Leucine	0.110 ± 0.009	0.323 ± 0.026	[27] [28]
Lysine	0.139 ± 0.032	0.409 ± 0.094	[27] [29,33]
Methionine	0.015 ± 0.006	0.044 ± 0.018	[27] [29,33]
Ornithine	0.120 ± 0.028	0.353 ± 0.082	[27] [29]
Phenylalanine	0.049 ± 0.006	0.144 ± 0.018	[27] [28,29,33]
Proline	0.137 ± 0.035	0.403 ± 0.103	[27] [28,29]
Serine	0.149 ± 0.032	0.438 ± 0.094	[27] [28]
Taurine	0.349 ± 0.057	1.026 ± 0.168	[27]
Threonine	0.116 ± 0.022	0.341 ± 0.065	[27] [28,29]
Tyrosine	0.059 ± 0.009	0.173 ± 0.026	[27] [28,29,33]
Valine	0.171 ± 0.028	0.503 ± 0.082	[27] [28,29,33]
Creatine	0.33 ± 0.11	1.00 ± 0.33	[39]
Creatinine	0.159	0.481	[38]
Cystine	0.016 ± 0.002	0.048 ± 0.006	[33]
Ergothioneine	0.355 ± 0.112	1.076 ± 0.339	[29]
Ethanolamine	0.007	0.021	[29]
Glutathione oxidized	0.0036 ± 0.0014	0.011 ± 0.004	[37]
Glutathione reduced	2.234 ± 0.354	6.57 ± 1.04	[12]
Tryptophan	0.024 ± 0.004	0.073 ± 0.009	[29] [32,33,36]
Uric acid	0.113	0.342	[38] [29]
Urea	4.121 ± 0.420	12.487 ± 1.273	[29]

* Measured in samples treated with sodium sulfite before analysis.
NOTE: The results are given as mean ± standard deviation.

TABLE 30-7   Human erythrocyte coenzyme and vitamins

Compound	$\mu mol/ml$ RBC	$\mu mol/g$ Hb	Reference
Ascorbic acid	0.0199 ± 0.0023	0.059 ± 0.0069	[40–42]
Choline (free)	Trace	Trace	[43]
Cocarboxylase	0.00021	0.00065	[44]
Coenzyme A	0.0027	0.0083	[45]
Nicotinic acid	0.105	0.318	[46]
Pantothenic acid	0.001 ± 0.00028	0.0032 ± 0.00083	[47]
Nicotinamide adenine dinucleotide	See Table 30-3		
Nicotinamide adenine dinucleotide phosphate	See Table 30-3		
Pyridoxine (pyridoxal, pyridoxamine)	1×10^{-5}	3×10^{-5}	[48]
Riboflavin	0.00059 ± 0.00021	0.00179 ± 0.000064	[49]
Flavin adenine dinucleotide	0.000398 ± 0.000042	0.0012 ± 0.00012	[50]
Thiamine	0.00027	0.00082	[51]

NOTE: The results are given as mean $\pm$ standard deviation.

TABLE 30-8   Human erythrocyte carbohydrates, organic acids, and metabolites

Compound	$\mu mol/ml$ RBC	$\mu mol/g$ Hb	Reference
Deoxyribonucleic acid	Trace	Trace	[52]
Dihydroxyacetone phosphate	0.0094 ± 0.0028	0.028 ± 0.008	[12]
2,3-Diphosphoglycerate	4.171 ± 0.636	12.270 ± 1.870	[12] [16,20,53,54]
Fructose-6-P	0.0093 ± 0.002	0.027 ± 0.006	[12] [15,20,55]
Fructose-1,6-diphosphate	0.0019 ± 0.0006	0.005 ± 0.0018	[12] [15,16,20,55]
Glucuronic acid	Trace	Trace	[56]
Glucose	In equilibrium with plasma		[57] [58]
Glucose-6-P	0.0278 ± 0.0075	0.082 ± 0.022	[12] [15,20,55]
Glucose-1,6-diphosphate	0.18–0.30	0.54–0.91	[59] [15]
Glyceraldehyde-3-P	Not detectable		[12]
Lactic acid	0.932 ± 0.211		[12] [60,61]
Mannose-1,6-diphosphate	0.150	0.459	[59]
Octulose-1,8-diphosphate	Trace	Trace	[62]
Pyruvate	0.0533 ± 0.0215		[12]
3-Phosphoglycerate	0.0449 ± 0.0051	0.132 ± 0.015	[12] [20]
2-Phosphoglycerate	0.0073 ± 0.0025	0.0215 ± 0.0073	[12] [20]
Phosphoenol pyruvate	0.0122 ± 0.0022	0.036 ± 0.006	[12]
Ribonucleic acid	1.355 mg	4.10 mg	[63]
Ribose-1,5-diphosphate	<0.02	<0.06	[66]
Ribulose-5-P	Trace	Trace	[64]
Sedoheptulose-7-P	Trace	Trace	[64]
Sedoheptulose diphosphate	Trace	Trace	[65]
Sialic acid	0.825 ± 0.028	2.426 ± 0.082	[66]
Uridine diphospho-N-acetylglucosamine	See Table 30-3		
Uridine diphosphoglucose	See Table 30-3		

NOTE: The results are given as mean $\pm$ standard deviation.

TABLE 30-9 Human erythrocyte electrolytes

Electrolyte	$\mu mol/ml$ RBC	$\mu mol/g$ Hb	Reference
Aluminum	0.0026	0.0078	[68]
Bromide	0.1225	0.3711	[69]
Chloride	78	236.34	[70]
Calcium	0.0089 ± 0.0030	0.0262 ± 0.0088	[71] [72]
Copper	0.018	0.054	[73] [74]
Cobalt	0.0002	0.0006	[75]
Fluoride	0.0131	0.0396	[76]
Iodine, protein-bound	0.00043	0.0013	[77]
Lead	0.0027	0.0082	[68] [80]
Sodium	6.2 ± 0.8	18.2 ± 2.4	[78] [79,81]
Potassium	102.4 ± 3.9	301.1 ± 11.5	[78] [79,81–83]
Magnesium	3.06	9.272	[74] [82]
Chromium	0.0004	0.0012	[74]
Zinc	0.153	0.463	[74] [85,86]
Nickel	0.0009	0.0027	[74]
Silicon	Trace	Trace	[44]
Silver	Trace	Trace	[68]
Sulphur	0.0044	0.0133	[87]
Tin	0.0022	0.0066	[68]
Manganese	0.0034	0.0103	[68] [88]
Phosphorus (acid soluble):			
Total P	13.2	40.00	[89]
Inorganic P	0.466	1.412	[89]
Lipid P	3.840	11.63	[90]
Unidentified P	0.955	2.894	[89]

NOTE: The results are given as mean.

References

1. Nichols, G., and Nichols, N.: Electrolyte equilibria in erythrocytes during diabetic acidosis. *J. Clin. Invest.* 32:113, 1953.
2. Ponder, E.: *Hemolysis and Related Phenomena.* Grune & Stratton, New York, 1948.
3. Behrendt, H.: *Chemistry of Erythrocytes.* Charles C Thomas, Springfield, Ill., 1957.
4. Guidotti, G.: The protein of human erythrocyte membranes. I. Preparation, solubilization and partial characterization. *J. Biol. Chem.* 243:1985, 1968.
5. Silverman, L., and Glick, D.: Measurement of protein concentration by quantitative electron microscopy. *J. Cell Biol.* 40:773, 1969.
6. Farquhar, J. W.: Human erythrocyte phosphoglycerides. I. Quantification of plasmalogens, fatty acids and fatty aldehydes. *Biochim. Biophys. Acta* 60:80, 1962.
7. Brun, G. C.: Cholesterol content of the red blood cells in man. *Acta Med. Scand. (Suppl.)* 99:237, 1939.
8. Kates, M., Allison, A. C., and James, A. T.: Phosphatides of human blood cells and their role in spherocytosis. *Biochim. Biophys. Acta* 48:571, 1961.
9. James, A. T., Lovelock, J. E., and Webb, J. P. W.: The lipids of whole blood, I: Lipid biosynthesis in human blood in vitro. *Biochem. J.* 73:106, 1959.
10. Kirk, E.: The concentration of lecithin, cephalin, ether-insoluble phosphatide, and cerebrosides in plasma and red blood cells of normal adults. *J. Biol. Chem.* 123:637, 1938.
11. Phillips, G. B., and Roome, N. S.: Quantitative chromatographic analysis of the phospholipids of abnormal human red blood cells. *Proc. Soc. Exp. Biol. Med.* 109:360, 1962.
12. Beutler, E.: *Red Cell Metabolism,* 2d ed. Grune & Stratton, New York, 1975.
13. Bishop, C., Rankine, D. M., and Talbott, J. H.: The nucleotides in normal human blood. *J. Biol. Chem.* 234:1233, 1959.
14. Mandel, P., Chambon, P., Karon, H., Kulic, I., and Serter, M.: Nucleotides libres des globules rouges et des reticulocytes. *Folia Haematol. (Leipz.)* 78:525, 1961–1962.
15. Bartlett, G. R.: Human red cell glycolytic intermediates. *J. Biol. Chem.* 234:449, 1959.
16. Gerlach, E., Fleckenstein, A., and Gross, E.: Der Intermediäre Phosphat-Stoffwechsel des Menschen-Erythrocyten. *Pfluegers Arch.* 266:528, 1958.
17. Löhr, G. W., and Waller, H. D.: The biochemistry of erythrocyte aging. *Folia Haematol. (Leipz.)* 78:384, 1961.
18. Yoshikami, H., Nakao, M., Miyamoto, K., and Tachibana, M.: Phosphorus metabolism in human erythrocyte. II. Separation of acid-soluble phosphorus compounds incorporating p32 by column chromatography with ion exchange resin. *J. Biochem.* 47:635, 1960.
19. Beutler, E., and Mathai, C. K.: A comparison of normal red cell ATP levels as measured by the firefly system and the hexokinase system. *Blood* 30:311, 1967.
20. Minakami, S., Suzuki, C., Saito, T., and Yoshikawa, H.: Studies on erythrocyte glycolysis. I. Determination of the glycolytic intermediates in human erythrocytes. *J. Biochem.* 58:543, 1965.
21. De Luca, C., Stevenson, J. H., Jr., and Kaplan, E.: Simultaneous multiple-column chromatography: Its application to the separation of the adenine nucleotides of human erythrocytes. *Anal. Biochem.* 4:39, 1962.
22. Jorgensen, S.: Adenine nucleotides and oxypurines in stored donor blood. *Acta Pharmacol. Toxicol. (Kbh.)* 13:102, 1957.
23. Patterson, W. D., Hardman, J. G., and Sutherland, E. W.: A comparison of cyclic nucleotide levels in plasma and cells of rat and human blood. *Endocrinology* 95:325, 1974.
24. Kirkman, H. N., Gaetani, G. D., Clemons, E. H., and Mareni, C.: Red cell NADP+ and NADPH in glucose-6-phosphate dehydrogenase deficiency. *J. Clin. Invest.* 55:875, 1975.
25. Overgard-Hansen, K., and Jorgensen, S.: Determination and concentration of adenine nucleotides in human blood. *Scand. J. Clin. Lab. Invest.* 12:10, 1960.
26. Mills, G. C.: Uridine diphosphate glucose and uridine diphosphate

N-acetyle-glucosamine in erythrocytes. *Texas Rep. Biol. Med. 18:*446, 1960.

27. Hagenfeldt, L., and Arvidsson, A.: The distribution of amino acids between plasma and erythrocytes. *Clin. Chim. Acta 100:*133, 1980.

28. Leighton, W. P., Rosenblatt, S., and Chanley, J. D.: Determination of erythrocyte amino acids by gas chromatography. *J. Chromatog. 164:*427, 1979.

29. McMenamy, R. H., Lund, C. C., Neville, G. J., and Wallach, D. F. H.: Studies of unbound amino acid distributions in plasma, erythrocytes, leukocytes and urine of normal human subjects. *J. Clin. Invest. 39:*1675, 1960.

30. Gutman, G. E., and Alexander, B.: Studies of amino acid metabolism blood glycine and alanine and their relationship to the total amino acids in normal subjects. *J. Biol. Chem. 168:*527, 1947.

31. Wiss, O., and Kruger, R.: Der Einfluss Enteral und Parenteral Verabreichter Glucose auf den Alaningehalt des Blutes. *Helv. Chim. Acta 31:*1774, 1948.

32. Hier, S. W., and Bergeim, O.: The microbiological determination of certain free amino acids in human and dog plasma. *J. Biol. Chem. 163:*129, 1946.

33. Johnson, C. A., and Bergeim, O.: The distribution of free amino acids between erythrocytes and plasma in man. *J. Biol. Chem. 188:*833, 1951.

34. Iyer, G. Y. N.: Distribution of glutamine, glutamic acid, and aspartic acid between erythrocytes and plasma. *Ind. J. Med. Res. 44:*201, 1956.

35. von Euler, H., and Heller, L.: Free histidine in the blood serum of normal and Jensen sarcoma-bearing rats. *Arkiv Mineral Geol. 24A:*23, 1947.

36. Steele, B. F., Reynolds, M. S., and Baumann, C. A.: Amino acids in the blood and urine of human subjects ingesting different amounts of the same proteins. *J. Nutr. 40:*145, 1950.

37. Srivastava, S. K., and Beutler, E.: Oxidized glutathione levels in erythrocytes of glucose-6-phosphate-dehydrogenase-deficient subjects. *Lancet, 2:*23, 1968.

38. Jellinek, E. M., and Looney, J. M.: Statistics of some biochemical variables on healthy men in the age range of twenty to forty-five years. *J. Biol. Chem. 128:*621, 1939.

39. Griffiths, W. J., and Fitzpatrick, M.: The effect of age on the creatine in red cells. *Br. J. Haematol. 13:*175, 1967.

40. Barkhan, P., and Howard, A. N.: Distribution of ascorbic acid in normal and leukaemic human blood. *Biochem. J. 70:*163, 1958.

41. Butler, A. M., and Cushman, M.: Distribution of ascorbic acid in the blood and its nutritional significance. *J. Clin. Invest. 19:*459, 1940.

42. Sargent, F.: A study of the normal distribution of ascorbic acid between the red cells and plasma of human blood. *J. Biol. Chem. 171:*471, 1947.

43. Luecke, R., and Pearson, P. B.: The microbiological determination of free choline in plasma and urine. *J. Biol. Chem. 153:*259, 1944.

44. Beerstecher, E., and Spangler, S.: In *Blood and Other Body Fluids*, edited by D. S. Dittmer. Fed. Am. Soc. Exp. Biol., Washington, 1961, p. 108.

45. Kaplan, N. O., and Lipmann, F.: The assay of distribution of coenzyme A. *J. Biol. Chem. 174:*37, 1948.

46. Klein, J. R., Perlzweig, W. A., and Handler, P.: Determination of nicotinic acid in blood cells and plasma. *J. Biol. Chem. 145:*27, 1942.

47. Pearson, P. B.: The pantothenic acid content of the blood of mammalia. *J. Biol. Chem. 140:*423, 1941.

48. Marsch, M. E., Greenberg, L. D., and Rinehart, J. F.: The relationship between pyridoxine ingestion and transaminase activity. *J. Nutr. 56:*115, 1955.

49. Burch, H. B., Bessey, O. A., and Lowry, O. H.: Fluorometric measurements of riboflavin and its natural derivatives in small quantities of blood serum and cells. *J. Biol. Chem. 175:*457, 1948.

50. Beutler, E.: Glutathione reductase: Stimulation in normal subjects by riboflavin supplementation. *Science 165:*613, 1969.

51. Burch, H. B., Bessey, O. A., Love, R. H., and Lowry, O. H.: The determination of thiamine and thiamine phosphates in small quantities of blood and blood cells. *J. Biol. Chem. 198:*477, 1952.

52. Metais, P., and Mandel, P.: Teneur en acide desoxypentosenucleique des leucocytes chez l'homme normal et a l'état pathologique. *C. R. Soc. Biol. (Paris) 144:*277, 1950.

53. Eaton, J. W., and Brewer, G. J.: The relationship between red cell 2,3-diphosphoglycerate and levels of hemoglobin in the human. *Proc. Natl. Acad. Sci. U.S.A. 61:*756, 1968.

54. Denis, P., Cazor, J. L., Feret, J., Weisang, E., Lefrancois, R.: 2,3-Diphosphoglycerate red cell concentration changes during the menstrual cycle in women. *Biomedicine 25:*144, 1976.

55. Lionetti, F. J., McLellan, W. L., Fortier, N. L., and Foster, J. M.: Phosphate esters produced from inosine in human erythrocyte ghosts. *Arch. Biochem. 94:*7, 1961.

56. Deichmann, W. B., and Dierker, M.: The spectrophotometric estimation of hexuronates (expressed as glucuronic acid) in plasma or serum. *J. Biol. Chem. 163:*753, 1946.

57. Jung, C. Y.: Carrier-mediated glucose transport across human red cell membranes, edited by D. M. Surgenor, in *The Red Blood Cell*, 2d ed. Academic, New York, 1975, pp. 705–751.

58. Lacko, L., Wittke, B., Geck, P.: The temperature dependence of the exchange transport of glucose in human erythrocytes. *J. Cell. Physiol. 82:*213, 1973.

59. Bartlett, G. R.: Glucose and mannose diphosphates in the red blood cell. *Biochim. Biophys. Acta 156:*231, 1968.

60. Behrendt, H.: *Chemistry of Erythrocytes.* Charles C Thomas, Springfield, Ill., 1957.

61. Johnson, R. E., Edward, H. T., Dill, D. B., and Wilson, J. W.: Blood as a physicochemical system. XIII. The distribution of lactate. *J. Biol. Chem. 157:*461, 1945.

62. Bartlett, G. R., and Bucolo, G.: Octulose phosphates from the human red blood cell. *Biochem. Biophys. Res. Commun. 3:*474, 1960.

63. Mandel, P., and Métals, P.: Les Acides nucléiques du plasma sanguin chez l'homme. *C. R. Soc. Biol. 142:*241, 1948.

64. Bruns, F. H., Noltmann, E., and Vahlhaus, E.: Über den Stoffwechsel von Ribose-5-phosphat in Hämolysaten I. Aktivitätsmessung und Eigenschaften der Phosphoribose-isomerase. II. Der Pentosephosphat-Cyclus in roten Blutzellen. *Biochem. Z. 330:*483, 1958.

65. Bucolo, G., and Bartlett, G. R.: Sedoheptulose diphosphate formation by the human red blood cell. *Biochem. Biophys. Res. Commun. 3:*620, 1960.

66. Aminoff, D., Anderson, J., Dabich, L., and Gathmann, W. D.: Sialic acid content of erythrocytes in normal individuals and patients with certain hematologic disorders. *Am. J. Hematol. 9:*381, 1980.

67. Vanderheiden, B. S.: Ribosediphosphate in the human erythrocyte. *Biochem. Biophys. Res. Commun. 6:*117, 1961.

68. Kehoe, R. A., Cholak, J., and Story, R. V.: A spectrochemical study of the normal ranges of concentration of certain trace metals in biological materials. *J. Nutr. 19:*579, 1940.

69. Hunter, G.: Micro-determination of bromide in body fluids. *Biochem. J. 60:*261, 1955.

70. Bernstein, R. E.: Potassium and sodium balance in mammalian red cells. *Science 120:*459, 1954.

71. Bernard, J. F., Bournier, O., and Boivin, P.: Human erythrocyte calcium concentration in hemolytic anemia. *Biomedicine 23:*431, 1975.

72. O'Rear, E. A., Udden, M. M., McIntire, L. V., and Lynch, E. C.: Problems in measurement of erythrocyte calcium. *Am. J. Hematol. 11:*283, 1981.

73. Lahey, M. E., Gubler, C. J., Cartwright, G. E., and Wintrobe, M. M.: Studies on copper metabolism. VI. Blood copper in normal human subjects. *J. Clin. Invest. 32:*322, 1953.

74. Herring, W. B., Leavell, B. S., Paixao, L. M., and Yoe, J. H.: Trace metals in human plasma and red blood cells: A study of magnesium, chromium, nickel, copper and zinc. I. Observations of normal subjects. *Am. J. Clin. Nutr. 8:*846, 1960.

75. Heyrovsky, A.: The biochemistry of cobalt. III. Amounts of cobalt in plasma, erythrocytes, urine, and feces of normal subjects. *Cas. Lek. Cesk. 91:*680, 1952.

76. Largent, E. J., and Cholak, J.: In *Blood and Other Body Fluids*, edited by D. S. Dittmer. Fed. Am. Soc. Exp. Biol., Washington, 1961.

77. McClendon, J. F., and Foster, W. C.: Protein-bound iodine in erythrocytes and plasma and elsewhere. *Am. J. Med. Sci. 207:*549, 1944.

78. Fortes Mayer, K. D., and Starkey, B. J.: Simpler flame photometric determination of erythrocyte sodium and potassium: The reference range for apparently healthy adults. *Clin. Chem. 23(2):*275, 1977.

79. Bernard, J. F., Bournier, O., Renoux, M., Charron, D., and Boivin, P.: Unclassified haemolytic anaemia with splenomegaly and erythro-

cyte cation abnormalities: A disease of the spleen? *Scand. J. Haematol.* 17:231, 1976.

80. Jensovsky, L., and Roth, Z.: Der normale Bleigehalt im menschlichen Blute. *Naturwissenschaften* 48:382, 1961.

81. Overman, R. R., and Davis, A. K.: The application of flame photometry to sodium and potassium determinations in biological fluids. *J. Biol. Chem.* 168:641, 1947.

82. McCance, R. A., and Widdowson, E. M.: The effect of development, anaemia, and undernutrition on the composition of the erythrocytes. *Clin. Sci.* 15:409, 1956.

83. Hald, P. M.: Notes on the determination and distribution of sodium and potassium in cells and serum of normal human blood. *J. Biol. Chem.* 163:429, 1946.

84. Streef, G. M.: Sodium and calcium content of erythrocytes. *J. Biol. Chem.* 129:661, 1939.

85. Vallee, B. L., and Gibson, J. G.: The zinc content of normal human whole blood, plasma, leucocytes, and erythrocytes. *J. Biol. Chem.* 176:445, 1948.

86. Zak, B., Nalbandian, R. M., Williams, L. A., and Cohen, J.: Determination of human erythrocyte zinc: Hemoglobin ratios. *Clin. Chim. Acta* 7:634, 1962.

87. Reed, L., and Denis, W.: On the distribution of the non-protein sulfur of the blood between serum and corpuscles. *J. Biol. Chem.* 73:623, 1927.

88. Miller, D. O., and Yoe, J. H.: Spectrophotometric determination of manganese in human plasma and red cells with benzohydroxamic acid. *Anal. Chim. Acta* 26:224, 1962.

89. Bartlett, G. R., Savage, E., Hughes, L., and Marlow, A. A.: Carbohydrate intermediates and related cofactors in the human erythrocyte. *J. Appl. Physiol.* 6:51, 1953–1954.

90. Ferranti, F., and Giannetti, O.: The microdetermination of phosphorus (inorganic, acid-soluble, lipoid and total) in the blood and excretions. *Diagn. Tec. Lab. Napoli Riv. Mens.* 4:664, 1933.

91. Friedeman, H., and Rapoport, S. M.: Enzymes of the red cell: A critical catalogue, edited by H. Yoshikawa and S. M. Rapoport, in *Cellular and Molecular Biology of Erythrocytes.* University Park Press, Baltimore, 1974, p. 181.

92. Pennell, R. B.: Comparison of normal human red cells, edited by D. M. Surgenor, in *The Red Blood Cell.* Academic, New York, 1974, p. 93.

CHAPTER *31*

Synthesis of heme

BARRY H. KAPLAN

The prosthetic groups of the hemoglobin molecule are the four heme moieties, one bound to each globin chain. Heme is also the prosthetic group of other proteins, such as myoglobin, catalase, peroxidase, and tryptophan pyrrolase. It is not surprising, therefore, that heme is synthesized by almost all organisms and in most tissues thus far studied.

Structure of heme

As shown in Fig. 31-1, heme is composed of an iron atom coordinated to four pyrrole rings through their substituent nitrogen atoms. Thus heme is a tetrapyrrole,

a group of compounds which includes chlorophyll and vitamin B_{12}. The β positions of the pyrrole rings of heme are fully substituted with a total of eight residues, four methyl groups, two propionate residues, and two vinyl groups. The pyrrole rings are joined to one another by methene bridges. These features characterize the porphyrins, and heme is classified as a metalloporphyrin. Reviews of the chemical properties of the porphyrins [1] and of their nomenclature [2] are available.

The methene bridges and pyrrole rings form an extended conjugated ring system, i.e., a sequence of alternating single and double bonds, involving 11 double bonds, which results in a high degree of resonance stabilization of the molecule. Conjugated double bonds readily absorb visible light and are responsible for the red color of hemoglobin. The absorption spectrum of oxyhemoglobin has two peaks in the visible region, at 576 nm and 540 nm, which are typical for metalloporphyrins, and an intense absorption peak at 412 to 415 nm, which is the Soret band found in tetrapyrroles with the conjugated ring structure [3].

In addition to its coordination with the pyrrole rings, the iron atom in heme may bind two other ligands, one above and one below the plane of the porphyrin ring. In hemoglobin, one of these ligands is a histidine residue of the globin chain which is firmly bound to the iron atom (see Chap. 37). The other coordination position of iron is unoccupied in deoxyhemoglobin and protected from oxidation by the nonpolar environment provided by the amino acid residues surrounding the heme moiety [4]. Oxygen readily binds to this coordination position, resulting in the formation of oxyhemoglobin.

The iron in hemoglobin must be in the ferrous state to permit this reversible combination with oxygen. If the iron is oxidized to the ferric form, hemoglobin is

FIGURE 31-1 Structure of heme.

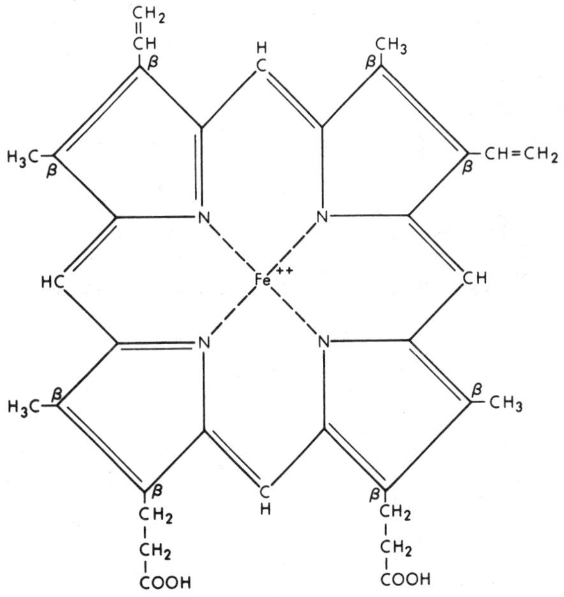

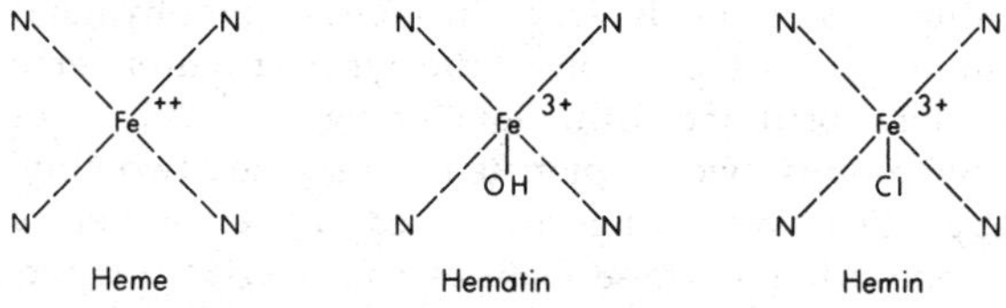

FIGURE 31-2 Forms of iron protoporphyrin.

converted to methemoglobin, which cannot serve as an oxygen carrier (see Chap. 81). Resolution of heme from globin in an aqueous medium results in immediate oxidation of the iron atom and the formation of hematin or, in the presence of chloride ion, the formation of hemin [5] (Fig. 31-2).

Pathway of heme synthesis

An important feature of the heme synthetic pathway (Fig. 31-3) is the intracellular localization of some steps in the reaction sequence. In higher organisms, the formation of δ-aminolevulinic acid (ALA) and the conver-

FIGURE 31-3 Pathway of heme synthesis. Pr = propionate; Ac = acetate; Me = methyl; and Vi = vinyl groups.

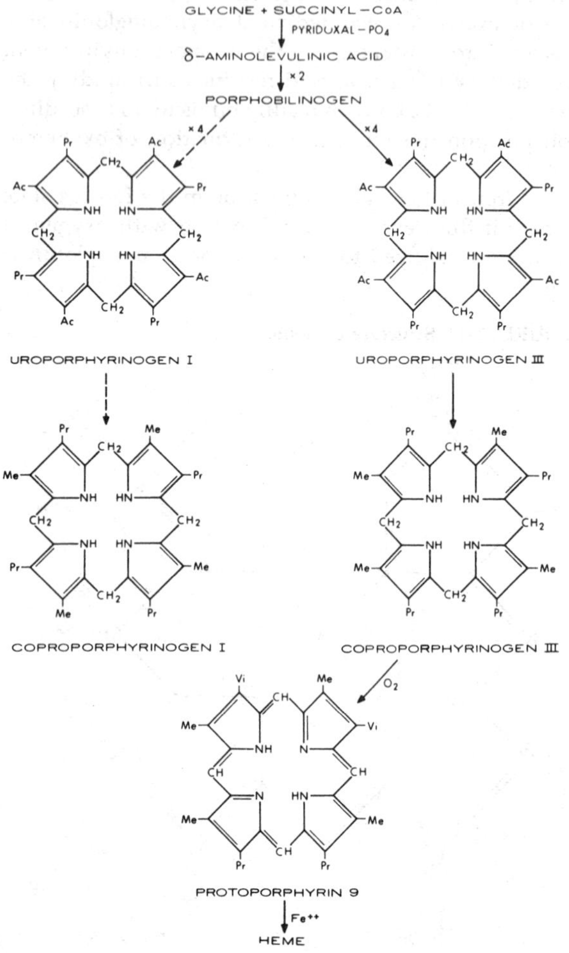

sion of coproporphyrinogen to protoporphyrin and heme take place in the particular cell fraction, whereas the reaction sequence from ALA to coproporphyrinogen is carried out in the soluble portion of the cell [6]. The particulate enzymes are contained within the mitochondria; heme synthesis does not occur in mature mammalian erythrocytes which lack mitochondria.

FORMATION OF δ-AMINOLEVULINIC ACID (ALA)
ALA is synthesized from succinyl CoA and glycine in the presence of pyridoxal phosphate and the enzyme δ-aminolevulinic acid synthase (ALA-S) [7,8].

Succinyl CoA is produced by the following reactions [4]:

$$\alpha\text{-Ketoglutarate} + CoA + NAD^+ \rightarrow$$
$$\text{succinyl CoA} + CO_2 + NADH + H^+ \tag{1}$$
$$\text{Succinate} + \text{nucleoside triphosphate} + CoA \rightleftharpoons$$
$$\text{succinyl CoA} + \text{nucleoside diphosphate} + P_i \tag{2}$$
$$\text{Succinate} + \text{acetoacetyl CoA} \rightleftharpoons$$
$$\text{succinyl CoA} + \text{acetoacetate} \tag{3}$$
$$\text{Methylmalonyl CoA} \rightleftharpoons \text{succinyl CoA} \tag{4}$$

Reaction 1 is part of the tricarboxylic acid (TCA) cycle, and intermediates of the TCA cycle are rapidly incorporated into ALA. In a guinea pig liver mitochondrial preparation, 85 percent of the succinyl CoA used for ALA synthesis is derived from reaction 1 with α-ketoglutarate, isocitrate, or citrate as substrates, but 60 percent is derived from reaction 2 with succinate as substrate [9]. Although methylmalonyl CoA can be incorporated into ALA via reaction 4, this reaction is not a major source of succinyl CoA for ALA synthesis [10].

The role of pyridoxal phosphate in heme synthesis was first suggested by studies in pyridoxine-deficient animals [11]. Subsequently the requirement for pyridoxal phosphate in ALA formation has been amply confirmed in cell-free systems.

ALA-S has been highly purified from bacterial sources [12,13], but not from mammalian tissue. The enzyme has a pronounced tendency to aggregate, and M_r has been reported to vary from 70,000 to 650,000 daltons. Purification and properties of the enzyme have been described [14–16].

Under normal conditions, ALA-S is localized within the particulate cell fraction, apparently in the matrix of mitochondria [17] A substantial increase of the amount of the enzyme in liver cytosol results from treatment of rats with allylisopropylacetamide, a drug which causes an overproduction of porphyrin precursors in these animals (see below). Cytoplasmic ALA-S has been purified to homogeneity from this source [18]. This enzyme appears to consist of two identical subunits with a subunit weight of 51,000 daltons. The K_m for succinyl CoA is 11 μM and the K_m for glycine is 7.5 mM. In embryonic chick liver [15], the enzyme appears to be synthesized on polyribosomes as a polypeptide of 75,000 daltons, which is then processed into mitochondria as an enzyme with a M_r of 65,000 daltons.

Glycine is activated by combining with pyridoxal

phosphate in Schiff's base linkage. This combination permits the formation of a stabilized carbanion of glycine for reaction with succinyl CoA [7] (Fig. 31-4).

An intermediate in the formation of ALA, α-amino-β-ketoadipic acid, has been postulated [19,20]. The mono- and diethyl esters of this proposed intermediate are rapidly incorporated into ALA. However, α-amino-β-ketoadipic acid is unstable and undergoes decarboxylation to ALA. It has been shown that the evolution of CO_2 parallels the formation of ALA [21], a finding that suggests that either no intermediate is present or, if any is present, it is extremely short-lived.

Although most studies indicate that in mammalian cells the reaction catalyzed by ALA-S is the major mechanism for the formation of ALA, in plants, ALA is formed from a five-carbon precursor derived from glutamic acid or α-ketoglutaric acid [22]. An enzyme capable of carrying out this alternative synthesis of ALA has been purified from bovine liver mitochondria [23]. The physiologic role of this alternative pathway is uncertain.

The important role of the formation of ALA in the control of heme biosynthesis will be discussed below.

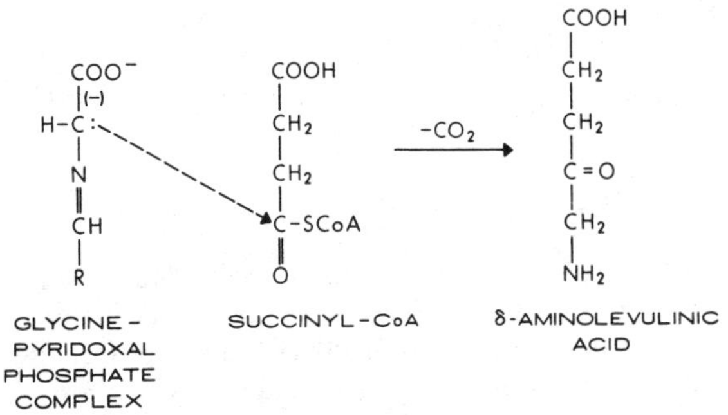

FORMATION OF PORPHOBILINOGEN

The combination of 2 mol ALA to form porphobilinogen (PBG) is catalyzed by ALA dehydratase. Investigations of the dehydratase have utilized preparations from a wide variety of sources ranging from *Rh. spheroides* [24] and *P. shermanii* [25] to liver [26] and erythrocytes [27,28] of higher organisms, including man. The enzyme requires a thiol reductant for activity, and the dehydratase from mammalian liver [29], rabbit reticulocytes [27], and soy bean callus [30] is inhibited by EDTA. Bovine liver ALA-D has been shown to require zinc ion for activity [31]; it has a M_r of about 285,000 daltons and is comprised of eight identical subunits [32]. It is exquisitely sensitive to inhibition by lead. Detailed studies of the mechanism of formation of PBG have been carried out with highly purified enzyme from *Rh. spheroides* [33]. The enzyme binds ALA through a Schiff's base intermediate which permits combination with a second molecule of ALA to form PBG (Fig. 31-5).

TETRAPYRROLE INTERMEDIATES

The structures of the tetrapyrrole intermediates of heme biosynthesis are shown in Fig. 31-3. The pyrrole rings in uroporphyrinogen and coproporphyrinogen are joined by methylene bridges in contrast to the methene bridges in protoporphyrin and heme. The porphyrinogens therefore lack an extended conjugated ring system and are colorless.

Uroporphyrin and coproporphyrin are formed by oxidation in the excreta and body tissues of the methylene bridges of the corresponding porphyrinogens to methene bridges. These compounds and protoporphyrin are colored, have typical porphyrin spectra, and fluoresce when exposed to ultraviolet irradiation. It had

FIGURE 31-4 Proposed mechanism of reaction for ALA synthesis. R represents the part of the pyridoxal phosphate molecule not included in the figure. (From B. H. Kaplan, The control of heme synthesis, in *Regulation of Hematopoiesis*, edited by A. S. Gordon. Appleton Century Crofts, New York, 1970, vol. 1, p. 677. Reprinted by permission of the editor and publisher.)

been thought that the porphyrins were intermediates in heme synthesis, but addition of uroporphyrin to systems capable of forming heme does not stimulate heme synthesis [34]. It became apparent that the porphyrinogens are the true intermediates and that uroporphyrin and coproporphyrin are by-products of heme formation.

Isomers of the porphyrins and porphyrinogens are classified according to the location of the groups in the β positions of the pyrrole rings. Of the four possible isomers of uroporphyrinogen and coproporphyrinogen, only types I and III shown in Fig. 31-3 are found in significant amounts in nature. Similarly, of 15 isomers of protoporphyrin, only type 9 is a natural compound. Uroporphyrinogen I can be converted to uroporphyrinogen III or to coproporphyrinogen I; its possible role as an intermediate in heme synthesis is discussed below. Coproporphyrinogen I appears to be a nonfunctional side product.

FIGURE 31-5 Mechanism for PBG formation. $E-NH_2$ represents ALA dehydrase with an amine group from an amino acid at the active site of the enzyme. (From B. H. Kaplan, The control of heme synthesis, in *Regulation of Hematopoiesis*, edited by A. S. Gordon. Appleton Century Crofts, New York, 1970, vol. 1, p. 677. Reprinted by permission of the editor and publisher.)

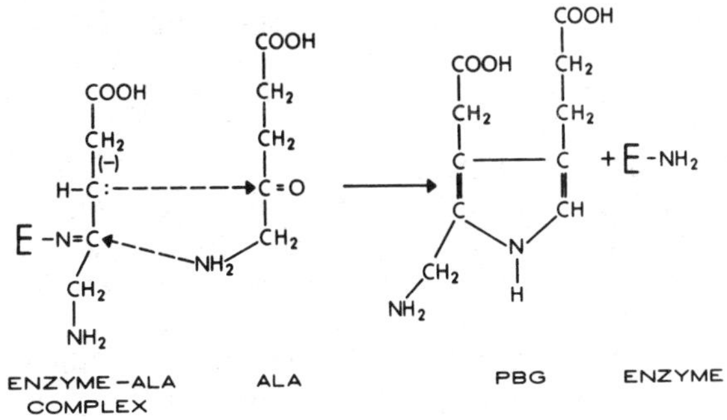

FORMATION OF UROPORPHYRINOGEN III

The conversion of 4 mol PBG to 1 mol uroporphyrinogen III requires two enzymes. *Uroporphyrinogen I synthase* (PBG deaminase) catalyzes reaction 5:

$$4 \text{ PBG} \xrightarrow{\text{PBG deaminase}} \text{uroporphyrinogen I} + 4\text{NH}_3 \qquad (5)$$

The presence of this enzyme is easily demonstrated because of its heat stability. When preparations which catalyze the overall reaction PBG to uroporphyrinogen III are heated, interfering enzymatic activities are destroyed but PBG deaminase remains intact. Inhibition of this enzyme with ammonium ion or hydroxylamine has no effect on the consumption of PBG, but a linear polypyrrole is formed instead of uroporphyrinogen I [35].

The second enzyme involved in the conversion of PBG to uroporphyrinogen III is *uroporphyrinogen III cosynthase* (uroporphyrinogen isomerase). This enzyme acts in the presence of uroporphyrinogen I synthase to convert PBG to uroporphyrinogen III:

$$4 \text{ PBG} \xrightarrow[\text{uroporphyrinogen isomerase}]{\text{PBG deaminase} +} \text{uroporphyrinogen III}$$

$$+ 4\text{NH}_3 \qquad (6)$$

The addition of varying quantities of the isomerase to the deaminase has no effect on the consumption of PBG or the total amount of uroporphyrinogen formed, but the amount of isomerase added determines the percentage of type III isomer synthesized. In the absence of the deaminase, uroporphyrinogen isomerase reacts with neither PBG nor uroporphyrinogen I [36].

The activity of PBG deaminase is quite low in liver [37], but it is higher in reticulocytes [38]. The deaminase has been purified from several sources [39]. Apparently homogeneous preparations from human [40,41] and bovine [41] erythrocytes separate into five or six isoenzymes on analytical polyacrylamide disc gel electrophoresis. The isoenzymes may represent different enzyme-substrate (none, mono-, di-, tri-, and tetrapyrrole) complexes; all have a M_r of about 40,000 daltons.

Uroporphyrinogen isomerase is unstable but has been partially purified [42,43]. The M_r of the isomerase from wheat germ is 62,000 daltons [43]. When the deaminase, the isomerase, and PBG are incubated together, a complex is formed. Since free mono-, di-, and tripyrroles compete poorly with PBG, it has been suggested that the conversion of PBG to uroporphyrinogen III occurs on the surface of the deaminase-isomerase complex, without free intermediates [42].

UROPORPHYRINOGEN DECARBOXYLASE

Uroporphyrinogen III is converted to coproporphyrinogen III by successive decarboxylation of its four acetate groups. Intermediates with seven, six, and five carboxyl groups can be demonstrated but do not accumulate to a significant extent under normal conditions. The overall reaction is carried out by a single enzyme,

uroporphyrinogen decarboxylase, which has been partially purified from rabbit [44] and chicken [45] erythrocytes and from mouse spleen [46]. The enzyme is stimulated by EDTA, GSH, and anaerobic conditions. It is inhibited by iron [47]. The decarboxylase is active with uroporphyrinogen III and with the subsequent intermediates with five to seven carboxyl groups. It will convert uroporphyrinogen I to coproporphyrinogen I, but at a much slower rate than the type III isomers. The porphyrin derivates do not act as substrates for the enzyme.

The stereochemistry of uroporphyrinogen III and related intermediates is maintained during the successive decarboxylations [48], an observation that suggests that the reactions take place on the surface of the enzyme, without free intermediates.

SYNTHESIS OF PROTOPORPHYRIN 9

Oxidative decarboxylation of two propionate groups to vinyl residues and oxidation of the methylene bridges to methene bridges result in the conversion of coproporphyrinogen III to protoporphyrin 9. This process occurs within mitochondria and requires molecular oxygen.

Coproporphyrinogen oxidase is the enzyme which catalyzes the formation of the vinyl groups. It has been purified to homogeneity from bovine liver [49]. It has a M_r of 74,000 daltons and is rich in aromatic amino acid residues. Neither sulfhydryl agents nor metal chelators have a significant effect on enzymic activity, and no metal is present in the purified enzyme. The oxidase is highly specific for coproporphyrinogen III; neither coproporphyrinogen I nor coproporphyrin III is a substrate for the enzyme.

Oxidative decarboxylation appears to require hydroxylation of the propionate residues to form β-hydroxypropionate groups, which are then decarboxylated and dehydrated. The propionate residue in the 2 position is oxidized to a vinyl group before the 4 position is altered [50]. The 2-vinylporphyrinogen harderoporphyrinogen was first isolated from the harderian gland of the rat; normally, it is not a free intermediate but remains bound to the enzyme [48].

Oxidation of the methylene bridges of protoporphyrinogen can occur spontaneously, but the process in vivo has been shown to be stereospecific [50], a finding that could result only from an enzymatic reaction. Such an enzyme, protoporphyrinogen oxidase, has been solubilized from yeast mitochondria and shown to be separate from coproporphyrinogen oxidase [51].

FERROCHELATASE

In the final step of the heme synthetic pathway, ferrous iron is inserted into protoporphyrin to form heme. Although this reaction occurs spontaneously at a slow rate under physiologic conditions, it is clear that the reaction is catalyzed in vivo by the enzyme ferrochelatase [52]. Ferrochelatase is a mitochondrial enzyme, most likely associated with the inner mitochondrial membrane [53]. Ferric ion is not utilized by the enzyme, and only dicarboxylic acid porphyrins can serve as substrates [54].

The enzymatic activity has been shown to be influenced by phospholipids. Extraction of an acetone-dried powder of chicken erythrocyte stroma with 0.4 M KCl results in a preparation with little enzymatic activity and only a small amount of lipid. Activity can be restored by the addition of egg-yolk phospholipids or crude phospholipid from chicken erythrocyte stroma. The effect of various phospholipids depends on the conditions employed in the enzymatic assay. In the absence of cholate, lysophospholipids are the most effective activators; when cholate is present, choline-containing phospholipids are most effective [55]. These observations may be important for eventual understanding of the role of membrane structure in heme synthesis.

Because of its particular nature and apparent instability, ferrochelatase has not been purified. The enzyme can be solubilized from bacterial cytoplasmic membranes with detergents [56], and sonication of mammalian hepatic mitochondria yields activity if copper ions are added [57].

The assay of ferrochelatase is fraught with difficulties. In addition to the impurity and instability of the enzyme, protoporphyrin 9, the substrate for the enzyme, is only sparingly soluble at physiologic pH; the reaction must be carried out under strictly anaerobic conditions or in the presence of thiols or other reducing agents to prevent oxidation of ferrous iron to ferric iron, and the product of the reaction, heme, is unstable under the assay conditions [58]. Some of these assay problems can be bypassed by using analogs or protoporphyrin 9, such as mesoporphyrin 9 [59], but in view of the difficulties with the assay, conclusions based on changes in ferrochelatase activity must be considered tentative.

Control of heme synthesis

Many of the steps in the pathway for heme synthesis involve decarboxylation or aromatization, which are strongly favored thermodynamically [60]. In addition, the formation of heme is different from its degradation, in which bilirubin is formed. These data suggest that the reaction sequence for heme biosynthesis is unidirectional and irreversible.

Control mechanisms for unidirectional biosynthetic pathways are commonly located at the first enzymatic step uniquely concerned with the synthesis of the end product [61]. Glycine and succinyl CoA are involved in numerous pathways in addition to heme biosynthesis; ALA, however, is utilized predominantly for heme formation. Although the δ carbon of ALA is incorporated into purines [62], this incorporation does not appear to be quantitatively significant under normal circumstances. ALA formation is, therefore, a likely site

for the control of heme synthesis, and, at least in the liver, there is no doubt that the synthesis of ALA is the single most important control point in the biosynthetic pathway. Data to be discussed below suggest that control in erythroid cells may be somewhat different. An excellent review of the regulation of heme synthesis is available [63].

ALA-S activity in normal liver is significantly lower than that of any other enzyme involved in heme synthesis, except for PBG deaminase, which has only slightly higher activity than ALA-S. The level of ALA-S activity in liver is reduced still further by the administration of heme. Three mechanisms for this effect of heme have been suggested: one is direct feedback inhibition of heme on ALA-S in mitochondria, the second is interference with the processing of the enzyme after its synthesis, and the third is the repression of the synthesis of new molecules of ALA-S.

Direct inhibition of partially purified ALA-S by heme has been demonstrated [14,16], but the concentration of heme required to inhibit the enzyme significantly is quite high—about 10 μM. This concentration is much higher than the level of free heme in the cell. It is possible that because ferrochelatase is in mitochondria close to ALA-S, high concentrations of heme can accumulate locally and inhibit the enzyme, but it seems unlikely that direct inhibition of ALA-S by heme plays an important role in control mechanisms.

ALA-S must be incorporated into mitochondria in order to function physiologically, since the enzyme requires succinyl CoA; however, the enzyme is synthesized on polyribosomes in the cytoplasm and then must be transported from the cytoplasm into mitochondria [15,18]. Heme can be shown to inhibit the transport process [18]. Whether this effect of heme is important physiologically remains to be established.

ALA-S turns over rapidly in liver, with an estimated half-life as short as 35 min [18]. This property allows for rapid changes in ALA-S activity by stimulating or inhibiting the rate of enzyme synthesis. Heme appears to act mainly by repressing the synthesis of ALA-S, while an increased demand for heme induces an increase in enzyme synthesis.

Data to support this hypothesis come from studies of the porphyrias, a group of disorders characterized by the accumulation and/or excretion of precursors of heme in amounts far in excess of normal. The porphyrias are discussed in detail in Chap. 76.

Patients with acute intermittent porphyria excrete increased quantities of PBG and ALA in the urine as a result of reduced levels of PBG deaminase [64]. Levels of hepatic ALA-S are markedly increased in these patients [65]. Drugs, the most notable of which are the barbiturates, and other stimuli associated with an increased requirement for heme synthesis exacerbate acute intermittent porphyria; the intravenous administration of hematin results in decreased ALA and PBG excretion [66] and clinical improvement [67]. Extensive studies of the mechanism of these effects have been car-

TABLE 31-1   Normal levels of porphyrins and porphyrin precursors

	Urine, $\mu g/24\ h$	Feces, $\mu g/g\ dry\ wt$	RBC, $\mu g/dl$	Plasma, $\mu g/dl$
ALA	2300 ± 400	—	31 ± 11	$5.6 + 0.02$
PBG	1500 ± 200	—	—	—
Uroporphyrin	<60	2.2 ± 0.9	Trace	—
Coproporphyrin	120 ± 50	20 ± 10	2.0 ± 1.5	—
Protoporphyrin	Trace	30 ± 20	25 ± 10	—
Total porphyrin	—	<150	—	0.35 ± 0.2

ried out on animal models of the porphyrias [68]. Experimental porphyria can be induced in animals by the administration of drugs such as those known to exacerbate acute intermittent porphyria. Similar biochemical changes can also be produced in chick embryo liver cells [69].

Studies in these model systems are in agreement with the findings in acute intermittent porphyria. Increased activity of ALA-S is uniformly observed, and the administration of heme blocks the development of the disorder. That the increased activity of ALA-S is due to induction rather than the absence of feedback inhibition is suggested by the observation that compounds which inhibit protein synthesis prevent increased ALA formation [70,71]. Immunologic studies have now confirmed that there is an increase in the number of ALA-S molecules present in experimental porphyria [72]. The amount of protein precipitable by a monospecific antibody against ALA-S in porphyric chick embryo liver correlates precisely with enzyme activity. As the activity rises in response to drugs which cause porphyria, so too does the amount of immunoprecipitable protein. The increase in ALA-S activity in this system can be prevented by hemin at a concentration of 0.1 μM, a concentration 100 times lower than the level required to inhibit the enzyme directly [73].

The activity of ALA-S in liver cells is regulated by the level of heme available for feedback control of enzyme synthesis. Any factor that decreases this level will result in increased ALA-S activity and cause or exacerbate experimental porphyria and acute intermittent porphyria. 2-Allyl-2-isopropyl-acetamide (AIA), for example, destroys free heme and heme in microsomal cytochromes, while 3,5-dicarboxy-1,4-dihydrocollidine (DDC) inhibits ferrochelatase; these compounds are the most potent inducers of experimental porphyria [63]. Certain steroids, glucose, cAMP, and other compounds have an effect on the induction of ALA-S in experimental porphyria and acute intermittent porphyria [68]. It is likely that these effects are indirect and result from changes in the utilization or synthesis of heme.

Control mechanisms for heme synthesis in erythroid cells may be different from those in liver cells. While heme levels in liver must change markedly in response to alterations in metabolic state, particularly drug administration, heme synthesis in erythroid cells is at a very high level, and the amount of heme required per red cell does not change significantly under normal conditions.

One system for studying the control of heme synthesis in erythroid cells is murine Friend virus transformed erythroleukemia cells. These cells can be made to synthesize heme when treated with dimethylsulfoxide (DMSO), but it has been shown that ALA-S has already been induced significantly before the increase in heme synthesis occurs [74]. This observation suggests that ALA is not rate-limiting in this system. Ferrochelatase has been identified as an alternate control site [75].

There remains considerable uncertainty as to the mechanism of regulation of heme synthesis in erythroid cells. It is clearly different quantitatively and probably qualitatively from that in hepatic tissue.

NATURAL OCCURRENCE OF HEME PRECURSORS

The normal levels for the intermediates of heme synthesis shown in Table 31-1 are a consensus drawn from several studies [76–78]. Porphyrinogens are customarily converted to the corresponding porphyrins and included in the determination of porphyrin levels. Considerable variation in the determinations from different laboratories has resulted from differences in methods of collection, storage, and assay and differences in the populations studied. Newer methods of studying porphyrins and porphyrin precursors have evolved [79,80] and are gradually supplanting the older methods.

Urinary excretion of ALA is normally less than 5 mg per day; marked increases have been observed in lead poisoning (80 to 150 mg per day) and in porphyria (see Chap. 76). Patients with hereditary tyrosinemia have significantly elevated urinary excretion of ALA (6 to 150 times normal) [81]. Plasma levels of ALA are increased in porphyria and lead poisoning [78]. PBG excretion in the urine, normally less than 3 mg per day, is markedly increased only in porphyria.

Urinary coproporphyrin concentration is somewhat higher in men than in women and is about 60 percent type III. Increased coproporphyrin excretion occurs in cirrhosis and other forms of liver disease (200 to 800 μg per day); nonalcoholic cirrhosis is accompanied by increased proportions of the type I isomer, but increased type III is observed in alcoholic cirrhosis [82]. Marked elevation of coproporphyrin excretion occurs in lead poisoning (1000 to 4000 μg per day) and porphyria. Significant increases are also observed in patients with anemia of varying causes (200 to 400 μg per day) and in toxicity due to gold, arsenic, benzene, carbon tetrachloride, barbiturates, etc. [83]. In lead poisoning and in anemias secondary to decreased production of erythrocytes, such as iron-deficiency anemia, most of the coproporphyrin excreted is type III; coproporphyrin I predominates in hemolytic anemia [82]. In the Dubin-Johnson syndrome, urinary excretion of coproporphyrin I increases and excretion of coproporphyrin III decreases. The change in the ratio of these isomers has been used for genetic studies of this syndrome [84].

Urinary uroporphyrin normally is predominantly type I. Excretion of uroporphyrin increases in porphyria, liver disease, and lead poisoning.

Fecal porphyrins are increased as a result of bleeding into the gastrointestinal tract, hemolysis, and in certain forms of porphyria. Coproporphyrin in the feces is 70 to 90 percent type I, even in lead poisoning when the urinary coproporphyrin is type III [85].

Erythrocyte protoporphyrin and coproporphyrin levels generally are proportional to the reticulocyte count, except that the level of protoporphyrin is elevated in iron deficiency anemia (150 to 1200 μg/dl), and erythrocyte porphyrins are significantly increased in lead poisoning and porphyria [83].

In children, urinary excretion of PBG and coproporphyrin, when corrected for body weight, is equivalent to adult levels, but ALA excretion is decreased [86,87]. Ninety percent of the coproporphyrin excreted in the urine is the type III isomer. Erythrocyte coproporphyrin and protoporphyrin levels are increased in childhood [87].

References

1. Adler, A. D. (ed.): The chemical and physical behavior of porphyrin compounds and related structures. *Ann. N.Y. Acad. Sci.* 206:5, 1973.
2. Merritt, J. E., and Leoning, K. L.: IUPAC-IUB Joint Commission on Biochemical Nomenclature, nomenclature of tetrapyrroles. *Eur. J. Biochem.* 108:1, 1980.
3. Lemberg, P., and Legge, J. W.: *Hematin Compounds and Bile Pigments.* Interscience, New York, 1949, chap. 6, p. 228.
4. Perutz, M. F.: The haemoglobin molecule, The Croonian Lecture, 1968. *Proc. R. Soc. Lond.* [Biol.] 113:1969.
5. Lascelles, J.: *Tetrapyrrole Biosynthesis and Its Regulation.* Benjamin, New York, 1964.
6. Sano, S., and Granick, S.: Mitochondrial coproporphyrinogen oxidase and protoporphyrin formation. *J. Biol. Chem.* 236:1173, 1961.
7. Kikuchi, G., Kumar, A., Talmage, P., and Shemin, D.: The enzymatic synthesis of δ-aminolevulinic acid. *J. Biol. Chem.* 233:1214, 1958.
8. Gibson, K. D., Laver, W. G., and Neuberger, A.: Initial stages in the biosynthesis of porphyrins. II. The formation of δμ-aminolaevulic acid from glycine and succinyl-coenzyme A by particles from chicken erythrocytes. *Biochem. J.* 70:71, 1958.
9. Granick, S., and Urata, G.: Increase in activity of δ-aminolevulinic acid synthetase in liver mitochondria induced by feeding of 3,5-dicarbethoxy-1,4-dihydrocollidine. *J. Biol. Chem.* 238:821, 1963.
10. Nakao, K., and Takaku, F.: Utilization of propionate for heme synthesis. *J. Lab. Clin. Med.* 72:958, 1968.
11. Schulman, M. P., and Richert, D. A.: Heme synthesis in vitamin B_6 and pantothenic acid deficiencies. *J. Biol. Chem.* 226:181, 1957.
12. Warnick, G. R., and Burnham, B. F.: Regulation of porphyrin biosynthesis: Purification and characterization of δ-aminolevulinic acid synthetase. *J. Biol. Chem.* 246:6880, 1971.
13. Fanica-Gaignier, M., and Clement-Metral, J.: δ-Aminolevulinic acid synthetase of *Rhodopseudomonas spheroides. Eur. J. Biochem.* 40:13, 1973.
14. Whiting, M. J., and Granick, S.: δ-Aminolevulinic acid synthetase

from chick embryo liver mitochondria. I. Purification and some properties. *J. Biol. Chem.* 251:1340, 1976.
15. Ades, I. Z., and Harpe, K. G.: Biogenesis of mitochondrial proteins. Identification of the mature and precursor forms of the subunit of δ-aminolevulinate synthetase from embryonic chick liver. *J. Biol. Chem.* 256:9329, 1981.
16. Kaplan, B. H.: δ-Aminolevulinic acid synthetase from the particulate fraction of liver of porphyric rats. *Biochim. Biophys. Acta* 235:381, 1971.
17. McKay, R., Druyan, R., Getz, G. S., and Rabinowitz, M.: Intramitochondrial localization of δ-aminolaevulate synthetase and ferrochelatase in rat liver. *Biochem. J.* 114:455, 1969.
18. Kikuchi, G., and Hayashi, N.: Regulation by heme of synthesis and intracellular translocation of δ-aminolevulinate synthase in the liver. *Mol. Cell Biochem.* 37:27, 1981.
19. Shemin, D., Russell, C. S., and Abramsky, T.: The succinate-glycine cycle. I. The mechanism of pyrrole synthesis. *J. Biol. Chem.* 215:613, 1955.
20. Neuberger, A., and Scott, J. J.: Aminolaevulinic acid and porphyrin biosynthesis. *Nature* 172:1093, 1953.
21. Shemin, D., Kikuchi, G., and Abramsky, T.: Enzymic studies of the synthesis of some intermediates in porphyrin biogenesis, in *Les Maladies du metabolisme des porphyrines: 2e Colloque International de Biologie* de Saclay. Presses Universitaires de France, Paris, 1962, p. 173.
22. Beale, S. I. and Castelfranco, P. A.: The biosynthesis of δ-aminolevulinic acid in higher plants. II. Formation of ^{14}C-δ-aminolevulinic acid from labeled precursors in greening plant tissues. *Plant Physiol.* 53:297, 1974.
23. Varticovski, L., Kushner, J. P., and Burnham, B. F.: Biosynthesis of porphyrin precursors: Kinetic studies on mammalian L-alanine: γ,δ-dioxovaleric acid aminotransferase. *Eur. J. Biochem.* 12:739, 1980.
24. Nandi, D. L., Baker-Cohen, K. F., and Shemin, D.: δ-Aminolevulinic acid dehydratase of *Rhodopseudomonas spheroides.* I. Isolation and properties. *J. Biol. Chem.* 243:1224, 1968.
25. Menon, I. A., and Shemin, D.: Concurrent decrease of enzymic activities concerned with the synthesis of coenzyme B_{12} and of propionic acid in propionibacteria. *Arch Biochem.* 121:304, 1967.
26. Batlle, A. M. del C., Ferramola, A. M., and Grinstein, M. V.: Purification and general properties of δ-aminolaevulate dehydratase from cow liver. *Biochem. J.* 104:244, 1967.
27. Granick, S., and Mauzerall, D.: Porphyrin biosynthesis in erythrocytes. II. Enzymes converting δ-aminolevulinic acid to coproporphyrinogen. *J. Biol. Chem.* 232:1119, 1958.
28. Vergnano, C., Cartasegna, C., and Bonsignore, D.: Regolazione allosterica della attività δ-aminolevulinco-deidratasica eritrocitaria: Nota I. *Boll. Soc. Ital, Biol. Sper.* 44:692, 1968.
29. Gibson, K. D., Neuberger, A., and Scott, J. J.: The purification and properties of δ-aminolaevulic acid dehydrase. *Biochem. J.* 61:618, 1955.
30. Tigier, H. A., Batlle, A. M. del C., and Locascio, G.: Porphyrin biosynthesis in soybean callus tissue system: Isolation, purification and general properties of δ-aminolaevulinate dehydratase. *Biochim. Biophys. Acta* 151:300, 1968.
31. Cheh, A., and Neilands, J. B.: Zinc, an essential metal ion for beef liver δ-aminolevulinate dehydratase. *Biochem. Biophys. Res. Commun.* 55:1060, 1973.
32. Shemin, D.: Porphyrin synthesis: Some particular approaches. *Ann. N.Y. Acad. Sci.* 244:348, 1975.
33. Nandi, D. L., and Shemin, D.: δ-Aminolevulinic acid dehydratase of *Rhodopseudomonas spheroides.* III. Mechanism of porphobilinogen synthesis. *J. Biol. Chem.* 243:1236, 1968.
34. Neve, R. A., Labbe, R. F., and Aldrich, R. A.: Reduced uroporphyrin III in the biosynthesis of heme. *J. Am. Chem. Soc.* 78:691, 1956.
35. Bogorad, L.: Enzymatic mechanisms in porphyrin synthesis: Possible enzymatic blocks in porphyrias. *Ann. N.Y. Acad. Sci.* 104:676, 1963.
36. Bogorad, L.: The enzymatic synthesis of porphyrins from porphobilinogen. II. Uroporphyrin III. *J. Biol. Chem.* 233:510, 1958.
37. Miyagi, K., Cardinal, R., Bassenmaier, I., and Watson, C. J.: The serum porphobilinogen and hepatic porphobilinogen deaminase in normal and porphyric individuals. *J. Lab. Clin. Med.* 78:683, 1971.
38. Sassa, S., and Bernstein, S. E.: Levels of δ-aminolevulinate dehy-

dratase, uroporphyrinogen I synthetase, and protoporphyrin IX in erythrocytes from anemic mutant mice. *Proc. Natl. Acad. Sci. U.S.A.* 74:1181, 1977.

39. Batlle, A. M. del C., and Rossetti, M. V.: Review-enzymic polymerization of porphobilinogen into uroporphyrinogens. *Int. J. Biochem.* 8:251, 1977.

40. Anderson, P. M., and Desnick, R. J.: Purification and properties of uroporphyrinogen I synthase from human erythrocytes, identification of stable enzyme-substrate intermediates. *J. Biol. Chem.* 255:1993, 1980.

41. Miyagi, K., Petryka, Z. J., Kaneshima, M., Kawakami, J., and Pierach, C. A.: Uroporphyrinogen I synthase isoenzymes from bovine and human erythrocytes. *Int. J. Biochem.* 12:769, 1980.

42. Frydman, B., Frydman, R. B., Valasinas, A., Levy, S., and Feinstein, G.: The mechanism of uroporphyrinogen biosynthesis. *Ann. N.Y. Acad. Sci.* 244:371, 1975.

43. Higuchi, M. and Bogorad, L.: The purification and properties of uroporphyrinogen I synthase and uroporphyrinogen III cosynthase: Interactions between the enzymes. *Ann. N.Y. Acad. Sci.* 244:401, 1975.

44. Mauzerall, D., and Granick, S.: Porphyrin biosynthesis in erythrocytes. III. Uroporphyrinogen and its decarboxylase. *J. Biol. Chem.* 232:1141, 1958.

45. DeViale, L. C., Garcia, R. C., DePisarev, D. K., Tomio, J. M., and Grinstein, M.: Studies on uroporphyrinogen decarboxylase from chicken erythrocytes. *FEBS Lett.* 5:149, 1969.

46. Romeo, G., and Levin, E. Y.: Uroporphyrinogen decarboxylase from mouse spleen. *Biochim. Biophys. Acta* 230:330, 1971.

47. Kushner, J. P., Steinmuller, D. P., and Lee, G. R.: The role of iron in pathogenesis of porphyria cutanea tarda II. Inhibition of uroporphyrinogen decarboxylase. *J. Clin. Invest.* 56:661, 1975.

48. Akhtar, M., Abboud, M. M., Barnard, G., Jordan, P., and Zaman, Z.: Mechanism and stereochemistry of enzymic reactions involved in porphyrin biosynthesis. *Philos. Trans. R. Soc. Lond.* [Biol.] 273:117, 1976.

49. Yoshinaga, T., and Sano, S.: Coproporphyrinogen oxidase. I. Purification, properties and activation by phospholipid. *J. Biol. Chem.* 255:472, 1980.

50. Jackson, A. H., and Games, D. E.: The later stages of porphyrin synthesis. *Ann. N.Y. Acad. Sci.* 244:591, 1975.

51. Poulson, R. and Polglase, W. J.: The enzymic conversion of protoporphyrinogen IX to protoporphyrin IX. *J. Biol. Chem.* 250:1269, 1975.

52. Goldberg, A., Ashenbrucker, H., Cartwright, G. E., and Wintrobe, M. M.: Studies on the biosynthesis of heme in vitro by avian erythrocytes. *Blood* 11:821, 1956.

53. Jones, M. S., and Jones, O. T. G.: Evidence for the location of ferrochelatase on the inner membrane of rat liver mitochondria. *Biochem. Biophys. Res. Commun.* 31:977, 1968.

54. Yoshikawa, H., and Yoneyama, Y.: Incorporation of iron in the haem moiety of chromoproteins, in *Iron Metabolism,* edited by F. Gross. Springer-Verlag, Berlin, 1964, p. 24.

55. Yoneyama, Y., Sawada, H., Takeshita, M., and Sugita, Y.: The role of lipids in heme synthesis. *Lipids* 4:321, 1969.

56. Dailey, H. A., Jr., and Lascelles, J.: Ferrochelatase activity in wild-type and mutant strains of *Spirillum tersoni. Arch. Biochem. Biophys.* 160:523, 1974.

57. Wagner, G. S. and Tephly, T. R.: A possible role of copper in the regulation of heme biosynthesis through ferrochelatase. *Adv. Exp. Med. Biol.* 58:343, 1975.

58. Porra, R. J., Vitols, K. S., Labbe, R. F., and Newton, N. A.: Studies on ferrochelatase: The effects of thiols and other factors on the determination of activity. *Biochem. J.* 104:321, 1967.

59. Porra, R. J.: A rapid spectrophotometric assay for ferrochelatase activity in preparations containing much endogenous hemoglobin and its application to soybean root-nodule preparations. *Anal. Biochem.* 68:289, 1975.

60. George, P.: Thermodynamic aspects of porphyrin synthesis and biosynthesis. *Am. N.Y. Acad. Sci.* 206:84, 1973.

61. Stadtman, E. R.: Allosteric regulation of enzyme activity. *Adv. Enzymol.* 28:41, 1966.

62. Shemin, D., and Russell, C. S.: δ-Aminolevulinic acid, its role in the biosynthesis of porphyrins and purines. *J. Am. Chem. Soc.* 75:4873, 1953.

63. Sassa, S., and Kappas, A.: Genetic, metabolic, and biochemical aspects of the porphyrias. *Adv. Human Genet.* 11:121, 1981.

64. Meyer, U. A., Strand, L. J., Doss, M., Rees, A. C., and Marver, H. S.: Intermittent acute porphyria: Demonstration of genetic defect in porphobilinogen metabolism. *N. Engl. J. Med.* 286:1277, 1972.

65. Tschudy, D. P., Perlroth, M. G., Marver, H. S., Collins, A., Hunter, G., Jr., and Rechcigl, M., Jr.: Acute intermittent porphyria: The first "overproduction disease" localized to a specific enzyme. *Proc. Natl. Acad. Sci. U.S.A.* 53:841, 1965.

66. Bonkowsky, et al.: Repression of the overproduction of porphyrin precursors in acute intermittent porphyria by intravenous infusion of hematin. *Proc. Natl. Acad. Sci. U.S.A.* 68:2725, 1971.

67. Dhar, G. J., Bossenmaier, I., Petryka, Z. J., Cardinal R., and Watson, C. J.: Effects of hematin in hepatic porphyria. *Ann. Int. Med.* 83:20, 1975.

68. Tschudy, D. P., and Lamon J. M.: Porphyrin metabolism and the porphyrias, in *Metabolic Control and Disease,* 8th ed., edited by P. K. Bondy and L. E. Rosenberg. Saunders, Philadelphia, 1980, pp. 939–1007.

69. Sassa, S. and Granick, S.: Induction of δ-aminolevulinate synthetase in chick embryo liver cells in culture. *Proc. Natl. Acad. Sci. U.S.A.* 67:517, 1970.

70. Granick, S.: The induction in vitro of the synthesis of δ-aminolevulinic acid synthetase in chemical porphyria: A response to certain drugs, sex hormones, and foreign chemicals, *J. Biol. Chem.* 241:1359, 1966.

71. Marver, H. S., Collins, A., Tschudy, D. P., and Rechcigl, M., Jr.: δ-Aminolevulinic acid synthetase. II. Induction in rat liver. *J. Biol. Chem.* 241:4323, 1966.

72. Whiting, M. J., and Granick, S.: δ-Aminolevulinic acid synthetase from chick embryo liver mitochondria. II. Immunochemical correlation between synthesis and activity in induction and repression. *J. Biol. Chem.* 251:1347, 1976.

73. Sinclair, P. R., and Granick, S.: Heme control of the synthesis of delta-aminolevulinic acid synthetase in cultured chick embryo liver cells. *Ann. N.Y. Acad. Sci.* 244:509, 1975.

74. Sassa, S.: Sequential induction of heme pathway enzymes during erythroid differentiation of mouse Friend leukemia virus-infected cells. *J. Exp. Med.* 143:305, 1976.

75. Rutherford, T., Thompson, G. G., and Moore, M. R.: Heme biosynthesis in Friend erythroleukemia cells: Control by ferrochelatase. *Proc. Natl. Acad. Sci. U.S.A.* 76:833, 1979.

76. von Goreczky, L., Roth, I., and Breckner, M.: Normalwerte der Porphyrine und Porphyrin-Vorstufen. *Z. Klin, Chem.* 6:489, 1968.

77. Eales, L., Levey, M. J., and Sweeney, G. D.: The place of screening tests and quantitative investigations in the diagnosis of the porphyrias, with particular reference to variegate and symptomatic porphyria. *S. Afr. Med. J.* 40:63, 1966.

78. Chisolm, J. J., Jr.: Determination of δ-aminolevulinic acid in plasma. *Anal. Biochem.* 22:54, 1968.

79. Jackson, A. H.: Modern spectroscopic and chromatographic techniques for the analysis of porphyrins on a microscale. *Semin. Hematol.* 14:193, 1977.

80. Elder, G. H.: The porphyrias: Clinical chemistry, diagnosis and methodology. *Clin. Haematol.* 9:371, 1980.

81. Gentz, J., Johnsson, S., Lindblad, B., Lindstedt, S., and Zetterstrom, R.: Excretion of δ-aminolevulinic acid in hereditary tyrosinemia. *Clin. Chim. Acta* 23:257, 1969.

82. von Clotten, R., and Doyen, A.: Über die Ausscheidung der Koproprophyrin-Isomere I und III bei Erkankungen der Leber und des Blutes. *Z. Klin. Chem.* 5:54, 1967.

83. McColl, K. E. L., and Goldberg, A.: Abnormal porphyrin metabolism in diseases other than porphyria. *Clin. Haematol.* 9:427, 1980.

84. Wolkoff, A. W., Cohen, L. E., and Arias, I. M.: Inheritance of the Dubin-Johnson syndrome. *N. Engl. J. Med.* 288:113, 1973.

85. Watson, C. J.: Porphyrin metabolism, in *Diseases of Metabolism,* 5th ed., edited by G. C. Duncan. Saunders, Philadelphia, 1964, p. 850.

86. Kaser, H. Koblet, H., and Riva, G.: Die Ausscheidung von Porphyrin-präkursoren im Urin bei Kindern verschiedenen Lebensalters. *Schweiz. Med. Wochenschr.* 93:1052, 1963.

87. Aldrich, R. A., Labbe, R. F., and Talman, E. L.: Review of porphyrin metabolism with special reference to childhood. *Am. J. Med.* 230:675, 1953.

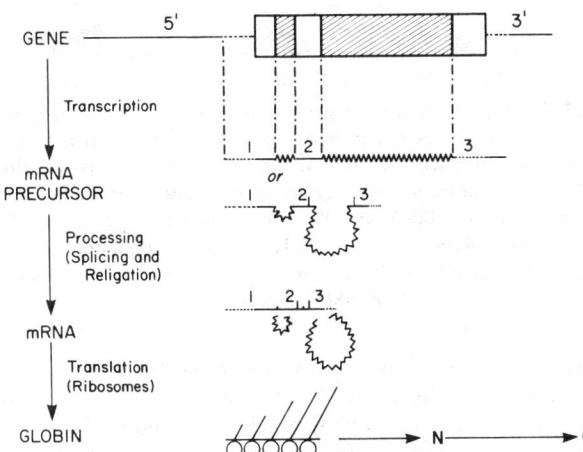

CHAPTER 32

The synthesis of globin

ARTHUR BANK

New methods have permitted detailed analysis of the structure and organization of the globin genes, and new levels of control of the expression of these genes have been discovered [1–3]. Direct nucleotide analysis of the globin genes in several species indicates that the biosynthesis of globin is a process that has been highly conserved throughout evolution. Certain nucleotide sequences within the coding regions in these genes as well as in those sequences flanking the globin genes have been largely unchanged over millions of years [4].

Regulation of expression of the globin genes can occur at the level of (1) globin gene transcription, (2) metabolism of nuclear RNA transcripts containing globin mRNA (globin mRNA processing), (3) globin mRNA stability, and (4) globin mRNA translation.

DNA to RNA to protein

The biosynthesis of human globin involves the usual pathway of information flow in eukaryotic cells from DNA to RNA to protein (Fig. 32-1). Recombinant DNA technology has led to a determination of the complete nucleotide sequence of most human globin structural genes [5–9]. A major feature of these genes is the so-called intervening sequences or "introns" [10–14]. These intervening sequences are stretches of DNA that interrupt the nucleotides used in coding for amino acids (coding sequences). These DNA sequences are initially transcribed into RNA together with the coding nucleotide sequences (Fig. 32-1). Subsequently, the intervening sequences are removed from the RNA precursors for globin messenger RNA (mRNA) and the coding sequences in the globin mRNA are rejoined (religated) by a process called *splicing*. This religated product is the mature globin mRNA found in abundance in the cytoplasm of the globin-synthesizing cell. It becomes associated with polyribosomes, and in the presence of activating enzymes; initiation, elongation, and termination factors; amino acids; and tRNAs, globin mRNA translation takes place. Hemin both stimulates globin mRNA translation and is added to the globin subunits after their synthesis and release from polyribosomes to form hemoglobin. As far as is known, the synthesis of α- and β-globin chains occurs independently, and the assembly of hemoglobin is directed solely by the physicochemical affinities of globin subunits and subsequently their interaction with hemin.

Globin gene structure

Restriction enzyme analysis of cellular DNA and cloning of human globin genes have led to characterization

FIGURE 32-1 Globin biosynthesis. The β-globin gene coding sequences *(clear areas of rectangle)* are interrupted by two intervening sequences *(hatched areas)*. Globin mRNA precursors include intervening sequences (〰〰) which are removed by splicing and religation.

of almost all the normal human globin structural genes. Restriction endonuclease mapping studies first demonstrated the organization of these genes with relation to each other and some of the detail of the intragenic structure of these genes [10,12–14]. In this technique, cellular DNA is treated with one of many available restriction endonucleases, enzymes which cleave DNA at specific nucleotide sequences. The DNA fragments generated by these enzymes are separated on an agarose gel, denatured, and transferred to nitrocellulose filters by a process known as "blotting" [15]. The detection of the appropriate globin gene within these fragments is achieved by hybridization with radioactive "probes." Such probes are unique strands of DNA whose globin gene sequence has been labeled with [32]P. Radiolabeled [32]P α, β, and γ complementary DNA (cDNA) probes were initially used for this analysis [16,17]. Such probes lack the intervening sequences, because they were originally prepared from "mature" messengers. More recently, cloned globin DNA fragments have become available as probes [5,18,19]. Under appropriate conditions of temperature and ionic strength and in the presence of formamide, the radioactive probe will attach firmly to strands of DNA with complementary sequences, namely, a globin gene. After such hybridization with ^{32}P-labeled DNA probes, the filters are washed and the fragments containing the globin genes identified by radioautography. By the use of multiple restriction endonucleases, the relationship of nucleotide sequences within and surrounding the human globin genes has been determined. More recently, each of the human globin genes has been cloned in bacteria using λ phages as vectors [19,20], and their organization and nucleotide sequences have been determined by restriction analysis of the clones [21–23] and by direct nucleotide sequencing techniques [5–9,21,24–26].

These studies have revealed certain features common to all of the human globin genes studied to date (Fig. 32-

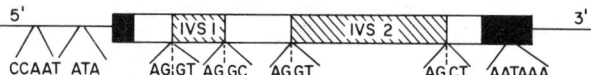

FIGURE 32-2 β-Globin gene structure. The β-globin gene coding sequences *(clear areas)* are interrupted by two intervening sequences *(hatched areas)*. The black areas are the 5' and 3' untranslated regions of the gene. The horizontal lines represent the 5' and 3' flanking regions. The nucleotide sequences shown are the largely conserved sequences in the 5' and 3' junctions of IVS 1 and IVS 2, in the 3' untranslated region, and in the 5' flanking region.

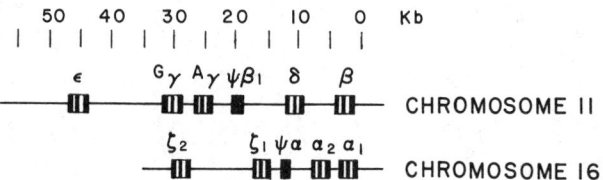

FIGURE 32-3 Organization of human globin genes. The ϵ, γ, δ, and β genes are on chromosome 11, and the ζ and α genes are on chromosome 16. The distance between the genes is shown in kilobases (kb) at the top. The black regions within each rectangle are coding regions of the genes, and the clear regions the intervening sequences.

2). First, each of these genes contains two intervening sequences: a small intervening sequence (IVS 1) located between codons 30 and 31 of all non-α genes, that is, ϵ, γ, δ, and β genes, and a larger intervening sequence (IVS 2) between codons 104 and 105 in each of these genes [4]. The location of IVS 1 and IVS 2 in the α and ζ genes is different only because of a change in total number of nucleotides from 146 to 141 in these genes as compared with non-α genes. Similarly placed IVS 1 and 2 have been identified in all functioning globin genes of all species studied to date, including mouse, rabbit, and goat. At the 3' end* of the structural gene there are an extra 75 to 100 untranslated (noncoding) nucleotides which include the sequence AATAAA [4,27]. This latter sequence identifies the site at which polyadenylation (poly A addition) of mRNA will occur. This polyadenylation usually takes place rapidly after RNA transcription in the nucleus [28], but it is clearly a posttranscriptional event (not coded for in the DNA).

The 5' end of the globin-gene transcript, the site on DNA at which transcription begins, is 50 to 60 nucleotides 5' to the AUG initiation codon and represents a 5' "untranslated region" of the globin mRNA (Fig. 32-2). At the 5' extremity of this 5' untranslated region is the so-called cap site; this is the 5' terminus of the globin mRNA precursor which is methylated and contains no free 5' phosphate and is found at the 5' end of most mRNAs. The structure at the 5' end of globin mRNA precursor in the nucleus as well as in mature cytoplasmic globin mRNA is 7-methyl, 5',5'-guanosine, 6 methyl adenine [29].

Two other regions of significant sequence conservation are found flanking the globin genes in the 5' direction and are also 5' to most other genes studied [4]. These are the so-called TATA or ATA box sequences approximately 30 to 40 base pairs 5' to the cap site and CAAT box sequences approximately 70 to 80 base pairs 5' to the cap site. These are regions identified by specific nucleotide homologies which appear to be of sig-

nificance in either RNA polymerase binding or for other as yet unknown interactions between globin genes and other nuclear proteins.

Organization of the globin genes

Studies of cellular DNA by restriction analysis and of the nucleotide content of a variety of clones by sequencing different globin genes have yielded the detailed organization of the globin genes (Fig. 32-3). The δ and β genes used in the synthesis of adult hemoglobins (hemoglobin A, $\alpha_2\beta_2$ and hemoglobin A_2, $\alpha_2\delta_2$) are linked approximately 5.5 kilobases (kb) apart at the 3' end of a single piece of DNA which also contains the γ and ϵ genes. Two γ genes, $^G\gamma$ and $^A\gamma$, are separated from each other by approximately 3.5 kb and from the δ gene by approximately 15 kb. The ϵ gene is 5' to the γ genes. The non-α genes are on chromosome 11. (See Chapters 37 and 50 for a discussion of hemoglobin gene expression during different phases of development.)

The α genes are linked on a single fragment of DNA of chromosome 16. These two genes are separated by approximately 2.5 kb. Two embryonic ζ genes are located in a position 5' to the α-globin genes. In the β-globin gene complex, there is one so-called pseudogene, a sequence of DNA which does not contain all of the structural features required for functionally intact globin genes but which has significant nucleotide homology with the β-like genes [23]. The so-called pseudogene $\psi\beta_1$ is located between $^A\gamma$ and δ genes (Fig. 32-3). Similarly, a pseudo-α ($\psi\alpha$) gene is located between the ζ genes and the α genes [30,31].

Another interesting structural feature of the globin gene complex is so-called inverted repeat sequences present in specific regions flanking the structural globin genes [23]. They are located 5' to the ϵ gene, 5' to the $^G\gamma$ gene, 3' to the $^A\gamma$ gene, 5' to the δ gene, and 3' to the β gene and are approximately 250 base pairs long. They occur in regions which may demarcate specific domains of globin transcription, since they are located at the boundaries of ϵ, γ, and $\delta\beta$ transcriptional complexes. These inverted repeats, such as 5'CCTT . . . AAGG3', are able to form intramolecular double-stranded struc-

---

*DNA and RNA are polymers of nucleotides in which the hydroxyl group attached to the third carbon (3'—OH) of each nucleotide pentose is joined to the hydroxyl group of the fifth carbon (5'—OH) of the adjacent nucleotide by a phosphate ester. All the 3' and 5'—OH groups are therefore joined by phosphate to another nucleotide except the pentoses at both ends of the polymer. At one end the 3'—OH is free; this end is designated the 3' end. At the other end the 5'—OH is free; this is designated the 5' end.

tures because of their complementary sequences; i.e., the TT can pair with AA and the CC with GG in the preceding example. In vitro transcription studies indicate that the repeat regions 5' to the γ and 5' to the δ genes can lead to specific RNA transcription in the presence of RNA polymerase III [32].

Globin gene transcription

Globin gene transcription requires RNA polymerase II, an appropriate chromatin configuration of the globin template, and soluble factors necessary for RNA synthesis, including nucleotides and energy-generating compounds. Accurate initiation of globin mRNA transcripts has been demonstrated using cloned globin genes as templates in both HeLa-cell and L-cell extracts [31,33]. In marrow cells in culture, high-molecular-weight RNA precursors are synthesized as the primary gene transcription products [34–36]. In the case of the β-globin gene, this transcript is approximately 15 S in size and, as indicated earlier, includes both the 5' and the 3' untranslated regions and the two intervening sequences (Fig. 32-2). The intervening sequences seem to be required for efficient expression of these genes [37,38]. The level at which the intervening sequences function is unclear; it may be the DNA or RNA level [39,40].

The primary RNA transcripts which include intervening sequences are subsequently cleaved at the junction of coding and intervening sequences in a highly specific way, presumably by splicing enzymes. Details of the process of religating the cleaved ends of the mRNA precursors are also unknown. Recently, another class of RNA, so-called small nuclear RNAs, or sn RNAs, have been implicated in the splicing process [41,42]. These RNAs may specifically interact with the nucleotide sequences at the borders of the intervening sequences and coding sequences and may facilitate splicing-enzyme action. The formation of base-paired structures more easily cleaved by splicing enzymes is suggested by the homologies between splice junctions and these small nuclear RNAs. It has not, however, been shown definitively that the small nuclear RNAs indeed do interact with globin mRNA precursors in this splicing process in vivo.

There also may be a stepwise set of splicing reactions between primary RNA transcription and the formation of mature globin. This is suggested by the presence of discrete globin mRNA containing RNA intermediates demonstrated in analyses of mouse and rabbit globin mRNA metabolism. In the mouse system [43], it can be shown that several size classes of globin mRNA precursors exist consistent with the presence of several different splices within the globin mRNA. In rabbit globin mRNA, a different set of intermediates has been found [44]. These include those with IVS 1 partially or completely removed and others with all of IVS 1 and part of IVS 2 lost. No intermediates containing IVS 1 but not IVS 2 were found.

Polyadenylation of globin mRNA precursors occurs at an extremely rapid rate in the nucleus, since little or no nuclear nonpolyadenylated RNA has thus far been isolated [28]. The 5' methylation and capping of globin mRNA precursors also occurs in the nucleus, but this process is apparently somewhat slower than polyadenylation, since some noncapped mRNA precursors are detectable.

Globin mRNA—structure and function

The structure of several human globin mRNAs has been determined by direct nucleotide sequencing of the globin genes, as well as by the nucleotide analysis of isolated globin mRNA [5–9,27]. These studies have shown great consistency in sequence analysis and indicate that mature globin mRNAs are generally composed of 600 to 700 nucleotides: approximately 50 nucleotides of 5' untranslated region, approximately 420 to 450 nucleotides of coding sequence, approximately 75 to 100 nucleotides of 3' untranslated sequence, and 100 to 150 adenine residues at the 3' end. The 5' end of the molecule contains an unusual methylated cap with nucleotides in 5',5' position with no free 5' phosphate [45–48]. A variety of secondary structures can be drawn for each of the globin mRNAs, which indicates a molecule composed of a series of stems and loops with differing stabilities. While secondary structures must be important in the in vivo configuration of globin mRNA, such models are difficult to define in detail because of the potential interactions of globin mRNA with polyribosome structures and with proteins in vivo [49,50]. The presence of poly A at the 3' end of the mRNA appears to be associated with increased globin mRNA stability [51–53].

Globin translation

In the process of translation in the cytoplasm of cells, polyadenylated globin mRNA becomes associated with a variety of proteins in the cytoplasm, including eukaryotic initiation factors (eIF), elongation factors, and termination factors, as well as with tRNAs (Fig. 32-4). The eIFs are all proteins of molecular weight from 15,000 to greater than 500,000 daltons; eIF-1 is the smallest at 15,000 daltons and eIF-3 the largest [54,55]. The initial event in globin mRNA translation is initiation. This requires the association of 40 S ribosomal subunits, eIF-2, an eIF-2 stimulating protein, methionine-bound initiator tRNA (met-tRNA$_f$) and GTP to give a 40 S met-tRNA$_f$ complex with GTP (Fig. 32-4). The met tRNA$_f$ is a specific initiator tRNA complementary in its anticodon sequence to the AUG at the first translated codon of globin mRNA. Another initiation factor, eIF-3, may also function at this step. At least three of the seven known eukaryotic initiation factors, eIF-3, eIF-4A, and eIF-4B, are required to bind mRNA to this complex (Fig. 32-4).

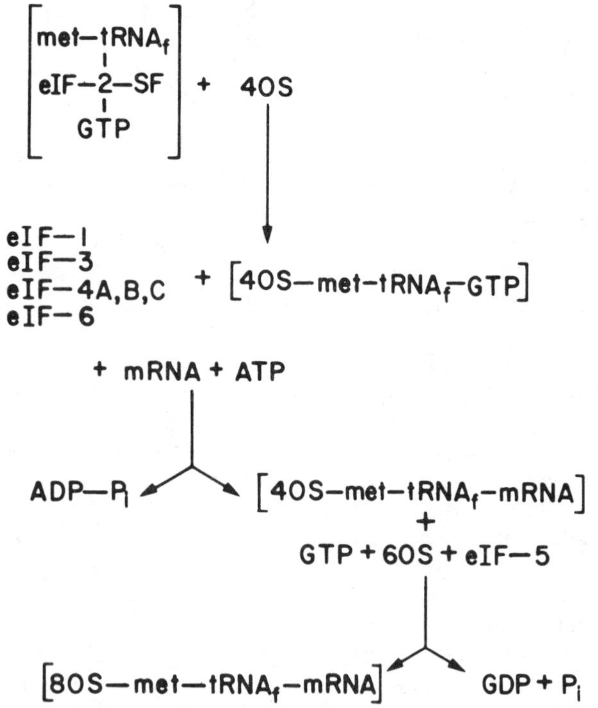

$$\begin{bmatrix} \text{met-tRNA}_f \\ | \\ \text{eIF-2-SF} \\ | \\ \text{GTP} \end{bmatrix} + 40S$$

$$\begin{matrix} \text{eIF-I} \\ \text{eIF-3} \\ \text{eIF-4A,B,C} \\ \text{eIF-6} \end{matrix} + [40S - \text{met-tRNA}_f - \text{GTP}]$$

$$+ \text{mRNA} + \text{ATP}$$

$$\text{ADP-P}_i \swarrow \searrow [40S - \text{met-tRNA}_f - \text{mRNA}] \\ + \\ \text{GTP} + 60S + \text{eIF-5}$$

$$[80S - \text{met-tRNA}_f - \text{mRNA}] \searrow \text{GDP} + \text{P}_i$$

FIGURE 32-4 Sequence of events in formation of the initiation complex between mRNA and ribosomes. The eIF are eukaryotic initiation factors; met-tRNA$_f$ is the methionine-bound initiator transfer RNA. SF is a recently described stimulatory factor.

This interaction of the 40 S met-tRNA$_f$ complex and globin mRNA occurs in the presence of ATP to form a 40 S met-tRNA$_f$–GTP-mRNA complex with the generation of ADP and inorganic phosphate (P$_i$). The final step in the formation of 80 S ribosomal subunits is the addition of 60 S ribosomal subunits in the presence of eIF-5 (Fig. 32-4) with the conversion of GTP to GDP and P$_i$.

After the 80 S initiation complex is complete, successive amino acids are added to the growing polypeptide chains by a series of interdependent reactions [56]. A new amino acyl-tRNA is positioned on the ribosome 3' to the methionine-bound initiator tRNA in the presence of elongation factor 1 (EF1) in a reaction that requires GTP. After the amino acid is correctly positioned, GTP is hydrolyzed to GDP and P$_i$; EF1 is released and a peptide bond formed between methionine and the amino acid associated with the incoming tRNA molecule. This reaction is catalyzed by a ribosomal protein, peptidyl transferase. Translocation of the ribosome along the mRNA is coupled with the ejection of the first tRNA, whose place will then be occupied by a second aminoacyl tRNA. This process requires the action of elongation factor 2 (EF2) and another molecule of GTP. The action of EF2 and GTP propels the ribosome three residues along the mRNA, where it is prepared to accept the next aminoacyl-tRNA brought in by EF1. This overall process preserves aminoacyl and peptidyl sites on the ribosome and ensures continued polypeptide chain elongation. Termination of the globin polypep-

tide chain is signaled by the presence of any one of three codons in the mRNA: UAA, UAG, or UGA. These sequences are recognized by "release" or "termination" protein factors, which cause the polypeptide chains to be released from the ribosomes and from tRNA [57].

The ribosome cycle

A process known as the *ribosome cycle* results from the mechanisms of globin-chain initiation and elongation described above and protects the mRNA molecules during globin-chain translation. It results in the production of many globin chains utilizing a single globin mRNA. In this cycle, initiation begins as described earlier as met-tRNA binds to the 40 S subunit and is joined to the 5' AUG codon of globin mRNA, and the addition of the 60 S subunit forms an 80 S ribosome complex. The 80 S ribosome moves toward the 3' end as the nascent polypeptide chain attached to the mRNA grows and folds. As the 5' end of the mRNA becomes available, new 40 S ribosomal subunits with met-tRNA$_f$ molecules become attached to it and initiate a new globin chain. As this process continues, up to five globin chains are initiated and elongated on a single mRNA-polyribosome complex. Each new initiation of a globin chain is accompanied by new 40 S and 60 S subunits binding to the mRNA.

At the 3' end of the mRNA, as the ribosome reaches a termination codon, the nascent globin chain and the ribosomal subunits are released. These subunits may either rejoin the mRNA or associate with each other to form inactive 80 S ribosomes. Under steady-state conditions, they are most likely to reinitiate protein synthesis on the mRNA.

The translation of human globin mRNA appears to require no specific protein or nucleic acid factors found uniquely in erythroid cells. In addition, no factors specific for the α- or β-globin mRNA translation are known. These conclusions are derived from the finding that cell-free systems from Krebs ascites tumor cells, rabbit reticulocytes, and wheat germ can all accurately translate human globin mRNA and produce relatively equal amounts of α- and β-globin. In addition, α-globin translation continues in the absence of β-globin biosynthesis, and the converse is also true [58–60]. The final assembly of hemoglobin tetramers appears to be a process in which α- and β-globin subunits associate with hemin and then combine to form dimers. Two dimers then associate spontaneously to form the functional hemoglobin tetramer.

Regulation of globin biosynthesis

Globin synthesis is primarily regulated in the nucleus. The amount of globin produced is almost always directly proportional to and dependent on the amount of globin mRNA present. Although translational control of globin production does exist, it is less important in determining the extent of globin biosynthesis than nuclear events. In the nucleus, regulation must occur at the level of globin mRNA transcription [61]. The molecular events triggering globin mRNA biosynthesis are not yet known, but they appear to involve interactions of nuclear proteins, presumably nonhistone proteins and histones, with the globin genes to uncover the globin genes preferentially and make them available for transcription. Studies in which nuclei and chromatin have been treated with nucleases indicate that the globin genes are in a different physicochemical configuration in globin-producing cells than in those cells which do not produce globin [62,63]. The precise binding sites for RNA polymerase II and the other protein factors required for the optimal initiation of globin mRNA transcription are undetermined.

The factors regulating expression of globin genes are largely unknown and are, in many cases, probably quite subtle. Although deletions of structural-gene sequences clearly can decrease globin-gene expression, this cannot explain most changes in gene expression, which are quantitative in extent. For example, the human δ and β genes differ by only 10 of 146 amino acids and yet differ significantly in their expression. The δ-globin gene product, δ-globin, is expressed at one-fortieth the rate of β-globin in normal cells. There are differences in the structure of δ- and β-globin genes in both the ATA box region 5′ to the gene, in IVS 1, and even greater divergence in IVS 2. These nucleotide sequences or others yet to be defined may be responsible for differences in globin-gene transcription. Additionally, the differences in expression of these genes may be reflected at the level of RNA processing rather than at the level of gene transcription. Either decreased δ-globin gene transcription, defective δ-globin mRNA precursor processing, or decreased stability of δ-globin mRNA can result in decreased amounts of δ-globin mRNA and δ-globin.

Events in processing of globin mRNA precursors can also control globin mRNA biosynthesis. Any change resulting in decreased cleavage or religation of globin mRNA precursors will diminish the amount of globin mRNA in the cytoplasm and will decrease globin synthesis. There is evidence that abnormal processing of globin mRNA precursors is responsible for some β^+ and β^0 thalassemias (see Chap. 52).

Hemin acts at several levels in globin mRNA translation and is clearly a factor required for the optimal globin mRNA translation [61]. In the absence of hemin, reticulocytes accumulate inhibitors of globin mRNA translation, which act primarily at the level of initiation. This effect is mediated by a hemin-controlled inhibitor, a cyclic AMP (cAMP)–independent protein kinase that inhibits chain initiation through phosphorylation of one of the subunits of eIF-2 [61]. Hemin-controlled inhibitor (HCI) is activated by phosphorylation by a cAMP-dependent protein kinase [61]. Addition of eIF-2 can reverse the effect of HCI. Hemin deficiency affects the binding of the 40 S met-tRNA complex to α mRNA

more than to β mRNA and a preferential decline in α synthesis is seen [64]. Hemin also increases polyribosome formation in globin-producing cells and in this way enhances globin biosynthesis.

References

1. Bunn, H. F., Forget, B. G., and Ranney, H. M.: The thalassemias and the molecular genetics of human hemoglobin synthesis, in *Hemoglobinopathies*, edited by L. H. Smith. Saunders, Philadelphia, 1977, pp. 28–94.
2. Bank, A., Mears, J. G., and Ramirez, F.: Disorders of human hemoglobin. *Science* 207:486, 1980.
3. Weatherall, D. J., and Clegg, J. B.: *The Thalassemia Syndromes*, 3d ed. Blackwell, Oxford, 1979.
4. Efstratiadis, A., et al.: The structure and evolution of the human β globin gene family. *Cell* 21:653, 1980.
5. Lawn, R. M., Efstratiadis, A., O'Connell, C., and Maniatis, T.: The nucleotide sequence of the human β globin gene. *Cell* 21:647, 1980.
6. Slightom, J., Blechl, A. E., and Smithies, S.: Human ᴳγ and ᴬγ globin genes: Complete nucleotide sequences suggest that DNA can be exchanged between these duplicated genes. *Cell* 21:627, 1980.
7. Spritz, R., deRiel, J. K., Forget, B. G., and Weissman, S.: Nucleotide sequence of the human δ globin gene. *Cell* 21:639, 1980.
8. Liebhaber, S. A., Goossens, M. J., and Kan, Y. W.: Cloning and complete nucleotide sequence of human 5′ α globin gene. *Proc. Natl. Acad. Sci. U.S.A.* 77:7054, 1980.
9. Baralle, F. E., Shoulders, C., and Proudfoot, N. J.: The primary structure of the human ε gene. *Cell* 21:621, 1980.
10. Jeffreys, A. J., and Flavell, R. A.: A physical map of the DNA regions flanking the rabbit β globin gene. *Cell* 12:429, 1977A.
11. Tilghman, S. M., et al.: Intervening sequence of DNA identified in the structural portion of a mouse β globin gene. *Proc. Natl. Acad. Sci. U.S.A.* 75:725, 1978.
12. Mears, J. G., Ramirez, F., Leibowitz, D., and Bank, A.: Organization of human δ and β globin genes in cellular DNA and the presence of intragenic inserts. *Cell* 15:15, 1978.
13. Flavell, R. A., Kooter, J. M., DeBoer, E., Little, P. F. R., and Williamson, R.: Analysis of the human βδ globin gene loci in normal and Hb Lepore DNA: Direct determination of gene linkage and intergene distance. *Cell* 15:25, 1978.
14. Little, P. F. R., Flavell, R. A., Kooter, J. M., Annison, G., and Williamson, R.: Structure of the human fetal globin gene locus. *Nature* 278:227, 1979.
15. Southern, E. M.: Detection of specific sequences among DNA fragments separated by gel electrophoresis. *J. Mol. Biol.* 98:503, 1975.
16. Smithies, O., et al.: Cloning human fetal γ globin and mouse α type globin DNA: Characterization and partial sequencing. *Science* 202:1284, 1978.
17. Wilson, J. T., et al.: Insertion of synthetic copies of human globin genes into bacterial plasmids. *Nucleic Acids Res.* 5:563, 1978.
18. Fritsch, E. P., Lawn, R. M., and Maniatis, T.: Characterization of deletions which affect the expression of fetal globin genes in man. *Nature* 279:598, 1979.
19. Blattner, F. R., et al.: Charon phages: Softer derivatives of bacteriophage λ for DNA cloning. *Science* 196:161, 1977.
20. Maniatis, T., et al.: The isolation of structural genes from libraries of eucaryotic DNA. *Cell* 15:687, 1978.
21. Lawn, R. M., Fritsch, E. F., Parker, R. C., Blake, G., and Maniatis, T.: The isolation and characterization of linked δ and β globin genes from a cloned library of human DNA. *Cell* 15:1157, 1978.
22. Ramirez, F., Burns, A. L., Mears, J. G., Spence, S., Starkman, D., and Bank, A.: Isolation and characterization of cloned human fetal globin genes. *Nucleic Acids Res.* 7:1147, 1979.
23. Fritsch, E. F., Lawn, R. M., and Maniatis, T.: Molecular cloning and characterization of the human β-like globin gene cluster. *Cell* 19:959, 1980.
24. Maxam, A. M. and Gilbert, W.: A new method for sequencing DNA. *Proc. Natl. Acad. Sci. U.S.A.* 74:560, 1977.
25. Sanger, F. E., Coulson, A. R., Barelle, B. G., Smith, A. J. H., and Roe,

B. A.: Cloning in single stranded bacteria phage as an aid to rapid cDNA sequencing. *J. Mol. Biol.* 143:161, 1981.

26. Sanger, F., Nicklen, S., and Coulson, A. R.: DNA sequencing with chain terminating inhibitors. *Proc. Natl. Acad. Sci. U.S.A.* 74:5463, 1977.

27. Marotta, C. A., Wilson, J. T., Forget, B. G., and Weissman, S. M.: Human β globin messenger RNA. III. Nucleotide sequences derived from complementary DNA. *J. Biol. Chem.* 252:5040, 1977.

28. Curtis, P. J., Mantei, N., and Weissman, C.: Characterization and kinetics of synthesis of 15S β globin RNA, a putative precursor of β globin mRNA. *Cold Spring Harbor Symp. Quant. Biol.* 42:971, 1977.

29. Revel, M. and Groner, Y.: Post-transcriptional and translational controls of gene expression in eukaryotes. *Ann. Rev. Biochem.* 47:1079, 1978.

30. Lauer, J., Shen, C.-K. J., and Maniatis, T.: The chromosomal arrangement of human α-like globin genes: Sequence homology and α globin gene deletions. *Cell* 20:119, 1980.

31. Proudfoot, N. J., Shander, M. H. M., Manley, J. L., Gelter, M. L., and Maniatis, T.: Structure and *in vitro* transcription of human globin genes. *Science* 209:1329, 1980.

32. Duncan, C., et al.: RNA polymerase III transcriptional units are interspersed among human non-α globin genes. *Proc. Natl. Acad. Sci. U.S.A.* 76:5095, 1980.

33. Weil, P. A., Luse, D. S., Segall, J., and Roeder, R. G.: Selective and accurate initiation of transcription at the AC2 major late promoter in a soluble system dependent on purified RNA polymerase II and DNA. *Cell* 18:469, 1979.

34. Maquat, L., et al.: Processing of the human β globin mRNA precursor to mRNA is defective in three patients with β⁺ thalassemia. *Proc. Natl. Acad. Sci. U.S.A.* 77:4287, 1980.

35. Kantor, J. A., Turner, P. H., and Nienhuis, A. W.: β Thalassemia: Mutations which affect processing of the β globin mRNA precursor. *Cell* 8:148, 1980.

36. Benz, E. J., Scarpa, A., and Tonkonow, B.: Metabolism of δ and γ globin mRNA in human erythroblasts. *Clin. Res.* 29:330A, 1981 (abstract).

37. Hamer, D. H., and Leder, P. Splicing and the formation of stable RNA. *Cell* 18:1299, 1979.

38. Mulligan, R. C., and Berg, P.: Expression of a bacterial gene in mammalian cells. *Science* 209:1422, 1980.

39. Bank, A., Burns, A. L., Baird, M., and Pergolizzi, R.: Globin gene pathology: Clues to gene function and hemoglobin switching, in *Globin Gene Organization and Expression*, edited by A. W. Nienhuis and G. Stamatoyannopoulos. Liss, New York, 1981.

40. Lazowska, J., Jacq, C., and Slonimski, P.: Sequence of introns and flanking exons in wild type and box 3 mutants of cytochrome b reveals an interlaced splicing protein coded by an intron. *Cell* 22:333, 1980.

41. Lerner, M. R., Boyle, J. A., Mount, S. M., Wolin, S. L., and Steitz, J. A.: Are snRNPs involved in splicing? *Nature* 283:220, 1980.

42. Rogers, J., and Wall, R.: A mechanism for RNA splicing. *Proc. Natl. Acad. Sci. U.S.A.* 77:1877, 1980.

43. Kinniburgh, A. J., and Ross, J.: Processing of the mouse β globin in RNA precursor: At least two cleavage-ligation reactions are necessary to excise the large intervening sequence. *Cell* 17:915, 1979.

44. Grosveld, G. C., Koster, A., and Flavell, R. A.: A transcription map for the rabbit β globin gene. *Cell* 23:573, 1981.

45. Shatkin, A. J.: Capping of eucaryotic mRNAs. *Cell* 9:645, 1976.

46. Both, G. W., Banerjee, A. K., and Shatkin, A. J.: Methylation-dependent translation of viral messenger RNAs *in vitro*. *Proc. Natl. Acad. Sci. U.S.A.* 72:1189, 1975.

47. Both, G. W., Furuichi, Y., Muthukrishnan, S., and Shatkin, A. J.: Ribosome binding to reovirus mRNA in protein synthesis requires 5' terminal 7-methylguanosine. *Cell* 6:185, 1975.

48. Furuichi, Y., LaFiandra, A., and Shatkin, A. J.: 5' terminal structure and mRNA stability. *Nature* 266:235, 1977.

49. Blobel, G.: A protein of molecular weight 78,000 bound to the polyadenylate region of eukaryotic messenger RNAs. *Proc. Natl. Acad. Sci. U.S.A.* 70:924, 1973.

50. Jeffrey, W. R., and Brawerman, G.: Association of the polyadenylate segment of messenger NRA with other polynucleotide sequences in mouse sarcoma 180 polyribosomes. *Biochemistry* 14:3445, 1975.

51. Soreq, H., Nudel, U., Salomon, Revel, M., and Littauer, U. Z.: *In vitro* translation of polyadenylic acid-free rabbit globin messenger RNA. *J. Mol. Biol.* 88:233, 1974.

52. Williamson, R., Crossley, J., and Humphries, S.: Translation of mouse globin messenger ribonucleic acid from which the polyadenylic acid sequence has been removed. *Biochemistry* 13:703, 1974.

53. Maniatis, G. M., Ramirez, F., Cann, A., Marks, P. A., and Bank, A.: Translation and stability of human globin mRNA in *Xenopus* oocytes. *J. Clin. Invest.* 58:1419, 1976.

54. Merrick, W. C., Peterson, D. T., Safer, B., Lloyd, M., and Kemper, W. M.: Eukaryotic initiation of protein synthesis, in *Gene Expression: FEBS Federation of European Biochemical Societies, 11th Meeting,* edited by F. C. Clark, H. Klenow, and J. Zeuthen. Pergamon, Oxford, 1977, pp. 17 and 43.

55. Trachsel, H., Erni, B., Schreier, M., and Staehelin, M.: Initiation of mammalian protein synthesis. II. The assembly of the initiation complex with purified initiation factors. *J. Mol. Biol.* 116:755, 1977.

56. Haselkorn, R., and Rothman-Denes, L. B.: Protein biosynthesis. *Ann. Rev. Biochem.* 42:397, 1973.

57. Beaudet, A. L., and Caskey, C. T.: Chain termination in the mechanism of protein synthesis and its regulation, in *The Mechanism of Protein Synthesis and Its Regulation,* edited by L. Bosch. Elsevier-North Holland, Amsterdam, 1972, p. 133.

58. Bank, A., and Marks, P. A.: Excess α chain synthesis relative to β chain synthesis in β thalassemia major and minor. *Nature* 212:1198, 1966.

59. Clegg, J. B., and Weatherall, D. J.: Hemoglobin synthesis in α thalassemia (haemoglobin H disease). *Nature* 215:1241, 1967.

60. Bank, A.: Critical review: The thalassemia syndromes. *Blood* 51:369, 1978.

61. Ochoa, S., and deHaro, C.: Regulation of protein synthesis in eukaryotes. *Ann. Rev. Biochem.* 48:549, 1979.

62. Weintraub, H., and Groudine, M.: Chromosomal subunits in active genes have an altered configuration. *Science* 93:848, 1976.

63. Weintraub, H., Larsen, A., and Groudine, M.: α Globin gene switching during the development of chicken embryos: Expression and chromosome structure. *Cell* 24:333, 1981.

64. Beuzard, Y., and London, I. M.: The effects of hemin and double stranded RNA on α and β synthesis in reticulocyte and Krebs II ascites cell-free system and the relationship of the effects to an initiation factor preparation. *Proc. Natl. Acad. Sci. U.S.A.* 71:2863, 1974.

CHAPTER *33*

Iron metabolism

VIRGIL F. FAIRBANKS
ERNEST BEUTLER

Iron is an essential element of all living cells and a participant in numerous metabolic pathways. The dependence of all forms of life on iron may relate to the ease with which iron is reversibly oxidized and reduced and to its abundant presence in virtually all soils and waters. It is the second most common metal in the earth's crust. Yet iron is not readily extracted from its insoluble oxides by living cells. This paradox of geologic abundance but biologic scarcity is mirrored in the abundance of iron (as hemoglobin) in erythrocytes, its minute concentration in other tissues, the tenacity with which the body conserves iron as if it were a trace element, and the extraordinary mechanisms that microorganisms have evolved to obtain the iron they need in competition with host tissues.

In living tissues iron does not exist, except transiently, as a free cation; instead it is bound by or incorporated into various proteins. The iron proteins which occur in man may be broadly grouped as heme proteins, iron flavoproteins, and a heterogeneous group of proteins which contain iron in a variety of molecular configurations. Among the heme proteins are hemoglobin, myoglobin, the cytochromes, cytochrome oxidase, homogentisic oxidase, peroxidases, and catalase. Iron flavoproteins include cytochrome c reductase, succinate dehydrogenase, NADH dehydrogenase, acyl coenzyme A dehydrogenase, and xanthine oxidase. Xanthine oxidase is a complex flavoprotein which contains, at the active site of the molecule, both iron and molybdenum in addition to a quinone-like group; it is thought that these internal structures constitute a chain of electron donors within the enzyme molecule. Iron is apparently a functional part of another important enzyme, aconitase. Iron can be removed from aconitase by dialysis, suggesting that it is quite loosely bound, but aconitase thereby becomes inactive [1]. Nearly half the enzymes and cofactors of the Krebs tricarboxylic acid cycle either contain iron or require its presence.

Iron compartments in man

On the basis of anatomic distribution, chemical characteristics, and function, six iron compartments can be described (Table 33-1).

HEMOGLOBIN
The largest of the compartments is hemoglobin iron, normally containing approximately 2 g iron. Hemoglobin contains 0.34 percent iron by weight. Thus 1 ml of packed erythrocytes contains approximately 1 mg of iron. The size of the hemoglobin compartment changes in anemia and polycythemia.

STORAGE COMPARTMENT
The iron in this compartment exists in two distinct forms: ferritin and hemosiderin. Ferritin is a water-soluble complex of ferric hydroxide and a protein, apoferritin. Apoferritin forms a shell within which ferric ions, hydroxyl ions, and oxygen are dispersed in a latticelike relationship [2–4]. The crystalline core of ferritin is formed principally of ferric oxyhydroxide, FeOOH, with small quantities of phosphate, perhaps at sites of breaks or irregularities in the structure of the $(FeOOH)_x$ crystal. The interior of the apoferritin shell can accommodate up to 4300 FeOOH molecules in the crystal. However, spatial constraints and kinetics of crystal growth result in ferritin molecules that predominantly contain 2000 iron atoms [5–7]. When maximally iron-saturated, a ferritin molecule should have an M_r of 800,000 daltons and would be 31 percent Fe by weight.

TABLE 33-1 Iron compartments in normal man*

Compartment	Iron content, mg	Total body iron, %
Hemoglobin iron	2000	67
Storage iron (ferritin, hemosiderin)	1000	27
Myoglobin iron	130	3.5
Labile pool	80	2.2
Other tissue iron	8	0.2
Transport iron	3	0.08

*These values represent estimates for an "average" person, that is, 70 kg, 177 cm (70 in.) in height. They are derived from data in several sources.

However, maximal saturation is rarely attained; the usual M_r is 620,000 daltons, 18 percent of which is iron. The apoferritin component is a shell of approximately 130-Å external diameter with an interior cavity of about 70-Å diameter and an M_r of 441,000 daltons [8,9]. The apoferritin shell is composed of 24 similar or identical subunits so arranged as to resemble a sphere or "snubbed cube" (a cube with rounded corners) (Fig. 33-1). Groups of four apoferritin monomers form each facet of the snubbed cube, and between these, centered on each cube facet, is a pore of about 10-Å diameter. Through these six pores Fe^{2+} and small molecules enter or leave the interior cavity of the ferritin molecule. The apoferritin monomers each have an M_r of 19,700 daltons [9–12]. Each is composed of a long protein strand which contains 174 amino acids [12]. The protein chain of each monomer is arranged in four nearly parallel, long, rodlike helical segments, designated A, B, C, and D, two very short helical segments, designated E and P, and connecting nonhelical strands [13,14]. The short helical E and P segments line each intermonomeric pore and may also be the site where binding

FIGURE 33-1 A scheme for the quaternary structure of apoferritin. Twenty-four subunits or apoferritin monomers are joined to form a rounded cube, thus approximating a hollow sphere. Six groups of four monomers lie in the planes of the cube facets. Centered on the cube facets, each surrounded by four monomers, are six pores through which Fe^{2+} and small molecules may pass to the interior cavity of the apoferritin shell. (Harrison [130], by permission of Academic Press.)

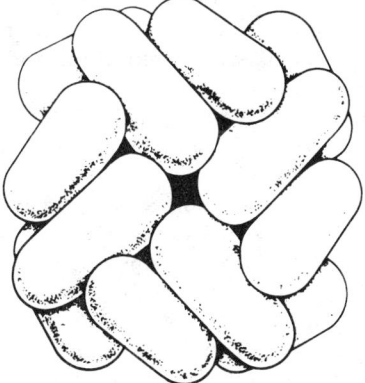

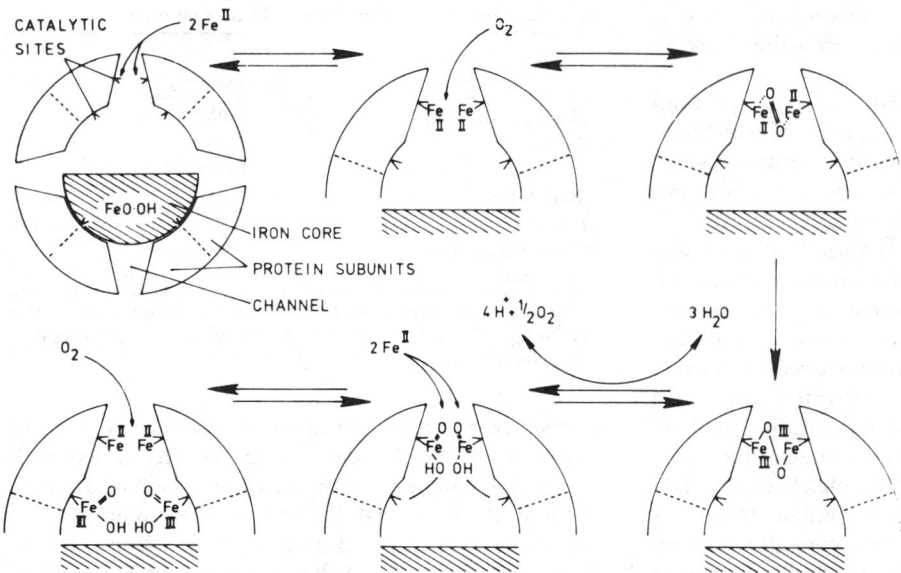

FIGURE 33-2 A scheme for the uptake and oxidation of Fe^{2+} by apoferritin. Two iron-binding sites are hypothesized within each pore channel. The outermost of these has a higher affinity for Fe^{2+}, and the innermost has a higher affinity for Fe^{3+}. As two ferrous ions enter the pore, they are bound, then oxidized, and the product $Fe^{3+}:::O—O:::Fe^{3+}$ forms. The iron is then displaced to the inner binding site, where FeOOH is formed, and this molecule is then released to be added to the growing $(FeOOH)_x$ crystal in the central cavity of apoferritin. Apoferritin thus acts as a ferroxidase in the oxidation of Fe^{2+} to Fe^{3+}. It is not clear whether release of iron from the crystal requires enzymatic action. Reduced flavin mononucleotide and other small reducing substances can enter passively through the pores into the cavity and reduce FeOOH directly to Fe^{2+}, which then passes out through the pores. (Crichton and Roman [131], by permission of the *Journal of Molecular Catalysis*.)

and oxidation occur as Fe^{2+} ions enter the ferritin interior cavity [8]. The complete amino acid sequence of the monomer protein chain has now been established for horse spleen ferritin [12]. Uptake and release of iron by ferritin is very rapid [5,6,15–17]. The ferritin molecule appears to function as a ferroxidase enzyme in binding and oxidizing Fe^{2+} ions and releasing the FeOOH formed to the growing crystalline core [15–17] (Fig. 33-2). Conversely, release of iron appears to be mediated by small reducing substances, particularly by reduced flavin mononucleotide, and to a lesser extent by ascorbic acid and other molecules small enough to traverse the 10-Å pores [6,18]. Of interest is that the molecular dimensions of desferrioxamine B are just below the 10-Å limit that would exclude entry to the interior of ferritin [19]. An enzymatic basis for reduction and release of iron from ferritin has been postulated but not proved [20]. Many authors have observed multiple "isoferritin" bands by isoelectric focusing of ferritin in polyacrylamide gel [21–27]. Despite a large literature on isoferritins, their significance is moot. Some workers regard isoferritins as laboratory artifacts [28,29].

Ferritin occurs in virtually all cells of the body and also in tissue fluids. In blood plasma ferritin is present in minute concentration. Nevertheless, the plasma (serum) ferritin concentration correlates with total-body iron stores, which makes this measurement im-

portant in the diagnosis of many disorders of iron metabolism (see Chaps. 40 and 52).

Hemosiderin, the other iron-storage compound, is found predominantly in cells of the monocyte-macrophage system (marrow, Kupffer cells of the liver, spleen). Under pathologic conditions, it may accumulate in large quantities in almost every tissue of the body. Ferritin granules have been found in hemosiderin by electron microscopy [30]. Immunologic studies have shown that the protein components of both storage compounds are antigenically identical [31]. Hemosiderin contains ferritin partially or completely stripped of the apoferritin protein shell; i.e., much of hemosiderin appears to consist of aggregates of $(FeOOH)_x$ core crystals [32,33].

Hemosiderin is water-insoluble and can be seen microscopically in unstained tissue sections or marrow films as clumps or granules of golden refractile pigment (Fig. 33-3). It contains approximately 25 to 30 percent iron by weight.

The size of the storage compartment is subject to the greatest variation both in normal circumstances and in disease. Normally in adult men it amounts to 800 to 1000 mg; in adult women it is a few hundred milligrams less. Depletion of the storage compartment occurs when iron loss exceeds iron absorption. The mobilization of storage iron involves the release from intracellular ferritin of iron in the divalent state. Ceruloplasmin in the plasma then oxidizes iron to the trivalent state.

MYOGLOBIN

Myoglobin is structurally similar to hemoglobin, but it is monomeric: each myoglobin molecule consists of a heme group nearly surrounded by loops of a long polypeptide chain containing approximately 150 amino acid residues. Its M_r is 17,000 daltons, and it contains 0.34 percent iron by weight. It is present in small amounts in all skeletal and cardiac muscle cells, in which it may serve as an oxygen reservoir to protect against cellular injury during periods of oxygen deprivation.

LABILE IRON POOL

The labile iron pool is a concept derived from studies of iron kinetics [34–36]. Iron leaves the plasma and enters the interstitial and intracellular fluid compartments. Here it may be bound to cell membranes or to intracellular proteins for a relatively brief period before it is incorporated into heme or storage compounds. Some of the iron returns to the plasma, and this reflux from a labile iron pool causes a deflection of the curve of plasma iron clearance, which is evident 1 to 2 days after injection of radioactive iron (^{59}Fe). The change in slope of the curve is a function of the size of the labile pool. The labile pool has been estimated to contain from 80 to 90 mg of iron in normal persons. Whether a single mechanism accounts for these kinetic findings is uncertain. It has been suggested that a widely distributed intracellular protein may be responsible for short-term binding and release of iron and therefore may represent the labile iron pool. This is an acetate-extractable ferroprotein (AEP) with an M_r of approximately 12,000 daltons. It has been found in lung, liver, intestine, erythrocytes, spleen, and kidney of rats. The Fe^{3+}-binding kinetics of AEP exhibits an exponential curve with $T_{1/2}$ of 30 h, which is similar to that of the labile iron pool [37].

TISSUE IRON COMPARTMENT

Parenchymal, or tissue, iron normally amounts to 6 to 8 mg. This comprises the cytochromes and a variety of enzymes. Although a small compartment, it is an extremely vital one. Some of the components of this compartment reflect changes in the total body iron content [38–43].

TRANSPORT COMPARTMENT

From the standpoint of its total iron content, normally about 3 mg, the transport compartment is the smallest of the iron compartments. Yet kinetically it is the most active because its iron is normally replaced, or "turned over," at least 10 times every 24 h. This represents a common intermediate pathway by which iron in the other compartments can be interchanged (Fig. 33-4). Transport iron is bound to the specific protein transferrin, a somewhat elongated glycoprotein that migrates

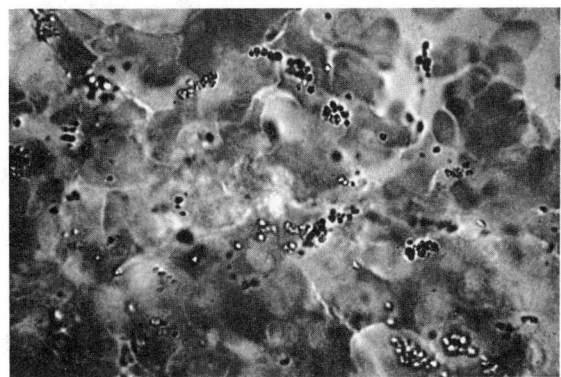

FIGURE 33-3 Hemosiderin granules in unstained marrow film from patient with idiopathic hemochromatosis.

electrophoretically with the β-globulins and has an M_r of 80,000 daltons. At each end of the molecule there are globular sialoprotein moieties, and at each of these sites one trivalent iron atom may be bound in association with a bicarbonate ion. Controversy has arisen over whether iron binds to these two sites in a completely random manner [44–51]. Probably the two sites are equivalent or practically equivalent [48,49]. Normally,

FIGURE 33-4 Scheme of major iron compartments and their relationships. In this scheme, the major flow of iron is clockwise (*heavy arrows*). The plasma (transferrin iron) pool (transport pool) serves as a common pathway of exchange. Destruction of senescent erythrocytes results in hemoglobin degradation by cells of the monocyte-macrophage (M-M) system. Kinetic studies suggest two functional iron compartments within the M-M system, here designated *I*, which exchanges rapidly with plasma transferrin iron, and *II*, a larger but more slowly exchanging compartment. Iron in M-M compartment I may be heme and in M-M compartment II may be ferritin or hemosiderin. However, the nature of iron in the M-M pools is conjectural. As indicated by the bracket, the M-M system is also part of the site of deposition of storage iron. The labile pool may represent iron bound to a protein in many or most cells of the body. Ineffective erythropoiesis (i.e.) normally occurs to a small extent and may represent a major pathway of hemoglobin catabolism in certain pathologic states. Rhopheocytosis (r.p.) may play a minor role in transport of iron to erythroblasts. (Based in part on observations of Dresch and Najean [129].)

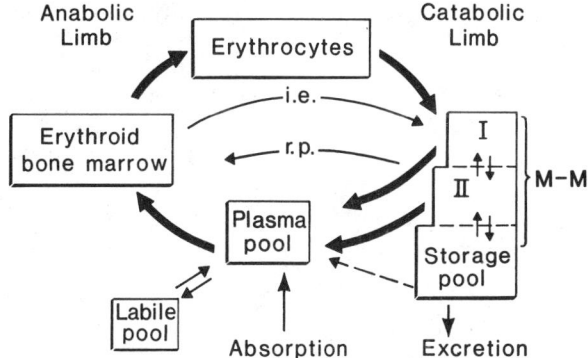

approximately one-third of the transferrin iron binding sites are occupied by iron. About 200 mg (2.5 μmol) of transferrin carrying about 100 μg (1.8 μmol) of iron per deciliter is normally contained in human plasma. This is subject to large diurnal fluctuations and also varies under different physiologic and pathologic conditions, as described below.

The transferrin-Fe^{2+} complex binds to erythroblasts or reticulocytes at specific receptor sites, and it has been suggested that the entire complex may be internalized [52]. Apotransferrin (transferrin devoid of iron) is synthesized by hepatocytes and by cells of the monocyte-macrophage system [53,54]. At least 19 genetically determined molecular variants of transferrin have been described [55]. Their iron-binding and kinetic properties seem to be identical.

Iron absorption

IRON REQUIREMENTS

To provide sufficient iron for normal synthesis of hemoglobin and other iron proteins, the body must absorb small amounts of iron through the intestinal mucosa. For a normal adult male, the amount of iron absorbed need only balance that small amount which is excreted, mostly in the stool, approximately 1 mg per day. A higher iron requirement exists during growth periods or when there is loss of blood. In women, iron absorbed must be sufficient to replace that lost through menstruation or diverted to the fetus during pregnancy (Table 33-2).

DIETARY IRON

The iron content of the diet is variable. The infant's diet is inadequate for its needs unless iron is added during preparation of the formula or unless feeding with iron-fortified cereals is begun early. The iron content of the average "well-balanced" American diet is 10 to 20 mg [56].

Appreciable amounts of iron may be contributed to food by cooking in iron pots and pans. This important source of dietary iron is being sacrificed as iron utensils are replaced with aluminum, stainless steel, or plastic-coated vessels [56]. The iron gained by food during cooking or other food processing is in the form of simple inorganic salts or, perhaps to some extent, in

iron-amino acid complexes. However, intrinsic food iron exists to a large extent as heme compounds such as hemoglobin and myoglobin. The mechanism for absorption of heme iron differs from that of simpler iron compounds [57–59]. Heme iron is better absorbed than is inorganic iron, especially in individuals who are iron-deficient [60].

SITE OF IRON ABSORPTION

Simple iron compounds may be absorbed from almost any level of the intestine. However, iron absorption is most efficient in the duodenum [61–63] and becomes progressively less so farther along the alimentary canal.

MECHANISMS OF IRON ABSORPTION

To enter the body, iron must traverse the mucosal epithelium and pass into the submucosal capillary network. There seems to be no lymphatic uptake of iron. In some mammalian species, heme or hemoglobin iron may pass directly through the epithelial cell [64]. In humans only a tiny fraction of the heme absorbed by mucosal cells passes directly into plasma [65,66]. Most of the heme taken up by mucosal cells is degraded to free iron and tetrapyrrole by a microsomal heme-splitting enzyme, *heme oxygenase*, which converts heme to bilirubin, CO, and inorganic iron [59,67]. Absorption of inorganic iron by the mucosal cell appears to be an active process; the mechanism may be by endocytosis, but this remains to be proved. Within the mucosal cell, transferrin may carry iron to the submucosal surface of the cell, where it passes through the cell membrane into the capillary network. Here it is again taken up by plasma transferrin, which transports the iron to hemopoietic and other tissues (Fig. 33-5). Ceruloplasmin is a plasma ferroxidase that effects the conversion from Fe^{2+} to Fe^{3+} as the iron is taken up by transferrin [68–71].

Since iron excretion is relatively fixed, the body must regulate its iron content by modulating the amount of iron absorbed. It does so through a poorly understood "mucosal intelligence," which provides increased iron absorption in iron deficiency and often decreased iron absorption when iron overload is present.

The rate of absorption of iron is influenced by many factors. One of these is the iron content of the intestinal mucosal cell. Much controversy has surrounded the mechanism of mucosal absorption and the possible regulatory role of the mucosal epithelium. Some studies

TABLE 33-2   Minimal daily iron requirements

	Amount which must be absorbed for hemoglobin synthesis, mg	Minimal amount which should be ingested daily, mg
Infants	1	10
Children	0.5	5
Young nonpregnant women	2	20
Pregnant women	3	30
Men and postmenopausal women	1	10

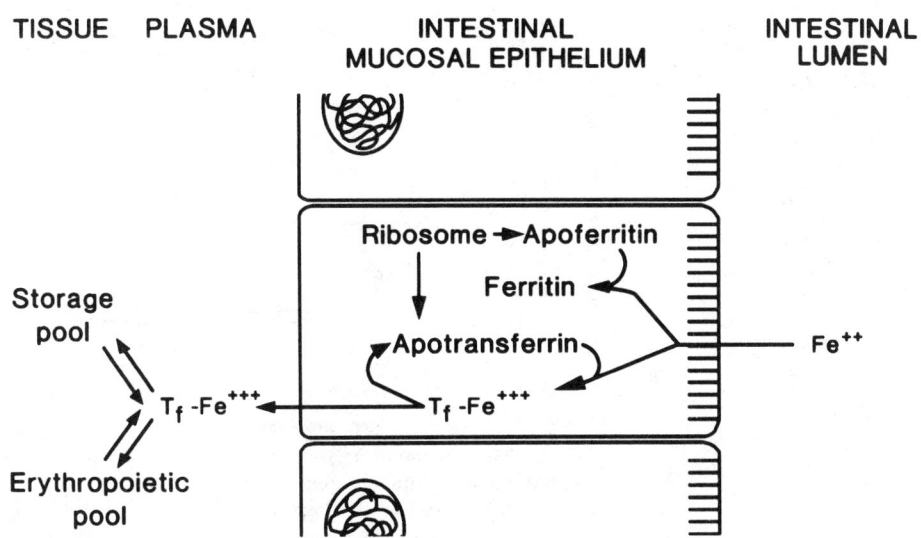

TISSUE   PLASMA   INTESTINAL   INTESTINAL
                    MUCOSAL EPITHELIUM   LUMEN

FIGURE 33-5   A concept of the mechanism of uptake of inorganic iron from the intestinal lumen by the mucosal cell. Ferritin and a transferrinlike protein and some less clearly defined iron-binding proteins have all been demonstrated in mucosal epithelial cells. Apoferritin may function as an iron trap in the cell, retaining iron in the mucosal cell when body iron stores are increased. Apotransferrin (or a similar protein), however, may facilitate iron uptake by endocytosis and may also serve as the cytosolic transport protein. Some features of this diagram are speculative; the complete details of this process of iron uptake by mucosal epithelium are still unknown (T_f = apotransferrin).

[72–75] seem to indicate that a physiologic mechanism exists within the mucosal cells for trapping iron when the level of body iron stores is high. If the level of iron stores is low, there is little or no trapping of iron, and it passes almost directly from the intestinal lumen through the cell and into the plasma. With the passage of time the mucosal cell advances from the base to the tip of the villus and is sloughed and lost in the feces, together with its retained iron (Fig. 33-6). In addition, some plasma iron may pass into the mucosal cell, become fixed there, and ultimately be lost. Some iron-laden macrophages may also find their way into the intestinal lumen. This flexible scheme also provides for intestinal excretion of iron, but such excretion is very limited. Ferritin is normally found within the intestinal mucosa, incorporated in cytoplasmic "F bodies" [73]. It has sometimes been assumed that ferritin is the substance which forms within the cell to prevent the passage of unneeded iron into the plasma. Transferrin or a transferrin-like protein is also present in intestinal mucosal epithelial cells [76,77]. Some evidence indicates that in iron deficiency, the amount of apotransferrin is increased and may therefore enhance iron absorption. The modulation of iron absorption may involve both ferritin and transferrin in the cytosol of mucosal epithelial cells.

The physiologic mechanism of regulation of iron absorption may play an important role when iron is present in the intestinal lumen at low concentration. It is easily overcome, however, by the higher concentration which may be imposed therapeutically or by accidental ingestion of iron compounds by a child. There is indeed no mechanism by which the intestinal mucosa can block the increased iron absorption which occurs as the concentration of iron in the intestinal lumen is increased. Numerous studies have shown unequivocally that for each increment in dose of an inorganic iron compound there is a corresponding increment in the amount of iron absorbed [78–81] (Fig. 33-7).

Other gastrointestinal mechanisms also influence iron absorption. Gastric secretions undoubtedly are important, but the mechanism is as yet poorly understood. Gastric juice in some manner stabilizes ionic iron, preventing its precipitation as insoluble ferric hydroxide [82,83]. This may be due to chelation of iron by small molecules in the gastric juice, such as amino acids and keto sugars [85,86]. Some studies have shown that a protein component of gastric juice (gastroferrin) binds iron and prevents its absorption [87]. Conversely, other studies seem to have shown a component of gastric juice which binds iron and facilitates its absorption [88]. While these observations are not necessarily incompatible, clearly the problem of the gastric factor(s) needs better resolution.

In the presence of chronic liver disease or chronic pancreatic disease iron absorption is enhanced [88–93]. How this is effected is unknown. Conflicting data have been reported regarding the effect of pancreatic secretions on iron absorption [94,95], and it is, in fact, quite doubtful that pancreatic disorders influence iron absorption at all [96,97]. Bile may play a limited role in facilitating iron absorption in iron-deficient dogs [98].

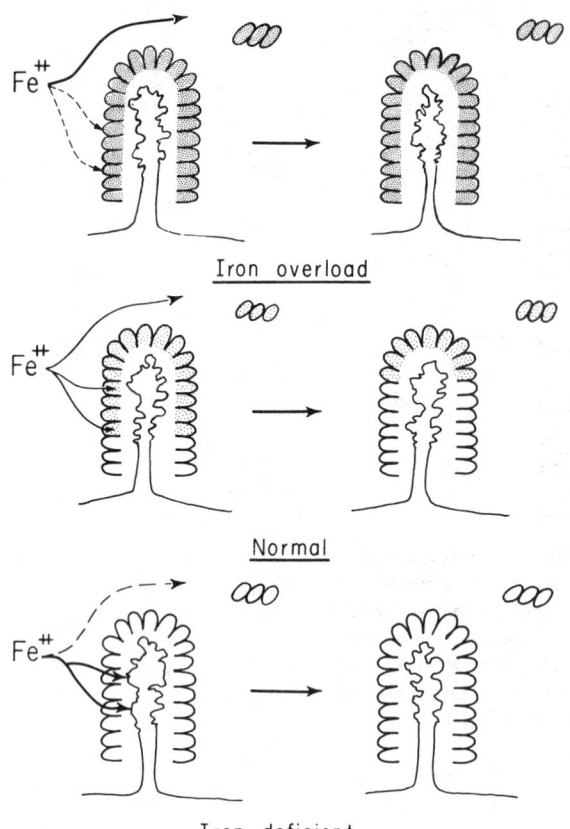

FIGURE 33-6 Mucosal regulation of iron absorption. Normally, some iron passes directly through the mucosal cell into the plasma and some is retained in the mucosal cell. As the cell ages, it advances toward the tip of the villus and is sloughed into the intestinal lumen; its retained iron is lost in feces. In states of iron overload, little iron is taken up by the mucosal epithelium, and most of this is retained and lost as the cell is sloughed. In iron deficiency, more iron traverses the mucosal cell and enters the plasma; little or none is trapped in mucosal epithelium. (Slightly modified from Conrad and Crosby [72].)

The ingestion of certain foods, reducing agents, or alcohol influences the rate of iron absorption; oxalates, phytates, and phosphates, for example, complex with iron and retard its absorption. Many simple reducing substances have been found to increase iron absorption. Among these are hydroquinone, ascorbate, lactate, pyruvate, succinate, fructose, cysteine, and sorbitol [99–101]. Ascorbate has also been shown to enhance iron absorption in an isolated segment of intestine. Although it was formerly believed that ingestion of alcohol enhances iron absorption [103], more recent careful studies indicate that this is not the case [104].

Among the factors operating outside the alimentary tract to increase iron absorption are hypoxia, anemia, depletion of iron stores, and increased erythropoiesis. Each of these factors appears to exert an independent effect, but the means by which they "instruct" the bowel to absorb more iron remains a mystery. The degree of

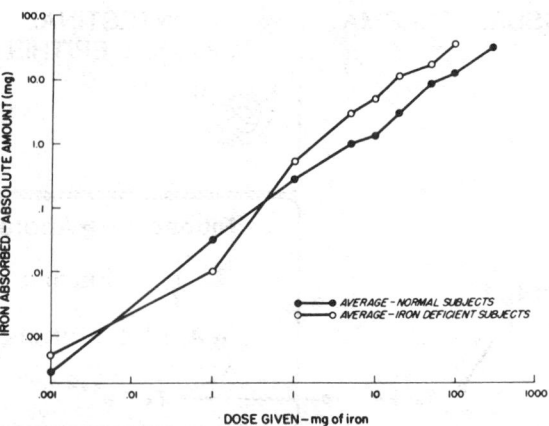

FIGURE 33-7   Relation between iron dosage and amount of iron absorbed in human beings. When the logarithm of the dose is plotted against the logarithm of the amount of iron absorbed, a straight line gives a remarkably good fit. It is apparent, therefore, that even at high dosage levels of iron, increasing iron dose gives greater iron absorption. (Drawn from data of Smith and Pannacciuli [78].)

transferrin saturation, the concentration of plasma iron, the rate of plasma iron clearance, and the plasma concentration of erythropoietin have been considered as humoral messengers. Evidence from numerous studies of this problem may be summarized briefly: Each of the factors enumerated may play a limited role, but none by itself adequately explains all the observations. It may be that the intestinal mucosa is responsive to more than one humoral mechanism for the fine control of the rate of iron absorption.

Transport of iron

Once an atom of iron enters the body, it is virtually in a closed system (Fig. 33-8) in which it cycles almost endlessly from the plasma to the developing erythroblast (where it is utilized in hemoglobin synthesis), thence into the circulating blood for about 4 months, and thence to phagocytic macrophages. Here it is removed from hemoglobin and released back into the plasma to repeat the cycle. Clearly the transport of iron in the plasma is of central importance to this process.

The major function of the transport protein transferrin is to provide the means of moving iron from wherever it enters the plasma (intestinal villi, splenic sinusoids) to the erythroblasts of the marrow. It binds briefly to the erythroblast membrane, where it delivers its burden of iron [105–107]. The binding of transferrin and release of iron are active processes which can be abolished by enzyme inhibitors [108]. Much of the evidence supporting this concept has been derived from studies of reticulocytes; although hemoglobin synthesis is nearly complete by this stage of erythrocyte maturation, the membrane of a reticulocyte can still bind from 25,000 to 50,000 iron-laden transferrin molecules per minute. Radioactive iron (^{59}Fe)-labeled transferrin binds to reticulocyte membranes, but not to the membranes of leukocytes, platelets, or mature erythrocytes [107]. Many studies have shown that the transferrin-Fe^{3+} complex actually enters the erythroid precursors by the process of endocytosis, and transferrin may play a role in the transport of iron across the cytosol to deliver iron to mitochondria [108–112].

The importance of transferrin in the delivery of iron to the erythroblast is emphasized by two other significant observations: (1) when transferrin is fully saturated, iron absorbed by the intestine is deposited in the liver [113], and (2) when transferrin is congenitally absent, iron is absorbed by the intestine and accumulates in the liver, pancreas, spleen, and other viscera, but little gets to the marrow and a severe hypochromic microcytic anemia results (see Chap. 49) [10].

Relatively small amounts of iron are transported to other tissues, especially in a slow exchange with the iron in ferritin and hemosiderin, and to a much lesser extent with other tissue forms of iron.

Iron in the erythroblast

Previously it was believed that transferrin binds only briefly to the erythroblast membrane, discharging its burden of iron and returning to the plasma. However, the transferrin-iron complex enters the erythroblast cytoplasm by endocytosis [108,110–112,115]. When transferrin labeled with ^{59}Fe is incubated with reticulocytes and the cytosol proteins are examined at intervals, radioactivity is found in cytosolic transferrin, ferritin, and another small protein tentatively called iron-binding protein I (IBP-I) [112]. Pulse-chase experiments have shown that ^{59}Fe remains briefly on cytosol transferrin, but persists on ferritin and IBP-I [112]. Presumably the ^{59}Fe is transferred from transferrin to mitochondria; ferritin and IBP-I may serve as intermediaries in this process. The transferrin which has thus given up its Fe^{3+} is presumed to be extruded from the erythroblast to recycle in the plasma. The Fe^{3+} must next cross the mitochondrial membrane to be incorporated into heme. The mechanism of this passage has not been elucidated. By electron microscopy, iron is visualized in mitochondria as amorphous aggregates called *ferruginous micelles* [116]. When heme synthesis is impaired, as in lead poisoning or in the sideroblastic anemias (see Chap. 54), the mitochondria accumulate excessive amounts of these amorphous iron aggregates. The mitochondria can then be stained by the Prussian blue reaction and are seen by light microscopy as a ring of large blue siderotic granules encircling the erythroblast nucleus (ringed sideroblast). In normal marrow, siderotic granules are also demonstrable in erythroblast cytoplasm. However, these are very small, usually only one to three in number, and randomly distributed in the cytoplasm. These normal siderotic granules appear to be ferritin aggregates and are not located in mitochondria [71].

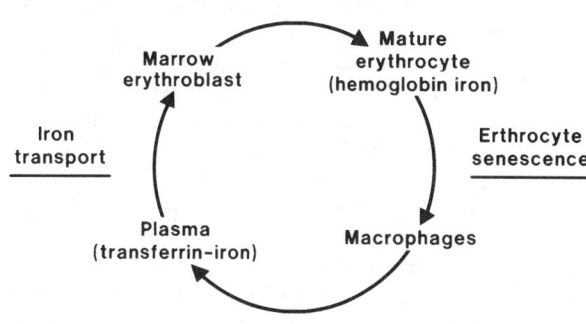

FIGURE 33-8 Internal iron cycle. Once an atom of iron enters the body, it is in a virtually closed system where it cycles repeatedly. A small quantity of iron atoms escapes each day, to other iron proteins or to the exterior of the body, and an equal number enter the system.

Erythroblasts containing these ferritin siderotic granules are designated *sideroblasts* and normally represent 20 to 50 percent of the erythrocyte precursors of the marrow. In iron deficiency, sideroblasts almost disappear from the marrow. Conversely, in some states of iron overload, they may become more numerous and contain more siderotic granules than normally.

Within the mitochondria, iron is inserted into protoporphyrin to become heme. This reaction requires the presence of heme synthetase (ferrochelatase). Heme has been shown to inhibit the release of iron from transferrin [117]. This may be an important feedback mechanism for adjusting the supply of iron to the rate of hemoglobin synthesis in the erythroblast.

Role of the monocyte-macrophage system

Destruction of aged erythrocytes and hemoglobin degradation occur within cells of the monocyte-macrophage system, chiefly in the liver and spleen. Digestion of phagocytized red cells proceeds at a rate sufficient to release approximately 20 percent of the hemoglobin iron within a few hours. The plasma iron derived by the action of the monocyte-macrophage system is bound to transferrin and is ultimately redistributed, approximately 80 percent being rapidly reincorporated into hemoglobin. Thus about 40 percent of the hemoglobin iron of nonviable erythrocytes reappears in circulating red cells in 12 days. The rate of reutilization varies considerably in normal subjects, for example, 19 to 69 percent reincorporation in 12 days, and is even more variable in the presence of disease. The remainder of the iron derived from hemoglobin degradation enters the storage pool as ferritin or hemosiderin and normally turns over very slowly. In normal subjects, approximately 40 percent of this iron remains in storage after 140 days. When there is an increased iron demand for hemoglobin synthesis, however, storage iron may be mobilized more rapidly [118]. Conversely, in the presence of infection or other inflammatory process or malignancy, iron derived from degradation of hemoglobin by the monocyte-macrophage system is reutilized in hemoglobin synthesis at a much slower than normal rate [118–120]. These perturbations in iron reutilization are believed to be due to changes in the rate of iron release by cells of the monocyte-macrophage system. Thus in the presence of chronic inflammatory disease there is a reduction in the rate of release of iron by the phagocytic cell and an increase in the storage of iron in the monocyte-macrophage system. The effect is a reduced rate of delivery of iron to the developing erythroblast, an accelerated rate of transport to the marrow of iron available in the plasma pool, a reduction in plasma iron concentration, and a less than optimal rate of erythropoiesis. Microcytic erythrocytes may result from the reduced flow of iron from the monocyte-macrophage system to the developing erythroblasts.

The release of iron from ferritin is accelerated in states of hypoxia or when erythropoiesis is increased. Iron release may be effected experimentally by various means, including a variety of reducing agents, such as dithionite, thioglycolate, cysteine, and ascorbate [18,19, 96]. Reduced flavin mononucleotide may be the physiologically important mediator of iron release from ferritin. Iron is released from ferritin as the ferrous ion and as such traverses the cytosol and cell membrane to enter plasma, where it is again oxidized by ceruloplasmin to Fe^{3+} and is taken up by transferrin. It has been suggested that in certain disorders poor reutilization of hemoglobin iron may be improved by testosterone therapy [122].

In addition to its role in regulating the size of iron stores, the monocyte-macrophage system appears to participate in regulation of the concentration of transferrin. Macrophages of this system have the capacity both to synthesize apotransferrin and to take up and degrade transferrin [123–126].

Iron excretion

The body conserves its hoard of iron with such remarkable efficiency that less than a thousandth of it is lost each day, an amount easily replaced if dietary sources are adequate. Almost all this iron loss occurs by way of the feces and normally amounts to about 1 mg per day. Exfoliation of skin and dermal appendages results in a much smaller loss, as does perspiration. Even in climates that stimulate marked perspiration, the loss of iron in sweat is minimal [127]. Iron is excreted also in urine, but in very small amounts. In humans, lactation may cause excretion of about 1 mg iron daily, thus doubling the overall rate of iron excretion. In addition, varying amounts of blood are lost by normal menstruation, as will be discussed in Chap. 48.

While total daily iron excretion is normally about 1 mg for males and about 2 mg for menstruating women, persons with marked iron overload, e.g., hemochromatosis, may lose as much as 4 mg of iron daily by these mechanisms, a quantity insufficient to prevent the accumulation of storage iron [128].

References

1. Beutler, E.: Iron enzymes in iron deficiency. VI. Aconitase activity and citrate metabolism. *J. Clin. Invest. 38*:1605, 1959.
2. Harrison, P. M., Fischbach, F. A., Hoy, T. G., and Haggis, G. H.: Ferric oxyhydroxide core of ferritin. *Nature 216*:1188, 1967.
3. Brady, G. W., et al.: The structure of an iron core analog of ferritin. *Biochemistry 7*:2185, 1968.
4. Hoy, T. G., Harrison, P. M., and Hoare, R. J.: Quarternary structure of apoferritin: The rotation function at 9 A resolution. *J. Mol. Biol. 84*:515, 1974.
5. Harrison, P. M., et al.: Ferritin iron uptake and release. *Biochem. J. 143*:445, 1974.
6. Hoy, T. G., Harrison, P. M., and Shabbir, M.: Uptake and release of ferritin iron. *Biochem. J. 139*:603, 1974.
7. Macara, I. G., Hoy, T. G., and Harrison, P. M.: The formation of ferritin from apoferritin. *Biochem. J. 126*:151, 1972.
8. Banyard, S. H., Stammers, D. K., and Harrison, P. M.: Electron density map of apoferritin at 2.8-Å resolution. *Nature 271*:282, 1978.
9. Bjork, I., and Fish, W. W.: Native and subunit molecular weights of apoferritin. *Biochemistry 10*:2844, 1971.
10. Crichton, R. R.: The subunit structure of apoferritin and other eicosamers. *Biochem. J. 126*:761, 1972.
11. Crichton, R. R., et al.: The subunit structure of horse spleen apoferritin: The molecular weight of the oligomer and its stability to dissociation by dilution. *Biochem. J. 131*:855, 1973.
12. Heusterspreute, M., Wustefeld, C., Mathijs, J. M., Mareschal, J. C., Charlier, G., and Crichton, R. R.: Comparative studies of ferritins. *Proceedings of the Peptides of the Biological Fluids Colloquium 28*:91, 1980.
13. Harrison, P. M., et al.: The structure and function of ferritin. *Ciba Found. Symp. 51*:19, 1976.
14. Clegg, G. A., Stansfield, R. F. D., Bourne, P. E., and Harrison, P. M.: Helix packing and subunit conformation in horse spleen apoferritin. *Nature 288*:298, 1980.
15. Crichton, R. R., and Paques, E. P.: A kinetic study of the mechanism of ferritin formation. *Biochem. Soc. Trans. 5*:1130, 1977.
16. Hoy, T. G., et al.: The release of iron from horse spleen ferritin to 1,10-phenanthroline. *Biochem. J. 137*:67, 1974.
17. Jones, T., Spence, R., and Walsh, C.: Mechanism and kinetics of iron release from ferritin by dihydroflavins and dihydroflavin analogues. *Biochemistry 17*:4011, 1978.
18. Dogin, J., and Crichton, R. R.: Mobilization of iron from ferritin fractions of defined iron content by biological reductants. *FEBS Lett. 54*:234, 1975.
19. Harrison, P. M.: Ferritin: An iron-storage molecule. *Semin. Hematol. 14*:55, 1977.
20. Crichton, R. R.: A role of ferritin in the regulation of iron metabolism. *FEBS Lett. 34*:125, 1973.
21. Adelman, T. G., Arosio, P., and Drysdale, J. W.: Multiple subunits in human ferritins: Evidence for hybrid molecules. *Biochem. Biophys. Res. Commun. 63*:1056, 1975.
22. Alahonai, Y., et al.: Electrofocusing analysis of isoferritins, in *Onco-Developmental Gene Expression*, edited by W. H. Fishman and S. Sell. Academic, New York, 1976, pp. 763–767.
23. Alfrey, C. P., Lynch, E. C., and Whitley, C. E.: Characteristics of ferritin isolated from human marrow, spleen, liver, and reticulocytes. *J. Lab. Clin. Med. 70*:419, 1967.
24. Alpert, E.: Characterization and subunit analysis of ferritin isolated from normal and malignant human liver. *Cancer Res. 35*:1505, 1975.

25. Arosio, P., Adelman, T. G., and Drysdale, J. W.: On ferritin heterogeneity. Further evidence for heteropolymers. *J. Biol. Chem.* 253:4451, 1978.

26. Asakawa, H., Taguchi, T., and Mori, W.: Immunological heterogeneity in human ferritinemia. *Gann.* 67:347, 1976.

27. Bomford, A., et al.: The iron content of human liver and spleen isoferritins correlates with their isoelectric point and subunit composition. *Biochem. Biophys. Res. Commun.* 83:334, 1978.

28. Bryce, C. F. A., Magnusson, C. G. M., and Crichton, R. R.: A reappraisal of the electrophoretic patterns obtained from ferritin and apoferritin in the presence of denaturants. *FEBS Lett.* 96:257, 1978.

29. Shingo, S., and Harrison, P. M.: Artifacts in ferritin isoelectric focusing profiles. *FEBS Lett.* 105:353, 1979.

30. Richter, G. W.: Electron microscopy of hemosiderin: Presence of ferritin and occurrence of crystalline lattices in hemosiderin deposits. *J. Biophys. Biochem. Cytol.* 4:55, 1958.

31. Wöhler, F.: Ferritin and haemosiderin. *Ger. Med. Mon.* 9:377, 1964.

32. Fischbach, F. A., Gregory, D. W., Harrison, P. M., et al.: On the structure of hemosiderin and its relationship to ferritin. *J. Ultrastruct. Res.* 37:495, 1971.

33. General discussion. I. Haemosiderin. *Ciba Found. Symp.* 51:69, 1976.

34. Greenberg, G. R., and Wintrobe, M. M.: A labile iron pool. *J. Biol. Chem.* 165:397, 1946 (letter to the editor).

35. Pollycove, M., and Mortimer, R.: The quantitative determination of iron kinetics and hemoglobin synthesis in human subjects. *J. Clin. Invest.* 40:763, 1961.

36. Hosain, F., Marsaglia, G., and Finch, C. A.: Blood ferrokinetics in normal man. *J. Clin. Invest.* 46:1, 1967.

37. Boulard, M., Delin, M., and Najean, Y.: Identification and purification of a new non-heme, non-ferritin iron protein. *Proc. Soc. Exp. Biol. Med.* 139:1379, 1972.

38. Beutler, E.: Iron enzymes in iron deficiency. I. Cytochrome C. *Am. J. Med. Sci.* 234:517, 1957.

39. Beutler, E., and Blaisdell, R. K.: Iron enzymes in iron deficiency. III. Catalase in rat red cells and liver with some further observations on cytochrome C. *J. Lab. Clin. Med.* 52:694, 1958.

40. Beutler, E., and Blaisdell, R. K.: Iron enzymes in iron deficiency. V. Succinic dehydrogenase in rat liver, kidney and heart. *Blood* 15:30, 1960.

41. Jacobs, A.: Iron-containing enzymes in the buccal epithelium. *Lancet* 2:1331, 1961.

42. Dallman, P. R., Sunshine, P., and Leonard, Y.: Intestinal cytochrome response with repair of iron deficiency. *Pediatrics* 39:863, 1967.

43. Srivastava, S. K., Sanwal, G. G., and Tewari, K. K.: Biochemical alterations in rat tissue in iron deficiency anemia and repletion with iron. *Indian J. Biochem.* 2:257, 1965.

44. Zapolski, E. J., Ganz, R., and Princiotto, J. V.: Biological specificity of the iron-binding sites of transferrin. *Am. J. Physiol.* 226:334, 1974.

45. Fletcher, J., and Huehns, E. R.: Significance of the binding of iron by transferrin. *Nature* 215:584, 1967.

46. Fletcher, J., and Huehns, E. R.: Function of transferrin. *Nature* 218:1211, 1968.

47. Morgan, E. H., Huebers, H., and Finch, C. A.: Differences between the binding sites for iron binding and release in human and rat transferrin. *Blood* 52:1219, 1978.

48. Morgan, E. H.: Studies of the mechanism of iron release from transferrin. *Biochim. Biophys. Acta.* 580:312, 1979.

49. Okada, S., Jarvis, B., and Brown, E. B.: In vivo evidence for the functional heterogeneity of transferrin bound iron. V. Isotransferrins: An explanation of the Fletcher-Huehns phenomenon in the rat. *J. Lab. Clin. Med.* 93:189, 1979.

50. Verhoef, N. J., et al.: Functional heterogeneity of transferrin bound iron. *Acta Haematol.* 60:210, 1978.

51. Verhoef, N. J., and Noordeloos, P. J.: Binding of transferrin and uptake of iron by rat erythroid cells in vitro. *Clin. Sci. Mol. Med.* 52:87, 1977.

52. Haurani, F. I., Meyer, A., and O'Brien, R.: Production of transferrin by the macrophage. *J. Reticuloendothel. Soc.* 14:309, 1973.

53. Thorbecke, G. J., Liem, H. H., Knight, S., Cox, K., and Muller-Eberhard, U.: Sites of formation of the serum proteins transferrin and hemopexin. *J. Clin. Invest.* 52:725, 1973.

54. Giblett, E. R.: *Genetic Markers in Human Blood.* Davis, Philadelphia, 1969, p. 135.

55. Aisen, P.: The transferrins, in *Iron in Biochemistry and Medicine,* edited by A. Jacobs and M. Worwood. Academic, New York, 1980, vol. 2, pp. 87–129.

56. Moore, C. V.: Iron nutrition and requirements. *Ser. Haematol.* 6:1, 1965.

57. Callender, S. T., Mallet, B. J., and Smith, M. D.: Absorption of haemoglobin iron. *Br. J. Haematol.* 3:186, 1957.

58. Hallberg, L., and Sölvell, L.: Absorption of hemoglobin iron in man. *Acta Med. Scand.* 181:335, 1967.

59. Conrad, M. E., Benjamin, B. I., Williams, H. L., and Foy, A. L.: Human absorption of hemoglobin-iron. *Gastroenterology* 53:5, 1967.

60. Hussain, R., Walker, R. B., Layrisse, M., Clark, P., and Finch, C. A.: Nutritive value of food iron. *Am. J. Clin. Nutr.* 16:464, 1965.

61. Moore, C. V., Arrowsmith, W. R., Welch, J., and Minnich, V.: Studies in iron transportation and metabolism. IV. Observations on the absorption of iron from the gastro-intestinal tract. *J. Clin. Invest.* 18:553, 1939.

62. Rhodes, J., Beton, D., and Brown, D. A.: Absorption of iron instilled into the stomach, duodenum, and jejunum. *Gut* 9:323, 1968.

63. Brown, E. B., Jr., and Justus, B. W.: In vitro absorption of radioiron by everted pouches of rat intestine. *Am. J. Physiol.* 194:319, 1958.

64. Schiffer, L. M., Price, D. C., and Cronkite, E. P.: Iron absorption and anemia. *J. Lab. Clin. Med.* 65:316, 1965.

65. Turnbull, A., Cleton, F., and Finch, C. A.: Iron absorption. IV. The absorption of hemoglobin iron. *J. Clin. Invest.* 41:1897, 1962.

66. Weintraub, L. R., Weinstein, M. B., Huser, H.-J., and Rafal, S.: Absorption of hemoglobin iron: The role of a heme-splitting substance in the intestinal mucosa. *J. Clin. Invest.* 47:531, 1968.

67. Raffin, S. B., Woo, C. H., Roost, K. T., Price, D. C., and Schmid, R.: Intestinal absorption of hemoglobin iron-heme cleavage by mucosal heme oxygenase. *J. Clin. Invest.* 54:1344, 1974.

68. Roeser, H. P., Lee, G. R., Nacht, S., and Cartwright, G. E.: The role of ceruloplasmin in iron metabolism. *J. Clin. Invest.* 49:2408, 1970.

69. Frieden, E.: The ferrous to ferric cycles in iron metabolism. *Nutr. Rev.* 31:41, 1973.

70. Osaki, S., Johnson, D. A., and Frieden, E.: The possible significance of the ferrous oxidase activity of ceruloplasmin in normal human serum. *J. Biol. Chem.* 241:2746, 1966.

71. Cartwright, G. E., and Deiss, A.: Sideroblasts, siderocytes, and sideroblastic anemia. *N. Engl. J. Med.* 292:185, 1975.

72. Conrad, M. E., Jr., and Crosby, W. H.: Intestinal mucosal mechanisms controlling iron absorption. *Blood* 22:406, 1963.

73. Hartman, R. S., Conrad, M. E., Jr., Hartman, R. E., Joy, R. J. T., and Crosby, W. H.: Ferritin containing bodies in human small intestinal epithelium. *Blood* 22:397, 1963.

74. Crosby, W. H., Conrad, M. E., Jr., and Wheby, M. S.: The rate of iron accumulation in iron storage disease. *Blood* 22:429, 1963.

75. Wheby, M. S., and Crosby, W. H.: The gastrointestinal tract and iron absorption. *Blood* 22:416, 1963.

76. Huebers, H., Huebers, E., and Rummel, W.: Mechanism of iron absorption: Iron-binding proteins and dependence of iron absorption on an elutable factor, in *Iron Metabolism and Its Disorders,* edited by H. Kief. American Elsevier, New York, 1975, pp. 13–21.

77. Huebers, H., et al.: Isolation ahd characterization of iron binding proteins from rat intestinal mucosa. *Eur. J. Biochem.* 66:447, 1976.

78. Smith, M. D., and Pannacciulli, I. M.: Absorption of inorganic iron from graded doses: Its significance in relation to iron absorption tests and the 'mucosal block' theory. *Br. J. Haematol.* 4:428, 1958.

79. Bonnet, J. D., Hagedorn, A. B., and Owen, C. A., Jr.: A quantitative method for measuring gastrointestinal absorption of iron. *Blood* 15:36, 1960.

80. Brown, E. B., Jr., Dubach, R., and Moore, C. V.: Studies in iron transportation and metabolism. XI. Critical analysis of mucosal block by large doses of inorganic iron in human subjects. *J. Lab. Clin. Med.* 52:335, 1958.

81. Beutler, E., Kelly, B. M., and Beutler, F.: The regulation of iron absorption. II. Relationship between iron dosage and iron absorption. *Am. J. Clin. Nutr.* 11:559, 1962.

82. Beutler, E., Fairbanks, V. F., and Fahey, J. L.: *Clinical Disorders of Iron Metabolism.* Grune & Stratton, New York, 1963.

83. Jacobs, A.: Gastric factor in iron absorption. *Lancet* 1:1313, 1968.

84. Van Campen, D.: Enhancement of iron absorption from ligated segments of rat intestine by histidine, cysteine, and lysine: Effects of removing ionizing groups and of stereoisomerism. *J. Nutr.* 103:139, 1973.

85. Davis, P. S., and Deller, D. J.: Prediction and demonstration of iron chelating ability of sugars. *Nature* 212:405, 1966.

86. Conrad, M. E., and Schade, S. G.: Ascorbic acid chelates in iron absorption: A role for hydrochloric acid and bile. *Gastroenterology* 55:35, 1968.

87. Davis, P. S., Luke, C. G., and Deller, D. J.: Reduction of gastric iron-binding protein in haemochromatosis: A previously unrecognized metabolic defect. *Lancet* 2:1431, 1966.

88. Murray, M. J., and Stein, N.: A gastric factor promoting iron absorption. *Lancet* 1:614, 1968.

89. Callender, S. T., and Malpas, J. S.: Absorption of iron in cirrhosis of liver. *Br. Med. J.* 2:1516, 1963.

90. Williams, R., Williams, H. S., Scheuer, P. J., Pitcher, C. S., Loiseau, E., and Sherlock, S.: Iron absorption and siderosis in chronic liver disease. *Q. J. Med.* 36:151, 1967.

91. Davis, A. E., and Badenoch, J.: Iron absorption in pancreatic disease. *Lancet* 2:6, 1962.

92. Smith, R. S.: Iron absorption in cystic fibrosis. *Br. Med. J.* 1:608, 1964.

93. Wissler, R. W., Bethard, W. F., Barker, P., and Mori, H. D.: Effects of polyoxyethylene sorbitan monolaurate (Tween 20) upon gastrointestinal iron absorption in hamsters. *Proc. Soc. Exp. Biol. Med.* 86:170, 1954.

94. Biggs, J. C., and Davis, A. E.: The exocrine pancreas and iron absorption. *Aust. Ann. Med.* 15:36, 1966.

95. Kavin, H., Charlton, R. W., Jacobs, P., Green, R., Torrance, J. D., and Bothwell, T. H.: Effect of the exocrine pancreatic secretions on iron absorption. *Gut* 8:556, 1967.

96. Murray, M. J., and Stein, N.: Does the pancreas influence iron absorption? A critical review of information to date. *Gastroenterology* 51:694, 1966.

97. Balcerzak, S. P., Peternel, W. W., and Heinle, E. W.: Iron absorption in chronic pancreatitis. *Gastroenterology* 53:257, 1967.

98. Wheby, M. S., Conrad, M. E., Hedberg, S. E., and Crosby, W. H.: The role of bile in the control of iron absorption. *Gastroenterology* 42:319, 1962.

99. Herndon, J. F., Rice, E. G., Tucker, R. G., Van Loon, E. J., and Greenberg, S. M.: Iron absorption and metabolism. III. The enhancement of iron absorption in rats by D-sorbitol. *J. Nutr.* 64:615, 1958.

100. Hallberg, L., and Sölvell, L.: Iron absorption studies: [1] Determination of the absorption rate of iron in man. [2] Absorption of a single dose of iron in man. [3] Iron absorption during constant intragastric infusion of iron in man. [4] Effect of iron and transferrin intravenously on iron absorption and turnover in man (Sölvell alone). *Acta Med. Scand. (Suppl. 358)* 168:1, 1960.

101. Pollack, S., Kaufman, R. M., and Crosby, W. H.: Iron absorption: Effects of sugars and reducing agents. *Blood* 24:577, 1964.

102. Jacobs, P., Bothwell, T. H., and Charlton, R. W.: Intestinal iron transport: Studies using a loop of gut with an artificial circulation. *Am. J. Physiol.* 210:694, 1966.

103. Charlton, R. W., Jacobs, P., Seftel, H., and Bothwell, T. H.: Effect of alcohol on iron absorption. *Br. Med. J.* 2:1427, 1964.

104. Celada, A., Rudolf, H., and Donath, A.: Effect of single ingestion of alcohol on iron absorption. *Am. J. Hematol.* 5:225, 1978.

105. Jandl, J. H., Inman, J. K., Simmons, R. L., and Allen, D. W.: Transfer of iron from serum iron-binding protein to human reticulocytes. *J. Clin. Invest.* 38:161, 1959.

106. Katz, J. H.: The delivery of iron to the immature red cell: A critical

107. Jandl, J. H., and Katz, J. H.: The plasma-to-cell cycle of transferrin. *J. Clin. Invest.* 42:314, 1963.

108. Sly, D. A., Grohlich, D., and Bezkorovainy, A.: Transferrin in the reticulocyte cytosol. *Biochim. Biophys. Acta* 385:36, 1975.

109. Hemmaplardh, D., and Morgan, E. H.: The mechanism of iron exchange between synthetic iron chelators and rabbit reticulocytes. *Biochim. Biophys. Acta* 373:84, 1974.

110. Morgan, E. H., and Appleton, T. C.: Autoradiographic localization of ^{125}I-labelled transferrin in rabbit reticulocytes. *Nature* 223:1371, 1969.

111. Martinez-Medellin, J., and Schulman, H. M.: The kinetics of iron and transferrin incorporation into rabbit erythroid cells and the nature of stromal-bound iron. *Biochim. Biophys. Acta* 264:272, 1972.

112. Nunez, M. T., Coles, E. S., and Glass, J.: Cytosol intermediates in the transport of iron. *Blood* 55:1051, 1980.

113. Fawwaz, R. A., Winchell, H. S., Pollycove, M., and Sargent, T.: Hepatic iron deposition in humans. I. First-pass hepatic deposition of intestinally absorbed iron in patients with low plasma latent iron-binding capacity. *Blood* 30:417, 1967.

114. Bessis, M., and Breton-Gorius, J.: L'Ilot érythroblastique et la rhophéocytose de la ferritine dans l'inflammation. *Nouv. Rev. Fr. Hematol.* 1:569, 1961.

115. Sullivan, A. L., Grasso, J. A., and Weintraub, L. R.: Micropinocytosis of transferrin by developing red cells: An electron-microscopic study utilizing ferritin-conjugated transferrin and ferritin-conjugated antibodies to transferrin. *Blood* 47:133, 1976.

116. Bessis, M., and Breton-Gorius, J.: Accumulation de granules ferrugineux dans les mitochondries des érythroblastes. *C. R. Acad. Sci.* 244:2846, 1957.

117. Ponka, P., Neuwirt, J., and Borova, J.: The role of heme in the release of iron from transferrin in reticulocytes. *Enzyme* 17:91, 1974.

118. Noyes, W. D., Bothwell, T. H., and Finch, C. A.: The role of the reticulo-endothelial cell in iron metabolism. *Br. J. Haematol.* 6:43, 1960.

119. Haurani, F. I., Burke, W., and Martinez, E. J.: Defective reutilization of iron in the anemia of inflammation. *J. Lab. Clin. Med.* 65:560, 1965.

120. Haurani, F. I., Young, K., and Tocantins, L. M.: Reutilization of iron in anemia complicating malignant neoplasms. *Blood* 22:73, 1963.

121. Sirivech, S., Frieden, E., and Osaki, S.: The release of iron from horse spleen ferritin by reduced flavins. *Biochem. J.* 143:311, 1974.

122. Haurani, F. I., and Green, D.: Primary defective iron reutilization: Response to testosterone therapy. *Am. J. Med.* 42:151, 1967.

123. MacSween, R. N. M., and MacDonald, R. A.: Iron metabolism by reticuloendothelial cells in vitro uptake of transferrin-bound iron by rat and rabbit cells. *Lab. Invest.* 21:230, 1969.

124. MacDonald, R. A., MacSween, R. N. M., and Pechet, G. A.: Iron metabolism by reticuloendothelial cells in vitro: Physical and chemical conditions, liprotrope deficiency, and acute inflammation. *Lab. Invest.* 21:236, 1969.

125. Hemmaplardh, D., and Morgan, E. H.: Transferrin and iron uptake by human cells in culture. *Exp. Cell Res.* 87:207, 1974.

126. O'Shea, M. J., Kershenobich, D., and Tavill, A. S.: Effects of inflammation on iron and transferrin metabolism. *Br. J. Haematol.* 25:707, 1973.

127. Green, R., Charlton, R., Seftel, H., Bothwell, T., Mayet, F., Adams, B., and Finch, C.: Body iron excretion in man: A collaborative study. *Am. J. Med* 45:336, 1968.

128. Crosby, W. H., Conrad, M. E., and Wheby, M. S.: The rate of iron accumulation in iron storage disease. *Blood* 22:429, 1963.

129. Dresch, C., and Najean, Y.: Hemoglobin iron kinetics in man. *Rev. Eur. Etudes Clin. Biol.* 17:930, 1972.

130. Harrison, P. M., Clegg, G. A., and May, K.: Ferritin structure and function, in *Iron in Biochemistry and Medicine,* edited by A. Jacobs and M. Worwood. Academic, New York, 1980, vol. 2, pp. 131–171.

131. Crichton, R. R., and Roman, F.: A novel mechanism for ferritin iron oxidation and deposition. *J. Mol. Catal.* 4:75, 1978.

CHAPTER 34

Metabolic aspects of vitamin B_{12} and folic acid

WILLIAM S. BECK

Vitaminology of vitamin B_{12}

Vitamin B_{12} (cobalamin) and folic acid (pteroylglutamic acid) have special significance for hematology for both historical and substantive reasons. To understand fully their clinical significance, one must comprehend what is known of their biochemistry and metabolism. Knowledge of both vitamins is expanding rapidly, and international symposia on both have taken place since the last edition of this book [1,2].

Vitamin B_{12} occupies a special place in the history of hematology. Thomas Addison's description of pernicious anemia is a classic of clinical medicine [3]. The discovery by Minot and Murphy of the beneficial effect of liver feeding in pernicious anemia [4] was a key introduction to the era of physiologic hematology. Castle's discovery of intrinsic factor [5] still stands as a model clinical investigation and a major biologic advance.

Studies of the treatment of pernicious anemia have led to much of our present knowledge of the biochemistry of vitamin B_{12} and folic acid [6,7]. The discovery and crystallization of vitamin B_{12} in 1948 by Rickes and associates [8,9] followed the astute observation by Shorb of proportionality between the nutrient activity of liver extracts in cultures of *Lactobacillus lactis* Dorner and their therapeutic activity in pernicious anemia [10]. Shortly thereafter, vitamin B_{12} was isolated from liver by Wijmenga and associates. Following the unwitting use of cyanide-activated papain as a proteolytic ferment, these workers found that the cyanide converted various forms of the vitamin to stable and readily crystallizable cyano derivatives [11]. Isolation was also achieved independently by Lester Smith in England in 1948 [12]. Hodgkin's elucidation of the three-dimensional structure followed [13], and Barker subsequently discovered one coenzyme function of vitamin B_{12} [14]. The history, chemistry, and biology of vitamin B_{12} have been extensively reviewed [15–31].

NUTRITIONAL ASPECTS

SOURCES

Vitamin B_{12} is synthesized only by certain microorganisms. Hence it is a unique vitamin. Wherever it occurs in nature, it can be traced to bacteria or other microorganisms growing in soil, sewage, water, intestine, or rumen. Animals depend ultimately on microbial synthesis for their vitamin B_{12} supply; foods in the human diet that contain vitamin B_{12} are essentially those of animal origin—liver, seafood, meat, eggs, and milk. Although the nitrogen-fixing bacteria associated with leguminous plants are vitamin B_{12}–dependent, vitamin B_{12} has not been found in plant tissues.

The most intensive natural synthesis of vitamin B_{12} occurs in rumen bacteria [30]. Of the microorganisms that synthesize the vitamin, many do so in quantities just sufficient for their needs [31]. However, organisms such as the rumen organism *Propionibacterium shermanii* and the antibiotic-producing molds *Streptomyces griseus* and *Streptomyces aureofaciens* synthesize amounts sufficient to make them feasible commercial sources. Some microorganisms that cannot synthesize vitamin B_{12} (e.g., *L. lactis, L. leishmanii,* etc.) require an exogenous supply and hence are useful organisms for the microbiological assay of vitamin B_{12}. Other microorganisms cannot synthesize vitamin B_{12} and appear not to require it (e.g., *Escherichia coli*).

DAILY REQUIREMENTS

The average daily diet in Western countries contains 5 to 30 μg of vitamin B_{12}. Of this, 1 to 5 μg is absorbed [32]. Less than 250 ng appears in the urine; the unabsorbed remainder appears in the feces. Long-term studies employing radioactive vitamin B_{12} suggested a total daily loss of 0.66 to 2.1 μg, with a mean of 1.3 μg [33]. Of an administered oral dose of 0.5 to 2 μg of pure vitamin B_{12}, 60 to 80 percent is absorbed. As the oral dosage increases, the percentage absorbed decreases; at a dose of 5 μg, 30 percent or less is absorbed.

Total-body content is 2 to 5 mg in an adult individual [34,35]. Of this, approximately 1000 μg is in the liver. Thus the concentration in adult liver is about 0.7 μg per gram wet weight. The kidneys are also rich in vitamin B_{12} [36].

Vitamin B_{12} has a daily rate of obligatory loss approximating 0.1 percent of the total body pool, irrespective of its size [32]. This conclusion implies (1) that the daily dietary requirement is 2 to 5 μg and (2) that a deficiency state will not develop for several years after cessation of vitamin B_{12} intake. The officially recommended daily allowance for adults is 5 μg [37]; for infants during the first year the recommended allowance is 1 to 2 μg. It had earlier been believed that the minimal daily requirement was 0.6 to 1.2 μg. However, this amount is adequate to maintain nutritional balance only in subjects with low body stores (i.e., in whom daily obligatory losses are proportionately low).

Growth, hypermetabolic states, and pregnancy increase daily requirements. Because of the prolonged buffering effects of body stores, it has been difficult to obtain precise nutritional data in these conditions. It is believed, however, that a diet containing 15 μg per day will gradually replenish depleted body stores [37]. Average U.S. diets appear to meet this requirement.

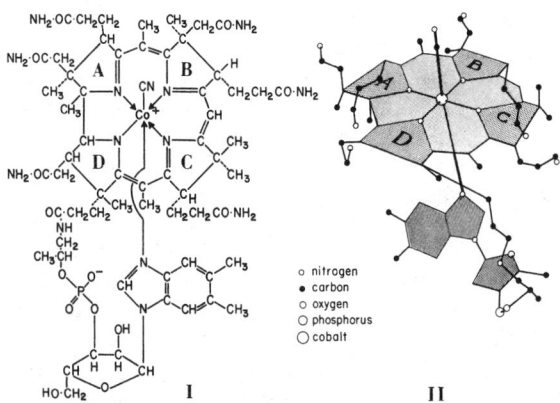

FIGURE 34-1 Formula I, chemical structure of vitamin B$_{12}$ (cyanocobalamin). Formula II, semidiagrammatic representation of three-dimensional structure showing relations of planar and nucleotide moieties. Hydrogen atoms and a number of oxygen atoms are omitted. (Beck [10].)

CHEMICAL ASPECTS

STRUCTURE AND NOMENCLATURE OF VITAMIN B$_{12}$ COMPOUNDS

The structure of vitamin B$_{12}$ has several unique features (formula I, Fig. 34-1). The cyanocobalamin molecule ($C_{63}H_{88}O_{14}N_{14}PCo$; M_r = 1355) has two major portions: a planar group, which bears a close but imperfect resemblance to the porphyrin macro ring, and a nucleotide, which lies nearly perpendicular to the planar group (formula II). The porphyrin-like moiety contains four reduced pyrrole rings (designated A through D) that link to a central cobalt atom, the two remaining coordination positions of which are occupied by a cyano group (above) and a 5,6-dimethylbenzimidazolyl moiety (below the planar group). With one exception, the pyrrole rings are connected to one another by methylene carbon bridges similar to those found in por-

FIGURE 34-2 Systematic nomenclature of vitamin B$_{12}$ and related compounds. Inset shows porphin structure for comparison. Note that pyrrole rings of the corrin macro ring are designated A through D. Substituent acetamide and propionamide groups are designated a through g. (Beck [10].)

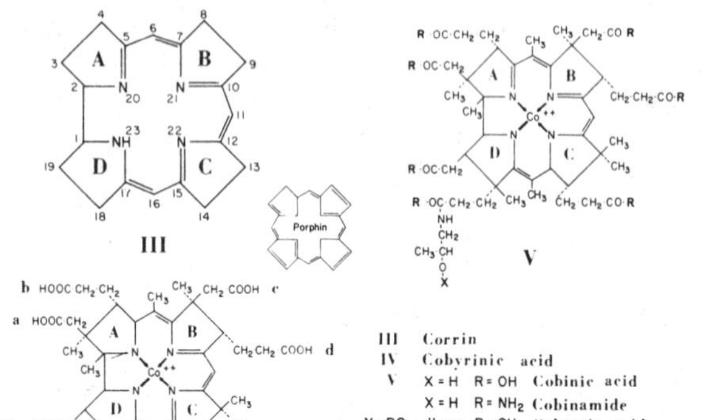

III   Corrin
IV   Cobyrinic acid
V   X=H   R=OH   Cobinic acid
     X=H   R=NH$_2$ Cobinamide
     X=PO$_3$-ribose R=OH   Cobamic acid
     X=PO$_3$-ribose R=NH$_2$ Cobamide

phyrin precursors (Fig. 34-2). The exception is the direct linkage between the α carbons of rings A and D. Another dissimilarity from the porphin structure is the relatively saturated or reduced character of the pyrrole rings, which are extensively substituted with methyl groups or longer acetamide and propionamide residues.

The macro ring of vitamin B$_{12}$ and related compounds is termed *corrin*; the major corrin derivatives are known as *corrinoid* compounds. Corrin and porphin macro rings are both synthesized from δ-aminolevulinic acid [38,39], and porphobilinogen, a precursor of uroporphyrin, coproporphyrin, and protoporphyrin, is incorporated into the corrin system by certain microorganisms.

Unusual features include a nucleotide, the base of which—5,6-dimethylbenzimidazole—had not previously been encountered in nature. Its base-ribose linkage is sterically an α glycoside unlike the β linkages typical of nucleic acid and coenzyme nucleotides. The ribose is phosphorylated at C-3, one of the few known naturally occurring ribose 3-phosphates. There are two connections between the planar and nucleotide moieties: (1) an ester linkage between the nucleotide phosphate and a 1-amino-2-propanol moiety that is joined in turn in amide linkage with a propionic side chain in ring D, and (2) the coordinate linkage between cobalt and the glyoxalinium nitrogen atom of benzimidazole.

Many corrinoid compounds are known. Some occur naturally; others have been prepared by chemical transformation or by manipulation of microbial biosynthetic systems. A systematic nomenclature is now available [19,40,41]. Numbering and ring designations of the corrin system are summarized in Fig. 34-2. Nucleotide derivatives of the corrinoids are named by adding -yl to the name of the nucleotide base; for example, α-(5,6-dimethylbenzimidazolyl) cyanocobamide is vitamin B$_{12}$. The semisystematic term *cobalamin*, introduced before its chemical structure was known, is now used to refer to the combining form of vitamin B$_{12}$ that lacks a ligand in the cobalt-β position (i.e., above the plane) and contains a 5,6-dimethylbenzimidazolyl moiety. As judged by recent symposia and reviews [18,19], cobalamin is now favored over the less precise term *vitamin B$_{12}$*.[1] In the chemical relatives of vitamin B$_{12}$ (i.e., cyanocobalamin), various ligands are covalently bound to cobalt above the plane. Such compounds include hydroxocobalamin (or the basic product of its combination with H$^+$, aquacobalamin) and nitritocobalamin. The ligand below the plane can also be replaced. In strong acid, a second H$_2$O$^-$ displaces the 5,6-dimethylbenzimidazolyl moiety to form diaquocobalamin. Pseudovitamin B$_{12}$, a cyanocobalamin analog containing adenine in place of 5,6-dimethylbenzimidazole, is active in some microorganisms but inert in higher animals.

[1] The term *corrin* was proposed originally to refer to the *core* of the vitamin B$_{12}$ molecule. The first two letters of corrin do not refer to the cobalt content of vitamin B$_{12}$. That fact is implied by the *cob* of cobalamin.

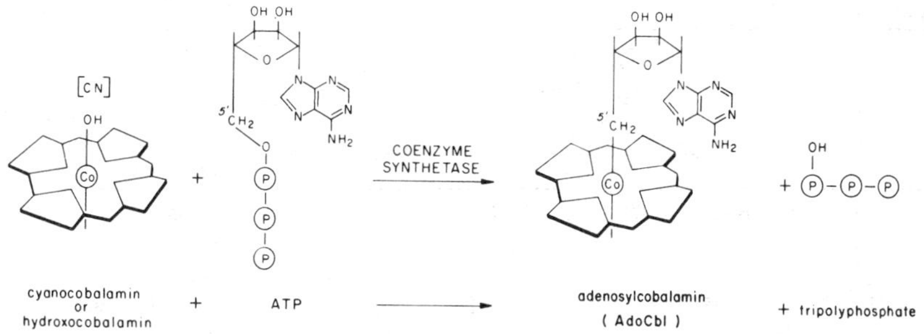

FIGURE 34-3   **The coenzyme synthetase reaction in which ATP adenosylates vitamin B$_{12}$ to form adenosylcobalamin.**

COBALAMINS IN BODY CELLS

Four cobalamins are of importance in animal cell metabolism. Two are the vitamin cyanocobalamin and its analog hydroxocobalamin. The other two are alkyl derivatives that are synthesized from the vitamin and serve as coenzymes. In one a 5'-deoxy-5'-adenosyl (or in short form, adenosyl) moiety replaces CN as the ligand of cobalt above the plane (Fig. 34-3). This compound is usually called *adenosylcobalamin*. Its new official abbreviation [41] is AdoCbl.[2] Awareness of this compound came from classic studies of Barker and associates on the conversion of glutamate to β-methylaspartate by extracts of *Clostridium tetanomorphum* [14,15]. In adenosylcobalamin the 5'-methylene carbon atom of the 5'-deoxy-5'-adenosyl moiety is linked directly to the cobalt atom [42].

In the second cobalamin with coenzyme activity, the ligand of cobalt is a methyl group [43]. Methylcobalamin is the major form of vitamin B$_{12}$ in human blood plasma [44,45]. In both coenzymes, adenosylcobalamin and methylcobalamin, the carbon-cobalt bond is labile to light, cyanide, and acid. It is likely that many of the cyanocorrinoids encountered in nature, including cyanocobalamin, arise in part from an attack on corrinoid compounds by cyanide.

Cyanocobalamin and hydroxocobalamin are readily converted to adenosylcobalamin in tissues by a "coenzyme synthetase" system (Fig. 34-3) [46,47]. The reaction requires ATP, a thiol or dithiol, and a reduced flavin. ATP is the biologic alkylating agent. The 5'-deoxy-5'-adenosyl moiety of ATP is transferred to the vitamin, and the three phosphates of ATP are released as inorganic triphosphate. Reducing agents are required in a preliminary step that converts the trivalent cobalt of vitamin B$_{12}$ [cyanocob(III)alamin] through the bivalent state [vitamin B$_{12r}$ or cob(II)alamin] to the univalent state [vitamin B$_{12s}$ or cob(I)alamin], which has nucleophilic properties.

METABOLIC ASPECTS

The advances in understanding of the metabolic functions of vitamin B$_{12}$ coenzymes have been extensively

[2] Approved abbreviations for the other three significant cobalamins are as follows: methylcobalamin, MeCbl; cyanocobalamin, CN-Cbl; and hydroxocobalamin, OH-Cbl.

surveyed [9–19,48,49]. Adenosylcobalamin-dependent methylmalonyl CoA mutase, methylcobalamin-dependent methyltetrahydrofolate-homocysteine methyltransferase, and leucine 2,3-aminomutase [50] are the only cobalamin-dependent enzymes known to be present in animal cells. All other well-studied systems have been derived from bacteria.

This section briefly surveys those few vitamin B$_{12}$–dependent enzyme reactions that have been proved or postulated to occur in human (or other animal) cells. The metabolic features of the vitamin B$_{12}$ deficiency syndromes are discussed below.

ADENOSYLCOBALAMIN-DEPENDENT REACTIONS

The apparent diversity of the several reactions requiring adenosylcobalamin was clarified with the recognition that (1) in all such reactions, the coenzyme is an acceptor-donor of hydrogen, the locus of the transfer being the 5'-deoxyadenosyl carbon atom next to the cobalt atom, and that (2) in some cobalamin-dependent reactions, hydrogen transfer occurs intramolecularly, while in one, hydrogen transfer occurs intermolecularly. As shown in Table 34-1, reactions in which there is a cobalamin-mediated intramolecular transfer of hydrogen form a new carbon-hydrogen bond. For example, the methylmalonyl CoA mutase reaction, a step in the catabolic pathway of propionate [51,52] (Fig. 34-4), occurs as follows:

$$\underset{\text{Methylmalonyl CoA}}{\overset{\overset{\displaystyle\text{COCoA}}{|}}{CH_3-CH-COOH}} \xrightarrow[\phantom{\text{adenosylcobalamin}}]{\text{adenosylcobalamin}} \underset{\text{Succinyl CoA}}{\overset{\overset{\displaystyle\text{COCoA}}{|}}{CH_2-CH_2-COOH}}$$

The one known cobalamin-dependent reaction in which hydrogen is transferred intermolecularly — hence it is a reduction — is the ribonucleoside triphosphate reductase reaction in which ribonucleotides are converted to deoxyribonucleotides [58–61]. In this reaction, so far demonstrated only in lactobacilli, *Euglena gracilis*, and other cobalamin-requiring protists, hydrogen for the reduction of the ribonucleotide substrate comes from a dithiol [62,63].

The strategic significance of the reductase reaction for the synthesis of DNA precursors in a vitamin B$_{12}$–requiring lactobacillus is suggested by the scheme in Fig. 34-5. In lactobacilli, the cobalamin-dependent reac-

TABLE 34-1   Adenosylcobalamin-dependent enzymes

Enzyme	Mode of hydrogen transfer	R^1	R^2	R^3	Biologic occurrence
Glutamate mutase [8]	Intramolecular	H	$CH(NH_2)COOH$	COOH	*Clostridia*
Methylmalonyl CoA mutase [51–53]	Intramolecular	H	COCoA	COOH	Animal cells, propionibacteria
Leucine 2,3-amino mutase [50]	Intramolecular	$(CH_3)_2CH$	NH_2	COOH	Animal cells, bacteria
Dioldehydrase [54]	Intramolecular	CH_3	OH	OH	*Aerobacter*
		H	NH_2	OH	
Glycerol dehydrase [55]	Intramolecular	CH_2OH	OH	OH	*Aerobacter*
Ethanolamine deaminase [56]	Intramolecular		NH_2	OH	*Clostridia*
β-Lysine mutase [57]	Intramolecular	–	NH_2	$CH_2CH(NH_2)CH_2COOH$	*Clostridia*
Ribonucleoside triphosphate reductase [58–61]	Intermolecular	Ribonucleotide $+ R(SH)_2 \rightarrow$ deoxyribonucleotide $+ R(S)_2$			Lactobacilli, protists

tion is the link between ribosyl and deoxyribosyl nucleotides. This explains the occurrence of unbalanced growth (i.e., impaired DNA synthesis and inability to divide, and unimpaired RNA and protein synthesis [64, 65]). The resulting forms are elongated filaments with elevated RNA/DNA ratios that are analogous to those of the megaloblasts of human vitamin B_{12} deficiency.

METHYLCOBALAMIN-DEPENDENT REACTIONS
Methylcobalamin participates in the cobalamin-dependent synthesis of methionine in bacteria [43,66] and animal cells [67] according to the scheme shown in Fig. 34-6 [15]. In humans this pathway, one of several means by which the body acquires methionine, serves also as a mechanism for converting N^5-methyltetrahydrofolate to tetrahydrofolate. The intracellular level of this enzyme appears related to the proliferative capacity of the cell [68,69]. Nitrous oxide (N_2O) impairs this enzyme by promoting the oxidation of cob(I)alamin (vitamin B_{12s})

to cob(III)alamin (vitamin B_{12a}) [70], thereby depleting the level of methylcobalamin and producing a vitamin B_{12}-deficiency-like state [71].

Methylcobalamin is an intermediary in the biosynthesis of methane by the several methane bacteria and of acetate by *C. aceticum* and other clostridia. Of the two known alkyl cobamide coenzyme forms of vitamin B_{12}, methylcobalamin acts by exchanging the entire alkyl group with the substrate and adenosylcobalamin acts by exchanging only certain of its hydrogen atoms.

OTHER POSSIBLE METABOLIC ASPECTS
Cyanide conversion Vitamin B_{12} may participate in the metabolism of cyanide in humans. Although the evidence is inconclusive, cobalamin has the capacity to bind cyanide, which is gaining metabolic importance because of increasing exposure from sources such as tobacco and certain foods (fruits, beans, and nuts) [72,73].

Ribonucleoside diphosphate reductase A role for cobalamin in the pathway of DNA synthesis was long ago postulated on the basis of evidence of impaired DNA synthesis in vitamin B_{12} deficiency. It is appropriate here to note those enzymatic steps in the pathway which have been shown by conclusive biochemical study to be cobalamin-independent.

It was assumed at first that the role of cobalamin in the pathway of DNA synthesis in animal cells was as cofactor for ribonucleotide reductase, in analogy with the situation in lactobacilli (see Fig. 34-4). However, it was early discovered that the pathway of DNA synthesis in *E. coli* [74] and Novikoff hepatoma [75] includes a ribonucleoside *di*phosphate reductase, which, unlike the ribonucleoside *tri*phosphate reductase of *L. leishmanii*, is cobalamin-independent. Marrow and other human cells contain a cobalamin-independent ribonucleoside diphosphate reductase.

FIGURE 34-4 Pathway of propionic acid metabolism. (Beck et al. [51,52].)

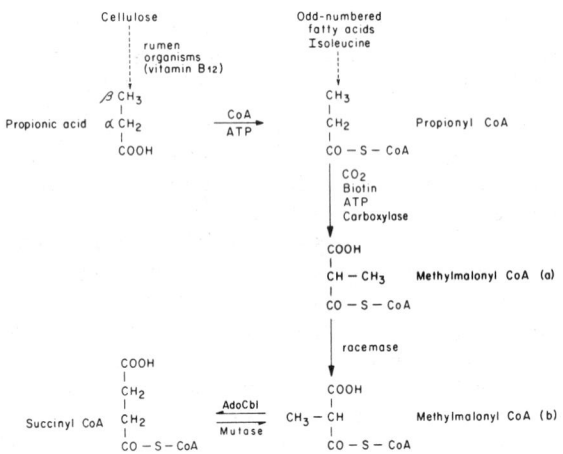

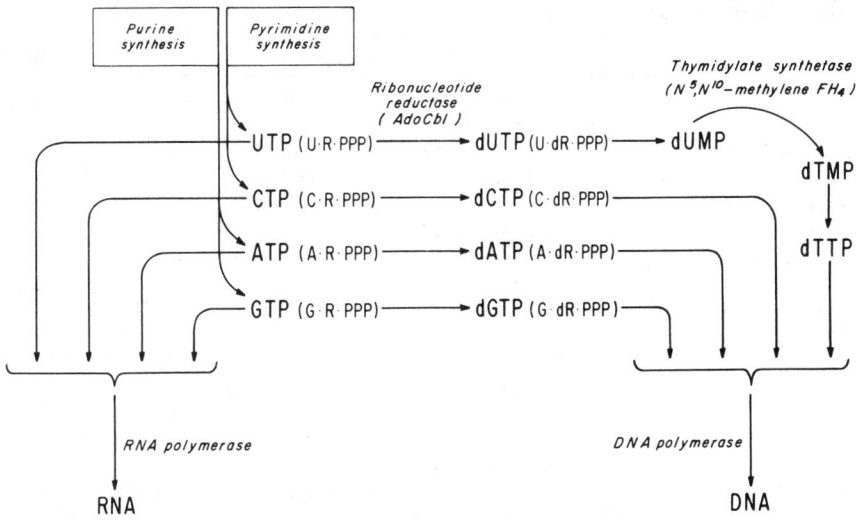

FIGURE 34-5 Pathways of nucleotide and nucleic acid synthesis in *Lactobaccilus leishmanii*.

Thymidylate synthetase It has been claimed that net conversion of deoxyuridylate (dUMP) to thymidylate (dTMP) is impaired in vitamin B_{12}–deficient cells. However, the enzyme thymidylate synthetase has no requirement for a cobalamin derivative [78]. The activity of this critical enzyme is dependent only on its substrate, dUMP, and a coenzyme, N^5,N^{10}-methylene-tetrahydrofolate, which serves as donor of methyl carbon and two hydrogens. As discussed below, decreased vitamin B_{12} availability appears to diminish thymidylate synthetase activity by diminishing the level of its folate coenzyme.

ROLE OF VITAMIN B_{12} IN ANIMAL CELL METABOLISM
As noted earlier, a partial explanation for the role of vitamin B_{12} in animal cell DNA synthesis is the so-called methylfolate trap theory [79]. Vitamin B_{12} deficiency slows the cobalamin-dependent pathway of methionine synthesis (see Fig. 34-6). As a result, folate is sequestered as N^5-methyltetrahydrofolate [80], a form that is unavailable to the critical thymidylate synthetase reaction. There is also evidence [81] that decreased synthesis of methionine results in decreased oxidation of methionine methyl to formate, a precursor of N^{10}-formyltetrahydrofolate.

It is now believed that the actual folate coenzymes in tissue are folylpolyglutamates. The enzyme converting folate (folylmonoglutamate) to folylpolyglutamate requires N^{10}-formyltetrahydrofolate or tetrahydrofolate as substrate and cannot act on N^5-methyltetrahydrofolate. When the latter form accumulates in vitamin B_{12} deficiency, it is unavailable for conversion to folylpolyglutamate, the active coenzymatic form, and thus the thymidylate synthetase reaction is further deprived of its folate cofactor.

Other evidence favoring this theory includes the following: (1) changes in folate metabolism that often occur in vitamin B_{12} deficiency [79] such as elevation of the N^5-methyltetrahydrofolate in serum [80], and increased urinary excretion of formiminoglutamic acid after an oral histidine loading dose [82]; (2) the presence of megaloblastosis in a patient with congenital methyltransferase deficiency [83]; (3) evidence of diminished methyltransferase activity in vitamin B_{12}–deficient rats [84]; and (4) claims of impaired conversion of dUMP to dTMP in marrow cells from vitamin B_{12}–deficient subjects, the so-called dU suppression test [85].

The following evidence tends to deny the validity of the methylfolate trap hypothesis: (1) clearance studies by some investigators [86] (but not by all [87]) showing

FIGURE 34-6 Methylcobalamin-dependent pathway of methionine synthesis, showing essential role of cobalamin-dependent methyltransferase in conversion of N^5-methyl FH_4 to FH_4. If folate is "trapped" as N^5-methyl FH_4, it cannot be converted to $N^{5,10}$-methylene FH_4, the cofactor of thymidylate synthetase.

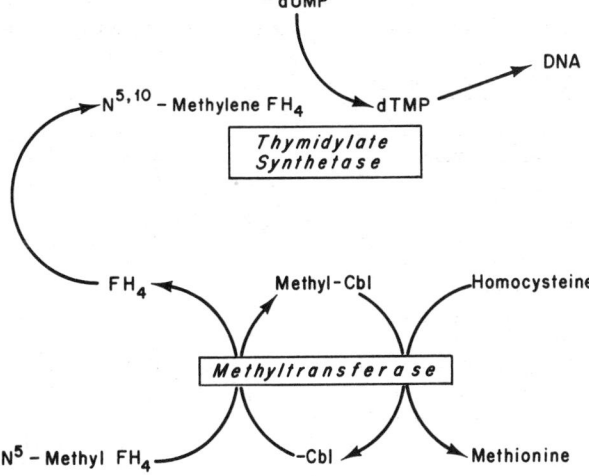

TABLE 34-2   Summary of major vitamin B_{12}–binding proteins

Source	Protein(s)	Function	Class*
Gastric juice	Intrinsic factor (IF)	Promotes absorption of vitamin B_{12} in ileum	S
Gastric juice	"Cobalophilin(s)"	May be involved in formation of IF-B_{12}; binds cobalamin analogs	R
Plasma	Transcobalamin I (TC I) ("cobalophilin")	May participate in plasma transport of vitamin B_{12}	R
Plasma	Transcobalamin II (TC II)	Promotes entry of vitamin B_{12} into cells	S
Plasma (and granulocytes)	Transcobalamin III (TC III) ("cobalophilin")	Unknown	R

*Based on electrophoretic mobility. R, rapid; S, slow.

normal rates of N^5-methyltetrahydrofolate utilization in vitamin B_{12} deficiency and suggesting that the rise in serum N^5-methyltetrahydrofolate is due to translocation rather than entrapment; (2) normal rates of $^{14}CO_2$ production from (^{14}C-methyl)-N^5-methyltetrahydrofolate in vitamin B_{12}–deficient rats [88]; (3) evidence of a cobalamin-independent pathway for the release of methyl groups from N^5-methyltetrahydrofolate in neural tissue [89,90] and blood cells [91]; (4) depression of total red cell folate content in vitamin B_{12} deficiency [90], which would not be predicted by the methylfolate trap hypothesis; (5) a disproportionate decrease in plasma methylcobalamin concentration [93,94] that seems surprising if N^5-methyltetrahydrofolate is present in abundance; (6) questions that have been raised about the validity of the so-called dU suppression test [95,96] which has been widely employed [97–101] without critical scrutiny; and (7) data from the study of three children with severe homocystinuria, cystathioninuria, hypomethioninemia, and methylmalonic aciduria [102–104] who displayed evidence of defective formation of both deoxyadenosylcobalamin and methylcobalamin, resulting perhaps from a defect in membrane transport of vitamin B_{12} or binding by an essential vitamin B_{12}–binding protein. Significantly, these children did not have megaloblastic anemia. Cultured fibroblasts from skin biopsies showed a depressed net level of methyltrans-

TABLE 34-3   Properties of human intrinsic factor

Property	Value	Reference
M_r (approximate)	44,000	[107]
$E_{1\ cm}^{1\%}$ at 279 nm	9.5	[109]
$S_{20,\ w}^0$	5.75	[109]
Cyanocobalamin-binding capacity, μg/mg	30.1	[107]
	18.6	[109]
Association constant for cyanocobalamin, M^{-1}	1.5×10^{10}	[107]
Composition:		
Carbohydrate content, %	15.0	[107]
Hexoses, including fucose, %	6.9	[109]
Hexosamine, residues/mol	4.1	[109]
Sialic acid, residues/mol	1.7	[109]

ferase activity and a correspondingly impaired conversion of homocysteine to methionine—precisely the defect envisioned in the methylfolate trap hypothesis.

In summary the two major metabolic systems requiring vitamin B_{12} coenzymes in humans are (1) methylmalonyl CoA isomerization, and thus propionate catabolism; and (2) methionine methyl synthesis, and thus tetrahydrofolate regeneration.

PHYSIOLOGIC ASPECTS

INTESTINAL ABSORPTION: THE INTRINSIC FACTOR MECHANISM

Intrinsic factor (IF) is the name given long ago by Castle [5,23] to a normal constituent of gastric juice that is necessary to complete the hemopoietic activity of the essential dietary ingredient (i.e., "extrinsic factor") now recognized as vitamin B_{12}. It is now known that IF is needed to facilitate the absorption in the ileum of cobalamins administered orally at physiologic dosage levels. We also know that IF is but one of a number of vitamin B_{12}–binding proteins (Table 34-2) and that indeed vitamin B_{12} in nature is always protein-bound [20,105].

After many difficulties [106], substantial purification of IF was finally achieved in 1973 [107–109] by the use of affinity chromatographic methods. Human IF has been revealed to be an alkali-stable glycoprotein that binds a molecule of cobalamin (cyano-, hydroxo-, or adenosyl-derivative) with a high affinity constant and in so doing forms dimers and oligomers [107]. Its properties are summarized in Table 34-3. Bound vitamin alters the conformation of IF, producing a more compact form that is resistant to proteolytic digestion. Human IF has been sequenced to a total of 84 amino acid residues out of 340 [110].

Gastric juice contains several vitamin B_{12}–binding proteins [111], some of which lack IF activity, such activity being defined as the capacity to promote intestinal absorption of vitamin B_{12}. At least two immunologically nonidentical binders or classes of binders are found in gastric juices, one with slow and one with rapid electrophoretic mobility. They are designated, respectively, S and R protein(s). These terms were originally invented to designate classes of vitamin B$_{12}$–binding proteins in human gastric juice. IF activity resides exclusively in an S protein. The term *R protein* was later applied to a large class of immunologically related proteins (perhaps a single protein) found in serum, leukocytes, saliva, and virtually all body cells. Saliva is a major source of the R protein(s) of gastric juice. The name *cobalophilin* has been proposed for all R proteins [112].

IF is secreted by the parietal cells of the fundic mucosa in humans, guinea pigs, cats, rabbits, and monkeys; by the chief cells in the rat; and by glandular cells of the pylorus and duodenum in the hog. Secretion of IF usually parallels that of HCl. It is enhanced by histamine, methacholine, and gastrin.

Vitamin B$_{12}$ derivatives in food are liberated in the stomach by peptic digestion and bound there to IF. Proteins or peptides bound to naturally occurring cobalamins are competitively displaced by IF at the low pH of gastric juice. The stable IF-B$_{12}$ complex encounters specific mucosal receptors on the microvilli of the ileum. The IF receptor has been isolated and purified [113–115]. It contains two subunits, and the similarity of its amino acid sequence to that of IF suggests that IF arose in evolution by gene duplication. A specific site on the IF molecule avidly attaches to a receptor. Attachment requires neutral pH, Ca^{2+}, or other divalent cations, but no energy [116]. The model in Fig. 34-7 has been proposed for the attachment of IF-B$_{12}$ complex to IF receptor [117]. The binding of IF-B$_{12}$ complex to receptor may be analogous to the formation of an IF oligomer.

Pancreatic secretions may contain a factor that promotes vitamin B$_{12}$ absorption [118]. In exocrine pancreatic deficiency, a substantial amount of vitamin B$_{12}$ in gastric juice is bound to R protein to yield an unabsorbable cobalamin complex [119]. The pancreatic factor appears to be a proteolytic enzyme that in normal subjects acts by selectively degrading R proteins and R-B$_{12}$ while sparing IF and IF-B$_{12}$ [120].

Following attachment of IF-B$_{12}$ to receptor, the vitamin either passes into the cell leaving IF behind or the complex enters a mucosal cell by pinocytosis and then dissociates. Unlike the rapid attachment of IF-B$_{12}$ to surface receptors, passage of vitamin into the mucosal cell is a slow, energy-requiring process [121]. Vitamin B$_{12}$ entering the ileal cell is bound to intracellular R protein [117]. In the guinea pig, vitamin B$_{12}$ in the ileal cell accumulates in mitochondria [122]. Within cells, R protein promotes the Ca^{2+}-dependent uptake of vitamin B$_{12}$ by mitochondria and other organelles [123]. Intracellular Ca^{2+} levels determine the number of R-B$_{12}$ receptors on organelles [123].

Vitamin B$_{12}$ (without IF) is eventually transferred to portal blood. After a small oral dose (10 to 20 μg), vitamin B$_{12}$ first appears in the blood in 3 to 4 h, reaching a peak level at 8 to 12 h. Larger oral doses are absorbed by simple diffusion that is not mediated by IF. In these instances, vitamin appears in blood within minutes.

At least two types of anti-IF antibodies are recognized: (1) blocking antibodies, which prevent binding of vitamin B$_{12}$ by IF; and (2) binding antibodies, which combine with IF-B$_{12}$ complex or with free IF without impairing its ability to bind vitamin B$_{12}$.

TRANSPORT OF VITAMIN B$_{12}$ IN PLASMA
Normal plasma contains 150 to 450 pg of vitamin B$_{12}$ per milliliter (the range of normal varying with the assay method and laboratory, as noted below). All the plasma vitamin B$_{12}$ is bound to transport proteins of unusual physiologic complexity.

Properties of transcobalamins   As shown in Table 34-2, plasma and extracellular fluids contain two major vi-

FIGURE 34-7   Scheme postulated to account for IF-mediated absorption of vitamin B$_{12}$ in ileum. The Cbl-IF complex tends to aggregate and forms a pseudo-oligomer with a related protein, the IF receptor. It is probably attached to the cobalamin-free subunit β, which upon binding Cbl-IF acquires an α conformation. Intracellular R protein accepts Cbl from α. (Adapted from Gräsbeck [117].)

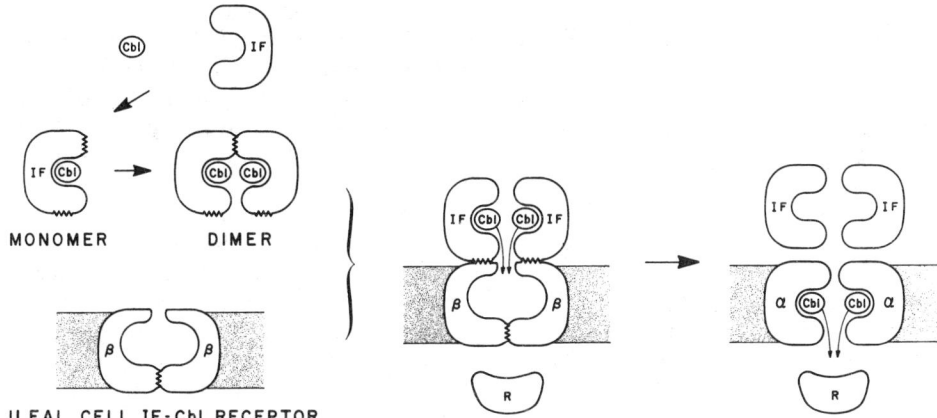

TABLE 34-4   Properties of the vitamin B_{12}–binding proteins of plasma

Property	TC I	TC II	TC III
Electrophoretic mobility (pH 8.6)	α_1	$\alpha_2\beta$	α_2
M_r (approximate)	120,000*	38,000*	120,000*
Cyanocobalamin-binding capacity, $\mu g/mg$	12.2	28.6	12.2
Protein type (R or S)	R	S	R
Composition:			
Carbohydrate content, %	33–40	0	33–40
Sialic acid, residues/mol	18	0	11
Fucose, residues/mol	9	0	20
Portion of plasma vitamin B_{12} bound, % (approximate)	75	25	
Portion of binder unsaturated, % (approximate)	50	98	98
$T_{1/2}$ of TC-B_{12} complex	9–12 days	60–90 min	<60 min
Reacts with:			
Anti-TC II	No	Yes	No
Anti-TC I	Yes	No	Yes
Anti-saliva R protein	Yes	No	Yes

*M_r is 150,000 daltons by gel filtration and 95,000 to 100,000 daltons by sodium dodecylsulfate electrophoresis.
SOURCE: Allen and Majerus [125], Schneider et al. [126], and Burger et al. [130].

tamin B_{12}–binding proteins—transcobalamin I (TC I) and transcobalamin II (TC II) [124–127]—and a minor protein (or class of proteins) that has been variously named and is now generally referred to as TC III [128–130]. Properties of these proteins are summarized in reviews [20,105,131–133] and in Table 34-4.

The nature and function of TC III was puzzling until recently. Many investigators have observed vitamin B_{12} binders other than TC I and TC II in association with myeloproliferative and other granulocytic diseases [128,133]. It is now recognized that so-called granulocyte binder and TC III are indistinguishable [130,134]. Like TC I, TC III is an R protein. All R proteins have the same amino acid sequence in their polypeptide portions but differ in carbohydrate content [135]. Probably TC III is an isoprotein of TC I that is unsaturated with vitamin B_{12} and therefore less charged. Both appear to arise from granulocytes [136–138], but R proteins also arise from salivary and gastric glands. Much of the plasma TC III appears to arise from granulocytes in vitro after blood has been collected—that is, during clotting [129,136]. Thus the content of R proteins differs in plasma and serum.

The source of human TC II is not known. Inconclusive data have suggested hepatic synthesis [139], but it appears also to be produced by many body cells, including fibroblasts, macrophages, marrow cells [140], and perhaps ileal enterocytes [20].

Functions of transcobalamins   TC I and TC II are present in plasma in trace quantities (about 60 and 20 μg/liter, respectively.) TC III is often undetectable. In fasting plasma, three-quarters of the circulating vitamin B_{12} is bound to TC I. Nevertheless, TC I has substantial unsaturated binding capacity, which may range from 79 to 939 pg per milliliter plasma (mean 330) [141]. Thus in

normal plasma more than half the binding capacity of TC I is saturated with vitamin B_{12}; the remaining 10 to 50 percent is free.

TC II binds only 10 to 25 percent of the total plasma vitamin B_{12} [130,142]. The unsaturated TC II–binding capacity of normal plasma is 611 to 1505 pg/ml (mean 986) [141]. Less than 2 percent of the TC II in plasma is saturated at a given moment, and at least two-thirds of the unsaturated vitamin B_{12}–binding power of plasma is due to TC II.

Known functions of the cobalamin binders include (1) prevention of loss of cobalamins in urine, sweat, and other body secretions and (2) transport of cobalamins through cell membranes. However, as noted below, they may have other functions. When a small dose of vitamin B_{12} (injected or orally administered) enters the blood, it is initially bound by TC II. Indeed, more than 90 percent of recently absorbed vitamin B_{12} is carried by TC II [143]. TC II–B_{12} complex is then cleared from plasma in minutes [132,144], vitamin and protein moiety disappearing at comparable rates [126]. In contrast, TC I, which carries most of the vitamin B_{12} in plasma, clears slowly from plasma [132,145], with a half-life of 9 to 10 days. Despite the rapid disappearance of most TC II-bound freshly absorbed vitamin B_{12}, a small portion of the circulating vitamin B_{12} continues to be carried by TC II long after its intestinal absorption [142]. Vitamin B_{12} evidently recirculates to an extent, and recycling vitamin is bound to TC II.

A puzzling feature is the failure of TC I to behave as an effective transport protein. Indeed, congenital absence of TC I is seemingly harmless [146]; in contrast, a severe, even lethal, megaloblastic anemia occurs in infants lacking TC II [147]. There are no other functional transport proteins. Only TC II has the capacity to promote cellular uptake of vitamin B_{12} [148]. Vitamin B_{12} is taken up by many cells, and liver cells have a selectively high affinity for TC II–bound vitamin B$_{12}$.

The following abnormalities of plasma vitamin B$_{12}$–binding proteins have been described in various disease states: (1) plasma TC III and TC I levels rise in myeloproliferative disorders, most notably in chronic myelogenous leukemia [131,149], in polycythemia vera [150], and occasionally in hepatocellular carcinoma [151,152] and other solid tumors [153]; (2) TC II levels increase in chronic myeloproliferative disorders, liver disease, and inflammatory disorders; (3) TC I is undersaturated in pernicious anemia and other vitamin B$_{12}$–deficiency states; (4) the sum of unsaturated TC I and TC II—sometimes referred to as serum unsaturated B$_{12}$–binding capacity, or UBBC—may be decreased in cirrhosis and infectious hepatitis [154], when serum vitamin B$_{12}$ is elevated, or increased when plasma TC I is elevated [155,156]; and (5) UBBC tends to rise in transient neutropenia [157].

Assay of serum vitamin B$_{12}$ The standard microbiological assay of serum vitamin B$_{12}$ usually employs the cobalamin-dependent organisms *L. leishmanii* ATCC 7830 [158,159], *E. gracilis* strain Z [160], and *E. coli* 113-3 [161]. Of these, the *L. leishmanii* method is simplest and fastest. However, these procedures were widely supplanted in the 1960s by the advent of a radioisotope dilution assay (RIDA) employing a vitamin B$_{12}$–binding protein [162,163]. The disturbing fact that this assay always gave higher results than the microbiological assay is explained [164] by the discovery in serum and tissue of a class of cobalamin analogs that are not recognized as vitamin B$_{12}$ by microorganisms but are assayed as vitamin B$_{12}$ by RIDA procedures when the binder is R protein but not when it is IF. This discovery led to the development of RIDA methods which use IF as binder and yield results in agreement with those of microbiological assays. The chemical nature and biologic significance of these analogs are unknown [165]. Conceivably, it is the role of R proteins in gastric juice to bind analogs of dietary origin in order to minimize their absorption in the intestine.

ENTEROHEPATIC CIRCULATION OF VITAMIN B$_{12}$
In humans, between 0.5 and 9 μg of the total cobalamin enters the intestine each day via the bile [166,167]. Of this, 65 to 75 percent is reabsorbed by IF-dependent mechanisms [168]. TC III contains less sialic acid than TC I (Table 34-3) [130], which may explain its low level in plasma, since asialoglycoproteins are cleared more rapidly from plasma by the liver than sialoglycoproteins [169,170].

In rabbits, vitamin B$_{12}$ bound to R-type proteins is processed by hepatocytes before reentering the plasma or being excreted in the bile [169]. If hepatocytes in humans also preferentially process vitamin B$_{12}$ bound to R proteins such as TC I and TC III [171,172], the liver may play an important role in clearing the circulation of cobalamin analogs by excreting them preferentially

into the bile. Since IF binds a narrow range of analogs [164,173,174], many may not be reabsorbed from the intestine.

Vitaminology of folic acid

In 1891 Sir Frederick Gowland Hopkins isolated xanthopterin and leucopterin, yellow and white pigments from butterflywings. These were not fully characterized until 1940, when Wieland and the Munich school showed them to be members of a novel group of heterobicyclic compounds, the pterins or pteridines [175]. The most important member of the group is folic acid, discovered in the late 1940s—an event that Gowland Hopkins lived to witness.

The converging lines of nutritional research that led to the recognition of folic acid and its related derivatives have been amply reviewed [176–180]. The first line of research, begun in 1931, described "Wills factor," an antianemia principle of yeast [181]. Subsequently reported unidentified factors included "vitamin M," an antianemia principle of liver and yeast [182]; "factor U," a growth factor for chicks from yeast and bran [183]; "vitamin B$_c$," a liver factor that prevents macrocytic anemia in chicks [184]; "Norit eluate factor," a factor that supports the growth of *L. casei* [185]; and, finally, "folic acid," the name given by Mitchell, Snell, and Williams to a substance from spinach leaves that promotes growth of *L. casei* and *S. lactis* R, later renamed *S. fecalis* R [186]. Each of these was subsequently identified as pteroylmonoglutamic acid or one of its derivatives. In 1948 crystalline folic acid was obtained from liver [187] and its structure confirmed by organic synthesis [188].

Although experimental folic acid deficiency was known to produce megaloblastic anemia, it was early recognized that folic acid is not the anti-pernicious anemia principle of liver [189]. Confusion arose because folic acid therapy in pernicious anemia produced notable reticulocyte responses. Hemoglobin regeneration was incomplete, however, and relapses and neurologic complications occurred during treatment. Liver extracts active against pernicious anemia were then found by direct assay to contain little or no folic acid. Thus it was recognized that vitamin B$_{12}$ deficiency is the basis of the megaloblastic anemia of pernicious anemia and that folic acid deficiency is a distinctive cause of megaloblastic anemia.

CHEMICAL ASPECTS
Folic acid is the useful trivial name for pteroylmonoglutamic acid, parent compound of the large family of compounds known collectively as *folate* or *folates*. Official rules of nomenclature have been published [190]. The molecule contains three structural moieties (Fig. 34-8*a*): (1) a pteridine derivative, (2) a *p*-aminobenzoic residue, and (3) an L-glutamic acid residue. The combination of the first two comprises *pteroic acid*, the systematic name

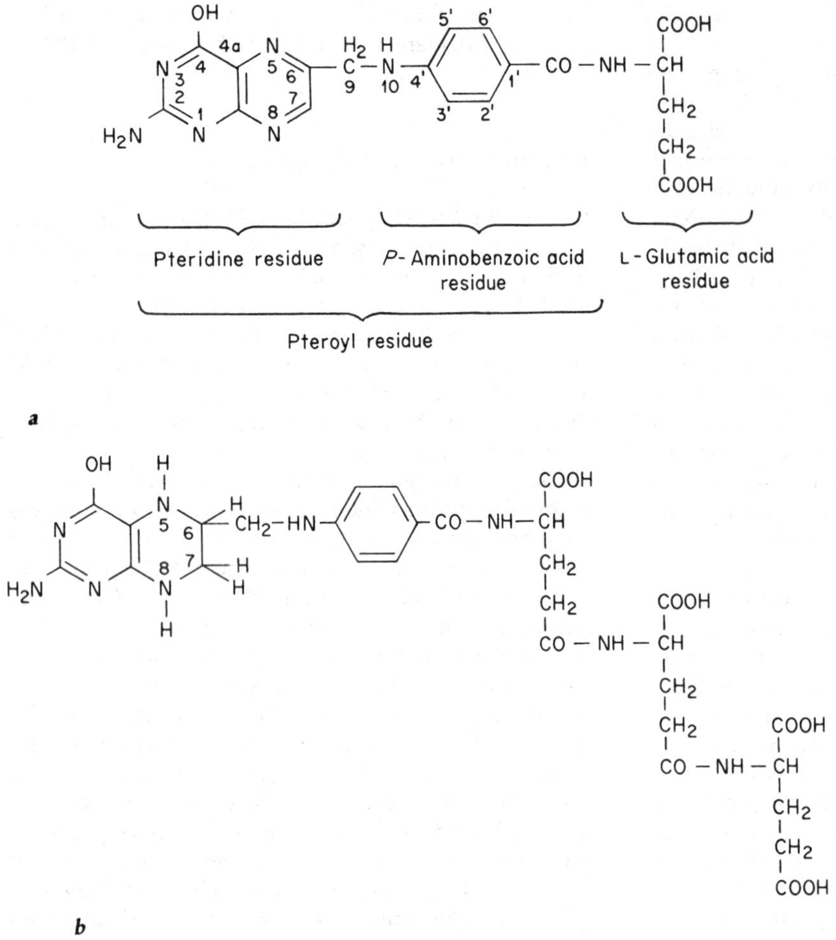

FIGURE 34-8   Folic acid. (*a*) Pteroylmonoglutamic acid, showing names of several components of the molecule. (*b*) 5,6,7,8-Tetrahydropteroyltriglutamic acid.

of which is *N*-(2-amino-4-hydroxypteridin-6-ylmethyl)-*p*-aminobenzoic acid. The corresponding acyl radical is termed *pteroyl*; hence folates are pteroylglutamates.

Folic acid occurs in nature largely as conjugates in which multiple glutamic acid residues are attached by peptide linkages to the γ-carboxyl group of the preceding glutamic acid residue (Fig. 34-8*b*). Pteroylmonoglutamate is often designated simply as *pteroylglutamate*. Higher conjugates are termed *pteroyldiglutamate, pteroyltriglutamate,* etc. Solubility decreases as the number of glutamic acid residues increases. The synthetic folic acid used therapeutically in ordinary circumstances is pteroylmonoglutamate.

Pteroylmonoglutamate may be indicated by the symbols PteGlu or F (for folic acid). For simplicity, the latter is used here, but alternative abbreviations are indicated where appropriate. The conversion of F to 5,6,7,8-tetrahydrofolic acid (FH$_4$, H$_4$PteGlu) is a necessary prerequisite to its participation in enzyme reactions (Fig. 34-8*b*). In the enzymatic synthesis of FH$_4$, F is first reduced to 7,8-dihydrofolic acid (FH$_2$); FH$_2$ is then reduced to FH$_4$ (sometimes termed *folacin*). In animal cells both reactions are catalyzed by a single NADPH-linked

enzyme, dihydrofolate reductase. A notable property of dihydrofolate reductase is its sensitivity to folate analogs containing a 4-amino group, e.g., Aminopterin and methotrexate, which are avidly bound and are inhibitory at concentrations of approximately 10^{-9} *M*. This is one basis of their chemotherapeutic action.

The folate family consists largely of FH$_4$ derivatives bearing a one-carbon substituent. Such a compound may be symbolized as ©-FH$_4$. The varieties of ©-FH$_4$ differ in the identity of the one-carbon unit and the site of its attachment of FH$_4$ (Fig. 34-9). Known one-carbon substituents of FH$_4$ are the following:

formyl	—CHO	methylene	—CH$_2$—
hydroxymethyl	—CH$_2$OH	methenyl	—CH=
methyl	—CH$_3$	formimino	—CHNH

Note that three oxidation levels of carbon are represented among the one-carbon units (formyl, hydroxymethyl, and methyl) and that only one unit (formimino) contains nitrogen. It is seen in Fig. 34-9 that one-carbon units attach to N^5 or N^{10} or both, and that specific enzymes interconvert many of these compounds.

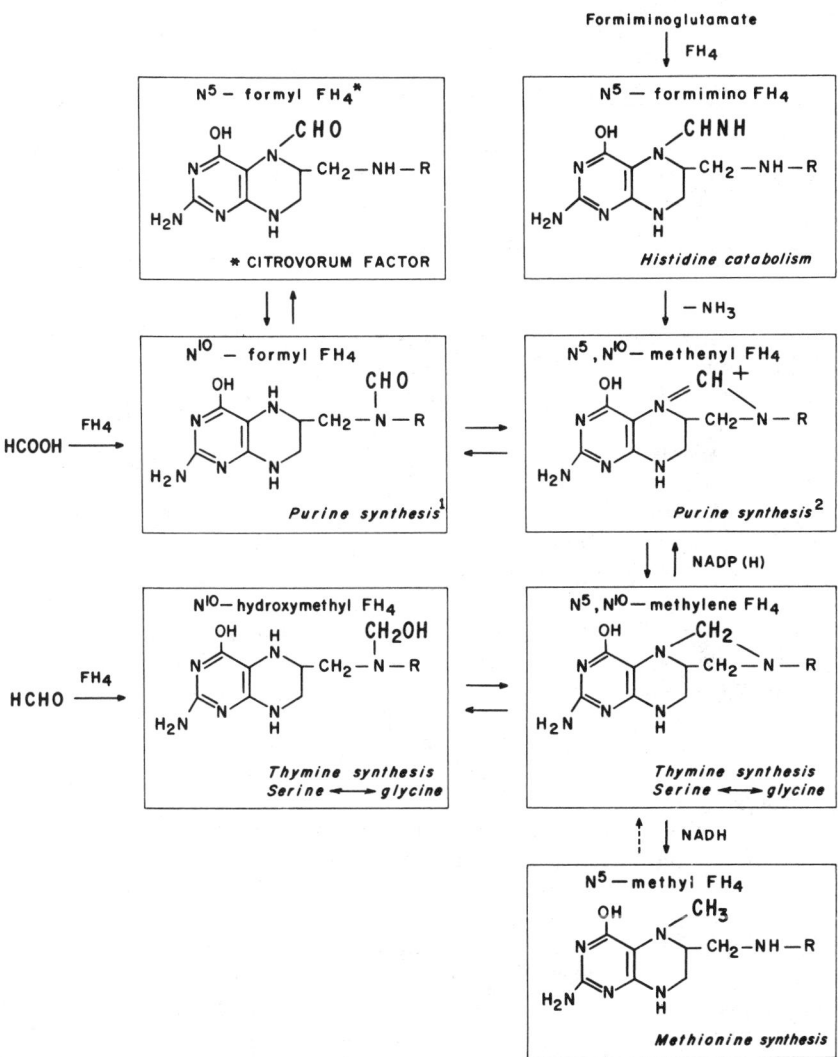

FIGURE 34-9   Derivatives of tetrahydrofolic acid (FH$_4$), their interconversions, and the metabolic pathways in which they participate. One-carbon substituents are shown in boldface. "Purine synthesis^{1}" refers to the step in purine synthesis in which 5-amino-4-imidazole carboxamide ribotide in converted to 5-formamido-4-imidazole carboxamide ribotide; "purine synthesis^{2}" refers to the conversion of glycinamide ribotide to formylglycinamide ribotide (see Table 34-6).

Reduced derivatives of folic acid are sensitive to oxidation in air and hence are unstable, especially under autoclave conditions. A notable exception is N^5-formyl FH$_4$, a compound isolated from liver and yeast soon after the discovery of folic acid [191]. It was first recognized as a growth factor for *Leuconostoc citrovorum* (later renamed *Pediococcus cerevisiae*) and thus was named *citrovorum factor* (other trivial names for it are *leucovorin* and *folinic acid*).

NUTRITIONAL ASPECTS

SOURCES

The many compounds of the folate group are of wide biologic distribution. Green leaves are rich in the vitamin and are presumed to be sites of active synthesis. The richest vegetable sources are asparagus, broccoli, endive, spinach, lettuce, and lima beans, each of which contains more than 1 mg of folate per 100 g dry weight. The best fruit sources are lemons, bananas, and melons. Folates are also found in liver, kidney, yeast, and mushrooms. The vitamin is synthesized by many bacteria. Sulfonamide drugs attack bacteria by interfering competitively with the incorporation of *p*-aminobenzoic into pteroic acid, an intermediate that reacts with glutamate in the presence of ATP to form pteroylglutamate. The major product of the natural synthetic pathway is 7,8-dihydrofolate.

Determination of food folate requires extraction procedures that prevent destruction of labile reduced forms. Since precautions have not always been observed, many published values of folate content in foods are unreliable. Results of folate determinations are influenced by the assay method used. *S. fecalis*, a com-

TABLE 34-5 Activity of various folic acid derivatives as bacterial nutrients

Folic acid derivative	Pediococcus cerevisiae*	Streptococcus fecalis	Lactobacillus casei
FH$_4$ and derivatives except N^5-methyl FH$_4$	+	+	+
F and pteroyl*di*glutamates	−	+	+
N^5-methyl FH$_4$, N^5-methyl FH$_2$, and pteroyl*tri*glutamates	−	−	+

* Formerly named *Leuconostoc citrovorum.*

monly used assay organism, does not utilize N^5-methyl FH$_4$ or short polyglutamates; *L. casei,* another assay organism, utilizes them as well as the forms available to *S. fecalis* (Table 34-5). Unless subjected to pretreatment with conjugases, higher polyglutamates are unavailable to all assay organisms. An average daily U.S. diet prepared without unusual precautions and treated with conjugases contains approximately 200 μg of folate by *S. fecalis* assay and an additional 400 to 600 μg of folate active only with *L. casei* [192,193]. Values are approximately one-fourth as high without conjugase treatment. The folate in some vegetables (broccoli, lettuce, and asparagus) is almost entirely conjugated. Unconjugated *L. casei*-active folate activity in cow's milk averages 55 μg/liter.

Excessive cooking, particularly with large amounts of water, can remove or destroy a high percentage of the folate in foods. Folate deficiency in England is said to be commonly due to the tendency there to overcook food.

DAILY REQUIREMENTS
The minimum daily requirement for folic acid, or its equivalent, in the normal adult is approximately 50 μg. As noted earlier, the average diet contains many times this amount in the form of various folate compounds, some of which may be unavailable. The officially recommended daily allowance of *food* folate for the adult is 0.4 mg [194]. The body is thought to contain approximately 5 mg of folate compounds; hence body reserves of folic acid are relatively much smaller than those of vitamin B$_{12}$. When a subject receiving a normal intake is switched to a daily intake of 5 μg per day, megaloblastic anemia develops in about 4 months [195].

Increased requirements for folic acid occur in hemo-

lytic anemia, leukemia, and other malignant diseases; during growth; and in pregnancy and lactation, which increase requirements threefold to sixfold [196].

METABOLIC ASPECTS

FOLATE-DEPENDENT ENZYMES
In metabolism, FH$_4$ is a catalytic self-regenerating acceptor-donor of one-carbon units in reactions involving one-carbon transfers from a carbon-containing donor compound, X-Ⓒ, to an acceptor, Y:

$$X—Ⓒ + FH_4 \rightarrow FH_4—Ⓒ + X$$
$$FH_4—Ⓒ + Y \rightarrow Y—Ⓒ + FH_4$$
$$\text{Sum:} \quad X—Ⓒ + Y \rightarrow Y—Ⓒ + X$$

The metabolic systems of animal tissues known to require folic acid coenzymes are summarized in Table 34-6. Biochemical aspects of these systems have been extensively reviewed [2,177,180,197–200].

The major clinical manifestations in human folate deficiency are probably produced by impairment of thymidylate synthesis. Methylation of deoxyuridylate to thymidylate, catalyzed by the enzyme thymidylate synthetase, is an essential preliminary step in the synthesis of DNA (Fig. 34-5). The coenzyme of this reaction, N^5,N^{10}-methylene FH$_4$, is unique among folate coenzymes because it transfers a one-carbon group and serves as hydrogen donor in reducing the transferred group to a methyl group [201]. The reaction generates FH$_2$ (Table 34-6), which must be reduced again to FH$_4$ by dihydrofolate reductase before it can again be utilized as a coenzyme. Thus the following "thymidylate

TABLE 34-6 Metabolic systems requiring folic acid coenzymes in animal cells

System	Related transformations of folic acid coenzymes
Serine $\rightleftarrows$ glycine	Serine + FH$_4$ $\rightleftarrows$ N^5,N^{10}-methylene FH$_4$ + glycine
Thymidylate synthesis	Deoxyuridylate (dUMP) + N^5, N^{10}-methylene FH$_4$ $\rightarrow$ FH$_2$ + thymidylate (dTMP)
Histidine catabolism	Formiminoglutamate + FH$_4$ $\rightarrow$ N^5-formimino FH$_4$ + glutamate
Methionine synthesis	Homocysteine + N^5-methyl FH$_4$ $\rightarrow$ FH$_4$ + methionine
Purine synthesis	Glycinamide ribotide + N^5,N^{10}-methenyl FH$_4$ $\rightarrow$ FH$_4$ + formylglycinamide ribotide
Purine synthesis	5-amino-4-imidazole carboxamide ribotide + N^{10}-formyl FH$_4$ $\rightarrow$ FH$_4$ + 5-formamido-4-imidazole carboxamide ribotide

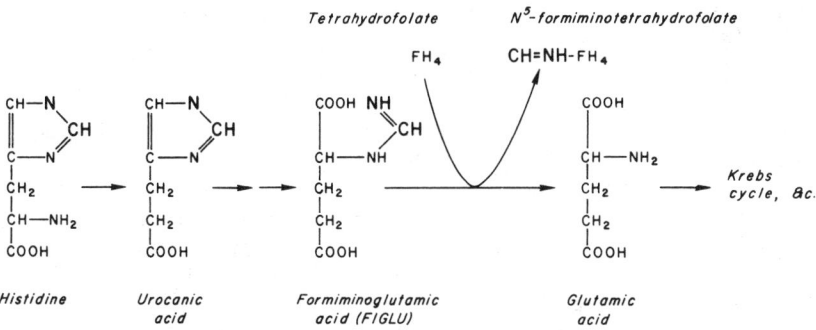

FIGURE 34-10 Pathway of histidine catabolism, showing synthesis and FH$_4$-dependent degradation of FIGlu.

synthesis cycle" exists, in which the hydroxymethyl carbon of serine is transformed into the methyl carbon of thymine as FH$_4$ is regenerated from FH$_2$ at the expense of NADPH:

$$\text{Serine} + \text{FH}_4 \rightleftharpoons N^5,N^{10}\text{-methylene FH}_4 + \text{glycine} + \text{H}_2\text{O}$$
$$\text{dUMP} + N^5,N^{10}\text{-methylene FH}_4 \rightarrow \text{FH}_2 + \text{dTMP}$$
$$\text{FH}_2 + \text{NADPH} + \text{H}^+ \rightarrow \text{FH}_4 + \text{NADP}^+$$

Limitation of thymidylate synthesis in folic acid deficiency impairs DNA synthesis, with resulting megaloblastic transformation.

Interference with the breakdown of histidine (Fig. 34-10) and its catabolic product, formiminoglutamic acid (FIGlu), in folic acid deficiency has no morbid effects, but it provides the basis for a test which can be used in the diagnosis of folic acid deficiency [202–204].

Deficiency of folate also diminishes the folate-dependent conversion of 5-amino-4-imidazole carboxamide ribotide (AICAR) to 5-formamido-4-imidazole carboxamide ribotide. AICAR accumulates and is excreted in the urine in excessive amounts in the partially degraded form, 5-amino-4-imidazole carboxamide (AICA). No clinical manifestations have thus far been related to the block in purine synthesis.

FIGlu and AICA are occasionally excreted in pure vitamin B$_{12}$ deficiency, possibly because lack of vitamin B$_{12}$ may depress the vitamin B$_{12}$–dependent pathway of methionine synthesis in which N^5-methyl FH$_4$ is converted to FH$_4$ [205–207].

NEW ROLES FOR FOLATE AND PTERIDINE DERIVATIVES

As noted earlier, N^5-methyl FH$_4$ homocysteine methyltransferase depends on a folate derivative and a cobalamin. Impairment of this reaction in vitamin B$_{12}$ deficiency has been considered to "trap" folate as N^5-methyl FH$_4$ because it appeared that N^5-methyl FH$_4$ can be converted to FH$_4$ only during the folate-dependent methylation of homocysteine. However, this reaction occurs to a small extent by a series of cobalamin-independent steps [208–212] circumventing the putative "trap."

One more unusual metabolic system merits comment.

The free pteridine tetrahydrobiopterin has been identified as the coenzyme of the enzymatic hydroxylation of phenylalanine to tyrosine, of the oxidation of long-chain alkyl ethers of glycerol to fatty acids, and perhaps of other reactions, e.g., the hydroxylation of tryptophan and the 17-α-hydroxylation of progesterone [198,213]. FH$_4$ is weakly active in these systems in vitro but appears to have no such functions in vivo. Sources of the pteridine and implications of possible deficiency states are unclear. It appears not to arise from dietary folate.

SIGNIFICANCE OF FOLYLPOLYGLUTAMATES

The folates of plant and animal cells exist primarily as polyglutamates [214–221] of various peptide chain lengths [222–224]. In chicken liver [225] and rat liver [221,226], about 70 percent of the folate present is in the form of N^5-methyl FH$_4$ derivatives that include several types of polyglutamates. About 80 percent of the folate compounds in human leukocytes are conjugated [227]. Human erythrocytes contain a total folate level (in nanograms per milliliter) that has been reported as 165 to 600 (mean 336) [228] and 135 to 569 (mean 289) [229]. The bulk of this folate has four or more glutamyl residues. The length of the polyglutamate chain of liver folates is inversely related to the total concentration of liver folates [230]. In other words, chains are shorter in folate deficiency.

Plasma folate consists exclusively of the monoglutamate N^5-methyl FH$_4$ [180]. Human plasma contains sufficient conjugase to convert polyglutamates containing more than three glutamyl residues to monoglutamates [231]. Cellular conjugase is a lysosomal enzyme. Synthesis of folylpolyglutamate from FH$_4$ is catalyzed by an ATP-dependent *synthetase* that occurs in liver and other body cells [232,233]. There is evidence that folylpolyglutamate synthetase is regulated within cells, activity closely paralleling rates of DNA synthesis [234].

Folylpolyglutamates and their reduced and substituted forms are the active coenzymes of folate-dependent enzyme reactions (e.g., thymidylate synthetase [235,236] and N^5-methyl FH$_4$-homocysteine methyltransferase [237]) and AICAR transformylase [238]. The interconversion of folymonoglutamates and folylpolyglutamates may provide a mechanism for the regulation of

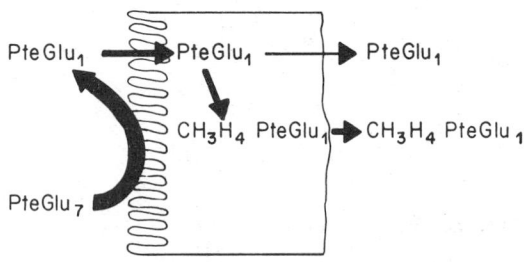

INTESTINAL   INTESTINAL   MESENTERIC
LUMEN   EPITHELIAL   CIRCULATION

FIGURE 34-11 Proposed schema of digestion and absorption of polyglutamyl folate by the intestine. Hydrolysis of pteroyl-heptaglutamate (PteGlu$_7$) to pteroylmonoglutamate (PteGlu$_1$) by intestinal enzymes is rapid, and the overall rate of transport into the mesenteric circulation is controlled by the movement of the monoglutamyl folate. Under appropriate conditions, a substantial portion of monoglutamate is reduced and methylated in the intestinal cell and appears in the circulation as 5-methyltetrahydrofolate (CH$_3$H$_4$PteGlu$_1$). (Rosenberg [246].)

folate-dependent metabolic systems, perhaps through the intervention of folate-binding proteins with a specificity for polyglutamates [239]. This hypothesis derives largely from the observations in vitamin B$_{12}$–deficient human beings and other animals of alterations in the normal ratio of polyglutamates to monoglutamates. Although total red cell folate is decreased in vitamin B$_{12}$ deficiency [240] and plasma N^5-methyl FH$_4$ is elevated [241,242], the relative concentration of polyglutamates is notably decreased [229,243,244]. This pattern has been interpreted to signify a failure of folylpolyglutamate synthesis in vitamin B$_{12}$ deficiency. Because folylpolyglutamate is synthesized from N^{10}-formyl FH$_4$ and FH$_4$, and not from N^5-methyl FH$_4$, the accumulation of the latter in vitamin B$_{12}$ deficiency may account for reduced polyglutamate synthesis rather than any direct effect of vitamin B$_{12}$ deficiency on folylpolyglutamate-synthetase [245]. Such observations support this view that polyglutamates are the active coenzymes.

PHYSIOLOGIC ASPECTS

INTESTINAL ABSORPTION

The mechanism of intestinal absorption of folate is imperfectly understood and controversial [246–248]. The proximal jejunum is the principal site of folate absorption. Absorption of an oral 1-mg dose of unconjugated folic acid begins within minutes, and peak values are reached in 1 to 2 h. When ^{3}H-folylmonoglutamic acid and synthetic ^{3}H-folylheptaglutamate are administered orally, both substances comparably increase plasma folate [249]. Whether synthetic or natural polyglutamate is administered [250], only folylmonoglutamate appears in plasma. Thus folylpolyglutamate is hydrolyzed during absorption across the intestine. Although such data

may not accurately reflect the disposition of food folate, which is largely conjugated, it does not appear that much of this folate is nutritionally available. Nonetheless, studies with ingested ^{14}C-polyglutamates indicate that fecal losses are greater as the length of the poly-γ-glutamyl side chain increases.

Conjugases play an important but not completely understood role in the intestinal absorption of folate [248,250]. Folylpolyglutamate may be hydrolyzed within the lumen of the intestine and the monoglutamate product is absorbed subsequently. Alternatively, as summarized in Fig. 34-11, hydrolysis may occur on or at the brush border of the intestinal cell, with subsequent transport, reduction, and methylation of the monoglutamate. A third theory is that polyglutamate enters the epithelial cell intact, hydrolysis occurring as an intracellular process followed by transport of the hydrolytic product. Existing data are insufficient to define the exact mechanism of folate absorption [246]. However, data showing the folate can be absorbed against a concentration gradient suggest the existence of an active transport mechanism [251,252]. Several investigators [247,253] have argued that passive transport may also occur.

Conjugases have been found in many tissues and organs of the rat, hog, dog, crow, rabbit, and chicken [254,255] and in an extract of the Portuguese man-of-war *Physalia physalis* [256]. Of these, only the enzymes from chicken and mouse tissues have been studied in detail. They are heat-labile carboxypeptidase with a pH optimum of around 8 [254,257].

METABOLISM

When a small dose of tritiated folylmonoglutamate (^{3}H-F) is administered intravenously, 60 percent is cleared from the plasma in one circulation time and 90 to 95 percent is removed in 3 min [258]. The rapidity of clearance suggests that folate is absorbed actively and bound intracellularly to a binding substance of high affinity. Studies with intravenously administered ^{3}H-F show that a large fraction of the original labeled material can be displaced from the cells and recovered unaltered in the urine several days later by administration of unlabeled folic acid in large doses [259]; hence intracellular conversion of assimilated folic acid to active coenzymes proceeds slowly. Indeed, nonhepatic tissue cells may not be a primary locus of folate reduction. Alternatively, F (in contrast to FH$_2$) may not be the primary natural substrate for dihydrofolate reductase.

Folates have been found in all body tissues analyzed. The principal form of the vitamin in serum, red blood cells, and liver appears to be N^5-methyl FH$_4$ [260–263], although some evidence suggests that one-third or more of the serum folate is N^5-methyl FH$_2$ [264]. After the oral ingestion of folic acid, blood emerging from the hepatic vein is rich in *L. casei*–active material and meager in *S. fecalis*–active material [265], presumably owing to the displacement of N^5-methyl FH$_4$ from the liver by incoming folic acid in portal blood. That such displacement occurs is also suggested by data showing that nonradioactive N^5-methyl FH_4 appears in the urine after parenteral administration of ^{3}H-F [266].

The role of red cell folate, most of which is conjugated, is unclear. Little more is known of leukocyte folate. Human liver contains 0.7 to 17 μg of folate per gram [267]. Nutritional data suggest that total-body folate is at least several milligrams.

A portion of the folate turned over each day is degraded to p-aminobenzoylglutamate and other cleavage products. Different folate compounds vary in their rate of breakdown. The fate of the pteridine moiety is unknown.

FOLATE-BINDING PROTEINS

Although serum folate is largely dialyzable [268], early attempts to demonstrate specific folate-binding proteins were only suggestive [269]. Conclusive data had to await the development of high-specific-activity ^{3}H-F and ^{3}H-methyl FH_4. In the course of efforts to develop a convenient radioassay for the measurement of serum folate [270], investigators found that folate is bound by a serum protein. Using tracer amounts of ^{3}H-F, they found that normal serum bound less than 10 percent (average 18 pg per 0.4 ml) and folate-deficient serum bound significantly greater amounts (average 133 pg per 0.4 ml). This elevation of serum-binding protein appeared early in the course of folate deficiency and fell promptly to normal range after treatment with folic acid. Such changes were not observed in vitamin B_{12} deficiency [271]. Elevations of folate-binding protein comparable to those found in folate-deficient serum have also been observed in sera from most patients with uremia, some women taking oral contraceptives, and some normal subjects [272,273].

The specific folate-binding protein from folate-deficient sera has a rapid association and slow dissociation rate for the binding of ^{3}H-F [271]. It appears to consist of two proteins (or classes of proteins), one with an M_r in excess of 200,000 daltons, the other with an M_r of 50,000 daltons. The macromolecular material is also found in human milk and lymphocyte membranes. The smaller protein behaves as a β-globulin and has the mobility of transferrin on polyacrylamide gel electrophoresis. It is immunologically distinguishable from transferrin. The protein(s) binds oxidized folylmonoglutamates and polyglutamates in preference to reduced folates. It retards the delivery and uptake of ^{3}H-F into HeLa cell monolayer cultures. As noted earlier, some evidence suggests that a membrane-derived intracellular folate-binding protein may be an important regulator of folate uptake into the cell and a storage site for folylpolyglutamates. The binding protein has many properties in common with β-lactoglobulin, the folate-binding protein of cow's milk. [274].

EXCRETION

Intact folates and their cleavage products are excreted by the kidney. Folates from food sources and administered folic acid in doses lower than 15 μg/kg are excreted in the urine in reduced forms and particularly as N^{10}-formyl FH_4. Normal urine also contains some N^5-methyl FH_4, free folic acid [275], and citrovorum factor (N^5-formyl FH_4) [276]. Filtered folic acid is actively reabsorbed by the renal tubule by a process that is blocked by methotrexate. At low concentrations folic acid is not transferred into the circulation but appears to remain in the tubule cells. It is the folate stored in tubule cells that is displaced into the urine by a large dose of unlabeled folic acid. After oral doses of folic acid greater than 15 μg/kg, large amounts are excreted unchanged.

A small percentage of parenterally administered ^{3}H-F is recoverable in the feces. Bile contains approximately 2 to 10 times the folate concentration of normal serum [227–279], biliary excretion accounting for up to 100 μg of folate per day. About half the bile folate is S. fecalis–active and a third is P. cerevisiae–active [279]. After folate ingestion, bile folate concentration increases rapidly. Loss of folate by biliary excretion may accelerate folate depletion in patients with folate malabsorption.

ASSAY OF SERUM FOLATE

The serum folate assay, a microbiologic procedure employing L. casei (ATCC 7469) or the technically superior nonagglutinating variant ATCC 7469a [280], is still the most reliable method for the definitive diagnosis of folic acid deficiency, although isotopic methods employing various folate binders have now achieved acceptable reliability. Since its introduction in 1959 [281], the microbiologic assay has undergone minor modifications [280,282–284] and its value has been extensively debated. Presently available methods are precise, although as in other microbiologic assays antimicrobial agents in serum may interfere [285]. This problem is easily controlled with the use of recovery studies [286]. Typical results in normal and folic acid–deficient subjects are summarized in Table 34-7.

TABLE 34-7   Folate content of serum and blood cells*

	Normal subjects	Folate deficiency (severe)	Vitamin B_{12} deficiency (severe)
Serum, ng/ml	9.8 (6.5 to 19.6)	1.7 (0.6 to 2.5)	11.4 (2.0 to 32)
White cells, ng/ml packed cells	92 (60 to 123)	20 (7.0 to 30)	82 (36 to 149)
Red cells, ng/ml packed cells	336 (165 to 600)	74 (24 to 135)	164 (66 to 244)

* Lactobacillus casei–active material.
SOURCE: Hoffbrand and Newcombe [228].

References

1. Zagalak, B., and Friedrich, W. (eds.): *Vitamin B_{12}. Proceedings of the Third European Symposium on Vitamin B_{12} and Intrinsic Factor. University of Zürich, March 5–8, 1979, Zürich, Switzerland*. Walter de Gruyter, New York, 1979.
2. Kisliuk, R. L., and Brown, G. M. (eds.): Chemistry and biology of pteridines, in *Proceedings of the Sixth International Symposium on the Chemistry and Biology of Pteridines, La Jolla, California, September 25–28, 1978*. Elsevier/North Holland, New York, 1979.
3. Wilks, S., and Bettany, G. T.: *Biographical History of Guy's Hospital*. Ward, Lock, Bowden, London, 1892.
4. Minot, G. R., and Murphy, W. P.: Treatment of pernicious anemia by a special diet. *JAMA* 87:470, 1926.
5. Castle, W. B.: Observations on the etiologic relationship of achylia gastrica to pernicious anemia. I. The effect of administration to patients with pernicious anemia of the contents of the normal human stomach recovered after the ingestion of beef muscle. *Am. J. Med. Sci.* 178:748, 1929; (reprint) 267:2, 1974.
6. Castle, W. B.: The history of corrinoids, in *Cobalamin: Biochemistry and Pathophysiology*, edited by B. M. Babior. Wiley-Interscience, New York, 1975, p. 1.
7. Castle, W. B.: The conquest of pernicious anemia, in *Blood, Pure and Eloquent*, edited by M. M. Wintrobe. McGraw-Hill, New York, 1980, p. 283.
8. Rickes, E. L., Brink, N. G., Koniuszy, F. R., Wood, T. R., and Folkers, K.: Crystalline vitamin B_{12}. *Science* 107:396, 1948.
9. West, R.: Activity of vitamin B_{12} in Addisonian pernicious anemia. *Science* 107:398, 1948.
10. Shorb, M. S.: Activity of vitamin B_{12} for growth of *Lactobacillus lactis*. *Science* 107:397, 1948.
11. Wijmenga, H. G., Lens, J., and Middlebeck, A.: Some properties of vitamin B_{12}. *Chem. Week* 45:342, 1949.
12. Smith, E. L.: Purification of anti-pernicious anemia factors from liver. *Nature (London)* 161:638, 1948.
13. Hodgkin, D. C., Kamper, J., Mackay, M., Pickworth, J., Trueblood, K. N., and White, J. G.: Structure of vitamin B_{12}. *Nature (London)* 178:64, 1956.
14. Barker, H. A., Weissbach, H., and Smyth, R. D.: A coenzyme containing pseudovitamin B_{12}. *Proc. Natl. Acad. Sci. U.S.A.* 44:1093, 1958.
15. Barker, H. A.: Biochemical functions of corrinoid compounds. *Biochem. J.* 105:1, 1967.
16. Beck, W. S.: Deoxyribonucleotide synthesis and the role of vitamin B_{12} in erythropoiesis. *Vitam. Horm.* 26:413, 1968.
17. Beck, W. S.: The metabolic functions of vitamin B_{12}. *N. Engl. J. Med.* 266:708, 765, 814, 1962.
18. Hogenkamp, H. P. C.: Enzymatic reactions involving corrinoids. *Annu. Rev. Biochem.* 37:225, 1968.
19. Smith, E. L.: *Vitamin B_{12}*, 3d ed. Wiley, New York, 1965.
20. Weissbach, H., and Dickerman, H.: Biochemical role of vitamin B_{12}. *Physiol. Rev.* 45:80, 1965.
21. Weissbach, H., and Taylor, R. T.: Metabolic role of vitamin B_{12}. *Vitam. Horm.* 26:395, 1968.
22. Stadtman, T. C.: Vitamin B_{12}. *Science* 171:859, 1971.
23. Barker, H. A.: Corrinoid-dependent enzymatic reactions. *Annu. Rev. Biochem.* 41:55, 1972.
24. Arnstein, H. R. V., and Wrighton, R. J., eds.: *The Cobalamins: A Glaxo Symposium*. Williams & Wilkins, Baltimore, 1971.
25. Babior, B. M., ed.: *Cobalamin: Biochemistry and Pathophysiology*, Wiley-Interscience, New York, 1975.
26. Castle, W. B.: The contributions of George Richards Minot to experimental medicine. *N. Engl. J. Med.* 247:585, 1952.
27. Jacob, E., Baker, S. J., and Herbert, V.: Vitamin B_{12}-binding proteins. *Physiol. Rev.* 60:918, 1980.
28. Dolphin, D. (ed): *B_{12}*. Wiley-Interscience, New York, in press.
29. Folkers, K.: Historical perspectives on the isolation of crystalline vitamin B_{12}, in *Vitamin B_{12}. Proceedings of the Third European Symposium on Vitamin B_{12} and Intrinsic Factor. University of Zürich, March 5–8, 1979, Zürich, Switzerland*, edited by B. Zagalak and W. Friedrich. Walter de Gruyter, New York, 1979, p. 7.
30. Perlman, D.: Microbial synthesis of cobamides, in *Advances in Applied Microbiology*, edited by W. W. Umbreit. Academic, New York, 1959, vol. 1, p. 87.
31. Beck, W. S.: Biological and medical aspects of vitamin B_{12}, in *B_{12}*, edited by D. Dolphin. Wiley-Interscience, New York, in press.
32. Heyssel, R. M., Bozian, R. C., Darby, W. J., and Bell, M. C.: Vitamin B_{12} turnover in man: The assimilation of vitamin B_{12} from natural foodstuff by man and estimates of minimal daily dietary requirements. *Am. J. Clin. Nutr.* 18:176, 1966.
33. Hall, C. A.: Long-term excretion of $Co^{57}B_{12}$ and turnover within the plasma. *Am. J. Clin. Nutr.* 14:156, 1964.
34. Adams, J. F.: Considerations governing the maintenance treatment of patients with pernicious anemia, in *Vitamin B12 und Intrinsic Faktor, 2d Europäisches Symposion*, edited by H. C. Heinrich. Enke, Stuttgart, 1962, p. 628.
35. Gräsbeck, R.: Calculations on vitamin B_{12} turnover in man. *Scand. J. Clin. Lab. Invest.* 11:250, 1959.
36. Hsu, J. M., Kawin, B., Minor, P., and Mitchell, J. A.: Vitamin B_{12} concentrations in human tissues. *Nature (London)* 210:1264, 1966.
37. Food and Nutrition Board, National Research Council: *Recommended Dietary Allowances*, 7th ed. publication 1964. National Academy of Sciences, Washington, 1968.
38. Corcoran, J. W., and Shemin, D.: Biosynthesis of the porphyrin-like moiety of vitamin B_{12}: Mode of utilization of δ-aminolevulinic acid. *Biochim. Biophys. Acta* 25:661, 1957.
39. Friedmann, H. C.: Biosynthesis of corrinoids, in *Cobalamin: Biochemistry and Pathophysiology*, edited by B. M. Babior. Wiley-Interscience, New York, 1975, p. 75.
40. IUPAC-IUB: Tentative rules. *J. Biol. Chem.* 241:2991, 1966.
41. IUPAC-IUB. The nomenclature of corrinoids. *Biochemistry* 13:1555, 1974.
42. Lenhert, P. G., and Hodgkin, D. C.: Structure of the 5,6-dimethylbenzimidazolylcobamide coenzyme. *Nature (London)* 192:937, 1961.
43. Guest, J. R., Friedman, S., Woods, D. D., and Smith, E. L.: A methyl analogue of cobamide coenzyme in relation to methionine synthesis by bacteria. *Nature (London)* 195:340, 1962.
44. Stahlberg, K. G.: Studies on methyl-B_{12} in man. *Scand. J. Haematol.* (Suppl. 1) 1, 1967.
45. Linnell, J. C.: The fate of cobalamins *in vivo*, in *Cobalamin: Biochemistry and Pathophysiology*, edited by B. M. Babior. Wiley-Interscience, New York, 1975, p. 287.
46. Peterkofsky, A., and Weissbach, H.: Release of inorganic tripolyphosphate from adenosine triphosphate during vitamin B_{12} coenzyme biosynthesis. *J. Biol. Chem.* 238:1491, 1963.
47. Ohta, H., and Beck, W. S.: Studies of the ribosome-associated vitamin B_{12} adenosylating enzyme of *Lactobacillus leichmannii*. *Arch. Biochem. Biophys.* 174:713, 1976.
48. Poston, J. M., and Stadtman, T. C.: Cobamides as cofactors: Methylcobamides and the synthesis of methionine, methane, and acetate, in *Cobalamin: Biochemistry and Pathophysiology*, edited by B. M. Babior. Wiley-Interscience, New York, 1975, p. 111.
49. Babior, B. M.: Cobamides as cofactors: Adenosylcobamide-dependent reactions, in *Cobalamin: Biochemistry and Pathophysiology*, edited by B. M. Babior. Wiley-Interscience, New York, 1975, p. 141.
50. Poston, J. M.: Leucine 2,3-aminomutase, an enzyme of leucine catabolism. *J. Biol. Chem.* 251:1859, 1976.
51. Beck, W. S., Flavin, M., and Ochoa, S.: Metabolism of propionic acid in animal tissues. III. Formation of succinate. *J. Biol. Chem.* 229:997, 1957.
52. Beck, W. S., and Ochoa, S.: Metabolism of propionic acid in animal tissues. IV. Further studies on the enzymatic isomerization of methylmalonyl coenzyme A. *J. Biol. Chem.* 232:931, 1958.
53. Retey, J., and Arigoni, D.: Coenzyme B_{12} als gemeinsamer Wasserstoffübertrager der Dioldehydrase- und der Methylmalonyl-CoA-Mutase-Reaktion. *Experientia* 22:783, 1966.
54. Abeles, R. H., and Lee, H. A., Jr.: An intramolecular oxidation-reduction requiring a vitamin B_{12} coenzyme. *J. Biol. Chem.* 236:2347, 1961.
55. Smiley, K. L., and Sobolov, M.: A cobamide-requiring glycerol dehydrase from an acrolein-forming lactobacillus. *Arch. Biochem. Biophys.* 97:538, 1962.
56. Kaplan, B. A., and Stadtman, E. R.: Ethanolamine deaminase, a

cobamide, coenzyme-dependent enzyme. II. Purification, assay, and properties of the enzyme. *J. Biol. Chem.* 243:1787, 1968.

57. Stadtman, T. C., and Renz, P.: Anaerobic degradation of lysine. V. Some properties of the cobamide-dependent β-lysine mutase of *Clostridium sticklandii*. *Arch. Biochem.* 125:226, 1968.

58. Blakley, R. L., and Barker, H. A.: Cobamide stimulation of the reduction of ribotides to deoxyribotides in *Lactobacillus leichmannii*. *Biochem. Biophys. Res. Commun.* 16:391, 1964.

59. Beck, W. S., and Hardy, J.: Requirement of ribonucleotide reductase for cobamide coenzyme: A product of ribosomal activity. *Proc. Natl. Acad. Sci. U.S.A.* 54:286, 1965.

60. Abrams, R., and Duraiswami, S.: Deoxycytidylate formation from cytidylate without glycosidic cleavage in *Lactobacillus leichmannii* extracts containing vitamin B$_{12}$ coenzyme. *Biochem. Biophys. Res. Commun.* 18:409, 1965.

61. Goulian, M., and Beck, W. S.: Purification and properties of cobamide-dependent ribonucleotide reductase from *Lactobacillus leichmannii*. *J. Biol. Chem.* 241:4233, 1966.

62. Gottesman, M. M., and Beck, W. S.: Transfer of hydrogen in the cobamide-dependent ribonucleotide reductase reaction. *Biochem. Biophys. Res. Commun.* 24:353, 1966.

63. Abeles, R. H., and Beck, W. S.: The mechanism of action of cobamide coenzyme in the ribonucleotide reductase reaction. *J. Biol. Chem.* 242:3589, 1967.

64. Beck, W. S., Hook, S., and Barnett, B. H.: The metabolic functions of vitamin B$_{12}$. I. Distinctive modes of unbalanced growth behavior in *Lactobacillus leichmannii*. *Biochim. Biophys. Acta* 55:455, 1962.

65. Beck, W. S.: The metabolic basis of megaloblastic erythropoiesis. *Medicine (Baltimore)* 43:715, 1964.

66. Taylor, R. T., and Weissbach, H.: N⁵-methyltetrahydrofolate-homocysteine transmethylase. *J. Biol. Chem.* 242:1502, 1967.

67. Loughlin, R. E., Elford, H. L., and Buchanan, J. M.: Enzymatic synthesis of the methyl group of methionine. VII. Isolation of a cobalamin-containing transmethylase (5-methyltetrahydrofolate homocysteine) from mammalian liver. *J. Biol. Chem.* 239:2888, 1964.

68. Sauer, H.-J., Wilms, K., Wilmanns, W., and Jaenicke, L.: Die Aktivität der methionin-synthetase (5-methyl-5,6,7,8-tetrahydrofolsäure: homocystein methyltransferase) als proliferationsparameter in wachsenden Zellen. *Acta Haematol. (Basel)* 49:200, 1973.

69. Peytremann, R., Thorndike, J., and Beck, W. S.: Studies on N⁵-methyltetrahydrofolate-homocysteine methyltransferase in normal and leukemic leukocytes. *J. Clin. Invest.* 56:1293, 1975.

70. Banks, R. G. S., Henderson, R. J., Pratt, J. M.: Reactions of gases in solution. III. Some reactions of nitrous oxide with transition-metal complexes. *J. Chem. Soc. (A):*2886, 1968.

71. Chanarin, I.: Cobalamins and nitrous oxide: A review. *J. Clin. Pathol.* 33:909, 1980.

72. Matthews, D. M., and Wilson, J.: Cobalamins and cyanide metabolism in neurological diseases, in *The Cobalamins: A Glaxo Symposium*, edited by H. R. V. Arnstein and R. J. Wrighton. Williams & Wilkins, Baltimore, 1971, p. 115.

73. Wokes, F., and Picard, C. W.: The role of vitamin B$_{12}$ in human nutrition. *Am. J. Clin. Nutr.* 3:383, 1955.

74. Larsson, A., and Reichard, P.: Enzymatic reduction of ribonucleotides. *Prog. Nucleic Acid Res.* 7:305, 1967.

75. Moore, E. C., and Reichard, P.: Enzymatic synthesis of deoxyribonucleotides. VI. The cytidine diphosphate reductase system from Novikoff hepatoma. *J. Biol. Chem.* 239:3453, 1964.

76. Fujioka, S., and Silber, R.: Ribonucleotide reductase in human bone marrow: Lack of stimulation by 5'-deoxyadenosyl B$_{12}$. *Biochem. Biophys. Res. Commun.* 35:759, 1969.

77. Hopper, S.: Ribonucleotide reductase of rabbit bone marrow. I. Purification properties, and separation into two protein fractions. *J. Biol. Chem.* 247:3336, 1972.

78. Friedkin, M.: Thymidylate synthetase. *Adv. Enzymol.* 38:235, 1972.

79. Norohna, J. M., and Silverman, M.: On folic acid, vitamin B$_{12}$ methionine and formiminoglutamic acid metabolism, in *Vitamin B$_{12}$ und Intrinsic Faktor, 2d Europäisches Symposion*, edited by H. C. Heinrich. Enke, Stuttgart, 1962.

80. Herbert, V., and Zalusky, R.: Interrelations of vitamin B$_{12}$ and folic

acid metabolism: Folic acid clearance studies. *J. Clin. Invest.* 41:1263, 1962.

81. Chanarin, I., Deacon, R., Perry, J., and Lumb, M.: How vitamin B$_{12}$ acts. *Br. J. Haematol.* 47:487, 1981.

82. Silverman, M., and Pitney, A. S.: Dietary methionine and the excretion of formiminoglutamic acid by the rat. *J. Biol. Chem.* 233:1179, 1958.

83. Arakawa, I.: Congenital defects in folate utilization. *Am. J. Med.* 48:594, 1970.

84. Kutzbach, C., Galloway, E., and Stokstad, E. L. R.: Influence of vitamin B$_{12}$ and methionine on levels of folic acid compounds and folate enzymes in rat liver. *Proc. Soc. Exp. Biol. Med.* 124:801, 1967.

85. Killman, S.-A.: Effect of deoxyuridine on incorporation of tritiated thymidine: Difference between normoblasts and megaloblasts. *Acta Med. Scand.* 175:483, 1964.

86. Nixon, P. F., and Bertino, J. R.: Impaired utilization of serum folate in pernicious anemia: A study with radiolabeled 5-methyltetrahydrofolate. *J. Clin. Invest.* 51:1431, 1972.

87. Herbert, V.: Recent developments in cobalamin metabolism, in *The Cobalamins*, edited by H. R. V. Arnstein and R. J. Wrighton. Churchill, Livingston, London, 1971, p. 20.

88. Thenen, S. W., Hawthorne, J. M., and Stokstad, E. L. R.: The oxidation of 5-methyl-¹⁴C-tetrahydrofolate and histidine-2-¹⁴C to ¹⁴CO$_2$ in vitamin B$_{12}$-deficient rats. *Proc. Soc. Exp. Biol. Med.* 134:199, 1970.

89. Laduron, P.: N-methylation of a dopamine to epinine in brain tissue using N-methyltetrahydrofolic acid as the methyl donor. *Nature [New Biol.]* 238:212, 1972.

90. Taylor, R. T., and Hanna, M. L.: 5-methyltetrahydrofolate aromatic alkylamine N-methyltransferase: An artefact of 5,10-methylenetetrahydrofolate reductase activity. *Life Sci.* 17:111, 1975.

91. Thorndike, J., and Beck, W. S.: Enzymatic production of formaldehyde from N⁵-methyltetrahydrofolate in normal and leukemic leukocytes. *Cancer Res.* 37:1125, 1977.

92. Cooper, B. A., and Lowenstein, L.: Relative folate deficiency of erythrocytes in pernicious anaemia and its correction with cyanocobalamin. *Blood* 24:502, 1964.

93. Linnell, J. C., Mackenzie, H. M., Wilson, J., and Matthews, D. M.: Patterns of plasma cobalamins in control subjects and in cases of vitamin B$_{12}$ deficiency. *J. Clin. Pathol.* 22:545, 1969.

94. Linnell, J. C., Hoffbrand, A. V., Peters, T. J., and Matthews, D. M.: Chromatographic and bioautographic estimation of plasma cobalamins in various disturbances of vitamin B$_{12}$ metabolism. *Clin. Sci.* 40:1, 1971.

95. Pelliniemi, T. T., and Beck, W. S.: Biochemical mechanisms in the Killmann experiment: Critique of the deoxyuridine suppression test. *J. Clin. Invest.* 65:449, 1980.

96. Van Der Weyden, M. B.: Deoxyuridine metabolism in human megaloblastic marrow cells. *Scand. J. Haematol.* 23:37, 1979.

97. Metz, J., Kelly, A., Sweth, V. C., Waxman, S., and Herbert, V.: Deranged DNA synthesis by bone marrow from vitamin B$_{12}$-deficient humans. *Br. J. Haematol.* 14:575, 1968.

98. Waxman, S., Mertz, J., and Herbert, V.: Defective DNA synthesis in human megaloblastic bone marrow: Effects of homocysteine and methionine. *J. Clin. Invest.* 48:284, 1969.

99. Stebbins, R., Scott, J., and Herbert, V.: Therapeutic trial in the test tube: The "dU suppression test" using "physiologic" doses of B$_{12}$ and folic acid to replace therapeutic trial in vivo for diagnosis of B$_{12}$ and folate deficiency. *Blood* 40:927, 1972.

100. Van der Weyden, M. B., Cooper, M., and Firkin, B. G.: Defective DNA synthesis in human megaloblastic bone marrow: Effects of hydroxy-B$_{12}$ 5'-deoxyadenosyl-B$_{12}$ and methyl-B$_{12}$. *Blood* 41:299, 1973.

101. Herbert, V. L.: Laboratory aids in the diagnosis of folic acid and vitamin B$_{12}$ deficiencies. *Ann. Clin. Lab. Sci.* 1:193, 1971.

102. Levy, H. L., Mudd, S. H., Schulman, J. D., Dreyfus, P. M., and Abeles, R. H.: A derangement in B$_{12}$ metabolism associated with homocystinemia, cystathioninemia, hypomethioninemia and methylmalonic aciduria. *Am. J. Med.* 48:390, 1970.

103. Mudd, S. H., Uhlendorf, B. W., Hinds, K. R., and Levy, H. L.: Deranged B$_{12}$ metabolism: Studies of fibroblasts grown in tissue culture. *Biochem. Med.* 4:215, 1970.

104. Goodman, S. I., Moe, P. G., Hammond, K. B., Mudd, S. H., and

Uhlendorf, B. W.: Homocystinuria with methylmalonic aciduria: Two cases in a sibship. *Biochem. Med. 4*:500, 1970.

105. Ellenbogen, L.: Absorption and transport of cobalamin: Intrinsic factor and the transcobalamins, in *Cobalamin: Biochemistry and Pathophysiology*, edited by B. M. Babior. Wiley-Interscience, New York, 1975, p. 215.

106. Castle, W. B.: Development of knowledge concerning the gastric intrinsic factor and its relation to pernicious anemia. *N. Engl. J. Med. 249*:614, 1953.

107. Allen, R. H., and Mehlman, C. S.: Isolation of gastric vitamin B₁₂-binding proteins using affinity chromatography. I. Purification and properties of human intrinsic factor. *J. Biol. Chem. 248*:3660, 1973.

108. Christensen, J. M., et al.: Purification of human intrinsic factor by affinity chromatography. *Biochim. Biophys. Acta 303*:319, 1973.

109. Visuri, K., and Gräsbeck, R.: Human intrinsic factor: Isolation by improved conventional methods and properties of the preparation. *Biochim. Biophys. Acta 310*:508, 1973.

110. Nexø, E., Olesen, H., Hansen, M. R., Bucher, D., and Thomsen, J.: Primary structure of human intrinsic factor: Progress report on cyanogen bromide fragmentation. *Scand. J. Lab. Clin. Invest. 38*:649, 1978.

111. Marcouillis, G., and Gräsbeck, R.: Vitamin B₁₂-binding proteins in human gastric mucosa: General pattern and demonstration of intrinsic isoproteins typical of mucosa. *Scand. J. Clin. Lab. Invest. 35*:5, 1975.

112. Stenman, U.-H.: Vitamin B₁₂-binding proteins of R-type cobalophilin: Characterization and comparison of cobalophilin from different sources. *Scand. J. Haematol. 14*:91, 1975.

113. Cotter, R., Rothenberg, S. P., Weiss, J. P.: Purification of the intestinal receptor for intrinsic factor by affinity chromatography. *Biochim. Biophys. Acta 490*:19, 1977.

114. Marcoullis, G., and Gräsbeck, R.: Isolation of the porcine ileal intrinsic factor receptor by sequential affinity chromatography. *Biochim. Biophys. Acta 499*:309, 1977.

115. Yamada, S., Itaya, H., Nazakawa, O., and Fukuda, M.: Purification of rat intestinal receptor for intrinsic factor. Vitamin B₁₂ complex by affinity chromotography. *Biochim. Biophys. Acta 496*:571, 1977.

116. Herbert, V., and Castle, W. B.: Divalent cation and pH dependence of rat intrinsic factor action in everted sacs and mucosal homogenates of rat small intestine. *J. Clin. Invest. 40*:1978, 1961.

117. Gräsbeck, R.: Soluble and membrane-bound vitamin B₁₂ transport proteins, in *Vitamin B₁₂. Proceedings of the Third European Symposium on Vitamin B₁₂ and Intrinsic Factor. University of Zürich, March 5–8, 1979, Zürich, Switzerland*, edited by B. Zagalak and W. Friedrich. Walter de Gruyter, New York, 1979, p. 743.

118. Toskes, P. P., Hansell, J., Cerda, J., and Deren, J. J.: Vitamin B₁₂ malabsorption in chronic pancreatic insufficiency. *N. Engl. J. Med. 284*:627, 1973.

119. Marcoullis, G., Parmentier, Y., Nicolas, J.-P., Jiminez, M., and Gerard, P.: Cobalamin malabsorption due to nondegradation of R proteins in the human intestine. Inhibited cobalamin absorption in exocrine pancreatic dysfunction. *J. Clin. Invest. 66*:430, 1980.

120. Allen, R. H., Seetharam, B., Podell, E., and Alpers, D. H.: Effect of proteolytic enzymes on the binding of cobalamin to R protein and intrinsic factor. *J. Clin. Invest. 61*:47, 1978.

121. Hines, J. D., Rosenberg, A., and Harris, J. W.: Intrinsic factor-mediated radio-B₁₂ uptake in sequential incubation studies using everted sacs of guinea pig small intestine: Evidence that IF is not absorbed into the intestinal cell. *Proc. Soc. Exp. Biol. Med. 129*:653, 1968.

122. Peters, T. J., and Hoffbrand, A. V.: Absorption of vitamin B₁₂ by the guinea pig. I. Subcellular localization of vitamin B₁₂ in the ileal enterocyte during absorption. *Br. J. Haematol. 19*:369, 1970.

123. Becker, C. M., and Beck, W. S.: Calcium dependencies in the bindings of transcobalamins to subcellular particles of liver cells, in *Vitamin B₁₂. Proceedings of the Third European Symposium on Vitamin B₁₂ and Intrinsic Factor. University of Zürich, March 5–8, 1979, Zürich, Switzerland*, edited by B. Zagalak and W. Friedrich. Walter de Gruyter, New York, 1979, p. 833. Calcium dependencies of R binder-[⁵⁷Co] rat cyanocobalamin receptors in rat liver cell fractions. *Arch. Biochem. Biophys.*, submitted for publication.

124. Hall, C. A., and Finkler, A. E.: A second vitamin B₁₂-binding substance in human plasma. *Biochem. Biophys. Acta 78*:233, 1963.

125. Allen, R. H., and Majerus, P. W.: Isolation of vitamin B₁₂-binding proteins using affinity chromatography. III. Purification and properties of human plasma transcobalamin II. *J. Biol. Chem. 247*:7709, 1972.

126. Schneider, R. J., Burger, R. L., Mehlman, C. S., and Allen, R. H.: The role and fate of rabbit and human transcobalamin II in the plasma transport of vitamin B₁₂ in the rabbit. *J. Clin. Invest. 56*:27, 1976.

127. Hall, C. A., and Finkler, A. E.: Function of transcobalamin II: A vitamin B₁₂ binding protein in human plasma. *Proc. Soc. Exp. Biol. Med. 123*:55, 1966.

128. Hall, C. A., and Finkler, A. E.: Abnormal transport of vitamin B₁₂ in plasma in chronic myelogenous leukemia. *Nature 204*:1207, 1964.

129. England, M. M., Clarke, H. G. M., Down, M. C., and Chanarin, I.: Studies on the transcobalamins. *Br. J. Haematol. 25*:737, 1973.

130. Burger, R. L., Mehlman, C. S., and Allen, R. H.: Human plasma R-type vitamin B₁₂-binding proteins. I. Isolation and characterization of transcobalamin I, transcobalamin III, and the normal granulocyte vitamin B₁₂-binding protein. *J. Biol. Chem. 250*:7700, 1975.

131. Gräsbeck, R.: Intrinsic factor and the other vitamin B₁₂ transport proteins. *Prog. Hematol. 6*:233, 1969.

132. Olesen, H.: Serum transcobalamins. *Scand. J. Gasteroenterol. 9 (Suppl. 29)*:13, 1974.

133. Allen, R. H.: Human vitamin B₁₂ transport proteins. *Prog. Hematol. 9*:57, 1975.

134. Stenman, U.-H., Simons, K., and Gräsbeck, R.: Vitamin B₁₂ binding proteins in normal and leukemic leukocytes and sera. *Scand. J. Clin. Lab. Invest. 21 (Suppl. 101)*:13, 1974.

135. Burger, R. L., and Allen, R. H.: Characterization of vitamin B₁₂-binding proteins isolated from human milk and saliva by affinity chromatography. *J. Biol. Chem. 249*:7220, 1974.

136. Scott, J. M., Bloomfield, F. J., Stebbins, R., and Herbert, V.: Studies of derivation of transcobalamin III from granulocytes: Enhancement by lithium and elimination by fluoride of in vitro increments in vitamin B₁₂-binding capacity. *J. Clin. Invest. 53*:228, 1974.

137. Gilbert, H. S.: Demonstration of the "PV" B₁₂-binding protein in leukocytes of normals and patients with myeloproliferative disorders (MPD). *Blood 38*:805, 1971.

138. Carmel, R.: Vitamin B₁₂-binding protein abnormality in subjects without myeloproliferative disease. II. The presence of a third vitamin B₁₂-binding protein in serum. *Br. J. Haematol. 22*:53, 1972.

139. Tan, C. H., and Hansen, H. J.: Studies on the site of synthesis of transcobalamin-II. *Proc. Soc. Exp. Biol. Med. 127*:740, 1968.

140. Fràter-Schröder, M., Nissen, C., Gmür, J., Kierat, L., and Hitzig, W. H.: Bone marrow participates in the biosynthesis of human transcobalamin II. *Blood 56*:560, 1980.

141. Hom, B. L., and Ahluwalia, B. K.: The vitamin B₁₂ binding capacity of transcobalamin I and II on normal human serum. *Scand. J. Haematol. 5*:64, 1968.

142. Benson, R. E., Rappazzo, M. E., and Hall, C. A.: Late transport of vitamin B₁₂ by transcobalamin II. *J. Lab. Clin. Med. 80*:488, 1972.

143. Hall, C. A.: Transcobalamins I and II as natural transport proteins of vitamin B₁₂. *J. Clin. Invest. 56*:1125, 1975.

144. Hom, B. L., and Olesen, H. A.: Plasma clearance of ⁵⁷Cobalt-labelled vitamin B₁₂ bound in vitro and in vivo transcobalamin. *Scand. J. Clin. Lab. Invest. 23*:201, 1969.

145. Gizis, E. J., Arkun, S. N., Miller, I. F., Choi, G., Dietrich, M. F., and Meyer, L. M.: Plasma clearance of transcobalamin I- and transcobalamin II-bound Co⁵⁷ and vitamin B₁₂. *J. Lab. Clin. Med. 74*:574, 1969.

146. Carmel, R., and Herbert, V.: Deficiency of vitamin B₁₂-binding alpha globulin in two brothers. *Blood 33*:1, 1969.

147. Hakami, N., Neiman, P. E., Canellos, G. P., and Lazerson, J.: Neonatal megaloblastic anemia due to inherited transcobalamin II deficiency in two siblings. *N. Engl. J. Med. 285*:1163, 1971.

148. Finkler, A. E., and Hall, C. A.: Nature of the relationship between vitamin B₁₂ binding and cell uptake. *Arch. Biochem. 120*:79, 1967.

149. Zittoun, J., Zittoun, R., Marquet, J., and Sultan, C.: The three transcobalamins in myeloproliferative disorders and acute leukemia. *Br. J. Haematol. 31*:287, 1975.

150. Hall, C. A., and Finkler, A. E.: Vitamin B$_{12}$-binding protein in polycythemia vera plasma. *J. Lab. Clin. Med.* 73:60, 1969.

151. Waxman, S., and Gilbert, H. S.: A tumor-related vitamin B$_{12}$ binding protein in adolescent hepatoma. *N. Engl. J. Med.* 289:1053, 1973.

152. Burger, R. L., Waxman, S., Gilbert, H. S., Mehlman, C. S., and Allen, R. H.: Isolation and characterization of a novel vitamin B$_{12}$-binding protein associated with hepatocellular carcinoma. *J. Clin. Invest.* 56:1262, 1975.

153. Carmel, R.: Extreme elevation of serum transcobalamin I in patients with metastatic cancer. *N. Engl. J. Med.* 292:282, 1975.

154. Jorgensen, F. S.: Vitamin B$_{12}$ and its binding proteins in cirrhosis and infectious hepatitis. *Scand. J. Haematol.* 7:322, 1970.

155. Rachmilewitz, M., Aronovitch, M. J., and Grossowicz, N.: Serum concentrations of vitamin B$_{12}$ in acute and chronic liver disease. *J. Lab. Clin. Med.* 48:339, 1956

156. Retief, R. P., Vandenplas, L., and Visser, H.: Vitamin B$_{12}$ binding proteins in liver disease. *Br. J. Haematol.* 16:231, 1969.

157. Carmel, R., Coltman, C. A., Jr., and Brubaker, L. H.: Serum vitamin B$_{12}$-binding proteins in neutropenia. *Proc. Soc. Exp. Biol. Med.* 148:1217, 1975.

158. Thompson, H. T., Dietrich, L. S., and Elvehjem, C. A.: The use of *Lactobacillus leichmannii* in the estimation of vitamin B$_{12}$ activity. *J. Biol. Chem.* 184:175, 1950.

159. *United States Pharmacopeia* 15:885, 1955.

160. Shinton, N. K.: Total serum vitamin B$_{12}$ concentration in normal human adult serum assayed by *Euglena gracilis*. *Clin. Sci.* 18:389, 1959.

161. Burkholder, P. R.: Determination of vitamin B$_{12}$ with a mutant strain of *Escherichia coli*. *Science* 114:459, 1951.

162. Kelly, A., and Herbert, V.: Coated charcoal assay of erythrocyte vitamin B$_{12}$ levels. *Blood* 29:139, 1967.

163. Raven, J. L., Walker, P. L., and Barkhan, P.: Comparison of the radioisotope dilution-coated charcoal method and a microbiological method *(L. leichmannii)* for measuring vitamin B$_{12}$ in serum. *J. Clin. Pathol.* 19:610, 1966.

164. Kolhouse, J. F., Kondo, H., Allen, N. C., Podell, E., and Allen, R. H.: Cobalamin analogues are present in human plasma and can mask cobalamin deficiency because current radioisotope dilution assays are not specific for true cobalamin. *N. Engl. J. Med.* 299:785, 1978.

165. Kondo, H., Kolhouse, J. F., and Allen, R. H.: Presence of cobalamin analogues in animal tissues. *Proc. Nat. Acad. Sci. U.S.A.* 77:817, 1980.

166. Gräsbeck, R., Nyberg, W., and Reizenstein, P.: Biliary and fecal vitamin B$_{12}$ excretion in man: An isotope study. *Proc. Soc. Exp. Biol. Med.* 97:780, 1958.

167. Reizenstein, P. G.: Excretion of non-labeled vitamin B$_{12}$ in man. *Acta. Med. Scand.* 165:313, 1959.

168. Booth, M. A., and Spray, G. H.: Vitamin B$_{12}$ activity in the serum and liver of rats after total gastrectomy. *Br. J. Haematol.* 6:288, 1960.

169. Burger, R. L., Schneider, R. J., Mehlman, C. S., and Allen, R. H.: Human plasma R-type vitamin B$_{12}$-binding proteins. II. The role of transcobalamin I, transcobalamin III, and the normal granulocyte vitamin B$_{12}$-binding protein in the plasma transport of vitamin B$_{12}$. *J. Biol. Chem.* 250:7707, 1975.

170. Ashwell, G., and Morell, A. G.: The role of surface carbohydrates in the hepatic recognition and transport of circulating glycoproteins. *Adv. Enzymol.* 41:99, 1974.

171. Simons, K.: Vitamin B$_{12}$ binders in human body fluids and blood cells. *Soc. Sci. Fenn. Comm. Biol.* 27 (Suppl. 1):1, 1964.

172. Simons, K., and Weber, T.: The vitamin B$_{12}$-binding protein in human leukocytes. *Biochim. Biophys. Acta* 117:201, 1966.

173. Hippe, E., Haber, E., and Olesen, H.: Nature of vitamin B$_{12}$ binding. II. Steric orientation of vitamin B$_{12}$ on binding and number of combining sites of human intrinsic factor and the transcobalamins. *Biochim. Biophys. Acta* 243:75, 1971.

174. Gottlieb, C. W., Retief, F. P., and Herbert, V.: Blockade of vitamin B$_{12}$-binding sites in gastric juice, serum and saliva by analogues and derivatives of vitamin B$_{12}$ and by antibody to intrinsic factor. *Biochim. Biophys. Acta* 141:560, 1967.

175. Wieland, H., Tartter, A., and Purrmann, R.: Uber die Flügelpigmente der Schmetterlinge. IX. "Anhydro-leukopterin" und "Purpuroflavin." *Liebig Ann. Chem.* 545:209, 1940.

176. Wagner, A. F., and Folkers, K.: Pteroylmonoglutamic acid and the folic acid coenzymes, in *Vitamins and Coenzymes*. Wiley, New York, 1964, p. 113.

177. Friedkin, M.: Enzymatic aspects of folic acid. *Annu. Rev. Biochem.* 32:185, 1963.

178. Rabinowitz, J. C.: Folic acid, in *The Enzymes*, 2d ed., edited by P. D. Boyer, H. Lardy, and K. Myrback. Academic, New York, 1960, vol. 2, p. 185.

179. Sebrell, W. H., Jr., and Harris, R. S.: Folic acid, in *The Vitamins*. Academic, New York, 1959, vol. 3.

180. Blakeley, R. L.: *The Biochemistry of Folic Acid and Related Pteridines*. American Elsevier, New York, 1969.

181. Wills, L., Contab, A., and Lond, B. S.: Treatment of "pernicious anaemia of pregnancy" and "tropical anaemia." *Br. Med. J.* 1:1059, 1931.

182. Day, P. L., Langston, W. C., and Darby, W. J.: Failure of nicotinic acid to prevent nutritional cytopenia in the monkey. *Proc. Soc. Exp. Biol. Med.* 38:860, 1938.

183. Stokstad, E. L. R., and Manning, P. D. V.: Evidence of a new growth factor required by chicks. *J. Biol. Chem.* 125:687, 1938.

184. Hogan, A. G., and Parrott, E. M.: Anemia in chicks due to vitamin deficiency. *J. Biol. Chem.* 128:46, 1939.

185. Snell, E. E., and Peterson, W. H.: Growth factors for bacteria. X. Additional factors required by certain lactic acid bacteria. *J. Bacteriol.* 36:273, 1940.

186. Mitchell, H. K., Snell, E. E., and Williams, R. J.: The concentration of "folic acid." *J. Am. Chem. Soc.* 63:2284, 1941.

187. Hutchings, B. L., Stokstad, E. L. R., Bohonos, N., Sloan, N. H., and SubbaRow, Y.: The isolation of *Lactobacillus casei* factor from liver. *J. Am. Chem. Soc.* 70:3, 1948.

188. Waller, C. W., et al.: Synthesis of pteroylglutamic acid (liver *L. casei* factor) and pteroic acid. I. *J. Am. Chem. Soc.* 70:19, 1948.

189. Watson, J., and Castle, W. B.: Nutritional macrocytic anemia, especially in pregnancy: Response to a substance in liver other than that effective in pernicious anemia. *Am. J. Med. Sci.* 211:513, 1946.

190. IUPAC-IUB Commission on Biochemical Nomenclature: Tentative rules: Nomenclature and symbols for folic acid and related compounds. *Biochim. Biophys. Acta* 107:11, 1965; *J. Biol. Chem.* 241:2291, 1966.

191. Sauberlich, H. E., and Baumann, C. A.: A factor required for the growth of *Leuconostoc citrovorum*. *J. Biol. Chem.* 176:165, 1948.

192. Butterworth, C. E., Jr., Santini, R., Jr., and Frommeyer, W. B., Jr.: The pteroylglutamate components of American diets as determined by chromatographic fractionation. *J. Clin. Invest.* 42:1929, 1963.

193. Butterworth, C. E., Jr.: The availability of food folate. *Br. J. Haematol.* 14:339, 1968.

194. Food and Nutrition Board, National Research Council: *Recommended Dietary Allowances*, 7th ed., publication 1694. National Academy of Sciences, Washington, 1968.

195. Herbert, V.: Minimal daily adult folate requirement. *Arch. Intern. Med.* 110:649, 1962.

196. Alperin, J. B., Hutchinson, H. T., and Levin, W. C.: Studies of folic acid requirements in megaloblastic anemia of pregnancy. *Arch. Intern. Med.* 117:681, 1966.

197. Huennekens, F. M., and Osborn, M. J.: Folic acid coenzymes and one-carbon metabolism. *Adv. Enzymol.* 21:369, 1959.

198. Kaufman, S.: Pteridine cofactors. *Annu. Rev. Biochem.* 36:171, 1967.

199. Stokstad, E. L. R., and Koch, J.: Folic acid metabolism. *Physiol. Rev.* 47:83, 1967.

200. Huennekens, F. M.: Folic acid coenzymes in the biosynthesis of purines and pyrimidines. *Vitam. Horm.* 26:375, 1968.

201. Wahba, A. J., and Friedkin, M.: The enzymatic synthesis of thymidylate. I. Early steps in the purification of thymidylate synthetase of *Escherichia coli*. *J. Biol. Chem.* 237:3794, 1962.

202. Silverman, M., and Pitney, A. J.: Dietary methionine and the excretion of formiminoglutamic acid by the rat. *J. Biol. Chem.* 233:1179, 1958.

203. Tabor, H., and Wyngarden, L.: The enzymatic formation of formiminotetrahydrofolic acid, 5,10-methenyltetrahydrofolic acid and

10-formiminohydrofolic acid in the metabolism of formiminoglu-tamic acid. *J. Biol. Chem.* 234:1830, 1959.

204. Luhby, A. L., Cooperman, J. M., Teller, D. N., and Donnenfeld, A. M.: Excretion of formiminoglutamic acid in folic acid deficiency states. *J. Clin. Invest.* 37:915, 1958.

205. Knowles, J. P., and Prankerd, T. A. J.: Abnormal folic acid metabolism in vitamin B₁₂ deficiency. *Clin. Sci.* 22:233, 1962.

206. Herbert, V.: Folic acid. *Annu. Rev. Med.* 16:359, 1965.

207. Spray, G. H., and Witts, J. J.: Excretion of formiminoglutamic acid as an index of folic acid deficiency. *Lancet* 2:702, 1959.

208. Taylor, R. T., and Hanna, M. L.: 5-Methyltetrahydrofolate aromatic alkylamine N-methyltransferase: An artefact of 5,10-methylene-tetrahydrofolate reductase activity. *Life Sci.* 17:111, 1975.

209. Pearson, A. G. M., and Turner, A. J.: Folate-dependent 1-carbon transfer to biogenic amines mediated by methylene-tetrahydrofolate reductase. *Nature (London)* 258:173, 1975.

210. Rosengarten, H., Meller, E., and Freidhoff, A. J.: Synthesis of tetrahydro-β-carbolines from indoleamines via enzymatic formation of formaldehyde from 5-methyltetrahydrofolic acid. *Biochem. Pharmacol.* 24:1759, 1975.

211. Thorndike, J., and Beck, W. S.: Enzymatic production of for-maldehyde from N⁵-methyltetrahydrofolate in normal and leuke-mic leukocytes. *Cancer Res.* 37:1125, 1977.

212. Banerjee, S. P. and Snyder, S. H.: Methyltetrahydrofolic acid medi-ates N- and O-methylation of biogenic amines. *Science* 182:74, 1973.

213. Kaufman, S.: The phenylalanine hydroxylating system from mam-malian liver. *Adv. Enzymol.* 35:245, 1971.

214. Binkley, S. B., et al.: On the vitamin B꜀ conjugate in yeast. *Science* 100:36, 1944.

215. Bird, O. D., Binkley, S. B., Bloom, E. S., Emmett, A. D., and Pfiffner, J. J.: On the enzymatic formation of vitamin B꜀ from its conjugate. *J. Biol. Chem.* 157:413, 1945.

216. Corrocher, R., Bhuyan, B. K., and Hoffbrand, A. V.: Composition of pteroylpolyglutamates (conjugated folates) in guinea-pig liver and their formation from folic acid. *Clin. Sci.* 43:799, 1972.

217. Shin, Y. S., Buehring, K. U., and Stokstad, E. L. R.: Separation of folic acid compounds by gel chromatography on Sephadex G-15 and G-25. *J. Biol. Chem.* 247:7266, 1972.

218. Curthoys, N. P., Scott, J. M., and Rabinowitz, J. C.: Folate coenzymes of *Clostridium acidi-urici*. The isolation of (1)-5-methenyltetrahydropteroyltriglutamate, its conversion to (1)-tetrahydropteroyltriglutamate and (1)-10[¹⁴C]formyltetra-hydropteroyltriglutamate, and the synthesis of (1)-10-formyl-[6,7³H₂] tetrahydropteroyltriglutamate and (1)-[6,7-³H₂]tetra-hydropteroyltriglutamate. *J. Biol. Chem.* 247:1959, 1972.

219. Houlihan, D. M., and Scott, J. M.: The identification of pteroylpen-taglutamate as the major folate derivative in rat liver and the dem-onstration of its biosynthesis from exogenous [³H]pteroylglu-tamate. *Biochem. Biophys. Res. Commun.* 48:1675, 1972.

220. Leslie, G. I., and Baugh, C. M.: The uptake of pteroyl-¹⁴C glutamic acid into rat liver and its incorporation into the natural pteroyl poly-γ-glutamates of the organ. *Biochemistry* 13:4957, 1974.

221. Lavoie, A., Tripp, E., Parsa, K., and Hoffbrand, A. V.: Polygluta-mate forms of folate in resting and proliferating mammalian tis-sues. *Clin. Sci. Mol. Med.* 48:67, 1975.

222. Rabinowitz, J. C., and Himes, R. H.: Folic acid coenzymes. *Fed. Proc.* 19:963, 1960.

223. Schlie, I., and Jaenicke, L.: Tetrazolium bioautography of pteroyl-glutamic acid conjugates. *Z. Naturforsch.* 26b:1260, 1971.

224. Baugh, C. M., Braverman, E., and Nair, M. G.: The identification of poly-γ-glutamyl chain lengths in bacterial folates. *Biochemistry* 13:4952, 1974.

225. Noronha, M. M., and Silverman, M.: Distribution of folic acid derivatives in natural materials. I. Chicken liver folates. *J. Biol. Chem.* 237:3299, 1962.

226. Bird, O. D., McGlohom, V. M., and Vaitkus, J. W.: Naturally occur-ring folates in the blood and liver of the rat. *Anal. Biochem.* 12:18, 1965.

227. Swendseid, M. E., Bethell, F. H., and Bird, O. D.: The concentration of folic acid in leukocytes: Observations on normal subjects and persons with leukemia. *Cancer Res.* 11:864, 1951.

228. Hoffbrand, A. V., and Newcombe, B. F. A.: Leukocyte folate in vi-tamin B₁₂ folate deficiency in leukemia. *Br. J. Haematol.* 13:954, 1967.

229. Chanarin, I., Perry, J., and Lumb, M.: The biochemical lesion in vi-tamin B₁₂ deficiency in man. *Lancet* 1:1251, 1974.

230. Cassady, I. A., Budge, M. M., Healy, M. J., and Nixon, P. F.: An in-verse relationship of rat liver folate polyglutamate chain length to nutritional folate sufficiency. *Biochim. Biophys. Acta* 633:258, 1980.

231. Wolff, R., Drouet, P. L., and Karlin, R.: Recherches sur la vitamin-B꜀-conjugase: Action de quelques effecteurs sur l'activité con-jugasique du plasma. *Bull. Soc. Chim. Biol.* 31:1439, 1949.

232. Ritari, S. J., Sakami, W., Black, C. W., and Rzepka, J.: The determi-nation of folylpolyglutamate synthetase. *Anal. Biochem.* 63:118, 1975.

233. McGuire, J. J., Hsieh, P., Coward, J. K., and Bertino, J. R.: Enzyma-tic synthesis of folylpolyglutamates. Characterization of the reac-tion and its products. *J. Biol. Chem.* 255:233, 1970.

234. Siddharth, R., and Beck, W. S.: Evidence that folylpolyglutamate synthetase is under regulatory control. *Clin. Res.* 29:522A, 1981.

235. Kisliuk, R. L., Gaumont, Y., and Baugh, C. M.: Polyglutamyl derivatives of folate as substrates and inhibitors of thymidylate synthetase. *J. Biol. Chem.* 249:4100, 1974.

236. Kisliuk, R. L., Gaumont, Y., Lafer, E., Baugh, C. M., and Mont-gomery, J. A.: Polyglutamyl derivatives of tetrahydrofolate as sub-strates of *Lactobacillus casei* thymidylate synthetase. *Biochemistry* 20:929, 1981.

237. Coward, J. K., Chello, P. L., Cashmore, A. R., Parameswaran, K. N., DeAngelis, L. M., and Bertino, J. R.: 5-Methyl-5,6,7,8-tetrahydro-pteroyloligo-γ-L-glutamates: Synthesis and kinetic studies with methionine synthetase from bovine brain. *Biochem.* 14:1548, 1975.

238. Baggot, J. E., and Krumdiek, C. L.: Folate poly-γ-glutamyl deriva-tives as cosubstrates for chicken liver AICAR transformylase, in *Chemistry and Biology of Pteridines*, edited by R. L. Kisliuk and G. M. Brown. Elsevier/North Holland, New York, 1979, p. 347.

239. Waxman, S., and Schrieber, C.: Folic acid binding protein (FABP) membrane function and role in intracellular folylpolyglutamate distribution. *Clin. Res.* 33:284A, 1975.

240. Cooper, B. A., and Lowenstein, L.: Relative folate deficiency of erythrocytes in pernicious anemia and its correction with cyano-cobalamin. *Blood* 24:502, 1964.

241. Waters, A. H., and Mollin, D. L.: Studies on the folic acid activity of human serum. *J. Clin. Pathol.* 14:335, 1961.

242. Waters, A. H., and Mollin, D. L.: Observations on the metabolism of folic acid in pernicious anaemia. *Br. J. Haematol.* 9:319, 1963.

243. Jeejeebhoy, K. N., Pathare, S. M., and Noronha, J. M.: Observations on conjugated and unconjugated blood folate levels in megalobla-stic anemia and the effects of vitamin B₁₂. *Blood* 26:354, 1965.

244. Smith, R. M., and Osborne-White, W. S.: Folic acid metabolism in vitamin B₁₂-deficient sheep: Depletion of liver folates. *Biochem. J.* 136:279, 1973.

245. Lavoie, A., Trippe, E., and Hoffbrand, A. V.: The effect of vitamin B₁₂ deficiency on methylfolate metabolism and pteroylpolyglu-tamate synthesis in human cells. *Clin. Sci. Mol. Med.* 47:617, 1974.

246. Rosenberg, I. H.: Folate absorption and malabsorption. *N. Engl. J. Med.* 293:1303, 1975.

247. Elsborg, L.: Folic acid: A new approach to the mechanism of its in-testinal absorption. *Dan. Med. Bull.* 21:1, 1974.

248. Rosenberg, I. H., and Godwin, H. A.: The digestion and absorption of dietary folate. *Gastroenterology* 60:445, 1971.

249. Godwin, H. A., and Rosenberg, I. H.: Comparative studies of the intestinal absorption of [³H]pteroylmonoglutamate and [³H]pteroylheptaglutamate in man. *Gastroenterology* 69:364, 1975.

250. Butterworth, C. E., Jr., Baugh, C. M., and Krumdieck, C.: A study of folate absorption and metabolism in man utilizing carbon-14-labeled polyglutamates synthesized by the solid phase method. *J. Clin. Invest.* 48:1131, 1969.

251. Hepner, G. W., Booth, C. C., Cowan, J., Hoffbrand, A. V., and Mollin, D. L.: Absorption of crystalline folic acid in man. *Lancet* 2:302, 1968.

252. Cohen, N.: Differential microbiological assay in study of folic acid absorption in vitro by everted intestinal sacs. *Clin. Res.* 13:252, 1965.

253. Yoshino, T.: The clinical and experimental studies on the metabolism of folic acid using tritiated folic acid. II. The experimental studies on the absorption site and mechanism of tritiated folic acid in rats. *J. Vitaminol. (Osaka)* 14:35, 1968.

254. Laskowski, M., Mims, V., and Day, P. L.: Studies on the enzyme which produces the *Streptococcus lactis* R-stimulating factor from inactive precursor substance in yeast. *J. Biol. Chem.* 157:731, 1945.

255. Bird, O. D., Bressler, B., Brown, R. A., Campbell, C. J., and Emmett, A. D.: The microbiological assay of vitamin B_c conjugate. *J. Biol. Chem.* 159:631, 1945.

256. Wittenberg, J. B., Noronha, J. M., and Silverman, M.: Folic acid derivatives in the gas gland of *Physalia physalis* L. *Biochem. J.* 85:9, 1962.

257. Kisheik, R. L.: Pteroylpolyglutamates. *Mol. Cell. Biochem.* 39:331, 1982.

258. Johns, D. G., Sperti, S., and Burgen, A. S. V.: The metabolism of tritiated folic acid in man. *J. Clin. Invest.* 40:1684, 1961.

259. Johns, D. G., and Bertino, J. R.: Folates and megaloblastic anemia: A review. *Clin. Pharmacol. Ther.* 6:372, 1965.

260. Donaldson, K. O., and Keresztesy, J. C.: Naturally occurring forms of folic acid. I. "Prefolic A": Preparation of concentrate and enzymatic conversion to citrovorum factor. *J. Biol. Chem.* 234:3235, 1959.

261. Donaldson, K. O., and Keresztesy, J. C.: Naturally occurring forms of folic acid. II. Enzymatic conversion of methylenetetrahydrofolic acid to prefolic A-methyltetrahydrofolate. *J. Biol. Chem.* 237:1298, 1962.

262. Larrabee, A. R., Rosenthal, S., Cathou, R. E., and Buchanan, J. M.: A methylated derivative of tetrahydrofolate as an intermediate of methionine biosynthesis. *J. Am. Chem. Soc.* 83:4094, 1961.

263. Herbert, V., Larrabee, A. R., and Buchanan, J. M.: Studies on the identification of a folate compound of human serum. *J. Clin. Invest.* 41:1134, 1962.

264. Whitehead, V. M., and Cooper, B. A.: Apparent identification of 5-methyldihydrofolate as a significant component of serum folate in man. *Clin. Res.* 16:544, 1968.

265. Whitehead, V. M., and Cooper, B. A.: Absorption of unaltered folic acid from the gastrointestinal tract in man. *Br. J. Haematol.* 13:679, 1967.

266. Chanarin, I., and McLean, A.: Origin of serum and urinary methyltetrahydrofolate in man. *Clin. Sci.* 32:57, 1967.

267. Chanarin, I., Hutchinson, M., McLean, A., and Moule, M.: Hepatic folate in man. *Br. Med. J.* 1:396, 1966.

268. Hampers, C. L., Streiff, R., Nathan, D. G., Snyder, D., and Merrill, J. P.: Megaloblastic hematopoiesis in uremia and in patients on long-term hemodialysis. *N. Engl. J. Med.* 276:551, 1967.

269. Markkanen, T., and Peltola, O.: Carriers of folic acid activity in human serum. *Acta Haematol.* 45:106, 1971.

270. Waxman, S., and Schrieber, C.: Measurement of serum folate levels and serum folic acid-binding protein by ^{3}HPGA radioassay. *Blood* 42:281, 1973.

271. Waxman, S.: Folate binding proteins. *Br. J. Haematol.* 29:23, 1975.

272. Hines, J. D., Kamen, B., and Caston, D.: Abnormal folate binding proteins in azotemic patients. *Blood* 42:997, 1973.

273. Eichner, E. R., Paine, C. J., Dickson, V. L., and Hargrove, M. D., Jr.: Clinical and laboratory observations on serum folate-binding protein. *Blood* 46:599, 1975.

274. Waxman, S., and Schrieber, C.: Characteristics of folic acid-binding protein in folate-deficient serum. *Blood* 42:291, 1973.

275. McLean, A., and Chanarin, I.: Urinary excretion of 5-methyltetrahydrofolate in man. *Blood* 27:386, 1966.

276. O'Brien, J. S.: Urinary excretion of folic and folinic acids in normal adults. *Proc. Soc. Exp. Biol. Med.* 104:354, 1960.

277. Basker, S. J., Kumar, S., and Swaminathan, S. P.: Excretion of folic acid in bile. *Lancet* 1:685, 1965.

278. Herbert, V.: Excretion of folic acid in bile. *Lancet* 1:913, 1965.

279. Pratt, R. F., and Cooper, B. A.: Folates in plasma and bile of man after feeding folic acid-^{3}H and 5-formyltetrahydrofolate (folinic acid). *J. Clin. Invest.* 50:455, 1971.

280. Goulian, M., and Beck, W. S.: Modifications in the *Lactobacillus casei* assay of serum folate activity. *Am. J. Clin. Pathol.* 46:390, 1966.

281. Baker, H., et al.: A microbiological method for detecting folic acid deficiency in man. *Clin. Chem.* 5:275, 1959.

282. Harper, T. A.: A modified "aseptic addition" assay procedure for the measurement of serum "folic-acid" activity. *Nature* 207:947, 1965.

283. Herbert, V.: Aseptic addition method for *Lactobacillus casei* assay of folate activity in human serum. *J. Clin. Pathol.* 19:12, 1966.

284. Cooperman, J. M.: Microbiological assay of serum and whole-blood folic acid activity. *Am. J. Clin. Nutr.* 20:1015, 1967.

285. Beard, M. E., and Allen, D. M.: Effect of antimicrobial agents on the *Lactobacillus casei* folate assay. *Am. J. Clin. Pathol.* 48:401, 1967.

286. Beck, W. S.: Unpublished results.

CHAPTER 35

Energy metabolism and maintenance of erythrocytes

ERNEST BEUTLER

The binding, transport, and delivery of oxygen do not require the expenditure of an appreciable amount of metabolic energy by the red blood cell. If the red cell is to perform its function efficiently, however, and to survive in the circulation for its full life-span of approximately 120 days, it must have a source of energy. This energy is needed to maintain (1) the iron of hemoglobin in the divalent form, (2) the high potassium and low calcium and sodium levels within the cell against a gradient imposed by the high plasma calcium and sodium and low plasma potassium levels, (3) the sulfhydryl groups of red cell enzymes and of hemoglobin in the active, reduced form, and (4) the biconcave shape of the cell. If it is deprived of a source of energy, the red cell shape changes from a biconcave disc to a sphere. It becomes sodium-logged and potassium-depleted. Such a cell is quickly removed from the circulation by the filtering action of the spleen and by a perceptive monocyte-macrophage system. Even if it survived, such an energy-deprived cell would gradually turn brown as hemoglobin is oxidized to methemoglobin by the very high concentrations of oxygen within the erythrocyte. The cell would then be unable to perform its function of oxygen and carbon dioxide transport.

The process of extracting energy from a substrate, such as glucose, and of utilizing this energy is carried out by a large number of enzymes. Since the red cell loses its nucleus before it enters the circulation and most of its ribonucleic acid (RNA) within 1 or 2 days of its release into the circulation (see page 265), it does not have the capacity to synthesize new enzyme molecules to replace those which may become worn out during its

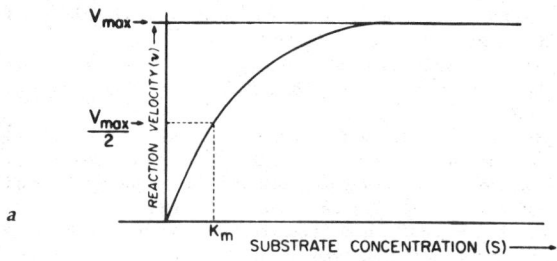

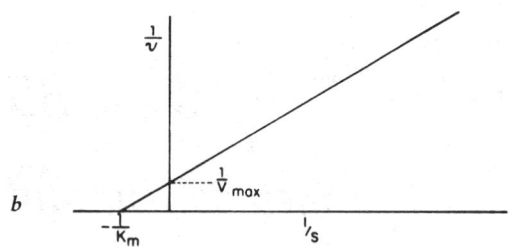

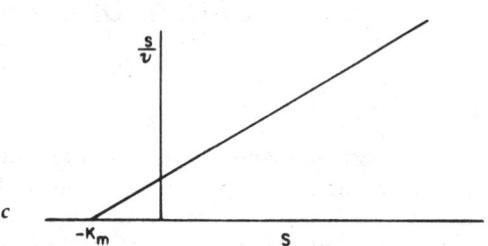

FIGURE 35-1 The relationship between enzyme velocity and substrate concentration: In (*a*) the substrate concentration (*S*) is plotted against the enzyme activity, or reaction velocity (*v*). The maximum velocity is designated as V_{max}. The Michaelis constant (K_m) is that substrate concentration at which the velocity is one-half the V_{max}. These parameters can be computed more readily by plotting the data in reciprocal form so that a straight line is obtained rather than the curve shown in (*a*). Two examples of this approach are given in (*b*) and (*c*). In (*b*) the reciprocal of the reaction rate, $1/v$, is plotted against the reciprocal of the substrate concentration, $1/s$. V_{max} and the K_m are obtained as reciprocals from the intercepts, as noted on the figure. In (*c*) the quotient of the substrate divided by the reaction velocity, s/v, is plotted against the substrate concentration. The K_m is obtained from the intercept with the abscissa, as noted on the figure.

life-span. The enzymes present in the red cells were formed by the nucleated marrow cell.

The rates at which glucose is catabolized to pyruvate or lactic acid, at which potassium is pumped into the cell, and at which methemoglobin or oxidized glutathione is reduced—indeed, the rates of all the metabolic processes of the cell—depend on the properties of the enzymes, the number of enzyme molecules present, the temperature, and the concentration of substrates, cofactors, activators, inhibitors, and hydrogen ions within the cell.

The activity of red cell enzymes is usually estimated

in the laboratory under conditions which permit maximal enzyme activity. In nature, most red cell enzymes do not operate under optimal conditions. They are rarely saturated with substrate, and various levels of inhibitors and activators may be present. The response of red cell enzymes to such inhibitors and activators plays an important role in the regulation of red cell metabolism, a role which is not understood in every instance.

It is customary to report enzyme activity under conditions of saturation with the substrate. Measurement of activity at lower substrate concentrations, however, provides information regarding the affinity of the enzyme for its substrate, expressed as its Michaelis constant (K_m) [1]. This constant represents the concentration of substrate which will permit the enzyme to function at one-half its maximal velocity (V_{max}), as illustrated in Fig. 35-1. The K_m of an enzyme depends on the conditions of assay, including concentration of other substrates, inhibitors, and activators.

Glucose metabolism

Glucose is the normal energy source of the red cell [2–4]. It is metabolized by the erythrocyte along two major pathways. The steps in these pathways are essentially the same as those found in other tissues and in other organisms, including even relatively simple ones such as *Escherichia coli* and yeast. Unlike most other cells, the red cell lacks a citric acid cycle. Only the reticulocytes maintain some capacity for the breakdown of pyruvate to CO_2 with the attendant highly efficient production of ATP. The mature red cell must content itself with extracting energy from glucose almost solely by anaerobic glycolysis. Before glucose can be metabolized by the red cell, it must pass through the membrane. The kinetics of glucose transfer are such as to preclude simple diffusion as the means by which the sugar gains entry into the cell. Rather, the membrane contains a carrier which can combine reversibly with glucose and other sugars at the cell surface and at the interior surface of the membrane. The protein component of this carrier migrates in the region designated as 4.5 when red cell membrane electrophoresis is performed by standard techniques (see Chap. 36) [5,6]. The red cell membrane contains insulin receptors [7,8], but the transport of glucose into red cells is independent of insulin [9].

THE DIRECT GLYCOLYTIC PATHWAY

In the Embden-Meyerhof direct glycolytic pathway (Fig. 35-2), glucose is catabolized anaerobically to pyruvate or lactate. Although 2 mol of high-energy phosphate in the form of adenosine triphosphate (ATP) is utilized in preparing glucose for its further metabolism, up to 4 mol of adenosine diphosphate (ADP) may be phosphorylated to ATP during the metabolism of each mole of glucose, giving a net yield of 2 mol of ATP per mole of glucose metabolized. The rate of glucose utilization is limited largely by the hexokinase and phosphofructo-kinase reactions. Both the enzymes catalyzing these reactions have a relatively high pH optimum; they have very little activity at pH levels lower than 7. For this reason, red cell glycolysis is very pH-sensitive, being stimulated by a rise in the pH. However, at higher-than-physiologic pH levels, the stimulation of hexokinase and phosphofructokinase activity merely results in the accumulation of fructose diphosphate and triose phosphates, because the glyceraldehyde phosphate dehydrogenase reaction becomes a limiting factor.

Branching of the metabolic stream after the formation of 1,3-diphosphoglycerate provides the red cell with flexibility in regard to the amount of ATP formed in the metabolism of each mole of glucose. 1,3-Diphosphoglycerate may be metabolized to 2,3-diphosphoglycerate (2,3-DPG), "wasting" the high-energy phosphate bond in position 1 of the glycerate. Removing the phosphate group at position 2 by diphosphoglycerate phosphatase results in the formation of 3-phosphoglycerate. Alternatively, 3-phosphoglycerate may be formed directly from 1,3-diphosphoglycerate through the phosphoglycerate kinase step, resulting in phosphorylation of a mole of ADP to ATP. While metabolism of glucose through the 2,3-DPG step occurs without any net gain of high-energy phosphate bonds in the form of ATP, metabolism of glucose through the phosphoglycerate kinase step results in the formation of two such bonds per mole of glucose metabolized. This portion of the direct glycolytic pathway has been called the "energy clutch" [10]. Regulation of metabolism at this branch point determines not only the rate of ADP phosphorylation to ATP, but also the concentration of 2,3-diphosphoglycerate, an important regulator of the oxygen affinity of hemoglobin (see Chap. 37). The concentration of 2,3-DPG depends on the balance between its rate of formation from 1,3-DPG by diphosphoglycerate mutase and its degradation by diphosphoglycerate phosphatase. Hydrogen ions inhibit the diphosphoglycerate mutase reaction and stimulate the phosphatase reaction. Thus red cell 2,3-DPG levels are exquisitely sensitive to pH: a rise in pH causes a rise in 2,3-DPG levels, while acidosis results in 2,3-DPG depletion.

It has been proposed that only ATP formed in the phosphoglycerate kinase step rather than that synthesized in the pyruvate kinase step is available for ion pumping [11,12]. This concept is based on indirect data which are subject to alternate interpretation, viz., that substrate entering below the phosphoglycerate kinase step wastes ATP in the reverse phosphoglycerate kinase reaction [13]. However, ATP labeled in the phosphoglycerate kinase step is equally as available for glucose phosphorylation as is ATP formed in the pyruvate kinase step [14]. This finding casts doubt on the concept that red cell ATP is compartmentalized. Metabolism of glucose by way of the Embden-Meyerhof pathway may also yield reducing energy in the form of NADH. The reduction of NAD^+ to NADH occurs in the glyceralde-

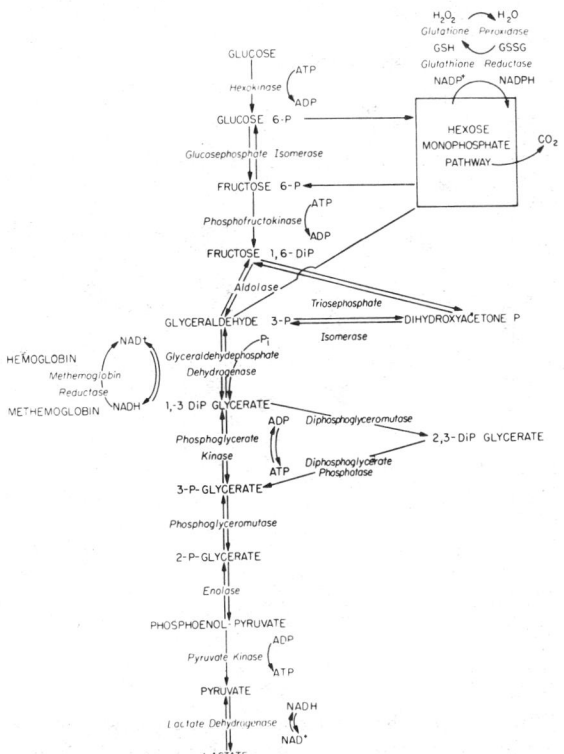

FIGURE 35-2 Glucose metabolism of the erythrocyte. The details of the hexose monophosphate pathway are shown in Fig. 35-3.

hyde phosphate dehydrogenase step. If NADH is reoxidized in reducing methemoglobin to hemoglobin, the end product of glucose metabolism is pyruvate. If NADH is not reoxidized by methemoglobin, however, pyruvate is reduced in the lactate dehydrogenase step, forming lactate as the final end product of glucose metabolism [15]. The lactate or pyruvate formed diffuses out of the red cell and is metabolized elsewhere in the body. Thus the erythrocyte has a flexible Embden-Meyerhof pathway which can adjust the amount of ADP phosphorylated per mole of glucose according to the requirement of the cell.

THE HEXOSE MONOPHOSPHATE SHUNT

Not all the glucose metabolized by the red cell passes through the direct glycolytic pathway. A direct oxidative pathway of metabolism, the hexose monophosphate shunt, is also available. In this pathway, glucose 6-phosphate is oxidized at position 1, yielding carbon dioxide. In the process of glucose oxidation, $NADP^+$ is reduced to NADPH. The pentose phosphate formed when glucose is decarboxylated undergoes a series of molecular rearrangements, eventuating in the formation of a triose, glyceraldehyde 3-phosphate, and a hexose, fructose 6-phosphate (Fig. 35-3). These are normal intermediates in anaerobic glycolysis and thus can rejoin that metabolic stream. Because the glucose phosphate isomerase reaction is freely reversible, so that fructose

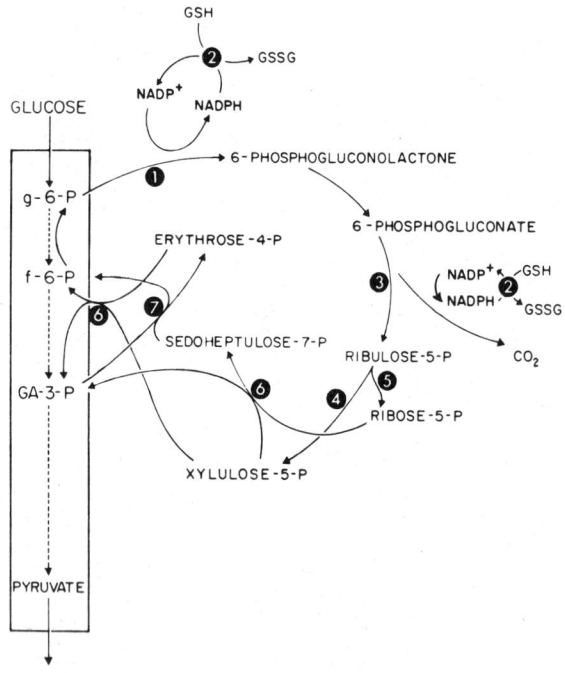

FIGURE 35-3   The hexose monophosphate pathway of the erythrocyte: (1) glucose-6-phosphate dehydrogenase, (2) glutathione reductase, (3) phosphogluconate dehydrogenase, (4) ribulosephosphate epimerase, (5) ribosephosphate isomerase, (6) transketolase, and (7) transaldolase.

6-phosphate can be converted to glucose 6-phosphate, recycling through the hexose monophosphate pathway is also possible. Unlike the anaerobic glycolytic pathway, the hexose monophosphate pathway does not generate any high-energy phosphate bonds. Its primary function appears to be the reduction of NADP+, and indeed, the amount of glucose passing through this pathway appears to be regulated by the amount of NADP+ that has been made available by the oxidation of NADPH. NADPH appears to function primarily as a substrate for the reduction of glutathione-containing disulfides in the erythrocyte (see page 338) through the mediation of the enzyme glutathione reductase, which catalyzes the conversion of glutathione (GSSG) to reduced glutathione (GSH) and the reduction of mixed disulfides of hemoglobin and GSH.

Enzymes of glucose metabolism

HEXOKINASE
Hexokinase catalyzes the phosphorylation of glucose in position 6 by ATP [16] (Fig. 35-2). It thus serves as the first step in the utilization of glucose, whether by the anaerobic or the hexose monophosphate pathway. Mannose or fructose may also serve as a substrate for this enzyme [17]. Red cell hexokinase appears to be devoid of

the capacity to phosphorylate galactose [18]. The average normal activity of this enzyme is about 1.3 IU per gram of hemoglobin (V_{max} at 37°C, pH 7.8) [19]. It is of interest that this is approximately 5 times the rate of glucose utilization by intact cells. Since young red cells contain much higher levels of hexokinase than do old cells [20–23], the level of activity of this enzyme has been used as an index of the average age of the red cell population.

Hexokinase has an absolute requirement for magnesium. It is strongly inhibited by its product, glucose 6-phosphate, and it has been reported that it is released from this inhibition by the inorganic phosphate ion [24]. Indeed, inorganic phosphate has a considerable stimulatory effect on the rate of glucose utilization by red cells. It has been suggested that this effect is not exerted through hexokinase, but rather through stimulation of the phosphofructose kinase reaction, resulting in a lowered glucose 6-phosphate concentration within the cell and thus releasing hexokinase from inhibition [25]. GSSG [26] and other disulfides [27] and 2,3-DPG [28,29] inhibit hexokinase.

Electrophoretically, the enzyme resolves into two major bands. These were originally thought to correspond to types I and II of liver hexokinase [30,31], but it has been found that both bands actually correspond to type I liver enzyme split into two fractions, types I_A and I_F [32,33]. The faster band, type I_F, is more prominent in cord blood, while the more slowly moving I_A band is more active in the red blood cells of adults. A small amount of type III hexokinase is also present in erythrocytes. Hexokinase deficiency is a rare cause of hereditary nonspherocytic hemolytic anemia [23] (see Chap. 59).

GLUCOSE PHOSPHATE ISOMERASE
Glucose-6-phosphate isomerase (GPI) catalyzes the interconversion of glucose 6-phosphate and fructose 6-phosphate [34]. The enzyme is highly active; normal hemolysates contain an average of about 61 IU per gram of hemoglobin (V_{max} at 37°C, pH 7.8) [19]. It is more active in young than in old erythrocytes [35]. Electrophoresis resolves the normal enzyme into three bands, all of which are products of the same gene [36]. There are reports of mutations of this enzyme that affect activity [34] and electrophoretic mobility [36]. Mutations producing GPI deficiency are one of the causes of hereditary nonspherocytic hemolytic anemia (see Chap. 59).

PHOSPHOFRUCTOKINASE
Phosphofructokinase is another enzyme which may be extremely important in regulating the rate of glucose consumption by intact erythrocytes [37]. This enzyme catalyzes the phosphorylation of the carbon 1 of fructose 6-phosphate by ATP. Its average normal activity is approximately 9 IU per gram of hemoglobin (V_{max} at 37°C, pH 7.8) [19]. It requires magnesium for activity and is

stimulated by both ADP and inorganic phosphate. Red cell phosphofructokinase exists as a series of tetramers comprised of muscle (M) and liver (L) subunits [38]. A platelet (P) subunit has also been identified. Deficiency of phosphofructokinase, which may be associated with mild hemolytic anemia and with type VII glycogen storage disease [39,40], is discussed in Chap. 59.

ALDOLASE

Aldolase reversibly cleaves fructose 1,6-diphosphate into two trioses. The "upper" half of the fructose 1,6-diphosphate molecule becomes dihydroxyacetone phosphate (DHAP) and the "lower" half becomes glyceraldehyde 3-phosphate (GAP). The average activity of aldolase is approximately 3 IU per gram of hemoglobin (V_{max} at 37°C, pH 7.8) [19]. Young red cells show a considerably higher level of activity than do old red cells [21,41]. Red cells contain aldolase A, as is found in muscle, and no aldolase B (liver aldolase). On isoelectric focusing of hemolysates, however, five isoenzymes can be resolved, as is the case with other tissues [42]. The isoenzymes presumably represent mixed tetramers of native α polypeptide chains and chains which have undergone posttranscriptional deamidation, α' chains. Young red cells contain more of the nondeamidated isoenzymes. Aldolase deficiency is a rare cause of hereditary nonspherocytic hemolytic anemia (see Chap. 59).

TRIOSEPHOSPHATE ISOMERASE

Triosephosphate isomerase (TPI) is the most active enzyme in the anaerobic glycolytic pathway. Its role is to catalyze interconversion of the two trioses formed by the action of aldolase—dihydroxyacetone phosphate (DHAP) and glyceraldehyde 3-phosphate (GAP) [43]. Although equilibrium is in favor of DHAP, GAP undergoes continued oxidation through the action of glyceraldehyde phosphate dehydrogenase and is thus removed from the equilibrium. The presence of TPI in red cells ensures the conversion of DHAP into GAP. The activity of TPI is approximately 2000 IU per gram of hemoglobin (v at 37°C, pH 7.8, with a DL-GAP concentration of 5.9 mM) [19], and it may be somewhat higher in young cells than in old cells [41]. A deficiency of this enzyme has been found in patients with hereditary nonspherocytic hemolytic anemia associated with a severe neuromuscular disorder [43] (see Chap. 59).

GLYCERALDEHYDE PHOSPHATE DEHYDROGENASE

Glyceraldehyde phosphate dehydrogenase (GAPD) performs the dual function of oxidizing and phosphorylating GAP, producing 1,3-diphosphoglycerate (1,3-DPG). In the process, NAD⁺ is reduced to NADH. This enzyme appears to be closely associated with the red cell stroma [44]. GAPD has an activity of approximately 225 IU per gram of hemoglobin (V_{max} at 37°C, pH 7.8, measured in the backward direction) [19]. It appears to be considerably more active in young than in old red cells [41,45], although conflicting evidence has been presented [21].

PHOSPHOGLYCERATE KINASE

Phosphoglycerate kinase (PGK) effects the transfer to ADP of the high-energy phosphate from the carbon 1 of 1,3-DPG to form ATP. The reaction is readily reversible. This enzyme is very active; hemolysates contain approximately 320 IU per gram of hemoglobin (V_{max} at 37°C, pH 7.8) [19]. PGK requires magnesium and is stimulated slightly by EDTA. Under appropriate conditions, electrophoresis of the enzyme discloses three bands of activity: one major band and two minor bands. These are resolved into a single band in the presence of ATP [46]. Electrophoretically detectable mutations of the enzyme have been described [47,48], and they confirm that the structural gene for PGK is sex-linked. The amino acid sequence of PGK has been determined in its entirety [49].

DIPHOSPHOGLYCEROMUTASE-
DIPHOSPHOGLYCERATE PHOSPHATASE

The same protein molecule is responsible for both diphosphoglycerate mutase and diphosphoglycerate phosphatase activities in the erythrocyte [50,51]. In its role as a diphosphoglyceromutase (DPGM) the enzyme competes with phosphoglycerate kinase for 1,3-diphosphoglycerate as a substrate. It changes 1,3-diphosphoglycerate to 2,3-diphosphoglycerate, thereby dissipating the energy of the high-energy acylphosphate bond [52]. It is inhibited by its product, 2,3-diphosphoglycerate, and by inorganic phosphate, and it is activated by 2-phosphoglycerate and by increased pH levels. It requires 3-phosphoglycerate for activity. Its average activity is 4.8 IU per gram of hemoglobin (v at 37°C, pH 7.8) [19].

Diphosphoglycerate phosphatase (DPGP) catalyzes the removal of the phosphate group from carbon 2 of 2,3-diphosphoglycerate [53,54]. It is inhibited by its product, 3-phosphoglycerate, and by sulfhydryl reagents. The unstimulated activity of the bifunctional enzyme is extremely low, approximately 0.02 IU per gram of hemoglobin (V_{max} at 37°C, pH 7) [53]. It is most active at a slightly acid pH and is strongly stimulated by bisulfite and phosphoglycolate. The latter substance is present in erythrocytes at very low concentrations [55], and an enzyme which hydrolyzes phosphoglycolate has also been documented in erythrocytes [56,57].

PHOSPHOGLYCEROMUTASE

An equilibrium is established between 3-phosphoglycerate and 2-phosphoglycerate by phosphoglyceromutase. 2,3-Diphosphoglycerate acts as an essential cofactor for the transformation. Activity of the enzyme is approximately 19 IU per gram of hemoglobin (V_{max} at 37°C, pH 7.8) [19].

ENOLASE

Enolase establishes an equilibrium between 2-phosphoglycerate and phosphoenolpyruvate (PEP). It has a requirement for and is stabilized by Mg²⁺ [58]. The activity of the enzyme is approximately 5.4 IU per gram of hemoglobin (V_{max} at 37°C, pH 7.8) and is similar in young and old cells [41]. Electrophoresis of red cell enolase gives three bands, supporting the suggestion that it is composed of two different subunits which associate randomly into dimers [59].

PYRUVATE KINASE

The transfer of phosphate from PEP to ADP, forming ATP and pyruvate, is catalyzed by pyruvate kinase [60]. This is one of the energy-yielding steps of glycolysis. The reaction is essentially irreversible. Pyruvate kinase is an allosteric enzyme, manifesting sigmoid kinetics with respect to PEP in the absence of fructose diphosphate. Hyperbolic kinetics are observed in the presence of even minute amounts of fructose diphosphate [61,62], so that at low concentrations of PEP the enzyme activity is greatly increased by fructose diphosphate. The average normal activity of pyruvate kinase is approximately 15 IU per gram of hemoglobin (V_{max} at 37°C, pH 7.8) [19]. The enzyme requires magnesium for activity. In addition, potassium markedly increases its affinity for ADP [63]. Electrophoresis of the enzyme reveals it to be similar to the main liver enzyme. While the liver and red cell enzyme are under common genetic control, they migrate differently on electrophoresis, probably because of posttranscriptional modification [62]. The red cell enzyme differs kinetically and electrophoretically from the white cell enzyme and is inherited through a different gene. A deficiency of red cell pyruvate kinase is an important cause of nonspherocytic congenital hemolytic disease (see Chap. 59) [64].

LACTATE DEHYDROGENASE

Lactate dehydrogenase (LDH) catalyzes the reversible reduction of pyruvate to lactate by NADH. The activity of the enzyme is approximately 200 IU per gram of hemoglobin (V_{max} at 37°C, pH 7.8) [19]. Little loss of activity is noted on aging of erythrocytes. On electrophoresis, all five LDH isoenzymes are found, but isoenzymes 1, 2, and 3 are the predominant forms [65], particularly in older red cells. Hereditary absence of red cell lactate dehydrogenase has been reported [66], but it seems to be a benign condition without clinical manifestations.

GLUCOSE-6-PHOSPHATE DEHYDROGENASE

Glucose-6-phosphate dehydrogenase (G-6-PD) is the most extensively studied erythrocyte enzyme [67]. It catalyzes the oxidation of glucose 6-phosphate to 6-phosphogluconolactone, which rapidly breaks down to 6-phosphogluconic acid. NADP+ is reduced to NADPH in the reaction. The enzyme has been purified to the crystalline state [68], and a large amount of information is available regarding substrate specificity, Michaelis constants, and pH optimum curves. The M_r of the highly purified enzyme has been reported to be 240,000 daltons [68], but in its natural state the M_r is probably approximately 105,000 daltons [69,70]. In the absence of NADP+, G-6-PD dissociates into subactive subunits of smaller size (40,000 or 50,000). The enzyme is strongly inhibited by physiologic amounts of NADPH [71–73] and, to a lesser extent, of ATP [74,75]. Its average normal activity is approximately 8.3 IU per gram of hemoglobin (V_{max} at 37°C, pH 7.8) [19]. Using the standard WHO assay [76], in which the activities of G-6-PD and 6-phosphogluconic dehydrogenase are measured together at 25°C, the average normal activity is 6.6 IU per gram of hemoglobin. The enzyme is much more active in young red cells than in older ones. In the presence of its coenzyme, NADP+, the enzyme moves electrophoretically as a single major band. Many electrophoretic mutations are known, as are others involving the activity, stability, and kinetic properties of the enzyme (see Chap. 58).

PHOSPHOGLUCONATE DEHYDROGENASE

Phosphogluconate dehydrogenase catalyzes the oxidation of phosphogluconate to ribulose 5-phosphate and CO_2 and the reduction of NADP+ to NADPH. The average normal activity of this enzyme is approximately 8.8 IU per gram of hemoglobin (V_{max} at 37°C, pH 7.8) [19]. Variability of electrophoretic mobility of the enzyme is common in humans and in various animal species [77]. Deficiency of the enzyme has been observed only rarely and appears to be essentially innocuous [78].

RIBOSEPHOSPHATE ISOMERASE

Ribosephosphate isomerase catalyzes the interconversion of ribulose 5-phosphate and ribose 5-phosphate [28,79]. It is an extremely active enzyme, with approximately 200 IU of activity per gram of hemoglobin (V_{max} at 37°C, pH 7.6) [79].

RIBULOSEPHOSPHATE EPIMERASE

Ribulosephosphate epimerase converts ribulose 5-phosphate to xylulose 5-phosphate [28]. The exact activity of this enzyme in human hemolysates has not been reported, but it seems to be less than that of ribosephosphate isomerase.

TRANSKETOLASE

Transketolase effects the transfer of two carbon atoms from xylulose 5-phosphate to ribose 5-phosphate, resulting in the formation of the 7-carbon sugar sedoheptulose 7-phosphate and the 3-carbon sugar glyceraldehyde 3-phosphate [28,80]. It can also catalyze the reaction between xylulose 5-phosphate and erythrose 4-phosphate, producing fructose 6-phosphate and glyceraldehyde 3-phosphate. Its activity is approximately 0.2 IU per gram of hemoglobin (V_{max} at 37°C, pH 7.6) [81]. Thiamine pyrophosphate is a coenzyme for transketolase, and the activity of this enzyme has been used as an index of the adequacy of thiamine nutrition [82].

TRANSALDOLASE

The conversion of sedoheptulose 7-phosphate and glyceraldehyde 3-phosphate into erythrose 4-phosphate and fructose 6-phosphate is catalyzed by transaldolase [79]. This is another one in the series of molecular rearrangements which eventuate in the conversion of the 5-carbon sugar formed in the phosphogluconate dehydrogenase step to metabolic intermediates of the Embden-Meyerhof pathway.

L-HEXONATE DEHYDROGENASE

Red cells contain an enzyme which has the capacity to reduce aldoses such as glucose, galactose, or glyceraldehyde to their corresponding polyol (i.e., glucose to sorbitol, galactose to dulcitol, and glyceraldehyde to glycerol). NADPH serves as a hydrogen donor for this reaction. Although it has been suggested that the enzyme responsible for this reaction is aldose reductase [83,84], it is probably a similar but distinct enzyme, L-hexonate dehydrogenase [85]. The activity of this enzyme is approximately 0.09 IU per gram of hemoglobin (V_{max} at 37°C, pH 7.4). The electrophoretic characteristics of L-hexonate dehydrogenase have not been studied. Deficiency of this enzyme is not known to occur.

The utilization of substrates other than glucose as energy sources

The red cell has the capacity to utilize several other substrates in addition to glucose as a source of energy. Among these are adenosine, inosine, fructose, mannose, galactose, dihydroxyacetone, and lactate. Although in the circulation red cells normally rely on glucose as their energy source, the utilization of other substrates, particularly during blood storage (see Chap. 164) and in certain experimental situations, is of interest.

ADENOSINE AND INOSINE

Adenosine is deaminated to inosine by the enzyme adenosine deaminase [86]:

$$\text{Adenosine} \xrightarrow{\text{adenosine deaminase}} \text{inosine} + NH_3$$

This enzyme normally has an activity of 1.1 IU per gram of hemoglobin (V_{max} at 37°C, pH 7.8) [19]. It apparently plays a regulatory role in the concentration of purine nucleotides in the red cell. Deficiency of adenosine deaminase is associated with severe combined immunodeficiency [87] (see Chap. 112). In this disorder, large quantities of deoxyadenine nucleotides, not normally present in erythrocytes, accumulate [88]. Increased activity of adenosine deaminase results in the depletion of red cell ATP and nonspherocytic hemolytic anemia [89].

Inosine formed in the adenosine deaminase reaction or added directly to red cells may enter the erythrocyte and undergo phosphorolysis to form hypoxanthine and ribose 1-phosphate (R-1-P) [86,90,91]:

$$\text{Inosine} + P_i \xrightarrow{\text{nucleoside phosphorylase}} \text{R-1-P} + \text{hypoxanthine}$$

Human red cells have approximately 359 IU of purine nucleoside phosphorylase activity per gram of hemoglo-

bin [92]. This reaction is of particular interest because it results in the introduction of a phosphorylated sugar, R-1-P, into the erythrocyte without the utilization of ATP. The R-1-P may then be further metabolized to yield high-energy phosphate. The nucleoside phosphorylase reaction appears to be the only practical means by which ATP may be formed in the cell without first expending ATP to prepare an unphosphorylated substrate for further metabolism. The use of inosine has therefore received much attention in the field of blood banking (see Chap. 164). A deficiency of nucleoside phosphorylase has been associated with immunodeficiency [93].

FRUCTOSE

Fructose is readily utilized by the erythrocyte, although at a rate somewhat slower than that of glucose [94]. Fructose undergoes phosphorylation at position 6 in the hexokinase reaction:

$$\text{Fructose} + ATP \xrightarrow[\text{Mg}^{2+}]{\text{hexokinase}} \text{fructose 6-P} + ADP$$

Since fructose 6-phosphate is a normal metabolic intermediate in the anaerobic glycolytic pathway, the fructose 6-phosphate formed may be presumed to be utilized in a manner entirely analogous to the utilization of glucose.

Fructose may also be metabolized by another red cell enzyme, sorbitol dehydrogenase [95,96]. This enzyme reduces fructose to its corresponding polyol, sorbitol, with NADH serving as a hydrogen donor. The reaction is reversible, and a pathway therefore exists for the formation of fructose from glucose through L-hexonate dehydrogenase and sorbitol dehydrogenase.

MANNOSE

Mannose is also phosphorylated in the hexokinase reaction [17]:

$$\text{Mannose} + ATP \xrightarrow[\text{Mg}^{2+}]{\text{hexokinase}} \text{mannose 6-P} + ADP$$

Mannose 6-phosphate must be isomerized to fructose 6-phosphate before it is further metabolized by erythrocytes. This is accomplished by phosphomannose isomerase (PMI) [97,98]:

$$\text{Mannose 6-P} \xrightleftharpoons{\text{PMI}} \text{fructose 6-P}$$

Phosphomannose isomerase of red cells has very low activity, even at its pH optimum of 5.9 [17]. The rate of mannose utilization is therefore limited by the activity of PMI. Young red cells have enhanced PMI activity and can therefore utilize mannose at a more rapid rate than can mature red cells.

GALACTOSE

The utilization of galactose by erythrocytes is more complex than that of most other substrates. At low concentrations of galactose, metabolism occurs by way of galactokinase, galactose-1-phosphate uridyl transferase, and phosphoglucomutase [18,99]. Unlike fructose, mannose, and glucose, galactose is phosphorylated at position 1:

$$\alpha\text{-Galactose} + ATP \xrightarrow[Mg^{2+}]{galactokinase} \alpha\text{-galactose 1-P} + ADP$$

The galactose 1-phosphate formed in the galactokinase reaction exchanges with the glucose-1-phosphate moiety of uridine diphosphoglucose (UDPG) in the galactose-1-phosphate uridyl transferase reaction:

$$\alpha\text{-Galactose-1-P} + UDPG \xrightleftharpoons{transferase} \alpha\text{-glucose 1-P} + UDP \text{ galactose}$$

The uridine diphosphogalactose (UDPgalactose) formed in this reaction is epimerized to UDPG:

$$UDP \text{ galactose} \xrightleftharpoons[NAD^+]{epimerase} UDPG$$

The α-glucose 1-phosphate in the transferase reaction is transformed to α-glucose 6-phosphate in the phosphoglucomutase (PGM) reaction [100], with glucose 1,6-diphosphate acting as coenzyme:

$$\alpha\text{-Glucose 1-P} \xrightleftharpoons[glucose\ 1,6\text{-diP}]{PGM} \alpha\text{-glucose 6-P}$$

The α-glucose 6-phosphate formed may join the direct metabolic stream after conversion by phosphoglucose isomerase to fructose 6-phosphate. It may also undergo anomerization to β-glucose 6-phosphate and enter the hexose monophosphate pathway if $NADP^+$ is available. Very high concentrations of galactose appear to be metabolized by way of another pathway, as yet poorly delineated. This pathway is known not to involve galactose-1-phosphate uridyl transferase or to have the capacity to reduce NAD^+ [18].

DIHYDROXYACETONE AND GLYCERALDEHYDE

As indicated earlier, glyceraldehyde can be reduced in erythrocytes to glycerol in the L-hexonate dehydrogenase reaction. In addition, glyceraldehyde and dihydroxyacetone can each be phosphorylated by ATP in the presence of the enzyme triokinase [101]. Like other kinases, this enzyme has a requirement for magnesium. With dihydroxyacetone serving as a substrate, the activity of the enzyme is approximately 0.15 IU per gram of hemoglobin [101]. A remarkable feature of this enzyme is its extraordinarily low K_m for dihydroxyacetone. It is one-half saturated with this substrate at a concentration of only 0.5 μM. The products of the triokinase reaction, DHAP or GAP, are normal metabolic intermediates and can be metabolized in the usual fashion. Because of its capacity to act as an alternate substrate for red cell energy metabolism and 2,3-DPG formation,

dihydroxyacetone had been studied as an experimental additive for blood storage [102,103].

Glycogen metabolism

Red cells have the capacity to form and to break down glycogen. They contain the enzymes UDPG-glycogen glucosyltransferase and α-1,4-glucan: α-1,4-glucan-6-glycosyltransferase (the brancher enzyme) for the formation of glycogen from glucose 1-phosphate. They contain the enzymes phosphorylase and amylo 1,6-glucosidase (the debrancher enzyme) for the breakdown of glycogen [104]. Only very little glycogen is present in normal red cells [105], and most of what was thought to be in red cells may actually be platelet and leukocyte glycogen [106]. The function of glycogen in red cell metabolism is not understood.

Glutathione metabolism of the erythrocyte

The red cell contains a high concentration (approximately 2 mM) of the sulfhydryl-containing tripeptide reduced glutathione (GSH) [71]. Red cell GSH appears to undergo a rapid turnover, with a $T_{1/2}$ of approximately 4 days [107]. Synthesis occurs in two steps:

$$\text{Glutamate} + \text{cysteine} + ATP \longrightarrow \gamma\text{-glutamyl cysteine} + ADP + P_i$$

$$\gamma\text{-Glutamyl cysteine} + \text{glycine} + ATP \longrightarrow GSH + ADP + P_i$$

Both steps have been shown to be catalyzed by red cell hemolysates [108–111]. The red cell requires a system for the synthesis of GSH because of the active transport of GSSG from the erythrocyte [112,113]. It has also been suggested that a requirement for GSH synthesis comes from function of the γ-glutamyl cycle [114]. However, this pathway is not present in red cells [115–117].

One important function of GSH in the erythrocyte appears to be the detoxification of low levels of hydrogen peroxide which may form spontaneously or as a result of drug administration. In either event, the superoxide radical may be formed first and then be converted to H_2O_2 by the action of the copper-containing enzyme superoxide dismutase [118]. Hydrogen peroxide is reduced to water through the mediation of the enzyme glutathione peroxidase [119,120]. Glutathione peroxidase is a selenium-containing enzyme [121,122]. In New Zealand, dietary selenium intake is extremely low, and glutathione peroxidase activities are much lower than are observed elsewhere [123]. An activity polymorphism most common in persons of Mediterranean descent [124,125] has also been described. The consequent decreases in enzyme activity are without clinical effect. An electrophoretic polymorphism has also been described [126].

GSH may also function in maintaining integrity of the erythrocyte by reducing sulfhydryl groups of hemoglobin, membrane proteins, and enzymes which may become oxidized [127].

In the process of reducing peroxides or oxidized-protein sulfhydryl groups, GSH is converted to oxidized glutathione (GSSG) or may form mixed disulfides. Glutathione reductase provides an efficient mechanism for the reduction of GSSG to GSH in the red cell. It is a flavin enzyme, and either NADPH or NADH may serve as a hydrogen donor [128–130]. In the intact cell, only the NADPH system appears to function [131–133]. The same enzyme system appears to have the capacity to reduce mixed disulfides of GSH and proteins [134]. Although genetic variation of the activity of this enzyme exists [125] and electrophoretic polymorphisms are known [135,136], the activity of red cell glutathione reductase is strongly influenced by the riboflavin content of the diet [137]. Activity of glutathione *S*-transferase, an enzyme which transfers glutathione to a suitable receptor forming a thioether bond, has been demonstrated in erythrocytes [138].

GSSG, like certain other disulfides, has the capacity to inhibit red cell hexokinase [26,139], although greater than physiologic levels appear to be needed for this effect. It may also complex with hemoglobin A to form hemoglobin A_3 [128]. There is a system which actively extrudes GSSG from the erythrocyte [112,113,140–142].

Methemoglobin reduction

The reduction of methemoglobin in normal red cells is achieved primarily through a NADH-linked system [15,143]. A methemoglobin reductase (known also as NADH diaphorase) utilizes NADH generated in the glyceraldehyde-phosphate dehydrogenase reaction to reduce the iron of methemoglobin from the trivalent to the divalent form. It has been suggested that two such NADH-linked enzymes are present. One, NADH diaphorase I, is a flavin enzyme responsible for approximately 90 percent of the methemoglobin-reducing capacity of the NADH-linked system. The other, NADH diaphorase II, is a nonflavin enzyme which accounts for the remaining 10 percent of the NADH-linked methemoglobin-reducing capacity [144]. Cytochrome b_5 is an intermediate in the enzymatic reduction of methemoglobin [145]. Red cells also contain a NADPH-linked methemoglobin-reducing system [15] which functions only in the presence of an artificial electron carrier, such as methylene blue. Nonenzymatic reduction of methemoglobin by GSH and ascorbic acid accounts for only a small portion of the total methemoglobin-reducing rate of red cells.

Other red cell enzymes

Erythrocytes contain a high concentration of carbonic anhydrase. In catalyzing the equilibrium between carbon dioxide and carbonic acid, this enzyme aids in oxygen and carbon dioxide transport of the erythrocyte.

This enzyme has been obtained from red cells in highly purified state and has been "fingerprinted" [146].

The red blood cell is a rich source of catalase, the enzyme which decomposes hydrogen peroxide to water and oxygen. Hereditary lack of catalase does not seem to cause any hematologic disorder [147,148]. This enzyme functions efficiently only when relatively high concentrations of peroxide are present. Low concentrations of peroxide are detoxified by the enzyme glutathione peroxidase (see page 338) [119,120].

The red cell membrane contains large amounts of acetylcholinesterase. Although the activity of this enzyme is diminished in paroxysmal nocturnal hemoglobinuria, this does not appear to play an etiologic role (see Chap. 21) [149,150]. Indeed, hereditary lack of red cell cholinesterase activity does not appear to be associated with any clinical hematologic effects [151].

Red cell membranes also contain protein kinase activities [152–156]. Several such enzymes catalyze the transfer of the terminal phosphate from ATP to various stromal receptors, primarily band 2 of spectrin and "band 3" (see Chap. 36). One is relatively insensitive to stimulation by cyclic adenosine 3',5'-monophosphate (cAMP) and unaffected by cyclic guanosine 3',5'-monophosphate (cGMP). It has the capacity to phosphorylate exogenous protein receptors, such as casein and histones, as well as endogenous stromal proteins. An abnormality in the phosphorylation of the red cell stromal proteins has been observed in hereditary spherocytosis [157], but this is neither specific for hereditary spherocytosis nor does it seem to represent a true decrease in the activity of protein kinase [158,159]. The role of this enzyme in the structural properties of the red cell membrane is not yet clear.

An aldehyde dehydrogenase of red cells makes it possible for erythrocytes to utilize aldehydes such as formaldehyde as substrates for methemoglobin reduction [160]. The presence of amino acid–activating enzymes [161], dipeptidases [162], formate-activating enzyme [163], glutamic-oxaloacetic transaminase [21], glyoxalase [164], pyridoxine kinase [165,166], uroporphyrinogen 1 synthase [167], pyrroline-5-carboxylate reductase [168], and numerous other enzymes [169] has been reported in erythrocytes.

Nucleotide synthesis

Most cells achieve the *de novo* synthesis of purine nucleotides by constructing the heterocyclic purine ring in a series of enzymatic reactions which begin with the synthesis of phosphoribosyl pyrophosphate (PRPP) from ribose 5-phosphate and ATP. Methyl groups are added through the mediation of folate coenzymes and nitrogens are supplied by glutamine, lysine, and aspartic acid. The initial product of the *de novo* pathway, inosine 5'-monophosphate (IMP) is then converted to AMP and to guanosine 5'-phosphate through further enzymatic transformations. Pyrimidine nucleotides are synthesized *de novo* through pathways beginning with

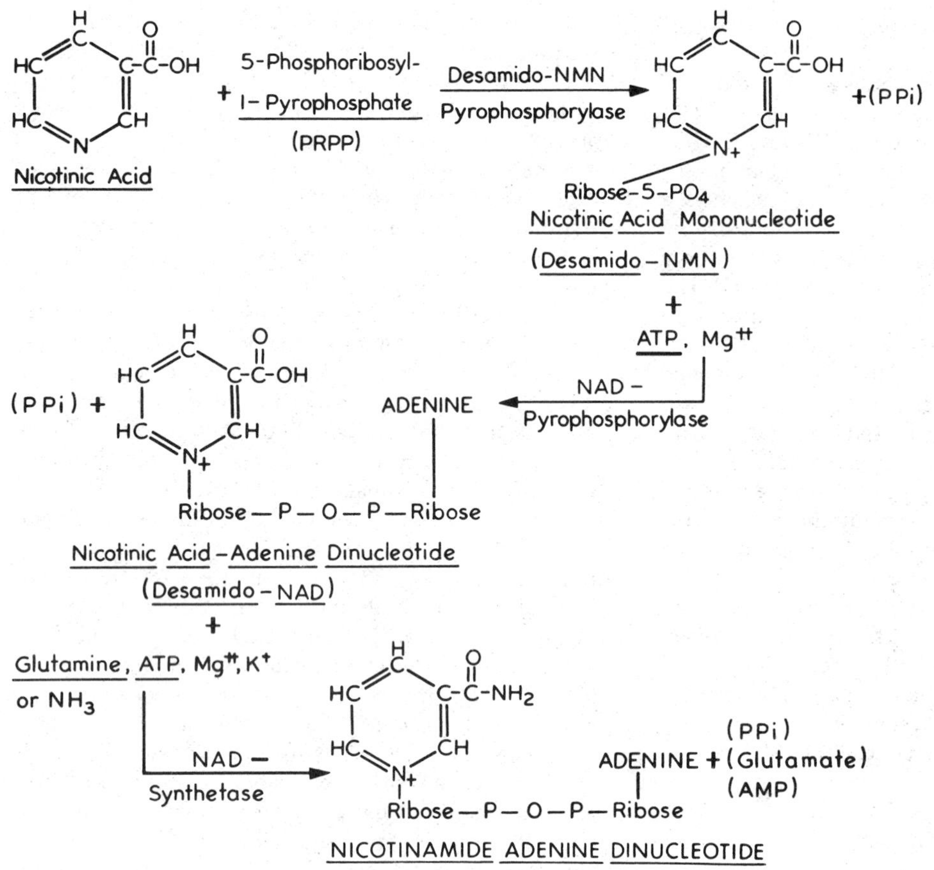

FIGURE 35-4   The nicotinic acid pathway for the biosynthesis of nicotinamide adenine dinucleotide.

the reaction of carbamyl phosphate and aspartic acid to form carbamyl aspartate. Further intermediates include dihydroorotate, orotate, and orotidine 5'-phosphate, which is finally converted to uridine 5'-phosphate.

Although all the reactions for synthesis of purine and pyrimidine nucleotides presumably occur in erythroid precursors, the mature erythrocyte depends on the so-called salvage pathway for its supply of purine nucleotides. The adenine phosphoribosyltransferase (APRT) and hypoxanthine-guanine phosphoribosyltransferase (HGPRT) reactions serve to incorporate adenine (in the case of APRT) or hypoxanthine or guanine (in the case of HGPRT) into nucleotides:

$$\text{Adenine} + \text{PRPP} \xrightarrow{\text{APRT}} \text{AMP}$$

$$\text{Guanine (or hypoxanthine)} + \text{PRPP} \xrightarrow{\text{HGPRT}} \text{GMP (or IMP)}$$

The first of these reactions is the basis for the use of adenine in blood preservatives (Chap. 164). Absence of APRT, inherited as an autosomal-recessive disorder, results in nephrolithiasis, deoxyadenine stones being deposited in the kidneys [170,171]. The function of HGPRT in red cells is unclear, since the role of guanine and inosine nucleotides remains undefined. Absence of this enzyme, inherited as a sex-linked disorder, results in hyperuricemia and a neurologic disorder characterized by self-mutilation, the so-called Lesch-Nyhan syndrome [172]. Red cells are also able to synthesize adenine nucleotides by phosphorylating adenosine. This reaction is catalyzed by adenosine kinase [173].

The bridge between ribonucleotides and deoxyribonucleotides is provided by the enzyme ribonucleotide reductase. All dividing cells require deoxyribonucleotides for DNA synthesis. Ribonucleotides are needed not only for the synthesis of RNA for protein synthesis, but also to perform many other functions. For example, ATP and GTP provide the energy for many biochemical processes and serve as precursors of cyclic nucleotides, the regulators of many enzymatic reactions. Uridine nucleotides are sugar carriers which serve as intermediates in various carbohydrate transformations and in the synthesis of glycoproteins and glycolipids.

The mature erythrocyte contains small quantities of pyrimidine nucleotides. Little is known of their function in this cell. The capacity of erythrocytes to metabolize galactose (see page 338) reflects one function of a pyrimidine nucleotide, UDPGlucose, in the erythrocyte. However, since the red cell is a trivial site of galactose metabolism in the body, this function of the pyrimidine nucleotide can hardly be considered to be of much physiologic importance. The enzyme pyrimidine 5'-nucleotidase specifically dephosphorylates pyrimidine mononucleotides and thus presumably plays a role in the catabolism of ribose polynucleotides in the red cell.

The nicotinic acid nucleotides NAD⁺ and NADP⁺ are also a vital component of the biochemical machinery of the cell, and pathways for their synthesis exist. NAD⁺ is synthesized from nicotinic acid as shown in Fig. 35-4. PRPP is attached to the nicotinic acid ring through the mediation of the enzyme desamido-NMN pyrophosphorylase, forming desamido nicotinic acid mononucleotide. After attachment of AMP through a pyrophosphate bond, glutamine provides an amino group for completion of the synthesis of NAD⁺ [174,175]. The only known pathway for the synthesis of NADP⁺ involves a phosphorylation of NAD⁺ by ATP in the presence of NAD kinase [162]. Large oral doses of nicotinic acid promote an increase in the concentration of red cell NAD⁺, but not of NADP⁺ [176]. NAD⁺ is degraded by the enzyme NADase, which hydrolyzes the pyridine nucleotides at the nicotinamide-ribose linkage. The enzymes can catalyze the exchange of free nicotinamide with pyridine nucleotide–bound nicotinamide [162]. A deficiency of this activity, apparently without significant effect, has been documented [177].

Reticulocyte metabolism

The energy metabolism of young red cells is in general more active than that of older erythrocytes, probably because the activity of enzymes which are important in regulating the rate of glycolysis is increased in young red cells. In addition to their capacity to carry out glycolysis at a relatively rapid rate, reticulocytes have mitochondria with a complete complement of mitochondrial enzymes [178]. This enables them to metabolize glucose not only through the Embden-Meyerhof pathway and hexose monophosphate shunt, but also through the Krebs cycle. The rate of oxygen consumption of reticulocytes is 60 times that of mature red cells; the rate of glucose consumption is 7.5 times as great [179]. This metabolic capacity provides these cells with the potential of phosphorylating ADP to ATP at a greatly accelerated rate and of providing succinate for the synthesis of heme.

References

1. Dixon, M., and Webb, E. C.: *Enzymes,* 2d ed. Academic, New York, 1964.
2. Beutler, E.: *Hemolytic Anemia in Disorders of Red Cell Metabolism.* Plenum, New York, 1978.
3. Beutler, E.: Disorders due to enzyme defects in the red blood cell. *Adv. Metab. Disord. 6:*131, 1972.
4. Jacobasch, G., Minakami, S., and Rapoport, S. M.: Glycolysis of the erythrocyte, in *Cellular and Molecular Biology of Erythrocytes,* edited by H. Yoshikawa and S. M. Rapoport. University Park Press, Baltimore, 1974, pp. 55–92.
5. Kahlenberg, A., and Zala, C. A.: Reconstitution of D-glucose transport in vesicles composed of lipids and intrinsic protein (zone 4.5) of the erythrocyte membrane. *J. Supramol. Struct. 7:*287, 1977.
6. Kondo, T., and Beutler, E.: Developmental changes in glucose transport of guinea pig erythrocytes. *J. Clin. Invest. 65:*1, 1980.
7. Herzberg, V., Boughter, J. M., Carlisle, S., and Hill, D. E.: Evidence for two insulin receptor populations on human erythrocytes. *Nature 286:*279, 1980.
8. Robinson, T. J., Archer, J. A., Gambhir, K. K., Hollis, V. W., Jr., Carter, L., and Bradley, C.: Erythrocytes: A new cell type for the evaluation of insulin receptor defects in diabetic humans. *Science 205:*200, 1979.
9. Eadie, G. S., MacLeod, J. J. R., and Noble, E. C.: Insulin and glycolysis. *Am. J. Physiol. 65:*462, 1923.
10. Keitt, A. S., and Bennett, D.C.: Pyruvate kinase deficiency and related disorders of red cell glycolysis. *Am. J. Med. 41:*762, 1966.
11. Feig, S. A., Segel, G. B., Shohet, S. B., and Nathan, D. G.: Energy metabolism in human erythrocytes. II. Effects of glucose depletion. *J. Clin. Invest. 51:*1547, 1972.
12. Proverbio, F., and Hoffman, J. F.: Membrane compartmentalized ATP and its preferential use by the Na, K-ATPase of human red cell ghosts. *J. Gen. Physiol. 69:*605, 1977.
13. Chillar, R. K., and Beutler, E.: Explanation for the apparent lack of ouabain inhibition of pyruvate production in hemolysates: The "backward" PGK reaction. *Blood 47:*507, 1976.
14. Beutler, E., Guinto, E., Kuhl, W., and Matsumoto, F.: Existence of only a single functional pool of adenosine triphosphate in human erythrocytes. *Proc. Natl. Acad. Sci. U.S.A. 75:*2825, 1978.
15. Gibson, Q. H.: The reduction of methemoglobin in red blood cells and studies on the cause of idiopathic methemoglobinemia. *Biochem. J. 42:*13, 1948.
16. De Verdier, C.-H., and Garby, L.: Glucose metabolism in normal erythrocytes. II. Factors influencing the hexokinase step. *Scand. J. Haematol. 2:*305, 1965.
17. Beutler, E., and Teeple, L.: Mannose metabolism in the human erythrocyte. *J. Clin. Invest. 48:*461, 1969.
18. Beutler, E., and Mathai, C. K.: Genetic variation in red cell galactose-1-phosphate uridyl transferase, in *Hereditary Disorders of Erythrocyte Metabolism,* edited by E. Beutler. Grune & Sratton, New York, 1968, City of Hope Symposium Series, vol. 1, pp. 66–86.
19. Beutler, E.: *Red Cell Metabolism. A Manual of Biochemical Methods,* 2d ed. Grune & Stratton, New York, 1975.
20. Brewer, C. J., and Powell, R. D.: Hexokinase activity as a function of age of the human erythrocyte. *Nature 199:*704, 1963.
21. Chapman, R. G., and Schaumburg, L.: Glycolysis and glycolytic enzyme activity of aging red cells in man. *Br. J. Haematol. 13:*665, 1967.
22. Brok, F., Ramot, B., Zwang, E., and Danon, D.: Enzyme activities in human red blood cells of different age groups. *Isr. J. Med. Sci. 2:*291, 1966.
23. Valentine, W. N., Oski, F. A., Paglia, D. E. Baughan, M. A., Schneider, A. S., and Naiman, J. L.: Hereditary hemolytic anemia with hexokinase deficiency. Role of hexokinase in erythrocyte aging. *N. Engl. J. Med. 276:*1, 1967.
24. Rose, I. A., Warms, J. V. B., and O'Connell, E. L.: Role of inorganic phosphate in stimulating the glucose utilization of human red blood cells. *Biochem. Biophys. Res. Commun. 15:*33, 1964.
25. Gerber, G., Kloppick, E., and Rapoport, S.: Über den Einfluss des Anorganisschen Phosphats auf die Glykolyse: Seine Unwirksamkeit auf die Hexokinase des Menschenerythrozyten. *Acta Biol. Med. Ger. 18:*305, 1967.
26. Beutler, E., and Teeple, L.: The effect of oxidized glutathione (GSSG) on human erythrocyte hexokinase activity. *Acta Biol. Med. Ger. 22:*707, 1969.
27. Eldjarn, L., and Bremer, J.: The inhibitory effect at the hexokinase level of disulphides on glucose metabolism in human erythrocytes. *Biochem. J. 84:*286, 1962.
28. Dische, Z.: The pentose phosphate metabolism in red cells, in *The Red Blood Cell,* edited by C. Bishop and D. M. Surgenor. Academic, New York, 1964, pp. 189–209.

29. Beutler, E.: 2,3-Diphosphoglycerate affects enzymes of glucose metabolism in red blood cells. *Nature* 232:20, 1971.

30. Holmes, E. W., Jr., Malone, J. I., and Oski, F. A.: Hexokinase isoenzymes in human erythrocytes: Association of type II with fetal hemoglobin. *Science* 156:646, 1967.

31. Malone, J. I., Winegrad, A. I., Oski, F. A., and Holmes, E. W., Jr.: Erythrocyte hexokinase isoenzyme patterns in hereditary hemoglobinopathies. *N. Engl. J. Med.* 279:1071, 1968.

32. Kaplan, J. C., and Beutler, E.: Hexokinase isoenzymes in human erythrocytes. *Science* 159:215, 1968.

33. Altay, C., Alper, C. A., and Nathan, D. G.: Normal and variant isoenzymes of human blood cell hexokinase and the isoenzyme patterns in hemolytic anemia. *Blood* 36:219, 1970.

34. Baughan, M. A., Valentine, W. N., Paglia, D. E., Ways, P. O., Simon, E. R., and De Marsh, Q. B.: Hereditary hemolytic anemia associated with glucosephosphate isomerase (GPI) deficiency — A new enzyme defect of human erythrocytes. *Blood* 32:236, 1968.

35. Marks, P. A., Johnson, A. B., and Hirschberg, E.: Effect of age on the enzyme activity in erythrocytes. *Proc. Natl. Acad. Sci. U.S.A.* 44:529, 1958.

36. Detter, J. C., et al.: Inherited variations in human phosphohexose isomerase. *Ann. Hum. Genet.* 31:329, 1968.

37. Minakami, S., Saito, T., Suzuki, C., and Yoshikawa, H.: The hydrogen ion concentrations and erythrocyte glycolysis. *Biochem. Biophys. Res. Commun.* 17:748, 1964.

38. Vora, S., Seaman, C., Durham, S., and Piomelli, S.: Isozymes of human phosphofructokinase: Identification and subunit structural characterization of a new system. *Proc. Natl. Acad. Sci. U.S.A.* 77:62, 1980.

39. Tauri, S., Kono, N., Nasu, T., and Nishikawa, M.: Enzymatic basis for the coexistence of myopathy and hemolytic disease in inherited muscle phosphofructokinase deficiency. *Biochem. Biophys. Res. Commun.* 34:77, 1969.

40. Waterbury, L., and Frenkel, E. P.P Hereditary nonspherocytic hemolysis with erythrocyte phosphofructokinase deficiency. *Blood* 39:415, 1972.

41. Löhr, G. W., Waller, H. D., Karges, O., Schlegel, B., and Müller, A. A.: Zur Biochemie der Alterung Menschlicher Erythrozyten. *Klin. Wochenschr.* 36:1008, 1958.

42. Beutler, E., Scott, S., Bishop, A., Margolis, N., Matsumoto, F., and Kuhl, W.: Red cell aldolase deficiency and hemolytic anemia: A new syndrome. *Trans. Assoc. Am. Physicians* 86:154, 1974.

43. Schneider, A. S., Valentine, W. N., Hattori, M., Heins, H. L., Jr.: Hereditary hemolytic anemia with triosephosphate isomerase deficiency. *N. Engl. J. Med.* 272:229, 1965.

44. Schrier, S. L.: Organization of enzymes in human erythrocyte membranes. *Am. J. Physiol.* 210:139, 1966.

45. Bartos, H. R., and Desforges, J. F.: Enzymes as erythrocyte age reference standards. *Am. J. Med. Sci.* 254:862, 1967.

46. Beutler, E.: Electrophoresis of phosphoglycerate kinase. *Biochem. Genet.* 3:189, 1969.

47. Chen, S.-H., Malcolm, L. A., Yoshida, A., and Giblett, E. R.: Phosphoglycerate kinase: An X-linked polymorphism in man. *Am. J. Hum. Genet.* 23:87, 1971.

48. Yoshida, A., Watanabe, S., Chen, S.-H., Giblett, E. R., and Malcolm, L. A.: Human phosphoglycerate kinase. II. Structure of a variant enzyme. *J. Biol. Chem.* 247:446, 1972.

49. Huang, I. Y., Rubinfein, E., and Yoshida, A.: Complete amino acid sequence of human phosphoglycerate kinase. Isolation and amino acid sequence of tryptic peptides. *J. Biol. Chem.* 255:6408, 1980.

50. Rosa, R., Gaillardon, J., and Rosa, J.: Diphosphoglycerate mutase and 2,3-diphosphoglycerate phosphatase activities of red cells: Comparative electrophoretic study. *Biochem. Biophys. Res. Commun.* 51:536, 1973.

51. Sasaki, R., Ikura, K., Sugimoto, E., and Chiba, H.: Purification of bisphosphoglyceromutase, 2,3-bisphosphoglycerate phosphatase and phosphoglyceromutase from human erythrocytes. *Eur. J. Biochem.* 50:581, 1975.

52. Rose, Z. B.: The purification and properties of diphosphoglycerate mutase from human erythrocytes. *J. Biol. Chem.* 243:4810, 1968.

53. Sauer, G., and Scholz, D.: Über die Reinigung und Charak-

54. Harkness, D. R., and Roth, S.: Purification and properties of 2,3-diphosphoglyceric acid phosphatase from human erythrocytes. *Biochem. Biophys. Res. Commun.* 34:849, 1969.

55. Rose, Z. B., and Salon, J.: The identification of glycolate-2-P as a constituent of normal red blood cells. *Biochem. Biophys. Res. Commun.* 87:869, 1979.

56. Badwey, J. A.: Phosphoglycolate phosphatase in human erythrocytes. *J. Biol. Chem.* 252:2441, 1977.

57. Beutler, E., and West, C.: An improved assay and some properties of phosphoglycolate phosphatase. *Anal. Biochem.* 106:163, 1980.

58. Hoorn, R. K. J., Filkweert, J. P., and Staal, G. E. J.: Purification and properties of enolase of human erythrocytes. *Int. J. Biochem.* 5:845, 1974.

59. Chen, S.-H., and Giblett, E. R.: Enolase: Human tissue distribution and evidence for three different loci. *Ann. Hum. Genet.* 39:277, 1976.

60. Rose, I. A., and Warms, J.: Control of glycolysis in the human blood cell. *J. Biol. Chem.* 241:4848, 1966.

61. Blume, K. G., Hoffbauer, R. W., Busch, D., Arnold, H., and Löhr, G. W.: Purification and properties of pyruvate kinase in normal and in pyruvate kinase deficient human red blood cells. *Biochim. Biophys. Acta* 227:364, 1971.

62. Kahn, A., Marie, J., Garreau, H. and Sprengers, E. D.: The genetic system of the L-type pyruvate kinase forms in man. Subunit structure, interrelation and kinetic characteristics of the pyruvate kinase enzymes from erythrocytes and liver. *Biochim. Biophys. Acta* 523:59, 1978.

63. Beutler, E., Matsumoto, F., and Guinto, E.: The effect of 2,3-DPG on red cell enzymes. *Experientia* 30:190, 1974.

64. Tanaka, K. R., Valentine, W. N., and Miwa, S.: Pyruvate kinase (PK) deficiency hereditary non-spherocytic hemolytic anemia. *Blood* 19:267, 1962.

65. Starkweather, W. H., Cousineau, L., Schock, H. K., and Sarafonetis, C. J.: Alterations of erythrocyte lactate dehydrogenase in man. *Blood* 26:63, 1965.

66. Miwa, S., Nishina, T., Kakehashi, Y., Kitamura, M., Hiratsuka, A., and Shizume, K.: Studies on erythrocyte metabolism in a case with hereditary deficiency of H-subunit of lactate dehydrogenase. *Acta Haematol. Jap.* 34:2, 1971.

67. Beutler, E.: Glucose-6-phosphate dehydrogenase deficiency, in *The Metabolic Basis of Inherited Disease*, 4th ed., edited by J. B. Stanbury, J. B. Wyngaarden, and D. S. Fredrickson. McGraw-Hill, New York, 1978, pp. 1430–1450.

68. Yoshida, A., Stamatoyannopoulos, G., and Motulsky, A.: Negro variant of glucose-6-phosphate dehydrogenase deficiency (A−) in man. *Science* 155:97, 1967.

69. Rattazzi, M. C.: Glucose-6-phosphate dehydrogenase from human erythrocytes: Molecular weight determination by gel filtration. *Biochem. Biophys. Res. Commun.* 31:16, 1968.

70. Kirkman, H. N., and Hendrickson, E. M.: Glucose-6-phosphate dehydrogenase from human erythrocytes. II. Subactive states of the enzyme from normal persons. *J. Biol. Chem.* 237:2371, 1962.

71. Balinsky, D., and Bernstein, R. E.: The purification and properties of glucose-6-phosphate dehydrogenase from human erythrocytes. *Biochim. Biophys. Acta* 67:313, 1963.

72. Luzzatto, L., and Afolayan, A.: Genetic variants of human erythrocyte glucose-6-phosphate dehydrogenase. II. In vitro and in vivo function of the A− variant. *Biochemistry* 10:420, 1971.

73. Yoshida, A.: Hemolytic anemia and G-6-PD deficiency. *Science* 179:532, 1973.

74. Avigad, G.: Inhibition of glucose-6-phosphate dehydrogenase by adenosine-5-triphosphate. *Proc. Natl. Acad. Sci. U.S.A.* 56:1543, 1966.

75. Ben-Bassat, I., and Beutler, E.: Inhibition by ATP of erythrocyte glucose-6-phosphate dehydrogenase variants. *Proc. Soc. Exp. Biol. Med.* 142:410, 1973.

76. Betke, K., et al.: Standardization of procedures for the study of glucose-6-phosphate dehydrogenase. Report of a WHO scientific group. *WHO Tech. Rep. Ser.* 366, 1967.

77. Shih, L., Justice, P., and Hsia, D. Y.: Purification and character-

terisierung der 2,3-P gase roter Blutzellen. *Folia Haematol. (Leipz.)* 83:271, 1964.

ization of genetic variants of 6-phosphogluconate dehydrogenase. *Biochem. Genet.* 1:359, 1968.

78. Parr, C. W., and Fitch, L. I.: Inherited quantitative variations of human phosphogluconate dehydrogenase. *Ann. Hum. Genet.* 30:339, 1967.

79. Bruns, F. H., Noltmann, E., and Valhaus, E.: Über den Stoffwechsel von Ribose-5-Phosphat in Haemolysaten. I. Aktivitätsmessung und Eigenschaften der Phosphoribose-isomerase. II. Der Pentosephosphate cyclus in roten Blutzellen. *Biochem. Z.* 330:483, 1958.

80. Brownstone, Y. S., and Denstedt, O. F.: The pentose phosphate metabolic pathway in the human erythrocyte. II. The transketolase and transaldolase activity of the human erythrocyte. *Can. J. Biochem.* 39:533, 1961.

81. Bruns, F. H., Dunwald, E., and Noltmann, E.: Über den Stoffwechsel von Ribose-5-phosphat in Haemolysatin III. Quantitative Bestimmung von Sedoheptulose-7-phosphat und einige Eigenschaften der Transketolase der Erythrocyten und des Blutserums. *Biochem. Z.* 330:497, 1958.

82. Wolfe, S. J., Brin, M., and Davidson, C. S.: The effect of thiamine deficiency on human erythrocyte metabolism. *J. Clin. Invest.* 37:1476, 1958.

83. Halder, A. B., Wolff, S., Ting, H. H., and Crabbe, M. J. C.: An aldolase reductase from the human erythrocyte. *Biochem. Soc. Trans.* 8:64, 1980.

84. Travis, S. F., Morrison, A. D., Clements, R. S., Jr., Winegrad, A. I., and Oski, F. A.: Metabolic alterations in the human erythrocyte produced by increases in glucose concentration. The role of the polyol pathway. *J. Clin. Invest.* 50:2104, 1971.

85. Beutler, E., and Guinto, E.: The reduction of glyceraldehyde by human erythrocytes. L-Hexonate dehydrogenase activity. *J. Clin. Invest.* 53:1258, 1974.

86. Gabrio, B. W., Finch, C. A., and Huennekens, F. M.: Erythrocyte preservation: A topic in molecular biochemistry. *Blood* 11:103, 1956.

87. Giblett, E. R., Anderson, J. E., Cohen, F., Pollara, B., and Meuwissen, H. J.: Adenosine deaminase deficiency in two patients with severely impaired cellular immunity. *Lancet* 2:1067, 1972.

88. Bakay, B., Telfer, M. A., and Nyhan, W. L.: Assay of hypoxanthineguanine and adenine phosphoribosyl transferases. A simple screening test for the Lesch-Nyhan syndrome and related disorders of purine metabolism. *Biochem. Med.* 3:230, 1969.

89. Valentine, W. N., Paglia, D. E., Tartaglia, A. P., and Gilsanz, F.: Hereditary hemolytic anemia with increased red cell adenosine deaminase (45- to 70-fold) and decreased adenosine triphosphate. *Science* 195:783, 1977.

90. Kim, B. K., Cha, S., and Parks, R. E., Jr.: Purine nucleoside phosphorylase from human erythrocytes. I. Purification and properties. *J. Biol. Chem.* 243:1763, 1968.

91. Kim, B. K., Cha, S., and Parks, R. E., Jr.: Purine nucleoside phosphorylase and human erythrocytes. II. Kinetic analysis and substrate-binding studies. *J. Biol. Chem.* 243:1771, 1968.

92. Oski, F. A., Sugarman, H. J., and Miller, L. D.: Experimentally induced alterations in the affinity of Hb for oxygen. I. In vitro restoration of erythrocyte 2,3-DPG and its relationship to erythrocyte purine nucleoside phosphorylase activity in a variety of species. *Blood* 39:522, 1972.

93. Giblett, E. R., Ammann, A. J., Wara, D. W., Sandman, R., and Diamond, L. K.: Nucleoside-phosphorylase deficiency in a child with severely defective T-cell immunity and normal B-cell immunity. *Lancet* 1:1010, 1975.

94. Valentine, W. N., Oski, F. A., Paglia, D. E., Baugham, M. A., Schneider, A. S., and Naiman, J. L.: Erythrocyte hexokinase and hereditary hemolytic anemia, in *Hereditary Disorders of Erythrocyte Metabolism*, edited by E. Beutler. Grune & Stratton, New York, 1968, City of Hope Symposium Series, vol 1.

95. Morsches, B., Holzmann, H., and Bettingen, C.: Zum Nachweis der Sorbit dehydrogenase in menschlichen Erythrocyten. *Klin. Wochenschr.* 47:672, 1969.

96. Barretto, O. C. D., and Beutler, E.: The sorbitol oxidizing enzyme of red blood cells. *J. Lab. Clin. Med.* 85:645, 1975.

97. Bruns, F. H., and Noltmann, E.: Phosphomannoisomerase, an SH-dependent metal-enzyme complex. *Nature* 181:1467, 1958.

98. Bruns, F. H., Noltmann, E., and Willemsen, A.: Phosphomannoseisomerase. I. Über die Aktivitätsmessung und die Sulfhydryl sowie die Metallabhängigkeit der Enzymwirkung in einigen tierischen Geweben. *Biochem. Z.* 330:411, 1958.

99. Isselbacher, K. J., Anderson, E. P., Kurahashi, E., and Kalckar, H. M.: Congenital galactosemia, a single enzymatic block in galactose metabolism. *Science* 123:635, 1956.

100. Noltmann,E., and Bruns, F. H.: Über die Phosphoglucomutase der Erythrocyten und des Serums. *Hoppe Seylers Z. Physiol. Chem.* 313:194, 1959.

101. Beutler, E., and Guinto, E.: Dihydroxyacetone metabolism by human erythrocytes: Demonstration of triokinase activity and its characterization. *Blood* 41:559, 1973.

102. Brake, J. M., and Deindoerfer, F. H.: Preservation of red blood cell 2 3-diphosphoglycerate in stored blood containing dihydroxyacetone. *Transfusion* 13:84, 1973.

103. Wood, L., and Beutler, E.: The effect of ascorbate and dihydroxyacetone on the 2,3-diphosphoglycerate and ATP levels of stored human red cells. *Transfusion* 14:272, 1974.

104. Moses, S. W., Chayoth, R., Levin, S., Lazarovitz, E., and Rubinstein, D.: Glucose and glycogen metabolism in erythrocytes from normal and glycogen storage disease type III subjects. *J. Clin. Invest.* 47:1343, 1968.

105. Sidbury, J. B., Jr., Cornblath, M., Fisher, J., and House, E.: Glycogen in erythrocytes of patients with glycogen storage disease. *Pediatrics* 27:103, 1961.

106. Bartels, H.: Untersuchungen zur Frage des Glykogen-gehaltes von Erythrocyten, in *Metabolism and Membrane Permeability of Erythrocytes and Thrombocytes*, edited by E. Deutsch, E. Gerlach, and K. Moser. Georg Thieme Verlag, Stuttgart, 1968, 1st International Symposium, Vienna, pp. 132–134.

107. Dimant, E., Landberg, E., and London, I. M.: The metabolic behavior of reduced glutathione in human and avian erythrocytes. *J. Biol. Chem.* 213:769, 1955.

108. Boivin, P., and Galand, C.: La Synthése du glutathion au cours de l'anémie hémolytique congénitale avec déficit en glutathion réduit. Déficit congénital en glutathion-synthétase érythrocytaire? *Nouv. Rev. Fr. Hematol.* 5:707, 1965.

109. Boivin, P., Galand, C., Andre, R., and Debray, J.: Anémies hémolytiques congénitales avec déficit isolé en glutathion reduit par déficit en glutathion synthétase. *Nouv. Rev. Fr. Hematol.* 6:859, 1966.

110. Sass, M. D.: Glutathione synthesis in cell-free preparations from erythrocytes of different ages. *Clin. Chim. Acta* 22:207, 1968.

111. Jackson, R. C.: Studies in the enzymology of glutathione metabolism in human erythrocytes. *Biochem. J.* 111:309, 1969.

112. Srivastava, S. K., and Beutler, E.: The transport of oxidized glutathione from human erythrocytes. *J. Biol. Chem.* 244:9, 1969.

113. Lunn, G., Dale, G. L., and Beutler, E.: Transport accounts for glutathione turnover in human erythrocytes. *Blood* 54:238, 1979.

114. Palekar, A. G., Tate, S. S., and Meister, A.: Formation of 5-oxoproline from glutathione in erythrocytes by the γ glutamyl-transpeptidase-cyclotransferase pathway. *Proc. Natl. Acad. Sci. U.S.A.* 71:293, 1974.

115. Board, P. G., and Smith, J. E.: Erythrocyte γ-glutamyl transpeptidase. *Blood* 49:667, 1977.

116. Srivastava, S. K., Awasthi, Y. C., Miller, S. P., Yoshida, A., and Beutler, E.: Studies on γ-glutamyl transpeptidase in human and rabbit erythrocytes. *Blood* 47:645, 1976.

117. Young, J. D., Ellory, J. C., and Wright, P. C.: Evidence against the participation of the γ-glutamyl transferase–γ-glutamylcyclotransferase pathway in amino acid transport by rabbit erythrocytes. *Biochem. J.* 152:713, 1975.

118. Winterbourn, C. C., Hawkins, R. E., Brian, M., and Carrell, R. W.: The estimation of red cell superoxide dismutase activity. *J. Lab. Clin. Med.* 85:337, 1975.

119. Mills, G. C., and Randall, H. P.: Hemoglobin catabolism II. The protection of hemoglobin from oxidative breakdown in the intact erythrocyte. *J. Biol. Chem.* 232:589, 1958.

120. Cohen, G., and Hochstein, P.: Glutathione peroxidase: The primary agent for the elimination of hydrogen peroxide in erythroyctes. *Biochemistry* 2:1420, 1963.

121. Rotruck, J. T., Pope, A. L., Ganther, H. E., Swanson, A. B., Hafeman, D. G., and Hoekstra, W. G.: Selenium: Biochemical role as a component of glutathione peroxidase. *Science* 179:588, 1973.

122. Awasthi, Y. C., Beutler, E., and Srivastava, S. K.: Purification and properties of human erythrocyte glutathione peroxidase. *J. Biol. Chem.* 250:5144, 1975.

123. Thomson, C. D., Rea, H. M., Doesburg, V. M., and Robinson, M. F.: Selenium concentrations and glutathione peroxidase activities in whole blood of New Zealand residents. *Br. J. Nutr.* 37:457, 1977.

124. Beutler, E., and Matsumoto, F.: Ethnic variation in red cell glutathione peroxidase activity. *Blood* 46:103, 1975.

125. Loos, H., Roos, D., Weening, R., and Houwerzijl, J.: Familial deficiency of glutathione reductase in human blood cells. *Blood* 48:53, 1976.

126. Beutler, E., West, C., and Beutler, B.: Electrophoretic polymorphism of gluthathione peroxidase. *Ann. Hum. Genet.* 38:163, 1974.

127. Jacob, H. S., and Jandl, J. H.: Effects of sulfhydryl inhibition of red blood cells. I. Mechanism of hemolysis. *J. Clin. Invest.* 41:779, 1962.

128. Huisman, T. H. J., and Dozy, A. M.: Studies on the heterogeneity of hemoglobin. V. Binding of hemoglobin with oxidized glutathione. *J. Lab. Clin. Med.* 60:302, 1962.

129. Scott, E. M., Duncan, I. W., and Ekstrand, V.: Purification and properties of glutathione reductase of human erythrocytes. *J. Biol. Chem.* 238:3928, 1963.

130. Icen, A.: Glutathione reductase of human erythrocytes. Purification and properties. *Scand. J. Clin. Lab. Invest.* 96:1, 1967.

131. Beutler, E., and Yeh, M. K. Y.: Erythrocyte glutathione reductase. *Blood* 21:573, 1963.

132. Rieber, E. E., Kosower, N. S., and Jaffé, E. R.: Reduced nicotinamide adenine dinucleotide and the reduction of oxidized glutathione in human erythrocytes. *J. Clin. Invest.* 47:66, 1968.

133. Smith, J. E., and Parks, P.: Glutathione reduction: Studies using deoxyribonucleosides as substrates. *Proc. Soc. Exp. Biol. Med.* 129:750, 1968.

134. Srivastava, S. K., and Beutler, E.: Glutathione metabolism of the erythrocyte. The enzymic cleavage of glutathione-haemoglobin preparations by glutathione reductase. *Biochem. J.* 119:353, 1970.

135. Long, W. K.: Glutathione reductase in red blood cells: Variant associated with gout. *Science* 155:712, 1967.

136. Kaplan, J. C., and Beutler, E.: Electrophoretic study of glutathione reductase in human erythrocytes and leucocytes. *Nature* 217:256, 1968.

137. Beutler, E.: Glutathione reductase: Stimulation in normal subjects by riboflavin supplementation. *Science* 165:613, 1969.

138. Marcus, C. J., Habig, W. H., and Jakoby, W. B.: Glutathione transferase from human erythrocytes. *Arch. Biochem. Biophys.* 188:287, 1978.

139. Magnani, M., Stocchi, V., Ninfali, P., Dacha, M., and Fornaini, G.: Action of oxidized and reduced glutathione on rabbit red blood cell hexokinase. *Biochim. Biophys. Acta* 615:113,1980.

140. Smith, J. E.: Relationship of in vivo erythrocyte glutathione flux to the oxidized glutathione transport system. *J.Lab. Clin. Med.* 83:444, 1974.

141. Prchal, J., Srivastava, S. K., and Beutler E.: Active transport of GSSG from reconstituted erythrocyte ghosts. *Blood* 46:111, 1975.

142. Kondo, T., Dale, G. L., and Beutler, E.: Glutathione transport by inside-out vesicles from human erythrocytes. *Proc. Natl. Acad. Sci. U.S.A.* 77:6359, 1980.

143. Jaffe, E. R.: Metabolic processes involved in the formation and reduction of methemoglobin in human erythrocytes, in *The Red Blood Cell*, edited by C. Bishop and D. M. Surgenor. Academic Press, New York, 1964, pp. 397–422.

144. Scott, E. M.: Congenital methemoglobinemia due to DPNH-diaphorase deficiency, in *Hereditary Disorders of Erythrocyte Metabolism.* Grune & Stratton, New York, 1968, City of Hope Symposium Series, vol. 1, pp. 102–113.

145. Hultquist, D. E., and Passon, P. G.: Catalysis of methaemoglobin reduction by erythrocyte cytochrome b$_5$ and cytochrome b$_5$ reductase. *Nature* [*New Biol.*] 229:252, 1971.

146. Tashian, R. E., Riggs, S. K., and Yu, Y. L.: Characterization of a mutant human erythrocyte carbonic anhydrase: Carbonic anhydrase 1c$_{GUAM}$. *Arch. Biochem. Biophys.* 117:320, 1966.

147. Takahara, S.: Acatalasemia in Japan, in *Hereditary Disorders of Erythrocyte Metabolism*, edited by E. Beutler. Grune & Stratton, New York, 1968, City of Hope Symposium Series, vol. 1, pp. 21–40.

148. Aebi, H., Bossi, E., Cantz, M., Matsubara, S., and Suter, H.: Acatalas(em)ia in Switzerland, in *Hereditary Disorders of Erythrocyte Metabolism*, edited by E. Beutler. Grune & Stratton, New York, 1968, City of Hope Symposium Series, vol. 1, pp. 41–65.

149. De Sandre, G., and Ghiotto, G.: An enzymic disorder in the erythrocytes of paroxysmal nocturnal haemoglobinuria: A deficiency in acetylcholinesterase activity. *Br. J. Haematol.* 6:39, 1960.

150. Auditore, J. V., Hartmann, R. C., Flexner, J. M., and Balchum, O. J.: The erythrocyte acetylcholinesterase enzyme in paroxysmal nocturnal hemoglobinemia. *Arch. Pathol.* 69:534, 1960.

151. Johns, R. J.: Familial reduction in red-cell cholinesterase. *N. Engl. J. Med.* 267:1344, 1962.

152. Boivin, P., and Galand, C.: Purification and characterization of an adenosine cyclic 3',5'-monophosphate–dependent protein kinase from human erythrocyte membrane. *Biochem. Biophys. Res. Commun.* 81:473, 1978.

153. Avruch, J., and Fairbanks, G.: Phosphorylation of endogenous substrates by erythrocyte membrane protein kinases. I. A monovalent cation-stimulated reaction. *Biochemistry* 13:5507, 1974.

154. Guthrow, C. E., Jr., Allen, J. E., and Rasmussen, H.: Phosphorylation of an endogenous membrane protein by an endogenous membrane-associated cyclic adenosine 3',5'-monophosphate–dependent protein kinase in human erythrocyte ghosts. *J. Biol. Chem.* 247:8145, 1972.

155. Imhof, B. A., et al.: Phosphorylation and dephosphorylation of spectrin from human erythrocyte ghosts under physiological conditions: Autocatalysis rather than reaction with separate kinase and phosphatase. *Proc. Natl. Acad. Sci. U.S.A.* 77:3264, 1980.

156. Avruch, J., and Fairbanks, G.: Demonstration of a phosphopeptide intermediate in the Mg^{++} dependent, Na$^+$- and K$^+$-stimulated adenosine triphosphatase reaction of the erythrocyte membrane. *Proc. Natl. Acad. Sci. U.S.A.* 69:1216, 1972.

157. Greenquist, A. C., and Shohet, S. B.: Defective protein phosphorylation in membranes of hereditary spherocytosis erythrocytes. *Febs. Lett.* 48:133, 1974.

158. Beutler, E., Guinto, E., and Johnson, C.: Human red cell protein kinase in normal subjects and patients with hereditary spherocytosis, sickle cell disease, and autoimmune hemolytic anemia. *Blood* 48:887, 1976.

159. Wolfe, L. C., and Lux, S. E.: Membrane protein phosphorylation of intact normal and hereditary spherocytic erythrocytes. *J. Biol. Chem.* 253:3336, 1978.

160. Matthies, H.: Untersuchungen über eine Aldehyd-dehydrogenase in kernlosen Erythrocyten. *Biochem. Z.*329:421, 1957.

161. Izak, G., Wilner, T., and Mager, J.: Amino acid activating enzymes in red blood cells of normal, anemic and polycythemic subjects. *J. Clin. Invest.* 39:1763, 1960.

162. Kaplan, N. O.: Metabolic pathways involving niacin and its derivatives, in *Metabolic Pathways*, edited by D. M. Greenberg. Academic, New York, 1961, p. 627.

163. Bertino, J. R., Simmons, B., and Donohue, D. M.: Purification and properties of the formate-activating enzyme from erythrocytes. *J. Biol. Chem.* 237:1314, 1962.

164. Valentine, W. N., and Tanaka, K. R.: The glyoxalase content of human erythrocytes and leukocytes. *Acta Haematol.* 26:303, 1961.

165. Anderson, B. B., and Mollin, D. L.: Red-cell metabolism of pyridoxine in sideroblastic and related anaemias. *Br. J. Haematol.* 23:159, 1972.

166. Chern, C. J., and Beutler, E.: Pyridoxal kinase: Decreased activity in red blood cells of Afro-Americans. *Science* 187:1084, 1975.

167. Magnussen, C. R., Levine, J. B., Doherty, J. M., Cheesman, J. O., and Tschudy, D. P.: A red cell enzyme method for the diagnosis of acute intermittent porphyria. *Blood* 44:857, 1974.

168. Yeh, G. C., and Phang, J. M.: The function of pyrroline-5-carboxylate reductase in human erythrocytes. *Biochem. Biophys. Res. Commun.* 94:450, 1980.

169. Friedemann, H., and Rapoport, S. M.: Enzymes of the red cell: A critical catalogue, in *Cellular and Molecular Biology of Erythrocytes*,

edited by H. Yoshikawa and S. M. Rapaport. University Park Press, Baltimore, 1974, pp. 181–259.

170. Cartier, P., and Hamet, M.: Une Nouvelle Maladie métabolique: Le Déficit complet en adenine-phosphoribosyltransferase avec lithiase de 2,8-dihydroxyadenine. *C. R. Acad. Sci. (Paris) 279,* 1974.

171. Van Acker, K. J., Simmonds, A., Potter, C., and Cameron, J. S.: Complete deficiency of adenine phosphoribosyltransferase. Report of a family. *N. Engl. J. Med. 297:*127, 1977.

172. Seegmiller, J. E., Rosenbloom, F. M., and Kelley. W. N.: Enzyme defect associated with a sex-linked human neurological disorder and excessive purine synthesis. *Science 155:*1682, 1967.

173. Kyd, J. M., and Bagnara, A. S.: Adenosine kinase from human erythrocytes: Determination of the conditions required for assay in crude hemolysates. *Clin. Chim. Acta 103:*145, 1980.

174. Preiss, J., and Handler, P.: Biosynthesis of diphosphopyridine nucleotide. I. Identification of intermediates. *J. Biol. Chem. 233:*488, 1958.

175. Preiss, J., and Handler, P.: Biosynthesis of diphosphopyridine nucleotide. II. Enzymatic aspects. *J. Biol. Chem. 233:*493, 1958.

176. Beutler, E.: Red cell metabolism. A. Defects not causing hemolytic disease. B. Environmental modification. *Biochemie 54:*759, 1972.

177. Ng, W. G., Donnell, G. N., and Bergren, W. R.: Deficiency of erythrocyte nicotinamide adenine dinucleotide nucleosidase (NADase) activity in the Negro. *Nature 217:*64, 1968.

178. Rapoport, S.: Reifung und Alterungsvorgange in Erythrozyten. *Folia Haematol. (Leipz.) 78,* 1961.

179. Rapoport, S., Rosenthal, S., Schewe, T., Schultze, M., and Miller, N.: The metabolism of the reticulocyte, in *Cellular and Molecular Biology of Erythrocytes,* edited by H. Yoshikawa and S. M. Rapoport. University Park Press, Baltimore, 1974.

CHAPTER 36

The red cell membrane

STEPHEN B. SHOHET
ERNEST BEUTLER

In 1839, Francois Magendie, describing his microscopic observations of red cells, wrote [1]:

It is possible (but I would not affirm that such is the case) that these bodies are provided within an investment which tears. Observers are, indeed, generally of the opinion that they are surrounded with a very delicate pellicle; and this idea receives some support from the fact that in the globules of dead subjects there is a sort of puckering visible, such as is presented by membranes of extreme thinness when they begin to dry; for instance, the outer skin on onions.

The membrane, or red cell ghost, as we now designate the "pellicle" which surrounds the erythrocyte, forms a boundary between the interior of the cell, containing its highly concentrated solution of hemoglobin, and the plasma surrounding it. The membrane serves as a barrier to help maintain in the interior of the red cell a concentration of various ions and metabolites which differs markedly from the concentrations found in the external environment. It must be insoluble in aqueous

solution; not surprisingly, then, approximately one-half of the mass of the human erythrocyte membrane consists of lipid [2], largely arranged as a bilayer.

In addition to serving as a barrier, the membrane contains pumps for the movement of sodium, potassium, calcium, and oxidized glutathione, and it facilitates the transport of glucose. It is also responsible for the biconcave shape of the erythrocyte. These functions are performed by membrane proteins.

Membrane lipids

All the lipids in the mature cell are contained within the membrane and are partially responsible for many of its physical characteristics. For example, both the passive cation permeability and the mechanical flexibility of the red cell can be significantly influenced by modifying the lipid composition of its membrane [3,4].

Lipid composition

Phospholipids and nonesterified cholesterol account for more than 95 percent of the total lipid within the membrane. Small amounts of glycolipids, glycerides, and free fatty acids are also present [5]. On a molar basis, the phospholipids and cholesterol are present in nearly equal amounts, and there is evidence that considerable interaction may occur between these major lipid classes within the membrane (e.g., cholesterol "condenses" and stabilizes bimolecular phosphatide leaflets [6,7]).

The phospholipids are divided into subclasses, distinguished, with the exception of sphingomyelin, by the base group which is in phosphodiester linkage to the third carbon atom of their glycerol backbone (Fig. 36-1). Usually, there are two esterified fatty acids on the 1 and 2 positions of the glycerol backbone, although vinyl ether linkages occur to a substantial extent on the 2 position in some acidic phosphatides, such as phosphatidylethanolamine. The major phospholipids, which are usually named after their bases, and their approximate concentration in human erythrocytes are as follows: phosphatidylcholine (PC), 30 percent; phosphatidylethanolamine (PE), 28 percent; phosphatidylserine (PS), 14 percent; and sphingomyelin (SM), 25 percent.

FIGURE 36-1 The acylation reaction basic to red cell membrane lipid renewal. A lysophosphatide is esterified with a free fatty acid to produce a complete phosphatide with profoundly different physical properties [36–38]. FA = fatty acid.

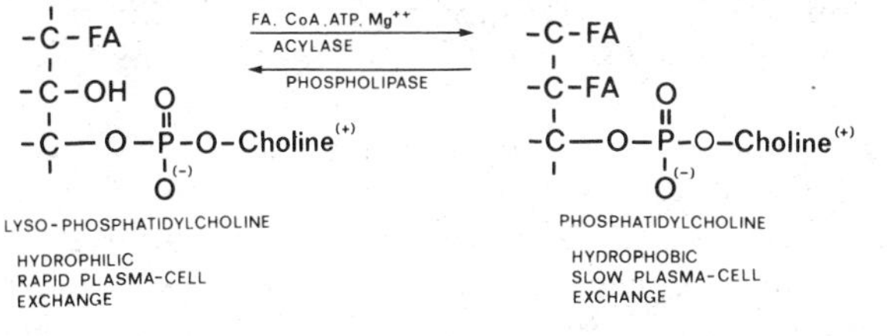

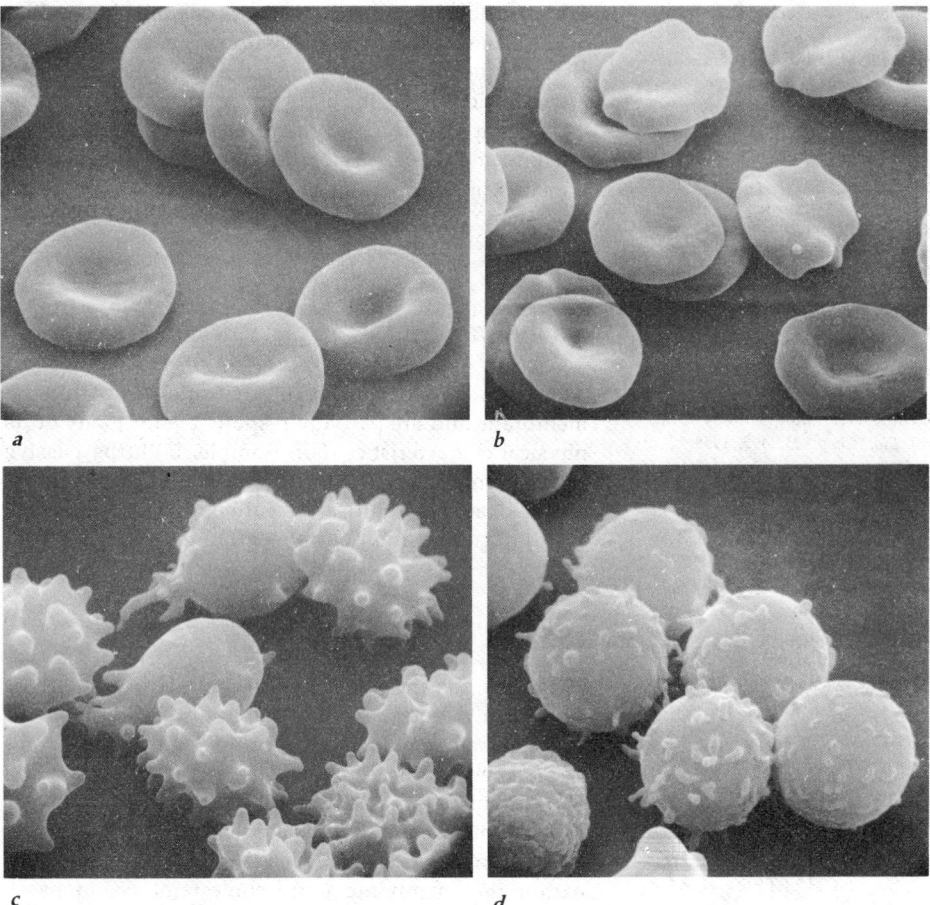

FIGURE 36-2 Scanning electron micrographs of erythrocytes subjected to increasing concentrations of membrane lysophosphatidylcholine (LPC). (*a*) Membrane LPC, 0.12 μmole per cm³ cells. (*b*) Membrane LPC, 0.15 μmole per cm³ cells. (*c*) Membrane LPC, 0.30 μmole per cm³ cells. (*d*) Membrane LPC, 0.50 μmole per cm³ cells. The bulk of the changes seen in (*a*) to (*c*) could be reversed by washing the cells with defatted albumin. The changes seen in the red cells in (*d*) are irreversible and represent, in part, membrane loss due to microvesiculation induced by the high LPC concentration.

Sphingomyelin is distinct structurally from the rest of the group (see Fig. 103-1) and does not appear to enter into many of the exchange, acyl transport, and renewal reactions described below. Small amounts of phosphatidic acid, phosphatidyl inositides, and polyglycerol phosphatides are also present in red cells [5]. There are characteristic patterns of the esterfied fatty acids within each phospholipid class, and these also serve to distinguish phosphatide subgroups.

Phospholipids containing only one fatty acid are known as lysophosphatides (Fig. 36-1). The absence of one of the acyl (fatty acid) groups profoundly influences the physical characteristics of the phospholipid. Although phospholipids with two fatty acids are highly lipophilic, the lysophosphatide compounds are nearly balanced in terms of lipophilic and hydrophilic characteristics. They tend to concentrate, therefore, at phase interfaces. This change in relative solubility increases both their detergent qualities and their rate of exchange between the cell membrane and the plasma [8,9]. Be-

cause of these properties, lysophosphatides in low concentrations ($2 \times 10^{-4}\,M$) can cause the lysis of red cell membranes—hence their trivial name. In even smaller concentrations, they can produce profound, eventually irreversible, shape changes ("echinocytogenesis") in the membrane (Fig. 36-2*a* through *d* and Chap. 29). Red cell membranes usually contain only small amounts of lysophosphatides. In normal cells, there are at least three mechanisms, which will be discussed below, for maintaining these potentially dangerous lyso- compounds at acceptably low levels.

Disposition of the lipids within the membrane

Although many structural relationships have been proposed, the precise anatomic localization of the lipids within the membranes is still unknown. There is, however, little doubt that a large percentage of the lipid is arrayed in bimolecular leaflet form [10,11]. In this bilayer disposition, the polar headgroups of each lipid layer face away from the center of the membrane into the hydrophilic environments of the cytoplasm and the plasma, while the long acyl tails of the lipids form a central hydrophobic core of the membrane. This hydrophobic core is in a liquid-crystalline state at normal temperatures and may facilitate the physiologically essential flexibility and deformability of the red cell membrane. It has been proposed that many of the protein elements of the membrane are inserted into this lipid matrix in much the same way as icebergs float in the ocean [12] (Fig. 36-3). In this model, some of the proteins and glycoproteins are confined to one leaflet, while others, especially those assumed to have transport and shape-mediating roles, span the entire membrane. In addition, both the inserted proteins and the lipids are relatively free to move laterally within the plane of the membrane at comparatively rapid rates. In contrast, motions across the bilayer from one leaflet to the other are much more restricted. Since it is reasonable to assume that the lipid composition partially determines membrane viscosity, any significant changes in lipid composition which affect the membrane's internal microviscosity (e.g., an increase in cholesterol) might be expected to have some effect on the flexibility of the whole cell. However, the protein constituents of the membrane are of major importance in this regard, and calculations of the physical forces involved suggest that lipid-protein interactions must be much more important than pure lipid effects [13]. However, membrane flexibility is not the only or even predominant requirement for whole-cell deform-ability. The cell must avoid reductions in surface area and increases in intracellular viscosity to maintain optimal deformability. In the latter case, it is likely that the physical characteristics of the membrane are subordinate to its permeability and water regulation characteristics in maintaining cell deformability [14].

The lipids are not symmetrically distributed between the inner and outer leaflets of the membrane. It appears that the majority of the phosphatidylethanolamine and the phosphatidylserine are contained within the inner or cytoplasmic leaflet of the membrane, while the majority of the phosphatidylcholine and the sphingomyelin are contained in the leaflet facing the plasma [15,16]. The biochemical basis of this asymmetry may be the combined result of the site specificity of the phospholipid exchange and renewal reactions described below and the sluggish lipid exchange rates between the inner and outer membrane leaflets. Although the full extent of the physiologic consequences of this asymmetry is not known, at the very least considerable transmembrane charge potential is induced by the excess of positive charges on the inner leaflet. This asymmetry is apparently disturbed in some abnormal states (e.g., sickled and irreversibly sickled cells) [17,18], and it has been speculated that such externalization of acidic red cell phospholipids may have thrombotic consequences [19]. The asymmetric distribution of the typical intramembranous particles seen on freeze-fracture electron microscopy [20], where the large majority of particles are found on the inner or A face of the cleaved membrane, may also be a consequence of lipid asymmetry.

FIGURE 36-3 A schematic representation of the Singer-Nicholson fluid mosaic model for the structure of cell membranes. Irregular proteins are seen penetrating both into and through the biomolecular leaflet composed of regular arrays of phospholipid molecules. The head groups of the phospholipids face the cytoplasmic and plasma environments, while their acyl tails are enmeshed to form the lipophilic membrane core [12].

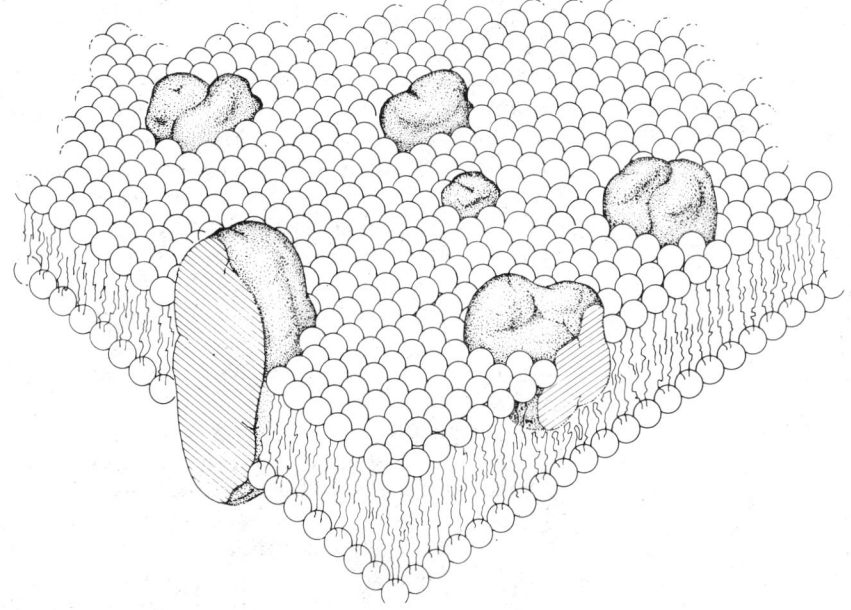

Another potential consequence of lipid asymmetry may involve coupling of the membrane bilayer to the so-called membrane skeleton. This structure consists primarily of spectrin, actin, and protein bands 2.1 (ankyrin) and 4.1. It appears to serve as a scaffolding for the lipid bilayer and to have a dominating role in influencing membrane stability and deformability [21,22]. Although elegant studies have established specific protein interactions between this "membrane skeleton" and protein components embedded in the lipid bilayer, such as bands 3 [23] and PAS 2' [24], spectrin:phosphatidylethanolamine and spectrin:phosphatidylserine interactions have also been observed [25,26]. However, it is not clear if the membrane asymmetry which places these acidic phospholipids in intimate contact with spectrin at the interface between the inner leaflet of the lipid bilayer and the membrane skeleton is a cause or a consequence of such interactions.

Erythrocyte lipid turnover and renewal pathways

There is no *de novo* synthesis of fatty acids in the mature erythrocyte [27]. However, the red cell continuously

FIGURE 36-4   Schema of the major exchange and metabolism pathways for lipids in the mature erythrocyte. Alb-FFA = albumin-bound free fatty acid; F1 = surface pool of freely exchangeable free fatty acid; F2 = "deeper" pool of free fatty acid used as a source of acyl groups for phosphatides within the membrane; PC_A = phosphatidylcholine actively synthesized within the membrane; PC_P = phosphatidylcholine passively acquired by exchange with the plasma by the membrane; PE = phosphatidylethanolamine; Alb-LPC = albumin-bound lysophosphatidylcholine, which, together with Alb-FFA = serves as the precursor for PC_A; GPC = glycerolphosphorylcholine; C = cholesterol; CE = cholesterol ester; LCAT = lecithin cholesterol acyltransferase. See text for further details.

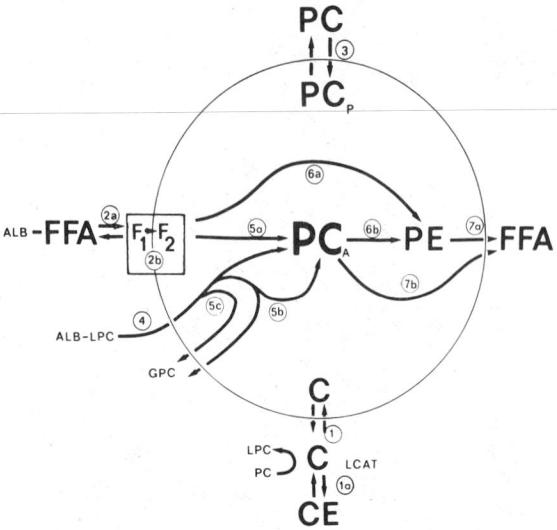

remodels its lipid and possesses mechanisms for lipid incorporation during its lifetime. The known lipid renewal and lipid turnover mechanisms in human erythrocytes are schematically outlined in Fig. 36-4.

PASSIVE EXCHANGE PATHWAYS
Red cell cholesterol is in comparatively rapid equilibrium with unesterified plasma cholesterol, but not with esterified plasma cholesterol. Hence the activity of the plasma enzyme lecithin-cholesterol acyltransferase, which helps to regulate the level of free cholesterol in plasma, indirectly influences the level of cholesterol in the cell (pathway 1, Fig. 36-4).

A portion of the phosphatides of the red cells is likewise in passive equilibrium with the plasma phosphatides [9,28,29] (pathway 3, Fig. 36-4). This reaction is confined primarily to phosphatidylcholine [29]. This may be because serum levels of phosphatidylethanolamine and phosphatidylserine are very low or because of the asymmetric disposition of these phosphatides within the two membrane leaflets, as previously noted. Apparently, the sphingomyelin in the membrane is tightly bound, since it, too, undergoes little exchange with plasma sphingomyelin. The exchange rates of phosphatidylcholine by this passive pathway are considerably less than those of cholesterol but still approach 1 percent per hour, so that approximately one-fourth of red cell phosphatidylcholine exchanges per day with plasma phosphatidylcholine. This exchange, however, is confined to a limited (~ 50 percent) fraction of the total phosphatidylcholine of the cell. Hence, the precise acyl group composition of the red cell phosphatidylcholine, though modulated by that of the plasma, is not identical with it [30].

Erythrocyte lysophosphatidylcholine is similarly involved in an exchange equilibrium with plasma lysophosphatidylcholine, which is primarily albumin-bound (pathway 4, Fig. 36-4) [31,32]. In this case, probably because of the surfactant qualities of this molecule, the equilibrium is obtained much more quickly than with the complete diacyl phosphatide [33].

Albumin-bound free fatty acid is also in rapid passive equilibrium with a small pool of erythrocyte-free fatty acid (pathway 2a, Fig. 36-4) [33,34]. The extent of this equilibrium may differ between species of fatty acids. Penetration of free fatty acid from the surface of the red cell to a "deeper," metabolically active location in the membrane (pathway 2b, Fig. 36-4) depends upon adenosine triphosphate [33]. Carnetine acyltransferase facilitates a similar translocation of fatty acids in other systems, but though present, is not required for this reaction in human erythrocytes [35].

ACTIVE INCORPORATION PATHWAYS
Free fatty acid and lysophosphatidylcholine within the membrane can undergo at least three subsequent reactions in addition to return-exchange to the plasma. The most important of these is acylation of the lysophosphatide with the free fatty acid to produce the complete

diacyl compound, phosphatidylcholine [36]. This is a two-stage reaction which requires adenosine triphosphate, coenzyme A, and magnesium [37,38]. It consists of the initial activation of fatty acid to form acyl coenzyme A and the subsequent transfer of the activated fatty acid to the lysophosphatidylcholine (pathway 5*a*, Fig. 36-4). The L-PC isomer which is preferentially used as substrate is the 1-acyl form [37], while the fatty acid used is the "deeper" fatty acid (F$_2$, Fig. 36-4) produced by pathway 2*b* [33]. The availability of membrane lysophosphatidylcholine for this reaction may be influenced by oxidant drugs or perhaps by antecedent peroxidation of the membrane [39]. Specific acyltransferases may exist for each fatty acid, and different rates and positional preferences for the acylation of each fatty acid have been observed [37]. An apparent loss of acyltransferase capacity has been noted in older erythrocytes [40], although the importance of this phenomenon as a proportional index of cell age has been questioned [41]. Whatever the mechanism, erythrocyte fatty acid composition is modified in the transformation from a reticulocyte to a mature cell [42,43].

The phosphatidylcholine assembled in the membrane by acylation is much less exchangeable with the plasma than either the free fatty acid or the lysophosphatide obtained from the plasma used for its production [9]. Hence, the cell, in effect, traps membrane phosphatide with a minimal expenditure of energy and without *de novo* synthesis, while at the same time reducing the levels of a potentially dangerous lyso- compound by means of this reaction [33,38]. The phosphatidylcholine produced by the active process is maintained in a metabolic pool distinct from the phosphatidylcholine obtained by passive exchange, and there is little mixing between these two pools [29]. The active pool of phosphatidylcholine may be contained primarily in the inner leaflet of the membrane, while the passive exchange pool of phosphatidylcholine appears to be contained within the outer leaflet [44].

Although in terms of the total energy economy of the cell, the metabolic requirements for this acylation pathway for the renewal of red cell lipids are modest, the pathway is sensitive to serious metabolic depletion of the whole cell. The "acylase" reaction has been estimated to consume no more than 5 percent of the total ATP generated by the cell [33]. The K_m for ATP for the acylation reaction has been estimated to be 0.3 to 0.8 mM [40], while the metabolically intact erythrocyte has an ATP concentration of 1.5 mM.

In vitro, however, when ATP levels in glucose-starved cells fall to below 0.1 to 0.2 mM, acylation of lysophosphatides ceases and cell lysophosphatidylcholine levels begin to rise. Gradually, as significant intramembranous lysophosphatidylcholine accumulates, cell shape distortion similar to that shown in Fig. 36-2 occurs, and echinocytes and spherocytes are produced, cell cation permeability increases, and finally, hemolysis ensues. These changes can be accelerated by artificially increasing the concentration of lysolecithin in the medium, which, by equilibration, increases the lysolecithin concentration in the membrane itself.

Lysophosphatidylcholine can also be used to form phosphatidylcholine without the addition of free fatty acid by a dismutation of two molecules of lysophosphatidylcholine to produce one molecule of phosphatidylcholine and one molecule of glycerophosphorylcholine (pathway 5*b*, Fig. 36-4). This reaction probably occurs preferentially at high lysophosphatidylcholine concentrations and at low pH, but is relatively less important under physiologic conditions [45].

Finally, membrane lysophosphatidylcholine can be directly detoxified by phospholipase B from the plasma, which can cleave the remaining fatty acid to produce free fatty acid and water-soluble glycerophosphorylcholine, which can rapidly return to the plasma (pathway 5*c*, Fig. 36-4) [31].

The acylation process described for the assembly of phosphatidylcholine from lysophosphatidylcholine and fatty acid (reaction 5*a*, Fig. 36-4) can also produce phosphatidylethanolamine from lysophosphatidylethanolamine (reaction 6*a*, Fig. 36-4). Since there is very little lysophosphatidylethanolamine in plasma, most of the precursor for this reaction must come from the cell itself. Some phosphatidylethanolamine is also produced by a transacylation of fatty acid from phosphatidylcholine to lysophosphatidylethanolamine (reaction 6*b*, Fig. 36-4) [46]. Both these reactions imply hydrolysis of a fatty acid from phosphatidylethanolamine and some findings suggest that there may be α-phospholipase activity in human red cells. Interestingly, this phospholipase activity may require the presence of the serum as well as the cells and hence may represent an incomplete enzyme which operates only at the surface of the cell. Alternatively, this process might operate only when the cell passes through an area of the microcirculation in which free phospholipase is present in the plasma (e.g., the spleen) [47,48].

Much of the free fatty acid incorporated into phosphatides can return to the plasma as free fatty acid (reactions 7*a* and 7*b*, Fig. 36-4) [29]. This process probably depends upon a membrane phospholipase of the type just noted or upon a plasma phospholipase that also operates at the surface of the red cell. The characterization of this process is presently incomplete.

Very small amounts of inorganic phosphates are directly incorporated into erythrocyte phospholipids. From studies with ^{32}P these appear to be primarily phosphatidic acid, phosphatidylserine, and phosphatidylinositol [49–51]. Incorporation of inorganic phosphate into phosphoethanolamine and other phospholipids has been found, but because of the extremely rapid incorporation of ^{32}P into white blood cells and platelets, the possibility that those results might be influenced by minor white cell or platelet contamination is very real. In any event, the extent of the exchange in acylation pathways is vastly in excess of any inorganic phosphorus incorporation [51], and it can be assumed that the great majority of lipid renewal is brought about by

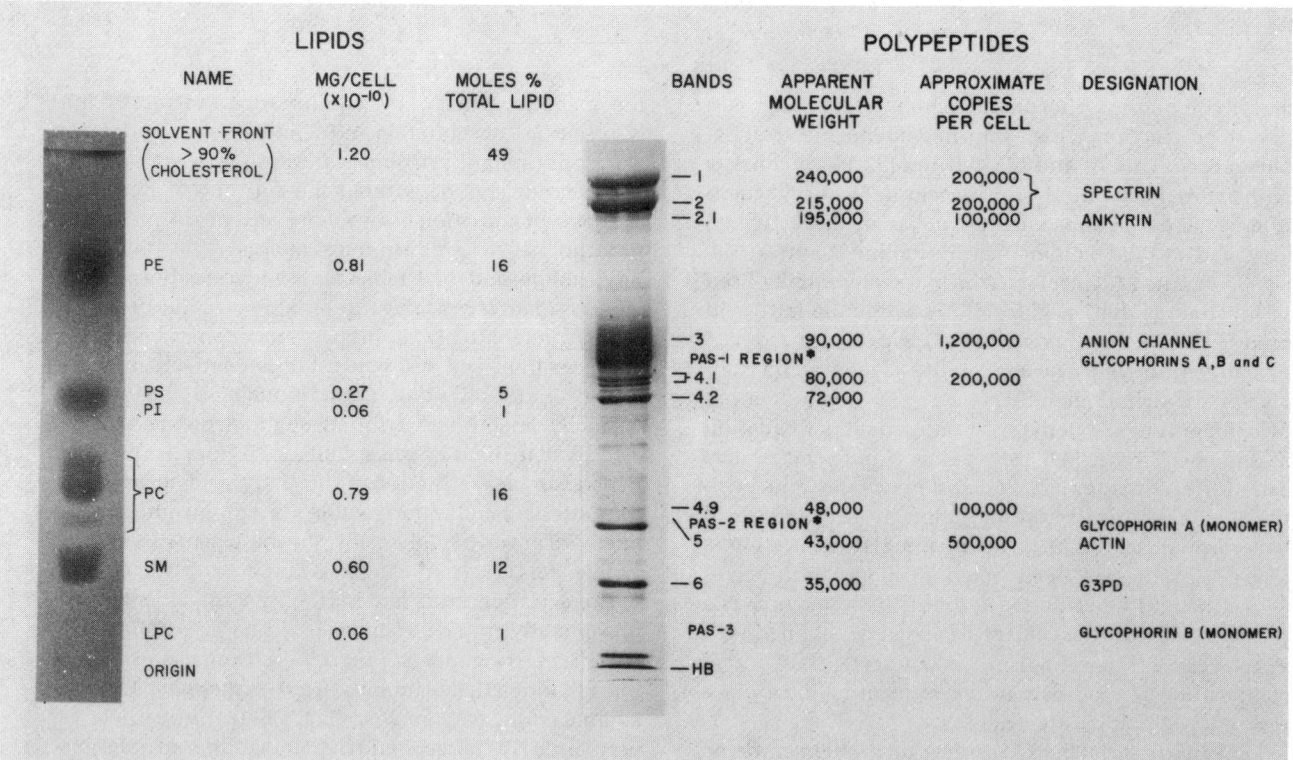

LIPIDS				POLYPEPTIDES			
	NAME	MG/CELL (×10⁻¹⁰)	MOLES % TOTAL LIPID	BANDS	APPARENT MOLECULAR WEIGHT	APPROXIMATE COPIES PER CELL	DESIGNATION
	SOLVENT FRONT (>90% CHOLESTEROL)	1.20	49	—1	240,000	200,000 ⎫	
				—2	215,000	200,000 ⎬	SPECTRIN
				—2.1	195,000	100,000	ANKYRIN
	PE	0.81	16				
				—3	90,000	1,200,000	ANION CHANNEL
				PAS-1 REGION*			GLYCOPHORINS A,B and C
	PS	0.27	5	⊐4.1	80,000	200,000	
	PI	0.06	1	—4.2	72,000		
	PC	0.79	16	—4.9	48,000	100,000	GLYCOPHORIN A (MONOMER)
				⟨PAS-2 REGION*			
				5	43,000	500,000	ACTIN
	SM	0.60	12	—6	35,000		G3PD
	LPC	0.06	1	PAS-3			GLYCOPHORIN B (MONOMER)
	ORIGIN			—HB			

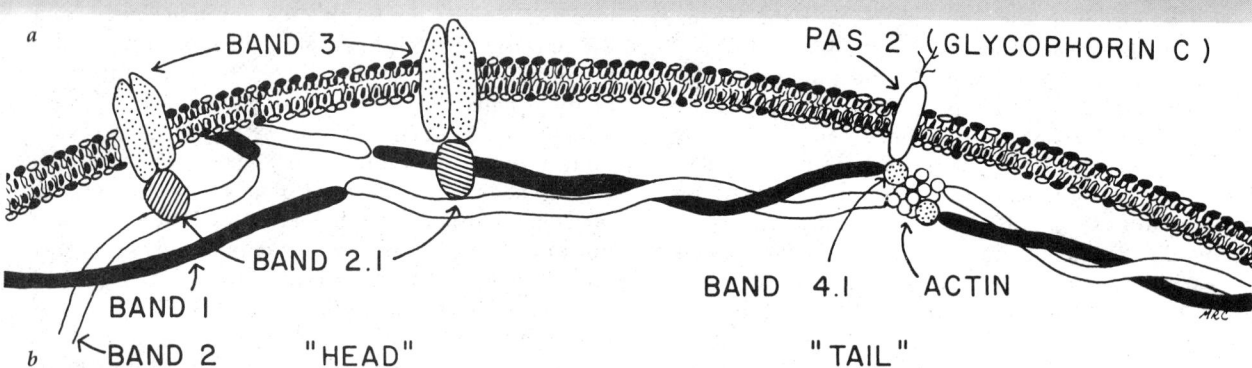

FIGURE 36-5 Current concepts of red cell membrane composition and organization. (*a*) Thin layer chromatogram of red cell membrane lipids (*left*) and Coomassie blue–stained SDS poly-acrylamide gel electrophoretogram of red cell membrane proteins (*right*). (*b*) Diagrammatic cross section of membrane bilayer and supporting "skeleton." The predominant protein of the membrane, spectrin, occurs as a heterodimer (bands 1 and 2) linked together into fibrous network. The linkage between the "tail," or amino, ends of the dimers appears to be mediated by actin (band 5) and band 4.1. Linkage between the "head," or carboxy, ends of the dimers occurs by direct contact between complimentary strands of the heterodimer. Attachment of the skeleton to the membrane is produced by a specific association between band 2 of spectrin and band 3 in the lipid bilayer via the spectrin-binding protein, band 2.1 (ankyrin), near the head end of the spectrin dimer. An additional association of the skeletal complex with the lipid bilayer may be provided by a connection between spectrin and another bilayer protein, PAS2 via band 4.1. Bands 2, 2.1, 3, and 4.1 can be phosphorylated, and some of that phosphorylation is cyclic AMP–dependent. The phosphorylation sites of spectrin band 2, which are not shown in this diagram, appear to be close to the end of the dimer. The outer leaflet of the bilayer is composed predominantly of choline-containing phospholipids (indicated by black head groups), and the inner leaflet is predominantly composed of acidic phospholipids, such as phosphatidylethanolamine and phosphatidylserine (indicated by white head groups). Cholesterol (indicated by black ovals) is shown embedded symmetrically in each leaflet among the fatty acid side groups of the phospholipid, although this has not yet been experimentally verified.

The PAS1 and PAS2 bands have been better defined by additional biochemical studies, including gel electrophoresis techniques with improved resolution. It is now known that the PAS1 region contains the dimer of the sialoglycopeptide glycophorin A and that the PAS2 region resolves into three bands: the dimer of glycophorin B ($M_r = 47,000$ daltons), the monomer of glycophorin A ($M_r = 38,000$ daltons), and glycophorin C, also called glyconnectin ($M_r = 35,000$ daltons). Unfortunately, there is not, as of yet, a universally accepted nomenclature for these PAS-staining sialoglycopeptides.

the two mechanisms of whole molecule exchange and fatty acid incorporation just described.

Thus, although the erythrocyte is incapable of *de novo* lipid synthesis, it is well endowed with mechanisms for lipid turnover and renewal, as well as mechanisms for lysophosphatide detoxification. These mechanisms are probably important for modulating red cell function and regulating red cell life-span.

Membrane proteins

Study of red cell membrane proteins has proved to be extraordinarily difficult because of their insolubility in aqueous media of physiologic ionic strength. Indeed, any membrane proteins which did not have such properties would be lost as membranes were washed in the course of preparing hemoglobin-free ghosts [52]. It is possible, however, to dissolve red cell membranes completely in sodium duodecyl sulfate and to accurately analyze protein subunits varying in size from the larger subunit of spectrin ($M_r = 240,000$ daltons) to traces of globin monomers ($M_r = 16,000$ daltons) with great sensitivity. The study of red cell membrane proteins has been appreciably advanced by the uniform numbering of such polypeptides [53] which most investigators now use (Fig. 36-5).

A variety of stratagems have been employed to deduce the relative positions of the various protein subunits in the membrane. For example, it has been possible to determine whether or not a human protein is exposed at the outer or the inner surface of the membrane by labeling membrane preparations on the inside or the outside with radioactive iodine using lactoperoxidase. Cross-linking studies have been employed to determine which proteins may be regarded as "neighbors." The fact that spectrin and actin (bands 1, 2, and 5) and band 4.1 play a major role in maintaining the shape of the erythrocyte may be deduced from the fact that ghosts of various poikilocytes extracted with nonionic detergents such as triton X100 maintain their initial shape [54]. These components of the membrane are sometimes designated as the "extrinsic" membrane proteins because they can be released from the membrane by treatment with very low ionic strength slightly alkaline solutions [53] without disrupting the lipid bilayer. In contrast, the "intrinsic" proteins of the membrane, those which are imbedded in the lipid bilayer, are removed only by detergent treatment.

Through these types of studies, the concept of a "membrane skeleton" of proteins which may have a role in modulating cell shape and deformability has emerged. This skeleton appears to be a moderately dense meshwork of interconnected extensive proteins immediately subjacent to the lipid bilayer. In this position it supports the bilayer and acts as a scaffolding for that otherwise weak and ephemeral structure. The strength of this skeleton appears to be primarily due to its predominant protein, spectrin, a long fiber-like molecule ideally suited to be the major structural element in

a network. The spectrin, which occurs as a heterodimer in solution and forms tetrameric or higher oligomeric associations in the membrane, is bound together into the network by two other proteins, red cell actin and band 4.1, which apparently facilitate its cross-linking. Importantly, the entire meshwork is then connected to the membrane bilayer by at least one additional linking protein, band 2.1, also called ankyrin or syndein. This protein, by binding to both spectrin and to the integral membrane protein, band 3, serves to "anchor" the membrane skeleton to the bilayer, forming the complete membrane unit. It has been proposed that this unique supporting structure may be responsible for some of the very unusual characteristics in the red cell membrane— in particular, its remarkable strength and flexibility.

The studies leading to this concept of a membrane skeleton have been reviewed [54,55], and the picture which has emerged is presented schematically in Fig. 36-5.

As might be expected, it now appears that a number of red cell morphologic abnormalities and hemolytic conditions may be associated with abnormalities in both the constituents of this newly defined structure and in their interactions. These abnormalities include deficiencies of particular proteins, such as spectrin, in a limited number of patients with hereditary spherocytosis [56] and perhaps in pyropoikilocytosis [57], as well as in murine models of spherocytosis [58,59]. In addition, deficiency of band 4.1 has been found in cases of severe, possibly homozygous, hereditary elliptocytosis [22,60,61], and deficiency of band 2.1, or ankyrin, has been found in a rare heat-sensitive fragmentation hemolytic anemia [62]. Possible conditions with qualitative abnormalities in the elements of this skeletal structure, or in their interactions, include abnormalities in spectrin:4.1 binding in other cases of hereditary spherocytosis [63,64] and probably abnormalities in spectrin:spectrin interactions in hereditary pyropoikilocytosis [57,65,66].

It seems likely that many additional abnormalities in the components and interactions of the membrane skeleton will be found when hemolytic disorders of the membrane are exhaustively examined. In fact, it may well be that the limited morphologic variations which we see in the clinical blood film in hemolytic anemia represent the final common pathway of many distinct and diverse biochemical abnormalities in this unusual membrane structure.

References

1. Magendie, F.: *Lectures on the Blood*. Haswell, Barrington, and Haswell, Philadelphia, 1839, p. 252.
2. Ways, P., and Hanahan, D. J.: Characterization and quantification of red cell lipids in normal man. *J. Lipid Res.* 5:318, 1964.
3. Kroes, J., and Ostwald, R.: Erythrocyte membranes: Effect of increased cholesterol content on permeability. *Biochim. Biophys. Acta* 249:647, 1971.
4. Cooper, R. A., Arner, E. C., Wiley, J. S., and Shattil, S.: Modification of red cell membrane structure by cholesterol-rich lipid dispersions: A model for the primary spur cell defect. *J. Clin. Invest.* 55:115, 1975.

5. Sweeley, C. C., and Dawson, G.: Lipids of the erythrocyte, in *Red Cell Membrane Structure and Function,* edited by G. A. Jamieson and T. J. Greenwalt. Lippincott, Philadelphia, 1969, p. 172.

6. McConnell, H. M., and McFarland, B. G.: The flexibility gradient in biological membranes. *Ann. N.Y. Acad. Sci.* 195:207, 1972.

7. Rothman, J. E., and Engleman, D. M.: Molecular mechanism for the interaction of phospholipid with cholesterol. *Nature [New Biol.]* 237:42, 1972.

8. Tarlov, A. R.: Lecithin and lysolecithin metabolism in rat erythrocyte membranes. *Blood* 28:990, 1966.

9. Reed, C. F.: Phospholipid exchange between plasma and erythrocytes in man and the dog. *J. Clin. Invest.* 47:749, 1968.

10. Gorter, E., and Grendel, F.: On biomolecular layer of lipoids on the chromocytes of the blood. *J. Exp. Med.* 41:439, 1925.

11. Danielli, J. F., and Davson, H.: A contribution to the theory of permeability of thin films. *J. Cell. Comp. Physiol.* 5:495, 1935.

12. Singer, S. J., and Nicolson, G. L.: The fluid mosaic model of the structure of cell membranes. *Science* 175:720, 1972.

13. Rand, R. P.: The structure of a model membrane in relation to the viscoelastic properties of the red cell membrane. *J. Gen. Physiol.* 52 (Suppl.):173, 1968.

14. Mohandas, N., Clark, M. R., Jacobs, M. S., and Shohet, S. B.: Analysis of factors regulating erythrocyte deformability. *J. Clin. Invest.* 66:563, 1980.

15. Bretscher, M.: Asymmetrical lipid bilayer structure for biological membranes. *Nature [New Biol.]* 236:11, 1972.

16. Gordesky, S. E., and Marinetti, G. V.: The asymmetric arrangement of phospholipids in the human erythrocyte membrane. *Biochem. Biophys. Res. Commun.* 50:1027, 1973.

17. Chiu, D., Lupin, B., and Shohet, S. B.: Erythrocyte membrane lipid reorganization during the sickling process. *Br. J. Haematol.* 41:223, 1979.

18. Lubin, B., Chiu, D., Bastacky, J., Roelofsen, B., and van Deenen, L. L. M.: Abnormalities in membrane phospholipid organization in sickled erythrocytes. *J. Clin. Invest.* 67:1643, 1981.

19. Zwaal, R. F., Comfurius, P., and van Deenen, L. L. M.: Membrane asymmetry and blood coagulation. *Nature* 268:358, 1977.

20. Pinto DaSilva, P.: Translational mobility of the membrane intercalated particles of human erythrocyte ghosts. *J. Cell. Biol.* 53:777, 1972.

21. Shohet, S. B.: Reconstitution of spectrin deficient spherocyte membranes. *J. Clin. Invest.* 64:483, 1979.

22. Tchernia, G., Mohandas, N., and Shohet, S. B.: Deficiency of skeletal protein band 4.1 in homozygous elliptocytosis: Implications for membrane stability. *J. Clin. Invest.* 68:454, 1981.

23. Bennett, V., and Stenbuck, P. J.: Identification and purification of ankyrin, the high affinity attachment site for human erythrocyte spectrin. *J. Biol. Chem.* 254:2533, 1979.

24. Mueller, T. J., and Morrison, M.: Glycoconnectin (PAS 2'), a component of the cytoskeleton of the human erythrocyte membrane. *J. Cell Biol.* 87:202a, 1980.

25. Haest, C. W. M., Plasa, G., Kamp, D., and Deutricke, B.: Spectrin as a stabilizer of the phospholipid asymmetry in the human erythrocyte membrane. *Biochim. Biophys. Acta* 509:21, 1978.

26. Mombers, C., De Gier, J., Demel, R. A., and van Deenen, L. L. M.: Spectrin-phospholipid interaction. A monolayer study. *Biochim. Biophys. Acta* 603:52, 1980.

27. Pittman, J. G., and Martin, D. B.: Fatty acid biosynthesis in human erythrocytes: Evidence in mature erythrocytes for an incomplete long chain fatty acid synthesizing system. *J. Clin. Invest.* 45:165, 1966.

28. Sakagami, T., Minari, O., and Orii, T.: Behavior of plasma lipoproteins during exchange of phospholipids between plasma and erythrocytes. *Biochim. Biophys. Acta* 98:111, 1965.

29. Shohet, S. B.: Release of phospholipid fatty acid from human erythrocytes. *J. Clin. Invest.* 49:1668, 1970.

30. De Gier, J., and van Deenan, L. L. M.: A dietary investigation on the variations in phospholipid characteristics of red-cell membranes. *Biochim. Biophys. Acta* 84:294, 1964.

31. Mulder, E., van den Berg, J. W. O., and van Deenen, L. L. M.: Metabolism of red-cell lipids. II. Conversions of lysophosphoglycerides. *Biochim. Biophys. Acta* 106:118, 1965.

32. Switzer, S., and Eder, H. A.: Transport of lysolecithin by albumin in human and rat plasma. *J. Lipid Res.* 6:506, 1965.

33. Shohet, S. B., Nathan, D. G., et al.: Stages in the incorporation of fatty acids into red blood cells. *J. Clin. Invest.* 47:1096, 1968.

34. Goodman, D. S.: The interaction of human erythrocytes with sodium palmitate. *J. Clin. Invest.* 37:1729, 1958.

35. McLeod, M. E., and Bressler, R.: Some aspects of phospholipid metabolism in the red cell. *Biochim. Biophys. Acta* 144:391, 1967.

36. Oliveira, M. M., and Vaughan, M.: Incorporation of fatty acids into phospholipids of erythrocyte membranes. *J. Lipid Res.* 5:156, 1964.

37. Waku, K., and Lands, W. E. M.: Control of lecithin biosynthesis in erythrocyte membranes. *J. Lipid Res.* 9:12, 1968.

38. Mulder, E., and van Deenen, L. L. M.: Metabolism of red-cell lipids. I. Incorporation *in vitro* of fatty acids into phospholipids from mature erythrocytes. *Biochim. Biophys. Acta* 106:106, 1965.

39. Lubin, B. H., Shohet, S. B., and Nathan, D. G.: Changes in fatty acid metabolism after erythrocyte peroxidation: Stimulation of a membrane repair process. *J. Clin. Invest.* 51:338, 1972.

40. Ferber, K., Krüger, J., Munder, P. G., Kohlschütter, A., and Fischer, H.: Acyltransferase und Lysophospholipase-Aktivität in Membranen von Erythrocyten während der Alterung *in vivo* und *in vitro*, in *Metabolism and Membrane Permeability of Erythrocytes and Thrombocytes*, edited by E. Deutch, E. Gerlach, and K. Moser. Thieme, Stuttgart, 1969, p. 393.

41. Winterbourn, C. C., and Batt, R. D.: The uptake of plasma fatty acids into human red cells and its relationship to cell age. *Biochim. Biophys. Acta* 202:9, 1970.

42. van Gastel, C., van den Berg, D., de Gier, H., and van Deenen, L. L. M.: Some lipid characteristics of normal red blood cells of different age. *Br. J. Haematol.* 11:193, 1965.

43. Phillips, G. B., Dodge, J. T., and Howe, C.: The effect of aging of human red cells *in vivo* on their fatty acid composition. *Lipids* 4:544, 1969.

44. Renooij, W., van Golde, L. M. G., Zwaal, R. F. A., Roelofsen, B., and van Deenen, L. L. M.: Preferential incorporation of fatty acids at the inside of human erythrocyte membranes. *Biochim. Biophys. Acta* 363:287, 1974.

45. Erbland, J. F., and Marinetti, G. V.: The enzymatic acylation and hydrolysis of lysolecithin. *Biochim. Biophys. Acta* 106:128, 1965.

46. Shohet, S. B.: The apparent transfer of fatty acid from phosphatidylcholine to phosphatidylethanolamine in human erythrocytes. *J. Lipid Res.* 12:139, 1971.

47. Gallai-Hatchard, J. J., and Thompson, R. H.: Phospholipase-A activity of mammalian tissue. *Biochim. Biophys. Acta* 98:128, 1965.

48. Weiss, L.: Personal communication.

49. Reed, C. F.: Incorporation of orthophosphate-^{32}P into erythrocyte phospholipids in normal subjects and in patients with hereditary spherocytosis. *J. Clin. Invest.* 47:2630, 1968.

50. Grossman, C. M., Horky, J., and Kohn, R.: *In vitro* incorporation of ^{32}P orthophosphate into phosphatidyl ethanolamine and other phosphatides by mature human erythrocyte ghosts. *Arch. Biochem. Biophys.* 117:18, 1966.

51. Shohet, S. B., and Nathan, D. G.: Incorporation of phosphatide precursors from serum into erythrocytes. *Biochim. Biophys. Acta* 202:202, 1970.

52. Dodge, J. T., Mitchell, C., and Hanahan, D. J.: The preparation and chemical characteristics of hemoglobin-free ghosts of human erythrocytes. *Arch. Biochem. Biophys.* 100:119, 1963.

53. Fairbanks, G., Steck, T. L., and Wallach, D. F. H.: Electrophoretic analysis of the major polypeptides of the human erythrocyte membrane. *Biochemistry* 10:2606, 1971.

54. Lux, S. E.: Spectrin-actin membrane skeleton of normal and abnormal red blood cells. *Semin. Hematol.* 16:21, 1979.

55. Branton, D., Cohen, C. M., and Tyler, J.: Interaction of cytoskeletal proteins on the human erythrocyte membrane. *Cell* 24:24, 1981.

56. Agre, P., Orringer, E. P., and Bennett, V.: Deficient red cell spectrin in severe, recessively inherited spherocytosis. *N. Engl. J. Med.* 306:1115, 1982.

57. Palek, J., Liu, S. C., Prchal, J., and Castleberry, R. P.: Altered assembly of spectrin in red cell membranes in hereditary pyropoikilocytosis. *Blood* 57:130, 1981.

58. Shohet, S. B.: Reconstitution of spectrin deficient spherocyte membranes. *J. Clin. Invest.* 64:483, 1979.

59. Lux, S. E., Pease, B., Tomaselli, M. B., John, K. M., and Bernstein, S. E.: Hemolytic anemias associated with deficient dysfunctional spectrin, in *Normal and Abnormal Red Cell Membranes*, edited by S. E. Lux, V. T. Marchesi, and C. G. Fox. Liss, New York, 1979, pp. 463–469.

60. Feo, C. J., Fischer, S., Piau, J. P., Grange, M. J., and Tchernia, G.: Première observation de l'absence d'une proteine de la membrane erythrocytaire (bande 4-1) dans un cas d'anémie elliptocytaire familiale. *Nouv. Rev. Fr. Hematol.* 22:315, 1980.

61. Mueller, T. J., and Morrison, M.: *Erythrocyte Membranes 2: Recent Clinical and Experimental Advances.* Liss, New York, 1981, pp. 95–112.

62. Agre, P., Orringer, E. P., Chui, D. H. K., and Bennett, V.: A molecular defect in two families with hemolytic poikilocytic anemia. *J. Clin. Invest.* 68:1566, 1981.

63. Goodman, S. R., Shiffer, K. A., Casoria, L. A., and Eyster, M. E.: Identification of the molecular defect in the erythrocyte membrane skeleton of some kindreds with hereditary spherocytosis. *Blood* 60:772, 1982.

64. Wolfe, L. C., John, K. M., Falcone, J., and Lux, S. E.: Identification of the molecular defect in some kindreds with hereditary spherocytosis (HS): Defective binding of protein 4.1 by HS spectrin. *Blood* (Suppl. 1):50a, 1981 (abstract).

65. Chang, K., Williamson, J. R., and Zarkowsky, H. S.: Altered circular dichroism of spectrin in hereditary pyropoikilocytosis. *J. Clin. Invest.* 64:326, 1979.

66. Knowles, W. J., and Marchesi, V. T.: Analysis of structural changes in human erythrocyte spectrin. *Fed. Proc.* 41:512, 1982 (abstract).

CHAPTER 37

Structure and function of hemoglobin

HELEN M. RANNEY
VIJAY S. SHARMA

Many of the properties of hemoglobin that make it an ideal oxygen transporter were defined at the beginning of this century by the physiologists Haldane, Krogh, Bohr, and Bancroft. It was not until the latter part of the century, however, that the structural basis of these properties began to be delineated. The development of protein chemistry, the all-important applications of the techniques of x-ray crystallography [1], and studies of the kinetics of reactions of hemoglobin with ligands [2] have not only defined the structure of hemoglobin but have also indicated the roles of different parts of the hemoglobin molecule in the oxygen-transport function [3]. The concentration of hemoglobin within human red cells is extraordinarily high (34 g/dl), and its efficiency as an oxygen carrier is enhanced by its packaging in flexible (red) cells of optimal shape for the diffusion of gases.

Structure of hemoglobin

Normal mammalian hemoglobins contain two pairs of chains: α-like and non-α (β, γ, or δ). The α-like chains of all the hemoglobins encountered after early embryogenesis are the same: in early embryos an embryonic chain, ζ, resembles the adult α chain. The non-α chains include the β chain of normal adult hemoglobin (Hb A = $\alpha_2\beta_2$), the γ chain of fetal hemoglobin (Hb F = $\alpha_2\gamma_2$), and the δ chain of hemoglobin A_2 (Hb A_2 = $\alpha_2\delta_2$), the minor component which accounts for 2.5 percent of the hemoglobin of normal adults. A β-like chain, the ϵ chain is found in early embryos.

The amino acid sequence determines the structure of hemoglobin, and some of the residues appear to be critical to the stability and function of the molecule. Such residues are likely to be the same (invariant residues) in chains of a given type (α or β). The NH_2-terminal valines of the β chains are important in 2,3-DPG interactions and the C-terminal residues are important in the salt bridges of the unliganded molecules. Areas of contact between chains and heme-globin contacts tend to contain invariant residues. Unlike many proteins, native hemoglobin contains no disulfide bonds. Of its six —SH groups (cysteine residues $\alpha104$, $\beta93$, and $\beta112$), two are buried and only $\beta93$ is free (available to the solvent).

PRIMARY STRUCTURE OF THE HEMOGLOBIN SUBUNITS (Table 37-1)

The α-polypeptide chain is 141 amino acids in length. The NH_2 termini are $\alpha1$ valine and $\alpha2$ leucine, and the C termini are $\alpha140$ tyrosine and $\alpha141$ arginine. The α and ζ chains lack the residues of the D helix (of the β chains) and are shorter by five residues than the β chain. While the locus determining the synthesis of α chains is duplicated, all α chains have the same amino acid sequence. Isolated α chains form monomers or dimers and are unstable. They are not found in appreciable quantities even in β thalassemia probably because as free chains they undergo proteolysis within red cells.

The β chain is 146 amino acids in length, beginning with valine and histidine at the NH_2 terminus. The C-terminal residues are $\beta145$ tyrosine and $\beta146$ histidine. The δ chain differs from the β chain in only 10 residues: the eight residues at the NH_2 terminus and C-terminal residues 127 to 146 are the same in δ or β chains. Tetramers of β chains (β_4 = Hb H) may be found in α thalassemia in amounts ranging from traces to 30 percent of the total hemoglobin.

The γ chain of fetal hemoglobin differs from the β chain by 39 residues. Unlike the other chains, its NH_2-terminus is glycine: the C-terminal residues (145 and 146), tyrosine and histidine, are the same as in β or δ chains. Appreciable quantities of γ chains are found in the red cells, particularly in those of infants with α thalassemia. The γ chains form tetramers, γ_4 or Hb$_{Bart's}$.

TABLE 37-1   Primary structure of human globin subunits

Helix	α	ζ	Helix	β	δ	γ	ε
NA1	1 Val		NA1	1 Val	Val	Gly	Val
			NA2	2 His	His	His	His
NA2	2 Leu		NA3	3 Leu	Leu	Phe	Phe
A1	3 Ser		A1	4 Thr	Thr	Thr	Thr
A2	4 Pro		A2	5 Pro	Pro	Glu	Ala
A3	5 Ala		A3	6 Glu	Glu	Glu	Glu
A4	6 Asp		A4	7 Glu	Glu	Asp	Glu
A5	7 Lys		A5	8 Lys	Lys	Lys	Lys
A6	8 Thr	(Thr	A6	9 Ser	Thr	Ala	Ala
A7	9 Asn	Ser	A7	10 Ala	Ala	Thr	Ala
A8	10 Val	Leu	A8	11 Val	Val	Ile	Val
A9	11 Lys	Lys)	A9	12 Thr	Asn	Thr	Thr
A10	12 Ala	(Asn	A10	13 Ala	Ala	Ser	Ser
A11	13 Ala	Ala	A11	14 Leu	Leu	Leu	Leu
A12	14 Try	Try	A12	15 Try	Try	Try	Try
A13	15 Gly	Gly	A13	16 Gly	Gly	Gly	Ser
A14	16 Lys	Lys)	A14	17 Lys	Lys	Lys	Lys
A15	17 Val	(Ile	A15	18 Val	Val	Val	Met
A16	18 Gly	Ser					
AB1	19 Ala	Thr					
B1	20 His	Asp	B1	19 Asn	Asn	Asn	Asn
B2	21 Ala	Thr	B2	20 Val	Val	Val	Val
B3	22 Gly	Thr	B3	21 Asp	Asp	Glu	Glu
B4	23 Glu	Glu	B4	22 Glu	Ala	Asp	Glu
B5	24 Tyr	Ile	B5	23 Val	Val	Ala	Ala
B6	25 Gly	Gly	B6	24 Gly	Gly	Gly	Gly
B7	26 Ala	Thr	B7	25 Gly	Gly	Gly	Gly
B8	27 Glu	Glu	B8	26 Glu	Glu	Glu	Glu
B9	28 Ala	Ala	B9	27 Ala	Ala	Thr	Ala
B10	29 Leu	Leu	B10	28 Leu	Leu	Leu	Leu
B11	30 Glu	Glu	B11	29 Gly	Gly	Gly	Gly
B12	31 Arg	Arg)	B12	30 Arg	Arg	Arg	Arg
B13	32 Met	(Leu	B13	31 Leu	Leu	Leu	Leu
B14	33 Phe	His	B14	32 Leu	Leu	Leu	Leu
B15	34 Leu	Leu	B15	33 Val	Val	Val	Val
B16	35 Ser	Ser	B16	34 Val	Val	Val	Val
C1	36 Phe	Phe	C1	35 Tyr	Tyr	Tyr	Tyr
C2	37 Pro	Pro	C2	36 Pro	Pro	Pro	Pro
C3	38 Thr	Thr	C3	37 Trp	Trp	Trp	Trp
C4	39 Thr	Gln	C4	38 Thr	Thr	Thr	Thr
C5	40 Lys	Lys)	C5	39 Gln	Gln	Gln	Gln
C6	41 Thr		C6	40 Arg	Arg	Arg	Arg
C7	42 Tyr		C7	41 Phe	Phe	Phe	Phe
CE1	43 Phe		CD1	42 Phe	Phe	Phe	Phe
CE2	44 Pro		CD2	43 Glu	Glu	Asp	Asp
CE3	45 His		CD3	44 Ser	Ser	Ser	Ser
CE4	46 Phe		CD4	45 Phe	Phe	Phe	Phe
			CD5	46 Gly	Gly	Gly	Gly
CE5	47 Asp	(Leu	CD6	47 Asp	Asp	Asn	Asn
CE6	48 Leu	Leu	CD7	48 Leu	Leu	Leu	Leu
CE7	49 Ser	Ser	CD8	49 Ser	Ser	Ser	Ser
CE8	50 His		D1	50 Thr	Ser	Ser	Ser
			D2	51 Pro	Pro	Ala	Pro
			D3	52 Asp	Asp	Ser	Ser
			D4	53 Ala	Ala	Ala	Ala
			D5	54 Val	Val	Ile	Ile
			D6	55 Met	Met	Met	Leu
CE9	51 Gly	Gly	D7	56 Gly	Gly	Gly	Gly
E1	52 Ser	Phe	E1	57 Asn	Asn	Asn	Asn
E2	53 Ala	Ala	E2	58 Pro	Pro	Pro	Pro
E3	54 Gln	His	E3	59 Lys	Lys	Lys	Lys
E4	55 Val	Val	E4	60 Val	Val	Val	Val

TABLE 37-1 **Primary structure of human globin subunits** *(Continued)*

Helix	α		ζ	Helix	β	δ	γ	ε
E5	56	Lys	Lys)	E5	61 Lys	Lys	Lys	Lys
E6	57	Gly	(Ala	E6	62 Ala	Ala	Ala	Ala
E7	58	His	His	E7	63 His	His	His	His
E8	59	Gly	Gly	E8	64 Gly	Gly	Gly	Gly
E9	60	Lys	Ser	E9	65 Lys	Lys	Lys	Lys
E10	61	Lys	Lys)	E10	66 Lys	Lys	Lys	Lys
E11	62	Val	(Val	E11	67 Val	Val	Val	Val
E12	63	Ala	Ala	E12	68 Leu	Leu	Leu	Leu
E13	64	Asp	Glu	E13	69 Gly	Gly	Thr	Thr
E14	65	Ala	Ala	E14	70 Ala	Ala	Ser	Ser
E15	66	Leu	Leu	E15	71 Phe	Phe	Leu	Phe
E16	67	Thr	Thr	E16	72 Ser	Ser	Gly	Gly
E17	68	Asn	Ser	E17	73 Asp	Asp	Asp	Asp
E18	69	Ala	Ile	E18	74 Gly	Gly	Ala	Ala
E19	70	Val	Leu	E19	75 Leu	Leu	Ile	Thr,Ile
E20	71	Ala	Gly	E20	76 Ala	Ala	Lys	Lys
EF1	72	His	Pro	EF1	77 His	His	His	Asn
EF2	73	Val	Val	EF2	78 Leu	Leu	Leu	Met
EF3	74	Asp	Asp	EF3	79 Asp	Asp	Asp	Asp
EF4	75	Asp	Ser	EF4	80 Asn	Asn	Asp	Asn
EF5	76	Met	Phe	EF5	81 Leu	Leu	Leu	Leu
EF6	77	Pro	Lys)	EF6	82 Lys	Lys	Lys	Lys
EF7	78	Asn	(Asn	EF7	88 Gly	Gly	Gly	Pro
EF8	79	Ala	Ala	EF8	84 Thr	Thr	Thr	Ala
F1	80	Leu	Val	F1	85 Phe	Phe	Phe	Phe
F2	81	Ser	Gly	F2	86 Ala	Ser	Ala	Ala
F3	82	Ala	Ala	F3	87 Thr	Gln	Gln	Lys
F4	83	Leu	Leu	F4	88 Leu	Leu	Leu	Leu
F5	84	Ser	Ser	F5	89 Ser	Ser	Ser	Ser
F6	85	Asp	Glu	F6	90 Glu	Glu	Glu	Glu
F7	86	Leu	Val	F7	91 Leu	Leu	Leu	Leu
F8	87	His	His	F8	92 His	His	His	His
F9	88	Ala	Ala	F9	93 Cys	Cys	Cys	Cys
FG1	89	His	Lys)	FG1	94 Asp	Asp	Asp	Asp
FG2	90	Lys	(Ile	FG2	95 Lys	Lys	Lys	Lys
FG3	91	Leu	Leu	FG3	96 Leu	Leu	Leu	Leu
FG4	92	Arg	Arg)	FG4	97 His	His	His	His
FG5	93	Val		FG5	98 Val	Val	Val	Val
G1	94	Asp		G1	99 Asp	Asp	Asp	Asp
G2	95	Pro		G2	100 Pro	Pro	Pro	Pro
G3	96	Val		G3	101 Glu	Glu	Glu	Glu
G4	97	Asn		G4	102 Asn	Asn	Asn	Asn
G5	98	Phe		G5	103 Phe	Phe	Phe	Phe
G6	99	Lys		G6	104 Arg	Arg	Lys	Lys
G7	100	Leu	(Ala	G7	105 Leu	Leu	Leu	Leu
G8	101	Leu	Leu	G8	106 Leu	Leu	Leu	Leu
G9	102	Ser	Ser	G9	107 Gly	Gly	Gly	Gly
G10	103	His	His	G10	108 Asn	Asn	Asn	Asn
G11	104	Cys	Cys	G11	109 Val	Val	Val	Val
G12	105	Leu	Leu	G12	110 Leu	Leu	Leu	Met
G13	106	Leu	Gly	G13	111 Val	Val	Val	Val
G14	107	Val	Lys)	G14	112 Cys	Cys	Thr	Ile
G15	108	Thr	(Ser	G15	113 Val	Val	Val	Ile
G16	109	Leu	Leu	G16	114 Leu	Leu	Leu	Leu
G17	110	Ala	Glx	G17	115 Ala	Ala	Ala	Ala
G18	111	Ala	Ala	G18	116 His	Arg	Ile	Thr
G19	112	His	His	G19	117 His	Asn	His	His
GH1	113	Leu	Leu	GH1	118 Phe	Phe	Phe	Phe
GH2	114	Pro	Tyr)	GH2	119 Gly	Gly	Gly	Gly
GH3	115	Ala	(Ala	GH3	120 Lys	Lys	Lys	Lys
GH4	116	Glu	Glx	GH4	121 Glu	Glu	Glu	Glu
GH5	117	Phe	Phe	GH5	122 Phe	Phe	Phe	Phe

TABLE 37-1   Primary structure of human globin subunits *(Continued)*

Helix	α	ζ	Helix	β	δ	γ	ε
H1	118 Thr	Thr	H1	123 Thr	Thr	Thr	Thr
H2	119 Pro	Ile	H2	124 Pro	Pro	Pro	Pro
H3	120 Ala	Gly	H3	125 Pro	Gln	Glu	Glu
H4	121 Val	Val	H4	126 Val	Met	Val	Val
H5	122 His	Asx	H5	127 Gln	Gln	Gln	Gln
H6	123 Ala	Ala	H6	128 Ala	Ala	Ala	Ala
H7	124 Ser	Ser	H7	129 Ala	Ala	Ser	Ala
H8	125 Leu	Leu	H8	130 Tyr	Tyr	Trp	Trp
H9	126 Asp	Asp	H9	131 Gln	Gln	Gln	Gln
H10	127 Lys	Lys)	H10	132 Lys	Lys	Lys	Lys
H11	128 Phe	(Phe	H11	133 Val	Val	Met	Leu
H12	129 Leu	Leu	H12	134 Val	Val	Val	Val
H13	130 Ala	Ala	H13	135 Ala	Ala	Thr	Ser
H14	131 Ser	Ser	H14	136 Gly	Gly	Gly,Ala	Ala
H15	132 Val	Val	H15	137 Val	Val	Val	Val
H16	133 Ser	Ser	H16	138 Ala	Ala	Ala	Ala
H17	134 Thr	Thr	H17	139 Asn	Asn	Ser	Ile
H18	135 Val	Val	H18	140 Ala	Ala	Ala	Ala
H19	136 Leu	Leu	H19	141 Leu	Leu	Leu	Leu
H20	137 Thr	Glx	H20	142 Ala	Ala	Ser	Ala
H21	138 Ser	Ser	H21	143 His	His	Ser	His
HC1	139 Lys	Lys)	HC1	144 Lys	Lys	Arg	Lys
HC2	140 Tyr	(Tyr	HC2	145 Tyr	Tyr	Tyr	Tyr
HC3	141 Arg	Arg)	HC3	146 His	His	His	His

SOURCE: Adapted from Bunn et al. [3]. Sequence of ε chain is taken from nucleotide sequence [6].

In addition to the different NH_2-terminal residue, several other differences in primary structure between the γ and the β chains are noteworthy: the γ chain is the only nonembryonic chain that contains isoleucine (residues γ11, γ54, γ75, and γ116). Both hemoglobin F ($\alpha_2\gamma_2$) and Hb$_{Bart's}$ (γ_4) are more resistant to denaturation by alkali than are Hb A or Hb H. The increased alkali resistance has been attributed to the absence in the γ chain of two β-chain residues readily ionized and hydrated by alkali (β112 Cys and β130 Tyr) [3]; in γ chains, threonine is found at 112 and tryptophan at 130. The additional tryptophan at γ130 is also responsible for the increased absorption of Hb F or γ chains at 294 nm. Normal γ chains differ at residue 136: some have glycine ($^G\gamma$), and others have alanine ($^A\gamma$) [4].

These two types of γ chains $^G\gamma$ and $^A\gamma$ are determined by duplicated closely linked genes. A common γ-chain variant, Hb F$_{Sardinia}$, contains threonine instead of isoleucine at position 75 of the $^A\gamma$ chain.

EMBRYONIC CHAINS AND HEMOGLOBINS

Hemoglobins recovered from small fetuses (gestational age less than 3 months) indicate that during the time when erythropoiesis occurs in the yolk sac, unique embryonic hemoglobin chains [5] are made; the α-like ζ chain lacks the D helix. An embryonic non-α or ε chain [6] is also found (Table 37-1). A hemoglobin in which one type of chain is exclusively synthesized in embryos (ζ or ε) is designated as *embryonic*. Hemoglobins containing these embryonic chains have been designated Gower 1 ($\zeta_2\epsilon_2$), Gower 2 ($\alpha_2\epsilon_2$), and Portland ($\zeta_2\gamma_2$). In rare individuals with chromosomal abnormalities, embryonic hemoglobins have been demonstrated after birth, and the synthesis of embryonic hemoglobins has been induced in a human cultured cell line (K 562). Embryonic hemoglobins appear to function as oxygen-transport proteins with high oxygen affinity.

In *secondary structure*, about 75 percent of the amino acids are arranged in an α helix with 3.6 amino acids per turn. All the chains of hemoglobin (as well as myoglobin) that have been studied have similar helical content by physical measurements and by x-ray crystallography (Fig. 37-1). Eight helical areas, lettered A to H, occur in the β chains: the residues connecting two helical segments have the letters of the helices they connect. Thus residue EF3 is the third residue of the segment connecting the E and F helices, while residue F8 is the eighth residue of the F helix. When the chains are aligned according to helical designators, as in Table 37-1, the homology is readily seen. Residue F8 is the proximal heme-linked histidine of all the chains, while residue E7 is the histidine at the distal side of the heme.

POSTTRANSLATIONAL MODIFICATION OF HEMOGLOBIN

Several posttranslational modifications of hemoglobin have been observed. The NH_2-terminal residues of 10 to 20 percent of the γ chains of hemoglobin F are acetylated [7]. Acetylation of NH_2 terminals, catalyzed by an acetyltransferase enzyme with acetyl CoA as a substrate, occurs in many proteins, but in human hemoglobins it has been demonstrated only in a small fraction of the γ chains. The acetylation occurs during the synthesis of hemoglobin F, either in particular subsets of erythropoietic cells or at particular steps of maturation of erythroid cells [8]. The chromatographic fraction containing acetylated hemoglobin F is designated F_1, while the nonacetylated fraction is designated F_0.

Another posttranslational modification of hemoglobin which has commanded considerable clinical attention is the nonenzymatic glycosylation of human hemoglobin. A chromatographically separate component of normal hemoglobin, designated Hb A_{1c} [9], was found to be increased in patients with diabetes mellitus [10]. This component, which generally amounts to 4 to 6 percent of the hemoglobin, accumulates during the life-span of the red cell as glucose reacts with the NH_2-terminal valines of the β chain [11]. The initial Schiff base linkage between N-termini and glucose undergoes a rearrangement to a ketoamine linkage [12]. The observed proportions of hemoglobin A_{1c} depend both on the concentration of glucose and on the life-span of the red cells. Increases in proportions of hemoglobin A_{1c} to 2 to 4 times normal may be found in uncontrolled diabetes mellitus; the observed levels of hemoglobin A_{1c} correlate with the levels of blood sugar during the several weeks preceding the determination. Nonenzymatic glycosylation occurs at other sites (differing in vivo and in vitro); an additional 8 to 10 percent of hemoglobin is glycosylated at the NH_2 termini of the α chains or the ϵ-amino groups of lysines [13]. The hemoglobin glycosylated at the latter sites is not separated from the main hemoglobin (HbA_0) on chromatography.

Proteins other than hemoglobin are glycosylated to a greater extent in poorly regulated diabetes than in normals. The potential significance of excessive glycosylation in the complications of diabetes has led to the use of Hb A_{1c} measurements as an indication of the control of the blood sugar in diabetes.

A third posttranslational modification of hemoglobin has been noted recently in the carbamylation of hemoglobin in patients with elevated levels of urea nitrogen [14]. The significance of this reaction is not known, but since carbamylated hemoglobin co-chromatographs with Hb A_{1c}, it may be a source of spurious elevation of Hb A_{1c} levels.

THE TERTIARY STRUCTURE OF α AND β CHAINS [15–17]

The prosthetic group of hemoglobin is ferroprotoporphyrin IX. Its structure is shown in Fig. 37-2a. The heme group is located in a crevice between the E and F helices in each subunit of the molecule. The highly polar propionate side chains of the heme are on the surface of the molecule and at the physiologic pH these groups are ionized. The rest of the heme is located inside the molecule, where it is surrounded by nonpolar residues except for two histidines. The iron atom is linked by a coordinate bond to the imidazole nitrogen (N_ϵ) of histidine at position F8, also known as the *proximal* histidine. A second histidine residue (E7), termed

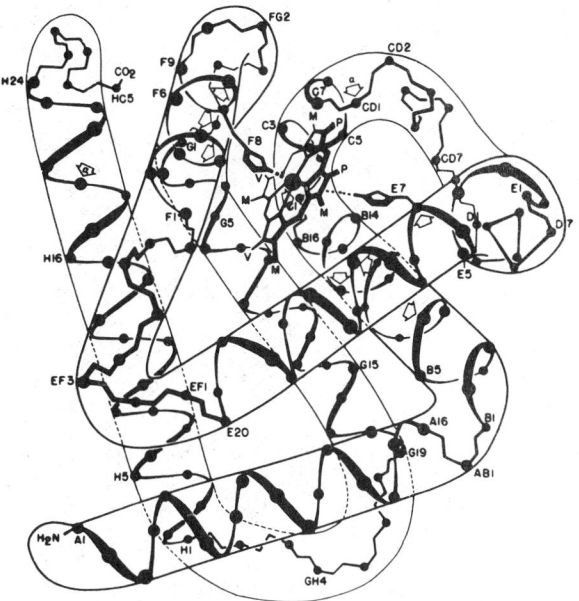

A

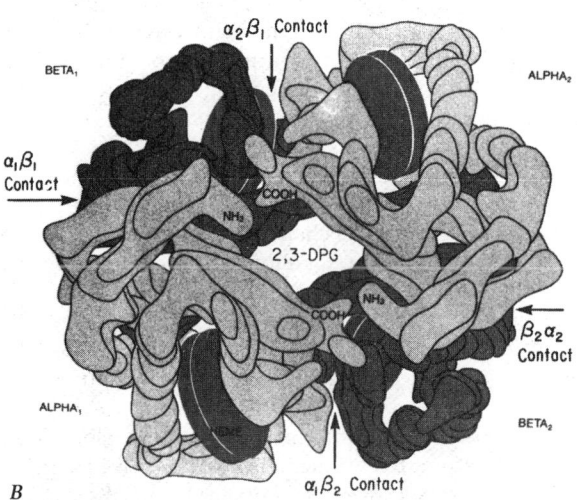

B

FIGURE 37-1 (*A*) The representation of the structure of β chains. Arrows indicate sites of substitutions in a number of unstable hemoglobins. (*B*) The hemoglobin molecule, as deduced from x-ray diffraction studies, shown from above. The molecule is comprised of four subunits: two identical α chains (*light blocks*) and two identical β chains (*dark blocks*). 2,3-DPG binds to the two β chains in the deoxyhemoglobin molecule.

the *distal* histidine, is located on the other side of the heme plane; this histidine is not bonded to Fe but is very close to the ligand-binding site.

The residues in contact with heme come from different segments of the linear sequence of amino acids: 42 to 136 in α chains and 41 to 141 in β chains. In both chains there is a preponderance of nonpolar residues in the immediate vicinity of heme. On the proximal side the important residues in contact with heme are Val

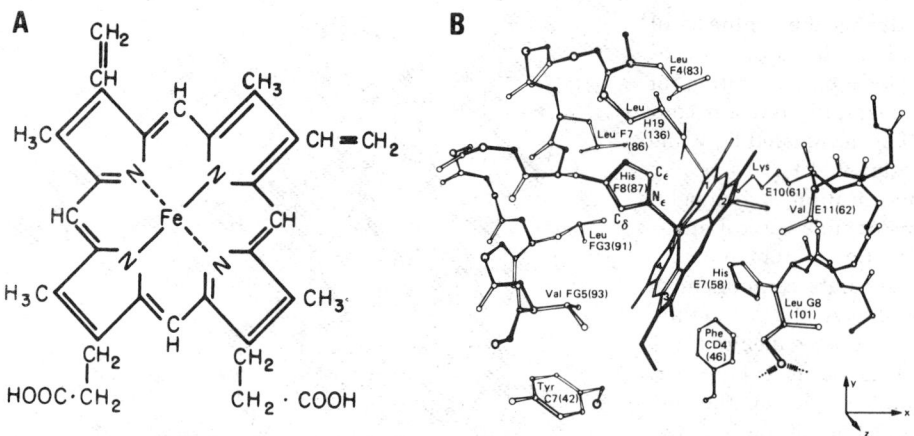

FIGURE 37-2 (*A*) Structure of heme (ferroprotoporphyrin IX). (*B*) Heme group and its environment in the unliganded α chain. Only selected side chains are shown: the heme 4-propionate is omitted. (Gelin and Karplus [18].)

FG5, Leu FG3, His F8, Leu F7, Leu H19, and Leu F4; on the distal side important heme-contacts are Phe CD4, His E7, Leu G8, Val E11, and Lys E10. The V produced by helices E and F provides the main walls of the heme pocket. Helices B, G, and H form the floor, and the segments C and CD guard the opening to this pocket. Important features of the heme pocket are:

1. The hydrophobic "cage" around the heme provides the main stabilizing force for the binding of heme to the protein. The side chains comprising the cage are closely packed and do not allow significant movement of the heme.

2. In a nonpolar environment it is much more difficult to oxidize Fe^{2+} to Fe^{3+}. This feature enables the heme to undergo reversible oxygenation without oxidation.

3. E11 Val. In β subunits of deoxyhemoglobin the methyl group of E11 valine is in van der Waal's contact with porphyrin. It overlaps the van der Waal's radii of heme ligand(s) (O_2, CO, and NO). This steric hindrance by E11 Val occurs to a much smaller extent in α chains [17].

4. Two atoms of the distal histidine (E7) are in van der Waal's contact with the porphyrin in both oxyhemoglobin and deoxyhemoglobin, and the imidazole N also overlaps with the heme-binding site. The histidine side chain also acts as a gate to the ligand-binding site, not allowing ligand to enter or leave unless it swings out of the way.

5. The hydrophobic residues in C and CD segments that guard the opening to the heme pocket effectively exclude polar ligands from entering the heme pocket.

6. The imidazole N of the proximal histidine is hydrogen-bonded to the carboxyl of Leu F4 and the OH of Ser F5. This hydrogen bonding and the neighboring side chains hold the proximal F8 His in position rather rigidly.

7. Both α and β hemes form about 75 contacts with 30 atoms in 16 globin residues in each heme pocket.

Although x-ray structure of deoxyhemoglobin is based on planar porphyrin with iron displaced 0.6 Å out of the plane in α chains and 0.63 Å in β chains, data on model compounds and considerations based on energy-minimized geometry suggest that the plane of pyrrole nitrogens might be displaced toward iron by 0.22 Å in α chains and by 0.17 Å in β chains as compared with the mean plane of the porphyrin carbons. The energy difference between the domed and the planar porphyrin structure is small. The iron atom in both deoxyhemoglobins and methemoglobins is high-spin, and it has been suggested that its ionic radius is too large to fit into the plane of the porphyrin ring. In both subunits of deoxyhemoglobin, the imidazole ring of the proximal histidine F8 is in an asymmetric position with respect to the porphyrin nitrogens of the heme, such that the atom C_ϵ is closer to porphyrin $N_{(1)}$ than C_δ is to $N_{(3)}$ [18] (Fig. 37-2*b*).

In both the α and β subunits of human deoxyhemoglobin, the ligand-binding site is blocked. In α subunits, a water molecule is attached to the distal histidine E7. There is no direct bond between the water molecule and the iron atom. In β chains, the methyl group of E11 lies within 1.8 Å of the ligand-binding site. Both these groups would have to move out of the way before the ligand could bind to iron [17].

THE QUATERNARY STRUCTURE [17]

In the deoxy state, the hemoglobin tetramer is held together by intersubunit salt bonds and intersubunit hydrophobic contacts, in addition to a certain number of hydrogen bonds.

1. The intersubunit salt bonds (Fig. 37-3). Four of these salt bonds involving Arg HC3(141) are between the two α chains. The two salt bonds involving His HC3(146) are between β and α chains. There are two intramolecular salt bonds in β chains [19].

2. The $\alpha_1\beta_1$ (or $\alpha_2\beta_2$) and $\alpha_1\beta_2$ (or $\alpha_2\beta_1$) subunit contacts (Fig. 37-1):

   a. $\alpha_1\beta_1$ Contact. This more extensive contact between α_1 and β_1 subunits involves 32 residues, including 126 atoms, 4 hydrogen bonds, and 1 solvent-mediated hydrogen bond.

   b. $\alpha_1\beta_2$ Contact. Slightly less extensive than the $\alpha_1\beta_1$ contacts, this contact involves 27 residues, including 107 atoms, 6 hydrogen bonds, and 3 solvent-mediated hydrogen bonds.

BINDING OF 2,3-DPG TO Hb TETRAMER (Fig. 37-1)

2,3-DPG is situated in the central cavity between the two β chains [20]. The phosphate groups form salt bonds with β N-terminal amino groups and the imidazoles of $\beta143$ histidine; the carboxyl groups bind to $\beta82$ lysine.

STRUCTURAL CHANGES THAT OCCUR ON LIGAND BINDING [21,22]

The changes that occur on going from the deoxy to the oxy structure are of two types: the tertiary structural changes within the subunits of $\alpha_1\beta_1$ (or $\alpha_2\beta_2$) dimer and a quaternary structure change in which the position of $\alpha_1\beta_1$ changes relative to $\alpha_2\beta_2$. The two structural changes are linked.

Iron-to-ligand bond formation would require moving the iron atom toward the heme plane. This would bring the C_ϵ atom of the proximal histidine too close to both porphyrin N_1 and C atoms in the pyrrole ring, producing large steric strain. The tertiary structural changes involving heme, proximal histidine, F helix, FG corner, and others all minimize the steric strain produced as a result of metal-to-ligand bond formation.

The most important of the tertiary structural changes seems to be the translation of the F helix approximately 1 Å across the heme plane, its tilting with respect to the heme, and the movement of heme and the FG corner toward the center of the molecule. This movement of the F helix takes the proximal histidine from its asymmetric position in deoxyhemoglobin to a more symmetric position in liganded hemoglobin. The motion of β hemes removes the ligand-binding site from the vicinity of Val $\beta E11$, which may hinder ligand binding in the deoxy state. These changes in the tertiary structure are linked to the quaternary changes through the motion of FG corners. The C helices and FG corners of the $\alpha_1\beta_1$ dimer are in contact with the FG corners and C helices of $\alpha_2\beta_2$ in both quaternary structures. The contacts between α_1FG and β_2C (and α_2FG and β_1C) act as "flexible joints" and undergo only small relative motions. The contacts between α_1C and β_2FG (and α_2C and β_1FG) act as switch regions that have two different stable positions. The change between the two stable positions involves a relative movement of approximately 6 Å.

QUATERNARY STRUCTURAL CHANGES [22]

The quaternary structural change that occurs on ligand binding to hemoglobin involves rotation of the $\alpha_2\beta_2$ dimer interface relative to the $\alpha_1\beta_1$ by 14.9 degrees and

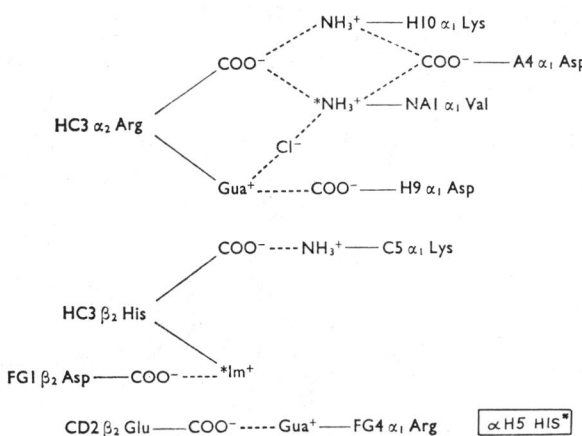

FIGURE 37-3   Salt bridges in deoxyhemogobin (* = ionizable group less protonated at pH 9.0 than at pH 7.0). These groups account for 60 percent of the alkaline Bohr effect. The remainder is due to α H5 HIS. (Perutz [19].)

translation of 0.8 Å. The overall number of intersubunit hydrogen bonds and intersubunit contacts may not change significantly, but they become less stringent.

The carboxy salt bridges involving Arg $\alpha141$(HC3) are not made in the quaternary liganded structure, because the space between $\alpha_1\beta_1$ and $\alpha_2\beta_2$ is too narrow for these residues to occupy the position they have in the deoxy quaternary state. The carboxy-terminal residues His $\beta146$(HC3) are separated from Lys $\alpha40$(C5), the group to which they are bonded in the deoxy state, by a 7-Å shift that occurs in these regions in the quaternary structural change.

The rotation and translation of the $\alpha_2\beta_2$ dimer with respect to the $\alpha_1\beta_1$ dimer mentioned earlier also renders the central cavity too small, especially the gap between the H helices of the β chains for the binding of 2,3-DPG of the two β chains. In addition, the distance between the α-amino groups increases from 16 to 20 Å, so they cannot bind to the phosphates of 2,3-DPG. All these structural changes cause expulsion of 2,3-DPG from the hemoglobin tetramer in the fully liganded hemoglobin (Fig. 37-1). The quaternary structures of unliganded and liganded hemoglobin are known as the *T-state* ("tense") and *R-state* ("relaxed") *structures*, respectively. The alternate terms are *low-affinity* and *high-affinity states* or *deoxy* and *oxy states*, respectively.

OXYGEN AFFINITY IN T AND R STRUCTURES

A recently proposed mechanism [22] takes into account the x-ray crystallographic data and calculations of energies associated with various structural changes that might occur at the heme on ligand binding [18,23,24]. The low affinity of deoxyhemoglobin for its first ligand appears to be due to the strain induced by the steric repulsion arising from the position of the F helix and, in particular, the position of the proximal histidine relative to the heme: the imidazole ring of each chain is tilted so that its interaction with porphyrin-ring carbons provides steric hindrance in iron-to-oxygen bond forma-

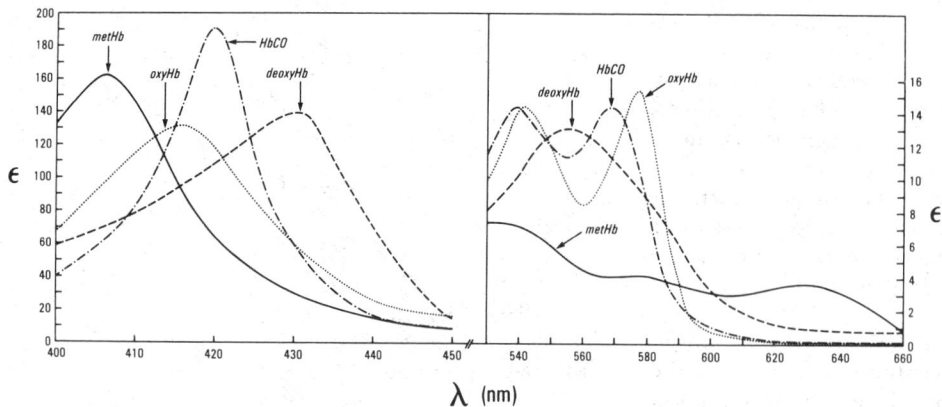

FIGURE 37-4   Spectra of some hemoglobin derivatives. Extinction coefficients plotted against wavelength (pH 7.4).

tion. Quaternary structural changes brought about by the tertiary structural changes via the changes at the intersubunit contacts (particularly at β_2FG-α_1C and β_1FG-α_2C) place the proximal histidine in a symmetric position with respect to the plane of the porphyrin ring and thus minimize the steric interaction between the imidazole (C_ϵ) and porphyrin N_1 and a carbon atom in the pyrrole-1 ring. In β subunits, an additional factor increases ligand affinities in the R state: the translational and rotational movements of β hemes remove the ligand-binding site from the vicinity of the E11 Val side chain.

Calculations [18,24] suggest that the geometry of the heme in deoxyhemoglobin may be very similar to that in isolated heme. If this is correct, then the iron atom in deoxyhemoglobin is in its optimal position for five coordinate high-spin Fe^{2+} ion, and there is little strain on the unliganded heme. Instead, the heme in the liganded subunit in the deoxy quaternary tetramer would be under strain.

THE TWO-STATE MODEL

The mechanisms of cooperative ligand binding by hemoglobin proposed by various workers must be regarded as tentative, since none of them is capable of explaining all physicochemical properties of hemoglobin even qualitatively. It is not clear in this mechanism at which point in ligation the transition from low-affinity (T) to high-affinity (R) structure takes place. An alternative approach is provided by a model [25] that considers the two species in equilibrium:

$$\mathrm{Hb}^T_4 \overset{LC^n}{\rightleftharpoons} \mathrm{Hb}^R_4$$

where n = number of ligands bound to Hb
$\quad L = (\mathrm{Hb}^T_4)/(\mathrm{Hb}^R_4)$
$\quad C = K_R/K_T$

K_R and K_T = the ligand-dissociation constants in the R and T state, respectively

Shift in the equilibrium between T and R species with fractional saturation could then account for the cooperative ligand binding and other features of the O_2 dissociation curve. The transitional point from T to R structure acquires a statistical meaning and is given by the equation

$$n_t = -\log L/\log C$$

where n_t = the number of ligands bound at the switchover point from T to R

Depending on the experimental conditions, the value of n_t for hemoglobin lies in the range of 2.3 to 3.0 [26].

METHEMOGLOBIN

Figure 37-4 shows the absorption spectra of deoxyhemoglobin, oxyhemoglobin, and carboxyhemoglobin. Hemoglobin with oxidized iron (i.e., Fe^{3+}) is known as *methemoglobin*. The spectra of O_2, CO, and deoxy derivatives are not affected by pH in the pH range from 6 to 9.5. The spectrum of methemoglobin is pH-dependent; at pH 7 and below, the spectrum of aquomethemoglobin with maximum at 630 nm is observed. At alkaline pH, the spectrum of hydroxymethemoglobin and disappearance of the λ maximum at 630 nm is seen. Methemoglobin solutions are believed to be equilibrium mixtures of quaternary R and T structures.

Oxygen equilibria of hemoglobin— the oxygen dissociation curve

Some of the important gas-transport properties of hemoglobin are evident from inspection of the oxygen dissociation curve (Fig. 37-5). First, the oxygen affinity increases with increasing oxygen saturation of the hemoglobin. Second, cooperative interactions describe the sigmoid shape of the oxygen dissociation curve, i.e., the change in oxygen affinity with increasing oxygen saturation. The term *heme-heme interaction* is also used to describe this increase in oxygen affinity. Third, the binding of more protons by deoxyhemoglobin than by oxyhemoglobin is known as the *Bohr effect*; it is reflected in the left shift of O_2 dissociation curves with increasing pH. These functional properties are interdependent or linked [28]; the O_2 affinity depends on the state of oxygenation (cooperative interactions) and on the pH (Bohr effect).

OXYGEN AFFINITY OF HEMOGLOBIN

The oxygen affinity of hemoglobin is usually expressed in terms of the P_{50}, the oxygen tension at which hemoglobin is half saturated. This value is 26 torr (mmHg) in normal red cells or concentrated hemolysates at 37°C and plasma pH of 7.4. (The pH of the interior of the red cell is about 0.2 units lower than the pH of the plasma.) The partial pressure of oxygen in room air is about 100 torr; in the pulmonary alveoli it is about 95 torr. Oxygen diffuses passively across the alveolar capillary membrane during the time (<1 s) that the red cell spends within the pulmonary vasculature. Desaturated blood from the bronchial (and other) veins returns to pulmonary veins, resulting in a P_{O_2} of about 90 torr in the left heart; i.e., systemic arterial blood is almost fully saturated with oxygen. As the blood traverses the systemic capillaries, the delivery of oxygen is determined by the P_{O_2} of the tissues. The steep portion of the oxygen dissociation curve allows a relatively large amount of oxygen to be unloaded for a small decrement in P_{O_2}. The P_{O_2} in the capillaries of different organs varies with oxygen consumption. Exercise, for example, leads to a marked decrease in P_{O_2} in muscles and in the blood of their efferent vessels.

The value of P_{50} is taken from the midpoint of the oxygen dissociation curve and does not reflect the shape of the curve. With increasing oxygen affinity, the value for P_{50} becomes smaller; i.e., the dissociation curve is "shifted to the left." High values for P_{50} indicates a lower oxygen affinity of the hemoglobin or red cells. Since hemoglobin is nearly fully saturated with oxygen at a P_{O_2} of 85 torr, a right shift in the dissociation curve will facilitate oxygen delivery: nearly full saturation will still occur in the lungs.

FACTORS THAT AFFECT OXYGEN AFFINITY

The three primary determinants of the value of P_{50} are temperature, pH, and red cell 2,3-DPG concentration. The increase in oxygen affinity with lower temperatures is observed in red cells or in hemoglobin solutions.

The Bohr effect, or the effect of hydrogen ions, is observed in red cells and hemoglobin solutions (see inset of Fig. 37-5). With increasing H^+ concentration (decreasing pH), P_{50} increases; i.e., oxygen affinity declines. Another way of looking at the Bohr effect is the observed increase in affinity of deoxyhemoglobin for protons, which makes a solution of oxyhemoglobin more acidic than a solution of deoxyhemoglobin. Pro-

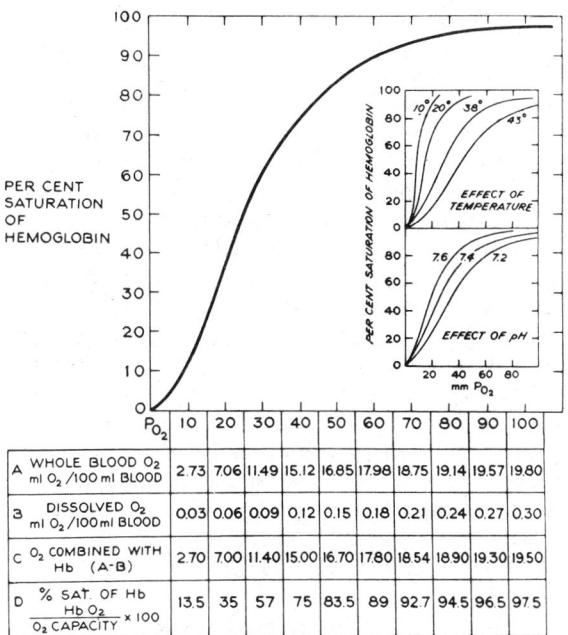

P_{O_2}		10	20	30	40	50	60	70	80	90	100
A	WHOLE BLOOD O_2 ml O_2 /100 ml BLOOD	2.73	7.06	11.49	15.12	16.85	17.98	18.75	19.14	19.57	19.80
B	DISSOLVED O_2 ml O_2/100 ml BLOOD	0.03	0.06	0.09	0.12	0.15	0.18	0.21	0.24	0.27	0.30
C	O_2 COMBINED WITH Hb (A-B)	2.70	7.00	11.40	15.00	16.70	17.80	18.54	18.90	19.30	19.50
D	% SAT. OF Hb $\frac{Hb\ O_2}{O_2\ CAPACITY} \times 100$	13.5	35	57	75	83.5	89	92.7	94.5	96.5	97.5

FIGURE 37-5 Oxygen dissociation curve of human hemoglobin. Inserts: Effect of temperature (*upper*) and Bohr effect (*lower*). (Comroe [27].)

tons stabilize the T state by stabilizing the intersubunit bonds and the bonds between the two β chains and 2,3-DPG; 2,3-DPG and other anions stabilize the T state by complexing preferentially with hemoglobin in this state. Both these factors shift T-to-R equilibrium toward the T (low-affinity) state.

The Bohr shift constitutes an important buffer system of the body. When blood reaches the tissues, where the oxygen tension is lower and the hydrogen ion concentration is increased by lactic acid or by carbon dioxide, the Bohr shift of the dissociation curve makes more oxygen available. As the hemoglobin loses its oxygen and the unliganded form binds protons, changes in hydrogen ion concentration are minimized. The proton binding of deoxyhemoglobin provides an important part of carbon dioxide transport: carbon dioxide diffuses into the red cell and its conversion there to bicarbonate is catalyzed by carbonic anhydrase. The bicarbonate ion leaves the red cell and the hydrogen ion is bound by deoxyhemoglobin. The ultimate effectiveness of this physiologic buffer system depends on the ease with which carbon dioxide or bicarbonate is retained or eliminated in the lungs and kidneys. The Bohr effect is also observed in the reactions of hemoglobin with ligands other than oxygen (e.g., carbon monoxide, ethyl isocyanide) and in the oxidation of hemoglobin to methemoglobin (the oxidation Bohr effect).

Carbon dioxide reacts with N-terminal residues of the β chains of hemoglobin to yield carbamino derivatives, a phenomenon separate from the Bohr effect. These carbamino derivatives are of minor importance in CO_2 transport by hemoglobins that bind DPG.

EFFECTS OF 2,3-DPG ON O_2 EQUILIBRIA

The usual P_{50} measurements are done under standard conditions of temperature, pH, and P_{CO_2}. Therefore, observed variations in the oxygen affinity are usually related to the concentration of 2,3-DPG [29] (normal value of 2,3-DPG is about 5 mmol/liter of packed red cells). The P_{50} of whole blood or of hemoglobin solutions increases with increasing concentrations of 2,3-DPG [29] (normal value of 2,3-DPG is about 5 mmol/liter of packed red cells). The relationship of 2,3-DPG and P_{50} is not linear—with higher concentrations, smaller increments in P_{50} are observed. In addition to its stabilization of the deoxy form of the tetramer, 2,3-DPG, because it is an impermeant anion, lowers intracellular pH relative to plasma pH. Other factors such as CO_2 in carbamino linkage and mean corpuscular hemoglobin concentration probably do not much affect the oxygen affinity under conditions encountered clinically, although the CO_2 effect is rather large when the P_{50} values at pH 7.2 are compared at P_{CO_2} ranging from 0 to 40.

Increases in P_{50} may be observed in acidosis, or in any state (anemia, hypoxia, ascent to high altitudes) in which 2,3-DPG is increased. A higher oxygen affinity (lower P_{50}) is seen in hemoglobins modified by treatment with a number of agents, including cyanate. The role of organic phosphates in regulating O_2 delivery to the tissues has provided an explanation for the finding that although the oxygen affinity of cord blood exceeds that of maternal blood, the O_2 affinity of "purified" Hb F does not differ greatly from that of Hb A. The oxygen affinity of phosphate-free Hb F is lower than that of Hb A, but the effect of 2,3-DPG on the O_2 affinity of Hb F is much less than that on adult hemoglobin [3]. The oxygen affinity of fetal blood is therefore higher than that of adult blood, permitting more complete extraction of oxygen from maternal blood in the placenta.

COOPERATIVE INTERACTIONS

The physiologic advantages which derive from the sigmoid shape of the oxygen dissociation curve are obvious from the data in Fig. 37-5. A fall in P_{O_2} from 100 to 60 torr results in a decline in O_2 saturation from 97.5 to 89 percent, while a fall from 60 to 20 torr will be accompanied by a decline in oxygen saturation from 89 to 35 percent and the release of more than 10 ml O_2 per 100 ml of blood to the tissues. The rather "flat" portion of the O_2 dissociation curve at P_{O_2} from 70 to 100 torr results in nearly complete saturation of hemoglobin, even at the lower partial pressures of oxygen found at high altitudes. The advantages of decreased oxygen affinity as a compensatory mechanism in hypoxemia obtain only if the sigmoid shape of the oxygen dissociation curve is preserved.

THE HILL PLOT

The plot of log $[y/(1-y)]$ against log P_{O_2} is known as the *Hill plot*. The Hill equation is:

$$\log [y/(1-y)] = \log K + n \log P_{O_2}$$

where y = fractional saturation with O_2

K = an empiric overall constant without physicochemical basis

The n value (the slope from the Hill plot at half saturation) is taken as a convenient measure of cooperativity. Values of n in noninteracting hemoglobins which exhibit hyperbolic oxygen dissociation curves (e.g., myoglobin or Hb H) are about 1. In a normal tetrameric hemoglobin with four oxygen-reactive sites, the maximum value for n would be 4.0; however, n values of 2.7 to 3.0 rather than 4.0 are encountered in normal hemoglobin.

KINETICS OF REACTIONS WITH LIGANDS

The reactions of hemoglobin with ligands are much faster than would be needed for reaction during transit in the microvasculature. The exception to this is the slow rate of dissociation of carbon monoxide and nitric oxide from hemoglobin, which results in the extremely high affinity of these ligands and prevents equilibration of CO- or NO-containing red cells with oxygen in the lungs. The O_2 dissociation curve does not reveal certain finer details of the overall reaction between hemoglobin and ligands (i.e., O_2, CO, or NO). These details can be observed when one considers the rates of ligand binding (the "on" rates) and the rates of ligand dissociation (the "off" rates) separately:

$$\text{Hb} + \text{L} \underset{\text{"off"}}{\overset{\text{"on"}}{\rightleftharpoons}} \text{HbL}$$

The stepwise binding of ligands to hemoglobin tetramer can be written in terms of the Adair four-step model [30]:

$$\text{Hb}_4 + \text{L} \underset{x_1}{\overset{x'_1}{\rightleftharpoons}} \text{Hb}_4\text{L} \qquad X_1 = \frac{x'_1}{x_1}$$

$$\text{Hb}_4\text{L} + \text{L} \underset{x_2}{\overset{x'_2}{\rightleftharpoons}} \text{Hb}_4\text{L}_2 \qquad X_2 = \frac{x'_2}{x_2}$$

$$\text{Hb}_4\text{L}_2 + \text{L} \underset{x_3}{\overset{x'_3}{\rightleftharpoons}} \text{Hb}_4\text{L}_3 \qquad X_3 = \frac{x'_3}{x_3}$$

$$\text{Hb}_4\text{L}_3 + \text{L} \underset{x_4}{\overset{x'_4}{\rightleftharpoons}} \text{Hb}_4\text{L}_4 \qquad X_4 = \frac{x'_4}{x_4}$$

The letter x (or x') in the preceding equations is a general symbol and is replaced by k, l, or j (or k', l', or j') when the ligand is O_2, CO, or NO, respectively. The letters K, L, and J are used for the corresponding equilibrium constants. The Adair reaction scheme contains eight constants: four stepwise "on" rate constants (x_1', ..., x_4') and four stepwise "off" rate constants (x_1, ..., x_4). The stepwise equilibrium and rate constants for the reactions of O_2, CO, and NO have been determined [31–33]. It should be noted, however, that because of the cooperative nature of reactions, the accurate determination of the intermediate equilibrium and rate constants is not easy, and therefore, constants for those two steps have a considerable degree of uncertainty.

The "on" reactions of O_2, CO, and NO with deoxyhemoglobin are strictly first-order in ligand and hemoglobin concentrations; hence, the overall reaction is second-order. The reaction rates accelerate as the reaction proceeds. The initial rates approximate the rate constant for the formation of the monoliganded species: Hb_4L [2]. Oxyhemoglobin and particularly carboxyhemoglobin are photosensitive, and each loses its ligand on exposure to light. This property has been used to study the rate constants for the formation of the fully liganded species. Five or less percent of ligand is removed from fully liganded hemoglobin using a flash of strong light, usually for 2 μs to 1.5 ms, and observing rates of subsequent ligand recombination with the triliganded species. As the percent photolysis of Hb_4L_4 is increased, the other intermediates, Hb_4L_2, Hb_4L, and Hb_4, are also formed and the reaction becomes heterogeneous. The CO recombination at 3°C and pH 9 after complete photolysis as a function of CO concentration has been found to occur as a biphasic reaction [34]. The fast component of this reaction is 40 times as rapid as that of ordinary deoxyhemoglobin. The hemoglobin responsible for the fast component has been designated Hb*, or the quickly reacting hemoglobin. It is proposed that Hb* is hemoglobin trapped in the high-affinity conformation. It was estimated that it decays into the regular deoxy conformation by a first-order process:

$$Hb^* \xrightarrow{200 \text{ s}^{-1}} Hb$$

At 20°C in pH 9 borate buffer, Hb* relaxes to normal deoxyhemoglobin at a rate of 6500 per second and much more quickly at pH 7 in phosphate buffer [2].

The ligand dissociation rates from $Hb_4(O_2)_4$ and $Hb_4(NO)_4$ also accelerate as the reaction proceeds and are strongly affected by phosphates. Carboxyhemoglobin, however, dissociates without any detectable acceleration of the reaction rate, and the reaction rates are not as much affected by phosphates.

The kinetic studies also bring out certain interesting features of ligand binding to hemoglobin that are not apparent from the ligand dissociation curve alone:

1. The cooperativity in the reactions of hemoglobin, if considered in terms of "off" and "on" rates, is highly dependent on the nature of ligand. Thus while CO shows cooperativity *mainly* in the ligand combination rates, oxygen and nitric oxide show cooperativity in the ligand dissociation rates [35]. These differences arise from the differences in the stereochemistry of these ligands. Oxygen prefers bent bonding (with respect to the axis perpendicular to the heme plane) with Fe in heme and avoids steric interaction with the residues on the distal side of heme. The variations in "off" rate constants, in this case, mainly reflect the tension on the Fe—O_2 bond owing to steric and/or electronic factors originating on the proximal side of heme. This should also be true for NO. Carbon monoxide, however, prefers linear bonding with Fe in heme. The residues on the distal side of heme in the heme pocket—particularly E7 His and Val E11 in β chains—are situated too close to the ligand-binding site and therefore provide steric hindrance in the formation of the Fe-to-ligand bond in this case. Variations in "on" rate constants for CO, therefore, reflect the variations in the steric hindrance from the distal residues. From the values of CO "off" rates it is also obvious that Fe—CO bond is too strong to respond to the same extent as the Fe—O_2 bond to the "tension" from the proximal side.

2. The "off" rates for oxyhemoglobin and the "on" rates for CO hemoglobin also favor a model in which there is strong interaction between pairs of heme in Hb tetramers; l_1' is approximately equal to l_3' and l_2' to l_4'. These observations cannot be explained by the two-state model [25] or the stereochemical mechanism for oxygen binding [1].

3. The effect of phosphates in oxyhemoglobin is due primarily to changes in the "off" rates rather than to changes in the "on" rates; species in the quaternary T state show larger enhancement in the dissociation rates [31]. Various equilibria and kinetic studies suggest that although phosphates bind to β chains, they affect the properties of α chains more.

4. Kinetic studies indicate that α and β chains in hemoglobin tetramers have different reactivity. These differences are shown in the reactions of deoxy-Hb_4 as well as in fully liganded hemoglobin [2].

Hemoglobin is believed to be the product of a billion years of evolutionary change [36]. It is only recently that the structural basis of its unique functional properties has begun to be elucidated. While our knowledge of that structural-functional relationship continues to expand, it is not yet complete.

References

1. Perutz, M. F.: Regulation of oxygen affinity of hemoglobin. *Ann. Rev. Biochem.* 48:327, 1979.
2. Parkhurst, L. J.: Hemoglobin and myoglobin ligand kinetics. *Ann. Rev. Phys. Chem.* 30:503, 1979.
3. Bunn, H. F., Forget, B. G., and Ranney, H. M.: *Human Hemoglobins.* Saunders, Philadelphia, 1977.
4. Schroeder, W. A., et al.: Evidence for multiple structural genes for γ chains of human fetal hemoglobin. *Proc. Natl. Acad. Sci. U.S.A.* 60:537, 1968.
5. Fantoni, A., Farace, M. G., and Gambari, R.: Embryonic hemoglobins in man and other mammals. *Blood* 57:623, 1981 (review).
6. Baralle, F. E., Shoulders, C. C., and Proudfoot, N. J.: The primary structure of the human ϵ-globin gene. *Cell* 21:621, 1980.
7. Schroeder, W. A., Cua, J. T., Matsuda, G., and Fenninger, W. D.: Hemoglobin F_1, an acetyl-containing hemoglobin. *Biochim. Biophys. Acta* 63:532, 1962.
8. Garlick, R. L., Schaeffer, J. R., Chapman, P. B., Kingston, R. E., Mazer, J. S., and Bunn, H. F.: Synthesis of acetylated human fetal hemoglobin. *J. Biol. Chem.* 256:1727, 1981.
9. Holmquist, W. R., and Schroeder, W. A.: A new N-terminal blocking group involving a Schiff base in hemoglobin A_{1c}. *Biochemistry* 5:2489, 1966.

10. Rahbar, S.: An abnormal hemoglobin in red cells of diabetes. *Clin. Chem. Acta* 22:296, 1968.

11. Bunn, H. F., et al.: Biosynthesis of human hemoglobin A_{1c}. Slow glycosylation of hemoglobin *in vivo*. *J. Clin. Invest.* 57:1652, 1976.

12. Bunn, H. F., Haney, D. N., Gabbay, K. H., and Gallop, P.: Further identification of the nature of linkage of the carbohydrate in hemoglobin A_{1c}. *Biochem. Biophys. Res. Commun.* 67:103, 1975a.

13. Shapiro, R., McManus, M. J., Zalut, C., and Bunn, H. F.: Sites of non-enzymatic glycosylation of human hemoglobin A. *J. Biol. Chem.* 255:3120, 1980.

14. Flückiger, R., Harmon, W., Meier, W., Loo, S., and Gabbay, K. H.: Hemoglobin carbamylation in uremia. *N. Eng. J. Med.* 304:823, 1981.

15. Stryer, L.: *Biochemistry*. Freeman, San Francisco, 1975.

16. Dickerson, R. E., and Geis, I.: *The Structure and Action of Proteins*. Harper & Row, New York, 1969.

17. Fermi, G.: Three-dimensional Fourier synthesis of human deoxy-haemoglobin at 2.5 Å resolution: Refinement of the atomic model. *J. Mol. Biol.* 97:237, 1975.

18. Gelin, B. R., and Karplus, M.: Mechanism of tertiary structural change in hemoglobin. *Proc. Natl. Acad. Sci. U.S.A.* 74:801, 1977.

19. Perutz, M. F.: Structure and mechanism of hemoglobin. *Br. Med. Bull.* 32:195, 1976.

20. Arnone, A.: X-ray diffraction study of binding of 2,3-diphosphoglycerate to human deoxyhemoglobin. *Nature* 237:146, 1972.

21. Baldwin, J. M.: The structure of human carbon-monoxyhaemoglobin at 2.7 Å resolution. *J. Mol. Biol.* 136:103, 1980.

22. Baldwin, J., and Chothia, C.: Haemoglobin: The structural changes related to ligand binding and its allosteric mechanism. *J. Mol. Biol.* 129:175, 1979.

23. Eisenberger, P., Shulman, R. G., Kincaid, B. M., Brown, G. S., and Ogawa, S.: Extended x-ray absorption fine structure determination of iron nitrogen distances in haemoglobin. *Nature* 274:30, 1978.

24. Warshel, A.: Energy-structure correlation in metalloporphyrins and the control of oxygen binding by hemoglobin. *Proc. Natl. Acad. Sci. U.S.A.* 74:1789, 1977.

25. Monod, J., Wyman, J., and Changeux, J. P.: On the nature of allosteric transitions: A plausible model. *J. Mol. Biol.* 12:88, 1965.

26. Imai, K.: Analyses of oxygen equilibria of native and chemically modified human adult hemoglobins on the basis of Adair's stepwise oxygenation theory and the allosteric model of Monod, Wyman, and Changeux. *Biochemistry* 12:798, 1973.

27. Comroe, J. H., Jr.: *Physiology of Respiration*. Yearbook, Chicago, 1965, p. 161.

28. Wyman, J., Jr.: Linked functions and reciprocal effects in hemoglobin: A second look, in *Advances in Protein Chemistry*, edited by C. B. Anfinsen, Jr., J. T. Edsall, M. C. Anson, and F. M. Richards. Academic, New York, 1964, vol. 19, pp. 223–286.

29. Benesch, R., and Benesch, R. E.: Effect of organic phosphate from human erythrocytes on allosteric properties of hemoglobin. *Biochem. Biophys. Res. Commun.* 26:162, 1967.

30. Adair, G. S.: The hemoglobin system. VI. The oxygen dissociation curve of hemoglobin. *J. Biol. Chem.* 63:529, 1925.

31. Gibson, Q. H.: The reaction of oxygen with hemoglobin and the kinetic basis of the effect of salt on binding of oxygen. *J. Biol. Chem.* 245:3285, 1970.

32. MacQuarrie, R., and Gibson, Q. H.: Use of a fluorescent analogue of 2,3-diphosphoglycerate as a probe of human hemoglobin conformation during carbon monoxide binding. *J. Biol. Chem.* 246:5832, 1971.

33. Cassoly, R., and Gibson, Q. H.: Conformation, co-operativity and ligand binding in human hemoglobin. *J. Mol Biol.* 91:301, 1975.

34. Gibson, Q. H.: The photochemical formation of a quickly reacting form of haemoglobin. *Biochem. J.* 71:293, 1959.

35. Sharma, V. S., Geibel, J. F., and Ranney, H. M.: "Tension" on heme by the proximal base and ligand reactivity: Conclusions drawn from model compounds for the reaction of hemoglobin. *Proc. Natl. Acad. Sci. U.S.A.* 75:3747, 1978.

36. Efstratiadis, A., et al.: The structure and evolution of the human β-globin gene family. *Cell* 21:653, 1980.

Erythrokinetics

CHAPTER 38

Production of erythrocytes

ALLAN J. ERSLEV

The morphologic keystone in erythropoiesis is the proerythroblast, a cell programmed both for proliferation and for production, packaging, and protection of hemoglobin molecules. The proerythroblast is derived from a pool of more primitive cells, so-called stem cells or progenitor cells capable of self-renewal and differentiation. It is believed that this pool consists of a core of pluripotential stem cells which replenish compartments of unipotential stem cells, each committed to a single cell line. The stem cells committed to the erythroid line are believed to proliferate and mature in the presence of a burst-promoting factor. Eventually they become receptive to erythropoietin and undergo transformation to proerythroblasts. Subsequent cellular multiplication and maturation appear to be almost autonomous, with the formation in 3 to 4 days of about 8 to 16 orthochromatic erythroblasts from each proerythroblast (Fig. 38-1). At this stage of maturation, the nucleus has become small and dense and presumably is incapable of further genetic transcription. It is extruded, leaving a reticulocyte containing enough stable messenger RNA for a few more days of synthetic activity. At some point during the final stage of maturation, the reticulocyte is released from the marrow, and it finishes its transformation from reticulocyte to mature red blood cell in the spleen and in the circulating blood.

Phylogeny of red cell production

Hemoglobin has been demonstrated in the most primitive animal forms, such as *Paramecium* and *Tetrahymena*, but the development of a cell especially designed to synthesize, carry, and protect respiratory pigments had to await the development of a circulatory system [1]. Until then, some crustaceans, such as the *Daphnia*, were capable of developing a fairly sophisticated oxygen transport system without circulating red cells [2]. The specific advantage derived from packaging hemoglobin in red cells is not related to viscosity, since the viscosity of blood is the same whether hemoglobin molecules are dissolved in plasma or concentrated in red cells [3]. It appears

more likely that the emergence of red cells is related to the protective and regulatory effect of intracellular compounds on hemoglobin and its oxygen affinity.

Circulating nucleated erythrocytes first appear in the worms of the phylum Nemertina and in the sessile marine creatures of the phylum Phoronida. Erythropoiesis in these primitive invertebrates takes place near or on the peritoneal surface, with endothelial cells acting as stem cells [1].

In the phylum Annelida, which is considerably further up on the evolutionary scale, nonnucleated red cells are observed for the first time. However, the evolutionary advantage derived from denucleation appears to be slight, and nucleated red cells are observed in much further advanced animals, such as reptiles and birds [4]. All mammalian erythrocytes are nonnucleated, even those in the most primitive forms such as the Australian duckbilled platypus [5].

In the premammalian species, the spleen in the fundamental erythropoietic organ. In some fish, the kidneys are also involved in red cell production [6,7], but it is questionable if this is related to the existence of a renal erythropoietic hormone. In the vertebrates, there is an evolutionary shift from the spleen to the liver and from the liver to the hollow bones. It appears that any organ with a relatively stagnant sinusoidal vascular system may serve as a site for red cell production, and the sinusoidal structure of the bone cavities in mammals renders these areas particularly well suited [8].

The homeostatic regulation of blood or hemoglobin production has been studied in *Daphnia* [2]. In these crustaceans, there is a balance between oxygen need and hemoglobin production. In the higher animals, this relationship is maintained by adjusting red cell production. Studies of birds [9], fish [10], and mammals [11] indicate that red cell production is controlled by a humoral substance, erythropoietin, which is capable of adjusting red cell production to the demands for oxygen in the tissues. Studies of erythropoietin isolated from a number of mammals indicate some biochemical variability, but still a considerable biologic similarity [12].

Ontogeny of red cell production

A number of tissues in the mammalian species can support red cell production, but the environment inside the bone apparently is optimal for cellular proliferation and maturation. However, bone cavities do not develop until the fifth fetal month, and other, presumably less favorable, sites are responsible for red cell production during early embryonic life. In the human, blood cells are first formed outside the embryo in the numerous blood islands of the yolk sac [13] (Fig. 12-1). The cells formed here are very large and remain nucleated throughout their functional life-span [14]. During the second gestational month, they are slowly replaced by smaller, nonnucleated cells derived from hepatic

ERYTHROPOIESIS

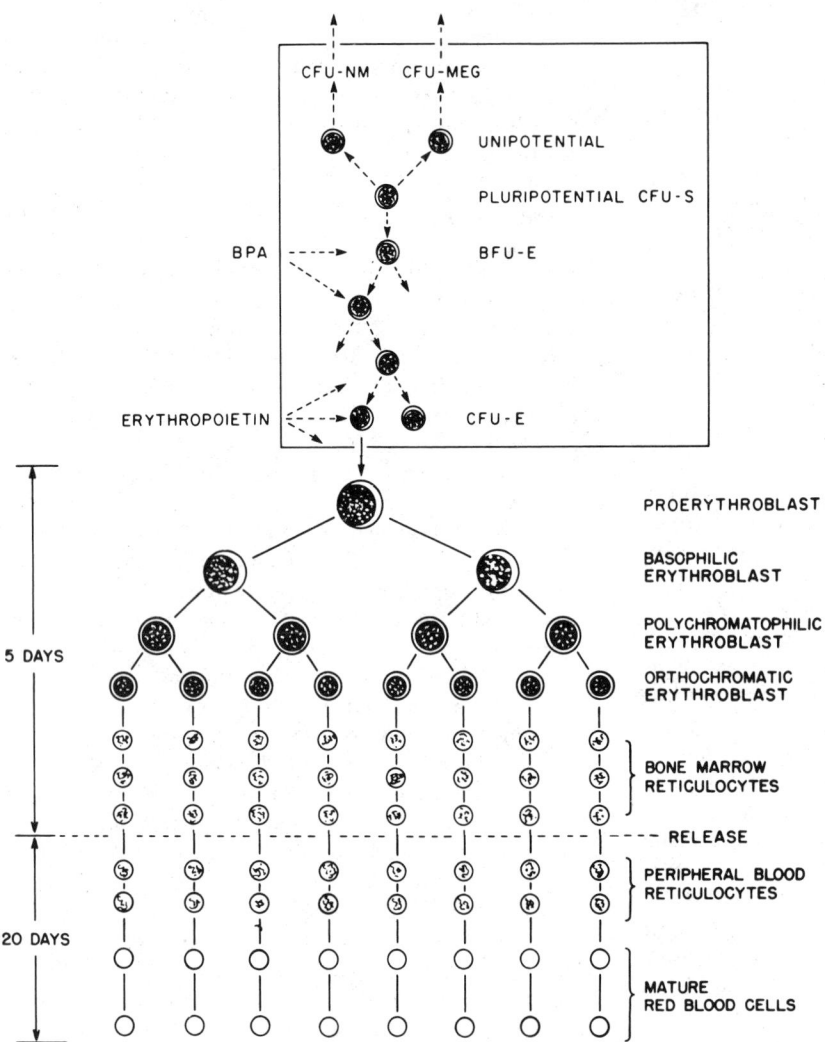

FIGURE 38-1   A model of the stem cell pool and its erythropoietic progeny.

erythropoiesis [15]. In the first 10 weeks of embryonic life, hemoglobins Gower 1 (ϵ_4), Gower 2 ($\alpha_2\epsilon_2$), and Portland ($\zeta_2\lambda_2$) are synthesized [16]. There is then a gradual replacement of hemoglobins containing ϵ and ζ chains with hemoglobins containing α and γ chains ($\alpha_2\gamma_2$), but whether or not the production of Gower and Portland hemoglobins is the prerogative of the yolk sac is not known [16]. Some studies suggest that the expression of hemoglobin genes follows a chronologic program built into the stem cells [17,18], but the immediate microenvironment may also be of importance, since stem cells from yolk sacs will produce adult hemoglobin in another setting [19].

During the next fetal months, the liver is the main red cell–producing organ. Splenic red cell production is presumed to be of importance between the third and the seventh fetal months. However, the spleen may sequester and destroy nucleated red cells formed else-where, and the presence of early erythroid cells in this organ does not conclusively indicate splenic erythropoiesis [20].

At about the fifth fetal month, granulopoietic cells can be recognized in the central cartilaginous region of the bones, but the bone cavities only slowly become capable of supporting erythropoiesis. At the time of birth, the hepatic phase of blood cell production is finished, and all bone cavities are actively engaged in erythropoiesis. Concomitantly, there is a gradual switch from γ to β hemoglobin chain synthesis, but the reason for or mechanism of this important biosynthetic change is still unknown [21]. During the neonatal period, the volume of available marrow space is almost the same as the total volume of hemopoietic cells [22]. This precarious balance continues for a few years until the growth of the bones and bone cavities outstrips the growth of the hemopoietic mass. During the early years, the lack of reserve space forces reactivation of extramedullary foci in the liver and spleen whenever the hemopoietic system is challenged by blood loss, hypoxia, or hemolysis [23].

During adult life, the expansion of marrow space continues, possibly by bone resorption, and there is a gradual increase in the amount of fatty tissue in all bone cavities. Because of the abundant marrow space, compensatory reactivation of extramedullary sites rarely takes place in later life, even during periods of prolonged and intense demand for additional blood cell formation. Extramedullary hemopoiesis during these years usually indicates inappropriate rather than compensatory blood formation [24].

During late fetal life, the physiologic control of red cell production is probably tied to tissue hypoxia and release of erythropoietin [25]. The fetus is under continuous hypoxic stimulation ("Everest in utero"), and erythropoietin has been demonstrated in the amniotic fluid of mothers with erythroblastotic babies. Erythropoietin can apparently not pass the placental barrier [26], and infants born of mothers with various hematologic disorders varying from severe anemia to secondary polycythemia are usually born with the same degree of normal postpartum erythrocytosis. Since bilateral nephrectomy of fetal sheep [27] fails to alter the rate of erythropoietin production, it appears that during fetal life this production is primarily extrarenal. At the time of birth, there is or has been [28] a switch to renal production of erythropoietin, and in the adult it is responsible for 90 to 95 percent of total production.

Kinetics of red cell production

STEM CELL POOL

Mammalian nucleated red cells are characterized biochemically and morphologically by their continuous synthesis and accumulation of hemoglobin molecules. Because of this condition of relentless maturation, nucleated red cells must be derived from a stable compartment of cells capable of both differentiation and self-renewal. The existence of such cells designated as stem cells was recognized and expressed in various ways by Ehrlich, Pappenheim, and Maximow at the turn of the century, but first supported experimentally by recent in vivo and in vitro studies [29]. In vivo studies on the effect of erythropoietin on an erythropoietically inactive spleen (Fig. 38-2) indicate the existence of cells morphologically distinct from nucleated red cells but capable of replenishing the erythroid compartment [30]. In vitro studies of marrow cultured on semisolid medium have similarly disclosed the presence of small mononuclear cells which in response to erythropoietin form colonies of nucleated red blood cells [31]. These colonies appear 1 to 2 days after marrow plating, grow to a final size of 32 to 64 hemoglobin-containing cells, and then disappear after 3 to 4 more days. They are derived from cells called CFU-E and only grow if erythropoietin is present in the

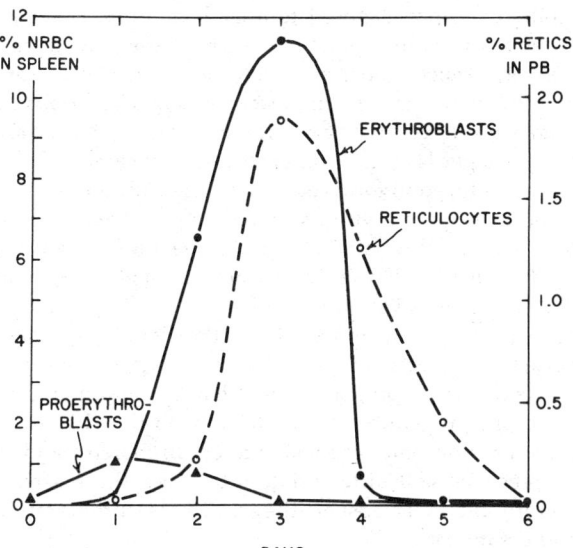

FIGURE 38-2 **The appearance of successive waves of erythropoietic cells in the spleen following the injection of erythropoietin to a hypertransfused mouse. Prior to the injection, the spleen did not contain cells which could be recognized morphologically as erythropoietic cells. (Filmanowicz and Gurney [30].)**

medium. Since CFU-E are present in increased numbers in anemias and decreased numbers in transfusion-induced polycythemias [32], they must be considered to be erythroid precursor cells rather than self-perpetuating stem cells. However, they appear to be recruited from true stem cells collectively called BFU-E [33] and present both in marrow and in the lymphocyte fraction of peripheral blood [34]. Colonies derived from these stem cells appear in the cultures several days after the disappearance of the CFU-E and in the presence of erythropoietin grow to huge clusters containing thousands of nucleated red cells. Studies of the growth and development of these colonies indicate that in the presence of crude erythropoietin, early BFU-Es proliferate and migrate for some distance in the semisolid medium. Simultaneously they mature until they become CFU-Es and capable of responding to erythropoietin with blast transformation to nucleated red cells [35]. Although the BFU-E in turn can be replenished from an earlier compartment of pluripotential stem cells [36], they are believed to be mainly self-perpetuating and only replenished intermittently if damaged or depleted.

How the BFU-E compartment controls the size of the red cell mass and how it responds to peripheral feedback signals are poorly understood. Recent studies indicate that the BFU-Es are surprisingly unresponsive to erythroid activity [37]. The total number of BFU-Es and their proliferative activity as measured by tritiated thymidine incorporation are little affected by major changes in the rate of red cell production and in the concentration of erythropoietin [38]. Indeed the BFU-Es will proliferate when exposed to a large number of agents unrelated to erythropoietin [37–39]. These agents, collectively called *burst-promoting activity* (BPA), are present in serum and tissue extracts and are derived from various cell types including T lymphocytes [40], macrophages [41], and monocytes [42]. Since BFU-E also can be induced to form colonies by the addition of large amounts of pure erythropoietin, it is possible that both BPA and erythropoietin regulate the rate of red cell production [43]. However, it seems more plausible that BPA is permissive while erythropoietin is regulatory. Such a concept would envision the BFU-E as a self-perpetuating compartment which in the presence of BPA provides a progeny of proliferating and maturing erythroid progenitor cells. After four to five divisions, these cells become responsive to erythropoietin and in its presence will differentiate into proerythroblasts. If erythropoietin is absent, they will cease proliferation and disappear.

In regard to hemoglobin synthesis by the BFU-E colonies, it appears that colonies derived from the earliest erythroid precursors contain more fetal hemoglobin than those derived from later stages [21]. These early progenitors are found in small numbers in peripheral blood and can be induced to produce large amounts of fetal hemoglobin when stimulated by BPA from T lymphocytes [44]. The later progenitors are found primarily in the marrow and produce exclusively adult hemoglobin, but whether these differences are due to age and maturity of the erythroid progenitors, to character of the BPA, or to some other cause is still unknown.

ERYTHROPOIETIC POOL

The creation of a normal red cell is the end result of an orderly transformation of a proerythroblast with a large nucleus and a volume of about 900 μl^3 to a red, anucleated disc with a volume of about 90 μl^3. Although the cytoplasmic maturation is continuous, the interposed mitotic divisions cause a stepwise reduction in volume, making it quite easy to recognize distinct stages [45,46]. A model outlining the stages in red cell production is presented in Fig. 38-1. This model is based on morphologic observations which suggest four stages of nucleated red cells separated by three mitotic divisions. These blast stages have been given the prefix *normo-* by

Wintrobe in his excellent textbooks on clinical hematology [47], but in this book will be designated as *proerythroblasts, basophilic erythroblasts, polychromatophilic erythroblasts,* and *orthochromatic erythroblasts.*

Clinical observations indicate that it takes about 5 days from an erythropoietic stimulation until new reticulocytes emerge from the marrow. Consequently, it seems permissible to assign a total intramedullary maturation time of 5 days to nucleated red cells and reticulocytes, or with a generation time of about 18 hours (see below), 3 days for erythroblasts and 2 days for reticulocytes. When these values and certain well-established red cell parameters are used, it is possible to make a rough assessment of the total size of the erythropoietic pool. The circulating blood volume averages 70 ml per kilogram of body weight, which, with a red blood cell count of 5×10^6 per microliter, equals 350×10^9 red cells per kilogram of body weight. With a red cell life-span of 120 days, the daily production must be $(350 \times 10^9)/120$, or 3×10^9 cells per kilogram. Although the intramedullary life-span is about 5 days, the earlier stages have fewer cells, so that the total intramedullary erythropoietic pool can be estimated to contain $3.3 \times (3 \times 10^9)$, or 10×10^9, cells per kilogram of body weight. It is reassuring that this rough calculation is consistent with more exact determinations. When marrow differential counts and ^{59}Fe incorporation have been used, the intramedullary erythropoietic pool (nucleated red cells plus marrow reticulocytes) has been determined to be 13×10^9 cells per kilogram of body weight [48,49] (Table 38-1). When marrow differential counts and mitotic indices have been used, the nucleated red cell pool has been determined to be 3.5×10^9 cells per kilogram of body weight [50]. If the values from Table 38-1 on the marrow reticulocytes are added, the total pool would be 11.5×10^9 cells per kilogram of body weight.

The total size of the adult marrow is traditionally equated with that of the liver or the red cell mass [51]. This size, about 30 ml/kg, may not be out of line with the preceding calculation, indicating that the erythropoietic pool contains one-thirtieth as many cells as the circulating red cell mass. The facts that only one of two or three marrow cells is erythroid, that the volume of some early erythroid cells may be 10 times the volume of mature red cells, and that at least 50 percent of the marrow volume is made up by fat must be taken into consideration.

Contemporary studies of the composition and kinetics of the erythropoietic pool employ measurements of nucleus size, mitotic activity, and isotope incorporation. The nucleus diameter decreases stepwise after each successive division and provides a reasonably clear separation between each maturation stage [45,46]. Nevertheless, studies with tritiated thymidine show that a very active synthetic phase precedes each division [52], and it is likely that the decrease in nucleus size represents histone condensation rather than DNA loss.

Studies on the mitotic activity of normal human marrow have shown that at any one time 2.5 percent of the

TABLE 38-1   Erythropoietic pool

Cell types	Number of cells × 10⁹ per kilogram of body weight
Proerythroblasts	0.10
Basophilic erythroblasts	0.48
Polychromatophilic erythroblasts	1.47
Orthochromatic erythroblasts	2.95
Marrow reticulocytes	8.20
Blood reticulocytes	3.10
Mature red blood cells	330.00

SOURCE: Adapted from Donohue et al. [48] and Finch et al. [49].

proerythroblasts, 5 percent of the basophilic erythroblasts, and 6 percent of polychromatophilic erythroblasts are dividing [53]. Since the number of mitoses observed depends on the time spent in the various phases of the cell cycle, it is possible to relate the mitotic index M^I (i. e., the fraction of cells present in mitosis) to generation time, the time from one mitosis to the next:

$$M^I = \frac{N^M \text{ (no. of cells in mitosis)}}{N \text{ (no. of cells in interphase)}}$$

$$= \frac{t^M \text{ (mitotic time)}}{t^G \text{ (generation time)}}$$

Since the mitotic time has been measured to be about 30 to 60 min, the generation time for proerythroblasts can be estimated to be about 20 to 40 h, and the generation time for basophilic and polychromatophilic erythroblasts, 10 to 20 h.

Similar consideration and calculations based on autoradiographic studies on marrow [54] can be used to estimate the generation time. If a DNA label, such as tritiated thymidine, is used, the labeling index L^I can be determined as follows:

$$L^I = \frac{N^S \text{ (no. of cells labeled)}}{N \text{ (no. of cells unlabeled)}}$$

$$= \frac{t^S \text{ (time in synthesis)}}{t^G \text{ (generation time)}}$$

The time spent in the synthetic (S) phase can be estimated by using a DNA label and a spindle-blocking agent, such as colchicine [54]. Generation times estimated in this manner are 11 h for proerythroblasts, 16 h for basophilic erythroblasts, and 26 h for polychromatophilic erythroblasts [55]—unfortunately quite different from the times estimated on the basis of the mitotic index. In the absence of more consistent data, it seems permissible to use 18 h as a practical approximation of the generation time for each maturation stage.

After about three cellular generations the nucleus of the erythroid cell has become dense or pyknotic and presumably incapable of replication, and it is either carried as inert baggage in the mature red cell or is extruded. Extrusion, which is the normal procedure in all adult mammalian species, is usually spontaneous but may be facilitated by mechanical forces dependent on the discrepancy between nuclear size and the size of the openings in the endothelial linings of marrow sinusoids [56]. The rigid nucleus cannot squeeze through and is extruded with a small amount of attached hemoglobin (Fig. 31-9). Consequently, the presence of nucleated red cells in tissue cultures of marrow, or in blood of patients with extramedullary erythropoiesis, may reflect lack of opportunities for pitting of the nucleus rather than accelerated erythropoiesis.

Cytoplasmic maturation and hemoglobin synthesis proceed uninterruptedly during the transitions from early to late nucleated red cells. After the nucleus has been extruded, eliminating further production of mRNA, there is a gradual disappearance of ribosomal particles, mitochondria, and binding sites for transferrin, and over a period of 2 to 4 days the reticulocyte transforms into a mature red cell [51]. This transition involves a moderate loss of surface and volume and a disappearance of the "stickiness" which glues immature cells together and is responsible for the frequent appearance of reticulocytes in clumps. It has been proposed that the stickiness is contributed by a surface coating of transferrin molecules discharging their cargo of iron to the cells [57]. As the binding sites for transferrin diminish, so does the stickiness, a possible explanation for the unmooring of marrow reticulocytes and their discharge into circulating blood. The final transformation of reticulocytes to mature red cells takes place in the circulation or in the spleen, which normally sequesters some of the more immature and sticky reticulocytes [57]. The varying patterns of reticulocyte release and splenic sequestration unfortunately render the reticulocyte count only a semiquantitative measure of the rate of red cell production.

REGULATION OF RED CELL PRODUCTION
FEEDBACK CONTROLS
Under physiologic conditions, the circulating red cell mass is maintained at an optimal size by appropriate adjustments in the rate of red cell production. Red cell destruction and red cell loss may influence the size of the red cell mass, but these are not physiologic variables, and the spleen of humans [58], unlike that of dogs [59] and race horses [60], does not serve as a reservoir of red cells. The feedback signals which adjust the rate of production of red cells to the need for red cells could be generated from tissues serviced by red cells (functional feedback) or from the red cells themselves (end-product feedback).

FUNCTIONAL FEEDBACK
The red cell mass is a large organ designed almost exclusively for the purpose of transporting oxygen to the tissues. It also promotes elimination of carbon dioxide from the tissues by means of red cell carbonic anhydrase, but this enzyme is present in such excess that the capacity of the red cell mass to process carbon dioxide has not been shown to be rate-limiting. Thus the size of the red cell mass and the rate of red cell production must be closely related to the supply and demand for oxygen in the tissues.

Studies on the rate of red cell production under conditions of low atmospheric oxygen pressure [61] were initiated by Jourdanet in 1863 [62] and climaxed 82 years later in a classic paper from Peru by Hurtado and coworkers [63]. The conclusion from these studies was that a low arterial oxygen tension stimulates red cell production. Arterial hypoxia caused by right-to-left shunt in congenital heart disease, or by pulmonary dysfunction, was likewise found to be associated with accelerated red cell production. However, erythropoietic

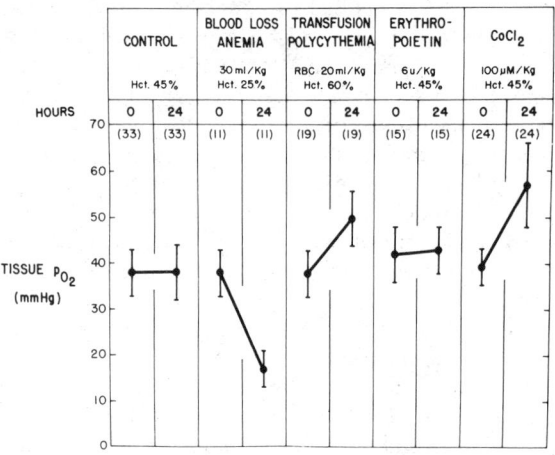

FIGURE 38-3 Oxygen tension of airpockets introduced subcutaneously in rats. The effects of bleeding, transfusion, erythropoietin, and cobalt on the oxygen tension are given. As expected, bleeding causes hypoxia, transfusion causes hyperoxia, and erythropoietin has no immediate effect. Cobalt causes tissue hyperoxia, presumably reflecting impaired oxygen utilization because of inhibited cellular oxidative metabolism.

stimulation was also found in blood loss anemia despite normal arterial oxygen pressure. Since the common denominator for these conditions is an inadequate supply of oxygen to the tissues, it was concluded that red cell production is stimulated by a low tissue tension of oxygen [64].

A high tissue tension of oxygen as induced by hypertransfusion [65] or by breathing air mixtures with high partial oxygen pressure [66] was conversely found to

FIGURE 38-4 The immediate (reticulocytes and marrow erythroblasts) and delayed (red blood cells and hematocrit) response in normal rabbits to the infusion of large amounts of plasma obtained from rabbits with blood loss anemia. (Erslev [71].)

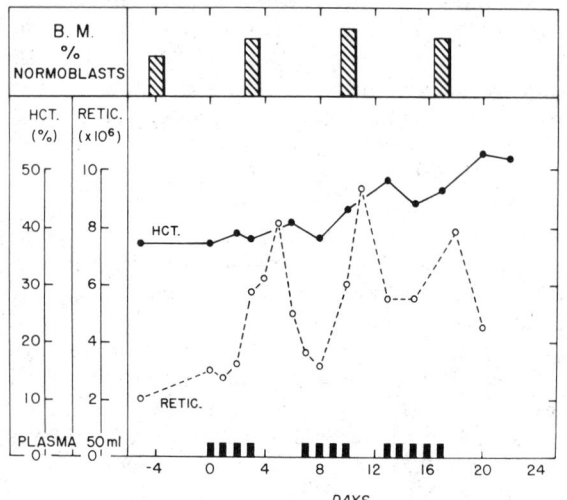

decrease the rate of red cell production. This reciprocal relationship between tissue tension of oxygen and red cell production has subsequently been found not to depend on the oxygen pressure per se but on its effect on the oxidative metabolism of tissue cells. Thus the administration of cobalt, a potent erythropoietic stimulant, is associated with an increase in the tissue tension of oxygen presumably caused by a cobalt-induced inhibition of oxidative processes in the tissues [67] (Fig. 38-3). Recent studies have clarified the mechanism which links intracellular aerobic metabolism and red cell production and suggest that it is mediated by a renal erythropoietic hormone, erythropoietin.

ERYTHROPOIETIN

In 1906, Carnot and Deflandre first suggested that arterial hypoxia generates a humoral factor capable of stimulating red cell production [68]. This attractive hypothesis was unfortunately not supported by acceptable experimental data, and it took almost 50 years before such data became available. In 1950, Reissmann, using parabiotic rats, showed that red cell production can be stimulated by a humoral factor [69]. A few years later, Stohlman and coworkers [70] reached the same conclusion, after having found the same degree of erythroid hyperplasia in marrow obtained from cyanotic and from normal areas of a patient with reverse blood flow through a patent ductus arteriosus. Direct evidence for the existence of an erythropoietic hormone was provided in 1953 (Fig. 38-4) [71], and since then there has been a rapid expansion in our knowledge of the character and metabolism of this hormone, appropriately named *erythropoietin*.

After the demonstration of a tangible erythropoietic substance, it was immediately suggested that this substance not only stimulates red cell production, but actually is responsible for the regulation of red cell production [64]. Subsequent studies strengthened this suggestion by demonstrating that erythropoietin is present in serum and urine from both anemic and hypoxic individuals and that its concentration is related to the degree of anemic hypoxia [72,73] (Figs. A17-2 and A17-3).

Erythropoietin has been characterized biochemically as a nondialyzable, relatively thermostable α-globulin. It contains sialic acid, and its biologic activity in vivo but not in vitro is destroyed by neuraminidase because of its rapid removal from the circulation [74]. The molecular size has been estimated to be about 40,000 daltons, and pure erythropoietin has been reported to have a specific activity of about 70,000 units per milligram of protein [75]. Erythropoietins obtained from various mammals are immulogically weakly cross-reactive but appear to have very similar biochemical and biologic properties [76,77].

PRODUCTION OF ERYTHROPOIETIN

Cellular hypoxia is obviously the initiating event in the production of erythropoietin, but the exact location and type of cells responsible for translating oxygen pressure into hormone synthesis are still unknown. Because of the compensatory redistribution of blood in anemia, some vital organs such as the heart, brain, or liver probably maintain a near-normal oxygen supply and must be quite insensitive to moderate variations in the oxygen-carrying capacity. However, organs providing blood for this redistribution, such as the subcutaneous tissue or the kidneys, would notice even mild anemia and would a priori be logical sites for an "oxygen stat" [64]. Of these two, the kidneys would appear less suitable because of their extensive blood supply and relatively small oxygen demand. Nevertheless, the classic study by Jacobson and coworkers in 1957 [78] has established the kidneys as the site of production of erythropoietin. These workers showed that "anephric" rats fail to respond to anemia with an increase in plasma erythropoietic activity, while "nephric" rats rendered equally uremic by ureteral ligation respond in a near-normal fashion.

These studies have been confirmed and extended [79], and the present working hypothesis is that renal hypoxia induces production and release of erythropoietin. A compromised blood supply to the kidneys, caused by partial renal artery ligation in experimental animals [80] or by arteriosclerotic plaques in humans [81,82], has been shown in some instances to lead to the release of erythropoietin and the induction of secondary polycythemia. Renal microinfarcts induced by the injection of plastic spheres into the renal artery may likewise cause an inappropriate release of erythropoietin and erythrocytosis [83]. A similar mechanism may explain the observation that rejection of a transplanted kidney frequently is heralded by the release of erythropoietin [84]. Nevertheless, the erythrocytosis observed in some patients with functioning transplants [85] is probably caused by inappropriate secretion of erythropoietin by the remnant kidney and not by the transplanted kidney [86]. Polycythemia occurs occasionally in patients with hypernephroma, and in some cases it is caused by an inappropriate secretion of erythropoietin by the neoplastic cells [87]. However, polycythemia has also been described in patients with Wilms' tumor, lymphosarcoma of the kidney, solitary cyst, polycystic disease, and hydronephrosis [88]. The common denominator for all these conditions appears to be compression of the remaining normal kidney tissue, possibly causing renal ischemia and erythropoietin release [89].

A reduction in the amount of functioning renal tissue gradually leads to a decrease in the capacity of the kidneys to respond to anemia with production of erythropoietin [90]. In patients with end-stage kidney disease, or in anephric patients, the production ceases altogether, but the marrow continues to make some red cells [91]. This base-line activity is responsive to tissue hypoxia [92] and probably is maintained by extrarenal production of erythropoietin [93].

About 5 to 10 percent of erythropoietin produced by the normal adult is extrarenal, and it appears that either hepatocytes or Kupffer cells in the liver are responsible for this production [94–96]. During fetal development, extrarenal erythropoietin may be of major importance for red cell production, since it has been shown that anephric fetal sheep [27] produce normal amounts of erythropoietin and red cells. At time of birth there is a gradual switch in sheep from hepatic to renal erythropoietin production [97], and attempts to restore hepatic synthesis have been unsuccessful. However, regenerating livers, such as those in rats after partial hepatectomy [98,99] and in humans after hepatitis [100], apparently synthesize more erythropoietin than normal. Erythropoietin produced in anephric individuals behaves immunologically and biologically like renal erythropoietin, but biochemical identity has not as yet been established [91,93,101].

Attempts to pinpoint the site of production of renal erythropoietin to a specific renal component have been unsuccessful. Erythropoietin antibodies tagged with fluorescein will concentrate in the glomeruli [102], but since erythropoietin is filtered here, this finding may reflect clearance rather than production. The juxtaglomerular apparatus has been proposed as a possible site of production [103], and many investigators have attempted to relate granule counts to erythropoietic activity [104]. So far the findings indicate the existence of a relationship between juxtaglomerular granularity and blood volume, but not between granularity, tissue oxygen tension [105], or erythropoietin production [106].

Bioassay of tissue homogenate would appear to be the most direct way to localize the site of production. Until recently, however, most bioassays of renal tissue failed to reveal erythropoietic activity, even when the kidneys were obtained from animals engaged in active erythropoietin production. As an explanation for this surprising finding it was proposed that the kidneys do not produce erythropoietin but rather release an enzyme, erythrogenin, which is capable of changing an inactive circulating erythropoietinogen produced by the liver into erythropoietin [107]. The existence of such a system of activation was supported by the observation that a renal subcellular fraction, renal erythropoietic factor, renders normal serum erythropoietically active after a brief period of incubation [108]. However, the fact that kidneys obtained from hypoxic animals and perfused in vitro with a serum-free medium continue to produce erythropoietin [109] made this hypothesis untenable. An alternate explanation for the difficulty in recovering erythropoietin from renal homogenates is that the kidney tissue contains several inhibitors which tend to inactivate erythropoietin during the preparation of renal homogenates [110,111]. In a recent reexamination of the extraction procedures it was found that extracts from carefully prepared homogenates of kidneys obtained from rats exposed to hypoxia are erythropoietically active [112]. Most of this activity resided in the cortex, but the exact cellular source has not as yet been identified.

METABOLISM OF ERYTHROPOIETIN

The rate of disappearance of erythropoietin in circulating blood has been measured after hypertransfusion, and the half-life has been estimated to be between 1 and 6 h in laboratory animals [113–116] and up to 1 to 2 days in human subjects [117]. There has been some reluctance to accept these values because of the concept that a large amount of erythropoietin may be "consumed" by erythropoietic tissue and that this consumption is proportional to the degree of erythropoietic activity [118]. This would mean that the rate of disappearance of endogenous erythropoietin following hypertransfusion or hyperoxia may have little relevance to the physiologic half-life of erythropoietin. The concept of marrow consumption of erythropoietin is based on the well-substantiated finding that the level of plasma erythropoietin, after reaching a peak 1 day after the induction of anemia or hypoxia [119], rapidly decreases toward normal values. Furthermore, the plasma erythropoietin titers and the urinary excretion of erythropoietin appear to be higher in aplastic anemia that in other types of anemia with corresponding hemoglobin concentration [120]. Other studies, however, have suggested that the early erythropoietin peak after acute anemic or hypoxic hypoxia is caused by a temporary hyperventilation alkalosis with a shift in the oxygen dissociation curve to the left [121,122] and that erythropoietin catabolism is independent of marrow activity [115,123]. It is difficult indeed to explain how red cell production can be regulated smoothly by the plasma concentration of erythropoietin if this concentration fluctuates according to marrow activity.

Measurements of erythropoietin excretion in the urine have established that from 1 to 4 units of erythropoietin are excreted per day at normal hemoglobin concentrations [73] and that the amount excreted is inversely proportional to the hemoglobin concentration. The amount excreted is probably only a fraction of the amount produced, since the renal clearance of erythropoietin has been found in dogs and human subjects to be only about 0.1 to 0.7 ml/min [117,124]. The liver [125] and the kidney [116] are possible sites for erythropoietin catabolism, but supporting data are not conclusive.

ACTION OF ERYTHROPOIETIN

To explain the capacity of the marrow to adjust its production of red cells from near zero to 10 or more times the normal rate, erythropoietic regulation must involve a stage which permits considerable cellular amplification. Additional mitotic divisions during the intramedullary maturation sequence of nucleated red cells would not be anticipated to cause more than a doubling or possibly quadrupling of red cell production. Furthermore, since most studies suggest that marrow overactivity is associated with a shortened erythroid transit time, it seems unlikely that extra divisions can be interposed. These considerations, as well as the fact that a brief erythropoietic stimulus results in an accelerated reticulocyte output 4 to 5 days later, led to the hypothesis that erythropoietin acts on stem cells [126]. This hypothesis has been supported by some in vivo observations [30,127] and subsequently by most in vitro studies of stem cell proliferation.

According to current concepts of stem cell kinetics, erythropoietin acts by transforming undifferentiated but erythroid-committed CFU-E to proerythroblasts. This transformation is associated with proliferation [128–130] and based on the activation of genes necessary for erythroid development.

As a polypeptide hormone it is assumed that erythropoietin acts via surface receptors and intracellular secondary messengers. The presence of surface receptors has not been established but has been inferred from studies of trypsinized stem cells [131] and from the fact that erythropoietin coupled with macromolecular aggregates is still capable of CFU-E differentiation [132]. Its presumed surface action is enhanced by agents known to activate adenylcyclase, such as adrenergic agonists [133] and possibly thyroid hormones [134], but these agents cannot by themselves induce erythroid differentiation. Androgens [135] can also enhance the in vitro action of erythropoietin, but the mechanism responsible is not known.

Although it is assumed that erythropoietin has an effect on DNA transcription, causing the production of specific erythroid messenger RNAs, experimental support for this assumption is not impressive. Early studies of marrow suspension indicated that erythropoietin caused the production of new messenger RNA minutes after its addition to the culture medium [136]. However, subsequent studies of fetal mouse erythropoiesis indicate that the RNA induced by erythropoietin is not messenger RNA but ribosomal and transfer RNA needed to support the stimulation of ongoing synthetic activities [137].

In addition to the various stem cell-directed actions of erythropoietin, in vitro studies have shown that the proliferation of proerythroblasts and basophilis erythroblasts is accelerated by erythropoietin [138]. This acceleration results in a short marrow transit time [139], with the production of large and immature reticulocytes [140]. During their subsequent maturation these so-called stress reticulocytes lose excess cytoplasm [141], but otherwise behave as normal reticulocytes. It has also been suggested [142] that the release of reticulocytes from the marrow is controlled by erythropoietin, but early release could merely reflect the rapid changes in metabolic demands and space requirements which take place in an erythropoietin-stimulated marrow [56].

NEUROHUMORAL STIMULI

Many old case reports have been cited in support of the hypothesis that part of the functional feedback control of red cell production is mediated by the hypothalamus. Some studies have shown that hypothalamic stimulation may result in the release of erythropoietin [143,144], possibly explaining the well-established relationship between cerebellar tumors and polycythemia. The carotid bodies have been claimed to be involved in the production of erythropoietin and the control of erythro-

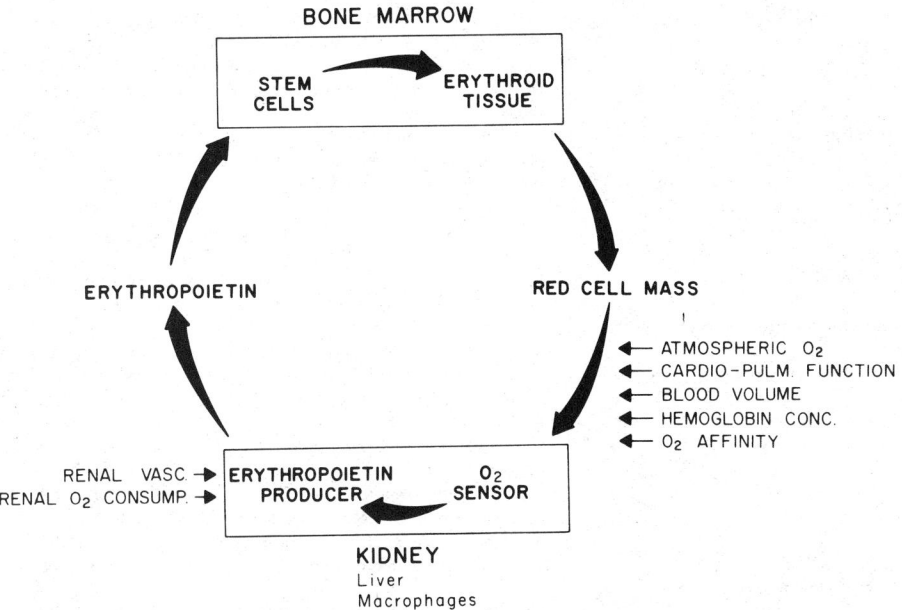

FIGURE 38-5 **Current model of the feedback circuit which regulates the rate of red blood cell production to the need for oxygen in the peripheral tissues.**

poiesis [145], but the data are neither convincing [146] nor reproducible [147].

The effect of pituitary hormones on red cell production has also been studied intensively, and it seems possible that the erythropoietic effect of various pituitary or pituitary-dependent hormones is accomplished by stimulating the release of renal erythropoietin [148].

END-PRODUCT FEEDBACK

Products released through the destruction of red cells have been thought to influence or even control the rate of red cell production. Supporting this hypothesis is the impression that anemia due to hemolysis is associated with a more pronounced erythroid hyperplasia and reticulocytosis than blood loss anemia of the same severity. Part of this difference may be related to the more chronic nature of many types of hemolytic anemia with the accompanying expansion of marrow and stem cell pools, to a selective destruction of nonreticulated red cells, to a shift of the reticulocyte pool from the marrow to the circulation [149], and to readily available iron from destroyed red cells [150]. Nevertheless, it is difficult to disregard this difference, and several investigators have now demonstrated that hemolysate may have a positive feedback effect on the rate of red cell production [151–153]. One study suggests that this effect is mediated via the release of renal erythropoietin [153].

It has been proposed that polycythemia exerts a negative feedback effect on red cell production by causing the release of an erythropoietic inhibitor [154,155]. Since hypertransfused animals are the preferred assay subjects for erythropoietin, it is difficult to imagine that these animals have an inhibited marrow. Furthermore, several investigators have been unable to repeat and confirm reports claiming the existence of erythropoietic

inhibitors in plasma from hypertransfused animals [156–158]. Although an inhibitor of erythropoietin has been demonstrated in renal homogenate [110,111], it is still too early to assign a physiologic role to this inhibitor.

Because of the sluggish blood flow in polycythemia, it has been reasoned that erythrocytosis must cause tissue hypoxia and erythropoietin release [159]. Since this obviously is contrary to the actual findings, it has been suggested that high blood viscosity per se suppresses marrow activity. So far no real experimental support for this suggestion has been provided. Furthermore, hemodynamic studies in polycythemia have shown clearly that polycythemia, with its increased blood volume and engorged vascular system, is associated with tissue hyperoxia rather than tissue hypoxia [160,161].

The observations and considerations discussed in this chapter in addition to new information about the adaptability of oxygen affinity (see Chap. 37) have led to the construction of a feedback circuit which appears capable of adjusting and maintaining the red cell mass at an optimal size for oxygen transport (Fig. 38-5). This circuit is based on a feedback between the marrow and the kidney mediated in one direction by oxygen and in the opposite by erythropoietin.

References

1. Scott, R. B.: Comparative hematology: The phylogeny of the erythrocyte. *Blut* 12:340, 1966.
2. Fox, H. M.: The hemoglobin of *Daphnia*. *Proc. Roy. Soc. Lond.* [*Biol.*] 135:195, 1948.
3. Schmidt-Nilsen, K., and Taylor, R. R.: The viscosity of hemoglobin inside and outside the red cells. *Science* 162:274, 1969.

4. Andrew, W.: *Comparative Hematology*. Grune & Stratton, New York, 1965.

5. Bolliger, A.: Observations on the blood of a monotreme *Tachyglossus aculeatus*. *Aust. J. Sci. 22:257*, 1959.

6. Jordan, H. E.: Comparative hematology, in *Handbook of Hematology*, edited by H. Downey. Hoeber-Harper, New York, 1938, p. 703.

7. Iorio, R. J.: Some morphologic and kinetic studies of the developing erythroid cells of the common gold fish, *Carassius auratus. Cell Tissue Kinet. 2(4):319*, 1969.

8. Robb-Smith, A. H. T.: *The Growth of Knowledge of the Functions of the Blood*, edited by R. G. Macfarlane and A. H. T. Robb-Smith. Academic, New York, 1961.

9. Rosse, W. F., and Waldmann, T. A.: Factors controlling erythropoiesis in birds. *Blood 27:654*, 1966.

10. Zanjani, E. D.: Humoral factors influencing erythropoiesis in the fish (Blud Gourami—*Trichogaster trichopterus*). *Blood 33:573*, 1969.

11. Erslev, A. J.: Control of red cell production. *Ann. Rev. Med. 11:315*, 1959.

12. Cotes, P. M., and Bangham, D. R.: The international reference preparation of erythropoietin. *Bull. WHO 35:751*, 1966.

13. Bloom, W., and Bartelmez, G. W.: Hemopoiesis in young human embryos. *Am. J. Anat. 67:21*, 1940.

14. Jones, O. P.: *Cytology of Pathologic Marrow Cells with Special Reference to Bone Marrow Biopsies*, edited by H. Downey. Hoeber-Harper, New York, 1938, p. 2043.

15. Knoll, W., and Pingel, E.: Der Gang der Erythropoese beim menschlichen Embryo. *Acta Haematol.* [Basel] *2:369*, 1949.

16. Fantoni, A., Farace, M. G., and Gambari, R.: Embryonic hemoglobins in man and other mammals. *Blood 57:623*, 1981.

17. Beaupain, D., Martin, C., and Dieterlen-Lièrre, F.: Are developmental hemoglobin changes related to the origin of stem cells and site of erythropoiesis? *Blood 53:212*, 1979.

18. Bunch, C., et al.: Hemoglobin synthesis by fetal erythroid cells in an adult environment. *Br. J. Haematol. 49:325*, 1981.

19. Moore, M. A. S., and Metcalf, D.: Ontogeny of the hematopoietic system. Yolk sac origin of in vivo and in vitro colony forming cells in the developing embryo. *Br. J. Haematol. 18:279*, 1970.

20. Rosenberg, M.: Fetal hematopoiesis: Case Report. *Blood 33:66*, 1969.

21. Stamatoyannopoulos, G., and Nienhuis, A. W.: *Cellular and Molecular Regulation of Hemoglobin Switching*. Grune & Stratton, New York, 1979.

22. Hudson, G.: Bone marrow volume in the human foetus and newborn. *Br. J. Haematol. 11:446*, 1965.

23. Brannon, D.: Extramedullary hematopoiesis in anemia. *Bull. Johns Hopkins Hosp. 41:104*, 1927.

24. Erslev, A. J.: Medullary and extramedullary blood formation. *Clin. Orthop. 52:25*, 1967.

25. Finne, P. H.: Erythropoietin production in fetal hypoxia and in anemic uremic patients. *Ann. N.Y. Acad. Sci. 149:497*, 1968.

26. Zanjani, E. D., and Gordon, A. S.: Erythropoietin production and utilization in fetal goats and sheep. *Isr. J. Med. Sci. 7:850*, 1971.

27. Zanjani, E. D., Peterson, E. N., Gordon, A. S., and Wasserman, L. R.: Erythropoietin production in the fetus: Role of the kidney and maternal anemia. *J. Lab. Clin. Med. 83:281*, 1974.

28. Caro, J., et al.: Erythropoietin production in response to anemia or hypoxia in the newborn rat. *Blood 60:984*, 1982.

29. Lajtha, L. G.: The common ancestral cell, in *Blood, Pure and Eloquent*, edited by M. M. Wintrobe. McGraw-Hill, New York, 1980, p. 81.

30. Filmanowicz, E., and Gurney, C. W.: Studies on erythropoiesis. XVI. Response to a single dose of erythropoietin in polycythemic mouse. *J. Lab. Clin. Med. 57:65*, 1961.

31. Stephenson, J. K., Axelrod, A. A., McLeod, D. L., and Shreeve, M. M.: Induction of hemoglobin-synthesizing cells by erythropoietin in vitro. *Proc. Natl. Acad. Sci. U.S.A. 65:1542*, 1971.

32. Hara, H., and Ogawa, M.: Erythropoietic precursors in mice under erythropoietic stimulation and suppression. *Exp. Hematol. 5:141*, 1977.

33. Axelrod, A. A., McLeod, D. L., Shreeve, M. M., and Heath, D. S.: Properties of cells that produce erythrocytic colonies in vitro, in

Hemopoiesis in Culture, edited by W. A. Robinson. DHEW Publ. No. (NIH)-74, 205, Washington, 1974, p. 226.

34. Ogawa, M., Grush, O. C., O'Dell, R. F., Hara, H., and MacEccheru, M. D.: Circulating erythropoietic precursors assessed in culture. *Blood 50:1081*, 1977.

35. Gregory, C. J., and Eaves, A. C.: Human marrow cells capable of erythropoietic differentiation in vitro: Definition of three erythroid colony responses. *Blood 49:855*, 1977.

36. Udupa, K. B., and Reissmann, K. R.: In vivo erythropoietin requirements of regenerating erythroid progenitors (BFU-E and CFU-E) in bone marrow of mice. *Blood 53:1164*, 1979.

37. Johnson, G. R., and Metcalf, D.: Erythropoietin independent erythroid colony formation in vitro by fetal mouse cells. *Exp. Hematol. 5:75*, 1977.

38. Iscove, N. N.: Erythropoietin independent stimulation of early erythropoiesis in adult marrow cultures by conditioned media from lectin-stimulated mouse spleen cells, in *Hematopoietic Cell Differentiation*, edited by D. W. Golde, M. J. Cline, D. Metcalf, and C. F. Fox. Academic, New York, 1978, p. 37.

39. Wagemaker, G., Peters, M. F., and Bol, S. J. L.: Induction of erythropoietin responsiveness in vitro by a distinct population of bone marrow cells. *Cell. Tiss. Kinet. 12:521*, 1979.

40. Nathan, D. G., et al.: Human erythroid burst forming unit (BFU-E); T cell requirement for proliferation in vitro. *J. Exp. Med. 147:324*, 1978.

41. Gordon, L. J., Wesley, J. M., Branda, R. F., Zanjani, E. D., and Jacob, H. S.: Regulation of erythroid colony formation by bone marrow macrophages. *Blood 55:1047*, 1980.

42. Zuckerman, K. S.: Human erythroid burst-forming units. Growth in vitro is dependent on monocytes, but not T lymphocytes. *J. Clin. Invest. 67:702*, 1981.

43. Iscove, N. N., and Guilbert, L. J.: Erythropoietin-independence of early erythropoiesis and a two-regulator model of proliferative control of the hemopoietic system, in *In Vitro Aspects of Erythropoiesis*, edited by M. J. Murphy et al. Springer-Verlag, New York, 1978, p. 3.

44. Clarke, B. J., Nathan, D. G., Alter, B. P., Forget, B. G., Hillman, D. G., and Housman, D.: Hemoglobin synthesis in human BFU-E and CFU-E-derived erythroid colonies. *Blood 54:805*, 1979.

45. Weicker, H.: Das Mass-, Mengen- und Zeitgefüge der Erythropoese unter physiologischen und pathologischen Bedingungen. *Schweiz. Med. Wochenschr. 87:1210*, 1957.

46. Marks, P. A., and Rifkind, R. A.: Protein synthesis in erythropoiesis. *Science 175:955*, 1972.

47. Wintrobe, M. M.: *Clinical Hematology*, eds. 1–8. Lea & Febiger, Philadelphia, 1942–1981.

48. Donohue, D. M., Reiff, R. H., Hanson, M. L., Betson, Y., and Finch, C. A.: Quantitative measurement of the erythrocytic and granulocytic cells of the marrow and blood. *J. Clin. Invest. 37:1571*, 1958.

49. Finch, C. A., Harker, L. A., and Cook J. D.: Kinetics of the formed elements of human blood. *Blood 50:699*, 1977.

50. Lajtha, L. G., and Oliver, R.: Studies on the kinetics of erythropoiesis: A model of the erythron, in *Ciba Foundation Symposium on Haemopoiesis*, edited by G. E. W. Wolstenholme and M. O'Connor. Little, Brown, Boston, 1960, p. 289.

51. Mechanik, N.: Untersuchungen über das Gewicht des Knochenmarkes des Menschen. *A. Ges. Anat. 79:58*, 1926. Summarized by R. E. Ellis, *Phys. Med. Biol. 5:255*, 1961.

52. Marks, P. A., and Kovach, J. S.: Development of mammalian erythroid cells, in *Current Topics in Developmental Biology*, edited by A. Moscona and A. A. Monroy. Academic, New York, 1966, p. 213.

53. Killmann, S. A., Cronkite, E. P., Fliedner, T. M., and Bond, V. P.: Mitotic indices of human bone marrow cells. I. Number and cytologic distribution of mitoses. *Blood 19:743*, 1962; and III. Duration of some phases of erythrocytic and granulocytic proliferation computed from mitotic indices. *Blood 24:267*, 1964.

54. LeBlond, C. P.: Classical techniques for the study of the kinetics of cellular proliferation, in *The Kinetics of Cellular Proliferation*, edited by F. Stohlman, Jr. Grune & Stratton, New York, 1959.

55. Skårberg, K. O.: Cellularity and cell proliferation rates in human bone marrow. II. Studies on generation times and radiothymidine

uptake of human red cell precursors. *Acta Med. Scand.* 195:301, 1974.

56. Lichtman, M. A., Chamberlain, J. K., and Santillo, P. A.: Factors thought to contribute to the regulation of egress of cells from marrow, in *The Year of Hematology*, edited by R. Silber, J. LoBue, and A. S. Gordon. Plenum, New York, 1978, p. 243.

57. Jandl, J. H.: Agglutination and sequestration of immature red cells. *J. Lab. Clin. Med.* 55:663, 1960.

58. Prankerd, T. A. J.: The spleen and anemia. *Br. Med. J.* 2:517, 1963.

59. Baker, C. H., and Remington, J. W.: Role of the spleen in determining total body hematocrit. *Am. J. Physiol.* 198:906, 1960.

60. Turner, A. W., and Hodgetts, V. E.: The dynamic red cell storage function of the spleen in sheep. II. Jugular hematocrit fall after some tranquilizing agents, particularly chlorpromazine. *Aust. J. Exp. Biol. Med. Sci.* 38:79, 1960.

61. Erslev, A. J.: Blood and mountains, in *Blood, Pure and Eloquent*, edited by M. M. Wintrobe. McGraw-Hill, New York, 1980, p. 257.

62. Jourdanet, D.: *De l'Anémie des altitudes et de l'anémie en général dans ses rapports avec la pression de l'atmosphère.* Bailliere, Paris, 1863.

63. Hurtado, A., Merino, C., and Delgado, E.: Influence of anoxemia on the hemopoietic activity. *Arch. Intern. Med.* 75:284, 1945.

64. Erslev, A. J.: Physiologic control of red cell production. *Blood* 10:954, 1955.

65. Birkhill, F. R., Maloney, M. A., and Levenson, S. M.: Effect of transfusion polycythemia upon bone marrow activity and erythrocyte survival in man. *Blood* 6:1021, 1951.

66. Tinsley, J. C., Moore, C. V., Dubach, R., Minnich, V., and Grinstein, M.: The role of oxygen in the regulation of erythropoiesis: Depression of the rate of delivery of new red cells to the blood by high concentrations of inspired oxygen. *J. Clin. Invest.* 28:1544, 1949.

67. Thorling, E. B., and Erslev, A. J.: The effect of some erythropoietic agents on the "tissue" tension of oxygen. *Br. J. Haematol.* 23:483, 1972.

68. Carnot, P., and Deflandre, C.: Sur l'activité hématopoietique des serum au cours de la régénération du sang. *Acad. Sci. M.* 3:384, 1906.

69. Reissman, K. R.: Studies on the mechanism of erythropoietic stimulation in parabiotic rats during hypoxia. *Blood* 5:372, 1950.

70. Stohlman, F., Jr., Rath, C. E., and Rose, J. C.: Evidence for a humoral regulation of erythropoiesis: Studies on a patient with polycythemia secondary to regional hypoxia. *Blood* 9:721, 1954.

71. Erslev, A. J.: Humoral regulation of red cell production. *Blood* 8:349, 1953.

72. Erslev, A. J., Caro, J., Miller, O., and Silver, R.: Plasma erythropoietin in health and disease. *Ann. Clin. Lab. Sci.* 10:250, 1980.

73. Adamson, J. W., Alexanian, R., Martinez, C., and Finch, C. A.: Erythropoietin excretion in normal man. *Blood* 28:354, 1966.

74. Goldwasser, E., Kung, C. K.-H., and Eliason, J. F.: On the mechanism of erythropoietin-induced differentiation. XIII. The role of sialic acid in erythropoietic action. *J. Biol. Chem.* 249:4202, 1974.

75. Hiyake, T., Kung, C. K.-H., and Goldwasser, E.: Purification of human erythropoietin. *J. Biol. Chem.* 252:5558, 1977.

76. Rioux, E., and Erslev, A. J.: Immunologic studies of a partially purified sheep erythropoietin. *J. Immunol.* 101:6, 1968.

77. Schooley, J. C., Garcia, J. F., Cantor, L. N., and Havens, V. W.: A summary of some studies on erythropoiesis using antierythropoietin immune serum. *Ann. N.Y. Acad. Sci.* 149:266, 1968.

78. Jacobson, L. O., Goldwasser, E., Fried, W., and Plzak, L.: Role of the kidney in erythropoiesis. *Nature* [*Lond.*] 179:633, 1957.

79. Reissmann, K. R., Nomura, T., Gunn, R. W., and Brosius, F.: Erythropoietic response to anemia or erythropoietic injection in uremic rats with or without functioning renal tissue. *Blood* 16:1411, 1960.

80. Hansen, P.: Polycythemia produced by constriction of the renal artery of the rabbit. *Acta Pathol. Microbiol. Scand.* 60:465, 1964.

81. Hudgson, P., Pearce, J. M., and Yeates, W. K.: Renal artery stenosis with hypertension and high hematocrit. *Br. Med. J.* 1:18, 1967.

82. Gallagher, N. I., and Donati, R. M.: Inappropriate erythropoietin elaboration. *Ann. N.Y. Acad. Sci.* 149:528, 1968.

83. Abbrecht, P. H., Malvin, R. L., and Vander, A. J.: Renal production of erythropoietin and renin after experimental infarction. *Nature* [*Lond.*] 211:1318, 1966.

84. Westerman, M. P., Jenkins, J. L., Dekker, A., Krentner, A., and Fisher, B.: Significance of erythrocytosis and increased erythropoietin secretion after renal transplantation. *Lancet* 755, 1967.

85. Nies, B. A., Cohn, R., and Schrier, S. L.: Erythremia after renal transplantation. *N. Engl. J. Med.* 273:785, 1965.

86. Dagher, F. J., Ramos, E., Erslev, A. J., Alonzi, S. V., Karmi, S. A., and Caro, J.: Are the native kidneys responsible for erythrocytosis in renal allorecipients? *Transplantation* 28:496, 1979.

87. Waldman, T. A., Rosse, W. F., and Swarm, R. L.: The erythropoiesis-stimulating factors produced by tumors. *Ann. N.Y. Acad. Sci.* 149:509, 1968.

88. Thorling, E. B.: Paraneoplastic erythrocytosis and inappropriate erythropoietin production: A review. *Scand. J. Haematol.*, suppl. 17, 1972.

89. Mitus, W. J., Galbraith, P., Gollerkeri, M., and Toyama, K.: Experimental renal erythrocytosis. I. Effects of pressure and vascular interference. *Blood* 24:343, 1964.

90. Brown, R.: Plasma erythropoietin in chronic uremia. *Br. Med. J.* 2:1036, 1965.

91. Erslev, A. J., McKenna, P. J., Capelli, J. P., Hamburger, R. J., Cohn, H. E., and Clark, J. E.: Erythropoiesis in nephrectomized patients. *Arch. Intern. Med.* 122:230, 1968.

92. Nathan, D. G., Schupak, E., Stohlman, F., Jr., and Merill, J. P.: Erythropoiesis in anephric man. *J. Clin. Invest.* 43:2158, 1964.

93. Fried, W., Kilbridge, R., Krantz, S., McDonald, I. P., and Lange, R. D.: Studies on extrarenal erythropoietin. *J. Lab. Clin. Med.* 73:244, 1969.

94. Fried, W.: The liver as a source of extrarenal erythropoietin production. *Blood* 40:671, 1972.

95. Naughton, B. A., Gordon, A. S., Piliero, S. J., and Liu, P.: Extrarenal erythropoietin, in *In Vitro Aspects of Erythropoiesis*, edited by M. J. Murphy et al. Springer-Verlag, New York, 1978, p. 194.

96. Erslev, A. J., Caro, J., Kansu, E., and Silver, R.: Renal and extrarenal erythropoietin production in anemic rats. *Br. J. Haematol.* 45:65, 1980.

97. Zanjani, E. D., Ascensao, J. L., McGlave, P. B., Banisadre, M., and Ash, R. C.: Studies on the liver to kidney switch of erythropoietin production. *J. Clin. Invest.* 67:1183, 1981.

98. Anagnostou, A., Schade, S., Barone, J., and Fried, W.: Effects of partial hepatectomy on extrarenal erythropoietin production in rats. *Blood* 50:457, 1977.

99. Naughton, B. A., Kaplan, S. M., Roy, M., Bardowsky, A. J., Gordon, A. S., and Piliero, J. J.: Hepatic regeneration and erythropoietin production in the rat. *Science* 196:301, 1977.

100. Brown, S., Caro, J., Erslev, A. J., and Murray, T.: Rise in erythropoietin and hematocrit associated with transient liver enzyme abnormalities in an anephric hemodialysis patient. *Am. J. Med.* 68:280, 1980.

101. Naets, J. P., and Wittek, M.: Erythropoiesis in anephric man. *Lancet* 941, 1968.

102. Busuttil, R. W., Roh, B. L., and Fisher, J. W.: Cytological localization of erythropoietin in the human kidney using the fluorescent antibody technique. *Proc. Soc. Exp. Biol. Med.* 137:327, 1971.

103. Mitus, W. J., Toyama, K., and Braner, M. J.: Erythrocytosis, juxtaglomerular apparatus (JGA) and erythropoietin in the course of experimental unilateral hydronephrosis in rabbits. *Ann. N.Y. Acad. Sci.* 149:107, 1968.

104. Demopoulos, H. B., Highman, B., Altland, P. D., Gerving, M. A., and Kaley, G.: Effects of high altitudes on granular juxtaglomerular cells and their possible role in erythropoietin production. *Am. J. Pathol.* 46:497, 1965.

105. Goldfarb, B., and Tobian, L.: Relationship of erythropoietin to renal juxtaglomerular cells. *Proc. Soc. Exp. Biol. Med.* 129:845, 1968.

106. Fisher, J. W., and Balcerzak, S. P.: Effect of exogenous erythropoietin on juxtaglomerular cells. *Proc. Soc. Exp. Biol. Med.* 132:367, 1969.

107. Gordon, A. S., Cooper, G. W., and Zanjani, E. D.: The kidney and erythropoiesis. *Semin. Hematol.* 4:337, 1967.

108. Zanjani, E. D., Contrera, J. F., Gordon, A. S., Cooper, G. W., Wong, K. K., and Katz, R.: The renal erythropoietic factor (R.E.F.). III. Enzymatic role in erythropoietin production. *Proc. Soc. Exp. Biol. Med.* 125:505, 1967.

109. Erslev, A. J.: In vitro production of erythropoietin by kidneys perfused with a serum-free solution. *Blood* 44:77, 1974.
110. Fisher, J. W., Hatch, F. E., Roh, B. L., Allen, R. C., and Kelley, B. J.: Erythropoietin inhibitor in kidney extracts and plasma from anemic uremic human subjects. *Blood* 31:440, 1968.
111. Erslev, A. J., and Kazal, L. A.: Inactivation of erythropoietin by tissue homogenates. *Proc. Soc. Exp. Biol. Med.* 129:845, 1968.
112. Fried, W., Barone-Varelas, J., and Berman, M.: Detection of high erythropoietin titers in renal extracts of hypoxic rats. *J. Lab. Clin. Med.* 85:82, 1981.
113. Erslev, A. J.: Observations on the nature of the erythropoietic factor. II. Erythropoietic activity of serum and bone marrow after time limited exposure to anemic and hypoxic anoxia. *J. Lab. Clin. Med.* 50:543, 1957.
114. Stohlman, F., Jr.: Observations on the physiology of erythropoietin and its role in the regulation of red cell production. *Ann. N.Y. Acad. Sci.* 77:710, 1959.
115. Naets, J. P., and Wittek, M.: Effect of erythroid hyperplasia on the disappearance rate of erythropoietin in the dog. *Acta Haematol.* [Basel] 39:42, 1968.
116. Naets, J. P., and Wittek, M.: Role of the kidney in the catabolism of erythropoietin in the rat. *J. Lab. Clin. Med.* 84:99, 1974.
117. Rosse, W. F., and Waldman, T. A.: The metabolism of erythropoietin in patients with anemia due to deficient erythropoiesis. *J. Clin. Invest.* 43:1348, 1964.
118. Stohlman, F., Jr., and Brecher, G.: Humoral regulation of erythropoiesis. V. Relationship of plasma erythropoietin level to bone marrow activity. *Proc. Soc. Exp. Biol. Med.* 100:40, 1959.
119. Stohlman, F., Jr.: Erythropoiesis. *N. Engl. J. Med.* 267:392, 1962.
120. Finne, P. H.: On the correspondence between red cell production and plasma erythropoietin level. *Scand. J. Clin. Lab. Invest.* 17:135, 1965.
121. Miller, M. E., et al.: The effects of acute bleeding on acid-base balance, erythropoietin (Ep) production and in vivo P50 in the rat. *Br. J. Haematol.* 33:379, 1976.
122. Miller, M. E., et al.: pH effect on erythropoietin response to hypoxia. *N. Engl. J. Med.* 288:706, 1973.
123. Alexanian, R.: Erythropoietin excretion in bone marrow failure and hemolytic anemia. *J. Lab. Clin. Med.* 82:438, 1973.
124. Weintraub, A. H., Gordon, A. S., Becker, E. L., Camiscoli, J. F., and Contrera, J. F.: Plasma and renal clearance of exogenous erythropoietin in the dog. *Am. J. Physiol.* 207:523, 1964.
125. Alpen, E. L.: The metabolic fate of erythropoietin, in *Erythropoiesis*, edited by L. O. Jacobson and M. Doyle. Grune & Stratton, New York, 1962, p. 134.
126. Erslev, A. J.: The effect of anemic anoxia on the cellular development of nucleated red cells. *Blood* 14:386, 1959.
127. Alpen, E. L., and Cranmore, A.: Observations on the regulation of erythropoiesis and on cellular dynamics by Fe59 autoradiography, in *Kinetics of Cellular Proliferation*, edited by F. Stohlman, Jr. Grune & Stratton, New York, 1959, p. 290.
128. Reissmann, K. F., and Samorapoompichit, S.: Effect of erythropoietin on proliferation of erythroid stem cells in the absence of transplantable colony-forming units. *Blood* 36:287, 1970.
129. Kennedy, W. L., Alpen, E. L., and Garcia, J. F.: Regulation of red blood cell production by erythropoietin: Normal mouse marrow in vitro. *Exp. Hematol.* 8:1114, 1980.
130. Roodman, G. D., Kaplan, J. M., Kaplan, M. E., and Zanjani, E. D.: Effects of shortened erythropoietin exposure on sheep marrow culture. *Br. J. Haematol.* 47:195, 1981.
131. Chang, S. C.-S., Sikkema, D., and Goldwasser, E.: Evidence for an erythropoietin receptor protein on rat bone marrow cells. *Biochem. Biophys. Res. Commun.* 57:399, 1974.
132. Roodman, G. D., Spivak, J. L., and Zanjani, E. D.: Stimulation of erythroid colony formation in vitro by erythropoietin immobilized on agarose-bound lectins. *J. Lab. Clin. Med.* 98:684, 1981.
133. Brown, J. E., and Adamson, J. W.: Modulation of in vitro erythropoiesis: The influence of β-adrenergic agonists on erythroid colony formation. *J. Clin. Invest.* 60:70, 1977.
134. Golde, D., Bersch, N., Chopra, J., and Cline, M. J.: Thyroid hormones stimulate erythropoiesis in vitro. *Br. J. Haematol.* 37:173, 1977.
135. Moriyama, Y., and Fisher, J. W.: Effects of testosterone and erythropoietin on erythroid colony formation in human bone marrow cultures. *Blood* 45:665, 1975.
136. Krantz, S. B., and Goldwasser, E.: On the mechanism of erythropoietin induced differentiation. II. The effect on RNA synthesis. *Biochim. Biophys. Acta* 103:325, 1965.
137. Rifkind, R. A., and Marks, P. A.: The regulation of erythropoiesis. *Blood Cells* 1:417, 1975.
138. Glass, J., Lavidor, L. M., and Robinson, S. H.: Use of Ficall separation and short-time culture techniques to study erythroid development. *Blood* 46:705, 1975.
139. Papayannopoulou, T., and Finch, C. A.: Radioiron measurements of red cell maturation. *Blood Cells* 1:535, 1975.
140. Brecher, G., and Stohlman, F., Jr.: The macrocytic response to erythropoietic stimulation. *Proc. Soc. Exp. Biol. Med.* 107:887, 1961.
141. Ganzoni, A., Hillman, R. S., and Finch, C. A.: Maturation of the macroreticulocyte. *Br. J. Haematol.* 16:119, 1969.
142. Chamberlain, J. K., LeBlond, P. F., and Weed, R. I.: Reduction of adventitial cell cover: An early direct effect of erythropoietin on bone marrow ultrastructure. *Blood Cells* 1:655, 1975.
143. Halvorsen, S.: The central nervous system in regulation of erythropoiesis. *Acta Haematol.* 35:65, 1966.
144. Feldman, S., Rachmilewitz, E. A., and Izak, G.: The effect of central nervous system stimulation of erythropoiesis in rats with chronically implanted electrodes. *J. Lab. Clin. Med.* 67:713, 1966.
145. Tramazzani, J. H., Morita, E., and Chiocchio, S. R.: The carotid body as a neuroendocrine organ involved in control of erythropoiesis. *Proc. Natl. Acad. Sci. U.S.A.* 68:52, 1971.
146. Erslev, A. J.: The search for erythropoietin. *N. Engl. J. Med.* 284:849, 1971 (editorial).
147. Lugliani, R., Whipp, B. J., Winter, B., Tanaka, K. R., and Wasserman, K.: The role of the carotid body in erythropoiesis in man. *N. Engl. J. Med.* 285:1112, 1971.
148. Meincke, H. A., and Crafts, R. C.: Further observations on the mechanisms by which androgens and growth hormone influence erythropoiesis. *Ann. N.Y. Acad. Sci.* 149:298, 1968.
149. Finch, C. A., Hanson, M. L., and Donohue, D. M.: Kinetics of erythropoiesis: A comparison of response to anemia induced by phenylhydrazine and by blood loss. *Am. J. Physiol.* 197:761, 1959.
150. Hillman, R. S., and Henderson, P. A.: The control of marrow production by the level of iron supply. *J. Clin. Invest.* 48:454, 1969.
151. Sanchez-Medal, L., and Labardini, J.: Hemolysis and erythropoiesis. II. The effect of hemolysis and hemolysates on erythropoiesis. *Ann. N.Y. Acad. Sci.* 149:377, 1968.
152. Labardini, J., Sanchez-Medal, L., Arriaga, L., Lopez, D., and Smyth, J. F.: Hemolysis and erythropoiesis. IV. Effect of hemolysates on the erythropoiesis of normal, starved, and polycythemic rats. *J. Lab. Clin. Med.* 72:419, 1968.
153. Erslev, A. J.: The effect of hemolysates on red cell production and erythropoietin release. *J. Lab. Clin. Med.* 78:1, 1971.
154. Whitcomb, W. H., and Moore, M. Z.: The inhibitory effect of plasma from hypertransfused animals on erythrocyte iron incorporation in mice. *J. Lab. Clin. Med.* 66:641, 1965.
155. Whitcomb, W. H., Moore, M. Z., and Rhodes, J. P.: Influence of polycythemic and anemic plasma on erythrocyte iron incorporation in the plethoric hypoxic mouse. *J. Lab. Clin. Med.* 73:584, 1969.
156. Erslev, A. J., and Thorling, E. B.: Effect of polycythemic serum on the rate of red cell production. *Ann. N.Y. Acad. Sci.* 149:173, 1968.
157. Matoth, Y., and Zaizor, R.: Absence of an inhibitor of erythropoiesis in postnatal plasma. *Isr. J. Med. Sci.* 3:477, 1967.
158. Necas, E., and Neuwirt, J.: Feedback regulation by red cell mass of the sensitivity of the erythropoietin-producing organ to hypoxia. *Blood* 36:754, 1970.
159. Erslev, A. J.: The erythropoietic effect of hematocrit variations in normovolemic rabbits. *Blood* 27:629, 1966.
160. Murrary, J. F., Gold, P., and Johnson, B. L., Jr.: The circulatory effects of hematocrit variations in normovolemic and hypervolemic dogs. *J. Clin. Invest.* 42:1150, 1963.
161. Thorling, E. B., and Erslev, A. J.: The "tissue" tension of oxygen and its relation to hematocrit and erythropoiesis. *Blood* 31:332, 1968.

CHAPTER *39*

Destruction of erythrocytes

RICHARD A. COOPER
JAMES H. JANDL

Although it is known that normal red blood cells live for 120 days, the mechanisms of their destruction are unclear, and our knowledge of red cell destruction has been derived almost exclusively from the study of cells with a shortened life-span. Abnormal red cells are removed from the circulation by three general mechanisms: (1) red cells manifesting mild and often subtle abnormalities are cleared by the exceedingly sensitive sequestering system of the spleen; (2) more severely injured red cells are removed by the liver; (3) red cells so severely damaged that their structural integrity is compromised are destroyed as they circulate, with the release of their intracellular contents into the plasma. This chapter will consider these mechanisms in greater detail and will examine the red cell changes that lead to premature destruction.

Sites of red cell destruction

Gross injuries to the red cell, such as those induced by trauma or by complement, result in red cell destruction in the intravascular space. However, most forms of red cell injury are not sufficiently severe to cause intravascular lysis. Rather, detection of the injury and trapping and destruction of the cell occur in the monocyte-macrophage system, primarily in the spleen and liver and secondarily in the marrow and other sites.

The spleen is particularly efficient in trapping and destroying red cells which have minimal defects, often so mild that they are undetectable by in vitro techniques. This unique ability of the spleen results from its unusual vascular anatomy [1–5]. Red cells flow from the small arterioles of the spleen into the "marginal zone" of the lymphatic white pulp. Although the cells which occupy this zone are not phagocytic, they serve as a mechanical filter that hinders the progress of damaged red cells. As they enter the red pulp, red cells flow either into the broad sinuses leading directly to splenic veins or into narrow cords which end blindly but which communicate with sinuses between sinus lining cells. These openings, which may be as small as 3 μm in diameter [6], stringently test the ability of red cells to deform (Fig. 39-1). Most splenic blood flows directly into the splenic sinuses, whereas only 1 to 2 percent of the red cells entering the spleen traverse the cordal system [7]. Hereditary spherocytes [8] and Heinz body–containing red cells [9] are retarded in their circulation through the splenic cords. In most hemolytic disorders the marginal zones, sinuses, and cords are diffusely filled with cells [10]. Erythrostasis in the spleen [11], enhanced by plasma skimming, exposes red cells to the unphysiologic conditions of glucose deprivation [7] and lowered pH [12], contributing to their final destruction.

The liver lacks the spleen's fine perception of red cell abnormalities. However, when red cell aberrations are

FIGURE 39-1 A splenic sinus. The left panel represents a diagram of an electron micrograph, part of which (*rectangle*) is shown on the right. Two macrophages seen in the left panel are in the cordal space surrounding the sinus. An erythrocyte (*arrow in left panel* and *E in right panel*) is seen squeezing between endothelial cells lining the sinus on its way from the splenic cord to sinus. Filamentous bands (FB) of the sinus endothelial cells arch between successive ring components of the basement membrane. Small arrows indicate cross sections of these bands. Above the filamentous bands is a leukocyte (*large arrow*) which is apparently moving toward the sinus. (Chen and Weiss [199].)

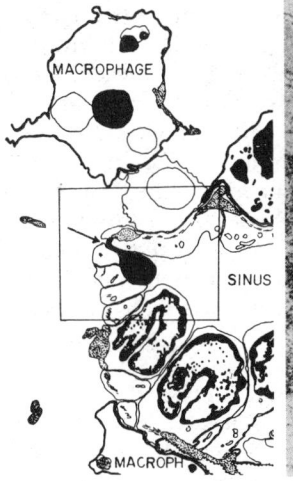 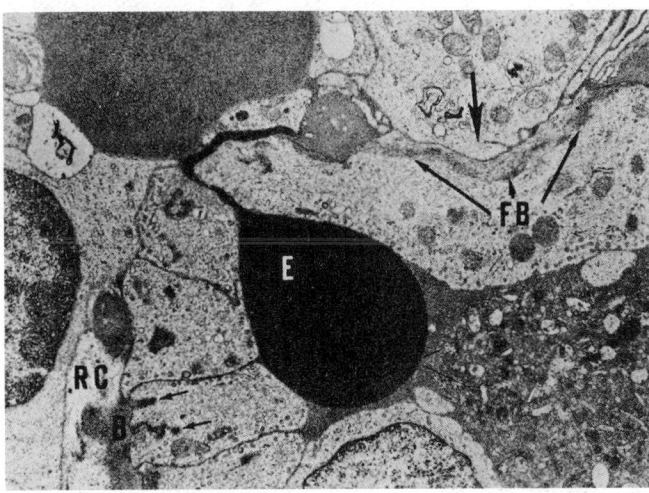

sufficiently gross to be detected by the liver, this organ efficiently clears them from the circulation. Thus, while the spleen senses red cells minimally affected by heat [13], sulfhydryl blocking compounds [14], or IgG antibodies [15], the liver detects and destroys red cells only after considerably more heat damage or exposure to larger amounts of sulfhydryl blocking reagents, complement-fixing antibodies, or very large amounts of IgG antibody [14–17]. In addition, the liver senses gross changes in the red cells, such as those produced by sickled hemoglobin. Because the spleen receives less than 5 percent of the cardiac output whereas the liver receives 35 percent or more, the liver may be more effective than the spleen in clearing red cells that it recognizes as abnormal [7]. Maximum clearance rates for these two organs correspond to their respective shares of the cardiac output. Although phagocytosis of red cells stimulates macrophage proliferation in both the spleen and the liver, the proliferative response of the spleen is far more dramatic, leading to marked hyperplasia, increased blood flow, and functional overactivity ("hypersplenism") [7,10,18,19]. Conversely, the spleen undergoes atrophy when, under experimental conditions, its phagocytic function is not exercised [18,19].

Destruction of senescent red cells

While considerable data exist describing the mode of destruction of abnormal red cells, relatively little is known about normal red cell aging and the mode of destruction of senescent red cells. A variety of changes have been described in the red cell as it ages, although their significance, if any, in the final destruction of the cell is unknown. It appears that older cells are smaller than younger cells, and they have an increase in density and mean corpuscular hemoglobin concentration (MCHC) [20–22]. Older red cells also have a decrease in sialic acid content and, therefore, in zeta potential [23,24]. Whereas red cells depleted of sialic acid enzymatically have a shortened survival [25], red cells in patients with acquired polyagglutinability due to a decreased amount of red cell sialic acid do not [26], and the

TABLE 39-1   Mechanisms of red cell destruction

1. Decreased surface-area/volume ratio
   a. Decreased surface area
   b. Increased volume
2. Structural modification of the red cell membrane
   a. Decreased fluidity of membrane lipids
   b. Decreased elasticity of membrane proteins
   c. Membrane modifications recognized by the reticuloendothelial system
   d. Disruption of membrane integrity
3. Increased internal viscosity
   a. Hemoglobin aggregation
   b. Decreased cell water
   c. Precipitated hemoglobin
4. Splenic hyperfunction

consequence of a decrease in sialic acid for senescent red cells is not totally resolved. It has been proposed that the IgG coating of red cells increases as they age [27], and decreased activity of several red cell enzymes has been described. Reticulocytes are rich in membrane lipids, and this excess lipid, present both in intracellular organelles and plasma membranes, is lost during reticulocyte maturation [28]. Data concerning a continued loss of membrane lipid during the life-span of mature red cells are difficult to interpret because of technical limitations in the separation of cells by age [20,29]; however, it appears that little or no lipid is lost from red cells during the final half of their life-span [30]. Senescent red cells are sequestered in the spleen [31], and their destruction presumably occurs because of a subtle abnormality detected by the spleen. However, splenectomy does not enhance red cell survival in otherwise normal people [32,33].

Mechanisms of premature red cell destruction

The exact cause of hemolysis in many hemolytic disorders remains obscure or incompletely established; however, it appears that the premature destruction of circulating red cells is caused by one or more of four general mechanisms: (1) a decrease in the surface-area/volume ratio, (2) a structural modification of the red cell membrane, (3) an increased internal viscosity, or (4) splenic hyperfunction (Table 39-1).

DECREASED SURFACE-AREA/VOLUME RATIO

DECREASED SURFACE AREA
As it flows through the microcirculation, the red cell is dependent for survival on its ability to undergo rapid changes in shape. Extreme deformations are required when red cells are packed at cell concentrations greater than 60% [34] or when they traverse orifices smaller than their own diameter [35,36]. Although the red cell membrane can be bent, it offers a high resistance to stretch [37]. Thus the demands of the circulation require that the red cell be deformable [38] (Fig. 39-2). Its discoid shape, providing a surface area that exceeds by 60 to 70 percent the minimum necessary to encompass its contents, allows considerable deformation. At the other extreme, a sphere possesses the least surface area to contain a given volume and cannot be deformed. The limits of deformability, therefore, depend on the surface-area/volume ratio of the red cell. Osmotic fragility is a useful test of this ratio (Chap. 55). Deformability may be assessed directly by observing the ease with which red cells pass through filters of small pore size [12,39] or pipettes with narrow orifices [37,40,41]. However, the most critical measure of deformability is the ability of red cells to traverse the spleen filter. The deformability of hereditary spherocytes is decreased because their surface area is decreased, and these cells are selectively

sequestered in the spleen. Through a process of conditioning [11], the spleen itself causes red cells to lose surface area under certain conditions. This occurs when red cells are predisposed to stagnation in the spleen (e.g., hereditary spherocytes [42] or spur cells [43]), when the spleen recognizes red cells as abnormal (e.g., in autoimmune hemolytic anemia [15] and possibly in oxidant hemolysis caused by lipophilic chemicals [44]), and when normal red cells become pooled in a hypertrophic [45] or congested [46] spleen. Whatever the cause, the result of a decreased surface area is a decreased ability to pass the spleen filter again, leading ultimately to irreversible trapping and destruction in the spleen.

INCREASED CELL VOLUME

The maintenance of red cell deformability requires regulation of cell volume. The relatively high concentration of impermeant molecules in the cell creates an osmotic force [47]. Normally the red cell prevents osmotic swelling by actively extruding the semipermeant cation sodium. For this it requires energy in the form of ATP. Under conditions of erythroconcentration and glucose deprivation [7], or in the presence of disordered energy metabolism, volume control is lost, the cell swells from the unopposed entry of sodium and water, and its essential regulation of shape and viscosity is disturbed. The membrane permeability to sodium is increased in certain disorders, such as hereditary spherocytosis [48,49], hereditary elliptocytosis [50], and hereditary stomatocytosis [51–53], and its permeability to potassium is increased by amphotericin B [54] and agents which react with membrane sulfhydryl groups [55]. To maintain volume control under these conditions, the red cell accelerates its rate of glycolysis and active cation transport. Although compensation for this "leakiness" is usually achieved, such cells are particularly susceptible to damage under conditions of metabolic deprivation [7].

STRUCTURAL MODIFICATION OF THE RED CELL MEMBRANE

DECREASED FLUIDITY OF MEMBRANE LIPIDS

Current concepts consider the red cell membrane to be largely composed of a lipid bilayer containing various membrane proteins [56]. Some of these proteins span the bilayer; others are present only on its inner surface [57]. A vital cytoskeletal component, *spectrin*, is thought to form a structural framework on the inner membrane surface [58]. Abnormalities of spectrin may be responsible for the abnormal shape and survival of red cells in hereditary elliptocytosis [59]. The bilayer is composed of approximately equal quantities of cholesterol and phospholipid [59]. Of the major phospholipids, lecithin and sphingomyelin are primarily on the outer surface and phosphatidylethanolamine and phosphatidylserine are primarily on the inner membrane surface [60]. The fluidity of membrane lipids is an expression of the amount of random motion which exists among the lipid

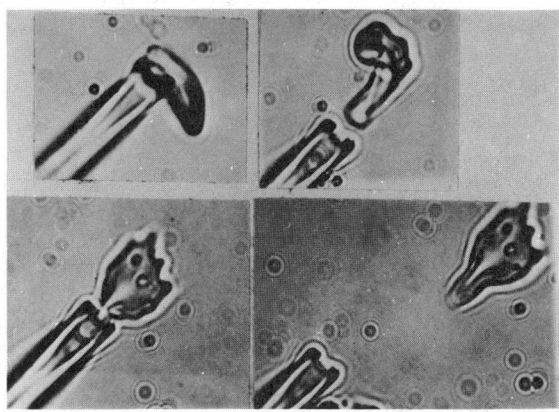

FIGURE 39-2   Red blood cell deformation. The extreme deformability and the viscoelastic properties of the red cell are demonstrated in this sequence, which depicts a normal red cell (*upper*) and a crenated red cell (*lower*) being first drawn into and then ejected from a micropipette. (From R. P. Rand, Ph.D. thesis, University of Western Ontario, 1964; reprinted in Burton [41].)

molecules in the hydrophobic core of the membrane bilayer [61]. Cholesterol restricts molecular motion in the hydrophobic core, thereby decreasing fluidity and making them more viscous [62], much as lowering temperature slows molecular motion in oils. Indeed, doubling the amount of cholesterol has the same effect as lowering the temperature of red cell membranes by 15°C. An increase in membrane cholesterol decreases the ability of red cells to traverse filters of small pore size in vitro [64], and it underlies the splenic pooling, conditioning, and destruction of cholesterol-rich spur cells in patients with cirrhosis and splenomegaly [43] (Chap. 57).

Of the phospholipids, sphingomyelin is more rigid than lecithin [64]. The acanthocytes of patients with abetalipoproteinemia (Chap. 57) are enriched with sphingomyelin at the expense of lecithin [65], leading to a decreased membrane fluidity [66], and a decreased red cell filterability [66,67]. However, splenomegaly is not an inherent feature of this disorder, and red cell survival is only mildly shortened [68].

Osmotically resistant target cells in patients with liver disease have an increased membrane surface area due to an excessive amount of membrane cholesterol and phospholipid (lecithin), with only a slight excess of cholesterol over phospholipid [79]. Therefore membrane fluidity is not distinctly abnormal. This excess of both lipid and surface area is acquired and reversible in mature red cells (Fig. 39-3). The life-span of target cells is normal in obstructive jaundice, but it is decreased in patients with splenomegaly due to cirrhosis. Alcoholic patients with acute fatty livers may have transient periods of hemolysis coincident with their active liver disease and acute portal hypertension. When it is also associated with hypertriglyceridemia, it has come to be known as *Zieve's syndrome* [70]. But hypertri-

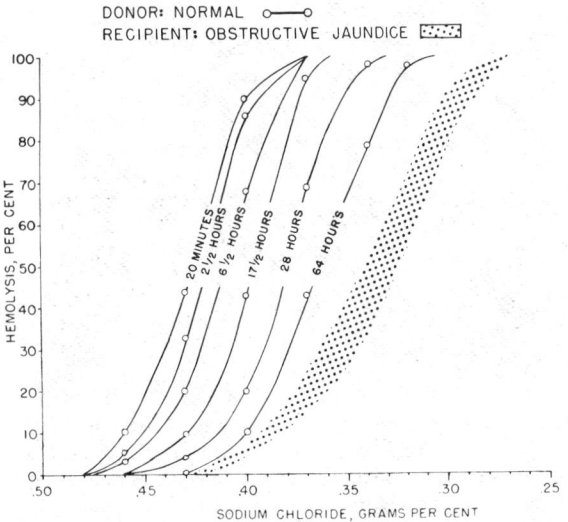

DONOR: NORMAL ○——○
RECIPIENT: OBSTRUCTIVE JAUNDICE ▨▨▨

FIGURE 39-3   The acquisition of membrane lipid and surface area in vivo. Normal radioactive-chromium–labeled (^{51}Cr-labeled) red blood cells acquire membrane lipid and surface area following their transfusion into patients with obstructive jaundice and osmotically resistant target cells. As shown, they become progressively more osmotically resistant with time. (Cooper and Jandl [200].)

glyceridemia per se does not cause hemolysis [71], and of the various features of this syndrome only portal hypertension and hemolysis appear to be related pathogenetically.

DECREASED ELASTICITY OF MEMBRANE PROTEINS
Membrane deformability (elasticity) is the property of the membrane which permits it to withstand a shear

FIGURE 39-4   Binding of antibody-coated red blood cells to a mononuclear cell. Normal human red cells coated with incomplete anti-D adhere to and are made spherical by a peripheral blood mononuclear cell. Fingerlike processes of the mononuclear cell invaginate some red cells (*upper left*), and periodic sites of attachment (*right*) appear to exist. (Abramson, LoBuglio, Jandl, and Cotran [85].)

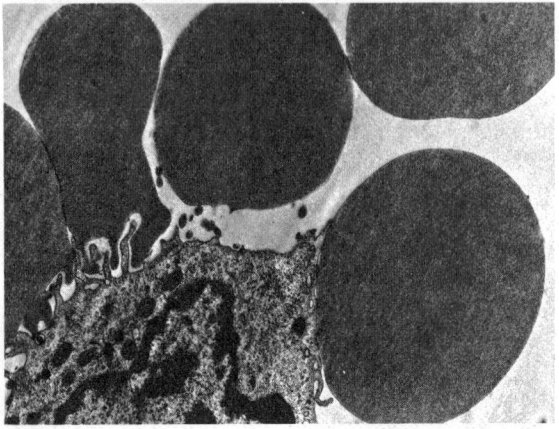

stress [72]. It should be differentiated from *red cell deformability,* which is related not only to the properties of the membrane but also to the properties of hemoglobin and to the surface-area/volume ratio [73,74]. The deforming energy is stored within the membrane, and it reestablishes cell shape when the deforming force has been removed. This elastic property of the red cell membrane appears to be due, in large part, to spectrin [72,74], and it is strongly influenced by the amount of calcium present [40,74]. Intracellular ATP is important as a source of phosphate for membrane proteins [75–77]. In addition, it is the fuel for the "pump" which extrudes calcium and competes with the membrane for calcium binding. As ATP levels decline, more calcium associates with the membrane, thus decreasing elasticity. Striking changes in red cell deformability occur when ATP is depleted [40], and this may underly the destruction of red cells deficient in enzymes of the Embden-Meyerhof pathway. ATP depletion and calcium accumulation may also occur under conditions of prolonged erythrostasis and glucose deprivation in the spleen. An increase in cell calcium in the absence of ATP depletion accompanies the deoxygenation of sickle cells, and it may play a role in the genesis of irreversible sickled forms [78].

MEMBRANE MODIFICATION RECOGNIZED BY THE MONOCYTE-MACROPHAGE SYSTEM
Attachment of IgG   Although spherocytosis is often a prominent feature of hemolysis in vivo, coating of normal red cells with IgG in vitro does not lead to spherocytosis. IgG antibodies are most active at 37°C and usually do not fix complement. Their presence on the surface of red cells does not interfere with cell metabolism [79]. The negative charge of red cells prevents agglutination by IgG antibodies unless the surface characteristics are changed, as when red cells are treated with trypsin or ficin [80], or unless close approximation of red cells is achieved by other factors, such as anisometric molecules [81]. Although clumps of agglutinated red cells are not normally seen in the peripheral blood of patients with IgG antibodies, their presence in the spleen suggests that the unusual conditions of cell packing and plasma dehydration in the spleen red pulp may induce the agglutination of IgG-coated cells [15]. However, this does not explain their initial trapping in the spleen, particularly since such trapping occurs both when red cells are coated with amounts of antibody undetectable by in vitro techniques [82] and when red cells are coated with IgG by nonimmunologic means [83].

In 1958 it was noted that normal red cells coated with IgG (incomplete anti-D) appeared spherocytic as they clustered around leukocytes in vitro [79]. In further studies of this phenomenon, it was demonstrated that red cells coated with IgG adhere to monocytes and to splenic and peritoneal macrophages [84–86] (Fig. 39-4). The ability to cause this red cell–leukocyte interaction is essentially a property of IgG subclasses 1 and 3 and is not shared by IgM, IgA, or albumin. Sphering of adherent red cells can be demonstrated by an increased osmotic fragility which persists after papain treatment releases them from the monocytes. It is assumed that the monocyte partially phagocytoses or digests a portion of the red cell membrane, thereby producing a cell with a decreased surface-area/volume ratio; however, little is known about this process. Attachment to monocytes occurs whether IgG is bound to the red cell immunologically or by nonimmunologic means, such as chronic chloride or cephalothin. This process of attachment is inhibited by corticosteroids [87].

The spleen is particularly efficient in trapping red cells which are coated with IgG antibodies, but these cells are ordinarily not detected by the liver. However, with large amounts of antibody, the liver shares in this process [16]. When the number of antibody-coated red cells is small, they are completely cleared from the circulation by the spleen. No spherocytosis is observed in the peripheral blood, although spherocytes can be demonstrated in the spleen [88]. When large numbers of red cells are coated with IgG, there appears to be a backup into the circulation of red cells made spherical and then released [89]. Such spherical red cells are in double jeopardy as they recirculate through the spleen: they risk being bound again by phagocytes, and they are hindered in their passage through the splenic circulation because of their spherocytic shape.

Attachment of C3 Antibodies of the IgM class are capable of agglutinating red cells. In human disease these antibodies have a thermal amplitude with greatest activity at 4°C and usually no significant activity above 32°C, although in some patients activity extends to body temperatures [90]. The monocyte-macrophage system does not appear to have receptors which recognize IgM [84]. Rather, the mode of destruction of red cells in cold agglutinin disease appears to relate to the ability of IgM antibodies to fix complement. Since complement is fixed at warm temperatures, whereas IgM antibodies dissociate from the cell at these temperatures, this is not an efficient process, and fixation of sufficient molecules of C1 to permit ultimate cell lysis occurs only very rarely. Rather, cells become coated with C3 and, to a smaller extent, C4. Monocytes [91] and liver Kupffer cells [92] have receptors for C3 in its biologically active form (C3b). Degradation of C3b on the red cell surface to a form which is immunologically recognizable but biologically inactive (C3d) results in the circulation of C3d-coated red cells which are not in jeopardy [93,94] and which are actually more resistant than normal to the effects of IgM antibodies [93]. Human monocytes bind and sphere human red cells coated with C3b in a fashion totally analogous to that observed with IgG, and the process is inhibited by corticosteroids [95]. However, spherocytosis in the peripheral blood is uncommon, possibly because Kupffer cells, which appear to predominate in the clearance of C3b-coated cells, do not release partially injured red cells as readily as splenic macrophages. Coating of red cells with C3 is not a unique property of IgM antibodies, but may also occur when a high concentration of IgG antibodies is present on the cell surface. In both conditions there is a general correlation between amount of C3 present on the cell surface and the cell survival [96].

Spherocytosis appears to be a constant feature of red cells brought into close contiguity with monocytes or macrophages. Thus it occurs when red cells are bound to monocytes immunologically by means of IgG or C3b. It also occurs when red cells are bound to monocytes by the plant lectin concanavalin A in vitro [97] or when concanavalin A is injected into animals in vivo [98]. It is generally thought that the spherocytosis caused by splenic pooling of red cells results from the adverse metabolic conditions which exist within spleen cords engorged with red cells. Such engorgement may also provide the necessary degree and duration of contiguity between red cell and macrophage to permit this same process to occur in the absence of bridging molecules such as IgG, C3b, or concanavalin A.

Oxidation of membrane proteins Interference with the functional capability of membrane sulfhydryl groups, either by their oxidation or by their blockade with sulfhydryl-reactive reagents, e.g., N-ethylmaleimide (NEM) or parahydroxymercuribenzoate (PMB), results in premature red cell destruction in vivo [14]. High concentrations of sulfhydryl-active agents in vitro interfere with membrane permeability to cations and lead ultimately to osmotic swelling and hemolysis [55]. With mild sulfhydryl group injury, transfused red cells are destroyed exclusively in the spleen. However, with greater damage, destruction occurs both in the spleen and in the liver [14]. In order to achieve hemolysis in vitro the red cell injury must be considerable, while destruction of red cells in vivo may be observed using amounts of sulfhydryl inhibitors lower than those capable of causing changes in vitro. Thus the spleen filter is able to perceive very subtle membrane injury, the precise nature of which is unknown. Once trapped in the spleen, sulfhydryl-inhibited red cells undergo a progressive increase in osmotic fragility [14].

Most oxidant drugs are substituted benzene derivatives which act as free-radical intermediates facilitating reactions between molecular oxygen and proteins within the red cell. In the presence of oxygen these compounds stimulate generation of highly reactive free-radical forms of oxygen (superoxide, peroxide, hydroxyl free radical, and singlet oxygen) [99]. While hemoglobin is the protein most frequently oxidized (resulting in Heinz body formation), membrane sulfhydryl groups are also oxidized, and those drugs which are lipophilic have the greatest tendency to cause membrane rather than globin oxidation [100]. The result is spherocytosis and hemolysis [44]. Although it had been suggested that Heinz bodies themselves could block membrane sulfhydryl groups by forming mixed disulfides [101], no evidence of such disulfide formation has been found [102]. Nonetheless, Heinz body–containing cells, as in hemoglobin Köln [101], and α-chain–containing cells in β thalassemia [103] have an increased potassium permeability, suggesting that precipitated hemoglobin interacts in some other way (perhaps by hydrophobic bonding [102]) with the membrane [104].

Red cell membrane phospholipids, phosphatidylethanolamine in particular, are subject to peroxidation [105,106]. Protection against this is usually provided by vitamin E, a lipid-soluble "antioxidant." A deficiency of this vitamin is responsible for the increased autohemolysis seen in acanthocytosis, although this deficiency does not apparently contribute to the mild degree of hemolysis seen in vivo [107]. However, a deficiency of vitamin E does not appear to be important in the genesis of hemolysis in pyknocytosis [108], a type of hemolytic anemia observed in premature infants [109,110]. Newborn infants may be particularly susceptible to this deficiency because of their decreased ability to detoxify H_2O_2 [111]. Vitamin E–deficient animals are subject to severe hemolytic anemia when exposed to hyperbaric oxygen [112], and hemolysis secondary to hyperbaric oxygen has been described in human beings [113]. Whether the formation of lipid peroxides is itself damaging to the membrane or whether damage results from the binding of lipid peroxides to membrane sulfhydryl groups is unclear [114].

Disruption of membrane integrity

Complement lysis   This occurs with antibodies which are able to induce the fixation of all complement components to the red cell membrane (Chap. 15). It has been inferred that complement causes a membrane defect which varies in size among species but which exceeds 32 Å in diameter in humans [115,116]. Moreover, electron microscopy has demonstrated what were thought to be membrane "holes," 100 Å in diameter, after complement lysis [117]. However, the membrane depressions created by globular clusters of activated components C5 through C9, while severely disturbing permeability properties, do not represent through-and-through holes.

Animal red cells vary in sensitivity to complement. For example, sheep red cells are particularly sensitive, the fixation of one molecule of activated C1 being capable of initiating a complement sequence resulting in cell lysis [118]. In contrast, lysis of human red cells requires more than 100 molecules of activated C1 per cell [119]. The efficiency of complement lysis may be diminished by naturally occurring inhibitors found in human serum [120,121]. Moreover, the antibodies which usually participate in complement fixation are of the IgM class with a thermal amplitude which is usually below body temperature. For these reasons, lysis by complement-fixing antibodies is uncommon in human hemolytic disorders. Isoantibodies of the ABO system are effective throughout the range of body temperature, so that hemolysis of incompatible transfused blood is often dramatic [122]. The ability of IgM antibodies to fix complement apparently relates to their subunit structure.

Complement fixation requires the attachment of antibody to two antigen sites in close proximity; in the case of IgM, these two antibody attachments are a part of the same molecule [123]. The fact that the Donath-Landsteiner (D-L) antibody of paroxysmal cold hemoglobinuria is a potent complement-fixing antibody despite its being of the IgG class [123,124] appears to be due to the binding of antibody to two related and adjacent antigenic determinants, P_1 and P_2, thereby creating a doublet of IgG [125,126].

Red cells in paroxysmal nocturnal hemoglobinuria (PNH) have an inordinate sensitivity to complement lysis [127]. Whereas antibodies activate the classic complement pathway (beginning with C1), complement activation in PNH may proceed via the alternate pathway without antibody [128,129]. Moreover, for a given amount of complement lysis, PNH cells require only one-third the amount of C3 necessary for equivalent lysis of normal red cells. In contrast, the sensitivity to lysis of red cells in HEMPAS (hereditary erythroblastic multinuclearity with positive acidified serum test) results from an inordinate fixation of C4 per molecule of C1 [130]. Since these components of complement are members of the classic (antibody-mediated) pathway, spontaneous fixation of complement with lysis in vivo is not a feature of this disorder.

Phospholipase   Although the phospholipids within the red cell membrane are subject to the action of some phospholipases, they appear to be unreactive with the serum phospholipase A of pancreatic origin [131]. Phospholipase C, produced by *Clostridium welchii*, is capable of cleaving the glycerolphosphoryl bond of lecithin and lysing human red cells. Infection with this organism is a rare cause of spherocytic hemolytic anemia [132]. However, bloodstream infection with *C. welchii* is commonly associated with profound hemolysis [133] (Chap. 66). Various cobra venoms differ in their ability to lyse red cells, and this lytic activity may be distinguishable from their phospholipase activity [131,134].

Heat   Although the red cell is a viscoelastic structure [135], disruption of the membrane occurs when its limited capacity to withstand strain is exceeded [37,136,137]. Red cell membranes are able to reseal following disruption, and under certain circumstances the red cell may be cleaved into two or more fragments with the loss of little or no hemoglobin [37]. This phenomenon was first described in the membrane instability induced in vitro by temperatures in excess of 49°C [138]. Disruption of the membrane at this temperature results from denaturation of spectrin [59]. It accounts for the spherocytosis in patients who have suffered from severe burns [139].

Trauma in the circulation   Red cells, probably in the cutaneous circulation, may lyse when exposed to trauma such as that associated with karate [140] or prolonged running or marching [141] (Chap. 62). The latter condition is alleviated by the use of sponge-rubber soles

[142]. Cleavage and resealing of red cells, usually with the loss of some hemoglobin into the plasma, occurs under conditions in the circulation which expose the red cell to inordinate physical stress. Red cells lacking a normal degree of intrinsic pliability—for example, HS red cells—are excessively susceptible to the mechanical stress of the long-distance runner [143]. The resulting red cell fragments assume a variety of shapes, including helmets, triangles, and spherocytes. Abnormalities of the heart valves, particularly aortic valve prostheses, may cause fragmentation and hemolysis by exposing red cells to excessive impact and turbulence [144–146] (Chap. 63).

The term *microangiopathic hemolytic anemia* has been used to describe traumatic hemolysis as it occurs, often with thrombocytopenia, in association with diseases diffusely involving arterioles [147], such as in malignant hypertension, polyarteritis, cancer, and renal cortical necrosis [147–150]. Red cell fragmentation and hemolysis characteristically occur when fibrin is diffusely deposited in small vessels, as in arteriolar disease, thrombotic thrombocytopenic purpura [151,152], the hemolytic-uremic syndrome [153], and various forms of disseminated intravascular coagulation. The cleavage of red cells as they flow through a loose fibrin mesh appears to be important in the pathogenesis of this form of hemolysis [154–156] (Chap. 64). Primary disorders of the red cell may increase its sensitivity to physical factors in the circulation, and fragmentation has been suggested in the pathogenesis of many types of hemolytic anemia [157].

Increased internal viscosity

Under certain conditions, the flow properties of red cells are altered because of altered intracellular constituents. The most striking example of this is seen in sickle cell anemia, wherein the molecular alignment of hemoglobin upon deoxygenation [158] markedly increased its viscosity [159]. Cells containing hemoglobin in this form are impeded in their transit through small pores in vitro [39] and through the microvasculature in vivo. Upon reoxygenation, sickle cell hemoglobin assumes a normal molecular configuration and red cells reacquire a normal shape and viscosity. However, prolonged maintenance of red cells in the sickled form causes permanent membrane distortion despite the subsequent reoxygenation and dispersion of the hemoglogin [160,161]. The low solubility and increased viscosity of hemoglobin C [162] appear to account for the increased viscosity and decreased deformability of red cells in this disorder [162,163]. Finally, an increased viscosity due to an increased MCHC may play a role in the destruction of red cells in hereditary spherocytosis [164] and in some variants of hereditary stomatocytosis [55,165]. This latter group encompasses a range of phenotypic expression of a familial disease characterized by increased permeability of red cells to both sodium and potassium with an increase in cell sodium and a decrease

in cell potassium. The net result of these changes in some patients is an increased cell ion and water content (true stomatocytosis). However, in most patients there is a net decrease in the cell content of sodium plus potassium and a decrease in cell water. On dried smears these cells appear as target cells rather than as stomatocytes [53,165–167]. Lecithin is more abundant than normal in the red cell membranes of these patients. Their decreased cell water increases internal viscosity, and this appears to contribute to the hemolytic process.

The most profound increase in hemoglobin viscosity is that resulting from the precipitation of hemoglobin. Hemoglobin precipitates as Heinz bodies when the globin thiols are oxidized. To prevent this from occurring, the red cell maintains a reservoir of reduced glutathione and an enzymatic system (the hexose monophosphate shunt) for purposes of maintaining reduced glutathione (Chap. 58). It appears that superoxide and other forms of activated oxygen play a central role in hemoglobin oxidation [100]. The spontaneous precipitation of certain "unstable" hemoglobins may result from a structural abnormality in the region of the heme pocket that allows the entry of water, which, together with heme and oxygen, generates superoxide [100]. Administration of oxidant drugs to patients with glucose-6-phosphate dehydrogenase deficiency is the most frequent cause of hemoglobin oxidation and Heinz body precipitation. Heinz bodies are not the only forms of precipitated hemoglobin. Excess α chains readily precipitate in β thalassemia [168,169], and tetramers of β chains (hemoglobin H) in α thalassemia are subject to precipitation [170]. Large aggregates of precipitated hemoglobin or precipitated globin chains impair the passage of red cells through the cordal circulation of the spleen [9]. The spleen is capable of removing Heinz bodies from some red cells without destroying the cell, and this may account for the morphologic finding of red cells with what appears to be bites taken from their periphery, a morphologic hallmark of Heinz body hemolytic anemias.

SPLENOMEGALY

The spleen plays some role in most forms of hemolysis and a dominant one in many. Although the normal spleen poses no threat to normal red cells, splenomegaly exaggerates the adverse conditions to which red cells are exposed. Splenic enlargement as a result of infiltrative diseases (such as chronic myelogenous leukemia and the lymphomas) and storage disease (such as Gaucher's disease) usually contribute little to the variable degree of anemia occurring in some patients with these disorders. A more consistent pattern of red cell injury and destruction occurs when the spleen hypertrophies in response to systemic inflammatory diseases [45] or when the red cell's passage through the spleen is retarded by an elevated, opposing splenic vein pressure, as in congestive splenomegaly [46]. In each case, spherocytosis and hemolysis result. Because red cell destruction in the spleen is itself a stimulus for splenic hyperplasia [19], hemolysis begets more hemolysis.

These anatomic and hemodynamic factors are particularly threatening to red cells with an intrinsic, mild abnormality. Thus patients with undiagnosed hereditary spherocytosis or hereditary elliptocytosis may appear to have an acute, acquired hemolytic anemia in the course of an inflammatory disease such as infectious mononucleosis [171]. Similarly, a mild abnormality of red cell membrane fluidity acquired in some patients with liver disease results in the formation of acanthocytes or spur cells which in turn may be hemolyzed because of the congestive splenomegaly which accompanies this disorder [43]. Thus a spectrum exists. At one extreme normal red cells are destroyed by an abnormal spleen, and at the other extreme abnormal red cells may survive normally if the spleen is absent. The hemolytic rate often reflects this interplay between the structure of the red cell and the status of the spleen through which it must circulate.

Destruction of immature red cells (ineffective erythropoiesis)

The factors which retain developing cells in the marrow cavity and those which permit their release at the appropriate time are not fully known. The membrane of reticulocytes has a protein coat, including transferrin, which causes them to be more sticky than more mature cells [172,173]. To leave the marrow, reticulocytes must traverse sinusoids [174] which contain phagocytes capable of destroying damaged red cells [175]. As marrow cells mature, they become more able to deform and traverse these sinusoids [176]. After leaving the marrow, some reticulocytes are temporarily sequestered in the spleen, from which they may be released after 1 to 2 days [172]. Gross abnormalities of the developing red cells, such as in thalassemia and pernicious anemia, result in red cell destruction within the marrow cavity [177,178]. Abnormal reticulocytes, produced under these conditions, may be released from the marrow but thereafter undergo destruction in the monocyte-macrophage system [179]. Earlier data suggesting that stress reticulocytes may also be short-lived [180] have been reinterpreted in light of newer information showing that reticulocytes survive normally but undergo a process of remodeling during which they lose hemoglobin [28,181,182]. The catabolism of hemoglobin derived from the destruction of immature red cells or the remodeling of stress reticulocytes appears as an early peak of labeled bile pigments following the administration of isotopically labeled heme precursors [177,178,183]. In disorders such as pernicious anemia and thalassemia in which maturation division is profoundly impaired, the vast majority of newborn cells fail to mature to a viable stage and die within the marrow. In such erythropoietic disorders, as many as 90 percent of the developing cells may suffer intramedullary hemolysis, thereby accounting for most of the net cell destruction and the pro-

nounced increase in the "early labeling peak" of bilirubin [183].

Repair of injured red cells in vivo

Relatively little is known about reparative processes that may occur in vivo to prevent the destruction of injured cells. Red cells made spherocytic in vitro by treatment with crude lecithin preparations [15] or by cholesterol depletion [184] undergo changes in vivo permitting most or all of them to survive normally. Similarly, membrane lesions induced by sulfhydryl-blocking agents are potentially reversible with time in vivo, permitting a portion of the red cells so treated in vitro to survive normally upon transfusion [14,157]. Red cells with a grossly altered cation content and diminished volume resulting from storage reconstitute their cations and volume over a period of several days after transfusion [185,186]. Evidence exists that all, or at least a portion, of their repair process in stored red cells [187] and cells treated with lecithin [15] occurs during a period of temporary sequestration in the spleen, a process which may be analogous to the temporary sequestration of reticulocytes in the spleen [172]. The spleen also functions to remove solid particles from the cytoplasm of red cells without destroying the red cell itself. This "pitting function" of the spleen has been most clearly demonstrated by the removal of siderotic granules [188]. In addition, the spleen also removes nuclear debris and Heinz bodies.

Mature red cells have a limited synthetic capacity. They are unable to synthesize new protein, and the protein of their membranes is a stable structural component [189]. They can lengthen fatty acid chains but cannot initiate fatty acid synthesis [190]. Through a process requiring ATP and coenzyme A (CoA), red cells are capable of reacylating lysophosphatides [191,192], but they are unable to carry out phospholipid synthesis *de novo* [193]. However, the lipids of the membrane, fatty acids, lecithin, and cholesterol in particular, are in an exchange equilibrium with lipids in serum, and the renewal of membrane lipids which this allows may be of importance in the repair of membrane injury [194–198].

References

1. Weiss, L.: The structure of fine splenic arterial vessels in relation to hemoconcentration and red cell destruction. *Am. J. Anat.* 111:131, 1962.
2. Weiss, L.: The structure of intermediate vascular pathways in the spleen of rabbits. *Am. J. Anat.* 113:51, 1963.
3. Weinberg, E., and Weiss, L.: The structure of the spleen and hemolysis. *Annu. Rev. Med.* 20:29, 1969.
4. Snook, T.: Studies on the perifollicular region of the rat's spleen. *Anat. Rec.* 148:149, 1964.
5. Galendo, B., and Freeman, J. A.: Fine structure of splenic pulp. *Anat. Rec.* 147:25, 1963.
6. Bjorkman, S. E.: The splenic circulation. *Acta Med. Scand.* [*Suppl.*] 191, 1947.

7. Jandl, J. H., and Aster, R. H.: Increased splenic pooling and the pathogenesis of hypersplenism. *Am. J. Med. Sci.* 253:383, 1967.

8. Whipple, A. O.: Recent studies on the circulation of the portal bed and of the spleen in relation to splenomegaly. *Trans. Stud. Coll. Physicians Phila.* 8:203, 1941.

9. Rifkind, R. A.: Heinz body anemia: An ultrastructural study. II. Red cell sequestration and destruction. *Blood* 26:433, 1965.

10. Jandl, J. H., Files, N. M., Barnett, S. B., and MacDonald, R. A.: Proliferative response of the spleen and liver to hemolysis. *J. Exp. Med.* 122:299, 1965.

11. Ham, T. H., and Castle, W. B.: Studies on destruction of red blood cells: Relation of increased hypotonic fragility and of erythrostasis to the mechanism of hemolysis in certain anemias. *Proc. Am. Philo. Soc.* 82:411, 1940.

12. Murphy, J. R.: The influence of pH and temperature on some physical properties of normal erythrocytes and erythrocytes from patients with hereditary spherocytosis. *J. Lab. Clin. Med.* 69:758, 1967.

13. Kimber, R. J., and Lander, H.: The effect of heat on human red cell morphology, fragility, and subsequent surivival in vivo. *J. Lab. Clin. Med.* 64:922, 1964.

14. Jacob, H. S., and Jandl, J. H.: Effects of sulfhydryl inhibition on red blood cells. II. Studies in vivo. *J. Clin. Invest.* 41:1514, 1962.

15. Jandl, J. H., Jones, A. R., and Castle, W. B.: The destruction of red cells by antibodies in man. I. Observations on the sequestration and lysis of red cells altered by immune mechanisms. *J. Clin. Invest.* 36:1428, 1957.

16. Jandl, J. H., and Kaplan, M. E.: The destruction of red cells by antibodies in man. III. Quantitative factors influencing the patterns of hemolysis in vivo. *J. Clin. Invest.* 39:1145, 1960.

17. Cutbush, M., and Mollison, P. L.: Relation between characteristics of blood-group antibodies in vitro and associated patterns of red-cell destruction in vivo. *Br. J. Haematol.* 4:115, 1958.

18. De Lagen, C. D.: Function of the spleen and blood. *Acta Med. Scand.* 115:271, 1943.

19. Jacob, H. S., MacDonald, R. A., and Jandl, J. H.: Regulation of spleen growth and sequestering function. *J. Clin. Invest.* 42:1476, 1963.

20. Danon, D., and Marikowsky, Y.: Determination of density distribution of red cell population. *J. Lab. Clin. Med.* 64:668, 1964.

21. Piomelli, S., Lurinsky, G., and Wasserman, L. R.: The mechanism of red cell aging. I. Relationship between cell age and specific gravity evaluated by ultra-centrifugation in a discontinuous density gradient. *J. Lab. Clin. Med.* 69:659, 1967.

22. Ganzoni, A. M., Oakes, R., and Hellman, R. S.: Red cell aging in vivo. *J. Clin. Invest.* 50:1373, 1971.

23. Walter, H., and Selby, F.: Counter-current distribution of red blood cells of slightly different ages. *Biochim. Biophys. Acta.* 112:146, 1966.

24. Aminoff, D., Anderson, J., Dabich, L., and Gathmann, W. D.: Sialic acid content of erythrocytes in normal individuals and patients with certain hematologic disorders. *Am. J. Hematol.* 9:381, 1980.

25. Durocher, J. R., Payne, R. C., and Conrad, M. E.: Role of sialic acid in erythrocyte survival. *Blood* 45:1, 1975.

26. Lalezari, P., and Al-Mondhiry, H.: Sialic acid deficiency of human red blood cells associated with red cell, leukocyte and platelet polyagglutinability. *Br. J. Haematol.* 25:399, 1973.

27. Kay, M. B.: Mechanism of removal of senescent cells by human macrophages in situ. *Proc. Natl. Acad. Sci. U.S.A.* 72:3521, 1975.

28. Shattil, S. J., and Cooper, R. A.: Maturation of macroreticulocyte membranes in vivo. *J. Lab. Clin. Med.* 79:215, 1972.

29. Westerman, M. P., Pierce, L. E., and Jensen, W. N.: Erythrocyte lipids: A comparison of normal young and normal old populations. *J. Clin. Med.* 62:394, 1963.

30. Winterbourn, C. C., and Batt, R. D.: Lipid composition of human red cells of different ages. *Biochim. Biophys. Acta* 202:1, 1970.

31. Finch, C. A., et al.: Iron metabolism: The pathophysiology of iron storage. *Blood* 5:983, 1950.

32. Singer, K., and Weiss, L.: The life cycle of the erythrocyte after splenectomy and the problems of splenic hemolysis and target cell formation. *Am. J. Med. Sci.* 210:301, 1945.

33. Gevirtz, N. R., Nathan, D. G., and Berlin, N. I.: Erythrokinetic studies in primary hypersplenism with pancytopenia. *Am. J. Med.* 32:148, 1962.

34. Chien, S., Dellenback, R. J., Usami, S., Seaman, G. V. F., and Gregersen, M. I.: Centrifugal packing of suspensions of erythrocytes hardened with acetaldehyde. *Proc. Soc. Exp. Biol. Med.* 127:982, 1968.

35. Rand, R. P., and Burton, A. C.: Area of volume changes in hemolysis of single erythrocytes. *J. Cell Comp. Physiol.* 61:245, 1963.

36. Gregersen, M. I., Bryant, C. A., Hammerle, W. E., Usami, S., and Chien, S.: Flow characteristics of human erythrocytes through polycarbonate sieves. *Science (Washington)* 157:825, 1967.

37. Rand, R. P., and Burton, A. C.: Mechanical properties of the red cell membrane. I. Membrane stiffness and intracellular pressure. *Biphys. J.* 4:115, 1964.

38. Weed, R. I.: The importance of erythrocyte deformability. *Am. J. Med.* 49:147, 1970.

39. Jandl, J. H., Simmons, R. L., and Castle, W. B.: Red cell filtration and the pathogenesis of certain hemolytic anemias. *Blood* 18:133, 1961.

40. Weed, R. I., La Celle, P. L., and Merrill, E. W.: Metabolic dependence of red cell membrane deformability. *J. Clin. Invest.* 48:785, 1969.

41. Burton, S. C.: Role of geometry, of size and shape, in the microcirculation. *Fed. Proc.* 25:1753, 1966.

42. Emerson, C. P., Jr., Shen, S. C., Ham, T. H., and Castle, W. B.: Studies on the destruction of red blood cells. IX. Quantitative methods for determining the osmotic and mechanical fragility of red cells in the peripheral blood and splenic pulp: The mechanism of increased hemolysis in hereditary spherocytosis (congenital hemolytic jaundice) as related to the functions of the spleen. *Arch. Intern. Med.* 97:1, 1956.

43. Cooper, R. A., Kimball, D. B., and Durocher, J. R.: Role of the spleen in membrane conditioning and hemolysis of spur cells in liver disease. *N. Engl. J. Med.* 290:1279, 1974.

44. Beutler, E.: Drug induced hemolytic anemia. *Pharmacol. Rev.* 21:73, 1969.

45. Jandl, J. H., Jacob, H. S., and Daland, G. A.: Hypersplenism due to infection: A study of five cases manifesting hemolytic anemia. *N. Engl. J. Med.* 264:1063, 1961.

46. Jandl, J. H.: The anemia of liver disease: Observations on its mechanism. *J. Clin. Invest.* 34:390, 1955.

47. Jandl, J. H.: Leaky red cells. *Blood* 26:367, 1965.

48. Bertles, J. F.: Sodium transport across the surface membrane of red blood cells in hereditary spherocytosis. *J. Clin. Invest.* 36:816, 1957.

49. Jacob, H. S., and Jandl, J. H.: Increased cell membrane permeability in the pathogenesis of hereditary spherocytosis. *J. Clin. Invest.* 43:1704, 1964.

50. Peters, J. C., Rowland, M., Israels, L. G., and Zipursky, A.: Erythrocyte sodium transport in hereditary elliptocytosis. *Can. J. Physiol. Pharmacol.* 44:817, 1966.

51. Zarkowsky, H. S., Oski, F. A., Sha'afi, R., Shohet, S. B., and Nathan, D. G.: Congential hemolytic anemia with high sodium, low potassium red cells. I. Studies of membrane permeability. *N. Engl. J. Med.* 278:573, 1968.

52. Oski, F. A., et al.: Congenital hemolytic anemia with high-sodium, low potassium red cells: Studies of three generations of a family with a new variant. *N. Engl. J. Med.* 280:909, 1969.

53. Wiley, J. S., Ellory, J. C., Shuman, M. A., Shaller, C. C., and Cooper, R. A.: Characteristics of the membrane defect in hereditary stomatocytosis syndrome. *Blood* 46:337, 1975.

54. Blum, S. F., Shohet, S. B., Nathan, D. G., and Gardner, F. H.: The effect of amphotericin B on erythrocyte membrane cation permeability: Its relation in vivo erythrocyte survival. *J. Lab. Clin. Med.* 73:980, 1969.

55. Jacob, H. S., and Jandl, J. H.: Effects of sulfhydryl inhibition on red blood cells. I. Mechanism of hemolysis. *J. Clin. Invest.* 41:779, 1962.

56. Singer, S. J., and Nicolson, G. L.: The fluid mosaic model of the structure of cell membranes. *Science (Washington)* 175:720, 1972.

57. Marchesi, V. T.: Functional properties of the human red blood cell membrane. *Semin. Hematol.* 16:3, 1979.

58. Lux, S. E.: Spectrin-actin membrane skeleton of normal and abnormal red blood cells. *Semin. Hematol.* 16:21, 1979.

59. Cooper, R. A.: Lipids of the human red cell membrane: Normal composition and variability in disease. *Semin. Hematol.* 7:296, 1970.

60. Verkleij, A. J., Zwall, R. F. A., Roelofsen, B., Comfurius, P., Kastelijn, D., and Van Deemen, L. L. M.: The asymmetric distribution of phospholipids in the human red cell membrane. *Biochim. Biophys. Acta* 323:178, 1973.

61. Shinitzky, M., Dianoux, A. C., Gitler, C., and Weber, G.: Microviscosity and order in the hydrocarbon region of micelles and membranes determined with fluorescent probes. *Biochemistry* 10:2106, 1971.

62. Vanderkooi, J., Fischkoff, S., Chance, B., and Cooper, R. A.: Fluorescent probe analysis of the lipid architecture of natural and experimental cholesterol-rich membranes. *Biochemistry* 13:1589, 1974.

63. Cooper, R. A., Arner, E. C., Wiley, J. S., and Shattil, S. J.: Modification of red cell membrane structure by cholesterol-rich lipid dispersions. *J. Clin. Invest.* 55:636, 1975.

64. Shinitzky, M., and Barenholz, Y.: Dynamics of the hydrocarbon layer in liposomes of lecithin and sphingomyelin containing diacetylphosphate. *J. Biol. Chem.* 249:2652, 1974.

65. Phillips, G. B.: Quantitative chromatographic analysis of plasma and red blood cell lipids in patients with acanthocytosis. *J. Lab. Clin. Med.* 59:357, 1963.

66. Cooper, R. A., Durocher, J. R., and Leslie, M. H.: Decreased fluidity of red cell membrane lipids in abetalipoproteinemia. *J. Clin. Invest.* 60:115, 1977.

67. McBride, J. A., and Jacob, H. S.: Abnormal kinetics of red cell membrane cholesterol in acanthocytosis: Studies of genetic and experimental abetalipoproteinemia and in spur cell anemia. *Br. J. Haematol.* 18:383, 1970.

68. Simon, E. R., and Ways, P.: Incubation hemolysis and red cell metabolism in acanthocytosis. *J. Clin. Invest.* 43:1311, 1964.

69. Cooper, R. A., Dilop-Puray, M., Lando, P., and Greenberg, M. S.: An analysis of lipoproteins, bile acids and red cell membranes associated with target cells and spur cells in patients with liver disease. *J. Clin. Invest.* 51:3182, 1972.

70. Zieve, L.: Hemolytic anemia in liver disease. *Medicine (Baltimore)* 45:497, 1966.

71. Bagdade, J. D., and Ways, P. O.: Erythrocyte membrane lipid composition in exogenous and endogenous hypertriglyceridemia. *J. Lab. Clin. Med.* 75:53, 1970.

72. Evans, E. A., and La Celle, P. L.: Intrinsic material properties of the erythrocyte membrane indicated by mechanical analysis of deformation. *Blood* 45:29, 1975.

73. Mohandas, N., Clark, M. R., Jacobs, M. S., and Shohet, S. V.: Analysis of factors regulating erythrocyte deformability. *J. Clin. Invest.* 66:563, 1980.

74. Palek, J., and Liu, S.-C.: Dependence of spectrin organization in red blood cell membranes on cell metabolism: implications for control of red cell shape, deformability, and surface area. *Semin. Hematol.* 16:75, 1979.

75. Jacob, H. S.: Tightening red cell membranes. *N. Eng. J. Med.* 294:1234, 1976.

76. Sheetz, M. P., and Singer, S.: On the mechanism of ATP-induced shape changes in human erythrocyte membrane. *J. Cell. Biol.* 73:638, 1977.

77. Nakashima, K., and Beutler, E.: Effect of anti-spectrin antibody and ATP on deformability of resealed erythrocyte membranes. *Proc. Natl. Acad. Sci. U.S.A.* 75:3823, 1978.

78. Eaton, J. W., Skelton, T. D., Swofford, H. S., Koklin, C. E., and Jacob, H. S. Elevated erythrocyte calcium in sickle cell disease. *Nature* 246:105, 1973.

79. Jandl, J. H., and Tomlinson, A. S.: The destruction of red cells by antibodies in man. II. Pyrogenic, leukocytic and dermal responses to immune hemolysis. *J. Clin. Invest.* 37:1202, 1958.

80. Jandl, J. H.: Mechanisms of antibody-induced red cell destruction. *Haematologica (Pavia)* 9:35, 1965.

81. Pollock, W., Hager, H. J., Rickel, R., Toren, D. A., and Singher, H. O.: A study of the forces involved in the second stage of hemagglutination. *Transfusion* 5:158, 1965.

82. Jandl, J. H., and Greenberg, M. S.: The selective destruction of transfused "compatible" normal red cells in two patients with splenomegaly. *J. Lab. Clin. Med.* 49:233, 1957.

83. Jandl, J. H., and Simmons, R. L.: The agglutination and sensitization of red cells by metallic cations: Interactions between mul-

tivalent metals and the red-cell membrane. *Br. J. Haematol.* 3:19, 1957.

84. LoBuglio, A. F., Cotran, R. S., and Jandl, J. H.: Red cells coated with immunoglobulin G: Binding and sphering by mononuclear cells in man. *Science (Washington)* 158:1582, 1967.

85. Abramson, N., LoBuglio, A. F., Jandl, J. H., and Cotran, R. S.: The interaction between human monocytes and red cells: Binding characteristics. *J. Exp. Med.* 132:1191, 1970.

86. Abramson, N., Gelfand, E. W., Jandl, J. H., and Rosen, F. S.: The interaction between human monocytes and red cells: Specificity for IgG subclasses and IgG fragments. *J. Exp. Med.* 132:1207, 1970.

87. Schreiber, A. D., Parsons, J., McDermott, P., and Cooper, R. A.: Effect of corticosteroids on the human monocyte receptors for IgG and complement. *J. Clin. Invest.* 56:1189, 1975.

88. Weisman, R., Jr., Ham, T. H., Hinz, C. F., Jr., and Harris, J. W.: Studies of the role of the spleen in the destruction of erythrocytes. *Trans. Assoc. Am. Physicians* 68:131, 1955.

89. Cooper, R. A.: Loss of membrane components in the pathogenesis of antibody-induced spherocytosis. *J. Clin. Invest* 51:16, 1972.

90. Schreiber, A. D., Herskovitz, B., and Goldwein, M.: Low titer cold hemagglutinin disease: Mechanism of hemolysis and response to corticosteroids. *N. Eng. J. Med.* 296:1490, 1977.

91. Huber, H., Polly, M. J., Linscott, W. D., and Müller-Eberhard, H. J.: Human monocytes: Distinct receptor sites for the third component of complement and for immunoglobulin G. *Science (Washington)* 162:1281, 1968.

92. Brown, D. L., and Nelson, D. A.: Surface microfragmentation of red cells as a mechanism for complement-mediated immune spherocytosis. *Br. J. Haematol.* 24:301, 1973.

93. Evans, R. S., Turner, E., Bingham, M., and Woods, R.: Chronic hemolytic anemia due to cold agglutinins. II. The role of C' in red cell destruction. *J. Clin. Invest* 47:691, 1968.

94. Atkinson, J. P., and Frank, M. M.: Studies on the in vivo effects of antibody: Interaction of IgM antibody and complement in the immune clearance and destruction of erythrocytes in man. *J. Clin. Invest.* 54:339, 1974.

95. Schreiber, A. D., Herskovitz, B., and Goldwein, M.: Low titer cold hemagglutinin disease: Mechanism of hemolysis and response to high dose corticosteroids. *Clin. Res.*, 24:319A, 1976.

96. Fischer, J. T., Petz, L. D., Garratly, G., and Cooper,, N. R.: Correlations between quantitative assay of red cell-bound C3 serologic reactions and hemolytic anemia. *Blood* 44:359, 1974.

97. Guerry, D., Kenna, M. A., Schreiber, A. D., and Cooper, R. A.: Concanavalin A mediated binding and sphering of human RBCs by homologous monocytes. *Proc. Am. Soc. Hematol.*, 1975.

98. Ham, T. H., and Castle, W. B.: Relation of increased hypotonic fragility and of erythrostasis to the mechanism of hemolysis in certain anemias. *Trans. Assoc. Am. Physicians* 55:127, 1940.

99. Carrell, R. W., Winterbourn, C. C., and Rachmilewitz, E. A.: Activated oxygen and hemolysis. *Br. J. Haematol.* 30:259, 1975.

100. Miller, A., and Smith, H. C.: The intracellular and membrane effects of oxidant agents on normal red cells. *Br. J. Haematol.* 19:417, 1970.

101. Jacob, H. S., Brain, M. C., and Dacie, J. V.: Altered sulfhydryl reactivity of hemoglobins and red blood cell membranes in congenital Heinz body hemolytic anemia. *J. Clin. Invest.* 47:2664, 1968.

102. Winterbourn, C. C., and Carrell, R. W.: The attachment of Heinz bodies to the red cell membrane. *Br. J. Haematol.* 25:585, 1973.

103. Nathan, D. G., and Shohet, S. B.: Erythrocyte ion transport defects and hemolytic anemia: "Hydrocytosis" and "desiccytosis." *Semin. Hematol.* 7:381, 1970.

104. Flynn, T. P., Johnson, G. J., and Allen. D. W.: Sucrose density gradient analysis of erythrocyte membranes in hemolytic anemias. *Blood* 57:59, 1981.

105. Dodge, J. T., Cohen, G., Kayden, H. J., and Phillips, G. B.: Peroxidative hemolysis of red blood cells from patients with abetalipoproteinemia (acanthocytosis). *J. Clin. Invest.* 46:357, 1967.

106. Jacob, H. S., and Lux, S. E.: Degradation of membrane phospholipids and thiols in peroxide hemolysis: Studies in vitamin E deficiency. *Blood* 32:549, 1968.

107. Kayden, H. J., and Silber, R.: The role of vitamin E deficiency in the abnormal autohemolysis of acanthocytosis. *Trans. Assoc. Am. Physicians* 78:334, 1965.

108. Oski, F. A., and Barness, L. A.: Vitamin E deficiency: A previously unrecognized cause of hemolytic anemia in the premature infant. *J. Pediatr.* 70:211, 1967.

109. Tuffy, P., Brown, A. K., and Zuelzer, W. W.: Infantile pyknocytosis: A common erythrocyte abnormality of the first trimester. *Am. J. Dis. Child.* 98:227, 1959.

110. Keimowitz, R., and Desforges, J. F.: Infantile pyknocytosis. *N. Engl. J. Med.* 273:1152, 1965.

111. Gross, R. T., Bracci, R., Rudolph, N., Schroeder, E., and Kochen, J. A.: Hydrogen peroxide toxicity and detoxification in the erythrocytes of newborn infants. *Blood* 29:481, 1967.

112. Mengel, L. E., Kann, H. E., Smith, W. W., and Horton, B. D.: Effects of in vivo hyperoxia on erythrocytes. I. Hemolysis in mice exposed to hyperbaric oxygenation. *Proc. Soc. Exp. Biol. Med.* 116:259, 1964.

113. Mengel, L. E., Kann, H. E., Heyman, A., and Metz, E.: Effects of in vivo hyperoxia on erythrocytes. II. Hemolysis in a human after exposure to oxygen under high pressure. *Blood* 25:822, 1965.

114. Lewis, S. E., and Wells, E. D.: The destruction of SH groups of proteins and amino acids by peroxides of unsaturated fatty acids. *Biochem. Pharmacol.* 11:901, 1962.

115. Scott, J. G., Weed, R. I., and Swisher, S. N.: Further studies on the mechanism of antibody-complement induced hemolysis: Specificity of complement. *J. Immunol.* 96:119, 1965.

116. Green, H., Barrow, P., and Goldberg, B.: Effect of antibody and complement on permeability control in ascites tumor cells and erythrocytes. *J. Exp. Med.* 110:699, 1959.

117. Rosse, W. F., Dourmashkin, R., and Humphrey, J.: Immune lysis of normal human and paroxysmal nocturnal hemoglobinuria (PNH) red blood cells. III. The membrane defects caused by complement lysis. *J. Exp. Med.* 123:969, 1966.

118. Colten, H. R., Borsos, T., and Rapp, H. J.: Efficiency of the first component of complement (C'1) in the hemolytic reaction. *Science (Washington)* 158:1390, 1967.

119. Rosse, W. F.: Quantitative antibody studies in autoimmune hemolytic anemia due to warm-reactive antibodies. *J. Clin. Invest.* 48:70a, 1969.

120. Donaldson, V. H., and Evans, R. R.: A biochemical abnormality in hereditary angioneurotic edema. *Am. J. Med.* 35:37, 1963.

121. Lachmann, P. J., and Müller-Eberhard, H. J.: The demonstration in human serum of "conglutinogen-activating factor" and its effects on the third component of complement. *J. Immunol.* 100:691, 1968.

122. Greenwalt, T. J.: Pathogenesis and management of hemolytic transfusion reactions. *Semin. Hematol.* 18:84, 1981.

123. Rosse, W. F.: Fixation of the first component of complement (C'1a) by human antibodies. *J. Clin. Invest.* 47:2430, 1968.

124. Dacie, J. V.: *The Haemolytic Anaemias.* Grune & Stratton, New York, 1962, vol. 2.

125. Race, R. R., and Sanger, R.: *Blood Groups in Man*, 6th ed. Blackwell, London, 1975.

126. Levine, P., Celano, M. J., and Falkowski, F.: Short communications: The specificity of the antibody in paroxysmal cold hemoglobinuria (PCH). *Transfusion* 3:278, 1963.

127. Rosee, W. F., and Dacie, J. V.: Immune lysis of normal human and paroxysmal nocturnal hemoglobinuria (PNH) red blood cells. I. The sensitivity of PNH red cells to lysis by complement and specific antibody. *J. Clin. Invest.* 45:736, 1966.

128. Götze, O., and Müller-Eberhard, H. J.: Paroxysmal nocturnal hemoglobinuria: Hemolysis initiated by the C3 activator system. *N. Engl. J. Med.* 286:180, 1972.

129. May, J. E., Rosse, W., and Frank, M. M.: Paroxysmal nocturnal hemoglobinuria: Alternate-complement-pathway–mediated lysis induced by magnesium. *N. Engl. J. Med.* 289:705, 1973.

130. Rosse, W. F., Logue, G. L., Adams, J., and Crookston, J. H.: Mechanisms of immune lysis of the red cells in hereditary erythroblastic multinuclearity with a positive acidified serum test and paroxysmal nocturnal hemoglobinuria. *J. Clin. Invest.* 53:31, 1974.

131. Ibrahim, S. A., and Thompson, R. H. S.: Action of phospholipase A on human red cell ghosts and intact erythrocytes. *Biochim. Biophys. Acta* 99:331, 1965.

132. Bennett, J. M., and Healy, P. J. M.: Spherocytic anemia and acute cholecystitis caused by *Clostridia welchii*. *N. Engl. J. Med.* 268:1070, 1963.

133. Dean, H. M., Decker, C. L., and Baker, L. D.: Temporary survival in clostridial hemolysis and absence of circulating red cells. *N. Engl. J. Med.* 277:700, 1967.

134. Condrea, E., Mammon, Z., Aloof, S., and De Vries, A.: Susceptibility of erythrocytes of various animal species to the hemolytic and phospholipid splitting action of snake venom. *Biochim. Biophys. Acta* 84:365, 1964.

135. Katchalsky, A., Kedem, O., Klibansky, C., and De Vries, A.: Rheological considerations of the haemolysing red blood cells, in *Flow Properties of Blood and Other Biological Systems*, edited by A. L. Copley and G. Stainsby. Pergamon Press, New York, 1960, p. 155.

136. Jay, A. W. L.: Visoelastic properties of the human red blood cell membrane. I. Deformation, volume loss and rupture of red cells in micropipettes. *Biophys. J.* 13:1166, 1973.

137. Rand, R. P.: Mechanical properties of the red cell membrane. II. Viscoelastic breakdown of the membrane. *Biophys. J.* 4:303, 1964.

138. Schultze, M.: Ein heizbarer objecttisch und seine Verwendung bei Untersuchungen des Blutes. *Arch. Mikroscop. Anat.* 1:1, 1865.

139. Ham, T. H., Shen, S. C., Fleming E. M., and Castle, W. B.: Studies on the destruction of red blood cells. IV. Thermal injury: Action of heat in causing increased spheroidicity, osmotic and mechanical fragilities and hemolysis of erythrocytes; observations on the mechanisms of destruction of such erythrocytes in dogs and in a patient with a fatal thermal burn. *Blood* 3:373, 1948.

140. Streeton, J. A., and Melb, M. B.: Traumatic haemoglobinuria caused by karate exercises. *Lancet* 2:191, 1967.

141. Gilligan, D. R., and Blumgart, H. L.: March hemoglobinuria: Studies of the clinical characteristics; blood metabolism and mechanism, with observations on three new cases, and review of literature. *Medicine (Baltimore)* 20:341, 1941.

142. Davidson, R. J.: Exertional haemoglobinuria: A report on three cases with studies on the haemolytic mechanism. *J. Clin. Pathol.* 17:536, 1964.

143. Godal, H. C., and Refsum, H. E.: Haemolysis in athletes due to hereditary spherocytosis. *Scand. J. Haematol.* 22:83, 1979.

144. Brodeur, M. T. H., Sutherland, D. W., Koler, R. D., Starr, A., Kimsey, J. A., and Griswold, H. E.: Red blood cells survival in patients with aortic valvular disease and ball-valve prosthesis. *Circulation* 32:70, 1965.

145. DeCesare, W., Roth, C., and Hufnagel, C.: Hemolytic anemia of mechanism origin with aortic valve prosthesis. *N. Engl. J. Med.* 272:1045, 1965.

146. Verdon, T. A., Jr., Forrester, R. H., and Crosby, W. H.: Hemolytic anemia after open-heart repair of ostium-primum defects. *N. Engl. J. Med.* 269:444, 1963.

147. Brain, M. C., Dacie, J. V., and Hourihane, D. O'B.: Microangiopathic haemolytic anaemia: The possible roles of vascular lesions in pathogenesis. *Br. J. Haematol.* 8:358, 1962.

148. Capelli, J. P., Wisson, L. B., Jr., and Erslev, A. J.: Malignant hypertension and red cell fragmentation syndrome: Report of a case. *Ann. Intern. Med.* 44:128, 1966.

149. Lynch, E. C., Bakken, C. L., Casey, T. H., and Alfrey, C. P.: Microangiopathic hemolytic anemia in carcinoma of the stomach. *Gastroenterology* 52:88, 1967.

150. Dacie, J. V.: *The Haemolytic Anaemias.* Grune & Stratton, New York, 1967, vol. 3.

151. Muirhead, E. E., Crass, G., and Hill, J. M.: Diffuse platelet thrombosis with thrombocytopenia and hemolytic anemia (thrombotic thrombocytopenic purpura). *Am. J. Clin. Pathol.* 18:523, 1948.

152. McCormack, P., O'Brien, D. J., and Oliver, R. A. M.: Two cases of thrombocytopenic purpura associated with changes in red cell morphology. *J. Clin. Pathol.* 16:436, 1963.

153. Allison, A. C.: Acute haemolytic anaemia with distortion and fragmentation of erythrocytes in children. *Br. J. Haematol.* 3:1, 1957.

154. Brain, M. C., and Hourihane, D. O'B.: Microangiopathic haemolytic anaemia: The occurrence of haemolysis in experimentally produced vascular disease. *Br. J. Haematol.* 13:135, 1967.

155. Rubenberg, M. L., Regoeczi, E., Bull, B. S., Dacie, J. V., and Brain, M. C.: Microangiopathic haemolytic anaemia: The experimental production of haemolysis and red-cell fragmentation by defibrination in vivo. *Br. J. Haematol.* 14:627, 1968.

156. Bull, B. S., Rubenberg, M. L., Dacie, J. V., and Brain, M. C.: Microangiopathic haemolytic anaemia: Mechanisms of red-cell fragmentation: In vitro studies. *Br. J. Haematol.* 14:643, 1968.

157. Weed, R. I., and Reed, C. F.: Membrane alterations leading to red cell destruction. *Am. J. Med. 41*:681, 1966.
158. Harris, J. W.: Studies on the destruction of red blood cells. VIII. Molecular orientation in sickle cell hemoglobin solutions. *Proc. Soc. Exp. Biol. Med. 75*:197, 1950.
159. Harris, J. W., Brewster, H. H., Ham, T. H., and Castle, W. B.: Studies on the destruction of red blood cells. X. The biophysics and biology of sickle cell disease. *Arch. Intern. Med. 97*:145, 1956.
160. Shen, S. C., Fleming, E. M., and Castle, W. B.: Studies on the destruction of red blood cells. V. Irreversible sickled erythrocytes: Their experiimental production in vitro. *Blood 4*:498, 1949.
161. Bertles, J. F., and Dobler, J.: Reversible and irreversible sickling: A distinction by electron microscopy. *Blood 33*:884, 1969.
162. Murphy, J. R.: Hemoglobin CC disease: Rheological properties of erythrocytes and abnormalities in cell water. *J. Clin. Invest. 47*:1483, 1968.
163. Charache, S., Conley, C. L., Waugh, D. F., Ugoretz, R. J., and Spurrell, J. R.: Pathogenesis of hemolytic anemia in homozygous hemoglobin C disease. *J. Clin. Invest. 46*:1795, 1967.
164. Erslev, A. J., and Atwater, J.: Effect of mean corpuscular hemoglobin concentration on viscosity. *J. Lab. Clin. Med. 62*:401, 1963.
165. Glader, B. E., Fortier, N., Alhala, M. M., and Nathan, D. G.: Congenital hemolytic anemia associated with dehydrated erythrocytes and increased potassium loss. *N. Engl. J. Med. 291*:491, 1974.
166. Jaffe, E. R., and Gottfried, E. L.: Hereditary monospherocytic hemolytic disease associated with an altered phospholipid composition of the erythrocytes. *J. Clin. Invest. 47*:1375, 1965.
167. Shohet, S. B., Nathan, D. G., Livermore, B. M., Feig, S. A., and Jaffe, E. R.: Hereditary hemolytic anemia assoicated with abnormal membrane lipid. II. Ion permeability and transport abnormalities. *Blood 42*:1, 1973.
168. Fessas, P.: Inclusions of hemoglobin in erythroblasts and erythrocytes of thalassemia. *Blood 21*:21, 1963.
169. Nathan, D. G.: Thalassemia. *N. Engl. J. Med. 286*:586, 1972.
170. Rigas, D. A., and Koler, R. D.: Decreased erythrocyte survival in hemolglobin H disease as a result of the abnormal properties of hemoglobin H: The benefit of splenectomy. *Blood 18*:1, 1961.
171. Taylor, J. J.: Hemolysis in infectious mononucleosis: Inapparent hereditary spherocytosis. *Br. Med. J. 4*:525, 1973.
172. Jandl. J. H.: The agglutination and sequestration of immature red cells. *J. Lab. Clin. Med. 55*:663, 1960.
173. Key, J. A.: Studies on erythrocytes, with special reference to reticulum, polychromatophilia and mitochondria. *Arch. Intern. Med. 28*:511, 1921.
174. Tavassoli, M.: The marrow-blood barrier. *Br. J. Haematol. 41*:297, 1979.
175. Keene, W. R., and Jandl, J. H.: Studies of the reticuloendothelial mass and sequestering function of rat bone marrow. *Blood 26*:157, 1965.
176. Leblonde, P. F., La Celle, P. L., and Weed, R. I.: Cellular deformability: A possible determinant of the normal release of maturing erythrocytes from the bone marrow. *Blood 37*:40, 1971.
177. London, I. M., and West, R.: The formation of bile pigment in pernicious anemia. *J. Biol. Chem. 184*:359, 1950.
178. Grinstein, M., Bannerman, R. M., Vavra, J. D., and Moore, C. V.: Haemoglobin metabolism in thalassemia: In vivo studies. *Am. J. Med. 29*:18, 1960.
179. Bailey, I. S., and Prankerd, T. A. J.: Studies in thalassaemia. *Br. J. Haematol. 4*:150, 1958.
180. Stohlman, F., Jr.: Humoral regulation of erythorpoiesis. VII. Shortened survival of erythrocytes produced by erythropoietin or severe anemia. *Proc. Soc. Exp. Biol. Med. 107*:884, 1961.
181. Ganzoni, A., Hellman, R. S., and Finch, C. A.: Maturation of the macroreticulocyte. *Br. J. Haematol. 16*:119, 1969.
182. Come, S. E., Shohet, S. B., and Robinson, S.: Surface remodeling of reticulocytes produced in response to erythroid stress. *Nature [New Biol.] 236*:157, 1972.
183. Robinson, S., Vanur, T., Desforges, J. F., and Schmid, R.: Jaundice in thalassemia minor: A consequence of "ineffective erythropoiesis." *N. Engl. J. Med. 267*:523, 1962.
184. Cooper, R. A., Jandl. J. H.: The selective and conjoint loss of red cell lipids. *J. Clin. Invest. 48*:906, 1969.
185. Maizels, M., and Paterson, J. H.: Survival of stored blood after transfusion. *Lancet 2*:417, 1940.
186. Crawford, H., and Mollison, P. L.: Reversal of electrolyte changes in stored red cells after transfusion. *J. Physiol. 129*:639, 1955.
187. Valeri, C. R., McCallum, L. E., and Danon, D.: Relationships between in vivo survival and (1) density distribution; (2) osmotic fragility of previously frozen autologous, agglomerated, deglycerolized erythrocytes. *Transfusion 6*:554, 1966.
188. Crosby, W. H.: Siderocytes and the spleen. *Blood 12*:165, 1957.
189. Morrison, M., Michaels, A. W., Phillips, D. R., and Choi, S.-I.: Life span of erythrocyte membrane protein. *Nature 248*:763, 1974.
190. Pittman, J. G., and Martin, D. B.: Fatty acid biosynthesis in human erythrocytes: Evidence in mature erythrocytes for an incomplete long chain fatty acid synthesizing system. *J. Clin. Invest. 45*:165, 1966.
191. Waker, K., and Lands, W. E. M.: Control of lecithin biosynthesis in erythrocyte membranes. *J. Lipid Res. 9*:12, 1968.
192. Mulder, E., Vandenberg, J. W. O., and Van Deenen, L. L. M.: Metabolism of red cell lipids. II. Conversion of lyophosphoglycerides. *Biochim. Biophys. Acta 106*:118, 1965.
193. Van Deenen, L. L. M., and de Gier, J.: Chemical composition and metabolism of lipids in red cells of various animal species, in *The Red Blood Cell*, edited by C. Bishop and D. M. Surgenor. Academic, New York, 1964, p. 285
194. Hagerman, J. S., and Gould, R. G.: The in vitro interchange of cholesterol between plasma and red cells. *Proc. Soc. Exp. Biol. Med. 78*:329, 1951.
195. Reed, C. F.: Phospholipid exchange between plasma and erythrocytes in man and the dog. *J. Clin. Invest. 47*:749, 1968.
196. Farquhar, J. W., and Ahrens, E. H.: Effects of dietary fats on human erythrocyte fatty acid patterns. *J. Clin. Invest. 42*:675, 1963.
197. Shohet, S. B., Nathan, D. G., and Karnovsky, M. L.: Stages in the incorporation of fatty acids into red blood cells. *J. Clin. Invest 47*:1096, 1968.
198. Cooper, R. A., and Jandl, J. H.: The role of membrane lipids in the survival of red cells in hereditary spherocytosis. *J. Clin. Invest. 48*:736, 1969.
199. Chen, L.-T., and Weiss, L.: Electron microscopy of the red pulp of the human spleen. *Am. J. Anat. 134*:425, 1972.
200. Cooper, R. A., and Jandl, J. H.: Bile salts and cholesterol in the pathogenesis of "target cells" in obstructive jaundice. *J. Clin. Invest. 47*:809, 1968.

CHAPTER 40

Degradation of hemoglobin

STEPHEN H. ROBINSON

The major pathways of heme degradation are shown schematically in Fig. 40-1. Most heme degradation and bilirubin production are related to erythrocyte senescence. The reasons that red blood cells normally die at about 120 days of age in humans are not well understood and the anatomic sites in which these cells are destroyed are known only imprecisely. Nevertheless, this process is presumed to take place in phagocytic cells of the monocyte-macrophage system in the spleen, liver, and marrow. When red blood cells are taken up by these phagocytic cells, the globin is hydrolyzed to its constituent amino acids, which mix with the general amino acid pool [2]. The iron liberated from heme is largely lost from the phagocytic cell and is transported by transferrin to early erythroid cells in the marrow, where it is reutilized for new hemoglobin synthesis. Some iron may remain in the cell in a storage form. The heme moiety is degraded to biliverdin and carbon monoxide, and the biliverdin is rapidly reduced to bilirubin, which is excreted into the bile. There are two additional sources of normal bilirubin production, one related to red cell development in the marrow and the other to turnover of nonhemoglobin hemes, primarily in the liver.

Increased rates of hemoglobin degradation take place with hemolysis, ineffective erythropoiesis, or the resorption of hematomas. There are two general forms of hemolytic anemia with regard to the major site of red cell destruction, intravascular and extravascular hemolysis. In the former there is considerable release of hemoglobin into plasma as the result of the destruction of red cells within the free circulation. Much of this plasma hemoglobin is bound to haptoglobin and carried to the liver, where it is converted to bilirubin. In the more common extravascular form of hemolysis, red cells are destroyed primarily within phagocytic cells, where the heme of hemoglobin is converted directly to bilirubin; there is also some liberation of free hemoglobin into the plasma as evidenced by the depletion of haptoglobin. Based on the kinetics of haptoglobin turnover, it has been surmised that perhaps 10 to 20 percent of normal red cell senescence also involves the release of hemoglobin into the plasma [3,4]. Thus, when evaluating either normal or abnormal red blood cell destruction, one must deal both with the metabolic disposition of plasma hemoglobin and with the production and excretion of bilirubin.

Disposition of plasma hemoglobin and heme

Hemoglobin liberated into the plasma is bound to the plasma protein haptoglobin [3,5]. The haptoglobin-hemoglobin complex is carried to the parenchymal cells of the liver, where the heme of the hemoglobin is converted to bilirubin [6]. This occurs very rapidly; the $T_{1/2}$ of disappearance of haptoglobin-hemoglobin from the plasma is 10 to 30 min [7], as compared with a $T_{1/2}$ of 5 days for haptoglobin alone. Haptoglobin is depleted during this process and plasma haptoglobin levels are usually low in both intravascular and extravascular hemolytic states because the liver fails to compensate with an increase in haptoglobin synthesis [8]. However, haptoglobin is an acute-phase reactant, levels of which rise in various conditions [9]. Thus haptoglobin concentration may be normal or even increased in patients with both hemolysis and a coexisting inflammatory, infectious, or neoplastic illness.

Haptoglobin is a glycoprotein which migrates as an

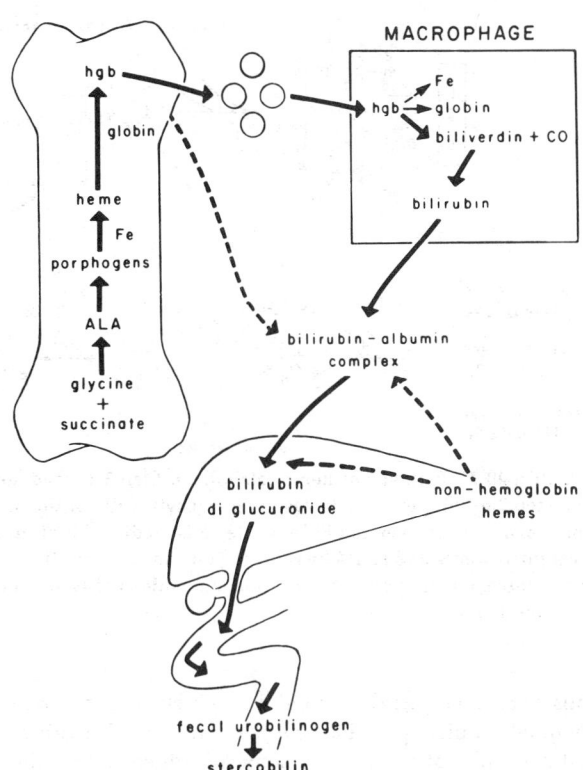

FIGURE 40-1 Schematic summary of heme degradation and bilirubin metabolism. The solid arrows show the major metabolic pathway. The dashed arrows indicate the two minor pathways related to erythropoiesis and turnover of nonhemoglobin hemes. Bilirubin derived from nonhemoglobin sources in the liver may be excreted directly into the bile or may first enter the plasma. ALA = δ-aminolevulinic acid; porphogens = porphobilinogen and the porphyrinogens. (Adapted from Robinson [1], with permission.)

α_2-globulin on electrophoresis [9]. Its plasma concentration is usually expressed in terms of its hemoglobin-binding capacity, the normal range being 50 to 200 mg/dl. Haptoglobin is composed of α and β polypeptide chains. Genetic variations in the α peptide chains are responsible for polymorphism and may be useful markers for genetic studies. These are described in Chap. 163. The haptoglobin-hemoglobin complex consists of one molecule of hemoglobin and one molecule of haptoglobin [10]. The binding is primarily between the β chains of haptoglobin and the α chains of hemoglobin [10] and is essentially irreversible.

The size of the haptoglobin-hemoglobin complex is too large to allow for filtration across the glomerulus. When plasma haptoglobin is depleted, however, hemoglobin readily passes into the glomerular filtrate in the form of α,β dimers [11]. These are reabsorbed by proximal tubular cells [12], and when a maximal rate of tubular reabsorption of about 1.4 mg/min is exceeded [13], hemoglobin is excreted in the urine. Whether or not there is hemoglobinuria, the presence of hemoglobin in the glomerular filtrate becomes manifest as he-

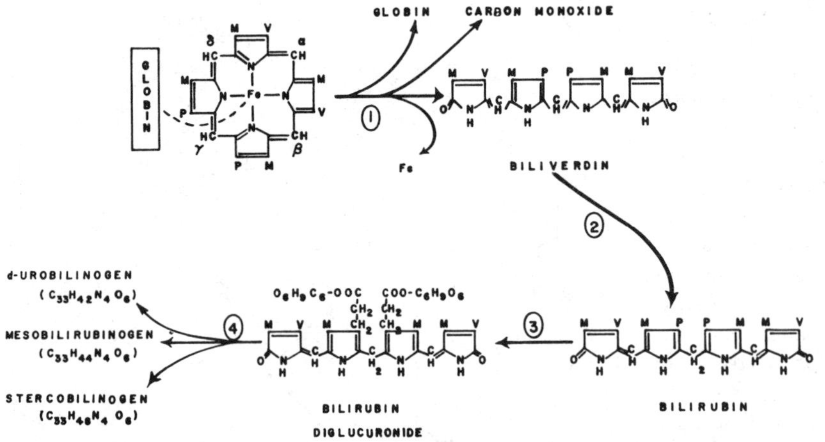

FIGURE 40-2   Pathway of heme catabolism. Step 1 is mediated by microsomal heme oxygenase and step 2 by biliverdin reductase in phagocytic cells of the monocyte-macrophage system or parenchymal cells of liver and kidney. Step 3 is mediated by bilirubin UDP-glucuronyltransferase in liver microsomes and step 4 by reducing enzymes in intestinal bacteria, leading to the formation of these three major types of urobilinogen. Side-chains on the pyrrole rings are M, methyl; P, propionyl; and V, vinyl.

mosiderinuria [14,15]. Hemoglobin which is reabsorbed by renal tubular epithelial cells is degraded to bilirubin, with the liberation of iron, some of which enters the plasma pool and some of which is complexed into the iron storage proteins ferritin and hemosiderin [11,14]. When the tubular cells eventually are sloughed into the urine, the presence of hemosiderin can be detected by staining the urine sediment with Prussian blue (see Chap. A3). Testing for hemosiderinuria is an easy and inexpensive means of detecting recent intravascular hemolysis.

With depletion of haptoglobin, not only is hemoglobin metabolized and excreted by the kidney, but some is probably cleared by direct uptake into other parenchymal organs such as the liver [6] and some is oxidized to methemoglobin. The oxidized heme moiety (hemin) is readily dissociated from methemoglobin [16] and is avidly bound to hemopexin, another plasma protein which is synthesized by the liver [17]. Hemopexin is a glycoprotein of the β-globulin class which binds hemin, but not hemoglobin, in a 1:1 molar ratio. This hemin-hemopexin complex is cleared by hepatic parenchymal cells relatively slowly as compared with the hemoglobin-haptoglobin complex, with a $T_{1/2}$ of 7 to 8 h [18]. As is the case with haptoglobin, hemopexin is usually depleted in patients with hemolysis. When hemopexin is depleted, free hemin is associated with albumin, also in 1:1 molar ratio, to form methemalbumin. Methemalbumin and hemopexin-hemin may impart a brownish color to the plasma and may be detected spectrophotometrically by the so-called Schumm test [19]. Clearance of methemalbumin from the plasma is quite slow and probably involves the transfer of hemin from albumin to newly synthesized hemopexin [17], by which the hemin is transported to the liver for conversion to bilirubin.

Enzymatic conversion of heme to bilirubin

Many cells contain the enzymatic apparatus for converting heme to bilirubin. These include phagocytic cells of the monocyte-macrophage system in the spleen, marrow, and liver and parenchymal cells in the liver and kidney. Schism of the α-carbon bridge of the tetrapyrrolic heme molecule (see Fig. 40-2) is mediated by an enzyme system in the microsomal fraction of these cells [20–23]. This enzyme system, known as *microsomal heme oxygenase*, utilizes molecular oxygen and NADPH which is regenerated through an NADPH-dependent cytochrome c reductase. Initially, it was thought that cytochrome P_{450} was involved as a terminal oxidase, but it now appears that catabolism of heme is an autooxidative process in which binding of heme to heme oxygenase provides the chemical microenvironment for activation and cleavage of the heme ring [20,24]. For every heme molecule thus degraded, one molecule of biliverdin and one molecule of carbon monoxide result [20–23]. The biliverdin is promptly converted to bilirubin by a second enzyme, biliverdin reductase, which is present in the soluble fraction of the same cells in which biliverdin is formed from heme [25]. Bilirubin reductase also requires NADPH, is specific for the α isomer of bilirubin which is produced by microsomal heme oxygenase, and is present in excess so that biliverdin is not detectable in the plasma, even when there is a marked increase in red blood cell destruction. Thus it is bilirubin which emerges into the plasma and is transported to the liver for excretion into the bile.

Cleavage of the heme ring with oxidation of its α-carbon bridge represents the only metabolic source of carbon monoxide production in mammals [26,27]. Carbon monoxide is carried in the blood in the form of carboxyhemoglobin and is excreted via the lungs [28].

Techniques for measuring the rate of carbon monoxide formation or bilirubin production can provide very useful information about the rate of red cell hemolysis, ineffective erythropoiesis, and the turnover of nonhemoglobin hemes [26,29–33].

Sources of bilirubin

When labeled glycine is used as a precursor of heme, several fractions of labeled bile pigment formation can be discerned [34–38] (Figs. 40-3 and 40-4). As expected, the major fraction is formed as senescent red blood cells are destroyed. In addition, there is an "early labeled" fraction which is formed before there is significant label in red cell hemoglobin [34,35]. This early fraction accounts for 15 to 20 percent of the total bilirubin produced under normal conditions and has been shown to consist of at least two subcomponents [36,37,40]. The first of these subcomponents is produced very rapidly and is derived from the turnover of nonhemoglobin hemes, primarily in the liver [41–44] but also in other tissues, including the kidney and the marrow [44,45]. It has been surmised [45] that the earliest phase of this nonhemoglobin bilirubin component may arise from the catabolism of a labile pool of free or unassigned heme which may have important regulatory functions and that later phases may be derived from the turnover of various hemoproteins such as cytochrome P_{450} [46]. Although studies with labeled glycine indicate that the entire early labeled fraction normally comprises 15 to 20 percent of the total labeled bilirubin, studies based on other techniques suggest that it is larger than this and that the hepatic nonhemoglobin subcomponent alone may account for 20 percent or more of the total pigment production [47,48].

The second subcomponent of early labeled bilirubin is related to erythropoiesis [36–38]. This component is enhanced when there is erythroid hyperplasia of the marrow and may be strikingly augmented in pathologic conditions associated with ineffective erythropoiesis [49]. In these pathologic states the excess of early labeled bilirubin is clearly derived from the destruction of defective red cell precursors in or soon after release from the marrow [50]. There may be a small degree of ineffective erythropoiesis during physiologic red cell production, and this may account for the small erythropoietic fraction produced under normal conditions. Another possible mechanism for erythropoietic bilirubin formation in normal individuals is that the extruded nucleus of maturing erythroid cells is accompanied by a rim of cytoplasm [51], the hemoglobin of which is degraded to early labeled bilirubin. Surface remodeling of reticulocytes, particularly of cells produced in response to erythroid stress, doubtless contributes to this bilirubin fraction as well [50,52].

Each of the three fractions of normal bilirubin production is a potential source of bilirubin overproduction and unconjugated hyperbilirubinemia. An increase

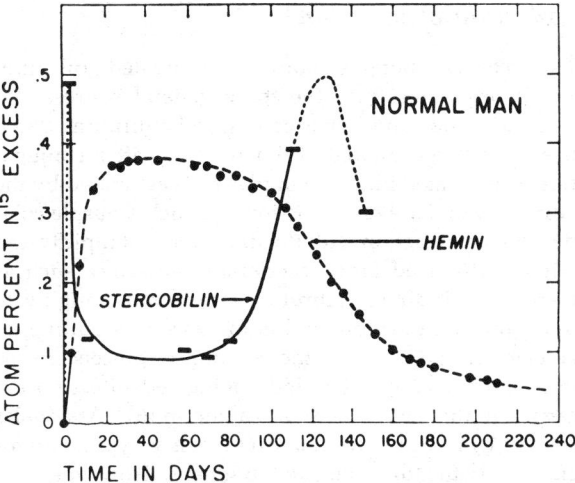

FIGURE 40-3 Labeling of blood hemoglobin heme and fecal bile pigment (stercobilin) in a human subject given ^{15}N-glycine. (London, et al. [34].)

in the rate of red cell destruction is certainly the most common cause of overproduction jaundice. An increase in the nonhemoglobin fraction of bilirubin formation has been described in animals and human beings with disorders affecting liver function [53–55]. It is not yet clear whether hyperbilirubinemia of substantial degree ever results from this mechanism. Bilirubin overproduction as the result of ineffective erythropoiesis largely accounts for the mild unconjugated hyperbilirubinemia that is characteristially observed in patients with pernicious anemia, thalassemia, refractory anemia, erythroleukemia, and more unusual instances of disordered erythropoiesis [30,56–60].

FIGURE 40-4 Sources of bilirubin production in humans based on studies with glycine-2-^{14}C. Measurements of bilirubin in plasma and bile have made it possible to observe the kinetics of labeled bilirubin formation more precisely than with studies of bile pigment in the feces. Note that there is some continuing bilirubin production from unknown sources between the early and late peaks. (Adapted from Robinson [39], with permission.)

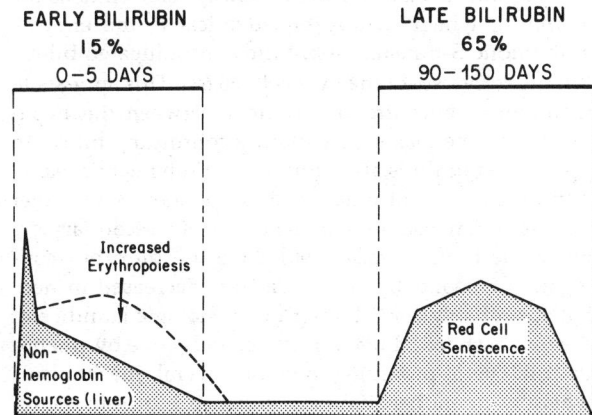

Excretion of bilirubin

The plasma contains both unconjugated bilirubin which originates from the three general sources described earlier and some conjugated bilirubin which has been "regurgitated" from the liver after conjugation. Conjugated bilirubin in plasma is estimated by the "direct" van den Bergh reaction in which a purple color develops on reaction with the diazo reagent rapidly and without the need for an accelerator substance such as methanol. "Indirect" bilirubin corresponds roughly to unconjugated bilirubin and is measured by adding an accelerator and allowing the reaction to proceed for 30 min. Both unconjugated and conjugated bilirubin are carried in the plasma bound to albumin [61]. At a molar ratio of 1:1 bilirubin to albumin there is very little dissociation of the unconjugated pigment. However, free bilirubin may be displaced from albumin by competing substances, including fatty acids, salicylates, and sulfa drugs, and by acidosis [62,63]. These are to be avoided in infants with severe unconjugated hyperbilirubinemia since lipid-soluble free bilirubin dissociated from albumin is available for transfer across the blood-brain barrier, with the risk of bilirubin toxicity to brain (kernicterus). The interaction between conjugated bilirubin and albumin is relatively weak, accounting for the fact that this water-soluble molecule gains access to the urine.

The excretion of bilirubin into the bile is mediated by the liver and is conventionally considered as occurring in three steps: hepatic uptake, conjugation, and secretion. Bilirubin uptake by the liver represents either simple diffusion or a carrier-mediated transport process [64] involving specific receptors on the liver cell membrane. Albumin is dissociated from bilirubin during the uptake process. A significant fraction, perhaps 40 percent, of the bilirubin taken up by the liver refluxes back into the plasma [64,65]. It is this bidirectional flux which accounts for the elevated plasma concentration of unconjugated bilirubin found in states of bilirubin overproduction. Otherwise the large excretory capacity of the liver would absorb virtually any increment in bilirubin production resulting from hemolytic anemia or ineffective erythropoiesis.

A protein called *ligandin*, previously referred to as the Y *protein*, which is probably identical to the enzyme glutathione S-transferase B, binds unconjugated bilirubin in the cytosol of the liver cell [66,67]. This appears to maintain a concentration gradient between the hepatocyte and the plasma, facilitating continuing bilirubin uptake. Ligandin is also important in the hepatic excretion of a variety of other anionic substances. Another protein, known as the Z *protein*, acts as a secondary cytoplasmic binding factor [66]. Like the bilirubin conjugating enzyme, ligandin levels are decreased in neonates, probably contributing to physiologic jaundice of the newborn [68]. Ligandin is also inducible by phenobarbital [69], providing one of several mechanisms whereby phenobarbital may enhance bilirubin excretion.

In the second step of hepatic bilirubin excretion, unconjugated bilirubin is conjugated with glucuronic acid by an enzyme, bilirubin UDP-glucuronyltransferase, which is located in the endoplasmic reticulum of the liver cell. This enzyme is a member of a family of transferases which mediate the biotransformation of a variety of substances, but there appears to be a specific glucuronyl transferase for bilirubin [70,71]. As a result of the action of this enzyme, the propionic acid side chains of bilirubin are esterified with glucuronic acid which is derived from uridine diphosphate glucuronic acid (UDPGA). Thus the nonpolar, lipid-soluble bilirubin molecule is converted to a polar, lipid-insoluble molecule which will be retained within the mucosal barrier of the biliary and intestinal excretory pathways [72].

There are both monoglucuronide and diglucuronide conjugates of bilirubin [73,74], and it has been suggested that the first molecule of glucuronic acid is added by the microsomal transferase enzyme and the second by a transglucuronidase enzyme associated with the canalicular membrane of the liver cell [75]. However, there is evidence that both these esterification steps are mediated by the microsomal transferase system [76]. It has recently been demonstrated that some bilirubin is conjugated with sugars such as xylose and glucose [77–79], but to a much smaller extent than with glucuronic acid.

Bilirubin glucuronyl transferase is entirely lacking in the rare congenital disorder Crigler-Najjar syndrome [80] and in a similar syndrome encountered in Gunn rats [81]. Both the humans and the rodents with this disorder suffer from severe unconjugated hyperbilirubinemia, usually with kernicterus. Partial deficiency of this enzyme has been described in a form of congenital unconjugated hyperbilirubinemia of intermediate severity [82,83] as well as in a common, mild form of unconjugated hyperbilirubinemia known as Gilbert's syndrome [84,85]. It is not clear whether the intermediate form of enzyme deficiency and Gilbert's syndrome are different disorders or represent parts of the spectrum of the same congenital disorder. It has been suggested that Gilbert's syndrome may not only be a deficiency of glucuronyl transferase, but that a defect in hepatic uptake of bilirubin may play a role as well [20]. The red cells of many patients with Gilbert's syndrome have a shortened life-span [86]. This is usually accounted for by the coexistence of common forms of hemolytic anemia such as hereditary spherocytosis or certain G-6-PD deficiencies. It has been suggested that since Gilbert's syndrome may occur in as much as 7 percent of the population [86], its presence is often brought to clinical light when there is superimposition of two relatively common causes of mild jaundice, the excretory defect of Gilbert's syndrome and the overproduction defect of mild hemolysis. In both Gilbert's syndrome and the syndrome resulting from an intermediate deficiency of bilirubin glucuronyl transferase, phenobarbital will reduce the level of jaundice [83,87,88] in part by inducing increased levels of the conjugating enzyme and in part by augmenting other aspects of the excretory pathway. By contrast, phenobarbital is without effect in patients with the Crigler-Najjar syndrome [83] and in Gunn rats [89] in which no enzyme substrate is available for induction.

In the third phase of hepatic bilirubin excretion, the conjugated pigment is secreted across the canalicular membrane into the bile. This is an active, energy-dependent transport process by which large concentration gradients are maintained across the liver cell membrane [64]. This is also the rate-limiting step in bilirubin excretion, and under conditions in which large amounts of bilirubin are being excreted, the amount of the pigment that reaches the bile is determined by saturation of the secretory apparatus [64,89]. This in turn leads to the regurgitation of some conjugated bilirubin from the liver cell back into the plasma. The secretory step is highly vulnerable to liver injury, and conjugated hyperbilirubinemia and the resulting bilirubinuria are common accompaniments of acquired liver damage. The Dubin-Johnson and related Rotor syndromes represent congenital disorders of the secretory mechanism [90,91].

After having been excreted into the bile, conjugated bilirubin traverses the intestinal tract and, on reaching the colon, is converted to a series of compounds collectively called *urobilinogen* [92] (see Fig. 40-2). These molecules are derived from bilirubin by a series of reductive steps mediated by the bacteria of the large intestine [93,94]. The glucuronic acid residues of bilirubin or urobilinogen are hydrolyzed by β-glucuronidase in the intestinal mucosa. The resulting deconjugated urobilinogen compounds are largely excreted in the feces, where they undergo oxidative reactions leading to the formation of a series of corresponding compounds known as *urobilin* or *stercobilin*. However, perhaps 20 percent of the total urobilinogen in the large intestine is reabsorbed and enters the portal circulation, through which it is delivered to the liver. Under normal conditions, the liver cell efficiently extracts virtually all this urobilinogen and excretes it into the bile, thus completing an enterohepatic circulation [95]. A small amount of urobilinogen escapes reexcretion by the liver cell and is eliminated in the urine. When there is hepatic cell dysfunction, an increased fraction of recirculated urobilinogen may escape hepatic extraction and be excreted in the urine; this may occur even when there is a decrease in urobilinogen excretion in the feces, e.g., during the so-called obstructive phase of infectious hepatitis.

Quantitative measurements of fecal urobilinogen may be used to estimate the total rate of bilirubin production [96]. However, approximately 40 percent of the bile pigment reaching the large intestine is degraded to unidentifiable products other than urobilinogen. Moreover, administration of antibiotics with the consequent alteration in fecal flora may reduce the conversion of bilirubin to urobilinogen. Fecal urobilinogen measurements are no longer used commonly to measure the rate of heme degradation. However, if they are, urobilinogen should be related to the blood hemoglobin concentration (the urobilinogen index) since, in an anemic pa-

tient, there is less hemoglobin substrate for conversion to bile pigment. Measurement of urinary urobilinogen excretion [97,98] is a still less accurate index of heme degradation. Not only is urinary excretion of urobilinogen affected by the status of the liver, but it is also influenced by variations in kidney function and urinary pH.

Alternate pathways of heme and bilirubin degradation

Alternate pathways of heme degradation that do not give rise to bilirubin are probably negligible under normal conditions. However, they may be observed clinically in patients with Heinz body formation as the result of an unstable hemoglobin or one of the thalassemic disorders. These patients may excrete in the urine a brownish pigment consisting of dipyrroles [99–101]. Similarly, much of the labeled heme in Heinz bodies produced experimentally in rats is converted to dipyrrolic compounds rather than bilirubin [102]. Small amounts of dipyrrolic substances are also produced by normal subjects; these are labeled rapidly after administration of glycine-^{14}C [103], and their metabolic source is unknown.

Just as heme may be degraded to unusual catabolites in certain pathologic conditions, the major catabolic product of heme, bilirubin, may be degraded to smaller pyrrolic moieties, especially when there is impairment of bilirubin excretion. With prolonged hyperbilirubinemia owing to impaired conjugation, as encountered in the Crigler-Najjar syndrome, bilirubin is degraded to polar catabolites which can be excreted into the bile without prior conjugation [104]. Photooxidation of bilirubin by light of wavelengths 410 to 460 nm also produces degradation products of bilirubin, and these too are readily excreted in the bile. This forms the basis of phototherapy [105,106] which is used commonly in the management of neonatal hyperbilirubinemia. In normal subjects, however, it appears that virtually all heme is eliminated as bilirubin and carbon monoxide and that little if any heme degradation is manifest in terms of these smaller catabolic products of heme or bilirubin metabolism.

References

1. Robinson, S. H.: Heme metabolism and the porphyrias, in *Hematology*, 2d ed., Harvard Pathophysiology Series, edited by W. S. Beck. M.I.T. Press, Cambridge, Mass., 1977, pp. 153–164.
2. Ehrenreich, B. A., and Cohn, Z. A.: Fate of hemoglobin pinocytosed by macrophages in vitro. *J. Cell Biol. 38*:244, 1968.
3. Giblett, E. R.: Haptoglobin. *Ser. Haematol. 1*:3, 1968.
4. Noyes, W. D., and Garby, L: Rate of haptoglobin synthesis in normal man. *Scand. J. Clin. Lab. Invest. 20*:33, 1967.
5. Hershko, C.: The fate of circulating hemoglobins. *Br. J. Haematol. 29*:199, 1975.
6. Bissell, D. M., Hammaker, L., and Schmid, R.: Hemoglobin and erythrocyte catabolism in rat liver: The separate roles of parenchymal and sinusoidal cells. *Blood 40*:812, 1972.

7. Garby, L., and Noyes, W. D.: Studies on hemoglobin metabolism. I. The kinetic properties of the plasma hemoglobin pool in normal man. *J. Clin. Invest.* 38:1479, 1959.

8. Nyman, M., Gydell, K., and Nosslin, B.: Haptoglobin und erythrokinetik. *Clin. Chim. Acta* 4:82, 1959.

9. Laurell, C. B., and Gronvall, C.: Haptoglobins. *Adv. Clin. Chem.* 5:135, 1962.

10. Nagel. R. L., and Gibson, Q. H.: The binding of hemoglobin to haptoglobin and its relation to subunit dissociation of hemoglobin. *J. Biol. Chem.* 246:69, 1971.

11. Bunn, H. F., Esham, W. T., and Bull, R. W.: The renal handling of hemoglobin. *J. Exp. Med.* 129:909, 1969.

12. Lathem, W., et al.: The renal excretion of hemoglobin. *J. Clin. Invest.* 38:652, 1959.

13. Lowenstein, J., et al.: The glomerular clearance and renal transport of hemoglobin in adult males. *J. Clin. Invest.* 40:1172, 1961.

14. Sears, D. A., Anderson, P. R., Fox, A. L., Williams, H. L., and Crosby, W. H.: Urinary iron excretion and renal metabolism of hemoglobin in hemolytic diseases. *Blood* 28:708, 1966.

15. Pimstone, N. R.: Renal degradation of hemoglobin. *Semin. Hematol.* 9:31, 1972.

16. Bunn, H. F., and Jandl, J. H.: Exchange of heme among hemoglobins and between hemoglobin and albumin. *J. Biol. Chem.* 243:465, 1968.

17. Muller-Eberhard, U.: Hemopexin. *N. Engl. J. Med.* 283:1090, 1970.

18. Sears, D. A.: Disposal of plasma heme in normal man and patients with intravascular hemolysis. *J. Clin. Invest.* 49:5, 1970.

19. Rosen, H., and Sears, D. A.: Spectral properties of hemopexin-heme: The Schumm test. *J. Lab. Clin. Med.* 74:941, 1969.

20. Schmid, R.: Hyperbilirubinemia, in *The Metabolic Basis of Inherited Disease*, 3d ed., edited by J. B. Stanbury, J. B. Wyngaarden, and D. S. Fredrickson. McGraw-Hill, New York, 1978, pp. 1221–1257.

21. Tenhunen, R. S., Marver, H. S., and Schmid, R.: Microsomal heme oxygenase. Characterization of the enzyme. *J. Biol. Chem.* 44:638, 1969.

22. Tenhunen, R.: The enzymatic degradation of heme. *Semin. Hematol.* 9:19, 1972.

23. Pimstone, N. R., et al.: The enzymatic degradation of hemoglobin to bile pigments by macrophages. *J. Exp. Med.* 133:1264, 1971.

24. Yoshida, T., Takahashi, S., and Kikuchi, G.: Partial purification and reconstitution of the heme oxygenase system from pig spleen microsomes. *J. Biochem.* 75:1187, 1974.

25. Tenhunen, R., et al.: Reduced nicotinamide-adenine dinucleotide phosphate dependent biliverdin reductase: Partial purification and characterization. *Biochemistry* 9:298, 1970.

26. Sjostrand, T.: Endogenous formation of carbon monoxide in man under normal and pathological conditions. *Scand. J. Clin. Lab. Invest.* 1:201, 1949.

27. Coburn, R. F., et al.: The production of carbon monoxide from hemoglobin in vivo. *J. Clin. Invest.* 46:346, 1967.

28. Loumanmaki, K., and Coburn, R. F.: Effects of metabolism and distribution of carbon monoxide on blood and body stores. *Am. J. Physiol.* 217:354, 1969.

29. Coburn, R. F., Williams, W. J., and Kahn, S. B.: Endogenous carbon monoxide production in patients with hemolytic anemia. *J. Clin. Invest.* 45:460, 1966.

30. White, P., et al.: Carbon monoxide production associated with ineffective erythropoiesis. *J. Clin. Invest.* 46:1986, 1967.

31. Landaw, S. A., Callahan, E. W., Jr., and Schmid, R.: Catabolism of heme in vivo: Comparison of the simultaneous production of bilirubin and carbon monoxide. *J. Clin. Invest.* 49:914, 1970.

32. Berk, P. D., et al.: Comparison of plasma bilirubin turnover and carbon monoxide production in man. *J. Lab. Clin. Med.* 83:29, 1974.

33. Lundh, B., Cavallin-Stahl, E., and Mercke, C.: Heme catabolism, carbon monoxide production and red cell survival in anemia. *Acta Med. Scand.* 197:161, 1975.

34. London, I. M., et al.: On the origin of bile pigment in normal man. *J. Biol. Chem.* 184:351, 1950.

35. Gray, C. H., Neuberger, A., and Sneath, P. H.: Incorporation of N^{15} in the stercobilin in the normal and the porphyric. *Biochem. J.* 47:87, 1950.

36. Israels, L. G., et al.: Shunt bilirubin: Evidence for two components. *Science* 139:1054, 1963.

37. Robinson, S. H., et al.: The sources of bile pigment in the rat: Studies of the "early-labeled" fraction. *J. Clin. Invest.* 45:1569, 1966.

38. Robinson, S. H., et al.: Early-labeled peak of bile pigment in man. Studies with glycine-C^{14} and delta-aminolevulinic acid-H^3. *N. Engl. J. Med.* 277:1323, 1967.

39. Robinson, S. H.: Ineffective erythropoiesis and the erythropoietic component of early-labeled bilirubin, in *Hemopoietic Cellular Proliferation*, edited by F. Stohman, Jr. Grune & Stratton, New York, 1970, pp. 180–188.

40. Yammamoto, T., et al.: The early appearing bilirubin: Evidence for two components. *J. Clin. Invest.* 44:31, 1965.

41. Robinson, S. H., et al.: Bilirubin formation in the liver from nonhemoglobin sources: Experiments with isolated, perfused rat liver. *Blood* 26:823, 1965.

42. Ibrahim, G. W., Schwartz, S., and Watson, C. J.: Early labeling of bilirubin from glycine and delta-aminolevulinic acid in bile fistula dogs, with special reference to stimulated versus suppressed erythropoiesis. *Metabolism* 15:1129, 1966.

43. Levitt, M., et al.: The non-erythropoietic component of early bilirubin. *J. Clin. Invest.* 47:1281, 1968.

44. Yannoni, C. Z., and Robinson, S. H.: Early-labelled haem in erythroid and hepatic cells. *Nature (London)* 258:330, 1975.

45. Yannoni, C. Z., and Robinson, S. H.: Early-labeled heme synthesis in normal rats and rats with iron deficiency anemia. *Biochim. Biophys. Acta* 428:533, 1976.

46. Schmid, R., Marver, H. S., and Hammaker, L.: Enhanced formation of rapidly labeled bilirubin by phenobarbital: Hepatic microsomal cytochromes as a possible source. *Biochem. Biophys. Res. Commun.* 24:319, 1966.

47. Berk, P. D., et al.: A new approach to quantitation of the various sources of bilirubin in man. *J. Lab. Clin. Med.* 87:767, 1976.

48. Kirshenbaum, G., Shames, D. M., and Schmid, R.: An expanded model of bilirubin kinetics: Effect of feeding, fasting, and phenobarbital in Gilbert's syndrome. *J. Pharmacokinet. Biopharm.* 4:115, 1976.

49. Robinson, S. H.: Formation of bilirubin from erythroid and non-erythroid sources. *Semin. Hematol.* 9:43, 1972.

50. Come, S. E., Shehet, S. B., and Robinson, S. H.: Surface remodelling versus whole-cell hemolysis of reticulocytes produced with erythroid stimulation or iron deficiency anemia. *Blood* 44:817, 1974.

51. Bessis, M, Breton-Gorius, J., and Thiery, J. P.: Rôle possible de l'hémoglobine accompagnant le noyau des erythroblastes dans l'origine de la stercobiline eliminée précocement. *C. R. Acad. Sci.* [D] (Paris) 252:2300, 1961.

52. Robinson, S. H., and Tsong, M.: Hemolysis of "stress" reticulocytes: A source of erythropoietic bilirubin formation. *J. Clin. Invest.* 49:1025, 1970.

53. Robinson, S. H.: Increased bilirubin formation from nonhemoglobin sources in rats with disorders of the liver. *J. Lab. Clin. Med.* 73:668, 1969.

54. Tarao, K., et al.: The effects of acute infectious hepatitis and cirrhosis of the liver on the nonerythropoietic component of early bilirubin. *J. Lab. Clin. Med.* 87:240, 1976.

55. Coburn, R. F.: Enhancement by phenobarbital and diphenylhydantoin of carbon monoxide production in normal man. *N. Engl. J. Med.* 283:512, 1970.

56. Robinson, S. H.: Increased formation of early-labled bilirubin in rats with iron deficiency anemia: Evidence for ineffective erythropoiesis. *Blood* 33:909, 1969.

57. London, I. M., et al.: Porphyrin formation and hemoglobin metabolism in congenital porphyria. *J. Biol. Chem.* 184:365, 1950.

58. London, I. M., and West, R.: The formation of bile pigment in pernicious anemia. *J. Biol. Chem.* 184:359, 1950.

59. Robinson, S. H., et al.: Jaundice in thalassemia minor: A consequence of "ineffective erythropoiesis." *N. Engl. J. Med.* 267:523, 1962.

60. Grinstein, M., et al.: Hemoglobin metabolism in thalassemia. *Am. J. Med.* 29:18, 1960.

61. Ostrow, J. D., and Schmid. R.: The protein-binding of C^{14}-bilirubin in human and murine serum. *J. Clin. Invest.* 42:1286, 1963.

62. Odell, G. B.: The distribution and toxicity of bilirubin. *Pediatrics* 45:16, 1970.

63. Thaler, M. M., and Schmid, R.: Drugs and bilirubin. *Pediatrics* 47:807, 1971.
64. Goresky, C. A.: The hepatic uptake process: Its implications for bilirubin transport, in *Jaundice*, edited by C. A. Goresky and M. M. Fisher. Plenum, New York, 1975, pp. 159–174.
65. Berk, P. D., et al.: Studies of bilirubin kinetics in normal adults. *J. Clin. Invest.* 48:2176, 1969.
66. Levi, A. J., Gatmaitan, Z., and Arias, I. M.: Two hepatic cytoplasmic protein factors, Y and Z, and their possible role in the hepatic uptake of bilirubin, sulfobromophthalein, and other anions. *J. Clin. Invest.* 48:2156, 1969.
67. Arias, I. M., and Jansen, P.: Protein binding and conjugation of bilirubin in the liver cell, in *Jaundice*, edited by C. A. Goresky and M. M. Fisher. Plenum, New York, 1975, pp. 175–188.
68. Levi, A. J., Gatmaitan, Z., and Arias, I. M.: Deficiency of hepatic organic anion-binding protein, impaired organic anion uptake, and "physiologic" jaundice in newborn monkeys. *N. Engl. J. Med.* 283:1136, 1970.
69. Reyes, H., et al.: Studies on Y and Z, two hepatic cytoplasmic organic anion-binding proteins: Effect of drugs, chemicals, hormones, and cholestasis. *J. Clin. Invest.* 50:2242, 1971.
70. Vessey, D. A., Goldenberg, J., and Zakim, D.: Differentiation of homologous forms of hepatic microsomal UDP-glucuronyltransferase. II. Characterization of the bilirubin conjugating form. *Biochim. Biophys. Acta* 309:75, 1973.
71. Jacobson, M. M., and Conney, A. H.: Studies on bilirubin and steroid glucuronidation by rat liver microsomes. *Biochem. Pharmacol.* 24:655, 1975.
72. Lester, R., and Schmid, R.: Intestinal absorption of bile pigments. II. Bilirubin absorption in man. *N. Engl. J. Med.* 269:178, 1963.
73. Jansen, P. L. M.: The enzyme-catalyzed formation of bilirubin diglucuronide by a solubilized preparation from rat liver microsomes. *Biochim. Biophys. Acta* 338:170, 1974.
74. Halac, E., Dipiazza, M., and Detwiler, P.: The formation of bilirubin mono- and diglucuronide by rat liver microsomal fractions. *Biochim. Biophys. Acta* 279:544, 1972.
75. Jansen, P. L. M., et al.: Enzymatic conversion of bilirubin monoglucuronide to diglucuronide by rat liver plasma membranes. *J. Biol. Chem.* 252:2710, 1977.
76. Blanckaert, N., Gollan, J., and Schmid, R.: Mechanism of bilirubin diglucuronide formation in intact rats: Bilirubin diglucuronide formation in vivo. *J. Clin. Invest.* 65:1332, 1980.
77. Billing, B. H., and Jansen, F. H.: Enigma of bilirubin conjugation. *Gastroenterology* 61:258, 1971.
78. Kuenzle, C. C.: Bilirubin conjugates of human bile: The excretion of bilirubin as the acyl glycosides of aldobiouronic acid, with a branched-chain hexuronic acid as one of the components of the hexuronosylhexuronide. *Biochem. J.* 119:411, 1970.
79. Fevery, J., et al.: Bilirubin conjugates in bile of man and rats in the normal state and in liver disease. *J. Clin. Invest.* 51:2482, 1972.
80. Crigler, J. F., and Najjar, V. A.: Congenital familial nonhemolytic jaundice with kernicterus. *Pediatrics* 10:169, 1952.
81. Carbone, J. V., and Grodsky, G. M.: Constitutional nonhemolytic hyperbilirubinemia in the rat: Defect of bilirubin conjugation. *Proc. Soc. Exp. Biol. Med.* 94:461, 1957.
82. Arias, I. M.: Chronic unconjugated hyperbilirubinemia without overt signs of hemolysis in adolescents and adults. *J. Clin. Invest.* 41:2233, 1962.
83. Arias, I. M., et al.: Chronic nonhemolytic unconjugated hyperbilirubinemia with glucuronyl transferase deficiency. *Am. J. Med.* 47:395, 1969.
84. Gilbert, A., Lereboullet, P., and Herscher, M.: Les Trois Cholemies congenitales. *Bull. Soc. Med. Hop. Paris* 24:1203, 1907.
85. Foulk, W. T., et al.: Constitutional hepatic dysfunction (Gilbert's disease): Its natural history and related syndromes. *Medicine (Baltimore)* 38:25, 1959.
86. Berk, P. D., Wolkoff, A. W., and Berlin, N. I.: Inborn errors of bilirubin metabolism. *Med. Clin. North. Am.* 59:803, 1975.
87. Yaffe, S. J., et al.: Enhancement of glucuronide-conjugating capacity in a hyperbilirubinemic infant due to apparent enzyme induction by phenobarbital. *N. Engl. J. Med.* 275:1461, 1966.
88. Black, M., and Sherlock, S.: Treatment of Gilbert's syndrome with phenobarbitone. *Lancet* 1:1359, 1970.
89. Robinson, S. H., Nagasawa, S., and Yannoni, C.: Bilirubin excretion in rats with normal and impaired bilirubin conjugation: Effect of phenobarbital. *J. Clin. Invest.* 50:2606, 1971.
90. Dubin, I. N.: Chronic idiopathic jaundice: A review of 50 cases. *Am. J. Med.* 24:268, 1958.
91. Wolkoff, A. W., et al.: Rotor's syndrome: A distinct inheritable pathophysiologic entity. *Am. J. Med.* 60:173, 1976.
92. Elder, G., Gray, C. H., and Nicholson, D. G.: Bile pigment fate in gastrointestinal tract. *Semin. Hematol.* 9:71, 1972.
93. Watson, C. J.: Recent studies of the urobilin problem. *J. Clin. Pathol.* 16:1, 1963.
94. Troxler, R. F., Dawber, N. H., and Lester, R.: Synthesis of urobilinogen by broken cell preparations of intestinal bacterial. *Gastroenterology* 54:568, 1968.
95. Lester, R., Schumer, W., and Schmid, R.: Intestinal absorption of bile pigments. IV. Urobilinogen absorption in man. *N. Engl. J. Med.* 272:939, 1965.
96. Bloomer, J. R., et al.: Comparison of fecal urobilinogen excretion with bilirubin production in normal volunteers and patients with increased bilirubin production. *Clin. Chim. Acta* 29:463, 1970.
97. Bourke, E., Milne, M. D., and Stokes, G. S.: Mechanisms of renal excretion of urobilinogen. *Br. Med. J.* 2:1510, 1965.
98. Levy, M., Lester, R., and Levinsky, N. G.: Renal excretion of urobilinogen in the dog. *J. Clin. Invest.* 47:2117, 1968.
99. Kreimer-Birnbaum, M., et al.: Dipyrrolic urinary pigments in congenital Heinz-body anaemia due to Hb Köln and in thalassemia. *Br. Med. J.* 2:396, 1966.
100. Lange, R. D., and Akeroyd, J. H.: Congenital hemolytic anemia with abnormal pigment metabolism and red cell inclusion bodies: A new clinical syndrome. *Blood* 13:950, 1958.
101. Schmid, R., Brecher, G., and Clemens, T.: Familial hemolytic anemia with erythrocyte inclusion bodies and a defect in pigment metabolism. *Blood* 14:991, 1959.
102. Goldstein, G. W., Hammaker, L., and Schmid, R.: The catabolism of Heinz bodies: An experimental model demonstrating conversion to non-bilirubin catabolites. *Blood* 31:388, 1968.
103. Gilbertsen, A. S., et al.: Studies of the dipyrrylmethene ("fuscin") pigments. I. The anabolic significance of the fecal mesobilifuscin. *J. Clin. Invest.* 38:1166, 1959.
104. Schmid, R., and Hammaker, L.: Metabolism and disposition of C^{14}-bilirubin in congenital nonhemolytic jaundice. *J. Clin. Invest.* 42:1720, 1963.
105. McDonagh, A. F.: Thermal and photochemical reactions of bilirubin IX-α. *Ann. N.Y. Acad. Sci.* 244:553, 1975.
106. Ostrow, J. D., Berry, C. S., and Zarembo, J. E.: Studies on the mechanism of phototherapy in the congenitally jaundiced rat, in *Phototherapy in the Newborn: An Overview*, edited by R. E. Behrman and A. Simopoulos. National Academy of Science, Washington, 1974.

CHAPTER *41*

Erythrokinetics

NATHANIEL I. BERLIN

The development of techniques for the quantitation of erythropoiesis has led to an understanding of the mechanisms leading to anemia and polycythemia. In principle, the circulating red cells can be regarded as an organ whose total volume is regulated by two factors: the rate of production of red cells and the life-span of red cells. To describe this organ quantitatively, three factors must be determined: volume, rate of production, and rate of destruction (red cell life-span). In the determination of these three factors, simpler techniques, such as reticulocyte count, marrow examination, and plasma unconjugated bilirubin concentration, have been supplemented by the more precise quantitation made possible by the use of radioisotopes.

Total red cell volume

RED CELL LABELS
The total circulating red cell volume is best measured by the use of labeled red cells. Isotopic labels utilizing ^{55}Fe [1], ^{59}Fe [2], ^{32}P [3], ^{42}K [4], ThB [5], ^{51}Cr [6], ^{11}CO (carbon monoxide) [7], and ^{99m}Tc [8] have been employed, but ^{51}Cr (as $Na_2^{51}CrO_4$) is the most widely used label [9]. Stable CO [10] can also be used to label red cells and to measure the total red cell volume. However, both CO and ^{11}CO overestimate the total red cell volume compared with other red cell labels [7,11].

Radioactive iron is one of the few labels that requires biosynthetic incorporation into the red cell, but this isotope is not currently used for measurement of total red cell volume. The radiation dose to the donor, requirements for cross-matching, and the hazards of transfusions of donor cells preclude its use in humans, and it has been almost totally supplanted by autologous or allogeneic ^{51}Cr-labeled red cells [9]. The labeling of red cells in vitro is accomplished during a short period (½ h or less) of incubation of the cells with the isotope, with subsequent return of the labeled red cells to the patient. The excess isotope, i.e., that which is not incorporated into red cells, may be removed by washing the cells. If the excess isotope is not removed by washing, a correction has to be applied for the isotope not fixed in red cells. When the white blood cell count is above 25,000 per microliter, it is desirable to remove the white cells and to wash the labeled red cells with saline prior to reinfusion.

The total red cell volume (TRCV) is calculated from the following equation:

$$TRCV = \frac{Q}{cpm/ml\ RBC_{(t)}}$$

where Q is the amount of isotope injected in labeled cells and cpm/ml $RBC_{(t)}$ is the amount of isotope in red blood cells at time t after administration of labeled cells. Sampling time t is generally 15 min, but for patients with splenomegaly, samples at $t = 20$, 30, and 45 min should be obtained to ensure "complete" mixing of the labeled cells [12].

There is no theoretical objection to measuring the total volume of red cells by using labeled red cells. It is independent of the hematocrit of the blood utilized to measure radioactivity. Replicate determinations can be made with a coefficient of variation of approximately 1.5 percent [13]. The principal precaution is the necessity

for complete administration of the labeled cells into the circulatory system.

There are four ways of reporting total red cell volume values: (1) as a volume (milliliters), (2) as volume per unit of body weight (milliliters per kilogram), (3) as volume related to body surface area (milliliters per square meter), and (4) as a function of fat and lean tissue. The most common method is to report the values in terms of milliliters per kilogram, although some workers utilize tables of height and weight to calculate the body surface area. Those who have studied the relationship of total red cell volume to body composition in terms of fat and lean tissue have provided some insight into the relationship between these factors, but measurements of lean tissue and body fat are not widely available [14,15]. In general, these studies indicate that red cell volume correlates better with lean body mass than with total body weight. Table 41-1 lists blood volume in normal adult men and women [14,16–19].

PLASMA LABELS
A number of dyes have been utilized for the measurement of plasma volume. In the 1920s, T-1824 (Evans blue dye) came into widespread use for the measurement of the plasma volume [20]. However, like most other "plasma" labels, it is bound to albumin and serves as a tracer for this plasma protein. The volume measured is the initial volume of distribution of albumin. When radioactive iodine (^{131}I) became available, it was utilized to label albumin and to measure volume, and it has virtually supplanted T-1824 [9]. Subsequently, other radioactive isotopes of iodine (^{125}I and ^{132}I) and technetium 99m have been used to label albumin and other plasma proteins.

After the albumin-dye complex or the isotopically labeled albumin has been injected, time is allowed for mixing, and a clearance curve is determined. Two problems influence the interpretation of these curves. The first problem is the continual loss of either dye or isotope from the plasma. To overcome this problem, some type of analysis of the data is required to determine what the concentration of the test substance would have been if mixing in the plasma volume had been instantaneous and there had been no loss of test substance from the plasma. Most workers have adopted one of two procedures to make this analysis. Some utilize a single point at 10 to 15 min after injecting the tracer, with the assumption that there has been little loss of the test substance from the plasma volume in that time [20]. Alternatively, and more commonly, a number of samples can be taken and the concentration extrapolated to the time of injection. If it is assumed that there was a constant rate of loss, then

$$Plasma\ volume = \frac{Q}{label/ml\ plasma_{(t)}}$$

where Q is the amount of dye or labeled protein administered, and label/ml plasma$_{(t)}$ is determined by ex-

TABLE 41-1 Blood volume in normal adult males and females

Number	Blood volume, ml/kg ± 1 SD	Total red cell volume, ml/kg ± 1 SD	Plasma volume,* ml/kg ± 1 SD	References
		MALES		
71	69.0	29.9	38.7	[16]
42	60.4 ± 8.1	27.8 ± 4.6	32.7 ± 4.3	[14]
10 (elderly)	70.5 ± 18.2†	27.5 ± 8.8		[17]
6 (young)	76.5 ± 11.6†	30.9 + 3.1		
201	62.4 ± 7.8	28.2 ± 4.0	34.2 ± 4.5	[18]
Mean, all cases (330)	67.8	28.9		
		FEMALES		
16	64.4 ± 7.6	27.0 ± 3.4	37.0 ± 4.8	[16]
20	58.3 ± 6.8	23.8 ± 2.8	34.4 ± 4.7	[14]
27 (elderly)	63.1 ± 18.9†	24.3 ± 7.5	24.3 ± 7.5	[17]
6 (young)	63.7 ± 16.0	23.0 ± 5.3		
101	61.9 ± 6.3	25.3 ± 3.0	36.6 ± 4.3	[19]
Mean, all cases (170)	62.3	24.7		

*Calculated from measured total red cell volume and peripheral hematocrit. As discussed in the text, when measured directly, the plasma volume varies with the labeled protein used. In general, the values in this table are of the order of 5 to 10 percent less than would be obtained with a labeled protein.

†Calculated from a measured (labeled cells) total red cell volume and the body hematocrit (not peripheral venous hematocrit) as determined by a formula, and for this reason higher than the other values listed.

trapolation to t_0, the time of injection, or alternatively, t is set at 10 to 15 min.

The second problem involved in the interpretation of these curves is the difficulty in defining the plasma volume itself, both physiologically and anatomically. In contrast to the total volume of red cells, which is easy to define and can be readily measured, the plasma volume is labile. Since it is approximately 90 percent water and there is a large exchange of water across the capillary bed, the plasma volume can change quickly. In reality, the plasma volume is defined in terms of the substance used to measure it and the method used in analyzing the data.

There is also the possibility that when albumin is injected intravenously, a fraction (on the order of 10 to 15 percent) exchanges with a small, rapidly exchanging pool and that this occurs during the mixing period and thus cannot be measured. The best evidence for this is the fact that in both dogs and humans, the plasma volume measured with labeled fibrinogen is smaller than that measured with labeled albumin [21,22]. Since a larger fraction remains in the intravascular space, fibrinogen can be considered a better test substance than albumin for measurement of the plasma volume.

Total-body hematocrit

When the total red cell volume as measured with labeled cells was compared with that calculated from a measured plasma volume (either iodine-labeled albumin or T-1824 Evans blue dye), it was found that the total red cell volume (red cell label) was 10 to 20 percent lower than that calculated from a measured plasma volume and peripheral vessel hematocrit [1,23]. Since the la-

beled red cell method yields a value that is without theoretical objection, there must be some error in the calculation of the total red cell volume from a measured plasma volume. If it is assumed that the plasma volume is correctly determined, the only factor remaining in the equation for the calculation of the total red cell volume is the peripheral venous hematocrit. Earlier, many workers noted that there appeared to be changes in the hematocrit in the smallest of vessels when viewed under the microscope. This led to the concept that the large-vessel hematocrit (LVH) was greater than the mean hematocrit of all the vessels (total-body hematocrit, or TBH), where TBH is defined as

$$\frac{\text{Red cell volume (labeled cells)}}{\text{Red cell volume (labeled cells)} + \text{plasma volume (labeled plasma)}}$$

Generally, as measured with labeled red cells and iodinated albumin, the ratio of total-body hematocrit to large-vessel hematocrit is approximately 0.92 [23]. If this correction is applied, the total red cell volume calculated from a measured plasma volume, using the following equation, is equal to the total red cell volume measured with labeled red cells:

$$\text{TRCV}_{(\text{alb})} = \text{PV}_{(\text{alb})}\left(\frac{1}{1 - \frac{\text{TBH}}{\text{LVH}}\text{LVH}} - 1\right)$$

where $\text{TRCV}_{(\text{alb})}$ = total red cell volume as calculated from a labeled-albumin plasma volume
$\text{PV}_{(\text{alb})}$ = plasma volume determined with labeled albumin
TBH = total-body hematocrit
LVH = large-vessel hematocrit

The ratio TBH/LVH is generally taken as being approximately 0.92.

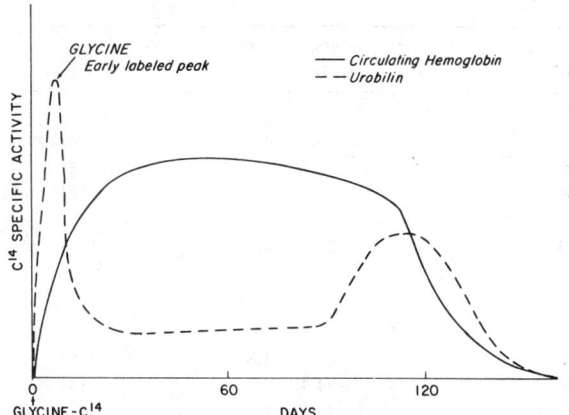

FIGURE 41-1   The ¹⁴C content of the hemoglobin of circulating red blood cells and fecal urobilin after administration of glycine-2-¹⁴C. The circulating hemoglobin-specific activity can be analyzed to yield the mean red cell life-span, either graphically or analytically. Graphically the mean red cell life-span can be considered as the time interval between the 50 percent of maximum value on the rising and descending portions of the curve. This is the common method of analysis.

Since studies with labeled fibrinogen, γ-globulin, and cold agglutinin [21,24,25] indicate that the plasma volume is smaller with these labels than that measured with labeled albumin, the discrepancy between total-body hematocrit and large-vessel hematocrit is smaller than previously suggested. Recommended procedures for the practical determination of blood volume have been developed by the ICSH Panel on Diagnostic Use of Radioisotopes in Hematology [9] and are outlined in Chap. A19.

Red cell production

Normal red cell production is extremely effective, and most red cells produced live, or have the potential to live, a normal life-span. Under certain conditions, however, a fraction of red cell production is ineffective, with destruction of nonviable red cells either within the marrow or shortly after the cells reach the blood [26].

Total erythropoiesis, i.e., the sum of effective and ineffective red cell production, can be estimated from the marrow examination. Films or sections from marrow aspirates are first examined for relative content of fat and hemopoietic tissue. This gives an estimate of overall hemopoietic activity within the marrow space. Then a differential count is performed with determination of a ratio between granulocytic and erythroid precursors (the M/E ratio). In a normal adult, the ratio is about 3:1 to 5:1, and it can be used to estimate whether erythropoiesis is normal, increased, or decreased (see Chap. 3). It is obviously only an approximation of total erythroid activity, since the ratio can be altered by changing the myeloid as well as the erythroid compo-

nents. However, when used in conjunction with determination of red blood cell count and reticulocyte count, it will under most circumstances provide qualitative information about the rate and effectiveness of the production of red blood cells. A more accurate quantitation of total erythropoiesis can be made by measuring the rate of synthesis of hemoglobin (ferrokinetics) or, in steady-state conditions, by measuring the rate of catabolism of hemoglobin (bilirubin production or carbon monoxide excretion).

Effective erythropoiesis is most simply estimated by determining the reticulocyte count. This count is usually expressed as the percentage of red cells which are reticulocytes, but it can also be expressed as the total number of circulating reticulocytes per cubic millimeter of blood. The usefulness of this latter figure can be further enhanced by using correction factors based on estimated life-span of the reticulocytes (see Chap. 72). Because of ease of performance, the reticulocyte count can be determined as frequently as desired and can provide rapid indication of a sudden change in the rate of red cell production. Effective erythropoiesis can also be calculated from measured total red cell volume, rate of red cell production, and/or red cell life-span. This demands steady-state conditions, during which red cell destruction equals red cell production, and is discussed below.

Ineffective erythropoiesis is suspected when the reticulocyte count is normal or only slightly increased despite erythroid hyperplasia of the marrow. It was first recognized as an entity from the study of incorporation of isotopes into fecal urobilin following the administration of labeled glycine, a precursor of heme [27,28]. Two peaks were observed: an early one at 3 to 5 days and a late one at 100 to 120 days (Fig. 41-1). It was suggested that one of the sources of early labeled peak was the hemoglobin of developing red cells that had never completed their development and had been catabolized either in the marrow or shortly after reaching the blood. Subsequent studies have revealed that in certain disorders, such as pernicious anemia, thalassemia, and sideroblastic anemia, ineffective erythropoiesis is a major component of total erythropoiesis. This component can be quantitated by measuring ¹⁵N-labeled glycine incorporation into the early bilirubin peaks [29], bilirubin turnover [30], or ferrokinetics [31,32]. The bilirubin turnover in milligrams per day includes the bilirubin derived from the catabolism of senescent red cells plus the bilirubin derived from ineffective erythropoiesis plus the bilirubin derived from the liver. Since the bilirubin derived from the catabolism of senescent red cells can be calculated from the measured total red cell volume and the red cell life-span, and since bilirubin derived from the liver can be taken as a constant, approximately 0.80 mg/kg per day, it is possible to calculate ineffective erythropoiesis. Under normal conditions, this is about 0.25 mg/kg per day, equivalent to the daily destruction of 1.5 ml red blood cells in a 70-kg person, or in other words, about 9 percent of total erythropoiesis. This value in normal subjects agrees well with the range of 4 to 12 percent found by measuring glycine incorporation into the early-labeled peak [29]. Using ferrokinetic methods, ineffective erythropoiesis is calculated as the difference between total plasma iron turnover and erythrocyte iron turnover plus storage iron turnover (see below). The values from such studies in normal subjects are somewhat higher, ranging from 14 to 34 percent [31]. However, these results probably are misleading, since none of the methods actually measure cell death but only the turnover of heme and iron. It is possible that there is little premature death of cells in normal subjects and that much of the early turnover of bilirubin and iron is derived from the rim of hemoglobin extruded during enucleation of erythroblasts [33]. Nevertheless, these methods provide useful information as to degree of ineffectiveness in patients with an accelerated rate of red cell production.

FERROKINETICS

In 1950, Huff and his associates first described a method for the measurement of the rate of production of red cells, utilizing a model of iron metabolism [34] (Fig. 41-2). In this method, radioactive iron complexed to transferrin in vitro was injected intravenously and the rate of clearance from the plasma (^{59}Fe plasma $T_{1/2}$) and the uptake in the red cells were measured. From these two measurements, and from measurements of the plasma iron concentration and the plasma volume, a calculation was made of the rate of formation of red cells, the red cell iron turnover, as follows:

$$RBC\ IT = (PIT)U$$

where RBC IT = red cell turnover in milligrams per day
U = fraction of radioactive iron corporated into circulating red cells at days 7 to 10
PIT = plasma iron turnover in milligrams per day

$$PIT = \frac{1000}{T_{1/2}} \times plasma\ volume\ (ml) \times plasma\ iron\ (mg/ml)$$

where $T_{1/2}$ is time, in minutes, for plasma radioactive iron content to decrease by one-half after intravenous administration. The RBC IT by this method was 20 to 40 percent greater than that calculated from a measured red cell life-span and total red cell volume. Table 41-2 provides examples for the qualitative interpretation of plasma radioactive iron clearance and red cell radioactive iron uptake data.

With more sensitive counting equipment and longer sampling periods (up to 14 days), it was shown that following an intravenous dose of ^{59}Fe, the plasma ^{59}Fe clearance was not a single exponential, but could be represented by three exponentials [35,36]. This led to the introduction of more complex models of iron kinetics [37–40]. These models provide for the plasma iron to exchange with other compartments, generally desig-

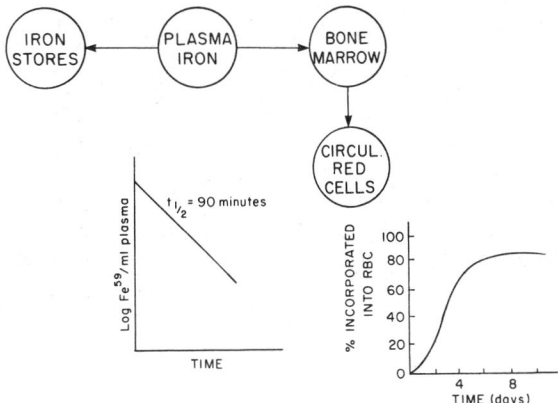

FIGURE 41-2 The single dynamic pool model of iron metabolism. Radioactive iron injected into the plasma iron pool is cleared from the plasma with a single exponential and approximately 80 percent is incorporated into circulating red blood cells.

nated as stores and marrow, respectively (Fig. 41-3). It should be pointed out that at days 3 to 5 after injection of iron there can be a transient increase in the plasma ^{59}Fe activity. This is thought to be due to ineffective erythropoiesis.

From the three-exponential plasma radioactive iron clearance equation, U (the circulating red cell radioac-

FIGURE 41-3 A complex model of iron metabolism. The marrow is depicted as a series of five compartments, with reflux to the plasma from the middle marrow compartment and reflux from the stores. In the normal state, there is a system delay in the return of radioactive iron from circulating red blood cells via the monocyte-macrophage system that amounts to about 90 days and reaches its peak at 120 days. The plasma iron clearance is described mathematically as

$$P_t = Ae^{-k_1t} + Be^{-k_2t} + Ce^{-k_3t}$$

where $P_t = \dfrac{\text{Cpm } ^{59}\text{Fe/ml plasma}}{\text{Cpm } ^{59}\text{Fe injected}} \times$ plasma volume

In effect, this is the fraction ^{59}Fe in the plasma at any given time, and it is normalized so that the sum of the intercepts ($A + B + C$) of the exponential components will be 1.

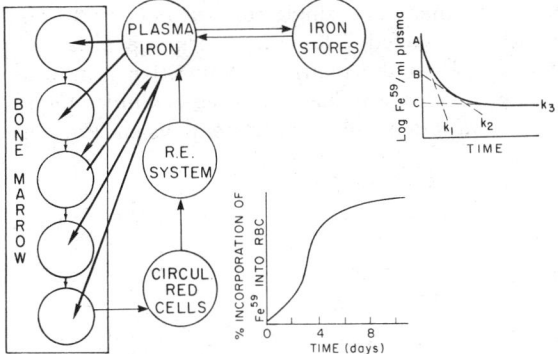

TABLE 41-2   Plasma radioactive iron clearance and red blood cell uptake

Condition	Plasma ^{59}Fe $T_{1/2}$	RBC uptake, %
Normal	90 min	80–90
Increased erythropoiesis	Rapid (10 to 40 min)	80–90
Hemolytic anemia	Rapid	20–90*
Ineffective erythropoiesis	Normal to rapid	10–30
Iron deficiency anemia	Normal to rapid	100
Decreased erythropoiesis	Slow (180 min or greater)	0–20

* This variability is due to variability in intensity of hemolysis and size of iron stores.

tive iron uptake at 10 to 14 days), plasma volume, and plasma iron concentration, the red cell iron turnover can be calculated as was done originally, but in this case the plasma iron turnover (PIT) is given by

$$\frac{1000}{\frac{A}{k_1}+\frac{B}{k_2}+\frac{C}{k_3}} \times \text{plasma volume (ml)} \times \text{plasma iron (mg/ml)}$$

where PIT is the plasma iron turnover in milligrams per day, and $A + B + C = 1$ represents the intercepts associated with the rate constants k_1, k_2, and k_3, respectively. When there is intense random destruction of red cells, U may be falsely low and in these situations should be considered to be 1.0 or to approach 1.0. When the three-exponential plasma iron clearance data are used, the value obtained for RBC IT in the normal subject is in good agreement with that predicted from a measured total red cell volume and the red cell life-span.

Complete analysis of plasma iron clearance curves has generated methods for calculating the degree and effectiveness of erythroid activity [32,41–43]. Although possibly more accurate than conventional methods, they appear to be too cumbersome for clinical use.

One of the difficulties in calculating the rate of erythropoiesis from plasma radioactive iron clearance and red cell radioactive iron incorporation data stems from the nonerythron iron turnover, i.e., turnover of storage iron, principally in the liver and spleen. If large doses of unlabeled iron are given after the radioactive iron, the effect of storage iron turnover can be reduced to some degree [44,45]. The calculated red cell iron turnover is lower than in the single-compartment model and approaches expected values. In effect, the unlabeled iron has blocked the return of radioactive iron from stores and in this way has converted a multicompartment system to a single-compartment system (see Fig. 41-2).

Red cell destruction

RED CELL LIFE-SPAN
The original method for the measurement of the red cell life-span consisted of the transfusion from one subject to another of cells that were compatible but identifiable immunologically—the Ashby technique [46]. During World War II and shortly after, this method was intensively studied, primarily from the standpoint of methodology and less from the standpoint of disease. In recent years the technique has been standardized [47] and has even become automated [48].

In 1946, Shemin and Rittenberg demonstrated that ^{15}N-labeled glycine could be utilized to measure the lifespan of the red cell [49]. Since then, a number of other isotopic methods have been developed [50]. These can be divided into three groups: (1) those which label a cohort of cells, (2) those which label cells randomly (that is, all the circulating cells are uniformly labeled), and (3) those which are indirect (that is, the red cell life-span is calculated from some other measurement, such as the rate of production of red cells or the rate of production of bilirubin or carbon monoxide). The first two classes yield information about the nature of the shortening of red cell life-span (age-dependent or random); the last group yields only mean values. In view of the widespread prevalence of hepatitis viruses, considerable caution should be used in studies of the red cell lifespan involving the transfusion of donor cells to recipients for other than therapeutic purposes. Less recognized is the potential hazard of sensitizing the recipient to foreign antigens in the transfused cells [51].

COHORT METHODS
The cohort methods depend on the biosynthetic incorporation, usually in vivo, of the label into the developing red cell. In these methods, a group of cells of approximately the same age is labeled. They generally represent a small fraction of the circulating red cells, on the order of 5 percent or less. The labels used are glycine containing labeled nitrogen (^{15}N) [49] or radioactive carbon (^{14}C) [52] and radioactive iron, either ^{55}Fe or ^{59}Fe [53]. Radioactive manganese (^{41}Mn) [54] and selenomethionine (^{75}Se) [55] have both been used as cohort labels, but not extensively. Neutron activation analysis has also been used to make measurements of ^{58}Fe [56], a stable isotope of iron which could be used as a cohort label. In the experimental animal [57], as well as in humans, administration of therapeutic doses of unlabeled iron has been found to decrease the percentage reutilization of the radioactive iron by red cells, so that a dis-

tinct decrease in red cell radioactive iron occurs at the end of the red cell life-span.

RANDOM-LABEL METHODS

The random-label methods are the Ashby differential agglutination technique, which uses an immunologic marker [46], and isotopic techniques employing chromium (^{50}Cr or ^{51}Cr) [58,59] or DFP labeled with ^{32}P [60], ^{3}H [61], or ^{14}C [62]. The precise localization of the DFP in the red cell is not known. The chromium method suffers from continuous elution of the isotope, i.e., loss of isotope from intact surviving red cells at a rate varying from 0.5 to 2.9 percent per day [63,64]. This poses problems in interpretation of the data. DFP is irreversibly bound in the red cell, but there is a limit to the binding capacity, and the excess is eluted within a period of from 3 to 5 days [65]. The ^{14}C cyanhemoglobin method has not been used extensively, but it appears to be excellent.

There are a number of difficulties in interpretation of the data from either class of method [50]. These difficulties stem principally from a requirement that the total red cell volume be constant or, if it is not constant, that the rate of change be known. The latter can be approximated by changes in the hematocrit, but precision requires repeated measurement of the total red cell volume. This is possible, but most workers have not been willing to make the additional measurements required.

Red cell survival has also been measured by the use of stable chromium (^{50}Cr) and activation analysis [58]. This offers the opportunity of studying the red cell life-span in those instances which would preclude the use of radioactive isotopes, e.g., in normal children, in pregnant women, and in women of childbearing age.

In the normal person, the red cell life-span is about 120 days [50]. However, there normally is some random destruction of red cells in humans. When shortened, the red cells either have approximately the same life-span or are randomly destroyed, i.e., without regard to their age. When the red cells have about the same life-span, the equation for survival of randomly labeled cells is

$$N_t = N_0 \left(1 - \frac{t}{T} \right) \tag{1}$$

where N_t = number of cells surviving to time t
  N_0 = number of cells administered
  T = red cell life-span

When the cells are randomly destroyed, and when the rate of destruction k is such that, for practical purposes, few if any cells survive to the potential life-span (120 days), then

$$N_t = N_0 e^{-kt} \tag{2}$$

and the mean red cell life-span is $T = 1/k$. In these equations, k equals the first-order rate constant describing random destruction of red cells. When the rate of random destruction is low in normal cells and when some cells survive to T,

$$N = N_0 \left(1 - \frac{t}{T} \right) e^{-kt} \tag{3}$$

Generally, DFP red cell survival data are fitted to either Eq. 1 or Eq. 2. Equation 3 has not been widely used, largely because it is necessary to have more data than are usually available in order to obtain a good estimate of T and k.

When ^{51}Cr is used as a label, each equation must be modified by a factor to provide for the elution of ^{51}Cr from intact surviving red cells. The equation corresponding to Eq. 1 is

$$N_t = N_0 \left(1 - \frac{t}{T} \right) e^{-k_e t} \tag{4}$$

where k_e is the first-order rate constant of ^{51}Cr elution from red cells. In the normal subject, k_e has a mean value of 0.0131, corresponding to a mean elution rate of 1.3 percent per day, with a range of 0.88 to 1.65 percent per day. Elution rates range from 0.5 to 2.9 percent per day in various disease states [63,64].

When ^{51}Cr is used, Eq. 2 is rewritten as

$$N_t = N_0 e^{-(k_e + k)t} \tag{5}$$

Similarly, Eq. 3 is written as

$$N_t = N_0 \left(1 - \frac{t}{T} \right) e^{-(k_e + k)t} \tag{6}$$

Most laboratories report ^{51}Cr survival times in terms of a red cell ^{51}Cr half-life. This is the time required for red cell ^{51}Cr content to decrease by one-half, starting usually 24 h after injection. The normal value of $T_{1/2}$ for ^{51}Cr varies from 27 to 35 days. It has not been customary to determine which of these three equations applies in any given situation in which a ^{51}Cr red cell survival time is computed. This would require sampling for much longer periods of time than is generally done, probably for 100 days.

It should be noted that N_t, as utilized here, is the total number of circulating labeled cells at time t. In practice, the amount of label per milliliter of red cells or per milliliter of blood at time t is determined. When the total red cell volume remains constant, label per milliliter of blood may be utilized. In either event, one or the other must be assumed to be constant, or repeated measurements of blood volume or total red cell volume must be made. In practice, it is advisable to utilize both label per milliliter of red cells and label per milliliter of blood, since a comparison provides a check on the assumptions of a constant total red cell volume or blood volume.

The amount of random destruction that occurs in the normal state is low in humans (0.06 to 0.4 percent per day [66]) and even lower in dogs [67]. It is 0.48 percent per day in rats [68] and 1.5 percent per day in pigs [69]. Red cell life-span data in a variety of species have been summarized elsewhere [50]. For humans, the generally accepted value is 120 days; in dogs, 100 to 110 days; in rats, 50 to 60 days; and in pigs, 86 days.

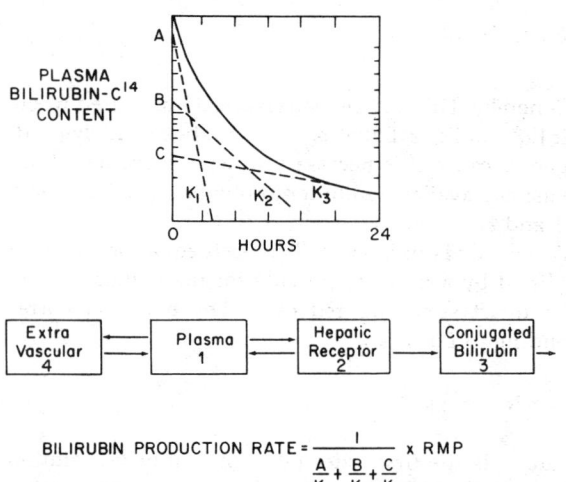

$$\text{BILIRUBIN PRODUCTION RATE} = \frac{1}{\dfrac{A}{K_1} + \dfrac{B}{K_2} + \dfrac{C}{K_3}} \times RMP$$

FIGURE 41-4   Four-compartment model of bilirubin metabolism and diagrammatic representation of a radioactive bilirubin plasma clearance curve. RMP = rapidly miscible bilirubin pool; it is calculated from RMP = Q/(Br/ml plasma t_0), where Q is the amount of labeled bilirubin administered (dpm); and Br/ml plasma t_0 is the amount of labeled bilirubin per ml plasma extrapolated at t_0, $A + B + C = 1$, and k_1, k_2, and k_3 are the rate constants for each of the exponentials depicted.

INDIRECT METHODS

There are two approaches to the calculation of the red cell life-span by indirect methods: from a measurement of the rate of production of red cells utilizing radioactive iron [70] or from a measurement of the rate of breakdown of hemoglobin to bilirubin and carbon monoxide [71,72]. In each instance it is necessary that at the time of study either the patient be in a steady state, i.e., the rate of production is the same as the rate of destruction and hence the total red cell volume is constant, or the rate of change from the steady state will require some assumptions. Nevertheless, in the normal individual, the calculated values are in good agreement either with measured values or with known values for humans, and in many instances the calculated values in disease are in good agreement with measured values.

BILIRUBIN METABOLISM

The two catabolic excretory products of the porphyrin moiety of hemoglobin are bilirubin and carbon monoxide [73,74]. In the gastrointestinal tract, bilirubin is converted to a series of products which can be measured and which are referred to as *fecal urobilins* [75]. The measurement of fecal urobilin has long been used as an indicator of the rate of catabolism of hemoglobin. However, it has been shown that conversion of bilirubin to excreted urobilinogen is not quantitative, and the conclusion has been drawn that measured fecal urobilinogen provides a lower limit to the amount of hemoglobin catabolized. Thus when the fecal urobilinogen is elevated, either increased catabolism of hemoglobin

derived from circulating red cells or ineffective erythropoiesis is present. A normal value, because of the variation in conversion of bilirubin to the urobilins, does not preclude hemolysis.

It is possible to estimate the rate of production of bilirubin by using isotopically labeled bilirubin [73]. This is done by measuring the rate of clearance from the plasma of a tracer dose of labeled bilirubin and the unconjugated serum bilirubin concentration. Figure 41-4 shows that the clearance of labeled bilirubin from the plasma can be described as the sum of three exponentials and lists the equation used to calculate the bilirubin production rate.

In the normal state, approximately 85 percent of the bilirubin produced per day results from the catabolism of the hemoglobin contained in senescent red cells. This value varies only slightly, except in patients with thalassemia, pernicious anemia, congenital erythropoietic porphyria, lead poisoning, and other forms of ineffective erythropoiesis; in such patients, the value may be much less than 85 percent. A measured bilirubin production can thus be used to calculate the mean red cell life-span in both the normal state and most disease states [71]. This method has the advantage of requiring samples for only 24 to 48 h, in contrast to 150 to 180 days for cohort methods and 20 to 40 days for random-label methods.

What has not been widely appreciated is that the plasma unconjugated bilirubin concentration and changes in the plasma unconjugated bilirubin concentration have substantial meaning for the hematologist [73]. The plasma unconjugated bilirubin concentration (BR) is determined by total red cell volume, red cell life-span, hepatic clearance of bilirubin, and to a small degree, the plasma volume and is calculated according to the following equation:

$$BR = k \frac{TRCV}{RBCLS \times CBR}$$

where k = a constant
   TRCV = total red blood cell volume
   RBCLS = red blood cell life-span
   CBR = hepatic clearance of bilirubin

This equation indicates that the plasma unconjugated bilirubin level relates linearly and directly with total red cell volume and inversely with red cell life-span and hepatic bilirubin clearance. It has also been shown that changes in unconjugated bilirubin may be the most rapid indication of a therapeutic effect in hemolytic anemia [73].

CARBON MONOXIDE EXCRETION

An early step in the catabolism of the iron-protoporphyrin of hemoglobin and heme enzymes is the opening of the protoporphyrin ring at the α-bridge carbon, which is then excreted as carbon monoxide (see Fig. 40-2). This is generally considered to be the sole source of endogenous carbon monoxide, but there is evidence of additional quantitatively minor sources [76]. At present, the methods for measurement of carbon monoxide production are somewhat cumbersome, since they require placing the patient's head in a gas-tight chamber and maintaining a constant partial pressure of oxygen within the chamber. The rate of production of carbon monoxide can be measured from the carbon monoxide concentration in the patient's blood as car-boxyhemoglobin or in the chamber air. The red cell life-span can be calculated from these data, in the same way as with labeled bilirubin, by assuming that 15 percent of the carbon monoxide does not originate from senescent red cells [72,74,77].

Alternatively, the red blood cell life-span (RBC LS) can be calculated as follows:

$$\text{RBC LS} = \frac{\text{T-heme}}{V_{\text{CO}}}$$

where T-heme is the total-body (marrow plus circulating) hemoglobin, and V_{CO} is the rate of CO production. T-heme is the volume distribution of carbon monoxide, determined by adding carbon monoxide to the gas phase of the rebreathing system, and V_{CO} is either the rate of rise of CO concentration in the rebreathing system or the rate of rise of carboxyhemoglobin.

T-heme overestimates total circulating hemoglobin by 5 to 15 percent, and V_{CO} includes the CO derived from ineffective erythropoiesis and hepatic bilirubin synthesis. These are compensating errors, and the red cell life-span obtained, with some exceptions, is a good approximation (98 days in normal subjects) [78], although significant differences between values obtained with DFP and CO have been reported [79]. The problems that remain include (1) difficulty in using this method in smokers and the possible effects of atmospheric pollution, (2) a significant difference in normal women during the menstrual cycle [80], and (3) increase in CO production as a result of caloric reduction [81].

In humans and in experimental animals, the excretion of radioactive carbon monoxide after the administration of ^{14}C-labeled glycine can be used to measure the red cell life-span. This is not a simple procedure [82,83], and theoretically, it would appear to be particularly difficult in cases in which there is intense random hemolysis because of continued availability of labeled glycine.

Localization of erythrokinetic activity

Two techniques have been developed for studying the localization of erythropoiesis using radioactive iron. The first, the *kinetic method*, consists of placing scintillation detectors over liver, spleen, and marrow and measuring the radioactivity in these organs at varous times after the intravenous administration of radioactive iron [84,85] (Fig. 41-5). The second method is *scintigraphic imaging* to record the anatomic localization of the radio-

active iron [86]. Since good imaging requires the use of the very short-lived isotope ^{52}Fe, it has almost been replaced by the use of ^{99m}Tc sulfur colloid. Although this isotope labels the monocyte-macrophage system, its distribution is similar to that of ^{52}Fe, and it can be used to estimate the distribution of erythroid tissue [87] (see Chap. 4).

The kinetic data can be analyzed either by making a correction for the amount of isotope contained in the blood (precordial reading) [85] (Fig. 41-5a) or by comparing the total organ isotope content to that at the time of injection [88] (Fig. 41-5b). Using either of these calculations, it is possible to determine whether the spleen is the site of red cell formation or destruction [84]. Production of red cells in the spleen is demonstrated by an increased uptake of radioactive iron in the spleen fol-

FIGURE 41-5 (*a*) The radioactive iron content of marrow (sacrum), liver, and spleen corrected for amount of isotope in blood after intravenous injection of radioactive iron-labeled transferrin. (*b*) The radioactive iron content of marrow (sacrum), liver, and spleen at time *t* after intravenous administration of radioactive iron-labeled transferrin, plotted as t/t_0. The data for the first 24 h are expanded graphically to show the detail of organ uptake.

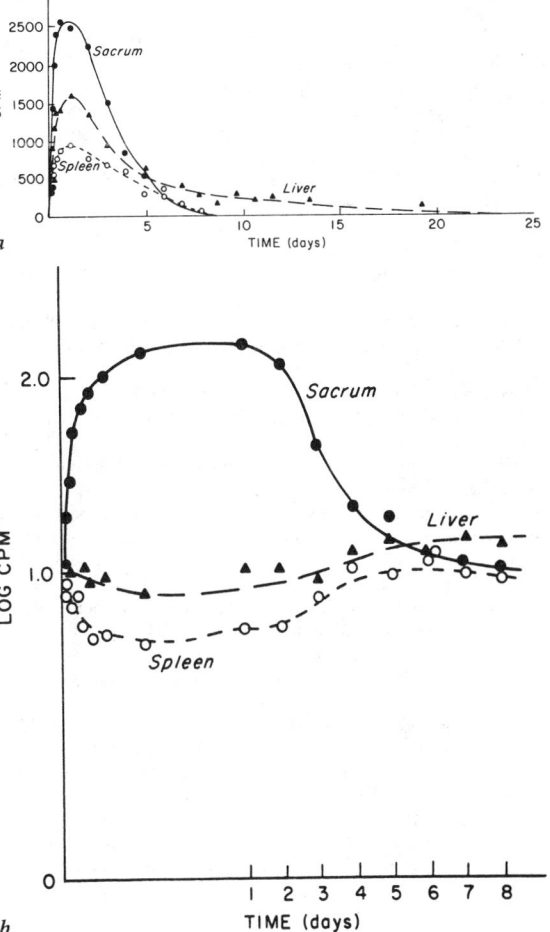

lowed by rapid discharge and release of the red cell–bound iron into peripheral blood. The entire curve for the spleen resembles that depicted for the marrow in the normal state (Fig. 41-5a). A late rise in spleen radioactive iron content or a persistent uptake at an increased level indicates splenic sequestration of circulating red blood cells (see Chap. A19, Fig. A19-3).

Red blood cell sequestration or destruction in the spleen is best elucidated by splenic scanning after administration of red cells labeled with ^{51}Cr [88]. A rise in splenic activity indicates splenic sequestration. Some investigators rely on absolute changes in radioactivity; others take the ratio of spleen to precordium or spleen to liver radioactivity to indicate splenic sequestration, i.e., splenic hemolysis [85,88,89] (see Chap. A19, Fig. A19-4). If the red cells are damaged, e.g., by heat [90], they will be taken up rapidly by the spleen, and if a scanner is used, the size of the spleen can be determined. However, this is done now much more effectively and accurately by the use of ^{99m}Tc (see Chap. 4).

References

1. Gibson, J. G., II, Peacock, W. C., Seligman, A. M., and Sack, T.: Circulating red cell volume measured simultaneously by the radioactive iron and dye methods. *J. Clin. Invest.* 25:838, 1946.
2. Peacock, W. C., et al.: The use of two radioactive isotopes of iron in tracer studies of erythrocytes. *J. Clin. Invest.* 25:605, 1946.
3. Hevesy, G., and Zerahn, K.: Determination of the red corpuscle content. *Acta Physiol. Scand.* 4:376, 1942.
4. Hevesy, G., and Nylin, G.: Application of ^{42}K labelled red corpuscles in blood volume measurements. *Acta Physiol. Scand.* 24:285, 1951.
5. Hevesy, G., and Nylin, G.: Application of "Thorium B" labelled red corpuscles in blood volume studies. *Circ. Res.* 1:102, 1953.
6. Sterling, K., and Gray, S. J.: Determination of the circulating red cell volume in man by radioactive chromium. *J. Clin. Invest.* 29:1614, 1950.
7. Glass, H. I., Brant, A., Clark, J. C., de Garetta, A. C., and Day, L. G.: Measurement of blood volume using red cells labeled with radioactive carbon monoxide. *J. Nucl. Med.* 9:571, 1968.
8. Jones, J., and Mollison, P. L.: A simple and efficient method of labelling red cells with ^{99m}Tc for determination of red cell volume. *Br. J. Haematol.* 38:141, 1978.
9. ICSH panel on diagnostic applications of radioisotopes in hematology: Standard techniques for the red cell and plasma volume. *Br. J. Haematol.* 25:797, 1973.
10. Sjöstrand, T.: A method for the determination of the total haemoglobin content of the body. *Acta Physiol. Scand.* 16:211, 1949.
11. Nomof, N., Hopper, J., Jr., Brown, E., Scott, K., and Wennesland, R.: Simultaneous determinations of the total volume of red blood cells by use of carbon monoxide and chromium^{51} in healthy and diseased human subjects. *J. Clin. Invest.* 33:1382, 1954.
12. Tizianello, A., and Pannacciulli, I.: The effect of splenomegaly on dilution curves of tagged erythrocytes and red blood cell volume. *Acta Haematol. [Basel]* 21:346, 1959.
13. Chaplin, H., Jr.: Precision of red cell volume measurement using P^{32} labeled cells. *J. Physiol.* 123:22, 1954.
14. Huff, R. L., and Feller, D. D.: Relation of circulating red cell volume to body density and obesity. *J. Clin. Invest.* 35:1, 1956.
15. Nathan, D. G.: Comments on the interpretation of measurements of total red cell volume in the diagnosis of polycythemia vera. *Semin. Hematol.* 3:216, 1966.
16. Berlin, N. I., Hyde, G. M., Parsons, R. J., and Lawrence, J. H.: Medical progress: The blood volume in various medical and surgical conditions. *N. Engl. J. Med.* 247:675, 1952.
17. Hurdle, A. D. F., and Rosin, A. J.: Red cell volume and red cell survival in normal aged people. *J. Clin. Pathol.* 15:343, 1962.
18. Wennesland, R., et al.: Red cell plasma and blood volume in healthy men measured by radiochromium (Cr^{51}) cell tagging and hematocrit: Influence of age, somatotype and habits of physical activity on the variance after regression of volume to height and weight combined. *J. Clin. Invest.* 38:1065, 1959.
19. Brown, E., Hopper, J., Jr., Hodges, J. L., Jr., Bradley, B., Wennesland, R., and Yamauchi, H.: Red cell, plasma, and blood volume in healthy women measured by radiochromium cell-labeling and hematocrit. *J. Clin. Invest.* 41:2182, 1962.
20. Gibson, J. G., II, and Evans, W. A., Jr.: Clinical studies on the blood volume. I. Application of a method employing the azo dye "Evans blue" and the spectrophotometer. *J. Clin. Invest.* 16:301, 1937.
21. Baker, C. H., and Wycoff, H. D.: Time-concentration curves and dilution spaces of T-1824 and I^{131}-labeled proteins in dogs. *Am. J. Physiol.* 201:1159, 1961.
22. Larsen, O. A.: Studies of the body hematocrit phenomenon: Dynamic hematocrit of large vessel and initial distribution space of albumin and fibrinogen in the whole body. *Scand. J. Clin. Lab. Invest.* 22:189, 1968.
23. Crispell, K. R., Porter, B., and Nieset, R. T.: Studies of plasma volume using human serum albumin tagged with radioactive iodine^{131}. *J. Clin. Invest.* 29:513, 1950.
24. Chaplin, H., Jr., Mollison, P. L., and Vetter, H.: The body venous hematocrit ratio: Its constancy over a wide hematocrit range. *J. Clin. Invest.* 32:1309, 1953.
25. Valeri, C. R., Cooper, A. G., and Pivacek, L. E.: Limitations of measuring blood volume with iodinated ^{125}J serum albumin. *Arch. Intern. Med.* 132:534, 1973.
26. Giblett, E. R., Coleman, D. H., Pirzio-Biroli, G., Donahue, D. M., Motulsky, A. G., and Finch, C. A.: Erythrokinetics: Quantitative measurements of red cell production and destruction in normal subjects and patients with anemia. *Blood* 11:291, 1956.
27. London, I. M., West, R., Shemin, D., and Rittenberg, D.: On the origin of bile pigment in normal man. *J. Biol. Chem.* 184:351, 1950.
28. Gray, C. H., Neuberger, A., and Sneath, P. H. A.: Incorporation of N^{15} in stercobilin in the normal and the porphyric. *Biochem. J.* 47:87, 1950.
29. Samson, D., Halliday, D., Nicholson, D. C., and Chanarin, I.: Quantitation of ineffective erythropoiesis from incorporation of [^{15}N] deltaaminolaevulinic acid in [^{15}N]glycine into early labelled bilirubin. *Br. J. Haematol.* 34:33, 1976.
30. Berk, P. D., Blaschke, T. F., Scharschmidt, B. F., Waggoner, J. G., and Berlin, N. I.: A new approach to the quantitation of the various sources of bilirubin in man. *J. Lab. Clin. Med.* 87:767, 1976.
31. Finch, C. A., et al.: Ferrokinetics in man. *Medicine* 49:17, 1970.
32. Ricketts, C., Jacobs, A., and Cavill, I.: Ferrokinetics and erythropoiesis in man. The measurement of effective erythropoiesis, ineffective erythropoiesis and red cell lifespan using ^{59}Fe. *Br. J. Haematol.* 31:65, 1975.
33. Bessis, M., Breton-Gorius, J., and Thiery, J.-P.: Rôle possible de l'hémoglobine accompagnant le noyan des érythroblastes dans l'origine de la stercobiline éliminée précocement. *Compte Rendy Hebdomedaise des Seances de l'Académie des Sciences* 252:2300, 1961.
34. Huff, R. L., Hennessey, T. G., Austin, R. E., Garcia, J. F., Roberts, B. M., and Lawrence, J. H.: Plasma and red cell iron turnover in normal subjects and in patients having various hematopoietic disorders. *J. Clin. Invest.* 29:1041, 1950.
35. Wasserman, L. R., et al.: Studies in iron kinetics. I. Interpretation of ferrokinetic data in man. *Mt. Sinai J. Med. N.Y.* 32:262, 1965.
36. Hosain, F., Marsaglia, G., and Finch, C. A.: Blood ferrokinetics in normal man. *J. Clin. Invest.* 46:1, 1967.
37. Huff, R. L., and Judd, O. J.: Kinetics of iron metabolism. *Adv. Biol. Med. Phys.* 4:223, 1956.
38. Pollycove, M., and Mortimer, R.: The quantitative determination of iron kinetics and hemoglobin synthesis in human subjects. *J. Clin. Invest.* 40:753, 1961.
39. Nooney, G. C.: Iron kinetics and erythron development. *Biophys. J.* 5:755, 1965.
40. Cook, J. D., Marsaglia, G., Eschbach, J. W., Funk, D. D., and Finch,

C. A.: Ferrokinetics: A biologic model for plasma iron exchange in man. *J. Clin. Invest.* 49:197, 1970.

41. Cavill, I., and Ricketts, C.: Erythropoiesis and iron kinetics. *Br. J. Haematol.* 38:433, 1978.

42. Ricketts, C., Cavill, I., Napier, J. A. F., and Jacobs, A.: Ferrokinetics and erythropoiesis in man: An evolution of ferrokinetic measurements. *Br. J. Haematol.* 35:41, 1977.

43. Cazzola, M., et al.: The use of ^{59}Fe for estimating red cell production and destruction: A comparative evaluation of two methods for the analysis of experimental data. *Haematologica* 64:696, 1979.

44. Lockner, D., and Skårberg, K. O.: Quantitation of erythropoiesis by a new method. III. The blocking effect of inactive iron on radioiron reutilization. *Acta. Med. Scand.* 195:319, 1974.

45. Lockner, D.: Quantitation of erythropoiesis by a new method. IV. Sudies using ^{59}Fe and DF^{32}P simultaneously in haematological disease. *Scand. J. Haematol.* 13:146, 1974.

46. Ashby, W.: Determination of length of life of transfusion blood corpuscles in man. *J. Exp. Med.* 29:267, 1919.

47. JCSH panel on standardization in haematology: Recommended method for radioisotope red-cell survival studies. *Br. J. Haematol.* 45:659, 1980.

48. Szymanski, I. O., Valeri, C. R., McCallum, L. E., Emerson, C. P., and Rosenfield, R. E.: Automated differential agglutination technic to measure red cell survival. I. Methodology. *Transfusion* 8:65, 1968.

49. Shemin, D., and Rittenberg, D.: Life span of human red blood cell. *J. Biol. Chem.* 166:627, 1946.

50. Berlin, N. I., and Berk, P. D.: The biological life of the red cell, in *The Red Blood Cell*, edited by D. Surgenor. Academic, New York, 1975, chap. 24.

51. Adner, P. L., Foconi, S., and Sjölin, S.: Immunization after intravenous injection of small amounts of ^{51}Cr-labelled red cells. *Br. J. Haematol.* 9:288, 1963.

52. Berlin, N. I., Meyer, L. M., and Lazarus, M.: Life span of the rat red blood cell as determined by glycine 2-C^{14}. *Am. J. Physiol.* 165:565, 1951.

53. Burwell, E. L., Brickley, B. A., and Finch, C. A.: Erythrocyte life span in small animals: Comparison of two methods employing radioiron. *Am. J. Physiol.* 172:718, 1953.

54. Borg, D. C., and Cotzias, G. C.: Incorporation of manganese into erythrocytes as evidence for a manganese porphyrin in man. *Nature* 182:1677, 1958.

55. Penner, J. A.: Investigation of erythrocyte turnover with selenium^{75} labeled methionine. *J. Lab. Clin. Med.* 67:427, 1966.

56. Lowman, J. T., and Krivit, W.: New in vivo tracer method with the use of nonradioactive isotopes and activation analysis. *J. Lab. Clin. Med.* 61:1042, 1963.

57. Finch, C. A., Wolff, J. A., Rath, C. E., and Fluharty, R. G.: Iron metabolism: Erythrocyte iron turnover. *J. Lab. Clin. Med.* 34:1480, 1949.

58. Donaldson, G. W. K., Johnson, P. F., Tothill, P., and Richmond, J.: Red cell survival time in man measured by ^{50}Cr and activation analysis. *Br. Med. J.* 2:585, 1968.

59. Ebaugh, F. G., Jr., Emerson, C. P., and Ross, J. F.: The use of radioactive chromium^{51} as an erythrocyte tagging agent for the determination of red cell survival in vivo. *J. Clin. Invest.* 32:1260, 1953.

60. Cohen, J. A., and Warringa, M. G. P. J.: The fate of P^{32} labeled diisopropyl-fluorophosphonate in human body and its use as a labeling agent in study of turnover of blood plasma and red cells. *J. Clin. Invest.* 33:459, 1954.

61. Cline. M. J., and Berlin. N. I.: Measurement of red cell survival with tritiated diisopropyl fluorophosphate. *J. Lab. Clin. Med.* 60:826, 1962.

62. Milner, P. F., and Charache, S.: Life span of carbamylated red cells in sickle cell anemia. *J. Clin. Invest.* 52:3161, 1973.

63. Cline, M. J., and Berlin, N. I.: The red cell chromium elution rate in patients with some hematologic diseases. *Blood* 21:63, 1963.

64. Bentley, S. A., Glass, H. I., Lewis, S. M., and Szur, L.: Elution correction in ^{51}Cr red cell survival studies. *Br. J. Haematol.* 26:179, 1974.

65. Cline, M. J., and Berlin, N. I.: Simultaneous measurement of the survival of two populations of erythrocytes with the use of labelled diisopropyl fluorophosphate. *J. Lab. Clin. Med.* 61:249, 1963.

66. Eadie, G. S., and Brown, I. W., Jr.: Potential life span and ultimate

67. survival of fresh red blood cells in normal healthy recipients as studied by simultaneous Cr^{51} tagging and differential hemolysis. *J. Clin. Invest.* 34:629, 1955.

67. Weissman, S. M., Waldmann, T. A., and Berlin, N. I.: Quantitative measurement of erythropoiesis in the dog. *Am. J. Physiol.* 198:183, 1960.

68. Belcher, E. H., and Harriss, E. B.: Studies of red cell life span in the rat. *J. Physiol.* 146:217, 1959.

69. Bush, J. A., Berlin, N. I., Jensen, W. N., Brill, A. B., Cartwright, G. E., and Wintrobe, M. M.: Erythrocyte life span in growing swine as determined by glycine-2-C^{14}. *J. Exp. Med.* 101:451, 1955.

70. Ricketts, C., Cavill, I., Napier, J. A. F.: The measurement of red cell lifespan using ^{59}Fe. *Br. J. Haematol.* 37:403, 1977.

71. Berk, P. D., Bloomer, J. R., Howe, R. B., Blaschke, T. F., and Berlin, N. I.: Bilirubin production as a measure of red cell life span. *J. Lab. Clin. Med.* 79:364, 1972.

72. Lundh, B., Cavallin-Stahl, E., and Mercke, C.: Haem catabolism, carbon monoxide production and red cell survival in anaemia. *Acta Med. Scand.* 197:161, 1975.

73. Berlin, N. I., and Berk, P. D.: Quantitative aspects of bilirubin metabolism for hematologists. *Blood* 57:983, 1981.

74. Coburn, R. F., Blakemore, W. S., and Forster, R. E.: Endogenous carbon monoxide production in man. *J. Clin. Invest.* 42:1172, 1963.

75. Gray, C. H.: *Bile Pigments in Health and Disease.* Thomas, Springfield, Ill., 1961.

76. Miyahara, S., and Takahashi, H.: Biological coevolution: Carbon monoxide evolution during auto and enzymatic oxidation of phenols. *J. Biochem.* 69:231, 1971.

77. Coburn, R. F., Williams, W. J., and Kahn, S. B.: Endogenous carbon monoxide production in patients with hemolytic anemia. *J. Clin. Invest.* 45:460, 1966.

78. Cohman, C. A., and Dudley, G. M., III: The relationship between endogenous carbon monoxide production and total heme mass in normal and abnormal subjects. *Am. J. Med. Sci.* 258:374, 1969.

79. Logue, G. L., Rosse, W. F., Smith, W. T., Saltzman, H. A., and Gutterman, L. A.: Endogenous carbon monoxide production measured by gas phase analysis: An estimation of heme catabolic rate. *J. Lab. Clin. Med.* 77:867, 1971.

80. Lynch, S. R., and Moede, A. L.: Variation in the rate of endogenous carbon monoxide production in normal human beings. *J. Lab. Clin. Med.* 79:85, 1972.

81. Egger, G., Kutz, K., Bachofen, H., and Preisig, R.: Bilirubin production in subjects with Gilbert's syndrome (GS), in *The Liver: Quantitative Aspects of Structure and Function*, edited by R. Preisig and A. Baumgartner. Karger, Basel, 1973, p. 194.

82. White, P., Coburn, R. F., Williams, W. J., Goldwein, M. I., Rother, M. L., and Shafer, B. C.: Carbon monoxide production associated with ineffective erythropoiesis. *J. Clin. Inves.* 46:1986, 1967.

83. Landaw, S. A., and Winchell, H. S.: Endogenous production of carbon-^{14} labeled carbon monoxide: An *in vivo* technique for the study of heme catabolism. *J. Nucl. Med.* 7:696, 1966.

84. Elmlinger, P. J., Huff, R. L., Tobias, C. A., and Lawrence, J. H.: Iron turnover abnormalities in patients having anemia: Serial blood and in vivo tissue studied with Fe^{59}. *Acta Haematol. (Basel)* 9:73, 1953.

85. ICSH panel on diagnostic applications of radioisotopes in hematology: Recommended methods for surface counting to determine sites of red cell destruction. *Br. J. Haematol.* 30:249, 1975.

86. Van Dyke, D., and Anger, H. O.: Patterns of marrow hypertrophy and atrophy in man. *J. Nucl. Med.* 6:109, 1965.

87. Fordham, E. W., and Ali, A.: Radionuclide imaging of bone marrow. *Semin. Hematol.* 18:222, 1981.

88. Jandl, J. H., Greenberg, M. S., Yonemoto, R. H., and Castle, W. B.: Clinical determination of the sites of red cell sequestration in hemolytic anemias. *J. Clin. Invest.* 35:842, 1956.

89. Najean, Y., Cacchione, R., Dresch, C., and Rain, J. D.: Methods of evaluating the sequestration site of red cells labelled with ^{51}Cr: A review of 96 cases. *Br. J. Haematol.* 29:495, 1975.

90. Winkleman, J. W., Wagner, H. N., McAfee, J. G., and Mozley, J. M.: Visualization of the spleen in man by radioisotope scanning. *Radiology* 75:465, 1960.

Erythrocyte disorders—classification

CHAPTER 42

Classification of erythrocyte disorders

ALLAN J. ERSLEV

Erythrocyte disorders are traditionally divided into two groups: (1) anemia and (2) polycythemia (erythrocytosis). Although this division is based on the presence of too few red cells or too many red cells, anemia is functionally best characterized by a hemoglobin concentration below normal and polycythemia by a hematocrit above normal. Clinical considerations suggest this use of two different erythroid parameters in the characterization of anemia and polycythemia. Anemia is a disorder in which the patient suffers from tissue hypoxia, the consequence of a low oxygen-carrying capacity of the blood. Polycythemia, however, is a disorder in which the clinical manifestations are related to increased whole blood viscosity and increased blood volume, both consequences of a high hematocrit.

On the basis of determinations of the red cell mass, both anemia and polycythemia can be classified as: (1) relative and (2) absolute.

Relative anemia and relative polycythemia are both characterized by a normal total red cell mass. Such conditions are usually not thought of as hematologic disorders but rather as disturbances in the regulation of the plasma volume. However, both dilution anemia and dehydration polycythemia are of considerable clinical and differential diagnostic importance for the hematologist.

Absolute anemia with a decreased red cell mass can be classified according to morphologic or pathophysiologic criteria. Each classification scheme has its own strengths and weaknesses, and a wholly satisfactory classification is not available.

The *morphologic classification* subdivides anemia as follows: (1) macrocytic anemia, (2) normocytic anemia, and (3) microcytic hypochromic anemia.

The main advantages of this classification are that it emphasizes the importance of direct microscopic observation of red cells and that it forces the physician always to consider the most important types of treatable anemia: vitamin B_{12}, folic acid, and iron deficiency anemia. Such practical considerations have led to a wide acceptance of this classification. However, a morphologic classification is by necessity static and does not adequately support the present dynamic and biochemical approach to red cell disorders.

The *pathophysiologic classification* appears to be best suited for relating disease processes to present concepts of their mechanisms. The great drawback is, of course, that some of the present concepts are tentative and not solidly established. When they are used as bases for classification, they may appear to indicate facts rather than hypotheses. However, a useful classification should be open-ended and should incorporate both established facts and current opinions; the obvious need for future modifications does not detract from its immediate value as a clinical tool and an intellectual challenge.

In the pathophysiologic classification presented here (Table 42-1), absolute anemia is first divided into two groups: (1) anemia due to decreased red cell production, and (2) anemia due to increased red cell destruction or loss.

Several kinds of anemia appear to be caused by both decreased production and increased destruction of red cells and must be pigeonholed according to which of the two defects predominates. For example, the life-span of the red cell in megaloblastic anemia, anemia of renal failure, and thalassemia is shorter than the life-span of red cells in normal persons. Nevertheless, a responsive marrow could easily compensate for the increased rate of red cell destruction by an appropriate increase in red cell production. When such compensation does not occur because of absolute or relative marrow failure, the resulting anemia is classified as being predominantly a result of decreased red cell production.

Anemia predominantly caused by decreased red cell production can be subdivided according to the cell type primarily involved. A defect of self-renewing pluripotential hemopoietic stem cells results in disturbed proliferation and may cause aplasia of the marrow (aplastic anemia) or hyperplasia with the production of numerous effective blood cells (polycythemia vera) or ineffective cells (dyshemopoietic anemia). Paroxysmal nocturnal hemoglobinuria is also believed to originate in a clone of defective pluripotential stem cells. These disorders are described separately in Part Three of this book under disorders of hemopoietic stem cells, but in Table 42-1 they are listed according to their erythroid manifestations.

Failure of the next cell type, the unipotential progenitor cells committed to the erythroid series, may be caused by a disturbance in the regulatory mechanisms or a defect in the cellular metabolism. Impaired erythropoietin production causes a subnormal erythroid response to a reduction in hemoglobin concentration and is in part responsible for the anemia of chronic renal failure, anemia of endocrine disorders, and anemia of

TABLE 42-1   Classification of erythrocyte disorders

I. Anemia
   A. Relative
      1. Macroglobulinemia
      2. Pregnancy
      3. Nutritional deficiency
      4. Splenomegaly
   B. Absolute
      1. Anemia predominantly caused by decreased red cell production.
        a. Disturbance of proliferation and differentiation of hemopoietic stem cells.
          (1) Aplastic anemia
          (2) Dyshemopoietic anemia
        b. Disturbance of proliferation and differentiation of erythroid progenitor or precursor cells.
          (1) Pure red cell aplasia
          (2) Anemia of chronic renal failure
          (3) Anemia of endocrine disorders
          (4) Congenital dyserythropoietic anemia
        c. Disturbance of DNA synthesis (megaloblastic anemia)
          (1) Vitamin B_{12} deficiency
          (2) Folic acid deficiency
          (3) Acquired and congenital defects in purine and primidine metabolism
        d. Disturbance of hemoglobin synthesis (hypochromic anemia)
          (1) Iron deficiency
          (2) Congenital atransferrinemia and idiopathic pulmonary hemosiderosis
          (3) Thalassemia
        e. Unknown or multiple mechanisms
          (1) Anemia of chronic disorders
          (2) Anemia associated with marrow infiltration
          (3) Anemia associated with nutritional deficiencies
          (4) Sideroblastic anemia
      2. Anemia caused predominantly by increased erythrocyte destruction or loss
        a. Intrinsic abnormality
          (1) Membrane defect
             (*a*) Hereditary spherocytosis
             (*b*) Hereditary elliptocytosis
             (*c*) Hereditary stomatocytosis
             (*d*) Acanthocytosis
          (2) Enzyme deficiency
             (*a*) Glucose-6-phosphate dehydrogenase deficiency
             (*b*) Pyruvate kinase (PK) and other enzyme deficiencies
             (*c*) Porphyria
          (3) Globin abnormality (hemoglobinopathy)
             (*a*) Sickle cell disease and related disorders
             (*b*) Unstable hemoglobins
             (*c*) Low oxygen-affinity hemoglobinopathies
          (4) Paroxysmal nocturnal hemoglobinuria
        b. Extrinsic abnormality
          (1) Mechanical
             (*a*) March hemoglobinuria
             (*b*) Traumatic cardiac hemolytic anemia
             (*c*) Microangiopathic hemolytic anemia
          (2) Chemical or physical
             (*a*) Hemolytic anemia due to chemical or physical agents
          (3) Infectious
             (*a*) Hemolytic anemia due to infection with microorganisms
          (4) Antibody-mediated
             (*a*) Acquired hemolytic anemia due to warm-reacting autoantibodies
             (*b*) Cryopathic hemolytic syndrome
             (*c*) Drug reaction involving antibodies reacting with erythrocytes
             (*d*) Alloimmune hemolytic disease of the newborn
          (5) Hyperactivity of the monocyte-macrophage system
             (*a*) Hypersplenism
          (6) Blood loss
             (*a*) Acute blood loss anemia
II. Polycythemia (erythrocytosis)
   A. Relative
      1. Dehydration
      2. Spurious (stress or smokers) erythrocytosis
   B. Absolute
      1. Primary
        a. Polycythemia vera
        b. Erythremia
      2. Secondary
        a. Appropriate
          (1) Altitude
          (2) Cardiopulmonary disorder
          (3) Increased affinity of hemoglobin for oxygen
        b. Inappropriate
          (1) Renal tumor and cyst
          (2) Hepatoma
          (3) Cerebellar hemangioblastoma

chronic disorders. Pure red cell aplasia and congenital dyserythropoietic anemia, however, are probably caused by defects in the target cells, the erythropoietin responsive stem cell.

Failure of normal proliferation and maturation of differentiated precursor cells can be caused by (1) disturbance of DNA synthesis, (2) disturbance of hemoglobin synthesis, or (3) unknown or multiple mechanisms. Whether the common anemia of chronic systemic disease belongs in a subgroup of disturbance of hemoglobin synthesis or in a subgroup of failure of unipotential stem cells is a moot question. Failure of iron reutilization undoubtedly plays a role in the development of this type of anemia, but its associated lack of compensatory erythroid hyperplasia has resulted in its tentative assignment to anemia caused by unknown or multiple mechanisms. The exact pathogenesis of sideroblastic anemia has not been established either, and this type has tentatively been assigned to the same section.

All types of anemia predominantly caused by increased red cell destruction—so-called hemolytic anemia—are characterized by an actual or potential shortening of the red cell life-span. In some conditions, the compensatory efforts of the marrow may prevent overt anemia (compensated hemolysis), and in others the red call defect is so minimal that it demands exposure to a drug or an infection in order to become manifest. Nevertheless, these conditions are classified with anemia and are further subdivided into (1) intrinsic abnormalities and (2) extrinsic abnormalities.

With the exception of paroxysmal nocturnal hemoglobinuria, all types of anemia due to intrinsic abnormalities are caused by hereditary defects in the formation or protection of the cellular constituents of the circulating red cells. Such defects may lead to abnormalities in (1) membranes, (2) red cell enzymes, (3) globins, and (4) heme.

Most of the hemolytic or potentially hemolytic inherited disorders can be assigned to one of these four groups. However, it must be emphasized that the pathogenetic mechanisms for many of these disorders are still quite obscure.

Abnormalities of the extrinsic environment may cause injury and destruction of red cells by means of (1) mechanical forces, (2) chemicals or microorganisms, (3) antibodies, and (4) sequestration in the monocyte-macrophage system.

Absolute polycythemia with an increased red cell mass can be classified as (1) primary and (2) secondary. Primary polycythemia is a purposeless, idopathic hyperplasia of pluripotential stem cells causing pancytosis (polycythemia vera) or, rarely, essential erythremia. The erythropoietin titer is low or absent and separates primary from secondary polycythemia, in which it is elevated.

Secondary polycythemia can be classified as (1) appropriate and (2) inappropriate. Secondary appropriate polycythemia should perhaps not be considered a hematologic disorder, since it represents a physiologic compensatory response to tissue hypoxia. Secondary inappropriate polycythemia is generally believed to be caused by an inappropriate secretion of erythropoietin.

Erythrocyte disorders—anemias related to disturbance of erythroid precursor cell proliferation or differentiation

CHAPTER *43*

Pure red cell aplasia

ALLAN J. ERSLEV

Pure red cell aplasia is a widely used name for a type of anemia caused and characterized by an isolated depletion of the erythroid tissue. Many terms have been applied to this marrow disorder, and names such as *erythroblastic hypoplasia, erythroblastopenia, erythroid hypoplasia,* or *red cell agenesis* are all as descriptive as *pure red cell aplasia.* Certain other names such as *hypoplastic anemia* or *aregenerative anemia* have been used, but may lead to confusion, since they also are used respectively to characterize the pancytopenia of aplastic anemia and the refractory anemia of chronic disorders. In this chapter, the term *pure red cell aplasia* has been chosen because it is vivid and noncommittal.

Pure red cell aplasia was first clearly separated from aplastic anemia in 1922 by Kaznelson [1]. Since then it has received steadily increasing attention because of its intriguing relation to autoimmunity and to thymic tumors. At the present time, it can be classified into three types: an acute self limited type and a chronic type, either constitutional or acquired.

Acute pure red cell aplasia

In 1942, Lyngar [2] recognized that the anemic crisis in children with hereditary spherocytosis was frequently caused by decreased production of red cells rather than by increased hemolysis. In. an outstanding paper in 1948, Owren [3] employed the term *aplastic crisis* for this temporary production defect and outlined its natural history from the onset of a mild infection, through total erythroid aplasia, to recovery with rebound erythroid hyperplasia (Figs. 43-1 and 43-2). The following year,

FIGURE 43-1 Hematologic findings in a 30-year-old man with hereditary spherocytosis who developed an aplastic crisis following a brief febrile illness of unknown cause. (Case 4 in Owren [3].)

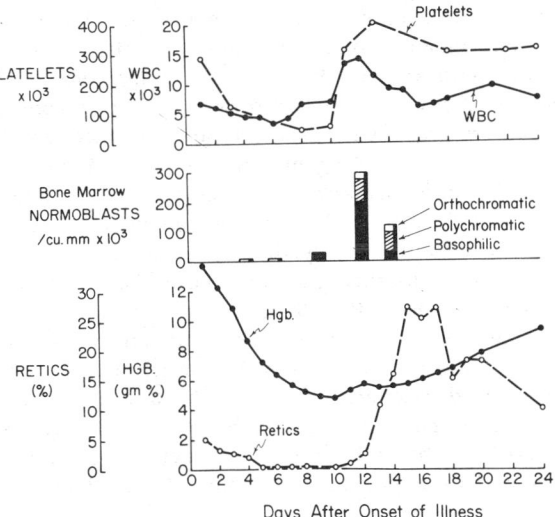

Days After Onset of Illness

FIGURE 43-2 Serial marrow samples from the patient whose course is outlined in Fig. 43-1. (Case 4 in Owren [3].)

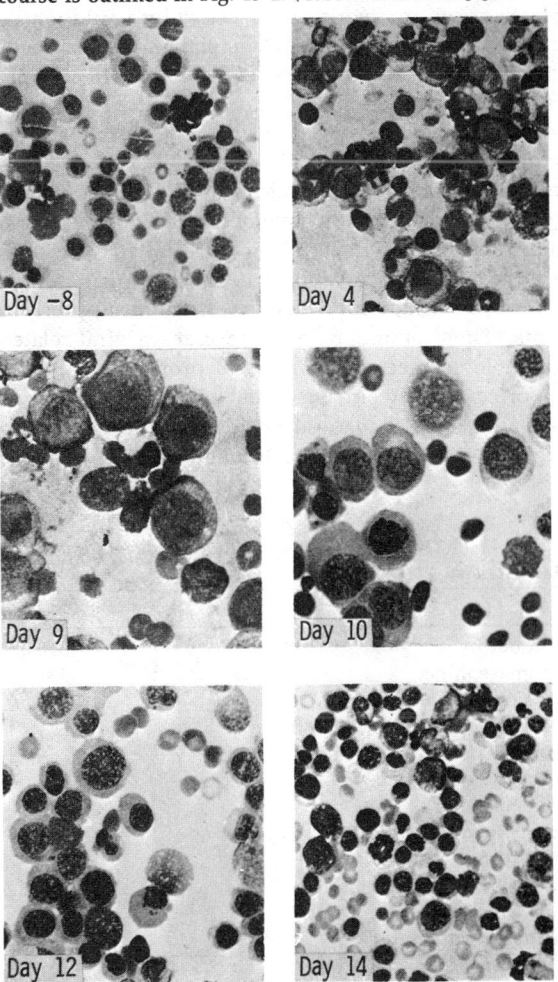

Gasser [4] described a similar type of self-limited erythroid aplasia in patients without hemolytic anemia, and since then, numerous instances of acute erythroid aplasia have been reported in both hematologically normal and abnormal individuals.

INCIDENCE

Most cases of self-limited aplastic crisis have been reported in patients with hereditary spherocytosis [5–8], acquired hemolytic anemia [9,10], paroxysmal nocturnal hemoglobinuria [11], or other hemolytic disorders [12–18]. Obviously, a brief period of erythroid aplasia in a patient with a short red cell life-span will have a far more noticeable effect on the hemoglobin concentration than the same period of aplasia would have in an individual with a normal red cell life-span. Consequently, it must be assumed that the cases of aplastic crisis reported in patients without underlying hemolytic disorders [4,12,15,19–28] represent merely a fraction of the actual occurrence of temporary erythroid aplasia. As a measure of its clinical significance for patients with hemolytic disorders, 9 of 89 hospitalized patients with sickle cell anemia in one series were admitted because of aplastic crisis [16].

ETIOLOGY AND PATHOGENESIS

Aplastic crises are frequently preceded by a mild febrile illness with upper respiratory complaints and gastroenteritis, and they may afflict several members of a family within a short period of time. Aplastic crises have specifically been observed in patients with primary atypical pneumonia [12,15], mumps [15], infectious mononucleosis [14], and viral hepatitis [29,30]. Specific erythropoietic inhibitors have only been observed in a single case [28], and the brief and self-limited course has precluded valid observations of the therapeutic effectiveness of glucocorticoids or immunosuppressive agents. Thus, although in some cases a viral-related immunologic mechanism appears probable, it is still supported only by circumstantial evidence.

Aplastic crises have also been related to toxicity to drugs [31–51] (Table 43-1). Although in some of these cases there may be an underlying immunologic mechanism, in others it appears that the isolated erythroid aplasia is merely the first manifestation of a general marrow suppression which is prevented by the immediate discontinuation of the drug.

Folic acid deficiency has been suspected to be a cause of aplastic crisis [52,53]. There is undoubtedly an increased requirement for folic acid in chronic hemolytic anemia [54], and folic acid deficiency or resistance can produce reticulocytopenia and erythroid hypoplasia [55,56]. In the few cases treated with folic acid, however, physiologic doses were ineffective [53].

Deficiencies of vitamin C and riboflavin and protein malnutrition have also been implicated in the etiology of aplastic crises. Although kwashiorkor may be associated with reticulocytopenia, erythroid hypoplasia, and "giant proerythroblasts" [57,58], the association between nutritional deficiencies and aplastic crises is still very tenuous.

CLINICAL AND LABORATORY FEATURES

The rapid onset of listlessness and increasing pallor in a patient with a chronic, well-adjusted hemolytic process should always raise the suspicion of an aplastic crisis. Characteristically, there is a history of a recent mild febrile illness with upper respiratory or intestinal symptoms, but aplastic crisis may occur without any preceding illness or in association with a variety of bacterial and inflammatory diseases. In patients without underlying hemolytic anemia, the associated illness is usually the event which leads to medical attention, while pallor and anemia are more incidental findings.

Apart from pallor, the physical examination does not contribute any significant clues unless a careful examiner detects decreased jaundice in a patient with chronic hemolytic anemia. The laboratory examination reveals anemia with red cell morphologic features characteristic of the underlying hematologic disorder, virtual absence of reticulocytes, and normal or low serum bilirubin. Moderate granulocytopenia and thrombocytopenia may be present, but granulocytes and platelets are frequently normal or even increased in number.

If examined early enough, the marrow will show complete depletion of all erythroid elements. However, most patients are seen during the early stage of spontaneous recovery when the marrow may display cohorts of early erythroid cells. These cells are often erroneously interpreted as reflecting maturation arrest or megaloblastosis, but serial marrow examinations usually show a normal maturation sequence followed by distinct reticulocytosis. Occasionally, there are large, intensely basophilic cells (so-called giant proerythroblasts). There is frequently some shift to the left in the myeloid series. The morphology of megakaryocytes is not measurably changed, and they are present in normal numbers.

The rapid recovery phase may be associated with severe bone pain, presumably because of marrow expansion, and by "rebound" reticulocytosis, granulocytosis, and thrombocytosis. In splenectomized patients

TABLE 43-1   Drugs associated with the development of aplastic crisis

Generic name	References
Azathioprine	[31,32]
Carbamazephine	[33]
Cephalothin	[34]
Chloramphenicol	[35–37]
Chlorpropamide	[38–40]
Co-Trimoxazole	[41]
D-Penicillamine	[42]
Diphenylhydantoin	[43–47]
Fenoprofen	[48]
Gamma-benzene hexachloride	[49]
Gold	[50]
Thiamphenicol	[51]

or in asplenic sickle cell anemia patients, the recovery phase may be characterized by an outpouring of nucleated red cells from the marrow, but this erythroblastic crisis probably reflects the absence of an extramedullary site for final maturation of immature erythroid cells.

Erythrokinetic analysis of red cell production and red cell destruction during the brief aplastic crisis is difficult to carry out because of the absence of steady-state conditions. During the crisis, serum iron is high, with almost complete saturation of iron-binding capacity, but it drops precipitously when erythroid activity commences. The erythropoietin titer is also high initially and decreases moderately during the recovery phase [59].

THERAPY

Therapy should include discontinuation, if possible, of all drug intake, maintenance of the hemoglobin at a level above that which causes symptoms, treatment of any associated illness, and the wait for spontaneous remission. Since red cell destruction continues throughout the period of erythroid aplasia, severe incapacitating anemia may develop rapidly, and preventive transfusions of 1 or 2 units of packed red cells may be advisable. Folic acid and multivitamins are usually given in addition, but their effectiveness in acute aplastic crises is at best uncertain.

Chronic pure red cell aplasia

CONSTITUTIONAL

A chronic form of isolated erythroid hypoplasia occurring early in childhood and believed to be congenital or inherited was first described in 1936 by Joseph [60] and 2 years later by Diamond and Blackfan [61]. Since then, many hundreds of cases have been reported of this condition, now best known as the *Diamond-Blackfan anemia* [62,63].

INCIDENCE

In a few infants, pallor and anemia are recognized at birth, but in most reported cases, a definite diagnosis of anemia is first made between the ages of 2 weeks and 1 year [63]. There is no characteristic sex preponderance and no consistent abnormality of the pregnancy or delivery. Minor physical aberrations such as short stature, thumb deformities, and eye changes are present in about 30 percent of patients, but they appear to be quite different from the major birth defects observed in Fanconi's aplastic anemia. In 10 percent of cases there are more than one affected family member, and the occasional reports of consanguinity suggest an autosomal recessive inheritance [63].

ETIOLOGY AND PATHOGENESIS

Recent studies of erythroid colony formation in vitro have suggested that the constitutional pure red cell aplasia is caused by the inheritance of a defective stem cell. Cultures of marrow CFU-E and marrow and blood BFU-E have disclosed that these erythroid-committed stem cells are markedly decreased in numbers [64,65] and also are quite insensitive to the action of erythropoietin [65]. Although there is some improvement in the number and erythropoietin sensitivity of stem cells after steroid-induced remissions, they remain abnormal. Chromosomal studies, however, have been unrewarding and actually have shown only nonspecific breaks and inversions in a few patients [63]. The progenies of these presumably defective stem cells are mature but definitely abnormal red cells. They are macrocytic, contain increased amounts of fetal hemoglobin, have i surface antigen and a fetal distribution of intracellular enzymes [63]. Although such changes could indicate a constitutional abnormality, they are also seen in normal individuals exposed to acute or chronic hemopoietic demands [66].

The therapeutic effectiveness of steroids in constitutional pure red cell aplasia as well as its morphologic kinship to the acquired autoimmune cases have led to a search for an immunologic pathogenesis. Such a search led to the finding of a circulating inhibitor of erythropoiesis in one case [67] and of erythroid suppressor lymphocytes in several more [68,69]. However, these patients had all received prior transfusions, and since studies in the majority of cases have failed to reveal evidence for a humoral or cellular immunologic mechanism, it appears that the observed suppressors probably relate to sensitizing transfusions rather than to the basic pathogenesis.

The appearance in some patients of nonmaturing proerythroblasts have led to the suggestion that the erythroid tissue is deficient in necessary metabolic components for maturation and hemoglobin synthesis. However, erythropoietin, vitamin B_{12}, folic acid, and pyridoxine do not appear to be lacking, and the report of excessive anthranilic acid excretion, suggesting a metabolic defect in the handling of tryptophan, although challenging, has not led to a constructive working hypothesis [70,71].

CLINICAL FEATURES

The presenting symptoms and signs reflect the severity of this type of anemia. Pallor, listlessness, and poor appetite are early manifestations, progressing into borderline congestive failure with breathlessness, hepatomegaly, and splenomegaly. These initial symptoms and signs respond readily to transfusions. Subsequently, however, hepatic changes may be induced by transfusion hemosiderosis, serum hepatitis, and cardiac cirrhosis, and irreversible hepatomegaly and splenomegaly may dominate the clinical picture.

A variety of minor associated congenital abnormalities have been reported, such as strabismus, inverted nipples, webbed neck, or bony abnomalities of fingers and ribs [63]. Major congenital abnormalities such as achondroplasia and double ureters with hydronephrosis have been observed in only a few cases [72]. Thymic hyperplasia or thymic tumors have not been found in children with constitutional pure red cell anemia.

LABORATORY FEATURES

Normochromic, macrocytic anemia with absolute reticulocytopenia is found in all cases. The white blood cell count is normal or only slightly decreased, but the platelet count is often mildly elevated. Secondary hypersplenism may lead to peripheral pancytopenia, but marrow examination readily separates this condition from the pancytopenia of marrow aplasia.

Marrow examination is mandatory for a diagnosis. Characteristically, it discloses a cellular marrow with a profound erythroid hypoplasia and a high myeloid/erythroid ratio. The few remaining erythroid cells are usually young and may display some nuclear changes suggestive of megaloblastosis. The morphology and maturation sequence of the myeloid cells and megakaryocytes are normal, and the plasma cells and mononuclear lymphoid cells also appear normal. Prior to the onset of hypersplenism, the red cell life-span, as estimated from transfusion requirements, bilirubin levels, and urobilinogen excretion, is probably normal. Erythropoietin titers in the serum are appropriately elevated [59], but the daily urinary excretion of erythropoietin is claimed to be higher than in other kinds of anemia.

Serum iron is at a high normal level with increased saturation of iron-binding protein, and folic acid and vitamin B_{12} serum levels are normal. Fetal hemoglobin, distributed unevenly among the red cells, is elevated in most cases, as is the concentration of i antigen on the red cell surface [63]. Hypogammaglobulinemia has been observed in several patients, but liver function tests are usually normal prior to the development of transfusion hemosiderosis.

THERAPY

Transfusions and adrenal corticosteroids are standard therapeutic agents and can maintain many patients in nearly normal health for many years. Hemosiderosis is an unavoidable complication of transfusions and will eventually lead to liver damage, portal hypertension, and hypersplenism (see Chap. 79). Hemosiderosis will also cause fibrosis of the pancreas, endocrine glands, and cardiac musculature. Failure of growth and sexual maturity may mar an otherwise successful therapeutic regimen, and myocardial failure is frequently responsible for death [73]. However, the recent introduction of intensive iron chelation by continuous infusions of desferrioxamine may ameliorate and postpone the effect of iron overload [74]. Splenectomy is a reasonable therapeutic approach to the hypersplenism which may occur secondary to hepatic fibrosis. Otherwise, splenectomy would not be expected to influence erythropoietic function of the marrow.

Adrenal corticosteroids have been used extensively and have been held responsible for temporary improvements, complete remissions, and cures [62,75]. Steroids must be given in large doses initially, 60 to 100 mg of prednisone or prednisone equivalents (1 to 2 mg/kg), and the therapeutic trial should not be abandoned until the end of 4 to 6 weeks of unsuccessful therapy. If a reticulocyte response occurs, the prednisone dosage should be reduced appropriately, and it is frequently possible to maintain adequate red cell production with almost "homeopathic" amounts of steroids. The most distressing complication has been growth retardation, but steroid-related viremia and gastroenteritis have also been encountered. Androgens have been used in refractory cases [62], but their use should be undertaken with great reluctance in the prepubertal child. Marrow transplantation has so far only been used occasionally [76], but it certainly should be considered in patients refractory to therapy and having HLA identical siblings.

COURSE AND PROGNOSIS

Transfusions and carefully adjusted steroid therapy have been successful in the long-term management of many patients. About one-third to one-half of the patients may develop prolonged unmaintained remissions, but many of these individuals will eventually need further therapy. The toll of therapy has been considerable, since almost all the deaths are related to therapeutic complications, possibly including the few patients who have developed acute leukemias [77,78].

ACQUIRED

Pure red cell aplasia in the adult is an unusual disease characterized by acquired, isolated erythroid hypoplasia and by a frequent association with thymic tumors. This association was first described by Opsahl in 1939 [79], and since then, about 30 to 50 percent of all reported patients have had thymomas, a relationship suggesting an immunologic pathogenesis. This suggestion has been supported by the observation that many patients with pure red cell aplasia have antibodies directed at erythroid cells and their precursors [80].

INCIDENCE

The disease is observed primarily in middle-aged adults. More than 200 cases have been reported in the literature, and among those there are almost as many cases with thymomas as without [80–83] (Fig. 43-3). This, however, may not reflect the true incidence of thymomas in pure red cell aplasia, since there undoubtedly is more of a tendency to publish cases with a challenging concurrence of two different disease processes than there would be to publish cases of either disease alone. In patients with thymomas, the incidence of pure red cell aplasia has been estimated to be about 7 percent, probably also an unrealistically high incidence. There appears to be a significant preponderance of females over males (2:1) in the group having pure red cell aplasia associated with thymoma, while males dominate in the group without thymoma [84]. It must be

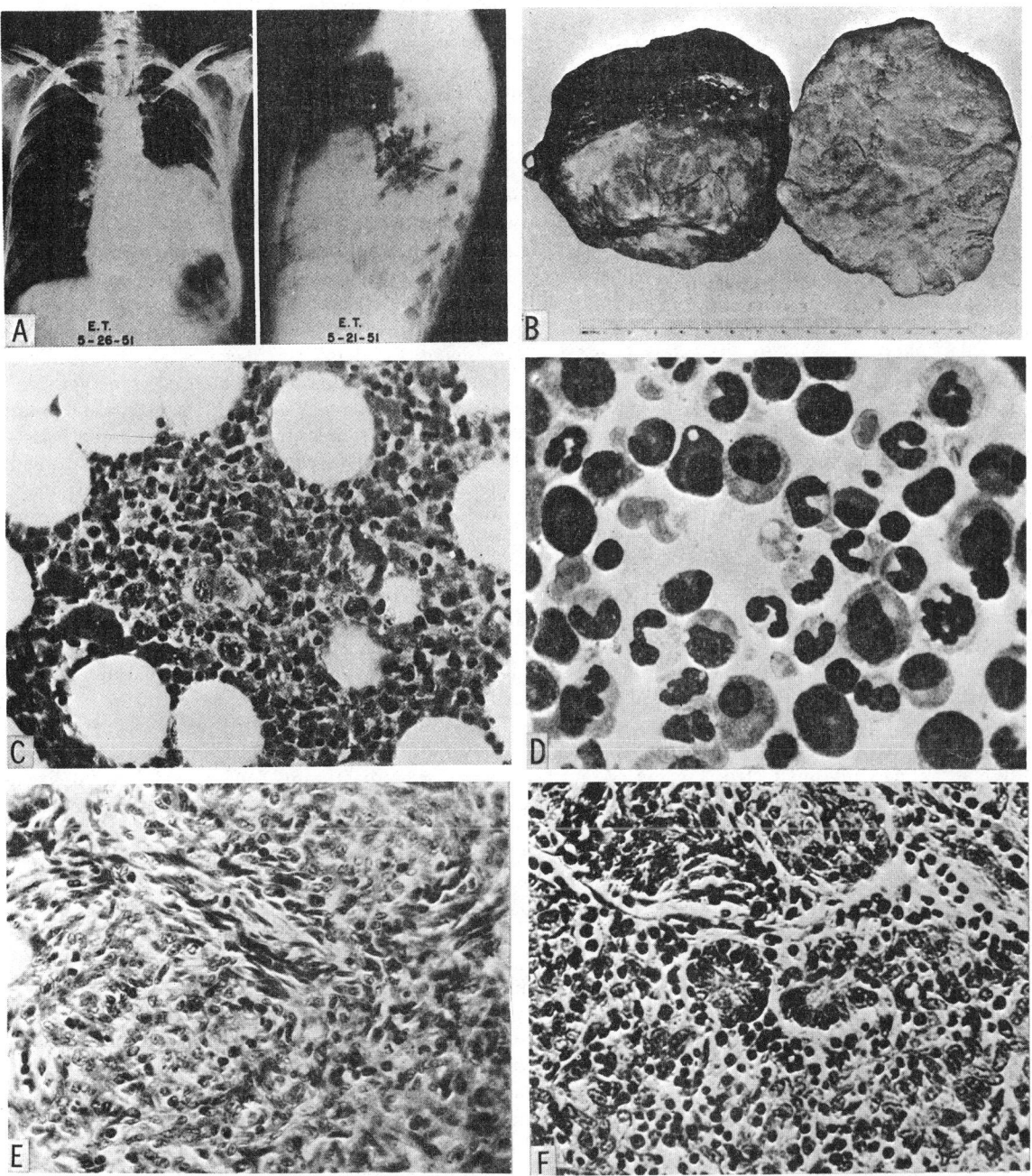

FIGURE 43-3   A 45-year-old woman with a dry cough and severe anemia. The chest x-ray revealed a large mediastinal mass (*A*), and marrow examination (C and D) disclosed pure red cell aplasia. Thymectomy was performed (*B*), and histologic examination of the tumor (*E* and *F*) showed spindle cells forming palisades and rosettes. Surgery did not change the marrow picture, and the patient continued to require regular transfusion therapy. (Case 2 in Ross et al. [83].)

emphasized that in some patients who appear to have pure red cell aplasia the condition is later found to be less than "pure," as leukopenia, thrombocytopenia, and generalized marrow aplasia develop.

ETIOLOGY AND PATHOGENESIS

The presence of a thymoma in about 30 to 50 percent of the reported cases strongly suggests that an im-

munologic mechanism is involved in the etiology or pathogenesis. The current concept of thymic function envisions the thymus as being involved in the conditioning of those lymphocytes responsible for delayed hypersensitivity and tissue rejection [85,86] (see Chaps. 105 and 106). Thymic aplasia is clearly related to distinct syndromes of immunologic incapacity, but thymic hyperplasia or thymomas are most often incidental and nonsymptomatic findings [87]. However, in a few cases, thymomas are found in association with apparently unrelated but immunologic-oriented diseases, such as myasthenia gravis, thyroiditis, hypogammaglobulinemia, and rheumatoid arthritis [88–91]. Similarly, chronic pure red cell aplasia without thymomas has also occurred in immunologic-oriented diseases, such as systemic lupus erythematosus [92–94] and chronic lymphocytic leukemia [95–97]. It is these relationships which have led to the hypothesis that pure red cell aplasia is caused by an immunologic rejection of the erythroid tissue. The striking erythropoietic response to adrenal steroid therapy observed occasionally and the reports of the therapeutic effectiveness of immunosuppressive agents have added support for this hypothesis.

The direct demonstration of antibodies which react with nucleated red cells have now been made in about 50 percent of patients with chronic pure red cell aplasia [98–101]. These antibodies inhibit in vitro heme synthesis by normal marrow cells and suppress the in vitro growth of both normal and the patient's own CFU-E. Some are complement-fixing and cytolytic, while others act in the absence of complement [102]. In contradistinction to constitutional pure red cell aplasia, the growth of erythroid colonies cultured in the absence of the patient's own serum are unaffected. In some cases it has been claimed that the antibodies are directed against erythropoietin [103], but in general the erythropoietin titers are high and apparently unaffected.

Toxic interference by drugs with the metabolism of nucleated red cells has been suspected in several cases (see Table 43-1). However, this type of anemia is either rapidly reversible after discontinuation of the drug or, if irreversible, gradually changes into a generalized marrow hypoplasia. So far it has not been possible to relate the erythroid hypoplasia in patients with chronic pure red cell anemia to metabolic deficiencies or inhibitory substances.

CLINICAL FEATURES
Pallor is usually the only physical finding of note on the initial examination. A thymoma, when present, is rarely large enough to be detected on physical examination, and congenital malformations are not part of the clinical picture. Later on, after prolonged transfusion and steroid therapy, there may be additional findings caused by secondary hemochromatosis and steroid-induced side effects.

LABORATORY FEATURES
The form of anemia accompanying this disease is normochromic and normo- or macrocytic and associated with absolute reticulocytopenia. The leukocyte and platelet counts are normal, and the marrow is cellular with normal myelopoiesis and megakaryocytopoiesis, but with profound erythroid hypoplasia. The remaining erythroid cells are immature but morphologically normal. In the marrow, there may be an increase in eosinophils and particularly in small, intensely stained lymphoid-like cells. In a few cases, granulocytes and platelet production appear to be affected, but characteristically there is a complete separation between hypofunctioning erythroid tissue and normofunctioning myeloid and megakaryocytic tissue.

The serum iron level is elevated with almost complete saturation of the iron-binding capacity, the half-life of radioactive iron is prolonged, and the iron utilization is low, conforming to the morphologic observation of erythroid hypoplasia. The red cell life-span is normal initially, but may become shortened owing to transfusion-induced hemochromatosis with congestive splenomegaly or to the presence of red cell antibodies. Immunologic studies have disclosed a great variety of findings. Both hypogammaglobulinemia and hypergammaglobulinemia have been described, although most patients have a normal protein electrophoretic pattern [90,104,106]. There have been frequent associations with many kinds of specific antibodies, such as cold and warm hemagglutinins, cold hemolysins, heterophile antibodies, false-positive serologic tests for syphilis, antinuclear antibodies and positive lupus erythematosus tests [88,90,92–94,106]. Folic acid and vitamin B_{12} metabolism are usually unimpaired, although in a few cases megaloblastosis and response to folic acid have suggested an abnormal handling or availability of these coenzymes [81].

Thymic enlargement, when present, is usually detected on routine chest x-ray examinations as a mass in the anterior mediastinum. Tomography, angled supraclavicular exposure, or even pneumomediastinography may be needed to demonstrate a small thymoma, but diagnostic surgery is rarely indicated if the radiologic examinations are negative. In one series of 56 cases of pure red cell anemia with thymoma [81], the thymomas in 46 cases were encapsulated and composed primarily of spindle cells. The germinal centers were absent, but there was diffuse scant infiltration with small lymphocytes. In 10 cases the thymomas were infiltrating and considered malignant. In these cases, the tissues were composed of lymphocytes and reticulum cells in a disorganized pattern. In the 7 cases in this series with associated myasthenia gravis, the gross or microscopic pattern did not differ significantly from the other cases.

THERAPY
Transfusion with packed red cells is the mainstay of symptomatic therapy. A hemoglobin concentration maintained at 8 to 10 g/dl is an attainable goal and demands transfusion of about 2 units of packed red cells every 2 weeks. Febrile reactions can be minimized by using washed or frozen red cells and antihistamine drugs. However, a gradual shortening of the effective life-span of transfused red cells because of hypersplenism or of red cell antibodies can make this therapy increasingly frustrating and ineffective.

The more definitive therapies include thymectomy, adrenal steroids, and immunosuppressive agents, and these should be instituted after proper consideration of potential benefits and potential side effects. The use of folic acid or riboflavin can hardly be condemned, but usually neither is of benefit in chronic acquired pure red cell aplasia. Cobalt has been used as a nonspecific erythropoietic agent [107], but there is little theoretic or practical justification for the use of this toxic chemical.

Thymectomy   Whenever thymic enlargement is found, it is advisable to perform a thymectomy in order to provide a diagnosis, to prevent possible malignant extension, and to promote reactivation of the marrow. In one series of 56 patients, 25 were treated by thymectomy and 16 appeared to benefit from the operation [81]. There was not a single good remission among patients not operated on. The benefit derived from thymectomy could not always be related directly to surgery, and it is still difficult to assess the benefits derived from thymectomy alone. However, in one case a serum inhibitor of the erythroid tissue apparently disappeared after thymectomy [108]. Irradiation of the thymus was completely unsuccessful in the 5 patients so treated [81]. The current consensus appears to be that removing a normal-sized thymus gland without a thymoma is of no help to a patient with pure red cell aplasia.

Steroids   Corticosteroids are frequently effective in reactivating red cell production [103,109–111]. Unfortunately, rather substantial doses may be needed, and side effects often preclude the continuous employment of these drugs. When small maintenance doses are effective, however, adrenal steroid treatment can eliminate transfusion dependence and be the treatment of choice. Androgens have been used for their potential erythropoietic effect and in an occasional patient may be a valuable adjunct to adrenal steroid therapy [83].

Immunosuppressive drugs   On the assumption that acquired red cell aplasia is an autoimmune disorder, therapy with cyclophosphamide or 6-mercaptopurine has been tried and has been successful in a number of cases [35,98,112–115]. It appears worthwhile to give these drugs a trial and to tailor subsequent therapy to the results of this trial.

Splenectomy   Splenectomy has been performed in many patients, but unless there is evidence for extravascular hemolysis [116], the therapeutic benefit derived has been minimal. Obviously, hypersplenic red cell destruction and excessive splenic antibody formation will be eliminated by splenectomy, but the underlying disease is not dependent on spleen function and will not be helped by splenectomy.

COURSE AND PROGNOSIS

Remissions have been induced in about 25 percent of patients both with and without thymomas, but only half of these have been sustained without further therapy. In most cases, maintenance therapy with transfusions and adrenal steroids has been responsible for both symptomatic control of the disease and for high mortality. In one series of 56 patients with thymomas, 17 died within 6 months of the date of diagnosis, and a total of 50 were dead at the time of the compilation of the report [81]. Of 16 cases without thymomas observed at the Mayo Clinic, 8 died 1 to 3 years after the onset of the disease [82]. The causes of death were hemosiderosis, steroid-induced hemorrhages or infections, and aplastic anemia. With the current use of experimental immunosuppressive drugs, it seems possible that the rate of both remissions and complications may increase, but it is also to be hoped that this treatment will lead to better understanding of the disease process and a more rational therapy.

References

1. Kaznelson, P.: Zur Enstehung der Blut Plattchen. *Verh. Dtsch. Ges. Inn. Med. Kong.* 34:557, 1922.
2. Lyngar, E.: Samtidig optreden av anemisk kriser hos 3 barn i en familie med hemolytisk ikterus. *Nord Med.* 14:1246, 1942.
3. Owren, P. A.: Congential hemolytic jaundice: The pathogenesis of the "hemolytic crisis." *Blood* 3:231, 1948.
4. Gasser, C.: Akute Erythroblastopenie: 10 Falle aplastischer Erythroblastenkrisen mit Riesen Proerythroblasten bei allergisch-taxischen Zustands bildern. *Helv. Paediatr. Acta* 4:107, 1949.
5. Dameshek, W., and Bloom, M. L.: The events of the hemolytic crisis of hereditary spherocytosis with particular reference to the reticulocytopenia, pancytopenia and abnormal splenic mechanism. *Blood* 3:1381, 1948.
6. Greig, H. B. W., Metz, J., Bradlow, B. A., Theron, J. J., and Morris, R. W.: The familial crisis in hereditary spherocytosis: Report of five cases. *S. Afr. J. Med. Sci.* 23:17, 1958.
7. Chanarin, I., Burman, D., and Bennett, M. C.: The familial aplastic crisis in hereditary spherocytosis: Urocanic acid and formiminoglutamic acid excretion studies in a case with megaloblastic arrest. *Blood* 20:33, 1962.
8. Bouroncle, B. A.: Familial crises in hereditary spherocytosis. *J. Am. Med. Wom. Assoc.* 19:1045, 1964.
9. Miesch, D. C., Baxter, R., and Levin, W. C.: Acute erythroblastopenia: Pathogenesis, manifestations and management. *Arch. Intern. Med.* 99:461, 1957.
10. Daris, L. J., Kennedy, A. C., Baikie, A. G., and Brown, A.: Hemolytic anemias of various types treated with ACTH and cortisone: Report of ten cases, including one of acquired type in which erythropoietic arrest occurred during crises. *Glasgow Med. J.* 33:263, 1952.
11. Crosby, W. H.: Paroxysmal nocturnal haemoglobinuria: Report of a case complicated by an aregenerative (aplastic) crisis. *Ann. Intern. Med.* 39:1107, 1953.
12. Singer, K., Motulsky, A. G., and Wile, S. A.: Aplastic crisis in sickle cell anemia: A study of its mechanism and its relationship to other types of hemolytic crisis. *J. Lab. Clin. Med.* 35:721, 1950.
13. Hilkowitz, G.: The "aplastic crisis" and erythroid maturation defect occurring simultaneously in three members of a family. *Arch. Intern. Med.* 105:100, 1960.
14. Chernoff, A. I., and Josephson, A. M.: Acute erythroblastopenia in sickle cell anemia and infectious mononucleosis. *Am. J. Dis. Child.* 82:310, 1951.
15. Gasser, C.: Aplasia of erythropoiesis: Acute and chronic erythroblastopenias or pure (red cell) aplastic anaemias in childhood. *Pediatr. Clin. North. Am.*, May 1957, p. 445.
16. Charney, E., and Miller, G.: Reticulocytopenia in sickle cell disease. *Am. J. Dis. Child.* 107:450, 1964.
17. Hurdle, A. D. F., and Walker, A. G.: Bone marrow hypoplasia in the course of haemolytic disease of the newborn. *Br. Med. J.* 1:518, 1963.
18. MacIver, J. E.: The aplastic crises in sickle cell anemia. *Lancet* 1:1086, 1961.
19. Bauman, A. W., and Swisher, S. N.: Hyporegenerative processes in hemolytic anemia. *Semin. Hematol.* 4:265, 1967.
20. Chanarin, I., Barkhan, P., Peacock, M., and Stamp, T. C. B.: Acute arrest of haemopoiesis. *Br. J. Haematol.* 10:43, 1964.

21. Wang, W. C., and Mentzer, W. C.: Differentiation of transient erythroblastopenia of childhood from congenital hypoplastic anemia. *J. Pediatr.* 88:784, 1976.

22. Wranne, L., Bonnevier, J. O., Killander, A., and Killander, J.: Pure red-cell anaemia with pro-erythroblast maturation arrest. *Scand. J. Haematol.* 7:73, 1970.

23. Wranne, L.: Transient erythroblastopenia in infancy and childhood. *Scand. J. Haematol.* 7:76, 1970.

24. Lovric, V. A.: Anaemia and temporary erythroblastopaenia in children. *Aust. Ann. Med.* 1:34, 1970.

25. Shah, N. R., Wolff, J. A., and Sitarz, A.: Transient acquired red blood cell (RBC) aplasia in children without hematologic disease. *Pediatr. Res.* 10:381, 1976.

26. Tillman, W., Prindull, G., and Schroter, W.: Severe anemia due to transient pure red cell aplasia in early childhood; arrest at the level of the committed stem cells? *Eur. J. Pediatr.* 123:51, 1976.

27. Clarke, B. J., et al.: Hemoglobin synthesis in human BFU-E and CFU-E derived colonies. *Blood*, in press.

28. Koenig, H. L., Lightsey, A. L., Nelson, D. L., and Diamond, L. K.: Immune suppression of erythropoiesis in transient erythroblastopenia of childhood. *Blood* 54:742, 1979.

29. Sears, D. A., George, J. N., and Gold, H. S.: Association of transient pure red cell aplasia (PRCA) with chronic viral hepatitis. *Clin. Res.* 22:67a, 1974.

30. Wilson, H. A., McLaren, G. D., Dworken, H. J., and Tebbi, K.: Transient pure red cell aplasia: Cell mediated suppression of erythropoiesis associated with hepatitis. *Ann. Intern. Med.* 92:196, 1980.

31. Declerck, Y. A., Ettenger, R. B., Ortega, J. A., and Pennisi, A. J.: Macrocytosis and pure RBC anemia caused by azathioprine. *Am. J. Dis. Child.* 134:377, 1980.

32. McGrath, B. P., et al.: Erythroid toxicity of azathioprine: Macrocytosis and selective marrow hypoplasia. *Am. J. Med.* 44:57, 1975.

33. Hirai, H.: Two cases of erythroid hypoplasia caused by carbamazephine. *Jpn. J. Clin. Hematol.* 18:33, 1977.

34. MacCulloch, D., Jackson, J. M., and Venerys, J.: Drug induced red cell aplasia. *Br. Med. J.* 4:163, 1974.

35. Vilan, J., Rhyner, K., and Ganzoni, A.: Pure red cell aplasia. Successful treatment with cyclophosphamide. *Blut* 26:27, 1973.

36. Yunis, A. A., and Bloomberg, G. R.: Chloramphenicol toxicity: Clinical features and pathogenesis, in *Progress in Hematology*, edited by C. B. Moore and E. B. Brown. Grune & Stratton, New York, 1964, vol. 4, p. 138.

37. Ozer, F. L., and Truax, W. E., and Levin, W. C.: Erythroid hypoplasia associated with chloramphenicol therapy. *Blood* 16:997, 1960.

38. Gill, M. J., Ratliff, D. A., and Harding, L. K.: Hypoglycemic coma, jaundice, and pure RBC aplasia following chlorpropamide therapy. *Arch. Intern. Med.* 140:714, 1980.

39. Planas, A. T., Kranwinkel, R. N., Soletsky, H. B., and Pezzimenti, J. F.: Chlorpropamide-induced pure RBC aplasia. *Arch. Intern. Med.* 140:707, 1980.

40. Recker, R. R., and Hymes, H. E.: Pure red cell aplasia associated with chlorpropamide therapy. *Arch. Intern. Med.* 123:445, 1969.

41. Stephens, M. E.: Transient erythroid hypoplasia in a patient on long-term co-trimoxazole therapy. *Postgrad. Med. J.* 50:235, 1974.

42. Bollan, J. L., Hussein, S., Hoffbrand, A. V., and Sherlock, S.: Red cell aplasia following prolonged D-penicillamine therapy. *J. Clin. Pathol.* 29:135, 1976.

43. Huijgens, P. C., Thijs, L. G., and Den Ottolander, G. J.: Pure red cell aplasia, toxic dermatitis and lymphadenopathy in a patient taking diphenyl-hydantoin. *Acta Haematol.* 59:31, 1978.

44. Hotta, T., Hirabayashi, N., Kobayashi, T., Nakamura, S., and Suzuki, Y.: Five cases showing hemoglobinuria and aplastic crisis following administration of diphenylhydantoin after craniotomy. *Rinsho Ketsueki* 21:536, 1980.

45. Brittingham, T. E., Lutcher, C. L., and Murphy, D. L.: Reversible erythroid aplasia induced by diphenylhydantoin. *Arch. Intern. Med.* 113:764, 1964.

46. Yune-Gill, J., Jung, Y., and River, G. L.: Pure RBC aplasia and diphenylhydantoin. *JAMA* 229:314, 1974.

47. Yunis, A. A., Arimura, G. K., Lutcher, C. L., Blasquez, J., and Halloran, M.: Biochemical lesion in dilantin-induced erythroid aplasia. *Blood* 30:587, 1967.

48. Weinberger, K. A.: Fenoprofen and red cell aplasia. *J. Rheumatol.* 6:475, 1979.

49. Vodopick, H.: Cherchez la chienne. I. Erythropoietic hypoplasia after exposure to gamma-benzene hexachloride *JAMA* 234:850, 1975.

50. Reid, G., and Patterson, A. C.: Pure red cell aplasia after gold treatment. *Br. Med. J.* 2:1457, 1977.

51. Cornet, A., et al.: A case of reversible erythroblastopenia due to thiamphenicol. *Sem. Hop. Paris* 50:1567, 1974.

52. Pierce, L. E., and Rath, C. E.: Evidence for folic acid deficiency in the genesis of anemic sickle cell crisis. *Blood* 20:19, 1962.

53. Alperin, J. B.: Folic acid deficiency complicating sickle cell anemia. *Arch. Intern. Med.* 120:398, 1967.

54. Shojania, A. M., and Gross, S.: Hemolytic anemia and folic acid deficiency in children. *Am. J. Dis. Child.* 108:53, 1964.

55. Jandl, J. H., and Greenberg, M. S.: Bone marrow failure due to relative nutritional deficiency in Cooley's hemolytic anemia. *N. Engl. J. Med.* 260:461, 1959.

56. Branda, R. F., Moldow, C. F., MacArthur, J. R., Wintrobe, M. M., Anthony, B. K., and Jacob, H. S.: Folate-induced remission in aplastic anemia with familial defect of cellular folate uptake. *N. Engl. J. Med.* 298:469, 1978.

57. Kho, L. K.: Erythroblastemia with giant pro-erythroblasts in kwashiorkor. *Blood* 12:171, 1957.

58. Zucker, J. M.: Tchernia, G., Vuylsteke, P., Becart-Michel, R., Giorgi, R., and Blot, J.: Acute and transitory erythroblastopenia in kwashiorkor under treatment. *Nouv. Rev. Fr. Hematol. Blood Cells* 11:131, 1971.

59. Hammond, D., Shore, N., and Movassaghi, N.: Production, utilization and excretion of erythropoietin. I. Chronic anemias. II. Aplastic crises. III. Erythropoietic effect of normal plasma. *Ann. N.Y. Acad. Sci.* 149:516, 1968.

60. Joseph, W. H.: Anemia of infancy and early childhood. *Medicine (Baltimore)* 15:307, 1936.

61. Diamond, L. K., and Blackfan, K. D.: Hypoplastic anemia. *Am. J. Dis. Child.* 56:464, 1938.

62. Diamond, L. K., Wang, W. C., and Alter, B. P.: Congenital hypoplastic anemia. *Adv. Pediatr.* 22:349, 1976.

63. Alter, B. P.: Childhood red cell aplasia. *Am. J. Pediatr. Hematol./Oncol.* 2:121, 1980.

64. Freedman, M. H., Amato, D., and Saunders, E. F.: Erythroid colony growth in congenital hypoplastic anemia. *J. Clin. Invest.* 57:673, 1976.

65. Nathan, D. G., et al.: Erythroid precursors in congenital hypoplastic (Diamond-Blackfan) anemia. *J. Clin. Invest.* 61:489, 1978.

66. Alter, B. P.: Fetal erythropoiesis in stress hematopoiesis. *Exp. Hematol.* 7:200, 1979.

67. Ortega, J. A., Shore, N. A., Dukes, P. P., and Hammond, D.: Congenital hypoplastic anemia inhibition of erythropoiesis by sera from patients with congenital hypoplastic anemia. *Blood* 45:83, 1975.

68. Hoffman, R., et al.: Diamond-Blackfan syndrome: Lymphocyte-mediated suppression of erythropoiesis. *Science* 193:899, 1976.

69. Steinberg, M. H., Coleman, M. F., and Pennebaker, J. B.: Diamond-Blackfan syndrome: Evidence for T-cell mediated suppression of erythroid development and a serum blocking factor associated with complete remission. *Br. J. Haematol.* 41:57, 1979.

70. Altman, K. I., and Miller, G.: A disturbance of tryptophan metabolism in congenital hypoplastic anaemia. *Nature* 172:868, 1953.

71. Hankes, L. V., Brown, R. R., Schiffer, L., and Schmaeler, M.: Tryptophan metabolism in humans with various types of anemias. *Blood* 32:649, 1968.

72. Hughes, D. W. O'G.: Hypoplastic anemia in infancy in childhood: Erythroid hypoplasia. *Arch. Dis. Child.* 36:349, 1961.

73. Sanyal, S. K., Johnson, W., Jayalakshmamma, B., and Green, A. A.: Fatal "iron heart" in an adolescent; biochemical and ultrastructural aspects of the heart. *Pediatrics* 55:336, 1975.

74. Cooper, B., et al.: Treatment of iron overload in adults with continuous parenteral desferrioxamine. *Am. J. Med.* 63:958, 1977.

75. Allen, D. M., and Diamond, L. K.: Congenital (erythroid) hypoplastic anemia: Cortisone treated. *Am. J. Dis. Child.* 102:416, 1961.

76. August, C. S., et al.: Establishment of erythropoiesis following

bone marrow transplantation in a patient with congenital hypoplastic anemia (Diamond-Blackfan syndrome). *Blood* 48:491, 1976.

77. Wasser, J. S., Yolken, R., Miller, D. R., and Diamond, L.: Congenital hypoplastic anemia (Diamond-Blackfan syndrome) terminating in acute myelogenous leukemia. *Blood* 51:991, 1978.

78. Kreshvan, E. U., Wegner, K., and Gara, S. K.: Congenital hypoplastic anemia terminating in acute promyelocytic leukemia. *Pediatrics* 61:898, 1978.

79. Opsahl, R.: Thymus-karcinom og aplastic anemia. *Nord. Med.* 2:1835, 1979.

80. Krantz, S. B., and Zaentz, S. D.: Pure red cell aplasia, in *The Year in Hematology*, edited by R. Silber, A. S. Gordon, and J. LoBue. Plenum, New York, 1977, p. 153.

81. Hirst, E., and Robertson, T. I.: The syndrome of thymoma and erythroblastopenic anemia. *Medicine (Baltimore)* 46:225, 1967.

82. Tsai, S. Y., and Levin, W. C.: Chronic erythrocytic hypoplasia in adults. *Am. J. Med.* 22:322, 1957.

83. Ross, J. F., Finch, S. C., Street, R. B., Jr., and Strieder, J. W.: The simultaneous occurrence of benign thymoma and refractory anemia. *Blood* 9:935, 1954.

84. Schmid, J. R., Kiely, J. M., Harrison, E. G., Jr., Bayrd, E. D., and Pease, G. L.: Thymoma associated with red cell agenesis: Review of literature and report of cases. *Cancer* 18:216, 1965.

85. Peterson, R. D. A., Cooper, M. D., and Good, R. A.: The pathogenesis of immunologic deficiency diseases. *Am. J Med.* 38:579, 1965.

86. Meuwissen, H. J., Stutman, O., and Good, R. A.: Functions of the lymphocytes. *Semin. Hematol.* 6:28, 1969.

87. Fisher, E. R.: Pathology of the thymus and its relation to human disease, in *The Thymus in Immunobiology*, edited by R. A. Good and A. E. Gabrielson. Hoeber-Harper, New York, 1964, p. 676.

88. Prasad, A. S., Berman, L., Tranchida, L., and Poulik, M. D.: Red cell hypoplasia, cold hemoglobinuria and M-type gamma G serum para-protein and Bence Jones proteinuria in a patient with lymphoproliferative disorders. *Blood* 31:151, 1968.

89. Dawson, M. A.: Thymoma associated with pancytopenia and Hashimoto's thyroiditis. *Am. J. Med.* 52:406, 1972.

90. Rogers, B. H. G., Manaligod, J. R., and Blazek, W. V.: Thymoma associated with pancytopenia and hypogammaglobulinemia. *Am. J. Med.* 44:154, 1968.

91. DeSevilla, E., Forrest, J. V., Zivnuska, F. R., and Sagel, S. S.: Metastatic thymoma with myasthenia gravis and pure red cell aplasia. *Cancer* 36:1154, 1975.

92. Doughaday, W. H.: Lupus erythematosus with severe anemia, selective erythroid hypoplasia and multiple red blood cell isoantibodies. *Am. J. Med.* 44:590, 1968.

93. Cassileth, P. A., and Myers, A. R.: Erythroid aplasia in systemic lupus erythematosus. *Am. J. Med.* 55:706, 1973.

94. MacKechnie, H. L. N., Squires, A. H., Platts, M., and Pruzanski, W.: Thymoma, myasthenia gravis, erythroblastopenic anemia, and systemic lupus erythematosus in one patient. *Can. Med. Assoc. J.* 109:733, 1973.

95. Battle, J. D., Hewlett, J. S., and Hoffman, G. C.: Prolonged erythroid aplasia in chronic lymphocytic leukemia. *Ann. Intern. Med.* 58:731, 1963.

96. Abeloff, M. D., and Waterbury, L.: Pure red cell aplasia and chronic lymphocytic leukemia. *Arch. Intern. Med.* 134:721, 1974.

97. Nagasawa, T., Abe, T., and Nagagawa, T.: Pure red cell aplasia and hypogammaglobulinemia associated with Tγ-cell chronic lymphocytic leukemia. *Blood* 57:1025, 1981.

98. Krantz, S. B., and Kao, V.: Studies on red cell aplasia. I. Demonstration of a plasma inhibitor to heme synthesis and an antibody to erythroblastic nuclei. *Proc. Natl. Acad. Sci. U.S.A.* 58:493, 1967.

99. Krantz, S. B., and Kao, V.: Studies on red cell aplasia. II. Report of a second patient with an antibody to erythroblast nuclei and a remission after immunosuppressive therapy. *Blood* 34:1, 1969.

100. Field, E. O., Caughi, M. N., Blackett, N. M., and Smithers, D. W.: Marrow-suppressing factors in the blood in pure red cell aplasia, thymoma and Hodgkin's disease. *Br. J. Haematol.* 15:101, 1968.

101. Krantz, S. B., Moore, W. H., and Zaentz, S. D.: Studies on red cell aplasia. V. Presence of erythroblast cytotoxicity in γG globulin fraction of plasma. *J. Clin. Invest.* 52:324, 1973.

102. Browman, G. P., Freedman, M. H., Blajchman, M. A., and McBride, J. A.: A complement independent erythropoietic inhibitor acting on the progenitor cell in refractory anemia. *Am. J. Med.* 61:572, 1976.

103. Peschle, C., et al.: Pure red cell aplasia: Studies on an IgG serum inhibitor neutralizing erythropoietin. *Br. J. Haematol.* 30:411, 1975.

104. Linsk, J. A., and Murray, C. K.: Erythrocyte aplasia and hypogammaglobulinemia: Response to steroids in a young adult. *Ann. Intern. Med.* 55:831, 1961.

105. Geary, C. G., Byron, P. R., Taylor, G., MacIver, J. E., and Zervas, J.: Thymoma associated with pure red cell aplasia, immunoglobulin deficiency, and an inhibitor of antigen-induced lymphocyte transformation. *Br. J. Haematol.* 29:479, 1975.

106. Dameshek, W., Brown, S. M., and Rubin, A. D.: "Pure" red cell anemia (erythroblastic hypoplasia) and thymoma. *Semin. Hematol.* 4:222, 1967.

107. Fountain, J. R., and Dales, M.: Pure red cell aplasia successfully treated with cobalt. *Lancet* 325:541, 1955.

108. Al-Mondhiry, H., Zanjani, E. D., Spivack, M., Zalusky, R., and Gordon, A. S.: Pure red cell aplasia and thymoma: Loss of serum inhibitor of erythropoiesis following thymectomy. *Blood* 38:576, 1971.

109. Finkel, H. E., Kimber, R. J., and Dameshek, W.: Corticosteroid responsive acquired pure red cell aplasia in adults. *Am. J. Med.* 43:771, 1967.

110. Haremann, V. K., Kuni, H., and Schmitz-Moormann, P.: Klinische und erythrokinetische Befunde bei isolierter Aplasie der Erythropoese vor und nach erfolgreicher Therapie mit Kortikosteroiden. *Blut* 26:193, 1973.

111. Mitchell, A. B. S., Pinn, G., and Pegrum, G. D.: Pure red cell aplasia and carcinoma. *Blood* 37:594, 1971.

112. Bottiger, L. E., and Rausing, A.: Pure red cell anemia: Immunosuppressive treatment. *Ann. Intern. Med.* 76:593, 1972.

113. Krantz, S. B.: Studies on red cell aplasia. III. Treatment with horse anti-human thymocyte gammaglobulin. *Blood* 39:347, 1972.

114. Zaetz, S. D., Krantz, S. B., and Brown, E. B.: Studies on pure red cell aplasia. VIII. Maintenance therapy with immunosuppressive drugs. *Br. J. Haematol.* 32:47, 1976.

115. Marmon, A., Peschle, C., Sanguineti, M., and Condorelli, M.: Pure red cell aplasia (PRCA): Response of three patients to cyclophosphamide and/or antilymphocyte globulin (ALG) and demonstration of two types of serum IgG inhibitors to erythropoiesis. *Blood* 45:247, 1975.

116. Eisemann, G., and Dameshek, W.: Splenectomy for pure red cell hypoplastic (aregenerative) anemia associated with hemolytic disease. *N. Engl. J. Med.* 251:1044, 1954.

CHAPTER *44*

Anemia of chronic renal failure

ALLAN J. ERSLEV

Anemia is one of the most characteristic and visible manifestations of chronic renal failure. In 1836, Richard Bright first commented on the pallor of patients with renal disease [1], and since then, numerous observers have attempted to characterize and explain the underlying anemia. The degree of anemia appears to be roughly proportional to the degree of uremia [2] (Fig. 44-1), but it is not surprising that a strict linear relationship does

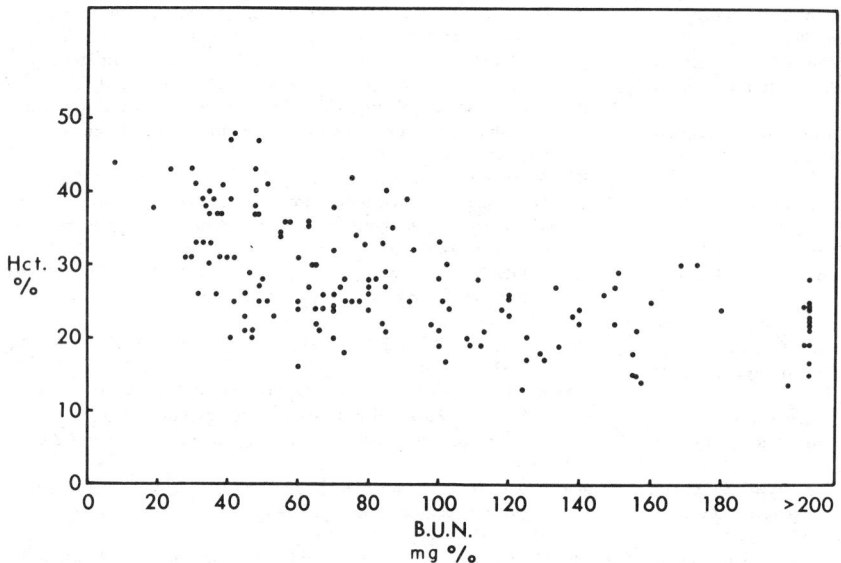

FIGURE 44-1   Relation between hematocrit and blood urea nitrogen in 152 patients with chronic renal disease. (Erslev and Shapiro [2].)

not exist. A reduction in the hematocrit may be caused by any one of a number of changes in the rate of red cell production and red cell destruction, and an increase in the blood urea nitrogen may be caused by a variety of infectious, neoplastic, allergic, metabolic, or hydrodynamic injuries to the renal parenchyma. However, Fig. 44-1 does illustrate that at blood urea nitrogen concentrations in excess of 100 mg per deciliter of plasma, the hematocrit is almost always below 30 percent.

Recent experimental and clinical observations on the effect of intensive dialysis and of bilateral nephrectomy have clarified some of the pathophysiologic mechanisms responsible for the anemia. It appears that it is caused both by failure of renal excretory function leading to hemolysis, blood loss, and marrow supression and by failure of renal endocrine function leading to impaired erythropoietin production.

Etiology and pathogenesis

FAILURE OF RENAL EXCRETORY FUNCTION

HYDREMIA

The hematocrit or the concentration of hemoglobin reflects both red cell mass and plasma volume. Since the plasma volume may vary widely in renal failure, it is important to know the extent of dehydration or hydremia before using these parameters as measures of red cell mass and red cell production. Conversely, because of this relationship, the hematocrit determination becomes an excellent short-term guide in the monitoring of peritoneal dialysis or hemodialysis.

HEMOLYSIS

The life-span of red cells in patients with chronic renal disease is usually shorter than normal. Since the red cells survive normally when injected into healthy recipients, and since normal red cells may have a shortened life-span in uremic recipients [3,4], it appears that the metabolic or mechanical environment is unfavorable to red cells. The presence of a metabolic defect is suggested by the linear relation found by some investigators between blood urea nitrogen and red cell life-span [5–8] and by the occasional normalization of the red cell life-span after intensive dialysis [9]. However, most red cell enzymes show normal or increased activity in uremia, and the intracellular level of ATP is high [10,11]. Only the levels of transketolase, active in the hexose monophosphate shunt [12], and ATPase, powering the Na^+-K^+ membrane pumps [13], are decreased. The decreased response of the hexose monophosphate shunt renders the hemoglobin and red cell membrane excessively sensitive to oxidant drugs or chemicals [14,15]. For example, tap water used for hemodialysis and purified with chloramine can cause the formation of Heinz bodies and hemolytic anemia [16]. The decreased activity of the Na^+-K^+ pumps could cause changes in red cell shape and rigidity and in turn in red cell life-span. The toxic substances responsible for these metabolic impairments are presumably dialyzable but have not been identified.

Despite these impressive data on a metabolic basis for hemolysis, there are a considerable number of investigators who have failed to find a clear-cut correlation between red cell life-span and degree of renal failure [2]. It has been suggested that red cell injury and premature destruction may be caused by mechanical trauma rather than by metabolic alterations [17]. Normal red cells exposed to strong shearing stress, especially at a fibrin interphase [18], will become deformed and vulnerable to monocyte-macrophage sequestration. In some cases of malignant hypertension, extensive red cell fragmentation occurs with the induction of severe hemolytic anemia [19], but in most cases of chronic renal disease the hemolysis as well as the morphologic changes are moderate. At the present, it appears reasonable to relate premature destruction of red cells in uremia to mechanical disruption of metabolically impaired cells.

The so-called hemolytic uremic syndrome is probably a distinct entity, the renal failure being a consequence of the hematologic disorder rather than a cause. It was first described in 1955 by Gasser and coworkers [20], who found hemolysis and uremia in infants and young children subsequent to episodes of gastrointestinal or upper respiratory infections. Since then the syndrome has been recognized in patients of all ages and associated with a variety of exogenous agents [21]. It appears to be initiated by damage to the endothelium of glomerular capillaries and renal arterioles. This leads to local intravascular coagulation and ischemic renal cortical necrosis. The clinical manifestations are pallor, purpura, jaundice, and oliguria, and the hematologic examinations reveal anemia with a blood film displaying many deformed and fragmented red cells (Fig. 44-2), increased number of reticulocytes, and occasional nucleated red cells [17,22]. Despite the uremia, the erythropoietin titer is elevated [23]. There is thrombocytopenia but many marrow megakaryocytes, and in some cases there is depletion of several coagulation proteins. The clinical, morphologic, and laboratory manifestations are similar to findings in patients with various microangiopathic disorders (see Chap. 64) or consumptive coagulopathy (see Chap. 158) and the differences between hemolytic uremic syndrome, thrombotic thrombocytopenic purpura, and endotoxin-induced Shwartzman phenomenon may be quantitative rather than qualitative [2,17].

IMPAIRED RED BLOOD CELL PRODUCTION

Marrow composition [24] and iron turnover [25–28] in patients with chronic renal failure are usually "normal" or, in other words, fail to show a compensatory erythroid response to the anemia. Since erythropoietin production also fails to increase in response to anemia (see below), the relative marrow failure has been related to a lack of stimulation. However, recent studies have suggested that in addition to this lack of stimulation azotemia per se causes suppression of erythroid stem cells and their offspring [29]. First, the response to exogenous erythropoietin is subnormal in uremic animals [30] and in the few uremic humans so tested [31,32]. Second, intensive hemodialysis and peritoneal dialysis [33–35] increase hematocrit and iron utilization without altering the level of circulating erythropoietin. These in vivo observations have been correlated with in vitro

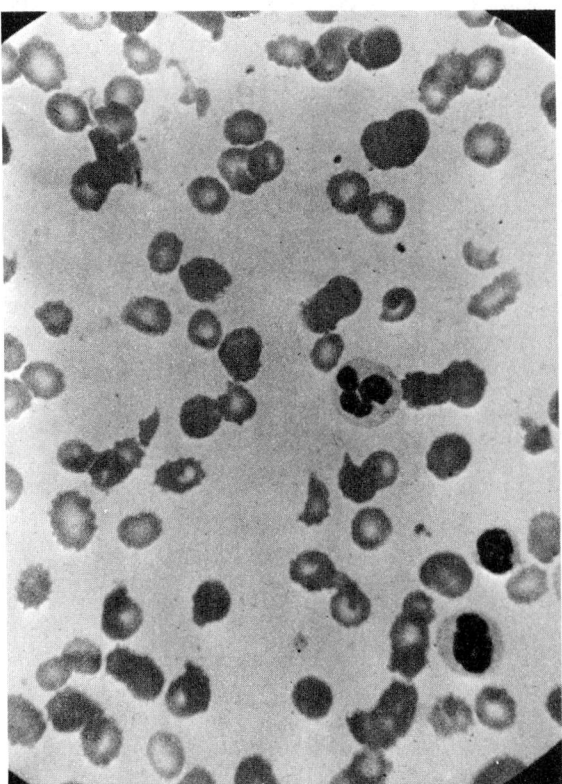

FIGURE 44-2   Peripheral blood film from a patient with the hemolytic uremic syndrome, showing fragmentation and distortion of red blood cells.

studies which have shown that plasma from uremic individuals has an inhibitory effect on heme synthesis [36,37] and erythroid stem cell proliferation [38,39]. Although spermine, a poorly dialyzed polyamine, is suspected [39], the responsible uremic inhibitor(s) has as yet not been identified.

Since parathyroidectomy in patients with chronic renal failure often is followed by an increase in hematocrit [40], the parathyroid hormones have also been suspected of being uremic toxins and causing erythroid suppression [41]. However, this relation is somewhat tenuous and, if it exists, is probably indirect and caused by postoperative changes in hemoglobin oxygen affinity [42] or in marrow sclerosis [43].

VARIOUS DEFICIENCIES

Patients with chronic renal failure should always be screened carefully for treatable deficiency syndromes. Iron may be in short supply because of blood lost from the gastrointestinal or female genital tract, in repeated laboratory tests, or in the discarded hemodialysis coils [44,45]. Renal inflammatory lesions may also lead to low serum iron levels because of defective reutilization of iron [46]. In a rare case of nephrosis, the urinary loss of transferrin has been reported to cause low iron-binding capacity, with impairment in the metabolic cycling of iron [47]. Folic acid deficiency should always be suspected and prevented in patients undergoing intensive dialysis, since folic acid is dialyzable and may be lost in the dialysis bath [48].

BLEEDING TENDENCY

Purpura, gastrointestinal, and gynecologic bleeding occur in one-third to one-half of all patients with chronic renal failure [49–51]. This loss of blood constitutes an additional erythropoietic demand and contributes significantly to the development of anemia. The pathogenesis of the bleeding tendency is poorly understood. Thrombocytopenia, when present, is rarely of sufficient magnitude to explain spontaneous blood loss [52]. However, platelet or vascular function, as evaluated from bleeding time, platelet adhesiveness and aggregation, clot retraction, prothrombin consumption, or prostacyclin production by vessel walls is abnormal in the majority of cases and may account for the bleeding tendency [49,50,53] (see Chap. 147). Dialysis has been found to correct or ameliorate both the laboratory test for platelet function and the clinical manifestations [50], but the dialyzable agent responsible has not been identified. Urea or creatinine is probably not involved [50], and although certain guanidine compounds are suspected [54], the responsible agent has not been identified.

FAILURE OF RENAL ENDOCRINE FUNCTION

In 1957, Jacobson and coworkers reported that nephrectomized and uremic rats fail to respond to blood loss with erythropoietin release, while ureter-ligated and equally uremic rats respond in an almost normal manner [55]. This extremely important observation led to the hypothesis that the kidney produces erythropoietin.

Numerous studies since then have supported this hypothesis and have suggested that renal tissue hypoxia causes the release of erythropoietin. Experimental [56,57] or pathologic [58,59] reduction in the supply of arterial blood to the kidneys has been shown to cause erythropoietin release and secondary erythrocytosis. Local ischemic injury of renal parenchyma induced experimentally by the injection of plastic microspheres into the renal artery [60] or by the exertion of cortical pressure [61] has also been observed to cause erythrocytosis. It seems likely that the erythrocytosis found in some patients with renal cysts, hydronephrosis, or renal tumors [62] may similarly be caused by pressure ischemia of normal renal tissue as well as inappropriate secretion of erythropoietin. It is also possible that the increase in erythropoietin titers, which occasionally heralds impending rejection of a transplanted kidney, is caused by local vascular injury and hypoxia [63].

The site of production of erythropoietin in the kidney appears to be the cortex. Fluorescent-labeled anti-erythropoietin tends to highlight the glomeruli [64], and there is a suggestive relationship between renin production and erythropoietin release [65,66]. Direct confirmation by tissue assays is supportive but not yet definitive [67]. Indeed, attempts to isolate erythropoietin from renal tissue extracts were generally unsuccessful, leading to the hypothesis that the kidney does not synthesize erythropoietin per se, but rather produces an enzyme (erythrogenin) capable of transforming an inactive circulating erythropoietin into active erythropoietin [68]. However, studies on isolated perfused kidneys have shown that the kidney in the absence of a serum substrate can synthesize erythropoietin [69]. Furthermore, recent successful extraction of erythropoietin from kidney homogenates [67] has shown that the kidney is capable of both sensing an oxygen deficit and producing erythropoietin [70].

In the anephric individual with complete absence of renal erythropoietin, the compensatory capacity of marrow is severely reduced, and marrow activity becomes stabilized at a subnormal level [71,72] (Fig. 44-3). The attainment and maintenance of this level appear to be

FIGURE 44-3   Hemoglobin concentration, corrected reticulocyte count, serum iron turnover, and erythropoietin titers in a female patient who was nephrectomized 7 months before renal transplantation. The patient was maintained on weekly hemodialysis, and the hemoglobin concentration was adjusted by transfusions from a low of 5 g/dl to a high of 16 g/dl. (Erslev et al. [72].)

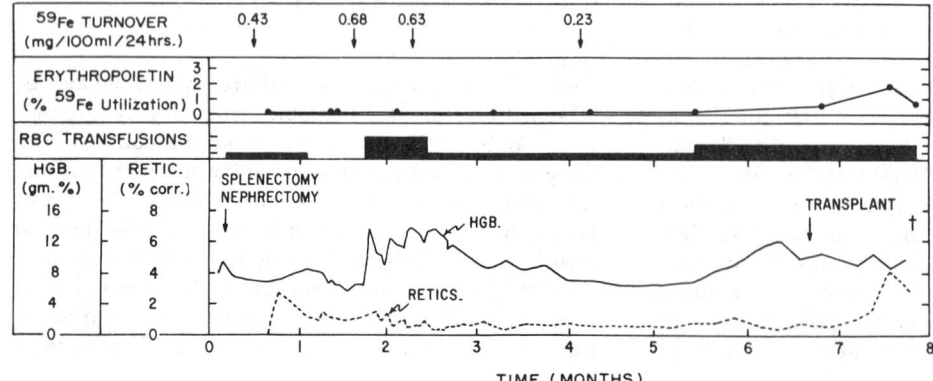

caused by the release of extrarenal erythropoietin, presumably produced by the liver [73,74].

In patients with chronic renal disease, the degree of impairment in erythropoietin release and marrow compensation vary widely [25,75–78]. In some cases, the rate of erythropoietin production is maintained at a fairly good level, possibly because of inappropriate secretion of erythropoietin by the injured kidneys [79]. In most cases, however, the production is substantially lower than that of normal individuals with intact kidneys at corresponding hematocrits (Fig. 44-4). Nevertheless, the amount of circulating erythropoietin should be sufficient for a normal rate of red cell production but obviously not for the higher rate needed to balance uremic blood loss, hemolysis, and marrow suppression. Intensive dialysis will not increase the production of erythropoietin, and the amelioration of anemia observed in patients on a chronic dialysis program [33] is probably caused by decreased hemolysis and bleeding and increased marrow effectiveness.

Clinical and laboratory features

The symptoms and physical manifestations of renal failure depend primarily on the underlying disorder. However, pallor and anemia are common manifestations and may become of major clinical concern.

The anemia is characteristically normocytic and normochromic and is associated with a normal or slightly decreased number of reticulocytes. On blood films, a few red cells appear deformed, some with multiple tiny spicules and others with grossly abnormal contour and loss of volume. The former cells, echinocytes or burr cells, were thought to be quite characteristic of chronic renal failure [80]. However, even normal cells will undergo a reversible transformation to spiculed, burr cell-like echinocytes when exposed to a glass surface or suspended in incubated plasma [81]. This suggests that the echinocytes in uremia at least in part are artifactual and do not circulate as such in blood.

Grossly deformed cells, however, such as acanthocytes with a few large spicules or fragmented schistocytes, are undoubtedly formed in the microcirculation in vivo [82]. They are found most abundantly in the hemolytic uremic syndrome (Fig. 44-2), but in small numbers can be recognized on blood films from most uremic patients.

The capacity of red cells to function as oxygen carriers in uremia does not appear to be impaired. The intracellular concentration of 2,3-diphosphoglycerate is appropriately increased in response to anemia and hyperphosphatemia [83–85] and the affinity of hemoglobin for oxygen is appropriately decreased [86]. In the presence of uremic acidosis, this decrease in oxygen affinity is augmented by a shift to the right in the oxygen dissociation curve (Bohr effect). However, acidosis will also tend to decrease glycolysis and decrease the concentration of intracellular organic phosphates, estab-

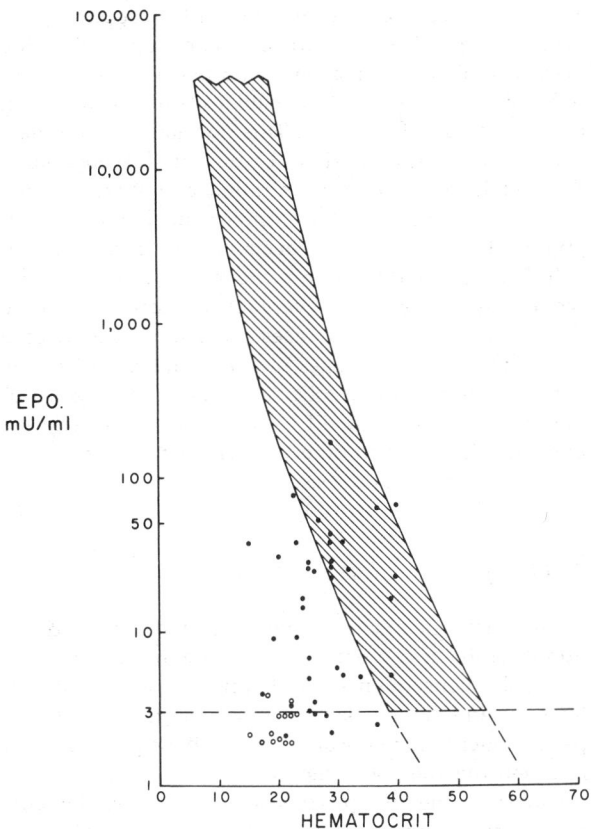

FIGURE 44-4   Erythropoietin titers in nephric and anephric uremic patients. The range of values for individuals with intact kidneys is indicated by the hatched area. The broken line indicates that erythropoietin levels below 3 mU/ml are not accurately measured by the method used. ● = nephrics; ○ = anephrics.

lishing a complex of opposing effects on the oxygen affinity of hemoglobin [85,87]. Intensive dialysis may initially cause a reduction in the concentration of intracellular organic phosphate compounds, possibly because of hypophosphatemia [88]. This would result in increased oxygen affinity of hemoglobin and a temporary aggravation of tissue hypoxia and may play a role in the so-called dialysis disequilibrium syndrome [89,90].

The total and differential leukocyte count and the platelet count are usually normal, but, as with all other hematologic parameters, the underlying disorder plays a modifying role. Furthermore, uremia and dialysis per se may have an effect on both leukocytes and platelets. The phagocytic activity of granulocytes may be reduced [91], and complement activation by the hemodialysis membrane may cause pulmonary leukostasis with temporary granulocytopenia [92]. Cell-mediated immunity is also depressed, resulting in both an increased incidence of infections and a prolonged graft survival [91]. Platelet function, as mentioned earlier, is abnormal and related to degree of uremia and dialysis [50]. The marrow may appear somewhat hypoplastic, and in acute renal failure, severe erythroid hypoplasia has been described [93]. However, characteristically, the marrow is almost normal with a normal appearance and maturation sequence of all cellular elements including the nucleated red cells [24]. This normality of the marrow is nevertheless spurious, because in the context of a reduced hemoglobin concentration a normal marrow should have displayed a compensatory increase in erythroid activity. The titer of circulating erythropoietin [77] (Fig. 44-4) and the iron turnover are also "normal," while iron utilization in severe renal failure is regularly decreased [27]. In many cases the underlying disease will cause specific changes in iron kinetics and in the serum concentration of folic acid, iron, and transferrin. These changes may modify and aggravate the relative marrow failure which otherwise characterizes the anemia of chronic renal disease.

Therapy

In the past, anemia was often considered a relatively minor problem for patients suffering from the many metabolic consequences of failing kidneys. Efficient hospital and home dialysis, however, have provided partial relief from many of these metabolic problems but have left the anemia unchecked.

Currently, the therapy consists of providing elements necessary for red cell production, transfusing with packed cells when necessary, and stimulating erythropoietin production [94].

Folic acid is often given routinely, but the most important supplement is undoubtedly iron. Iron deficiency is present because of blood loss from capillary bleedings and from blood removed in discarded hemodialyzer membranes and laboratory studies. The most useful test for assessing iron stores is serum ferritin, and a value of less than 30 μg/liter is an indication for iron supplementation [95]. The use of parenteral iron is rec-

ommended if the stores are severely depleted. Otherwise, and despite conflicting reports on intestinal iron absorption [96], oral iron preparations should suffice.

Splenectomy as a means of prolonging red cell life-span in patients with splenomegaly and excessive red cell destruction has been performed occasionally [97]. The results are rarely spectacular and the decision to operate should not be taken lightly.

Transfusion of patients with severe anemia of chronic renal failure is often necessary and may even be desirable. Until recently, exposure to tissue antigens in the transfused leukocytes and platelets was believed to jeopardize the success of a possible future kidney transplant. However, the opposite appears to be the case, and transfusions have been found to improve kidney graft survival [98]. The immunologic mechanism responsible for this observation remains elusive, but transfusion pretreatment has become routine in some kidney transplantation centers. Excessive blood loss associated with prolonged bleeding time has empirically but successfully been managed by the infusion of cryoprecipitate [99]. Reduction in the concentration of the still unknown uremic marrow toxins and in turn an increase in hematocrit are to a certain extent accomplished by hemodialysis [33]. Continuous ambulatory peritoneal dialysis appears to remove such toxins even more efficiently and has been reported to cause a striking increase in the hematocrit of some patients [35].

Stimulation of erythropoietin production has been achieved in patients with chronic renal disease by the administration of cobalt [100] or androgens [101–105]. Cobalt, however, causes cellular hypoxia, and any increase in erythropoietin production is probably achieved at the expense of generalized tissue hypoxia [106]. Androgen administration may be associated with some unpleasant side effects, such as fluid retention, hirsutism, skin infections, and cholestasis, but the erythropoietic effect has so far not been related to the induction of tissue hypoxia. The effect is somewhat capricious, but in most nephric uremic patients and in some anephric patients, androgens cause a moderate increase in erythropoietin release and red cell production. Since even a small increase may remove the patients from the transfusion-dependent ranks, androgens are being used extensively in most dialysis centers (Fig. 44-5). The mechanism of action is not clear, but in addition to a stimulation of renal and extrarenal erythropoietin release, it seems likely that androgens also have a direct stimulating action of erythroid tissue [104]. Fluoxymesterone and oxymetholone are given by mouth in doses of 10 to 20 mg per day and 1 to 4 mg per kilogram of body weight per day, respectively, while parenteral preparations, presumed to be more effective [105], such as nandrolone decanoate or testosterone propionate or enanthate, are given in doses of 1 to 4 mg per kilogram of body weight once a week. Replacement therapy with erythropoietin, the most rational approach to the treatment of the anemia of chronic renal failure, unfortunately still lies in the future [107].

FIGURE 44-5 **Hematocrit and transfusion requirements before and after treatment with fluoxymesterone in 14 patients on maintenance hemolysis. (Eschbach et al. [101].)**

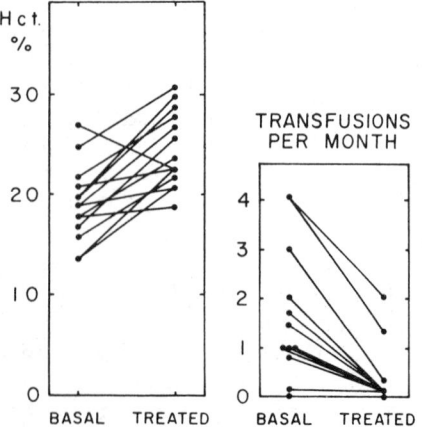

References

1. Bright, R.: Cases and observations, illustrative of renal disease accompanied with the secretion of albuminous urine. *Guys Hosp. Rep.* 1:340, 1836.
2. Erslev, A. J., and Shapiro, S. S.: Hematologic aspects of renal failure, in *Diseases of the Kidney*, edited by L. E. Earley and C. W. Gottschalk. Little, Brown, Boston, 1979, p. 277.
3. Ragen, P. A., Hagedorn, A. B., and Owen, C. A.: Radioisotope study of anemia in chronic renal disease. *Arch. Intern. Med.* 105:518, 1960.
4. Desforges, J. F., and Dawson, J. P.: The anemia of renal failure. *Arch. Intern. Med.* 101:326, 1958.
5. Joske, R. A., McAllister, J. M., and Prankerd, T. A. J.: Isotope investigations of red cell production and destruction in chronic renal disease. *Clin. Sci.* 15:511, 1956.
6. Kuroyanagi, T.: Anemia associated with chronic renal failure with special reference to kinetics of the erythron. *Acta Haematol. Jap.* 24:156, 1961.
7. Shaw, A. B.: Haemolysis in chronic renal failure. *Br. Med. J.* 2:213, 1967.
8. Adamson, J. W., Eschbach, J., and Finch, C. A.: The kidney and erythropoiesis. *Am. J. Med.* 44:725, 1968.
9. Berry, E. R., Rambach, W. A., Alt, H. L., and Del Greco, F.: Effect of peritoneal dialysis on erythrokinetics and ferrokinetics of azotemic anemia. *Trans. Am. Soc. Artif. Intern. Organs* 10:415, 1965.
10. Mansell, M., and Grimes, A. J.: Red and white cell abnormalities in chronic renal failure. *Br. J. Haematol.* 42:169, 1979.
11. Wallas, C. H.: Metabolic studies on the erythrocytes from patients with chronic renal disease on haemodialysis. *Br. J. Haematol.* 27:145, 1974.
12. Lonergan, E. T., et al.: Erythrocyte transketolase activity in dialyzed patients. A reversible metabolic lesion of uremia. *N. Eng. J. Med.* 284:1399, 1971.
13. Cole, C. H.: Decreased ouabain-sensitive adenine triphosphatase activity in the erythrocyte membrane of patients with chronic renal disease. *Clin. Sci.* 45:775, 1973.
14. Yawata, Y., Howe, R., and Jacob, H. S.: Abnormal red cell metabolism causing hemolysis in uremia: A defect potentiated by tap water hemodialysis. *Ann. Intern. Med.* 79:362, 1973.
15. Rosenwund, A., Binswanger, U., and Straub, P. W.: Oxidative injury to erythrocytes, cell rigidity, and splenic hemolysis in hemodialyzed uremic patients. *Ann. Intern. Med.* 82:460, 1975.
16. Eaton, J. W., Kolpin, C. F., Swofford, H. S., Kjellstrand, C. M., and Jacob, H. S.: Chlorinated urban water: A cause of dialysis-induced hemolytic anemia. *Science* 181:463, 1973.
17. Brain, M. C.: The haemolytic-uremic syndrome. *Semin. Hematol.* 6:162, 1969.
18. Bull, B. S., Rubenberg, M. L., Dacie, J. V., and Brain, M. C.: Microangiopathic hemolytic anemia: Mechanisms of red cell fragmentation. *Br. J. Haematol.* 14:643, 1968.
19. Capelli, J. P., Wesson, L. G., and Erslev, A. J.: Malignant hypertension and red cell fragmentation syndrome. *Ann. Intern. Med.* 64:128, 1966.
20. Gasser, C., Gautier, E., Steck, A., Siebenmann, R. E., and Oechslin, R.: Hämolytisch-urämische Syndrome. Bilaterale Nierenrindennekrosen bei akuten erworbenen hämolytischen Anämien. *Schweiz. Med. Wocehnschr.* 85:906, 1955.
21. Kaplan, B. S., and Drummond, K. N.: The hemolytic-uremic syndrome is a syndrome. *N. Engl. J. Med.* 298:964, 1978.
22. Lieberman, E., Heuser, E., Donnell, G. N., Landing, B. H., and Hammond, G. D.: Hemolytic-uremic syndrome: Clinical and pathological considerations. *N. Engl. J. Med.* 275:277, 1966.
23. Miller, R. P., and Denny, W. F.: Hemolytic anemia during acute renal failure: Observations on plasma erythropoietin levels. *South. Med. J.* 61:29, 1968.
24. Callen, J. R., and Limarzi, L. R.: Blood and bone marrow studies in renal disease. *Am. J. Clin. Pathol.* 20:3, 1950.
25. Loge, J. P., Lange, R. D., and Moore, C. V.: Characterization of the anemia associated with chronic renal insufficiency. *Am. J. Med.* 24:4, 1958.
26. Magid, E., and Hilden, M.: Ferrokinetics in patients suffering from chronic renal disease and anemia. *Scand. J. Haematol.* 4:33, 1967.
27. Finch, C. A., et al.: Ferrokinetics in man. *Medicine (Baltimore)* 49:17, 1970.
28. Lawson, D. H., Boddy, K., King, P. C., Linton, A. L., and Will, G.: Iron metabolism in patients with chronic renal failure on regular dialysis treatment. *Clin. Sci.* 41:345, 1971.
29. Fisher, J. W.: Mechanism of the anemia of chronic renal failure. *Nephron* 25:106, 1980.
30. Bozzini, C. E., Devoto, F. C. H., and Tomio, J. M.: Decreased responsiveness of hematopoietic tissue to erythropoietin in acutely uremic rats. *J. Lab. Clin. Med.* 68:411, 1966.
31. Van Dyke, D., Keighley, G., and Lawrence, J.: Decreased responsiveness to erythropoietin in a patient with anemia secondary to chronic uremia. *Blood* 22:838, 1963.
32. Larsen, O. A., Josephsen, P., and Lassen, N. A.: Nefrogen anaemi behandlet med erythropoietin. *Ugeskr. Laeger,* 125:435, 1963.
33. Eschbach, J. W., Funk, D., Adamson, J. W., Kuhn, I., Scribner, B. H., and Finch, C. A.: Erythropoiesis in patients with renal failure undergoing chronic dialysis. *N. Engl. J. Med.* 276:653, 1967.
34. Koch, K. M., Patyna, W. D., Shaldon, S., and Werner, E.: Anemia of the regular hemodialysis patient and its treatment. *Nephron* 12:405, 1974.
35. Zappacosta, A. R., Caro, J., and Erslev, A.: The normalization of hematocrit in end-stage renal disease patients on continuous ambulatory peritoneal dialysis: The role of erythropoietin. *Am. J. Med.* 72:53, 1982.
36. Fisher, J. W., Hatch, F. E., Roh, B. L., Allen, R. C., and Kelley, B. J.: Erythropoietin inhibitor in kidney extracts and plasma from anemic uremic human subjects. *Blood* 31:440, 1968.
37. Wallner, S. F., Kurnick, J., Ward, H., Vautrin, R., and Alfrey, A. C.: The anemia of chronic renal failure and chronic diseases: In vitro studies of erythropoiesis. *Blood* 47:561, 1976.
38. Ohno, Y., Rege, A. B., Fisher, J. W. and Barona, J.: Inhibitors of erythroid colony forming cells (CFU-E and BFU-E) in sera of azotemic patients with anemia of renal disease. *J. Lab. Clin. Med.* 92:916, 1978.
39. Radtke, H. W., et al.: Identification of spermine as an inhibitor of erythropoiesis in patients with chronic renal failure. *J. Clin. Invest.* 67:1623, 1981.
40. Barbour, G. L.: Effect of parathyroidectomy on anemia in chronic renal failure. *Arch. Intern. Med.* 139:889, 1979.
41. Massry, S. G.: Is parathyroid hormone a uremic toxin? *Nephron* 19:125, 1977.
42. Connelly, T. J., Caro, J., Erslev, A. J., and Silver, R.: The effect of a low phosphate diet on hematocrit and oxygen transport in uremic rats. *Am. J. Hematol.* 12:55, 1982.
43. Weinberg, S. G., Lubin, A., Wiener, S. N., Decras, M. P., Ghose, M. K., and Kopelman, R. C.: Myelofibrosis and renal osteodystrophy. *Am. J. Med.* 65:757, 1977.
44. Holken, A. G., and Marwah, P. K.: Iatrogenic contribution to anemia of renal failure. *Lancet* 1:164, 1971.
45. Eschbach, J. W., Cook, J. D., Scribner, B. H., and Finch, C. A.: Iron balance in hemodialysis patients. *Ann. Intern. Med.* 87:710, 1977.
46. Bock, H. F., Nieth, N., and Solth, K.: Anemia in renal failure. *Dtsch. Med. Wochenschr.* 87:573, 1962.
47. Rifkind, D., Kravetz, H. M., Knight, V., and Schade, A. L.: Urinary excretion of iron-binding protein in the nephrotic syndrome. *N. Engl. J. Med.* 265:115, 1961.
48. Hampers, C. L., Streiff, R., Nathan, D. K., Snyder, D., and Merrill, J. P.: Megaloblastic hematopoiesis in uremia and in patients on long-term hemodialysis. *N. Engl. J. Med.* 276:551, 1967.
49. Castaldi, P. A., Rozenberg, M. C., and Stewart, J. H.: The bleeding disorder of uremia: A qualitative platelet defect. *Lancet* 2:66, 1966.
50. Rabiner, S. F., and Drake, R. F.: Platelet function as an indicator of adequate dialysis. *Kidney Int.* [Suppl.] 2:5, 1975.
51. Rabiner, S. F.: Uremic bleeding, in *Progress in Hemostatis and Thrombosis*, edited by T. H. Spaet. Grune & Stratton, New York, 1972, p. 233.
52. Stewart, J. H.: Platelet numbers and life span in acute and chronic renal failure. *Thromb. Diath. Haemorrh.* 17:532, 1967.

53. Remuzzi, G., Cavenaghi, A. E., Mecca, G., Donati, M. B., and Gaetano, G.: Prostacyclin-like activity and bleeding in renal failure. *Lancet* 2:1195, 1977.

54. Horowitz, H. J., Stein, J. M., Cohen, B. D., and White, J. M.: Further studies on the platelet-inhibitory effect of guanidino succinic acid and its role in uremic bleeding. *Am. J. Med.* 49:336, 1970.

55. Jacobson, L. O., Goldwasser, E., Fried, W., and Plzak, L.: Role of the kidney in erythropoiesis. *Nature* 179:633, 1957.

56. Hansen, P.: Polycythemia produced by constriction of the renal artery of the rabbit. *Acta Pathol. Microbiol. Scand.* 60:465, 1964.

57. Fisher, J. W., and Samuels, A. J.: Relationship between renal blood flow and erythropoietin production. *Proc. Soc. Exp. Biol. Med.* 125:482, 1967.

58. Hudgson, P., Pearce, J. M., and Yeates, W. K.: Renal artery stenosis with hypertension and high hematocrit. *Br. Med. J.* 1:18, 1967.

59. Luke, R. G., Kennedy, A. C., Stirling, W. B., and McDonald, G. A.: Renal artery stenosis, hypertension and polycythemia. *Br. Med. J.* 1:164, 1965.

60. Abbrecht, P. H., Malvin, R. L., and Vander, A. J.: Renal production of erythropoietin and renin after experimental infarction. *Nature* 211:1318, 1966.

61. Mitus, W. J., Galbraith, P., Gallerken, M., and Toyana, K.: Experimental renal erythrocytosis. I. Effects of pressure and vascular interference. *Blood* 24:343, 1964.

62. Thorling, E. B.: Paraneoplastic erythrocytosis and inappropriate erythropoietin production. *Scand. J. Haemol. Suppl.* 17, 1972.

63. Westerman, M. P., Jenkins, J. L., Dekker, A., Kreutner, A., and Fisher, B.: Significance of erythrocytosis and increased erythropoietin secretion after renal transplantation. *Lancet* 2:755, 1967.

64. Busuttil, R. W., Roh, B. L., and Fisher, J. W.: Cytological localization of erythropoietin in the human kidney using the fluorescent antibody technique. *Proc. Soc. Exp. Biol. Med.* 137:327, 1971.

65. Mitus, W. J., Toyama, K., and Braner, M. J.: Erythrocytosis, juxtaglomerular apparatus (JGA) and erythropoietin in the course of experimental unilateral hydronephrosis in rabbits. *Ann. N.Y. Acad. Sci.* 149:107, 1968.

66. Gould, A. B., Goodman, S., DeWolf, R., Onesti, G., and Swartz, C.: Interrelations of the renin system and erythropoietin in rats. *J. Lab. Clin. Med.* 96:523, 1980.

67. Fried, W., et al.: Detection of high erythropoietin titers in renal extract from hypoxic rats. *J. Lab. Clin. Med.* 97:82, 1981.

68. Gordon, A. S., Cooper, G. W., and Zanjani, E. D.: The kidney and erythropoiesis. *Semin. Hematol.* 4:337, 1967.

69. Erslev, A. J.: In vitro production of erythropoietin by kidneys perfused with a serum-free solution. *Blood* 44:77, 1974.

70. Erslev, A. J.: Renal biogenesis of erythropoietin. *Am. J. Med.* 58:25, 1975.

71. Nathan, D. G., Schupack, E., Stohlman, F., Jr., and Merrill, J. P.: Erythropoiesis in anephric man. *J. Clin. Invest.* 43:2158, 1964.

72. Erslev, A. J., McKenna, P. J., Capelli, J. P., Hamburger, R. J., Cohen, H. E., and Clark, J. E.: Erythropoiesis in nephrectomized patients. *Arch. Intern. Med.* 122:230, 1968.

73. Mirand, E. A., Murphy, G. P., Steeves, R. A., Groenewald, J. M., and DeKlerk, J. N.: Erythropoietin activity in anephric, allotransplanted, unilaterally nephrectomized and intact man. *J. Lab. Clin. Med.* 73:121, 1969.

74. Fried, W., and Anagnostou, A.: Extrarenal erythropoietin production, in *Kidney Hormones*, edited by J. W. Fisher. Academic, New York, 1977, vol. 2, p. 231.

75. Naets, J. P., and Hense, A. F.: Measurement of erythropoietin stimulating factor in anemic patients with and without renal lesions. *J. Lab. Clin. Med.* 60:365, 1962.

76. Gral, T., Schroth, P., and Maxwell, M. H.: Plasma erythropoietic activity in patients on chronic dialysis with or without kidneys. *Trans. Am. Soc. Artif. Intern. Organs* 18:291, 1972.

77. Caro, J., Brown, S., Miller, O., Murray, T., and Erslev, A. J.: Erythropoietin levels in uremic and anephric patients. *J. Lab. Clin. Med.* 93:449, 1979.

78. Radtke, H. W., Claussner, A., Erbes, P. M., Scheuerman, E. H., Schoeppe, W., and Koch, K. M.: Serum erythropoietin concentration in chronic renal failure: Relationship to degree of anemia and excretory function. *Blood* 54:877, 1979.

79. Dagher, F. J., Ramas, E., Erslev, A. J., Alongi, S. V., Karmi, S. A., and Caro, J.: Are the native kidneys responsible for erythrocytosis in renal allorecipients. *Transplantation* 28:496, 1979.

80. Schwartz, S. O., and Motto, S. A.: The diagnostic significance of "burr" red blood cells. *Am. J. Med. Sci.* 218:563, 1949.

81. Brecher, G., and Bessis, M.: Present status of spiculed red cells and their relationship to the discocyte-echinocyte transformation: A critical review. *Blood* 40:333, 1972.

82. Weed, R.: The red membrane in hemolytic disorders: Plenary papers. *XII Congr. Int. Soc. Hematol.*, 1968, p. 81.

83. Torrance, J., Jacobs, P., Restrepo, A., Eschbach, J., Lenfant, C., and Finch, C. A.: Intraerythrocytic adaptation to anemia. *N. Engl. J. Med.* 283:165, 1970.

84. Blumberg, A., Scherrer, M., Marti, H. R., and Meyer, M.: Red cell organic phosphate levels and in vivo oxygen-hemoglobin dissociation in patients on maintenance dialysis with anaemia. *Blut* 22:109, 1971.

85. Chillar, R. K., and Desforges, J. F.: Red cell organic phosphates in patients with chronic renal failure on maintenance haemodialysis. *Br. J. Haematol.* 26:549, 1974.

86. Mitchell, T. R., and Pegrum, G. D.: The oxygen affinity of haemoglobin in chronic renal failure. *Br. J. Haematol.* 21:463, 1971.

87. Lichtman, M. A., Murphy, M. S., Whitbeck, A. A., and Kearney, E. A.: Oxygen binding to haemoglobin in subjects with hypoproliferative anaemia, with and without chronic renal disease: Role of pH. *Br. J. Haematol.* 27:439, 1974.

88. Lichtman, M. A., Miller, O. R., and Freeman, R. B.: Erythrocyte adenosine triphosphate depletion during hypophosphatemia in a uremic subject. *N. Engl. J. Med.* 280:240, 1969.

89. Torrance, J. D., Milne, F. J., Hurwitz, S., Zwi, S., and Rabkin, R.: Changes in oxygen delivery during hemodialysis. *Clin. Nephrol.* 3:53, 1975.

90. Hirszel, P., Maher, J. F., Tempel, G. E., and Mengel, C. E.: Effect of hemodialysis on factors influencing oxygen transport. *J. Lab. Clin. Med.* 85:978, 1975.

91. Goldblum, S. E., and Reed, W. P.: Host defenses and immunologic alterations associated with chronic hemodialysis. *Ann. Intern. Med.* 93:597, 1980.

92. Craddock, P. R., Fehr, J., Brigham, K. L., Kronenberg, R. S., and Jacob, H. S.: Complement and leukocyte-mediated pulmonary dysfunction in hemodialysis. *N. Engl. J. Med.* 296:769, 1977.

93. Pasternack, A., and Wahlberg, P.: Bone marrow in acute renal failure. *Acta. Med. Scand.* 181:505, 1967.

94. Erslev, A. J.: Management of the anemia of chronic renal failure. *Clin. Nephrol.* 2:174, 1974.

95. Birgegård, G., Nilsson, P., and Wide, L.: Regulation of iron therapy by S-ferritin estimations in patients on chronic hemodialysis. *Scand. J. Nephrol.* 15:59, 1981.

96. Lawson, D. H., Boddy, K., King, P. C., Linton, A. L., and Will, G.: Iron metabolism in patients with chronic renal failure on regular dialysis treatment. *Clin. Sci.* 41:345, 1971.

97. Hartley, R. A., Morgan, T. O., Innis, M. D., and Climie, G. J. A.: Splenectomy for anemia in patients on regular dialysis. *Lancet* 2:1343, 1971.

98. Opelz, G., and Terasaki, P. J.: Dominant effect of transfusions on kidney graft survival. *Transplantation* 29:153, 1980.

99. Janson, P. A., Jubelirer, S. J., Weinstein, M. J., and Deykin, D.: Treatment of the bleeding tendency in uremia with cryoprecipitate. *N. Engl. J. Med.* 303:1318, 1980.

100. Gardner, F. H.: The use of cobaltous chloride in the anemia associated with chronic renal disease. *J. Lab. Clin. Med.* 41:46, 1953.

101. Eschbach, J. W., and Adamson, J. W.: Improvement in the anemia of chronic renal failure with fluoxymesterone. *Ann. Intern. Med.* 78:527, 1973.

102. Hendler, E. D., Goffinet, J. A., Ross, S., Longnecker, R. E., and Bakovic, V.: Controlled study of androgen therapy in anemia of patients on maintenance hemodialysis. *N. Engl. J. Med.* 291:1046, 1975.

103. Buchwald, D., et al.: Effect of nandrolone decanoate on the anemia of chronic hemodialysis patients. *Nephron* 18:232, 1977.

104. Shahidi, N. T.: Anabolic androgenic hormones. *Am. J. Med.* 62:546, 1977.

105. Neff, M. S., et al.: A comparison of androgens for anemia in patients on hemodialysis. N. Engl. J. Med. 304:871, 1981.
106. Dameshek, W., (ed.): Panels in therapy. V. The use of cobalt and cobalt-iron preparations in the therapy of anemia. Blood 10:852, 1955.
107. Essers, U., Müller, W., and Brunner, E.: Zur Wirkung von Erythropoietin bei Gesunden und bei Patienten mit chronischer Urämie. Klin. Wochenschr. 51:1005, 1973.

CHAPTER *45*

Anemia of endocrine disorders

ALLAN J. ERSLEV

Many hormones are involved in the regulation and function of the erythropoietic tissue, and patients lacking such hormones frequently exhibit erythroid hypoplasia and anemia. In the first place, red blood cell production is controlled by the renal hormone erythropoietin, and the characteristic anemia of renal disease (see Chap. 44) is caused in part by impaired renal endocrine function. Second, the production of renal erythropoietin is controlled by the tissue tension of oxygen, which in turn is influenced by the hormonal equilibrium of the body. Third, in addition to enzymes and metabolic building blocks, certain hormones are essential for the synthesis of hemoglobin and other red cell constituents.

The endocrine glands most often involved in the development of erythroid hypoplasia are the pituitary, the thyroid, the adrenals, and the gonads.

Anemia of pituitary deficiency

Hypophysectomy in the experimental animal is regularly followed by the development of a moderately severe erythroid hypoplasia and anemia [1,2]. In rats, the selective removal of the posterior or intermediate lobe does not cause anemia [3], and it is generally assumed that the pathogenesis of this form of anemia is related to the absence of anterior lobe hormones, which in turn modulate renal erythropoietin production [4]. Of these, the thyroid-stimulating hormone (TSH) is probably of most importance, since the anemia of hypophysectomy is very similar to the anemia of thyroidectomy [5]. Nevertheless, it is claimed that the rate of red cell production in hypophysectomized animals is restored to normal only if the administration of TSH is supplemented by ACTH [6] or if the administration of thyroid hormone is supplemented by both corticosteroids and androgens [1]. It has been proposed repeatedly that the pituitary gland produces a specific erythropoietic hormone [7,8], but the therapeutic effectiveness of target organ hormones alone is not in accord with such a possibility.

Growth hormone [9–11] has been shown to be capable of stimulating red cell production, but whether or not this effect is of physiologic significance remains unclear [12]. The same holds true for the hypothetical effect of the hypothalamus on red cell production. It has been claimed that hypothalamic injury may affect either erythropoietin release [13], the rate of red cell production [14], or both [15], and it has been proposed that these effects are mediated via the hypophysis. However, the experimental data provided in support of this hypothesis are somewhat conflicting and need confirmation.

In human subjects, hypophyseal dysfunction or hypophyseal ablation is often associated with a leukopenia and regularly accompanied by a normochromic and normocytic anemia. The red cell life-span is normal, but marrow examination and ferrokinetic studies disclose moderate hypoplasia and relative marrow failure [16,17]. Replacement therapy with a combination of thyroid, adrenal, and gonadal hormones usually corrects the anemia [18,19].

Anemia of thyroid dysfunction

In 1881, Charcot [20] first recognized that cretins and patients with myxedema were anemic. At about the same time, the great Swiss surgeon Kocher [21] reported that thyroidectomy also is followed by a reduction in the red cell count. The character of this type of anemia has been a source of debate ever since, and it has been variously described as normocytic, microcytic, or macrocytic [22]. Recent studies have clarified the pathogenesis by separating the component caused by a lack of thyroid hormone from the components caused by complicating deficiencies of iron, vitamin B_{12}, or folic acid [23–25].

Animal studies have shown that the rate of red cell production increases after the administration of thyroxin, triiodothyronine, or desiccated thyroid [26,27] and decreases after thyroidectomy [28,29]. These erythropoietic responses appear to be quite appropriate, since the need for circulating red cells depends on the cellular requirements for oxygen, which in turn are influenced by thyroid hormones [27,30].

Although studies of the response of hypertransfused and nephrectomized animals to thyroid hormone indicate that the effect is related to aerobic cellular metabolism and to the release of renal erythropoietin [31], it has also been proposed that the thyroid hormones have a noncalorigenic effect on red cell production [32]. Recent studies of the influence of thyroid hormones on in vitro erythropoiesis have shown that both calorigenic T_3 and T_4 and noncalorigenic rT_3 potentiate the effect of erythropoietin on the formation of erythroid colonies [33,34]. This effect appears to be mediated by receptors with β_2-adrenergic properties [34]. Anemia observed in thyroidectomized animals conforms to both mechanisms by being normochromic and normocytic and associated with reticulocytopenia and hypoplasia of the erythropoietic tissue in the marrow. The red cell lifespan is normal, and ferrokinetic studies indicate the existence of a hypofunctioning but effective marrow [35].

Anemia observed in human subjects with myxedema or other hypothyroid conditions is not always this clearcut, since the condition may be complicated by nutritional deficiencies. However, many hypothyroid patients have a hypoplastic anemia which is unresponsive to therapy with iron, vitamin B_{12}, or folic acid and is very similar to the form of anemia observed in thyroidectomized animals [22,23]. The degree of anemia is mild to moderate, with a hemoglobin concentration rarely less than 8 to 9 g/dl. The corresponding decrease in erythroid marrow activity is frequently too small to be morphologically demonstrable [36]. Ferrokinetic studies show a decrease in the turnover of plasma and red cell iron, a decrease which also may be so small that it is first recognized when compared with values obtained after thyroid replacement therapy [37,38]. As in hypothyroid animals, the red cell life-span and the rate of red cell utilization are normal. The degree of anemia does not always reflect the reduction in marrow activity and the size of the red cell mass, since the plasma volume is decreased in hypothyroid patients [39]. This may result in a temporary aggravation of apparent anemia after thyroid replacement therapy, since the plasma volume will be restored to normal before the red cell mass.

Although normochromic and normocytic anemia must be considered the characteristic form of anemia of hypothyroidism, the most frequent type of anemia observed is a microcytic, hypochromic anemia caused by iron deficiency [22,40]. In hypothyroid women, menorrhagia is a frequent complication and may explain adequately the lack of iron. However, even in men, iron is in short supply either because of the histamine refractory achlorhydria, which is present in about 50 percent of anemic patients [41], or possibly because of intestinal malabsorption of iron [42,43].

Macrocytosis is frequently identified with anemia of hypothyroidism [22]. However, a true increase in the mean corpuscular volume occurs in less than 10 percent of the patients, and in these cases it is usually caused by a megaloblastic erythropoiesis owing to vitamin B_{12} or folic acid deficiency [23]. In hypothyroid patients, the incidence of true pernicious anemia with gastric atrophy and intrinsic factor deficiency has been claimed to be unusually high. This has led to interesting but still inconclusive speculations on the effect of cross-reacting antibodies against thyroglobulins and intrinsic factor or gastric parietal cells [44–46]. However, in a study of eight patients with coexisting megaloblastic anemia and hypothyroidism, it was concluded that all eight, rather than having vitamin B_{12} deficiency, had folic acid deficiency, from either poor dietary intake of folic acid or intestinal malabsorption [25].

Despite the direct and indirect erythropoietic effect of thyroid hormones, patients with hyperthyroidism or thyrotoxicosis rarely have elevated hemoglobin concentrations or hematocrit percentages [39,47,48]. This absence of an expected secondary polycythemia has been explained by assuming that an increased cardiac output and rate of tissue perfusion meet the increased tissue requirements for oxygen. Conflicting data have been presented as to the effect of thyroid hormone in vitro on the intracellular concentration of 2,3-diphosphoglycerate and in turn the oxygen affinity of hemoglobin [49,50]. So far, however, direct studies of hyperthyroid patients do not suggest the presence of enhanced oxygen transport to the tissues [51]. It actually seems more likely that the absence of an overt secondary polycythemia is due to hemodilution. Direct measurements of the size of the red cell mass [39], the erythroid activity of the marrow [36], and the turnover of plasma and red cell iron [47] find them above normal, and if it was not for the concomitant increase in plasma volume, these patients would have elevated hemoglobin and hematocrit levels. Studies of the red cell-life span in patients with thyrotoxicosis suggest a moderate shortening in red cell survival [52], a result in curious conflict with animal studies indicating that the thyroid hormones have no effect on red cell life-span [53]. In a few cases, severe hyperthyroidism has been found to be associated with anemia and abnormal iron utilization, apparently reflecting ineffective red cell production [40]. The institution of radioiodine therapy results in a reduction in the size of the red cell mass to normal but only a slight change in the hematocrit percentage.

Anemia of adrenal dysfunction

Adrenalectomy in experimental animals causes a mild anemia responsive to therapy with adrenal corticoids or erythropoietin [16,28,54]. A similar type of normochromic, normocytic anemia has been observed in Addison's disease [16,55], but because of the concomitant reduction in plasma volume, the hemoglobin concentration and the hematocrit percentage do not reflect the true decrease in red cell mass. The character of this type of anemia and the erythropoietic effect of physiologic amounts of ACTH or adrenal cortical hormones are still unclear, possibly because the changes involved are too small for adequate study. When administered in pharmacologic amounts, these hormones appear to cause mild erythrocytosis [56] of about the same magnitude as that observed in Cushing's disease [57,58]. However, whether this is mediated via release of renal erythropoietin or by direct action on the erythropoietic cells in the marrow is unknown.

Anemia of gonadal dysfunction

The erythropoietic effect of androgens in both physiologic and pharmacologic dosages is well recognized and extensively utilized in the treatment of patients with various types of refractory anemia.

Castration of the male experimental animal causes a decrease in the rate of red cell production until the hemoglobin concentration and the red cell mass become stabilized at levels approximately the same as those of the normal female [59,60]. In sexually mature human males, the hemoglobin is 1 to 2 g/dl higher than the level observed in males during childhood, advanced age, or gonadal hypofunction. Under those circumstances, the hemoglobin level is similar to that of the normal human female [61–63].

In pharmacologic doses, androgens have been shown to stimulate red cell production [64] by increasing the production of erythropoietin [65,66] and by enhancing the effect of erythropoietin on the marrow [67]. These actions have been attributed to two isomeric metabolites formed by the reduction of a $4{=\!=}5$ double bond. The 5α-H isomer is androgenic and believed to cause a release of erythropoietin from the kidney [68]. The 5β-H isomer is not androgenic or erythropoietinogenic but is believed to cause inactive marrow stem cells to enter an erythropoietin-responsive phase [69].

Studies on the effect of physiologic doses of estrogens suggest that these hormones cause a slight suppression of red cell production [70]. In large doses, estrogens have been shown to cause the development of moderately severe anemia [71,72], but it has not been resolved whether this is caused by suppressed erythropoietin production [72] or inhibition of the stem cell action of erythropoietin [73].

Human placental lactogen and sheep prolactin have been shown to have erythropoietic activity in the mouse [74], but the physiologic significance of these observations is still unknown [75].

Anemia of pregnancy

Although pregnancy obviously cannot be classified as an endocrine disorder, some aspects of anemia in pregancy have been attributed to changes in the hormonal environment.

Studies of pregnant mice have shown that despite a progressive decrease in hematocrit, the erythropoietin secretion, the rate of red cell production, and the total red cell mass increase during pregnancy [74,75]. It has been suggested that placental lactogen, which is erythropoietically active in the mouse [76], may in part be responsible for the erythropoietic stimulation, but the exact hormonal mechanisms underlying both the increase in red cell mass and the even more pronounced increase in plasma volume are unknown. It is possible that the increase in plasma volume is the initiating event causing hypervolemia and the establishment of a new oxygen transport curve [77] (see Fig. 8-5). Although the red cell mass may be adequate in terms of oxygen transport, the hypervolemia will establish it as suboptimal, and the rate of red cell production will be adjusted upward in order to approach the optimal level for the blood volume [77].

In human subjects, anemia in pregnancy is most often caused or aggravated by a concomitant iron deficiency [78,79]. In a smaller number of cases, folic acid deficiency may also play a pathogenetic role [80], and it seems appropriate to give every pregnant woman preventive iron and folic acid supplements. However, even in the well-cared-for pregnant woman, anemia becomes manifest at about the eighth week of pregnancy, progresses slowly until the thirty-second to thirty-fourth week, and is then stable until it rather suddenly improves just before delivery [81,82]. It is moderate in severity, with hemoglobin concentrations rarely below 10 g/dl, and careful studies of the red cell mass have shown conclusively that it is a dilution anemia [81,82]. The red cell volume actually increases during pregnancy by about 20 percent, but the average increase in plasma volume is approximately 30 percent. The red cell lifespan has been found to be normal, and the increase in red cell mass is a reflection of increased marrow erythropoiesis, as demonstrated by plasma and red cell iron turnover studies [83]. Although the hemoglobin concentration is decreased, the hypervolemic state ensures the tissues, and particularly the uterus, of excellent blood perfusion and oxygen supply.

Anemia of parathyroid dysfunction

Primary hyperparathyroidism is occasionally (12 of 57 patients in one series [84]) associated with anemia which disappears after parathyroidectomy [85,86]. Similarly, it has been reported that parathyroidectomy in chronic renal disease often results in some improvement in the anemia [87,88], and it has been suggested that the parathyroid hormone may be a toxin which can suppress normal red cell production [88]. It appears more likely, however, that primary or secondary hyperparathyroidism, when associated with suppressed red cell production, acts by causing either renal calcification with reductions in erythropoietin formation or marrow sclerosis with reduction in erythroid proliferation [89].

References

1. Crafts, R. C., and Meineke, H. A.: The anemia of hypophysectomized animals. *Ann. N.Y. Acad. Sci.* 77:501, 1959.
2. Gordon, A. S.: Endocrine influences upon the formed elements of blood and blood forming organs. *Progn. Hormone Res.* 10:339, 1954.
3. Van Dyke, D. C., Garcia, J. F., Simpson, M. E., Huff, R. L., Contopoulos, A. N., and Evans, H. M.: Maintenance of circulating red cell volume in rats after removal of the posterior and intermediate lobes of the pituitary. *Blood* 7:1017, 1952.

4. Peschle, C., et al.: Role of hypophysis in erythropoietin production during hypoxia. *Blood* 51:1117, 1978.

5. Crafts, R. C.: The similarity between anemia induced by hypophysectomy and that induced by a combined thyroidectomy and adrenalectomy in adult female rats. *Endocrinology* 53:465, 1953.

6. Fisher, J. W., and Crook, J. J.: Influence of several hormones on erythropoiesis and oxygen consumption in the hypophysectomized rat. *Blood* 19:557, 1962.

7. Contopoulos, A. N., Simpson, M. E., Van Dyke, D. C., Ellis, S., Lawrence, J. H., and Evans, H. M.: The pituitary erythropoietic factor. *Anat. Rec.* 118:290, 1954.

8. Lindeman, R., Trygstad, O., and Halvorsen, S.: Pituitary control of erythropoiesis. *Scand. J. Haematol.* 6:77, 1969.

9. Fruhman, G. J., Gerstner, R., and Gordon, A. S.: Effects of growth hormone upon erythropoiesis in the hypophysectomized rat. *Proc. Soc. Exp. Med.* 85:93, 1954.

10. Meineke, H. A., and Crafts, R. C.: Further observations on the mechanism by which androgens and growth hormone influence erythropoiesis. *Ann. N.Y. Acad. Sci.* 149:298, 1968.

11. Jepson, J. H., and McGarry, E. E.: Hemopoiesis in pituitary dwarfs treated with human growth hormone and testosterone. *Blood* 39:238, 1972.

12. Halvorsen, S.: Effects of growth hormone on erythropoiesis in the intact rabbit and the polycythemic mouse. *Acta Physiol. Scand.* 66:203, 1966.

13. Halvorsen, S.: Effect of hypothalamic stimulation on erythropoiesis and on the production of erythropoiesis-stimulating factors in intact and nephrectomized rabbits. *Ann. N.Y. Acad. Sci.* 149:88, 1968.

14. Feldman, S., Rachmilewitz, E. A., and Izak, G.: The effect of central nervous system stimulation on erythropoiesis in rats with chronically implanted electrodes. *J. Lab. Clin. Med.* 67:713, 1966.

15. Mirand, E. A., Grace, J. T., Johnston, G. S., and Murphy, G. P.: Effect of hypothalamic stimulation on the erythropoietic response in the rhesus monkey. *Nature* 204:1163, 1964.

16. Daughaday, W. H., Williams, R. H., and Daland, G. A.: The effect of endocrinopathies on the blood. *Blood* 3:1342, 1948.

17. Degrossi, O. J., Houssay, A. B., Varela, J. E., and Capalbo, E. E.: Erythrokinetic studies in the anemia of thyroid and pituitary insufficiency, in *Advance in Thyroid Research.* Pergamon, New York, 1961, p. 410.

18. Ferrari, E., Ascari, E., Bossoto, P. A., and Barosi, G.: Sheehan's syndrome with complete bone marrow aplasia: Long term results of substitution therapy with hormones. *Br. J. Haematol.* 33:575, 1976.

19. Daughaday, W. H.: The adeno hypophysis, in *Textbook of Endocrinology*, 4th ed., edited by R. H. Williams, Saunders, Philadelphia, 1968, p. 59.

20. Charcot, M.: Myxedéme, cachexie pachydermique ou état cretinoide. *Gaz. Hop. Paris* 54:73, 1881.

21. Kocher, T.: Ueber Kropfexstirpation und Ihre Folgen. *Arch. Klin. Chir.* 29:254, 1883.

22. Bomford, R.: Anemia in myxoedema and the role of the thyroid gland in erythropoiesis. *Q. J. Med.* 7:495, 1938.

23. Tudhope, G. R., and Wilson, G. M.: Anemia in hypothyroidism incidence, pathogenesis and response to treatment. *Q. J. Med.* 29:513, 1960.

24. Carpenter, J. T., Mohler, D. N., Jr., Thorup, O. A., Jr., and Leavell, B. S.: Anemia in myxedema, in *Current Concepts in Hypothyroidism*, edited by K. R. Crispell. Macmillan, New York, 1963, p. 147.

25. Hines, J. D., Halsted, C. H., Griggs, R. C., and Harris, J. W.: Megaloblastic anemia secondary to folate deficiency associated with hypothyroidism. *Ann. Intern. Med.* 68:792, 1968.

26. Donati, R. M., Warnecke, M. A., and Gallagher, N. J.: Effect of triiodothyronine administration on erythrocyte radio iron incorporation in rats. *Proc. Soc. Exp. Biol. Med.* 115:405, 1964.

27. Chalet, M., Coe, D., and Reissmann, K. R.: Mechanisms of erythropoietic action of thyroid hormone. *Proc. Soc. Exp. Biol. Med.* 123:443, 1966.

28. Crafts, R. C.: The effect of endocrines on the formed elements of the blood. I. The effects of hypophysectomy, thyroidectomy and adrenalectomy on the blood of the adult female rat. *Endocrinology* 29:596, 1941.

29. Gordon, A. S., Kadow, P. C., Finkelstein, G., and Charipper, H. A.: The thyroid and blood regeneration in the rat. *Am. J. Med. Sci.* 212:385, 1946.

30. Jacobson, L. O., Goldwasser, E., Gurney, C. W., Fried, W., and Plzak, L.: Studies on erythropoietin: The hormone regulating red cell production. *Ann. N.Y. Acad. Sci.* 77:551, 1959.

31. Lucarelli, G., et al.: The effect of triiodothyronine on the erythropoiesis: Assay in the normal, starved, polycythemic and nephrectomized rat. *Biochim. Biol. Sper.* 5:475, 1966.

32. Meineke, H. A., and Crafts, R. C.: Evidence for a noncalorigenic effect of thyroxin on erythropoiesis as judged by radio iron utilization. *Proc. Soc. Exp. Biol. Med.* 117:520, 1964.

33. Golde, D. W., Bersch, N., Chopra, J. J., and Cline, M. J.: Thyroid hormones stimulate erythropoiesis in vitro. *Br. J. Haematol.* 37:173, 1977.

34. Popovic, W. J., Brown, J. E., and Adamson, J. W.: The influence of thyroid hormones on in vitro erythropoiesis. Mediation by a receptor with beta adrenergic properties. *J. Clin. Invest.* 60:907, 1977.

35. Cline, M. J., and Berlin, N. I.: Erythropoiesis and red cell survival in the hypothyroid dog. *Am. J. Physiol.* 204:415, 1963.

36. Axelrod, A. R., and Berman, L.: The bone marrow in hyperthyroidism and hypothyroidism. *Blood* 6:436, 1951.

37. Kiely, J. M., Purnell, D. C., and Owen, C. A., Jr.: Erythrokinetics in myxedema. *Ann. Intern. Med.* 67:533, 1967.

38. Finch, C. A., et al.: Ferrokinetics in man. *Medicine (Baltimore)* 49:17, 1970.

39. Muldowney, F. P., Crooks, J., and Wayne, E. J.: The total red cell mass in thyrotoxicosis and myxoedema. *Clin. Sci.* 16:309, 1957.

40. Larsson, S. D.: Anemia and iron metabolism in hypothyroidism. *Acta. Med. Scand.* 157:349, 1967.

41. Lerman, J., and Means, J. H.: The gastric secretion in exophthalmic goiter and myxoedema. *J. Clin. Invest.* 11:167, 1932.

42. Pirzio-Biroli, G., Bothwell, T. H., and Finch, C. A.: Iron absorption. II. The absorption of radio iron administered with standard meal. *J. Lab. Clin. Med.* 51:37, 1958.

43. Donati, R. M., Fletcher, J. W., Warnecke, M. A., and Gallagher, N. J.: Erythropoiesis in hypothyroidism. *Proc. Soc. Exp. Biol. Med.* 144:78, 1973.

44. Irvine, W. J., Davies, S. H., Delamore, J. W., and Williams, A. W.: Immunologic relationship between pernicious anemia and thyroid disease. *Br. Med. J.* 2:454, 1962.

45. Markson, J. L., and Moore, J. M.: Thyroid antibodies in pernicious anemia. *Br. Med. J.* 2:1352, 1962.

46. Ardeman, S., Chanarin, I., Krafchik, B., and Singer, W.: Addisonian pernicious anemia and intrinsic factor antibodies in thyroid disorders. *Q. J. Med.* 35:421, 1966.

47. Donati, R. M., Warnecke, M. A., and Gallagher, N. J.: Ferrokinetics in hyperthyroidism. *Ann. Intern. Med.* 63:945, 1963.

48. Rivlin, R. S., and Wagner, H. N.: Anemia in hyperthyroidism. *Ann. Intern. Med.* 70:507, 1969.

49. Beutler, E., and West, C.: The effect of thyroid hormones, sodium sulfite and other compounds on red cell 2,3-DPG levels in vitro. *Int. Res. Comm. Sys.* 1973.

50. Miller, W. W., Delivoria-Papadopoulos, M., Miller, L. D., and Oski, F. A.: Oxygen releasing factor in hypothyroidism. *JAMA* 211:1824, 1970.

51. Zaroulis, C. G., Kourides, J. A., and Valeri, C. R.: Red cell 2,3-diphosphoglycerate and oxygen affinity of hemoglobin in patients with thyroid disorders. *Blood* 52:181, 1978.

52. McClellan, J. E., Donegan, C., Thorup, O. A., and Leavell, B. S.: Survival time of the erythrocyte in myxedema and hyperthyroidism. *J. Lab. Clin. Med.* 51:91, 1958.

53. Waldman, T. A., Weissman, S. M., and Levin, E. H.: Effect of thyroid administration on erythropoiesis in the dog. *J. Lab. Clin. Med.* 59:926, 1962.

54. Van Dyke, D. C., Contopoulos, A. N., Williams, B. S., Simpson, M. E., Lawrence, J. H., and Evans, M. H.: Hormonal factors influencing erythropoiesis. *Acta Haematol. (Basel)* 11:203, 1954.

55. Báez-Villasenor, J., Rath, C. E., and Finch, C. A.: The blood picture in Addison's disease. *Blood* 3:769, 1948.

56. Fisher, J. W.: Increase in circulating red cell volume of normal rats

after treatment with hydrocortisone or cortico-sterone. *Proc. Soc. Exp. Biol. Med.* 97:502, 1958.

57. Thompson, K. W., and Eisenhardt, L.: Further consideration of the Cushing's syndrome. *J. Clin. Endorcinol. Metab.* 3:445, 1943.
58. Platz, C. M., Knowlton, A. J., and Ragan, C.: The natural history of Cushing's syndrome. *Am. J. Med.* 13:597, 1952.
59. Steinglass, P., Gordon, A. S., and Charipper, H. A.: Effect of castration and sex hormones on blood of the rat. *Proc. Soc. Exp. Biol. Med.* 48:169, 1941.
60. Crafts, R. C.: Effect of hypophysectomy, castration and testosterone propionate on hemopoiesis in the adult male rat. *Endocrinology* 39:401, 1946.
61. Hawkins, W. W., Speck, E., and Leonard, V. G.: Variation of the hemoglobin level with age and sex. *Blood* 9:999, 1954.
62. Leichenring, J. M., Norris, L. M., Lamison, S. A., and Halbert, M. L.: Blood cell values for healthy adolescence. *Am. J. Dis. Child.* 90:159, 1955.
63. McCullagh, E. P., and Jones, T. R.: Effects of androgens on the blood count of man. *J. Clin. Endocrinol.* 2:243, 1942.
64. Shahidi, N. T.: Androgens and erythropoiesis. *N. Engl. J. Med.* 289:72, 1973.
65. Rishpon-Meyerstein, N., Kilbridge, T., Simone, J., and Fried, W.: The effect of testosterone on erythropoietin levels in anemic patients. *Blood* 31:453, 1968.
66. Alexanian, R.: Erythropoietin and erythropoiesis in anemic man following androgens. *Blood* 33:564, 1969.
67. Naets, J. P., and Wittek, M.: The mechanism of action of androgens on erythropoiesis. *Ann. N.Y. Acad. Sci.* 149:366, 1968.
68. Paulo, L. G., Fink, G. D., Roh, B. L., Fisher, J. W.: Effects of several androgens and steroid metabolites on erythropoietin production in the isolated perfused dog kidney. *Blood* 43:39, 1974.
69. Gorshein, D., Hait, W. N., Besa, E. C., Jepson, J. H., and Gardner, F. H.: Rapid stem cell differentiation induced by 19-nortestosterone decanoate. *Br. J. Haematol.* 26:215, 1974.
70. Dukes, P. P., and Goldwasser, E.: Inhibition of erythropoiesis by estrogens. *Endocrinology* 69:21, 1961.
71. Tyslowitz, R., and Dingemanse, E.: Effect of large doses of estrogen on the blood picture of dogs. *Endocrinology* 29:817, 1941.
72. Piliero, S. J., Medici, P. T., and Haber, C.: The interrelationships of the endocrine and erythropoietic systems in the rat with special reference to the mechanism of action of estradiol and testosterone. *Ann. N.Y. Acad. Sci.* 149:336, 1968.
73. Jepson, J. H., and Lowenstein, L.: Inhibition of the stem-cell action of erythropoietin by estradiol. *Proc. Soc. Exp. Biol. Med.* 123:457, 1966.
74. Jepson, J. H., and Lowenstein, L.: Hormonal control of erythropoiesis during pregnancy in the mouse. *Br. J. Haematol.* 14:555, 1968.
75. Fruhman, G. J.: Blood formation in the pregnant mouse. *Blood* 31:242, 1968.
76. Jepson, J. H., and Lowenstein, L.: The effect of testosterone, adrenal steroids and prolactin on erythropoiesis. *Acta Haematol. (Basel)* 38:292, 1970.
77. Thorling, E. B., and Erslev, A. J.: The "tissue" tension of oxygen and its relation to hematocrit and erythropoiesis. *Blood* 31:332, 1968.
78. Benjamin, F., Bassen, F. A., and Meyer, L. M.: Serum levels of folic acid, vitamin B_{12} and iron in anemia of pregnancy. *Am. J. Obstet. Gynecol.* 96:310, 1966.
79. Pritchard, J. A., and Hunt, C. F.: A comparison of the hematologic responses following the routine prenatal administration of intramuscular and oral iron. *Surg. Gynecol. Obstet.* 106:516, 1958.
80. Alperin, J. B., Hutchinson, H. T., and Levin, W. C.: Studies of folic acid requirements in megaloblastic anemia of pregnancy. *Arch. Intern. Med.* 117:681, 1966.
81. Low, J. A., Johnston, E. E., and McBride, R. L.: Blood volume adjustments in the normal obstetric patient with particular reference to the third trimester of pregnancy. *Am. J. Obstet. Gynecol.* 91:356, 1965.
82. Pritchard, J. A.: Changes in the blood volume during pregnancy and delivery. *Anesthesiology* 26:393, 1965.
83. Pritchard, J. A., and Adams, R. H.: Erythrocyte production and destruction during pregnancy. *Am. J. Obstet. Gynecol.* 79:750, 1960.
84. Malette, L. E., Bilezikian, J. P., Heath, D. A., and Aurbach, G. D.: Primary hyperparathyroidism: Clinical and biochemical features. *Medicine (Baltimore)* 53:127, 1974.
85. Boxer, H., Ellman, L., Geller, R., and Wang, Chi-An.: Anemia in primary hyperparathyroidism. *Arch. Intern. Med.* 137:588, 1977.
86. Falco, J. M., Guy, J. T., Smith, R. E., and Mazzaferri, E. L.: Primary hyperthyroidism and anemia. *Arch. Intern. Med.* 136:887, 1976.
87. Zingraff, J., et al.: Anemia and secondary hyperparathyroidism. *Arch. Intern. Med.* 138:1650, 1978.
88. Massey, S. G.: Is parathyroid hormone a uremic toxin? *Nephron* 19:125, 1977.
89. Slackman, N., Green, A. A., and Naiman, J. L.: Myelofibrosis in children with chronic renal insufficiency. *J. Pediatr.* 87:720, 1975.

CHAPTER 46

The congenital dyserythropoietic anemias

WILLIAM N. VALENTINE

The term *congenital dyserythropoietic anemia* (CDA) has been applied [1–3] to a group of hereditary refractory anemias characterized by ineffective erythropoiesis, erythroid multinuclearity, and secondary tissue siderosis. The ineffective erythropoiesis has been documented in terms of increased plasma iron turnover, diminished incorporation of tracer iron into circulating red cells, elevated fecal stercobilin level, increased endogenous carbon monoxide production (presumably derived from heme catabolism), intense marrow erythroid hyperplasia, and normal or at most slightly elevated absolute reticulocyte counts. Mild increases in indirect-reacting serum bilirubin, splenomegaly, and variably severe anemia are present. The life-span of circulating erythrocytes may be normal to moderately shortened, but dyserythropoiesis with a large component of intramedullary cell death is the dominant factor in pathogenesis. The term *dyserythropoiesis* broadens the concept of "ineffective erythropoiesis" [4]. The latter implies intramedullary cell destruction, a decrease in the number of circulating erythrocytes derived from each progenitor, with a discrepancy between red cells discharged into the blood and the erythroid content of marrow. *Dyserythropoiesis* expands on these kinetic features and incorporates data relative to abnormalities in morphology, membrane characteristics, antigenic makeup, serologic reactions, and enzymatic activities occurring as a result of the dysplastic marrow erythroid cells. The causes of these syndromes are unknown. It has been proposed that three types of CDA can be distinguished [5] (Table 46-1).

TABLE 46-1   Congenital dyserythropoietic anemia, types I, II, III — marrow and serologic features

| | Marrow | | |
CDA Type	Light microscopy	Electron microscopy	Serology
I	Most erythroid cells abnormal: megaloblastoid changes; large cells with incompletely divided nuclear segments; double nuclei; internuclear chromatin bridges	Widened nuclear pores, cytoplasmic invasion of nucleus, disaggregation of ribosomes, and presence of cytoplasmic microtubules	No serologic abnormalities
II "HEMPAS"	Late polychromatophilic and orthochromic erythroblasts often contain 2 to 7 normal-appearing nuclei	Excess endoplasmic reticulum appearing as a double cell membrane	Cell possess unique "HEMPAS" antigen and are lysed by 30% of acidified normal sera; increased agglutination by anti-i, increased lysis by anti-I
III	Giant erythroblasts, up to 50 μm in diameter, with up to 12 nuclei; prominent basophilic stippling	Clefts and blebs within nuclear region, autolytic areas in cytoplasm, some iron-filled mitochondria, and myelin figures	Data inadequate: a single case showed increased agglutination by anti-i and increased lysis by anti-I, but a negative acidified serum test

CDA type I [2,3,6–16]

This rare disorder of hematopoiesis, first manifested in infancy or adolescence, is characterized by slight hyperbilirubinemia, moderate anemia (hematocrit usually 25 to 36 percent), and commonly, splenomegaly. The level of serum haptoglobin is low; that of serum iron is normal or high. The red cell morphologic picture is characterized by well-marked aniso- and poikilocytosis and slight to moderate macrocytosis. The intensely cellular erythroid marrow shows megaloblastoid features [2,3,6]. By light microscopy, the majority of erythroblasts are seen to have varying degrees of abnormality. In particular, three forms of morphologic aberrations have been regarded as typical [6]: (1) very large cells containing an irregularly shaped nuclear mass with two nuclear segments suggesting incomplete nuclear division (1 to 2 percent of erythroblasts), (2) double nucleated cells in which the two nuclei differ in size, structure, and stainability (0.3 to 0.8 percent of erythroblasts), and (3) pairs of erythroblasts connected by thin chromatin bridges of different lengths (0.8 to 2.3 percent of erythroblasts). The erythroid series alone shows significant abnormalities by electron and light microscopy. The normal pores of the nuclear envelope of the erythroid cells become abnormally numerous and wide with progressive maturation. Later, in many cells, the cytoplasm has invaded between the nuclear chromatin strands and there is intense clumping of the dense chromatin. In even more severely affected cells, the cytoplasm separates the chromatin fragments and gives the nucleus a spongy appearance [6–9,11–13]. The persistence of cytoplasmic microtubules has also been demonstrated [12]. Some mitochondria show deposition of ferruginous micelles, causing a loss of normal structure, but these changes are quantitatively much less severe than in the sideroblastic anemias (Chap. 54). In other studies, hypertetraploid DNA values were found in a high proportion of erythroblasts, and RNA synthesis was markedly reduced, leading to impaired hemoglobin synthesis [13,14]. Serologic abnormalities, such as will be described in CDA type II, have usually not been present. No effective treatment is available, but, although anemic, most subjects do not require transfusion. The latter is to be avoided if at all possible, since iron overload is often present [6]. Cautious phlebotomy or administration of iron-chelating agents to help prevent tissue siderosis has been suggested but not adequately evaluated. The mode of genetic transmission is autosomal recessive.

CDA type II (HEMPAS)[1]

The type of CDA which now seems to be the most common [24–27] was first described in 1962 [17,18]. In 1966 and later, the unusual serologic abnormalities characterizing this disorder were defined [1,19]. HEMPAS is characterized by anemia varying widely from mild to severe. The circulating red cells exhibit moderate to marked aniso- and poikilocytosis and anisochromia. There are also a few irregularly contracted spherocytes. Ferrokinetic studies document the ineffective erythropoiesis [19,24]. Reticulocyte counts are normal or slightly elevated. Body iron stores and serum iron are usually increased. From 10 to 30 percent of the erythro-

[1] Hereditary Erythroblastic Multinuclearity associated with a Positive Acidified Serum test [1,17–32].

blasts, chiefly the more mature stages, have two or more nuclei or lobulated nuclei (Fig. 46-1). Gaucher-like cells may develop due to phagocytosis of erythroblasts by macrophages. Ringed sideroblasts are not conspicuous. A characteristic feature of HEMPAS is the behavior of the patient's cells in serologic tests. HEMPAS cells are lysed by certain group-compatible sera at pH 6.8, resembling in this respect cells of paroxysmal nocturnal hemoglobinuria (PNH) [1,19,24,27] (see Chap. 22). However, HEMPAS differs from PNH in several important respects [24,27]. The sucrose hemolysis test (see Chap. A14) is negative [24], and the cells are not lysed by their own acidified serum. Only about 30 percent of group-compatible sera lyse HEMPAS cells. Unlike PNH, HEMPAS cells behave as a "single population" in quantitative lysis tests. The lysis of HEMPAS cells appears due to a naturally occurring IgM complement-binding antibody which can be removed by absorption with HEMPAS but not with normal or PNH cells. The antibody is not directed against any presently defined antigen. A constant finding in HEMPAS is the strong reactivity with anti-i, in which respect the cells resemble those of newborn infants [19,24,27]. HEMPAS cells are agglutinated and lysed more readily than normal by cold-reacting antibodies (anti-I and anti-i), and it appears that this is largely explained by increased antibody binding rather than by increased sensitivity to complement [22]. By electron and light microscopy, multinuclearity and karyorrhexis have been observed in 15 to 20 percent of late erythroblasts, and by autoradiography these are no longer synthesizing DNA. Other abnormalities have also been observed [24,25,29], including an excess of endoplasmic reticulum perceived as a "double membrane" at the periphery of the cell. HEMPAS is not exceedingly rare [1,17–32]. In 1975, the clinical and hematologic features in 84 patients in 55 families were reviewed [29]. Their geographic distribution suggests a higher frequency of the HEMPAS gene in northwest Europe, in Italy, and in North Africa. Both sexes are affected; the mode of genetic transmission is autosomal recessive. No satisfactory treatment is available, but partial benefit has been reported with splenectomy [24].

CDA type III [10,17,33–37]

A third type of CDA was described in a woman and all three of her children, in whom 16 to 22.7 percent of marrow erythroblasts were multinucleated [33]. Giant-sized erythrocytes were present in the peripheral blood, and giant erythroblasts with coarse basophilic stippling and up to 12 nuclei were present in the marrow. All patients were asymptomatic, with absent or minimal anemia. The reticulocyte count was below 3 percent. A similar, dominantly transmitted disorder has also been described in 15 members of a large Swedish family [34] under the name of *hereditary benign erythroreticulosis*. In 1972, a case of dyserythropoietic anemia with marrow

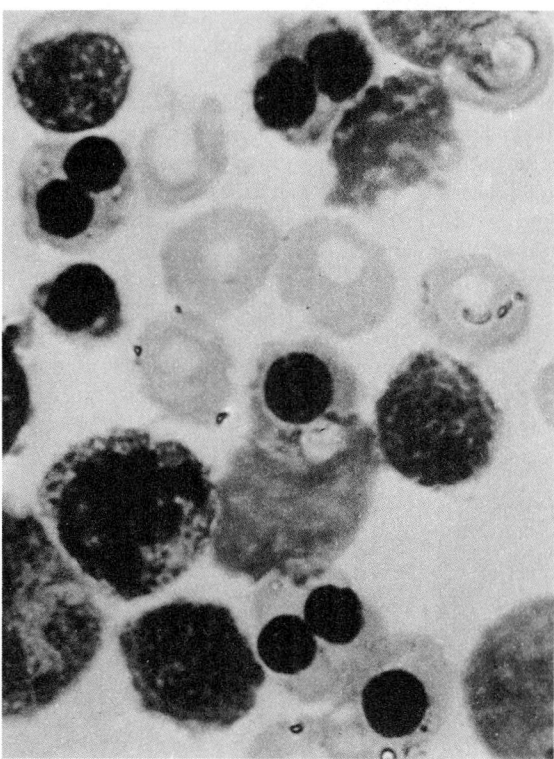

FIGURE 46-1   Multinuclearity of the erythroblasts in the marrow of a patient with HEMPAS.

multinucleated gigantoblasts believed to be consistent with CDA type III was studied. It was unlike the disorder in the first reported family, in that moderately severe anemia was present. There was striking variability in DNA content per erythroblast nucleus, and increased agglutination and lysis by anti-i and anti-I antibodies were noted. No documentation of a dominant type of inheritance was presented [35].

Other forms of CDA and similar disorders [38–42]

A number of cases of CDA clearly at variance from types I, II, and III have been reported. The salient features of these have recently been summarized [41]. In some, marrow erythroid multinuclearity resembled that of HEMPAS, but the acidified serum lysis test was negative. In two kindreds, CDA was clearly inherited in dominant fashion. Unbalanced globin-chain synthesis with excess production of α chains was documented in several patients. In one such kindred, a disorder with features of both thalassemia and hereditary erythroid multinuclearity was dominantly transmitted [40]. In variant syndromes, there were also differences in the degree of agglutination by anti-i serum and in the concentrations of Hb F and A_2. In one case of CDA, the acidified serum lysis test was positive, but erythroid multinuclearity was absent.

Still other ill-defined forms of CDA undoubtedly exist. Several cases of apparently lifelong anemia, thought to be hereditary, have been described. These were characterized by marked aniso- and poikilocytosis and occasional teardrop and fragmented erythrocytes in the peripheral blood. Hyperplastic marrows showed megaloblastoid features without multinuclearity or ringed sideroblasts [42, cases 6–9]. Neutropenia was present in all, and thrombocytopenia in some. Cytogenetic studies of marrow revealed no chromosomal abnormalities. Reticulocyte response to anemia was absent or inappropriately low in all. Studies of parents failed to reveal abnormalities, suggesting an autosomal recessive mode of transmission. High-dose androgen therapy appeared to benefit two subjects partially.

Enzyme abnormalities in CDA

In both CDA types I and II, as well as in certain less well defined but apparently hereditary dyserythropoietic anemias, a diversity of abnormalities of individual red cell enzyme activities and of activity ratios has been clearly present [28,42]. Enzyme patterns differ strikingly from those of either normal red cells or reticulocyte-rich blood. They resemble closely, however, patterns observed in a variety of disorders characterized by ineffective erythropoiesis, including certain acquired and congenital sideroblastic anemias, certain preleukemic states, and certain refractory, nonsideroblastic anemias with cellular marrow [42]. It is not known why the enzymatic aberrations which characterize a variety of dyserythropoietic states fail to differentiate among the obviously very heterogenous entities in which a large component of ineffective erythropoiesis is a common denominator.

Differential diagnosis

CDA may be confused with the thalassemic syndromes because of the frequent presence of well-marked aniso- and poikilocytosis, hypochromia, and evidence of ineffective erythropoiesis. The readily evident erythroid multinuclearity of CDA type II and the marrow gigantocytes of the rarer CDA type III point toward the correct diagnosis in these conditions. The marrow changes in CDA type I are, however, more subtle and more easily missed. Family studies and evaluation of hemoglobin A_2 levels indicate that thalassemia is not present. The megaloblastoid marrow structure may cause some confusion with other disorders associated with abnormalities of vitamin B_{12}, folic acid, and nucleic acid metabolism. Some forms of CDA also bear resemblances to certain of the acquired and hereditary sideroblastic anemias, but sideroblastosis is not prominent and the other marrow features described earlier point to the correct diagnosis. The abnormal serologic tests observed with HEMPAS are of obvious major diagnostic importance.

Otherwise, indirect hyperbilirubinemia and splenomegaly may suggest a hemolytic process, but low reticulocyte counts, the marrow features, and findings of ineffective erythropoiesis should point to the correct diagnosis.

References

1. Crookston, J. H., et al.: Congenital dyserythropoietic anaemia. XIth Congr. Int. Soc. Haemat., Sydney, August 1966. *Abstracts of Papers.* AB 8, 1966, p. 18.
2. Wendt, F., and Heimpel, H.: Kongenitale dyserythropoietische Anamie bei einem sweieiigen Zwillingsparr. *Med. Klin.* 62:172, 1967.
3. Heimpel, H., Wendt, F., Klemm, D., Schubothe, H., and Heilmeyer, L.: Kongenitale dyserythropoietische Anämie. *Arch. Klin. Med.* 215:174, 1968.
4. Lewis, S. M., and Verwilghen, R. L.: Dyserythropoiesis: Definition, diagnosis, and assessment, in *Dyserythropoiesis*, edited by S. M. Lewis and R. L. Verwilghen. Academic, London, 1977, pp. 3–20.
5. Heimpel, H., and Wendt, F.: Congenital dyserythropoietic anaemia with karyorrhexis and multinuclearity of erythroblasts. *Helv. Med. Acta* 34:103, 1968.
6. Heimpel, H., Forteza-Vila, J., Queisser, W., and Spiertz, E.: Electron and light microscopic study of the erythroblasts of patients with congenital dyserythropoietic anemia. *Blood* 37:299, 1971.
7. Keyserlingk, D. G., Boll, I., and Meuret, G.: Ultrastruktur der gestörten Erythropäiese bei einer kongenitalen dysertythropoietischen. Anämie. *Klin. Wochenschr.* 48:728, 1970.
8. Maldonado, J. E., and Taswell, H. F.: Type I dyserythropoietic anemia in an elderly patient. *Blood* 44:495, 1974.
9. Breton-Gorius, J., Daniel, M. T., Clauvel, J. P., and Dreyfus, B.: Anomalies ultrastructurales des érythroblastes et des érythrocytes dans six cas de dysérythropoïèse congénitale. *Nouv. Rev. Fr. Hematol.* 13:23, 1973.
10. Faille, A., Najean, Y., and Dresch, C.: Cinétique de l'érythropoïèse dans 14 cas "d'erythropoïèse inéfficase" avec anomalies morphologiques des érythroblastes et polynucléarité. *Nouv. Rev. Fr. Hematol.* 12:631, 1972.
11. Clauvel, J. P., et al.: Dysérthropoïèse congénitale (étude de 6 observations). *Nouv. Rev. Fr. Hematol.* 12:653, 1972.
12. Lewis, S. M., Nelson, D. A., and Pitcher, C. S.: Clinical and ultrastructural aspects of congenital dyserythropoietic anaemia Type I. *Br. J. Haematol.* 23:113, 1972.
13. Meuret, V. G., Boll, I., Keyserlingk, D. G., and Heissmeyer, H.: Morphologische und kinetische Befinde bei einer kongenitalen dyserythropoietischen Anämie. *Blut* 21:341, 1970.
14. Meuret, G., Tschan, P., Schlüter, G., Graf Keyserlingk, D. G., and Boll, I.: DNA-, histone-, RNA-, hemoglobin-content and DNA-synthesis in erythroblasts in a case of congenital dyserythropoietic anemia type I: *Blut* 24:32, 1972.
15. Heimpel, H.: Congenital dyserythropoietic anaemia type I: Clinical and experimental aspects, in *Congenital Disorders of Erythropoiesis*, Ciba Foundation Symposium 37 (new series). Elsevier/Excerpta Medica/North Holland, Amsterdam, 1976, pp. 135–149.
16. Heimpel, H.: Congenital dyserythropoietic anaemia, type I, in *Dyserythropoiesis*, edited by S. M. Lewis and R. L. Verwilghen. Academic, London, 1977, pp. 55–70.
17. De Lozzio, C. B., Valencia, J. I., and Accame, E.: Chromosomal study in erythroblastic endopolyploidy. *Lancet* 1:1004, 1962.
18. Roberts, P. D., Wallis, P. G., and Jackson, A. D. M.: Haemolytic anaemia with multinucleated normoblasts in the marrow. *Lancet* 1:1186, 1962 (letter).
19. Crookston, J. H., et al.: Hereditary erythroblastic multinuclearity associated with a positive acidified-serum test: A type of congenital dyserythropoietic anaemia. *Br. J. Haematol.* 17:11, 1969.
20. Schärer, K., Marti, H. R., and Baumann, Th.: Konstitutionelle Anämie mit Kernteilungsstörung der Erythroblasten. *Schweiz. Med. Wochenschr.* 95:1511, 1965.
21. Accame, E., de Lozzio, C. G., and Valencia, J. I.: Polyploidie

erythroblastique familiale bénigne avec anémia hémolytique et splénomegalie. *Blut 18*:348, 1969.

22. Lewis, S. M., Grammaticos, P., and Dacie, J. V.: Lysis by anti-I in dyserythropoietic anaemias: Role of increased uptake of antibody. *Br. J. Haematol. 18*:465, 1970.

23. Verwilghen, R. L., Verhaegen, H., Waumans, P., and Beert, J.: Inefficient erythropoiesis with morphologically abnormal erythroblasts and unconjugated hyperbilirubinaemia. *Br. J. Haematol. 17*:27, 1969.

24. Crookston, M. C.: HEMPAS: Congenital dyserythropoietic anemia (type II). *Q. J. Med. 166*:257, 1973.

25. Hug, G., Wong, K. Y., and Lampkin, B. C.: Congenital dyserythropoietic anemia type II. Ultrastructure of erythroid cells and hepatocytes. *Lab. Invest. 26*:11, 1972.

26. Murphy, S., and Oski, F.: Congenital dyserythropoietic anemia. Type II: Report of two cases and a review of the literature. *Pediatrics 50*:858, 1972.

27. Crookston, J. H., and Crookston, M. C.: Hereditary anemia with multinuclear erythroblasts ("HEMPAS"), in *Birth Defects, Original Article Series, Clinical Delineation of Birth Defects*, edited by D. Bergsma. Williams & Wilkins, Baltimore, 1972, vol. 8, p. 15.

28. Valentine, W. N., Crookston, J. H., Paglia, D. E., and Konrad, P. N.: Erythrocyte enzymatic abnormalities in HEMPAS (hereditary erythroblastic multinuclearity with a positive acidified-serum test). *Br. J. Haematol. 23*:107, 1972.

29. Verwilghen, R. L.: Congenital dyserythropoietic anaemia, type II (HEMPAS), in *Congenital Disorders of Erythropoiesis*, Ciba Foundation Symposium 37 (new series). Elsevier/Excerpta Medica/North Holland, Amsterdam, 1976, pp. 151–170.

30. Punt, K., Borst-Eilers, E., and Nijessen, J. G.: Congenital dyserythropoietic anaemia, type II (HEMPAS), in *Dyserythropoiesis*, edited by S. M. Lewis and R. L. Verwilghen. Academic, London, 1977, pp. 71–81.

31. Veltore, L., DeSandre, G., DiJorio, E. E., Winterhalter, K. H., Lang, A., and Lehmann, H.: A new abnormal hemoglobin O Padova, $\alpha 30$ (B11) Glu $\rightarrow$ Lys and a dyserythropoietic anemia with erythroblastic multinuclearity coexisting in the same patient. *Blood 44*:869, 1974.

32. Crookston, J. H., and Crookston, M. C. Personal communication.

33. Wolff, J. A., and von Hofe, F. H.: Familial erythroid multinuclearity. *Blood 6*:1274, 1951.

34. Bergström, I., and Jacobsson, L.: Hereditary benign erythroreticulosis. *Blood 19*:296, 1962.

35. Goudsmit, R., et al.: Congenital dyserythropoietic anaemia, type III, *Br. J. Haematol. 23*:97, 1972.

36. Goudsmit, R.: Congenital dyserythropoietic anaemia, type III, in *Dyserythropoiesis*, edited by S. M. Lewis and R. L. Verwilghen. Academic, London, 1977, pp. 83–92.

37. Björksten, P., Holmgren, G., Roos, G., and Stenling, R.: Congenital dyserythropoietic anaemia, type III: An electron microscope study. *Br. J. Haematol. 38*:37, 1978.

38. McBride, J. A., Wilson, W. E., and Baille, N.: Congenital dyserythropoietic anaemia-type IV. *Blood 38*:837, 1971.

39. Hruby, M. A., Mason, R. G., and Honig, G. R.: Unbalanced globin chain synthesis in congenital dyserythropoietic anemia. *Blood 42*:843, 1973.

40. Weatherall, D. J., Clegg, J. B., Knox-Macaulay, H. H. M., Bunch, C., Hopkins, C. R., and Temperley, I. J.: A genetically determined disorder with features both of thalassemia and congenital dyserythropoietic anemia. *Br. J. Haematol. 24*:681, 1973.

41. David, G., and Van Dorpe, A.: Aberrant congenital dyserythropoietic anaemias, in *Dyserythropoiesis*, edited by S. M. Lewis and R. L. Verwilghen. Academic, London, 1977, pp. 93–100.

42. Valentine, W. N., Konrad, P. N., and Paglia, D. E.: Dyserythropoiesis, refractory anemia, and "preleukemia": Metabolic features of the erythrocytes. *Blood 41*:857, 1973.

Erythrocyte disorders—anemias related to disturbance of DNA synthesis (megaloblastic anemias)

CHAPTER *47*

The megaloblastic anemias

WILLIAM S. BECK

Megaloblastic anemia is a widely used although imprecise term that designates a group of disorders having in common a characteristic pattern of morphologic and functional abnormalities in the blood and marrow. The pattern is a result of impairment of DNA synthesis, a phenomenon that may have many causes.

The term is imprecise for two reasons. First, "megaloblastic anemia" is sometimes diagnosed when anemia is not present. Second, through common usage, the adjective *megaloblastic* and the noun *megaloblast* have acquired different connotations. *Megaloblastic* denotes an abnormal pattern of morphologic change in any of the cell lines in marrow. The normal antithesis of the pattern is *normoblastic*. Thus one speaks of megaloblastic erythropoiesis, granulopoiesis, or thrombopoiesis. However, *megaloblast* has come to refer only to cells of the erythroid series.

In 1880, Ehrlich gave the name *megaloblast* to the abnormal erythroid precursors found in pernicious anemia [1]. These cells, whatever their stage of maturation, were thought to belong to a series separate and distinct from that of normal erythroid precursors, which were termed *normoblasts*. Later workers, especially Downey [2], Jones [3], Naegeli [4], and Fieschi and Astaldi [5], concurred and spoke of a megaloblast series (i.e., promegaloblast, basophilic megaloblast, polychromatophilic megaloblast, and orthochromatic megaloblast) that parallels the normoblast (erythroblast) series. Other workers, notably Sabin [6] and Doán [7], viewed the megaloblast as an early maturation stage of normal erythropoiesis, occurring between the primitive endothelial cell and the erythroblast.

Current workers, in disagreement with both early schools, regard megaloblasts as functionally and mor-

phologically abnormal erythroblasts. The abnormality frequently is reversible by therapy. The current view rests in part on the rapidity with which megaloblasts can be converted to erythroblasts in vivo [8–10] and in vitro [11] and erythroblasts to megaloblasts in vitro [12].

Though some contemporary hematologists reserve the term *megaloblast* for the large, colorful promegaloblast, in the following discussion the unqualified term *megaloblast* denotes any maturation stage of the megaloblastic erythroid series. Specific maturation stages will be referred to by their full names (i.e., promegaloblast, orthochromatic megaloblast, etc.). The term *megaloblastic* refers to morphologic and functional patterns in erythrocyte, granulocyte, and platelet precursors. Indeed, the term *megaloblastic* may be usefully applied to certain abnormal cells of the buccal and vaginal mucosa and other tissues. The process wherein erythroblastic cells become megaloblastic is termed *megaloblastic transformation*. The term *megaloblastosis* refers to disorders caused by defective DNA synthesis whether or not anemia is present

Biologic nature of megaloblastic cells

MORPHOLOGY

The collective appearance and characteristics of aspirated marrow in the several types of megaloblastic anemia are described later. The following description deals with the morphology of individual megaloblastic cells in conventional Wright's-stained films of marrow aspirates.

Megaloblastic erythrocyte precursors at all stages of development appear larger than corresponding erythroblastic cells and often have a higher than normal ratio of cytoplasmic area to nuclear area. Promegaloblasts, the most immature of the series and the most easily recognized, display a brilliantly colored, deeply basophilic, granule-free cytoplasm and a lavender-tinted chromatin with a characteristic open and fine-grained, or particulate, texture that contrasts decidedly with the ground-glass texture of the fibrous or strand-like proerythroblast chromatin (see Plate 3). Large blue nucleoli and a prominent perinuclear halo may be present. As the cell matures, the chromatin retains its granular texture and is slow to form coarse, deeply basophilic clumps. Development of a dense pyknotic nucleus like that of an orthochromatic erythroblast either fails to occur or is delayed. As hemoglobin synthesis accelerates, the apparent maturity of the cytoplasm contrasts with the apparent immaturity of the nucleus—a feature termed *nuclear-cytoplasmic asynchronism* or *dissociation*. Sometimes the chromatin adherent to the nuclear membrane displays a distinctive configuration in the basophilic, polychromatophilic, and orthochromatic megaloblasts of vitamin B_{12} or folic acid deficiency. This chromatin may appear separated from other chromatin, thus giving the nuclear border the appearance of a clock face.

In mild or incipient megaloblastic anemia or in megaloblastic anemia associated with iron deficiency and other conditions to be described later, the marrow may contain partially developed or "intermediate" or "megaloblastoid" megaloblasts [13]. These cells reveal less striking features than fully developed megaloblasts and may present diagnostic difficulties.

Megaloblastic granulocyte precursors, when present, also display nuclear-cytoplasmic asynchronism and apparent enlargement, the most striking enlargement occurring at the metamyelocyte stage. A "giant metamyelocyte" has a relatively large "horseshoe" nucleus, sometimes bizarre in shape, with a characteristic ragged or uneven chromatin pattern. The nucleus takes stain poorly and in rare instances may appear pinched off in several places, an apparent early sign of the hypersegmentation of the mature neutrophil. The cytoplasm appears more immature (i.e., more basophilic and freer of granules) than that of a normal metamyelocyte. Comparable changes may be found in myelocytes and in band forms. The characteristic hypersegmented neutrophil of blood is described below.

Megaloblastic megakaryocytes do not always display distinctive morphologic features. Occasionally they are abnormally large. Granulation of the cytoplasm may be deficient. In severe megaloblastosis, the nucleus may be more bizarre than usual, showing numerous distinct and unattached lobes that give the cell an exploded appearance [14,15].

MECHANISM OF MEGALOBLASTIC TRANSFORMATION

Biochemical study of megaloblasts has established that (1) megaloblasts contain a substantially increased amount of RNA and a normal or slightly increased amount of DNA per cell [16,17], the former presumably accounting for the cytoplasmic basophilia; and (2) labeled thymidine can be incorporated into the DNA of megaloblasts and thus DNA synthesis can occur [18]. In addition, results from the Killmann experiment [19], later termed the deoxyuridine (or dU) suppression test by other workers [20], suggest that megaloblastosis is associated with impaired conversion of dUMP to dTMP.

The megaloblast appears to be in a state of unbalanced growth, owing to impaired synthesis of one or more deoxyribonucleotides [21,22]. The notion that megaloblastosis is due only to diminution of DNA synthesis seems simplistic in view of evidence that (1) megaloblastic cells contain short DNA fragments [23,24] that are probably breakdown products rather than biosynthetic intermediates of the Okazaki types, and (2) inhibition of thymidylate synthesis leads not only to decreased DNA synthesis, but to accumulations within cells of dUMP and dUTP, uracil misincorporation into DNA [25,26], excision of misincorporated uracils from DNA by uracil-DNA-glycosylase [27], failure of repair of DNA strand breaks owing to lack of dTTP and failure of repair systems, leakage of DNA fragments from cells [28,29], and cell death. This tentative model accounts for

the chromosome breaks known to occur in megaloblastic cells [30–32]. Since cell lines differ in their capacity to exclude uracil from DNA [28], this may account for differences among cell lines in their susceptibility to megaloblastic transformation.

As in the unbalanced growth pattern observed in *E. coli* [33] and other species, DNA replication and cell division are blocked, while synthesis of cytoplasm (RNA and protein) proceeds normally. Studies of the unbalanced growth state in bacteria [33–35] and in animal cells [36], whether resulting from lack of an essential nutrient or exposure to an inhibitor of DNA synthesis, indicate that prolongation of unbalanced growth results in permanent loss of the capacity for mitosis and in eventual cell death. Such loss of cell viability occurs in animal cells in culture following exposure to an inhibitor of DNA synthesis for a period corresponding to about one generation [37]. In megaloblastic marrow, the degree of impairment of DNA synthesis varies from cell to cell, ranging from complete inhibition to none, and from cell series to cell series, being usually more evident among erythrocyte precursors than among granulocyte precursors.

Many data support the conclusion that megaloblastic cells are in a state of unbalanced growth. These include evidence that the maturation time of the promegaloblast is prolonged [38–41] and that DNA synthesis is impaired, as demonstrated by isotopic methods [20,42–45]. Until the chain of events in megaloblastic transformation is understood in greater detail, we would simply state that in this disorder defective DNA synthesis blocks or delays cell division, and the resulting state of unbalanced growth predisposes to premature cell death or abnormal cell division with resulting dysplasia.

CLINICAL FEATURES

The major clinical manifestations of the several types of megaloblastic anemia are common to all of them. Anemia may be mild or severe, but because it develops slowly, it may produce few symptoms until the hematocrit is severely depressed. When symptoms appear, they are the usual symptoms of anemia—weakness, palpitation, fatigue, light-headedness, and shortness of breath. Congestive heart failure may supervene. Patients characteristically demonstrate severe pallor and slight jaundice, producing the often-described lemon-yellow tint.

LABORATORY FEATURES

APPEARANCE OF BLOOD CELLS

All formed elements can be affected. Erythrocytes display striking variations in size and shape and, in severe cases, inclusions such as stippling, Howell-Jolly bodies, and Cabot rings; the last reportedly contain arginine-rich histone and nonhemoglobin iron [46]. The anemia is normochromic (unless iron deficiency coexists) and macrocytic, with mean corpuscular volumes ranging

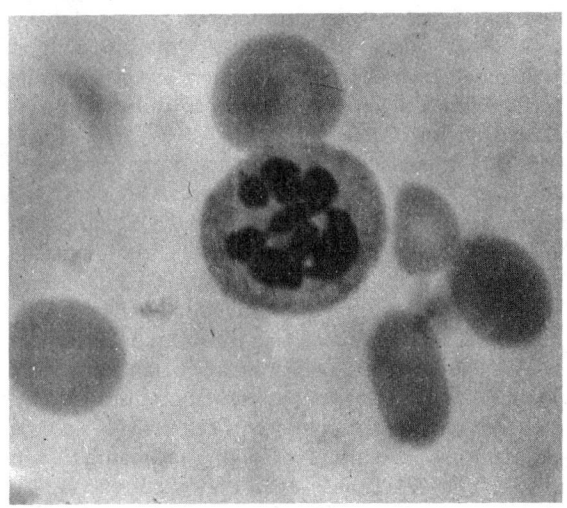

FIGURE 47-1 Megaloblastic hypersegmented granulocyte (×1500).

from 100 to more than 150 μm^3. Macroovalocytes, up to 14 μm in diameter, are characteristically present. The reticulocyte count is lower than normal, both in absolute and in percentage terms. In general, the more severe the anemia, the more severe the erythrocyte changes. When the hematocrit is low (i.e., <20 percent), nucleated red cells may appear in the blood. Such cells show typical megaloblastic features—indeed, well-developed promegaloblasts are occasionally found. In such instances, a diagnosis of megaloblastic anemia may be made with certainty from the blood film.

Many neutrophils have more than the usual three to four segments (Fig. 47-1). The number of segments may average 5 to 6, although some cells may have up to 16 segments. The presence of hypersegmented neutrophils (or macropolycytes) may be an early sign of megaloblastosis [47,48]. These macropolycytes may be quite large (Plate 1). Typically, more than 5 percent of the neutrophils have five or more segments. Such cells are often said to be older than normal, but hypersegmentation is more likely a result of abnormalities of nuclear division or of chromatin itself. Chromosomes in megaloblastic anemia are reportedly elongated or broken, and these changes disappear after specific therapy [44,50]. However, the significance of these changes is in doubt.

APPEARANCE OF MARROW

Aspirated marrow is cellular and often hyperplastic. Striking megaloblastic changes may be seen in the erythrocyte, granulocyte, and platelet precursors, although frequently the major changes are seen in the erythroid series. The M/E ratio (i.e., the ratio of myeloid precursors to erythroid precursors) typically drops to 1:1. Megaloblastic granulocytopoiesis is more evident when situations coexist such as infection, in which increased granulocyte production is being called forth. Granulocyte reserves are decreased in megaloblastic anemia [51].

In typical severe megaloblastic anemia, many of the erythroid cells are promegaloblasts. An unusually large number of mitotic figures are found among them. Unless iron deficiency is present, iron in reticulum cells is commonly increased, but ring sideroblasts are usually absent. Electron micrographs suggest that the macrophages ingest and catabolize megaloblasts of various ages [52]. The liberated iron appears as dense granules in membranous vesicles.

Before the marrow is aspirated, a patient may have received small amounts of vitamin B_{12} or folic acid, the latter perchance in the form of nutritious hospital food taken after prolonged malnutrition. Anemia may persist, or may be slightly improved, but megaloblastic changes in the marrow are obscured. Prior transfusion therapy [53] or coexisting infection or other disease may have similar results. In such circumstances, recognition of the underlying megaloblastic character of the morphologic pattern may tax the most experienced observer.

CHEMICAL CHANGES IN BODY FLUIDS

Plasma bilirubin and iron levels are slightly to moderately increased; serum lactic dehydrogenase level (isozymes 1 and 2) is markedly elevated in rough proportion to the severity of the anemia [54–56]. It is of interest that in normal erythrocytes and in those of various nonmegaloblastic anemias, the level of lactic dehydrogenase isozyme 2 (LDH-2) activity exceeds that of LDH-1 [57]. In the erythrocytes of megaloblastic anemia, however, LDH-1 exceeds LDH-2. This reversal of the LDH isozyme pattern also occurs in the serum in megaloblastic anemia.

Elevations are also found in the levels of serum muramidase [58–60], malic dehydrogenase, 6-phosphogluconic dehydrogenase [61], and thymidine kinase [62]. Serum glutamic oxaloacetic transaminase is normal [61]. Serum alkaline phosphatase [63] and cholinesterase [64] are decreased. Aminoaciduria reportedly occurs [65–67], but observers differ on its frequency and significance. Perhaps it is related to the rise in serum β-leucine recently discovered in vitamin B_{12} deficiency but not in folic acid deficiency [68].

CYTOKINETICS

ERYTHROKINETICS

Whatever its cause, megaloblastic anemia is associated with two pathophysiologic abnormalities: an abnormal degree of ineffective erythropoiesis and moderate hemolysis of circulating erythrocytes. The presence of increased ineffective erythropoiesis is indicated by (1) a marked increase in the number of erythroid precursors in marrow and in the ratio of erythroid precursors to released erythrocytes (reticulocytes); (2) an increase in plasma iron turnover to 3 to 5 times the normal level, with normal iron uptake by individual erythroid precursors [69,70]; (3) a decreased rate of reappearance of labeled plasma iron in blood erythrocytes [70]; and (4) indirect evidence of intramedullary destruction of megaloblasts, the main elements of which are (a) high serum levels of erythrocyte-type lactic dehydrogenase isozymes that almost certainly reflect intramedullary destruction of erythroid cells containing higher than normal levels of lactic dehydrogenase per cell [71,72]; (b) striking increases in production of "early-labeled" bilirubin, which exceeds that which can be attributed to destruction of circulating red cells [73]; (c) increased production of endogenous carbon monoxide [74]; (d) the ease with which megaloblasts undergo autohemolysis in vitro compared with erythroblasts [75]; and finally, (e) the fact noted earlier that marrow macrophages actively devour erythroid precursors in megaloblastic anemia.

Ineffective erythropoiesis is synonymous with intramedullary hemolysis. That a substantial degree of extramedullary hemolysis also occurs in megaloblastic anemia is suggested by life-span studies of circulating erythrocytes [76,77]. Life-span is moderately decreased (to one-half to one-third normal), whether erythrocytes are tested in the patient or in a normal subject. Thus an intracorpuscular defect is present. However, decreased survival of normal erythrocytes in untreated patients suggests the existence of an extracorpuscular defect.

LEUKOKINETICS

It had been generally assumed that inadequate marrow production or delivery of leukocytes accounted for their decreased numbers in peripheral blood. Studies have suggested that the increased level of serum muramidase in megaloblastic anemia is attributable to an increased rate of granulocyte turnover [58-60]. Although these data leave it uncertain whether the increased turnover occurs in the marrow, in which case the mechanism would be ineffective leukopoiesis, or in the peripheral blood or tissues, in which case the mechanism would be granulocytolytic leukopenia, it seems reasonable to suppose that defective DNA synthesis causes ineffective leukopoiesis as it does ineffective erythropoiesis. This conclusion is compatible with the morphologic evidence of active but abnormal leukopoiesis in marrow aspirates. Disintegrating giant metamyelocytes and band forms are the probable sources of the elevated serum muramidase.

THROMBOKINETICS

Ineffective thrombopoiesis may also occur in patients with megaloblastic anemia [78]. This state is characterized by an increased megakaryocyte mass in the marrow but a decreased rate of platelet turnover. Hence the pathophysiology of ineffective thrombopoiesis parallels that of ineffective erythropoiesis and leukopoiesis. The term *ineffective thrombopoiesis* should probably be restricted to situations in which daily platelet production per nuclear megakaryocyte unit is less than half that expected [78]. In subjects with vitamin B_{12} deficiency, platelet production was actually found to be only 10 percent of that expected from the megakaryocyte mass [78].

The platelets in the megaloblastosis of severe vitamin B_{12} deficiency appear to be functionally abnormal [79].

DIAGNOSIS

MAJOR CAUSES
Table 47-1 summarizes the major categories of megaloblastic anemia and their specific etiologic mechanisms. Vitamin B_{12} deficiency and folic acid deficiency are by far the most common causes, although each deficiency has many underlying causes, common and rare. In both categories, the defect is a tissue coenzyme deficiency that is readily correctable by repletion of the lacking vitamin. Repletion is rapidly followed by reversion of megaloblastic hematopoiesis to normal. The various types of megaloblastic anemia resulting from causes other than vitamin B_{12} and folate deficiencies are unresponsive to therapy with these vitamins. Of these, the ones associated with pyridoxine-responsive anemia, inhibitors of DNA synthesis, and hereditary orotic aciduria are reversible with appropriate therapy. The rest are grimly refractory.

GENERAL APPROACH
Beyond the routine history and physical examination, the approach to the average patient should be to complete the following sequence: (1) recognize the presence of anemia, (2) determine whether it is caused by marrow failure, (3) determine whether it is megaloblastic anemia, (4) elucidate the broad etiologic category (i.e., vitamin B_{12} deficiency, folate deficiency, etc., as outlined in Table 47-1), (5) elucidate the specific etiologic mechanism, and (6) treat and observe the response to treatment.

The so-called deoxyuridine suppression test has been widely recommended in the diagnosis of megaloblastosis [80-82], but in the view of some critics [45,83], this test is influenced by too many variables to serve as a reliable diagnostic test.

Megaloblastic anemia of vitamin B_{12} deficiency

ETIOLOGY AND PATHOGENESIS
Deficiency of vitamin B_{12}, as of all vitamins, may result from inadequate dietary intake, defective intestinal absorption, abnormally increased requirements, or impaired utilization in the tissues. The disorders in these several categories that lead to vitamin B_{12} deficiency are summarized in Table 47-1.

CAUSES OF VITAMIN B_{12} DEFICIENCY
Deficiency of vitamin B_{12} results from *poor diet* only rarely. Reported instances have occurred mainly in vegetarians who also avoid all dairy products and eggs. Occasionally it is associated with severe general malnutrition.

TABLE 47-1   Etiologic classification of the megaloblastic anemias

Category	Etiologic mechanisms
I. *Vitamin B₁₂ deficiency*	
A. Decreased intake	Poor diet, lack of animal products, strict vegetarianism
	Impaired absorption
	Intrinsic factor deficiency
	Pernicious anemia
	Gastrectomy (total and partial)
	Destruction of gastric mucosa by caustics
	Anti-IF antibody in gastric juice
	Abnormal intrinsic factor molecule
	Intrinsic intestinal disease
	Familial selective malabsorption (Imerslund's syndrome)
	Ileal resection, ileitis
	Sprue, celiac disease
	Infiltrative intestinal disease (lymphoma, scleroderma, etc.)
	Drug-induced malabsorption
	Competitive parasites
	Fish tapeworm infestations (*Diphyllobothrium latum*)
	Bacteria in diverticula of bowel, blind loops
	Chronic pancreatic disease
B. Increased requirement	Pregnancy
	Neoplastic disease
	Hyperthyroidism
C. Impaired utilization	Enzyme deficiencies
	Abnormal serum vitamin B₁₂–binding protein
	Lack of TC II; abnormal TC II
	Nitrous oxide administration
II. *Folate deficiency*	
A. Decreased intake	Poor diet, lack of vegetables
	Alcoholism
	Infancy
	Hemodialysis
	Impaired absorption
	Intestinal short circuits
	Steatorrhea
	Sprue, celiac disease
	Intrinsic intestinal disease
	Anticonvulsants, oral contraceptives, other drugs
B. Increased requirement	Pregnancy; infancy
	Hyperthyroidism
	Hyperactive hematopoiesis
	Neoplastic disease; exfoliative skin disease
C. Impaired utilization	Folic acid antagonists: MTX, triamterene, trimethoprim
	Enzyme deficiencies
III. *Unresponsive to vitamin B₁₂ or folate therapy*	Metabolic inhibitors
	Purine synthesis: 6-mercaptopurine, 6-thioguanine, azathioprine
	Pyrimidine synthesis: 6-azauridine
	Thymidylate synthesis: 5-fluorouracil
	Deoxyribonucleotide synthesis: hydroxyurea, cytosine arabinoside, severe iron deficiency
	Inborn errors
	Lesch-Nyhan syndrome
	Hereditary orotic aciduria
	Deficiency of formiminotransferase, methyltransferase, etc.
	Unexplained disorders
	Pyridoxine-responsive megaloblastic anemia
	Thiamine-responsive megaloblastic anemia
	Erythroleukemia (Di Guglielmo syndrome)

Vitamin B_{12} deficiency is most often the result of *diminished intestinal absorption*. The most common cause is pernicious anemia, in which a gastric mucosal defect decreases intrinsic factor (IF) synthesis. Other and less common causes include (1) total (occasionally subtotal) gastrectomy; (2) pancreatic disease, in which lack of proteases in the duodenum appears to interfere with formation of the IF-B_{12} complex; (3) overgrowth of intestinal bacteria that occurs in the "blind loop" syndrome, strictures, anastomoses, diverticula, and other conditions producing intestinal stasis; (4) parasitic infestation with the vitamin B_{12}–utilizing fish tapeworm *Diphyllobothrium latum;* and (5) organic disease of the ileum that interferes with vitamin B_{12} absorption despite the presence of adequate IF. The large vitamin B_{12} reserve must be depleted before clinical signs of the deficiency syndrome develop. Hence several years may pass after total gastrectomy or cessation of treatment in pernicious anemia before the appearance of deficiency symptoms. Vitamin B_{12} deficiency due to *increased requirements* occurs mainly in pregnancy, presumably arising from the superimposition of fetal demands on a background of poor nutrition. No examples are known in which a tissue deficiency of vitamin B_{12} arises from failure of activation or from antimetabolites.

PERNICIOUS ANEMIA: ETIOLOGY AND PATHOGENESIS
Pernicious anemia is of special interest in the history of medicine [84]. Addison's description in 1855 of an invariably fatal "idiopathic anemia" has been considered the classic description of pernicious anemia. However, important features of the disease were not described for some years. The name *pernicious anemia* was introduced by Biermer in 1872. Critics agree that Biermer's description is superior to that of the great clinician of Guy's.

Flint in 1860 and Fenwick in 1880 suggested that inadequate assimilation of food is the fundamental cause. William Hunter in 1907, observing excess iron in the tissues, believed the basic process to be hemolytic, resulting from infection. The regularity with which achylia gastrica antedates clinical symptoms was recognized in the early part of the century. Whipple's classic studies on the effect of liver feeding on the rate of hemoglobin regeneration after hemorrhage then led to the epoch-making discoveries by Minot and Murphy in 1926 of the effect of liver feeding in pernicious anemia [85] and by Castle in 1929 of intrinsic factor [86]. As pointed out by Castle [84], the key to the achievement of Minot and Murphy was their appreciation of the reticulocyte crisis as an index of therapeutic response. It is also of interest that the data of Whipple were successfully misinterpreted, since the dogs he studied undoubtedly suffered from iron deficiency rather than vitamin B_{12} deficiency.

The old name pernicious anemia (PA) is now reserved for the once fatal condition resulting from defective secretion of IF by the gastric mucosa. Modern therapy makes it quite "unpernicious." It is important to use it only for the distinctive type of gastropathy described below. The name is often used wrongly as a synonym for vitamin B_{12} deficiency, of which pernicious anemia is one cause, or for megaloblastic anemia, of which vitamin B_{12} deficiency is one cause. As a partial though inadequate clarification, the term Addisonian pernicious anemia is sometimes used to distinguish true pernicious anemia from non-Addisonian pernicious anemia, i.e., vitamin B_{12} deficiency from other causes, or in some writings, megaloblastic anemia of any type.

Etiology The conclusion that pernicious anemia is genetically determined rests on the following evidence: (1) the relatively high incidence of the disease in Scandinavians, an unusually inbred population, and in certain regions, e.g., central Sweden [87], New England, and the Great Lakes regions; (2) the recently recognized high incidence in American blacks [88–90], a group in which the disease occurs at an earlier age, often affects women, and is often severe; (3) a higher incidence of blood group A in pernicious anemia patients and their relatives [91,92]; and (4) the occurrence of pernicious anemia [93,94] or immunologic abnormalities, achlorhydria, or decreased serum vitamin B_{12} levels [95–98] in the families of patients. Despite these hints, the mode of inheritance remains unknown.

It is also not known how a genetic predisposition is translated into fully developed pernicious anemia. Findings suggesting an autoimmune mechanism are the following [99–102]: (1) Serum autoantibodies to gastric parietal cell cytoplasm are found in about 90 percent of patients with pernicious anemia; however, they occur in 5 to 8 percent of a random 30- to 60-year-old population, in 14 percent of women over 60, in 60 percent of patients with simple atrophic gastritis, and in a variable but significant percentage of patients with thyroid disease [103]. (2) Blocking and binding antibodies to IF or IF-B_{12} complex can be detected in the serum [104,105], gastric juice [106–108], or saliva [109] in a variable, though large, percentage of patients with pernicious anemia, especially affected black women [90]. (3) Thyroid autoantibodies occur in the serum of many patients with pernicious anemia; pernicious anemia occurs with increased frequency in patients with thyrotoxicosis, hypothyroidism, and Hashimoto's thyroiditis; and many patients with these thyroid disorders have serum autoantibodies to gastric parietal cells and, in rare cases, to IF [110,111].

Although provocative, the evidence is inconclusive. Nor is it clear how or if the process is instigated by genetic determinants. The presence of certain antibodies is undoubtedly of importance. For example, autoantibodies to IF in gastric juice may inhibit IF-mediated absorption of vitamin B_{12} in the ileum and thereby hasten the onset of vitamin B_{12} deficiency. Some evidence suggests that antibodies to IF in serum may inhibit the synthesis or release of gastric IF. In two reports [112,113], infants subjected in utero to transplacentally transferred maternal antibody to IF had no detectable gastric IF at birth. IF appeared as circulating autoantibody disappeared. A third study [114] revealed adequate IF at birth despite prenatal exposure to maternal anti-IF.

Since the antiparietal cell antibody seemingly does no injury to the cell containing its antigen, it appears to have no role in the pathogenesis of PA. The antibody may have diagnostic value, however. In the presence of a megaloblastic anemia, the presence of serum antiparietal cell antibody makes the diagnosis of PA likely; its presence *and* the presence of anti-IF antibodies makes the diagnosis almost certain.

Glucocorticoids are apparently able to reverse the histologic and laboratory evidence of pernicious anemia [115–117]. Atrophic gastric mucosa appears to regenerate and IF production to increase. Steroids decrease the levels of serum autoantibodies to IF, but the reappearance of IF in gastric juice antedates the decrease of serum autoantibodies. Also, the beneficial effect of steroids has been observed in patients without detectable antibodies to IF. Discontinuance of steroid therapy results in recurrence of mucosal atrophy with absent IF production. The mechanism of these responses is unknown.

Pathology Biopsy specimens of the gastric mucosa reveal no pathognomonic changes. The mucosa is thin and atrophic, with moderate infiltration by inflammatory cells (i.e., atrophic gastritis) that decreases as atrophy progresses. Mononuclear inflammatory cells in gastric biopsy specimens sometimes contain antibody to IF-B_{12} complex [118]. There is a striking deficiency of IgA-containing mononuclear cells compared with normal controls [119]. Atrophy is not reversed by vitamin B_{12} therapy.

Surface cells recovered by gastric lavage are large, i.e., megaloblastic, as are epithelial cells throughout the body [120]. Many exfoliated gastric cells display cytologic abnormalities suggestive of early malignant transformation [121].

Biopsy of the small intestine reveals decreased mitoses in crypts, shortening of villi, megaloblastic changes in epithelial cells, and cellular infiltration in the lamina propria in untreated pernicious anemia [122,123]. Conceivably these changes account for occasional instances of D-xylose and carotene malabsorption in pernicious anemia [124]. The changes are reversed by vitamin B_{12} therapy.

"JUVENILE PERNICIOUS ANEMIA"
So called juvenile pernicious anemia is now thought to include four entities [125,126]: (1) true pernicious anemia with failure of IF secretion, an exceedingly rare occurrence [127,128], (2) selective malabsorption of vitamin B_{12} (i.e., absorption of other nutrients is normal) with normal secretion of IF and HCl in the stomach, (3) congenital lack of gastric IF secretion without other apparent abnormality of the stomach or its secretions, and (4) production of a biologically inert IF [129,130].

Selective malabsorption of vitamin B_{12} This rare disorder, sometimes called *Imerslund's syndrome* [131], is characterized by a genetically determined defect of vitamin B_{12} absorption and persistent proteinuria [131–

134]. IF and HCl secretion are normal, as are the gastric histologic findings. Antibodies to IF are absent. The intestinal defect for vitamin B_{12} malabsorption is obscure, as is the cause for the proteinuria. In one study, ileal homogenate bound vitamin B_{12} normally [135]. Hence ileal receptors were intact. Other congenital abnormalities (e.g., duplication of the renal pelvis and ureter) have been reported in these patients.

Congenital IF deficiency This disorder resembles true pernicious anemia in that defective vitamin B_{12} absorption is correctable with orally administered IF [136]. The histologic findings in the gastric mucosa have been found to be normal in reported cases many years after the onset of liver or vitamin B_{12} therapy. Hence the condition is not merely early pernicious anemia. Acid secretion remains normal. There is no associated endocrinopathy or proteinuria. Antibodies to IF and parietal cells have not been found. Conceivably, these patients might have been producing functionally abnormal IF.

GASTRECTOMY SYNDROMES
Surgical removal of all or part of the stomach without subsequent nutritional supplementation frequently leads to anemia. The character and rapidity of onset of anemia depend on the degree of impairment of the receptacle, food-mixing, and secretory functions of the stomach. Often the resulting form of anemia is one with multiple etiologic mechanisms. Most common by far is hypochromic, microcytic anemia, which results from iron deficiency [137,139].

Megaloblastic anemia due to vitamin B_{12} deficiency is inevitable after total gastrectomy if the patient survives the operation for 5 to 6 years and vitamin B_{12} therapy is omitted [140,141]. The delay reflects the time needed for exhaustion of vitamin B_{12} stores after loss of IF and subsequent cessation of vitamin B_{12} absorption. Vitamin B_{12} deficiency is rare, however, after operations in which a portion of the stomach remains, and most large series of patients with partial gastrectomy reveal few cases— usually less than 1 percent of the surveyed populations [139,140,142–145]. Although frank vitamin B_{12} deficiency is rare, studies reveal that 2 to 6 percent of partially gastrectomized patients have intermediate megaloblastic transformation, 14 to 60 percent have depressed serum vitamin B_{12} levels, and many have decreased IF secretion as measured by the Schilling test [144,146,147], though often this test gives normal results in the postgastrectomy state even when the serum vitamin B_{12} level is depressed [148]. It has been speculated that such patients have more difficulty absorbing protein-bound food vitamin B_{12} than the purified vitamin. When Schilling test results are depressed, they are correctable with administered IF. Calcium by mouth is without effect. Achlorhydria, not present before gastrectomy, is regularly found some years afterward. Postgastrectomy patients with depressed serum vitamin B_{12} levels usually have low serum iron levels as well, in contrast to the hyperferremia associated with vitamin B_{12}

deficiency of other etiologies. To an extent, coexisting iron deficiency may mask the morphologic features of postgastrectomy megaloblastic anemia. A marrow aspirate after treatment with iron often reveals enhanced megaloblastic changes.

Vitamin B_{12} deficiency after partial gastrectomy is attributable to partial extirpation of IF-producing cells with subsequent atrophy of the remaining gastric mucosa and loss of residual IF-producing cells [149,150]. The atrophy, demonstrably absent before surgery, is believed to be a result of iron deficiency, although only occasionally is it reversible by iron therapy. Intestinal malabsorption of fat, protein, calcium, and folic acid may also follow partial gastrectomy. As noted below, folic acid deficiency resulting from reduced dietary intake accounts for somewhat more of the instances of postgastrectomy megaloblastic anemia than vitamin B_{12} deficiency. Often it accompanies vitamin B_{12} deficiency.

Vitamin B_{12} should be administered prophylactically to all patients after total gastrectomy. Although a similar policy in patients undergoing partial gastrectomy would be of value [151], many consider it needlessly conservative. An optimal approach might be to administer vitamin B_{12} to patients with demonstrated depression of serum vitamin B_{12} level or vitamin B_{12} absorption.

INTESTINAL DISORDERS

A rare intestinal disorder leading to vitamin B_{12} deficiency was referred to earlier — selective malabsorption of vitamin B_{12}, presumably due to defective receptor sites for the IF-B_{12} complex. Other intestinal disorders predisposing to deficiency include (1) extensive resection of the ileum [152], (2) regional ileitis [153], (3) vitamin B_{12} malabsorption associated with hypothyroidism [154], administration of colchicine [155], *p*-aminosalicylic acid [156,157], and other drugs, (4) effects of vitamin B_{12} deficiency itself [158,159], and (5) tropical sprue [160], which is discussed later. In each of these, administered IF fails to correct an abnormal Schilling test result.

COMPETITIVE PARASITES

"Blind loop syndrome" The association of megaloblastic anemia with various anatomic lesions of the small intestine — stricture, diverticula, anastomoses, and blind loops due to short-circuiting operations — has been long recognized [161]. Newer diagnostic procedures have revealed these disorders to be associated with normal IF secretion, decreased vitamin B_{12} absorption not correctable with administered IF, and low serum vitamin B_{12} levels. This type of anemia is relieved by surgical correction of the abnormality or vitamin B_{12} therapy. Interestingly, this kind of anemia is reversible, in many cases, by tetracycline therapy, an observation that gave rise to the thesis that decreased vitamin B_{12} absorption in these disorders is a result of proliferation of colonic bacteria in stagnant areas of the bowel.

The syndrome that is caused by localized stasis of intestinal contents is conveniently termed the *blind loop*

syndrome, whether it is caused by surgically formed intestinal blind loops, stricture, or diverticulae. Colonic bacteria, not normally found above the terminal ileum, proliferate actively in the small intestine. Although decisive proof is lacking, competition of bacteria with host for vitamin B_{12} and IF-B_{12} complex in the intestinal lumen seems the most likely mechanism of the deficiency [162,163]. Although wild-type *E. coli* utilizes and contains vanishingly small amounts of vitamin B_{12} [164], other strains of *E. coli* as well as a wide variety of enteric organisms bind significant amounts of vitamin B_{12} [165,166]. Little evidence exists for toxic depression by bacteria of vitamin B_{12} absorption by intestinal mucosa.

Steatorrhea, another manifestation of the blind loop syndrome, is caused by malabsorption of dietary fat, a result of the effect of bacteria on bile salts, and by direct inhibition by bile acids of the mucosal uptake and esterification of fats.

Fish tapeworm infestation One of the more intriguing causes of vitamin B_{12} deficiency is infestation with the broad tapeworm *Diphyllobothrium latum*, a cestode indigenous to areas near the Baltic Sea, the Great Lakes, and certain Swiss lakes near the French border (Fig. 47-2). *D. latum* attacks humans only as final host (Fig. 33-2). It inhabits the intestine, growing to a length of 10 m, with 3000 to 4000 proglottids. Eggs but not segments are passed in the feces. Egg embyronate only in cool fresh water. Embryonation takes 2 or more weeks. The ciliated embryos (coracidia) swim actively, die in 24 h, or are swallowed by freshwater crustacea, especially "water fleas" (*Cyclops*), which become the first intermediate host. The embryo minus its ciliated cover burrows into the body cavity and transforms itself in 2 or 3 weeks

FIGURE 47-2 Life cycle of *Diphyllobothrium latum*. Inner circle represents developmental stages of parasite. 1, adult worm; 2, egg; 3, embryonated egg (coracidium); 4, procercoid larva; 5, plerocercoid larva. Outside circle shows first intermediate host (*Cyclops*), second intermediate host (fish), and definitive host (man). (Adapted from Wirth and Farrow [167].)

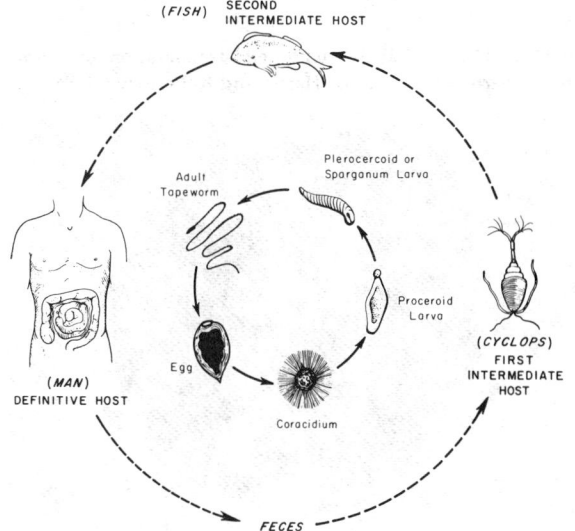

into a mature first larval stage, a hooklet-bearing procercoid. The first intermediate host is swallowed by the second intermediate host, a freshwater fish—commonly a pike, pickerel, perch, or trout. Procercoids migrate into the fish's flesh and after 3 or 4 days encyst as the second larval stage, plerocercoids, between muscle fibers. Large, edible fish may become infected by eating their infected young. Human subjects become infected by eating infected fish roe or insufficiently cooked fish muscle. In the human intestine an adult worm develops from a plerocercoid in 5 to 6 weeks. Egg laying then begins. The worm may live for years.

Vitamin B_{12} deficiency in human *D. latum* infestation is caused by competition between the worm and the host for the vitamin B_{12} in ingested food [168–174]. One reason for the frequency of infestation in Scandinavian countries is the habit of tasting raw fish during the preparation of fishkefrikadeller, a popular fish dish. The clinical picture of *D. latum* infestation ranges from no morbidity to mild macrocytosis (in carriers) to full-blown megaloblastic anemia with neurologic changes. Only about 3 percent of persons harboring the parasite become anemic. *D. latum* rarely produces a severe vitamin B_{12} deficiency state in areas outside the high-incidence district of eastern Finland [174]. The difference may be a result of differences in the biologic nature of *D. latum* in other areas of the world or, more likely, to the higher number (and mass) of plerocercoids in the fish of Finland and of worms in infested Finns.

Diagnosis of fish tapeworm infestation depends on the demonstration of tapeworm ova in feces. Treatment consists of expelling the worms by administration of niclosamide, paromomycin, or atabrine with saline purgations.

OTHER DISORDERS
Dietary deficiency   Because of the adequacy of vitamin B_{12} reserves and the high concentrations of vitamin B_{12} in foods of animal origin, deficiency rarely results from poor diet. Vegetarianism does not lead to vitamin B_{12} deficiency unless the diet is lacking in milk, eggs, and

FIGURE 47-3   Subacute combined degeneration of spinal cord in pernicious anemia. (Harris and Kellermeyer [186].)

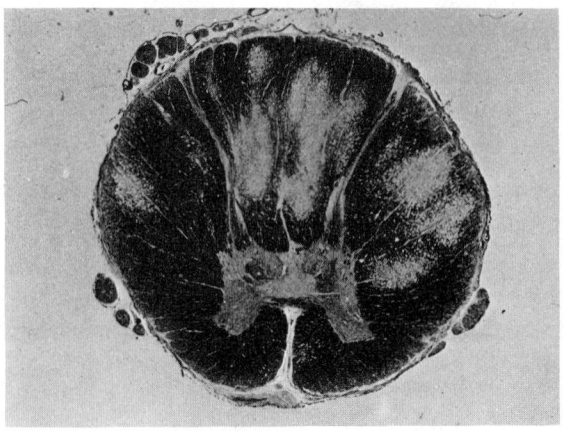

other animal products. Members of the "vegans" sects and many modern-day vegetarians do ingest such a diet, and vitamin B_{12} deficiency, along with mild megaloblastic anemia, glossitis, and neurologic disturbances, is common among them [175–178]. Occasional reports note deficiencies in psychotic or eccentric individuals on similar diets [179,180]. The serum iron is depressed in veganism, possibly owing to the large quantity of phytic acid in the whole-meal bread ingested. Vitamin B_{12} deficiency does not accompany the type of megaloblastic anemia associated with kwashiorkor or marasmus [181].

Increased requirements   Vitamin B_{12} reserves are adequate to buffer against the demands of pregnancy, hyperthyroidism, and hyperactive erythropoiesis, and these conditions rarely cause vitamin B_{12} deficiency, though they frequently cause folic acid deficiency. Neoplastic growth only occasionally causes vitamin B_{12} deficiency (see Table 47-1). Plasma cell dyscrasias and myeloproliferative disorders are among the more common causes [182–184].

CLINICAL FEATURES
The clinical picture of human vitamin B_{12} deficiency includes the nonspecific manifestations of megaloblastic anemia—glossitis, elevated serum LDH, weight loss, etc.—*plus* the following features specifically due to vitamin B_{12} deficiency: (1) neurologic abnormalities, (2) characteristic response to vitamin B_{12} therapy and lack of response to therapy with physiologic doses of folic acid, and (3) decreased serum vitamin B_{12} levels and methylmalonic aciduria.

NEUROLOGIC ABNORMALITIES
Classically, the neurologic syndrome of vitamin B_{12} deficiency consists of symmetric paresthesias in feet and fingers, with associated disturbances of vibratory sense and proprioception, progressing to spastic ataxia resulting from degenerative changes of the dorsal and lateral columns, the so-called subacute combined system disease. In fact, the picture is more often chronic than subacute and more varied and complex. Early pathologic changes in the cord consist of swelling of individual myelinated nerve fibers in small foci. Later the lesions coalesce into large foci involving many fiber systems (Fig. 47-3), but not in a systematic manner [185]. Signs of cerebral involvement are electroencephalographic changes with slowed wave frequency, irritability, somnolence, and perversion of taste, smell, and vision with central scotomata and occasional optic atrophy. There are also reports of severe psychologic and mental derangements (including "megaloblastic madness" [187]) in vitamin B_{12} deficiency [188–190], but they do not all withstand critical scrutiny. As noted earlier, tobacco amblyopia, a curious visual disorder in vitamin B_{12}–deficient smokers, has been attributed to the tendency of cyanide in tobacco smoke to convert a meager supply of vitamin B_{12} coenzyme to metabolically inert cyanocobalamin [191].

The neurologic syndrome of vitamin B$_{12}$ deficiency may occur and progress in the absence of megaloblastic anemia [192]. The neurologic syndrome is now seen infrequently, perhaps because of earlier diagnosis and treatment. An explanation of the neurologic consequences of vitamin B$_{12}$ deficiency has not been provided. Animal models have been unavailable, although neurologic lesions have been produced in vitamin B$_{12}$–deficient fruit bats [193] and monkeys [194]. It is generally considered that the major neuropathologic feature is "demyelination." It is not clear, however, whether this comes about through impairment of myelin synthesis, abnormal destruction of existing myelin, or some other process [195].

Two general hypotheses have sought to connect known enzymologic functions of coenzymes with postulated mechanisms of neurologic involvement [20]. One envisions abnormalities in the metabolism of myelin lipids as a consequence of impairment of the methylmalonyl-CoA mutase reaction [196–198]. The second postulates inactivation of vitamin B$_{12}$ by chronic cyanide intoxication.

The idea of lipid abnormalities is based on the role of methylmalonyl-CoA as an intermediate in the catabolism of a short fatty acid, propionyl-CoA (see Fig. 34-4). Conceivably, accumulated methylmalonyl-CoA either inhibits the synthesis of myelin lipids or is incorporated into the lipids synthesized, which thereby become abnormal. The resulting myelin is defective, and "demyelination" follows. Evidence against this concept is the relatively low level of propionate metabolism in humans and the lack of correlation between the degree of methylmalonic aciduria and the severity of neurologic disease.

The hypothesis that neurologic lesions occur in vitamin B$_{12}$ deficiency as a consequence of occult chronic cyanide intoxication rests on fragmentary evidence that includes (1) the relatively high incidence of so-called tobacco amblyopia, retrobulbar neuritis, and optic atrophy in vitamin B$_{12}$–deficient tobacco smokers and in vitamin B$_{12}$–deficient males [199]; (2) the relatively elevated cyanocobalamin fraction reported in the plasma vitamin B$_{12}$ of smokers [200], a claim not confirmed as yet [165]; and (3) the reported association of neurologic disorders with chronic cyanide exposure or abnormalities of cyanide metabolism. Conceivably, an exogenous cyanide load tends to convert cobalamin coenzymes to cyanocobalamin, which is metabolically inactive and less firmly bound to plasma proteins and hence more readily lost to renal excretion than other forms of vitamin B$_{12}$. Any such theory would have to rest on the assumption that the nervous system is more vulnerable to such effects than is the marrow.

It has generally been held that impairment of DNA synthesis accounts for megaloblastic erythropoiesis and related phenomena in vitamin B$_{12}$ deficiency, but not for neurologic damage, since it was believed that affected nerve cells were nondividing and thus not engaged in DNA synthesis. However, the cells that make myelin do divide, and recent preliminary evidence has implicated

impairment of N^5-methyl-FH$_4$-homocysteine methyltransferase (an enzyme related to DNA synthesis) in the neuropathy resulting from N$_2$O exposure [202].

RESPONSE TO TREATMENT

The clinical response to vitamin B$_{12}$ therapy is another useful diagnostic datum. Following parenteral administration of vitamin B$_{12}$ to deficient subjects, elevated plasma bilirubin, iron, and lactic dehydrogenase levels fall promptly (Fig. 47-4). Decreasing plasma iron turnover and fecal urobilinogen excretion reflect cessation of ineffective erythropoiesis. Within 8 to 12 h, the appearance of a marrow aspirate begins to convert from megaloblastic to erythroblastic. Transformation is complete in 48 to 72 h. The population of accumulated megaloblasts is probably converted to erythroblasts ineffectively; that is, a majority of the megaloblasts die within the marrow or soon after delivery into the circulation. Abrupt reticulocytosis begins on the third to fifth day, reaching a climax on the fourth to tenth day. Cells released at this time apparently come from new erythroblasts, not from converted megaloblasts. The intensity of the reticulocyte crisis is roughly proportional to the severity of the anemia.

FIGURE 47-4   Effect of cyanocobalamin on reticulocyte count, serum iron, serum bilirubin, stool urobilinogen, and plasma iron turnover. (Adapted from Finch et al. [203].)

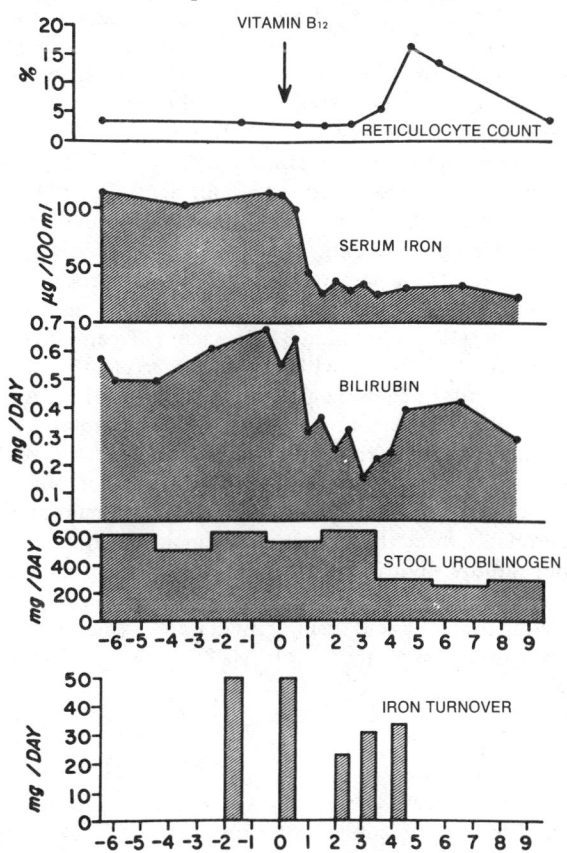

Hemoglobin levels begin to rise, though the increase during the reticulocyte crisis is relatively smaller than the increase in circulating red cells as judged by the reticulocyte count. The discrepancy is attributable to the fact that the unusually young reticulocytes delivered after sudden remission of a megaloblastic process undergo prolonged maturation in the blood [204]. Hence the count at a given moment reflects the accumulated reticulocyte output of several days.

When maturation delay in the marrow is corrected by vitamin B_{12}, a new condition is established in which a still severe anemia elicits an intensive erythropoietin-mediated stimulation of erythropoiesis. In later stages of hemoglobin restoration, hypochromia and other signs of iron deficiency may appear. In such instances the plasma iron level decreases as the vitamin B_{12} level becomes normal. A second reticulocyte response may then be produced by iron administration.

Other changes produced by repletion of vitamin B_{12} deficiency include the following: (1) striking and prompt improvement in sense of well-being; (2) rise in serum alkaline phosphatase (which is often depressed in vitamin B_{12} deficiency [205]); (3) positive nitrogen balance; (4) sharp rise in serum and urine uric acid (variably depressed in vitamin B_{12} deficiency) within 24 h of the start of therapy (a peak occurs 24 h before the peak of the reticulocyte crisis) [206]; (5) decrease in serum folate; (6) decrease in urine phosphorus after vitamin B_{12} administration, increase during reticulocytosis, and then normal [207]; (7) rise in serum vitamin B_{12} [208]; and (8) sharp drop in serum potassium, in some cases severe enough to warrant replacement therapy [209]. Failure to provide such replacement has occasionally led to sudden death during the therapy of vitamin B_{12} deficiency [210].

A patient with pure vitamin B_{12} deficiency fails to respond to a physiologic dose of folic acid, e.g., 100 to 400 μg per day, that is capable of producing a maximal response in folic acid deficiency [211]. However, a larger dose of folic acid, e.g., 5 to 15 mg per day, can produce a sizable reticulocyte response and suboptimal hemoglobin regeneration in vitamin B_{12} deficiency. Treatment of vitamin B_{12} deficiency with folate also accelerates the development of neurologic abnormalities [212]. Although this phenomenon has not yet been explained, one may conjecture that stimulation of DNA synthesis by excess folic acid (perhaps by direct stimulation of the thymidylate synthetase reaction) somehow translocates vitamin B_{12} from the nervous system to marrow and other rapidly dividing cells. Although this hypothesis remains to be tested, it finds some support in data showing that folic acid therapy in vitamin B_{12} deficiency depresses serum vitamin B_{12} levels [213,214].

LABORATORY FEATURES

SERUM VITAMIN B_{12} LEVEL

The assay of serum vitamin B_{12} is discussed in Chap. 34. Satisfactory radioisotope dilution methods are now available [215]. As noted in Chap. 34, the normal range in the author's laboratory is 150 to 450 pg/ml.[1] Signs and symptoms appear when the serum level is below about 80 to 100 pg/ml. Serum folate is often elevated when serum vitamin B_{12} is depressed, unless folate deficiency is also present.

METHYLMALONIC ACIDURIA

Methylmalonic aciduria is a reliable index of vitamin B_{12} deficiency [217,218], except in the rare cases in which it is due to an inborn metabolic error [219,220]. Urinary methylmalonate may be assayed by paper [221], gas [222], or thin-layer chromatography [223]. Normal subjects excrete only trace amounts of methylmalonate: 0 to 3.5 mg per 24 h. Levels vary in vitamin B_{12} deficiency but are elevated, sometimes to 300 mg or more per 24 h. Vitamin B_{12} therapy restores excretion patterns to normal in several days, though an occasional patient continues to excrete abnormal amounts of methylmalonate following vitamin repletion. In practice, the determination of urinary methylmalonate excretion is rarely necessary as a diagnostic tool.

ASSAY OF VITAMIN B_{12} ABSORPTION AND INTRINSIC FACTOR

Following the observation that a large parenteral dose (1 mg) of nonradioactive vitamin B_{12} increases excretion of radioactive vitamin B_{12}, presumably by blocking vitamin B_{12}–binding sites in plasma and liver [224,225], it became feasible to assess vitamin B_{12} absorption by studies of urinary excretion following oral administration. The so-called Schilling test procedure is as follows: After voiding, a fasting patient takes 0.5 μCi (0.5 to 2.0 μg) ^{60}Co- or ^{57}Co-cyanocobalamin in water by mouth at time zero. A 24-h urine collection is begun. At 2 h, 1 mg of nonradioactive cyanocobalamin is administered intramuscularly. This is the "flushing" dose. The patient may then take food. An adequate sample of pooled urine is assayed for radioactivity and the percentage of administered radioactivity excreted in the first 24 h is calculated. With a 1-μg dose of labeled vitamin B_{12}, normal subjects excrete 7 percent or more of the administered radioactivity in the first 24 h. A greater percentage is excreted when a smaller dose is given. It is important that laboratories performing this procedure establish a range of normal in suitable control subjects.

If excretion of radioactivity is slow, the second part of the Schilling test is performed in no less than 5 days. The procedure is the same except that 60 mg of demonstrably active hog IF (equivalent to 1 N.F. unit) is given orally with the radioactive vitamin B_{12}. If poor excretion in the first part was due to IF deficiency, the result in the second part should be normal. If excretion in the second part is still abnormal, other explanations must be found for malabsorption of vitamin B_{12}.

The kidneys excrete cyanocobalamin and inulin in a similar manner. Indeed, radioactive vitamin B_{12} is useful in measurement of the glomerular filtration rate

---

[1] Expressed in the SI system [216], these values are equivalent to 110 to 330 pmol/l.

[226]. Renal disease associated with impaired glomerular filtration may delay excretion of radioactivity in the Schilling test [227]. In order to circumvent that difficulty, various modifications have been proposed—for example, a 72-h urine collection with flushing doses of vitamin B_{12} every 24 h. Whole-body counting may be the only satisfactory technique in severe renal insufficiency [228]. In this procedure, the flushing dose is omitted. Normal subjects retain 45 to 80 percent of administered radioactivity following an oral dose of radioactive vitamin B_{12}. In one such procedure [229], the plasma of normal subjects 8 h after an oral dose of ^{57}Co vitamin B_{12} contained 1.4 to 4.1 percent of administered radioactivity per liter of plasma, with a mean of 2.3 percent. The pernicious anemia group had a range of 0.0 to 0.6 percent, with a mean of 0.2 percent.

Certain precautions are necessary in using the Schilling test. Cobalamin in food is protein-bound and cannot be absorbed until it is released from the binding protein and then bound by gastric intrinsic factor. The Schilling test measures the absorption of unbound cobalamin and thus does not detect patients whose only defect is malabsorption of dietary cobalamin. Such situations have been reported after partial gastrectomy [230], after vagotomy [231], among patients with gastric ulcer [232], and during cimetidine therapy [233]. Indeed, the anemia of vitamin B_{12} deficiency is occasionally associated with normal Schilling test results and malabsorption of protein-bound cobalamin [234].

A major source of error in the performance of the test is incomplete urine collection. Completeness of urine collection may be assessed by a determination of total creatinine content in a 24-h urine specimen. The lower limit of normal is 15 mg per kilogram of body weight per day. Other occasional difficulties with the Schilling test are apparent malabsorption due to renal dysfunction or inadequate flushing with nonradioactive cyanocobalamin, apparent normal absorption due to a previous Schilling test or administration of other isotopes, and inappropriate low results when the test is repeated with an oral intrinsic factor supplement due to high concentrations of intrinsic factor antibodies in the patient's gastric juice or to a "macrocytic" distal ileum in untreated patients.

When these hazards are avoided, the Schilling test is an indispensable diagnostic tool in the assessment of vitamin B_{12} absorption. It may also be used to assay IF on the basis of its functional attributes. Assays of IF in gastric juice can also be based on IF-mediated (1) enhancement of vitamin B_{12} uptake by intestinal cell preparations in vitro [235–238], (2) inhibition of an AdoCbl-dependent enzyme [239], and (3) various immunologic parameters [240,241]. The use of such techniques led to discovery of a physiologically inert IF molecule in a child with vitamin B_{12} malabsorption [129]. Studies of the abnormal IF molecule isolated by affinity chromatography [130] directly demonstrated nonidentity of the vitamin B_{12} and ileum receptor binding sites on the IF molecule. The genetic abnormality was confined to the latter site.

PERNICIOUS ANEMIA: CLINICAL FEATURES AND DIAGNOSIS

Pernicious anemia occurs typically in a 40- to 80-year-old Northern European of fair complexion. The traditional description of a typical patient—gray or white-haired, blue-eyed, long-eared, and of characteristic habitus—long ago passed into the mythology of hematology. Such patients are seen in Scandinavian countries where pernicious anemia is common. However, many patients do not fit the description and many healthy Scandinavians do. Moreover, the disease is being recognized with increasing frequency in peoples of other races and ethnic groups [88–90], although it is still relatively uncommon in Orientals.

The main clinical manifestations are the features of megaloblastic anemia (pancytopenia, glossitis, elevated serum lactic dehydrogenase, etc.) and the specific features of vitamin B_{12} deficiency (low serum vitamin B_{12} level, neurologic disorder, methylmalonic aciduria, response to vitamin B_{12} therapy, etc.) described above. In addition, there is depressed parietal cell function, as expressed by achlorhydria after histamine stimulation and decreased vitamin B_{12} absorption in the first part of the Schilling test with correction by oral IF in the second part.

Over the years, diagnostic criteria have changed with the advent of newer diagnostic tests. In practice it is unnecessary to perform all such tests before diagnosing pernicious anemia. The physician is quite justified in making the diagnosis in a typical patient who demonstrates megaloblastic anemia, achlorhydria after histamine stimulation, and response to vitamin B_{12} therapy. Increasingly, the serum vitamin B_{12} assay and the Schilling test have replaced gastric analysis and careful monitoring of the reticulocyte response.

The Schilling test is often something of a luxury in a practice setting. It is of course reassuring to have consonant results in a typical case. In an atypical case the test is indispensable. Several considerations should govern the use of the Schilling test. Since the test involves the administration of a large flushing dose of vitamin B_{12}, performance of the test early in the diagnostic workup initiates specific therapy. However, the Schilling test can be performed at any time, even after full repletion of a vitamin B_{12} deficiency and correction of anemia. An IF deficiency, if present, will still be present.

There is an understandable tendency in many institutions to neglect the gastric analysis in favor of the Schilling test. The early technique of assaying gastric acid following a gruel test meal has been replaced by better methods. Secretion of gastric juice is now stimulated by histamine or betazole (Histalog) and all the juice secreted over a given time period withdrawn. An improved version of the test, the "augmented histamine test" [242], permits measurement of maximal gastric acid production under standard conditions. Previously, achlorhydria was defined according to the reaction with Töpfer's reagent, which changes color at pH 3 (i.e., at a HCl concentration of 10^{-3} M). Absence of color change with Töpfer's reagent was interpreted to mean "no free acid.'' It was later recognized that in this procedure substantial amounts of gastric HCl can be overlooked, and it became customary to measure the pH of gastric juice with a pH meter. Achlorhydria is now said to be present when the pH of gastric juice is never less than 3.5 and does not decrease by more than one pH unit following maximal stimulation with histamine. When the pH drop after histamine is more than one pH unit, though the initial pH is above 3.5, the condition is termed hypochlorhydria.

The use of this technique has shown that achlorhydria is less common than was formerly believed and is always to be considered pathologic. Though not of itself diagnostic of pernicious anemia—it occurs as well in iron deficiency—its absence interdicts that diagnosis, and its presence, along with the other elements of the clinical picture, supports it. The gastric juice of pernicious anemia reveals, in addition to achlorhydria, decreased volume and diminished pepsin and rennin levels. In many instances, achlorhydria precedes by many years the development of symptoms [243] and the loss of IF secretion. Fasting plasma gastrin levels measured by radioimmunoassay are elevated in about 75 percent of patients with PA [244]. However, gastrin levels are also high in achlorhydria with adequate vitamin B_{12} absorption [245,246].

Pernicious anemia is often overlooked or misdiagnosed [247] because of its insidious onset; its tendency to be masked by the uncritical use of multivitamin preparations containing folic acid [248]; its many presenting pictures, e.g., bleeding owing to thrombocytopenia [249] or thrombocytopathy [250], neurologic disorder, constipation, etc.; and its association with other disease states, e.g., hypothyroidism [251], hyperthyroidism [252], hypogammaglobulinemia [253], hypergammaglobulinemia with positive antiglobulin test [254], endocrine disorders [255], ulcerative colitis [256], gastric carcinoma [257,258], vitiligo [259], and others. Perhaps the only clinical state that is notably rare in association with pernicious anemia is pregnancy. Indeed, female patients under 40 may suffer from infertility [260], as do male patients from hypospermia and sterility [261]. The frequent absence of macrocytosis in blacks with pernicious anemia has also led to misdiagnosis [262]. This phenomenon may be caused by the high incidence in blacks of α thalassemia, which would tend to mask macrocytic expression of pernicious anemia [263].

THERAPY OF VITAMIN B_{12} DEFICIENCY

Therapy consists in the parenteral administration of vitamin B_{12} (cyanocobalamin or hydroxocobalamin) in amounts sufficient to provide the 2 to 5 μg needed for the daily requirement and to replete liver stores and other reservoirs, which normally contain 2 to 5 mg of vitamin B_{12}. Because of its low cost and lack of toxicity, doses larger than those actually needed are generally administered. As noted above, parenterally administered vitamin B_{12} is bound to plasma proteins and cellular binding sites. If much more than 100 μg is given parenterally in a single dose, delay in encountering vacant

binding sites leads to rapid renal excretion of unbound vitamin.

Since hydroxocobalamin is bound more tightly by binding proteins than cyanocobalamin [264], it is less rapidly excreted by the kidney and more effective in achieving high serum vitamin B_{12} levels [265]. In practice, these theoretical advantages are of questionable value. Moreover, variations of response in different patients exceed the small differences in the behavior of hydroxocobalamin and cyanocobalamin [266]. It also appears [165] that many (or all) commercial hydroxocobalamin preparations are contaminated with several unidentified cobalamin analogs in varying amounts.

Many regimens are used for the administration of vitamin B_{12} according to these guiding principles. Indeed, if enough vitamin B_{12} is given, it is difficult to misuse it. The following treatment schedule is used in the author's clinic: (1) 1000 μg intramuscularly daily for 1 to 2 weeks, (2) the same dose weekly for an additional 4 weeks or until the hematocrit is normal, and (3) the same dose once monthly for the lifetime of the patient. Larger amounts are not harmful; a dosage schedule of 1000 μg every 2 weeks for 6 months is recommended for patients with neurologic manifestations.

Liver extracts are no longer used. None is listed in U.S.P. XVI. Depot preparations of vitamin B_{12} once found favor but are now little used because they may elicit antibodies to TC II [267]. Oral vitamin B_{12}–IF preparations are not recommended, since patients often become refractory to therapy owing to the development of IF antibodies [268,269]. Oral therapy with large amounts of vitamin B_{12} is effective, but because of unpredictable absorption should be reserved for the occasional patient who for some reason cannot receive parenteral therapy. Patients receiving oral medication who feel well often stop their medication. The patient with pernicious anemia should understand that he or she must be treated for life.

Transfusion is rarely necessary in pernicious anemia, though it may be indicated when the hemoglobin level is below 5 g/dl or when the patient is debilitated, infected, or in heart failure. In such instances, packed erythrocytes should be administered slowly under supervision. Since the response to vitamin B_{12} occurs within 48 to 72 h, it is seldom necessary to subject the patient to the risks, discomfort, and expense of blood transfusion.

There is no need for iron therapy in pernicious anemia unless there is evidence of associated iron deficiency or reason to expect that tissue iron reserves are deficient—as, for example, in women of early middle age who may have had heavy menstrual losses or several pregnancies. In such cases, hemoglobin and erythrocyte regeneration are delayed until iron is given. There is no need to administer folic acid or ascorbic acid in addition to the vitamin B_{12}, provided that the patient takes an adequate diet.

Infections, which occur frequently—especially in the genitourinary tracts of patients with neurologic involvement—must be treated vigorously with appropriate antibiotics, else they may impair the response to vitamin B_{12} therapy.

Many multivitamin preparations are available containing vitamin B_{12} and folic acid (and often iron). These "shot-gun" preparations, or so-called hematinics, have been repeatedly condemned by authorities, yet they continue to be used. The vitamin B_{12} content is usually too small to be important, but with the inclusion in some preparations of IF substance, sufficient vitamin B_{12} may be absorbed to obscure a clinical diagnosis.

With the exception of hereditary methylmalonic aciduria [219,220], vitamin B_{12} deficiency is the only valid indication for vitamin B_{12} therapy. It has been recommended, nevertheless, for many disorders in which there is no evidence of deficiency, especially for the various types of neuropathy, liver disease, dermatologic disorders, allergies, and as a "tonic" or appetite stimulant. The usefulness of vitamin B_{12} in these circumstances has not been proved, and its use for such purposes is not recommended. The administration of vitamin B_{12} to stimulate growth in underdeveloped children is also of dubious value in the light of the evidence.

Megaloblastic anemia of folic acid deficiency

ETIOLOGY AND PATHOGENESIS

The major causes of folic acid deficiency, summarized in Table 47-1, are (1) decreased intake of folate caused by poor nutrition, (2) decreased intake caused by impaired absorption, (3) increased folate requirements, and (4) impaired utilization.

DECREASED INTAKE CAUSED BY POOR NUTRITION

The amount of folic acid in the diet is not greatly in excess of the nutritional requirement. Because body folate reserves are relatively meager, folic acid deficiency develops rapidly in persons taking an inadequate diet [270]. Such persons, common in every medical practice, include familiar archetypes: the elderly widower who is too weary, anorectic, or uninterested to buy and prepare food properly; the ailing old woman who subsists on tea and toast; the chronic alcoholic who rarely eats or who picks at food. Less well recognized victims of inadequate folic acid intake are young infants (especially those with infection or diarrhea) who drink cow's or goat's milk and whose diets lack vegetables, eggs, and meat [271]; premature infants whose reserves are small [272]; children on a synthetic diet for phenylketonuria [273], maple syrup urine disease, or other inborn errors; subjects undergoing hyperalimentation therapy [274]; and patients on maintenance hemodialysis, in whom anorexia prevents repletion of the folic acid lost by dialysis [275,276].

As mentioned in Chap. 34, loss of food folate through excessive cooking often accounts for folic acid deficiency, especially among disadvantaged peoples who live on finely divided foods such as rice. Folic acid deficiency is said to be more common in India than in China or Malaya because the Indian diet contains little meat, consisting largely of well-cooked gourds and nonleafy vegetables that are cooked for many hours [277]. The relative infrequency of folic acid deficiency among the Chinese is attributable to their custom of eating leafy vegetables prepared at mealtime by scalding rather than prolonged cooking [278,279]. In modern China, northerners have poorer access to green vegetables than southerners [280] and apparently for that reason more commonly have megaloblastic anemia, presumably owing to folic acid deficiency.

Megaloblastic anemia occurring in chronic liver disease is usually caused by folic acid deficiency [281,282] resulting from poor diet and impaired hepatic storage of folic acid. Therapy consists of treatment of the cirrhosis, control of alcoholism, and repletion of folic acid. Although folic acid deficiency is an important cause of anemia in malnourished alcoholics, acute alcoholic intoxication may itself suppress the levels of serum folate [283] and of circulating reticulocytes, platelets, and granulocytes [284–286]. Alcoholic intoxication also interferes with the metabolism and interconversion of the various folate derivatives [287,288]. In addition, reversible vacuolation of red cell and white cell precursors in the marrow like that seen in chloramphenicol toxicity [289] and functional impairment of granulocytes [290] are common in acute alcoholism. These changes occur even when pharmacologic doses of folic acid are administered concomitantly [291]. Although alcohol ingestion accelerates megaloblastic transformation, the critical factor in determining the time of onset of tissue folate deficiency is the state of body folate stores [292].

Unlike the rare pure vitamin B_{12} deficiency of strict vegetarians, nutritional folic acid deficiency is often associated with multiple vitamin deficiencies. In such patients, a significant history of gross dietary inadequacy is usually easy to obtain. The typical spongy gums, muscular hemorrhages, and perifollicular petechiae of scurvy are commonly associated with folic acid deficiency resulting from malnutrition. Latent deficiencies of other vitamins may become overt during recovery, when metabolism is increased. Although folic acid therapy facilitates utilization of other vitamins, they should be provided in adequate supply early in the illness.

It is of interest that the frequency of nutritional folic acid deficiency was not appreciated until the assay procedures for serum folate and vitamin B_{12} became widely available in the early 1960s. Prior to that time, many such patients were considered to have pernicious anemia, particularly since vitamin B_{12} therapy produced partial therapeutic responses [293,294].

DECREASED INTAKE CAUSED BY IMPAIRED ABSORPTION

Diagnosis The importance of intestinal malabsorption as a cause of folic acid deficiency has been firmly established by investigators using test procedures that assess by microbiologic or isotopic techniques the concentration of folate in the serum, urine, or stool following an oral test dose of the vitamin. The following routine and research procedures permit assessment of the intestinal absorption of folic acid:

1. Comparison of the microbiologically assayed time course of urinary folic acid activity after parenteral and oral administration of 5 mg of folic acid. An "excretion index" (excretion after oral dosage divided by excretion after parenteral dosage) of less than 75 percent constitutes evidence of malabsorption [295]. This test initiates therapy with folic acid, precludes later assay of serum folate, and may vary with the level of renal functions.

2. Microbiologic determinations of serum folate activity after an oral dose of folic acid [296–298]. The patient must first be saturated with folic acid to prevent rapid plasma clearance of folic acid and spuriously low serum levels. In one protocol [298], the patient receives 5 mg of folic acid parenterally for 3 consecutive days and, 36 h after the last dose, 40 μg of folic acid per kilogram of body weight orally. In normal subjects, serum levels reach peak values of greater than 40 ng/ml 1 to 2 h later. In malabsorption, no peak is observed.

3. Determination of urinary radioactivity after an oral dose of ^{3}H-F (40 μg per kilogram of body weight) accompanied by a parenteral flushing dose of 15 mg of unlabeled folic acid [299,300]. Under test conditions, normal subjects excrete 26 to 58 percent of the test dose, with a mean of 41 percent. Patients with malabsorption excrete less than 26 percent [299]. As in the test just described, preliminary saturation with folic acid is necessary.

4. Fecal radioactivity after an oral dose of ^{3}H-F may be determined by a variety of techniques [300]. Normal subjects excrete 9.2 to 59 percent (mean, 21.3 percent) of a test dose of 200 μg ^{3}H-F. Fecal excretion in excess of 60 percent is observed in malabsorption. This test does not require preliminary saturation with folic acid and hence does not require initiation of therapy. Collections are difficult, however.

In using these tests in the diagnosis of malabsorption, it is important to distinguish the problem of diagnosing folic acid deficiency from that of diagnosing folic acid malabsorption, which is but one cause of folic acid deficiency. The serum folate assay establishes the presence of a deficiency but gives no clue to its mechanism. If malabsorption is already known to be present (from clinical evidence, the xylose excretion test, etc.), serum folate may be assayed to determine if malabsorption has led to folate deficiency. If it has—i.e., if the serum folate level is low—it is seldom necessary to perform the tests decribed above to document the presence of folate malabsorption. Such tests are used occasionally because experience has taught that in some cases folic acid may be malabsorbed without other signs of malabsorption. Conversely, severe malabsorption may be present without malabsorption of folic acid. In general, however, the tests for folic acid malabsorption are too unwieldy for routine clinical use.

Subtotal gastrectomy   As noted earlier, malabsorption of vitamin B_{12} occurs occasionally in patients who have undergone subtotal gastrectomy. Folic acid deficiency may also occur in such patients. These deficiencies are usually mild and do not lead to megaloblastic anemia. Serum folate levels are depressed in 12 to 50 percent of patients selected randomly after subtotal gastrectomy and in from 54 to 67 percent of those who develop megaloblastic anemia [301–303]. Red cell folate is also depressed in many partially gastrectomized patients [304].

The cause of folic acid deficiency after subtotal gastrectomy is not entirely clear. Decreased dietary intake may be a factor. Jejunal morphology was normal in one series of folic acid-deficient patients following subtotal gastrectomy [302], and folic acid absorption was normal in tests employing crystalline folic acid.

Nontropical sprue (gluten-induced enteropathy; celiac disease)   The old term *sprue* referred originally to a chronic wasting disorder that is common in the tropics and is associated clinically with glossitis, diarrhea, and the passage of light-colored, bulky, and frothy stools.

A condition similar to tropical sprue occurs in persons who have never been in the tropics. Nontropical sprue—also called *idiopathic steatorrhea*, to distinguish it from steatorrhea resulting from pancreatic insufficiency—is often associated with hypoferremia, hypocalcemia, osteroporosis, and osteomalacia. The disease in adults is considered an extension of "celiac disease" of childhood [305]; hence *adult celiac disease* and *celiac sprue* are commonly used synonyms.

Nontropical sprue is now recognized as a generalized disorder of absorption that may be related to the ingestion of wheat protein (i.e., gluten) or its glutamine-rich polypeptide components [306–308]. The mechanism of toxicity is not known. Since certain peptidases can convert toxic peptides to nontoxic dipeptides or amino acids, the picture may result from a specific peptidase deficiency.

The diagnosis rests on (1) clinical evidence of folic acid deficiency, (2) a response to therapy with a gluten-free diet, (3) a jejunal biopsy specimen showing subtotal villous atrophy, crypt elongation, change in surface epithelium from columnar to cuboid, and mucosal infiltration by mononuclear cells—a picture that is characteristic but not pathognomonic—and (4) steatorrhea.

Steatorrhea may be detected by simple microscopic estimation of fat droplets in the stool. Quantitative chemical measurements of stool fat are more desirable but not widely available. A rough screening test for malabsorption of fat is the determination of fasting serum carotene. Normal subjects have levels above 100 μg/dl. Lower levels suggest malabsorption and warrant further investigation. The most commonly used screening test for malabsorption is the D-xylose excretion test. D-Xylose is only partially metabolized; the remainder is excreted in the urine in proportion to the amount absorbed. Excretion of less than 1.5 g of xylose within 5 h of a 5-g dose is presumptive evidence of malabsorption.

Malabsorption of folic acid is demonstrably present in most patients with this disorder [295,298–300,309]. Studies with ^{3}H-F show a correlation between the severity of jejunal villous atrophy and the degree of impairment of folic acid absorption. Serum folate levels are also depressed in most patients [310], although not all have megaloblastic anemia. Gluten-free diets reverse the abnormality of folic acid absorption [309].

Tropical sprue   Tropical sprue, in many ways similar to nontropical sprue, is a malabsorptive disorder of unknown etiology with a wide spectrum of clinical manifestations. It occurs frequently and endemically in the tropics—notably in the West Indies, the Indian subcontinent, and southeast Asia—and can be acquired by residents of temperate climates who go to the tropics; it persists for many years after a return from the tropics. Thus it has been found in North Americans returning from the Caribbean area [312], British servicemen returning from India [277,313], and Puerto Ricans who have moved to New York City [314].

Although tropical sprue is now known to occur in overt and subclinical forms and to vary in its manifestations from area to area, its hallmark is the rapid responsiveness of intestinal malabsorption to folic acid therapy. Indeed, such responsiveness is now considered as much a diagnostic criterion as responsiveness to a gluten-free diet is for nontropical sprue. Gluten intolerance is not a factor in the etiology of tropical sprue. The dramatic therapeutic effect of folic acid administration is puzzling, especially since nutritional folic acid deficiency does not lead to tropical sprue. Indeed, the disease can occur in well-nourished individuals.

The relations between tropical sprue and folic acid metabolism are complex, and many theories have been proposed to account for the disorder [315], among them (1) a deficiency [316] (or lack [317]) of intestinal conjugase, (2) a defect in folic acid absorption that is remediable by folic acid therapy, (3) an inborn error of folate metabolism, (4) the presence in the bowel of a naturally occurring folate antagonist such as pteroic acid, and (5) the effects of pathogenic enteric microorganisms. An infectious etiology is suggested by the beneficial effect of broad-spectrum antibiotics [318,319], the acquisition of the disease by travelers, and the occasional epidemic behavior of the disease, especially in India, where "sprue houses" are recognized [320].

The clinical picture of tropical sprue has been well described [321,322]. In brief, there occur defective absorptions of fat and carbohydrates (and D-xylose), hypoalbuminemia, hypocalcemia, folic acid and often (in the later stages) vitamin B$_{12}$ deficiency [323], and characteristic though not diagnostic morphologic changes in the small intestine. The degree of folate malabsorption varies in different studies.

Conventional therapy consists of the daily oral administration of 1 to 3 mg of folic acid, though physiologic doses are effective. Vitamin B$_{12}$–deficient patients require repletion with this vitamin. Patients with tropical sprue seem to need more folic acid than is available in the diet, and since they tend to relapse without supplementation, maintenance therapy is recommended for at least 2 years. Antibiotic therapy is a useful adjunct to folic acid therapy. Alone, it fails to correct abnormalities of jejunal morphology. During the acute phase, when glossitis is present, a bland diet is desirable. After remission has been achieved, dietary restrictions are unnecessary, although the diet should contain adequate protein and green vegetables.

Other intestinal disorders   Malabsorption of folic acid commonly occurs in regional enteritis [324,325], after resections of the small intestine in which all but a few feet of jejunum are removed [326], in lymphomatous or leukemic infiltration of the small intestine [327,328], in Whipple's disease [328], in scleroderma and amyloidosis [329], and in diabetes mellitus [330,331]. Systemic bacterial infections also impair folate absorption [332].

Ingestion of anticonvulsant and other drugs   Many reports indicate an association between anticonvulsant drug ingestion and depressed serum folate levels and in some cases megaloblastic anemia [333–342]. All three major anticonvulsant drugs (diphenylhydantoin, phenobarbital, and primidone) have been implicated. Most patients taking these agents for prolonged periods have subnormal serum folate levels, normal serum vitamin B$_{12}$ levels, and normal marrow morphology. Overt megaloblastic anemia occurs only occasionally—probably when drug ingestion is associated with inadequate dietary intake of folic acid.

The mechanism of production of folate deficiency by anticonvulsant drugs is uncertain. Although folic acid absorption was demonstrably normal in several series of patients with diphenylhydantoin-associated megaloblastic anemia [297,333], most workers believe that the drug somehow impairs intestinal absorption. Subnormal folic acid absorption has been reported in several nonanemic patients taking diphenylhydantoin [340,341], and others on the drug have a defect in the absorption of D-xylose [335] and vitamin B$_{12}$ that is reversed by folic acid treatment. Evidence that anticonvulsant-induced megaloblastic anemia responds to dietary folate [338,342,343] has suggested that the drug impairs intestinal deconjugation of polyglutamate forms of folic acid, but this view has been challenged [344]. The chemical similarities between the major anticonvulsants and the folic acid molecule raise the possibility that these drugs are mild competitive inhibitors of folate metabolism. It has been suggested that folate metabolism may be involved in the anticonvulsant actions of these drugs and, indeed, in the seizure mechanism itself [339]. Physicians treating convulsive disorders should be aware of the effects of anticonvulsant drugs and administer folic acid as necessary.

Other drugs have been associated with depressed

serum folate levels and megaloblastic anemia, among them glutethimide [345], isoniazid and cycloserine [346], and oral contraceptives containing mestranol [347–349]. Oral contraceptives interfere with folic acid absorption in a small percentage of women taking them, possibly by inhibiting deconjugation of polyglutamates. It is possible that affected women have a defect of the conjugase system.

INCREASED FOLATE REQUIREMENTS

Pregnancy   Anemia, perhaps the commonest complication of pregancy, is difficult to diagnose because the physiologic hydremia accompanying gestation decreases hemoglobin concentration by a few grams per deciliter despite concurrent increase in total hemoglobin mass [350–352]. A survey of pregnant women in a large clinic population in New York City [353] revealed significant individual deficiencies of iron, vitamin B_{12}, and folate and various combined deficiencies. Though only 9 percent were deficient in folate alone, about two-thirds of the anemic women were deficient in folate plus another nutrient during pregnancy. The incidence of folic acid deficiency is even higher when studies are performed at term. In England, 95 percent of women at term had low serum folate levels [354]; in Australia, 60 percent [355] had similar levels. Frank megaloblastic anemia of pregnancy is less frequent, though not uncommon. Of 3199 obstetric patients near London, 474 had hemoglobin levels below 9.5 g/dl, of whom 90 had megaloblastic anemia [356].

Many data [357–361] indicate that folic acid deficiency is the major cause of megaloblastic anemia of pregnancy. Its frequency is attributable to low body reserves of folic acid and the fact that pregnancy increases daily requirements for folic acid fivefold to tenfold, especially in the last trimester [362,363]. The presence of multiple fetuses, poor diet (a frequent result of anorexia or nausea), infection, coexisting hemolytic anemia, or anticonvulsant medication may further increase requirements. Lactation also severely aggravates folic acid deficiency [364–366]. A curious phenomenon is the capacity of the fetus to take up folic acid (and other nutrients) at the expense of the mother, even when the available supply is severely reduced.

Controversy has surrounded the questions of whether folic acid supplementation should be given routinely to all pregnant women and, if so, in what dose [367]. Concern that uncritical administration of folic acid could harm a patient with undiagnosed pernicious anemia led several years ago to the deletion of folic acid from multivitamin preparations intended for antenatal therapy. Although pregnancy in a patient with pernicious anemia is so rare as to be a curiosity, it does occur [368]. Nonetheless, reformulation of multivitamin capsules did lead to a rise in the incidence of megaloblastic anemia of pregnancy in many communities.

Most workers agree that routine folic acid supplementation is desirable during pregnancy not only because folic acid requirements are increased, but also because clinical evidence suggests an association between severe folic acid deficiency and complications of pregnancy other than anemia, e.g., abruptio placentae, embryopathology, spontaneous abortion, and bleeding [360,361,369–372]. However, in one study [373], folate supplementation did not alter the incidence of such complications. Nonetheless, dietary folate deficiency [374] and folate antagonists [375,376] do cause fetal abnormalities in experimental animals.

The amount of folic acid necessary to produce distinct evidence of hematologic response during pregnancy exceeds the amount required immediately after delivery by nearly 0.5 mg per day [363]. Since a uniform dose of 1 mg per day of folic acid is effective treatment for megaloblastic anemia of pregnancy, supplementation at this level has been recommended for all pregnant women [363]. Others [377,378] have recommended 0.5 mg as a safe routine daily dosage.

Hyperactive hemopoiesis   The requirement for folic acid rises sharply in hemolytic anemia associated with chronic overactivity of the marrow [379–382], such as sickle cell anemia, hereditary spherocytosis, thalassemia, the various types of hemolytic hemoglobinopathy, immunohemolytic anemia, and paroxysmal nocturnal hemoglobinuria. Indeed, megaloblastic changes may appear in the marrow almost simultaneously with the onset of a severe acute hemolytic process.

The conclusion that folic acid requirements are abnormally high in these disorders rests not only on the frequency of associated megaloblastic anemia (and the resulting decrease in reticulocyte percentage), but also on the fact that therapy with folic acid is successful only if unusually large doses (up to 25 mg per day) are given [379,381].

Skin diseases   Folic acid deficiency occurs in a substantial percentage of patients with chronic exfoliative dermatitis [383–385]. Direct measurements of folate content of exfoliated skin indicate daily losses of 5 to 20 μg of folic acid [385]. Interestingly, the folate content of exfoliated skin is 4 to 6 times that of normal skin. No evidence of intestinal malabsorption of folate has been found in this group of patients.

Since psoriasis may be treated with methotrexate [386], these patients have an added reason for becoming deficient in folate coenzymes. It has been suggested that pretreatment of such patients with folic acid prior to methotrexate therapy might prevent the hematologic manifestation of folic acid deficiency without impairing the therapeutic effect of methotrexate [385].

Neoplastic disease   Megaloblastic anemia, fully developed or intermediate in character, and depressed serum folate level (or elevated FIGlu excretion) are frequently observed in patients with neoplastic disease [387–389], especially metastatic cancer [390] and leukemia [391–393].

Because of the early (unjustified) suspicion that supplementation with folic acid in patients with acute lymphocytic leukemia may accelerate the disease [394]—an observation that led to the development of antifolate drugs for the treatment of this disease—some physicians have been reluctant to correct the folic acid deficiency associated with leukemia and other malignant disorders. There is in fact no evidence that folic acid therapy accelerates malignant growth.

The deficiency of folic acid that accompanies tumor growth is presumed to reflect utilization of the vitamin by tumor cells, a phenomenon that resembles the preemption of maternal nutrients by a fetus. However, other explanations for deficiency in a given patient may be valid, among them poor diet, cachexia, malabsorption, and hepatic insufficiency [395].

IMPAIRED UTILIZATION
Folic acid antagonists The 4-aminopteroyl glutamates (Aminopterin and methotrexate) are powerful inhibitors of dihydrofolate reductase that can cause deficiency of folate coenzymes in tissues within hours [396–398]. Other enzymes of folic acid metabolism are inhibited only weakly [399], and probably not at all when drugs are administered in conventional dosages.

The pharmacology and clinical applicability of the folic acid antagonists have been reviewed [400,401] and are discussed elsewhere in this book. Methotrexate, the most widely used of these agents, is employed in the therapy of acute leukemia in children, psoriasis, and various neoplastic disease. The drug may be administered by diverse routes and is rapidly excreted by the kidney. If renal function is impaired, effects and toxicity are prolonged and enhanced. Citrovorum factor effectively blocks the actions of methotrexate, but only if it is given simultaneously or after a short time interval [402].

Major toxic effects are necrotic mouth lesions; ulcerations of the esophagus, small intestine, and colon, with abdominal pain, vomiting, and diarrhea; megaloblastic anemia and subsequent marrow hyperplasia and pancytopenia; and a miscellany of effects including alopecia, increased sensitivity to infection, and hyperpigmentation.

Pyrimethamine (Daraprim), a drug used in the treatment of chloroquine-resistant malaria and ocular toxoplasmosis, and its relative trimethoprim (Trimpex, Bactrim, and Septra), used in the treatment of urinary tract infections, are folic acid antagonists that are more toxic to the parasite than to the host [403,404]. They occasionally produce in the host mild megaloblastosis that is relieved by administration of citrovorum factor or withdrawal of the drug [405]. It is of interest that citrovorum factor does not protect the parasite against the effects of these drugs [406].

CLINICAL FEATURES
The clinical picture of human folic acid deficiency includes all the nonspecific manifestations of megaloblastic anemia that were described earlier—glossitis, cytologic abnormalities in various types of epithelium

[407,409], elevated serum LDH, etc.—that occur in vitamin B_{12} deficiency as well *plus* the following specific features that make possible the diagnosis of folic acid deficiency, irrespective of the underlying cause: (1) a history of circumstances likely to lead to folic acid deficiency, e.g., poor diet, frank malabsorption, alcoholism, etc.; (2) lack of neurologic changes of the type seen in vitamin B_{12} deficiency; (3) full clinical response to therapy with physiologic doses of folic acid; and (4) laboratory features to be described below (i.e., decreased serum folate level, decreased red cell folate level, elevated excretion of FIGlu after a loading dose of histidine, abnormally rapid disappearance from the serum of an intravenously injected standard dose of folic acid, decreased urinary excretion of radioactivity following a standard oral dose of ^{3}H-F, and normal serum vitamin B_{12} and urine methylmalonate levels).

The occurrence of a full therapeutic response following administration of a physiologic dose of folic acid (i.e., 200 μg daily) distinguishes folic acid deficiency from vitamin B_{12} deficiency, in which a response to folic acid occurs only after pharmacologic doses (e.g., 5 mg daily) [409]. The practical usefulness of this procedure is limited by the many necessary precautions described earlier. It should be noted that vitamin B_{12} therapy may produce a partial therapeutic response in folic acid deficiency [293,294].

LABORATORY FEATURES
When folate intake is abruptly decreased, the serum folate level falls many weeks before megaloblastic anemia appears [410]. Hence low serum folate (i.e., below about 3 ng/ml) may signify an actual deficiency of body folate but only an imminent deficiency of tissue coenzymes.

Folic acid deficiency may be diagnosed and treated with reasonable safety without a serum folate assay or the other diagnostic tests to be described. Such tests are necessary, however, when the diagnosis is in doubt or when accurate information is essential. As with the assay for serum vitamin B_{12}, serum should be taken early in the course of hospitalization and saved in the freezer in case later assay is necessary. This procedure is more important for the serum folate than for the serum vitamin B_{12} assay, because hospital food is likely to begin the early repletion of a deficient patient, especially one whose deficiency is caused by malnutrition.

Serum folate may be elevated in vitamin B_{12} deficiency, although frequently it is not. The rise in serum folate is most striking in vitamin B_{12}–deficient individuals who are replete in folic acid. Vitamin B_{12}–deficient individuals who are also folic acid-deficient have serum folate levels in the normal or low range—although their levels would be even lower were it not for the coexisting vitamin B_{12} deficiency.

Although assay of red cell folate is said to provide a better assessment of the level of folate coenzymes in tissues than serum folate (see Table 34-7), this assay is not yet widely used. The test exploits the observation, noted earlier, that serum folate decreases well before red cell folate decreases and megaloblastic anemia appears. Several methods are available [411–415].

The FIGlu excretion test [416,417], although a useful and simple test for folate deficiency, is less specific than the serum folate assay. It becomes abnormal later than the serum folate and thus gives a better measure of tissue coenzyme levels. Its greatest usefulness is in subjects taking antifolate drugs—or drugs stimulating their actions—in whom serum folate levels may be normal and tissue coenzyme level drastically reduced.

Descriptions of other tests, including the plasma clearance of an injected dose of folic acid [418–420], the urinary excretion of an orally administered dose of ^{3}H-F [300], and the assay of folate activity in lymphocytes by quantifying the incorporation of ^{14}C-formate into serine [421], may be found in the original publications.

THERAPY OF FOLIC ACID DEFICIENCY
Folic acid is usually administered orally in 1-mg tablets. Oral therapy is satisfactory for most needs. Even in the presence of intestinal malabsorption, the relatively large doses used ordinarily permit sufficient absorption to achieve repletion.

The usual dose is 1 to 5 mg daily, although doses in excess of 1 mg are probably unnecessary. Folic acid in these doses also partially corrects the hemopoietic and gastrointestinal manifestations of vitamin B_{12} deficiency. Neurologic abnormalities, however, may progress with disastrous results. This is the principal danger in the uncritical use of folic acid.

A parenteral preparation containing 15 mg/ml of the sodium salt may be used in severely ill patients, in certain cases of malabsorption, or in patients incapable of taking oral medication. Citrovorum factor (leucovorin, folinic acid, N^5-formyl FH_4) is available as a parenteral therapeutic preparation. Its main clinical indication is severe intoxication by folic acid antagonists that block folate reduction. In the absence of such inhibition, little is accomplished by treating folic acid deficiency with this compound instead of folic acid. The usual dose of citrovorum factor is 3 to 6 mg per day administered intramuscularly.

Toxicity from folic acid has not been observed even with doses many times higher than the usual therapeutic level. The sole indication for folic acid therapy is folic acid deficiency (or, as in pregnancy, anticipated folic acid deficiency). All therapeutic effects are attributable to reversal of the deficiency state.

Megaloblastic anemias unresponsive to vitamin B_{12} or folic acid

Megaloblastic anemia is occasionally not accompanied by evidence of vitamin B_{12} or folic acid deficiency and fails to respond to therapy with either vitamin. In other cases, the serum folate or vitamin B_{12} level is depressed, but vitamin repletion corrects the serum level without affecting the megaloblastosis. In these cases, the vitamin deficiency coexists with the megaloblastic anemia but is not responsible for it.

It is convenient to consider these occurrences under three headings: (1) megaloblastic anemia occurring in patients receiving an antimetabolite drug that interferes with DNA synthesis by a process that would not be reversed by simultaneously administered folic acid or citrovorum factor, (2) megaloblastic anemia resulting from demonstrated inborn errors of metabolism, and (3) refractory megaloblastic anemia of undetermined etiology.

Except for certain dysplastic features to be described, the megaloblasts in these marrows generally resemble those in the vitamin-deficiency megaloblastic types of anemia, and it is assumed here that the fundamental defect in all is an inability to duplicate DNA at a normal rate.

ANTIMETABOLITE DRUGS
The lengthening list of antimetabolites employed in the chemotherapy of leukemia, lymphoma, sarcoma, and carcinoma or for the purpose of immunosuppression includes many agents that block the synthesis of DNA, either as a solitary effect or in concert with similar effects on RNA or protein synthesis. Agents that block DNA synthesis inhibit either single or multiple steps in the biosynthetic pathway.

The following discussion considers only major examples of each class of agents and summarizes only their biochemical loci of action and effects on the marrow. Discussions of their chemotherapeutic applications and general pharmacology will be found in other chapters. Considerations of agents (such as methotrexate) that block DNA synthesis by mechanisms that are neutralized by simultaneously administered folic acid or citrovorum factor were discussed earlier.

INHIBITORS OF PURINE SYNTHESIS
The most commonly employed purine analogs are the thiopurines, 6-mercaptopurine (6-MP), thioguanine (6-TG), and azathioprine (Imuran) (Fig. 47-5). Multiple sites of action have been demonstrated for the thiopurines and their nucleotide derivatives (Fig. 47-6) [422–424]. For example, 6-MP competes with hypoxanthine for a binding site on hypoxanthine guanine phosphoribosyl transferase and is itself converted to thioinosinic acid (TIMP). This in turn inhibits the conversions of inosinic acid (IMP) to xanthylic acid (XMP) and adenylic acid (AMP) via adenylosuccinate (SAMP) and is enzymatically converted to ribonucleoside diphosphate and triphosphate. It is not certain that thioinosine triphosphate is incorporated into nucleic acids [422]. Incorporation of 6-TG into RNA and DNA has been demonstrated. In addition, TIMP simulates AMP and GMP as a feedback inhibitor of the first step of purine synthesis, in which phosphoribosylamine is formed from glutamine and phosphoribosylpyro-

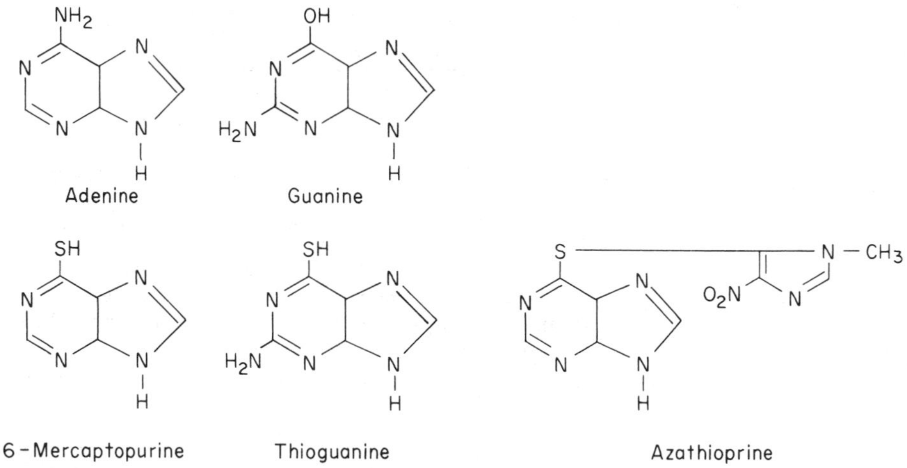

Adenine

Guanine

6-Mercaptopurine

Thioguanine

Azathioprine

FIGURE 47-5   Several inhibitors of purine synthesis. Formulas of parent compounds, adenine and guanine, are shown for comparison.

phosphate. Thus there are several significant loci of action for 6-MP in addition to those shown in Fig. 47-6. These considerations suggest that the thiopurines and their congeners can inhibit RNA and DNA synthesis, both early in the *de novo* synthesis of purines and late in the purine nucleotide interconversion step. They can be incorporated into both nucleic acids, thereby causing chromosome breaks and possible malfunctions of the several forms of nucleic acid. They can also inhibit coenzyme formation and function, thereby interfering with diverse aspects of cell metabolism.

The main toxic effects of 6-MP and other thiopurines is marrow depression with resulting leukopenia, anemia, and thrombocytopenia. Long before hypoplasia occurs, the marrow regularly displays megaloblastic transformation [425]. Serum folate and vitamin B_{12} levels are normal, and vitamin therapy is unavailing. The megaloblastic process, usually a mild one, disappears when the antimetabolite is withdrawn.

INHIBITORS OF PYRIMIDINE SYNTHESIS

Two categories of chemotherapeutic agents block the synthesis of pyrimidine nucleotides: those which block the methylation of deoxyuridylate to deoxythymidylate

and those which block the *de novo* synthesis of the pyrimidine ring.

The first category includes 5-fluoro-2'-deoxyuridine (FUdR), the deoxyribonucleoside of 5-fluorouracil [426]. In part its chemotherapeutic action rests on the thymine deficiency produced by the inhibitory action of FUdR (or its in vivo product, 5-fluorodeoxyuridylate) on thymidylate synthetase. The result is a classic form of the "thymineless" syndrome that originally led to recognition of the unbalanced growth state [33,427]. A large portion of administered FUdR is degraded to free 5-fluorouracil (FU), some of which is incorporated into RNA, presumably after conversion to the corresponding ribonucleoside and ribonucleotide, and much of which is catabolized and excreted. Interestingly, 5-fluorodeoxyuridine 5'-triphosphate is absent from cells (owing to the action of dUTPase), and 5-fluorouracil is absent from DNA (owing to uracil-DNA-glycosylase) [428,429]. Neither 5-fluorouridine nor free FU inhibits thymidylate synthetase.

Other 5-halogenodeoxyuridines (bromodeoxyuridine, iododeoxyuridine, etc.) are also converted to deoxynucleoside triphosphates that are extensively incorporated into DNA in place of dTTP. The heavier

FIGURE 47-6   Pathways of nucleotide interconversions in which 6-MP or its nucleotide derivatives (TIMP, TIDP, TITP) act as inhibitors. Dashed lines denote inhibition. Active inhibitors are in rectangles. (Modified from Hitchings and Elion [424].)

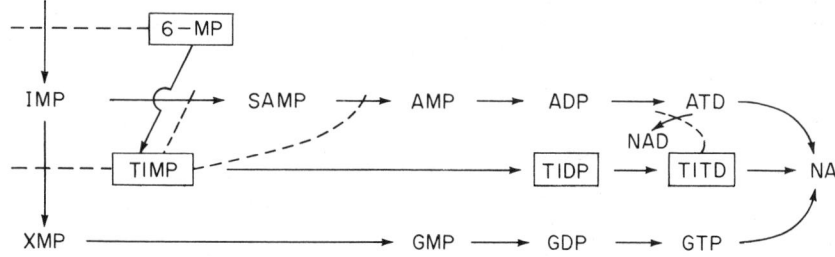

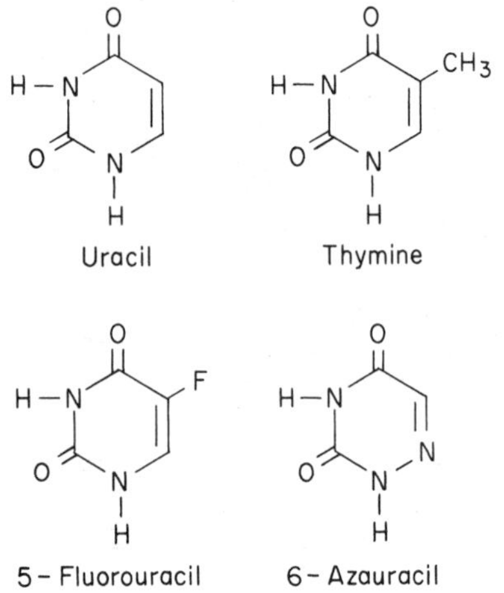

FIGURE 47-7 **Two inhibitors of pyrimidine synthesis. Formulas of parent compounds, uracil and thymine, are shown for comparison.**

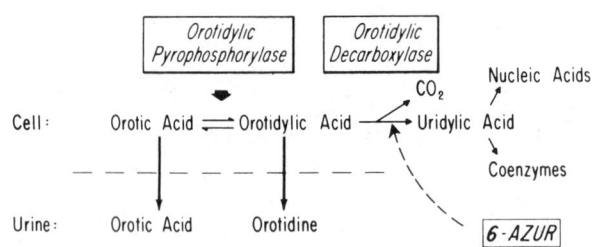

FIGURE 47-8 **Terminal portion of *de novo* pathway of pyrimidine synthesis, showing locus of action of 6-AzUR (6-azauridylic acid, competitive inhibitor of orotidylic decarboxylase). Dashed line indicates inhibition.**

halogen atoms more resemble the methyl group of thymine and presumably for this reason elude excision by uracil-DNA-glycosylase.

Administration of FUdR produces mild megaloblastic anemia [430] along with other toxic effects in rapidly proliferating tissues—glossitis, diarrhea, etc. Marrow eventually becomes hypoplastic. Although the other fluorinated pyrimidines differ in mechanism of action, their clinical and toxic effects are similar.

The second category of inhibitors of pyrimidine synthesis is exemplified by 6-azauridine (6-AzUR), the ribonucleoside of the triazine analog of uracil, 6-azauracil [430,431] (Fig. 47-7). The central nervous system disturbance caused by free 6-azauracil precludes its use in therapy; 6-AzUR does not produce these side ef-

fects when given intravenously. The drug is a powerful inhibitor of orotidylic decarboxylase; thus it blocks the conversion of orotidylic acid to uridylic acid (Fig. 47-8). It may occasionally produce megaloblastosis associated with the accumulation and renal excretion of orotic acid and orotidine.

INHIBITORS OF DEOXYRIBONUCLEOTIDE SYNTHESIS

Two antitumor agents in widespread use appear to act by inhibiting ribonucleotide reductase, the enzyme that catalyzes the reductive conversion of ribonucleotides to deoxyribonucleotides. The agents are 1-β-D-arabinofuranosylcytosine (ara-C, cytosine arabinoside) and hydroxyurea (Fig. 47-9). Ara-C is a nucleoside in which the sugar component is arabinose, an analog of both ribose and deoxyribose [433,434]. Studies of ascites tumor and tissue culture preparations have suggested that it blocks the conversion of cytidylate (at the diphosphate or triphosphate level) to deoxycytidylate [435–437]. However, this conclusion was not substantiated in in vitro studies with purified ribonucleotide reductase

FIGURE 47-9 **Two inhibitors of deoxyribonucleotide synthesis. Insets show structure of ribosyl and deoxyribosyl moieties for comparison.**

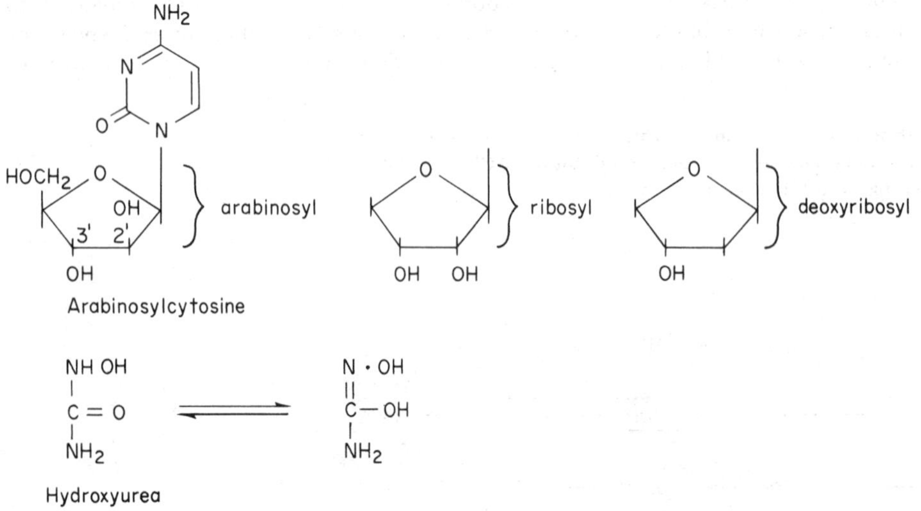

from Novikoff and Ehrlich tumor cells [438], and evidence has appeared that ara-C (or its triphosphate derivative) may inhibit DNA polymerase [439]. Incorporation of ara-C nucleotide into DNA has not been proved. The effects of ara-C are readily reversible by administration of deoxycytidine, but not by thymidine, deoxyuridine, or cytidine.

Megaloblastosis unresponsive to vitamin therapy regularly accompanies ara-C administration [440–442]. Phase microscopy has revealed that the megaloblasts appearing during ara-C therapy differ from typical megaloblasts in that their nuclei have irregular borders and little internal detail [443]. These abnormalities appear as early as 6 h after the initial dose of ara-C, reach a peak on the fifth day, and subside in 2 weeks.

Hydroxyurea (Fig. 47-9), known to chemists for over a century, was introduced into cancer chemotherapy following discovery of its activity against mouse leukemia L 1210 [444,445]. Its main area of usefulness is in the treatment of chronic granulocytic leukemia [446]. Marked megaloblastic changes are found in marrow within 24 to 48 h of the initiation of hydroxyurea therapy [445]. Hydroxyurea inhibits the reductive conversion of CDP (or CTP) to dCDP (or dCTP) [447–449], apparently by chelating an essential nonheme iron in ribonucleoside diphosphatase reductase [450–452]. This effect may account for the occurrence of megaloblastic transformation, but it is not entirely clear whether it is the basis for the cytotoxicity of hydroxyurea. Some data [453,454] showing that exogenous deoxyribonucleosides incompletely reverse the effect of hydroxyurea on DNA synthesis suggest that the drug interferes with DNA synthesis at multiple loci.

A number of drugs have been shown to inhibit DNA synthesis, among them daunomycin [455] and Adriamycin [456–458], and others. It may be anticipated that these agents will also be found to have a propensity for causing megaloblastic transformation of greater or lesser degree.

INBORN ERRORS

HEREDITARY OROTIC ACIDURIA
Hereditary orotic aciduria is a rare disorder of pyrimidine metabolism manifested by megaloblastic anemia refractory to vitamin therapy, growth impairment, and the renal excretion of orotic acid in large quantities. The disease was first described [459] in a 9-month-old boy with severe megaloblastic anemia who failed to respond to conventional therapy but did respond to an orally administered yeast extract containing uridylic and cytidylic acids with improvement in the clinical manifestations and reduction of the urinary orotic aciduria. The child died of varicella at age 2. It was postulated that a defect in the conversion of orotic acid to uridylic acid would explain the picture, and subsequent studies in the parents and siblings (who were clinically well) revealed reduced activities of orotidylic pyrophos-

phorylase and orotidylic decarboxylase (Fig. 47-8) in the red cells [460]. The living family members also exhibited a partial defect in the metabolism of orotic acid by intact leukocytes, reduced levels or orotidylic decarboxylase activity in disrupted leukocyte preparations [461], and increased urinary excretion of orotic acid [462]. No evidence could be found of vitamin B_{12} or folic acid deficiency.

The original patient with orotic aciduria was assumed to be homozygous for this genetic disorder because of the pattern of partial enzyme defects within the immediate family and because of the consanguinity of the parents. Further investigation of the mode of transmission of the defect within the family established it as an autosomal trait with asymptomatic heterozygotes [463]. These results were confirmed in subsequent case reports [464–468]. However, it now appears that several biochemical patterns can produce the picture. The majority (termed *type I* [468]) are grossly deficient in both orotidylic decarboxylase and pyrophosphorylase and excrete only orotic acid. Type II patients [467,468] are deficient only in decarboxylase (pyrophosphorylase is, in fact, increased) and excrete orotic acid and orotidine. The dual enzyme deficiency and the finding in heterozygotes of enzyme levels below half of the normal levels suggest that the mutation in hereditary orotic aciduria resembles a regulator gene mutation in bacteria.

INBORN ERRORS OF FOLATE METABOLISM
A number of cases have been reported of diverse congenital errors in folate metabolism [469,470]. All or most have demonstrated neurologic impairment. Some have responded to folate therapy. Thus far, congenital deficiencies have been observed of dihydrofolate reductase [471], methenyltetrahydrofolate cyclohydrolase [472], methylenetetrahydrofolate reductase [473], glutamate formiminotransferase [474–476], and methyltetrahydrofolate-homocysteine methyltransferase [477].

The diagnosis of possible inborn error of folate metabolism should be considered when vitamin B_{12} deficiency is not present and a patient displays (1) low serum folate and poor response to oral folic acid; (2) unexplained mental retardation, especially if the serum folate level is elevated; (3) elevated urinary formiminoglutamic acid, with or without an oral histidine load, unresponsive to physiologic doses of folic acid; or (4) megaloblastic anemia in infancy, unresponsive to physiologic doses of folic acid but responsive to pharmacologic doses of folic acid or physiologic doses of reduced folate (i.e., citrovorum factor).

Another metabolic error produces the Lesch-Nyhan syndrome, a sex-linked disorder of purine metabolism that is characterized by hyperuricemia, hyperuricosuria, and a neurologic disease with self-mutilation. It is caused by a deficiency of hypoxanthine–guanine phosphoribosyltransferase. In one case, the patient had megaloblastic anemia that responded to the administration of adenine [478].

UNEXPLAINED DISORDERS

There remains to be described a small group of disorders associated with megaloblastic transformation, sometimes of severe degree, which do not respond to therapy with vitamn B_{12} or folic acid and which have not yet been associated with an enzyme defect (but which may nevertheless result from such a defect).

PYRIDOXINE-RESPONSIVE MEGALOBLASTIC ANEMIA

The rare disorder of hemoglobin synthesis known as pyridoxine-responsive anemia is discussed elsewhere in this book (Chap. 53). It is mentioned also in this summary of the types of megaloblastic anemia not associated with vitamin B_{12} or folic acid deficiency because a small percentage of cases are associated with megaloblastosis [479–481]. The mechanism of megaloblastic transformation in these cases is unknown. Since pyridoxine and folic acid both participate in the serine-glycine interconversion (Table 34–6), it is conceivable that a defect of this enzyme induces a requirement for pharmacologic doses of pyridoxine in the absence of which folic acid metabolism is impaired.

THIAMINE-RESPONSIVE MEGALOBLASTIC ANEMIA

Two extraordinary cases have been reported. In one, a 6-year-old girl had megaloblastic anemia refractory to folic acid and vitamin B_{12} but responsive to oral therapy with thiamine [482,483]. Withdrawal of thiamine was followed by a relapse in 16 weeks. Despite this provocative evidence that a thiamine-dependent enzyme participates in DNA synthesis, it remains to be identified. Presumably, a defect of the postulated enzyme causes it to require thiamine in an abnormally high concentration. Both cases were associated with sensorineural deafness and diabetes mellitus.

REFRACTORY ANEMIA

The perplexing subject of refractory forms of anemia has been diligently reviewed by a number of students [484–487] and is discussed elsewhere in this book (Chap. 54). These disorders are characterized by ringed sideroblasts, excess iron, mast cell hyperplasia, and a mixture of erythroblastic and megaloblastic erythropoiesis in the marrow [483,484]. All are presumably due to metabolic errors—some hereditary and sex-linked, others apparently acquired—and all are variably associated with megaloblastic changes that are unresponsive to therapy with vitamin B_{12}. Some patients respond to folic acid therapy, but responses, when present, do not restore a normal hemoglobin level [488,489]. Usually megaloblastic changes are atypical, with dysplastic features confined to the erythroid series. Serum lactic dehydrogenase is only moderately elevated [490,491]. When megaloblastic transformation is severe and extensive, the disorder becomes indistinguishable from erythremic myelosis.

ERYTHROLEUKEMIA (DI GUGLIELMO'S SYNDROME)

Erythroleukemia is· also considered elsewhere in this book (Chap. 30). It is mentioned here briefly because it is associated with severe megaloblastic anemia that is refractory to therapy with vitamin B_{12} or folic acid.

The nature and pathogenesis of erythroleukemia are as unclear as those of the other types of refractory megaloblastic anemia. The author suspects that in all these disorders the marrow has acquired a hardy clone of somatically mutated cells in which the defect is loss of one or another of the enzymes in the pathway of DNA synthesis. Whether or not the chromosomal abnormalities found in this disorder [492,493] support such a view is a moot question. In any event, this theory, earlier intimated by a number of writers [487,494], would account for the failure of these megaloblasts to respond to vitamin therapy or to therapy aimed at blocking DNA synthesis (e.g., methotrexate, 6-MP, etc.). DNA synthesis, presumably, is already blocked. Any of several enzymes could be deleted, among them ribonucleotide reductase, thymidylate synthetase, DNA polymerase, a deoxyribonucleotide kinase, etc. Clearly, it is a hypothesis that will be tested only by careful enzymologic studies on normal and diseased marrow cells.

References

1. Ehrlich, P.: *Farbenanalytische Untersuchungen zur Histologie und Klinik des Blutes.* Hirschwald, Berlin, 1891.
2. Downey, H.: *Handbook of Hematology.* Hoeber, New York, 1938.
3. Jones, O. P.: The origin of megaloblasts and normoblasts in biopsied human marrow and the difference between the two series. *Anat. Rec. (Suppl.)* 58:23, 1934.
4. Naegeli, O.: *Blutkrankheiten und Blutdiagnostic.* Springer, Berlin, 1931.
5. Fieschi, A., and Astaldi, G.: *La Cultura in vitro del midollo osseo: Problemi di fisiopatologia ematologica studiati con la tecnica della cultura dei tessuti.* Tipografia del Libro, Pavia, 1946.
6. Sabin, F. R., Miller, F. R., Smithburn, K. C., Thomas, R. M., and Hummel, L. E.: Changes in the bone marrow and blood cells of developing rabbits. *J. Exp. Med.* 64:97, 1936.
7. Doan, C. A.: Current views on the origin and maturation of the cells of the blood. *J. Lab. Clin. Med.* 17:887, 1932.
8. Davidson, L. S. P., Davis, L. J., and Innes, J.: Effect of liver therapy on erythropoiesis as observed by serial sternal punctures in twelve cases of pernicious anemia. *Q. J. Med.* 11:19, 1942.
9. Tasker, P. W. G.: The direct action of folic acid, folinic acid and vitamin B_{12} on megaloblasts in vivo. *Br. J. Haematol.* 2:205, 1956.
10. Stasney, J., and Pizzolato, P.: Serial bone marrow studies in pernicious anemia. *Proc. Soc. Exp. Biol. Med.* 51:335, 1943.
11. Pendl, I., and Franz, W.: Transformation of megaloblasts to normoblasts by cultivating human bone marrow in presence of vitamin B_{12} and vitamin B_{12}-binding protein. *Nature (London)* 181:488, 1958.
12. Lajtha, L. G.: Culture of human bone marrow in vitro. *J. Clin. Pathol.* 5:67, 1952.
13. Fudenberg, H., and Estren, S.: The intermediate megaloblast in the differential diagnosis of pernicious and related anemias. *Am. J. Med.* 25:198, 1958.
14. Epstein, R. D.: Cells of the megakaryocyte series in pernicious anemia. *Am. J. Pathol.* 25:239, 1949.
15. Queisser, U., Queisser, W., and Spiertz, B.: Polyploidization of megakaryocytes in normal humans, in patients with idiopathic thromobcytopenic purpura and with pernicious anaemia. *Br. J. Haematol.* 20:489, 1971.
16. Glazer, H. S., Mueller, J. F., Jarrold, T., Sakurai, K., Will, J. J., and Vilter, R. R.: Effect of vitamin B_{12} and folic acid on nucleic acid composition of the bone marrow of patients with megaloblastic anemia. *J. Lab. Clin. Med.* 43:905, 1954.

17. White, J. C., Leslie, I., and Davidson, J. N.: Nucleic acids of bone marrow cells, with special reference to pernicious anemia. *J. Pathol. Bacteriol.* 66:291, 1953.

18. Lessner, H. E., and Friedkin, M.: The in vitro incorporation of deoxyuridine and thymidine into the deoxyribonucleic acid of human megaloblastic and normoblastic bone marrow. *Clin. Res.* 7:207, 1959.

19. Killman, S.-A.: Effect of deoxyuridine on incorporation of tritiated thymidine: Difference between normoblasts and megaloblasts. *Acta Med. Scand.* 175:483, 1964.

20. Beck, W. S.: Metabolic features of cobalamin deficiency in man, in *Cobalamin: Biochemistry and Pathophysiology*, edited by B. M. Babior. Wiley-Interscience, New York, 1975, p. 403.

21. Beck, W. S.: The metabolic functions of vitamin B_{12}. *N. Engl. J. Med.* 266:708, 814, 1962.

22. Beck, W. S.: The metabolic basis of megaloblastic erythropoieses. *Medicine (Baltimore)* 43:715, 1964.

23. Pelliniemi, T.-T., and Beck, W. S.: Prevention of uracil misincorporation into DNA in megaloblastic cells. *Blood 54 (Suppl. 1):*43a, 1979.

24. Wickremasinghe, R. G., and Hoffbrand, A. V.: Defective DNA synthesis in megaloblastic anaemia. *Biochim. Biophys. Acta* 563:46, 1979.

25. Goulian, M., Bleile, B., and Tseng, B. Y.: Methotrexate-induced misincorporation of uracil into DNA. *Proc. Natl. Acad. Sci. U.S.A.* 77:1956, 1980.

26. Goulian, M., Bleile, B., and Tseng, B. Y.: The effect of methotrexate on levels of dUTP in animal cells. *J. Biol. Chem.* 255:10630, 1980.

27. Lindahl, T.: New class of enzymes acting on damaged DNA. *Nature* 259:64, 1976.

28. Beck, W. S., and Vilpo, J. A.: Unpublished results.

29. Rogers, J. C.: Characterization of DNA excreted from phytohemagglutinin-stimulated lymphocytes. *J. Exp. Med.* 143:1249, 1976.

30. Heath, C. W., Jr.: Cytogenetic observations in vitamin B_{12} and folate deficiency. *Blood* 27:800, 1966.

31. Menzies, R. C., Crossen, P. E., Fitzgerald, P. H., and Gunz, F. W.: Cytogenetic and cytochemical studies on marrow cells in B_{12} and folate deficiency. *Blood* 28:581, 1966.

32. Jensen, M. K., and Friis-Møller, A.: Chromosome studies in pernicious anemia. *Acta Med. Scand.* 181:571, 1967.

33. Cohen, S. S., and Barner, H. D.: Studies on unbalanced growth in *Escherichia coli. Proc. Natl. Acad. Sci. U.S.A.* 40:885, 1954.

34. Freifelder, D., and Maaløe, O.: Energy requirement for thymineless death in cells of *Escherichia coli. J. Bacteriol.* 88:987, 1964.

35. Beck, W. S., Hook, S., and Barnett, B. H.: The metabolic functions of vitamin B_{12}. I. Distinctive modes of unbalanced growth behavior in *Lactobacillus leichmannii. Biochim. Biophys. Acta* 55:455, 1962.

36. Ruekert, R. R., and Mueller, G. C.: Studies on unbalanced growth in tissue culture. I. Induction and consequence of thymidine deficiency. *Cancer Res.* 20:1584, 1960.

37. Kim, J. H., Perez, A. G., and Djordjevic, B.: Studies on unbalanced growth in synchronized HeLa cells. *Cancer Res.* 28:2443, 1968.

38. Myhre, E.: Studies on megaloblasts in vitro. *Scand. J. Clin. Lab. Invest.* 16:307, 320, 1964.

39. Nathan, D. G., and Gardner, F. H.: Erythroid cell maturation and hemoglobin synthesis in megaloblastic anemia. *J. Clin. Invest.* 41:1086, 1962.

40. Rondanelli, E. G., Gorini, P., Magliulo, E., and Fiori, G. P.: Differences in proliferative activity between normoblasts and pernicious anemia megaloblasts. *Blood* 24:542, 1964.

41. Wickramasinghe, S. N., Chalmers, D. G., and Cooper, E. H.: Disturbed proliferation of erythropoietic cells in pernicious anemia. *Nature (London)* 215:189, 1967.

42. Williams, A. M., Chosy, J. J., and Schilling, R. F.: Effect of vitamin B_{12} in vitro on incorporation of nucleic acid precursors by pernicious anemia bone marrow. *J. Clin. Invest.* 42:670, 1963.

43. Bock, H. E., Hartje, J., Müller, D., and Wilmanns, W.: Thymin-nucleotid-Synthese und Proliferation von Knochenmarkzellen bei megaloblastären Anämien unter dem Einwirkung von Vitamin B_{12}. *Klin. Wochenschr.* 45:176, 1967.

44. Waxman, S., Metz, J., and Herbert, V.: Defective DNA synthesis in human megaloblastic bone marrow: Effects of homocysteine and methionine. *J. Clin. Invest.* 48:284, 1969.

45. Pelliniemi, T.-T., and Beck, W. S.: Biochemical mechanisms in the Killmann experiment. Critique of the deoxyuridine suppression test. *J. Clin. Invest.* 65:449, 1980.

46. Kass, L.: Origin and composition of Cabot rings in pernicious anemia. *Am. J. Clin. Pathol.* 64:53, 1975.

47. Herbert, V.: Expermental nutritional folate deficiency in man. *Trans. Assoc. Am. Physicians* 75:307, 1962.

48. Lindenbaum, J., and Nath, B. J.: Megaloblastic anemia and neutrophil hypersegmentation. *Br. J. Haematol.* 44:511, 1980.

49. Keller, R., Lindstrand, K., and Nordén, Å.: Disappearance of chromosomal abnormalities in megaloblastic anemia after treatment. *Scand. J. Haematol.* 7:478, 1970.

50. Lawler, S. D., Roberts, P. D., and Hoffbrand, A. V.: Chromosome studies in megaloblastic anemia before and after treatment. *Scand. J. Haematol.* 8:309, 1971.

51. Liu, Y. K., and Sullivan, L. W.: Marrow granulocyte reserve in pernicious anemia. *Clin. Res.* 14:321, 1966.

52. Goodman, J. R., Wallerstein, R. O., and Hall, S. G.: The ultrastructure of bone marrow histiocytes in megaloblastic anaemia and the anaemia of infection. *Br. J. Haematol.* 14:471, 1968.

53. Davidson, C. S., Murphy, J. C., Watson, R. J., and Castle, W. B.: Comparison of the effects of massive blood transfusions and of liver extract in pernicious anemia. *J. Clin. Invest.* 25:858, 1946.

54. Hess, B., and Gehm, E.: Uber die Milchsäuredehydrogenase in Menschlichen Serum. *Klin. Wochenschr.* 33:91, 1955.

55. Anderssen, N.: The activity of lactic dehydrogenase in megaloblastic anaemia. *Scand. J. Haematol.* 1:212, 1964.

56. Emerson, P. M., and Wilkinson, J. H.: Lactate dehydrogenase in the diagnosis and assessment of response to treatment of megaloblastic anemia. *Br. J. Haematol.* 12:678, 1966.

57. Winston, R. M., Warburton, F. G., and Stott, A.: Enzymatic diagnosis of megaloblastic anaemia. *Br. J. Haematol.* 19:587, 1970.

58. Perillie, P. E., Kaplan, S. S., and Finch, S. C.: Significance of changes in serum muramidase activity in megaloblastic anemia. *N. Engl. J. Med.* 277:10, 1967.

59. Catovsky, D., Galton, D. A. G., Griffin, C., Hoffbrand, A. V., and Szur, L.: Serum lysozyme and vitamin B_{12}-binding capacity in myeloproliferative disorders. *Br. J. Haematol.* 21:661, 1971.

60. Hansen, N. E., and Karle, H.: Blood and bone marrow lysozyme in neutropenia: An attempt towards pathogenetic classification. *Br. J. Haematol.* 21:261, 1971.

61. Heller, P., Weinstein, H. G., West, M., and Zimmerman, H. J.: Glycolytic, citric acid cycle, and hexosemonophosphate shunt enzymes of plasma and erythrocytes in megaloblastic anemia. *J. Lab. Clin. Med.* 55:425, 1960.

62. Ellims, P. H., Hayman, R. J., and Van Der Weyden, M. B.: Plasma thymidine kinase in megaloblastic anaemia. *Br. J. Haematol.* 44:167, 1980.

63. van Dommelen, C. K. V., and Klassen, C. H. L.: Cyanocobalamin-dependent depression of the serum alkaline phosphatase level in patients with pernicious anemia. *N. Engl. J. Med.* 271:541, 1964.

64. Meyer, L. M., Sawitsky, A., Ritz, N., and Fitch, H. W.: A study of cholinesterase activity of the blood of patients with pernicious anemia. *J. Lab. Clin. Med.* 33:1068, 1948.

65. Keeley, K. J., and Politzer, W. M.: Aminoaciduria in the megaloblastic anaemias. *J. Clin. Pathol.* 9:142, 1956.

66. Todd, D.: Observations on the amino-aciduria in megaloblastic anaemia. *J. Clin. Pathol.* 12:238, 1959.

67. Fowler, D., Cox, E. V., Cooke, W. T., and Meynell, M. J.: Aminoaciduria and megaloblastic anaemia. *J. Clin. Pathol.* 13:230, 1960.

68. Poston, J. M.: Cobalamin-dependent formation of leucine and β-leucine by rat and human tissue. Changes in pernicious anemia. *J. Biol. Chem.* 255:10067, 1980.

69. Finch, C. A., Coleman, D. H., Motulsky, A. G., Donohue, D. M., and Reiff, R. H.: Erythrokinetics in pernicious anemia. *Blood* 11:807, 1956.

70. Myhre, E.: Studies on the erythrokinetics in pernicious anemia. *Scand. J. Clin. Lab. Invest.* 16:391, 1964.

71. Heller, P., Weinstein, H. G., West, M., and Zimmerman, H. J.: Enzymes in anemia: A study of abnormalities of several enzymes of carbohydrate metabolism in the plasma and erythrocytes in patients with anemia, with preliminary observations of bone marrow enzymes. *Ann. Intern. Med.* 53:898, 1960.

72. Libnoch, H. A., Yakulis, V. J., and Heller, P.: Lactate dehydrogenase in megaloblastic bone marrow. *Am. J. Clin. Pathol.* 45:302, 1966.

73. London, I. M., and West, R.: The formation of bile pigment in pernicious anemia. *J. Biol. Chem.* 184:359, 1950.

74. White, P., Coburn, R. F., Williams, W. J., Goldwein, M. I., Rother, M. L., and Shafer, B. C.: Carbon monoxide production associated with ineffective erythropoiesis. *J. Clin. Invest.* 46:1986, 1967.

75. Lynch, E. C., and Alfrey, C. P., Jr.: Studies in vitro on the autohemolysis of normoblastic and megaloblastic marrow cells. *Tex. Rep. Biol. Med.* 24:180, 1966.

76. Singer, K., King, J., and Robin, S.: The life span of the megalocyte and the hemolytic syndrome of pernicious anemia. *J. Lab. Clin. Med.* 33:1068, 1948.

77. Hamilton, H. E., Sheets, R. F., and DeGowin, E. L.: Studies with inagglutinable erythrocyte counts. VII. Further investigation of the hemolytic mechanism in untreated pernicious anemia and the demonstration of a hemolytic property in the plasma. *J. Lab. Clin. Med.* 51:942, 1958.

78. Harker, L. A., and Finch, C. A.: Thrombokinetics in man. *J. Clin. Invest.* 48:963, 1969.

79. Levine, P. H.: A qualitative platelet defect in severe vitamin B_{12} deficiency. *Ann. Intern. Med.* 78:533, 1973.

80. Herbert, V., Tisman, G., Go, L. T., and Brenner, L.: The dU suppression test using ^{125}I-UdR to define biochemical megaloblastosis. *Br. J. Haematol.* 24:713, 1973.

81. Van der Weyden, M. B., Cooper, M., and Firkin, B. G.: Defective DNA synthesis in human megaloblastic bone marrow: Effects of hydroxy-B_{12}, 5'-deoxyadenosyl-B_{12} and methyl-B_{12}. *Blood* 41:299, 1973.

82. Wickramasinghe, S. N., and Longland, J. E.: Assessment of deoxyuridine suppression test in diagnosis of vitamin B_{12} or folate deficiency. *Br. Med. J.* 487:148, 1974.

83. Van der Weyden, M. B.: Deoxyuridine metabolism in human megaloblastic marrow cells. *Scand. J. Haematol.* 23:37, 1979.

84. Castle, W. B.: The conquest of pernicious anemia, in *Blood, Pure and Eloquent*, edited by M. M. Wintrobe. McGraw-Hill, New York, 1980, p. 283.

85. Minot, G. R., and Murphy, W. P.: Treatment of pernicious anemia by a special diet. *JAMA* 87:470, 1926.

86. Castle, W. B.: Observations on the etiologic relationship of achylia gastrica to pernicious anemia. I. The effect of administration to patients with pernicious anemia of the contents of the normal human stomach recovered after the ingestion of beef muscle. *Am. J. Med. Sci.* 178:748, 1929; (reprint) 267:2, 1974.

87. Nordenson, N. G., Segerdahl, E., Strandell, B., and Wallman-Carlsson, C.: Die Frequenz und geographische Verbreitung der pernizösen Anämie in Schweden. *Acta Med. Scand.* 97:222, 1938.

88. Carmel, R., and Johnson, C. S.: Racial patterns in pernicious anemia; early age of onset and increased frequency of intrinsic factor antibody in black women. *N. Engl. J. Med.* 298:647, 1978.

89. Metz, J., Randal, T. W., and Kniep, C. H.: Addisonian pernicious anemia in young Bantu females. *Br. Med. J.* 1:178, 1961.

90. Solanki, D. L., Jacobson, R. J., Green, R., McKibbon, J., and Berdoff, R.: Pernicious anemia in blacks. *Am. J. Clin. Pathol.* 75:96, 1981.

91. Creger, W. P., and Sortor, A. T.: The incidence of blood group A in pernicious anemia. *Arch. Intern. Med.* 98:136, 1956.

92. Hoskins, L. C., Loux, H. A., Britten, A., and Zamcheck, N.: Distribution of ABO blood groups in patients with pernicious anemia, gastric carcinoma and gastric carcinoma associated with pernicious anemia. *N. Engl. J. Med.* 273:633, 1965.

93. Callender, S. T., and Denborough, M. A.: A family study of pernicious anemia. *Br. J. Haematol.* 3:88, 1957.

94. Ardeman, S., Chanarin, I., Jacobs, A., and Griffiths, L.: Family study in Addisonian pernicious anemia. *Blood* 27:599, 1966.

95. Whittingham, S., Mackay, I. R., Ungar, B., and Mathews, J. D.: The genetic factor in pernicious anemia. *Lancet* 1:95, 1969.

96. Te Velde, K., Abels, J., Anders, G. J. P. A., Arends, A., Hoedemaeker, P. J., and Nieweg, H. O.: A family study of pernicious anemia by an immunologic method. *J. Lab. Clin. Med.* 64:177, 1964.

97. Wangel, A. G., Callender, S. T., Spray, G. H., and Wright, R.: A family study of pernicious anaemia. I. Autoantibodies, achlorhydria, serum pepsinogen and vitamin B_{12}. *Br. J. Haematol.* 14:161, 1968.

98. Wangel, A. G., Callender, S. T., Spray, G. H., and Wright, R.: A family study of pernicious anemia. II. Intrinsic factor secretion, vitamin B_{12} absorption and genetic aspects of gastric autoimmunity. *Br. J. Haematol.* 14:183, 1968.

99. Irvine, W. J.: Immunologic aspects of pernicious anemia. *N. Engl. J. Med.* 273:432, 1965.

100. Roitt, I. M., Doniach, D., and Shapland, C.: Autoimmunity in pernicious anemia and atrophic gastritis. *Ann. N.Y. Acad. Sci.* 124:644, 1965.

101. Goldberg, L. S., and Fudenberg, H. H.: The autoimmune aspects of pernicious anemia. *Am. J. Med.* 46:489, 1969.

102. Fisher, J. M., and Taylor, K. B.: Annotation: The significance of gastric antibodies. *Br. J. Haematol.* 20:1, 1971.

103. Irvine, W. J., Davies, S. H., Teitelbaum, S., Delamore, I. W., and Williams, A. W.: The clinical and pathological significance of gastric parietal cell antibody. *Ann. N.Y. Acad. Sci.* 124:657, 1965.

104. Ardeman, S., and Chanarin, I.: A method for the assay of human gastric intrinsic factor and for the detection and titration of antibodies against intrinsic factor. *Lancet* 2:1350, 1963.

105. Schade, S. G., Abels, J., and Schining, R. F.: Studies on antibody to intrinsic factor. *J. Clin. Invest.* 46:615, 1967.

106. Fisher, J. M., Rees, C., and Taylor, K. B.: Intrinsic factor antibodies in gastric juice of pernicious anaemia patients. *Lancet* 2:88, 1966.

107. Bardhan, K. D., Hall, J. R., Spray, G. H., and Callender, S. T. E.: Blocking and binding autoantibody to intrinsic factor. *Lancet* 2:62, 1968.

108. Schade, S. G., Feick, P., Muckerheide, M., and Schilling, R. F.: Occurrence in gastric juice of antibody to a complex of intrinsic factor and vitamin B_{12}. *N. Engl. J. Med.* 275:528, 1966.

109. Carmel, R., and Herbert, V.: Intrinsic factor antibody in the saliva of a patient with pernicious anemia. *Lancet* 1:80, 1967.

110. Doniach, D., Roitt, I. M., and Taylor, K. B.: Autoimmunity in pernicious anemia and thyroiditis: A family study. *Ann. N.Y. Acad. Sci.* 124:605, 1965.

111. Ardeman, S., Chanarin, I., Krafchik, B., and Singer, W.: Addisonian pernicious anaemia and intrinsic factor antibodies in thyroid disorders. *Q. J. Med.* 35:421, 1966.

112. Bar-Shany, S., and Herbert, V.: Transplacentally acquired antibody to intrinsic factor with vitamin B_{12} deficiency. *Blood* 30:777, 1967.

113. Goldberg, L. S., Barnett, E. V., and Desai, R.: Effect of transplacental transfer to antibody to intrinsic factor. *Pediatrics.* 40:851, 1967.

114. Charache, P., Hodkinson, B. A., Lambiotte, B., and McIntyre, P. A.: Genetic and auto-immune features of pernicious anemia. II. Effect of transplacental tranfer of antibody to intrinsic factor. *Johns Hopkins Med. J.* 122:184, 1968.

115. Frost, J. W., and Goldwein, M. I.: Observations on vitamin B_{12} absorption in primary pernicious anemia during administration of adrenocortical steroids. *N. Engl. J. Med.* 258:1096, 1958.

116. Ardeman, S., and Chanarin, I.: Steroids and Addisonian pernicious anemia. *N. Engl. J. Med.* 273:1352, 1965.

117. Rødbro, P., Dige-Petersen, H., Schwartz, M., and Dalggard, O. Z.: Effect of steroids on gastric mucosal structure and function in pernicious anemia. *Acta Med. Scand.* 181:445, 1967.

118. Baur, S., Fisher, J. M., Strickland, R. G., and Taylor, K. B.: Autantibody-containing cells in the gastric mucosa in pernicious anaemia. *Lancet* 2:887, 1968.

119. Odgers, R. J., and Wangel, A. G.: Abnormalities in IgA-containing mononuclear cells in the gastric lesion of pernicious anemia. *Lancet* 2:846, 1968.

120. Boddington, M. M., and Spriggs, A. I.: The epithelial cells in megaloblastic anaemias. *J. Clin. Pathol.* 12:228, 1969.

121. Nieburgs, H. E., and Glass, G. B. J.: Gastric-cell maturation disorders in atrophic gastritis, pernicious anemia, and carcinoma. *Am. J. Dig. Dis.* 8:135, 1963.

122. Sauli, S., Astaldi, G., and Malossini, L.: Histopathology of intestinal mucosa obtained by Crosby's biopsy in pernicious anemia before and after vitamin B_{12} treatment. *Acta Vitaminol. (Milano)* 4:143, 1963.

123. Foroozan, P., and Trier, J. S.: Mucosa of the small intestine in pernicious anemia. *N. Engl. J. Med.* 277:553, 1967.

124. Bezman, A., Kinnear, D. G., and Zamcheck, N.: D-Xylose and potassium iodide absorption and serum carotene in pernicious anemia. *J. Lab. Clin. Med.* 53:226, 1959.

125. Spurling, C. L., Sacks, M. S., and Jiji, R. M.: Juvenile pernicious anemia. *N. Engl. J. Med.* 271:995, 1964.
126. Lillibridge, C. B., Brandborg, L. L., and Rubin, C. E.: Childhood pernicious anemia: Gastrointestinal secretory, histological and electron microscopic aspects. *Gastroenterology* 52:792, 1967.
127. Lambert, H. P., Prankerd, T. A. J., and Smellie, J. M.: Pernicious anaemia in childhood: A report of two cases of one family and their relationship to the etiology of pernicious anemia. *Q. J. Med.* 30:71, 1960.
128. McIntyre, O. R., Sullivan, L. W., Jeffries, G. J., and Silver, R. H.: Pernicious anemia in childhood. *N. Engl. J. Med.* 272:981, 1965.
129. Katz, M., Lee, S. K., and Cooper, B. A.: Vitamin B_{12} malabsorption due to a biologically inert intrinsic factor. *N. Engl. J. Med.* 287:425, 1972.
130. Katz, M., Mehlman, C. S., and Allen, R. H.: Isolation and characterization of an abnormal human intrinsic factor. *J. Clin. Invest.* 53:1274, 1974.
131. Imerslund, O., and Bjornstad, P.: Familial vitamin B_{12} malabsorption. *Acta Haematol. (Basel)* 30:1, 1963.
132. Waters, A. H., and Murphy, M. E. B.: Familial juvenile pernicious anaemia: A study of the hereditary basis of pernicious anaemia. *Br. J. Haematol.* 9:1, 1963.
133. Mohamed, S. D., McKay, E., and Galloway, W. H.: Juvenile familial megaloblastic anaemia due to selective malabsorption of vitamin B_{12}. *Q. J. Med.* 35:433, 1966.
134. Goldberg, L. S., and Fudenberg, H. H.: Familial selective malabsorption of vitamin B_{12}: Re-evaluation of an *in vivo* intrinsic factor inhibitor. *N. Engl. J. Med.* 279:405, 1968.
135. Mackenzie, I. L., Donaldson, R. M., Trier, J. S., and Mathan, V. I.: Ileal mucosa in familial selective vitamin B_{12} malabsorption. *N. Engl. J. Med.* 286:1021, 1972.
136. Miller, D. R., Bloom, G. E., Streiff, R. R., LoBuglio, A. F., and Diamond, L. K.: Juvenile "congenital" pernicious anemia: Clinical and immunologic studies. *N. Engl. J. Med.* 275:978, 1966
137. Morley, J., and Roberts, M.: The technique and results of partial gastrectomy for chronic gastric ulcer. *Br. J. Surg.* 16:239, 1928.
138. Gordon-Taylor, G., Hudson, R. V., Dodds, E. C., Warner, J. L., and Whitby, L. E. H.: The remote results of gastrectomy. *Br. J. Surg.* 16:641, 1929.
139. Lyngar, E.: Blood changes after partial gastrectomy for ulcer. *Acta Med Scand.* 138 (Suppl. 247):1, 1950.
140. Paulson, M., and Harvey, J. C.: Haematological alterations after total gastrectomy: Evolutionary sequences over a decade. *JAMA* 156:1556, 1954.
141. MacLean, L. D., and Sunberg, R. D.: Incidence of megaloblastic anemia after total gastrectomy. *N. Engl. J. Med.* 254:885, 1956.
142. Wells, C., and McPhee, I. W.: Partial gastrectomy: Ten years later. *Br. Med. J.* 2:1128, 1954.
143. Badenoch, J., Evans, J. R., Richards, W. C. D., and Witts, L. J.: Megaloblastic anemia following partial gastrectomy and gastroenterostomy. *Br. J. Haematol.* 1:339, 1955.
144. Deller, D. J.: Megaloblastic and transitional megaloblastic anemia following parital gastrectomy: Study of 27 cases. *Aust. Ann. Med.* 2:235, 1969.
145. MacLean, L. D.: Incidence of megaloblastic anemia after subtotal gastrectomy. *N. Engl. J. Med.* 257:262, 1957.
146. Deller, D. J., and Witts, L. J.: Changes in the blood after partial gastrectomy with special reference to vitamin B_{12}. I. Serum vitamin B_{12}, haemoglobin, serum iron, and bone marrow. *Q. J. Med.* 31:71, 1962.
147. Deller, D. J., Perry, S. W., and Witts, L. J.: Radioactive vitamin B_{12} after partial gastrectomy. *Lancet* 2:162, 1963.
148. Mahmud, K., Ripley, D., and Doscherholmen, A.: Vitamin B_{12} absorption tests: Their unreliability in postgastrectomy states. *JAMA* 216:1167, 1971.
149. Joske, R. A., Finckh, E. S., and Wood, I. J.: Gastric biopsy. *Q. J. Med.* 24:269, 1955.
150. Badenoch, J., Evans, J. R., and Richards, W. C. D.: The stomach in hypochromic anaemia. *Br. J. Haematol.* 3:175, 1957.
151. Waters, A. H.: The haematological management of patients following partial gastrectomy. *Br. J. Haematol.* 15:423, 1968.
152. Allcock, E.: Absorption of vitamin B_{12} in man following extensive resection of the jejunum, ileum and colon. *Gastroenterology* 40:81, 1961.
153. Steinberg, F.: The megaloblastic anemia of regional ileitis. *N. Engl. J. Med.* 264:186, 1961.
154. Tudhope, G. R., and Wilson, G. M.: Deficiency of vitamin B_{12} in hypothyroidism. *Lancet* 1:703, 1962.
155. Webb, D. I., Chodos, R. B., Mahar, C. Q., and Faloon, W. W.: Mechanism of vitamin B_{12} malabsorption in patients receiving colchicine. *N. Engl. J. Med.* 279:845, 1968.
156. Heinivaara, O., and Palva, I. P: Malabsorption and deficiency of vitamin B_{12} caused by treatment with para-aminosalicylic acid. *Acta Med. Scand.* 177:337, 1965.
157. Bleifeld, W., and Gehrmann, G.: Imperfect absorption of vitamin B_{12} during treatment with PAS. *Ger. Med. Mon.* 11:12, 1966 (*Deutsch. Med. Wochenschr.* 90:1765, 1965).
158. Haurani, F. I., Sherwood, W., and Goldstein, F.: Intestinal malabsorption of vitamin B_{12} in pernicious anemia. *Metabolism* 13:1342, 1964.
159. Goldberg, L. S., Bickel, Y. B., and Fudenberg, H. H.: Immunologic approaches to malabsorption of vitamin B_{12}. *Arch Intern. Med.* 123:397, 1969.
160. Sheehy, T. W., Perez-Santiago, E., and Rubini, M. E.: Tropical sprue and vitamin B_{12}. *N. Engl. J. Med.* 265:1232, 1961.
161. Cameron, D. G., Watson, G. M., and Witts, L. J.: The clinical association of macrocytic anemia with intestinal stricture and anastomosis. *Blood* 4:793, 1949.
162. Dellipiani, A. W., Samson, R. R., and Girdwood, R. H.: The uptake of vitamin B_{12} by *E. coli*: Possible significance in relation to the blind loop syndrome. *Am. J. Dig. Dis.* 13:718, 1968.
163. Donaldson, R. M., Corrigan, H., and Natsios, G.: Malabsorption of Co^{60}-labeled cyanocobalamin in rats with intestinal diverticula. II. Studies on contents of the diverticula. *Gastroenterology* 43:282, 1962.
164. Beck, W. S.: Unpublished results.
165. Donaldson, R. M.: Malabsorption of Co^{60}-labeled cyanocobalamin in rats with intestinal diverticula. I. Evaluation of possible mechanisms. *Gastroenterology* 43:271, 1962.
166. Giannella, R. A., Broitman, S. A., and Zamcheck, N.: Vitamin B_{12} uptake by intestinal microorganisms: Mechanism and relavance to syndromes of bacterial overgrowth. *J. Clin. Invest.* 50:1100, 1971.
167. Wirth, W. A., and Farrow, C. C.: Human sparganosis. *JAMA* 177:76, 1961.
168. von Bonsdorf, B., and Gordin, R.: Antianemic activity of dried fish tapeworm: *Diphyllobothrium latum* and pernicious anemia. *Acta Med. Scand.* 142 (Suppl. 266):283, 1952.
169. von Bondsdorf, B., and Gordin, R.: Treatment of pernicious anemia with intramuscular injections of tapeworm extracts. XIV. *Diphyllobothrium latum* and pernicious anemia. *Acta Med. Scand.* 144:263, 1953.
170. Nyberg, W.: Microbiological investigations on antipernicious anemia factors in the fish tapeworm. *Acta Med. Scand.* 144 (Suppl. 271):1, 1952.
171. Nyberg, W.: Absorption and excretion of vitamin B_{12} in subjects infected with *Diphyllobothrium latum* and in non-infected subjects following oral administration of radioactive B_{12}. *Acta Haematol. (Basel)* 19:90, 1958.
172. Scudmore, H. H., Thompson, J. H., and Owen, C. A.: Absorption of Co^{60}-labeled vitamin B_{12} in man and uptake by parasites, including *Diphyllobothrium latum*. *J. Lab. Clin. Med.* 57:240, 1961.
173. Nyberg, W., Grasbeck, R., and Sippola, V.: Urinary excretion of radiovitamin B_{12} in carriers of *Diphyllobothrium latum*. *N. Engl. J. Med.* 259:216, 1958.
174. Nyberg, W.: *Diphyllobothrium latum* and human nutrition with particular reference to vitamin B_{12} deficiency. *Proc. Nutr. Soc.* 22:8, 1963.
175. Smith, A. D. M.: Veganism: A clinical survey with observations of vitamin B_{12} metabolism. *Br. Med. J.* 1:1655, 1962.
176. Hines, J. D.: Megaloblastic anemia in an adult vegans. *Am. J. Clin. Nutr.* 19:260, 1969.
177. Harrison, R. J., Booth, C. C., and Mollin, D. L.: Vitamin B_{12} deficiency due to defective diet. *Lancet* 1:727, 1956.
178. Wokes, F., Badenoch, J., and Sinclair, H. M.: Human dietary deficiency of vitamin B_{12}. *Am. J. Clin. Nutr.* 3:375, 1955.
179. Pollycove, M., Apt. L., and Colbert, M.: Pernicious anemia due to dietary deficiency of vitamin B_{12}. *N. Engl. J. Med.* 255:164, 1956.

180. Forshaw, J., Moorhouse, E. H., and Harwood, L.: Megaloblastic anemia due to dietary deficiency. *Lancet* 1:1004, 1964.

181. Adams, E. G., and Scragg, J. N.: Serum vitamin B_{12} concentrations in megaloblastic anemia associated with kwashiokor and marasmus. *J. Pediatr.* 60:580, 1962.

182. van Dommelen, C. K., Olie, R. J., and Slagboom, G.: B_{12} lack ("pernicious anemia"), possibly caused by "parasitization" (consumption by a neoplasm), in a case of Waldenstrom's macroglobulinaemia. *Acta Med. Scand.* 176:611, 1964.

183. Wellington, M. S., and Whitcomb, J.: Association of cyanocobalamin deficiency with myeloproliferative states: Report of three cases. *Am. J. Med. Sci.* 239:750, 1960.

184. Hippe, E., Paaske Hansen, O., and Drivholm, A.: Decreased serum cobalamin in multiple myeloma without signs of vitamin B_{12} deficiency: A preliminary report. *Scand. J. Gastroenterol. 9 (Suppl. 29)*:85, 1974.

185. Pant, S. S., Asbury, A. K., and Richardson, E. P.: The myelopathy of pernicious anemia: A neuropathologic reappraisal. *Acta Neurol. Scand. 44(Suppl. 35)*:7, 1968.

186. Harris, J. W., and Kellermeyer, R. W.: *The Red Cell: Production, Metabolism, Destruction: Normal and Abnormal*, rev. ed. Harvard, Cambridge, Mass., 1970.

187. Smith, A. D. M.: Megaloblastic madness. *Br. Med. J.* 2:1840, 1960.

188. Fraser, T. N.: Cerebral manifestations of Addisonian pernicious anemia. *Lancet* 2:458, 1960.

189. Stracham, R. W., and Henderson, J. G.: Psychiatric syndromes due to avitaminosis B_{12} with normal blood and marrow. *Q. J. Med.* 34:303, 1965.

190. Shulman, R.: Psychiatric aspects of pernicious anaemia. *Br. Med. J.* 3:266, 1967.

191. Smith, A. D. M., and Duckett, S.: Cyanide, vitamin B_{12}, experimental demyelination and tobacco amblyopia. *Br. J. Exp. Pathol.* 46:615, 1965.

192. Victor, M., and Lear, A.: Subacute combined degeneration of the spinal core: Current concepts of the disease process: Value of serum vitamin B_{12} determinations in clarifying some of the common clinical problems. *Am. J. Med.* 20:896, 1956.

193. Green, R., van Tonder, S. V., Oettle, G. J., Cole, G., and Metz, J.: Neurological changes in fruit bats deficient in vitamin B_{12}. *Nature* 254:148, 1975.

194. Goodman, A. M., and Harris, J. W.: Studies in B_{12}-deficient monkeys with combined system disease. I. B_{12}-deficient patterns in bone marrow deoxyuridine suppression tests without morphologic or functional abnormalities. *J. Lab. Clin. Med.* 96:722, 1980.

195. Davison, A. N.: Myelination and diseases of the nervous system: Abnormalities of myelin composition, in *Myelination*, edited by A. N. Davison and A. Peters. Thomas, Springfield, 1970, p. 162.

196. Cardinale, G. J., Carty, T. J., and Abeles, R. H.: Effect of methylmalonyl coenzyme A, a metabolite which accumulates in vitamin B_{12} deficiency, on fatty acid synthesis. *J. Biol. Chem.* 247:4270, 1972.

197. Barley, F. W., Sato, G. H., and Abeles, R. H.: An effect of vitamin B_{12} deficiency in tissue culture. *J. Biol. Chem.* 247:4270, 1972.

198. Frenkel, E. P.: Abnormal fatty acid metabolism in peripheral nerves of patients with pernicious anemia. *J. Clin. Invest.* 52:1237, 1973.

199. Wokes, F.: Tobacco amblyopia. *Lancet* 2:526, 1958.

200. Linnell, J. C.: The fate of cobalamin *in vivo*, in *Cobalamin: Biochemistry and Pathophysiology*, edited by B. M. Babior. Wiley-Interscience, New York, 1975, p. 287.

201. Matthews, D. M., and Wilson, J.: Cobalamins and cyanide metabolism in neurological diseases, in *The Cobalamins: A Glaxo Symposium*, edited by H. R. V. Arnstein and R. J. Wrighton. Williams & Wilkins, Baltimore, 1971, p. 115.

202. Green, R., Jacobsen, D. W., and Sommer, C.: Effect of nitrous oxide on methionine synthetase activity in brain and kidney of vitamin B_{12} deficient fruit bats. *Proc. 18th Congr. Int. Soc. Hematol.*, Montreal, 1980, p. 148.

203. Finch, C. A., Colman, D. H., Motulsky, A. G., Donohue, D. M., and Reiff, R. H.: Erythrokinetics in pernicious anemia. *Blood* 11:807, 1956.

204. Hillman, R. S., Adamson, J., and Burka, E.: Characteristics of vitamin B_{12} correction of the abnormal erythropoiesis of pernicious anemia. *Blood* 31:419, 1968.

205. van Dommelen, C. K. V., and Klaassen, C. H. L.: Cyanocobalamin-dependent depression of the serum alkaline phosphatase level in patients with pernicious anemia. *N. Engl. J. Med.* 271:541, 1964.

206. Riddle, M. C.: Endogeneous uric acid metabolism in pernicious anemia. *J. Clin. Invest.* 8:69, 1929.

207. James, G. W., III, and Abbott, L. D., Jr.: Nitrogen and phosphorus metabolism during vitamin B_{12}-induced remission. *Metabolism* 1:259, 1952.

208. Adams, J. F., Hume, R., Kennedy, E. H., Pirrie, T. G., and Whitelaw, J. W.: Metabolic responses to low doses of cyanocobalamin in patients with megaloblastic anaemia. *Br. J. Nutr.* 22:575, 1968.

209. Lawson, D. H., Murray, R. M., Parker, J. L. W., and Hay, G.: Hypokalemia in megaloblastic anaemias. *Lancet* 2:588, 1970.

210. Lawson, D. H., Murray, R. M., Parker, J. L. W.: Early mortality in megaloblastic anaemias. *Q. J. Med.* 41:1, 1972.

211. Marshall, R. A., and Jandl, J. H.: Responses to "physiologic" doses of folic acid in the megaloblastic anemias. *Arch. Intern. Med.* 105:352, 1960.

212. Vilter, C. F., Vilter, R. W., and Spies, T. D.: The treatment of pernicious and related anemias with synthetic folic acid. I. Observations on the maintenance of a normal hematologic status and on the occurrence of combined system disease at the end of one year. *J. Lab. Clin. Med.* 32:262, 1947.

213. Bok, J., Faber, J. G., DeVries, J. A., Kroese, W. F. S., and Nieweg, H. O.: Effect of pteroylglutamic acid administration on the serum vitamin B_{12} concentration in pernicious anemia in relapse. *J. Clin. Med.* 51:667, 1958.

214. Lear, A. A.: Effect of folic acid on serum vitamin B_{12} concentrations in pernicious anemia. *J. Clin. Invest.* 34:948, 1955.

215. Beck, W. S.: On the assay of serum vitamin B_{12}. *Ligand Q.* 2:10, 1979.

216. Young, D. S.: Normal laboratory values in SI units. *N. Engl. J. Med.* 292:795, 1975.

217. Cox, E. V., and White, A. M.: Methylmalonic acid excretion: An index of vitamin B_{12} deficiency. *Lancet* 2:853, 1962.

218. Kahn, S. B., et al.: Methylmalonic acid excretion: A sensitive indicator of vitamin B_{12} deficiency in man. *J. Lab. Clin. Med.* 66:75, 1965.

219. Mudd, S. H., Levey, H. L., and Abeles, R. H.: A derangement in B_{12} metabolism leading to homocystinemia, cystathioninemia, and methylmalonic aciduria. *Biochem. Biophys. Res. Commun.* 35:121, 1969.

220. Rosenberg, L. E., Lilljeqvist, A-C., and Hsia, Y. E.: Methylmalonic aciduria: An inborn error leading to metabolic acidosis, long-chain ketonuria and intermittent hyperglycinemia. *N. Engl. J. Med.* 278:1319, 1969.

221. Giorgio, A. J., and Plaut, G. W. E.: A method for the colorimetric determination of urinary methylmalonic acid in pernicious anemia. *J. Lab. Clin. Med.* 62:667, 1965.

222. Hoffman, N. E., and Barboriak, J. J.: Gas chromatographic determination of urinary methylmalonic acid. *Anal. Biochem.* 18:10, 1967.

223. Bashir, H. V., Hinterberger, H., and Jones, B. P.: Methylmalonic acid excretion in vitamin B_{12} deficiency. *Br. J. Haematol.* 12:704, 1966.

224. Conley, C. L., Krevans, J. R., Chow, B. F., Barrows, C., and Lang, C. A.: Observations on the absorption, utilization, and excretion of vitamin B_{12}. *J. Lab. Clin. Med.* 38:84, 1951.

225. Schilling, R. F.: Intrinsic factor studies. II. The effect of gastric juice on the urinary excretion of radioactivity after the oral administration of radioactive vitamin B_{12}. *J. Lab. Clin. Med.* 42:860, 1953.

226. Nelp, W. B., Wagner, H. N., Jr., and Reba, R. C.: Renal excretion of vitamin B_{12} and its use in measurements of glomerular filtration rate in man. *J. Lab. Clin. Med.* 63:480, 1964.

227. Rath, C. E., McCurdy, P. R., and Duffy, B. J.: Effect of renal disease on the Schilling test. *N. Engl. J. Med.* 256:111, 1956.

228. Callender, S. T., Witts, L. J., Warner, G. T., and Oliver, R.: The use of a simple whole-body counter for haematological investigations. *Br. J. Haematol.* 12:276, 1966.

229. Akun, S. N., Miller, I. F., and Meyer, L. M.: Vitamin B_{12} absorption test. *Acta Haematol. (Basel)* 41:341, 1969.

230. Mahmud, K., Ripley, D., and Doscherholmen, A.: Vitamin B_{12} absorption tests: Their unreliability in postgastrectomy states. *JAMA* 216:1167, 1971.

231. Streeter, A. M., Duraippah, B., Boyle, R., O'Neil, B. J., and Pheils, M. T.: Malabsorption of vitamin B_{12} after vagotomy. *Am. J. Surg.* 128:340, 1974.

232. Streeter, A. M., Duncombe, V. M., Boyle, R., and Pheils, M. T.: A simple method of measuring the absorption of protein-bound vitamin B_{12}. *Aust. N.Z. J. Med.* 5:382, 1975.

233. Steinberg, W. M., King, C. E., and Toskes, P. P.: Malabsorption of protein-bound cobalamin but not unbound cobalamin during cimetidine administration. *Dig. Dis. Sci.* 25:188, 1980.

234. Streeter, A. M., Shu, H. Y., Duncombe, V. M., Hewson, J. W., and Thorpe, M. E. C.: Vitamin B_{12} malabsorption associated with a normal Schilling test result. *Med. J. Aust.* 1:54, 1976.

235. Ellenbogen, L.: Absorption and transport of cobalamin: Intrinsic factor and the transcobalamins, in *Cobalamin: Biochemistry and Pathophysiology*, edited by B. M. Babior. Wiley-Interscience, New York, 1975, p. 215.

236. Herbert, V., and Castle, W. B.: Divalent cation and pH dependence of rat intrinsic factor action in everted sacs and mucosal homogenates of rat small intestine. *J. Clin. Invest.* 40:1978, 1961.

237. Strauss, E. W., and Wilson, T. H.: Factors controlling B_{12} uptake by intestinal sacs in vitro. *Am. J. Physiol.* 198:103, 1960.

238. Schjönsby, H., and Peters, T. J.: The estimation of intrinsic factor using guinea pig intestinal brush borders. *Scand. J. Gastroenterol.* 65:441, 1971.

239. Ellenbogen, L., Highley, D. R., Barker, H. A., and Smyth, R. D.: Inhibition of cobamide coenzyme activity by intrinsic factor. *Biochem. Biophys. Res. Commun.* 3:178, 1960.

240. Gottlieb, C., Lau, K. S., Wasserman, L. R., and Herbert, V.: Rapid charcoal assay for intrinsic factor (IF), gastric juice unsaturated B_{12} binding capacity, antibody to IF, and serum unsaturated B_{12} binding capacity. *Blood* 25:875, 1965.

241. Rødbro, P., Christiansen, P. M., and Schwartz, M.: Intrinsic factor secretion in stomach diseases. *Lancet* 2:1200, 1965.

242. Kay, A. W.: Effect of large doses of histamine on gastric secretion of HCl and an augmented histamine test. *Br. Med. J.* 2:77, 1953.

243. Wilkinson, J. F.: Gastric secretions in pernicious anemia. *Q. J. Med.* 1:361, 1932.

244. McGuigan, J. E., and Trudeau, W. L.: Serum gastric concentrations in pernicious anemia. *N. Engl. J. Med.* 282:358, 1970.

245. Ganguli, P. C., Cullen, D. R., and Irvine, W. J.: Radioimmunoassay of plasma-gastrin in pernicious anemia, achlorhydria without pernicious anemia, hypochlorhydria, and in controls. *Lancet* 1:155, 1971.

246. Walsh, J. H., and Grossman, M. I.: Gastrin. *N. Engl. J. Med.* 292:1377, 1975.

247. Hall, C. A.: The nondiagnosis of pernicious anemia. *Ann. Intern. Med.* 63:951, 1965.

248. Ellison, A. B.: Pernicious anemia masked by multivitamins containing folic acid. *JAMA* 173:240, 1960.

249. Smith, M. D., Smith, D. A., and Fletcher, M.: Haemorrhage associated with thrombocytopenia in megaloblastic anemia. *Br. Med. J.* 1:982, 1962.

250. Stefanini, M., and Karaca, M.: Acquired thrombocytopathy in patients with pernicious anemia. *Lancet* 1:400, 1966.

251. Comin, D. B., Hines, J. D., and Wieland, R. G.: Coexistent pernicious anemia and idiopathic hypoparathyroidism in a woman. *JAMA* 207:1147, 1969.

252. Sharpstone, P., and James, D. G.: Pernicious anaemia and thyrotoxicosis in a family. *Lancet* 1:246, 1965.

253. Conn, H. O., Binder, H., and Burns, B.: Pernicious anemia and immunologic deficiency. *Ann. Intern. Med.* 68:603, 1968.

254. Pirofsky, B., and Vaughn, M.: Addisonian pernicious anemia with positive antiglobulin tests: A multiple autoimmune disease syndrome. *Am. J. Clin. Pathol.* 50:459, 1968.

255. Witts, L. J.: Pernicious anemia and endocrine disease. *Isr. Med. J.* 22:294, 1963.

256. Perillie, P. E., and Nagler, R.: Development of pernicious anemia in a young patient with chronic ulcerative colitis. *N. Engl. J. Med.* 261:1175, 1959.

257. Zamchek, N., Grable, E., Ley, A., and Norman, L.: Occurrence of gastric cancer among patients with pernicious anemia at the Boston City Hospital. *N. Engl. J. Med.* 252:1103, 1955.

258. Elsborg, L., and Mosbech, J.: Gastric cancer as a risk factor in pernicious anemia, in Vitamin B_{12}. *Proceedings of the Third European Symposium on Vitamin B_{12} and Intrinsic Factor. University of Zürich, March 5–8, 1979, Zürich, Switzerland*, edited by B. Zagalak and W. Friedrich. Walter de Gruyter, New York, 1979, p. 1119.

259. Howitz, J., and Schwartz, M.: Vitiligo, achlorhydria, and pernicious anemia. *Lancet* 1:1331, 1971.

260. Jackson, I., Doig, W. B., and McDonald, G.: Pernicious anaemia as a cause of infertility. *Lancet* 2:1159, 1967.

261. Watson, A. A.: Seminal vitamin B_{12} and sterility. *Lancet* 2:644, 1962.

262. Solanki, D. L., et al.: Pernicious anemia in blacks. *Am. J. Clin. Pathol.* 75:96, 1981.

263. Green, R., et al.: Masking of macrocytosis by alpha-globin chain deletions in blacks with pernicious anemia. *N. Engl. J. Med.* 307:1322, 1982.

264. Boddy, K., King, P., Mervyn, L., Macleod, A., and Adams, J. F.: Retention of cyanocobalamin, hydroxocobalamin, and coenzyme B_{12} after parenteral administration. *Lancet* 2:710, 1968.

265. Chalmers, J. N. M., and Shinton, N. K.: Comparison of hydroxocobalamin and cyanocobalamin in the treatment of pernicious anemia. *Lancet* 2:1305, 1965.

266. Tudhope, G. R., Swan, H. T., and Spray, G. H.: Patient variation in pernicious anemia, as shown in a clinical trial of cyanocobalamin, hydroxocobalamin and cyanocobalamin-zinc tannate. *Br. J. Haematol.* 13:216, 1967.

267. Olesen, H., Hom, B. L., and Schwartz, M.: Antibody to transcobalamin II in patients treated with long acting vitamin B_{12} preparations. *Scand. J. Haematol.* 5:5, 1968.

268. Schwartz, M., Lous, P., and Meulengracht, E.: Reduced effect of heterologous intrinsic factor after prolonged oral treatment in pernicious anemia. *Lancet* 1:751, 1957.

269. Lowenstein, L., Cooper, B. A., Brunton, L., and Gartha, S.: An immunologic basis for acquired resistance to oral administration of hog intrinsic factor and vitamin B_{12} in pernicious anemia. *J. Clin. Invest.* 40:1656, 1961.

270. Gough, K. R., Read, A. E., McCarthy, C. F., and Waters, A. H.: Megaloblastic anaemia due to nutritional deficiency of folic acid. *Q. J. Med.* 32:243, 1963.

271. Luhby, A. L.: Megaloblastic anaemia in infancy. III. Clinical considerations and analysis. *J. Pediatr.* 54:617, 1959.

272. Strelling, M. K., Blackledge, G. D., Goodall, H. B., and Walker, C. H. M.: Megaloblastic anaemia and whole-blood folate levels in premature infants. *Lancet* 1:898, 1966.

273. Royston, N. J. W., and Parry, T. E.: Megaloblastic anaemia complicating dietary treatment of phenylketonuria in infancy. *Arch. Dis. Child.* 37:430, 1962.

274. Ballard, H. S., and Lindenbaum, J.: Megaloblastic anemia complicating hyperalimentation therapy. *Am. J. Med.* 56:740, 1974.

275. Hampers, C. L., Streiff, R., Nathan, D. G., Snyder, D., and Merrill, J. P.: Megaloblastic hematopoiesis in uremia and in patients with long-term hemodialysis. *N. Engl. J. Med.* 276:551, 1967.

276. Whitehead, V. M., Comty, C. H., Posen, G. A., and Kaye, M.: Homeostasis of folic acid in patients undergoing maintenance hemodialysis. *N. Engl. J. Med.* 279:970, 1968.

277. O'Brien, W.: Acute military tropical sprue in Southeast Asia. *Am. J. Clin. Nutr.* 21:1007, 1968.

278. Todd, D., and Kan, D. S.: Anaemia, in pregnancy in Hong Kong. *J. Obstet. Gynaec. Br. Commonw.* 72:738, 1965.

279. Herbert, V.: Folic acid deficiency in man. *Vitam. Horm.* 26:525, 1969.

280. Li, R.-S.: Personal communication, 1982.

281. Jandl, J. H.: Anemia of liver disease: Observations on its mechanism. *J. Clin. Invest.* 34:390, 1955.

282. Jandl, J. H., and Lear, A. A.: The metabolism of folic acid in cirrhosis. *Ann. Intern. Med.* 45:1027, 1956.

283. Jarrold, T., Will, J. J., and Davies, A. R.: Bone marrow erythroid morphology in alcoholic patients. *Am. J. Clin. Nutr.* 20:716, 1967.

284. McFarland, W., and Libre, E. P.: Abnormal leukocyte response in alcoholism. *Ann. Intern. Med.* 59:865, 1963.

285. Post, R. M., and Desforges, J. F.: Thrombocytopenia and alcoholism. *Ann. Intern. Med.* 68:1230, 1968.

286. Lindenbaum, J.: Folate and vitamin B_{12} deficiencies in alcoholics. *Semin. Hematol.* 17:119, 1980.

287. Sullivan, L. W., and Herbert, V.: Suppression of hematopoiesis by ethanol. *J. Clin. Invest.* 43:2048, 1964.
288. Lieber, C. S.: Metabolism and metabolic effects of alcohol. *Semin. Hematol.* 17:85, 1980.
289. McCurdy, P. R., Pierce, L. E., and Rath, C. E.: Abnormal bone-marrow morphology in acute alcoholism. *N. Engl. J. Med.* 266:505, 1962.
290. Liu, Y. K.: Effects of alcohol on granulocytes and lymphocytes. *Semin. Hematol.* 17:130, 1980.
291. Lindenbaum, J., and Lieber, C. S.: Hematological effects of alcohol in man in the absence of nutritional deficiency. *N. Engl. J. Med.* 281:333, 1969.
292. Eichner, E. R., Pierce. H. I., and Hillman, R. S.: Folate balance in dietary-induced megaloblastic anemia. *N. Engl. J. Med.* 284:933, 1971.
293. Zalusky, R., Herbert, V., and Castle, W. B.: Cyanocobalamin therapy effect in folic acid deficiency. *Arch. Intern. Med.* 109:545, 1962.
294. Alperin, J. B.: Effect of vitamin B_{12} therapy in a patient with folic acid deficiency. *Am. J. Clin. Nutr.* 15:117, 1964.
295. Doig, A., and Girdwood, R. H.: Absorption of folic acid and labeled cyanocobalamin in intestinal malabsorption. *Q. J. Med.* 29:333, 1960.
296. Spray, G. H., and Witts, L. J.: Utilization of folic acid given by mouth. *Clin. Sci.* 11:273, 1952.
297. Chanarin, I., Mollin, D. L., and Anderson, B. B.: Folic acid deficiency and the megaloblastic anaemias. *Proc. R. Soc. Med.* 51:757, 1958.
298. Chanarin, I., Anderson, B. B., and Mollin, D. L.: Absorption of folic acid. *Br. J. Haematol.* 4:156, 1958.
299. Anderson, B., Belcher, B. H., Chanarin, I., and Mollin, D. L.: Urinary and faecal excretion of radioactivity after oral doses of H^3-folic acid. *Br. J. Haematol.* 6:439, 1960.
300. Klipstein, F. A.: The urinary excretion of orally administered tritium-labeled folic acid as a test of folic acid absorption. *Blood* 21:626, 1963.
301. Mollin, D. L., and Hines, J. D.: Observations on the nature and pathogenesis of anaemia following partial gastrectomy. *Proc. R. Soc. Med.* 57:575, 1964.
302. Gough, K. R., Thirkettle, J. L., and Read, A. E.: Folic acid deficiency in patients after gastric resection. *Q. J. Med.* 34:1, 1965.
303. Deller, D. J., Begley, M. D., Edwards, R. G., and Addison, M.: Metabolic effects of gastrectomy with special reference to calcium and folic acid. II. The contribution of folic acid deficiency to the anaemia. *Gut* 5:218, 1964.
304. Mahmud, K., Kaplan, M. E., Ripley, D., Swaim, W. R., and Doscherholmen, A.: The importance of red cell B_{12} and folate levels after partial gastrectomy. *Am. J. Clin. Nutr.* 27:51, 1974.
305. Cooke, W. T., Peeney, A. L. P., and Hawkins, C. F.: Symptoms, signs and diagnostic features of idiopathic steatorrhea. *Q. J. Med.* 22:59, 1953.
306. Benson, G. D., Kowlessar, O. D., and Sleisenger, M. H.: Adult celiac disease with emphasis upon response to gluten-free diet. *Medicine (Baltimore)* 43:1, 1964.
307. Kowlessar, O. D., and Sleisenger, M. H.: The role of gliadin in the pathogenesis of adult celiac disease. *Gastroenterology* 44:357, 1963.
308. Jeffries, G. H., Weser, E., and Sleisenger, M. H.: Malabsorption. *Gastroenterology* 56:777, 1969.
309. Kinnear, D. G., Johns, D. G., McIntosh, P. C., Burgen, A. S. V., and Cameron, D. G.: Intestinal absorption of tritium-labeled folic acid in idiopathic steatorrhea: Effect of a gluten-free diet. *Can. Med. Assoc. J.* 89:957, 1963.
310. Dormandy, K. M., Waters, A. H., and Mollin, D. L.: Folic acid deficiency in coeliac disease. *Lancet* 1:632, 1963.
311. Collins, J. R., and Isselbacher, K. J.: Treatment of adult celiac disease (nontropical sprue). *N. Engl. J. Med.* 271:1153, 1964.
312. Sheehy, T. W., Cohen, W. C., Wallace, D. K., and Legters, L. J.: Tropical sprue in North Americans. *JAMA* 194:1069, 1965.
313. O'Brien, W., and England, N. W. J.: Military tropical sprue from Southeast Asia. *Br. Med. J.* 2:1157, 1966.
314. Klipstein, F. A.: Tropical sprue in New York City. *Gastroenterology* 47:457, 1964.
315. Butterworth, C. E.: Tropical sprue: A consideration of some possible aetological mechanisms, in *Malabsorption*, edited by R. H.

Girdwood and A. N. Smith. Pfizer Medical Monographs 4, University of Edinburgh Press, Edinburgh, 1969, p. 238.
316. Klipstein, F. A.: Intestinal folate conjugase activity in tropical sprue. *Am. J. Clin. Nutr.* 20:1004, 1967.
317. Corcino, J. J., Reisenauer, A. M., and Halsted, C. H.: Jejunal perfusion of simple and conjugated folates in tropical sprue. *J. Clin. Invest.* 58:298, 1976.
318. Guerra, R., Wheby, M. S., and Bayless, T. M.: Long term antibiotic therapy in tropical sprue. *Ann. Intern. Med.* 63:619, 1965.
319. Klipstein, F. A., Schenk, E. A., and Samloff, I. M.: Folate repletion associated with oral tetracycline therapy in tropical sprue. *Gastroenterology* 51:317, 1966.
320. Mathan, V. I., Ignatius, M., and Baker, S. J.: A household epidemic of tropical sprue. *Gut* 1:490, 1966.
321. Gardner, F. H.: Tropical sprue. *N. Engl. J. Med.* 258:791, 835, 1958.
322. Klipstein, F. A.: Progress in gastroenterology: Tropical sprue. *Gastroenterology* 54:275, 1968.
323. Sheehy, T. W., Perez-Santiago, E., and Rubini, M. E.: Tropical sprue and vitamin B_{12}. *N. Engl. J. Med.* 265:1232, 1961.
324. Cox, E. V., Meynell, M. J., Cooke, W. T., and Gaddie, R.: Folic acid excretion test in the steatorrhea syndrome. *Gastroenterology* 35:390, 1958.
325. Chanarin, I., and Bennett, M. C.: Absorption of folic acid and D-xylose as tests of small intestinal function. *Br. Med. J.* 1:985, 1962.
326. Booth, C. C.: Metabolic effects of intestinal resection in man. *Postgrad. Med. J.* 37:725, 1961.
327. Sleisenger, M. H., Almy, P. T., and Barr, D. P.: The sprue syndrome secondary to lymphoma of the small bowel. *Am. J. Med.* 15:666, 1953.
328. Pitney, W. R., Joske, R. A., and Mackinnon, N. L.: Folic acid and other absorption tests in lymphosarcoma, chronic lymphocytic leukemia and some related conditions. *J. Clin. Pathol.* 13:440, 1960.
329. Hoskins, L. C., Norris, T. H., Gottlieb, L. S., and Zamchek, N.: Functional and morphologic alterations of the gastrointestinal tract in progressive systemic sclerosis (scleroderma). *Am. J. Med.* 33:459, 1962.
330. Wruble, L. D., and Kalser, M. H.: Diabetic steatorrhea: A distinct entity. *Am. J. Med.* 37:118, 1964.
331. Vinnik, I. E., Kern, F., Jr., and Struthers, J. E., Jr.: Malabsorption and the diarrhea of diabetes mellitus. *Gastroenterology* 43:507, 1962.
332. Cook, G. C., Morgan, J. O., and Hoffbrand, A. V.: Impairment of folate absorption by systemic bacterial infections. *Lancet* 2:1417, 1974.
333. Ryan, G. M. S., and Forshaw, J. W. B.: Megaloblastic anemia due to phenytoin sodium. *Br. Med. J.* 2:242, 1955.
334. Klipstein, F. A.: Subnormal serum folate and macrocytosis associated with anticonvulsant drug therapy. *Blood* 23:68, 1964.
335. Reynolds, E. H., Hallpike, J. F., Phillips, B. M., and Matthews, D. M.: Reversible absorptive defects in anticonvulsant megaloblastic anemia. *J. Clin. Pathol.* 18:593, 1965.
336. Kiorboe, E., and Plum, C. M.: Megaloblastic anaemia developing during treatment of epilepsy. *Acta Med. Scand. (Suppl.)* 445:349, 1966.
337. Reynolds, E. H., Milner, G., Matthews, D. M., and Chanarin, I.: Anticonvulsant therapy, megaloblastic haemopoiesis and folic acid metabolism. *Q. J. Med.* 35:521, 1966.
338. Druskin, M. S., Wallen, M. H., and Bonagura, L.: Anticonvulsant-associated anemia. *N. Engl. J. Med.* 267:483, 1962.
339. Reynolds, E. H.: Anticonvulsants, folic acid, and epilepsy. *Lancet* 1:1376, 1973.
340. Klipstein, F. A.:Folate deficiency secondary to disease of the intestinal tract. *Bull. N.Y. Acad. Med.* 42:638, 1966.
341. Dahlke, M. B., and Mertens-Roster, E.: Malabsorption of folic acid due to diphenylhydantoin. *Blood* 30:341, 1967.
342. Rosenberg, I. H., Godwin, H. A., Streiff, R. R., and Castle, W. B.: Impairment of intestinal deconjugation of dietary folate: Possible explanation of megaloblastic anaemia associated with phenytoin therapy. *Lancet* 2:530, 1968.
343. Hoffbrand, A. V., and Necheles, T. F.: Mechanism of folate deficiency in patients receiving phenytoin. *Lancet* 2:528, 1968.
344. Baugh, C. M., and Krumdieck, C. L.: Effects of phenytoin on folic acid conjugases in man. *Lancet* 2:519, 1969.

345. Pearson, D.: Megaloblastic anemia due to glutethimide. *Lancet* 1:110, 1965.
346. Klipstein, F. A., Berlinger, F. G., and Reed, L. J.: Folate deficiency associated with drug therapy for tuberculosis. *Blood* 29:697, 1967.
347. Shojania, A. M., Hornady, G., and Barnes, P. H.: Oral contraceptives and serum-folate level. *Lancet* 1:1376, 1968.
348. Streiff, R. R.: Malabsorption of polyglutamic folic acid secondary to oral contraceptives. *Clin. Res.* 17:345, 1969.
349. Pietarinen, G. J., Leichter, J., and Pratt, R. F.: Dietary folate intake and concentration of folate in serum and erythrocytes in women using oral contraceptives. *Am. J. Clin. Nutr.* 30:275, 1977.
350. Tysoe, F. W., and Lowenstein, L.: Blood volume and hematologic studies in pregnancy and the puerperium. *Am. J. Obstet. Gynec.* 60:1187, 1950.
351. Verloop, M. C., Blokhuis, E. W. M., and Bos, C. C.: Causes of the "physiological" anemia of pregnancy. *Acta Haematol. (Basel)* 22:158, 1959.
352. Low, J. A., Johnston, E. E., and McBride, R. L.: Blood volume adjustments in the normal obstetric patient with particular reference to the third trimester of pregnancy. *Am. J. Obstet. Gynec.* 91:356, 1965.
353. Benjamin, F., Bassen, F. A., and Meyer, L. M.: Serum levels of folic acid, vitamin B_{12} and iron in anemia of pregnancy. *Am. J. Obstet. Gynec.* 96:310, 1966.
354. Ball, E. W., and Giles, C.: Folic acid and vitamin B_{12} levels in pregnancy and their relation to megaloblastic anaemia. *J. Clin. Pathol.* 17:165, 1964.
355. Whiteside, M. G., Ungar, B., and Cowling, D. C.: Iron, folic acid and vitamin B_{12} levels in normal pregnancy, and their influence on birth-weight and the duration of pregnancy. *Med. J. Aust.* 1:338, 1968.
356. Giles, C., and Shuttleworth, E. M.: Megaloblastic anaemia of pregnancy and the puerperium. *Lancet* 2:1341, 1958.
357. Bethell, F. H., Meyers, M. C., and Neligh, R. B.: Vitamin B_{12} in pernicious anemia and puerperal macrocytic anemia. *J. Lab. Clin. Med.* 33:1477, 1948.
358. Lowenstein, L., Pick, C. A., and Philpott, N. W.: Megaloblastic anemia of pregnancy and puerperium. *Am. J. Obstet. Gynec.* 70:1309, 1955.
359. Chanarin, I., MacGibbon, B. M., O'Sullivan, W. J., and Mollin, D. L.: Folic acid deficiency in pregnancy: Pathogenesis of megaloblastic anemia of pregnancy. *Lancet* 2:634, 1959.
360. Stone, M. L., Luhby, A. L., Feldman, R., Gordon, M., and Cooperman, J. M.: Folic acid metabolism in pregnancy. *Am. J. Obstet. Gynec.* 99:638, 1967.
361. Streiff, R. R., and Little, A. B.: Folic acid deficiency in pregnancy. *N. Engl. J. Med.* 276:776, 1967.
362. Willoughby, M. L. N.: An investigation of folic acid requirements in pregnancy. II. *Br. J. Haematol.* 13:503, 1967.
363. Pritchard, J. A., Scott, D. E., and Whalley, P. J.: Folic acid requirements in pregnancy-induced megaloblastic anemia. *JAMA* 208:1163, 1969.
364. Osler, W.: Observations on the severe anemias of pregnancy and the post-partum state. *Br. Med. J.* 1:1, 1919.
365. Badenoch, J., Callender, S. T., Evans, J. R., Turnbull, A. L., and Witts, L. J.: Megaloblastic anemia of pregnancy and the puerperium. *Br. Med. J.* 1:1245, 1955.
366. Shapiro, J., Alperts, H. W., Welch, P., and Metz, J.: Folate and vitamin B_{12} deficiency associated with lactation. *Br. J. Haematol.* 11:498, 1965.
367. Editorial: Anaemia during pregnancy. *Lancet* 2:1429, 1974.
368. Hibbard, E. D., and Spencer, W. S.: Low serum B_{12} levels and latent Addisonian anaemia in pregnancy. *J. Obstet. Gynaec. Br. Commonw.* 77:52, 1970.
369. Hibbard, B. M.: The role of folic acid in pregnancy. *J. Obstet. Gynaec. Br. Commonw.* 71:529, 1964.
370. Hibbard, E. D., and Smithells, R. W.: Folic acid metabolism and human embryopathy. *Lancet* 1:1254, 1965.
371. Martin, R. H., Harper, T. A., and Kelso, W.: Serum-folic acid in recurrent abortions. *Lancet* 1:670, 1965.
372. Hourihane, B., Coyle, C. V., and Drury, M. I.: Megaloblastic anemia of pregnancy. *J. Irish Med. Assoc.* 47:1, 1960.
373. Fletcher, J., Gurr, A., Fellingham, F. R., Prankerd, T. A. J., Brant, H. A., and Menzies, D. N.: The value of folic acid supplements in pregnancy. *J. Obstet. Gynaec. Br. Commonw.* 78:781, 1971.
374. Asling, C. N., Nelson, M. M., Dougherty, H. L., Wright, H. V., and Evans, H. M.: The development of cleft palate resulting from maternal pteroylglutamic (folic) acid deficiency during the latter half of gestation in rats. *Surg. Gynec. Obstet.* 111:19, 1960.
375. Nelso, M. M., Asling, C. W., and Evans, H. M.: Production of multiple congenital abnormalities in young by maternal pteroylglutamic acid deficiency during gestation. *J. Nutr.* 48:61, 1952.
376. Thiersch, J. B.: Therapeutic abortions with a folic acid antagonist, 4-amino-pteroyl-glutamic acid (4-amino PGA) administered by the oral route. *Am. J. Obstet. Gynecol.* 63:1298, 1952.
377. Lawrence, C., and Klipstein, F. A.: Megaloblastic anemia of pregnancy in New York City. *Ann. Intern. Med.* 66:25, 1967.
378. WHO Tech. Rep. Ser 503, 1972.
379. Jandl, J. H., and Greenberg, M. S.: Bone marrow failure due to relative nutritional deficiency in Cooley's hemolytic anemia. *N. Engl. J. Med.* 260:461, 1959.
380. Cox, E. V., Meynell, M. J., Cooke, W. T., and Gaddie, R.: Folic acid activity during blood regeneration. *Clin. Sci.* 19:219, 1960.
381. Lindenbaum, J., and Klipstein, F. A.: Folic acid deficiency in sickle cell anemia. *N. Engl. J. Med.* 269:875, 1963.
382. Oliner, H. L., and Heller, P.: Megaloblastic erythropoiesis and acquired hemolysis in sickle-cell anemia. *N. Engl. J. Med.* 261:19, 1959.
383. Knowles, J. P., Shuster, S., and Wells, G. C.: Folic acid deficiency in patients with skin disease. *Lancet* 1:1138, 1963.
384. Shuster, S., Marks, J., and Chanarin, I.: Folic acid deficiency in patients with skin disease. *Br. J. Dermatol.* 79:398, 1967.
385. Hild, D.: Folate losses from the skin in exfoliative dermatitis. *Arch. Intern. Med.* 123:51, 1969.
386. Van Scott, E. J., Auerback, R., and Weinstein, G. D.: Parenteral Methotrexate in psoriasis. *Arch. Dermatol.* 89:550, 1964.
387. Noeypatimanond, S., Watson-Williams, E. J., and Israëls, M. C. G.: Excretion of formiminoglutamic acid in reticulosis and carcinoma. *Lancet* 1:454, 1966.
388. Carey, R. W., Brena, G. P., and Krant, M. J.: Urinary formiminoglutamic acid excretion in patients with neoplastic disease. *Cancer* 17:713, 1964.
389. Rama Rao, P. B., Lagerlöf, B., Einhorn, J., and Reizenstein, P. G.: Folic acid activity in leukemia and cancer. *Cancer Res.* 25:221, 1965.
390. Magnus, E. M.: Folate activity in serum and red cells of patients with cancer. *Cancer Res.* 27:490, 1967.
391. Pitney, R. W., Joske, R. A., and Mackinnon, N. L.: Folic acid and other absorption tests in lymphosarcoma, chronic lymphocytic leukaemia and some related conditions. *J. Clin. Pathol.* 13:440, 1960.
392. Rose, D. P.: Folic acid deficiency in leukaemia and lymphomas. *J. Clin. Pathol.* 19:29, 1966.
393. Hoogstraten, B., Baker, H., and Gilbert, H. S.: Serum folate and serum vitamin B_{12} in patients with malignant hematologic diseases. *Cancer Res.* 25:1933, 1965.
394. Farber, S.: Some observations of the effect of folic acid antagonists on acute leukemia and other forms of incurable cancer. *Blood* 4:160, 1949.
395. Spector, I., and Hutter, A. M.: Folic acid deficiency in neoplastic disease. *Am. J. Med. Sci.* 252:419, 1966.
396. Bertino, J. R., Boothe, B. A., Bieber, A. L., and Sartorelli, A. C.: Studies on the inhibition of dihydrofolate reductase by the folate antagonists. *J. Biol. Chem.* 239:479, 1964.
397. Osborn, M. J., Freeman, M., and Huennekens, F. M.: Inhibition of dihydrofolate reductase by aminopterin and amethopterin. *Proc. Soc. Exp. Biol. Med.* 97:429, 1958.
398. Werkheiser, W. C.: Specific binding of 4-amino folic acid analogues by folic acid reductase. *J. Biol. Chem.* 236:888, 1961.
399. Slavikova, V., Slavik, K., and Pristoupilova, K.: Metabolism of folic acid. VIII. Mechanism of biochemical action of some 4-amino analogues of folic acid and their dibromo derivatives. *Coll. Czech. Chem. Commun.* 27:1955, 1962.
400. Werkheiser, W. C.: Biochemical, cellular and pharmacological action and effects of the folic acid antagonists. *Cancer Res.* 23:1227, 1963.

401. Rosenfelt, F.: Methotrexate and the need for continued research. *Yale J. Biol. Med. 48:*97, 1975.

402. Groff, J. P., and Blakley, R. L.: Rescue of human lymphoid cells from the effects of methotrexate *in vitro. Cancer Res. 38:*3847, 1978.

403. Falco, E. A., Hitchings, G. H., Russell, P. B., and VanderWerff, H.: Antimalarials as antagonists of purines and pteroylglutamic acid. *Nature 164:*107, 1949.

404. Hitchings, G. H., Falco, E. A., VanderWerff, H., Russell, P. B., and Elion, G. B.: Antagonists of nucleic acid derivatives. VII. 2,4-diaminopyrimidines. *J. Biol. Chem. 199:*43, 1952.

405. Waxman, S., and Herbert, V.: Mechanism of pyrimethamine-induced megaloblasts in human bone marrow. *N. Engl. J. Med. 280:*1316, 1969.

406. Giles, C. L., Jacobs, L., and Melton, M. L.: Experimental use of folic acid in treatment of toxoplasmosis with pyrimethamine. *Arch. Ophthalmol. 72:*82, 1964.

407. Gardner, F. H.: Observations on the cytology of gastric epithelium in tropical sprue. *J. Lab. Clin. Med. 47:*529, 1956.

408. van Niekerk, W. A.: Cervical cytological abnormalities caused by folic acid deficiency. *Acta Cytol. (Baltimore) 10:*67, 1966.

409. Marshall, R. A., and Jandl, J. H.: Responses to "physiologic" doses of folic acid in the megaloblastic anemias. *Arch. Intern. Med. 105:*353, 1960.

410. Herbert, V.: Minimal daily adult folate requirement. *Arch. Intern. Med. 110:*649, 1962.

411. Hoffbrand, A. V., Newcombe, B. F. A., and Mollin, D. L.: Method of assay of red cell folate activity and the value of the assay as a test for folate deficiency. *J. Clin. Pathol. 19:*17, 1966.

412. Spray, G. H.: Estimation of red cell folate activity. *J. Clin. Pathol. 22:*212, 1969.

413. Rothenberg, S. P., DaCosta, M., and Rosenberg, Z.: A radioassay for serum folate: Use of a two-phase sequential incubation ligand-binding system. *N. Engl. J. Med. 286:*1335, 1972.

414. Liu, Y. K.: Microbiologic assay of erythrocytic folate content by the aseptic addition method. *Am. J. Clin. Pathol. 62:*688, 1974.

415. Schreiber, C., and Waxman, S.: Measurement of red cell folate levels by ³H-pteroylglutamic acid (³H-PteGlu) radioassay. *Br. J. Haematol. 27:*551, 1974.

416. Johns, D. G., and Bertino, J. R.: Folates and megaloblastic anemia: A review. *Clin. Pharmacol. Ther. 6:*372, 1965.

417. Johnstone, J. M., Kemp, J. H., and Hibbard, E. D.: A colorimetric method for the estimation of urinary formiminoglutamic acid. *Clin. Chim. Acta 12:*440, 1965.

418. Chanarin, I., Mollin, D. L., and Anderson, B. B.: The clearance from the plasma of folic acid injected intravenously in normal subjects and patients with megaloblastic anaemia. *Br. J. Haematol. 4:*435, 1958.

419. Metz, J., Stevens, K., Krawitz, S., and Brandt, V.: The plasma clearance of injected doses of folic acid as an index of folic acid deficiency. *J. Clin. Pathol. 14:*622, 1961.

420. Sheehy, T. W., Santini, R., Jr., Guerra, R., Angel, R., and Plough, I. C.: Tritiated folic acid as a diagnostic acid in folic acid deficiency. *J. Lab. Clin. Med. 61:*650, 1963.

421. Ellegaard, J., and Esmann, V.: Folate activity of human lymphocytes determined by measurement of serine synthesis. *Scand. J. Clin. Lab. Invest. 31:*9, 1973.

422. Elion, G. B.: Biochemistry and pharmacology of purine analogues. *Fed. Proc. 26:*898, 1967.

423. Elion, G. B., and Hitchings, G. H.: Metabolic basis for the action of analogs of purines and pyrimidines. *Adv. Chemother. 2:*91, 1965.

424. Hitchings, G. H., and Elion, G. B.: Purine analogues, in *Metabolic Inhibitors,* edited by R. M. Hochster and J. H. Quastel. Academic, New York, 1963, vol. 1, p. 215.

425. Bethell, F. H., and Thompson, D. S.: Treatment of leukemia and related disorders with 6-mercaptopurine. *Ann. N.Y. Acad. Sci. 60:*436, 1954.

426. Heidelberger, C., and Ansfield, F. J.: Experimental and clinical use of fluorinated pyrimidines in cancer chemotherapy. *Cancer Res. 23:*1226, 1963.

427. Cohen, S. S., Flaks, J. G., Barner, H. D., Loeb, M. R., and Lichtenstein, J.: The mode of action of 5-fluorouracil and its derivatives. *Proc. Natl. Acad. Sci. U.S.A. 44:*1004, 1958.

428. Ingraham, H. A., Tseng, B. Y., and Goulian, M.: Mechanism for exclusion of 5-fluorouracil from DNA. *Cancer Res. 40:*998, 1980.

429. Williams, M. V., and Cheng, Y.: Human deoxyuridine triphosphate nucleotidohydrolase: Purification and characterization of the deoxyuridine triphosphate nucleotidohydrolase from acute lymphocytic leukemia. *J. Biol. Chem. 254:*2897, 1979.

430. Brennan, M. J., Vaitkevicius, V. K., and Rebuck, J. W.: Megaloblastic anemia associated with inhibition of thymine synthesis: Observations during 5-fluorouracil therapy. *Blood 16:*1535, 1960.

431. Jaffe, J. J., Handschumacher, R. E., and Welch, A. D.: Studies on the carcinostatic activity in mice of 6-azauracil riboside (Azauridine) in comparison with that of 6-azauracil. *Yale J. Biol. Med. 30:*168, 1957.

432. Sorm, F., and Keilova, H.: The anti-tumor activity of 6-azauracil riboside. *Experientia 14:*215, 1958.

433. Cohen, S. S.: Sponges, cancer chemotherapy, and cellular aging. *Perspect. Biol. Med. 6:*215, 1963.

434. Cohen, S. S.: Introduction to the biochemistry of D-arabinosyl nucleosides. *Proc. Nucl. Acid Res. Mol. Biol. 5:*1, 1966.

435. Ho, D. H. W., and Freireich, E. J.: Clinical pharmacology of arabinosylcytosine, in *Antineoplastic and Immunosuppressive Agents,* edited by A. C. Sarterelli and D. G. Johus. Springer-Verlag, Berlin, 1975, part II, p. 257.

436. Kim, J. H., and Eidinoff, M. L.: Action of 1-β-arabinofuranosylcytosine on the nucleic acid metabolism and viability of HeLa cells. *Cancer Res. 25:*698, 1965.

437. Creasey, W. A., Deconti, R. C., and Kaplan, S. R.: Biochemical studies with 1-β-D-arabinofuranosylcytosine in human leukemic leukocytes and normal bone marrow cells. *Cancer Res. 28:*1074, 1968.

438. Moore, E. C., and Cohen, S. S.: Effects of arabinonucleotides on ribonucleotide reduction by an enzyme system from rat tumor. *J. Biol. Chem. 242:*2116, 1967.

439. Furth, J. J., and Cohen, S. S.: Inhibition of mammalian DNA polymerase by the 5'-triphosphate of 1-β-D-arabinofuranosylcytosine and the 5'-triphosphate of 9-β-D-arabinofuranosylcytosine. *Cancer Res. 28:*2061, 1968.

440. Talley, R. W., and Vaitkevicius, V. K.: Megaloblastosis produced by a cytosine antagonist 1-β-D-arabinofuranosylcytosine. *Blood 21:*352, 1963.

441. Block, J. B., Bell, W., Whang, J., and Carbone, P. P.: Hematological and cytogenetic abnormalities during cytosine arabinoside therapy. *Proc. Am. Assoc. Cancer Res. 6:*6, 1965.

442. Papac, R. J.: Clinical and hematologic studies with 1-β-D-arabinosylcytosine. *J. Natl. Cancer Inst. 40:*997, 1968.

443. Bell, W. R., Whang, J. J., Carbone, P. P., Brecher, G., and Block, J. B.: Cytogenetic and morphologic abnormalities in the human bone marrow cells during cytosine arabinoside therapy. *Blood 27:*771, 1966.

444. Stearns, B., Losee, K. A., and Berstein, J.: Hydroxyurea: A new type of potential antitumor agent. *J. Med. Chem. 6:*201, 1963.

445. Krakoff, J. H.: Clinical and physiologic effects of hydroxyurea, in *Antineoplastic and Immunosuppressive Agents,* edited by A. C. Sarterelli and D. G. Johus. Springer-Verlag, Berlin, 1975, part II, p. 789.

446. Fishbein, W. N., Carbone, P. P., Freireich, E. J., Misra, D., and Frei, E., III: Clinical trials of hydroxyurea in patients with cancer and leukemia. *Clin. Pharmacol. Ther. 5:*574, 1964.

447. Young, C. W., and Hodas, S.: Hydroxyurea: Inhibitory effects on DNA metabolism. *Science 146:*1172, 1964.

448. Frenkel, E. P., Skinner, W. N., and Smiley, J. D.: Studies on a metabolic defect induced by hydroxyurea (NSC-32065). *Cancer Chemother. Rep. 40:*19, 1964.

449. Frenkel, E. P., and Arthur, C.: Induced ribotide reductive conversion by hydroxyurea and its relationship to megaloblastosis. *Cancer Res. 27:*1016, 1967.

450. Brown, N. D., Eliasson, R., Reichard, P., and Thelander, L.: Non-heme iron as a cofactor in ribonucleotide reductase from *E. coli. Biochem. Biophys. Res. Commun. 30:*522, 1968.

451. Moore, E. C.: The effects of ferrous ion and dithioerythritol on inhibition by hydroxyurea of ribonucleotide reductase. *Cancer Res. 29:*291, 1969.

452. Lewis, W. H., and Wright, J. A.: Altered ribonucleotide reductase activity in mammalian tissue culture cells resistant to hydroxyurea. *Biochem. Biophys. Res. Commun.* 60:926, 1974.

453. Young, C. W., Schochetman, G., and Karnofsky, D. A.: Hydroxyurea-induced inhibition of deoxyribonucleotide synthesis: Studies in intact cells. *Cancer Res.* 27:526, 1967.

454. Yarbro, J. W.: Further studies on the mechanism of action of hydroxyurea. *Cancer Res.* 28:1082, 1968.

455. Kim, J. H., Gelbard, A. S., Djordjevic, B., Kim, S. H., and Perez, A. G.: Action of daunomycin on the nucleic acid metabolism and viability of HeLa cells. *Cancer Res.* 28:2437, 1968.

456. Chabner, B. A., et al.: The clinical pharmacology of antineoplastic agents. *N. Engl. J. Med.* 292:1107, 1975.

457. Goodman, M. F., Bessman, M. J., and Bachur, N. R.: Adriamycin and daunorubicin inhibition of mutant T4 DNA polymerases. *Proc. Natl. Acad. Sci. U.S.A.* 71:1193, 1974.

458. Schwartz, H. S., and Kanter, P. M.: Cell interactions: Determinants of selective toxicity of adriamycin (NSC-123127) and daunorubicin (NSC-82151). *Cancer Chemother. Rep.* 6:107, 1975.

459. Huguley, C. M., Jr., Bain, J. A., Rivers, S. L., and Scoggins, R. B.: Refractory megaloblastic anemia associated with excretion of orotic acid. *Blood* 14:615, 1959.

460. Smith, L. H., Jr., Sullivan, M., and Huguley, C. M., Jr.: Pyrimidine metabolism in man. IV. Enzymatic defect of orotic aciduria. *J. Clin. Invest.* 40:656, 1961.

461. Fallon, H. J., Lotz, M., and Smith, L. H., Jr.: Congenital orotic aciduria: Demonstration of enzyme defect in leukocytes and comparison with drug-induced orotic aciduria. *Blood* 20:700, 1962.

462. Lotz, M., Fallon, H. J., and Smith, L. H., Jr.: Excretion of orotic acid and orotidine in heterozygotes of congenital orotic aciduria. *Nature* 197:194, 1963.

463. Fallon, H. J., Smith, L. H., Graham, J. B., and Burnett, C. H.: A genetic study of hereditary orotic aciduria. *N. Engl. J. Med.* 270:878, 1964.

464. Becroft, D. M. O., and Phillips, L. I.: Hereditary orotic aciduria and megaloblastic anaemia: A second case with response to uridine. *Br. Med. J.* 1:547, 1965.

465. Haggard, M. E., and Lockhart, L. H.: Megaloblastic anemia and orotic aciduria: A hereditary disorder of pyrimidine metabolism responsive to uridine. *Am. J. Dis. Child.* 113:733, 1967.

466. Rogers, L. E., Warford, L. R., Patterson, R. B., and Porter, F. S.: Hereditary orotic aciduria. I. A new case with family studies. *Pediatrics* 42:415, 1968.

467. Fox, R. M., O'Sullivan, W. J., and Firkin, B. G.: Orotic aciduria: Differing enzyme patterns. *Am. J. Med.* 47:332, 1969.

468. Fox, R. M., Wood, M. H., Royse-Smith, D., and O'Sullivan, W. J.: Hereditary orotic aciduria: Types I and II. *Am. J. Med.* 55:791, 1973.

469. Arakawa, T.: Congenital defects in folate utilization. *Am. J. Med.* 48:594, 1970.

470. Erbe, R. W.: Inborn errors of folate metabolism. *N. Engl. J. Med.* 293:753, 807, 1975.

471. Walters, T.: Congenital megaloblastic anemia responsive to N⁵-formyltetrahydrofolic acid administration. *J. Pediatr.* 70:686, 1967.

472. Arakawa, T., et al.: Mental retardation with hyperfolic-acidemia not associated with formiminoglutamic-aciduria: Cyclohydrolase deficiency syndrome. *Tohoku J. Exp. Med.* 88:341, 1966.

473. Freeman, J. M., Finkelstein, J. D., and Mudd, S. H.: Folate responsive homocystinuria and "schizophrenia": A defect in methylation due to deficient 5,10-methylene-tetrahydrofolate reductase activity. *N. Engl. J. Med.* 292:491, 1975.

474. Arakawa, T., et al.: Formiminotransferase-deficiency syndrome: A new inborn error of folic acid metabolism. *Ann. Pediatr.* 205:1, 1965.

475. Arakawa, T., Fujii, M., and Hirono, H.: Tetrahydrofolate-dependent enzyme activities in formiminotransferase deficiency syndrome. *Tohoku J. Exp. Med.* 88:305, 1966.

476. Arakawa, T., et al.: Formiminotransferase deficiency syndrome associated with megaloblastic anemia responsive to pyridoxine or folic acid. *Tohoku J. Exp. Med.* 94:3, 1968.

477. Mudd, S. H.: Homocystinuria and homocystein metabolism: Selected aspects, in *Heritable Disorders of Amino Acid Metabolism*, edited by W. L. Nyhan. Wiley, New York, 1974, p. 429.

478. van der Zee, S. P. M.: Megaloblastic anemia in the Lesch-Nyhan syndrome. *Lancet* 1:1427, 1968.

479. Harris, J. W., and Horrigan, D. L.: Pyridoxine-responsive anemia: Prototype and variations on the theme. *Vitam. Horm.* 22:721, 1964.

480. Horrigan, D. L., and Harris, J. W.: Pyridoxine-responsive anemia: Analysis of 62 cases. *Adv. Intern. Med.* 12:103, 1964.

481. Horrigan, D. L., and Harris, J. W.: Pyridoxine-responsive anemias in man. *Vitam. Horm.* 26:549, 1968.

482. Rogers, L. E., Porter, F. S., and Sidbury, J. B., Jr.: Thiamine-responsive megaloblastic anemia. *J. Pediatr.* 74:494, 1969.

483. Viana, M. B., and Carvalho, R. I.: Thiamine-responsive megaloblastic anemia, sensorineural deafness and diabetes mellitus: A new syndrome. *J. Pediatr.* 93:235, 1978.

484. Vilter, R. W., Jarrold, T., Wills, J. J., Mueller, J. F., Friedman, B. L., and Hawkins, V. R.: Refractory anemia with hyperplastic bone marrow. *Blood* 15:1, 1960.

485. Dacie, J. V., Smith, M. D., White, J. C., and Mollin, D. C.: Refractory normoblastic anaemia: A clinical and hematological study of seven cases. *Br. J. Haematol.* 5:56, 1959.

486. Bjorkman, S. E.: Chronic refractory anemia with sideroblastic bone marrow: A study of four cases. *Blood* 11:250, 1956.

487. Heller, P., and Fried, W.: Refractory anemias. *D. M.*, April, 1967.

488. MacGibbon, B. H., and Mollin, D. L.: Sideroblastic anaemia in man: Observations on seventy cases. *Br. J. Haematol.* 11:59, 1965.

489. Dacie, J. V., and Mollin, D.: Siderocytes, sideroblasts, and sideroblastic anaemia. *Acta Med. Scand. (Suppl. 445):* 237, 1966.

490. Hoffbrand, A. V., Kremenchozky, S., and Butterworth, P. J.: Serum lactic dehydrogenase activity and folate deficiency in myelosclerosis and other hematological diseases. *Br. Med. J.* 1:577, 1966.

491. Rosenthal, D. S., Skarin, A. T., and Moloney, W. C.: Serum lactic dehydrogenase activity in refractory anemia. *Acta Haematol. (Basel)* 40:187, 1969.

492. Castoldi, G., Yam, L. T., Mitus, W. J., and Crosby, W. H.: Chromosomal studies in erythroleukemia and chronic erythremic myelosis. *Blood* 31:202, 1968.

493. Heath, C. W., Jr., Bennett, J. M., Whang-Peng, J., Berry, E. W., and Wiernick, P. H.: Cytogenetic findings in erythroleukemia. *Blood* 33:453, 1969.

494. Dameshek, W.: Pernicious anemia, megaloblastosis, and the DiGuglielmo syndrome. *Blood* 13:1085, 1958.

Erythrocyte disorders—anemias related to disturbances of hemoglobin synthesis

CHAPTER *48*

Iron deficiency

VIRGIL F. FAIRBANKS
ERNEST BEUTLER

Iron deficiency is the state in which the content of iron in the body is less than normal. It occurs in varying degrees of severity which merge imperceptibly into one another. The term *iron depletion* has been applied to the earliest stage of iron deficiency, in which storage iron is decreased or absent but serum iron concentration and blood hemoglobin and hematocrit levels are normal [1]. The designation *iron deficiency without anemia* describes a somewhat more advanced stage of iron deficiency, characterized by decreased or absent storage iron, usually low serum iron concentration and transferrin saturation, without frank anemia. A still more advanced stage of iron deficiency is termed *iron deficiency anemia.* It is characterized by decreased or absent iron stores, low serum iron concentration, low transferrin saturation, and low hemoglobin concentration or hematocrit value.

Iron deficiency anemia is a more advanced state of iron deficiency than is iron depletion. However, in certain rare disorders, such as pulmonary hemosiderosis (see Chap. 49) or paroxysmal nocturnal hemoglobinuria (see Chap. 21), iron deficiency anemia may occur without iron depletion.

The clinical manifestations of iron deficiency anemia appear to have been recognized in earliest times. A disease characterized by pallor, dyspnea, and edema was described in about 1500 B.C. in the *Papyrus Ebers*, an Egyptian manual of therapeutics believed to be the oldest complete manuscript extant [2]. Medical historians have attributed this ancient disease to ancylostomal anemia, a form of iron deficiency anemia. Chlorosis, or "green sickness," was well known to European physicians after the middle of the sixteenth century. In France by the middle of the seventeenth century, iron salts were used along with many other remedies (including, oddly enough, phlebotomy) in the treatment of chlorosis. Not long thereafter, iron was recommended by Sydenham as a specific remedy for chlorosis. For the 100 years between 1830 and 1930, iron was used in treatment of chlorosis, often in ineffective doses, although the mechanism of action or iron and the appropriateness of its use were highly controversial.

By the beginning of the twentieth century, it had been established that chlorosis was characterized by a decrease in the iron content of the blood and by the presence of hypochromic erythrocytes. Most of the fundamental work on iron metabolism and iron deficiency has been carried out during this century [3].

Etiology and pathogenesis

ETIOLOGY
Iron deficiency may occur as a result of inadequate dietary iron intake, malabsorption of iron, chronic blood loss, diversion of iron to fetal and infant erythropoiesis during pregnancy and lactation, intravascular hemolysis with hemoglobinuria, or a combination of these factors.

DIETARY IRON DEFICIENCY
In infants, iron deficiency is most often a result of the use of unsupplemented milk diets which contain an inadequate amount of iron. During the first year of life, the full-term infant requires approximately 160 mg iron for erythropoiesis; the premature infant requires about 240 mg. About 50 mg of this need is met by the destruction of erythrocytes, which occurs physiologically during the first week of life. The rest must come from the diet. Milk products are very poor sources of iron, and prolonged breast- or bottle-feeding of infants frequently leads to iron deficiency anemia unless there is iron supplementation. This is especially true of premature infants. Table 48-1 lists the iron content of several widely used infant foods.

In older children, an iron-poor diet may contribute to the development of iron deficiency anemia, but other

TABLE 48-1 Iron content of infant foods

Food	Iron content, mg/oz
Breast milk	0.03
Evaporated milk	0.05
Whole milk	0.02
Similac*	Trace
SMA, reconstituted*	0.24
Cereals:*	
Pablum	9.0
Gerber	14.0
Purées:*	
Vegetable	0.2
Meat	0.8

*Based on statement of commercial producer or processor.

factors, such as intestinal parasitism or bleeding gastrointestinal lesions, may be present.

Since the adult male needs to absorb only about 1 mg iron daily from his diet in order to maintain normal iron balance, iron deficiency in men is only very rarely caused by dietary iron deficiency alone. Exceptions to this rule are known, such as the case of a man who remained on a nearly iron-free diet for 27 years [4].

MALABSORPTION OF IRON

Intestinal malabsorption of iron is an uncommon cause of iron deficiency except after gastrointestinal surgery and in malabsorption syndromes. As many as 50 percent of patients who have had subtotal gastric resection develop iron deficiency anemia years later. Many such patients have impaired absorption of food iron, caused in part by more rapid gastrojejunal transit and in part by partially digested food bypassing some of the duodenum as a result of the location of the anastomosis. However, medicinal iron is well absorbed. Only a very small proportion of such patients have folic acid or vitamin B_{12} deficiency. However, gastrointestinal blood loss may also play an important role in anemia following gastric resection. In malabsorption syndromes, absorption of iron may be so limited that iron deficiency anemia develops over a period of years.

BLEEDING

Gastrointestinal In adult males and in postmenopausal women, iron deficiency is most commonly caused by chronic bleeding from the gastrointestinal tract. A partial list of causes of such blood loss is presented in Table 48-2. In the adult, the commonest causes of gastrointestinal bleeding are peptic ulcer, hiatal hernia, gastritis (including that due to alcohol or salicylate ingestion), hemorrhoids, and neoplasms.

The frequent association of diaphragmatic (hiatal) hernia with gastrointestinal bleeding has long been recognized [5]. In large, representative series of patients with hiatal hernia, the frequency of anemia ranged from 8 to 38 percent [6–8]. Bleeding is more likely to occur with large hernias than with small ones [9]. Mucosal changes cannot always be demonstrated by esophagoscopy or gastroscopy in patients who have had blood loss from hiatus hernia. Anemia accompanying hiatal hernia may be severe and is three times as common in patients with paraesophageal hernias as in those with sliding hernias [7]. It has been suggested [7] that hemorrhage follows mucosal injury at the neck of the sac, where the hernia rides to and fro over the crus of the diaphragm during respiration.

Gastritis due to drug ingestion is another common cause of bleeding. Salicylate ingestion seems as likely to cause bleeding in patients without preexisting ulcer as in those with peptic ulcer [10]. Other medicaments (such as adrenocortical steroids, indomethacin, and phenylbutazone) may also cause bleeding by inducing gastric or duodenal ulcers. Use of enteric-coated medications containing potassium chloride has led to

TABLE 48-2 Causes of gastrointestinal blood loss

Esophagus	Biliary tract
Varices	Trauma
Hiatal hernia	Cholelithiasis
Stomach	Neoplasm
Varices	Aberrant pancreas
Ulcer	Ruptured aneurysm
Carcinoma	Intrahepatic bleeding
Gastritis	*Colon*
Leiomyoma	Ulcerative colitis
Small intestine	Amebiasis
Ulcer	Carcinoma
Aberrant pancreas	Telangiectasia
Meckel's diverticulum	Diverticulum
Telangiectasia	*Rectum*
Polyp	Hemorrhoids
Carcinoma (ampulla of Vater)	Ulceration
Regional enteritis	Carcinoma
Helminthiasis	
Vascular occlusion	
Intussusception	
Volvulus	
Leiomyoma	

serious bleeding from enteric ulcerations. Gastritis due to alcohol ingestion may also cause significant blood loss.

A malignancy was the cause of gastrointestinal bleeding in 2 percent of cases in one large series [11]. However, in 100 cases in which the site of bleeding could not be established by any means short of laparotomy, a malignancy was found to be the cause in 10 percent [12]. Enteritis after therapeutic irradiation of abdominal viscera may also be a cause of gastrointestinal bleeding leading to iron deficiency anemia [13]. Leiomyomas, adenomas, and other benign neoplasms of the intestine may also result in chronic blood loss.

Chronic blood loss from esophageal or gastric varices may lead to iron deficiency anemia. In hereditary hemorrhagic telangiectasia (Chap. 151), characteristic lesions commonly occur on fingertips, nasal septum, tongue, lips, margins (helices) of ears, oral and pharyngeal mucosa, palms and soles, and other epithelial and cutaneous surfaces throughout the body. Tortuous, dilated sublingual venous structures, the cherry hemangiomas commonly seen in the elderly, and the spider telangiectases of chronic liver disease are usually easily distinguished from the lesions of hereditary hemorrhagic telangiectasia. Furthermore, lesions of the skin and oral and nasal mucous membranes may be rather inconspicuous in hereditary hemorrhagic telangiectasia. Bleeding from intestinal telangiectases has also been observed in diffuse systemic sclerosis (scleroderma) [13] and in Turner's syndrome [14]. Chronic blood loss is often the cause of anemia in rheumatoid arthritis (perhaps a result of the salicylate or steroid therapy), ulcerative colitis, and regional enteritis. Hemorrhoidal bleeding may lead to severe iron deficiency anemia. Hemorrhage into the gallbladder is a rare cause of chronic iron deficiency anemia [15]. Chronic blood loss may result from diffuse gastric mucosal hypertrophy (Ménétrier's disease) [16].

Anemia which follows subtotal gastrectomy has usually been attributed to reduced absorption of dietary iron [17–19], but the possibility that chronic, intermittent, occult gastrointestinal bleeding may also be a contributory factor is suggested by a careful study of eight patients whose erythrocytes were labeled with $Na_2^{51}CrO_4$ to permit precise quantitation of daily fecal blood loss [20]. Seven were shown to lose from 3.2 to 6.5 ml of blood per day. This is a very slight but significant increase in daily fecal blood loss which, over a span of several years, could well lead to iron deficiency anemia. Chemical tests for fecal blood loss are usually insensitive to a daily loss of less than 5 to 10 ml of blood, although this depends to some extent on the site of bleeding within the gastrointestinal tract.

Gastrointestinal bleeding may also play a significant role in the development of iron deficiency anemia in infants. There is a substance in fresh cow's milk which, unless inactivated by heating, may induce protein-losing enteropathy and gastrointestinal bleeding in infants [21–23], probably on the basis of hypersensitivity or allergy [24–26]. However, since most infant-feeding formulas derived from cow's milk are subjected to heat treatment at some stage, this factor should rarely play an important role. Anemia itself may increase the amount of blood lost in the infant's feces, perhaps because of an adverse effect of iron deficiency on the intestinal mucosa [27]. Intrinsic lesions of the gastrointestinal tract, such as are listed above, may cause bleeding in infants and in older children as well. In infants or small children, peptic ulcer is an uncommon cause of gastrointestinal bleeding. Meckel's diverticulum usually causes gross gastrointestinal bleeding, manifested as hematochezia. Since Meckel's diverticulum is usually not demonstrated by gastrointestinal x-ray examination, it is easily overlooked as a cause of gastrointestinal hemorrhage.

Intestinal parasitism, particularly by hookworms, is a major cause of gastrointestinal blood loss in many parts of the world.

Defects in coagulation may lead to gastrointestinal bleeding, but this is more likely to be associated with thrombocytopenia than with deficiency of coagulation factors. Gastrointestinal bleeding is common in von Willebrand's disease (Chap. 155). When a patient with a disorder of hemostasis suffers from gastrointestinal bleeding, it is important to consider the possibility that the bleeding may not be caused by a hemostatic defect alone, but that an anatomic lesion of the gastrointestinal tract, such as listed above, may also be present.

Respiratory tract Recurrent hemoptysis, from any cause, may lead to iron deficiency anemia. In such cases, hemoptysis may be due to congenital anomalies of the respiratory tract, endobronchial vascular anomalies, chronic infections, neoplasms, or valvular heart disease.

Severe iron deficiency anemia is a characteristic manifestation of idiopathic pulmonary hemosiderosis and of Goodpasture's syndrome (progressive glomerulonephritis with intrapulmonary hemorrhage) (see Chap. 49). In some of these disorders, hemoptysis may not be observed, but blood-laden sputum may be swallowed in amounts sufficient to result in positive tests for occult blood in the stools.

Genitourinary tract Menstrual bleeding is a very common cause of iron deficiency. The amount of blood lost with menstruation varies markedly from one woman to another and is often difficult to evaluate by questioning the patient. Accurate measurement has shown that the volume of blood lost in the course of one menstrual cycle may be as high as 495 ml in apparently healthy, nonanemic women who regard their menstrual flow as not excessive [29]. Several studies have shown the average menstrual blood loss to be about 40 ml per cycle [29–32]. Blood loss exceeds 80 ml (equivalent to about 30 mg of iron) per cycle in only 10 percent of women [32]. The amount of menstrual blood lost does not seem to vary markedly from one cycle to another for any given individual [33]. The use of an intrauterine coil for contraception has been shown [34] to increase menstrual blood loss, especially during the first year of use. Since the absorption of 1 mg of iron per day requires a dietary intake of between 10 and 20 mg of iron, it is easy to understand why, with an average dietary iron intake of approximately 10 mg per day, iron balance in many menstruating women is precarious.

Excessive bleeding also may be caused by uterine fibroids and malignant neoplasms. Neoplasms, stones, or inflammatory disease of the kidney, ureter, or bladder may cause enough chronic blood loss to produce iron deficiency.

PREGNANCY

In pregnancy, the average iron loss resulting from diversion of iron to the fetus for erythropoiesis, blood loss at delivery (equivalent to an average of 150 to 200 mg of iron), and lactation is altogether about 900 mg; in terms of iron content, this is equivalent to the loss of over 2 liters of blood. Approximately 30 mg of iron may be expended monthly in lactation. Since many or most women begin pregnancy with their iron reserves already depleted, it is not surprising that these additional demands frequently result in iron deficiency anemia. In fact, iron depletion has been reported in some 85 to 100 percent of pregnant women. This was also true, although to a lesser degree, in women who took oral iron supplementation [35]. The clear implication is that all pregnant women should receive prophylactic oral iron. Fortunately, this seems currently to be a nearly universal practice of obstetricians.

INTRAVASCULAR HEMOLYSIS AND HEMOGLOBINURIA

Iron deficiency anemia may occur in paroxysmal nocturnal hemoglobinuria (Chap. 21) and in hemolysis resulting from mechanical erythrocyte trauma from intracardiac myxomas [36–38], valvular prostheses, or patches [39–41] (Chap. 63). In these disorders, iron is lost in the urine in the forms of hemosiderin, ferritin, and hemoglobin [41].

DIALYSIS TREATMENT OF CHRONIC RENAL DISEASE
The use of extracorporeal dialysis for treatment of chronic renal disease has often resulted in marked iron deficiency, which may be superimposed upon the anemia of chronic renal disease. The genesis of iron deficiency in these cases is the trapping of blood in the dialyzing equipment. This problem usually can be avoided by returning as much blood as possible to the patient after each dialysis [42].

PATHOGENESIS
Figure 48-1 shows the changes which take place in various iron compartments as iron deficiency progresses from a state of mild iron depletion to one of advanced iron deficiency anemia.

As the body becomes depleted of iron, changes occur in many tissues. Hemosiderin and ferritin virtually disappear from marrow and other storage sites. There is a decreased activity of many other important iron proteins: cytochrome c [44,45], cytochrome oxidase [46–50], succinic dehydrogenase [51], aconitase [49,52,53], xanthine oxidase [54], and myoglobin [55]. Reduced activity has also been reported for some enzymes which do not contain or require iron [54,56–59]. Thus disturbances in cellular metabolism and function may occur in many tissues in iron deficiency. The capacity of the gastric mucosa to secrete hydrochloric acid is often reduced [60–63]. Histamine-fast achlorhydria has been found in as many as 43 percent of patients with iron deficiency [13,63–65]. In many cases, gastric function has improved after correction of the iron deficiency, although in persons over the age of 30 the achlorhydria is usually irreversible [63–67]. Furthermore, when atropic gastritis coexists with iron deficiency, no improvement in gastric secretory function has followed iron therapy [66].

That dysfunction of the nervous system may also occur in iron deficiency is suggested by the fact that some iron-deficient patients complain of paresthesias, and approximately 40 instances of papilledema and other neurologic manifestations have been described [3].

Iron deficiency may also lead to gross anatomic changes in various organs. The rapidly proliferating cells of the upper part of the alimentary tract seem particularly susceptible to the effect of iron deficiency. There may be atrophy of the mucosa of the tongue and esophagus [68], stomach [69,70], and small intestine [48,71]. Buccal mucosa has shown thinning and keratinization of epithelium and increased mitotic activity [72,73]. In the laryngopharynx, mucosal atrophy may lead to web formation in the postcricoid region, thereby giving rise to dysphagia (Plummer-Vinson syndrome) [74–77]. If these alterations are of long duration, they

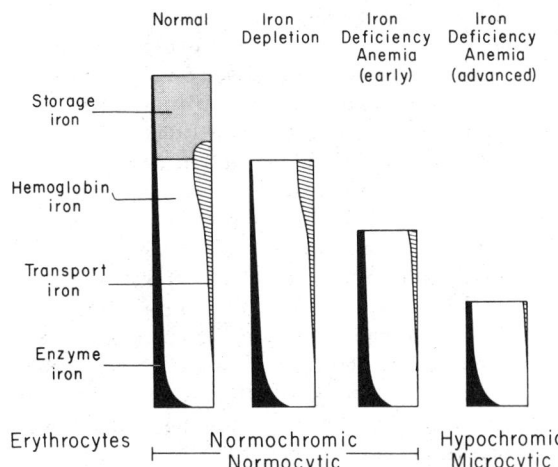

FIGURE 48-1 Stages in the development of iron deficiency. Early iron deficiency (iron depletion) is usually not accompanied by any abnormalities in blood; at this stage, serum iron concentration is occasionally below normal values and storage iron is markedly depleted. As iron deficiency progresses, development of anemia precedes appearance of morphologic changes in blood, although some cells may be smaller and paler than normal; serum iron concentration is usually low at this time, but it may be normal [43]. With advanced iron depletion, classic changes of hypochromic, microcytic, hypoferremic anemia become manifest.

may lead to pharyngeal carcinoma [78]. Although it has been generally thought that these changes are secondary to long-standing iron deficiency, this mechanism is not universally accepted [79]. Widening of diploic spaces of bones, particularly those of the skull and hands [80–82], may be a consequence of chronic iron deficiency beginning in infancy. In the skull, this is of the same character as in thalassemia [81–87], except that in β thalassemia major there is maxillary hypertrophy, whereas in severe iron deficiency anemia maxillary growth and pneumatization are normal [87]. The sella turcica may be abnormally small in iron-deficient children, and it has been suggested, but not proved, that this implies reduction in pituitary hormonal secretion in long-standing iron deficiency anemia [86]. In iron deficiency anemia resulting from "idiopathic pulmonary hemosiderosis," characteristic pathologic changes are found in the lungs, including intense deposition of iron in the littoral cells of the alveoli (Chap. 49). The possibility that iron deficiency may be a cause of atrophic rhinitis [88–90] has been suggested, but conflicting evidence has been presented [91,92].

Incidence

Iron deficiency is widespread throughout the world. It afflicts persons of all ages and economic groups, although it is more common among the very young, among those on poor diets, and among women. It is likely that iron deficiency is the most common chronic organic malady of humankind. Based on reported studies of the frequency of iron deficiency in persons of various age and sex groups [1,35,93–101], an estimate might be made that at least 20 million persons in the United States are iron-deficient.

Iron deficiency anemia is common in infants and is nearly universal in premature infants unless iron supplements are administered [93]. In a careful study [94] of school children in New York City, iron deficiency anemia was rare in families of favorable economic status; among economically deprived groups, the frequency of anemia was about 3 percent. Other studies have confirmed that in low-income families in the United States, anemia occurs in about 3 percent (0.6 to 7.7 percent) of children over the age of 4 years [95]. A frequency of microcythemia (mean corpuscular volume < 77 fl) of 5.5 percent was found in inner-city (i.e., poor, predominantly black) children of ages 5 to 8, after exclusion of β thalassemia [96]. Not known at the time of these studies was the high prevalence of α thalassemia in American blacks, of whom at least 2 percent are homozygous for a chromosome region with deletion of a single α-chain structural gene locus (α thalassemia 2) with resulting microcytosis [102]. Earlier studies which related the prevalence of iron deficiency to the prevalence of microcytosis in blacks must be reinterpreted in this context.

It has been shown by various techniques that 35 to 58 percent of young, apparently healthy women have evidence of iron depletion [97–100], and some degree of iron deficiency seems to be nearly universal during pregnancy [33]. Even with iron supplementation, iron stores may remain depleted [33], although iron deficiency anemia is thereby prevented. The approximate frequencies of iron deficiency in four high-risk groups are given in Table 48-3.

In parts of the world where there is a high frequency of intestinal helminthiasis and the population subsists on an iron-poor diet, iron deficiency anemia may be almost the norm.

TABLE 48-3 Approximate frequency of iron depletion or iron deficiency with or without anemia (in four high-risk groups)

Group	Frequency, %* Of iron depletion or iron deficiency without anemia	Of iron deficiency anemia
Infants	50	25
Children	Data inadequate	0–6
Women:		
Premenopausal	50	15
Pregnant	90	30†

*Percentages are based on data from several sources; they may be considered as representative of recent studies.
†In women not receiving iron supplementation during pregnancy.

Clinical features

In iron deficiency, symptoms may be due to (1) the clinical manifestations of the primary disorder when there is an anatomic lesion leading to bleeding, (2) the presence of anemia, or (3) impaired function of cells as a result of reduced activity of iron proteins (enzymes) other than hemoglobin. The first of these causes of symptoms will not be discussed. The general symptoms of anemia are presented in Chap. 8.

When anemia develops slowly, as it usually does in patients with chronic iron deficiency resulting from occult bleeding, homeostatic mechanisms provide remarkable adaptation even to severe anemia; it is not unusual to find patients with marked iron deficiency anemia who stoutly deny any degree of fatigue, weakness, or palpitation. Very often, such patients will admit to improved work tolerance after treatment, but this may be, in part, a response to the interest and attention given such patients by physicians. The symptoms of anemia are more likely to reflect the rate of progression of anemia rather than its severity. In fact, the traditionally accepted relationship between symptoms and anemia has been questioned. In an evaluation of the correlation between symptoms and hemoglobin concentration in 295 persons (including 56 who were mildly anemic), there was poor correlation between presence or severity of symptoms and hemoglobin concentration of the peripheral blood [103]. Iron therapy in patients with iron deficiency anemia produced no statistically significant improvement in symptom scores. Such results may only emphasize the difficulty in evaluating the subtle symptoms associated with this disorder when anemia is mild.

Fatigue, irritability, and headaches are common complaints in women with iron deficiency. In iron deficiency, depletion of storage iron and, to some extent, of tissue iron precedes the appearance of anemia; these observations raised the possibility [104] that many of these symptoms may be caused by impaired function of iron enzymes or iron proteins other than hemoglobin. In a few studies of this problem, patients received either iron therapy or placebos in random double-blind series. In one of these investigations, patients with iron deficiency had greater symptomatic improvement with iron medication than with placebos [104]; in other studies with a somewhat different experimental design, this was not true [105,106]. Objective measurements of work performance and studies using O_2 consumption as an index of work performance have also given contradictory results [107–110]. In subjects rendered iron-depleted but not anemic by repeated blood donation, iron-supplemented and untreated groups showed the same O_2 consumption during exercise [107]. However, rats rendered iron-deficient but not anemic exhibited diminished exercise tolerance and evidence of irritability [111–113]. Iron-deficient humans have, in most studies, demonstrated diminished maximal exercise tolerance [109,110,114–120], although some reports have been contradictory [107,108].

Headache, paresthesias, and a burning sensation of the tongue are symptoms of iron deficiency which are not attributed to anemia and which seem most likely to be caused by deficiency of iron within tissue cells (Chap. 33). An increase in volume of menstrual blood loss has been considered to be a result as well as a cause of iron deficiency [121,122], but this interpretation has been disputed [29]. Pica, the craving to eat unusual substances such as dirt, clay, ice, and laundry starch, is a classic manifestation of iron deficiency and is usually cured by iron therapy.

The overt manifestations of iron deficiency anemia include, in approximate order of frequency: pallor, glossitis (smooth, red tongue), stomatitis, and angular cheilitis. Koilonychia, once found in some 18 percent of patients with iron deficiency anemia, is now encountered rarely (Fig. 48-2). As in any type of anemia, retinal hemorrhages and exudates may be seen in severely anemic patients (e.g., hemoglobin concentration of 5 g/dl or less). In the 1930s, splenomegaly was found in about one-third of patients with hypochromic anemia [123]. In a study begun in 1938, splenomegaly was found in 11 percent of patients with hypochromic anemia [11]. In contrast, of 100 patients with iron deficiency anemia seen at the Mayo Clinic during recent years, the tip of the spleen could be palpated in only 3. The reason for these discordant observations is not altogether clear. Hypochromic anemia as defined in the earlier studies [11,123] embraced other disorders besides iron deficiency anemia. For example, the prevalence and clinical features of β thalassemia minor were not well delineated until 1947, and the extraordinarily high prevalence of α thalassemia in black Americans was not recognized until 1979 [102]. Undoubtedly, the earlier series included patients with unrecognized thalassemic disorders. Anemia was more severe, and perhaps of longer duration, in the series begun in the 1930s. The mean hemoglobin concentration in one of these [11] was 7.6 g/dl; in contrast, in the Mayo Clinic series, mean hemoglobin concentration was 9.5 g/dl. In the latter series, the three patients with palpable spleens had hemoglobin concentrations below 7.5 g/dl. In the context of current practice in the United States, splenomegaly must be regarded as an unusual manifestation of iron deficiency anemia: the presence of an enlarged spleen should lead the physician to question the diagnosis of iron deficiency anemia.

Laboratory features

In severe uncomplicated iron deficiency anemia, the erythrocytes are hypochromic and microcytic, the plasma iron concentration is diminished, the iron-binding capacity increased, the plasma ferritin level is low, the free erythrocyte protoporphyrin concentration is increased, and the marrow is depleted of stainable iron. Unfortunately, this classic combination of laboratory

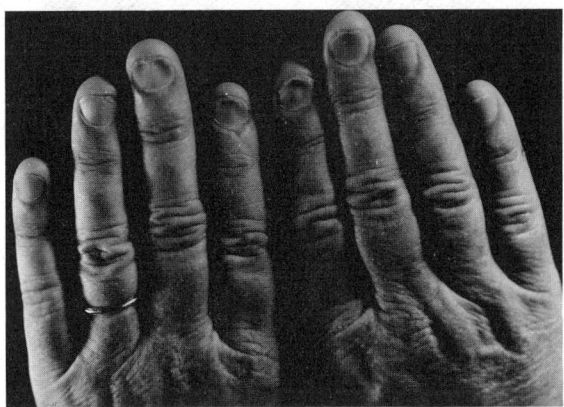

FIGURE 48-2 Koilonychia. Note the ridging, thinning, and splitting, as well as spoonlike concavity of the fingernails. (Courtesy of Dr. Wayne Rundles.)

findings occurs consistently only when iron deficiency anemia is far advanced, when there are no complicating factors such as superimposed infection or malignant neoplasms, and when there has not been previous therapy with transfusions or parenteral iron.

BLOOD CELLS

The earliest and most consistent finding in the blood is anemia [124,125]. In adults, when iron deficiency is of only moderate severity, anemia is likely to be slight and the erythrocytes are usually normochromic and normocytic (Fig. 48-3). Often there is considerable anisocytosis and poikilocytosis. Anisocytosis may, in fact, be the earliest recognizable morphologic change of erythrocytes in iron deficiency anemia [126].

As the degree of iron deficiency increases, the hemoglobin concentration decreases further, and microcytosis and hypochromia appear. The changes in erythrocyte volume and hemoglobin content which will accompany severe iron deficiency may be expressed quanitatively in the erythrocyte corpuscular indices. Except when iron deficiency anemia is moderate or severe (e.g., in males with hemoglobin concentrations less than 12 g/dl or in women with hemoglobin concentrations less than 10 g/dl) these indices are usually normal (Fig. 48-4). Measurement of the mean corpuscular hemoglobin concentration (MCHC) is of little diagnostic value except when iron deficiency anemia is severe [125,127–131]. In infants and children, hypochromia may occur earlier in the course of iron deficiency, and erythrocyte counts in excess of 5,500,000 per microliter are sometimes encountered.

In a review of 100 cases of iron deficiency anemia observed at the Mayo Clinic, 14 percent were found to have leukocyte counts between 3000 and 4400 per microliter. Leukopenia was unrelated to severity of anemia and could not be ascribed to any other condition. In these cases, differential leukocyte counts were normal. Thrombocytopenia and thrombocytosis have been attributed to iron deficiency. Thrombocytosis has been

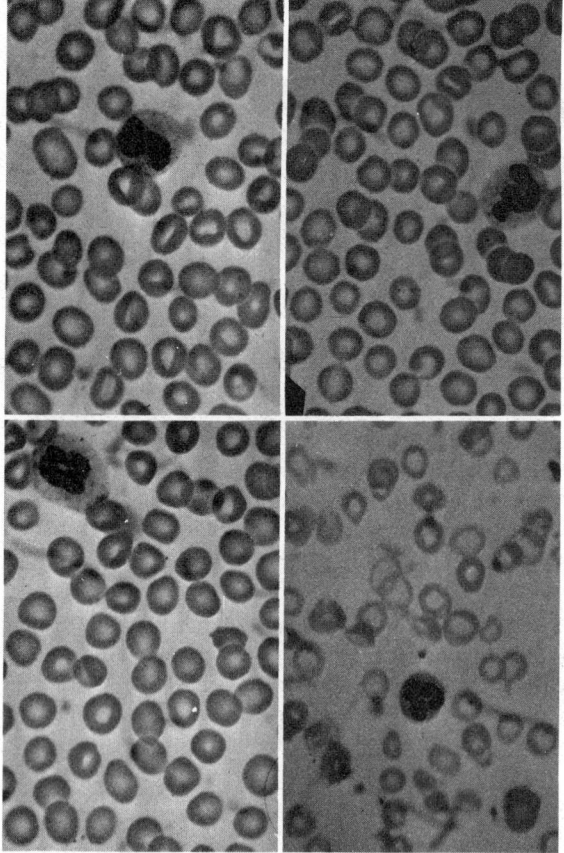

FIGURE 48-3 Variability in morphologic diagnosis of iron deficiency anemia from blood film. Interpret and compare them with those of nine experienced hematologists who reviewed the original slides. The slides were part of a coded series which contained blood films from normal subjects and from iron deficiency anemia patients in random order. The fields reproduced here were typical for each slide. ×600. (From Fairbanks [127]; by permission of the J. B. Lippincott Company.)

(Upper left) From a young woman with iron deficiency anemia due to excessive menstrual bleeding; hemoglobin 10.1 g/dl; serum iron, 36 μg/dl (6.4 μmol/liter). After treatment with ferrous gluconate, hemoglobin concentration increased to 13.1 g/dl. On 13 examinations of this slide by nine hematologists, 11 opinions were that there was no evidence to suggest iron deficiency.

(Upper right) From a normal woman. Hemoglobin, 14.6 g/dl; MCHC, 34 percent; serum iron, 77 μg/dl (13.8 μmol/liter); total iron-binding capacity, 300 μg/dl (53.7 μmol/liter). Three of nine hematologists who reviewed this film thought the erythrcytes were morphologically abnormal and consistent with iron deficiency anemia.

(Lower left) From a normal young man. Hemoglobin, 15.8 g/dl; MCHC, 34 percent; serum iron, 141 μg/dl (25.2 μmol/liter); total iron-binding capacity, 278 μg/dl (49.8 μmol/liter). Nine hematologists made a total of 13 examinations of this slide; one examiner reported the slide as showing evidence of iron deficiency.

(Lower right) From a 56-year-old man with anemia due to bleeding from paraesophageal hiatus hernia. Hemoglobin, 4.0 g/dl; erythrocyte count, 2.24 × 10¹² per liter; reticulocyte count, 2.5 percent; serum iron, 2 μg/dl (0.4 μmol/liter); total iron-binding capacity, 387 μg/dl (69.3 μmol/liter). Hypochromia was marked, and all observers agreed that morphologically the cells suggested iron deficiency anemia.

reported in 50 to 75 percent of adults with classic hypochromic anemia due to chronic blood loss [132,133]. However, it has been suggested that thrombocytosis may be found only in those patients who are actively bleeding [134]. In infants and children, thrombocytopenia occurred almost as frequently (28 percent) as did thrombocytosis (35 percent); thrombocytopenia was associated with more severe anemia [135].

Characteristically, the reticulocyte count is normal or decreased in iron deficiency, but a reticulocyte count of 2 to 3 percent occasionally may be noted.

MARROW

In iron deficiency anemia, there is variability both in the degree of cellularity of the marrow and in the relative proportion of erythroid to myeloid cells. There is poor correlation between severity of anemia and degree of erythroid hyperplasia. In severe iron deficiency, erythroblasts of the marrow may be smaller than normal, with narrow, ragged rims of cytoplasm containing little hemoglobin. However, the morphologic changes in the marrow are not sufficiently distinctive to be of any diagnostic value.

Decreased or absent hemosiderin in the marrow is an almost invariable characteristic of iron deficiency. Hemosiderin, if present, appears in the unstained marrow film as golden refractile granules, but its identification is subject to error. The hemosiderin content of the marrow film is more readily and more reliably evaluated after staining by the simple Prussian blue method. Stored iron (see Chap. A3) in the macrophages of the marrow can be seen in marrow spicules on the marrow section, or in marrow films. It can be distinguished from artifacts which may occur with the Prussian blue–stained sections because it either is clearly intracellular or is seen to conform to the cellular structure of the marrow. In the particles on marrow films, hemosiderin has a granular appearance, while artifacts are often globular or filamentous in appearance. In addition, enumeration of sideroblasts in the marrow is of diagnostic value. Siderotic granules, normally found in 10 percent or more of erythroblasts, become rare but may not be entirely absent. Although, in general, the evaluation of marrow iron stores is a sensitive and reliable means for the diagnosis of iron deficiency anemia, misleading results may be obtained in patients who have been transfused or who have been treated with parenteral iron. The marrow of such patients may contain normal, or even increased, quantities of stainable iron in the face of typical iron-responsive iron deficiency anemia. Apparently, in such patients, the artificially created iron stores which are perceived on marrow examination are not readily available for erythropoiesis. Further, the ability of marrow to store iron seems to be impaired in some patients with chronic myelogenous leukemia and possibly in those with myelofibrosis. In such patients, absence of marrow iron is often observed without other evidence of iron deficiency, and such patients do not respond to iron therapy.

Because of the ease and rapidity with which the iron stain can be performed and interpreted and the diagnostic value of the information thus obtained, staining the marrow for iron should be a routine part of every diagnostic marrow study. As an example of the information which can thus be obtained, in a study [136] of 1332 consecutive routine marrow aspirates, one-third contained no stainable iron; in the majority of these cases (55 percent), iron deficiency was unsuspected on the basis of other clinical or laboratory data; and in almost one-fourth of these cases, the serum iron concentration was normal.

SERUM IRON CONCENTRATION

The serum iron concentration is usually low in untreated iron deficiency anemia; however, it may be normal [136,137]. The normal range depends to some extent on the assay method used. In most laboratories, the normal range for males is between 75 and 175 μg/dl (13 and 31 μmol/liter); for women, it is about 10 μg/dl (2 μmol/liter) lower. The measurement of serum iron concentration is subject to many variables, which may introduce substantial errors into results. Such variables include inadequately processed glassware, contamination of reagents with small amounts of iron, turbidity, and entrapment of iron in plasma proteins during their precipitation. The reagents used in some techniques may not be entirely specific for iron. The presence of free hemoglobin in concentrations too small to be detected visually may give erroneously high results by the atomic absorption method unless a protein-free extract of serum is used.

The serum iron concentration also is influenced by many pathologic and physiologic states. Physiologically, the serum iron concentration has a diurnal rhythm; it decreases in late afternoon and evening, reaching a nadir near 9 P.M., and increases to its maximum between 7 and 10 A.M. [138–140]. It decreases at about the time of menstrual bleeding either when menses are under normal hormonal control [141,142] or when bleeding occurs after withdrawal of oral contraceptive agents [143,144]. The serum iron concentration is reduced in the presence of either acute or chronic inflammatory processes [145–147] or malignancy [148] and following acute myocardial infarction [149,150]. The serum iron concentration under these circumstances may be decreased sufficiently to suggest iron deficiency.

Normal or high concentrations of serum iron are commonly observed even in patients with iron deficiency anemia if such patients receive iron medication before blood is drawn for these measurements. Even multiple vitamin preparations that commonly contain 18 mg of elemental iron can result in this effect. A physician who is unaware that a patient is taking such a vitamin pill may be misled by results. Oral iron medication must be withheld for 24 h. Parenteral injection of iron dextran may result in a very high serum iron concentration (e.g., 500 to 1000 μg/dl) for several weeks.

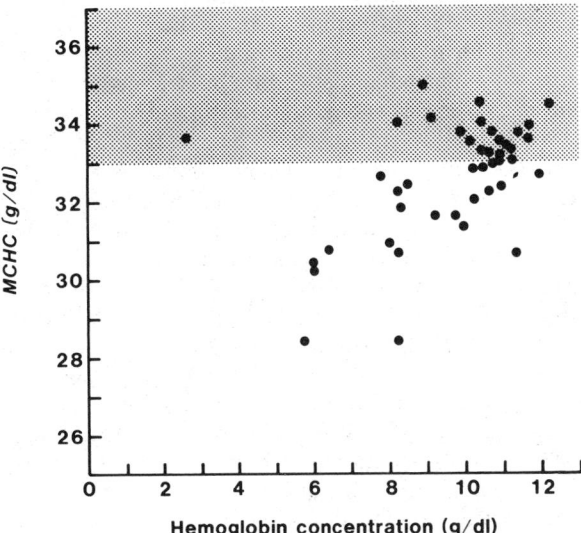

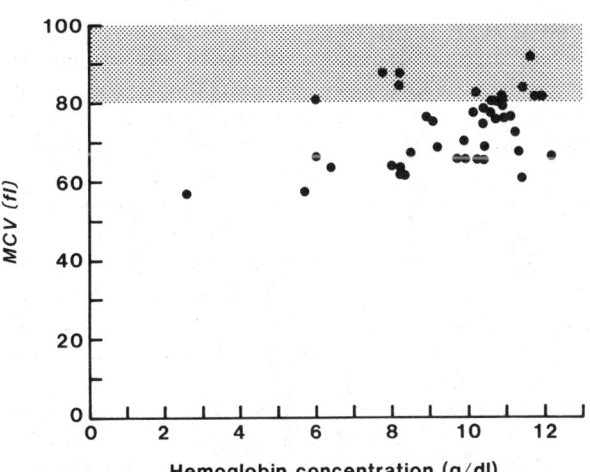

FIGURE 48-4 Erythrocyte indices in iron deficiency anemia of adults, data obtained with Coulter counter, model S. Normal ranges of indices observed in approximately 500 healthy adults [249] using the same instrument are indicated by stippling. (*Upper*) Correlation between venous blood hemoglobin concentration and mean corpuscular hemoglobin concentrations (MCHC). More than half of 62 patients with iron deficiency anemia had MCHC values clearly in the normal range. (*Lower*) Correlation between venous blood hemoglobin concentrations and mean corpuscular volume (MCV). Nearly 70 percent of cases exhibited distinct microcytosis. Thus when indices are determined by automated cell-counting methods, the MCV is much more sensitive than is the MCHC in detecting changes of iron deficiency. However, at least 30 percent of cases of iron deficiency anemia will be misdiagnosed if physicians rely on the erythrocyte indices. (From Beutler and Fairbanks [250]; by permission of Academic Press.)

IRON-BINDING CAPACITY AND TRANSFERRIN SATURATION

The iron-binding capacity is a measure of the amount of transferrin in circulating blood. There are several methods for measuring iron-binding capacity, and results vary somewhat, depending on the method used. Normally, there is enough transferrin present in 100 ml serum to bind 250 to 450 μg of iron (44 to 80 μmol/liter); since the normal serum iron concentration is about 100 μg/dl (18 μmol/liter), transferrin may be found to be about one-third "saturated" with iron; i.e., one-third of the binding sites are occupied. The "unsaturated" or "latent" iron-binding capacity (UIBC) is easily measured with radioactive iron or by spectrophotometric techniques. The sum of the UIBC and the plasma iron represents total iron-binding capacity (TIBC). TIBC may also be measured directly. In iron deficiency anemia, UIBC and TIBC are often increased. Transferrin is normally 20 to 50 percent saturated with iron. A transferrin saturation of 15 percent or less is often found in iron deficiency anemia. A normal value for transferrin saturation often accompanies a low serum iron concentration in "chronic disorders" such as inflammation or malignancy. However, exceptions are so common as to detract considerably from the diagnostic value of measuring transferrin saturation [43].

SERUM FERRITIN

Several methods are now available for measurement of serum ferritin concentration [151]. Commercially available kits make it possible for most clinical laboratories to perform a reliable assay. Serum ferritin concentration correlates with total-body iron stores, although the correlation is not a rectilinear relationship, as is sometimes asserted [152–154]. Serum ferritin concentrations of less than 10 μg/liter are characteristic of iron deficiency anemia. Values of 10 to 20 μg/liter should be regarded as presumptive, but not diagnostic of iron deficiency. Moderate increase in serum ferritin concentration occurs in inflammatory disorders, such as rheumatoid arthritis, in chronic renal disease, and in malignancies [155–159]. When one of these conditions coexists with iron deficiency, as they often do, the serum ferritin concentration is commonly in the normal range; interpretation of results of this assay then become difficult. Moderate increases in serum ferritin concentrations are also characteristic of some hematologic malignancies and may closely reflect remissions and relapses [158]. Marked increases in serum ferritin concentration occur in patients with hepatitis [154,160,161]. Oral or parenteral iron administration also results in increased serum ferritin concentration [162–165]. This appears to be particularly a problem in infants given oral iron. In adults with iron deficiency anemia who were given oral iron in a dose of 60 mg of elemental iron thrice daily, the serum ferritin concentration remained below 10 μg/liter for 2 to 3 weeks [164]. However, for adults who have taken oral iron medication for more than 3 weeks, the serum ferritin assay would be of no value to confirm a diagnosis of iron deficiency. Parenteral administration of iron dextran results in a rise in serum ferritin concentration to normal or supranormal values within 24 h, and this effect persists for at least a month [164].

ERYTHROCYTE PROTOPORPHYRIN

Free erythrocyte protoporphyrin (FEP) is increased in disorders of heme synthesis, including iron deficiency, lead poisoning, and sideroblastic anemias, as well as other conditions. The measurement of FEP has been proposed as a screening procedure for iron deficiency [166,167]. Since this procedure requires small blood samples, it may be practical for large-scale screening programs designed to identify children with either iron deficiency or lead poisoning. It does not differentiate between iron deficiency and the anemia which accompanies inflammatory or malignant processes.

^{57}Co ABSORPTION

Several metals, e.g., cobalt, which are chemically similar to iron appear to be absorbed by the same mechanism as iron [168,169]. The absorption of ^{57}Co is enhanced in iron deficiency. However, since the absorbed cobalt is not incorporated into any heme compound, it is promptly excreted in the urine. Thus the urinary excretion of ^{57}Co, following an oral dose, is greater in iron-deficient subjects than in normal subjects [169,170]. This appears to be a very sensitive index of increased iron absorption, as occurs in iron deficiency, in iron-loading states (e.g., hemochromatosis), or following recent blood loss. It is not specific for iron deficiency. Furthermore, the results of this test may be misleading in clinical disorders more complex than simple blood loss [170].

ERYTHROCYTE SURVIVAL

Accelerated hemoglobin catabolism was first demonstrated in iron deficiency anemia in 1937 [145]. Subsequent studies have also demonstrated slight to moderate shortening of erythrocyte survival [171–173].

FERROKINETICS

A study of the movement of iron atoms between various iron compartments (such as plasma pool, labile pool, and hemoglobin compartment) may be performed by intravenous injection of radioactive iron (^{59}Fe) followed by measurement of the rate of clearance of ^{59}Fe from plasma and of its incorporation into the hemoglobin of circulating erythrocytes. The principles underlying such "ferrokinetic" studies are discussed in Chaps. 41 and A19.

In iron deficiency, plasma iron clearance is rapid and is closely correlated with the serum iron concentration. The plasma iron transport rate may be normal or increased.

The percentage of iron utilized in hemoglobin synthesis is normal or increased. Some studies have shown evidence of ineffective erythropoiesis (see Chap. 41).

IRON TOLERANCE TESTS

In an iron tolerance test [174–176], the patient receives an oral dose of an inorganic iron compound, and the subsequent change in the serum iron concentration is measured. In iron deficiency, there is an increased rate of absorption of the test dose, and this is often reflected in a more rapid increase and a higher plateau than in normal subjects. The test has been modified in recent years by incorporating a small amount of radioactive iron (^{59}Fe) in the test dose. Then the rate of change in plasma radioactivity can be measured. Although this test has been widely used for the diagnosis of iron deficiency, we do not recommend it because of the large number of factors which may influence results in unpredictable ways and because of the inconvenience imposed by the number of blood samples required.

TESTS USING IRON-CHELATING AGENTS

Several investigators [177–182] have devised methods for assessment of iron stores based on the injection of iron-chelating agents and measurement of the amount of iron which is thereby mobilized from storage and excreted in the urine. The synthetic iron-chelating substance DTPA (diethylenetriaminopentaacetic acid) and the microbially synthesized iron chelator deferoxamine (desferrioxamine) have been used for this purpose. A differential feroxamine test which uses ^{59}Fe-labeled feroxamine has been devised [181].

When iron stores are increased, the effect of these compounds is to remove iron from storage pools, thus increasing the urinary excretion of iron. Conversely, when iron stores are depleted, only small increments in urinary iron excretion can be obtained. However, a strong negative correlation ($r = 0.93$) has been found between the logarithm of the amount of iron excreted after a dose of DTPA and the UIBC, suggesting that measurement of the UIBC gives much the same information as is given by the more complex chelation procedures. Furthermore, review of published data suggests that with chelation methods there is appreciable overlap among iron-deficient, normal, and iron-overloaded groups. In some iron-deficient patients, administration of a chelating agent has paradoxically resulted in excretion of more iron than when normal control subjects received the chelating agent [179].

Differential diagnosis

When iron deficiency anemia is severe, there is usually little difficulty in recognizing the disorder. A history of excessive blood loss is sometimes easily obtained. Pallor may be readily apparent. The peripheral blood film may display marked hypochromia, poikilocytosis, and microcytosis without polychromatophilia and other signs of erythrocyte regeneration which might suggest a different cause. Under such circumstances, it is reasonable to start iron therapy immediately and to begin a search for the site of blood loss. However, it must be borne in mind that even those morphologic findings considered classic for iron deficiency anemia may also occur in other conditions, particularly in chronic disorders and in thalassemias: the morphologic diagnosis of iron deficiency must always be regarded as tentative and subject to confirmation by other means, including the response to therapy. Early in the course of iron deficiency, changes in the blood may be imperceptible, and the differential diagnosis of anemia may then be more difficult.

DIFFERENTIATION OF IRON DEFICIENCY ANEMIA FROM OTHER FORMS OF ANEMIA

The forms of anemia which must be distinguished from iron deficiency anemia include those which occur with thalassemia minor, chronic inflammatory disease, malignancy, chronic liver disease, chronic renal disease, hemolytic anemia, and aplastic anemia. It is the microcytic anemias which are most likely to be confused with iron deficiency. Such anemias are summarized in Table 48-4. Each of these types of anemia is discussed elsewhere in this book. Attention will be directed here primarily to laboratory aids for differentiating iron deficiency anemia from the frequently occurring disorders which may have similar manifestations.

1. *Thalassemia minor.* In many parts of the world, and in many communities of North America, the frequency of β thalassemia minor is second only to that of iron deficiency as a cause of hypochromic microcytic anemia (Chap. 50). In black Americans, as indicated earlier, homozygosity for the α thalassemia 2 gene (containing a single α-locus deletion) is a very common cause of

TABLE 48-4 Microcytic disorders which may be confused with iron deficiency

1. Thalassemias and hemoglobinopathies

   β Thalassemia major
   β Thalassemia minor
   δβ Thalassemia minor
   α Thalassemia minor
   Hemoglobin Lepore trait
   Hemoglobin E trait
   Hemoglobin H disease
   Combination of above (double heterozygotes)
   Homozygous hemoglobin E

2. Blockade of heme synthesis caused by chemicals

   Lead
   Pyrazinamide
   Isoniazid

3. Disorders of obscure cause

   Sideroblastic anemias
   Hereditary sex-linked
   Idiopathic acquired
   Other

4. Chronic inflammatory states
5. Neoplasms, benign or malignant

microcytosis since it occurs in about 2 to 3 percent of persons of this ethnic group [102]. It is usually not associated with anemia [252]. Hemoglobin Lepore-Boston trait occurs predominantly in persons of Mediterranean origin. Among persons of Italian ancestry who appear to have thalassemia minor on the basis of erythrocyte morphology, approximately 1 of every 40 have hemoglobin Lepore trait [183,184]; probably 10,000 to 20,000 Americans have hemoglobin Lepore trait as a cause of mild microcytosis unassociated with anemia. Among the nearly 600,000 Southeast Asians resettled in the United States during the late 1970s and early 1980s, α thalassemia minor, β thalassemia minor, hemoglobin E trait, and iron deficiency all occur frequently. These conditions are characterized by microcytosis, and none can be distinguished reliably from the others on the basis of erythrocyte morphology or erythrocyte indices alone. In each of these conditions there may be only mild to moderate microcytosis without any other distinctive changes. However, in nearly 85 percent of patients with α or β thalassemia minor, the erythrocyte count is greater than 5×10^6 per microliter, despite low hemoglobin concentration. Similar findings are typical of hemoglobin Lepore trait and of hemoglobin E trait [185–187].

In contrast, only about 3 percent of adults with iron deficiency anemia have erythrocyte counts of 5×10^6 per microliter or higher [113]. Paradoxic erythrocytosis may be seen in children with iron deficiency anemia or in polycythemia vera patients who have become anemic following hemorrhage or therapeutic phlebotomy.

The mean corpuscular volume (MCV) is almost always reduced in α and β thalassemia minor and in homozygous hemoglobin E, with values of 55 to 70 fl being the rule. Values this low are seen only in severe iron deficiency anemia. In hemoglobin Lepore trait and hemoglobin E trait, only minimal microcytosis is observed [185–187]. The MCV is now commonly measured directly, by an automated technique, together with the erythrocyte count and hemoglobin concentration. This widespread adoption of the routine measurement of MCV has lead to proposals that criteria for differentiation of iron deficiency from thalassemia minor might be based, in part, on the values of the erythrocyte count and the MCV [131]. Some proposed rules [130][1] could separate iron deficiency from thalassemia minor with 90

percent accuracy when groups of iron deficiency and thalassemic patients were of nearly equal numbers. However, in a population in which iron deficiency is more prevalent than thalassemia minor, use of these criteria would result in an excessive number of diagnostic errors. None of these and other proposed rules seems completely reliable for distinguishing iron deficiency from thalassemia [188]. Anisocytosis seems to be more pronounced in iron deficiency than in thalassemias [126], but most observers may find this a criterion difficult to apply.

Reticulocytosis of a mild degree is more likely to be encountered in β thalassemia minor, $\delta\beta$ thalassemia minor, and hemoglobin Lepore trait than in iron deficiency anemia, but may be absent in these disorders [189]. The same is true of polychromatophilia and basophilic stippling. In contrast, the serum iron concentration is usually normal or increased in these thalassemia minor syndromes and is usually low in iron deficiency anemia. Similarly, examination of marrow iron stores will help to differentiate these disorders. The presence of thalassemia minor syndromes is substantiated by the demonstration of increased proportions of hemoglobin A_2 or F, or by the presence on electrophoresis of hemoglobin H or Lepore (see Chaps. 50 and A7 through A9).

The diagnosis of α thalassemia minor is usually made at present on the basis of exclusion of other causes of microcytosis, since no specific diagnostic test has yet proved practical. In the evaluation of results of hemoglobin studies, it is important to remember that iron deficiency may mask concurrent thalassemia. The amounts of both hemoglobin A_2 and hemoglobin H are reduced disproportionately to the reduction in hemoglobin A in the presence of iron deficiency (Chap. 50). Thus when a patient with proved iron deficiency (and normal hemoglobin studies) continues to exhibit microcytosis and hypochromia after adequate therapy, the concentration of hemoglobin A_2 should be measured again and electrophoresis performed to determine whether hemoglobin H is present.

Hemoglobin H disease is an α thalassemia with the features both of thalassemia minor and of an unstable hemoglobin (Chap. 50). Milder α thalassemias may also have all the features described for thalassemia minor without electrophoretic abnormalities and may be easily mistaken for iron deficiency on the basis of erythrocyte morphology.

In thalassemia major, although erythrocyte morphologic changes are usually pronounced, evidence of enhanced erythropoiesis (polychromatophilia and reticulocytosis) may be absent [189]. The serum iron concentration is normal or increased, and marrow aspirates contain increased amounts of hemosiderin. The demonstration of high concentrations (30 to 80 percent) of hemoglobin F in the blood, together with appropriate family studies, confirms the diagnosis of thalassemia major or intermedia.

2. *Anemia of chronic inflammatory disease and malignancy.* Any malignant neoplasm, infectious disease, or

---

[1] The formulas and criteria which have been examined are the following:

1. D.F.$'$ = [MCV − (5 × hemoglobin concentration) − erythrocyte count − K]. K = 3.4 if the hematocrit is corrected for plasma trapping; otherwise K = 8.4. D.F.$'$ is said to be ≥ 1.0 in iron deficiency anemia, ≤ -1.0 in thalassemia minor. Values between −1.0 to +1.0 are indeterminate.

2. The ratio of MCV to erythrocyte count (in millions per microliter) is greater than 14 in iron deficiency anemia, 14 or less in thalassemia minor.

3. The ratio of MCH to erythrocyte count (in millions per microliter) is greater than 4.4 in iron deficiency anemia, 4.4 or less in thalassemia minor.

4. The erythrocyte count is less than 5×10^6 per microliter in iron deficiency anemia, 5×10^6 per microliter or greater in thalassemia minor.

other inflammatory condition which persists for more than a few weeks may result in anemia (Chap. 51). Usually this type of anemia is normochromic and normocytic, but it may be hypochromic and microcytic. Hypochromic anemia occurs in 20 to 30 percent of patients with chronic infections or malignancies [146,147]. Thus these disorders cannot be distinguished from iron deficiency anemia on the basis of the peripheral blood film. Furthermore, the serum iron concentration is usually decreased in these disorders [146,148], sometimes severely. Measurement of the serum iron concentration and TIBC is of some help. In iron deficiency, the TIBC is usually increased, whereas in inflammatory and neoplastic diseases it is commonly decreased. However, there is considerable overlap among TIBC values of normal subjects, those with iron deficiency anemia, and those with chronic inflammatory diseases. Among the neoplasms that may lead to erroneous diagnosis of iron deficiency, particularly to be noted are hypernephromas, atrial myxomas, and angiofollicular lymphoid hyperplasia (sometimes called *lymphoid hamartoma*). Patients with these latter disorders frequently are erroneously treated for iron deficiency for long intervals of time before the correct diagnoses are made. It is important to identify these tumors early, because surgical removal often results in complete and permanent cure.

In iron deficiency anemia, transferrin saturation is usually less than 15 percent and may be 5 percent or less, whereas in chronic diseases it is usually more than 15 percent. However, this widely used criterion is actually quite unreliable. Transferrin saturation may be normal in iron deficiency anemia, and conversely, low saturation is sometimes observed in chronic disease [147]. Thus measurement of serum iron and TIBC and calculation of transferrin saturation can sometimes be misleading in the study of patients with anemia in the presence of chronic inflammatory or neoplastic disease. The plasma ferritin level is useful in differentiating between iron deficiency and the anemia of chronic disease. While the ferritin level is usually diminished in iron deficiency, it is generally increased in chronic inflammatory and neoplastic disorders. Examination of the marrow for stainable iron is particularly helpful. It will be decreased in amount in iron deficiency anemia and normal or increased in the other disorders.

3. *Anemia of chronic liver disease.* The erythrocytes in the blood film in chronic liver disease may be normochromic and normocytic, macrocytic, or hypochromic, with target cells being frequent. Since the blood film in iron concentration deficiency anemia may also display these features, differential diagnosis must be based on other observations. Determination of serum iron concentration is helpful. In acute chemically induced liver injury and in hepatitis, the serum iron concentration is usually modestly increased [160,190], possibly owing to release of ferritin into the plasma [160,161]. In cirrhosis, the serum iron concentration is likely to be increased unless there has been blood loss [191]. The TIBC may be normal or decreased. Thus the

percentage transferrin saturation is likely to be increased. The quantity of hemosiderin is normal or increased in marrow aspirates.

4. *Anemia of chronic renal disease.* Changes in small renal blood vessels may cause marked distortions in erythrocyte structure, such as schizocytes and burr cells. However, these morphologic changes, when present, are nonspecific. Unless there is distinct microcytosis and hypochromia, iron deficiency anemia cannot be differentiated from anemia resulting from chronic renal disease (Chap. 44) on the basis of the blood film. The serum iron concentration may be normal or decreased, depending on the cause of the renal disease. Measurement of the TIBC may be of no help in this circumstance. Iron deficiency may complicate the anemia of chronic renal disease in patients who are subjected to repeated extracorporeal hemodialysis, possibly as a result of loss of blood into the dialyzing apparatus [42]. When the mechanism of anemia is uncertain or appears to be complex, examination of marrow aspirates for iron content may clarify the pathogenesis.

5. *Anemia of hemolytic disease.* Hemolytic disease can usually be distinguished from iron deficiency anemia on the basis of the peripheral blood film. The marked poikilocytosis, polychromatophilia, and other morphologic features characteristic of hemolysis usually are not seen in iron deficiency anemia. Furthermore, reticulocytosis is usually marked in hemolytic disorders but minimal or absent in iron deficiency anemia. However, there are some outstanding exceptions to these generally valid principles.

In unstable hemoglobin syndromes, such as hemoglobin H disease or hemoglobin Köln disease, erythrocytic hypochromia may be quite pronounced. In these disorders, there is moderate reticulocytosis, which helps to differentiate them from iron deficiency anemia. The serum iron concentration is normal or increased. Unstable hemoglobins are easily precipitated by heating or by mixing hemolysates with dilute isopropanol. These measures of molecular instability are the basis of simple diagnostic tests (Chaps. 61 and A6).

When there is severe intravascular hemolysis, the erythrocytes in peripheral blood may display marked morphologic abnormalites, such as burr cells and schizocytes. Yet, because of loss of iron by hemoglobinuria, iron deficiency may be the dominant cause of the resulting anemia. Measurement of serum iron concentration and TIBC or, better, evaluation of iron content marrow aspirates may clarify the mechanism of this form of anemia. An increase in serum lactic dehydrogenase activity often occurs in iron deficiency anemia secondary to intravascular hemolysis. Studies of erythrocyte survival or of iron kinetics may sometimes help in investigation of the mechanism of anemia in these cases. However, these are time-consuming, expensive procedures which do not, in general, add any diagnostically useful information beyond that which can be obtained by the simpler techniques already indicated. Furthermore, iron deficiency anemia alone may result in shortened erythrocyte survival and in some degree of ineffective erythropoiesis. If bleeding occurs during studies of erythrocyte survival, the results are usually indistinguishable from those which are considered to be characteristic of hemolysis.

6. *Hypoplastic and aplastic anemia* (Chap. 20). In their early phases, these disorders cannot reliably be differentiated from mild iron deficiency anemia on the basis of erythrocyte morphology alone. The presence of neutropenia and thrombocytopenia suggests a diagnosis of aplastic anemia, but mild neutropenia may also occur in iron deficiency anemia. The serum iron concentration is usually increased in aplastic anemia; the percentage transferrin saturation may be high. Marrow aspiration may produce scant material for cytologic study, and marrow biopsy may be necessary: iron stain usually reveals increased amounts of hemosiderin in aplastic or hypoplastic anemia. However, if chronic bleeding has occurred—e.g., due to thrombocytopenia—iron stores may be depleted.

7. *Myeloproliferative diseases.* In polycythemia vera, erythrocytes may be small and hypochromic (Chap. 23). Even in the absence of distinctive morphologic changes in erythrocytes, the serum iron concentration is usually decreased [192–194], the TIBC is normal or increased, and marrow aspirates show little or no hemosiderin. Ferrokinetic studies show accelerated plasma iron incorporated in the hemoglobin of circulating erythrocytes [195]. These findings simply reflect iron deficiency, which is almost always present in this disease, as a result primarily of increased gastrointestinal blood loss, therapeutic phlebotomy, or marked expansion in total hemoglobin mass. Possibly for the same reason, the serum iron concentration and marrow hemosiderin content are often decreased in other myeloproliferative disorders.

8. *Sideroblastic (iron-loading) anemia.* In this heterogeneous group of disorders (Chap. 54), the peripheral blood findings often simulate those of iron deficiency anemia. Reticulocytosis is usually absent, and the serum iron concentration is generally normal or increased. Diagnosis requires examination of marrow aspirate films stained for iron; the films display increased amounts of both storage and sideroblastic iron.

9. *Congenital dyserythropoietic anemia.* In the rare congenital dyserythropoietic anemias (CDA), erythrocyte morphologic abnormalities may resemble those of iron deficiency or thalassemia (Chap. 46). In general, in CDA, poikilocytosis is very striking and occurs with less reduction in MCV than in iron deficiency or thalassemias. Often, however, such cases are believed to be thalassemic until the marrow is examined.

10. *Megaloblastic anemia.* In pernicious anemia and other types of megaloblastic anemia (Chap. 47), the blood film usually shows changes sufficiently distinctive that there is little difficulty in differential diagnosis. One potential source of error is the change in serum iron concentration which occurs after therapy. In the untreated patient with pernicious anemia or folic acid deficiency, the serum iron concentration is normal or increased. However, on treatment the serum iron concentration decreases markedly as iron is utilized rapidly for hemoglobin synthesis [145,196]. Thus the finding of a low serum iron concentration in such circumstances should not be taken as evidence of iron deficiency. Iron deficiency anemia and anemia due to folic acid or vitamin B_{12} deficiency may coexist. During the course of treatment, with the rapid increase in the number of red cells, the typical manifestations of severe iron deficiency may develop.

11. *Anemia of myxedema* (Chap. 45). The anemia of myxedema is usually normochromic and normocytic and may be accompanied by mild to moderate depression of serum iron concentration. Ferrokinetic studies may show a decreased rate of plasma iron transport but normal iron utilization. Marrow examination may be required to determine whether iron deficiency is present, especially since iron deficiency often complicates myxedema because of menorrhagia, which is common in this disorder.

SPECIAL STUDIES

The procedures discussed up to this point are those primarily related to the diagnosis of the hematologic disorder. However, it must be stressed again that the physician who establishes a diagnosis of iron deficiency resulting from blood loss has the obligation to determine the site and cause of hemorrhage. Sometimes this is an easy task, but often it is not. Many additional diagnostic studies may be required. Examination of the stools for the presence of blood is particularly helpful in determining what additional studies should be carried out. Specimens should be examined on several days, because bleeding may be intermittent. Occasionally, it is helpful to label the patient's erythrocytes with ^{51}Cr and to determine quantitatively the amount of blood lost daily in feces (or during menstrual flow). When there is reason to believe that bleeding is from the gastrointestinal tract, proctoscopic and roentgenographic studies are indicated, and gastroscopy and esophagoscopy may also be required.

Percutaneous retrograde angiography of celiac or mesenteric arteries has proved valuable in localizing sites of active gastrointestinal bleeding [197–199]. The method appears to be capable of demonstrating sites of bleeding when rate of blood flow into the intestinal lumen is 0.5 ml/min or greater [197]. This procedure should be contemplated in any patient actively bleeding from the gastrointestinal tract, in whom the site of blood loss has not been established and for whom surgery is contemplated. Angiography should be carried out prior to barium contrast studies. The rate of bleeding may be increased following angiography [200].

Meckel's diverticulum is one of the most common causes of obscure gastrointestinal bleeding in children.

The diverticula often contain ectopic gastric mucosa, which will concentrate pertechnetate following intravenous injection for scintigraphic study; such scintigrams have been useful in identifying Meckel's diverticulum as the cause of gastrointestinal blood loss [201–203].

When other diagnostic measures have failed to disclose the site of occult gastrointestinal bleeding, exploratory laparotomy may be warranted [12], because 10 percent of adults with unexplained occult bleeding have gastrointestinal malignancies. There may be an even stronger indication for laparotomy in children and infants with unexplained gastrointestinal bleeding, since Meckel's diverticulum may not be detectable otherwise [204,205].

An iron stain of sputum may reveal hemosiderin-laden macrophages when there is intrapulmonary bleeding.

THERAPEUTIC TRIAL

In the final analysis, the response to iron therapy is the proof of correctness of diagnosis of iron deficiency anemia. Furthermore, some physicians or patients may not have access to all the techniques described for diagnosis of iron deficiency anemia. In this event, the patient's response to therapy may become a primary diagnostic measure. Iron administration in such a therapeutic trial should be by the oral route only. A therapeutic trial under any circumstances should be followed carefully. If the cause of anemia is iron deficiency, adequate iron therapy should result in reticulocytosis with a peak occurring between the seventh and tenth days of therapy, although if anemia is mild, the reticulocyte response may be minimal. A significant increase in the hemoglobin concentration of the blood should be evident 3 to 4 weeks later, and the hemoglobin concentration should attain a normal value within 2 months. Unless there is evidence of continued, substantial blood loss, the absence of these changes must be taken as evidence that iron deficiency is not the cause of anemia. Iron therapy should be discontinued and another mechanism sought.

Therapy

Once it has been established that a patient is deficient in iron, replacement therapy should be instituted. Although further diagnostic studies will often be indicated to determine the cause of bleeding and permit, when possible, its elimination, this is no justification for delaying institution of replacement therapy.

Iron may be administered in one of several forms—orally, as simple iron salts, or parenterally, as an iron-carbohydrate complex or as a blood transfusion. In general, the oral route is preferred. Iron can be administered most economically, in the highest dosage, and in the most readily assimilated form as simple iron compounds. Table 48-5 compares the cost to the patient of

TABLE 48-5   Comparison of oral and parenteral iron therapy

Therapy	Cost, $/g Fe*	Response rate	Toxicity
Oral:			
Ferrous sulfate	0.30	Rapid	Gastrointestinal symptoms
Steak	250.00	Slow	None
Parenteral:			
Iron dextran	120.00	Rapid	Pain, fever, arthralgia, anaphylactic shock
Transfusion	300.00	Immediate	Fever, hepatitis, renal failure, death

*Incorporated in these numbers are 1981 estimates of charges for procuring, processing, and administering the blood or for office visits for injection. Since such charges may vary from one community to another, the costs indicated in the table must be regarded only as approximations.

each gram of iron administered in each of several forms, as well as the comparative rates of response and possible toxic effects. Clearly, treatment by the oral route is safer and also less expensive than parenteral therapy. Conversely, transfusion is both the most expensive and the most hazardous means of therapy. In most patients, iron deficiency anemia is a disorder of long duration and slow progression. Precipitous measures to restore a normal hemoglobin concentration overnight by transfusing the patient are never warranted and are, indeed, hazardous. There is time to wait for normal mechanisms of erythropoiesis to respond to the body's needs and for gradual adjustment of the cardiovascular system to reexpansion of the total circulating erythrocyte volume.

ORAL IRON THERAPY

DIETARY THERAPY

The patient should be encouraged to eat a diversified diet supplying all nutritional requirements. Nonetheless, it must be emphasized that neither meat nor any other dietary article contains enough iron to be useful therapeutically. Meat contains small amounts of myoglobin and hemoglobin (blood trapped in capillaries) and insignificant amounts of iron in other proteins. In fact, an average (3-oz) serving of steak provides only about 3 mg iron. Provision of sufficient dietary iron to permit a maximal rate or recovery from iron deficiency anemia might require a daily intake of at least 10 lb of steak. For these and other reasons, medicinal iron is much superior to dietary iron in the therapy of iron deficiency.

IRON PREPARATIONS

The pharmaceutical market is glutted with iron preparations in nearly every conceivable form, each promoted to appeal to physician or patient for one reason or another. The following simple principles may help the physician to find a way through this chaos.

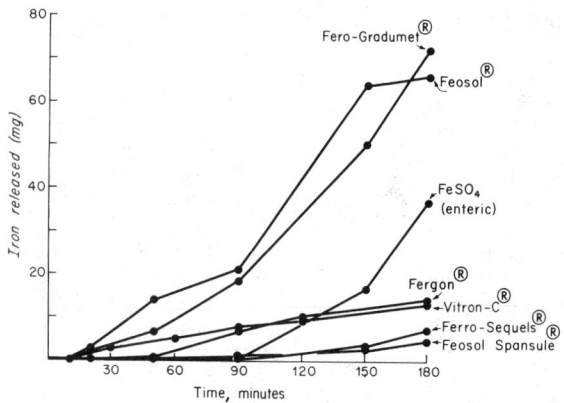

FIGURE 48-5 Dissolution rates of various commercially available oral iron preparations in acidic (pH 2 or less) gastric juice. Very similar results were obtained in achlorhydric gastric juice and in fluid obtained by perfusion of normal human duodenum. In each, release of iron from Feosol Spansule, Ferro-Sequels, Vitron-C, and enteric-coated ferrous sulfate was poor with up to 3 h of incubation. Other preparations had released 80 to 100 percent of their iron content within 3 h in each of these media. Although iron release from Fergon was poor in acidic gastric juice, it was relatively rapid in other media tested.

1. Each tablet or capsule of an iron preparation for an adult should contain between 50 and 100 mg iron. Numerous carefully controlled clinical studies have demonstrated that single doses of this magnitude infrequently cause unpleasant side effects [206,207]. Smaller doses have been popular in the past, but these may result in a slower recovery of the patient or no recovery at all.

2. The iron should be readily released in acidic or neutral gastric juice or duodenal juice (usually pH 5 to 6), because maximal absorption occurs when iron is presented to the duodenal mucosa. Enteric-coated and prolonged-release preparations dissolve slowly in any of these fluids (Fig. 48-5). Thus with such preparations the iron which eventually is released may be presented to a portion of the intestinal mucosa in which absorption is least efficient. Some patients who have been treated unsuccessfully with enteric-coated or prolonged-release iron preparations respond quite promptly to the administration of non-enteric-coated ferrous salts (Fig. 48-6).

3. The iron, once released, should be readily absorbed. Iron is absorbed in the ferrous form; consequently, only ferrous salts should be used.

4. Side effects should be infrequent. This seems not to be a particular problem of any of the common commercially available iron compounds. Despite the claims of pharmaceutical companies, there is no convincing evidence that any one effective preparation is superior in this respect to any other.

5. The cost to the patient should be small.

6. The use of preparations containing several hematinics is to be condemned.

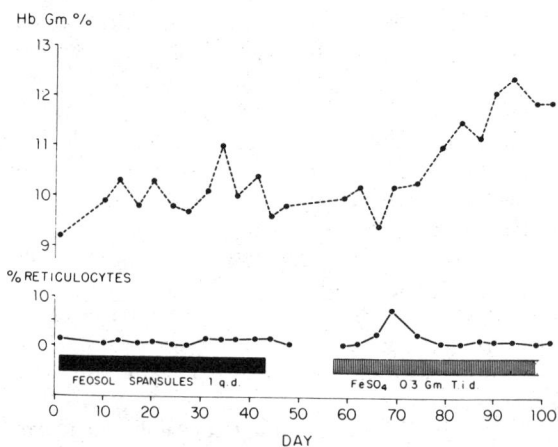

FIGURE 48-6 Rate of response of patient with iron deficiency anemia to 43 days of treatment with prolonged-release Feosol Spansules (containing 225 mg ferrous sulfate), one capsule daily, the dosage recommended by the manufacturer, followed by 43 days of treatment with nonenteric ferrous sulfate (0.3 g three times daily). Clearly, 225 mg of ferrous sulfate daily in prolonged-release form failed to elicit any significant hemopoietic response in this case. The rapid response subsequently elicited with conventional ferrous sulfate may be taken as a typical response to effective therapy in adequate dosage, whether by oral or parenteral route. (From Beutler and Meerkreebs [251]; by permission of the Massachusetts Medical Society.)

Table 48-6 compares a few of the commonly used iron preparations.

Physicians should be aware that if ferrous sulfate is prescribed generically, the choice of preparation is left to the pharmacist and many will dispense enteric-coated tablets. It is advisable to specify "nonenteric" or to prescribe by brand name a compound which is not enteric-coated.

Although substances such as ascorbic acid, succinate, and fructose have been shown to enhance iron absorption, the gain is offset to a large extent by the increase in frequency of side effects or cost of therapy, or both. There is no convincing evidence to support the use of chelated forms of iron or of iron in combination with wetting agents.

Dosage   For the therapy of iron deficiency in adults, the dosage should be sufficient to provide between 150 and 200 mg elemental iron daily. The iron may be taken orally in three or four doses 1 h before meals. Infants may be given 50 to 100 mg daily in divided doses for therapy or 10 to 20 mg daily for prophylaxis of iron deficiency (Table 48-7).

Side effects   Mild gastrointestinal side effects occur occasionally in the form of pyrosis, constipation, or looseness of stools. A metallic taste may be experienced. In some patients these side effects may be psychologic in origin. One should avoid suggesting to patients that ad-

TABLE 48-6   Comparison of some oral iron preparations

Preparations	Iron content, mg/pill	Approximate cost to patient, dollars/month of treatment*
Single agents:		
Ferrous sulfate	60	$ 1.70
Ferrous gluconate	37	2.50
Ferrous fumarate	66	1.70
Prolonged release or enteric-coated:		
Ferrous sulfate Enseals	66	2.90
Fero-Gradumet	105	7.40
Feosol Spansule	45	5.30
Ferro-Sequels	50	16.20
Ferronord	75	11.90
Mol-Iron Chronosule	78	10.90
Combination hematinics:		
Geritol	50	11.30
Iberol	105	10.40
Perihemin	55	19.30
Trinsicon	90	10.70
Simron	10	59.40
Vitron-C	66	5.70
Fero-Grad-500	105	8.80

*On the basis of dose adequate to provide 180 to 230 mg elemental iron per day. Costs quoted for single agents are based on the lowest priced non-enteric-coated generic preparations. Each cost entry in the right column is an estimation of the over-the-counter price to the patient for equivalent therapeutic iron dosage. The cost entries include the customary retail markup calculated from the wholesale cost to the pharmacy times 1.5. Since the price markup may vary somewhat from one pharmacy to another, the prices quoted should be regarded as approximations. They are based on wholesale price quotations cited in the *American Druggist Redbook*, 1981. Prices were essentially the same in 1982.

verse effects are to be expected. In truth, they are not: the majority of patients tolerate this dose of iron without the least side effect, and many tolerate much larger doses well. However, there is no doubt that some patients, perhaps 1 or 2 out of 10, experience symptoms which may be ascribed to the iron preparation and may be related in part to the size of the dose [206,207]. In such cases, reduction of the frequency of administration to one tablet a day for a few days may alleviate the symptoms; later, the patient may be able to tolerate treatment in full dosage. It may also be useful to change to another iron preparation, especially one with a different external appearance.

Acute iron poisoning   Acute iron poisoning is a serious problem in infants or small children. It is usually a consequence of the accidental ingestion of iron-containing medications intended for use by adults. Ingestion of less than half a dozen tables of ferrous sulfate by a child has led to serious iron poisoning. Any potent oral preparation may cause acute iron poisoning.

The earliest manifestation of iron poisoning is vomiting, usually within an hour of the ingestion. There may be hematemesis or melena. Restlessness, hypotension, tachypnea, and cyanosis may develop soon thereafter and may be followed within a few hours by coma and death. So inexorable a course is not the rule, however. Usually, medical aid is sought early and, with proper treatment, most iron-poisoned children should survive.

The initial treatment is prompt evacuation of the stomach. In the home this may be induced by digital stimulation of the pharyngeal gag reflex. Oral administration of a tepid solution of baking soda serves two useful purposes: it may provoke emesis, and the bicarbonate ion complexes with the iron and retards absorption. When a child who has ingested more than a few iron pills is seen in a hospital emergency room, gastric intubation and lavage should be performed promptly, preferably with a solution containing 4 g sodium bicarbonate (or 3.6 g disodium phosphate and 0.8 g monosodium phosphate) per deciliter. Before the tube is withdrawn, a solution containing 5 to 10 g deferoxamine, or approximately 60 ml of the bicarbonate or phosphate solution,

TABLE 48-7   Iron preparations for pediatric use*

Chemical designation	Iron content, mg/ml	Commercial (proprietary) designation	Therapeutic dosage
Ferrous sulfate solution, USP	8		1 tsp, 2 or 3 times daily
Ferrous sulfate solution, concentrated	25	Fer-In-Sol	1 ml, 3 or 4 times daily
Ferrous sulfate elixir (5% ethanol)	9	Feosol elixir	1 tsp, 2 or 3 times daily

*This is not a complete list of preferred iron preparations, nor does it imply endorsement of these products; other commercially available iron preparations may be equally efficacious.

should be introduced into the stomach.[2] Supportive measures should be used as needed for shock or for metabolic acidosis should these develop. Deferoxamine is presently the agent of choice for specific therapy of hyperferremia. It usually should be administered intramuscularly in an initial dose of 1 g, followed by 0.5 g intramuscularly 4 and 8 h later and therefore at 12-h intervals as the clinical status warrants. If the child is hypotensive, the dose may be administered intravenously at a rate not exceeding 15 mg/kg/h for a total initial dose of 1 g, with repetition of this dosage started every 4 to 12 h as the clinical status of the patient seems to warrant [208]. Parenteral administration of deferoxamine should not exceed 6 g in any 24-h period. Improvement often appears several hours to a few days after onset of iron poisoning. This improvement may be permanent, but it may also be misleading, because pneumonitis or severe hepatic or neurologic decompensation may soon supervene. There may be seizures, coma, hyperreflexia, jaundice, and bilirubinemia. Children who survive for 3 or 4 days usually recover without sequelae. However, gastric strictures and fibrosis or intestinal stenosis may occur as late complications. These have been reported as early as 6 weeks after acute iron poisoning. More detailed information concerning acute iron poisoning is provided in several extensive reviews of this subject [209–212].

PARENTERAL IRON THERAPY

INDICATIONS

Occasionally it becomes necessary to administer iron by the parenteral route. The indications are malabsorption, intolerance to iron taken orally, iron need in excess of an amount which can be taken orally, and uncooperativeness of the patient. In rare instances, inability of the patient to follow instructions or to return for follow-up may justify use of parenteral iron. However, in view of the significantly greater hazards of parenteral therapy, the indications must be carefully considered. Routine use of parenteral iron therapy is rarely justified.

PREPARATIONS

Iron dextran   At present, iron dextran is the only compound commercially available in the United States for parenteral iron therapy.

CHEMISTRY   Iron dextran is a colloidal suspension in which the iron-dextran complex exists as micro-

spherules of approximately 5 nm diameter and an average mass equivalent to 73,000 daltons. Electron microscopy reveals that each particle has an electron-dense ferric oxyhydroxide (FeOOH) core surrounded by an electron-lucent shell believed to consist of chains of dextran extending radially from the core [213]. The commercial preparation is marketed as a stable, dark brown, slightly acidic (pH 6) solution containing 50 mg elemental iron per ml.

METABOLISM   After intramuscular injection, iron dextran is slowly absorbed, approximately 72 h being required for 50 percent of a dose to move out of the injection site [214,215]. It is slowly cleared from plasma. Peak plasma concentrations of thousands of micrograms of iron per deciliter are found even 10 days after intramuscular injection; the plasma iron concentration decreases slowly, reaching normal values after 3 to 4 weeks [214,216]. Iron dextran is cleared from plasma by the macrophages, and ultimately the iron is used in hemoglobin synthesis. Mobilization of iron dextran from an intramuscular site is relatively slow and incomplete; 20 to 35 percent of the dose may remain at the injection site 1 month later [217,218]. Furthermore, the rate of incorporation of iron dextran into hemoglobin is somewhat slower than that for simpler ferric hydroxide colloids [218,219]. It appears that the iron dextran complex is only slowly dissociated in macrophages. Studies in phlebotomized subjects have established that the hemopoietic response to iron dextran is less than would be predicted on the basis of the amount of iron administered. At most, approximately 70 percent of the iron is readily utilized in hemoglobin synthesis, the remainder being very slowly liberated from macrophages despite persistent iron deficiency anemia [220].

DOSAGE AND ROUTE OF ADMINISTRATION   Iron dextran is usually administered by deep intramuscular injection. It is given in divided doses of 2.0 ml (100 mg) per dose intramuscularly or intravenously. Total dose infusion has also been employed, but is not approved in the United States [216,220–225]. The rate of intravenous injection of undiluted iron dextran should not exceed 1 ml/min. If any adverse effect is noted, injection must be terminated at once and appropriate countermeasures taken.[3]

For either intramuscular or intravenous administration, the manufacturer recommends, for adults, test doses of 0.5 and 2.0 ml at 2- to 3-day intervals and thereafter, if no adverse effect is manifested, daily doses of not more than 2.0 ml by either intravenous or intramuscular route. Smaller doses are indicated for children, proportional to weight.

Various formulas have been used for estimating total

---

[2] These solutions are slightly hypertonic and slightly alkaline (pH 7.2 to 7.8). The specified volume and concentrations are recommended for children 1 to 2 years of age and are adequate to bind temporarily the iron released from approximately 10 ferrous sulfate tablets. Larger volumes may be used with older children. Although phosphate may bind iron more efficiently, the universal availability of sodium bicarbonate may, in most emergencies, favor the use of bicarbonate solutions when deferoxamine is not available.

[3] A syringe containing a solution of epinephrine should be immediately accessible for treatment of anaphylaxis should this occur. The patient must be attended during the course of intravenous therapy by a physician who is acquainted with the manifestations and treatment of anaphylactic reactions.

dose required for treatment. Since total blood volume is *approximately* 65 ml/kg and the iron content of hemoglobin is 0.34 percent by weight, the simplest formula for estimating the total dose required *for correction of anemia only* can be derived as follows:

$$D_{Fe}(g) = (D_h \div 100) \times W_{kg} \times 65 \times 0.0034$$
$$D_{Fe}(mg) = D_h \times W_{kg} \times 2.2$$
$$D_{Fe}(mg) = D_h \times W_{lb}$$

where D_{Fe} = total hemoglobin iron deficit
$\quad\quad D_h$ = whole blood hemoglobin deficit, g/dl
$\quad\quad W_{kg}$ = body weight, kg
$\quad\quad W_{lb}$ = body weight, lb

Assuming normal mean hemoglobin concentration of 16 g/dl, a male weighing 170 lb, whose hemoglobin concentration is 7 g/dl, would require $170 \times (16 - 7) = 1530$ mg iron to correct this anemia. To this should be added a sufficient quantity of iron to replete iron stores, approximately 1000 mg for men and approximately 600 mg for women. Thus a 170-lb male with a hemoglobin concentration of 7 g/dl should receive 2530 mg iron, equivalent to 50 ml of iron dextran.

SIDE EFFECTS   Intramuscular administration of iron dextran causes a moderate degree of pain at the injection site and a dark stain in the skin which may remain for as long as 1 to 2 years. "Z-track" and other techniques of injection recommended by the manufacturer reduce but do not eliminate the discoloration of the skin.

Intravenous administration also may cause local side effects, in the form of thrombophlebitis. This occurs most commonly when iron dextran is diluted with 5% glucose solution, less frequently when diluted with isotonic saline solution, and infrequently when iron dextran is injected undiluted. Thrombophlebitis at the injection site appears to be unusual with the technique of total-dose infusion, and other adverse effects appear to be no more frequent than with the intramuscular route. In one study from which patients with a history of any antecedent allergy were excluded, more than 124 patients were treated by total-dose infusion with a singular absence of reactions [225]. To prevent local thrombophlebitis, venipuncture was performed with a needle that was free of iron dextran on either the inner or outer surface.

The frequency of systemic reactions of iron dextran therapy has been markedly variable in different series, ranging from near 0 [216,225,226] to nearly 50 percent of patients given iron dextran [227,228]. Arthralgias and fever are of relatively common occurrence and may be experienced by as many as one-third of patients. Other systemic reactions are infrequent and include hypotension, bradycardia, myalgia, headache, abdominal pain, nausea and vomiting, dizziness, lymphadenopathy, pleural effusion, and urticaria. Generalized gray discoloration of the skin has been reported following total-dose injection [224]. The discoloration per-

sisted for 3 months. Regional lymph nodes may become enlarged and tender for a few weeks after injection. Generalized lymphadenopathy has been reported [229,230]. In one case [231], fever (temperature up to 41°C persisted for 10 days and was accompanied by tachycardia, inguinal lymphadenopathy, increased erythrocyte sedimentation rate, and leukocytosis (15,000 per microliter) with neutrophilia. Seven cases have been observed in which iron dextran infusion was followed by an acute febrile illness accompanied by tender lymphadenopathy and splenomegaly lasting 10 to 14 days [232]. Pleocytosis of the cerebrospinal fluid has been observed [233] during a febrile reaction to iron dextran; in this case there was also a peripheral blood leukocyte count of 88,000 per microliter. Acute, severe exacerbation of arthritis has been observed following iron dextran therapy in patients with rheumatoid arthritis [234] and ankylosing spondylitis [235].

In 1981–1982 an unusually high frequency of side effects was reported following a change in manufacturing procedure. This led the manufacturer to recall all ampules of lot No. 3511ML. The manufacturer also discontinued production of 5.0-ml ampules. Iron dextran is now available in 2.0-ml ampules and 10.0-ml multiple-dose vials. The manufacturer urges that not more than 2.0 ml of iron dextran be administered at one time, that it be given only with caution to patients with abnormal liver function, and that it not be given to pregnant women, in view of a single report of stillbirth occurring a few weeks after a toxic reaction to iron dextran administration.

Intramuscular deposition of iron dextran has led to malignancy in some experimental animals [236,237]. Fibrosarcoma and undifferentiated pleomorphic sarcoma have developed at the site of injection in several human subjects following repeated or protracted iron dextran therapy [238–240]. This appears to be an extremely rare phenomenon and may in some cases have been coincidental rather than causally related. However, the time required for iron dextran induction of neoplasia in humans may be as long as 20 years.

The most dangerous complication of iron dextran therapy is anaphylactic reaction [241,242]. This occurs in less than 1 percent of patients treated by either the intramuscular or intravenous route. It is not dose-dependent and may follow the infusion of only a few drops of diluted iron dextran solution or a fraction of a milliliter of intramuscularly injected iron dextran. Characteristically, during the first few minutes of infusion, the patient complains of difficulty breathing, or a choking or smothering sensation, becomes sweaty and anxious, may complain of nausea, and may vomit. Respiratory stridor may be observed, followed by apnea. The blood pressure may drop abruptly; stupor and coma may quickly supervene. At the first evidence of this reaction, the infusion must be terminated immediately, and epinephrine should immediately be injected subcutaneously (0.5 ml of 1:1000 aqueous epinephrine). Other measures to combat shock and anaphylaxis are appropriate. These may include lowering the head, ventilatory assistance (positive-pressure breathing), and intravenous administration of adrenocortical steroids (e.g., cortisol, 100 mg). With these countermeasures, most patients survive. However, at least six deaths are ascribed to iron dextran–induced anaphylactic shock [242–245], in some cases despite appropriate treatment of this complication. Hemiparesis and myocardial infarction have followed an anaphylactic reaction to iron dextran infusion [246].

Freshly opened vials of iron dextran have been found to contain as much as 100 mg divalent iron per deciliter. This has raised the possibility that the hypotension, which occasionally occurs, might be a result of the presence of divalent iron which forms only a weak and easily dissociable complex with dextran. Iron dextran causes hypotension when administered intravenously to cats, and the hypotensive effect correlates to some extent with the amount of divalent iron in the solution [247].

Administration of iron dextran does not interfere with blood cross-matching or cause abnormalities of coagulation [222].

COMMERCIAL SOURCES AND COSTS FOR IRON DEXTRAN   Iron dextran has long been marketed in the United States as Imferon. Generic preparations of iron dextran are available at considerably lower cost.

Course and prognosis

If therapy is adequate, the correction of iron deficiency anemia is usually quite gratifying. Symptoms such as headache, fatigue, paresthesias, and burning sensation of the oropharyngeal mucosa may abate within a few days. In the blood, the reticulocyte count begins to increase after a few days, usually reaches a maximum at about 7 to 12 days, and thereafter decreases. When anemia is mild, little or no reticulocytosis may be observed. Little change in hemoglobin concentration or hematocrit value is to be expected for the first 2 weeks, but then the anemia is corrected rapidly. The hemoglobin concentration in the blood may be halfway back to normal after 4 to 5 weeks of therapy. By the end of 2 months of therapy, and often much sooner, the hemoglobin concentration should have reached a normal level. There is little difference in the rate of response whether iron is administered by the oral or the parenteral route, except in patients with intestinal malabsorption [248].

When the cause of the iron deficiency is a benign disorder, the prognosis is excellent, provided bleeding is controlled or can be compensated for by continual iron therapy. Too often, therapy is interrupted as soon as anemia has been corrected, and iron stores are not replenished. Such inadequately treated patients are likely to have recurrent anemia. For this reason, and because iron therapy brings about replenishment of iron stores very slowly, oral therapy should be con-

tinued for at least 12 months after anemia has been corrected. If there is a benign cause of recurrent bleeding which is not an indication for surgical correction, such as hiatal hernia, menorrhagia, or hereditary hemorrhagic telangiectasia, oral iron therapy may be continued indefinitely; if the bleeding is especially brisk, supplementation with parenterally administered iron or, rarely, with transfusion may be needed. Continuous iron administration may also be required in patients with iron deficiency secondary to intravascular hemolysis with hemoglobinuria.

Appropriate therapy of iron deficiency anemia may add much to the patient's comfort even in the presence of an incurable disease.

If the diagnosis of iron deficiency anemia is correct, anemia and other manifestations of iron deficiency will respond to adequate therapy. However, the physician is occasionally disappointed in the results of treatment of patients who seem to have iron deficiency anemia. In some cases this apparent failure of therapy is a result of treatment of patients with iron preparations which are virtually insoluble, which are enteric-coated, or which contain iron in only minute amounts. Careful inquiry into the nature, duration, and regularity of iron therapy may reveal a reason for the failure of therapy and permit a gratifying response to be elicited with adequate therapy. Other questions which should be asked in evaluation of such a case are these: (1) Has bleeding been controlled? (2) Has the patient been on therapy long enough to show a response? (3) Has the dose been adequate? (4) Are there other factors—inflammatory disease, neoplastic disease, hepatic or renal disease, concomitant deficiencies (vitamin B_{12}, folic acid, thyroid)—which might retard response? (5) Is the diagnosis correct?

References

1. Finch, C. A., et al.: Iron deficiency in the United States. *JAMA* 203:407, 1968.
2. Bryan, C. P.: *The Papyrus Ebers*. Appleton-Century-Crofts, New York, 1931.
3. Fairbanks, V. F., Fahey, J. L., and Beutler, E.: *Clinical Disorders of Iron Metabolism*, 2d ed. Grune & Stratton, New York, 1971.
4. Rosenbaum, E., and Leonard, J. W.: Nutritional iron deficiency anemia in an adult male: Report of a case. *Ann. Intern. Med.* 60:683, 1964.
5. Moersch, H. J.: Hiatal hernia. *Ann. Otol.* 47:754, 1938.
6. Murphy, W. P., and Hay, W. E.: Symptoms and incidence of anemia in hernia at the esophageal hiatus. *Arch. Intern. Med.* 72:58, 1943.
7. Windsor, C. W. O., and Collis, J. L.: Anaemia and hiatus hernia: Experience in 450 patients. *Thorax* 22:73, 1967.
8. Phear, D.: Hiatus hernia. *Lancet* 1:708, 1957.
9. Holt, J. M., Mayet, F. G., Warner, G. T., Callender, S. T., and Gunning, A. J.: Iron absorption and blood loss in patients with hiatus hernia. *Br. Med. J.* 3:22, 1968.
10. Roth, W. A., Waldes-Dapena, A., Pieses, P., and Buchman, E.: Topical action of salicylates in gastrointestinal erosion and hemorrhage. *Gastroenterology* 44:146, 1963.
11. Beveridge, B. R., Bannerman, R. M., Evanson, J. M., and Witts, L. J.: Hypochromic anaemia: A retrospective study and followup of 378 in-patients. *Q. J. Med.*, n.s., 34:145, 1965.
12. Retzlaff, J. A., Hagedorn, A. B., and Bartholomew, L. G.: Ab-

dominal exploration for gastrointestinal bleeding of obscure origin. *JAMA* 177:104, 1961.

13. Holt, J. M., and Wright, R.: Anaemia due to blood loss from the telangiectases of scleroderma. *Br. Med. J.* 3:537, 1967.

14. Rosen, K. M., Sirota, D. K., and Marinoff, S. C.: Gastrointestinal bleeding in Turner's syndrome. *Ann. Intern. Med.* 67:145, 1967.

15. Fitzpatrick, T. J.: Hemocholecyst: A neglected cause of gastrointestinal hemorrhage. *Ann. Intern. Med.* 55:1008, 1961.

16. Singh, A. K., Cumaraswang, R. C., and Corrin, B.: Diffuse hypertrophy of gastric mucosa (Ménétrier's disease) and iron-deficiency anaemia. *Gut* 10:735, 1969.

17. Moeschlin, S., and Schmid, J. R.: Anaemien nach Gastrektomie. *Bibl. Gastroenterol.* 6:199, 1964.

18. Hines, J. D., Hoffbrand, A. V., and Mollin, D. L.: The hematologic complications following partial gastrectomy: A study of 292 patients. *Am. J. Med.* 43:555, 1967.

19. Hallberg, L. Sölvell, L., and Zederfeldt, B.: Iron absorption after partial gastrectomy: A comparative study on the absorption from ferrous sulphate and hemoglobin. *Acta Med. Scand. 179 (Suppl. 445):*269, 1966.

20. Kimber, C., Patterson, J. F., and Weintraub, L. R.: The pathogenesis of iron deficiency anemia following partial gastrectomy: A study of iron balance. *JAMA* 202:935, 1967.

21. Wilson, J. F., Heiner, D. C., and Lahey, M. E.: Milk induced gastrointestinal bleeding in infants with hypochromic microcytic anemia. *JAMA* 189:568, 1964.

22. Wilson, J. F., and Lahey, M. E.: A unifying concept for the pathogenesis of the syndrome of iron deficiency anemia, hypocupremia, and hypoproteinemia in infants. *J. Clin. Invest.* 44:1112, 1965 (abstract).

23. Lahey, M. E., and Wilson, J. F.: The etiology of iron deficiency anemia in infants: A reappraisal. *J. Pediatr.* 69:339, 1966.

24. Heiner, D. C., Wilson, J. F., and Lahey, M. E.: Sensitivity to cow's milk. *JAMA* 189:563, 1964.

25. Woodruff, C. W., and Clark, J. L.: The role of fresh cow's milk in iron deficiency. *Am. J. Dis. Child.* 124:18, 1972.

26. Woodruff, C. W., Wright, S. W., and Wright, R. P.: The role of fresh cow's milk in iron deficiency. *Am. J. Dis. Child.* 124:26, 1972.

27. Guha, D. K., and Rashmi, A.: Occult blood loss in iron deficiency anemia in children. *Indian J. Pediatr.* 34:1, 1967.

28. Rankin, G. L. S., Veall, N., Huntsman, R. G., and Liddell, J.: Measurement with ^{51}Cr of red-cell loss in menorrhagia. *Lancet* 1:567, 1962.

29. Jacobs, A., and Butler, E. B.: Menstrual blood-loss in iron deficiency anemia. *Lancet* 2:407, 1965.

30. Hagedorn, A. B., Kiely, J. M., Tauxe, W. N., and Owen, C. A., Jr.: The clinical value of radioisotopic quantitation of blood loss. *Proc. VIII Cong. Int. Soc. Hematol.,* vol. 1, p. 249, 1962.

31. Barer, A. P., and Fowler, W. M.: The blood loss during normal menstruation. *Am. J. Obstet. Gynecol.* 31:979, 1936.

32. Halberg, L., Högdahl, A.-M., Nilsson, L., and Rybo, G.: Menstrual blood loss: A population study. *Acta Obstet. Gynecol. Scand.* 45:320, 1966.

33. Hallberg, L., and Nilsson, L.: Constancy of individual menstrual blood loss. *Acta Obstet. Gynecol. Scand.* 43:352, 1964.

34. Zadeh, J. A., Kaabus, C. D., and Fielding, J.: Haemoglobin concentration and other values in women using an intrauterine device or taking corticosteroid contraceptive pills. *Br. Med. J.* 4:708, 1967.

35. De Leeuw, N. K. M., Lowenstein, L., and Hsieh, Y.: Iron deficiency and hydremia in normal pregnancy. *Medicine (Baltimore)* 45:291, 1966.

36. Goodwin, J. F.: Diagnosis of left atrial myxoma. *Lancet* 1:464, 1963.

37. Goodwin, J. F., et al.: Clinical features of left atrial myxoma. *Thorax* 17:19, 1962.

38. Vuopio, P., and Nikkilä, E. A.: Hemolytic anemia and thrombocytopenia in a case of left atrial myxoma associated with mitral stenosis. *Am. J. Cardiol.* 17:585, 1966.

39. Eyster, E., Mayer, K., and McKenzie, S.: Traumatic hemolysis with iron deficiency anemia in patients with aortic valve lesions. *Ann. Intern. Med.* 68:995, 1968.

40. Reynolds, R. D., Coltman, C. A., Jr., and Beller, B. M.: Iron treatment in sideropenic intravascular hemolysis due to insufficiency of Starr-Edwards valve prostheses. *Ann. Intern. Med.* 66:659, 1967.

41. Sears, D. A., Anderson, Pearl R., Foy, A. L., Williams, H. L., and Crosby, W. H.: Urinary iron excretion and renal metabolism of hemoglobin in hemolytic diseases. *Blood* 28:708, 1966.

42. Adamson, J. W., Eschbach, J., and Finch, C. A.: The kidney and erythropoiesis. *Am. J. Med.* 44:725, 1968.

43. Beutler, E., Robson, M. J., and Buttenwieser, E.: A comparison of the plasma iron, iron-binding capacity, sternal marrow iron and other methods in the clinical evaluation of iron stores. *Ann. Intern. Med.* 48:60, 1958.

44. Beutler, E.: Iron enzymes in iron deficiency. I. Cytochrome C. *Am. J. Med. Sci.* 234:517, 1957.

45. Beutler, E., and Blaisdell, R. K.: Iron enzymes in iron deficiency. III. Catalase in rat red cells and liver with some further observations on cytochrome C. *J. Lab. Clin. Med.* 52:694, 1958.

46. Beutler, E.: Iron enzymes in iron deficiency. IV. Cytochrome oxidase in rat kidney and heart. *Acta Haematol. (Basel)* 21:371, 1959.

47. Beutler, E.: Iron enzymes in iron deficiency states. *Illinois Med. J.* 116:16, 1959.

48. Dallman, P. R., Sunshine, P., and Leonard, Y.: Intestinal cytochrome response with repair of iron deficiency. *Pediatrics* 39:863, 1967.

49. Masuya, T.: Pathophysiological studies in sideropenic symptoms: Biological consideration. *Isr. J. Med. Sci.* 1:733, 1965.

50. Dagg, J. H., Jackson, J. M., Curry, B., and Goldberg, A.: Cytochrome oxidase in latent iron deficiency (sideropenia) *Br. J. Haematol.* 12:331, 1966.

51. Beutler, E., and Blaisdell, R. K.: Iron enzymes in iron deficiency. V. Succinic dehydrogenase in rat liver, kidney and heart. *Blood* 15:30, 1960.

52. Beutler, E.: Iron enzymes in iron deficiency. VI. Aconitase activity and citrate metabolism. *J. Clin. Invest.* 38:1605, 1959.

53. Swarup, S., Ghosh, S. K., and Chatterjea, J. B.: Aconitase activity in iron deficiency. *Acta Haematol. (Basel)* 37:53, 1967.

54. Srivastava, S. K., Sanwal, G. G., and Tewari, K. K.: Biochemical alterations in rat tissue in iron deficiency anaemia and repletion with iron. *Indian J. Biochem.* 2:257, 1965.

55. Gubler, C. J., Cartwright, G. E., and Wintrobe, M. M.: Studies on copper metabolism. XX. Enzyme activities and iron metabolism in copper and iron deficiencies. *J. Biol. Chem.* 224:533, 1957.

56. Srivastava, S. K., Zaheer, N., and Krishnan, P. S.: Specific inhibition of hepatic glucose-6-phosphate dehydrogenase in iron deficiency anemia in albino rats. *Arch. Biochem.* 105:446, 1964 (letter to the editor).

57. Macdougall, L. G.: Red cell metabolism in iron deficiency anemia. *J. Pediatr.* 72:303, 1968.

58. Jacobs, A.: Leucocyte oxygen consumption in iron deficiency anaemia. *Br. J. Exp. Pathol.* 46:545, 1965.

59. Jacobs, A., and Cavill, I.: The oral lesions of iron deficiency anaemia: Pyridoxine and riboflavin status. *Br. J. Haematol.* 14:291, 1968.

60. Shearman, D. J. C., Delamore, I. W., and Gardner, D. L.: Gastric function and structure in iron deficiency. *Lancet* 1:845, 1966.

61. Dagg, J. H., Goldberg, A., Gibbs, W. N., and Anderson, J. R.: Detection of latent pernicious anaemia in iron deficiency anaemia. *Br. Med. J.* 2:619, 1966.

62. Voigt, D., and Brüschke, G.: Magenschleimhaut und Eisenmangel. *Deutsch. Med. Wochenschr.* 1:1082, 1967.

63. Leonard, B. J.: Gastric acid in iron-deficiency anaemia. *Lancet* 2:440, 1966.

64. Jacobs, A., Lawrie, J. H., Entwistle, C. C., and Campbell, H.: Gastric acid secretion in chronic iron-deficiency anaemia. *Lancet* 2:190, 1966.

65. Stone, W. D.: Gastric secretory response to iron therapy. *Gut* 9:99, 1968.

66. Davidson, W. M. B., and Markson, J. L.: The gastric mucosa in iron-deficiency anaemia. *Lancet* 2:639, 1955.

67. Lees, F., and Rosenthal, F. D.: Gastric mucosal lesions before and after treatment in iron deficiency anaemia. *Q. J. Med.,* n.s., 27:19, 1958.

68. Baird, I. M., Dodge, O. G., Palmer, F. J., and Wawman, R. J.: The tongue and oesophagus in iron-deficiency anaemia and the effect of iron therapy. *J. Clin. Pathol.* 14:603, 1961.

69. Cheli, R., Dodero, M., Celle, G., and Vassalotti, M.: Gastric biopsy and secretory findings in hypochromic anaemias: comparison of

the gastric mucosa with tongue and esophageal mucosa. *Acta Haematol. (Basel)* 22:1, 1959.

70. Lees, F., and Rosenthal, F. D.: Gastric mucosal lesions before and after treatment in iron deficiency anaemia. *Q. J. Med.*, n.s., 27:19, 1958.

71. Naiman, J. L., Oski, F. A., Diamond, L. K., Vawter, G. F., and Schwachman, H.: The gastrointestinal effects of iron-deficiency anemia. *Pediatrics* 33:83, 1964.

72. Boddington, M. M.: Changes in buccal cells in the anaemias. *J. Clin. Pathol.* 12:222, 1959.

73. Jacobs, A.: The buccal mucosa in anaemia. *J. Clin. Pathol.* 13:463, 1960.

74. Suzman, M. M.: Syndrome of anemia, glossitis, and dysphagia: Report of eight cases, with special reference to observations at autopsy in one instance. *Arch. Intern. Med.* 51:1, 1933.

75. Kelly, A. B.: Spasm at the entrance to the oesophagus. *J. Laryngol.* 34:285, 1919.

76. Paterson, D. R.: A clinical type of dysphagia. *J. Laryngol.* 34:289, 1919.

77. Vinson, P. P.: Hysterical dysphagia. *Minn. Med.* 5:107, 1922.

78. Ahlbom, H. E.: Simple achlorhydric anaemia, Plummer-Vinson syndrome, and carcinoma of the mouth, pharynx, and oesophagus in women: Observations at Radiumhemmet, Stockholm. *Br. Med. J.* 2:331, 1936.

79. Jacobs, A., and Kilpatrick, G. S.: The Paterson-Kelly syndrome. *Br. Med. J.* 2:79, 1964.

80. Rajasuriya, K., Nagaratnam, N., and Somasundram, M.: Bone changes in iron deficiency anaemia. *J. Trop. Med. Hyg.* 66:83, 1963.

81. Shahidi, N. T., and Diamond, L.,K.: Skull changes in infants with chronic iron-deficiency anemia. *N. Engl. J. Med.* 262:137, 1960.

82. Lanzkowsky, P.: Radiological features of iron deficiency anemia. *Am. J. Dis. Child.* 116:16, 1968.

83. El-Najjar, M. Y., Lozoff, B., and Ryan, D. J.: The paleoepidemiology of porotic hyperostosis in the American southwest: Radiological and ecological consideration. *Am. J. Roentgenol.* 125:189, 1975.

84. El-Najjar, M. Y., and Robertson, A. L., Jr.: Spongy bones in prehistoric America. *Science* 193:141, 1976.

85. Reimann, F., and Kuran, S.: Ursache, Entstehung und Wesen des "Bürstensymptoms" am Schädel bei schweren Erkrankungen des Blutes. VI. Untersuchungen über die Veränderungen des Skeletsystems bei schweren Bluterkrankungen. *Virchows Arch. [Pathol. Anat.]* 358:173, 1973.

86. Reimann, V. F., Berker, F., Gökmen, E., and Kücükackirlar, T.: Das Verhalten der Sella turcica bei jugendlichen Patienten mit schwerer Eisenmangelkrankheit. *Fortschr. Röntgenstr.* 129:598, 1978.

87. Moseley, J. E.: Skeletal changes in the anemias. *Semin. Roentgenol.* 9:170, 1974.

88. Bernát, I.: Die Bedeutung der Hyposiderose in der Pathogenese der Ozaena. *Folia Haematol. (Leipz.)* 80:153, 1963.

89. Bernát, I.: *Ozaena: A Manifestation of Iron Deficiency* (translated by P. Fenyö). Pergamon, New York, 1965.

90. Bernát, I., and Valló, J.: Ozaena: The causes of its familial occurrence. *Acta Med. Acad. Sci. Hung.* 20:89, 1964.

91. Mros, B., Brüschke, G., and Voigt, D.: Eisenmangel als ätiologischer Faktor der Ozaena. *Dtsch. Gesundheitsw.* 21:2216, 1966.

92. Barkve, H., and Djupesland, G.: Ozaena and iron deficiency. *Br. Med. J.* 2:336, 1968.

93. Lundström, U., Siimes, M. A., and Dallman, P. R.: At what age does iron supplementation become necessary in low-birth-weight infants? *J. Pediatr.* 91:878, 1977.

94. Christakis, G., et al.: A nutritional epidemiologic investigation of 642 New York City children. *Am. J. Clin. Nutr.* 21:107, 1968.

95. Pearson, H. A., Abrams, I., Fernback, D. J., Gyland, S. P., and Hahn, D. A.: Anemia in preschool children in the United States of America. *Pediatr. Res.* 1:169, 1967.

96. Karp, R. J., Haaz, W. S., Starke, K., and Gorman, J. M.: Iron deficiency in families of iron-deficient inner-city school children. *Am. J. Dis. Child.* 128:18, 1974.

97. Fielding, J., O'Shaughnessy, M. C., and Brunström, G. M.: Iron deficiency without anaemia. *Lancet* 2:9, 1965.

98. Monsen, E. R., Kuhn, I. N., and Finch, C. A.: Iron status of menstruating women. *Am. J. Clin. Nutr.* 20:842, 1967.

99. Elwood, P. C., Rees, G., and Thomas, J. D. R.: Community study of

100. Scott, D. E., and Pritchard, J. A.: Iron deficiency in healthy young college women. *JAMA* 199:897, 1967.

menstrual iron loss and its association with iron deficiency anaemia. *Br. J. Prev. Soc. Med.* 22:127, 1968.

101. Fairbanks, V. F.: Nutrient deficiencies in man: Iron, in *CRC Handbook. Series in Nutrition and Food.* Section E: *Nutritional Disorders,* vol. 3, edited by M. Rechcigl, Jr. CRC Press, West Palm Beach, Fla., 1978.

102. Dozy, A. M., et al.: Alpha globin gene organization in blacks precludes the severe form of α-thalassemia. *Nature* 280:605, 1979.

103. Wood, M. M., and Elwood, P. C.: Symptoms of iron deficiency anaemia: A community survey. *Br. J. Prev. Soc. Med.* 20:117, 1966.

104. Beutler, E., Larsh, S. E., and Gurney, C. W.: Iron therapy in chronically fatigued, nonanemic women: A double-blind study. *Ann. Intern. Med.* 52:378, 1960.

105. Cochrane, A. L., and Elwood, P. C.: Iron deficiency without anaemia. *Lancet* 1:591, 1968.

106. Morrow, J. J., Dagg, J. H., and Goldberg, A.: A controlled trial of iron therapy in sideropenia. *Scot. Med. J.* 13:78, 1968.

107. Lieden, G., and Adolfsson, L.: Physical work capacity in blood donors. *Scand. J. Clin. Lab. Invest.* 34:37, 1974.

108. Vellar, O. D., and Hermansen, L.: Physical performance and hematological parameters. *Acta Med. Scand.* 519–525S:11, 1971.

109. Andersen, H. T., and Barkve, H.: Iron deficiency and muscular work performance. *Scand. J. Clin. Lab. Invest.* 114S:7, 1970.

110. Ericsson, P.: The effect of iron supplementation on the physical work capacity in the elderly. *Acta Med. Scand.* 188:361, 1970.

111. Edgerton, V. R., Bryant, S. L., Gillespie, C. A., and Gardner, G. W.: Iron deficiency anemia and physical performance and activity of rats. *J. Nutr.* 102:381, 1972.

112. Glover, J., and Jacobs, A.: Activity pattern of iron-deficient rats. *Br. Med. J.* 2:627, 1972.

113. Finch, C. A., et al.: Iron deficiency in the rat. Physiological and biochemical studies of muscle dysfunction. *J. Clin. Invest.* 58:447, 1976.

114. Andersen, H. T., and Stavem, P.: Iron deficiency anaemia and the acid-base variations of exercise. *Nutr. Metab.* 14:129, 1972.

115. Viteri, F. E., and Torún, B.: Anaemia and physical work capacity. *Clin. Haematol.* 3:609, 1974.

116. Davies, C. T. M., Chukweumeka, A. C., and Van Haaren, J. P. M.: Iron-deficiency anaemia: Its effect on maximum aerobic power and responses to exercise in African males aged 17–40 years. *Clin. Sci.* 44:555, 1973.

117. Davies, C. T. M., and Van Haaren, J. P. M.: Effect of treatment on physiological responses to exercise in East African industrial workers with iron deficiency anaemia. *Br. J. Ind. Med.* 30:335, 1973.

118. Davies, C. T. M.: The physiological effects of iron deficiency anaemia and malnutrition on exercise performance in East African school children. *Acta Paediatr. Belg.* 28 (Suppl.):253, 1974.

119. Gardner, G. W., Edgerton, V. R., Senewiratne, B., Barnard, R. J., and Ohira, Y.: Physical work capacity and metabolic stress in subjects with iron deficiency anemia. *Am. J. Clin. Nutr.* 30:910, 1977.

120. Charlton, R. W., et al.: Anaemia, iron deficiency, and exercise: Extended studies in human subjects. *Clin. Sci. Mol. Med.* 53:537, 1977.

121. Taymor, M. L., Sturgis, S. H., and Yahia, C.: The etiological role of chronic iron deficiency in production of menorrhagia. *JAMA* 187:323, 1964.

122. Samuels, A. J.: Studies in patients with functional menorrhagia: The antihemorrhagic effect of the adequate repletion of iron stores. *Isr. J. Med. Sci.* 1:851, 1965.

123. Wintrobe, M. M., and Beebe, R. T.: Idiopathic hypochromic anemia. *Medicine (Baltimore)* 12:187, 1933.

124. Conrad, M. E., and Crosby, W. H.: The natural history of iron deficiency induced by phlebotomy. *Blood* 20:173, 1962.

125. Beutler, E.: The red cell indices in the diagnosis of iron-deficiency anemia. *Ann. Intern. Med.* 50:313, 1959.

126. Bessman, J. D., and Feinstein, D. I.: Quantitative anisocytosis as a discriminant between iron deficiency and thalassemia minor. *Blood* 53:288, 1979.

127. Fairbanks, V. F.: Is the peripheral blood film reliable for the diagnosis of iron deficiency anemia: *Am. J. Clin. Pathol.* 55:447, 1971.

128. England, J. M., Walford, D. M., and Waters, D. A. W.: Re-assess-

ment of the reliability of the hematocrit. *Br. J. Haematol. 23:*247, 1972.

129. Rose, M. S.: Epitaph for the M.C.H.C. *Br. Med. J. 4:*169, 1971.
130. Klee, G., Fairbanks, V. F., Pierre, R. V., and O'Sullivan, M. B.: Use of electronic erythrocyte measurements in the diagnosis of iron deficiency and thalassemia trait. *Am. J. Clin. Pathol. 66:*870, 1976.
131. England, J. M., and Fraser, P. M.: Differentiation of iron deficiency from thalassemia trait by routine blood count. *Lancet 1:*449, 1973.
132. Schloesser, L. L., Kipp, M. A., and Wenzel, F. J.: Thrombocytosis in iron-deficiency anemia. *J. Lab. Clin. Med. 66:*107, 1965.
133. Kasper, C. K., Whissel, D. Y. E., and Wallerstein, R. O.: Clinical aspects of iron deficiency. *JAMA 191:*359, 1965.
134. Dinol, K., and Aksoy, M.: On the platelet levels in chronic iron deficiency anemia. *Acta Haematol. (Basel) 41:*135, 1969.
135. Gross, S., Keefer, V., and Newman, A. J.: The platelets in iron-deficiency anemia. I. The response to oral and parenteral iron. *Pediatrics 34:*315, 1964.
136. Ellis, L. D., Jensen, W. N., and Westerman, M. P.: Marrow iron: An evaluation of depleted stores in a series of 1,322 needle biopsies. *Ann. Intern. Med. 61:*44, 1964.
137. Garby, L., Irnell, L., and Werner, I.: Iron deficiency in women of fertile age in a Swedish community. II. Efficiency of several laboratory tests to predict the response to iron supplementation. *Acta Med. Scand. 185:*107, 1969.
138. Hamilton, L. D., Gubler, C. J., Cartwright, G. E., and Wintrobe, M. M.: Diurnal variation in the plasma iron level of man. *Proc. Soc. Exp. Biol. Med. 75:*65, 1950.
139. Hoyer, K.: Physiologic variations in the iron content of human blood serum. I. The variations from week to week, from day to day and through twenty-four hours. II. Further studies of the intra diem variations. *Acta Med. Scand. 119:*562, 1944.
140. Speck, B.: Diurnal variation of serum iron and the latent iron binding capacity in normal adults. *Helv. Med. Acta 34:*231, 1968.
141. Zilva, J. F., and Patston, V. J.: Variations in serum-iron in healthy women. *Lancet 1:*459, 1966.
142. Fujino, M., Dawson, E. B., Holeman, T., and McGanity, W. J.: Interrelationships between estrogenic activity, serum iron and ascorbic acid levels during the menstrual cycle. *Am. J. Clin. Nutr. 18:*256, 1966.
143. Mardell, M., and Zilva, J. F.: Effect of oral contraceptives on the variations in serum-iron during the menstrual cycle. *Lancet 2:*1323, 1967.
144. Burton, J. L.: Effect of oral contraceptives on haemoglobin, packed-cell volume, serum-iron, and total iron-binding capacity in healthy women. *Lancet 1:*978, 1967.
145. Heilmeyer, L., and Plötner, K.: *Das Serumeisen und die Eisenmangelkrankheit (Pathogenese, Symptomatologie und Therapie).* Gustav Fischer Verlag, Jena, 1937, p. 92.
146. Cartwright, G. E.: The anemia of chronic disorders. *Semin. Hematol. 3:*351, 1966.
147. Bainton, D. F., and Finch, C. A.: The diagnosis of iron deficiency anemia. *Am. J. Med. 37:*62, 1964.
148. Banerjee, R. N., and Narang, R. M.: Haematological changes in malignancy. *Br. J. Haematol. 13:*829, 1967.
149. Handjani, A. M., Banihashemi, A., Rafiee, R., and Tolou, H.: Serum iron in acute myocardial infarction. *Blut 23:*363, 1971.
150. Syrkis, I., and Machtey, I.: Hypoferremia in acute myocardial infarction. *J. Am. Geriatr. Soc. 21:*28, 1973.
151. Fairbanks, V. F., and Klee, G. G.: Ferritin, in *Progress in Clinical Pathology,* vol. 8, edited by M. Stefanini. Grune & Stratton, New York, 1981.
152. Jacobs, A., Miller, F., Worwood, M., Beamish, M. R., and Wardrop, C. A.: Ferritin in the serum of normal subjects and patients with iron deficiency and iron overload. *Br. Med. J. 4:*206, 1972.
153. Jacob, R. A., Sandstead, H. H., Klevay, L. M., and Johnson, L. K.: Utility of serum ferritin as a measure of iron deficiency in normal males undergoing repetitive phlebotomy. *Blood 56:*786, 1980.
154. Lipschitz, D. A., Cook, J. D., and Finch, C. A.: A clinical evaluation of serum ferritin as an index of iron stores. *N. Engl. J. Med. 290:*1213, 1974.
155. Ali, M. A. M., Luxton, A. W., and Walker, W. H. C.: Serum ferritin concentration and bone marrow iron stores: A prospective study. *Can. Med. Assoc. J. 118:*945, 1978.

156. Aljama, P., et al.: Serum ferritin concentration: A reliable guide to iron overload in uremic and hemodialyzed patients. *Clin. Nephrol. 10:*101, 1978.
157. Jacobs, A., et al.: Serum ferritin concentration in untreated Hodgkin's disease. *Br. J. Cancer 34:*162, 1976.
158. Matzner, Y., Konijn, A. M., and Hershko, C.: Serum ferritin in hematologic malignancies. *Am. J. Hematol. 9:*13, 1980.
159. Bieber, C. P., and Bieber, M. M.: Detection of ferritin as a circulating tumor-associated antigen in Hodgkin's disease. *Natl. Cancer Inst. Monogr. 36:*147, 1973.
160. Eckey, P.: Die Kinetik des Serumeisenspiegels im Verlauf der Hepatitis. *Z. Gesamte Inn. Med. 19:*433, 1964.
161. Prieto, J., Barry, M., and Sherlock, S.: Serum ferritin in patients with iron overload and with acute and chronic liver diseases. *Gastroenterology 68:*525, 1975.
162. Heinrich, H. C.: Serum-Ferritin ungeeignet als Kontrollparameter der oralen Eisentherapie. *Dtsch. Med. Wochenschr. 102:*1788, 1977.
163. Siimes, M. A., Addiego, J. E., and Dallman, P. R.: Ferritin in serum: Diagnosis of iron deficiency and iron overload in infants and children. *Blood 43:*581, 1974.
164. Thomas, W. J., et al.: Free erythrocyte porphyrin: Hemoglobin ratios, serum ferritin, and transferrin saturation levels during treatment of infants with iron-deficiency anemia. *Blood 49:*455, 1977.
165. Wheby, M. S.: Effect of iron therapy on serum ferritin levels in iron-deficiency anemia. *Blood 56:*138, 1980.
166. Piomelli, S.: A micromethod for free erythrocyte porphyrins: The FEP test. *J. Lab. Clin. Med. 81:*932, 1973.
167. Stockman, J. A., Weiner, L. S., Simon, G. E., Stuart, M. J., and Oski, F. A.: The measurement of free erythrocyte porphyrin (FEP) as a simple means of distinguishing iron deficiency from beta-thalassemia trait in subjects with microcytosis. *J. Lab. Clin. Med. 85:*113, 1975.
168. Pollack, S., George, J. N., Reba, R. C., et al.: The absorption of nonferrous metals in iron deficiency. *J. Clin. Invest. 44:*1470, 1965.
169. Valberg, L. S., Sorbie, J., Corbett, W. E. N., and Ludwig, J.: Cobalt tests for the detection of iron deficiency anemia. *Ann. Intern. Med. 77:*181, 1972.
170. Wahner-Roedler, D. L., Fairbanks, V. F., and Linman, J. W.: Cobalt excretion test as index of iron absorption and diagnostic test for iron deficiency. *J. Lab. Clin. Med. 85:*253, 1975.
171. Huser, H.-J., Rieber, E. E., and Berman, A. R.: Experimental evidence of excess hemolysis in the course of chronic iron deficiency anemia. *J. Lab. Clin. Med. 69:*405, 1967.
172. Loría, A., Sanchez-Medal, L., Lisker, R., de Rodriguez, E., and Labardini, J.: Red cell life span in iron deficiency anaemia. *Br. J. Haematol. 13:*294, 1967.
173. Pollycove, M.: Iron metabolism and kinetics. *Semin. Hematol. 3:*235, 1966.
174. Hauge, B. N.: The iron absorption test: Clinical investigation and evaluation. *Acta Med. Scand. 168:*109, 1960.
175. Verloop, M. C., Meeuwissen, J. E. T., and Blokhuis, E. W. M.: Comparison of the "iron absorption test" with the determination of the iron-binding capacity of serum in the diagnosis of iron deficiency. *Br. J. Haematol. 4:*70, 1958.
176. Wiltink, W. F., Ybema, H. J., Leijnse, B., and Gerbrandy, J.: The iron tolerance test: Measurement of absorption and utilization of a therapeutic dose of iron. *Clin. Chim. Acta 13:*701, 1966.
177. Balcerzak, S. P., Westerman, M. P., Heinle, E. W., and Taylor, F. H.: Measurement of iron stores using deferoxamine. *Ann. Intern. Med. 68:*518, 1968.
178. Wardle, E. N., and Israëls, M. C.: The differential ferrioxamine test in rheumatoid disease, neoplastic and other haematological disorders. *Br. J. Haematol. 14:*5, 1968.
179. Powell, L. W., and Thomas, M. J.: Use of diethylenetriamine pentaacetic acid (D.T.P.A.) in the clinical assessment of total body iron stores. *J. Clin. Pathol. 20:*896, 1967.
180. Singh, A. K.: Measurement of a labile iron store. *Br. J. Haematol. 14:*411, 1968.
181. Fielding, J.: Differential ferrioxamine test for measuring chelatable body iron. *J. Clin. Pathol. 18:*88, 1965.
182. Losowsky, M. S.: Effects of desferrioxamine in patients with iron-loading with a simple method for estimating urinary iron. *J. Clin. Pathol. 19:*165, 1966.

183. Quattrin, N., and Ventruto, V.: Hemoglobin Lepore: Its significance for thalassemia and clinical manifestations. *Blut* 28:327, 1974.
184. Fairbanks, V. F.: *Hemoglobinopathies and Thalassemias.* Thieme-Stratton, New York, 1980.
185. Gerald, P. S., and Diamond, L. K.: A new hereditary hemoglobinopathy (the Lepore trait) and its interaction with thalassemia trait. *Blood* 13:835, 1958.
186. Duma, H., et al.: Study of nine families with haemoglobin-Lepore. *Br. J. Haematol.* 15:161, 1968.
187. Fairbanks, V. F., Gilchrist, G. S., Brimhall, B., Jereb, J. A., and Goldston, E. C.: Hemologin E trait reexamined: A cause of microcytosis and erythrocytosis. *Blood* 53:109, 1979.
188. Klee, G. G.: Role of morphology, and erythrocyte indices in screening and diagnosis, in *Hemoglobinopathies and Thalassemias,* edited by V. F. Fairbanks. Thieme-Stratton, New York, 1980.
189. Wallerstein, R. O., and Aggeler, P. M.: Differentiating between thalassemia minor and iron deficiency. *Calif. Med.* 84:176, 1956.
190. Klavins, J. V., Kinney, T. D., and Kaufman, N.: Serum iron changes due to ethionine: Resemblance to some aspects of idiopathic hemochromatosis. *Arch. Pathol.* 81:67, 1966.
191. Chiandussi, L., Bianco, A., Massaro, A., Mazza, V., and Cesano, L.: The quantitative determination of iron kinetics and hemoglobin synthesis in anemia of cirrhosis studies with ^{59}Fe. *Blut* 10:120, 1964.
192. Pollycove, M., Winchell, H. S., and Lawrence, J. H.: Classification and evolution of patterns of erythropoiesis in polycythemia vera as studied by iron kinetics. *Blood* 28:807, 1966.
193. Brodsky, I., Kahn, S. B., and Brady, L. W.: Polycythaemia vera: Differential diagnosis by ferrokinetic studies and treatment with busulphan (Myleran). *Br. J. Haematol.* 14:351, 1968.
194. Kiely, J. M., Stroebel, C. F., Hanlon, D. G., and Owen, C. A., Jr.: Clinical value of plasma-iron turnover rate in diagnosis and management of polycythemia. *J. Nucl. Med.* 2:1, 1961.
195. Ellis, L. S., Westerman, M. P., and Balcerzak, S. P.: The effect of iron stores on ferrokinetics in polycythemia. *Br. J. Haematol.* 13:892, 1967.
196. Hilal, H., and McCurdy, P. R.: A pitfall in the interpretation of serum iron values. *Ann. Intern. Med.* 66:983, 1967.
197. Baum, S., Nusbaum, M., Blakemore, W. S., and Finkelstein, A. K.: The preoperative radiographic demonstration of intraabdominal bleeding from undetermined sites by percutaneous selective celiac and superior mesenteric arteriography. *Surgery* 58:797, 1965.
198. Koehler, P. R., and Salmon, R. B.: Angiographic localization of unknown acute gastrointestinal bleeding sites. *Radiology* 89:244, 1967.
199. Casarella, W. J., Kanter, I. E., and Seaman, W. B.: Right-sided colonic diverticula as a cause of acute rectal hemorrhage. *N. Engl. J. Med.* 286:450, 1972.
200. Chait, A., and Dann, R. H.: G-I bleed after angiography. *N. Engl. J. Med.* June 29, 1972.
201. Jewett, T. C., Jr., Duszynski, D. O., and Allen, J. E.: The visualization of Meckel's diverticulum with ^{99m}Tc-pertechnetate. *Surgery* 68:567, 1970.
202. Kilpatrick, Z. M., and Aseron, C. A., Jr.: Radioisotope detection of Meckel's diverticulum causing acute rectal hemorrhage. *N. Engl. J. Med.* 289:653, 1972.
203. Berquist, T. H., Nolan, N. G., Adson, M. A., and Schutt, A. J.: Diagnosis of Meckel's diverticulum by radioisotope scanning. *Mayo Clin. Proc.* 48:98, 1973.
204. Brayton, D.: Gastrointestinal bleeding of "unknown origin": A study of cases in infancy and childhood. *Am. J. Dis. Child.* 107:288, 1964.
205. Shandling, B.: Laparotomy for rectal bleeding. *Pediatrics* 35:787, 1965.
206. O'Sullivan, D. J., Higgins, P. G., and Wilkinson, J. F.: Oral iron compounds: A therapeutic comparison. *Lancet* 2:482, 1955.
207. Hallberg, L., Ryttinger, L., and Sölvell, L.: Side-effects of oral iron therapy: A double-blind study of different iron compounds in tablet form. *Acta Med. Scand. (Suppl.)* 459:3, 1966.
208. Westlin, W. F.: Deferoxamine in the treatment of acute iron poisoning: Clinical experiences with 172 children. *Clin. Pediatr. (Phila.)* 5:531, 1966.
209. Greengard, J., and McEnery, J. T.: Iron poisoning in children. *G. P.* 37:88, 1968.
210. Whitten, C. F., and Brough, A. J.: The pathophysiology of acute iron poisoning. *Clin. Toxicol.* 4(4):585, 1971.
211. McEnery, J. T.: Hospital management of acute iron ingestion. *Clin. Toxicol.* 4(4):603, 1971.
212. Fairbanks, V. F., Fahey, J. L., and Beutler, E.: *Clinical Disorders of Iron Metabolism,* 2d ed. Grune & Stratton, New York, 1971.
213. Cox, J. S. G., Kennedy, G. R., King, J., Marshall, P. R., and Rutherford, D.: Structure of an iron-dextran complex. *J. Pharm. Pharmacol.* 24:513, 1972.
214. Muranda, M., et al.: Experiencias con el uso del fierro-dextran marcado con Fe-59. *Rev. Med. Chile* 93:134, 1965.
215. Will, G.: The absorption, distribution and utilization of intramuscularly administered iron-dextran: A radio-isotope study. *Br. J. Haematol.* 14:395, 1968.
216. Marchasin, S., and Wallerstein, R. O.: The treatment of iron-deficiency anemia with intravenous iron dextran. *Blood* 23:354, 1964.
217. Grimes, A. J., and Hutt, M. S. R.: Metabolism of ^{59}Fe-dextran complex in human subjects. *Br. Med. J.* 2:1074, 1957.
218. Garby, L., and Sjölin, S.: Some observations on the distribution kinetics of radioactive colloidal iron (Imferon and ferric hydroxide). *Acta Med. Scand.* 157:319, 1957.
219. Henderson, P. A., and Hillman, R. S.: Characteristics of iron dextran utilization in man. *Blood* 34:357, 1969.
220. Olsson, K. S., and Weinfeld, A.: Availability of iron dextran for hemoglobin synthesis. *Acta Med. Scand.* 192:543, 1972.
221. Will, G., and Groden, B. M.: The treatment of iron deficiency anaemia by iron-dextran infusion: A radioisotope study. *Br. J. Haematol.* 14:61, 1968.
222. Groden, B. M., Whitelaw, J., and Will, G.: The treatment of iron-deficiency anaemia by iron-dextran infusion, with special reference to the effect on blood-grouping, coagulation, sedimentation and haemolysis. *Postgrad. Med. J.* 44:433, 1968.
223. Rhyner, K., and Ganzoni, A. M.: Die therapeutische Infusion von Eisen-III-Hydroxyd-Kohlenhydrat-Komplexen. *Schweiz. Med. Wochnschr.* 102:561, 1972.
224. Mehta, B. C., and Patel, J. C.: Iron-dextran total dose infusion in the treatment of iron deficiency anemia. *Indian. J. Med. Sci.* 22:1, 1968.
225. Loriá, A., Cordourier, E., Arroyo, P., Piedras, J., and Medal, S.: Anemia nutricional. IV. Hierro dextran en dosis intravenosa úrica en la profilaxis de la anemia hipoferrémica del embarazo. *Rev. Invest. Clin.* 24:113, 1972.
226. Wallerstein, R. O.: Intravenous iron-dextran complex. *Blood* 32:690, 1968.
227. Mehta, B. C., Ambani, L. M., Pawaskar, M., and Patel, J. C.: Iron-dextran total dose injection (I.V. undiluted) in the treatment of iron deficiency anemia. *Indian J. Med. Sci.* 22:20, 1968.
228. Kanakaraddi, V. P., Hoskatti, C. G., Nadig, V. S., Patil, C. K., and Yaiya, M.: Comparative therapeutic study of T.D.I. & I.M. injections of iron dextran complex in anaemia. *J. Assoc. Physicians India* 21:849, 1973.
229. Theodoropoulos, G., Makkous, A., and Constantoulakis, M.: Lymph node enlargement after a single massive infusion of iron dextran. *J. Clin. Pathol.* 21:492, 1968.
230. Solanki, S. V., and Kabrawala, V. N.: Lymphadenopathy due to parenteral iron therapy. *J. Indian Med. Assoc.* 51:22, 1968.
231. Helsel, E. V., Jr.: Severe febrile reaction to intramuscular administration of iron-dextran. *Am. J. Obstet. Gynecol.* 91:582, 1965.
232. Ruiz, Reyes, G., Tamayo-Pérez, R., and Mendoza-López, M.: Fiebre, adenomegalia y esplenomegalia, consecutiva a la aplicación de dosis única total de hierro-dextran en anemia por uncinariasis, in *Memorias de la X Jornada Anual de la Agrupación Mexicana para el Estudio de la Hematologia.* México, D. F., 1969.
233. Forristal, T., and Witt, M.: Pleocytosis after iron dextran injection. *Lancet* 1:1428, 1968.
234. Reddy, P. S., and Lewis, M.: The adverse effect of intravenous iron-dextran in rheumatoid arthritis. *Arthritis Rheum.* 12:454, 1969.
235. Cantor, R. I., Downs, G. E., and Abruzzo, J. L.: Acute exacerbation of ankylosing spondylitis after an iron dextran infusion. *Ann. Intern. Med.* 77:933, 1972.
236. Richmond, H. G.: Induction of sarcoma in the rat by iron-dextran complex. *Br. Med. J.* 1:947, 1959.

237. Carter, R. L., Mitchley, C. V., and Roe, F. J. C.: Induction of tumours in mice and rats with ferric sodium gluconate and iron dextran glycerol glycoside. *Br. J. Cancer* 22:521, 1968.
238. Robinson, C. E. G., Bell, D. N., and Sturdy, J. H.: Possible association of malignant neoplasm with iron-dextran injection: A case report. *Br. Med. J.* 2:648, 1960.
239. MacKinnon, A. E., and Bancewicz, J.: Sarcoma after injection of intramuscular iron. *Br. Med. J.* 2:277, 1973.
240. Greenberg, G.: Sarcoma after intramuscular iron injection. *Br. Med. J.* 1:1508, 1976.
241. Lane, R. S.: Intravenous infusion of iron-dextran complex for iron-deficiency anaemia. *Lancet* 1:852, 1964.
242. Becker, C. E., MacGregor, R. R., Walker, K. S., and Jandl, J. H.: Fatal anaphylaxis after intramuscular iron-dextran. *Ann. Intern. Med.* 65:745, 1966.
243. Clay, B., Rosenberg, B., Sampson, N., and Samuels, S. I.: Reactions to total dose intravenous infusion of iron dextran (Imferon). *Br. Med. J.* 1:29, 1965.
244. Callender, S. T., and Smith, M. D.: Intramuscular iron (letter to editor). *Br. Med. J.* 2:1487, 1954.
245. Jacobs, J.: Death due to iron parenterally. *South. Med. J.* 62:216, 1969.
246. Mitchell, A. B. S., and Gill, A. M.: Choice of iron therapy. *Practitioner* 213:370, 1974.
247. Cox, J. S. G., and King, R. E.: Valency investigations of iron dextran (Imferon). *Nature (Lond.)* 207:1202, 1965.
248. McCurdy, P. R.: Oral and parenteral iron therapy: A comparison. *JAMA* 191:859, 1965.
249. Klee, G. G.: "Decision Rules for Accelerated Hematology Laboratory Investigation." Thesis, University of Minnesota, 1974.
250. Beutler, E., and Fairbanks, V. F.: The effects of iron deficiency, in *Iron in Biochemistry and Medicine*, vol. 2, edited by A. Jacobs and M. Worwood. Academic, New York, 1980.
251. Beutler, E., and Meerkreebs, G.: Doses and dosing. *N. Engl. J. Med.* 274:1152, 1966 (correspondence).
252. Johnson, C. S., Tegos, C., and Beutler, E.: α-Thalassemia. Prevalence and hematologic findings in American Blacks. *Arch. Intern. Med.* 142:1280, 1982.

CHAPTER *49*

Congenital atransferrinemia and idiopathic pulmonary hemosiderosis

VIRGIL F. FAIRBANKS
ERNEST BEUTLER

Congenital atransferrinemia

In 1961, Heilmeyer and coworkers [1] described a young girl with severe congenital hypochromic anemia in whose plasma no transferrin could be demonstrated. The condition has been called *congenital atransferrinemia*. Additional cases have been reported from Czechoslovakia [2], Mexico [3], and Japan [4,5].

ETIOLOGY AND PATHOGENESIS
In the absence of transferrin, the primary system for the delivery of iron to the marrow cannot function. Thus hemoglobin synthesis is severely impaired, and hypochromic anemia results.

MODE OF INHERITANCE
The pattern of inheritance is that of an autosomal recessive trait. Transferrin concentrations of half-normal values without associated anemia were observed in siblings and parents in each of the families reported, and in one family [3], hypochromic anemia and atransferrinemia occurred in siblings.

CLINICAL FEATURES
Pallor and fatigue are characteristic. A systolic ejection cardiac murmur has been present in most cases. Some patients have mild hepatomegaly. Heilmeyer's patient [1] died at the age of 7 years from refractory congestive heart failure and showed, at necropsy, marked hemosiderosis and fibrosis of liver, pancreas, thyroid, myocardium, and kidneys, but no iron in the marrow. (This patient had received numerous transfusions.) Additionally, Heilmeyer's patient suffered from recurrent infections, a feature lacking in subsequent cases.

LABORATORY FEATURES
As shown in Table 49-1, the degree of anemia has been variable. Total iron-binding capacity has ranged from 24 to 81 μg/dl (4.1 to 14.0 μmol/liter), and transferrin concentration has been 0 to 39 mg/dl (0 to 5 μmol/liter) [normal value 200 to 300 mg/dl (25 to 40 μmol/liter)]. Measurement of transferrin in these cases has been by a radial immunodiffusion method. The absence or small diameter of the precipitin ring in reported cases strongly suggests a quantitative deficiency of transferrin rather than the presence of a functionally abnormal protein. It seems likely, on the basis of analogy with other genetic disorders, that deficiency of transferrin in these cases is due either to a reduced rate of synthesis of transferrin or to its accelerated destruction, possibly due to structural instability. Studies of iron metabolism in several of these cases [3–5] have demonstrated normal to enhanced iron absorption from the gastrointestinal tract, normal to moderately accelerated plasma iron clearance, and diminished incorporation of iron into hemoglobin (ranging from 7 to 55 percent; normal 30 to 100 percent). It has been shown that the infusion of either normal plasma or purified transferrin is followed in 10 to 14 days by reticulocytosis and then by a rise in hemoglobin concentration [4,5].

DIFFERENTIAL DIAGNOSIS
Congenital atransferrinemia may be differentiated from other causes of hypochromic anemia by the profound depression of the total iron-binding capacity. It must be considered, however, that atransferrinemia has also been described in association with the nephrotic syndrome [6]. In that situation, loss of transferrin presum-

TABLE 49-1   Laboratory findings in congenital atransferrinemia

Author	Case	Hemoglobin concentration, g/dl	Serum iron concentration, μg/dl	Total iron-binding, μg/dl	Transferrin concentration, mg/dl
Heilmeyer et al. [1]	1	9.1	10	33	4.4
Cáp et al. [2]	2	4.8	30	30	0
Loperena et al. [3]	3	4.1	19	24	0
	4	7.9	38	69	6.0
Sakata[4]	5	3.2	16	81	39
Goya et al. [5]	6	6.4	12	46	"Trace"

ably occurs through the kidney. A perplexing combination of atransferrinemia and persistence of fetal hemoglobin has been described in a case of erythroleukemia [7]. In another reported case [8] the total iron-binding capacity was 75 μg/dl (12.9 μmol/liter), and severe normochromic anemia required repeated transfusions. It is possible that chronic urinary tract infection may have been responsible for the decreased transferrin levels in the plasma of this patient, since chronic infection is usually associated with diminished transferrin levels. A syndrome with many features similar to those described in congenital atransferrinemia has been reported. Two unrelated pairs of siblings were found to have hypochromic microcytic anemia with absent or diminished marrow iron in spite of hemosiderosis of the liver [9–11]. These cases were different from congenital atransferrinemia in that the plasma iron was increased (ranging from 170 to 250 μg/dl or 29 to 43 μmol/liter) and the total iron-binding capacity was normal. One case has been described of a functional disorder of transferrin due to transferrin-IgG-transferrin immune complexes [12]. This patient had clinical and laboratory features of hemochromatosis, marked elevation in serum iron concentration, and absence of stainable iron in marrow.

THERAPY
Promising results have been achieved with infusion of normal human plasma or of purified transferrin [3–5,13]. Unfortunately, the rise in plasma transferrin concentration which can be so attained does not persist beyond a week. However, the cohort of erythroblasts which will take up iron during this time will mature to circulate for as long as 4 months. Therefore it may suffice to infuse normal plasma or transferrin at intervals of 2 to 4 months. Two patients have been given 1 to 2 g of highly purified transferrin intravenously every 3 to 4 months for 4 to 7 years with good effect and without the development of antitransferrin antibodies [13]. Use of purified transferrin (or Cohn fraction IV-7) considerably reduces the risk of hepatitis that would attend infusion of whole plasma. The need for erythrocyte transfusion and the consequent long-term risk of hemochromatosis are also obviated by use of transferrin infusion.

COURSE AND PROGNOSIS
Of six reported cases, one patient died at age 7, apparently of complications of iron overload. Five were living at the time of their case reports; the long-term prognosis is uncertain.

Idiopathic pulmonary hemosiderosis

Idiopathic pulmonary hemosiderosis is a disease in which there is marked hemosiderosis of the lungs and the blood picture of iron deficiency anemia. It was first recognized in a living patient by Anspach [12] in 1939, and approximately 200 cases have been described since then [15–58].

ETIOLOGY AND PATHOGENESIS
The cause of the disorder is unknown, although it has been suggested that it may be a result of allergy to unspecified inhaled substances, to ingestion of cow's milk [25–29], that it may be a form of autoimmune disease, or that it may be caused by the formation of abnormal pulmonary alveolar epithelium or elastic fibers. In some cases, idiopathic pulmonary hemosiderosis has occurred in association with or prior to the manifestations or autoimmune disorders, including systemic lupus erythematosus [30], Wegener's granulomatosis, and rheumatoid arthritis [16,31,32]. Although renal involvement is not usually considered part of the clinical picture of idiopathic hemosiderosis, several cases have now been reported with this association. In one there was focal glomerulitis, as in Goodpasture's syndrome [31]. In three cases, a deposition of immunoglobulin was demonstrated along the glomerular basement membranes, although in two of these cases no renal manifestations were described [33,34]. Renal amyloidosis with nephrotic syndrome has also been described in idiopathic pulmonary hemosiderosis [35]. These associations suggest an immunologic aberration as the cause of idiopathic pulmonary hemosiderosis. The clinical manifestations are due to repeated spontaneous intrapulmonary hemorrhage, with the consequent appearance of hemosiderin-laden macrophages in the lung. The iron in these macrophages is not readily available for erythropoiesis and may, to a considerable extent, be lost

in the sputum. Thus the anemia is essentially that of chronic blood loss.

Histologic changes in the lungs have consisted of degeneration, hyperplasia, and desquamation of the epithelial cells of pulmonary alveoli, capillary proliferation and dilatation, vasculitis, and thrombosis and embolism. Interstitial fibrosis, degeneration of interstitial and alveolar elastic fibers, sclerosis of pulmonary arteries and veins, muscular hypertrophy of bronchial arteries, and hyaline membranes may be present. Unfortunately, these histologic changes are nonspecific, being found in any disorder accompanied by recurrent hemoptysis. Earlier electron microscopy showed nonspecific changes [36,39]. More recent ultrastructural studies of lungs have shown piling up and splitting of alveolar capillary basement membranes and deposition of fibrillar material between layers of basement membrane [40,41]. Immunoglobulins, complement components, or fibrinogen are not usually demonstrated in lung [39,41]. Hemosiderosis affects predominantly the interstitial phagocytic cells. Although marrow iron is absent, hemosiderosis of the spleen and liver has been reported to occur in some cases of idiopathic pulmonary hemosiderosis [15]. Changes in the renal glomeruli have been noted in some instances, suggesting that the distinction between this disorder and Goodpasture's syndrome may be artificial. In one case, an antibody to glomerular basement membrane was demonstrated in the patient's serum, as in Goodpasture's syndrome [33]. This patient also exhibited linear deposits of immunoglobulin along both the pulmonary alveolar basement membrane and the renal glomerular basement membrane.

MODE OF INHERITANCE AND INCIDENCE

Almost all reported cases of idiopathic pulmonary hemosiderosis have been sporadic and nonfamilial. However, occurrence in siblings has been reported twice [42,43], raising the possibility of an autosomal recessive mode of inheritance. It has also been reported in mother and son [44], an observation consistent with autosomal dominant or X-linked mode of inheritance. It seems premature to ascribe a hereditary transmittance until more family studies have been reported. Idiopathic pulmonary hemosiderosis is predominantly a disease of children, only about one patient in five being over the age of 16 years. It has been reported in a 6-week-old child [29]. Few cases have been reported in persons 50 years of age or older. In children the disease does not appear to affect one sex more than the other, but two-thirds of adults with idiopathic pulmonary hemosiderosis are males.

CLINICAL FEATURES

The most consistently present manifestations of idiopathic pulmonary hemosiderosis are cough, failure to gain weight, fatigue, and pallor. Copious amounts of blood may be produced on coughing, or only slight

streaks of blood in the sputum may be observed. Indeed, hemoptysis may be absent during the course of the disease [17,19]. Signs of pulmonary dysfunction, such as dyspnea and clubbing of the fingers, develop as the disease progresses. Pulmonary hypertension may develop and be followed by cardiac failure.

LABORATORY FINDINGS

The findings are those of chronic iron deficiency anemia. The blood displays the classic changes of severe iron depletion: anisocytosis, poikilocytosis, microcytosis, and hypochromia. Eosinophilia of moderate degree occurs in about 12 percent of the cases. The serum iron concentration is low, and iron-binding capacity is increased. The serum bilirubin concentration and urobilinogen excretion may be increased by the increased porphyrin catabolism. Radioisotope studies of erythrocyte survival and of ferrokinetics show the features commonly associated with chronic blood loss. Serum antibodies to bovine milk protein were found in one of three cases tested [28].

Urinalysis has shown microscopic hematuria in some cases. Gross hematuria occurs infrequently. Stools may contain occult blood as a result of swallowed blood-laden sputum.

Sputum stained for hemosiderin shows iron-laden macrophages, a finding of considerable diagnostic value in those patients without gross hemoptysis. Pulmonary-function tests have been carried out in a few cases and have revealed reduction in vital capacity and maximal breathing capacity, impairment of oxygen diffusion, and decreased lung compliance. Results of such studies may suggest either obstructive or restrictive lung disease or normal pulmonary function, and these findings correlate with the severity of clinical manifestations. Cardiac catheterization reveals marked pulmonary hypertension. Early in the course of the disease, x-ray examination of the lungs usually reveals patchy evanescent pulmonary infiltrates, due to blood in alveoli. These infiltrates clear rapidly as blood is reabsorbed. Progression of the disease is accompanied by miliary stippling of the lung and perihilar fibrosis. There may be hilar lymphadenopathy. The radiographic findings are nonspecific; identical roentgenograms may be seen in pneumonitis due to tuberculosis, *Pneumoncystis carinii*, *Mycoplasma pneumoniae*, or other infections [45]. Following intravenous injection of ^{59}Fe, there is accumulation of radioactivity in the lungs during the ensuing 10 to 30 days [20,46].

DIFFERENTIAL DIAGNOSIS

The syndrome of idiopathic pulmonary hemosiderosis should be considered when iron deficiency anemia is associated with pulmonary symptoms and signs. It is closely related to Goodpasture's syndrome, in which recurrent pulmonary hemorrhage is associated with glomerulonephritis [47–52]. Goodpasture's syndrome is predominantly a disease of young adult males, but it has also been reported in a 78-year-old woman [48]. Hemoptysis is a frequent manifestation of this disease but is rarely massive [15]. Unlike idiopathic pulmonary hemosiderosis, progressive glomerulonephritis tends to dominate the clinical course of Goodpasture's syndrome. Azotemia appears early and commonly leads to death from uremia within a few weeks to a few years. Many of the clinical, roentgenologic, and histologic features of idiopathic pulmonary hemosiderosis are the same as those of Goodpasture's syndrome, and these may be varying expressions of a single disorder [15,33,34,50–52]. Indeed, since the pulmonary manifestations and renal glomerular basement membrane changes may long precede overt signs of renal disease, it has been urged that renal biopsy be done in cases that appear to be idiopathic pulmonary hemosiderosis in order to detect renal lesions early and permit therapy before significant renal injury occurs [34].

In one case of idiopathic pulmonary hemosiderosis, despite absence of any renal manifestations, renal biopsy showed dense mesangial and paramesangial deposits of immunoglobulins IgG and IgA and of C3, a picture typical of the recently recognized disorder called *IgA nephropathy* [53].

COURSE AND PROGNOSIS

The course of pulmonary hemosiderosis is variable, and survival from onset may range from a little more than a week to many years. Prolonged remissions have been described, but whether a permanent remission or cure may occur is as yet uncertain. Some evidence indicates that intrapulmonary bleeding continues during apparent clinical remission [19]. Death results from cardiac decompensation or from massive pulmonary hemorrhage. Myocarditis has been reported to occur [17,18] and was the cause of death in one case.

TREATMENT

The anemia responds to iron therapy (see Chap. 48). Immunosuppressive therapy with cyclophosphamide, azathioprine, or adrenocortical steroids appears to have been of benefit in most cases [22,31,41–44,54,56–58] but not in all [55]. Some cases have remitted on the avoidance of cow's milk and milk products [25–29]. It is difficult to interpret apparent therapeutic responses in this disorder, which is characterized by spontaneous remissions and exacerbations.

References

1. Heilmeyer, L. Keller, W., Vivell, O., Betke, K., Wöhler, F., and Keiderling, W.: Die kongenitale Atransferrinämie. *Schweiz. Med. Wochenschr. 91*:1203, 1961.
2. Cáp, J., Lehotská, V., and Mayerová, A.: Kongenitálna atransferinémia u 11-mesačného dietäta. *Cesk. Pediatr. 23*:1020, 1968.
3. Loperena, L., et al.: Atransferrinemia hereditaria. *Bol. Med. Hsop. Infant. Mex. 31*:519, 1974.
4. Sakata, T.: A case of congenital atransferrinemia. *Shonika Shinryo 32*:1523, 1969.
5. Goya, N., Miyazaki, S., Kodate, S., and Ushio, B.: A family of congenital atransferrinemia. *Blood 40*:239, 1972.
6. Oliva, G., Dominici, G., Latini, P., and Cozzolino, G.: Sindrome nefrosica atransferrinemica. *Minerva Med. 59*:1297, 1968.
7. Hitzig, W. H., Schmid, M., Betke, K., and Rothschild, M.: Erythroleukämie mit Hämoglobinopathie und Eisenstoffwechselstörung. *Helv. Paediatr. Acta 15*:203, 1960.
8. Riegel, C., and Thomas, D.: Absence of beta-globulin fraction in the serum protein of a patient with unexplained anemia: Report of a case. *N. Engl. J. Med. 255*:434, 1956.
9. Shahidi, N. T.: Anémie hypochrome par un trouble du métabolisme du fer. *Schweiz. Med. Wochenschr. 94*:1385, 1964.
10. Shahidi, N. T., Nathan, D. G., and Diamond, L. K.: Iron deficiency anemia associated with an error of iron metabolism in two siblings. *J. Clin. Invest. 43*:510, 1964.
11. Stavem, P., Saltvedt, E., Elgjo, K., and Rootwelt, K.: Congenital hypochromic microcytic anaemia with iron overload of the liver and hyperferraemia. *Scand. J. Haematol. 10*:153, 1973.
12. Westerhausen, M., and Meuret, G.: Transferrin-immune complex disease. *Acta Haematol. 57*:96, 1977.
13. Schwick, H. G., Cap, J., and Goya, N.: Therapy of atransferrinemia with transferrin. *J. Clin. Chem. 16*:73, 1978.
14. Anspach, W. E.: Pulmonary hemosiderosis. *Am. J. Roentgenol. 41*:592, 1939.
15. Soergel, K. H., and Sommers, S. C.: Idiopathic pulmonary hemosiderosis and related syndromes. *Am. J. Med. 32*:499, 1962.
16. Ognibene, A. J., and Johnson, D. E.: Idiopathic pulmonary hemosiderosis in adults: Report of case and review of literature. *Arch. Intern. Med. 111*:503, 1963.
17. Kennedy, W. P., Shearman, D. J. C., Delamore, I. W., Simpson, J. D., Black, J. W., and Grant, I. W. B.: Idiopathic pulmonary haemosiderosis with myocarditis: Radio-isotope studies in a patient treated with prednisone. *Thorax 21*:220, 1966.
18. Murphy, K. J.: Pulmonary haemosiderosis (apparently idiopathic) associated with myocarditis, with bilateral penetrating corneal ulceration, and with diabetes mellitus. *Thorax 20*:341, 1965.
19. Aledort, L. M., and Lord, G. P.: Idiopathic pulmonary hemosiderosis: Severe anemia without hemoptysis: One year follow-up of pulmonary function. *Arch. Intern. Med. 120*:220, 1967.
20. DeGowin, R. L., Sorensen, L. B., Charleston, D. B., Gottschalk, A., and Greenwald, J. H.: Retention of radioiron in the lungs of a woman with idiopathic pulmonary hemosiderosis. *Ann. Intern. Med. 69*:1213, 1968.
21. Matsaniotis, N., Karpouzas, J., Apostolopoulou, E., and Messaritakis, J.: Idiopathic pulmonary haemosiderosis in children. *Arch. Dis. Child. 43*:307, 1968.
22. Steiner, B., and Nabrady, J.: Immunoallergic lung purpura treated with azathioprine. *Lancet 1*:140, 1965.
23. Fuleihan, F. J. D., Abboud, R. T., and Hubaytar, R.: Idiopathic pulmonary hemosiderosis: Case report with pulmonary function tests and review of the literature. *Am. Rev. Respir. Dis. 98*:93, 1968.
24. McPherson, J. R., Bernatz, P. E., and Holley, K. E.: Anemia, chest pain, dyspnea, and hemoptysis in a 26-year-old-man. *Mayo Clin. Proc. 43*:592, 1968.
25. Archer, J. M.: Idiopathic pulmonary haemosiderosis treated with a milk-free diet. *Proc. Roy. Soc. Med. 64*:53, 1971.
26. Boat, T. F., Polmar, S. H., Whitman, V., Kleinerman, J. I., Stern, R. C., and Doershuk, C. F.: Hyperreactivity to cow milk in young children with pulmonary hemosiderosis and cor pulmonale secondary to nasopharyngeal obstruction. *J. Pediatr. 87*:23, 1975.
27. Lee, S. K., Kniker, W. T., Cook, C. D., and Heiner, D. C.: Cow's milk–induced pulmonary disease in children. *Adv. Pediatr. 25*:39, 1978.
28. Stafford, H. A., Polmar, S. H., and Boat, T. F.: Immunologic studies in cow's milk induced pulmonary hemosiderosis. *Pediatr. Res. 11*:898, 1977.
29. Opitz, J. C.: Idiopathic pulmonary hemosiderosis (Report of a six-week-old infant who is now in clinical remission). *Wis. Med. J. 79*:43, 1980.
30. Byrd, R. B., and Trunk, G.: Systemic lupus erythematosus presenting as pulmonary hemosiderosis. *Chest 64*:128, 1973.

31. O'Donohue, W. J.: Idiopathic pulmonary hemosiderosis with manifestations of multiple connective tissue and immune disorders. *Am. Rev. Respir. Dis.* 109:473, 1974.

32. Perelman, R., Nathanson, M., Danis, F., Hayem, F., Gesnu, M., and Goudal, M.: Hémosiderose pulmonaire associée a une arthrite rheumatoide avec cellules LE. *Sem. Hop. Paris* 55:1129, 1979.

33. Wilson, C. B., and Dixon, F. J.: Diagnosis of immunopathologic renal disease. *Kidney Int.* 5:389, 1974.

34. Mathew, T. H., Hobbs, J. B., Kalowski, S., Sutherland, P. W., and Kincaid-Smith, P.: Goodpasture's syndrome: Normal renal diagnostic findings. *Ann. Intern. Med.* 82:215, 1975.

35. Douglas, N. L., Psimenos, G., Vlachos, P., and Liakokos, D.: Renal amyloidosis with nephrotic syndrome in a child suspected of having idiopathic pulmonary hemosiderosis. *Helv. Paediatr. Acta* 32:383, 1977.

36. Bässler, R.: Elektronenmikroskopische Befunde bei essentieller Lungenhämosiderose. *Z. Pathol.* 71:259, 1961.

37. Hyatt, R. W., Adelstein, E. R., Halazun, J. F., and Lukens, J. N.: Ultrastructure of the lung in idiopathic pulmonary hemosiderosis. *Am. J. Med.* 52:822, 1972.

38. Roberts, L. N., Montessori, G., and Patterson, J. G.: Idiopathic pulmonary hemosiderosis. *Am. Rev. Respir. Dis.* 106:904, 1972.

39. Irwin, R. S., Cottrell, T. S., Hsu, K. C., Griswold, W. R., and Thomas, H. M.: Idiopathic pulmonary hemosiderosis: An electron microscopic and immunofluorescent study. *Chest* 65:41, 1974.

40. Gonzalez-Crussi, F., Hull, M. T., and Grosfeld, J. L.: Idiopathic pulmonary hemosiderosis: Evidence of capillary basement membrane abnormality. *Am. Rev. Respir. Dis.* 114:689, 1976.

41. Yeager, H., Powell, D., Weinberg, R. M., Bauer, H., Bellanti, J. A., and Katz, S.: Idiopathic pulmonary hemosiderosis. *Arch. Intern. Med.* 136:1145, 1976.

42. Beckerman, R. C., Taussig, L. M., and Pinnas, J. L.: Familial idiopathic pulmonary hemosiderosis. *Am. J. Dis. Child.* 133:609, 1979.

43. Breckenridge, R. L., and Ross, J. S.: Idiopathic pulmonary hemosiderosis: A report of familial occurrence. *Chest* 75:636, 1979.

44. Thaell, J. F., Greipp, P. R., Stubbs, S. E., and Siegal, G. P.: Idiopathic pulmonary hemosiderosis: Two cases in a family. *Mayo Clin. Proc.* 53:113, 1978.

45. Seidl, G., Hofner, W., Korn, P., Küster, W., and Stummvoll, H. K.: Das Lungenbild bei genuiner Haemosiderose und Goodpasture-Syndrom. *Radiologe* 17:52, 1977.

46. Dutau, G., Ghisolfi, J., Rochiccioli, P., Boneu, A., Corberand, J. J., and Dalous, A.: Hemosiderose pulmonaire idiopathique. *Pediatrie*, 27:647, 1972.

47. Goodpasture, E. W.: The significance of certain pulmonary lesions in relation to the etiology of influenza. *Am. J. Med. Sci.*, 158:863, 1919.

48. Parkin, T. W., Rusted, I. E., Burchell, H. B., and Edwards, J. E.: Hemorrhagic and interstitial pneumonitis with nephritis. *Am. J. Med.* 18:220, 1955.

49. Freeman, R. M., Vertel, R. M., and Easterling, R. E.: Goodpasture's syndrome: Prolonged survival with chronic hemodialysis. *Arch. Intern. Med.* 117:643, 1966.

50. MacGregor, C. S., Johnson, R. S., and Turk, K. A.: Fatal nephritis complicating idiopathic pulmonary haemosiderosis in young adults. *Thorax* 15:198, 1960.

51. Proskey, A. J., Weatherbee, L., Easterling, R. E., Greene, J. A., Jr., and Weller, J. M.: Goodpasture's syndrome: A report of five cases and review of the literature. *Am. J. Med.* 48:162, 1970.

52. Lange, H. P., and Röttger, P.: Die "Goodpasture-Glomerulonephritis," eine Herdnephritis mit erkennbarer Spezifität. *Virchows Arch.* [*Pathol. Anat.*] 358:61, 1973.

53. Yum, M. N., Lampton, L. M., Bloom, P. M., and Edwards, J. L.: Asymptomatic IgA nephropathy associated with pulmonary hemosiderosis. *Am. J. Med.* 64:1056, 1978.

54. Schöck, V.: Kasuistik: Intermittierende immunesuppressive Behandlung bei idiopathischer Lungenhämosiderose. *Monatsschr. Kinderheilkd.* 122:81, 1974.

55. Allue, X., Wise, M. B., and Beaudry, P. H.: Pulmonary function studies in idiopathic pulmonary hemosiderosis in children. *Am. Rev. Respir. Dis.* 107:410, 1973.

56. Gutteberg, T. J., Moe, P. J., and Noren, C. E.: Diagnosis and therapeutic studies in idiopathic pulmonary hemosiderosis. *Acta Paediatr. Scand.* 68:913, 1979 (short communication).

57. Martinez-Vazquez, J. M., Bernardo, L., Pahissa, A., and Bacardi, R.: Evolución clínico-radiológica de 4 casos de hemasiderosis pulmonar idiopática. *Rev. Clin. Esp.* 148:307, 1978.

58. Carnelli, V., Biraghi, V., Zurlo, M. G., Rossi, M. R., and Parziani, V.: Efficacia della terapia con ciclofosfamide in un caso di emosiderosi polmonare idiopatica. *Minerva Pediatr.* 31:893, 1979.

CHAPTER *50*

The thalassemias

DAVID J. WEATHERALL

Definitions and history

A form of severe anemia occurring early in life and associated with splenomegaly and bone changes was first described by Cooley and Lee in 1925 [1]. The condition was later named *thalassemia*, from θαλασσα, "the sea," since early cases were all of Mediterranean background. It was only after 1940 that the true genetic character of this disorder was fully appreciated. It became clear that the disease described by Cooley and Lee is the homozygous state for a partially dominant autosomal gene, for which the heterozygous state is associated with much milder hematologic changes. The severe homozygous condition became known as *thalassemia major*, while the heterozygous states were designated according to their severity, *thalassemia minor* or *minima* [2–4].

More recently it has been established that thalassemia is not a single disease but a group of disorders, each of which results from an inherited abnormality of globin production [4]. These conditions form part of the spectrum of disorders known collectively as the *hemoglobinopathies*. The latter can be classified broadly into two types. First, there are those, such as sickle cell anemia, which result from an inherited structural alteration in one of the globin chains. Although such abnormal hemoglobins may be synthesized less efficiently or broken down more rapidly than normal adult hemoglobin, the associated clinical abnormalities result from the physical properties of the abnormal hemoglobin. The second major subdivision of the hemoglobinopathies, the thalassemias, results from inherited defects in the rate of synthesis of one or more of the globin chains. This causes ineffective erythropoiesis, hemolysis, and a variable degree of anemia.

Since the structural hemoglobin variants and the thalassemias occur with a high frequency in some populations, the two types of genetic defect may be found in the same individual. The different genetic varieties of thalassemia and their combinations with the genes for abnormal hemoglobins produce a series of disorders known collectively as the *thalassemia syndromes* [4]. There are several monographs and reviews which describe the historical aspects of this subject in detail [2,4,5].

Etiology and pathogenesis

THE GENETIC CONTROL AND SYNTHESIS OF HEMOGLOBIN

The genetic control of hemoglobin structure and the mechanisms which govern its rate of synthesis are reviewed in Chaps. 32 and 37, and only those aspects with particular reference to the thalassemia problem will be restated here.

Human adult hemoglobin is a heterogeneous mixture of proteins consisting of a major component, hemoglobin A, and a minor component, hemoglobin A_2, constituting about 2.5 percent of the total. In intrauterine life, the main hemoglobin is hemoglobin F. The structure of these hemoglobins is similar. Each consists of two separate pairs of identical globin chains. Except for some of the embryonic hemoglobins (see below), all the normal human hemoglobins have one pair of α chains: in hemoglobin A these are combined with β chains ($\alpha_2\beta_2$), in hemoglobin A_2 with δ chains ($\alpha_2\delta_2$), and in hemoglobin F with γ chains ($\alpha_2\gamma_2$).

Human hemoglobin shows further heterogeneity, particularly in fetal life, and this has important implications for an understanding of the thalassemias and for possible approaches to the prenatal diagnosis of these disorders. Hemoglobin F is a mixture of molecular species with the formulas $\alpha_2\gamma_2^{136\text{Gly}}$ and $\alpha_2\gamma_2^{136\text{Ala}}$. The γ chains containing glycine as position 136 are designated $^G\gamma$ *chains*, and those which contain alanine at this position are called $^A\gamma$ *chains* [6]. At birth the ratio of molecules containing $^G\gamma$ chains to those containing $^A\gamma$ chains

is about 3:1; this ratio varies widely in the trace amounts of Hb F present in normal adults.

Before the eighth week of intrauterine life there are three embryonic hemoglobins present, hemoglobins Gower 1 ($\zeta_2\epsilon_2$), Gower 2 ($\alpha_2\epsilon_2$), and Portland ($\zeta_2\gamma_2$). The ζ and ϵ chains are the embryonic counterparts of the adult α and β and γ and δ chains, respectively [7–9]. ζ-Chain synthesis persists beyond the embryonic stage of development in some of the α thalassemias; so far, persistent ϵ-chain production has not been found in any of the thalassemia syndromes.

During fetal development there is an orderly switch from ζ- to α- and ϵ- to γ-chain production, followed by β-and δ- chain production after birth [7]. β-Chain synthesis is activated by about the eighth week of intrauterine life, and hemoglobin A makes up about 10 percent of the total hemoglobin from the eighth to the thirty-fourth week, after which β-chain synthesis increases and γ-chain synthesis gradually declines. The switch from γ- to β-chain production is synchronized throughout all the fetal organs [10], and the early activation of the β-chain locus offers an opportunity for the intrauterine diagnosis of disorders of β-chain production (see "Prevention," below).

Pedigree analyses have shown that the α- and non-α-globin genes are genetically unlinked. Furthermore, these studies indicate that there are two α-globin genes per haploid genome and that the non-α genes lie in a linked cluster in the order $^G\gamma$-$^A\gamma$-δ-β [4]. These observations have been confirmed by restriction endonuclease analysis [11,12]. Somatic-cell fusion analyses using human and mouse fibroblasts have provided unequivocal evidence that the two α-globin genes are on chromosome 16 and that the γ-δ-β gene cluster is on chromosome 11 [13,14]. The organization of the genetic control of human hemoglobin is summarized in Fig. 50-1.

The fine structure and arrangement of the α-like and β-like globin genes have been analyzed using recombinant clones of genomic DNA [11,12] (see Fig. 32-3). The linked α genes lie "upstream" from an inactive α-globin locus ($\psi\alpha$) and two ζ-chain loci. The linked δ and β loci are separated from the $^G\gamma$ and $^A\gamma$ loci by 13.9 kilobases (kb), which contain a β-like gene called $\psi\beta1$. The ϵ loci lie 13.3 kb to the left of the γ loci. The loci designated $\psi\alpha$, $\psi\beta1$, and $\psi\beta2$ are pseudogenes; i.e., they have sequence homology with the α and β genes but have mutations that prevent their expression. It is possible that they represent evolutionary remnants of what may have once been functional loci. An unexpected outcome of these gene-mapping studies has been that the hemoglobin genes, like most other mammalian genes that have been analyzed in this way to date, contain one or more noncoding inserts or intervening sequences (*introns*) at the same position along their length. Thus the β, γ, δ, and ϵ genes each contain two introns of 122 to 130 and 850 to 900 base pairs between codons 30 and 31 and 104 and 105, respectively [11,12]. Similar, although smaller, noncoding segments occur in the mouse and human α-globin genes.

FIGURE 50-1   The genetic control of human hemoglobin.

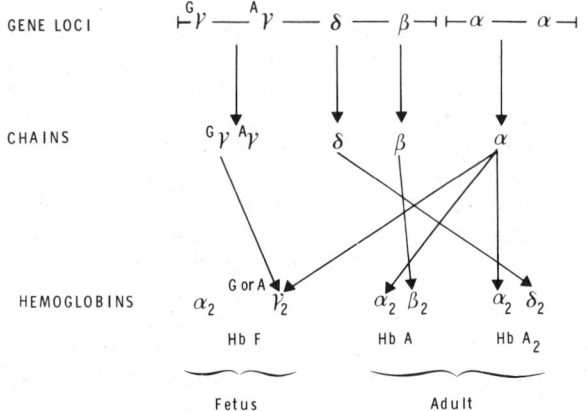

TABLE 50-1   The main forms of β thalassemia*

β-Thalassemia type	Homozygote	Heterozygote	Molecular defect
β^0	Thalassemia major Hb A absent Hb F 97–98% Hb A$_2$ 1–3%	Thalassemia trait Hb A$_2$ 3.5–7% Hb F 0.5–3%	Heterogeneous Partial gene deletions Premature chain termination Defective splicing of β mRNA
β^+ (severe)	Thalassemia major Hb F 60–90% Hb A$_2$ 1–5% Hb A present	As above	Heterogeneous Defective transcription of β mRNA Defective splicing of β mRNA
β^+ (mild; Negro)	Thalassemia intermedia Hb F 30–60% Hb A$_2$ 2–6%	As above	Unknown
β^+ (normal Hb A$_2$ type 1; "silent" β thalassemia)	Thalassemia intermedia Hb F 15–25% Hb A$_2$ 4–6%	Normal blood picture and Hb A$_2$ level	Unknown
β^+ or β^0 (normal Hb A$_2$ type 2)†	Not described	Thalassemia trait Normal Hb A$_2$ level	Unknown

* The other less well defined varieties such as the Ferrara and Dutch forms are described in the text.
†These conditions may represent the heterozygous states for either β^+ or β^0 thalassemia in association with δ-thalassemia determinants.

The complete sequences of the five non-α-globin genes and the two α genes have now been determined and compared with those of other mammals [15–18]. Some interesting homologies have been found. At the 5' side of the β genes there are two blocks of sequence homology which are present at analogous positions in many eukaryotic genes [15]. The first is AT-rich (A = adenine; T = thymine), a sequence originally found in the histone-gene cluster of *Drosophila* and called the *Hogness box*. The second region of homology, called the *CCAAT box* (C = cytosine), is found about 70 base pairs to the 5' end of the gene. These regions may be involved in transcription initiation or RNA processing, or both. Another unexpected finding arising from these structural studies is that in the gene clusters there are nonglobin repeat sequences, some of which are reiterated up to 300,000 times in the total human genome. Their function is unknown.

The first step in the production of globin messenger RNA (mRNA) is the transcription of the entire coding and noncoding sequences in the form of a giant RNA precursor molecule that belongs to the general class of RNAs called *heterogeneous nuclear RNA* (HnRNA) [4,11,12]. This initial precursor molecule is then modified at its 5' end by establishing a 5'ppp5' linkage through TTP to form a so-called CAP structure, and at the 3' end by attaching a string of adenylic acid residues [poly(A)]. The noncoding intervening sequences (introns) are then removed by successive excision and ligation reactions (splicing), and the coding parts of the molecule (exons) are joined together to form the mature mRNA. The structures of all the globin mRNAs have now been determined in detail.

There is increasing evidence that during its time in the nucleus and for much of its time in the cytoplasm,

HnRNA and mRNA are associated with various protein molecules which may serve to stabilize and protect them from nuclease attack. The interaction of these proteins with RNA may be of considerable importance in the regulation of RNA metabolism.

The processes of globin-chain initiation, elongation, and termination seem to follow the general patterns of protein synthesis in other cells (see Chap. 32). Each of the steps in globin synthesis has been analyzed in detail in both normal and thalassemic individuals (see later section). Heme is synthesized in an independent pathway, and it is probably inserted into its pocket in the globin chains while they are still on the ribosomes or immediately after release. Once the synthesis of the chains is complete, they associate with partner chains to form a stable tetramer.

Virtually nothing is known about the regulation of human hemoglobin synthesis or about the factors involved in the switch from fetal to adult hemoglobin production during development. Several recent reviews deal with these problems in detail [4,7,19,20].

The preceding account of the molecular genetics of hemoglobin indicates that there are many levels at which a genetic defect might operate to reduce the output of a globin gene.

THE DIFFERENT FORMS OF THALASSEMIA

Thalassemias are classified according to which globin chain (or chains) is synthesized at a reduced rate [4]. The main subtypes which have now been defined with certainty are the α, β, δβ, δ, and γδβ thalassemias.

The β thalassemias (Table 50-1) are characterized by persistent synthesis of fetal hemoglobin beyond the neonatal period (Fig. 50-2). They can be divided into

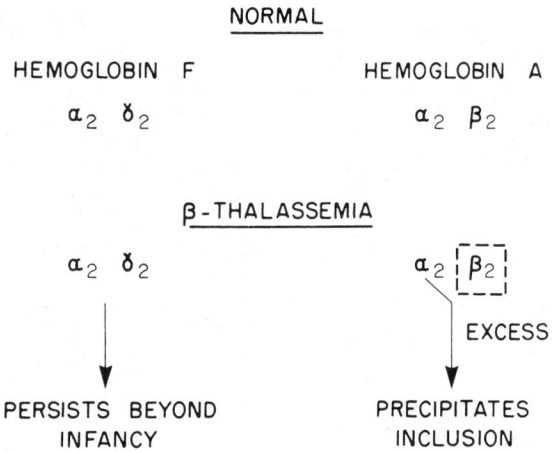

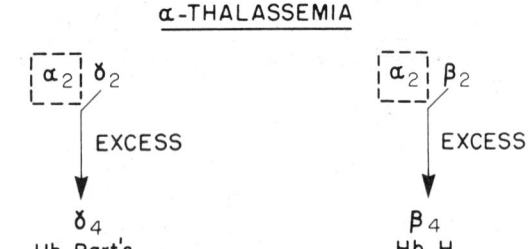

FIGURE 50-2   **The main groups of thalassemias with their pathophysiologic mechanisms.**

two main varieties: in one form there is a total absence of β-chain production, β^0 thalassemia, and in the other there is a partial deficiency of β-chain production, β^+ thalassemia. β^+ thalassemia is further subdivided into the common type, in which there is an elevated level of hemoglobin A_2 in heterozygotes, and a series of less-common forms, in which heterozygotes have normal

TABLE 50-2   **Inherited disorders of δ- and β- chain production.**

Hemoglobin Lepore:
  Hb Lepore Boston $(\delta\beta)^+$
  Hb Lepore Baltimore $(\delta\beta)^+$
  Hb Lepore Hollandia $(\delta\beta)^+$
  ?Others with same charge as Hb A or A_2
δβ Thalassemia:
  $^G\gamma^A\gamma$ $(\delta\beta)^0$ thalassemia
  $^G\gamma^A\gamma$ $(\delta\beta)^0$ thalassemia (Sardinian type)
  $^G\gamma$ $(\delta\beta)^0$ thalassemia
  ?Other δβ or γδβ thalassemias with partial or total suppression of δβ-chain synthesis without increased Hb F
$^G\gamma^A\gamma$ and $^G\gamma$ hereditary persistence of fetal hemoglobin:
  Classified in Table 50-7

NOTE: The whole group of δβ-chain production defects form a continuum of conditions, the clinical severity of which seems to depend mainly on the degree of compensation by γ-chain synthesis.
SOURCE: Weatherall and Clegg [4].

levels of hemoglobin A_2. In addition, there are some rare variants of β^+ and β^0 thalassemia associated with unusually high levels of hemoglobin F in heterozygotes. Both β^+ and β^0 thalassemia are extremely heterogeneous at the molecular level.

The δβ thalassemias are also heterogeneous (Table 50-2). In some cases, no δ or β chains are synthesized. These disorders can be subdivided according to the structure of the hemoglobin F which is produced into $^G\gamma^A\gamma(\delta\beta)^0$ and $^G\gamma(\delta\beta)^0$ thalassemia. In other forms of δβ thalassemia, an abnormal hemoglobin is produced which has normal α chains combined with non-α chains that consist of the N-terminal residues of the δ chain fused to the C-terminal residues of the β chain. These fusion variants, called the *Lepore hemoglobins,* also show structural heterogeneity.

The δ thalassemias are characterized by a reduced output of δ chains with reduced levels of hemoglobin A_2 in heterozygotes and an absence of hemoglobin A_2 in homozygotes. They are of no clinical significance.

A disorder characterized by defective γ-, δ-, and β-chain synthesis has been defined at the clinical and molecular level. This condition, γδβ *thalassemia,* is associated with neonatal anemia and the clinical picture of heterozygous β thalassemia with normal hemoglobin A_2 levels in adult life.

Since α chains are present in both fetal and adult hemoglobins, a deficiency of α-chain production will affect hemoglobin synthesis in fetal as well as in adult life (Fig. 50-2). A reduced rate of α-chain synthesis in fetal life results in an excess of γ chains, which form γ_4 tetramers or hemoglobin Bart's. In adult life, a deficiency of α chains results in an excess of β chains, which form β_4 tetramers or hemoglobin H. At least three groups of α-thalassemia determinants have been defined (Table 50-3). These are α^0 thalassemia (also called α thalassemia 1), in which no α chains are produced; α^+ thalassemia (also called α thalassemia 2), in which there is a reduced output of α chains; and hemoglobin Constant Spring and related abnormal hemoglobins, structural variants which are associated with a reduced output of α chains. The interaction of these three different α-thalassemia determinants produces the different clinical forms of α thalassemia. Each of these types of α thalassemia is heterogeneous at the molecular level.

Since it is possible to inherit genes for α or β thalassemia together with those for α- or β-globin-chain structural variants, the thalassemia syndromes are made up of a bewilderingly complex series of different genetic entities.

THE MOLECULAR BASIS OF THE THALASSEMIAS

Knowledge about the molecular defects in thalassemia has stemmed largely from the introduction of technology, such as that devised for the isolation and assay of human mRNA, the use of complementary DNA (cDNA) copies of mRNA for demonstrating the presence or absence of gene loci and determining levels of mRNA in thalassemic cells, and the use of restriction enzyme analysis and recombinant DNA technology to investigate the structure of the globin genes in detail.

THE β, $\delta\beta$, AND $\gamma\delta\beta$ THALASSEMIAS (Tables 50-1 and 50-2)

β^+ thalassemia β-Chain initiation, elongation, and termination are normal in some of these disorders [4]. β^+-Thalassemic reticulocytes have a reduced activity of β-chain mRNA [21,22], and this is due to a reduction in the amount of β-chain mRNA rather than reduced activity of normal amounts of β-chain mRNA [23–25]. In some cases the reduced amount of β-chain mRNA may result from a defect in processing of the nuclear mRNA precursor [26,27]. The entire β-globin genes and their flanking regions from two patients with β^+ thalassemia have been completely sequenced and a single base change has been found in the small intervening sequence. This change may have created a new splice site and interfere with posttranscriptional processing of β-globin mRNA precursors [28,29]. β^+ thalassemia may also result from single base substitutions in the regulatory regions to the left of the β genes; presumably these interfere with initiation of transcription [193].

β^0 thalassemia   There is no β-globin-chain synthesis in the reticulocytes of patients with β^0 thalassemia, and globin mRNA isolated from these cells promotes no detectable β-chain synthesis in a cell-free system [30,31]. Using the technique of cDNA/DNA hybridization, it has been found that the β-globin genes are intact in this disorder [32], but using cDNA/RNA hybridization, it has been found that in some cases there is no detectable β-chain mRNA while in others inactive β-chain mRNA can be demonstrated [34,35]. These studies indicate that the β^0 thalassemias are heterogeneous at the molecular level.

In most cases, globin-gene mapping shows no abnormalities of the globin genes of patients with β^0 thalassemia. An exception has been found in DNA obtained from several Afro-Asian patients. Although these individuals all appeared to be homozygous for β^0 thalassemia, in fact, they were compound heterozygotes for a β^0 thalassemia determinant associated with a normal β-globin gene map and one in which there was a 0.6-kb deletion at the 3' end of the β-globin gene [36,37]. In one patient [38], the deletion removed the terminal third of the large intron, the entire 3' coding block, and about 150 bases past the end (upstream) of the β-globin gene. This small group of β^0 thalassemics are the only patients in whom any major structural abnormality of the β-globin genes has been found by restriction endonuclease mapping.

Another type of molecular defect underlying β^0 thalassemia has been defined in a Chinese patient. Determining the nucleotide sequence of the non-functional β-globin mRNA revealed that the AAG codon for lysine at position $\beta17$ had changed to the chain-termination codon UAG, leading to premature chain termination

TABLE 50-3   General classification of α thalassemia

α^0 Thalassemia
α^+ Thalassemia:
Deletion
Nondeletion
Chain-termination mutations

with the production of a short, 16-residue N-terminal fragment of the β chain [39]. These findings were confirmed by translating the defective β-globin mRNA in a cell-free system using a UAG tyrosine suppressor tRNA; full-length β-globin chains were synthesized [40]. It seemed likely that further "nonsense" mutations of this type would be defined, since there are 25 different single-base mutations in the β-globin gene which could result in the production of new termination codons [41]. Recently this prediction has been proved correct [193].

Finally, there is a form of β^0 thalassemia which occurs in the Ferrara region of Italy in which it appears that β-globin mRNA is present but β-globin chain synthesis occurs only in the presence of a factor obtained from a soluble cell fraction from normal cells [42,43]. This condition has not been found in any other racial group, and these findings still require confirmation.

In summary, although the DNA of many patients with β^0 thalassemia has been analyzed by restriction endonuclease mapping, to date only a small group of Afro-Asian patients have been found to have a β-globin gene deletion. A premature chain-termination mutation has been found in the β-globin mRNA of one Chinese patient. In the majority of β^0 thalassemias, the underlying molecular defect awaits clarification. There is some very recent evidence that some of these conditions may result from nucleotide changes in the splice junction of the large intron [194] or in the TATA box to the left of the β globin gene [195].

The $\delta\beta$ thalassemias   Soluble hybridization analysis of DNA prepared from $^G\gamma^A\gamma$ $\delta\beta$ thalassemia homozygotes has shown that there is a major deletion involving the δ- and β-globin genes [44,45]. These findings have been confirmed and extended by globin gene-mapping analysis, which shows that this disorder results from a gene deletion which leaves the 5' end of the δ-globin gene intact but extends right through the β-globin gene and some distance beyond its 3' end [46–48]. $^G\gamma$ $\delta\beta$ thalassemia is heterogeneous at the molecular level. In DNA from a Turkish $^G\gamma$ $\delta\beta$ thalassemia homozygote there is a long deletion involving the δ-,β- , and $^A\gamma$-globin genes [49]. $^G\gamma$ $\delta\beta$ thalassemia can also result from a major disruption of the γ-δ-β–globin gene cluster comprising an inversion of most of the DNA between the δ and $^A\gamma$ genes together with two deletions involving the $^A\gamma$ and the δ and β genes [50]. It seems, therefore, that at least some of the $\delta\beta$ thalassemias have arisen from a series of deletions and inversions involving the γ-δ-β–globin gene cluster (Fig. 50-3), or from frame-shift mutations in the β-globin gene exons [193].

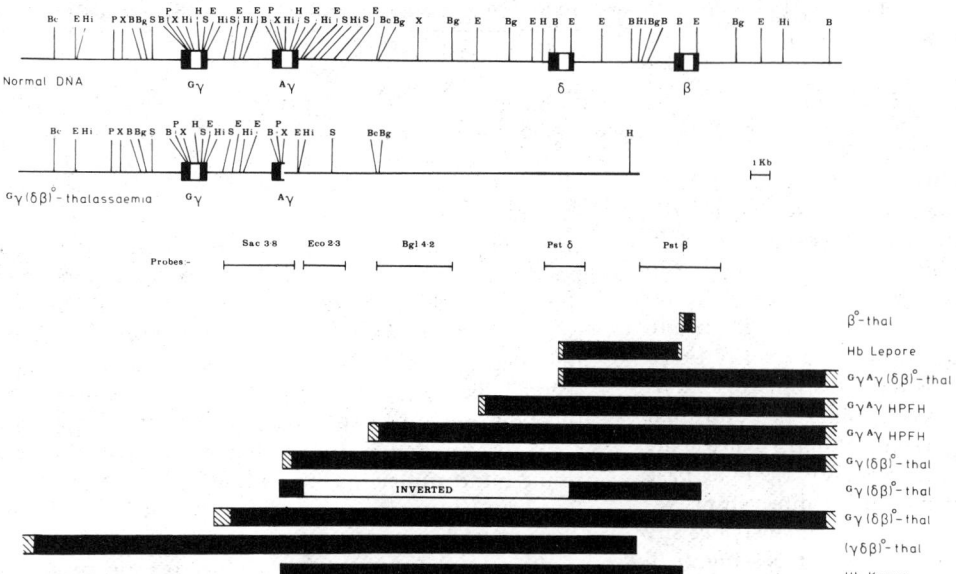

FIGURE 50-3   Some of the different deletions and inversions responsible for δβ thalassemia and hereditary persistence of fetal hemoglobin. The upper part of the figure shows the various restriction sites and the position of the probes which were used to define the inversion responsible for one form of ᴳγ δβ thalassemia [50].

The Lepore hemoglobins consist of normal α chains combined with δβ chains. It is thought that the latter are the product of δβ fusion genes which have arisen by unequal crossing-over between the δ- and β-globin loci during meiosis [51–53]. The Lepore hemoglobins show structural heterogeneity which depends on the precise site of the normal crossing-over (Figs. 50-4 and 16-3 and 16-4). Three variants, Lepore Washington [53], Hollandia [54], and Baltimore [55], have been defined. The δβ fusion chains are inefficiently synthesized, at least in part because of instability of δβ-globin mRNA [56]. Hence the Lepore hemoglobins are associated with the clinical phenotype of δβ thalassemia.

The abnormal crossing-over which gives rise to the Lepore hemoglobins also produces a chromosome which, in addition to having normal δ- and β-globin-chain loci, contains a δβ fusion gene (Fig. 50-4). The products of the latter combine with α chains to produce anti-Lepore hemoglobins, such as hemoglobins Miyada and P Congo [57,58]. Although these variants are not as-

FIGURE 50-4   The mechanisms for the production of the Lepore hemoglobins and hemoglobin Kenya.

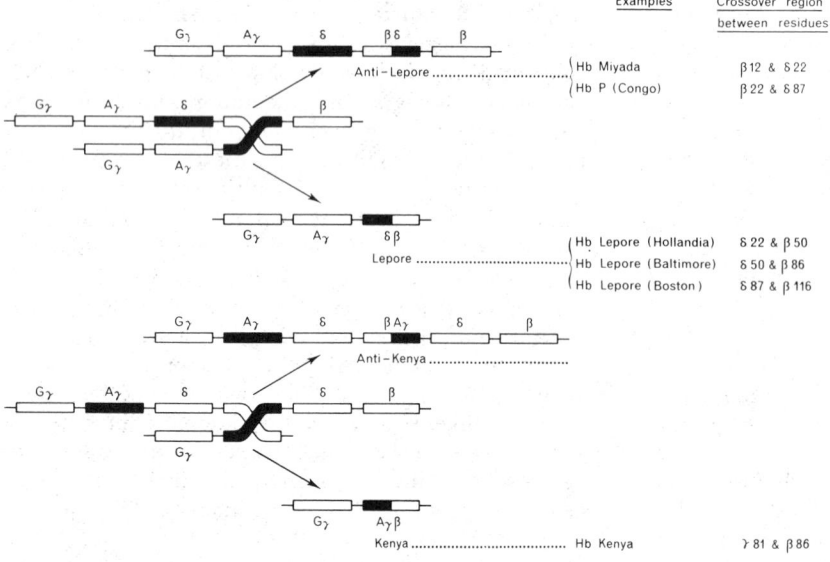

sociated with the clinical phenotype of thalassemia, the $\beta\delta$ fusion gene seems to reduce the capacity for increasing the output of the β-globin genes *in cis*, i.e., on the same chromosome. Thus, if an individual inherits an anti-Lepore hemoglobin from one parent and a β-thalassemia gene from the other, she or he would have more globin-chain imbalance than occurs in heterozygous β thalassemia alone [59].

$\gamma\delta\beta$ *thalassemia*   The molecular basis for this condition is a long deletion involving both the $^{G}\gamma$ and $^{A}\gamma$ loci and the δ locus [60]. The β locus may be intact, and yet affected individuals have a marked reduction in β-chain production. It appears that a long deletion "upstream" from the β locus can affect its output without altering its structure.

THE α THALASSEMIAS

Both α^0 thalassemia (α thalassemia 1) and α^+ thalassemia (α thalassemia 2) are due to a very heterogeneous series of molecular defects which cause correspondingly heterogeneous clinical disorders, i.e., the hemoglobin Bart's hydrops syndrome and hemoglobin H disease.

Nomenclature   It is difficult to formulate a suitable nomenclature for all the different molecular forms of α thalassemia. The most convenient approach is to describe these disorders by their particular haplotype. Normal individuals have two α genes per haploid genome, and hence their α-globin gene haplotype is written $\alpha\alpha/$, and their full genotype is $\alpha\alpha/\alpha\alpha$. Deletion of one or both α-globin genes gives the haplotyes $-\alpha/$ or $--/$, respectively. Sometimes there is a partial deletion of an α-globin gene together with a complete deletion of the other. Because on gene mapping these partially deleted and nonfunctional genes produce a band or bands with an α-globin gene probe, they have been called *dysfunctional α-globin genes* and are represented as (α). Finally, some types of α thalassemia are associated with no gene deletions. Since it is uncertain whether the activity of one or both of the linked α-chain loci is depressed, these disorders are represented as $\alpha\alpha^T$.

α^0-*Thalassemia determinants* (Table 50-4)   The α^0-thalassemia determinant results from the loss of both the linked α-globin genes on chromosome 16 [61,62]. The extent of these deletions has been determined by restriction endonuclease analysis of DNA from homozygotes for α^0 thalassemia or from individuals with hemoglobin H disease.

The two α genes are linked to two ζ genes with an inactive α locus, the $\psi\alpha$ gene, in between (see Fig. 34-3). The deletion which causes the α^0-thalassemia phenotype in Southeast Asian (SEA) patients involves both the α-globin genes but leaves both ζ genes intact [63]. However, the α^0-thalassemia determinant in Mediterranean (MED) populations results from a deletion of about 17.4 kb, which involves both α-globin genes, the $\psi\alpha$ gene, and the 3′ ζ-globin gene [63–65]. These deletions

TABLE 50-4   The α^0-thalassemia haplotypes

The approximate size of the deletions (in kilobases) is shown for each variety. SEA denotes Southeast Asian and MED denotes Mediterranean patients. The dysfunctional forms (α) are the result of deletions which leave part of one α-globin gene intact. It is likely that the homozygous state for the $-(\alpha)^{25}/$ lesion is incompatible with fetal survival; that for the other three defects causes the hemoglobin Bart's hydrops syndrome.

Normal haplotype:
$\alpha\alpha/$
Complete deletions
$--^{SEA17.5}/$
$--^{MED17.4}/$
Partial deletions (dysfunctional)
$-(\alpha)^{5.2}/$
$-(\alpha)^{25}/$

are represented as $--^{SEA}/$ and $--^{MED}/$. Another variety of deletion of about 5.2 kb which involves the loss of a piece of one α-globin gene and all of the other has been found in the Mediterranean population [66]. This deletion starts within the 3′ (right hand) α gene and extends downstream to involve the 5′ gene but not the two ζ genes. Finally, there is yet another deletion of about 25 kb which starts at codon 57 of the 5′ α-globin gene, extends right through the 3′ gene, and involves the $\psi\alpha$ gene and both ζ-globin genes [66,67]. These different deletions are illustrated in Fig. 50-5.

It seems likely that these different-sized deletions of the α-globin genes have resulted from unequal crossing-over similar to that which is responsible for the Lepore hemoglobins (see above). The precise determination of the site of crossing-over will require detailed analysis of the affected regions of the genome obtained by cloning of DNA fragments from appropriate patients.

α^+ *thalassemia* (Table 50-5)   The α^+ thalassemias can result either from loss of one of the linked α-globin-chain genes, from nondeletion defects which involve either one or both of the linked genes, or from globin-chain termination mutations.

If the normal α-globin-gene haplotype (i.e., gene complement on a single chromosome) is written $\alpha\alpha$, the deletion of a single α-globin gene can be written $-\alpha$ [68,69]. Gene-mapping analysis has shown that at least two different molecular events have given rise to the deletion forms of α^+ thalassemia. The commonest seems to have been unequal crossing-over between misaligned α-globin genes, which has resulted in the loss of parts of both the 5′ and 3′ genes (3.7 kb in all) with the production of a single α gene [66,70] (Fig. 50-6). In some Chinese α^+-thalassemia carriers, the crossover seems to have involved loss of 4.2 kb, including all of the 5′ α-globin gene [70]. A consequence of unequal crossing-over between mispaired α-chain genes is that one of the chromosomes produced should have three α genes on it, just as the anti-Lepore chromosome has three non-α

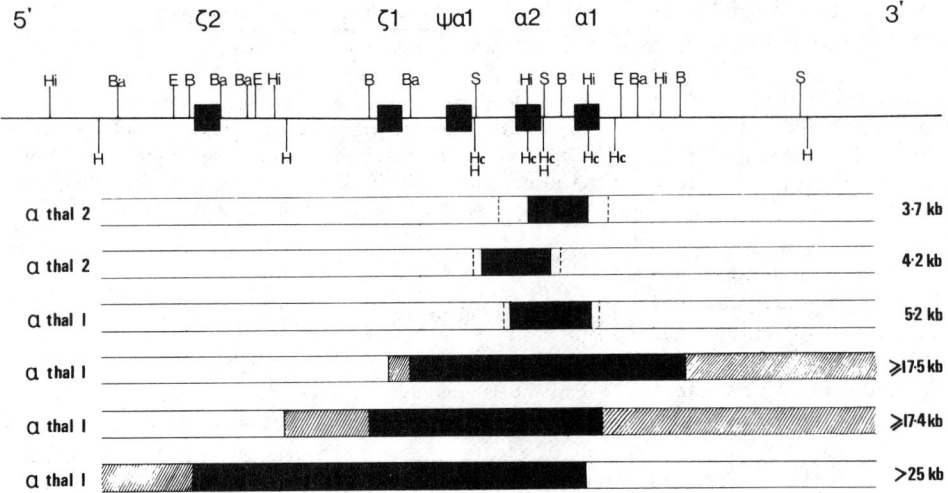

FIGURE 50-5   Some deletions responsible for the α^0 (α thal 1) and α^+ (α thal 2) thalassemias.

genes (Fig. 50-6). Examples of the $\alpha\alpha\alpha/$ haplotype have been discovered [71,72]. The clinical consequences of having five α-globin genes, i.e., chromosomes with the arrangement $\alpha\alpha$ and $\alpha\alpha\alpha$, seem to be minimal.

The nondeletion α^+ thalassemias are characterised by a reduced output of α-globin chains and α-globin mRNA in the presence of two intact α-globin genes. At least three types have been defined which vary in the relative reduction of α-globin mRNA output [73]. The molecular basis for nondeletion α thalassemia is still uncertain, although at least one form appears to result from pentanucleotide (TGAGG) deletion within the 5' splice

junction of the α2-globin gene [174] and another from a single base change in the α2 gene which gives rise to a highly unstable α chain [196].

Hemoglobin Constant Spring   Hemoglobin Constant Spring has an elongated α chain with 31 extra residues attached to the C-terminal end. The first of these additional residues is glutamine at position 142. This finding suggested that hemoglobin Constant Spring might have arisen from a single-base change in the terminating codon, normally UAA, to CAA, which codes for glutamine [75,76]. Thus the α chain, instead of ending at

FIGURE 50-6   The abnormal crossover responsible for the production of the deletion form of α^+ thalassemia and a chromosome carrying three α-globin genes. The positions of the various restriction enzyme sites which are used to map the α-globin genes and to determine the site of these crossovers are shown.

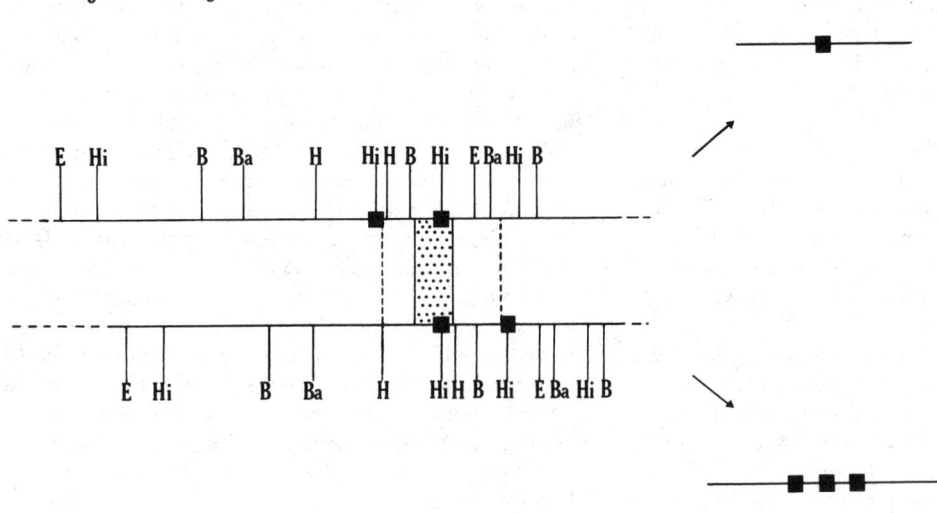

TABLE 50-5 The α^+-thalassemia haplotypes and main hematologic features

Haplotype	Homozygous state	Heterozygous state
Normal:		
$\alpha\alpha/$	Normal	Normal
Deletion:		
$-\alpha^{3.7}/$	Thalassemia trait 5–10% Hb Bart's at birth	Normal blood picture 0–2% Hb Bart's at birth
$-\alpha^{4.2}/$	—	—
Nondeletion:		
$\alpha\alpha^{T(LM)}/$	?Thalassemia trait ?10–20% Hb Bart's at birth	?Normal blood picture ~ 5% Hb Bart's at birth
$\alpha\alpha^{T(LM, Saudi)}/$	Hemoglobin H disease	
$\alpha\alpha^{T(HM)}/$	—	—
Chain termination:		
$\alpha^{CS}\alpha/$	Mild hemolytic anemia 6–7% Constant Spring	Normal blood picture 1–2% Hb Bart's at birth 0.5% Hb Constant Spring
$\alpha^{Ic}\alpha/$	—	Normal blood picture 0.5% Hb Icaria
$\alpha^{KD}\alpha/$	—	Normal blood picture 0.5% Hb Koya Dora
$\alpha^{SR}\alpha/$	—	Normal blood picture 0.5% Hb Seal Rock

NOTE: The size of the deletions is shown in kilobases. The nondeletion forms ($\alpha\alpha^T$) are divided into low (LM) and high (HM) α-globin messenger RNA varieties. The molecular base for one form of HM variety has been determined recently [196]. The Saudi Arabian form seems to be a specific entity. The chain-termination mutants are classified according to the associated elongated α-chain variant, i.e., CS = Constant Spring, Ic = Icaria, KD = Koya Dora, and SR = Seal Rock.

position 141, has glutamine at position 142. In addition it appears that there is mRNA after the terminating codon which is not normally translated. In the case of hemoglobin Constant Spring this is translated until another stop codon is reached. This hypothesis has gained strong support from the discovery of hemoglobin Wayne [77], which also has an elongated α chain but which appears to have resulted from a frame-shift mutation. The UAA → CAA change apparently involves the 5' (α2) gene, as deduced from the fact that the sequence of the 3' untranslated regions of the α1 and α2 genes are different [193].

A single-base change in the codon UAA could result in other amino acid substitutions, and the model for the production of hemoglobin Constant Spring predicted that there would be other hemoglobin variants with different substitutions at position 142 but with the same additional amino acid residues in their elongated α chains [75,76]. This prediction has been borne out by the discovery of hemoglobins Icaria [78], Koya Dora [79], and Seal Rock [80]. A summary of the substitutions in these chain-terminating mutant hemoglobins and other theoretical variants of this type which remain to be discovered is given in Fig. 50-7.

It is still not clear why the chain-termination mutant hemoglobins are synthesized slowly. The αCS chains are synthesized only in nucleated red cells, and there is no synthesis at the reticulocyte stage of development [75,76]. This suggests that the αCS mRNA is relatively unstable, possibly because parts of the mRNA at the

usually untranslated 3' end are translated in the case of the αCS mRNA. This may alter its stability, possibly by affecting its steric properties.

Interactions of the different molecular forms of α thalassemia It has been estimated recently that there are at least 105 possible α-thalassemia genotypes which could arise from interactions of the determinants defined so

FIGURE 50-7 The chain-termination mutant hemoglobins in man. Of the theoretical single-base substitutions in a chain-terminating codon, UAA, hemoglobins Constant Spring (CS), Koya Dora, Icaria, and Seal Rock have already been discovered. One substitution would produce hemoglobin A, since it would be another terminating codon, and two substitutions remain to be discovered.

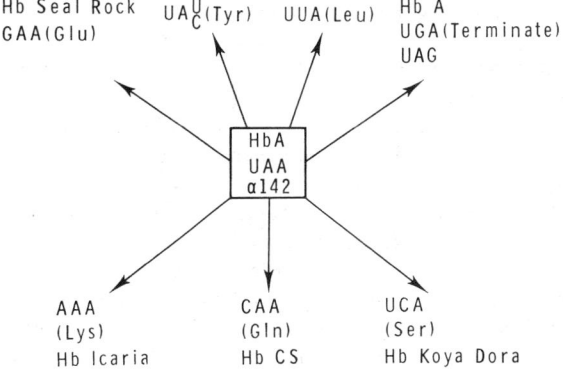

TABLE 50-6   Some hemoglobin H disease genotypes.

α^0-Thalassemia interactions	Dysfunctional α-thalassemia interactions
$-\,-^{\text{SEA}}/-\alpha^{3.7}*$	$-(\alpha)^{5.2}/-\alpha^{3.7}*$
$-\,-^{\text{SEA}}/-\alpha^{4.2}*$	$-(\alpha)^{25}/-\alpha^{3.7}*$
$-\,-^{\text{MED}}/-\alpha^{3.7}*$	$-(\alpha)^{25}/-\alpha^{4.2}$
$-\,-^{\text{SEA}}/\alpha\alpha^{\text{T(LM)}}*$	$-(\alpha)^{25}/\alpha\alpha^{\text{T(LM)}}$
$-\,-^{\text{SEA}}/\alpha\alpha^{\text{T(HM)}}*$	$-(\alpha)^{25}/\alpha\alpha^{\text{T(HM)}}$
$-\,-^{\text{SEA}}/\alpha^{\text{CS}}\alpha*$	
$-\,-^{\text{MED}}/\alpha\alpha^{\text{T(LM)}}*$	
$-\,-^{\text{MED}}/\alpha\alpha^{\text{T(HM)}}$	
$\alpha\alpha^{\text{T(LM, Saudi)}}/\alpha\alpha^{\text{T(LM, Saudi)}}*$	

NOTE: The various haplotypes are defined in Tables 50-4 and 50-5.
*Already encountered; the remainder are potential genotypes.

far. To date, about 30 of these have been encountered [73].

The homozygous state for the different forms of α^0 thalassemia results in the hemoglobin Bart's hydrops syndrome, a disorder in which there is a complete absence of α-chain production. Presumably, affected fetuses survive because they produce ζ chains, thus allowing them to synthesize hemoglobin Portland ($\zeta_2\gamma_2$). Unlike hemoglobin Bart's, this hemoglobin shows normal heme/heme interaction. Hence it appears that when there is a major deletion involving the α-globin genes, ζ-chain synthesis persists beyond the embryonic stage of development, thus allowing affected fetuses to survive nearly until term. Presumably, the α^0 thalassemias, caused by the longer deletions which remove both the α- and ζ-globin loci, are incompatible with survival in their homozygous states [63,64].

Hemoglobin H disease results from a variety of different interactions (Table 50-6). The commonest and best defined, is the interaction between α^0 thalassemia and α^+ thalassemia [4,66,81]. Affected individuals inherit one chromosome 16 with no α-globin genes ($-\,-/$) and another with a single α-globin gene ($-\alpha/$; their genotype is thus $-\,-/-\alpha$. Hemoglobin H disease can also result from the inheritance of an α^0-thalassemia determinant from one parent and a nondeletion α-thalassemia determinant from the other ($-\,-/\alpha\alpha^{\text{T}}$) [73,82]. It can also result from the inheritance of α^0 thalassemia together with hemoglobin Constant Spring ($-\,-/\alpha^{\text{CS}}\alpha$) [76] and, in certain Saudi Arabian populations, from the homozygous state for a more severe form of nondeletion α thalassemia ($\alpha\alpha^{\text{T}}/\alpha\alpha^{\text{T}}$) [83] (Table 50-6).

Clearly, the clinical spectrum of the different α-thalassemia interactions will depend very much on the types of determinants present in any particular population. For example, the hemoglobin Bart's hydrops syndrome and hemoglobin H disease will be very rare in populations in which the α^0-thalassemia determinants do not occur at a high frequency, such as in West African populations. Individuals of this racial background who are apparently α^0-thalassemia heterozygotes are, in fact, homozygotes for the deletion form of α^+ thalassemia ($-\alpha/-\alpha$) [68,69]. The hematologic findings in persons who have two missing α-globin genes are the same whether the missing loci are on the same chromosome ($-\,-/\alpha\alpha$) or on different chromosomes ($-\alpha/-\alpha$).

Gene-mapping analysis has also clarified some of the interactions between α thalassemia and α-chain hemoglobin variants. For example, it has been found that at least one form of hemoglobin Q is due to a mutation of an α-chain gene which is on a chromosome in which the other α-chain locus is deleted ($-\alpha^{\text{Q}}$). Thus individuals who inherit this chromosome from one parent and an α^0-thalassemia determinant from the other have hemoglobin QH disease ($-\,-/-\alpha^{\text{Q}}$), in which the hemoglobin consists of Q and H only, with no hemoglobin A [84,85].

THE PATHOPHYSIOLOGY OF THE ANEMIA OF THE THALASSEMIAS

β THALASSEMIA

In vitro studies of globin-chain synthesis in β thalassemia have clarified the mechanism of the anemia of this disorder [88–90]. In all patients studied, α-chain synthesis exceeds severalfold that of the combined synthesis of β, γ, and δ chains (Fig. 50-8). This suggests that an excess of free α chains is released into the red cells of patients with β thalassemia. In some experiments, β-chain synthesis appears to be completely deficient, only hemoglobins F and A_2 and free α chain being synthesized [90]. Similar studies on the cells of patients with hemoglobin E thalassemia and sickle cell thalassemia [90] confirm that these disorders are of two types: those in which hemoglobin A is produced and those in which there is a total deficiency of β chains. These correspond to β^+ thalassemia and β^0 thalassemia, respectively.

Free α chains can be isolated from the cells of patients with β thalassemia [89,90]. Excess α chains are unstable and almost certainly give rise to the inclusion bodies found in the red cell precursors in this disorder.

Thalassemic erythrocytes have several well-defined metabolic abnormalities. The membrane is more permeable to potassium, and there is a reduced ability to regenerate ATP [91,92]. This "leakiness" of the red cell membrane has also been found in patients with various unstable hemoglobin disorders, such as hemoglobin Köln. It seems probable that the inclusion bodies resulting from the precipitated α chains are in some way responsible for this change in membrane physiology. Probably damage results from mechanical trauma as the inclusion bodies are "pitted out" of the red cells during passage through the splenic sinusoids. Membrane damage might also be caused by lipid peroxidation resulting from free-radical generation in red cells which are poorly hemoglobinized, contain excess iron, and are exposed to oxidant stress caused by hemoglobin subunit precipitation [93]. The abnormal membrane function occurs to a greater degree in cell populations with greatest chain imbalance; cells with a relatively greater number of γ chains (i.e., hemoglobin F) have less membrane damage and a longer survival [4,94,95]. This has been proved both in labeling experiments in vivo and in differential centrifugation studies, which have shown higher fetal hemoglobin levels in the older cell populations. Presumably, cells with a relatively greater γ-chain production will have the smallest excess of α chains and accordingly the smallest number of inclusions. There is also strong evidence that the poor hemoglobinization of thalassemic cells may contribute to the associated changes in membrane function [96].

Defective heme synthesis has been clearly demonstrated in β thalassemia [2]. Heme inhibits ALA synthetase and thus controls the rate of heme synthesis by "feedback" inhibition. The defect in heme production is probably the result of accumulation of heme due to defective globin-chain synthesis. Some of this heme will be combined with free α chain and be degraded in the red cell precursors. Degradation of this heme is probably responsible for the large "early labeled bilirubin" peak found in iron kinetic studies of patients with homozygous β thalassemia [2], as well as for the increase in the urinary dypyrroles described in this disorder [97].

In addition to the accumulation of heme as a result of defective globin-chain synthesis, there appears to be an increased amount of iron within the red cell precursors. Excess iron loading of the mitochondria may be responsible for at least some of the metabolic changes, such as diminished ATP regeneration, in the red cell precursors. All these observations point to the importance of the excess of α-chain production in the pathogenesis of both the hemolytic and ineffective erythropoietic component of β thalassemia.

There is good evidence of ineffective erythropoiesis with considerable intramedullary breakdown of hemoglobin in all forms of thalassemia [98]. It seems probable that cells with relatively little γ-chain production, and hence with a relatively large excess of α chains, may never leave the marrow. This cell population, with its free α chains with heme attached, may be the main source of the early labeled bile peak and increased production of urinary dypyrroles referred to above. An abnormal pattern of proliferation, with arrest of the red cell precursors in the G_1 phase of the cell cycle, has been demonstrated in the marrow of β-thalassemic patients [99]. It seems likely that the abnormal cell division is related to excess α-chain production [100]; indeed, α-chain precipitates can be seen in the nuclei of erythroblasts in this disorder [101].

The marked degree of ineffective erythropoiesis combines with the shortened peripheral red cell survival to produce a severe degree of anemia in β-thalassemia homozygotes. This in turn combines with the relatively high oxygen affinity of the red cells, which contain large amounts of fetal hemoglobin, to produce considerable tissue anoxia and hence a strong stimulus to erythropoietin production. Marked expansion of the marrow results, and the total erythron in β thalassemia

FIGURE 50-8 Globin-chain synthesis in homozygous β thalassemia. The red cells were incubated with [³H]leucine and the chains separated by CM cellulose chromatography in 8 M urea. The broken line represents radioactivity and shows quite clearly the excess of counts incorporated into the α chains as compared with the non-α chains.

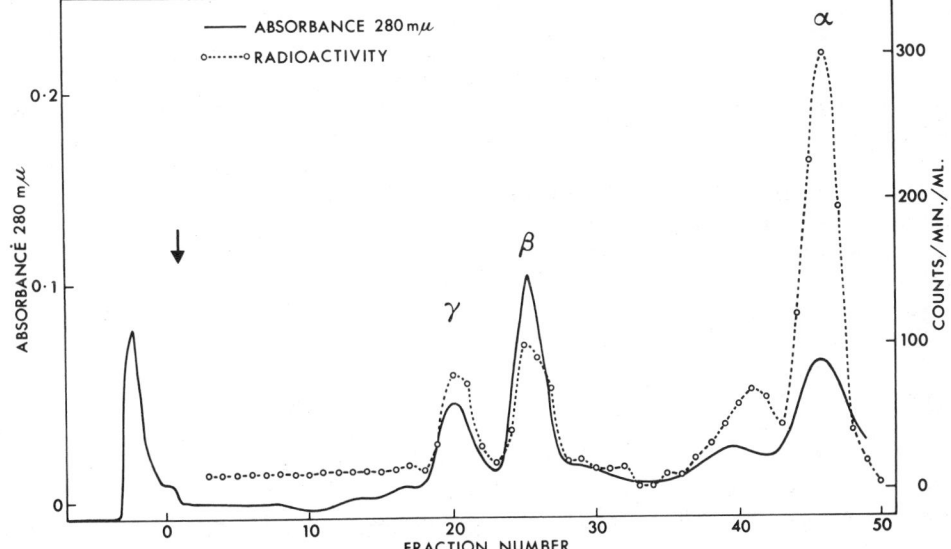

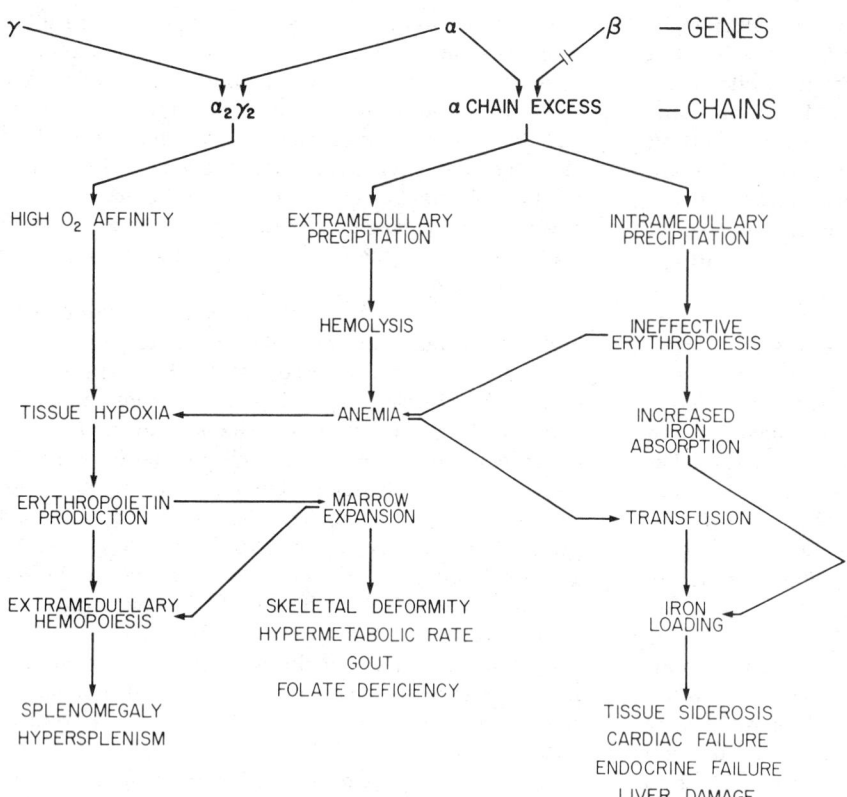

FIGURE 50-9   The pathophysiology of β thalassemia.

may be hypertrophied as much as fortyfold [102]. The hypermetabolic state which results causes wasting, growth retardation, hyperuricemia, fever, and increased folate requirements. The marked erythroid hyperplasia and ineffective erythropoiesis are probably responsible for increased iron absorption, and this, together with regular blood transfusion, results in the marked iron overload which causes the death of these patients. It is thus possible to relate all the clinical findings observed in β-thalassemia homozygotes to the basic defect in β-chain production (Fig. 50-9).

α THALASSEMIA

The pathophysiology of the anemia of α thalassemia is quite different from that of β thalassemia [4,91]. In conditions such as hemoglobin H disease, in which there is a marked deficit of α-chain production, excess β chains are produced. However, unlike the excess α chains of β thalassemia, unpaired β chains do not precipitate significantly in the marrow, but form $β_4$ tetramers. Similarly, during intrauterine life, excess γ chains form $γ_4$ tetramers, which are also relatively stable. Thus the α thalassemias are not associated with any significant degree of ineffective erythropoiesis. However, the $β_4$ molecule is relatively unstable, and as red cells age, inclusion bodies are formed which are removed in the spleen and other parts of the monocyte-macrophage system. This causes mechanical damage to the red cells

during their passage through the microcirculation and hence leads to a shortened red cell survival time and to a hemolytic anemia. The red cells are hypochromic owing both to removal of denatured hemoglobin and to a reduction in the overall amount of hemoglobin synthesized. Thus the α thalassemias are characterized by hypochromic, microcytic red cells, and if there is a significant degree of globin-chain imbalance, there is an additional hemolytic component.

Another important factor in the pathophysiology of the severe α thalassemias is that hemoglobins H and Bart's show no heme/heme interaction and therefore are relatively inefficient as oxygen carriers. Indeed, it is not clear how infants with the hemoglobin Bart's hydrops syndrome survive to term unless the hemoglobin Portland which most of them synthesize acts as their principal oxygen carrier. Similarly, adults with large amounts of hemoglobin H have left-shifted oxygen dissociation curves and therefore are not able to adapt appropriately to the level of anemia caused by shortened red cell survival and ineffective hemoglobin synthesis.

Population genetics of thalassemia [2–4]

The β thalassemias are distributed widely in Mediterranean populations, the Middle East, parts of India and Pakistan, and throughout Southeast Asia. The disease occurs widely in the southern parts of the USSR and in the People's Republic of China. The β thalassemias are rare in Africa, except for some isolated pockets in West Africa, notably Liberia, and in parts of North Africa. It should be remembered, however, that β thalassemia occurs sporadically in all racial groups and has been observed in the homozygous state in persons of pure Anglo-Saxon stock. Thus a patient's racial background does not preclude the diagnosis. The reasons for the maintenance of the thalassemia polymorphisms are still unknown; some evidence relates the high gene frequency to the previous existence of *Plasmodium falciparum* malaria. However, the cellular mechanism for this protective effect has not yet been determined.

The $\delta\beta$ thalassemias have been observed sporadically in many racial groups, although no high-frequency populations have been defined. Similarly, the hemoglobin Lepore syndromes have been found in many populations, but with the possible exception of central Italy and Yugoslavia, these disorders have not been found to occur with a high frequency in any particular region.

The α thalassemias occur widely throughout Africa, the Mediterranean countries, the Middle East, and Southeast Asia. The α^0 thalassemias are found most commonly in the Mediterranean and Oriental populations and are extremely rare in Africa and the Middle East. However, the deletion forms of α^+ thalassemia occur with a high frequency throughout West Africa, the Mediterranean, the Middle East, and Southeast Asia. Up to 40 percent of the population of some parts of West Africa are carriers for the deletion form of α^+ thalassemia. At the moment it is uncertain how common the nondeletion forms of α^+ thalassemia are in any particular populations, but they have been well defined in some of the Mediterranean island populations and also in parts of the Middle East and Southeast Asia. Because the hemoglobin Bart's hydrops syndrome and hemoglobin H disease require the action of an α^0-thalassemia determinant, these disorders are only found at a high frequency in Southeast Asia and in parts of the Mediterranean region. The α-chain termination mutants such as hemoglobin Constant Spring seem to be particularly common in Southeast Asia, and in Thailand approximately 4 percent of the population are hemoglobin Constant Spring carriers.

Clinical and laboratory features

THE β AND $\delta\beta$ THALASSEMIAS

The characteristics of the β thalassemias are summarized in Table 50-1. The group is composed of two main varieties, β^+ thalassemia and β^0 thalassemia, in which there is a partial or total deficiency, respectively, of β-chain synthesis. In addition, there are several disorders resulting from both defective δ-chain and β-chain production, the $\delta\beta$ thalassemias. Finally, there are the conditions arising from heterozygosity for one of these forms of β thalassemia and α thalassemia or α-chain or β-chain structural hemoglobin variants.

HOMOZYGOUS β THALASSEMIA [4,102,103]

The homozygous state for β thalassemia, *thalassemia major*, produces the clinical picture first described by Thomas Cooley in 1925. Affected infants are well at birth. Anemia usually develops during the first few months of life and becomes progressively severe. The infants fail to thrive and may have feeding problems, bouts of fever, and diarrhea and other gastrointestinal symptoms. The majority of infants who are going to develop transfusion-dependent homozygous β thalassemia will present with these symptoms within the first year of life. A later onset suggests that the condition may develop into one of the intermediate forms of β thalassemia (see later section).

The course of the disease in childhood depends almost entirely on whether or not the child is maintained on an adequate transfusion program. The classical textbook picture of Cooley's anemia describes the disease as it was seen before these children could be maintained with relatively normal hemoglobin levels by regular blood transfusions. If transfusions are possible, the affected children grow and develop normally and have no abnormal physical signs. Few of the complications of the disorder occur during childhood, and the disease only presents a problem when the effects of iron loading resulting from ineffective erythropoiesis and from repeated blood transfusions begin to become apparent at the end of the first decade.

However, the inadequately transfused child develops the typical features of Cooley's anemia. Growth is stunted, and with bossing of the skull and overgrowth of the maxillary region, the whole face gradually assumes a "mongoloid" appearance. These changes are associated with a characteristic radiologic appearance of the skull, long bones and hands (Fig. 50-10). There is widening of the diploë, with a "hair on end" or "sunray" appearance and a lacy trabeculation of the long bones and phalanges, and there may be gross skeletal deformities. The liver and spleen are enlarged, and the pigmentation of the skin increases. Many features of a hypermetabolic state with fever, wasting, and hyperuricemia may develop.

The clinical course is one of severe anemia with frequent complications. These children are particularly prone to infection, which is a common cause of death. Because of increased folate utilization by the hypertrophied marrow, folic acid deficiency occurs frequently. Spontaneous fractures occur commonly as a result of the expansion of the marrow cavities with thinning of the long bones and skull. Maxillary deformities often lead to dental problems from malocclusion. The formation of massive deposits of extramedullary hemopoietic tissue may cause complications such as spinal neoplasms on chest x-ray. With the gross splenomegaly which may occur, a secondary thrombocytopenia and leukopenia frequently develop, leading to a

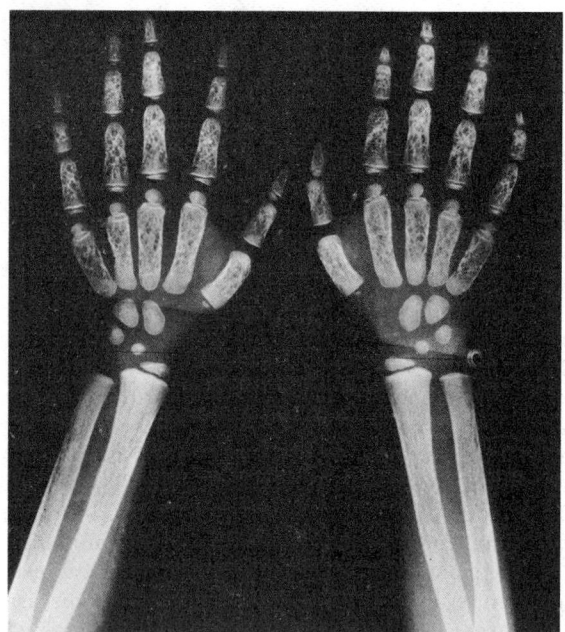

FIGURE 50-10 X-rays of the hands of a child with homozygous β thalassemia.

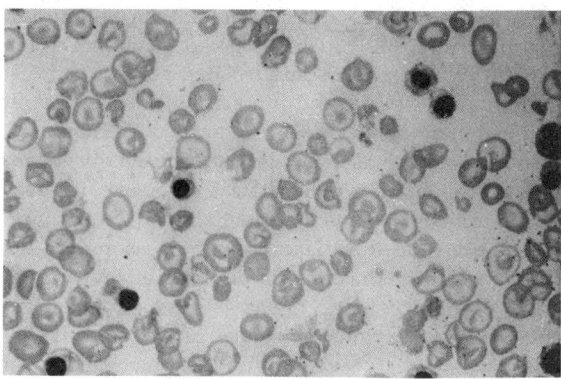

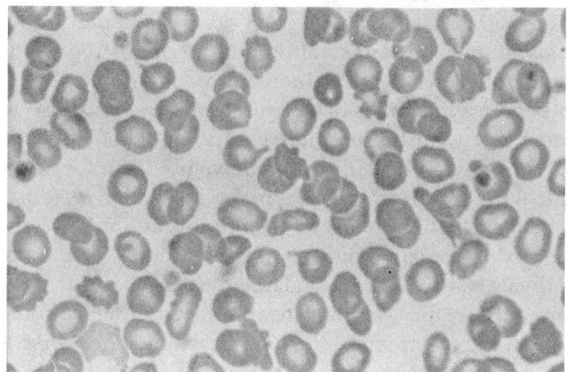

FIGURE 50-11 The blood in β thalassemia. (*Top*) A postsplenectomy film from a patient homozygous for β thalassemia. (*Bottom*) The blood in heterozygous β thalassemia.

further tendency to infection and bleeding. There may be a bleeding tendency in the absence of thrombocytopenia. Epistaxis is particularly common. These hemostatic problems are associated with poor liver function in some cases. Chronic leg ulceration may occur, although it is more common in thalassemia intermedia (see later section).

Children who have grown and developed normally throughout the first 10 years of life as a result of regular blood transfusion start to develop the symptoms of iron overload as they enter puberty. The first indication of iron loading is usually absence of the puberal growth spurt and a failure of the menarche. Over the succeeding years, a variety of endocrine disturbances may develop, in particular diabetes mellitus and adrenal insufficiency. Toward the end of the second decade cardiac complications arise, and death usually occurs in the second or third decades as a result of cardiac siderosis. This may cause an acute cardiac death with arrhythmia or intractable cardiac failure. Both these complications may be precipitated by intercurrent infection [4,103].

Some children who appear to have homozygous β thalassemia do not require regular blood transfusions and although puberty may be delayed, they develop normally and, despite many of the stigmata of β thalassemia, survive to adult life. The problem of this type of disorder, called *thalassemia intermedia*, will be considered in a later section.

In thalassemia major, hemoglobin levels may be in the 2 to 3 g/dl range or even lower. The red cells show marked aniso-poikilocytosis, with hypochromia, target cell formation, and a variable degree of basophilic stippling (Fig. 50-11). The appearance of the blood film

varies somewhat, depending on whether or not the spleen is intact [4,91]. In nonsplenectomized patients, large poikilocytes are common, whereas after splenectomy, large, flat macrocytes and small, deformed microcytes are frequently seen. The reticulocyte count is moderately elevated, and there are nearly always nucleated red cells in the blood. The latter may reach very high levels after splenectomy. The white cell and platelet counts are slightly elevated unless there is secondary hypersplenism. Staining of the blood with methyl violet, particularly in splenectomized subjects, reveals stippling or ragged inclusion bodies in the red cells [104]. These inclusions can nearly always be found in the red cell precursors in the marrow (Fig. 50-12). The marrow usually shows erythroid hyperplasia with morphologic abnormalities of the erythroblasts such as striking basophilic stippling and increased iron deposition. In some cases there may be an increase of "ringed" sideroblasts, but these changes are not so marked as those in the primary sideroblastic anemias (see Chap. 54). Iron kinetic studies indicate the presence of markedly ineffective erythropoiesis, and red cell survival is usually shortened. There are populations of cells with very short survival and also a longer-lived population of cells; the latter contain relatively more fetal hemoglobin.

An increased level of fetal hemoglobin, ranging from less than 10 percent to over 90 percent, is characteristic of homozygous β thalassemia. In some instances there may be a total deficiency of hemoglobin A synthesis. This represents a specific type of β thalassemia (β^0 thalassemia), since other affected family members also show a similar absence of hemoglobin A. The acid elution test (Chap. A9) shows that the fetal hemoglobin is quite heterogeneously distributed among the red cells. Hemoglobin A_2 levels in homozygous β thalassemia may be low, normal, or high. If expressed as a proportion of hemoglobin A, however, the hemoglobin A_2 level is almost invariably elevated. Differential centrifugation studies indicate some heterogeneity of hemoglobin F and A_2 distribution among thalassemic red cells, and their level in the whole blood gives little indication of their total rates of synthesis [4,95]. In some instances, alkaline starch gel electrophoresis of hemolysates prepared by high-speed centrifugation reveals traces of free α chains in the region of the origin.

In vitro hemoglobin synthesis studies indicate a marked degree of globin-chain imbalance; there is always a marked excess of α- over β- and γ-chain production (see Fig. 50-8). This approach has confirmed that the β thalassemias may be divided into β^+ and β^0 varieties [88–90].

HETEROZYGOUS β THALASSEMIA [4]
The heterozygous state for β thalassemia is not usually associated with any clinical disability except in periods of stress, such as pregnancy or during severe infection, when a moderate degree of anemia may be present. Hemoglobin values are usually in the 9 to 11 g/dl range. The most striking and consistent finding is small, poorly hemoglobinized red cells (MCH values of 20 to 22 pg and MCV values of 50 to 70 fl). The red cell indices are particularly useful in screening for heterozygous carriers of thalassemia in population surveys. Although reports of cases of apparent heterozygous β thalassemia with severe anemia and splenomegaly have appeared, these cases have not been subjected to full genetic and hemoglobin synthetic characterization. Therefore, symptomatic β-thalassemia carriers must be very rare, if indeed such a condition exists.

The marrow in heterozygous β thalassemia shows slight erythroid hyperplasia with rare red cell inclusions. Occasional cases of megaloblastic transformations due to folic acid deficiency occur, particularly during pregnancy. There is a mild degree of ineffective erythropoiesis, but the red cell survival is normal or nearly so.

The hemoglobin A_2 level is increased to 3.5 to 7 percent in carriers of β thalassemia. The level of fetal hemoglobin is elevated in about half the patients, usually to 1 to 3 percent and rarely to more than 5 percent. The hemoglobin A_2 value may be artificially depressed in patients with β thalassemia who have coexistent iron deficiency, and it may rise into the β-thalassemia range with the institution of iron therapy [105].

In vitro hemoglobin synthesis studies indicate that in heterozygous β thalassemia, α-chain production is about twice that of β chains [106].

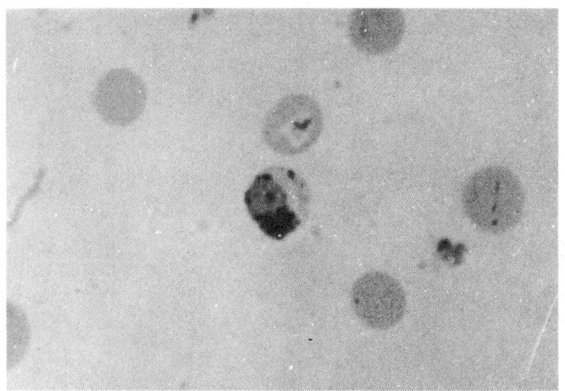

FIGURE 50-12 Inclusion bodies in the marrow of a patient homozygous for β thalassemia. An erythroblast is shown with a dense inclusion body on the periphery of the cell which is quite distinct from the nucleus. Methyl violet stain, ×600.

$\delta\beta$ THALASSEMIA
The homozygous state for $\delta\beta$ thalassemia has been observed in only a few patients [107–110]. It is clinically milder than Cooley's anemia and is one form of thalassemia intermedia. Only hemoglobin F is present; hemoglobins A and A_2 are absent. Analysis of the structure of the hemoglobin F enables the condition to be classified into $^G\gamma$ and $^G\gamma^A\gamma$ forms. The homozygous state for $^G\gamma$ $\delta\beta$ thalassemia may be more severe than that for $^G\gamma^A\gamma$ $\delta\beta$ thalassemia [110].

Heterozygous $\delta\beta$ thalassemia is hematologically similar to β thalassemia minor [4]. The fetal hemoglobin level is higher, being in the 5 to 20 percent range, and the hemoglobin A_2 value is normal or slightly reduced. As in β thalassemia, the fetal hemoglobin is heterogeneously distributed among the red cells, thus distinguishing this disorder from hereditary persistence of fetal hemoglobin (Fig. 50-13).

Heterozygosity for both β thalassemia and $\delta\beta$ thalassemia results in a condition clinically similar to but slightly milder than classical Cooley's anemia; the hemoglobin consists largely of hemoglobin F, with a small amount of hemoglobin A_2. This occurs because the associated β-thalassemia gene has always been the β^0 variety. $\delta\beta$ thalassemia has also been observed in individuals heterozygous for hemoglobins S or C [4].

THE HEMOGLOBIN LEPORE THALASSEMIAS [4,111]
In 1958, Gerald and Diamond [112] noted that one parent of a child with Cooley's anemia had the hematologic picture of thalassemia minor with the presence of a hemoglobin variant which migrated to the position of hemoglobin S. This variant, which made up about 8 percent of the total hemoglobin, was called *Lepore* after the family name of the patient. The first definitive chemical studies of hemoglobin Lepore were carried out on a sample from a patient from Washington, but the complete analysis of the variant was worked out on a sample from a patient from Boston, and hence the common form of hemoglobin Lepore is correctly designated

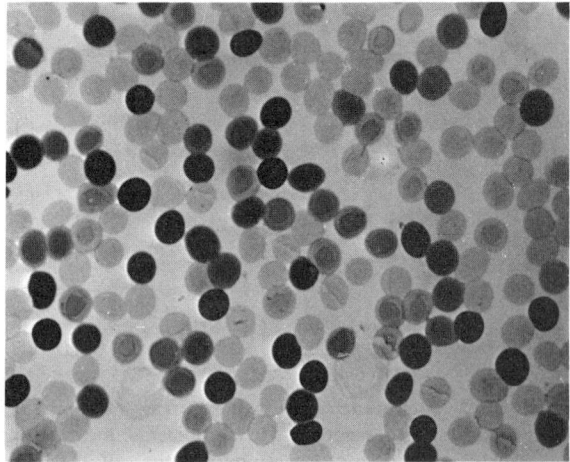

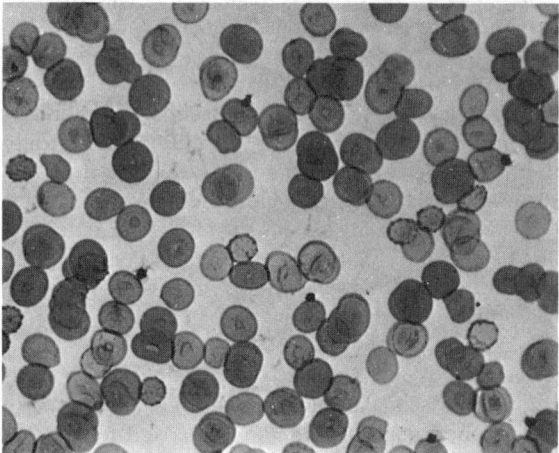

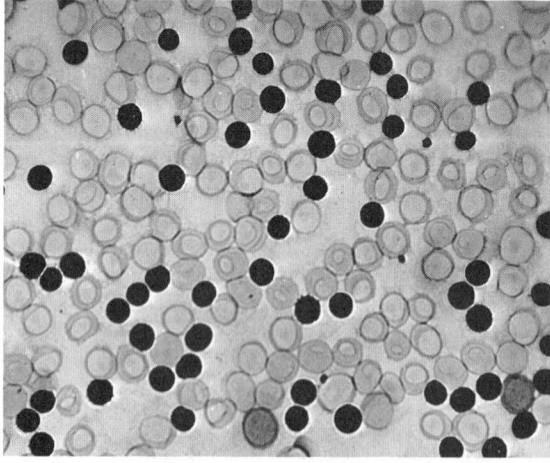

FIGURE 50-13   Acid elution preparations from the blood of patients with δβ thalassemia and hereditary persistence of fetal hemoglobin. (*Top*) Heterozygous δβ thalassemia. (*Middle*) Heterozygous hereditary persistence of fetal hemoglobin. (*Bottom*) An artificial mixture of fetal and adult erythrocytes.

hemoglobin Lepore$_{Boston}$. There are two other types of Lepore hemoglobins, hemoglobin Lepore$_{Hollandia}$ [54] and hemoglobin Lepore$_{Baltimore}$ [55], which differ from hemoglobin Lepore$_{Boston}$ only in the composition of the δβ chain (see Fig. 50-4). It has been suggested that

other hemoglobin Lepore-like variants may exist which, because of the site of the unequal crossing-over between δ- and β-globin-chain genes, have charges identical to those of either hemoglobin A or A$_2$ [111]; no examples of variants of this type have yet been encountered.

The hemoglobin Lepore disorders have been described in the homozygous state and in the heterozygous state either alone or in association with β or δβ thalassemia, hemoglobin S, or hemoglobin C. In the homozygous state, approximately 20 percent of the hemoglobin is of the Lepore type and 80 percent is fetal hemoglobin; hemoglobins A and A$_2$ are absent. The clinical picture is variable, some cases being identical to transfusion-dependent homozygous β thalassemia, others being associated with the clinical picture of thalassemia intermedia. In the heterozygous state, the findings are of β thalassemia minor, the hemoglobin consisting of about 8 percent hemoglobin Lepore, with a reduced level of hemoglobin A$_2$ and a slight increase in the level of fetal hemoglobin. The Lepore hemoglobins have been found sporadically in most racial groups. In the majority of cases, chemical analysis has shown that they are identical to hemoglobin Lepore$_{Boston}$, and hemoglobin Lepore$_{Hollandia}$ and Lepore$_{Baltimore}$ have only been observed in a few patients [4,111].

HEREDITARY PERSISTENCE OF FETAL HEMOGLOBIN (HPFH)

Hereditary persistence of fetal hemoglobin (HPFH) is the term used to describe a heterogeneous group of inherited conditions in which fetal hemoglobin production continues into adult life in the absence of any major hematologic abnormalities. There is increasing evidence that at least some of these disorders represent extremely mild forms of δβ thalassemia in which the absence of δ- and β-chain production is almost but not entirely compensated for by persistent γ-chain synthesis [110].

It is current practice to classify HPFH into two main groups; *pancellular* and *heterocellular*, in which the intercellular distribution of hemoglobin F is either uniform or uneven [113] (see Fig. 50-13). Since the latter may depend on such factors as the sensitivity of the method used, this division may be artificial [110]. As mentioned earlier, it is also possible to divide these conditions into deletion and nondeletion forms. Again, this may not be entirely satisfactory, since even those disorders in which gene mapping shows no abnormality may result from deletions which are too small to be defined by currently available methods. Hence we shall use the pancellular/heterocellular classification here.

Pancellular HPFH is subdivided according to the structure of the hemoglobin F into $^G\gamma$, $^G\gamma^A\gamma$, and $^A\gamma$ forms [4,114,115]. The condition is further classified depending on whether there is any β- or δ-chain synthesis *cis* to its genetic determinant. For example, $^G\gamma$ HPFH can be further classified into $^G\gamma$ β$^+$ and $^G\gamma$ (γβ)$^+$ forms; the latter condition is characterized by the presence of a hemoglobin variant, hemoglobin Kenya, which consists of normal α chains combined with non-α chains which are made up of the N-terminal residues of the $^A\gamma$ chains fused to the C-terminal residues of β chain [116]. It has arisen in exactly the same way as hemoglobin Lepore, only in this case there has been a crossover between the $^A\gamma$- and β-globin-chain genes with exclusion of the C-terminal end of the $^A\gamma$ gene, the whole of the δ-chain gene, and the N-terminal end of the β-chain gene (see Fig. 50-4). A classification of the different forms of pancellular HPFH is shown in Table 50-7.

The only form of pancellular HPFH which has been found in the homozygous state is the classical $^G\gamma^A\gamma$ African form of the condition [4,110]. Homozygotes have 100 percent hemoglobin F and their blood shows mild thalassemic changes with reduced MCH and MCV values. Hemoglobin synthesis studies show that such persons have imbalanced globin-chain synthesis with α/non-α globin-chain synthesis ratios similar to those of heterozygous β thalassemia [117]. Heterozygotes for this condition have approximately 20 to 30 percent hemoglobin F with slightly reduced hemoglobin A_2 values and completely normal blood pictures. Thus it appears that $^G\gamma^A\gamma$ HPFH is an extremely well compensated form of $\delta\beta$ thalassemia in which the output of γ chains almost entirely compensates for the complete absence of β and δ chains. The $^G\gamma^A\gamma$ HPFH determinant has been found in association with hemoglobins S and C or with β thalassemia. These compound heterozygous states are associated with little clinical disability [4].

The other forms of HPFH have only been observed in the heterozygous state or in the compound heterozygous state with β thalassemia or hemoglobins S or C. Heterozygotes for $^G\gamma \beta^+$ HPFH or hemoglobin Kenya have 5 to 20 percent $^G\gamma$ hemoglobin F and completely normal hematologic findings. Hemoglobin Kenya heterozygotes have, in addition, about 5 to 15 percent hemoglobin Kenya as well as increased hemoglobin F. In the common form of HPFH in Greece, heterozygotes have approximately 15 percent hemoglobin F, which consists of about 90 percent $^A\gamma$ chains with a small but significant amount of $^G\gamma$ chains [118,119]. Compound heterozygotes for the Greek form of pancellular HPFH and β thalassemia have a mild form of β thalassemia intermedia.

Heterocellular HPFH also appears to be heterogeneous, although so far the various subgroups are ill-defined [4]. Small amounts of hemoglobin F are found in most normal adults; it is confined to a few red cells, which are called *F cells* [120]. The number of F cells in normal adults appears to be under genetic control [121]. There is a condition in which there appears to be an inherited increase in the number of F cells; this was first observed in Swiss Army personnel and hence is called the *Swiss form* of HPFH [122], although it is found in 1 to 2 percent of most populations [4]. Recent work indicates that its genetic determinant is linked to the γ-δ-β-globin gene cluster [123]. The only hematologic importance of Swiss HPFH is that when it is inherited together with a β-thalassemia determinant, the level of hemoglobin F is usually significantly increased above that found in heterozygous β thalassemia alone [124,125]. Similarly, individuals with homozygous β thalassemia who have inherited a gene for the Swiss form of HPFH have particularly high levels of hemoglobins F and appear to run an unusually mild course [126].

Other forms of heterocellular HPFH are usually named after the place of origin of the affected family. In the British form of heterocellular HPFH, for example, both homozygous and heterozygous individuals have been defined [127]. Homozygotes have approximately 20 percent hemoglobin F unevenly distributed among their red cells, whereas heterozygotes have, on average, about 8 percent hemoglobin F. Again the genetic determinant for this condition is linked to the γ-δ-β-globin gene cluster [123]. Several other varieties of heterocellular HPFH have been reported, including the Seattle [127] and Atlanta [128] forms; heterozygotes have 2 to 5 percent hemoglobin F, and the conditions have been further classified according to its $^G\gamma/^A\gamma$ composition.

β THALASSEMIA ASSOCIATED WITH β STRUCTURAL HEMOGLOBIN VARIANTS

The combination of β thalassemia with β structural hemoglobin variants of most clinical importance are sickle cell thalassemia, hemoglobin C thalassemia, and hemoglobin E thalassemia [4].

Sickle cell thalassemia [129,130] occurs in parts of Africa and in the Mediterranean population, particularly in Greece and Italy. The clinical results of carrying one gene for hemoglobin S and one gene for β thalassemia depend mainly on the type of β-thalassemia gene. Where no normal β chain is synthesized, the hemoglobin pattern consists of hemoglobin S with an increase in hemoglobins F and A_2. The associated clinical findings are similar to those of sickle cell anemia, with severe anemia and recurrent sickle crises (see Chap. 60). Where the β-thalassemia gene only partly depresses β-chain production, the hemoglobin consists of about 70 percent hemoglobin S and 10 to 25 percent hemoglobin A. The associated clinical findings tend to be less severe than in sickle cell anemia, with mild anemia and few sickle crises. The relationship between the hemoglobin pattern and the clinical findings in sickle cell thalassemia is not invariable, and some patients with hemoglobin A–producing type of sickle cell thalassemia (β^+ thalassemia) have had a relatively severe clinical course [130].

Hemoglobin C thalassemia is a mild hemolytic disorder associated with splenomegaly [4]. The hemoglobin pattern is variable, depending on whether the thalassemia gene is of the β^+ or β^0 type. In the latter instance, the hemoglobin consists of hemoglobin C only, and the clinical impact tends to be more severe. This disorder has been recorded mainly in North Africa but has been observed in the American Negro population [4]. Where some hemoglobin A is produced, the hemolytic disorder is extremely mild and may present only during pregnancy as a refractory anemia or with folic acid deficiency.

TABLE 50-7   Some of the better-defined types of HPFH*

Type	Homozygotes			Heterozygotes				Output of linked genes in cis		Molecular defect	Other comments
	Hb F, %	Gly 136‡	Hb A₂, %	Hb F, %	Gly 136‡	Hb A₂, %	Distribution of Hb F	β	δ		
Negro $^G\gamma^A\gamma (\delta\beta)^0$	100	0.5–0.6	0	17–36†	0.3–0.5†	1.2–2.7	Pancellular	0	0	Deletion of β and δ genes	—
Negro $^G\gamma (\delta\beta)^+$	—	—	—	15–20	1.0	1.6–2.2	Pancellular	+	?0	?	Preliminary experiments indicate gene map is normal
Negro $^G\gamma (\delta\beta)^+$ (Kenya)	—	—	—	4.5–10.5 (Hb Kenya 5.5–27)	1.0	1.0–2.1	Pancellular	0	?0	βγ fusion gene Deletion of parts of $^A\gamma$ and β genes	—
Negro $^G\gamma (\delta\beta)^0$	—	—	—	15–25	1.0	1.5–2.5	Pancellular	?0	?0	?	—
Greek $^G\gamma^A\gamma (\delta\beta)^+$	—	—	—	10–20	0.07–0.13	1.6–2.8	Pancellular	?+	?+	?	Normal gene map
British	19–21	0.1	1.5–1.6	4–12	0.1	2.0–2.5	Heterocellular	+	+	?	Normal gene map
Georgia	—	—	—	2.6–6	0.1	2.0–2.5	Heterocellular	+	+	?	—
Swiss	—	—	—	?1–5	—	2.0–3.0	Heterocellular	+	+	?	Normal gene map
Atlanta	—	—	—	2.3–3.8	1.0	2.0–3.0	Heterocellular	+	+	?	—
Seattle	—	—	—	3.7–7.8	0.4–0.5	2.8–3.3	Heterocellular	+	+	?	—

* The heterocellular forms are named according to their place of discovery—it is not clear whether they are separate entities.

† May be several subclasses based on percent hemoglobin F and glycine/alanine composition.

‡ The proportions of $^G\gamma$ and $^A\gamma$ chains in hemoglobin F are determined by analyzing peptides which include residue 136, such as the tryptic peptide γ15 (residues 133 to 144) or the cyanogen bromide peptide γCB3 (residues 134 to 146). Alternatively the $^G\gamma/^A\gamma$ ratio can be determined directly by methods such as reverse-phase high-performance liquid chromatography or chromatography or electrophoresis in buffers containing non-ionic detergents, which separate the $^G\gamma$ and $^A\gamma$ globin chains [4].

Hemoglobin E thalassemia is a severe public health problem in Southeast Asia and the Indian subcontinent [4,131]. Recent work has shown that hemoglobin E is synthesized at a reduced rate and hence produces the clinical phenotype of a mild form of β thalassemia [132]. Hence when it is inherited together with a β-thalassemia gene, and usually this is a β^0-thalassemia variety in Southeast Asia and India, there is a marked deficit of β chains and hence the clinical picture of severe β thalassemia. In fact, hemoglobin E thalassemia shows a remarkable variability in clinical expression, ranging from a mild form of thalassemia intermedia to a transfusion-dependent condition clinically identical to homozygous β thalassemia. The reasons for this variability of expression are considered in a later section which deals with thalassemia intermedia.

In the more severe forms of hemoglobin E thalassemia, the clinical picture is similar to that of Cooley's anemia, with severe anemia, growth retardation, bone deformity, marked tendency to infection, iron loading, and variable splenomegaly and hypersplenism. The hematologic features are indistinguishable from homozygous β thalassemia, but the hemoglobin consists of hemoglobins E, F, and A_2, with no hemoglobin A. Occasional cases of the interaction of hemoglobin E and β^+ thalassemia have been reported; the hemoglobin pattern consists of hemoglobins E and F, with about 10 percent hemoglobin A [4].

LESS WELL DEFINED DISORDERS OF β-, δ-, OR γ-CHAIN SYNTHESIS

β thalassemia with normal hemoglobin A_2 levels In some Mediterranean populations there are forms of β thalassemia in which heterozygotes have normal hemoglobin A_2 levels [133]. There are two main varieties which are called *normal hemoglobin A_2 β thalassemia types 1 and 2*. It seems likely that type 1 is a genuine form of β thalassemia, while type 2 may represent the compound heterozygous state for β thalassemia and δ thalassemia.

Normal hemoglobin A_2 β thalassemia type 1 is characterized by almost no hematologic changes in heterozygotes, and it can only be identified with certainty by globin-chain synthesis studies which show mild chain imbalance and α/β globin-chain synthesis ratios of approximately 1.2:1.3. The disorder is also called *silent β thalassemia* [134]. The homozygous state has been defined in Turkey [135] and is a mild thalassemia-like disorder in which there is approximately 20 percent hemoglobin F and an elevated level of hemoglobin A_2. Compound heterozygotes for normal hemoglobin A_2 β thalassemia type 1 and β thalassemia have a mild form of thalassemia intermedia [133] (see later section).

Normal hemoglobin A_2 β thalassemia type 2 in heterozygotes is indistinguishable from typical β thalassemia with elevated hemoglobin A_2 levels [133]. The homozygous state for this condition has not been described. The compound heterozygous state for this gene and β thalassemia with raised hemoglobin A_2 levels is associated with the clinical picture of severe transfusion-dependent homozygous β thalassemia [133].

Family data obtained in Italy suggest that this condition may, in fact, represent the compound heterozygous state for both β thalassemia and δ thalassemia [136]. The practical importance of identifying this form of β thalassemia is that it may be mistaken for the heterozygous form of α^0 thalassemia, and hence incorrect genetic counseling may be given to parents affected with this variant (see later section).

Other β-thalassemia variants Several other β-thalassemia-like disorders have been reported. In the so-called Dutch form of β thalassemia, heterozygotes have unusually high levels of hemoglobin F in the 5 to 15 percent range [137]. They also have an elevated level of hemoglobin A_2, which distinguishes this condition from heterozygous $\delta\beta$ thalassemia. This disorder has so far been found only in Holland [137] and Thailand [138].

An unusually severe heterozygous β thalassemia exists in which affected patients have anemia, splenomegaly, jaundice, and relatively severe dyserythropoiesis and hemolysis [4]. At least some of these conditions appear to be the result of highly unstable variants, such as hemoglobin Indianapolis [139]. However, in several other well-defined families with this type of disorder, extremely careful analysis has disclosed no evidence for an unstable hemoglobin variant [4]. These conditions require further definition.

δ THALASSEMIA

This condition causes an absence of hemoglobin A_2 in homozygotes [140] and a reduction in the level of hemoglobin A_2 heterozygotes. Apart from its effect on β thalassemia in reducing hemoglobin A_2 levels to normal (see previous section), it is of no clinical significance.

γ-δ-β THALASSEMIA

This condition has been observed in the heterozygous state in two families [60,141]. It is characterized by neonatal hemolysis and, in adult life, by the hematologic picture of heterozygous β thalassemia with normal hemoglobin A_2 levels.

THALASSEMIA INTERMEDIA

Some patients who are apparently homozygous for β thalassemia manage to survive with either occasional or no blood transfusions [4]. In some cases no transfusions are required during early childhood, but the patient becomes transfusion-dependent when hypersplenism develops in later life. The clinical picture of apparent homozygous β thalassemia which is not transfusion-dependent from early life is called *β thalassemia intermedia*. This descriptive term covers a very broad spectrum of clinical severity ranging from the clinical picture of transfusion-dependent homozygous β thalassemia to disorders which are only slightly more severe than the heterozygous carrier state for β thalassemia.

The mechanisms which reduce the severity of homozygous β thalassemia are only partly understood. Some cases seem to result from the homozygous state for an unusually mild form of β^+ thalassemia. This disorder is

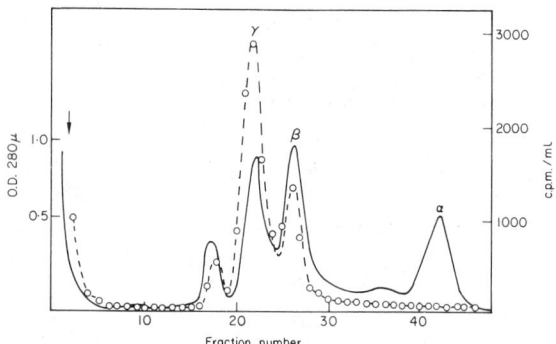

FIGURE 50-14 Hemoglobin synthesis in the blood of an infant with the hemoglobin Bart's hydrops syndrome. The experiment was carried out exactly in the same way as that shown in Fig. 50-8. The broken line shows the radioactivity eluting from the column and indicates that there is a complete absence of α-chain synthesis.

particularly common in black populations and has been well defined in Africa and the United States [4]. Many cases of homozygous β thalassemia intermedia in the Mediteranean region and Southeast Asia result from the inheritance of a form of α thalassemia in addition to the β-thalassemia genes [4,131,142,143]. Individuals who are homogyzous for β⁺ thalassemia have an extremely mild disease if they also inherit a deletion form of α⁺ thalassemia [144]. The effect of the α-thalassemia determinant is to reduce globin-chain imbalance and hence the amount of ineffective erythropoiesis which usually occurs in homozygous β thalassemia. However, it is as yet uncertain how many cases of homozygous β⁰ or β⁺ thalassemia intermedia result from the interaction with α-thalassemia determinants.

The more severe forms of β thalassemia intermedia are associated with a variety of complications, including bone deformity, folate deficiency, hypersplenism, iron overload due to increased gastrointestinal absorption of iron, and an increased susceptibility to infection [4,131,145]. Chronic leg ulceration and severe deforming bone and joint disease seem to be particularly common in this form of thalassemia.

THE α THALASSEMIAS

THE HEMOGLOBIN BART'S HYDROPS FETALIS SYNDROME

This disorder is a frequent cause of stillbirth in Southeast Asia [146,147]. Affected infants are either stillborn between 34 and 40 weeks gestation or are liveborn but die within the first few hours. There is pallor, edema, and hepatosplenomegaly, and the clinical picture resembles that of hydrops fetalis due to Rh blood group incompatibility. The blood film is that of severe thalassemia with many nucleated red cells. At autopsy there is massive extramedullary hemopoiesis and enlargement of the placenta.

The hemoglobin in this disorder consists mainly of

hemoglobin Bart's, with small amounts of hemoglobins H and Portland. There is no hemoglobin A or F, and biosynthetic studies have confirmed a total absence of α-chain synthesis in affected infants [4] (Fig. 50-14).

The parents of such infants have a thalassemic blood picture with low MCH and MCV values and a normal hemoglobin electrophoresis. Biosynthetic studies indicate a marked reduction in α-chain synthesis, with α/β production ratios of approximately 0.7. These findings are diagnostic of the carrier state for an α⁰-thalassemia determinant.

This condition is associated with a high incidence of maternal toxemia of pregnancy and difficulties at the time of delivery because of the massive placenta [147]. The reason for the placental hypertrophy is unknown, although, because a similar phenomenon is observed in hydropic infants with Rh incompatibility, it may reflect severe intrauterine hypoxia.

HEMOGLOBIN H DISEASE

Hemoglobin H disease was described independently in the United States and in Greece in 1955 [148,149]. The clinical findings are variable, some patients being almost as severely affected as those homozygous for β thalassemia, while many have a much milder course [4,131,147]. There is lifelong anemia with variable splenomegaly and bone changes. The blood film shows hypochromia and aniso-poikilocytosis. The reticulocyte count is usually in the 5 percent range. Incubation of the red cells with brilliant cresyl blue results in ragged inclusion bodies in practically all the cells. These form because of precipitation of hemoglobin H in vitro as a result of redox action of the dye (Chap. A6). After splenectomy, large, single Heinz bodies are observed in some cells (Fig. 50-15). These are formed by the in vivo precipitation of the unstable hemoglobin H molecule and are seen only after splenectomy.

In hemoglobin H disease, hemoglobin A always constitutes the major component, while the level of hemoglobin H varies from 5 to 30 percent. In addition, there is sometimes a small amount of hemoglobin Bart's. Hemoglobins H and Bart's are unique among the hemoglobin variants in their anodal migration at pH 6.5 to 7.0 and therefore are easily identified. In about 40 percent of cases of hemoglobin H disease in Southeast Asia, trace amounts of hemoglobin Constant Spring can be observed on alkaline starch-gel electrophoresis [76,131,147].

α⁰-THALASSEMIA AND α⁺-THALASSEMIA TRAITS

The α⁰-thalassemia trait is characterized by the presence of 5 to 15 percent hemoglobin Bart's at birth [4,131,147]. This hemoglobin disappears during maturation and is not replaced by a similar amount of hemoglobin H. An occasional cell with hemoglobin H inclusion bodies may appear after incubation with brilliant cresyl blue, and this phenomenon is often used as a diagnostic test for α-thalassemia trait. However, it is difficult to standardize and needs much experience to be useful, and its

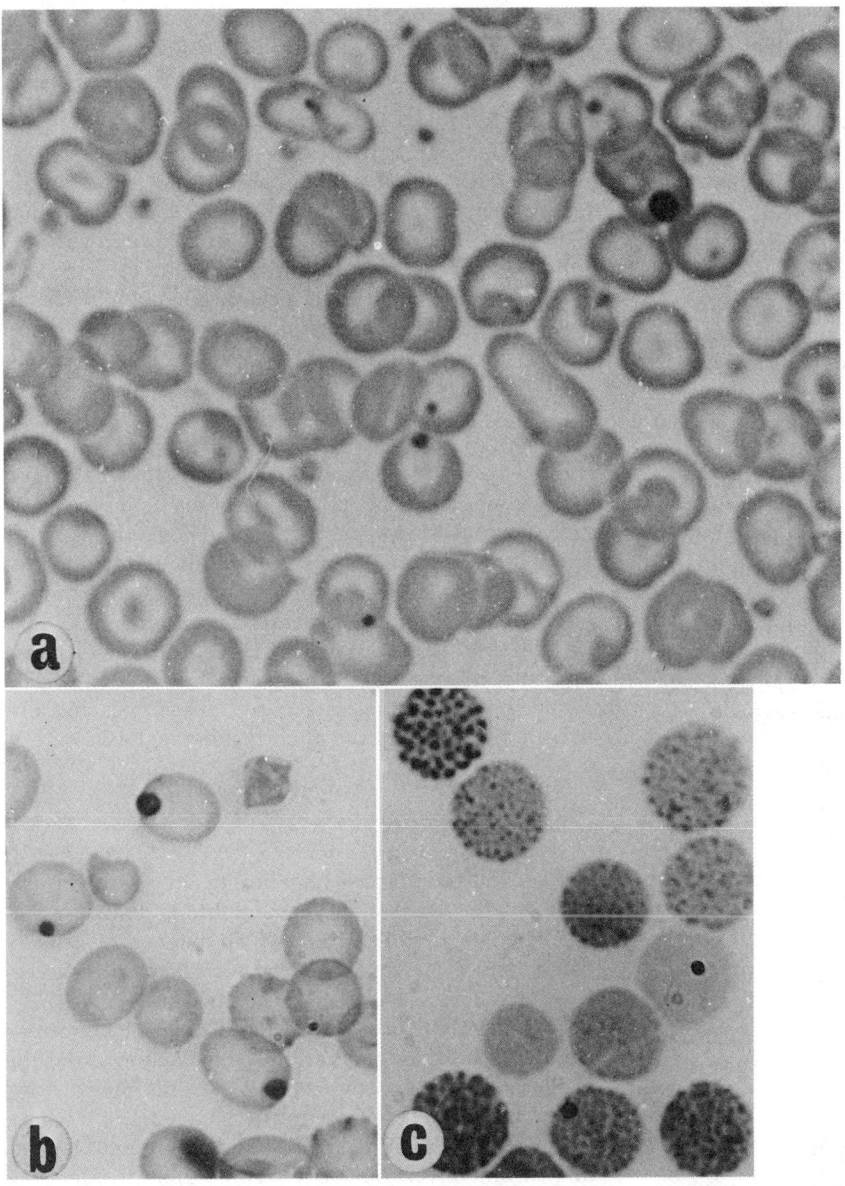

FIGURE 50-15   Hematologic changes in hemoglobin H disease. (*a*) Blood. (*b*) Single inclusions found in the blood after splenectomy (methyl violet stain). (*c*) Multiple inclusion bodies generated after incubating the blood with brilliant cresyl blue.

reliability must be considered quite uncertain. In adult life, the red cells of heterozygotes have morphologic changes of heterozygous thalassemia with low MCH and MCV values. The electrophoretic pattern is normal, and globin synthesis studies indicate a deficit of α-chain production, with an α/β chain production ratio of approximately 0.7 [4,150]. The α^+-thalassemia trait is characterized by minimal hematologic changes, traces of hemoglobin Bart's at birth in some cases, and a slightly reduced α/β chain production ratio of approximately 0.8. This ratio can be distinguished from normal only by studying relatively large numbers of samples and comparing the mean α/β ratio with normal controls.

This approach is not reliable for diagnosing individual cases of the α^+-thalassemia trait, and unfortunately there is no really reliable way of making the diagnosis in adults.

Recent studies using restriction endonuclease analysis indicate that there is a marked overlap between the different α-thalassemia carrier states with regard to the hematologic and globin synthesis findings [151,152]. In addition, they show that many α^+-thalassemia carriers do not have elevated levels of hemoglobin Bart's at birth. These studies confirm that short of gene-mapping analysis, there is no way of identifying specific α-thalassemia carrier states with certainty.

HEMOGLOBIN CONSTANT SPRING

Hemoglobin Constant Spring is an α-chain variant which has an elongated α chain with 31 extra residues attached to its C-terminal end [75,76]. It is synthesized inefficiently and produces the clinical picture of α thalassemia [76].

In the homozygous state for hemoglobin Constant Spring, the blood picture is that of a mild thalassemic disorder with normal-sized red cells [138,153,154]. There is usually mild splenomegaly, icterus, and a raised reticulocyte count. The disorder is thus more severe than the homozygous state for α^+ thalassemia for reasons which are not yet clear [138]. There is about 5 to 6 percent hemoglobin Constant Spring, normal levels of hemoglobin A_2, and trace amounts of hemoglobin Bart's. The remainder is hemoglobin A.

The heterozygous state for hemoglobin Constant Spring shows no hematologic abnormality. The hemoglobin pattern consists of normal levels of hemoglobins A and A_2 with approximately 0.5 percent hemoglobin Constant Spring [75,76]. The latter can be observed on alkaline starch-gel electrophoresis as a faint band migrating between hemoglobin A_2 and the origin. It is seen best on heavily loaded starch gels and is easily missed if other electrophoretic techniques are used (Fig. 50-16).

The heterozygous state for hemoglobin Constant Spring and α^0 thalassemia produces hemoglobin H disease.

HOMOZYGOUS STATE FOR α^+ THALASSEMIA

This condition is found in 2 to 3 percent of West Africans and quite commonly in Southeast Asia. It is characterized by a thalassemic blood picture with 5 to 15 percent hemoglobin Bart's at birth and hematologic findings similar to those of α^0-thalassemia heterozygotes in adult life [151,152].

α THALASSEMIA IN ASSOCIATION WITH α- OR β-CHAIN HEMOGLOBIN VARIANTS

Several α structural variants are due to single amino acid substitutions at α-chain loci on chromosomes which carry only a single α-chain gene. Individuals who inherit variants of this type together with an α^0-thalassemia determinant have a form of hemoglobin H disease in which the hemoglobin consists of the α-chain variant hemoglobin and hemoglobin H. Well-documented examples and the associated genotypes include hemoglobin QH disease $(- -/-\alpha^Q)$ [155,156], $G_{Philadelphia}H$ disease $(- -/\alpha^G)$ [157,158], and hemoglobin Hasharon H disease $(- -/-\alpha^{Hash})$ [159]. There are many examples of the coexistence of the homozygous or heterozygous states for β-chain hemoglobin variants and different α-thalassemia determinants [4]. Particularly well characterized disorders include the various interactions of α^0 and α^+ thalassemia with hemoglobin E [131,147] and hemoglobin S [151,152]. Carriers for these hemoglobin variants who also have the α^0- or α^+-thalassemia traits have thalassemic red cell indices and unusually low levels of the abnormal hemoglobin.

Differential diagnosis

The clinical and hematologic findings in cases of homozygous β thalassemia and hemoglobin H disease are so characteristic that little difficulty in diagnosis is usually encountered. A simple flowchart for laboratory investigations of a suspected case is shown in Fig. 50-17.

In early childhood, difficulty may occasionally be encountered in distinguishing the thalassemias from the congenital sideroblastic anemias, but the marrow appearances in the latter are quite characteristic. Because of the high levels of hemoglobin F encountered in juvenile chronic myelogenous leukemia, this disorder may superficially resemble β thalassemia. However, the finding of primitive cells in the marrow and, on hemoglobin electrophoresis, the absence of elevated Hb A_2 levels and the decrease in carbonic anhydrase in juvenile chronic myelogenous leukemia readily differentiate this disorder from β thalassemia.

Prevention, treatment, and prognosis

PREVENTION

In those parts of the world where the incidence is high, the economic burden placed on society by thalassemia is immense. For example, it has been estimated that if all the thalassemic children who are born in Cyprus over the next few years are treated by regular blood transfusions and iron-chelation therapy, within 15 years the total medical budget of the island will be required to

FIGURE 50-16 The electrophoretic pattern of patients with hemoglobin Constant Spring. (*Left to right*) (1) hemoglobin Constant Spring carrier; (2) normal adult; (3 and 4) hemoglobin H disease with hemoglobin Constant Spring; (5) hemoglobin H disease without hemoglobin Constant Spring; and (6) hemoglobin Constant Spring carrier. (Vertical descending starch-gel electrophoresis, pH 8.5, benzidine stain.) Hemoglobin Constant Spring breaks into multiple bands, presumably because of the action of proteolytic enzymes on the native hemoglobin.

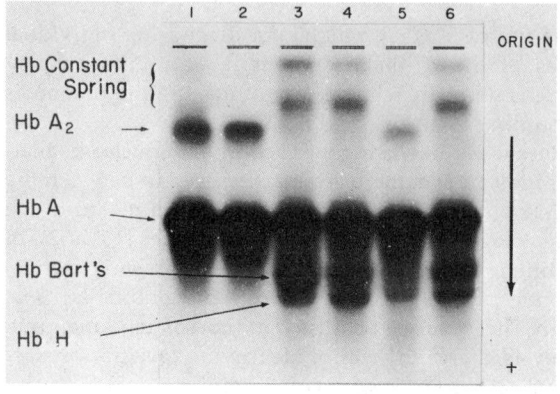

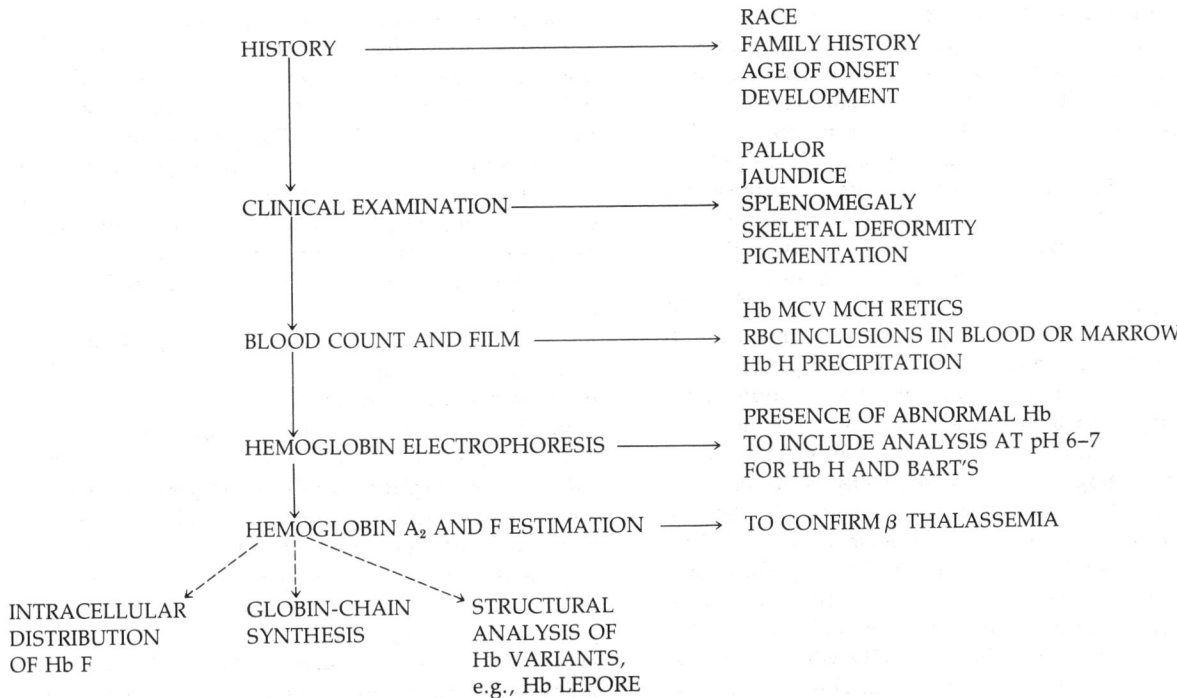

FIGURE 50-17   A flowchart showing approach to the diagnosis of the thalassemia syndromes.

treat this single disease [103]. Clearly, this approach is not always feasible, and hence there is considerable current interest in the development of programs for prevention of the different forms of thalassemia.

There are two ways in which this could be achieved. The first is by prospective genetic counseling, i.e., screening total populations while still at school and warning carriers about the potential risks of marriage to another carrier. There are few data available about the value of programs of this type; a pilot study in Greece was unsuccessful [160], and the results of large-scale studies being carried out in parts of Italy [161] are not yet available. Because it is felt that this approach is unlikely to be very successful in many populations, much more effort has been put into developing the other major method of prevention of thalassemia, i.e., prenatal diagnosis [162–166].

Prenatal diagnosis programs for the prevention of thalassemia entail screening of mothers at their first prenatal visit, screening the fathers in cases in which the mother is a thalassemia carrier, and offering the couple the possibility of prenatal diagnosis and therapeutic abortion if they are both carriers of a gene for a severe form of thalassemia. Currently, these programs are devoted mainly to prenatal diagnosis of the severe transfusion-dependent forms of homozygous β^+ or β^0 thalassemia. Some experience has been gained in prenatal diagnosis of mothers at the risk of having a fetus with the hemoglobin Bart's hydrops syndrome because of the distress caused by a long and difficult pregnancy and the obstetric problems which result from the birth of a hydropic infant with a massive placenta.

The methods used for prenatal diagnosis of β thalassemia have been extensively reviewed [162–166] and will only be outlined here. Fetal blood samples are obtained between 15 and 20 weeks' gestation, either by placental aspiration or by direct-vision fetoscopy. The fetal cells are incubated with radioactive amino acids and the relative rates of α-, β-, and γ-chain synthesis determined. In normal fetuses at this stage of gestation, the β/γ globin-chain synthesis ratio is approximately 0.10, while in fetuses homozygous for β thalassemia, it ranges from 0 to 0.020. Intermediate values are found in heterozygous fetuses. If the fetal blood samples are heavily contaminated with maternal red cells, it is necessary to carry out a preliminary separation to isolate the fetal cells before analyzing the radioactivity incorporation into the globin chains.

The results of over 500 attempts at prenatal diagnosis for β thalassemia [167] indicate a gradual improvement in the technology over the last 2 years. At the time of this writing, fetal mortality is less than 5 percent, and the error rate is in a similar range. The technique has been successfully applied on a large scale in Sardinia [168], Greece [169], the United States [167], and Great Britain [170]. Data from Sardinia [168] indicate that it has been widely accepted by the population and that already it may be causing a genuine decrease in the number of homozygous β thalassemics born into the population.

Clearly, it would be better if it were possible to carry out prenatal diagnosis of thalassemia by examination of amniotic fluid rather than fetal blood. Amniotic fluid cells are mainly of fetal origin, and it is relatively simple to isolate DNA and to analyze the globin genes by restriction endonuclease mapping. Using this approach, it has been possible to diagnose the deletion forms of α thalassemia in utero [171], but unfortunately, most of the β thalassemias are associated with normal β-globin gene maps. However, there are polymorphisms of DNA sequences adjacent to the globin genes, and these can be used for prenatal diagnosis in appropriate cases. For instance, the enzyme Hpa 1 cleaves DNA at the sequence GTTAAC. When normal DNA is digested with this enzyme, the β-globin genes are found on a DNA fragment about 7.6-kb long. However, in some individuals, the DNA fragment containing the β-globin genes is lengthened to 13 kb as a result of a mutation in the Hpa recognition site at the 3' side of the β-globin gene. It turns out that in many black populations the variant 13-kb Hpa 1 fragment is very frequently associated with the sickle cell mutation, and this linkage can be used for prenatal diagnosis of sickle cell anemia [172,173]. This finding has led to a search for similar polymorphisms related to the thalassemia genes. The problem is much more difficult in the case of thalassemia because of the considerable molecular heterogeneity which underlies the different forms of the condition. However, a polymorphism of the DNA sequence close to the β-globin gene has been found in Sardinia and promises to be useful for the prenatal diagnosis of β^0 thalassemia in that population, at least in up to 30 percent of cases [174]. Furthermore, polymorphisms involving the γ-globin genes and other polymorphisms in the γ-δ-β-globin gene cluster have been identified and can be used in appropriate cases to determine whether an infant is homozygous for β^+ or β^0 thalassemia [175]. As more polymorphisms of this type are discovered, it may be possible to identify homozygous fetuses in many different forms of thalassemia using this approach [176]. The recent development of fetal DNA analysis by trophoblast biopsy in the first trimester promises to revolutionize the prenatal diagnosis of the common forms of β thalassemia [197].

SYMPTOMATIC TREATMENT
The only forms of treatment available for thalassemic children are regular blood transfusions, iron-chelation therapy in an attempt to prevent iron overload, the judicious use of splenectomy in cases complicated by hypersplenism, and a good standard of general pediatric care.

If children with homozygous β thalassemia are maintained at a hemoglobin level of 10 to 14 g/dl, they grow and develop normally and develop none of the distressing skeletal complications of thalassemia [177–179]. Hence if blood is available, an attempt should be made to maintain these children at a normal hemoglobin level throughout childhood. The transfusion program should not be started too early, but only when it is quite clear that the hemoglobin level is too low to be compatible with normal development. If transfusion is started too early, cases of thalassemia intermedia may be missed and the child may be transfused unnecessarily. Usually

blood transfusions are given every 6 to 8 weeks on an outpatient basis. To avoid transfusion reactions it is important to use washed red cells or frozen cells so that the majority of the white cells and plasma-protein components are removed [4,103,179]. More ambitious programs using separated, young erythrocyte populations ("neocytes") for transfusion, together with the removal of the patients' older cells, have been described [180], but their use is restricted to only a few centers because of the difficulty and expense of these procedures (see Chap. 164).

Since every child maintained on a high-transfusion regimen will ultimately develop iron overload and die of siderosis of the myocardium, it is vital, where possible, to start these children on a program of iron chelation some time within the first 5 years of life. Despite extensive searches for an oral chelating agent, desferrioxamine remains the only drug of real value for the treatment of thalassemia. It is best administered by a 12-h overnight infusion into the subcutaneous tissues of the anterior abdominal wall [181–184]. When this program is being started, the child should be admitted to hospital and a dose-response curve established, starting at 0.5 g desferrioxamine and increasing until maximum iron excretion is achieved; this varies considerably among children [183]. Once the appropriate dose of desferrioxamine has been determined, the child's parents should be taught to administer the drug on 5 nights a week using a small infusion pump. Regular assessments of the urinary iron should be carried out. Recent work suggests that at least as much iron (or even more) as is excreted in the urine may be removed through the feces on this regime [185]. Because of the small but significant risk of cataract formation from desferrioxamine therapy, the children should be kept under close ophthalmologic surveillance [179]. The amount of iron excreted is considerably greater if the patients are maintained on doses of 50 to 100 mg of ascorbic acid daily [182–184]. Higher doses should be avoided because of potential cardiac toxicity [186]. If the child or its parents cannot manage the subcutaneous desferrioxamine regimen, it is still worthwhile giving the drug as a single daily injection of the largest dose that the child can tolerate [4,179]. This is usually about 25 mg/kg. The drug is dissolved in 2 to 4 ml of water for injection and is given intramuscularly.

There is increasing evidence that children maintained at a high hemoglobin level do not develop hypersplenism [4,103,178,179]. However, in patients who have been kept at a lower hemoglobin level, enlargement of the spleen with increased transfusion requirements occurs commonly. Splenectomy should be carried out if there is a dramatic increase in the transfusion requirements [103], or if thrombocytopenia or neutropenia, or pain develops because of the size of the spleen. Because of the risk of overwhelming pneumococcal infection [187,188], this should not be done in the first 5 years of life. Whenever it is carried out, some physicians prefer to maintain children on prophylactic oral penicillin after the operation (see Chap. 71).

Apart from the measures just outlined, the management of thalassemia requires a high standard of general pediatric care. Infection should be treated early. If the diet is inadequate in folate, supplements should be given; this is probably unnecessary in children maintained on a high-transfusion regimen. Particular attention should be paid to the ear, nose, and throat of these children because of the problems of chronic sinus infection and middle-ear diseases resulting from bone deformity of the skull. Similarly, regular dental surveillance is essential, since poorly transfused thalassemic children have a variety of deformities of the maxilla and poorly developed teeth. In the later stages of the illness, when iron loading becomes the major feature, endocrine replacement therapy may be necessary together with symptomatic treatment for cardiac failure.

Finally, a few points must be mentioned about the management of specific forms of thalassemia. Hemoglobin H disease usually requires no specific therapy, although splenectomy may be of value in cases associated with severe anemia and splenomegaly [4,147]. There is increasing evidence that this may be followed by a higher incidence of thromboembolic disease than occurs in splenectomized children with β thalassemia [4,189], and therefore the spleen should be removed only in cases of extreme anemia and splenomegaly. Oxidant drugs should be avoided in patients with hemoglobin H disease. The management of symptomatic sickle cell thalassemia follows the lines described for sickle cell anemia (see Chap. 60). Thalassemia intermedia presents a particularly complex therapeutic problem. It is difficult to be certain whether a child with a steady-state hemoglobin level of 6 to 7 g/dl should be transfused. Probably the best compromise is to watch these children very closely during the first years of life, and if they are growing and developing normally and there are no signs of bone changes, they should be maintained without transfusion. If, however, their early growth pattern is retarded or their activity is limited due to their anemia, they should go on a regular transfusion regimen. It is especially important to determine whether hypersplenism is playing a role in their anemia as they get older and to carry out a splenectomy if this is the case. Since many of these patients have significant iron loading from the gastrointestinal tract, regular estimations of serum iron and ferritin should be carried out and chelation therapy instituted where appropriate [145].

PROGNOSIS

In a survey of the entire thalassemic population of the United Kingdom, standard actuarial analysis indicated that there was a sharp increase in the death rate in homozygous β thalassemics after the age of 15 and that it is unlikely that any transfusion-dependent adolescent could expect to survive much after the age of 25 years [190]. The patients in this study had received bolus injections of desferrioxamine but in a random and sporadic way. However, recent analysis of the small group of patients who formed part of a controlled trial of the value of bolus desferrioxamine [191] indicated that even

if the drug is given in this inadequate way, survival may be prolonged [190]. It is too early to say whether the use of regular subcutaneous desferrioxamine will prolong the life of a transfusion-dependent child, although this seems likely. Information on this critically important topic should become available in the next 5 to 10 years. The prognosis for an inadequately transfused thalassemic child is extremely poor, and few of them reach the end of the second decade.

The outlook for other forms of thalassemia is much better. Recent studies on adults with homozygous β thalassemia intermedia suggest that many of them develop symptoms of iron loading and severe crippling bone disease in the third and fourth decades [4,192]. The mechanism of the bone disease is uncertain; it seems likely that at least one factor is the marked marrow hyperplasia which occurs in many patients with thalassemia intermedia. Furthermore, there appears to be a high incidence of diabetes secondary to iron loading of the pancrease in this group. Despite these problems, the outlook for a patient who has received no blood transfusion or who has been sporadically transfused during periods of infection, or when hypersplenism occurs, is good, and such patients can expect to live at least until middle age.

References

1. Cooley, T. B., and Lee, P.: A series of cases of splenomegaly in children with anemia and peculiar bone changes. *Trans. Am. Pediatr. Soc.* 37:29, 1925.
2. Bannerman, R. M.: *Thalassemia. A Survey of Some Aspects.* Grune & Stratton, New York, 1961.
3. Chernoff, A. I.: The distribution of the thalassemia gene: A historical review. *Blood* 14:899, 1959.
4. Weatherall, D. J., and Clegg, J. B.: *The Thalassemia Syndromes*, 3d ed. Blackwell Scientific, Oxford, 1981.
5. Weatherall, D. J.: Toward an understanding of the molecular biology of some common inherited anemias: The story of thalassemia, in *Blood, Pure and Eloquent*, edited by M. M. Wintrobe. McGraw-Hill, New York, p. 373.
6. Schroeder, W. A., et al.: Evidence for multiple structural genes for the γ-chain of human fetal hemoglobin. *Proc. Natl. Acad. Sci. U.S.A.* 60:537, 1968.
7. Wood, W. G., Clegg, J. B., and Weatherall, D. J.: Developmental biology of human hemoglobins. *Prog. Hematol.* 10:43, 1977.
8. Huehns, E. R., and Farooqui, A. M.: Oxygen dissociation properties of human embryonic red cells. *Nature* 254:335, 1975.
9. Gale, R. E., Clegg, J. B., and Huehns, E. R.: Human embryonic haemoglobins Gower 1 and Gower 2. *Nature* 280:162, 1979.
10. Wood, W. G., and Weatherall, D. J.: Haemoglobin synthesis during human foetal development. *Nature* 244:162, 1973.
11. Proudfoot, N. J., Shander, M. H. M., Lanley, J. L., Gefter, M. L., and Maniatis, T.: Structure and in vitro transcription of human globin genes. *Science* 209:1329, 1980.
12. Maniatis, T., Fritsch, E. F., Lauer, J., and Lawn, R. M.: The molecular genetics of human hemoglobins. *Ann. Rev. Genet.* 14:145, 1980.
13. Deisseroth, A., Nienhuis, A., Lawrence, J., Riles, R., Turner, P. and Ruddle, F.: Chromosomal localization of human β globin gene on chromosome 11 in somatic cell hybrids. *Proc. Natl. Acad. Sci. U.S.A.* 75:1456, 1978.
14. Deisseroth, A., et al.: Localization of the human α-globin structural gene to chromosome 16 in somatic cell hybrids by molecular hybridization. *Cell* 12:205, 1977.

15. Lawn, R. M., Efstratiadis, A., O'Conell, C., and Maniatis, T.: The nucleotide sequence of the human β-globin gene. *Cell* 21: 647, 1980.

16. Lauer, J., Shen, C.-K. J., and Maniatis, T.: The chromosomal arrangement of human α-like globin genes: Sequence homology and α-globin gene deletions. *Cell* 20:119, 1980.

17. Spritz, R. A., de Riel, J. K. Forget, B. G., and Weissman, S. M.: Complete nucleotide sequence of the human δ-globin gene. *Cell* 21:639, 1980.

18. Slightom, J. L., Blechl, A. E., and Smithies, O.: Human fetal ᴳγ- and ᴬγ-globin genes: Complete nucleotide sequences suggest that DNA can be exchanged between these duplicated genes. *Cell* 21:627, 1980.

19. Nienhuis, A. W., and Stamatoyannopoulos, G.: Hemoglobin switching. *Cell* 15:307, 1978.

20. Wood, W. G., and Jones, R. W.: Erythropoiesis and hemoglobin production: A unifying model involving sequential gene activation, in *Proceedings of the Second Conference on Hemoglobin Switching*, edited by G. Stamatoyannopoulos and A. W. Niehuis. Airlie House, Virginia, 1980. Alan R. Liss, New York.

21. Benz, E. J., and Forget, B. G.: Defect in messenger RNA for human hemoglobin synthesis in beta thalassemia. *J. Clin. Invest.* 50:2755, 1971.

22. Nienhuis, A. W., and Anderson, W. F.: Isolation and translation of hemoglobin messenger RNA from thalassemia, sickle cell anemia, and normal human reticulocytes. *J. Clin. Invest.* 50:2458, 1971.

23. Kacian, D. L., et al.: Decreased globin messenger RNA in thalassemia detected by molecular hybridization. *Proc. Natl. Acad. Sci. U.S.A.* 70:1886, 1973.

24. Housman, D., Forget, B. G., Skoultchi, A., and Benz, E. J.: Quantitative deficiency of chain specific messenger ribonucleic acids in the thalassemia syndromes. *Proc. Natl. Acad. Sci. U.S.A.* 70:1809, 1973.

25. Housman, D., Skoultchi, A., Forget, B. G., and Benz, E. J.: Use of globin cDNA as a hybridisation probe for globin mRNA. *Ann. N.Y. Acad. Sci.* 241:280, 1974.

26. Maquat, L. E., et al.: Processing of human β-globin mRNA precursor mRNA is defective in three patients with β⁺ thalassemia. *Proc. Natl. Acad. Sci. U.S.A.* 77:4287, 1980.

27. Kantor, J. A., Turner, P. H., and Nienhuis, A. W.: Beta thalassemia: Mutations which affect processing of the β-globin mRNA precursor. *Cell* 21:149, 1980.

28. Spritz, R. A., et al.: Base substitution in an intervening sequence of a β⁺ thalassemic human globin gene. *Proc. Natl. Acad. Sci. U.S.A.* 78:2455, 1981.

29. Westway, D., and Williamson, R.: An intron nucleotide sequences variant in a cloned β⁺-thalassemia globin gene. *Nucleic Acids Res.*, 9:1777, 1981.

30. Weatherall, D. J., Clegg, J. B., Na-Nakorn, S., and Wasi, P.: The pattern of disordered haemoglobin synthesis in homozygous and heterozygous β-thalassemia. *Br. J. Haematol.* 16:251, 1969.

31. Pritchard, J., Clegg, J. B., Weatherall, D. J., and Longley, J.: The translation of human globin messenger RNA in heterologous assay systems. *Br. J. Haematol.* 28:141, 1974.

32. Tolstoshev, P., et al.: Presence of gene for β globin in homozygous β₀ thalassemia. *Nature* 260:95, 1976.

33. Ramirez, F., et al.: Abnormal or absent β mRNA in β⁰ Ferrara and gene deletions in δβ thalassemia. *Nature* 263:471, 1976.

34. Benz, E. J., Forget, B. G., Hillman, D. G., Cohen-Solal, M., Pritchard, J., and Cavellesco, C.: Variability in the amount of β globin mRNA in β⁰ thalassemia. *Cell* 14:299, 1978.

35. Old, J. M., Proudfoot, N. J., Wood, W. G., Longley, J. I., Clegg, J. B., and Weatherall, D. J.: Characterization of β-globin mRNA in the β⁰ thalassemias. *Cell* 14:289, 1978.

36. Orkin, S. H., Old, J. M., Weatherall, D. J., and Nathan, D. G.: Partial deletion of β-globin gene DNA in certain patients with β⁰ thalassemia. *Proc. Natl. Acad. Sci.* 76:2400, 1979.

37. Flavell, R. A., et al.: The structure of the human β-globin gene in β-thalassemia. *Nucleic Acids Res.* 6:2749, 1979.

38. Orkin, S. H., Kolonder, R., Michelson, A., and Husson, R.: Cloning and direct examination of a structurally abnormal human β⁰ thalassemia globin gene. *Proc. Natl. Acad. Sci. U.S.A.* 77:3586, 1980.

39. Chang, J. C., and Kan, Y. W.: β⁰ thalassemia, a nonsense mutation in man. *Proc. Natl. Acad. Sci. U.S.A.* 76:2886, 1979.

40. Chang, J. C., Temple, G. F., Trecartin, R. F., and Kan, Y. W.: Suppression of the nonsense mutation in homozygous β⁰ thalassaemia. *Nature* 281:602, 1979.

41. Chang, J. C., Kan, Y. W., Trecartin, R. F., and Temple, G. F.: Nonsense mutation as a cause of β⁰ thalassemia. *Ann. N.Y. Acad. Sci.* 344:113, 1980.

42. Conconi, F., et al.: Appearance of beta globin synthesis in erythroid cells of Ferrara beta⁰-thalassemia patients following blood transfusion. *Nature* 254:256, 1975.

43. Conconi, F., and del Senno, L.: The molecular defect of Ferrara β-thalassemia. *Ann. N.Y. Acad. Sci.* 232:54, 1974.

44. Ottolenghi, S., et al.: δβ thalassemia is due to a gene deletion. *Cell* 9:71, 1976.

45. Ottolenghi, S., Lanyon, W. G., Williamson, R., Weatherall, D. J., Clegg, J. B., and Pitcher, C. S.: Human globin gene analysis for a patient with β⁰/δβ⁰-thalassemia. *Proc. Natl. Acad. Sci. U.S.A.* 72:2294, 1975.

46. Mears, J. G., et al.: Changes in restricted human cellular DNA fragments containing globin gene sequences in thalassemias and related disorders. *Proc. Natl. Acad. Sci. U.S.A.* 75:1222, 1978.

47. Bernards, R., Kooter, J. M., and Flavell, R. A.: Physical mapping of the globin gene deletion in (δβ)⁰ thalassemia. *Gene* 6:265, 1979.

48. Fritsch, E. F., Lawn, R. M., and Maniatis, T.: Characterisation of deletions which affect the expression of fetal globin genes in man. *Nature* 279:598, 1979.

49. Orkin, S. H., Alter, B. P., and Altay, C.: Deletion of the ᴬγ globin gene in ᴳγ δβ-thalassemia. *J. Clin. Invest.* 64:866, 1979.

50. Jones, R. W., Old, J. M., Trent, R. J., Clegg, J. B., and Weatherall, D. J.: A major rearrangement in the human β-globin gene cluster. *Nature* 291:39, 1981.

51. Baglioni, C.: The fusion of two peptide chains in hemoglobin Lepore and its interpretation as a genetic deletion. *Proc. Natl. Acad. Sci. U.S.A.* 48:1880, 1962.

52. Flavell, R. A., Kooter, J. M., de Boer, E., Little, P. F. R., and Williamson, R.: Analysis of the β-δ-globin gene loci in normal and Hb Lepore DNA: Direct determination of gene linkage and intergene distance. *Cell* 15:25, 1978.

53. Baglioni, C.: Abnormal human hemoglobins. X. A study of hemoglobin Lepore (Boston). *Biochim. Biophys. Acta* 97:37, 1965.

54. Barnabas, J., and Muller, C. J.: Haemoglobin Lepore_Hollandia. *Nature* 194:931, 1962.

55. Ostertag, W., and Smith, E. W.: Hemoglobin Lepore Baltimore, a third type of δβ crossover (δ⁵⁰, β⁸⁶). *Eur. J. Biochem.* 10:371, 1969.

56. Wood, W. G., Old, J. M., Roberts, A. V. S., Clegg, J. B., Weatherall, D. J., and Quattrin, N.: Human globin gene expression: Control of β, δ and δβ chain production. *Cell* 15:437, 1978.

57. Yanase, T., et al.: Molecular basis or morbidity from a series of studies of haemoglobinopathies in Western Japan. *Jpn. J. Hum. Genet.* 13:40, 1968.

58. Lehmann, H., and Charlesworth, D.: Observations on haemoglobin P (Congo type). *Biochem. J.* 119:43, 1970.

59. Abu-Sin, A., et al.: Hb P-Nilotic in association with β⁰-thalassemia: Cis mutation of a hemoglobin βᴬ chain regulatory determinant. *J. Lab. Clin. Med.* 93:973, 1979.

60. Van der Ploeg, L. H. T., Konings, A., Oort, M., Roos, D., Bernini, L., and Flavell, R. A.: γ-β-Thalassaemia: Studies showing that deletion of the γ- and δ-gene influences β-globin gene expression in man. *Nature* 283:637, 1980.

61. Ottolenghi, S., et al.: The severe form of α thalassemia is caused by a haemoglobin gene deletion. *Nature* 251:389, 1974.

62. Taylor, J. M., et al.: Genetic lesion in homozygous α thalassaemia (hydrops fetalis). *Nature* 251:392, 1974.

63. Pressley, L., Higgs, D. R., Clegg, J. B., and Weatherall, D. J.: Gene deletions in α thalassaemia prove that the 5' ζ-locus is functional. *Proc. Natl. Acad. Sci. U.S.A.* 77:3586, 1980.

64. Kattamis, C., et al.: The haemoglobin Bart's hydrops syndrome in Greece. *Br. Med. J.* 281:268, 1980.

65. Sophocleous, T., et al.: The molecular basis for the haemoglobin Bart's hydrops fetalis syndrome in Cyprus. *Br. J. Haematol.* 47:153, 1981.

66. Orkin, S. H., et al.: The molecular basis of α-thalassemias: Frequent occurrence of dysfunctional α loci among non-Asians with Hb H disease. *Cell* 17:33, 1979.

67. Orkin, S. H., and Michelson, A.: Partial deletion of the α globin structural gene in human α thalassaemia. *Nature 286:*538, 1980.
68. Higgs, D. R., et al.: Negro α-thalassaemia is caused by a deletion of a single α-gene. *Lancet 2:*272, 1979.
69. Dozy, A. M., et al.: Alpha globin gene organization in blacks precludes the severe form of α thalassaemia. *Nature 280:*605, 1979.
70. Embury, S. H., Lebo, R. V., Dozy, A. M., and Kan, Y. W.: Organization of the α-globin genes in the Chinese α-thalassaemia syndromes. *J. Clin. Invest. 63:*1307, 1979.
71. Goossens, M., et al.: Triplicated α-globin loci in humans. *Proc. Natl. Acad. Sci. U.S.A. 77:*518, 1980.
72. Higgs, D. R., Old, J. M., Pressley, L., Clegg, J. B., and Weatherall, D. J.: A novel α globin gene arrangement in man. *Nature 284:*632, 1980.
73. Higgs, D. R., et al.: Genetic and molecular diversity in non-deletion Hb H disease. *Proc. Natl. Acad. Sci. U.S.A. 78:*5833, 1981.
74. Orkin, S. H., Goff, S. C., and Hechtman, R. L.: An intervening sequence splice junction mutation in man. *Proc. Natl. Acad. Sci. U.S.A. 78:*5041, 1981.
75. Clegg, J. B., Weatherall, D. J., and Milner, P. F.: Haemoglobin Constant Spring—A chain termination mutant? *Nature 234:*337, 1971.
76. Weatherall, D. J., and Clegg, J. B.: The α chain termination mutants and their relationship to the α thalassaemias. *Philos. Trans. R. Soc. Lond. [Biol.] 271:*411, 1975.
77. Seid-Akhaven, M., Winter, W. P., Abramson, R. K., and Rucknagel, D. L.: Hemoglobin Wayne: A framesift mutation detected in human hemoglobin alpha chains. *Proc. Natl. Acad. Sci. U.S.A. 73:*882, 1976.
78. Clegg, J. B., Weatherall, D. J., Contopolou-Griva, I., Caroutsos, K., Poungouras, P., and Tsevrenis, H.: Haemoglobin Icaria, a new chain termination mutant which causes α-thalassaemia. *Nature 251:*245, 1974.
79. Bernini, L. F., de Jong, W. W. W., and Khan, P. M.: Haemoglobin variants in the tribal population of Andhra Pradesh. Evidence for duplication of the α Hb locus in man. *Atti Assoc. Genet. 15:*191, 1970.
80. Bradley, T. B., Wohl, R. C., and Smith, G. J.: Elongation of the α chain in a black family: Interaction with Hb G Philadelphia. *Clin. Res. 23:*131, 1975.
81. Kan, Y. W., et al.: Deletion of α globin genes in haemoglobin H disease demonstrates multiple α structural loci. *Nature 255:*255, 1975.
82. Kan, Y. W., Dozy, A. M., Trecartin, R., and Todd, D.: Identification of a non-deletion defect in α thalassaemia. *N. Engl. J. Med. 297:*1081, 1977.
83. Pressley, L., Higgs, D. R., Pembrey, M. E., Clegg, J. B., and Weatherall, D. J.: A new genetic basis for hemoglobin H disease. *New. Engl. J. Med. 303:*1383, 1980.
84. Lie-Injo, L. E., Dozy, A. M., Kan, Y. W., Lopes, M., and Todd, D.: The α-globin gene adjacent to the gene for Hb Q-α 30 Asp→His is deleted, but not that adjacent to the gene for Hb G-α 30 Glu→Gln; three fourths of the α-globin genes are deleted in Hb Q-α-thalassemia. *Blood 54:*1407, 1979.
85. Higgs, D. R., Hunt, D. M., Drysdale, C. D., Clegg, J. B., Pressley, L., and Weatherall, D. J.: The genetic basis of Hb Q-H disease. *Br. J. Haematol. 46:*387, 1980.
86. Surrey, S., Chambers, J. S., Muni, D., and Schwartz, E. C.: Restriction endonuclease analysis of human globin genes in cellular DNA. *Biochem. Biophys. Res. Commun. 83:*1125, 1978.
87. Sancar, G. B., Cedeno, M. H., and Rieder, R. F.: The varied arrangements of the alpha globin genes in alpha thalassemia and Hb H disease in American blacks. *Johns Hopkins Med. J. 146:*264, 1980.
88. Weatherall, D. J., Clegg, J. B., and Naughton, M. A.: Globin synthesis in thalassaemia: An in vitro study. *Nature 208:*1061, 1965.
89. Bank, A., and Marks, P. A.: Excess α chain synthesis relative to β chain synthesis in thalassaemia major and minor. *Nature 212:*1198, 1966.
90. Bargellesi, A., Pontremoli, S., Menini, C., and Conconi, F.: Excess of alpha globin synthesis in homozygous beta-thalassemia and its removal from the red blood cell cytoplasm. *Eur. J. Biochem. 3:*364, 1968.
91. Nathan, D. G., and Gunn, R. B.: Thalassemia: The consequence of unbalanced hemoglobin synthesis. *Am. J. Med. 41:*815, 1966.
92. Nathan, D. G., Stossel, T. B., Gunn, R. B., Zarkowsky, H. S., and

Laforet, M. T.: Influence of hemoglobin precipitation on erythrocyte metabolism in alpha and beta thalassemia. *J. Clin. Invest. 48:*33, 1969.
93. Rachmilewitz, E. A.: The role of intracellular hemoglobin precipitation, low MCHC and iron overload on red blood cell membrane peroxidation in thalassemia. *Birth Defects 12:*123, 1976.
94. Gabuzda, T. G., Nathan, D. G., and Gardner, F. H.: The turnover of hemoglobins A, F and A₂ in the peripheral blood of three patients with thalassemia. *J. Clin. Invest 42:*1678, 1963.
95. Loukopoulos, D., and Fessas, P.: The distribution of hemoglobin types in thalassemic erythrocytes. *J. Clin. Invest. 44:*231, 1965.
96. Knox-Macaulay, H. H. M., Weatherall, D. J., Clegg, J. B., Bradley, J., and Brown, M. J.: Clinical and biosynthetic characterization of αβ-thalassaemia. *Br. J. Haematol. 22:*497, 1972.
97. Kreimer-Birnbaum, M., Rusnak, P. A., Bannerman, R. M., and Glass, U.: Urinary pyrrole pigments in thalassemia and unstable hemoglobin diseases. *Ann. N.Y. Acad. Sci. 232:*283, 1974.
98. Finch, C. A., et al.: Ferrokinetics in man. *Medicine (Baltimore) 49:*17, 1970.
99. Wickramasinghe, S. N., Letsky, E., and Moffatt, B.: Effect of α-chain precipitates on bone marrow function in homozygous β-thalassaemia. *Br. J. Haematol. 25:*123, 1973.
100. Wickramasinghe, S. N., Hughes, M., Hollan, S. R., Horanyi, M., and Szelenyi, J.: Electron microscopic and high resolution autoradiographic studies of the erythroblasts in haemoglobin H disease. *Br. J. Haematol. 45:*401, 1980.
101. Wickramasinghe, S. N.: The morphology and kinetics of erythropoiesis in homozygous β-thalassaemia. Congenital disorders of erythropoiesis. *Ciba Found. Symp.*, p. 221, 1976.
102. Fessas, P., and Loukopoulos, D.: The β thalassaemias. *Clin. Haematol. 3:*411, 1974.
103. Modell, C. B., and Berdoukas, V. A.: *The Clinical Approach to Thalassemia.* Grune & Stratton, New York, 1982, in press.
104. Fessas, P.: Inclusions of hemoglobin in erythroblasts and erythrocytes of thalassemia. *Blood 21:*21, 1963.
105. Wasi, P., Disthasongchan, P., and Na-Nakorn, S.: The effect of iron deficiency on the levels of hemoglobins A₂ and E. *J. Lab. Clin. Med. 71:*85, 1968.
106. Chalevelakis, G., Clegg, J. B., and Weatherall, D. J.: Imbalanced globin chain synthesis in heterozygous β-thalassemic bone marrow. *Proc. Natl. Acad. Sci. U.S.A. 72:*3853, 1975.
107. Silvestroni, E., Bianco, I., and Reitano, G.: Three cases of homozygous δβ-thalassemia (or microcythemia) with high haemoglobin F in a Sicilian family. *Acta Haematol. (Basel) 40:*220, 1968.
108. Ramot, B., Ben-Bassat, I., Garni, D., and Zaanoon, R.: A family with three βδ-thalassemia homozygotes. *Blood 35:*158, 1970.
109. Tsistrakis, G. A., Amarantos, S. P., and Konkouris, L. L.: Homozygous βδ-thalassemia. *Acta Haematol. (Basel) 51:*185, 1974.
110. Wood, W. G., Clegg, J. B., and Weatherall, D. J.: Hereditary persistence of fetal haemoglobin (HPFH) and δβ thalassemia. *Br. J. Haematol. 43:*509, 1979 (annotation).
111. Efremov, G. D.: Hemoglobin Lepore and anti-Lepore. *Hemoglobin 2:*197, 1978.
112. Gerald, P. S., and Diamond, L. K.: The diagnosis of thalassemia trait by starch block electrophoresis of the hemoglobin. *Blood 13:*61, 1958.
113. Boyer, S. H., et al.: Inheritance of F cell frequency in heterocellular hereditary persistence of fetal hemoglobin: An example of allelic exclusion. *Am. J. Hum. Genet. 29:*256, 1977.
114. Huisman, T. H. J., et al.: Evidence for multiple structural genes for the γ-chain of human fetal hemoglobin in hereditary persistence of fetal hemoglobin. *Ann. N.Y. Acad. Sci. 165:*320, 1969.
115. Huisman, T. H. J., et al.: The present status of the heterogeneity of fetal hemoglobin in β-thalassemia: An attempt to unify some observations in thalassemia and related conditions. *Ann. N.Y. Acad. Sci. 232:*107, 1974.
116. Huisman, T. H. J., Wrightstone, R. N., Wilson, J. B., Schroeder, W. A., and Kendall, A. G.: Hemoglobin Kenya, the product of fusion of γ and β polypeptide chains. *Arch. Biochem. Biophys. 153:*850, 1972.
117. Charache, S., Clegg, J. B., and Weatherall, D. J.: The Negro variety of hereditary persistence of fetal haemoglobin is a mild form of thalassaemia. *Br. J. Haematol. 34:*527, 1976.

118. Fessas, P., and Stamatoyannopoulos, G.: Hereditary persistence of fetal hemoglobin in Greece. A study and a comparison. *Blood* 24:223, 1964.

119. Clegg, J. B., Metaxatou-Mavromati, A., Kattamis, C., Sofroniadou, K., Wood, W. G., and Weatherall, D. J.: Occurrence of ᴳγ Hb F in Greek HPFH: Analysis of heterozygotes and compound heterozygotes with β thalassemia. *Br. J. Haematol.* 43:521, 1979.

120. Wood, W. G., Stamatoyannopoulos, G., Lim, G., and Nute, P. E.: F cells in the adult: Normal values and levels in individuals with hereditary and acquired elevations of Hb F. *Blood* 46:671, 1975.

121. Zago, M. A., Wood, W. G., Clegg, J. B., Weatherall, D. J., O'Sullivan, M., and Gunson, H.: Genetic control of F-cells in human adults. *Blood* 53:977, 1979.

122. Marti, H. R.: *Normale und anormale menschliche Hamoglobine.* Springer, Berlin, 1963, p. 81.

123. Old, J. M., Ayyub, H., Wood, W. G., Clegg, J. B., and Weatherall, D. J.: Linkage analysis of non-deletion hereditary persistence of fetal haemoglobin. *Science* 215:981, 1982.

124. Wood, W. G., Weatherall, D. J., Clegg, J. B., Hamblin, T. J., Edwards, J. H., and Barlow, A. M.: Heterocellular hereditary persistence of fetal haemoglobin (heterocellular HPFH) and its interaction with β thalassaemia. *Br. J. Haematol.* 36:461, 1977.

125. Wood, W. G., Weatherall, D. J., and Clegg, J. B.: Interaction of heterocellular hereditary persistence of foetal haemoglobin with β thalassaemia and sickle cell anaemia. *Nature* 264:247, 1976.

126. Cappellini, M. D., Fiorelli, G., and Bernini, L. F.: Interaction between homozygous β⁰ thalassaemia and the Swiss type of hereditary persistence of fetal haemoglobin. *Br. J. Haematol.* 48:139, 1981.

127. Stamatoyannopoulos, G., Wood, W. G., Papayannopoulou, T., and Nute, P. E.: A new form of hereditary persistence of fetal hemoglobin in Blacks and its association with sickle cell trait. *Blood* 46:683, 1975.

128. Altay, C., Huisman, T. H. J., and Schroeder, W. A.: Another form of hereditary persistence of fetal hemoglobin (the Atlanta type)? *Hemoglobin* 1:125, 1976.

129. Silvestroni, E., and Bianco, I.: *La Malattia Microdrepanocitica.* Il Pensiero Scientifico, Editore, Roma, 1955.

130. Serjeant, G. R., Ashcroft, M. T., Serjeant, B. E., and Milner, P. F.: The clinical features of sickle-cell β thalassaemia in Jamaica. *Br. J. Haematol.* 24:19, 1973.

131. Wasi, P., et al.: Alpha- and beta- thalassemia in Thailand. *Ann. N.Y. Acad. Sci.* 165:60, 1969.

132. Traeger, J., Wood, W. G., Clegg, J. B., Weatherall, D. J., and Wasi, P.: Defective synthesis of Hb E is due to reduced levels of βᴱ mRNA. *Nature* 288:497, 1980.

133. Kattamis, C., Mataxatou-Mavromati, A., Wood, W. G., Nash, J. R., and Weatherall, D. J.: The heterogeneity of normal Hb A₂ β thalassaemia in Greece. *Br. J. Haematol.* 42:109, 1979.

134. Schwartz, E.: The silent carrier of beta thalassemia. *N. Engl. J. Med.* 281:1327, 1969.

135. Aksoy, M., Dinçol, G., and Erdem, S.: Different types of beta-thalassaemia intermedia. *Acta Haematol. (Basel)* 59:178, 1978.

136. Bianco, I., Graziani, B., and Carboni, C.: Genetic patterns in thalassemia intermedia (constitutional microcytic anemia). Familial, hematologic and biosynthetic studies. *Hum. Hered.* 27:257, 1977.

137. Schokker, R. C., Went, L. N., and Bok, J.: A new genetic variant of beta-thalassaemia. *Nature* 209:44, 1966.

138. Wasi, P., Pootrakul, S., Pootrakul, P., Pravatmuang, P., Winichagoon, P., and Fucharoen, S.: Thalassemia in Thailand. *Ann. N.Y. Acad. Sci.* 344:352, 1980.

139. Adams, J. G., Boxer, L. A., Baehner, R. L., Forget, B. G., Tsistrakis, G. A., and Steinberg, M. H.: Hemoglobin Indianapolis (β112[G14]arginine). An unstable β-chain variant producing the phenotype of severe β thalassemia. *J. Clin. Invest.* 63:931, 1979.

140. Ohta, Y., Yamaoka, K., Sumida, I., Fujita, S., Fujimura, T., and Yanase, T.: Homozygous delta-thalassemia first discovered in a Japanese family with hereditary persistence of fetal hemoglobin. *Blood* 37:706, 1971.

141. Kan, Y. W., Forget, B. G., and Nathan, D. G.: Gamma-beta thalassemia: A cause of hemolytic disease of the newborn. *N. Engl. J. Med.* 286:129, 1972.

142. Kan, Y. W., and Nathan, D. G.: Mild thalassemia: The result of interactions of alpha and beta thalassemia genes. *J. Clin. Invest.* 49:635, 1970.

143. Loukopoulos, D., Loutradi, A., and Fessas, P.: A unique thalassaemia syndrome: Homozygous α-thalassaemia + homozygous β-thalassaemia. *Br. J. Haematol.* 39:377, 1978.

144. Weatherall, D. J., et al.: The clinical and molecular heterogeneity of the thalassaemia syndromes. *Ann. N.Y. Acad. Sci.* 344:83, 1980.

145. Pippard, M. J., Callender, S. T., Warner, G. T., and Weatherall, D. J.: Iron absorption and loading in beta-thalassaemia intermedia. *Lancet* 2:819, 1979.

146. Lie-Injo, L. E., and Jo, B. H.: A fast moving haemoglobin in hydrops foetalis. *Nature* 185:698, 1960.

147. Wasi, P., Na-Nakorn, S., and Pootrakul, S.: The α thalassaemias. *Clin. Haematol.* 3:383, 1974.

148. Gouttas, A., Fessas, P., Tsevrenis, H., and Xefteri, E.: Déscription d'une nouvelle variété d'anaemie hemolytique congenitale. (Étude hematologique, éléctrophoretique et genetique.) *Sang* 26:911, 1955.

149. Rigas, D. A., Koler, R. D., and Osgood, E. E.: Haemoglobin H. Clinical, laboratory and genetic studies of a family with a previously undescribed haemoglobin. *J. Lab. Clin. Med.* 47:51, 1956.

150. Schwartz, E., Kan, Y. W., and Nathan, D. G.: Unbalanced globin chain synthesis in alpha-thalassemia heterozygotes. *Ann. N.Y. Acad. Sci.* 165:288, 1969.

151. Higgs, D. R., Pressley, L., Clegg, J. B., Weatherall, D. J., and Serjeant, G. R.: α Thalassemia in black populations. *Johns Hopkins Med. J.* 146:300, 1980.

152. Higgs, D. R., Pressley, L., Serjeant, G. R., Clegg, J. B., and Weatherall, D. J.: The genetics and molecular basis of α thalassaemia in association with Hb S in Jamaican Negroes. *Br. J. Haematol.* 47:43, 1981.

153. Lie-Injo, L. E., Ganesan, J., Clegg, J. B., and Weatherall, D. J.: Homozygous state for Hb Constant Spring (slow moving Hb X components). *Blood* 43:251, 1974.

154. Lie-Injo, L. E., Ganesan, J., and Lopez, C. G.: The clinical, hematological, and biochemical expression of hemoglobin Constant Spring and its distribution, in *Abnormal Haemoglobins and Thalassaemia,* edited by R. M. Schmidt. Academic, New York, p. 275.

155. Vella, F., Wells, R. H. C., Ager, J. A. M., and Lehmann, H.: A haemoglobinopathy involving haemoglobin H and a new (Q) haemoglobin. *Br. Med. J.* 1:752, 1958.

156. Lie-Injo, L. E., Pillay, R. P., and Thuraisingham, V.: Further cases of Hb-Q-H disease (Hb Q-α-thalassemia). *Blood* 28:830, 1966.

157. Milner, P. F., and Huisman, T. H. J.: Studies of the proportion and synthesis of haemoglobin G Philadelphia in red cells of heterozygotes, a homozygote and a heterozygote for both haemoglobin G and alpha thalassaemia. *Br. J. Haematol.* 34:207, 1976.

158. Rieder, R. F., Woodbury, D. H., and Rucknagel, D. L.: The interaction of α-thalassaemia and haemoglobin G Philadelphia. *Br. J. Haematol.* 32:159, 1976.

159. Pich, P., et al.: Interaction between Hb Hasharon and α-thalassemia: An approach to the problem of the number of human α loci. *Blood* 51:339, 1978.

160. Stamatoyannopoulos, G.: Problems of screening and counseling in the hemoglobinopathies. *Proceedings of the IVth International Conference on Birth Defects, Vienna,* 1973, p. 268.

161. Silvestroni, E., Bianco, I., Graziani, B., Carboni, C., and D'Arca, S. U.: First premarital screening of thalassaemia carriers in intermediate schools in Latium. *J. Med. Genet.* 15:202, 1978.

162. Alter, B. P.: Prenatal diagnosis of hemoglobinopathies and other hematologic diseases. *J. Pediatr.* 95:501, 1979.

163. Alter, B. P., Orkin, S. H., and Nathan, D. G.: Prenatal diagnosis of the hemoglobinopathies, in *Laboratory Investigation of Fetal Disease,* edited by A. J. Barson. Wright and Sons, London, 1979.

164. Alter, B. P., and Nathan, D. G.: Antenatal diagnosis of haematological disorders—1978. *Clin. Haematol.* 7:19, 1978.

165. Kan, Y. W., Trecartin, R. F., and Dozy, A. M.: Prenatal diagnosis of hemoglobinopathies. *Ann. N.Y. Acad. Sci.* 344:141, 1980.

166. Furbetta, M., et al.: Prenatal diagnosis of β-thalassaemia by fetal red cell enrichment with NH₄Cl-NH₄HCO₃ differential lysis of maternal cells. *Br. J. Haematol.* 44:441, 1980.

167. Alter, B. P., Orkin, S. H., Forget, B. G., and Nathan, D. G.: Prenatal

diagnosis of hemoglobinopathies. The New England approach. *Ann. N.Y. Acad. Sci.* 344:151, 1980.

168. Cao, A., Furbetta, M., Angius, A., Ximenes, A., Angioni, G., and Caminiti, F.: Prenatal diagnosis of β thalassemia: Experience with 133 cases and effect of fetal blood sampling on child development. *Ann. N.Y. Acad. Sci.* 344:165, 1980.

169. Aleporou-Marinou, V., Sakarelou-Papepetrou, N., Antsaklis, A., Fessas, P., and Loukopoulos, D.: Prenatal diagnosis of thalassemia major in Greece. Evaluation of the first large series of attempts. *Ann. N.Y. Acad. Sci.* 344:181, 1980.

170. Matsakis, M., et al.: Haematological aspects of antenatal diagnosis for thalassaemia in Britain. *Br. J. Haematol.* 46:185, 1980.

171. Koenig, H. M., Vedvick, T. S., Dozy, A. M., Globus, H. S., and Kan, Y. W.: Prenatal diagnosis of hemoglobin H disease. *J. Pediatr.* 92:278, 1978.

172. Kan, Y. W., and Dozy, A. M.: Polymorphisms of DNA sequence adjacent to human β-globin structural gene: Relation to sickle mutation. *Proc. Natl. Acad. Sci. U.S.A.* 75:5631, 1978.

173. Kan, Y. W., and Dozy, A. M.: Antenatal diagnosis of sickle cell anaemia by DNA analysis of amniotic-fluid cells. *Lancet* 2:910, 1978.

174. Kan, Y. W., Lee, K. Y., Furbetta, M., Angius, A., and Cao, A.: Polymorphism of DNA sequences in the beta globin gene region. Application to prenatal diagnosis of β⁰ thalassaemia in Sardinia. *N. Engl. J. Med.* 302:185, 1980.

175. Little, P. F. R., Annison, G., Darling, S., Williamson, R., Camba, L., and Modell, B.: Model for antenatal diagnosis of β-thalassaemia and other monogenic disorders by molecular analysis of linked DNA polymorphisms. *Nature* 285:144, 1980.

176. Kazazian, H. H., Phillips, J. A., Boehm, C. D., Vik, T. A., Mahoney, M. J., and Ritchey, A. K.: Prenatal diagnosis of β-thalassemias by amniocentesis: Linkage analysis using multiple polymorphic restriction endonuclease sites. *Blood* 56:926, 1980.

177. Wolman, I. J.: Transfusion therapy in Cooley's anemia: Growth and health as related to long-range hemoglobin levels, a progress report. *Ann. N.Y. Acad. Sci.* 119:736, 1964.

178. Piomelli, S., et al.: Hypertransfusion regimen in patients with Cooley's anemia. *Ann. N.Y. Acad. Sci.* 232:186, 1974.

179. Modell, C. B.: Total management in thalassaemia major. *Arch. Dis. Child.* 52:489, 1977.

180. Propper, R. D.: Current concepts in the overall management of thalassemia. *Ann. N.Y. Acad. Sci.* 344:375, 1980.

181. Propper, R. D., Shurin, S. B., and Nathan, D. G.: Reassessment of the use of desferrioxamine B in iron overload. *N. Engl. J. Med.* 294:1421, 1976.

182. Propper, R. D., et al.: Continuous subcutaneous administration of deferoxamine in patients with iron overload. *N. Engl. J. Med.* 297:418, 1977.

183. Pippard, M. J., Callender, S. T., and Weatherall, D. J.: Intensive iron-chelation therapy with desferrioxamine in iron loading anaemias. *Clin. Sci. Mol. Med.* 54:99, 1978.

184. Hussain, M. A. M., Green, N., Flynn, D. M., and Hoffbrand, A. V.: Effect of dose, time and ascorbate in iron excretion after subcutaneous desferrioxamine. *Lancet* 1:977, 1977.

185. Pippard, M. J., Callender, S. T., and Finch, C. A.: Ferrioxamine excretion in iron-loaded man. *Blood* 60:288, 1982.

186. Nienhuis, A. W.: Safety of intensive chelation therapy. *N. Engl. J. Med.* 296:114, 1977.

187. Smith, C. H., Erlandson, M. E., Stern, G., and Hilgartner, H.: Postsplenectomy infection in Cooley's anemia. *Ann. N.Y. Acad. Sci.* 119:748, 1964.

188. Bullen, A. W., and Losowsky, M. S.: Consequences of impaired splenic function. *Clin. Sci.* 57:129, 1979.

189. Hirsh, J., and Dacie, J. V.: Persistent post-splenectomy thrombocytosis and thrombo-embolism. A consequence of continuing anaemia. *Br. J. Haematol.* 12:44, 1966.

190. Modell, B., Letsky, E. A., Flynn, D. M., Peto, R., and Weatherall, D. J.: Survival and desferrioxamine in thalassemia major. *Brit. Med. J.* 284:1081, 1982.

191. Barry, M., Flynn, D. N., Letsky, E. A., and Risdon, R. A.: Long-term chelation therapy in thalassaemia major: Effect on liver iron concentration, liver histology and clinical progress. *Br. Med. J.* 1:16, 1974.

192. Weatherall, D. J.: The iron loading anemias, in *Development of Iron Chelators for Clinical Use*, edited by A. E. Martell, W. F. Anderson, and D. G. Badman. Elsevier, North Holland, 1981, p. 3.

193. Orkin, S. H., et al.: Linkage of β-thalassemia mutations and β-globin gene polymorphisms with DNA polymorphisms in human β-globin gene cluster. *Nature* 296:627, 1982.

194. Baird, M., et al.: A nucleotide change at a splice junction in the human β-globin gene is associated with β⁰-thalassaemia. *Proc. Natl. Acad. Sci.* 78:4218, 1981.

195. Poncz, M., Ballantine, M., Solowiejczyk, D., Barak, I., Schwartz, E., and Surrey, S.: β-Thalassemia in a Kurdish Jew. *J. Biol. Chem.* 257:5994, 1982.

196. Goossens, M., Lee, K. Y., Liebhaber, S. A., and Kan, Y. W.: Globin structural mutant $\alpha^{125Leu \rightarrow Pro}$ is a novel cause of α-thalassaemia. *Nature* 296:864, 1982.

197. Old, J. M., Ward, R. H. T., Petrou, M., Karagozlu, F., Modell, B., and Weatherall, D. J.: First trimester diagnosis for haemoglobinopathies; a report of 3 cases. *Lancet* 2:1413, 1982.

Erythrocyte disorders—anemias related to unknown or multiple mechanisms

CHAPTER *51*

Anemia of chronic disorders

ALLAN J. ERSLEV

History and definition

Weakness, weight loss, and pallor have been recognized as hallmarks of chronic illness as far back as we have medical and literary records. Yet, despite the preoccupation with blood and bloodlettings, it apparently was not recognized until the early nineteenth century that the common pallor of tuberculosis ("consumption") was associated with a lack of blood. In their classic review, "The Anemia of Infection" [1], Cartwright and Wintrobe mention that French investigators in 1842 demonstrated that blood from patients with typhoid fever and smallpox contained a smaller mass of red cells than normal blood. The development of methods for the counting of red cells and for measuring hemoglobin concentration led to the realization that the common infections which ravaged the world, such as pneumonia, syphilis, tuberculosis, and typhoid fever, were all associated with an anemia appropriately designated as the *anemia of infection*. During the last 20 years, it has become recognized that noninfectious disorders, such as rheumatoid arthritis, Hodgkin's disease, or metastatic carcinoma, are associated with a similar anemia, and the names *simple chronic anemia* and *anemia of chronic disorders* have been introduced.

These anemias are usually moderate, with hemoglobin concentrations ranging from 7 to 11 g/dl, and are rarely symptomatic or in need of therapy. The anemias are indeed so commonplace and innocuous that hemoglobin concentrations in this range often are considered "normal" for patients with chronic disorders. Studies of thyroid metabolism actually support this concept by showing that many patients with chronic disease have low levels of calorigenic T_3 and therefore should need less oxygen-carrying capacity than normal persons [3,4].

The reason for assuming that the anemias observed in a variety of chronic clinical disorders are related is that these anemias have certain common features. They are associated with a low serum iron, a low iron-binding capacity, increased tissue iron stores, and relative bone marrow failure. Indeed these features are so characteristic that the name *sideropenic anemia with reticuloendothelial siderosis* has been suggested [2], a reasonable but not a very happy addition to our collection of hematologic tongue twisters. Consequently, it appears justifiable to retain the name *anemia of chronic disorders* until further clarification of the pathogenesis leads to a more appropriate designation.

Incidence

The spectacular change wrought by antibiotics on the ecology of disease has led to a decrease in the incidence of chronic, incapacitating infections and true anemia of infection. However, numerous past reports on tuberculosis, lung abscess, subacute bacterial endocarditis, chronic osteomyelitis, and chronic mycotic infections attest that almost all chronic suppurative infections are associated with anemia [1,2,5–13] and that the severity of the anemia is roughly proportional to the severity of symptoms such as fever, weight loss, and general debility. It requires about 1 to 2 months of sustained infection for anemia to develop, after which a new balance is established between red cell production and red cell destruction, and the hemoglobin level becomes stabilized [2].

The anemia complicating chronic inflammatory diseases behaves functionally like the anemia complicating infections but has assumed greater importance because of the less effective therapies available for these diseases. The collagen diseases, with rheumatoid arthritis [14–18] as the most prominent member, are regularly associated with anemia. Regional enteritis, ulcerative colitis, and a variety of poorly understood inflammatory syndromes may also be complicated by the anemia of chronic disorders [1,2,19,20]. Of particular contemporary importance is the anemia found in patients with metastatic or necrotizing carcinoma, with Hodgkin's disease, and with malignant lymphoma [21–26].

Etiology and pathogenesis

The anemia of chronic disorders is characterized by a slightly shortened red cell life-span, a disturbed iron metabolism, and an impaired compensatory increase in the rate of red cell production. Because of the moderate degree of the anemia and the modifying influence of underlying disorders, it has been difficult to relate these observations and establish a firm pathogenetic mechanism. However, it has been suggested that the anemia is part of a "hematological stress syndrome" [27] caused by the mobilization of cellular and metabolic defense mechanisms. In this view stimulation of the monocyte-macrophage system could lead to excessive macrophage sequestration of iron and iron-binding protein, increased splenic destruction of red cells, and suppression of erythroid stem cells. Furthermore, associated protein and caloric malnutrition causing a decrease in transformation of T_4 to T_3 could lead to a protective functional hypothyroidism [28] and a physiologic decrease in erythropoietin production [29].

RED CELL LIFE-SPAN

Cross-transfusion studies have convincingly established that extracorpuscular factors are responsible for the reduction of red cell life-span [2]. A single extracorpuscular factor shared by infections, sterile inflammations, and neoplastic diseases is difficult to envision, unless tissue breakdown is the common denominator. It is possible that red cells are damaged by passing through injured tissue or that injured tissues release membrane-active factors. However, such mechanisms have not been easy to establish, since even a subtle injury to red cells may cause a reduction in red cell life-span. Another possibility is that the monocyte-macrophage system, as part of a general defense mechanism, becomes hyperplastic, resulting in a slight but sustained premature sequestration and destruction of normal red cells [30,31].

IRON METABOLISM

A low serum iron level despite adequate iron stores indicates a profound disturbance of iron metabolism. The rate of gastrointestinal absorption of iron has been measured in a number of patients with chronic disorders [2,17,32–35], but the results have been difficult to interpret. In general, however, it appears that the intestinal absorption is impaired [2,32], as shown in dogs with turpentine-induced abscesses [1]. Since the uptake of iron into intestinal cells and its subsequent incorporation into intracellular ferritin are normal [36], the defect apparently lies in the subsequent release of iron, possibly akin to the defective iron release from the monocyte-macrophage system and hepatic cells in patients with chronic diseases.

Nevertheless, enough iron must have been released from intestinal cells to stock the iron stores, and it seems most likely that the low serum iron level is caused by impaired release of iron from the monocyte-macrophage system to circulating transferrin, or in other words by impaired reutilization of iron. Direct evidence for such a monocyte-macrophage block was provided by experiments which showed that dogs with sterile turpentine-induced abscesses failed to reutilize iron from senescent red blood cells labeled with radioactive iron [37]. This observation was confirmed in patients with infections [38], and similar studies employing labeled hemoglobin solutions rather than intact labeled red cells revealed poor reutilization of hemoglobin iron in patients with infection, cancer, Hodgkin's disease, and rheumatoid arthritis [23,39] (Fig. 51-1). Since intact red cells are degraded in the monocyte-macrophage system and free hemoglobin is degraded in

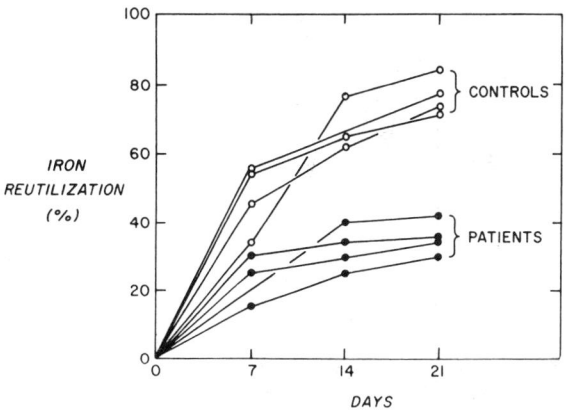

FIGURE 51-1 Reutilization of ^{59}Fe-tagged hemoglobin solution in patients with anemia of inflammation and in normal controls. (Haurani, Burke, and Martinez [39].)

hepatic parenchymal cells [40], these studies suggest the presence of a basic but still unexplained disturbance in the cellular mobilization of iron from ferritin or hemosiderin to circulating transferrin. This disturbance occurs rapidly after almost all kinds of infectious or inflammatory injuries [41,42], and significant hypoferremia can be observed within 24 h after both major and minor surgery [41–45] (Fig. 51-2) and after pyrogen-induced fever [46].

A reduced concentration of transferrin is character-

FIGURE 51-2 Mean serum iron and iron-binding capacity ±1 standard deviation of nine patients undergoing cholecystectomy. (Erslev and McKenna [45].)

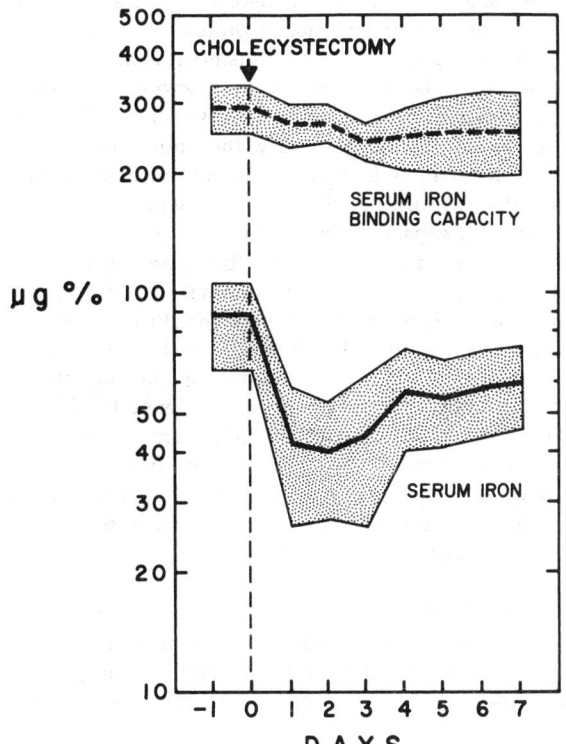

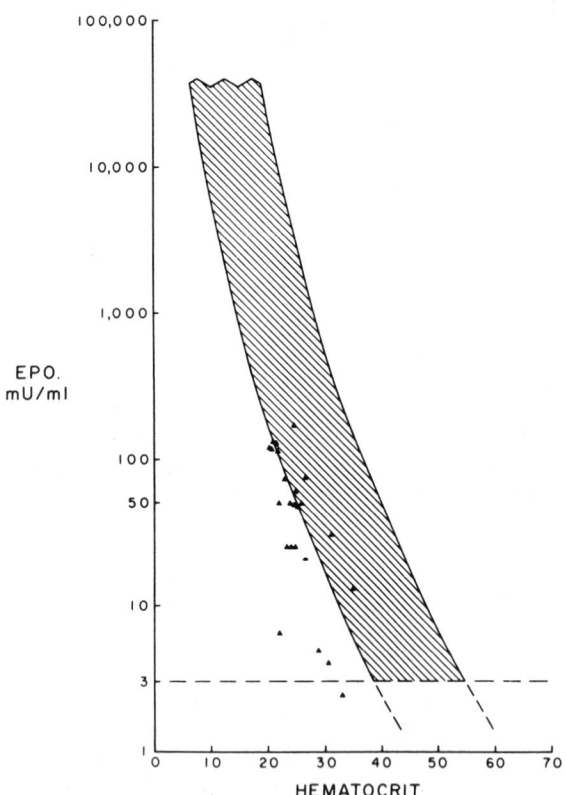

FIGURE 51-3 Plasma erythropoietin titers in patients with anemia of chronic disorders. The range of values for control subjects is given by the hatched area. The broken line indicates that erythropoietin levels below 3 mU/ml are not accurately measured by the method used.

istic of the anemia of chronic disorders. Turnover studies indicate a decreased rate of production [47], but it has also been suggested that transferrin is absorbed to iron-loaded cells of the monocyte-macrophage system [48] or is sequestered in inflammatory foci [49]. Because of the low iron-binding capacity, the amount of unsaturated transferrin is less in the anemia of chronic disorders than in iron-deficiency anemia with its elevated iron-binding capacity. Since it has been shown [50] that there is a competition for iron between unsaturated transferrin and the membrane of immature red cells, the transfer of iron to erythroid cells should be more efficient in chronic disorders than in iron deficiency. This may explain the fact that although the anemia of chronic disorders shows features of iron deficiency (such as a reduced number of sideroblasts [51], increased erythrocyte protoporphyrin [52], and red cell hypochromia), the degree of anemia and the extent of hypochromia or microcytosis are rarely as pronounced as in true iron-deficiency anemia.

MARROW FUNCTION

Since a normal marrow easily could compensate for the moderately shortened red cell life-span, a relative marrow failure must exist. It has been proposed that this failure is caused by decreased release of, or decreased response to, erythropoietin. Studies of the release of erythropoietin in patients with chronic disorders have produced conflicting results. In some studies, the release is markedly decreased in patients with rheumatoid arthritis [53] and chronic infections and malignancies [54,55]; in others it is only decreased in patients with infections and malignancies [56]; and in still others the decrease is erratic [57–59] (Fig. 51-3).

Studies of the response to erythropoietin are equally conflicting, but, as expected, there is no absolute block of erythropoietic function. The marrow of rats with abscesses, for example, is capable of responding to exogenous erythropoietin [60]. Furthermore, cobalt, which presumably acts via the production of cellular hypoxia and the release of erythropoietin, will ameliorate the anemia of infection in dogs [61] and humans [62].

However, erythrokinetic and stem cell studies have shown that the marrow is relatively resistant to erythropoietin. In mice with turpentine-induced abscesses nucleated red cells, erythroid stem cells [63], and marrow stromal cells [64] are all decreased in number, and in humans with chronic disease but adequate erythropoietin levels the erythroid response in subnormal. The production of cellular and humoral inhibitors has been invoked to explain these findings. Coculture of normal marrow with cancer cells [65] or macrophages from chronically infected patients [66] has resulted in suppression of normal erythroid stem cells, and circulating inhibitors of erythroid stem cells have been isolated from patients with disseminated lupus and rheumatoid arthritis [67]. Furthermore the low serum iron level may also be responsible for suppressed erythropoiesis. Iron is a necessary component not only of the hemoglobin molecule but also of several crucial enzymes, such as cytochrome c, catalase, cytochrome oxidase, and succinic dehydrogenase [68]. Consequently it is possible that iron deficiency impairs the proliferative response to erythropoietin in addition to depriving nucleated red cells of a component necessary for hemoglobin synthesis [45,69]. These observations and considerations have led to the conclusion that relative marrow failure plays a major, if not *the* major, role in the development of anemia of chronic disease.

Clinical and laboratory features

The clinical manifestations of the mild to moderate anemia complicating chronic disorders are usually overshadowed by the symptoms of the underlying disease. Under physiologic conditions, a reduction in hemoglobin concentration to 7 to 11 g/dl, the level usually observed in the anemia of chronic disorders, need not be symptomatic. However, in patients with severe pulmonary impairment, fever, or physical debility, a moderate reduction in the oxygen-carrying capacity of the blood may aggravate preexisting symptoms. On physical examination there are no findings characteristic of this anemia, and the diagnosis hinges on the laboratory findings.

The anemia is traditionally described as normocytic and normochromic [1]. However, the majority of patients actually have hypochromic red cells with a mean corpuscular hemoglobin concentration (MCHC) below 31 percent, and many patients have microcytic cells with a mean corpuscular volume (MCV) of less than 80 μm^3 [2].

The absolute reticulocyte count is within the normal range or slightly elevated. Changes in the white blood cell count or platelet count are not consistent and depend almost exclusively on the underlying disorders.

A reduction in serum iron concentration (hypoferremia) is a *sine qua non* for the diagnosis of anemia of chronic disorders (Table 51-1). It occurs promptly after the onset of an infection or injury, and precedes the development of anemia [45,70]. The concentration of the iron-binding protein, transferrin, is moderately decreased [1,2], resulting in a higher iron saturation than would be the case if the transferrin concentration were normal or, as for patients with iron deficiency anemia, were increased (Table 51-1). This relative "protection" of iron saturation may be of benefit by enhancing the transfer of iron from a reduced pool of circulating iron to immature erythroid cells [51]. The reduction in transferrin after injury occurs more slowly than the reduction in serum iron (Fig. 51-2), presumably because of a longer half-life of transferrin (8 to 12 days) [71] than that of iron (90 min), and because of different metabolic functions [48].

Measurements of serum ferritin levels have been found useful in assessing marrow iron stores in patients with low serum iron concentrations [72]. In most instances there is no overlap between levels in patients with chronic disease and increased body stores of iron and patients with iron deficiency [73]. However, depleted iron stores in patients with chronic disease may not be as readily detected by ferritin measurements since fever and infections increase synthesis of ferritin and produce inappropriately high serum levels [79].

Marrow aspirates may be difficult to interpret because the underlying disorders can be responsible for alterations in cellular patterns and structure. However, in general, the marrow is normal. The myeloid/erythroid ratio is about 3:1 or 4:1, and there is little evidence of compensatory erythroid hyperplasia. The most important information derived from a marrow examination pertains to its iron content. Iron in a marrow preparation can be found as storage iron in the cytoplasm of macrophages or as functional iron in nucleated red cells. In normal individuals a few Prussian blue–staining particles can be found inside or adjacent to many macrophages, and about one-third of nucleated red cells contain blue inclusion bodies and are therefore called *sideroblasts* [75]. In iron deficiency there is an absence of both sideroblasts and macrophage iron. However, in the anemia of chronic disorders only sideroblasts are decreased in number; macrophage iron is increased

TABLE 51-1   Iron metabolism

	Normal range	Iron deficiency mean	Chronic disease mean
Plasma iron, μg/dl	70–190	30	30
Iron-binding capacity, μg/dl	250–400	450	200
Percent saturation	30	7	15
Macrophage iron in marrow	2+	0	3+
Serum ferritin, ng/ml	20–220	10	150

[51,76,77]. This increase in storage iron in the face of a decreased level of circulating iron and a decreased number of sideroblasts is characteristic of the anemia of chronic disorders and is found in no other diseases.

The results of red cell survival studies have varied, as would be expected when one considers the great diversity of the underlying disorders, but, in general, normal cells have displayed a slightly shortened survival when injected into patients with chronic disorders [16,78–81], and red cells from such patients have had a normal survival in normal recipients [16,79,80]. These findings indicate an extracorpuscular destruction of red cells, presumably caused by infectious or inflammatory foci.

The observation that the patient's cells, after appropriate labeling, appear to survive for a normal length of time when injected into his or her own circulation has been somewhat disturbing [23,39,81–84]. One explanation given is that the labeled cells, because of premature extracorpuscular destruction, are somewhat younger than normal cells and will live relatively longer [81]. However, it must also be remembered that the reduction in red cell life-span is small and is quite difficult to quantitate accurately.

In accordance with the morphologic appearance of the marrow, measurements of plasma and red cell iron-turnover rates have disclosed a normal or only slightly increased rate of effective red cell production [16,22,23,33,79,85]. The half-life of intravenously injected radioactive iron is very short, but, when adjusted for the low level of circulating iron, the calculated plasma iron turnover is only slightly higher than normal. Since 70 percent or more of the injected radioactive iron can be accounted for in circulating red cells, erythropoiesis is mostly effective with the production and release of viable cells [86,87]. When these normal values are correlated with the fact that the marrow maintains a red cell mass of less than normal size, they support the direct measurements of a shortened red cell life-span.

Differential diagnosis

Most patients with chronic infections, inflammations, or neoplastic disorders are anemic, but such anemias should be designated as anemias of chronic disorders only if the anemia is moderate, the cellular pattern in the marrow is nearly normal, the serum iron and iron-binding capacity are low, the iron content of the marrow macrophages is normal or increased, and the serum ferritin is elevated. Since the underlying diseases can predispose the patients to many other hematologic disturbances, a final diagnosis of anemia of chronic disorders should first be made after having ruled out other etiologic mechanisms. The following causes for anemia may, in particular, aggravate or obscure the anemia of chronic disorders:

1. Dilution anemia. The incidence of a relative anemia in patients with chronic illnesses, especially in patients with far-advanced neoplastic diseases, have been discussed extensively. High plasma volumes have been reported in such patients [88–90], but the problems involved in relating plasma volume to body weight in emaciated individuals have led other investigators to question these results [22]. However, the anemia in some patients with myeloma and macroglobulinemia may in part be caused by a selective increase in plasma volume [91,92].

2. Drug-induced marrow suppression or drug-induced hemolysis should always be considered. As a general rule, the serum iron will tend to be high in marrow suppression as a reflection of reduced erythroid maturation. Reticulocyte counts, haptoglobin level, bilirubin determination, Coombs' test, and determination of glucose-6-phosphate dehydrogenase activity should be done to rule out a hemolytic component.

3. Chronic blood loss or iron malabsorption will eliminate the characteristic macrophage siderosis, and one has to rely heavily on the level of transferrin in order to distinguish between iron deficiency anemia and the anemia of chronic disorders. The simplest diagnostic approach to a patient with anemia and low or absent iron in the bone marrow is a therapeutic trial of iron followed by reevaluation.

4. Renal impairment causes both a shortened red cell life-span and a relative marrow failure. Although the serum iron level is either normal or high in the so-called anemia of uremia, the diagnosis rests on the finding of an increased blood urea nitrogen or creatinine. The diagnosis of anemia of uremia should not be made unless there is biochemical evidence of azotemia, and, on the other hand, the diagnosis of anemia of chronic disorders cannot be made in the face of overt uremia.

5. Metastatic replacement of the marrow by carcinomas or lymphomas will aggravate or mimic anemia of chronic disorders. The serum iron concentration is usually normal or increased, and there may be telltale signs of marrow involvement in the peripheral blood such as poikilocytes, teardrop-shaped red cells, normoblasts, or immature myeloid cells. Serum alkaline phosphatase determinations and x-ray studies of bone may help establish a diagnosis of myelophthisic anemia.

In short, the diagnosis of anemia of chronic disorders has to rest not only on the demonstration of certain characteristic features of this anemia but also on the elimination of other causes for a reduction in the hemoglobin concentration.

Therapy

Any anemia occurring in a patient with chronic debilitating disease should be thoroughly investigated in order to rule out specific deficiencies or complications. If the anemia after such studies can be designated as an anemia of chronic disorders, it rarely demands therapy. A hemoglobin level between 7 and 11 g should be of concern, but it has not been definitely shown that it is detrimental to health or impedes reparative processes. Similarly, a low serum iron concentration, especially when associated with a near-normal percent saturation of transferrin, has not been proved to be harmful. To the contrary, it has even been proposed that a low iron level may be an adapative defense mechanism against iron-dependent bacteria [93,94]. Nevertheless, it still seems reasonable to believe that if both serum iron and hemoglobin concentrations could be restored to normal it would be of some benefit to a chronically ill patient.

Attempts to provide iron by mouth or parenterally have had little or no effect on the iron or hemoglobin concentration [95,96]. Iron dextran will release small amounts (about 1 to 3 percent) of iron directly to transferrin [97], but the bulk of iron will first be released after ingestion of the compound by the monocyte-macrophage system [98]. This release, however, is blocked in anemia of chronic disorders in the same way as the release of intestinal iron or hemoglobin iron [99]. It has been suspected that the few patients who were helped by oral or parenteral iron had, in addition to the anemia of chronic disorder, an iron deficiency which contributed to the anemia [2].

Erythropoietin, if available in a therapeutic form, would undoubtedly increase the rate of red cell production, but it could aggravate the hypoferremia and thereby be of very questionable therapeutic benefit. Cobalt, presumably acting by releasing renal erythropoietin, has been shown to ameliorate the anemia of chronic disorders [62,100]. However, its toxic side effects, as well as its suppressive action on oxidative metabolism, render it an unacceptable treatment for a fairly benign condition. Androgens likewise should probably not be used therapeutically in this condition [101]. In summary, it appears that the drug therapy of the anemia of chronic disorders should be avoided and that transfusions of packed red cells be used in the few patients in whom the anemia has become symptomatic.

References

1. Cartwright, G. E., and Wintrobe, M. M.: The anemia of infection, in *Advances in Internal Medicine*, edited by W. Dock and J. Snapper. Year Book, Chicago, 1952, vol. 5, p. 165.

2. Cartwright, G. E.: The anemia of chronic disorders. *Semin. Hematol.* 3:351, 1966.
3. Carter, J. N., Eastman, C. J., Corcoran, J. M., and Lazarus, L.: Effect of severe chronic illness on thyroid function. *Lancet II:*971, 1974.
4. Chapra, J. J., Solomon, D. H., Hepner, G. W., and Morgenstein, A. A.: Misleadingly low free thyroxine index and usefulness of reverse triiodothyronine measurement in nonthyroidal illnesses. *Ann. Intern. Med.* 90:905, 1979.
5. Braverman, M. M.: The anemia of pulmonary tuberculosis. *Am. Rev. Tuberc.* 38:466, 1938.
6. Miescher, P., Gsell, O., and Fust, B.: Pathogenesis of anemia of tuberculosis. *Schweiz. Med. Wochenschr.* 85:917, 1955.
7. Parson, W. B., Jr., Cooper, T., and Scheifley, C. H.: Anemia in bacterial endocarditis. *JAMA* 133:14, 1953.
8. Hemmeler, G.: *L'Anemia infectieuse.* Benno Schwabe, Basel, 1946.
9. James, G. W., Riblet, L. A., Robinson, J. G., Johnson, R. E., and Kark, R. M.: Studies on prolonged suppurative infection in man. *J. Lab. Clin. Med.* 33:1607, 1948.
10. Saiti, M. F., and Vaughan, J. M.: The anemia associated with infection. *J. Pathol. Bacteriol.* 56:189, 1955.
11. Vaughan, J. M.: Anemia associated with trauma and sepsis. *Br. Med. J.* 1:35, 1948.
12. Adams, E. B., and Mayet, F. G. H.: Hypochromic anemia in chronic infections. *S. Afr. Med. J.* 40:738, 1966.
13. Glasser, R. M.: The significance of hematologic abnormalities in patients with tuberculosis. *Arch. Intern. Med.* 125:69, 1970.
14. Nilsson, F.: Anemia problems in rheumatoid arthritis. *Acta Med. Scand. (Suppl.)* 130:210, 1948.
15. Jeffrey, M. R.: Some observations on anemia in rheumatoid arthritis. *Blood* 8:502, 1953.
16. Ebaugh, F. G.: The anemia of rheumatoid arthritis, in *Iron in Clinical Medicine,* edited by Wallerstein and Methier. University of California Press, Berkeley, 1958, p. 261.
17. Roberts, F. D., Hagedorn, A. B., Slocumb, C. H., and Owen, C. A.: Evaluation of the anemia of rheumatoid arthritis. *Blood* 21:470, 1963.
18. Strandberg, O.: Anemia of rheumatoid arthritis. *Acta Med. Scand. (Suppl.)* 454:1, 1966.
19. Garvin, R. O., and Bargen, J. A.: Hematologic picture of chronic ulcerative colitis. *Am. J. Med. Sci.* 193:744, 1937.
20. Ormerod, T. P.: Observations on the incidence and cause of anaemia in ulcerative colitis. *Gut* 8:107, 1967.
21. Price, V. E., and Greenfield, R. E.: Anemia in cancer. *Adv. Cancer Res.* 5:199, 1958.
22. Hyman, G. A.: Anemia in malignant neoplastic disease. *J. Chron. Dis.* 16:645, 1963.
23. Haurani F. I., Young, K., and Tocantins, L. M.: Reutilization of iron in anemia complicating malignant neoplasms. *Blood* 22:73, 1963.
24. Friedell, G. H.: Anaemia in cancer. *Lancet* 1:356, 1965.
25. Barkhan, P.: Hematological aspects of Hodgkin's disease. *Guys Hosp. Rep.* 115:319, 1966.
26. Chatterjee K., and MacLe'lan, G. E.: Sideropenic anaemia with reticu'oendothelial siderosis in a case of hypernephroma. *Postgrad. Med. J.* 44:259, 1968.
27. Reizenstein P.: The hematological stress syndrome. *Br. J. Haematol.* 43:329, 1979.
28. Utiger R. D.: Decreased extrathyroidal triiodothyronine production in nonthyroidal illness: Benefit or harm? *Am. J. Med.* 69:807 1980.
29. Caro, J., Silver R., Erslev, A. J., Mi'ler, O. P., and Birgegård, G.: Erythropoietin production in fasted rats. *J. Lab. Clin. Med.* 98:860, 1981.
30. Jandl, J. H., Jacob H. S., and Daland, G. A.: Hypersplenism due to infection: Study of five cases manifesting hemolytic anemia. *N. Engl. J. Med.* 264:1063 1961.
31. Mackaness, G. B.: The monocyte in cellular immunity. *Semin. Hematol.* 7:172 1970.
32 Haurani F. I., Green D., and Young, K.: Iron absorption in hypoferremia. *Am. J Med. Sci* 249:537, 1965.
33. Weinstein I. M.: A correlative study of the erythrokinetics and disturbances in iron metabolism associated with the anemia of rheumatoid arthritis. *Blood* 14:950, 1959.
34. Jeffrey, M. R., Freundlish, H. F., Jackson, E. B., and Watson, D.: The absorption and utilization of radioiron in rheumatoid disease. *Clin. Sci.* 14:395, 1955.
35. Vas, M. R., and DeLeeuw, N. K. M.: Iron absorption in patients with rheumatoid arthritis and in normal subjects. *Med. Assoc. J.* 97:504, 1967.
36. Schade, S. G.: Normal incorporation of iron into intestinal ferritin in inflammation. *Proc. Soc. Exp. Biol. Med.* 139:620, 1972.
37. Freireich, E. M., Miller, A., Emerson, C. P., and Ross, J. F.: The effect of inflammation on the utilization of erythrocyte and transferrin-bound radio-iron for red cell production. *Blood* 12:972, 1957.
38. Noyes, W. D., Bothwell, T. H., and Finch, C. A.: The role of the reticuloendothelial cell in iron metabolism. *Br. J. Haematol.* 6:43, 1960.
39. Haurani, F. I., Burke, W., and Martinez, E. J.: Defective reutilization of iron in the anemia of inflammation. *J. Lab. Clin. Med.* 65:560, 1965.
40. Hershko, C., Cook, J. D., and Finch, C. A.: Storage iron kinetics. II. The uptake of hemoglobin iron by hepatic parenchymal cells. *J. Lab. Clin. Med.* 80:624, 1972.
41. Handjani, A. M., Banihashemi, A., Rafie, R., and Tolan, H.: Serum iron in acute myocardial infarction. *Blut* 23:263, 1971.
42. Cartwright, G. E., Hamilton, L. D., Gubler, C. J., Fellows, N. M., Ashenbrucker, H., and Wintrobe, M. M.: The anemia of infection. XIII. Studies on experimentally produced acute hypoferremia in dogs and the relationship of the adrenal cortex to hypoferremia. *J. Clin. Invest.* 30:161, 1951.
43. Feldthusen, U., Larsen, V., and Lassen, N. A.: Serum iron and operative stress. *Acta Med. Scand.* 147:311, 1953.
44. Baird, J. M., Padmore, D. A., and Wilson, G. M.: Changes in iron metabolism following gastrectomy and other surgical operations. *Clin. Sci.* 16:463, 1957.
45. Erslev, A. J., and McKenna, P. J.: Effect of splenectomy on red cell production. *Ann. Intern. Med.* 67:5, 1967.
46. Elin, R. J., Wolff, S. M., and Finch, C. A.: Effect of induced fever on serum iron and ferritin concentrations in man. *Blood* 49:147, 1977.
47. Jarnum, S., and Lassen, N. A.: Albumin and transferrin metabolism in infectious and toxic diseases. *Scand. J. Clin. Lab. Invest.* 13:357, 1961.
48. Bothwell, T. H., and Finch, C. A.: *Iron Metabolism.* Little, Brown, Boston, 1962.
49. Umeda, T.: Pathophysiological studies on iron metabolism. II. Transferrin (siderophilin) metabolism in infection. *J. Kyushu Hematol. Soc.* 15:153, 1965.
50. Jandl, J. H., and Katz, J. H.: The plasma to cell cycle of transferrin. *J. Clin. Invest.* 42:314, 1963.
51. Bainton, D. F., and Finch, C. A.: The diagnosis of iron deficiency anemia. *Am. J. Med.* 37:62, 1964.
52. Kramer, A., Cartwright, G. E., and Wintrobe, M. M.: The anemia of infection. XIX. Studies on free erythrocyte coproporphyrin and protoporphyrin. *Blood* 9:183, 1954.
53. Ward, H. P., Gordon, B., and Pickett, J. C.: Serum levels of erythropoietin in rheumatoid arthritis. *J. Lab. Clin. Med.* 74:93, 1969.
54. Ward, H. P., Kurnick, J. E., and Pisarczyk, M. J.: Serum level of erythropoietin in anemias associated with chronic infection, malignancy and primary hematopoietic disease. *J. Clin. Invest.* 50:332, 1971.
55. Wallner, S. F., Kurnick, J. E., Vautrin, R. M., White, M. J., Chapman, R. G., and Ward, H. P.: Levels of erythropoietin in patients with the anemias of chronic diseases and liver failure. *Am. J. Haematol.* 3:37, 1977.
56. Zucker, S., Friedman, S., and Lysck, R. M.: Bone marrow erythropoiesis in the anemia of infection, inflammation and malignancy. *J. Clin. Invest.* 53:1132, 1974.
57. Alexanian, R.: Erythropoietin excretion in hemolytic anemia and in the hypoferremia of chronic disease. *Blood* 40:946, 1972 (abstract).
58. Douglas, S. W., and Adamson, J. W.: The anemia of chronic disorders: Studies of marrow regulation and iron metabolism. *Blood* 45:55, 1975.
59. Erslev, A. J., Caro, J., Miller, O., and Silver, R.: Plasma erythropoietin in health and disease. *Ann. Clin. Lab. Sci.* 10:250, 1980.
60. Lukens, J. N.: Control of erythropoiesis in rats with adjuvant-induced chronic inflammation. *Blood* 41:37, 1973.

61. Wintrobe, M. M., Grinstein, M., Dubash, J. J., Humphrey, S. R., Ashenbrucker, H., and Worth, W.: The anemia of infection. VI. The influence of cobalt on the anemia associated with inflammation. *Blood* 2:323, 1947.

62. Robinson, J. C., James, G. W., III, and Kark, R. M.: The effect of oral therapy with cobaltous chloride on the blood of patients suffering with chronic suppurative infection. *N. Engl. J. Med.* 240:749, 1949.

63. Reissmann, K. R., and Udupa, K. B.: Effect of inflammation on erythroid precursors (BFU-E and CFU-E) in bone marrow and spleen of mice. *J. Lab. Clin. Med.* 92:22, 1978.

64. Werts, E. D., Gibson, D. P., and Degowin, R. L.: Chronic inflammation suppresses bone marrow stromal cells and medullary erythropoiesis. *J. Lab. Clin. Med.* 93:995, 1979.

65. Zucker, S., Lysik, R. M., and DiStefano, J. F.: Cancer cell inhibition of erythropoiesis. *J. Lab. Clin. Med.* 96:770, 1980.

66. Zanjani, E. D., McGlave, P. B., Davies, S. F., Banisadre, M., Kaplan, M. E., and Sarosi, G. A.: In vitro suppression of erythropoiesis by bone marrow adherent cells from some patients with fungal infection. *Br. J. Haematol.* 50:479, 1982.

67. Dainiak, N., Hardin, J., Floyd, V., Callahan, M., and Hoffman, R.: Humoral suppression of erythropoiesis in systemic lupus and rheumatoid arthritis. *Am. J. Med.* 69:537, 1980.

68. Beutler, E.: Tissue effects of iron deficiency. *Scand. J. Haematol. (Ser. Haematol.)* 6:41, 1965.

69. Hillman, R. A., and Henderson, D. A.: The control of marrow production by the level of iron supply. *J. Clin. Invest.* 48:454, 1969.

70. Cartwright, G. E., Lauritsen, M. A., Humphreys, S., Jones, P. J., Merill, J. M., and Wintrobe, M. M.: The anemia of infection. II. The experimental production of hypoferremia and anemias in dogs. *J. Clin. Invest.* 25:81, 1946.

71. Awai, M., and Brown, E. B.: Studies of the metabolism of 1[131]-labeled human transferrin. *J. Lab. Clin. Med.* 61:363, 1963.

72. Lipschitz, D. A., Cook, J. D., and Finch, C. A.: A clinical evaluation of serum ferritin as an index of iron stores. *N. Engl. J. Med.* 290:1213, 1974.

73. Bentley, C. P., and Williams, P.: Serum ferritin concentrations as an index of iron storage in rheumatoid arthritis. *J. Clin. Path.* 27:786, 1974.

74. Birgegård, G., Hallgren, R., Killander, A., Stromberg, A., Venge, P., and Wide, L.: Serum ferritin during infection. *Scand. J. Haematol.* 21:333, 1978.

75. Cartwright, G. E., and Deiss, A.: Sideroblasts, siderocytes and sideroblastic anemia. *N. Engl. J. Med.* 292:185, 1975.

76. Ellis, L. D., Jensen, W. N., and Westerman, M. D.: Marrow iron: An evaluation of depleted stores in a series of 1,332 needle biopsies. *Ann. Intern. Med.* 61:44, 1964.

77. Gardner, D. L., and Roy, L. M. H.: Tissue iron and the reticuloendothelial system in rheumatoid arthritis. *Ann. Rheum. Dis.* 20:258, 1961.

78. Alexander, W. R. M., Richmond, J., Roy, L. H. M., and Duthie, J. J. R.: Nature of anemia in rheumatoid arthritis. II. Survival of transfused erythrocytes in patients with rheumatoid arthritis. *Ann. Rheum. Dis.* 15:12, 1956.

79. Freireich, E. J., Ross, J. F., Bayles, T. B., Emerson, D. P., and Finch, S. C.: Radioactive iron metabolisms and erythrocyte survival studies of the mechanisms of the anemia associated with rheumatoid arthritis. *J. Clin. Invest.* 36:1043, 1951.

80. Hyman, G. A., Gellhorn, A., and Harvey, J. L.: Studies on the anemia of disseminated malignant neoplastic disease. II. Study of the life-span of the erythrocytes. *Blood* 11:618, 1956.

81. Richmond, J., Alexander, W. R. M., Potter, J. L., and Duthie, J. J. R.: The nature of anemia in rheumatoid arthritis. V. Red cell survival measured by radioactive chromium. *Ann. Rheum. Dis.* 20:133, 1961.

82. Biechi, A., Stapleton, J. E., Woodbury, J. F. L., and Reed, H. C.: Anemia in rheumatoid arthritis. I. Red cell survival studies. *Can. Med. Assoc. J.* 86:401, 1962.

83. Hollingsworth, J. W., and Hollingsworth, D. R.: Study of total red cell volume and erythrocyte survival using radioactive chromium in patients with advanced pulmonary tuberculosis. *Ann. Intern. Med.* 42:810, 1955.

84. Lewis, S. M., and Porter, I. H.: Erythrocyte survival in rheumatoid arthritis. *Ann. Rheum. Dis.* 19:54, 1960.

85. Bush, J. A., Ashenbrucker, H., Cartwright, G. E., and Wintrobe, M. M.: The anemia of infection. XX. The kinetics of iron metabolism in the anemia associated with chronic infection. *J. Clin. Invest.* 35:89, 1956.

86. Cavill, I., Ricketts, L., and Napier, J. A. F.: Erythropoiesis in the anaemia of chronic disease. *Scand. J. Haematol.* 19:509, 1977.

87. Dinant, H. J., and deMaat, C. E. M.: Erythropoiesis and mean red-cell life span in normal subjects and in patients with the anaemia of active rheumatoid arthritis. *Brit. J. Haematol.* 39:437, 1978.

88. Kelly, K. H., Bierman, H. R., and Shimkin, M. B.: Blood volume, body water, and circulation time in patients with advanced neoplastic disease. *Cancer Res.* 12:814, 1952.

89. Berlin, N. J., Hyde, G. M., Parsons, R. J., and Lawrence, J. H.: The blood volume in cancer. *Cancer* 8:796, 1955.

90. Reilly, W. A., Helwig, H. L., and Scott, K. G.: Blood volume measurements in cancer using the Cr[51] red blood cell tagging method. *Cancer* 9:273, 1956.

91. Kopp, W. L., MacKinney, A. A., Jr., and Wasson, G.: Blood volume and hematocrit value in macroglobulinemia and myeloma. *Arch. Intern. Med.* 123:394, 1969.

92. Alexanian, R.: Blood volume in monoclonal gammopathy. *Blood* 49:301, 1977.

93. Bullen, J. J.: Iron binding proteins and infection. *Br. J. Haematol.* 23:389, 1972.

94. Weinberg, E. D.: Iron and susceptibility to infectious disease. *Science* 184:952, 1974.

95. Richmond, J., Roy, L. M. H., Gardner, D. L., Alexander, W. R. M., and Duthie, J. J. R.: Nature of anemia of rheumatoid arthritis. IV. Effects of intravenous administration of saccharated oxide of iron. *Ann. Rheum. Dis.* 17:406, 1958.

96. Hume, R., Currie, W. J. C., and Tennant, M.: Anemia of rheumatoid arthritis and iron therapy. *Ann. Rheum. Dis.* 24:451, 1965.

97. Szilagyi, G., and Erslev, A. J.: Effect of organic iron compounds on the iron uptake of reticulocytes in vitro. *J. Lab. Clin. Med.* 75:275, 1970.

98. Kornfeld, S., Chipman, B., and Brown, E. B.: Intracellular catabolism of hemoglobin and iron dextran by the rat liver. *J. Lab. Clin. Med.* 73:181, 1969.

99. Beamish, M. R.: The measurement of reticuloendothelial iron release using iron dextran. *Br. J. Haematol.* 21:617, 1971.

100. Weinsaft, P. P., and Bernstein, L. H. T.: Cobaltous chloride in the treatment of certain refractory anemias. *Ann. J. Med. Sci.* 230:246, 1955.

101. Gardner, F. H., and Pringle, J. C.: Androgens and erythropoiesis. *Arch. Intern. Med.* 107:846, 1961.

CHAPTER *52*

Anemia associated with marrow infiltration

JOHN LASZLO

Definition and classification

Myelophthisic anemia describes the hematologic consequences of marrow infiltration. The blood findings are characterized by a mild to moderate anemia and mild thrombocytopenia, although leukocytosis or even thrombocytosis may be present. The red cells are deformed, showing marked anisocytosis, poikilocytosis, and teardrop shapes. Giant platelets are usually found on blood films, in addition to a moderate number of nucleated red cells and immature granulocytes. When the latter are present in large numbers, the blood films have been described as showing leukoerythroblastosis [1–4].

The most frequent causes of marrow infiltration and damage to normal hemopoietic cells are the lymphoid malignancies and metastatic carcinoma. Less common causes of marrow replacement are lipid storage diseases, tuberculosis and fungus infections, and granulomatous disorders (see Table 52-1). The microenvironment of the red marrow seems to be a particularly hospitable site for the implantation of blood-borne carcinoma cells. *Marrow metastasis* is usually a more correct term than the clinical cliché "bone metastasis." Phagocytic cells are abundant in the marrow and actively engulf bacteria, fungi, lipid particles, chylomicrons, and cellular debris of all kinds. Organisms that are "contained" but not killed may grow slowly and produce the tissue changes associated with myelophthisic anemia.

Pathogenesis

Except in the case of the myeloproliferative disorders, which are reviewed elsewhere (see Chaps. 23 to 28), the severity of the associated systemic illness often so overshadows the hematologic manifestations that detailed studies of the exact mechanism(s) of myelophthisic anemia are not considered to be especially relevant. It is well recognized that the severity of the anemia is not quantitatively related to the extent of clinically detectable infiltration; indeed, anemia need not be present at first [1,2,6]. It is also known that moderate degrees of anemia, even with misshapen red cells, may be found in patients with cancer that has not invaded the marrow [3,7,8,9]. Since the anemia in these patients may be associated with ineffective red cell production, shortened red cell survival, intrinsic, red cell abnormalities, or blood loss, there is every reason to expect that these mechanisms for producing anemia are also operative in those whose marrow is invaded by tumor cells. Furthermore, chemotherapy may be expected to modify blood counts and to cause morphologic abnormalities such as large hypersegmented polymorphonuclear leukocytes with Döhle bodies, giant platelet forms, etc. [10].

Despite these complicating factors, certain pathophysiologic mechanisms can be identified. The release of normal cellular elements from the marrow appears to require egress through sinus endothelial cells [11]. Marrow egress thus depends on membrane distensibility and the deformability of cells maturing in the marrow [12], and premature release of granulocytic and erythroid elements would be expected from mechanical disruption of the microarchitecture. When the marrow-blood barrier is disrupted, even poorly deformable cells such as myeloblasts, promyelocytes, and erythroblasts are able to enter the circulation.

In some patients, "crowding-out" of normal marrow elements by tumor elements is quite obvious—indeed,

TABLE 52-1   Causes of marrow infiltration

Tumors: primary (hematologic)
  Leukemias, acute and chronic
  Malignant lymphomas—Hodgkins and non-Hodgkins entities
  Plasma cell myeloma
  Hairy cell leukemia
Tumors: metastatic carcinomas
  Breast, prostate, lung, gastrointestinal, etc.
  Neuroblastoma
Myelofibrosis (myelosclerosis)
  Primary, acute and chronic
  Secondary to toxins, occlusive vascular disease, cancer
Metabolic abnormalities
  Gaucher and other lipid storage diseases
Infections
  Bacterial (e.g., staphylococcus, typhoid)
  Fungus (e.g., mucormycosis)
  Miliary tuberculosis
Granulomas
  Sarcoid
  Histiocytosis

one may find total replacement of the marrow by viable tumor cells or mixtures of living cells and tumor debris [13]. In less advanced cases, areas of hyperplastic erythropoiesis and granulopoiesis may surround tumor foci [14]. The remaining or adjacent marrow appears to be stimulated or "irritated" into an excessive but ineffective localized activity, resulting in breakdown of normal marrow growth patterns. Occasionally, marrow metastases may be associated with significant degrees of myelofibrosis and sclerosis, together with splenomegaly and myeloid metaplasia, so that the hematologic picture resembles that of a primary myeloproliferative disorder [15–17]. It is also quite possible that, in addition to the marrow-suppressive effects of chronic disease, tumor cells growing in the marrow compete for nutritional or other factors required from normal hemopoietic development.

Pancytopenia may be caused in part by slowly progressive hypersplenism, which may result from myeloid metaplasia in the spleen, from massive accumulation of lipids in phagocytes or histiocytes, or in response to infection. Although tumors and granulomas frequently involve the spleen, this type of involvement rarely produces clinical evidence of hypersplenism. In patients with malignant lymphomas or with lymphocytic or plasma cell proliferative diseases, abnormal proteins may be produced which function as physical, mechanical, or immunologic agents interfering with marrow function and leading to accelerated red cells hemolysis.

Clinical features and diagnosis

The clinical features associated with infiltrative marrow disorders are usually related to the underlying disease, although occasionally anemia or bleeding from thrombocytopenia or disseminated intravascular coagulation may be presenting features. Some enlargement of the

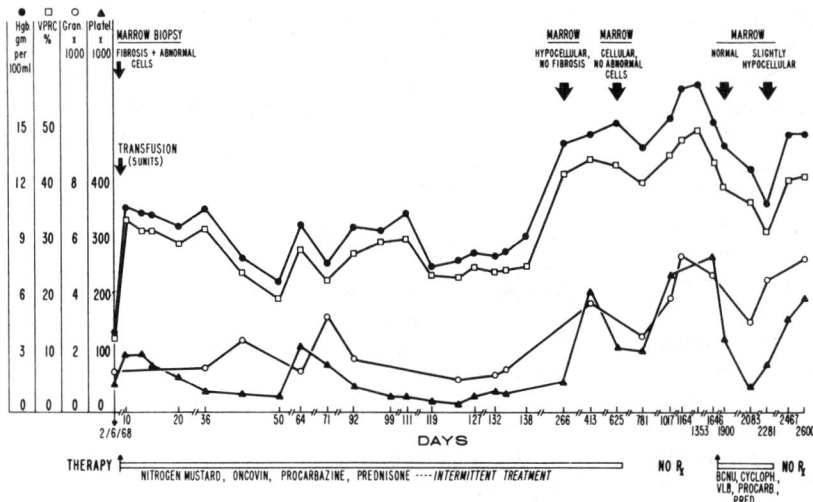

FIGURE 52-1   Myelophthisic anemia due to Hodgkin's disease. This graph illustrates the clinical course of a 46-year-old laborer who had generalized adenopathy, hepatosplenomegaly, severe anemia with pancytopenia, and abnormal liver function tests. Lymph node biopsy showed Hodgkin's disease, subsequently classified as nodular sclerosing type. A marrow aspirate was unsuccessful, and marrow biopsy showed extensive fibrosis and abnormal cells. After initial transfusion he was treated with an intermittent MOPP program, with judicious use of nitrogen mustard because of pancytopenia. The intermittent courses of treatment were discontinued in March 1970, with the patient in clinical remission. In December 1972 (day 1646) the patient was still asymptomatic but had enlarging cervical and para-aortic nodes without demonstrable liver or marrow involvement; node biopsy confirmed recurrent Hodgkin's disease. Eleven courses of BCNU, cyclophosphamide, vinblastine, procarbazine, and prednisone were given through day 2200, and he remains in remission without further therapy for over 10 years' follow-up.

VPRC = packed red cell volume; Gran. = granulocyte count (cells per microliter); Platel. = platelet count (platelets per microliter).

liver and spleen or lymph nodes is frequent. Increased bone pain in one or many areas, bone destruction, and symptoms and signs related to hypercalcemia are symptoms or signs which may bring patients to medical attention.

Myelophthisic anemia should be considered whenever nucleated red cells (often without an increased number of reticulocytes) or immature white cells are found in the blood of patients who appear to have atypical hemolytic anemia. If a patient is known to have a malignant disease, the presence of immature cells in the circulation probably signals marrow invasion. Although leukoerythroblastic anemia has generally been regarded as having a dire prognosis, some carcinomas respond well to treatment, and furthermore, leukoerythroblastosis may be encountered in a variety of conditions more or less benign from the hematologic standpoint. A group of 215 patients with leukoerythroblastosis was found in a survey of approximately 50,000 patients who had had routine total and differential white counts: 136 had malignant disease, including hematologic, nonhematologic, and myeloproliferative disorders; 17 had hemolytic diseases; and 62 had various other conditions [18]. Conversely, about one-half of patients with marrow metastases manifest a leukoerythroblastic blood picture [19–21]. Some patients with abnormalities such as marrow metastases or Gaucher disease may have pancytopenia with few or no

immature cells in the circulating blood to signify marrow replacement.

When leukoerythroblastosis does occur with marrow infiltration, the erythrocytes may show marked anisocytosis and poikilocytosis. Teardrop forms are particularly suggestive of myelofibrosis. On rare occasions, granulocytosis with cellular immaturity and large platelets or circulating megakaryocyte nuclei may be so striking as to suggest the possibility of chronic myelogenous leukemia [22]. In such instances an intensely positive leukocyte alkaline phosphatase stain and lack of the Ph1 chromosome are useful, although not absolute, indications of a leukemoid reaction. Patients with miliary tuberculosis may have pancytopenia with considerable myeloid immaturity. This infection may coexist with acute leukemia and present a most difficult diagnostic problem [23].

Although bone scintiphotographic studies are often positive in patients with marrow metastases, a negative scan does not exclude marrow involvement [19]. The diagnosis of marrow infiltration usually depends on marrow biopsy. Although aspiration of marrow from tender bones is a useful way to demonstrate tumor cells in suitable candidates [24–27], the marrow may be involved in a spotty manner or may be so solidly packed that aspiration is impossible. Moreover, interpretation of marrow aspirates has frequently been found to be misleading [28]. Indeed, inability to aspirate marrow from a tender bone is highly suggestive of marrow infiltration. The yield may be higher with one or more core needle biopsies than with aspiration alone [1,6]. The yield of positive findings on marrow biopsy will vary considerably in different hands, depending on such factors as the selection of patients, number and type of biopsies, stage of disease, and type of tumor.

The diagnosis of marrow necrosis should also be considered in patients who show leukoerythroblastosis and anemia, since the hematologic manifestations may be quite similar [29–33]. Indeed, aside from marrow necrosis associated with sickle cell disease, extensive marrow involvement by cancer (e.g., lymphoma, leukemia) appears to be the most common cause. Generalized infection with gram-positive or gram-negative bacteria and with fungus may also give rise to marrow necrosis. This is often not recognized during life, occurring as it does in fulminating infections. If patients are cured of their underlying disease, the marrow may either recover or be subsequently involved with focal or widespread myelofibrosis and with myeloid metaplasia.

The hematologic manifestations seen in patients with advanced anorexia nervosa may at first be confused with the infiltrative marrow disorders that occur in cachectic patients with pancytopenia. However, leukoerythroblastosis is not a feature of this condition, and the marrow is hypocellular and contains a background of gelatinous material which appears to consist of acid mucopolysaccharides [34].

Treatment and prognosis

The goal of treatment is generally to improve the underlying disease which is responsible for marrow infiltration. Short of that goal, however, gratifying improvement can be expected after splenectomy in those disorders in which hypersplenism is a major contributing factor, even though there is no improvement in marrow production. Some patients with myelofibrosis or other types of marrow disease will show partial improvement in anemia after androgen or corticosteroid therapy [35]. Patients with marrow replacement due to leukemia, myeloma, lymphoma, or breast or prostate cancer may show a remarkable and prompt improvement with successful chemotherapy. An example of the clinical response of one such patient is shown in Fig. 52-1. Caution must be observed in treating patients having pancytopenia, however, in that the starting dosage of marrow-suppressive drugs should be reduced by one-half or two-thirds. Unfortunately, despite all known therapeutic measures, most patients with cancers metastatic to the marrow rapidly deteriorate and die.

References

1. Contreras, E., Ellis, L. D., and Lee, R. E.: Value of the bone marrow biopsy in the diagnosis of metastatic carcinoma. *Cancer* 29:778, 1972.
2. Abasov I. T.: The state of the peripheral blood in cancer metastases to bone marrow. *Haematologia* 2:381, 1968.
3. Kremer, W. B., and Laszlo, J.: Hematologic effects of cancer, in *Cancer Medicine*, edited by J. F. Holland and E. Frei. Lea & Febiger, Philadelphia, 1973. p. 1085.
4. Vaughan, J. M.: Leuco-erythroblastic anaemia. *J. Pathol. Bacteriol.* 42:541, 1936.
5. Laszlo, J.: Myeloproliferative disorders. *Semin. Hematol.* 12:409, 1975.
6. Hansen, H. H., Muggia, F. M., and Selawry O. S.: Bone-marrow examination in 100 consecutive patients with bronchogenic carcinoma. *Lancet* 2:443, 1971.
7. Hyman G. A.: Anemia in malignant neoplastic disease. *J. Chron. Dis.* 16:645, 1963.
8. Berlin, N. I.: Anemia of cancer. *Ann. N.Y. Acad. Sci.* 230:209, 1974.
9. Morrison, M.: An analysis of the blood picture in 100 cases of malignancy. *J. Lab. Clin. Med.* 17:1071, 1932.
10. Laszlo, J, and Kremer, W. B.: Hematologic effects of chemotherapeutic drugs and radiation, in *Cancer Medicine*, edited by J. F. Holland and E. Frei. Lea & Febiger, Philadelphia, 1973, p. 1085.
11. Weiss, L.: The histophysiology of bone marrow. *Clin. Orthop.* 52:13, 1967.
12. Lichtman, M. A.: Cellular deformability during maturation of the myeloblast: Possible role in marrow egress. *N. Engl. J. Med.* 283:943, 1970.
13. Brittin, G. M., and Brecher, G.: Appearance of bone marrow smears with necrotic tumor cells. *Blood* 38:229, 1971.
14. Britton, C. J. C.: The leukemias, in *Disorders of the Blood*, 9th ed., edited by L. E. H. Whitby and C. J. C. Britton. Blackston, Philadelphia, 1950 p. 531.
15. Kiely, J. M., and Silverstein, M. N.: Metastatic carcinoma simulating agnogenic myeloid metaplasia and myelofibrosis. *Cancer* 24:1041, 1969.
16. Blummer, H., Aronoff, A., Chartier, J., and Shapiro, L.: Carcinoma of the stomach with myelosclerosis: Presentation of a case and review of the literature. *Can. Med. Assoc. J.* 84:1254, 1961.
17. Hennekeuser, H. H., and Fischer, R.: Extramedulläre Blutbildung und leukemoide Reaktion bei bösartige Tumoren. *Deutsch. Med. Wochenschr.* 92:479, 1967.
18. Weick, J. K., Hagedorn, A. B., and Linman, J. W.: Leukoerythroblastosis: Diagnostic and prognostic significance. *Mayo Clin. Proc.* 49:111, 1974.
19. Broghamer, Jr., W. L., and Keeling, M. M.: The bone marrow biopsy, osteoscan, and peripheral blood in non-hematopoietic cancer. *Cancer* 40:836, 1977.
20. Chernow, B., and Wallner, S. F.: Variables predictive of bone marrow metastasis. *Cancer* 42:2373 1978.
21. Delsol, G., Guiu-Godfrin, B., Guiu, M., Pris, J., Corberand, J., and Fabre, J.: Leukoerythroblastosis and cancer frequency, prognosis, and physiopathologic significance. *Cancer* 44:1009, 1979.
22. Chen, H. P., and Walz D. V.: Leukemoid reaction in the bone marrow, associated with malignant neoplasms. *Am. J. Clin. Pathol.* 29:345, 1958.
23. Glasser, R. M., Walker, R. I., and Herion, J. C.: The significance of hematologic abnormalities in patients with tuberculosis. *Arch. Intern. Med.* 125:691 1970.
24. Rohr, K., and Hegglin, R.: Tumorzellen in sternalpunktat. *Deutsch. Arch. Klin. Med.* 179:61, 1936.
25. Rundles, R. W., and Jonsson, U.: Metastases in bone marrow and myelophthisic anemia from carcinoma of the prostate. *Am. J. Med. Sci.* 218:241, 1949.
26. Jonsson, U., and Rundles, R. W.: Tumor metastases in bone marrow. *Blood* 6:16, 1951.
27. Garrett, T. J., Gee, T. S., Lieberman, P. H., McKenzie, S., and Clarkson, B. D.: The role of bone marrow aspiration and biopsy in detecting marrow involvement by nonhematologic malignancies. *Cancer* 38:2401, 1976.
28. Emerson, C. P., and Finkel H. E.: Problem of tumor cell identification in the bone marrow. *Cancer* 19:1527, 1966.
29. Brown, C. H., III.: Bone marrow necrosis. A study of seventy cases. *Johns Hopkins Med. J.* 131:189, 1972.
30. Crail, H. W., Alt, H. L., and Nadler, W. H.: Myelofibrosis associated with tuberculosis: Report of 4 cases. *Blood* 3:1426, 1948.
31. Caraveo, J., et al.: Bone marrow necrosis associated with a mucor infection. *Am. J. Med.* 62:404, 1977.

32. Kiraly, J. F., and Wheby. M. S.: Bone marrow necrosis. *Am. J. Med.* 60:361, 1976.
33. Norgard, M. J., Carpenter, J. T., and Conrad, M. E.: Bone marrow necrosis and degeneration. *Arch. Intern. Med.* 139:905, 1979.
34. Kubanek, B., Heimpel, H., Paar, G., and Schoengen, A.: Hämatologische Veränderungen bei Anorexia Nervosa. *Blut* 35:115, 1977.
35. Kennedy, B. J.: Effect of androgenic hormone in myelofibrosis. *JAMA.* 182:116, 1962.

CHAPTER 53

Anemia related to nutritional deficiencies other than vitamin B₁₂ and folic acid

FRANK A. OSKI

Anemia may result from nutritional deficiencies of a variety of vitamins and trace minerals. Vitamin deficiencies that have been implicated as causes of anemia in humans, in addition to folic acid and vitamin B_{12}, include vitamins A, C, and E, and pyridoxine and riboflavin, members of the B group. Copper, as well as iron, is recognized as a mineral essential for optimal erythropoiesis. Complex nutritional disturbances such as those observed in starvation, protein-deficiency malnutrition, and alcoholism are also associated with anemia.

Vitamin-deficiency anemias

VITAMIN A DEFICIENCY
Chronic deprivation of vitamin A results in an anemia similar to that observed in iron deficiency [1–4]. Mean red cell volume (MCV) and mean red cell hemoglobin concentration (MCHC) are reduced. Anisocytosis and poikilocytosis may be present, and serum iron levels are low. Unlike iron-deficiency anemia, however, in this type of anemia liver and marrow iron stores are increased, the serum transferrin concentration is usually normal or decreased, and the administration of medicinal iron does not correct the anemia.

Experimentally induced vitamin A deficiency in otherwise well-nourished adult males produces an anemia with a mean hemoglobin concentration of 12 g/dl. Following vitamin A repletion the hemoglobin concentration promptly rises to a mean of 15 g/dl [1].

Nutritional surveys conducted in developing countries have demonstrated a strong relationship between serum levels of vitamin A and blood hemoglobin concentration [5]. Subjects with serum vitamin A concentrations in the range of 20 to 30 μg/dl had a mean hemoglobin concentration of 6 g/dl as contrasted with a mean hemoglobin level of 16 g/dl in subjects in whom the serum vitamin A concentration exceeded 60 μg/dl. Vitamin A deficiency may be as common a cause of anemia as iron deficiency in developing countries. Although vitamin A deficiency is recognized to occur in the United States [6], the relation between it and anemia is not known.

Experimentally induced vitamin A deficiency in the rat produces an initial fall in hemoglobin concentration followed by a return to normal or polycythemic levels [7]. This "masked anemia" appears to be a result of severe hemoconcentration that usually accompanies profound vitamin A deficiency in rodents [8]. However, marrow hypoplasia and fibrosis has been observed at autopsy in animals [9] and infants [4] with severe vitamin A deficiency.

DEFICIENCIES OF MEMBERS OF THE VITAMIN B GROUP
Isolated nutritional deficiencies of members of the vitamin B group, with the exception of folic acid and vitamin B_{12}, are apparently very uncommon in humans, and evidence linking isolated nutritional deficiencies of pyridoxine, riboflavin, pantothenic acid, and niacin to anemia in such patients is inconclusive. Deficiency states experimentally induced in animals are more commonly associated with hematologic abnormalities.

VITAMIN B₆ DEFICIENCY
Vitamin B_6 includes pyridoxal, pyridoxine, and pyridoxamine. These are converted to pyridoxal 5-phosphate, which acts as a coenzyme in the decarboxylation and transamination of amino acids and in the synthesis of δ-aminolevulinic acid, the porphyrin precursor. Vitamin B_6 deficiency induced in two infants was associated with a hypochromic, microcytic anemia [10]. A malnourished patient with a hypochromic anemia who failed to respond to iron therapy but did subsequently respond to the administration of vitamin B_6 has been described [11]. Occasionally, patients receiving therapy with antituberculosis agents, such as isoniazid, which interfere with vitamin B_6 metabolism, develop a microcytic anemia that can be corrected with large doses of pyridoxine [12,13]. Some patients with sideroblastic anemias (see Chap. 58) will respond to the administration of pyridoxine, but these patients are not deficient in this vitamin. Swine maintained on a vitamin B_6–deficient diet do become anemic [14].

RIBOFLAVIN DEFICIENCY
Riboflavin deficiency will result in a decrease in red cell glutathione reductase activity, since this enzyme requires flavin adenine dinucleotide for activation. The glutathione reductase deficiency induced by riboflavin deficiency is not associated with a hemolytic anemia or

increased susceptibility to oxidant-induced injury [15]. Human volunteers maintained on a semisynthetic riboflavin-deficient diet and fed the riboflavin antagonist, galactoflavin, develop pure red cell aplasia [16]. Vacuolated erythroid precursors are evident prior to the development of aplasia. This anemia is reversed specifically by the administration of riboflavin.

PANTOTHENIC ACID DEFICIENCY

Pantothenic acid deficiency, when artificially induced in humans, is not associated with anemia [17], although swine deficient in this vitamin develop a normocytic anemia in conjunction with the neuronal degeneration of colitis [18].

NIACIN DEFICIENCY

Niacin deficiency in dogs results in the appearance of a macrocytic anemia [19], although evidence for anemia in human subjects with pellagra, which can be specifically ascribed to the niacin deficiency, has not been reported.

VITAMIN C (ASCORBIC ACID) DEFICIENCY

It is still unclear whether vitamin C has a direct role in hemopoiesis or if the anemia observed in subjects with vitamin C deficiency (scurvy) is a result of the interactions of ascorbic acid with folic acid and iron metabolism.

Although approximately 80 percent of individuals with scurvy [20] are anemic, attempts to induce anemia in human volunteers by severe restriction of dietary ascorbic acid have been unsuccessful [21,22].

Confusion arises because the anemia observed in subjects with scurvy may be normocytic, macrocytic, or hypochromic; and the marrow may be hypocellular, normocellular, or hypercellular. In about 10 percent of patients the marrow is obviously megaloblastic [20]. Human subjects with scurvy and megaloblastic anemia fail to respond hematologically to vitamin C as long as they are kept on a folic acid–deficient diet. When folic acid is given to these subjects, in a dose of 50 μg per day, a prompt hematologic response is observed [23].

Ascorbic acid is required for the maintenance of folic acid reductase in its reduced, or active, form. Impaired folic acid reductase activity results in an inability to form tetrahydrofolic acid, the metabolically active form of folic acid. Patients with scurvy and megaloblastic anemia excrete 10-formylfolic acid as the major urinary folate metabolite. Following ascorbic acid therapy, 5-methyltetrahydrofolic acid becomes the major urinary folate metabolite. This observation has led to the suggestion [24] that ascorbic acid serves to prevent the irreversible oxidation of methyltetrahydrofolic acid to formylfolic acid. Failure to synthesize tetrahydrofolic acid or to protect it from oxidation ultimately results in the appearance of a megaloblastic anemia. Under these circumstances, ascorbic acid therapy will produce a hematologic response only if sufficient folic acid is present to interact with the ascorbic acid [25].

Dietary iron deficiency in children often occurs in association with dietary ascorbic acid deficiency. Scurvy itself may cause iron deficiency as a consequence of external bleeding. Iron balance may be further compromised by the ascorbic acid deficiency because this vitamin serves to facilitate intestinal iron absorption. Patients with scurvy, particularly children, often require both iron and vitamin C to correct a hypochromic, microcytic anemia [26].

In patients with iron overload from repeated blood transfusions, the level of vitamin C in leukocytes is often decreased because of rapid conversion of ascorbate to oxalate [27]. Desferrioxamine-induced iron excretion is diminished when stores of vitamin C are reduced, but excretion returns to expected values with vitamin C supplementation [28]. The presence of scurvy in patients with iron overload may protect them from tissue damage [29]. Both in scorbutic guinea pigs and in Bantu subjects with nutritional vitamin C deficiency and dietary hemosiderosis, iron accumulates in the monocyte-macrophage system rather than in the parenchymal cells of the liver [30,31].

Despite the evidence linking ascorbic acid deficiency to alterations in either folic acid or iron metabolism, many patients with scurvy do have a normocytic, normochromic anemia accompanied by a persistent reticulocytosis of 5 to 10 percent. Administration of vitamin C produces an initial increase in reticulocyte count followed by a rise in hemoglobin concentration and an ultimate correction of all hematologic abnormalities [32]. In such circumstances the deficiency of ascorbic acid may result in anemia by compromising cellular antioxidant defense mechanisms [33].

VITAMIN E DEFICIENCY

Vitamin E, α-tocopherol, is a fat-soluble vitamin that appears to serve as an antioxidant in humans and not as an essential cofactor in any recognized reactions. Nutritional deficiency of vitamin E in humans is extremely uncommon because of the widespread occurrence of α-tocopherol in food. The daily requirement for adults is in the range of 5 to 7 mg of d-α-tocopherol, but the requirement varies with the polyunsaturated fatty acid content of the diet and the content of peroxidizable lipids in tissues. Hematologic manifestations of vitamin E deficiency in humans are virtually limited to the neonatal period and to pathologic states associated with chronic fat malabsorption. In a variety of nonhematologic conditions, vitamin E in pharmacologic amounts has been claimed to be helpful [34].

Low-birth-weight infants are born with low serum and tissue concentrations of vitamin E. When these infants are fed a diet unusually rich in polyunsaturated fatty acids and inadequate in vitamin E, a hemolytic anemia will develop by 4 to 6 weeks of age, particularly if iron is also present in the diet [35,36]. The anemia is often associated with morphologic alterations of the erythrocytes [37], thrombocytosis, and edema of the dorsum of the feet and pretibial area [38]. Treatment with vitamin E produces a prompt increase in hemoglobin, a decrease in the elevated reticulocyte count, a normalization of the red cell life-span, and a disappearance of the thrombocytosis and edema.

Vitamin E deficiency is common in patients with cystic fibrosis if they are not receiving daily supplements of the water-soluble form of the vitamin. Red cell life-span has been found to be shortened in such patients to an average ^{51}Cr half-life of 19 days. After vitamin E therapy the red cell half-life increased to 27.5 days [39]. These patients, with a modest decrease in red cell life-span, are not anemic.

Pharmacologic doses of vitamin E have been employed, with apparent success, in the absence of vitamin deficiency, to compensate for genetic defects that limit the erythrocytes' defense against oxidant injury. Chronic administration of 400 to 800 units of vitamin E per day lengthened the red cell life-span of patients with hereditary hemolytic anemias associated with glutathione synthetase deficiency and glucose-6-phosphate dehydrogenase deficiency [40] and in subjects with the Mediterranean-type glucose-6-phosphate dehydrogenase deficiency [41].

The administration of 450 units of vitamin E per day for 6 to 36 weeks to patients with sickle cell anemia has been found to produce a significant reduction in the number of irreversibly sickled erythrocytes [42].

Mineral deficiencies other than iron

COPPER DEFICIENCY
Copper is present in a number of metalloproteins. Among the cuproenzymes are cytochrome c oxidase, dopamine β-hydroxylase, urate oxidase, tyrosine and lysyl oxidase, ascorbic acid oxidase, and superoxide dismutase (erythrocuprein). More than 90 percent of the copper in the blood is carried bound to ceruloplasmin, an α_2-globulin with ferroxidase activity. Copper appears to be required for the absorption and utilization of iron. It has been proposed [43] that copper, in the form of a ferroxidase, converts and maintains iron in the Fe^{3+} state for its transport by transferrin.

Copper deficiency in swine results in macrocytic, hypochromic anemia, hypoferremia, and connective tissue abnormalities producing fragmentation of the elastic lining of blood vessels, dissecting aneurysms, and rupture of the myocardium [44].

Copper deficiency has been described in malnourished children [45] and in both infants [46] and adults [47] receiving parenteral alimentation. Copper deficiency in humans is characterized by a microcytic anemia that is unresponsive to iron therapy, hypoferremia, neutropenia, and, usually, the presence of vacuolated erythroid precursors in the marrow. In infants and young children with copper deficiency, radiologic abnormalities are generally present. These abnormalities include osteoporosis, flaring of the anterior ribs with spontaneous rib fractures, cupping and flaring of long-bone metaphyses with spur formation and submetaphyseal fractures, and epiphyseal separation. These radiologic changes have frequently been misinterpreted as signs of scurvy.

The diagnosis of copper deficiency can be established by the demonstration of a low serum ceruloplasmin or serum copper level. Adequate normal values for the first 2 to 3 months have not been well defined and are normally lower than those observed later in life. Despite these limitations, a serum copper level of less than 40 μg/dl or a ceruloplasmin value of less than 15 mg/dl after 1 or 2 months of age can be regarded as evidence of copper deficiency. In later infancy, childhood, and adulthood, serum copper values should normally exceed 70 μg/dl.

Low serum copper values may be observed in hypoproteinemic states such as exudative enteropathies and nephrosis, as well as in Wilson's disease. In these circumstances a diagnosis of copper deficiency cannot be established by serum measurements alone, but instead requires analysis of liver copper content or clinical response after a therapeutic trial of copper supplementation.

The anemia and neutropenia are quickly corrected by administration of copper. Therapy in a dose of 0.2 mg per kilogram of body weight will cause a prompt reticulocytosis and rise in the leukocyte count. This can be given as a 10% solution of copper sulfate ($CuSO_4 \cdot 5H_2O$), which contains about 25 mg copper per milliliter.

ZINC DEFICIENCY
Zinc is required for approximately 20 zinc metalloenzymes and zinc-activated enzymes [48]. Zinc deficiency occurs in a variety of pathologic states in humans [49], including hemolytic anemias such as thalassemia [50] and sickle cell anemia [51]. Although human zinc deficiency may produce growth retardation, impaired wound healing, impaired taste perception, immunologic abnormalities, and acrodermatitis enteropathica, there is no evidence, at present, that isolated zinc deficiency produces anemia.

Anemia of starvation

Studies conducted during World War II among prisoners of war and conscientious objectors demonstrated that semistarvation for 24 weeks resulted in a mild to moderate normocytic normochromic anemia [52]. Marrow cellularity was usually reduced and was accompanied by a decrease in the erythroid/myeloid ratio. Measurements of red cell mass and plasma volume suggested that dilution was a major factor responsible for the reduction in hemoglobin concentration.

In persons subjected to complete starvation, either for experimental purposes or to treat severe obesity, anemia was not observed during the first 2 to 9 weeks of fasting [53]. Starvation for 9 to 17 weeks produced a fall in hemoglobin and marrow hypocellularity [54].

Resumption of a normal diet was accompanied by a reticulocytosis and disappearance of anemia. It has been suggested that the anemia of starvation is a response to a hypometabolic state with its attendant decrease in oxygen requirements.

Anemia of protein deficiency (kwashiorkor)

From the study of the anemia of protein deficiency in rats [55] it was deduced that oxygen consumption and, therefore, erythropoietin production are reduced. Other studies confirmed this observation but related the reductions to calorie deprivation with its associated decrease in the blood levels of T$_3$ and T$_4$ [56]. As a result, erythropoiesis decreases and the reticulocyte count falls. The plasma iron turnover and red cell uptake of radioactive iron are markedly reduced, and the red cell mass gradually declines [57]. Protein deficiency also produces a maturation block at the erythroblast level and a slight decrease in the erythropoietin-sensitive stem cell pool [58]. If exogenous erythropoietin is provided, normal erythropoiesis is restored despite protein depletion [59], an observation which has explained the empirical but successful use of starved rats in the bioassay for erythropoietin.

In infants and children with protein-calorie malnutrition, the hemoglobin concentration may fall to 8 g per deciliter of blood [60,61], but some children with kwashiorkor are admitted to the hospital with normal hemoglobin levels, probably because of a decreased plasma volume. The anemia is normocytic and normochromic, but there is a considerable variation in size and shape of the red cells on the blood film. The white blood cells and the platelets are usually normal. The marrow is most often normally cellular or slightly hypocellular, with a reduced erythroid/myeloid ratio. Erythroblastopenia, reticulocytopenia, and a marrow containing a few giant pronormoblasts may be found, particularly if these children have an infection. With treatment of the infection, erythroid precursors may appear in the marrow and the reticulocyte count may rise. When nutrition is improved by feeding high-protein diets (powdered milk or essential amino acids), there is reticulocytosis, a slight fall in hematocrit due to hemodilution, and then a rise in hemoglobin, hematocrit, and red blood cell count. Improvement is very slow, however, and during the third or fourth week when the children are clinically improved and the serum proteins are approaching normal, another episode of erythroid marrow aplasia devoid of giant pronormoblasts may develop. This relapse is not associated with infection, does not respond to antibiotics, and does not remit spontaneously. It does respond either to riboflavin or to prednisone, and, unless treated with these agents, children who develop this complication may die suddenly. It has been suggested [62] that the erythroblastic aplasia is a manifestation of riboflavin deficiency.

Although the plasma volume is reduced to a variable degree in children with kwashiorkor, the total circulating red cell mass decreases in proportion to the decrease in lean body mass as protein deprivation reduces metabolic demands [60].

During repletion, an increase in plasma volume may occur before an increase in red cell mass, and the anemia may seem to become more severe, despite reticulocytosis. The erythropoietin level increases [63] as the hemoglobin concentration falls and, more importantly, as oxygen demand increases. This may in part account for the reticulocytosis. Also during the repletion period, occult deficiencies of iron and folic acid and occasionally of riboflavin, vitamin E, and vitamin B$_{12}$, may become manifest unless these essential nutrients are supplied in adequate amounts.

Alcoholism

Chronic alcohol ingestion is often associated with anemia. The anemia may be nutritional in origin, a result of chronic gastrointestinal bleeding, secondary to hepatic dysfunction, or a direct toxic effect of alcohol on erythropoiesis. Quite commonly all these factors work in concert to produce anemia. The myriad hematologic complications of alcoholism have been extensively reviewed [64].

Macrocytosis is common in chronic alcoholics and is often associated with a megaloblastic anemia. Among hospitalized, malnourished alcoholics, it is the most common type of anemia, occurring alone or in combination with ringed sideroblasts in approximately 40 percent of all patients [65,66]. In contrast, megaloblastic anemia is rarely observed in nonhospitalized chronic alcoholics or relatively well nourished subjects admitted to the hospital for purposes of alcohol withdrawal [67]. Anemia, when associated with megaloblastic marrow changes in alcoholics, is almost always due to folate deficiency.

Iron deficiency is often associated with folate deficiency in alcoholics [67]. In patients with both nutritional deficiencies the blood film will be "dimorphic" with macrocytes, hypersegmented neutrophils, and hypochromic microcytes.

Although liver disease is frequently present in alcoholics with megaloblastic anemia, it is not responsible for the folate deficiency. Megaloblastic anemia occurs almost exclusively in alcoholics who have been eating poorly. It is seen more commonly in heavy drinkers of wine and whiskey, substances which contain little or no folate, than in drinkers of beer, a rich source of the vitamin. Although decreased dietary folate intake appears to be a necessary factor in the etiology of the megaloblastic anemia, ethanol itself interferes with folate metabolism [68,69] by an unknown mechanism.

Macrocytosis is quite common among alcoholics but does not always indicate the presence of a megaloblastic anemia [70]. Macrocytosis in alcoholics may be due to one of at least four causes: (1) folate deficiency, with macroovalocytes observed in association with hyper-segmentation of the neutrophils; (2) reticulocytosis, usually as a consequence of hemolysis, gastrointestinal bleeding, or ethanol withdrawal; (3) the macrocytosis of liver disease; and (4) the macrocytosis of alcoholism [71]. In the latter the degree of macrocytosis is usually mild, with MCVs in the 100 to 110 range. As many as 82 to 96 percent of chronic alcoholics will exhibit this macrocytosis, which is unrelated to the presence of liver disease or folate deficiency. Anemia is usually absent. In the blood smear, the macrocytes are typically round rather than oval, and neutrophil hypersegmentation is not present. The macrocytosis persists until the patient abstains from alcohol. Even then, the MCV does not become completely normal for periods of 2 to 4 months [72].

Alcohol ingestion, for 5 to 7 days, will produce vacuolation of early red cell precursors [73]. These changes disappear promptly when alcohol ingestion is discontinued. Vacuolation of a similar appearance occurs in subjects fed a phenylalanine-deficient diet, on chloramphenicol or pyraziname medication, in hyperosmolar coma, or deficient in copper or riboflavin [74]. No recognized nutritional explanation has been found for this morphologic change in subjects with ethanol abuse.

References

1. Hodges, R. E., et al.: Hematopoietic studies in vitamin A deficiency. Am. J. Clin. Nutr. 31:876. 1978.
2. Mohanram, M., Kulkarni K. A., and Reddy, V.: Hematological studies in vitamin A deficient children. Int. J. Vitam. Nutr. Res. 47:389, 1977.
3. Majia, L. A., Hodges, R. E., Arroyave, G., Viteri, F., and Torun, B.: Vitamin A deficiency and anemia in Central American children. Am. J. Clin. Nutr. 30:1175, 1977.
4. Blackfan, K. D., and Wolbach, S. B.: Vitamin A deficiency in infants, a clinical and pathological study. J. Pediatr. 3:679, 1933.
5. Nutrition Survey of Paraguay, May-August, 1965. Nutrition Program, National Center for Chronic Disease Control, U.S. Dept. of Health, Education and Welfare. U.S. Government Printing Office, Washington, D.C., 1967.
6. Ten-State Nutrition Survey of the United States. Center for Disease Control, Atlanta, Ga. DHEW Pub. (HSM) 72-8130-8133. Reports I–V, 1972.
7. Mejia, L. A., Hodges, R. E., and Rucker, R. B.: Clinical signs of anemia in vitamin A-deficient rats. Am. J. Clin. Nutr. 32:1439, 1979.
8. Mahant, L., and Eaton, H. D.: Effects of chronic hypovitaminosis A on water metabolism of the weanling rat. J. Nutr. 106:1817, 1976.
9. Findlay, G. M., and MacKenzie, R. D.: The bone marrow in deficiency diseases. J. Pathol. 25:402, 1922.
10. Snyderman, S. E., Holt, L. E., Jr., Carretero, R., and Jacobs, K.: Pyridoxine deficiency in the human infant. J. Clin. Nutr. 1:200, 1953.
11. Foy, H., and Kondi, A.: Hypochromic anemias of the tropics associated with pyridoxine and nicotinic acid deficiencies. Blood 13:1054, 1958.
12. McCurdy, P. R., Donohoe, R. F., and Magovern, M.: Reversible sideroblastic anemia caused by pyrazinoic acid (pyrazinamide). Ann. Intern. Med. 63:1280, 1966.
13. Frimpter, G. W.: Pyridoxine (B6) dependency syndrome. Ann. Intern. Med. 68:1131, 1968.
14. Wintrobe, M. M., et al.: Pyridoxine deficiency in swine. Bull. Johns Hopkins Hosp. 72:1, 1943.
15. Beutler, E., and Srivastava, S. K.: Relationship between glutathione

16. Lane, M., and Alfrey, C. P.: The anemia of human riboflavin deficiency. Blood 22:811, 1963.
17. Hodges, R. E., Bean, W. B., Ohlson, M. A., and Bleiler, R. E.: Human pantothenic acid deficiency produced by omegamethylpantothenic acid. J. Clin. Invest. 38:1421, 1959.
18. Wintrobe, M. M., Follis, R. H., Jr., Alcoyaga, R., Paulson, M., and Humphreys, S.: Pantothenic acid deficiency in swine. Bull. Johns Hopkins Hosp. 73:313, 1943.
19. Handler, P., and Featherston, W. P.: The biochemical defect in nicotinic acid deficiency. J. Biol. Chem. 151:395, 1943.
20. Vilter, R. W., Woolford, R. M., and Spies, T. D.: Severe scurvy, a clinical and hematological study. J. Lab. Clin. Med. 31:609, 1946.
21. Crandon, J. H., Lund, C. C., and Dill, D. B.: Experimental human scurvy. N. Engl. J. Med. 223:353, 1940.
22. Hodges, R. E., Baker, E. M., Hood, J., Sauberlich, H. E., and March, S. C.: Experimental scurvy in man. Am. J. Clin. Nutr. 22:535, 1969.
23. Zalusky, R., and Herbert, V.: Megaloblastic anemia in scurvy with response to 50 micrograms of folic acid daily. N. Engl. J. Med. 265:1033, 1961.
24. Stokes, P. L., Melikian, V., Leeming, R. L., Portman-Graham, H., Blair, J. S., and Cooke, W. T.: Folate metabolism in scurvy. Am. J. Clin. Nutr. 28:126, 1975.
25. Cox, E. V., Meynell, M. J., Northham, B. E., and Cooke, W. T.: The anemia of scurvy. Am. J. Med. 42:220, 1966.
26. Zuelzer, W. W., Hutnoff, L., and Apt, L.: Relationship of anemia and scurvy. Am. J. Dis. Child. 77:128, 1949.
27. Wapnick, A. A., Lynch, S. R., Krawitz, P., Seftel, H. C., Charlton, R. W., and Bothwell, T. H.: Effects of iron overload on ascorbic acid metabolism. Br. Med. J. 3:704, 1968.
28. Wapnick, A. A., Lynch, S. R., Charlton, R. W., Seftel, H. C., and Bothwell, T. H.: The effect of ascorbic acid deficiency on desferrioxamine-induced urinary iron excretion. Br. J. Haematol. 17:563, 1969.
29. Cohen, A., Cohen, I. J., and Schwartz, E.: Scurvy and altered iron stores in thalassemia major. N. Engl. J. Med. 304:158, 1981.
30. Lipschitz, D. A., Bothwell, T. H., Seftel, H. C., Wapnick, A. A., and Charlton, R. W.: The role of ascorbic acid in the metabolism of storage iron. Br. J. Haematol. 20:155, 1971.
31. Bothwell, T. H., Abrahams, C., Bradlow, B. A., and Charlton, R. W.: Idiopathic and Bantu hemochromatosis. Arch. Pathol. 79:163, 1965.
32. Cox, E. V.: The anemia of scurvy, in International Symposium on Vitamin-related Anemias. Vitamins and Hormones, Advances in Research and Applications, edited by R. S. Harris, I. G. Wool, and J. A. Loraine. Academic, New York, 1968, vol. 26, p. 635.
33. Chow, C. K.: Nutritional influence on cellular antioxidant defense systems. Am. J. Clin. Nutr. 32:1066, 1979.
34. Horwitt, M. K.: Therapeutic uses of vitamin E in medicine. Nutr. Rev. 38:105, 1980.
35. Melhorn, D. K., and Gross, S.: Vitamin E dependent anemia in premature infant. I. Effect of large doses of medicinal iron. J. Pediatr. 79:569, 1971.
36. Williams, M. L., Shott, R. J., O'Neal, P. L., and Oski, F. A.: Role of dietary iron and fat on vitamin E deficiency anemia of infancy. N. Engl. J. Med. 292:887, 1975.
37. Oski, F. A., and Barness, L. A.: Hemolytic anemia in vitamin E deficiency. Am. J. Clin. Nutr. 21:45, 1968.
38. Ritchie, J. H., Fish, M. B., McMasters, V., and Grossman, M.: Edema and hemolytic anemia in premature infants: Vitamin E deficiency. N. Engl. J. Med. 279:1185, 1968.
39. Farrell, P. M., Bieri, J. G., Fratantoni, J. F., Wood, R. E., and di Sant' Agnese, P. A.: The occurrence and effects of vitamin E deficiency: A study in patients with cystic fibrosis. J. Clin. Invest. 60:233, 1977.
40. Spielberg, S. P., Boxer, L. A., Corash, L. M., and Schulman, J. D.: Improved erythrocyte survival with high-dose vitamin E in chronic hemolyzing G6PD and glutathione synthetase deficiencies. Ann. Intern. Med. 90:53, 1979.
41. Corash, L., et al.: Reduced chronic hemolysis during high-dose vitamin E administration in Mediterranean-type glucose-6-phosphate dehydrogenase deficiency. N. Engl. J. Med. 303:416, 1980.
42. Natta, C. L., Machlin, L. J., and Brin, M.: A decrease in irreversibly

reductase activity and drug-induced haemolytic anaemia. Nature 226:759, 1970.

sickled erythrocytes in sickle cell anemia patients given vitamin E. *Am. J. Clin. Nutr. 33*:968, 1980.

43. Frieden, E.: The ferrous to ferric cycles in iron metabolism. *Nutr. Rev. 31*:41, 1973.

44. Shields, G. S., Carlson, W. F., Kimball, D. A., Carnes, W. H., Cartwright, G. E., and Wintrobe, M. M.: Studies on copper metabolism. XXII. Cardiovascular lesions in copper deficient swine. *Am. J. Pathol. 41*:603, 1952.

45. Graham, G. G., and Cordano, A.: Copper depletion and deficiency in the malnourished infant. *Johns Hopkins Med. J. 124*:139, 1969.

46. Joffe, G., Etzioni, A., Levy, J., and Benderly, A.: A patient with copper deficiency anemia while on prolonged intravenous feeding. *Clin. Pediatr. 20*:226, 1981.

47. Dunlop, W. M., James, G. W., III, and Hume, D. M.: Anemia and neutropenia caused by copper deficiency. *Ann. Intern. Med. 80*:470, 1974.

48. Parisi, A. F., and Vallee, B. L.: Zinc metalloenzymes: Characteristics and significance in biology and medicine. *Am. J. Clin. Nutr. 22*:1222, 1969.

49. Sandstead, H. H.: Zinc, in *Present Knowledge in Nutrition*, 4th ed. The Nutrition Foundation, Inc., Washington, D.C., 1976, p. 290.

50. Prasad, A. S., Diwany, M., Gabr, M., Sandstead, H. H., Mokhtar, N., and El Hefney, A.: Biochemical studies in thalassemia. *Ann. Intern. Med. 62*:87, 1965.

51. Prasad, A. S., Schoomaker, E. B., Ortega, J., Brewer, G. J., Oberleas, D., and Oelshlegel, F. J., Jr.: Zinc deficiency in sickle cell disease. *Clin. Chem. 21*:582, 1975.

52. Keys, A., Brozek, J., Henschel, A., Nichelsen, D., and Taylor, H. L.: *The Biology of Semistarvation.* University of Minnesota Press, Minneapolis, 1950, vol. 1, p. 245.

53. Thomson, T. J.: Treatment of obesity by total fasting for up to 249 days. *Lancet 2*:992, 1966.

54. Drenick, E. J., Swendseid, M. E., Blahd, W. H., and Tuttle, S. G.: Prolonged starvation as treatment for severe obesity. *JAMA 187*:100, 1964.

55. Delmonte, L., Aschenasy, A., and Eyquem, A.: Studies on the hemolytic nature of protein-deficiency anemia in the rat. *Blood 24*:49, 1964.

56. Caro, J., Silver, R., Erslev, A. J., Miller, O. P., and Birgegård, G.: Erythropoietin production in fasted rats: Effects of thyroid hormones and glucose supplementation. *J. Lab. Clin. Med. 98*:860, 1981.

57. Reissmann, K. R.: Protein metabolism and erythropoiesis. I. The anemia of protein deprivation. *Blood 23*:137, 1964.

58. Naets, J. P.: Effect of starvation on the response to erythropoietin in the rat. *Acta Haematol. (Basel) 52(3)*:141, 1974.

59. Ito, K., and Reissmann, K. R.: Quantitative and qualitative aspects of steady state erythropoesis induced in protein starved rats by long term erythropoietin injection. *Blood 27*:343, 1966.

60. Viteri, R. E., Alvaredo, J., Luthringer, D. G., and Wood, R. P.: II. Hematological changes in protein-calorie malnutrition, in *International Symposium on Vitamin-related Anemias. Vitamins and Hormones, Advances in Research and Applications*, edited by R. S. Harris, I. G. Wool, and J. A. Loraine. Academic, New York, 1968, vol. 26, p. 573.

61. Adams, E. B., Scragg, J. N., Naidoo, B. T., Liljestrand, S. K., and Cockram, V. J.: Observations on the aetiology and treatment of anaemia in kwashiorkor. *Br. Med. J. 3*:451, 1967.

62. Foy, H., and Kondi, A.: Comparison between erythroid aplasia in marasmus and kwashiorkor and the experimentally induced erythroid aplasia in baboons by riboflavin deficiency, in *International Symposium on Vitamin-related Anemias. Vitamins and Hormones, Advances in Research and Applications*, edited by R. S. Harris, I. G. Wool, and J. A. Loraine. Academic, New York, 1968, vol. 26, p. 653.

63. McKenzie, D., Friedman, R., Katz, B., and Lanzkowsky, P.: Erythropoietin levels in anemia of kwashiorkor. *S. Afr. Med. J. 41*:1044, 1967.

64. Herbert, V. (ed.): Hematologic complications of alcoholism. *Sem. Hematol.* vol. 17, nos. 1 and 2, 1980.

65. Eichner, E. R., and Hillman, R. S.: The evolution of anemia in alcoholic patients. *Am. J. Med. 50*:218, 1971.

66. Hines, J. D., and Cowan, D. H.: Anemia in alcoholism, in *Drugs and Hematologic Reactions*, edited by N. V. Dimitrov and J. H. Nodine. Grune & Stratton, New York, 1974, p. 141.

67. Eichner, E. R., Buchanan, B., and Smith, J. W.: Variations in the hematologic and medical status of alcoholics. *Am. J. Med. Sci. 263*:35, 1972.

68. Sullivan, L. W., and Herbert, V.: Suppression of hematopoiesis by ethanol. *J. Clin. Invest. 43*:2048, 1964.

69. Eichner, E. R., and Hillman, R. S.: Effect of alcohol on serum folate level. *J. Clin. Invest. 52*:584, 1973.

70. Lindenbaum, J.: Folate and vitamin B_{12} deficiencies in alcoholism. *Sem. Hematol. 17*:119, 1980.

71. Wu, A., Chanarin, I., and Levi, A. J.: Macrocytosis of chronic alcoholism. *Lancet 1*:829, 1974.

72. Myrhed, M., Berglund, L., and Bottiger, L. E.: Alcohol consumption and hematology. *Acta Med. Scand. 202*:11, 1977.

73. McCurdy, P. R., Pierce, L. E., and Rath, C. E.: Abnormal bone marrow morphology in acute alcoholism. *N. Engl. J. Med. 266*:505, 1962.

74. McCurdy, P. R., and Rath, C. E.: Vacuolated nucleated bone marrow cells in alcoholism. *Sem. Hematol 17*:100, 1980.

CHAPTER *54*

Sideroblastic anemias

WILLIAM N. VALENTINE

Definition and history

Sideroblastic anemias [1–41] are a heterogeneous group of disorders which have as a common feature the presence of large numbers of ringed sideroblasts in the marrow (Fig. 54-1a and Plates 3-D4 and 3-D5), ineffective erythropoiesis, usually increased levels of tissue iron, and varying proportions of hypochromic erythrocytes in the peripheral blood (Fig. 54-1b). They may be acquired or hereditary (Table 54-1). The former may be primary or secondary to the administration of certain drugs, to toxins, or to neoplastic or inflammatory disease [5]. The primary acquired sideroblastic anemias may or may not be pyridoxine-responsive. Hereditary sideroblastic anemias include both X chromosome–linked [3,17,33–39] and autosomally linked [40] entities. The sideroblastic anemias are normocytic or slightly macrocytic. The marrow structure often exhibits dyserythropoietic features such as megaloblastoid maturation or, at times, some increases in numbers of binucleated erythroblasts. Despite intense marrow hyperplasia, the reticulocyte response to anemia is inappropriately low. Many erythroid precursors undergo intramedullary destruction, resulting in increased production of bile pigment apparently derived in substantial part from the hemoglobin of these destroyed cells.

NORMAL SIDEROBLASTS
Sideroblasts are erythroblasts containing one or more Prussian blue–positive granules demonstrable on light microscopy, representing aggregates of nonheme iron [42–47]. The morphology of these cells in normal and abnormal states is discussed in detail in Chap. 29. In

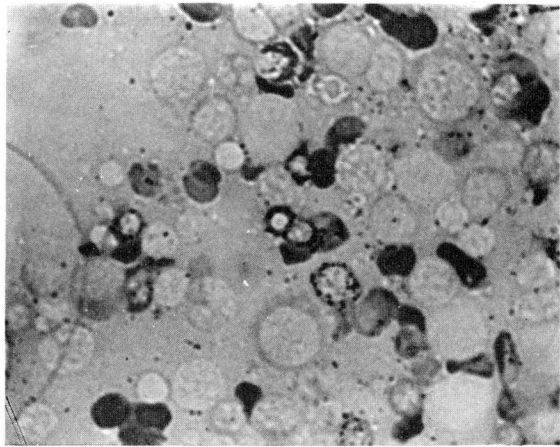

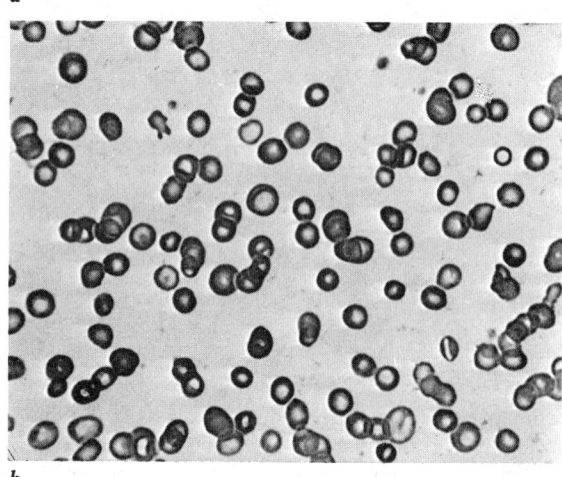

FIGURE 54-1 (a) Ringed sideroblasts in iron stains of bone marrow. (b) Peripheral blood from a patient with sideroblastic anemia. Note the variation in size and shape and the dimorphism. Some of the cells are well hemoglobinized, while many are hypochromic. (Courtesy of D. Mollin.)

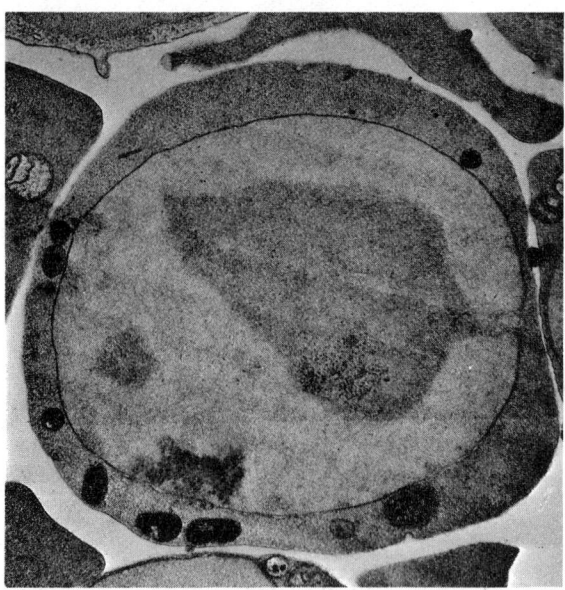

FIGURE 54-2 Electron-microscopic view of ringed sideroblast showing the ferruginous micelles in mitochondria. (Courtesy of Dr. M. Bessis.)

ondary lysosomes [50,55]. Under conditions of marrow stress, some red cells may fully mature before siderotic granules are eliminated. Such cells—now called *siderocytes*—are unable to excrete ferritin, and the granules must be "pitted" by a process dependent upon the spleen.

PATHOLOGIC SIDEROBLASTS
In contrast to the normal cytoplasmic location of siderotic granules, the cells in the sideroblastic anemias exhibit large amounts of iron deposited as dust or plaque-like ferruginous micelles between the cristae of mitochondria (Fig. 54-2) [50,56]. The iron-loaded mitochondria are distorted and swollen, their cristae are indistinct, and the identification of mitochondria may itself be difficult. The mitochondrial iron, viewed by electron microscopy, fails to display the ultrastructural characteristics of ferritin, although aggregates of ferritin may be present in the cytoplasm. Energy-dispersive x-ray analysis [57] of mitochondria has also demonstrated that mitochondrial deposits have an elemental composition different from that of ferritin or hemosiderin. Iron and phosphate were present in all, suggesting that deposits may largely be insoluble ferric phosphate. Iron in the ferric form can not be inserted into the protoporphyrin ring. In humans, the mitochondria of the erythroblast are distributed perinuclearly [11], and this accounts for the distinctive "ringed" sideroblast identified by Prussian blue staining when mitochondrial iron overload is present (Fig. 54-1a and Plates 3-D4 and 3-D5).

Though the perinuclear distribution of siderotic granules in the nucleated red blood cells of patients with various types of anemia was described in 1947 [58,59], the concept of sideroblastic anemia as a generic desig-

normal subjects without iron deficiency, 30 to 50 percent of marrow erythroblasts contain such granules, which, when viewed by electron microscopy, are seen to be neither within mitochondria nor associated with other cytoplasmic organelles [48–50]. Transferrin-bound iron attaches to specific receptors in the membranes of immature erythroid cells, and is transferred to the cell by means of an energy-requiring transport system [51,52]. There it combines with molecules of *de novo* synthesized apoferritin to form ferritin [53,54]. Initially, ferritin is diffusely distributed, but gradually granular aggregates large enough to be seen by light microscopy are formed. With the loss of its nucleus, the sideroblast may become a reticulated siderocyte (R-S cell—a reticulocyte with mitochondria and polyribosomes, which still contains Prussian blue-staining granules [47]). The R-S cells are metabolically active and are able to dispose of siderotic granules by a process of active excretion, the ferritin being eliminated in ruptured vesicles or in sec-

nation was not generally accepted until the last two decades. The publications of Björkman [1], Dacie et al. [2], Heilmeyer and his associates [3,4], Bernard et al. [12], and Mollin [5] were chiefly responsible for the current focus and orientation. After description of the primary adult form of refractory sideroblastic anemia [1,2], the similarity of the morphologic and erythrokinetic changes in hereditary (sex-linked) hypochromic anemia was recognized. It then became evident that similar abnormalities were associated with a wide variety of diseases [6], with pyridoxine-responsive anemia [5,7–9], with treatment with antituberculous drugs in occasional patients[10,24], and with lead intoxication [11,31,32,60]; these "secondary" acquired disorders were then incorporated into the classification.

Acquired sideroblastic anemia

PRIMARY SIDEROBLASTIC ANEMIA
This designation includes chronic refractory anemia with sideroblastic bone marrow, refractory erythroblastic anemia, sideroachrestic anemia, and refractory sideroblastic anemia.

ETIOLOGY AND PATHOGENESIS
The pathogenesis of primary acquired idiopathic sideroblastic anemia may be viewed from three standpoints: the pathogenesis of the anemia itself, the etiology of the ringed sideroblast, and the underlying biochemical lesions.

Mechanism of anemia The dominant factor producing anemia is clearly ineffective erythropoiesis; the rate of red call destruction is usually near normal, but it may be accelerated moderately to levels for which a normally functioning marrow could easily compensate [2,14,15,61,63]. The half-time of disappearance of intravenously injected tracer doses of radioactive iron may be normal, but it usually is rapid (25 to 50 min; normal mean, 90 to 100 min). The plasma iron turnover tends to be increased (1.5 to 5.9 mg per deciliter of whole blood per day; normal, approximately 0.6 ± 0.2 mg) but incorporation of the radioactive iron into heme and its delivery to the blood as newly synthesized hemoglobin are depressed (15 to 30 percent of tracer dose; normal, 80 to 90 percent). Red cell survival, as determined by the ^{51}Cr technique, varies from a half-time of 15 days to normal, corresponding to a mean erythrocyte life-span of approximately 40 to 120 days. As in other kinds of anemia characterized by ineffective erythropoiesis, the total fecal stercobilin excreted per day may be greater than can be accounted for by the daily catabolism of circulating hemoglobin.

Abnormalities of heme synthesis Except when due to iron deficiency, impairment of heme biosynthesis at the iron-protoporphyrin step results in mitochondrial iron overload and eventually in sideroblastic anemia. The

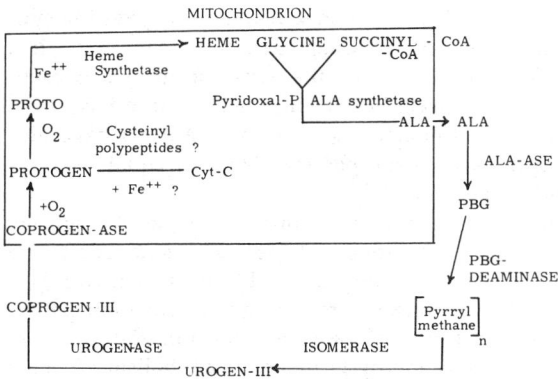

FIGURE 54-3 Biosynthetic pathway of heme synthesis; reactions thought to occur within mitochondria are enclosed in the box. Pyridoxal-P = pyridoxal phosphate; ALA = aminolevulinic acid; ALA-ASE = ALA dehydrogenase; PBG = porphobilinogen; UROGEN = uroporphyrinogen; COPROGEN = coproporphyrinogen; PROTOGEN = protoporphyrinogen; PROTO = protoporphyrin.

final insertion of iron into the porphyrin ring is an intramitochondrial process, is dependent upon an intact electron transport system, and is mediated by the enzyme heme synthetase (ferrochelatase) (Fig. 54-3) [64,65]. However, the primary defect resulting in failure of the final common pathway may lie in the inadequate synthesis of protoporphyrin, in a deficiency of heme synthetase, and also in defective synthesis of globin. The latter must progress in a balanced fashion with heme synthesis for optimal production of hemoglobin [48,66–68]. The iron may damage the mitochondria by peroxidation of mitochondrial lipids and perhaps by other mechanisms. In any event, the deterioration of mitochondrial function and loss of crucial mitochondrial-mediated activities per se could contribute to ineffective erythropoiesis and to the premature destruction of marrow erythroid precursors.

In the search for the basic biochemical lesions responsible for the development of sideroblastic anemia, attention has been focused upon an intramitochondrial defect in heme synthesis or on a disturbance in pyridoxine metabolism. This has been fostered by the clear demonstration that pyridoxine deficiency in animals is a prototype of sideroblastic anemia [28,56,69]. Moreover, certain sideroblastic disorders, though clearly not due to pyridoxine deficiency in a conventional sense, are nonetheless responsive to pharmacologic doses of pyridoxine [7–9,19]. Pyridoxal phosphate is a necessary coenzyme for the initial reaction of protoporphyrin synthesis, the condensation of glycine and succinyl CoA to form δ-aminolevulinic acid (ALA), mediated by ALA synthetase. Sideroblastic anemia with deficiency of ALA synthetase of marrow erythroid cells has been documented in five subjects with the congenital disorder, and a limited group with the acquired disease [70,71]. In one or more additional patients a deficiency of uroporphyrinogen decarboxylase [72,73] and heme synthetase [74–76], enzymes also necessary for the synthesis of heme (see Chap. 31), has been identified. Pyridoxal 5'-phosphate, the active form of the coenzyme, must itself be enzymatically synthesized from pyridoxine. Deficiencies in its biosynthesis have also been invoked as the possible cause of certain sideroblastic anemias [9,77].

Since iron-loaded mitochondria are morphologically and functionally abnormal [46], and since defective heme synthesis is unquestionably present in the sideroblastic anemias, it is tempting to define their pathogenesis in terms of passive mitochondrial iron accumulation secondary to defective anabolism of heme and hemoglobin. In this connection, electron microscope autoradiography of ringed sideroblasts in two patients with primary acquired sideroblastic anemia demonstrated that depressed DNA, RNA, and protein synthesis, as well as ultrastructural abnormalities, were largely confined to a small proportion of erythroblasts with the largest deposits of intramitochondrial iron [78]. It appeared that iron accumulation could arrest the progress of early polychromatic erythroblasts through the cell cycle. By inference, the death of the most iron-laden cells contributed most greatly to ineffective erythropoiesis. This viewpoint may suffice for those sideroblastic anemias in which there are defined hereditary or acquired molecular lesions, or in those reversible syndromes secondary to drugs or toxins with known sites of action. However, it is too simplistic for extrapolation to the sideroblastic anemias as a whole. Indeed, the cause of most cases of acquired sideroblastic anemia remains obscure, and in some the mitochondrial lesion may well be only one manifestation of wide-ranging, more fundamental, and undefined disturbances in metabolism of erythroid and, in some instances, other marrow elements. In many instances, no abnormalities in the protoporphyrin synthetic pathway have been demonstrable [79]. Heme synthetase activity has only rarely been observed to be reduced [23,79]. Free erythrocyte protoporphyrin has been usually increased, not decreased [23,25]. Further, a simple defect in heme synthesis fails to explain adequately certain commonly encountered features such as megaloblastoid and other dyserythropoietic features, the frequently low serum folate levels, and, at times, partial responses to folate administration. It must be remembered, however, that both pyridoxal phosphate and folate are cofactors in the enzymatic conversion of serine to glycine (see Chap. 50). This reaction generates a form of folate coenzyme necessary for the formation of thymidylate, an important step in DNA synthesis.

Other abnormalities   There are additional abnormalities which are difficult to rationalize in terms of defects in heme synthesis or other mitochondrial dysfunction. For example, the activity of glyceraldehyde-3-phosphate dehydrogenase is greatly increased in some, but not all, patients. Dramatically altered activity ratios of a wide diversity of enzymes, many of which are thought to be unrelated to mitochondrial function, have been de-

scribed. There are alterations in red cell antigen patterns, and, in some instances, a variety of metabolic abnormalities [80–85]. Similar findings occur in certain hereditary and acquired refractory anemias with cellular marrows but *without ringed sideroblasts* [80,83]. Such dyscrasias are also characterized by ineffective erythropoiesis, and except for the lack of ringed sideroblasts, may in some instances be virtually indistinguishable from their sideroblastic counterparts [86]. Such unexplained observations suggest that a metabolic disturbance resulting in mitochondrial iron overload may be too simplistic an explanation for the pathogenesis of the sideroblastic anemias. In the acquired primary forms of sideroblastic anemia, the presence in some patients of two morphologically distinct populations of red cells suggests the concept of a somatic mutation, giving rise to a dominant, metabolically abnormal clone of cells, but the existence of such a mechanism has not been proved.

CLINICAL FEATURES

Primary acquired sideroblastic anemia occurs most frequently in patients over 50 years of age, but cases have been recognized in younger subjects. The disorder is uncommon, but not rare. Heilmeyer [25] was able to study 18 patients in continental Europe, and MacGibbon and Mollin [6], 22 patients in Great Britain. In one large hematology clinic [23], idiopathic acquired sideroblastic anemia constituted about 1 percent of referred cases. Both sexes may be affected [23], and, although varying from series to series, the sex ratio is probably close to unity. Symptoms of weakness, dyspnea, angina of effort, and occasionally anorexia develop insidiously, and have sometimes been present for several years when the patient first seeks medical attention. The skin and mucous membranes tend to be pale, but in some instances a light lemon-yellow hue is evident or the skin of the hands and arms has a dusky pigmentation. Purpura and other bleeding manifestations are unusual [15]. In roughly half the patients, the firm edge of the spleen can be felt at or just below the left costal margin, and the liver may be palpated several centimeters below the right costal margin. Splenic and hepatic enlargement do not necessarily occur together, and marked increase in the size of either organ is rare. Peripheral lymph node enlargement is unusual. Findings on neurologic examination are normal. Dermal photosensitivity has been reported in one patient whose free erythrocyte protoporphyrin was markedly increased [75].

LABORATORY FEATURES

The anemia is normocytic or slightly macrocytic. The hemoglobin level may be as low as 3 g/dl, but more commonly it is in the range of 7 to 10 g/dl. The most striking morphologic change in the erythrocytes is dimorphism. Some of the cells have a normal amount of hemoglobin, others are hypochromic. The hypochromic cells vary markedly in size and shape (Fig. 54-1*b*). A few target cells, fragmented cells, siderocytes, and erythroblasts may be seen. The reticulocyte count is usually normal but may be slightly increased. Osmotic fragility tends to be decreased. The white blood cell count varies from normal to leukopenic levels; when present, leukopenia is accompanied by neutropenia. Values below 2000 cells per microliter are rare. Neutrophils may be deficient in granules. The neutrophil alkaline phosphatase score is reduced in about one-half the patients. An occasional myelocyte may be found in the peripheral blood film. Lymphocytes and monocytes are morphologically normal, but the proportion of monocytes may be moderately increased. The platelet count is usually normal, but thrombocytopenia or thrombocytosis occurs in a minority of patients. Serum folate levels have been reported to be low in 80 percent of cases in one series from Great Britain [6].

The marrow is characterized by intense erythroid hyperplasia, often associated with a shift to younger forms, particularly polychromatophilic erythroblasts, some of which show megaloblastic nuclear changes. Other nuclear abnormalities include binucleated cells and pyknosis. The cytoplasm of many of the cells may appear foamy, vacuolated, and poorly hemoglobinized. The amount of PAS-positive material in the erythroblastic cytoplasm is usually normal or low [23]. Iron stains show many abnormal ringed sideroblasts and increased amounts of hemosiderin (Fig. 54-1a and Plates 3-D4 and 3-D5). Granulocyte precursors frequently are normal in appearance, but modest increases in the number of promyelocytes and myeloblasts may be seen. At times the changes are sufficient to make the most experienced morphologist wonder whether they might be those of early leukemia. Megakaryocytes are usually normal, but their number may be depressed in patients who have thrombocytopenia.

The quantity of free erythrocyte protoporphyrin is almost always moderately increased, and rarely it is markedly so [23]. Somewhat conflicting values have been noted for free erythrocyte coproporphyrin concentrations. Heilmeyer [25] reported marked elevations, but others have noted normal, or only occasionally increased, levels [23]. A deficiency of heme synthetase, a mitochondrial enzyme catalyzing the incorporation of iron into protoporphyrin to form heme, could account both for defective hemoglobin production and the accumulation of free protoporphyrin. However, convincing data indicate that both heme synthetase activity [23,79] and indeed the entire heme biosynthetic pathway [79] are often not demonstrably defective. Heme synthetase deficiency appears documented in a few subjects, however [74–76].

Erythrokinetic studies demonstrate ineffective erythropoiesis (see "Etiology and Pathogenesis" earlier in this chapter). Much of the erythropoietic activity of the marrow fails to achieve normal fruition in terms of production of viable, circulating erythrocytes. The ineffective erythropoiesis is accompanied by hemosiderosis of marrow, liver, and spleen, and usually by a high degree of saturation of serum transferrin. Despite iron overload, secondary severe dysfunction of liver, pancreas, or heart has not been common.

Finally, the acquired idiopathic sideroblastic anemias share a profusion of other abnormalities with a variety of heterogeneous dyserythropoietic states. These include striking departures from normal values and enzyme activity ratios in the case of glycolytic and nonglycolytic enzymes of the erythrocyte, variations from normal isoenzyme patterns, increases at times in the amount of fetal hemoglobin, and unusual anomalies in the antigen composition of the erythrocytes [80–85]. Similar abnormalities occur in other refractory anemias, both hereditary and acquired, sideroblastic as well as nonsideroblastic [80,83]. These diverse syndromes have in common ineffective erythropoiesis and cyto- and karyokinetic abnormalities associated with abnormal cell maturation and division.

DIFFERENTIAL DIAGNOSIS

The forms of anemia most likely to be confused with primary acquired sideroblastic anemia are those in which the erythrocytes are also hypochromic. Iron-deficiency anemia should present no problem, since the serum iron level is low, the iron-binding capacity is elevated, the marrow contains essentially no stainable iron, sideroblasts are absent, and the serum ferritin level is diminished. In spite of these differences, patients are sometimes erroneously assumed to have iron deficiency because of the evident hypochromia, and may be treated with iron for variable lengths of time. Differentiation from thalassemia minor can be more difficult; it depends on estimations of the concentrations of hemoglobins F and A_2 (see Chap. 50), the family history, and sometimes hematologic evaluation of other members of the family. Ringed sideroblasts are usually few in number in thalassemia minor. Thalassemia major is less of a problem, since it becomes manifest early in life. Differentiation of primary from secondary forms of sideroblastic anemia depends on careful clinical evaluation to ascertain possible exposure to antituberculosis drugs, lead, and the other agents listed in Table 54-1 and

TABLE 54-1   Classification of sideroblastic anemias

I. Acquired
   A. Primary sideroblastic anemia
      [1,2,5,6,11,12,14,15,22–25,46,47,74,75,77,79]
   B. Sideroblastic anemia secondary to:
      1. Certain drugs: isoniazid [10.22.24,28];
         pyrazinamide [24,28]; cycloserine [24,28];
         chloramphenicol [24,29,30,88]
      2. Ethanol [20,24,26,27,91–93]
      3. Lead [11,22,31,32,60,96]
      4. Chronic neoplastic and inflammatory disease
         [5,6,16,24,80,83]
II. Hereditary
   A. X chromosome-linked
      1. Pyridoxine-responsive [17,33–36]
      2. Pyridoxine-refractory [3,25,37]
   B. Autosomal: pyridoxine-refractory [40]
III. Pyridoxine-responsive anemia [7,8,19,34,77]
   A. "Classical"
   B. Variant forms

the detection of those diseases that may cause sideroblastic changes. At times, the nucleated erythroid elements in the marrow bear enough resemblance to megaloblasts to suggest the diagnosis of pernicious anemia [2] or other disorders of vitamin B_{12} or folate metabolism. Differentiation from preleukemia or the early stages of acute myelogenous leukemia (AML) can be the most difficult of all, and has led to the suggestion that primary acquired sideroblastic anemia is simply an early stage of AML with erythroid features [13]. When leukocyte immaturity is a feature of the sideroblastic anemia, it is difficult to be certain that leukemia will not develop, even after several years. Differentiation from other syndromes with ineffective erythropoiesis, such as certain congenital dyserythropoietic anemias (Chap. 46) and certain refractory anemias without sideroblastosis, may occasion difficulty if only the peripheral blood and clinical findings are considered. Here the crucial diagnostic procedure is bone marrow examination, since prominent sideroblastosis is absent, and other differential features such as erythroid multinuclearity may be evident.

THERAPY

Most patients are refractory to all forms of therapy, including liver extracts, vitamin B_{12}, folic acid, pyridoxine, corticosteroids, and androgens. Hemoglobin levels of 8 g/dl or more can usually be tolerated. If anemia becomes more severe, or if symptoms of hypoxia, cardiac failure, or angina occur in elderly patients, transfusions must be given even though iron overload and sensitization to minor blood groups or to platelet and leukocyte antigens usually occur. Such sensitization may be delayed by the use of packed or washed red cells. Viral hepatitis is also a hazard. Patients who have subnormal serum folate levels may show a partial response to the administration of folic acid (1 to 3 mg daily, orally); the hemoglobin level does not return to normal but may rise enough so that transfusions become unnecessary [6,23]. Not all patients with low serum folate and megaloblastic changes are benefited. A few patients will also show enough hematologic improvement after the administration of pharmacologic doses of pyridoxine (100 to 200 mg per day orally for at least 3 months) to obviate the need for further transfusions [15]. Some ringed sideroblasts and hypochromia apparently always persist. A more detailed description of the therapeutic response is given below under the heading "Pyridoxine-Responsive Sideroblastic Anemia" (Fig. 54-4). A therapeutic trial with folic acid and pyridoxine is worthwhile, even though only a small percentage of patients are helped by it. Occasionally, androgen therapy (oxymetholone, 50 to 150 mg per day, orally, or testosterone enanthate, 50 to 600 mg per week by injection), either alone or in combination with prednisone, for at least 3 months may cause enough improvement to decrease or eliminate the necessity for transfusion. Splenectomy fails to bring about improvement.

COURSE AND PROGNOSIS

The course in most patients is protracted, lasting for 1 to 10 years or more, until death results from pneumonia, myocardial infarction, cardiac failure, or one of the other diseases to which elderly patients are susceptible. Increased susceptibility to infection is usually not a problem, and hemorrhagic manifestations tend to occur only in those unfortunate patients who develop severe thrombocytopenia. When transfusions are necessary, the prognosis is worse and complications are frequent. Hemosiderosis may develop, and a few patients manifest clinical features commonly associated with hemochromatosis: diabetes mellitus, cirrhosis, and cardiac arrhythmias. A variable number of patients develop acute myelogenous leukemia, sometimes after only a few months but usually after several years [1,3,15,16,23]. The course is then rapidly fatal. Whether the incidence of leukemia is definitely higher in these patients than in those with other forms of marrow failure is not yet clear. In this minority of patients, it is difficult to say whether leukemia evolved as a separate disorder, or whether the refractory anemia represented a "preleukemic" state irrevocably destined to become overt leukemia.

FIGURE 54-4 Therapeutic response to pyridoxine in a patient with primary acquired sideroblastic anemia. Only a minority of these patients are pyridoxine-responsive; erythrocyte values do not return to normal. If therapy is stopped, relapse occurs within 2 to 3 months. By contrast, a patient with the "classic" form of pyridoxine-responsive anemia will often respond to smaller doses and will have a return of red blood cell values to normal or near normal.

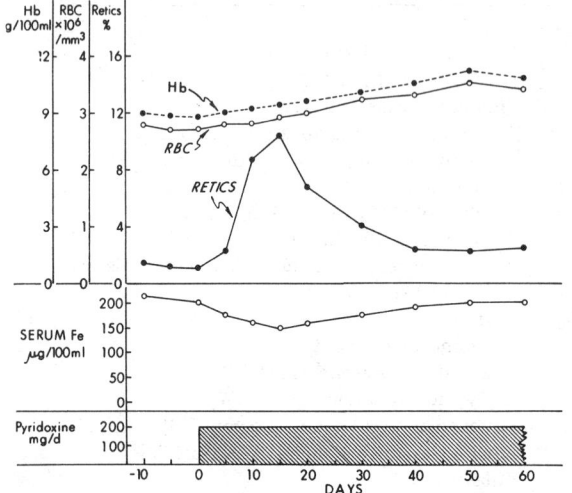

Secondary sideroblastic anemias

Sideroblastic anemia has been reported to coexist with hemolytic anemia, erythremic myelosis, leukemia, myeloma, and myeloproliferative disease, as well as with such nonhemopoietic disorders as hypothyroidism, thyrotoxicosis, carcinoma, uremia, rheumatoid arthritis, porphyria cutanea tarda, and polyarteritis nodosa [5,6,29]. Why it occurs in some patients with chronic diseases and not in others remains a mystery. In some instances, there may be chance association of two disease processes in the same patient; in others, the chronic underlying disease may be associated with either nutritional inadequacies or with unknown metabolic abnormalities.

Sideroblastic anemia has also been observed after administration of the drugs isoniazid [10,22,24,28], cycloserine [24,28], pyrazinamide [24,28], and chloramphenicol [24,29,30,88]. All these agents impair ALA synthetase activity. The first three inhibit a variety of pyridoxal-5'-phosphate-catalyzed reactions [87] whereas chloramphenicol inhibits mitochondrial protein synthesis in general, including synthesis of cytochrome oxidase [88], ALA synthetase [89], and heme synthetase [90]. Some patients with chronic alcoholism also develop sideroblastic anemia. Alcohol is believed to inhibit pyridoxal kinase and hence the synthesis of pyridoxal 5'-phosphate from nonphosphorylated precursors, or alternatively to accelerate its degradation by enhancing pyridoxal phosphate phosphatase activity [91,92]. Serum pyridoxal-5'-phosphate levels have been reported to be low in patients with sideroblastic anemia secondary to alcoholism [26,93], and it has also been reported that pyridoxal 5'-phosphate is more effective than pyridoxine in reversing the anemia [24]. However, earlier studies [92] indicating that pyridoxine kinase activity is diminished in patients with alcoholic sideroblastic anemia have not been confirmed [93–95], nor could evidence of diminished concentrations of pyridoxal 5'-phosphate within erythrocytes of patients with idiopathic or alcohol-induced sideroblastic anemia be documented [95].

Lead intoxication may also produce sideroblastosis, particularly in children, who tend to have more severe anemia than adults. The pathogenesis is complex, since lead interferes at many points in heme biosynthesis, including the inhibition of both ALA synthetase and heme synthetase [96]. Lead overburden may be directly diagnosed when blood levels are greater than 70 μg/dl (normal = 10 to 40). It may be suggested indirectly by increased red cell–free erythrocyte protoporphyrin levels or increased urinary excretion of ALA and coproporphyrin. The latter are not entirely specific for lead intoxication. The anemia of lead intoxication is discussed in Chap. 65.

The treatment of secondary acquired sideroblastic anemias depends on the nature of the underlying pathogenetic process. Those cases associated with neoplastic or inflammatory disease should be given a trial of pyridoxine (100 to 200 mg per day, orally) and folic acid (1 to 3 mg per day, orally), general nutrition should be optimized, and, when possible, the underlying disease itself should be treated. While some cases achieve partial responses to folic acid and pyridoxine, results are unpredictable and remissions rarely complete.

Drug-induced sideroblastic anemia ordinarily responds to withdrawal of the offending agent, the administration of folic acid and pyridoxine, and improvement in general nutrition [10]. Though reversibility may occur when supplementary pyridoxine is given and INH and cycloserine are continued [21], discontinuation of the drug has usually been necessary for achievement of full hematologic remission. Patients with alcoholism usually have megaloblastic marrows. They tend to respond rapidly to alcohol withdrawal, normal diets, and folic acid supplements. Where lead overburden is involved, it is necessary to remove the patient from lead exposure and, in selected cases, to mobilize lead through administration of chelating agents such as calcium EDTA and penicillamine.

Hereditary sideroblastic anemia

Like the acquired disorders, the hereditary forms of sideroblastic anemia are heterogeneous. Nearly 100 congenital or familial cases have now been recorded [71]. Apparently the X chromosome–linked varieties are most common, although in many reports there are insufficient data to determine conclusively the genetic pattern of transmission, or firmly to rule out environmental factors in the pathogenesis of the disorder. Support for hereditary transmission and X chromosome linkage is found, however, in several well-documented family studies [3,17,24,33–39]. In one, two sisters with erythrocyte mosaicism—one red cell population being normal and a second hypochromic and microcytic—were heterozygous for the X-linked Xg^a red cell antigen. In both, the hypochromic red cells were Xg^a-positive, expressing an X chromosome inherited from the mother, while the normal populations were Xg^a-negative and determined by the X chromosome of the father [38]. Additional support has been derived from a study of X-linked sideroblastic anemia and G-6-PD deficiency in nine black patients from a family of 29 [35]. In accordance with expectations based on the phenomenon of random X chromosome inactivation in females, all affected males had a severe disorder, whereas females exhibited dimorphic erythrocyte populations but were otherwise normal. In six cases called *anemia hypochromica sideroachrestica hereditaria*, the sideroblastic anemia was pyridoxine-refractory and characterized by increased red cell coproporphyrin and decreased free protoporphyrin [4]. The hereditary cases, even when sex-linked, appear to be of diverse pathogenesis. Some are pyridoxine-responsive and some are not. In pyridoxine-responsive cases, hematologic improvement is partial and less complete than in the "classic" cases of pyridoxine-response anemia initially described [7,8,19]. Abnormal marrow and erythrocyte structures persist after pyridoxine therapy. In certain pedigrees, the mode of inheritance of sideroblastic anemia appears to be autosomal [40].

Pyridoxine-responsive sideroblastic anemia

Pyridoxine-responsive sideroblastic anemia is classified separately because it occurs in both the primary and secondary forms of sideroblastic anemia. Since 1946 more than 100 cases have been described [7,8,17,19,33–36,40,76]. A variety of pathogenic mechanisms is probably involved; clinical and hematologic manifestations as well as the derangements in iron metabolism are similar to those for other patients with sideroblastic anemia. Diagnosis is dependent on a significant hematologic response to large (pharmacologic) doses of pyridoxine. What determines this therapeutic responsiveness in certain sideroblastic anemias and not in others is not known. It has most often been thought that massive pyridoxine dosage in some way facilitates a pyridoxal-dependent reaction such as ALA biosynthesis or, alternatively, partially corrects defects in the biosynthesis of pyridoxal 5-phosphate from pyridoxine. The distinction between pyridoxine responsiveness and pyridoxine deficiency is not always sharp [97,98]. The hematologic manifestations are similar except that in pyridoxine deficiency ringed sideroblasts may be less prominent [28]; manifestations are completely corrected by small (nutritional) amounts of pyridoxine; and enlargement of the liver and spleen is not a feature. By contrast, in pyridoxine-responsive anemia, evidences of body-wide deficiency of pyridoxine (convulsions, neuropathy, glossitis, dermatitis) are, with rare exceptions, strikingly absent; large doses of pyridoxine (50 to 200 mg per day, orally) are required for a therapeutic response (Fig. 54-4); complete return of erythrocyte values to normal are rare; erythrocyte morphologic abnormalites (abnormal variations in size and shape, hypochromia, ringed sideroblasts) almost invariably persist; and relapse commonly occurs if therapy is interrupted. These considerations suggest that pyridoxine responsiveness may be engrafted upon other more primary hematologic or biochemical abnormalities. In a single case, however, primary pyridoxine-responsive sideroblastic anemia treated with repeated phlebotomy to relieve iron overload, with pyridoxine, and with folic acid exhibited essentially complete reversal of all abnormalities [99]. Normal levels of hemoglobin were restored, as were normal ferrokinetic values. Histopathologic abnormalities in liver reverted to normal, as did marrow morphology. A significant reduction in numbers of ringed sideroblasts also occurred [99]. Precise definition, however, is made difficult by the great variability among reported cases. For instance, some patients with sideroblastic anemia will excrete increased amounts of xanthurinic acid in response to a loading dose of L-tryptophan, as if they were pyridoxine-deficient, and may show hematologic improvement with a daily dose of pyridoxine as small as 1 to 5 mg [19].

Pyridoxine-responsive anemia has been divided into classic and variant types [8,19]. The "classic" form comprises about 20 percent of reported cases, resembles the hematologic disorder found in pyridoxine-deficient animals, and usually occurs in young adult or early middle-aged males in families where more than one male is often affected. The hematologic abnormalities are those already described for primary sideroblastic anemia except that this type of anemia tends to be more severe, the red cells are most frequently microcytic, and megaloblastoid changes are less common. The administration of pyridoxine is followed by a prompt reticulocyte response, fall in the serum iron level, a sense of well-being, and a rise in hemoglobin values to normal or near-normal, even though variations in the size and shape of the red corpuscles and some hypochromicity persist. If pyridoxine therapy is discontinued, hematologic relapse tends to occur within 8 to 10 weeks. The remaining approximately 80 percent of the pyridoxine-responsive types of anemia constitute a diverse group which cannot at present be separated from the other forms of primary and secondary sideroblastic anemia except for the pyridoxine responsiveness. Megaloblastoid changes may be found in the bone marrow; the therapeutic response to pyridoxine is less dramatic and less complete than in the classic form.

References

1. Björkman, S. E.: Chronic refractory anemia with sideroblastic bone marrow: A study of four cases. *Blood 11*:250, 1956.
2. Dacie. J. V., Smith, M. D., White J. C., and Mollin, D. L.: Refractory normoblastic anaemia: A clinical and haematologic study of seven cases. *Br. J. Haematol. 5*:56, 1959.
3. Heilmeyer, L., Keiderling. W., Bilger, R., and Bernauer. H.: Über chronische refractare Anämien mit sideroblastischen Knochenmark (anaemia refractoria sideroblastica). *Folia Haematol. (Frankfurt) 2*:49, 1958.
4. Heilmeyer. L., Emmrich, J., Hennemann, H. H., Keiderling, W., Lee. M., Bilger, R., and Schubothe, H.: Über eine chronische hypochrome Anämie bei zwei Geschwistern auf der Grundlage einer Eisenverwertungs-störung (anaemia hypochromica sideroachrestica hereditaria). *Folia Haematol. (Frankfurt) (N.F.) 2*:61, 1958.
5. Mollin, D. L.: Sideroblasts and sideroblastic anaemia. *Br. J. Haematol. 11*:41, 1965.
6. MacGibbon, B. H., and Mollin, D. L.: Sideroblastic anaemia in man: Observations on seventy cases. *Br. J. Haematol. 11*:59, 1965.
7. Harris, J. W., Whittington, R. M., Weisman, R. J., and Horrigan, D. L.: Pyridoxine responsive anemia in the human adult. *Proc. Soc. Exp. Biol. Med. 91*:427, 1956.
8. Horrigan D. L., and Harris, J. W.: Pyridoxine-responsive anemia in man. in *Vitamins and Hormones, Advances in Research and Applications.* Academic, New York, 1968, vol. 26, p. 549.
9. Gehrmann. G.: Pyridoxine responsive anaemias. *Br. J. Haematol. 11*:86, 1965.
10. Verwilghen, R., Reybrouch, G., Callens, L., and Cosemans, J.: Antituberculous drugs and sideroblastic anaemia. *Br. J. Haematol. 11*:92, 1965.
11. Bessis, M. C., and Jensen, W. N.: Sideroblastic anaemia, mitochondria and erythroblastic iron. *Br. J. Haematol. 11*:49, 1965.
12. Bernard, J., Lortholary, P., Levy, J. P., Bonon, M., Najean, Y., and Tanzer, J.: Les Anémies normochromes sidéroblastiques primitives. *Nouv. Rev. Fr. Hematol. 3*:723, 1963.
13. Dameshek, W.: Sideroblastic anaemia: Is this a malignancy? *Br. J. Haematol. 11*:52, 1965.
14. Bell. R. E., and Schewchuk, H. W.: Refractory normoblastic anemia with sideroblasts in the bone marrow. *Am. J. Clin. Pathol. 35*:338, 1961.

15. Barry, W. E., and Day, H. J.: Refractory sideroblastic anemia: Clinical and hematologic study of ten cases. *Ann. Intern. Med. 61:*1029, 1964.

16. Hayhoe, F. G. J., and Quaglino, D.: Refractory sideroblastic anaemia and erythremic myelosis: Possible relationship and cytochemical observations. *Br. J. Haematol. 6:*381, 1960.

17. Rundles, R. W., and Falls, H. F.: Hereditary (?sex-linked) anemia. *Am. J. Med. Sci. 211:*641, 1946.

18. Losowsky, M. S., and Hall, R.: Hereditary sideroblastic anaemia. *Br. J. Haematol. 11:*70, 1965.

19. Horrigan, D. L., and Harris, J. W.: Pyridoxine-responsive anemia: Analysis of 62 cases, in *Advances in Internal Medicine,* edited by W. Dock and I. Snapper. Year Book, Chicago, 1964, vol. 12, p. 103.

20. Hines, J. D.: Reversible megaloblastic and sideroblastic marrow abnormalities in alcoholic patients. *Br. J. Haematol. 16:*87, 1969.

21. Haden, H. T.: Pyridoxine-responsive sideroblastic anemia due to antituberculous drugs. *Arch. Intern. Med. 120:*602, 1967.

22. Dacie, J. V., and Mollin, D. L.: Siderocytes, sideroblasts, and sideroblastic anaemia. *Acta Med. Scand, 179* (Suppl.) 445:237, 1966.

23. Kuschner, J. P., Lee, G. R., Wintrobe, M. M., and Cartwright, G. E.: Idiopathic refractory sideroblastic anemia: Clinical and laboratory investigation of 17 patients and review of the literature. *Medicine 50:*139, 1971.

24. Hines, J. D., and Grasso, J. A.: The sideroblastic anemias. *Semin. Hematol. 7:*86, 1970.

25. Heilmeyer, L.: *Disturbances in Heme Synthesis.* Charles C Thomas, Springfield, Ill., 1966, p. 103.

26. Hines, J. D., and Cowan, D. H.: Studies on the pathogenesis of alcohol-induced bone marrow abnormalities. *N. Engl. J. Med. 283:*441, 1970.

27. Eichner, E. R., and Hillman, R. S.: The evolution of anemia in alcoholic patients. *Am. J. Med. 50:*218, 1971.

28. Harris, E. B., MacGibbon, B. H., and Mollin, D. L.: Experimental sideroblastic anemia. *Br. J. Haematol. 11:*99, 1965.

29. Goodman, J. R., and Hall, S. G.: Accumulation of iron in mitochondria of erythroblasts. *Br. J. Haematol. 13:*335, 1967.

30. Beck, E. A., Ziegler, G., Schmid, R., and Lüdin, H.: Reversible sideroblastic anemia caused by chloramphenicol. *Acta Haematol. (Basel) 38:*1, 1967.

31. Jensen, W. N., and Moreno, G.: Les Ribosomes et les ponctuations basophiles des érythrocytes dans l'intoxication par le plomb. *C. R. Acad. Sci. (Paris) 258:*3596, 1964.

32. Jensen, W. N., Moreno, G. D., and Bessis, M. C.: An electron microscopic description of basophilic stippling in red cells. *Blood 25:*933, 1965.

33. Bishop, R. C., and Bethell, F. H.: Hereditary hypochromic anemia with transfusion siderosis treated with pyridoxine. *N. Engl. J. Med. 261:*486, 1959.

34. Harris, J. W., and Horrigan, D. L.: Pyridoxine responsive anemia: The prototype and variations on the theme. *Vitam. Horm. 22:*721, 1964.

35. Prasad, A. S., et al.: Hereditary sideroblastic anemia and glucose-6-phosphate dehydrogenase deficiency in a Negro family. *J. Clin. Invest. 47:*1415, 1968.

36. Vogler, W. R., and Mingioli, E. S.: Heme synthesis in pyridoxine responsive anemia. *N. Engl. J. Med. 273:*347, 1965.

37. Garby, L. S., Sjolin, S., and Vahlquist, B.: Chronic refractory hypochromic anemia with disturbed haem metabolism. *Br. J. Haematol. 3:*55, 1957.

38. Lee, G. R., MacDiarmid, W. D., Cartwright, G. E., and Wintrobe, M. M.: Hereditary X-linked sideroachrestic anemia: The isolation of two erythrocyte populations differing in Xg^a blood type and porphyrin content. *Blood 32:*59, 1968.

39. Weatherall, D. J., Pembrey, M. E., Hall, E. G., Sanger, R., Tippett, P., and Gavin, J.: Familial sideroblastic anemia: Problem of Xg and X chromosome inactivation. *Lancet 2:*744, 1970.

40. Cottom, H. B., and Harris, J. W.: Familial pyridoxine-responsive anemia. *J. Clin. Invest. 41:*1352, 1962.

41. Hoffbrand, A. V.: Sideroblastic anemia, in *Dyserythropoiesis,* edited by S. M. Lewis and R. L. Verwilghen. Academic, London, 1977, p. 139.

42. Grüneberg, H.: Siderocytes: A new kind of erythrocytes. *Nature (Lond.) 148:*114, 1941.

43. Pappenheimer, A. M., Thompson, W. P., Parker, D. D., and Smith, K. E.: Anaemia associated with unidentified erythrocyte inclusions, after splenectomy. *Q. J. Med. 14:*75, 1945.

44. Case, R. A. M.: Siderocytes in haemolytic diseases: A new index of severity and progress. *J. Pathol. Bacteriol. 57:*271, 1945.

45. McFadzean, A. J. S., and Davis, I. J.: Iron-staining erythrocyte inclusions with especial reference to acquired haemolytic anaemia. *Glasgow Med. J. 28:*237, 1947.

46. Douglas, A. S., and Dacie, J. V.: The incidence and significance of iron-containing granules in human erythrocytes and their precursors. *J. Clin. Pathol. 6:*307, 1953.

47. Cartwright, G. E., and Deiss, A.: Sideroblasts, siderocytes, and sideroblastic anemia. *N. Engl. J. Med. 292:*185, 1975.

48. Bessis, M. C., and Breton-Gorius, J.: Ferritin and ferruginous micelles in normal erythroblasts and hypochromic hypersideremic anemias. *Blood 14:*423, 1959.

49. Bessis, M. C., and Breton-Gorius, J.: Iron metabolism in the bone marrow as seen by electron microscopy: A critical review. *Blood 19:*635, 1962.

50. Bessis, M. C.: *Living Blood Cells and Their Ultrastructure,* translated by R. I. Weed. Springer-Verlag, New York, 1973.

51. Jandl, J. H., and Katz, J. H.: The plasma-to-cell cycle of transferrin. *J. Clin. Invest. 42:*314, 1963.

52. Morgan, E. H., and Baker, E.: The effect of metabolic inhibitors on transferrin and iron uptake and transferrin release from reticulocytes. *Biochim. Biophys. Acta 184:*442, 1969.

53. Zail, S. S., Charlton, R. W., Torrance, J. D., and Bothwell, T. H.: Studies on the formation of ferritin in red cell precursors. *J. Clin. Invest. 43:*670, 1964.

54. Primosigh, J. V., and Thomas, E. D.: Studies on the partition of iron in bone marrow cells. *J. Clin. Invest. 47:*1473, 1968.

55. Kent, G., Minick, O. T., Volini, F. I., and Urfei, E.: Autophagic vacuoles in human red cells. *Am. J. Pathol. 48:*831, 1966.

56. Hammond, E., Deiss, A., Carnes, W. H., and Cartwright, G. E.: Ultrastructural characteristics of siderocytes in swine. *Lab. Invest. 21:*292, 1969.

57. Grasso, J. A., Myers, T. J., Hines, J. D., and Sullivan, A. L.: Energy-dispersive x-ray analysis of mitochondria of sideroblastic anemia. *Br. J. Haematol. 46:*57, 1980.

58. Dacie, J. V., and Doniach, I.: The basophilic property of the iron-containing granules in siderocytes. *J. Pathol. Bacteriol. 59:*684, 1947.

59. McFadzean, A. J. S., and Davis, L. J.: Iron-staining erythrocyte inclusions with special reference to acquired haemolytic anaemia. *Glasgow Med. J. 28:*237, 1947.

60. Griggs, R. C.: Lead poisoning: Hematologic aspects, in *Progress in Hematology,* edited by C. V. Moore and E. B. Brown. Grune & Stratton, New York, 1964, vol. 4, p. 117.

61. Bernard, J., Bessis, M., Boiron, M., Mallassenet, R., and Caroli, J.: Anémie hypochromie hypersidérémique sans anomalie de l'hémoglobine. Etude du métabolisme du fer. Effet de la pyridoxine. *Nouv. Rev. Fr. Hematol. 15:*318, 1960.

62. Wickramsinghe, W. N., Chalmers, D. G., and Cooper, E. H.: A study of ineffective erythropoiesis in sideroblastic anemia. *Cell Tissue Kinet. 1:*43, 1968.

63. Singh, A. K., Shinton, N. K., and Williams, J. D. F.: Ferrokinetic abnormalities and their significance in patients with sideroblastic anaemia. *Br. J. Haematol. 18:*67, 1970.

64. Barnes, R., Connelly, J. L., and Jones, O. T. G.: The utilization of iron and its complexes by mammalian mitochondria. *Biochem. J. 128:*1043, 1972.

65. Williams, D. M., Lee, G. R., and Cartwright, G. E.: Mitochondrial iron metabolism. *Fed. Proc. 32:*924, 1973.

66. Heller, P., Stone, J. V., Apple, D., and Coleman, R. D.: Defective globin synthesis in hypochromic hypersideremic anemia (α-thalassemia?) *Blood 25:*635, 1965.

67. Kramer, S., Viljoen, E., Becker, D., Zail, S. S., and Meta, J.: The relationship between haem and globin synthesis by erythroid precursors in refractory normoblastic anaemia. *Scand. J. Haematol. 6:*293, 1969.

68. White, J. M., Brain, M. C., and Ali, M. A. M.: Globin synthesis in sideroblastic anaemia. I. α and β peptide chain synthesis. *Br. J. Haematol. 20:*263, 1971.

69. Deiss, A., Kurth, D., Cartwright, G. E., and Wintrobe, M. M.: Experimental production of siderocytes. *J. Clin. Invest.* 45:353, 1966.

70. Aoki, Y., Urata, G., Wada, O., and Takaku, F.: Measurement of Δ-aminolevulinic acid synthetase activity in human erythroblasts. *J. Clin. Invest.* 53:1326, 1974.

71. Buchanan, G. R., Bottomly, S. S., and Nitschke, R.: Bone marrow delta-aminolaevulinate synthase deficiency in a female with congenital sideroblastic anemia. *Blood* 55:109, 1980.

72. Goodman, J. R., and Hall, S. G.: Accumulation of iron in mitochondria of erythroblasts. *Br. J. Haematol.* 13:335, 1967.

73. Kuschner, J. P., and Barbuto, A. J.: Decreased activity of hepatic uroporphyrinogen decarboxylase (Urodecarb) in porphyria cutanea tarda (PCT). *Clin. Res.* 22:178, 1974.

74. Lee, G. R., Cartwright, G. E., and Wintrobe, M. M.: The response of free erythrocyte protoporphyrin to pyridoxine therapy in a patient with sideroachrestic (sideroblastic) anemia. *Blood* 27:557, 1966.

75. Rothstein, G., Lee, G. R., and Cartwright, G. E.: Sideroblastic anemia with dermal photosensitivity and greatly increased erythrocyte protoporphyrin. *N. Engl. J. Med.* 280:587, 1969.

76. Vogler, W. R., and Mindioli, E. S.: Porphyrin synthesis and heme synthetase activity in pyridoxine-responsive anemia. *Blood* 32:979, 1968.

77. Mason, D. Y., and Emerson, P. M.: Primary acquired sideroblastic anaemia: Response to treatment with pyridoxal-5-phosphate. *Br. Med. J.* 1:389, 1973.

78. Wickramasinghe S. N., and Hughes, M.: Capacity of ringed sideroblasts to synthesize nucleic acids and protein in patients with primary acquired sideroblastic anaemia. *Br. J. Haematol.* 38:345, 1978.

79. Vavra, J. D., and Poff, S. A.: Heme and porphyrin synthesis in sideroblastic anemia. *J. Lab. Clin. Med.* 69:904, 1967.

80. Rochant, H., Dreyfus, B., Bouguerra, M., and Hoi Tant-Hot: Hypothesis: Refractory anemias, preleukemic conditions, and fetal erythropoiesis. *Blood* 39:721, 1972.

81. Boivin, P., Galand, C., and Audollent, M.: Erythroenzymopathies acquises. I. Anomalies quantitatives observées dans 100 cas d'hémopathies diverses. *Pathol. Biol. (Paris)* 18:175, 1970.

82. Boivin, P., Galand, C., and Dreyfus, B.: Activités enzymatiques érythrocytaires au cours des anémies réfractaires. *Nouv. Rev. Fr. Hematol.* 9:105, 1969.

83. Valentine, W. N., Konrad, P. N., and Paglia, D. E.: Dyserythropoiesis, refractory anemia, and "preleukemia": Metabolic features of the erythrocytes. *Blood* 41:857, 1973.

84. Dreyfus, B., Rochant, H., Sultan, C., Clauvel, J.-P., Yvart, J., and Chesneau, A. M.: Anomalies of blood group antigens and erythrocyte enzymes in two types of chronic refractory anaemia. *Br. J. Haematol.* 16:303, 1969.

85. Salmon, C., et al.: Étude des modifications des antigènes des groupes sanguins dans 11 cas "d'anémies réfractaires." *Nouv. Rev. Fr. Hematol.* 9:113, 1969.

86. Geschke, W., and Beutler, E.: Refractory sideroblastic and non-sideroblastic anemia. A review of 27 cases. *West. J. Med.* 127:85, 1977.

87. Holtz, P., and Palm, D.: Pharmacologic aspects of vitamin B_6. *Pharmacol. Rev.* 16:113, 1969.

88. Firkin, F. C.: Mitochondrial lesions in reversible erythropoietic depression due to chloramphenicol. *J. Clin. Invest.* 51:2085, 1972.

89. Rosenberg, A., and Marcus, O.: Effect of chloramphenicol on reticulocyte Δ-aminolaevulinic acid synthetase in rabbits. *Br. J. Haematol.* 26:79, 1974.

90. Manyan, D. R., Arimura, G. K., and Yunis, A. A.: Chloramphenicol-induced erythroid suppression and bone marrow ferrochelatase activity in dogs. *J. Lab. Clin. Med.* 79:137, 1972.

91. Anderson, B. B., Fulford-Jones, C. E., Child, J. A., Beard, E. J., and Bateman, C. J. T.: Conversion of vitamin B_6 compounds to active forms in the red blood cell. *J. Clin. Invest.* 50:1901, 1971.

92. Hines. J. D.: Altered phosphorylation of vitamin B_6 in alcoholic patients induced by oral administration of alcohol. *J. Lab. Clin. Med.* 74:882, 1969.

93. Lumeng, L., and Li, T.-K.: Vitamin B_6 metabolism in chronic alcohol abuse: Pyridoxal phosphate levels in plasma and the effects of acetaldehyde on pyridoxal phosphate synthesis and degradation in human erythrocytes. *J. Clin. Invest.* 53:693, 1974.

94. Solomon, L., and Hillman, R. S.: Vitamin B_6 metabolism in the anemia of alcoholism. *Clin. Res.* 24:442, 1976.

95. Chillar, R. E., Johnson, C. G., and Beutler, E.: Erythrocyte pyridoxine kinase levels in patients with sideroblastic anemia. *N. Engl. J. Med.* 295:881, 1976.

96. Goldberg, A.: Lead poisoning as a disorder of heme synthesis. *Semin. Hematol.* 5:424, 1968.

97. Snyderman, S. E., Holt, L. E., Jr., Carretero, R., and Jacobs, K. G.: Pyridoxine deficiency in the human infant. *Am. J. Clin. Nutr.* 1:200, 1953.

98. Vilter, R. W., et al.: The effect of vitamin B_6 deficiency induced by desoxy-pyridoxine in human beings. *J. Lab. Clin. Med.* 42:335, 1953.

99. Hines, J. D.: Effect of pyridoxine plus chronic phlebotomy on the function and morphology of bone marrow and liver in pyridoxine-responsive sideroblastic anemia. *Semin. Hematol.* 13:133, 1976.

Erythrocyte disorders—anemias due to increased destruction of erythrocytes with abnormal shape and normal hemoglobin (membrane defects?)

CHAPTER *55*

Hereditary spherocytosis

JAMES H. JANDL
RICHARD A. COOPER

Definitions and history

Hereditary spherocytosis (HS), or congenital hemolytic jaundice, is a disease of autosomal dominant inheritance in which premature destruction of intrinsically abnormal erythrocytes occurs in the spleen. An increased osmotic fragility of spherocytes seen in this disorder was described 80 years ago by Minkowski [1] and was confirmed soon after by others. This characteristic was shown by Castle and Daland [2] to indicate a decreased surface area/volume ratio. The osmotic fragility of HS red blood cells further increases during prolonged static incubation with metabolic depletion in vitro [3–5]. This vulnerability to erythrostasis led to an intensive search for an intrinsic metabolic abnormality in HS erythrocytes. The importance of the spleen, which is almost invariably enlarged, and the curative role of splenectomy in this disorder were recognized from the early studies of Heilmeyer [6], Dacie [7], and others and emphasized by the detailed observations of Emerson et al. [8] and Young and coworkers [9]. The nature of the structural and metabolic red cell defects in HS and the ability of the spleen to recognize this defect have dominated the thinking about this disease up to the present time.

Etiology and pathogenesis

THE CELL DEFECT IN HEREDITARY SPHEROCYTOSIS

The survival of red cells in the circulation is critically dependent on the maintenance of a smooth biconcave shape and the possession of sufficient membrane surface area to permit cells to undergo the extremes of deformation which the circulation demands. In their repetitive passage through the filtering systems of the body, of which the spleen is the most exacting, slight alterations in the surface area/volume ratio of red cells may lead to their trapping and eventual destruction. HS red cells are deficient in membrane surface area, and the magnitude of this deficiency correlates quite well with the shortening of their life-span in vivo [10]. Indeed, experimentally increasing the surface area of HS cells prolongs their survival in vivo despite the presence of a normally functioning spleen [11]. Thus their spheroidal shape causes hereditary spherocytes to be trapped in the spleen, where they are subject to hemoconcentration and erythrostasis, conditions which lead to their demise [12].

MEMBRANE STRUCTURE

The molecular nature of the presumed membrane defect in HS is not yet defined. Because lipids determine many properties of the membrane, attention has been directed to the possibility that the primary defect resides in membrane lipids. Although young cell populations tend to have increased lipid values [15], total lipid content is decreased in HS cells in patients who have spleens and are actively hemolyzing [11,13,14]. The total lipid content of HS red cells after splenectomy is similar to that found in red cells from normal subjects with spleens [11,13]. However, normal red cells have an increased lipid content following splenectomy [11], and HS red cells after splenectomy are actually deficient in cholesterol and phospholipid. The relative proportions of cholesterol, total phospholipid, and the various phospholipid fractions are normal [13,16,17]. Furthermore, membrane lipids are structurally stable in HS as long as cellular metabolism is unimpaired [11,18]. Although one report describes abnormal fatty acid composition of HS membrane phospholipids [19], this has not been confirmed [20].

Fluidity is a characteristic which reflects the organization of lipid in cell membranes [21]. It is influenced by factors such as the length and saturation of membrane fatty acids, the composition of phospholipids, the presence of lysophosphatides, and the relative amounts of cholesterol and phospholipid. Controversy still exists concerning whether membrane fluidity is normal or abnormal in HS [22–24].

Thus, although a number of issues concerning membrane lipids in HS remain unresolved, two findings appear to be established. These are that HS red cells have less lipid per cell than normal both before and after splenectomy [11,13] and that they have less surface area per unit lipid [11]. However, it is important to note that the decrease in membrane lipid alone is insufficient to account for the cell's spheroidal shape, suggesting that an abnormality of lipid-protein association may be of fundamental importance. This is further suggested by the fact that, when depleted of glucose in vitro, HS cell membranes lose both cholesterol and phospholipid at a more rapid rate than is observed with normal cells [13,18].

Many attempts have been made to demonstrate a discrete abnormality of membrane protein in HS [25]. The results obtained with HS red cell membranes have been quite variable [26–30] and seem best explained in terms of differences in the solubility of certain proteins of HS cell membranes as compared with normal red cells. No distinct deficiency has been observed. The phosphoproteins of HS membranes have been reported to be both normal [31] and abnormal [28]. A number of observations suggest that spectrin may be functionally abnormal in HS. For example, solubilized membrane proteins aggregate abnormally in the presence of cations and vinblastine [32], probably representing a property of spectrin. Similarly, there is an impairment of drug-induced endocytosis in HS red cells [33], possibly also representing an abnormality of the membrane cytoskeleton. Membrane cytoskeletons prepared by the triton extraction of red cell membranes fragment and associate at concentrations of urea which, for HS cell membranes, are lower than those required to dissociate normal membrane skeletons [34]. Recent studies indicate that, in some HS families, the defect may involve a portion of the spectrin molecule important in the association of spectrin with band 4.1 [35,36]. Another study indicates that spectrin is normal in many patients with HS, but an abnormality exists in bands 2.1 or 4.1, with which spectrin associates [37]. Thus, the putative protein abnormality has been elusive, but it appears to involve the cytoskeleton. Moreover, it appears that a number of mutations involving the cytoskeleton lead to the formation of spherocytes.

MEMBRANE PERMEABILITY AND CELL METABOLISM
Red cell membranes must not only preserve their physical properties, such as viscosity, shape, and smoothness, but their viability depends upon volume control and osmotic homeostasis. Red cells are freely permeable to the plasma anions, chloride and bicarbonate, and to water. However, the cations, sodium and potassium, traverse the normal membrane at an extremely slow, limited rate. In order to regulate its volume and to maintain osmotic balance in the face of the osmotic pressure of its impermanent constituents (principally hemoglobin, glutathione, and the glycolytic intermediates, particularly 2,3-DPG), the red cell sustains an energy-dependent system of active ion transport. In human red cells, most sodium enters by passive transfer along a steep electrochemical gradient, and is actively "pumped" out; most potassium is actively transported into the cell against a comparably steep gradient, and passively diffuses out.

The mature red cell contains no glycogen and is dependent on glucose, adenine, and phosphate as substrates for the generation of ATP. After incubation without glucose for several hours, normal red cells begin to undergo progressive structural and chemical changes. Within about 12 h of glucose depletion the red cell levels of 2,3-DPG and ATP fall, and in the near absence of ATP, volume control is lost. During the first 24 h the cells swell because of an influx of sodium which exceeds the potassium efflux. This swelling is associated with an increase in osmotic fragility [3,38]. At first these changes are reversible, but with longer periods of glucose deprivation and erythrostasis the cells have a diminished viability when reinjected into the circulation [39]. After 24 to 48 h of incubation, the membrane permeability barrier to cations is entirely lost and the intracellular and extracellular cations approach equilibrium. Potassium loss is prominent [4] and is accompanied by the loss of phosphate and a number of glycolytic intermediates [40], resulting in a reduction in cell volume. Concomitantly, membrane is lost from the red cells [13,18], decreasing the cells' critical hemolytic volume [8,41]. Within 48 h of incubation, normal red cells have become nonviable and are permeable to hemoglobin, and "autohemolysis" commences [4,42].

Early evidence that cell metabolism plays a role in the abnormality of hereditary spherocytosis red cells was the finding that these cells undergo an inordinately rapid increase in osmotic fragility upon sterile incubation [3,43]. Two findings relate directly to this. First, HS red cells manifest an increased glycolytic rate as determined by glucose consumption and lactate formation [39,44]. When glucose is limiting, this hypermetabolism leads to a rapid and premature decline in ATP and 2,3-DPG [44,45]. This occurs even in red cells from patients with hereditary spherocytosis who have undergone splenectomy and represents an acceleration of anaerobic glycolysis, since there is no acceleration in the oxidative (hexose monophosphate) pathway [39]. Second, the rate of sodium flux is increased [39,46–50] and there is a concomitant increase in sodium-potassium ATPase (Na^+-K^+ ATPase) activity [51]. It appears that the metabolic rate results from an increased passive sodium influx, necessitating a more rapid than normal active sodium efflux. This is consistent with the increased metabolic rate of red cells in other clinical [52,53] and experimental [54,55] conditions in which the rate of active flux is increased. Thus it appears that HS red cells depend for their preservation on a sustained and somewhat accelerated glycolysis to compensate for an abnormality of cell membrane permeability. This does not put the cell in jeopardy when the spleen is absent, but it does place it at an added disadvantage when it is trapped in the spleen and exposed to conditions of erythroconcentration and glucose deprivation.

From the foregoing, it is evident that the HS cell membrane does not lack a specific component demonstrable by currently available techniques. Rather, the membrane defect appears to be a functional modification of membrane proteins which are (1) important in determining cell surface area, (2) in close association with lipids, and (3) intimately involved with the permeability properties of the cell membrane and transport processes across the cell membrane. Most of the features of HS red cells can be mimicked by experimental exposure of normal red cells to low concentrations of membrane-reactive thiol blocking agents: impermeable sulfhydryl inhibitors cause an increase in sodium influx, stimulation of outward active transport of sodium, an increase in glycolysis and spherocytosis, and extreme susceptibility of the treated cells to splenic sequestration [55]. However suggestive these findings are, there is no evidence that HS cells are abnormal with regard to surface thiol reactivity. Spin label studies of maleimide binding groups, in membranes from HS cells, have failed to demonstrate differences from normal in the depth or mobility of sulfhydryl groups [56]. The adenylate cyclase and cAMP levels of membranes from splenectomized HS patients are normal, and in actively hemolytic, unsplenectomized patients the enzyme activity is appropriately elevated [57].

THE ROLE OF THE SPLEEN

Hereditary spherocytes have a diminished life-span in the patient or in a normal subject when the spleen is present [58,59], but their survival is almost normal in patients or normal subjects after splenectomy [59–61]. They are sequestered in the spleen but not elsewhere [62], and prior to actual sequestration the circulation time through the spleen is abnormally slow [63]. Normal red cells survive normally when transfused into patients with hereditary spherocytosis [64]. Thus the erythrocyte defect is intrinsic, is nontransferable, and causes significant destruction of the cell only in the presence of the spleen.

Within the splenic circulation red cells that enter the blind-end splenic cords must escape by traversing slit-like spaces between the endothelial cells lining the splenic sinuses, spaces claimed to be as small as 3 μm across [65]. The spheroidal shape of HS cells, particularly at the lower pH of the spleen [66], decreases their ability to deform sufficiently to traverse such small orifices. This difficulty is compounded by an increased internal viscosity of HS cells [67]. Consequently, during transit through the cordal compartment of the spleen, HS cells are selectively detained; the duration of erythrostasis lengthens on each passage until, after an estimated 20 or 30 passages, the repetitive, cumulative damage to these metabolically fragile cells proves lethal [68]. Direct observations of splenic blood in hereditary spherocytosis have shown that the erythrocytes in the splenic pulp are more nearly spherical than those in the peripheral circulation [3,8]. Spherocytes are selectively retained in the pulp of spleen, as determined after transfusion in vivo [3,8,69] and after splenic perfusion in vitro [7,9]. Moreover, spherocytes can be partially separated from normal erythrocytes by passage through

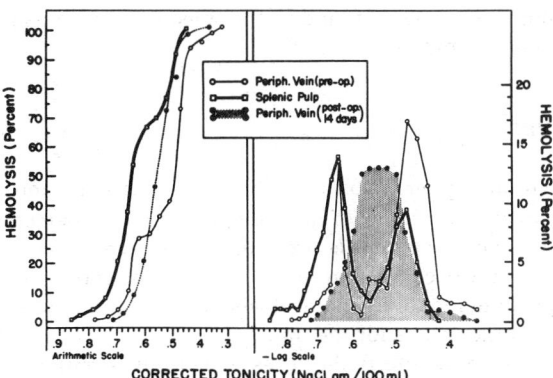

FIGURE 55-1 Osmotic fragility of red blood cells from the splenic pulp compared with that of peripheral blood before and after splenectomy in a case of hereditary spherocytosis. The proportion of red cells with an increased osmotic fragility was approximately 30 percent in the peripheral blood and 70 percent in the splenic pulp, as estimated from the first phase of the biphasic summation curves. The maximum osmotic fragility of red cells from the splenic pulp exceeded significantly that observed in the peripheral blood. These observations suggest conditioning of red cells in the spleen and release of some to the peripheral blood. The asymmetry of the curve of osmotic fragility before splenectomy was extreme. (Emerson et al. [8] with permission of the publisher.)

mechanical filters in vitro [70]. Sequential studies in vivo demonstrated that HS red cells undergo several days of repetitive "conditioning" while circulating through the spleen before they acquire the "hyperspheroidal" shape that precedes their removal from the circulation [70]. Thus a minor population of very spheroidal "conditioned" cells is produced [68,71] that adds a "tail" to the osmotic fragility curve (Fig. 55-1). This population continually gains newly conditioned cells and loses older cells. After splenectomy there may be a transient pile-up in the circulation of very spheroidal cells, but shortly thereafter this population disappears. The osmotic fragility curve then indicates that the bimodal population of cells characteristic of untreated hereditary spherocytosis is replaced by a uniform population of cells, often of intermediate fragility [3,5,59]. Thus spherocytosis persists after splenectomy, but excessive destruction of the spherocytes ceases. So specific is the spleen in detecting this red cell defect that splenectomy is almost invariably curative clinically.

At operation the spleen is darkly congested with blood and usually weighs from 500 to 2000 g. Some of this weight is accounted for by red cells which are pooled in the spleen, but at least 80 to 90 percent of the spleen weight represents hyperplasia of the monocyte-macrophage system. After an initial gush of large-vessel blood, the incised or cut surface of the spleen does not bleed despite its engorged appearance.

Histologically the spleen pulp cords are congested with red cells, while the sinuses are often dilated and empty. The splenic components are hyperplastic, particularly the perifollicular reticulum cells. Although foci of hemopoiesis may be found in the spleen, they are usually not prominent.

Genetics

Hereditary spherocytosis is inherited as an autosomal dominant character [72,73], although in 15 to 20 percent of cases neither parent is affected. The incidence among siblings is close to 50 percent [73]. There is no certain example of hereditary spherocytosis in which the parents were homozygous for the trait.

This disease affects the sexes equally. It is clinically apparent often in early infancy, but sometimes escapes detection until late adult life. It occurs in all races but is most common in people of European origin. Among those of Northern European descent it is the most common of the hereditary hemolytic disorders. Its incidence in the United States is approximately 220 per million [73].

Linkage analyses of HS have not shown a relationship to blood group loci, but there is some evidence that the HS locus is on or near the short arm of either chromosome 8 or chromosome 12 and that it belongs to the Gm-Pi linkage group [74]. Evidence that HS is linked to Gm and is a homogeneous disorder is quite strong.

Clinical features [5,48]

The major clinical manifestations of HS are anemia, jaundice, and splenomegaly. The prominence of jaundice in this disease accounts for its prior designation, "congenital hemolytic jaundice." The severity of these manifestations varies greatly from family to family and may be so mild that they are only discovered through routine examination in adult life. Compensatory erythroblastic hyperplasia of the marrow occurs, with the extension of red marrow into the midshafts of long bones and occasionally with extramedullary erythropoiesis. Paravertebral masses made up by extension of marrow may be visible on chest x-ray. Because the marrow capacity to increase erythropoiesis by six- to tenfold exceeds the usual rate of hemolysis in this disease, anemia is only mild or moderate and often absent in an otherwise healthy individual. However, destruction of red cells is sometimes extremely rapid, and occasionally life-threatening. Whether or not HS is associated with anemia, there is usually some degree of jaundice without bile in the urine (acholuric jaundice). This may be variable or intermittent and tends to be less pronounced in early childhood [55]. Because of the increased bile pigment metabolism, gallstones of the pigment type are common even in childhood [75]. Patients having little or no anemia but with disproportionately severe icterus and reticulocytosis are said to have a "compensated" form of hemolytic anemia [76]. Compensation may be temporarily interrupted by episodes of bone marrow failure, often referred to as *aplastic crises*, associated

with erythroid hypoplasia and reticulocytopenia [77]. These are most commonly precipitated by infections, and the aplastic crisis may be the most profound manifestation of the infection. If communicable, these infections may cause an "epidemic" of aplastic crises in an affected family.

Aplastic crises of a more gradual onset may result from folic acid deficiency [78]. It appears that in patients with chronic hemolytic disorders folic acid utilization is accelerated, presumably in relation to a net increase in the rate of deoxyribonucleic acid synthesis [78]. This is particularly striking during pregnancy [79,80]. Anemia may also occur because of an accelerated rate of hemolysis (*hemolytic crises*). These are less common than aplastic crises in hereditary spherocytosis. Hemolytic crises associated with acute or subacute infection may result from the splenic hypertrophy which occurs in response to infection [81]. In some instances track and field performers with symptomless, latent HS have developed clinically significant hemolytic anemia during vigorous exercise [82].

Chronic leg ulcers, similar in appearance to those observed in sickle cell anemia, are occasionally observed in patients with active hemolysis.

Laboratory features

The laboratory findings are those which are common to all hemolytic processes: anemia, an increased concentration of reticulocytes, a slight to moderate rise in serum indirect-reacting (nonglucuronide) bilirubin, and an elevated fecal excretion of urobilinogen. Because the site of erythrocyte destruction is extravascular, and because hemoglobin is catabolized to bilirubin at the site of destruction, hemoglobin is not ordinarily released into the plasma, and hemoglobinemia is uncommon. However, haptoglobin levels are commonly depressed. Thrombocytopenia of mild to moderate degree is observed occasionally and remits upon splenectomy [83].

The characteristic erythrocyte abnormality of this type of hereditary hemolytic anemia is the spherocyte. Similar cells may be observed in acquired immune hemolytic anemias, in hemolysis due to certain oxidant drugs, and in patients with increased erythrocyte destruction secondary to a large spleen. However, the cells in HS are generally more uniformly spheroidal than in these other disorders. The mean corpuscular volume is usually normal or slightly decreased, but because of the cell's spheroidal shape, cell diameter is substantially decreased, leading to the descriptive term *microspherocyte*. These are cells which appear dark and rounded on smear and lack a pale center. The mean corpuscular hemoglobin concentration (MCHC) of hereditary spherocytes is usually elevated, and may be as high as 40 g/dl [67].

Spheroidicity may be quantitatively assessed in terms of osmotic fragility (Fig. 55-1) [8]. In the osmotic fragility test, erythrocytes are suspended in aqueous solutions containing various concentrations of sodium chloride (see Chap. A12). Since there is almost no exchange of cations during the relatively short duration of the test, osmotic equilibrium is achieved by the rapid movement of water across the red cell membrane. In hypotonic solution the red cell swells until it approaches a sphere. Any further uptake of water renders the cell membrane porous and permits leakage of intracellular contents, of which hemoglobin is the most easily measured. Accordingly, assuming that the blood has a normal osmolarity, the pH is kept constant, and the duration of the test is sufficiently short to obviate significant transmembrane movement of cations, the osmotic fragility test is a precise measure of how nearly spherical a cell is at the time of exposure to the hypotonic medium [2]. Usually most of the red cells, including newly formed reticulocytes, of patients with hereditary spherocytosis have an increase in osmotic fragility; i.e., they become spheroidal and lyse at higher concentrations of sodium chloride than is the case with normal red cells.

On microscopic examination spherocytes are usually detected even when present in very small numbers. However, as ordinarily executed, the osmotic fragility test will not reveal spherocytes unless they constitute at least 1 to 2 percent of the total cell population. Thus it is not uncommon in mild forms of the disease to find some spherocytes on smear and yet a normal osmotic fragility. In such cases the incubated fragility is of particular diagnostic importance [8]. This test measures the osmotic fragility of red cells following the sterile incubation of whole blood for 24 h at 37°C. Under these conditions the osmotic fragility of erythrocytes from both normal subjects and those with hereditary spherocytosis is increased, but, for reasons discussed above, this occurs to an inordinate degree in hereditary spherocytosis. An extension of the incubation fragility test is the autohemolysis test (Chap. A13), which measures the spontaneous lysis of red cells incubated at 37°C for 48 h [4,42]. In hereditary spherocytosis blood autohemolysis ranges from 10 to 50 percent, whereas in normal blood it rarely exceeds 4 percent. The addition of glucose prior to incubation of HS cells causes a substantial decrease in the degree of autohemolysis in most patients before or after splenectomy. However, in the reticulocyte-rich blood of some untreated HS patients, the addition of glucose may not protect against the stress of protracted static incubation, and, in part because of the Crabtree effect (i.e., inhibition of oxidative phosphorylation by excess glucose), glucose fortification may actually enhance autohemolysis of red cells from patients with severe HS and marked reticulocytosis. Autohemolysis of HS cells is inhibited by addition of osmotically active impermeable molecules such as sucrose or ATP [84]. Autohemolysis is also increased in the immune spherocytic anemias and in the hereditary hemolytic anemias because of enzymatic defects. In the former the addition of glucose is usually not protective, and in the latter the response to glucose is variable. For example, glucose increases autohemolysis in pyruvate kinase deficiency.

Differential diagnosis

Hereditary spherocytosis must be distinguished from the spherocytic hemolytic anemias associated with erythrocyte antibodies. Family history and examination of family members will usually be helpful. The diagnosis of immune spherocytosis is usually readily made by use of the Coombs' test. Spherocytes, often in considerable numbers, are seen associated with hemolysis in patients with hypersplenism due to cirrhosis or chronic infections [75] and a few spherocytes are seen in the course of a wide variety of hemolytic anemias. In contrast with other disorders in which spherocytes are seen, the MCHC in HS is usually greater than 35 g/dl.

Therapy

Splenectomy almost invariably causes a cessation of hemolysis, although the red cell defect persists [8,9]. However, a mild decrease in red cell survival has been demonstrated in some patients following splenectomy [61]. Rare relapses have been reported and are probably attributable to the postoperative growth of splenic autotransplants ("splenosis") [85] or to hyperplasia of splenunculi that were overlooked at operation [86–88]. Because of the potential for gallstones and for episodes of aplastic or hemolytic crises, splenectomy should be considered in children and young adults with HS, even if anemia is only mild. In patients diagnosed in later life in whom complications from HS have not occurred, splenectomy is rarely indicated. The incidence of pyogenic infections, particularly with pneumococcus, is increased after splenectomy. Immunization with polyvalent pneumococcal vaccine should be carried out in all patients, preferably before splenectomy. Because of the risks of infection, splenectomy in children should be postponed until the age of 3 years, if possible, although it may be performed at any age. Because of the increased requirement for folic acid in patients with hemolysis [78], a deficiency of this vitamin may exist, and folic acid supplement may result in an improved hematocrit.

Course and prognosis

The course of HS is usually that of mild anemia or no anemia at all. Fluctuating degrees of jaundice occur, and intermittent episodes of increased anemia accompany aplastic or hemolytic crises. Gallstones are common, and they frequently serve to identify patients who are unaware that they have HS. Because the spleen plays such a central role in red cell destruction, splenectomy is almost invariably "curative." The operative mortality from splenectomy approaches that of anesthesia alone. When viewed in large groups of patients, splenectomy leads to a clear, statistically significant increase in the risk of acquiring serious infections. This is most striking in young children, thus forming the basis for delaying splenectomy in early childhood. The incidence of severe infection in the older age group is approximately 0.5 percent [89]. Although no specific data exist, it is the impression of most hematologists that HS after splenectomy is consistent with a normal life expectancy.

References

1. Minkowski, O.: Uber eine hereditäre, unter dem Bilde eines chronischen Icterus mit Urobilinurie, Splenomegalie und Nierensiderosis verlaufende Affection. *Verh. Cong. Inn. Med. Wiesbaden* 18:316 1900.

2. Castle, W. B., and Daland G. A.: Susceptibility of erythrocytes to hypnotic hemolysis as a function of discoidal form. *Am. J. Physiol.* 120:371, 1937.

3. Emerson, C. P., Jr., Shen, S. C., Ham. T. H., and Castle, W. B.: The mechanism of blood destruction in congenital hemolytic jaundice. *J. Clin. Invest.* 26:1180, 1947.

4. Selwyn, J. G., and Dacie, J. V.: Autohemolysis and other changes resulting from the incubation in vitro of red cells from patients with congenital hemolytic anemia. *Blood* 9:414, 1954.

5. Young, L. E., Izzo, M. J., and Platzer, R. F.: Hereditary spherocytosis. I. Clinical, hematologic and genetic features in 28 cases, with particular reference to the osmotic and mechanical fragility of incubated erthrocytes. *Blood* 6:1073, 1951.

6. Heilmeyer, L.: Spherocytosis as a manifestation of pathological spleen function. *Dtsch. Arch. Klin. Med.* 179:292, 1940.

7. Dacie, J. V.: Familial haemolytic anaemia (acholuric jaundice), with particular reference to changes in fragility produced by splenectomy. *Q. J. Med.* 36:101, 1943.

8. Emerson, C. P., Jr., Shen, S. C., Ham, T. H., Fleming, E. M., and Castle, W. B.: Studies on the destruction of red blood cells. IX. Quantitative methods for determining the osmotic and mechanical fragility of red cells in the peripheral blood and splenic pulp: The mechanism of increased hemolysis in hereditary spherocytosis (congenital hemolytic jaundice) as related to the functions of the spleen. *Arch. Intern. Med.* 97:1, 1956.

9. Young, L. E., Platzer, R. F., Ervin, D. M., and Izzo, M. J.: Hereditary spherocytosis. II. Observations on the role of the spleen. *Blood* 6:1099, 1951.

10. Wiley, J. S.: Red cell survival studies in hereditary spherocytosis. *J. Clin. Invest.* 49:666, 1970.

11. Cooper, R. A., and Jandl, J. H.: Role of membrane lipids in the survival of red cells in hereditary spherocytosis. *J. Clin. Invest.* 48:736, 1969.

12. Ham, T. H., and Castle, W. B.: Studies on destruction of red blood cells: Relation of increased hypotonic fragility and of erythrostasis to the mechanism of hemolysis in certain anemias. *Proc. Am. Phil. Soc.* 82:411, 1940.

13. Reed, C. F., and Swisher. A. N.: Erythrocyte lipid loss in hereditary spherocytosis. *J. Clin. Invest.* 45:777, 1966.

14. Cooper, R. A., and Jandl, J. H.: The role of membrane lipids in the survival of red cells in hereditary spherocytosis. *J. Clin. Invest.* 48:736. 1969.

15. van Gastel, C., van Den Berg, D., De Gier, J., van Deenen, L. L. M.: Some lipid characteristics of normal red blood cells of different age. *Br. J. Hematol.* 11:193, 1965.

16. De Gier, J., van Deenen, L. L. M., Verloop, M. D., and van Gastel, C.: Phospholipid and fatty acid characteristics of erythrocytes in some cases of anaemia. *Br. J. Haematol.* 10:246, 1964.

17. Bradlow, B. A., Lee, J., and Rubenstein, R.: Erythrocyte phospholipids: Quantitative thin layer chromatography in paroxysmal nocturnal haemoglobinuria and hereditary spherocytosis. *Br. J. Hematol.* 11:315, 1965.

18. Cooper, R. A., and Jandl, J. H.: The selective and conjoint loss of red cell lipids. *J. Clin. Invest.* 48: 06, 1969.

19. Kuiper, J. C. P., and Livne, A.: Differences in fatty acid composition between normal erythrocytes and hereditary spherocytosis affected cells. *Biochim. Biophys. Acta* 260:755, 1972.

20. Zail, S. S., and Pickering, A.: Fatty acid composition of erythrocytes in hereditary spherocytosis. *Br. J. Haematol.* 42:399, 1979.

21. Cooper, R. A.: Abnormalities of cell membrane fluidity in the pathogenesis of disease. *N. Engl. J. Med.* 297:371, 1977.

22. Aloni, B., Shinitzky, M., Moses, S., and Livne, A.: Elevated microviscosity in membranes of erythrocytes affected by hereditary spherocytosis. *Br. J. Haematol.* 31:117, 1975.

23. Jansson, S. E., Johnsson, R., Gripenberg, J., and Vuopio, P.: The fluidity gradient in erythrocyte membranes in hereditary spherocytosis: A spin label study. *Br. J. Haematol.* 46:73, 1980.

24. Cooper, R. A.: Normal fluidity of red cell membranes in hereditary spherocytosis. *Br. J. Haematol.* 46:299, 1980.

25. Steck, T. L.: The organization of proteins in the human red blood cell membrane. *J. Cell Biol.* 62:1, 1974.

26. Zail, S. S., and Joubert, S. M.: Starch gel electrophoresis of erythrocyte membranes in hereditary spherocytosis. *Br. J. Haematol.* 14:57, 1957.

27. Limber, G. K., Davis, R. F., and Bakerman, S.: Acrylamide gel electrophoresis studies of human erythrocyte membrane. *Blood* 36;111, 1970.

28. Gomperts, E. D., Metz, J., and Zail, S. S.: A red cell membrane protein abnormality in hereditary spherocytosis. *Br. J. Haematol.* 23:363, 1972.

29. Nozawa, Y., Noguchi, T., Lida, H., Fuckushima, H., Sekiya, T., and Ito, Y.: Erythrocyte membrane of hereditary spherocytosis: Alteration in surface ultrastructure and membrane protein as inferred by scanning electron microscopy and SDS-disc gel electrophoresis. *Clin. Chim. Acta* 55:81, 1974.

30. Hayashi, S., et al.: Abnormality of a specific protein in the erythrocyte membrane in hereditary spherocytosis. *Biochem. Biophys. Res. Commun.* 57:1038, 1974.

31. Zail, S. S., and van den Hoek, A. K.: Studies on protein kinase activity and the binding of adenosine 3'5-monophosphate by membranes of hereditary spherocytosis erythrocytes. *Biochem. Biophys. Res. Comm.* 66:1078, 1975.

32. Jacob, H. S., Ruby, A., Overland, E. S., and Mazia, D.: Abnormal membrane protein of red blood cells in hereditary spherocytosis. *J. Clin. Invest.* 50:1800, 1971.

33. Schrier, S. L., Ben-Bassat, I., Bensch, K., Seeger, M., and Junga, I.: Erythrocyte vacuole formation in hereditary spherocytosis. *Br. J. Haematol.* 26:59, 1974.

34. Lux, S. E.: Spectrin-actin membrane skeleton of normal and abnormal red blood cells. *Semin. Hematol.* 16:21, 1979.

35. Wolfe, L. C., John, K. M., Falcone, J., and Lux, S. E.: Identification of the molecular defect in some kindreds with hereditary spherocytosis (HS): Defective binding of protein 4.1 by HS spectrin. *Blood* 58 (Suppl. 1):50A, 1981.

36. Goodman, S. R., and Eyster, M. E.: Alteration of the spectrin-protein 4.1 interaction in hereditary spherocytosis. *Blood* 58 (Suppl. 1):42A, 1981.

37. Hill, J. S., Sawyer, W. H., Howlett, G. J., and Wiley, J. S.: Hereditary spherocytosis: Altered binding of the cytoskeleton to the red cell membrane. *Blood* 58 (Suppl. 1):43A, 1981.

38. Ham, T. H., and Castle, W. B.: Relation of increased hypotonic fragility and of erythrostasis to the mechanisms of hemolysis in certain anemias. *Tr. Assoc. Am. Physicians* 55:127, 1940.

39. Jacob, H. S., and Jandl, J. H.: Increased cell membrane permeability in the pathogenesis of hereditary spherocytosis. *J. Clin. Invest.* 43:1704, 1964.

40. Robinson, M. A., Loder, P. B., and DeGruchy, G. C.: Red-cell metabolism in non-spherocytic congenital haemolytic anaemia. *Br. J. Haematol.* 7:327, 1961.

41. Weed, R. I., and Bowdler, A. J.: Metabolic dependence of critical hemolytic volume of human erythrocytes: Relationship to osmotic fragility and autohemolysis in hereditary spherocytosis and normal red cells. *J. Clin. Invest.* 45:1137, 1966.

42. Young, L. E., Izzo, M. J., Altman, K. I., and Swisher, S. N.: Studies on spontaneous in vitro autohemolysis in hemolytic disorder. *Blood* 11:977, 1956.

43. Emerson, C. P., Jr., Shen, S. C., and Castle, W. B.: The osmotic fragility of the red cells of the peripheral and splenic blood in patients with congenital hemolytic jaundice transfused with normal red cells. *J. Clin. Invest.* 25:922, 1946.

44. Mohler, D. N.: Adenosine triphosphate metabolism in hereditary spherocytosis. *J. Clin. Invest.* 44:1417, 1965.

45. Prankerd, T. A. J.: Studies on the pathogenesis of haemolysis in hereditary spherocytosis. *Q. J. Med.* 53:199, 1960.

46. Harris, E. J., and Prankerd, T. A. J.: The rate of sodium extrusion from human erythrocytes. *J. Physiol.* 121:470, 1953.

47. Bertles, J. F.: Sodium transport across the surface membrane of red blood cells in hereditary spherocytosis. *J. Clin. Invest.* 36:816, 1957.

48. Zipursky, A., and Israels, L. G.: Significance of erythrocyte sodium flux in the pathophysiology and genetic expression of hereditary spherocytosis. *Pediatr. Res.* 5:614, 1971.

49. Mayman, D., and Zipursky, A.: Hereditary spherocytosis: The metabolism of erythrocytes in the peripheral blood and in the splenic pulp. *Br. J. Haematol.* 27:201, 1974.

50. Johnsson, R., and Salminen, S.: Effect of ouabain on osmotic resistance and monovalent cation transport of red cells in hereditary spherocytosis. *Scand. J. Haematol.* 25:323, 1980.

51. Wiley, J. S.: Co-ordinated increase of sodium leak and sodium pump in hereditary spherocytosis. *Br. J. Haematol.* 22:529, 1972.

52. Oski, F. A., et al.: Congenital hemolytic anemia with high-sodium, low-potassium red cells. *N. Engl. J. Med.* 280:909, 1969.

53. Zarkowsky, H., Oski, F., Sha'afi, R., Shohet, S. B., and Nathan, D. G.: Congenital hemolytic anemia with high-sodium low-potassium red cells. *N. Engl. J. Med.* 278:573, 1968.

54. Whittam, R., and Ager, M. E.: The connection between active cation transport and metabolism in erythrocytes. *Biochem. J.* 97:214, 1965.

55. Jacob, H. S., and Jandl, J. H.: Effects of sulfhydryl inhibition on red cells. I. Mechanism of hemolysis. *J. Clin. Invest.* 41:779, 1962.

56. Janssen, S.-E., Johnsson, R., Gripenberg, J., and Vuopio, P.: The fluidity gradient in erythrocyte membranes in hereditary spherocytosis: A spin label study. *Br. J. Haematol.* 46:73, 1980.

57. Piau, J. P., Delauney, J., Fisher, S., Tortolero, M., and Schapiro, G.: Human red cell membrane adenylate cyclase in normal subjects and patients with hereditary spherocytosis, sickle cell disease, and **unidentified hemolytic anemias**. *Blood* **56:963, 1980.**

58. Dacie, J. V.: The congenital anaemias, in *The Haemolytic Anaemias, Congenital and Acquired*. Grune & Stratton, New York, 1960. part I, chap. 2.

59. Emerson, C. P.: The influence of the spleen on the osmotic behavior and the longevity of red cells in hereditary spherocytosis (congenital hemolytic jaundice): A case study. *Boston Med. Q.* 5:65, 1954.

60. Schrumph, A.: Durée de vie des globules rouges dans la sphérocytose héréditaire. *Rev. Hematol.* 11:140, 1956.

61. Chapman R. G.: Red cell life span after splenectomy in hereditary spherocytosis. *J. Clin. Invest.* 47:2263, 1968.

62. Jandl, J. H., Greenberg, M. S., Yonemoto, R. H., and Castle, W. B.: Clinical determination of the sites of red cell sequestration in hemolytic anemias. *J. Clin. Invest.* 35:842, 1956.

63. Harris, I. M., McAlister, J. M., and Prankerd, T. A. J.: The relationship of abnormal red cells to the normal spleen. *Clin. Sci.* 16:233 1957.

64. Dacie J. V., and Mollison, P. L.: Survival of normal erythrocytes after transfusion to patients with familial haemolytic anaemia (acholuric jaundice). *Lancet* 1:550, 1943.

65. Björkman, S. E.: The splenic circulation. *Acta Med. Scand. [Suppl.]* 191, 1947.

66. Murphy, J. R.: The influence of pH and temperature on some physical properties of normal erythrocytes and erythrocytes from patients with hereditary spherocytosis. *J. Lab. Clin. Med.* 69:758, 1967.

67. Erslev, A. J., and Atwater, J.: Effect of mean corpuscular hemoglobin concentration on viscosity. *J. Lab. Clin. Med.* 62:401, 1963.

68. Jandl, J. H., and Aster R. H.: Increased splenic pooling and the pathogenesis of hypersplenism. *Am. J. Med. Sci.* 253:383. 1967.

69. Weisman R., Jr., Hurley. T. H., Harris, J. W., and Ham, T. H.: Studies of the function of the spleen in the hemolysis of red cells in hereditary spherocytosis and sickle cell disorders. *J. Lab. Clin. Med.* 42:965, 1953.

70. Jandl, J. H., Simmons, R. S., and Castle, W. B.: Red cell filtration and the pathogenesis of certain hemolytic anemias. *Blood* 18:133. 1961.

71. Griggs, R. C., Weisman R., Jr., and Harris, J. W.: Alterations in osmotic and mechanical fragility related to in vivo erythrocyte aging and splenic sequestration in hereditary spherocytosis. *J. Clin. Invest.* 39:89, 1960.

72. Race, R. R.: On the inheritance and linkage relations of acholuric jaundice. *Ann. Eugenics* 11:365, 1942.

73. Morton, N. E., MacKinney, A. A., Kosower N., Schilling, R. F., and Gray. M. P.: Genetics of spherocytosis. *Am. J. Hum. Genet.* 14:170, 1962.

74. Klimberling, W. J., Taylor, R. A., Chapman, R. G., and Tubs, H. A.: Linkage and gene localization of hereditary spherocytosis (HS). *Blood* 52:859, 1978.

75. Gairdner, D.: The association of gallstones with acholuric jaundice in children. *Arch. Dis. Child.* 14:109, 1963.

76. Fernandez, L. A., and Erslev. A. J.: Oxygen affinity and compensated hemolysis in hereditary spherocytosis. *J. Lab. Clin. Med.* 80:780, 1972.

77. Owren, P. A.: Congenital hemolytic jaundice. The pathogenesis of the "hemolytic crisis." *Blood* 3:231, 1948.

78. Jandl, J. H., and Greenberg, M. S.: Bone-marrow failure due to relative nutritional deficiency in Cooley's hemolytic anemia: Painful "erythropoietic crises in response to folic acid." *N. Engl. J. Med.* 260:461, 1959.

79. Delamore, I. W., Richmond, J., and Davies, S. H.: Megaloblastic anaemia in congenital spherocytosis. *Br. Med. J.* 1:543, 1961.

80. Kohler, H. G., Meynell, M. J., and Cooke, W. T.: Spherocytic anaemia, complicated by megaloblastic anaemia of pregnancy. *Br. Med. J.* 1:779, 1960.

81. Jandl, J. H., Jacob, H. S., and Daland, G. A.: Hypersplenism due to infection: A study of five cases manifesting hemolytic anemia. *N. Engl. J. Med.* 264:1063, 1961.

82. Godal, H. C., and Refsum, H. E.: Haemolysis in athletes due to hereditary spherocytosis. *Scand. J. Haematol.* 22:83, 1979.

83. Krueger, H. C., and Burgert, E. O.: Hereditary spherocytosis in 100 children. *Mayo Clin. Proc.* 41:821, 1966.

84. Mohler, D. N.: Reduction of in vitro autohemolysis in hereditary spherocytosis by impermeant molecules. *Blood* 30:449, 1967.

85. Stobie, G. H.: Splenosis. *Can. Med. Assoc.* 56:374, 1947.

86. Jones, N. C., Barkhan, P., and Mollison, P. L.: Relapse in hereditary spherocytosis with proven splenunculus. *Lancet* 1:1102, 1962.

87. Bart, J. B., and Appel, M. F.: Recurrent hemolytic anemia secondary to accessory spleens. *South Med. J.* 17:608, 1978.

88. Merrill, K. S., Abbott, O. D., and Rubin, R. N.: Recurrence of hemolysis in hereditary spherocytosis: A case due to leukemic infiltration of an accessory spleen. *Milit. Med.* 146:55, 1981.

89. Weed, R. I.: Hereditary spherocytosis. *Arch. Intern. Med.* 135:1316, 1975.

CHAPTER *56*

Hereditary elliptocytosis and related disorders

RICHARD A. COOPER

Hereditary elliptocytosis

Red blood cells of oval or elliptical shape are normally found in birds, reptiles, camels, and llamas, but in humans they occur in appreciable numbers only in hereditary elliptocytosis (HE). This disorder, first described by Dresbach in 1904 [1], is transmitted as an autosomal dominant trait [2,3] and affects 0.02 to 0.05 percent of the population [4]. It has in the past also been designated *hereditary ovalocytosis*. Lux and Wolfe [5] have analyzed the range of manifestations of HE among various families and have designated five subgroups: mild HE with little or no hemolysis; mild HE with transient poikilocytosis and pyknocytosis in infancy; HE with sporadic hemolysis; HE with hemolysis and spherocytosis; and homozygous HE with severe hemolysis associated with butting and fragmentation of red cells. In addition, as noted below, an autosomal recessive disorder is associated with stomatocytic elliptocytes.

PATHOGENESIS

Unlike the elliptocyte of the llama, cytoplasmic constituents in hereditary elliptocytosis of humans exhibit polarization [6]. Ghosts of mature red cells are elliptic [7], as are the membrane protein cytoskeletons prepared by triton extraction of red cell ghosts [8]; however, nucleated precursors are round [9]. Studies of the membrane structural defect in HE indicate that it involves spectrin and/or the proteins with which spectrin closely associates. These membrane studies also emphasize the diversity of the disease known as HE. In one study an abnormal response of spectrin to heat denaturation was demonstrated in the red cells from some kindred, whereas it was normal in others [8]. Most patients have normal membrane proteins on polyacrylamide gel electrophoresis, but membrane protein band 4.1 is absent in some families [10,11]. Of four unrelated patients studied, one was shown to have an increased susceptibility of spectrin to tryptic digestion [12]. Defective spectrin dimer-dimer association has been observed in a subset of HE patients [13]. Thus, there are probably a number of mutations involving the red cell cytoskeleton that lead to elliptocytosis. The glycolytic enzymes are normal [14], and, except in sporadic cases, hemoglobin is normal. A more rapid than normal decline in cellular ATP and 2,3-DPG upon sterile incubation of hereditary elliptocytes occurs in vitro [15], and a 40 to 50 percent increase in the ouabain-inhibitable sodium efflux has been observed [16]. However, neither the degree of ATP instability nor the rate of sodium efflux has correlated with the hemoglobin level or reticulocyte count. Thus the hereditary elliptocyte appears to share many features with the hereditary spherocyte: an abnormal cell shape associated with destruction in the spleen and a membrane permeability defect necessitating an increased rate of ATP utilization. Those factors which differentiate the hemolytic variety of this disorder from the asymptomatic condition remain unknown. In some families the gene for elliptocytosis is linked with the RH blood type [17,18], whereas in other families such linkage has not been demonstrated [4,14,17,19]. It appears that the hemolytic variety of elliptocytosis occurs most commonly in those families shown not to possess linkage with the Rh blood type [14,19]; however, there is often great variability in the degree of hemolysis among family members [20,21]. Severe hemolysis has been reported in several patients who were thought to be homozygous for this disease [22–24].

CLINICAL AND LABORATORY FEATURES

In normal subjects, up to 15 percent of red cells in the blood may be slightly oval or elliptic [9,25], whereas in patients with hereditary elliptocytosis, at least 25 percent [4] and commonly more than 75 percent of the red cells are elliptic, with an axial ratio of less than 0.78 [22]. The great majority of patients with this disorder manifest only mild hemolysis, with hemoglobin levels above 12 g/dl, reticulocyte counts of less than 4 percent, depressed haptoglobin levels, and red cell survival times within or just under the normal range [19,20,26–28]. In 10 to 15 percent of patients the rate of hemolysis is substantially increased, with radioactive chromium (^{51}Cr) red cell half-survival times as short as 5 days and reticulocytosis ranging to 20 percent [14,20,26,28]. Hemoglobin levels rarely fall below 9 to 10 g/dl. Red cell destruction occurs predominantly in the spleen, and hemolysis is prevented by splenectomy [14,20,22,29].

In both the anemic and nonanemic varieties of this disorder the red cells are normochromic and normocytic. Patients with hemolysis frequently have microelliptocytes, bizarre-shaped red cells, and red cell fragments, and these increase in number following splenectomy [20,22,29]. The degree of hemolysis does not correlate with the percentage of elliptocytes [20]. Osmotic fragility is usually normal but may be increased in patients with overt hemolysis, and the incubation fragility follows the same pattern. Similarly, autohemolysis is usually normal in patients without overt hemolysis but may be increased when overt hemolysis is present. A palpable spleen is common in patients with increased hemolysis. Jaundice may intermittently be present and gallstones may develop [30]. Transient splenomegaly, for example with acute infections, causes an increased rate of hemolysis [31], and overt hemolysis may for the first time become manifest as a result of intercurrent infection [20].

DIFFERENTIAL DIAGNOSIS

Other disorders in which elliptic cells occur include thalassemia, iron deficiency, myelophthisic anemias, and sickle cell disease. Macroelliptocytes are common in megaloblastic anemias. Associated features usually permit these disorders to be distinguished readily from hereditary elliptocytosis. When elliptocytes are few in number, hereditary elliptocytosis may be confused with the hereditary nonspherocytic hemolytic anemias [20].

TREATMENT AND PROGNOSIS

In most patients hereditary elliptocytosis represents a benign disorder with no overt hemolysis and no increase in pigment metabolism, which, when present, leads to the formation of gallstones. No therapy is required in such patients, and the presence of this genetic abnormality poses no threat. When an increased hemolytic rate is present, splenectomy is advisable and, as in hereditary spherocytosis, is curative for the hemolytic process, thus protecting the patient from the complications of the disorder.

Hereditary pyropoikilocytosis

A rare hemolytic disorder, termed *hereditary pyropoikilocytosis* (HPP), has been described in children. The morphologic hallmark is tiny, distorted microspherocytes, often only 2 to 3 μm in diameter [32,33]. They appear to result from the spontaneous disruption of the membrane cytoskeleton in a fashion similar to that induced in normal red cells by heating to 49°C [34]. In contrast, red cells from patients with HPP fragment when heated to 45°C [32]. Analysis of membrane proteins using circular dichroism has demonstrated that the midpoint of structural transition is displaced from the normal 49 to 44°C in HPP cells [35]. Since it has been shown that the heat-denatured protein is spectrin [36], it has been assumed that the structural basis for HPP resides in the spectrin molecule. Evidence supporting this has been obtained in studies of spectrin extracted from red cell membranes. Normally the spectrin so extracted exists as tetramers, whereas the spectrin extracted from membranes of HPP red cells contains a substantial proportion of dimers [37].

A relationship between HPP and HE appears to exist. This syndrome was included as a variant of HE by Dacie [38]. On morphologic grounds it is similar to homozygous HE [5], and several reported cases of HPP have occurred in families in which either the parents or siblings had HE [32]. Splenectomy is the treatment of choice for patients with this disorder, but it only partially ameliorates the hemolytic process.

Hereditary stomatocytosis

The syndrome of hereditary stomatocytosis encompasses what must be a heterogeneous group of red cell membrane disorders which have in common a greatly increased membrane permeability to both sodium and potassium as well as greatly accelerated rates of sodium and potassium transport. In all cases there is a decrease in cell potassium and an increase in cell sodium. If the sodium gain exceeds the potassium loss, there is a net increase in sodium + potassium (and of water, as well), resulting in overhydrated cells with a decreased MCHC [39–43]. On dried films these cells take on the characteristic appearance of stomatocytes; i.e., they have slitlike pale centers. These cells have also been referred to as *hydrocytes*.

More commonly, the result of the membrane permeability abnormality is a net decrease in sodium + potassium (and water), resulting in underhydrated cells with an increased MCHC. On dried smears these cells take on the appearance of target cells [44–49]. If these cells are overhydrated by suspension in hypotonic media, they appear morphologically identical to overhydrated stomatocytes [47]. In one family the red cell morphologic abnormality consisted of stomatocytic elliptocytes [50]. Because of their decreased water content, they have also been called *desiccocytes*, and recently the term *xerocy-*

tosis has been used to designate this disorder. The structural basis for this membrane abnormality is poorly understood, although in several reports an increase in the membrane content of phosphatidylcholine has been noted [47,48].

Like HE and HS, hereditary stomatocytosis appears to follow an autosomal dominant inheritance pattern. The degree of hemolysis is usually moderate, similar in magnitude to most patients with HS. However, unlike both HS and HE, splenectomy leads to a variable amelioration of hemolysis. In some patients the accelerated rate of red cell destruction is totally prevented, but in most patients splenectomy decreases but does not fully correct the hemolytic process.

References

1. Dresbach, M.: Elliptical human red corpuscles. *Science 19:*469, 1904.
2. Hunter, W. C., and Adams, R. B.: Hematologic study of three generations of a white family showing elliptical erythrocytes. *Ann. Intern. Med. 2:*1162, 1929.
3. Cheney, G.: Elliptic human erythrocytes. *JAMA. 98:*878, 1932.
4. Bannerman, R. M., and Renwick, J. H.: The hereditary elliptocytoses: Clinical and linkage data. *Ann. Hum. Genet. 26:*23, 1962.
5. Lux, S. E., and Wolfe, L. C.: Inherited disorders of the red cell membrane skeleton. *Pediatr. Clin. North Am. 27:*463, 1980.
6. Rebuck, J. W., and van Slyck, E. J.: An unsuspected ultrastructural fault in human elliptocytes. *Am. J. Clin. Pathol. 49:*19, 1968.
7. Rebuck, J. W., Appelhot, W. H., and Meier, F. W.: Electron microscopy of elliptocytes in man and llama. *Anat. Rec. 130:*362, 1958 (abstract).
8. Tomaselli, M. B., John, K. M., and Lux, S. E.: Elliptical erythrocyte membrane skeletons and heat-sensitive spectrin in hereditary elliptocytosis. *Proc. Natl. Acad. Sci. U.S.A. 78:*1911, 1981.
9. Florman, A. L., and Wintrobe, M. M.: Human elliptical red corpuscles. *Johns Hopkins Med. J. 63:*209, 1938.
10. Feo, C. J., Fischer, S., Piau, J. P., Grange, M. J., and Tchernia, G.: Première observation de l'absence d'une proteine de la membrane erythrocytaire (Bande 4-1) dans un cas d'anemie elliptocytaire familiale. *Nouv. Rev. Fr. Hematol. 23:*in press, 1980.
11. Mueller, T. J., Wilimas, J., Wang, W. C., and Morrison, M.: Cytoskeletal alterations in hereditary elliptocytosis. *Blood 58 (Suppl. 1):*47A, 1981.
12. Coetzer, T., and Zail, S. S.: Tryptic digestion of spectrin in variants of hereditary elliptocytosis. *J. Clin. Invest. 67:*12, 1981.
13. Liu, S. C., Lawler, J., Prchal, J., and Palek, J.: Defective dimer-dimer association and altered tryptic digestion of spectrin (Sp) in variants of hereditary elliptocytosis (HE). *Blood 58 (Suppl. 1):*45A, 1981.
14. Cutting, H. O., McHugh, W. J., Conrad, F. G., and Marlow, A. A.: Autosomal dominant hemolytic anemia characterized by ovalocytosis. *Am. J. Med. 39:*21, 1965.
15. DeGruchy, G. C., Loder, P. B., and Hennessy, I. V.: Haemolysis and glycolytic metabolism in hereditary elliptocytosis. *Br. J. Haematol. 8:*168, 1962.
16. Peters, J. C., Rowland, M., Israels, L. G., and Zipursky, A.: Erythrocyte sodium transport in hereditary elliptocytosis. *Can. J. Physiol. Pharmacol. 44:*817, 1966.
17. Morton, N. E.: The detection and estimation of linkage between the genes for elliptocytosis and the Rhesus blood type. *Am. J. Hum. Gent. 8:*80, 1956.
18. Goodall, H. B., Hendry, D. W. W., Lawler, S. D., and Stephen, S. A.: Data on linkage in man: Elliptocytosis and blood groups. II. Family 3. *Ann. Eugen. 17:*272, 1953.
19. Geerdink, R. A., Helleman, P. W., and Verloop, M. C.: Hereditary elliptocytosis and hyperhaemolysis: A comparative study of 6 families with 145 patients. *Acta Med. Scand. 179:*715, 1966.

20. Dacie, J. V.: The congenital hemolytic anemias. 2. Hereditary ellip-tocytosis, in *The Hemolytic Anemias Congenital and Acquired*. Part I. *The Congenital Anemias*. Grune & Stratton, New York, 1960.

21. Pearson, H. A.: The genetic basis of hereditary elliptocytosis with hemolysis. *Blood* 32:972, 1968.

22. Lipton, E. L.: Elliptocytosis with hemolytic anemia: The effects of splenectomy. *Pediatrics* 15:67, 1955.

23. Wyandt, H., Bancroft, P. M., and Winship, T. O.: Elliptic erythro-cytes in man. *Ann. Intern. Med.* 68:1043, 1941.

24. Pryor, D. S., and Pitney, W. R.: Hereditary elliptocytosis: A report of two families from New Guinea. *Br. J. Haematol.* 13:126, 1967.

25. Hedenstedt, S.: Elliptocyte transfusions as a method in studies of blood destruction, blood volume and peritoneal resorption. *Acta Chir. Scand.* [Suppl.] 128, 194

26. Kirkegaard, A., and Larsen, K.: Elliptische erythrocyten in einer danischen familie und einige untersuchungen uber die natur der elliptocytose. *Acta Med. Scand.* 110:521, 1942.

27. Penfold, J. B., and Lipscomb, J. M.: Elliptocytosis in man, associated with hereditary hemorrhagic telangiectasia. *Q. J. Med.* 36:157, 1943.

28. Torlontano, G., Tonietti, G., Centurelli, G., and Conti, C.: Incidence, hematological, enzymological findings and hemolysis in hereditary elliptocytosis: Study of fifty-four cases. *Rass. Esiopatol. Clin. Ter.* 37:1, 1965.

29. Wilson, H. E., and Long, M. H.: Hereditary ovalocytosis (elliptocy-tosis) with hypersplenism. *Arch. Inter. Med.* 95:438, 1955.

30. Motulsky, A. G., Singer, K., Crosby, W. H., and Smith, V.: The life-span of the elliptocyte: Hereditary elliptocytosis and its relationship to other familial hemolytic diseases. *Blood* 9:57, 1954.

31. McCurdy, P. R.: Clinical, genetic and physiological studies in hered-itary elliptocytosis. *Proc. Int. Soc. Hematol. IX Congress* 1:155, 1962.

32. Zarkowsky, H. S., Mohandas, N., Speaker, C. B., and Shohet, S. B.: A congenital haemolytic anaemia with thermal sensitivity of the erythrocyte membrane. *Br. J. Haematol.* 29:537, 1975.

33. Wiley, J. S., and Gill, F. M.: Red cell calcium leak in congenital hemo-lytic anemia with extreme microcytosis. *Blood* 47:197, 1976.

34. Ham, T. H., Shen, S. C., Fleming, E. M., and Castle, W. B.: Studies of the destruction of red blood cells. IV. Thermal injury: Action of heat in causing increased spheroidicity, osmotic and mechanical fragili-ties and hemolysis of erythrocytes; observations on the mechanisms of destruction of such erythrocytes in dogs and in a patient with a fatal thermal burn. *Blood* 3:373, 1948.

35. Chang, K., Williamson, J. R., and Zarchowsky, H. S.: Effect of heat on the circular dichroism of spectrin in hereditary pyropoikilocy-tosis. *J. Clin. Invest.* 64:326, 1979.

36. Lux, S. E.: Spectrin-actin membrane skeleton of normal and abnor-mal red blood cells. *Semin. Hematol.* 16:21, 1979.

37. Liu, S.-C., Palek, J., Prchal, J., and Castleberry, P.: Altered spectrin dimer-dimer association and instability of erythrocyte membrane skeletons in hereditary pyropoikilocytosis. *J. Clin. Invest.* 68:597, 1981.

38. Dacie, J. V.: The congenital hemolytic anemias. Hereditary ellipto-cytosis. The hemolytic anemias. Part I. Grune & Stratton, New York, 1960, p. 151.

39. Lock, S. P., Smith, R. S., and Hardisty, R. M.: Stomatocytosis: A he-reditary red cell anomaly associated with haemolytic anaemia. *Br. J. Haematol.* 7:303, 1961.

40. Zarkowsky, H. S., Oski, F. A., Sha'afi, R., Shohet, S. B., and Nathan, D. G.: Congenital hemolytic anemia with high sodium, low potas-sium red cells. I. Studies of membrane permeability. *N. Engl. J. Med.* 278:577, 1968.

41. Mentzer, W. C., Jr., Smith, W. B., Goldstone, J., and Shohet, S. B.: Hereditary stomatocytosis membrane and metabolism studies. *Blood* 46:659, 1975.

42. Bienzle, J., Bhadki, S., Knufermann, H., Niethammer, D., and Klei-hauer, E.: Abnormality of erythrocyte membrane protein in a case of congenital stomatocytosis. *Klin. Wochenschr.* 55:569, 1977.

43. Alki, F. A., et al.: Congenital hemolytic anemia with high-sodium, low-potassium red cells. Studies of three generations of a family with a new variant. *N. Engl. J. Med.* 280:909, 1969.

44. Glader, B. E., Fortier, N., Albala, M. M., and Nathan, D. G.: Congeni-tal hemolytic anemia associated with dehydrated erythrocytes and increased potassium loss. *N. Engl. J. Med.* 291:491, 1974.

45. Snyder, L. M., Lutz, H. U., Sauberman, N., Jacobs, J., and Fortier, N. L.: Fragmentation and myelin formation in hereditary xerocy-tosis and other hemolytic anemias. *Blood* 52:750, 1978.

46. Miller, D. R., Rickles, F. R., Lichtman, M. A., LaCelle, P. L., Bates, J., and Weed, R. I.: A new variant of hereditary hemolytic anemia with stomatocytosis and erythrocyte cation abnormality. *Blood* 38:184, 1971.

47. Wiley, J. S., Ellory, J. C., Shuman, M. A., Shaller, C. C., and Cooper, R. A.: Characteristics of the membrane defect in the hereditary stomatocytosis syndrome. *Blood* 46:337, 1975.

48. Jaffe, E. R., and Gottfried, E. L.: Hereditary nonspherocytic hemo-lytic disease associated with an altered phospholipid composition of the erythrocytes. *J. Clin. Invest.* 47:1375, 1968.

49. Lande, W., Cerrone, K., and Mentzer, W.: Congenital anemia with abnormal cation permeability and cold hemolysis in vitro. *Blood* 54:29a, 1979.

50. Honig, G. R., Lacson, P. S., and Maurer, H. S.: A new familial disorder with abnormal erythrocyte morphology and increased per-meability of the erythrocytes to sodium and potassium. *Pediatr. Res.* 5:159, 1971.

CHAPTER *57*

Acanthocytosis

RICHARD A. COOPER
JAMES H. JANDL

Acanthocytes are mature red cells with multiple, ir-regularly arranged, spiny or blunt projections (Fig. 57-1*a*). They were first described by Bassen and Kornzweig in a young girl suffering from malabsorption, diffuse nervous system involvement, and retinitis pigmentosa [1], a syndrome subsequently found to result from the congenital absence of β-lipoprotein. Cells of similar structure occur in normolipidemic patients with an inherited neuromuscular disorder. Red cells with spiny projections are observed in some patients with severe liver disease; the term *spur cells* has been applied to the cells in this latter condition, although they have also been designated as acanthocytes. In addition, small numbers of red cells which resemble acanthocytes have been observed after splenectomy, in malnutrition, in myxedema, and occasionally in other conditions less well defined.

Abetalipoproteinemia

This autosomal recessive inherited disease usually presents with diarrhea and steatorrhea within the first 2 years of life. It differs from celiac disease in that fat ab-sorption alone is impaired, and the absorption of other nutrients such as xylose and vitamin B_{12} is usually nor-mal [2]. The mucosal cells of the small intestine contain lipid droplets which are composed almost entirely of triglyceride. Neuromuscular manifestations include profound weakness, ataxia, intention tremors, nystagmus, and hyporeflexia. Degenerative changes in the retina, usually in association with an atypical retinitis pigmentosa, often result in blindness.

Plasma lipid abnormalities are prominent. The plasma levels of triglyceride, which is normally transported in association with the B protein (the protein moiety of β-lipoprotein), approach zero. Plasma cholesterol is usually less than 50 mg/dl, and phospholipid less than 100 mg/dl [3,4]. Sphingomyelin accounts for a greater than normal proportion of plasma phospholipid, and there is a reciprocal decrease in the percentage of lecithin [3,5]. The fatty acids esterified to plasma phospholipids contain one-third to one-half the normal content of linoleic acid [5]. Attempts to demonstrate the B protein immunologically have been unsuccessful, and the question of whether a B protein of altered antigenicity exists remains unsettled [6,7].

The cholesterol content of acanthocytes is normal [4,9–11] or slightly increased [12,13], and the phospholipid content is normal or slightly decreased. Red cell phospholipid and fatty acid composition reflect that of serum [3], and this is more striking in old red cells than in young red cells [14]. Attempts to induce or reverse the red cell morphologic abnormality in vitro have been unsuccessful [15,16]. On the other hand, normal red cells transfused into patients with acanthocytosis become morphologically abnormal [17]. Autohemolysis [8,18] and peroxidative hemolysis [19] are increased but are corrected by the addition of vitamin E in vitro or in vivo. Vitamin E does not alter the lipid composition or structure of acanthocytes. However, it does serve as an antioxidant, and the beneficial effects of adding vitamin E reflect a deficiency state for this vitamin induced by malabsorption. Acanthocytes have normal rates of glycolysis [8] and of cation permeability [20] and a normal osmotic fragility [8].

Anemia, when present, is usually mild, and ^{51}Cr red cell half-survival times are only slightly shortened [3,8]. Reticulocytes may be normal or slightly increased in number. Red cells are normochromic and normocytic. The slightly increased rate of red cell destruction in this disease appears to be due to an increase in membrane rigidity. At the molecular level this is manifested by a decrease in the fluidity of acanthocyte membranes [21], probably due to the relative increase in sphingomyelin (a rigid lipid) over lecithin (a more fluid lipid) [22]. At a macroscopic level, rigidity is manifested as a decreased deformability of red cells [12,21]. Neither the abnormal fluidity nor the abnormal deformability is as marked as the acanthocytes of patients with cirrhosis. Whereas the splenic congestion characteristic of cirrhosis combined with the membrane structural abnormality of acanthocytes is sufficient to cause substantial hemolysis, the milder abnormality of acanthocytes coupled with a spleen of normal size is well tolerated in abetalipoproteinemia.

Acanthocytosis associated with neurologic disorders

A wide spectrum of neuronal abnormalities occurs in affected patients, including muscular atrophy of the Charcot-Marie-Tooth type, neck and shoulder girdle atrophy, choreiform movement similar to that in Huntington's chorea, dementia, and nonfocal grand mal seizures [23–27]. Multiple tics were described in one patient [24]. Unlike the defect in abetalipoproteinemia, the neurologic abnormalities do not involve long tracks, nor do they cause retinitis pigmentosa.

Red cells have the typical acanthocytic appearance. Chromium red cell half-survival times are decreased slightly, to 18 to 20 days [23,25]. Plasma lipoproteins are normal or only slightly decreased. No abnormalities have been observed in plasma or red cell cholesterol or phospholipid content or in the relative amounts of the various phospholipids and fatty acids [23,25]. The nature of the red cell and neuron abnormality remains unexplained. The inheritance pattern is not clear, and in some families the disorder appears to be an autosomal dominant trait, whereas in others it appears to be an autosomal recessive trait.

Spur cells (acanthocytes) in liver disease

Hemolytic anemia with bizarre-shaped red cells (Fig. 57-1a) occurs in some patients with severe hepatocellular disease, usually alcoholic cirrhosis [28–31], although it has also been described in neonatal hepatitis. Hemoglobin levels are between 5.5 and 10.0 g, and reticulocytes are 5 to 15 percent. Chromium red cell half-survival times are decreased and may be as short as 6 days. Osmotic fragility is within normal limits; however, both a "tail" of cells with increased fragility and a "shoulder" of osmotically resistant cells are present [29]. Splenomegaly and jaundice are constant features, and red cell destruction is localized to the spleen.

The surface membrane of spur cells is enriched with cholesterol by 50 to 70 percent, but its total phospholipid content is normal [30]. In this way, spur cells are distinct from the more usual "target" red cells in liver disease, which possess an excess of both cholesterol and phospholipid [30,32]. Among the phospholipids, there is relatively more lecithin and less sphingomyelin, a characteristic of both target cells and spur cells in patients with liver disease [30,32]. Excessive cholesterol relative to phospholipid in the membrane of spur cells decreases the fluidity of lipids within the membrane bilayer [33], and there is an associated decrease in red cell deformability [12,29,34].

Normal red cells acquire the spur abnormality when incubated in vitro in serum from affected patients [29] (Fig. 57-2) or when transfused in vivo [29,31], limiting the utility of transfusion therapy [34]. This results from

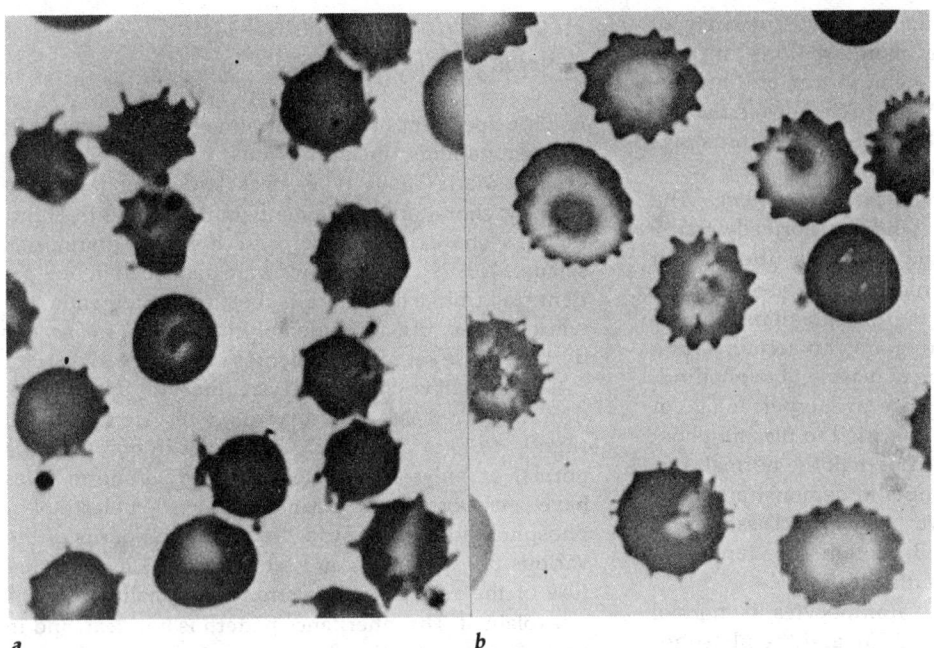

FIGURE 57-1 (*a*) Left panel depicts the characteristic appearance of acanthcytes when viewed on stained smears. Those shown were obtained from a patient with cirrhosis and spur cells. (*b*) Same patient after splenectomy, demonstrating the effect of added membrane cholesterol per se without subsequent conditioning in the spleen. (Cooper et al. [34] with permission of the publisher.)

the presence in plasma of an abnormal low-density lipoprotein with an increased molar ratio of free (or unesterified) cholesterol to phospholipid [30]. The pathologic condition can be mimicked by incubation of normal red cells in normal serum in which the free cholesterol/phospholipid ratio has been increased by the addition of sonicated dispersions of cholesterol and phospholipid [35]. In contrast to circulating spur cells in patients, normal red cells which have acquired cholesterol in vitro have an increased surface area and a decreased osmotic fragility, and they have a regular pat-

FIGURE 57-2 Sequence of events leading to the formation and destruction of spur cells in patients with cirrhosis. (Cooper et al. [34] with permission of the publisher.)

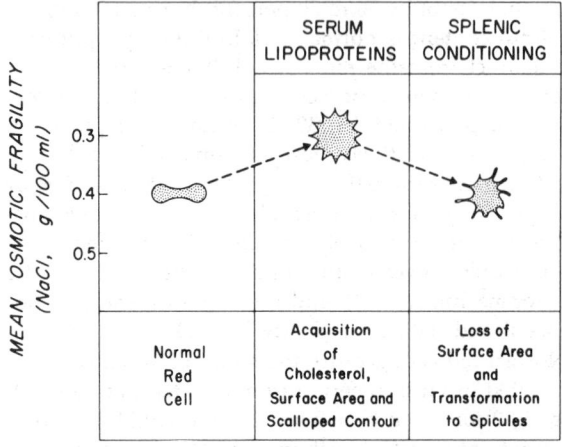

tern of spicule deformity (Fig. 57-2). This is also true in vivo both for normal transfused red cells during their initial 24 h in the circulation of a patient with spur cells [29] and for spur cells in patients following splenectomy [34] (Fig. 57-1*b*).

Thus, spur cells in patients with liver disease are innocent bystanders. The excess amount of cholesterol imposed on them by equilibration with lipoproteins of abnormal lipid composition causes their membranes to have rigid physical properties. These are of sufficient magnitude that they are detected by the filtering system of the spleen, aided by congestive splenomegaly in cirrhosis. During circulation in vivo in the presence of the spleen, cholesterol-rich spur cells lose surface area and transform to an increasingly irregular pattern of spiculation. This process of membrane "conditioning" by the spleen is progressive, and the cell is destroyed in the spleen. Attempts to influence red cell cholesterol by the use of various lipid-lowering drugs have been unsuccessful. Although splenectomy is effective in ameliorating the hemolysis of spur cells [34], it carries a high risk in patients with severe liver disease who also have coagulation defects, and it must be reserved for selected patients in whom hemolysis is a major clinical problem and who are good surgical risks.

Other causes of acanthocytosis

Patients with anorexia nervosa [39] and infants with malnutrition [12,37] have small numbers of irregularly shaped red cells. Little is known about these cells, although in one infant red cell cholesterol was slightly increased [12]. In one male patient with anorexia nervosa, red cell lipids were normal in total amount, but there was an increased proportion of the long-chain polyunsaturated fatty acids associated with starvation [36]. Normal red cells do not acquire this abnormality upon incubation in serum from affected patients [36]. However, the phenomenon is reversible when a normal nutritional status is reestablished [39]. Its effect on cell survival is unknown.

Small numbers of irregularly shaped red cells have also been noted in 50 to 60 percent of patients with myxedema [38] and in patients with panhypopituitarism. These disappear with effective endocrine therapy. Red cell lipids are normal in all these patients [40].

Irregularly shaped red cells are seen in association with the McLeod phenotype, a red cell membrane abnormality characterized by the absence of the Kx antigenic substance, which is necessary for the normal expression of Kell antigens [41–43]. This has been reported to affect only the red cells of some patients [41,42] and to affect both the red cells and the granulocytes of some boys with X-linked chronic granulomatous disease (CGD) [43]. The red cell abnormality leads to a shortened red cell survival and reticulocytosis. Membrane lipid composition and fluidity are normal [44], and the morphologic abnormality appears to be due to a structural defect in membrane proteins.

Over the past few years there have been reports of patients whose red cells are peculiarly shaped and resemble pieces of a picture puzzle. One reported patient had hemolysis in association with carcinoid metastatic to the liver [45]. In another the trait was familial, involving the patient and three children, and was named the *Woronets trait* [46]. We have seen seven other patients with hematocrit readings ranging from 30 to 39 with reticulocyte counts of 2 percent or less. This phenomenon was familial in four patients, involving a parent and child in each instance. A small increase in the ratio of membrane cholesterol to phospholipid was observed in this group of patients, and there was a correspondingly small decrease in membrane fluidity. The structural basis for this disorder remains unknown.

Acanthocytes should be distinguished from regularly scalloped crenated red cells (echinocytes) [48]. Echinocytes are a frequent artifact on blood films and should be considered as significant only when present on multiple films prepared with alcohol-washed slides. It is wise to confirm their presence by examining wet preparations by phase microscopy. Echinocytes ("burr cells") occur in patients with uremia, apparently because of the action of the plasma factor [49–51]. Small, dense crenated spheres (*spheroechinocytes*) are occasionally seen in small numbers in patients with congenital nonspherocytic hemolytic anemia due to an enzyme deficiency in the Embden-Meyerhof pathway. They may represent ATP-depleted red cells just prior to their destruction.

References

1. Bassen, F. A., and Kornzweig, A. L.: Malformation of the erythrocytes in a case of atypical retinitis pigmentosa. *Blood* 5:381, 1950.
2. Isselbacher, K. J., Scheif. R., Plotkin, G. R., and Caulfield J. B.: Congenital β-lipoprotein deficiency: An hereditary disorder involving a defect in the absorption and transport of lipids. *Medicine* 43:347, 1964.
3. Ways, P., Reed, C. F., and Hanahan, D. J.: Red-cell and plasma lipids in acanthocytosis. *J. Clin. Invest.* 42:1248, 1963.
4. Levy R. I., Fredrickson, D. S., and Laster, L.: The lipoproteins and lipid transport in abetalipoproteinemia. *J. Clin. Invest.* 45:531, 1966.
5. Jones, J W., and Ways, P.: Abnormalities of high density lipoproteins in abetalipoproteinemia. *J. Clin. Invest.* 46:1151, 1967.
6. Lees, R. S.: Immunological evidence for the presence of B protein (apoprotein of β-lipoprotein) in normal and abetalipoproteinemic plasma. *J. Lipid Res.* 8:396, 1967.
7. Gotto, A. M , Levy, R. I., Birnbaumer. M. E., and Fredrickson, D. S.: Application of optical and immunologic techniques to the question of circulating β-apoprotein in normals and patients with abetalipoproteinemia. *Clin. Res.* 37:383. 1969 (abstract).
8. Simon, E. R., and Ways, P.: Incubation hemolysis and red cell metabolism in acanthocytosis. *J. Clin. Invest.* 43:1311, 1964.
9. Phillips, G. B.: Quantitative chromatographic analysis of plasma and red blood cell lipids in patients with acanthocytosis. *J. Lab. Clin. Med.* 59:357, 1962.
10. Frederickson, D. S.: Familial high-density lipoprotein deficiency: Tangier disease, in *The Metabolic Basis of Inherited Disease*, 2d ed., edited by J. B. Stanbury, J. B. Wyngaarden and D. S. Frederickson. McGraw-Hill, New York, 1966, p. 486.
11. Cooper, R. A., and Gulbrandson, C. A.: The relationship between plasma lipoproteins and red cell membranes in abetalipoproteinemia: Deficiency of lecithin: cholesterol acyltransferase. *J. Lab. Clin. Med.* 78:323 1971.
12. McBride, J. A., and Jacob, H. S.: Abnormal kinetics of red cell membrane cholesterol in acanthocytosis: Studies in genetic and experimental abetalipoproteinemia and in spur cell anemia. *Br. J. Hematol.* 18:383, 1970.
13. Shacklady. M. M., Djardjouras, E. M., and Lloyd, J. K.: Red-cell lipids in familial alphalipoprotein deficiency (Tangier disease). *Lancet* 2:151, 1968.
14. Ways, P., and Song, D.: Etiology of the RBC phospholipid abnormalities in abetalipoproteinemia. *Clin. Res.* 13:283, 1965.
15. Salt, H. B., Wolff, O. H., Lloyd, J. K., Fosbrooke, A. S., Cameron, A. H., and Hubble, D. V.: On having no betalipoprotein: A syndrome comprising abetalipoproteinemia, acanthocytosis, and steatorrhoea. *Lancet* 2:325, 1960.
16. Schwartz, J. F., et al.: Bassen-Kornzweig syndrome: Deficiency of serum beta-lipoprotein. A neuromuscular disorder resembling Friedreich's ataxia, associated with steatorrhea, acanthocytosis, retinitis pigmentosa, and a disorder of lipid metabolism. *Arch. Neurol.* 8:438, 1963.
17. Frezal, J., Rey, J., Polonovski, J., Levy, G., and Lamy, M.: L'Absence congénitale de β-lipoprotéins: Étude de l'absorption des graisses après exsanguino-transfusion mesure de la demi-vie des β-lipoprotéines injecteés. *Rev. Fr. Clin. Biol.* 6:677, 1961.
18. Kayden. H. J., and Silber, R.: The role of vitamin E deficiency in the abnormal autohemolysis of acanthocytosis. *Trans. Assoc. Am. Physicians* 78:334, 1965.
19. Dodge, J. T., Cohen, G., Kayden. H. J., and Phillips, G. B.: Peroxidative hemolysis of red blood cells from patients with abetalipoproteinemia (acanthocytosis). *J. Clin. Invest.* 46:357, 1967.
20. Hoffman J. F.: Cation transport and structure of the red cell plasma membrane. *Circulation* 26:1201, 1962.
21. Cooper, R. A , Durocher J. R., and Leslie, M.: Decreased fluidity of red cell membrane lipids in abetalipoproteinemia. *J. Clin. Invest.* 60:115, 1977.
22. Shinitzky. M., and Barenholz Y.: Dynamics of the hydrocarbon layer in liposomes of lecithin and sphingomyelin containing dicetylphosphate. *J. Biol. Chem.* 249:2652, 1974.
23. Estes, J. W., Morley, T. J., Levine, I. M., and Emerson, C. P.: A new

hereditary acanthocytosis syndrome. *Am. J. Med. 42*:868, 1967.

24. Critchley, E. M. R., Betts, J. J., Nicholston, J. T., and Weatherall, D. J.: Acanthocytosis, normolipidemia and multiple tics. *Postgrad. Med. J. 46*:698, 1970.

25. Critchley, E. M. R., Clark, D. B., and Wikler, A.: Acanthocytosis and a neurological disorder without abetalipoproteinemia. *Arch. Neurol. 18*:134, 1968.

26. Aminoff, M. J.: Acanthocytosis and neurological disease. *Brain 95*:749, 1972.

27. Bird, T. D., Cederbaum, S., Valpey, R. W., and Stahl, W. L.: Familial degeneration of the basal ganglia with acanthocytosis: A clinical, neuropathological, and neurochemical study. *Ann. Neurol. 3*:253, 1978.

28. Smith, J. A., Lonergan, E. T., and Sterling, K.: Spur-cell anemia: Hemolytic anemia with red cells resembling acanthocytes in alcoholic cirrhosis. *N. Engl. J. Med. 271*:396, 1964.

29. Cooper, R. A.: Anemia with spur cells: A red cell defect acquired in serum and modified in the circulation. *J. Clin. Invest. 48*:1820, 1969.

30. Cooper, R. A., Diloy-Puray, M., Lando, P., and Greenberg, M. S.: An analysis of lipoproteins, bile acids and red cell membranes associated with target cells and spur cells in patients with liver disease. *J. Clin. Invest. 51*:3182, 1972.

31. Silber, R., Amorosi. E., Lhowe, J., and Kayden, H. J.: Spur-shaped erythrocytes in Laënnec's cirrhosis. *N. Engl. J. Med. 275*:639, 1966.

32. Neerhout, R. C.: Abnormalities of erythrocyte stromal lipids in liver disease. *J. Lab. Clin. Med. 71*:438, 1968.

33. Vanderkooi, J., Fischkoff, S., Chance, B., and Cooper, R. A.: Fluorescent probe analysis of the lipid architecture of natural and experimental cholesterol-rich membranes. *Biochemistry 13*:1589, 1974.

34. Cooper, R. A., Kimball, D. B., and Durocher, J. R.: The role of the spleen in membrane conditioning and hemolysis of spur cells in liver disease. *N. Engl. J. Med. 290*:1279, 1974.

35. Cooper, R. A., Arner, E. C., Wiley, J. S., and Shattil, S. J.: Modification of red cell membrane structure by cholesterol-rich lipid disper-

sions. *J. Clin. Invest. 55*:115, 1975.

36. Cooper, R. A., and Gabuzda, T.: Unpublished observations.

37. Gracey, M., and Hilton, H. B.: Acanthocytosis and hypobetalipoproteinemia. *Lancet 1*:679, 1973.

38. Wardrop, C., and Hutchisen, H. E.: Red cell shape in hypothyroidism. *Lancet 1*:1243, 1969.

39. Mant, M. J., and Faragher, B. S.: The hematology of anorexia nervosa. *Br. J. Hematol. 23*:737, 1972.

40. Neerhout, R. C.: Red cell lipids in hypothyroidism. *Clin. Chim. Acta 41*:347. 1972.

41. Allen, F. H., Krabbe, S. M. R., and Corcoran, P. A.: A new phenotype (McLoed) in the Kell blood group system. *Vox Sang 6*:555, 1961.

42. Taswell, H. F., Lewis, J. C., Marsh, W. L., Wimer, B. M., Pineda, A. A., and Brzica, S. M.: Erythrocyte morphology in genetic defects of the Rh and Kell blood group systems. *Mayo Clin. Proc. 52*:157, 1977.

43. Marsh, W. L., Oyen, R., Nichols, M. E., and Allen, F. H.: Chronic granulomatous disease and Kell blood groups. *Br. J. Haematol. 29*:247, 1975.

44. Galey. W. R., Evan, A. P., Van Nice, P. S., Dail, W. G., Wimer, E. M., and Cooper, R. A.: Morphology and physiology of the McLoed erythrocyte. *Vox Sang 34*:152, 1978.

45. Abramson, N., and Cooper, R. A.: Unpublished observation.

46. Keller, J. W., Majerus, P. W., and Finke, B. S.: An unusual type of spiculated erythrocytes in metastatic liver disease and hemolytic anemia. *Ann. Intern. Med. 74*:732, 1971.

47. Brecher, G., and Bessis, M.: Present status of spiculed red cells and their relationship to the discocyte-echinocyte transformation: A critical review. *Blood 40*:333, 1972.

48. Cooper, R. A.: Pathogenesis of burr cells in uremia. *J. Clin. Invest. 49*:22a, 1974.

49. Schwartz, S. O., and Motto, S. A.: The diagnostic significance of "burr" red blood cells. *Am. J. Med. Sci. 218*:563, 1949.

50. Stewart, J. H.: Haemolytic anemia in acute and chronic renal failure. *Q. J. Med. 36*:85, 1967.

Erythrocyte disorders—anemias due to increased destruction of erythrocytes with enzyme deficiencies

Glucose-6-phosphate dehydrogenase deficiency

ERNEST BEUTLER

Definition and history

Glucose-6-phosphate dehydrogenase (G-6-PD) deficiency is a hereditary abnormality in which the activity or stability of the enzyme G-6-PD is markedly diminished. Erythrocytes are most severely affected, and G-6-PD deficiency may result in hemolytic anemia, particularly after the administration of drugs, during infections and diabetic acidosis, and in the neonatal period.

The discovery of G-6-PD deficiency was the direct result of investigations of the hemolytic effect of the antimalarial drug primaquine, carried out in the early 1950s. It has long been known that 8-aminoquinoline antimalarial compounds have the capacity to produce hemolytic anemia in certain susceptible individuals. Hemolytic anemia due to the administration of these drugs was first reported in Panamanian plantation workers [1]. Subsequently, cases of 8-aminoquinoline-induced hemolysis were observed all over the world [2]. Attempts were made to determine why some individuals were uniquely sensitive to the hemolytic effect of these drugs, but these attempts were generally unsuccessful. During the Korean war, with the development of a more effective 8-aminoquinoline antimalarial, primaquine, it first became feasible to study this hemolytic reaction under carefully controlled conditions. By use of the then-new technique of labeling red blood cells with radioactive chromium (^{51}Cr), it was possible to show that the sensitivity to the hemolytic effect of this drug was due to an intrinsic abnormality of the red blood cell [3].

It was learned that the hemolytic anemia induced by primaquine was self-limited: after the initial hemolytic episode, the hemoglobin level returned to normal even when the same dose of primaquine which had initially induced the hemolytic reaction was continued [4]. Transfusion of red cells from subjects who had undergone hemolysis and were still receiving drugs showed that these cells were now insensitive to hemolysis even when challenged with drug in a volunteer who had never before received primaquine [4]. Conversely, when red cells from a primaquine-sensitive subject were transfused into an individual who had been pretreated with primaquine, they were rapidly destroyed. It appeared, therefore, that red cells of primaquine-sensitive individuals were heterogeneous with respect to their sensitivity to drugs. A sensitive population was quickly destroyed on administration of drug, while an insensitive population remained. Cohort labeling studies with radioactive iron (^{59}Fe) revealed that sensitivity to the drug was a function of red cell age [5]. This finding focused attention upon the metabolism of red cells, since it was well known that the activities of certain enzymes and metabolic processes of red cells decline on aging. It was found that the level of reduced glutathione (GSH) in primaquine-sensitive cells was diminished [6] and that the cells were unable to protect the GSH that was present against oxidative stress [7,8]. Examination of the pathways of GSH reduction within the red cells of primaquine-sensitive individuals then revealed that there was a deficiency of G-6-PD [9].

It soon became apparent that G-6-PD deficiency was a heterogeneous disorder. Not only was the defect more severe among Mediterranean subjects than among American black subjects [10], but significant differences were found between the biochemical properties of the residual enzymes in the red cells of black and Mediterranean G-6-PD–deficient subjects. Extensive variability was discovered within the Mediterranean population which was originally designated G-6-PD Mediterranean [11,12]. Furthermore, it was found that some patients with nonspherocytic congenital hemolytic anemia also were deficient in G-6-PD [13] and that their enzyme was different from the enzyme found in normal subjects, deficient black subjects, or deficient Mediterranean subjects [14]. The gene for G-6-PD deficiency was found to be sex-linked and has served as an important genetic marker both for population studies and for studies of the mechanism of genetic inactivation of the X chromosome (see Chap. 16).

Etiology and pathogenesis

PROPERTIES OF THE ENZYMES
G-6-PD deficiency results from the inheritance of any one of a large number of abnormalities of the structural gene which codes the amino acid sequence of the enzyme G-6-PD. In the case of the common deficient Afri-

can A— mutation the abnormal enzyme formed may be synthesized in normal quantity, but has decreased stability in vivo [15,16]. The mutations encountered in the Mediterranean region appear to result in the formation of enzyme molecules with decreased enzyme activity [17] and with altered kinetic properties such as lowered K_m for glucose-6-phosphate and NADP+ [18,19]. Some alterations of the kinetic properties of G-6-PD variants may render them functionally inadequate. Some variants (e.g., G-6-PD Oklahoma [20]) show a marked decrease in affinity for the substrates glucose-6-phosphate and NADP; some (e.g., G-6-PD Manchester and Tripler [21]) are abnormally sensitive to the inhibitory effect of NADPH. Various combinations of these properties may also occur, and over 150 variants of this enzyme have been described (Table 58-1). Their detailed biochemical characteristics have been tabulated in several reviews [138,144]. Figure 58-1 presents, semischematically, the biochemical properties of two of the more common variants.

The "normal" is designated as G-6-PD B. It represents the most common type of enzyme encountered in all the population groups which have been studied. Among Africans another variety of normally active enzyme is also very prevalent. This is known as G-6-PD A. It migrates electrophoretically more rapidly than the normal B enzyme and may be associated with slight reduction of red cell enzyme activity, but otherwise appears to be identical to the normal enzyme. Fingerprinting of G-6-PD A has been achieved, and it differs from the B enzyme only by a single amino acid substitution [145]. Approximately 16 percent of American black males carry this variant allele [146].

The A— type of G-6-PD is the most common clinically significant type of abnormal G-6-PD among the American black population. Eleven percent of black American males are affected by this abnormality. Their red cells contain only 5 to 15 percent of the normal amount of enzyme activity. The mobility of the enzyme present is rapid and is indistinguishable from that of the A variant in conventional electrophoretic systems. However, it can clearly be shown to differ from the G-6-PD A variant by chromatography [147].

Among Caucasian populations the most common variant enzyme was originally designated G-6-PD Mediterranean [18,19]. It is now apparent that many similar but distinct variants exist in that region [11,12,78,148]. The frequency of G-6-PD deficiency among Caucasian populations ranges from less than 1 in 1000 among northern European populations to 50 percent of the males among Kurdish Jews. The enzyme activity of the red cells of individuals who have inherited this abnormal gene is very low, often less than 1 percent of normal.

G-6-PD deficiency is also found among certain Chinese populations and in southeast Asia. Several variants appear to be common in Asian populations [67,149].

The distribution of G-6-PD deficiency among various population groups has been presented in detail elsewhere [137].

MECHANISM OF HEMOLYSIS

The life-span of G-6-PD–deficient red cells is shortened under many circumstances, such as during drug administration, the neonatal period, diabetic acidosis, or infections. The exact reason for this is not known.

Drug-induced hemolysis in G-6-PD–deficient cells is generally accompanied by the formation of Heinz bodies, particles of denatured hemoglobin and stromal protein (see Chap. 29), formed only in the presence of oxygen [150,151]. The mechanism by which Heinz bodies are formed and become attached to red cell stroma has been the subject of considerable investigation and speculation. Exposure of red cells to certain drugs results in the formation of low levels of hydrogen peroxide as the drug interacts with hemoglobin [152]. In addition, some drugs may form free radicals which oxidize GSH without the formation of peroxide as an intermediate [153]. The formation of free radicals of GSH through the action of peroxide or by the direct action of drugs may be followed either by oxidation of glutathione (GSH) to the disulfide form (GSSG) or complexing of the glutathione with hemoglobin to form a mixed disulfide. Such mixed disulfides are believed to form initially with the sulfhydryl group of the β-93 position of hemoglobin [154,155]. The mixed disulfide of GSH and hemoglobin is probably unstable and undergoes conformational changes exposing interior sulfhydryl groups to oxidation and mixed disulfide formation. Chain separation into free α and β chains has also been found to occur [156]. Phenylhydrazine-like drugs have also been shown to form a hemochromogen directly with hemoglobin, a complex forming between the iron of ferriheme and the nitrogen bound to the benzene ring [157]. Once such oxidation has occurred, hemoglobin is irreversibly denatured and will precipitate as Heinz bodies. Normal red cells can defend themselves to a considerable extent against such changes by reducing GSSG to GSH and by reducing the mixed disulfides of GSH and hemoglobin through the glutathione reductase reaction [158]. However, the reduction of these disulfide bonds requires a source of NADPH. Since G-6-PD–deficient red cells are unable to reduce NADP+ to NADPH at a normal rate, they are unable to reduce hydrogen peroxide or the mixed disulfides of hemoglobin and GSH. When such cells are challenged by drugs, they form Heinz bodies more readily than do normal cells. Cells containing Heinz bodies encounter difficulty in traversing the splenic pulp [160] and are relatively rapidly eliminated from the circulation. The metabolic events which may lead to red cell damage and eventually destruction are summarized in Fig. 58-2.

The formation of methemoglobin frequently accompanies the administration of drugs which have the capacity to produce hemolysis of G-6-PD–deficient cells [161]. The heme groups of methemoglobin become detached from the globin more readily than do the heme groups of oxyhemoglobin [162]. It is possible that methemoglobin formation represents an important step in the oxidative degradation of hemoglobin to Heinz bod-

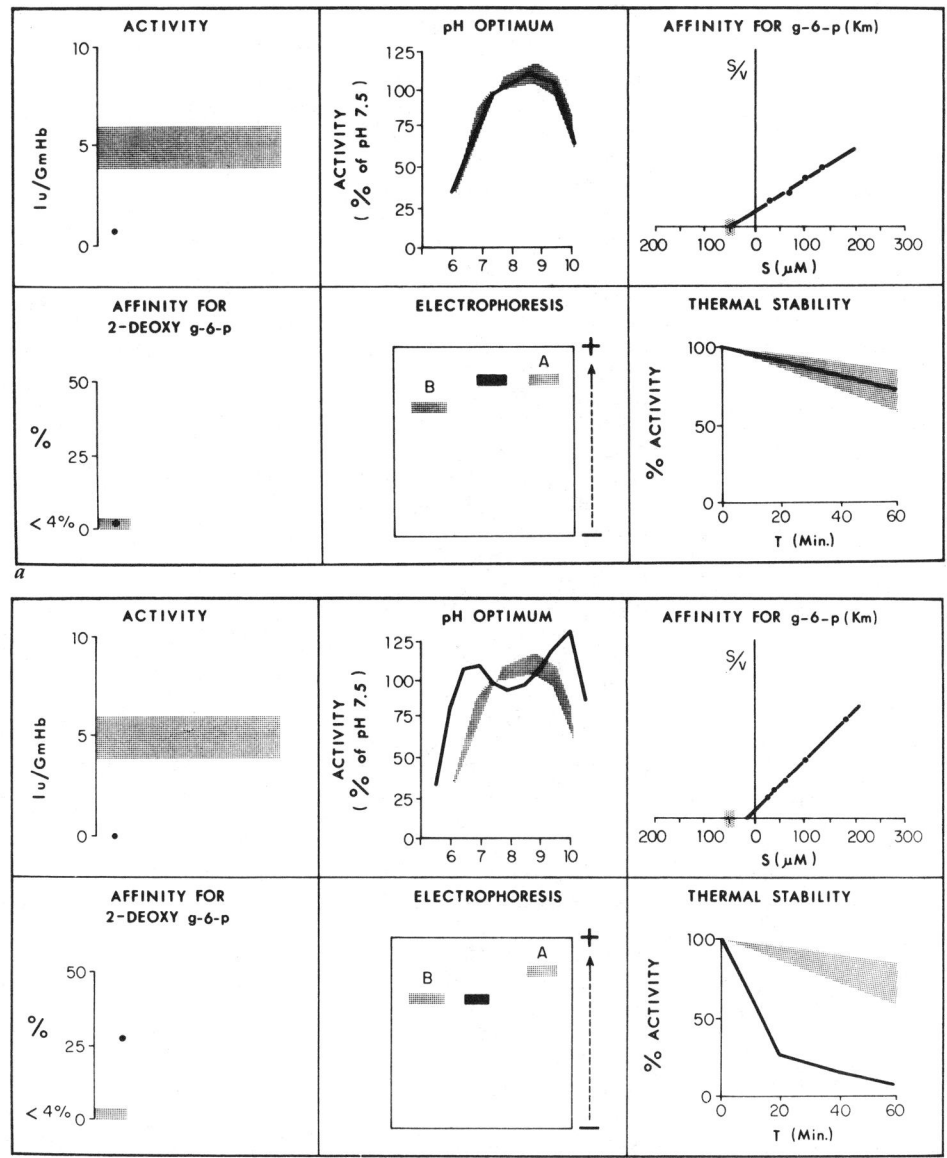

FIGURE 58-1   The biochemical properties of two common variants of G-6-PD. (*a*) **The biochemical characteristics of G-6-PD A−.** (*b*) **The biochemical characteristics of G-6-PD Mediterranean. In each panel the characteristics of the normal enzyme (types A and B) are indicated by the shaded areas.**

ies [163], but it is equally likely that the formation of methemoglobin is merely an incidental side effect of oxidative drugs [164].

Unusual susceptibility to icterus neonatorum of G-6-PD–deficient infants may represent the result of the coincidence of a lack of G-6-PD with the relative enzymatic immaturity of the newborn erythrocyte and with undefined stresses which may be present in the neonatal period.

The mechanism of hemolysis induced by infection or occurring spontaneously in G-6-PD–deficient subjects is even less well understood. It has been suggested that the generation of hydrogen peroxide by phagocytizing leukocytes may play a role in this type of hemolytic reaction [165].

Substances capable of destroying red cell GSH have been isolated from fava beans [165,166]. Favism occurs only in G-6-PD–deficient subjects, but not all individuals in a particular family may be sensitive to the hemolytic effect of the beans. Nonetheless, some tendency toward familial occurrence has suggested the possibility that an additional, genetic factor may be active [167]. The observation of increased excretion of glucaric acid [168] has led to the suggestion that a defect in glucuronide formation might be present. Immunologic factors do not seem to play a role in favism [169].

TABLE 58-1 Variants of glucose-6-phosphate dehydrogenase

CLASS 1 VARIANTS (Associated with nonspherocytic hemolytic anemia)	
Electrophoretically fast variants	Helsinki[b,d,g,i,o,u] [46]
St. Louis[c,h,j,q,u] [22]	Kremenchug[b,e,h,k,o,u] [47]
Baudelocque[b,h,j,q,u] [23]	Ogikubo[b,d,h,j,q,u] [48]
Lincoln Park[b,f,h,j,p,x] [24]	Yokohama[a,f,g,k,p,u] [48]
Hotel Dieu[b,f,h,k,p,v] [25]	Akita[b,d,g,i,p,u] [48]
Linda Vista[b,f,h,k,q,v] [26]	Dothan[a,f,g,j,q,u] [49]
Charleston[b,f,h,k,q] [27]	Dublin[a,e,h,q,u] [50]
San Diego[b,g,o,u] [28]	Sapporo[a,d,h,k,p,u] [51]
Guadalajara[b,f,h,k,o,u] [29]	*Electrophoretically slow variants*
East Harlem[c,f,g,j,p] [30]	Long Prairie[b,d,h,k,q,x] [52]
Jackson[b,f,g,k,o,u] [31]	Grand Prairie[b,d,g,k,q,u] [53]
Pea Ridge[a,f,g,j,q,u] [32]	Chicago[a,d,g,q,u] [32,54]
Barcelona[b,f,h,i,o,u] [33]	Panama[b,e,h,k,p,v] [55]
Gilgore[b,d,g,k,p,v] [34]	Arlington Heights[c,f,g,j,q,x] [56]
Electrophoretically normal variants	Rotterdam[b,d,h,o,v] [42]
Chinese[a,g,i,o,u] [35]	Minneapolis[c,f,h,j,q,x] [57]
Bat-Yam[b,h,q,v] [36]	Tripler[b,g,k,q,v] [58]
Albuquerque[c,f,g,q,x] [37]	Alhambra[a,e,g,p,x] [59]
Bangkok[a,f,h,q,x] [38]	Hong Hong Pokfulam[a,g,k,o,u] [35]
Oklahoma[c,f,g,p,x] [20]	Santa Barbara[a,f,g,j,q,w] [60]
Duarte[a,f,h,q,w] [39]	Ashod[c,h,p,v] [36]
Hong Kong[b,f,h,o,u] [40]	Ramat Gan[b,h,q,v] [36]
Boston[b,e,h,k,p,w] [41]	Manchester[a,f,g,k,p,v] [61]
Englewood[a,e,h,p,v] [42]	West Town[a,f,h,k,q,u] [24]
New York[a,d,h,p,w] [42]	Atlanta[a,f,g,j,q,u] [62]
Hawaii[b,f,g,j,q,v] [43]	Worcester[b,f,g,j,q,w] [63]
Tokushima[a,f,g,j,q,u] [44]	San Francisco[c,f,g,k,q,u] [64]
Hayem[b,h,k,p,u] [22]	Tokyo[a,f,g,i,q,u] [44]
Aarau[b,f,h,k,q,v] [45]	Kobe[c,f,h,k,q,w] [51]

CLASS 2 VARIANTS (Severely deficient, less than 10% residual activity)	
Electrophoretically fast variants	*Electrophoretically normal variants*
Hualien-Chi[b,h,o,v] [65]	Indonesia[b,f,h,p,v] [75]
San Jose[a,d,h,j,o,u] [66]	Campbellpore[b,h,q,v] [76]
Taipei-Hakka[b,d,h,p,v] [67]	Mediterranean[b,e,h,k,p,v] [18]
Union[b,d,h,k,p,v] [68]	Corinth[b,e,h,i,p,v] [77]
N-Sawan[b,e,g,k,q,v] [69]	El Fayoum[b,h,k,p,v] [78]
Ankara[a,f,g,k,p,v] [70]	Bagdad[c,f,h,q,v] [79]
Ferrara[b,d,h,k,q,u] [71]	Matam[b,e,h,k,p,v] [80]
Padrew[b,f,h,k,p,v] [69]	Abrami[b,f,h,k,p,v] [81]
Lublin[b,f,g,o] [72]	Hamm[b,f,h,k,q,x] [82]
Taiwan-Hakka[b,h,o,v] [67]	Tarsus[b,f,h,k,p,x] [82]
Markham[b,h,p,v] [73]	Bielefeld[b,f,h,k,o] [83]
Haad Yai[c,h,k,p,u] [69]	Petrich[b,h,k,p,v] [84]
Long Xuyen[b,h,k,p,v] [74]	Gotze Delchev[b,h,k,q,v] [84]
Hualien[b,h,q,v] [65]	Nukus[c,e,g,j,o,w] [85]
Teheran[b,g,o,v] [65]	Tashkent[b,e,g,o,u] [85]
	Blida[b,h,j,p,w] [86]
	Ogori[b,f,g,k,o,u] [87]

[a] Normal K_m G-6-P (50 to 70 μM).
[b] Low K_m G-6-P.
[c] High K_m G-6-P.
[d] Normal K_m NADP (2.9 to 4.4 μM).
[e] Low K_m NADP.
[f] High K_m NADP.
[g] Normal 2-deoxy G-6-P utilization (<4% of G-6-P).
[h] High 2-deoxy G-6-P utilization.
[i] Normal deamino NADP utilization (55 to 60% of NADP).
[j] Low deamino NADP utilization.
[k] High deamino NADP utilization.
[l] Normal K_i NADPH (19.22 ± 5.82).
[m] Low K_i NADPH.
[n] High K_i NADPH.
[o] Heat-stable (normal).
[p] Labile.
[q] Very labile.
[u] Normal pH optimum.
[v] pH-activity curve biphasic.
[w] pH-activity curve monophasic with optimum 8.
[x] pH-activity curve monophasic with optimum over 8.

564

TABLE 58-1 Variants of glucose-6-phosphate dehydrogenase (Continued)

Eletrophoretically slow variants	Kurume[b,f,h,k,q,v] [95]
Jammu[a,f,g,i,o,u] [88]	Zhitomir[b,e,h,k,p,v] [96]
Chainat[a,f,q,k,q,u] [69]	Lifta[b,h,q,w] [36]
Toulouse[a,e,h,k,q,v] [89]	West Bengal[b,f,g,o,u] [97]
Panay[b,f,g,p,v] [90]	Alger[b,h,j,q,v] [86]
Zakataly[b,d,h,k,p,v] [91]	Bideiz[b,d,h,k,q,v] [91]
Salata[c,f,h,i,o,u] [92]	Fukushima[b,f,g,j,p,u] [95]
Poznan[b,e,h,p,v] [93]	Wakayama[b,f,g,k,q,u] [95]
Okhut I[b,d,h,k,p,v] [91]	Shekii[b,e,h,k,q,v] [91]
Aachen[a,f,g,j,q,u] [94]	Yamaguchi[b,f,h,k,q,x] [95]
Shirin-Bulakh[b,e,h,k,q,x] [91]	

CLASS 3 VARIANTS (Moderately deficient, 10–60% residual activity)

Electrophoretically fast variants	*Electrophoretically slow variants*
Puerto Rico[b,g,p] [98]	Intanon[a,e,g,j,o,v] [116]
A-[a,d,g,i,o,u] [99–101]	Athens[b,f,h,k,p,v] [117]
Debrousse[b,e,h,o,u] [102]	Siwa[b,h,k,p,v] [78]
Muret[b,e,h,k,o,x] [103]	Bogia[a,f,h,k,o,u] [92]
Lozere[b,f,g,j,p,v] [104]	Kaluan[c,f,h,j,q,u] [92]
Ube[a,f,g,i,o,u] [105]	Vientiane[b,f,h,k,o,u] [118]
Castilla[a,f,h,k,p,u] [87]	Washington[a,g,o,u] [65]
Konan[b,f,g,i,o,u] [106]	Colomiers[b,e,h,k,o,w] [103]
Chibuto[b,f,g,p,u] [105]	Benevento[b,h,p,v] [98]
Chiapas[b,e,g,i,p,w] [107]	Los Angeles[b,f,h,j,o,v] [119]
San Juan[b,h,q,v] [98]	Titteri[b,h,j,o,x] [86]
Kabyle[a,g,o,u] [108]	Napoli[b,e,h,k,o,v] [120]
Laghouat[b,h,j,o,u] [86]	Ferrara II[b,e,h,k,o,v] [120]
Toronto[b,f,h,k,p,v] [109]	Agrigento[b,d,g,k,p,u] [121]
Canton[b,h,p,v] [110]	Trinacria[b,e,h,k,p,v] [122]
Bukitu[c,f,h,k,p,u] [92]	Okhut II[b,f,h,k,p,u] [91]
Tahta[b,g,o,u] [78]	Camperdown[b,e,h,k,o,v] [123]
Velletri[c,d,h,k,q,v] [111]	Thenia[a,q,j,o,v] [86]
Gallura[b,f,g,k,p,u] [112]	Mexico[b,e,h,o,u] [124]
Electrophoretically normal variants	Ciudad de la Habana[b,d,h,k,p,v] [125]
Mahidol[b,g,i,o,u] [113]	Seattle[b,e,h,o,v] [126]
El Morro[b,h,k,p,v] [98]	Kerala[b,e,h,o,v] [97]
Siriraj[b,h,k,p,v] [114]	Tel-Hashomer[b,g,o,v] [127]
Hofu[b,f,h,k,o,u] [115]	Carswell[b,f,g,o,u] [128]
El Kharga[a,h,j,p,x] [78]	Capetown[b,e,h,k,o,v] [129]
Kamiube[b,d,g,j,o,u] [106]	Anant[b,g,k,o,u] [130]

CLASS 4 VARIANTS (Normal activity, 60–150%)

Electrophoretically fast variants	*Electrophoretically slow variants*
Inhambane[b,f,g,o,v] [131]	Alexandra[b,d,g,j,o,u] [77]
Luz-Saint-Sauveur[b,d,g,o,u] [132]	Baltimore-Austin[a,d,g,o,u] [139]
A[a,d,g,i,o,u] [100,101,133]	Manjacase[c,d,g,o,u] [105]
Steilacom[a,d,g,o,u] [134]	Pinar Del Rio[b,d,g,p,v] [140]
Laurenzo Marquez[a,d,g,o,u] [105]	Port Royal[b,h,j,p] [141]
Kiwa[b,f,h,k,o,u] [106]	Ibadan-Austin[a,d,g,o,u] [139]
Electrophoretically normal variants	Porbandar[b,e,h,k,o,u] [142]
B[a,d,g,i,o,u] [135–138]	

CLASS 5 VARIANTS (Increased activity)

Electrophoretically fast veriants	
Hektoen[a,d,g,j,o,u] [143]	

---

[a] Normal K_m G-6-P (50 to 70 μM).	[m] Low K_i NADPH.
[b] Low K_m G-6-P.	[n] High K_i NADPH.
[c] High K_m G-6-P.	[o] Heat-stable (normal).
[d] Normal K_m NADP (2.9 to 4.4 μM).	[p] Labile.
[e] Low K_m NADP.	[q] Very labile.
[f] High K_m NADP.	[u] Normal pH optimum.
[g] Normal 2-deoxy G-6-P utilization (<4% of G-6-P).	[v] pH-activity curve biphasic.
[h] High 2-deoxy G-6-P utilization.	[w] pH-activity curve monophasic with optimum 8.
[i] Normal deamino NADP utilization (55 to 60% of NADP).	[x] pH-activity curve monophasic with optimum over 8.
[j] Low deamino NADP utilization.	
[k] High deamino NADP utilization.	
[l] Normal K_i NADPH (19.22 ± 5.82).	

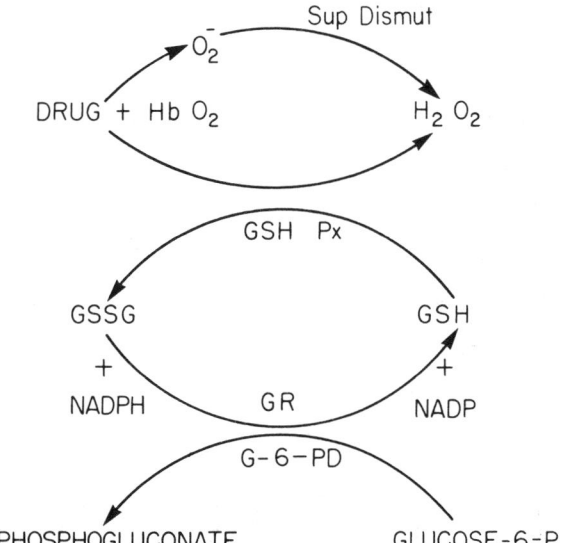

FIGURE 58-2 Reactions through which hydrogen peroxide is generated and detoxified in the erythrocyte. In G-6-PD deficiency inadequate generation of NADPH results in accumulation of GSSG and probably of H_2O_2. GR = glutathione reductase; GSH Px = glutathione peroxide; Sup Dismut = superoxide dismutase; GSSG = glutathione disulfide (oxidized glutathione).

Mode of inheritance

The gene determining the structure of G-6-PD is carried on the X chromosome; inheritance of G-6-PD deficiency is therefore sex-linked [170]. For this reason, the defect is fully expressed in affected males and is never transmitted from father to son, but only from mother to son. In females, only one of the two X chromosomes in each cell is active (see Chap. 16). Consequently, female heterozygotes for G-6-PD deficiency have two populations of red cells: deficient cells and normal cells [171]. The proportion of deficient to normal cells may vary greatly. Some heterozygous females appear to be entirely normal; others appear to be fully affected. The marked variability of expression of G-6-PD deficiency of heterozygotes is the result of certain features of the X-inactivation process. Because the process of inactivation is random, in some instances more of the maternally derived or more of the paternally derived X chromosomes may escape inactivation. More important, perhaps, is the fact that the clones of cells in which the maternally derived X is active, on the one hand, or in which the paternally derived X is active, on the other, may have a proliferative advantage. In the many cell generations between the time of X inactivation and maturity, even a small selective advantage of one set of clones over the other would result in marked disparity between the number of normal and deficient cells [172,173]. The marked variability of the ratio of G-6-PD deficient to normal red cells in the circulation of female heterozygotes, then, accounts for the marked differences in expression of the deficiency in such individ-

uals. G-6-PD deficiency seems to confer some degree of resistance to infection with the falciparum malaria parasite [174,175]. It has been suggested [176,177] that the incidence of G-6-PD deficiency is higher in individuals with sickle cell disease than in the general black population, reflecting a favorable effect of the enzyme deficiency on the clinical course of the sickling disorders. However, it seems that the increase of G-6-PD deficiency in patients with sickle disease may merely result from the markedly heterogeneous genetic composition of American blacks; those with more African genes are more likely to inherit sickle hemoglobin and G-6-PD A— [178,179].

Clinical features

Most G-6-P–deficient persons never suffer any clinical manifestations of this common genetic trait. When they do occur, the only clinical manifestation of G-6-PD deficiency, with rare exceptions, is hemolytic anemia. Usually the anemia is episodic, but some of the unusual variants of G-6-PD may cause nonspherocytic congenital hemolytic disease (see below). In general, hemolysis is associated with stress, most notably drug administration, infection, diabetic acidosis, the newborn period, and, in certain individuals, exposure to fava beans.

DRUG-INDUCED HEMOLYTIC ANEMIA
A large number of drugs and other chemicals that may have the capacity to precipitate hemolytic reactions in G-6-PD–deficient individuals are listed in Table 58-2. Some drugs, such as chloramphenicol, may induce mild hemolysis in a person with severe, Mediterranean-type G-6-PD deficiency [180] but not in those with the milder A- or Canton [181] type of deficiency. There appears, furthermore, to be a difference in the severity of the reaction of different individuals with the same G-6-PD variant to the same drug; for example, red cells from a single G-6-PD–deficient individual were hemolyzed in the circulation of some recipients who were given thiazolsulfone, but their survival was normal in the circulation of others [182]. Undoubtedly, individual differences in the metabolism and excretion of drugs influence the extent to which G-6-PD–deficient red cells are destroyed.

Typically, an episode of drug-induced hemolysis in G-6-PD–deficient individuals begins 1 to 3 days after drug administration is initiated [4]. Heinz bodies appear in the red cells, and the hemoglobin concentration begins to decline rapidly [183]. As hemolysis progresses, Heinz bodies disappear from the circulation, presumably as they or the erythrocytes which contain them are removed by the spleen. In severe cases abdominal or back pain may occur. The urine may turn dark— even black. Within 4 to 6 days, there is generally an increase in the reticulocyte count, except in instances in which the patient has received the drug in treatment of an active infection. Because of the tendency of infections and certain other stressful situations to precipitate hemolysis in G-6-PD–deficient individuals, many drugs have been incorrectly implicated as a cause. Other drugs, such as aspirin, have appeared on many lists of proscribed medications because very large doses had the capability of slightly reducing the red cell life-span. It is important to recognize that such drugs, listed in Table 58-3, do not produce clinically significant hemolytic anemia. Advising patients not to ingest these drugs may not only deprive patients of potentially helpful medications, but will also weaken their confidence in the advice which they have received. Most G-6-PD–deficient patients, after all, have taken aspirin without untoward effect and are likely to distrust an advisor who counsels them that the ingestion of aspirin would have catastrophic effects.

In the A– type of G-6-PD deficiency, the hemolytic anemia is self-limited [4]. This is true because the young red cells produced in response to hemolysis have nearly normal G-6-PD levels and are relatively resistant to hemolysis [5]. The hemoglobin level may return to normal even while the same dose of drug which initially precipitated hemolysis is administered. In contrast, hemolysis is not necessarily self-limited in the more severe Mediterranean type of deficiency [184,185].

In the common variants of G-6-PD, such as G-6-PD A– and Mediterranean, and even in most of the severely deficient variants, there is usually no demonstrated defect in leukocyte number or function. However, there have been reports of isolated instances of leukocyte dysfunction associated with rare, severely deficient variants of G-6-PD [33,186,187]. Patients with G-6-PD deficiency do not have a bleeding tendency, and studies of platelet function have yielded conflicting results [188,189]. Occasionally, cataracts have been observed in patients with variants of G-6-PD which produce nonspherocytic hemolytic anemia [190–192], and it has even been suggested that the incidence of senile cataracts may be increased in G-6-PD deficiency [193,194].

HEMOLYTIC ANEMIA OCCURRING DURING INFECTION

Anemia has often developed rather suddenly in G-6-PD–deficient individuals within a few days of onset of a febrile illness [195,196]. The anemia is usually relatively mild, with a decline in the hemoglobin concentration of 3 or 4 g/dl. Hemolysis has been noted particularly in patients suffering from pneumonia and in those with typhoid fever. Jaundice is not a prominent part of the clinical picture, except where hemolysis occurs in association with infectious hepatitis [197–201]. In that case it can be quite intense. Presumably because of the effect of the infection, reticulocytosis is usually absent, and recovery from the anemia is generally delayed until after the active infection has abated.

FAVISM

Favism is potentially one of the gravest clinical consequences of G-6-PD deficiency. It occurs much more commonly in children than in adults. The onset of

TABLE 58-2   Drugs and chemicals which have clearly been shown to cause clinically significant hemolytic anemia in G-6-PD deficiency*

Acetanilid	Primaquine
Methylene blue	Sulfacetamide
Nalidixic acid (NeGram)	Sulfamethoxazole (Gantanol)
Naphthalene	Sulfanilamide
Niridazole (Ambilhar)	Sulfapyridine
Nitrofurantoin (Furadantin)	Thiazolesulfone
Pamaquine	Toluidine blue
Pentaquine	Trinitrotoluene (TNT)
Phenylhydrazine	

* References given in Beutler [138].

hemolysis may be quite sudden, having been reported to occur within the first hours after exposure to fava beans. More commonly the onset is gradual, hemolysis being noticed 1 to 2 days after ingestion of the beans [202]. The urine becomes red or quite dark, and in severe cases shock may develop within a short time.

NEONATAL ICTERUS

Icterus neonatorum with no evidence of immunologic incompatibility occurs in some infants with G-6-PD deficiency. The jaundice may be quite severe and, if untreated, may result in kernicterus. An increased incidence of neonatal icterus has been observed in Mediterranean infants with G-6-PD deficiency [203] and among the Chinese [204]. It seems to occur quite rarely among neonates with the A– type of enzyme deficiency [205] in the United States, but some cases have been reported in G-6-PD–deficient infants [206–208] in Africa. The cause of the difference is unknown, but it may be related to some environmental factor such as vitamin E intake.

HEREDITARY NONSPHEROCYTIC HEMOLYTIC ANEMIA

Some of the rare types of G-6-PD deficiency are associated with hereditary nonspherocytic hemolytic anemia. Occasionally, patients with the common, Mediterranean type of defect have also been found to have this disorder [37,209]. The reason some individuals with the Mediterranean type of enzyme deficiency have chronic hemolysis while the majority have hemolysis only under conditions of stress is not clear; it is possible that hemolysis is due to some as yet undefined associated abnormality.

Hereditary nonspherocytic hemolytic anemia due to G-6-PD deficiency is usually first noted during infancy or childhood. In some instances, neonatal jaundice has been present. Hemolysis is often exacerbated by febrile illnesses or by the administration of drugs. Splenomegaly is commonly present. Splenectomy is generally ineffective, although some improvement has occasionally been reported [137,209] following removal of the spleen. In most cases the anemia is not very severe, but in some instances frequent transfusions have been necessary [37].

Laboratory features

In the absence of hemolysis, the light-microscopic morphology of G-6-PD–deficient red cells appears to be normal [183]. Differences in the texture of the stroma have been observed under the electron microscope [210]. Even during hemolytic episodes, morphologic changes are not striking. When a hemolytic drug has been administered, Heinz bodies (Chap. 29) develop in the erythrocytes immediately preceding and in the early phases of hemolysis. If the hemolytic anemia is very severe, spherocytosis and red cell fragmentation may be seen in the stained film. Although "bite cells" have been noted in the blood of some patients undergoing drug-induced hemolysis, they were *not* G-6-PD–deficient [211,212]. Varying degrees of hyperbilirubinemia may be evident. As the hemoglobin level of blood falls, reticulocytosis occurs, and polychromasia is seen on the stained smear. No consistent changes occur in platelet or white cells.

Diagnosis of G-6-PD deficiency depends on the demonstration of decreased enzyme activity either through a quantitative assay or a screening test. Assay of the enzyme is generally carried out by measuring the rate of reduction of $NADP^+$ to NADPH in an ultraviolet spectrophotometer [213]. Several acceptable visual screening tests have been described [214–218], and the prepared reagents for carrying out some of these procedures are commercially available. The fluorescent procedure described in Chap. A11 is the most satisfactory screening test. Although detection of enzyme deficiency in the healthy, fully affected (hemizygous) male presents no problem and can be achieved readily through either assay or screening tests, difficulties arise when a patient with G-6-PD deficiency of the A— type has undergone a hemolytic episode. As the older, more enzyme-deficient cells are removed from the circulation and are replaced by young cells, the level of the enzyme begins to increase toward normal. Under such circumstances, suspicion that the patient may be G-6-PD–deficient should be raised by the fact that enzyme activity is not increased, even though the reticulocyte count is elevated. Centrifugation of the blood followed by testing of the most dense (oldest) red cells has been employed as a means for the detection of G-6-PD deficiency in persons with the A— defect who have recently undergone hemolysis [219,220]. It is helpful to carry out family studies or to wait until the circulating red cells have aged sufficiently to betray their lack of enzyme.

Even greater difficulties are encountered in attempting to diagnose the heterozygous enzyme deficiency state [221]: the presence of a population of normal red cells coexisting with the deficient cells (see Chap. 16) may mask the enzyme deficiency when screening tests are used. Even enzyme assays on heterozygous females may frequently be in the normal range. Here methods which depend upon histochemical demonstration of individual red cell enzyme activity may be useful [222]. In addition, the ascorbate-cyanide test [215], in which screening is carried out on a whole cell population rather than on a lysate, may be more sensitive than the other screening procedures.

The classification of G-6-PD deficiency by subtype (that is, A—, Mediterranean, Canton, etc.) requires the use of relatively sophisticated biochemical techniques. The enzyme must be partially purified, and then its K_m for $NADP^+$ and glucose 6-phosphate, utilization of substrate analogs, pH optima, and electrophoretic mobility must be determined in standard systems [213]. Detailed characterization of G-6-PD variants is of value chiefly in appraising the role of G-6-PD deficiency in the etiology of nonspherocytic hemolytic anemia. For example, if a black male with chronic hemolysis is found to have a common A— variant of G-6-PD, it is necessary to seek elsewhere for a source of hemolysis. On the other hand, if an unusual, thermolabile variant is found, it is more likely that the G-6-PD deficiency plays an etiologic role in the hemolytic process.

Differential diagnosis

Drug-induced hemolytic anemia due to G-6-PD deficiency is similar in its clinical features and in certain laboratory features to drug-induced hemolytic anemia associated with unstable hemoglobins (see Chap. 61). Other enzyme defects affecting the pentose-phosphate shunt, such as a deficiency of γ-glutamyl cysteine synthetase or GSH synthetase, may also mimic G-6-PD deficiency (see Chap. 59). The hemoglobinopathies can be ruled out by performing a stability test and hemoglobin electrophoresis (see Chaps. A6 and A7). Both of these are normal in G-6-PD deficiency. Some of the screening tests, particularly the ascorbate-cyanide test [215], may give positive results in the above-named disorders, but a G-6-PD assay or the fluorescent screening test will be positive only in G-6-PD deficiency.

Therapy

G-6-PD–deficient individuals should avoid drugs which might induce hemolytic episodes (see Table 58-2). If hemolysis occurs as a result of drug ingestion or infection, particularly in the milder A— type of deficiency, transfusion is not usually required. If, however, the rate of hemolysis is very rapid, as may occur, for example, in favism, transfusions of whole blood or packed cells may be useful. Good urine flow should be maintained in patients with hemoglobinuria to avert renal damage. Infants with neonatal jaundice due to G-6-PD deficiency may require exchange transfusion; in areas where G-6-PD deficiency is prevalent, care must be taken not to give G-6-PD–deficient blood to such newborns. Patients with hereditary nonspherocytic hemolytic anemia usually do not require any therapy. Splenectomy has occasionally been reported to be of some benefit [63] but is usually not helpful. The antioxidant properties of vi-

TABLE 58-3   Drugs which can probably safely be given in normal therapeutic doses to G-6-PD-deficient subjects without nonspherocytic hemolytic anemia*

Acetaminophen (paracetamol, Tylenol, Tralgon, hydroxyacetanilide)	*p*-Aminobenzoic acid
	Phenylbutazone
Acetophenetidin (phenacetin)	Phenytoin
Acetylsalicylic acid (aspirin)	Probenecid (Benemid)
Aminopyrine (Pyramidon, amidopyrine)	Procain amide hydrochloride (Pronestyl)
Antazoline (Antistine)	
Antipyrine	Pyrimethamine (Daraprim)
Ascorbic acid (vitamin C)	Quinidine
Benzhexol (Artane)	Quinine
Chloramphenicol	Streptomycin
Chlorguanidine (Proguanil, Paludrine)	Sulfacytine
Chloroquine	Sulfadiazine
Colchicine	Sulfaguanidine
Diphenhydramine (Benadryl)	Sulfamerazine
Isoniazid	Sulfamethoxypyridazine (Kynex)
L-Dopa	Sulfisoxazole (Gantrisin)
Menadione sodium bisulfite (Hykinone)	Trimethoprim
	Tripelennamine (Pyribenzamine)
Menapthone	Vitamin K

* References given in Beutler [138]

tamin E have been tested in G-6-PD–deficient subjects, and it has been reported that a slight but statistically significant reduction in hemolysis was observed [223,224].

Course and prognosis

Hemolytic episodes in the A– type of deficiency are usually self-limited, even if drug administration is continued. This may not be the case in the more severe Mediterranean type of deficiency. In patients with hereditary nonspherocytic hemolytic anemia due to G-6-PD deficiency, gallstones may occur. During periods of infections or drug administration anemia may increase in severity. Otherwise, the hemoglobin level of affected subjects remains relatively stable.

Nearly all patients with drug- or infection-induced hemolysis recover uneventfully. Favism must be considered, by comparison, a relatively dangerous disease. Prior to the institution of modern hospital therapy, fatalities from favism were not uncommon.

In one large population study, a decreasing incidence of G-6-PD deficiency was noted with increasing age of the population [225]. While this might represent evidence of a shorter life-span for individuals with the A– deficiency, other factors are more likely explanations. For example, in black American society the more economically deprived segment of the population manifests both a higher incidence of African genes and a shorter life-span. This would cause a decreasing incidence of G-6-PD deficiency with advancing age, but there would be no cause-and-effect relation between G-6-PD deficiency and life-span. Examination of the health records of over 65,000 U.S. Veterans Administration males failed to reveal any higher frequency of any illness in G-6-PD–

deficient compared with nondeficient subjects [226]. In view of the benign nature of the common types of G-6-PD deficiency, community-based population screening is not to be recommended. However, screening for G-6-PD deficiency of all patients admitted to the hospital may be useful in anticipating hemolytic reactions and in understanding them if they occur.

References

1. Cordes, W.: Experiences with plasmochin in malaria. United Fruit Co. (Med. Dept.) 15th Annual Report, Boston, 1926, pp. 66–71.
2. Beutler, E.: The hemolytic effect of primaquine and related compounds. A review. *Blood 14:*103, 1959.
3. Dern, R. J., Weinstein, I. M., Le Roy, G. V., Talmage, D. W., and Alving, A. S.: The hemolytic effect of primaquine. I. The localization of the drug-induced hemolytic defect in primaquine-sensitive individuals. *J. Lab. Clin. Med. 43:*303, 1954.
4. Dern, R. J., Beutler, E., and Alving, A. S.: The hemolytic effect of primaquine. II. The natural course of the hemolytic anemia and the mechanism of its self-limited character. *J. Lab. Clin. Med. 44:*171, 1954.
5. Beutler, E., Dern, R. J., and Alving, A. S.: The hemolytic effect of primaquine. IV. The relationship of cell age to hemolysis. *J. Lab. Clin. Med. 44:*439, 1954.
6. Beutler, E., Dern, R. J., Flanagan, C. L., and Alving, A. S.: The hemolytic effect of primaquine. VII. Biochemical studies of drug-sensitive erythrocytes. *J. Lab. Clin. Med. 45:*286, 1955.
7. Beutler, E.: The glutathione instability of drug-sensitive red cells. A new method for the in vitro detection of drug-sensitivity. *J. Lab. Clin. Med., 49:*84, 1957.
8. Beutler, Robson, M., and Buttenwieser, E.: The mechanism of glutathione destruction and protection in drug-sensitive and non-sensitive erythrocytes. In vitro studies. *J. Clin. Invest. 36:*617, 1957.
9. Carson, P. E., Flanagan, C. L., Ickes, C. E., and Alving, A. S.: Enzymatic deficiency in primaquine-sensitive erythrocytes. *Science 124:*484, 1956.
10. Marks, P. A., and Gross, R. T.: Erythrocyte glucose-6-phosphate dehydrogenase deficiency: Evidence of differences between Negroes and Caucasians with respect to this genetically determined trait. *J. Clin. Invest. 38:*2253, 1959.

11. Testa, U., Meloni, T., Lania, A., Battistuzzi, G., Cutillo, S., and Luzzatto, L.: Genetic heterogeneity of glucose 6-phosphate dehydrogenase deficiency in Sardinia. *Hum. Genet.* 56:99, 1980.

12. Kirkman, H. N., Doxiadis, S. A., Valaes, T., Tassopoulos, N., and Brinson, A. G.: Diverse characteristics of glucose-6-phosphate dehydrogenase from Greek children. *J. Lab. Clin. Med.* 65:212, 1965.

13. Newton, W. A., Jr., and Bass, J. C.: Glutathione sensitive chronic non-spherocytic hemolytic anemia. *Am. J. Dis. Child.* 96:501, 1958.

14. Kirkman, H. N., Riley, H. D., Jr., and Crowell, B. B.: Different enzymic expressions of mutants of human glucose-6-phosphate dehydrogenase. *Proc. Natl. Acad. Sci. U.S.A.* 46:938, 1960.

15. Marks, P. A., and Gross, R. T.: Further characterization of the enzymatic defect in erythrocyte glucose-6-phosphate dehydrogenase deficiency. A genetically determined trait. *J. Clin. Invest.* 38:1023, 1959.

16. Piomelli, S., Corash, L. M., Davenport, D. D., Miraglia, J., and Amorosi, E. L.: In vivo lability of glucose-6-phosphate dehydrogenase in Gd^A and Gd^{Mediterranean} deficiency. *J. Clin. Invest.* 47:940, 1968.

17. Kahn, A., Cottreau, D., and Boivin, P.: Molecular mechanism of glucose-6-phosphate dehydrogenase deficiency. *Humangenetik* 25:101, 1974.

18. Kirkman, H. N., Schettini, F., and Pickard, B. M.: Mediterranean variant of glucose-6-phosphate dehydrogenase. *J. Lab. Clin. Med.* 63:726, 1964.

19. Soldin, S. J., and Balinsky, D.: The kinetic properties of human erythrocyte glucose-6-phosphate dehydrogenase. *Biochemistry* 7:1077, 1968.

20. Kirkman, H. N., and Riley, H. D., Jr.: Congenital nonspherocytic hemolytic anemia. *Am. J. Dis. Child.* 102:313, 1961.

21. Yoshida, A.: Hemolytic anemia and G-6-PD deficiency. *Science* 179:532, 1973.

22. Kahn, A., Boulard, M., Hakim, J., Schaison, G., Boivin, P., and Bernard, J.: Anémie hémolytique congénitale non sphèrocytaire par deficit en glucose-6-phosphate-deshydrogenase erythrocytaire. Description de deux nouvelles variantes: GD (−) Saint Louis (Paris) et GD (−) Hayem. *Nouv. Rev. Fr. Hematol.* 14:587, 1974.

23. Junien, C., Kaplan, J.-C., Meienhofer, M. C., Maigret, P., and Sender, A.: G-6-PD Baudelocque: A new unstable variant characterized in cultured fibroblasts. *Enzyme* 18:48, 1974.

24. Honig, G. R., Habacon, E., Vida, L. N., Matsumoto, F., and Beutler, E.: Three new variants of glucose-6-phosphate dehydrogenase associated with chronic nonspherocytic hemolytic anemia: G-6-PD Lincoln Park, G-6-PD Arlington Heights, and G-6-PD West Town. *Am. J. Hematol.* 6:353, 1979.

25. Kahn, A., Dao, C., Cottreau, D., and Bilski-Pasquier, G.: "GD (−) Hotel Dieu": A new G-6-PD variant with chronic hemolysis in a negro patient for Senegal. *Hum. Genet.* 39:353, 1977.

26. Smith, J. W., and Beutler, E.: Unpublished. 1981.

27. Beutler, E., Grooms, A. M., Morgan, S. K., and Trinidad, F.: Chronic severe hemolytic anemia due to G-6-PD Charleston: A new deficient variant. *J. Pediatr.* 80:1005, 1972.

28. Howell, E. B., Nelson, A. J., and Jones, O. W.: A new G-6-PD variant associated with chronic non-spherocytic haemolytic anaemia in a Negro family. *J. Med. Genet.* 9, 160, 1972.

29. Vaca, G., Ibarra, B., Romero, F., Olivares, N., Cantu, J. M., and Beutler, E.: G-6-PD Guadalajara: A new mutant associated with chronic non-spherocytic hemolytic anemia. *Hum. Genet.*, 1982, in press.

30. Feldman, R., Gromisch, D. S., Luhby, A. L., and Beutler, E.: Congenital nonspherocytic hemolytic anemia due to glucose-6-phosphate dehydrogenase East Harlem: A new deficient variant. *J. Pediatr.* 90:89, 1977.

31. Thigpen, J. T., Steinberg, M. H., Beutler, E., Gillespie, G. T., Jr., Dreiling, B. J., and Morrison, F. S.: Glucose-6-phosphate dehydrogenase Jackson. A new variant associated with hemolytic anemia. *Acta Haematol.* 51:310, 1974.

32. Fairbanks, V. F., Nepo, A. G., Beutler, E., Dickson, E. R., and Honig, G.: Glucose-6-phosphate dehydrogenase variants: Reexamination of G6PD Chicago and Cornell and a new variant (G6PD Pea Ridge) resembling G6PD Chicago. *Blood* 55:216, 1980.

33. Vives-Corrons, J. L., Feliu, E., Pujades, M. A., Rozman, C., Carreras, A., and Vallespi, M. T.: Severe glucose-6-phosphate dehydrogenase (G6PD) deficiency associated with chronic hemolytic anemia, granulocyte dysfunction and increased susceptibility to infections. Description of a new molecular variant (G6PD Barcelona). *Blood* 59:428, 1982.

34. Alperin, J. B., and Mills, G. C.: New variants of glucose-6-phosphate dehydrogenase: G6PD Kilgore and G6PD Galveston. *Tex. Rep. Biol. Med.* 31:727, 1973.

35. Chan, T. K., and Lai, M. C. S.: Glucose 6-phosphate dehydrogenase: Identity of erythrocyte and leukocyte enzyme with report of a new variant in Chinese. *Biochem. Genet.* 6:119, 1972.

36. Ramot, B., Ben-Bassat, I., and Shchory, M.: New glucose-6-phosphate dehydrogenase variants observed in Israel and their association with congenital nonspherocytic hemolytic disease. *J. Lab. Clin. Med.* 74:895, 1969.

37. Beutler, E., Mathai, C. K., and Smith, J. E.: Biochemical variants of glucose-6-phosphate dehydrogenase giving rise to congenital nonspherocytic hemolytic disease. *Blood* 31:131, 1968.

38. Talalak, P., and Beutler, E.: G-6-PD Bangkok: A new variant found in congenital nonspherocytic hemolytic disease (CNHD). *Blood* 33:772, 1969.

39. Nance, W. E.: Turner's syndrome, twinning, and an unusual variant of glucose-6-phosphate dehydrogenase. *Am. J. Hum. Genet.* 16:380, 1964.

40. Wong, P. W. K., Shih, L.-Y., and Hsia, D. Y. Y.: Characterization of glucose-6-phosphate dehydrogenase among Chinese. *Nature* 208:1323, 1965.

41. Necheles, T. F., Snyder, L. M., and Strauss, W.: Glucose-6-phosphate dehydrogenase Boston. A new variant associated with congenital nonspherocytic hemolytic disease. *Humangenetik* 13:218, 1971.

42. Rattazzi, M. C., Corash, L. M., Van Zanen, G. E., Jaffe, E. R., and Piomelli, S.: G6PD deficiency and chronic hemolysis: Four new mutants: Relationships between clinical syndrome and enzyme kinetics. *Blood* 38:205, 1971.

43. Beutler, E., and Matsumoto, F.: Unpublished. 1975.

44. Miwa, S., et al.: Two new glucose 6-phosphate dehydrogenase variants associated with congenital nonspherocytic hemolytic anemia found in Japan: Gd(−) Tokushima and Gd(−) Tokyo. *Am. J. Hematol.* 1:433, 1976.

45. Gahr, M., Schroeter, W., Sturzenegger, M., Bornhalm, D., and Marti, H. R.: Glucose-6-phosphate dehydrogenase (G-6-PD) deficiency in Switzerland. *Helv. Paediatr. Acta* 31:159, 1976.

46. Vuopio, P., Harkonen, R., Johnsson, R., and Nuutinen, M.: Red cell glucose-6-phosphate dehydrogenase deficiency in Finland. *Ann. Clin. Res.* 5:168, 1973.

47. Chernyak, N. B., Batischev, A. I., Lamzina, N. V., Tokarev, Y. N., and Alexeev, G. A.: Electrophoretic and kinetic properties of glucose-6-phosphate dehydrogenase from erythrocytes or patients with hemolytic anemia, related to deficiency of the enzyme activity. *Vopr. Med. Khim.* 23:166, 1977.

48. Miwa, S., et al.: Three new electrophoretically normal glucose-6-phosphate dehydrogenase variants associated with congenital nonspherocytic hemolytic anemia found in Japan: G6PD Ogikubo, Yokohama, and Akita. *Hum. Genet.* 45:11, 1978.

49. Prchal, J., Moreno, H., Conrad, M., and Vitek, A.: G-6-PD Dothan: A new variant associated with chronic hemolytic anemia. *IRCS* 7:348, 1979.

50. McCann, S. R., Smithwick, A. M., Temperley, I. J., and Tipton, K.: G6PD (Dublin): Chronic non-spherocytic haemolytic anaemia resulting from glucose-6-phosphate dehydrogenase deficiency in an Irish kindred. *J. Med. Genet.* 17:191, 1980.

51. Fujii, H., et al.: Glucose-6-phosphate dehydrogenase variants: A unique variant (G6PD Kobe) showed an extremely increased affinity for galactose 6-phosphate and a new variant (G6PD Sapporo) resembling G6PD Pea Ridge. *Hum. Genet.* 58:405, 1981.

52. Johnson, G. J., Kaplan, M. E., and Beutler, E.: G-6-PD Long Prairie: A new mutant exhibiting normal sensitivity to inhibition by NADPH and accompanied by nonspherocytic hemolytic anemia. *Blood* 49:247, 1977.

53. Cederbaum, A. I., and Beutler, E.: Nonspherocytic hemolytic anemia due to G-6-PD Grand Prairie. *IRCS* 3:579, 1975.

54. Kirkman, H. N., Rosenthal, I. M., Simon, E. R., Carson, P. E., and Brinson, A. G.: "Chicago I" variant of glucose-6-phosphate dehydrogenase in congenital hemolytic disease. *J. Lab. Clin. Med.* 63:715, 1964.

55. Beutler, E., Matsumoto, F., and Daiber, A.: Nonspherocytic hemolytic anemia due to G-6-PD Panama. *IRCS* 2:1389, 1974.

56. Honig, G. R., Habacon, E., Vida, L. N., Matsumoto, F., and Beutler, E.: Three new variants of glucose-6-phosphate dehydrogenase associated with Arlington Heights, and G-6-PD West Town. *Am. J. Hematol.* 6:353, 1979.

57. Johnson, G. J., and Beutler, E.: Unpublished. 1980.

58. Engstrom, P. F., and Beutler, E.: G-6-PD Tripler: A unique variant associated with chronic hemolytic disease. *Blood* 36:10, 1970.

59. Beutler, E., and Rosen, R.: Nonspherocytic congenital hemolytic anemia due to a new G-6-PD variant: G-6-PD Alhambra. *Pediatrics* 45:230, 1970.

60. Kidder, W. R., and Beutler, E.: Unpublished. 1979.

61. Milner, G., Delamore, I. W., and Yoshida, A.: G-6-PD Manchester: A new variant associated with chronic nonspherocytic hemolytic anemia. *Blood* 43:271, 1974.

62. Beutler, E., Keller, J. W., and Matsumoto, F.: A new glucose-6-P dehydrogenase (G-6-PD) variant associated with nonspherocytic hemolytic anemia: G-6-PD Atlanta. *IRCS* 4:579, 1976.

63. Snyder, L. M., Necheles, T. F., and Reddy, W. J.: G-6-PD Worcester: A new variant, associated with X-linked optic atrophy. *Am. J. Med.* 49:125, 1970.

64. Mentzer, W. C., Jr., Warner, R., Addiego, J., Smith, B., and Walter, T.: G6PD San Francisco: A new variant of glucose-6-phosphate dehydrogrenase associated with congenital nonspherocytic hemolytic anemia. *Blood* 55:195, 1980.

65. McCurdy, P. R.: Unpublished. 1975.

66. Castro, G. A. M., and Snyder, L. M.: G6PD San Jose: A new variant characterized by NADPH inhibition studies. *Humangenetik* 21:361, 1974.

67. McCurdy, P. R., Blackwell, P. Q., Todd, D., Tso, S. C., and Tuchinda, S.: Further studies on glucose-6-phosphate dehydrogenase deficiency in Chinese subjects. *J. Lab. Clin. Med.* 75:788, 1970.

68. Yoshida, A., Baur, E. W., and Motulsky, A. G.: A Philippino glucose-6-phosphate dehydrogenase variant (G6PD Union) with enzyme deficiency and altered substrate specificity. *Blood* 35:506, 1970.

69. Panich, V., and Na-Nakorn, S.: G-6-PD variants in Thailand. *J. Med. Assoc. Thai.* 63:537, 1980.

70. Kahn, A., North, M. L., Messer, J., Boivin, P.: G-6-PD "Ankara", a new G-6-PD variant with deficiency found in a Turkish family. *Humangenetik* 27:247, 1975.

71. Carandina, G., Moretto, E., Zecchi, G., and Conighi, C.: Glucose-6-phosphate dehydrogenase Ferrara. A new variant of G-6-PD identified in Northern Italy. *Acta Haematol.* 56:116, 1976.

72. Pawlak, A. L., Zagorski, Z., Roxynkowa, D., and Horst, A.: Polish variant of glucose-6-phosphate dehydrogenase (G-6-PD Lublin). *Humangenetik* 10:340, 1970.

73. Kirkman, H. N., Kidson, C., and Kennedy, M.: Variants of human glucose-6-phosphate dehydrogenase. Studies of samples from New Guinea, in *Hereditary Disorders of Erythrocyte Metabolism*, edited by E. Beutler. City of Hope Symposium Series, Grune & Stratton, New York, 1968, vol. I, pp. 126–145.

74. Panich, V., et al.: Glucose-6-phosphate dehydrogenase deficiency in South Vietnamese. *Hum. Hered.* 30:361, 1980.

75. Kirkman, H. N., and Luan, Eng, L.-I.: Variants of glucose 6 phosphate dehydrogenase in Indonesia. *Nature* 221:959, 1969.

76. McCurdy, P. R., and Mahmood, L.: Red cell glucose-6-phosphate dehydrogenase deficiency in Pakistan. *J. Lab. Clin. Med.* 76:943, 1970.

77. Yoshida, A.: Unpublished. 1975.

78. McCurdy, P. R., Kamel, K., and Selim, O.: Heterogeneity of red cell glucose-6-phosphate dehydrogenase (G-6-PD) deficiency in Egypt. *J. Lab. Clin. Med.* 84:673, 1974.

79. Geerdink, R. A., Horst, R., and Staal, G. E. J.: An Iraqi Jewish family with a new red cell glucose-6-phosphate dehydrogenase variant (Gd-Bagdad) and kernicterus. *Isr. J. Med. Sci.* 9:1040, 1973.

80. Kahn, A., Hakim, J., Cottreau, D., and Boivin, P.: Gd (−) Matam,

and African glucose-6-phosphate dehydrogenase variant with enzyme deficiency. Biochemical and immunological properties in various hemopoietic tissues. *Clin. Chim. Acta* 59:183, 1975.

81. Kahn, A., Bernard, J.-F., Cottreau, D., Marie, J., and Boivin, P.: Gd(−) Abrami. A deficient G-6PD variant with hemizygous expression in blood cells of a woman with primary myelofibrosis. *Humangenetik* 30:41, 1975.

82. Gahr, M., Bornhalm, D., and Schroeter, W.: Haemolytic anaemia due to glucose-6-phosphate dehydrogenase (G6PD) deficiency; Demonstration of two new biochemical variants, G6PD Hamm and G6PD Tarsus. *Br. J. Haematol.* 33:363, 1976.

83. Gahr, M., Bornhalm, D., and Schroeter, W.: Biochemische Eigenschaften einer neuen Variante des Glucose-6-Phosphatdehydrogenase (G-6-PD)-Mangels mit Favismus: G-6-PD Bielefeld. *Klin. Wochenschr.* 55:379, 1977.

84. Shatskaya, T. L., Krasnopolskaya, K. D., Tzoneva, M., Mavrudieva, M., and Toncheva, D.: Variants of erythrocyte glucose-6-phosphate dehydrogenase (G6PD) in Bulgarian populations. *Hum. Genet.* 54:115, 1980.

85. Yermakov, N., et al.: New stable mutant Gd(−) variants: G6PD Tashkent and G6PD Nucus. Molecular basis of hereditary enzyme deficiency. *Acta Biol. Med. Ger.* 40:559, 1981.

86. Banabadji, M., et al.: Heterogeneity of glucose-6-phosphate dehydrogenase deficiency in Algeria. *Hum. Genet.* 40:177, 1978.

87. Lisker, R., Briceno, R. P., Zavala, C., Navarrete, J. I., Wessles, M., and Yoshida, A.: A glucose 6-phosphate dehydrogenase Gd(−) Castilla variant characterized by mild deficiency associated with drug induced hemolytic anemia. *J. Lab. Clin. Med.* 90:754, 1977.

88. Beutler, E.: Glucose-6-phosphate dehydrogenase deficiency: A new Indian variant. G 6 PD Jammu, in *Trends in Haematology*, edited by N. N. Sen and A. K. Basu. N. N. Sen, Calcutta, India, 1975, pp. 279–283.

89. Vergnes, H., Yoshida, A., Gourdin, D., Gherardi, M., Bierme, R., and Ruffie, J.: Glucose-6-phosphate dehydrogenase Toulouse. A new variant with marked instability and severe deficiency discovered in a family of Mediterranean ancestry. *Acta Haematol.* 51:240, 1974.

90. Fernandez, M., and Fairbanks, V. F.: Glucose-6-phosphate dehydrogenase deficiency in the Phillipines: Report of a new variant— G 6 PD Panay. *Mayo Clin. Proc.* 43:645, 1968.

91. Krasnopolskaya, K. D., et al.: Genetic heterogeneity of G 6 PD deficiency: Study of mutant alleles in Shekii district of Azerbaijan. *Genetika* 13:1455, 1977.

92. Chockkalingan, K., and Board, P. G.: Further evidence for heterogeneity of glucose-6-phosphate dehydrogenase deficiency in Papua New Guinea. *Hum. Genet.* 56:209, 1980.

93. Pawlak, A. L., Mazurkiewicz, C. A., Ordynski, J., Rozynkowa, D., and Horst, A.: G-6-PD Poznan, variant with severe enzyme deficiency. *Humangenetik* 28:163, 1975.

94. Kahn, A., Esters, A., and Habedank, M.: Gd(−) Aachen, a new variant of deficient glucose-6-phosphate dehydrogenase. *Hum. Genet.* 32:171, 1976.

95. Miwa, S., et al.: Four new electrophoretically slow-moving glucose 6-phosphate dehydrogenase variants associated with congenital nonspherocytic hemolytic anemia found in Japan: Gd(−) Kurume, Gd(−) Fukushima, Gd(−) Yamaguchi and Gd(−) Wakayama. *Am. J. Hematol.* 5:131, 1978.

96. Shatskaya, T. L., Krasnopolskaya, K. D., and Idelson, L. J.: Mutant forms of erythrocyte glucose-6-phosphate dehydrogenase in Ashkenazi. Description of two new variants: G6PD Kirovograd and G6PD Zhitomir. *Hum. Genet.* 33:175, 1976.

97. Azevedo, E., Kirkman, H. N., Morrow, A. C., and Motulsky, A. G.: Variants of red cell glucose-6-phosphate dehydrogenase among Asiatic Indians. *Ann. Hum. Genet.* 31:373, 1968.

98. McCurdy, P. R., Maldonado, N., Dillon, D. E., and Conrad, M. E.: Variants of glucose-6-phosphate dehydrogenase (G-6-PD) associated with G-6-PD deficiency in Puerto Ricans. *J. Lab. Clin. Med.* 82:432, 1973.

99. Yoshida, A., Stamatoyannopoulos, G., and Motulsky, A.: Negro variant of glucose-6-phosphate dehydrogenase deficiency (A−) in man. *Science* 155:97, 1967.

100. Kirkman, H. N., McCurdy, P. R., and Naiman, J. L.: Functionally

abnormal glucose-6-phosphate dehydrogenases. *Cold Spring Harbor Symp. Quant. Biol.* 29:391, 1964.

101. Kirkman, H. N., and Hendrickson, E. M.: Sex-linked electrophoretic difference in glucose-6-phosphate dehydrogenase. *Am. J. Hum. Genet.* 15:241, 1963.

102. Kissin, C., and Cotte, J.: Étude d'un variant de glucose-6-phosphate deshydrogenase: Le type Constantine. *Enzyme* 11:277, 1970.

103. Vergnes, H., Riber, A., Bommelaer, G., Amadieu, J., and Brun, H.: Gd(−) Muret and Gd(−) Colomiers, two new variants of glucose-6-phosphate dehydrogenase associated with favism. *Hum. Genet.* 57:332, 1981.

104. Vergnes, H., Gherardi, M., and Yoshida, A.: G6PD Lozere and Trinacrialike. Segregation of two nonhemolytic variants in a French family. *Hum. Genet.* 34:293, 1976.

105. Nakashima, K., Ono, J., Abe, S., Miwa, S., and Yoshida, A.: G6PD Ube, a glucose-6-phosphate dehydrogenase variant found in four unrelated Japanese families. *Am. J. Hum. Genet.* 29:24, 1977.

106. Nakatsuji, T., and Miwa, S.: Incidence and characteristics of glucose-6-phosphate dehydrogenase variants in Japan. *Hum. Genet.* 51:297, 1979.

107. Lisker, R., Briceno, R. P., Agrilar, L., and Yoshida, A.: A variant glucose-6-phosphate dehydrogenase Gd (−) Chiapas. Associated with moderate enzyme deficiency and occasional hemolytic anemia. *Hum. Genet.* 43:81, 1978.

108. Kaplan, J. C., Rosa, R., Seringe, P., and Hoeffel, J. C.: Le Polymorphisme génétique de la glucose-6-phosphate deshydrogenase erythrocytaire chez l'homme. *Enzyme* 8:332, 1967.

109. Crookston, J. H., Yoshida, A., Lin, M., and Booser, D. J.: G 6 PD Toronto. *Biochem. J.* 8:259, 1973.

110. McCurdy, P. R., Kirkman, H. N., Naiman, J. L., Jim, R. T. S., and Pickard, B. M.: A Chinese variant of glucose-6-phosphate dehydrogenase. *J. Lab. Clin. Med.* 67:374, 1966.

111. Mandelli, F., Amadori, S., De Laurenzi, A., Kahn, A., Isacchi, G., and Papa, G.: Glucose-6-phosphate dehydrogenase Velletri. *Acta Haematol.* 57:121, 1977.

112. Sansone, G., Perroni, L., and Yoshida, A.: Glucose-6-phosphate dehydrogenase variants from Italian subjects associated with severe neonatal jaundice. *Br. J. Haematol.* 31:159, 1975.

113. Panich, V., Sungnate, T., Wasi, P., and Na Nakorn, S.: G-6-PD Mahidol. The most common glucose-6-phosphate dehydrogenase variant in Thailand. *J. Med. Assoc. Thai.* 55:576, 1972.

114. Panich, V., Sungnate, T., and Na Nakorn, S.: Acute intravascular hemolysis and renal failure in a new glucose-6-phosphate dehydrogenase variant: G-6-PD Siriraj. *J. Med. Assoc. Thai.* 55:726, 1972.

115. Miwa, S., Nakashima, K., Ono, J., Fujii, H., and Suzuki, E.: Three glucose 6-phosphate dehydrogenase variants found in Japan. *Hum. Genet.* 36:327, 1977.

116. Panich, V.: G-6-PD Intanon. A new glucose-6-phosphate dehydrogenase variant. *Humangenetik* 21:203, 1974.

117. Stamatoyannopoulos, G., Yoshida, A., Bacopoulos, C., and Motulsky, A.: Athens variant of glucose-6-phosphate dehydrogenase. *Science* 157:831, 1967.

118. Kahn, A., North, M. L., Cottreau, D., Giron, G., and Lang, J. M.: G6PD Vientiane: A new glucose-6-phosphate dehydrogenase variant with increased stability. *Hum. Genet.* 43:85, 1978.

119. Beutler, E., and Matsumoto, F.: A new glucose-6-phosphate dehydrogenase variant: G-6-PD (−) Los Angeles. *IRCS* 5:89, 1977.

120. De Flora, A., et al.: G6PD Napoli and Ferrara II: Two new glucose-6-phosphate dehydrogenase variants having similar characteristics but different intracellular lability and specific activity. *Br. J. Haematol.* 48:417, 1981.

121. Sansone, G., Perroni, L., and Yoshida, A.: Glucose-6-phosphate dehydrogenase variants from Italian subjects associated with severe neonatal jaundice. *Br. J. Haematol.* 31:159, 1975.

122. Sansone, G., Perroni, L., Yoshida, A., and Dave, V.: A new glucose-6-phosphate dehydrogenase variant (Gd Trinacria) in two unrelated families of Sicilian ancestry. *Ital. J. Biochem.* 26:44, 1977.

123. Yoshida, A.: Unpublished. 1975.

124. Lisker, R., Linares, C., and Motulsky, A. G.: Glucose-6-phosphate dehydrogenase Mexico. A new variant with enzyme deficiency, abnormal mobility and absence of hemolysis. *J. Lab. Clin. Med.* 79:788, 1972.

125. Gonzalez, R., Estrada, M., Garcia, M., and Guttierrez, A.: G6PD Ciudad de La Habana: A new slow variant with deficiency found in a Cuban family. *Hum. Genet.* 55:133, 1980.

126. Kirkman, H. N., Simon, E. R., and Pickard, B. M.: Seattle variant of glucose-6-phosphate dehydrogenase. *J. Lab. Clin. Med.* 66:834, 1965.

127. Kirkman, H. N., Ramot, B., and Lee, J. T.: Altered aggregational properties in a genetic variant of human glucose-6-phosphate dehydrogenase. *Biochem. Genet.* 3:137, 1969.

128. Siegel, N. H., and Beutler, E.: Hemolytic anemia caused by G-6-PD Carswell, a new variant. *Ann. Intern. Med.* 75:437, 1971.

129. Botha, M. C., Dern, R. J., Mitchell, M., West, C., and Beutler, E.: G6PD Capetown, a variant of glucose-6-phosphate dehydrogenase. *Am. J. Hum. Genet.* 21:547, 1969.

130. Panich, V., and Sungnate, T.: Characterization of glucose-6-phosphate dehydrogenase in Thailand. *Humangenetik* 18:39, 1973.

131. Reys, L., Manso, C., and Stamatoyannopoulos, G.: Genetic studies on Southeastern Bantu of Mozambique. I. Variants of glucose-6-phosphate dehydrogenase. *Am. J. Hum. Genet.* 22:203, 1970.

132. Vergnes, H., Gherardi, M., Quilici, J. C., Yoshida, A., and Giacardy, R.: G6PD Luz-Saint-Sauveur: A new variant with abnormal electrophoretic mobility, mild enzyme deficiency and absence of haematological disorders. *IRCS* 73:3-1-14, 1973 (abstract).

133. Boyer, S. H., Porter, I. H., and Weilbacher, R. G.: Electrophoretic heterogeneity of glucose-6-phosphate dehydrogenase and its relationship to enzyme deficiency in man. *Proc. Natl. Acad. Sci. U.S.A.* 48:1868, 1962.

134. Yoshida, A., Baur, E., and Voigtlander, B.: Unpublished. 1975.

135. Yoshida, A.: Glucose-6-phosphate dehydrogenase of human erythrocytes. I. Purification and characterization of normal (B+) enzyme. *J. Biol. Chem.* 241:4966, 1966.

136. Kirkman, H. N., and Hendrickson, E. M.: Glucose-6-phosphate dehydrogenase from human erythrocytes. II. Subactive states of the enzyme from normal persons. *J. Biol. Chem.* 237:2371, 1962.

137. Boyer, S. H., Porter, I. H., and Weilbacher, R. G.: Electrophoretic heterogeneity of glucose-6-phosphate dehydrogenase and its relationship to enzyme deficiency in man. *Proc. Natl. Acad. Sci. U.S.A.* 48:1868, 1962.

138. Beutler, E.: *Hemolytic Anemia in Disorders of Red Cell Metabolism.* Plenum, New York, 1978.

139. Long, W. K., Kirkman, H. N., and Sutton, H. E.: Electrophoretically slow variants of glucose-6-phosphate dehydrogenase from red cells of Negroes. *J. Lab. Clin. Med.* 65:81, 1965.

140. Gonzalez, R., Wade, M., Estrada, M., Svarch, E., and Colombo, B.: G6PD Pinar Rio: A new variant discovered in a Cuban family. *Biochem. Genet.* 15:909, 1977.

141. Kaplan, J. C., Hanzlickova Leroux, A., Nicholas, A. M., Rosa, R., Weiler, C., and Lepercq, G.: A new glucose-6-phosphate dehydrogenase variant (G6PD Port-Royal). *Enzyme* 12:25, 1970.

142. Cayanis, E., Lane, A. B., Jenkins, T., Nurse, G. T., and Balinsky, D.: Glucose-6-phosphate dehydrogenase Probandar: A new slow variant with slightly reduced activity in a South African family of Indian descent. *Biochem. Genet.* 15:765, 1977.

143. Dern, R. J., Mc Curdy, P. R., and Yoshida, A.: A new structural variant of glucose-6-phosphate dehydrogenase with a high production rate (G6PD). *J. Lab. Clin. Med.* 73:283, 1969.

144. Yoshida, A., and Beutler, E.: G-6-PD variants: Another up-date. *Ann. Hum. Genet.* 47:27, 1983.

145. Yoshida, A.: A single amino acid substitution (asparagine to aspartic acid) between normal (B+) and the common Negro variant (A+) of human glucose-6-phosphate dehydrogenase. *Proc. Natl. Acad. Sci. U.S.A.* 57:835, 1967.

146. Porter, I. H., Boyer, S. H., Watson-Williams, E. J., Adam, A., Szeinberg, A., and Siniscalco, M.: Variation of glucose-6-phosphate dehydrogenase in different populations. *Lancet* 1:895, 1964.

147. Luzzatto, L., and Allan, N. C.: Different properties of glucose-6-phosphate dehydrogenase from human erythrocytes with normal and abnormal enzyme levels. *Biochem. Biophys. Res. Commun.* 21:547, 1965.

148. Stamatoyannopoulos, G., Voigtlandger, V., Kotsakis, P., and Akrivakis, A.: Genetic diversity of the "Mediterranean" glucose-6-phosphate dehydrogenase deficiency phenotype. *J. Clin. Invest.* 50:1253, 1971.

149. Chan, T. K., and Todd, D.: Characteristics and distribution of

glucose-6-phosphate dehydrogenase-deficient variants in South China. *Am. J. Hum. Genet. 24*:475, 1972.

150. Beutler, E., Dern, R. J., and Alving, A. S.: The hemolytic effect of Primaquine. VI. An in vitro test for sensitivity of erythrocytes to Primaquine. *J. Lab. Clin. Med. 45*:40, 1955.

151. Fertman, M. H., and Fertman, M. D.: Toxic anemias and Heinz bodies. *Medicine (Baltimore) 34*:131, 1955.

152. Cohen, G., and Hochstein, P.: Generation of hydrogen peroxide in erythrocytes by hemolytic agents. *Biochemistry 3*:895, 1964.

153. Kosower, N. S., Song, K.-R., Kosower, E. M., and Correa, W.: Glutathione. II. Chemical aspects of azoester procedure for oxidation to disulfide. *Biochim. Biophys. Acta 192*:8, 1969.

154. Allen, E. W., and Jandl, J. H.: Oxidative hemolysis and precipitation of hemoglobin. II. Role of thiols in oxidant drug action. *J. Clin. Invest. 40*:454, 1961.

155. Birchmeier, W., Tuchschmid, P. E., and Winterhalter, H.: Comparison of human hemoglobin A carrying glutathione as a mixed disulfide with the naturally occurring human hemoglobin A3. *Biochemistry 12*:3667, 1973.

156. Rachmilewitz, E. A., Harari, E., and Winterhalter, K. H.: Separation of α and β chains of hemoglobin A by acetylphenylhydrazine. *Biochim. Biophys. Acta 371*:402, 1974.

157. Itano, H. A., Hosokawa, K., and Hirota, K.: Induction of haemolytic anaemia by substituted phenylhydrazines. *Br. J. Haematol. 32*:99, 1976.

158. Srivastava, S. K., and Beutler, E.: Glutathione metabolism of the erythrocyte. The enzymic cleavage of glutathione-haemoglobin preparations by glutathione reductase. *Biochem. J. 119*:353, 1970.

159. Rifkind, R. A.: Heinz body anemia: An ultrastructural study. II. Red cell sequestration and destruction. *Blood 26*:433, 1965.

160. Harley, J. D., and Mauer, A. M.: Studies on the formation of Heinz bodies. I. Methemoglobin production and oxyhemoglobin destruction. *Blood 16*:1722, 1960.

161. Bunn, H. E. F., and Jandl, J. H.: Exchange of heme among hemoglobin molecules. *Proc. Natl. Acad. Sci. U.S.A. 56*:974, 1966.

162. Jandl, J. H.: The Heinz body hemolytic anemias. *Ann. Intern. Med. 58*:702, 1963.

163. Beutler, E.: Abnormalities of glycolysis (HMP shunt). *Bibl. Haematol. 29*:146, 1968.

164. Baehner, R. L.: Nathan, D. G., and Castle, W. B.: Oxidant injury of Caucasian glucose-6-phosphate dehydrogenase-deficient red blood cells by phagocytosing leukocytes during infection. *J. Clin. Invest. 50*:2466, 1971.

165. Mager, J., Glaser, G., Razin, A., Izak, G., Bien, S., and Noam, M.: Metabolic effects of pyrimidines derived from fava bean glycosides on human erythrocytes deficient in glucose-6-phosphate dehydrogenase. *Biochem. Biophys. Res. Commun. 20*:235, 1965.

166. Beutler, E.: L-Dopa and Favism. *Blood 36*:523, 1970.

167. Stamatoyannopoulos, G., Fraser, G. R., Motulsky, A. G., Fessas, P. Akrivakis, A., and Papayannopoulou, T.: On the familial predisposition to favism. *Am. J. Hum. Genet. 18*:253, 1966.

168. Cassimos, C. H. R., Malaka Zafiriu, K., and Tslures, J.: Urinary D-glucaric acid excretion in normal and G-6-PD deficient children with Favism. *J. Pediatr. 84*:871, 1974.

169. Fiorelli, G., Podd, M., Corrias, A., and Fargion, S.: The relevance of immune reactions in acute Favism. *Acta Haematol. 51*:211, 1974.

170. Childs, B., Zinkham, W., Browne, E. A., Kimbro, E. L., Torbert, J. V.: A genetic study of a defect in glutathione metabolism of the erythrocyte. *Johns Hopkins Med. J. 102*:1958.

171. Beutler, E., and Baluda, M. C.: The separation of glucose-6-phosphate dehydrogenase-deficient erythrocytes from the blood of heterozygotes for glucose-6-phosphate dehydrogenase deficiency. *Lancet 1*:189, 1964.

172. Gartler, S. M., and Linder, D.: Developmental and evolutionary implications of the mosaic nature of the G-6-PD system. *Cold Spring Harbor Symp. Quant. Biol. 29*:253, 1964.

173. Beutler, E.: The distribution of gene products among populations of cells in heterozygous humans. *Cold Spring Harbor Symp. Quant. Biol. 29*:261, 1964.

174. Motulsky, A. G.: Metabolic metamorphisms and the role of infectious diseases in human evolution. *Hum. Biol. 32*:28, 1960.

175. Luzzatto, L., Usanga, E. A., and Reddy, S.: Glucose 6-phosphate dehydrogenase deficient red cells: Resistant to infection by malarial parasites. *Science 164*:839, 1969.

176. Piomelli, S., Reindorf, C. A., Arzanian, M. T., and Corash, L. M.: Clinical and biochemical interactions of glucose-6-phosphate dehydrogenase deficiency and sickle-cell anemia. *N. Engl. J. Med. 287*:213, 1972.

177. Lewis, R. A., and Hathorn, M.: Correlation of S hemoglobin with glucose-6-phosphate dehydrogenase deficiency and its significance. *Blood 26*:176, 1965.

178. Steinberg, M. H., and Dreiling, B. J.: Glucose-6-phosphate dehydrogenase deficiency in sickle cell anemia. *Ann. Intern. Med. 80*:217, 1974.

179. Beutler, E., Johnson, C., Powars, D., and West, C.: Prevalence of glucose-6-phosphate dehydrogenase deficiency in sickle cell disease. *N. Engl. J. Med. 290*:826, 1974.

180. McCaffrey, R. P.: Halsted, C. H., Wahab, M. F. A., and Robertson, R. P.: Chloramphenicol-induced hemolysis in Caucasian glucose-6-phosphate dehydrogenase deficiency. *Ann. Intern. Med. 74*:722, 1971.

181. Chan, T. K., Chesterman, C. N., McFadzean, A. J. S., and Todd, D.: The survival of glucose-6-phosphate dehydrogenase-deficient erythrocytes in patients with typhoid fever on chloramphenicol therapy. *J. Lab. Clin. Med. 77*:177, 1971.

182. Dern, R. J., Beutler, E., and Alving, A. S.: The hemolytic effect of Primaquine. V. Primaquine sensitivity as a manifestation of a multiple drug sensitivity. *J. Lab. Clin. Med. 45*:40, 1955.

183. Beutler, E., Dern, R. J., and Alving, A. S.: The hemolytic effect of Primaquine. III. A study of primaquine-sensitive erythrocytes. *J. Lab. Clin. Med. 44*:177, 1954.

184. Salvidio, E., Pannacceulli, I., and Tizianello, A.: La capacità eritropoietica dei soggetti con deficienza di g 6 PD eritrocitaria. *Atti. Accad. Med. Lomb. 22*:16, 1967.

185. George, J. N., Sears, D. A., McCurdy, P., and Conrad, M. E.: Primaquine sensitivity in Caucasians: Hemolytic reactions induced by primaquine in G-6-PD deficient subjects. *J. Lab. Clin. Med. 70*:80, 1967.

186. Gray, G. R., et al.: Neutrophil dysfunction, chronic granulomatous disease, and nonspherocytic haemolytic anaemia caused by complete deficiency of glucose-6-phosphate dehydrogenase. *Lancet 2*:530, 1973.

187. Cooper, M. R., De Chatelet, L. R., McCall, C. E., La Via, J. F., Spurr, C. L., and Baehner, R. L.: Complete deficiency of leukocyte glucose-6-phosphate dehydrogenase with defective bactericidal activity. *J. Clin. Invest. 51*:769, 1972.

188. Schwartz, J. P., Cooperberg, A. A., and Rosenberg, A.: Platelet-function studies in patients with glucose-6-phosphate dehydrogenase deficiency. *Br. J. Haematol. 27*:273, 1974.

189. Gray, G. R., Naiman, S. C., and Robinson, G. C. F.: Platelet function and G-6-PD deficiency. *Lancet 1*:997, 1974.

190. Harley, J. D., Agar, N. S., and Yoshida, A.: Glucose-6-phosphate dehydrogenase variants: Gd (+) Alexandra associated with neonatal jaundice and Gd (−) Camperdown in a young man with lamellar cataracts. *J. Lab. Clin. Med. 91*:295, 1978.

191. Harley, J. D., Agar, N. S., and Gruca, M. A.: Cataracts with a glucose-6-phosphate dehydrogenase variant. *Br. Med. J. 2*:86, 1975.

192. Westring, D. W., and Pisciotta, A. V.: Anemia, cataracts, and seizures in patient with glucose-6-phosphate dehydrogenase deficiency. *Arch. Intern. Med. 118*:385, 1966.

193. Panich, V., and Na Nakorn, S.: G-6-PD deficiency in senile cataracts. *Hum. Genet. 55*:123, 1980.

194. Orzalesi, N., Sorcinelli, R., and Guiso, G.: Increased incidence of cataract in male subjects deficient in glucose-6-phosphate dehydrogenase. *Arch. Ophthalmol. 99*:69, 1981.

195. Beutler, E.: Glucose-6-phosphate dehydrogenase deficiency and non-spherocytic congenital hemolytic anemia. *Semin. Hematol. 2*:91, 1965.

196. Burka, E. R., Weaver, Z., III, and Marks, P. A.: Clinical spectrum of hemolytic anemia associated with G 6 PD deficiency. *Ann. Intern. Med. 64*:817, 1966.

197. Salen, G., Goldstein, F., Haurani, F., and Wirts, C. W.: Acute hemolytic anemia complicating viral hepatitis in patients with glucose-6-phosphate dehydrogenase deficiency. *Ann. Intern. Med. 65*:1210, 1966.

198. Phillips, S. M., and Silvers, N. P.: Glucose-6-phosphate dehydrogenase deficiency, infectious hepatitis, acute hemolysis, and renal failure. *Ann. Intern. Med.* 70:99, 1969.

199. Clearfield, H. R., Brody, J. I., and Tumen, H. J.: Acute viral hepatitis, glucose-6-phosphate dehydrogenase deficiency, and hemolytic anemia. *Arch. Intern. Med.* 123:689, 1969.

200. Kattamis, C. A., and Tjortjatou, F.: The hemolytic process of viral hepatitis in children with normal or deficient glucose-6-phosphate dehydrogenase activity. *J. Pediatr.* 77:422, 1970.

201. Boon, W. H.: Viral hepatitis in G-6-PD deficiency. *Lancet* 1:882, 1966.

202. Kattamis, C. A., Kyriazakou, M., and Chaidas, S.: Favism. Clinical and biochemical data. *J. Med. Genet.* 6:34, 1969.

203. Doxiadis, S. A., Fessas, P., Valaes, T., and Mastrokalos, N.: Glucose-6-phosphate dehydrogenase deficiency. *Lancet* 1:297, 1961.

204. Smith, G., and Vella, F.: Erythrocyte enzyme deficiency in unexplained kernicterus. *Lancet* 1:1133, 1960.

205. Zinkham, W. H.: Peripheral blood and bilirubin values in normal full-term primaquine-sensitive Negro infants: Effect of vitamin K. *Pediatrics* 31:983, 1963.

206. Ifekwunigwe, A. E., and Luzzatto, L.: Kernicterus in G-6-PD deficiency. *Lancet* 1:667, 1966.

207. Eshaghpour, E., Oski, F. A., and Williams, M.: The relationship of erythrocyte glucose-6-phosphate dehydrogenase deficiency to hyperbilirubinemia in Negro premature infants. *J. Pediatr.* 70:595, 1967.

208. Lopez, R., and Cooperman, J. M.: Glucose-6-phosphate dehydrogenase deficiency and hyperbilirubinemia in the newborn. *Am. J. Dis. Child.* 122:66, 1971.

209. Ben-Bassat, J., and Ben-Ishay, D.: Hereditary hemolytic anemia associated with glucose-6-phosphate dehydrogenase deficiency (Mediterranean type). *Isr. J. Med. Sci.* 5:1053, 1969.

210. Danon, D., Sheba, C., and Ramot, B.: The morphology of glucose 6 phosphate dehydrogenase deficient erythrocytes: Electron-microscopic studies. *Blood* 17:229, 1961.

211. Greenberg, M. S.: Heinz body hemolytic anemia. *Arch. Intern. Med.* 136:153, 1976.

212. Nathan, D. M., Siegel, A. J., and Bunn, H. F.: Acute methemoglobinemia and hemolytic anemia with phenazopyridine. *Arch. Intern. Med.* 137:1636, 1977.

213. Betke, K., et al.: Standardization of procedures for the study of glucose-6-phosphate dehydrogenase. Report of a WHO Scientific Group. *WHO Tech. Rep. Ser. No. 366*, 1967.

214. Beutler, E.: Glucose-6-phosphate dehydrogenase deficiency, diagnosis, clinical and genetic implications. *Am. J. Clin. Pathol.* 47:303, 1967.

215. Jacob, H., and Jandl, J. H.: A simple visual screening test for G-6-PD deficiency employing ascorbate and cyanide. *N. Engl. J. Med.* 274:1162, 1966.

216. Beutler, E., and Mitchell, M.: Special modifications of the fluorescent screening method for glucose-6-phosphate dehydrogenase deficiency. *Blood* 32:816, 1968.

217. Brewer, G. J., Tarlov, A. R., and Alving, A. S.: The methemoglobin reduction test for Primaquine-type sensitivity of erythrocytes. *JAMA* 180:386, 1962.

218. Fairbanks, V. F., and Beutler, E.: A simple method for detection of erythrocyte glucose-6-phosphate dehydrogenase deficiency (G-6-PD spot test). *Blood* 20:591, 1962.

219. Herz, F., Kaplan, E., and Scheye, E. S.: Diagnosis of erythrocyte glucose-6-phosphate dehydrogenase deficiency in the Negro male despite hemolytic crisis. *Blood* 35:90, 1970.

220. Ringelhahn, B.: A simple laboratory procedure for the recognition of A− (African type) G6PD deficiency in acute haemolytic crisis. *Clin. Chim. Acta* 36:272, 1972.

221. Fairbanks, V. F., and Lampe, L. T.: A tetrazolium-linked cytochemical method for estimation of glucose-6-phosphate dehydrogenase activity in individual erythrocytes: Applications in the study of heterozygotes for glucose-6-phosphate dehydrogenase deficiency. *Blood* 31:589, 1968.

222. Beutler, E.: G-6-PD activity of individual erythrocytes and X-chromosomal inactivation, in *Biochemical Methods in Red Cell Genetics*, edited by J. J. Yunis. Academic, New York, 1969, pp. 95–113.

223. Spielberg, S. P., Boxer, L. A., Corash, L. M., and Schulman, J. D.: Improved erythrocyte survival with high dose vitamin E in chronic hemolyzing G6PD and glutathione synthetase deficiencies. *Ann. Intern. Med.* 90:53, 1978.

224. Corash, L., et al.: Reduced chronic hemolysis during high-dose vitamin E administration in Mediterranean-type glucose-6-phosphate dehydrogenase deficiency. *N. Engl. J. Med.* 303:416, 1980.

225. Petrakis, N. L., Wiesenfeld, S. L., Sams, B. J., Collen, M. F., Cutler, J. L., and Siegelaub, A. B.: Prevalence of sickle-cell trait and glucose-6-phosphate dehydrogenase deficiency. *N. Engl. J. Med.* 282:767, 1970.

226. Heller, P., Best, W. R., Nelson, R. B., and Becktel, J.: Clinical implications of sickle-cell trait and glucose-6-phosphate dehydrogenase deficiency in hospitalized black male patients. *N. Engl. J. Med.* 300:1001, 1979.

CHAPTER *59*

Hereditary nonspherocytic hemolytic anemia — pyruvate kinase deficiency and other abnormalities

ERNEST BEUTLER

Definition

Although in the previous two decades other patients fitting this description had been documented, the designation *hereditary nonspherocytic hemolytic anemia* was first introduced by Crosby [1] in 1950. Dacie and his colleagues [2] subsequently reported several families in which affected members manifested hemolytic anemia from an early age and in whom the osmotic fragility of the red cells was normal. The latter finding, and the fact that most of the affected individuals failed to benefit from splenectomy, distinguished this disorder from hereditary spherocytosis. Thus defined essentially by exclusion as a hereditary hemolytic anemia that is not hereditary spherocytosis, it is not at all surprising that hereditary nonspherocytic hemolytic anemia has proved to be extremely heterogeneous, both in etiology and in clinical manifestations. Sometimes this disorder is also designated *congenital nonspherocytic hemolytic anemia*, but the name *hereditary* is more accurate, and is therefore preferable. While hereditary ovalocytosis, pyropoikylocytosis, stomatocytosis, and even sickle cell disease and thalassemia major are hereditary hemolytic anemias that are not spherocytic, they are not included. Rather, the diagnosis of hereditary nonspherocytic hemolytic anemia is reserved for those patients who have no major aberrations of red cell morphology.

In 1954 Selwyn and Dacie [3] studied the autohemolysis (spontaneous lysis of red cells after sterile incubation of 24 to 48 h at 37°C) of four patients with hereditary nonspherocytic hemolytic anemia and found that in two of them lysis was only slightly increased and was prevented by glucose; these patients were designated as *type 1*. Autohemolysis of the red cells of the other two patients was more marked and was not corrected by glucose; these patients were classified as *type 2*. It is remarkable that the autohemolysis test and the classification of patients with hereditary nonspherocytic hemolytic anemia into types 1 and 2 has occupied center stage in the differential diagnosis of this type of anemia for the past quarter century, although the test is of little or no value [4–6]. The test does have historical significance, however. The fact that autohemolysis was modified by the addition of ATP, a substance that we now recognize does not penetrate the red cell membrane, suggested to De Gruchy et al. [7,8] that patients with type 2 autohemolysis suffered from a defect in ATP generation. This suggestion, born of a misunderstanding of red cell metabolism, turned out to be correct: one of the major causes of hereditary nonspherocytic hemolytic anemia has proved to be a deficiency of the ATP-generating enzyme pyruvate kinase (PK). This enzyme deficiency was first demonstrated in 1961 by Valentine et al. [9]. A deficiency of glucose-6-phosphate dehydrogenase (G-6-PD) had been found a few years earlier by Newton and Bass [10] to be responsible for hemolysis in other patients. These were only the first of a large number of enzyme defects that have been shown to account for this heterogeneous syndrome [11,12].

Etiology and pathogenesis

Hereditary nonspherocytic hemolytic anemia defined in the broad clinical sense may be caused by (1) an enzyme deficiency, (2) a hemoglobinopathy, or (3) a defect in membrane structure. In the majority of patients the underlying lesion cannot be identified. The enzyme deficiencies which have been shown to cause hereditary nonspherocytic hemolytic anemia are listed in Table 59-1. How a deficiency of any one of these enzymes results in shortening of red cell life-span remains unknown, although it has been the object of much experimental work and of speculation. It is often believed that ATP depletion is a common pathway in producing damage to the cell, leading to its destruction [46], but the evidence that this is the case is not always compelling [47]. It is possible that, at least in some cases, distortion of the pattern of red cell intermediate metabolites interferes with synthesis of cell components in early stages of development of the cell.

Not all deficiencies of red cell enzymes lead to hemolytic disease [48]. Red cell enzyme deficiencies which do not produce hemolytic disease are summarized in Table 59-2. Thus, acatalasemia, the virtually total absence of red cell catalase, is devoid of hemato-

logic manifestations. Similarly, red cells without cholinesterase [73,74] and those without lactate dehydrogenase [75] seem to survive normally. Although deficiencies of phosphoglycerate kinase and of glutathione synthetase are usually associated with hereditary nonspherocytic hemolytic anemia, cases have been reported in which these deficiencies were unassociated with any hematologic manifestations [76,77]. Although it has at times been suggested that moderate decreases in the activity of glutathione reductase and of glutathione peroxidase caused hemolytic anemia, the best available evidence indicates that these enzymes are not ordinarily rate-limiting in erythrocyte metabolism and are not associated with hemolytic anemia [12]. Even the total absence of glutathione reductase in the red cells of members of one family were associated with only rare episodes of hemolysis, possibly caused by fava beans, in otherwise hematologically normal individuals [32].

Patients with unstable hemoglobins may present with the clinical picture of hereditary nonspherocytic hemolytic anemia. The mechanism of destruction of the red cells in these disorders is probably related to changes in deformability of the cell and to abnormalities of the membrane induced by attachment of denatured globin precipitates. Lacking normal deformability characteristics, such cells presumably encounter difficulty in negotiating the tortuous course through the spleen. The unstable hemoglobins are discussed in Chap. 61.

It is not known precisely why cells with abnormal membrane composition may have a shortened life-span, but since it is the membrane of the cell which comes into contact with the macrophages, altered recognition is probably an important factor. It is often assumed that impaired membrane deformability also plays a major role in cell destruction. However, this has not clearly been shown to be the case.

Mode of inheritance

The modes of inheritance of the various enzyme abnormalities leading to hereditary nonspherocytic hemolytic anemia are summarized in Table 59-1.

Examples of all of the ordinary types of Mendelian inheritance are to be found. Glucose-6-phosphate dehydrogenase deficiency and phosphoglycerate kinase deficiency are inherited as sex-linked disorders. The other deficiencies of glycolytic enzymes are inherited as autosomal recessive disorders. In most instances heterozygotes manifest partial enzyme deficiencies, but this is not always true; in aldolase deficiency both parents were normal [19]. Autosomal dominant inheritance is characteristic of the unstable hemoglobins and in patients with increased adenosine deaminase. The only membrane abnormality which has been clearly identified as producing hereditary nonspherocytic hemolytic anemia is an abnormality in lipid composition encountered in a single family [78]. The inheritance in this family seemed to be autosomal dominant.

TABLE 59-1 Red cell enzyme abnormalities leading to hematologic disease

Enzyme	Clinical features*	Inheritance*	Red cell morphology	Diagnosis — Screening test	Diagnosis — Assay	Response to splenectomy†	Approximate frequency‡	Reference
Hexokinase	HNSHA	AR	Unremarkable	–	[13]	++	Rare	[12,14]
Glucose phosphate isomerase	HNSHA	AR	Unremarkable	[15]	[13]	+++	Unusual	[12,16]
Phosphofructokinase	HNSHA and/or muscle glycogen storage disease	AR	Unremarkable	–	[13]	0	Rare	[12,17,18]
Aldolase	HNSHA and mild liver glycogen storage; ? mental retardation	AR	Unremarkable	–	[13]	?	Very rare	[19,89]
Triosephosphate isomerase	HNSHA and severe neuromuscular disease	AR	Unremarkable	[20,21]	[13]	0	Rare	[22]
Phosphoglycerate kinase	HNSHA; mild behavioral disturbances	SL	Unremarkable	–	[13]	++	Rare	[12,23,24]
Diphosphoglycerate mutase	HNSHA; polycythemia	AR	Unremarkable	–	[13]		Rare	[12,25,26]
Pyruvate kinase	HNSHA	AR	Usually unremarkable; occasionally contracted echinocytes	[27]	[13]	++	Unusual	[9,12,28]
Glucose-6-phosphate dehydrogenase	HNSHA; drug or infection-induced hemolysis; favism	SL	Usually unremarkable; rarely "bite cells"	[29]	[13]	±	Very common in some populations	[10,12,30,31]
Glutathione reductase (complete)	Drug sensitive hemolytic anemia and favism		Unremarkable	[27]	[13]	?	Very rare	[32]
γ-Glutamyl cysteine synthetase	HNSHA; drug- or infection-induced hemolysis	AR	Unremarkable	[33]	[34]	?	Very rare	[12,35]
Glutathione synthetase	HNSHA; drug- or infection-induced hemolysis; neurologic defect and 5-oxoprolinuria in some cases	AR	Usually unremarkable	[33]	[34]	++	Rare	[12,36,37]

TABLE 59-1   Red cell enzyme abnormalities leading to hematologic disease (*Continued*)

Enzyme	Inheritance*	Clinical features	Red cell morphology	Diagnosis		Response to splenectomy†	Approximate frequency‡	Reference
				Screening test	Assay			
Pyrimidine-5'-nucleotidase	AR	HNSHA; ? mental retardation in some cases	Prominent stippling	[38]	[39]	+	Rare	[38,40]
Adenosine deaminase (increased activity)	AR	HNSHA	Unremarkable		[13]		Very rare	[40,41]
Adenosine deaminase (decreased activity)	AR	Immunodeficiency	Unremarkable		[13]		Rare	[42]
Adenylate kinase	AR	HNSHA			[13]	?	Very rare	[43,90]
NADH-diaphorase (cytochrome b_5 reductase)	AR	Methemoglobinemia; sometimes with mental retardation	Unremarkable	[44]	[13]		Unusual	[45]

* AR = autosomal recessive; AD = autosomal dominant; SL = sex linked.
† On a scale of 0 to 4+, where 4+ is complete response. In many cases data are meager.
‡ Very common if incidence is greater than 5%. Unusual if more than 100 cases reported. Rare if 10 to 100 cases reported. Very rare if less than 10 cases reported.

TABLE 59-2   Red cell enzyme abnormalities not leading to hematologic disease

Enzyme	Clinical features	Inheritance‡	Diagnosis assay	Estimated frequency*	Reference
Glutathione reductase (partial deficiency)	None	Usually not inherited	[13]	Very common	[12,49]
Glutathione peroxidase (partial deficiency)	None	AR and AD	[13]	Very common	[12,50]
Catalase	Oral ulcers in some types	AR	[13]	Rare	[51,52]
Hypoxanthine-guanine phosphoribosyl transferase (HGPRT)	Lesch-Nyhan syndrome (neurologic symptoms and gout)	SL	[53]	Rare	[54]
Adenine phosphoribosyl transferase	Kidney stones	AR	[55]	Rare	[56]
Galactokinase	Cataracts	AR	[57,58]	Rare	[59]
Galactose-1-P-uridyl transferase	Cataracts; mental retardation; liver disease	AR	[60]	Rare	[61]
Lactate dehydrogenase	None	AR	[13]	Rare	[62]
Phosphoglucomutase	None	AR	[13]	Rare	[63]
Uroporphyrinogen 1 synthase	Acute intermittent porphyria	AD	[64]	Unusual (common in selected populations)	[65]
Glyceraldehyde phosphate dehydrogenase (partial defect)	None	AD	[13]	Unusual	[66]
6-Phosphogluconate dehydrogenase (complete deficiency)	None	AR	[13]	Unusual	[67]
NADPH diaphorase	None	AR	[13]	Rare	[68]
Carbonic anhydrase I	None	AR	[69]	Rare	[70]
ITPase	None	AR	[71]		[72]
Glyoxalase I	None	AR		Rare	[91]
Acetyl-cholinesterase	None	AR			
δ-ALA dehydrase	None	AD			

* Very common if incidence is greater than 5%, common if 1 to 5%, unusual if 0.01 to 1%, rare if less than 0.01%.
‡ See Table 59-1 for definition of abbreviations.

Clinical features

Most of the patients with hereditary nonspherocytic hemolytic anemia manifest only the usual clinical signs and symptoms of chronic hemolysis. The degree of anemia in this group of disorders varies widely, and steady-state hemoglobin levels as low as 5 g/dl may be encountered in some patients, while others may manifest compensated hemolysis with a normal steady-state hemoglobin concentration. Chronic jaundice is a common finding, and splenomegaly is often present. Gallstones are common. When hemolysis is due to an abnormal hemoglobin, unusual pyrrole pigments may be excreted in the urine.

In the case of some enzyme defects characteristic nonhematologic systemic manifestations may be present, and these may be the only sign of the enzyme deficiency. For example, patients with phosphofructokinase deficiency may have type VII muscle glycogen storage disease without any evidence of hemolysis. In some patients with this defect hemolysis is present without muscle manifestations [79,80], and in other patients both muscle abnormalities and hemolysis occur [18]. Similarly, glutathione synthetase deficiency may be associated with 5-oxoprolinuria and neuromuscular disturbances, and such abnormalities may occur either with [81] or without hematologic abnormalities [77]. On the other hand, some patients with glutathione synthetase deficiency manifest only the hematologic abnormalities [37]. Patients with triosephosphate isomerase deficiency nearly always manifest serious neuromuscular disease, and most of the patients who inherit this abnormality die in the first decade of life [82–84]. The various clinical features of enzyme deficiencies causing nonspherocytic hemolytic anemia are summarized in Table 59-1.

Laboratory features

Varying degrees of anemia and reticulocytosis represent the main, routine hematologic laboratory features of hereditary nonspherocytic hemolytic anemia. Basophilic stippling of the erythrocytes is prominent in most patients with pyrimidine-5'-nucleotidase deficiency, but may no longer be apparent in blood that has been collected in EDTA anticoagulant. Heinz bodies are often found in the erythrocytes of splenectomized patients with unstable hemoglobins, but are usually not seen in the unsplenectomized state. The presence of small, densely staining cells has often been noted in the blood films of patients with hereditary nonspherocytic hemolytic anemia. Particularly when manifesting an echinocytic appearance, such cells have been thought to be common in pyruvate kinase deficiency. In one reported case [85] spectacular numbers of such cells were observed. However, cells of this type are seen in many blood films both from patients with glycolytic enzyme deficiencies and from those with other disorders, and it

is hazardous to attempt to make an enzymatic diagnosis on the basis of such findings. Leukopenia is occasionally observed in patients with hereditary nonspherocytic hemolytic anemia, possibly secondary to splenic enlargement. Other laboratory stigmata of increased hemolysis may include increased levels of serum bilirubin, decreased haptoglobin levels, and increased serum lactic dehydrogenase activity.

Differential diagnosis

Physicians often attempt to establish the cause of hereditary nonspherocytic hemolytic anemia on the basis of the appearance of red cells on a blood film and the results of the autohemolysis test (see Chap. A13). In reality, red cell morphology is helpful only in the diagnosis of pyrimidine-5'-nucleotidase deficiency (Table 59-1). After splenectomy, the appearance of Heinz bodies points to the possible presence of an unstable hemoglobin. Autohemolysis tests provide no diagnostic information of value, except occasionally in the confirmation of the presence of hereditary spherocytosis.

Since the laboratory diagnosis of these disorders may entail considerable expenditure of time and effort, it is prudent to perform the simplest tests for the most common causes of hereditary nonspherocytic hemolytic anemia first. Accordingly, it is useful to carry out screening tests for G-6-PD [29] and PK [27] activity and an isopropanol stability test [86] to detect an unstable hemoglobin. The characteristically elevated red cell 2,3-diphosphoglycerate level is also helpful in the diagnosis of PK deficiency. If the levels of 2,3-diphosphoglycerate are normal, it is extremely unlikely that the patient has PK deficiency. If prominent stippling of erythrocytes is present, examination of the ultraviolet spectrum of a perchloric extract of the erythrocytes may help to establish diagnosis of pyrimidine-5'-nucleotidase deficiency [87] (see Chap. A20). Beyond these relatively simple procedures it is probably rarely profitable to pick and choose individual enzyme assays on the basis of family history of clinical manifestations. Rather, it is usually appropriate to submit a blood sample to a reference laboratory which has a capability of performing all the enzyme assays listed in Table 59-1.

The estimation of the proportion of various red cell membrane lipids to one another and the study of membrane proteins are usually carried out only in research laboratories.

Therapy

The principal decision which the physician must make regarding patients with hereditary nonspherocytic hemolytic anemia is whether or not they require a splenectomy. This decision is not made easily, and should be based upon the following considerations: (1) severity of the disease; (2) family history of response to splenectomy; (3) the underlying defect; (4) whether cholecystectomy is needed. Since it is unusual to obtain more than a partial response to splenectomy, this procedure should probably be reserved for patients whose normal function is impaired by their anemia. The operation needs to be considered especially for patients who require frequent transfusion and for those who require gallbladder surgery, in which splenectomy might be carried out as part of the same procedure. The best guide to the therapeutic efficacy of splenectomy is probably response of other family members who may have undergone the operation. Unfortunately, such information is only occasionally available. The physician must therefore rely upon the experience of other patients with hereditary nonspherocytic hemolytic anemia of similar etiology to serve as a guide. However, even as the large group of patients with hereditary nonspherocytic hemolytic anemia represents a heterogeneous population, so individuals with a single enzymatic lesion, such as PK deficiency, are heterogeneous. Each family is likely to be afflicted with a distinct mutant enzyme, and the various mutants may differ both with respect to clinical manifestations and with respect to response to splenectomy. Some of the available information regarding response to splenectomy of patients with hereditary nonspherocytic hemolytic anemia has been reviewed [12] and is summarized in Table 59-1. Relatively little is known of the response of patients with unstable hemoglobins to splenectomy, but in the instance of patients with unstable hemoglobins with a high oxygen affinity the results may be disastrous, with the development of thromboembolic complications probably because of the occurrence of secondary polycythemia after the spleen has been removed [88].

Steroids are of no known value in this group of disorders. Folic acid is often given, as it is in other patients with increased marrow activity, but without proven hematologic benefit. In the absence of iron deficiency, iron is probably contraindicated, although overload is not a frequent complication in this group of disorders.

Course and prognosis

The diagnosis of hereditary nonspherocytic hemolytic anemia has been made as late as the seventh decade [48], and the disease can be fatal in the first few years of life. Triosephosphate isomerase deficiency appears to have the worst prognosis of all the known defects that cause this disorder. With few exceptions patients with this deficiency have died by the fifth or sixth year of life, usually of cardiopulmonary failure. Pyruvate kinase deficiency, too, can be fatal in early childhood; the gene prevalent among the Amish of Pennsylvania produces particularly severe disease [89]. Unless the affected homozygous children are splenectomized, they generally perish. In general, however, hereditary nonspherocytic

hemolytic anemia is a relatively mild disease, and most affected individuals lead a relatively normal life, apparently without much compromise of life-span.

References

1. Crosby, W. H.: Hereditary nonspherocytic hemolytic anemia. *Blood* 5:233, 1950.
2. Dacie, J. N.: *The Haemolytic Anaemias. 1. The Congenital Anaemias.* Grune & Stratton, New York, 1960, p. 171.
3. Selwyn, J. G., and Dacie, J. F.: Autohemolysis and other changes resulting from the incubation in vitro of red cells from patients with congenital hemolytic anemia. *Blood* 9:414, 1954.
4. Dacie, J. V.: The hereditary non-spherocytic haemolytic anaemias. *Acta Haematol.* 31:177, 1964.
5. Beutler, E.: Why has the autohemolysis test not gone the way of the cephalin flocculation test? *Blood* 51:109, 1978.
6. Keitt, A. S.: Diagnostic strategy in a suspected red cell enzymopathy. *Clin. Haematol.* 10:3, 1981.
7. Robinson, M. A., Loder, P. B., and De Gruchy, G. C.: Red cell metabolism in non-spherocytic congenital haemolytic anaemia. *Br. J. Haematol.* 7:327, 1961.
8. De Gruchy, G. C., Santamaria, J. N., Parsons, I. C., and Crawford, H.: Nonspherocytic congenital hemolytic anemia. *Blood* 16:1371, 1960.
9. Valentine, W. N., Tanaka, K. R., and Miwa, S.: A specific erythrocyte glycolytic enzyme defect (pyruvate kinase) in three subjects with congenital non-spherocytic hemolytic anemia. *Trans. Assoc. Am. Physicians* 74:100, 1961.
10. Newton, W. A., Jr., and Bass, J. C.: Glutathione sensitive chronic non-spherocytic hemolytic anemia. *Am. J. Dis. Child.* 96:501, 1958.
11. Dacie, J. C.: Life and death of the red cell, in *Blood, Pure and Eloquent,* edited by M. M. Wintrobe. McGraw-Hill, New York, 1980, p. 211.
12. Beutler, E.: *Hemolytic Anemia in Disorders of Red Cell Metabolism.* Plenum, New York, 1978.
13. Beutler, E.: *Red Cell Metabolism. A Manual of Biochemical Methods,* 2d ed. Grune & Stratton, New York, 1975.
14. Valentine, W. N., Oski, F. A., Paglia, D. E., Baughan, M. A., Schneider, A. S., and Naiman, J. L.: Hereditary hemolytic anemia with hexokinase deficiency. Role of hexokinase in erythrocyte aging. *N. Eng. J. Med.* 276:1, 1967.
15. Blume, K. G., and Beutler, E.: Detection of glucose-phosphate isomerase deficiency by a screening procedure. *Blood* 39:685, 1972.
16. Baughan, M. A., Valentine, W. N., Paglia, D. E., Ways, P. O., Simon, E. R., and De Marsh, Q. B.: Hereditary hemolytic anemia associated with glucosephosphate isomerase (GPI) deficiency — A new enzyme defect of human erythrocytes. *Blood* 32:236, 1968.
17. Vora, S., Corash, L., Engel, W. K., Durham, S., Seamn, C., and Piomelli, S.: The molecular mechanism of the inherited phosphofructokinase deficiency associated with hemolysis and myopathy. *Blood* 55:629, 1980.
18. Tarui, S., Kono, N., Nasu, T., and Nishikawa, M.: Enzymatic basis for the coexistence of myopathy and hemolytic disease in inherited muscle phosphofructokinase deficiency. *Biochem. Biophys. Res. Commun.* 34:77, 1969.
19. Beutler, E., Scott, S., Bishop, A., Margolis, N., Matsumoto, F., and Kuhl, W.: Red cell aldolase deficiency and hemolytic anemia: A new syndrome. *Trans. Assoc. Am. Physicians* 86:154, 1974.
20. Kaplan, J. C., Shore, N., and Beutler, E.: The rapid detection of triose phosphate isomerase deficiency. *Am. J. Clin. Pathol.* 50:656, 1968.
21. Lowe, M. L., and Gin, J. B.: Modification in a screening test for triosephosphate isomerase deficiency. *Clin. Chem.* 18:1551, 1972.
22. Schneider, A. S., Valentine, W. N., Hattori, M., and Heins, H. L., Jr.: Hereditary hemolytic anemia with triosephosphate isomerase deficiency. *N. Engl. J. Med.* 272:229, 1965.
23. Kraus, A. P., Langston, M. F., Jr., and Lynch, B. L.: Red cell phosphoglycerate kinase deficiency. *Biochem. Biophys. Res. Commun.* 30:173, 1968.
24. Valentine, W. N., et al.: Hereditary hemolytic anemia associated

with phosphoglycerate kinase deficiency in erythrocytes and leukocytes. *N. Engl. J. Med. 280*:528, 1969.

25. Rosa, R., Pewhu, M.-O., Beuzard, Y., and Rosa, J.: The first case of a complete deficiency of diphosphoglycerate mutase in human erythrocytes. *J. Clin. Invest. 62*:907, 1978.
26. Cartier, P., Labie, D., Leroux, J. P., Najman, A., and Demaugre, F.: Déficit familial en diphosphoglycerate-mutase: Étude hematologique et biochimique. *Nouv. Rev. Fr. Hematol. 12*:269, 1972.
27. Beutler, E.: A series of new screening procedures for pyruvate kinase deficiency, glucose-6-phosphate dehydrogenase deficiency, and glutathione reductase deficiency. *Blood 28*:553, 1966.
28. Kahn, A., Kaplan, J.-C., and Dreyfus, J.-C.: Advances in hereditary red cell enzyme anomalies. *Hum. Genet. 50*:1, 1979.
29. Beutler, E., and Mitchell, M.: Special modifications of the fluorescent screening method for glucose-6-phosphate dehydrogenase deficiency. *Blood 32*:816, 1968.
30. Carson, P. E., Flanagan, C. L., Ickes, C. E., and Alving, A. S.: Enzymatic deficiency in primaquine-sensitive erythrocytes. *Science 124*:484, 1956.
31. Luzzatto, L., and Testa, U.: Human erythrocyte glucose-6-phosphate dehydrogenase: Structure and function in normal and mutant subjects, in *Current Topics in Hematology*, edited by S. Piomelli and S. Yachnin. Alan R. Liss, New York, 1978.
32. Loos, H., Roos, D., Weening, R., and Houwerzijl, J.: Familial deficiency of glutathione reductase in human blood cells. *Blood 48*:53, 1976.
33. Beutler, E., Duron, O., and Kelly, B. M.: Improved method for the determination of blood glutathione. *J. Lab. Clin. Med. 61*:882, 1963.
34. Minnich, V., Smith, M. B., Brauner, M. J., and Majerus, P. W.: Glutathione biosynthesis in human erythrocytes. I. Identification of the enzymes of glutathione synthesis in hemolysates. *J. Clin. Invest. 50*:507, 1971.
35. Konrad, P. N., Richards, F., II, Valentine, W. N., and Paglia, D. E.: Gamma-glutamyl-cysteine synthetase deficiency. *N. Engl. J. Med. 286*:557, 1972.
36. Boivin, P., and Galand, C.: La Synthèse du glutathion au cours de l'anémie hémolytique congénitale avec déficit en glutathion réduit. Déficit congénital en glutathion-synthètase erythrocytaire? *Nouv. Rev. Fr. Hematol. 5*:707, 1965.
37. Mohler, D. N., Majerus, P. W., Minnich, V., Hess, C. E., and Garrick, M. D.: Glutathione synthetase deficiency as a cause of hereditary hemolytic disease. *N. Engl. J. Med. 283*:1253, 1970.
38. Valentine, W. N., Fink, K., Paglia, D. E., Harris, S. R., and Adams, W. S.: Hereditary hemolytic anemia with human erythrocyte pyrimidine 5'-nucleotidase deficiency. *J. Clin. Invest. 54*:886, 1974.
39. Torrance, J., West, C., and Beutler, E.: A simple rapid radiometric assay for pyrimidine-5'-nucleotidase. *J. Lab. Clin. Med. 90*:563, 1977.
40. Paglia, D. E., and Valentine, W. N.: Haemolytic anaemia associated with disorders of the purine and pyrimidine salvage pathways. *Clin. Haematol. 10*:81, 1981.
41. Valentine, W. N., Paglia, D. E., Tartaglia, A. P., and Gilsanz, F.: Hereditary hemolytic anemia with increased red cell adenosine deaminase (45-to-70 fold) and decreased adenosine triphosphate. *Science 195*:783, 1977.
42. Giblett, E. R., Anderson, J. E., Cohen, F., Pollara, B., and Meuwissen, H. J.: Adenosine deaminase deficiency in two patients with severely impaired cellular immunity. *Lancet 2*:1067, 1972.
43. Boivin, P., Galand, C., and Demartial, M. C.: Erythroenzymopathies acquises. II. Déficit en adenylate-kinase au cours des hémopathies. *Pathol. Biol. (Paris) 20*:781, 1972.
44. Kaplan, J., Nicolas, A., Hanzlickova Leroux, A., and Beutler, E.: A simple spot screening test for fast detection of red cell NADH-diaphorase deficiency. *Blood 36*:330, 1970.
45. Gibson, Q. H.: The reduction of methemoglobin in red blood cells and studies on the cause of idiopathic methemoglobinemia. *Biochem. J. 42*:13, 1948.
46. Valentine, W. N., and Paglia, D. E.: The primary cause of hemolysis in enzymopathies of anaerobic glycolysis: A viewpoint. *Blood Cells 6*:819, 1980.
47. Beutler, E.: A commentary on "The primary cause of hemolysis in enzymopathies of anaerobic glycolysis: A viewpoint." *Blood Cells 6*:827, 1980.

48. Beutler, E.: Red cell enzyme defects as non-diseases and as diseases. *Blood 54*:1, 1979.
49. Beutler, E.: Effect of flavin compounds on glutathione reductase activity: In vivo and in vitro studies. *J. Clin. Invest. 48*:1957, 1969.
50. Beutler, E., and Matsumoto, F.: Ethnic variation in red cell glutathione peroxidase activity. *Blood 46*:103, 1975.
51. Takahara, S.: Acatalasemia and hypocatalasemia in the Orient. *Semin. Hematol. 8*:397, 1971.
52. Aebi, H., Bossi, E., Cantz, M., Matsubara, S., and Suter, H.: *Acatalasemia in Switzerland. Hereditary Disorders of Erythrocyte Metabolism. City of Hope Symp. Series.* Edited by E. Beutler. Grune & Stratton, New York, 1968, vol. I, p. 41.
53. Johnson, L. A., Gordon, R. B., and Emmerson, B. T.: Hypoxanthine-guanine phosphoribosyltransferase: A simple spectrophotometric assay. *Clin. Chim. Acta 80*:203, 1977.
54. Seegmiller, J. E., Rosenbloom, F. M., and Kelley, W. N.: Enzyme defect associated with a sex-linked human neurological disorder and excessive purine synthesis. *Science 155*:1682, 1967.
55. Johnson, L. A., Gordon, R. B., and Emmerson, B. T.: Adenine phosphoribosyltransferase: A simple spectrophotometric assay and the incidence of mutation in the normal population. *Biochem. Genet. 15*:265, 1977.
56. Cartier, P., and Hamet, M.: Une Nouvelle Maladie métabolique: Le Déficit complet en adenine-phosphoribosyltransferase avec lithiase de 2,8-dihydroxyadenine. *C. R. Acad. Sci. (Paris) 279*:883, 1974.
57. Beutler, E., and Matsumoto, F.: A rapid simplified assay for galacto-kinase activity in whole blood. *J. Lab. Clin. Med. 82*:818, 1973.
58. Stocchi, V., Dacha, M., Bossu, M., and Fornaini, G.: Modification of the radioactive method for erythrocyte galactokinase assay. *Clin. Chim. Acta 89*:371, 1978.
59. Gitzelmann, R.: Hereditary galactokinase deficiency, a newly recognized cause of juvenile cataracts. *Pediatr. Res. 1*:14, 1967.
60. Beutler, E., and Mitchell, M.: New rapid method for the estimation of red cell galactose-1-phosphate uridyl transferase activity. *J. Lab. Clin. Med. 72*:527, 1968.
61. Kalckar, H. M., Kinoshita, J. H., and Donnell, G. N.: Galactosemia: Biochemistry, genetics, pathophysiology, and developmental aspects. *Biol. Brain Dysfunction 1*:31, 1972.
62. Miwa, S., Nishina, T., Kakehashi, Y., Kitamura, M., Hiratsuka, A., and Shizume, K.: Studies on erythrocyte metabolism in a case with hereditary deficiency of H-subunit of lactate dehydrogenase. *Acta Haematol. Jap. 34*:2, 1971.
63. Kaplan, J.-C., Alexandre, Y., and Dreyfus, J.-C.: Déficit sélectif d'un des loci génétiques de la phosphoglucomutase dans les globules rouges. *C. R. Acad. Sci. (D) (Paris) 270*:1060, 1070.
64. Chamberlain, B. R., and Buttery, J. E.: Reappraisal of the uroporphyrinogen I synthase assay, and a proposed modified method. *Clin. Chem. 26*:1346, 1980.
65. Strand, L. J., Meyer, U. A., Felsher, B. F., Redeker, A. G., and Marver, A. S.: Decreased red cell uroporphyrinogen I synthetase activity in intermittent acute porphyria. *J. Clin. Invest. 51*:2530, 1972.
66. McCann, S. R., Finkel, B., Cadman, S., and Allen, D. W.: Study of a kindred with hereditary spherocytosis and glyceraldehyde-3-phosphate dehydrogenase deficiency. *Blood 47*:171, 1976.
67. Parr, C. W., and Fitch, L. I.: Inherited quantitative variations of human phosphogluconate dehydrogenase. *Ann. Hum. Genet. 30*:339, 1967.
68. Sass, M. D., Caruso, C. J., and Farhangi, M.: TPNH-methemoglobin reductase deficiency: A new red-cell enzyme defect. *J. Lab. Clin. Med. 70*:760, 1967.
69. Armstrong, J. M., Myers, D. V., Verpoorte, J. A., and Edsall, J. T.: Purification and properties of human erythrocyte carbonic anhydrases. *J. Biol. Chem. 241*:5137, 1966.
70. Kendall, A. G., and Tashian, R. E.: Erythrocyte carbonic anhydrase. I. Inherited deficiency in humans. *Science 197*:471, 1977.
71. Holmes, S. L., Turner, B. M., and Hirschhorn, K.: Human inosine triphosphatase catalytic properties and population studies. *Clin. Chim. Acta 97*:143, 1979.
72. Vanderheiden, B. S.: Genetic studies of human erythrocyte inosine triphosphatase. *Biochem. Genet. 3*:289, 1969.
73. Johns, R. J.: Familial reduction in red-cell cholinesterase. *N. Engl. J. Med. 267*:1344, 1962.

74. Shinohara, K., and Tanaka, K. R.: Hereditary deficiency of erythrocyte acetylcholinesterase. *Am. J. Hematol.* 7:313, 1979.

75. Kitamura, M., Iijima, N., Hashimoto, F., and Hiratsuka, A.: Hereditary deficiency of subunit H of lactate dehydrogenase. *Clin. Chim. Acta* 34:419, 1971.

76. Rosa, R., George, C. L., and Rosa, J.: Severe deficiency of red cell phosphoglycerate kinase (PGK) without concomitant hemolysis. *Blood 54 (Suppl. 1)*:35A, 1979, (abstract).

77. Marstein, S., Jellum, E., Halpern, B., Eldjarn, L., and Perry, T. L.: Biochemical studies of erythrocytes in a patient with pyroglutamic acidemia (5-oxoprolinemia). *N. Engl. J. Med.* 295:406, 1976.

78. Jaffe, E. R., and Gottfried, E. L.: Hereditary nonspherocytic hemolytic disease associated with an altered phospholipid composition of the erythrocyte. *J. Clin. Invest.* 47:1375, 1968.

79. Waterbury, L., and Frenkel, E. P.: Hereditary nonspherocytic hemolysis with erythrocyte phosphofructokinase deficiency. *Blood 39*:415, 1972.

80. Vora, S.: Isozymes of phosphofructokinase, in *Isozymes: Current Topics in Biological and Medical Research,* edited by M. C. Rattazzi, J. G. Scandalios, and G. S. Whitt. Liss, New York, 1982, vol. 6, pp. 119–167.

81. Wellner, V. P., Sekura, R., Meister, A., and Larsson, A.: Glutathione synthetase deficiency, an inborn error of metabolism involving the gamma-glutamyl cycle in patients with 5-oxoprolinuria (pyroglutamic aciduria). *Proc. Natl. Acad. Sci. U.S.A.* 71:2505, 1974.

82. Skala, H., Dreyfus, J. C., Vives-Corrons, J. L., Matsumoto, F., and Beutler, E.: Triose phosphate isomerase deficiency. *Biochem. Med.* 18:226, 1977.

83. Valentine, W. N., Schneider, A. S., Baughan, M. M., Paglia, D. E., and Heins, H. L., Jr.: Hereditary hemolytic anemia with triosephosphate isomerase deficiency. *Am. J. Med.* 41:27, 1966.

84. Schneider, A. S., Valentine, W. N., Baughan, M. A., Paglia, D. E., Shore, N. A., and Heins, J. L., Jr.: Triosephosphate isomerase deficiency. A multisystem inherited enzyme disorder: Clinical and genetic aspects, in *Hereditary Disorders of Erythrocyte Metabolism. City of Hope Symp. Series.* Edited by E. Beutler. Grune & Stratton, New York, 1968, vol. I, p. 265.

85. Oski, F. A., Nathan, D. G., Sidel, V. W., and Diamond, L. K.: Extreme hemolysis and red-cell distortion in erythrocyte pyruvate kinase deficiency. *N. Engl. J. Med.* 270:1023, 1964.

86. Carrell, R. W., and Kay, R.: A simple method for the detection of unstable haemoglobins. *Br. J. Haematol.* 23:615, 1972.

87. Valentine, W. N., Paglia, D. E., Fink, K., and Madokoro, G.: Lead poisoning. Association with hemolytic anemia, basophilic stippling, erythrocyte pyrimidine 5′-nucleotidase deficiency, and intraerythrocytic accumulation of pyrimidines. *J. Clin. Invest.* 58:926, 1976.

88. Beutler, E., Lang, A., and Lehmann, H.: Hemoglobin Duarte: ($\alpha_2\beta_2^{62}$ (E6)Ala→Pro): A new unstable hemoglobin with increased oxygen affinity. *Blood* 43:527, 1974.

89. Bowman, H. S., McKusick, V. A., and Dronamraju, K. R.: Pyruvate kinase deficient hemolytic anemia in an Amish isolate. *Am. J. Hum. Genet.*, 17:1, 1965.

90. Beutler, E., et al.: Red cell adenylate kinase deficiency: Another non-disease? *Blood 60 (Suppl. 1)*, 1982 (abstract), in press.

91. Valentine, W. N., Paglia, D. E., Neerhout, R. C., and Konrad, P. N.: Erythrocyte glyoxalase II deficiency with coincidental hereditary elliptocytosis. *Blood* 36:797, 1970.

Erythrocyte disorders— anemias related to abnormal globin

CHAPTER 60

The sickle cell diseases and related disorders

ERNEST BEUTLER

History

James Herrick, the astute Chicago physician who was credited with description of the clinical syndrome of coronary thrombosis, was the first to observe sickled cells in the blood of an anemic black medical student[1] (Fig. 60-1). Emmel [2] demonstrated that red cells sickled when blood from such patients was sealed under glass and allowed to stand at room temperature for several days, but the fact that the transformation to sickled cells occurs in response to a fall in oxygen tension was not recognized until the classic studies of Hahn and Gillespie in 1927 [3]. In 1923 the sickling phenomenon was shown to be inherited as an autosomal dominant trait [4]. Much later Neel [5] and Beet [6] clarified the genetic basis of sickle cell anemia by demonstrating that heterozygosity for the sickle cell gene resulted in sickle cell trait without significant clinical symptoms, while homozygosity resulted in sickle cell anemia.

In 1949 Pauling and his colleagues [7] found that all the hemoglobin in patients with sickle cell anemia showed an abnormally slow rate of migration on electrophoresis, while the parents of these patients showed evidence of normal as well as abnormal hemoglobin. Soon after, other abnormal hemoglobins were discovered by subjecting hemoglobin to electrophoresis. The biochemical nature of the defect in sickle cell anemia was elucidated by Ingram [8], who digested hemoglobin with trypsin and separated the resulting peptides on paper by electrophoresis in one direction and chromatography in the other. This technique ("fingerprinting") demonstrated that one of the digestion products of sickle hemoglobin migrated differently from that of normal hemoglobin. Determination of the amino acid com-

position of this peptide indicated that sickle cell anemia was the result of the replacement of a glutamic acid residue by valine. This discovery established that the substitution of a single amino acid in a polypeptide chain can alter the function of the gene product sufficiently to produce widespread clinical effects. Conley has chronicled the fascinating history of sickle cell disease [9].

Nomenclature of the hemoglobinopathies

After the discovery that sickle hemoglobin, or hemoglobin S (Hb S), was electrophoretically altered, additional variants were assigned letters of the alphabet—C, D, E, etc. The letters of the alphabet were rapidly exhausted, however, and subsequent abnormal hemoglobins were named after the geographic location in which they were found (e.g., hemoglobin Memphis, hemoglobin Mexico). If the hemoglobin had the physical characteristics of one previously described by a letter, the geographic designation was added as a subscript (e.g., hemoglobin $M_{Saskatoon}$). In this case the M indicates an amino acid substitution resulting in a methemoglobin. In a fully characterized hemoglobin the amino acid substitution is designated by a superscript to the globin chain involved, as, for example, hemoglobin S, $\alpha_2\beta_2^{6\ Glu \to Val}$ and hemoglobin $G_{Norfolk}$, $\alpha_2^{35\ Asp \to Asn}\beta_2$.

FIGURE 60-1 Peculiar elongated and sickle-shaped red corpuscles in a case of severe anemia. (Herrick [1], by permission.)

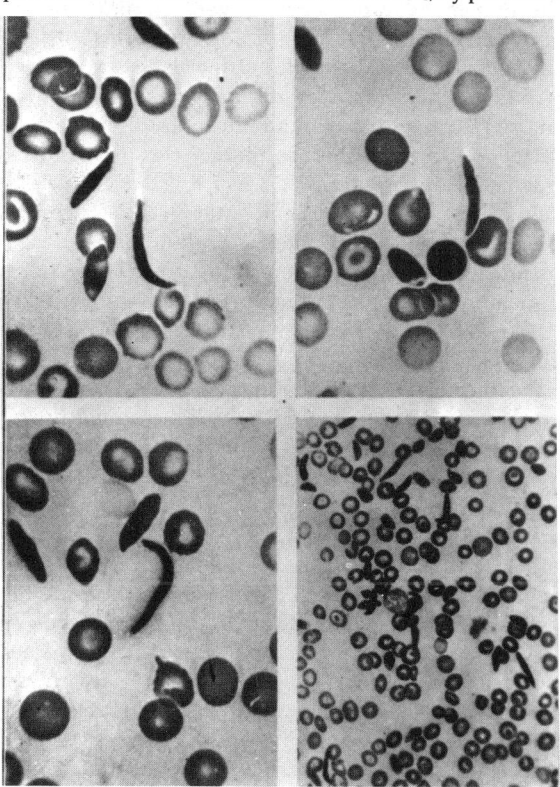

The term *sickling disorder* refers to states in which the red cell undergoes sickling when it is deoxygenated. The *sickle cell diseases* are those disorders in which sickling produces prominent clinical manifestations. Included are sickle cell-hemoglobin C disease, sickle cell–hemoglobin D disease, sickle cell β thalassemia, and *sickle cell anemia*. The latter term is reserved for the homozygous state for the sickle cell gene.

Etiology and pathogenesis

BIOCHEMICAL BASIS OF SICKLING

There are few diseases of man whose etiology can be traced to as basic a level as sickle cell disease. Sickle cell anemia is due to the substitution of thymine for adenine in the glutamic acid DNA codon (GAG→GTG), which results, in turn, in substitution of β6 valine for glutamic acid. The exact reason why this amino acid substitution causes sickling of the red cell is not known. As discussed in Chap. 37, hemoglobin exists in two conformations, designated the oxy (relaxed, R) and deoxy (tense, T) states. Deoxygenation of hemoglobin shifts this equilibrium toward the T conformation. Molecules of deoxyhemoglobin S have a strong tendency to aggregate, and such aggregation requires the substitution of valine for glutamic acid in the β6 position, since only those hemoglobin variants with this substitution (e.g., S and Harlem) undergo sickling. Certain other structural features of the molecule are also of importance [10].

Electron micrographs of deoxygenated sickle hemoglobin show the presence of multiple microtubules [11,12] consisting of hemoglobin molecules stacked on top of each other. A number of arrangements have been proposed [10]. It is thought that the molecules do not lie directly over one another, so that a helical structure is formed. The distorted sickled red cell is the visible end result of this molecular aggregation. The process is time-dependent. Initially there is a rate-limiting nucleation process in which, contrary to earlier suggestions, the membrane does not seem to play a significant role [13]. When a cell sickles and unsickles repeatedly, the membrane is affected and the cell becomes irreversibly sickled; it remains so even when the oxygen pressure is increased. An irreversibly sickled cell has a high hemoglobin concentration and a high calcium and low potassium content and may be ATP-depleted [14]. It has a short intravascular life-span, and the severity of the hemolytic process is directly related to the number of these cells in a patient's circulation [15]. Although the primary defect in sickle cell disease is clearly in the hemoglobin, secondary alterations in red cell metabolism and membrane structure and function have also been described. Rapid potassium loss occurs early in the sickling process [16]. Abnormalities of sickle cell membrane phosphorylation have been documented [17–19]. The calcium pump is abnormal [20], and the calcium content of sickle cell membranes, particularly of those cells that are irreversibly sickled, is increased [14,21].

VARIABILITY IN SEVERITY OF SICKLING

Because a large number of inherited and acquired factors influence the pathogenesis of clinical symptoms, the sickling disorders vary in clinical severity from the virtually symptomless sickle cell trait to the potentially lethal state characteristic of sickle cell anemia. Wide variation in the severity of clinical manifestations also occurs among patients with sickle cell anemia. Some die within the first few years of life, while others have been discovered late in life as a result of a chance survey.

Both intracellular and extracellular factors influence sickling. The nature of the hemoglobins, and to a considerable extent the activity of the red cell enzymes and levels of metabolites, is inherited and largely invariant. The variability of extracellular factors probably accounts for the natural pattern of this group of diseases—periods of comparative well-being interspersed with periods of clinical deterioration (crises). Although such factors may account for the development of sickle crises, it is unusual for individual factors to be clearly implicated in the development of crises. Of those events which appear to be associated with the appearance of crises, infections are probably among the most common.

INHERITED FACTORS

Amount of hemoglobin S in the red cell   A correlation exists between the concentration of sickle hemoglobin within a red cell and its susceptibility to sickling. The red cells of the sickle cell carrier, who is virtually symptom-free, always contain less than 50 percent Hb S; the remainder is largely normal adult hemoglobin. The exact proportions vary from one individual to another. It was proposed many years ago that the distribution of sickle hemoglobin in the red cells of subjects with the sickle cell trait was bimodal [22]. More recent studies have confirmed the existence of more than a single mode and, indeed, suggest that the distribution might actually be trimodal [23]. The reason for such a discontinuous distribution has become apparent with the recognition of the very high frequency of α thalassemia in persons of African ancestry. Individuals carrying α-thalassemic genes have a higher ratio of hemoglobin A to hemoglobin S than those who have four normal copies of the α locus [24,25]. Interaction of the α-thalassemic gene and the sickle gene may also influence the course of sickle cell disease: the lower corpuscular hemoglobin concentration in α-thalassemics would be expected to tend to protect against sickling. It has been suggested that such an interaction may influence the severity of sickle cell disease in American blacks [26,27] and that it may play an important role in producing the very mild clinical manifestation of sickle cell anemia in Saudi Arabia [28]. However, a recent study of the severity of the clinical manifestations of sickle cell anemia in 214 patients showed no relationship between clinical manifestations and the mean corpuscular hemoglobin concentration [29].

Nature of other hemoglobins in the red cell Other hemoglobins present in a red cell containing sickle hemoglobin need not be inert bystanders in the sickling process [30]. Two common abnormal hemoglobins, Hb C and Hb D, and the relatively rare hemoglobin O$_{Arab}$ readily become involved in the formation of the sickling tubule. The interaction of these hemoglobins with sickle hemoglobin increases the propensity of red cells to sickle. It is this ability of hemoglobins to interact that accounts for the fact that their presence in the red cell along with hemoglobin S usually results in symptoms.

Other hemoglobins do not appear to play an active role in the sickling process, and their presence in the red cell can greatly reduce the clinical severity of sickle cell anemia. Fetal hemoglobin, for example, protects the red cell from sickling [31]. It is distributed heterogeneously in the red cells of an SS homozygote [32,33], and those cells with the largest amount are least susceptible to sickling [32,34]. The remarkably mild clinical manifestations of patients in the Middle East with sickle cell anemia has been ascribed, at least in part, to the high level of fetal hemoglobin present in their red cells [35,36]. In the United States, however, no significant correlation exists between fetal hemoglobin levels and the severity of the clinical manifestations of sickle cell anemia [29]. In adults, hemoglobin S constitutes more than 50 percent of the hemoglobin of persons who are heterozygotes for hemoglobin S and hereditary persistence of hemoglobin F. However, because each cell contains a considerable amount of hemoglobin F, such persons experience a benign clinical course [37–39]. The presence of the abnormal hemoglobin Memphis ($\alpha_2^{23Glu \rightarrow Gln}\beta_2$) also decreases the clinical severity of sickle cell disease [40], presumably by inhibiting the formation of the sickle tubule.

Interaction of sickling and thalassemia (see Chap. 50) The interaction of β thalassemia with sickling is discussed on page 509. Patients with sickle cell anemia who are carriers of α thalassemia appear to have a relatively benign clinical course [26,27,41], and the percentage of sickle hemoglobin is distinctly less in persons with the sickle cell trait who also have α thalassemia [24,25].

Glucose-6-phosphate dehydrogenase deficiency It has been suggested that G-6-PD deficiency may have a beneficial effect on the clinical course of sickle cell anemia [42,43], but this correlation has not been confirmed [44–47]. While it has also been proposed that hemolytic crises are more common in patients with sickle cell diseases who are also G-6-PD–deficient [48], it seems unlikely that the G-6-PD–deficient cells of such a patient would be particularly sensitive in hemolytic stress; because the erythrocytes are young, they have relatively normal G-6-PD activity. In Jamaica G-6-PD deficiency did not influence hemoglobin concentration, reticulocyte count, hemoglobin F concentration, irreversibly sickled cell counts, or plasma hemoglobin concentration, and there was no relationship between clinical severity and presence or absence of G-6-PD deficiency [49].

ACQUIRED (VARIABLE) FACTORS
Deoxygenation Deoxygenation for a sufficient period of time is the most important factor determining the occurrence of sickling in a red cell containing hemoglobin S. The degree of deoxygenation required to produce sickling varies with the percentage of hemoglobin S in the cells. Sickle trait cells will sickle at an oxygen tension of about 15 mmHg, whereas those from a patient with sickle cell anemia will begin to sickle at an oxygen tension of about 40 mmHg [50–52]. Changes that impair adequate oxygenation of the blood may be deleterious to any person with sickle hemoglobin.

An arterial oxygen tension of about 66 mmHg is found at about 10,000 ft (3048 m). Hypoxia may result from flying in unpressurized aircraft; most commercial aircraft, however, maintain an atmospheric pressure in the cabin equivalent to that encountered at an altitude of 5000 to 7000 ft (1524 to 2134 m). Occasional patients with sickle cell anemia or sickle cell–hemoglobin C disease have been reported to experience painful crises or splenic infarctions under such circumstances. However, there is no evidence that the person with sickle trait is at risk in a pressurized airplane [53]. The oxygen content of the air may also be reduced during anesthesia or when using an artificial breathing apparatus, as in scuba diving. If pulmonary or cardiac function deteriorates (e.g., in pneumonia or in cardiac failure), any resulting reduction in arterial oxygen tension may prove hazardous to the patient with sickle cell disease. In severe cyanotic congenital heart disease, such as the tetralogy of Fallot, even patients with sickle cell trait may show signs of hemolysis [54].

Vascular stasis The P$_{O_2}$ level producing in vitro sickling of cells containing Hb S bears little direct relationship to clinical measurements of arterial and venous P$_{O_2}$. This is because the P$_{O_2}$ in the larger peripheral vessels does not accurately reflect the oxygen tension in areas of vascular stasis, such as the sinusoids of the spleen, in which hypoxia is common and sickling is likely to occur. Although a period of 2 to 4 min is required for the development of marked red cell distortion [55], the red cells normally remain within the venous circulation for only about 10 to 15 s. For this reason, red cells in areas of vascular stasis are more vulnerable to sickling. Once sickling has occurred, increased blood viscosity [55,56] results in further vascular stasis, further sickling, possible vascular obstruction, and infarction. This course of events leads to tissue death, manifested clinically as a painful crisis.

While no organ of the body is immune to infarction due to in vivo sickling, certain sites notorious for circulatory stasis are characteristically affected. Splenic and marrow infarctions due to vascular stasis are particularly frequent, and priapism may occur in the male. The role of vascular stasis in the development of leg ulcers and of retinal and renal lesions is discussed below under "Clinical Features." The reason for the increased tendency of patients with sickle cell anemia to develop duodenal ulcers is obscure, but mucosal hypoxia due to sickling may be a causative factor.

Temperature   Low temperatures tend to precipitate sickle crises, presumably because of the accompanying vasoconstriction.

Acidosis   Hydrogen ions produce a right shift in the oxygen dissociation curve (the Bohr effect), presumably by displacing the equilibrium between the high-affinity oxy conformation and the low-affinity deoxy conformation toward the deoxy conformation of hemoglobin. Since it is sickle hemoglobin in the deoxy conformation which aggregates, the lowered pH profoundly affects the sickling of red cells, even when the percent oxygenation is maintained at a constant level [57,58]. Alkalosis, on the other hand, by shifting the equilibrium toward the oxy conformation, tends to retard sickling but impairs oxygen release to tissue.

Corpuscular hemoglobin concentration   The tendency of hemoglobin S solutions to aggregate is very strongly concentration-dependent [34]. Accordingly, sickling of red cells is markedly influenced by the concentration of sickle hemoglobin in the cells. Suspending sickle cells in a hyperosmolar medium increases the intracellular hemoglobin concentration as the cell is dehydrated. This phenomenon may account in part for sickling in renal papillae [57,59]. Conversely, any agent which causes increased red cell volume will retard the sickling process. Marked dehydration results in both vascular stasis and hypertonicity and can precipitate a crisis.

Vascular endothelium   Little is known of the role of variations in the vascular endothelium in the sickling process. It has been proposed that the adherence of sickle cells to endothelial cells may vary, and that the degree of adherence may play a role in the development of sickle crises [60].

Infections   It is a common clinical observation that infarctive crises may be precipitated by infections. In many cases the mechanism by which infection increases sickling is easily discernible: fever, vomiting, and diarrhea may produce dehydration; lack of food intake may produce acidosis; and hypoxia may result from pneumonia. It is quite possible that other, more subtle mechanisms may also be responsible for precipitation of crises in patients with sickle diseases.

HEMOGLOBIN C
In hemoglobin C, glutamic acid in the sixth position from the N terminal of the β chain has been replaced by lysine [61]. Red cells containing principally hemoglobin

C are more rigid than normal, and their fragmentation in the circulation may result in the formation of microspherocytes. Red blood cell life-span is shortened to a mean of 30 to 55 days [62]. The rate of hemoglobin production in hemoglobin C disease has been reported to be 2.5 to 3 times normal [63]. However, the erythroid marrow response is generally suboptimal, resulting in the presence of a mild chronic anemia. This is probably related to the fact that erythrocytes from patients with hemoglobin C disease have a low oxygen affinity, possibly due to a reduction, for unknown reasons, of the intracellular pH [64].

HEMOGLOBIN D
In his early studies of the hemoglobinopathies Itano [65] encountered a white family with an abnormal hemoglobin which migrated at the same rate as hemoglobin S but did not sickle. Its solubility in the reduced state resembled that of hemoglobin A, and this new abnormal hemoglobin was designated hemoglobin D. Subsequently, this name was given to any hemoglobin variant which manifested the same electrophoretic properties as hemoglobin S at an alkaline pH but had normal solubility properties. With the exact chemical analysis of hemoglobin variants, it became apparent that hemoglobin $D_{Los Angeles}$ was identical to hemoglobin D_{Punjab}, both manifesting a substitution of glutamate for lysine at the one hundred twenty-first position in the β chain. Another "D" hemoglobin $G_{Philadelphia}$ is, on the other hand, an α-chain variant with a substitution of asparagine for lysine at the sixty-eighth position.

HEMOGLOBIN E
Hemoglobin E is a β-chain mutation, $\alpha_2\beta_2^{26\ Glu\rightarrow Lys}$ [66], which is somewhat unstable when subjected to oxidative stress [67], perhaps because of weakening of the bonds between the monomers constituting the hemoglobin tetramer.

Geographic distribution of abnormal hemoglobins

Hemoglobin S occurs with greatest prevalence in tropical Africa; the heterozygote frequency is usually about 20 percent, but in some areas it reaches 40 percent. The sickle cell trait has a frequency of about 8 percent in American black populations. The sickle cell gene is found to a lesser extent in the Middle East, in Greece, and in aboriginal tribes in India (Fig. 60-2). On occasion sickle cell disease is found in Caucasians in many other areas, especially where racial admixture has occurred over the centuries [69].

The high prevalence of sickle cell trait in areas of the world where malaria has been common has strongly suggested that persons with sickle cell trait have a selective advantage over normal individuals when they con-

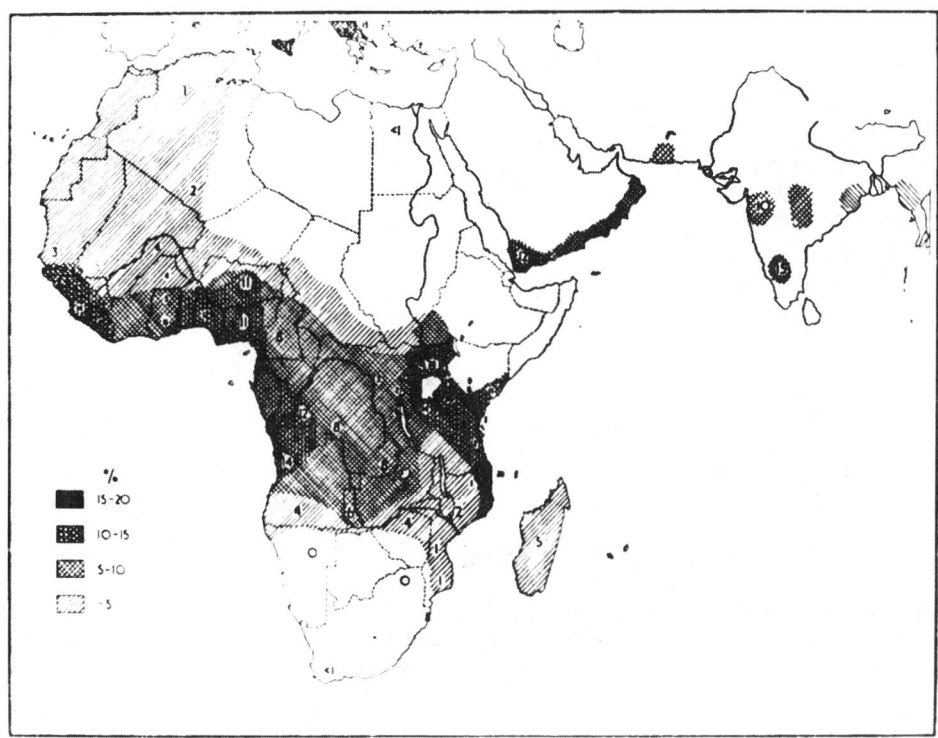

FIGURE 60-2   Distribution of sickle cell gene in Africa and Asia. (Allison [68], by permission.)

tract this disease [70,71]. This advantage seems to be restricted to young children with *Plasmodium falciparum* infection. Although children with sickle cell trait are readily infected by *P. falciparum*, the parasite counts remain low. It may be that the infected red cell is preferentially sickled and destroyed, probably in the vascular system of the liver or spleen, where oxygen tensions are low and phagocytic cells abound. Whatever the mechanism, the result is that the infection is of short duration and the incidence of cerebral malaria and death is low.

Until recently one could only speculate as to whether the sickle cell mutation had arisen only once and had gradually gained a worldwide distribution or whether the same mutation had arisen independently in various populations and then had been subject of selection, presumably through a protective effect against malaria. The ability to detect mutations in nontranscribed portions of DNA adjacent to the β-globin gene (see Chap. 16 page 115) has now provided insight into this problem. Such mutations are so close to the β-globin gene that the probability of a crossover (see Chap. 16) is vanishingly small. Thus the relationship of the two mutations to one another will persist through hundreds of generations, permitting one to trace population movements. When the DNA of most humans is digested with the restriction endonuclease Hpa I, the β-globin gene is found in a DNA fragment which is 7.6 kilobases (kb) long. Two variants have been found, however. In one of these the Hpa I site is closer to the β globin gene, and in one it is farther away. Digestion of DNA carrying these muta-

tions gives rise to β-globin gene-containing fragments of 7.0 and 13.0 kb, respectively. In West Africa the sickle gene apparently arose in a β-globin gene adjacent to the mutation, giving the 13.0-kb Hpa I site [72]. Population studies in the United States show that a very high proportion of sickle genes are associated with the 13-kb mutation, and in limited studies this appears to be the case also in subjects with the sickle gene in Sicily and Cyprus. However, in East Africa the sickle gene is associated with the 7.6-kb Hpa I site, and the same is true of the sickle gene in Saudi Arabia and India [72]. One may conclude from these findings that the sickle gene(s) in those parts of the world arose independently of the mutation which traveled from West Africa to the Mediterranean and to the United States.

Hemoglobin C is found in 17 to 28 percent of West Africans, particularly in the vicinity of North Ghana [73]. The selective factors which account for this high incidence are unknown at present. The incidence among blacks in the United States is 2 to 3 percent [74]. Sporadic cases have also been reported in other populations, including Italian [75] and Dutch [76] populations.

Hemoglobin E, like hemoglobin S and hemoglobin C, occurs with sufficient frequency to be considered a polymorphism. The distribution of the gene for this β-chain mutation is illustrated in Fig. 60-3. It is found principally in Burma, Thailand, Cambodia, Malaysia, and Indonesia, and in some areas is found with a prevalence of 30 percent [77]. On the other hand, it is not prevalent among the Chinese.

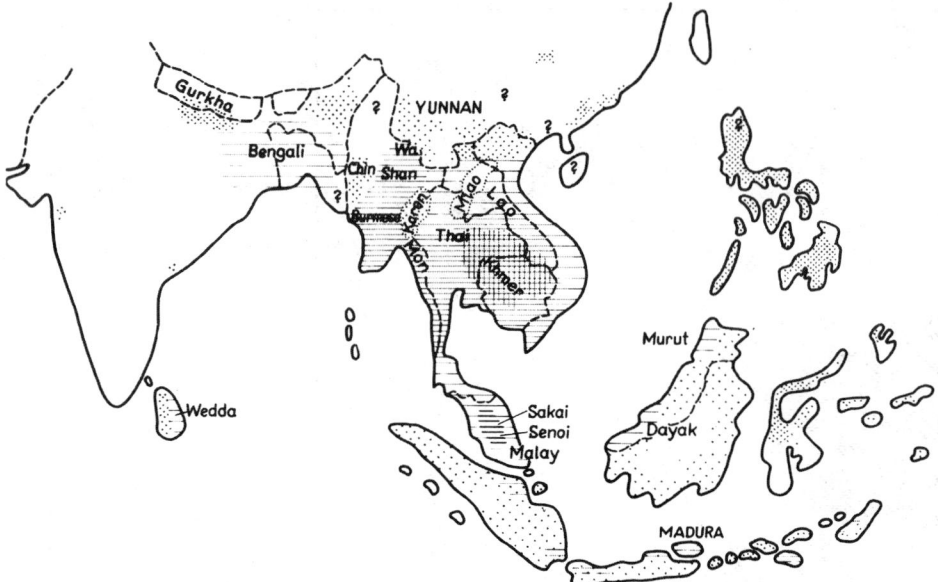

FIGURE 60-3   Distribution of hemoglobin E in Southeast Asia. Gene frequencies: cross-hatching indicates >0.2 percent; narrow hatching indicates 0.1 to 0.2 percent; wide hatching indicates 0.02 to 0.1 percent; dotted area indicates <0.02 percent and sporadic occurrence. (Flatz [77], by permission.)

Sickle cell trait

The most benign of the sickling disorders, sickle cell trait is also one of the most misunderstood. Affecting some 8 percent of American blacks, and an even higher percentage of the population in Africa, sickle cell trait does not produce any abnormalities of the blood counts and is an exceedingly rare cause of morbidity. Red cell life-span is normal in sickle cell trait [78]. Not only patients, but even physicians [79] often appear to believe that sickle cell trait represents a mild type of sickle cell disease. Cerebral thrombosis, mishaps during anesthesia, and sudden death attract little notice when occurring in a person who does not have a known genetic variant, but the same occurrence in the 1 of 12 American blacks who happen to have carried this trait immediately raises the question of a cause-and-effect relationship. Thus, there is a legion of anecdotal reports suggesting that sickle cell trait contributed to a patient's illness [80]. In reality, the morbidity and possible mortality associated with sickle cell trait is very low and therefore difficult to document accurately. It seems to be limited largely to hematuria that is otherwise unexplained and possibly to thromboembolic episodes involving the lung. In a massive study, encompassing over 65,000 consecutively admitted black male patients in 13 U.S. Veterans Administration hospitals [81], slightly higher incidences only of hematuria of unspecified cause (2.5 percent versus 1.3 percent) and pulmonary embolism (2.2 percent versus 1.5 percent) were found. No age stratification was found, indicating that the life-span of patients with sickle cell trait is normal.

Surgical patients with sickle cell trait had no greater perioperative mortality, no longer postoperative stay, and no greater mortality than those with normal hemoglobin. Similar conclusions have been drawn in other studies [82].

Sudden death resulting from rhabdomyolysis has been reported in several subjects with sickle cell trait following severe exercise [83,84]. It is indeed conceivable that dehydration resulting from severe exertion in a subject with an abnormal renal concentrating mechanism [85] may on rare occasions lead to a catastrophic result under severe stress. Therefore, anecdotal reports of this type are somewhat disturbing, but there is no clearly documented excess mortality in persons with sickle trait, and if sickle trait does ever cause death, the incidence must be exceedingly low. It has not been possible to document any differences from normal in cardiovascular function of sickle cell trait subjects subjected to maximum exercise [86].

Because of reports of episodes of splenic infarction in individuals thought to have sickle cell trait who were flying in an unpressurized aircraft [87,88] or who ascended to very high altitudes [89], there has been concern about the safety of permitting persons with sickle cell trait to fly. Since commercial aircraft maintain a cabin pressure equivalent to that encountered at 5000 to 7000 feet (1524 to 2134 m), this concern is unwarranted [53].

The diagnosis of sickle cell trait depends upon demonstration of the presence of hemoglobin S and hemoglobin A in the affected individual. The amount of hemoglobin S is always less than the concentration of hemoglobin A. In contrast, in sickle cell β^+ thalassemia the amount of hemoglobin S exceeds that of hemoglobin A.

The sickle cell diseases

Sickle cell anemia (SS disease) may be considered the prototype of the sickle cell diseases, and in general the clinical features and treatment of all these disorders are the same. The homozygous state, sickle cell anemia, is the most severe of these disorders, with sickle cell–hemoglobin C disease and sickle cell β thalassemia tending to be somewhat milder and sickle cell–hemoglobin D disease being the mildest of the group. However, there is a great deal of overlap in the severity of the clinical manifestations of these disorders. Some patients with sickle cell thalassemia or sickle cell–hemoglobin C disease may be more anemic and have more severe and frequent crises than some mildly affected patients with homozygous sickle cell anemia. Attempts have been made to delineate clinical features of these disorders [90], but in reality the principal difference between these diseases is in their laboratory diagnosis.

INHERITANCE
A patient with sickle cell anemia is homozygous for the gene for sickle hemoglobin, and has therefore inherited one abnormal gene from each parent. If 7.8 percent of a population are sickle cell trait carriers [81], as in the American black population, there is a 1:164 chance that two carriers will marry, and the chances that an offspring of such a marriage will have sickle cell anemia is 1:4. In such a population, about 1 in 650 will have sickle cell anemia.

Similarly, persons with hemoglobin SC disease must have one parent with a sickle hemoglobin gene and another with a hemoglobin C gene. Since these genes are allelic β-chain mutations, persons with hemoglobin SC disease have no normal β-polypeptide-chain gene and therefore have no hemoglobin A. The carrier rate for hemoglobin C in American blacks is about 2.3 percent [81]. If 7.8 percent of a population carries the hemoglobin S gene, then the probability of a sickle cell trait and hemoglobin C trait mating is about 1 in 280, and therefore 1 in about 1120 newborns will inherit hemoglobin SC disease. The same principles apply for inheritance of sickle cell β thalassemia, since the β-thalassemia gene is also allelic to the gene for sickle hemoglobin. In black Americans the frequency of β thalassemia is approximately 0.8 percent [91], so that the expected birth frequency of sickle cell β thalassemia is about 1 per 3200.

Hemoglobin D$_{Punjab}$, now recognized to be identical with hemoglobin D$_{Los Angeles}$, both having the structure $\alpha_2\beta_2^{21\,Glu\rightarrow Gln}$ also interacts with hemoglobin S in forming aggregates in the deoxy conformation. Hemoglobin SD disease is a relatively mild sickle cell disease. This he-

moglobin is found in frequencies of approximately 3 percent in Northwest India; however, it is relatively rare in populations of African origin, and hemoglobin SD disease is therefore very uncommon.

Although we regard sickle cell anemia as the prototype of the sickle cell diseases, in the American black population only about one-half of the patients with sickle cell diseases have sickle cell anemia (homozygous SS disease). This fact is important from the point of view of genetic counseling (see page 596): about half of all children with sickle cell disease arise from matings in which only one of the parents carries the sickle cell gene.

CLINICAL FEATURES
The newborn infant is protected by the high level of fetal hemoglobin in the red cells during the first few months of life. As the level declines, the clinical manifestations of sickle cell disease will appear.

CRISES
Many patients with sickle cell anemia are in reasonably good health much of the time, achieving a steady-state level of fitness. This state of relative well-being is periodically interrupted by a crisis [92,93], which may have a sudden onset and, occasionally, a fatal outcome. The early recognition and subsequent clinical assessment of sickle crises are greatly facilitated by familiarity with the patient's steady state.

Various types of crises occur, and these may be classified as follows: infarctive (painful) crisis, aplastic and megaloblastic crises, sequestration crisis, and hemolytic crisis.

Infarctive crisis The infarctive crisis is the most common form of crisis and is the hallmark of the patient with sickle cell disease. The infarctive crises result from obstruction of blood vessels by rigid, sickled red cells. Tissue hypoxia occurs and ultimately leads to tissue death; pain is the chief clinical manifestation. It is important to distinguish the pain of an infarctive crisis from the pain caused by other, sometimes more treatable disorders. Fever is often present, even in the absence of demonstrable infection. Sickle cell crisis is, to a large extent, a diagnosis by exclusion [94]. Infarctive crises may affect any tissue, but the pain occurs especially in bones, chest, and abdomen. Infarctions in the spleen are so common in sickle cell anemia that after childhood the spleen usually becomes very small because of scarring (autosplenectomy).

Aplastic and megaloblastic crises Aplastic and megaloblastic crises in sickle cell disease are of the type familiar in patients with other hemolytic disorders. Depression of erythropoiesis is generally associated with infections, especially those of viral origin. Because of the short red cell life-span in sickle cell disease, even in the steady state, a temporary depression of marrow activity can cause a catastrophic fall in hemoglobin level manifesting as an aplastic crisis. Marrow output failure may also result from a deficiency of folic acid, especially during late pregnancy (megaloblastic crisis). The very high maternal mortality reported some years ago in Africa was greatly reduced by folic acid supplements given during pregnancy to patients with hemoglobin SC disease [95].

Sequestration crisis   The sequestration crisis occurs particularly in infants and young children [96]. It is characterized by sudden massive pooling of red cells, especially in the spleen. Such crises are probably responsible for the majority of deaths that occur in the first years of life in patients with sickle cell disease.

Hemolytic crisis   The red cell life-span is shortened in all the varieties of sickle cell disease. It may suddenly be further reduced, probably for a variety of reasons. This increased rate of hemolysis is designated a *hemolytic crisis*. The resulting increase in jaundice is associated with a falling hemoglobin and an elevated reticulocyte count. Such crises are very rare; in most instances changes regarded as due to increased hemolysis represent some other complication of sickle cell disease [97]. It has been suggested that concurrent G-6-PD deficiency may be a factor leading to hemolytic crises [48], but it is not at all clear that this is actually the case. An increase in the level of jaundice is not necessarily an indication of increased hemolysis. Other causes for jaundice, such as hepatitis, cirrhosis, and gallstones, should be sought. Patients with a chronic hemolytic anemia are especially likely to form bilirubin stones, which may cause extrahepatic biliary obstruction (page 592). Intrahepatic cholestasis with extremely high levels of circulating bilirubin also appears to be a feature of sickle cell anemia.

OTHER CLINICAL MANIFESTATIONS
Growth   Young children with sickle cell anemia tend to be shorter than normal. Puberty is delayed, but consid-

FIGURE 60-4   **Sickle cell dactylitis (hand-foot syndrome). Note the swelling of the right hand involving the thumb and first and second fingers. (Diggs [92], by permission.)**

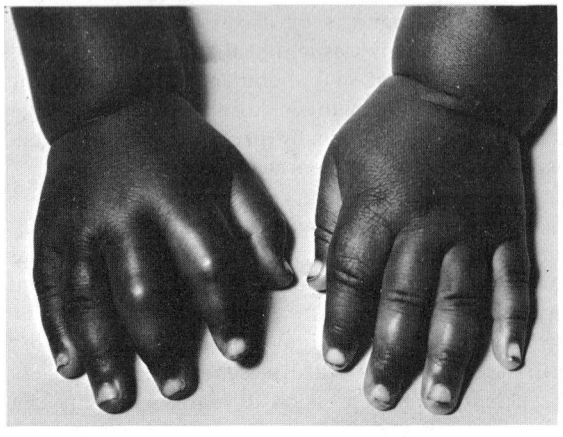

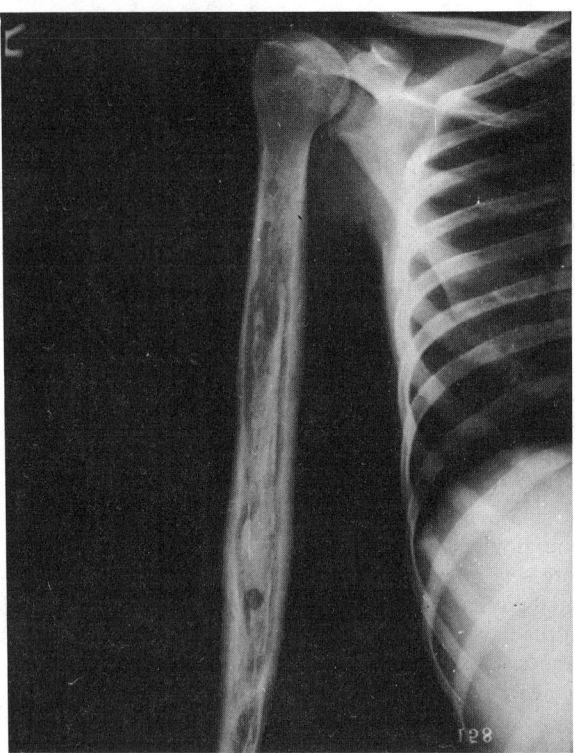

FIGURE 60-5   *Salmonella typhimurium* **osteomyelitis in a patient with hemoglobin SC disease. (River, Robbins, and Schwartz [100], by permission.)**

erable growth occurs in late adolescence, so that the adult with sickle cell anemia is as tall as or taller than normal.

Bony abnormalities   The chronic hemolytic anemia with erythroblastic hyperplasia will result in widening of the medullary spaces, thinning of the cortices, and a sparseness of the trabecular pattern [98]. Although these changes are recognizable in the skull, they are usually not as marked as the typical "hair-on-end" appearance characteristic of patients with β thalassemia major. The vertebral bodies may show biconcavities of the upper and lower surfaces (codfish spine). Pressure from the nucleus pulposus into an area of bony infarction may result in steplike depressions—as if a coin had been pushed into the vertebral body. These depressions are highly suggestive of sickle cell disease.

Crises with bone pain may be followed by the appearance of periosteal reaction, and irregular areas of osteosclerosis may be seen, representing areas of bone infarction. Bone scans with ^{99m}Tc are not helpful in delineating areas involved in painful crises [99]. Sickle cell dactylitis resulting in painful swelling of the dorsal surfaces of the hands and feet is found in infancy (Fig. 60-4). In later life, necrosis of the head of the femur due to infarction of the nutrient artery is common, especially in sickle cell–hemoglobin C disease, and may be responsible for serious disturbances of gait. The bone manifestations of sickle cell disease may closely mimic osteomyelitis or arthritis.

The presence of necrotic marrow may favor the development of infection, especially with *Salmonella* (Fig. 60-5) [101,102]. Necrotic marrow may later detach and produce pulmonary emboli and sometimes sudden death [103,104].

Genitourinary system   The renal medulla is an area which is particularly susceptible to damage in sickle cell disease. The unique renal environment, characterized by stasia and anoxia, hyperosmolality, and low pH, predisposes to sickling. Indeed, the kidney appears to be so susceptible to the effects of the sickling phenomena that it is only this organ which is commonly affected in the generally benign sickle cell trait. The ability to concentrate urine is lost not only in patients with sickle cell disease, but even in those with sickle cell trait [85]. Infarctions may occur, with renal papillary necrosis (Fig. 60-6). Hematuria is frequently present [85]. Priapism is a serious complication of sickle cell disease. It often requires surgical decompression and results in permanent impotence. Underdeveloped genitalia and hypogonadism may occur.

Spleen   Splenomegaly is prominent in early childhood, but splenic function is impaired [106]. In adults spleno-

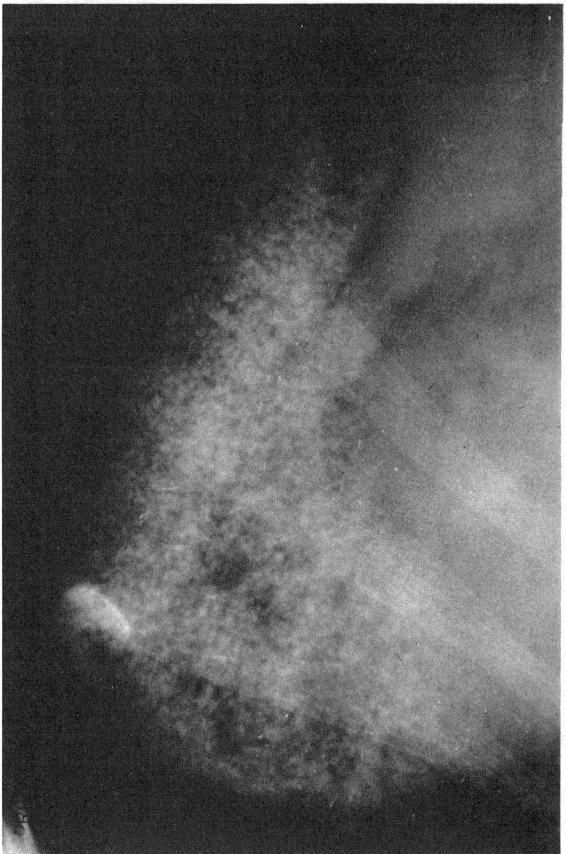

FIGURE 60-7   Punctate calcifications in the spleen of a 19-year-old male with sickle cell anemia. (Hemley, Mellins, and Finby [107], by permission.)

FIGURE 60-6   Renal papillary necrosis in a patient with sickle cell trait. Note the small medullary cavities in the upper three calices of the left kidney (arrows). (Harrow, Sloane, and Liebman [105], by permission.)

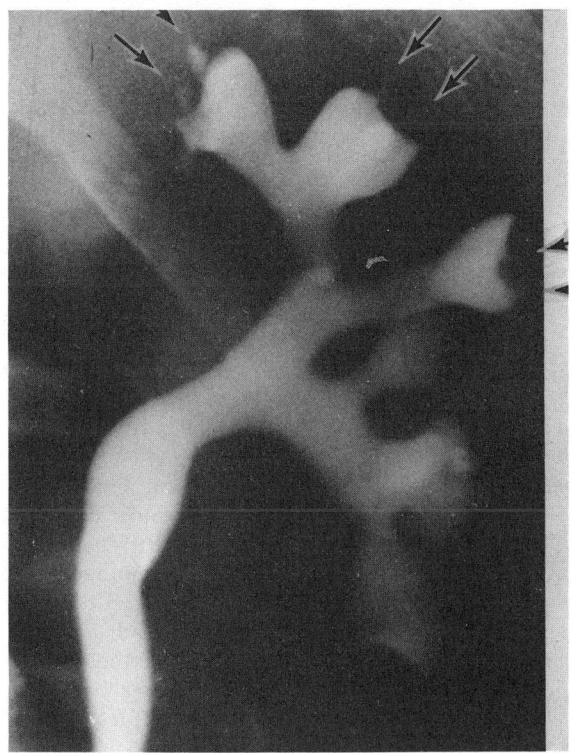

megaly is rare because of splenic fibrosis and calcifications secondary to repeated infarctions (Fig. 60-7). This shrinkage is called *autosplenectomy*. The finding of a palpable spleen in an adult with sickle cell anemia suggests an unusually mild clinical state. However, in sickle cell diseases other than SS disease, i.e., sickle cell thalassemia or sickle cell–hemoglobin C disease, splenomegaly commonly persists into adult life.

Liver   Jaundice and hepatomegaly are common in sickle cell anemia. The liver is occasionally massively enlarged, extending to the iliac crest, particularly in young children and again in middle age, at which time there may be evidence of hepatic dysfunction [108]. Histologic study shows dilated sinusoids lined by a foamlike reticulum, which spreads into the lumen. The small number of sickled cells found in the hepatic vein after passage through the liver suggests that the cells most susceptible to sickling are trapped by their rigidity and engulfed by phagocytes during their passage through the hepatic sinusoids, where the oxygen content of the blood is extremely low. The liver may transiently increase in size during a painful crisis [108]. In sickle cell disease excretion of urobilinogen is usually greater than normal. Some 50 percent of adult patients

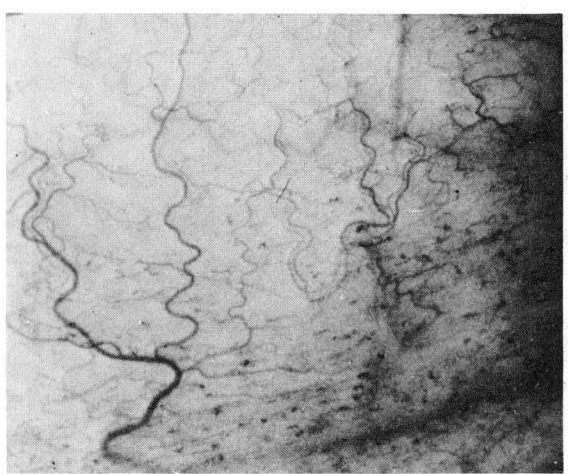

FIGURE 60-8   Lower bulbar conjunctiva in a patient with sickle cell anemia, showing many segmentations. (Paton [115], by permission.)

may have bilirubin gallstones, but cystic and common duct obstruction secondary to pigment stones is quite rare [109]. Although more common in the adult, gallstones have been found in children as young as 6 years of age [110]. Patients who have received transfusions may develop hepatitis, which is sometimes mistaken for a hemolytic crisis (see page 590).

Cardiopulmonary system   The heart is frequently the site of some of the most prominent physical findings in sickle cell disease [111]. During crises, striking tachycardia may occur because of the combination of fever and anemia. The precordium demonstrates the overactivity similar to that seen with marked hyperthyroidism. The point of maximal impulse is usually forceful and pounding in nature, and the heart is frequently enlarged to both the left and the right. Systolic and diastolic flow murmurs are usually heard.

Pulmonary infarctions are common in persons with sickle cell disease and may lead to repeated episodes of chest pain, unexplained dyspnea, "atypical pneumonia." A combination of fever, chest pain, rise in the white count, and appearance of a pulmonary infiltrate in patients with sickle cell diseases has been designated the *acute chest syndrome.* The clinical and roentgenologic features observed in these patients do not aid in differentiating pulmonary infarction from pulmonary infection. It has been recommended that if a normal flora is seen on Gram-stained sputum in a patient who is not seriously ill, no antibiotics should be used, if gram-positive cocci in clumps predominate, a penicillinase-resistant penicillin should be given, and if a predominance of gram-negative cocci bacillary forms are present, the use of ampicillin or tetracycline would be appropriate [112]. In adults, in contrast to children, such pulmonary events appear to be rarely due to infection with pneumococci [112]. The combination of increased flow rate and pulmonary vascular occlusions may result

in increased pulmonary pressure and eventually cor pulmonale [113].

Eye   Retinal vessel obstruction is followed by neovascularization with arteriovenous aneurysms. These may eventually result in hemorrhage, scarring, retinal detachment, and blindness [114]. These changes occur at the periphery and may initially be difficult to visualize through an ophthalmoscope, even with a fully dilated pupil. At the early stage of retinal disease, vision is therefore not impaired. Examination of the conjunctiva may reveal multiple, short, comma-shaped capillary segments which often appear isolated from the vascular network because the afferent and efferent lumens are empty [115,116]. These transient sites of tightly clumped intravascular erythrocytes are found on the bulbar conjunctiva underneath the eyelids (see Fig. 60-8). They occasionally disappear during the course of a lengthy examination because of the warmth of the light.

Central nervous system   Cerebrovascular accidents are one of the most devastating complications of sickle cell disease [23]. They occur particularly in children and usually cause severe disability. Patients with sickle cell anemia have approximately an 8 percent risk of developing a stroke, while the incidence among patients with hemoglobin SC disease is significantly lower, at approximately 2 percent. No predictive factors have been found to identify patients who are particularly at risk to develop this complication. However, recurrence of strokes in patients who have suffered one is a prominent feature of this complication; at least 67 percent of patients who have one stroke will suffer at least one more. Such episodes were particularly common within the first 36 months after a stroke [23].

Many other neurologic symptoms have been described, including drowsiness, coma, convulsions, headache, temporary or permanent blindness, cranial nerve palsies, and paresthesias of the extremities [117].

Leg ulcers   Although encountered in patients with other types of hemolytic disease, ulcers around the ankles are a particularly common feature of sickle cell disease [118]. They are unusual in the younger child, and stasis clearly plays some part in their formation.

Pregnancy   Pregnancy in women with sickle cell anemia is accompanied by an increased incidence of pyelonephritis, pulmonary infarctions, pneumonia, antepartum hemorrhage, prematurity, and fetal death [119]. Megaloblastic anemia responsive to folic acid, especially in late pregnancy, also occurs with increased frequency. The birth weight of infants of mothers with sickle cell anemia is below average [120], and the fetal wastage is high. The cause of neonatal death is somewhat obscure: the postmortem findings are those of intrapartum anoxia [121]. On occasion, maternal bone disease may lead to pelvic deformity and malpresentation [57] complications which could affect the delivery of mothers with sickle cell disease [122]. The maternal mortality in sickle cell disease was formerly prohibitively high, with rates averaging 33 percent, but is now very low, averaging 1.6 percent in various series [123].

Laboratory findings and diagnosis

The steady-state hemoglobin level of patients with sickle cell anemia is usually between 5 and 11 g/dl. The anemia is normochromic and normocytic in spite of the elevated reticulocyte count [124]. In comparison with patients with a similarly increased reticulocyte count these patients may be considered to have a "microcytic" anemia. The anemia is accompanied by laboratory signs of hemolysis with increased indirect-reacting serum bilirubin, with reticulocytosis, and often with circulating nucleated red cells. Sickled erythrocytes are often evident on inspection of the blood film. Target cells may be present, particularly in sickle cell–hemoglobin C disease and in sickle cell β thalassemia. Examination of the red cells by inference phase-contrast microscopy reveals surface indentations in approximately 20 percent of the cells [106]. A modest polymorphonuclear leukocytosis with a left shift is common even in the steady state [125,126] and may be due in part to redistribution of leukocytes from the marginal to the circulating granulocyte pool [125]. It does not necessarily signify an infection. Thrombocytosis is also common, but evidence of intravascular coagulation with thrombocytopenia has been noted during crisis [127]. The marrow shows erythroid hyperplasia. Immunoglobulin levels are frequently increased. IgA levels are particularly elevated in all forms of sickle cell disease. Elevations of IgG levels are also sometimes seen, while IgM levels appear to be elevated particularly in patients with sickle cell thalassemia and in individuals with other combinations such as sickle cell–hemoglobin C disease [128]. A decreased number of T lymphocytes and increased β lymphocytes in the blood have been reported [129]. A defect in the alternative complement pathway has been detected in some patients [130]. Plasma tocopherol [131] and zinc [132,133] levels are often low. Serum ferritin levels are normal in the first two decades of life but tend to rise in older patients. Modest elevations in plasma iron content are also frequently encountered [134].

Diagnosis depends upon documentation of the presence of sickle hemoglobin. This can be achieved by demonstration of its insolubility in the deoxygenated form and by its characteristic electrophoretic mobility. In the classic sickling test intact red cells are suspended in an oxygen-poor environment and transformation to the sickled form is observed [135]. This test is by no means as easy to interpret as one might imagine, with errors arising from the presence of poikylocytosis, from the use of metabisulfite which has aged, and from solutions that are too concentrated [136]. An alternative approach is to recognize the presence of sickle hemoglobin by demonstrating the turbidity which occurs in solutions of high salt concentrations because of the insolubility of hemoglobin S. Many such tests have been described, and these are usually reliable [137–139] and may be automated [140] (see Chap. A10).

Hemoglobin electrophoresis is routinely carried out at an alkaline pH. Hemoglobin S moves more slowly than hemoglobin A under these conditions, occupying a position approximately midway between hemoglobin A and hemoglobin A_2. However, the common nonsickling hemoglobin D_{Punjab} occupies a position identical to hemoglobin S under these conditions, and the demonstration of decreased solubility of the putative hemoglobin S is mandatory. Differentiation of Hb S from Hb D can also be achieved by agar gel electrophoresis at acid pH (see Chap. A7). At alkaline pH hemoglobin C moves more slowly than hemoglobin S, occupying the same position as the normal minor hemoglobin, hemoglobin A_2. Hemoglobins O_{Arab} and E both have a mobility which is similar to hemoglobin C at an alkaline pH. Agar gel electrophoresis at acid pH will distinguish these variants (see Chap. A7). Because there are no normal β-polypeptide-chain genes, patients with sickle cell anemia or sickle cell–hemoglobin C disease have no normal adult hemoglobin. In the heterozygote for the sickle cell gene and that for β° thalassemia no hemoglobin A is found, but small amounts of normal hemoglobin are present in the heterozygote for the sickle cell and β⁺-thalassemia genes. The concentration of fetal hemoglobin is usually increased in sickle cell β thalassemia and is heterogeneously distributed among the red cells. The quantitation of hemoglobin A_2 is of value in differentiating sickle cell anemia from sickle cell β° thalassemia; hemoglobin A_2 levels tend to be increased in the latter condition. Family studies are particularly helpful if sickle cell β° thalassemia is to be clearly differentiated from sickle cell anemia.

Sickle cell anemia can be diagnosed at birth by subjecting cord blood samples to electrophoresis [141–144]. Agar gel at acid pH or cellulose acetate with tris-EDTA-borate buffer [145] may be used to separate the relatively small amounts of normal adult hemoglobin and hemoglobin S from the large amounts of fetal hemoglobin (about 70 percent) in the hemolysate (Fig. 60-9). Ideally, all babies of ethnic groups with a high frequency of the sickle cell gene should be screened at birth. Screening is particularly desirable if the mother has sickle cell trait.

The diagnosis of sickle cell anemia in the unborn fetus is more difficult and should be made by about the eighteenth week in order to consider a therapeutic abortion. Sampling fetal blood is relatively hazardous, with a loss of over 10 percent of the fetuses being reported by an experienced group in 1977 [146]. Studies of globin-chain synthesis requires a high degree of technical skill, although some simplifications in the procedure [147] may make the technique more generally applicable.

The fortuitous linkage relationship between the sickle gene and the 13-kb Hpa I fragment (see page 115) makes possible accurate prenatal detection of sickle cell disease in appropriate families without the necessity of obtaining fetal blood. Restriction enzyme analysis can be carried out using amniotic fluid cells, a cell type which

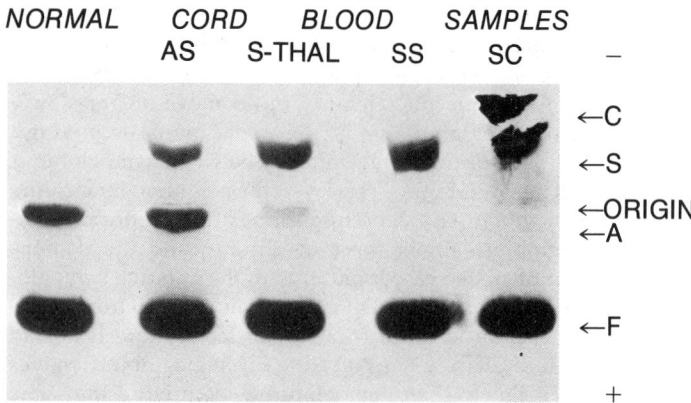

FIGURE 60-9 Acid agar gel electrophoresis of cord blood hemolysates. This electrophoretic system has the capacity to separate fetal hemoglobin from the other hemoglobins present.

is much more easily and safely obtained than is fetal blood. If both parents, heterozygous for the sickling gene, are also heterozygotes for the 13.0-kb fragment, it may be assumed that only infants homozygous for the 13.0-kb fragment will prove to have inherited sickle cell anemia [148,149]. There are restriction endonucleases which recognize the altered nucleotide sequence at the site of the mutation which produces sickle cell disease. Restriction mapping with such enzymes provides a more specific means for the prenatal diagnosis of sickle cell disease. Amniotic fluid cell DNA may be subjected to digestion by the restriction endonucleases Dde I or Mst II, which recognize the normal nucleotide sequence [229,230].

TREATMENT

USE OF ANTISICKLING AGENTS

For a number of years, attempts have been made to treat sickle cell disease by modifying the hemoglobin S molecule either directly or indirectly in a manner that will suppress the sickling process. Examples of this approach have included conversion of hemoglobin to carboxyhemoglobin [150–152] or methemoglobin [153], acetylation of the hemoglobin molecules with aspirin [154,155] or succinyldisalicylate [156], cross-linking hemoglobin molecules with dimethyladipimidate [157,158], and use of carbonic anhydrase inhibitors to reduce the formation of H_2CO_3 [159]. Distilled water has been given intravenously to lower the mean corpuscular hemoglobin concentration (MCHC) [160]. Other antisickling agents that have been studied for a possible therapeutic effect include urea [161], cyanate [162], procaine [163], zinc [164], pyridoxine [165] and its derivatives [166,167], phenothiazines [168], steroids [157], nitrogen mustard [169], glyceraldehyde [170], hexamethylenetetramine [171], vitamin E [172], and cetiedil [173].

Most of these agents have been tested only in in vitro model systems, but a few have had clinical trials. The induction of methemoglobinemia [153] by the admin-

istration of sodium nitrite or p-aminopropiophenone lengthened the life-span of sickle cells, and the inhalation of carbon monoxide [152] was found to have a similar effect. Pyridoxine [165], in contrast, did not influence red cell life-span. The use of alkali to counteract the Bohr effect (the reduction of the oxygen affinity of hemoglobin at acid pH) [174] has been thought to have some therapeutic value, but no beneficial effect could be demonstrated in controlled trials [175]. The rationale for the use of urea was the ability of this chemical to dissociate hydrophobic molecular bonds and thus interfere with the sickling process. The concentration required to achieve such an effect cannot be reached in vivo, and clinical trials have proved disappointing [176]. Carbamylation of the hemoglobin molecule by cyanate increases the affinity of the hemoglobin for oxygen [177]. Because the sickling process requires the hemoglobin to be in the deoxy conformation, any agent capable of affecting the equilibrium between the oxy and deoxy conformations and thereby increasing the avidity of hemoglobin for oxygen must have an antisickling effect [58]. Unfortunately, in clinical trials cyanate provoked polyneuropathy [178], retinal changes [178], and cataracts [179] and therefore appears to be too toxic for systemic use. However, extracorporeal treatment with removal of excess cyanate by washing the red cells before returning them to the patient may overcome this problem [180–182].

Because sickling is highly concentration-dependent, efforts to treat the disorder by swelling the red cells have been made. These have included the administration of distilled water intravenously [160] and the lowering of serum sodium by the administration of a long-acting vasopressin derivative and vigorous hydration [183]. The effectiveness and safety of the latter treatment has been questioned [184,231]. Such treatment must still be regarded as experimental.

GENERAL MEASURES

The modification of sickle hemoglobin molecule chemically has not yet become clinically useful, and physicians must therefore concentrate their therapeutic efforts in the direction of continuous and effective general medical care and appropriate management of complications as they arise. High social status appears to improve the survival of children with sickle cell anemia [185], suggesting that favorable environmental influences may improve the outlook in this disorder. Current therapy emphasizes the prevention of crises by removing as completely as is feasible the factors that encourage the sickling phenomenon.

Folic acid supplementation is probably desirable, and particularly so in pregnancy. Personal and community hygiene should be maintained at a satisfactory level. The administration of antipneumococcal vaccine has been recommended [186]. However, a number of failures of the vaccine to protect children with sickle cell disease against infection with the pneumococcus have been reported, and it has been suggested that children with sickle disease should receive both penicillin prophylaxis and pneumococcal vaccine until the age of 6, at which time penicillin prophylaxis may no longer be necessary [187]. Antimalarial medication is essential in areas where this disease is endemic [188]. Infections should be treated vigorously with antibiotics. A patient with sickle cell anemia is unable to concentrate urine adequately, and dehydration therefore represents a special risk. Sudden exposure to cold and high altitudes should be avoided.

Because of "autosplenectomy" hypersplenism is seldom a problem in sickle cell anemia. Hypersplenism may be suspected in other forms of sickle disease if a long-term transfusion program becomes necessary to maintain life or if leukopenia and thrombocytopenia are associated with a palpable spleen. Under these circumstances, splenectomy may very occasionally be warranted. It has been recommended that all adolescent and adult sickle cell anemia patients be examined for the presence of gallstones, and that elective cholecystectomy be performed when stones are present [189].

Special vocational training of patients with sickle cell anemia for suitable occupations is useful. It is important that these patients live as normal a life as possible. Their performance in occupations which do not require heavy manual labor and in which occasional absences from work are practical can be excellent and may make them useful both to themselves and to society.

MANAGEMENT OF CRISES
Infarctive crisis Once a small blood vessel is totally obstructed by sickled cells the obstruction is probably irreversible. Yet the function of neighboring blood vessels in the area containing sludged cells may be preserved by a number of therapeutic measures. The patient should be kept warm, and adequate hydration should be maintained by the oral or intravenous route. The role of oxygen therapy in the treatment of infarctive crises is poorly defined. Although the administration of oxygen was once considered to be contraindicated because of a putative negative effect on erythropoiesis, it seems doubtful that it does any harm. Even in the adequately

oxygenated patient, the presence of a small amount of additional dissolved oxygen in the plasma may conceivably be of some help. In attempting to cope with the situation for which no specific therapy is available, we sometimes administer nasal oxygen to patients in sickle cell crises, but do so, admittedly, without conviction or enthusiasm. Hyperbaric oxygen usually fails to benefit the patient [190], although occasional success using this treatment has been claimed [191]. Small transfusions have been advocated for the termination of painful crises [192,193].

Anticoagulants (e.g., dicumarol [194] and Arvin [195]) have been tried without success. Intravenous administration of magnesium sulfate [196] has been reported to be beneficial, particularly in the treatment of priapism, although a therapeutic effect has not been confirmed [197]. The administration of urea for sickle cell crises has been advocated but is dangerous and ineffective [198]. Oral sodium bicarbonate or sodium citrate therapy has been tried in the treatment of an established infarctive crisis, as well as in its prevention [197], but its efficacy could not be confirmed in a controlled study [198].

Management of the pain of infarctive crises represents a particularly difficult problem for the physician. Nonnarcotic analgesics such as aspirin or propoxyphene should be used whenever they provide effective pain relief. Sedation may be accomplished with agents such as chlorpromazine, barbiturates, diazepam, or chlordiazepoxide. However, it is often necessary to use narcotics. As in many other diseases associated with chronic or recurrent pain, many patients with sickle cell disease have become addicted to narcotics, and those who have not may become so. It is impossible to judge how much pain a patient is having, since there are no objective measurements which are helpful. The anxiety which usually accompanies an infarctive crisis may make the patient's perception of it more severe. But this is of no matter: from the patient's point of view the pain is severe. Thus, it is often necessary to use narcotics in pain management. When they are used, the dose and frequency should, of course, be as low as commensurate with obtaining adequate pain relief. Since it is essential to maintain good oxygenation, the doses of narcotics given should never be sufficient to significantly impair respiration.

Occasionally a patient may develop serious complications, and such patients may respond to prompt exchange transfusion [199,200].

In most instances the manifestations of infarctive crises gradually disappear over a period of hours or days on symptomatic management.

CONTRACEPTION AND PREGNANCY
Oral contraception may offer some additional hazard of thromboembolism to a patient with sickle hemoglobin [203], but the risk is probably small compared to the risk of the pregnancy itself.

Although very high maternal mortality rates have been greatly reduced with good prenatal care, pregnancy and the postpartum period are still potentially hazardous for a mother with sickle cell disease [123]. The patient should be closely supervised during pregnancy. Although prophylactic blood transfusions have been given to some pregnant patients with what appear to be satisfactory results [204,205], the effectiveness of this type of therapy is not considered to be proven, and further studies are required [123,206].

ANESTHESIA

The patient with sickle cell disease is at greater risk than normal subjects during anesthesia, although the magnitude of the excess risk is debatable [207–209]. If surgery is indicated, scrupulous care is needed to avoid factors known to precipitate crisis, including hypoxia, dehydration, circulatory stasis, acidosis, cold, and infections.

SURGERY

Preoperative transfusion with packed red cells may help to avoid complications in patients with sickle cell disease undergoing surgery. Although partial exchange transfusion has been advocated [210], this more complex procedure probably has little if any advantage over simple transfusion, particularly if surgery is elective, as might be the case with patients requiring cholecystectomy or hip replacement. Elevation of the hemoglobin level of the blood will markedly reduce the production of sickle cells by the marrow and, in view of the short life-span of the patient's own circulating erythrocytes, the patient should be amply protected by the administration of 10 to 15 ml of normal red blood cells per kilogram of body weight in the week before surgery.

LEG ULCERS

Leg ulcers may respond to conservative treatment such as bed rest, elevation of the affected limb, and zinc sulfate pressure dressings. Maintenance transfusion is very helpful. It has been claimed that oral zinc sulfate hastens healing [211]. Skin grafting may give gratifying results but often proves disappointing.

RETINAL CHANGES

Hemorrhage and subsequent blindness may be the end result of the neovascularization that follows retinal infarction. Close supervision and intraocular coagulation of new vessels may have a role in the management of patients with retinal changes [212–214].

COURSE AND PROGNOSIS

For a number of years it was unclear why sickle cell anemia was relatively common in the North American black and yet appeared to be a rare disease in Central Africa. Subsequently it was recognized that the early mortality associated with sickle cell anemia in Central Africa [215–217] was responsible for its apparent rarity: the surveys of the distribution of sickle hemoglobin in Africa did not include the afflicted who had died. With good medical care, patients with sickle cell anemia usually survive to middle age [218–220]. Assessment of the overall mortality of sickle cell anemia must take into ac-

count the fact that cases first diagnosed in late childhood, adolescence, or adult life are likely to result in a preponderance of the clinically more benign patients. In order to obtain a true natural history of the disease, it is essential to diagnosis sickle cell anemia at birth and follow babies with the disease and suitably matched controls in a longitudinal study [221].

The manifestations of sickle cell disease vary with age [222]. Acute manifestations are often associated with severe infections in childhood, while in the adult, symptoms are characteristically chronic and organ-related, albeit still potentially life-threatening. Until more data on the disease in infancy become available, it is not possible to predict whether the sudden death syndrome in infants with sickle cell anemia is a common or a rare event. In the meantime, the diagnosis must be considered in cases of acute general illness and unexplained death, especially in ethnic groups where the sickle cell gene is known to occur commonly.

PREVENTION

The occurrence of sickle cell disease can theoretically be prevented by detection of those who may transmit this disorder. They may then be provided with genetic counseling and educated about the options of not having children or of having pregnancies monitored for the occurrence of a sickle cell disease in the fetus followed by selective abortion. Since approximately half of the children with sickle cell diseases have only one parent with sickle hemoglobin (see page 589), effective screening programs must do more than merely detect the presence of this abnormal hemoglobin. They must also use means which will permit detection of hemoglobin C and of β thalassemia trait. Because of the benign clinical nature of these three genetic traits, no useful purpose other than that of genetic counseling seems to be served by screening populations for these carrier states. Indeed, misunderstandings concerning the significance of the carrier states has led to unwarranted harm to individuals who are detected as carriers in screening programs [223].

Although many screening programs have been implemented, there are not data permitting assessment of the actual effect of screening programs on birth frequency of infants with sickling disorders. It is clear, however, that if screening programs are to perform a useful function it is important for them to be established only with adequate laboratory backup and expert counseling.

Hemoglobin C disease

Hemoglobin C disease (CC disease) is the homozygous state for hemoglobin C. The heterozygous state, hemoglobin C trait, is entirely asymptomatic. The pathogenesis of this disorder has been described earlier. Splenomegaly is a fairly constant feature of hemoglobin C disease, and may be associated with fleeting abdominal pain.

The anemia in hemoglobin C disease is mild, with the hemoglobin level ranging from 8 to 12 g/dl. There is a marked increase in the number of target cells in the blood film (Fig. 60-10). Some target cells may also be observed in the trait. Occasionally, intraerythrocytic hemoglobin crystals may be seen on the blood film, and these may appear in larger numbers if the red cells have been dehydrated either by drying or by suspension in a hypertonic solution (see Chap. 29). The osmotic fragility of the red cells may be decreased.

The diagnosis of homozygous hemoglobin C disease is achieved by electrophoresis, hemoglobin C moving in the same position as hemoglobin A_2, hemoglobin E, and hemoglobin O_{Arab} at an alkaline pH. These hemoglobins are readily distinguished from hemoglobin C by acid agar gel electrophoresis (see Chap. A7).

No specific therapy is available or required for patients with hemoglobin C disease. Anemia may become more severe following infections, but the overall prognosis is considered to be excellent.

Hemoglobin D disease

The heterozygous state for hemoglobin D is entirely asymptomatic [225]. The abnormal hemoglobin constitutes between 35 and 50 percent of the total hemoglobin. Homozygous hemoglobin D disease is very rare, and some patients originally believed to be homozygous for hemoglobin D [226] subsequently were found to be heterozygous for hemoglobin D and β thalassemia. We know of no reports of firmly established homozygous hemoglobin D disease, but presumably the clinical manifestations of such a disorder would be quite mild.

Hemoglobin E disease

Homozygosity for hemoglobin E results in a relatively mild anemia characterized by microcytosis and targeting of the red cells [227]. The osmotic fragility is decreased. In the hemoglobin E carrier state, 30 to 45 percent of the hemoglobin is hemoglobin E [227], and such carriers are asymptomatic but do manifest microcytosis [228]. Although the prevalence of the gene for hemoglobin E is quite high in Southeast Asia (Fig. 60-3), relatively few patients with homozygous E disease, as distinguished from hemoglobin E β thalassemia, have been described. When homozygous hemoglobin E disease is encountered, it is apparently associated with marked microcytosis and hypochromia but little or no anemia. Splenomegaly is unusual, and the red cell lifespan is normal. Clinically, the state closely resembles β thalassemia minor.

The clinical manifestations of the heterozygous state between hemoglobin E and β thalassemia are somewhat more severe, with moderate anemia and splenomegaly representing the usual manifestation.

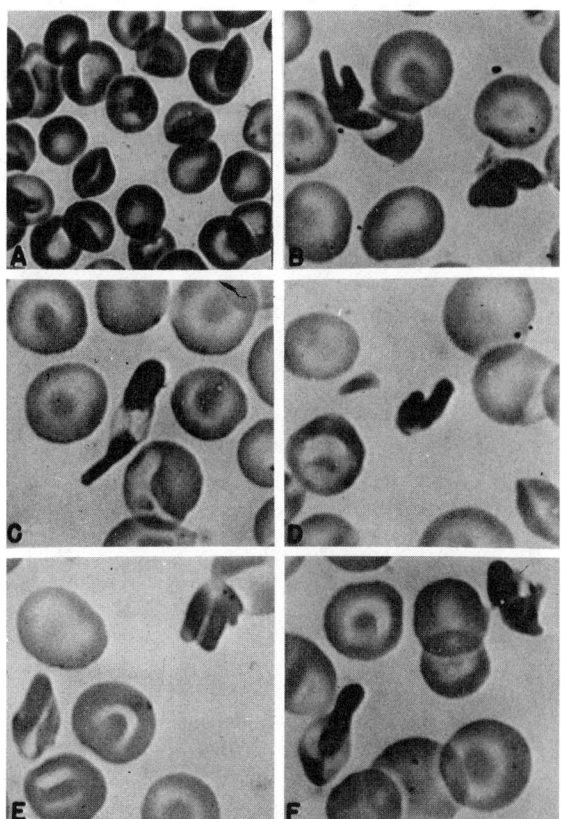

FIGURE 60-10 Bizarre-shaped erythrocytes in the blood film of patients with hemoglobin SC disease. (*A*) "Fat sickle cells." (*B*) Crescent-shaped erythrocyte with three deep-hued crystals (center left). Two bizarre condensed hemoglobin masses in a red blood cell (lower right). (*C*) Elongated red corpuscle with concentration of hemoglobin at each end and hemoglobin-free central area (center). (*D*) Red cell with two parallel, dark, crystal-like structures of different lengths, terminating in a pyramid tip (center). (*E*) Erythrocyte with two parallel formations separated by a clear area (upper right). Red cell with one elongated mass (lower left). (*F*) Erythrocyte with densely stained hemoglobin masses (upper right). Red cell with one dark, elongated, rounded bulge and one small triangular hemoglobin mass, leaving two areas relatively free of hemoglobin (lower left). (Diggs and Bell [224], by permission.)

Other hemoglobinopathies

In comparison with hemoglobins S, C, D, and E, other abnormal hemoglobins are rare. Some, such as the unstable hemoglobins discussed in Chap. 61 and hemoglobins producing erythrocytosis (Chap. 75) and those producing cyanosis (Chap. 78), are of clinical importance. Many of the other hemoglobins do not produce significant clinical alterations but have, nonetheless, been important in clarifying the role of amino acid substitutes at specific sites on the structure and function of the hemoglobin molecule. A list of the abnormal hemoglobins which have been characterized up to the early part of 1981 is presented in Table 60-1.

TABLE 60-1   Known hemoglobin variants

Amino acid (sequential number)	Amino acid substitution	Name	Major abnormal property*	Reference
		α-CHAIN VARIANTS		
5	Ala–Asp	J Toronto		Nature 208:1059, 1965
6	Asp–Ala	Sawara	(1)	Biochim. Biophys. Acta 322:23, 1973
6	Asp–Asn	Dunn		Hemoglobin 3:137, 1979
11	Lys–Glu	Anantharaj		Biochim. Biophys. Acta 405:161, 1975
12	Ala–Asp	J Paris		Nouv. Rev. Fr. Hematol. 6:423, 1966
15	Gly–Asp	J Oxford		Nature 204:269, 1964
				Acta Haematol. 32:9, 1964
15	Gly–Arg	Ottawa		Biochim. Biophys. Acta 336:25, 1974
				Hum. Genet. 23:199, 1974
16	Lys–Glu	I		J. Lab. Clin. Med. 68:940, 1966
18	Gly–Arg	Handsworth		FEBS Lett. 75:93, 1977
19	Ala–Asp	J Kurosh		Biochim. Biophys. Acta 427:119, 1976
20	His–Tyr	Necker Enfants-Malades		Hemoglobin 4:177, 1980
21	Ala–Asp	J Nyanza		Biochim. Biophys. Acta 310:357, 1973
22	Gly–Asp	J Medellin		Fed. Proc. 23:172, 1964
23	Glu–Gln	Memphis		J. Lab. Clin. Med. 66:886, 1965
23	Glu–Val	G Audhall		Nature 219:1164, 1968
23	Glu–Lys	Chad		Am. J. Hum. Genet. 20:570, 1969
27	Glu–Val	Spanish Town		Biochim. Biophys. Acta 427:530, 1976
27	Glu–Gly	G Fort Worth		Biochim. Biophys. Acta 243:164, 1971
29	Leu–Val	Lapin		Clinical Hematology, 7th ed.
				Lea & Febiger, Philadelphia, p. 798, Table 24-1
30	Glu–Gln	G Chinese		J. Biol. Chem. 237:1517, 1962
30	Glu–Lys	Opadova		Blood 44:869, 1974
30	Glu–Lys	O Padua		Blood 44:869, 1974
31	Arg–Ser	Prato		Science 6:234, 1978
43	Phe–Leu	Hirosaki		Biochim. Biophys. Acta 405:155, 1975
43	Phe–Val	Torino	(3)(2)	Nature 217:1016, 1968
44	Pro–Leu	Milledgeville		Biochim. Biophys. Acta 626:424, 1980
45	His–Arg	Fort de France	(1)	Biochim. Biophys. Acta 493:228, 1977
45	His–Gln	Bari		Biochim. Biophys. Acta 622:315, 1980
47	Asp–Gly	L Ferrara		Nature 198:395, 1963
				J. Med. Genet. 2:48, 1965
47	Asp–Asn	Arya	(3)	Biochim. Biophys. Acta 386:525, 1975
47	Asp–His	Hasharon	(3)	Isr. J. Med. Sci. 3:827, 1967
47	Asp–Gly	Umi		Jpn. J. Hum. Genet. 19:343, 1975
48	Leu–Arg	Montgomery		Biochim. Biophys. Acta 379:28, 1975
49	Ser–Arg	Savaria		Hemoglobin 4:27, 1980
50	His–Asp	J Sardegna		Nature 218:470, 1968
51	Gly–Arg	Russ		Biochim. Biophys. Acta 130:541, 1966
51	Gly–Asp	J Abidjan		Nouv. Rev. Fr. Hematol. 12:289, 1972
53	Ala–Asp	J Rovigo	(3)	Biochim. Biophys. Acta 342:1, 1974
54	Gln–Arg	Shimonoseki		Acta Haematol, Jp. 26:531, 1963
54	Gln–Glu	Mexico		Clin. Res. 11:105, 1963
56	Lys–Thr	Thailand		Hemoglobin 1:781, 1977
	Lys–Glu	Shaare Zedek		FEBS Lett. 113:235, 1980
57	Gly–Asp	Norfolk		J. Biol. Chem. 237:69, 1962
57	Gly–Arg	L Persian Gulf		Acta Haematol. 42:169, 1969
58	His–Tyr	M Boston	(2)	Proc. Natl. Acad. Sci. 47:1758, 1961
60	Lys–Asn	Zambia		Br. Med, J, 4:595, 1969
60	Lys–Glu	Dagestan		Hemoglobin 5:133, 1981
61	Lys–Asn	J Buda		Biochim. Biophys. Acta 336:344, 1974
63	Ala–Asp	Pontoise		Biochim. Biophys. Acta 491:16, 1977
64	Asp–His	Q India		J. Med. Genet. 9:436, 1972
64	Asp–Asn	Aida		W.H.O. Tech. Rep. Ser. No. 509, Geneva, 1972
64	Asp–Tyr	Persepolis		Biochim. Biophys. Acta 322:27, 1973
68	Asn–Lys	G Philadelphia		Biochim. Biophys. Acta 48:253, 1961

* (1) ↑ O₂ affinity; (2) ↓ O₂ affinity; (3) unstable; (4) ↑ dissociation; (5) sickling; (6) methemoglobin.

TABLE 60-1   Known hemoglobin variants *(Continued)*

Amino acid (sequential number)	Amino acid substitution	Name	Major abnormal property*	Reference
		α-CHAIN VARIANTS *(Continued)*		
68	Asn–Asp	Ube II		*Clin. Chim. Acta 16:347, 1967*
71	Ala–Glu	J Habana		*Biochim. Biophys. Acta 351:1, 1974*
72	His–Arg	Daneshgag-Tehran		*Nature [New Biol.] 245:268, 1973*
74	Asp–His	Q		*Biochim. Biophys. Acta 200:70, 1970*
				Can. J. Biochem. 48:1066, 1970
				Br. J. Haematol. 19:117, 1970
74	Asp–Asn	G Pest		*Biochim. Biophys. Acta 336:344, 1974*
74	Asp–His	Mahidol		*Can. J. Biochem. 48:1066, 1970*
	Asp–Gly	Chapel Hill		*FEBS Let. 65:297, 1976*
75	Asp–His	Q Iran		*Br. J. Haematol. 19:117, 1970*
75	Asp–Tyr	Winnipeg		*Clin. Biochem. 6:66, 1973*
75	Asp–Gly	Mizushi		*Hemoglobin 4:209, 1980*
78	Asn–Lys	Stanleyville II		*Br. Med J. 4:92, 1968*
78	Asn–Asp ⎞			
79	Ala–Gly ⎠	J Singapore		*Biochim. Biophys. Acta 278:482, 1972*
80	Leu–Arg	Ann Arbor	(3)	*Proc. 1st Inter-Am. Symp. Hemoglobins, Caracus, 1969*
				Karger, Basel, 1971, p. 53
81	Ser–Cys	Nigeria		*Blood 52 (Suppl. 1):113, 1978*
82	Ala–Asp	Garden State		*Clin. Res. 26:122A, 1978*
84	Ser–Arg	Etobicoke	(1)	*Can. J. Biochem. 47:143, 1969*
85	Asp–Tyr	Atago		*Int. J. Protein Res., 3:35, 1971*
85	Asp–Asn	G Norfolk		*Biochim. Biophys. Acta 379:22, 1975*
85	Asp–Val	Inkster		*Br. J. Haematol. 26:475, 1974*
86	Leu–Arg	Moabit	(3)(2)	*Acta Haematol. 61:121, 1979*
87	His–Tyr	M Iwate	(2)	*Acta Haematol. Jpn. 26:538, 1963*
90	Lys–Asn	Broussais		*C. R. Soc. Biol., 160:2270, 1966*
90	Lys–Thr	J Rajappen		*Biochim. Biophys. Acta 243:515, 1971*
91	Leu–Pro	Port Phillip	(3)	*FEBS Lett. 81:115, 1977*
92	Arg–Leu	Chesapeake	(1)	*J. Molec. Biol. 19:91, 1966*
92	Arg–Gln	J Capetown	(1)	*Nature 212:792, 1966*
94	Asp–Tyr	Setif	(3)	*FEBS Lett. 27:298, 1972*
94	Asp–Asn	Titusville	(2)(4)	*Biochim. Biophys. Acta 393:195, 1975*
94	Asp–His	Sunshine Seth		*Hemoglobin 3:145, 1979*
95	Pro–Leu	G Georgia	(4)(1)	*Biochim. Biophys. Acta 200:578, 1970*
95	Pro–Ser	Rampa	(4)(1)	*Biochim. Biophys. Acta 236:197, 1971*
95	Pro–Ala	Denmark Hill	(1)	*Biochim. Biophys. Acta 278:459, 1972*
95	Pro–Arg	St. Luke's	(4)	*Eur. J. Biochem. 29:301, 1972*
102	Ser–Arg	Manitoba	(3)	*Can. J. Biochem. 48:911, 1970*
109	Leu–Arg	Suan-Dok	(3)	*Hemoglobin 3:161, 1979*
112	His–Asp	Hopkins-2	(3)(1)	*Blood 36:852, 1970*
112	His–Arg	Serbia		*FEBS Lett. 58:226, 1975*
				Biochim. Biophys. Acta 412: 81, 1975
112	His–Gln	Dakar		*12th Congr. Int. Soc. Haematol. New York, 1968, p. 73*
114	Pro–Arg	Chiapas		*Biochim. Biophys. Acta 154:488, 1968*
115	Ala–Asp	J Tongariki		*J. Med. Genet. 4:1, 1967*
116	Glu–Lys	O Indonesia		*Nature 196:229, 1962*
116	Glu–Ala	Ube-4		*Hemoglobin 2:181, 1978*
112	His–Asp ⎞			
114	Pro–Ser ⎬	Hopkins-2-II		*Nature [New Biol.]237:90, 1972*
118	Thr–Gly ⎠			
118	Glu, Phe, Thr	Grady		*Proc. Natl. Acad. Sci. U.S.A. 71:3270, 1974*
119	inserted			
120	Ala–Glu	J Birmingham		*Ann. Clin. Biochem. 11:53, 1974*
				Biochim. Biophys. Acta 351:7, 1974
122	His–Gln	Westmead		*Hemoglobin 4:39, 1980*
126	Asp–Asn	Tarrant	(1)	*Biochim. Biophys. Acta 490:443, 1977*
127	Lys–Thr	St. Claude		*Biochim. Biophys. Acta 365:318, 1974*
127	Lys–Asn	Jackson		*Am. J. Clin. Pathol. 66:453, 1976*

* (1) ↑ O₂ affinity; (2) ↓ O₂ affinity; (3) unstable; (4) ↑ dissociation; (5) sickling; (6) methemoglobin.

TABLE 60-1   Known hemoglobin variants *(Continued)*

Amino acid (sequential number)	Amino acid substitution	Name	Major abnormal property*	Reference
			α-CHAIN VARIANTS *(Continued)*	
136	Leu–Pro	Bibba	(3)(4)	*Biochim. Biophys. Acta 154:220, 1968*
141	Arg–Pro	Singapore		*Nature 222:379, 1969*
141	Arg split off on hemolysis in plasma	Koellicker		*Acta Haematol. 37:174, 1967*
141	Arg–His	Suresnes	(1)	*FEBS Lett. 69:103, 1976*
	Arg–Ser	J Cubujuqui		*Biochim. Biophys. Acta 494:48, 1977*
	Arg–Leu	Legnano	(1)	*Hemoglobin 2:249, 1978*
	Arg–Gly	J Camaguey		*Hemoglobin 2:47, 1978*
		β-CHAIN VARIANTS		
1	Val–Ala	Raleigh	(2)(4)	*Biochem. 16:4872, 1979*
2	His–Arg	Deer Lodge		*Clin. Biochem. 5:46, 1972*
6	Glu–Val	S	(5)	*Biochim. Biophys. Acta 36:402, 1959*
6	Glu–Lys	C		*Biochim. Biophys. Acta 42:409, 1960*
6	Glu–Ala	G Makassar		*Biochim. Biophys. Acta 214:396, 1970*
6 or 7	Glu deleted	Leiden		*Nature 220:788, 1968*
7	Glu–Gly	G San Jose		*J. Biol. Chem. 235:3182, 1960*
7	Glu–Lys	Siriraj		*Br. Med. J. 1:1583, 1965*
9	Ser–Cys	Porto Alegre		*Science (NY) 158:800, 1967*
10	Ala–Asp	Ankara		*FEBS Lett. 42:121, 1974*
14	Leu–Arg	Sogn		*Scand. J. Haematol. 5:353, 1968*
14	Leu–Pro	Saki	(3)	*Biochim. Biophys. Acta 393:182, 1975*
15	Trp–Arg	Belfast	(3)(1)	*Br. Med. J. 4:324, 1974*
16	Gly–Asp	J Baltimore		*Biochim. Biophys. Acta 78:637, 1963*
16	Gly–Arg	D Bushman		*Nature 216:688, 1967*
17	Lys–Glu	Nagasaki		*Int. J. Protein Res. 2:147, 1970*
17–18	Lys, Val deleted	Lyon		*Biochim. Biophys. Acta 351:306, 1074*
19	Asn–Lys	D Ouled Rabah		*Biochim. Biophys. Acta 310:360, 1973*
19	Asn–Asp	Alamo		*Hemoglobin 1:703, 1977*
20	Val–Met	Olympia	(1)	*J. Clin. Invest. 52:342, 1973*
20	Val–Asp	Strasbourg		*FEBS Lett. 72:1, 1976*
21	Asp–Gly	Connecticut		W. F. Moo-Penn; personal communication
22	Glu–Lys	E Saskatoon		*Can. J. Biochem. 45:1385, 1967*
22	Glu–Ala	G Coushatta		*Biochem. Biophys. Res. Commun. 26:466, 1967*
22	Glu–Gly	G Taipei		*Biochim. Biophys. Acta 175:237, 1969*
22	Glu–Gln	D Iran		*Br. J. Haematol. 24:31, 1973*
23	Val deleted	Freiburg		*Science (NY) 154:1024, 1966*
24	Gly–Arg	Riverdale-Bronx	(3)	*Biochem. Biophys. Res. Commun. 33:1004, 1968*
24	Gly–Val	Savannah	(3)	*J. Clin. Invest. 50:650, 1971*
24	Gly–Asp	Moscva	(3)(2)	*Nature 249:768, 1974*
25	Gly–Arg	G Taiwan-Ami		*Biochem. Biophys. Res. Commun. 30:690, 1968*
26	Glu–Lys	E		*Biochim. Biophys. Acta 49:520, 1961*
26	Glu–Val	Henri Mondor	(3)	*FEBS Lett. 72:5, 1976*
27	Ala–Asp	Volga	(3)	*FEBS Lett. 58:122, 1975*
28	Leu–Pro	Genova	(3)(1)	*Nature 214:877, 1967*
28	Leu–Gln	St. Louis	(3)(6)(1)	*FEBS Lett. 33:37, 1973*
29	Gly–Asp	Lufkin		*Hemoglobin 1:700, 1977*
30	Arg–Ser	Tacoma	(3)	*Biochemistry (NY) 8:2125, 1969*
32	Leu–Pro	Perth	(3)	*Br. J. Haematol. 25:607, 1973*
32	Leu–Arg	Castilla	(3)	*Biochim. Biophys. Acta 405:161, 1975*
34	Val–Phe	Pitie-Salpetriere		
35	Tyr–Phe	Philly	(3)(1)	*J. Clin. Invest 48:1627, 1969*
37	Trp–Ser	Hirose	(1)	*Blood 38:730, 1971*
37	Trp–Arg	Rothchild		*FEBS Lett. 82:243, 1977*
39	Gln–Lys	Alabama		*Biochim. Biophys. Acta 379:28, 1975*
39	Gln–Glu	Vaasa		*Hemoglobin 1:292, 1977*

* (1) ↑ O₂ affinity; (2) ↓ O₂ affinity; (3) unstable; (4) ↑ dissociation; (5) sickling; (6) methemoglobin.

TABLE 60-1   Known hemoglobin variants *(Continued)*

Amino acid (sequential number)	Amino acid substitution	Name	Major abnormal property*	Reference
		β-CHAIN VARIANTS *(Continued)*		
40	Arg–Ser	Austin	(1)(4)	*Arch. Biochem. Biophys.* 179:86, 1977
40	Arg-Lys	Athens-Georgia	(1)	*Biochim. Biophys. Acta* 439:70, 1976
41	Phe–Tyr	Mequon		*Clin. Res.* 22:176A, 1974
42	Phe–Leu	Louisville	(3)(2)	*J. Clin. Invest.* 50:2395, 1971
42	Phe–Leu	Bucuresti	(3)(2)	*Biochim. Biophys. Acta* 251:1, 1971
42	Phe–Ser	Hammersmith		*Nature* 216:633, 1967
43	Glu–Ala	G Galveston		*Blood* 23:193, 1964
43	Glu–Gln	Hoshida		*Hemoglobin* 2:235, 1978
42–44 or 43–45	Phe, Glu, Ser deleted	Niteroi		*Archivo "Casa Sollievo Della Sofferanza,"* Med. Ed. no. 2, 1972, p. 11
46	Gly–Glu	K Ibadan		*Nature* 208:658, 1965
47	Asp–Asn	G Copenhagen		*Biochim. Biophys. Acta* 140:231, 1967
47	Asp–Gly	Gavello		*Hemoglobin* 1:771, 1977
	Asp–Ala	Avicenna		*Biochim. Biophys. Acta* 576:466, 1979
48	Leu–Arg	Okaloosa	(3)(2)	*J. Clin. Invest.* 52:2858, 1973
50	Thr–Lys	Edmonton		*Clin. Biochem.* 4:114, 1971
51	Pro–Arg	Williamette	(1)	*Hemoglobin* 1:45, 1976
52	Asp–Asn	Osu Christianborg		*J. Med. Genet.* 8:302, 1971
52	Asp–Ala	Ocho Rios		*J. Med. Genet.* 9:151, 1972
52	Asp–His	Summer Hill		*Biochim. Biophys. Acta* 623:360, 1980
56	Gly–Asp	J Bangkok		*J. Molec. Biol.* 19:91, 1966
56	Gly–Arg	Hamadan		*Biochim. Biophys. Acta* 379:645, 1975
57	Asn–Lys	G Ferrara	(3)	*IRCS* 2:1553, 1974
6 58	Glu–Val Pro–Arg	C Ziguinchor		*FEBS Lett.* 58:149, 1975
58	Pro–Arg	Dhofar		*Biochim. Biophys. Acta* 168:58, 1968
59	Lys–Glu	I High Wycombe		*Br. J. Haematol.* 20:671, 1971
59	Lys–Asn	J Lome		*FEBS Lett.* 84:372, 1977
59	Lys–Thr	J Kaoshiung		*Biochim. Biophys. Acta* 229:343, 1971
56–59	Gly, Asn, Pro, Lys deleted	Tochigi		*Proc. Jpn. Acad.* 46:440, 1970
60	Val–Leu	Yatsushiro		*Biochim. Biophys. Acta* 532:195, 1978
61	Lys–Asn	Hikari		*Clin. Chim. Acta* 10:101, 1064
61	Lys–Glu	N Seattle		*Biochim. Biophys. Acta* 154:278, 1968
62	Ala–Pro	Duarte	(3)(1)	*Blood* 43:527, 1974
63	His–Arg	Zurich	(3)(1)	*Biochim. Biophys. Acta* 50:595, 1961
63	His–Pro	Bicetre	(3)	*J. Mol. Med.* 1:187, 1976
63	His–Tyr	M Saskatoon	(1)	*Proc. Natl. Acad. Sci. U.S.A.* 47:1758, 1961
64	Gly–Asp	J Cosenza	(3)	*Int. Symp. Abnormal Hemoglobins and Thalassemia, Istanbul,* Abstr. no. 68, 1974
65	Lys–Asn	J Sicilia		*FEBS Lett.* 39:200, 1974
65	Lys–Gln	J Cairo		*Biochim. Biophys. Acta* 420:97, 1976
66	Lys–Glu	I Toulouse	(3)(6)	*Nature* 223:190, 1969
67	Val–Glu	M Milwaukee	(2)(6)	*Proc. Natl. Acad. Sci. U.S.A.* 47:1758, 1961
67	Val–Ala	Sydney	(3)	*Nature* 215:626, 1967
67	Val–Asp	Bristol	(3)	*Br. J. Haematol.* 18:435, 1970
68	Leu–Pro	Mizuho	(3)	*Hemoglobin* 1:467, 1977
68	Leu–His	Great Lakes		*Blood* 58:813, 1981
69	Gly–Asp	J Cambridge		*Biochim. Biophys. Acta* 140:231, 1967
70	Ala–Asp	Seattle	(2)	*Nature* [New Biol.] 243::275, 1973
71	Phe–Ser	Christchurch	(3)	*Biochim. Biophys. Acta* 236:507, 1971
73	Asp–Asn	Korle Bu		*J. Med. Genet.* 5:107, 1968
73	Asp–Val	Mobile	(2)	*Biochem. Genet.* 13:411, 1975
6 73	Glu–Val Asp–Asn	C Harlem		*Biochem. Biophys. Res. Commun.* 23:122, 1966
73	Asp–Tyr	Vancouver	(2)	*J. Mol. Evol.* 9:37, 1976

* (1) ↑ O_2 affinity; (2) ↓ O_2 affinity; (3) unstable; (4) ↑ dissociation; (5) sickling; (6) methemoglobin.

TABLE 60-1   Known hemoglobin variants *(Continued)*

Amino acid (sequential number)	Amino acid substitution	Name	Major abnormal property*	Reference
		β-CHAIN VARIANTS *(Continued)*		
74	Gly–Asp	Shepherds Bush	(3)(1)	*Nature 225:939, 1970*
74	Gly–Val	Bushwick		*Nature 254:725, 1975*
74–75	Gly, Leu deleted	St. Antoine		*Biochim. Biophys. Acta 295:495, 1973*
75	Leu–Pro	Atlanta	(3)	*Biochim. Biophys. Acta 386:538, 1975*
75	Leu–Arg	Pasadena	(3)(1)	*Biochim. Biophys. Acta 623:360, 1980*
76	Ala–Asp	J Chicago		*Blood 45:387, 1975*
77	His–Asp	J Iran		*Br. Med. J. 1:674, 1967*
79	Asp–Gly	G Hsi-Tsou	(1)	*Biochim. Biophys. Acta 257:49, 1972*
79	Asp–Tyr	Tampa		*Biochim. Biophys. Acta 623:119, 1980*
80	Asn–Lys	G Szuhu		*Biochim. Biophys. Acta 188:59, 1969*
81	Leu–Arg	Baylor	(1)(3)	*Hemoglobin 1:85, 1976*
82	Lys–Met	Helinski	(1)	*Acta Haematol. 56:257, 1976*
82	Lys–Asn	Providence	(2)	*Blood 46:1030, 1975*
82	Lys–Thr	Rahere	(1)	*Br. Med. J. 4:200, 1975*
83	Gly–Cys	Ta-Li		*Biochim. Biophys. Acta 243:467, 1971*
83	Gly–Asp	Pyrgos		*Abstr., Mtg. Am. Soc. Hematol. Abstr. no, 168, 1972*
85	Phe–Ser	Buenos Aires	(3)(1)	*Acta Haematol. 50:357, 1973* *Blood 40:947, 1975*
87	Thr–Lys	D Ibadan		*Nature 205:1273, 1965*
87	Thr deleted	Tours		*Biochim. Biophys. Acta 295:495, 1973*
88	Leu–Pro	Santa Ana	(3)	*J. Med. Genet. 5:292, 1968*
88	Leu–Arg	Boras	(3)	*Nature 222:953, 1969*
89	Ser–Asn	Creteil	(1)	*FEBS Lett. 43.93, 1974*
89	Ser–Arg	Vanderbilt		*Br. J. Haematol. 39:249, 1978*
90	Glu–Lys	Agenogi	(2)	*Clin. Chim. Acta 14:624, 1966*
91	Leu–Arg	Caribbean	(3)(2)	*Biochim. Biophys. Acta 69:99, 1976*
91	Leu–Pro	Sabine	(3)	*N. Engl. J. Med. 280:739, 1969*
92	His–Tyr	M Hyde Park		*J. Clin. Invest. 45:1021, 1966*
92	His–Pro	Newcastle		*FEBS Lett. 60:435, 1975*
92	His–Gln	Saint Etienne	(3)(1)(4)	*FEBS Lett. 27:76, 1972*
92	His–Asp	J Altgeld Gardens		*Clin. res. 23:487, 1975*
95	Lys–Asn	Detroit		*Biochim. Biophys. Acta 536:283, 1978*
95	Lys–Glu	N Baltimore		*Nature 207:945, 1965*
95 / 6	Lys–Glu / Glu–Lys	Arlington Park		*Blood 42:1973*
91–95 or 92–96 or 93–97	Leu, His, Cys, Asp deleted	Gun Hill		*Science (NY) 157:1581, 1967*
97	His–Gln	Malmö	(1)	*Biochem. J. 119:68P, 1970*
97	His–Leu	Wood	(1)	*Biochim. Biophys. Acta 400:348, 1975*
98	Val–Met	Köln	(3)(1)	*Nature 210:915, 1966*
98	Val–Gly	Nottingham	(3)(1)	*Proc. R. Soc. Med. 66:507, 1973*
98	Val–Ala	Djelfa	(3)(1)	*FEBS Lett. 58:238, 1975*
99	Asp–His	Yakima	(1)	*J. Clin. Invest. 46:1840, 1967*
99	Asp–Asn	Kempsey	(1)	*Blood 31:623, 1968*
99	Asp–Ala	Radcliffe	(1)	*Br. J. Haematol. 35:177, 1977*
99	Asp–Tyr	Ypsi	(1)	*Ann. Rev. Med. 22:221, 1971*
99	Asp–Gly	Hotel-Dieu	(1)	*Hemoglobin 5:19, 1981*
100	Pro–Leu	Brigham	(1)	*J. Clin. Invest. 52:2060, 1973*
101	Glu–Gln	Rush	(3)	*Blood 43:261, 1974*
101	Glu–Lys	British Columbia	(1)	*Hemoglobin 1:171, 1976*
	Glu–Gly	Alberta	(1)	*Hemoglobin 1:183, 1976-77*
	Glu–Asp	Potomac	(1)	*Blood 51:331, 1978*
102	Asn–Ser	Beth Israel	(2)	*Abstr. Mtg. Am. Soc. Haematol. Dallas, 1975*

* (1) ↑ O₂ affinity; (2) ↓ O₂ affinity; (3) unstable; (4) ↑ dissociation; (5) sickling; (6) methemoglobin.

TABLE 60-1   Known hemoglobin variants *(Continued)*

Amino acid (sequential number)	Amino acid substitution	Name	Major abnormal property*	Reference
		β-CHAIN VARIANTS *(Continued)*		
102	Asn–Thr	Kansas	(2)(4)	*J. Biol. Chem.* 243:980, 1968
102	Asn–Lys	Richmond		*J. Biol. Chem.* 244:6105, 1969
130	Phe–Leu	Heathrow	(1)	*Br. Med. J.* 3:665, 1973
104	Arg–Ser	Camperdown	(3)	*Biochim. Biophys. Acta* 393:195, 1975
104	Arg–Thr	Sherwood Forest		*FEBS Lett.* 83:260, 1977
106	Leu–Gln	Tübingen	(3)(1)	*FEBS Lett.* 64:443, 1976
106	Leu–Pro	Casper	(1)(3)	*Am. J. Med.* 55:549, 1973
107	Gly–Arg	Burke	(2)	*16th Int. Congr. Hematology,* Sept. 1976
108	Asn–Asp	Yoshizuka	(2)	*J. Clin. Invest.* 48:2341, 1969
108	Asn–Lys	Presbyterian	(2)	*FEBS Lett.* 92:53, 1978
109	Val–Met	San Diego	(1)	*J. Clin. Invest.* 53:230, 1974
111	Val–Phe	Petersborough	(3)(2)	*Br. J. Haematol.* 22:125, 1972
112	Cys–Arg	Indianapolis	(3)	*Clin. Res.* 26:501A, 1978
113	Val–Glu	New York		*Nature* 213:876, 1967
115	Ala–Pro	Madrid	(3)	*Acta Haematol.* 52:53, 1974
117	His–Arg	P		*J. Lab Clin. Med.* 73:616, 1969
119	Gly–Asp	Fannin-Lubbock	(3)	*Biochim. Biophys. Acta* 453:472, 1976
119	Gly–Val	Bougardiery-Mali		*Hemoglobin* 3:253, 1979
120	Lys–Glu	Hijiyama		*Science (NY)* 159:204, 1968
120	Lys–Asn	Riyadh		*Hemoglobulin* 1:59, 1977
120	Lys–Gln	Takamatsu		*Hemoglobin* 4:165, 1980
121	Glu-Gln	D Punjab	(1)	*Biochim. Biophys. Acta* 59:437, 1962
121	Glu-Lys	O Arab		*Nature* 196:229, 1962
121	Glu-Val	Beogard		*Biochim. Biophys. Acta* 328:81, 1973
124	Pro–Arg	Khartoum	(3)	*Nature* 222:379, 1969
124	Pro–Glu	Ty Gard	(1)	*FEBS Lett.* 88:155, 1978
126	Val–Glu	Hofu		*Nature* 217:89, 1968
127	Gln–Glu	Hacettepe		*Biochim. Biophys. Acta* 434:1, 1976
128	Ala–Asp	J Guantanamo	(3)	*Biochim. Biophys. Acta* 491:1, 1977
129	Ala–Asp	J Taichung		*Biochim. Biophys. Acta* 194:1, 1969
129	Ala-Pro	Crete		*Blood* 54:54, 1979
130	Tyr–Asp	Wien	(3)	*Acta Haematol.* 51:351, 1974
131	Gln–Glu	Camden		*Nature [New Biol.]* 243:467, 1973
131	Gln deleted	Leslie		*Biochim. Biophys. Res. Commun.* 65:8, 1975
132	Lys–Gln	K Woolwich		*Nature* 208:658, 1965
134	Val–Glu	North Shore	(3)	*FEBS Lett.* 80:261, 1977
135	Ala–Pro	Altdorf	(3)(1)	*FEBS Lett.* 63:193, 1976
136	Gly–Asp	Hope	(3)	*Blood* 25:830, 1965
138	Ala–Pro	Brockton	(3)	*Hemoglobin* 4:347, 1980
141	Leu–Arg	Olmsted		*Biochem. J.* 119:68P, 1970
141	Leu deleted	Coventry†		*Br. J. Haematol.* 33:143, 1976
142	Ala–Pro	Toyoake	(3)(1)	*Hemoglobin* 4:307, 1980
142	Ala–Asp	Ohio	(1)	*Hemoglobin* 4:347, 1980
143	His–Arg	Abruzzo	(1)	*Clin. Chim. Acta* 38:258, 1972
143	His–Gln	Little Rock	(1)	*Nature [New Biol.]* 243:117, 1973
143	His–Pro	Syracuse	(1)	*J. Clin. Invest.* 55:469, 1975
144	Lys–Asn	Andrew-Minneapolis	(1)	*Blood* 44:543, 1974
145	Tyr–Cys	Rainier	(1)	*Nature [New Biol.]* 230:264, 1971
145	Tyr–Term.	McKees Rocks	(1)	*J. Clin. Invest.* 57:772, 1976
145	Tyr–His	Bethesda	(1)	*Nature [New Biol.]* 230:264, 1971
145	Tyr–Asp	Fort Gordon		*FEBS Lett.* 56:39, 1975
				Biochim. Biophys. Acta 400:343, 1975
				Johns Hopkins Med. J. 136:132, 1975
146	His–Asp	Hiroshima	(1)	*Nature [New Biol.]* 232:147, 1971
146	His–Arg	Cochin–Port Royal		*Biochim. Biophys. Acta* 400:354, 1975
146	His–Pro	York	(1)	*Nature* 259:155, 1976
146	His–Leu	Cowtown	(1)	*Am. J. Clin. Pathol.* 72:1028, 1979

* (1) ↑ O$_2$ affinity; (2) ↓ O$_2$ affinity; (3) unstable; (4) ↑ dissociation; (5) sickling; (6) methemoglobin.
† Chemically β chain but genetically βδ chain.

TABLE 60-1 Known hemoglobin variants *(Continued)*

Amino acid (sequential number)	Amino acid substitution	Name	Major abnormal property*	Reference
		γ-CHAIN VARIANTS		
1	Gly–Cys	Malaysia (136 Gly)		*J. Med. Genet. 11:25, 1974*
5	Glu–Lys	F Texas I		*Br. J. Haematol. 13:252, 1967*
		(136 Ala)		*Biochim. Biophys. Acta 271:61, 1972*
6	Glu–Lys	F Texas II		*Br. J. Haematol. 14:233, 1968*
7	Asp–Asn	F Auckland		*Biochim. Biophys. Acta 365:323, 1974*
12	Thr–Lys	F Alexandra		*Biochim. Biophys. Acta 200:70, 1970*
16	Gly–Arg	F Melbourne (136 Gly)		*Biochim. Biophys. Acta 490:452, 1977*
22	Asp–Gly	F Kuala Lumpur (136 Ala)		*Biochim. Biophys. Acta 322:224, 197*
61	Lys–Glu	F Jamaica (136 Ala)		*Br. J. Haematol. 18:369, 1970*
63	His–Tyr	F M Osaka		*Hemoglobin 4:47, 1980*
75	Ile–Thr	F Sardinia (136 Gly)		*Acta Haematol. 53:347, 1975*
80	Asp–Tyr	F Victoria Jubilee		*Biochim. Biophys. Acta 393:188, 1975*
97	His–Arg	F Dickinson		*Proc. XIII Int. Cong. Haematol. Munich, 1970*
108	Asn–Lys	F Ube		*Chem. Abstr. 83:266, 1975*
117	His–Arg	F Malta (136 Gly)		*Nature 223:311, 1969*
121	Glu–Lys	F Hull (136 Ala)		*Br. Med. J. 3:531, 1967*
				New Aspects of the Structure, Function and Synthesis of Hemoglobins, CRC Press, 1971, p. 54
121	Glu–Lys	F Carlton (136 Gly)		*Biochim. Biophys. Acta 490:452, 1977*
125	Glu–Ala	F Port Royal		*Br. J. Haematol. 27:313, 1974*
130	Trp–Gly	F Poole (136 Gly)		*J. Clin. Pathol. 28:317, 1975*
		δ-CHAIN VARIANTS		
2	His–Arg	A₂ Sphakia		*Science (NY) 151:1406, 1966*
12	Asn–Lys	NYU		*J. Clin. Invest. 48:2057, 1969*
16	Gly–Arg	A'₂		*Nature 209:1217, 1966*
20	Val–Glu	A₂ Roosevelt		*Biochim. Biophys. Acta 439:581, 1976*
22	Ala–Glu	A₂ Flatbush		*Clin. Res. 14:168, 1966*
43	Glu–Lys	A₂ Melbourne		*Biochim. Biophys. Acta 359:233, 1974*
51	Pro–Arg	A₂ Adria		*XIII Meeting Gruppo di Studio Dell'Entrocita, Torino, 1977*
69	Gly–Arg	A₂ Indonesia		*Biochim. Biophys. Acta 229:335, 1971*
116	Arg–His	A₂ Coberg		*Biochim. Biophys. Acta 393:379, 1975*
136	Gly–Asp	A₂ Babinga		*Nature 219:1360, 1968*

Name	Reference
FUSION HEMOGLOBINS	
Lepore Hollandia	*Nature 194:931, 1962*
Lepore Baltimore	*Eur. J. Biochem. 10:371, 1969*
Lepore Boston	*Proc. Natl. Acad. Sci. U.S.A. 48:1880, 1962*
Miyada	*Jpn. J. Hum. Genet. 13:40, 1968*
P Congo	*Biochem. J. 119:43P, 1970*
P Nilotic	*Nature [New Biol.]242:107, 1973*
STOP CODON MUTATIONS	
Constant Spring	*Nature 234:337, 1971*
Icaria	*Nature 251:245, 1974*
Koya Dora	*Am. J. Hum. Genet. 27:81, 1975*
Seal Rock	*Clin. Res 23:131A, 1975*
FRAMESHIFT MUTATION	
Lys, Tyr, Arg replaced by Asn, Thr, Val, Lys, Leu, Glu, Pro, Arg	
Wayne	*Blood 40:927, 1975*

* (1) ↑ O₂ affinity; (2) ↓ O₂ affinity; (3) unstable; (4) ↑ dissociation; (5) sickling; (6) methemoglobin.

NOTE: See H. Lehmann and P. A. M. Kynoch, *Human Haemoglobin Variants and Their Characteristics*, North-Holland Publishing Company, Amsterdam, 1976.

References

1. Herrick, J. B.: Peculiar elongated and sickle-shaped red corpuscles in a case of severe anemia. *Arch. Intern. Med. 6*:517, 1910.

2. Emmel, V. E.: A study of the erythrocytes in a case of severe anemia with elongated and sickle-shaped red blood corpuscles. *Arch. Intern. Med. 20*:586, 1917.

3. Hahn, E. V., and Gillespie, E. B.: Report of a case greatly improved by splenectomy: Experimental study of sickle cell formation. *Arch. Intern. Med. 39*:233, 1927.

4. Taliaferro, W. H., and Huck, J. G.: The inheritance of sickle-cell anemia in man. *Genetics 8*:594, 1923.

5. Neel, J. V.: The inheritance of sickle cell anemia. *Science 110*:64, 1949.

6. Beet, E. A.: The genetics of the sickle-cell trait in a Bantu tribe. *Ann. Eugen. (Lond.) 14*:279, 1949.

7. Pauling, L., Itano, H. A., Singer, S. J., and Wells, I. C.: Sickle cell anemia, a molecular disease. *Science 110*:543, 1949.

8. Ingram, V. M.: Gene mutations in human hemoglobin: The chemical difference between normal and sickle cell hemoglobin. *Nature 180*:326, 1957.

9. Conley, C. L.: Sickle-cell anemia—The first molecular disease, in *Blood, Pure and Eloquent*, edited by M. M. Wintrobe, McGraw-Hill, New York, 1980, p. 319.

10. Dean, J., and Schechter, A. N.: Sickle-cell anemia: Molecular and cellular bases of therapeutic approaches. *N. Engl. J. Med. 299*:752, 1978.

11. Murayama, M.: A molecular mechanism of sickled erythrocyte formation. *Nature 202*:258, 1964.

12. Murayama, M.: Molecular mechanisms of red cell "sickling." *Science 153*:145, 1966.

13. Goldberg, M. A., Lalos, A. T., and Bunn, H. F.: The effect of erythrocyte membrane preparations on the polymerization of sickle hemoglobin. *J. Biol. Chem. 256*:193, 1981.

14. Eaton, J. W., Jacob, H. S. and White, J. G.: Membrane abnormalities of irreversibly sickled cells. *Semin. Hematol. 16*:52, 1979.

15. Serjeant, G. R., Serjeant, B. E., and Milner, P. F.: The irreversibly sickled cell: A determinant of haemolysis in sickled-cell anaemia. *Br. J. Haematol. 17*:527, 1969.

16. Tosteson, D. C., Carlsen, E., and Dunham, E. T.: The effects of sickling on ion transport. I. Effect of sickling on potassium transport. *J. Gen. Physiol. 39*:31, 1955.

17. Dzandu, J. K., and Johnson, R. M.: Membrane protein phosphorylation in intact normal and sickle cell erythrocytes. *J. Biol. Chem. 255*:6382, 1980.

18. Beutler, E., Guinto, E., and Johnson, C.: Human red cell protein kinase in normal subjects and patients with hereditary spherocytosis, sickle cell disease, and autoimmune hemolytic anemia. *Blood 48*:887, 1976.

19. Hosey, M. M., and Tao, M.: Altered erythrocyte membrane phosphorylation in sickle cell disease. *Nature 263*:424, 1976.

20. Bookchin, R. M., and Lew, V. L.: Progressive inhibition of the Ca pump and Ca: Ca exchange in sickle red cells. *Nature 284*:561, 1980.

21. Steinberg, M. H., Eaton, J. W., Berger, E., Coleman, M. B., and Oelshlegel, F. J.: Erythrocyte calcium abnormalities and the clinical severity of sickling disorders. *Br. J. Haematol. 40*:533, 1978.

22. Itano, H. A.: Qualitative and quantitive control of adult hemoglobin synthesis: A multiple allele hypothesis. *Am. J. Hum. Genet. 5*:34, 1953.

23. Huisman, T. H. J.: Sickle cell anemia as a syndrome: A review of diagnostic features. *Am. J. Hematol. 6*:173, 1979.

24. Embury, S. H., and Dozy, A. M.: Correlation of alpha-globin genotype with hematologic parameters in sickle cell trait. *Blood 54 (Suppl. 1)*:53A, 1979.

25. Brittenham, G., Lozoff, B., Harris, J. W., Kan, Y. W., Dozy, A. M., and Nayudu, N. V. S.: Alpha globin gene number: Population and restriction endonuclease studies. *Blood 55*:706, 1980.

26. Mears, J. G., Lachman, H., Patel, P., Gross, B., Labie, D., and Nagel, R. L.: Alpha gene deletions are beneficial to sickle cell (SS) patients. *Blood 58 (Suppl. 1)*:62A, 1981.

27. Embury, S. H., Clark, M. R., Hoesch, R., and Mohandas, N.: Alpha

28. El Hazmi, M. A. F.: On the nature of sickle-cell disease in the Arabian peninsula. *Hum. Genet. 52*:323, 1979.

29. Powars, D. R., Schroeder, W. A., Weiss, J. N., Chan, L. S., and Azen, S. P.: Lack of influence of fetal hemoglobin levels or erythrocyte indices on the severity of sickle cell anemia. *J. Clin. Invest. 65*:732, 1980.

30. Bookchin, R. M., and Nagel, R. L.: Interactions between human hemoglobins: Sickling and related phenomena. *Semin. Hematol. 11*:577, 1974.

31. Jackson, J. F., Odom, J. L., and Bell, W. N.: Amelioration of sickle cell disease by persistent fetal hemoglobin. *JAMA 17*:867, 1961.

32. Bradley, T. B., Jr., Brawner, J. N., III, and Conley, C. L.: Further observations on an inherited anomaly characterized by persistence of fetal hemoglobin. *Johns Hopkins Med. J. 108*:242, 1962.

33. Shepherd, M. K., Weatherall, D. J., and Conley, C. L.: Semiquantitative estimation of fetal hemoglobin in red cell populations. *Johns Hopkins Med. J. 110*:293, 1962.

34. Singer, K., and Singer, L.: Studies on abnormal hemoglobins. VIII. The gelling phenomenon of sickle cell hemoglobin: Its biologic and diagnostic significance. *Blood 8*:1008, 1953.

35. Ali, S. A.: Milder variant of sickle-cell disease in Arabs in Kuwait associated with unusually high levels of foetal haemoglobin. *Br. J. Haematol. 19*:613, 1970.

36. Perrine, R. P., Pembrey, M. E., John, P., Perrine, S., and Shoup, F.: Natural history of sickle cell anemia in Saudi Arabs. *Ann. Intern. Med. 88*:1, 1978.

37. Jacob, G. F., and Raper, A. B.: Hereditary persistence of foetal haemoglobin production and its interaction with the sickle cell trait. *J. Haematol. 4*:1368, 1958.

38. Mac Iver, J. E., Went, L. N., and Irvine, R. A.: Hereditary persistence of foetal haemoglobin: A family study suggesting allelism of the F gene to the S and C haemoglobin genes. *Br. J. Haematol. 7*:373, 1961.

39. Conley, C. L., Weatherall, D. J., Richardson, S. N., Shepherd, M. K., and Charache, S.: Hereditary persistence of fetal hemoglobin: A study of 79 affected persons in 15 Negro families in Baltimore. *Blood 21*:261, 1963.

40. Kraus, L. M., Miyaji, T., Iuchi, I., and Kraus, A. P.: Characterization of α 23 Glu NH2 in hemoglobin Memphis. Hemoglobin Memphis/ S, a new variant of molecular disease. *Biochemistry 5*:3701, 1966.

41. Van Enk, H., Lang, A., White, J. M., and Lehmann, H.: Benign obstetric history in women with sickle-cell anaemia associated with alpha thalassemia. *Br. Med. J. 4*:524, 1972.

42. Lewis, R. A., and Hathorn, M.: Glucose-6-phosphate dehydrogenase deficiency correlated with S Hemoglobin. *Ghana Med. J. 2*:131, 1963.

43. Piomelli, S., Reindorf, C. A., Arzanian, M. T., and Corash, L. M.: Clinical and biochemical interactions of glucose-6-phosphate dehydrogenase deficiency and sickle-cell anemia. *N. Engl. J. Med. 287*:213, 1972.

44. Naylor, J., Rosenthal, I., Grossman, A., Schulman, I., and Hsia, D. Y. Y.: Activity of glucose-6-phosphate dehydrogenase in erythrocytes of patients with various abnormal hemoglobins. *Pediatrics 26*:285, 1960.

45. Milner, P. F., and Serjeant, G. R.: Laboratory studies in sickle cell anaemia. *Blood 34*:729, 1969.

46. Lewis, R. A.: Glucose-6-phosphate dehydrogenase electrophoresis in Ghanaians with AA and SS haemoglobin. *Acta Haematol. 50*:105, 1973.

47. Beutler, E., Johnson, C., Powars, D., and West, C.: Prevalence of glucose-6-phosphate dehydrogenase deficiency in sickle cell disease. *N. Engl. J. Med. 290*:826, 1974.

48. Smits, H. L., Oski, F. A., and Brody, J. I.: The hemolytic crisis of sickle cell disease: The role of glucose-6-phosphate dehydrogenase deficiency. *J. Pediatr. 74*:544, 1969.

49. Gibbs, W. N., Wardle, J., and Serjeant, G. R.: Glucose-6-phosphate dehydrogenase deficiency and homozygous sickle cell disease in Jamaica. *Br. J. Haematol. 45*:73, 1980.

50. Lange, R. D., Minnich, V. and Moore, C. V.: Effect of oxygen ten-

thalassemia regulates the determinants of hemolysis and vaso-occlusion in sickle cell anemia (SCA). *Blood 58 (Suppl. 1)*:59A, 1981.

sion and of pH on the sickling and mechanical fragility of erythrocytes from patients with sickle cell anemia and sickle cell trait. *J. Lab. Clin. Med.* 37:789, 1951.

51. Allison, A. C.: Observations on the sickling phenomenon and on the distribution of different hemoglobin types in erythrocyte populations. *Clin. Sci.* 15:497, 1956.

52. Harris, J. W., Brewster, H. H., Ham, T. H., and Castle, W. B.: Studies on the destruction of red blood cells. X, The biophysics and biology of sickle-cell disease. *Arch. Intern. Med.* 97:145, 1956.

53. Green, R. L., Huntsman, R. G., and Sergeant, G. R.: The sickle-cell and altitude. *Br. Med. J.* 2:593, 1971.

54. Smith, E. W., and Conley, C. L.: Clinical manifestations of sickle-cell disease. *N.A.S.N.R.C. Publ.* 554:276, 1958.

55. Charache, S., and Conley, C. L.: Rate of sickling of red cells during deoxygenation of blood from persons with various sickling disorders. *Blood* 24:25, 1964.

56. Diggs, L. W., and Bibb, J.: The erythrocyte in sickle cell anemia. *JAMA* 112:695, 1939.

57. Akinla, O.: Pregnancy and the skeletal complications of sickle cell disease. *Postgrad. Med. J.* 49:255, 1973.

58. Beutler, E.: Hypothesis: Changes in the O_2 dissociation curve and sickling: A general formulation and therapeutic strategy. *Blood* 43:297, 1974.

59. Perillie, P. E., and Epstein, F. H.: Sickling phenomenon produced by hypertonic solutions: A possible explanation for the hyposthenuria in sicklemia. *J. Clin. Invest.* 42:570, 1963.

60. Hebbel, R. P., Boogaerts, M. A. B., Eaton, J. W., and Steinberg, M. H.: Erythrocyte adherence to endothelium in sickle-cell anemia. *N. Engl. J. Med.* 302:992, 1980.

61. Hunt, J. A., and Ingram, V. M.: Allelomorphism and the chemical differences of the human hemoglobins A, S, and C. *Nature* 181:1062, 1958.

62. Thomas, E. D., Motulsky, A. G., and Walters, D. H.: Homozygous hemoglobin C disease. *Am. J. Med.* 18:832, 1955.

63. Movitt, E. R., Pollycove, M., Mangum, J. F., and Porter, W. R.: Hemoglobin C disease: Quantitative determination of iron kinetics and hemoglobin synthesis. *Am. J. Med. Sci.* 247:558, 1964.

64. Murphy, J. R.: Hemoglobin CC erythrocytes: Decreased intracellular pH and decreased O_2 affinity-anemia. *Semin. Hematol.* 13:177, 1976.

65. Itano, H. A.: A third abnormal hemoglobin associated with hereditary hemolytic anemia. *Proc. Natl. Acad. Sci. U.S.A.* 37:775, 1951.

66. Hunt, J. A., and Ingram, V. M.: Abnormal human haemoglobins. VI. The chemical difference between hemoglobins A and E. *Biochim. Biophys. Acta* 49:520, 1961.

67. Frischer, H., and Bowman, J.: Hemoglobin E, an oxidatively unstable mutation. *J. Lab. Clin. Med.* 85:531, 1975.

68. Allison, A. C.: *Genetical Variations in Human Populations*, edited by G. A. Harrison. Pergamon, New York, 1961, p. 16.

69. Dunston, T., Rowland, R., Huntsman, R. G., and Yawson, G. I.: Sickle-cell haemoglobin C disease and sickle-cell β thalassemia in white South Africans. *S. Afr. Med. J.* 46:1423, 1972.

70. Allison, A. C.: Parasitological reviews. Malaria in carriers of the sickle-cell trait and in newborn children. *Exp. Parasitol.* 6:418, 1957.

71. Luzzatto, L.: Genetics of red cells and susceptibility to malaria. *Blood* 54:961, 1979.

72. Kan, Y. W., and Dozy, A. M.: Evolution of the hemoglobin S and C genes in world populations. *Science* 209:388, 1980.

73. Edington, G. N., and Lehmann, H.: A case of sickle cell hemoglobin C disease in a survey of hemoglobin C incidence in West Africa. *Trans. R. Soc. Trop. Med. Hyg.* 48:332, 1954.

74. Schneider, R. G.: Incidence of hemoglobin C trait in 505 normal Negroes: A family with homozygous hemoglobin C and sickle-cell trait union. *J. Lab. Clin. Med.* 44:133, 1954.

75. Diggs, L. W., Kraus, A. P., Morrison, D. B., and Rudnicki, R. P. T.: Intraerythrocytic crystals in a white patient with hemoglobin C in the absence of other types of hemoglobin. *Blood* 9:1172, 1954.

76. Dunston, T., Rowland, R., Huntsman, R. G., and Yawson, G.: Sickle-cell haemoglobin C disease and sickle-cell β thalassaemia in white South Africans. *S. Afr. Med. J.* 46:1423, 1972.

77. Flatz, G.: Hemoglobin E: Distribution and population dynamics. *Humangenetik* 3:189, 1967.

78. Barbedo, M. M. R., and McCurdy, P. R.: Red cell life span in sickle cell trait. *Acta Haematol.* 51:339, 1974.

79. Kellon, D. B., and Beutler, E.: Physician attitudes about sickle cell. *JAMA* 227:71, 1974.

80. Sears, D. A.: The morbidity of sickle cell trait. *Am. J. Med.* 64:1021, 1978.

81. Heller, P., Best, W. R., Nelson, R. B., and Becktel, J.: Clinical implications of sickle-cell trait and glucose-6-phosphate dehydrogenase deficiency in hospitalized black male patients. *N. Engl. J. Med.* 300:1001, 1979.

82. Atlas, S. A.: The sickle cell trait and surgical complications. *JAMA* 229:1078, 1974.

83. Jones, S. R., Binder, R. A., and Donowho, E. M., Jr.: Sudden death in sickle cell trait. *N. Engl. J. Med.* 282:323, 1970.

84. Koppes, G. M., Daley, J. J., Coltman, Jr., C. A., and Butkus, D. E.: Exertion-induced rhabdomyolysis with acute renal failure and disseminated intravascular coagulation in sickle cell trait. *Am. J. Med.* 63:313, 1977.

85. Schlitt, L. E., and Keitel, H. G.: Renal manifestations of sickle cell disease: A review. *Am. J. Med. Sci.* 239:773, 1960.

86. Francis, C. K., and Bleakley, D. W.: The risk of sudden death in sickle cell trait: Noninvasive assessment of cardiac response to exercise. *Cathet. Cardiovasc. Diagn.* 6:73, 1980.

87. O'Brien, R. T., Pearson, H. A., Godley, J. A., and Spencer, R. P.: Splenic infarct and sickle (cell) trait. *N. Engl. J. Med.* 287:720, 1972.

88. Nichols, S. D.: Splenic and pulmonary infarction in a Negro athlete. *Rocky Mount Med. J.* 65:49, 1968.

89. Rywlin, A. M., and Benson, J.: Massive necrosis of the spleen with formation of a pseudocyst: Report of a case in a white man with sickle cell trait. *Am. J. Clin. Pathol.*, 36:142, 1961.

90. Smith, E. W., and Conley, C. L.: Clinical features of the genetic variants of the sickle cell disease. *Johns Hopkins Med. J.* 94:289, 1954.

91. Goldstein, M. A., Patpongpanij, N., and Minnich, V.: The incidence of elevated hemoglobin A_2 levels in the American Negro. *Ann. Intern. Med.* 60:95, 1964.

92. Diggs, L. W.: Sickle-cell crises. *Am. J. Clin. Pathol.* 44:1, 1965.

93. Song, J.: *Pathology of Sickle-Cell Disease.* Charles C Thomas, Springfield, Ill., 1971.

94. Charache, S.: The treatment of sickle cell anemia. *Arch. Intern. Med.*, 133:698, 1974.

95. Fullerton, W. T., and Watson-Williams, E. J.: Haemoglobin SC disease and megaloblastic anaemia of pregnancy. *J. Obstet. Gynaecol. Br. Commonw.*, 69:729, 1962.

96. Seeler, R. A., and Shwiaki, M. Z.: Acute splenic sequestration crises (ASSC) in young children with sickle-cell anemia. *Clin. Pediatr.* 1:701, 1972.

97. Diggs, L. W.: Crises in sickle cell anemia. *Am. J. Clin. Pathol.* 26:1109, 1956.

98. Moseley, J. E.: *Bone Changes in Hematologic Disorders (Roentgen Aspects).* Grune & Stratton, New York, 1963.

99. Sain, A., Sham, R., and Silver, L.: Bone scan in sickle cell crisis. *Clin. Nuclear Med.*, 3:85, 1978.

100. River, G. L., Robbins, A. B., and Schwartz, S. O.: SC hemoglobin: A clinical study. *Blood* 18:385, 1961.

101. Hook, E. W., Campbell, C. G., Weens, H. S., and Cooper, G. R.: Salmonella osteomyelitis in patients with sickle-cell anemia. *N. Engl. J. Med.* 257:403, 1957.

102. Roberts, A. R., and Hillburg, L. E.: Sickle cell disease with Salmonella osteomyelitis. *J. Pediatr.* 52:170, 1958.

103. Vance, B. M., and Fisher, R. C.: Sickle cell disease: Two cases presenting fat embolism as a fatal complication. *Arch. Pathol.* 32:378, 1941.

104. Shelley, W. M., and Curtis, E. M.: Bone marrow and fat embolism in sickle-cell anemia and sickle-cell hemoglobin C disease. *Johns Hopkins Med. J.* 103:8, 1958.

105. Harrow, B. R., Sloane, J. A., and Lieberman, N. C.: Roentgenologic demonstration of renal papillary necrosis in sickle-cell trait. *N. Engl. J. Med.* 268:969, 1963.

106. Pearson, H. A., McIntosh, S., Ritchey, A. K., Lobel, J. S., Rooks, Y., and Johnston, D.: Developmental aspects of splenic function in sickle cell diseases. *Blood* 53:358, 1979.

107. Hemley, S. D., Mellins, H. Z., and Finby, N.: Punctate calcification of the spleen in sickle cell anemia. *Am. J. Med.* 34:483, 1963.

108. Green, T. W., Conley, C. L., and Berthrong, M.: The liver in sickle cell anemia. *Johns Hopkins Med. J.* 92:99, 1953.
109. Song, Y. S.: Hepatic lesions in sickle anemia. *Am. J. Pathol.* 33:331, 1957.
110. Mintz, A. A., and Pugh, D. P.: Choledocholithiasis in sickle cell anemia. *South Med. J., 63, 1498, 1970.*
111. Miller, G. J., Serjeant, G. R., Sivapragasam, S., and Petch, M.: Cardiopulmonary responses and gas exchange during exercise in adults with homozygous sickle cell disease. *Clin. Sci.* 44:113, 1973.
112. Charache, S., Scott, J. C., and Charache, P.: Acute chest syndrome in adults with sickle cell anemia. Microbiology, treatment and prevention. *Arch. Intern. Med.* 139:67, 1979.
113. Moser, K. M., and Shea, J. G.: The relationship between pulmonary infarction, cor pulmonale and the sickle cell states. *Am. J. Med.* 22:561, 1957.
114. Condon, P. L., and Serjeant, G. R.: Ocular findings in homozygous sickle-cell anemia in Jamaica. *Am. J. Ophthalmol.* 73:533, 1972.
115. Paton, D.: Conjunctival sign of sickle cell disease. *Arch. Ophthalmol.* 68:627, 1962.
116. Comer, P. B., and Fred, H. L.: Diagnosis of sickle cell disease by ophthalmoscopic inspection of the conjunctiva. *N. Engl. J. Med.* 271:344, 1964.
117. Baird, R. L.: Studies in sickle cell anemia. XXI. Clinicopathological aspects of neurological manifestations. *Pediatrics* 34:92, 1964.
118. Cummer, C. L., and Larocco, C. G.: Ulcers on the legs in sickle cell anemia. *Arch. Dermatol.* 42:1015, 1940.
119. Mc Curdy, P. R.: Abnormal hemoglobins and pregnancy. *Am. J. Obstet. Gynecol.* 90:891, 1964.
120. Anderson, M., Went, L. N., Mac Iver, J. E., and Dixon, H. G.: Sickle cell disease in pregnancy. *Lancet* 2:516, 1960.
121. Anderson, M. F.: The foetal risks in sickle cell anemia. *West Indian Med. J.* 2:288, 1971.
122. Hendrickse, J. P. D., and Watson-Williams, E. J.: Influence of haemoglobinopathies on reproduction. *Am. J. Obstet. Gynecol.* 94:739, 1966.
123. Charache, S., Scott, J., Niebyl, J., and Bonds, D.: Management of sickle cell disease in pregnant patients. *Obstet. Gynecol.* 55:407, 1980.
124. Glader, B. E., Propper, R. D., and Buchanan, G. R.: Microcytosis associated with sickle cell anemia. *Am. J. Clin. Pathol.* 72:63, 1979.
125. Boggs, D. R., Hyde, F., and Strodes, C.: An unusual pattern of neutrophil kinetics in sickle cell anemia. *Blood* 41:59, 1973.
126. Buchanan, G. R., and Glader, B. E.: Leukocyte counts in children with sickle cell disease. Comparative values in the steady state, vaso-occlusive crisis and bacterial infection. *Am. J. Dis. Child.* 132:396, 1978.
127. Corvelli, A. I., Binder, R. A., and Kales, A.: Disseminated intravascular coagulation in sickle cell crisis. *South. Med. J.* 72:23, 1979.
128. Ballas, S. K., Burka, E. R., Lewis, C. N., and Krasnow, S. H.: Serum immunoglobulin levels in patients having sickle cell syndromes. *Am. J. Clin. Pathol.* 73:394, 1980.
129. Glassman, A. B., Deas, D. V., Berlinsky, F. S., and Bennett, C. E.: Lymphocyte blast transformation and peripheral lymphocyte percentages in patients with sickle cell disease. *Ann. Clin. Lab. Sci.* 10:9, 1980.
130. Corry, J. M., Polhill, R. B., Jr., Edmonds, S. R., and Johnston, R. B., Jr.: Activity of the alternative complement pathway after splenectomy: Comparison to activity in sickle cell disease and hypogammaglobulinemia. *J. Pediatr.* 95:964, 1979.
131. Natta, C., and Machlin, L.: Plasma levels of tocopherol in sickle cell anemia subjects. *Am. J. Clin. Nutr.* 32:1359, 1979.
132. Karayalcin, G., Lanzkowsky, P., and Kazi, A. B.: Zinc deficiency in children with sickle cell disease. *Am. J. Ped. Hematol./Onc.* 1:283, 1979.
133. Niell, H. B., Leach, B. E., and Kraus, A. P.: Zinc metabolism in sickle cell anemia. *JAMA* 242:2686, 1979.
134. O'Brien, R. T.: Iron burden in sickle cell anemia. *J. Pediatr.* 92:579, 1978.
135. Daland, G. A., and Castle, W. B.: A simple and rapid method for demonstrating sickling of the red blood cells: The use of reducing agents. *J. Lab. Clin. Med.* 33:1082, 1948.
136. Schneider, R. G., Alperin, J. B., and Lehmann, H.: Sickling tests: Pitfalls in performance and interpretation. *JAMA* 202:419, 1967.
137. Itano, H. A.: Solubilities of naturally occurring mixtures of human hemoglobin. *Arch. Biochem. Biophys.* 47:148, 1953.
138. Canning, D. M., and Huntsman, R. G.: An assessment of Sickledex as an alternative to the sickling test. *J. Clin. Pathol.* 23:736, 1970.
139. Serjeant, B. E., and Serjeant, G. R.: A whole blood solubility and centrifugation test for sickle-cell hemoglobin. *Am. J. Clin. Pathol.* 58:11, 1972.
140. Canning, D. M., Crane, R. S., Huntsman, R. G., and Yawson, G. I.: An automated screening technique for the detection of sickle-cell haemoglobin. *J. Clin. Pathol.* 25:330, 1972.
141. VanBaelen, H., Vandepitte, J., and Eeckels, R.: Observations on sickle cell anaemia and haemoglobin Bart's in Congolese neonates. *Ann. Soc. Belge Med. Trop.* 49:157, 1969.
142. Yawson, G. I., Huntsman, R. G., and Metters, J. S.: An assessment of techniques suitable for the diagnosis of sickle-cell disease and haemoglobin C disease in cord blood samples. *J. Clin. Pathol.* 23:533, 1970.
143. Schneider, R. G., Gustavson, L. P., Haggard, M. E., Brimhall, B., and Jones, R. T.: The incidence of genetically determined hemoglobin abnormalities in 11,427 cord blood samples. *Abstr. XIII, Int. Soc. Haematol.* J. F. Lehmanns, Verlag, Munich, 1970, p. 356.
144. Pearson, H. A., O'Brien, R. T., McIntosh, S., Aspnes, G. T., and Yang, M. M.: Routine screening of cord blood for sickle cell disease. *JAMA* 227:420, 1974.
145. Schneider, R. G.: *Developments in Laboratory Diagnosis in Sickle Cell Disease,* edited by H. Abramson, J. F. Bertles, and D. L. Wethers. Mosby, St. Louis, 1973.
146. Kan, Y. W., Golbus, M. S., Trecartin, R. F., and Filly, R. A.: Prenatal diagnosis of beta-thalassaemia and sickle-cell anaemia. Experience with 24 cases. *Lancet* 1:269, 1977.
147. Tegos, C., and Beutler, E.: A simplified method for studies of haemoglobin biosynthesis. *Clin. Lab. Haematol.* 2:191, 1980.
148. Kan, Y. W., and Dozy, A. M.: Antenatal diagnosis of sickle-cell anaemia by DNA analysis of amniotic-fluid cells. *Lancet* 2:910, 1978.
149. Kan, Y. W., and Dozy, A. M.: Polymorphism of DNA sequence adjacent to human beta-globin structural gene: Relationship to sickle mutation. *Proc. Natl. Acad. Sci. U.S.A.* 75:5631, 1978.
150. Sirs, J. A.: The use of carbon monoxide to prevent sickle-cell formation. *Lancet* 1:971, 1963.
151. Puruggganan, H. B., and McElfresh, A. E.: Failure of carbonmonoxy sickle-cell haemoglobin to alter the sickle state. *Lancet* 1:79, 1964.
152. Beutler, E.: The effect of carbon monoxide on red cell life span in sickle cell disease. *Blood* 46:253, 1975.
153. Beutler, E.: The effect of methemoglobin formation in sickle cell disease. *J. Clin. Invest.* 40:1856, 1961.
154. Paniker, N. V., Ben-Bassat, I., and Beutler, E.: Evaluation of sickle hemoglobin and desickling agents by falling ball viscometry. *J. Lab. Clin. Med.* 80:282, 1972.
155. Shamsuddin, M., Mason, R. G., Ritchey, J. M., Honig, G. R., and Klotz, I. M.: Sites of acetylation of sickle cell hemoglobin by aspirin. *Proc. Natl. Acad. Sci. U.S.A.* 71:4693, 1974.
156. Zaugg, R. H., King, L. C., and Klotz, I. M.: Acylation of hemoglobin by succinyldisalicylate, a potential crosslinking reagent. *Biochem. Biophys. Res. Commun.* 64:1192, 1975.
157. Isaacs, W. A., and Hayhoe, F. G. J.: Steroid hormones in sickle cell disease. *Nature* 215:1139, 1967.
158. Waterman, M. R., Yamaoka, K., Chuang, A. H., and Cottam, G. L.: Antisickling nature of dimethyl adipimidate. *Biochem. Biophys. Res. Commun.* 63:580, 1975.
159. Hilkowitz, G.: Sickle cell disease: New method of treatment: Preliminary report. *Br. Med. J.* 2:266, 1957.
160. Knochel, J. P.: Hematuria in sickle cell trait. *Arch. Intern. Med.* 123:160, 1969.
161. Nalbandian, R. M., Shulta, G., Lusher, J. M., Anderson, J. W., and Henry, R. L.: Sickle cell crisis terminated by intravenous urea in sugar solutions: A preliminary report. *Am. J. Med. Sci.* 261:309, 1971.
162. Gillette, P. N., Manning, J. M., and Cerami, A.: Increased survival of sickle cell erythrocytes after treatment in vitro with sodium cyanate. *Proc. Natl. Acad. Sci. U.S.A.* 68:2791, 1971.

163. Baker, R., Powars, D., and Haywood, J.: Restoration of the deformability of "irreversibly" sickled cells by procaine hydrochloride. *Biochem. Biophys. Res. Commun.* 59:548, 1974.

164. Brewer, G. J., Brewer, L. F., and Prasad, A. S.: Suppression of irreversibly sickled erythrocytes by zinc therapy in sickle cell anemia. *J. Lab. Clin. Med.* 90:549, 1977.

165. Beutler, E., Paniker, N. V., and West, C. J.: Pyridoxine administration in sickle cell disease: An unsuccessful attempt to influence the properties of sickle hemoglobin. *Biochem. Med.* 6:139, 1972.

166. Kark, J. A., et al.: Inhibition of erythrocyte sickling in vitro by pyridoxal. *J. Clin. Invest.* 62:888, 1978.

167. Benesch, R., Benesch, R. E., Edalji, R., and, Suzuki, T.: 5'-Deoxypyridoxal as a potential anti-sickling agent. *Proc. Natl. Acad. Sci. U.S.A.* 74:1721, 1977.

168. Bounameaux, Y.: Action inhibitrice de la nivaquine et de divers anti-histaminiques sur la formation d'nématies en faciles dans l'anémie drepanocytaire. *C. R. Soc. Biol. (Paris)* 155:425, 1961.

169. Fung, L. W. M., Ho, C., Roth, E. F., Jr., and Nagel, R. L.: The alkylation of hemoglobin S by nitrogen mustard: High resolution proton nuclear magnetic resonance studies. *J. Biol. Chem.* 250:4786, 1975.

170. Nigen, A. M., and Manning, J. M.: Inhibition of erythrocyte sickling in vitro by DL-glyceraldehyde. *Proc. Natl. Acad. Sci. U.S.A.* 74:367, 1977.

171. Ross, P. D., and Subramanian, S.: Hexamethylenetetramine: A powerful and novel inhibitor of gelation of deoxyhemoglobin S. *Arch. Biochem. Biophys.* 190:736, 1978.

172. Natta, C. L., Machlin, L. J., and Brin, M.: A decrease in irreversibly sickled erythrocytes in sickle cell anemia patients given vitamin E. *Am. J. Clin. Nutr.* 33:968, 1980.

173. Asakura, T., et al.: Effect of cetiedil on erythrocyte sickling: New type of antisickling agent that may affect erythrocyte membranes. *Proc. Natl. Acad. Sci. U.S.A.* 77:2955, 1980.

174. Greenberg, M. S., and Kass, E. H.: Studies on the destruction of red blood cells. XIII. Observations on the role of pH in the pathogenesis and treatment of painful crisis in sickle cell disease. *Arch. Intern. Med.* 101:355, 1958.

175. Rhodes, R. S., Revo, L., Hara, S., Hartmann, R. C., and Van Eys, J.: Therapy for sickle cell vaso-occlusive crises, controlled clinical trials and cooperative clinical study of intravenously administered alkali. *JAMA* 228:1129, 1974.

176. Bensinger, T. A., Mahmood, L., Conrad, M. E., and McCurdy, P. R.: The effect of oral urea administration on red cell survival in sickle cell disease. *Am. J. Med. Sci.* 264:283, 1972.

177. Kilmartin, J. V., and Rossi-Bernardi, L.: The binding of carbon dioxide by horse haemoglobin. *Biochem. J.* 124:31, 1971.

178. Peterson, C. M., et al.: Sodium cyanate induced polyneuropathy in patients with sickle-cell disease. *Ann. Intern. Med.* 81:152, 1974.

179. Nicholson, D. H., Harkness, D. R., Benson, W. E., and Peterson, C. M.: Cyanate-induced cataracts in patients with sickle-cell hemoglobinopathies. *Arch. Ophthalmol.* 94:927, 1976.

180. Langer, E. E., et al.: Extracorporeal treatment with cyanate in sickle cell disease: Preliminary observations in four patients. *J. Lab. Clin. Med.* 87:462, 1976.

181. Charache, S., Dreyer, R., Zimmerman, I., and Hsu, C. K.: Evaluation of extracorporeal alkylation of red cells as a potential treatment for sickle cell anemia. *Blood* 47:481, 1976.

182. Diederich, D. A., Trueworthy, R. G., Gill, P., Crader, A. M., and Larsen, W. E.: Hematologic and clinical responses in patients with sickle cell anemia after chronic extracorporeal red cell carbamylation. *J. Clin. Invest.* 58:642, 1976.

183. Rosa, R. M., et al.: A study of induced hyponatremia in the prevention and treatment of sickle-cell crisis. *N. Engl. J. Med.* 303:1138, 1980.

184. Leary, M., and Abramson, N.: Induced hyponatremia for sickle-cell crisis. *N. Engl. J. Med.* 304:844, 1981.

185. Konotey-Ahula, F. I. D.: Effect of environment on sickle cell disease in West Africa: Epidemiologic and clinical considerations, in *Sickle Cell Disease: Diagnosis, Management, Education and Research*, edited by H. Abramson, J. F. Bertles, and D. L. Wethers. Mosby, St. Louis, 1973, p. 20.

186. Ammann, A. J., Addiego, J., Wara, D. W., Lubin, B., Smith, W. B., and Mentzer, W. C.: Polyvalent pneumococcal-polysaccharide immunization of patients with sickle-cell anemia and patients with splenectomy. *N. Engl. J. Med.* 297:897, 1977.

187. Ahonkhai, V. I., et al.: Failure of pneumococcal vaccine in children with sickle-cell disease. *N. Engl. J. Med.* 301:26, 1979.

188. Konotey-Ahulu, F. I. D.: Treatment and prevention of sickle cell crisis. *Lancet* 2:1255, 1971.

189. Solanki, D. L., and McCurdy, P. R.: Cholelithiasis in sickle cell anemia: A case for elective cholecystectomy. *Am. J. Med. Sci.* 277:319, 1979.

190. Laszlo, J., Obenour, W., and Saltzman, H. A.: Effects of hyperbaric oxygenation on sickle syndromes. *South. Med. J.* 62:453, 1969.

191. Reynolds, J. D. H.: Painful sickle cell crisis: Successful treatment with hyperbaric oxygen therapy. *JAMA* 216:1977, 1971.

192. Brody, J. I., Goldsmith, M. H., Park, S. K., and Soltys, H. D.: Symptomatic crises of sickle cell anemia treated by limited exchange transfusion. *Ann. Intern. Med.* 72:327, 1970.

193. Sommer, A., Kontras, S. B., and Craenen, J. M.: Partial exchange transfusion in sickle cell anemia complicated by heart disease. *JAMA* 215:483, 1971.

194. Henderson, A. B.: Sickle cell disease: Studies "in vivo" sickling and the effect of certain pharmacological agents. *Am. J. Med. Sci.* 221:628, 1951.

195. Mann, J. R., Deeble, T. J., Breeze, G. R., and Stuart, J.: Ancrod in sickle cell crisis. *Lancet* 1:934, 1972.

196. Hugh-Jones, K., Lehmann, H., and McAlister, J. M.: Some experiences in managing sickle cell anaemia in children and young adults using alkalis and magnesium. *Br. Med. J.* 2:226, 1964.

197. Barreras, L., and Diggs, L. W.: Sodium citrate orally for painful sickle cell crises. *JAMA* 215:762, 1971.

198. Cooperative Urea Trials Group.: Clinical trials of therapy for sickle cell vaso-occlusive crises. *JAMA* 228:1120, 1974.

199. Green, M., Hall, R. J. C., Huntsman, R. G., Lawson, A., Pearson, T. C., and Wheeler, P. C. G.: Sickle cell infarctive crises treated by exchange transfusion. *JAMA* 231:948, 1975.

200. Davey, R. J., Esposito, D. J., Jacobson, R. J., and Corn, M.: Partial exchange transfusion as treatment for hemoglobin SC disease in pregnancy. *Arch. Intern. Med.* 138:937, 1978.

201. Bellingham, A. J., and Huehns, E. R.: Compensation in haemolytic anaemias caused by abnormal haemoglobins. *Nature* 218:924, 1968.

202. May, A., and Huehns, E. R.: The concentration dependence of the oxygen affinity of haemoglobin S. *Br. J. Haematol.* 30:317, 1975.

203. Greenwald, J. G.: Stroke, sickle cell trait and oral contraceptives. *Ann. Intern. Med.* 72:960, 1970.

204. Morrison, J. C., Schneider, J. M., Whybrew, W. D., Bucovaz, E. T., and Menzel, D. M.: Prophylactic transfusions in pregnant patients with sickle hemoglobinopathies: Benefit versus risk. *Obstet. Gynecol.* 56:274, 1980.

205. Cunningham, F. G., and Pritchard, J. A.: Prophylactic transfusions of normal red blood cells during pregnancies complicated by sickle cell hemoglobinopathies. *Am. J. Obstet. Gynecol.* 135:994, 1979.

206. Morrison, J. C., and Foster, H.: Transfusion therapy in pregnant patients with sickle-cell disease. A National Institute of Health Consensus Development Conference. *Ann. Intern. Med.* 91:122, 1979.

207. Searle, J. F.: Anaesthesia in sickle cell states. *Anaesthesia* 28:48, 1973.

208. Oduro, K. A., and Searle, J. F.: Anaesthesia in sickle cell states: A plea for simplicity. *Br. Med. J.* 4:596, 1972.

209. Howells, T. H., Huntsman, R. G., Boys, J. E., and Mahmood, A.: Anaesthesia and sickle cell haemoglobin. *Br. J. Anaesth.* 44:975, 1972.

210. Morrison, J. C., Whybrew, W. D., and Bucovaz, E. T.: Use of partial exchange transfusion preoperatively in patients with sickle cell hemoglobinopathies. *Am. J. Obstet. Gynecol.* 132:59, 1978.

211. Serjeant, G. R., Galloway, R. E., and Gueri, M.: Oral zinc sulphate in sickle cell ulcers. *Br. Med. J.* 1:820, 1970.

212. Goldberg, M. F.: Treatment of proliferative sickle retinopathy. *Trans. Am. Acad. Ophthalmol. Otolaryngol.* 75:532, 1971.

213. Goldberg, M. F., and Acacio, I.: Argon laser photocoagulation of proliferative sickle retinopathy. *Arch. Ophthalmol.* 90:35, 1973.

214. Condon, P. I., and Serjeant, G. R.: Photocoagulation and diathermy in the treatment of proliferative sickle retinopathy. *Br. J. Ophthalmol.* 58:650, 1974.

215. Lambotte-Legrand, J., and Lambotte-Legrand, C.: Le Prognostic de

l'anémie drepanocytaire au Congo Belge (à propos de 300 cas et de 150 décès). *Ann. Soc. Belge Med. Trop.* 35:53, 1955.

216. Vandepitte, J. M.: Present day aspects of the sickle cell problem. *Doc. Med. Geogr. Trop. (AMST)* 7:154, 1955.

217. Trowell, H. C., Raper, A. B., and Welbourn, H. F.: The natural history of homozygous sickle cell anaemia in Central Africa. *Q. J. Med.* 25:401, 1957.

218. Sydenstricker, V. P., Kemp., J. A., and Metts, J. C.: Prolonged survival in sickle cell disease. *Am. Pract.* 13:584, 1962.

219. Miall, W. E., Milner, P. F., Lovell, H. G., and Standard, K. L.: Haematological investigations of population samples in Jamaica. *Br. J. Prev. Soc. Med.* 21:45, 1967.

220. Serjeant, G. R., Richards, R. R., Barbor, P. H. H., and Milner, P. F.: Relatively benign sickle cell anaemia in 60 patients over 30 in the West Indies. *Br. Med. J.* 2:86, 1968.

221. Serjeant, B. E., Forbes, M., and Williams, L. L.: Screening cord bloods for detection of sickle cell disease in Jamaica. *Clin. Chem.* 20:666, 1974.

222. Powars, D. R.: Natural history of sickle cell disease—The first ten years. *Semin. Hematol.* 12:267, 1975.

223. Beutler, E., Boggs, D. R., Heller, P., Maurer, A., Motulsky, A. G., and Sheehy, T. W.: Hazards of indiscriminate screening for sickling. *N. Engl. J. Med.* 285:1485, 1971.

224. Diggs, L. W., and Bell, A.: Intraerythrocytic hemoglobin crystals in sickle cell hemoglobin C disease. *Blood* 25:218, 1958.

225. Chernoff, A. I.: Hgb D syndromes. *Blood* 13:116, 1958.

226. Bird, G. W. G., and Lehmann, H.: Haemoglobin D in India. *Br. Med. J.* 1:514, 1956.

227. Chernoff, A. I., Minnich, V., Na Nakorn, S., Tuchinda, S., Kashemsant, C., and Chernoff, R. R.: Studies on hemoglobin E. I. The clinical, hematologic and genetic characteristics of the hemoglobin E syndromes. *J. Lab. Clin. Med.* 47:455, 1956.

228. Fairbanks, V. F., Gilchrist, G. S., Brimhall, B., Jereb, J. A., and Goldston, E. C.: Hemoglobin E trait reexamined: A cause of microcytosis and erythrocytosis. *Blood* 52:109, 1979.

229. Wilson, J. T., et al.: Use of restriction endonucleases for mapping the allele for β S-globin. *Proc. Natl. Acad. Sci. U.S.A.* 79:3628, 1982.

230. Chang, J. C., and Kan, Y. W.: Antenatal diagnosis of sickle cell anaemia by direct analysis of the sickle mutation. *Lancet* 2:1127, 1981.

231. Charache, S., and Walker, W. G.: Failure of desmopressin to lower serum sodium or prevent crisis in patients with sickle cell anemia. *Blood* 58:892, 1981.

CHAPTER *61*

Hemoglobinopathies associated with unstable hemoglobin

ERNEST BEUTLER

The sporadic occurrence of hemolytic anemia with the appearance of inclusion bodies in the red cells was occasionally observed in the 1940s and 1950s [1–3], but it was not until 1962 [4,5] that it was recognized that such patients had abnormal hemoglobins which spontaneously denatured within the circulating red cell. The unstable hemoglobins which will be discussed in this chapter are those which result from a mutation that changes the amino acid sequence of one of the globin chains. Homotetramers of normal β chains (hemoglobin H) or normal γ chains (hemoglobin Barts) are also unstable hemoglobins. These unstable hemoglobins occur in patients with α thalassemia and are discussed in Chap. 50.

Etiology and pathogenesis

The tetrameric hemoglobin molecule has evolved so that a variety of noncovalent forces maintain the structure of each subunit and bind the subunits to each other. The delicate balance which allows the molecule to change from one state to another, facilitating its oxygen-binding function while maintaining its structural integrity, has been discussed in Chap. 37. It is not surprising that a variety of amino acid substitutions or deletions will weaken the forces which maintain the structure of hemoglobin. When this occurs, the hemoglobin molecule denatures and precipitates as insoluble globins. These precipitates often attach to the cell membrane together with heme and with denatured membrane proteins and are called Heinz bodies.

Instability of hemoglobin can arise from any one of the following processes:

1. Replacement of an amino acid which contacts the heme group often results in an unstable molecule with a tendency to lose heme from the abnormal globin chains. $Hb_{Hammersmith}$ is an example of this type of unstable hemoglobin.

2. Replacement of nonpolar by polar residues in the interior of the molecule results in gross distortion of the protein, particularly if the new polar residue remains in the interior portion of the molecule. $Hb_{Bristol}$ and Hb_{Volga} are examples of this type of mutation.

3. Deletions or insertions of additional amino acids, particularly when critical helical regions of the sequence are involved, create instability. $Hb_{Niteroi}$ is an example of this type of mutation.

4. Replacements at intersubunits contacts, particularly those between the α_1 and β_1 chain, create instability so that dissociation into monomers may occur. Hb_{Philly} and Hb_{Tacoma} are mildly unstable for this reason. Replacements at the contact between the α_1- and β_2-globin monomers usually result in hemoglobins with a high oxygen affinity.

5. If proline is introduced into an α helix beyond the third residue, distortion of the helix results in instability [6]. Variants in which proline substitution results in instability include Hb_{Duarte} and $Hb_{Santa\ Ana}$.

6. In areas of the hemoglobin molecule in which atoms are very tightly packed, substitution of amino acids with larger side chains for glycine may produce marked changes in stability. In particular, at the points where the B and E helices approach each other there is no room for the substitution of larger amino acids for glycine at B6 and E8. $Hb_{Riverdale-Bronx}$, $Hb_{Savannah}$, and Hb_{Moscva} arise in such a fashion.

Many unstable hemoglobins have an increased susceptibility to oxidation to methemoglobin. However, the exact sequence of events which leads to the precipitation of hemoglobin is not fully understood, and very likely varies in the case of different unstable hemoglobins. The formation of hemichromes may be involved. These are compounds in which heme has been removed from its normal binding site and has become bonded to another part of the globin molecule [7–9]. These pigments can be shown to form during in vitro denaturation of some abnormal hemoglobins [10], and they are present in hemoglobin H inclusion bodies [11]. The release of activated oxygen in the form of superoxide radicals with the subsequent formation of peroxide and the hydroxyl radicals [12,13] may also play a role. The attachment of Heinz bodies to the cell membrane impairs the deformability of the erythrocyte and impedes its ability to negotiate the narrow spaces between the endothelial cells lining the splenic sinuses. The "pitting" of Heinz bodies from the erythrocyte results in loss of membrane and ultimately in destruction of the red cells. Although Heinz bodies are formed, their presence in the blood does not become a prominent feature except in patients who have been splenectomized (see "Laboratory Features").

Mode of inheritance

Unstable hemoglobins are inherited as autosomal dominant disorders. Affected individuals are heterozygotes who have usually inherited the defect from one of their parents and who on the average will transmit it to one-half of their offspring. Since unstable hemoglobins produce a disease state, genes for these disorders are subjected to negative selection, and the persistence of the unstable hemoglobinopathies in the population is the result of new mutations. Thus, it is not rare to encounter a patient with an unstable hemoglobin neither of whose parents had the abnormality. While the homozygous state for an unstable hemoglobin has not been observed, a homozygous-like state can occur when an unstable β-chain mutation is inherited together with a β^0-thalassemic gene. This has been observed in the case of Hb$_{Duarte}$. The index patient had red cells which contained exclusively the abnormal hemoglobin because he had inherited the gene for the unstable hemoglobin from one parent and the β^0-thalassemic gene from the other [14].

Over 80 percent of unstable hemoglobins which have been characterized affect the β chain. This probably reflects the fact that the normal genome contains four copies of the α chain, so that inheritance of a single unstable α-chain mutant might well produce subclinical results.

Although most patients with unstable hemoglobins have been found to have a combination of hemoglobin A and unstable hemoglobin in their red cells, there are a number of reports of the inheritance of unstable hemoglobins with other hemoglobinopathies [14–19].

Clinical features

A broad spectrum of clinical manifestations is induced by unstable hemoglobins. In most cases, hemolysis is well compensated. Indeed, when the unstable hemoglobin also has a left-shifted oxygen dissociation curve, i.e., a raised O_2 affinity (see Table 61-1), the hemoglobin level may be in the upper portion of the normal range. Episodes of infection and treatment with "oxidant" drugs are likely to precipitate hemolytic episodes in persons whose anemia is well compensated under ordinary circumstances. It is at this juncture that the diagnosis is often first made. In the case of patients who have particularly unstable variants, such as Hb$_{Hammersmith}$, Hb$_{Bristol}$, Hb$_{Santa Ana}$, or Hb$_{Madrid}$, a chronic hemolytic anemia may become evident during the first year of life as γ-chain production is replaced by production of the mutant β chain. In contrast, in the rare instances where the γ chain bears the abnormality [131] the hemolytic anemia is evident at birth and disappears as normal β chains are formed.

The physical findings include jaundice, splenomegaly, and, when the anemia is severe, pallor. In some patients, dark urine has been observed, probably as a result of the excretion of dipyrrole pigments derived from the catabolism of free heme groups or of Heinz bodies [150]. In some instances methemoglobulinemia may develop, and cyanosis may then be evident.

Laboratory features

The hemoglobin concentration of the blood may be normal or decreased. The mean corpuscular hemoglobin is usually diminished because of the loss of hemoglobin from the red cells as a result of its denaturation and subsequent pitting from the erythrocytes. The blood film may show slight hypochromia, and, in addition, poikilocytosis, polychromasia, anisocytosis, and some basophilic stippling may be evident. Reticulocytosis is often out of proportion to the severity of the anemia, particularly when the abnormal hemoglobin has a high oxygen affinity. After splenectomy many Heinz bodies may be found in the circulation.

Diagnosis of this disorder depends upon the demonstration of the presence of an unstable hemoglobin. Three tests are used for this purpose (see Chap. A6). The most convenient is the isopropanol stability test. The heat stability test is also useful, but is somewhat more difficult to interpret. Finally, incubation of blood with brilliant cresyl blue generates Heinz bodies in the unstable hemoglobinopathies. Further identification of unstable hemoglobins is aided by procedures such as hemoglobin electrophoresis (see Chap. A7); however, the electrophoretic pattern is often normal, and the diagnosis of the hemoglobinopathy cannot be ruled out in this way. The oxygen affinity of unstable hemoglobins is often altered, and the determination of the P_{50} may help further in detecting and characterizing the unstable hemoglobin. In the final analysis unstable

TABLE 61-1 The unstable hemoglobins*

Hemoglobin	Substitution	Helical notation	Hemoglobin, g%	% Variant	Reticulocytes, %	Comments	References
Leiden	β6 or β7 Glu deleted	A3 or A4	11.3–13.6	25–30	3–6	Excess α-chain production in the heterozygote	[20,21]
Sogn	β14 Leu→Arg	A11	12–13	30	0–4	No clinical abnormality	[22,23]
Saki	β14 Leu→Pro	A11	12.2	41	—	Found with Hb S	[18]
Belfast	β15 Trp→Arg	A12	10.6–13.7	28	4	Normal synthesis; raised O_2 affinity	[24]
Lyon	β17–18 Lys-Val deleted	A14–15	11.0	37	—	Raised O_2 affinity; decreased cooperativity	[25]
Freiburg	β23 Val deleted	B5	13.1	27–32	9	Raised O_2 affinity	[26,27]
Riverdale-Bronx	β24 Gly→Arg	B6	11–12	30	10	Defective synthesis; raised O_2 affinity	[28–30]
Savannah	β24 Gly→Val	B6	3.7–7.0	15–30	20–50	Dissociates more readily into dimers than Hb A	[31]
Moscva	β24 Gly→Asp	B6	10.7	17	3.2	Reduced O_2 affinity	[30,32]
Henri Mondor	β26 Glu→Val	B8	7.5	37.5	0.5		[33]
Volga	β27 Ala→Asp	B9	11–12	15–20	20–30	Charge on the new Asp side chain suppressed in the tetramer	[34]
Geneva	β28 Leu→Pro	B10	10–11	15–25	9–16	Normal synthesis; raised O_2 affinity; reduced cooperativity	[35–37]
St. Louis	β28 Leu→Gln	B10	—	30	—	β hemes in permanent Fe^{3+} state; increased O_2 affinity; decreased cooperativity; normal synthesis	[38,39]
Tacoma	β30 Arg→Ser	B12	13–14	42–43	0.4	$\alpha_1\beta_1$ contact; Bohr effected reduced above pH 7.4	[40–43]
Castilla	β32 Leu→Arg	B14	9.6	22	Elevated	Free α chains detected; βB helix distorted	[44]
Perth† (Abraham Lincoln)	β32 Leu→Pro	B14	7–14	33	17–75	Slight heme loss; decreased synthesis	[45–47]
Philly	β35 Tyr→Phe	C1	12.6–14.6	30–35	2–8	$\alpha_1\beta_1$ contact; increased dissociation into monomers	[48]
Hammersmith	β42 Phe→Ser	CD1	6.0–6.2	30	46–71	Heme contact; normal synthesis; reduced O_2 affinity; no cooperativity	[8,49,50]
Bucuresti† (Louisville)	β42 Phe→Leu	CD1	11.5–13.9	35–50	3–10	Heme contact; reduced O_2 affinity and cooperativity	[51,52]
Niteroi	β42–44, or β43–45 Phe, Glu, Ser deleted	CD1–3 or CD2–4	—	28	—	Loses heme; raised O_2 affinity	[53,54]
Okaloosa	β48 Leu→Arg	CD7	13–17.9	32–36	1.8–4.3	Decreased O_2 affinity	[55]
Tochigi	β56–59 Gly-Asn-Pro-Lys deleted	D7–E3	6.5–13.0	20–25	7.3–18.0	Loses heme	[56,57]
G-Ferrara	β57 Asn→Lys	E1	—	94	—		[58]

* Some hemoglobins M (see Chap. 11) also give positive instability tests but are not included in this list.
† The parentheses indicate alternative names for these variants but are not intended to suggest that one or the other name is to be preferred.
NOTE: N = normal; — = not reported.

TABLE 61-1 The unstable hemoglobins* (Continued)

Hemoglobin	Substitution	Helical notation	Hemoglobin, g%	% Variant	Reticulo- cytes, %	Comments	References
Duarte	β62 Ala→Pro	E6	15.1–16.8	–	0.6–10.4	Raised O_2 affinity; found with β° thalassemia	[14]
Bicêtre	β63 His→Pro	E7	–	20–25	–	^{51}Cr half-life 2 days	[59]
Zürich	β63 His→Arg	E7	11.0–14.7	25–30	5–13	Heme contact; raised O_2 affinity; normal synthesis	[5,60,61]
J Calabria	β64 Gly→Arg	E8	–	–	–	Found with β^+ thalassemia	[19]
Toulouse	β66 Lys→Glu	E10	12–14	40	1–4	Readily forms metHb	[62,63]
Bristol	β67 Val→Asp	E11	7–8	36	37	Normal synthesis; heme contact; reduced O_2 affinity and cooperativity	[1,64]
Sydney	β67 Val→Ala	E11	11.8–13.2	30	4–10	Heme contact; normal synthesis; found with Hb Coventry	[16,65,66]
Mizuho	β68 Leu→Pro	E12	5.2–8.5	5.9	–		[67]
Seattle	β70 Ala→Asp	E14	9.5–10.4	39–43	3	Heme contact; reduced O_2 affinity	[68–70]
Christchurch	β71 Phe→Ser	E15	5.5–10.5	22	8–15	Heme contact	[71]
Shepherd's Bush	β74 Gly→Asp	E18	13	24	5–8	Normal synthesis; raised O_2 affinity due to diminished 2,3-DPG binding	[72,73]
Bushwick	β74 Gly→Val	E18	10.5–14.1	1–2	2.0–5.7	Loses heme; rapid postsynthetic destruction	[74]
St. Antoine	β74–75 Gly-Leu deleted	E18–19	–	–	–	Only slightly unstable	[75]
Atlanta	β75 Leu→Pro	E19	9.6–11.6	30	3.4–7.5	Only mildly unstable	[76]
Pasadena	β75 Leu→Arg	E19	16.1	31–32	10.2	Raised O_2 affinity	[77]
Baylor	β81 Leu→Arg	EF5	15.8	20	4.0	Raised O_2 affinity	[78]
Buenos Aires† (Bryn Mawr)	β85 Phe→Ser	F1	12.6–14.0	45–50	3.5–9.0	Raised O_2 affinity; reduced cooperativity	[79,80]
Tours	β87 Thr deleted	F3	–	25	–	Loses heme; raised O_2 affinity, no cooperativity	[75]
Santa Ana	β88 Leu→Pro	F4	7.6–14.0	10	3–28	Heme contact; loses heme; raised O_2 affinity; reduced cooperativity	[81–83]
Boras	β88 Leu→Arg	F4	8.1–12.6	10	–	Raised O_2 affinity; no cooperativity	[84,85]
Sabine	β91 Leu→Pro	F7	8.5–10.5	7–10	35–67	Heme contact; loses heme; raised O_2 affinity, reduced cooperativity, no Bohr effect; normal synthesis	[86,87]
Caribbean	β91 Leu→Arg	F7	9.7–10.3	39	1.2	Lowered O_2 affinity	[88]
Newcastle	β92 His→Pro	F8	7–9.3	26	11–18	Heme contact; loses heme	[89]
St. Etienne† (Istanbul)	β92 His→Gln	F8	9.1–15.0	15–25	1.6–4.0	Heme contact; loses heme; raised O_2 affinity, reduced cooperativity, no Bohr effect	[90–92]
Gun Hill	β91–95 or 92–96 or 93–97 Leu, Cys, Asp, His deleted	F7–FG2 or F8–FG3 or F9–FG4	12.6–13.5	30	4–10	Loses heme; increased synthesis	[93–95]
Köln† (Ube I)	β98 Val→Met	FG5	9.0–14.3	10–20	4–16	Normal synthesis, loses heme; raised O_2 affinity, reduced cooperativity	[96–104]
Djelfa	β98 Val→Ala	FG5	–	15	–	Increased O_2 affinity	[105]
Nottingham	β98 Val→Gly	FG5	5.2–7.2	–	50	Loses heme; raised O_2 affinity, reduced co-operativity	[106]

Name	Substitution	Position				Properties	References
Rush	β101 Glu→Gln	G3	11.5–11.9	33.9–35.1	3.7–4.3	Forms hybrid tetramers	[107]
Camperdown	β104 Arg→Ser	G6	11.1–18.8	—	—	Only slightly unstable	[108]
Caspart (Southampton)	β106 Leu→Pro	G8	4.5–14.0	20–40	2–94	Heme contact	[109–111]
Tübingen	β106 Leu→Gln	G8	15.5	22.9–41.2	1.6–4.0	Heme contact; free α chains detected; raised O2 affinity	[112,113]
Burke	β107 Gly→Arg	G9	11.5	30	8.1–14.7		[152]
Peterborough	β111 Val→Phe	G13	11.9	33–67	4	Reduced O2 affinity; found in combination with 26% Hb Lepore	[15]
Indianapolis	β112 Cys→Arg	G14	—	—	—		[114]
Madrid	β115 Ala→Pro	G17	9.7	23	33.5	α1β1 contact	[115]
Fannin-Lubbock	β119 Gly→Asp	GH2	11.6–14.2	41–45	1.0–2.2		[116]
Khartoum	β124 Pro→Arg	H2	—	30	—	α1β1 contact	[117]
J-Guantanamo	β128 Ala→Asp	H6	10–11	36–38	3–4		[118]
Wien	β130 Tyr→Asp	H8	9.5–10.6	10	15	Charge internally compensated	[119,120]
Leslie† (Deaconess)	β131 Gln deleted	H9		29–85	—	Found with β° thalassemia, Hb C, and Hb S	[17,121]
North Shore	β134 Val→Glu	H12	10.4	35	—		[122]
Altdorf	β135 Ala→Pro	H13	—	10–20	—	Raised O2 affinity	[123]
Brockton	β138 Ala→Pro	H16	4.8–5.8	5–10	7–8		[124]
Olmsted	β141 Leu→Arg	H19	8.5–10.6	10	8–30	Heme contact	[83,125]
Coventry	β141 Leu deleted	H19	12–13	35–36	<1	Found with Hb Sydney	[16]
Tak	Elongation of β-chain C-terminus					Raised O2 affinity; defective synthesis; only slightly unstable	[126,127]
Toyoake	β142 Ala→Pro	H20		7.9		Raised O2 affinity	[128]
Cranston	Elongation of β-chain C-terminus		14.4–17.1	25–40	7.1–9.4	Only slightly unstable; raised O2 affinity	[129,130]
Poole	γ130 Trp→Gly	H8	10.4–13.1	—	—	Unstable γ chain; Gγ locus affected	[131]
Torino	α43 Phe→Val	CD1	7–13	8	4–16	Heme contact; reduced O2 affinity	[132,133]
Hirosaki	α43 Phe→Leu	CD1	7.9–14.2	—	2.9–17.6	α-Chain homolog of Hb Bucuresti	[134,135]
Hasharon† (Sinai, Sealy)	α47 Asp→His	CD5	N	14–20	1–5	Only slightly unstable	[136–138]
Rovigo	α53 Ala→Asp	E2	N	35–50	N	Only slightly unstable	[139]
Tottori	α59 Gly→Val	E8	12.5	3–11	10.9		[153]
Ann Arbor	α80 Leu→Arg	F1	12	2–14	10	Rapid postsynthetic destruction of abnormal α chains	[140]
Etobicoke	α84 Ser→Arg	F5	11.4–14.1	15	1–3	Only slightly unstable	[141]
Moabit	α86 Leu→Arg	F7	12.4–14.0	15	6–10	Reduced O2 affinity	[142]
Port Phillip	α91 Leu→Pro	FG3	10.7	5–7	3–4		[143]
Suan-Dok	α109 Leu→Arg	G16	12.3	9	—		[144]
Hopkins II	α112 His→Asp	G19	normal	22	normal	Slightly raised O2 affinity, decreased heme-heme interaction	[145,146]
Dakar	α112 His→Gln	G19	10	10	—		[147]
Bibba	α136 Leu→Pro	H19	6.5–7.5	5–11	6–16	Heme contact; dissociates more readily into dimers than Hb A	[148,149]

* Some hemoglobins M (see Chap. 11) also give positive instability tests but are not included in this list.

† The parentheses indicate alternative names for these variants but are not intended to suggest that one or the other name is to be preferred.

NOTE: N = normal; — = not reported.

hemoglobins can be identified only by physical separation of the abnormal hemoglobin from the normal hemoglobin, globin chain separation, and peptide analysis.

Differential diagnosis

The possibility that an unstable hemoglobin is present should be considered in all patients who present the clinical picture of hereditary nonspherocytic hemolytic anemia (Chap. 59), particularly when hypochromia of the red cells is present and when the extent of the reticulocytosis is out of keeping with the degree of anemia. However, not all patients with a positive test for unstable hemoglobins should be classified as having this disorder. The stability of methemoglobin, hemoglobin F, and sickle hemoglobin is appreciably less than that of hemoglobin A, and false-positive isopropanol stability tests may be obtained in patients with increased quantities of these hemoglobins. Hemoglobin H (β_4) and hemoglobin Barts (γ_4) are unstable. These fast-moving hemoglobins can be detected on electrophoresis (see Chap. A7). Patients whose red cells contain these hemoglobins are diagnosed as having α thalassemia (see Chap. 50).

Course and prognosis

Most patients with unstable hemoglobins follow a relatively benign course. As with other hemolytic states gallstones are common and cholecystectomy may be required. Hemolytic episodes may be precipitated by infection or by the ingestion of "oxidative" drugs. Sulfonamides have been particularly prominent in inducing hemolysis, and derivatives which do not produce hemolysis in G-6-PD deficiency have been shown to precipitate hemolysis in patients with some unstable hemoglobins. A few deaths believed to have been directly related to unstable hemoglobins have been reported. A patient with Hb$_{Hirosaki}$ is thought to have died following a hemolytic crisis precipitated by a common cold [134]. Two sisters with Hb$_{Duarte}$ [14] died of thromboembolic complications less than a year following splenectomy. This unstable variant has an increased oxygen affinity, and it is likely that a combination of postsplenectomy erythrocytosis and thrombocytosis led to the demise of the patients.

Treatment

Treatment is not usually required. As in the case of other hemolytic disorders, folic acid in a dose of 1 mg per day is often given, but its usefulness has not been established. "Oxidant" drugs such as those listed in Table 58-2 should be avoided. In addition, the use of all sulfonamides should be eschewed, particularly in the case of those variants which have been associated with drug-induced hemolysis. Splenectomy has proved to be useful in some patients with splenomegaly and severe hemolysis [151], while others have enjoyed little benefit. In view of the fact that a few patients with high-oxygen-affinity unstable hemoglobin have died after a splenectomy, it is probably best to avoid this operation in such patients.

References

1. Cathie, I. A. B.: Apparent idiopathic Heinz body anaemia. *Great Ormond St. J.* 3:43, 1952.
2. Lange, R. D., and Akeroyd, J. H.: Congenital hemolytic anemia with abnormal pigment metabolism and red cell inclusion bodies: A new clinical syndrome. *Blood* 13:950, 1958.
3. Schmid, R., Brecher, G., and Clemens, T.: Familial hemolytic anemia with erythrocyte inclusion bodies and a defect in pigment metabolism. *Blood* 14:991, 1959.
4. Grimes, A. J., and Meisler, A.: Possible cause of Heinz bodies in congenital Heinz-body anaemia. *Nature* 194:190, 1962.
5. Frick, P. G., Hitzig, W. H., and Betke, K.: Hemoglobin Zürich: A new hemoglobin anomaly associated with acute hemolytic episodes with inclusion bodies after sulfonamide therapy. *Blood* 20:261, 1962.
6. Perutz, M. F., Kendrew, J. C., and Watson, H. C.: Structure and function of haemoglobin. II. Some relations between polypeptide chain configuration and amino acid sequence. *J. Mol. Biol.* 13:669, 1965.
7. Rachmilewitz, E. A., Peisach, J., and Blumberg, J. E.: Studies on the stability of oxyhemoglobin A and its constituent chains and their derivatives. *J. Biol. Chem.* 246:3356, 1971.
8. Dacie, J. V., Shinton, N. K., Gaffney, P. J., Carrell, R. W., and Lehmann, H.: Haemoglobin Hammersmith (β42(CD1)Phe→Ser). *Nature* 216:663, 1967.
9. Brunori, M., Falcioni, G., Fioretti, E., Giardina, B., and Rotilio, G.: Formation of superoxide in the autoxidation of the isolated α and β chains of human hemoglobin and its involvement in hemichrome precipitation. *Eur. J. Biochem.* 53:99, 1975.
10. Rachmilewitz, E. A., and White, J. M.: Haemichrome formation during the *in vitro* oxidation of haemoglobin Köln. *Nature [New Biol.]* 241:115, 1973.
11. Rachmilewitz, E. A., Peisach, J., Bradley, T. B., and Blumberg, W. E.: Role of haemichromes in the formation of inclusion bodies in haemoglobin H disease. *Nature* 222:248, 1969.
12. Carrell, R. W., Winterbourn, C. C., and Rachmilewitz, E. A.: Activated oxygen and haemolysis. *Br. J. Haematol.* 30:259, 1975.
13. Winterbourn, C. C., McGrath, B. M., and Carrell, R. W.: Reactions involving superoxide and normal and unstable haemoglobins. *Biochem. J.* 155:493, 1976.
14. Beutler, E., Lang, A., and Lehmann, H.: Hemoglobin Duarte ($\alpha_2\beta_2^{62(E6)Ala→Pro}$): A new unstable hemoglobin with increased oxygen affinity. *Blood* 43:527, 1974.
15. King, M. A. R., Wiltshire, B. G., Lehmann, H., and Morimoto, H.: An unstable haemoglobin with reduced oxygen affinity: Haemoglobin Peterborough β111 (G13) valine→phenylalanine, its interaction with normal haemoglobin and haemoglobin Lepore. *Br. J. Haematol.* 22:125, 1972.
16. Casey, R., Lang, A., Lehmann, H., and Shinton, N. K.: Double heterozygosity for two unstable haemoglobins: Hb Sydney β67(E11)Val→Ala and Hb Coventry β141(H19) Leu deleted. *Br. J. Haematol.* 33:143, 1976.
17. Lutcher, C. L., and Huisman, T. H. J.: Hemoglobin Leslie, an unstable variant due to deletion of Gln β131 occurring in combination with β-thalassemia, Hb S and Hb C. *Clin. Res.* 23:278A, 1975.
18. Beuzard, Y., et al.: Haemoglobin Saki $\alpha_2\beta_2^{Leu→Pro(A11)}$ structure and function. *Biochim. Biophys. Acta* 393:182, 1975.
19. Tentori, L.: Three examples of double heterozygosis: Beta-thalas-

semia and rare hemoglobin variant. *Abstracts, International Symposium on Abnormal Hemoglobin and Thalassemia.* Istanbul, 1974, p. 68.

20. De Jong, W. W. W., Went, L. N., and Bernini, L. F.: Haemoglobin Leiden: Deletion of β6 or 7 glutamic acid. *Nature* 220:788, 1968.

21. Rieder, R. F., and James, G. W.: Imbalance in α and β globin synthesis associated with a hemoglobinopathy. *J. Clin. Invest.* 54:948, 1974.

22. Monn, E., Gaffney, P. J., and Lehmann, H.: Hb Sogn (β14 Arginine): A new haemoglobin variant. *Scand. J. Haematol.* 5:353, 1968.

23. Monn, E., and Bjark, P.: Hb Sogn (β14 Arginine): Haematological and genetical studies. *Scand. J. Haematol.* 7:455, 1970.

24. Kennedy, C. C., Blundell, G., Lorkin, P. A., Lang, A., and Lehmann, H.: Haemoglobin in Belfast β15 (A12) tryptophan→arginine: A new unstable haemoglobin variant. *Br. Med. J.,* 4:324, 1974.

25. Cohen-Solal, M., et al.: Haemoglobin Lyon β17-18 (A14-15)Val-Lys 0: Determination by sequenator analysis. *Biochim. Biophys. Acta* 351:306, 1974.

26. Jones, R. T., Brimhall, B., Huisman, T. H. J., Kleihauer, E., and Betke, K.: Hemoglobin Freiburg: Abnormal hemoglobin due to deletion of a single amino acid residue. *Science* 154:1024, 1966.

27. Betke, K., and Kleihauer, E.: Hämoglobinanomalien in der deutschen Bevolkerung. *Schweiz. Med. Wochenschr.* 92:1316, 1962.

28. Ranney, H. M., Jacobs, A. S., Udem, L., and Zalusky, R.: Hemoglobin Riverdale-Bronx, an unstable hemoglobin resulting from the substitution of arginine for glycine at helical residue B6 of the β polypeptide chain. *Biochem. Biophys. Res. Commun.* 33:1004, 1968.

29. Bank, A., O'Donnell, J. V., and Braverman, A. S.: Globin chain synthesis in heterozygotes for β chain mutants. *J. Lab. Clin. Med.* 76:616, 1970.

30. Idelson, L. I., Didkowsky, N. A., Casey, R., Lorkin, P. A., and Lehmann, H.: New unstable haemoglobin Hb Moscva, β24(B6) Gly→Asp found in the U.S.S.R. *Nature* 249:768, 1974.

31. Huisman, T. H. J., et al.: Hemoglobin Savannah (B6 (24) β glycine→valine): An unstable variant causing anemia with inclusion bodies. *J. Clin. Invest.* 50:650, 1971.

32. Idelson, L. I., Didkovsky, N. A., Lehmann, H., Casey, R., and Lorkin, P. A.: New unstable haemoglobin Moskva β24 (B6) glycine→aspartic acid. *Probl. Gematol. Pereliv. Krovi* 19:21, 1974.

33. Blouquit, Y., Arous, N., Machado, P. E. A., and Carel, M. C.: Hb Henri Mondor: β²⁶(B8) Glu→Val: A variant with a substitution localized at the same position as that of Hb E β²⁶ ᴳˡᵘ→ᴸʸˢ. *FEBS Lett.* 72:5, 1976.

34. Idelson, L. I., Didkovsky, N. A., Filippova, A. V., Casey, R., Kynoch, P. A. M., and Lehmann, H.: Haemoglobin Volga, β27 (B9) Ala→Asp: A new highly unstable haemoglobin with a suppressed charge. *FEBS Lett.* 58:122, 1975.

35. Sansone, G., Carrell, R. W., and Lehmann, H.: Haemoglobin Genova: β28 (B10) leucine→proline. *Nature* 214:877, 1967.

36. Wrightstone, R. N., Wilson, J. B., Reynolds, C. A., Huisman, T. H. J., Padmanabh, S., and Vella, F.: Hb Genova (α₂β₂²⁸⁽ᴮ¹⁰⁾ᴸᵉᵘ→ᴾʳᵒ): Methods for detection and analysis of unstable hemoglobins. *Clin. Chim. Acta* 44:217, 1973.

37. Cohen-Solal, M., and Labie, D.: A new case of hemoglobin Genova α₂β₂²⁸⁽ᴮ¹⁰⁾ᴸᵉᵘ→ᴾʳᵒ: Further studies on the mechanism of instability and defective synthesis. *Biochim. Biophys. Acta* 295:67, 1973.

38. Cohen-Solal, M., Seligmann, M., Thillet, J., and Rosa, J.: Haemoglobin Saint Louis β28 (B10) Leucine→Glutamine: A new unstable haemoglobin only present in a ferri form. *FEBS Lett.* 33:37, 1973.

39. Cohen-Solal, M., Lebeau, M., and Rosa, J.: *In vitro* normal biosynthesis of an unstable ferri-hemoglobin: Hemoglobin Saint Louis B10(β28) leu→gln. *Nouv. Rev. Fr. Hematol.* 14:621, 1974.

40. Baur, E. W., and Motulsky, A. G.: Hemoglobin Tacoma: A β-chain variant associated with increased HbA₂. *Humangenetik* 1:621, 1965.

41. Brimhall, B., Jones, R. T., Bauer, E. W., and Motulsky, A. G.: Structural characterization of hemoglobin Tacoma. *Biochemistry* 8:2125, 1969.

42. Idelson, L. I., Didkowsky, N. A., Casey, R., Lorkin, P. A., and Lehmann, H.: Structure and function of haemoglobin Tacoma (β30 Arg→Ser) found in a second family. *Acta Haematol.* 52:303, 1974.

43. Hayashi, A., Suzuki, T., and Stamatoyannopoulos, G.: Electro-phoretic and functional abnormalities of haemoglobin Tacoma β30 (B12) Arg→Ser. *Bichim. Biophys. Acta* 351:453, 1974.

44. Garel, M. C., Blouquit, Y., Rosa, J., and Romero-Garcia, C.: Hemoglobin Castilla β32 (B14) Leu→Arg: A new unstable variant producing severe hemolytic disease. *FEBS Lett.* 58:145, 1975.

45. Honig, G. R., et al.: Hemoglobin Abraham Lincoln, β32 (B14) leucine→proline: An unstable variant producing severe hemolytic disease. *J. Clin. Invest.* 52:1746, 1973.

46. Jackson, J. M., Yates, A., and Huehns, E. R.: Haemoglobin Perth β32 (B14) Leu→Pro: An unstable haemoglobin causing haemolysis. *Br. J. Haematol.* 25:607, 1973.

47. Honig, G. R., Mason, R. G., Vida, L. N., and Shamsuddin, M.: Synthesis of hemoglobin Abraham Lincoln (β32 Leu→Pro). *Blood* 43:657, 1974.

48. Rieder, R. F., Oski, F. A., and Clegg, J. B.: Hemoglobin Philly (β35 tyrosine→phenylalanine): Studies in the molecular pathology of hemoglobins. *J. Clin. Invest.* 48:1627, 1969.

49. White, J. M., and Dacie, J. V.: *In vitro* synthesis of Hb Hammersmith (CD1 Phe→Ser). *Nature* 225:860, 1970.

50. May, A., and Huehns, E. R.: The oxygen affinity of haemoglobin Hammersmith. *Br. J. Haematol.* 30:185, 1975.

51. Keeling, M. M., et al.: Hemoglobin Louisville β42 (CD1) Phe→Leu: An unstable variant causing mild hemolytic anemia. *J. Clin. Invest.* 50:2395, 1971.

52. Bratu, V., Lorkin, P. A., Lehmann, H., and Predescu, C.: Haemoglobin Bucuresti β42 (CD1) Phe→Leu: A cause of unstable haemoglobin haemolytic anaemia. *Biochim. Biophys. Acta* 251:1, 1971.

53. Praxedes, H., Wiltshire, B. G., and Lehmann, H.: Cited by H. Lehmann in *Proceedings of the International Symposium on Standardization in Haematology and Clinical Pathology, Medical Edition Archivio,* "Casa Sollievo della Sofferenza" medical edition no. 2, p. 11. C.I.S.M.E.L. publication, S. Giovanni Rotondo, Foggia, Italy, 1972.

54. Kynoch, P. A. M., and Lehmann, H.: Unpublished data.

55. Charache, S., Brimhall, B., and Milner, P. F.: Hemoglobin Okaloosa β48 (CD7) leucine→arginine: An unstable hemoglobin with low oxygen affinity. *J. Clin. Invest.* 52:2858, 1973.

56. Shibata, S., et al.: Hemoglobin Tochigi (β56-59 deleted): A new unstable hemoglobin discovered in a Japanese family. *Proc. Jpn. Acad.* 46:400, 1970.

57. Yamada, K., et al.: Hemoglobin Tochigi disease: A new unstable hemoglobin hemolytic anemia found in a Japanese family. *Acta Haematol. Jpn.* 34:484, 1971.

58. Giardina, B., Brunori, M., Antonini, E., and Tentori, L.: Properties of hemoglobin G Ferrara (β₅₇(E1) Asn→Lys). *Biochim. Biophys. Acta* 534:1, 1978.

59. Wajcman, H., Gacon, F., and Labie, D.: A new haemoglobin variant involving rhe distal histidine: Hb Bicetre β63 (E7) His→Pro. Abstract 30:01, Int. Soc. Haematol., European and African Division, 3d meeting, London, 1975.

60. Muller, C. J., and Kingma, S.: Haemoglobin Zürich: α₂ᴬβ₂⁶³ ᴬʳᵍ. *Biochim. Biophys. Acta* 50:595, 1961.

61. Rieder, R. F., Zinkham, W. H., and Holtzman, N. A.: Hemoglobin Zürich: Clinical chemical and kinetic studies. *Am. J. Med.* 39:4, 1965.

62. Rosa, J., et al.: Haemoglobin I Toulouse β66 (E10) Lys→Glu: A new abnormal haemoglobin with a mutation localized on the E10 porphyrin surrounding zone. *Nature* 223:190, 1969.

63. Labie, D., Rosa, J., Belkhodja, J., and Bierme, R.: Hemoglobin Toulouse α₂β₂66 (E10) Lys→Glu: Structure and consequences in molecular pathology. *Biochim. Biophys. Acta* 236:201, 1971.

64. Steadman, J. H., Yates, A., and Huehns, E. R.: Idiopathic Heinz body anaemia: Hb Bristol (β67 (E11) Val→Asp). *Br. J. Haematol.* 18:435, 1970.

65. Carrell, R. W., Lehmann, H., Lorkin, P. A., Raik, E., and Hunter, E.: Haemoglobin Sydney: β67(E11) valine→alanine: An emerging pattern of unstable haemoglobins. *Nature* 215:626, 1967.

66. Raik, E., and Hunter, E. G.: Compensated hereditary haemolytic disease resulting from an unstable haemoglobin fraction. *Med. J. Aust.* 1:955, 1967.

67. Ohba, Y., Miyaji, T., Matsuoka, M., Sugiyama, K., Suzuki, T., and Sugiura, T.: Hemoglobin Mizuho or β68(E12) leucine→proline, a new unstable variant associated with severe hemolytic anemia. *Hemoglobin* 1:467, 1977.

68. Stamatoyannopoulos, G., Parer, J. T., and Finch, C. A.: Physiologic implication of a hemoglobin with decreased oxygen affinity (hemoglobin Seattle). *N. Engl. J. Med.* 281:915, 1969.

69. Huehns, E. R., Hecht, F., Yoshida, A., Stamatoyannopoulos, G., Hartman, J., and Motulsky, A.: Hemoglobin Seattle ($\alpha_2^A\beta_2^{76 \text{ Glu}}$): An unstable hemoglobin causing chronic hemolytic anemia. *Blood* 36:209, 1970.

70. Kurachi, S., Hermodson, M., Hornung, S., and Stamatoyannopoulous, G.: Structure of haemoglobin Seattle. *Nature [New Biol.]* 243:275, 1973.

71. Carrell, R. W., and Owen, M. D.: A new approach to haemoglobin variant identification: Haemoglobin Christchurch β71 (E15) phenylalanine serine. *Biochim. Biophys. Acta* 236:507, 1971.

72. White, J. M.: The synthesis of abnormal haemoglobins. *Ser. Haematol.* 4:116, 1971.

73. White, J. M., Brain, M. C., Lorkin, P. A., Lehmann, H., and Smith, M.: Mild "unstable haemoglobin haemolytic anaemia" caused by haemoglobin Shepherd's Bush β74(E18)Gly→Asp. *Nature* 225:939, 1970.

74. Rieder, R. F., Wolf, D. J., Clegg, J. B., and Lee, S. L.: Rapid post-synthetic destruction of unstable haemoglobin Bushwick. *Nature* 254:725, 1975.

75. Wajcman, H., Labie, D., and Schapira, G.: Two new hemoglobin variants with deletion: Hemoglobin Tours Thr β87 (F3) deleted and hemoglobin St. Antoine Gly-Leu β74-75 (E18-19) deleted: Consequences for oxygen affinity and protein stability. *Biochim. Biophys. Acta* 295:495, 1973.

76. Hubbard, M., et al.: Hemoglobin Atlanta or $\alpha_2\beta_2^{75 \text{Leu}\rightarrow\text{Pro(E 19)}}$: An unstable variant found in several members of a Caucasian family. *Biochim. Biophys. Acta* 386:538, 1975.

77. Johnson, C. S., Moyes, D., Schroeder, W. A., Shelton, J. B., Shelton, J. R., and Beutler, E.: Hemoglobin Pasadena, $\alpha_2\beta_2$ 75(E19) Leu→Arg: Identification by high performance liquid chromatography of a new unstable variant with increased oxygen affinity. *Biochim. Biophys. Acta* 623:360, 1980.

78. Schneider, R. G., Hettig, R. A., Bilunos, M., and Brimhall, B.: Hemoglobin Baylor ($\alpha_2\beta_2$ 81 (EF5) Leu→Arg): An unstable mutant with high oxygen affinity. *Hemoglobin* 1:85, 1976.

79. Bradley, T. B., Wohl, R. C., Murphy, S. B., Oski, F. A., and Bunn, H. F.: Properties of hemoglobin Bryn Mawr, β85 Phe→Ser: A new spontaneous mutation producing an unstable hemoglobin with high affinity. *Blood* 40:947, 1972.

80. De Weinstein, B. I., White, J. M., Wiltshire, B. G., and Lehmann, H.: A new unstable haemoglobin: Hb Buenos Aires, β85 (F1) Phe→Ser. *Acta Haematol.* 50:357, 1973.

81. Opfell, R. W., Lorkin, P. A., and Lehmann, H.: Hereditary non-spherocytic haemolytic anaemia with post-splenectomy inclusion bodies and pigmenturia caused by an unstable haemoglobin Santa Ana β88 (F4) leucine→proline. *J. Med. Genet.* 5:292, 1968.

82. Hollan, S. R., Szelenyi, J. G., Miltenyi, M., Charlesworth, D., Lorkin, P. A., and Lehmann, H.: Unstable haemoglobin disease caused by Hb Santa Ana β88 (F4) Leu→Pro. *Haematologia* 4:141, 1970.

83. Fairbanks, V. F., Opfell, R. W., and Burgert, E. O.: Three families with unstable hemoglobinopathies (Köln, Olmsted and Santa Ana) causing hemolytic anemia with inclusion bodies and pigmenturia. *Am. J. Med.* 46:344, 1969.

84. Svensson, B., and Straud, L.: A Swedish family with haemolytic anaemia, Heinz bodies and an abnormal haemoglobin. *Scand. J. Haematol.* 4:241, 1967.

85. Hollender, A., Lorkin, P. A., Lehmann, H., and Svensson, B.: New unstable haemoglobin Boras: β88 (F4) leucine→arginine. *Nature* 222:953, 1969.

86. Schneider, R. G., Ueda, S., Alperin, J. B., Brimhall, B., and Jones, R. T.: Hemoglobin Sabine β91 (F7) Leu→Pro: An unstable variant causing severe anemia with inclusion bodies. *N. Engl. J. Med.* 280:739, 1969.

87. Schaeffer, J. R., and Prostie, P.: *Abstr. Am. Soc. Hum. Genet.*, Indianapolis, 13, 12a, 1970, cited in R. G. Schneider, B. Brimhall, R. T. Jones, R. Bryant, C. B. Mitchell, and A. I. Goldsberg: Hb Ft Worth α27 Glu→Gly (B8): A variant present in unusually low concentration. *Biochim. Biophys. Acta* 243:164, 1971.

88. Ahern, E., et al.: Haemoglobin Caribbean β91(F7) Leu→Arg: A mildly unstable haemoglobin with low oxygen affinity. *FEBS Lett.* 69:99, 1976.

89. Walker, W., Casey, R., Lehmann, H., and Finney, R.: Hb Newcastle: β92 (F8) His→Pro. *FEBS Lett.* 60:435, 1975.

90. Aksoy, M., Erdem, S., and Efremov, G. D.: Hemoglobin Istanbul: Substitution of glutamine for histidine in a proximal histidine (F8(92))β. *J. Clin. Invest.* 51:2380, 1972.

91. Rosa, J., et al.: L'hemoglobine Saint-Etienne: $\alpha_2^A\beta_2$ His→Gln (F8): Une Nouvelle Variété d'hémoglobine instable avec absence d'héme sur les chaines β. *Nouv. Rev. Fr. Hematol.* 12:691, 1972.

92. Beuzard, Y., et al.: Structural studies of hemoglobin Saint-Etienne β92 (F8) His Gln: A new abnormal hemoglobin with loss of β proximal histidine and absence of heme on the β chains. *FEBS Lett.* 27:76, 1972.

93. Bradley, T. B., Wohl, R. C., and Rieder, R. F.: Hemoglobin Gun Hill: Deletion of five amino acid residues and impaired hemoglobin binding. *Science* 157:1581, 1967.

94. Rieder, R. F., and Bradley, T. B.: Hemoglobin Gun Hill: An unstable protein associated with chronic hemolysis. *Blood* 32:355, 1968.

95. Rieder, R. F.: Synthesis of hemoglobin Gun Hill: Increased synthesis of the heme-free β^{GH} globin chain and subunit exchange with a free α-chain pool. *J. Clin. Invest.* 50:388, 1971.

96. Carrell, R. W., and Lehmann, H.: The unstable haemoglobin haemolytic anaemias. *Semin. Hematol.* 6:116, 1969.

97. Carrell, R. W., Lehmann, H., and Hutchison, E.: Haemoglobin Köln (β98 valine→methionine): An unstable protein causing inclusion body anaemia. *Nature* 210:915, 1966.

98. Hutchison, H. E., Pinkerton, P. H., Waters, P., Douglas, A. S., Lehmann, H., and Beale, D.: Hereditary Heinz-body anaemia, thrombocytopenia and haemoglobinopathy (Hb Köln) in a Glasgow family. *Br. Med. J.* 2:1099, 1964.

99. Pribilla, W., Klesse, P., Betke, K., Lehmann, H., and Beale, D.: Hämoglobin Köln-Krankheit: Familiare hypochrome hämolytische Anämie mit Hämoglobin-anomalie. *Klin. Wochenschr.* 43:1049, 1965.

100. Vaughan-Jones, R., Grimes, A. J., Carrell, R. W., and Lehmann, H.: Köln haemoglobinopathy: Further data and a comparison with other hereditary Heinz body anaemias. *Br. J. Haematol.* 13:394, 1967.

101. Kreimer-Birnbaum, M., Pinkerton, P. H., Bannerman, R. M., and Hutchison, H. E.: Metabolism of haemoglobin Köln, an unstable haemoglobin. *Nature* 219:494, 1968.

102. White, J. M., and Brain, M. C.: Defective synthesis of an unstable haemoglobin: Haemoglobin Köln (β98 Val→Met). *Br. J. Haematol.* 18:195, 1970.

103. Huehns, E. R., and Steadman, J. H.: Peptide chain synthesis in unstable haemoglobin diseases, in *Proc. XIII Congr. Int. Soc. Haematol.* Lehmann-Verlag, Munich, 1970, p. 7.

104. Jackson, J. M., Way, B. F., and Woodliff, H. J.: A West Australian family with a haemolytic disorder associated with haemoglobin Köln. *Br. J. Haematol.* 13:474, 1967.

105. Gacon, G., Wajcman, H., Labie, D., and Cosson, A.: A new unstable hemoglobin mutated in β98 (FG5) Val→Ala: Hb Djelfa. *FEBS Lett.*, 58:238, 1975.

106. Gordon-Smith, E. C., Dacie, J. V., Blecher, T. E., French, E. A., Wiltshire, B. G., and Lehmann, H.: Haemoglobin Nottingham β FG5 (98) Val→Gly: A new unstable haemoglobin producing severe haemolysis. *Proc. R. Soc. Med.* 66:507, 1973.

107. Adams, J. G., Winter, W. P., Tausk, K., and Heller, P.: Hemoglobin Rush β101 (G3) glutamine: A new unstable hemoglobin causing mild hemolysis. *Blood* 43:261, 1974.

108. Wilkinson, T., et al.: Haemoglobin Camperdown β104 (G6) arginine→serine. *Biochim. Biophys. Acta* 393:195, 1975.

109. Koler, R. D., et al.: Hemoglobin Caspar β106 (G8) Leu→Pro: A contemporary mutation. *Am. J. Med.* 55:549, 1973.

110. Jones, R. T., Koler, R. D., Duerst, M., and Stocklen, Z.: Hemoglobin Caspar, G8 β106 Leu→Pro: Further evidence that hemoglobin mutations are not random. *Adv. Exp. Med. Biol.* 28:79, 1972.

111. Hyde, R. D., Hall, M. D., Wiltshire, B. G., and Lehmann, H.: Haemoglobin Southampton, β106 (G8) Leu→Pro: An unstable variant causing severe haemolysis. *Lancet* 2:1170, 1972.

112. Kleihauer, E., Waller, H. D., Benohr, H. C., Kohne, E., and Gelinsky, P.: Eine neue β-Kettenvariante (βTp10-12) mit erhöhter Spontanoxydation. *Klin. Wochenschr.* 49:651, 1971.

113. Kohne, E., Kley, H. P., Kleihauer, E., Versmold, H., Benöhr, H. C., and Braunitzer, G.: Structural and functional characteristics of Hb Tübingen: β 106 (G8) Leu-Gln. *FEBS Lett.* 64:443, 1976.

114. Adams, J. G., Boxer, L. A., Baehner, R. L., Forget, B. G., Tsistrokis, G. A., and Steinberg, M. H.: Hemoglobin Indianapolis: Posttranslational degradation of an unstable β-chain variant producing a phenotype of severe heterozygous β-thalassemia. *Clin. Res.* 26:501A, 1978.

115. Outeirino, J., Casey, R., White, J. M., and Lehmann, H.: Haemoglobin Madrid β115 (G17) alanine→proline: An unstable variant associated with haemolytic anaemia. *Acta Haematol.* 52:53, 1974.

116. Schneider, R. G., Berkman, N. L., Brimhall, B., and Jones, R. T.: Hemoglobin Fannin-Lubbock ($\alpha_2\beta_2^{119(GH2)}$Gly→Asp): A slightly unstable mutant. *Biochim. Biophys. Acta* 453:478, 1976.

117. Clegg, J. B., Weatherall, D. J., Boon, W. H., and Mustafa, D.: Two new human haemoglobin variants involving proline substitutions. *Nature* 222:379, 1969.

118. Martinez, G., Lima, F., and Colombo, B.: Haemoglobin J-Guantanamo ($\alpha_2\beta_2$ 128 (H6) Ala→Asp). A new fast unstable haemoglobin found in a Cuban family. *Biochim. Biophys. Acta* 491:1, 1977.

119. Lorkin, P. A., Pietschmann, H., Braunsteiner, H., and Lehmann, H.: Structure of haemoglobin Wien β130 (H8) tyrosine-aspartic acid: An unstable haemoglobin variant. *Acta Haematol.* 51:351, 1974.

120. Braunsteiner, H., Dienstl, F., Sailer, S., and Sandhofer, F.: Angeborene hämolytische Anämie mit Mesobilifuscinurie und Innenkörperbildung nach Splenectomie. *Acta Haematol.* 32:314, 1964.

121. Moo-Penn, W. F., et al.: Hemoglobin Deaconess: A new deletion mutant β131 (H9) glutamine deleted. *Biochem. Biophys. Res. Commun.* 65:8, 1975.

122. Arends, T., Lehmann, H., Plowman, D., and Stathopoulou, R.: Haemoglobin North Shore-Caracas β134 (H12) Valine→Glutamic acid. *FEBS Lett.* 80:261, 1977.

123. Marti, H. R., Winterhalter, K. H., Dilorio, E. E., Lorkin, P. A., and Lehmann, H.: Hb Altdorf $\alpha_2\beta_2$135(H13) Ala→Pro: A new electrophoretically silent unstable haemoglobin variant from Switzerland. *FEBS Lett.* 63:193, 1976.

124. Moo-Penn, W. F., Jue, D. L., Johnson, M. H., Bechtel, K. C., and Patchen, L. C.: Hemoglobin variants and methods used for their characterization during 7 years of screening at the Center for Disease Control. *Hemoglobin* 4:347, 1980.

125. Lorkin, P. A., Lehmann, H., and Fairbanks, V. F.: The amino acid substitution in Hb Olmsted: β141(H19) leucine→arginine. *Biochim. Biophys. Acta* 386:256, 1975.

126. Flatz, G., Kinderlerer, J. L., Kilmartin, J. V., and Lehmann, H.: Haemoglobin Tak: A variant with additional residues at the end of the β-chains. *Lancet* 2:732, 1971.

127. Lehmann, H., et al.: Haemoglobin Tak: A β-chain elongation. *Br. J. Haematol.* 31 (Suppl.):119, 1975.

128. Ohba, Y., Miyaji, T., Hattori, Y., Fuyuno, K., and Matsuoka, M.: Unstable hemoglobins in Japan. *Hemoglobin* 4:307, 1980.

129. Bunn, H. F., Schmidt, G. J., Muss, H., and Dluhy, R. G.: Hemoglobin Cranston, an unstable variant having an elongated β-chain due to unequal crossover between two normal genes. *Clin. Res.* 23:401A, 1975.

130. Bunn, H. F., Schmidt, G. J., Haney, D. N., and Dluhy, R. G.: Hemoglobin Cranston, an unstable variant having an elongated β chain due to non-homologous crossover between two normal β chain genes. *Proc. Natl. Acad. Sci.* 72:3609, 1975.

131. Lee-Potter, J. P., Deacon-Smith, R. A., Simpkiss, M. J., Kamuzora, H., and Lehmann, H.: A new cause of haemolytic anaemia in the newborn: A description of an unstable fetal haemoglobin F Poole, $\alpha_2^G\gamma_2$130 tryptophan→glycine. *J. Clin. Pathol.* 28:317, 1975.

132. Beretta, A., Prato, V., Gallo, E., and Lehmann, H.: Haemoglobin Torino α43 (CD1) phenylalanine→valine. *Nature* 217:1016, 1968.

133. Prato, V., Gallo, E., Ricco, G., Mazza, V., Bianco, G., and Lehmann, H.: Haemolytic anaemia due to haemoglobin Torino. *Br. J. Haematol.* 19:105, 1970.

134. Ohba, Y., et al.: Hemoglobin Hirosaki (α43 (CD1) Phe→Leu): A new unstable variant. *Biochim. Biophys. Acta* 405:155, 1975.

135. Yokoyama, M., Numakura, H., Nagata, K., and Takebe, Y.: Hereditary nonspherocytic hemolytic anemia with high activity of erythrocyte ATP-ase. *Acta Paediatr. Jpn.* 13:40, 1971.

136. Halbrecht, I., Isaacs, W. A., Lehmann, H., and Ben-Porat, F.: Hemoglobin Hasharon (α47 aspartic acid→histidine). *Isr. J. Med. Sci.* 3:827, 1967.

137. Schneider, R. G., Ueda, S., Alperin, J. B., Brimhall, B., and Jones, R. T.: Hemoglobin Sealy ($\alpha_2^{47His}\beta_2$): A new variant in a Jewish family. *Am. J. Hum. Genet.* 20:151, 1968.

138. Charache, S., Mondzac, A. M., and Gessner, U.: Hemoglobin Hasharon α_2^{47His}(CD5)β_2: A hemoglobin found in low concentration. *J. Clin. Invest.* 48:834, 1969.

139. Alberti, R., Mariuzzi, G. M., Artibani, L., Bruni, E., and Tentori, L.: A new haemoglobin variant: J Rovigo α53(E-2)alanine→aspartic acid. *Biochim. Biophys. Acta* 342:1, 1974.

140. Adams, J. G., Winter, W. P., Rucknagel, D. L., and Spencer, H. H.: Biosynthesis of hemoglobin Ann Arbor: Evidence for catabolic and feedback regulation. *Science* 176:1427, 1972.

141. Crookston, J. H., Farquarson, H. A., Beale, D., and Lehmann, H.: Hemoglobin Etobicoke: α84 (F5) Serine replaced by arginine. *Can. J. Biochem.* 47:143, 1969.

142. Knuth, A., Pribilla, W., Marti, H. R., and Winterhalter, K. H.: Hemoglobin Moabit: Alpha 86 (F7) Leu→Arg. A new unstable abnormal hemoglobin. *Acta Haemat.* 61:121, 1979.

143. Brennan, S. O., Tauro, G. P., Melrose, W., and Carrell, R. W.: Haemoglobin Port Phillip α91 (FG3) Leu→Pro. A new unstable haemoglobin. *FEBS Lett.* 81:115, 1977.

144. Sanguansermsri, T., Matragoon, S., Changloah, L., and Flatz, G.: Hemoglobin Suan-Dok ($\alpha_2$109 (G16) Leu→Arg β_2): An unstable hemoglobin associated with α-thalassemia. *Hemoglobin* 3:161, 1979.

145. Charache, S., and Ostertag, W.: Hemoglobin Hopkins-2 ((α112 Asp) 2 β2): "Low output" protects from potentially harmful effects. *Blood* 36:852, 1970.

146. Clegg, J. B., and Charache, S.: The structure of hemoglobin Hopkins-2. *Hemoglobin* 2:85, 1978.

147. Rosa, J., Oudart, J. C., Paynier, J., Belkhodja, O., Boigne, J. M., and Labie, D.: A new abnormal haemoglobin: $\alpha_2^{112His-Gln}\beta_2$ Hb Dakar. *Abstr. XII Congr. Int. Soc. Haematol.*, New York, 1968, p. 72.

148. Kleihauer, E. F., et al.: Hemoglobin Bibba or $\alpha_2^{136Pro}B_2$: An unstable α chain abnormal hemoglobin. *Biochim. Biophys. Acta* 154:220, 1968.

149. Smith, L. L., Barton, B. P., and Huisman, T. H. J.: Subunit dissociation of the unstable hemoglobin Bibba α_2^{136Pro}(H19)β_2. *J. Biol. Chem.* 245:2185, 1970.

150. Kreimer-Birnbaum, M., Pinkerton, P. H., Bannerman, R. M., and Hutchison, H. E.: Dipyrrolic urinary pigments in congenital Heinz-body anaemia due to Hb Köln and thalassaemia. *Br. Med. J.* 2:396, 1966.

151. Vichinsky, E. P., and Lubin, B. H.: Unstable hemoglobins, hemoglobins with altered oxygen affinity, and M-hemoglobins. *Pediatr. Clin. North Am.* 27:421, 1980.

152. Turner, J. W., Jr., Jones, R. T., Brimhall, B., DuVal, M. C., and Koler, R. D.: Characterization of hemoglobin Burke [β107 (G9) Gly→Arg] *Biochem. Genet.* 14:577, 1976.

153. Nakatsuji, T., Miwa, S., Ohba, Y., Miyaji, T., Matsumoto, N., and Matsuoka, I.: Hemoglobin Tottori (α59[E8] Glycine→Valine). A new unstable hemoglobin. *Hemoglobin* 5:427, 1981.

Erythrocyte disorders—anemias related to mechanical damage to erythrocytes

CHAPTER 62

March hemoglobinuria

WENDELL F. ROSSE

Definitions and history

March hemoglobinuria is the development of hemoglobinuria following exercise, especially walking or running. The first clinical description of this disorder was by Fleischer [1] in 1881, who reported the case of a young German soldier who complained of passing dark urine following a "strenuous field march." Even though the event occurred during the month of March, Fleischer noted that this form of hemoglobinuria differed from the well-described paroxysmal hemoglobinuria due to cold. He showed that it could not be brought about by drinking beer or by the ingestion of acid or alkali, and he suspected the accumulation of a toxic material. During the next 70 years, many case reports of hemoglobinuria following exercise were noted [2], but it was not until 1965 that the logical explanation was brought forth.

Pathogenesis

March hemoglobinuria had been observed to follow only certain types of exercise, usually walking long distances or running, and specifically not following swimming and bicycle riding [3]. Unusual causes of this type of hemoglobinuria were beating of the head against the wall [4], hand-strengthening exercises in a practitioner of karate [5], and playing the conga drum [6]. All the forms of exercise resulting in hemoglobinuria involved forceful contact of a portion of the body against a hard surface.

Two track runners who complained of this symptom were noted to have a particularly forceful, stamping gait, and it was hypothesized that the red cells were destroyed in the soles of the feet during running. When blood was placed in plastic tubes and put in the soles of their shoes, it was demonstrated that these runners brought about the hemolysis of a larger percentage of red blood cells in the tubes than control subjects running the same course. It was noted, furthermore, that blood from the control subjects was lysed to the same extent as that of the two runners. When the runners changed their stride or wore softer linings in their shoes, hemoglobinuria disappeared [7]. This finding has been substantiated by more recent reports [8], and it now seems almost certain that the cause of the hemoglobinuria is the traumatic disruption of the red cells by pressure on the soles during running or walking.

The disruption of red cells by this process is more common in young men but also occurs in athletic women [9]. Two-thirds of 26 runners in the Boston marathon of 1941 showed increases in plasma hemoglobin levels, and four of these developed hemoglobinuria [10]. It often occurs early in training and disappears as training progresses. The reasons that the same amount of exercise produces more severe hemolysis in some than in others are not apparent.

Clinical and laboratory features

The results of physical examination are entirely normal in patients with march hemoglobinuria. Neither splenomegaly nor hepatomegaly is present, and scleral icterus is rare.

The blood may occasionally show slight reticulocytosis, especially if episodes are frequent, but in most instances, even shortly after the run, the number and morphology of the red cells is normal. Fragmented forms (schizocytes) have not been observed. The level of plasma hemoglobin may be markedly elevated and serum haptoglobin decreased, particularly with repeated episodes. The urine shows hemoglobinuria and often hemoglobin casts. The second urine specimen following a bout of exercise usually contains less hemoglobin than the first, and within 6 to 12 h the urine is completely free of hemoglobin.

Differential diagnosis

March hemoglobinuria must be distinguished from other forms of hemoglobinuria and from myoglobinuria. The hemoglobinuria in this disorder follows exercise rather than chilling or sleep. However, the tests for paroxysmal nocturnal hemoglobinuria (acidified serum lysis test or sucrose lysis test) and paroxysmal cold hemoglobinuria (Donath-Landsteiner test) should be performed if any question arises. The hemoglobinuria in paroxysmal nocturnal hemoglobinuria can apparently be exacerbated by exercise [11].

Myoglobinuria can be distinguished from hemoglobinuria by chemical tests of the urine (Chap. A15). Most patients with myoglobinuria have muscle pain during the exercise episode, whereas this is not necessarily true for patients with hemoglobinuria.

Therapy

The treatment of march hemoglobinuria consists primarily of reassuring the patient that nothing is seriously wrong. Adding rubberized insoles to the shoes and changing the gait will ameliorate the condition [7]. Alkalinization of the urine to prevent precipitation of hemoglobin appears unnecessary, and no instances of renal failure have been reported.

References

1. Fleischer, R.: Über eine neue Form von Hämoglobinurie beim Menschen. *Berlin. Klin. Wochenschr. 18:*691, 1881.
2. Dacie, J. V.: *The Haemolytic Anemias,* pt. III, 2d ed. Grune & Stratton, New York, 1967, p. 966.
3. Gilligan, D. R., and Blumgart, H. L.: March hemoglobinuria: Studies of the clinical characteristics, blood metabolism and mechanisms with observations on three new cases and review of literature. *Medicine (Baltimore) 20:*314, 1941.
4. Ensor, C. W., and Barnett, J. O. W.: Paroxysmal haemoglobinuria of traumatic origin. *Med.-Chir. Trans. 86:*165, 1903.
5. Streeton, J. A.: Traumatic haemoglobinuria caused by karate exercises. *Lancet 2:*191, 1967.
6. Furie, B., and Penn, A. S.: Pigmenturia from conga drumming: Hemoglobinuria and myoglobinuria. *Ann. Intern. Med. 80:*727, 1974.
7. Davidson, R. J. L.: Exertional haemoglobinuria: A report on three cases with studies on the haemolytic mechanism. *J. Clin. Pathol. 17:*536, 1964.
8. Buckle, R. M.: Exertional (march) haemoglobinuria: Reduction of haemolytic episodes by use of sorbo-rubber insoles in shoes. *Lancet i:*1136, 1965.
9. Gilligan, D. R., and Altschule, M. D.: March hemoglobinuria in a woman. *N. Engl. J. Med. 243:*944, 1950.
10. Gilligan, D. R., Altschule, M. D., and Katersky, E. M.: Psychologic intravascular hemolysis of exercise: Hemoglobinemia and hemoglobinuria following cross-country runs. *J. Clin. Invest. 22:*859, 1943.
11. Strübing, P.: Paroxysmale Hämoglobinurie. *Dtsch. Med. Wochenschr. 8:*1, 17, 1882.

CHAPTER *63*

Traumatic cardiac hemolytic anemia

WENDELL F. ROSSE

Patients who have had intracardiac corrective surgery, especially surgery involving placement of prostheses, may develop a hemolytic anemia with hemoglobinuria. This complication of cardiac surgery was first noted in patients in whose aorta a Hufnagel valve had been inserted [1]. However, the characteristics of the anemia were not well studied until 1961, when hemolytic anemia due to red blood cell fragmentation was described following the repair of an endocardial cushion defect with Teflon [2]. Since then many instances of intravascular hemolysis with red cell fragmentation have been observed in patients with prosthetic cardiac valves [3–5].

Pathogenesis

Hemolysis following cardiac surgery appears to be due to the forceful interaction of normal red cells and an abnormal environment. Intrinsic abnormalities of the red cells are not present, and in some patients correction of the blood flow pattern by reparative surgery has corrected the hemolytic anemia.

The hemolysis is the result of the traumatic rupture of the erythrocyte membrane. The red cell membrane appears to be able to withstand shear-stress forces to 3000 dyn/cm² [6]. Forces exceeding the critical level can be generated during the cardiac cycle if the flow of blood is impeded by a small aperture or an abnormal surface.

In a model system, a jet velocity exceeding 2000 cm/s was required to produce sufficient shear stress to produce significant hemolysis of red cells. However, interaction of red cells with a wall of a vessel was found to play an important role in hemolysis [7].

The majority of instances of cardiac traumatic hemolysis involve the aortic valve. Mild hemolysis may be present in some patients with aortic [8] or subaortic [9] stenosis prior to the insertion of a prosthesis, particularly if the pressure gradient across the valve is greater than 50 mmHg [10]. Mild hemolysis is present in many patients with uncomplicated valvular replacement [4,5]. This is usually greater with aortic than mitral valves, and most patients with both valves replaced have significant hemolysis [4,10].

Thus the nature of the surface offered by the prosthesis may play a role in cardiac traumatic hemolysis. Homografts or xenografts cause hemolysis less often than do plastic valves [11,12]. Hemolysis frequently follows insertion of a prosthetic patch in the repair of an endocardial cushion (ostium primum) defect [13]. When the bisected mitral valve is not fully repaired and forceful regurgitation of blood through the mitral valve persists, the regurgitant jet is directed at the patch, which may remain unendothelialized. The plastic prosthesis offers a roughened surface upon which red cells may be caught and fragmented by the force of the ventricular impulse. More hemolysis is seen with Beall valves with cloth-covered struts [15], particularly when the cloth tears [16]. The prostheses used in aortofemoral bypasses also may cause hemolysis [17].

Trauma due to the impact of one part of the prosthesis against another has been implicated in fragmentation hemolysis. The Lucite tube comprising the outer portion of the Hufnagel ball valve did not, by itself, cause hemolysis when inserted into the aorta [18]. Hemolysis occurred when the ball was included in the tube, suggesting that striking of the ball against the tube was responsible for breaking the cells.

Several complications may give rise to increased hemolysis. More severe hemolysis is commonly associated with regurgitation of blood through or around a prosthesis, often as a result of faulty placement of the valve in the aortic root [19]. The blood may flow through a passage created by the separation of the valve from the root, and hemolysis may, in part, be due to the flow of blood across an unendothelialized surface. Regurgitation through a prosthetic mitral valve may also result in hemolysis [20]. Hemolysis may result if the outlet of the valve is too constricted because too small a valve was used or because of "ball variance" in which the plastic ball used in some prostheses takes up lipids, swells, and does not move freely in the cage, resulting in stenosis or insufficiency of the valve [21].

Clinical features

The severity of the anemia is highly variable in patients with hemolytic anemia secondary to heart valve prostheses. A mild, completely compensated hemolysis is usually present, although some patients may have such severe anemia that frequent transfusions are required. The anemia itself may be a greater detriment to the cardiac patient than it would be to patients not having cardiac abnormalities, since congestive heart failure has been ascribed to anemia and has been alleviated by transfusions. Reduction in erythropoiesis and an inability to compensate for the increased hemolysis may result from the "postperfusion syndrome" or from bacterial endocarditis.

The amount of cardiac output may have some influence on the amount of hemolysis in patients with traumatic cardiac hemolysis. Hemolysis is said to be greater during the day and when the patient exercises than when the patient is maintained at bed rest [22]. The presence of anemia itself may increase the hemolysis by increasing the cardiac output, thus initiating a cycle of increasing hemolysis and increasing anemia. However, quantitative data relating cardiac output to hemolytic rate are not available. No specific abnormalities are found on physical examination except those related to hemolysis and to the cardiac lesion and prosthesis.

Laboratory features

ERYTHROCYTES
Hemoglobin levels may be very low and the reticulocyte count considerably elevated. Schizocytes consisting of helmet cells, triangle cells, and other fragmented forms having sharp points are nearly always present on the blood film. Microspherocytes may also be present. In addition to fragmented forms, the red cells may also show hypochromia if iron deficiency due to urinary loss of hemoglobin or hemosiderin is present.

The plasma hemoglobin level is elevated, and the serum haptoglobin concentration is diminished or absent. Hemosiderinuria is a constant finding, but the hemoglobinuria may vary from none to large amounts. The serum lactic acid dehydrogenase activity may be elevated.

LEUKOCYTES
The leukocyte count may be normal or slightly elevated.

PLATELET AND CLOTTING FACTORS
The platelet count may be diminished. The degree of reduction has been correlated with the surface area of plastic exposed to the blood, implying that platelets are caught and destroyed on the surface of the prosthesis [23]. However, decrease in the levels of plasma clotting factors is not recorded, and the turnover of fibrinogen is normal [24].

URINE AND RENAL FUNCTION
Although 80 percent of all patients have hemosiderinuria, with or without hemoglobinuria, renal function is normal [25]. Marked hemosiderosis of the kidney is frequently found at postmortem examination [26].

Differential diagnosis

The presence of fragmented red cells and other evidence of intravascular hemolysis and the history of cardiac disease or surgery suggest that this form of hemolytic anemia is present. One must be certain that the anemia is not due to autoimmune disease. In addition, bacterial endocarditis on occasion may imitate or complicate the syndrome but by itself does not cause fragmented erythrocytes or intravascular hemolysis.

Treatment

If the anemia is sufficiently severe, the most effective treatment for schizocytic hemolysis secondary to cardiac prostheses consists of reoperation and replacement of the prosthesis.

IRON REPLACEMENT
Most patients with valvular prosthesis should be given iron because iron deficiency is a frequent complication of the insertion of artificial valves and can complicate the patient's course by imposing a limit on erythropoiesis.

TRANSFUSION
Transfusion may be necessary to maintain an adequate hemoglobin level when the marrow is unable to compensate for the hemolysis, as during intercurrent febrile illnesses. It may also be required when hemolysis is very rapid. However, in the latter case reoperation should be considered.

GLUCOCORTICOIDS

Glucocorticoids do not seem to be beneficial in most instances of cardiac hemolysis.

Course and prognosis

Hemolysis due to cardiac abnormalities rarely improves spontaneously. Hence the course and prognosis are determined largely by the severity of the primary cardiac lesion.

References

1. Rose, J. C., Hufnagel, C. A., Fries, E. D., Harvey, W. P., and Partenope, E. A.: The hemodynamic alterations produced by plastic valvular prosthesis for severe aortic insufficiency in man. *J. Clin. Invest.* 33:891, 1954.
2. Sayed, H. M., Dacie, J. V., Handley, D. A., Lewis, S. M., and Cleland, W. P.: Haemolytic anaemia of mechanical origin after open heart surgery. *Thorax* 16:356, 1961.
3. Marsh, G. W., and Lewis, S. M.: Cardiac haemolytic anaemia. *Semin. Hematol.* 6:133, 1969.
4. Brodeur, M. T. H., Sutherland, D. W., Koler, R. D., Starr, A., Kinsey, J. A., and Griswold, H. E.: Red blood cell survival in patients with aortic valvular disease and ball valve prostheses. *Circulation* 32:570, 1965.
5. Marsh, G. W.: Intravascular haemolytic anaemia after aortic-valve replacement. *Lancet* 2:986, 1964.
6. Nevaril, C. G., Lynch, E. C., Alfrey, C. P., and Hellums, J. D.: Erythrocyte damage and destruction induced by shearing stress. *J. Lab. Clin. Med.* 71:784, 1968.
7. Bernstein, E. F., Blackshear, P. L., and Keller, K. H.: Factors influencing erythrocyte destruction in artificial organs. *Am. J. Surg.* 114:126, 1967.
8. Miller, D. S., Mengel, C. E., Kremer, W. B., Gutterman, J., and Senningen, R.: Intravascular hemolysis in a patient with valvular heart disease. *Ann. Intern. Med.* 65:210, 1966.
9. Solanki, D. L., and Sheikh, M. U.: Fragmentation of hemolysis in idiopathic hypertrophic subaortic stenosis. *South Med. J.* 71:599, 1978.
10. Jacobson, A. J., Rath, C. E., and Perloff, S. K.: Intravascular hemolysis and thrombocytopenia in left ventricular outflow obstruction. *Br. Heart J.* 35:49, 1973.
11. Myers, T. J., Hild, D. H., and Rihaldi, M. J.: Hemolytic anemia associated with heterograft replacement of the mitral valve. *J. Thorac. Cardiovasc. Surg.* 76:214, 1978.
12. Febres-Roman, P. R., Bovry, W. C., Crone, R. A., Davis, R. C., Jr., and Williams, T. H.: Chronic intravascular hemolysis after aortic valve replacement with Ionescu-Shiley xenograft: Comparative study with Bjork-Shiley prosthesis. *Am. J. Cardiology* 46:735, 1980.
13. Sigler, A. T., Forman, E. N., Zinkham, W. H., and Neill, C. A.: Severe intravascular hemolysis following surgical repair of endocardial cushion defects. *Am. J. Med.* 35:407, 1963.
14. Crexells, C., Aerichide, N., Bonny, Y., Lepage, C., and Campeau, L.: Factors influencing hemolysis in valve prosthesis. *Am. Heart J.* 84:161, 1972.
15. Santinga, J. T., Flora, J. D., Batsakis, J., and Kirsch, M. M.: Hemolysis in patients with the cloth-covered aortic valve prosthesis. *Am. J. Cardiol.* 34:533, 1974.
16. Shah, A., Dolgin, M., Tice, D., and Trehan, N.: Complications due to cloth wear in cloth-covered Starr-Edwards aortic and mitral valve prostheses—and their management. *Am. Heart J.* 96:407, 1978.
17. Manny, J., et al.: Traumatic hemolysis after aortofemoral bypass. *Isr. J. Med. Sci.* 13:50, 1977.
18. Rodgers, B. M., and Sabiston, D. C., Jr.: Hemolytic anemia following prosthetic valve replacement. *Circulation* 39:155, 1969.
19. Kastor, J. A., Akburian, M., and Buckley, M. J.: Paravalvular leaks and hemolytic anemia following Starr-Edwards aortic and mitral valves. *J. Thorac. Cardiovasc. Surg.* 56:279, 1968.
20. Eyster, E.: Traumatic hemolysis with hemoglobinuria due to ball variance. *Blood* 33:391, 1969.
21. Stohlman, F., Jr., Sarnoff, S. J., Case, R. B., and Ness, A. T.: Hemolytic syndrome following the insertion of a lucite ball valve prosthesis into the cardiovascular system. *Circulation* 13:586, 1956.
22. Sears, D. A., Anderson, P. R., Foy, A. L., Williams, H. L., and Crosby, W. H.: Urinary iron excretion and renal metabolism of hemoglobin in hemolytic diseases. *Blood* 28:708, 1966.
23. Harker, L. A., and Slichter, S. J.: Studies of platelet and fibrinogen kinetics in patients with prosthetic heart valves. *N. Engl. J. Med.* 283:1302, 1970.
24. Baker, L. R. I., Rubenberg, M. L., Dacie, J. V., and Brain, M. C.: Fibrinogen catabolism in microangiopathic haemolytic anaemia. *Br. J. Haematol.* 14:617, 1968.
25. Slater, S. D., Rahman, M., and Lindsay, R. M.: Renal function in chronic intravascular haemolysis associated with prosthetic cardiac valves. *Clin. Sci.* 44:511, 1973.
26. Roberts, W. C.: Renal hemosiderosis (blue kidney) in patients with valvular heart disease. *Am. J. Pathol.* 48:409, 1966.

CHAPTER *64*

Microangiopathic hemolytic anemia

WENDELL F. ROSSE

Hemolytic anemia due to intravascular fragmentation of red cells is characterized by the presence of distinctive abnormal red blood cells (schizocytes), intravascular hemolysis, and, in some instances, deficiency of platelets and of the clotting factors. The major causes of intravascular red cell fragmentation have been described: (1) abnormalities of the vascular endothelium, especially of the arterioles, or the presence of disseminated intravascular coagulation; (2) the insertion of prosthetic devices in the heart and major vessels (see Chap. 63). In both instances, the fundamental cause of hemolysis is the traumatic disruption of the red cell by the force of the blood pushing cells through blood vessels which have been narrowed by disease or which are partially obstructed by fibrin strands. The disorders causing schizocytic hemolytic anemia are listed in Table 64-1.

Etiology and pathogenesis

Most of the diseases characterized by fragmentation hemolytic anemia involve abnormalities of the arteriolar and precapillary endothelium. Hence, in 1962, Brain, Dacie, and Hourihane [1] coined the term

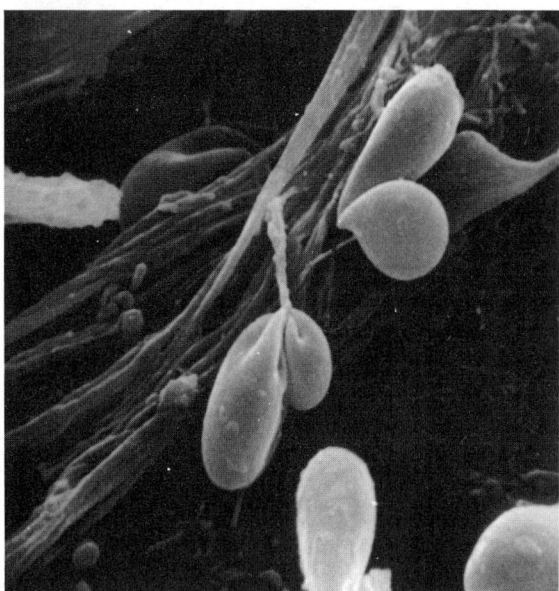

FIGURE 64-1 Hanged red cell. Dense fibrin band in background formed from accumulations of finer strands, some of which are still evident. It is only these denser, more amorphous structures that typically persist postmortem. × 2100 in vitro model, scanning electron microscope. (From B. S. Bull and I. N. Kuhn, The production of schistocytes by fibrin strands: A scanning electron microscope study. *Blood* 35:104, 1970. By permission.)

microangiopathic hemolytic anemia to describe this syndrome. They found that uremia was often present in the patients but that the morphologic abnormalities were not related to its presence alone.

Intravascular coagulation may play a major role in bringing about intravascular fragmentation hemolysis in many, if not most, instances. The induction of intravascular coagulation by thrombin or snake venom results in elevated plasma hemoglobin levels and formation of schizocytes [2]. Elevation of the plasma hemoglobin concentration parallels the rapidity of the defibrination (coagulation) process. The hemolytic reaction can be suppressed if coagulation is suppressed and enhanced if fibrinolysis is inhibited with ε-aminocaproic acid.

The mechanics of fragmentation of blood were studied in vitro in a system in which blood could be circulated and clotting induced on a filter bed [3]. Hemolysis resulted when coagulation occurred if the flow rate within the system was sufficiently high. Typical schizocytic forms appeared to develop as the result of the folding of cells over fibrin strands, apposing the inner surface of the membrane (Fig. 64-1). If sufficient force was supplied by the flow of blood, the membrane was torn at the fibrin strand, the membrane around one or both of the pieces was resealed, and the fragments floated free. The composition of the strand was of little impor-

tance so long as it was small enough to permit folding over; glass or nylon could be substituted for fibrin.

In nearly all instances of fragmentation hemolytic anemia, except for that caused by prosthetic heart valves, the turnover rate of plasma fibrinogen is increased [4]. This suggests that even in those instances in which depletion of the clotting factors does not occur, intravascular coagulation is probably still an important event in bringing about schizocytic hemolytic anemia. Abnormalities of the vascular endothelium, when present, appear to provide a site for the propagation of intravascular coagulation. If this occurs in the arterioles where sufficient force can be applied to the red cells caught upon fibrin strands, fragmentation results.

Fragmentation hemolysis plays an important role in the pathogenesis of the anemia seen in thrombotic thrombocytopenic purpura [5,6] and its pediatric variant, the hemolytic uremic syndrome [7]. In patients with these illnesses, an abnormality in the arteriolar wall results in the deposition of platelets and fibrin with the production of red cell fragmentation and hemolysis. If the lesions are widespread, severe disturbances of the affected organ, especially the kidney or the brain, may be demonstrated [8]. These syndromes are described in greater detail in Chap. 142.

Illnesses characterized by vasculitis, with disturbances resembling the Shwartzman phenomenon, may also exhibit disseminated intravascular coagulation and fragmentation anemia. Similar phenomena are thought to occur in certain illnesses such as Rocky Mountain spotted fever [9], purpura fulminans [10], and some forms of septicemia [11]. Arteriolar necrosis or arteriolar vasculitis resulting in schizocytosis may also occur in malignant hypertension (usually only when severe renal involvement is present), renal cortical necrosis, acute glomerulonephritis, polyarteritis, and allergic vasculitis [1]. Widespread malignant neoplasms, such as adenocarcinoma of the breast or stomach, may cause fragmentation hemolysis [1,12]. The fragmentation is thought to be due to coagulation about the tumor or tumor emboli [13]. Rare vascular anomalies such as cavernous giant capillary hemangiomata (Kasabach-Merritt syndrome) [14] (see Chap. 142) and traumatic arteriovenous fistulae [15] may also result in intravascular fragmentation of the red cells and intravascular coagulation. Fragmentation hemolysis may occur in the absence of primary vascular disease in disseminated intravascular coagulation occurring in patients with abruptio placentae [16], after certain snake bites [2], and perhaps with clostridial infections [17].

Clinical features

The clinical syndrome in patients with fragmentation hemolytic anemia will depend largely on the primary disease causing the vascular lesions or on the degree, site, and duration of the intravascular coagulation. The hemolysis may be sudden and profound. Splenomegaly is occasionally present.

Laboratory features

Diagnosis of fragmentation hemolytic anemia can often be made by finding the fragmented forms on the blood film. These forms consist of cells with one or more, commonly two, points. Such erythrocytes have been called *helmet cells, schizocytes* (or *schistocytes*), or *keratocytes (horn cells)* (see Chap. 29). Microspherocytes with a slightly irregular outline may be seen.

True schizocytes must be distinguished from other abnormally shaped red cells. Unlike acanthocytes (burr cells and "spur" cells), they usually have no more than two or three points, which are sharp, as if drawn out like molten glass. Sometimes in other hemolytic diseases, especially in the absence of the spleen, cells may be seen which appear to be fragments, but the points are usually not as sharp as those of true schizocytes.

The reticulocyte count is usually elevated, often even despite severe uremia, and nucleated red cells may be present in the blood. The leukocyte count is often mildly to moderately elevated. No distinctively abnormal forms are seen. The platelet count may or may not be decreased, depending on the degree of intravascular coagulation. The marrow usually shows erythrocytic and perhaps megakaryocytic hyperplasia. Megakaryocytes often appear somewhat young. Intravascular hemolysis is reflected by markedly elevated plasma hemoglobin, absence of haptoglobin, and occasional presence of urine hemoglobin and hemosiderin. Abnormalities of clotting factors may be demonstrated in those patients in whom the defibrination syndrome is present. In particular, fibrinogen, prothrombin, factor V, and factor VIII levels may be diminished (see Chap. 158). Evidence of the activation of the fibrinolytic system, including the presence of fibrin split products in the plasma, may aid in the diagnosis. On the other hand, if the defibrination process is mild, coagulation abnormalities can only be inferred from special studies [17].

Differential diagnosis

Microangiopathic hemolytic anemia must be distinguished from other forms of intravascular hemolysis. However, the clinical manifestations of the primary disease usually make differentiation simple. If any doubt exists, tests for immune hemolysis and paroxysmal nocturnal hemoglobinuria should be performed. Once the presence of microangiopathic hemolytic anemia has been established, the primary cause of the vascular changes or intravascular clotting should be determined (Table 64-1).

TABLE 64-1   The causes of schizocytic hemolytic anemia

I. Abnormalities of heart and large vessels
   A. Without surgery
      1. Aortic stenosis
      2. Ruptured sinus of Valsalva
      3. Ruptured chordae tendineae
      4. Coarctation of aorta
      5. Aortic aneurysm
   B. Following surgery
      1. "Patching" operations
        a. Ostium primum repair, especially if mitral regurgitation present
        b. Aortic aneurysm repair (aortofemoral bypass)
      2. Valvular replacement
        a. Uncomplicated
          (1) Outflow too small
          (2) Large area of exposed plastic
          (3) Cloth-covered struts
          (4) Two or more valves replaced
          (5) Xenograft
        b. Complicated
          (1) Ball variance
          (2) Regurgitation around seating of valve
          (3) Rupture of cloth or cloth-covered strut
II. Microvascular abnormalities (often accompanied by localized intravascular coagulation)
   A. Congenital
      1. Kasabach-Merritt syndrome
      2. Hepatic hemangioendothelioma
      3. Arteriovenous
   B. "Primary" acquired
      1. Thrombotic thrombocytopenic purpura
      2. Hemolytic uremic syndrome
   C. Associated with immunologic phenomena
      1. Acute glomerulonephritis
      2. Polyarteritis involving small vessels
      3. Scleroderma, especially involving kidney
      4. Wegener's granulomatosis
      5. Renal allograft rejection, particularly if hyperacute
      6. Allergic vasculitis
      7. Rocky Mountain spotted fever
   D. Associated with hypertension
      1. Malignant hypertension with fibrinoid necrosis
      2. Pulmonary hypertension
      3. Eclampsia and preeclampsia
   E. Associated with malignancy
      1. Adenocarcinoma
      2. Lymphoma
III. Disseminated intravascular coagulation
   A. Primary activation of fluid-phase procoagulants
      1. Abruptio placentae
      2. Administration of "activated" factor IX preparations
      3. Promyelocytic leukemia
      4. Snake bite (vipers and rattlesnakes)
      5. Shunting of ascites fluid through La Veen shunt
   B. Infections of inflammatory process
      1. Sepsis
      2. Purpura fulminans
      3. Acute hemolytic transfusion reactions
      4. Adult respiratory distress syndrome
      5. Pancreatitis
      6. Heat stroke
      7. Immunologic reactions to drugs

Treatment

Treatment of the intravascular clotting syndrome in microangiopathic hemolytic anemia consists of treatment of the primary disease, treatment of the intravascular coagulation, and treatment of the anemia. Treatment of the primary disease may at times be difficult, and the therapy of the most dramatic causes of the syndrome, thrombotic thrombocytopenic purpura (and hemolytic uremia syndrome), is discussed in Chap. 142. The treatment of malignant hypertension with antihypertensive drugs, when successful, may result in a decrease in the hemolytic process. Vascular anomalies such as cavernous hemangiomata may be irradiated [14], and obliteration of traumatic arteriovenous fistulae brings about cessation of intravascular coagulation and fragmentation hemolysis [15].

The prevention of coagulation should ameliorate the process of intravascular fragmentation. Intravenous heparin in moderately large doses (35,000 or 40,000 to 50,000 units per day) has been given [17]. When the primary disease is refractory to treatment, amelioration of the intravascular coagulation and fragmentation may not affect the ultimate outcome. Heparinization has been unsuccessful in the treatment of microangiopathic hemolytic anemia complicating metastatic carcinoma of the breast [14].

Treatment of the anemia usually consists of transfusion as necessary.

Prognosis

The prognosis in microangiopathic hemolytic anemia depends on the cause.

References

1. Brain, M. C., Dacie, J. V., and Hourihane, D. O'B.: Microangiopathic haemolytic anaemia: The possible role of vascular lesions in pathogenesis. Br. J. Haematol. 8:358, 1962.

2. Rubenberg, M. L., Regoeczi, E., Bull, B. S., Dacie, J. V., and Brain, M. C.: Microangiopathic haemolytic anaemia: The experimental production of haemolysis and red cell fragmentation by defibrination in vivo. Br. J. Haematol. 14:627, 1968.

3. Bull, B. S., Rubenberg, M. L., Dacie, J. F., and Brain, M. C.: Microangiopathic haemolytic anaemia: Mechanisms of red cell fragmentation: In vitro studies. Br. J. Haematol. 14:643, 1968.

4. Baker, L. R. I., Rubenberg, M. L., Dacie, J. V., and Brain, M. C.: Fibrinogen catabolism in microangiopathic haemolytic anaemia. Br. J. Haematol. 14:617, 1968.

5. Adelson, E., Heitzman, E. J., and Fennessey, J. F.: Thrombohemolytic thrombocytopenic purpura. Arch. Intern. Med. 94:42, 1954.

6. Gasser, W. C., Gautier, E., Steck, A., Siebenmann, R. E., and Oechslin, R.: Hämolytisch-urämische Syndrome: Bilaterale Nierenrindennekrosen bei alkuten erworbenen Hämolytischen Anämien. Schweiz. Med. Wochenschr. 85:905, 1955.

7. Brain, M. C.: The haemolytic-uremic syndrome. Semin. Hematol. 6:162, 1959.

8. Amorosi, E. L., and Ultmann, J. E.: Thrombotic thrombocytopenic purpura: Report of 16 cases and review of the literature. Medicine 45:139, 1966.

9. Trigg, J. W.: Hypofibrinogenemia in Rocky Mountain spotted fever. N. Engl. J. Med. 270:1042, 1964.

10. Hollingsworth, J. H., and Mohler, D. N.: Microangiopathic hemolytic anaemia caused by purpura fulminans. Ann. Intern. Med. 68:1310, 1968.

11. McGehee, W. G., Rapaport, S. I., and Hyort, P. F.: Intravascular coagulation in fulminant meningococcemia. Ann. Intern. Med. 67:250, 1967.

12. Antman, K. H., Skarin, A. T., Mayer, R. J., Hargreaves, H. K., and Canellos, G. P.: Microangiopathic hemolytic anemia and cancer: A review. Medicine 58:377, 1979.

13. Helgard, P., and Gordon-Smith, E.: Microangiopathic haemolytic anaemia in experimental tumor cell emboli. Br. J. Haematol. 26:651, 1974.

14. Propp, R. P., and Scharfman, W. B.: Hemangiomathrombocytopenia syndrome associated with microangiopathic hemolytic anemia. Blood 28:623, 1966.

15. Chamberlain, J. K., O'Brien, F., Christ, L. M., and Breckenridge, R. T.: Intravascular hemolysis with traumatic arteriovenous fistula. N.Y. State. J. Med. 74:686, 1974.

16. Pritchard, J. A., and Brekken, A. L.: Clinical and laboratory studies on severe abruptio placentae. Am. J. Obstet. Gynecol. 97:681, 1967.

17. Dean, H. M., Decker, C. L., and Baker, L. D.: Temporary survival in clostridial hemolysis with absence of circulating red cells. N. Engl. J. Med. 277:700, 1967.

18. Brain, M. C., Baker, L. R. I., McBride, J. A., Rubenberg, M. L., and Dacie, J. V.: Treatment of patients with microangiopathic haemolytic anaemia with heparin. Br. J. Haematol. 15:603, 1968.

Erythrocyte disorders—anemias related to erythrocyte damage mediated by chemicals, physical agents, or microorganisms

CHAPTER 65

Hemolytic anemia due to chemical and physical agents

ERNEST BEUTLER

Many drugs and a variety of toxins have been associated with red blood cell destruction. In some instances the mechanism that produces the hemolytic response is fairly well understood. For example, hemolysis may result from the interaction of an environmental influence (a toxin) with a hereditary defect of the erythrocyte, as is the case when certain drugs are administered to patients deficient in glucose-6-phosphate dehydrogenase or glutathione or to those with an unstable hemoglobin. This type of hemolytic anemia has been described in Chaps. 58, 59, and 61. "Oxidative" drugs which cause hemolysis in individuals with such red cell defects (see Table 58-2) will produce hemolysis also in those with normal red blood cells if given in sufficient dosage. The mechanism of hemolysis of normal red cells is probably the same as that in persons with intrinsic red cell defects: even the defense mechanisms of normal cells can be overcome when exposed to sufficiently severe stresses. Immune mechanisms may also play a role in drug- or toxin-induced hemolytic anemias. These are discussed in Chap. 69. Various other drugs and chemicals have also been implicated in the development of hemolysis.

Arsenic hydride

The inhalation of arsine gas (arsenic hydride, AsH_3) is a well-recognized cause of hemolytic anemia [1]. Arsine is formed in the course of many industrial processes. In most cases it results from the reaction of nascent hydrogen, generated by the action of acid on metal, with arsenic compounds. The arsenic is usually present as a contaminant of either the acid or the metal, so that the contact with arsenic compounds may not be apparent from the history. Exposure to sufficient amounts of the gas will lead to severe anemia, jaundice, and hemoglobinuria. The mechanism of hemolysis is not clearly understood, although the well-known reactions of arsenic compounds with sulfhydryl groups in the cell membrane may play an important role.

Lead

Lead poisoning has been recognized since antiquity. The ingestion of beverages containing lead leached from highly soluble lead glazes or earthenware containers has been blamed for the extinction of the Roman aristocracy and is even now an occasional cause of lead intoxication [2]. The distillation of alcohol in leaded flasks is another rare cause of plumbism in certain areas, although the practice was prohibited in 1723 by the Massachusetts Bay Colony after it was noticed that consumption of rum so distilled resulted in abdominal pain known as the "dry gripes" [2]. Among the earliest published descriptions of lead poisoning is a letter written in 1786 by Benjamin Franklin [3,4], who had learned, as a printer, that working over small furnaces of melted metal or drying racks of wet type in front of a fire might cause pain in the hands. Today, lead intoxication in children generally results from ingestion of flaking lead paint or from chewing lead-painted articles. In adults, it occurs primarily as the result of inhalation of lead compounds used or produced in industrial processes.

Most patients with lead poisoning manifest some degree of anemia, although anemia is only rarely the predominant clinical manifestation [5]. However, examination of the blood often provides the key diagnostic clue, and thus the hematologic findings are of special interest. Modest shortening of red cell life-span is a relatively constant feature of the disorder [6,7]. In vitro treatment of red cells with lead produces measurable membrane damage. Lead interferes with the cation pump [8], possibly in inhibiting membrane ATPase [9,10]. It is not at all clear, however, that the hemolysis observed in lead poisoning is due to these changes. In some children with lead poisoning, an abnormal hemoglobin indistinguishable from hemoglobin A_3 comprises approximately 15 percent of the total pigment [11].

The anemia of lead intoxication is not usually due primarily to hemolysis. Lead apparently interferes with the normal production of erythrocytes, probably through a combination of mechanisms. Heme synthesis is markedly abnormal in patients with lead poisoning. Several enzymes of heme synthesis are inhibited, including δ-aminolevulinic acid (ALA) synthetase, ALA dehydrase, heme synthetase, porphyrinogen deaminase, uroporphyrinogen decarboxylase, and coproporphyrinogen oxidase [5,6,12]. ALA dehydrase appears to be particularly sensitive to inhibition, showing decreased activity in erythrocytes at blood lead levels in the upper portions of the normal range [9]. Increased amounts of δ-aminolevulinic acid and coproporphyrin are found in the urine [12], and the free protoporphyrin levels of the erythrocytes are strikingly increased, presumably as a result of inhibition of the heme biosynthetic enzymes. Marked inhibition of the enzyme pyrimidine 5'-nucleotidase is also observed [13]. In the absence of this enzyme pyrimidine nucleotides accumulate in the red cells and normal depolymerization of reticulocyte ribosomal RNA does not occur. In hereditary pyrimidine 5'-nucleotidase deficiency, basophilic stippling of erythrocytes is a characteristic finding (Chap. 59), and it has been suggested that its inhibition by lead may be responsible for the basophilic stippling of erythrocytes which occurs in plumbism (see below). Synthesis of α- and β-globin chains seems to be defective in lead poisoning [14], and this may play a contributory role in the anemia of lead poisoning.

The anemia of chronic lead poisoning is usually mild in the adult but is frequently more severe in children. The red cells are normocytic and slightly hypochromic. Basophilic stippling of the erythrocytes may be fine or coarse, and the number of granules seen in each cell may be quite variable. When blood is collected in ethylenediaminetetraacetic acid (EDTA), the stippling may disappear [15]. Young polychromatophilic cells are most likely to be stippled. Electron microscopic studies [16] have demonstrated that the basophilic granules represent abnormally aggregated ribosomes. In the marrow, ringed sideroblasts are frequently found (see Chap. 54). Iron-laden mitochondria are present [16] but do not appear to contribute to the basophilic stippling which is observed on light microscopy. It may be presumed that iron which has entered the developing erythroblast fails to be incorporated into heme at a normal rate either because of lead-induced impairment of heme synthesis or because of the direct effect of lead on mitochondria.

Remarkably complete observations of the hematologic changes occurring after the intravenous injection of lead in an attempt to treat malignant disease were published in 1928 [17]. Distortion of red cells was observed both in blood films and in wet preparations made immediately after infusion of lead.

Copper

Hemolysis has also resulted from ingestion of copper sulfate in suicide attempts and from accumulation of toxic amounts from hemodialysis fluid contaminated by copper pipes [18,19]. Hemolysis in Wilson's disease has been attributed to the elevated plasma copper levels which are characteristic of that disorder [20,21]. The pathogenesis of this hemolytic anemia may be related to oxidation of intracellular GSH, hemoglobin, and NADPH and inhibition of glucose-6-phosphate dehydrogenase (G-6-PD) by copper [22]. However, the amount of copper required to inhibit G-6-PD is large, and copper in much lower concentrations inhibits pyruvate kinase [23], hexokinase, phosphogluconate dehydrogenase, phosphofructokinase, and phosphoglycerate kinase [24].

Chlorates

Sodium and potassium chlorate are oxidative drugs which have been known to produce methemoglobinemia, Heinz bodies, and hemolytic anemia. While it might be presumed that the mechanism of hemolysis is similar to that resulting from other oxidative drugs, no cases have been observed in patients deficient in glucose-6-phosphate dehydrogenase. The rare instances of chlorate poisoning which have been reported usually resulted from prescription errors in which sodium chlorate was dispensed instead of sodium chloride [25]. Hemolytic anemia with Heinz body formation has also occurred in patients undergoing dialysis when the tap water used contained a substantial amount of chloramines. Oxidative damage of the red cells of these patients was demonstrated by the presence of Heinz bodies, a positive ascorbate-cyanide test, and methemoglobinemia [26]. Leaching of formaldehyde from plastic used in a water filter employed for hemodialysis is also a cause of hemolytic anemia. It was suggested that the effect of the low levels of formaldehyde found in the water were not mediated through its fixative effect but rather by inducing metabolic changes in the red cells [27].

Miscellaneous chemicals

There are also isolated reports of hemolytic anemia occurring after the administration of resorcin [28], apiol [29], nitrobenzene [30], zinc ethylene bisdithiocarbamate [31], aniline [32], mephenesin [33], salicylazosulfapyridine (Azulfidine) [34], phenazopyridine (Pyridium) [35,36], and cisplatin [37]. When large amounts of distilled water gain access to the systemic circulation, either by intravenous injection or when used as an irrigating solution during surgery, hemolysis will occur [38]. Severe hemolysis may also result from water inhalation in near-drowning.

Hyperbaric oxygen

Hemolytic anemia has been observed in astronauts exposed to 100 percent oxygen. In at least one patient, hyperbaric oxygenation was associated with acute hemolysis [39]. It was suggested that hemolysis in this instance may have been due to abnormal peroxidation of lipids in the erythrocytes, but evidence supporting this view is indirect and equivocal. Hemolysis occurs in vitamin E–deficient mice exposed to hyperbaric oxygenation [40]. However, there is no known relationship between vitamin E and hyperoxic hemolysis in humans.

Insect venoms

Bee [41] and wasp [42] stings have been associated with severe hemolysis, and spider or scorpion bites have occasionally been followed by hemolytic anemia and hemoglobinuria [43–45]. The spiders usually thought to be responsible are *Loxosceles loeta* and *Loxosceles reclusus.* The reasons some patients suffer hemolysis after insect bites while others do not are not known. Although snake venom is known to cause hemolysis in vitro by converting lecithin to lysolecithin (see Chap. 38), hemolysis does not often result from snake bites [46].

Heat

It has been known for over a hundred years that heating blood to temperatures above 47°C rapidly produces visible damage to erythrocytes. The sequence of events has been defined in detail [47]. Cells damaged by heating not only show morphologic changes and increases in osmotic and mechanical fragility but are also removed rapidly after reinjection into the circulation [48]. These observations are apparently quite relevant to the severe hemolytic anemia which occurs in patients with extensive burns. Spherocytosis and increased osmotic fragility are found in many patients, and blood films may show fragmentation, budding, spherocytosis, and severe microspherocytosis. These changes are particularly evident if films are made promptly after the burn occurs. Gross hemoglobinemia was observed in 11 of 40 patients with second- and third-degree burns involving 15 to 65 percent of the body surface [49]. It seems likely that the acute hemolytic anemia occurring within the 24 h following a burn is due to the direct effect of heat on circulating erythrocytes. Hemolysis occurring more than 24 h after the burn may sometimes be due to the infusion of isoagglutinins (particularly anti-A) in pooled plasma, when this has been administered to the patient as part of treatment [50].

Radiation

Although reduced red cell survival is a part of the complex series of events occurring after administration of large doses of total body radiation [51], erythrocytes appear to be very resistant to the direct effects of radiation [52]. It seems likely, therefore, that such shortened red cell survival as may occur after radiation is related

largely to red cell loss through internal bleeding and to various secondary events such as infection.

References

1. Jenkins, G. C., Ind, J. E., Kazantzis, G., and Owen, R.: Arsine poisoning: Massive haemolysis with minimal impairment of renal function. *Br. Med. J.* 2:78, 1965.
2. Klein, M., Namer, R., Harpur, E., and Corbin, R.: Earthenware containers as a source of fatal lead poisoning. *N. Engl. J. Med.* 283:669, 1970.
3. *The Complete Works of Benjamin Franklin,* edited by J. Bigelow. Knickerbocker Press, Putnam, New York, 1888, vol. 9, p. 329.
4. Andreasen, N. J. C.: Benjamin Franklin: Physicus et medicus. *JAMA* 236:57, 1976.
5. Harris, M. W., and Kellermeyer, R. W.: Acquired abnormality: Porphyrinuria, in *The Red Cell.* Harvard, Cambridge, Mass., 1970, chap. 35.
6. Waldron, H. A.: The anaemia of lead poisoning: A review. *Br. J. Ind. Med.* 23:83, 1966.
7. Westerman, M. P., Pfitzer, E., Ellis, L. D., and Jensen, W. N.: Concentrations of lead in bone in plumbism. *N. Engl. J. Med.* 273:1246, 1965.
8. Vincent, P. C., and Blackburn, C. R. B.: The effects of heavy metal ions on the human erythrocyte. I. Comparisons of the action of several heavy metals. *Aust. J. Exp. Biol. Med. Sci.* 36:471, 1958.
9. Hernberg, S., and Nikkanen, J.: Enzyme inhibition by lead under normal urban conditions. *Lancet* 1:63, 1970.
10. Hasan, J., Vihko, V., and Hernberg, S.: Deficient red cell membrane (Na$^+$ + K$^+$)-ATPase in lead poisoning. *Arch. Environ. Health* 14:313, 1967.
11. Charache, S., and Weatherall, D. J.: Fast hemoglobin in lead poisoning. *Blood* 28:377, 1966.
12. Goldberg, A.: Annotation: Lead poisoning and haem biosynthesis. *Br. J. Haematol.* 23:521, 1972.
13. Paglia, D. E., Valentine, W. N., and Dahlgren, J. G.: Effects of low-level lead exposure on pyrimidine 5′-nucleotidase and other erythrocyte enzymes. *J. Clin. Invest.* 56:1164, 1975.
14. White, J. M., and Harvey, D. R.: Defective synthesis of α and β globin chains in lead poisoning. *Nature* 236:71, 1972.
15. White, J. M., and Selhi, H. S.: Lead and the red cell. *Br. J. Haematol.* 30:133, 1975.
16. Jensen, W. N., Moreno, G. D., and Bessis, M. C.: An electron microscopic description of basophilic stippling in red cells. *Blood* 25:933, 1965.
17. Brookfield, R. W.: Blood changes occurring during the course of treatment of malignant disease by lead, with special reference to punctate basophilia and the platelets. *J. Pathol.* 31:277, 1928.
18. Klein, W. J., Jr., Metz, E. N., and Price, A. R.: Acute copper intoxication: A hazard of hemodialysis. *Arch. Intern. Med.* 129:578, 1972.
19. Manzler, A. D., and Schreiner, A. W.: Copper-induced acute hemolytic anemia: A new complication of hemodialysis. *Ann. Intern. Med.* 73:409, 1970.
20. McIntyre, N., Clink, H. M., Levi, A. J., Cumings, J. N., and Sherlock, S.: Hemolytic anemia in Wilson's disease. *N. Engl. J. Med.* 276:439, 1967.
21. Deiss, A., Lee, G. R., and Cartwright, G. E.: Hemolytic anemia in Wilson's disease. *Ann. Intern. Med.* 73:413, 1970.
22. Fairbanks, V. F.: Copper sulfate-induced hemolytic anemia. *Arch. Intern. Med.* 120:428, 1967.
23. Blume, K. G., Hoffbauer, R. W., Löhr, G. W., and Rüdiger, H. W.: Genetische und biochemische Aspekte der pyruvatkinase menschlicher Erythrozyten (E.C.2.7.1.40). *Verh. Dtsch. Ges. Inn. Med.* 75:450, 1969.
24. Boulard, M., Blume, K., and Beutler, E.: The effect of copper on red cell enzyme activities. *J. Clin. Invest.* 51:459, 1972.
25. Jackson, R. C., Elder, W. J., and McDonnell, H.: Sodium-chlorate poisoning complicated by acute renal failure. *Lancet* 2:1381, 1961.
26. Eaton, J. W., Kopin, C. F., Swofford, H. S., Kjellstrand, C.-M., and Jacob, H. S.: Chlorinated urban water: A cause of dialysis-induced hemolytic anemia. *Science* 181:463, 1973.

27. Orringer, E. P., and Mattern, W. D.: Formaldehyde-induced hemolysis during chronic hemodialysis. *N. Engl. J. Med.* 294:1416, 1976.

28. Gasser, V. C.: Perakute hämolytische Innenkörperanämie mit Methämoglobinamie nach Behandlung eines Säuglingsekzems mit Resorcin. *Helv. Paediatr. Acta* 9:285, 1954.

29. Lowenstein, and Ballew, D. H.: Fatal acute haemolytic anaemia, thrombocytopenic purpura, nephrosis and hepatitis resulting from ingestion of a compound containing apiol. *Can. Med. Assoc. J.* 78:195, 1958.

30. Hunter, D.: Industrial toxicology. *Q. J. Med.* 12:185, 1943.

31. Pinkhas, J., Djaldetti, M., Joshua, H., Resnick, C., and De Vries, A.: Sulfhemoglobinemia and acute hemolytic anemia with Heinz bodies following contact with a fungicide—zinc ethylene bisidithiocarbamate—in subject with glucose-6-phosphate dehydrogenase deficiency and hypo-catalasemia. *Blood* 21:484, 1963.

32. Lubash, G. D., Phillips, R. E., Shields, J. D., and Bonsnes, R. W.: Acute aniline poisoning treated by hemodialysis. *Arch. Intern. Med.* 114:530, 1964.

33. Pugh, J. I., and Enderby, G. E. H.: Haemoglobinuria after intravenous myanesin. *Lancet* 253:387, 1947.

34. Kaplinsky, N., and Frankl, O.: Salicylazosulphapyridine-induced Heinz body anemia. *Acta Haematol.* 59:310, 1978.

35. Adams, J. G., Heller, P., Abramson, R. K., and Vaithianathan, T.: Sulfonamide-induced hemolytic anemia and hemoglobin Hasharon. *Arch. Intern. Med.* 137:1449, 1971.

36. Greenberg, M. S.: Heinz body hemolytic anemia. *Arch. Intern. Med.* 136:153, 1976.

37. Getaz, E. P., Beckley, S., Fitzpatrick, J., and Dozier, A.: Cisplatin-induced hemolysis. *N. Engl. J. Med.* 302:334, 1980.

38. Landsteiner, E. K., and Finch, C. A.: Hemoglobinemia accompanying transurethral resection of the prostate. *New Eng. J. Med.* 237:310, 1947.

39. Mengel, C. E., Kann, H. E., Jr., Heyman, A., and Metz, E.: Effects of in vivo hyperoxia on erythrocytes. II. Hemolysis in a human after exposure to oxygen under high pressure. *Blood* 25:822, 1965.

40. Mengel, C. E., Kann, H. E., Jr., Smith, W. W., and Horton, B. D.: Effects of in vivo hyperoxia on erythrocytes. I. Hemolysis in mice exposed to hyperbaric oxygenation. *Proc. Soc. Exp. Biol. Med.*, 116:259, 1964.

41. Dacie, J. V.: *The Haemolytic Anaemias,* 2d ed. Grune & Stratton, New York, 1967, p. 1091.

42. Monzon, C., and Miles, J.: Hemolytic anemia following a wasp sting. *J. Pediatr.* 96:1039, 1980.

43. Nance, W. E.: Hemolytic anemia of necrotic arachnidism. *Am. J. Med.* 31:801, 1961.

44. Madrigal, G. C., Ercolani, R. L., and Wenzl, J. E.: Toxicity from a bite of the brown spider (*Loxosceles reclusus*), skin necrosis, hemolytic anemia, and hemoglobinuria in a nine-year-old child. *Clin. Pediatr.* 11:641, 1972.

45. Chadha, J. S., and Leviav, A.: Hemolysis, renal failure, and local necrosis following scorpion sting. *JAMA* 241:1038, 1979.

46. Reid, H. A.: Cobra-bites. *Br. Med. J.* 2:540, 1964.

47. Ham, T. H., Shen, S. C., Fleming, E. M., and Castle, W. B.: Studies on the destruction of red blood cells, IV. *Blood* 3:373, 1948.

48. Wagner, H. N., Jr., Razzak, M. A., Gaertner, R. A., Caine, W. P., Jr., and Feagin, O. T.: Removal of erythrocytes from the circulation. *Arch. Intern. Med.* 110:90, 1962.

49. Shen, S. C., Ham, T. H., and Fleming, E. M.: Studies on the destruction of red blood cells. III. Mechanism and complications of hemoglobinuria in patients with thermal burns: Spherocytosis and increased osmotic fragility of red blood cells. *N. Engl. J. Med.* 229:701, 1943.

50. Topley, E., Bull, J. P., Maycock, W. D., Mourant, A. E., and Parkin, D.:The relation of the isoagglutinins in pooled plasma to the haemolytic anaemia of burns. *J. Clin. Pathol.* 16:79, 1963.

51. Stohlman, F., Jr., Brecher, G., Schneiderman, M., and Cronkite, E. P.: The hemolytic effect of ionizing radiations and its relationship to the hemorrhagic phase of radiation injury. *Blood* 12:1061, 1957.

52. Davis, W., Dole, N., Izzo, M. J., and Young, L. E.: Hemolytic effect of radiation: Observation on renal bile fistula dogs subjected to total body radiation and on human blood irradiated in vitro. *J. Lab. Clin. Med.* 35:528, 1950.

CHAPTER 66

Hemolytic anemia due to infections with microorganisms

ERNEST BEUTLER

Shortening of erythrocyte life-span occurs commonly in the course of inflammatory and infectious diseases. This may occur particularly in patients with glucose-6-phosphate dehydrogenase (G-6-PD) deficiency (Chap. 58). Many infections are associated with splenomegaly (Chaps. 71 and 108), which may result in accelerated removal of erythrocytes from the circulation. In some infections, however, rapid destruction of erythrocytes represents a prominent part of the overall clinical picture (Table 66-1). This chapter deals only with the latter states.

Malaria

Known since antiquity, malaria is the world's most common cause of hemolytic anemia. Transmitted by the bite of an infected female *Anopheles* mosquito, the sporozoites invade the liver and possibly other internal organs in the asymptomatic tissue stage of malaria. Merozoites emerging at first from the tissues and later from previously parasitized red cells enter the erythrocyte and grow intracellularly, nourished by the cell's contents (Chap. A5). Osmotic fragility is increased in nonparasitized cells as well as cells containing plasmodia [16]. The erythrocyte cation permeability is altered in monkeys with malaria [17]. Positive Coombs' tests have been reported to occur, but their role in the etiology of the anemia is not clear [18]. *Plasmodium falciparum*–infected red cells have a highly irregular surface defect. This may be produced by the intracellular growth of the plasmodium, or it could represent the site of parasite entry. Nonparasitized cells often have similar surface defects [19], suggesting a phenomenon known to occur in simian malaria [20], the "pitting" of parasites from an infected cell.

Destruction of parasitized red cell appears to be largely splenic, and splenomegaly is typically present in chronic malarial infection. The fever associated with malaria is characteristically cyclic, varying in frequency according to the malaria type. Although classic periodicity is often absent, febrile paroxysms of *P. vivax* malaria tend to occur every 48 h, those of *P. malariae* infection occur each 72 h, and those of *P. falciparum* malaria, daily. Falciparum malaria is occasionally associated with particularly severe hemolysis and may result in the passage of dark, almost black, urine. This disorder, also called *blackwater fever,* is no longer common. At one time, it was seen frequently among Europeans in Africa and in India, usually after quinine was given in treatment of malaria. The relative roles of the malarial infection and of the drug have never been clarified [21].

Diagnosis of malaria depends upon demonstration of the parasites on the blood film (Chap. A5). Eradication of blood forms is achieved with quinine, chloroquine, or various sulfones or sulfonamides given together with pyrimethamine. Tissue stages of vivax malaria are effectively treated with primaquine. This drug, as well as certain sulfones used in the treatment of malaria, produces severe hemolysis in patients with G-6-PD deficiency (Chap. 58).

When acute, unusually severe hemolysis occurs in the course of falciparum malaria (blackwater fever), the physician should be certain that a hemolytic drug is not being administered to a G-6-PD-deficient individual. Transfusions may be needed in blackwater fever, and if renal failure occurs, extracorporeal dialysis may be required.

With early institution of therapy the prognosis in malaria is excellent. However, when treatment is delayed or the strain is resistant to the administered agent, falciparum malaria may follow a rapid fatal course.

Bartonellosis

In 1885, Daniel A. Carrión, a medical student, inoculated himself with blood obtained from a verrucous node of the skin of a patient with verruca peruviana. He developed a fatal hemolytic anemia with the characteristics of Oroya fever, a disease which had first been observed some years earlier among workers in a railroad construction project near the city of Oroya in the Peruvian Andes. This fatal self-experiment established the identity of the verrucous form and the hemolytic phase of human bartonellosis, an infection which now bears the name *Carrión's disease* [5]. Human bartonellosis is transmitted by the sand fly. The red blood cells become infected with *Bartonella bacilliformis,* and it is believed that the organism does not grow within the red cell but rather adheres to its exterior surface: when infected red cells are washed with citrated plasma, free organisms are found but the red cells are not hemolyzed. In hanging-drop cultures masses or organisms are clearly seen outside the erythrocytes, while the cells themselves are intact [22]. The osmotic fragility of the red cells is normal [5]. They are rapidly removed from the circulation, apparently both by liver and spleen. Normal red cells transfused into patients with bartonellosis meet a similar fate [4].

As demonstrated by Carrión's experiment, bartonellosis has two clinical stages. The acute hemolytic anemia, Oroya fever, represents the early, invasive stage of a chronic granulomatous disorder designated

TABLE 66-1   Organisms causing hemolytic anemia

Aspergillus [1]
Atypical pneumonia virus [2]
Babesia microti and *Babesia divergens* [3]
Bartonella bacilliformis [4,5]
Clostridium welchii [6]
Coxsackie virus [2]
Cytomegalovirus [7,8]
Diplococcus pneumoniae [9]
Epstein-Barr virus [10]
Escherichia coli [9]
Hemophilus influenzae [9]
Herpes simplex virus [2]
Influenza A virus [2]
Leishmania donovani [11]
Mycobacterium tuberculosis [9]
Mycoplasma pneumoniae [12]
Neisseria intracellularis (meningococci) [9]
Plasmodium falciparum [9]
Plasmodium malariae [9]
Plasmodium vivax [9]
Rubeola virus [2]
Salmonella [9]
Shigella [13,14]
Streptococcus [9]
Toxoplasma [9]
Varicella virus [2]
Vibrio cholerae [9]
Yersinia enterocolitica [15]

verruca peruviana. Most patients manifest no clinical symptoms during this phase, but when anemia does occur, its onset is dramatic. It has been stated that the anemia "develops so rapidly that it can be compared only with the anemia occurring in acute hemorrhage" [5]. In one series of 13 uncomplicated cases of Carrión's disease the recorded nadir of the red cell count averaged 994,000. In addition to symptoms of anemia, patients manifest thirst, anorexia, sweating, and generalized lymphadenopathy. Spleen and liver enlargement is unusual. Large numbers of nucleated red cells appear in the blood smear, and reticulocytosis is often striking. The white cell count is variable. Diagnosis is established by demonstrating the presence of the organism B. bacilliformis on the erythrocytes. Giemsa-stained smears reveal red-violet rods varying in length from 1 to 3 μm and in width from 0.25 to 0.2 μm.

The mortality rate among untreated patients is very high, but those who do survive undergo a sudden transitional period in which the bartonellae change from an elongated to a coccoid form, the number of parasitized cells decreases, and the red cell count increases. Lymphocytosis and a right shift in the granulocyte series is observed with disappearance of the fever and abatement of other symptoms. Oroya fever responds well to treatment with penicillin, streptomycin, chloramphenicol, and the tetracyclines. The second stage of *Bartonella* infection, verruca peruviana, is a nonhematologic disorder characterized by an eruption over the face and extremities developing into bleeding warty tumors.

Clostridium welchii

Clostridium welchii sepsis is most likely to occur in patients who have undergone septic abortion. The α toxin of *Clostridium welchii* is a lecithinase which may react with lipoprotein complexes at cell surfaces, liberating potently hemolytic substances, lysolecithins (Chap. 36). Severe, often fatal hemolysis occurs in patients with *C. welchii* septicemia. Striking hemoglobinemia and hemoglobinuria occur. The serum may become a brilliant red, and the urine is a dark-brown mahogany color. Microspherocytosis is prominent, and leukocytosis with a left shift as well as thrombocytopenia is often present. Acute renal and hepatic failure usually develops, and the prognosis is grave; more than half of the patients die, even with intensive treatment [23].

Babesiosis

Babesia are intraerythrocytic protozoa transmitted by ticks which may infect many species of wild and domestic animals. Rarely humans have become infected with the *Babesia microti* or *Babesia divergens*, species which normally parasitize rodents and cattle, respectively [3]. While the disease is usually tick-borne in man, it is also thought to have been transmitted by transfusion [24]. The disease generally has a gradual onset with malaise, anorexia, fatigue, followed by fever, often sweats and muscle and joint pains. Parasites can be seen in the red cells in Giemsa-stained thin blood films. Serologic tests for antibodies to *Babesia* have been described. The disease is believed to be more severe in individuals who have been splenectomized. It has responded to chemotherapy with clindamycin and quinine [31]. In one critically ill patient whole-blood exchange was used with a marked improvement [24].

Other infections

A variety of other infections have occasionally been associated with hemolytic anemia. The mechanisms involved vary. Some organisms, among them such common pathogens as *Hemophilus influenzae*, *Escherichia coli*, and *Salmonella* species can produce red cell agglutination in vitro, but it is not known whether this phenomenon is important in initiating in vivo hemolysis [25]. Bacteria may also produce destruction of red cells indirectly when bacterial polysaccharides are adsorbed onto erythrocytes. Action of an antibody directed against the antigen-coated cells results in their agglutination. Although demonstrated in vitro, it is not certain whether this mechanism is active in vivo [26]. The unmasking of T-type antigens by bacteria renders the cell polyagglutinable. This may be a rare cause of hemolysis occurring in the course of bacterial infections [27].

Many different types of microorganisms may play a role in precipitating autoimmune hemolytic disease (see Chap. 67). In one study of 234 patients [2], 55 were found to have an antecedent bacterial infection, 18 of these exhibiting an "unequivocal etiologic relationship" of infection to anemia. However, the principal evidence for such a relationship was a temporal one. A number of viral agents, including measles, cytomegalovirus (CMV), varicella, herpes simplex, influenza A, Epstein-Barr, and coxsackie virus have also been associated with autoimmune hemolytic disease [2]. Various mechanisms have been postulated, including absorption of immune complexes and complement, cross-reacting antigen, and a true autoimmune state with possible loss of tolerance secondary to the infectious organism [2]. Histopathologic and sometimes virologic evidence of infection with cytomegalovirus has been reported in a high percentage of children with lymphadenopathy and hemolytic anemia [7]. A positive antiglobulin reaction was demonstrated in some of these patients. Others, however, showed no evidence of autoantibodies, an observation supporting the view that their appearance represents a secondary phenomenon and that many cases of "idiopathic autoimmune hemolytic anemia" are in fact due to cytomegalovirus infection [7].

The high cold agglutinin titer which may develop in the course of atypical viral pneumonia (*Mycoplasma pneumoniae* pneumonia) may occasionally result in hemolytic anemia [2,12], although most patients with high cold agglutinin titers do not become anemic. The red cells of a number of patients with a kala azar were found to be agglutinated with anticomplement and anti-non-γ-globulin serum [11]. Both splenic and hepatic sequestration of red cells appears to occur in this disease [10].

Microangiopathic hemolytic anemia is discussed in detail in Chap. 64. This disorder may be triggered by a variety of infections, some of which are caused by well-characterized organisms such as species of *Shigella* [13,14] or *Aspergillus* [1]. The suggestion that this type of anemia may be due to bartonella-like organism [28] has not been confirmed [29,30].

References

1. Robboy, S. J., Salisbury, K., Ragsdale, B., Bobroff, L. M., Jacobson, B. M., and Colman, R. W.: Mechanism of *Aspergillus*-induced microangiopathic hemolytic anemia. *Arch. Intern. Med.* 128:790, 1971.
2. Pirofsky, B: *Infectious Disease and Autoimmune Hemolytic Anemia: Autoimmunization and the Autoimmune Hemolytic Anemias.* Waverly, Baltimore, 1969, chap. 7, p. 147.
3. Ruebush II, T. K., et al.: Human babesiosis on Nantucket Island. *Ann. Intern. Med.* 86:6, 1977.
4. Reynafarje, C., and Ramos, J.: The hemolytic anemia of human bartonellosis. *Blood* 17:562, 1961.
5. Ricketts, W. E.: *Bartonella bacilliformis* anemia (Oroya fever): A study of thirty cases. *Blood* 3:1025, 1948.
6. Suzuki, A., Yamada, A., and Maruyama, H.: A case of acute hemolytic anemia due to *Clostridium perfrigens* A septicemia. *Jap. J. Clin. Hematol.* 13:850, 1972.
7. Zuelzer, W. W., Stulberg, C. S., Page, R. H., Teruya, J., and Brough,

A. J.: The Emily Cooley lecture: Etiology and pathogenesis of acquired hemolytic anemia. *Transfusion 6*:438, 1966.

8. Franklin, A. J.: Cytomegalovirus infection presenting as acute haemolytic anaemia in an infant. *Arch. Dis. Child. 47*:474, 1972.

9. Dacie, J. V. (ed.): *Secondary or Symptomatic Hemolytic Anemias: The Haemolytic Anaemias.* Grune & Stratton, New York, 1967, pt. III, chap. 15, p. 908.

10. Tonkin, A. M., Mond, H. G., Alford, F. P., and Hurley, T. H.: Severe acute haemolytic anaemia complicating infectious mononucleosis. *Med. J. Aust. 2*:1048, 1973.

11. Woodruff, A. W., Topley, E., Knight, R., and Downie, C. G. B.: The anaemia of kala azar. *Br. J. Haematol. 22*:319, 1972.

12. Fiala, M., Myhre, B. A., Chinh, L. T., Territo, M., Edgington, T. S., and Kattlove, H.: Pathogenesis of anemia associated with *Mycoplasma pneumoniae. Acta Haematol. (Basel) 51*:297, 1974.

13. Ullis, K. C., and Rosenblatt, R. M.: Shiga bacillus dysentery complicated by bacteremia and disseminated intravascular coagulation. *J. Pediatr. 83*:90, 1973.

14. Chesney, R., and Kaplan, B. S.: Hemolytic-uremic syndrome with shigellosis. *J. Pediatr. 84*:312, 1974 (letter).

15. Van Knorring, J., and Pettersson, T.: Haemolytic anaemia complicating *Yersinia enterocolitica* infection: Report of a case. *Scand. J. Haematol. 9*:149, 1972.

16. George, J. N., Wicker, D. J., Fogel, B. J., Shields, C. E., and Conrad, M. E.: Erythrocytic abnormalities in experimental malaria. *Proc. Soc. Exp. Biol. Med. 124*:1086, 1967.

17. Overman, R. R.: Reversible cellular permeability alterations in disease: In vivo studies on sodium, potassium and chloride concentrations in erythrocytes of the malarious monkey. *Am. J. Physiol. 152*:113, 1948.

18. LeFrancais, G., Bras, J. L., Simonneau, M., Bouvet, E., Vroklans, M., and Vachon, F.: Anti-erythrocyte autoimmunisation during chronic falciparum malaria. *Lancet 2*:661, 1981.

19. Balcerzak, S. P., Arnold, J. D., and Martin, D. C.: Anatomy of red cell damage by *Plasmodium falciparum* in man. *Blood 40*:98, 1972.

20. Conrad, M. E.: Pathophysiology of malaria: Hematologic observations in human and animal studies. *Ann. Intern. Med. 70*:134, 1969.

21. Zuckerman, A.: Autoimmunization and other types of indirect damage to host cells as factors in certain protozoan diseases. *Exp. Parasitol. 15*:138, 1964.

22. Aldana, L.: Bacteriologia de la enfermedad de Carrión. *Cron. Med. 46*:235, 1929.

23. Mahn, H. E., and Dantuono, L. M.: Postabortal septicotoxemia due to *Clostridium welchii. Am. J. Obstet. Gynecol.* 604, 1955.

24. Jacoby, G. A., et al.: Treatment of transfusion-transmitted babeiosis by exchange transfusion. *N. Engl. J. Med. 303*:1098, 1980.

25. Neter, E.: Bacterial hemagglutination and hemolysis. *Bacteriol. Rev. 20*:166, 1956.

26. Ceppellini, R., and De Gregorio, M.: Crisi emolitica in animali batterioimmuni transfusi con sangue omologo sensibilizzato in vitro mediante l'antigene batterico specifico. *Bull. 1st. Sieroter. Milan 32*:445, 1953.

27. Dausset, J., Moullec, J., and Bernard, J.: Acquired hemolytic anemia with polyagglutin ability of red blood cells due to a new factor. *Blood 14*:1079, 1959.

28. Mettler, N. E.: Isolation of a microtatobiote from patients with hemolytic-uremic syndrome and thrombotic thrombocytopenic purpura and from mites in the United States. *N. Engl. J. Med. 281*:1023, 1969.

29. Lieberman, E.: Hemolytic-uremic syndrome. *J. Pediatr. 80*:1, 1972.

30. Van Wieringen, P. M. V., Monnens, L. A. H., and Schretlen, E. D. A.: Haemolytic-uraemic syndrome: Epidemiological and clinical study. *Arch. Dis. Child. 49*:432, 1974.

31. Wittner, M., et al.: Successful chemotherapy of transfusion babesiosis. *Ann. Int. Med. 96*:601, 1982.

Erythrocyte disorders—anemias due to increased erythrocyte destruction mediated by antibodies

CHAPTER 67

Acquired hemolytic anemia due to warm-reacting autoantibodies

CHARLES H. PACKMAN
JOHN P. LEDDY

Among the most important acquired hemolytic disorders are those mediated directly or indirectly by the patient's own immunologic mechanisms. Chapters 67 to 69 are devoted to the major classes of acquired immune hemolytic disorders associated with erythrocyte autoantibodies (autoimmune hemolytic anemia, AHA) or with antibodies to drugs. The present chapter focuses on the commonest form of AHA—that mediated by warm-reacting autoantibodies. However, many of the observations and principles concerning historical, pathophysiologic and clinical aspects of warm antibody AHA developed below apply also to AHA generally. Those features which are distinctive for the cryopathic and drug-associated hemolytic syndromes will be presented in the succeeding chapters.

Definitions and history

The two essential features of immune hemolytic disease are (1) shortened red cell survival in vivo and (2) evidence of an immune response directed toward autologous red cells, most frequently demonstrated by a positive direct antiglobulin reaction (Coombs' test). Reticulocytosis, evidence of increased marrow production of red cells, is present in nearly all patients, but it is not essential to the diagnosis. Some patients may be unable to mount an adequate marrow response because of unrelated marrow-suppressive factors such as infection, renal failure, iron or folate deficiency. Anemia is present in most patients, but an occasional patient is able to maintain a normal hemoglobin by increasing marrow erythrocyte production to a high level (compensated AHA). Such patients should have elevated reticulocyte counts.

During the first third of this century, clinicians experienced considerable difficulty in differentiating acquired from congenital hemolytic disorders. The distinction between AHA and hereditary spherocytosis caused particular confusion since both are characterized by the presence of spherocytes. Two major advances in immunohematology helped to sharpen the distinction between congenital and acquired hemolytic anemias: (1) the concept of intracorpuscular and extracorpuscular defects, and (2) the development of the direct antiglobulin test. The distinction between intracorpuscular and extracorpuscular defects depends upon measurement of in vivo survival of labeled red cells. Red cells from patients with congenital hemolytic anemias were found to be intrinsically defective, i.e., incapable of surviving for normal periods either in the patient or in a normal recipient. Such cells are said to possess an intracorpuscular defect. In contrast, in patients with acquired hemolytic anemia, destruction of red cells appeared to be mediated by an extracorpuscular mechanism because survival of such red cells was improved in normal recipients.

The second important development, the antiglobulin test, is one of the most useful tools in immunohematology. It had been recognized earlier that the sera of some patients with acquired hemolytic anemia could agglutinate saline suspensions of normal or autologous human red cells. These serum factors, later shown to be specific antibodies (largely of the IgM class), were termed *direct* or *saline agglutinins*. In a smaller proportion of cases, the patients' sera could mediate lysis of the test red cells in the presence of fresh serum as a complement source. The heat-stable factors necessary for such in vitro complement-mediated lysis were called *hemolysins*. However, in the majority of cases of acquired hemolytic anemia, neither direct agglutinins nor hemolysins could be demonstrated in the patients' sera. In 1945 Coombs, Mourant, and Race [1] reported that red cells coated with nonagglutinating Rh isoantibodies (now known to be the IgG class) could be agglutinated by rabbit antiserum to human globulin. That is, the rabbit antiglobulin serum cross-linked antibody-coated red cells to produce visible agglutination. Subsequently, it was found that the direct antiglobulin test (Coombs' test) was positive in many patients with acquired hemolytic anemia, including cases lacking saline agglutinins or hemolysins [2,3]. In congenital hemolytic disorders, on the other hand, a positive antiglobulin test is exceedingly rare. By analogy to the observations of Coombs and coworkers on Rh isoantibodies [1], the positive antiglobulin reactions in acquired hemolytic anemia [2,3] gave important impetus to the study of immune mechanisms in the path-

TABLE 67-1   Classification of autoimmune hemolytic anemia

I. On basis of serologic characteristics of involved autoimmune process
   A. Warm autoantibody type—autoantibody maximally active at body temperature, 37°C
   B. Cold autoantibody type—autoantibody active at temperatures below 37°C
II. On basis of presence or absence of underlying or significantly associated disorder
   A. Primary or idiopathic AHA
   B. Secondary AHA
      1. Associated with lymphoproliferative disorders
      2. Associated with rheumatic disorders, particularly systemic lupus erythematosus
      3. Associated with certain infections
      4. Associated with certain nonlymphoid neoplasms, e.g., ovarian tumors
      5. Associated with certain chronic inflammatory diseases, e.g., ulcerative colitis
      6. Associated with ingestion of certain drugs, e.g., α-methyldopa

ogenesis of this disorder. Subsequent studies have established that positive antiglobulin reactions in acquired hemolytic anemia are attributable to coating of the red cells with immunoglobulins and/or complement proteins.

AHA may be classified in two complementary ways (Table 67-1). Whereas the majority of cases (80 to 90 percent) are mediated by warm-active autoantibodies [4–10], a smaller proportion are attributable to autoantibodies exhibiting greater affinity for the red cell at temperatures below 37°C (cold-active autoantibodies) (Chap. 68). This distinction is useful because of differences in the pathophysiology of red cell injury mediated by these two types of antibody.

It is also useful to classify cases based on presence or absence of underlying diseases (Table 67-1). When no recognizable underlying disease is present, the AHA is termed *primary* or *idiopathic.* When AHA appears to be one manifestation of an underlying disorder of the immune system, the term *secondary* AHA is applied. Lymphocytic malignancies, particularly chronic lymphocytic leukemia and lymphomas, account for about half of secondary cases of AHA of both warm and cold antibody types. Systemic lupus erythematosus and other rheumatic diseases account for a lesser but considerable proportion of the warm antibody cases. Infectious mononucleosis [11,12] and mycoplasma pneumonia [13] have occasionally been associated with cryopathic AHA. Other associated diseases, less commonly reported, are listed in Table 67-1. The etiologic and pathogenetic significance of these associations is known, but most of these associated diseases are now recognized to involve components of the immune system, either by neoplasia or by aberrant immunopathologic responses.

Estimations of the incidence of idiopathic AHA vary from 20 to 80 percent of all types of AHA [5–10]. In an individual clinical practice, the frequency of secondary AHA will be influenced by the makeup of the patient group and by the diligence with which the physician pursues clues to an associated disease. Careful follow-up is essential since hemolytic anemia may be the presenting finding in a patient who subsequently develops overt evidence of underlying lymphoproliferative or rheumatic disease.

Etiology and pathogenesis

The etiology of AHA, as with other autoimmune diseases, is unknown [14,15]. In many patients with idiopathic AHA, erythrocyte autoantibodies are the only recognizable evidence of immunologic aberrations. In such cases AHA resembles other "selective" autoimmune disorders in which the autoantibodies appear to be reactive, in the main, with a single target tissue, e.g., idiopathic thrombocytopenic purpura, nephritis associated with antibody to glomerular basement membrane, and several antireceptor autoimmune disorders including myasthenia gravis. In other patients, AHA is associated with more gross disturbances of the immune system: systemic lupus erythematosus (SLE) or other rheumatic diseases with autoantibodies reactive with a variable array of target tissues, several kinds of lymphoproliferative diseases and, paradoxically, primary hypogammaglobulinemia. It is easier to visualize a fairly general derangement in immunoregulation in the latter group than in the more selective autoimmune disorders, even though a selective AHA may prove ultimately to be a harbinger of SLE, lymphoma, or chronic lymphocytic leukemia.

A still unexplained observation is that the drug α-methyldopa can induce in apparently immunologically normal persons the production of warm-type IgG red cell autoantibodies which cannot be distinguished from those arising in many cases of "spontaneous" AHA (see Chap. 69). Since these antibodies eventually subside when the drug is discontinued, this abnormal response does not imply a permanent dysfunction of the immune system. Rather, a prolonged stimulus is suggested, but one which we do not yet understand.

Autoantibodies from patients with warm antibody AHA show reactivity with native structures present on the patients' own and other human red cells. These autoantibodies may exhibit specificity for a defined blood group antigen (see below), and, in such cases, the corresponding antigen is invariably present on the patients' own red cells. Furthermore, autoantibodies in patients' sera or red cell eluates kept in frozen storage during active disease react strongly with patient (autologous) red cells after complete remission of the hemolytic process has occurred [16,17]. This indicates the stability of the relevant autoantigen(s).

Erythrocyte autoantibodies are clearly pathogenetic. In patients whose autoantibodies are directed against an identifiable red cell antigen, prolonged survival of red cells lacking that antigen has been observed, in contrast to rapid clearance of cells possessing the antigen [5,18,19]. Furthermore, there is, in general, an inverse relationship between quantity of red cell–bound IgG autoantibody and red cell survival, particularly when serial studies are made on a given patient [20–25].

The decreased survival of red cells in warm antibody AHA is largely due to their progressive trapping by macrophages in the Billroth cords of the spleen and to a lesser extent by Kupffer cells in the liver [18,20,21,23–29]. This process leads to sphering, fragmentation, and ingestion of the trapped cells [28,30,31]. In warm antibody AHA, red cells are typically coated with IgG autoantibodies, with or without complement proteins. The macrophage plasma membrane has receptors for the Fc region of IgG [30–33], primarily IgG1 and IgG3 [33–35], and for an opsonic fragment of C3 (C3b) [32,36,37]. When present together on the red cell surface, IgG and C3b appear to act cooperatively as opsonins to enhance trapping and phagocytosis [23,24,32,37–41]. Although red cell sequestration in warm antibody AHA occurs primarily in the spleen [18,25–27], very large quantities of red cell–bound IgG [20,22,29] or the presence of C3b on the red cell [20,23,24] may favor trapping in the liver as well.

Interaction of a trapped red cell with splenic macrophages may result in phagocytosis of the entire cell. More commonly, a type of partial phagocytosis occurs, resulting in spherocyte formation. As red cells adhere to macrophages via the Fc receptors, portions of red cell membrane are internalized by the macrophage. Since membrane is lost in excess of contents, the noningested portion of the red cell assumes the geometric shape with the lowest surface area/volume ratio, a sphere [30,31,41]. Spherical red cells are more rigid and less deformable than normal red cells and are thus further fragmented and ultimately destroyed in future passages through the microvasculature, particularly in the spleen. Spherocytosis is a consistent and diagnostically important hallmark of AHA [42]. The degree of spherocytosis correlates well with severity of hemolysis [12].

Direct complement-mediated hemolysis with hemoglobinuria is unusual in warm antibody AHA despite the fact that many warm antibodies fix complement, as evidenced by the detection of red cell–bound C4 and C3 in the direct antiglobulin test. The failure of C3-coated red cells to be hemolyzed by the terminal complement cascade has been attributed, at least in part, to the ability of plasma C3b/C4b inactivator and β 1H-globulin to alter the hemolytic function of cell-bound C3b and C4b [43,44].

Although phagocytic mechanisms have been emphasized in the destruction of red cells in warm antibody AHA, cytotoxic properties of effector cells, principally macrophages and lymphocytes, may be important as well. Monocytes can lyse IgG-coated red cells in vitro, independently of phagocytosis [45,46]. Cell-bound complement is neither necessary nor sufficient for such cytotoxicity, but bound C3b/C3d can potentiate the effects of IgG [46]. In one study [45], cytoxicity but not phagocytosis was inhibited by hydrocortisone. Lymphocytes are also able to lyse IgG antibody-coated red cells in vitro [46–49]. The pathogenetic importance in vivo of antibody-dependent monocyte- and lymphocyte-mediated cytotoxicity in warm antibody AHA is not known.

In experimental settings, antibody-*independent* cytotoxicity has been demonstrated with cells thought to be cytotoxic T lymphocytes. There is thus far no evidence for destruction of autologous red cells by such a mechanism, but this process could possibly explain certain cases of "Coombs-negative" acquired hemolytic anemia.

Incidence

AHA is uncommon but not rare. The annual incidence of AHA is estimated at about 1 case per 80,000 population [50,51]. AHA has been diagnosed in people of all ages—from infants to the elderly [50,52]. The majority of patients are over age 40, with peak incidence around the seventh decade. This age distribution probably reflects, in part, the increased frequency of lymphoproliferative malignancies in the elderly. No racial predisposition has been uncovered. Familial occurrence of AHA is rare but has been documented [50,53–56]. Such cases tend to be associated with other autoimmune or lymphoproliferative disorders.

Clinical features

Warm antibody AHA exhibits a highly variable spectrum in onset, clinical characteristics, and course. Presenting complaints are usually referable to the anemia itself, although occasionally jaundice is the immediate cause for seeking medical advice. Symptoms are usually slow and insidious in onset over several months, but an occasional patient may note sudden onset of symptoms of severe anemia and jaundice over a period of a few days. In secondary AHA, the hemolytic anemia and associated features may be obscured by the more dramatic symptoms and signs of the underlying disease.

In idiopathic AHA with only mild anemia, the physical examination may be normal. Hepatosplenomegaly of modest degree may be present in patients with moderately severe hemolytic anemia. In very severe cases, particularly with acute onset of hemolysis, patients may exhibit fever, pallor, jaundice, hepatosplenomegaly hyperpnea, tachycardia, and heart failure. Other physical findings may be contributed by associated disorders in secondary AHA. Massive splenomegaly or lymphadenopathy is suggestive of an underlying lymphoproliferative disorder.

A variety of common events are known to precipitate episodes of increased red cell destruction in patients with AHA, but by unknown mechanisms. These include infection, pregnancy, surgery, and physical trauma. AHA has occurred following treatment of lymphoma with either alkylating agents or x-ray therapy, but no causal relationship has been uncovered [57].

Laboratory features

GENERAL

The anemia varies from mild to severe, with hematocrits occasionally as low as 10 percent or less. As mentioned earlier, some patients have compensated hemolytic anemia, in which case the diagnosis is suspected because of splenomegaly, supportive laboratory data (described below), or the presence of an associated disease.

Important diagnostic features are found on examination of the blood film. Polychromasia indicates the presence of reticulocytes, reflecting an increased rate of egress of red cells from marrow.

Spherocytes are seen in patients with moderate to severe hemolytic anemia and such cells are fragile in the osmotic fragility test. Autohemolysis is usually also increased, but in contrast to hereditary spherocytosis it is not corrected by the addition of glucose. The presence of many spherocytes is strongly suggestive of immune hemolytic anemia provided hereditary spherocytosis can be ruled out. Red cell fragments, nucleated red cells, and occasionally erythrophagocytosis by monocytes may be seen. The reticulocyte count is usually elevated, and the reticulocyte index may be greater than 3, and sometimes as high as 6 or 7 (see Chap. 72). Reticulocytopenia has occasionally been noted in patients with normal or hyperplastic erythroid marrow [58–60]. The mechanism is unknown, although it has been speculated that autoantibodies directed against antigens on reticulocytes may lead to their selective destruction [58]. Reticulocytopenia may also be seen in patients with marrow function compromised by an underlying disease, toxic chemicals, or nutritional deficiency. The need for prompt transfusion of reticulocytopenic patients in this situation has been emphasized [59]. Marrow examination usually reveals erythroid hyperplasia, and may also provide evidence for an underlying lymphoproliferative disorder. Most patients exhibit mild leukocytosis and neutrophilia, but leukopenia and neutropenia are occasionally seen [12,61]. Platelet counts are typically normal. Rarely, severe immune thrombocytopenia is associated with warm antibody AHA; this constellation is termed *Evans' syndrome* [62].

Hyperbilirubinemia (chiefly unconjugated) is highly suggestive of hemolytic anemia, although its absence does not exclude the diagnosis. Total bilirubin is only modestly increased, up to 5 mg/dl, and with rare exceptions [63,64] the conjugated (direct) fraction constitutes less than 15 percent of the total [64,65]. Urinary urobilinogen is regularly increased, but bile is not detected in the urine unless serum conjugated bilirubin is increased. The historical term *acholuric jaundice* was applied to the situation in hemolytic anemia when clinical jaundice was encountered without bilirubinuria. Serum haptoglobin levels are usually low. Hemoglobinuria is encountered in rare patients with hyperacute hemolysis who develop significant hemoglobinemia. Fecal urobilinogen levels and increased respiratory excretion of carbon monoxide are both sensitive indicators of increased red cell destruction, but are mainly research tools.

The study of in vivo survival and site of destruction of ^{51}Cr-labeled (radioactive chromium–labeled) red cells have been very useful in clinical investigation of AHA. Both patient red cells and normal donor red cells show abnormally rapid clearance from the circulation, and the cells are sequestered primarily in spleen and liver. However, such studies are rarely necessary to diagnose hemolytic anemia, and the presence or absence of splenic sequestration should have no bearing on a decision for or against splenectomy [15,65].

SEROLOGIC FEATURES

The diagnosis of AHA is dependent on the demonstration of immunoglobulin and/or complement bound to the patient's red cells. As a screening procedure, it is customary to use a broad-spectrum antiglobulin (Coombs') reagent, i.e., one which contains antibodies directed against human immunoglobulin as well as complement components (principally C3). If agglutination is noted with a broad-spectrum reagent, antisera reacting selectively with immunoglobulins (the gamma Coombs') or with complement components (the so-called non-gamma Coombs') may be used to define the specific pattern of red cell sensitization. Monospecific antisera to IgG, IgM, IgA, C3, and C4 have also been employed, mainly for investigation. By the use of such specific antisera, three major patterns of direct antiglobulin reaction have been noted in warm antibody AHA: (1) coating of red cells with IgG alone, (2) coating of red cells with IgG plus complement components, and (3) coating with complement components in the absence of detectable immunoglobulin. In patterns 2 and 3, the complement components usually detected are C3 and C4 because of the relatively large numbers of these molecules bound to red cells during complement activation. These patterns of red cell autosensitization occur with variable frequencies among reported series [11,15,66,67]. All three patterns have been associated with accelerated red cell destruction. Positive antiglobulin reactions with anti-IgA or anti-IgM are encountered less commonly, usually in association with bound IgG and/or complement [68–71]. Positive direct antiglobulin tests may rarely be found in otherwise healthy individuals serving as blood donors (1 or 2 per 10,000 donors) [72,73].

The autoantibody in patients with warm antibody

AHA exists in a reversible, dynamic equilibrium between red cells and plasma [74,75]. Thus, autoantibody may sometimes be detected in the plasma or serum of these patients by means of the *indirect* antiglobulin test. In the indirect antiglobulin test, the patient's serum (plasma) is incubated with normal donor erythrocytes at the appropriate temperature (in this case, 37°C). The cells are then washed, resuspended in saline, and tested for agglutination with antiglobulin serum. The presence of such unbound autoantibody in plasma depends upon the total amount of antibody being produced and the binding affinity of the antibody for red cell antigens. In general, patients with heavily sensitized red cells are more likely to exhibit plasma autoantibody. Protease-modified red cells are more sensitive than native red cells in detecting plasma antibody, but such data must be interpreted with caution, since isoantibodies, natural antibodies, and other serum components may interact with enzyme-modified red cells. Patients with a positive indirect antiglobulin test due to a warm-reactive autoantibody should also have a positive direct antiglobulin test. The occasional patient who exhibits a serum anti-red cell antibody (indirect antiglobulin reaction) in the presence of a negative direct antiglobulin reaction probably does not have an autoimmune process but rather an alloantibody stimulated by prior transfusion or pregnancy.

Figure 67-1 relates the intensity of the direct an-

FIGURE 67-1   Comparison of direct antiglobulin reactions (with anti-IgG serum) with molecules of red cell–bound IgG determined by a quantitative antibody consumption assay (method in Ref. 76). The two assays were conducted concurrently on the same blood samples. The antiglobulin reactions were performed manually and read macroscopically.

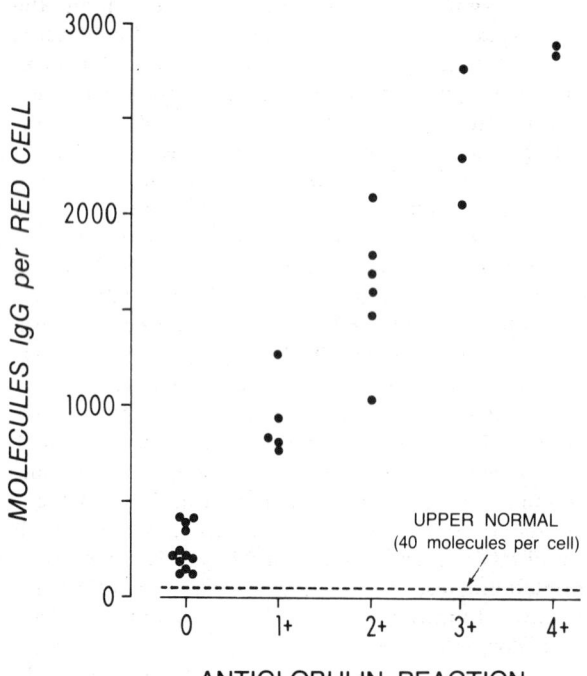

tiglobulin reaction, using specific anti-IgG serum, to the number of IgG molecules per red cell. The latter was determined by a sensitive antibody consumption method [76]. A trace-positive antiglobulin reaction (read macroscopically) detects 300 to 400 molecules of IgG per cell [76,77]. In another laboratory, a trace-positive antiglobulin reaction with anti-C3 was obtained with 60 to 115 molecules C3 per cell [45].

The newer methods for quantifying red cell–bound IgG have allowed better definition of a group of patients who have all the usual hallmarks of warm antibody AHA but negative antiglobulin reactions with antiimmunoglobulin and anticomplement reagents [76–79]. In many such patients, the red cells are coated with quantities of IgG autoantibody which are too low to give a positive antiglobulin reaction (subthreshold IgG). However, the specialized methods (e.g., anti-IgG consumption assays or automated enhanced agglutination techniques) do detect very small quantities of cell-bound IgG [down to 10 to 40 molecules per cell]. In such cases, studies with concentrated red cell eluates confirm that these IgG molecules are warm-reacting anti-red cell autoantibodies [76]. These patients generally exhibit relatively mild hemolysis and often respond favorably to corticosteroid therapy. By these specialized methods, subthreshold IgG may also be detected in a significant number of patients who exhibit the "complement alone" pattern of direct antiglobulin reaction, in the absence of drug sensitivity or cold agglutinins. In such cases, studies with concentrated red cell eluates have suggested that these subthreshold IgG antibodies are capable of fixing larger quantities of C3 to the cell membrane [76].

As mentioned earlier, in most but not all patients there is a rough correlation between the strength of the antiglobulin reaction (IgG molecules per cell) and the rate of red cell destruction. The IgG subclass composition of warm autoantibodies may have an important influence on the ability of these antibodies to shorten red cell survival. IgG1 is the most commonly encountered subclass, either alone or in combination with other IgG subclasses. IgG1 and IgG3 autoantibodies appear to be more effective in decreasing red cell life-span than those of the IgG2 and IgG4 subclasses [68,80]. The explanation for these findings is thought to reside in (1) the preferential affinity of macrophage Fc receptors for IgG1 and IgG3 subclasses, and (2) a greater complement-fixing capacity of antibodies belonging to the IgG1 or IgG3 subclasses [40,41,81,82].

In warm antibody AHA, the autoantibodies eluted from patient red cells, or present in the plasma, usually bind to all the common types of human red cells in the test panels used by blood banks. Though this universal type of reactivity has been termed *nonspecific*, the antibody is probably recognizing one or more antigens common to all human red cells. When tested against the rare human Rh-null red cell, which lacks all known determinants of the Rh complex, the warm autoantibodies of some patients exhibit no reaction or a reduced reaction compared with the common types of human red cells [15,70,83–85]. This has been interpreted as evidence that such autoantibodies possess at least partial specificity for the core structural unit of the Rh complex [86]. Warm antibodies from many other patients exhibit equally strong reactions with Rh-null and normal human red cells of common phenotype [15,83,85]. The latter autoantibodies may comprise a heterogenous group of specificities [70,71]. An occasional patient may possess autoantibodies with clear serologic specificity for a defined blood group antigen which is also present on the patient's own red cells. Usually these autoantibodies of defined specificity are directed toward Rh system antigens such as e or c [12]. More commonly, autoantibodies with defined specificity in the Rh system are accompanied by the above-described antibodies reactive with all human red cells except Rh-null (anti-Rh core). Knowledge of the nature and diversity of the relevant red cell antigens, which is now in a crude state, will undoubtedly be advanced in coming years by the application of immunochemical and monoclonal (hybridoma) antibody techniques.

In some series, those autoantibodies which are fully reactive with Rh-null cells tend to be associated with complement binding to the patient's red cells in vivo, as determined by a positive direct antiglobulin test with anticomplement reagents [15,70,85]. Conversely, autoantibodies which show specificity for Rh antigens or fail to react with Rh-null cells are often found in patients in whom the anti-complement Coombs' reaction is negative [15,85]. These associations, for which there are exceptions [15,70,84,85,87], may be related to the fact that two closely adjacent IgG antibody molecules are required to fix C1 and activate the complement cascade [88,89]. Thus, antigen distribution on the red cell surface, i.e., sparse versus dense or clustered, or the multiplicity of specificities included in a given patient's autoantibody population may be important determinants of complement fixation, beyond the effects of IgG subclass.

Differential diagnosis

Certain hemolytic anemias are likely to be confused with AHA because of the presence of spherocytes, splenomegaly, or other common characteristics. Hereditary spherocytosis, Zieve's syndrome, clostridial sepsis, and the hemolytic anemia which precedes Wilson's disease each have spherocytosis as a dominant morphologic feature. The most important discriminating feature in differential diagnosis is the positive direct antiglobulin reaction, present only in AHA.

Among the congenital hemolytic anemias, hereditary spherocytosis most closely resembles AHA because it may present in adulthood with little antecedent history of anemia or familial incidence. Spherocytosis and splenomegaly are prominent in both diseases. However, in hereditary spherocytosis, in addition to a negative antiglobulin reaction, the autohemolysis test shows a marked abnormality which is corrected by addition of glucose to the blood. Family studies at this point usually identify other affected individuals.

In hemolytic anemia accompanied by a positive antiglobulin reaction, serologic characterization of the autoantibody will help to distinguish warm antibody AHA from cold-reacting autoantibody syndromes (see Chap. 68). Diagnosis of a drug-related immune hemolytic anemia depends upon a history of appropriate drug intake, supported by compatible serologic findings (see Chap. 69). In patients who have recently been transfused, a positive direct antiglobulin reaction may in reality reflect the binding of a newly formed alloantibody to circulating donor red cells. This result could lead to a false impression of an autoimmune process.

Other acquired types of hemolytic anemia are less easily confused with AHA because spherocytes are not prominent on the blood film, and the direct antiglobulin reaction is negative. Patients with paroxysmal nocturnal hemoglobinuria (PNH) may complain of dark urine (hemoglobinuria), which is unusual in warm antibody AHA but can occur in the cold antibody syndromes (Chap. 68). The reticulocyte count is only mildly elevated in PNH in contrast to uncomplicated AHA, which typically exhibits marked reticulocytosis. The acidified serum test and sucrose hemolysis test are usually both positive in paroxysmal nocturnal hemoglobinuria and are negative in AHA. Microangiopathic hemolytic disorders, such as thrombotic thrombocytopenic purpura and hemolytic uremic syndrome, are further distinguished by examination of the blood smear, which reveals marked red blood cell fragmentation and minimal spherocytosis, the converse of what is seen in warm antibody AHA. Microangiopathic hemolytic anemia is frequently associated with thrombocytopenia, whereas in warm antibody AHA such an association is rare (Evans' syndrome).

Therapy

TRANSFUSION

The clinical consequences of any anemia are related to both the severity and the rapidity with which the anemia develops. Most patients with AHA are in little danger of circulatory failure since the anemia, although often severe, develops over a sufficient period of time to allow cardiovascular compensation to occur. Thus, in most patients it is not necessary to institute transfusion therapy. However, in patients with concurrent underlying disorders, such as coronary artery disease with angina, or in patients who suddenly develop severe anemia and exhibit signs and symptoms of circulatory failure, transfusion may prove lifesaving.

Transfusion of red cells in AHA presents two sets of difficulties: the problem of cross-matching and the rapid in vivo destruction of transfused cells. It is nearly always impossible to find truly serocompatible donor blood except in rare cases in which the autoantibody can be shown to have specificity for a defined blood group antigen (see "Serologic Features," above). If such specificity cannot be defined by testing of serum or eluted autoantibodies against standard cell panels, donor red cells should be chosen on the basis of least incompatibility with the patient's serum in cross-match testing. It is also important to test the patient's serum carefully for an alloantibody which could cause a severe hemolytic transfusion reaction against donor red cells [90,91]. The risk of an alloantibody is greatest in patients with a history of pregnancy or prior transfusion. Once selected, the packed red cells should be transfused very slowly as the patient is monitored for signs of a hemolytic transfusion reaction (see Chap. 164). The transfused cells may be destroyed as rapidly as the patient's own cells, or perhaps more so. However, the increased oxygen-carrying capacity provided by the transfused cells may be sufficient to maintain the patient for the few days required for other modes of therapy to become effective.

GLUCOCORTICOIDS

The introduction of glucocorticoid therapy for idiopathic warm antibody AHA has greatly improved the management and reduced the mortality of this disease [11,15,63]. First used for this disorder about 30 years ago [92], these drugs can cause dramatic cessation or marked slowing of hemolysis in about two-thirds of patients. About 20 percent of treated patients with warm antibody AHA undergo complete remission. About 10 percent show minimal or no response to glucocorticoids [15]. The best responses are seen in idiopathic cases and in those related to lupus erythematosus [12,70,93].

In most patients, treatment is initiated with large doses of oral prednisone, 60 to 100 mg daily, rather than starting at a lower level and having to escalate the dose when there is no response. Critically ill patients with rapid hemolysis should receive intravenous therapy equivalent to at least 400 mg hydrocortisone over the first 24 h. High doses of prednisone may be required for 10 to 14 days. When the hematocrit stabilizes or begins to increase, the prednisone dose may be tapered to 45 and then 30 mg per day. With continued improvement in hematocrit, the prednisone may be further tapered at a rate of 5 mg per day every week, to a dose of 15 to 20 mg daily. These doses should be administered for 2 to 3 months after the acute hemolytic episode has subsided, after which the patient may be tapered off the drug over 1 to 2 months, or switched to an alternate-day schedule, e.g., 20 to 40 mg every other day. Alternate-day therapy minimizes glucocorticoid side effects, but should be attempted only after the patient has achieved stable remission on daily prednisone in the range of 15 to 20 mg per day. Though many patients achieve full remission of their first hemolytic episode, relapses are not infrequent after discontinuation of glucocorticoids. Therefore, these patients should be followed for at least several

years after treatment. Relapse may necessitate further glucocorticoid therapy, splenectomy, or immunosuppression. Occasional patients who present with only a positive direct antiglobulin test, minimal hemolysis, and stable hematocrit may require no treatment initially, but careful observation of these patients is important since the rate of red cell destruction may increase spontaneously.

Glucocorticoids may influence hemolysis in warm antibody AHA by several mechanisms. Earlier investigators noted that hematologic improvement was often, though not always, accompanied by reduction in the strength of the direct antiglobulin test [12]. The subsequent observation of a decrease in cell-bound and/or free serum autoantibody during stable glucocorticoid-induced remission [74,94] suggests that a decrease in synthesis of autoantibody may ultimately be important in improving red cell survival. However, reduction in autoantibody synthesis cannot explain the rapid improvement seen in many patients within 24 to 72 h after starting glucocorticoid therapy. There is substantial clinical and experimental evidence that the most important early effect of glucocorticoids is to suppress sequestration of opsonized red cells by splenic macrophages [31,32,46,95]. Another proposed early effect of glucocorticoid therapy may be a reduction in binding affinity of autoantibody for the patient's red cells [29].

SPLENECTOMY

Perhaps one-third of patients with warm antibody AHA require prednisone in doses greater than 15 mg daily to maintain an acceptable red cell mass, and are thus candidates for splenectomy. A patient's clinical data currently constitute the best selection criteria for splenectomy. Attempts to select responders by ^{51}Cr red cell sequestration studies have been disappointing because of poor correlation with results of splenectomy [15,63,96]. In most cases, it is reasonable to continue corticosteroids for 1 to 2 months while waiting for a favorable response. However, if the patient's condition deteriorates or the anemia is very severe, splenectomy should be done sooner. Results of splenectomy vary widely, but approximately two-thirds of splenectomized patients will have a partial or complete remission [63,97,98]. The relapse rate, however, is disappointingly high. Many patients require further glucocorticoid therapy to maintain acceptable hemoglobin levels [11,12,63], although often at lower dosage than required prior to splenectomy [97,99].

Splenectomy may effect improvement in warm antibody AHA by several mechanisms. The simplest rationale is removal of the primary site of red cell trapping. Investigations in humans [29] and in animals [31] confirm that maintenance of a given rate of red cell destruction requires 6 to 10 times as much red cell–bound IgG in splenectomized subjects compared with nonsplenectomized subjects. The continuation of hemolysis after splenectomy is partly related to persisting high levels of autoantibody, favoring red cell destruction in the liver [29,31,36].

Several investigators have noted disappearance of antibody from the red cells of warm antibody AHA patients following splenectomy [6,12,63], possibly because of removal of a primary site of antibody production. However, a significant proportion of patients show no change in cell-bound antibody following splenectomy. The processes which determine the rate of autoantibody production are poorly understood, and any beneficial effect of splenectomy is likely to be related to several factors interacting in complex fashion [98].

The immediate mortality and morbidity from splenectomy depends upon the presence of underlying disease and the preoperative clinical status but in general is quite low [100]. There is a slightly increased risk of pneumococcal sepsis, more in children than in adults [101]. It is reasonable to give pneumococcal vaccine, though efficacy is not yet proved in this setting. Prophylactic penicillin (250 to 500 mg daily) is probably of value in children.

IMMUNOSUPPRESSIVE DRUGS
Cytotoxic drugs such as cyclophosphamide, 6-mercaptopurine, azathioprine, or 6-thioguanine were first tried in AHA with the idea that they may inhibit synthesis of autoantibody. Though there is little direct evidence for such an effect [102], beneficial responses to immunosuppressive drugs may be observed in some patients who fail to respond to glucocorticoids [102,103]. It must be emphasized that the majority of patients with warm antibody AHA respond to glucocorticoids and/or splenectomy and are usually not candidates for immunosuppressive therapy. At present, immunosuppressive therapy should be reserved primarily for those patients who have failed to respond to glucocorticoids and splenectomy, or those patients who are poor surgical risks [102]. The drugs of choice are cyclophosphamide 60 mg/m² or azathioprine 80 mg/m², given daily. If the drug is tolerated by the patient, it is reasonable to continue treatment for up to 6 months while waiting for a response. When response occurs, the drug may be slowly tapered. If there is no response, the alternative drug may be similarly tried. Both cyclophosphamide and azathioprine cause marrow suppression, and patients' blood counts must be monitored during therapy. Both agents are associated with increased risk of subsequent neoplasia, and cyclophosphamide may also cause severe hemorrhagic cystitis.

OTHER THERAPIES
Plasma exchange or plasmapheresis has been attempted in warm antibody AHA. Improvement has been reported in a few cases [104,105], but not in others [106]. Thymectomy has been reported as useful in a few children who are refractory to corticosteroids and splenectomy [102]. In the older literature, responses to heparin have been reported [102]. Selective injury to splenic macrophages by administration of vinblastine-loaded, IgG-sensitized platelets has been undertaken in two patients with AHA, with a preliminary report of success [107]. All of these latter forms of therapy should be considered experimental and reserved for those patients who have failed to respond to established forms of treatment.

Course and prognosis

Idiopathic warm antibody AHA pursues an unpredictable course characterized by relapses and remissions. No particular feature of the illness has consistently been a good predictor of outcome. In spite of a rather high initial rate of response to glucocorticoids and splenectomy, the overall mortality rate has been significant (up to 46 percent) in several older series, but appears to be improving in recent years [12,15,16,63,108,109]. The actuarial survival at 10 years is reported to be 73 percent [108]. Thromboembolic episodes, infection, and severe anemia are causes of death. The prognosis in secondary warm antibody AHA is largely dependent on the course of the underlying disease.

In children, warm antibody AHA frequently follows an acute infection or immunization [110,111]. The majority of patients exhibit an acute self-limited course and respond rapidly to corticosteroids. Those who recover from the initial hemolytic episode have a good prognosis and are unlikely to relapse, although exceptions are known. The overall mortality rate is lower than in adults, ranging from 10 to 30 percent [6,110–112].

References

1. Coombs, R. R. A., Mourant, A. E., and Race, R. R.: A new test for the detection of weak and incomplete Rh agglutinins. *Br. J. Exp. Pathol.* 26:255, 1945.
2. Boorman, K. E., Dodd, B. E., and Loutit, J. F.: Haemolytic icterus (acholuric jaundice), congenital and acquired. *Lancet* 1:812, 1946.
3. Loutit, J. F., and Mollison, P. L.: Haemolytic icterus (acholuric jaundice), congenital and acquired. *J. Pathol. Bacteriol.* 58:711, 1946.
4. Eyster, M. E., and Jenkins, D. E., Jr.: Erythrocyte coating substances in patients with positive direct antiglobulin reactions. Correlation of γG globulin and complement coating with underlying diseases, overt hemolysis and response to therapy. *Am. J. Med.* 46:360, 1969.
5. Dacie, J. V.: *The Haemolytic Anaemias, Congenital and Acquired. II. The Autoimmune Haemolytic Anaemias,* 2d ed. Grune & Stratton, New York, 1962.
6. Evans, R. S., and Weiser, R. S.: The serology of autoimmune hemolytic disease: Observations on forty-one patients. *Arch. Intern. Med.* 100:371, 1957.
7. Bell, C. A., Zwicker, H., and Sacks, H. J.: Autoimmune hemolytic anemia: Routine serologic evaluation in a general hospital population. *Am. J. Clin. Pathol.* 60:903, 1973.
8. Dacie, J. V., and Worlledge, S. M.: Auto-immune hemolytic anemias. *Prog. Hematol.* 6:82, 1969.
9. Dausett, J., and Colombani, J.: The serology and the prognosis of 128 cases of autoimmune hemolytic anemia. *Blood* 14:1280, 1959.
10. Dacie, J. V.: *The Haemolytic Anaemias, Congenital and Acquired. III. Secondary or Lymptomatic Haemolytic Anaemias,* 2d ed. Grune & Stratton, New York, 1967.

11. Worlledge, S. M., and Dacie, J. V.: Haemolytic and other anaemias in infectious mononucleosis, in *Infectious Mononucleosis*, edited by H. G. Carter and R. L. Penman. Blackwell Scientific, Oxford, 1969.

12. Wilkinson, L. S., Petz, L. D., and Garratty, G.: Reappraisal of the role of anti-i in haemolytic anaemia in infectious mononucleosis. *Br. J. Haematol.* 25:715, 1973.

13. Jacobson, L. B., Longstreth, G. F., and Edington, T. S.: Clinical and immunologic features of transient cold agglutinin hemolytic anemia. *Am. J. Med.* 54:514, 1973.

14. Rose, N. R.: Autoimmune diseases, in *Principles of Immunology*, 2d ed., edited by N. R. Rose, F. Milgrom, and C. J. van Oss. Macmillan, New York, 1979, p. 436.

15. Talal, N.: Tolerance and autoimmunity, in *Clinical Immunology*, edited by C. W. Parker. Saunders, Philadelphia, 1980, p. 86.

16. Leddy, J. P.: Reactivity of human γG erythrocyte autoantibodies with fetal, autologous and maternal red cells. *Vox Sang.* 17:525, 1969.

17. Witebsky, E.: Acquired hemolytic anemia. *Ann. N.Y. Acad. Sci.* 124:462, 1965.

18. Mollison, P. L.: Measurement of survival and destruction of red cells in haemolytic syndromes. *Br. Med. Bull.* 15:59, 1959.

19. Holländer, L.: Erythrocyte survival time in a case of acquired haemolytic anaemia. *Vox Sang.* 4:164, 1954.

20. Mollison, P. L., Crome, P., Hughes Jones, N. C., and Rochna, E.: Rate of removal from the circulation of red cells sensitized with different amounts of antibody. *Br. J. Haematol.* 11:461, 1965.

21. Mollison, P. L., and Hughes Jones, N. C.: Clearance of Rh-positive red cells by low concentration of Rh antibody. *Immunology* 12:63, 1967.

22. Rosse, W. F. Quantitative immunology of immune hemolytic anemia. II. The relationship of cell-bound antibody to hemolysis and the effect of treatment. *J. Clin. Invest.* 50:734, 1971.

23. Schreiber, A. D., and Frank, M. M.: Role of antibody and complement in the immune clearance and destruction of erythrocytes. 1. In vivo effects of IgG and IgM complement-fixing sites. *J. Clin. Invest.* 51:575, 1972.

24. Atkinson, J. P., Schreiber, A. D., and Frank, M. M.: Effects of corticosteroids and splenectomy on the immune clearance and destruction of erythrocytes. *J. Clin. Invest.* 52:1509, 1973.

25. Atkinson, J. P., and Frank, M. M.: Complement independent clearance of IgG sensitized erythrocytes: Inhibition by cortisone. *Blood* 44:629, 1974.

26. Jandl, J. H.: Sequestration by the spleen of red cells sensitized with incomplete antibody and with metallo-protein complexes. *J. Clin. Invest.* 34:912, 1955.

27. Jandl, J. H., Richardson-Jones, A., and Castle, W. B.: The destruction of red cells by antibodies in man. I. Observations on the sequestration and lysis of red cells altered by immune mechanisms. *J. Clin. Invest.* 36:1428, 1957.

28. Jandl, J. H., and Tomlinson, A. S.: The destruction of red cells by antibodies in man. II. Pyrogenic, leukocytic and dermal responses to immune hemolysis. *J. Clin. Invest.* 37:1202, 1958.

29. Jandl, J. H., and Kaplan, M. E.: The destruction of red cells by antibodies in man. III. Quantitative factors influencing the pattern of hemolysis in vivo. *J. Clin. Invest.* 39:1145, 1960.

30. Abramson, N., LoBuglio, A. F., Jandl, J. H., and Cotran, R. S.: The interaction between human monocytes and red cells: Binding characteristics. *J. Exp. Med.* 132:1191, 1970.

31. LoBuglio, A. F., Cotran, R. S., and Jandl, J. H.: Red cells coated with immunoglobulin G: Binding and sphering by mononuclear cells in man. *Science* 158:1582, 1967.

32. Huber, H., Polley, M. J., Linscott, W. D., Fudenberg, H. H., and Müller-Eberhard, H. J.: Human monocytes: Distinct receptor sites for the third component of complement and for immunoglobulin G. *Science* 162:1281, 1968.

33. Abramson, N., Geifand, E. W., Jandl, J. H., and Rosen, F. S.: The interaction between human monocytes and red cells: Specificity for IgG subclasses and IgG fragments. *J. Exp. Med.* 132:1207, 1970.

34. Huber, H., Douglas, S. D., Nusbacher, J., Kochwa, S., and Rosenfield, R. E.: IgG subclass specificity of human monocyte receptor sites. *Nature* 229:419, 1971.

35. Huber, H., and Fudenberg, H. H.: Receptor sites of human monocytes for IgG. *Int. Arch. Allergy Appl. Immunol.* 34:18, 1968.

36. Gigli, I., and Nelson, R. A.: Complement-dependent immune phagocytosis: I. Requirements for C1, C4, C2, C3. *Exp. Cell Res.* 51:45, 1968.

37. Lay, W. H., and Nussenzweig, V.: Receptors for complement on leukocytes. *J. Exp. Med.* 128:991, 1968.

38. Fischer' J. T., Petz, L. D., Garratty, G., and Cooper, N. R.: Correlations between quantitative assay of red cell bound C3, serologic reactions, and hemolytic anemia. *Blood* 44:359, 1974.

39. Schreiber, A. D., Parsons, J., McDermott, P., and Cooper, R. A.: Effect of corticosteroids on the human monocyte IgG and complement receptors. *J. Clin. Invest.* 56:1189, 1975.

40. Ehlenberger, A. G., and Nussenzweig, V.: The role of membrane receptors for C3b and C3d in phagocytosis. *J. Exp. Med.* 145:357, 1977.

41. Rosse, W. F., de Boisfleury, A., and Bessis, M.: The interaction of phagocytic cells and red cells modified by immune reactions. Comparison of antibody and complement coated red cells. *Blood Cells* 1:345, 1975.

42. Dameshek, W., and Schwartz, S. O.: Acute hemolytic anemia (acquired hemolytic icterus, acute type). *Medicine (Baltimore)* 19:231, 1940.

43. Carlo, J. R., Ruddy, S., Studer, E. J., and Conrad, D. H.: Complement receptor binding of C3b-coated cells treated with C3b inactivator, β 1H globulin and trypsin. *J. Immunol.* 123:523, 1979.

44. Atkinson, J. P., and Frank, M. M.: Complement, in *Clinical Immunology*, edited by C. W. Parker, Saunders, Philadelphia, 1980, p. 219.

45. Fleer, A., Van Schaik, M. L. J., Borne, A. E. G. Kr. von dem, and Engelfriet, C. P.: Destruction of sensitized erythrocytes by human monocytes in vitro. Effects of cytochalasin B, hydrocortisone and colchicine. *Scand. J. Immunol.* 8:515, 1978.

46. Kurlander, R. J., Rosse, W. F., and Logue, W. L.: Quantitative influence of antibody and complement coating of red cells on monocyte-mediated cell lysis. *J. Clin. Invest.* 61:1309, 1978.

47. Urbaniak, S. J.: Lymphoid cell dependent (K-cell) lysis of human erythrocytes sensitized with rhesus alloantibodies. *Br. J. Haematol.* 33:409, 1976.

48. Handwerger, B. S., Kay, N. W., and Douglas, S. D.: Lymphocyte-mediated antibody-dependent cytolysis: Role in immune hemolysis. *Vox Sang.* 34:276, 1978.

49. Milgrom, H., and Shore, S. L.: Lysis of antibody-coated human red cells by peripheral blood mononuclear cells. Altered effector cell profile after treatment of target cells with enzymes. *Cell. Immunol.* 39:178, 1978.

50. Pirofsky, B.: *Autoimmunization and the Autoimmune Hemolytic Anemias*. Williams & Wilkins, Baltimore, 1969.

51. Swisher, S. N.: Acquired hemolytic disease. *Postgrad. Med.* 40:378, 1966.

52. Habibi, B., Homberg, J. C., Schaison, G., and Salmon, C.: Autoimmune hemolytic anemia in children: A review of 80 cases. *Am. J. Med.* 56:61, 1974.

53. Pirofsky, B.: Hereditary aspects of autoimmune hemolytic anemia: A retrospective analysis. *Vox Sang.* 14:334, 1968.

54. Dobbs, C. E.: Familial auto-immune hemolytic anemia. *Arch. Intern. Med.* 116:273, 1965.

55. Cordova, M. S., Baez-Villasenor, J., Mendez, J. J., and Campos, E.: Acquired hemolytic anemia with positive antiglobulin (Coombs' test) in mother and daughter. *Arch. Intern. Med.* 117:692, 1966.

56. Shapiro, M.: Familial autohemolytic anemia and runting syndrome with Rh_0-specific autoantibody. *Transfusion* 7:281, 1967.

57. Lewis, F. B., Schwartz, R. S., and Dameshek, W.: X-radiation and alkylating agents as possible "trigger" mechanisms in the autoimmune complications of malignant lymphoproliferative disease. *Clin. Exp. Immunol.* 1:3, 1966.

58. Hegde, U. M., Gordon-Smith, E. C., and Worlledge, S. M.: Reticulocytopenia and absence of red cell autoantibodies in immune haemolytic anaemia. *Br. Med. J.* 2:1444, 1977.

59. Conley, C. L., Lippman, S. M., and Ness, P.: Autoimmune hemolytic anemia with reticulocytopenia. A medical emergency. *JAMA* 244:1688, 1980.

60. Greenberg, J., Curtis-Cohen, M., Gill, F. M., and Cohen, A.: Prolonged reticulocytopenia in autoimmune hemolytic anemia of childhood. *J. Pediatr. 97:*784, 1980.

61. Evans, R. S., and Duane, R. T.: Acquired hemolytic anemia. I. The relation of erythrocyte antibody production to activity of the disease. II. The significance of thrombocytopenia and leukopenia. *Blood 4:*1196, 1949.

62. Evans, R. S., Takahashi, K., Duane, R. T., Payne, R., and Lui, C. K.: Primary thrombocytopenic purpura and acquired hemolytic anemia: Evidence for a common etiology. *Arch. Intern. Med. 87:*48, 1951.

63. Tisdale, W. A., Klatskin, G., and Kinsella, E. D.: The significance of the direct-reacting fraction of serum bilirubin in hemolytic jaundice. *Am. J. Med. 26:*214, 1959.

64. Maldonado, J. E., Kyle, R. A., and Schoenfield, L. J.: Increased serum conjugated bilirubin in hemolytic anemia. *Clin. Gastroenterol. 55:*183, 1974.

65. Allgood, J. W., and Chaplin, H., Jr.: Idiopathic acquired autoimmune hemolytic anemia: A review of forty-seven cases treated from 1955 through 1965. *Am. J. Med. 43:*254, 1967.

66. Leddy, J. P.: Immunological aspects of red cell injury in man. *Semin. Hematol. 3:*48, 1966.

67. Engelfriet, C. P., Borne, A. E. G., Vander Giessen, M., Beckers, D., and Van Loghem, J. J.: Autoimmune haemolytic anaemias. I. Serological studies with pure anti-immunoglobulin reagents. *Clin. Exp. Immunol. 3:*605, 1968.

68. Engelfriet, C. P., von dem Boerne, A. E. G. Kr., Beckers, D., and van Loghem, J. J.: Autoimmune haemolytic anaemia: Serological and immunochemical characteristics of the autoantibodies; mechanisms of cell destruction. *Ser. Haematol. 7:*328, 1974.

69. Hsu, T. C. S., Rosenfield, R. E., Burkart, P., Wong, K. Y., and Kochwa, S.: Instrumented PVP-augmented antiglobulin tests. II. Evaluation of acquired hemolytic anemia. *Vox Sang. 26:*305, 1974.

70. Dacie, J. V.: Autoimmune hemolytic anemia. *Arch. Intern. Med. 135:*1293, 1975.

71. Issitt, P. D., et al.: Anti-Wr^b, and other autoantibodies responsible for positive direct antiglobulin test in 150 individuals. *Br. J. Haematol. 34:*5, 1976.

72. Worlledge, S. M.: The interpretation of a positive direct antiglobulin test. *Br. J. Haematol. 39:*157, 1978.

73. Gorst, D. W., Rawlinson, V. I., Merry, A. H., and Stratton, F.: Positive direct antiglobulin test in normal individuals. *Vox Sang. 38:*99, 1980.

74. Evans, R. S., Bingham, M., and Boehni, P.: Autoimmune hemolytic disease: Antibody dissociation and activity. *Arch. Intern. Med. 108:*338, 1961.

75. Evans, R. S., Bingham, M., and Turner, E.: Autoimmune hemolytic disease: Observations of serological reactions and disease activity. *Ann. N.Y. Acad. Sci. 124:*422, 1965.

76. Gilliland, B. C., Leddy, J. P., and Vaughan, J. H.: The detection of cell-bound antibody on complement-coated human red cells. *J. Clin. Invest. 49:*898, 1970.

77. Gilliland, B. C., Baxter, E., and Evans, R. S.: Red-cell antibodies in acquired hemolytic anemia with negative antiglobulin serum tests. *N. Engl. J. Med. 285:*252, 1971.

78. Rosse, W. F.: The detection of small amounts of antibody on the red cell in autoimmune hemolytic anemia. *Ser. Haematol. 7:*3, 1974.

79. Gilliland, B. C.: Coombs-negative immune hemolytic anemia. *Semin. Hematol. 13:*267, 1976.

80. von dem Borne, A. E. G. Kr., Beckers, D., van der Meulen, W., and Engelfriet, C. P.: IgG4 autoantibodies against erythrocytes, without increased hemolysis: A case report. *Br. J. Haematol. 37:*137, 1977.

81. Yasmeen, D., Ellerson, J. R., Dorrington, K. J., and Painter, R. M.: Evidence for the domain hypothesis: Location of the site of cytophilic activity toward guinea pig macrophages in the C_H3 homology region of human immunoglobulin G. *J. Immunol. 110:*1706, 1973.

82. Müller-Eberhard, H. J.: Complement. *Annu. Rev. Biochem. 44:*697, 1975.

83. Weiner, W., and Vos, G. H.: Serology of acquired hemolytic anemia. *Blood 22:*606, 1963.

84. Eyster, M. E., and Jenkins, D. E., Jr.: γG erythrocyte autoantibodies: Comparison of in vivo complement coating and in vitro "Rh" specificity. *J. Immunol. 105:*221, 1970.

85. Leddy, J. P., Peterson, P., Yeaw, M. A., and Bakemeier, R. F.: Patterns of serologic specificity of human γG erythrocyte autoantibodies. *J. Immunol. 105:*677, 1970.

86. Wiener, A. S., Gordon, E. B., and Gallop, C.: Studies on autoantibodies in human sera. *J. Immunol. 71:*58, 1953.

87. Vos. G. H., Petz, L. D., and Fudenberg, H. H.: Specificity and immunoglobulin characteristics of autoantibodies in acquired hemolytic anemia. *J. Immunol. 106:*1172, 1971.

88. Borsos, T., and Rapp, H. J.: Complement fixation on cell surfaces by 19S and 7S antibodies. *Science 150:*505, 1965.

89. Rosse, W. F.: Fixation of the first component of complement (C'1a) by human antibodies. *J. Clin. Invest. 47:*2430, 1968.

90. Issitt, P. D.: Autoimmune hemolytic anemia and cold hemagglutinin disease: Clinical disease and laboratory findings. *Prog. Clin. Pathol. 7:*137, 1978.

91. Petz, L. D., and Garrity, G.: *Acquired Immune Hemolytic Anemias.* Churchill Livingstone, London, 1980.

92. Dameshek, W., Rosenthal, M. C., and Schwartz, S. O.: The treatment of acquired hemolytic anemia with adrenocorticotrophic hormone (ACTH). *N. Engl. J. Med. 244:*117, 1951.

93. Pirofsky, B.: Immune haemolytic disease: The autoimmune hemolytic anemias. *Clinics Haematol. 4:*167, 1975.

94. Leddy, J. P., and Swisher, S. N.: Acquired immune hemolytic disorders (including drug-induced immune hemolytic anemia), in *Immunological Diseases,* edited by M. Samter. Little, Brown, Boston, 1978, p. 1025.

95. Greendyke, R. M., Bradley, E. B., and Swisher, S. N.: Studies of the effects of administration of ACTH and adrenal corticosteroids on erythrophagocytosis. *J. Clin. Invest. 44:*746, 1965.

96. Parker, A. C., MacPherson, A. I. S., and Richmond, J.: Value of radiochromium investigation in autoimmune haemolytic anemia. *Br. Med. J. 1:*208, 1977.

97. Christensen, B. E.: The pattern of erythrocyte sequestration in immunohaemolysis: Effects of prednisone treatment and splenectomy. *Scand. J. Haematol. 10:*120, 1973.

98. Bowdler, A. J.: The role of the spleen and splenectomy in autoimmune hemolytic disease. *Semin. Hematol. 13:*335, 1976.

99. Chaplin, H., and Avioli, L. V.: Autoimmune hemolytic anemia. *Arch. Intern. Med. 137:*346, 1977.

100. Schwartz, S. I., Bernard, R. P., Adams, J. T., and Bauman, A. W.: Splenectomy for hematologic disorders. *Arch. Surg. 101:*338, 1970.

101. Eichner, E. R.: Splenic function: Normal, too much and too little. *Am. J. Med. 66:*311, 1979.

102. Murphy, S., and LoBuglio, A. F.: Drug therapy of autoimmune hemolytic anemia. *Semin. Hematol. 13:*323, 1976.

103. Skinner, M. D., and Schwartz, R. S.: Immunosuppressive therapy. *N. Engl. J. Med. 287:*221, 1972.

104. Branda, R. F., Moldow, C. F., McCullough, J. J., and Jacob, H. S.: Plasma exchange in the treatment of immune disease. *Transfusion 15:*570, 1975.

105. Pattern, E., Reuter, F. P., Castle, R., and Mercer, C.: Evan's syndrome: Benefit from plasma exchange. *Transfusion 18:*383, 1978.

106. Rosenfield, R. E., and Jagathambal: Transfusion therapy for autoimmune hemolytic anemia. *Semin. Hematol. 13:*311, 1976.

107. Ahn, Y. S., and Harrington, W. J.: Clinical uses of macrophage inhibition. *Adv. Intern. Med. 25:*453, 1980.

108. Silverstein, M. N., Gomes, M. R., Elveback, L. R., ReMine, W. H., and Linman, J. W.: Idiopathic acquired hemolytic anemia. Survival in 117 cases. *Arch. Intern. Med. 129:*85, 1972.

109. Worlledge, S. M.: Immune haemolytic anaemias, in *Blood and Its Disorders,* edited by R. M. Hardisty and D. J. Weatherall. Blackwell, Oxford, 1974, p. 714.

110. Buchanan, G. R., Boxer, L. A., and Nathan, D. G.: The acute and transient nature of idiopathic immune hemolytic anemia in childhood. *J. Pediatr. 88:*780, 1976.

111. Zupanska, B., et al.: Autoimmune haemolytic anaemia in children. *Br. J. Haematol. 34:*511, 1976.

112. Carapella de Luca, E., Casadei, A. M., di Piero, G., Midulla, M., Bisdomini, C., and Purpura, M.: Autoimmune haemolytic anaemia in childhood. Followup in 29 cases. *Vox Sang. 36:*13, 1979.

CHAPTER 68

Cryopathic hemolytic syndromes

CHARLES H. PACKMAN
JOHN P. LEDDY

Cryopathic hemolytic syndromes are autoimmune disorders in which the autoantibodies have enhanced activity at temperatures below 37°C and usually below 31°C. These disorders are encountered much less commonly than autoimmune hemolytic anemia (AHA) due to warm autoantibodies. One form of "cold antibody" AHA is mediated by cold agglutinins as either an acute or chronic process. The second and much rarer cold antibody–mediated hemolytic disorder is paroxysmal cold hemoglobinuria in which the responsible antibody (the Donath-Landsteiner antibody) is not an agglutinin but a potent hemolysin (for discussion of these terms, see the introductory section of Chap. 67). Both cryopathic syndromes require the complement system for red cell injury, and have a much greater potential for direct intravascular hemolysis than warm antibody AHA. It must be emphasized that the laboratory temperatures (e.g., 0 to 5°C) commonly used to demonstrate these cold antibodies in vitro are far below the temperatures required for these antibodies to produce pathologic effects in vivo.

Cold antibody autoimmune hemolytic anemia

DEFINITIONS AND HISTORY

Cold agglutinins were first described by Landsteiner in 1903 [1]. However, recognition of the connection between cold agglutinins, hemolytic anemia, and Raynaud-like peripheral vascular phenomena evolved slowly. In 1918 Clough and Richter detected cold agglutinins in a patient with pneumonia [2]. In 1925 and 1926, Iwai and Mei-Sai [3,4] reported two cases with cold agglutinins and Raynaud's phenomenon and showed that flow of blood through capillary tubes in vitro or in superficial capillaries in vivo was impeded at low temperatures. During the late 1940s and early 1950s, the observations of many workers gradually established the pathogenetic importance of cold agglutinins in red cell injury. Schubothe introduced the term *cold agglutinin disease* in 1953 and clearly distinguished this disorder from other acquired hemolytic syndromes [5].

In current usage, cold agglutinin disease pertains to that minority of patients with chronic autoimmune hemolytic anemia in which the autoantibody directly agglutinates human red cells at temperatures below body temperature, maximally at 0 to 5°C. Fixation of complement to red cells by cold agglutinins occurs at higher temperatures but generally below 37°C (see below). Affected patients exhibit varying combinations of hemolytic anemia, episodic hemoglobinuria, and acrocyanosis or other peripheral vaso-occlusive phenomena, all initiated or intensified by cold exposure.

Cold agglutinin disease is traditionally considered to occur in primary (idiopathic) and secondary forms. The most common settings for the secondary form are (1) an acute, self-limited hemolytic process occasionally complicating *Mycoplasma pneumoniae* infections or infectious mononucleosis and occuring mainly in adolescents or young adults; and (2) a chronic disorder occurring in older patients with known malignant lymphoproliferative diseases. *Idiopathic* chronic cold agglutinin disease, with no identifiable underlying disorder at the time of diagnosis, has its peak incidence after age 50. Some cases in this group gradually develop features of a lymphoproliferative disorder resembling Waldenström's macroglobulinemia. Thus, the distinction between primary and secondary types of chronic cold agglutinin disease is not absolute.

ETIOLOGY AND PATHOGENESIS

ORIGIN OF COLD AGGLUTININS
The stimulus or immunoregulatory defect leading to the chronic production of high-titered monoclonal cold agglutinins remains enigmatic. This problem must be viewed against the background knowledge that cold-reactive autoantibodies with apparently similar specificity for I/i antigens of the red cell are induced *transiently* in many otherwise healthy humans during infections with *M. pneumoniae* or Ebstein-Barr virus. Cold agglutinins arising during *M. pneumoniae* infection do not react with the intact mycoplasma organism itself [6,7]; however, a cross-reaction with a crude lipopolysaccharide fraction of mycoplasma has been reported [7]. I/i antigens or structurally related analogues occur widely in nature: (1) in human saliva, milk, amniotic fluid, or hydatid cyst fluid [8]; (2) on rabbit (I-like) or sheep (i-like) erythrocytes [9,10]; and (3) on human lymphocytes, neutrophils, and monocytes [11]. The presence of i antigen on lymphocytes could be pertinent to the formation of anti-i cold agglutinins in infectious mononucleosis; i.e., the immunogen could be lymphocyte-derived and related to the marked lymphocytic stimulation and destruction occurring in this disease.

PATHOGENETIC EFFECTS OF COLD AGGLUTININS
Most cold agglutinins are unable to agglutinate red cells at temperatures above 30°C. The highest temperature at which agglutination is detected is termed the *thermal amplitude*. This property, which varies considerably from one case to another, appears to have an important influence on the clinical picture. Thermal amplitude is

generally correlated with the magnitude of the cold agglutinin titer [5], but important exceptions occur.

Cold agglutinins are typically IgM. The potential of a given patient's IgM cold agglutinins to produce a hemolytic anemia appears to be determined by the capacity of these antibodies to activate and bind complement components to host red cells at temperatures occurring in the superficial microvasculature [12–18]. Although in vitro agglutination of the red cells is maximal at 0 to 5°C, complement fixation by these antibodies occurs optimally at 20 to 25°C and may be pathogenetically significant at higher temperatures, even at 37°C [13,19]. Thus, agglutination is not required for complement fixation to take place. Temperatures of 28 to 31°C occur in superficial vessels of acral body parts, depending upon ambient temperature. Lower temperatures are probably achieved during severe chilling. These cooler areas of the microvasculature are thought to be the major sites for in vitro binding of cold agglutinins and complement to red cells [15].

The critical temperatures for the above reactions occur at ordinary room temperatures in those patients with high-titer, high-thermal-amplitude cold antibodies. These patients tend to have a sustained hemolytic process and acrocyanosis [9]. Other patients with antibodies of lower thermal amplitude require significant chilling to initiate complement-mediated injury of red cells. This sequence often results in a burst of hemolysis with hemoglobinuria [9]. Combinations of these clinical patterns also occur. Active hemolytic anemia has been observed in patients with cold agglutinins of modest titer (e.g., 1:256) but high thermal amplitude [19]. IgA cold agglutinins, which do not fix complement, cause acrocyanosis but not hemolysis [20–22]. Thus, hemolysis and/or impeded red cell flow producing acrocyanosis are variable, depending on the properties and quantity of the cold agglutinins in a given patient.

Complement may injure red cells by two major mechanisms: (1) direct lysis and (2) opsonization for sequestration by hepatic and splenic macrophages. Red cell injury probably occurs by both mechanisms in most patients. Direct lysis requires propagation of the full C1-C9 sequence on the cell membrane. If this occurs to a significant degree, the patient may experience massive hemolysis, manifested by hemoglobinemia and hemoglobinuria. More commonly, the complement sequence on many red cells is completed only through the early stages, leaving opsonic fragments of C3 (C3b) on the cell surface (see Chap. 67 for discussion of opsonization of red cells). Red cells heavily coated with C3b are subject to removal from the circulation by hepatic and, to a lesser extent, splenic macrophages [13,14,17,23,24]. Some of these trapped red cells may undergo phagocytosis or partial membrane ingestion, producing spherocytosis. Although red cells coated with C3b alone provide a relatively weak stimulus for phagocytosis by monocytes in vitro [25,26], other studies have shown that *activated* macrophages do ingest C3b-coated particles [27]. In vivo studies on the fate of ^{51}Cr-labeled

C3b-coated red cells in humans and animal models [14,17,18,28] have revealed that a substantial portion of the erythrocytes initially trapped in the liver and spleen gradually reenter the circulation. These released cells were found to be coated with the opsonically inactive C3 fragment, C3d. Conversion of cell-bound C3b to C3d presumably results from the action of the naturally occurring complement inhibitors (C3b inactivator, β1H, and an undefined protease [29]). These surviving C3d-coated red cells circulate with a near-normal life-span [13,14,17,18,28,30] and are resistant to further uptake of cold agglutinins or complement [13,17,31,32], but they react to anticomplement (anti-C3) serum. Thus, a major portion of the antiglobulin-positive red cells in a patient's circulation appear to be "survivors" of the two types of complement-mediated destruction.

INCIDENCE

All forms of cold agglutinin disease are relatively rare and occur considerably less frequently than cases of warm antibody AHA. In several series on AHA of all types, cold agglutinin–mediated AHA accounted for approximately 10 to 20 percent of cases [12,33–35], with women more commonly affected [12,36]. No genetic or racial factors are known.

Although the majority of patients with mycoplasma pneumonia have significant cold agglutinin titers, the development of AHA on this basis is uncommon [37–39]. However, subclinical red cell injury may occur. In one series of *M. pneumoniae* infections, weakly positive direct antiglobulin reactions and/or mild reticulocytosis were noted in a substantial number of cases, in the absence of anemia [37]. Cold agglutinins occur in over 60 percent of patients with infectious mononucleosis, but again hemolytic anemia is rare [40–42].

CLINICAL FEATURES

In some patients with cold agglutinin AHA, the clinical picture may be that of chronic hemolytic anemia with or without jaundice. In other patients, the principal feature is episodic, acute hemolysis with hemoglobinuria induced by chilling. Combinations of these clinical features may occur. Acrocyanosis and other cold-mediated, vaso-occlusive phenomena affecting the fingers, toes, nose, and ears are associated with sludging of red cells in the cutaneous microvasculature. Skin ulceration and necrosis are distinctly unusual complications. Hemolysis occurring in *M. pneumoniae* infections is acute in onset, typically appearing as the patient is recovering from pneumonia and coincident with peak titers of cold agglutinins. The hemolysis is self-limited, lasting 1 to 3 weeks [33]. Hemolytic anemia in infectious mononucleosis develops either at the onset of symptoms or within the first 3 weeks of illness [33,41].

Physical findings are variable, depending upon the presence of an underlying disease. Splenomegaly, which is a characteristic finding in lymphoproliferative processes and infectious mononucleosis, may also be observed in idiopathic cold agglutinin disease.

LABORATORY FEATURES

GENERAL

In classic chronic cold agglutinin disease the anemia is fairly stable, and in most cases mild to moderate in degree. However, hemoglobin levels as low as 5 to 6 g/dl may be encountered. In addition to polychromasia, the blood film may show spherocytosis, but the latter is usually less marked than in typical cases of warm antibody AHA. Clumps of red cells, characteristic of autoagglutination, may be noted on the blood film. Autoagglutination may also be evident in anticoagulated blood at room temperature. This phenomenon may be intensified by cooling the blood to 4°C, and reversed by warming to 37°C, a property which distinguishes cold autoagglutination from rouleaux formation. Occasionally, erroneous red cell indices are recorded because of autoagglutintation in electronic cell counters. As clumps of red cells pass through the counting orifice, the mean cell volume is read as falsely high and the red cell count and derived hematocrit are falsely low. A very high mean corpuscular hemoglobin and mean corpuscular hemoglobin concentration are important clues to this artifact [43]. Mild to moderate leukocytosis is often seen during active hemolysis, e.g., following exposure of the patient to chilling. The platelet count is usually normal. Mild hyperbilirubinemia is common. Hemosiderinuria is seen in patients who have had episodes of hemoglobinuria.

SEROLOGIC FEATURES

As noted above, cold agglutinins are characteristically 19 S IgM globulins. IgA or IgG cold agglutinins have been reported in a few cases [8,20–22,44,45]. Cold agglutinins are distinguished by their ability to agglutinate saline-suspended human red cells at low temperature, maximally at 0 to 5°C. This reaction is reversible by warming. Low titers of cold agglutinins (1:32 or less) are found normally in most human sera [46]. In cold agglutinin AHA the serum titers are commonly 1:1000 or higher, and may reach 1:100,000 or more.

The direct antiglobulin test is positive with anticomplement (anti-C3 or anti-C4) reagents. The antibody itself is not detected by antiglobulin reactions with antisera to human immunoglobulins, nor by specific anti-IgM, anti-IgA or anti-IgG. This is because the cold agglutinins, unlike the more firmly bound complement proteins, dissociate from the red cells, e.g., during the washing steps of the antiglobulin procedure.

The majority of cold agglutinins are reactive with human erythrocyte antigens of the I/i system, which is closely related to the major ABO blood groups. Both I and i appear to be antigenic mosaics containing multiple oligosaccharide determinants bound to the major red cell glycoprotein, glycophorin [8,47–50]. Both anti-I and anti-i cold agglutinins bind well to solubilized red cell glycoproteins (bearing I/i antigens) at 37°C, suggesting that the temperature dependence of cold agglutination may be a function of temperature-related conformational effects on the red cell surface [47,48]. The I antigen complex is expressed strongly on adult red cells but weakly on neonatal (cord) red cells. The converse is true of the i antigen complex. Thus, cold agglutinin titers performed with adult red cells may underestimate anti-i titers.

Anti-I is the predominant specificity of cold agglutinins associated with idiopathic disease, with mycoplasma pneumonia, and in some cases with lymphoma. Cold agglutinins with anti-i specificity are found in patients with infectious mononucleosis and in some patients with lymphoma. A small percentage of cold agglutinin–containing sera, largely, but not entirely, in patients with chronic cold agglutinin disease, display equally strong reactions with adult and neonatal red cells. These antibodies appear to recognize antigens outside the I/i system such as the Pr group [8].

In hemolytic anemia associated with infectious mononucleosis, the patient's serum may contain IgM anti-i antibodies or cold-reactive nonagglutinating IgG anti-i plus IgM cold-reactive anti-IgG antibodies ("rheumatoid factors") which cross-link the IgG-coated red cells to produce agglutination [44,51].

In idiopathic or lymphoma-associated cold agglutinin disease the cold agglutinins display monoclonal characteristics, including electrophoretic homogeneity. Occasionally the cold agglutinin is present in sufficient concentration to produce an abnormal peak in the serum electrophoretic pattern [52]. The majority of anti-I cold agglutinins are IgMκ molecules with homogeneous electrophoretic mobility, whereas monoclonal anti-i molecules may possess either kappa or lambda light chains [8,53–56]. With rare exceptions, the transiently occurring postinfectious cold agglutinins with anti-I specificity are of polyclonal origin, including both κ and λ molecules [57,58].

DIFFERENTIAL DIAGNOSIS

The clinical and laboratory features of cold agglutinin AHA are sufficiently distinctive that the differential diagnostic possibilities are limited. In general, cold agglutinins of high titer (>1:256) together with a direct antiglobulin test positive for complement (but not IgG) point strongly toward a diagnosis of cold agglutinin AHA. Warm antibody AHA, congenital hemolytic disorders, and paroxysmal nocturnal hemoglobinuria (PNH) should be ruled out in cases exhibiting primarily a chronic hemolytic anemia. The pattern of the antiglobulin reaction, family history, and the acid or sucrose hemolysis test provide additional help in difficult cases. When the hemolysis is episodic in nature, one should also consider paroxysmal cold hemoglobinuria and march hemoglobinuria, as well as PNH. When cold-induced peripheral vaso-occlusive symptoms are predominant, the differential diagnosis should include cryoglobulinemia and Raynaud's phenomenon with or without an associated rheumatic disease. Infectious mononucleosis, *M. pneumoniae* infection, or lymphoma may be considered in appropriate clinical settings.

THERAPY

Keeping the patient warm, particularly the extremities, provides moderately effective symptomatic relief. This may be the only measure required in patients with mild chronic hemolysis. Chlorambucil or cyclophosphamide therapy has been helpful in some patients, and deserves consideration in difficult cases [5,59–61]. Splenectomy [12,62–64] and corticosteroids [12,36,59,65] have generally been disappointing, although exceptions have been reported [12,19]. There is some experimental [23] and clinical [19] basis for considering very high doses of corticosteroids in seriously ill patients. Plasma exchange may provide temporary amelioration of hemolysis [15,66], but no long-term benefit can be expected [67]. Red cell transfusions should be reserved for those patients with severe anemia of rapid onset and in danger of cardiorespiratory complications. Because reduction in serum complement levels in such cases may limit the hemolytic rate, administration of washed red cells is preferred, to avoid replenishing depleted complement components and thus reactivating the hemolytic sequence.

COURSE AND PROGNOSIS

Patients with idiopathic cold agglutinin disease often have a relatively benign course and survive for many years [5,12,59,61]. Occasionally death results from infection or severe anemia, or in the case of secondary cold agglutinin disease, from the underlying lymphoproliferative process.

The postinfectious forms of cold agglutinin AHA are typically self-limited. Recovery generally occurs in a few weeks. A few cases with massive hemoglobinuria have been complicated by acute renal failure, requiring a period of hemodialysis.

Paroxysmal cold hemoglobinuria

DEFINITIONS AND HISTORY

Paroxysmal cold hemoglobinuria (PCH) is a very rare form of AHA characterized by acute episodes of massive hemolysis following cold exposure. The disease was well recognized during the latter half of the nineteenth century [68] and was probably more common then because of its association with congenital or tertiary syphilis. With present-day control of syphilis, this cause of PCH has almost disappeared. Now PCH occurs in a chronic idiopathic form and in an acute transient form following several types of viral syndromes, including the childhood exanthems [12,69]. In 1904, Donath and Landsteiner first described the cold-reactive autoantibody which now bears their names and is responsible for the complement-mediated hemolysis.

ETIOLOGY AND PATHOGENESIS

The cause of autoantibody production in PCH is unknown. However, the mechanism of episodic hemolysis probably parallels events which are observable in vitro (see below). During severe chilling, blood flowing through skin capillaries is exposed to low temperatures. The Donath-Landsteiner antibody and early-acting complement components apparently bind to red cells at these lowered temperatures. Upon return of the cells to 37°C in the central circulation, the cells are rapidly lysed by propagation of the terminal complement sequence through C9. The Donath-Landsteiner antibody dissociates from the red cells at body temperature.

INCIDENCE

Medical centers that receive many referrals report that PCH comprises 2 to 5 percent of all cases of AHA [33,59]. There are no known racial or genetic predispositions, although familial occurrence has been reported [12]. The disease occurs at all ages. Years ago more cases were reported in young children, reflecting the high incidence of congenital syphilis [12]. Now most childhood cases appear following specific viral infections or upper respiratory infections of undefined etiology [12,33].

CLINICAL FEATURES

Constitutional symptoms are prominent during a paroxysm. A few minutes to several hours after cold exposure, the patient develops aching pains in the back or legs, abdominal cramps, and perhaps headaches. Chills and fever usually follow. The first urine passed after onset of symptoms typically contains hemoglobin. The constitutional symptoms and hemoglobinuria generally last a few hours. Raynaud's phenomenon and cold urticaria sometimes occur during an attack, and jaundice may follow.

LABORATORY FEATURES

GENERAL

The hemoglobin level often drops rapidly during a severe attack. Chronic anemia, reticulocytosis, hemoglobinemia, and hyperbilirubinemia may be present, depending on the frequency and severity of attacks. Serum complement titers are usually depressed during an acute episode because of consumption in the hemolytic reaction. Spherocytosis and erythrophagocytosis by monocytes and neutrophils are typically found on the blood film during an attack. Leukopenia is often seen early in the attack, followed by neutrophilic leukocytosis. The urine may be dark red or brown due to the presence of hemoglobin and methemoglobin.

SEROLOGY

The direct antiglobulin reaction is usually positive during and briefly following a paroxysm, but remains negative between attacks. The positive reaction is due to coating of surviving red cells with complement, primarily C3 fragments. The Donath-Landsteiner antibody is a nonagglutinating IgG which binds only in the cold, and readily dissociates from the red cell at room temperature and above. The antibody is detected in vitro by the biphasic Donath-Landsteiner test in which the patient's fresh serum is incubated initially with red cells at 4°C and the mixture then warmed to 37°C [12,33]. Intense hemolysis occurs. It may be necessary to add fresh guinea pig serum or ABO-compatible human serum as a source of fresh complement if the patient's serum has been stored or is complement-depleted. Antibody titers rarely exceed 1:16. The Donath-Landsteiner antibody typically has specificity for the P blood group antigen [69,70] which is found not only on red cells but also on lymphocytes and skin fibroblasts [71]. The latter finding might be related in some way to the occurrence of cold urticaria in PCH, a phenomenon which has been passively transferred by serum to normal skin [12].

DIFFERENTIAL DIAGNOSIS
PCH must be distinguished from the subset of cases with chronic cold agglutinin disease which manifest episodic hemolysis and hemoglobinuria. This distinction is made primarily in the laboratory. In general, patients with PCH lack high titers of cold agglutinins. Furthermore, the Donath-Landsteiner antibody is a potent in vitro hemolysin, in contrast to most cold agglutinins, which are weak hemolysins. Warm antibody AHA, march hemoglobinuria, myoglobinuria, and paroxysmal nocturnal hemoglobinuria may be distinguished by history and by appropriate serologic studies.

THERAPY
Acute attacks in both chronic and transient PCH may be prevented by avoidance of cold. Corticosteroid therapy and splenectomy have not been useful. When PCH is associated with syphilis, effective treatment of the latter may interrupt the hemolytic process. Antihistaminic and adrenergic agents may relieve symptoms of cold urticaria.

COURSE AND PROGNOSIS
Postinfectious forms of PCH terminate spontaneously within a few days to weeks after onset, though the Donath-Landsteiner antibody may persist in low titer for several years [12]. Most patients with chronic idiopathic PCH survive for many years in spite of occasional paroxysms of hemolysis.

References

1. Landsteiner, K.: Über Beziehungen zwischen dem Blutserum und den Körperzellen. *Munch. Med. Wochenschr.* 50:1812, 1903.
2. Clough, M. C., and Richter, I. M.: A study of an autoagglutinin occurring in a human serum. *Johns Hopkins Hosp. Bull.* 29:86, 1918.
3. Iwai, S., and Mei-Sai, N.: Etiology of Raynaud's disease: A preliminary report. *Jpn. Med. World* 5:119, 1925.
4. Iwai, S., and Mei-Sai, N.: Etiology of Raynaud's disease. *Jpn. Med. World* 6:345, 1926.
5. Schubothe, H.: The cold hemagglutinin disease. *Semin. Hematol.* 3:27, 1966.
6. Liu, C., Eaton, M. D., and Heyl, J. T.: Studies on primary atypical pneumonia. II. Observations concerning the development and immunological characteristics of antibody in patients. *J. Exp. Med.* 109:545, 1959.
7. Costea, N., Yakulis, V. J., and Heller, P.: Inhibition of cold agglutinins (anti-I) by *M. pneumoniae* antigens. *Proc. Soc. Exp. Biol. Med.* 139:476, 1972.
8. Roelcke, D.: Cold agglutination: Antibodies and antigens. *Clin. Immunol. Immunopathol.,* 2:266, 1974.
9. Evans, R. S., Turner, E., and Bingham, M.: Studies with radioiodinated cold agglutinins of ten patients. *Am. J. Med.* 38:378, 1965.
10. Tönder, O., and Harboe, M.: Heterogeneity of cold haemagglutinins. *Immunology* 11:361, 1966.
11. Pruzanski, W., and Shumak, K. H.: Biologic activity of cold-reacting autoantibodies. *N. Engl. J. Med.* 297:583, 1977.
12. Dacie, J. V.:*The Haemolytic Anaemias, Congenital and Acquired. II. The Autoimmune Haemolytic Anaemias,* 2d ed. Grune & Stratton, New York, 1962.
13. Evans, R. S., Turner, E., Bingham, M., and Woods, R.: Chronic hemolytic anemia due to cold agglutinins. II. The role of C' in red cell destruction. *J. Clin. Invest.,* 47:691, 1968.
14. Brown, D. L., Lachmann, P. J., and Dacie, J. V.: The in vivo behaviour of complement-coated red cells: Studies in C6-deficient, C3-depleted and normal rabbits. *Clin. Exp. Immunol.* 7:401, 1970.
15. Logue, G. L., Rosse, W. F., and Gockerman, J. P.: Measurement of the third component of complement bound to red blood cells in patients with the cold agglutinin syndrome. *J. Clin. Invest.* 52:493, 1973.
16. Fischer, J. T., Petz, L. D., Garratty, G., and Cooper, N. R.: Correlations between quantitative assay of red cell bound C3, serologic reactions, and hemolytic anemia. *Blood* 44:359, 1974.
17. Jaffe, C. J., Atkinson, J. P., and Frank, M. M.: The role of complement in the clearance of cold agglutinin-sensitized erythrocytes in man. *J. Clin. Invest.* 58:942, 1976.
18. Atkinson, J. P., and Frank, M. M.: Studies on in vivo effects of antibody: Interaction of IgM antibody and complement in the immune clearance and destruction of erythrocytes in man. *J. Clin. Invest.* 54:339, 1974.
19. Schreiber, A. D., Herskovitz, B. S., and Goldwein, M.: Low-titer cold-hemagglutinin disease. *N. Engl. J. Med.* 296:1490, 1977.
20. Angevine, C. D., Andersen, B. R., and Barnett, E. V.: A cold agglutinin of the IgA class. *J. Immunol.* 96:578, 1966.
21. Roelcke, D., and Dorow, W.: Besonderheiten der Reaktionsweise mit Plasmacytom-γA-Paraprotein identischen Kälteagglutinins. *Klin. Wochenschr.* 46:126, 1968.
22. Tonthat, H., Rochant, H., Henry, A., Leporrier, M., and Dryfus, B.: A new case of monoclonal IgA kappa cold agglutinin with anti-PrId specificity in a patient with persistent HB antigen cirrhosis. *Vox Sang.* 30:464, 1976.
23. Atkinson, J. P., Schreiber, A. D., and Frank, M. M.: Effects of corticosteroids and splenectomy on the immune clearance and destruction of erythrocytes. *J. Clin. Invest.* 52:1509, 1973.
24. Brown, D. L., and Nelson, D. A.: Surface microfragmentation of red cells as a mechanism for complement-mediated immune spherocytosis. *Br. J. Haematol.* 24:301, 1973.
25. Mantovani, B., Rabinovitch, M., and Nussenzweig, V.: Phagocytosis of immune complexes by macrophages: Different roles of the macrophage receptor sites for complement (C3) and for immunoglobulin (IgG). *J. Exp. Med.* 135:780, 1972.
26. Ehlenberger, A. G., and Nussenzweig, V.: The role of membrane receptors for C3b and C3d in phagocytosis. *J. Exp. Med.* 145:357, 1977.
27. Silverstein, S. C., Steinman, R. M., and Cohn, Z. A.: Endocytosis. *Annu. Rev. Biochem.* 46:669, 1977.
28. Schreiber, A. D., and Frank, M. M.: Role of antibody and complement in the immune clearance and destruction of erythrocytes. I. In vivo effects of IgG and IgM complement-fixing sites. *J. Clin. Invest.* 51:575, 1972.
29. Carlo, J. R., Ruddy, S., Studer, E. J., and Conrad, D. H.: Complement receptor binding of C3b-coated cells treated with C3b inactivator, β1H globulin and trypsin. *J. Immunol.* 123:523, 1979.
30. Lewis, S. M., Dacie, J. V., and Szur, L.: Mechanism of haemolysis in the cold-haemagglutinin syndrome. *Br. J. Haematol.* 6:154, 1960.
31. Boyer, J. T.: Complement and cold agglutinins. II. Interactions of the

components of complement and antibody within the haemolytic complex. *Clin. Exp. Immunol.* 2:241, 1967.

32. Evans, R. S., Turner, E., and Bingham, M.: Chronic hemolytic anemia due to cold agglutinins. I. The mechanism of resistance of red cells to C' hemolysis by cold agglutinins. *J. Clin. Invest.* 46:1461, 1967.

33. Petz, L. D., and Garrity, G.: *Acquired Immune Hemolytic Anemias.* Churchill, Livingstone, New York, 1980.

34. Swisher, S. N.: Acquired hemolytic disease. *Postgrad. Med.* 40:378, 1966.

35. Eyster, M. E., and Jenkins, D. E., Jr.: Erythrocyte coating substances in patients with positive direct antiglobulin reactions. Correlation of γG globulin and complement coating with underlying diseases, overt hemolysis and response to therapy. *Am. J. Med.* 46:360, 1969.

36. Dausset, J., and Colombani, J.: The serology and the prognosis of 128 cases of autoimmune hemolytic anemia. *Blood* 14:1280, 1959.

37. Feizi, T.: Cold agglutinins, the direct Coombs' test and serum immunoglobulins in *Mycoplasma pneumoniae* infection. *Ann. N. Y. Acad. Sci., 143:801, 1967.*

38. Jacobson, L. B., Longstreth, G. F., and Edington, T. S.: Clinical and immunologic features of transient cold agglutinin hemolytic anemia. *Am. J. Med.* 54:514, 1973.

39. Murray, H. W., Masur, H., Senterfit, L. B., and Roberts, R. B.: The protean manifestations of *Mycoplasma pneumoniae* infection in adults. *Am. J. Med.* 58:229, 1975.

40. Rosenfield, R. E., Schmidt, P. J., Calvo, R. C., and McGinniss, M. H.: Anti-i, a frequent cold agglutinin in infectious mononucleosis. *Vox Sang.* 10:631, 1965.

41. Worlledge, S. M., and Dacie, J. V.: Haemolytic and other anaemias in infectious mononucleosis, in *Infectious Mononucleosis*, edited by R. L. Carter and H. G. Penman. Blackwell Scientific, Oxford, 1969, p. 82.

42. Hossaini, A. A.: Anti-i in infectious mononucleosis. *Am. J. Clin. Pathol.* 53:198, 1970.

43. Hattersley, P. G., Gerard, P. W., Caggiano, V., Nash, D. R.: Erroneous values on the model S Coulter counter due to high titer cold autoagglutinins. *Am. J. Clin. Pathol.* 55:442, 1971.

44. Goldberg, L. S., and Barnett, E. V.: Mixed γG-γM cold agglutinin. *J. Immunol.* 99:803, 1967.

45. Ambrus, M., and Bajtai, G.: A case of IgG-type cold agglutinin disease. *Haematologia* 3:225, 1969.

46. Adinolfi, M.: Anti-I antibody in normal human newborn infants. *Immunology* 9:43, 1965.

47. Rosse, W. F., and Lauf, P. K.: Reaction of cold agglutinins with I antigen solubilized from human red cells. *Blood* 36:777, 1970.

48. Lau, F. O., and Rosse, W. F.: The reactivity of red blood cell membrane glycophorin with "cold-reacting" antibodies. *Clin. Immunol. Immunopathol.* 4:1, 1975.

49. Roelcke, D., Ebert, W., Metz, J., and Weicher, H.: I-, MN-, and Pr1/Pr2-activity of human erythrocyte glycoprotein fractions obtained by ficin treatment. *Vox Sang.* 21:352, 1971.

50. Feizi, T., Kabat, E. A., Vicari, G., Anderson, B., and Marsh, W. L.: Immunochemical studies on blood groups. XLVII. The I antigen complex precursors in the A, B, H, Le^a and Le^b blood group system: Hemagglutination inhibition studies. *J. Exp. Med.* 133:39, 1971.

51. Capra, J. D., Dowling, P., Cook, S., and Kunkel, H. G.: An incomplete cold-reactive γG antibody with i specificity in infectious mononucleosis. *Vox Sang.* 16:10, 1969.

52. Christenson, W. N., Dacie, J. V., Croucher, B. E. E., and Charlwood, P. A.: Electrophoretic studies on sera containing high-titre cold haemagglutinins: Identification of the antibody as the cause of an abnormal γ₁ peak. *Br. J. Haematol.* 3:153, 1957.

53. Harboe, M., van Furth, R., Schubothe, H., Lind, K., and Evans, R. S.: Exclusive occurrence of κ chains in isolated cold haemagglutinins. *Scand. J. Haematol.* 2:259, 1965.

54. Wollheim, F. A., Williams, R. C., Jr., and Polesky, H. F.: Studies on the macroglobulins of human serum. III. Quantitative aspects related to cold agglutinins. *Blood* 29:203, 1967.

55. Cooper, A. G.: Purification of cold agglutinins from patients with chronic cold haemagglutinin disease. Evidence of their homogeneity from starch gel electrophoresis of isolated light chains. *Clin. Exp. Immunol.* 3:691, 1968.

56. Roelcke, D., Ebert, W., and Feizi, T.: Studies on the specificities of two IgM lambda cold agglutinins. *Immunology* 27:879, 1974.

57. Harboe, M., and Lind, K.: Light chain types of transiently occurring cold haemagglutinins. *Scand. J. Haematol.* 3:269, 1966.

58. Feizi, T.: Monotypic cold agglutinins in infection by *Mycoplasma pneumoniae*. *Nature* 215:540, 1967.

59. Dacie, J. V., and Worlledge, S. M.: Auto-immune hemolytic anemias. *Prog. Hematol.* 6:82, 1969.

60. Hippe, E., Jensen, K. B., Olesen, H., Lind, K., and Thomsen, P. E. B.: Chlorambucil treatment of patients with cold agglutinin syndrome. *Blood* 35:68, 1970.

61. Evans, R. S., Baxter, E., and Gilliland, B. D.: Chronic hemolytic anemia due to cold agglutinins: A 20-year history of benign gammopathy with response to chlorambucil. *Blood* 42:463, 1973.

62. McCurdy, P. R., and Rath, C. E.: Splenectomy in hemolytic anemia: Results predicted by body scanning after injection of Cr⁵¹-tagged red cells. *N. Engl. J. Med.* 259:459, 1958.

63. Pirofsky, B.: *Autoimmunization and the Autoimmune Hemolytic Anemias.* Williams & Wilkins, Baltimore, 1969.

64. Bell, C. A., Zwicker, H., and Sacks, H. J.: Autoimmune hemolytic anemia. *Am. J. Clin. Path.* 60:903, 1973.

65. Pisciotta, A. V.: Cold hemagglutination in acute and chronic hemolytic syndromes. *Blood* 10:295, 1955.

66. Taft, E. G., Propp, R. P., and Sullivan, S. A.: Plasma exchange for cold agglutinin hemolytic anemia. *Transfusion* 17:173, 1977.

67. Rosenfield, R. E., and Jagathambal: Transfusion therapy for autoimmune hemolytic anemia. *Semin. Hematol.* 13:311, 1976.

68. Götze, L.: Beitrag zur Jehre von der parorysmalen Hämaglobinurie. *Berlin Klin. Wochenschr.* 21:716, 1884.

69. Worlledge, S. M., and Rousso, C.: Studies of the serology of paroxysmal cold haemoglobinuria (P.C.H.) with special reference to its relationship with P blood group system. *Vox Sang.* 10:293, 1965.

70. Levine, P., Celano, M. J., and Falkowski, F.: The specificity of the antibody in paroxysmal cold hemaglobinuria (PCH). *Transfusion* 3:278, 1963.

71. Fellous, M., Gerbal, A., Tessier, C., Frezal, J., Dausett, J., and Salmon, C.: Studies of the biosynthetic pathway of human P erythrocyte antigens using somatic cells in culture. *Vox Sang.* 26:518, 1974.

CHAPTER **69**

Drug-related immunologic injury of erythrocytes

CHARLES H. PACKMAN
JOHN P. LEDDY

Definitions and history

Drug-related immune injury to red cells has been recognized for almost 30 years. This group of disorders must be distinguished from spontaneous forms of autoimmune hemolytic anemia (AHA) and from other drug-induced, nonimmune hemolytic reactions which occur upon exposure of inherently defective red cells to a drug or its metabolites (see Chap. 58). These distinctions are important because drug-induced immune hemolytic

TABLE 69-1 The association between drugs and positive red cell antiglobulin tests, with or without increased red cell destruction

Mechanism (see text)	Drugs	References
Hapten	Penicillin	[4–8]
	Cephalosporins	[9]
	Tetracycline	[10]
	Carbromal	[11]
Immune complex deposition	Quinine	[12]
	Quinidine	[13,14]
	Stibophen	[3]
	Chlorpropamide	[15]
	Rifampicin	[16]
	Antazoline	[17]
Autoantibody induction	Alpha-methyldopa	[18–21]
	L-Dopa	[22–26]
	Mefenamic acid	[27–29]
Nonimmunologic protein adsorption	Cephalothin	[29,30]
Mechanism of immune injury uncertain	Mesantoin	[2]
	Phenacetin	[12]
	Insecticides	[31]
	Chlorpromazine	[37]
	Melphalan	[33]
	Isoniazid	[34]
	p-Aminosalicylic acid	[35]
	Acetaminophen	[36]
	Thiazides	[37]
	Streptomycin	[38]
	Ibuprofen	[39]
	Procainamide	[40]
	Triamterene	[41]
	Erythromycin	[42]

anemia is usually a relatively benign process which, once recognized, is easily treated or prevented.

The first example of drug-related immune blood cell destruction was Ackroyd's description of "Sedormid purpura" in 1949 [1]. Shortly thereafter, descriptions of drug-induced immune red cell injury appeared. In 1953, Snapper and coworkers described a case of immune hemolysis and pancytopenia in a patient treated with mephenytoin (Mesantoin) [2]. The hemolysis ceased upon withdrawal of the drug. In 1956, Harris reported what are now classical studies of a patient who developed immune hemolytic anemia during a second course of stibophen for schistosomiasis [3]. Since then, many drugs have been implicated in the production of positive direct antiglobulin tests and/or accelerated red cell destruction.

Table 69-1 lists important drugs implicated in immune red cell injury, with selected references. In reviewing the literature, it is not always possible to assign the probable mechanism of immune injury or even to be certain the cited drug is unequivocally involved in the pathogenesis of the hemolytic anemia. However, it is important for the clinician to be aware of these potential associations as part of a careful evaluation of the possible role of drugs in patients with immune hemolytic anemia.

Etiology and pathogenesis

It is a well-established immunologic principle that low-molecular-weight substances such as drugs are not immunogenic in their own right. Stimulation of the formation of antidrug antibody is thought to require firm chemical coupling of the drug (as a haptenic group) to a protein carrier. The protein(s) serving such a carrier function in this inductive phase may or may not be a component of the target tissue (e.g., red cell) which the antidrug antibody may ultimately damage during the effector phase of this process.

Four distinct mechanisms of drug-mediated immunologic injury to red cells have been recognized (Table 69-2).

HAPTEN MECHANISM
This mechanism applies to drugs which bind firmly to proteins, including those on the red cell surface. Penicillin is the prime example [4–8]. Most individuals who have received penicillin therapy develop IgM antibodies directed against the benzylpenicilloyl determinant of penicillin, but this antibody plays no role in penicillin-related immune injury to red cells. The antibody responsible for hemolytic anemia is of the IgG class, occurs less frequently than the IgM antibody, and

TABLE 69-2 Characteristics of positive direct antiglobulin tests and hemolytic anemia related to drug ingestion

Mechanism	Hapten	Immune complex	Autoantibody induction	Nonimmunologic protein adsorption
Prototype drug	Penicillin	Quinidine	α-Methyldopa	Cephalothin
Role of drug	Binds to red cell membrane	Forms immune complex with antibody	Induces formation of antibody to native red cell antigens	? Alters red cell membrane
Drug affinity to red cell	Strong	Weak	None demonstrated	Strong
Antibody to drug	Present	Present	Absent	Absent
Antibody class predominating	IgG	IgM	IgG	None
Proteins detected by direct antiglobulin test	IgG, rarely complement	Complement	IgG, rarely complement	Multiple plasma proteins
Dose of drug associated with positive antiglobulin test	High	Low	High	High
Presence of drug required for indirect antiglobulin test	Yes (coating test red cells)	Yes (added to test medium)	No	Yes (added to test medium)
Mechanism of red cell destruction	Splenic sequestration of IgG-coated cells	Direct lysis by complement sequence plus clearance of C3b-cells	Splenic sequestration	None

may be directed against the benzylpenicilloyl [7] or, more commonly, nonbenzylpenicilloyl determinants [4–6,8]. Other manifestations of penicillin sensitivity are usually not present.

Patients receiving high doses of penicillin develop substantial coating of their red cells with penicillin. This penicillin coating itself is not injurious. If the dose of penicillin is very high (10 to 30 million units per day, or less in the setting of renal failure) and if the patient has an IgG antipenicillin antibody, the antibody binds to the red cell–bound penicillin molecules and the direct antiglobulin test with anti-IgG becomes positive [5,7, 8,13,43,44]. Antibody eluted from such patients' red cells, or present in the serum, reacts (in indirect antiglobulin tests) only against penicillin-coated red cells.

Destruction of red cells coated with penicillin and IgG anti-penicillin antibody occurs mainly through splenic sequestration [6,45], as with IgG autoantibodies (Chap. 67). Importantly, not all patients receiving high-dose penicillin develop a positive direct antiglobulin reaction or hemolytic anemia, since only a small proportion of such individuals produce the requisite antibody. Hemolytic anemia due to penicillin is subacute in onset, occurs typically only after the patient has received the drug for 7 to 10 days, and ceases a few days to weeks after discontinuation of the drug.

Cephalosporins have antigenic cross-reactivity with penicillin [46–48] and also bind firmly to red cell membranes. Hemolytic anemia, similar to that seen with penicillin, has been ascribed to cephalothin administration [9], but this is rare. Tetracycline may also cause hemolysis by this mechanism [10]. Carbromal causes positive IgG antiglobulin reactions by a similar mechanism [11], but hemolytic anemia has not been described.

IMMUNE COMPLEX MECHANISM

This mechanism can mediate immune injury of red cells, platelets, and probably of leukocytes. Although not yet fully understood, the immune complex mechanism differs from the hapten mechanism in three important ways. First, the drugs themselves exhibit only weak affinity for blood cell membranes. Second, only a small dose of drug is required to trigger hemolysis. Third, red cell injury is mediated chiefly via the complement system. In common with penicillin-induced hemolytic anemia, the relevant antibodies can interact with red cells only in the presence of the offending drug.

The pathogenesis of the immune complex mechanism has been extensively studied in drug-induced thrombocytopenia. A very analogous mechanism appears to be operative in immune red cell destruction by these drugs [49–51]. In well-studied examples (e.g., quinidine antibodies), complexes consisting of IgM antibodies and drug have been implicated in red cell destruction [13,51], whereas drug–IgG antibody complexes have been correlated with platelet injury [51]. Exceptions to these examples have been noted [15,17,52]. Preferential platelet injury by IgG complexes probably relates to the presence of IgG Fc receptors on human platelets [53]. Human red cells lack Fc receptors but possess a small number of C3b receptors [54] which may facilitate uptake of complement-bearing IgM complexes.

Hemolysis by this mechanism is believed to occur when the offending drug combines with preformed antibody in the plasma. The resulting immune complexes appear to bind reversibly to red cells (or platelets) and induce activation and binding of complement components to the cell membrane. The immune complexes can migrate from cell to cell, fixing complement at each stop. This may partially explain why small quantities of drug, and therefore of drug-antidrug complexes, are able to damage a large number of blood cells. Cell destruction may occur intravascularly after completion of the whole complement sequence. Some destruction of C3b-coated (but unlysed) red cells may be mediated by splenic and liver sequestration via the C3b receptors on macrophages. The direct antiglobulin test is positive only with anticomplement reagents. Since the responsible antibodies have little or no affinity for the red cell itself, and the immune complexes interact only transiently with the red cell membrane, this type of immune injury has also been termed the *innocent bystander* mechanism.

AUTOANTIBODY INDUCTION

The principal offender is α-methyldopa [18–21]. L-Dopa and an unrelated drug used for treatment of arthritis, mefenamic acid, have also been incriminated in the mechanism [22–28]. Positive direct antiglobulin reactions (with anti-IgG reagents) in patients taking α-methyldopa vary in frequency from 8 to 36 percent. Patients taking higher doses of the drug develop antiglobulin positivity with greater frequency [18,20,21]. There is a lag period of 3 to 6 months between the start of therapy and development of a positive antiglobulin test. This delay is not shortened when the drug is readministered to patients who previously had positive antiglobulin tests while taking α-methyldopa [20].

In contrast to the frequent observation of positive antiglobulin reactions, less than 1 percent of patients taking α-methyldopa exhibit hemolytic anemia [19,55]. Development of hemolytic anemia does not seem to depend upon drug dosage. The hemolysis is usually mild to moderate and occurs chiefly by splenic sequestration of IgG-coated red cells.

The direct antiglobulin reaction is usually positive only for IgG [52,56]. Occasionally, weak anticomplement reactions are encountered as well [56]. Patients who have immune hemolytic anemia due to α-methyldopa therapy typically have strongly positive direct an-

tiglobulin reactions as well as serum antibody, evidenced by the indirect antiglobulin reaction [56]. (See Chap. 67 for explanation of direct and indirect antiglobulin tests.) Antibodies in the serum or eluted from red cell membranes react optimally at 37°C with unaltered autologous or homologous red cells *in the absence of drug* [19,21,57]. The antibodies frequently show evidence of specificity for determinants of the Rh complex [19,21,57].

In this form of drug-induced immune injury, the antibodies appear to be true autoantibodies reactive with native red cell antigens. It is not possible to distinguish these antibodies from similar warm-reacting autoantibodies in idiopathic AHA. Thus, the mechanism by which these methyldopa-associated autoantibodies arise is of special interest for students of autoimmune diseases. The radiolabeled drug does not appear to react directly with human red cells [21]. A recent study suggests that α-methyldopa may interact with human T lymphocytes, resulting in loss of suppressor cell function and formation of autoantibodies by B lymphocytes [58].

NONIMMUNOLOGIC PROTEIN ADSORPTION

A small proportion (less than 5 percent) of patients receiving cephalosporin antibiotics develop positive antiglobulin reactions [56,59] due to nonspecific adsorption of plasma proteins to red cell membranes [29,30,60]. This may occur within a day or two after the drug is instituted. Multiple plasma proteins, including immunoglobulins, complement, albumin, fibrinogen, and others, may be detected on red cell membranes in such cases [60,61]. Hemolytic anemia due to this mechanism has not been reported. The main clinical importance of this phenomenon is its potential to produce difficulties in cross-match procedures unless the drug history is taken into account. As noted above, cephalosporin antibiotics may also induce red cell injury by the hapten mechanism, but this appears to occur much less frequently than the nonimmunologic reaction.

Clinical features

A careful history of drug exposure should be obtained in all patients with hemolytic anemia or a positive direct antiglobulin test. As in idiopathic AHA (Chaps. 67 and 68), the clinical picture in drug immune hemolytic anemia is quite variable. The severity of symptoms is largely dependent upon the rate of hemolysis. In general, patients with hapten (e.g., penicillin) and autoimmune (e.g., α-methyldopa) types of drug-induced hemolytic anemia exhibit mild to moderate red cell destruction with insidious onset of symptoms developing over a period of days to weeks. In contrast, patients with immune complex hemolysis (e.g., quinine or quinidine) may have sudden onset of severe hemolysis with hemoglobinuria. In the latter setting, hemolysis can occur after only one dose of the drug if the patient has been previously exposed to the drug. Acute renal failure may accompany severe hemolysis by the immune complex mechanism [52].

Laboratory features

The hematologic findings are similar to those described for spontaneously occurring AHA (Chaps. 67 and 68). Most patients exhibit anemia and reticulocytosis, as evidence of increased red cell turnover. Leukopenia and thrombocytopenia may be noted in cases of immune complex–mediated hemolysis. The serological features are summarized above and in Table 69-2.

Differential diagnosis

Immune hemolysis due to drugs must be distinguished from (1) the warm and cold antibody types of idiopathic AHA, (2) congenital hemolytic anemias such as hereditary spherocytosis, and (3) drug-mediated hemolysis due to disorders of red cell metabolism such as G-6-PD deficiency. Patients with drug-related immune hemolytic anemia exhibit a positive direct antiglobulin test. This feature would generally make the disorders in groups 2 and 3 less likely.

In the hapten mechanism of immune injury associated with penicillin, the patient's red cells are coated with IgG or, rarely, with both IgG and complement components. Such cases could have superficial resemblance to warm antibody AHA. The key serological difference is that in penicillin-related immune hemolytic anemia the antibodies in the patient's serum or eluted from the patient's red cells react *only* with penicillin-coated red cells. In contrast, the IgG antibodies in warm-type AHA react with unmodified human red cells and may show preference for certain known blood groups (e.g., within the Rh complex). Such serological distinction plus the history of exposure to high blood levels of penicillin should be decisive.

In immune complex–mediated hemolysis, the direct antiglobulin test is positive with anticomplement serum. Immunoglobulins are not detectable on the patient's red cells. This pattern is similar to that encountered in AHA mediated by cold agglutinins. Moreover, the brisk type of hemolysis in the drug-immune complex mechanism is also seen in certain cases of cold antibody AHA (Chap. 68). In the drug-induced cases, however, the cold agglutinin titer and the Donath-Landsteiner test are normal, and the demonstration of serum antibody acting on human red cells is dependent upon the presence of the drug in the test system. For example, the indirect antiglobulin reaction with anticomplement serum may be positive if the incubation mixture permits the interaction of (1) normal red cells, (2) antidrug antibody from the patient's serum, (3) the relevant drug, either still in the patient's serum or added in vitro in appropriate concentration, and (4) a source of complement, i.e., fresh normal serum or the patient's own serum if freshly obtained. A negative result does not necessarily absolve the suspected drug because the critical haptenic group could be a metabolic derivative of the drug in question.

In patients with autoimmune hemolytic anemia due to α-methyldopa, the direct antiglobulin reaction is strongly positive for IgG but only rarely is complement detected on the patient's red cells. Anti-red cell autoantibody is regularly present in the serum of these patients and mediates a positive indirect antiglobulin reaction with unmodified human red cells, often showing specificity related to the Rh complex. There is, however, no presently available specific serological test to separate idiopathic warm-reacting IgG autoantibodies with Rh-related specificities from those induced by methyldopa administration. The evidence must be circumstantial, with the helpful knowledge that discontinuation of α-methyldopa, without any form of immunosuppressive therapy, has consistently permitted a slow but definite recovery from anemia and a gradual disappearance of anti-red cell antibodies.

It should be recognized that in recently transfused patients, a positive "direct" antiglobulin test might really reflect the binding of newly formed *allo*antibodies to transfused donor red cells. Neither the drugs the patient is receiving nor autoantibodies may be involved.

Finally, helpful information may be gained by stopping any drug that is suspect. The patient is then monitored for improvement in hematocrit level, decrease in reticulocytosis, and gradual disappearance of the positive antiglobulin reaction. Rechallenge with the suspected drug may confirm the diagnosis, but this measure is seldom necessary in patient management, and may be unsafe.

Therapy

Discontinuation of the offending drug is often the only treatment needed. This measure is essential, and may be lifesaving, in patients with severe hemolysis mediated by the immune complex mechanism. In some cases of mild hemolytic anemia due to penicillin, it may be possible and advisable to continue the drug in certain clinical settings (see below). Glucocorticoids are generally unnecessary, and their efficacy is questionable. Transfusions should be given in the unusual circumstance of severe, life-threatening anemia. Problems with cross-matching, similar to those encountered in warm antibody AHA, may occur in patients with a strongly positive indirect antiglobulin test, e.g., in α-methyldopa–related cases. Patients with hemolytic anemia due to the drug hapten mechanism should have a compatible cross-match because the plasma antibody reacts only with the drug-coated cells. However, if therapy with the offending drug is still in progress, transfused cells may be destroyed at an increased rate as they become coated with drug in vivo.

In patients taking α-methyldopa, antiglobulin testing should be performed at 4- to 6-month intervals, or with the development of anemia. The drug should be discontinued in patients who develop hemolytic anemia. In the absence of anemia, a positive direct antiglobulin test is not necessarily an indication for stopping the drug. Since a positive *indirect* antiglobulin reaction (due to autoantibody in the patient's serum) may interfere with cross-matching procedures, it may be prudent to consider alternative antihypertensive therapy for such patients. This would apply particularly to patients who are anemic for reasons unrelated to α-methyldopa therapy and who may subsequently require blood transfusion.

High-dose penicillin is the treatment of choice in several life-threatening infections. If alternative antibiotic regimens are clearly inferior to penicillin, the drug need not be discontinued because of a positive direct antiglobulin reaction alone. A change in therapy is indicated only in the presence of overt hemolytic anemia. Lowering the penicillin dose, e.g., by using a combination of antibiotics, may allow continuation of the drug in some cases, particularly if hemolysis is not severe.

Course and prognosis

Immune hemolysis due to drugs is usually mild, and the prognosis good. Occasional episodes of exceptionally severe hemolysis and death have been reported, usually due to drugs operating through the immune complex mechanism [52]. In hemolysis due to immune complex or hapten mechanisms, the direct antiglobulin test becomes negative within a short time after the drug is discontinued, i.e., soon after the drug is cleared from the circulation. In cases of autoantibody formation due to α-methyldopa, a positive direct antiglobulin test (of gradually diminishing intensity) may remain for weeks or months, although the hemolysis usually ceases promptly after cessation of the drug.

References

1. Ackroyd, J. F.: The pathogenesis of thrombocytopenic purpura due to hypersensitivity to Sedormid (allylisopropyl-acetylcarbamide). *Clin. Sci. 7:249,* 1949.
2. Snapper, I., Marks, D., Schwartz, L., and Hollander, L.: Hemolytic anemia secondary to Mesantoin. *Ann. Intern. Med. 39:619,* 1953.
3. Harris, J. W.: Studies on the mechanism of drug-induced hemolytic anemia. *J. Lab. Clin. Med. 47:760,* 1956.
4. VanArsdel, P. P., Jr., and Gilliland, B. C.: Anemia secondary to penicillin treatment: Studies on two patients with non-allergic serum hemagglutinins. *J. Lab. Clin. Med. 65:277,* 1965.
5. Petz, L. D., and Fudenberg, H. H.: Coombs-positive hemolytic anemia caused by penicillin administration. *N. Engl. J. Med. 274:171,* 1966.
6. Swanson, M. A., Chanmougan, D., and Schwartz, R. S.: Immunohemolytic anemia due to antipenicillin antibodies. *N. Engl. J. Med. 274:178,* 1966.
7. Levine, B., and Redmond, A.: Immunochemical mechanisms of penicillin induced Coombs positivity and hemolytic anemia in man. *Int. Arch. Allergy Appl. Immunol. 1:594,* 1967.
8. White, J. M., Brown, D. L., Hepner, G. W., and Worlledge, S. M.: Penicillin induced hemolytic anaemia. *Br. Med. J. 3:26,* 1968.
9. Gralnick, H. R., McGinnis, M. H., Elton, W., and McCurdy, P.: Hemolytic anemia associated with cephalothin. *JAMA 217:1193,* 1971.
10. Wenz, B., Klein, R. L., and Lalezari, P.: Tetracycline-induced immune hemolytic anemia. *Transfusion 14:265,* 1974.
11. Stefanini, M., and Johnson, N. L.: Positive antihuman globulin test in patients receiving carbromal. *Am. J. Med. Sci. 259:49,* 1970.
12. Muirhead, E. E., Halden, E. R., and Granes, M.: Drug dependent Coombs (antiglobulin) test and anemia: Observations on quinine and acetophenetidine (phenacetin). *Arch. Intern. Med 101:827,* 1958.
13. Croft, J. D., Jr., Swisher, S. N., Gilliland, B. C., Bakemeier, R. F., Leddy, J. P., and Weed, R. I.: Coombs test positivity induced by drugs: Mechanisms of immunologic reactions and red cell destruction. *Ann. Intern. Med 68:176,* 1968.
14. Freedman, A. L., Barr, P. S., and Brody, E.: Hemolytic anemia due to quinidine: Observations on its mechanism. *Am. J. Med. 20:806,* 1956.
15. Logue, G. L., Boyd, A. E., and Rosse, W. F.: Chlorpropamide-induced immune hemolytic anemia. *N. Engl. J. Med. 283:900,* 1970.
16. Lakshminarayan, S., Sahn, S. A., and Hudson, L. D.: Massive hemolysis caused by rifampicin. *Br. Med. J. 2:282,* 1973.
17. Bengtsson, U., Staffan, A., Aurell, M., and Kaijser, B.: Antazoline-induced immune hemolytic anemia, hemoglobinuria and acute renal failure. *Acta Med. Scand. 198:223,* 1975.
18. Carstairs, K. C., Breckenridge, A., Dollery, C. T., and Worlledge, S. M.: Incidence of a positive direct Coombs test in patients on alpha-methyldopa. *Lancet 2:133,* 1966.
19. Worlledge, S. M., Carstairs, K. C., and Dacie, J. V.: Autoimmune haemolytic anaemia associated with α-methyldopa therapy. *Lancet 2:133,* 1966.
20. Breckenridge, A., Dollery, C. T., Worlledge, S. M., Holborow, E. J., and Johnson, G. D.: Positive direct Coombs tests and antinuclear factors in patients treated with methyldopa. *Lancet 2:1265,* 1967.
21. Lo Buglio, A. F., and Jandl, J. H.: The nature of alpha-methyldopa red cell antibody. *N. Engl. J. Med. 276:658,* 1967.
22. Cotzias, G. C., and Papavasiliou, P. S.: Autoimmunity in patients treated with levodopa. *JAMA 207:1353,* 1969.
23. Henry, R. E., Goldberg, L. S., Sturgeon, P., and Ansel, R. D.: Serologic abnormalities associated with L-dopa therapy. *Vox Sang. 20:306,* 1971.
24. Joseph, C.: Occurrence of positive Coombs test in patients treated with levodopa. *N. Engl. J. Med. 286:1400,* 1972.
25. Gabor, E. P., and Goldberg, L. S.: Levodopa induced Coombs positive haemolytic anaemia. *Scand. J. Haematol. 11:201,* 1973.
26. Territo, M. C., Peters, R. W., and Tanaka, K. R.: Autoimmune hemolytic anemia due to levodopa therapy. *JAMA 226:1347,* 1973.
27. Scott, G. L., Myles, A. B., and Bacon, P. A.: Autoimmune haemolytic anaemia and mefenamic acid therapy. *Br. Med. J. 3:543,* 1968.
28. Robertson, J. H., Kennedy, C. C., and Hill, C. M.: Haemolytic anaemia associated with mefenamic acid. *Br. Med. J. 140:226,* 1971.
29. Gralnick, H. R., Wright, L. D., and McGinnis, M. H.: Coombs' positive reactions associated with sodium cephalothin therapy. *JAMA 199:725,* 1967.
30. Molthan, L., Reidenberg, M. M., and Eichman, M. F.: Positive direct Coombs' tests due to cephalothin. *N. Engl. J. Med. 277:123,* 1967.
31. Muirhead, E. E., Groves, M., Guy, R., Halden, E. R., and Bass, R. K.: Acquired hemolytic anemia, exposures to insecticides and positive Coombs' test dependent on insecticide preparations. *Vox Sang. 4:277,* 1959.
32. Lindberg, L. G., and Norden, A.: Severe hemolytic reaction to chlorpromazine. *Acta Med. Scand. 170:195,* 1961.
33. Eyster, M. E.: Melphalan (Alkeran) erythrocyte agglutinin and hemolytic anemia. *Ann. Intern. Med. 66:573,* 1967.
34. Robinson, M. G., and Foadi, M.: Hemolytic anemia with positive Coombs' test: Association with isoniazid therapy. *JAMA 208:656,* 1969.
35. Mueller-Eckhardt, C., Kretschmer, V., and Coburg, K. H.: Allergic, immunohemolytic anemia due to para-aminosalicylic acid (PAS). Immunohematologic studies of three cases. *Dtsch. Med. Wochenschr. 97:234,* 1972.
36. Manor, E., Marmor, A., Kaufman, S., and Leiba, H.: Massive hemolysis caused by acetaminophen. *JAMA 236:2777,* 1976.

37. Vila, J. M., Blum, L., and Dosik, H.: Thiazide-induced immune hemolytic anemia. *JAMA* 236:1723, 1976.
38. Martinez, L., et al.: Immune haemolytic anaemia and renal failure induced by streptomycin. *Br. J. Haematol.* 35:561, 1977.
39. Korsager, S.: Hemolysis complicating ibuprofen treatment. *Br. Med. J.* 1:79, 1978.
40. Jones, G. W., George, T. L., and Bradley, R. D.: Procainamide-induced hemolytic anemia. *Transfusion* 18:224, 1978.
41. Takahaski, H., and Tsukada, T.: Triamterine-induced immune hemolytic anemia with acute intravascular hemolysis and acute renal failure. *Scand. J. Haematol.* 23:169, 1979.
42. Wong, K. Y., Boose, G. M., and Issitt, C. H.: Erythromycin-induced hemolytic anemia. *J. Pediatr.* 98:647, 1981.
43. Kerr, R. O., Cardamone, J., Dalmasso, A. P., and Kaplan, M. E.: Two mechanisms of erythrocyte destruction in penicillin-induced hemolytic anemia. *N. Engl. J. Med.* 287:1322, 1972.
44. Ries, C. A., Rosenbaum, T. J., Garratty, G., Petz, L. D., and Fudenberg, H. H.: Penicillin-induced immune hemolytic anemia. Occurrence of massive intravascular hemolysis. *JAMA* 233:432, 1975.
45. Nesmith, L. W., and Davis, J. W.: Hemolytic anemia caused by penicillin. *JAMA* 203:27, 1968.
46. Brandriss, M. W., Smith, J. W., and Steinman, H. G.: Common antigenic determinants of penicillin G, cephalothin and 6-aminopenicillanic acid in rabbits. *J. Immunol.* 94:696, 1965.
47. Abraham, G. N., Petz, L. D., and Fudenberg, H. H.: Immunohematological cross-allergenicity between penicillin and cephalothin in humans. *Clin. Exp. Immunol.* 3:343, 1968.
48. Petz, L. D.: Immunologic cross reactivity between penicillins and cephalosporins: A review. *J. Infect. Dis.* 137:S74, 1978.
49. Ackroyd, J. F.: The immunological basis of purpura due to drug hypersensitivity. *Proc. R. Soc. Med.* 55:30, 1962.
50. Shulman, N. R.: Mechanism of blood cell damage by adsorption of antigen-antibody complexes, in *Immunopathology, III International Symposium*, edited by P. Grabar and P. A. Miescher. Schwabe, Basel, 1963, p. 388.
51. Schulman, N. R.: A mechanism of cell destruction in individuals sensitized to foreign antigens and its implications in autoimmunity. *Ann. Intern. Med.* 60:506, 1964.
52. Worlledge, S. M.: Immune drug-induced hemolytic anemias. *Semin. Hematol.* 10:327, 1973.
53. Fearon, D. T.: Identification of the membrane glycoprotein that is the C3b receptor of the human erythrocyte, polymorphonuclear leukocyte, B lymphocyte and monocyte. *J. Exp. Med.* 152:20, 1980.
54. Henson, P. M., and Spiegelberg, H. L.: Release of serotonin from human platelets induced by aggregated immunoglobulins of different classes and subclasses. *J. Clin. Invest.* 52:1282, 1973.
55. Worlledge, S. M.: Immune drug-induced haemolytic anaemias. *Semin. Hematol.* 6:181, 1969.
56. Petz, L. D., and Garrity, G. (eds.): *Acquired Immune Hemolytic Anemia.* Churchill Livingstone, New York, 1980.
57. Bakemeier, R. F., and Leddy, J. P.: Erythrocyte autoantibody associated with alpha-methyldopa: Heterogeneity of structure and specificity. *Blood* 32:1, 1968.
58. Kirtland, H. H., III, Mohler, D. N., Horwitz, D. A.: Methyldopa inhibition of suppressor-lymphocyte function. A proposed cause of autoimmune hemolytic anemia. *N. Engl. J. Med.* 302:825, 1980.
59. Swisher, S. N.: Antibiotics and red blood cells, in *Drugs and Hematologic Reactions,* edited by N. V. Dimitrov and J. H. Nodine. Grune & Stratton, New York, 1974, p. 123.
60. Spath, P., Garratty, G., and Petz, L. D.: Studies on the immune response to penicillin and cephalothin in humans. II. Immunohematologic reactions to cephalothin administration. *J. Immunol.* 107:860, 1971.
61. Garraty, G., and Petz, L.: Drug-induced hemolytic anemia. *Am. J. Med.* 58:398, 1975.

CHAPTER 70

Alloimmune hemolytic disease of the newborn

JOHN M. BOWMAN

Definition and history

Alloimmune hemolytic disease of the newborn (erythroblastosis fetalis) is a disease of the fetus and newborn infant characterized by hemolytic anemia, extramedullary erythropoiesis, and hyperbilirubinemia. Anasarca (hydrops fetalis) with fetal or neonatal death occurs in 20 to 25 percent of cases. Severe neonatal jaundice (icterus gravis) with risk of brain damage (kernicterus) occurs in another 25 to 30 percent.

Hydrops fetalis and kernicterus were described in a set of twins as early as 1608, and exchange transfusion was carried out for this disease as early as 1925 [1]. However elucidation of the etiology and pathogenesis of hemolytic disease had to await the epoch-making rhesus monkey red cell studies of Landsteiner and Wiener in 1940 [2].

In the 40 years since their work, the complexities of the Rh blood group system have been unraveled and many other blood group systems have been discovered. Sensitive manual and automated methods of screening maternal blood for blood group antibodies and measuring their strength have been developed [3,4]. The pathogenesis of icterus gravis, kernicterus, and hydrops fetalis have been defined clearly. Methods of diagnosing hemolytic disease after birth (the direct antiglobulin or Coombs' test [5]), of determining severity of hemolytic disease in utero (amniocentesis [6]), and of managing the affected fetus and newborn infant (early delivery [7], intrauterine fetal transfusion [8], exchange transfusion [9]) have been introduced. Finally, prevention of Rh immunization by the administration of Rh antibody in the form of Rh immune globulin (Rh IgG) has been developed and implemented [10–12].

Etiology and pathogenesis

THE Rh BLOOD GROUP SYSTEM

Although other blood group antigens may cause alloimmunization and hemolytic disease of the newborn, D antigen in the Rh blood group system is by far the most important [13]. According to the CDE nomenclature and theories of inheritance of Fisher and Race [14], there are three pairs of genetically determined antigens: Cc, D(d), Ee. The presence or absence of D determines the Rh-positive or Rh-negative status of the individual. Since no antibody with the specificity anti-d has ever been found, the antigen (d) is hypothetical. It is the production of anti-D in the Rh(D)-negative woman and the transplacental passage of anti-D into the circulation of the Rh-positive fetus that causes hemolytic disease of the newborn. Each parent transmits a set of the three antigens [CDe, c(d)e, cDE are the commonest] to the fetus, who may therefore be Rh(D)-negative (dd), Rh-positive heterozygous for D (Dd), or homozygous for D (DD). The zygosity for D of the Rh-positive husband of the Rh-negative woman is important. If he is homozygous, all of their children will be D-positive; if heterozygous, in each pregnancy the chances are equal that the fetus will be D-positive or D-negative. Only the D-positive fetus can provoke Rh immunization, and only the D-positive fetus will be affected by the anti-D produced.

About 15 percent of Caucasians are D-negative, and almost half of those who are D-positive are homozygous for D. The incidence of D-negativity in other races is much less, ranging from about 8 percent in North American blacks to less than 1 percent in the oriental races. The incidence in Basques is more than twice that of other Caucasians.

Blood transfusion remains a common cause of atypical alloimmunization to antigens of potential clinical importance such as c, Kell, C, and E. Only when there is a hospital or laboratory error is transfusion now a cause of Rh(D) immunization. Transplacental passage of fetal D-positive red cells, postulated by Wiener in 1948 [15] and proved by Chown in 1954 [16], is now the way in which the Rh-negative mother becomes Rh-immunized. As demonstrated by the Kleihauer technique [17], it occurs in at least 50 percent of pregnancies, increasing in frequency and size as pregnancy progresses and reaching a maximum at the time of delivery. In the majority of instances transplacental hemorrhage amounts to less than 0.1 ml of red cells but can occasionally be greater than 12 to 15 ml of red cells [18].

Following exposure to D-positive red cells, the development of a primary immune response is slow, requiring weeks or even months, and initially may consist of IgM, which does not cross the placenta. Sensitization occurs in 7 to 8 percent of women at risk within 6 months after delivery of an ABO-compatible fetus, and in 2 percent after delivery of an ABO-incompatible fetus. An equal number demonstrate that they were sensitized by mounting a secondary immune response in the next Rh-positive pregnancy. In addition, sensitive enzyme screening tests have shown that about 2 percent of women at risk undergo primary Rh sensitization during pregnancy [19,20].

The dose of Rh antigen influences the risk of immunization. As little as 0.1 ml of ABO-compatible D-positive red cells will provoke a primary immune response in 3 percent of women [21]; a dose in excess of 5 ml will provoke a response in 60 percent. The overall risk of Rh immunization is 17 percent if the D-positive fetus is ABO-compatible [22]. Spontaneous or therapeutic abortion carries with it a 2 to 4 percent risk of Rh im-

munization. Complications such as preeclampsia and obstetrical procedures such as amniocentesis, external version, cesarean section, and manual removal of the placenta increase the risk of transplacental passage of fetal red cells and the risk of Rh immunization. The secondary immune response which may be evoked by a very small amount of fetal red cells (< 0.1 ml) is rapid in onset, strong, and predominantly IgG in nature.

IgG anti-D traverses the placenta and coats fetal Rh-positive red cells. The coated red cells form rosettes around macrophages primarily in the spleen. Phagocyte pseudopodia invaginate the red cell membrane, causing membrane loss, sphering, erythrophagocytosis, and ultimately lysis. Hemolysis produces anemia, erythropoietin production, compensatory medullary and extramedullary erythropoiesis, and hepatosplenomegaly with an outpouring of immature nucleated red cells. In the most severe cases portal and umbilical venous pressures rise and ascites occurs. Further anemia and intrahepatic circulatory obstruction cause hepatocellular damage, hypoalbuminemia, and generalized anasarca. The fetus, now hydropic, either dies in utero or if born alive frequently cannot be saved.

In utero the toxic product of hemolysis (unconjugated bilirubin) is for the most part cleared across the placenta. It is conjugated by the maternal liver to bilirubin diglucuronide and is excreted. Despite placental clearance, total bilirubin levels in the severely affected fetus at birth may be as high as 8 to 10 mg per deciliter of plasma (137 to 171 μmol/liter), a significant portion of which may be direct-acting conjugated bilirubin due to hepatocellular damage. After birth the infant's immature hepatic Y-transport and glucuronyl transferase mechanism is unable to conjugate the large amounts of bilirubin produced by red cell hemolysis. If left untreated, the bilirubin-binding capacity of albumin is rapidly exceeded. Free, lipid-soluble, unconjugated bilirubin traverses the lipid cell membrane of the neurons, interferes with vital intracellular metabolic processes, and causes neuron cell death. At autopsy, cerebellar tonsils, hippocampal gyrus, midbrain, and medullary nuclei are stained bright yellow (kernicterus).

Thrombocytopenia is common in severely affected babies, and with hypoxia, which causes capillary endothelial damage, it aggravates the hemorrhagic tendency of the neonate.

ABO erythroblastosis serologically is much more common than Rh erythroblastosis and often occurs in first pregnancies. It never produces severe anemia but may produce hyperbilirubinemia severe enough to require treatment. ABO disease usually occurs in type A or B babies born of type O mothers who are more prone to produce IgG anti-A or anti-B than type A or B mothers with ABO-incompatible fetuses. The disease is milder because most anti-A and anti-B are IgM and do not cross the placenta; A and B antigens are ubiquitous and present in many fetal tissues and body fluids. However, they are relatively poorly developed in the red cell at birth.

Hemolytic disease due to anti-c or anti-Kell is much rarer than hemolytic disease due to anti-D but does not differ in degree of severity or outlook. Disease due to anti-C or anti-E is usually but not invariably very mild. Other blood group antibodies as a general rule produce minimal, if any, hemolytic disease.

Clinical features

Fifty percent of erythroblastotic infants are mildly affected, develop only mild hyperbilirubinemia and/or anemia, and recover without treatment. Twenty-five to thirty percent are born in good condition but with mild to moderate pallor. If examined carefully, they appear slightly jaundiced at birth or within an hour or two after birth. Varying degrees of hepatosplenomegaly are present, but edema is absent. If these infants are not treated, jaundice progresses rapidly and within 2 to 4 days of birth they show evidence of brain damage. Initially they become hypotonic and refuse to suck; then they lose their neurovegetative reflexes. They become spastic, lie in a position of opisthotonus, and may convulse. Respiratory failure supervenes, and most of these infants die. The 10 percent who survive have devastating brain damage, characterized by choreoathetosis, severe nerve deafness, and some degree of mental retardation. Prematurity and complications of prematurity such as asphyxia and acidosis lower the blood-brain barrier and interfere with albumin binding, and thus increase the risk of kernicterus at bilirubin levels which would not be hazardous in a full-term, nonasphyxiated, nonacidotic infant. Similarly, the presence of salicylate, benzoate, or sulfonamide radicals will reduce reserve albumin-binding capacity and increase the risk of kernicterus. Heparin may also increase the risk by raising the levels of nonesterified free fatty acids.

The most severely affected 20 to 25 percent of fetuses are grossly hydropic. Half become so between 34 and 40 weeks' gestation, the other half between 22 and 34 weeks' gestation. The majority die in utero. The occasional hydropic infant born alive presents with extreme pallor, gross ascites, and generalized edema. Pleural effusions and pulmonary compression frequently thwart all resuscitative attempts. Contrary to what was once believed, hepatic obstruction and hepatocellular damage rather than heart failure are the primary causes of hydrops fetalis [23,24]. Moderate disease and hydrops fetalis grade one into the other. Intermediate prehydropic or early hydropic babies present with severe pallor, marked hepatosplenomegaly, petechiae, and moderate edema. Although heart failure is usually not present at birth, therapeutic measures frequently precipitate heart failure.

Anti-c and anti-Kell erythroblastosis do not differ in their clinical expression from anti-D erythroblastosis. Anti-C and anti-E rarely if ever produce hydrops, and anti-A and anti-B never do. Jaundice and the risk of ker-nicterus are the only clinical problems in anti-A, anti-B, anti-C, and anti-E hemolytic disease.

Mothers carrying severely affected erythroblastotic fetuses not infrequently present with polyhydramnios and a preeclampsia-like syndrome. If the disease is ameliorated by intrauterine fetal transfusion, the maternal syndrome disappears.

Laboratory features

MATERNAL
Maternal blood group antibody screening during pregnancy is essential. Only if alloimmunization is diagnosed early and followed carefully will optimal clinical management be possible. At the first prenatal visit the Rh group of maternal blood should be determined and the plasma screened for alloantibodies. Antibody screening tests such as the enzyme method [3] must be used since indirect antiglobulin tests are not sufficiently sensitive. Testing of the unimmunized Rh-negative mother should be repeated at 24 to 26 weeks' gestation and thereafter every 6 to 8 weeks until delivery. She is a candidate for Rh prophylaxis at 28 weeks' gestation and after delivery if she remains unimmunized. At the time of delivery, Kleihauer fetal cell testing [17], if available, should be carried out to determine the presence and size of transplacental hemorrhage, if any.

If the mother is found to be alloimmunized, the specificity of the antibody and its titer should be determined by either an albumin or indirect antiglobulin method. Repeat antibody titration should be carried out at 20 weeks' gestation and every 2 to 4 weeks thereafter until delivery. Since hydrops may develop as early as 22 weeks' gestation and intrauterine fetal transfusions may be successful as early as 22 weeks' gestation, the antibody titer upon which further laboratory tests will be based must be known by 20 weeks' gestation.

FETAL
The determination of the risk of hydrops and fetal death is based partially upon history and antibody titer. The disease is usually but not always as severe or more severe than in previously affected siblings. Antibody titers of 1:16 to 1:32 are usually the levels at which there is a risk of hydrops. History and antibody titer by themselves will predict severity of hemolytic disease accurately in only 62 percent of cases [7]. They do, however, allow the determination of the woman at risk who requires an amniocentesis to define degree of severity of hemolytic disease accurately [6,7].

Serial measurements of the optical density of the amniotic fluid at 450 nm provide information about the severity of hemolytic disease. They predict severity of hemolytic disease with 94 percent accuracy [18] and should be started as early as 20 weeks' gestation. Although amniocentesis carries no risk to the mother, traversing the placenta can be hazardous to the fetus and may increase the severity of alloimmunization. Amniocentesis should be carried out with careful ultrasound placental localization, which minimizes the risk of placental trauma. It should only be performed when maternal history and/or antibody titer indicate that the fetus is at significant risk.

Serial amniotic fluid ΔOD 450 readings rising into the upper 80 percent of Liley's zone 2 before 30 weeks' gestation or into zone 3 after 30 weeks' gestation indicate severe fetal disease, impending hydrops and fetal death, and the need for prompt therapeutic intervention [18].

NEONATAL

At the time of delivery, cord blood findings taken in conjunction with the clinical appearance of the infant will determine the need for, and the type of, treatment. A direct antiglobulin (Coombs') test should be done. The Coombs test is invariably positive in all forms of erythroblastosis with the exception of ABO sensitization. Even in this condition cord red cells are usually weakly positive if a sensitive Coombs test is used. Cord hemoglobin and unconjugated bilirubin estimations reflect severity of disease. Prompt treatment is indicated if the cord hemoglobin is less than 11 to 11.5 g/dl or the indirect bilirubin level is greater than 4.5 to 5 mg/dl (77 to 86 μmol/liter). If the infant is premature or has been asphyxiated, prompt treatment should be carried out at hemoglobin levels of less than 12.5 g/dl and bilirubin levels greater than 3.5 mg/dl (60 μmol/liter). Reticulocyte counts, although elevated, are not in themselves of much value in management; nucleated red cell counts are more helpful in assessing the degree of disease and the need for prompt treatment. The presence of conjugated bilirubin in cord blood or more than 2.5 mg/dl (43 μmol/liter) or heme (red-brown discoloration) is always indicative of severe hemolytic disease.

Whether treatment has been required initially or not, serial hemoglobin and unconjugated bilirubin measurements at 8- to 12-h intervals help determine further management. Unconjugated bilirubin levels rising at greater than 0.4 to 0.5 mg/dl (7 to 8 μmol/liter) per hour or absolute levels per deciliter of 8 to 10 mg (137 to 171 μmol/liter) at 12 h, 12 to 14 mg (205 to 239 μmol/liter) at 24 h, 15 to 16 mg (256 to 274 μmol/liter) at 36 h, 17 to 18 mg (291 to 308 μmol/liter) at 48 h, or 20 mg (342 μmol/liter) or more thereafter are indications for prompt therapeutic intervention. These criteria may be modified somewhat if measurements of free bilirubin [25] or reserve albumin-binding capacity [26] are available. If the reserve albumin-binding capacity is greater than 50 percent and the infant is mature and not acidotic, there is little if any risk of kernicterus and therapeutic intervention may be delayed until indirect bilirubin levels are over 20 mg/dl (342 μmol/liter).

In severely affected infants, thrombocytopenia is a frequent finding. Platelet counts should be done at frequent intervals if thrombocytopenia is present. Levels below 30,000 per microliter carry a risk of cerebral, pulmonary, or gastrointestinal hemorrhage.

Persistent elevations of conjugated bilirubin to levels as high as 20 to 30 mg/dl (342 to 543 μmol/liter) are due to hepatocellular damage. Although they indicate severe disease which may have a poor outcome, they are in themselves benign. If the infant survives, the conjugated bilirubin levels subside over the first few weeks or months, leaving no residual hepatic damage [18].

Following recovery from the acute phase of erythroblastosis fetalis, transient marrow inactivity with anemia is universal. Hemoglobin estimations should be made every 7 to 14 days until the infant is 6 to 8 weeks of age. The anemia is well tolerated, and no treatment should be undertaken unless the hemoglobin drops below 7 g/dl. After 6 to 8 weeks, marrow activity returns and the hemoglobin rises without treatment.

Differential diagnosis

Anasarca due to α thalassemia or cardiac, renal, hepatic, or idiopathic causes, so-called atypical hydrops, is differentiated from alloimmune hydrops fetalis by the lack of any blood group antibodies in the mother's blood and the failure of her serum to react with the father's red blood cells.

Other types of associated anemia and jaundice in the newborn (hereditary spherocytosis, enzyme-deficient hemolysis, sepsis, extravasated blood, etc.) may be differentiated also by the absence of maternal antibodies and the negative direct Coombs test of the infant's red cells. Other forms of indirect hyperbilirubinemia due to glucuronyl transferase inhibition or delayed development are not associated with anemia or a positive direct Coombs test. The conjugated hyperbilirubinemia of hepatitis, biliary atresia, galactosemia, etc., may also be differentiated from the conjugated hyperbilirubinemia of severe erythroblastosis by the absence of anemia and a negative direct Coombs test.

On occasion ABO erythroblastosis may be hard to differentiate from hereditary spherocytosis and enzymopathies if the direct Coombs test is negative. Anti-A or anti-B red cell elution studies may be helpful, as may be studies of red cell enzyme and red cell morphology.

Treatment

FETAL THERAPY

Management of a fetus who, according to amniotic fluid ΔOD 450 measurements, has impending hydrops depends upon fetal maturity. If past 33 weeks' gestation and amniotic fluid lecithin/sphingomyelin and phosphatidyl glycerol measurements indicate pulmonary maturity, prompt delivery is indicated either vaginally or, in the presence of fetal distress, by immediate cesarean section.

If the fetus is immature, i.e., between 21½ and 32 weeks' gestation, or if it is over 32 weeks' gestation without evidence of pulmonary maturity, intrauterine intraperitoneal fetal transfusion should be carried out. This procedure has revolutionized the outlook for the 10 percent of affected fetuses doomed to become hydropic before 34 weeks' gestation [8]. In tertiary-level perinatal care settings, survival rates are as high as 80 percent [18] when the fetus is not hydropic, 21 percent when the fetus is hydropic at first intrauterine transfusion [18], and 76 percent when the fetus is hydropic at second intrauterine transfusion [18]. In another series, salvage rates of 29 percent for hydropic fetuses and 60 percent for nonhydropic fetuses were reported [27]. To achieve optimal salvage of these very severely affected fetuses [18], a team approach with careful ultrasound monitoring is necessary during and after intrauterine transfusion. The second transfusion is given 10 to 12 days after the first. Subsequent transfusions are given at 3½- to 4-week intervals, and the last transfusion is given 4 weeks before the fetus is mature enough to be delivered.

NEONATAL THERAPY

EXCHANGE TRANSFUSION
Exchange transfusion after delivery is the cornerstone of management [9,28,29]. A two blood volume exchange transfusion removes about 85 to 90 percent of coated hemolysing red cells, preventing anemia and further bilirubin overproduction [30]. It removes only 25 to 30 percent of preformed bilirubin. Bilirubin removal may be increased by addition of 5 to 6 g of human albumin to each unit of blood used [31]. Prior to transfusion, a volume of plasma equivalent to the volume of citrate anticoagulant or citrate plus the added albumin should be removed from the blood unit to restore the hemoglobin concentration to normal.

The blood should be group O or group-specific if mother and baby are ABO-compatible and negative for the red cell antigen to which the mother is immunized. It must be cross-matched against maternal serum for the initial exchange and against the previous post-exchange transfusion blood sample for subsequent exchange transfusions. The blood should be not more than 96 h old, and less if the infant is prehydropic, severely anemic, and/or thrombocytopenic. The exchange transfusion should be carried out in 10- to 20-ml aliquots. Careful attention should be paid to the venous pressure, with production of a suitable volume deficit if the venous pressure is elevated, thereby reducing the likelihood of heart failure. Repeated exchange transfusions should be carried out for the indications outlined under laboratory features.

PHOTOTHERAPY
Visual light in the blue spectrum causes a physical disruption of the bilirubin molecule, converting it to water-soluble dipyrroles which are excreted without requiring the glucuronyl transferase conjugation mechanism. Phototherapy [32] is a valuable adjunct in the management of all forms of neonatal hyperbilirubinemia, reducing the need for repeated exchange transfusions and sometimes avoiding the need for exchange transfusion altogether. Since it does not prevent hemolysis, the hemoglobin level of the erythroblastotic infant treated with phototherapy must be followed carefully.

ALBUMIN
Albumin administration (1 g per kilogram body weight per day) raises reserve albumin-binding capacity [31,33]. It reduces the risk of kernicterus and reduces the need for exchange transfusion. Albumin should not be given to the severely anemic infant who may be in borderline heart failure.

PHENOBARBITAL
Phenobarbital induces enzyme maturation and when given to the mother (30 mg tid) or to the infant (4 mg/kg per day) after birth, enhances glucuronyl transferase formation and lowers peak bilirubin levels [34]. Since there is a 48-h latent interval, phenobarbital is not very effective once hyperbilirubinemia has developed.

AGAR
Agar has been administered with equivocal results in an attempt to bind bilirubin diglucuronide in the bowel, thereby preventing its conversion back to bilirubin by β-glucuronidase and reabsorption into the circulation [35].

OTHER ANCILLARY MEASURES
Optimal management of the very sick hydropic or prehydropic premature erythroblastotic infant may tax all the resources of a neonatal intensive care unit. Abdominal and pleural paracentesis, mechanical ventilation, and treatment of congestive heart failure, thrombocytopenia, patent ductus arteriosus, and necrotizing enterocolitis may all be required. Throughout the management of these very sick infants every effort must be made to prevent hypoxia and acidosis, which if present materially increase the risk of kernicterus, cerebral hemorrhage, and heart and renal failure.

Whether the affected infant has required intrauterine and/or exchange transfusion, progressive anemia in the first 6 to 10 weeks of life may require treatment. In the infants whose hemoglobin levels drop below 7 g/dl, 20 ml per kilogram of body weight of compatible packed red cells should be transfused by scalp vein.

SUPPRESSION OF Rh IMMUNIZATION
Promethazine hydrochloride [36] interferes with antibody-coated red cell phagocyte rosette formation but also interferes with fetal and neonatal T-lymphocyte function [37], which may be hazardous to the neonate. The reported success of orally administered Rh-positive red cell stroma in reducing severity of Rh disease by altering the immunocyte Rh-antibody immune response from IgG to IgA and IgM [38] awaits confirmation. Plasma exchange, first carried out in 1967 [39], is costly,

and its benefits are equivocal [40,41,42,43]. It should be reserved for the pregnant woman with a history of hydropic fetal death before 26 weeks' gestation. Fifteen to twenty liters of plasma should be exchanged weekly, starting at 14 to 16 weeks' gestation, in an effort to postpone the need for intrauterine transfusions until 25 to 28 weeks' gestation, when the hazards are less.

PREVENTION OF Rh IMMUNIZATION

Whereas the ability to suppress Rh immunization once it has developed is doubtful, there can be no question about the ability to prevent Rh immunization from developing. Von Dungern in 1900 [44] was the first to demonstrate that the administration of passive antibody to an antigen prevented active immunization to the antigen. This information was used 65 years later [10,11,12] to develop a practical method of preventing Rh immunization. Experimental work and clinical trials have shown that Rh antibody administered in the form of Rh immune globulin (Rh IgG) to the Rh-negative, unimmunized woman carrying an Rh-positive fetus or delivered of an Rh-positive baby, and therefore at risk of Rh immunization, prevents Rh immunization. To be effective it must be given prior to the beginning of the primary Rh immune response and it must be given in adequate dose.

Systematic administration of Rh IgG in doses of from 100 to 300 μg IM after delivery has reduced the incidence of Rh immunization by about 80 to 85 percent. In order to reduce Rh immunization to the smallest possible level, Rh immune globulin must be given in situations during pregnancy where there is an increased risk of transplacental hemorrhage and Rh immunization, such as after amniocentesis and following obstetrical procedures such as external version. It must be given to the Rh-negative woman after therapeutic or spontaneous abortion. If massive transplacental hemorrhage is diagnosed [17], or in the rare event of Rh-incompatible blood transfusion, it should be given in doses in excess of 20 μg for every milliliter of Rh-positive red cells in the maternal circulation. It must also be administered routinely (240- to 300-μg dose) at 28 weeks' gestation [19,43] if Rh immunization is to be prevented in the 1.5 to 2.0 percent of women at risk of becoming Rh-immunized during pregnancy.

Most Rh immune globulin used in Europe and North America is prepared by the Cohn cold ethanol process. Column ion-exchange methods [45,46] produce an Rh immune globulin which is purer and can be given intravenously. Rh IgG given intravenously is twice as effective, conserving a vital human plasma resource which may, in the near future, be in short supply.

Course and prognosis

With modern management, the perinatal mortality from alloimmune hemolytic disease has been reduced from 12 to 13 percent in the mid-1960s to 1 to 2 percent in the late 1970s [18]. With successful Rh prevention programs embodying antenatal, postnatal, and postabortion prophylaxis, the numbers of severely affected Rh erythroblastotic fetuses at risk of hydrops fetalis and neonatal death will continue to diminish. The small incidence of severely affected anti-c, anti-Kell, and other antibody-related erythroblastotic fetuses and infants will not change but will become of relatively greater importance as anti-D immunization becomes more and more infrequent.

References

1. Hart, A. P.: Familial icterus gravis of the newborn and its treatment. *Can. Med. Assoc. J.* 15:1008, 1925.
2. Landsteiner, K., and Weiner, A. S.: An agglutinable factor in human blood recognized by immune sera for rhesus blood. *Proc. Soc. Exp. Biol. Med.* 43:223, 1940.
3. Lewis, M., and Chown, B.: A short albumin method for the determination of isohemagglutinins, particularly incomplete Rh antibodies. *J. Lab. Clin. Med.* 50:494, 1957.
4. Rosenfield, R. E., and Haber, G. V.: Detection and measurement of homologous human hemagglutinins. *Automation in Analytical Chemistry-Technicon Symposia*, 1965, p. 503.
5. Coombs, R. R. A., Mourant, A. E., and Race, R. R.: A new test for the detection of weak and "incomplete" Rh agglutinins. *Br. J. Exp. Pathol.* 26:255, 1945.
6. Liley, A. W.: Liquor amnii analysis in management of pregnancy complicated by rhesus immunization. *Am. J. Obstet. Gynecol.* 82:1359, 1961.
7. Bowman, J. M., and Pollock, J. M.: Amniotic fluid spectrophotometry and early delivery in the management of erythroblastosis fetalis. *Pediatrics* 35:815, 1965.
8. Liley, A. W.: Intrauterine transfusion of fetus in hemolytic disease. *Br. Med. J.* 2:1107, 1963.
9. Wallerstein, H.: Treatment of severe erythroblastosis by simultaneous removal and replacement of blood of the newborn. *Science* 103:583, 1946.
10. Clarke, C. A., et al.: Further experimental studies in the prevention of Rh-haemolytic disease. *Br. Med. J.* 1:979, 1963.
11. Freda, V. J., Gorman, J. G., and Pollack, W.: Successful prevention of experimental Rh sensitization in man an anti-Rh gamma 2-globulin antibody preparation: A preliminary report. *Transfusion* 4:26, 1964.
12. Chown, B., et al.: Prevention of primary Rh immunization: First report of the Western Canadian Trial. *Can. Med. Assoc. J.* 100:1021, 1969.
13. Wiener, A. S., and Wexler, I. B.: *Heredity of the Blood Groups.* Grune & Stratton, New York, 1958.
14. Race, R. R.: The Rh genotype and Fisher's theory. *Blood 3 (special issue No. 2)*:27, 1948.
15. Wiener, A. S.: Diagnosis and treatment of anemia of the newborn caused by occult placental hemorrhage. *Am. J. Obstet. Gynecol.* 56:717, 1948.
16. Chown, B.: Anemia from bleeding of the fetus into the mother's circulation. *Lancet* 1:1213, 1954.
17. Kleihauer, E., Braun, H., and Betke, K.: Demonstration von Fetalem Haemoglobin in den Erythrozyten eines Blutausstriches. *Klin. Wochenschr.* 35:637, 1957.
18. Bowman, J. M.: Management of Rh-isoimmunization. *Obstet. Gynecol.* 52:1, 1978.
19. Bowman, J. M., et al.: Rh-immunization during pregnancy: Antenatal prophylaxis. *Can. Med. Assoc. J.* 118:623, 1978.
20. Blajchman, M., Zipursky, A. (Hamilton), Bartsch, F. R., Hermann, M. (Sweden): McMaster Conference on Prevention of Rh Immunization. *Vox Sang.* 36:50, 1979.
21. Zipursky, A., and Israels, L. G.: The pathogenesis and prevention of Rh immunization. *Can. Med. Assoc. J.* 97:1245, 1967.

22. Woodrow, J. C.: Rh immunization and its prevention. *Ser. Haematol. III(3):*33, 1970.

23. James, L. S.: *International Symposium on the Management of the Rh Problem*, edited by J. G. Robertson and F. Dambrosio. Milan, Italy, *Ann. Ostet. Ginec. Spec. No. 193*, 1970.

24. Phibbs, R. H., Johnson, P., and Tooley, W. H.: Cardio-respiratory status of erythroblastotic infants. II. Blood volume, hematocrit and serum albumin concentration in relation to hydrops fetalis. *Pediatrics 53:*13, 1974.

25. Kaufmann, N. A., Kapitulnik, J., and Blondheim, S. H.: The absorption of bilirubin by sephadex and its relation to the criteria for exchange transfusion. *Pediatrics 44:*543, 1969.

26. Porter, E. G., and Waters, W. J.: A rapid micro-method for measuring the reserve albumin binding capacity in serum from newborn infants with hyperbilirubinemia. *J. Lab. Clin. Med. 67:*660, 1966.

27. Frigoletto, F. D., Jr., et al.: Intrauterine fetal transfusion in 365 fetuses during fifteen years. *Am. J. Obstet. Gynecol. 139:*781, 1981.

28. Diamond, L. K., et al.: Erythroblastosis fetalis: Round table discussion. *Pediatrics 10:*337, 1952.

29. Bowman, J. M.: *Neonatal Management in Modern Management of the Rh Problem*, 2d ed., edited by J. T. Queenan. Harper & Row, Hagerstown, Md., 1977, p. 209.

30. Veall, N., and Mollison, P. L.: The rate of red cell exchange in replacement transfusions. *Lancet 2:*792, 1950.

31. Waters, W. J., and Porter, E. G.: Indications for exchange transfusion based upon the role of albumin in the treatment of hemolytic disease of the newborn. *Pediatrics 33:*749, 1964.

32. Lucey, J. F.: Neonatal jaundice and phototherapy. *Pediatr. Clin. North Am. 19:*827, 1972.

33. Odell, G. B., and Cohen, S. N.: Albumin priming in the management of hyperbilirubinemia by exchange transfusion. *Am. J. Dis. Child. 102:*699, 1961.

34. Trolle, D.: Decrease of total serum bilirubin concentration in newborn infants after phenobarbitone treatment. *Lancet 2:*705, 1968.

35. Maurer, H. M., Shumway, C. N., Draper, D. A., and Hossaini, A. A.: Controlled trial comparing agar, intermittent phototherapy and continuous phototherapy for reducing neonatal hyperbilirubinemia. *J. Pediatr. 82:*73, 1973.

36. Gusdon, J. P., Jr., et al.: Phagocytosis and erythroblastosis. I. Modification of the neonatal response by promethazine hydrochloride. *Am. J. Obstet Gynecol. 125:*224, 1976.

37. Rubinstein, A., et al.: Possible effect of maternal promethazine therapy on neonatal immunologic functions. *J. Pediatr. 89:*136, 1976.

38. Bierme, S. J., Blanc, M., Abbal, M., and Fournie, A.: Oral Rh treatment for severely immunized mothers. *Lancet 1:*604, 1979.

39. Bowman, J. M., Peddle, L. J., and Anderson, C.: Plasmapheresis in severe Rh-isoimmunization. *Vox Sang. 15:*272, 1968.

40. Barclay, G. R., Ayoub Greiss, M., and Urbaniak, S. J.: Adverse effect of plasma exchange on anti-D production in rhesus immunization owing to removal of inhibitory factors. *Br. Med. J. 1:*1569, 1980.

41. Graham-Pole, J., Barr, W., and Willoughby, M. L. N.: Continuous flow plasmapheresis in management of severe Rhesus disease. *Br. Med. J. 1:*1185, 1977.

42. Isbister, J. P., Ting, A., and Seeto, K. M.: Development of Rh-specific maternal autoantibodies following intensive plasmapheresis for Rh immunization during pregnancy. *Vox Sang. 33:*353, 1977.

43. Bowman, J. M.: Suppression of Rh isoimmunization: A review. *Obstet. Gynecol. 52:*385, 1978.

44. Von Dungern, F.: Beitrage zur Immunitatslehr. *Munch. Med. Wochenschr. 47:*677, 1900.

45. Hoppe, H. H., et al.: Prevention of Rh-immunization: Modified production of IgG Anti-Rh for intravenous application by ion exchange chromatography (IEC). *Vox Sang. 25:*308, 1973.

46. Bowman, J. M., Friesen, A. D., Pollock, J. M., and Taylor, W. E.: WinRho: Rh Immune globulin prepared by ion exchange for intravenous use. *Can. Med. Assoc. J. 123:*1121, 1980.

Erythrocyte disorders—anemias related to hyperactivity of the monocyte-macrophage system

CHAPTER *71*

Hypersplenism

WILLIAM H. CROSBY

Background and definition

Many attempts have been made to define *hypersplenism* [1]. Chauffard, who must have coined the word [2], employed it as a description of the spleen's hemolytic activity in hereditary spherocytosis. Yet it has been argued that splenic destruction of red cells in hereditary spherocytosis is not an example of hypersplenism, because the spleen is not functioning abnormally. Hemolysis in hereditary spherocytosis is merely the consequence of normal splenic action against abnormal red cells. We may ask, Is the destruction of platelets in idiopathic thrombocytopenic purpura (ITP) hypersplenic? Although the spleen participates in antibody production against autogenous platelets [3], its primary action is in destroying sensitized platelets, a normal splenic function. Thus it is argued that ITP is not a good example of hypersplenism.

As a result of such disputation, hypersplenism has been divided into two varieties: primary, where the spleen per se behaves abnormally and causes disease, and secondary, where the spleen is involved because of an extrasplenic disorder. This classification seems artificial if one suspects that all hypersplenism is probably secondary. In another argument it has been suggested that the concept of hypersplenism is unnecessary. Logically it may be, but clinically it remains a useful designation. How, then, does one define hypersplenism?

Dameshek proposed a tetralogy [4] whereby the syndrome of hypersplenism might be recognized: (1) a lack of one or more cellular elements in the blood; (2) a marrow hyperplasia corresponding to that lack, e.g., megakaryocytic hyperplasia in thrombocytopenia; (3) splenomegaly; (4) correction of the disorder following splenectomy. While this definition does fit most cases,

there are a few important exceptions to the first three rules. First, hypersplenism may be almost completely compensated for by increased cellular production; for example, patients with the hypersplenism of hereditary spherocytosis may have no anemia despite a shortened red cell life-span [5]. Second, patients with hypocellular disease of the marrow may also have hypersplenism [6]. Third, patients with ITP uncommonly have splenomegaly [7], and even autoimmune hemolytic anemia may be associated with a spleen of normal size [8]. The fourth rule, improvement or cure after splenectomy, remains inviolable and suggests a simplified, although post hoc, operational definition: "When a person is hematologically better off without his spleen, he had hypersplenism" [1].

Pathogenesis

Several years ago a famous dispute took place about the mechanism of hypersplenism [2]. One faction believed the spleen caused anemia, leukopenia, or thrombocytopenia by destroying blood cells at a rate exceeding what a hypercellular, maximally active marrow could compensate for [9]. The opposing faction believed that hypersplenism resulted from inhibition of the marrow by splenic humoral factors [4]. Investigators now agree that the filtering and phagocytic actions of the spleen are responsible for most of the phenomena of hypersplenism [10]. However, a few additional actions are recognized: (1) In immunologic hypersplenism, e.g., ITP and autoimmune hemolytic anemia, the spleen is a source of pathogenic antibody. (2) In some patients the spleen appears to inhibit marrow hemopoiesis, and splenectomy results in recovery of marrow function. (3) In a few disorders, such as thrombotic thrombocytopenic purpura, splenectomy may be followed by remission with healing of damage in organs remote from the spleen.

Implicit in our understanding of the function of the spleen (Chap. 14) is the fact that normal functions of a normal-size spleen may become hematologically harmful. The filtering and phagocytic function of the spleen removes blood cells altered by age, by congenital abnormalities in shape or hemoglobin structure, by oxidative injury to the membrane, or by antibody coating; they are removed despite the fact that these cells may be functionally normal and useful for the body [11]. The spleen may also produce antibodies to minimally altered blood cells and thereby contribute to their destruction. These functions are further exaggerated when the spleen is enlarged. In addition, an enlarged spleen may mechanically sequester normal blood cells and withhold them temporarily from the circulation [12]. Thus up to 90 percent of the total platelets of the body may be sequestered in an enlarged spleen (see Chap. 143), and from 10 to 45 percent of the total red cell mass may be similarly isolated [13,14].

Further, in patients with splenomegaly not associated with immunologic or hereditary disease of the red cells, as many as 4 percent of the red cells may be destroyed daily in the spleen [14]. Granulocytes may be retained in the spleen of hypersplenic granulocytopenia. Splenomegaly due to portal hypertension (Banti's syndrome) may be especially detrimental to circulating cells because of the slow blood flow, which enhances the effectiveness of the splenic filtering and phagocytic action [15].

Enlargement of the spleen may contribute to cytopenia by a dilutional effect [16,17]. When the spleen is greatly enlarged, the plasma volume and total blood volume are significantly expanded. Many such patients have low hemoglobin concentrations, while the red cell mass is normal or greater than normal. The apparent anemia is probably due to a combination of splenic sequestration of red cells and dilution of circulating red cells in the expanded plasma volume. In the dilution anemia of splenomegaly, the concentration of plasma albumin is normal, suggesting increased synthesis of albumin. Removal of the enlarged spleen partially corrects the dilutional anemia, but it may take 6 months or more before the plasma volume returns to normal [18].

Splenomegaly and hypersplenism

The causes of splenomegaly are many and various (Table 71-1), but truly massive enlargement of the spleen occurs in relatively few diseases (Table 71-2).

Not all big spleens are bad spleens, but "the greater the increase in splenic tissue, the greater, usually, is the degree of hypersplenism" [4]. The importance of spleen size in the pathogenesis of hypersplenism is discussed above.

Accessory spleens overlooked at splenectomy provide corroboration of the importance of splenic size. Because they are usually quite small, they rarely cause recurrence of hematologic disease [1]. Splenunculi weighing 20 to 50 g have been believed to cause recurrent thrombocytopenia in previously splenectomized patients with ITP. Although remissions have occurred following removal of such splenunculi, in some cases this may have been coincidental. Recurrence of nonimmunologic hypersplenism demands the presence of a large mass of splenic tissue which may develop with double spleens, retroperitoneal spleens, or splenosis [1]. A small accessory spleen cannot function as an effective filter for 5 liters of blood. Even an accessory spleen weighing about 100 g was reported not to produce a recurrence in a previously splenectomized patient with hereditary spherocytosis [19]. On the other hand, a patient with hereditary spherocytosis who relapsed after an ordinary splenectomy was cured by removal of a 220-g retroperitoneal spleen [20]. The presence of Howell-Jolly bodies in circulating red cells after splenectomy is substantial evidence for lack of splenic function, and they should be sought when the question of recurrent hypersplenism is moot [21].

While there is no pathognomonic characteristic of hypersplenism, the cause of splenomegaly is often evi-

TABLE 71-1   A classification of causes of splenomegaly

Infections
  Acute, subacute, chronic
Inflammatory diseases
  Rheumatoid arthritis, sarcoid, lupus, amyloid
Neoplasms
  Leukemia, lymphoma, polycythemia vera, myeloid metaplasia
  Primary tumors, metastases, cysts
Hemolytic diseases
  Hereditary, acquired: acute, chronic
Deficiency diseases
  Severe iron deficiency anemia, pernicious anemia
Storage diseases
  Gaucher, Niemann-Pick
Splenic vein hypertension
  Cirrhosis, splenic and portal vein thrombosis and stenosis
Idiopathic
  With or without hypersplenism

dent [22]. Microscopic examination of the spleen in leukemia may demonstrate that much of the splenic volume is occupied by neoplastic cells produced there or in transit [23]. Actually, careful examination of the blood of patients with leukemia sometimes reveals evidence of hyposplenism, suggesting that the spleen has been incapacitated by the cellular overload [1]. The same phenomenon develops in children with sickle cell disease, where abnormal red cells glut the splenic machinery. As a result, Howell-Jolly bodies and pitted red cells appear in the blood, and splenic uptake of labeled colloid is reduced [24,25].

Abrupt sequestration of massive numbers of red cells in the spleen may reduce the circulating blood volume so quickly that the patient develops shock and may die. This catastrophe, referred to as the *acute pooling syndrome* or *acute splenic sequestration crisis*, has been de-

TABLE 71-2   Causes of truly massive splenomegaly*

Chronic:
  Chronic granulocytic leukemia
  Myeloid metaplasia
  Polycythemia vera (end-stage)
  Primary thrombocythemia (uncommon)
  Malignant reticuloendotheliosis
  Malignant lymphoma
  Hairy-cell leukemia
  Hodgkin's disease (rare)
  Gaucher's disease
  Cooley's anemia
  Sicklemia (rare)
  Kala azar
  Malaria in combination with, e.g., cirrhosis
  Sarcoid (rare)
  Felty's syndrome (rare)
Acute:
  Malaria: splenic crisis with blackwater fever
  Sicklemic splenic crisis

*The spleen extends into one or both lower quadrants of the abdomen or weighs > 3000 g.

scribed in sickle cell disease [26] and in blackwater fever [27].

Dilution studies with radioactive red cells in patients with greatly enlarged spleens indicate that a large proportion of the total red cell mass may be sequestered in the spleen [13,14,28]. This extensive accumulation of red cells in the spleen is accompanied by a corresponding proliferation of functional spleen cells (adventitial cells, lymphocytes, macrophages) [29].

In acute infections with antibody production, the spleen enlarges modestly and temporarily because of lymphocyte-plasma cell hyperplasia [30]. When acute infections involve parasitization of red cells (e.g., malaria and bartonellosis), the splenic enlargement, even the growth of splenunculi, may be rapid and painful [31]. Splenic hypertrophy in these situations is associated with massive macrophage activity. The cords are expanded by a honeycomb of overstuffed erythrophagocytes [32].

In cirrhosis the splenomegaly is termed congestive because of high splenic vein pressure and engorged sinuses. However, portacaval shunt does not always reduce the spleen to normal size [33], and it has been demonstrated that splenomegaly can develop in cirrhosis independently of increased splenic vein pressure [34].

Indications for splenectomy in hypersplenism

Hypersplenism is defined as a state in which an individual would be hematologically better off without the spleen. However, anticipated benefit must be weighed against risk (Table 71-3). In proposing splenectomy, the

TABLE 71-3   Considerations regarding splenectomy for hypersplenism

1. Severity of hypersplenism. Is the anemia incapacitating, requiring transfusion? Is the purpura life threatening? Is the neutropenia associated with infections?
2. Chronicity of hypersplenism. Has enough time passed to establish that the disease (e.g., ITP or hemolytic anemia) is not self-limited? What risk is involved in waiting?
3. Progression of hypersplenism. Will spleen size increase and anemia become more severe? Will increasing debility of the patient ultimately contraindicate splenectomy? Can a massive spleen be shrunken by chemotherapy prior to splenectomy?
4. Age of patient. If the patient is a young child, can splenectomy be deferred without risk to safety or development? In elderly patients when should splenectomy be ruled out because of old age?
5. Other illness. When do coexistent diseases (e.g., cardiac, pulmonary, renal, or hematologic) rule out splenectomy for correctable hypersplenism? In pregnancy should splenectomy be done early, late, or after?
6. Alternatives. Is splenectomy a greater risk than corticosteroid administration, immunosuppression, transfusion, or doing nothing at all?

physician must first be assured of the quality of surgical skill available to the patient. Second, some possibility of benefit must be expected from the correction of hypersplenism. Third, a grave risk sometimes may be acceptable when the alternative is death or severe debility. The following are some varieties of hypersplenism in which the decision for or against splenectomy requires special consideration.

Granulocytopenia   Granulocytopenia unassociated with anemia or thrombocytopenia is not often due to hypersplenism, and hypersplenism rarely destroys granulocytes so effectively as to cause clinical trouble. The granulocyte count may be low, even in the range of 1 percent, but if the patients can make pus they usually are not subject to septic disease, so characteristic of agranulocytosis caused by marrow failure. In hypersplenism the marrow produces granulocytes, and although the spleen may destroy what it receives, enough granulocytes are available wherever needed. It is evident that such patients do not require splenectomy to live a normal life, and splenectomy may even fail to improve the low leukocyte count [36]. It is from this perspective that the hematologist should make a decision concerning splenectomy in obviously healthy patients with granulocytopenia.

Felty's syndrome [37]   The association of splenomegaly and leukopenia, especially granulocytopenia, in patients with rheumatoid arthritis is of clinical importance because the syndrome is often associated with episodes of severe infection or indolent ulcers, especially on the legs. Anemia and thrombocytopenia may be present as well. Splenectomy has been recommended because granulocytopenia was assumed to be the cause of the infections. However, the granulocytes are adequate as indicated by the capacity to form purulent foci. The cause of the susceptibility to infection is really unknown. Following splenectomy the propensity to develop infections is frequently lost, the leg ulcers heal, and coincident anemia and thrombocytopenia are improved [38,39]. Yet the granulocyte counts may or may not be improved. The indication for splenectomy in Felty's syndrome should be frequent infections or indolent ulcers. Asymptomatic granulocytopenia is not an indication. Rarely has rheumatoid arthritis per se been improved after splenectomy [40].

Congestive splenomegaly (Banti's syndrome)   The hypersplenism of hepatic cirrhosis is rarely, if ever, so severe as to require splenectomy. Although splenectomy usually corrects the mild to moderate granulocytopenia and thrombocytopenia and usually improves the anemia, the patient is not substantially benefited [41]. Pancytopenia is one of the patient's lesser problems.

Gaucher's disease   Pancytopenia, and especially thrombocytopenia, are often found in patients with splenomegaly due to Gaucher's disease. If marrow examination has established that the cytopenia is due to hypersplenic destruction rather than marrow replacement, the patient is usually considered a candidate for splenectomy. However, it should be remembered that the spleen acts as the primary sump for the undigestible glucocerebrosides, and that splenectomy often is followed by an accelerated and symptomatic infiltration of Gaucher's cells in the marrow and liver [42]. Consequently, splenectomy should not be performed until the cytopenia has become life-threatening, and it may be advisable to leave a small amount of splenic tissue for future splenic restoration [43].

Thrombotic thrombocytopenic purpura (Moschcowitz's syndrome)   This savage disease, involving injury to arterioles in many organs, is often rapidly fatal. Splenectomy and large doses of corticosteroids have been reported to be of therapeutic benefit [44,45]. Since the prognosis is grave, it has been suggested that surgical intervention should be decided upon early and carried out regardless of the seriousness of the patient's condition. However, the glowing reports on the successful use of plasma transfusion, plasmapheresis, or exchange transfusion, with or without antiplatelet-aggregation agents, have made these therapeutic interventions the initial choice in most cases (see Chap. 142).

Chronic aplastic anemia   As would be expected, splenectomy is rarely followed by a dramatic improvement or cure of marrow failure [46]. Nevertheless, in perhaps 25 percent of patients there is a modest sustained improvement of hemoglobin or platelet count, possibly because of absent splenic sequestration [47]. Splenectomy should be considered when a modest improvement in the platelet count from, for example, 5000 to 20,000 per microliter, or in the hemoglobin levels from 6 to 9 g/dl can be expected to be beneficial.

Idiopathic thrombocytopenic purpura   Because ITP in children is often a brief, self-limited disorder and because chronic ITP can often be controlled with corticosteroids, the decision for splenectomy may be difficult. In chronic ITP, steroid treatment should be used first, but if the patient's platelet count has not responded to steroids in about 4 weeks, it probably will never respond, and splenectomy should be considered (see Chap. 142). If spontaneous bleeding is present ("wet purpura"), the situation is apparently more critical than if there are only petechiae and ecchymoses ("dry purpura") [48]. If the thrombocytopenia responds to steroids but the improved platelet count remains steroid-dependent, splenectomy should be considered after 2 to 3 months of steroid therapy. Splenectomy may be a lesser risk than permanent treatment with steroid drugs (see Chap. 142).

Remote effects of splenectomy

The removal of a large spleen has certain predictable hemodynamic and immunologic effects:

1. From 10 to 55 percent of cardiac output may be shunted through a large spleen [49]. Removing this shunt immediately reduces the cardiac workload. In portal hypertension, splenectomy may reduce significantly the volume of blood flowing through the portal circulation [15], resulting in less ascites and less bleeding from esophageal varices [50].

2. Many patients with massive splenomegaly have a greatly increased blood volume. The plasma volume may exceed 100 ml/kg [51]. The red cell mass may be normal or increased, while the hemoglobin concentration is low [17,51]. Immediately following splenectomy the plasma volume is somewhat diminished, and correction to normal levels occurs over a period of months [18].

3. After splenectomy serum IgM levels fall. This may be the consequence of removal of a major immunoglobulin-producing lymphoid organ. IgG and IgA levels remain unchanged [52].

In addition to these predictable effects, splenectomy may be followed by unanticipated and unexplained remissions of disorders in organs remote from the spleen. In most reports showing such remote effects, the cause-effect relationship is conjectural, but in some the circumstances indicate that coincidence is an unlikely explanation. However, the spleen is an immunologic organ; more and more obscure disorders seem to have an autoimmune pathogenesis and could, at least in theory, be helped by the removal of an antibody-producing organ.

As noted above, purulent infections and leg ulcers may disappear after splenectomy in patients who have been ill for years with Felty's syndrome. In thrombotic thrombocytopenia purpura, lesions in arterioles of the brain, myocardium, kidney, and other organs may also subside after splenectomy and corticosteroid therapy. In addition, the following conditions have been claimed to respond to splenectomy:

Aregenerative disorders of the marrow   A deficiency of proliferating marrow elements has on rare occasions been restored after splenectomy. This has been observed in patients with pure red cell aplasia [53], a condition that now is recognized as being caused by an autoimmune reaction against nucleated red blood cells [54]. Deficiencies in plasma cells [55], megakaryocytes [56], and marrow precursor cells have also been reported to respond to splenectomy on rare occasions [44].

Indolent ulcer   Ulcers, especially on the lower leg, may be found in a number of hematologic disorders associated with splenomegaly. They have been reported especially in sickle cell anemia in children but also in homozygous hemoglobin C disease, hemoglobin SC disease in adults, thalassemia, hereditary spherocytosis, Felty's syndrome, tropical splenomegaly, and other splenomegalic disorders [1]. Ulcers have persisted as long as 40 years, with prompt healing following splenectomy, even when the associated hematologic disease was unimproved. Corneal ulceration and even chronic non-union of a fracture have been reported to respond to splenectomy [58,59].

Pulmonary hemosiderosis In this syndrome an abnormal fragility of pulmonary vessels results in the loss of red cells into lung parenchyma. Pulmonary macrophages ingest the red cells and trap large amounts of iron. The patient develops iron deficiency anemia while the lungs become siderotic, which ultimately causes pulmonary insufficiency. In some cases, splenectomy has been followed by improvement in the pulmonary disease [60,61].

Splenogenital syndrome Delayed sexual maturation has been described in some children with splenomegaly [62]. No recent reports support the existence of such a syndrome, however.

Complications of splenectomy

Thromboembolic disease This is a threat in the immediate postoperative weeks and months. It is a special danger when myeloproliferative disease causes excess production of platelets [63], as well as in paroxysmal nocturnal hemoglobinuria [64]. The postsplenectomy surge of circulating platelets even following removal of a normal spleen is cause for concern, especially if the patient is bedridden because of postoperative complications. If the platelet count reaches 1 million per microliter or the patient is immobilized, consideration should be given to anticoagulant and antiplatelet-aggregation therapy after splenectomy [65,66]. Where possible, and indicated, preoperative myelosuppressive therapy should be given to patients with myeloid metaplasia and chronic granulocytic leukemia. Primary thrombocytosis is a proliferative disease in which splenectomy is contraindicated, except for a catastrophe such as rupture or massive infarction.

Infection After splenectomy the remaining macrophages of the monocyte-macrophage system require increased amounts of antibody to accomplish clearance of opsonized, intravascular particles [67]. This requirement may place an asplenic patient at serious risk when intravascular infections occur.

Overwhelming postsplenectomy infection is usually caused by an encapsulated organism, most often a pneumococcus. The onset is abrupt, and death is often rapid [68,69]. The risk is greatest, perhaps 1 in 10, among the very young whose debilitating hematologic disease e.g., thalassemia major, has required splenectomy. Among older, healthy children whose spleens have been removed for curable disease, e.g., hereditary spherocytosis or immune thrombocytopenic purpura, the risk may be of the order of 1 in 100. Even healthy adults with congenital asplenia or whose normal, ruptured spleens have been removed are at some risk [70].

Prevention Awareness of this complication has made abdominal surgeons more concerned about performing a casual splenectomy. Torn spleens are sometimes repaired, and inconveniently located spleens are being shown a new deference during left upper quadrant operations [71].

Immunization with polyvalent pneumococcus vaccine is done before splenectomy, when feasible, and, under present recommendations, every 3 years thereafter. The precise value of the immunization is not known. Some types of pneumococcus are not represented, and cases of septicemia have occurred after immunization against the infecting type [72].

Some pediatricians prescribe penicillin prophylactically for every asplenic child [73]. Other physicians tell all asplenic persons that no febrile infection should be considered trivial and instruct them to take penicillin immediately upon onset of symptoms and not to wait for culture results or office visits.

In malarious areas, splenectomy may diminish resistance of the host to malarial attack. This has been demonstrated in the monkey [74], and clinical experience has suggested that human susceptibility may also be increased [75]. Infections with other intraerythrocyte organisms such as *Bartonella* [76] and *Babesia* [77] may be more severe in the absence of the spleen.

Ischemic heart disease A long-term follow-up of 740 servicemen splenectomized because of injuries during World War II showed a significant excess mortality from pneumonia and from ischemic heart disease during the period 1946–1974. The risk of cancer and the risk of thromboembolism were not increased [78].

Acceleration of disease As mentioned above, splenectomy in Gaucher's disease may accelerate the involvement of marrow and liver [42]. In some patients with myeloid metaplasia, marked hepatomegaly has developed after splenectomy because of increased metaplastic involvement of the liver [79].

References

1. Crosby, W. H.: Hypersplenism, *Annu. Rev. Med.* 13:127, 1962.
2. Crosby, W. H.: The spleen, in *Blood, Pure and Eloquent*, edited by M. M. Wintrobe, McGraw-Hill, New York, 1980, p. 96.
3. McMillan, R., Longmire, R. L., Yelenosky, R., Donnell, R. L., and Armstrong, S.: Quantitation of platelet-binding IgG produced in vitro by spleens from patients with idiopathic thrombocytopenic purpura. *N. Engl. J. Med. 291:812,* 1974.
4. Dameshek, W.: Hypersplenism. *Bull. N.Y. Acad. Med. 31:113,* 1955.
5. Crosby, W. H., and Conrad, M. E.: Hereditary spherocytosis: Observations on hemolytic mechanisms and iron metabolism. *Blood 15:662,* 1960.
6. Loeb, V., Moore, C. V., and Dubach, R.: The physiologic evaluation and management of chronic bone marrow failure. *Am. J. Med. 15:499,* 1953.
7. Orringer, E., Lewis, M., Silverberg, J., and Rosenbach, L.: Splenectomy in chronic thrombocytopenic purpura. *J. Chronic Dis. 23:117,* 1970.
8. Allgood, J. W., and Chaplin, H.: Idiopathic acquired autoimmune hemolytic anemia: A review of 47 cases treated from 1955 to 1965. *Am. J. Med. 43:254,* 1967.

9. Doan, C. A.: Hypersplenism. *Bull. N.Y. Acad. Med.* 25:625, 1949.
10. Crosby, W. H.: Is hypersplenism a dead issue? *Blood* 20:94, 1962.
11. Weiss, L., and Tavassoli, M.: Anatomical hazards to the passage of erythrocytes through the spleen. *Semin. Hematol.* 7:372, 1970.
12. Aster, R. H.: Pooling of platelets in the spleen: Role in the pathogenesis of "hypersplenic thrombocytopenia." *J. Clin. Invest.* 45:645, 1966.
13. Nightingale, D., Prankerd, T. A. J., Richards, J. D. M., and Thompson, D.: Splenectomy in anaemia. *Q. J. Med.* 41:261, 1972.
14. Christensen, B. E.: Quantitative determination of splenic red blood cell destruction in patients with splenomegaly. *Scand. J. Haematol,* 14:294, 1975.
15. Koyama, K.: Hemodynamics of the spleen in Banti's syndrome. *Tohoku J. Exp. Med.* 93:199, 1967.
16. McFadzean, A. J. S., Todd, D., and Tsang, K. C.: Observations on the anemia of crytogenic splenomegaly. II. Expansion of the plasma volume. *Blood* 13:524, 1958.
17. Blendis, L. M., Ramboer, C., and Williams, R.: Studies on the hemodilutional anemia of splenomegaly. *Eur. J. Clin. Invest.* 1:54, 1970.
18. Hess, C. E., Ayers, C. R., Sandusky, W. R., Carpenter, M. A., Wetzel, R. A., and Mohler, D. N.: Mechanisms of dilutional anemia in massive splenomegaly. *Blood* 47:629, 1976.
19. Edward, H. C.: Observations on splenectomy in disorders of the blood. *Proc. R. Soc. Med.* 48:55, 1955.
20. Mackenzie, F. A. F., Elliot, D. H., Eastcott, H. H. G., Hughes-Jones, N. C., Barkhan, P., and Mollison, P. L.: Relapse in hereditary spherocytosis with proven splenunculus. *Lancet* 1:1102, 1962.
21. Lipson, R. L., Bayrd, E. D., and Watkins, C. H.: The postsplenectomy blood picture. *Am. J. Clin. Pathol.* 32:526, 1959.
22. Blaustein, A. U., and Diggs, L. W.: Pathology of the spleen, in *The Spleen*, edited by A. U. Blaustein. McGraw-Hill, New York, 1963, p. 45.
23. Turner, A., and Kjeldsberg, C. R.: Hairy cell leukemia: A review. *Medicine (Baltimore)* 57:477, 1978.
24. Pearson, H. A., Cornelius, E. A., Schwartz, A. D., Zelson, J. H., Wolfson, S. L., and Spencer, R. P.: Transfusion-reversible functional asplenia in young children with sickle-cell anemia. *N. Engl. J. Med.* 283:334, 1970.
25. Casper, J. T., Koethe, S., Rodey, G. E., and Thatcher, L. G.: A new method for studying splenic reticuloendothelial dysfunction in sickle cell disease patients and its clinical application: A brief report. *Blood* 47:183, 1976.
26. Jenkins, M. E., Scott, R. B., and Baird, R. L.: Studies in sickle cell anemia. XVI. Sudden death during sickle cell anemia crisis in young children. *J. Pediatr.* 56:30, 1960.
27. Maegraith, B.: The spleen and bone marrow, in *Pathological Processes in Malaria and Blackwater Fever.* Charles C Thomas, Springfield, Ill., 1948, chap. 10, p. 290.
28. Toghill. P. J.: Red cell pooling in enlarged spleens. *Br. J. Haematol.* 10:347, 1964.
29. Jandl. J. H., Files, N. M., Barnett, S. B., and MacDonald, R. A.: Proliferative response of the spleen and liver to hemolysis. *J. Exp. Med.* 122:299, 1965.
30. Langevoort, H. L.: The histophysiology of the antibody response. I. Histogenesis of the plasma cell reaction in rabbit spleen. *Lab. Invest.* 12:106, 1963.
31. Gill, A. J.: Traumatic autograft of splenic tissue in the body wall. *J. Lab. Clin. Med.* 29:247, 1944.
32. Crosby, W. H., and Benjamin, N. R.: Frozen spleen reimplanted and challenged with Bartonella. *Am. J. Pathol.* 39:119, 1961.
33. Macpherson, A. I. S., and Innes, J.: Peripheral blood picture after operation for portal hypertension. *Lancet* 1:1120, 1953.
34. Cameron, G. R., and de Saram, G. S. W.: Method for permanently dissociating spleen from portal ciculation ("marsupialized" spleen) and its use in study of experimental liver cirrhosis. *J. Pathol.* 48:41, 1939.
35. Crosby, W. H.: How many "polys" are enough? *Arch. Intern. Med.* 123:722, 1969.
36. Kyle, R. A., and Linman, J. W.: Chronic idiopathic neutropenia. *N. Engl. J. Med.* 279:1015, 1968.
37. Crosby. W. H.: What to treat in Felty's syndrome. *JAMA* 225:1114, 1973.
38. Laszlo, J., Jones, J., Silberman, H. R., and Banks, P. M.: Splenectomy for Felty's syndrome: Clinicopathologic study of 27 patients. *Arch. Intern. Med.* 138:597, 1978.
39. Logue. G. L., Huang, A. T., and Shimm, D. S.: Failure of splenectomy in Felty's syndrome: The role of antibodies supporting granulocyte lysis by lymphocytes. *N. Engl. J. Med.* 304:580, 1981.
40. Hanrahan, E. M., and Miller, S. R.: Effect of splenectomy in Felty's syndrome. *JAMA.* 99:1274, 1932.
41. Walker, R. M., Shaldon, C., and Vowles, K. D. J.: Late results of portacaval anastamosis. *Lancet* 2:727, 1961.
42. Silverstein, M. N., and Kelley, P. J.: Osteoarticular manifestations of Gaucher's disease. *Am. J. Med. Sci.* 253:569, 1967.
43. Jacob, H. S.: Born again to work again. *N. Engl. J. Med.* 198:1415, 1978.
44. Bernard, R. P., Bauman, A. W., and Schwartz, S. I.: Splenectomy for thrombotic thrombocytopenic purpura. *Ann. Surg.* 169:616, 1969.
45. Cuttner, J.: Splenectomy, steroids and dextran 70 in thrombotic thrombocytopenic purpura. *JAMA.* 227:397, 1974.
46. Koch, J. L.: Aplastic anemia and splenectomy. *Arch. Intern. Med.* 119:305, 1967.
47. Scott, J. L., Cartwright, G. E., and Wintrobe, M. M.: Acquired aplastic anemia: An analysis of 39 cases and review of the pertinent literature. *Medicine* 38:119, 1959.
48. Crosby. W. H.: Wet purpura, dry purpura. *JAMA.* 232:744, 1975.
49. Garnett, E. S., Goddard, B. A., Markby, D., and Webber, C. E.: The spleen as an arteriovenous shunt. *Lancet* 1:386, 1969.
50. Rosenbaum, D. L., Murphy, G. W. and Swisher, S. N.: Hemodynamic studies of the portal circulation in myeloid metaplasia. *Am. J. Med.* 41:360, 1966.
51. Pryor, D. S.: Splenectomy in tropical splenomegaly. *Br. Med. J.* 3:825, 1967.
52. Bischel. M. D., Neiman, R. S., Berne, T. V., Telfer, N., Lukes, R. J., and Barbour, B. H.: Hypersplenism in the uremic dialyzed patient, the effect of splenectomy: Effect on transplantation and proposed mechanisms. *Nephron* 9:146, 1972.
53. Zaentz, S. D., Krantz, S. B., and Sears, D. A.: Studies on pure red cell aplasia. VII. Presence of proerythroblasts and response to splenectomy: A case report. *Blood* 46:261, 1975.
54. Krantz, S, B.: Pure red cell aplasia. *Br. J. Haematol.* 25:1, 1973.
55. O'Brien, J. S., and Walsh, J. R.: Hypogammaglobulinemia and hypersplenism associated with lymphosarcoma of the spleen. *Am. J. Med.* 30:813, 1961.
56. Strawitz, J. G., Sokal, J. E., Grace, J. T., Mukhtar, F., and Moore, G. E.: Surgical aspects of hypersplenism in lymphoma and leukemia. *Surgery* 112:89, 1961.
57. Korbitz, B. C., Reiquam, C. W., and Palmer, H. D.: Splenic myelosuppressive syndrome. *Cancer* 22:1185, 1968.
58. Hutt, M. S. R., Richardson, J. S., and Staffurth, J. S.: Felty's syndrome. *Q. J. Med.* 20:57, 1951.
59. Doan, C. A., Wiseman, B. K., and Erf, L. A.: Studies in hemolytic jaundice. *Ohio State Med. J.* 30:493, 1934.
60. Steiner, B.: Essential pulmonary hemosiderosis as immunohematologic problem: Improvement following splenectomy. *Arch. Dis. Child.* 29:391, 1954.
61. Cooper, A. S.: Idiopathic pulmonary hemosiderosis. *N. Engl. J. Med.* 263:1100, 1960.
62. Schellen, T. M. C. M.: Relation between the spleen and the gonads: Splenogenital syndrome. *Fertil. Steril.* 11:590, 1960.
63. Crosby, W. H., Whelan, T. J., and Heaton, L. D.: Splenectomy in the elderly. *Med. Clin. North Am.* 50:1533, 1966.
64. Crosby, W. H.: Paroxysmal nocturnal hemoglobinuria: Relation of the clinical manifestations to underlying pathogenic mechanisms. *Blood* 8:769, 1953.
65. Neuschatz, J., and Crosby, W. H.: The prevention of postoperative thrombosis: A simple, safe approach. *Arch. Intern. Med.* 130:966, 1972.
66. Preston, F. E., Hastin, J. F., Stewart, R. M., and Davies-Jones, G. A. B.: Thrombocytosis, circulating platelet aggregates and neurologic dysfunction. *Br. Med. J.* 2:1561, 1979.
67. Hosea, S. W., Brown, E. J., Hamburger, M. I., and Frank, M. M.: Opsonic requirements for intravascular clearance after splenectomy. *N. Engl. J. Med.* 304:245, 1981.
68. Erakalis, A. J., Kevy, S. V., Diamond, L. K., and Gross, R. E.: Hazard

of overwhelming infection after splenectomy in childhood. *N. Engl. J. Med.* 276:1225, 1967.

69. Torres, J., and Bisno, A. L.: Hyposplenism and pneumococcemia. *Am. J. Med.* 55:851, 1973.
70. Gopal, V., and Bisno, A. L.: Fulminant pneumococcal infections in "normal" asplenic hosts. *Arch. Intern. Med.* 137:1526, 1977.
71. Abramowicz, M.: Prevention of serious infections after splenectomy. *Med. Lett.* 19:2, 1977.
72. Austrian, R., et al.: Prevention of pneumococcal pneumonia by vaccination. *Clin. Res.* 24:483A, 1976.
73. Horan, M., and Colebatch. J. H.: Relation between splenectomy and subsequent infections: A clinical study. *Arch. Dis. Child.* 37:398, 1962.
74. Conrad, M. E., and Dennis, L. H.: Splenic function in experimental malaria. *Am. J. Trop. Med. Hyg.* 17:170, 1968.
75. Watson-Williams, E. J., Allan, N. C., and Fleming, A. F.: "Big spleen" disease. *Br. Med. J.* 2:416, 1967.
76. Reynafarje, C., and Ramos, J.: The hemolytic anemia of human bartonellosis. *Blood* 17:562, 1961.
77. Ruebush, T. K., Cassaday, P. B., Marsh, H. J., et al.: Human babesiosis on Nantucket Island: Clinical features. *Ann. Intern. Med.* 86:6, 1977.
78. Robinette, C. D., and Fraumini, J. F.: Splenectomy and subsequent mortality in veterans of the 1939–45 war. *Lancet* 2:127, 1977.
79. Silverstein, M. N.: *Agnogenic Myeloid Metaplasia.* Publishing Sciences Group, Acton, Mass., 1975.

Erythrocyte disorders—anemias due to acute blood loss

CHAPTER *72*

Acute blood loss anemia

ROBERT S. HILLMAN

Acute blood loss anemia may occur after trauma or when a disease process damages vascular integrity sufficiently to allow red blood cells to escape from the intravascular space. A rapid hemorrhage of major proportions actually represents a double threat to the homeostasis of the organism. First, severe blood loss can acutely decrease the total blood volume to the point of cardiovascular collapse, irreversible shock, and death. In this situation, the loss of circulating red cells is of far less importance than the sudden depletion of the total blood volume. Second, when blood loss is more gradual and the total blood volume is restored by expansion of the plasma volume, the circulating red cell mass may be so depleted as to impair oxygen delivery to peripheral tissues. In each case, the human organism responds in a characteristic manner, trying to compensate for the abnormality and maintain a normal total blood volume and oxygen supply. This involves the interaction of a number of physiologic mechanisms, including adjustments in cardiovascular dynamics, blood volume, red cell production, and oxygen transport by adult erythrocytes [1]. A sound understanding of these adaptive mechanisms is extremely important both for accurate diagnosis and proper management. This is especially true when the clinical manifestations of blood loss are greatly modified by the characteristics of the underlying disease process or when hemorrhage is internal, in a body cavity, internal organ, or muscle mass.

Volume loss and replacement

CLINICAL MANIFESTATIONS

Regardless of the cause of an acute, severe hemorrhage, the immediate clinical manifestations are essentially the same and depend on the volume of blood lost. In the initial evaluation of the magnitude of an acute blood loss, the hematocrit may fail to reflect the quantity of blood lost and the physician must use clinical signs and symptoms to estimate blood volume depletion. As outlined in Table 72-1, a normal person can rapidly lose up to 20 percent of the total blood volume without noticeable signs or symptoms of anemia or cardiovascular collapse. However, once the hemorrhage exceeds 1000 ml, signs of cardiovascular distress appear. At first, this is limited to tachycardia with exercise and postural hypotension in some individuals. When the blood loss exceeds 30 to 40 percent of the original blood volume, there is a measurable fall in cardiac output and the gradual onset of shock; the patient becomes immobile and exhibits air hunger; a rapid, thready pulse; and cold, clammy skin. Unless further hemorrhage is prevented and effective therapy begun, organ damage and death ensue. A very rapid blood loss which exceeds 50 percent of the patient's blood volume carries a high mortality unless immediate volume replacement therapy is initiated.

This sequence of events is true for instance of very rapid hemorrhage where physiologic mechanisms for replacing lost volume have had no opportunity to be effective. The clinical manifestations of acute volume loss reflect adjustments in cardiac output and vascular tone which help prevent circulatory collapse and maintain oxygen supply to vital organs. With more gradual blood loss, sufficient restoration of plasma volume can occur to permit a loss of even larger volumes of blood without the onset of shock. However, unless the physician intercedes with volume replacement therapy, plasma volume expansion is a relatively slow process. Following a sudden loss of 20 percent of the total vol-

TABLE 72-1 Reaction to acute blood loss of increasing severity

Volume lost up to		Clinical signs
%TBV	ml*	
10	500	None. Rarely see vasovagal syncope in blood bank donors [1].
20	1,000	With the patient at rest it is still impossible to detect volume loss. Tachycardia is usual with exercise, and a slight postural drop in blood pressure may be evident [2,3].
30	1,500	Neck veins are flat when supine. Postural hypotension and exercise tachycardia are generally present, but the resting, supine blood pressure and pulse still can be normal.
40	2,000	Central venous pressure, cardiac output, and arterial blood pressure are below normal even when the patient is supine and at rest [4,5]. The patient usually demonstrates air hunger; a rapid, thready pulse; and cold, clammy skin.
50	2,500	Severe shock, death.

* For a normal 70-kg person with a 5000-ml total blood volume.

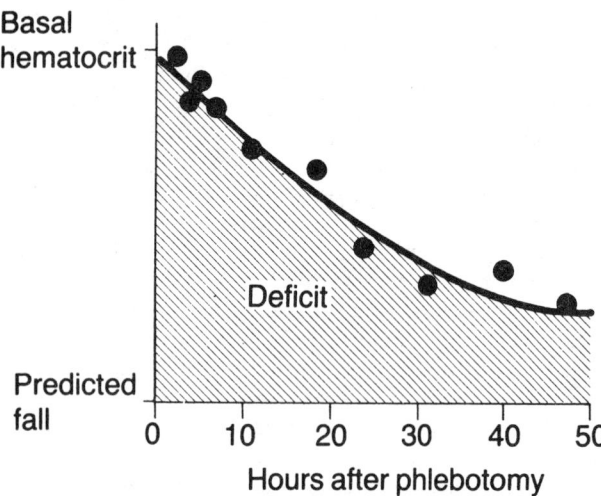

FIGURE 72-1   After a sudden loss of whole blood, the fall in hematocrit is a gradual process which depends on the rate of mobilization of albumin from extravascular sites [7]. Full expansion of the blood volume and the lowest hematocrit value may not be appreciated for up to 72 h.

ume, it takes 20 to 60 h to restore a normal blood volume by endogenous plasma replacement [2,6,7]. In humans, this is accomplished by mobilizing albumin from extravascular sites and not by an immediate increase in albumin production [7]. For this reason, the hematocrit falls gradually over a period of 2 to 3 days after a sudden, single hemorrhagic event (Fig. 72-1). This fact must be kept in mind in the evaluation of the bleeding patient, for overreliance on hematocrit values can lead to a misinterpretation of the severity of the hemorrhage.

REPLACEMENT THERAPY

In the initial management of the patient with acute hemorrhage, little attention need be given to the red cell mass; the first requirement is to maintain an adequate blood volume and prevent shock. This may be accomplished by intravenous infusion of crystalloid (electrolyte) solutions; colloid solutions of plasma protein, albumin, or dextran; or fresh whole blood. For the emergency situation, albumin, dextran, and electrolyte solutions are preferred. Albumin solutions containing 5% albumin in normal saline have the advantage of giving a known volume expansion in the hypovolemic patient [8–10].

The most important of the currently used dextran solutions are a 6% solution of high-molecular-weight dextran (dextran 70, average M_r 70,000 daltons) and a 10% solution of low-molecular-weight dextran (dextran 40 with an average M_r of 40,000 daltons). Infusions of dextran 70 in hypovolemic individuals produce an initial volume effect which is slightly more than the amount infused. The material is then gradually cleared over the next 24 to 48 h so that the blood volume support continues until normal, physiologic mechanisms have

replaced the volume lost. With dextran 40 the initial volume effect is nearly twice the amount infused. However, because of the low molecular weight, the material is more rapidly cleared into the urine and extravascular compartments so that by 3 to 4 h after infusion the volume effect is no greater than the amount infused. Without additional therapy over the next 24 h, hypovolemia may recur before normal volume replacement mechanisms can replace the volume lost [11]. A number of clinical studies confirm the fact that dextran solutions are satisfactory for the treatment of acute blood loss. It should be recognized, however, that dextran solutions may interfere with platelet adhesiveness and coagulation mechanisms when given in amounts exceeding 1000 ml.

Crystalloid solutions, normal saline and Ringer's lactate, may also be used for blood volume support in the emergency situation. Since crystalloid solutions are rapidly distributed between the intravascular and extravascular compartments, a greater volume must be infused for a measured effect. Rapid infusion of Ringer's lactate or normal saline in a volume of two or three times the estimated blood loss is probably the most widely used fluid therapy for hemorrhagic shock, and in the younger patient may be the preferred form of initial treatment [12]. When large volumes of crystalloid fluids are given, patients usually develop peripheral edema, and, in the case of the elderly individual, may have more difficulty with pulmonary edema. However, the debate as to whether colloid solutions are better than crystalloid solutions in supporting the blood volume without causing pulmonary edema has not been resolved [13]. Proponents of crystalloid therapy suggest that pulmonary edema in the hemorrhagic shock patient can be made worse by vascular overload and a leak of the infused albumin into the interstitial space of the lungs. Advocates of colloid replacement counter with the argument that the increased intravascular oncotic pressure which results from colloid transfusion should help to keep fluids from entering lung tissue. An extension of this thinking has led to the development of the HALFD (hypertonic albuminated fluid demand) regimen. This involves transfusing the patient with a fluid containing 120 meq of sodium lactate, 120 meq of sodium chloride, and 12.5 g of albumin per liter of solution. The oncotic pressure of this fluid is felt to prevent an interstitial fluid leak while providing reliable blood volume support. However, its success may require careful monitoring of arterial and central venous pressures to avoid fluid overload.

Complete reliance on fresh whole blood for the treatment of acute blood loss should be discouraged. Its use requires that large amounts of type O Rh-negative whole blood be available. If typing and cross-match procedures are carried out prior to transfusion, an unnecessary and possibly dangerous delay in therapy is introduced. In addition, fresh whole blood cannot always be relied upon to produce adequate volume expansion. A reaction to allergenic substances within the plasma or cells in whole blood can restrict volume expansion or even produce plasma volume contraction [14]. Therefore, transfusion of whole blood or red blood cells should be reserved for specific treatment of a low red cell mass where tissue hypoxia is a potential threat.

Red cell loss and replacement

CLINICAL MANIFESTATIONS

With precipitous hemorrhage the immediate effects of volume depletion are more important than the loss of circulating red blood cells. Only when blood loss is relatively slow and the total blood volume is maintained by natural or artificial means does anemia become a problem. How much of a problem depends on a number of variables, including the patient's general physical condition, the nature of the complicating illness, the ability of the cardiovascular system to compensate, and the flow characteristics of vital vascular pathways [1]. Whereas a normal, healthy young adult can tolerate a loss of up to 50 to 60 percent of the red cell mass, a patient with advanced arteriosclerotic cardiovascular disease may experience organ ischemia with as little as a 30 percent fall in the number of circulating red blood cells.

As previously mentioned (Fig. 72-1), the depletion of the red cell mass which occurs with blood loss cannot be appreciated from the hematocrit until the total blood volume has been returned to normal by expansion of the plasma volume. While the change in the hematocrit is relatively slow, there is often a rapid increase in the number of circulating polymorphonuclear leukocytes and platelets during the hemorrhage. The leukocyte count can rise to levels between 10,000 and 30,000 within a few hours, as a result of a shift of marginated leukocytes into the circulation and a release of white cells from the marrow granulocyte pool. Similarly, the platelet count can rise to levels approaching 1 million. In severe hemorrhage, more immature elements—metamyelocytes, myelocytes, and nucleated red blood cells—may enter the circulation. This is most commonly seen in those instances of severe blood loss which are accompanied by shock and tissue hypoxia.

Inasmuch as there is no ready reserve of mature red cells available to replace the lost red cell mass, oxygen supply to peripheral tissues must initially be maintained by adjustments in cardiovascular dynamics. Immediately after a hemorrhage, this is accomplished by arteriolar constriction in certain oxygen-insensitive areas such as skin and kidneys and a decrease in vascular resistance in sensitive organs where oxygen delivery is essential. Over the next several days, other physiologic mechanisms become important. Plasma levels of erythropoietin increase within 6 h of the appearance of an anemia in the bled patient. The magnitude of this increase correlates with the severity of the anemia, and

a linear fall in the hematocrit is accompanied by a logarithmic rise in the amount of erythropoietin excreted in the urine [15]. This hormone is then responsible for the subsequent increase in red cell production by the erythroid marrow. In addition, oxygen delivery by circulating erythrocytes may improve by means of a shift in the oxygen dissociation curve. Studies of human subjects subjected to high-altitude anoxia have demonstrated a significant shift of the hemoglobin oxygen dissociation curve within 24 h of the onset of anoxia [1,16]. This is an adaptive response of the circulating, adult erythrocytes and is associated with an increase in the intracellular levels of 2,3-diphosphoglycerate (2,3-DPG). Although this mechanism may be of importance in high-altitude hypoxia and in chronic anemias [17], its effectiveness as a compensatory mechanism immediately after a hemorrhage remains to be defined.

RED CELL REPLACEMENT

Replacement of the red cell mass by increased red cell production is a gradual process. In response to erythropoietin stimulation, marrow stem cells must first proliferate and then mature over a period of 2 to 5 days prior to their delivery to the circulation as effective adult red cells. There is, therefore, a considerable time lag before red cell production can appreciably increase the red cell mass.

The first response of the erythroid marrow to an acute hemorrhage is the erythropoietin-related shift of marrow reticulocytes into circulation. This may be assessed from the appearance of polychromatophilic macrocytes in the peripheral smear [18–20]. By the second to third day, erythroid hyperplasia is visible on a marrow aspirate. At this time, the reticulocyte production index will not have changed since more time is required for intramarrow precursor maturation. By the tenth day the marrow erythroid/myeloid (E/M) ratio and the reticulocyte production index will be comparable. These events are summarized in Table 72-2.

Erythropoietin has specific effects on both the stem cell and the reticulocyte pool of the marrow. A rising tide of erythropoietin not only initiates marrow proliferation and maturation of erythroblasts but also results in the premature delivery of marrow reticulocytes to the circulation [18–20]. The latter event may be seen within 6 to 12 h of the onset of a hemorrhagic anemia by the simple technique of examining a peripheral smear stained with Wright's stain [20]. Because of their imma-

TABLE 72-2   Response to acute hemorrhage

	6 h	*1 day*	*2–3 days*	*5 days*	*10 days*
Polychromasia	±	+	+	++	+++
Marrow E/M ratio	1/3	1/3	1/2–1/1	1/1	1/1
Reticulocyte index	1.0	1.0	1.0	2.0	3.0–5.0

turity and increased content of ribonucleic acid and ribosomes, the marrow reticulocytes appear as poly-chromatophilic macrocytes with this stain. At first, only a few such cells may be visible. However, as marrow production increases over the next several days, the polychromasia increases in intensity. This fact should be recognized in the interpretation of the reticulocyte count. In order to obtain an accurate estimate of the daily production of red cells, the observed reticulocyte percentage must be corrected both for the reduction in hematocrit and for premature delivery of reticulocytes, which then require more than 1 day to lose their reticulum.[1]

The proliferative response of the erythroid marrow may be recognized as early as the second day by examination of a marrow aspirate. After 5 days, erythroid hyperplasia is readily apparent; the E/M ratio is 1:1 or higher. Since these new red cell precursors must mature for a period of 2 to 5 days prior to delivery to circulation, the reticulocyte count does not immediately reflect the increase in marrow production. Although the observed reticulocyte count may appear to increase soon after the onset of the anemia, the reticulocyte production index does not actually increase for 3 to 5 days. A full level of marrow production as estimated from the reticulocyte production index occurs only after 8 to 10 days, at which time the erythroid hyperplasia of the marrow and the reticulocyte index are of the same magnitude [21]. Unless this disparity is recognized, an evaluation of a patient during the first week after a hemorrhage can lead to an error in diagnosis. Specifically, there will be a noticeable discrepancy between the marrow E/M ratio and the reticulocyte production index which will resemble the pattern seen with ineffective erythropoiesis where the death of red cell precursor during maturation precludes delivery of appropriate numbers of reticulocytes. The erythroid hyperplasia observed on the marrow aspirate is not accompanied by an equivalent level of reticulocytosis (Table 71-2).

The maximum rate of red cell production observed by the tenth day after a hemorrhage is determined by the integrity of the marrow, the level of the anemic stimu-

---

[1] A corrected reticulocyte count (i.e., a reticulocyte production index) is a more accurate measurement of effective red cell production than the observed reticulocyte count. It is obtained by making appropriate corrections both for variations in the hematocrit and premature delivery of marrow reticulocytes [20]. For example, an observed reticulocyte count of 9 percent in a patient with a hematocrit of 30 percent and erythropoietin-induced polychromasia on smear should be corrected as follows:

$$9\% \times \frac{30 \text{ (observed hematocrit)}/45 \text{ (normal hematocrit)}}{2}$$

$$= \text{reticulocyte production index of 3 times normal}$$

Once the observed reticulocyte count is corrected for the lower hematocrit, it is divided by 2 to correct for the longer maturation time of prematurely delivered marrow reticulocytes so as to give an index of production (basal production = 1) [18,20].

lus, and the iron supply to the marrow. In humans, the response to a hemorrhagic anemia does not involve the development of new marrow beds; the available marrow syncytium is uniquely designed to provide the blood supply and space necessary for a rapid increase in red cell production to better than five times normal. However, any disorder of marrow structure such as tumor invasion, a defect in vasculature, or a fibrosis of supporting elements can severely limit the capacity of the marrow to produce red cells.

The severity of the anemia is also important in determining the degree of marrow response. As long as the marrow structure is intact and iron supply to the red cell precursors is not rate-limiting, the observed increase in red cell production will usually reflect the severity of the anemia. However, damage to the kidneys, inflammation, or a hypometabolic state can markedly interfere with the response [22,23]. A normal individual with an intact erythropoietin mechanism will increase marrow production by a factor of two to three times normal after red cell mass depletions of 10 to 20 percent. When the hematocrit falls below 30 percent, indicating a loss of more than 25 percent of the red cell mass, plasma erythropoietin levels rise even higher, and marrow production will increase to levels of three to five times normal or more if iron supply is sufficient [21].

In the majority of individuals where marrow structure and erythropoietin response mechanisms are normal, the amount of iron available to the erythroid marrow is the prime determinant of the level of marrow production (Fig. 72-2) [21–23]. With increasing anemia, the level of marrow response directly reflects the number of available iron supply pools and the rate of iron delivery from these pools [21]. For example, following a gastrointestinal hemorrhage, a normal individual is able to deliver sufficient iron to support a marrow production level of no greater than three times normal despite increasingly severe anemia. This reflects the maximum rate of mobilization and delivery of storage iron from the monocyte-macrophage system. Moreover, if these iron stores are exhausted, the subject is unable to increase the red cell production even to this level, and the proliferative response of the marrow is severely restricted. This effect on marrow production is the earliest sign of absolute iron deficiency. It antedates by weeks or months the typical microcytosis and hypochromia of long-standing iron deficiency. In contrast, when additional iron supply pools are available, as in the subject who bleeds internally and then mobilizes iron from the degraded red cells or who receives large supplements of oral iron in the presence of normal hemosiderin iron stores, marrow production may attain levels of four to five times normal. When large amounts of red cells are continually destroyed by the monocyte-macrophage system, as with a hemolytic anemia, the iron recovered from the degraded hemoglobin is even more rapidly returned to the erythroid marrow so as to permit marrow production levels exceeding five times normal at low hematocrit levels. These characteristics of marrow production must be recognized in order to predict the rate of recovery of the patient's hematocrit and plan proper therapy.

Although transfusions of whole blood or red blood cells are the obvious immediate therapy for a blood loss anemia of major severity, it is always to the patient's benefit to take full advantage of the normal mechanisms of compensatory red cell production. With prolonged bleeding episodes and nonemergency situations every effort should be made to evaluate the adequacy of the patient's marrow production response and institute appropriate therapy to maximize the body's own red cell output. Primarily, this is an evaluation of iron supply, i.e., the number and adequacy of various iron pools and the level of iron delivery from these pools as determined from the serum iron and marrow proliferative response. Therapy may then concentrate on developing new iron supply pools and improving the rate of iron delivery from these sites. At least, the exhaustion of iron stores and onset of iron-deficient erythropoiesis should be anticipated and avoided. In the patient with blood loss anemia this really amounts to a decision between the use of oral and parenteral iron preparations.

Basically, there is very little difference between oral iron and parental iron preparations in regard to the rate and amount of iron supplied to the marrow. Studies of the rate of hemoglobin regeneration in iron-deficient patients given either oral or parenteral iron have shown no significant advantage for either form of iron [24,25]. Marrow production studies [21,26] do show a greater increase in red cell production immediately after intravenous infusions of large amounts of iron dextran than is seen with oral iron. However, this is sustained for only 10 to 14 days; the major portion of the injected iron dextran is made available by the action of the macrophages at a rate no greater than the level of iron absorbed from 4 to 8 oral iron tablets per day. Therefore, in the final analysis a single source of iron, whether normal macrophage storage iron, oral iron, or parenteral iron injections, will provide approximately the same iron supply, enough for a maximum red cell production level of three times normal. In order to exceed this limit, it is necessary to provide several sources of iron at one time. Thus, a combination of an oral iron supplement and macrophage or parenchymal iron deposits may improve iron delivery and permit marrow production to increase to levels of four to five times normal.

In the majority of situations, these differences in red cell production are of minor importance. Once hemorrhage has ceased, the recovery of the red cell mass to normal is usually accomplished gradually without inconvenience to the patient. Serious attempts at increasing iron supply by combination therapy should therefore be reserved for those situations where a rapid maximum response is essential, as in preparation of the patient for surgery or in treatment of prolonged, continuous hemorrhage. Blood transfusion may then be reserved for those instances where normal response mechanisms and iron supplementation are insufficient

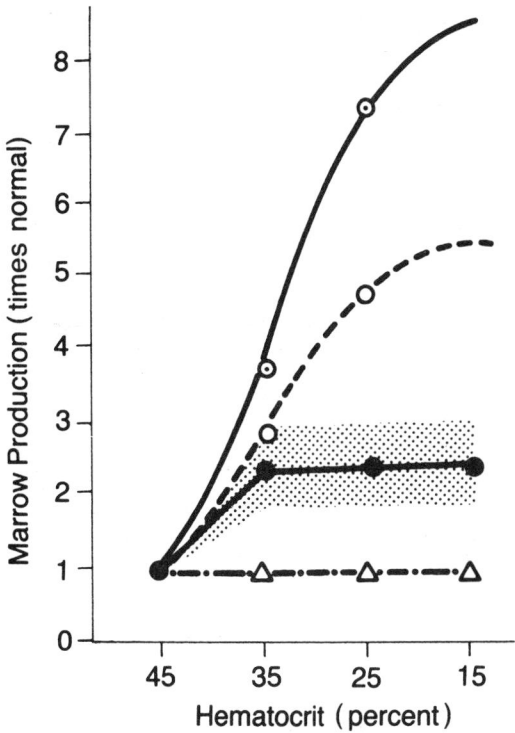

FIGURE 72-2 The rate of red blood cell production after hemorrhage reflects both the severity of the anemia and the rate of iron delivery from various sources. With red cell mass depletions of 20 percent or less, marrow production will increase to two to three times normal regardless of the source of iron. However, at lower hematocrit levels, production reflects the type of iron supply. A normal individual who must rely on hemosiderin stores in the monocyte-macrophage system is unable to increase production further (solid dots, shaded area). In contrast, in patients with a hemolytic process (circled dots) or with more than one source of iron supply (open circles), production can increase to levels of four to seven times normal when the hematocrit falls to 25 percent. Iron-deficient patients fail to show a marrow production increase at either hematocrit level (triangles).

to sustain an adequate red cell mass or the acuteness of the situation demands an immediate response.

References

1. Finch, C. A., and Lenfant, C.: Oxygen transport in man. *N. Engl. J. Med.* 286:407, 1972.
2. Ebert, R. V., Stead, E. A., Jr., and Gibson, J. G.: II. Response of normal subjects to acute blood loss. *Arch. Intern. Med.* 68:578, 1941.
3. Theyl, R. A., and Tuohy, G. F.: Hemodynamics and blood volume during operation with ether anesthesia and unreplaced blood loss. *Anesthesiology* 25:6, 1964.
4. Howarth, S., and Sharpey-Schafer, E. P.: Low blood pressure phases following hemorrhage. *Lancet* 1:19, 1947.
5. Tovey, G. H., and Lennon, G. G.: Blood volume studies in accidental hemorrhage. *J. Obstet. Gynaecol. Br. Commonw.* 5:749, 1962.
6. Lister, J., McNeill, I. F., Marshall, V. C., Plzak, L. F., Dagher, F. J., and Moore, F. D.: Transcapillary refilling after hemorrhage in normal man: Basal rates and volumes; effect of norepinephrine. *Ann. Surg.* 158:698, 1963.

7. Adamson, J., and Hillman, R. S.: Blood volume and plasma protein replacement following acute blood loss in normal man. *JAMA* 205:609, 1968.

8. Rieger, A.: Blood volume and plasma protein. *Arch. Chir, Scand. Suppl. 379*, 1967.

9. Bertrand, J. J., et al.: Clinical investigations with a heat-treated plasma protein fraction—plasmanate. *Vox Sang. 4*:385, 1959.

10. Hillman, R. S.: Pooled human plasma as a volume expander. *N. Engl. J. Med. 271*:1027, 1964.

11. Gruber, U. F.: *Blood Replacement*. Springer-Verlag, Berlin, 1969.

12. Shires, G. T.: Current status of the shock problem, in *Current Problems in Surgery*, edited by M. M. Ravitch. Year Book, Chicago, 1966, p. 1.

13. Shine, K. I., Kuhn, M., Young, L. S., and Tillisch, J. H.: Aspects of the management of shock. *Ann. Intern. Med. 93*:723, 1980.

14. Hutchison, J. L., Freedman, J. O., Richards, B. A., and Burgen, A. S. V.: Plasma volume expansion and reactions after infusion of analogous plasma in man. *J. Lab. Clin. Med. 56*:734, 1960.

15. Adamson, J. W.: The erythropoietin/hematocrit relationship in normal and polycythemic man: Implications of marrow regulation. *Blood 32*:597, 1968.

16. Eaton, J. W., Brewer, G. J., and Grover, R. F.: Role of red cell 2,3-diphosphoglycerate in the adaption of man to altitude. *J. Lab. Clin. Med. 73*:603, 1969.

17. Torrance, J., Jacobs, P., Restrepo, A., Eschbach, J., Lenfant, C., and Finch, C.: Intraerythrocytic adaptation to anemia. *N. Engl. J. Med. 283*:165, 1970.

18. Hillman, R. S.: Characteristics of marrow production and reticulocyte maturation in normal man in response to anemia. *J. Clin. Invest. 48*:443, 1969.

19. Gordon, A. S., LoBue, J., Dornfest, B. S., and Cooper, G. W.: Reticulocyte and leukocyte release from isolated perfused rat legs and femurs, in *Erythropoiesis*. Grune & Stratton, New York, 1962, p. 321.

20. Hillman, R. S., and Finch, C. A.: Erythropoiesis: Normal and abnormal. *Semin. Hematol. 4*:327, 1967.

21. Hillman, R. S., and Henderson, P. A.: Control of marrow production by the level of iron supply. *J. Clin. Invest. 48*:454, 1969.

22. Hillman, R. S.: The importance of iron supply in thalassemic erythropoiesis. *Ann. N.Y. Acad. Sci. 165*:100, 1969.

23. Erslev, A. J., and McKenna, P. J.: Effect of splenectomy on red cell production. *Ann. Intern. Med. 67*:990, 1967.

24. Cope, W., Gillhespy, R. O., and Richardson, R. W.: Treatment of iron-deficiency anemia: Comparisons of methods. *Br. Med. J. 2*:638, 1956.

25. Bothwell, T. H., Charlton, R. W., Cook, L. D., and Finch, C. A.: *Iron Metabolism in Man*. Blackwell Scientific, Oxford, 1979.

26. Henderson, P. A., and Hillman, R. S.: Characteristics of iron dextran utilization in man. *Blood 34*:357, 1969.

Erythrocyte disorders— erythrocytosis

CHAPTER *73*

Secondary polycythemia (erythrocytosis)

ALLAN J. ERSLEV

Definitions and history

Secondary polycythemia is an absolute erythrocytosis caused by an enhanced stimulation of red blood cell production. Since erythropoietin has been either demonstrated or suspected as the responsible stimulus in most cases, it seems reasonable to consider all cases of secondary polycythemia as caused by excessive release of erythropoietin. In most instances this release is appropriate and part of a compensatory effect to minimize a threatening tissue hypoxia. However, in a few cases the release appears inappropriate since the resulting increase in oxygen-carrying capacity is of no discernible benefit to the patient.

In his famous monograph on barometric pressure published in 1878 [1], Paul Bert showed that the physiologic impairment observed at high altitude was due to a reduction in the oxygen content of air. A few years earlier his friend and mentor Dennis Jourdanet had observed an increase in the number of red corpuscles in the blood of the highlanders of Mexico [2], and Bert recognized that such an increase would tend to ameliorate the effect of atmospheric hypoxia. However, neither he nor Jourdanet suspected a cause-effect relationship. It was actually not until Viault [3] in 1890 observed a prompt increase in the number of his own red corpuscles after having traveled from Lima, Peru, at sea level to Morococha at 15,000 ft (4570 m) that altitude erythrocytosis was accepted as a compensatory adaptation to hypoxia [4].

At about the same time, it was observed that many patients with cyanosis were also polycythemic. Both the cardiacos negros [5] with severe pulmonary failure and arterial oxygen unsaturation, and the children with morbus caeruleus, or right-to-left shunt through a congenital cardiac malformation, were found to have increased red cell counts [6]. Mechanical or neurogenic hypoventilation as a cause for cyanosis and polycythe-

mia was first popularized in 1956 with the classic description of the Pickwickian syndrome by Burwell et al. [7]. Recently, there has been an increasing interest in the polycythemia associated with arterial hypoxia due to carbon monoxide or with tissue hypoxia due to inherited abnormal hemoglobins with high oxygen affinity. Polycythemia has also been described in patients without demonstrable tissue hypoxia, and in some of these an inappropriate section of erythropoietin from various cysts and tumors has been demonstrated.

In this chapter secondary polycythemia will be divided into appropriate, compensatory types and inappropriate, pathologic types. Although the term *erythrocytosis* is more descriptive than polycythemia or erythremia, *secondary polycythemia* is a time-honored name and will be used here.

Appropriate secondary polycythemia

ERYTHROCYTOSIS DUE TO LOW ATMOSPHERIC PRESSURE

PHYSIOLOGY OF HIGH-ALTITUDE ACCLIMATIZATION
The enormous human capacity for physiologic adaptation is no better demonstrated than at high altitudes. Human beings and most domesticated animals can readily adjust to atmospheric pressures of about two-thirds of normal (14,000 ft, or 4270 m). Although exact medical statistics are sparse, the inhabitants of mining towns in the high Andes, such as Morococha, Peru, at 14,900 ft (4540 m), appear to be as healthy and have as long a life-span as their compatriots at sea level [8]. Permanent settlements above 15,000 ft (4570 m) are few, the highest one probably being Aucanquilcha in the Chilean Andes at 17,500 ft (5330 m), presumably the upper limit of long-term human endurance [9]. Members of an expedition led by Sir Edmund Hillary attempted gallantly to achieve acclimatization by staying for 5 months at 18,750 ft (5720 m), or at slightly less than one-half normal atmospheric pressure, but failed [10]. The mountain climbers experienced a steady physical deterioration, and severe thrombotic complications occurred in at least two members of the party. A few birds, insects, and spiders inhabit the Himalayas between 18,000 (5480 m) and 20,000 ft (6100 m), but above this level only transient visits are possible [9]. Such visits culminated in the first scaling of Mount Everest in 1953, but it was not until 1978 that Messner and Habeler, in a heroic climb, reached the summit at 29,028 ft (8850 m) without the use of supplementary oxygen [11]. One cannot fail to share the marvel of the British mountain climber George Lowe when he watched from the slopes of Mount Everest a flock of bar-headed geese flying in effortless echelon directly over the summit. It is known that the bar-headed geese start from the lakes of India at sea level and complete their spring migration to Tibet in a single majestic flight, but their mechanism of adaptation is entirely unknown [9].

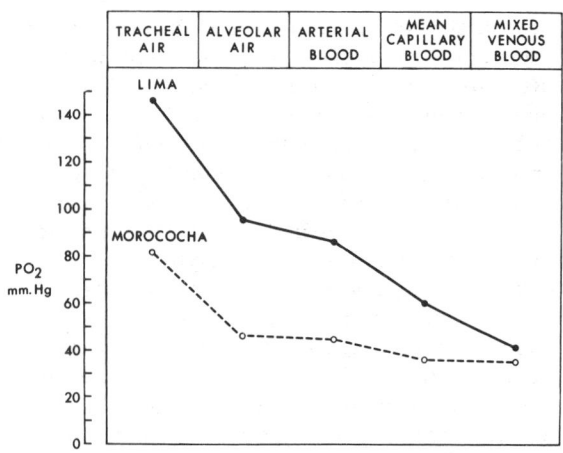

FIGURE 73-1 The oxygen gradient from atmospheric air to the tissues in individuals living at sea level and in Morococha, Peru, at 14,900 ft (4540 m) above sea level. (Redrawn from Hurtado [15].)

The first human adaptive adjustment described was that of polycythemia. However, polycythemia is not a particularly efficient way to enhance oxygen transport [12], and mammals, such as the llama, with a longer evolutionary exposure to high altitudes, do not use polycythemia as a compensatory device [13]. In a series of classic papers, Hurtado and coworkers have described the various adaptive changes which permit people living at 14,900 ft (4540 m) in Morococha to maintain a normal tissue tension oxygen [8,14,15] (Fig. 73-1).

The initial oxygen gradient between atmospheric air and alveolar air can be reduced by means of hyper-

FIGURE 73-2 Oxygen dissociation curves at sea level and in Morococha at 14,900 ft (4540 m) above sea level. (Redrawn from Hurtado [15].)

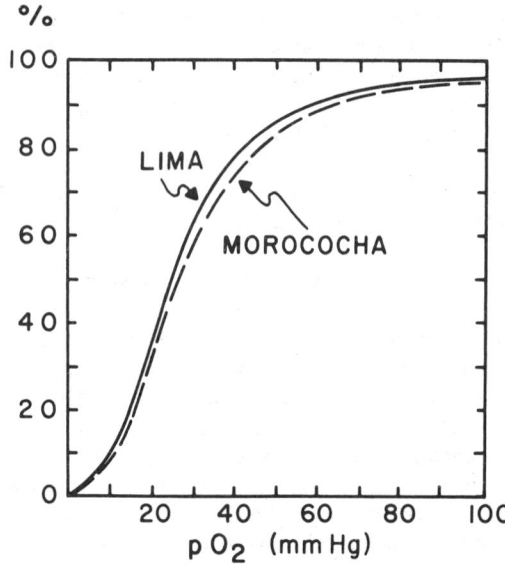

ventilation. Unfortunately, the dead space and the water vapor pressure are quite constant, and the gradient is reduced only from about 51 mm at sea level to about 37 mm at Morococha. Some further reduction can be achieved when needed, but the metabolic cost of increased ventilatory activity is excessive.

At high altitudes the chronic ventilatory stress leads to so-called altitude emphysema with increased vital capacity [16]. This pulmonary "stretch" may be responsible for an increase in the alveolocapillary diffusing area and a decrease in the alveoloarterial gradient from about 9 mm to an almost imperceptible 1.5 mm.

In addition to the alveolar oxygen tension, the amount of oxygen taken up by the arterial blood in the lungs also depends on the oxygen dissociation curve. Since the oxygen dissociation curve in well-acclimatized individuals is shifted slightly to the right (Fig. 73-2), there is a moderate impairment in the oxygen attachment to hemoglobin as well as a moderate increase in the capacity of hemoglobin to release oxygen in the capillaries.

In the capillaries the arteriovenous oxygen gradient is kept at a minimum in order to maintain a high pressure head of oxygen throughout the length of the capillary. After oxygen molecules have reached the cells, no further kinetic energy is needed, since the intracellular transport is determined by the distribution of biochemical electron carriers. The maintenance of a high mean capillary oxygen pressure is made possible by a slight shift in the oxygen dissociation curve to the right and by an increase in the oxygen-carrying capacity of blood. An increase in cardiac output will also minimize the arteriocapillary gradient. However, the added workload on a vital organ is probably less desirable than induced changes in the oxygen dissociation curve or in the rate of red cell production, and, in the well-adapted individual, the cardiac output at high altitudes is somewhat lower than at sea level [17]. A reduction in oxygen consumption would tend to reduce the arteriovenous oxygen gradient, but all studies indicate that the cellular oxygen consumption is not influenced by altitude [18] and that whole-body oxygen consumption may even be somewhat increased because of excessive ventilatory work.

A shift in the oxygen dissociation curve to the right may be of benefit for short-term high-altitude acclimatization [19], but its usefulness for chronic acclimatization has probably been exaggerated [20]. In the unacclimatized subject exposed acutely to high altitude, hyperventilation alkalosis leads initially to a shift of the oxygen dissociation curve to the left and to additional tissue hypoxia [21]. The alkalosis and the hypoxia will in turn promote red cell synthesis of 2,3-diphosphogylcerate (2,3-DPG) and ATP and cause the oxygen dissociation curve to shift back to a normal or even a right-shifted position [22]. In chronic acclimatization, the blood pH is usually normal, and the curve is shifted only slightly to the right (Fig. 73-2). It actually seems very questionable if a shift to the right would be to the best advantage of high-altitude dwellers [23]. Such a shift would significantly impair the loading of oxygen onto hemoglobin in the lungs, a potentially dangerous effect when the ambient pressure is greatly reduced. It is of interest that animals indigenous to high altitudes such as the llamas and vicuñas have oxygen dissociation curves positioned far to the left [24]. This would suggest that the loading of oxygen in the lungs is of more importance for the sustained acclimatization than the unloading in the tissues. A similar suggestion was made in an intriguing study of two patients with the high-oxygen-affinity hemoglobin Andrew-Minneapolis [25]. These individuals when tested immediately after arriving at 9950 ft (3100 m) were found to be pre-adapted and were able to carry out physical tests with less mobilization of cardiac, pulmonary, and erythroid reserves than normal controls. The question is how the tissues obtain oxygen from hemoglobin with a high oxygen affinity. There may be more capillaries per gram of tissue, or the intracellular electron chain may be set for a lower oxygen pressure. In any case polycythemia does not appear to be needed, since llamas do not develop a compensatory erythrocytosis [13].

In the less well adapted mammals, polycythemia is the primary compensatory device for high-altitude living. High altitudes will cause some tissue hypoxia leading to the release of erythropoietin (Fig. 73-3), an increase in the rate of red cell production, and eventually a polycythemia with an enhanced oxygen-carrying capacity. Unfortunately, the associated increase in blood viscosity tends to reduce blood flow and negates some of the advantage derived from the higher hemoglobin concentration.

Possibly the major benefit derived from an increase in red cell production is not the increase in oxygen-carrying capacity but is the concomitant expansion in total blood volume [27,28]. Such expansion could lead to the opening of new capillaries with a shortening of the mean distance between capillary and tissue cell, which in turn permits even a low mean capillary oxygen pressure to provide enough oxygen to the tissues [29].

In addition to these mechanisms, there are adaptive changes in the myoglobin content of the muscles, in the distribution of blood flow, and in the biosynthesis and biodegradation of a variety of enzymes that are directly or indirectly involved in intracellular oxygen metabolism [30]. The overall result appears to be that the fully acclimatized individual exposed of air of two-thirds to one-half of normal atmospheric pressure experiences no more tissue hypoxia than that needed to mobilize and maintain the mechanisms of acclimatization.

CLINICAL AND LABORATORY FEATURES OF HIGH-ALTITUDE POLYCYTHEMIA

Ruddy cyanosis and physiologic emphysema are the two characteristic features of human beings living at high altitudes. Venous and capillary engorgement can be observed readily in the conjunctiva, mucous membranes, and skin, and may contribute to the remarkable

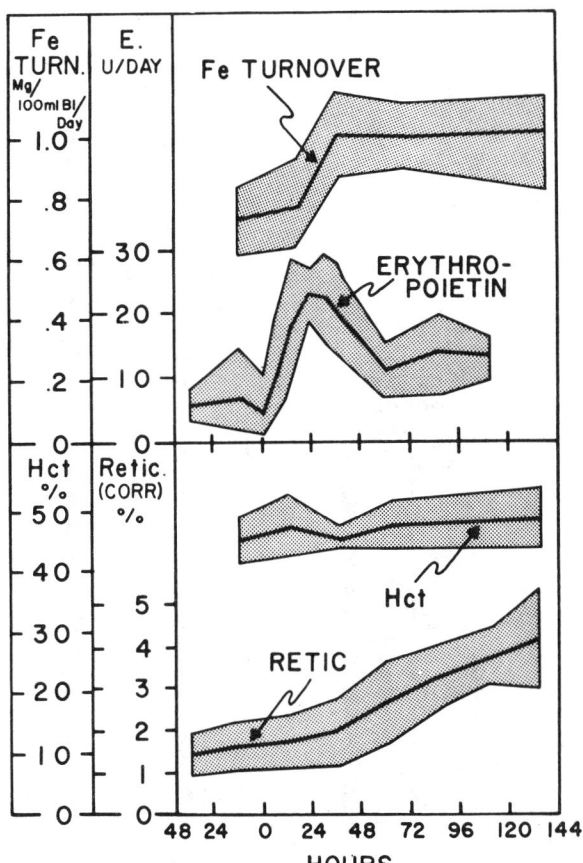

FIGURE 73-3 Mean plasma iron turnover and reticulocyte, hematocrit, and erythropoietin levels following exposure of seven subjects to high altitudes. Shaded area indicates 1 standard deviation. (Redrawn from Faura et al. [26].)

capacity of Sherpas to walk barefoot and sleep on ice and snow [10]. Splenomegaly and jaundice are unusual, although a sustained erythrocytosis obviously is associated with an increased rate of red cell destruction and bilirubin generation.

The laboratory studies reveal a normocytic, normochromic erythrocytosis with an increase in the absolute reticulocyte count and in the iron turnover [23].

The blood volume is increased primarily by the expansion in red cell mass (Fig. 73-4). The iron concentration and iron-binding capacity are usually normal, but the iron absorption may be increased [31,32]. The cellular composition of the marrow is not significantly changed. This can be attributed to the fact that an erythrocytosis can be maintained by a fairly small increase in the rate of red cell production as long as the red cell life-span is normal. A small increase, even a doubling, of red cell production may be difficult to ascertain from an examination of a marrow film, and a marrow examination is actually of very limited assistance in the diagnosis of secondary polycythemia. The white blood cell count and differential count are consistently normal. The platelet count decreases temporarily after arrival at

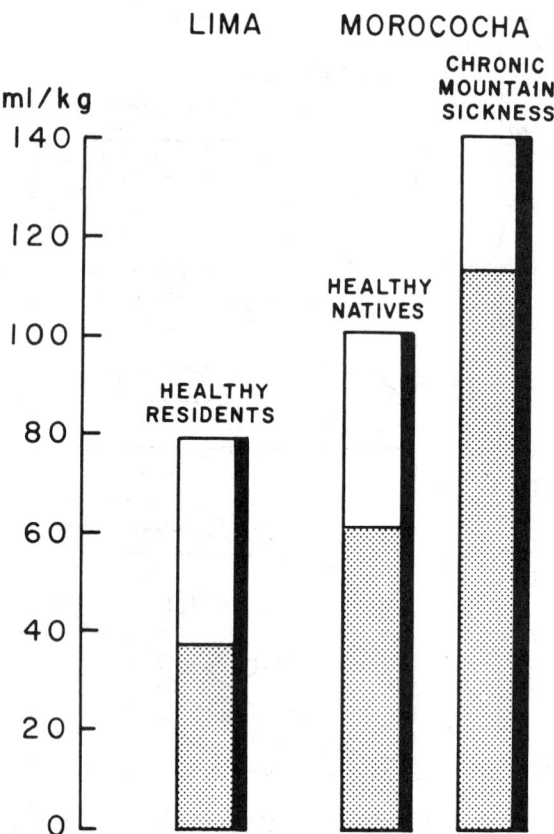

FIGURE 73-4 Red blood cell mass (stippled), and plasma volume (white), in normal individuals, in individuals well acclimatized to high altitudes, and in individuals suffering from chronic mountain sickness. (Redrawn from Hurtado [15].)

high altitude [25], but the moderate reduction observed in acclimatized individuals is probably a measuring artifact. Platelet counts are expressed per unit of whole blood rather than per unit of plasma, and the expanded red cell mass decreases the number of platelets per microliter of whole blood without changing the total number or the number per microliter of plasma [33]. The arterial gas studies reflect the fact that the individual is exposed to ambient air at low pressure.

PATHOLOGY OF HIGH-ALTITUDE ACCLIMATIZATION
Acute mountain sickness Tolerance to high altitudes varies greatly, but most normal individuals have no discomfort at altitudes of up to 7000 ft (2130 m). Above this level some manifestations of cerebral hypoxia are common. Headaches, sleeplessness, and palpitations are frequently encountered, and weakness, nausea, vomiting, and mental dullness may be present, constituting the syndrome of acute mountain sickness [34,35]. It appears that some of these symptoms are related to emotional attitudes toward high altitudes, because in the early days of the Pikes Peak railroad almost all passengers became violently ill at the summit, a relatively rare event today.

A characteristic feature of acute mountain sickness is Cheyne-Stokes respiration, especially at sleep, and many symptoms may be related to a temporary unresponsiveness of the respiratory center and may be prevented by the use of acetazolamide [36]. However, the more severe complications such as pulmonary edema and cerebral edema may be the consequence of abnormal fluid retention [34,37]. The normal response to altitudes is a *Höhen diurese* [34]; diuretics, acetazolamide, and oxygen or the return to lower altitudes are effective therapeutic remedies.

Chronic mountain sickness (Monge's disease) In 1937 Monge described a syndrome characterized by a slowly developing altitude decompensation [38]. Characteristically it occurs in individuals after prolonged exposure to high altitudes, and it is manifested by physical and emotional deterioration and by marked cyanosis and plethora. Clubbing of the fingers may be seen, and there are signs of right ventricular failure such as venous distention, edema, hepatomegaly, and even ascites. The hematocrit and red cell mass are far higher than usually seen in acclimatized subjects [15] (Fig. 73-4), and the resulting high blood viscosity may be responsible for many of the clinical manifestations [39].

Chronic mountain sickness appears to be caused by alveolar hypoventilation leading to excessive tissue hypoxia [40]. Carbon dioxide tension and content are elevated, and the respiratory center apparently has become refractory both to low oxygen tension and high carbon dioxide tension. In addition, it has been found that some of the patients with excessive erythrocytosis have abnormally high levels of red cell 2,3-DPG [41]. This would tend to shift the oxygen dissociation curve farther to the right, impair hemoglobin oxygenation in the lungs, and further aggravate tissue hypoxia. Therapeutic venesections provide symptomatic relief, but cure cannot be expected until some time after return to sea level.

ERYTHROCYTOSIS DUE TO PULMONARY DISEASE
Chronic pulmonary disease is frequently associated with cyanosis, clubbing, and arterial oxygen unsaturation but not always with an increase in hematocrit [42] (Fig. 73-5). This has been attributed to a concomitant increase in plasma volume [43–45], but in many studies of patients with chronic pulmonary disease and arterial oxygen unsaturation the increase in the red cell mass, although pronounced in some [46], has usually fallen far short of expectations [47–49]. The reason for the erythropoietic unresponsiveness to arterial hypoxia is not clear. The release of erythropoietin appears appropriate to the degree of arterial hypoxia [42,49], and there is no convincing evidence to support the idea that low oxygen tension or high carbon dioxide tension in marrow blood causes erythroid suppression. A shift to the right in the oxygen dissociation curve because of arterial hypoxemia and excessive production of 2,3-DPG

and ATP may be present but probably is no greater than the shift observed at high altitudes [41].

A decrease in iron reutilization because of chronic infection or chronic debility could provide an explanation [42,48]. The absence of a compensatory erythrocytosis in chronic pulmonary disease would then be comparable to the inability of patients with chronic illnesses to maintain a normal hemoglobin concentration. However, it must be conceded that the serum iron in chronic pulmonary disease usually is normal or high [49] and that many patients with emphysema show no evidence of chronic infection.

Therapeutic venesection in patients with high hematocrits is believed to be of doubtful value [50]. However recent studies in patients with secondary polycythemia have shown that venesection increases cerebral blood flow materially and may prevent cerebrovascular complications [51].

ERYTHROCYTOSIS DUE TO CARDIOVASCULAR DISEASE

Right-to-left shunt in congenital heart disease can cause profound arterial oxygen unsaturation, cyanosis, clubbing of fingers, and extreme erythrocytosis [52]. The hematocrit may reach levels of 75 to 85 percent and the red cell mass more than 100 ml/kg. The plasma volume is usually not changed significantly. Despite the high hematocrit, the patients rarely suffer from high-viscosity symptoms. However, dehydration due to acute illness or summer heat can rapidly cause a further increase in hematocrit and viscosity with circulatory stagnation and thrombosis. It has been questioned whether the extreme secondary polycythemia is of benefit to the patients or whether the associated increase in viscosity leads to a Pyrrhic compensation. Recent studies indicate that the increase in blood volume induced by the large red cell mass is of definite benefit in terms of tissue oxygenation and offsets the potentially hypoxic effect of sluggish blood flow [27,28]. Judicious venesections may be indicated if hematocrits are above 60 percent [51], especially prior to cardiac surgery, but many clinicians are reluctant to interfere actively in the homeostatic adjustment provided by nature [53].

Arterial hypoxemia and secondary polycythemia have been observed in patients with cirrhosis of the liver [54,55]. The hypoxemia is probably caused by pulmonary arteriovenous shunts or direct right-to-left vascular communications between portal and pulmonary veins. A similar syndrome has been described in patients with hereditary hemorrhagic telangiectasia [56] or with idiopathic pulmonary arteriovenous aneurysms [57].

Acquired heart disease with chronic decompensation is usually not associated with an erythrocytosis. However, careful determinations of total red cell mass before and after successful cardiac therapy indicate that there may be an increased rate of red cell production during periods of congestive failure, but that the ensuing erythrocytosis is obscured by a concomitant increase in plasma volume [58,59]. The responsible stimulus for in-

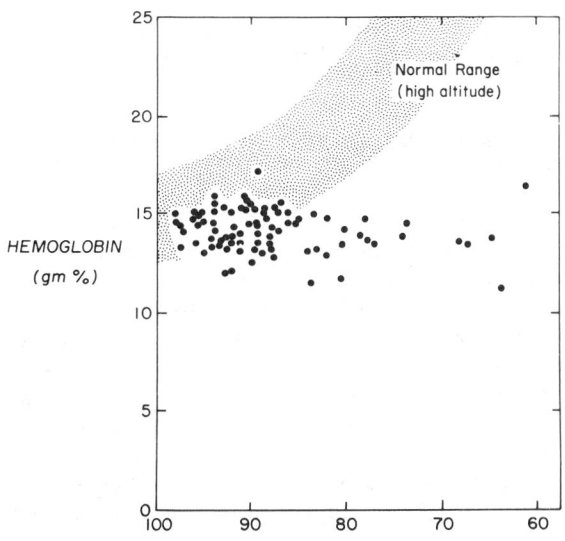

FIGURE 73-5 Hemoglobin concentration in patients with chronic pulmonary disease related to arterial oxygen saturation. The cross-hatched area represents the range of hemoglobin concentration attained at low arterial oxygen saturation caused by high altitudes [12]. (Redrawn from Gallo et al. [42].)

creased erythropoietic activity is probably tissue hypoxia secondary to thickening and edema of the pulmonary alveolar walls or to decrease in tissue perfusion.

ERYTHROCYTOSIS SECONDARY TO ALVEOLAR HYPOVENTILATION

Intermittent alveolar hypoventilation frequently observed in normal males during sleep [60] can, if severe, cause arterial hypoxemia and hypercapnia, cyanosis, somnolence, and secondary polycythemia [7,61]. Central alveolar hypoventilation due to an impaired respiratory center has been reported following cerebral thrombosis, parkinsonism, encephalitis, and barbiturate intoxication [62,63]. Peripheral alveolar hypoventilation due to mechanical impairment of the chest may be seen in patients with myotonic dystrophy, poliomyelitis, or severe spondylitis [64,65]. In the colorful Pickwickian syndrome, characterized by extreme obesity and somnolence, the associated erythrocytosis appears to be caused by a combination of central and peripheral hypoventilation. At the level of the medulla, there is a vicious circle involving somnolence, hypercapnia, and hypoventilation [63]. This leads to a respiratory unresponsiveness which becomes aggravated by the ventilatory burden of obesity and the excess CO_2 to be removed.

It is frequently difficult to demonstrate actual arterial hypoxemia and hypercapnia. Some fat patients who, like Mr. Wardle's proverbial boy, Joe, are always half asleep will be very much awake when exposed to arterial punctures and ventilatory testing, and their apprehensive hyperventilation will cause the disappearance of all abnormalities in arterial gas composition. As soon as they return to bed, however, they will go to sleep again and display the characteristic somnolent cyanosis.

ERYTHROCYTOSIS DUE TO DEFECTIVE OXYGEN TRANSPORT

CYANOTIC GROUP

Cyanosis is usually considered a reliable clinical sign of arterial hypoxemia. However, even alarming degrees of cyanosis may be seen in various methemoglobinemias or sulfhemoglobinemias without significant arterial hypoxemia. It takes about 4 to 5 g of reduced hemoglobin per deciliter of blood to produce cyanosis, but as little as 1.5 g/dl of methemoglobin [66] or 0.5 g/dl of sulfhemoglobin will cause the same degree of cyanosis.

Secondary polycythemia in patients with acquired or congenital methemoglobinemia is uncommon, but when it occurs, it may be caused less by reduced oxygen-carrying capacity and more by an associated shift of the oxygen dissociation curve to the left [67]. Chronic carbon monoxide poisoning is an important but generally unappreciated cause of mild polycythemia. Nervous chain smokers with increased hematocrits have been designated as having "stress polycythemia." However the presence of from 5 to 15 percent of carboxyhemoglobin in the blood of heavy smokers is not unusual and coupled with a moderate increase in the oxygen affinity of the remaining oxyhemoglobin [68] could provide the necessary hypoxic stimulus for erythropoietin formation [69,70].

In patients with methemoglobinopathy due to the presence of hemoglobin M, oxygen affinity depends on the specific site of amino acid substitution [71]. In the hemoglobin M with a substitution in the α chain, such as hemoglobin M_{Boston} or hemoglobin M_{Iwate}, there is a low oxygen affinity and consequently very rarely a compensatory erythrocytosis. On the other hand, in the hemoglobin $M_{Saskatoon}$ or hemoglobin $M_{Hyde Park}$, the oxygen affinity is increased and should lead to secondary polycythemia. However, the β variants are somewhat unstable, and mild hemolysis often prevents development of an erythrocytosis.

NONCYANOTIC GROUPS

It has been demonstrated that the hemoglobin in a number of patients with familial secondary polycythemia has an increased affinity for oxygen [72] (see Chap. 75). This abnormal affinity appears to be caused by amino acid substitutions in the contact area between the α and β chains. Such substitutions may prevent the normal conformational or allosteric changes which take place during deoxygenation and thereby interfere with the release of oxygen to the tissues. Both α variants such as $Hb_{Chesapeake}$ and $Hb_{Capetown}$ and β variants such as Hb_{Yakima}, $Hb_{Kempsey}$, $Hb_{Rainier}$, and $Hb_{Hiroshima}$ have been described. All are characterized by well-oxygenated blood, a shift to the left in the oxygen dissociation curve, and a compensatory erythrocytosis.

The heme deletions found in $Hb_{Gun Hill}$ would theoretically lead to a noncyanotic decrease in oxygen-carrying capacity and a secondary increase in hematocrit. However, the instability of the abnormal hemoglobin has made hemolysis rather than erythrocytosis the main clinical manifestation [73].

It has obviously become mandatory to include determinations of oxygen affinity in the evaluation of any patient with unexplained erythrocytosis. Such determinations have disclosed electrophoretically silent abnormal hemoglobins [74] and polycythemias caused by congenital deficiency of diphosphoglycerate mutase [75].

ERYTHROCYTOSIS DUE TO TISSUE HYPOXIA

A number of chemicals have been suspected of causing histotoxic anoxia and secondary polycythemia, but the only chemical with a predictable capacity to cause erythrocytosis is cobalt.

This erythropoietic effect has led to the therapeutic administration of 60 to 150 mg of cobalt chloride to patients with refractory anemias such as anemia of chronic infection, cancer, or uremia [76,77]. In many cases, there have been gratifying increases in the hemoglobin concentration, but side effects such as anorexia, nausea, and vomiting or, more seriously, deafness and thyroid hyperplasia have led to a general disuse of cobalt for therapeutic purposes [78]. Although the clinical disenchantment with cobalt has come from its side effects, the real contraindication to its use should come from its mode of action. Since cobalt administration will increase the oxygen tension in subcutaneous air pockets in rats [79] (Fig. 38-3) as well as increase erythropoietin production [80], it seems likely that it acts by inhibiting oxidative metabolism. Consequently, in the treatment of anemias, an agent which causes histotoxic anoxia is not much better than a trip to the top of Pikes Peak.

Inappropriate secondary polycythemia

Inappropriate secondary polycythemia is an absolute polycythemia characterized by increased erythropoietin production in the absence of generalized tissue hypoxia. The diagnosis can be difficult to establish clinically and should not be made until elevated concentrations of erythropoietin in plasma and urine have ruled out early polycythemia vera and cardiovascular and hemoglobin studies have ruled out defective oxygen transport. Although other erythropoietic agents or mechanisms may exist, so far all cases of inappropriate secondary polycythemia, in whom the source of stimulation has been identified, have been found to be caused either by renal erythropoietin released in response to structural or functional kidney abnormalities or by extrarenal erythropoietin from liver, cerebellum, or other organs [81] (Table 73-1). In cases in which erythropoietin cannot be identified as the cause, it has to be realized that the lower level of sensitivity of the routine bioassay for erythropoietin is 50 mU per milliliter of plasma. More sensitive assays have now disclosed that titers less than 50 mU/ml but higher than the normal titer of about 10 mU/ml can cause pronounced erythrocytosis [82,83]. Consequently, it seems likely that cases of inappropriate secondary polycythemia which in the past could not be related to excessive production of erythropoietin would have been found to be so with today's more accurate methods.

ERYTHROCYTOSIS DUE TO RENAL VASCULAR IMPAIRMENT

A partial obstruction of the renal artery should cause renal tissue hypoxia and a physiologic stimulation of erythropoietin production. Nevertheless, it has proved quite difficult to induce an erythrocytosis in laboratory animals by inserting a Goldblatt clamp on the renal arteries [84,85], and only a few patients with arteriosclerotic narrowing of the renal arteries have developed erythrocytosis [86,87]. However, it has been reported [88] that patients with renal hypertension have higher hematocrits than those with essential hypertension. Furthermore, in one case of inappropriate secondary polycythemia, a renal biopsy revealed thickened and tortuous interlobular and afferent arteries in the kidney [89]. The rarity of clear-cut polycythemic values in patients with impaired renal perfusion [90,91] can probably be attributed to the fact that decreased blood flow may cause structural damage and impaired erythropoietin production.

Some observations have suggested that kidney transplants may release an inappropriate amount of erythropoietin, presumably in response to intrarenal vascular obstruction by inflammatory cells [92]. The appearance of nucleated red cells and reticulocytes in circulating blood and an increase in erythropoietin titer have even been suggested as useful signs of impending rejection of the transplant [93]. Erythrocytosis, however, has been found in a significant number of transplanted patients with well-tolerated grafts [94,95]. In almost all such cases, the native kidneys are still in place, and it has been determined that the native, rather than the transplanted, kidneys are the source of inappropriate erythropoietin production [96].

ERYTHROCYTOSIS DUE TO RENAL CYSTS AND HYDRONEPHROSIS

Absolute erythrocytosis has by now been observed in a considerable number of patients with solitary renal cysts, polycystic renal disease, or hydronephrosis [97,98]. In most of these cases erythropoietin assays on cyst fluid, serum, or urine have disclosed the presence of erythropoietic material [99,100]. This material is inactivated by erythropoietin antibody and appears to be identical with normal physiologic renal erythropoietin [99]. Similar concentrations of erythropoietin have been found in cyst fluid from patients without overt erythrocytosis [101,102]. This may reflect a compensatory erythropoietic inactivity of the contralateral kidney or a concomitant renal injury reducing the overall mass of erythropoietin-producing tissue.

In general, however, it appears that patients with

TABLE 73-1 Inappropriate secondary polycythemia*

Location	Pathologic condition	Number of case reports until 1970
Kidney	Hypernephroma	118
	Other tumors	13
	Hydronephrosis	14
	Cystic disease	35
	Renal artery stenosis	2
	Transplantation rejection	7
	Bartter's syndrome	1
Liver	Hepatoma	64
Uterus	Leiomyoma	24
Cerebellum	Hemangioblastoma	50
Adrenal gland	Pheochromocytoma	5

*Data from Thorling [81].

polycystic disease have a hematocrit value slightly higher than normal and definitely higher than would have been expected of patients with uremia [97].

Since both cystic disease and hydronephrosis are associated with excessive erythropoietin production, it has been suggested that pressure on the remaining normal kidney causes tissue hypoxia, which in turn triggers erythropoietin secretion [103]. Experimentally, it has been found that renal pressure induced by subcapsular injection of plastic or by ligation of the ureters regularly produces some degree of erythrocytosis in the rabbit [104]. However, direct demonstration of an increased content of erythropoietin in the renal tissue has not been achieved.

ERYTHROCYTOSIS DUE TO RENAL TUMORS

It has been estimated that about 1 to 3 percent of all patients with hypernephromas have erythrocytosis [105]. In many of these, erythropoietin assays of serum and urine have disclosed higher than normal titers, and the erythrocytosis is most likely caused by excessive erythropoietin secretion [106]. Despite early equivocal results of tumor tissue assays, it has become generally accepted that hypernephroma cells can produce erythropoietin [107]. However, the presence of erythropoietin and of erythrocytosis in some patients with Wilms' tumor [108–110] and even in an occasional patient with benign adenoma [111] suggests that pressure-induced hypoxia in the adjoining normal parenchyma may also be of importance.

Successful extirpation of renal tumors in patients with erythrocytosis has in many cases been followed by hematologic remission [112]. Subsequent relapses have been described in patients developing metastatic recurrence of the tumors in the contralateral kidney [102].

ERYTHROCYTOSIS DUE TO UTERINE MYOMAS

The occasional association of erythrocytosis with large uterine myomas has been commented on for the last 20 years. In most cases, the tumor has been huge, and extirpation has routinely been followed by a hematologic "cure" [113]. It has been suggested that the tumor may

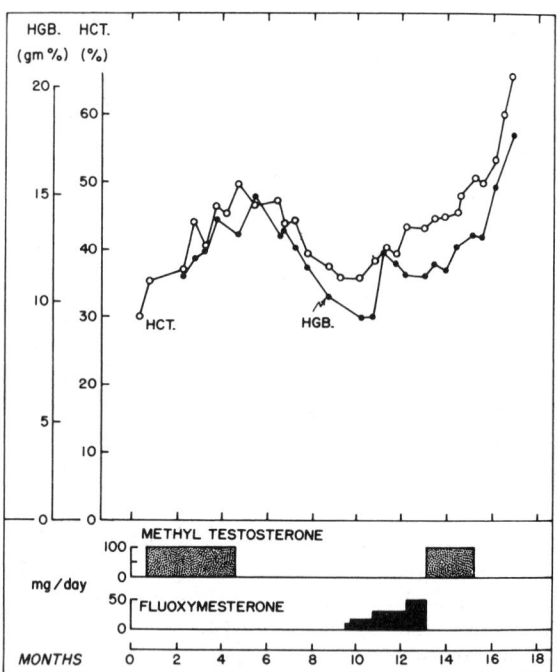

FIGURE 73-6 Erythropoietic response to testosterone derivatives in a patient with myelofibrosis. (Redrawn from Gardner and Pringle [149].)

interfere with pulmonary ventilation [114], but arterial gas findings have been normal in the few patients so studied [113]. Another possible mechanism is that the large abdominal mass causes mechanical interference with the blood supply to the kidneys, resulting in renal hypoxia and erythropoietin production [115]. Inappropriate erythropoietin secretion by smooth muscle cells has been demonstrated both in uterine myomas [116–118] and in one case of cutaneous leiomyoma [119].

ERYTHROCYTOSIS DUE TO CEREBELLAR HEMANGIOMAS

Erythrocytosis and inappropriate secretions of erythropoietin may be found in patients with cerebellar hemangiomas [120] (Table 73-1). Cyst fluid from the tumor has been shown to contain erythropoietic material [121], and careful immunologic, biochemical, and biophysical studies have demonstrated identity of this material with renal erythropoietin [99]. It has been assumed that the tumor cells secrete erythropoietin, but the many case reports of nonneoplastic neurogenic polycythemia [122] and the proximity of the tumor to the respiratory center and to the hypothalamus suggest alternative explanations. A neurogenic hypoventilation, however, is not a likely causative mechanism, since arterial gas studies have been normal in the cases adequately studied [123]. Some studies have indicated that hypothalamic stimulation will increase the rate of red cell production [124], and it is possible that cerebellar hemangioblastomas exert their erythropoietic action via a hypothalamo-renal connection [125].

ERYTHROCYTOSIS DUE TO HEPATOMAS

In 1958, McFadzean and coworkers reported that almost 10 percent of patients in Hong Kong with hepatocarcinoma developed erythrocytosis [126]. Since then this association has been recognized as an important clinical clue in the diagnostic consideration of patients with liver disease [127–129].

The cause of the erythrocytosis is unknown. An inappropriate extrarenal production of erythropoietin by the neoplastic cells is the most favored explanation, and in some cases erythropoietic material has actually been demonstrated in serum and tissue extract [87,130,131]. In support of this explanation is the fact that the normal liver is a source of physiologic extrarenal erythropoietin [132,133]. Since no erythropoietin could be demonstrated in tissue extracts in other cases [134,135], it has also been proposed that impaired hepatic function may lead to an excessive accumulation of potentially erythropoietic hormones such as androgens or even of erythropoietin itself.

ERYTHROCYTOSIS DUE TO ENDOCRINE DISORDERS

Pheochromocytomas, aldosterone-producing adenomas, and Bartter's syndrome have been described in causal association with erythrocytosis [136–138]. Erythropoietin titers were found elevated in the serum and returned to normal after extirpation of the tumors. A number of pathogenetic mechanisms have been suggested, including mechanical interference with renal blood supply, hypertensive damage to renal parenchyma, functional interaction between aldosterone, renin, and erythropoietin, and inappropriate secretion of erythropoietin by the tumors. The mild polycythemia frequently observed in patients with Cushing's syndrome [139] is probably caused by an excessive release of steroid hormones. Hydrocortisone and its steroid equivalents have been shown to cause a mild general marrow stimulation [140,141], and the polycythemia of Cushing's syndrome often involves white blood cells and platelets as well as red blood cells.

Many case reports, especially in the older literature, describe erythrocytosis in patients with various disorders of the brain and autonomic nervous system [122,142]. These cases of neurogenic polycythemia may be related to an excessive stimulation of the hypothalamus and the pituitary [124,143]. Many pituitary and pituitary-dependent hormones such as growth hormone [144], prolactin [145], and thyroxine [146] have been shown experimentally to have erythropoietic properties, but their capacity to cause clinical erythrocytosis is still unsettled. Of potential interest is a recent report of an erythropoietin-containing dermoid cyst of the ovary [160].

Of considerably more practical importance has been the proved erythropoietic effect of androgens. For many years, it was assumed that the higher red cell count in males was caused by androgens, but it was not until pharmacologic doses of testosterone were administered to women with carcinoma of the breast [147] that the erythropoietic potency of androgens was appreciated [148]. Since then various androgen preparations have been used in the treatment of refractory anemias [149], occasionally causing dramatic overshoots into the polycythemic range (Fig. 73-6).

The erythropoietic effect of androgens appears to be caused both by their capacity to stimulate erythropoietin production [150,151] and by their capacity to induce differentiation of marrow stem cells directly [152]. Recent studies indicate that these two effects have specific structural requirements. Androgens with the 5α-H configuration stimulate renal and extrarenal erythropoietin production, while androgens with the 5β-H configuration enhance the differentiation of stem cells [153,154].

ERYTHROCYTOSIS DUE TO ESSENTIAL OVERPRODUCTION OF ERYTHROPOIETIN

A number of reports have described children and young adults with severe but asymptomatic erythrocytosis associated with high erythropoietin titers. In some of these, family studies have suggested a genetic tendency to overproduction of erythropoietin [155,156]. In others, no family history was obtained but the erythrocytosis was present at a very early age [157–159]. It has been assumed that the excessive erythropoietin production is caused by intrarenal hypoxia, but in only one case has kidney biopsies suggested renal vascular changes [89]. A puzzling feature found in several cases has been autonomous CFU-E production in vitro in the absence of erythropoietin [157]. This is a feature thought to be specific for polycythemia vera or essential erythrocytosis, and it has been difficult to fit it into our current concepts of erythropoietin-induced erythrocytosis.

References

1. Bert, P.: *La Pression barometrique*. Masson, Paris, 1878.
2. Jourdanet, D.: *De l'anemie des altitudes et de l'anemie en general dans ses rapports avec la pression de l'atmosphere*. Bailliere, Paris, 1863.
3. Viault, F.: Sur l'augmentation considerable du nombre des globules rouges dans le sang chez les habitant des haut plateaux de l'Amerique du Sud. *C. R. Acad. Sci.* 111:917, 1890.
4. Erslev, A. J.: Blood and mountains, in *Blood, Pure and Eloquent*, edited by M. M. Wintrobe. McGraw-Hill, New York, 1980, p. 257.
5. Leopold, S. S.: The etiology of pulmonary arteriolosclerosis (Ayerza's syndrome). *Am. J. Med. Sci.* 219:152, 1950.
6. Abbott, M. E.: *Atlas of Congenital Heart Disease*. American Heart Association, New York, 1936.
7. Burwell, C. S., Robin, E. D., Whaley, R. D., and Bickelman, A. G.: Extreme obesity associated with alveolar hypoventilation: A Pickwickian syndrome. *Am. J. Med.* 21:811, 1956.
8. Hurtado, A.: Some clinical aspects of life at high altitudes. *Ann. Intern. Med.* 53:247, 1960.
9. Swan, L. W.: The ecology of the high Himalayas. *Sci. Am.* 205:68, 1961.
10. Bishop, B. C.: Wintering in the high Himalayas. *Natl. Geographic* 122:503, 1962.
11. Rennie, D.: High science: Present and future. *N. Engl. J. Med.* 301:1343, 1979.
12. Houston, C. S., and Riley, R. L.: Respiratory and circulatory changes during acclimatization to high altitude. *Am. J. Physiol.* 149:565, 1947.
13. Reynafarje, C., Faura, R. J., Villavicencio, D., and Vallenas, E.: Erythrokinetics in altitudes camelides. *Proc. XIII Cong. Int. Soc. Hematol.*, 1968, p. 79.
14. Hurtado, A., Merino, C., and Delgado, E.: Influence of anoxemia on the hematopoietic activity. *Arch. Intern. Med. 75*:287, 1945.
15. Hurtado, A.: Acclimatization to high altitudes, in *Physiological Effects of High Altitude*, edited by W. H. Weihe. Macmillan, New York, 1964, p. 1.
16. Frisancho, A. R.:Functional adaptation to high altitude hypoxia. *Science 187*:313, 1975.
17. Klausen, K.: Cardiac output in man in rest and work during and after acclimatization to 3800 m. *J. Appl. Physiol. 21*:609, 1966.
18. Grover, R. F.: Basal oxygen uptake of man at high altitude. *J. Appl. Physiol. 18*:909, 1963.
19. Moore, L. G., and Brewer, G. J.: Beneficial effect of rightward hemoglobin – oxygen dissociation curve shift for short-term high-altitude adaptation. *J. Lab. Clin. Med. 98*:145, 1981.
20. Finch, C. A., and Lenfant, C.: Oxygen transport in man. *N. Engl. J. Med. 286*:407, 1972.
21. Miller, M. E., et al.: pH effect on erythropoietin response to hypoxia. *N. Engl. J. Med. 288*:706, 1973.
22. Lenfant, C., et al.: Effect of altitude on oxygen binding by hemoglobin and on organic phosphate levels, *J. Clin. Invest. 47*:2652, 1968.
23. Eaton, J. W., Skelton, T. D., and Berger, E.: Survival at extreme altitude: Protective effect of increased hemoglobin-oxygen affinity. *Science 183*:743, 1974.
24. Hall, F. G., Dill, D. B., and Barron, E. S. G.: Comparative physiology in high altitudes. *J. Cell. Comp. Physiol. 8*:301, 1936.
25. Hebbel, R. P., Eaton, J. W., Kronenberg, R. S., Zanjani, E. D., Moore, L. G., and Berger, E. M.: Human llamas. Adaptation to altitude in subjects with high hemoglobin oxygen affinity. *J.Clin. Invest. 62*:593, 1978.
26. Faura, J., Ramos, J., Reynafarje, C., English, E., Finne, P., and Finch, C.A.: Effect of altitude on erythropoiesis. *Blood 33*:668, 1969.
27. Thorling, E. B., and Erslev, A. J.: The "tissue" tension of oxygen and its relation to hematocrit and erythropoiesis. *Blood 31*:332, 1968.
28. Smith, E. E., and Crowell, J. W.: Role of increased hematocrit in altitude acclimatization. *Aerosp. Med. 38*:39, 1967.
29. Tenney, S. M., and Ou, L. C.: Physiological evidence for increased tissue capillarity in rats acclimatized to high altitudes. *Respir. Physiol. 8*:137, 1970.
30. Robin, E. D.: Of men and mitochondria: Coping with hypoxic dysoxia. *Am. Rev. Respir. Dis. 122*:517, 1980.
31. Hathorn, M. V. S.: The influence of hypoxia on iron absorption in the rat. *Gastroenterology 60*:76, 1971.
32. Reynafarje, C., Lozano, R., and Valdivieso, J.: The polycythemia of high altitudes: Iron metabolism and related aspects. *Blood 14*:433, 1959.
33. Shaikh, B., and Erslev, A. J.: Thrombocytopenia in polycythemic mice. *J. Lab. Clin. Med. 92*:765, 1978.
34. Singh, I., Khanna, P. K., Srivastava, M. C., Lal, M., Roy, S. B., and Subramanyam, C. S. V.: Acute mountain sickness. *N. Engl. J. Med. 280*:175, 1969.
35. Hackett, P. H., Rennie, D., and Levine, N. D.: The incidence, importance and prophylaxis of acute mountain disease. *Lancet 2*:1149, 1976.
36. Sutton, J. R., et al.: Effect of acetazolamide on hypoxemia during sleep at high altitude. *N. Engl. J. Med. 301*:1329, 1979.
37. Hultgren, H. N., Spickard, W. B., Hellriegel, K., and Houston, C. S.: High altitude pulmonary edema. *Medicine 40*:289, 1961.
38. Monge, C.: High altitude disease. *Arch. Intern. Med. 59*:32, 1937.
39. Dintenfass, L.: A preliminary outline of the blood high viscosity syndromes. *Arch. Intern. Med. 118*:427, 1966.
40. Penaloza, D., and Sime, F.: Chronic cor pulmonale due to loss of altitude acclimatization (chronic mountain sickness.) *Am. J. Med. 50*:728, 1971.
41. Eaton, J. W., Brewer, G. J., and Grover, R. F.: Role of red cell 2,3-diphosphoglycerate in the adaptation of man to altitude. *J. Lab. Clin. Med. 73*:603, 1969.
42. Gallo, R. C., Fraimow, W., Cathcart, R. T., and Erslev, A. J.: Erythropoietic response in chronic pulmonary disease. *Arch. Intern. Med. 113*:559, 1964.

43. Lertzman, M., Israels, L. G., and Chermiack, R. M.: Erythropoiesis and ferrokinetics in chronic respiratory disease. *Ann. Intern. Med.* 56:821, 1962.

44. Shaw, D. B., and Simpson, T.: Polycythemia in emphysema. *Am. J. Med.* 30:135, 1961.

45. Murray, J. F.: Arterial oxygen studies in primary and secondary polycythemic disorders. *Am. Rev. Respir. Dis.* 92:435, 1965.

46. Harrison, B. D. W.: Polycythemia in a selected group of patients with chronic airway obstruction. *Clin. Sci.* 33:563, 1973.

47. Hammerstein, J. F., Whitcomb, W. H., Johnson, P. C., and Lowell, J. R.: The hematological adaptation of patients with hypoxia due to pulmonary emphysema. *Am. Rev. Tuberc.* 78:391, 1958.

48. Tura, S., Pollycove, M., and Gelpi, A. P.: Erythrocyte and iron-kinetics in patients with chronic pulmonary emphysema. *J. Nucl. Med.* 3:110, 1962.

49. Vanier, T., Dulfano, M. J., Wu, C., and Desforges, J. F.: Emphysema, hypoxia and the polycythemic response. *N. Engl. J. Med.* 269:169, 1963.

50. Dayton, L. M., McCollough, R. E., Weil, J. V., Scheinhorn, D. F., and Filley, G. F.: The effects of phlebotomy on lung function in secondary polycythemia. *Am. Rev. Resp. Dis.* 107:1112, 1973.

51. York, E. L., Jones, R. L., Menon, D., and Sproule, B. J.: Effects of secondary polycythemia on cerebral blood flow in chronic obstructive pulmonary disease. *Am. Rev. Resp. Dis.* 121:813, 1980.

52. Bing, R. J., Vandam, L. D., Handelsman, J. C., Campbell, J. A., Spencer, R., and Griswold, H. E.: Physiological studies in congenital heart disease. VI. Adaptations to anoxia in congenital heart disease with cyanosis. *Bull. Johns Hopkins Hosp.* 83:439, 1948.

53. Castle, W. B., and Jandl, J. H.: Blood viscosity and blood volume: Opposing influences upon oxygen transport in polycythemia. *Semin. Hematol.* 3:193, 1966.

54. Hutchison, D. C. S., Sapru, R. P., Sumerling, M. D., Donaldson, G. W. K., and Richmond, J.: Cirrhosis, cyanosis and polycythemia: Multiple pulmonary arteriovenous anastomoses. *Am. J. Med.* 45:139, 1968.

55. Wolfe, J. D., Toshkin, D. P., Holly, F. E., Brachman, M. B., and Genovesi, M. G.: Hypoxemia of cirrhosis: Detection of abnormal small pulmonary vascular channels by a quantitative radionuclide method. *Am. J. Med.* 63:746, 1977.

56. Saunders, W. H.: Hereditary hemorrhagic telangiectasia. *Arch. Otolaryngol.* 76:245, 1962.

57. Rodes, C. B.: Cavernous hemangiomas of the lung with seconary polycythemia. *JAMA.* 110:1914, 1938.

58. Hedlund, S.: Studies on erythropoiesis and total red cell volume in congestive heart failure. *Acta Med. Scand.* 146:1, 1953.

59. Chodos, R. B., Wells, R., Jr., and Chaffee, W. R.: A study of ferrokinetics and red cell survival in congestive heart failure. *Am. J. Med.* 36:553, 1964.

60. Block, A. J., Boysen, P. G., Wynne, J. W., and Hunt, L. A.: Sleep apnea, hypopnea and oxygen desaturation in normal subjects: A strong male predominance. *N. Engl. J. Med.* 300:513, 1979.

61. Cayler, G., Mays, T., and Riley, H. D.: Cardio-respiratory syndrome of obesity (Pickwickian syndrome) in children. *Pediatrics* 27:237, 1961.

62. Rodman, T., and Close, H. P.: The primary hypoventilation syndrome. *Am. J. Med.* 26:808, 1959.

63. Zwillich, C. W., Sutton, F. D., Pierson, D. J., Creagh, E. M., and Weil, J. V.: Decreased hypoxic ventilatory drive in the obesity-hypoventilation syndrome. *Am. J. Med.* 59:343, 1975.

64. Fishman, A. P., Turino, G. O., and Bevgofsky, E. F.: The syndrome of alveolar hypoventilation. Editorial. *Am. J. Med.* 23:333, 1957.

65. Alexander, J. K., Amad, K. H., and Cole, V. W.: Observations on some clinical features of extreme obesity with particular reference to cardio-respiratory effects. *Am. J. Med.* 32:512, 1962.

66. Jaffe, E. R.: Hereditary methemoglobinemias associated with abnormalities in the metabolism of erythrocytes. *Am. J. Med.* 41:786, 1966.

67. Darling, R. C., and Roughton, F. J. W.: The effect of methemoglobin on the equilibrium between oxygen and hemoglobin. *Am. J. Physiol.* 137:56, 1942.

68. Brody, J. S., and Coburn, R. F.: Carbon monoxide-induced arterial hypoxemia. *Science* 164:1297, 1969.

69. Sagone, A. L., Jr., and Balcerzak, S. P.: Smoking as a cause of erythrocytosis. *Ann. Intern. Med.* 82:512, 1975.

70. Smith, J. R., and Landaw, S. A.: Smokers' polycythemia. *N. Engl. J. Med.* 298:6, 1978.

71. Heller, P.: Hemoglobin M: An early chapter in the saga of molecular pathology. Editorial. *Ann. Intern. Med.* 70:1038, 1969.

72. Weatherall, D. J.: Polythemia resulting from abnormal hemoglobins. *N. Engl. J. Med.* 280:604, 1969.

73. Bradley, T. B., Wohl, R. C., and Rieder, R. F.: Hemoglobin Gun Hill: Detection of five amino acid residues and impaired hemoglobin binding. *Science* 157:1581, 1967.

74. Nute, P. E., Stamatoyannopoulos, G., Hermodson, M. A., and Roth, D.: Hemoglobinopathic erythrocytosis due to a new electrophoretically silent variant, Hemoglobin San Diego [β 109 (Gll) Val → Met]. *J. Clin. Invest.* 53:320, 1974.

75. Rosa, R., Prehu, M. O., Bengard, Y., and Rosa, J.: The first case of a complete deficiency of diphosphoglycerate mutase in human erythrocytes. *J. Clin. Invest.* 62:907, 1978.

76. Robinson, J. C., James, G. W., III, and Kark, R. M.: The effect of oral therapy with cobaltous chlorides on the blood of patients suffering with chronic suppurative infection. *N. Engl. J. Med.* 240:749, 1949.

77. Gardner, F. H.: The use of cobaltous chloride in the anemia associated with chronic renal disease. *J. Lab. Clin. Med.* 41:56, 1953.

78. Dameshek, W.: Panels in therapy. V. The use of cobalt and cobalt-iron preparations in the therapy of anemia. *Blood* 10:852, 1955.

79. Thorling, E. B., and Erslev, A. J.: The effect of some erythropoietic agents on the "tissue" tension of oxygen. *Br. J. Haematol.* 23:483, 1972.

80. Goldwasser, E., Jacobson, L. O., Fried, W., and Plzak, L. F.: Studies on erythropoiesis. V. The effect of cobalt on the production of erythropoietin. *Blood* 13:55, 1958.

81. Thorling, E. B.: Paraneoplastic erythrocytosis and inappropriate erythropoietin production. *Scand. J. Haematol. Suppl.* 17, 1972.

82. Erslev, A. J., Caro, J., Kansu, E., Miller, O., and Cobbs, E.: Plasma erythropoietin in polycythemia. *Am. J. Med.* 66:243, 1979.

83. Koeffler, H. P., and Goldwasser, J.: Erythropoietin radioimmunoassay in evaluating patients with polycythemia. *Ann. Intern. Med.* 94:44, 1981.

84. Hansen, P.: Polycythemia produced by constriction of the renal artery of the rabbit. *Acta Pathol. Microbiol. Scand.* 60:465, 1964.

85. Fischer, J., and Samuels, A. J.: Relationship between renal blood flow and erythropoietin production. *Proc. Soc. Exp. Biol. Med.* 125:482, 1967.

86. Hudgson, P., Pearce, J. M., and Yeates, W. K.: Renal artery stenosis with hypertension and high hematocrit. *Br. Med. J.* 1:18, 1967.

87. Luke, R. G., Kennedy, A. C., and Stirling, W. B.: Renal artery stenosis, hypertension and polycythemia. *Br. Med. J.* 1:164, 1965.

88. Tarazi, R. C., Frohlish, E. D., Dunstan, H. P., Gifford, R. W., and Page, I. H.: Hypertension and high hematocrit. *Am. J. Cardiol.* 18:855, 1966.

89. Maezawa, M., Takaku, F., Muto, Y., Mizoguchi, H., and Miura, Y.: A case of intrarenal artery stenosis associated with erythrocytosis. *Scand. J. Haematol.* 21:278, 1978.

90. Hoppin, E. C., Depner, T., Yamuchi, H.' and Hopper, J., Jr.: Erythrocytosis associated with diffuse parenchymal lesions of the kidney. *Br. J. Haematol.* 32:557, 1976.

91. Myers, D. I., Ciuffo, A. A., and Cooke, C. R.: Focal glomerulosclerosis and erythrocytosis. *Johns Hopkins Med. J.* 145:192, 1979.

92. Hoffman, G. C.: Human erythropoiesis following kidney transplantation. *Ann. N.Y. Acad. Sci.* 149:504, 1968.

93. Westerman, M. P., Jenkins, J. L., Dekker, A., Krentner, A., and Fisher, B.: Significance of erythrocytosis and increased erythropoietin secretion after renal transplantation. *Lancet* 755, 1967.

94. Nies, B. A., Cohn, R., and Schrier, S. L.: Erythremia after renal transplantation. *N. Engl. J. Med.* 273:785, 1965.

95. Nallan, R., Otis, P., and Martin, D. C.: Polycythemia following renal transplantation. *Urology* 6:158, 1975.

96. Dagher, F. J., Ramos, E., Erslev, A. J., Alonzi, S. V., Karmi, S. A., and Caro, J.: Are the native kidneys responsible for erythrocytosis in renal allorecipients? *Transplantation* 28:496, 1979.

97. Friend, D., Hoskins, R. G., and Kirkin, M. W.: Relative erythrocythemia (polycythemia) and polycystic kidney disease with uremia.

Report of a case with comments on frequency of occurrence. *N. Engl. J. Med.* 264:17, 1961.

98. Rosse, W. F., Waldmann, T. A., and Cohen, P.: Renal cysts, erythropoietin and polycythemia. *Am. J. Med.* 34:76, 1963.

99. Waldmann, T. A., Rosse, W. F., and Swarm, R. L.: The erythropoiesis-stimulating factors produced by tumors. *Ann. N.Y. Acad. Sci.* 149:509, 1968.

100. Hammond, D., and Winnick, S.: Paraneoplastic erythropoiesis and ectopic erythropoietin. *Ann. N.Y. Acad. Sci.* 230:219, 1974.

101. Plzak, L. F., Jr.: Erythropoietin and renal cyst fluid. *Clin. Res.* 13:281, 1965.

102. Murphy, G. P., Kenny, G. M., and Mirand, E. A.: Erythropoietin levels in patients with renal tumors or cysts. *Cancer* 26:191, 1970.

103. Toyama, L., and Mitus, W. J.: Experimental renal erythrocytosis. III. Relationship between the degree of hydronephrotic pressure and the production of erythrocytosis. *J. Lab. Clin. Med.* 68:740, 1966.

104. Mitus, W. J., Toyama, K., and Braner, M. J.: Erythrocytosis, juxtaglomerular apparatus (J.G.A.) and erythropoietin in the course of experimental unilateral hydronephrosis in rabbits. *Ann. N.Y. Acad. Sci.* 149:107, 1968.

105. Ways, P., Huff, J. W., Kosmaler, C. H., and Young, L. E.: Polycythemia and histologically proven renal disease. *Arch. Intern. Med.* 107:154, 1961.

106. Toyama, K., Fujiama, N., Suzuki, H., Chen, T. P., Tamaoki, N., and Neyama, Y.: Erythropoietin levels in the course of a patient with erythropoietin-producing renal cell carcinoma and transplantation of this tumor in nude mice. *Blood* 54:245, 1979.

107. Kazal, L. A., and Erslev, A. J.: Erythropoietin production in renal tumors. *Ann. Clin. Lab. Sci.* 5:98, 1975.

108. Thurman, W. G., Grabstald, H., and Lieberman, P. H.: Elevation of erythropoietin levels in association with Wilms' tumor. *Arch. Intern. Med.* 117:280, 1966.

109. Shalet, M. F., Holder, T. M., and Walters, T. R.: Erythropoietin-producing Wilms' tumor. *J. Pediatr.* 70:615, 1967.

110. Kenny, G. M., Mirand, E. A., Stanbitz, W. J., Allen, J. E., Trudel, P. J., and Murphy, G. P.: Erythropoietin levels in Wilms' tumor patients. *J. Urol.* 104:758, 1970.

111. DeMarsh, A. B., and Warmington, W. J.: Polycythemia associated with renal tumor. *Northwest Med.* 54:976, 1955.

112. Damon, A., Holub, D. A., Melicow, M. M., and Uson, A. C.: Polycythemia and renal carcinoma: Report of 10 new cases, two with long hematologic remission following nephrectomy. *Am. J. Med.* 25:182, 1958.

113. Morton, E. D., Evans, E. F., and Daines, W. P.: Polycythemia and uterine myomata. *JAMA.* 200:149, 1967.

114. VandenBerg, A. R., and Vasu, C. M.: Polycythemia associated with uterine fibroma. *JAMA.* 185:249, 1963.

115. Horwitz, A., and McKelway, W. P.: Polycythemia associated with uterine myomas. *JAMA.* 158:1360, 1955.

116. Wrigley, P. F. M., Malpas, J. S., Turnbull, A. L., Jenkins, G. C., and McArt, A.: Secondary polycythemia due to a uterine fibromyoma producing erythropoietin. *Br. J. Haematol.* 21:551, 1971.

117. Ossias, A. L., Zanjani, E. D., Zalusky, R., Estren, S., and Wasserman, L. R.: Case report: Studies on the mechanism of erythrocytosis associated with a uterine fibromyoma. *Br. J. Haematol.* 25:179, 1973.

118. Naets, J. P., Wittek, M., Delwiche, F., and Kram, I.: Polycythemia and erythropoietin producing uterine fibromyoma. *Scand. J. Haematol.* 19:75, 1977.

119. Eldor, A., Even-Paz, Z., and Polliack, A.: Erythrocytosis associated with multiple cutaneous leiomyomata: Report of a case with demonstration of erythropoietic activity in the tumour. *Scand. J. Haematol.* 16:245, 1976.

120. Donati, R. M., McCarthy, J. M., Lange, R. D., and Gallagher, N. J.: Erythrocythemia and neoplastic tumors. *Ann. Intern. Med.* 58:47, 1963.

121. Hennessy, T. G., Stern, W. E., and Herrick, S. E.: Cerebellar hemangioblastoma: Erythropoietic activity by radio-iron assay. *J. Nucl. Med.* 8:601, 1967.

122. Gilbert, H. S., and Silverstein, A.: Neurogenic polycythemia: Report of a case with transient erythrocytosis associated with occlu-

123. Waldman, T. A., Levin, E. H., and Baldwin, M.: The association of polycythemia with a cerebellar hemangioblastoma. *Am. J. Med.* 31:318, 1961.

124. Halvorsen, S.: The central nervous system in regulation of erythropoiesis. *Acta Haematol.* 35:65, 1966.

125. Erslev, A. J.: Hypothalamic control of red cell production. *Ann. Intern. Med.* 65:862, 1966.

126. McFadzean, A. J. S., Todd, D., and Tsang, K. C.: Polycythemia in primary carcinoma of the liver. *Blood* 13:427, 1958.

127. Browstein, M. H., and Ballard, H.: Hepatoma associated with erythrocytosis: Report of eleven new cases. *Am. J. Med.* 40:204, 1966.

128. Lizzi, F. A., Tartaglia, A. P., and Adamson, J. W.: Hemochromatosis, hepatoma, erythrocytosis and erythropoietin. *N.Y. State J. Med.* 73:1098, 1973.

129. Davidson, C. S.: Hepatocellular carcinoma and erythrocytosis. *Semin. Hematol.* 13:115, 1976.

130. Eppstein, S.: Primary carcinoma of the liver. *Am. J. Med. Sci.* 247:137, 1964.

131. Nakao, K., Kimura, K., Miura, Y., and Takaku, F.: Erythrocytosis associated with carcinoma of the liver (with erythropoietin assay of tumor extract). *Am. J. Med. Sci.* 251:161, 1966.

132. Gordon, A. S., Zanjani, E. D., and Zalusky, R.: A possible mechanism for the erythrocytosis associated with hepatocellular carcinoma in man. *Blood* 35:151, 1970.

133. Fried, W.: The liver as a source of renal erythropoietin production. *Blood* 40:671, 1972.

134. Kan, Y. W., McFadzean, A. J. S., Todd, D., and Tso, S. C.: Further observations on polycythemia in hepatocelular carcinoma. *Blood* 18:592, 1961.

135. Lehman, A. J., Erslev, A. J., and Myerson, R. M.: Erythrocytosis associated with hepatocellular carcinoma. *Am. J. Med.* 35:439, 1963.

136. Bradly, J. E., Young, J. D., and Lentz, G.: Polycythemia secondary to pheochromocytoma. *J. Urol.* 86:1, 1961.

137. Mann, D. L., Gallagher, N. J., and Donati, R. M.: Erythrocytosis and primary aldosteronism. *Ann. Intern. Med.* 66:335, 1967.

138. Erkeleus, D. W., and vanEps, L. W. S.: Bartter's syndrome and erythrocytosis. *Am. J. Med.* 55:711, 1973.

139. Platz, C. M., Knowlton, A. J., Ragan, C.: The natural history of Cushing's syndrome. *Am. J. Med.* 13:597, 1952.

140. Fisher, J. W.: Increase in circulatory red cell volume of normal rats after treatment with hydrocortisone or corticosterone. *Proc. Soc. Exp. Biol. Med.* 97:502, 1958.

141. Bishop, C., Athens, J. W., Boggs, D. R., and Cartwright, G. E.: The mechanism of cortisol induced granulocytosis. *Clin. Res.* 15:130, 1967.

142. Grant, W. C., and Root, W. S.: Fundamental stimulus for erythropoiesis. *Physiol. Rev.* 32:449, 1952.

143. Lindeman, R., Trygstad, O., and Halvorsen, S.: Pituitary control of erythropoiesis. *Scand. J. Haematol.* 6:77, 1969.

144. Jepson, J. H.: Effect of growth hormone on erythropoiesis and erythropoietin excretion of pituitary dwarfs. *Ann. Intern. Med.* 68:1169, 1968.

145. Jepson, J. H., and Lowenstein, L.: The effect of testosterone, adrenal steroids and prolactin on erythropoiesis. *Acta Haematol.* 38:292, 1967.

146. Meineke, H. A., and Crafts, R. C.: Evidence for non-caloriengic effect of thyroxin on erythropoiesis as judged by radio-iron utilization. *Proc. Soc. Exp. Biol. Med.* 117:520, 1964.

147. Kennedy, B. J., and Gilbertson, A. S.: Increased erythropoiesis induced by androgenic-hormone therapy. *N. Engl. J. Med.* 256:719, 1957.

148. Gardner, F. H., Nathan, D. G., Piomelli, S., and Cummins, J. F.: The erythrocythaemic effects of androgens. *Br. J. Haematol.* 14:611, 1968.

149. Gardner, F. H., and Pringle, J. C., Jr.: Androgens and erythropoiesis. II. Treatment of myeloid metaplasia. *N. Engl. J. Med.* 264:103, 1961.

150. Fried, W., and Gurney, C. W.: The erythropoietic-stimulating effects of androgens. *Ann. N.Y. Acad. Sci.* 149:356, 1968.

123. — sion of middle cerebral artery, and review of the literature. *Am. J. Med.* 38:807, 1965.

151. Alexanian, R.: Erythropoietin and erythropoiesis in anemic man following androgens. *Blood* 33:564, 1969.
152. Naets, J. P., and Wittek, M.: The mechanism of action of androgens on erythropoiesis. *Ann. N.Y. Acad. Sci.* 149:366, 1968.
153. Levere, R. D., Gordon, A. S., Zanjani, E. D., and Kappas, A.: Stimulation of mammalian erythropoiesis by metabolites of steroid hormones. *Trans. Assoc. Am. Physicians* 83:150, 1970.
154. Shahidi, N. T.: Androgens and erythropoiesis. *N. Engl. J. Med.* 289:72, 1973.
155. Adamson, J. W., Stamatoyannopoulos, G., Kontras, S., Lascari, A., and Detter, J.: Recessive familial erythrocytosis: Aspects of marrow regulation in two families. *Blood* 41:641, 1973.
156. Yonemitsu, H., Yamaguchi, K., Shigeta, H., Okuda, K., and Takaku, F.: Two cases of familial erythrocytosis with increased erythropoietin activity in plasma and urine. *Blood* 42:793, 1973.
157. Daniak, N., Hoffman, R., Lebowitz, A. J., Solomon, L., Maffei, L., and Ritchey, K.: Erythropoietin-dependent primary pure erythrocytosis. *Blood* 53:1076, 1979.
158. Davies, S. A., Goolden, A. W. G., Lewis, S. M., and Zaafran, A.: Autonomous erythropoietin induced erythrocytosis. *Scand. J. Haematol.* 22:105, 1979.
159. Whitcomb, W. H., Peschle, C., Moore, M., Nitschke, R., and Adamson, J. W.: Congenital erythrocytosis: A new form associated with an erythropoietin-dependent mechanism. *Br. J. Haematol.* 44:17, 1980.
160. Ghio, R. et al.: Erythrocytosis associated with a dermoid cyst of the ovary and erythropoietic activity of the tumour fluid. *Scand. J. Haematol.* 27:70, 1981.

CHAPTER 74

Relative polycythemia (erythrocytosis)

ALLAN J. ERSLEV

Relative polycythemia, or rather relative erythrocytosis, is a condition characterized by an elevated hematocrit despite a normal or decreased total red cell mass. Among patients with this combination, two groups can be clearly distinguished. Patients in the first group have a diminished plasma volume as a result of obvious dehydration. The elevated hematocrit level in these patients serves as a useful measure of the extent of their fluid imbalance but does not reflect a hematologic dysfunction. The patients in the second, more controversial group, have no definite manifestation of hemoconcentration, but in general they are asymptomatic middle-aged males with a long history of hypertension, obesity, or excessive smoking. Their medical problems seem no different from nonpolycythemic individuals with the same immoderate middle-age life-style, but some investigators have reported an increased incidence of thromboembolic disorders and cardiac complications.

Early investigators, whose methods for blood volume determination were, to say the least, imprecise, were aware that an elevated red cell count or hematocrit reading did not necessarily signify a true increase in the red cell mass. Thus, Osler wrote of "relative" polycythemia as a result of chronic fluid loss [1], and Keith and coworkers described cases of "polycythemia hypovolemia" in which elevation of the hematocrit level was attributed to a decrease in plasma volume [2]. In 1905, Gaisbock reported that a number of hypertensive patients had plethora and an elevated red cell count but no splenomegaly, a condition he termed *polycythemia hypertonica* [3] and we now tend to call *Gaisbock syndrome* [4]. In 1952, direct measurements of the red cell mass in patients with polycythemia led Lawrence and Berlin to identify a subgroup of patients with a normal red cell mass but with a reduced plasma volume [5]. Although some members of this group were hypertensive, the authors were more impressed by their tense and anxious behavior and coined the term *stress polycythemia*. Numerous reports since then have emphasized the correlation between relative polycythemia and either hypertension or stress [6,7]. Recently it has been demonstrated that excessive smoking causes both a moderate increase in red cell mass and a decrease in plasma volume [8,9], and the term *smoker's polycythemia* has been introduced [9]. However, many patients with elevated hematocrit levels appear merely to exhibit the combined effect of a high-normal red cell mass and a low-normal plasma volume and consequently should not be considered abnormal but only as having *spurious polycythemia* [10,11].

Etiology and pathogenesis

The main cause of relative polycythemia appears to be a chronically reduced plasma volume. The size of the red cell mass, however, may not always be normal or low. Its absolute size can be determined accurately by measuring the dilution of labeled red cells (see Chap. 41), but it is not easy to express this size in a meaningful manner. It probably should be expressed in relation to lean body weight as determined by complex equations using height and weight [12,13]. In practice, however, the red cell mass is usually expressed merely in terms of body weight. Such expression is useful and convenient but in obese patients not very accurate. Fatty tissue is relatively avascular, and an increased red cell mass in an obese patient may lie within normal limits when expressed per kilogram of body weight. Since polycythemia often occurs in overweight patients, many patients with absolute polycythemia undoubtedly are erroneously designated as having relative polycythemia.

The common association of hypertension and relative polycythemia has led to a number of convoluted hypotheses as to why hypertension should cause a contracted plasma volume. Decreased aldosterone secretion, decreased antidiuretic hormone secretion, increased hypostatic pressure, and the effect of antidiuretic therapy have been invoked [7], but no really satisfactory explanation has been forthcoming. Similarly, the pathogenetic effect of stress on plasma volume has not been well explained. Anxious and stressed individuals often attempt to alleviate their problems by chain smoking, and it may be smoking rather than stress which causes an increase in the hematocrit [9]. Heavy smoking will indeed cause both an increase in red cell mass and a decrease in plasma volume. Smoking, especially cigar smoking with deep inhalation, results in the formation of carboxyhemoglobin [8,14], which does not transport oxygen, and possibly also in an increase in the oxygen affinity of the remaining normal hemoglobin [9]. This would cause tissue hypoxia and a stimulation of red cell production. The resulting increase in the red cell mass may be too slight to be recognized by the usual measurements, especially when related to body weight in obese patients. The simultaneous decrease in plasma volume after heavy tobacco smoking appears to be an empirical fact, so far not readily explained. The association between heavy smoking and relative polycythemia is indeed impressive, with the hematocrit being higher among smokers than nonsmokers in general [15,16] and with the great majority of patients with relative polycythemia also having a history of heavy smoking [3,9]. Finally, there is a small group of polycythemic patients who are not obese, are not hypertensive, and are nonsmokers and in whom there merely seem to be a fortuitous combination of a high-normal red cell mass with a low-normal plasma volume, so-called spurious polycythemia [10,11].

Clinical features

Most patients with relative polycythemia are middle-aged white males who are often tense, anxious, and under "psychologic stress." In general they are mildly overweight, moderately hypertensive, and compulsive smokers. Although believed to have more than their share of thromboembolic problems [7,17] especially coronary thrombosis [18], they are in general asymptomatic and identified primarily through routine examinations.

Laboratory findings

With the exception of elevated hematocrit levels, hemoglobin concentrations, and red blood cell counts, the hematologic workup is within normal limits. The hematocrit in males is by definition above 53 percent (upper limit of normal) and in females above 50 percent, but in the majority of cases, the hematocrit does not exceed 60 percent. The viscosity of whole blood is elevated and increases logarithmically in relation to the hematocrit level. Carboxyhemoglobin levels are increased in heavy smokers and may in many cases provide an explanation for the development of erythrocytosis. In nonsmokers the level is between 0 and 2 percent, but may reach 20 percent in cigar smokers who habitually inhale the

smoke. Since the half-life of carbon monoxide in the body is 3 to 5 h [9], there is a progressive rise of carboxyhemoglobin during the day in smokers and a falloff at night. Consequently, blood samples for the determination of carboxyhemoglobin should preferably be obtained in the afternoon or evening. The red cell mass as measured by ^{51}Cr-labeled red cells is within normal limits when expressed per kilogram of body weight, while the plasma volume is usually moderately decreased. Hyperuricemia, hypercholesterolemia, and elevation in serum triglyceride levels are observed but possibly no more frequently than in a similar nonpolycythemic, middle-aged, obese, and hypertensive population. Ferrokinetic data and erythropoietin levels lie as expected within normal range.

Differential diagnosis

In the presence of overt dehydration, no further hematologic studies are needed, and the attention should be directed at restoring fluid balance. In patients with asymptomatic elevation of the hematocrit level and normal levels of carboxyhemoglobin the size of the red cell mass should be measured in order to rule out absolute polycythemia due either to autonomous overproduction of red cells (polycythemia vera) or to increased erythropoietin production [secondary polycythemic (erythrocytosis)].

Therapy

In most cases, specific therapy is not indicated except for attempts to persuade the patients to stop smoking and lose weight. Since an elevated hematocrit with its associated increase in viscosity has been shown to reduce cerebral blood flow [19] and possibly increase thromboembolic disease [17], it seems justified to keep the hematocrit level below 50 percent by phlebotomies. It may at least reduce anxiety and benefit the blood donor program.

Course and prognosis

The course and prognosis in these patients is ultimately determined by associated cardiovascular disease, which in turn has been claimed to be aggravated by a high hematocrit level, an increased whole-blood viscosity and a reduction in plasma volumes. However, this is still a moot point and at the present does not justify measures beyond those of judicious phlebotomies.

References

1. Osler, W.: Chronic cyanosis with polycythemia and enlarged spleen: A new clinical entity. *Am. J. Med. Sci.* 126:187, 1903.
2. Keith, N. M., Rountree, L. G., and Geraghty, J. T.: A method for the

determination of plasma and blood volume. *Arch. Intern. Med.* 16:547, 1915.

3. Gaisbock, F.: Die Bedeutung des Blutdruckmessung für die ärztlichen Praxis. *Dtsch. Arch. Klin. Med.* 83:363, 1905.

4. Yousef, M. K., and Bakewell, W. E., Jr.: The Gaisbock syndrome. *JAMA* 220:864, 1972.

5. Lawrence, J. H., and Berlin, N. I.: Relative polycythemia—The polycythemia of stress. *Yale J. Biol. Med.* 24:498, 1952.

6. Russell, R. P., and Conley, C. L.: Benign polycythemia: Gaisbock's syndrome. *Arch. Intern. Med.* 114:734, 1964.

7. Chrysant, S. G. et al.: Pathologic significance of "stress" or relative polycythemia in essential hypertension. *Am. J. Card.* 37:1069, 1976.

8. Sagove, A. L., and Balcerzak, S. P.: Smoking as a cause of erythrocytosis. *Ann. Intern. Med.* 82:512, 1975.

9. Smith, J. R., and Landaw, S. A.: Smokers' polycythemia. *N. Engl. J. Med.* 298:6, 1978.

10. Brown, S. M., Gilbert, H. S., Krauss, S., and Wasserman, L. R.: Relative polycythemia: A non-existent disease. *Am. J. Med.* 50:200, 1971.

11. Weinreb, N. J., and Shih, C.-F.: Spurious polycythemia. *Semin. Hematol.* 12:397, 1975.

12. Bentley, S. A., and Lewis, S. M.: The relationship between total red cell volume, plasma volume and venous hematocrit. *Br. J. Haematol.* 33:301, 1976.

13. Pearson, T. C., Glass, U. H., and Wetherley-Mein, G.: Interpretation of measured red cell mass in the diagnosis of polycythaemia. *Scand. J. Haematol.* 21:153, 1978.

14. Freedman, A. L.: Hypercarboxyhemoglobinemia from inhalation of cigar smoke. *Ann. Intern. Med.* 82:537, 1975.

15. Isager, H., and Hagerup, L.: Relationship between cigarette smoking and high packed cell volume and hemoglobin levels. *Scand. J. Haematol.* 8:241, 1971.

16. Stewart, R. D., et al.: Carboxyhemoglobin levels in anemic blood donors. *JAMA* 229:1187, 1974.

17. Burge, P. S., Johnson, W. S., and Prankerd, T. A. J.: Morbidity and mortality in pseudopolycythaemia. *Lancet* 1:1266, 1975.

18. Burch, G. E., and Depasquale, N. P.: Hematocrit, blood viscosity, and myocardial infarction. *Am. J. Med.* 32:161, 1962.

19. Humphrey, P. R. D., et al.: Cerebral blood-flow and viscosity in relative polycythaemia. *Lancet* 2:873, 1979.

CHAPTER 75

Hemoglobinopathies producing erythrocytosis

ALLAN J. ERSLEV

Definition and history

The capacity of hemoglobin to bind oxygen avidly in the lungs and then readily release it to the tissues is made possible by a complex series of intramolecular levers which link structure and function of the four heme groups [1]. (See Chap. 37.) It is not surprising, therefore, that among the many mutational changes which can occur in the hemoglobin molecule, some affect the operation of these levers and may produce molecules which do not release oxygen to the tissues as readily as normal hemoglobin does. Such high-oxygen-affinity hemoglobins would be expected to cause tissue

hypoxia and compensatory erythrocytosis. In 1966 Charache, Weatherall, and Clegg [2] described a family with this combination of an abnormal high-affinity hemoglobin, named $Hb_{Chesapeake}$, and a secondary erythrocytosis. Since then many other similar cases have been reported, and the identification and analysis of the mutational change in their hemoglobins have greatly enhanced our understanding of heme-heme interactions and their importance for oxygen transport.

Etiology

Oxygen transport by the normal hemoglobin molecule involves the sequential oxygenation and deoxygenation of four separate heme pockets. The kinetics of this process is usually depicted by the oxygen dissociation curve which relates oxygen pressure to hemoglobin saturation. Without interaction between the heme pockets the dissociation curve would be hyperbolic, as found for myoglobin with only one heme pocket or for hemoglobins with four identical chains such as Hb H (β_4) or $Hb_{Bart's}$ (γ_4). However, the dissociation curve for normal hemoglobin is sigmoid, indicating a progressive change in oxygen affinity of the heme pockets during oxygenation and deoxygenation. In the deoxygenated state the molecule has a low oxygen affinity. This affinity increases as the heme pockets become oxygenated. Fully oxygenated hemoglobin has an affinity that is almost 100 times higher than that of deoxyhemoglobin [1]. The overall oxygen affinity of hemoglobin is usually expressed in terms of P_{50}, the partial oxygen pressure at which hemoglobin is 50 percent deoxygenated.

In structural terms, the transition of hemoglobin from a deoxygenated low-affinity state (T for tense) to an oxygenated high-affinity state (R for relaxed) involves movements of many amino acids with the formation and breakage of numerous intramolecular bonds. These movements are triggered by the attachment of oxygen molecules to the iron atoms in the porphyrin rings. In the T state the heme irons are positioned above the plane of the porphyrin ring (see Fig. 37-2b). When oxygen enters the first heme pocket, the iron is drawn toward the plane of the porphyrins, pulling with it attached amino acids. The resulting molecular reorientation turns the relatively rigid α,β dimers at their α_1-β_2 interface, shrinks the central cavity between the β chains so it no longer can contain a 2,3-DPG molecule and breaks the stabilizing salt bridges between the C terminal and penultimate residues of the α and β chains. These allosteric changes in the hemoglobin structure lead to the formation of a less tense R state with a high oxygen affinity. They also cause the release of protons, produced by the CO_2 transformation to carbonic acid in the tissues and attached to hemoglobin in its more alkaline T state. The attachment and release of these protons are important for CO_2 transport and are responsible for the Bohr effect on oxygen affinity.

For proper heme-heme interaction there must be a balance in the relative stabilities of the oxy and deoxy structures. Factors which disturb the balance, by making the oxy structure more stable or the deoxy structure less stable, tend to shift the oxygenation curve nearer to that of the R state, with a consequent increase in affinity and decrease in P_{50} (Fig. 75-1) [3]. This is the problem with the high-affinity hemoglobins which are listed in Table 75-1 according to the sites of responsible mutations.

Mutations affecting the amino acids at the α_1-β_2 contact affect the normal rotational transition from a T to an R state and tend to lock the hemoglobin into its high-affinity R state. $Hb_{Chesapeake}$ [2] was the first hemoglobin to be recognized as having an abnormality in the α_1-β_2 interface, but many more have been identified subsequently.

Mutations affecting the C-terminal and penultimate amino acids will affect the salt bridges which stabilize the T state and tend to keep the hemoglobins in the high-affinity R state. This is the case for $Hb_{Rainier}$ [16], $Hb_{Bethesda}$ [17], and Hb_{Osler} [18], among many others. In some of these, for example, $Hb_{Hiroshima}$ [21] and $Hb_{Andrew-Minneapolis}$ [22], proton binding is also impaired, resulting in a reduced Bohr effect.

Changes in amino acids lining the pocket which contains 2,3-DPG will also destabilize the deoxy form. Hb_{Rahere} [24] and $Hb_{Little Rock}$ [27] are examples of such high-affinity hemoglobins. Finally heme pocket mutations may in some cases result in high-oxygen-affinity hemoglobins. However, most of these are unstable and are associated with hemolytic anemia or cyanosis. One exception is $Hb_{Heathrow}$ [30], which causes tissue hypoxia and secondary erythrocytosis.

Pathogenesis

Abnormal hemoglobins locked into the high-oxygen-affinity R state will only reluctantly release their oxygen to the tissues. This will cause relative tissue hypoxia until it is offset by an increase in the oxygen-carrying capacity of blood or, in others words, by a secondary polycythemia (erythrocytosis). (See Chap. 73.) Erythropoietin production is appropriately increased, but the increase may be too small to be detected by the routine in vivo assay. However, if the hemoglobin concentration is reduced towards normal by phlebotomy, the resulting tissue hypoxia will increase erythropoietin production and provide easily measurable levels in blood [36].

It has been suggested that women with high-oxygen-affinity hemoglobins have increased fetal losses because their hemoglobin would be less capable than normal hemoglobin of transferring oxygen to the fetus [10]. Experimental studies of pregnant rats indicate that this may be the case [37]. However, no increase in fetal losses has been detected in a number of families with high-oxygen-affinity hemoglobins [15].

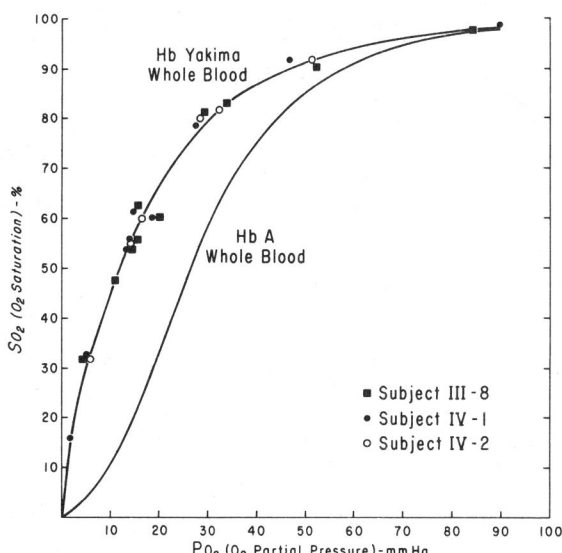

FIGURE 75-1 Oxygen-hemoglobin equilibrium of normal whole blood and whole blood from a patient with hemoglobin Yakima. Note the hyperbolic rather than sigmoid shape of the curve for hemoglobin Yakima. (Novy, Edwards, and Metcalfe [3], by permission of the *Journal of Clinical Investigation*.)

An important feature of the high-oxygen-affinity hemoglobins is that they are more completely oxygenated at low oxygen pressure than is normal hemoglobin. Nevertheless, the normal hemoglobin response of humans to the low oxygen pressure at high altitude is a moderate decrease in oxygen affinity, which enhances the oxygen delivery to the tissues but further impairs the oxygen loading in the lungs [38]. Since animals indigenous to high altitude, such as llamas and vicuñas have hemoglobins with high oxygen affinity [39], it has been suggested that the human response is inappropriate. Indeed two children with high-oxygen-affinity hemoglobin ($Hb_{Andrew-Minneapolis}$) were found to adapt immediately to an altitude of 3100 m without a significant change in heart rate, oxygen consumption, or erythropoietin level [40]. They appeared to be preadapted to high altitude, and apparently the ease with which oxygen was extracted from the rarefied atmosphere more than made up for problems in the release of oxygen to the tissues.

Mode of inheritance

Inheritance of these disorders is autosomal dominant. Only heterozygotes with about 50 percent abnormal hemoglobin have been observed; the homozygous state may be incompatible with survival. The largest family studied has had 20 affected individuals in four generations ($HB_{Brigham}$ [12]). In several cases, identical variants have been found in unrelated families in different parts of the world. $Hb_{Malmö}$ has been found in

TABLE 75-1 Hemoglobinopathies producing erythrocytosis

Hemoglobin	Substitution	Hct, %	References
α_1-β_2 contact:			
Chesapeake	α92(FG4)Arg $\rightarrow$ Leu		[2]
J Capetown	α92(FG4)Arg $\rightarrow$ Glu		[4]
Malmö	β97(FG4)His $\rightarrow$ Glu	51–60	[5–7]
Wood	β97(FG4)His $\rightarrow$ Leu	52–67	[8]
Kempsey	β99(G1)Asp $\rightarrow$ Asn	52–64.5	[9]
Yakima	β99(G1)Asp $\rightarrow$ His		[3,10]
Ypsilanti	β99(G1)Asp $\rightarrow$ Tyr	42–63	[11]
Brigham	β100(G2)Pro $\rightarrow$ Leu	43–59	[12]
Alberta	β101(G3)Glu $\rightarrow$ Gly	58	[13]
Radcliffe	β99(G1)Asp $\rightarrow$ Ala	62	[14]
Potomac	β101(G3)Glu $\rightarrow$ Asp	59	[15]
C terminal and penultimate:			
Rainier	β145(HC2)Tyr $\rightarrow$ Cys	44–60	[16]
Bethesda	β145(HC2)Tyr $\rightarrow$ His	52–56	[17]
Osler	β145(HC2)Tyr $\rightarrow$ Asp	47–67	[18]
Fort Gordon	β145(HC2)Tyr $\rightarrow$ Asp	58	[19]
Nancy	β145(HC2)Tyr $\rightarrow$ Asp	48	[20]
Hiroshima	β146(HC2)His $\rightarrow$ Asp	45–53	[21]
Andrew-Minneapolis	β144(HC1)Lys $\rightarrow$ Asn	57	[22]
McKees Rocks	β145(HC2)Tyr $\rightarrow$ Term	44–64	[23]
2,3-DPG binding:			
Rahere	β82(EF6)Lys $\rightarrow$ Thr	57	[24]
Helsinki	β82(EF6)Lys $\rightarrow$ Met	41–54	[25]
Providence	β82(EF6)Lys $\rightarrow$ Asn	45–47	[26]
Little Rock	β143(H21)His $\rightarrow$ Glu	70	[27]
Syracuse	β143(H21)His $\rightarrow$ Pro	48–60	[28]
Ohio	β142(H20)Ala $\rightarrow$ Asp	54–58	[29]
Heme pocket:			
Heathrow	β103(G5) Phe $\rightarrow$ Leu	48–64	[30]
Great Lakes	β68(E12)Leu $\rightarrow$ His	46–53	[31]
Others:			
San Diego	β109(G11)Val $\rightarrow$ Met	46–52	[32,33]
Olympia	β20(B2)Val $\rightarrow$ Met	56–62	[34]
Cretail	β89(F5)Ser $\rightarrow$ Asn		[35]

families in Sweden [5] and the United States [6,7], the family from the United States being of English ancestry. Hb$_{Osler}$ and Hb$_{Fort Gordon}$, which have the same substitution, β145 Tyr$\rightarrow$Asp, have been found in two black Americans [18,19], and the same variant has also been found in France as Hb$_{Nancy}$ [20]. Hb$_{San Diego}$ has been found in a Filipino family [32] and an Englishman [33], and Hb$_{Little Rock}$ has been found in one American man [27] and a Canadian family unrelated to him. Some of these are presumably genuine cases of the same mutation appearing independently in different parts of the world. Hb$_{Bethesda}$ appears to be a new mutation, as it was present in the propositus but absent in the parents [17].

Clinical features

Plethora, with occasional symptoms of headache and facial fullness, are the only clinical manifestations. Physical endurance does not appear to be reduced.

Laboratory features

Hemoglobin concentration, hematocrit percentage, and red cell mass are regularly increased above normal. The extent of increase is moderate and depends on individual homeostatic response to tissue hypoxia [41]. In some patients pulmonary and cardiovascular compensations are very efficient, and they only have a slight increase in red cell mass; in others the compensation is inefficient, and the patients may have pronounced erythrocytosis. Erythropoietin titers are slightly increased, reflecting the presence of enough remaining tissue hypoxia to sustain an increased rate of red cell production [42].

The P_{50} is decreased, but in only about half the cases can an abnormal hemoglobin be demostrated by starch gel electrophoresis. In the others it is demonstrable only by agar gel electrophoresis or by isoelectric focusing. In a few cases the mutation is electrophoretically silent and is first suspected by its high oxygen affinity.

Although the Bohr effect is often decreased, carbon dioxide transport is not affected.

Differential diagnosis

Every patient with erythrocytosis and absence of the characteristic features of either polycythemia vera (splenomegaly, increased granulocyte and platelet counts, high leukocyte alkaline phosphatase, elevated vitamin B_{12} concentrations in serum, and absent serum erythropoietin) or cardiopulmonary secondary polycythemia (decreased arterial oxygen saturation) should be examined for the presence of an abnormal hemoglobin with high oxygen affinity [43].

Therapy

Phlebotomy can be used for the symptomatic treatment of high-viscosity manifestations. However, the erythrocytosis is rarely severe enough to cause problems, and the patient is best left alone.

Course and prognosis

Patients with high-oxygen-affinity hemoglobins and erythrocytosis appear to live normal and uncomplicated lives.

References

1. Perutz, M. F.: Hemoglobin structure and respiratory transport. *Sci. Am.* 239:92, 1978.
2. Charache, S., Weatherall, D. J., and Clegg, J. B.: Polycythemia associated with a hemoglobinopathy. *J. Clin. Invest.* 45:813, 1966.
3. Novy, M. J., Edwards, M. J., and Metcalfe, J.: Hemoglobin Yakima. II. High blood oxygen affinity associated with compensatory erythrocytosis and normal hemodynamics. *J. Clin. Invest.* 46:1848, 1967.
4. Botha, M.C., Beale, D., Isaacs, W. A., and Lehmann, H.: Haemoglobin J Cape Town: α_2 92 Arginine→glutamine β_2. *Nature* 212:792, 1966.
5. Berglund, S.: Erythrocytosis associated with haemoglobin Malmö, accompanied by pulmonary changes occurring in the same family. *Scand. J. Haematol.* 9:35, 1972.
6. Fairbanks, V. F.: Familial erythrocytosis due to an electrophoretically undetectable haemoglobin with impaired oxygen dissociation (hemoglobin Malmö) $\alpha_2\beta_2$97 Gln. *Mayo Clin. Proc.* 46:721, 1971.
7. Boyer, S. H., Charache, S., Fairbanks, V. F., Maldonado, J. E., Noyes, A., and Gayle, E. E.: Hemoglobin Malmö (β-97 (FG4) histidine→glutamine): A cause of polycythemia. *J. Clin. Invest.* 51:666, 1972.
8. Taketa, F., Huang, Y. P., Liboch, J. A., and Dessel, B. H.: Hemoglobin Wood (β97 (FG4) His→Leu): A new high-oxygen-affinity hemoglobin associated with familial erythrocytosis. *Biochim. Biophys. Acta* 400:348, 1975.
9. Reed, C. S., et al.: Erythrocytosis secondary to increased oxygen affinity of a mutant hemoglobin, hemoglobin Kempsey. *Blood* 31:632, 1968.
10. Jones, R. T., et al.: Hemoglobin Yakima. I. Clinical and Biochemical studies. *J. Clin. Invest.* 46:1840, 1967.
11. Glynn, K. P., Penner, J. A., Smith, J. R., and Rucknagel, D. L.: Familial erythrocytosis: A description of three families, one with hemoglobin Ypsilanti. *Ann. Intern. Med.* 69:797, 1968.
12. Lokich, J. J., Moloney, W. C., Bunn, H. F., Bruckheimer, S. H., and

Ranney, H. M.: Hemoglobin Brigham ($\alpha_2^A\beta_2$100 Pro → Leu): Hemoglobin variant associated with familial erythrocytosis. *J. Clin. Invest.* 52:2060, 1973.
13. Mant, M. J., et al.: $Hb_{Alberta}$ or $\alpha_2\beta_2$ (101 (G3) Glu → Gly), a new high-oxygen-affinity hemoglobin variant causing erythrocytosis. *Hemoglobin* I:183, 1976-77.
14. Weatherall, D. J., et al.: Haemoglobin Radcliffe ($\alpha_2\beta_2^{99(GJ)\,Ala}$): A high oxygen-affinity variant causing familial polycythaemia. *Br. J. Haematol.* 35:177, 1977.
15. Charache, S., et al.: $Hb_{Potomac}$ (101 Glu → Asp): Speculations on placental oxygen transport in carriers of high-affinity hemoglobins. *Blood* 51:331, 1978.
16. Stamatoyannopoulos, G., Yoshida, A., Adamson, J. W., and Heinenberg, S.: Hemoglobin Rainier (β145 tyrosine-histidine): Alkali-resistant hemoglobin with increased oxygen affinity. *Science* 159:741, 1968.
17. Bunn, H. F., et al.: Structural and functional studies on hemoglobin Bethesda ($\alpha_2\beta_2^{145His}$): A variant associated with compensatory erythrocytosis. *J. Clin. Invest.* 51:2299, 1972.
18. Charache, S., Brimhall, B., and Jones, R. T.: Polycythemia produced by hemoglobin Osler (β145 (HC_2) Tyr→Asp). *Johns Hopkins Med. J.* 136:132, 1975.
19. Kleckner, H. B., et al.: Hemoglobin Fort Gordon or $\alpha_2\beta_2$ 145 Tyr→Asp: A new high-oxygen affinity variant. *Biochim. Biophys. Acta* 400:343, 1975.
20. Gacon, G., Wayman, H., Labie, D., and Vigneron, C.: Structural and functional study of Hb Nancy (β145 (HC2) Tyr→Asp): A high oxygen affinity hemoglobin. *FEBS Lett.* 56:39, 1975.
21. Perutz, M.F., et al.: Haemoglobin Hiroshima and the mechanism of the alkaline Bohr effect. *Nature [New Biol.]* 232:147, 1971.
22. Zak, S. J., Brimhall, B., Jones, R. T., and Kaplan, M. E.: Hemoglobin Andrew-Minneapolis ($\alpha_2\,\beta_2$ 144 Lys→Asn): A new high-oxygen affinity mutant human hemoglobin. *Blood* 44:543, 1974.
23. Winslow, R. M., Swenberg, M.-L., Gross, E., Chervenick, P. A., Buchman, R. R., and Anderson, W. F.: Hemoglobin McKees Rocks ($\alpha_2\beta_2^{145Tyr→Term}$). A human "nonsense" mutation leading to a shortened β-chain. *J. Clin. Invest.* 57:772, 1976.
24. Lorkin, P. A., Stephens, A. D., Beard, M. E. J., Wrigley, P. F. M., Adams, L., and Lehmann, H.: Haemoglobin Rahere (β82 (EF6) Lys→Thr): A new high affinity haemoglobin associated with decreased 2,3-DPG binding and relative polycythaemia. *Br. Med. J.* 4:200, 1975.
25. Ikkala, E., et al.: Haemoglobin Helsinki: A high oxygen affinity variant with a substitution at a 2,3-DPG binding site: β82 (EF6) lysine→methionine. *Acta Haematol. (Basel)* 56:257, 1976.
26. Charache, S., McCurdy, P., and Fox, J.: Hemoglobin Providence (Hb Prov): A fetal-like hemoglobin. *Blood* 46:1030, 1975.
27. Bromberg, P. A., et al.: High oxygen affinity variant of haemoglobin Little Rock with unique properties. *Nature [New Biol.]* 243:177, 1973.
28. Jensen, M., Bunn, H. F., Nathan, D. G., and Oski, F. A.: Hemoglobin Syracuse ($\alpha_2\beta_2$ 143 (H21) His→Pro): A new high-affinity variant detected by special electrophoretic methods. *J. Clin. Invest.* 55:469, 1975.
29. Moo-Penn, W. F., et al.: Hemoglobin Ohio (β142 Ala→Asp): A new abnormal hemoglobin with high oxygen affinity and erythrocytosis. *Blood* 56:246, 1980.
30. White, J. M., Szur, L., Gillies, I. D. E., Lorkin, P. A., and Lehmann, H.: Familial polycythaemia caused by a new haemoglobin variant Hb Heathrow, β103 (G5) phenylalanine→leucine. *Br. Med. J.* 3:665, 1973.
31. Rahbar, S., et al.: Hemoglobin Great Lakes (β68 [E12] Leucine→Histidine): A new high-affinity hemoglobin. *Blood* 58:813, 1981.
32. Nute, P. E., Stamatoyannopoulos, G., Hermodson, M. A., and Roth, D.: Hemoglobinopathic erythrocytosis due to a new electrophoretically silent variant: Hemoglobin San Diego (β109 (G11) Val→Met). *J. Clin. Invest.* 53:320, 1974.
33. Chanarin, I., Samson, D., Lang, A., Casey, R., Lorkin, P. A., and Lehmann, H.: Erythraemia due to haemoglobin San Diego. *Br. J. Haematol.* 30:167, 1975.
34. Stamatoyannopoulos, G., Nute, P. E., Adamson, J. W., Bellingham,

A. J., Funk, D., and Hornung, S.: Hemoglobin Olympia (β20 valine$\rightarrow$methionine): An electrophoretically silent variant associated with high oxygen affinity and erythrocytosis. *J. Clin. Invest.* 52:342, 1973.

35. Garel, M. C., Cohen-Solal, M., Blouquit, Y., and Ross, J.: A method for isolation of abnormal haemoglobins with high oxygen affinity due to frozen quaternary R structure: Application to Hb Creteil ($\alpha_2^{AB2(F5)89\ Asn}$). *FEBS Lett.* 43:93, 1974.

36. Adamson, J. W., Parer, J. T., and Stamatoyannopoulos, G.: Erythrocytosis associated with hemoglobin Rainier: Oxygen equilibria and marrow regulation. *J. Clin. Invest.* 48:1376, 1969.

37. Hebbel, R. P., Berger, E. M., and Eaton, J. W.: Effect of increased maternal hemoglobin oxygen affinity on fetal growth in the rat. *Blood* 55:969, 1980.

38. Finch, C. A., and Lenfant, C.: Oxygen transport in man. *N. Engl. J. Med.* 286:407, 1972.

39. Monge, C., and Whittembury, J.: High altitude adaptation of the whole animal, in *Environmental Physiology of Animals,* edited by J. Bligh, J. K. Cloudsley-Thompson, and A. G. MacDonald. Blackwell Scientific Publications, London, 1976, p. 289.

40. Hebbel, R. P., Eaton, J. W., Kronenberg, R. S., Zanjani, E. D., Moore, L. G., and Berger, E. M.: Human Llamas. Adaptation to altitude in subjects with high hemoglobin oxygen affinity. *J. Clin. Invest.* 62:593, 1978.

41. Charache, S., Achuff, S., Winslow, R., Adamson, J., and Chervenick, P.: Variability of the homeostatic response to altered P50. *Blood* 52:1156, 1978.

42. Erslev, A. J., et al.: Plasma erythropoietin in polycythemia. *Am. J. Med.* 66:243, 1979.

43. Lichtman, M. A., Murphy, M. S., and Adamson, J. W.: Detection of mutant hemoglobins with altered affinity for oxygen. A simplified technique. *Ann. Intern. Med.* 84:517, 1976.

Erythrocyte disorders—diseases related to abnormal heme or porphyrin metabolism

CHAPTER *76*

The porphyrias

DONALD P. TSCHUDY

The porphyrias [1–3] are diseases that result from mutations affecting enzymes of the heme biosynthetic pathway. Only one type, porphyria cutanea tarda, can occur as either a genetic or acquired toxic disorder [4]. These disorders should be distinguished from secondary porphyrinuria, in which increased urinary excretion of porphyrin, usually coproporphyrin, occurs in well-defined disorders [5–8].

Heme biosynthesis in normal and porphyric states

The heme biosynthetic pathway (Fig. 76-1) [1,2,9–11] consists of eight steps. In step 1, glycine, activated by reaction with pyridoxal phosphate, condenses with succinyl coenzyme A to form δ-aminolevulinic acid (ALA). The mitochondrial enzyme which catalyzes this reaction is inducible in liver. Its level is controlled mainly through the operation of a closed negative feedback loop, in which heme, the end product of the pathway, is involved in repression of the synthesis of the enzyme. When the pool of "repressor heme" is diminished as a result of decreased synthesis, increased turnover, or increased binding of heme to certain proteins, hepatic ALA synthase production is augmented in an attempt to restore the repressor heme pool size toward normal. As a result of increased levels of hepatic ALA synthase, there is a change in the pool sizes of substrates in the pathway. The tissue concentrations of substrates are functions of the levels of the various enzymes of the pathway and their affinity for substrate (K_m's) [12,13]. Each of the porphyrias is characterized by a specific pat-

tern of tissue levels and excretion of metabolites that results from (1) the genetically mediated decrease of a particular enzyme and (2) the magnitude of induction of ALA synthase in response to decreases of repressor heme concentrations. The effect of number 2 is seen in those hepatic porphyrias (see Table 76-1 for classifications) that are sometimes accompanied by acute attacks of neurological dysfunction. When these patients are asymptomatic, there may be no increase of urinary porphyrin precursor (ALA and porphobilinogen) excretion, indicating little or no induction of hepatic ALA synthase. During acute attacks, porphyrin precursor excretion increases in response to a presumed decrease of hepatic repressor heme.

The second step of the pathway involves the condensation by ALA dehydratase of two molecules of ALA to form porphobilinogen (PBG), the monopyrrole precursor of porphyrins and heme. This compound is excreted in the urine in increased quantities during acute attacks of acute intermittent, variegate, and hereditary coproporphyria, and the detection of a pronounced increase of urinary PBG excretion is diagnostic of the acute attack type of porphyria. Urinary ALA excretion is usually increased along with PBG in the acute attack type of porphyria. However, detection of an increased concentration of urinary ALA alone is not specific for this type of porphyria, since increases of urinary ALA (without increases of PBG) have been described in porphyria cutanea tarda [14], lead intoxication [15], and hereditary tyrosinemia [16,17]. Slight increases in excretion of urinary ALA have been described in the third trimester of pregnancy [18,19] and in diabetic ketosis [20]. Pronounced increases of urinary PBG are readily detected by qualitative tests such as the Watson-Schwartz [21] and Hoesch [22] tests. These are based on the production of a pink or red derivative when an acid solution of p-dimethylaminobenzaldehyde (Ehrlich's aldehyde reagent) reacts with PBG.

Steps 3 and 4 of Fig. 76-1 involve the polymerization of PBG to form uroporphyrinogen I or III. The porphyrinogens are the reduced (hexahydro) forms of porphyrins and are the intermediates utilized for protoporphyrin synthesis. They are readily oxidized in the presence of oxygen and light to the corresponding porphyrins. Production of the physiologically utilized asymmetric type III isomer requires the action of both uroporphyrinogen I synthase (PBG deaminase) and uroporphyrinogen III cosynthase. When acting alone, the former enzyme produces the symmetrical, but physiologically unutilized, type I isomer. The greatly increased excretion of uroporphyrin I in congenital erythropoietic porphyria results from a decreased ratio of the uroporphyrinogen III cosynthase to uroporphyrinogen I synthase.

The four acetic acid side chains of uroporphyrinogen undergo sequential decarboxylation, catalyzed by uroporphyrinogen decarboxylase, to form the methyl groups of coproporphyrinogen. Coproporphyrinogen

TABLE 76-1   Classification of porphyrias based on enzyme deficiency

Enzyme number in heme pathway (see Fig. 76-1)	Name of enzyme	Product of enzyme	Disease produced by mutation affecting enzyme	Type of genetic transmission	Major clinical manifestations
2	ALA dehydratase	Porphobilinogen	Not yet named		
3	Uroporphyrinogen I synthase		Acute intermittent porphyria	Dominant	Acute attacks of neurological dysfunction
	+	Uroporphyrinogen III			
4	Uroporphyrinogen III cosynthase		Congenital erythropoietic porphyria	Recessive	Severe cutaneous lesions and hemolysis
5	Uroporphyrinogen decarboxylase	Coproporphyrinogen	Porphyria cutanea tarda	Dominant	Cutaneous lesions
6	Coproporphyrinogen oxidase	Protoporphyrinogen	Hereditary coproporphyria	Dominant	Acute attacks of neurological dysfunction
7	Protoporphyrinogen oxidase	Protoporphyrin	Variegate porphyria	Dominant	Acute attacks of neurological dysfunction and/or cutaneous lesions
8	Ferrochelatase	Heme	Erythropoietic protoporphyria (erythrohepatic porphyria)	Dominant	Cutaneous symptoms and occasionally fatal liver disease

oxidase (step 6) converts the two propionic acid side chains on pyrrole rings A and B, through oxidation and decarboxylation, to vinyl groups. The resulting protoporphyrinogen is then converted by protoporphyrinogen oxidase to protoporphyrin (step 7). Ferrochelatase (heme synthase) forms heme through chelation of ferrous iron by protoporphyrin.

The function of hemoproteins can be divided into five categories: (1) transport of molecular oxygen (hemoglobins), (2) transport of electrons (mitochondrial cytochromes), (3) activation of oxygen (cytochrome oxidase, mixed function oxidases such as microsomal cytochromes, and tryptophan pyrrolase), (4) activation of hydrogen peroxide (peroxidases), and (5) decomposition of hydrogen peroxide (catalases).

Physiology of porphyrins and porphyrin precursors

PHOTOSENSITIVITY

Porphyrins are photosensitizing agents, and those wavelengths that are most effective in producing reactions in the presence of porphyrins (action spectrum) correspond to the wavelengths absorbed by porphyrins (absorbtion spectrum) [23–25]. Porphyrins exhibit a strong absorbtion in the region of 400 nm (Soret band), which is near the junction of the visible and ultraviolet portions of the electromagnetic spectrum. In contrast to the shorter ultraviolet wavelengths, which cause ordinary sunburn reactions, the radiation that causes skin damage in porphyria can pass through glass. All of the porphyrias, except for acute intermittent porphyria, may be accompanied by photosensitivity reactions, but the exact nature and the severity of the cutaneous reaction is not identical in all types of porphyria.

Photosensitivity reactions also occur in a group of disorders which have been categorized as polymorphous light eruptions [26] and sometimes as a complication of therapy with certain drugs, such as sulfonamides, chlorpromazine, nalidixic acid, isoniazid, demeclocycline, and rarely, other tetracyclines [26]. Cutaneous complications of light exposure can also occur in many other disorders, including pellagra, Hartnup syndrome, and the carcinoid syndrome [26].

Possible role of metabolites in neurological manifestations

While it is clear that photosensitivity reactions in the porphyrias are caused by porphyrins, the mechanism that produces neurological dysfunction in some porphyrias is not yet elucidated. The two most widely considered theories postulate neurotoxicity of porphyrin precursors [1,27] and nervous system heme deficiency [28]. Both theories provide a rationale for the use of intravenous hematin therapy for acute attacks of porphyria, since hematin has been shown to repress hepatic ALA synthase in animals [29,30], lower porphyrin precursor excretion in patients with acute attack types of porphyria [31,32], and correct hepatic heme deficiency [33].

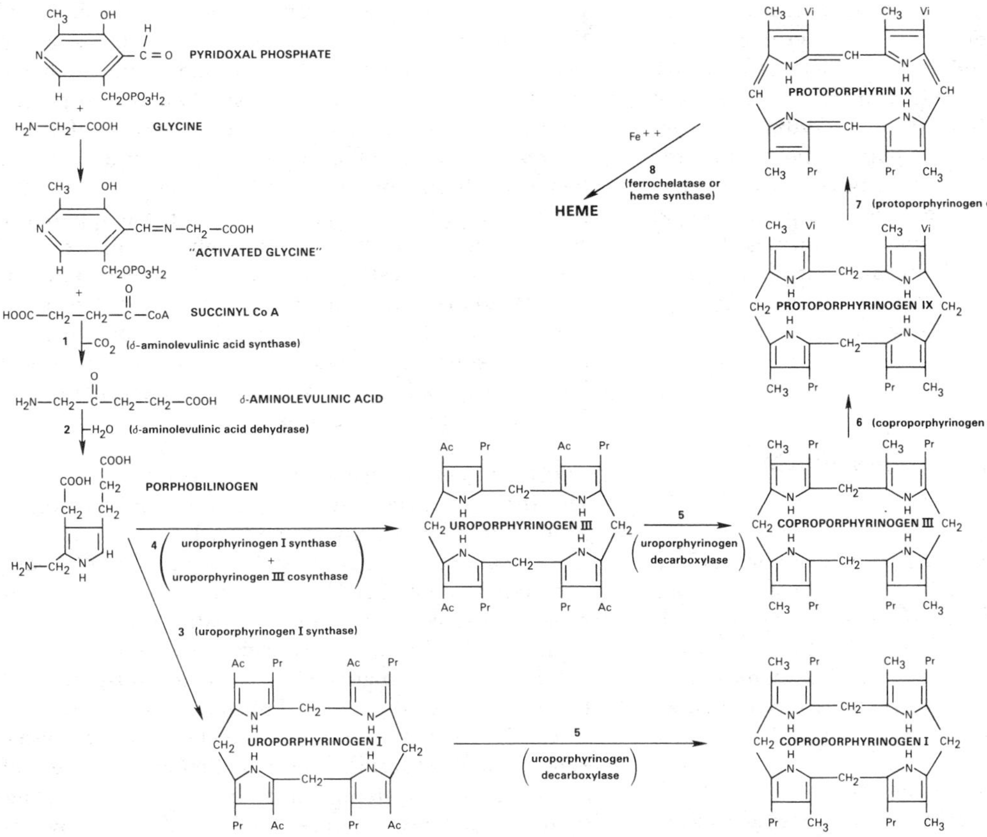

FIGURE 76-1 The heme biosynthetic pathway. The names of substrates and products are printed in capital letters. The names of the enzymes are presented in lowercase letters in parentheses. The boldface numbers identify the steps in the synthesis of heme and are used in the text and tables for this purpose. The side chains on the porphyrin molecules are identified by the following abbreviations: Pr = propionic acid; Ac = acetic acid; CH_3 = methyl; Vi = vinyl.

Classification of the porphyrias

The porphyrias can be classified on the basis of (1) the specific enzyme deficiencies, (2) the organs from which excess metabolites originate, or (3) the clinical manifestations. A classification based on number 1 is presented in Table 76-1. It contains a disorder not included in the older classifications based on numbers 2 or 3, i.e., ALA dehydratase deficiency [34,35]. In heterozygous form this defect appears to be asymtomatic in the few individuals studied thus far. However, two young men whose erythrocyte ALA dehydratase levels were less than 1 percent of normal had acute attacks similar to those of acute intermittent porphyria [35]. The acute attacks were characterized by abdominal colic, tachycardia, hypertension, and peripheral motor neuropathy. Lead intoxication and tyrosinemia were ruled out. The tremendous increase of urinary ALA with only a slight increase of PBG and increased urinary coproporphyrin in this disorder more closely resembles the chemical findings in lead intoxication than in the other acute attack types of porphyria. Classifications based on criteria 2 and 3 are presented in Table 76-2. Classification of the

TABLE 76-2 Other classifications of porphyrias

CLASSIFICATION BY RESPONSIBLE ORGAN
Erythropoietic:
  Congenital erythropoietic porphyria
  (Günther's disease)
Eythrohepatic porphyria (erythropoietic protoporphyria)
Hepatic:
  Acute intermittent porphyria
  Variegate porphyria (mixed porphyria)
  Hereditary coproporphyria
  Porphyria cutanea tarda

CLASSIFICATION BY CLINICAL MANIFESTATIONS
Porphyrias that produce cutaneous manifestations without neurological disease:
  Congenital erythropoietic porphyria
  Erythrohepatic porphyria (erythropoietic protoporphyria)
  Porphyria cutanea tarda
Porphyria that produces neurological disease, but no cutaneous manifestations:
  Acute intermittent porphyria
Porphyrias that can produce cutaneous and neurological disease:
  Variegate porphyria
  Hereditary coproporphyria

porphyrias into two groups, erythropoietic and hepatic, depending on the porphyrin or porphyrin precursor content of the marrow and liver is widely used [36,37], but it should be emphasized that the enzyme defects in these disorders are not limited to the erythron or liver. In the acute attack types of hepatic porphyria, the greatly increased excretion of porphyrin precursors during acute attacks results from the overproduction of these compounds as a consequence of increased levels of hepatic ALA synthase. Significant overproduction of the precursors does not occur in other tissues apparently because ALA synthase is only inducible to high levels in the liver.

Congenital erythropoietic porphyria (Günther's disease)

This very rare disease was the first type of porphyria to be described, undoubtedly because its manifestations of red urine and severe cutaneous lesions are so obvious. There are probably less than 100 authentic cases in the world literature. Günther described the clinical findings in 1911 [38] and 1922 [39], and more recent reviews have presented this disorder in detail [2,40].

ETIOLOGY AND PATHOGENESIS
In contrast to the other porphyrias, this disease is transmitted as an autosomal recessive disorder [2]. The great increase of urinary excretion of uroporphyrin I indicates an imbalance in the activities of uroporphyrinogen I synthase (PBG deaminase, enzyme 3 of the heme biosynthetic pathway) (Fig. 76-1) and uroporphyrinogen III cosynthase (enzyme 4 of the pathway). A decrease in cosynthase activity to levels about one-tenth to one-third of normal has been found in both bovine [41] and human disease [42]. The decreased activity in fibroblasts [43] indicates that the defect is not restricted to erythrocytes. However, the presence of a primary defect of uroporphyrinogen cosynthase has been questioned because the capacity for synthesis of type III isomers and heme, both in vivo and in vitro, is not deficient [44,45], and it has been proposed that the greatly increased excretion of uroporphyrin I resulted from a primary increase of ALA synthase or uroporphyrinogen I synthase [45]. Nevertheless, studies on erythrocytes [46,47] and fibroblasts [47] of patients and on the bovine disease [48] have shown considerable decreases of cosynthase activity. Such decrease of cosynthase activity was accompanied by an increase of uroporphyrinogen I synthase activity [46,48]. Synthesis of protoporphyrin from ALA in fibroblasts was not impaired [47], but the increased levels of ALA synthase in leukocytes [46] suggest a compensatory response in these cells to impaired heme synthesis.

It appears that mutation in the structural gene for uroporphyrinogen cosynthase is the fundamental defect. This enzyme is normally present in excess when compared with ALA synthase and uroporphyrinogen I synthase. Moderate decreases of the cosynthase as in heterozygotes would not be expected to impair heme synthesis. In the patients with congenital erythropoietic porphyria (homozygous for the defect), the greater, but variable, decrease of the cosynthase may tend to impair heme synthesis, but the moderate increase of ALA synthase and uroporphyrinogen I synthase apparently compensates sufficiently to maintain type III tetrapyrrole isomer synthesis at normal levels. This disease, in contrast to the acute attack types of porphyria, does not appear to involve a significant deficiency of heme. All the cutaneous manifestations result from the increased levels of circulating porphyrins, but the mechanism of hemolysis is not entirely clear.

CLINICAL AND LABORATORY FINDINGS
The disease causes cutaneous lesions and hemolytic anemia. It is almost always evident between birth and age 5 years, but three cases with onset after age 50 have been reported [49–51]. Vesicles and bullae occur on exposed portions of the body. Repeated ulceration and healing of these lesions may lead to severe scarring and deformity of the fingers, eyes, ears, and nose. Loss of the nails or even the terminal phalanges occurs in some cases. Ocular complications may include conjunctivitis, keratitis, and ectropion. The skin often exhibits areas of pigmentation and depigmentation, and while scarring in the scalp may produce areas of alopecia, hypertrichosis is often evident on the face and limbs.

Hemolysis is present in most of these patients, and while some develop normochromic anemia, others compensate adequately by increased erythrocyte production. Shortened red cell life-span, reticulocytosis, erythroblastic hyperplasia of the marrow, circulating erythroblasts, and increased fecal urobilinogen are demonstrable in some patients. Splenomegaly is often present, and the occasionally observed thrombocytopenia has been attributed to hypersplenism. Ineffective erythropoiesis may also contribute to anemia [2,49]. Photohemolysis of red cells from patients with erythropoietic protoporphyria has been demonstrated in vitro [52,53], but it is not thought to occur significantly in vivo in that disorder.

The diagnosis is easily made in children who have bullous or vesicular lesions on exposed areas of skin and who also excrete red urine. The teeth should be examined for erythrodontia, and if a brown or reddish discoloration is not obvious, fluorescence may still be demonstrable. The affinity of calcium phosphate for uroporphyrin explains the deposition of porphyrin in the bones and teeth. Quantitative measurement of urinary uroporphyrin and coproporphyrin should be performed to document the great increase of urinary uroporphyrin and lesser increase of coproporphyrin. Further confirmation is obtained by fluorescence microscopy, which demonstrates fluorescence of a variable fraction of circulating erythrocytes and erythroblasts in the marrow [37].

THERAPY AND PROGNOSIS

Since light causes the cutaneous manifestations, it is important to protect the skin from light as much as possible by the use of protective clothing. Topically applied agents that are ordinarily used for sunburn protection do not absorb the longer wavelengths that cause skin damage in the porphyrias and are of little value in these disorders. β-Carotene has been used widely as a photoprotective agent in erythropoietic protoporphyria (see below), but with questionable results here and in Günther's disease [40,54,55].

Hemolysis stimulates erythropoiesis, which augments porphyrin production and hence photosensitivity. Splenectomy has been performed to control hemolysis and porphyrin excretion in some cases and has been of variable value [54,56]. In some instances there has been a prolonged improvement in photosensitivity. Small doses of chloroquine in one case diminished erythrocyte rigidity and caused a transient increase of urinary porphyrin excretion [57]. Transfusions cause a decrease of erythropoiesis and porphyrin excretion [58,59] and a decrease of plasma ALA synthase [60]. Intravenous hematin caused a decrease of red cell, plasma, and urinary porphyrins [60]. While transfusions and intravenous hematin may prove useful on a short-term basis, they pose problems, such as iron overload, in long-term management.

Patients with severe mutilation in their twenties or earlier usually do not survive beyond age 40. Cirrhosis, renal failure, and bleeding have been some of the causes of death.

Erythropoietic protoporphyria (erythrohepatic protoporphyria)

This disorder, while far more common than congenital erythropoietic porphyria, was the last of the porphyrias to be described, and was only defined as a specific clinical entity in 1961 [61,62]. The delayed recognition undoubtedly resulted from the fact that this is the only type of porphyria in which there is no increase of urinary porphyrin precursors or porphyrins. The disease is characterized by the early onset of acute photosensitivity reactions and elevated erythrocyte protoporphyrin levels.

ETIOLOGY AND PATHOGENESIS

Numerous studies have indicated a Mendelian dominant mode of inheritance [1], but with variable penetrance [63–65]. However, this mode of inheritance has been questioned by some [64,65]. Profound decreases of ferrochelatase (enzyme 8 in the heme biosynthetic pathway) activity to levels in the range of 8 to 25 percent of normal have been demonstrated in marrows [66], reticulocytes [66], total blood cells [67], fibroblasts [66,68–70], and liver homogenates [70]. The affinity of the enzyme for porphyrin in this disorder is significantly lower than that in normals [69], indicating that the residual activity

is not normal enzyme. It has been suggested that the enzyme is unstable in this disease [67,71], and that sufficient levels of ferrochelatase activity are present in erythroblasts to allow hemoglobin synthesis to proceed at normal rates.

The disease was originally named *erythropoietic protoporphyria*, but excess protoporphyrin can also originate from the liver [1,2], and it has been suggested that the disease be named *erythrohepatic protoporphyria* [72].

CLINICAL AND LABORATORY FINDINGS

Clinical manifestations involve the skin and occasionally the liver. The mean age of onset in one series was 4.3 years, with the latest onset at 13 years [73]. Patients report burning, swelling, itching, and redness of the skin [74]. There may be only subjective symptoms such as itching and burning, without objective findings such as swelling, redness, and scarring. Symptoms may develop not only outdoors, but also from exposure to light passing through window glass. Burning may be mild or severe, and may occur after exposures of only a few minutes or after several hours. It can persist for days. Erythema and edema may occur in the involved areas. Solar urticaria occurs occasionally. Vesicles, bullae, and purpura may be seen in children and occasionally in adults. Thickening and scarring of the skin of the fingers, back of the hand, nose, and cheeks is evident in some patients. With extensive light exposure papular thickening of the skin may produce a "cobblestone" appearance. Erythrodontia and fluorescence of the teeth have not been reported in this disease, and hirsutism and hyperpigmentation occur only rarely.

Hepatobiliary complications relate to the low aqueous solubility of protoporphyrin. There appears to be an increased incidence of gallstones [1] that contain high levels of protoporphyrin [73,75,76]. At least 11 fatalities from rapidly progressive liver disease have been reported [1]. Liver function tests are normal in most patients [69,73] and are also usually normal in the fatal cases until shortly before liver failure becomes evident. During liver failure, findings have included increased serum transaminase, jaundice, hepatosplenomegaly, hepatic encephalopathy, and portal hypertension with bleeding esophageal varices.

A mild microcytic and hypochromic anemia is evident in some patients [77], but this is usually not a major problem. In contrast to congenital erythropoietic porphyria, hemolytic anemia is uncommon and usually not very significant. Iron utilization is normal in vivo [78,79] and in marrow cells studied in vitro [80].

Patients or asymptomatic relatives may exhibit any of three chemical patterns: (1) increased levels of free erythrocyte, plasma, and fecal protoporphyrin; (2) increased free erythrocyte protoporphyrin levels with no increase of fecal protoporphyrin excretion; and rarely (3) increased fecal protoporphyrin excretion with no increase of free erythrocyte protoporphyrin concentration. Pattern 3 has been seen in a few asymptomatic relatives of symptomatic patients and is not diagnostic of this disease, since increased fecal protoporphyrin levels occur in variegate porphyria. Pattern 2 appears to be the most common one in erythropoietic protoporphyria [69,73]. There are no abnormalities in the urine.

Fluorescence of a variable fraction of marrow erythroblasts and circulating erythrocytes is seen, but marrow morphology is normal [61,81]. In the liver, a brown pigment is deposited, which on fluorescence and polarization microscopy [82] exhibits the properties of protoporphyrin. It is thought that protoporphyrin deposition causes the liver disease.

The diagnosis requires both a typical history and the demonstration of increased free erythrocyte protoporphyrin levels. Neither of these findings alone is sufficient, since a typical history may be elicited in nonporphyric types of polymorphous light eruption and increased free erythrocyte protoporphyrin levels also occur in other disorders such as lead intoxication and iron deficiency. Fluorescence microscopy of red cells and erythroblasts is useful as a screening procedure, but the presence of fluorescence must be confirmed by chemical measurement of free erythrocyte protoporphyrin.

THERAPY AND PROGNOSIS
β-Carotene (Solatene) has been used as a photoprotective agent in this disease, with most patients reporting an increased tolerance to light [83–85] while taking oral doses in the range of 15 to 180 mg per day. Beneficial effects are usually evident after 1 to 2 months of therapy. In preliminary trials dosage should be sufficient to produce blood levels of at least 400 to 600 μg/dl. If this proves inadequate therapeutically, 180 mg of β-carotene per day can be administered for 3 months before discontinuing this agent as a failure. The latter dose should produce blood levels in the range of 800 μg/dl. Failure of β-carotene to produce a clear-cut therapeutic effect in one controlled study [86] has been attributed to a relatively low dose (100 mg per day) and other factors, including duration of treatment. The only significant side effect that has been reported is the yellowish discoloration of the skin produced by β-carotene. Canthaxanthin, another carotenoid, has also been used in the treatment of this disease [85,87].

The prophylaxis and treatment of the serious liver disease that may occur in erythropoietic protoporphyria are unsolved problems. Since the liver disease appears to result from protoporphyrin crystallization in the liver, attempts to diminish hepatic protoporphyrin production and interrupt the enterohepatic circulation of protoporphyrin are worthy of further study. Fecal protoporphyrin excretion in this disease was decreased by a high carbohydrate intake [88] and intravenous hematin administration [89], both of which are known to repress hepatic ALA synthase, and thereby diminish protoporphyrin production. Chronic intravenous hematin administration is an impractical and untested procedure. Whether a prolonged high carbohydrate intake

would have prophylactic value in preventing liver disease is unknown. Agents that bind protoporphyrin in the gut, such as cholestyramine [90], or bind it in vitro [91], have been studied. Recovery from hepatic decompensation in this disease has been reported after intensive therapy, including the use of exchange transfusions [92].

Acute intermittent porphyria

This disease can exist in latent form indefinitely, but sometimes produces attacks of neurological dysfunction with a variety of clinical manifestations, the most common of which is abdominal pain. The attacks are associated with increased porphyrin precursor (ALA and PBG) excretion. It is the one type of porphyria that does not produce photosensitivity. The first recorded case is probably that of Stokvis, who in 1889 described a woman who excreted red urine after ingestion of sulfonmethane (Sulfonal), and later died. Ranking and Pardington reported two cases in 1890 [1,2].

ETIOLOGY AND PATHOGENESIS
The disease is transmitted as an autosomal dominant disorder [93]. The fundamental defect involves a 50 percent decrease in the level of uroporphyrinogen I synthase (enzyme 3 of the heme biosynthetic pathway in Fig. 76-1) in a variety of tissues [1,2,94,95], including liver, red cells, fibroblasts, amniotic fluid cells, and lymphocytes. The lack of photosensitivity in this disease is explained by the fact that the partial block in the pathway exists prior to the production of porphyrinogens (and their oxidative products, porphyrins). Neurotoxicity of porphyrin precursors or heme deficiency is believed to be responsible for the acute attacks.

CLINICAL AND LABORATORY FINDINGS
Four groups of precipitating factors can convert the latent disease to active disease. These include certain drugs, certain sex hormones, starvation (or "crash" dieting), and infections. Since acute attacks of porphyria can produce severe and sometimes fatal illness, it is important to warn all patients of the known precipitating factors. The most widely discussed agents that are considered to be dangerous include barbiturates (particularly sodium thiopental used in dental and other surgical procedures), sulfonamides, phenytoin, griseofulvin, meprobamate, glutethimide, antipyrine, methyprylon, imipramine, ergot preparations, and ethanol [96].

Both endogenous and exogenous female sex hormones have been suspected of playing a role in the precipitation of acute attacks [1,2,97]. Endogenous hormones have been suspected because (1) the biochemical and clinical manifestations rarely occur before puberty, (2) acute attacks of porphyria are more common in females, (3) some women with this disorder experience a cyclic pattern of attacks that occur in relation to menstrual periods (attacks usually beginning about 3 days before menses), and (4) there are a number of reports of attacks of the disease during pregnancy. Exogenous estrogens augment porphyrin precursor excretion in this disease [98].

The fact that a high carbohydrate intake can prevent experimental porphyria [99] and decrease porphyrin precursor excretion in acute intermittent porphyria [100,101], suggests a role of diet in both the etiology of some acute attacks and in the therapy and prophylaxis of attacks. Furthermore, pronounced restriction of dietary intake by some patients has caused acute attacks.

The symptoms of the acute attack result from damage in the nervous system. Although any part of the nervous system may be involved, autonomic manifestations are seen most frequently. Abdominal pain occurs in most attacks, and is thought to result from autonomic neuropathy that causes imbalance in the innervation of the gut, with resultant areas of spasm and dilatation. The pain may be mild or severe and localized or general. It has been mistaken for a number of other abdominal problems, with the performance of unnecessary surgery in some cases, particularly when there is mild leukocytosis and low-grade fever. Vomiting and constipation (but occasionally diarrhea) often accompany the pain, which may be constant or colicky. Other autonomic manifestations include tachycardia, labile hypertension, postural hypotension, sweating, vascular spasm in the retina and extremities, and urinary retention.

Sensory neuropathy is often manifested as pain in the back and/or legs, but objective sensory findings are often absent. Any motor nerve can be affected. Motor involvement can be symmetrical or asymmetrical and can progress at highly variable rates over days, weeks, or months. Aphonia, inability to swallow or breathe, and quadriplegia may occur. The most frequent serious psychiatric manifestations are depression and an organic brain syndrome.

Profound hyponatremia occurs in some attacks and can result from gastrointestinal loss of sodium, inappropriate release of antidiuretic hormone, or primary renal sodium loss [102]. With the exception of BSP (sulfobromophthalein) retention [103] liver function tests are usually normal. Hypercholesterolemia occurs frequently in both experimental [104] and acute attack types of porphyria [104,105], but not in porphyria cutanea tarda [104]. Abnormalities of thyroid function [1,105] are seen in some patients, but no single pattern of disordered thyroid function is seen. Hyperamylasemia, without pancreatitis [106], may occur in both asymptomatic and active phases of the disease. Serum lipases have been normal in these cases. The metabolism of drugs by the heme-containing P_{450} enzyme system appears to be impaired [107,108].

During asymptomatic periods porphyrin precursor excretion is often, but not always, increased. When the disease becomes active, precursor excretion increases above its previous levels. The diagnosis should be suspected in patients with abdominal pain of obscure etiology, particularly if neurological manifestations develop. Since the porphyrin precursors are colorless, freshly voided urine may appear normal. However, PBG polymerizes readily in acid to form porphyrins and other pigments such as porphobilin. If this has occurred in acid urine, the urine may appear dark. This is the basis of the old test that involved placing a urine sample in light for a few days to see if pigment was generated. During acute attacks and sometimes during asymptomatic periods the Watson-Schwartz [21] and Hoesch [22] tests are positive, but these qualitative tests should be confirmed by quantitative measurement of porphyrin precursors. A number of methods have been devised for the measurement of erythrocyte uroporphyrinogen I synthase [109,110], which are useful in making the diagnosis during both asymptomatic and active phases of the disease. The range of normal and porphyric values overlap somewhat, and hence some values may not be diagnostic. Although the differential diagnosis involves a number of disorders that can produce abdominal pain, the one that most closely resembles acute porphyria is lead intoxication, which can produce abdominal pain, neurological manifestations, and abnormalities of porphyrin and porphyrin precursor metabolism. Since it inhibits ALA dehydratase, it causes increased excretion of ALA without significant increase of PBG, as seen in acute attacks of porphyria. The increased free erythrocyte protoporphyrin levels seen in lead intoxication are not seen in acute attack types of porphyria.

THERAPY AND PROGNOSIS

Therapeutic considerations involve (1) prevention of acute attacks, (2) treatment of symptoms and complications, and (3) treatment directed at the fundamental disease process. Since half the siblings and children of a patient with acute intermittent porphyria would be expected on statistical grounds to bear the defect, it is important to examine genetic relatives for the defect and warn them of the precipitating factors. Abdominal pain can sometimes be controlled with phenothiazines, presumably through their inhibition of autonomic activity. If these prove inadequate meperidine can be used. The lists of dangerous and presumed safe drugs in this disease [1,96,111] should be consulted before institution of pharmacologic therapy of the various complications (infections, hypertension, seizures, etc.) that can occur. The management of chronic seizure problems is difficult, sometimes requiring the use of bromides [112,113]. Propranolol has been used to treat autonomic manifestations of the acute attack, such as tachycardia and hypertension [114–116], but some have reported more profound effects of large doses of propranolol on the fundamental disease process, including decreases of porphyrin precursor excretion [117–119].

All patients experiencing an acute attack of porphyria should be given a high carbohydrate intake. The response varies from no effect to spectacular recovery. Furthermore, the dose at which a response occurs varies, since some patients show a decrease of porphyrin precursor excretion and clinical improvement with an intake of 300 g per day of carbohydrate, whereas others may require 500 g per day or more. Oral and parenteral supplementation of meals is indicated. A high carbohydrate intake blocks the induction of hepatic ALA synthase in experimental porphyria [120] and has been shown to decrease leukocyte ALA synthase in patients with acute intermittent porphyria [121].

The rationale for hematin therapy was presented above. Hematin in doses of 3 to 4 mg/kg has been given intravenously once or twice a day for periods of 3 to 8 days, but occasionally longer [122–124]. In almost all patients there was a pronounced decrease of porphyrin precursor excretion, and clinical improvement was evident within 48 h in many patients. When given once a week, intravenous hematin prevented the predictable monthly attacks that had occurred in relation to menses in one patient [125]. Some patients, particularly those whose attacks had progressed to respiratory insufficiency before hematin therapy was initiated, have died despite full courses of therapy. It has been recommended that hematin therapy, therefore, be initiated early in the attack [123]. Although 12 mg/kg of intravenous hematin produced reversible renal insufficiency [126], the usual doses produced no clinical side effects in this disease, except for local phlebitis in some patients.

Hormone prophylaxis has been successful in a small series of patients in preventing the cyclic attacks that occurred every month in relation to menses [127]. Oral contraceptives have been used, but currently available preparations are so low in estrogen content that some degree of estrogen supplementation may be necessary. These agents should not be given to women with porphyria who are not experiencing the cyclic attacks, since there is some risk of precipitating attacks with estrogen therapy.

Death in acute attacks may result from a variety of causes, including respiratory paralysis, arrythmias related to increased serum catecholamines, and hypertensive complications. The prognosis for affected individuals has improved in recent years, mainly through examination of relatives of known patients and by warning individuals with the latent disease to avoid the known precipitating factors. Prognosis has improved also through the newer methods of therapy that have been developed.

Variegate porphyria

This disease can produce acute attacks of neurological dysfunction similar to those of acute intermittent porphyria, but can also produce cutaneous lesions that resemble those of porphyria cutanea tarda. The acute attacks and cutaneous lesions may occur separately or simultaneously.

ETIOLOGY AND PATHOGENESIS
This disease is transmitted as an autosomal dominant disorder [102,128]. There is some difference of opinion concerning the enzyme defect in this disease. A decrease of ferrochelatase has been reported in leukocytes [129], erythroblasts [71], and fibroblasts [130], but no decrease was found in skeletal muscle [131]. In another study [132] ferrochelatase levels in skin fibroblasts were found to be normal by both direct and indirect assays, but protoporphyrinogen oxidase (enzyme 7 of the heme biosynthetic pathway) was found to be 43 percent of the normal level. Proponents of a ferrochelatase deficiency as the cause of this disease are faced with the paradox of two completely different diseases (erythropoietic protoporphyria and variegate porphyria) resulting from deficiencies of the same enzyme. Attempts to rationalize this apparent contradiction have included the suggestion [71,133] that the 50 percent decrease of ferrochelatase activity in variegate porphyria is caused by a dominant structural gene mutation resulting in an inactive ferrochelatase, whereas the greater than 50 percent decrease of ferrochelatase that appears to be well documented in erythropoietic protoporphyria is the result of a mutation that produces a "variant enzyme" of decreased stability [65,71]. A deficiency of protoporphyrinogen oxidase obviates the need to deal with the above paradox.

CLINICAL AND LABORATORY FINDINGS
The clinical manifestations of variegate porphyria [102,128,134] are acute attacks of neurological dysfunction and/or cutaneous lesions. Since the disease can produce features of both acute intermittent porphyria and cutanea tarda porphyria, it has sometimes been designated as *mixed porphyria*. The precipitating factors and manifestations of the acute attack are the same as in acute intermittent porphyria, but in addition to the hyponatremia, azotemia and hypokalemic alkalosis may be more frequent in variegate porphyria. Cutaneous manifestations result mainly from increased fragility of sun-exposed skin of the face and back of the hands. Minor trauma can lead to the formation of blisters or denuded oozing areas. Secondary infection can lead to scarring with pigmentation or depigmentation. Hypertrichosis may develop in exposed skin. In contrast to erythropoietic protoporphyria, acute photosensitivity reactions are uncommon in variegate porphyria, but may occur when hepatic impairment causes a deviation of porphyrin excretion from the feces to the urine.

During asymptomatic or cutaneous phases there is usually no significant increase of porphyrin precursors in the urine, but coproporphyrin and uroporphyrin excretion are increased, with the former usually exceeding the latter. During acute attacks urinary porphyrin precursors increase markedly, and the polymerization of porphobilinogen (PBG) in urine contributes to the great increase of urinary uroporphyrin that occurs. Fecal protoporphyrin is increased during both symptomatic and asymptomatic periods. Differentiation of the acute attack from those of acute intermittent or hereditary coproporphyria is somewhat academic, since prophylaxis and treatment of the acute attack is the same in all three disorders. The high fecal protoporphyrin distinguishes variegate from these two other acute attack types of porphyria. Lead intoxication causes an increase of urinary ALA without the increase of PBG seen in acute attacks and also causes an increase of free erythrocyte protoporphyrin, which is not seen in variegate porphyria. When cutaneous lesions are the only manifestation, variegate porphyria can be confused with cutanea tarda porphyria. The latter is characterized by frequent evidence of hepatic malfunction, freedom from acute attacks, a high urinary uroporphyrin that usually exceeds coproporphyrin, a normal or only slightly increased fecal porphyrin, and the presence of increased amounts of isocoproporphyrins [135] in the feces, a finding specific for cutanea tarda porphyria. Variegate porphyria has been distinguished from the other porphyrias by the specific fluorescence emission maximum (626 nm) exhibited by saline-diluted plasma from patients with this disease [136].

THERAPY AND PROGNOSIS
The prophylaxis and treatment of the acute attack is the same as that described for acute intermittent porphyria. Care to prevent even minor trauma to exposed skin and avoidance of sunlight as much as possible are the major measures to prevent cutaneous lesions. It is not known whether carotenoid therapy, as described for erythropoietic protoporphyria, will have prophylactic value for the cutaneous lesions in this disease. In a preliminary study canthaxanthin caused some decrease in the frequency of blisters and erosions in two of five patients, but no change in skin fragility [87].

In South Africa, where there are estimated to be at least 10,000 individuals with variegate porphyria, the prognosis has improved greatly in recent years [102]. There have been only three deaths in the last 18 years, and none in the last 9 years. This can be attributed to effective detection and prophylaxis of the disease as well as improved treatment of acute attacks.

Hereditary coproporphyria

This dominantly transmitted disorder results from a 50 percent decrease of coproporphyrinogen oxidase [137,138]. The clinical manifestations [95,139] involve acute attacks similar to those of acute intermittent porphyria and bullous lesions that can occur on exposed areas. Although fatalities can occur, acute attacks tend to be somewhat milder than those of acute intermittent porphyria, with less frequent occurrence of vomiting, paralysis, psychological symptoms, hypertension, and tachycardia. The cutaneous lesions do not occur without acute attacks, and in this regard hereditary coproporphyria differs from variegate porphyria, in which cutaneous lesions may occur independently or with acute attacks. During asymptomatic periods, urinary coproporphyrin is usually, but not always, increased. The urine may, therefore, not reveal any abnormalities when

examined in asymptomatic patients, and even when urinary coproporphyrin is increased, it is necessary to distinguish this disorder from those that can produce secondary coproporphyrinuria. Fecal coproporphyrin excretion is increased during both symptomatic and asymptomatic periods. During acute attacks there is an increase of urinary porphyrin precursor excretion. The prophylaxis and treatment in this disease are the same as for acute intermittent and variegate porphyria.

Porphyria cutanea tarda

This disease is characterized by cutaneous lesions on exposed portions of the body, uroporphyrinuria, and, frequently, liver disease.

ETIOLOGY AND PATHOGENESIS
Porphyria cutanea tarda can occur as an inherited or acquired disease. Studies of porphyrin excretion patterns of blood relatives of patients with porphyria cutanea tarda [1,140] have shown that some families have multiple members with abnormal excretion patterns whereas many other families have only one member in whom abnormalities were detected. This indication that the disease can be of genetic origin or acquired has been supported by multiple pieces of evidence. A toxic form of the disease occurred in thousands of individuals in Turkey who inadvertently ingested hexachlorobenzene [4]. The genetic basis for the disease was first demonstrated in 1976 by the finding of a 50 percent decrease of uroporphyrinogen decarboxylase in erythrocytes of patients with cutanea tarda porphyria [141]. Further studies of the enzyme aspects of this disease, however, have produced confusing findings [142]. Some patients have a decrease of both the erythrocyte and hepatic enzyme activities, whereas others have only a decrease of the hepatic enzyme activity. The former situation is clearly of genetic origin, but it is not certain whether the latter situation represents a second type of genetic defect or results from chemicals that selectively inhibit the liver enzyme.

CLINICAL AND LABORATORY FINDINGS
This disease does not produce acute attacks of neurological dysfunction that are seen in the other hepatic porphyrias, but is restricted to cutaneous manifestations [143,144]. Skin lesions are primarily on exposed areas and usually occur in response to minor trauma. They begin with erythema and either vesicles or bullae, which can be hemorrhagic. Erosions, scabs, and scarring occur later in the evolution of the lesions. Areas of pigmentation and depigmentation, hirsutism, milia, and sometimes scleroderma-like changes develop as chronic lesions. Although acute photosensitivity reactions are uncommon in this disease, cutaneous lesions tend to develop more frequently during sunny weather and often become evident during late summer or autumn.

Many reports have emphasized the coexistence of liver disease with cutanea tarda porphyria [1]. Abnormal serum levels were found for 1 or more of the 12 enzymes of hepatic origin examined in 161 patients with cutanea tarda porphyria [145]. γ-Glutamyl transferase was elevated in all 34 cases studied in another series [146]. A variety of hepatic abnormalities occur [145,147], and have been classified as chronic persistent hepatitis, chronic active hepatitis, and cirrhosis. Hepatitis-associated antigen was found in less than 4 percent of those studied. The liver changes in this disease have been said to have features that are distinct from other types of liver disease [147], including that related to alcoholism, a problem often encountered in these patients. With proper technique [148] needle-like inclusions in hepatocytes and fluorescence can be demonstrated. Porphyrin-producing hepatomas are rare causes of cutanea tarda porphyria [149], but non-porphyrin-producing primary hepatomas have been reported in as many as 6 percent of patients with alcohol-associated cutanea tarda porphyria [150]. The exact relationship between the liver disease and the porphyria is not clear. Excessive alcohol intake and the iron overload [151] characteristic of this disease play a role in activating the porphyria and undoubtedly contribute to the liver damage, but clearly porphyria cutanea tarda does not develop in all patients with excessive alcohol intake or iron overload.

Estrogen can precipitate the disease in both men (treated for prostatic cancer) and women (oral contraceptives) [152]. A bullous dermatosis resembling that of cutanea tarda porphyria has been reported in 1.2 to 18 percent of various hemodialysis series, but only four cases have been shown to have significant abnormalities of porphyrin metabolism [153]. Chloroquine can produce a severe systemic reaction in patients with cutanea tarda porphyria [1]. This includes high fever, abdominal pain, malaise, headache, and sometimes vomiting. The urine becomes red as a result of a great increase of urinary uroporphyrin that is mobilized from the liver. Serum transaminases increase, and mild jaundice may develop. A febrile and sometimes fatal reaction to quinidine has also been reported [102].

Urinary excretion of uroporphyrin and coproporphyrin is increased, with uroporphyrin usually exceeding coproporphyrin. In some patients there is a slight to moderate increase of urinary ALA, but PBG excretion is not increased and the Watson-Schwartz and Hoesch tests are negative. Fecal protoporphyrin excretion is not increased as in variegate porphyria. A chemical finding specific for cutanea tarda porphyria is the demonstration of fecal isocoproporphyrins [135]. Serum iron is elevated in some patients.

THERAPY AND PROGNOSIS
Phlebotomy has proved to be effective therapy for this disease [1,154]. After determining that there is no contraindication to phlebotomy, 500 ml of blood is removed every 2 or 3 weeks, and hemoglobin concentration and

urine porphyrins are monitored. If hemoglobin concentration should decline below 11 g/dl before there is a profound decrease of urinary uroporphyrin, further phlebotomy can be delayed until the hemoglobin rises to adequate levels. Therapy should be continued until urine uroporphyrin excretion is below 600 μg per day. Skin fragility and ulcers usually disappear when urinary uroporphyrin is less than 1 mg per day, and this clinical improvement is often evident within 6 months of initiation of therapy. Hyperpigmentation and hypertrichosis improve more slowly. In one series the mean amount of blood removed in order to produce a remission was 6.8 liters (range 2 to 14 liters) [154]. Remissions usually last for years, and recurrences can be retreated successfully with phlebotomy. Phlebotomy produces remission by removal of iron, since administration of iron after phlebotomy-induced remission activates the disease again [155,156].

Because chloroquine can mobilize the excess hepatic porphyrins in this disease, it has been used successfully to treat cutanea tarda porphyria by administration of doses low enough to avoid severe systemic reactions [157]. Patients in this study were given 125 mg chloroquine twice a week for 8 to 18 months, and therapy was discontinued when urinary uroporphyrin was less than 100 μg per day. In some patients the dose had to be doubled after 1 year in order to achieve satisfactory results. Hydroxychloroquine has also been used successfully in the treatment of this disease [158]. If there are no contraindications, phlebotomy is considered the treatment of choice.

The prognosis for the cutaneous disease is excellent, since treatment can produce a remission. However, neither phlebotomy [147] nor chloroquine therapy [159] caused significant improvement of hepatic morphology. The prognosis, therefore, is dependent on the course of the liver disease.

References

1. Tschudy, D. P., and Lamon, J. M.: Porphyrin metabolism and the porphyrias, in *Metabolic Control and Disease*, edited by P. K. Bondy and L. E. Rosenberg, 8th ed. Saunders, Philadelphia, 1980, p. 939.
2. Meyer, U. A., and Schmid, R.: The porphyrias, in *The Metabolic Basis of Inherited Disease*, edited by J. B. Stanbury, J. B. Wyngaarden, and D. S. Fredrickson, 4th ed. McGraw-Hill, New York, 1978, p. 1166.
3. With, T. K.: A short history of porphyrins and the porphyrias. *Int. J. Biochem.* 11:189, 1980.
4. Cripps, D. J., Gocmen, A., and Peters, H. A.: Porphyria turcica: Twenty years after hexachlorobenzene intoxication. *Arch. Dermatol.* 116:46, 1980.
5. Watson, C. J.: Porphyrin metabolism, in *Diseases of Metabolism*, edited by G. C. Duncan, 5th ed. Saunders, Philadelphia, 1964, p. 850.
6. McColl, K. E., and Goldberg, A.: Abnormal porphyrin metabolism in diseases other than porphyria. *Clin. Haematol.* 9:427, 1980.
7. Elder, G. H: Acquired disorders of haem synthesis. *Essays Med. Biochem.* 2:75, 1976.
8. Eales, L., Grosser, Y., and Levy, M.: Coproporphyrinuria and heart transplantation: Its significance. *S. Afr. Med. J.* 44:1023, 1970.

9. Burnham, B. F.: Metabolism of porphyrins and corrinoids, in *Metabolic Pathways*, edited by D. M. Greenberg. Academic, New York, 1969, vol. III, p. 403.

10. Granick, S., and Beale, S. I.: Hemes, chlorophylls and related compounds: Biosynthesis and metabolic regulation. *Adv. Enzymol.* 46:33, 1978.

11. Moore, M. R.: The biochemistry of the porphyrins. *Clin. Haematol.* 9:227, 1980.

12. Tschudy, D. P., and Bonkowsky, H. L.: A steady state model of sequential irreversible enzyme reactions. *Mol. Cell. Biochem.* 2:55, 1973.

13. Tschudy, D. P.: Enzyme aspects of acute intermittent porphyria. *Mol. Cell. Biochem.* 2:63, 1973.

14. Taddeini, L., and Watson, C. J.: The clinical porphyrias. *Semin. Hematol.* 5:335, 1968.

15. Haeger-Aronsen, B.: Studies on urinary excretion of δ-aminolaevulinic acid and other heme precursors in lead workers and lead-intoxicated rabbits. *Scand. J. Lab. Invest. 12 (Suppl. 47):9*, 1960.

16. Genz, J., Johansson, S., Lindblad, B., Lindstedt, S., and Zetterström, R.: Excretion of δ-aminolevulinic acid in hereditary tyrosinemia. *Clin. Chim. Acta* 23:257, 1969.

17. Lindblad, B., Lindstedt, S., and Steen, G.: On the enzymic defects in hereditary tyrosinemia. *Proc. Natl. Acad. Sci. U.S.A.* 74:4641, 1977.

18. Krupa, B.: The δ-aminolevulinic acid and porphobilinogen excretion in the course of gestation with consideration of the anemia of pregnancy. *Pol. Med. J.* 5:1261, 1969.

19. De Klerk, M., Weidman, A., Malan, C., and Shanley, B. C.: Urinary porphyrins and porphyrin precursors in normal pregnancy. Relationship to total estrogen excretion. *S. Afr. Med. J.* 49:581, 1975.

20. Czyzyk, A., and Gregor, A.: Urinary excretion of 5-aminolevulinate and porphobilinogen in diabetes. *Diabetologica* 7:152, 1971.

21. Watson, C. J., Taddeini, L., and Bossenmaier, I.: Present status of the Ehrlich aldehyde reaction for urinary porphobilinogen. *J. Am. Med. Assoc.* 190:501, 1964.

22. Lamon, J. M., Frykholm, B. C., and Tschudy, D. P.: Screening tests in acute porphyria. *Arch. Neurol.* 304:709, 1977.

23. Harber, L. C., Fleischer, A. S., and Baer, R. L.: Erythropoietic protoporphyria and photohemolysis. *J. Am. Med. Assoc.* 189:191, 1964.

24. Rimington, C., Magnus, I., Ryan, A., and Cripps, D.: Porphyria and photosensitivity. *Q. J. Med.* 36:29, 1967.

25. Magnus, I. A., Roe, D. A., and Bhutani, L. K.: Factors affecting the induction of porphyria in the laboratory rat. Biochemical and photobiological studies with diethyl-1,4-dihydro-2,4,6-trimethyl-pyridine-3,5-dicarboxylate (DDC) as a porphyrinogenic agent. *J. Invest. Dermatol.* 53:400, 1969.

26. Parrish, J. A., White, H. A. D., and Pathak, M.: Photomedicine, in *Dermatology in General Medicine*, edited by T. B. Fitzpatrick, A. Z. Eisen, K. Wolff, I. M. Freedberg, and K. F. Austen, 2d ed. McGraw-Hill, New York, 1979, p. 942.

27. Müller, W. E., and Snyder, S. H.: Delta-aminolevulinic acid: Influences on synaptic GABA receptor binding may explain CNS symptoms of porphyria. *Ann. Neurol.* 2:340, 1977.

28. Bissell, D. M., Liem, H. H., and Müller-Eberhard, U.: Secretion of haem by hepatic parenchymal cells. *Biochem. J.* 184:689, 1979.

29. Waxman, A. D., Collins, A., and Tschudy, D. P.: Oscillations of hepatic δ-aminolevulinic acid synthetase produced in vivo by heme. *Biochem. Biophys. Res. Commun.* 24:675, 1966.

30. Schacter, B. A., Yoda, B., and Israels, L. G.: Cyclic oscillations in rat hepatic heme oxygenase and δ-aminolevulinic acid synthetase following intravenous heme administration. *Arch. Biochem. Biophys.* 173:11, 1976.

31. Lamon, J. M., Frykholm, B. C., Hess, R. A., and Tschudy, D. P.: Hematin therapy in acute porphyria. *Medicine* 58:252, 1979.

32. Pierach, C. A., Bossenmaier, I., Cardinal, R., Weimer, M., and Watson, C. J.: Hematin therapy in porphyric attacks. *Klin. Wochenschr.* 58:829, 1980.

33. Correia, M. A., Farrell, G. C., Schmid, R., de Montellano, P. R. O., Yost, G. S., and Mico, B. A.: Incorporation of exogenous heme into hepatic cytochrome P-450 in vivo. *J. Biol. Chem.* 254:15, 1979.

34. Bird, T. D., Hamernyik, P., Nutter, J. Y., and Labbe, R. F.: Inherited deficiency of delta-aminolevulinic acid dehydratase. *Am. J. Hum. Genet.* 31:662, 1979.

35. Doss, M., von Tiepermann, R., and Schneider, J.: Acute hepatic porphyria syndrome with porphobilinogen synthase defect. *Int. J. Biochem.* 12:823, 1980.

36. Watson, C. J., Lowry, P. T., Schmid, R., Hawkinson, V. E., and Schwartz, S.: The manifestations of the different forms of porphyria in relation to chemical findings. *Trans. Assoc. Am. Physicians* 64:345, 1951.

37. Schmid, R., Schwartz, S., and Watson, C. J.: Porphyrin content of bone marrow and liver in the various forms of porphyria. *A.M.A. Arch. Intern. Med.* 93:167, 1954.

38. Günther, H.: Die Haematoporphyrie, *Dtsch. Arch. Klin. Med.* 105:89, 1911.

39. Günther, H.: Die Bedeutung der Haematoporphyrine in Physiologie and Pathologie. *Ergeb. Allg. Pathol. Anat.* 20:608, 1922.

40. Ippen, H., and Fuchs, T.: Congenital porphyria. *Clin. Haematol.* 9:323, 1980.

41. Levin, E. Y.: Uroporphyrinogen III cosynthetase in bovine erythropoietic porphyria. *Science* 161:907, 1968.

42. Romeo, G., and Levin, E. Y.: Uroporphyrinogen III cosynthetase in human congenital erythropoietin porphyria. *Proc. Natl. Acad. Sci. U.S.A.* 63:856, 1969.

43. Romeo, G., Kaback, M. M., and Levin, E. Y.: Uroporphyrinogen III cosynthetase activity in fibroblasts from patients with congenital erythropoietic porphyria. *Biochem. Genet.* 4:659, 1970.

44. Watson, C. J., Bossenmaier, I., and Cardinal, R.: Formation of porphyrin isomers from porphobilinogen by various hemolysates of red cells from bovine and human subjects with erythropoietic (uro-) porphyria. *Z. Klin. Chem. Klin. Biochem.* 7:119, 1969.

45. Miyagi, K., Petryka, Z. J., Bossenmaier, I., Cardinal, R., and Watson, C. J.: The activities of uroporphyrinogen synthetase and cosynthetase in congenital erythropoietic porphyria (CEP). *Am. J. Hematol.* 1:3, 1976.

46. Moore, M. R., Thompson, G. G., Goldberg, A., Ippen, H., Seubert, A., and Seubert, S.: The biosynthesis of haem in congenital erythropoietic porphyria. *Int. J. Biochem.* 9:933, 1978.

47. Grandchamp, B., Deybach, J. C., Grelier, M., De Verneuil, H., and Nordmann, Y.: Studies of porphyrin synthesis in fibroblasts of patients with congenital erythropoietic porphyria and one patient with homozygous coproporphyria. *Biochim. Biophys. Acta* 629:577, 1980.

48. Del Battle, A. M., De Xifra, E. A. W., Stella, A. M., Bustos, N., and With, T. K.: Studies on porphyrin biosynthesis and enzymes involved in bovine congenital erythropoietic porphyria. *Clin. Sci. Mol. Med.* 57:63, 1979.

49. Kramer, S., Viljoen, E., Mayer, A. M., and Metz, J.: The anemia of erythropoietic porphyria with the first description of the disease in an elderly patient. *Br. J. Haematol.* 11:666, 1965.

50. Pain, R. W., Welch, F. W., Woodroffe, A. J., Handley, D. A., and Lockwood, W. H.: Erythropoietic uroporphyria of Günther first presenting at 58 years with positive family studies. *Br. Med. J.* 3:621, 1975.

51. Weston, M. J., et al.: Congenital erythropoietic uroporphyria (Günther's disease) presenting in a middle aged man. *Int. J. Biochem.* 9:921, 1978.

52. Peterka, E. S., Runge, W. J., and Fusaro, R. M.: Erythropoietic protoporphyria. III. Photohemolysis. *Arch. Dermatol.* 94:282, 1966.

53. Hsu, J., Goldstein, B. D., and Harber, L. C.: Photoreactions associated with in vitro hemolysis in erythropoietic protoporphyria. *Photochem. Photobiol.* 13:67, 1971.

54. Eriksen, L., and Seip, M.: The effect of various therapeutic trials of the porphyrin excretion in a case of congenital erythropoietic porphyria. *Acta Pediatr. Scand.* 64:287, 1975.

55. Sneddin, I. B.: Beta carotene in congenital porphyria. *Arch. Dermatol.* 114:1242, 1978.

56. Varadi, S.: Haematological aspects in a case of erythropoietic porphyria. *Br. J. Haematol.* 4:270, 1958.

57. Ippen, H., Tillman, W., Seubert, S., and Seubert, A.: Porphyria erythropoetica congenita Günther und chloroquin. *Klin. Wochenschr.* 56:623, 1978.

58. Haining, R. G., Cowger, M. L., Labbe, R. L., and Finch, C. A.: Con-

genital erythropoietic porphyria. II. The effects of induced poly-cythemia. *Blood* 36:297, 1970.

59. Watson, C. J., Bossenmaier, I., Cardinal, R., and Petryka, Z. J.: Repression by hematin of porphyrin biosynthesis in erythrocyte precursors in congenital erythropoietic porphyria. *Proc. Natl. Acad. Sci. U.S.A.* 71:278, 1974.

60. Miyagi, K., and Watson, C. J.: δ-Aminolevulinic acid synthetase activity in human plasma: Relation to erythropoiesis and evidence of induction in erythropoietic porphyria. *Blood* 39:13, 1972.

61. Magnus, I. A., Jarrett, A., Prankerd, T. A. J., and Rimington, C.: Erythropoietic protoporphyria—A new porphyria syndrome with solar urticaria due to protoporphyrinemia. *Lancet* 2:448, 1961.

62. Langhof, H., Müller, H., and Rietschel, L.: Untersuchungen zur familiären protoporphyrinämischen Lichturticaria. *Arch. Klin. Exp. Dermatol.* 212:506, 1961.

63. Reed, W. B., Wuepper, K. D., Epstein, J. H., Redeker, A., Simonson, R. J., and McKusick, V. A.: Erythropoietic protoporphyria. *JAMA* 214:1060, 1970.

64. Schmidt, H., Snitker, G., Thomsen, K., and Lintrup, J.: Erythropoietic protoporphyria. A clinical study based on 29 cases in 14 families. *Arch. Dermatol.* 110:58, 1974.

65. Magnus, I. A.: Cutaneous porphyria. *Clin. Haematol.* 9:273, 1980.

66. Bottomley, S. S., Tanaka, M., and Everett, M. A.: Diminished erythroid ferrochelatase activity in protoporphyria. *J. Lab. Clin. Med.* 86:126, 1975.

67. De Goeij, A. F., Christianse, K., and von Steveninck, J.: Decreased heme synthetase activity in blood cells of patients with erythropoietic protoporphyria. *Eur. J. Clin. Invest.* 5:397, 1975.

68. Bloomer, J. R., Bonkowsky, H. L., Ebert, P. S., and Mahoney, M. J.: Inheritance in protoporphyria. Comparison of haem synthetase activity in skin fibroblasts with clinical features. *Lancet* 2:226, 1976.

69. Bloomer, J. R.: Characterization of deficient heme synthase activity in protoporphyria with cultured skin fibroblasts. *J. Clin. Invest.* 65:321, 1980.

70. Bonkowsky, H. L., Bloomer, J. R., Ebert, P. S., and Mahoney, M. J.: Heme synthetase deficiency in human protoporphyria. Demonstration of the defect in liver and cultured skin fibroblasts. *J. Clin. Invest.* 56:1139, 1975.

71. Becker, D. M., Viljoen, J. D., Katz, J., and Kramer, S.: Reduced ferrochelatase activity: A defect common to porphyria variegata and protoporphyria. *Br. J. Haematol.* 36:171, 1977.

72. Scholnick, P., Marver, H. S., and Schmid, R.: Erythropoietic protoporphyria: Evidence for multiple sites of excess protoporphyrin formation. *J. Clin. Invest.* 50:203, 1971.

73. De Leo, V. A., Poh-Fitzpatrick, M., Mathews-Roth, M., and Harber, L. C.: Erythropoietic protoporphyria. Ten years' experience. *Am. J. Med.* 60:8, 1976.

74. Mathews-Roth, M.: Erythropoietic protoporphyria—Diagnosis and treatment. *N. Engl. J. Med.* 297:98, 1977.

75. Cripps, D. J., and Scheuer, P. J.: Hepatobiliary changes in erythropoietic protoporphyria. *Arch. Pathol.* 80:500, 1965.

76. Goerz, G., Krieg, Th., Bolsen, K., Seubert, S. and Ippen, H.: Porphyrinuntersuchungen eines Gallensteines bei der erythropoietischen Protoporphyrie. *Arch. Dermatol. Res.* 256:283, 1976.

77. Mathews-Roth, M.: Anemia in erythropoietic protoporphyria. *JAMA* 230:824, 1974.

78. Clark, K. G. A., and Micholson, D. C.: Erythrocyte protoporphyrin and iron uptake in erythropoietic protophyria. *Clin. Sci.* 41:363, 1971.

79. Turnbull, A., Baker, H., Vernon-Roberts, B., and Magnus, I. A.: Iron metabolism in porphyria cutanea tarda and in erythropoietic protoporphyria. *Q. J. Med.* 42:341, 1973.

80. Porter, F. S.: Congenital erythropoietic protoporphyria. II. An experimental study. *Blood* 22:532, 1963.

81. Haeger-Aronsen, B.: Erythropoietic protoporphyria. A new type of inborn error of metabolism. *Am. J. Med.* 35:450, 1963.

82. Klatskin, G., and Bloomer, J. R.: Birefringence of hepatic pigment deposits in erythropoietic protoporphyria. Specificity of polarization microscopy in the identification of hepatic protoporphyrin deposits. *Gastroenterology* 67:294, 1974.

83. Mathews-Roth, M. M.: Carotenoid pigments and the treatment of erythropoietic protoporphyria. *J. Infect. Dis.* 138:924, 1978.

84. Haeger-Aronsen, B., Krook, G., and Abdulla, M.: Oral carotenoids for photohypersensitivity in patients with erythrohepatic protoporphyria, polymorphous light eruptions and lupus erythematosis discoides. *Int. J. Dermatol.* 18:73, 1979.

85. Thomsen, K., Schmidt, H., and Fischer, A.: Beta carotene in erythropoietic protoporphyria: 5 years' experience. *Dermatologica* 159:82, 1979.

86. Corbett, M. F., Herxheimer, A., Magnus, I. A., Ramsay, C. A., and Kobza-Black, A.: The long term treatment with β-carotene in erythropoietic protoporphyria: A controlled trial. *Br. J. Dermatol.* 97:655, 1977.

87. Eales, L.: The effects of canthaxanthin—A beta-carotene analogue on the photocutaneous manifestations of EHP, VP and SP. *S. Afr. Med. J.* 54:1050, 1978.

88. Redeker, A. G., and Sterling, R. E.: The "glucose effect" in erythropoietic protoporphyria. *Arch. Intern. Med.* 121:446, 1968.

89. Lamon, J. M., Poh-Fitzpatrick, M. B., and Lamola, A. A.: Hepatic protoporphyrin production in human protoporphyria: Effects of intravenous hematin and analysis of erythrocyte protoporphyrin distribution. *Gastroenterology* 79:115, 1980.

90. Kniffen, J. C.: Protoporphyrin removal in intrahepatic porphyrastasis. *Gastroenterology* 58:1027, 1970.

91. Eales, L.: Liver involvement in erythropoietic protoporphyria. *Int. J. Biochem.* 12:915, 1980.

92. Conley, C. L., and Chisholm, J. J.: Recovery from hepatic decompensation in protoporphyria. *Johns Hopkins Med. J.* 145:237, 1979.

93. Waldenström, J., and Haeger-Aronsen, B.: The porphyrias: A genetic problem. *Prog. Med. Genet.* 5:58, 1967.

94. Civin, W. H., and Epstein, E.: Enzyme defects in hereditary porphyria. *Ann. Clin. Lab. Sci.* 10:395, 1980.

95. Brodie, M. J., and Goldberg, A.: Acute hepatic porphyrias. *Clin. Haematol.* 9:253, 1980.

96. Moore, M. R.: International review of drugs in acute porphyria—1980. *Int. J. Biochem.* 12:1089, 1980.

97. Zimmerman, T. S., McMillin, J. M., and Watson, C. J.: Onset of manifestations of hepatic porphyria in relation to the influence of female sex hormones. *Arch. Intern. Med.* 118:229, 1966.

98. Welland, F. H., Hellman, E. S., Collins, A., Hunter, G. W., Jr., and Tschudy, D. P.: Factors affecting the excretion of porphyrin precursors by patients with acute intermittent porphyria. II. The effect of ethinyl estradiol. *Metabolism* 13:251, 1964.

99. Rose, J. A., Hellman, E. S., and Tschudy, D. P.: Effect of diet on the induction of experimental porphyria. *Metabolism* 10:514, 1961.

100. Welland, F. H., Hellman, E. S., Gaddis, E. M., Collins, A., Hunter, G. W., Jr., and Tschudy, D. P.: Factors affecting the excretion of porphyrin precursors by patients with acute intermittent porphyria. I. The effect of diet. *Metabolism* 13:232, 1964.

101. Felsher, B. F., and Redeker, A. G.: Acute intermittent porphyria: Effect of diet and griseofulvin. *Medicine* 46:217, 1967.

102. Eales, L., Day, R. S., and Belkkenhorst, G. H.: The clinical and biochemical features of variegate porphyria: An analysis of 300 cases studied at Groote Schuur hospital, Cape Town. *Int. J. Biochem.* 12:837, 1980.

103. Stein, J. A., Bloomer, J. R., Berk, P. D., Corcoran, P. L., and Tschudy, D. P.: The kinetics of organic anion excretion by the liver in acute intermittent porphyria. *Clin. Sci.* 38:677, 1970.

104. Taddeini, L., Nordstrom, K. L., and Watson, C. J.: Hypercholesterolemia in experimental and human hepatic porphyria. *Metabolism* 13:691, 1964.

105. Hollander, C. S., Scott, R. L., Tschudy, D. P., Perlroth, M. G., Waxman, A., and Sterling, K.: Increased protein-bound iodine and thyroxine-binding globulin in acute intermittent porphyria. *N. Engl. J. Med.* 277:995, 1967.

106. Hedger, R. W., and Hardison, W. G. M.: Transient macroamylasemia during an exacerbation of acute intermittent porphyria. *Gastroenterology* 60:903, 1971.

107. Song, C. S., Bonkowsky, H. L., and Tschudy, D. P.: Salicylamide metabolism in acute intermittent porphyria. *Clin. Pharmacol. Ther.* 15:431, 1974.

108. Anderson, K. E., Alvares, A. P., Sassa, S., and Kappas, A.: Studies in porphyria. V. Drug oxidation rates in hereditary hepatic porphyria. *Clin. Pharmacol. Ther.* 19:47, 1976.

109. Elder, G. H.: The porphyrias: Clinical chemistry, diagnosis and methodology. *Clin. Haematol. 9:*371, 1980.
110. Kreimer-Birnbaum, M., Bonkowsky, H. L., and Bottomley, S. S.: Experience with the red cell uroporphyrinogen synthase (Uro-S) assay in kindreds with acute intermittent porphyria (AIP). *Int. J. Biochem. 12:*807, 1980.
111. Eales, L.: Porphyria and the dangerous life-threatening drugs. *S. Afr. Med. J. 56:*914, 1979.
112. Magnussen, C. R., Doherty, J. M., Hess, R. A., and Tschudy, D. P.: Grand mal seizures and acute intermittent porphyria: The problem of differential diagnosis and treatment. *Neurology 25:*1121, 1975.
113. Bonkowsky, H. L., Sinclair, P. R., Emery, S., and Sinclair, J. F.: Seizure management in acute hepatic porphyria: Risks of valproate and clonazepam. *Neurology 30:*588, 1980.
114. Flacks, L. M.: Propranolol in acute porphyria. *Lancet 1:*363, 1970.
115. Beattie, A. D., Moore, M. R., Goldberg, A., and Ward, R. L.: Acute intermittent porphyria: Response of tachycardia and hypertension to propranolol. *Br. Med. J. 3:*257, 1973.
116. Menawat, A. S., Panwar, R. B., Kochar, D. K., and Joshi, C. K.: Propranolol in acute intermittent porphyria. *Postgrad. Med. J. 55:*546, 1979.
117. Blum, I., and Atsmon, A.: Reduction of porphyrin excretion in porphyria variegata by propranolol. *S. Afr. Med. J. 50:*898, 1976.
118. Douer, D., Weinberger, A., Pinkhas, J., and Atsmon, A.: Treatment of acute intermittent porphyria with large doses of propranolol. *JAMA 240:*766, 1978.
119. Brezis, M., Ghanem, J., Weider-Ravell, D., Epstein, O., and Morris, D.: Hematin and propranolol in acute intermittent porphyria. Full recovery from quadriplegic coma and respiratory failure. *Eur. J. Neurol. 18:*289, 1979.
120. Tschudy, D. P., Welland, F. H., Collins, A., and Hunter, G., Jr.: The effect of carbohydrate feeding on the induction of δ-aminolevulinic acid synthetase. *Metabolism 13:*396, 1964.
121. Brodie, M. J., Moore, M. R., Thompson, G. G., and Goldberg, A.: The treatment of acute intermittent porphyria with laevulose. *Clin. Sci. Mol. Med. 53:*365, 1977.
122. Lamon, J. M., Frykholm, B. C., Hess, R. A., and Tschudy, D. P.: Hematin therapy in acute porphyria. *Medicine 58:*252, 1979.
123. Pierach, C. A., Bossenmaier, I., Cardinal, R., Weimer, M., and Watson, C. J.: Hematin therapy in porphyric attacks. *Klin. Wochenschr. 58:*829, 1980.
124. McColl, K. E. L., Moore, M. R., Thompson, G. G., and Goldberg, A.: Treatment with haematin in acute hepatic porphyria. *Q. J. Med. 50:*161, 1981.
125. Lamon, J. M., Bennett, M., Frykholm, B., and Tschudy, D. P.: Prevention of acute porphyric attacks by intravenous hematin. *Lancet 2:*492, 1978.
126. Dhar, G. J., Bossenmaier, I., Petryka, Z. J., Cardinal, R., and Watson, C. J.: Effects of hematin in hepatic porphyria. Further studies. *Ann. Intern. Med. 83:*20, 1975.
127. Perlroth, M. G., Marver, H. S., and Tschudy, D. P.: Oral contraceptive agents and the management of acute intermittent porphyria. *JAMA 194:*1037, 1965.
128. Kramer, S., Porphyria variegata. *Clin. Haematol. 9:*303, 1980.
129. Brodie, M. J., Thompson, G. G., Moore, M. R., and Goldberg, A.: The enzyme abnormalities of the hereditary hepatic porphyrias. *Gut 17:*823, 1978.
130. Viljoen, D. J., Cayanis, E., Becker, D. M., Kramer, S., Dawson, B., and Bernstein, R.: Reduced ferrochelatase activity in fibroblasts from patients with porphyria variegata. *Am. J. Hematol. 6:*185, 1979.
131. Pimstone, N. R., Blekkenhorst, G., and Eales, L.: Enzymatic defects in hepatic porphyria. Preliminary observations in patients with porphyria cutanea tarda and variegate porphyria. *Enzyme 16:*354, 1973.
132. Brenner, D. A., and Bloomer, J. R.: The enzymatic defect in variegate porphyria. Studies with human cultured skin fibroblasts. *N. Engl. J. Med. 302:*765, 1980.
133. Kramer, S., and Viljoen, J. D.: Erythropoietic protoporphyria: Evidence that it is due to a variant ferrochelatase. *Int. J. Biochem. 12:*925, 1980.
134. Mustajoki, P.: Variegate porphyria. Twelve years' experience in Finland. *Q. J. Med. 49:*191, 1980.
135. Elder, G. H.: Differentiation of porphyria cutanea tarda symptomatica from other types of porphyria by measurement of isocoproporphyrin in faeces. *J. Clin. Pathol. 28:*601, 1975.
136. Poh-Fitzpatrick, M. B.: A plasma porphyrin fluorescence marker for variegate porphyria. *Arch. Dermatol. 116:*543, 1980.
137. Elder, G. H., Thomas, N., Evans, J. O., Cox, R., Brodie, M. J., and Goldberg, A.: The primary enzyme defect in hereditary coproporphyria. *Lancet 2:*1217, 1976.
138. Nordmann, Y., Grandchamp, B., Phung, N., De Verneuil, H., Grelier, M., and Noire, J.: Coproporphyrinogen-oxidase deficiency in hereditary coproporphyria. *Lancet 1:*140, 1977.
139. Brodie, J. J., Thompson, G. G., Moore, M. R., Beattie, A. D., and Goldberg, A.: Hereditary coproporphyria. Demonstration of the abnormalities in haem biosynthesis in peripheral blood. *Q. J. Med. 46:*229, 1977.
140. de Salamanca, R. E., Catalan, T., Cruces, M. J., Peña, M. L., Olmos, A., and Mas, V.: The inheritance of porphyria cutanea tarda. *Int. J. Biochem. 12:*869, 1980.
141. Kushner, J. P., Barbuto, A. J., and Lee, G. R.: An inherited enzymatic defect in porphyria cutanea tarda. *J. Clin. Invest. 58:*1089, 1976.
142. Elder, G. H., Sheppard, D. M., De Salamanca, R. E., and Olmos, A.: Identification of two types of porphyria cutanea tarda by measurement of erythrocyte uroporphyrinogen decarboxylase. *Clin. Sci. 58:*477, 1980.
143. Grossman, M. E., and Poh-Fitzpatrick, M. B.: Porphyria cutanea tarda. Diagnosis and management. *Med. Clin. North Am. 64:*807, 1980.
144. Magnus, I. A.: Cutaneous porphyria. *Clin. Haematol. 9:*273, 1980.
145. Topi, G. C., and D'Alessandro Gandolfo, L.: Liver in porphyria cutanea tarda, in *Porphyrins in Human Diseases,* edited by M. Doss. S. Karger, New York, 1976, p. 312.
146. Adjarov, D., and Ivanov, E.: Clinical value of serum gamma-glutamyl transferase estimation in porphyria cutanea tarda. *Br. J. Dermatol. 102:*541, 1980.
147. Cortés, J. M., Oliva, H., Paradinas, F. J., and Hernandez-Guio, C.: The pathology of the liver in porphyria cutanea tarda. *Histopathology 4:*471, 1980.
148. James, J. R., Cortés, J. M., and Paradinas, F. J.: Demonstration of intracytoplasmic needle-like inclusions in hepatocytes of patients with porphyria cutanea tarda. *J. Clin. Pathol. 33:*899, 1980.
149. Keczkes, K., and Barker, D. J.: Malignant hepatoma associated with acquired hepatic cutaneous porphyria. *Arch. Dermatol. 112:*78, 1976.
150. Eales, L., Grosser, Y., and Sears, W. G.: The clinical biochemistry of the human hepatocutaneous porphyrias in the light of recent studies of newly identified intermediates and porphyrin derivatives. *Ann. N.Y. Acad. Sci. 244:*441, 1975.
151. Lundvall, O., Weinfeld, A., and Lundin, P.: Iron storage in porphyria cutanea tarda. *Acta Med. Scand. 188:*37, 1970.
152. Taylor, J. S., and Roenigk, H. H., Jr.: Estrogen-induced porphyria cutanea tarda symptomatica, in *Porphyrins in Human Diseases,* edited by M. Doss. S. Karger, New York, 1976, p. 328.
153. Poh-Fitzpatrick, M. B., Masullo, A. S., and Grossman, M. E.: Porphyria cutanea tarda associated with chronic renal disease and hemodialysis. *Arch. Dermatol. 116:*191, 1980.
154. Lundvall, O.: The effect of phlebotomy therapy in porphyria cutanea tarda. *Acta Med. Scand. 189:*33, 1971.
155. Lundvall, O.: The effect of replenishment of iron stores after phlebotomy therapy in porphyria cutanea tarda. *Acta Med. Scand. 189:*51, 1971.
156. Felsher, B. F., Jones, M. L., and Redeker, A. G.: Iron and hepatic uroporphyrin synthesis. Relation in porphyria cutanea tarda. *JAMA 226:*663, 1973.
157. Kordač, V., Papežova, R., and Semrádova, M.: Chloroquine in the treatment of porphyria cutanea tarda. *N. Engl. J. Med. 296:*949, 1977.
158. Malkinson, F. D., and Levitt, L.: Hydroxychloroquine treatment of porphyria cutanea tarda. *Arch. Dermatol. 116:*1147, 1980.
159. Chlumska, A., Chlumsky, J., and Malina, L.: Liver changes in porphyria cutanea tarda patients treated with chloroquine. *Br. J. Dermatol. 102:*261, 1980.

Erythrocyte disorders— diseases with cyanosis

CHAPTER *77*

Methemoglobinemia and sulfhemoglobinemia

ERNEST BEUTLER

Definitions and history

Methemoglobinemia describes that clinical situation in which more than 1 percent of the hemoglobin of the blood has been oxidized to the ferric form. This condition may arise as a result of a hereditary deficiency of NADH-diaphorase, referred to as *congenital methemoglobinemia due to NADH-diaphorase deficiency*. This disorder is characterized by elevated levels of methemoglobin in the blood, in the absence of drug administration and without the existence of any abnormality of the globin portion of hemoglobin. The work of Gibson [1] clearly pointed to the site of the enzyme defect, and since enzyme assays have been available for the detection of the disorder [2], many cases have been described.

Toxic methemoglobinemia occurs when various drugs or toxic substances either oxidize hemoglobin directly in the circulation or facilitate its oxidation by molecular oxygen.

Methemoglobinemias due to inheritance of an abnormality in the structure of the globin portion of the hemoglobin molecule are known as *hemoglobin M diseases* and are discussed in Chap. 78.

Sulfhemoglobinemia refers to the presence in the blood of hemoglobin derivatives which are poorly characterized chemically but can be defined by their characteristic absorption of light at 620 nm in the presence of cyanide.

Etiology and pathogenesis

Hemoglobin is continuously oxidized in vivo from the ferrous to the ferric state. The rate of such oxidation is accelerated by many drugs and toxic chemicals, including sulfonamides, lidocaine and other aniline derivatives, and nitrites. A vast number of chemical substances have been found to cause methemoglobinemia [2,3]. NADH-diaphorase catalyzes a step in the major pathway for methemoglobin reduction (page 339). This enzyme reduces cytochrome b_5, using NADH as a hydrogen donor. The reduced cytochrome b_5 reduces, in turn, methemoglobin to hemoglobin. (See page 339.) A steady-state methemoglobin level is achieved when the rate of methemoglobin formation equals the rate of methemoglobin reduction either through the NADH-diaphorase system or through auxiliary mechanisms such as ascorbate and GSH [4]. Either a marked diminution in the activity of this enzyme, as in NADH-diaphorase deficiency, or a marked increase in the rate of formation of methemoglobin, as after exposure to toxic drugs or chemicals [2,3], will result in the accumulation of the brown pigment in circulating erythrocytes.

A combination of both factors may also occur. Since the activity of NADH-diaphorase is normally low in newborn infants [5], they are particularly susceptible to the development of methemoglobinemia. Thus serious degrees of methemoglobinemia have been observed as a result of toxic materials, such as aniline dyes used on diapers [6], and the ingestion of nitrate-contaminated water [7]. Nitrates in water are reduced to nitrites by bacterial action in the intestinal tract and may, therefore, cause methemoglobinemia. Heterozygotes for NADH-diaphorase deficiency are not usually clinically methemoglobinemic. However, under the stress of administration of drugs which normally induce only slight, clinically unimportant, methemoglobinemia, such persons may become severely cyanotic because of methemoglobinemia [8].

Sulfhemoglobin derives its name from the fact that it can be produced in vitro from the action of hydrogen sulfide on hemoglobin [9] and that the feeding of elemental sulfur to dogs has been associated with sulfhemoglobulinemia [10]. It has been claimed that sulfhemoglobin contains one excess sulfur atom [9,11]. However, the role of sulfur or sulfur compounds in the formation of the abnormal pigments which are called sulfhemoglobin is not clearly defined, although it seems that the sulfur may be bound to the heme ring [11]. Sulfhemoglobinemia has been associated with the administration of various drugs, particularly sulfonamides, phenacetin, and acetanilid [12,13]. It also occurs in some persons who have not received drugs, and has been thought to be related to chronic constipation or to purging [14]. Some patients with sulfhemoglobinemia or a past history of this disorder appear to have increased levels of red blood cell GSH [13]. The reason for this and its relationship to sulfhemoglobinemia is not clearly understood, but it may be of significance that some of the types of drugs which have been associated with sulfhemoglobinemia cause an elevation of red cell GSH levels [15,16], probably by activating the enzyme glutathione synthetase [17] or by increasing intracellular glutamate levels.

Mode of inheritance

Congenital methemoglobinemia is inherited in an autosomal recessive fashion [18]. In some instances the deficient enzyme appears to be electrophoretically normal, but several electrophoretic variants have been described [19–21].

Evidence for the occurrence of hereditary sulfhemoglobinemia [22] is not convincing, and it is likely that the single family reported represents a hemoglobin M hemoglobinopathy.

Clinical features

The major clinical feature of congenital methemoglobinemia is cyanosis, which is primarily of cosmetic importance. In some cases mild polycythemia is also present. In a few instances congenital methemoglobinemia has been associated with mental retardation. Such patients have NADH-diaphorase deficiency which affects not only the erythrocytes but also other tissues [23].

Toxic methemoglobinemia may be chronic or acute. In the case of chronic drug administration leading to an increased steady-state concentration of methemoglobin, the patient will have asymptomatic cyanosis. The same will be the case with sulfhemoglobinemia. Severe acute methemoglobinemia will produce symptoms of anemia, since methemoglobin lacks the capacity to transport oxygen. Acutely developing levels of methemoglobin exceeding 60 to 70 percent of the total pigment may be associated with vascular collapse, coma, and death.

Laboratory features

In congenital methemoglobinemia due to NADH-diaphorase deficiency, examination of the blood reveals that between 8 and 40 percent of the hemoglobin is in the oxidized (methemoglobin) form. The blood may have a chocolate-brown color. Assay of NADH-diaphorase either by the dichloroindophenol-linked method or, preferably, using the ferrocyanide-methemoglobin complex as receptor [24] reveals that enzyme activity is less than 20 percent of normal. For unknown reasons, glutathione reductase activity is usually also diminished [25,26].

In toxic methemoglobinemia an elevated level of methemoglobin is also found, but the activity of NADH-diaphorase is normal.

Sulfhemoglobin is detected in the lysate of blood treated with ferricyanide, cyanide, and ammonia by comparing the optical density at 620 nm with that at 540 nm. Details of procedures for the detection of methemoglobin and sulfhemoglobin are given in Chap. A16.

Differential diagnosis

Cyanosis due to methemoglobinemia or sulfhemoglobinemia must be differentiated from cyanosis due to cardiac or pulmonary disease and from congenital methemoglobinemia due to abnormal hemoglobins (see page 706). A family history is helpful in differentiating congenital methemoglobinemia due to NADH-diaphorase deficiency from hemoglobin M disease. The former has a recessive mode of inheritance, the latter a dominant mode. In NADH-diaphorase deficiency, incubation of the blood with small amounts of methylene blue will result in rapid reduction of the methemoglobin; in hemoglobin M disease, such reduction does not take place. The absorption spectra of methemoglobin and its derivatives are normal in NADH-diaphorase deficiency; they are abnormal in hemoglobin M disease.

In the case of toxic methemoglobinemia, cyanosis is usually of relatively recent origin, and a history of exposure to a drug or toxin may usually be obtained; in congenital methemoglobinemia a history of lifelong cyanosis may usually be elicited. Cyanosis due to an increased quantity of reduced hemoglobin in the blood, such as is seen in a right-to-left cardiac shunt, may also cause confusion. Blood from a patient with cyanosis due to a right-to-left shunt promptly becomes bright red upon being shaken with air. In addition, these causes of cyanosis are readily differentiated by carrying out quantitative blood methemoglobin and sulfhemoglobin levels.

Therapy

Congenital methemoglobinia due to NADH-diaphorase deficiency or toxic methemoglobinemia is readily treated by the administration of ascorbic acid, 300 to 600 mg orally daily divided into three or four doses, or methylene blue either intravenously (1 mg per kilogram body weight) or orally (60 mg three or four times daily). Presumably because it is a naturally occurring dietary substance, ascorbic acid has been used most frequently in treating congenital methemoglobinemia.

In patients with acute toxic methemoglobinemia who are symptomatic or whose methemoglobin level is rising rapidly, intravenous methylene blue is the preferred treatment because of its very rapid action. An exception exists in those patients who are glucose-6-phosphate dehydrogenase–deficient (see Chap. 62). In these subjects methylene blue would not only fail to give the desired effect on methemoglobin levels but might compound the patient's difficulty by inducing an acute hemolytic episode [27].

There is no treatment for sulfhemoglobinemia except for withdrawal of the offending drug.

Course and prognosis

The course of congenital methemoglobinemia is benign, but patients with this disorder should be shielded from exposure to aniline derivates, nitrites, and other agents which may, even in normal persons, induce methemoglobinemia.

Acute toxic methemoglobinemia, on the other hand, may represent a serious medical emergency. Because of the loss of oxygen-carrying capacity of the blood and because of the shift in the oxygen dissociation curve which occurs when methemoglobin is present in high concentrations [28], acute methemoglobinemia may be life-threatening when the level of the pigment exceeds half of the total circulating hemoglobin.

Sulfhemoglobin appears to be an essentially benign disorder. It tends to recur repeatedly in the same persons after exposure to drugs but does not generally appear to exert any important influence on their overall health. Unlike methemoglobin, sulfhemoglobin cannot be converted back to hemoglobin. Thus sulfhemoglobinemia, once it occurs, will persist until the erythrocytes carrying the abnormal pigment reach the end of their life-span.

References

1. Gibson, A. H.: The reduction of methemoglobin in red blood cells and studies on the cause of idiopathic methemoglobinemia. *Biochem. J. 42*:13, 1948.
2. Bodansky, O.: Methemoglobinemia and methemoglobin-producing compounds. *Pharmacol. Rev. 3*:144, 1951.
3. Kiese, M.: The biochemical production of ferrihemoglobin-forming derivatives from aromatic amines and mechanisms of ferrihemoglobin formation. *Pharmacol. Rev. 18*:1091, 1966.
4. Scott, E. M.: Congenital methemoglobinemia due to DPNH-diaphorase deficiency, in *Hereditary Disorders of Erythrocyte Metabolism*, edited by E. Beutler. Grune & Stratton, New York, 1968, p. 102.
5. Ross, J. D.: Deficient activity of DPNH-dependent methemoglobin diaphorase in cord blood erythrocytes. *Blood 21*:51, 1963.
6. Graubarth, J., Bloom, C. J., Coleman, F. C., and Solomon, H. N.: Dye poisoning in the nursery: A review of seventeen cases. *JAMA 128*:1155, 1945.
7. Comly, H. H.: Cyanosis in infants caused by nitrates in well water. *JAMA 129*:112, 1945.
8. Cohen, R. J., Sachs, J. R., Wicker, D. J., and Conrad, M. R.: Methemoglobinemia provoked by malarial chemoprophylaxis in Vietnam. *N. Engl. J. Med. 279*:1127, 1968.
9. Lemberg, R., and Legge, J. A.: *Hematin Compounds and Bile Pigments*. Interscience, New York, 1949, p. 492.
10. Harrop, G. A., Jr., and Waterfield, R. L.: Sulphemoglobinemia. *JAMA 95*:647, 1930.
11. Morell, D. B., Chang, Y., and Clezy, P. S.: The structure of the chromophore of sulphmyoglobin. *Biochim. Biophys. Acta 136*:121, 1967.
12. Finch, C. A.: Methemoglobinemia and sulfhemoglobinemia. *N. Engl. J. Med. 239*:470, 1948.
13. McCutcheon, A. D.: Sulphaemoglobinaemia and glutathione. *Lancet 2*:240, 1960.
14. Discombe, G.: Sulphaemoglobinaemia and glutathione. *Lancet 2*:371, 1960.
15. Bockris, L., and Smith, R. S.: Effect of methylene blue on red cell glutathione. *Nature 196*:278, 1962.
16. Paniker, N. V., and Beutler, E.: The effect of methylene blue and diaminodiphenysulfone on red cell reduced glutathione synthesis. *J. Lab. Clin. Med. 80*:481, 1972.
17. Paniker, N. V., and Beutler, E.: The effect of methylene blue and aminodiphenylsulfone on red cell reduced glutathione synthesis. *J. Lab. Clin. Med. 80*:481, 1972.
18. Jaffé, E. R.: Hereditary methemoglobinemias associated with abnormalities in the metabolism of erythrocytes. *Am. J. Med. 41*:786, 1966.
19. Kaplan, J.-C., and Beutler, E.: Electrophoresis of red cell NADH and NADPH-diaphorases in normal subjects and patients with congenital methemoglobinemia. *Biochem. Biophys. Res. Commun. 29*:605, 1967.
20. West, C. A., Gomperts, B. D., Huehns, E. R., Kessel, I., and Ashby, J. R.: Demonstration of an enzyme variant in a case of congenital methaemoglobinaemia. *Br. Med. J. 4*:212, 1967.
21. Hsieh, S.-S. and Jaffé, E. R.: Electrophoretic and functional variants of NADH-methemoglobin reductase in hereditary methemoglobinemia. *J. Clin. Invest. 50*:196, 1971.
22. Miller, A. A.: Congenital sulfhemoglobinemia. *J. Pediatr. 51*:233, 1957.
23. Leroux, A., Junien, C., and Kaplan, J.-C.: Generalized deficiency of cytochrome b₅ reductase in congenital methaemoglobinaemia with mental retardation. *Nature 258*:619, 1975.
24. Hegesh, E., Calmanovici, N., and Avron, M.: New method for determining ferrihemoglobin reductase (NADH-methemoglobin reductase) in erythrocytes. *J. Lab. Clin. Med. 72*:339, 1968.
25. Marti, H. R., Dorta, T., and Deubelbeiss, K. A.: Familiére Methämoglobinämie durch diaphorasemangel: Eine dritte Schweizer Sippe. *Schweiz. Med. Wochenschr. 96*:355, 1966.
26. Beutler, E.: The effect of flavin compounds on glutathione reductase activity. *In vivo* and *in vitro* studies. *J. Clin. Invest. 48*:1957, 1969.
27. Rosen, P. J., Johnson, C., McGehee, W. C., and Beutler, E.: Failure of methylene blue treatment in toxic methemoglobinemia: Association with glucose-6-phosphate dehydrogenase deficiency. *Ann. Intern. Med. 75*:83, 1971.
28. Darling, R. C., and Roughton, F. J. W.: The effect of methemoglobin on the equilibrium between oxygen and hemoglobin. *Am. J. Physiol. 137*:56, 1942.

CHAPTER *78*

Hemoglobinopathies producing cyanosis

ERNEST BEUTLER

Definition and history

A bluish discoloration of the skin and mucous membrane, designated *cyanosis*, has been recognized since antiquity to be a manifestation of lung or heart disease. Cyanosis occurring as a result of drug administration has also been recognized since before 1890 [1]. In 1912 Sloss and Wybauw reported a case of a patient with idiopathic methemoglobinemia [2]. Later Hitzenberger [3] suggested that hereditary familial methemoglobinemia might exist, and subsequently numerous such cases were reported [4]. In 1948 Hörlein and Weber [5] described a family in which eight members over four generations manifested cyanosis. The red cells of affected individuals had diaphorase activity, but the absorption spectrum of methemoglobin was abnormal. They demonstrated that the defect must reside in the globin portion of the molecule. In 1955 Singer suggested that such abnormal hemoglobins be given the designation *hemoglobin M* [6]. Separation of hemoglobin M from hemoglobin A by starch-block electrophoresis [7] made it possible to demonstrate more than one such hemoglobin by detecting differences in absorption spectra.

The existence of abnormal hemoglobins which lead to

cyanosis through quite another mechanism was first recognized in 1968 with the description of hemoglobin Kansas [8]. Here the cyanosis was not due to methemoglobin, as occurs in hemoglobin M, but rather to an abnormal oxygen affinity of the mutant hemoglobin. Thus, at normal oxygen tensions a large amount of deoxygenated hemoglobin is present.

Mode of inheritance

Methemoglobinemia due to hemoglobin M and cyanosis due to hemoglobins with altered oxygen affinities are inherited as autosomal dominant disorders.

Etiology and pathogenesis

The molecular mechanisms by which hemoglobin binds oxygen and releases it are discussed in detail in Chap. 37. Heme is held in a hydrophobic "heme pocket" between the E and F α-helices of each of the four globin chains. The iron atom in the heme forms four bonds with the pyrrole nitrogen atoms of the porphyrin ring and a fifth covalent bond with the imidazole nitrogen of a histidine residue in the nearby F α-helix (Fig. 78-1) [9]. This histidine, representing the eighty-seventh residue in the α chain and the ninety-second residue in the β chain, is designated as the *proximal histidine.* On the opposite side of the porphyrin ring the iron atom lies adjacent to another histidine residue to which, however, it is not covalently bonded. This *distal histidine* occupies position 58 in the α chain and position 63 in the β chain. Under normal circumstances oxygen is occasionally discharged from the heme pocket as a superoxide anion, removing an electron from the iron and leaving it in the ferric state. The enzymatic machinery of the red cell efficiently reduces the iron to the divalent form, converting the methemoglobin to hemoglobin (see Chaps. 35 and 77). In most of the hemoglobins M tyrosine has been substituted for either the proximal or the distal histidine. Tyrosine can form an iron-phenolate complex which resists reduction to the divalent state by the normal metabolic systems of the erythrocyte. Four hemoglobins M are a consequence of substitution of tyrosine for histidine in the proximal and distal sites of the α and β chains. As shown in Table 78-1 these four hemoglobins M have been designated by the geographic names Boston, Saskatoon, Iwate, and Hyde Park. The details of conformational changes which result from the substitution of tyrosine for histidine in these hemoglobins have been determined [48,49].

The fifth hemoglobin M, Hb $M_{Milwaukee}$, is formed by substitution of glutamic acid for valine in the sixty-seventh residue of the β chain, rather than substitution of tyrosine for histidine. The glutamic acid side chain points toward the heme group, and its γ-carboxyl group interacts with the iron atom, stabilizing it in the ferric state.

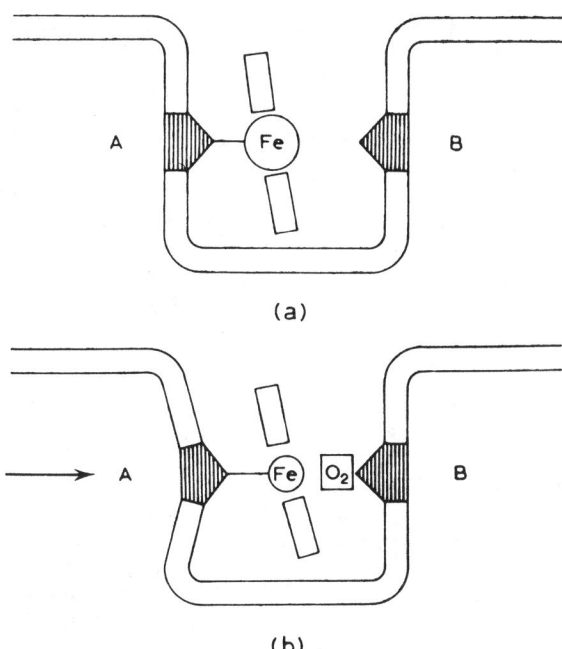

FIGURE 78-1 Diagrammatic representation of the heme group inserted into the heme pocket. *A* designates the proximal histidine while *B* is the distal histidine. (*a*) In the deoxygenated form the larger ferrous atom lies out of the plane of the porphyrin ring. (*b*) In the oxygenated form the now smaller "ferric-like" atom can slip into the plane of the porphyrin ring. As a result, the proximal histidine, and helix F into which it is incorporated, are displaced. (Lehmann and Huntsman [9] by permission.)

In some hemoglobin variants the deoxy conformation of the hemoglobin molecule is favored because the angle of the heme is altered from that found normally in deoxyhemoglobin. Such changes occur in Hb$_{Hammersmith}$, Hb$_{Bucuresti}$, Hb$_{Torino}$, and Hb$_{Peterborough}$. In other instances the quaternary conformation is changed by mutations involving the $\alpha_1\beta_2$ contact (Hb$_{Kansas}$, Hb$_{Titusville}$, and Hb$_{Yoshizuka}$). Properties of abnormal hemoglobins associated with low oxygen affinity are summarized in Table 78-1.

The "oxygen sensor" [50] of the body responds to the improved tissue oxygen supply brought about by a right-shifted oxygen dissociation curve by decreasing the output of erythropoietin [51]. As a result, the steady-state level of hemoglobin is diminished; mild anemia is characteristic of patients with hemoglobins with a decreased oxygen affinity.

Clinical features

Patients with hemoglobins M or with low-oxygen-affinity hemoglobin manifest cyanosis. In the case of α-chain variants, the dusky color of the infants will be noted at birth, but the clinical manifestations of β-chain variants become apparent only after β chains have largely replaced the γ chains at 6 to 9 months of age. In

TABLE 78-1 Properties of abnormal hemoglobins associated with cyanosis or low oxygen affinity of blood

Hemoglobin	Amino acid substitution	Oxygen dissociation properties, etc.	Clinical effect	Comment	Reference
HEMOGLOBINS M					
Hb M$_{Boston}$ (Hb M$_{Osaka}$)	α58(E7)His→Tyr	Very low O$_2$ affinity, almost nonexistent heme-heme interaction, no Bohr effect	Cyanosis due to formation of methemoglobin		[10,12]
Hb M$_{Saskatoon}$	β63(E7)His→Tyr	Increased O$_2$ affinity, reduced heme-heme interaction, normal Bohr effect, slightly unstable	Cyanosis due to methemoglobin formation, mild hemolytic anemia exacerbated by ingestion of sulfonamides	Phenol group of tyrosine forms iron-phenolate complex with iron atom (see text) stabilizing it in the Fe^{3+} (ferric) state	[10,13,14]
Hb M$_{Iwate}$ Hb M$_{Kankakee}$ (Hb M$_{Oldenburg}$)	α87(F8)His→Tyr	Low O$_2$ affinity, negligible heme-heme interaction, no Bohr effect	Cyanosis due to formation of methemoglobin		[10,15–17]
Hb M$_{Hyde\ Park}$	β92(F8)His→Tyr	Increased O$_2$ affinity, reduced heme-heme interaction, normal Bohr effect, slightly unstable	Cyanosis due to formation of methemoglobin, mild hemolytic anemia		[18–20]
Hb M$_{Milwaukee}$	β67(E11)Val→Glu	Low O$_2$ affinity, reduced heme-heme interaction, normal Bohr effect, slightly unstable	Cyanosis due to methemoglobin formation		[10,21,22]
OTHER ABNORMAL HEMOGLOBINS ASSOCIATED WITH CYANOSIS OR LOW OXYGEN AFFINITY					
Hb$_{Torino}$	α43(CE1)Phe→Val	Unstable hemoglobin (O$_2$ affinity?)	Cyanosis due to formation of methemoglobin, hemolytic crisis following ingestion of sulfonamides		[23]
Hb$_{Moabit}$	α86(F7)Leu→Arg	Slightly decreased O$_2$ affinity, unstable hemoglobin	Mild Heinz body hemolytic anemia and splenomegaly		[24]
Hb$_{Titusville}$	α94(G1)Asp→Asn	Very low O$_2$ affinity, low heme-heme interaction, dissociates into $\alpha\beta$ dimers in ligand form	Not visible; propositus is black American	$\alpha_1\beta_2$ contact involving same residues as Hb$_{Kansas}$	[25]
Hb$_{Raleigh}$	β1(NA1)Val→AcAla	Decreased O$_2$ affinity due to reduced number of cationic groups, normal Bohr effect and ligand binding	No clinical symptomatology	Affects the organic phosphate binding site	[26]
Hb$_{Freiburg}$	β23(B5)Val deleted	Increased O$_2$ affinity, unstable hemoglobin	Mild cyanosis due to methemoglobin formation	Deletion distorts corner between A and B helix, displacing invariant β24 (B6) glycine	[27]
Hb$_{Moscva}$	β24(B6)Gly→Asp	Decreased O$_2$ affinity, unstable hemoglobin, normal Bohr effect and heme-heme interaction			[28]
Hb$_{St.\ Louis}$	β28(B10)Leu→Gln	Increased O$_2$ affinity, reduced heme-heme interaction, normal Bohr effect, unstable hemoglobin, existing methemoglobin	Chronic hemolytic anemia associated with cyanosis	Side chain Gln may form H bond with carbonyl oxygen and NH group of distal histidine	[29]

TABLE 78-1   Properties of abnormal hemoglobins associated with cyanosis or low oxygen affinity of blood *(Continued)*

Hemoglobin	Amino acid substitution	Oxygen dissociation properties, etc.	Clinical effect	Comment	Reference
Hb$_{Louisville}$	β42(CD1)Phe→Leu	Decreased O$_2$ affinity, marked decrease in heme-heme interaction, normal Bohr effect, increased dissociation in presence of sulfhydryl blocking agents, unstable hemoglobin	Mild hemolytic anemia	Weakening of $\alpha_1\beta_2$ contact	[30]
Hb$_{Hammersmith}$ (Hb$_{Chiba}$)	β42(CD1)Phe→Ser	Decreased O$_2$ affinity, unstable hemoglobin	Heinz bodies, severe anemia unrelieved by splenectomy		[31]
Hb$_{Okaloosa}$	β48(CD7)Leu→Arg	Slightly decreased O$_2$ affinity, normal Bohr effect, unstable hemoglobin	Very mild or no clinical symptoms		[32]
Hb$_{Seattle}$	β70(E14)Ala→Asp	Decreased O$_2$ affinity, normal heme-heme interaction	Mild chronic anemia associated with reduced urinary erythropoietin; physiologic adaption to more efficient oxygen release to tissues	Heme contact	[33]
Hb$_{Vancouver}$	β73(E17)Asp→Tyr	Decreased O$_2$ affinity, normal subunit and heme-heme interaction, slightly increased Bohr effect	No clinical symptoms (hemolytic anemia in association with β thalassemia)	(Indirect effect on heme pocket by configurational change?)	[34]
Hb$_{Mobile}$	β73(E17)Asp→Val	Decreased O$_2$ affinity, normal heme-heme interaction, slight increase in Bohr effect	No clinical symptoms	(Same as above)	[34,35]
Hb$_{Providence}$	β82(EF6)Lys→Asn Asp	Decreased O$_2$ affinity at neutral pH, normal cooperative interactions, but reduced pH and anion interactions, reduced Bohr effect due to shift in pK			[36,37]
Hb$_{Agenogi}$	β90(F6)Glu→Lys	Decreased O$_2$ affinity, normal heme-heme interaction	None	Surface of molecule Lys may form salt bridge with C-terminal carboxyl of same chain	[38,39]
Hb$_{Caribbean}$	β91(F7)Leu→Arg	Decreased O$_2$ affinity, mildly unstable	No clinical symptoms	Weakened heme contact	[40]
Hb$_{Beth\ Israel}$	β102(G4)Asn→Ser	Decreased O$_2$ affinity, normal Bohr effect	No anemia or clinical symptoms except cyanosis, striking right-shifted O$_2$ equilibrium; increased 2,3-DPG	$\alpha_1\beta_2$ contact weakened	[41]
Hb$_{Kansas}$	β102(G4)Asn→Thr	Very low O$_2$ affinity, low heme-heme interaction, dissociates into dimers in ligand form	Cyanosis due to deoxy hemoglobin, mild anemia	$\alpha_1\beta_2$ and heme contact	[8,42,43]

TABLE 78-1 Properties of abnormal hemoglobins associated with cyanosis or low oxygen affinity of blood *(Continued)*

Hemoglobin	Amino acid substitution	Oxygen dissociation properties, etc.	Clinical effect	Comment	Reference
Hb$_{Burke}$	β107(G9)Gly$\rightarrow$Arg				[44]
Hb$_{Presbyterian}$	β108(G10)Asn$\rightarrow$ Lys	Decreased O_2 affinity, cooperative interaction; normal, slight increase in Bohr effect	Mild anemia	$\alpha_1\beta$ contact weakened	[45]
Hb$_{Yoshizuka}$	β108(G10)Asn$\rightarrow$ Asp	Decreased O_2 affinity, normal heme-heme interaction	Mild anemia, possibly in response to decreased oxygen affinity	$\alpha_1\beta_1$ contact	[46]
Hb$_{Peterborough}$	β111(G13)Val$\rightarrow$ Phe	Decreased O_2 affinity, normal heme-heme interaction, and normal Bohr effect	Mild anemia	Affects $\alpha_1\beta_1$ contact	[47]

FIGURE 78-2 Absorption spectra at pH 7.0. *A.* Methemoglobin A. *B.* Methemoglobin M$_{Boston}$. *C.* Methemoglobin M$_{Saskatoon}$. *D.* Methemoglobin A fluoride complex. For purposes of comparison all the optical densities have been made equal to 0.61 at 500 nm. (Gerald and George [52], by permission of the American Association for the Advancement of Science.)

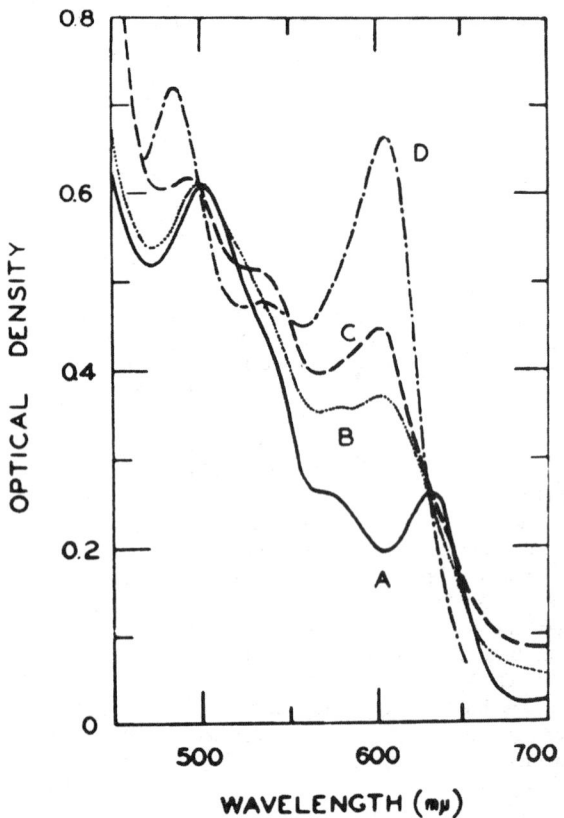

spite of the impaired hemoglobin function no cardiopulmonary symptoms are observed and there is no clubbing. In the case of Hb M$_{Saskatoon}$ and Hb M$_{Hyde Park}$ hemolytic anemia with jaundice may be present. The hemolytic state may be exacerbated by administration of sulfonamides [14].

Laboratory features

SPECTROSCOPY
The spectrum of normal methemoglobin A at pH 7.0 is illustrated in Fig. 78-1 [52]. Hemoglobins M may be differentiated from methemoglobin formed from hemoglobin A by measuring the absorption spectrum in the range of 450 to 750 nm. Since only some 20 to 35 percent of the total hemoglobin will ordinarily be the hemoglobin M, the mixed spectra of methemoglobin A and the hemoglobin M may be difficult to interpret. Therefore, it is preferable to isolate the hemoglobin M by electrophoretic or chromatographic means and to perform these spectral studies on the purified pigment [9].

ELECTROPHORESIS
All hemoglobin M samples should be converted to methemoglobin so that any differences found in electrophoresis will be due to the amino acid substitution and not to the different charge of the iron atom. Electrophoresis at pH 7.1 is most useful for separation of hemoglobins M since the imidizole groups of histidine have a net positive charge at this pH while at higher pH levels the histidines and the substituting tyrosines are both neutral. Details of procedures for performing electrophoresis of hemoglobins are presented in Chap. A7.

OTHER STUDIES
The hemoglobins M differ in their reactivity to cyanide and to azide ions [53,54]. This property may help to

identify the subunit affected, since the iron-phenolate bonds are stronger in the α-chain variants than in the β-chain variants. However, definitive identification of the variant depends upon peptide analysis.

Hemoglobins which cause cyanosis because of a diminished oxygen affinity may be detected by determining the oxygen dissociation curve of blood, being certain that the 2,3-DPG level is normal, or by estimating the oxygen dissociation curve of hemoglobin which has been stripped of 2,3-DPG by extensive dialysis against bis-tris buffer.

Differential diagnosis

Chronic cyanosis due to the hemoglobins M must be distinguished from other causes. When cyanosis is due to increased amounts of reduced hemoglobin, whether due to cardiac or pulmonary disease, on the one hand, or to an abnormal hemoglobin with low oxygen affinity, on the other, the blood will turn bright red when exposed to air. This is most easily done by placing a small amount of the blood in a flask or beaker and gently rotating the vessel so that the blood can spread out thinly on the surface of the glass. When this is done, methemoglobin and sulfhemoglobin do not change color. More precise investigation consists of measuring the absorption spectrum of the blood after diluting in a dilute phosphate buffer, pH 7.0. Reduced hemoglobin will become oxygenated in the buffer, and the spectrum will be that of oxyhemoglobin (see Fig. 78-2) [52]. If normal methemoglobin is present, a characteristic absorption band will be found in the 620- to 630-nm range. This band disappears immediately after the addition of a small amount of cyanide. The effect of cyanide on hemoglobins M is more variable, but they can be distinguished from normal methemoglobin by the abnormal position of the absorption bands. Sulfhemoglobin A, in contrast to methemoglobin, does not undergo a spectral change upon the addition of cyanide. Methods for the quantitation of methemoglobin and sulfhemoglobin are presented in Chap. A16.

The family history is quite useful in differentiating methemoglobinemia due to the hemoglobins M from that caused by NADH diaphorase deficiency (Chap. 77). Methemoglobins M are transmitted as autosomal dominant disorders. Although new mutations do occur with some frequency, most patients with cyanosis due to a hemoglobin M will have an affected parent and may have an affected child. As in other autosomal dominant defects, the incidence of consanguinity in patients with hemoglobin M disease is not increased over that found in the general population. In contrast, the parents and children of patients with NADH diaphorase deficiency do not have methemoglobinemia; this abnormality is inherited as an autosomal recessive disorder. The incidence of consanguinity in parents of patients with this enzyme deficiency is therefore increased. Diagnosis of

hereditary methemoglobinemia due to NADH diaphorase deficiency is made by enzyme assay (Chap. 77).

Course and prognosis

The hemoglobin M disorders and hemoglobins that decrease oxygen affinity do not appear to produce health problems. Their effect is chiefly cosmetic, and there is no indication that inheritance of these mutations shorten life-span.

Therapy

The iron-phenolate complex which exists in the hemoglobins M prevents the reduction of ferric to ferrous iron. For these reasons the methemoglobinemia does not respond to administration of ascorbic acid or of methylene blue. No effective treatment of the methemoglobinemia is known.

References

1. Hsieh, H.-S., and Jaffé, E. R.: The metabolism of methemoglobin in human erythrocytes, in *The Red Blood Cell*, 2d ed., edited by D. M. Surgenor. Academic, New York, 1975, pp. 799–824.
2. Sloss, A., and Wybauw, R.: Un Cas de methémoglobinémie idiopathique. *Ann. Soc. R. Sci. Med. Nat. Bruxettes* 70:206, 1912.
3. Hitzenberger, K.: Autotoxische Zyanose: Intraglobulare Methämoglobinämie. *Wien. Arch. Inn. Med.* 23:85, 1932.
4. Jaffé, E. R.: Hereditary methemoglobinemias associated with abnormalities in the metabolism of erythrocytes. *Am. J. Med.* 41:786, 1966.
5. Hörlein, H., and Weber, G.: Über chronische familiäre Methämoglobinämie und eine neue Modificazation des Methämoglobins. *Dtsch. Med. Wochenschr.* 73:476, 1948.
6. Singer, K.: Hereditary hemolytic disorders associated with abnormal hemoglobins. *Am. J. Med.* 18:633, 1955.
7. Gerald, P. S.: The electrophoretic and spectroscopic characterisation of Hgb M. *Blood* 13:939, 1958.
8. Bonaventura, J., and Riggs, A.: Hemoglobin Kansas, a human hemoglobin with a neutral amino acid substitution and an abnormal oxygen equilibrium. *J. Biol. Chem.* 243:980, 1968.
9. Lehmann, H., and Huntsman, R. G.: *Man's Hemoglobins*. Lippincott, Philadelphia, 1974.
10. Gerald, P. S., and Efron, M. L.: Chemical studies of several varieties of Hb M. *Proc. Natl. Acad. Sci. U.S.A.* 47:1758, 1961.
11. Shimizu, A., Hayashi, A., Yamamura, Y., Tsugita, A., and Kitayama, K.: Structural study of a new hemoglobin variant, Hb M Osaka. *Biochim. Biophys. Acta* 97:472, 1965.
12. Suzuki, T., Hayashi, A., Yamamura, Y., Enoki, Y., and Tyuma, I.: Functional abnormality of hemoglobin M Osaka. *Biochem. Biophys. Res. Commun.* 19:691, 1965.
13. Suzuki, T., Hayashi, A., Shimizu, A., and Yamamura, Y.: The oxygen equilibrium of hemoglobin M Saskatoon. *Biochim. Biophys. Acta* 127:280, 1966.
14. Stavem, P., Ströme, J., Lorkin, P. A., and Lehmann, H.: Haemoglobin M Saskatoon with slight constant haemolysis, markedly increased by sulphonamides. *Scand. J. Haematol.* 9:566, 1972.
15. Miyaji, T., Iuchi, I., Shibata, S., Takeda, I., and Tamura, A.: Possible amino acid substitution in the α chain (α87 Tyr) of Hb M Iwate. *Acta Haematol. Jpn.* 26:538, 1963.

16. Jones, R. T., Coleman, R., and Heller, P.: The chemical structure of hemoglobin M Iwate. *Fed. Proc.* 23 (Pt. 1):173, 1964.

17. Hayashi, N., Motokawa, Y., and Kikuchi, G.: Studies on relationships between structure and function of hemoglobin M Iwate. *J. Biol. Chem.* 241:79, 1966.

18. Heller, P., Coleman, R. D., and Yakulis, V.: Hemoglobin M Hyde Park: A new variant of abnormal methemoglobin. *J. Clin. Invest.* 45:1021, 1966.

19. Shibata, S., Miyaji, T., Iuchi, I., Ohba, Y., and Yamamoto, K.: Amino acid substitution in hemoglobin M Akita. *J. Biochem.* 63:193, 1968.

20. Hayashi, A., et al.: Some observations on the physiological properties of hemoglobin M Hyde Park. *Arch. Biochem. Biophys.* 125:895, 1968.

21. Hayashi, A., Suzuki, T., Imai, K., Marimoto, H., and Watari, H.: Properties of hemoglobin M, Milwaukee-1 variant and its unique characteristics. *Biochim. Biophys. Acta* 194:6, 1969.

22. Udem, L., Ranney, H. M., Bunn, H. F., and Pisciotta, A. V.: Some observations on the properties of hemoglobin M Milwaukee-1. *J. Mol. Biol.* 48:489, 1970.

23. Beretta, A., Prato, V., Gallo, E., and Lehmann, H.: Haemoglobin Torino-α43 (CD1) phenylalanine→valine. *Nature (London)* 217:1016, 1968.

24. Knuth, A., Pribilla, W., Marti, H. R., and Winterhalter, K. H.: Hemoglobin Moabit: Alpha 86 (F7) Leu→Arg. A new unstable abnormal hemoglobin. *Acta Haematol.* 61:121, 1979.

25. Schneider, R. G., et al.: Haemoglobin Titusville: α94 Asp→Asn: A new haemoglobin with a lowered affinity for oxygen. *Biochim. Biophys. Acta* 400:365, 1975.

26. Moo-Penn, W. F., et al.: Hemoglobin Raleigh (β1 valine→acetylalanine). Structural and functional characterization. *Biochemistry,* 16:4872, 1977.

27. Jones, R. T., Brimhall, B., Huisman, T. H. J., Kleihauer, E., and Betke, K.: Hemoglobin Freiburg: Abnormal hemoglobin due to a deletion of a single amino acid residue. *Science* 154:1024, 1966.

28. Idelson, L. I., Didkowsky, N. A., Casey, R., Lorkin, P. A., and Lehmann, H.: New unstable haemoglobin (Hb Moscva, β24(B6) Gly→Asp) found in the U.S.S.R. *Nature* 249:768, 1974.

29. Cohen-Solal, M., Seligmann, M., Thillet, J., and Rosa, J.: Haemoglobin Saint Louis β28(β10) leucine-glutamine. *FEBS Lett.* 33:37, 1973.

30. Keeling, M. M., et al.: Hemoglobin Louisville (β42(CD1) Phe→Leu): An unstable variant causing mild hemolytic anemia. *J. Clin. Invest.* 50:2395, 1971.

31. Dacie, J. V., Shinton, N. K., Gaffney, P. J., Jr., Carrell, R. W., and Lehmann, H.: Haemoglobin Hammersmith, (β42(CD1) Phe→Ser). *Nature (London)* 216:663, 1967.

32. Charache, S., Brimhall, B., Milner, P., and Cobb, L.: Hemoglobin Okaloosa (β48(CD7) Leucine→Arginine). An unstable hemoglobin with decreased oxygen affinity. *J. Clin. Invest* 52:2858, 1973.

33. Stamatoyannopoulos, G., Parer, J. T., and Finch, C. A.: Physiological implications of a hemoglobin with decreased oxygen affinity (hemoglobin Seattle). *N. Engl. J. Med.* 281:915, 1969.

34. Jones, R. T., Brimhall, B., Pootrakul, S., and Gray, G.: Hemoglobin Vancouver [α₂β₂ 73(E17) Asp→Tyr]: Its structure and function. *J. Mol. Evol.* 9:37, 1976.

35. Schneider, R. G., Hosty, T. S., Tomlin, G., Atkins, R., Brimhall, B., and Jones, R. T.: Hb Mobile [α2β2 73(E17) Asp→Val]: A new variant. *Biochem. Genet.* 13:411, 1975.

36. Moo-Penn, W. F., et al.: Hemoglobin Providence. A human hemoglobin variant occurring in two forms *in vivo. J. Biol. Chem.* 251:7557, 1976.

37. Bonaventura, J., et al.: Hemoglobin Providence. Functional consequences of two alterations of the 2,3-diphosphoglycerate binding site at position β82. *J. Biol. Chem.* 251:7563, 1976.

38. Miyaji, T., Suzuki, H., Ohta, Y., and Shibata, S.: Haemoglobin Agenogi (α₂β₂⁹⁰ˡʸˢ): A slow moving haemoglobin of a Japanese family resembling Hb-E. *Clin. Chim. Acta* 14:624, 1966.

39. Imai, K., Morimoto, H., Kolani, M., Shibata, S., Miyaji, T., and Matsumoto, K.: Studies on the function of abnormal haemoglobins Shimoneski, Ube II, Hikari, Gigu, and Agenogi. *Biochim. Biophys. Acta* 200:197, 1970.

40. Ahern, E., et al.: Haemoglobin Caribbean β91 (F7) Leu→Arg: A mildly unstable haemoglobin with low oxygen affinity. *FEBS Lett* 69:99, 1976.

41. Nagel, R. L., Joshua, L., Johnson, J., Landau, L., Bookchin, R. M., and Harris, M. B.: Hemoglobin Beth Israel: A mutant causing clinically apparent cyanosis. *N. Engl. J. Med.* 295:125, 1976.

42. Reissmann, K. R., Ruth, W. E., and Namura, T.: A human hemoglobin with lowered oxygen affinity and impaired heme-heme interactions. *J. Clin. Invest.* 40:1826, 1971.

43. Greer, J.: Three-dimensional structure of abnormal human hemoglobins Kansas and Richmond. *J. Mol. Biol.* 59:99, 1971.

44. Jones, R. T., and Koler, R. D.: Functional studies of seven new abnormal hemoglobins. 16th Inter. Congress in Hematology. September 1976, Abstract No. 1-21.

45. Moo-Penn, W. F., Wolff, J. A., Simon, G., Vacek, M., Jue, D. L., and Johnson, M. H.: Hemoglobin Presbyterian: β108(G10) asparagine→lysine. A hemoglobin variant with low oxygen affinity. *FEBS Lett.* 92:53, 1978.

46. Imamura, T., Fujita, S., Ohta, Y., Hanada, M., and Yanase, T.: Hemoglobin Yoshizuka (G10(108)β asparagine-aspartic acid): A new variant with a reduced oxygen affinity from a Japanese family. *J. Clin. Invest.* 48:2341, 1969.

47. King, M. A. R., Wiltshire, B. G., Lehmann, H., and Morimoto, H.: An unstable haemoglobin with reduced oxygen affinity: Haemoglobin Peterborough, β111(G13) valine→phenylalanine, its interaction with normal haemoglobin and with haemoglobin Lepore. *Br. J. Haematol.,* 22:125, 1972.

48. Pulsinelli, P. D., Perutz, M. F., and Nagel, R. L.: Structure of hemoglobin M Boston, a variant with a five co-ordinated ferric heme. *Proc. Natl. Acad. Sci. U.S.A.* 70:3870, 1973.

49. Greer, J.: Three dimensional structure of abnormal human haemoglobins, M Hyde Park and M Iwate. *J. Mol. Biol.* 59:107, 1971.

50. Beutler, E.: "A shift to the left" or "A shift to the right" in the regulation of erythropoiesis. *Blood* 33:496, 1969.

51. Stamatoyannopoulos, G., Parer, J. T., and Finch, C. A.: Physiologic implications of a hemoglobin with decreased oxygen affinity (hemoglobin Seattle). *N. Engl. J. Med.* 281:915, 1969.

52. Gerald, P. S., and George, P.: A second spectroscopically abnormal methemoglobin associated with hereditary cyanosis. *Science* 129:393, 1959.

53. Hayashi, A., Shimizu, A., Suzuki, T., and Yamamura, Y.: The properties of methemoglobin M to cyanide, azide and fluoride. *Biochim. Biophys. Acta* 140:25, 1967.

54. Hayashi, A., Suzuki, T., Shimizu, A., and Yamamura, Y.: Properties of hemoglobin M: Unequivalent nature of the α and β subunits in the hemoglobin molecule. *Biochim. Biophys. Acta* 168:262, 1968.

Disorders of iron metabolism

CHAPTER 79

Hemochromatosis

CLEMENT A. FINCH

Hemochromatosis is a systemic disease in which tissue iron overload is associated with pigmentation of the skin, cirrhosis and neoplastic change of the liver, diabetes, arthritis, gonadal failure in the male, and cardiopathy. The condition was first recognized at the necropsy table as pigmentary cirrhosis and was given the name *hemochromatosis* by von Recklinghausen in 1889 [1]. By 1935 it had been recognized as a clinical syndrome embracing the triad of pigmentation of the skin, hepatomegaly, and diabetes [2]. Because of the changes in skin color and the presence of diabetes, the term *bronzed diabetes* was often employed. By 1955 the role of iron in the pathogenesis of the disease had become more apparent, and hemochromatosis was referred to as an *iron-storage disease* [3]. Other diseases, such as alcoholic cirrhosis, have similarities to and interrelationships with this syndrome, but confusion can be largely avoided if hemochromatosis is considered in a physiologic context as a disorder of parenchymal iron overload [4]. The term *hemosiderosis* has been widely employed to indicate deposition of varying quantities of hemosiderin in the tissues, with or without associated tissue damage. Since it has no specific clinical meaning, it will not be used here.

Pathogenesis

The metabolism of iron and the regulation of iron absorption have been described in Chap. 35. An absolute increase in body iron content may arise in different ways. The most frequent increase in body iron is that seen with chronic inflammatory processes where the excess iron contained within the macrophage is quite innocuous. Of those conditions producing parenchymal iron overload, one of the two most prominent is *idiopathic hemochromatosis*. This hereditary disorder is an outstanding example of a regulatory abnormality involving both the intestinal mucosa and the macrophage. An excessive absorption of dietary iron permits the accumulation of 15 to 50 g of body iron over a period of 25 to 50 years [4]. During this time, the macrophage does not hold the excessive iron which then accumulates in the plasma and from there enters the parenchymal cells of the liver and other tissues. Consequently, it is possible to observe normal or only slightly increased iron content of macrophages at a time when parenchymal iron levels are very high.

Disorders of erythropoiesis (erythropoietic hemochromatosis) form a second group of conditions associated with increased iron absorption and overload [5]. In animals, increased erythropoiesis causes iron absorption to rise [6]. In humans, such increased absorption occurs mainly where erythropoiesis is at very high levels and is ineffective, such as in thalassemia major and sideroblastic anemias. In these conditions, too, iron storage in macrophages is limited and parenchymal overload predominates.

Other conditions that have been associated with some degree of parenchymal overload include liver disease, particularly cutaneous porphyria, the ingestion of alcoholic beverages containing excessive amounts of iron, exposure to large numbers of blood transfusions, and possibly the ingestion of large amounts of oral iron over prolonged periods of time [7]. Of these various conditions, the best documented is iron overload in the South African black, produced by drinking large amounts of home brew fermented in iron pots [8,9]. The beer prepared in this fashion contains fermentation products which lead to excessive iron absorption and deposits of iron both in macrophages and in parenchymal sites. Iron overload is obligatory in the individual who is repeatedly transfused and who is not at the same time bleeding, since iron excretion is limited to about 2 mg per day. Such parenteral iron must undergo processing in macrophages before it becomes available to other body tissues, and the usual iron deposition in transfused patients is predominantly in macrophages. However, those individuals with hyperplastic erythroid marrows show much greater movement of iron from macrophages to the liver parenchyma.

The site of iron storage may be predicted from the plasma iron level. When the plasma iron level is within normal limits, excessive iron localizes mainly in the macrophages. If, on the other hand, the plasma iron level is elevated and transferrin is more than 60 percent saturated (normal is 20 to 50 percent), iron is deposited in parenchymal cells, although many years may be required for such an accumulation to be of clinical significance. During the early stages of idiopathic hemochromatosis, increased iron absorption leads to an elevated plasma iron level, which decreases if the individual is placed on a diet low in iron content. Parenchymal iron may be only slightly increased at this time, and stores in macrophages may not be increased even after parenchymal iron deposits are large [10]. Eventually, both sites of iron storage are involved [11]. In erythropoietic hemochromatosis, the plasma iron level is also high, and both macrophage and parenchymal storage systems are usually overloaded.

The relationship between parenchymal iron overload and tissue iron damage became apparent when improvement was observed in cardiac and hepatic function on removal of iron by phlebotomy from patients with idiopathic hemochromatosis. Until then there had been a reluctance to accept this relationship, largely because of the difficulty in producing similar tissue damage in animals loaded with iron. However, there are major species differences in iron metabolism, and it has been difficult to produce the same degree of parenchymal iron overload in experimental animals as occurs in humans. Other evidence of iron toxicity in humans is observed in patients with thalassemia major. With the greater longevity resulting from more ample transfusion therapy, it is evident that most patients with thalassemia now die with the cardiomyopathy of iron overload.

Mode of inheritance

Idiopathic hemochromatosis is a hereditary disease in which the mutant gene is closely linked to the HLA locus of chromosome 11 [12,13]. The heterozygous form occurs in approximately one of 50 people but is not expressed by any change in iron stores. The clinical disorder is found in only a portion of the individuals with the homozygous abnormality. In most instances the disease is latent, and the course depends on such factors as sex and dietary iron intake as well as the presence of hepatoxins, especially alcohol. Clinical manifestations are found 5 to 10 times as frequently in men as in women [14]. This male vulnerability can be explained, at least in part, by the fact that women ingest less iron than men and lose iron through menstruation. The disease is exceedingly rare before the age of 20 and reaches a peak frequency in the fifth decade, at which time the damage from the gradually accumulated iron becomes apparent.

Clinical features

The cardinal manifestations of hemochromatosis are arthritis, loss of libido, pigmentation of the skin, hepatic cirrhosis, abdominal pain, diabetes, and cardiac dysfunction. In general, skin pigmentation, heart disease, and loss of libido occur at an earlier age, whereas abdominal pain, diabetes, and hepatoma are usually manifest after the patient is over 50 years. In perhaps one-third of patients with symptomatic iron overload, alcoholism is an associated feature. In these cases it is virtually impossible to differentiate the toxic effects of iron overload from those of the more potent toxin, alcohol.

The most frequent presenting symptoms are weakness, lassitude, and weight loss related to the onset of diabetes [3,14]. Diabetes may be mild or severe and is occasionally resistant to insulin. Associated vascular complications are usually mild. At the time of diagnosis, about 90 percent of symptomatic patients have excessive skin pigmentation, which is generally due to increased melanin deposition and thus has a bronze hue. When iron deposits are also present, the skin has a metallic gray color. The liver is the first organ damaged in idiopathic hemochromatosis. It is almost always firm and enlarged, having an average weight of 2500 g. Spider angiomas are frequent, but severe portal hypertension is much less common than with Laennec's cirrhosis. Hepatoma formerly occurred in 10 to 20 percent of older patients [3], but now that life has been extended by treatment, the frequency of hepatoma is greater. Loss of libido and the accompanying testicular atrophy are considered to be more prominent features of hemochromatosis than of Laennec's cirrhosis; gonadotropic hormones have been reported to be depressed in hemochromatosis but not consistently so [15,16]. Evidence of other endocrine involvement is occasionally present, and the clinical picture is sometimes that of hypopituitarism. Cardiac disease occurs in only about 15 percent of patients with idiopathic hemochromatosis, and is associated with arrhythmias and severe progressive congestive heart failure refractory to the usual therapeutic measures. Arthropathy involving both large and small joints of the extremities has been described in some detail [17]. An outstanding feature in many cases is chondrocalcinosis, which is associated with heavy iron deposits in the synovium. About a quarter of the patients complain of abdominal pain as part of the initial symptom complex. The cause of the pain is unknown. Occasionally, patients with hemochromatosis develop profound shock associated with some other illness such as pneumonia.

In other types of iron overload, the symptom complex may be similar but is influenced by the rate and amount of iron loading and the nature of the associated disease. For example, when excessive iron accumulation is due to thalassemia, cardiac manifestations are particularly prominent. However, this usually occurs at an iron load of about 1 g/kg, which is three to four times that found in idiopathic hemochromatosis. When hepatic iron overload is complicated by hepatitis, liver damage may be severe and account for most of the clinical problems. Recently, demineralization and vertebral collapse have been described in the Bantu, among whom iron overload is frequently associated with ascorbic acid depletion, presumably caused by oxidative effects of body iron [18,19].

LABORATORY DIAGNOSIS

The diagnosis of hemochromatosis begins with demonstration of parenchymal iron loading by appropriate laboratory tests [14]. For initial screening, the *plasma iron* and *iron-binding capacity* are determined. The average level of plasma iron in idiopathic hemochromatosis is 250 μg/dl (43μM), with a range most commonly extending from 225 to 325 μg/dl (39 to 56 μM); the transferrin saturation (plasma iron divided by total iron-binding capacity) is ordinarily from 70 to 100 percent. Somewhat lower plasma iron levels [150 to 250 μg/dl (26 to 43 μM)] resulting from the lower transferrin concentration may be seen when iron overload occurs in the alcoholic patient. The plasma iron level and percentage saturation in patients with overload may fall during inflammation or with development of a malignant neoplasm such as a hepatoma. A *plasma ferritin concentration* of over 500 ng/ml in the absence of advanced liver disease or inflammation or parenteral iron administration is also indicative of increased body iron stores, although it does not differentiate between macrophage and parenchymal storage [20]. Marrow examination for hemosiderin is not useful, since patients with idiopathic hemochromatosis may not have increased macrophage iron. However, when present the distribution of iron in marrow macrophages is often characteristic, consisting of many small spherical deposits scattered throughout the cell.

To obtain information concerning the degree of iron overload, the patient may be given 200 mg ascorbic acid daily for 1 week, and then the 24-h urinary iron excretion is determined after intramuscular injection of 10 mg/kg of the chelating agent deferoxamine [14,21,22]. This deferoxamine test reflects the amount of liver parenchymal iron, providing that renal function is normal and ascorbic acid deficiency is not present. Normally, less than 2 mg iron is excreted, but in idiopathic hemochromatosis the amount is usually more than 5 mg. If the test is positive, a liver biopsy specimen should be obtained in order to determine the amount and distribution of iron within the liver as well as the presence or absence of cirrhosis [23]. Other procedures useful in evaluating the extent of tissue damage include liver function tests, glucose tolerance test to determine whether diabetes is present, and an electrocardiogram. The blood should be examined for anemia and for red cell hypochromia and poikilocytosis, the presence of which would suggest that disturbed erythropoiesis is the cause of overload.

Of particular importance is the investigation of other family members when either idiopathic or erythropoietic hemochromatosis is suspected. Again, the most useful procedures are measurement of plasma iron and transferrin saturation (which may be elevated even when iron stores are not greatly increased) and plasma ferritin determinations [24,25]. Affected siblings frequently have a nearly saturated transferrin and elevated ferritin, but may or may not have increased deferoxamine excretion. These measurements should be performed on all family members over the age of 10, but they probably should not be regarded as definitive in excluding idiopathic hemochromatosis until the middle of the third decade. HLA typing has been shown useful in identifying sibling homozygotes, whose HLA profile is identical to that of the proband [26].

DIFFERENTIAL DIAGNOSIS
Since iron overload of macrophages does not, in itself, cause tissue damage, it must be differentiated from parenchymal iron overload. Increased iron storage in macrophages is usually not associated with an elevated plasma iron concentration, and excretion of iron after administration of deferoxamine does not exceed 3 mg. Those conditions which produce a consistently elevated plasma iron level and therefore a parenchymal loading state distinct from idiopathic hemochromatosis, are usually self-evident and include aplastic anemia, ineffective erythropoiesis, and liver disease. Porphyria cutanea tarda deserves special attention because this hepatic disorder is associated with a high plasma iron level and predominantly parenchymal loading, but the amount of storage iron is not great. The proper diagnosis is suspected by the presence of skin lesions typical of cutaneous porphyria and is confirmed by urinary porphyrin studies (see Chap. 76).

Hemochromatosis should also be suspected when any combination of the clinical manifestations described above is present. The effects of alcohol, in particular, including liver, pancreatic, and cardiac disease and pigmentation of the skin, mimic those of chronic iron overload. Even the liver biopsy may show excess iron deposits as in idiopathic hemochromatosis. The distinction can often be made from the smaller amount of parenchymal iron actually present, as reflected in a deferoxamine excretion of less than 3 mg, the heavier reticuloendothelial deposits in the liver biopsy, and the lack of evidence of iron overload in other family members.

Therapy

Definitive therapy is directed toward the removal of excess iron deposits from the body. In the patient with idiopathic hemochromatosis, as in any other patient with normal marrow function, it is possible to mobilize iron stores by repeated phlebotomies [27]. If 500 ml of blood, containing about 200 mg iron, is removed weekly, there is an initial fall in the hematocrit of about 6 percent by the second week; thereafter the hematocrit stabilizes. Since the average patient with idiopathic hemochromatosis has 20 to 40 g of stored iron, this weekly schedule must usually be continued for 2 to 3 years. During this period the plasma iron concentration remains high and falls only when available iron stores are depleted. At that time, longer intervals between phlebotomies are indicated, but bleeding should be continued as required to keep the ferritin level below 100, usually four to six times per year. Anemic patients, for example, those with sideroblastic anemia with hematocrit levels as low as 30 percent, may be treated successfully by phlebotomy. In alcoholic patients with poor diets, it may be necessary to replace plasma protein in order to prevent hypoproteinemia; however, patients who continue to consume alcohol are likely to benefit little from iron removal. Chelating agents, especially deferoxamine, have had extensive trial as a substitute method for iron removal in patients whose anemia is severe enough to preclude phlebotomy [28]. At present the most effective way to use deferoxamine is by the continuous intravenous or subcutaneous infusion of 2 g or more of the drug throughout the night. Depending on the iron load, amounts exceeding 50 mg per night may be mobilized and excreted in urine and stool. The administration of 1.5 g ascorbate per day together with deferoxamine has been shown to increase iron excretion in patients with thalassemia [29] and presumably has a similar effect in idiopathic hemochromatosis. It has been suggested [30] that ascorbate administration may aggravate the cardiomyopathy associated with iron storage disease by rapidly mobilizing iron from storage sites, but definitive evidence for such an effect is not available. Nonetheless, if ascorbate is given, it may be safer to administer it in small doses and only after infusion of deferoxamine has been started. Indications for chelation therapy in thalassemia major and sideroblastic anemias with equivalent overload are well founded, but those for elderly patients with aplastic or refractory anemia are less clearly established.

Various forms of supportive therapy are required in hemochromatosis, depending on the manifestations in the individual patient. Most important is the control of diabetes, the management of which does not differ from that conventionally employed. The loss of libido and changes in secondary sex characteristics in males may be reversed by testosterone therapy. Cirrhosis of the liver and cardiac complications are also treated in standard fashion.

Course and prognosis

Iron overload is tolerated by many individuals without clinical manifestations. The reason for its expression may be related to the amount and rapidity of parenchymal loading, the presence of associated liver disease of other etiology, and possibly as yet unidentified differences between individuals. In 1935 when treatment was limited to the usual management of diabetes, liver disease, and cardiac failure, the mean survival was 4.4 years after organ damage was manifest and the diagnosis made [2]. In 1968, a group of 28 patients treated by phlebotomy during the preceding 20 years was found to have a 5-year survival of 89 percent [27], and similar data have been presented more recently [14]. It is likely that the disease may be prevented in individuals whose tissues are not yet damaged, if excess iron is removed and future accumulation prevented. If tissue damage is present, further progression is prevented by iron removal, and some improvement may occur. Pigmentation of the skin decreases, and cardiac failure is reversed. Liver function may be improved and fibrosis arrested. Diabetes appears to be ameliorated in about one-third of the patients. Loss of libido and arthritis are not affected. Hepatoma emerges as the late complication of significance, occurring in perhaps 30 percent of patients with idiopathic hemochromatosis who had hepatic fibrosis at the time of the original diagnosis.

In thalassemia, there is evidence that hepatic damage may be arrested by chelation therapy [31]. It is also quite likely that fatal iron toxicity will be delayed or prevented.

References

1. von Recklinghausen: Über Haemochromatose, *Tageblatt der (62) Versammlung deutscher Naturforscher und Arzte in Heidelberg*, 1889, p. 324.
2. Sheldon, J. H.: *Haemochromatosis.* Oxford, London, 1935.
3. Finch, S. C., and Finch, C. A.: Idiopathic hemochromatosis, an iron storage disease. *Medicine (Baltimore)* 32:381, 1955.
4. Bothwell, R. H., Charlton, R. W., Cook, J. D., Finch, C. A.: *Iron Metabolism in Man.* Blackwell Scientific Publications, Oxford, London.
5. Byrd, R. B., and Cooper, T.: Hereditary iron-loading anemia with secondary hemochromatosis. *Ann. Intern. Med. 55:*103, 1961.
6. Conrad, M. E., Weintraub, L. R., and Crosby, W. H.: Iron metabolism in rats with phenylhydrazine-induced hemolytic disease. *Blood,* 25:990, 1965.
7. Johnson, B. F.: Hemochromatosis resulting from prolonged oral iron therapy. *N. Engl. J. Med.* 278:1100, 1968.
8. Hofvander, Y.: Hematological investigations in Ethiopia with special reference to a high iron intake. *Acta. Med. Scand. (Suppl.)* 494:1, 1968.
9. Bothwell, T. H., Seftel, H., Jacobs, P., Torrance, J. D., and Baumslag, N.: Iron overload in Bantu subjects. *Am. J. Clin. Nutr.* 14:47, 1964.
10. Bothwell, T. H., Cohen, I., Abrahams, O. L., and Perold, S. M.: A familial study in idiopathic hemochromatosis. *Am. J. Med.* 27:730, 1959.
11. Bothwell, R. H., Abrahams, C., Bradlow, B. A., and Charlton, R. W.: Idiopathic and Bantu hemochromatosis: Comparative histological study. *Arch. Pathol.* 79:1963, 1965.
12. Cartwright, G. E., et al.: Hereditary hemochromatosis: Phenotypic expression of the disease. *N. Engl. J. Med. 301:*4, 1979.
13. Simon, M., et al.: Idiopathic hemochromatosis: A study of biochemical expression in 247 heterozygous members of 63 families: Evidence for a single major HLA-linked gene. *Gastroenterology 78:*703, 1980.
14. Milder, M. S., Cook, J. D., Stray, S., and Finch, C. A.: Idiopathic hemochromatosis: An interim report. *Medicine* 59:34, 1980.
15. Stocks, A. E., and Powell, L. W.: Carbohydrate intolerance in idiopathic haemochromatosis and cirrhosis of the liver. *Q. J. Med., New Series XLII (168):*733, 1973.
16. Walker, R. J., and Williams, R.: Haemochromatosis and iron overload, in *Iron in Biochemistry and Medicine,* edited by A. Jacobs. Academic, London, 1974.
17. Hamilton, E., Williams, R., Barlow, K. A., and Smith, P. M.: The arthropathy of idiopathic haemochromatosis. *Q. J. Med.* 37:171, 1968.
18. Seftel, H. C., et al.: Osteoporosis, scurvy and siderosis in Johannesburg Bantu. *Br. Med. J.* 1:642, 1966.
19. Hankes, L. V., Jansen, C. R., and Schmaeler, M.: Ascorbic acid catabolism in Bantu with hemosiderosis (scurvy). *Biochem. Med.,* 9:244, 1974.
20. Halliday, J. W., Cowlishaw, J. L., Russo, A. M., Powell, L. W.: Serum-ferritin in diagnosis of haemochromatosis. *Lancet,* September 1977, p. 621.
21. Harker, L. A., Funk, D. D., and Finch, C. A.: Evaluation of storage iron by chelates. *Am. J. Med.* 45:105, 1968.
22. Saddi, R., Feingold, J., Degrese, C. H., and Fagard, R.: Desferrioxamine utilisation for the quantitation of iron excess: Study of 24 patients having idiopathic haemochromatosis. *Biomedicine* 23:41, 1978.
23. Kent, G., and Popper, H.: Liver biopsy in diagnosis of hemochromatosis. *Am. J. Med.* 44:837, 1968.
24. Edwards, C. Q., Carroll, M., Bray, P., Cartwright, G. E.: Hereditary hemochromatosis: Diagnosis in siblings and children. *N. Engl. J. Med.,* 297:1, 1977.
25. Bassett, M. L., Halliday, J. W., Powell, L. W.: Hemochromatosis—Newer concepts: Diagnosis and management, *DM,* January 1980.
26. Bassett, M. L., Halliday, J. W., Powell, L. W., Doran, T., Bashir, H.: Early detection of idiopathic haemochromatosis: Relative value of serum-ferritin and HLA typing. *Lancet,* 1979, p. 4.
27. Williams, R., Smith, P. M., Spicer, E. J. F., Barry, M., and Sherlock, S.: Venesection therapy in idiopathic haemochromatosis. *Q. J. Med.* 38:1, 1969.
28. Modell, B.: Advances in the use of iron-chelating agents for the treatment of iron overload, *Prog. Hematol.* 11:267, 1979.
29. O'Brien, R. T.: Ascorbic acid enhancement of desferrioxamine-induced urinary iron excretion in thalassemia major. *Ann. N.Y. Acad. Sci.* 232:221, 1974.
30. Nienhuis, A. W.: Vitamin C and iron. *N. Engl. J. Med.* 304:170, 1981.
31. Barry, M., et al.: Long-term chelation therapy in thalassaemia major: Effect on liver iron concentration, liver histology, and clinical progress. *Br. Med. J.* 2:16, 1974.

PART FIVE

Neutrophils, eosinophils, and basophils

Morphology of neutrophils

CHAPTER *80*

Morphology of neutrophils and neutrophil precursors

JOHN LASZLO
R. WAYNE RUNDLES

Many elaborate and ingenious microscopic, biochemical, and histochemical methods have been proposed to identify the various types of mature and immature leukocytes, but relatively simple morphologic procedures remain the standard for clinical purposes.

Total and differential counts of blood leukocytes are an essential part of the diagnostic study of nearly every sick person, and evaluation of granulocyte morphology is especially important in patients with leukocytosis or leukopenia. Examination of the blood frequently should be supplemented by study of the marrow and occasionally by special histochemical or cytologic procedures to differentiate the leukocytosis of infection from leukemoid reactions, drug- or toxin-induced granulocytopenia, and primary disorders of the marrow. The morphologic features of mature and immature granulocytes vary from patient to patient, particularly in those with leukemia, and cells cannot be identified simply by matching even the best photographs or drawings. Morphology has its limitations but carefully prepared and stained blood and marrow films provide information that is indispensable in the solution of a large number of clinical problems.

General morphologic features

The earliest recognizable granulocyte precursors, myeloblasts and related precursor cells, are large cells with dense basophilic cytoplasm. On dried films the nuclei are 12 to 15 μm in diameter and have prominent nucleoli which disappear during cell maturation. As the cells grow older, they usually become smaller, with the cytoplasm less basophilic and more abundant than the nucleus. In the older cells the nuclear chromatin becomes condensed and appears clumped when stained by polychrome (Wright's or Giemsa's) stain.

Granules become prominent in the cytoplasm of maturing cells in this series. Two major types of granules develop: the nonspecific (azurophilic, "A" granule) and the specific (secondary, "B" granule). The staining reactions of the specific granules lead to the classification of granulocytes as neutrophils, eosinophils, or basophils. Neutrophilic granules are tan or yellowish pink. They appear first in the early myelocyte stage and are located at the Golgi apparatus, close to the nucleus in deep blue cytoplasm. The number of granules increases rapidly and fills the cytoplasm by the late neutrophilic myelocyte stage. Eosinophilic granules appear in the basophilic cytoplasm of promyelocytes. These granules are ovoid refractile bodies, 0.2 to 0.3 μm in diameter and so packed that they resemble fish roe. They stain bright orange or red and remain uniform in size and distinctly refractile even in mature cells. Basophilic granules are nearly twice as large as eosinophilic, fewer in number, and stain bluish black. Description of eosinophil and basophil morphology is provided in Chaps. 90 and 91.

The features that are most useful in identifying the various types of cells and their stage of maturation relate therefore to size, relative area of the nucleus, prominence of nucleoli, granulation, and color of the cytoplasm. The ultrastructure of cells of interest to investigators will be described briefly in this chapter, although in clinical practice electron microscopic studies usually contribute little information beyond that obtained by light microscopy.

Normal granulocyte development

MYELOBLAST STAGE
The most immature cells which can be identified with certainty as belonging to the granulocytic series are myeloblasts (see Plate 2). More primitive progenitors are very infrequent and structurally uncharacterized and thus are difficult to identify in normal marrow.

Myeloblasts constitute about 1 percent of normal marrow cells and are never present in blood of healthy subjects. Myeloblasts vary in size from 15 to 20 μm in diameter. Myeloblasts are about 8 μm in diameter when in suspension, at which time they are approximately spherical. They are characterized by a relatively large, round nucleus with only a scanty amount of cytoplasm. The nuclear chromatin is finely dispersed and shows little condensation or clumping. In dealing with single cells, it is very difficult to distinguish myeloblasts from lymphoblasts. Neither type of cell contains cytoplasmic granules. The myeloblast usually has two morphologic features: (1) There are generally two or more pale blue nucleoli indistinctly outlined by the surrounding chromatin, whereas the lymphoblast commonly has but a single nucleolus with a sharp nucleolar border. (2) The cytoplasm is deeply basophilic and generally has no clear zone about the nucleus, whereas the lymphoblast has a prominent clear zone.

Study of myeloblast ultrastructure (Fig. 80-1) reveals

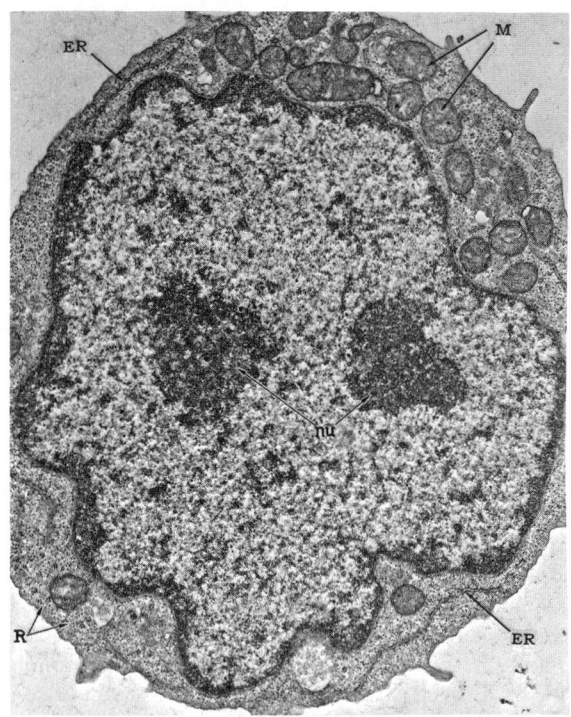

FIGURE 80–1   Myeloblast from acute granulocytic leukemia. Key to abbreviations for electron micrographs: b = basophilic body; ER = endoplasmic reticulum; G = Golgi; Gly = glycogen; M = mitochondrion; N = nucleus; nu = nucleolus; R = ribosome; S = small granule with subunits; L = large granule. (×10,000.) (All electron micrographs in this chapter are by courtesy of Dr. Douglas R. Anderson and Academic Press, New York.)

numerous round or oval mitochondria, 0.4 to 0.8 μm in diameter. The Golgi zone contains a centriole, vesicles, and sacs. There are many free ribosomes in the cytoplasm and scattered rough endoplasmic reticulum [1]. A few polyribosomal structures can be seen by electron microscopy [2].

PROMYELOCYTE STAGE

Promyelocytes (see Plate 2) develop from myeloblasts. The nucleus has the same chromatin pattern and prominent nucleoli. The mark of the promyelocyte is the presence in the cytoplasm of coarse blue or violet granules which may appear dense, homogeneous, or floccular. The nucleus is eccentric in position, and azurophilic granules are prominent in the cytoplasm of the cell. These granules are darker and more basophilic than those present in more mature cells. It has been demonstrated by studies of rabbit blood and marrow that *azurophilic granules* are distinct from the *specific granules* of the later granulocytic series with respect to size and enzyme composition [3–7]. Azurophilic granules measuring approximately 0.8 μm are formed in promyelocytes and represent the predominant granule of that stage of cell maturation. The granules are ovoid or irregularly spherical, have a homogeneous density, and

are surrounded by a typical unit membrane. Electron microscopic studies of these granules suggest that the condensation of this secretory material takes place within the inner Golgi cisternae. Lysosomal enzymes such as acid phosphatase, myeloperoxidase, indoxylesterase, and β-glucuronidase are found in the azurophilic granules of promyelocytes. Histochemically the granules of promyelocytes are positive for myeloperoxidase and negative for alkaline phosphatase. Synthesis of azurophilic granules is thought to cease during the promyelocyte stage. The granules are distributed between daughter cells when a late promyelocyte divides and matures into a myelocyte.

Promyelocytes have fewer mitochondria than myeloblasts, and the endoplasmic reticulum is more fully developed. This reticulum may be in the form of cisternae or as rounded sacs with ribosomes along the outer surface. In acute leukemia these cells may replicate or fail to mature, and the granules may form abnormal needlelike crystalloid inclusions called *Auer rods*, or plumper phi bodies. When basophils and eosinophils differentiate, their granules seem to condense en masse throughout the whole cell, and there is no well-defined promyelocyte stage.

MYELOCYTE STAGE

This phase (see Plate 2) encompasses the period of most extensive morphologic alteration in granulocyte development. Substages (e.g., early and late myelocytes) are sometimes described, but this is probably unnecessary. In blood films myelocytes vary in diameter from 16 to 24 μm and have a distinct cytoplasmic border. Clumping of nuclear chromatin first becomes evident in the myelocyte stage, and the nucleoli are less distinct. The nucleus is frequently eccentric, and even in thin films there are superimposed cytoplasmic granules. A pink cytoplasmic blush, which represents the synthesis of specific neutrophilic granules by the Golgi cisternae, first appears in the perinuclear region and subsequently expands to fill the cytoplasm. The neutrophilic granules vary somewhat in optical density. This variation is the result of the presence of two distinct types of particles, residual azurophilic granules, and the neutrophilic granules. The latter are 0.5 μm in diameter, and have a distinct limiting membrane and a finely granular interior somewhat less dense than that of the larger azurophilic granules. At this stage alkaline phosphatase is first detected histochemically.

In the myelocyte stage neutrophilic, basophilic, and eosinophilic granules are most prominent. Mitochondria decrease in number, and the dilated sacs of endoplasmic reticulum change to cisternae (Fig. 80-2). Seen by light microscopy, the chromatin pattern approaches that of mature cells.

METAMYELOCYTE (JUVENILE) STAGE

During this stage (see Plate 2) the cytoplasm assumes the characteristics of mature granulocytes. The background cytoplasm becomes uniformly pink. Neu-

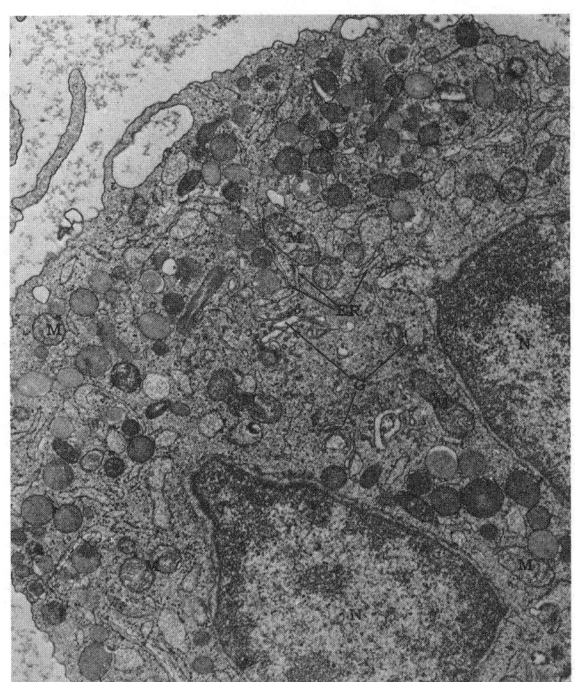

FIGURE 80–2 Myelocyte from granulocytic leukemia. (For key to abbreviations, see Fig. 80–1.) (×10,000.)

trophilic granules are smaller, fine blue-black or like graphite smudge, and diffusely scattered throughout the cytoplasm. In the eosinophils and basophils the characteristic granules stand out in stark relief around the nucleus. The nuclear chromatin becomes coarsely clumped and condensed peripherally, while the nucleus often becomes indented or bean-shaped, foretelling the first steps in nuclear segmentation. The metamyelocyte has lost the capacity for cell division, and further maturation consists predominantly of nuclear elongation and segmentation.

BAND (STAB) STAGE
Bands (see Plates 1 and 2) are similar to mature neutrophilic granulocytes in having the pink cytoplasm with fine azure or bluish granules. The nucleus is elongated like a sausage or folded over upon itself, and the nuclear chromatin is coarsely clumped. The band is found in the blood of normal persons and comprises 3 to 5 percent of the differential leukocyte count.

Morphology of the mature cell

POLYMORPHONUCLEAR NEUTROPHILS
These cells (see Plate 1) are fully mature granulocytes (Fig. 80-3). The cells tend to be fairly uniform in size (12 to 15 μm) with cytoplasm and granules similar to that of bands. The nucleus is coarsely clumped and segmented into two to five, most frequently three, lobes which are connected by thin chromatin strands. Should the lobes overlap, however, these strands may not be visible, and

the polymorphonuclear leukocyte becomes virtually indistinguishable from a band. In such instances it is acceptable arbitrarily to consider these cells as mature polymorphonuclear neutrophils. Some 5 to 10 percent of normal granulocytes contain nuclear irregularities such as pockets, bridges, appendices, and fibrillar bodies; these are accentuated in granulocytes from people with Down's syndrome and leukemia [8].

Mature polymorphonuclear leukocytes have predominance of the specific granules (80 to 90 percent) but retain some of the azurophilic granules (10 to 20 percent), suggesting that specific granules are formed during the myelocyte stage at a time when the formation of azurophilic granules has ceased. The azurophilic granules containing lysosomal enzymes are progressively diluted by cell division subsequent to their formation at the promyelocyte stage and by the continued formation of specific granules through the late myelocyte stage. By contrast, alkaline phosphatases are not found in the azurophilic granules of promyelocytes, but they begin to appear in myelocytes and are clearly demonstrable in all subsequent maturation stages. These enzymes appear to be restricted to the specific neutrophilic granules, which are thought to be a special type of secretory granule. Granulocytes have also been characterized with regard to their histochemical reactivity. For example, in normal granulocytes glycogen is stained red by the periodic acid–Schiff (PAS) technique, a reaction which is negated by amylase digestion. Normal granules may be stained for lipid with Sudan black B, for peroxidase by *o*-toluidine or benzidine, and for alkaline

FIGURE 80–3 Neutrophil in normal blood. The arrow at the top of the micrograph indicates vesicle formation by infolding of the plasma membrane. (For key to abbreviations, see Fig. 80–1.) (×7500.)

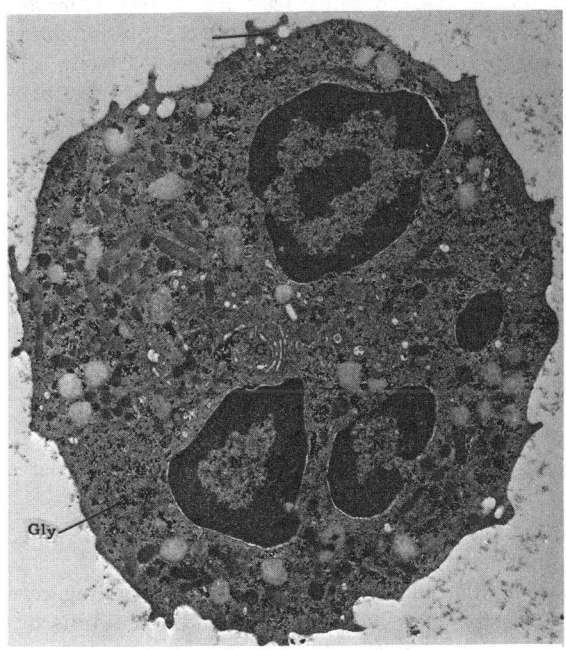

phosphatase by a dye-coupling reaction [9] (see Chaps. A22 to A24). These tinctorial characteristics are sometimes useful in the differential diagnosis of myeloproliferative syndromes, leukemoid reactions, and other conditions, as will be discussed in subsequent chapters. There are immunocytochemical stains, such as monospecific antisera to myeloperoxidase and lactoferrin, which permit simultaneous and selective visualization of azurophil and specific granules in single cells [10]. To date these have mainly been used for the study of the interaction of bacteria with granules during the process of phagocytosis. Finally, the ability of normal granulocyte plasma membranes to resist staining by merocyanine 540 appears to contrast them to leukemic granulocytes which are permeable to this fluorescent stain [11].

Motility is also characteristic of all granulocyte precursors studied under supravital conditions and is most prominent in mature cells. At 37°C they are constantly in motion. Pseudopodia of clear cytoplasmic membrane are projected in advance of the cell and pull the cytoplasm-containing granules and finally the nucleus (see Chap. 83).

DEVELOPMENT OF GRANULES

The histochemical evidence for the appearance of two different types of granules, one at the promyelocyte stage (peroxidase–positive) and the other at the myelocyte stage (alkaline phosphatase–positive), has largely been confirmed by zonal centrifugation methods. The granule population of mature granulocytic cells are heterogeneous, both physically and biochemically. In rabbit granulocytes [12,13], the enzyme myeloperoxidase and the cationic proteins are exclusively associated with a very heavy particle (primary, azurophilic granule) that is completely separable from the alkaline phosphatase–containing granules (specific granules) of intermediate density and size. These particles are, in turn, separable from additional, small, vesicular, acid phosphatase–containing particles (tertiary granules). Certain enzymes such as lysozyme [12], ribonuclease, and cathepsins [14,15], however, are distributed in both azurophilic granules and specific granules.

The enzyme-carrying granules of human granulocytes manifest analogous heterogeneity [16,17–20]. Myeloperoxidase and cationic proteins are associated with the heaviest particle (azurophilic granule) which is separable from an intermediate-sized lysozyme-carrying particle (specific granule). Alkaline phosphatase in human cells, however, in contrast to that in the rabbit, is largely microsomal and not associated with specific granules [18–20]. In human chronic myelogenous leukemia, alkaline phosphatase is not detectable in microsomes, in other subcellular elements, or in solution [20].

SEX DETERMINATION BY LEUKOCYTE MORPHOLOGY

Study of the cellular basis of sex in nondividing cells had its impetus in 1949 when Barr and Bertram discov-

ered at the periphery of the nucleus of nerve cells of the female cat a sex chromatin body which was absent in nuclei of male cells. In human beings, the Barr body is readily demonstrable in fixed and stained buccal scrapings from a female. In 1954, Davidson and Smith [18] described a unique "drumstick" appendage in a small percentage of polymorphonuclear leukocytes (see Plate 1) in females—a simple laboratory determination of genetic sex.

The drumstick is an oval mass of dense chromatin, 1.5 μm in size, attached to a nuclear lobe by a single slender filament. Found in approximately 3 percent of the polymorphonuclear leukocytes of normal females, they should be distinguished from nonspecific nodules lacking chromatin, from sessile nodules, and from those irregular in shape or attached to the nucleus in a nonfilamentous manner.

Practical applications of these tests and their relation to the X chromosome have been amply documented in chromosomal disorders. When sex identification by nuclear examination became available, it was found that men with Klinefelter's syndrome have Barr bodies and drumsticks—later to be correlated with the 47 chromosomes (XXY) characteristic of this condition. In a variety of other disorders, including those having four X chromosomes (XXXX or XXXXY), there will be one less Barr body and one less drumstick per cell than the number of X chromosomes.

Acquired abnormalities of granulocyte morphology

DÖHLE BODIES

Among the most frequent and easily recognizable abnormalities of neutrophil cytoplasm are Döhle bodies. Originally described in patients having scarlet fever [22], they are frequently found in a variety of infections, burns, trauma, pregnancy, and cancer. Induction of Döhle bodies follows the administration of cytoxic agents such as cyclophosphamide [23]. These are pale blue (Wright's stain, pH 7) cyst-like inclusion bodies usually located in the periphery of the cytoplasm and often protruding outside the normal cellular contour. They may be single or multiple and are delineated by the pink color of the surrounding cytoplasm and granules. Though most commonly encountered in mature neutrophils, they may be observed in earlier myeloid forms and sometimes in lymphocytes and monocytes. Döhle bodies are formed by parallel arrays of rough endoplasmic reticulum with bound ribosomes, which stain with basic dyes.

Other morphologic changes usually accompany the finding of Döhle bodies. Decreased nuclear segmentation in neutrophils, coarse leukocyte granules, and abnormally large platelets attest to the more general nature of the metabolic disturbance [23]. These abnormalities taken individually or in various combinations also constitute the major morphologic features of the Alder-Reilly and May-Hegglin inherited anomalies described below.

MACROPOLYCYTES

The average mature neutrophil is approximately 12 to 15 μm in diameter and contains two to five lobes per nucleus with an average of approximately three lobes. Macropolycytes (see Plate 1) are abnormally large (15 to 25 μm) neutrophils seen in patients having deficiencies of folic acid or of vitamin B_{12} and are frequently noted before the macrocytosis of red cells develops. The cell enlargement is not limited to neutrophils, since it is due to a general metabolic defect. All the granulocyte precursors in the marrow are enlarged, as are erythroid cells, megakaryocytes, and other rapidly dividing cells, such as epithelial cells from the bowel, bladder, and vagina.

Macropolycytes are occasionally present in other conditions, e.g., chronic infection [24], and myeloproliferative disorders, as well as following the use of certain antimetabolites, such as 6-mercaptopurine, methotrexate, hydroxyurea, and cytosine arabinoside. Macropolycytes may also be inherited as a dominant characteristic [25–27] in which the frequency of drumstick structures is also increased [28]. The hereditary existence of anomalous nuclear appendages has been reported [29,30].

OTHER ACQUIRED MORPHOLOGIC ALTERATIONS

Neutrophils of patients having infection may show nuclear pyknosis, toxic granulation, degranulation, and vacuolation [31,32]; the extent of these changes is possibly related to the severity of the disease [24]. Particles staining for iron may be present in mature neutrophils from patients having infections [33]. A high degree of correlation of vacuolation with septicemia and its usefulness in diagnosis have been demonstrated [34]. In a study of 3500 blood films, 122 showed vacuolated neutrophils, and bacterial infection was evident in 119 of these cases. In a prospective study of 21 consecutive patients with septicemia, 19 had vacuolation, and this was often recognized prior to knowledge of the blood culture findings.

Vacuolated and degranulated neutrophils are also frequently found in joint fluid from patients having various forms of joint disorders, particularly rheumatoid arthritis [35,36]. The cellular basis of degranulation is discussed in Chap. 83.

In cases of acute myelogenous leukemia, the slender rod-shaped structures called Auer rods or phi bodies may be found in the cytoplasm of myeloblasts and promyelocytes. By electron microscopy, they appear to be laminated homogeneous crystals, and probably represent a malformation of cytoplasmic azurophilic granule development [37–42]. The presence of these rods is useful in distinguishing acute myelogenous leukemia or preleukemia from acute lymphocytic leukemia or leukemoid reactions in which they do not occur.

Inherited abnormalities of granulocyte morphology

HEREDITARY HYPERSEGMENTATION OF NEUTROPHILS AND HEREDITARY MACROPOLYCYTES

Neutrophil hypersegmentation and macropolycytes have been found to exist not only as acquired abnormalities, such as those described above, but also as inherited conditions. Neutrophil hypersegmentation is inherited as an autosomal dominant trait; no other associated clinical abnormalities have been described [25,26,43]. Homozygotes with this condition have a mean nuclear index exceeding four lobes per cell as opposed to the normal of slightly less than three. A similar condition involving hypersegmentation of eosinophils rather than neutrophils has also been described [25].

Giant neutrophils may be inherited as an autosomal dominant trait not associated with specific blood groups, secretory state, or other disorders [27]. The giant neutrophils have a mean diameter of 16.9 μm (normal 12 to 15 μm) and a volume double that of normal neutrophils. These cells are also hypersegmented with 6 to 10 lobes per neutrophil, due perhaps to a failure of cytoplasmic division following nuclear division [30].

PELGER-HUËT ANOMALY

This anomaly is characterized by failure of normal lobe development in cells of the granulocytic series. Typically, these mature neutrophils and eosinophils have one or two lobes per nucleus and take on a round, dumbbell, or peanut shape. Originally described by Pelger in 1928 [44], the condition was considered to be one of the hematologic features of tuberculosis. Huët [45,46] showed the genetic nature of this anomaly, and it has since been found to be transmitted as a simple autosomal dominant trait occurring in at least 1 out of every 6000 people. This abnormal nuclear development is not associated with any other congenital abnormality and does not appear to affect neutrophil function [47]. A similar morphologic abnormality was discovered in rabbits, and in this species the homozygous state was either lethal or accompanied by skeletal or other anomalies [48]. The defect is demonstrable in human heterozygotes, in whom nearly all the mature neutrophils have a bilobed appearance. In the homozygous state mature neutrophils have round nuclei with clumped chromatin, nuclear bridging and appendices, diminished numbers of granules, and large secondary granules [49,50].

The morphology of the granulocytes in individuals having the Pelger-Huët anomaly may be further modified by conditions which cause leukocytosis. In these instances, the nuclei may have a rounded instead of a bilobed appearance. The morphologic features of the Pelger-Huët anomaly may be acquired by individuals who have severe infections, leukemia, and cancer metastatic to bone [51]. The changes can also be produced in some patients who are being treated with drugs such as colchicine and the sulfonamides. In these instances, the granulocytes become normal again when the infection or tumor is controlled or administration of the toxic agent suspended.

ALDER-REILLY ANOMALY
Described separately by Alder [52] and Reilly [53] to consist of giant granules in neutrophils in association with other hereditary defects such as gargoylism, this condition was later discovered [54] to be part of a general metabolic disorder of polysaccharides. The defect may be completely expressed with abnormally prominent granules in other granulocytes, monocytes, and lymphocytes [55], or it may be incompletely expressed with only one leukocyte type affected.

MAY-HEGGLIN ANOMALY
The inheritable combination of leukopenia with Döhle bodies in all neutrophils and giant platelet forms was described by May [56] and Hegglin [57]. Almost all the individuals known to have this disorder have been in good health despite mild leukopenia, thrombocytopenia, and bizarre platelets. Occasionally hemorrhagic manifestations have been reported in affected individuals. Ultrastructural studies of the leukocyte inclusion bodies show dense fibrils 50 Å in diameter, thought to be messenger RNA [58].

It is interesting to note that the findings in May-Hegglin anomaly have striking similarities to alterations acquired following infections or the use of cytotoxic drugs [23,29]. Although the morphologic features may be indistinguishable, the clinical setting is readily recognizable. It has been suggested that a common metabolic disorder may exist transiently in acquired conditions and permanently in some inherited disorders.

CHÉDIAK-HIGASHI ANOMALY
This is discussed in Chap. 89.

References

1. Anderson, D. R.: Ultrastructure of normal and leukemic leukocytes in human peripheral blood. *Ultrastruct. Res. Suppl. 9,* 1966.
2. Tryfiates, G. P., and Laszlo, J.: Human leukemic polyribosomes. *Proc. Soc. Exp. Biol. Med.* 124:1125, 1967.
3. Bainton, D. F., Ullyot, J. L., and Farquhar, M. G.: The development of neutrophilic polymorphonuclear leukocytes in human bone marrow: Origin and content of azurophil and specific granules. *J. Exp. Med.* 134:907, 1971.
4. Wetzel, B.K., Spicer, S. S., and Horn, R. G.: Fine structural localization of acid and alkaline phosphatases in cells of rabbit blood and bone marrow. *J. Histochem. Cytochem.* 15:311, 1967.
5. Bainton, D. F., and Farquhar, M. G.: Origin of granules in polymorphonuclear leukocytes: Two types derived from opposite faces of the Golgi complex developing granulocytes. *J. Cell Biol.* 28:277, 1966.
6. Bainton, D. F., and Farquhar, M. G.: Differences in enzyme content of azurophil and specific granules of polymorphonuclear leukocytes. I. Histochemical staining of bone marrow smears. *J. Cell Biol.* 39:286, 1968.
7. Bainton, D. F., and Farquhar, M. G.: Differences in enzyme content of azurophil and specific granules of polymorphonuclear leukocytes.
II. Cytochemistry and electron microscopy of bone marrow cells. *J. Cell Biol.* 39:299, 1968.
8. Ojaldetti, M., Bessler, H., Fishman, P., van der Lyn, E., and Joshua, H.: Ultrastructural features of the granulocytes in Down's syndrome. *Scand. J. Haematol.* 12:104, 1974.
9. Kaplow, L. S.: Cytochemistry of leukocyte alkaline phosphatase. *Am. J. Clin. Pathol.* 39:439, 1963.
10. Pryzwansky, K. B., MacRae, E. K., Spitznagel, J. K., and Cooney, M. H.: Early degranulation of human neutrophils: Immunocytochemical studies of surface and phagocytic events. *Cell* 18:1025, 1979.
11. Valinsky, J. E., Easton, T. G., and Reich, E.: Merocyanine 540 as a fluorescent probe of membranes: Selective staining of leukemic and immature hematopoietic cells. *Cell* 13:487, 1978.
12. Baggiolini, M. J., Hirsch, G., and De Duve, C.: Resolution of granules from rabbit heterophil leukocytes into distinct populations by zonal sedimentations. *J. Cell Biol.* 40:529, 1969.
13. Zeya, H. I., and Spitznagel, J. K.: Cationic protein bearing granules of polymorphonuclear leukocytes: Separation from enzyme rich granules. *Science* 163:1069, 1969.
14. Zeya, H. I., and Spitznagel, J. K.: Isolation of polymorphonuclear leukocyte granules from rabbit bone marrow. *Lab. Invest.* 24:237, 1971.
15. Zeya, H. I., and Spitznagel, J. K.: Characterization of cationic protein bearing granules of polymorphonuclear leukocyte. *Lab. Invest.* 24:229, 1971.
16. West, B. C., Rosenthal, A. S., Gebb, N. A., and Kimball, H. R.: Separation and characterization of human neutrophil granules. *Am. J. Pathol.* 77:41, 1974.
17. Olsson, I.: Isolation of human leukocyte granule using colloidal silica polysaccharide density gradient. *Exp. Cell Res.* 54:325, 1969.
18. Spitznagel, J. K., et al.: Character of azurophil and specific granules purified from human polymorphonuclear leukocytes. *Lab. Invest.* 30:775, 1974.
19. Bertz, U., and Baggiolini, M.: Biochemical and morphological characterization of azurophil and specific granules of human neutrophilic leukocytes. *J. Cell Biol.* 63:251, 1974.
20. Zeya, H. I., and Laszlo, J.: Granule assembly in precursors of human leukemia granulocytes. *Am. J. Pathol.* 71:467, 1973.
21. Davidson, W. M., and Smith, D. R.: A morphological sex difference in the polymorphologic leukocytes. *Br. Med. J.* 2:6, 1954.
22. Döhle, H.: Leukocyteneinschluesse bei Scharlach. *Zentralbl. Bakteriol.* 61:63, 1911.
23. Itoga, T., and Laszlo, J.: Döhle bodies and other granulocytic alterations with cyclophosphamide. *Blood* 20:668, 1962.
24. Ponder, E., and Ponder, R. van O.: The cytology of the polymorphonuclear leukocyte in toxic conditions. *J. Lab. Clin. Med.* 28:316, 1942.
25. Undritz, E.: Les Malformations héréditaires des éléments figurés du sang. *Sang* 25:296, 1954.
26. Undritz, E.: Eine neue Sippe mit erblich-konstitutioneller Hochsegmentierung der Neutrophilenkerne. *Schweiz. Med. Wochenschr.* 88:1000, 1958.
27. Davidson, W. M., Milner, R. D. G., and Lawler, S. D.: Giant neutrophil leukocytes: An inherited anomaly. *Br. J. Haematol.* 6:339, 1960.
28. Lüers, T.: Das numerische Verhalten der geschlechtsspezifischen Kernanhänge bei der erblich-konstitutionellen Hochsegmentierung der Neutrophilenkerne Undritz. *Schweiz. Med. Wochenschr.* 90:246, 1960.
29. Davidson, W. M.: Inherited variations in leukocytes. *Br. Med. Bull.* 17:190, 1960.
30. Davidson, W. M.: Inherited variations in leukocytes. *Semin. Hematol.* 5:255, 1968.
31. Metchnikoff, E.: *Lectures on the Comparative Pathology of Inflammation,* translated by F. A. Starling and E. H. Starling. Kegan Paul, Trench, Trübner, London, 1893.
32. Ewing, J.: *Clinical Pathology of the Blood.* Lea Brothers, Philadelphia, 1901.
33. Koszewski, B. J., Bahabzdadeh, H., and Willrodt, S.: Hemosiderin content of leukocytes in animals and man and its significance in the physiology of granulocytes. *Am. J. Clin. Pathol.* 48:474, 1967.

34. Zieve, P. D., Haghshenass, M., and Krevans, J. R.: Vacuolization of the neutrophil. *Arch. Intern. Med.* 118:356, 1966.
35. Malinin, T. I., Pekin, T. J., Bauer, H., and Zvaifler, N. J.: Vacuoles in synovial fluid leukocytes. *Am. J. Clin. Pathol.* 45:728, 1966.
36. Bodel. P. T., and Hollingsworth, J. W.: Comparative morphology, respiration and phagocytic function of leukocytes from blood and joint fluid in rheumatoid arthritis. *J. Clin. Invest.* 45:580, 1966.
37. Freeman, J. A.: The ultrastructure and genesis of Auer bodies. *Blood* 15:449, 1960.
38. White, J. G.: Fine structural demonstration of acid phosphatase activity in Auer bodies. *Blood* 29:667, 1967.
39. McDuffie, N. G.: Crystalline patterns in Auer bodies and specific granules of human leukocytes. *J. Microsc. (Oxf.)* 6:321, 1967.
40. Huhn, D., and Borchers, H.: Elektronenmikroskopischzytochemische Untersuchungen der Auer-Stäbchen bei akuter Paramyeloblasten-Leukämie. *Blut* 17:70, 1968.
41. Bessis, M., and Breton-Gorius, J.: Pathologie et asynchronisme de développement des organelles cellulaires au cours des leucemies aigues granulocytaires: Étude au microscope électronique. *Nouv. Rev. Hematol.* 9:245, 1969.
42. Hanker, J. S., Laszlo, J., and Moore, J. O.: The light microscopic demonstration of hydroperoxidase-positive phi bodies and rods in leukocytes in acute myeloid leukemia. *Histochemistry* 58:241, 1978.
43. Undritz, E., and Schali, H.: Eine neue Sippe mit erblichkonstitutioneller Hochsegmentierung der Neutrophilenkerne und das Knochenmarkbild beim homozygoten Träger dieser Anomalie. *Schweiz. Med. Wochenschr.* 94:1365, 1964.
44. Pelger, K.: Demonstratie van een paar zeldzaam voorkomende typhen van bloedlichaampjes en bespreking der patienten. *Discuss. Med. Tijdschr. Geneesk.* 72:1178, 1928.
45. Huët, G. J.: Familial anomaly of leukocytes. *Discuss. Med. Tijdschr. Geneesk.* 75:5956, 1931.
46. Huët, G. J.: Über eine bisher unbekannte Familiare Anomalie der Leukocyten. *Klin. Wochenschr.* 11:1264, 1932.
47. Undritz, E., and de Sepibus, C.: Results of recent examination of a family from Wallis, in which was found 25 years ago the first Swiss case of Pelger-Huëtscher nuclear anomaly: Present status of studies on this abnormality. *Schweiz. Med. Wochenschr.* 87:1258, 1957.
48. Harm, H.: Beiträge zur Morphologie und Genetik der Pelger-Anomalie bei Mensch und Kaninchen. *Z. Menschl. Vererb.* 30:501, 1952.
49. Begemann, W. H., and Campagne, A. van L.: Homozygous form of Pelger-Huët's nuclear anomaly in man. *Acta Haematol. (Basel)* 7:295, 1952.
50. Djeldetti, M., Weiss, S., and Gafter, V.: Ultrastructural features of the blood cells in a patient with Pelger-Hüet anomaly. *J. Clin. Pathol.* 65:942, 1976.
51. Dorr, A. D., and Moloney, W. C.: Acquired pseudo-Pelger anomaly of granulocytic leukocytes. *N. Engl. J. Med.* 261:742, 1959.
52. Alder, A.: Über Konstitutionell bedingte Granulationsveränderungen der Leukocyten. *Dtsch. Arch. Klin. Med.* 183:372, 1939.
53. Reilly, W. A.: The granules in the leukocytes in gargoylism. *Am. J. Dis. Child.* 62:489, 1941.
54. Reilly, W. A., and Lindsay, S.: Gargoylism (lipochondrodystrophy): A review of clinical observation in eighteen cases. *Am. J. Dis. Child.* 75:595, 1948.
55. Fricker-Alder, H.: Die Aldersche Granulationsanomalie: Nachuntersuchung des erstbeschriebenen Falles und Überblick über den heutigen Stand der Kenntnisse. *Schweiz. Med. Wochenschr.* 88:989, 1958.
56. May, R.: Leukocyten Einschlüsse. *Dtsch. Arch. Klin. Med.* 96:1, 1909.
57. Hegglin, R.: Gleichzeitige Konstitutionelle Veränderungen an Neutrophilen und Thrombozyten. *Helv. Med. Acta* 12:439, 1945.
58. Jordan, S. W., and Larsen. W. E.: Ultrastructure studies of the May-Hegglin anomaly. *Blood* 25:921, 1965.

Biochemistry and function of neutrophils

CHAPTER 81

Composition of neutrophils

ROBERT SILBER
CHARLES F. MOLDOW

The development of techniques for isolating blood leukocytes that are relatively free of contaminating platelets and erythrocytes has permitted biochemical studies of these cells [1,2]. Initially, glass-bead columns were used to separate polymorphonuclear leukcoytes from blood [3,4], but this method has been largely replaced by density gradient techniques for removal of lymphocytes and monocytes from granulocytes [5,6]. Methods are also available for the separation of eosinophils from polymorphonuclear neutrophils. Pure populations of granulocyte precursors have not yet been obtained [7]. Information concerning the composition of developing granulocyte forms in the marrow or blood has been derived from histochemical, ultrastructural, and radioautographic procedures, in which individual cell types can be identified.

The polymorphonuclear neutrophil (PMN) in blood is a fully differentiated cell in transit to tissues. Its primary function is phagocytosis. Digestion within the cell is facilitated by lysosome-like granules [8], the contents of which are discharged into vacuoles containing phagocytized microbes or other particulate matter. The release of these substances can also have deleterious effects on surrounding tissues, some of which can be counteracted and prevented by plasma inhibitors.

The structure and composition of leukocyte granules [9–15], as well as the recognition, ingestion, and killing of microorganisms by neutrophils, have been studied extensively. Significant progress has been made in recognizing plasma membrane-bound receptors and enzymes. The partial purification of plasma membrane from human neutrophils has been accomplished [16].

Composition of cytoplasmic granules

Light microscopy, histochemical staining, and electron microscopy reveal two types of granules, azurophilic and specific, in mature polymorphonuclear neutrophils. The azurophilic "primary" granules are lysosomes, membrane-bound particles storing acid hydrolases in a latent form [8], similar in structure and content to those in other vertebrate cells. Azurophilic granules are first seen in the promyelocyte. Since they are not formed after that stage of granulocyte maturation, their number per cell diminishes with subsequent divisions. During the myelocyte stage, a second population of granules, the specific "secondary" granules, is formed. In the mature neutrophil these are twice as numerous as the azurophilic granules. The content of enzymes and other proteins in neutrophil granules is given in Table 81-1. Many of the substances listed in this table have antibacterial properties and play a role in the phagocytic process. Studies of these enzymes during the maturation of granulocytes indicate that myeloperoxidase, acid hydrolases, neutral proteases, including a nonspecific collagenase, and bactericidal cationic proteins appear early in PMN development [10,11], as expected from their association with azurophilic granules. In contrast, lysozyme, a specific collagenase, a vitamin B_{12}–binding protein, and lactoferrin appear late in granulocyte development [10,17], in association with the development of specific granules. Unlike rabbit granulocytes, alkaline phosphatase in human neutrophils is not localized to either type of granule [13].

The peroxidase activity of blast cells has been used as an aid in the differential diagnosis of the leukemias. If present, this activity indicates that the cells belong to the granulocytic or monocytic series. Further differentiation between these types is aided by esterase cytochemistry. Promyelocytes and other granulocytes have a higher content of naphthol-AS-D-chloroacetate esterase than do monocytes, which in turn have a higher level of the α-naphthyl acetate and fluoride-sensitive naphthol-AS-D-acetate esterase activities [18]. The greenish color of unstained granulocytes is imparted by myeloperoxidase [19].

The neutrophil granules contain a wide array of enzymes, most of which catalyze catabolic reactions. The cell is endowed with the ability to degrade proteins, nucleic acids, carbohydrates, and lipids. Many of these lysozomal enzymes have been purified, some to homogeneity. The cationic proteins, originally considered to be a single substance called phagocytin [20,21], may be complexed to anionic glycosaminoglycans [22]. They include myeloperoxidase [19], which participates in oxygen-dependent bactericidal processes; lysozyme or muramidase [23], an enzyme catalyzing cell wall carbohydrate degradation; and lactoferrin, a regulatory protein that may inhibit colony-stimulating-activity production [24]. This iron-binding glycoprotein, which competes with bacteria for iron, may also play a role in inflammation independent of its chelating function through its ability to promote the adherence of neutrophils to endothelial cells [25] and enhance the hydroxyl radical production by neutrophils [26]. A bactericidal permeability-enhancing protein binds to the outer membrane of gram-negative organisms and activates a bacterial phospholipase A_1, resulting in a net loss of bacterial phospholipids [27]. The close association of this activity with a cellular phospholipase A_2 also suggests a functional relationship with neutrophil lipolytic activity for this oxygen-independent microbicidal system.

The extrusion of lysosomal contents may also result in damage to surrounding tissues [28,29]. Elastase is among the best characterized enzymes with possible involvement in connective tissue diseases [30]. This serine protease has been obtained in pure form and constitutes 5 percent of the cell's dry weight. Its broad specificity allows it to use elastin, insoluble collagen, bacterial cell walls, and cartilage proteoglycans as substrates. Collagenase is a metalloenzyme that cleaves only soluble collagen, showing preference for type I collagen found in bone and tendon [30–32]. Among the lysosomal proteases, cathepsin G resembles pancreatic chymotrypsin in specificity [33]. Like elastase, this enzyme attaches to insoluble collagen and is inhibited by α-antitrypsin inhibitor and by a neutrophil cytosol inhibitor. While elastase and cathepsin G can be distinguished immunologically, the stimulation of elastolytic activity by leukocyte cathepsin G suggests a functional interrelationship between this enzyme and elastase. Another lysosomal proteinase, cathepsin D, is an acid protease that may play a role in intracellular degradation of heterologous and perhaps autologous proteins [33]. This enzyme may also function in the generation of leukokinin in inflammatory exudates [34]. Kinin-forming and kinin-destroying proteases are found in human neutrophils [34]. These four proteases (elastase, collagenase, cathepsin G, and cathepsin D) are optimally active at acid pH, and all have relatively low molecular weights of under 100,000 [35]. Cationic proteins from granules of leukocytes are also pyrogenic [36,37]. They may have fibrinolytic activity [38,39] and cause tissue damage [35]. Phagocytosing human neutrophils inactivate their own lysosomal enzymes [40]. In addition, several plasma proteins have been shown to neutralize or inactivate neutrophil products [14]. The α_1-antitrypsin inhibitor inhibits elastase and nonspecific collagenase, while the α_2-macroglobulin inhibitor also inhibits such neutral proteases as cathepsin G. Ceruloplasmin, while not specifically a protease inhibitor, has a superoxide dismutase activity that functions as an effective extracellular scavenger for free radicals generated by neutrophils during the phagocytic process [41].

Electron microscopic studies of Auer bodies, the eosinophilic rods found in the cytoplasm of blast cells of some patients with acute myelogenous leukemia, indicate that they contain lysosomal enzymes, in particular acid phosphatase and peroxidase. These bodies may therefore be abnormal lysosomes [42–43]. Phi bodies, a morphologic variant of Auer bodies, are detected by a positive-staining reaction with peroxidase and have been described in the blast cells of patients with acute and chronic myelogenous leukemia [44].

TABLE 81-1   Major constituents of neutrophil granules

	Azurophil (primary)	Specific (secondary)
Acid phosphatase	+	−
Aminodipeptidase	+	−
α-Amylase	+	−
Cathepsin D	+	−
Cathepsin G	+	−
Cationic proteins		−
Collagenases:		
Specific	−	+
Nonspecific	+	−
Dextranase	+	−
Elastase	+	−
α-Fucosidase	+	−
α- and β-galactosidase	+	−
N-Acetyl-β-galactosaminidase	+	−
α- and β-glucosidase	+	−
N-Acetylglucosaminidase	+	−
β-Glucuronidase	+	−
Glycosyl aminoglycans	+	−
Lactoferrin	−	+
Laminaranase	+	−
Lysozyme	+	−
α-Mannosidase	+	−
Myeloperoxidase	+	−
Permeability-increasing protein	+	−
Vitamin B_{12}–binding protein	−	+

SOURCE: Adapted from Smolen and Weissman [35] and Olsson and Venge [14]. The substances whose presence has been detected are designated by a plus sign, those that have not been demonstrated in a given granule by a minus sign.

Plasma membrane receptors and cytoskeletal proteins

Neutrophils have receptors for the Fc portion of IgG molecules [45]. Binding sites are also found for the chemotactic peptide N-formylmethionyl-leucylphenylalanine [46] and for the C3b and C5a components of complement [47]. The C3b receptor is present on 90 percent of neutrophils and is sensitive to trypsin, while the IgG receptor is not affected by this enzyme. The presence of β-adrenergic receptors [48] and insulin-binding sites [49] have been demonstrated, although these receptors have not been purified. These receptors increase in number during the course of granulocyte maturation.

Mature neutrophils contain glycoproteins on their surface, and one that may play a role in neutrophil adherence has been found to be missing in a patient with multiple infections [50]. A number of disorders of phagocytosis have directed attention to a role of internal cytoskeletal proteins in this process. The decreased bactericidal activity of granulocytes in the Chédiak-Higashi syndrome has been attributed to defective polymerization of tubulin leading to impaired chemotaxis and degranulation [51]. However, the precise mechanism responsible in this disorder for the large azurophilic granules, which fail to fuse with phagosomes, remains to be elucidated.

The major cytoskeletal proteins actin and myosin have been purified and characterized from chronic myelogenous leukemia (CML) granulocytes [52]. Like its counterpart in skeletal muscle, CML granulocyte actin polymerized in the presence of potassium salts and activated the Mg^{2+}-ATPase activity of rabbit skeletal muscle myosin. The CML granulocyte myosin consists of heavy- and light-chain subunits. The ATPase activity of CML myosin can be stimulated by rabbit skeletal muscle actin. CML granulocytes also contain a high-molecular-weight actin-binding protein. These three proteins interact in the temperature-dependent gelation process of cytoplasmic extracts. An inhibitor of actin polymerization has been isolated from normal human granulocytes [53]. This inhibitor may be responsible for the unpolymerized condition of a large proportion of granulocyte actin. A single clinical example of a neutrophil actin dysfunction has been reported in an infant, with recurrent infections, whose granulocytes were defective in locomotion, ingestion, and regulation of granule secretion. When compared with normal neutrophil actin, incomplete polymerization of the patient's actin was observed [54]. The granulocyte content of other contractile elements such as tubulin and intermediate filament protein(s) remains unknown.

Oxidative killing of bacteria by polymorphonuclear leukocytes is a complex process involving the interaction of lysosomal plasma membrane and cytosol enzymes [55]. A plasma membrane–bound NADPH oxidase has been solubilized and characterized [56]. This enzyme catalyzes the production of superoxide O_2^- and hydroxyl radical $OH\cdot$, a key event in the respiratory burst manifested by neutrophils upon exposure to a variety of particulate or soluble stimuli. The enzyme system shows a preference for NADPH as a physiological electron donor, has flavin adenine dinucleotide as an essential bound cofactor, and may be regulated by ATP [55]. The O_2^--forming oxidase is partially buried in the lipid bilayer of the plasma membrane with a portion protruding into the cytoplasm [57]. The role played by this enzyme in its interaction with myeloperoxidase and a halide ion in microbicidal killing is discussed elsewhere. A b-type cytochrome may also be involved in the O_2^- production. The abnormal function of the NADPH oxidase and a decrease of the b-type cytochrome have been described in chronic granulomatous disease [58]. This b-type cytochrome appears to have a dual localization. While it is present in the plasma membrane fraction, it may be mainly localized in specific granules [16]. Two superoxide dismutases that convert O_2^- to H_2O_2 and O_2 have also been associated with neutrophil membranes, perhaps localized to the outside surface of the cell [59]; these are a dimeric enzyme of $M_r = 33,000$ daltons containing copper and zinc and a tetramer of $M_r = 85,000$ daltons containing manganese. Catalase is also present in neutrophils but functions predominantly during heavy external oxidative stress [60]. A glutathione peroxidase is also found that probably consumes much of the H_2O_2 produced in neutrophils. This selenium-containing enzyme catalyzes the reduction of H_2O_2 and of the hydroperoxide products of polyunsaturated fatty acid oxidation.

DNA and RNA content

As might be expected, the DNA content of normal mature granulocytes and immature marrow leukocytes is identical at 0.7×10^{-12} g of DNA phosphorus per cell [61,62]. DNA content is sometimes used as an alternate method of quantitating cell numbers [63]. The DNA content of acute leukemia cells is variable but usually somewhat higher than that of normal leukocytes [64–69]. This is almost certainly due to the frequency of abnormal chromosome numbers found in this disease, with "hyperdiploid" cells often noted [70,71]. Several tantalizing observations have been made that suggest that DNA isolated from chronic myelogenous leukemia (CML) cells differs chromatographically from DNA isolated from normal leukocytes [72–74]. Confirmation and extension of these studies with more modern extraction techniques would be most desirable, since the possibility has not been excluded that the reported alterations may reflect the presence of different nucleases in the normal and the leukemic cells. Furthermore, the extraction procedures used in some of the earlier studies may have yielded partially degraded DNA, making differences between normal and leukemic material difficult to interpret. DNA extracted from leukemic cells contains an increased proportion of 5-methylcytosine [75]. The presence of circular and catenated dimers of mitochondrial DNA has been reported in human leukocytes [76]. The circular dimer form was found in material isolated from the leukocytes of 14 patients with CML [77]. This structure could not be found in mitochondrial DNA from patients with leukemoid reactions, whereas the catenated dimer and circular monomers (rather than dimers) were present in both normal and leukemic cells. Serial study of cells from the same patient revealed that treatment with cytotoxic drugs lowered the frequency of the circular dimer. The presence of circular dimers in normal thyroid tissue [78] suggests that this form of DNA is not limited to malignant tissues.

Maturation of granulocytes is associated with a decrease in cytoplasmic basophilia as a reflection of the lower RNA content found in more mature forms [79,80]. In accord with this finding, blast cells from patients with acute leukemia have higher RNA/DNA ratios than mature granulocytes [66,80]. Granulocytes contain soluble (4 S) RNA and ribosomal RNA with sedimentation velocities of 28 S to 16 to 18 S [81,82]. A rapidly labeled RNA that has several characteristics of messenger RNA is also found in granulocytes. This material is predominantly localized in the nucleus and appears polydispersed on sucrose gradient-density ultracentrifugation [82,83]. It has been suggested that the rapidly labeled

RNA in human leukocytes is heterogeneous and that stable and unstable templates for protein synthesis may be found. Double-stranded RNA has been observed in blasts isolated from patients with acute granulocytic leukemia (AML) [84]. Polyribosomes have been isolated from normal and leukemic granulocytes [85].

Amino acids

Leukocytes readily incorporate and concentrate amino acids [86–88] and as a result the granulocyte contains several times higher concentrations of most amino acids than are found in plasma or erythrocytes [89,90], except for arginine, which is low in concentration in granulocytes [89,91]. The significance of the low levels of intracellular arginine is not known, but it may be a result of the presence of the enzyme arginase in these cells [92–94]. Leukemia cells appear to have higher levels of *o*-phosphoethanolamine, glutamic acid, and proline, but lower levels of ornithine, than normal granulocytes [91,95]. Only low levels of glycerate-3-phosphate dehydrogenase are found in normal and CML granulocytes. Since this enzyme is in the serine biosynthetic pathway, the rate of synthesis of this amino acid may be limited, giving rise to a serine requirement shown by leukocytes [95]. High levels of taurine and aminoethyl phosphate, two of the less common amino acids, have been found in leukocytes [95,97]. Increased levels of glutamic acid dehydrogenase occur in the blasts of acute leukemia or CML granulocytes [98]. Glutathione and other nonprotein sulfhydryl constituents are also present in leukocytes [99–101].

Glycogen

Blood glycogen has been found to be derived primarily from granulocytes [102]. The glycogen content of leukocytes is comparable to that in liver and muscle [103]. Methodologic differences in estimating glycogen content and the instability of this compound during leukocyte isolation [104,105] probably account for the discrepancies that are found in the literature concerning intracellular levels in various conditions. For example, sedimentation at 4°C or phagocytosis [106] may result in a decrease in leukocyte glycogen, while incubation at 37°C may result in a net increase [103].

Myeloid blast cells have little or no measurable glycogen; glycogen appears at the myelocyte stage and increases during further differentiation [102,106].

A decreased amount of leukocyte glycogen has been measured in patients with CML as compared with normal, while increased levels have been found in granulocytes of patients with myeloid metaplasia, polycythemia vera, and leukocytosis [104,107,108]. Treatment of CML patients with busulfan results in normalization of the glycogen levels [109]. Granulocyte glycogen is decreased in patients with poorly controlled diabetes [110]. Since

lymphoblasts, unlike myeloblasts, frequently have sufficient glycogen to give a positive periodic acid–Schiff reaction, this histochemical test is sometimes useful in distinguishing between acute lymphocytic leukemia (ALL) and AML [111].

Lipids

Considerable information is available on the types and quantities of lipids in rabbit [112] and human granulocytes [113,114]. About 5 percent of the wet weight of human granulocytes is lipid. Approximately 35 percent of the total lipid is phospholipid, while another one-third consists of neutral lipid, primarily triglyceride (20 percent) and free cholesterol (10 percent). Substantial amounts of glycolipid, mainly ceramide dihexoside (lactosyl ceramide), are also found, constituting about one-sixth of the total lipid content [115,116].

About two-thirds of the phospholipid content is phosphatidylcholine and phosphatidylethanolamine [114], 15 percent is sphingomyelin, and 15 percent is phosphatidylinositol. The fatty acid composition of human granulocytes differs from that of lymphocytes and shows a predominance of linoleic, palmitic, oleic, and stearic acids. In addition, small quantities of cardiolipin and lysolecithin, as well as traces of phosphatidic acid, are detectable [114]. Cholesterol is present mainly in the nonesterified form. In addition to triglycerides, small amounts of diglycerides and traces of monoglycerides have been found [114]. The methylation of phospholipids may be an early event in membrane perturbation [117]. Recent evidence suggests that two membrane methyl transferases catalyze the transfer of methyl groups from *S*-adenosylmethionine in the synthesis of phosphatidylcholine from phosphatidylethanolamine. It has been suggested that this relatively minor pathway is coupled to Ca^{2+} influx and arachidonic acid release. It may involve the transduction of membrane surface–directed stimuli to activate intracellular pathways of cyclic nucleotide and prostaglandin synthesis related to chemotaxis. Further studies, especially in the granulocyte, are needed to evaluate this interesting hypothesis. Polymorphonuclear leukocytes have about five times the lipid content of an erythrocyte but have 400 times the glycolipid content. This high concentration, coupled with the granulocyte's short life-span, accounts for the genesis of Gaucher cells, phagocytic cells laden with the glycolipid, glucocerebroside, in CGL [117] (see Chap. 99). The total lipid content of leukocytes from both CML and chronic lymphocytic leukemia (CLL) is as much as 40 percent less than that of normal mature cells of similar morphology, owing to a decrease in neutral lipid content [113]. CLL patients and CGL patients showed similar patterns. A recent report of a 50-fold increase in cholesterol synthesis in AGL over normal cells [118] requires further exploration to explain the apparent accelerated synthesis in a cell with a lower cholesterol content [119,120].

Vitamins and coenzymes

FOLIC ACID AND VITAMIN B₁₂

Leukocytes contain 60 to 123 ng of folates per milliliter of cells, as measured by microbiologic assay with *Lactobacillus casei* [121]. Decreased levels of leukocyte folates have been reported in patients with nutritional macrocytic anemia, megaloblastic anemia of pregnancy, and in some pernicious anemia patients [121,122]. In megaloblastic anemia patients, leukocyte levels correlate well with erythrocyte levels and urinary formiminoglutamic acid excretion [121]. Elevated levels of reduced folates, as measured by *Pediococcus cervisiae* and *L. casei* mcrobiologic assays, have been found in leukocytes of patients with leukemia as compared with normal leukocytes [122–129]. An intracellular folate-binding protein is found in the leukocytes from some patients with CML [130]. This high-molecular-weight protein binds folate and prevents its reduction by the enzyme dihydrofolate reductase [131].

Relatively few studies of granulocyte vitamin B₁₂ content have been performed [132,133]. The mean cell vitamin B₁₂ level in normal leukocytes is 400 pg per 10⁸ cells; no significant differences in content or binding were found in the cells of subjects with leukemia [132]. Higher ^{60}Co-vitamin B₁₂ binding was found in mature neutrophilic granulocytes than in immature granulocytes or eosinophils [106]. A high content of vitamin B₁₂–binding protein is found in the granule fraction [134].

Measurement of leukocyte levels of vitamin C is the most reliable measure of the tissue content of this vitamin [135,136]. Low levels have been observed in patients with and without clinical evidence of scurvy [137–140]. The function of ascorbic acid in the leukocyte is not known, but impaired phagocytosis and increased leukocyte fragility were noted in peritoneal guinea pig leukocytes obtained from scorbutic animals [141]. Human leukocytes take up dehydroascorbate and promptly reduce it to ascorbic acid. The reduction of dehydroascorbate results in a stimulation of hexose monophosphate shunt activity [142].

Riboflavin has been measured by microbial assay in normal and leukemic leukocytes [143]. In one study, lymphocytic leukemia cells contained only one-third to one-half as much vitamin as did granulocytic leukemia cells [144]. Levels did not correlate with leukocyte maturity. Lower levels of leukocyte riboflavin levels were measured by fluorometric methods [144–146]. Red cell riboflavin content, but not plasma or leukocyte levels, was found to decrease in experimental subjects placed on long-term riboflavin-deficient diets [145]. However, a decrease in riboflavin levels in white cells was measured in rats fed a riboflavin-deficient diet [144].

Thiamine levels of leukocytes from patients with granulocytic or lymphocytic leukemia were almost three times as high as those of normal leukocytes [147]. Decreased thiamine levels were found in both leukocytes and erythrocytes of patients with evidence of thiamine deficiency, and increased levels in these blood cells were noted after administration of the vitamin to normal persons [147].

The leukocyte pyridoxal phosphate level has been reported to be 0.30 ng per 10⁶ cells [148–151]. Lower concentrations were found in leukocytes of pregnant women at term than in nonpregnant controls [151,152]; cord-blood leukocytes showed the highest levels, indicating that the fetus can successfully compete with the mother for this important vitamin. Rats fed a diet deficient in vitamin B₆ were found to have low levels of this vitamin in tissues and leukocytes [150]. Lower-than-normal levels of pyridoxine have also been reported in patients with chronic and acute leukemia [153].

Pyridine nucleotides

The levels of oxidized and reduced pyridine nucleotides were similar in normal and leukemic cells, except that NAD levels were higher than normal in cells from patients with acute leukemia and with CGL [154].

Heparin and histamine

The metachromatic staining of the basophil and its tissue counterpart, the mast cell, is due to its heparin content [155–157]. The basophil also contains large quantities of histamine, and in normal blood it has been estimated that one-half the whole-blood histamine content is derived from the basophil, about one-third from the eosinophil, and the remaining one-sixth from all other elements [158]. Markedly elevated blood histamine levels have been measured in patients with CML; the increase is usually proportional to the basophil count [159,160]. Increased levels of histidine decarboxylase have been found in subjects with CML; some evidence also indicates that this enzyme is found primarily in the basophil [161,162]. Histamine may be released from blood cells by allergens, probably by reacting with IgE antibodies in or on the leukocyte [163]. In vitro binding of IgE to basophil receptor has been shown to stimulate phospholipid methylation, Ca²⁺ influx, and ultimately production of leukotrienes via the lipoxygenase pathway [117]. These are identical to the "slow-reacting substances" in anaphylaxis and may prove clinically relevant. Basophils lack acid hydrolases but contain the following enzymes: succinic dehydrogenase, malic dehydrogenase, lactic dehydrogenase, glucose-6-phosphate dehydrogenase, isocitric dehydrogenase, β-hydroxybutyric dehydrogenase, glutamic dehydrogenase, and NADH and NADPH diaphorase [15]. The relationship of histamine to the polymorphonuclear granulocyte is less clear, but added histamine will block granulocyte release of β-glucuronidase [164], perhaps acting via the H₂ receptors.

In addition, granulocytes contain histaminase, and this may be released following exposure of the granulocyte to the particle-bound C3b [165].

Trace metals

Leukocytes contain high levels of zinc, comparable to zinc levels in pancreatic tissue. A protein of unknown function containing 0.3 percent zinc has been extracted from leukocytes [166]. Neutrophil alkaline phosphatase contains zinc, but the level of this enzyme bears no relationship to the leukocyte zinc level. Low levels of zinc have been found in leukocytes from patients with chronic anemias and with acute and chronic leukemia, but levels were normal in subjects with polycythemia vera [166].

Copper, magnesium, cobalt, and iron have also been identified in leukocytes. The amount of iron present varied considerably from one species to another in one study [167]; human leukocytes contained very little iron. Some evidence has been presented to support the idea that the toxic granulations present in polymorphonuclear leukocytes of patients with infection are composed of hemosiderin, a consequence of active uptake of iron by leukocytes [167]. Leukocytes in AML were found to have five times the normal granulocyte ferritin content [168].

References

1. Bertino, J. R., et al.: Studies on normal and leukemic leukocytes. IV. Tetrahydrofolate-dependent enzyme systems and dihydrofolic reductase. *J. Clin. Invest.* 42:1899, 1963.
2. Fallon, M. J., Frei, E., III, Davidson, J. D., Trier, J. S., and Burke, D.: Leukocyte preparations from human blood: Evaluation of their morphologic and metabolic state. *J. Lab. Clin. Med.* 59:779, 1962.
3. Rabinowitz, Y.: Separation of lymphocytes, polymorphonuclear leukocytes and monocytes on glass columns, including tissue culture observations. *Blood* 23:811, 1964.
4. Rabinowitz, Y.: Adherence and separation of leukemic cells on glass bead columns. *Blood* 26:100, 1965.
5. Boyum, A.: Isolation of mononuclear cells and granulocytes from human blood. *Scand. J. Clin. Lab. Invest.* 21 (Suppl. 97):77, 1968.
6. Pertoft, H., Johnsson, A., Warmegard, B., and Seljelid, R.: Separation of human monocytes on density gradients of Percoll. *J. Immunol. Methods* 33:221, 1980.
7. Evans, W. H., Wolf, M. M., and Chabner, B. A.: Concentration of mature and immature granulocytes from human bone marrow. *Proc. Soc. Exp. Biol. Med.* 146:526, 1974.
8. deDuve, C., and Wattiaux, R.: Function of lysosomes. *Annu. Rev. Physiol.* 28:435, 1966.
9. Cohn, Z. A., and Hirsch, J. B.: Isolation and properties of specific cytoplasmic granules of rabbit polymorphonuclear leukocytes. *J. Exp. Med.* 112:983, 1960.
10. Bainton, D. F., and Farquhar, M. G.: Differences in enzyme content of azurophil and specific granules of polymorphonuclear leukocytes. I. Histochemical staining of bone marrow smears. *J. Cell Biol.* 39:286, 1968.
11. Bainton, D. F., and Farquhar, M. G.: Differences in enzyme content of azurophil and specific granules of polymorphonuclear leukocytes. II. Cytochemistry and electron microscopy of bone marrow cells. *J. Cell Biol.* 39:299, 1968.
12. Bainton, D. F.: Differentiation of human neutrophilic granulocytes: Normal and abnormal, in *The Granulocyte: Function and Clinical Utilization*, edited by T. J. Greenwalt and G. A. Jamieson. Alan R. Liss, New York, 1977, p. 1.
13. Baggiolini, M.: The Neutrophil, in *The Cell Biology of Inflammation*, edited by C. Weissmann. Elsevier, North-Holland, New York, 1980, p. 163.
14. Olsson, I., and Venge, P.: The role of the human neutrophil in the inflammatory reaction. *Allergy* 35:1, 1980.
15. Cline, M. J.: *The White Cell.* Harvard, Cambridge, Mass., 1975.
16. Sloan, E. P., Crawford, D. R., and Schneider, D.: Isolation of plasma membrane from human neutrophils and determination of cytochrome b and quinone contents. *J. Exp. Med.* 153:1316, 1981.
17. Pryzwansky, K. B., Martin, L. E., and Spitznagel, J. K. Immunocytochemical localization of myeloperoxidase, lactoferrin, lysozyme and neutral proteases in human monocytes and neutrophilic granulocytes. *J. Reticuloendothel. Soc.* 24:295, 1978.
18. Hayhoe, F. G. J., and Quaglino, D.: *Haematological Cytochemistry.* Churchill Livingstone, Edinburgh, 1980.
19. Schultz, J., Corlin, R., Oddi, F., Kanninker, K., and Jones, W.: Myeloperoxidase of the leukocyte of normal blood. III. Isolation of the peroxidase granule. *Arch. Biochem. Biophys.* 111:73, 1965.
20. Hirsch, J. G.: Further studies on preparation and properties of phagocytin. *J. Exp. Med.* 111:323, 1960.
21. Zeya, H. I., and Spitznagel, J. K.: Characterization of cationic protein bearing granules of polymorphonuclear leukocytes. *Lab. Invest.* 24:229, 1971.
22. Olsson, I., and Jardell, S.: Isolation and characterization of glycosaminoglycans from human leukocytes and platelets. *Biochim. Biophys. Acta* 141:348, 1967.
23. Bretz, U., and Baggiolini, M.: Biochemial and morphological characterization of azurophil and specific granules of human neutrophilic polymorphonuclear leukocytes. *J. Cell Biol.* 63:251, 1974.
24. Broxmeyer, H. E., Smithyman, A., Eger, R. R., Myers, P. A., and DeSousa, M.: Identification of lactoferrin as the granulocyte-derived inhibitor of colony-stimulating activity production. *J. Exp. Med.* 148:1052, 1978.
25. Oseas, R., Yang, H. H., Baehner, R. L., and Boxer, L. A.: Lactoferrin: A promoter of polymorphonuclear adhesiveness. *Blood* 57:939, 1981.
26. Ambruso, D. R., and Johnston, R. B., Jr.: Lactoferrin hydroxyradical production by human neutrophils, neutrophil particulate fractions, and an enzymatic generating system. *J. Clin. Invest.* 67:352, 1981.
27. Elsbach, P., Weiss, J., Franson, R. S., Beckerdite-Quagliata, S., Schneider, A., and Harris, L.: Separation and purification of the potent bactericidal/permeability increasing protein and a closely associated phospholipase A_2 from rabbit polymorphonuclear leukocytes. *J. Biol. Chem.* 254:11000, 1979.
28. Golub, E. S., and Spitznagel, J. K.: The role of lysosomes in hypersensitivity reactions: Tissue damage by PMN neutrophil lysosomes. *J. Immunol.* 95:1060, 1966.
29. Weissmann, G., Spilberg, I., and Krakauer, K.: Arthritis induced in rabbits by lysates of granulocyte lysosomes. *Arthritis Rheum.* 12:103, 1969.
30. Bieth, J.: Elastases: Structure, function and pathological role, in *Cyclic AMP and the Skin*, vol. 6: *Frontiers of Matrix Biology*, edited by J. Bieth, G. M. Collin-Lapinet, and L. Robert. Karger, Basel, 1978, p. 1–82.
31. Murphy, G., et al.: Collagenase is a component of the specific granules of human neutrophil leucocytes. *Biochem. J.* 162:195, 1977.
32. Lazarus, G. S., et al.: Role of granulocyte collagenase in collagen degradation. *Am. J. Pathol.* 68:565, 1972.
33. Ishikawa, I., and Cimason, G.: Isolation of cathepsin D from human leukocytes. *Biochim. Biophys. Acta* 480:228, 1977.
34. Wasi, S., Movat, H. Z., Pass, E., and Chan, J. Y. C.: Production, conversion and destruction of kinins by human neutrophil leukocyte proteases, in *Neutroproteases of Human Polymorphonuclear Leukocytes*, edited by K. Havemann and A. Janoff. Urban Schwarzenberg, Munich, 1978, p. 245.
35. Smolen, J. Z., and Weissmann, G.: Polymorphonuclear leukocytes, in *Arthritis*, edited by D. J. McCarthy, Lea & Fegiber, Philadelphia, 1979, p. 282.

36. Herion, J. C., Spitznagel, J. K., Walker, R. I., and Zeya, H. I.: Pyrogenicity of granulocyte lysosomes. *Am. J. Physiol. 211:*693, 1966.

37. Bodel, P. T., Wechsler, A., and Atkins, E.: Comparison of endogenous pyrogens from human and rabbit leukocytes utilizing sephadex filtration. *Yale J. Biol. Med. 41:*376, 1969.

38. Opie, E. L.: Experimental pleurisy. Resolution of a fibrinous exudate. *J. Exp. Med. 9:*391, 1967.

39. Prokopowicz, J., and Strmorken, H.: Fibrinolytic activity of leukocytes in smears of bone marrow and peripheral blood. *Scand. J. Haematol. 5:*29, 1968.

40. Zeya, H. I., and Spitznagel, J. K.: Cationic protein-bearing granules of polymorphonuclear leukocytes: Separation from enzyme-rich granules. *Science 163:*1069, 1969.

41. Goldstein, I. M., Kaplan, H. B., Edelson, H. S., and Weissmann, G.: Ceruloplasmin: A scavenger of superoxide anion radicals. *J. Biol. Chem. 254:*4040, 1979.

42. White, J. G.: Fine structural demonstration of acid phosphatase activity in Auer bodies. *Blood 29:*667, 1967.

43. Freeman, J. A.: Origin of Auer bodies. *Blood 27:*499, 1966.

44. Hanker, J. S., Laszlo, J., and Moore, J. O.: The light microscopic demonstration of hydroperoxidase-positive phi bodies and rods in leukocytes in acute myeloid leukemia. *Histochemistry 58:*241, 1978.

45. Messner, R. P., and Jelinek, J.: Receptors for human G globulin on human neutrophils. *J. Clin. Invest. 49:*2165, 1970.

46. Williams. L. T., Snyderman, R., Pike, M. C., and Lefkowitz, R. J.: Specific receptor sites for chemotactic peptides on human polymorphonuclear leukocytes. *Proc. Natl. Acad. Sci. U.S.A. 74:*1024, 1977.

47. Chenoweth, D. E., and Hugli, T. E.: Demonstration of specific C5a receptor on intact human polymorphonuclear leukocytes. *Proc. Natl. Acad. Sci. U.S.A. 75:*943, 1978.

48. Dulis, B. H., and Wilson, I. B.: The β-adrenergic receptor of line human polymorphonuclear leukocytes. *J. Biol. Chem. 255:*1043, 1980.

49. Fussganger, R. D., Kahn, R., Roth, J., and DeMeyts, P.: Binding and degradation of insulin by human peripheral granulocytes. *J. Biol. Chem. 251:*2761, 1976.

50. Crowley, C. A., et al.: An inherited abnormality of neutrophil adhesion. *N. Engl. J. Med. 302:*1163, 1980.

51. Spicer, S. S., Sato, A., Vincent, R., Eguchi, M., and Poon, K. C.: Lysosome enlargement in the Chediak-Higashi syndrome. *Fed. Proc. 40:*1451, 1980.

52. Boxer, L., and Stossel, T. P.: Interactions of actin, myosin and an actin-binding protein of chronic myelogenous leukemia leukocytes. *J. Clin. Invest. 57:*964, 1956.

53. Southwick, F. S., and Stossel, T. P.: Isolation of an inhibitor of actin polymerization from human polymorphonuclear leukocytes. *J. Biol. Chem. 256:*3030, 1981.

54. Boxer, L. A., Hedly-Whyte, E. T., and Stossel, T. P.: Neutrophil actin dysfunction and abnormal neutrophil motility. *N. Engl. J. Med. 293:*1093, 1974.

55. Babior, B. M., and Crowley, C.: Chronic granulomatous disease and other disorders of oxidative killing by phagocytes, in *The Metabolic Basis of Inherited Disease,* 5th ed., edited by J. B. Stanbury. McGraw-Hill, New York, 1981.

56. Babior, B. M., and Peters, W.: The O_2^--producing enzyme of human neutrophils. *J. Biol. Chem. 256:*2321, 1981.

57. Babior, G. L., Rosin, R. E., McMurrich, B. J., Peters, W. A., and Babior, B. M.: Arrangement of the respiratory burst oxidase in the plasma membrane of the neutrophi, *J. Clin. Invest. 67:*1724, 1981.

58. Segal, A. W., Webster, D., Jones, T. G., and Allison, A. C.: Absence of newly described neutrophils of patients with cytochrome b from chronic granulomatous disease. *Lancet 2:*446, 1978.

59. Salin, M. L., and McCord, J. M.: Superoxide dismutase in polymorphonuclear leukocytes. *Blood 54:*1005, 1974.

60. Roos, D., Weening, R. S., Syss, S. R., and Aebi, H. E. Protection of human neutrophils by endogenous catalase. *J. Clin. Invest. 65:*1515, 1980.

61. Elmes, P. C., Smith, J. D., and White, J. C.: The composition of human deoxyribonucleic acid isolated from hematopoietic and other tissues. II. *Congr. Int. Biochimie, Resume Commun.,* 1952, p. 7.

62. Garcia, A. M., and Iorio, R.: Studies on DNA in leukocytes and related cells of mammals. V. The fast green histone and the fuelgen-DNA content of rat leukocytes. *Acta Cytol. 12:*46, 1968.

63. Tedesco, T. A., and Mellman, W. J.: DNA assay as a measure of cell number in preparations from monolayer cell cultures and blood leukocytes. *Exp. Cell Res. 45:*230, 1967.

64. Mandel, P., and Metais, P.: Sur la constance de l'acide deoxy-pentose-nucleique des leukocytes chez l'homme. *Bull. Acad. Nat. Med. (Paris) 134:*449, 1950.

65. Hale, A. J., and Wilson, S. J.: The deoxyribonucleic acid content of the nucleus of leukemic leukocytes. *Lancet 1:*577, 1960.

66. Gahrton, G., and Foley, G. E.: Cytochemical population analyses of the DNA, RNA and protein content of human leukemic cells. *Acta Med. Scand. 180:*485, 1966.

67. Davidson, J. N., Leslie, J., and White, J. C.: Quantitative studies on the content of nucleic acid in normal and leukemic cells from blood and bone marrow. *J. Pathol. Bact. 63:*471, 1951.

68. Kit, S.: The nucleic acids of normal tissues and tumors, in *Amino Acids, Proteins and Cancer Biochemistry,* edited by John T. Edsall. Academic, New York, 1960, p. 147.

69. Muller, D.: Deoxyribonucleic acid determinations in the leukocytes of normal and leukemic granulopoiesis. *Klin. Wochenschr. 42:*224, 1964.

70. Sandberg, A. A., Ishihara, T., Nikuchi, Y., and Crosswhite, L. H.: Chromosomal differences among the acute leukemias. *Ann. N.Y. Acad. Sci. 113:*663, 1964.

71. Gunz, F. W., and Fitzgerald, P. H.: Chromosomes and leukemia. *Blood 23:*394, 1964.

72. DiMayorca, G., Rosenkranz, H. S., Polli, E. E., Korngold, G. C., and Bendich, A.: A chromatographic study of the deoxyribonucleic acids from normal and leukemic human tissues. *J. Natl. Cancer Inst. 24:*309, 1960.

73. Polli, E. E., Rosoff, M., DiMayorca, G., and Cavalieri, L. F.: Physico-chemical characterization of deoxyribonucleic acids from human leukemic leukocytes. *Cancer Res. 19:*159, 1959.

74. Corneo, G., Bianchi, P., Ginelli, E., and Polli, E.: Heterogeneity of base composition of DNA extracted from human leukemic leukocytes. *Eur. J. Cancer 2:*307, 1966.

75. Desai, L. S., Wulff, V. C., and Foley, G.: Human leukemic cells: Abnormal amount of methylated base in DNA. *Exp. Cell Res. 65:*260, 1971.

76. Clayton, D. A., and Vinograd, J.: Circular dimer and catenate forms of mitochondrial DNA in human leukemic leukocytes. *Nature 216:*652, 1967.

77. Clayton, D. A., and Vinograd, J.: Complex mitochondrial DNA in leukemic and normal human myeloid cells. *Proc. Natl. Acad. Sci. U.S.A. 62:*1077, 1969.

78. Paoletti, C., Riou, G., and Pairault, J.: Circular oligomers in mitochondrial DNA of human and beef non-malignant thyroid glands. *Proc. Natl. Acad. Sci. U.S.A. 69:*847, 1972.

79. Rigas, D., Duerst, M. L., Jamp, M. E., and Osgood, E. E.: The nucleic acids and other phosphorus compounds of human leukemic leukocytes: Relation to cell maturity. *J. Lab. Clin. Med. 48:*356, 1956.

80. Will, J. J., Glazon, H. S., and Vilter, R. W.: Nucleic acids, nucleases and nuclease inhibitors in leukemia, in *The Leukemias,* edited by J. W. Rebuck, F. H. Bethell, and R. W. Monto. Academic, New York, 1957, p. 417.

81. Cline, M. J: Isolation and characterization of RNA from human leukocytes. *J. Lab. Clin. Med. 68:*33, 1968.

82. Silber, R., Unger, K. W., and Ellman, L.: RNA metabolism in normal and leukaemic leukocytes: Further studies on RNA synthesis. *Br. J. Haematol. 14:*261, 1968.

83. Cline, M. J.: Ribonucleic acid biosynthesis in human leukocytes: The fate of rapidly labeled RNA in normal and abnormal leukocytes. *Blood 28:*650, 1966.

84. Torelli, V., Torelli, G., and Cadossi, R.: Double stranded ribonucleic acid in human leukemic blast cells. *Eur. J. Cancer 11:*117, 1975.

85. Tryfiates, G. P., and Laszlo, J.: Human leukemic polyribosomes. *Proc. Soc. Exp. Biol. Med. 124:*1125, 1967.

86. Baker, W. H., Zamecnik, P. C., and Stephenson, M. L.: In vitro incorporation of C^{14}DL leucine into normal and leukemic white cells. *Blood 12:*822, 1957.

87. Nadler, S. B., Hansen, H. J., Sprague, C. C., and Sherman, H.: The effect of 6-mercaptopurine on the incorporation of labelled amino acids into cellular protein of chronic granulocytic leukemia leukocytes. *Blood* 18:336, 1961.

88. Weisberger, A. S., and Levine, B.: Incorporation of radioactive L-cystine by normal and leukemic leukocytes in vitro. *Blood* 9:1082, 1954.

89. McMenamy, R. H., Lund, C. C., Neville, G. J., and Wallach, D. F. H.: Studies of unbound amino acid distribution in plasma, erythrocytes, leukocytes and urine of normal human subjects. *J. Clin. Invest.* 39:1675, 1960.

90. Okada, S., and Hayashi, T.: Studies on the amino-acid nitrogen content of the blood. *J. Biol. Chem.* 51:121, 1922.

91. McMenamy, R. H., Lund, C. C., and Wallach, D. F. H.: Unbound amino acid concentrations in plasma, erythrocytes, leukocytes and urine of patients with leukemia. *J. Clin. Invest.* 39:1688, 1960.

92. Borghetti, A., and Scarpioni, L.: Altivata arginasica dei leucocitici umani. *Enzymologia* 17:338, 1956.

93. Reynolds, J., Follette, J. H., and Valentine, W. H.: The arginase activity of erythrocytes and leukocytes with particular reference to pernicious anemia and thalassemia major. *J. Lab. Clin. Med.* 50:78, 1957.

94. Tanaka, K. R., and Valentine, W. N.: The arginase activity of human leukocytes. *J. Lab. Clin. Med.* 56:754, 1960.

95. Iyer, G. Y. N.: Free amino acids in leukocytes from normal and leukemic subjects. *J. Lab. Clin. Med.* 54:229, 1959.

96. Pizer, L. I., and Regan, J. D.: Basis for the serine requirements in leukemic and normal leukocytes: Reduced levels of the enzymes in the phosphorylated pathway. *J. Natl. Cancer Inst.* 48:1897, 1972.

97. Nour-Eldin, F., and Wilkinson, J. F.: Amino acid content of white blood cells in human leukemias. *Br. J. Haematol.* 1:358, 1955.

98. Waisman, H. A.: Some aspects of amino acid metabolism in leukemia, in *The Leukemias,* edited by J. W. Reduck, F. H. Bethell, and R. W. Monto. Academic, New York, 1957, p. 339.

99. Hardin, E. B., Valentine, W. N., Follette, J. H., and Lawrence, J. S.: Studies on the sulfhydryl content of human leukocytes and erythrocytes. *Am. J. Med. Sci.* 228:73, 1954.

100. Green, R., and Martin, S. P.: The non-protein soluble sulfhydryl content of human leukocytes and erythrocytes in infection and leukemia. *J. Lab. Clin. Med.* 45:119, 1955.

101. Contopoulos, A. N., and Anderson, H. H.: Sulfhydryl content of blood in dyscrasias. *J. Lab. Clin. Med.* 36:929, 1950.

102. Wagner, R.: The estimation of glycogen in whole blood and white blood cells. *Arch. Biochem.* 11:249, 1946.

103. Esman, V.: The glycogen content of leukocytes from diabetic and nondiabetic subjects. *Scand. J. Lab. Invest.* 13:134, 1961.

104. Valentine, W. N., Follette, J. H., and Lawrence, J. S.: The glycogen content of human leukocytes and various disease states. *J. Clin. Invest.* 32:251, 1953.

105. Bazin, S., and Avice, C.: Le Metabolisme glycogenique des polynucleases au cours de la phagocytases in vitro. *C. R. Soc. Biol. (Paris)* 147:1025, 1953.

106. Wagner, R.: Studies on the physiology of the white blood cell: The glycogen content of leukocytes in leukemia and polycythemia. *Blood* 2:235, 1947.

107. Wachstein, M.: The distribution of histochemically demonstrable glycogen in human blood and bone marrow cells. *Blood* 4:54, 1949.

108. Gahrton, G.: Glycogen synthesis in normal, leukemic and polycythemic leukocytes. *Acta Med. Scand.* 180:497, 1966.

109. Gahrton, G.: The periodic acid–Schiff reaction in neutrophil leukocytes in untreated and myleran treated chronic myelocytic leukemia: A quantitative microspectrophotometric study. *Blood* 28:554, 1966.

110. Esman, V.: The glycogen content of leukocytes from diabetic and nondiabetic patients. *Scand. J. Clin. Lab. Invest.* 13:134, 1961.

111. Quaglino, D., and Hayhoe, F. G.: Observations on the periodic acid–Schiff reaction in lymphoproliferative diseases. *J. Pathol. (London)* 78:521, 1969.

112. Elsbach, P.: Consumption and synthesis of lipids in resting and phagocytizing leukocytes. *J. Exp. Med.* 110:969, 1959.

113. Gottfried, E. L.: Lipids of human leukocytes: Relation to cell type. *J. Lipid Res.* 8:321, 1967.

114. Gottfried, E. L.: Lipid patterns of leukocytes in health and disease. *Semin. Hematol.* 9:241, 1972.

115. Miras, C. J., Mantzos, J. D., and Levis, G. M.: The isolation and partial characterization of glycolipids of normal human leukocytes. *Biochem. J.* 98:782, 1966.

116. Hildebrand, J., Stryckmans, P., and Stoffun, P.: Neutral glycolipids in leukemic and non-leukemic leukocytes. *J. Lipid Res.* 12:361, 1971.

117. Hirata, F., and Axelrod, J.: Phospholipid methylation and biological signal transmission. *Science* 209:1082, 1980.

118. Kattlove, H. E., Williams, S. C., Gaynor, E., Spivack, M., Bradley, R. M., and Brady, R. U.: Gaucher cells in chronic myelocytic leukemia, an acquired abnormality. *Blood* 33:379, 1969.

119. Heiniger, H. J., Chen, H. W., Applegate, O L., Jr., Schacter, L. P., Schacter, B. Z., and Anderson, P. N.: Elevated synthesis of cholesterol in human leukemic cells. *J. Mol. Med.* 1:109, 1976.

120. Gigante, D., Magalini, S. I., Dell'Amore, M., Mascioli, G., and Ghiucini, F.: Studies on components of normal and leukemic leukocytes. *Acta Haematol. (Basel)* 47:203, 1962.

121. Chiaroni, T., Nardi, E., and Valentine, P.: Gas-chromatography of leukocyte lipids in myeloid and lymphoid leukaemia. *Ital. J. Biochem.* 15:443, 1966.

122. Hoffbrand, A. V., and Newcomb, B. F. A.: Leukocyte folate in vitamin B_{12} and folate deficiency in leukemia. *Br. J. Haematol.* 13:954, 1967.

123. Butterworth, C. E., Nadel, H., Perez-Santiago, E., Santini, R., and Gardner, F. H. J.: Folic acid absorption, excretion and leukocyte concentration in tropical sprue. *J. Lab. Clin. Med.* 50:673, 1957.

124. Swenseid, M. E., Bethell, F. H., and Bird, O. D.: The concentration of folic acid in leukocytes: Observations on normal subjects and persons with leukemia. *Cancer Res.* 11:864, 1951.

125. Allison, R. R., and Hutchinson, D. J.: Metabolism of folic acid and citrovorum factor in leukemic cells, in *The Leukemias,* edited by J. N. Rebuck, F. H. Bethell, and R. W. Monto. Academic, New York, 1957, p. 467.

126. Bethell, F. H. and Swenseid, M. E.: The folic acid content of leukocytes: Observations on normal subjects and persons with leukemia. *J. Clin. Invest.* 25:194, 1946.

127. Rao, P. B. R., Lagerlof, B., Einhorn, J., and Reizenstein, P. G.: Folic acid activity in leukemia and cancer. *Canc. Res.* 25:221, 1967.

128. O'Brien, J. S., and Walsh, J. R.: Folinic acid activity in leukocytes. *Proc. Soc. Exp. Biol. Med.* 109:843, 1962.

129. Rosner, F., and Gabriel, F. D.: Leukocyte folate activity in patients with leukemia. *N.Y. State J. Med.* 71:2292, 1971.

130. Rothenberg, S. P.: A macromolecular factor in some leukemic cells which binds folic acid. *Proc. Soc. Exp. Biol. Med.* 133:428, 1970.

131. Rothenberg, S. P., and DaCosta, M.: Further observations on the folate-binding factor in some leukemic cells. *J. Clin. Invest.* 50:719, 1971.

132. Kidd, H. M., and Thomas, J. W.: The level of vitamin B_{12} in circulating leukemic leukocytes. *Br. J. Haematol.* 8:64, 1962.

133. Mollin, D. L., and Ross, G. I. M.: Serum vitamin B_{12} concentrations in leukemia and in some other hematological conditions. *Br. J. Haematol.* 1:155, 1955.

134. Corcino, J., Krauss, S., Waxman, S., and Herbert, V.: Release of vitamin B_{12}-binding protein by human leukocytes in vitro. *J. Clin. Invest.* 49:2250, 1970.

135. Crandon, J. H., Lennikan, R., Jr., Mikal, S., and Reif, A. E.: Ascorbic acid economy in surgical patients. *Ann. N.Y. Acad. Sci.* 92:246, 1961.

136. Crandon, T. H., Lund, C. C., and Dell, C. B.: Experimental human scurvy. *N. Engl. J. Med.* 223:353, 1940.

137. Butler, A. M., and Cushman, M.: Distribution of ascorbic acid in the blood and its nutritional significance. *J. Clin. Invest.* 19:459, 1941.

138. Lowry, O. H., Bessey, O. A., Brock, M. J., and Lopez, J. A.: The interrelationship of dietary, serum, white blood cell and total blood ascorbic acid. *J. Biol. Chem.* 166:111, 1946.

139. Steele, B. F., Liner, F. R., Pierce, Z. H., and Williams, H. H.: Content of ascorbic acid in the white cells of human subjects receiving controlled low intakes of the vitamin. *Fed. Proc.* 12:430, 1953.

140. Williamson, J. M., Goldberg, A., and Moore, F. M. L.: Leukocyte ascorbic acid levels in patients with malabsorption of previous gastric surgery. *Br. J. Med.* 2:23, 1967.

141. Nangester, W. J., and Ames, A. M.: The relationship between ascorbic acid and phagocytic activity. *J. Infect. Dis. 83:*50, 1948.

142. Bigley, R. H., and Stankota, L.: Uptake and reduction of oxidized and reduced ascorbate by human leukocytes. *J. Exp. Med. 139:*1084, 1974.

143. Prager, M. D., Malicky, M., Goemer, M., and Hill, H. M.: Riboflavin activity in normal and leukemic human leukocytes and nuclei. *J. Lab. Clin. Med. 53:*926, 1959.

144. Burch, H. B., Bessey, O. A., and Lowry, O. H.: Fluorometric measurements of riboflavin and its natural derivatives in small quantities of blood serum and cells. *J. Biol. Chem. 175:*457, 1948.

145. Bessey, O. A., Howitt, M. K., and Love, R. H.: Dietary deprivation of riboflavin and blood riboflavin levels in man. *J. Nutr. 58:*367, 1956.

146. Fujita, A., and Yamadori, M.: Distribution of thiamine and riboflavin in components of blood. *Arch. Biochem. Biophys. 28:*94, 1950.

147. Gorham, A. T., Abels, J. C., Robins, A. L., and Rhoads, C. P.: The measurement and metabolism of thiamin and of a pyrimidine stimulating yeast fermentation found in the blood cells and urine of normal individuals. *J. Clin. Invest. 21:*161, 1942.

148. Donald, E. A., and Ferguson, R. F.: A micromethod for determination of pyridoxal phosphate in leukocytes and liver. *Ann. Biochem. 7:*335, 1964.

149. Boxer, G.-E., Pruss, M. P., and Goodhart, R. S.: Pyridoxal 5-phosphoric acid in whole blood and isolated leukocytes of man and animals. *J. Nutr. 63:*623, 1957.

150. Wachstein, M., and Moore, C.: Pyridoxal phosphate levels in organs, leukocytes and blood of rats with developing vitamin B_6 deficiency. *Proc. Soc. Exp. Biol. Med. 97:* 905, 1958.

151. Wachstein, M., Moore, C., and Graffeo, L. W.: Pyridoxal phosphate levels of circulating leukocytes in maternal and cord blood. *Proc. Soc. Exp. Biol. Med. 96:*326, 1957.

152. Wachstein, M., Kellner, J. D., and Ortiz, J. M.: Pyridoxal phosphate in plasma and leukocytes of normal and pregnant subjects following B_6 load tests. *Proc. Soc. Exp. Biol. Med. 103:*350, 1960.

153. Wachstein, M., Kellner, J. D., and Ortiz, J. M.: Pyridoxal phosphate in patients with leukemia and other diseases. *Proc. Soc. Exp. Biol. Med. 105:*563, 1960.

154. Silber, R., Gabrio, B. W., and Huennekens, F. M.: Studies on normal and leukemic leukocytes. III. Pyridine nucleotides. *J. Clin. Invest. 41:*230, 1962.

155. Jorpes, E., Odelblad, E., and Bostrom, H.: An autoradiographic study on the uptake of S^{35}-labelled sodium sulphate in the mast cells. *Acta Haematol. 9:*273, 1953.

156. Mauri, C., and Soldati, M.: Les Caractéristiques cytochimiques des granulations cellulaires, de Alder. *Schweiz, Med. Wochenschr. 88:*992, 1958.

157. Parekh, A. C., and Glick, D.: Heparin and hexosamine in isolated mast cells: Determination, intracellular distribution and effects of biological state. *J. Biol. Chem. 237:*280, 1962.

158. Graham, H. T., Lowry, O. H., Wheelright, F., Lenz, M. A., and Parish, H. H., Jr.: Distribution of histamine among leukocytes and platelets. *Blood 10:*467, 1955.

159. Valentine, W. N., Pearce, M. L., and Lawrence, J. S.: Studies on the histamine content of blood with special reference to leukemia, leukemoid reactions and leukocytosis. *Blood 5:*623, 1950.

160. Valentine, W. N., Lawrence, J. S., Pearce, M. L., and Beck, W. S.: The relationship of the basophil to blood histamine in man. *Blood 10:*154, 1955.

161. Gingold, N.: The blood histamine level in the differential and early diagnosis of chronic myeloid leukemia. *Wien. Z. Inn. Med. 49:*180, 1968.

162. Hartman, W. J., Clark, W. G., and Cyr, S. S.: Histidine decarboxylase activity of basophils from chronic myelogenous leukemia patients: Origin of blood histamine. *Proc. Soc. Exp. Biol. Med. 107:* 123, 1961.

163. Ishizaka, T., Ishizaka, K., Johansson, S. G. O., and Bennich, H.: Histamine release from human leukocytes and anti-αE antibodies. *J. Immunol. 102:*884, 1969.

164. Busse, W. W., and Sosman, J., Histamine inhibition of neutrophil lysosomal enzyme release: An H-2 histamine receptor response. *Science 194:*737, 1976.

165. Herman, J. J., Rosner, I. K., Davis A. E., III, Zeigler, R. S., Arnaout, M. A., and Lolten, M. R.: Complement-dependent histaminase release from human granulocytes. *J. Clin. Invest. 63:*1195, 1979.

166. Fredricks, R. E., Tanaka, R. K., and Valentine, W. N.: Variations of human blood cell zinc in disease. *J. Clin. Invest. 43:*304, 1964.

167. Koszewski, B. J., Vahabzedeh, H., and Willrodt, B. S.: Hemosiderin content of leukocytes in animals and man and its significance in the physiology of granulocytes. *Am. J. Clin. Pathol. 48:*474, 1967.

168. Worwood, M., Summers, M., Miller, F., Jacobs, A., and Whittaker, J. A.: Ferritin in blood cells from normal subjects and patients with leukaemia. *Br. J. Haematol. 28:*27, 1974.

CHAPTER 82

Metabolism of neutrophils

ROBERT SILBER
CHARLES F. MOLDOW

The metabolism of granulocytes has been of interest to investigators since the beginning of the twentieth century. Human blood leukocytes have been used to verify biochemical pathways that had been discovered in microbial or animal systems. Granulocyte metabolism has been studied also to explore differences between normal and leukemic cells that could be exploited in chemotherapy or that might aid in the identification of cell types. The granulocytic series of leukemic subjects has been a source of homogeneous populations of precursor cells with which to compare intermediate or fully mature forms. Such comparison has yielded some information about the sequence in which pathways are activated and disappear as the myeloblast matures to the segmented granulocyte. Finally, the granulocyte can be used for enzyme assay to detect defects that may identify genetic disorders.

Biosynthetic reactions in granulocyte cell replication

DNA SYNTHESIS

The polymerization of deoxyribonucleotides into DNA is catalyzed by DNA polymerase. This enzyme is most active in immature forms of leukocytes [1]. Activity diminishes with cell maturation and is barely detectable in mature granulocytes. The increased DNA polymerase activity in granulocytes from patients with chronic myelogenous leukemia (CML) [2] is expected in view of the immaturity of leukemic cells. The DNA polymerase level of circulating CML cells is about tenfold that of marrow cells from patients with benign granulocytic hyperplasia. Two distinct types of DNA-dependent DNA-polymerase, α and β, with M_r 50,000 and 200,000 daltons, respectively, have been demonstrated in human granulocytes [3]. The high-molecular-weight cytoplasmic enzyme is 10 to 20 times as active in myeloblasts as in mature granulocytes. No significant increase in the activity of the low-molecular-weight nuclear enzyme in myeloblasts has been found. An increased rate of methylation of RNA and DNA has been found in acute leukemia (AL) and CML cells [4]. This may be correlated with an increased level of S-adenosylmethionine, which is the methyl donor for this reaction [5].

The results of studies utilizing tritiated thymidine [6,7] are consistent with the decline in DNA polymerase activity observed during granulocyte maturation. The myelocyte is the most mature granulocyte precursor that can still incorporate thymidine into DNA and undergo mitosis [6,7]. It is uncertain what changes result in the decreased mitotic potential.

Terminal deoxynucleotidyltransferase is an enzyme that catalyzes the polymerization of deoxyribonucleotides on the 3' hydroxyl ends of oligo- or polydeoxyribonucleotides in the absence of a DNA template. This enzyme has been detected and characterized in some leukemic cells [8,9], and high levels of activity, normally unique to the thymus, have been detected in cells from patients with acute lymphoblastic leukemia (ALL) [8] and from patients in the lymphoblastic phase of CML [9]. The finding of this enzyme in these disorders provides some biochemical support for the suggestion that thymus-derived lymphoid cells proliferate in these disorders. Very low levels of terminal deoxynucleotidyltransferase are found in normal marrow and in other leukemias with definite myeloid markers.

The biochemical mechanisms underlying the life cycle of RNA tumor viruses have been extensively documented in animal systems and involve the following enzymatic reactions: The information from tumor virus 70 S RNA is transcribed into complementary DNA by reverse transcriptase, an enzyme present in RNA tumor viruses [10,11]. The low-molecular-weight DNA is first found in a double-stranded form [12] as a DNA-RNA hybrid in which the newly formed complementary DNA is covalently linked to the primer RNA. Another enzyme, ribonuclease H, hydrolyzes the RNA strand of the hybrid. The remaining DNA strand is converted to a double-stranded DNA form by cellular polymerases and is incorporated as a stable heritable component of the cellular genome that codes for the synthesis of more virus. Certain biochemical properties of human leukemic leukocytes suggest that infection with RNA tumor viruses may have occurred. Reverse transcriptase has been detected in leukocytes of patients with acute and chronic leukemias [13–15]. The enzyme has been purified from leukocytes of patients with acute myelogenous leukemia (AML) and from the spleen of a patient with chronic lymphocytic leukemia (CLL) [14,16].

It has a molecular weight of 70,000 daltons and can be distinguished from normal DNA polymerases by its catalytic properties. Immunologic studies suggest an antigenic relationship to the reverse transcriptase of woolly monkey and gibbon tumor virus [17,18]. Reverse transcriptase activity had not been detected in normal marrow, blood leukocytes, or phytohemagglutinin-stimulated cells, but more recent studies suggest the need for a very critical interpretation of these results [19].

The data showing retrovirus-associated activities in malignant tissue must be regarded cautiously, since these viruses code for a transformation or sarcoma-specific protein that is a protein kinase capable of phosphorylating tyrosine residues of cellular proteins [20]. Analysis of noninfected mammalian cells reveals the presence of cellular DNA and mRNA that code for this protein [21]. In addition, low levels of a cellular protein with this same activity may be found in normal cells [22]. Therefore, genetic information responsible for the transformed phenotype is present in normal cells and may serve developmental function(s).

A cytoplasmic particulate fraction that sediments with the buoyant density of RNA tumor viruses containing 70 S RNA has been detected in leukemic cells [15]. The reverse transcriptase activity in this fraction is associated with a high-molecular-weight 70 S RNA like that characteristic of RNA tumor viruses [13]. With the technique of molecular hybridization, it has been possible to show that the RNA from human leukemic cells but not from normal cells contains sequences related to simian RNA tumor virus and also to a lesser extent to murine RNA tumor viruses [23,24]. Such "leukemia-specific" sequences have also been detected in DNA from leukocytes of leukemic patients but not from those of normal subjects [25]. The absence of these sequences from the DNA of leukocytes from the healthy identical twin of a leukemic patient suggested an acquired nature of the lesion [26]. The presence of a p30 protein that is associated with RNA tumor virus in animal systems was detected by radioimmunoassay of the leukocytes from five patients with AML. The protein is generally a constituent of RNA tumor viruses and is coded for by viral RNA [27].

Evidence for the persistence of the reverse transcriptase template complex in the circulating leukocytes of most patients with acute leukemia in remission has been reported [28]. Two RNA tumor viruses containing reverse transcriptase with characteristics similar to that of woolly monkey and baboon viruses have been isolated from human leukemic marrow cultures [29,30]. Similar particles have also been found in nonleukemic tissues [31]. To date, conclusive evidence for a human leukemia virus is lacking. Recent "virus-like" isolates from leukocytes obtained from a patient with cutaneous T-cell lymphoma have rekindled hopes for the identification of a retrovirus specific for human neoplasia [32] (see Chap. 120).

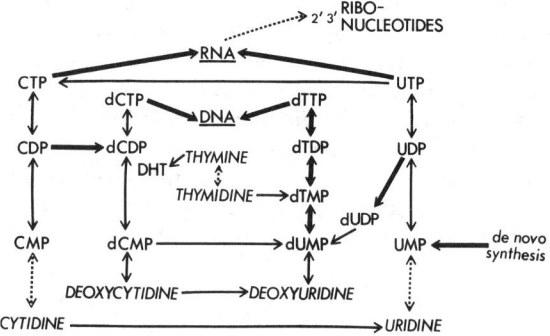

FIGURE 82-1   Pyrimidine interconversions in human granulocytes. The reactions that have been demonstrated to be increased in immature (leukemic) cells are indicated with heavy arrows, while reactions whose rates are diminished are shown with broken arrows. The salvage pathways that include nucleosides and free bases are also shown. Abbreviations and their meanings are as follows: CTP, cytidine triphosphate; CDP, cytidine diphosphate; CMP, cytidine monophosphate; dCTP, deoxycytidine triphosphate; dCDP, deoxycytidine diphosphate; dCMP, deoxycytidine monophosphate; DHT, dihydrothymine; dTTP, deoxythymidine triphosphate; dTDP, deoxythymidine diphosphate; dTMP, deoxythymidine monophosphate; dUMP, deoxyuridine monophosphate; dUDP, deoxyuridine diphosphate; UTP, uridine triphosphate; UDP, uridine diphosphate; UMP, uridine monophosphate; RNA, ribonucleic acid; DNA, deoxyribonucleic acid.

RNA SYNTHESIS

Despite the numerous technical difficulties that complicate the isolation of RNA from human granulocytes [30,33–37], the following evidence indicates that RNA synthesis is directed by DNA in normal leukocytes: (1) annealing experiments indicate a significant degree of complementarity between leukocyte RNA and DNA [35]; (2) the synthesis of RNA is sensitive to inhibition by low concentrations of actinomycin D; and (3) the RNA of human leukocytes, unlike the double-stranded product of RNA-directed RNA synthesis, is sensitive to the hydrolytic action of ribonuclease [37]. Double-stranded RNA has been reported to be present in human leukocytes, but confirmation of this potentially important finding is needed [38].

The rate of RNA synthesis has been explored by a variety of approaches. Early studies relied heavily on radioautography after incubation of cells with tritium-labeled nucleosides. More recently, the incorporation of radioactivity into RNA has been determined after sucrose density-gradient ultracentrifugation, a procedure that separates ribosomal and soluble RNA. Cells from patients with CML, CLL, and AML manifested ¹⁴C-uridine incorporation up to five times that of normal granulocytes or lymphocytes [37]. However, considerable heterogeneity was found among leukemic cells, with appreciable overlap into the normal range. It seems likely that the increase in RNA synthesis reflects cell immaturity and is not specific for leukemia, since similar increases have been found in infectious mononucleosis

cells [35]. Efforts to document RNA-directed RNA synthesis in human leukemic cells have thus far been unsuccessful.

PROTEIN SYNTHESIS

Mature granulocytes and granulocyte precursors incorporate labeled amino acids into protein. Leukocytes in AL and CML exhibit a more rapid incorporation of radioactive amino acids than do normal leukocytes [38–41]. The in vitro incorporation of ¹⁴C-leucine or ¹⁴C-alanine into the leukocyte proteins was about six times greater in blasts from patients with acute leukemia than in normal circulating leukocytes; circulating CML and CLL cells have intermediate values [42]. A reduction in the uptake of tritiated leucine appears to occur with maturation of normal marrow elements [43]. This observation suggests that the persistence of a high level of amino acid incorporation in the leukemic cells may be a reflection of their failure to mature.

NUCLEOTIDE BIOSYNTHESIS

PYRIMIDINES

Leukocytes are capable of *de novo* biosynthesis of pyrimidines. Aspartate carbamyltransferase, dihydroorotase, dihydroorotic dehydrogenase, and orotidylic decarboxylase, enzymes catalyzing pyrimidine biosynthesis, are found in normal leukocytes (predominantly granulocytes) [44]. A two- to tenfold increase in the activities of the first three of these enzymes was found in CML. In general, the increased activity paralleled morphologic immaturity [45]. As shown in Fig. 82-1, in addition to *de novo* synthesis, ribo- and deoxyribonucleotides can also be formed via the "salvage" pathway through the kinase-catalyzed interaction of ATP with nucleosides and deoxynucleosides (cytidine, uridine, deoxycytidine, deoxyuridine, and thymidine). CML granulocytes show a striking increase of thymidine kinase activity in comparison with normal leukocytes [46]. This reaction is competitively inhibited by dTMP, dTDP, dTTP, and dCTP to the same extent as with enzyme preparations obtained from normal or leukemic cells [47]. The activity of dTMP kinase is higher than that of thymidine kinase [48]. A pyrimidine deoxyribosyltransferase in granulocytes catalyzes the transfer of a deoxyribosyl group to the base thymine [49]. The activity of this enzyme in CML leukocytes is approximately 50 percent of normal, even when patients are in hematologic remission with a normal proportion of mature granulocytes in the peripheral blood [50]. The nucleotides undergo a number of enzymatic interconversions that are subject to feedback regulation by the end products. The activity of many, but not all, of the enzymes catalyzing these reactions is greater in immature leukemic granulocytes. Thymidylate synthase activity, for instance, is markedly increased in CML cells [51], while the level of deoxycytidylate deaminase in CML and AML cells is comparable to that in normal leukocytes. Thymidylate synthase is present in normal marrow, suggesting that its detection in leukemia is only a manifestation of cell immaturity [52]. Deoxycytidylate deaminase is subject to allosteric regulation by dCTP, which acts as a positive effector, and dTTP, which functions as a negative effector [53]. This enzyme is distinct from the cytidine and deoxycytidine deaminase activities found in granulocytes [53]. Cytidine deaminase catalyzes the deamination of the drug, cytosine arabinoside [54]. Deoxycytidine kinase activity has also been detected and purified from granulocytes. The activity of this enzyme decreases and that of cytidine deaminase increases with maturation of granulocytes [55]. There is a lower level of adenosine deaminase in myeloblasts than in lymphoblasts. This enzyme is inhibited by deoxycoformycin, an agent that has been used in the treatment of AL.

The conversion of ribonucleotides to deoxyribonucleotides takes place at an extremely low rate in hemopoietic tissue. The enzyme that catalyzes this reaction has not been detected in normal granulocytes, but low levels of activity have been found in cells from patients with CML and CL [56]. The ribonucleotide diphosphates serve as the preferred substrate for the reduction. There appears to be no stimulation by 5'-deoxyadenosyl B_{12} [57]. In this respect, the human system resembles its counterpart in *Escherichia coli* rather than the vitamin B_{12}–dependent enzyme in *Lactobacillus leichmannii*. The ribonucleotide reductase is subjected to a complex interplay of ribonucleotides and deoxyribonucleotides, which function as positive or negative allosteric effectors to regulate the deoxyribonucleotide levels in cells. Hydroxyurea, a drug that rapidly lowers the white blood cell count in AL and CML, is an inhibitor of ribonucleotide reductase. The concentration of the four deoxyribonucleotide triphosphates in the marrow of patients with AML or CML was found to be three times that in normal marrow [58].

PURINES

The early failure to demonstrate glycine-^{14}C incorporation into the acid-insoluble nucleotide pool in normal or leukemic leukocytes suggested that, in contradistinction to their ability to carry on pyrimidine biosynthesis *de novo*, these cells are incapable of the earlier steps of purine synthesis [59]. Other reports, however, indicate that some *de novo* synthesis of purine nucleotides occurs in human blood leukocytes [60]. The capacity of the human leukocyte to incorporate preformed adenine and guanine into acid-soluble nucleotides and nucleic acids may offer an additional source of purines. Each of these bases can be converted into the other [61]. Purine precursors may be synthesized in the liver and transported to marrow in the blood [62]. Enzymes of the purine salvage pathway are present in granulocytes. Significant elevations of the adenine and of the hypoxanthine-guanine phosphoribosyltransferase activities have been described in AL [63]. An altered ratio of this transferase and adenine phosphoribosyltransferase, which may impair thiopurine nucleotide synthesis, has been reported

in 23 percent of patients resistant to this type of antimetabolite [64]. This may be an example of drug resistance resulting from deletion of an enzyme.

FOLATE METABOLISM

Coenzyme forms of folic acid donate the 1-carbon units that are incorporated into the 2 and 8 positions of the purine skeleton. A folate coenzyme also participates in the formation of the methyl group of thymine. These biosynthetic functions, and the use of folate antagonists in the chemotherapy of leukemia, have stimulated many investigations of folic acid metabolism in leukocytes. Several folate-dependent enzymes are present in granulocytes. These include (1) formate-activating enzymes, (2) N^5,N^{10}-methylene tetrahydrofolate dehydrogenase, and (3) serine hydroxymethylase. The activities of the first two enzymes are somewhat elevated in CGL and AL leukocytes [65]. A fourth enzyme, dihydrofolate reductase, which catalyzes the reduction of folate to the coenzyme form, tetrahydrofolate, is of particular interest since it is the target protein for the folic acid antagonists. Only a trace of dihydrofolate reductase activity is detectable in normal granulocytes or lymphocytes, while higher levels are found in CGL or CLL cells. Paradoxically, the administration of folic acid antagonists to patients with leukemia or normal subjects results in a striking increase in the activity of dihydrofolate reductase [66]. This "induction" was originally thought to be related to stabilization of the enzyme by the inhibitor, but according to recent evidence, it results from amplifaction of the dihydrofolate reductase gene [67]. The selective amplification of this gene leads to an increased level of specific messenger RNA and the elevated enzyme content. Other mechanisms of resistance to folic antagonists that have been found are a decrease in the transport of methotrexate and the formation of an enzyme with an altered K_m [68]. Recently, the presence of methionine synthetase, which catalyzes the vitamin B_{12}–dependent transfer of the methyl group from 5-methyl tetrahydrofolate to homocysteine has been demonstrated in AML, ALL, and CLL cells [69,70]. Only trace levels of this enzyme were found in normal granulocytes or lymphocytes. The activity or methylmalonyl-CoA mutase is diminished in leukocytes from patients with pernicious anemia [71] but can be restored to normal by the addition of vitamin B_{12}.

CATABOLISM OF NUCLEIC ACIDS AND PROTEINS

Although the role of nucleases in the physiologic degradation of nucleic acids has not been fully clarified, the presence of ribonuclease and deoxyribonuclease in lysosomal granules of leukocytes [72,73] suggests that these organelles are involved in the breakdown of exogenous or, perhaps, endogenous nucleic acids. Ribonuclease has been quantitated and characterized in human leukocytes [74]. The enzyme activity is 10 times higher in mature granulocytes than in blast forms. Intermediate levels of activity are found in CML cells. A ribonuclease specific for the RNA strand of RNA-DNA hybrid molecules has been purified from AML leukocytes [75]. In addition, nucleotidases [76], several isoenzymes of acid phosphatase [77], and a nucleoside deaminase have been described [53]. Unlike lymphocytes, mature granulocytes contain only very low levels of 5'-nucleotidase and adenosine deaminase activity. The catabolic reduction of thymine to dihydrothymine also occurs in granulocytes. While dihydrothymine may be converted to β-ureidoisobutyric acid by granulocytes, it is probable that the subsequent steps in pyrimidine degradation occur in liver or kidney [78].

One of the most extensively investigated granulocyte enzymes is leukocyte alkaline phosphatase (LAP). Although the in vivo function of LAP remains uncertain, the assay of this activity has found many clinical applications. The marked decrease in LAP activity observed in patients with CML has been thoroughly documented [79]. Histochemical studies show that this decrease is found even more in the mature granulocytes in this disorder. The striking elevation in activity observed in normal granulocytes after the administration of glucocorticoids does not occur in CML granulocytes. Although a decrease in LAP activity is one of the hallmarks of CML, exceptions have been found in patients with otherwise classic CML. During remission, the LAP activity usually returns toward normal. Lower levels of LAP have also been described in paroxysmal nocturnal hemoglobinuria, idiopathic thrombocytopenic purpura, infectious mononucleosis, aplastic anemia, and in some patients with sarcoidosis, granulocytopenia, and myeloid metaplasia [80]. Low levels of LAP are also found in some patients with AML [81] or with monocytic leukemia [82].

LAP is a phosphomonoesterase with a pH optimum near 10 [83]. It catalyzes the hydrolysis of a wide variety of phosphoester substrates. The enzyme contains zinc [84]. LAP activity is limited to the neutrophilic granulocyte series. LAP activity first appears in myelocytes and rapidly increases with maturation of the cell to the segmented polymorphonuclear granulocyte [85]. Glucocorticoids markedly increase the activity in normal leukocytes, probably by induction of the enzyme, which may explain the high LAP activity observed during infections [86].

A report that the LAP in CML cells differed in electrophoretic mobility from that in normal granulocytes [87] was not confirmed in a subsequent study [88]. The results of the latter study, which combined enzymatic and immunologic methods, suggested that the enzyme protein present in CML cells had a lower specific activity than that in normal cells. A more recent investigation, however, found no evidence that CML granulocytes contain a large amount of antigenically reactive but enzymatically defective alkaline phosphatase [89]. The conclusion was reached that CML granulocytes have a decreased enzyme content rather than a catalytically defective enzyme. The mechanism of reduction of LAP activity in CML cells is still not clear but may reflect the impaired synthesis in the leukemic cell.

ENERGY METABOLISM

CARBOHYDRATE METABOLISM
Granulocyte energetics have attracted considerable interest because of their bearing on the phagocytic progress, and glycolysis has been intensively investigated, since an abnormal response in this pathway is a key feature of Warburg's theory of neoplasia (see below) [90,91].

GLYCOLYSIS AND RESPIRATION
Early in vitro studies on isolated leukocytes demonstrated that polymorphonuclear granulocytes utilize oxygen [92]. Oxygen consumption by granulocytes is influenced by a wide variety of physiologic and pathologic stimuli [93]. In addition to phagocytosis (see next chapter), these include thyroid hormone [94], CO_2 tension [95], glucose concentration [96], serum [97], pyrogens [98], complement components, chemotactic peptides, and immune complexes [99]. A number of chemicals depress granulocyte respiration, including saponin, thiouracil, chloramphenicol, cyanide, fluoracetate, malonate, and p-hydroxymercuribenzoate. Other compounds, such as ascorbic acid and dinitrophenol, increase O_2 consumption [93]. The main energy-producing pathway in the granulocyte is glycolysis, resulting in the conversion of glucose to lactate. In normal or leukemic leukocytes, glycolysis is only slightly decreased in the presence of oxygen, suggesting that the Pasteur effect is not fully operative in these cells. Warburg [100] had observed that the Pasteur effect—the inhibition of glycolysis under aerobic conditions—was greatly diminished in tumor tissue, and he postulated that the absence of a Pasteur effect was an essential characteristic of tumors. Normal granulocytes constituted the first exception to this theory. Although it was suggested that the high rate of aerobic glycolysis observed in leukocytes stemmed from injuries incurred during their isolation and that therefore the cell's behavior did not constitute an exception to the theory, no conclusive evidence for such injury was supplied. Other normal tissues that do not manifest the Pasteur effect have since been found [90].

When intact or homogenized leukocytes are incubated with glucose uniformly labeled with ^{14}C, about 80 percent of the radioactivity is recovered in lactic acid. Lactic acid production by mature leukocytes (mainly granulocytes) is more than three times that of CML cells. Hexokinase is the rate-limiting enzyme of glycolysis in both normal and leukemic cells [101]. The specific activity of the enzymes catalyzing the individual reactions is roughly proportional to the levels of aerobic glycolysis in leukemic and normal cells, with three exceptions: the activities of phosphohexose isomerase, aldolase, and triose phosphate isomerase are similar in CML and normal cells. The activity of the remainder of the enzymes (hexokinase, phosphofructokinase, glyceraldehyde-3-phosphate dehydrogenase, pyruvate kinase, and lactic dehydrogenase) is significantly reduced in CML cells.

Studies of maximum velocities, Michaelis constants, and pH responses revealed no differences between the enzymes isolated from normal and from leukemic cells. In both cell types, the glucose metabolized via the hexose monophosphate shunt amounted to less than 5 percent of the total glucose consumed. In CML leukocytes, the activity of several enzymes in this pathway, glucose-6-phosphate dehydrogenase, 6-phosphogluconate dehydrogenase, and transketolase, is about two-fifths that in normal leukocytes, while the phosphopentose isomerase level is identical in both.

Cyclic 3',5'-adenosine monophosphate (cAMP) is present in the human granulocyte. This "second messenger" is involved in the activation of leukocyte glycogen phosphorylase. The synthesis of cAMP is catalyzed by adenyl cyclase and its degradation by cAMP phosphodiesterase, both of which are found in normal granulocytes [102]. The accumulation of cAMP in the leukocyte is stimulated by epinephrine, prostaglandin E, and adenyl cyclase [103]. The cytosol of granulocytes contains a protein kinase that is stimulated by cAMP. These cells also contain histone phosphatases, which dephosphorylate the product of the protein kinase reaction [104]. A reduced responsiveness of β-receptor function for isoproterenol (Isuprel) in leukocytes of patients suffering from acute bronchial asthma has been reported [105,106]. In asthmatic patients in remission, this response was within normal limits [107].

OTHER PATHWAYS OF CARBOHYDRATE METABOLISM
Few mitochondria are found in mature granulocytes [108]. The tricarboxylic acid cycle and oxidative phosphorylation, therefore, although present [109], may play only a minor part in granulocyte energy production. This concept is supported by the finding that intracellular ATP levels are more sensitive to inhibitors of glycolysis than to inhibitors of respiration [110]. Although less than 5 percent of the glucose carbon chain is oxidized to CO_2 by the citric acid cycle, the following tricarboxylic acid cycle enzymes have been detected in leukocytes: isocitric dehydrogenase, aconitase, fumarase, and malic dehydrogenase [111–113]. The activities of isocitric dehydrogenase, aspartate aminotransferase, and alanine aminotransferase in blasts from AML are twice as high as those in normal granulocytes [114]. In general, the activity of these enzymes is higher in the immature leukemic cells. Definitive evidence bearing on the relative contributions of glycolysis and oxidative respiration to the production of ATP in vivo is not available. The four enzymes necessary for gluconeogenesis were not detected in leukocytes.

Granulocytes contain the bulk of the glycogen found in leukocytes [115]. Most of the glycogen arises from glucose. There is little net synthesis from substrates at the triose phosphate level. Galactose, mannose, and fructose can be metabolized by leukocytes [116]. Glycogen content decreases when these cells are deprived of glucose, but resynthesis occurs when adequate glucose is added [117]. Glycogen first appears in myelocytes and increases with cell maturation [118]. Cell glycogen is low in CML leukocytes but high in the leukocytes of granulocytosis due to infection and polycythemia vera [119]. Leukocytes metabolize propionate via propionyl-CoA carboxylase and methylmalonyl-CoA isomerase. An alternative metabolic route involving acrylyl-CoA has been described in leukocytes from patients with pernicious anemia [120]. Glycogen synthesis and glycolysis are diminished in leukocytes from diabetic subjects [121]. Galactose 1-phosphate uridylyltransferase activity was high in leukocytes from patients with ALL and somewhat elevated in cells from patients with CML [122].

Mucopolysaccharides have been identified in human leukocytes [123]. Their biosynthesis and degradation have not been studied in detail. Sulfation of mucopolysaccharide was about 50 percent of the normal level in cells from CML and approximately 15 percent of normal in AML or CML cells in blast crisis [124]. Lysozyme, also known as muramidase, a low-molecular-weight enzyme that depolymerizes certain polysaccharides, is found in granulocytes and monocytes. Markedly increased quantities of lysozyme are found in the plasma and urine of patients with acute monocytic or myelomonocytic leukemia. Moderate elevations are found in CML, while normal levels are found in AML [125]. The activity in ALL may actually be subnormal. Lysozyme activity increases with cellular maturity. Most of the enzyme in plasma and urine is the result of leukocyte breakdown and hence may provide some indication of leukocyte turnover [126]. It has been suggested that the serum lysozyme level in leukemia may correlate with the clinical activity of the disease [127], but some studies have failed to note this relationship [128]. Alterations in the catalase pattern of leukemia granulocytes have been reported: an abnormal antigen (α) with anodal migration appears in CML leukocytes, and the β antigen, which has a cathodal migration and is found in leukocytes from patients with inflammatory disease, is not detectable [129]. The levels of glutathione peroxidase in CML are comparable to those in normal granulocytes.

LIPID METABOLISM
Early studies revealed that lipid biosynthesis, as indicated by the incorporation of ^{14}C-acetate, occurs in normal and leukemic granulocytes. Two-thirds of the radioactivity is incorporated into the neutral lipids and the remainder into phospholipids [130]. Recent investigations using purer cell preparations have shown that PMN, unlike mononuclear cells, incorporated [2-^{14}C]-acetate or [2-^{14}C]mevalonate into squalene but not into sterols [131]. When ^{32}P was administered therapeutically to patients with CML, it was rapidly incorporated into lecithin, phosphatidylethanolamine, phosphatidylserine, inositol phosphatide, and sphingomyelin [132]. The phosphatidic acid pathway incorporating fatty acids into neutral lipids is operative in these cells [133]. The major phospholipids are also synthesized by the

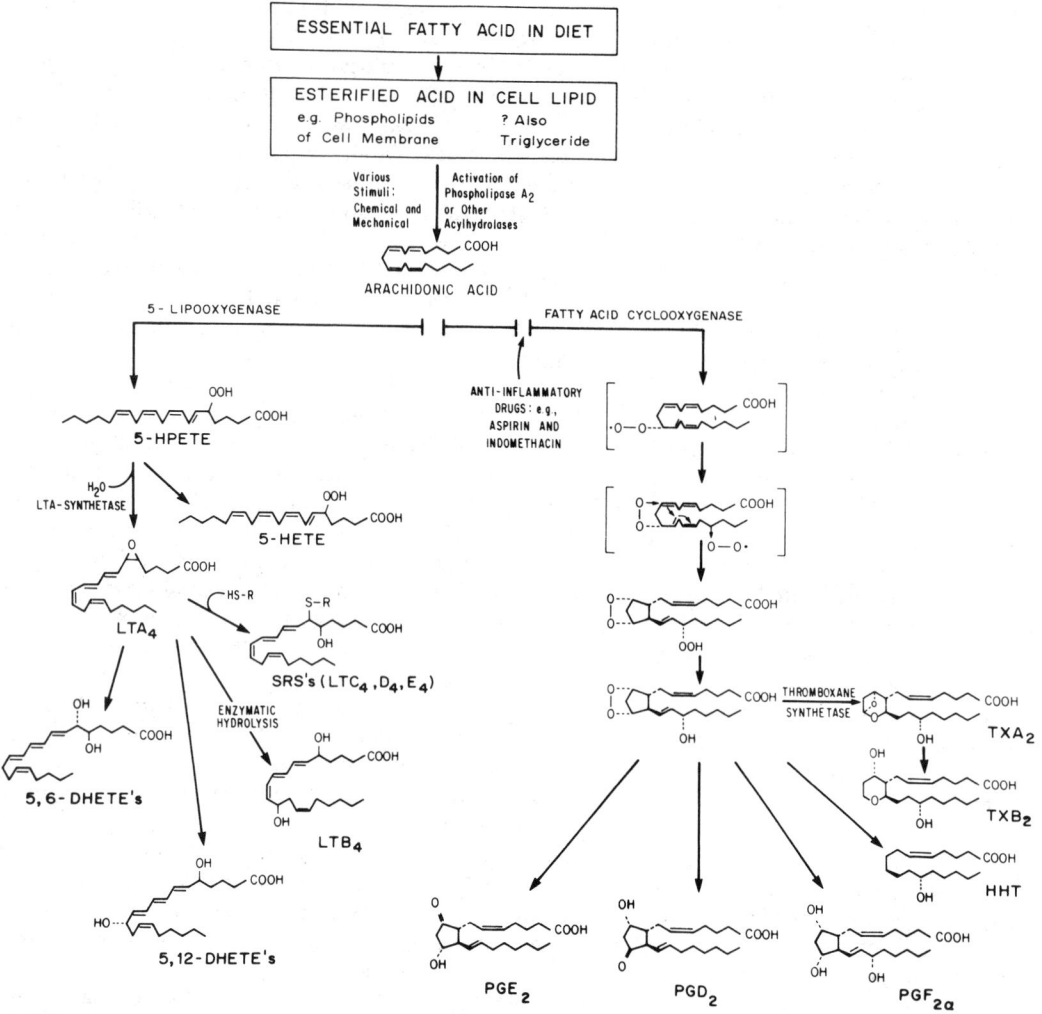

FIGURE 82-2 Biosynthesis of prostaglandins, thromboxanes, and leukotrienes. The two major pathways of arachidonic acid metabolism shown are initiated either via the cyclooxygenase or lipooxygenase reaction. Abbreviations and their meanings are as follows: 5-HPETE, 5-hydroperoxy-6,8,11,14-eicosatetraenoic acid; DHETE, dihydroxyeicosatetraenoic acid; 5-HETE, 5-hydroxyeicosatetraenoic acid; LT, leukotriene; SRS, slow-reacting substances; PG, prostaglandin; TX, thromboxane. (Hsia [160] and Bokoch and Reed [161].)

acylation of monoacyl derivatives, leading to the formation of diacylglyceryl phosphocholine and diacylglyceryl phosphoethanolamine [134]. Phagocytosis is accompanied by a threefold increase in the acylation of exogenous lysolecithin, leading to a net addition of phospholipid. The rate of lipid synthesis in cells from patients with acute leukemia and CGL is greater than that of normal granulocytes, while the leukocytes of patients with polycythemia vera showed normal or low rates of synthesis [135,136]. Acetyl CoA carboxylase, the first enzyme needed for the synthesis of long-chain fatty acids, is found in myeloblasts but not in mature granulocytes. The latter cells, however, retain the capability of elongating the chains of preformed fatty acids [137]. Increased activities of glucocerebroside-cleaving and sphingomyelin-cleaving enzymes in the leukocytes in AGL and CGL have been described [138].

A number of lipolytic activities are present in human granulocytes. One of these, a tricycloglycerol acylhydrolase acting on lipoprotein and chylomicron substrates, has been purified [139]. A cholesterylesterase activity is also associated with this enzyme. Fatty acid ester hydrolases have been described [140]. Several phospholipases are found in granulocytes [141]. Phospholipase A_2, associated with primary and secondary granules, is Ca^{2+}-dependent [142]. Activation of this enzyme may be an early event in phagocytosis, leading to changes in membrane fluidity and releasing polyunsaturated fatty acids needed as substrate for prostaglandin synthesis. Recent studies have described synthesis of a protein by rabbit peritoneal leukocytes, exposed to corticosteroids, that inhibits phospholipase A_2 [144]. The exact role of this substance during inflammatory events needs further exploration.

Prostaglandins and thromboxanes [145]

The biosynthetic pathways in PMNs for these potent modulators of the inflammatory response have been elucidated. Arachidonic acid, a polyunsaturated C_{20} fatty acid derived mainly from dietary linoleic acid, is a precursor for prostaglandin and thromboxane synthesis. Exposure of human neutrophils to such stimuli as opsonized zymosan, calcium ionophore, or chemotactic factors results in the generation of arachidonic acid [146]. The release of this compound from membrane phospholipids is mediated by phospholipase A_2. Arachidonic acid, which can induce neutrophil degranulation, is a precursor in neutrophils of either a cyclooxygenase or a lipoxygenase type of reaction (Fig. 82-2). It appears that in this cell metabolism via the lipoxygenase pathway is greater than that via the cyclooxygenase pathway [146–149]. The enzyme fatty acid cyclooxygenase (prostaglandin synthetase) catalyzes the formation of the fatty acid prostaglandin endoperoxides PGG_2 and PGH_2. The latter compound will be converted by isomerases to PGE_2, PGD_2, and PGF_2. Among these compounds, PGE_2 is a major mediator of the inflammatory process leading to edema and erythema [150]. PGH_2 is converted to the unstable vasoconstrictor thromboxane A_2 and its inactive form, thromboxane B_2 [151]. The latter compound is chemotactic. The initial product of the lipoxygenase reaction is 5-hydroperoxy-6,8,11,14-eicosatetraenoic acid (5-HPETE). This compound is reduced to form a major product, 5-hydroxyeicosatetraenoic acid (5-HETE) [152], an isomer of 12,L-hydroxy-5,8,10,14-eicosatetraenoic acid (12-HETE), a minor lipoxygenase product. Both 5- and 12-HETE have chemotactic properties and release lysozyme from neutrophils [153]. In addition, 5-HPETE is converted to a recently described series of metabolites, the leukotrienes. The formation of leukotriene A_4 [154], an unstable intermediate, is catalyzed by leukotriene A synthetase. Leukotriene A_4 is hydrolyzed to generate leukotriene B_4, a major mediator of the inflammatory process that has been reported to be chemotactic, and aggregates PMNs [155]. In addition, glutathionyl derivatives, leukotriene C_4, and the cyteinyl glycine derivative leukotriene D_4 have been isolated from human PMNs. These compounds correspond to the activity long known as the slow-reactivity substance of anaphylaxis (SRS) [156–159].

Study of the metabolic pathways in the leukocyte has been useful for detecting enzyme defects in genetic disorders. A wide variety of systemic disorders of carbohydrate, lipid, nucleic acid, or amino acid metabolism can be diagnosed by assaying the granulocytes [160].

During maturation, the PMN gradually loses its mitotic potential and develops a microbicidal armamentarium. Since the last edition of this book, the intriguing relationships of foreign substances and plasma factors modulating the response of an individual cell have been partially elucidated through the study of the enzymology of human PMNs. Much progress has also been made in understanding the pathways by which membrane receptors can transduce external stimuli into intracellular responses. There is still a lack of information concerning the differentiation process leading to the formation of PMNs.

References

1. Rabinowitz, Y.: DNA polymerase and carbohydrate metabolizing enzyme content of normal and leukemic glass column separated leukocytes. *Blood* 27:470, 1966.
2. Ove, P., Kremer, W. B., and Laszlo, J.: Increased DNA polymerase activity in human leukaemic cells. *Nature* 220:713, 1968.
3. Coleman, M. S., Hutton, J. J., and Bollum, F. J.: DNA polymerases in normal and leukemic human hematopoietic cells. *Blood* 44:19, 1974.
4. Silber, R., Berman, E., Goldstein, B., Stein, H., Farnham, G., and Bertino, J. R.: Methylation of nucleic acids in normal and leukemic leukocytes. *Biochim. Biophys. Acta* 123:638, 1966.
5. Baldessarini, R. J., and Carbone, P.: Adenosyl methionine elevation in leukemic white blood cells. *Science* 149:644, 1965.
6. Bond, V. P., Fliedner, T. M., Cronkite, E. P., Rubini, J. R., Brecher, G., and Schork, P. K.: Proliferative potentials of bone marrow and blood cells studied by in vitro uptake of H^3-thymidine. *Acta Haematol.* 21:1, 1959.
7. Rubini, J. R., Cronkite, E. P., Bond, V. P., and Fliedner, T.: The metabolism and fate of tritiated thymidine in man. *J. Clin. Invest.* 39:909, 1960.
8. McCaffrey, R., Smoler, D. F., and Baltimore, D.: Terminal deoxynucleotidyl transferase in a case of childhood acute lymphoblastic leukemia. *Proc. Natl. Acad. Sci.* 70:521, 1973.
9. Sarin, P. S., and Gallo, R. C.: Terminal deoxynucleotidyl transferase in chronic myelocytic leukemia. *J. Biol. Chem.* 249:8051, 1974.
10. Temin, H. M., and Mizutani, S.: RNA-dependent DNA polymerase in virions of Rous sarcoma virus. *Nature* 226:1211, 1970.
11. Baltimore, D.: Viral RNA-dependent DNA polymerase in virions of RNA tumour viruses. *Nature* 226:1209, 1970.
12. Spiegelman, S., et al.: Characterization of the products of RNA-directed DNA polymerases in oncogenic RNA viruses. *Nature.* 227:563, 1970.
13. Gallo, R. C., Yang, S. S., and Ting, R. C.: RNA-dependent DNA polymerase of human acute leukaemia cells. *Nature* 228:927, 1970.
14. Sarnagadharan, M. G., Sarin, P. S., Reitz, M. S., and Gallo, R. C.: Reverse transcriptase activity of human acute leukaemic cells: Purification of enzyme, response to AMV 70S RNA, and characterization of DNA product. *Nature* [*New Biol.*] 240:67, 1972.
15. Baxt, W., Hehlmann, R., and Spiegelman, S.: Human leukaemic cells contain reverse transcriptase associated with a high molecular weight virus-related RNA. *Nature* [*New Biol.*] 240:72, 1972.
16. Witkin, S., Ohno, T., and Spiegelman, S.: Purification of RNA-instructed DNA polymerase from human leukemic spleens. *Proc. Natl. Acad. Sci. U.S.A.* 72:4133, 1975.
17. Gallo, R. C., Miller, N. R., Saxinger, W. C., and Gillespie, D.: Primate RNA tumor virus-like particles from fresh human acute leukemic blood cells. *Proc. Natl. Acad. Sci. U.S.A.* 70:3219, 1973.
18. Todaro, G. J., and Gallo, R. C.: Immunological relationship of DNA polymerase from human acute leukaemia cells and primate and mouse leukaemia virus reverse transcriptase. *Nature* 244:206, 1973.
19. Kiessling, A. A., and Gouilan, M.: Detection of reverse transcriptase activity in human cells. *Cancer Res.* 39:2062, 1979.
20. Bishop, J. M.: The molecular biology of RNA tumor viruses: A physician's guide. *N. Engl. J. Med.* 303:675, 1980.
21. Cooper, G. M., Okenquist, S., and Silverman, L.: Transforming activity of DNA of chemically transformed and normal cells. *Nature* 284:417, 1980.
22. Opperman, H., Levinson, A. D., Varmus, M. E., Lenindow, L., and

Bishop, J. M.: Uninfected vertebrate cells contain a protein that is closely related to the product of the avian sarcoma virus transforming gene (src). *Proc. Natl. Acad. Sci. U.S.A.* 76:1804, 1979.

23. Gallagher, R. E., Todaro, G. J., Smith, R. G., Livingston, D. M., and Gallo, R. C.: Relationship between RNA-directed DNA polymerase (reverse transcriptase) from human acute leukemic blood cells and primate type-C viruses. *Proc. Natl. Acad. Sci. U.S.A.* 71:1309, 1974.

24. Hehlmann, R., Kufe, D., and Spiegelman, S.: RNA in human leukemic cells related to the RNA of a mouse leukemia virus. *Proc. Natl. Acad. Sci. U.S.A.* 69:435, 1972.

25. Baxt, W. G., and Spiegelman, S.: Nuclear DNA sequences present in human leukemic cells and absent in normal leukocytes. *Proc. Natl. Acad. Sci. U.S.A.* 69:3737, 1972.

26. Baxt, W., Yates, J. W., Wallace, H. J., Jr., Holland, J. F., and Spiegelman, S.: Leukemia-specific DNA sequences in leukocytes of the leukemic member of identical twins. *Proc. Natl. Acad. Sci. U.S.A.* 70:2629, 1973.

27. Sherr, C. J., and Todaro, G. J.: Primate type C virus p30 antigen in cells from humans with acute leukemia. *Science* 187:855, 1975.

28. Viola, M. V., Frazier, M., Wiernik, P., McCredie, K. B., and Spiegelman, S.: Reverse transcriptase in leukocytes of leukemic patients in remission. *N. Engl. J. Med.* 294:75, 1976.

29. Mak, T. W., Mamaster, J., Howatson, A. F., McCulloch, E. A., and Till, J. E.: Particles with characteristics of leukoviruses in cultures of marrow cells from leukemic patients in remission and relapse. *Proc. Natl. Acad. Sci. U.S.A.* 71:4336, 1974.

30. Gallagher, R. E., and Gallo, R. C.: Type C RNA tumor virus isolated from cultured human acute myelogenous leukemia cells. *Science* 197:350, 1975.

31. Pane, M., Prochownik, V., Reale, F. R., and Kirstein, W. H.: Isolation of type C virions from a normal human fibroblast strain. *Science* 189:297, 1975.

32. Reitz, M. S., Poiesz, B. J., Ruscetti, F. W., and Gallo, R. C.: Characterization and distribution of nucleic acid sequences of a novel type retrovirus isolated from neoplastic human T lymphocytes. *Proc. Natl. Acad. Sci. U.S.A.* 78:1887, 1981.

33. Marks, P. A., Willson, C., Kruh, J., and Gros, F.: Unstable ribonucleic acid in mammalian blood cells. *Biochem. Biophys. Res. Commun.* 8:9, 1962.

34. Silber, R., Unger, K. W., and Grooms, R.: RNA synthesis in normal leukocytes, leukaemia and macroglobulinaemia. *Nature* 205:1211, 1965.

35. Cline, M. J.: Isolation and characterization of RNA from human leukocytes. *J. Lab. Clin. Med.* 68:33, 1966.

36. Cline, M. J.: Ribonucleic acid biosynthesis in human leukocytes: The fate of rapidly labeled RNA in normal and abnormal leukocytes. *Blood* 28:650, 1966.

37. Silber, R., Unger, K. W., and Ellman, L.: RNA metabolism in normal and leukaemic leukocytes: Further studies on RNA synthesis. *Br. J. Haematol.* 14:261, 1968.

38. Torelli, V., Torelli, G., and Cadossi, R.: Double stranded ribonucleic acid in human blast cells. *Eur. J. Cancer* 11:117, 1975.

39. Weisberger, A. S., Suhrland, L. C., and Griggs, R. C.: Incorporation of radioactive L-cystine and L-methionine by leukemic leukocytes in vitro. *Blood* 9:1095, 1954.

40. Weisberger, A. S., and Levine, B.: Incorporation of radioactive L-cystine by normal and leukemic leukocytes in vivo. *Blood* 9:1082, 1954.

41. Baker, W. H., Zamecnik, P. C., and Stephenson, M. L.: In vitro incorporation of C14-DL-leucine into normal and leukemic white cells. *Blood* 12:822, 1957.

42. Nadler, S. H., Hansen, H. J., Sprague, C. C., and Sherman, H.: The effect of 6-mercaptopurine on the incorporation of labelled amino acids into cellular protein of chronic granulocytic leukemia leukocytes. *Blood* 18:336, 1961.

43. Gavosto, F., Pileri, A., and Maraini, G.: Protein metabolism in bone marrow and peripheral blood cells: Evaluation of H3-DL-leucine uptake by high resolution autoradiographic technique, in *Proc. VII Eur. Congr. Haematol.*, London, 1959, pt. ii, p. 380.

44. Smith, L. H., Jr., and Baker, F. A.: Pyrimidine metabolism in man. I. The biosynthesis of orotic acid. *J. Clin. Invest.* 38:798, 1959.

45. Smith, L. H., Jr., Baker, F. A., and Sullivan, M.: Pyrimidine metabolism in man. II. Studies of leukemic cells. *Blood* 15:360, 1960.

46. Wilmanns, W.: Die Thymidin-kinase in Normalen und Leukämischen Myeloischen Zellen. *Klin. Wochenschr.* 45:505, 1967.

47. Bresnick, E., and Karjala, R. J.: End-product inhibition of thymidine kinase activity in normal and leukemic human leukocytes. *Cancer Res.* 24:841, 1964.

48. Bianchi, P. A.: Thymidine phosphorylation and deoxyribonucleic acid synthesis in human leukaemia cells. *Biochim. Biophys. Acta* 55:547, 1962.

49. Marsh, J. C., and Perry, S.: Thymidine catabolism by normal and leukemic human leukocytes. *J. Clin. Invest.* 43:267, 1964.

50. Gallo, R. C., and Perry, S.: Enzyme abnormality in human leukaemia. *Nature* 218:465, 1968.

51. Silber, R., Gabrio, B. W., and Huennekens, F. M.: Studies on normal and leukemic leukocytes. VI. Thymidylate synthetase and deoxycytidylate deaminase. *J. Clin. Invest.* 42:1913, 1963.

52. Wilmanns, W., and Neef, V.: Thymidylate synthetase in white blood cells and bone marrow under normal and pathological conditions. *Klin. Wochenschr.* 49:755, 1971.

53. Silber, R.: Regulatory mechanisms in human leukocyte. I. Feedback control of deoxycytidylate deaminase. *Blood* 29:896, 1967.

54. Chabner, B. A., Jolins, D. G., Coleman, C. N., Drake, J. C., and Evans, W. H.: Purification and properties of cytidine deaminase from normal and leukemic leukocytes. *J. Clin. Invest.* 53:922, 1974.

55. Coleman, C. N., Stoller, R. G., and Chabner, B. A.: Properties of cytidine kinase enzyme from human leukemic granulocytes. *Blood* 46:791, 1975.

56. Fujioka, S., and Silber, R.: Leukocyte ribonucleotide reductase: Studies in normal subjects and a subject with leukemia and pernicious anemia. *J. Lab. Clin. Med.* 77:59, 1971.

57. Fujioka, S., and Silber, R.: Ribonucleotide reductase in human bone marrow: Lack of stimulation by 5'-deoxyadenosyl B₁₂. *Biochem. Biophys. Res. Commun.* 35:759, 1969.

58. Tattersall, M. H. N., Lavoie, A., Ganeshagura, K., Tripp, E., and Hoffbrand, A. V.: Deoxyribonucleoside triphosphates in human cells: Changes in disease and following exposure to drugs. *Eur. J. Clin. Invest.* 5:191, 1975.

59. Scott, J. L.: Human leukocyte metabolism in vitro. I. Incorporation of adenine-8-C¹⁴ and formate C¹⁴ into the nucleic acids of leukemic leukocytes. *J. Clin. Invest.* 41:67, 1962.

60. Brosh, S., Boer, P., Kupfer, D., DeVries, A., and Sperling, O.: De novo synthesis of purine nucleotides in human peripheral blood leukocytes: Excessive activity of the pathway in hypoxanthine-guanine phosphoribosyl-transferase deficiency. *J. Clin. Invest.* 58:289, 1976.

61. Shapira, J., Bornstein, I., Wells, W., and Winzler, R. J.: Metabolism of human leukocytes in vitro. IV. Incorporation and interconversion of adenine and guanine. *Cancer Res.* 21:265, 1961.

62. Lajtha, L. G., and Vane, J. R.: Dependence of bone marrow cells on the liver for purine supply. *Nature* 182:191, 1958.

63. Rosman, M., Lee, M. H., Creasey, W. A., and Sartorelli, A. C.: Mechanisms of resistance to 6-thiopurines in human leukemia. *Cancer Res.* 34:1052, 1974.

64. Rosman, M., and Williams, H. E.: Leukocyte purine phosphoribosyl-transferase in human leukemias sensitive and resistant to 6-thiopurines. *Cancer Res.* 33:1202, 1973.

65. Bertino, J. R., et al.: Studies on normal and leukemic leukocytes. IV. Tetrahydrofolate-dependent enzyme systems and dihydrofolic reductase. *J. Clin. Invest.* 42:1899, 1963.

66. Bertino, J. R., et al.: Increased dihydrofolic reductase level in leukocytes of patients treated with amethopterin. *Nature* 193:140, 1962.

67. Nunberg, J. H., Kaufman, R. J., Schimke, R. T., Urlaub, G., and Chasin, L. A.: Amplified dihydrofolate reductase genes are localized to a homogeneously staining region of a single chromosome in methotrexate-resistant Chinese hamster ovary cell line. *Proc. Natl. Acad. Sci. U.S.A.* 75:5553, 1978.

68. Bertino, J. R., and Skeel, R. T.: On natural and acquired resistance to folate antagonists in man, in *Pharmocological Basis of Cancer Chemotherapy*. Williams & Wilkins, Baltimore, 1975.

69. Sauer, H., Wilms, K., Wilmanns, W., and Jaenicke, C.: Die Aktivität der Methionin-synthetase als Proliferations Parameter in Wächsenden Zellen. *Acta Haematol.* 49:200, 1973.

70. Peytremann, R., Thordike, J., and Beck, N. S.: Studies on N⁵-

methyltetrahydrofolate in normal and leukemic leukocytes. *J. Clin. Invest.* 56:1293, 1975.

71. Contreras, E.: Leukocyte methyl malonyl CoA mutase. I. Vitamin B_{12} deficiency. *Am. J. Clin. Nutr.* 25:695, 1972.

72. Barnes, J. M.: The enzymes of lymphocytes and polymorphonuclear leucocytes. *Br. J. Exp. Pathol.* 21:261, 1940.

73. Cohn, Z. A., and Hirsch, J. G.: The isolation and properties of the specific cytoplasmic granules of rabbit polymorphonuclear leukocytes. *J. Exp. Med.* 112:983, 1960.

74. Silber, R., Unger, K. W., Keller, J., and Bertino, J. R.: RNA metabolism of normal and leukemic leukocytes. II. Ribonuclease. *Blood* 29:57, 1967.

75. Sarngadharan, M. G., Leis, J. P., and Gallo, R. C.: Isolation and characterization of a ribonuclease from human leukemic blood cells specific for ribonucleic acid of ribonucleic acid–deoxyribonucleic acid hybrid molecules. *J. Biol. Chem.* 250:365, 1975.

76. Swenseid, M. E., Wright, P. D., and Bethell, F. H.: Variations in nuclotidase activity of leukocytes: Studies with leukemia patients. *J. Lab. Clin. Med.* 40:515, 1952.

77. Li, C. Y., Yam, L. T., and Lam, K. W.: Acid phosphatase isoenzymes in human leukocytes in normal and pathologic conditions. *J. Histochem. Cytochem.* 18:473, 1970.

78. Marsh, J. C., and Perry, S.: The reduction of thymine by human leukocytes. *Arch. Biochem. Biophys.* 104:146, 1968.

79. Wachstein, M.: Alkaline phosphatase activity in normal and abnormal human blood and bone marrow. *J. Lab. Clin. Med.* 31:1, 1946.

80. Cline, M. J.: Metabolism of the circulation leukocyte. *Physiol. Rev.* 45:674, 1965.

81. Hayhoe, F. G. J., Quaglino, D., and Doll, R.: *The Cytology and Cytochemistry of Acute Leukemias.* H. M. Stationery Office, London, 1964.

82. Garg, S., and Silber, R.: Decreased leukocyte alkaline phosphatase in monocytic leukemia. *Am. J. Clin. Pathol.* 58:668, 1972.

83. Follette, J. H., Valentine, W. N., Hardin, E. B., and Lawrence, J. S.: A comparison of human phosphatase activity toward sodium beta-glycerophosphate, adenosine 5'-phosphate, and glucose-1-phosphate. *Blood* 14:415, 1959.

84. Trubowitz, S., Feldman, D., Morgenstern, S. W., and Hunt, V. M.: The isolation, purification and properties of the alkaline phosphatase of human leukocytes. *Biochem. J.* 80:369, 1961.

85. Valentine, W. N., and Beck, W. S.: Biochemical studies on leukocytes. I. Phosphatase activity in health, leukocytosis, and myelocytic leukemia. *J. Lab. Clin. Med.* 38:39, 1951.

86. Valentine, W. N., Folette, J. H., Solomon, D. H., and Reynolds, J.: The relationship of leukocyte alkaline phosphatase to "stress," to ACTH, and to adrenal 17-OH-corticosteroids. *J. Lab. Clin. Med.* 49:723, 1957.

87. Robinson, J. C., Pierce, J. E., and Goldstein, D. P.: Leukocyte alkaline phosphatase: Electrophoretic variants associated with chronic myelocytic leukemia. *Science* 150:58, 1965.

88. Bottomley, R. H., Lovig, C. A., Holt, R., and Griffin, M. J.: Comparison of alkaline phosphatase from human normal and leukemic leukocytes. *Cancer Res.* 29:1866, 1969.

89. Rosenblum, D., and Petzold, S.: Neutrophil alkaline phosphatase: Comparison of enzymes from normal subjects and patients with polycythemia vera and chronic myelogenous leukemia. *Blood* 45:335, 1975.

90. Beck, W. S.: Biochemical properties of normal and leukemic leukocytes, in *Proceedings of the International Conference on Leukemia-Lymphoma.* Lea & Febiger, Philadelphia, 1968, p. 245 (review).

91. Beck, W. S.: The control of leukocyte glycolysis. *J. Biol. Chem.* 232:251, 1958.

92. Grafe, E.: Die Steigerung des Stoffwechsels bei chronisher Leukamie und ihre Ursachen (Zugleich ein Beitrag zur Biologie der Weissen Blutzellen). *Dtsch. Arch. Klin. Med.* 102:406, 1911.

93. Cline. M. J.: *The White Cell.* Harvard, Cambridge, Mass., 1975.

94. Bisset, S. K., and Alexander, W. D.: The effect of intravenous injections of triiodoacetic acid and 1-triiodothyronine on the oxygen consumption of circulating human leukocytes. *Q. J. Exp. Physiol.* 46:50, 1961.

95. Bicz, W.: The influence of carbon dioxide tension on the respiration of normal and leukemic leukocytes. I. Influence on endogenous respiration. *Cancer Res.* 20:184, 1960.

96. McKinney, G. R., Martin, S. P., Rundles, R. W., and Green, R.: Respiration and glycolytic activities of human leukocytes in vitro. *J. Appl. Physiol.* 5:355, 1953.

97. MacLeod, J., and Rhoads, C.: Metabolism of leukocytes in Ringer-phosphate and in serum. *Proc. Soc. Exp. Biol. Med.* 41:268, 1939.

98. Cline, M. J., Melmon, K. L., Davis, W. C., and Williams, H. E.: Mechanism of endotoxin interaction with human leukocytes. *Br. J. Haematol.* 15:539, 1968.

99. Strauss, B. S., and Stetson, C. A., Jr.: Studies on the effect of certain macromolecular substances on the respiratory activity of the leucocytes of peripheral blood. *J. Exp. Med.* 112:653, 1960.

100. Warburg, O.: Über den Stoffwechsels der Tumoren. Springer-Verlag, Berlin, 1926.

101. Beck, W. S.: A kinetic analysis of the glycolytic rate and certain glycolytic enzymes in normal and leukemic leukocytes. *J. Biol. Chem.* 216:333, 1955.

102. Bourne, H. R., Lehrer, R. I., Cline, M. J., and Melmon, K. L.: Cyclic 3',5'-adenosine monophosphate in the human leukocyte: Synthesis, degradation, and effects on neutrophil candidacidal activity. *J. Clin. Invest.* 59:920, 1971.

103. Scott, R. E.: Effects of prostaglandins, epinephrine and NaF on human léukocyte, platelet and liver adenyl cyclase. *Blood* 35:514, 1974.

104. Tsung, P. K., Sakamoto, T., and Weissman, G.: Protein kinase and phosphatases from human polymorphonuclear leukocytes. *Biochem. J.* 143:437, 1975.

105. Parker, C. W.: Alterations in cyclic AMP metabolism in human bronchial asthma. II. Leukocyte and lymphocyte response to prostaglandins. *J. Clin. Invest.* 52:1336, 1973.

106. Parker, C. W.: Alterations in cyclic AMP metabolism in human bronchial asthma. III. Leukocyte and lymphocyte responses to steroids. *J. Clin. Invest.* 53:1342, 1973.

107. Alston, W. C., Patel, K. R., and Kerr, J. W.: Response of leukocyte adenyl cyclase to isoprenaline and effects of alpha blocking drugs in extrinsic bronchial asthma. *Br. Med. J.* 1:90, 1974.

108. Bessis, M.: *Cytology of the Blood and Blood-Forming Organs.* Grune & Stratton, New York, 1956.

109. Foster, J. M., and Terry, M. L.: Studies on the energy metabolism of human leukocytes. I. Oxidative phosphorylation by human leukocyte mitochondria. *Blood* 30:168, 1967.

110. Alleyasine, H., and Frei, J.: Origine de l'énergie chimique du polynucléaire neutrophile d'exudats péritoneaux de cobayes. *Helv. Physiol. Pharmacol. Acta* 22:C6, 1964.

111. Tanaka, K. R., and Valentine, W. N.: Aconitase activity of human leukocytes. *Acta Haematol.* 26:12, 1961.

112. Tanaka, K. R., and Valentine, W. N.: Fumarase activity of human leukocytes and erythrocytes. *Blood* 17:328, 1961.

113. Borel, C., Frei, J., Horvath, G., Montri, S., and Vanotti, A.: Ètude comparée du métabolisme du polynucléaire et de la cellule mononucléi chez l'homme. *Helv.Med. Acta* 26:785, 1959.

114. Belfiore, F., Borzi, V., LoVecchio, L., Napoli, E., and Rabuazzo, A. M.: Enzyme activities of NADPH forming metabolic pathways in normal and leukemic leukocytes. *Clin. Chem.* 21:880, 1925.

115. Gibb, R. P., and Stowell, R. E.: Glycogen in human blood cells. *Blood* 4:569, 1949.

116. Stjernholm, R. L., Burns, C. P., and Hohnadel, J. H.: Carbohydrate metabolism by leukocytes. *Enzyme* 13:7, 1972.

117. Scott, R. B.: Glycogen in human peripheral blood leukocytes. I. Characteristics of the synthesis and turnover of glycogen in vitro. *J. Clin. Invest.* 47:344, 1968.

118. Wachstein, M.: The distribution of histochemically demonstrable glycogen in human blood and bone marrow cells. *Blood* 4:54, 1949.

119. Valentine, W. N., Follette, J. H., and Lawrence, J. S.: The glycogen content of human leukocytes in health and various disease states. *J. Clin. Invest.* 32:251, 1953.

120. Stjernholm, R. L., Noble, E. P., Dimitrov, N. V., Kellermeyer, R. W., and Falor, W. H.: Differentiation of normal and leukemic leukocytes into three groups by propionate metabolism. *J. Reticuloendothel. Soc.* 8:446, 1970.

121. Esmann, V.: The diabetic leukocyte. *Enzyme (Basel)* 13:32, 1972.

122. Moretti, G., Staeffen, J., Ballan, P., Roques, J. C., and Beylot, J.: L'Activité galactose-1-phosphate uridylyl transférasique des leukocytes humains au cours des leucoses. *Ann. Biol. Clin. (Paris)* 30:261, 1972.

123. Kerby, G. P.: The occurrence of acid mucopolysaccharides in human leukocytes. *J. Clin. Invest. 34:*944, 1955.

124. Lau, P., Gottlieb, A. J., and Williams, W. J.: Mucopolysaccharide sulfation in normal and leukemic leukocytes. *Blood 40:*725, 1972.

125. Osserman, E. F., and Lawlor, D. P.: Serum and urinary lysozyme (muramidase) in monocytic and monomyelocytic leukemia. *J. Exp. Med. 124:*921, 1966.

126. Fink, M. E., and Finch, S. C.: Serum muramidase and granulocyte turnover. *Proc. Soc. Exp. Biol. Med. 127:*365, 1968.

127. Wiernik, P. H., and Serpick, A. A.: Clinical significance of serum and urinary muramidase activity in leukemia and other hematologic malignancies. *Am. J. Med. 46:*330, 1969.

128. Zucker, S., Hanes, D. J., Vogler, W. R., and Eanes, R. Z.: Plasma muramidase: A study of methods and clinical applications. *J. Lab. Clin. Med. 75:*83, 1970.

129. Mishimura, E. T., Hokama, Y., and Jim, R.: Appearance of abnormal catalase antigen and concurrent deletion of normal antigen in leukocytes of myelogenous leukemia. *Cancer Res. 32:*2353, 1972.

130. Marks, P. A., Gellhorn, A., and Kidson, C.: Lipid synthesis in human leukocytes, platelets and erythrocytes. *J. Biol. Chem. 235:*2579, 1960.

131. Fogelman, A. M., Seager, J., Edwards, P. A., Hokom, M., and Popjak, G.: Cholesterol biosynthesis in human lymphocytes, monocytes, and granulocytes. *Biochem. Biophys. Res. Commun. 76:*167, 1977.

132. Firkin, B. G., and Williams, W. J.: The incorporation of radioactive phosphorus into the phospholipids of human leukemic leukocytes and platelets. *J. Clin. Invest. 40:*423, 1961.

133. Elsbach, P.: Lipid metabolism by phagocytes. *Semin. Hematol. 9:*227, 1972.

134. Wang, P., Waite, M., and de Chatelet, L. R.: Membrane lipid metabolism of bacillus Calmette Guérin–induced rabbit alveolar macrophages. *Biochim. Biophys. Acta 487:*163, 1977.

135. Kidson, C.: Lipid synthesis in human leukocytes in acute leukemia. *Aust. Ann. Med. 10:*282, 1961.

136. Kidson, C.: Leukocyte lipid metabolism in myeloproliferative states. *Aust. Ann. Med. 11:*50, 1962.

137. Majerus, P. W., and Lastra, R.: Fatty acid biosynthesis in human leukocytes. *J. Clin. Invest. 46:*1596, 1967.

138. Kampine, J. P., Brady, R. O., Yankee, R. A., Kanfer, J. N., Shapiro, D., and Gal, A. E.: Sphingolipid metabolism in leukemic lymphocytes. *Cancer Res. 27:*1312, 1967.

139. Elsbach, P., and Kayden, H. J.: Chylomicron lipid-splitting activity in homogenates of rabbit polymorphonuclear leukocytes. *Am. J. Physiol. 209:*765, 1965.

140. Dienstle, F., Sailer, S., Sandhager, F., and Braunsteiner, H.: Lipid activity in leucocytes and macrophage. *Blood 24:*607, 1964.

141. Elsbach, P., and Weiss, J.: *Lipid Metabolism by Phagocytic Cells in the Reticuloendothelial System,* edited by A. J. Sbarra and R. R. Strauss. Plenum, New York, 1980, vol. 2, p. 91.

142. Elsbach, P., Weiss, J., Franson, R. C., Beckerdite-Quagliata, S., Schneider, A., and Harris, L.: Separation and purification of a potent bactericidal permeability increasing protein and a closely associated phospholipase A₂ from rabbit polymorphonuclear leukocytes. *J. Biol. Chem. 254:*11000, 1979.

143. Kampine, J. P., Brady, R. O., Kanfer, J. N., Feld, K., and Shapiro, D.: Diagnosis of Gaucher's disease and Niemann-Pick disease with small samples of venous blood. *Science 155:*86, 1967.

144. Hirata, F., et al.: Presence of autoantibody for phospholipase inhibitory protein, lipomodulin, in patients with rheumatic diseases. *Proc. Natl. Acad. Sci. U.S.A. 78:*3190, 1981.

145. Samuelsson, B., Goldyne, M., Granstrom, E., Hamberg, M., Hammarstrom, S., and Malmsten, C.: Prostaglandins and thromboxanes. *Annu. Rev. Biochem. 47:*997, 1978.

146. Walsh, C. E., Waite, B. M., Thomas, M. J., and de Chatelet, L. R.: Release and metabolism of arachidonic acid in human neutrophils. *J. Biol. Chem. 256:*7228, 1981.

147. Borgeat, P., and Samuelsson, B.: Transformation of arachidonic acid by rabbit polymorphonuclear leukocytes. Formation of a novel dihydroxyeicosatetraenoic acid. *J. Biol. Chem. 254:*2643, 1979.

148. Borgeat, P., and Samuelsson, B.: Metabolism of arachidonic acid in polymorphonuclear leukocytes. Structural analysis of novel hydroxylated compounds. *J. Biol. Chem. 254:*7865, 1979.

149. Bokoch, G. M., and Reed, P. W.: Stimulation of arachidonic acid metabolism in the polymorphonuclear leukocytes by an N-formylated peptide. *J. Biol. Chem. 255:*10223, 1980.

150. Moncada, S., Ferreira, S. H., and Vane, J. R.: Prostaglandins, aspirin-like drugs and the oedema of inflammation. *Nature 246:*217, 1973.

151. Goldstein, I. M., Malmsten, C. L., Kindahl, H. B., Radmark, O., Samuelsson, B., and Weisman, G.: Thromboxane generation by human peripheral blood polymorphonuclear leukocytes. *J. Exp. Med. 148:*787, 1978.

152. Borgeat, P., Hamberg, M., and Samuelsson, B.: Transformation of arachidonic acid and homo-δ-linoleic acid by rabbit polymorphonuclear leukocytes. *J. Biol. Chem. 252:*8772, 1977.

153. Stenson, W. F., and Parker, S. W.: Monohydroxyeicosatetraenoic acids (HETEs) induce degranulation of human neutrophils. *J. Immunol. 124:*2100, 1980.

154. Radmark, O., Malmsten, C., Samuelsson, B., Goto, G., Marfat, A., and Corey, E. J.: Leukotriene A, isolation from human polymorphonuclear leukocytes. *J. Biol. Chem. 255:*11828, 1980.

155. Ford-Hutchinson, A. W., Bray, M. A., Cunningham, F. M., Davidson, E. M., and Smith, M. J. H.: Isomers of leukotriene B4 possess different biological potencies. *Prostaglandins 21:*143, 1981.

156. Orning, L., Hammarstrom, S., and Samuelsson, B.: Leukotriene D: A slow reacting substance from rat basophilic leukemia cells. *Proc. Natl. Acad. Sci. U.S.A. 77:*2014, 1980.

157. Bach, M. K., Brashler, J. R., Hammarstrom, S., and Samuelsson, B.: Identification of leukotriene C-1 as a major component of slow-reacting substance from rat mononuclear cells. *J. Immunol. 125:*115, 1980.

158. Bach, M. K., Brashler, J. R., Hammarstrom, S., and Samuelsson, B.: Identification of a component of rat mononuclear cell SRS as leukotriene D. *Biochem. Biophys. Res. Commun. 93:*1121, 1980.

159. Samuelsson, B., Hammarstrom, S., Murphy, R. C., and Borgeat, P.: Leukotrienes and slow-reacting substance of anaphylaxis (SRS-A). *Allergy 35:*375, 1980.

160. Hsia, D. Y.: Utilization of leukocytes for the study of inborn errors of metabolism. *Enzyme 13:*161, 1972.

161. Bokoch, G. M., and Reed, P. W.: Evidence for inhibition of leukotriene A4 synthesis by 5,8,11,14-eicosatetraynoic acid in guinea pig polymorphonuclear leukocytes. *J. Biol. Chem. 256:*4156, 1981.

162. Moncada, S., Flower, R. J., and Vane, J. R.: Prostaglandins, prostacyclin, and thromboxane A₂, in *The Pharmacological Basis of Therapeutics,* 6th ed., edited by L. S. Goodman and A. Gilman. Macmillan, New York, 1980.

CHAPTER 83

Functions of neutrophils

THOMAS P. STOSSEL
LAURENCE A. BOXER

The neutrophil protects the host against pyogenic infection. Its function is closely integrated with that of lymphocytes and macrophages, cells also involved in the response to infection (Fig. 83-1) [1–4]. Neutrophils in the blood are attracted to sites of infection by chemotactic factors, which are generated by the interaction of plasma proteins with antigens or pathogens. The diffusion of these factors creates a chemical gradient that influences the direction of neutrophil migration, the neutrophil moving toward the source of the chemotactic factor. Plasma, in addition to elaborating chemical attractants, provides antibodies and complement that coat microorganisms, rendering them capable of ingestion by neutrophils. This process of antibody and complement coating has been called opsonization, from the Greek word for "providing victuals." The pathogenicity of microorganisms results from their ability to prevent opsonization. Neutrophils ingest the opsonized microorganisms by surrounding them with moving pseudopodia. These pseudopodia fuse to enclose the microbe within a vesicle called the *phagosome*. The cytoplasmic granules of the neutrophil fuse with the phagosome and discharge their contents into it, a process called *degranulation*. The neutrophil reduces oxygen enzymatically to generate "activated" metabolites such as hydrogen peroxide which, together with material discharged into the phagosome by the granules, can kill ingested microbes. Granule contents and oxygen metabolites may leak from the neutrophil into extracellular fluid, where they can injure tissue as well as microbes. The leakage results from secretion and from partially closed phagosomes (Fig. 83-2). This side effect of the attack of neutrophils against antigens or pathogens may be an important cause of tissue inflammation and in certain locations may be detrimental to the host.

Signal mechanisms for neutrophils—chemotactic factors and opsonins

CHEMOTACTIC FACTORS

Bacterial invasion or tissue necrosis initiates the elaboration of chemoattractants. One general mechanism is the activation of protein cascade systems in plasma which generate these factors. These systems, the complement system, the kinin-generating system, and to a lesser extent the clotting system, interact with one another also [5] (see Chap. 15). Chemotactic factors also can be derived from cells, especially from lymphocytes (lymphokines) and monocytes [6,7]. Within this category, the monocyte chemotactic factor plays a pivotal role in initiating delayed-type hypersensitivity reactions. Other lymphokines present in small concentrations have chemotactic activity for neutrophils and basophils.

Complement-mediated generation of chemotactic factors may be initiated by the combination of antibody with antigen followed by activation of the early classic complement proteins to cleave C1, C4, and C2 (see Chap. 15). The major cleavage fragments of C4, C4b, and of C2, C2a, associate to form a new enzyme called C3 convertase [8,9]. C3 is central to complement function and $\overline{C42}$ enzyme cleaves C3 into a small fragment, C3a ($M_r = 8900$ daltons), and a large fragment, C3b ($M_r =$

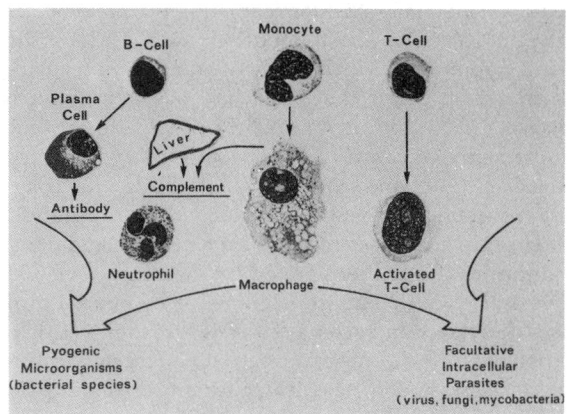

FIGURE 83-1   Cells involved in host defense against infection.

175,000 daltons). With a major cleavage fragment of C3 (C3b) added to the complex, a C5 convertase is formed, which is capable of cleaving C5 into two fragments, C5a and C5b ($M_r = 160,000$ daltons). C5b creates a complex with the later-acting components C6, C7, C8, and C9, of which $\overline{C567}$ has documented chemotactic power.

The same cleavage of C3 can be achieved by activation of the alternative complement pathway. The alternative pathway C3 and C5 convertases ($\overline{c3bBb}$) consist of a complex of C3b with the major cleavage fragment of factor B, Bb. Factor B is split and thereby activated by factor D when B is loosely complexed with C3b. In turn the alternative complement pathway can be activated by bacterial polysaccharides and antigen-antibody com-

FIGURE 83-2   Activities of the neutrophil.

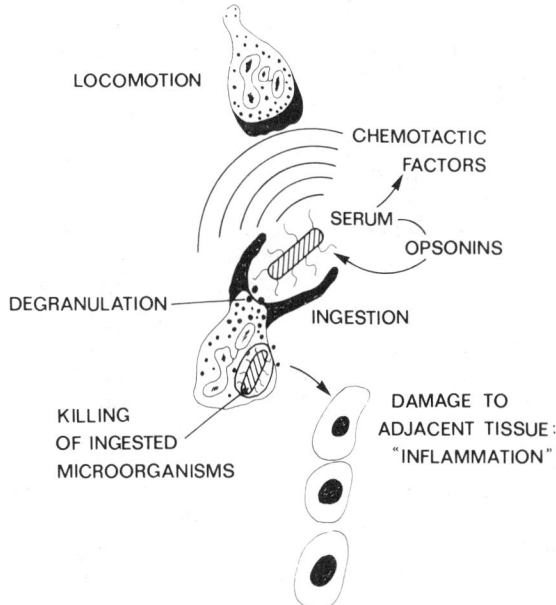

plexes. Mechanisms exist for regulating the biologic activity of C3b. The most important of these are the plasma proteins, β1H, C3b inactivator, and a trypsin-like enzyme [9]. This complex behaves as an enzyme to inactivate C3b. Not only can C3b be generated by the complement pathways, it can be formed by directed cleavage of C3 by thrombin activated through the coagulation system, by plasmin activated via the fibrinolytic system, or by proteases released from bacteria and damaged tissue. C5a is then formed by the activity of C3b convertase or can be generated like C3a by neutral proteases derived from bacteria or tissue lysosomes [10]. In the neutrophil, this enzymatic activity is largely attributable to elastase and, to a lesser extent, chymotrypsin [11]. The C5a fragment, like C4a and C3a, is an anaphylatoxin causing smooth muscle contraction and is also the most potent of the chemotactic factors [12] (human C3a is now thought to have relatively little chemotactic activity)[13,14]. C5a contains 74 amino acid residues, is highly cationic, has an M_r of 11,200 daltons and a single oligosaccharide at position 64 [15]. C5a is active at a concentration of approximately 1 nM. A carboxypeptidase B–type enzyme in plasma converts C5a to C5a desArg, leading to a loss of biological activity. However, the chemotactic activity can be largely restored by the addition of an unidentified cofactor which is also in plasma [14].

Bacterial products, especially endotoxin, activate Hageman factor (factor XII), which initiates the coagulation and fibrinolytic systems. In addition, activated Hageman factor (factor XIIa) catalyzes the conversion of prekallikrein to kallikrein, which may be chemotactic [16]. Fibrinopeptide B split from fibrin by plasmin activity and plasminogen activator also exerts chemotactic activity [17,18]. Bacteria release newly synthesized peptides and proteins which are chemotactic [19]. Neutrophils during ingestion release low levels of chemotactic factors [20]. Most factors released by bacteria, damaged tissue, and neutrophils are not well defined but may include neutral proteases [21–24]. Endotoxin, peptides generated by the action of collagenase on collagen, and oxidized lipids, which include 12-hydroxy-5,8,10,14-eicosatetraenoic acid (HETE), a product of the lipoxygenase-prostaglandin system, and 12-L-hydroxy-5,8,10-hepadecatrienoic acid (HHT), a product of the cyclooxygenase-prostaglandin pathway, possess chemotactic activity, although these products are less potent than C5a [25–27]. Leukotriene B (5,12-dihydroxy-6,8,10,14-eicosatetraenoic acid) is more chemotactic by several orders of magnitude than the other lipoxygenase products, which suggests that this is a truly relevant product in inflammation [28,29].

Another group of chemotactic factors includes the synthetic N-formylated di-, tri-, and tetrapeptides [30]. These peptides can be used as probes for studying neutrophil responses to chemotactic peptides. Chemotactic activity of the peptides [31] is related to the sequential order and stereospecificity of their amino acid chains and their hydrophobicity. Furthermore, there is a rela-

tionship between chemotactic activity of a peptide and its ability to elicit granule enzyme release [32]. C5a and the synthetic peptides bind to specific surface receptors on the neutrophil [33–35]. This membrane binding relates closely to the biological activity of peptide. There is a direct correlation between chemotactic activity and the ability of the neutrophil to hydrolyze the peptide. Protease inhibitors will suppress the chemotactic response of the neutrophil, and ectoenzymes may exist in proximity to the chemotactic receptor, providing a mechanism to clear the receptor of bound peptide. The neutrophil interiorizes the bound peptides, and the peptides become exposed to lysosomal proteases in endocytic vacuoles, which may also lead to their inactivation.

INHIBITORS OF CHEMOTACTIC FACTORS

The plasma chemical cascade reactions are controlled by chemical antagonists. The activation of the classic complement pathway is modulated by the C1 inhibitor [36]. Another blood protein, the C3b inactivator, inhibits activation of the classic pathway by degrading C4 in the presence of the C4b-binding protein and also inactivates C3b by the alternative pathway convertase when a protein called β1H is present [36]. Inhibitors of the coagulation and fibrinolytic systems are discussed in detail in Chaps. 136 and 138. Agents that influence the generation of chemotactic factors can themselves be inactivated. Human C5a is rapidly converted to C5a desArg by a potent carboxypeptidase in plasma, and in the absence of other plasma components C5a desArg is virtually devoid of chemotactic activity [14,15]. Complement factor inactivators (CFI) in normal serum inhibit fragments of C5 as well as other complement and noncomplement-derived chemotactic factors [37,38]. One of the CFI, a heat-labile α-globulin, specifically inactivates C5-derived chemotactic fragments. CFI inactivates bacterial chemotactic factors and synthetic peptides by an aminopeptidase-like activity [39]. A heat-stable inhibitor of C5a is found in the serum of patients with systemic lupus erythematosus [40] and correlates with increased disease activity and susceptibility to infection.

Surfaces which promote neutrophil recognition The neutrophil must recognize what it should attack. The surface charge, hydrophobicity, and chemical composition may influence the uptake of bacteria [41] or other particles. Neutrophils prefer particles with a strong net surface charge, whether positive or negative [42]. Neutrophils ingest an enormous variety of particles, but with a different avidity. Natural particles with modified surfaces and synthetic particles coated with normal proteins are poorly ingested, while natural particles whose surface has not been modified are more readily ingested [43].

Before ingestion, objects attach to the surface of the neutrophil [43]. If the surface chemistry is right, nonspecific attachment may occur. Nonspecific attachment may be a dead end or may gradually increase membrane adhesiveness, leading to recognition [44]. Thus attachment is not always a prelude to ingestion. If ingestion proceeds, pseudopodia begin to form at the contact point and extend around the object. Propagation requires that some recognition factor be distributed around the object [45], body temperature be maintained, and cellular energy be expended [46]. If these criteria are not fulfilled, ingestion may stop. This configuration resembles a "rosette" and occurs when erythrocytes sensitized with concanavalin surround a neutrophil [47,48].

Some bacteria can be ingested by neutrophils without further modification, but encapsulated virulent pathogens such as streptococci, *Escherichia coli, Staphylococcus aureus,* pneumococci, *Hemophilus influenzae,* and meningococci are not ingested unless first opsonized by plasma antibody [49]. The resistance of a microorganism to recognition varies with its species or with environmental influences [49,50]. The surfaces of most unencapsulated gram-negative bacteria are rich in lipopolysaccharide. In the absence of antibody, the lipopolysaccharide activates the complement pathway, leading to the deposition of C3b onto the bacterial surface, which promotes ingestion [51]. In contrast, capsulated *E. coli* resist ingestion because the capsule blocks complement fixation by masking surface lipopolysaccharide [52]. The capsules of gram-positive organisms are also determinants of virulence. The outer surface of the unencapsulated gram-positive bacteria, a cell wall containing peptidoglycan, promotes complement activation, whereas the capsule of *S. aureus* hinders ingestion by masking the underlying peptidoglycan layer [53,54]. Virulent gonococci fail to interact with plasma and are not ingested by neutrophils but attach to the surface of the neutrophil, while a nonvirulent variety is opsonized and rapidly ingested [55]. The neutrophil's failure to enclose the virulent gonococci within the phagosome contributes to its survival [56].

OPSONINS
The complement-mediated reactions which generate chemotactic factors in plasma also produce by-products which coat microbes and opsonize them. The products are C3b and a fragment of C3b [57]. This opsonic fragment of C3 is bound extremely tightly to the surface of a particle by both hydrophobic and covalent interactions [57,58]. It is not known how C3 binds to the particle surface or how it elicits recognition by the neutrophil. Antibody participation, especially IgM, in the activation of the complement components results in the deposition of C3 on the surface of microbes and initiates complement-dependent opsonization of encapsulated virulent pathogens. In some circumstances IgG antibody can opsonize particles. Opsonizing antibodies develop in the plasma of humans or animals chronically infected with the corresponding microbes [59], and opsonization is potentiated by complement. Serum from individuals with autoimmune thrombocytopenia or with antineutrophil isoantibodies can opsonize platelets or neu-

trophils for ingestion by neutrophils [60,61]. The Fab region of opsonically active antibody is the binding site for the target particle. Cleavage of the Fc region from antibody destroys its opsonic activity [60,61], indicating that the effector site for activation of the neutrophil resides in the Fc domain. Opsonic activity is mainly limited to antibody of the IgG class.

A vast number of particle surfaces can stimulate recognition by neutrophils, and substances in plasma or other body fluids can coat particles and enhance their ingestion [62,63]. One such is fibronectin, a glycoprotein found in plasma and in outer membrane of fibroblasts and endothelial cells [64].

CONTROL OF OPSONIC EXPRESSION
The C3b inactivator enzyme of plasma also has the capacity to remove opsonically active C3 from particles. Trypsin also removes opsonically active C3 from particles, and proteolytic activity in inflammatory lesions may have the same effect [56].

Sensory mechanisms of neutrophils — the membrane response complex

The neutrophil is "nonspecifically excitable." Chemotactic factors, ingested particles, and other substances produce metabolic and morphologic effects (Table 83-1). Ligand binding to the neutrophil surface activates the following series of events: The cell membrane becomes hyperpolarized [89,95]. Immediately following this membrane potential change, calcium ion is lost from the plasma membrane, calcium fluxes increase, and cyclic AMP rises transiently [92,96–98]. After a lag period of less than a minute, metabolic products are released and a condensation of subplasmalemmal microfilaments and assembly of microtubules occurs [92,99]. The neutrophil membrane has components that are mobile [99,100], some of which are receptors that bind ligands such as chemotactic factors or opsonins [101,102]. A soluble receptor preparation which retains binding affinity for the desired ligand has been obtained for the Fc receptor of macrophages [103] but not for neutrophils. The identification of distinct receptors on the surface of the neutrophil by affinity radiolabeling and analysis of labeled proteins has been achieved [104], and the formyl peptide chemotactic receptor present on human neutrophils has been identified as a polypeptide of M_r about 60,000 daltons. The results of many studies are compatible with the presence of specific receptors for the Fc fragment of IgG and for the C3b fragment of complement on the surface of the neutrophil. However, the evidence is indirect in that activity, not receptor molecules, is measured [46,105,106].

Ligands to receptors on the external surface of the membrane enhance the fluidity of the membrane [107]. Enhanced membrane fluidity activates two methyltransferase systems, which combines to catalyze methylation of phosphatidylethanolamine to phospha-

TABLE 83-1   Effect of various agents on neutrophils

Agent	Altered ion permeability	Directed locomotion	Vesiculation	Granule secretion	Activated O_2 metabolism	Phosphoinositide turnover increased	Lysophosphatide acylation increased	Arachidonic acid oxidation	References
Chemotactic factors	+	+	+	+	+	+		+	[27,65–73]
Ingestible particles			+	+	+	+	+	+	[74–80]
Endotoxins			+	+	+	+			[77,78,81]
Concanavalin A			+	+	+				[82,83]
NaF				+	+				[77]
Phorbol myristate acetate			+	+	+				[84,85]
Cytochalasin E					+				[86]
Digitonin	+				+	+			[77]
Deoxycholate					+	+			[77]
Leukocidin				+					[87]
Vitamin A				+					[88]
Antineutrophil antibodies					+				[61]
A23187	+			+	+	+			[70,89–91]
Immune complexes				+	+			+	[92]
Pyrogen									[93,94]

tidylcholine and translocate it from the internal to the external plasmalemma [108,109]. The cell surface negative charge decreases, and this may be the result of the choline group (positive charge) moving to the surface. Changes in lipid metabolism and an optimal cholesterol/phospholipid ratio are associated with chemotaxis [110]. There are still many gaps in our knowledge of how chemotactic factors or particles activate the membrane.

Chemotactic factors polarize the locomotion of neutrophils as if acting differentially on multiple sensory sites on the cell [111]. Chemotactic factors alter the net surface negative charge and calcium movement of neutrophils, but it is not known how these changes affect locomotion [112,113]. Neutrophils can orient and locomote in media devoid of calcium but require exogenous magnesium for adherence and locomotion [114]. Nevertheless, changes in free endogenous calcium may be essential for cell activation. The calcium ionophore (A23187), in the presence of extracellular calcium, causes monovalent cation permeability and a redistribution of intracellular calcium along with membrane potential changes, transient elevations in cyclic AMP, superoxide generation, and granule enzyme release [89]. Since the neutrophil has no obvious reservoirs for calcium in the cell cortex, it may acquire calcium through release from

the plasma membrane into the cytoplasm; but there are no data concerning the calcium-storage capacity of the plasma membrane [98]. Alternatively, based on studies with erythrocytes, calcium may enter the neutrophil very slowly by a passive leak [115]. Calcium could also be taken up by endocytosis (phagocytosis and pinocytosis). In the cell, calcium stores may be in mitochondria and endoplasmic reticulum. In an equilibrium state, calcium levels may be highest around those organelles which tend to be in the center of the cell. If the plasma membrane pumps actively drive calcium out of the cell, they might maintain a low calcium level near the inner surface of the plasma membrane. Phagolysosomes isolated from macrophages have an ATP-activated calcium pump, suggesting the existence of such a pump on the inner surface of the plasma membrane [116]. Perturbation of membrane receptors could directly or indirectly vary the activity of these enzymes. Alternatively, clustering of the pumps by such perturbation could concentrate pumping in a given region, thereby causing the free calcium beneath that area to change without increasing the activity of a given pump.

Once exposed to a chemotactic agent, the neutrophil loses its ability to respond a second time, a phenomenon called *deactivation* [117]. The binding of ligands to the cell surface receptor causes internalization of receptors, reducing the number available and thus the responsiveness to that ligand [118–120].

MOTILE CYTOPLASMIC RESPONSES OF THE NEUTROPHIL

MORPHOLOGY OF LOCOMOTION, INGESTION, AND DEGRANULATION

The similarity of the locomotion of neutrophils to that of amebas was noted long ago [121–124]. During locomotion toward a chemotactic source, neutrophils acquire a characteristic asymmetric shape (Figs. 83-2 and 83-3). In the front of the cell is a pseudopodium which advances before the body of the cell containing the nucleus and the cytoplasmic granules. At the rear of the moving cell is a knoblike tail. The anterior pseudopodium undulates or "ruffles" as the neutrophil moves, at a rate of up to 50 μm/min. The pseudopodium, which is very thin, forms immediately when the cell encounters a gradient of chemotactic factor. As the cell moves, the cytoplasm behind the anterior pseudopodium streams forward, almost obliterating the pseudopodium. At this point some granules appear to contact the cell periphery, and the release of lysosomal contents, a recognized response to chemotactic agents [70,72], occurs at this time. The pseudopodium extends again and the process repeats itself.

As the neutrophil meets a particle, the pseudopodium flows around the particle, its extensions fuse, and it thereby encompasses the particle [125]. The ingestion phase can be said to extend from recognition to the end of pseudopodium fusion. The particle thus becomes enclosed within a phagosome into which granules are rapidly discharged, as illustrated in Fig. 83-3 [126,127]. Locomotion is not a prerequisite for ingestion: if neutrophils collide with a particle not secreting a chemotactic substance, pseudopodia form abruptly at the contact point and envelop the particle. Ingested particles gradually move toward the cell interior, where they tumble about with the nucleus and cytoplasmic granules as the cell moves off.

The formation of a pseudopodium is essential for neutrophil locomotion. The interior cytoplasm is squeezed in the direction of the lamellopodium, possibly by the peripheral cytoplasm in the rear of the cell. The pseudopodium is also required for ingestion. When dissolution of the pseudopodium occurs, and the interior contents of the cell are allowed to contact the cell membrane, the granule discharge may occur. Fusion of membranes is a common feature of (1) ingestion, where pseudopodia fuse; (2) degranulation, where granules fuse with the phagosome; and possibly, (3) locomotion, where some granules may fuse with the plasma membrane. Pseudopodia form whether neutrophils are suspended in liquid medium or are attached to a surface, but the cell can only move translationally when fixed to a surface; thus it crawls but does not swim. Such "stickiness" is also a phase of ingestion. The neutrophil membrane adheres firmly to particles it ingests, presumably

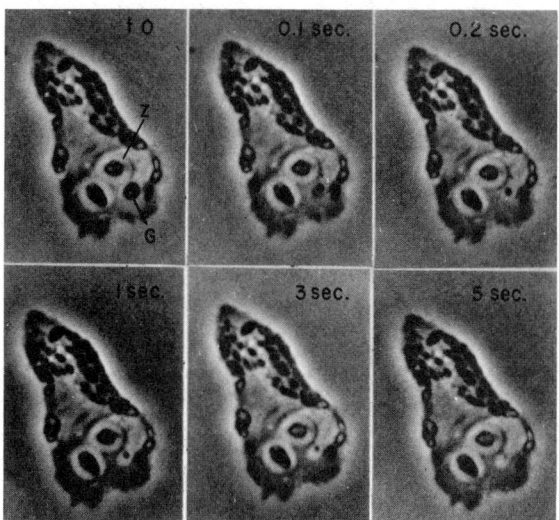

FIGURE 83-3 Cinemicrophotographic observation of granule lysis of a chicken neutrophil following phagocytosis of zymosan particles. Note the lysis of the cytoplasmic granule (G) against one of two ingested zymosan particles (Z). The dense body of the granule disappears from view in the interval of 5 s ($\times$1200). (From J. G. Hirsch, *J. Exp. Med.* **116:**827, 1962.)

to provide the frictional force needed to move pseudopodia around the particles [128]. Thus, the formation of pseudopodia, membrane fusion, and membrane adhesiveness are all characteristics associated with the functional responses of neutrophils.

Cytoskeleton biochemistry affords insight into the basis of neutrophil locomotion, particle ingestion, and digestion. The hyaline pseudopodia of the neutrophil contain filament networks (Fig. 83-4) [129] which are polymers of actin [130]. Actin comprises 10 percent of the protein of the neutrophil and exists in two states: a globular monomer or a double helical polymer. The distribution of the two is unknown, but many actin fibers, oriented in a random fashion, populate the neutrophil's peripheral cytoplasm and exist in a gel state [131]. Myosin represents about 1 percent of the cytoplasmic protein of neutrophils [131] and, like striated muscle myosin, is a hexamer composed of two heavy polypeptide chains and four light chains. By analogy with muscle myosin, the globular domain of neutrophil myosin heavy chains near the C terminus, called the head region, is associated with the light chains and is capable of forming repetitive cross-links with actin monomers into filaments. The cyclic cross-bridge formation requires ATP hydrolysis and results in movement of the actin filament relative to the myosin molecule(s)—the "sliding-filament" mechanism [132]. Actin in the pseudopodia exists as a gel, because actin-binding protein (M_r = 54,000 daltons) cross-links actin filaments [131]. Actin-binding protein, an asymmetrical dimer composed of two very flexible chains [133], comprises 1 percent of the total cell protein, and is concentrated at the cell periphery along with myosin during phagocytosis

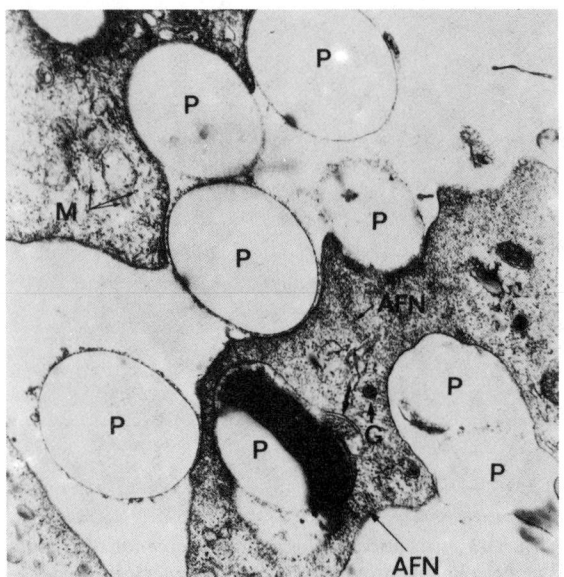

FIGURE 83-4 Thin-section electron micrograph of human neutrophils extending pseudopodia around polystyrene particles. Array of actin filament networks (AFN) and microtubules (MT) are visible and appear to insert into the plasma membrane. Granules (G) have fused with phagosomes (*arrow*).

[134–136]. Calcium concentrations greater than 0.2 μM dissolve the actin gel by activating the protein gelsolin [137], which shortens actin filaments between the cross-linking points [138]. When the calcium concentration falls below the critical level, gelsolin becomes inactive and reannealing and gelation of actin filaments occurs [138].

Myosin-catalyzed hydrolysis of ATP provides energy for the contraction of the actin gel [139,140]. The interaction between actin and myosin can explain the force generation for movement and the dependence of phagocytosis on metabolic energy [134], but not the directionality of the force which is required for purposeful movement. The explanation for this directionality lies in reversible gel-sol transformation of peripheral cytoplasm of phagocytes. Directionality is then provided by two factors which relate to alterations in gel resistance occurring from more highly gelled to less-gelled regions of the actin network. Although each contractile unit in the active lattice consisting of actin and myosin filaments theoretically can generate tension, this tension requires that the actin filaments interacting with myosin be tethered to each other; otherwise they would simply slip past one another. When the Ca^{2+}-gelsolin complex dissolves a region of an actin lattice, both the viscosity and rigidity of actin filaments in this domain decrease and movement occurs away from this area to the region where the lattice is more cross-linked. Control of directional movement arises from regulation of the network consistency of actin by gelsolin and Ca^{2+} [141]. Cytochalasin B, a fungal metabolite, severs actin filaments, leading to dissolution of actin gels, and is a potent inhibitor of phagocytosis [142,143]. In neutrophil actin dysfunction (see Chap. 89) only a fraction of actin forms filaments and phagocytosis is impaired [130].

Phagocytosis represents a sequential translocation of cortical cytoplasm and membrane about an object. A particle could increase calcium efflux at the site of membrane attachment and lead to a local decrease in cytoplasmic calcium concentration [46]. Actin filaments become gelled and subject to tension because of the action of myosin. Strengthening of the gel at the site of contact causes the cytoplasm to bulge lateral to the contact point, where the cortex is relatively weaker, and these bulges become incipient pseudopodia. New membrane-particle contacts propagate cross-linking, moving filaments from adjacent "sol" regions of the cortex near the original contact site into the more highly formed gelled region. As calcium leaks back into the cell cortex from the medium, and by diffusion from the interior of the cell, the calcium content is restored. The restoration of calcium content at the base of the pseudopodium causes the actin gel at the pit of the forming phagocytic vacuole and lateral to the original site of contact of particle and membrane to dissolve. With solution of cortical actin gel by the action of gelsolin and Ca^{2+} at the base of the forming phagocytic vacuole, and the dissipation of actin filaments into the gelated region at the top of the pseudopodium, lysosomes are able to approach the plasma membrane with which they eventually fuse. The thin tip of the pseudopodium is furthest from the cell center and, therefore, the last region to equilibrate its calcium content by diffusion. This region is easiest to clear of calcium by efflux and to maintain calcium concentrations low enough to promote gelation.

The low calcium concentration in the pseudopodium tip keeps a gradient of gel in the tip that recruits sol from the pseudopodium base, the same principle that moved cortical material in from the sides of the original forming pseudopodium. This sequence of events must occur in seconds to conform with the rate that pseudopodia form.

The neutrophil becomes more adhesive during chemotaxis or phagocytosis. It has been suggested that this may be caused by secretion of fibronectin by neutrophils [144]. Membrane fusion during phagosome formation or fusion of granules with the pseudopodium may require the movement of membrane proteins so that the lipid portions of the membrane fuse [145,146]. When neutrophils are in suspension, they aggregate if stimulated with chemotactic factors [147,148]. Aggregation may be sustained by the release of specific granule products and binding to the plasma membrane of "sticky" proteins from these granules, such as acidic proteins and lactoferrin [149,150].

AGENTS WHICH INFLUENCE NEUTROPHIL RESPONSES

Compounds which have been employed to probe the basis of neutrophil function are listed in Table 83-2. These agents can have pronounced, consistent effects on

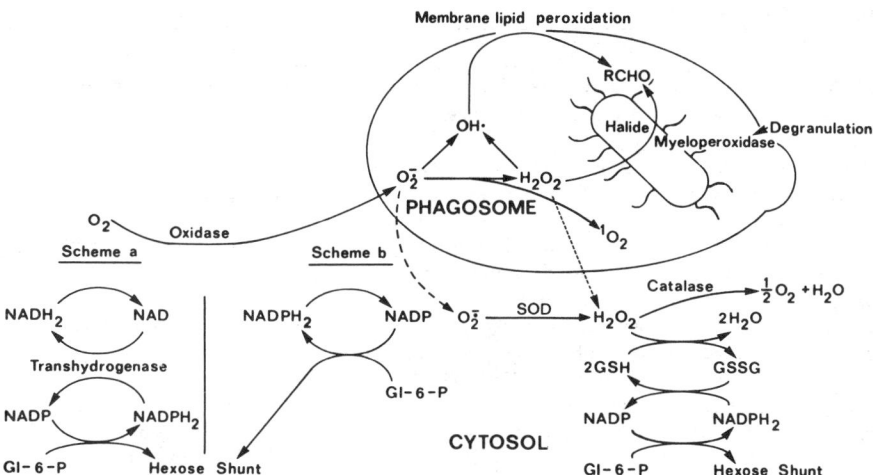

FIGURE 83-5   Possible mechanisms for the production, action, and detoxification of peroxides in polymorphonuclear leukocytes. Oxygen is reduced to superoxide (O_2^-) by an oxidase. Some investigators believe that NADH, regenerated from NADPH by a transhydrogenase or by other mechanisms, is the hydrogen donor for this oxidase (*scheme a*), whereas others favor direct reduction of oxygen by NADPH (*scheme b*). NADPH is regenerated from NADP by the hexose shunt. Superoxide may spontaneously decompose to hydrogen peroxide and singlet oxygen $^1O_2$. Hydrogen peroxide can react with superoxide to form hydroxyl radicals (OH) or generate bactericidal aldehydes by oxidizing bacterial constituents in the presence of halide ions and myeloperoxidase delivered to the phagosome by degranulation. Hydroxyl radicals may peroxidize unsaturated fatty acids of the phagosomal membrane and thereby yield potentially bactericidal aldehydes. Superoxide leaking out of the phagosome may be rapidly converted to hydrogen peroxide by superoxide dismutase (SOD). Hydrogen peroxide in the cytosol is destroyed by catalase or reduced glutathione (GSH). Reduced glutathione is regenerated by coupled reactions that stimulate the flow of glucose 6-phosphate (G-6-P) into the hexose shunt.

various neutrophil functions, but the mechanism of their action is often not fully explained.

Antimicrobial mechanisms of neutrophils

Membrane perturbation results in the formation of oxygen metabolites and the discharge of granule constituents into phagosomes and into the medium, resulting in bactericidal effects on microbes in the phagosome and in the vacinity of the neutrophil [4].

NEUTROPHIL OXYGEN METABOLISM AND ANTIMICROBIAL ACTIVITY

Simulated neutrophils convert oxygen to a series of reduction products [173,174] (Fig. 83-5) by mechanisms that are not entirely clear. It appears that a metal-dependent enzyme system associated with the external surface of the plasma membrane is activated by the stimuli outlined in Table 83-1 and transfers electrons from reduced pyridine nucleotides to molecular oxygen, reducing it to superoxide anion and hydrogen peroxide [173,182]. At an acid pH, superoxide spontaneously dismutates to hydrogen peroxide and generates a species of oxygen with reversed electron spins called singlet oxygen [173]. The decay of singlet oxygen to the ground state is associated with the emission of chemiluminescence. Superoxide and hydrogen peroxide permeate cell

membranes, and both substances are toxic to bacterial and animal cells [183]. The fate of these molecules varies with their location in the neutrophil.

The putative localization of the oxygen-reducing enzyme on the external surface of the plasma membrane provides a topological means of limiting or concentrating production of toxic oxygen metabolites either outside the cell or within the phagosome, and hydrogen peroxide is largely localized to the sites [180,184]. Since the pH of the phagosome falls during ingestion [185], superoxide in the phagosome is converted spontaneously to hydrogen peroxide. This reaction may be responsible for the fact that phagocytizing neutrophils produce chemiluminescence [186,187]. Hydrogen peroxide in the phagosome is degraded by the heme-containing enzyme myeloperoxidase, which enters the phagosome during degranulation. Superoxide anion, which has a low oxidizing potential, condenses with hydrogen peroxide to form a hydroxyl radical via the iron-catalyzed Haber-Weiss reaction. Iron for this reaction may be provided by the granule-associated iron-binding protein, lactoferrin [188]. Superoxide anion, hydrogen peroxide, hydroxyl radicals, singlet oxygen, and myeloperoxidase-mediated hydrogen peroxide degradation all have microbicidal activity [4,172,189]. The myeloperoxidase reaction requires a halide, either chloride or iodide, to kill microorganisms, but the mechanism of action is not entirely clear. The enzyme may

TABLE 83-2 Agents which alter neutrophil responses

Agent	Effects	Interpretation
Divalent cations: manganese magnesium, calcium	Enhance or in some instances required for chemotaxis, adhesiveness, ingestion, degranulation, oxygen metabolism [49,112,114,151]	Site of action unknown
Colchicine, vinca alkaloids, GSSG-forming oxidants	Inhibits chemotaxis and ingestion (in some instances), degranulation, oxygen metabolism; alter mobility of membrane receptors, impair adherence [99,152,153]	Interfere with stability microtubules
β-active amines, prostaglandin E_1, PGI_2	Increase cyclic AMP levels of neutrophils; inhibit adherence chemotaxis, ingestion, degranulation, oxygen metabolism [151,153–157]	Site of action unknown
Parasympathomimetic agents	Increase cyclic 3′,5′-guanosine monophosphate levels of neutrophils; enhance chemotaxis and degranulation; antagonize some effects of colchicine [153,158,159]	Site of action unknown
Organophosphorus compounds	Inhibit chemotaxis, ingestion, degranulation if present together with eliciting stimulus and superoxide anion generation	Inhibit activatable serine esterase of neutrophil [160] or some other site [161]
Inhibitors of glycolysis	Inhibit chemotaxis, adhesiveness, ingestion, degranulation	Prevent ATP formation [147]
Cytochalasin B	Depending on dose, enhances or inhibits chemotaxis; inhibits ingestion; enhances superoxide anion release, hexose transport [143,162–166]	Acts on glucose transport and fragments fibrillar actin [142]
Inhibitors of lipoxygenase activity	Inhibit chemotaxis	Deplete endogenous concentrations of HETE [167]
Glucocorticoids	Inhibit locomotion and phagocytosis (high doses and/or sustained administrations), inhibit phospholipase A_2 [168–170]	Site of action unknown
Local anesthetic agents	Inhibit adhesion, spreading, locomotion	Act on membrane; inhibit reactions mediated by calcium and calmodulin [171,172]

catalyze oxidation of a vital component of microbes, it may produce toxic halide oxidation products such as hypochlorous acid, or it may generate bactericidal aldehydes [4,173]. Superoxide which escapes from the phagosome may be converted rapidly to hydrogen peroxide by the enzyme superoxide dismutase [190,191]. The hydrogen peroxide thus formed in the cytosol is scavenged by the enzyme catalase and by a series of coupled reactions involving reduced glutathione and the hexose monophosphate shunt [192,193]. Hexose monophosphate shunt activation accompanies the general activities of stimulated neutrophils, is required for detoxification of hydrogen peroxide, and is also involved in the regeneration of reduced pyridine nucleotides, which serve to reduce oxygen to superoxide and hydrogen peroxide [194].

OTHER ANTIMICROBIAL PROCESSES
The increase in glycolytic rate accompanying ingestion generates lactic acid, which lowers the pH of the contents of the phagosome. Acid itself has some antibacterial action, and it optimizes the antimicrobial power of the oxygen-dependent and other enzymatic systems of the neutrophil. Degranulation, which occurs rapidly [195], delivers to the phagosome substances with antimicrobial activity (Table 83-3). These substances are apportioned among the primary (azurophil) and specific

granules of the neutrophil, and their function in the absence of oxygen metabolites is unknown. The weak antibacterial action of some of these agents may be potentiated by other processes. For example, the bacteriolytic action of lysozyme has been reported to be enhanced by complement and by ascorbic acid in the presence of metal ions [196,197]. The neutrophil can accumulate large quantities of ascorbate, although the reason for this is not known [207].

The neutrophil in immunity and inflammation

IMMUNITY
The determination of the neutrophil's role in immunity is based on observations of its function in animal models or in human disease. Interpretation of the results, particularly in human beings, is hampered by the complexity of susceptibility to infection. Infections associated with neutropenic states generally involve the superficial tissues and lungs and are usually caused by *S. aureus* and gram-negative enteric microorganisms. Mucosal ulcerations can occur. Clinical observations indicate that the neutrophil maintains control of the "frontier outposts" which interface with microbial pop-

TABLE 83-3 Antimicrobial agents associated with neutrophil granules

Granule class	Agent	Possible mechanism of action
Primary, or azurophilic granule	Myeloperoxidase	Potentiates microbicidal activity of hydrogen peroxidase [4]
	Lysozyme	Hydrolyzes glycosidic linkage between acetylmuramic acid and acetylglucosamine in the cell wall polymer of susceptible bacteria. Ascorbic acid, complement, or other agents may increase this susceptibility [196,197]
	Neutral and acid hydrolases	Limited degradation of microbial macromolecules [198,199]
	Cationic proteins [200–202]	Bactericidal to rough strains of gram-negative bacteria by causing alterations in permeability to macromolecular constituents [203]
Secondary, or specific (neutrophilic), granule	Lysozyme	
	Collagenase	Digests microbial macromolecules [204]
	Lactoferrin	Chelates iron required for microbial growth causing bacteriostasis [189,205,206]; catalyzes formation of hydroxyl radical

ulations. A steady flow of neutrophils into these areas is necessary to maintain this control, although the host appears able to tolerate prolonged periods of markedly diminished rates in this flow. Findings similar to those observed in patients with severe neutropenia were described [208] in an infant with a defect in neutrophil migration and in animals rendered neutropenic with antineutrophil serum [209].

INFLAMMATION

The discharge of neutrophil granule contents and of toxic oxygen metabolites into the surrounding tissues may be triggered by many mechanisms: (1) chemotactic factors activate degranulation and oxygen metabolism; (2) during ingestion, granule contents and oxygen metabolites may leak out of partially closed phagosomes or may be secreted directly; (3) cell death and dissolution may occur after an encounter with antigens or microbes. The antimicrobial agents of neutrophils are known to have deleterious effects on animal cells, including the neutrophil itself [210]. Hydrogen peroxide and myeloperoxidase plus a halide kill mammalian cells as well as bacteria [211]. The proteolytic enzymes of neutrophils are capable of digesting cartilage mucopolysaccharide [212] and lung tissue in α_1-antitrypsin deficiency [213], and oxidizing radicals can damage synovial tissue [214]. Products of the lipoxygenase pathway are chemotactic and can recruit more neutrophils to sites of inflammation [29]. Leukotriene (the slow-reacting substance of anaphylaxis) may constrict bronchioles, producing asthma.

The role of neutrophils in inflammatory states has been demonstrated in a number of diseases. Depletion of neutrophils protects the guinea pig from passive cutaneous anaphylaxis [215] and the rat from the inflammatory changes of homograft rejection [216]. Granule extrusion has been demonstrated ultrastructurally in experimental models of endothelial damage and urate crystal–induced inflammatory disease [217,218]. Urate crystal ingestion by neutrophils may be a cause of inflammatory changes in synovial tissues. The pathogen-

esis of diseases in which immune complexes are filtered by vascular organs, such as the kidney in acute glomerulonephritis, or appear in distinct tissues, such as in synovia in rheumatoid arthritis, or are incited by preformed complexes deposited into the lungs of animals can be explained by postulating that the complexes activate the complement and other cascades to produce chemotactic fragments. These fragments attract neutrophils which ingest the complexes, degranulate extracellularly, and generate toxic oxygen metabolites which injure the surrounding tissue. The proteases released from the neutrophils, in turn, create more chemotactic factors by direct breakdown of C3 and C5, thereby propagating the inflammatory cycle. Diseases such as acute glomerulonephritis, arthritis, or pneumonitis may result [219–221].

References

1. Bellanti, J. A., and Dayton, D. H. (eds.): _The Phagocytic Cell in Host Resistance._ Raven Press, New York, 1975.

2. Stossel, T. P.: Phagocytosis. _N. Engl. J. Med._ 290:717, 1974.

3. Cline, M. J., Craddock, C. G., Gale, R. P., Golde, D. W., and Lehrer, R. I.: Granulocytes in human disease. _Ann. Intern. Med._ 81:801, 1974.

4. Klebanoff, S. J., and Clark, R. A.: _The Neutrophil: Function and Clinical Disorders._ Elsevior North-Holland, New York, 1978, chaps. 1–7, p. 1.

5. O'Flaherty, J. T., and Ward, P. A.: Chemotactic factors and the neutrophil. _Semin. Hematol._ 16:163, 1979.

6. Cohen, S., and Ward, P. A.: _In vitro_ and _in vivo_ activity of a lymphocyte and the immune complex-dependent chemotactic factor for eosinophils. _J. Exp. Med._ 133:133, 1971.

7. Ward, P. A., Remold, H. G., and David, J. R.: The production by antigen-stimulated lymphocytes of a leukotactic factor distinct from migration inhibitory factor. _Cell. Immunol._ 2:162, 1970.

8. Alper, C. A., and Rosen, F. S.: Complement deficiencies in humans, in _Clinical Immunology Update, 1981,_ edited by E. A. Franklin. Elsevior North-Holland, New York, 1981, p. 59.

9. Muller-Eberhard, H. J.: Complement. _Annu. Rev. Biochem._ 44:697, 1975.

10. Hill, J. H., and Ward, P. A.: The phlogistic role of C5 leukotactic fragments in myocardial infarcts of rats. _J. Exp. Med._ 133:885, 1971.

11. Brozna, J. P., Senior, R. M., Kreutzer, D. L. and Ward, P. A.: Chemotactic factor inactivator of human granulocytes. *J. Clin. Invest.* 60:1280, 1977.

12. Hugli, T. E., and Muller-Eberhard, H. J.: Anaphylatoxins: C3a and C5a. *Adv. Immunol.* 26:1, 1978.

13. Taylor, J. C., Crawford, I., and Hugli, T. E.: Limited degradation of the third component (C3) of human complement by human leukocyte elastase (HLE): Partial characterization of C3 fragments. *Biochemistry* 16:3390, 1977.

14. Fernandey, H. N., Henson, P. M., Otani, A., and Hugli, T. E.: Chemotactic response to human C3a and C5a anaphylatoxins. I. Evaluation of C3a and C5a leukotaxis in vitro and under stimulated in vivo conditions. *J. Immunol.* 120:109, 1977.

15. Fernandez, H., and Hugli, T. E.: Primary structural analysis of the polypeptide portion of human C5a anaphylatoxin. *J. Biol. Chem.* 253:6955, 1979.

16. Kaplan, A. P., Kay, A. B., and Austen, K. F.: The prealbumin activator of prekallikrein. III. Appearance of chemotactic activity for human neutrophils by the conversion of human prekallikrein to kallikrein. *J. Exp. Med.* 135:81, 1972.

17. Stecher, V. J., and Sorkin, E.: The chemotactic activity of fibrinolysis products. *Int. Arch. Allergy Appl. Immunol.* 43:879, 1972.

18. Kaplan, A. P., Goetzl, E. J., and Austen, K. F.: The fibrinolytic pathway of human plasma. II. The generation of chemotactic activity by activation of plasminogen proactivator. *J. Clin. Invest.* 52:2591, 1973.

19. Ward, P. A., Lepow, I. H., and Newman, L. J.: Bacterial factors chemotactic for polymorphonuclear leukocytes. *Am. J. Pathol.* 52:725, 1968.

20. Goldstein, I. M., and Weissmann, G.: Generation of C5-derived lysosomal enzyme-releasing activity (C5a) by lysates of leukocyte lysosomes. *J. Immunol.* 113:1588, 1974.

21. Ward, P. A., Chapitis, J., Conroy, M. C., and Lepow, I. H.: Generation by bacterial proteinases of leukotactic factors from human serum and C3 and C5. *J. Immunol.* 110:1003, 1973.

22. Phelps, P.: Polymorphonuclear leukocyte motility *in vitro*. III. Possible release of a chemotactic substance after phagocytosis of urate crystals by polymorphonuclear leukocytes. *Arthritis Rheum.* 12:197, 1969.

23. Zigmond, S. H., and Hirsch, J. G.: Leukocyte locomotion and chemotaxis: New methods for evaluation and demonstration of a cell-derived chemotactic factor. *J. Exp. Med.* 137:387, 1973.

24. Spilberg, I., Gallacher, A., and Mandell, B.: Studies on crystal-induced chemotactic factors. II. Role of phagocytosis. *J. Lab. Clin. Med.* 85:631, 1975.

25. Sorkin, E., Stecher, V. J., and Borel, J. E.: Chemotaxis of leukocytes and inflammation. *Ser. Haematol.* 3:131, 1970.

26. Turner, S. R., Campbell, J. A., and Lynn, W. S.: Polymorphonuclear leukocyte chemotaxis toward oxidized lipid components of cell membranes. *J. Exp. Med.* 141:1437, 1975.

27. Goetzl, E. J., Woods, J. M., and Gorman, R. R.: Stimulation of human eosinophil and neutrophil polymorphonuclear leukocyte chemotaxis and random migration by 12-L-hydroxy-5,8,10,14-eicosatetraenoic acid. *J. Clin. Invest.* 59:179, 1977.

28. Ford-Hutchinson, A. W., Bray, M. A., Dois, M. V., Shipley, M. E., and Smith, N.: Leukotriene B, a potent chemokinetic and aggregating substance released from polymorphonuclear leukocytes. *Nature (London)* 286:264, 1980.

29. Kuehl, F. A., Jr., and Eagan, R. W.: Prostaglandins, arachidonic acid, and inflammation. *Science* 210:978, 1980.

30. Schiffmann, E., Cocoran, B. A., and Wahl, S. N.: N-formyl-methionyl peptides as chemoattractants for leucocytes. *Proc. Natl. Acad. Sci. U.S.A.* 72:1059, 1975.

31. Wilkinson, P. C.: Surface and cell membrane activities of leukocyte chemotactic factors. *Nature* 252:58, 1974.

32. Showell, H. J.: The structure-activity relations of synthetic peptides as chemotactic factors and inducers of lysosomal enzyme secretion for neutrophils. *J. Exp. Med.* 143:1154, 1976.

33. Schiffmann, E., and Aswanikumar, S.: *Molecular Events in the Response of Neutrophils to Synthetic N-f MET Chemotactic Peptides: Demonstration of a Specific Receptor*, edited by J. I. Gallin and P. G. Quie. Raven Press, New York, 1978, p. 97.

34. Synderman, R., and Pike, M. C.: *Pathophysiologic Aspects of Leuko-cyte Chemotaxis: Identification of a Specific Chemotactic Factor Binding Site on Human Granulocytes and Defects of Macrophage Function Associated with Neoplasia,* edited by J. I. Gallin and P. G. Quie. Raven Press, New York, 1978, p. 357.

35. Chenoweth, D. E., and Hugli, T. E.: Demonstration of specific C5a receptor an intact human polymorphonuclear leukocytes. *Proc. Natl. Acad. Sci. U.S.A.* 75:3943, 1978.

36. Ruddy, S., Gigli, I., and Austen, K. F.: The complement system of man. *N. Engl. J. Med.* 287:489, 1972.

37. Ward, P. A., Data, R., and Till, G.: Regulatory control of complement-derived chemotactic and anaphylatoxin mediators. *Prog. Immunol.* 2:209, 1974.

38. Goldstein, I. M.: Endogenous regulation of complement (C5)-derived chemotactic activity: Fine-tuning of inflammation. *J. Lab. Clin. Med.* 93:13, 1979.

39. Ward. P. A., and Ozols, J: Characterization of the protease activity in the chemotactic factor inactivator. *J. Clin. Invest.* 58:123, 1976.

40. Perez, H. D., Lipton, M., and Goldstein, I. M.: A specific inhibitor of complement (C5)-derived chemotactic activity in serum from patients with systemic lupus erythematosus. *J. Clin. Invest.* 63:29, 1979.

41. Van Oss, C. J., and Gillman, C. F.: Phagocytosis as a surface phenomenon. I. Contract angles and phagocytosis of nonopsonized bacteria. *J. Reticuloendothel. Soc.* 12:292, 1972.

42. Stossel, T. P., Mason, R. J., Hartwig, M., and Vaughan, M.: Quantitative studies of phagocytosis by polymorphonuclear leukocytes: Use of emulsions to measure the initial rate of phagocytosis. *J. Clin. Invest.* 51:615, 1972.

43. Rabinovitch, M.: Phagocytosis: The engulfment stage. *Semin. Hematol.* 5:134, 1968.

44. Jones, T. C., and Hirsch, J. G.: The interaction in vitro of *Mycoplasma pulmonis* with mouse peritoneal macrophages and L-cells. *J. Exp. Med.* 133:231, 1971.

45. Griffin, F. M., Griffin, J. A., and Silverstein, S. C.: Studies on the mechanism of phagocytosis. II. The interaction of macrophages with anti-immunoglobulin IgG-coated bone marrow–derived lymphocytes. *J. Exp. Med.* 144:788, 1976.

46. Silverstein, S. C., Steinman, R. M., and Cohn, Z. A.: Endocytosis. *Annu. Rev. Biochem.* 46:669, 1977.

47. Guerry, D., Kenna, M. A., Schreiber, A. D., and Cooper, R. A.: Concanavalin A–mediated binding and sphering of human red cells by homologous monocytes. *J. Exp. Med.* 144:1695, 1976.

48. Scribner, D. J., and Fahrney, D.: Neutrophil receptors for IgG and complement: Their roles in the attachment and ingestion phases of phagocytosis. *J. Immunol.* 116:892, 1976.

49. Stossel, T. P.: Phagocytosis: Recognition and ingestion. *Semin. Hematol.* 14:83, 1975.

50. Rottini, G., Dri, P., Soranzo, M. R., and Patriarca, P.: Correlation between phagocytic activity and metabolic response of polymorphonuclear leukocytes toward different strains of *Escherichia coli. Infect. Immun.* 11:417, 1975.

51. Repine, J. E., Clawson, C. C., and Friend, P. S.: Influence of a deficiency of the second component of complement on the bactericidal activity of neutrophils in vitro. *J. Clin. Invest.* 59:802, 1977.

52. Horwitz, M. A., and Silverstein, S. G.: Influence of the *Escherichia coli* capsule on complement fixation and on phagocytosis and killing by human phagocytes. *J. Clin. Invest.* 65:82, 1980.

53. Winkelstein, J. A., and Tomasz, A.: Activation of the alternative pathway by pneumococcal cell wall. *J. Immunol.* 118:451, 1977.

54. Wilkinson, B. J., Kim, Y., Peterson, P. K., Quie, P. G., and Michael, A. F.: Activation of complement by cell surface components of *Staphylococcus aureus. Infect. Immun.* 20:388, 1978.

55. Gibbs, D. L., and Roberts, R. B.: The interaction *in vitro* between human polymorphonuclear leukocytes and *Neisseria gonorrhorea* cultivated in the chick embryo. *J. Exp. Med.* 141:155, 1975.

56. Densen, P., and Mandell, G. L.: Gonococcal interactions with polymorphonuclear neutrophils. Importance of the phagosome for bactericidal activity. *J. Clin. Invest.* 62:1161, 1978.

57. Stossel, T. P., Field, R. J., Gitlin, J. D., Alper, C. A., and Rosen, F. S.: The osponic fragment of the third component of human complement (C3). *J. Exp. Med.* 141:1329, 1975.

58. Law, S. K., Lichtenberg, N. A., and Levine, R. P.: Evidence for an

ester linkage between the labile binding site of C3b and receptive surfaces. *J. Immunol. 123*:1388, 1979.

59. Quie, P. G., Messner, R. P., and Williams, R. C., Jr.: Phagocytosis in subacute bacterial endocarditis: Localization of the primary opsonic site to Fc fragment. *J. Exp. Med. 128*:553, 1968.

60. Handin, R. I., and Stossel, T. P.: Phagocytosis of antibody-coated platelets by human granulocytes. *J. Exp. Med. 290*:989, 1974.

61. Boxer, L. A., and Stossel, T. P.: Effects of anti-neutrophil antibodies in vitro: Quantitative studies. *J. Clin. Invest. 53*:1534, 1974.

62. Tullis, J. L., and Surgenor, D. M.: Phagocytosis-promoting factor of plasma and serum. *Ann. N.Y. Acad. Sci. 66*:386, 1956.

63. Kindmark, C.-O.: Stumulating effect of C-reactive protein on phagocytosis of various species of pathogenic bacteria. *Clin. Exp. Immunol. 8*:941, 1971.

64. Moser, D. F., and Procter, R. A.: Binding and factor XIIIa-mediated cross-linking of a 27-kilodalton fragment of fibronectin to *Staphylococcus aureus. Science 209*:927, 1980.

65. Boucek, M. M., and Synderman, R.: Calcium influx requirement for human neutrophil chemotaxis: Inhibition by lanthanum chloride. *Science 193*:905, 1976.

66. Naccache, P. H., Showell, H. J., Berker, E. L., and Sha'afi, R. I.: Transport of sodium, potassium, and calcium across rabbit polymorphonuclear leukocyte membranes: Effect of chemotactic factor. *J. Cell Biol. 75*:606, 1977.

67. Goldstein, I. M., et al.: Thromboxane generation by human peripheral blood polymorphonuclear leukocytes. *J. Exp. Med. 148*:787, 1978.

68. Borgeat, P., Hamberg, M., and Samuelsson, B.: Transformation of arachidonic acid and homo-γ-linoleic acid by polymorphonuclear leukocytes. *J. Biol. Chem. 251*:7816, 1976.

69. Bokoch, G. M., and Reed, P. W.: Stimulation of arachidonic acid and metabolism in the polymorphonuclear leukocyte by an N-formylated peptide: Comparison with ionophore A23187. *J. Biol. Chem. 255*:10223, 1980.

70. Becker, E. L., Showell, H. J., Henson, P. M., and Hsu, L. S.: The ability of chemotactic factors to induce lysosomal enzyme release. I. The characteristics of the release, the importance of surfaces and the relation of enzyme release to chemotactic responsiveness. *J. Immunol. 112*:2047, 1974.

71. Goetzl, E. J., and Austen, K. F.: Stimulation of human neutrophil leukocyte aerobic glucose metabolism by purified chemotactic factors. *J. Clin. Invest. 53*:591, 1974.

72. Goldstein, I., Hoffstein, S., Gallin, J., and Weissman, G.: Mechanisms of lysosomal enzyme release from human leukocytes: Microtubule assembly and membrane fusion induced by a component of complement. *Proc. Natl. Acad. Sci. U.S.A. 70*:2916, 1973.

73. Stenson, W. F., and Parker, C. W.: Monohydroyeicosatetraenoic acids (HETES) induce degranulation of human neutrophils. *J. Immunol. 124*:2100, 1980.

74. Naccache, P. H., Showell, H. J., Becker, E. L., and Sha'afi, R. I.: Changes of ionic movement across polymorphonuclear leukocyte membranes during lysosomal enzyme release. Possible ionic basis for lysosomal enzyme release. *J. Cell Biol. 75*:635, 1977.

75. Barthelemy, A., Paridaens, R., and Schell-Frederick, E.: Phagocytosis-induced ⁴⁵calcium efflux in polymorphonuclear leukocytes. *FEBS Lett. 82*:283, 1977.

76. Davidson, E. M., Doig, V., Ford-Hutchinson, A. W., and Smith, M. J. H.: Prostaglandin and thromboxane production of rabbit polymorphonuclear leukocytes and rat macrophages. *Adv. Prostaglandin Thromboxane Res. 8*:1661, 1980.

77. Karnovsky, M. L.: The metabolism of leukocytes. *Semin. Hematol. 5*:156, 1968.

78. Michell, R. H.: Inositol phospholipids and cell surface receptor function. *Biochim. Biophys. Acta 415*:81, 1975.

79. Ryan, G. B., Borysenko, J. Z., and Karnovsky, M. J.: Factors affecting the redistribution of surface-bound concanavalin A on human polymorphonuclear leukocytes. *J. Cell Biol. 65*:351, 1974.

80. Elsbch, P.: Lipid metabolis by phagocytes. *Semin. Hematol. 9*:227, 1972.

81. Simberkoff, M. S., and Elsbach, P.: The interaction *in vitro* between polymorphonuclear leukocytes and mycoplasma. *J. Exp. Med. 134*:1417, 1971.

82. Hoffstein, S., Soberman, R. B., Goldstein, I., and Weissman, G.: Concanavalin A induces microtubule assembly and specific granule discharge in human polymorphonuclear leukocytes. *J. Cell Biol. 68*:781, 1976.

83. Romeo, D., Zabucchi, G., and Rossi, F.: Reversible metabolic stimulation of polymorphonuclear leukocytes and macrophages by concanavalin A. *Nature (New. Biol.) 243*:111, 1973.

84. Repine, J. E., White, J. G., Clawson, C. C., and Holmes, B. M.: The influence of phorbol myristate acetate on oxygen consumption by polymorphonuclear leukocytes. *J. Lab. Clin. Med. 83*:911, 1974.

85. White, J. G., and Estensen, R. D.: Selective labilization of specific granules in polymorphonuclear leukocytes by phorbol myristate acetate. *Am. J. Pathol. 75*:45, 1974.

86. Nakagawara, A., Takeshige, K., and Minikami, S.: Induction of a phagocytosis-like metabolic pattern in polymorphonuclear leukocytes by cytochalasin E. *Exp. Cell. Res. 87*:392, 1974.

87. Woodin, A. M.: The extrusion of protein from the rabbit polymorphonuclear leukocyte treated with staphylococcal leucocidin. *Biochem. J. 82*:9, 1962.

88. Davies, P., Allison, A. C., and Haswell, A. D.: Selective release of lysosomal hydrolases from phagocytic cells by cytochalasin B. *Biochem. J. 134*:33, 1973.

89. Simchowitz, L., Spillberg, I., and Atkinson, J. P.: Superoxide generation and granule enzyme release induced by ionophore A23187: Studies on the early events of neutrophil activation. *J. Lab. Clin. Med. 96*:408, 1980.

90. Borgeat, P., and Samuelsson, B.: Arachidonic acid metabolism in polymorphonuclear leukocytes: Effects of ionophore A23187. *Proc. Natl. Acad. Sci. U.S.A. 76*:2148, 1979.

91. Stenson, W. F., and Parker, C. W.: Metabolism of arachidonic acid in ionophore stimulated neutrophils. Esterification of a hydroxylated metabolite into phospholipids. *J. Clin. Invest. 64*:1457, 1979.

92. Smolen, J. E., Korchak, H. M., and Weissmann, G.: Increased levels of cyclic adenosine-3',5'-monophosphate in human polymorphonuclear leukocytes after surface stimulation. *J. Clin. Invest. 65*:1077, 1980.

93. Klempner, M. S., Dinarello, C. A., and Gallin, J. I.: Human leukocyte pyrogen induces release of specific granule contents from human neutrophils. *J. Clin. Invest. 61*:1330, 1978.

94. Klempner, M. S., Dinarello, C. A., Henderson, W. R., and Gallin, J. I.: Stimulation of neutrophil oxygen-dependent metabolism by human leukocyte pyrogen. *J. Clin. Invest. 64*:996, 1979.

95. Korchak, H. M., and Weissmann, G.: Changes in membrane potential of human granulocytes antecede the metabolic responses to surface stimulation. *Proc. Natl. Acad. Sci. U.S.A. 75*:3818, 1978.

96. Whitin, J. C., Chapman, C. E., Simons, E. R., Chovaniec, M., and Cohen, H. J.: Correlation between membrane potential changes and superoxide production in human granulocytes stimulated by phorbol myristate acetate. *J. Biol. Chem. 255*:1874, 1980.

97. Seligmann, B. E., and Gallin, J. I.: Use of lipophilic probes of membrane potential to assess human neutrophil activation. Abnormality in chronic granulomatous disease. *J. Clin. Invest. 66*:493, 1980.

98. Nacchache, P. H., Volpi, M., Showell, H. J., Becker, E. L., and Sha'afi, R. I.: Chemotactic factor-induced release of membrane calcium in rabbit neutrophils. *Science 203*:461, 1979.

99. Baehner, R. L., and Boxer, L. A.: Disorders of polymorphonuclear leukocyte function related to alterations in the integrated reactions of cytoplasmic constituents with the plasma membrane. *Semin. Hematol. 16*:148, 1979.

100. Singer, S. J., and Nicolson, G. L.: The fluid mosaic model of the structure of membranes. *Science 1975*:720, 1972.

101. Anderson, C. L., and Grey, H. M.: Solubilization and partial characterization of cell membrane Fc receptors. *J. Immunol. 118*:819, 1977.

102. Fearson, D. T.: Identification of the membrane glycoprotein that is the C3b receptor of the human erythrocyte, polymorphonuclear leukocyte, B lymphocyte, and monocyte. *J. Exp. Med. 152*:20, 1980.

103. Kulcycki, A., Jr., Krause, V., Killon, C. C., and Atkinson, J. P.: Purification of Fcγ receptor from rabbit alveolar macrophages that retains ligand binding activity. *J. Immunol. 124*:2772, 1980.

104. Niedel, J. Davis, J., and Cuatrecasas, P: Covalent affinity labeling of

the formyl peptide chemotactic receptor. *J. Biol. Chem.* 255.7063, 1980.

105. Newman, S. L., and Johnston, R. B., Jr.: Role of binding through C3b and IgG in polymorphonuclear neutrophil function: Studies with trypsin-generated IgG. *J. Immunol.* 123:1839, 1979.

106. Messner, R. P., and Jelinek, J.: Receptors for human γ-globulin on human neutrophils. *J. Clin. Invest.* 49:2165, 1970.

107. Kimelberg, H. K.: The influence of membrane fluidity on the activity of membrane-bound enzymes, in *Dynamic Aspects of Cell Surface Organization*, edited by G. Poste and G. L. Nicolson. Elsevier North-Holland, New York, 1977, vol. 3, p. 205.

108. Hirata, F., and Axelrod, J.: Enzymatic synthesis and rapid translocation of phosphatidyl choline by two methyltransferases in erythrocyte membranes. *Proc. Natl. Acad. Sci. U.S.A.* 75:2348, 1978.

109. Pike, M. C., Kredich, N. M., and Synderman, R.: Requirement of S-adenosyl-L-methionine mediated methylation for human monocyte chemotaxis. *Proc. Natl. Acad. Sci. U.S.A.* 75:3928, 1978.

110. Pike, M. C., and Synderman, R.: Lipid requirements for leukocyte chemotaxis and phagocytosis: Effects of inhibitors of phospholipid and cholesterol synthesis. *J. Immunol.* 124:1963, 1980.

111. Zigmond, S. H.: Mechanisms of sensing chemical gradients by polymorphonuclear leukocytes. *Nature* 249:450, 1974.

112. Gallin, J. I., and Rosenthal, A. S.: The regulatory role of divalent cations in human granulocyte chemotaxis: Evidence for an association between calcium exchanges and microtubule assembly. *J. Cell Biol.* 62:594, 1974.

113. Gallin, J. I., Durocher, J. R., and Kaplan, A. P.: Interaction of leukocyte chemotactic factors with the cell surface. I. Chemotactic factor-induced changes in human granulocyte surface charge. *J. Clin. Invest.* 55:967, 1975.

114. Marasio, W. A., Becker, E. L., and Oliver, J. M.: The ionic basis of chemotaxis. Separate cation requirements for neutrophil orientation and locomotion in a gradient of chemotactic peptide. *Am. J. Pathol.* 98:749, 1980.

115. Schatzman, H. J., and Burgin, H.: Calcium in human red cells. *Ann. N.Y. Acad. Sci.* 307:125, 1978.

116. Lew. P. D., and Stossel, T. P.: Calcium transport by macrophage plasma membrane. *J. Biol. Chem.* 255:5841, 1980.

117. Ward, P. A., and Becker, E. L.: The deactivation of rabbit neutrophils by chemotactic factor and the nature of the activatable esterase. *J. Exp. Med.* 127:693, 1968.

118. Sullivan, S. J., and Zigmond, S. H.: Chemotactic peptide receptor modulation in polymorphonuclear leukocytes. *J. Cell Biol.* 85:703, 1980.

119. Niedel, J. E., Kahane, I., and Cvatrecasas, P.: Receptor-mediated internalization of fluorescent chemotactic peptide by human neutrophils. *Science* 205:1412, 1979.

120. Zigmond, S. H.: The ability of polymorphonuclear leukocytes to orient in gradient of chemotactic factor. *J. Cell Biol.* 75:606, 1977.

121. Lewis, W. H.: On the locomotion of the polymorphonuclear neutrophils of the rat in autoplasma cultures. *Bull. Johns Hopkins Hosp.* 55:273, 1934.

122. Dixon, H. M., and McCutcheon, M.: Chemotropism of leukocytes in relation to their rate of locomotion. *Proc. Soc. Exp. Biol. Med.* 34:173, 1936.

123. Debruyn, P. P. H.: The amoeboid movement of the mammalian leukocyte in tissue culture. *Anat. Res.* 95:177, 1946.

124. Zigmond, S. H.: Chemotaxis by polymorphonuclear leukocytes. *J. Cell Biol.* 77:269, 1978.

125. Mudd, E. B. H., and Mudd, S.: The process of phagocytosis. The agreement between direct observation and deductions from theory. *J. Gen. Physiol.* 16:625, 1933.

126. Hirsch, J. G., and Cohn, Z. A.: Degranulation of polymorphonuclear leukocytes following phagocytosis of microorganisms. *J. Exp. Med.* 112:1005, 1960.

127. Zucker-Franklin, D., and Hirsch. J. G.: Electron microscope studies on the degranulation of rabbit peritoneal leukocytes during phagocytosis. *J. Exp. Med.* 120:569, 1964.

128. Garvin, J. E.: Factors affecting the adhesiveness of human leukocytes and platelets in vitro. *J. Exp. Med.* 114:51, 1961.

129. Keyserlingk, D. G.: Elektronenmikroskopische Untersuchung uber

die Differzierungsvorgange im Cytoplasma von Segmentierten Neutrophilen Leukozyten wahrend der Zellbewegung. *Exp. Cell Res.* 51:79, 1968.

130. Boxer, L. A., Hedley-Whyte, E. T., and Stossel, T. P.: Neutrophil actin dysfunction and abnormal neutrophil motility. *N. Engl. J. Med* 293:1093, 1974.

131. Boxer, L. A., and Stossel, T. P.: Interactions of actin, myosin and an actin-binding protein of chronic myelogenous leukemic leukocytes. *J. Clin. Invest.* 57:964, 1976.

132. Adelstein, R. S., and Pollard, T. D.: Platelet contractile proteins, in *Progress in Hemostasis*, edited by T. H. Spaet, Grune & Stratton, New York, 1978, vol. 4. p. 37.

133. Hartwig, J. H., and Stossel, T. P.: Structure of actin-binding protein molecule in solution and interacting with actin filaments. *J. Mol. Biol.* 145:563, 1981.

134. Davies, W. A., and Stossel, T. P.: Peripheral hyaline blebs (podosomes) of macrophages. *J. Cell Biol.* 75:941, 1977.

135. Boxer, L. A., Richardson, S., and Floyd, A.: Identification of actin-binding protein in membrane of polymorphonuclear leukocytes. *Nature* 263:259, 1976.

136. Stendahl, O. I., Hartwig, J. H., Brotschi, E. A., and Stossel, T. P.: Distribution of actin-binding protein in macrophages during spreading and phagocytosis. *J. Cell Biol.* 84:215, 1980.

137. Yin, H., and Stossel, T. P.: Control of cytoplasmic actin gel-sol transformation by gelsolin, a calcium-dependent regulatory protein. *Nature* 281:583, 1979.

138. Yin, H. L., Zaner, K. S., and Stossel, T. P.: Ca^{2+} control of actin gelation. Interaction of gelsolin with actin filaments and regulation of actin gelation. *J. Biol. Chem.* 255:9494, 1980.

139. Stossel, T. P., and Pollard, T. D.: Myosin in polymorphonuclear leukocytes. *J. Biol. Chem.* 248:8288, 1973.

140. Shibata, H., Tatsumi, N., Tanaka, K., Okamura, Y., and Senda, N.: A contractile protein processing Ca^{2+} sensitivity (natural actomyosin) from leukocytes: Its extraction and some of its properties. *Biochim. Biophys. Acta* 256:565, 1972.

141. Stendahl, O. I., and Stossel, T. P.: Actin-binding protein amplifies actomyosin contraction and gelsolin confers calcium control on the direction of contraction. *Biochem. Biophys. Res. Commun.* 92:675, 1980.

142. Hartwig, J. H., and Stossel, T. P.: Cytochalasin B and the structure of actin gels. *J. Mol. Biol.* 134:539, 1979.

143. Malawista, S. E., Gee, J. B. L., and Bensch, K. G.: Cytochalasin B reversibly inhibits phagocytosis: Functional, metabolic and ultrastructural effects in human blood leukocytes and rabbit alveolar macrophages. *Yale J. Biol. Med.* 44:286, 1971.

144. Weissmann, G., et al.: Neutrophils synthesize and deposit fibronectin on surfaces to which they attach. *Clin. Res.* 28:552A, 1980.

145. Berlin, R. D., and Oliver, J. M.: Analogous ultrastructure and surface properties during capping and phagocytosis in leukocytes. *J. Cell Biol.* 77:789, 1978.

146. Chi, E. Y., Lagunoff, D., and Koehler, J. K.: Freeze-fracture study of mast cell secretion. *Proc. Natl. Acad. Sci. U.S.A.* 73:2823, 1976.

147. O'Flaherty, J. I., and Ward, P. A.: Leukocyte aggregation induced by chemotactic factors: A review. *Inflammation* 3:177, 1978.

148. Craddock, P. R., Hammerschmidt, D. E., Moldow, C. F., Yamado, O., and Jacob, H. S.: Granulocyte aggregation as a manifestation of membrane interactions with complement: Possible role in leukocyte margination, microvascular occlusion and endothelial damage. *Semin. Hematol.* 16:140, 1979.

149. Bockenstedt, L. K., and Goetzl, E. J.: Constituents of human neutrophils that mediate enhanced adherence to surfaces. Purification and identification of acidic proteins of the specific granules. *J. Clin. Invest.* 63:1372, 1980.

150. Oseas, R., Yang, H.-H., Baehner, R. L., and Boxer, L. A.: Lactoferrin: A promoter of polymorphonuclear leukocyte adhesiveness. *Blood* 57:939, 1981.

151. Becker, E. L., and Henson, P. M.: In vitro studies of immunologically induced secretion of mediators from cells and related phenomena. *Adv. Immunol.* 17:93, 1973.

152. Berlin, R. D., Oliver, J. M., Ukena, T. E., and Yin, H. H.: The cell surface. *N. Engl. J. Med.* 292:515, 1975.

153. Bandmann, U., Norberg, B., and Rydgren, L.: Polymorphonuclear leukocyte chemotaxis in Boyden chambers: Effect of low concentrations of vinblastine. *Exp. Cell Res.* 13:305, 1974.

154. Ignarro, L. J., Lint, T. F., and George, W. J.: Hormonal control of lysosomal enzyme release from human neutrophils: Effects of autonomic agents on enzyme release, phagocytosis, and cyclic nucleotide levels. *J. Exp. Med.* 139:1395, 1974.

155. Bourne, H. R., et al.: Modulation of inflammation and immunity by cyclic AMP. *Science* 184:19, 1974.

156. Boxer, L. A., Allen, J. M., and Baehner, R. L.: Diminished polymorphonuclear leukocyte adherence. Function dependent on release of cyclic AMP by endothelial cells after stimulation of B-receptors by epinephrine. *J. Clin. Invest.* 66:268, 1980.

157. Boxer, L. A., Allen, M. J., Schmidt, M., Yoder, M., and Baehner, R. L.: Inhibition of polymorphonuclear leukocyte adherence by tacyclin. *J. Lab. Clin. Med.* 95:672, 1980.

158. Estensen, R. D., Hill, H. R., Quie, P. G., Hogan, N., and Goldberg, N. D.: Cyclic GMP and cell movement. *Nature* 245:458, 1973.

159. Oliver, J. M., Zurier, R. B., and Berlin, R. D.: Concanavalin A cap formation on polymorphonuclear leukocytes of normal and beige (Chediak-Higashi) mice. *Nature* 253:471, 1975.

160. Woodin, A. M., and Harris, A.: The inhibition of locomotion of the polymorphonuclear leukocyte by organophosphorus compounds. *Exp. Cell Res.* 77:41, 1973.

161. Kitagawa, S., Takaku, F., and Sakamoto, S.: Serine protease inhibitors inhibit superoxide production by human polymorphonuclear leukocytes and monocytes stimulated by various surface active agents. *FEBS Lett.* 107:331, 1979.

162. Hawkins, D.: Neutrophilic leukocytes in immunologic reactions in vitro: Effect of cytochalasin B. *J. Immunol.* 110:294, 1973.

163. Davis, A. T., Estensen, R., and Quie, P. G.: Cytochalasin B. III. Inhibition of human polymorphonuclear leukocyte phagocytosis. *Proc. Soc. Exp. Biol. Med.* 137:161, 1970.

164. Davies, P., Allison, A. C., and Haswell, A. D.: Selective release of lysosomal hydrolases from phagocytic cells by cytochalasin B. *Biochem. J.* 134:33, 1973.

165. Skosey, J. L., Damgaard, E., Chow, D., and Sorensen, L. B.: Modification of zymosan-induced release of lysosomal enzymes from human polymorphonuclear leukocytes by cytochalasin B. *J. Cell Biol.* 62:625, 1974.

166. Boxer, L. A. et al.: Effects of a chemotactic factor, N-formyl-methionyl peptide, on adherence, superoxide anion generation, phagocytosis, and microtubule assembly of human polymorphonulcear leukocytes. *J. Lab. Clin Med.* 93:506, 1979.

167. Goetzl, E. J.: A rule for endogenous mono-hydroxy-eicosatetraenoic acids (HETEs) in the regulation of human neutrophil migration. *Immunology* 40:709, 1980.

168. Boggs, D. R., Athens, J. W., Cartwright, G. E., and Wintrobe, M. M.: The effect of adrenal glucocorticoids on the cellular composition of inflammatory exudates. *Am. J. Pathol.* 44:763, 1964.

169. Ward, P. A.: Leukotactic factors in health and disease. *Am. J. Pathol.* 54:121, 1971.

170. Hirata, F., Schiffmann, E., Venkatasubramaniain, K., Salomon, D., and Axelrod, J.: A phospholipase A₂ inhibitory protein in rabbit neutrophils induced by glucocorticoids. *Proc. Natl. Acad. Sci. U.S.A.* 77:2533, 1980.

171. MacGregor, R. R., Thorner, R. E., and Wright, D. N.: Lidocaine inhibits granulocyte adherence and prevents granulocyte delivery to inflammatory sites. *Blood* 56:203, 1980.

172. Cohen, H. J., Chovaniec, M. E., Ellis, S. E.: Chlorpromazine inhibition of granulocyte superoxide production. *Blood* 56:23, 1980.

173. Babior, B. M.: Oxygen-dependent microbial killing by phagocytes. *N. Engl. J. Med.* 298:659, 1978.

174. Badwey, J. A., and Karnovsky, M. L.: Active oxygen species and the functions of phagocytic leukocytes. *Ann. Rev. Biochem.* 49:695, 1980.

175. Cohen, H. J., Newburger, P. E., and Chovaniec, M. E.: NAD(P)H-dependent superoxide production by phagocytic versicles from guinea pig and human granulocytes. *J. Biol. Chem.* 255:6584, 1980.

176. Tauber, A. I., and Goetzl, E. J.: Structural and catalytic properties of the solubilized superoxide-generating activity of human polymor-phonuclear leukocytes. Solubilization, stabilization in solution, and partial characterization. *Biochemistry* 18:5576, 1979.

177. Patriarca, P., Basford, R. E., Cramer, R., Dri, P., and Rossi, F.: Studies on the NADPH oxidizing activity in polymorphonuclear leukocytes. *Biochim. Biophys. Acta* 362:221, 1974.

178. Curnutte, J. T., and Babior, B. M.: Biological defense mechanisms: The effect of bacteria and serum on superoxide production by granulocytes. *J. Clin. Invest.* 53:1662, 1974.

179. Root, R. L., Metcalf, J., Oshino, N., and Chance, B.: H₂O₂ release from human granulocytes during phagocytosis. I. Documentation, quantitation, and some regulating factors. *J. Clin. Invest.* 55:945, 1975.

180. Briggs, R. T., Karnovsky, M. L., and Karnovsky, M. J.: Cytochemical demonstration of hydrogen peroxide in polymorphonuclear leukocyte phagosomes. *J. Cell Biol.* 64:254, 1975.

181. Weening, R. S., Wever, R., and Roos, D.: Quantitative aspects of the production of superoxide radicals by phagocytizing human granulocytes. *J. Lab. Clin. Med.* 85:245, 1975.

182. Dewald B., Baggiolini, M., Curnutte, J. T., and Babior, B. M.: Subcellular localization of the superoxide-forming enzyme in human neutrophils. *J. Clin. Invest.* 63:21, 1979.

183. Baehner, R. L., Boxer, L. A., and Ingraham, L. M.: Reduced oxygen byproducts and white blood cells, in *Free Radicals in Biology*, edited by W. A. Pryor. Academic, New York, 1982, p. 91.

184. Root, R. K., and Stossel, T. P.: Myeloperoxidase-mediated iodination by granulocytes: Intracellular site of operation and some regulating factors. *J. Clin. Invest.* 53:1207, 1974.

185. Jensen, M. S., and Bainton, D. F.: Temporal changes in pH within the phagocytic vacuole of the polymorphonuclear leukocyte. *J. Cell Biol.* 56:379, 1973.

186. Allen, R. C., Yevich, S. J., Orth, R. W., and Steele, R. H.: The superoxide anion and singlet molecular oxygen: Their role in the microbicidal activity of the polymorphonuclear leukocyte. *Biochem. Biophys. Res. Commun.* 60:909, 1974.

187. McPhail, L. C., DeChatelet, L. R., and Johnston, R. B., Jr.: Generation of chemiluminescence by a particulate fraction isolated from human neutrophils. *J. Clin. Invest.* 63:648, 1979.

188. Ambruso, D. R., and Johnston, R. B., Jr.: Lactoferrin enhances hydroxyl radical production by human neutrophils, neutrophil particulate fractions, and an enzymatic generating system. *J. Clin. Invest.* 67:352, 1981.

189. Johnston, R. B., Jr., et al.: The role of superoxide anion generation in phagocytic bactericidal activity: Studies with normal and chronic granulomatous disease. *J. Clin. Invest.* 55:1357, 1975.

190. Patriarca, P., Dri, P., and Rossi, F.: Superoxide dismutase in leukocytes. *FEBS Lett.* 43:247, 1974.

191. Salin, M., and McCord, J. M.: Superoxide dismutases in polymorphonuclear leukocytes. *J. Clin. Invest.* 54:1005, 1974.

192. Baehner, R. L., Gilman, N., and Karnovsky, M. L.: Respiration and glucose oxidation in human and guinea pig leukocytes: Comparative studies. *J. Clin. Invest.* 49:692, 1970.

193. Reed, P. W.: Glutathione and the hexosemonophosphate shunt in phagocytizing and hydrogen peroxide-treated rat leukocytes. *J. Biol. Chem.* 244:2459, 1969.

194. Baehner, R. L., Johnston, R. B., Jr., and Nathan, D. G.: Comparative study of the metabolic and bactericidal characteristics of severely glucose-6-phosphate dehydrogenase-deficient polymorphonuclear leukocytes and leukocytes from children with chronic granulomatous disease. *J. Reticuloendothel. Soc.* 12:150, 1972.

195. Segal, A. W., Dorling, J., and Coade, S.: Kinetics of fusion of the cytoplasmic granules with phagocytic vacuoles in human polymorphonuclear leukocytes. *J. Cell Biol.* 85:42, 1980.

196. Wilson, L. A., and Spitznagel, J. K.: Molecular and structural damage to *Escherichia coli* produced by antibody complement and lysozyme systems. *J. Bacteriol.* 98:949, 1969.

197. Drath, D. B., and Karnovsky, M. L.: Bactericidal activity of metal-mediated peroxide-ascorbate systems. *Infect. Immunol.* 10:1077, 1974.

198. Janoff, A., and Blondin, J.: The effect of granulocyte elastase on bactericidal suspension. *Lab. Invest.* 29:454, 1973.

199. Elsbach, P.: On the interaction between phagocytes and microorga-

nisms. *N. Engl. J. Med. 289*:846, 1973.

200. Odeberg, H., and Olsson, I.: Antibacterial activity of cationic proteins from human granulocytes. *J. Clin. Invest. 56*:1118, 1975.

201. Spitznagel, J. K., et al.: Character of azurophil and specific granules purified from human polymorphonuclear leukocytes. *Lab. Invest. 30*:774, 1974.

202. Olsson, I., and Venge, P.: Cationic proteins of human granulocytes. II. Separation of the cationic proteins of the granules of leukemic myeloid cells. *Blood 44*:235, 1974.

203. Weiss, J., Beckerdite-Quagbata, S., and Elsbach, P.: Resistance of gram-negative bacteria to purified bactericidal leukocyte proteins. Relation to binding and bacterial lipopolysaccharide structure. *J. Clin. Invest. 65*:619, 1980.

204. Murphy, G., Reynolds, J. J., Brettz, U., and Baggioline, M.: Collagenase as a component of specific granules of human neutrophil leukocytes. *Biochem. J. 162*:195, 1977.

205. Masson, P. L., Heremans, J. F., and Schonne, E.: Lactoferrin: An iron-binding protein in neutrophilic leukocytes. *J. Exp. Med. 130*:643, 1969.

206. Arnold, R. R., Cole, M. F., and McGhee, J. R.: A bactericidal effect of human lactoferrin. *Science 197*:263, 1977.

207. Bigley, R. H., and Stankova, L.: Uptake and reduction of oxidized and reduced ascorbate by human leukocytes. *J. Exp. Med. 139*:1084, 1974.

208. Pincus, S. H., Boxer, L. A., and Stossel, T. P.: Chronic neutropenia in childhood: Analysis of 16 cases and a review of the literature. *Am. J. Med. 61*:849, 1976.

209. Simpson, D. M., and Ross, R.: The neutrophilic leukocyte in wound repair: A study with antineutrophil serum. *J. Clin. Invest. 51*:2009, 1972.

210. Baehner, R. L., Boxer, L. A., Allen, J. M., and Davis, J.: Autooxidation as a basis for altered function of polymorphonuclear leukocytes. *Blood 50*:327, 1977.

211. Edelson, P. J., and Cohn, Z. A.: Peroxidase-mediated mammalian cell cytoxicity. *J. Exp. Med. 138*:318, 1973.

212. Janoff, A., Feinstein, G., Malemud, C. J. and Elias, J. M.: Degradation of a cartilage proteoglycan by human leukocyte granule neutral proteases—A model of joint injury. I. Penetration of enzyme into rabbit articular cartilage and release of $^{35}SO_4$-labelled material from the tissue. *J. Clin. Invest. 57*:615, 1976.

213. Lieberman, J.: Elastase, collagenase, emphysema and alpha 1-antitrypsin deficiency. *Chest 70*:62, 1976.

214. McCord, J.: Free radicals and inflammation: Protection of synovial fluid by superoxide dismutase. *Science 185*:529, 1974.

215. Taichman, N. S., Movat, H. Z., Glynn, M. F., and Broder, I.: Further studies on the role of neutrophils in passive cutaneous anaphylaxis of the guinea pig. *Immunology 21*:623, 1971.

216. Winn, H. J., Baldamus, C. A., Jooste, S. V., and Russell, P. S.: Acute destruction by humoral antibody of rate skin grafted to mice: The role of complement and polymorphonuclear leukocytes. *J. Exp. Med. 137*:893, 1973.

217. Stewart, G. J., Ritchie, W. G. M., and Lynch, P. R.: Venous endothelial damage produced by massive sticking and emigration of leukocytes. *Am. J. Pathol. 74*:507, 1974.

218. Weissmann, G., and Rita, G.: Molecular basis of gouty inflammation: Interaction of nonosodium urate crystals with lysosomes and liposomes. *Nature (New Biol.) 240*:167, 1972.

219. Cochrane, C. G., Unanue, E. R., and Dixon, F. J.: A role of polymorphonuclear leukocytes and complement in nephrotoxic nephritis. *J. Exp. Med. 122*:99, 1965.

220. Henson, P. M.: Interaction of cells with immune complexes: Adherence, release of constituents, and tissue injury. *J. Exp. Med. 134*:144s, 1971.

221. Desai, U., Kretzer, D. L., Showell, H., Arroyave, C. V., and Ward, P. A.: Acute inflammatory pulmonary reactions induced by chemotactic factors. *Am. J. Pathol. 96*:71, 1979.

Neutrophil kinetics

CHAPTER 84

Production, distribution, and fate of neutrophils

DAVID W. GOLDE

Granulocytes are normally produced in the marrow, where they arise from precursor cells by a process of cellular proliferation and maturation. The formal sequence of development of neutrophils is myeloblast → promyelocyte → myelocyte → metamyelocyte → band (stab) neutrophil → segmented neutrophil (PMN, polymorphonuclear leukocyte). The term *granulocyte* is often loosely used to refer to neutrophils but strictly speaking encompasses the eosinophil and basophil series as well. Eosinophilic and basophilic granulocytes develop from myeloblasts in a manner analogous to the neutrophils, although commitment to neutrophilic, eosinophilic, or basophilic development is probably established at an early progenitor stage.

The normal human neutrophil production rate is 0.85 to 1.6×10^9 cells per kilogram per day. The mature neutrophils are stored in the marrow before release into the blood, where they circulate for about 6 h. These cells then enter the tissues and probably function for a few days before their death or loss from mucosal surfaces.

The granulopoietic system has a high production volume, yet it is finely modulated in the steady state and has a great capacity to increase production in response to inflammatory stimuli. This chapter outlines current concepts of neutrophil production, distribution, and survival. For detailed data and methods, the reader is referred to primary articles and reviews on granulocyte kinetics and granulopoiesis [1–16].

Stem and progenitor cells

A stem cell is defined by two characteristics: self-replication and differentiation. Stem cell replication permits maintenance of pool size without influx from a more primitive compartment. The differentiation potentials of stem cells are variable. A multipotential hemopoietic stem cell has the capacity to produce blood cells of more than one line, and a primitive stem cell exists which gives rise to cells of both the lymphoid and hemopoietic cells.

There is compelling evidence in mice and human beings for the existence of a stem cell common to the erythrocyte, megakaryocyte, mononuclear phagocyte, and granulocyte lines [9,13,15,17]. For example, when mouse marrow cells are injected into irradiated recipients, they form hemopoietic colonies in the spleen. These colonies derive from single stem cells and may contain mixtures of erythroid, megakaryocytic, and granulocytic elements [17–19]. The spleen colony assay is used to measure the multipotential hemopoietic stem cell, or CFU-S (colony-forming unit, spleen), in mice [9,17–19]. In humans, there is no definitive assay for the multipotential stem cell, but the distribution of the Philadelphia chromosome in chronic myelogenous leukemia provides strong evidence for the existence of such a cell. This abnormal chromosome is found in precursors of neutrophils, eosinophils, erythroblasts, and megakaryocytes, but not fibroblasts or lymphocytes dividing in response to phytohemagglutinin (PHA) [20]. Similar evidence has been adduced from the distribution of glucose-6-phosphate dehydrogenase phenotypes among cell lines [21]. Recently a technique has been developed in which multipotential human hemopoietic stem cells may be stimulated to give rise to colonies of erythroblasts, granulocytes, and megakaryocytes [22].

In addition more restricted progenitor cells exist with the capacity for differentiation along only a single cell line. This unipotential, or committed, cell is the antecedent of the earliest morphologically recognizable cells of each hemopoietic series. Most evidence suggests that cells of the mononuclear-phagocyte sytem (monocytes and macrophages) share a committed progenitor cell with granulocytes [13,23] (Fig. 84-1).

Regulation of neutrophilic granulopoiesis

Relatively little is known about the mechanisms which regulate cellular differentiation from the multipotential to the unipotential cell compartments [9]. Several factors are probably important. Multipotential stem cells may "sense" through cell-to-cell interactions the utilization of unipotential granulocytic progenitor cells, thereby signaling further differentiation in this direction [24]. The stromal environment of the marrow and spleen exerts important regulating influences on differentiating cells. These stromal elements have collectively been referred to as the *hemopoietic inductive microenvironment* (HIM) [25]. In mice, the microenvironment of the marrow is more conducive to granulopoiesis than that of the spleen, and in the spleen the medulla is more conducive than the cortex. In human adults, marrow appears to be the only tissue which normally supports granulopoiesis. Multipotential hemopoietic stem cells may also be regulated by humoral factors, in particular those derived from T lymphocytes [9,14].

In addition to short-range environmental influences,

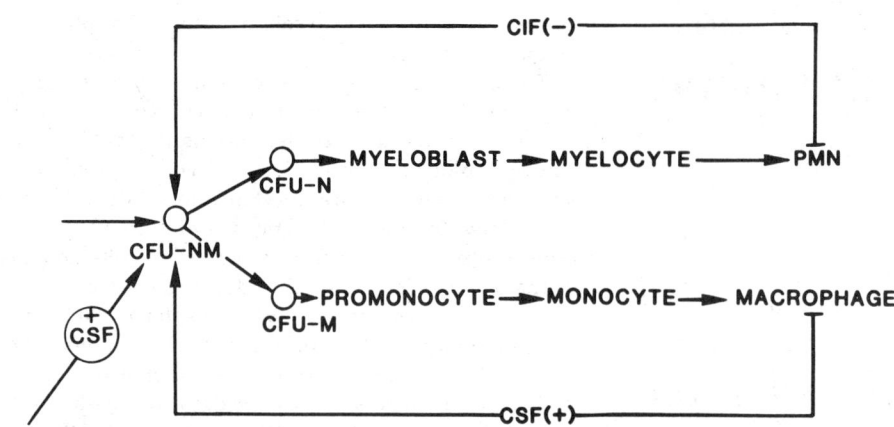

FIGURE 84-1   Neutrophils and monocytes are derived from a progenitor cell, which can be identified in culture as a cell that gives rise to colonies containing neutrophils and monocytes or macrophages. This cell, the CFU-NM, differentiates into CFU-N and CFU-M, which give rise to fully differentiated neutrophils and monocytes/macrophages, respectively. Stimulating factors which cause proliferation of these progenitors are referred to as CSF and are elaborated by stimulated lymphocytes, macrophages, and endothelial cells. CIF or colony-inhibiting factors are putative hormones which prevent the proliferation of neutrophil and macrophage progenitors and may be derived from mature neutrophils. The physiologic relevance of these factors is controversial, and their regulation is incompletely understood.

many humoral substances have been described as stimulators of granulopoiesis (granulopoietins or leukopoietins) [12–16]. There is also evidence for the existence of marrow granulocyte-releasing factors as well as granulopoietins. For example, when bacterial endotoxin is injected into humans or animals, a substance appears in the plasma which, when reinfused at a later time, causes leukocytosis and the release of young neutrophils from the marrow [26]. This neutrophil-releasing factor is probably identical with a material referred to as *leukocytosis-inducing factor* [27]. The releasing factors do not stimulate the production of granulocytes directly. However, they may have an important function in regulating acute changes in numbers of circulating neutrophils and their distribution between the marrow and blood.

The best evidence for a granulopoietin derives from in vitro marrow culture studies. The system most widely used employs agar or methylcellulose as a supporting matrix for the growth of hemopoietic cells. Under appropriate stimulation, cells believed to be committed to neutrophil and macrophage development undergo a series of proliferative and maturational steps culminating in the production of a colony of 50 to more than 2000 cells [12–16]. The in vitro colony-forming cell is referred to as CFU-NM (colony-forming unit, neutrophil, monocyte).

The stimulus to proliferation is a humoral factor (or factors) referred to as colony-stimulating factor (CSF) [12–15,28]. Colony-stimulating factor has been identified in many murine and human tissues; however, the prominent sources of human CSF are cells of the mononuclear phagocyte series, activated T lymphocytes, and endothelial cells [9,16,28–34]. The colony-stimulating factors are glycoprotein hormones containing sialic acid and having an M_r of about 30,000 daltons [28]. A macrophage-stimulating factor (MSF) closely related to the CSF for mouse granulocyte progenitors has been described [35]. MSF has been purified from murine L cells and stimulates the proliferation of mouse mononuclear phagocytes in vitro [36]. This material has been purified to homogeneity, and both a radioimmunoassay and a radioreceptor assay have been developed [28,37]. A murine CSF capable of stimulating granulocytic progenitors has been purified from lung-conditioned medium [28,38]; however, to date no human CSF has been purified to homogeneity. Highly purified human CSF, which stimulates human marrow progenitor cell growth and differentiation, has been obtained from certain tumor cell lines, including those derived from a carcinoma, a monocytic malignancy, and a T-lymphocyte tumor [39–41].

One of the most potent sources of human CSF is blood mononuclear cells [30,31]. The pulmonary, peritoneal, marrow, and hepatic macrophages (Kupffer cells) also produce CSF [14,16,42]. Lymphocytes responding to antigen or mitogen release a CSF [14,43,44]. There is limited information regarding the factors influencing the release of CSF, but endotoxin is known to increase CSF elaboration [45–48]. In addition, phagocytosis of bacteria enhances the elaboration of CSF by mononuclear cells [49]. Although CSF acts as a granulopoietin in vitro, there is only indirect evidence for its role as a physiologic regulator of neutrophilic granulopoiesis. Serum and urine CSF levels do correspond with the cycles of cyclic neutropenia, and purified urinary CSF preparations increase granulocyte production when injected into mice [15,16,50].

Many biologic systems involve negative feedback mechanisms whereby the end product of a process has an inhibitory effect on its further production. Investigators have searched extensively for a granulopoietic inhibitor. Tissue-specific inhibitors are referred to as *chalones,* and a granulocytic chalone elaborated by mature neutrophils has been reported [51,52]. This inhibitory material is believed to be of low molecular weight and to operate by inhibiting DNA synthesis in a committed progenitor stem cell [51]. Considerable data have been obtained concerning such inhibitors, and there is also other evidence that mature neutrophils inhibit granulopoiesis [15,16]. Lactoferrin produced by neutrophils may limit neutrophil production by inhibiting the release of CSF [53,54]. However, recent observations cast doubt on the significance of these in vitro findings [55,56]. Prostaglandins of the E series released by monocytes and macrophages have also been thought to be physiologic inhibitors of granulopoiesis [57,58], but probably act as selective inhibitors of monocyte-macrophage progenitors [54,59]. Therefore, while the prostaglandins may be important in regulating monocytopoiesis, they do not appear to have a major role in neutropoiesis. In summary, negative feedback of granulopoiesis has not been definitively demonstrated. Figure 84-1 outlines postulated schemes of humoral regulation of neutropoiesis based on a system of positive and negative feedback.

Techniques for studying neutrophil kinetics

Many methods have been used to study granulocyte kinetics. The major techniques may be summarized under the following categories: (1) granulocyte depletion or destruction to determine the size and rate of mobilization of reserves and compensatory increased granulopoiesis; (2) radioisotopic labels to study distribution, production rates, and survival times; (3) mitotic indices of marrow granulocytic cells to assess proliferative activity and cell cycle times; (4) induced inflammatory lesions to study the type and rate of cell movement into tissue sites. Of these approaches, radioisotope-labeling techniques are of widest applicability in studies of the production, destruction, and fate of granulocytes. The most frequently used radioactive materials are ^{3}H-thymidine, diisopropyl fluorophosphate (DF^{32}P), and radioactive chromium (^{51}Cr).

Tritiated thymidine is selectively incorporated into the DNA of dividing cells and provides a highly stable label which is ideal for radioautography [60,61]. Isotopically labeled DF^{32}P binds to granulocytes and mono-

cytes and does not appreciably label other leukocyte types. DF^{32}P may be used as either an in vivo or in vitro label [2,62,63]. ^{51}Cr is also used as a leukocyte label [64,65]. Although it has the advantage that its γ emissions permit surface monitoring, it indiscriminately labels most blood cell types and elutes readily from the cell. All the granulocyte-labeling methods have important limitations, and therefore data derived from comparative studies utilizing several techniques yield the most reliable estimates of cell kinetics. Important data are frequently derived by using several techniques in combination. For example, ^{3}H-thymidine labeling of marrow cells in combination with a determination of labeled mitoses provides considerable information as to cell cycle times and numbers of divisions involved in the various phases of granulocyte differentiation. Clinical approaches to the assessment of granulopoiesis are discussed in Chap. 85.

Neutrophil kinetics

It is conventional to analyze neutropoiesis and neutrophil kinetics by describing neutrophil movement through a number of interconnected compartments. These compartments may be arranged in three major groups: the marrow, the blood, and the tissue (Fig. 84-2).

FIGURE 84-2 A scheme of maturation of neutrophil precursor cells. The myeloblast (M.B.) is the first recognizable precursor of neutrophils. Myeloblasts undergo division and maturation into promyelocytes (Prom.) and thereafter into neutrophilic myelocytes (Myelocyte), after which stage mitotic capability is lost. The myeloblast, promyelocyte, and early myelocyte undergo a total of five divisions, and thus the myeloblast gives rise to 32 polymorphonuclear neutrophils (PMN).

The major compartments for granulocyte proliferation and distribution are indicated across the top of the figure: marrow, blood, and tissues. The marrow compartment is made up of the proliferating compartment (myeloblasts through myelocytes) and the maturation and storage compartment [metamyelocytes (Meta.) to mature PMN neutrophils]. Under normal conditions, there is no return of cells from the tissue compartment to the blood or marrow.

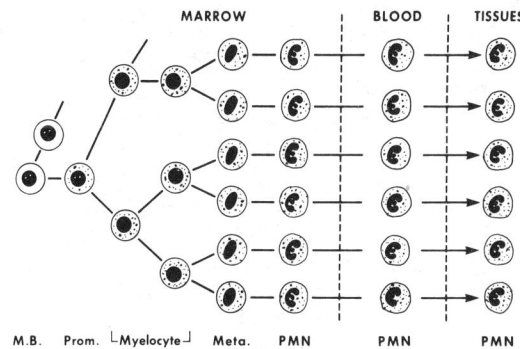

TABLE 84-1   Marrow neutrophil kinetics

	Fraction in mitosis (mitotic index)	Fraction in DNA synthesis (S phase)	Transit time range, h	Total cells × 10⁹/kg
Mitotic compartment:				
Myeloblast	0.025	0.85	23	0.14
Promyelocyte	0.015	0.65	26–78	0.51
Myelocyte	0.011	0.33	17–126	1.95
Maturation-storage compartment:				
Metamyelocyte			8–108	2.7
Band			12–96	3.6
PMN			0–120	2.5

SOURCE: Cronkite and Fliedner [7] and Donohue et al. [101].

The marrow

Marrow neutrophils may be divided into the mitotic, or the proliferative, compartment and the maturation-storage compartment (Fig. 84-2). Myeloblasts, promyelocytes, and myelocytes are capable of replication and constitute the mitotic compartment. Earlier progenitor cells are few in number, not morphologically identifiable, and usually neglected in kinetic studies. Metamyelocytes and mature PMNs are nonreplicating and constitute the maturation and storage compartment.

The number of cell divisions from the myeloblast to the myelocyte stage in the proliferative compartment has been estimated at between four and five [66]. Data obtained using DF³²P suggest that there are three divisions at the myelocyte stage, but the number of cell divisions at each step may not be constant. The major increase in neutrophil number most likely occurs at the myelocyte level, since the myelocyte pool is at least four times the size of the promyelocyte pool. Because of the difficulties in measuring human intramarrow neutrophil kinetics, a precise model of the dynamics of the mitotic compartment is not available. Estimates of the size of the marrow neutrophil compartments, transit times, and proliferative kinetics are given in Table 84-1. Precise studies have measured a postmitotic pool of 5.59 ± 0.9 × 10⁹ cells per kilogram and a mitotic pool (promyelocytes and myelocytes) of 2.11 ± 0.36 × 10⁹ cells per kilogram. These studies have led to a calculated normal marrow neutrophil production of 0.85 × 10⁹ cells per kilogram per day [10].

The maturation-storage compartment of the marrow contains the nonreplicating neutrophils. Evidence from radioautographic studies with ³H-thymidine support the concept of an orderly progression from metamyelocytes to mature PMN neutrophils within this compartment. Data from these studies also suggest a "first in, first out" pattern for cells leaving the storage compartment and entering the blood. By comparing data obtained with different labeling techniques, the myelocyte-to-blood transit time has been estimated at 5 to 7 days [8,67]. Previous studies with DF³²P gave a range of 8 to 14 days [5,66]. The myelocyte-to-blood transit time, however, may be as short as 48 h during infections [68].

It is not known with certainty whether the production of neutrophils in the mitotic compartment exactly equals the neutrophil turnover rate. It has been suggested that there is death of some immature neutrophils ("ineffective neutropoiesis") in the marrow of the dog [69]. Studies in human beings, however, have not confirmed these findings [10,70]. Ineffective neutropoiesis occurs in some pathologic states in a manner analogous to ineffective erythropoiesis. In the preleukemic syndromes [71] there is probably substantial intramedullary cell death, as may occur also in myelofibrosis and perhaps some of the idiopathic neutropenic disorders. At present, however, there is no convenient means to quantitate ineffective neutropoiesis.

With the completion of maturation, the PMN leukocytes are stored in the marrow and are referred to as the *mature neutrophil reserve*. At any time, this reserve contains many more cells than are normally circulating in the blood. Comparative data on the characteristics of the maturation-storage compartment are given in Table 84-2. Under certain stress conditions (1) maturation time may be shortened, (2) divisions may be skipped, and (3) release into the blood may occur prematurely.

Blood neutrophil kinetics

Neutrophils leave the marrow storage compartment and enter the blood without significant reentry into the marrow. The total blood neutrophil pool (TBNP) consists of all neutrophils in the vascular spaces. Some of these neutrophils do not circulate freely but adhere to the endothelium of small vessels. These adherent cells constitute the marginated neutrophil pool (MNP). When cells labeled with DF³²P are injected into normal subjects, approximately one-half can be accounted for in the circulating neutrophil pool (CNP); the remainder enter the marginated neutrophil pool (MNP) [1–3]. Cells readily move from the MNP to the CNP with exercise, epinephrine injection, or stress but eventually leave the blood and enter the tissues. Once they have entered the tissues, they do not normally return to the blood; the flow of cells is unidirectional.

Studies of neutrophil disappearance from the circula-

TABLE 84-2   Comparative data on marrow maturation-storage compartment

Size, cells × 10⁹ kg	Transit time, days	Measurement technique	References
6.5–13	4–8	³H-thymidine, in vitro DF³²P	[3]
3–23	8–14	In vivo and in vitro DF³²P	[66]
5.6	6.6	⁵⁹Fe and neutrophil/erythroid ratio	[10]

TABLE 84-3   Definitions and calculations relating to blood neutrophil kinetics

Circulating neutrophil pool (CNP) = blood neutrophil concentration × blood volume

Total blood neutrophil pool (TBNP) = all neutrophils in the circulation

Marginal neutrophil pool (MNP) = total blood neutrophil pool less circulating pool (MNP = TBNP = CNP)

Blood clearance half-time ($T_{1/2}$) = the disappearance time of half the labeled neutrophils from the circulation

Neutrophil turnover rate (NTR) = $\dfrac{0.693 \times \text{TBNP}}{T_{1/2}}$

tion measured with DF³²P yield a mean disappearance time ($T_{1/2}$) of 6.7 h [3,62,72]. These data are supported by the finding that over one-half of Pelger-Huët cells infused into a normal individual disappeared after 6 to 8 h [73]. Data obtained with ⁵¹Cr labeling of separated neutrophils, however, give substantially longer disappearance times [74].

The exponential disappearance of cells from the blood suggests that they leave in a random manner. Thus, neutrophils newly released from the marrow are as likely to leave the blood as neutrophils that have been circulating for several hours. Certain senescent neutrophils, however, may be removed in a nonrandom fashion and are probably disposed of by the macrophage system [68].

Assuming a random neutrophil loss from the blood, the neutrophil turnover rate (NTR) can be calculated from knowledge of the total neutrophil pool and the half-disappearance time ($T_{1/2}$): NTR = 0.693 × TBNP/$T_{1/2}$. In the steady state, the neutrophil turnover rate may be the measure of the rate of effective neutropoiesis. Definitions and calculations relating to blood neutrophil kinetics are given in Table 84-3 and data for normal human beings in Table 84-4. The high production rate of neutrophils under normal conditions is remarkable, especially since it may increase severalfold in response to inflammatory stimuli.

Glucocorticoids increase the total blood neutrophil pool. Five hours after administration of a single pharmacologic dose of cortisol or its congener prednisone [75–77] the neutrophils increase by about 4000 per microliter. The increase in the blood neutrophil pool is the result of increased influx of neutrophils from the marrow and decreased egress of neutrophils from the circulation. The $T_{1/2}$ of circulating neutrophils is increased from 6 to 10 h after glucocorticoids. There is also an increase in the proportion of cells in the circulating pool and a decrease in the proportion in the marginated pool. However, this shift does not alter the total circulating pool.

The decrement in neutrophil egress after administration of glucocorticoids is reflected in a marked reduction in accumulation at induced sites of skin inflammation [78]. Dexamethasone has been reported to produce a contrariwise effect, increasing mobilization from the circulation and accumulation in inflammatory sites [79].

When alternate-day, single-dose prednisone is used, neutrophil counts and kinetics are normal 24 hours after administration and during the day on which the drug is not administered [78].

Tissues

The activities of the mature neutrophil after it leaves the circulation are poorly documented. The migration of neutrophils into areas of inflammation has been widely studied, but little is known of the fate of granulocytes in normal tissues. Neutrophils normally migrate into the lung, oral cavity, gastrointestinal tract, liver, and spleen [80]. They may be lost from mucosal surfaces, die in the tissues, or be sequestered by the macrophage system. The life-span of the mature neutrophil is probably very short, since these cells survive only 2 or 3 days in tissue culture. Their life-span is even briefer if they encounter and ingest a substantial number of particles such as bacteria. Chemotactic stimuli draw neutrophils to areas of infection, where they may die in large numbers.

TABLE 84-4   Data for human blood neutrophil kinetics

Pool	Mean pool size × 10⁷ kg	95% limits
TBNP	70	14–160
CNP	31	11–46
MNP	39	0–85

	Mean value	95% limits
Blood clearance $T_{1/2}$	6.7 h	4–10 h
NTR	163 × 10⁷ kg/day	50–340 × 10⁷ kg/day

SOURCE: Athens et al. [2,3].

References

1. Cline, M. J.: *The White Cell.* Harvard, Cambridge, Mass., 1975.
2. Athens, J. W., et al.: Leukokinetic studies. III. The distribution of granulocytes in the blood of normal subjects. *J. Clin. Invest.* 40:159, 1961.
3. Athens, J. W., et al.: Leukokinetic studies. IV. The total blood, circulating and marginal granulocyte pools and the granulocyte turnover rate in normal subjects. *J. Clin. Invest.* 40:989, 1961.
4. Boggs, D. R.: The kinetics of neutrophilic leukocytes in health and in disease. *Semin. Hematol.* 4:359, 1967.
5. Cartwright, G. E., Athens, J. W., Boggs, D. R., and Wintrobe, M. M.: The kinetics of granulopoiesis in normal man. *Ser. Haematol.* 1:1, 1965.
6. Cronkite, E. P.: Kinetics in granulocytopoiesis. *Clin. Haematol.* 8:351, 1979.
7. Cronkite, E. P., and Fliedner, T. M.: Granulocytopoiesis. *N. Engl. J. Med.* 270:1347, 1964.
8. Vincent, P. C.: The measurement of granulocyte kinetics. *Br. J. Haematol.* 36:1, 1977.
9. Quesenberry, P., and Levitt, L.: Hematopoietic stem cells. *N. Engl. J. Med.* 301:755, 819, 868, 1979.
10. Dancey, J. T., Deubelbeiss, K. A., Harker, L. A., and Finch, C. A.: Neutrophil kinetics in man. *J. Clin. Invest.* 58:705, 1976.
11. Dresch, C., Faille, A., Rain, J. D., and Najean, Y.: Granulopoïèse: Étude comparative de différentes méthodes de mesure de la production et de la richesse médullaire. *Nouv. Rev. Fr. Hematol.* 15:31, 1975.
12. Robinson, W. A., and Mangalik, A.: The kinetics and regulation of granulopoiesis. *Semin. Hematol.* 12:7, 1975.
13. Metcalf, D., and Moore, M. A. S.: Haemopoietic cells, in *Frontiers in Biology,* edited by A. Neuberger and E. L. Tatum. North-Holland Publishing Company, Amsterdam, 1971.
14. Cline, M. J., and Golde, D. W.: Cellular interactions in haematopoiesis. *Nature* 277:177, 1979.
15. Golde, D. W., and Cline, M. J.: Regulation of granulopoiesis. *N. Engl. J. Med.* 291:1388, 1974.
16. Brennan, J. K., Lichtman, M. A., DiPersio, J. F., and Abboud, C. N.: Chemical mediators of granulopoiesis: A review. *Exp. Hematol.* 8:441, 1980.
17. Abramson, S., Miller, R. G., and Phillips, R. A.: The identification in adult bone marrow of pluripotent and restricted stem cells of the myeloid and lymphoid systems. *J. Exp. Med.* 145:1567, 1977.
18. Till, J. E., and McCulloch, E. A.: A direct measurement of the radiation sensitivity of normal mouse bone marrow cells. *Radiat. Res.* 14:213, 1961.
19. Wu, A. M., Till, J. E.: Siminovitch, L., and McCulloch, E. A.: A cytological study of the capacity for differentiation of normal hemopoietic colony-forming cells. *J. Cell. Physiol.* 69:177, 1967.
20. Koeffler, H. P., and Golde, D. W.: Chronic myelogenous leukemia: New concepts. *N. Engl. J. Med.* 304:1201, 1269, 1981.
21. Fialkow, P. J., Jacobson, R. J., and Papayannopoulou, T.: Chronic myelocytic leukemia: Clonal origin in a stem cell common to the granulocyte, erythrocyte, platelet and monocyte/macrophage. *Am. J. Med.* 63:125, 1977.
22. Fauser, A. A., and Messner, H. A.: Identification of megakaryocytes, macrophages, and eosinophils in colonies of human bone marrow containing neutrophilic granulocytes and erythroblasts. *Blood* 53:1023, 1979.
23. Metcalf, D.: Transformation of granulocytes to macrophages in bone marrow colonies in vitro. *J. Cell. Physiol.* 77:277, 1971.
24. Lajtha, L. G., Oliver, R., and Gurney, C. W.: Kinetic model of a bone-marrow stem-cell population. *Br. J. Haematol.* 8:442, 1962.
25. Trentin, J. J.: Determination of bone marrow stem cell differentiation by stromal hemopoietic inductive microenvironments (HIM). *Am. J. Pathol.* 65:621, 1971.
26. Boggs, D. R., Marsh, J. C., Chervenick, P. A., Cartwright, G. E., and Wintrobe, M. M.: Neutrophil releasing activity in plasma of normal human subjects injected with endotoxin. *Proc. Soc. Exp. Biol. Med.* 127:689, 1968.
27. Broxmeyer, H., Van Zant, G., Zucali, J. R., LoBue, J., and Gordon, A. S.: Mechanisms of leukocyte production and release. XII. A comparative assay of the leukocytosis-inducing factor (LIF) and the colony-stimulating factor (CSF). *Proc. Soc. Exp. Biol. Med.* 145:1262, 1974.
28. Burgess, A. W., and Metcalf, D.: The nature and action of granulocyte-macrophage colony stimulating factors. *Blood* 56:947, 1980.
29. Stanley, E. R., Hansen, G., Woodcock, J., and Metcalf, D.: Colony stimulating factor and the regulation of granulopoiesis and macrophage production. *Fed. Proc.* 34:2272, 1975.
30. Chervenick, P. A., and LoBuglio, A. F.: Human blood monocytes: Stimulators of granulocyte and mononuclear colony formation in vitro. *Science* 178:164, 1972.
31. Golde, D. W., and Cline, M. J.: Identification of the colony-stimulating cell in human peripheral blood. *J. Clin. Invest.* 51:2981, 1972.
32. Knudtzon, S., and Hertz, W.: Human tissues as source of colony-stimulating factor in human bone marrow cultures. *Scand. J. Haematol.* 19:482, 1977.
33. Quesenberry, P. J., and Gimbrone, M. A., Jr.: Vascular endothelium as a regulator of granulopoiesis: Production of colony-stimulating activity by cultured human endothelial cells. *Blood* 56:1060, 1980.
34. Nicola, N. A., Metcalf, D., Johnson, G. R., and Burgess, A. W.: Preparation of colony stimulating factors from human placental conditioned medium. *Leukemia Res.* 2:313, 1978.
35. Stanley, E. R., Cifone, M., Heard, P. M., and Defendi, V.: Factors regulating macrophage production and growth: Identity of colony-stimulating factor and macrophage growth factor. *J. Exp. Med.* 143:631, 1976.
36. Stanley, E. R.: Colony-stimulating factor (CSF) radioimmunoassay: Detection of a CSF subclass stimulating macrophage production. *Proc. Natl. Acad. Sci. U.S.A.* 76:2969, 1979.
37. Guilbert, L. J., and Stanley, E. R.: Specific interaction of murine colony-stimulating factor with mononuclear phagocytic cells. *J. Cell Biol.* 85:153, 1980.
38. Burgess, A. W., Camakaris, J., and Metcalf, D.: Purification and properties of colony-stimulating factor from mouse lung-conditioned medium. *J. Biol. Chem.* 252:1998, 1977.
39. Lusis, A. J., Quon, D. H., Golde, D. W.: Purification and characterization of a human T-lymphocyte-derived granulocyte-macrophage colony-stimulating factor. *Blood* 57:13, 1981.
40. DiPersio, J. F., Brennan, J. K., Lichtman, M. A., Abboud, C. N., and Kirkpatrick, F. H.: The fractionation, characterization, and subcellular localization of colony-stimulating activities released by the human monocyte-like cell line, GCT. *Blood* 56:717, 1980.
41. Wu, M.-c., and Yunis, A. A.: Common pattern of two distinct types of colony-stimulating factor in human tissues and cultured cells. *J. Clin. Invest.* 65:772, 1980.
42. Golde, D. W., Finley, T. N., and Cline, M. J.: Production of colony-stimulating factor by human macrophages. *Lancet* 2:1397, 1972.
43. Parker, J. W., and Metcalf, D.: Production of colony-stimulating factor in mitogen-stimulated lymphocyte cultures. *J. Immunol.* 112:502, 1974.
44. Cline, M. J., and Golde, D. W.: Production of colony-stimulating activity by human lymphocytes. *Nature* 248:703, 1974.
45. Eaves, A. C., and Bruce, W. R.: In vitro production of colony-stimulating activity. I. Exposure of mouse peritoneal cells to endotoxin. *Cell Tissue Kinet.* 7:19, 1974.
46. Ruscetti, F. W., and Chervenick, P. A.: Release of colony-stimulating factor from monocytes by endotoxin and polyinosinic-polycytidylic acid. *J. Lab. Clin. Med.* 83:64, 1974.
47. Quesenberry, P., Morley, A., Stohlman, F., Jr., Rickard, K., Howard, D., and Smith, M.: Effect of endotoxin on granulopoiesis and colony-stimulating factor. *N. Engl. J. Med.* 286:227, 1972.
48. Golde, D. W., and Cline, M. J.: Endotoxin-induced release of colony-stimulating activity in man. *Proc. Soc. Exp. Biol. Med.* 149:845, 1975.
49. Robinson, W. A., Entringer, M. A., Bolin, R. W., and Stonington, O. G., Jr.: Bacterial stimulation and granulocyte inhibition of granulopoietic factor production. *N. Engl. J. Med.* 297:1129, 1977.
50. Metcalf, D., and Stanley, E. R.: Haematological effects in mice of partially purified colony stimulating factor (CSF) prepared from human urine. *Br. J. Haematol.* 21:481, 1971.
51. Rytömaa, T.: Role of chalone in granulopoiesis. *Br. J. Haematol.* 24:141, 1973 (annotation).
52. Lozzio, B. B.: Regulators of cell division: A review. I. Endogenous mitotic inhibitors of hematopoietic cells. *Exp. Hematol.* 1:309, 1973.

53. Broxmeyer, H. E., Smithyman, A., Eger, R. R., Meyers, P. A., and de Sousa, M.: Identification of lactoferrin as the granulocyte-derived inhibitor of colony-stimulating activity production. *J. Exp. Med.* 148:1052, 1978.

54. Pelus, L. M., Broxmeyer, H. E., Kurland, J. I., and Moore, M. A. S.: Regulation of macrophage and granulocyte proliferation. Specificities of prostaglandin E and lactoferrin. *J. Exp. Med.* 150:277, 1979.

55. Winton, E. F., Kinkade, J. M., Jr., Vogler, W. R., Parker, M. B., and Barnes, K. C.: In vitro studies of lactoferrin and murine granulopoiesis. *Blood* 57:574, 1981.

56. Breton-Gorius, J., Mason, D. Y., Buriot, D., Vilde, J.-L., and Griscelli, C.: Lactoferrin deficiency as a consequence of a lack of specific granules in neutrophils from a patient with recurrent infections. *Am J. Pathol.*, 99:413, 1980.

57. Kurland, J. I., Bockman, R. S., Broxmeyer, H. E., and Moore, M. A. S.: Limitation of excessive myelopoiesis by the intrinsic modulation of macrophage-derived prostaglandin E. *Science* 199:552, 1978.

58. Kurland, J. I., Pelus, L. M., Ralph, P., Bockman, R. S., and Moore, M. A. S.: Induction of prostaglandin E synthesis in normal and neoplastic macrophages: Role for colony-stimulating factor(s) distinct from effects on myeloid progenitor cell proliferation. *Proc. Natl. Acad. Sci., U.S.A.* 76:2326, 1979.

59. Williams, N., and Jackson, H.: Limitation of macrophage production in long-term marrow cultures containing prostaglandin E. *J. Cell. Physiol.* 103:239, 1980.

60. Cleaver, J. E.: *Thymidine Metabolism and Cell Kinetics.* Wiley, New York, 1967.

61. Hughes, W. L., et al.: Cellular proliferation in the mouse as revealed by autoradiography with tritiated thymidine. *Proc. Natl. Acad. Sci. U.S.A.* 44:476, 1958.

62. Mauer, A. M., Athens, J. W., Ashenbrucker, H., Cartwright, G. E., and Wintrobe, M. M.: Leukokinetic studies. II. A method for labeling granulocytes in vitro with radioactive diisopropylfluorophosphate (DFP³²). *J. Clin. Invest.* 39:1481, 1960.

63. Athens, J. W., Mauer, A. M., Ashenbrucker, H., Cartwright, G. E., and Wintrobe, M. M.: Leukokinetic studies. I. A method for labeling leukocytes with diisopropylfluorophosphate (DFP³²). *Blood* 14:303, 1959.

64. Dresch, C., and Najean, Y.: Étude de la cinétique des polynucléaires après marquage "in vitro" par le radiochrome. *Nouv. Rev. Fr. Hematol.* 7:27, 1967.

65. Eyre, H. J., Rosen, P. J., and Perry, S.: Relative labeling of leukocytes, erythrocytes and platelets in human blood by ⁵¹chromium. *Blood* 36:250, 1970.

66. Warner, H. R., and Athens, J. W.: An analysis of granulocyte kinetics in blood and bone marrow. *Ann. N. Y. Acad. Sci.* 113:523, 1964.

67. Dresch, C., Faille, A., Bauchet, J., and Najean, Y.: Granulopoïèse: Comparison de différentes méthodes d'étude de la durée de maturation et des réserves médullaires. *Nouv. Rev. Fr. Hematol.* 13:5, 1973.

68. Fliedner, T. M., Cronkite, E. P., and Robertson, J. S.: Granulocytopoiesis. I. Senescence and random loss of neutrophilic granulocytes in human beings. *Blood* 24:402, 1964.

69. Patt, H. M., and Maloney, M. A.: Kinetics of neutrophil balance, in *The Kinetics of Cellular Proliferation,* edited by F. Stohlman, Jr. Grune & Stratton, New York, 1959, p. 201.

70. Cronkite, E. P.: Enigmas underlying the study of hemopoietic cell proliferation. *Fed. Proc.* 23:649, 1964.

71. Koeffler, H. P., and Golde, D. W.: Human preleukemia. *Ann. Intern. Med.* 93:347, 1980.

72. Bishop, C. R., Rothstein, G., Ashenbrucker, H. E., and Athens, J. W.: Leukokinetic studies. XIV. Blood neutrophil kinetics in chronic, steady-state neutropenia. *J. Clin. Invest.* 50:1678, 1971.

73. Rosse, W. F., and Gurney, C. W.: The Pelger-Huët anomaly in three families and its use in determining the disappearance of transfused neutrophils from the peripheral blood. *Blood* 14:170, 1959.

74. Dresch, C., Najean, Y., and Bauchet, J.: Kinetic studies of ⁵¹Cr and DF³²P labelled granulocytes. *Br. J. Haematol.* 29:67, 1975.

75. Bishop, C. R., Athens, J. W., Boggs, D. R., Warner, H. R., Cartwright, G. E., and Wintrobe, M. M.: Leukokinetic studies. XIII. A nonsteady-state kinetic evaluation of the mechanism of cortisone-induced granulocytosis. *J. Clin. Invest.* 47:249, 1968.

76. Dale, D. C., Fauci, A. S., DuPont, G., IV, and Wolff, S. M.: Comparison of agents producing a neutrophilic leukocytosis in man: Hydrocortisone, prednisone, endotoxin and etiocholanolone. *J. Clin. Invest.* 56:808, 1975.

77. Stausz, I., Barcsak, J., Kekes, E., and Szebeni, A.: Prednisone-induced acute changes in circulating neutrophil granulocytes. I. In cases of normal granulocyte reserves. *Haematologia* 1:319, 1967.

78. Dale, D. C., Fauci, A. S., and Wolff, S. M.: Alternate-day prednisone. Leukocyte kinetics and susceptibility to infections. *NEJM* 291:1154, 1974.

79. Peters, W. J., Holland, J. F., Senn, H., Rhomberg, W., and Banerjee, T.: Corticosteroid administration and localized leukocyte mobilization in man. *NEJM* 286:342, 1972.

80. Osgood, E. E.: Number and distribution of human hemic cells. *Blood* 9:1141, 1954.

CHAPTER *85*

Clinical evaluation of neutrophil kinetics

DAVID W. GOLDE

Many techniques are available for the assessment of neutrophil production, distribution, and utilization. The time-honored hematologic approach of gauging the cellularity of marrow clot sections or biopsies, quantitating the white blood cells, and doing differential counts is relatively simple and practical, but yields only crude estimates of cellular kinetics. Conversely, radioisotopic labeling methods often give precise information about the production and distribution of white cells, but are too cumbersome for routine clinical use. Table 85-1 presents available techniques for assessing neutrophil kinetics and summarizes their advantages and limitations. Techniques such as neutrophil depletion [1,2], which are of historical rather than practical clinical interest, are not included.

The white cell count and marrow cellularity

The white blood count and absolute neutrophil counts are the most widely used guides to the status of neutrophil production. They are useful in evaluating the effects of cytotoxic chemotherapy [3], although they do not provide quantitative information as to the rate of neutrophil production or destruction, the status of marrow reserves, or the presence of abnormalities in cell distribution.

Gauging neutrophilic granulopoiesis by the appearance of marrow films, clot sections, or biopsies also suffers from the limitations of sampling error and relatively poor correlation with kinetics as measured by other techniques [4]. For example, the morphologic

TABLE 85-1   Evaluation of granulocyte kinetics

Method	Advantages	Limitations
Blood white cell and differential counts	Simplicity	Not well correlated with reserves; yields no information on production vs. destruction
Marrow cellularity	Simplicity	Sampling problem; poor correlation with kinetic data
^{3}H-thymidine	Accurate assessment of cell proliferation in sample	Sampling errors; radioactive burden; time consuming
Mitotic index	Gives rough estimate of proliferation	Laborious; wide range of normal values
DFP labeling	Accurate assessment of cell proliferation and distribution	Complex and cumbersome
^{51}Cr labeling	Surface monitoring	Elution of label; question of validity
Endotoxin glucocorticoid, and epinephrine stimulation	Simple	Untoward reactions; not well standardized against kinetic studies
Lysozyme and vitamin B_{12}–binding protein	Noninvasive procedures; no radioactivity	Relatively poor correlation with kinetics except at extremes of production
Rebuck skin windows	Simplicity; assesses inflammatory response	Semiquantitative; does not evaluate kinetics
Skin blister and chambers	Simplicity; assesses inflammatory response	Semiquantitative; no information on production or distribution; infectious complications
^{99}Tc scanning	Simplicity	Poor correlation with granulopoiesis
In vitro culture	Measures committed stem cells; assesses cell differentiation	Information on concentration but not total numbers; technically demanding

findings in the marrow of a "maturation arrest," with little neutrophil development beyond the promyelocyte or myelocyte stage, does not distinguish between a true defect in cellular maturation and rapid mobilization of cells from the marrow. Similarly, it is often difficult to distinguish by purely morphologic means neutropenic conditions due to ineffective neutrophilic granulopoiesis from those caused by peripheral destruction of neutrophils. However, despite these limitations, when the absolute neutrophil count and marrow cellularity are used together, they provide a practical and useful guide in most clinical settings. If the absolute neutrophil count is less than 1000 per microliter and multiple marrow aspirations and/or biopsies are hypocellular, the patient almost invariably has impaired production of neutrophils. Low neutrophil counts correlate reasonably well with a higher incidence of infection, which becomes more striking as the neutrophil count falls below 500 per microliter. Unfortunately, the converse is not true; that is, the finding of a cellular marrow and a neutrophil count greater than 1000 per microliter does not mean that production is normal. Nevertheless, when marrow cellularity and absolute neutrophil count are considered together, they provide the most practical and clinically useful assessment of neutrophil production.

Newer techniques of marrow biopsy section preparation and staining have allowed for more accurate assessment of cellularity and differential cell counts [5]. When an accurate neutrophil-erythroid ratio is obtained, total neutrophil cellularity in the marrow may be derived from an estimate of total erythroblasts based on measurement of the erythroid iron turnover with ^{59}Fe [5].

Studies of this nature in conjunction with ^{3}H-TdR radioautography can provide detailed information on neutrophil kinetics. The laborious nature of these investigations, however, limits their clinical utility.

^{3}H-Thymidine (^{3}H-TdR) labeling and DNA measurement

A great deal of information can be obtained with ^{3}H-TdR as a DNA synthetic label, and much of our knowledge of the proliferative compartment within the marrow has come from the use of this labeled compound [6,7]. ^{3}H-TdR has the advantage of selective DNA labeling, rapid degradation of unincorporated material, low reutilization of label with cell death, and a weak β-particle emission that is ideal for radioautography. The major use of this DNA marker in the study of neutrophil kinetics is to label cells in DNA synthesis (S phase) in the pool of dividing cells. The subsequent movement of labeled cells can be followed sequentially as they progress to more mature compartments. For example, from the use of this label we know that myelocytes are the most mature cells of the neutrophil series that are capable of division.

Unfortunately, administration of ^{3}H-TdR in vivo is associated with an unreasonable body burden of radioactivity for routine human use. Studies in which marrow is incubated with ^{3}H-TdR in vitro can provide useful information about initial pulse labeling and generation times of neutrophil precursors in vitro. The studies have the limitation that cell proliferation in vitro may not be equivalent to that in the intact subject. In vitro ^{3}H-TdR–labeling studies may be useful in acute leukemia, where such data may be of therapeutic and prognostic significance. Pulse cytophotometry is a technique that can provide rapid information on the cell cycle and proliferative status of normal and leukemic cells [8,9]. Since cytophotometry measures the DNA content of stained cells in an automated fashion, it may have wide application in the future.

Mitotic index

The mitotic index (MI) for any morphologically homogeneous cell pool, such as the promyelocyte, is determined from the ratio of cells in mitosis to the total cells of the pool. Used alone, the MI provides little information on cell kinetics; however, when combined with ^{3}H-TdR–labeling studies, it can give valuable information on neutrophil precursor proliferation.

There are many limitations to the use of the MI, including the definition of the limits of the morphologic pool, the wide range of the MI in humans (from about 7 to 43 per 1000 nucleated marrow cells), and the labors involved in determination. These limitations have restricted the clinical utility of the MI alone or in combination with ^{3}H-TdR–labeling studies.

Explanations of the use of the MI and other methods of measuring neutrophil kinetics are presented in several reviews [10–12].

Diisopropyl fluorophosphate (DFP) and radioactive chromium (^{51}Cr)

DFP, containing either radioactive phosphate (^{32}P) or tritium, was introduced as a granulocyte marker in the late 1950s [13,14]. This radioactively labeled chemical binds to reactive groups on or in the granulocytes and monocytes. It also binds to erythrocytes, which must be eliminated when the isotope is counted. DFP may be used as either an in vivo or an in vitro label and may be used in non-steady-state conditions of granulopoiesis [15]. Contrary to previous concepts, it is now thought that ^{32}P may elute from a labeled cell and be reused by previously unlabeled cells [5,11,16]. DFP may also be toxic for the tagged cells. Nevertheless, the DFP label can be applied in vitro, and the radioisotope-labeled cells can be used to determine the total blood neutrophil pool by the isotope dilution method [13,17]. Intravenously administered DFP permits measurement of marrow transit times, neutrophil reserves, and marrow myelocyte turnover rates [13–15,17,18].

^{51}Cr also is a leukocyte label [16,19–22]. Although it has the advantage that its radioactive emission permits surface monitoring to ascertain the distribution of label, it also has the disadvantages that it labels leukocytes other than neutrophils, that a large fraction of the labeled cells never circulates, and that the label elutes from the cells. The agreement between DFP and ^{51}Cr studies of leukocyte kinetics has been variable [16,22, 23].

Although these labeling studies have given valuable information about normal and deranged neutrophil kinetics, they are too cumbersome for routine clinical use.

Endotoxin and other stimulatory substances

Endotoxin administered to human subjects causes a prompt neutropenia as a result of cell margination and sequestration, followed in 2 to 4 h by a rebound neutrophilia as a result of cell release from the marrow. The degree of neutrophilic response correlates fairly well with morphologic assessments of marrow cellularity and of functional marrow reserves [24–27]. Fever and malaise are unpleasant side effects.

Etiocholanolone administration produces neutrophilia without a preceding phase of neutropenia. There is a latent phase of 6 to 8 h before leukocytosis begins. Etiocholanolone stimulation is similar to that of endotoxin in assessing marrow reserves [28–30], but the steroid has been less widely used clinically. As a general rule, the endotoxin and etiocholanolone tests are probably not of practical use in monitoring cancer chemotherapy [31]. More recent studies showed that intravenous hydrocortisone (200 mg) or oral prednisone (40 mg) could be used as agents equivalent to endotoxin and etiocholanolone for measuring the neutrophil reserve response [31]. The glucocorticoids are the preferred agents as they are more convenient to administer and they do not cause fever and pain.

After administration of epinephrine, a peak leukocytosis occurs in 5 to 10 min and rarely lasts more than 20 min. This reflects a shift of cells from the marginated to the circulating pool, and the epinephrine stimulation test can be used to assess abnormalities of cell distribution in these pools.

Lysozyme and vitamin B_{12}–binding protein and other leukocyte products

Lysozyme and transcobalamins I and III are neutrophil constituents. Lysozyme (muramidase) is an enzyme contained in the granules of the neutrophil but not in those of the eosinophil and basophil. Measurement of serum and marrow lysozyme have been used to assess neutrophil production [32,33]. Unfortunately, despite optimistic reports to the contrary, the correlation with cell kinetics is disappointing, and the measurement of lysozyme for clinical purposes is not particularly useful in assessing neutrophil production [34]. This is not surprising, since there are many tissue sources of lysozyme, including mononuclear phagocytes and certain epithelial cells. The clearance of the enzyme from the serum is also variable, depending primarily on the proximal renal tubule cells. It should be noted, however, that serum lysozyme is almost invariably elevated in monocytic leukemia, and serial measurements may be useful in this disease [32,35].

Transcobalamin I appears to be a product of neutrophils. It may be found in cells as immature as promyelocytes, but is probably more abundant in mature cells [32,36]. Serum levels tend to be high in patients with chronic myelogenous leukemia, polycythemia vera, or inflammatory leukocytosis [36]. At extremely high granulocyte counts there is a reasonable correlation with serum concentration of this protein. Measurement of total vitamin B_{12}–binding capacity in combination with serum lysozyme determination can provide useful information, particularly in myeloproliferative disorders [32].

Accumulation in inflammatory sites

Several techniques have been used to study the type of cell migrating from the circulation into areas of inflammation and the rate of that migration. The Rebuck window technique, utilizing the adherence of leukocytes to sterile cover slips overlying areas of superficially abraded skin, was introduced in 1955 [37]. Because this method is qualitative and does not assess nonadherent cells, attempts have been made to introduce more quantitative techniques by producing and examining skin blisters [38] and skin chambers [39]. None of these methods, however, is wholly satisfactory, and all are at best semiquantitative.

Technetium 99 (^{99}Tc) scanning

^{99}Tc in its colloidal form is taken up by the phagocytic cells of the monocyte-macrophage system in the marrow as well as the liver, the spleen, and occasionally the lungs. Unfortunately, the distribution of macrophages does not correlate well with neutropoietic and erythropoietic marrow.

In vitro marrow culture

The cell that forms a neutrophil and macrophage colony in in vitro semisolid agar culture (CFU-NM) is usually regarded as the committed progenitor of these cell lines [40–42]. The number of colonies formed in agar from marrow aspirates should therefore reflect the number of CFU-NM in vivo. Unfortunately, in human subjects the technique can give information only about the relative concentration of CFU-NM among all the nucleated marrow cells; it does not give data about the total number of these progenitors. The technique therefore suffers from problems with sampling and determining absolute cell numbers. The in vitro culture method does permit assessment of abnormalities of granulocytic development in various hematologic disorders and may be of

particular use in preleukemia and the acute leukemias [42,43]. Inhibition of CFU-NM growth has also been used to identify antineutrophil antibodies [44,45].

A number of techniques are available for evaluation of granulocyte kinetics. Each method has advantages and limitations that can be balanced in the assessment of the state of neutropoiesis in the individual patient. With a firm knowledge of the physiology of normal neutropoiesis and its potential derangements, the hematologist can obtain much useful information from a neutrophil count and evaluation of marrow cellularity and morphology. Precise evaluation of kinetics requires the application of techniques not readily available to the clinician.

References

1. Bierman, H. R., Kelly, K. H., Byron, R. L., Jr., and Marshall, G. J.: Leucopheresis in man. I. Hematological observations following leucocyte withdrawal in patients with nonhematologic disorders. *Br. J. Haematol. 7*:51, 1961.
2. Thomas, E. D., Plain, G. L., and Thomas, D.: Leukocyte kinetics in the dog studied by cross circulation. *J. Lab. Clin. Med. 66*:64, 1965.
3. Cline, M. J., and Haskell, C. M.: *Cancer Chemotherapy*, 3d ed., Saunders, Philadelphia, 1980.
4. Bishop, C. R., Rothstein, G., Ashenbrucker, A. G., and Athens, J. W.: Leukokinetic studies. XIV. Blood neutrophil kinetics in chronic steady-state neutropenia. *J. Clin. Invest. 50*:1678, 1971.
5. Dancey, J. T., Deubelbeiss, K. A., Harker, L. A., and Finch, C. A.: Neutrophil kinetics in man. *J. Clin. Invest. 58*:705, 1976.
6. Cleaver, J. E.: *Thymidine Metabolism and Cell Kinetics.* Wiley, New York, 1967.
7. Hughes, W. L., et al.: Cellular proliferation in the mouse as revealed by autoradiography with tritiated thymidine. *Proc. Natl. Acad. Sci. U.S.A. 44*:476, 1958.
8. Hillen, H., Wessels, J., and Haanen, C.: Bone-marrow-proliferation patterns in acute myeloblastic leukaemia determined by pulse cytophotometry. *Lancet 1*:609, 1975.
9. Pulse cytophotometry. *Lancet 1*:435, 1975 (editorial).
10. LoBue, J.: Analysis of normal granulocyte production and release, in *Regulation of Hematopoiesis*, edited by A. S. Gordon. Appleton Century Crofts, New York, 1970, p. 1167.
11. Vincent, P. C.: The measurement of granulocyte kinetics. *Br. J. Haematol. 36*:1, 1977.
12. Dresch, C., Faille, A., Rain, J. D., and Najean, Y.: Granulopoïèse: Étude comparative de différentes méthodes de mesure de la production et de la richesse médullaire. *Nouv. Rev. Fr. Hematol. 15*:31, 1975.
13. Athens, J. W., Mauer, A. M., Ashenbrucker, H., and Cartwright, G. E.: Leukokinetic studies. I. A method for labeling leukocytes with diisopropylfluorophosphate (DFP^{32}). *Blood 14*:303, 1959.
14. Athens, J. W., Haab, O. P., et al.: Leukokinetic studies. IV. The total blood, circulating and marginal granulocyte pools and the granulocyte turnover rates in normal subjects. *J. Clin. Invest. 40*:989, 1961.
15. Rothstein, G., Bishop, C. R., Athens, J. W., and Ashenbrucker, H. E.: A method for leukokinetic study in the nonsteady state. *Blood 38*:302, 1971.
16. Dresch, C., Najean, Y., and Bauchet, J.: Kinetic studies of ^{51}Cr and DF^{32}P labelled granulocytes. *Br. J. Haematol. 29*:67, 1975.
17. Mauer, A. M., Athens, J. W., Ashenbrucker, H., Cartwright, G. E., and Wintrobe, M. M.: Leukokinetic studies. II. A method for labeling granulocytes in vitro with radioactive diisopropylfluorophosphate (DFP^{32}). *J. Clin. Invest. 39*:1481, 1960.
18. Kurth, D., Athens, J. W., Cronkite, E. P., Cartwright, G. E., and Wintrobe, M. M.: Leukokinetic studies. V. Uptake of tritiated di-

isopropylfluorophosphate by leukocytes. *Proc. Soc. Exp. Biol. Med. 107:*422, 1961.

19. McCall, M. S., Sutherland, D. A., Eisentraut, A. M., and Lanz, H.: The tagging of leukemic leukocytes with radioactive chromium and measurement of the in vivo cell survival. *J. Lab. Clin. Med. 45:*717, 1955.

20. Eyre, H. J., Rosen, P. J., and Perry, S.: Relative labeling of leukocytes, erythrocytes, and platelets in human blood by ⁵¹chromium. *Blood 36:*250, 1970.

21. MacMillan, R., and Scott, J. L.: Leukocyte labeling with ⁵¹chromium. I. Technique and results in normal subjects. *Blood 32:*738, 1968.

22. Spivak, J. L., and Perry, S.: Evaluation of ⁵¹Cr as a leukocyte label. *Br. J. Haematol. 25:*321, 1973.

23. Meuret, G., et al.: Neutrophil kinetics in man: Studies using autotransfusion of ³H-DFP labeled blood cells and autoradiography. *Blut 26:*97, 1973.

24. Craddock, C. G., Perry, S., Ventyke, L., and Lawrence, J. S.: Evaluation of marrow granulocyte reserves in normal and disease states. *Blood 15:*840, 1960.

25. Marsh, J. C., and Perry, S.: The granulocyte response to endotoxin in patients with hematologic disorders. *Blood 23:*581, 1964.

26. DeConti, R. C., Kaplan, S. R., and Calabresi, P.: Endotoxin stimulation in patients with lymphoma: Correlation with the myelosuppressive effects of alkylating agents. *Blood 39:*602, 1972.

27. Korbitz, B. C., Toren, F. A., Davis, H. L., Ramirez, G., and Ausfield, F. J.: The Piromen test: A useful assay of bone marrow granulocyte reserves. *Curr. Ther. Res. 11:*491, 1969.

28. Wolff, S. M., Kimball, H. R., Perry, S., Root, R., and Kappas, A.: The biological properties of etiocholanolone. *Ann. Intern. Med. 67:*1268, 1967.

29. Vogel, J. M., Kimball, H. R., Wolff, S. M., and Perry, S.: Etiocholanolone in the evaluation of marrow reserves in patients receiving cytotoxic agents. *Ann. Intern. Med. 67:*1226, 1967.

30. Karjalainen, J., and Wasastjerna, M. D.: The etiocholanolone test for prediction of the leukopenic effect of cytotoxic drugs. *Scand. J. Haematol. 11:*337, 1973.

31. Dale, D. C., Fauci, A. S., Guerry, D. P., IV, and Wolff, S. M.: Comparison of agents producing a neutrophilic leukocytosis in man.

Hydrocortisone, prednisone, endotoxin, and etiocholanolone. *J. Clin. Invest. 56:*808, 1975.

32. Catovsky, D., Galton, D. A. G., Griffin, C., Hoffbrand, A. V., and Szur, L.: Serum lysozyme and vitamin B₁₂ binding capacity in myeloproliferative disorders. *Br. J. Haematol. 21:*661, 1971.

33. Hansen, N. E.: The relationship between the turnover rate of neutrophilic granulocytes and plasma lysozyme levels. *Br. J. Haematol. 25:*771, 1973.

34. Levi, J. A., Macqueen, A., and Vincent, P. C.: Assessment of the value of lysozyme assay in neutropenia. *Br. J. Haematol. 25:*757, 1973.

35. Ohta, H., and Nagase, H.: Serial estimation of serum, urine, and leukocyte muramidase (lysozyme) in monocytic leukemia. *Acta Haematol. (Basel) 46:*257, 1971.

36. Rachmilewitz, B., Rachmilewitz, M., Moshkowitz, B., and Gross, J.: Serum transcobalamin in myeloid leukemia. *J. Lab. Clin. Med. 78:*276, 1971.

37. Rebuck, J. W., and Crowley, J. H.: A method of studying leukocyte functions in vivo. *Ann. N.Y. Acad. Sci. 59:*757, 1955.

38. Boggs, D. R., Athens, J. W., Cartwright, G. E., and Wintrobe, M. M.: The effect of glucocorticosteroids upon the cellular composition of inflammatory exudates. *Am. J. Pathol. 44:*763, 1964.

39. Mass, M. F., Dean, P. B., Weston, W. L., and Humbert, J. R.: Leukocyte migration in vivo: A new method of study. *J. Lab. Clin. Med. 86:*1040, 1975.

40. Quesenberry, P., and Levitt, L.: Hematopoietic stem cells. *N. Engl. J. Med. 301:*755, 819, and 868, 1979.

41. Brennan, J. K., Lichtman, M. A., Di Persio, J. F., and Abboud, C. N.: Chemical mediators of granulopoiesis: A review. *Exp. Hematol. 8:*441, 1980.

42. Golde, D. W., and Cline, M. J.: Regulation of granulopoiesis. *N. Engl. J. Med. 291:*1388, 1974.

43. Metcalf, D.: In-vitro cloning techniques for hemopoietic cells: Clinical applications. *Ann. Intern. Med. 87:*483, 1977.

44. Kelton, J. G., Huang, A. T., Mold, N., Logue, G., and Rosse, W. F.: The use of in vitro technics to study drug-induced pancytopenia. *N. Engl. J. Med. 301:*621, 1979.

45. van Brummelen, P., Willemz, R., Tan, W. D., and Thompson, J.: Captopril-associated agranulocytosis. *Lancet,* no. 8160, p. 150, 1980.

Neutrophil disorders— general considerations

CHAPTER 86

Classification of neutrophil disorders

MARSHALL A. LICHTMAN

Many disorders that involve multiple cell lines, such as the hemopoietic stem cell diseases, are frequently associated with neutropenia or neutrophilia. Anticancer drugs and infiltrative diseases of the marrow often lead to neutropenia, also. In this classification and in this section of the text, we consider those diseases in which the neutrophil concentration is solely affected or is the dominant cell line affected. Two examples in which several cell lines may be involved but neutropenia is the most constant and striking feature are Felty's syndrome and cyclic neutropenia.

A pathophysiologic classification of neutrophil disorders has proved elusive. Techniques to measure mechanisms of impaired production or accelerated destruction of neutrophils are much more difficult and complex than those used for red cells or platelets. The concentration of blood neutrophils is low in healthy subjects when compared with red cells or platelets, a situation accentuated in neutropenic states, and thus radioactive labeling techniques to study the circulation time of autologous cells are often impractical. The two compartments of neutrophils in the blood, the random disappearance of neutrophils from the circulation, the extremely short circulation time compared with platelets and red cells, the inability to measure the size of the tissue neutrophil compartment, and the disappearance of neutrophils by death or excretion from the tissue compartment make multicompartment kinetic analysis

TABLE 86-1 Classification of neutrophil disorders

I. Quantitative disorders of neutrophils
  A. Neutropenia
    1. Decreased neutrophilic granulopoiesis
      a. Congenital hypoplastic neutropenia (Kostmann's syndrome) [1,2]
      b. Reticular dysgenesis (congenital aleukocytosis) [3]
      c. Neutropenia and exocrine pancreas dysfunction (Shwachman-Diamond syndrome) [4,5]
      d. Neutropenia and immunoglobulin abnormality [6]
      e. Neutropenia and disordered cellular immunity [7]
      f. Chronic hypoplastic neutropenia
        (1) Drug-induced [8]
        (2) Cyclic
          (a) Sporadic [9]
          (b) Familial [10]
        (3) Idiopathic
          (a) Sporadic [11]
          (b) Familial [11]
      g. Acute hypoplastic neutropenia
        (1) Drug-induced [8]
        (2) Infectious [12,13]
      h. Chronic idiopathic neutropenia
        (1) Benign
          (a) Familial [14]
          (b) Sporadic [15]
        (2) Symptomatic [16,17]
    2. Accelerated neutrophil destruction
      a. Alloimmune neonatal neutropenia [18]
      b. Autoimmune neutropenia
        (1) Idiopathic [19,20]
        (2) Drug-induced [8]
        (3) Felty's syndrome [21,22]
        (4) Lupus erythematosus [22,23]
    3. Maldistribution of neutrophils
      a. Pseudoneutropenia [24]

  B. Neutrophilia
    1. Increased neutrophilic granulopoiesis
      a. Hereditary neutrophilia [25]
      b. Chronic idiopathic neutrophilia [26]
        (1) Asplenia [27]
      c. Neutrophilic leukemoid reactions [28]
        (1) Inflammation [28]
        (2) Infection [29]
        (3) Cancer [30]
        (4) Drugs (e.g., glucocorticoids, lithium) [31,32]
    2. Decreased neutrophil circulatory egress
      a. Drugs (e.g., glucocorticoids) [31]
    3. Maldistribution of neutrophils
      a. Pseudoneutrophilia [33]
II. Qualitative disorders of neutrophils [34,35]
  A. Defective adhesion of neutrophils
    1. Drug-induced [36]
  B. Defective locomotion [37]
    1. Lazy leukocyte syndrome [38]
    2. Actin polymerization abnormalities [39]
  C. Defective phagocytosis [34,35]
  D. Defective microbial killing [40,41]
    1. Chronic granulomatous disease [40,41]
    2. Myeloperoxidase deficiency [42,43]
    3. Job's syndrome [44]
    4. Glucose-6-phosphate dehydrogenase deficiency [45]
  E. Multiple or mixed disorders [34]
  F. Abnormal structure of the nucleus or of an organelle
    1. Hereditary macropolycytes [46]
    2. Hereditary hypersegmentation [47]
    3. Pelger-Huët anomaly [48]
    4. Alder-Reilly anomaly [49]
    5. May-Hegglin anomaly [50]
    6. Chédiak-Higashi disease [51,52]

exceedingly difficult. Also, neutropenic disorders are uncommon, and few laboratories are able, or prepared, to do all the studies necessary to define the mechanisms of development in sporadic cases. Therefore, efforts to understand the pathophysiology of neutropenia have had limited success. The classification of neutrophil disorders, thus, is partly pathophysiologic and partly descriptive (Table 86-1). Although imperfect, classification does provide a language for communication and a basis for rectification as knowledge of the cause and mechanism of disease advances.

The classification is self-explanatory except for two areas. First, certain childhood syndromes have been set off in the first five listings under decreased neutrophilic granulopoiesis. They could have been listed under chronic hypoplastic or idiopathic neutropenia; however, they seem to hold special interest, and their pathogenesis is still disputed.

A second area requiring explanation is the chronic idiopathic neutropenias. This group includes (1) cases with normocellular marrows but an inadequate compensatory increase in granulopoiesis for the degree of neutropenia and (2) cases with hyperplastic granulopoiesis which is apparently ineffective. Unlike hypoplastic neutropenias in which granulocyte precursors are markedly reduced or absent, in the idiopathic neutropenias precursors are present in marrow, but the extent of effective granulopoiesis is probably low.

References

1. Kostmann, R.: Infantile genetic agranulocytosis. *Acta Pediatr. 45* (Suppl. 105):1, 1956.
2. Chusid, M. J., Pisciotta, A. V., Duquesnoy, R. J., Camitta, B. M., and Tomasulo, P. A.: Congenital neutropenia: Studies of pathogenesis. *Am. J. Hematol.* 8:315, 1980.
3. Gitlin, D., Vawter, G., and Aaig, J. M.: Thymic alymphoplasia and congenital aleukocytosis. *Pediatrics* 33:184, 1964.
4. Shwachman, H., et al.: The syndrome of pancreatic insufficiency and bone marrow dysfunction. *J. Pediatr.* 65:645, 1964.
5. Saunders, E. F., Gall, G., and Freedman, M. H.: Granulopoiesis in Shwachman's syndrome (Pancreatic insufficiency and bone marrow dysfunction). *Pediatrics* 64:515, 1979.
6. Lonsdale, D., Deodhar, S. D., and Mercer, R. D.: Familial granulocytopenia associated with immunoglobulin abnormality. *J. Pediatr.* 71:760, 1967.
7. Lux, S. D., et al.: Chronic neutropenia and abnormal cellular immunity in cartilage-hair hypoplasia. *N. Engl. J. Med.* 282:231, 1970.
8. Hartl, P. W.: Drug-induced agranulocytosis in *Blood Disorders Due to Drugs and Other Agents*, edited by R. H. Girdwood. Excerpta Medica, Amsterdam, 1974, pp. 147–186.
9. Wright, D. G., Dale, D. C., Fauci, A. S., and Wolff, S. M.: Human cyclic neutropenia: Clinical review and long-term follow-up of patients. *Medicine* 60:1, 1981.
10. Morley, A. A., Carew, J. P., and Baikie, A. G.: Familial cyclic neutropenia. *Br. J. Haematol.* 13:719, 1967.
11. Spaet, T. H., and Dameshek, W.: Chronic hypoplastic neutropenia. *Am. J. Med.* 13:35, 1952.
12. Murdock, J. M. C., and Smith, C. C.: Haematologic aspects of systemic disease—Infection. *Clin. Haematol.* 1:619, 1972.
13. Olson, J. P., and Lichtman, M. A.: Neutropenia, in *Hematology for Practitioners*, edited by M. A. Lichtman. Little, Brown, Boston, 1978, pp. 105–120.
14. Cutting, H. O., and Lange, J. E.: Familial-benign chronic neutropenia. *Ann. Intern. Med.* 61:876, 1964.
15. Kyle, R. A.: Natural history of chronic idiopathic neutropenia. *N. Engl. J. Med.* 302:908, 1970.
16. Pincus, S. H., Boxer, L. A., and Stossel, T. P.: Chronic neutropenia in childhood. *Am. J. Med.* 61:849, 1976.
17. Dale, D. C., Guerry, D., IV, Wewerka, J. R., Bull, J. M., and Chusid, M. J.: Chronic neutropenia. *Medicine* 58:128, 1979.
18. Boxer, L. A., Yokoyama, M., and Lalezari, P.: Isoimmune neonatal neutropenia. *J. Pediatr.* 80:783, 1972.
19. Lalezari, P.: Neutrophil antigens: Immunology and clinical implications, in *The Granulocyte: Function and Clinical Utilization*, edited by T. J. Greenwalt and G. A. Jamieson. Alan R. Liss, New York, pp. 209–226.
20. Boxer, L. A., Greenberg, M. S., Boxer, G. J., and Stossel, T. P.: Autoimmune neutropenia. *N. Engl. J. Med.* 293:748, 1975.
21. Felty, A. R.: Chronic arthritis in the adult associated with splenomegaly and leucopenia. *Bull. Johns Hopkins Hosp.* 35:16, 1924.
22. Drew, S. I., and Terasaki, P. I.: Autoimmune cytotoxic granulocyte antibodies in normal persons and various diseases. *Blood* 52:941, 1978.
23. Dubois, E. L.: *Lupus Erythematosus.* McGraw-Hill, New York, 1966.
24. Joyce, R. A., Boggs, D. R., Hasiba, U., and Srodes, C. H.: Marginal neutrophil pool size in normal subjects and neutropenic patients as measured by epinephrine infusion. *J. Lab. Clin. Med.* 88:614, 1976.
25. Herring, W. B., Smith, L. G., Walker, R. I., and Herion, J. C.: Hereditary neutrophilia. *Am. J. Med.* 56:729, 1974.
26. Ward, H. N., and Reinhard, E. H.: Chronic idiopathic leukocytosis. *Ann. Intern. Med.* 75:193, 1971.
27. Joyce, R. A., O'Donnell, J., Sanghvi, J., and Westerman, M. P.: Asplenia and abnormal neutrophil kinetics in chronic idiopathic neutrophilia. *Am. J. Med.* 69:633, 1980.
28. Hilts, S. V., and Shaw, C. C.: Leukemoid blood reactions. *N. Engl. J. Med.* 249:343, 1953.
29. Marsh, J. C., Boggs, D. R., Cartwright, G. E., and Wintrobe, M. M.: Neutrophil kinetics in acute infection. *J. Clin. Invest.* 46:1943, 1967.
30. Norcross, J. W.: Hematologic manifestations of malignant disease. *Med. Clin. North Am.* 47:345, 1963.
31. Bishop, C. R.: Leukokinetic studies. XIII. A non-steady state kinetic evaluation of the mechanism of cortisone-induced granulocytosis. *J. Clin. Invest.* 47:249, 1968.
32. Murphy, D. L., Goodwin, F. K., and Bunney, W. E.: Leukocytosis during lithium treatment. *Am. J. Psychiatry* 127:135, 1971.
33. Athens, J. W., et al.: Leukokinetic studies. IV. The total blood, circulating and marginal granulocyte pools and the granulocyte turnover rate in normal subjects. *J. Clin. Invest.* 40:989, 1961.
34. Tauber, A. I.: Current views of neutrophil dysfunction. *Am. J. Med.* 70:1237, 1981.
35. Klebanoff, S. J., and Clark, R. A.: The neutrophil: Function and clinical disorders. North-Holland, Amsterdam, 1978.
36. MacGregor, R. R., Spagnulo, P. J., and Lentnek, A. L.: Inhibition of granulocyte adherence by ethanol, prednisone, and aspirin, measured with an assay system. *N. Engl. J. Med.* 291:642, 1974.
37. Clark, R. A.: Disorders of granulocyte chemotaxis: An analytical review. *Clin. Immunol. Immunopathol.* 15:52, 1980.
38. Miller, M. E., Oski, F. A., and Harris, M. B.: Lazy-leucocyte syndrome. A new disorder of neutrophil function. *Lancet* 1:665, 1971.
39. Boxer, L. A., Hedley-White, E. T., and Stossel, T. P.: Neutrophil actin dysfunction and abnormal neutrophil behavior. *N. Engl. J. Med.* 291:1043, 1974.
40. Quie, P. G.: Pathology of bactericidal power of neutrophils. *Semin. Hematol.* 12:143, 1975.
41. Babior, B. M.: Oxygen-dependent microbial killing by phagocytes. *N. Engl. J. Med.* 298:659, 1978.
42. Lehrer, R. I., and Cline, M. J.: Leukocyte myeloperoxidase deficiency and disseminated candidiasis: The role of myeloperoxidase in resistance to candida infection. *J. Clin. Invest.* 48:1478, 1969.
43. Lehrer, R. I., Hanifin, J., and Cline, M. J.: Defective bactericidal activity in myeloperoxidase-deficient human neutrophils. *Nature* 223:78, 1969.
44. Bannatyne, R. M., et al.: Job's syndrome—A variant of chronic granulomatous disease. *J. Pediatr.* 75:236, 1969.

45. Cooper, M. R., et al.: Complete deficiency of leukocyte G-6-P-D with defective bactericidal activity. *J. Clin. Invest. 51:*769, 1972.

46. Davidson, W. M., Milner, R. D. G., and Lawlor, S. D.: Giant neutrophil leukocytes: An inherited anomaly. *Br. J. Haematol. 6:*339, 1960.

47. Undritz, V. E.: Eine neue Sippe mit Erblich—Konstitutioneller Hochsegmentierung der Neutrophilenkerne. *Schweiz. Med. Wochenschr. 94:*1365, 1964.

48. Rebuck, J. W., Barth, C. L., and Petz, A. J.: New leucocytic dysfunction at the inflammatory sites in Hegglins, Hurler's, and Pelger-Huet anomalous states. *Fed. Proc. 22:*427, 1963.

49. Reilly, W. A., and Lindsay, S.: Gargoylism (lipochondrodystrophy): A review of clinical observations in eighteen cases. *Am. J. Dis. Child. 75:*595, 1948.

50. Oski, F. A., Naiman, J. L., Allen, D. M., and Diamond, L. K.: Leukocytic inclusions—Döhle bodies-associated with platelet abnormality (The May-Hegglin anomaly): Report of a family and review of the literature. *Blood 20:*657, 1962.

51. Clawson, C. C., White, J. G., and Repine, J. E.: The Chediak-Higashi syndrome. Evidence that defective leukotaxis is primarily due to an impediment by giant granules. *Am. J. Pathol. 92:*745, 1978.

52. Clawson, C. C., Repine, J. E., and White, J. G.: The Chediak-Higashi syndrome. Quantitation of a deficiency in maximal bactercidial capacity. *Am. J. Pathol. 94:*539, 1979.

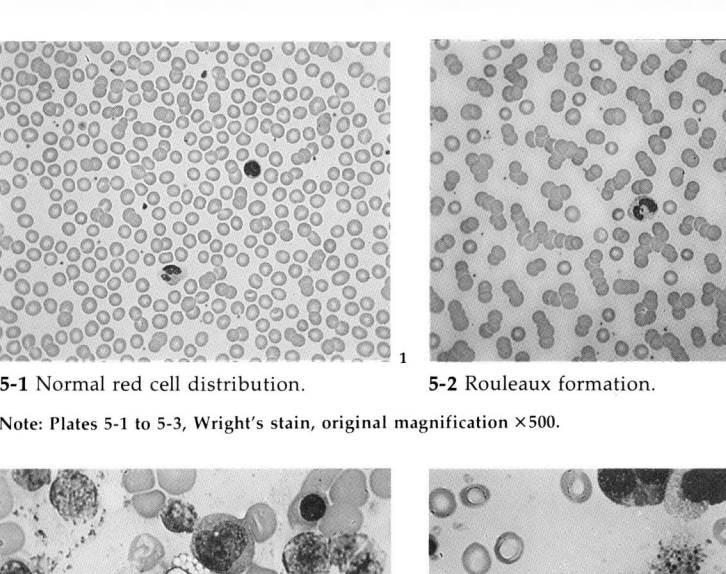

5-1 Normal red cell distribution.

5-2 Rouleaux formation.

5-3 Erythrocyte agglutination.

Note: Plates 5-1 to 5-3, Wright's stain, original magnification ×500.

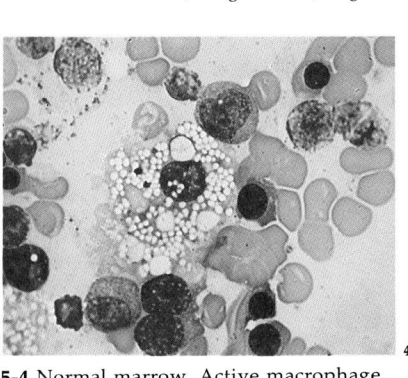

5-4 Normal marrow. Active macrophage.

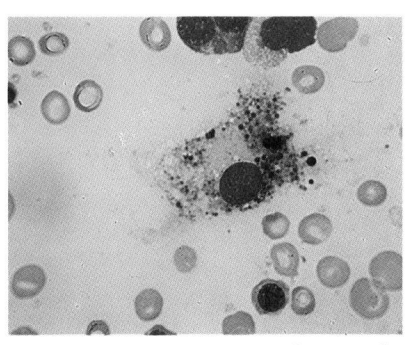

5-5 Normal marrow. Macrophage with iron particles, Wright's stain.

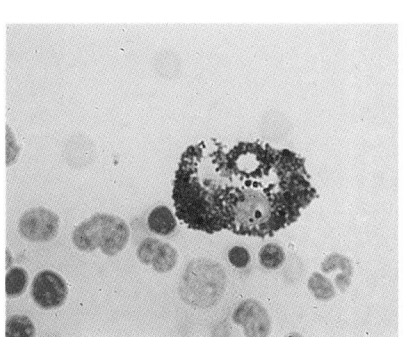

5-6 Normal marrow. Macrophage with iron particles, Prussian blue stain.

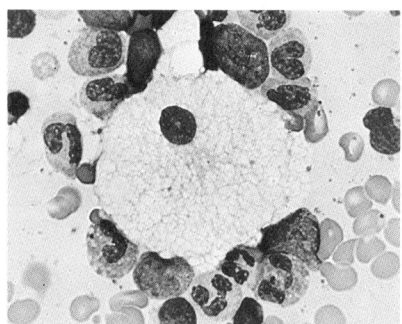

5-7 Niemann-Pick cell.

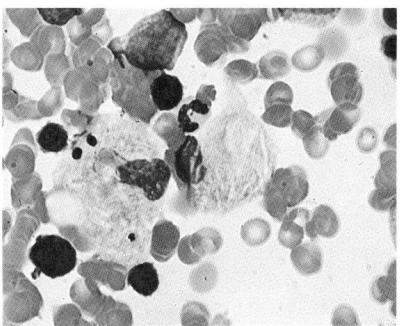

5-8 Gaucher cells in the adult form of Gaucher disease.

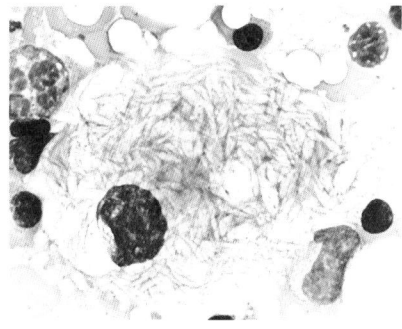

5-9 Pseudo-Gaucher cell in a patient with chronic myelogenous leukemia.

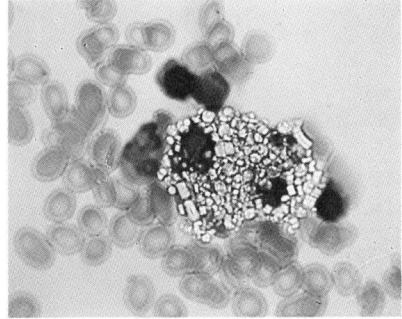

5-10 Cystine crystals in a macrophage.

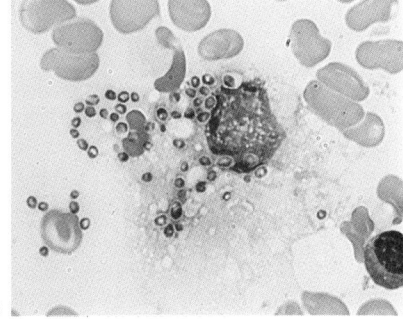

5-11 *Histoplasma capsulatum* in a marrow macrophage.

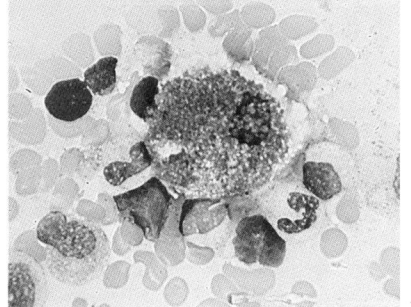

5-12 Macrophage in sea blue histiocytosis.

Note: Plates 5-4 to 5-12, Wright's stain, except as noted, original magnification ×500.

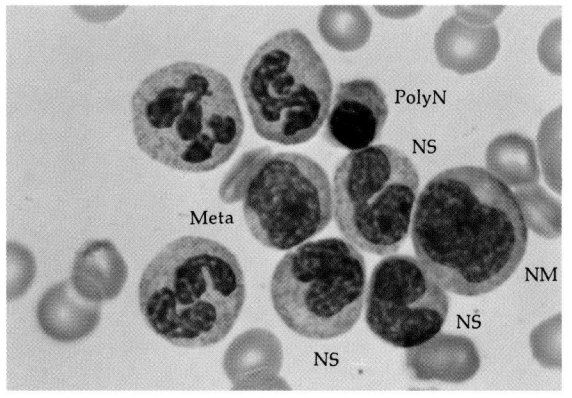 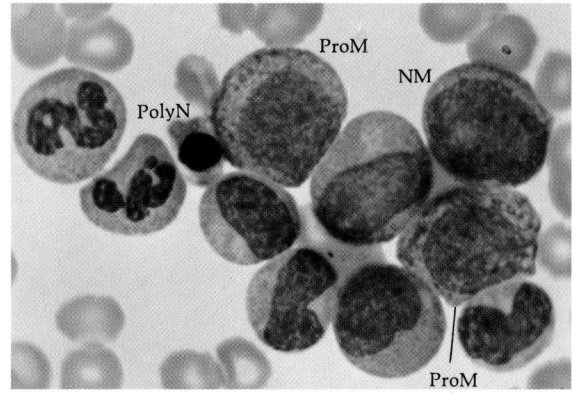

6-1 Blood film from a patient with chronic myelogenous leukemia, showing moderate immaturity but a predominance of bands and segmented forms of neutrophils. Present are neutrophilic myelocytes (NM), metamyelocytes (Meta), nonsegmented (band or stab) forms (NS), polychromatophilic erythroblasts (PolyN), and mature neutrophils (not labeled). **6-2** Blood film from a patient with chronic myelogenous leukemia. Cells show greater immaturity than those in Plate 6-1. Present are promyelocytes (ProM), myelocyte (NM), and a nucleated red cell precursor (PolyN). The remaining cells are metamyelocytes, bands, and mature polymorphonuclear neutrophils.

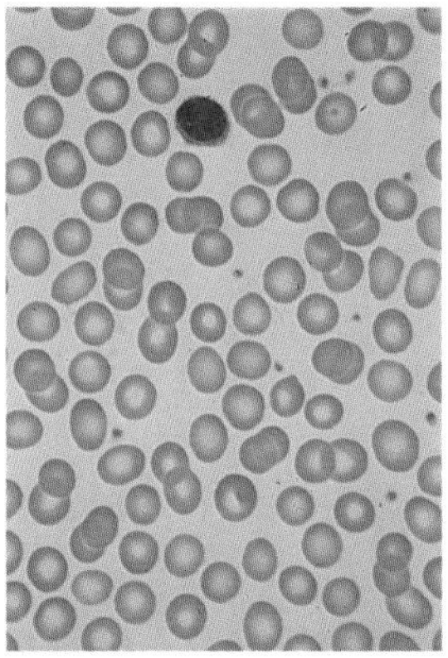

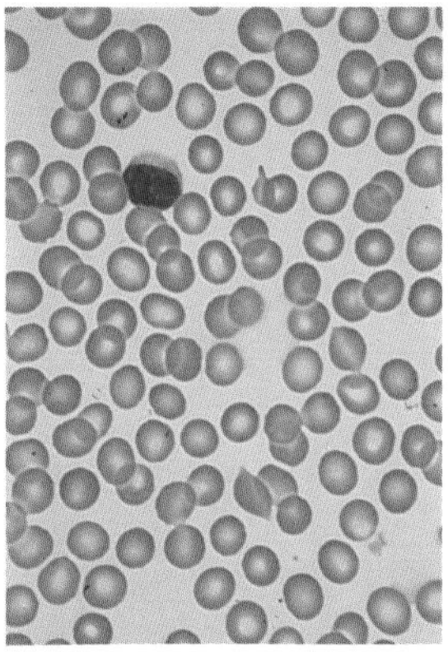

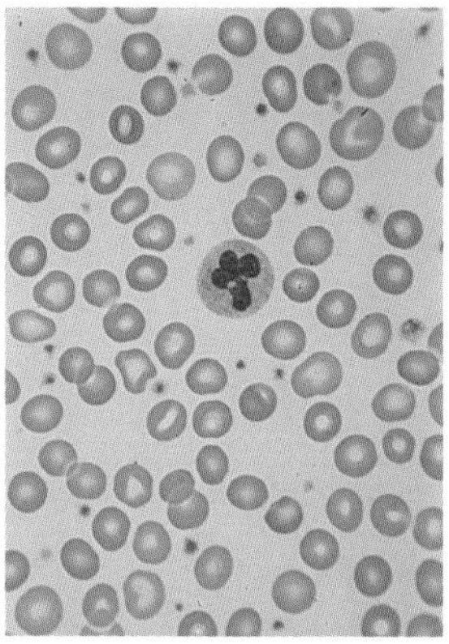

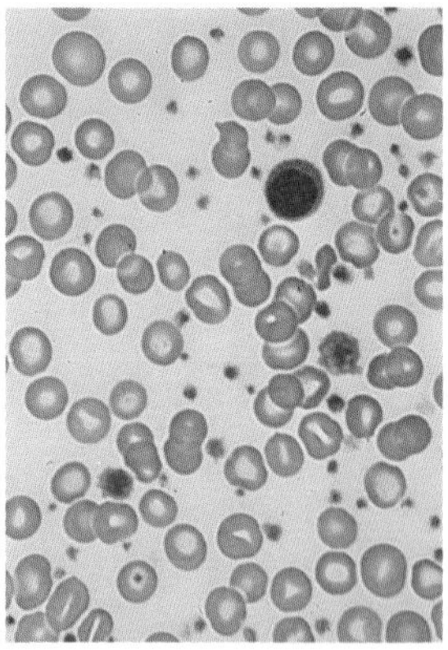

6-3 Blood film showing normal platelets. **6-4** Blood film showing thrombocytopenia. **6-5** Blood film showing reactive thrombocytosis. **6-6** Blood film showing thrombocythemia. Note the increased number of platelets, and the large abnormal platelets. **6-7** A megathrombocyte in normal blood. **6-8** Giant platelets. All of the blue-staining elements in the illustration are platelets. **6-9** Dwarf megakaryocytes in blood. **6-10** A megakaryocyte nucleus in the blood.

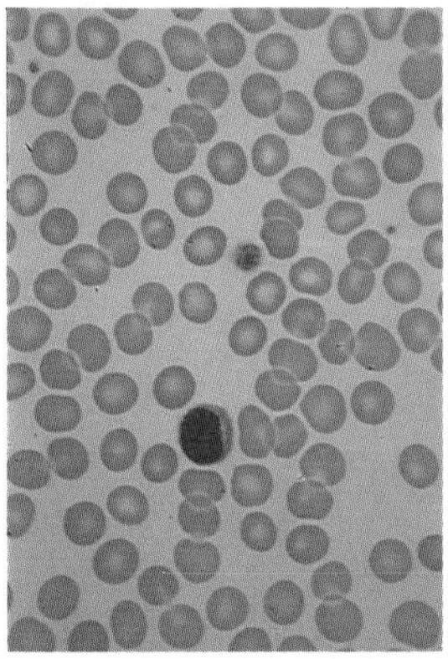

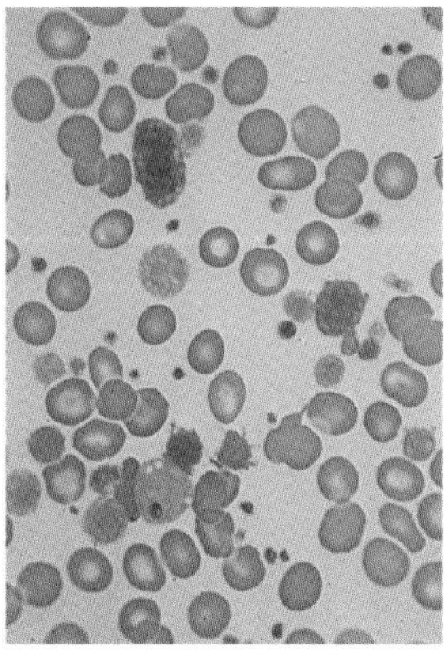

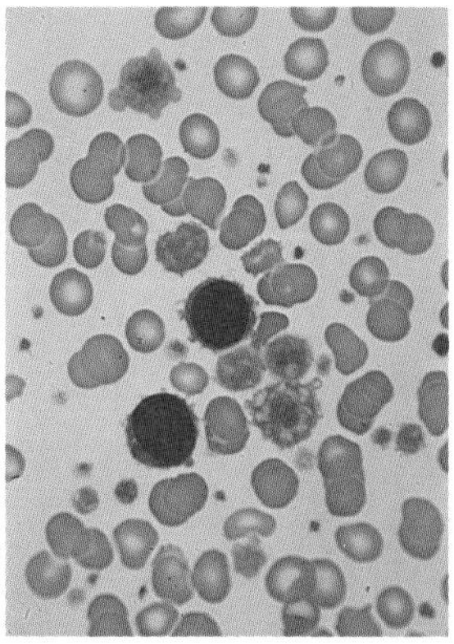

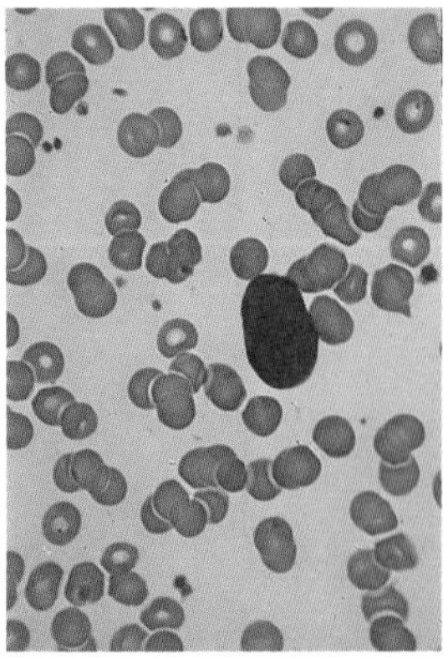

Note: Plates 6-1 to 6-10, Wright's stain, original magnification ×1000.

PLATE 6 Myeloproliferative diseases

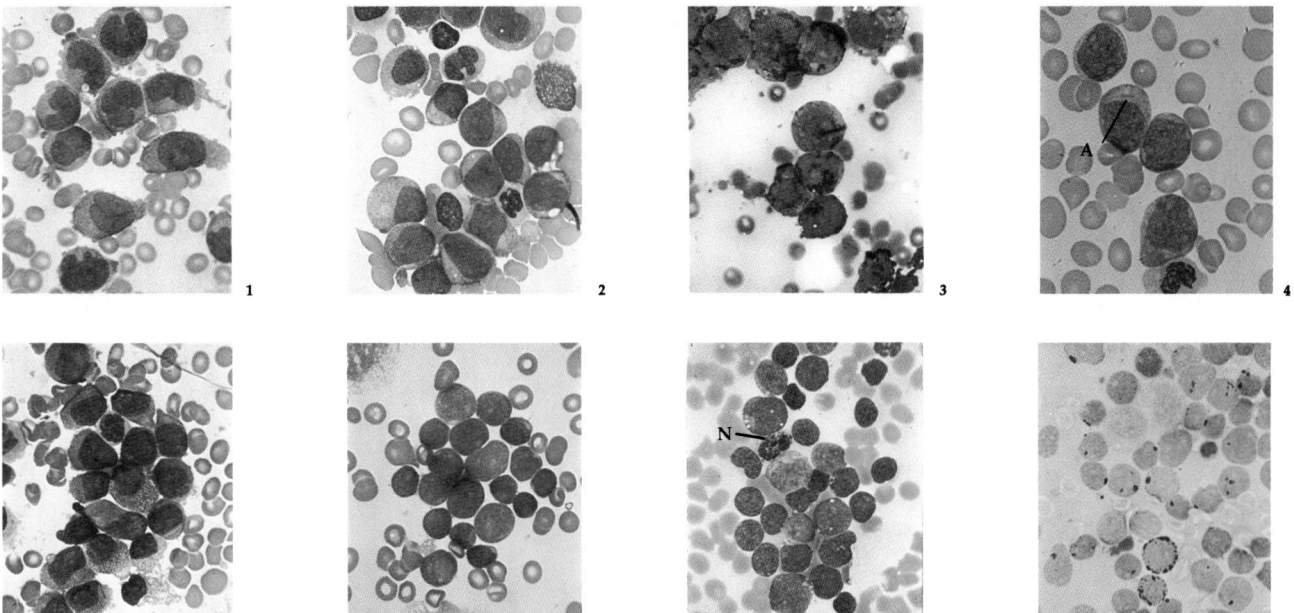

7-1 Acute monocytic leukemia. 7-2 Acute myelogenous leukemia. 7-3 Acute myelogenous leukemia. Blast cells stained for peroxidase. 7-4 Acute myelogenous leukemia. Blast cells, one containing an Auer rod (A). 7-5 Acute promyelocytic leukemia. 7-6 Acute lymphocytic leukemia. 7-7 Acute lymphocytic leukemia. Blast cells stained for peroxidase. The blast cells do not stain, but the neutrophil on this slide is positive (N). 7-8 Acute lymphocytic leukemia. Blast cells stained with periodic acid–Schiff (PAS) technique. Note the large masses of PAS-staining material in the blast cells.

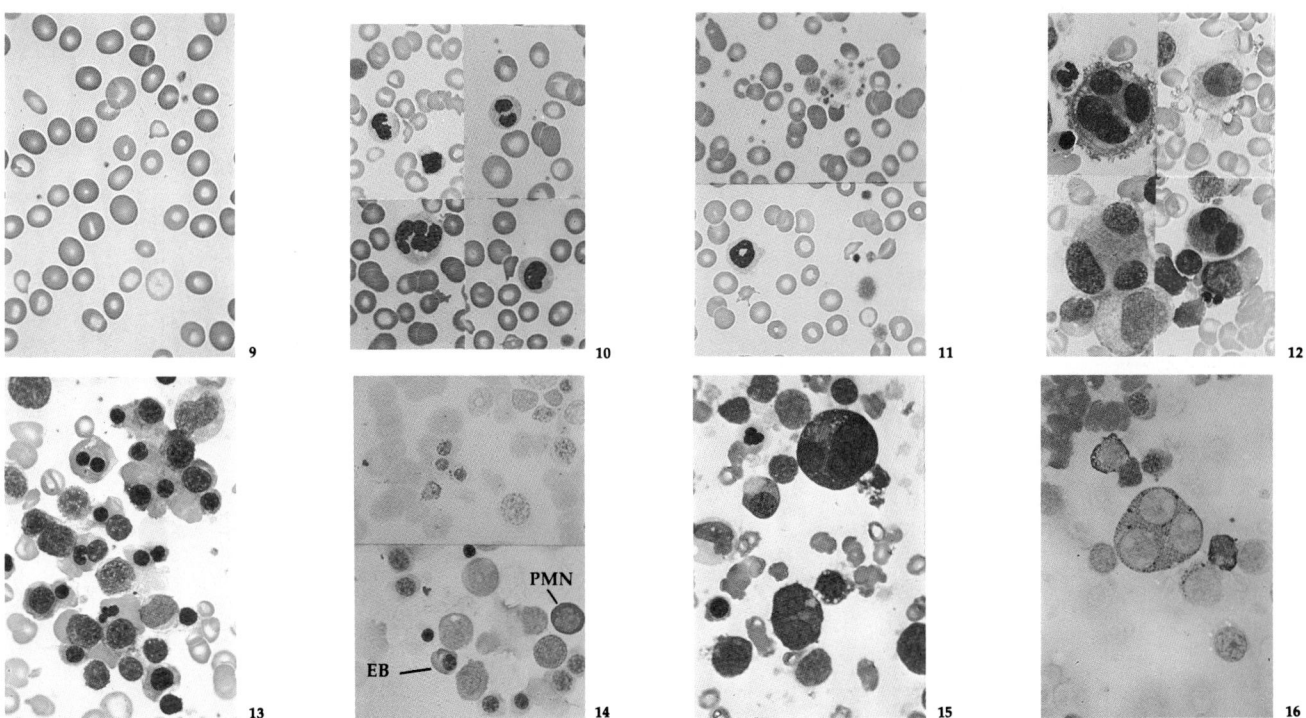

7-9 Preleukemia. Erythrocyte abnormalities in preleukemia. 7-10 Preleukemia. Acquired Pelger-Huët cells in preleukemia. 7-11 Preleukemia. Giant platelets in preleukemia. 7-12 Preleukemia. Abnormal megakaryocytes in preleukemia. 7-13 Preleukemia. Dyserythropoiesis in preleukemia. 7-14 Preleukemia. Sideroblasts in preleukemia. Stained for iron (Prussian blue) in the upper panel and by the PAS technique in the lower. PAS-positive erythroblasts are indicated by EB, and a positive polymorphonuclear neutrophil is designated by PMN. 7-15 Dyserythropoiesis in erythroleukemia. Wright's stain. 7-16 Dyserythropoiesis in erythroleukemia. PAS stain.

Note: Unless otherwise noted, all films were stained with Wright's stain, original magnification ×1000.

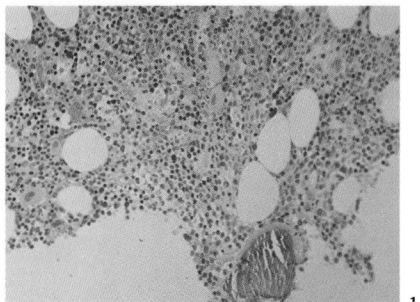 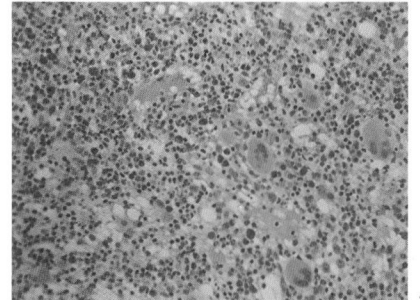 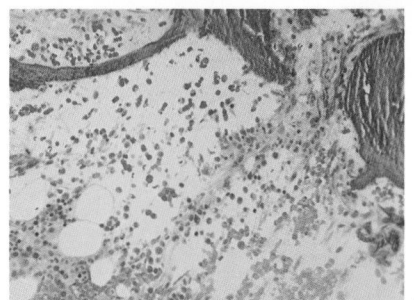

8-1 Normal marrow (×200). **8-2** Hypercellular marrow (×200). **8-3** Hypocellular marrow (×200).

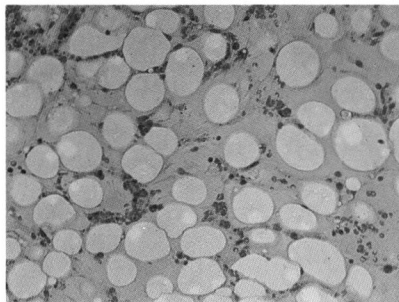 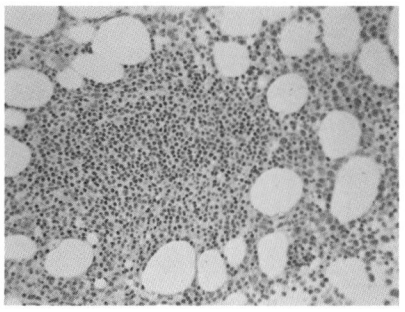 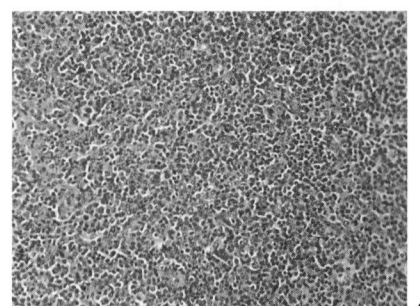

8-4 Aplastic marrow (×200). **8-5** Benign lymphoid follicle in normal marrow (×200). **8-6** Lymphoma involving the marrow (×200).

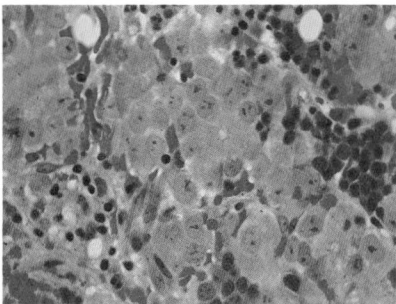 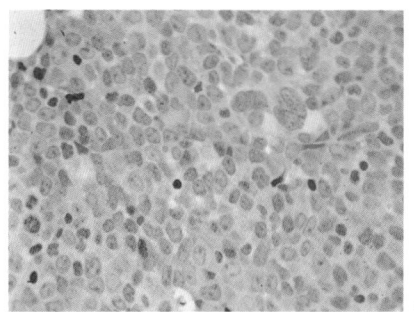 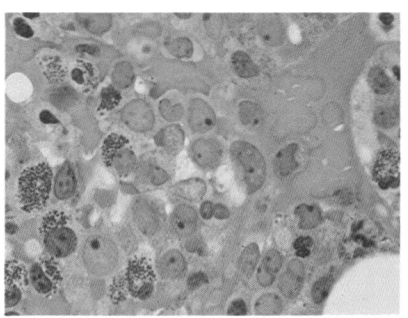

8-7 Metastatic carcinoma in the marrow (×500). **8-8** Acute myelogenous leukemia (×500). **8-9** Acute myelogenous leukemia with marked increase in eosinophils (×500).

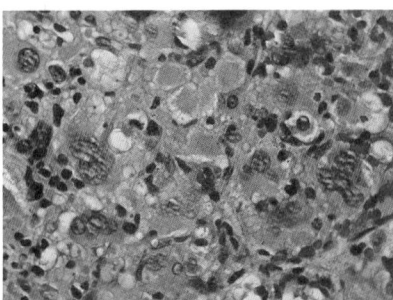 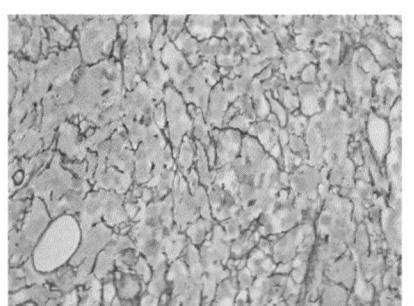 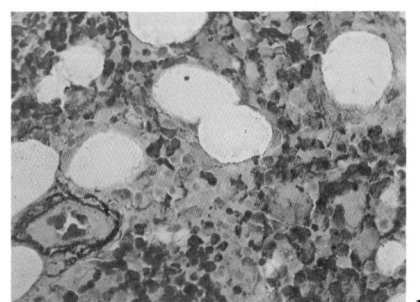

8-10 Myelofibrosis showing increased numbers of megakaryocytes and decreased marrow cellularity (×500). **8-11** Myelofibrosis. Silver stain showing increased reticulin. **8-12** Normal marrow stained by the silver method showing little reticulin except surrounding a blood vessel (×500).

Note: Plates 8-1 to 8-9 are thin plastic sections stained with Giemsa stain. Plates 8-10 to 8-12 are paraffin sections. Plate 8-10 was stained with Giemsa stain; Plates 8-11 and 8-12 were stained for reticulin. The original magnifications are given in parentheses.

PLATE 8   Marrow sections

Neutrophil disorders — benign, quantitative abnormalities of neutrophils

CHAPTER *87*

Neutropenia

STUART C. FINCH

Definition of neutropenia

The term *neutropenia* refers to a blood neutrophil concentration that is below the normal range. Frequently it is used interchangeably with the term *granulocytopenia*, although granulocytopenia refers to a reduction in all blood granulocytes (neutrophils, eosinophils, and basophils). The term *agranulocytosis* implies a complete absence of all granulocytes, but it is generally used to indicate very severe neutropenia. Neutrophil counts in adults below 500 per microliter are referred to as agranulocytosis.

Normal neutrophil levels should be stratified for age, race, and other factors. The lower normal limit of neutrophils for adult Caucasians (two standard deviations below the mean) is about 1500 per microliter (total leukocyte count per microliter × percent neutrophils) [1,2]. On the other hand, the average neutrophil count for a premature baby during the first day of life is 6000 ± 1000 per microliter, whereas the average neutrophil count for birth at gestational ages of 32 to 36 weeks or at 37 weeks or more is 8000 ± 1300 per microliter and 12,000 ± 1400 per microliter, respectively [3]. Thereafter, the neutrophils drop to a mean of about 4100 ± 2700 per microliter in the course of the next few days. They gradually reach levels that are carried through adult life [1–4]. Many blacks and Yemenite Jews have average neutrophil counts that are significantly lower than those for white Americans [5–11]. These relatively low counts probably are due to a redistribution of neutrophils within the vascular compartment [12–14].

Clinicians should be aware of conditions that produce spurious neutropenia. Neutrophils and platelets may adhere to erythrocytes in EDTA-anticoagulated blood [15]. Other causes of erroneously low counts include excessive leukocyte clumping in the presence of certain paraproteins, counts done long after blood is drawn, or excessive disintegration of abnormally fragile cells [16–17].

INFECTION AND NEUTROPENIA

The important clinical consequence of neutropenia is the risk of increased bacterial infection. There is a rough correlation between the degree of neutropenia and the risk of bacterial infection. Generally, the risk is slightly increased if the absolute neutrophil count is in the range of 500 to 1000 per microliter. Serious bacterial infections almost invariably occur if the neutrophil count is less than 500 per microliter, especially if the neutropenia persists for more than a few days. Endogenous bacteria are the most frequent invaders, but colonization with a variety of organisms of nosocomial origin is also common.

Susceptibility to bacterial infection, even with severe neutropenia, is quite variable. Some adult patients with neutrophil counts of 200 or less per microliter over a period of many years have not experienced serious infections [18,19]. Most patients with chronic neutropenia have normal or increased numbers of circulating monocytes [19,20]. In some instances there is evidence that the monocytes are moderately effective in protecting against bacterial infections [19,21], but in other instances the frequency of infection has had little relationship to the presence of adequate numbers of monocytes [19]. Monocytes are less efficient scavengers of bacteria than are neutrophils [21,22], and usually they migrate slowly to sites of infection, but in neutropenic patients then tend to move more rapidly into areas of focal infections [19]. Severe chronic neutropenia associated with monocytopenia without frequent infections has been reported [23,24]. It is very likely that the integrity of the humoral and cell-mediated immune systems and tissue macrophages play critical roles in the prevention of infection in the severely neutropenic individual.

The most frequent types of pyogenic infection in adults and children with significant neutropenia are cutaneous cellulitis, superficial or deep cutaneous abscesses, furunculosis, pneumonia, and septicemia [19, 20,25,26]. Otitis media frequently is observed in children. Stomatitis, gingivitis, and proctitis occur at all ages. The incidence of bacterial meningitis and viral, fungal, and parasitic infections does not appear to be increased in patients with chronic neutropenia. The most commonly isolated organisms from neutropenic patients are *Staphylococcus aureus*, *Pseudomonas aeruginosa*, *Escherichia coli*, and *Klebsiella* spp. [19,20,25,26]. The most common symptoms of infection are fever, malaise, chills, and diaphoresis. The usual symptoms and signs of local infection such as exudates, fluctuation, ulceration, fissure formation, local heat, swelling, and regional adenopathy are much less evident in neutropenic patients than they are in nonneutropenic individuals [27]. Erythema and pain or tenderness, however, are present at local sites of infection in practically all patients, irrespective of site infected or the neutrophil count [27].

Classification of the neutropenias

Current nomenclature for the identification of most of the neutropenic states, especially those that occur in childhood, is confusing [19,20,28–32]. A kinetic classification of the disorders presents many problems [19,28–31]. Leukocyte study techniques are difficult because there are no substances that provide a specific in vivo label for neutrophils and because of the paucity of neutrophils in circulation available for labeling. Some understanding of the neutrophil kinetics in neutropenic disorders is helpful for diagnosis and management.

Classification of drug-induced neutropenias also presents a difficult challenge. Major problems pertain to inconsistent clinical reporting, the inherent dangers of testing potentially harmful drugs in humans, the absence of reliable animal models, and the frequent use of multiple drugs. Susceptibility to the adverse or toxic effects of drugs is extremely variable in humans.

The clinical neutropenic disorders considered in this chapter are grouped according to etiology or clinical characteristics and are defined in terms of kinetic mechanisms, whenever possible. (See Table 87-1.) The identification of subtypes of chronic neutropenia, many of which may represent variations of a single genetic disorder, are maintained in order to provide useful clinical reference information. A kinetic classification of non-drug-induced (Table 87-2) and drug-induced (Table 87-3) neutropenic disorders has been developed in accordance with many clinical and experimental observations (Fig. 87-1).

Types of neutropenic disorders

HEREDITARY OR CONSTITUTIONAL STEM CELL DISORDERS

RETICULAR DYSGENESIS WITH CONGENITAL ALEUKOCYTOSIS

This is a rare immunologic deficiency disease of early fetal life associated with pluripotential stem cell failure [33–35]. The disorder is present at birth and is characterized by decreased or absent serum immunoglobulin levels, severe neutropenia with greatly reduced or absent hemopoietic precursors in the marrow, lymphopenia, and thymic aplasia. The neutropenia is presumably due to a failure of hemopoietic stem cells to develop. The few patients described with this disorder have had a severe, rapidly fatal illness. Defects in immunologic development in later fetal life may lead to thymic aplasia with considerably less involvement of the reticular system. This milder but also fatal form is characterized by reduced levels of immunoglobulins

TABLE 87-1 Kinetic classification of neutropenic disorders*

Type I *Reduced neutrophilic granulocytopoiesis*
Characterized by marrow granulocytic hypoplasia. There is a reduction in both total and effective neutrophilic granulocytopoiesis.

Ia *Predictable (chemotherapy) drug-induced neutrophilic granulocytopenia*
Reactions are slow in onset and are dose-dependent. Damage to stem cells and proliferating granulocytic progenitor cells is incurred through a variety of mechanisms (alkylating agents, antibiotics, etc.).

Ib *Idiosyncratic (chemotherapy) drug-induced neutrophilic granulocytopenia*
Reactions are slow in onset and dose-dependent, but there is wide variation in individual susceptibility (e.g., phenothiazine derivatives).

Ic *Idiosyncratic (hypersensitivity) drug-induced neutrophilic granulocytopenia*
Reactions are time-variable in onset and usually are dose-independent. The mechanism of impaired granulocytopoiesis is unknown. Reactions may be *acute*, lasting from days to weeks, or *chronic*, lasting from months to years.

Type II *Increased ineffective neutrophilic granulocytopoiesis*
Increased intramedullary destruction of granulocytes associated with variable total neutrophilic granulocytopoiesis. Marrow granulocyte cellularity is variable.

IIa *Predictable ineffective drug-induced granulocytopenia*
Reactions are slow in onset and are dose-dependent with wide individual susceptibility. The early marrow may be megaloblastic due to folic acid deficiency (e.g., methotrexate, diphenylhydantoin) and later may be hypoplastic.

Type III *Reduced neutrophil survival*
Granulocytopenia is due to increased destruction or utilization of neutrophils (e.g., sepsis, hypersplenism, antibody).

IIIa *Idiosyncratic (drug-hapten-antibody) neutropenia*
Reactions usually are extremely rapid in onset and are dose-independent in sensitized persons (e.g., aminopyrine).

Type IV *Combination (type I or II and type III) neutropenia*
Diminished effective granulocytopoiesis combined with increased peripheral destruction or utilization may result in severe neutropenia (e.g., sepsis, antineutrophil-antibody).

IVa *Drug-induced (combination) neutropenia*
Drug-activated antibody may accelerate peripheral granulocyte survival and eventually cause marrow myeloid damage (e.g., aminopyrine).

Type V *Pseudoneutropenia*
Total neutrophilic granulocyte pool is of normal size, but apparent neutropenia is due to reduced release from marrow storage pool or shift of neutrophils from the circulating to the marginal pool.

Va *Drug-induced pseudoneutropenia*
Reactions usually are secondary to vasomotor changes (e.g., histamine).

*Note that a small letter following a Roman numeral designates the subgroup class of drug-induced neutropenia.

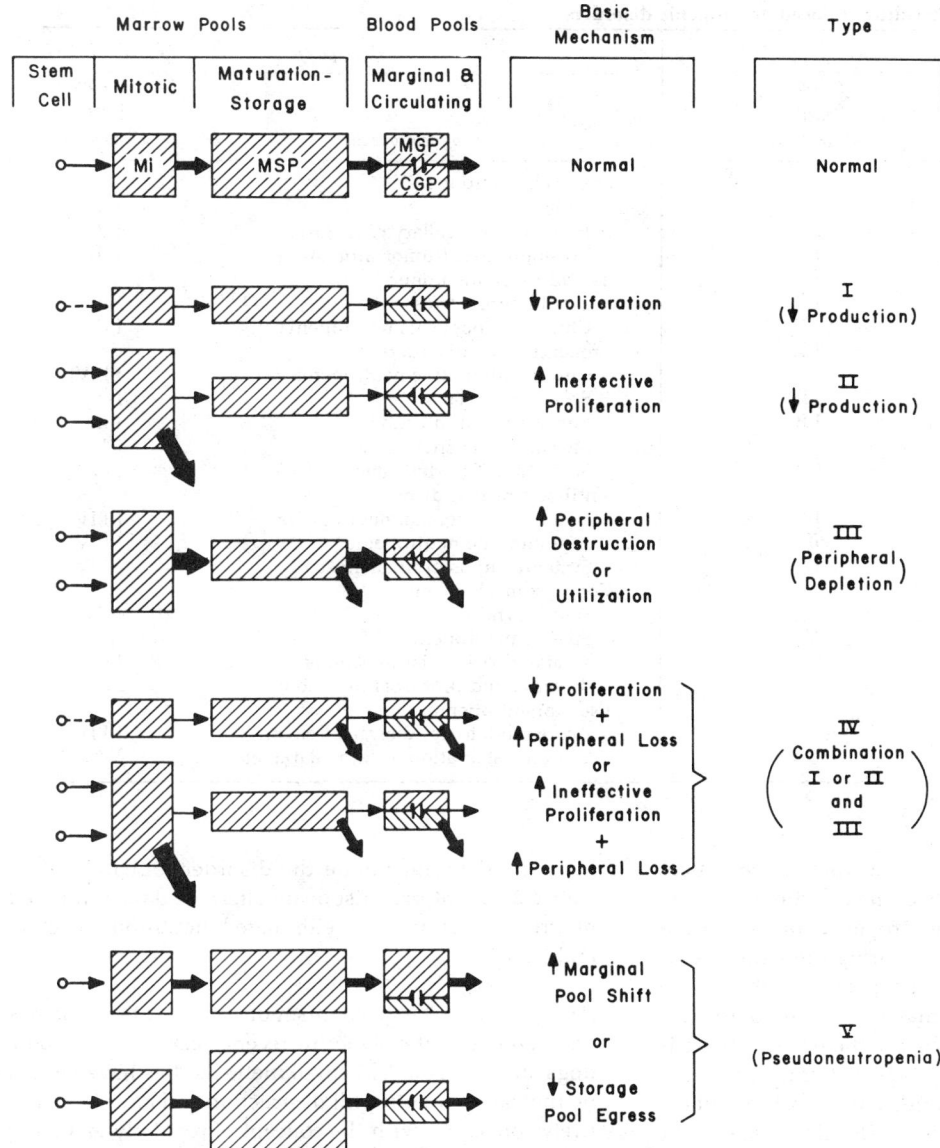

FIGURE 87-1   Neutropenic mechanisms. The types of neutropenia refer to those described in Table 87-1. The size of each granulocyte pool [stem cell, mitotic (Mi) maturation and storage pool (MSP), marginal neutrophilic granulocyte pool (MGP), and circulating neutrophilic granulocyte pool (CGP)] is schematically represented by the size of each cross-hatched area. The rate of cell flow into and out of each compartment is proportional to the size of the arrow.

and circulating granulocytes [36–39]. Two of the patients with neutropenia, lymphopenia, and abnormal cellular immunity have had cartilage-hair hypoplasia [39]. None has had splenomegaly. Marrow examinations have shown either complete absence of hemopoietic cells [33,34] or apparent arrest with vacuolization in some of the immature granulocytic elements [39]. The usual cause of death is bacterial [33–36] or viral infection [37,39].

CYCLIC NEUTROPENIA
This disorder is attributed to periodic pluripotential stem cell failure. Leale probably reported the first case

in 1910 [40], but the disorder was not well defined until about 1930 [41]. Genetic transmission is thought to be autosomal dominant with variable expression. The onset is most frequently in infancy or childhood, but it may occur at any age [42–49]. At intervals of about 21 days, rarely at intervals ranging from 15 to 35 days, the patient has a few days of fever and profound neutropenia associated with various combinations of stomatitis, pharyngitis, cervical adenitis, and skin infection. Concomitant with the development of profound neutropenia, some patients also may experience recurrent ulceration of vaginal or rectal mucosa. Occasionally, severe upper respiratory infections or recurrent ab-

TABLE 87-2 Classification of non-drug-induced neutropenic disorders

Hereditary or constitutional		Acquired	
Type of neutropenia	Possible kinetic mechanism(s)*	Type of neutropenia	Possible kinetic mechanism(s)*
Stem cell disorders:		Stem cell disorders:	
Reticular dysgenesis with congenital aleukocytosis	I	Preleukemia	I,II
Cyclic neutropenia	I	Histocytic medullary reticulosis	I,II
Dyskeratosis congenita with familial pancytopenia	I	Myelophthisis (tumor, fibrosis, etc.)	I,II
T- and B-cell disorders:		T- and B-cell disorders:	
Dysgammaglobulinemias	I	T-cell lymphocytes	I,II
Progenitor cell disorders:		Chronic hypoplastic neutropenia	I,II
Infantile genetic agranulocytosis	I,II	Progenitor cell disorders:	
Familial (severe) agranulocytosis	I,II	Chronic idiopathic neutropenia	I,II,V
Chronic neutropenia with constitutional defects	I,II	Severe bacterial sepsis	I–IV
Chronic (benign) neutropenia of childhood	I,II	Mycobacterial infections	I,II
Myelokathexis	II	Megaloblastic anemia	IV
Chédiak-Higashi syndrome	II	Starvation (Cu) deficiency	I,IV,V
Pseudoneutropenia:		Antibody-related disorders:	
Benign familial neutropenia	V	Isoimmune neonatal neutropenia	III,IV
Lazy leukocyte syndrome	V	Autoimmune neutropenia	III,IV
		Systemic lupus erythematosus	III,IV
		Complex mechanisms:	
		Felty's syndrome	I–IV
		Splenic neutropenia	III,IV
		Viral and rickettsial infections	I,IV,V
		Bacterial and protozoal infections	I,IV,V
		Pseudoneutropenia:	
		Acute (endotoxin, dialysis, C5a, etc.)	III,IV
		Chronic (starvation, cold, malaria, etc.)	V

*Refers to classification in Table 87-1.

dominal pain occur as a result of gastrointestinal mucosal ulceration [50]. The severity of the infections tends to parallel the severity of the neutropenia, but some patients escape infection entirely during the neutropenic period, which lasts for 3 to 4 days. During the leukopenic phase the neutrophils may disappear completely from the blood, and in about half of the patients there is a compensatory monocytosis [42]. Patients who have severe neutropenia without infection almost invariably have a significant monocytosis. Usually some cyclic variation occurs in all types of leukocytes as well as reticulocytes and platelets [30]. Marrow aspirates obtained during periods of granulocytopenia have shown either hypoplasia or an apparent arrest in maturation at the myelocyte stage. Between attacks, the patients are in good health, but mild splenomegaly may be present. There is a distinct tendency for the illness to become milder with time, and it may disappear completely within a span of 5 to 10 years [46]. Many mild cases probably are not detected [42], since oscillations in neutrophil counts frequently are observed in normal subjects and in patients with other types of blood dyscrasia [51].

A variety of treatment modalities for cyclic neutropenia have been employed [30,43–45,47,48,52]. An infusion of normal plasma has resulted in a significant neutrophil response in a child [49]. About 35 to 50 percent of patients have shown objective and subjective improvement following splenectomy [43,45], and some reports indicate that testosterone has been beneficial [47,48]. In many instances, ACTH and glucocorticoids

have failed to ameliorate the disorder, but in one instance 25 mg of prednisone on alternate days improved neutrophil counts and eliminated neutrophil cycling [52].

Pathogenesis The mechanism of cyclic neutropenia has been studied intensively in recent years in gray collie dogs and in humans. Leukokinetic studies have shown no increase in neutrophil destruction and have been entirely consistent with the concept of regularly recurring marrow failure [53–56]. The replacement of marrow in dogs having cyclic neutropenia with normal marrow has restored normal granulocytopoiesis [57,58]. Conversely, replacement of normal dog marrow with marrow from animals with cyclic neutropenia has induced cyclic neutropenia in the recipient [59]. Lithium has been shown to correct the cyclic neutropenia in dogs through a direct effect on proliferation and differentiation of granulocyte progenitor cells (CFU-c) [60]. These and other studies indicate that the disorder is the result of periodic pluripotential stem cell failure, possibly related to a disturbance of normal feedback mechanisms [56,61,62].

DYSKERATOSIS CONGENITA WITH FAMILIAL PANCYTOPENIA

This poorly defined sex-linked recessive disorder is associated with disturbances of the integument [63]. In most instances the only hematologic abnormality is mild neutropenia. Associated hematologic complica-

TABLE 87-3   Classification of common (idiosyncratic) drug-induced neutropenia

Drug	Possible kinetic mechanism(s)*	References	Drug	Possible kinetic mechanism(s)*	References
Analgesics:			Cardiovascular preparations:		
Aminopyrine	IIIa	[251,284,302–305]	Ajamaline	–	[313]
Dipyrone	IIIa	[251,284,364]	Aprindine	Ib,Ic	[312–314]
Noraminopyrine	IIIa	[365]	Captopril	Ib	[318,377]
Antibiotics:			Disopyramide	IIIa	[312,313,378]
Ampicillin	Ic	[267]	Methyldopa	Ic	[319]
Carbenicillin	Ib	[260]	Phenytoin	–	[313]
Cephalothin	Ib,IIIa	[262,263]	Procainamide	Ib,Ic	[284,313,316,317]
Chloramphenicol	Ia,Ib,Ic,IIa	[251,270,271]	Propranolol	Ic,IIIa	[379]
Clindamycin	Ic	[269]	Quinidine	Ic	[315]
Cloxacillin	Ib,Ic	[257,258]	Diuretics:		
Dicloxacillin	Ib,Ic	[258,259]	Acetazolamide	Ic	[381]
Ethambutol	Ib	[282]	Chlorthalidone	Ic	[382]
Gentamicin	Ic	[268]	Chlorothiazide	Ic	[332]
Griseofulvin	Ib	[367]	Ethacrynic acid	Ic	[333]
Isoniazid	Ib,Ic	[281,282,284,370]	Hydrochlorothiazide	Ic	[332]
Methicillin	Ib,Ic	[256,258]	Mercurials	Ic,IIIa	[331]
Nafcillin	Ib,Ic	[256,258,259]	Hypoglycemic agents:		
Nitrofurantoin	Ic	[265]	Chlorpropamide	Ic,IIIa	[284,330]
Novobiocin	Ib	[264]	Tolbutamide	–	[284,330]
Oxacillin	Ib,Ic	[258,259]	Phenothiazines and other antianxiety drugs:		
PAS	Ib,IIIa	[368]	Chlorpromazine	Ib,IIIa	[284,285,384]
Penicillin	Ic,IIIa	[255,366]	Mepazine	Ib	[251,284]
Rifampin	Ia	[282,284,369]	Methotrimeprazine	Ib	[251,383]
Ristocetin	Ia,Ib	[261]	Prochlorperazine	Ib	[251,284,285]
Steptomycin	Ib,IIIa	[266]	Promazine	Ib	[284,285]
Vancomycin	Ib,Ic	[261]	Thioridazine	Ib	[251,284,285,384]
Anticonvulsants:			Triflupromazine	Ib	[284,285,384]
Diphenylhydantoin	Ib,IIIa	[293,364]	Trimeprazine	Ib	[251]
Ethosuximide	Ib	[371]	Sedatives and neuropharmacologic agents:		
Mephenytoin	Ib	[284,372]	Chlordiazepoxide	Ib	[290]
Primidone	IIa	[292]	Clozapine	Ib	[385]
Trimethadione	Ib	[372,373]	Desipramine	Ib	[251,288]
Antihistamines:			Diazepam	Ib	[289]
Brompheniramine	–	[327]	Imipramine	Ib	[286,287]
Cimetidine	Ib	[328,329]	Meprobamate	Ib	[251,291]
Methaphenilene	Ib	[324]	Sulfonamide antibiotics:		
Pyribenzamine	Ib	[326,374]	Salicylazosulfapyridine	Ic,IIIa	[251,277]
Thenalidine	Ib	[325]	Sulfachlorpyridazine	–	[386]
Anti-inflammatory agents:			Sulfadiazine silver	Ib,IIIa	[276]
Aspirin	–	[294]	Sulfadimethoxine	Ic,IIIa	[387]
Gold salts	Ic,IIIa	[294,298–300]	Sulfaguanidine	Ic	[388]
Ibufen	–	[294]	Sulfamethoxypyridazine	Ic	[278]
Ibuprofen	–	[294]	Sulfapyridine	Ic,IIa	[254,272]
Indomethacin	Ib	[294,298]	Sulfasalazine	Ib,Ic	[279]
Oxyphenbutazone	Ib	[275,294,297]	Sulfisoxazole	Ib,Ic	[280]
Phenylbutazone	Ib	[275,294–297]	Sulfathiazole	Ib,Ic	[389]
Antimalarial agents:			Trimethoprim-sulfamethoxazole	Ib,Ic	[251,273,274,275]
Amodiaquine	–	[321]	Miscellaneous:		
Dapsone	–	[320]	Allopurinol	Ic	[251,284,334]
Hydrochloroquine	Ib	[323]	Benzene	Ia,Ic	[291]
Quinine	Ic	[322]	DDT	–	[392]
Pyrimethamine	IIa	[375]	Dinitrophenol	Ib,Ic	[251,393]
Antithyroid agents:			Ethanol	Ia,IIa	
Carbimazole	Ib,Ic	[251,284]	Levamisole	Ib,IIIa	[335–338]
Methimazole	Ib	[259,308,311]	Nitrous oxide	Ia	[394]
Methylthiouracil	Ib,IIIa	[376]	Penicillamine	Ib,Ic	[251,294,395]
Propylthiouracil	Ib,Ic,IIIa	[306–308,310]	Phenindione	Ic	[251,284,396]
Thiouracil	Ib	[284,309]			

*Refers to classification in Table 87-1.

tions in some patients have been mild, and most of those affected have reached adulthood. The combination of marrow granulocytic hypoplasia, sporadic thrombocytopenia and anemia, and resemblence to Fanconi's familial pancytopenia suggests that this may represent another stem cell disorder.

HEREDITARY OR CONSTITUTIONAL T- AND B-CELL DISORDERS

NEUTROPENIA WITH DYSGAMMAGLOBULINEMIA
This disease has been observed in a number of infants and children [64–72]. About half of the cases reported have been familial [66,67,69,70]. Both autosomal dominant [69,70] and sex-linked recessive [67] modes of transmission have been suggested. Clinical manifestations have been variable, but usually there is a history of frequent bacterial infections, failure to thrive, enlargement of the liver and spleen, impairment of humoral and cell-mediated immunity, and death during the first few years of life. Three children in one family died from infection before the age of 3 years [67]. The neutropenia has been moderate to severe and associated with monocytosis in some patients. Usually the neutropenia is persistent, but intermittent or cyclic fluctuations have been reported [64,66]. Marrow aspirations have demonstrated an abundance of early granulocytic forms with little maturation beyond the myelocyte stage. Abnormal vacuolization of the marrow granulocytic precursors has been reported [70]. Abnormalities have included absent or low levels of γ-globulins [64–67,70,71], sometimes associated with increased levels of IgM [65–67,71]. In some instances γ-globulins have been elevated as a result of increased levels of IgA [68,69]. The prognosis for patients with dysgammaglobulinemia is poor, with little or no benefit being reported from prednisone, thymectomy, or splenectomy [67]. Neutropenia disappeared transiently in a 6-year-old boy following an injection of γ-globulin [66], which suggests the possibility that a plasma factor deficiency may be responsible for the neutropenia. Neutrophilia in response to infection has been observed in several patients [69,72].

HEREDITARY OR CONSTITUTIONAL PROGENITOR (COMMITTED STEM) CELL NEUTROPENIC DISORDERS
A large and heterogenous group of neutropenic disorders of childhood involving progenitor (committed stem) cells may be considered subtypes of *chronic neutropenia* [18–20]. These neutropenias are thought to result from reduced effective granulopoiesis resulting from a variety of poorly defined mechanisms [28,30,31,73]. In many instances defective granulopoiesis has been attributed to diminished marrow microenvironment colony-stimulating activity [74–77].

INFANTILE GENETIC AGRANULOCYTOSIS
This disease was described by Kostmann in 1956 [78]. A number of closely related disorders that have been identified as various types of congenital or genetic neu-

tropenia probably represent variations of Kostman's disease [79]. Autosomal recessive transmission [78] with relationship to a specific histocompatibility antigen has been proposed [81]. Associations with consanguinity and congenital abnormalities are common [78,82,83].

The onset is marked by the development of frequent episodes of fever, skin infection, boils, aphthous stomatitis, and other similar problems early in life [19,20,78,84,85]. The blood neutrophil counts usually are extremely low and frequently are accompanied by a moderate eosinophilia or monocytosis [78,85–88]. Hyperglobulinemia is common [84,85,87]. Marrow findings have been variable, but usually there is normal granulocytic maturation up to the promyelocyte or myelocyte stage [78,85]. Chromosome structural abnormalities have been observed in the marrow granulocytic cells of some children with this disorder [89]. The growth of the marrow in tissue culture is variable. Most investigators have reported a normal number of colony-forming units associated with impairment of maturation [74–77,80,90–93]. The bulk of evidence suggests that the marrow maturation abnormalities are related to defective marrow microenvironment [74–77,94,95] or possibly to intrinsic cell maturation defects [80,92,93]. Neutrophil survival is normal [91].

The severe neutropenia of this disorder usually leads to fatal infection, but in a few instances it has remitted or has been relatively mild with prolonged survival [87,91]. Transition to leukemia has occurred [87,96]. Splenectomy, glucocorticoids, and androgens have had little therapeutic value [86,87], and in several instances splenectomy has been followed by fatal sepsis [84]. The use of antibiotics may prolong life for several years [78,85]. Marrow transplantation has resulted in partial [90] and complete [97] correction of the agranulocytosis.

FAMILIAL (SEVERE) NEUTROPENIA
This neutropenia of infancy was first described by Hitzig in 1959 and is probably transmitted as an autosomal dominant trait [63,98–100]. Bacterial infections of any type may develop, but particularly common are oral infections [98]. Splenomegaly is uncommon [98], but some monocytosis occurs in virtually all the patients. The marrow has generally been normocellular, with an apparent deficiency of granulocytes more mature than myelocytes. Hypergammaglobulinemia, thought to be compensatory, also has been noted [63,100]. Splenectomy in one patient did not correct the neutropenia [99]. Plasma transfusion transiently restored the blood neutrophils in a 13-year-old boy with this disorder and produced an equivocal response in his brother [100].

CHRONIC BENIGN NEUTROPENIA OF CHILDHOOD
This abnormality usually starts within the first 2 years of life, with frequent recovery within 1 or 2 years [20,32,101–106]. No genetic pattern of inheritance has been described. Most patients with this diagnosis have had little or no decrease in resistance to infection [20,101–106]. The condition is so poorly defined that it may not justify separate identification [20].

MYELOKATHEXIS

This term has been applied to describe a neutropenic disorder in a 9-year-old girl with frequent infections for 7 years [107–108]. Slight splenomegaly was present. Most of her blood neutrophils had cytoplasmic vacuoles and abnormal nuclei, with very thin filaments connecting the nuclear lobes. The marrow was hyperplastic and contained degenerating, hypersegmented granulocytes. Leukokinetic and morphologic studies were consistent with both the diminished survival of mature neutrophils and increased intramedullary neutrophil death. The cause of the neutropenia in a second patient with a similar clinical picture was thought to be impaired release of neutrophils from the marrow [109].

NEUTROPENIA WITH EXOCRINE PANCREAS DEFICIENCY (SHWACHMAN-DIAMOND SYNDROME)

Several types of childhood chronic neutropenia with constitutional defects have been described. Best recognized is the combination of neutropenia with exocrine pancreatic insufficiency [110–121]. There is good evidence for genetic transmission [111,114,117], possibly autosomal recessive, of this type of neutropenia [120]. The disorder is usually manifest during the first year of life, but it may appear anytime during the first decade. The initial symptoms may resemble those of fibrocystic disease with failure to thrive, steatorrhea, and frequent episodes of pneumonia or other infection. The sweat test is negative. Some children have other abnormalities such as metaphyseal dysostosis, Hirchsprung's disease, short stature, epiphyseal dysplasia, mental retardation, mild diabetes mellitus, galactosuria, hepatic dysfunction, and immunoglobulin abnormalities [110, 111,114,115–120]. Splenomegaly is noted occasionally. Secretion of pancreatic enzymes are diminished or absent. Fecal fat is increased, and D-xylose absorption is normal. In contrast to fibrocystic disease, chronic pulmonary disease is absent, and the prognosis is considerably better [111]. Steatorrhea tends to diminish with time, although pancreatic insufficiency persists. Histologic studies of the pancreas have shown acinar degeneration with fatty replacement. The degree of neutropenia is variable, with granulocyte counts averaging around 200 to 400 per microliter. Neutrophil counts tend to be constant and with no reciprocal monocytosis. A modest polymorphonuclear neutrophil leukocytosis may develop with bacterial infections [115]. A significant defect in neutrophil motility has been demonstrated in both patients with the disorder and in their parents [120]. In a few instances a cyclic tendency has been reported [112,113,119]. Marrow studies have generally shown granulocytic hyperplasia. A globulin factor cytotoxic for neutrophils has been present in the sera of several patients [131]. In vitro studies, however, have demonstrated no evidence of serum inhibitors against colony-forming units in culture (CFU-c) or colony-stimulating activity (CSA) [121]. The possibility of underlying defects in the marrow microenvironment or stem cells has been suggested [121].

DISORDERS OF METABOLISM AND NEUTROPENIA

Several children with *hyperglycinemia, hyperglycinuria,* and *ketoacidosis* have had significant neutropenia [122,123]. A 9-month-old male with *orotic aciduria* had megaloblastic marrow and neutropenia [124], and an 8-month-old male with *methylmalonic aciduria* developed transient neutropenia shortly after correction of his ketoacidosis [125].

CHÉDIAK-HIGASHI SYNDROME

The mechanism of the neutropenia is ineffective granulopoiesis (see Chap. 89) [126]. The basic defect leading to intramedullary destruction of proliferative granulocytic cells is related to defective cell granules [127].

HEREDITARY OR CONSTITUTIONAL PSEUDONEUTROPENIA

BENIGN FAMILIAL NEUTROPENIA

This condition was first reported by Huber in 1939 [128] and Gansslen in 1941 [128]. The disorder is characterized by slight to moderate lifetime neutropenia [128–132]. Autosomal dominant transmission has been demonstrated [129–131]. Marrow examinations usually are within normal limits. Leukoagglutinins are not present, and the leukocyte alkaline phosphatase score is usually normal, although this enzyme activity was absent in three members of one family [132]. Affected individuals are healthy, there is no progression, and therapy is unnecessary. A familial relationship to Fanconi's anemia has been suggested [133].

BENIGN ETHNIC NEUTROPENIA

In recent years the definition of benign familial neutropenia has been broadened to include several large ethnic groups with similar degrees of neutropenia. The most striking examples are the African and West Indian blacks who have average neutrophil counts in the range of 2100 to 2600 per microliter [6] in comparison to levels of 3000 to 4000 per microliter for American blacks [7,8] and 4400 to 4600 per microliter for white Americans [1,2,7]. A similar form of benign neutropenia affects a significant number of Yemenite Jews [9–11]. Most reports favor genetic transmission of the disorder for both groups [5,7–11], but an acquired etiology also has been suggested for the blacks [6,8]. The absence of increased bacterial infections [5,7–10], normal neutrophil response to pregnancy and hydrocortisone administration [12,13], and normal numbers of marrow granulocyte colony-forming cells [14] give strong support for the neutropenia being an abnormality in the marrow release mechanism [12–14].

LAZY LEUKOCYTE SYNDROME

This disorder has been described in two children with recurrent stomatitis, gingivitis, and other infections [134] (see Chap. 89). A profound neutropenia was present, although the marrow appeared to be normally cellular without granulocyte abnormalities. Recently a transient form of the lazy syndrome has been described [135].

ACQUIRED STEM CELL DISORDERS
Neutropenia may be a manifestation of *preleukemia* [136,137] (see Chap. 22). Its association with excessive leukophagocytosis has been observed in patients with *histiocytic medullary reticulosis* [138,139] (see Chap. 100). Neutropenia alone may also develop from *myelophthisis* due to the presence of marrow lymphoma, myeloma, carcinoma, or fibrosis [140] (see Chap. 52).

ACQUIRED T-CELL NEUTROPENIC DISORDERS
Neutropenia in chronic lymphocytic leukemia of T-cell origin has been described [141–143]. This has been further defined as an indolent form of *chronic T-cell lymphocytosis* or *T-cell lymphoproliferative disorder* with neutropenia secondary to the presence of increased numbers of cytotoxic suppressor T cells in the marrow [143,144]. Two patients with severe granulocytopenia and recurrent infections associated with excessive numbers of T cells with killer-cell but not suppressor-cell activity have been reported [145]. In some respects these chronic T-cell-induced forms of neutropenia resemble the few patients with *thymoma and agranulocytosis* [146,147] and possibly those with *chronic hypoplastic neutropenia* who have been reported [148,149].

ACQUIRED PROGENITOR (COMMITTED STEM) CELL DISORDERS

IDIOPATHIC NEUTROPENIA
Many of the previously described chronic neutropenic disorders of childhood and acquired chronic neutropenic disorders of adulthood have been referred to simply as *chronic idiopathic neutropenia* [18,30] or *chronic neutropenia* [20,31]. The clinical course of many patients with adult forms of chronic neutropenia is benign, despite blood neutrophil counts of 200 or less per microliter. It appears much more related to the capability of mobilizing neutrophils at sites of infection than other clinical features [18,19,20,30]. Most of the patients have moderate monocytosis and normocellular or hypercellular marrows with reduced late granulocytic forms [19,30,73]. Spontaneous clinical remissions occasionally occur during adulthood [30]. Defective or ineffective neutrophilic granulopoiesis, altered marrow release mechanisms, and increased vascular margination have been incriminated as possible mechanisms [19,30,31, 73,77].

BACTERIAL INFECTIONS
Profound neutropenia associated with marrow granulocytic degenerative changes may occur with severe *bacterial sepsis* [150]. This is particularly likely to develop in infants and old or debilitated patients, and its occurrence carries a grave prognosis. Severe and protracted neutropenia due to overwhelming bacterial sepsis probably is due mostly to direct endotoxin and bacterial damage to marrow granulocyte precursors, although

other mechanisms contribute. Staphylococcal, pneumococcal, and *Klebsiella* sepsis are most likely to be associated with this type of myelotoxicity. Neutropenia associated with *disseminated mycobacterial infection* [150–155] has been reported due to altered immunologic mechanisms [154] such as T-lymphocyte depression of granulopoiesis [155]. A severe and frequently fatal form of neutropenic enterocolitis characterized by malaise, fever, and abdominal pain with localizing signs has been described [156]. Prompt recognition and surgical intervention are prerequisites for survival.

VIRAL INFECTIONS
Severe and protracted neutropenia occasionally is observed with infectious hepatitis [157], infectious mononucleosis [158–160], and Kawasaki disease [161]. Direct marrow damage has been variously ascribed to possible toxic effects or autoantibody [157–160]. An acute, transient neutropenic disorder called *leukopenic infectious monocytosis* was believed, in past years, to be due to infection. Most, if not all, of the cases are due to drug toxicity [162].

MEGALOBLASTIC HEMOPOIESIS
Neutropenia associated with megaloblastic anemias, due to either folic acid deficiency or vitamin B_{12} deficiency, is probably the result of ineffective myelopoiesis [163,164], but diminished granulocyte survival [165] may contribute. Diminished marrow granulocyte reserves also have been demonstrated [166] (see Chap. 47). Protracted and moderate to severe neutropenia has been observed in marasmic infants [167–169] and malnourished adults on parenteral feedings [170,171]. Marrow megaloblastosis has been observed, and some of these patients have been thought to have copper deficiency since they have responded promptly to copper therapy [167,170,171].

IMMUNE NEUTROPENIAS

NEUTROPHIL ANTIBODY-ASSOCIATED NEUTROPENIC DISORDERS
Antibody with specificity for the neutrophil has been demonstrated in a number of different neutropenic disorders [30,32,172,173]. In some instances, however, the antibody may not be important in the pathogenesis of the neutropenia, and in others antibody has not been consistently detected. Interpretation of these discordant findings is difficult since the antibody detection tests employed have been unreliable. Experimentally, heterologous neutrophil-specific antibody will produce neutropenia by accelerated removal of circulating neutrophils and by increased intramedullary destruction of neutrophil precursors [174]. The clinical characteristics of some antineutrophil antibody-associated neutropenic disorders differ little from those in which antineutrophil antibody is absent [19]. It has been speculated that the paucity of late granulocyte precursors in many patients with chronic neutropenia could be due to

antibody against neutrophil precursors, a mechanism similar to that observed in antibody-induced pure red cell aplasia [175]. These analogies provide the basis for classifying these disorders in a separate category.

ISOIMMUNE NEONATAL NEUTROPENIA

This moderate to severe neutropenia in newborn infants lasts for several weeks and has been attributed to the transplacental passage of maternal IgG antineutrophil antibody [176–179]. The pathogenesis of this disorder first involves the movement of fetal granulocytes containing specific antigens into the maternal circulation during pregnancy [180–181]. The neutrophil-specific antigens then stimulate maternal production of antibody, which subsequently enters the fetal circulation. It is thought that the antibody agglutinates circulating neutrophils during the neonatal period [177]. The antibody reacts with the neutrophils of the patient and the father, but not the mother. The condition is very similar to Rh-induced hemolytic anemia of the newborn and provides the most convincing evidence of any antineutrophil antibody–induced disorder in humans [32,182]. Neutrophil-specific antigens NA and NB play an important role in the development of isoantibodies which are the basis of this disorder [182–184].

Infants with isoimmune neonatal neutropenia may be asymptomatic during the first few days of life. The disease becomes apparent with the appearance of bacterial infection. Cutaneous infections with common bacterial pathogens predominate, but respiratory tract and urinary tract infections may develop, and sepsis has resulted in death [178]. Affected infants with mild neutropenia remain asymptomatic and undiagnosed. The usual hematologic picture consists of severe neutropenia, moderate monocytosis, and normal concentrations of red cells and platelets. Marrow cellularity usually is normal or increased with reduced numbers of mature neutrophils. Diagnosis may be difficult in the presence of sepsis, since sepsis per se may induce severe neutropenia in infants [185]. The duration of the neutropenia coincides with survival of the maternal IgG antibody in the infant, usually a period of 6 to 12 weeks. Antibiotics should be used for infections [186]. Glucocorticoids are of little value in reversing the neutropenia. Plasmapheresis and leukocyte transfusions have been suggested for extreme situations [30,32].

The role of antineutrophil antibody in the pathogenesis of isoimmune neonatal neutropenia has been questioned since maternal leukoagglutinins are common in mutiparous females without deleterious effects on the infant [187,188]. This may be due to the fact that these leukoagglutinins are directed against HLA rather than neutrophil-specific antigens, are absorbed by many tissues, and do not accumulate in sufficient amounts on the neutrophils to produce neutropenia [30,32,182].

AUTOIMMUNE NEUTROPENIA

It has been speculated for many years that leukocyte autoantibody accelerates removal of granulocytes from the blood and eventually produces marrow exhaustion [189,190]. Only in recent years, however, with the development of improved techniques for antibody detection, has it been possible to document a few examples of probable autoimmune neutropenia [172,191–194]. Autoantibody specificity for the neutrophil-specific antigens NA_2 [192] and ND_1 [195] provide the most compelling evidence for the existence of autoimmune neutropenia. Severe neutropenia in association with granulocyte-specific cytotoxic antibody has been reported [196]. Response to steroids [197] and association with idiopathic thrombocytopenic purpura [198] have provided additional evidence for the probable existence of antibody-mediated autoimmune neutropenia. Direct evidence that autoimmune antineutrophil antibody results in accelerated granulocyte destruction or impaired granulopoiesis is fragmentary [172,191,199]. There are few unique clinical features of autoimmune neutropenia [30,32]. The age range has been wide, and females have dominated. About half of the patients have had slight to moderate splenomegaly. Neutropenia has been moderate to severe, and usually there is a moderate monocytosis.

Marrow granulocytic cellularity usually is normal or increased with a paucity of late granulocytic forms. The risk of bacterial infection is increased in relationship to the severity of the neutropenia. Bacterial infections are managed as they are for any chronic neutropenic state. Neutropenia is treated only if it is responsible for increased bacterial infections. Prednisone in a dose of 1 to 2 mg/kg per day has been effective in improving the neutropenia in about half of the patients treated [32]. Glucocorticoid therapy should be undertaken with extreme caution because of its ability to mask infections and possibly to impede the migration of neutrophils to sites of infection. Splenectomy has only been transiently effective and is not uniformly recommended because of subsequent increased risk of infection. Plasmapheresis and immunosuppressive therapy are of potential value.

SYSTEMIC LUPUS ERYTHEMATOSUS

The neutropenia that occurs in about half of the patients with systemic lupus erythematosus (SLE) is thought possibly to be due to antineutrophil antibody [173,200,201]. High levels of neutrophil-specific IgG have been demonstrated in the serums of several neutropenic patients with SLE who subsequently have corrected the neutropenia in response to therapy with glucocorticoids alone or in combination with immunosuppressive agents [201–203]. A significant shortening of granulocyte survival time has been demonstrated in some neutropenic patients [201]. Less than 5 percent of patients have neutropenia severe enough to increase their susceptibility to infection, but on rare occasions this becomes a major problem. Compensatory monocytosis is unusual. The effect of splenectomy is transient and should be reserved only for emergencies. There is evidence that splenectomy may be followed by increased cutaneous vasculitis and more frequent severe infections [204].

ACQUIRED NEUTROPENIC DISORDERS DUE TO COMPLEX MECHANISMS

FELTY'S SYNDROME

The triad of rheumatoid arthritis, splenomegaly, and neutropenia is referred to as *Felty's syndrome* [30,205–207]. It is a rare complication of advanced rheumatoid disease that usually predisposes the individual to frequent bacterial infections. Spleen size may vary from minimal to massive enlargement. Neutropenia is usually moderate to extreme without good relationship to either spleen size or susceptibility to infection. Impaired neutrophil chemotaxis and hypocomplementemia may contribute to increased susceptibility to infection [205,207]. Marrow neutrophilic granulopoiesis is usually normocellular or hypercellular, but may be hypocellular [207]. The pathophysiology of Felty's syndrome is poorly understood. Recent kinetic studies suggest that shortened neutrophil survival is associated with accelerated release of marrow neutrophils and an inadequate granulopoietic response [208]. Reduced granulopoiesis has been confirmed [209,210] and may be due to serum inhibitory factors [211,212] or increased suppressor T-cell activity [213–215]. Antineutrophil antibody [173,216–219] or immune complexes [205,207] may inhibit granulopoiesis and be responsible for impaired neutrophil function [205,207]. Other studies have failed to demonstrate shortening of neutrophil survival time and indicate that neutropenia is due to increased neutrophil margination [210] or impaired release of neutrophils from the marrow [219].

No specific therapy is recommended for the asymptomatic patient with Felty's syndrome. The most successful form of therapy for patients with an increased frequency of infections has been splenectomy. About 65 percent of patients following splenectomy will maintain satisfactory neutrophil levels, and in over 75 percent frequent infections will stop [220,221]. A high serum IgG granulocyte-binding protein concentration has been found to be the best predictor of a good response to splenectomy [222]. Reduction in spleen size and improvement in the number of neutrophils in the circulation has been reported following the administration of 500 to 1000 mg of gold salts intramuscularly [223,224]. Favorable responses to therapy with testosterone [225], penicillamine [226], and lithium [227] have also been reported.

HYPERSPLENISM

In 1942 Wiseman and Doan described a disorder known as *primary splenic neutropenia* [228]. The mechanism of the neutropenia was stated to be a selective splenic affinity for neutrophils. A variety of underlying disorders was probably responsible for this disorder. The most common causes are congestive splenomegaly secondary to liver disease, various autoimmune disorders, Felty's syndrome, sarcoid, hairy-cell leukemia, and lymphoma. Much less common causes of secondary hypersplenism are tuberculosis, kala-azar, malaria, and Gaucher's dis-

ease [229]. The usual picture is moderate leukopenia, which may be accompanied by moderate thrombocytopenia and anemia. Reduced neutrophil suvival correlates with spleen size, and the extent of neutropenia is dependent on marrow compensatory mechanisms [230]. In some patients with chronic active hepatitis and splenomegaly [231] immune mechanisms may contribute to the development of neutropenia [157].

INFECTIOUS AGENTS

Many types of acute systemic *viral* and *rickettsial infections* produce leukopenia or neutropenia [150,232]. The characteristic pattern is similar to that which occurs with acute infectious hepatitis [233] and infectious mononucleosis [234]. Leukopenia develops during the first 24 or 48 h of the illness and may persist for 3 to 5 days. This corresponds to the period of acute viremia and virus-induced leukocyte damage that probably results in increased neutrophil utilization, margination, or sequestration [235]. Toxic granulation and Döhle bodies in the cytoplasm of the neutrophil frequently accompany the neutropenic phase of infectious mononucleosis, which has been noted to occur in virtually all patients with this disorder when they are carefully followed [234]. Other viral infections frequently associated with neutropenia are dengue fever, yellow fever, influenza, poliomyelitis, psittacosis, sand-fly fever, chickenpox, smallpox, measles, and rubella [150,232].

Significant neutropenia may occur during certain *bacterial* and *protozoal infections*. The most commonly recognized have been brucellosis, bacillary dysentery, typhoid and paratyphoid, malaria, and kala-azar [150]. The mechanisms responsible for neutropenia with these disorders are poorly understood.

ACQUIRED PSEUDONEUTROPENIA

Acute pseudoneutropenia may develop during endotoxemia, hypersensitivity reactions, and antigen-antibody reactions. It may be caused by activation of the complement system, through either the alternate or conventional pathways, leading to the generation of C5a, which induces neutrophil aggregation and adhesion to endothelial surfaces [236,237]. Pulmonary capillary bed complement-mediated leukostasis may cause acute cardiopulmonary complications [238]. C5a-induced neutropenia transiently occurs during hemodialysis and continuous-flow leukopheresis [239,240]. More severe reactions may result from the transfusion of incompatible antibodies [32].

Chronic pseudoneutropenia may develop secondary to C5a generation in response to certain complex polysaccharides, soluble immune complexes, and paroxysmal nocturnal hemoglobinuria [208,241,242]. The neutropenias of prolonged fasting [243], anorexia nervosa [244], vivax malarial infection [245], certain types of splenomegaly [246], and chronic exposure to cold [247] are probably due to redistribution of neutrophils within the vascular pools.

DRUG-INDUCED NEUTROPENIA

The kinetic classification of most drug-induced neutropenic disorders continues to be difficult, but distinct patterns are suggested for some drugs (Table 87-2). Most common are the dose-related, drug-induced neutropenias of the chemotherapy type, which are due to drugs that interfere with cell proliferation. Their actions are not selective and probably involve the pluripotential stem cells. The phenothiazines and many other drugs behave much like some of the antimetabolic agents, but tend to act on an idiosyncratic basis. The second type of drug-induced neutropenia is usually not dose-related and is thought to be immunologic in origin. Some of these develop following a few days of drug exposure and behave like hypersensitivity reactions. Others are due to drug-activated antibody, and many occur within minutes to days after the initiation of drug therapy. These reactions tend to be quite selective, which suggests that activity is confined to the committed stem cell.

Patients with connective tissue diseases, allergy, or a previous history of adverse drug reaction are prone to develop drug-induced hypersensitivity reactions. Idiosyncratic reactions tend to develop more frequently in women than in men, and more often in older than in younger persons. Susceptibility to idiosyncratic drug-induced agranulocytosis may be related to the genotype of the individual [248]. Genetic variants of essential drug-detoxifying enzymes may lead to persistence of unusually high serum and tissue drug concentrations. The increased incidence of adverse effects with sulfasalazine in individuals who are slow acetylators as compared with those who rapidly acetylate the intermediate metabolites of this drug is an example of one type of genetic susceptibility [249]. There is now evidence that persons of the HLA-B27 genotype with rheumatoid arthritis may be at increased risk for agranulocytosis from levamisole [250].

Drug-induced agranulocytosis is a serious disorder with mortality rates reported at 20 percent or greater during the past decade [251–253]. Mortality, however, should be 5 percent or less if proper therapy of infections is initiated promptly. Patients with agranulocytosis are asymptomatic in the absence of bacterial infection. The diagnosis is suspected in anyone on any medication who develops sudden fever, chills, malaise, or objective evidence of infection. The blood neutrophil count is moderately to severely reduced. The marrow will range from moderate granulocytic hypocellularity with preferential reduction in late granulocytic forms to a virtual absence of all granulocytic cells or reduction in all hemopoietic cells. In early acute antibody-mediated neutropenia there may be granulocytic hyperplasia with predominance of early granulocytic forms. Hematologic recovery frequently commences a few days following cessation of drug therapy with the development of immature marrow granulocytic hyperplasia. This is followed in a few days with the appearance of a few monocytes and immature granulocytes in the blood.

During the next few days the neutrophil count rises rapidly to levels that often exceed the normal range for several more days before returning to normal. During recovery the transient combination of neutrophilia with immature cells in the blood and hyperplasia of immature granulocytic cells in the marrow closely resembles the picture of acute leukemia [254].

Antimicrobial agents constitute one of the leading causes of drug-induced agranulocytosis [255–282]. Penicillin has been responsible possibly for only a handful of cases and, then, only when administered in high doses [255]. On the other hand, the five semisynthetic penicillins currently in use (oxacillin, cloxacillin, dicloxacillin, nafcillin, and methicillin) frequently have been reported to induce agranulocytosis [256–258]. Almost all patients reported have received high-dose parenteral therapy for more than 2 to 3 weeks, but a few have received moderate doses for less than 10 days. The high-dose incidence rates for methicillin are estimated at about 8 percent [256]. Direct marrow granulocytic suppression probably is responsible for most cases of agranulocytosis with the semisynthetic penicillins, but some may be due to hypersensitivity or antibody reactions [258,259]. Carbenicillin [260] and vancomycin [261] also have caused reversible neutropenia following intensive therapy for several weeks or more. Either immune or marrow-inhibited types of reversible agranulocytosis occurs in about 0.1 percent of all patients treated with a cephalosporin [262,263]. Other antimicrobial agents that rarely produce significant neutropenia are novobiocin [264], nitrofurantoin [265], streptomycin [266], ampicillin [267], gentamicin [268], and clindamycin [269]. Chloramphenicol inhibits marrow granulocyte colony growth in therapeutic amounts [270]. About 9 percent of the blood dyscrasias attributed to chloramphenicol have been selective neutropenia, with about 50 percent mortality [271].

Many of the reactions to sulfonamides probably are the result of direct marrow depression, but others may involve immunologic mechanisms [259,272]. Trimethoprim-sulfamethoxazole currently is the sulfonamide preparation associated with the highest risk of neutropenia induction [252]. Prolonged use of this drug combination has resulted in mild to moderate neutropenia in 10 percent or more of patients treated [273,274]. In England patients who take co-trimoxazole have been found to be at high risk for the occurrence of fatal agranulocytosis [275]. Other neutropenia-inducing sulfonamide preparations include sulfadiazine silver [276], salicylazosulfapyridine [277], sulfamethoxypyridazine [278], sulfasalazine [279], and sulfisoxazole [280]. Isoniazid-, rifampicin-, and ethambutol-induced neutropenias have occurred during the treatment of tuberculosis [281,282].

The *phenothiazine derivatives* are probably the leading class of drugs that cause drug-induced neutropenia in the United States despite their recent moderate decline in use [283,284]. Individual susceptibility is extemely variable and depends on the ability of the marrow to compensate for phenothiazine inhibition of DNA synthesis [283–285]. Phenothiazine-induced agranulocytosis has a predilection for older white females, especially if they also are obese and have chronic disease [283–285]. It rarely occurs before 2 weeks or after 8 weeks of drug administration, or until the cumulative dose of phenothiazine is more than 5 g [284]. It is most frequently observed in mental hospitals where patients are on large doses of phenothiazines. The characteristic marrow picture is that of severe aplasia with preservation of only a few scattered lymphocytes. Hematologic recovery begins a few days after the cessation of drug therapy and is usually complete within a period of about 2 weeks. All piperidine and chlorpromazine-model phenothiazines have caused agranulocytosis. The prevalence of chlorpromazine- and promazine-induced agranulocytosis is estimated at about 1 in 250,000 treated patients [285]. The various preparations cross-react, with the risk of agranulocytosis in direct relationship to the amount of phenothiazine administered.

The mechanism of agranulocytosis with the *tricyclic antidepressant* drugs is similar to that of the phenothiazines [286]. The principal tricyclic and other antianxiety drus that may induce neutropenia are imipramine [287], desipramine [288], diazepam [289], chlordiazepoxide [290], and meprobamate [291]. Neutropenia may accompany the megaloblastic anemia produced by certain *anticonvulsant drugs* [292,293].

The nonsteroidal *anti-inflammatory drugs*, phenylbutazone and oxyphenbutazone, are common causes of agranulocytosis [251,294]. The clinical characteristics of agranulocytosis development in most instances resemble those of the phenothiazines. Older persons tend to be most susceptible, and usually agranulocytosis develops between 3 and 12 weeks of drug administration [295]. A rash frequently precedes the development of agranulocytosis occurring during the first month of therapy. An immune mechanism may be operative in such instances. There is evidence that these compounds directly suppress myelopoiesis and that susceptibility is related to an underlying marrow abnormality which is under genetic control [296,297]. Indomethacin and gold therapy occasionally cause selective agranulocytosis [251,294,298,299]. Children with early-onset rheumatoid arthritis may be at particular risk for the development of severe gold-induced neutropenia [298]. Some gold-induced neutropenia has the characteristics of a hypersensitivity reaction [299], but there also is evidence that the neutropenia in some patients is related to abnormal metabolism of gold salts leading to high marrow concentration and direct myelosuppression [300]. Rare instances of agranulocytosis have been reported with aspirin, ibufen, and ibuprofen [294].

Aminopyrine and its derivatives (dipyrone and noraminopyrine) are *analgesics* that continue to be an important cause of agranulocytosis throughout the world, despite the ban on its sale in many countries. Dipyrone preparations continue to be produced by many countries, including the United States, and are available in some over-the-counter preparations [301,302]. The in-

cidence of aminopyrine-induced agranulocytosis is estimated to be about 8 per thousand individuals who use the drug [251,303]. It now provides us with the classical example of a drug-antibody–mediated acute neutropenia due to rapid destruction of circulating neutrophils [304] and inhibition of granulopoiesis [305]. The mechanism of the agranulocytosis was established by showing that the administration of a mixture of aminopyrine and serum from a sensitized person will induce neutropenia in a normal recipient, and that the serum of the sensitized donor is totally inactive in the absence of the sensitizing drug [304].

Individuals susceptible to aminopyrine may develop adverse reactions within 7 to 10 days after beginning the drug for the first time. If they have used the drug previously, the reaction may occur immediately and precipitously. The usual history is that shortly after taking the medication there is a sudden onset of chilliness, fever, tachycardia, anxiety, and headache. The neutrophil count falls rapidly, and some patients develop mild shock. Ulceration in the mouth and throat, necrotizing tonsillitis, pharyngeal abscess, and bacteremia may develop. The marrow initially may show mild granulocytic hyperplasia, but with continued administration of the drug, granulocyte precursors disappear from the marrow. Suspension of drug therapy early in the course will be followed by prompt restoration of granulopoiesis, and in 6 to 8 days the granulocyte count again becomes normal. The recovery time is directly related to the duration of the drug-produced agranulocytosis.

The *antithyroid drugs* are responsible for neutropenia in from 6 to 12 percent of adults and possibly over 15 percent of children who are treated [306–311]. The incidence of agranulocytosis for propylthiouracil and methimazole is in the range of 0.2 to 2.0 percent [308]. Most agranulocytosis develops between the third and twelfth weeks of therapy, but it may occur as early as the first or second week of therapy [308,309]. The high incidence of neutropenia and its temporal occurrence in relation to therapy suggest drug depression of the marrow. On the other hand, immune mechanisms also must be considered since it occasionally occurs early in therapy with hypersensitivity characteristics in association with antineutrophil antibodies [307,310]. Most antithyroid compounds have been reported to produce neutropenia [251,284,303].

The *cardiac antiarrhythmic drugs* which are likely to cause agranulocytosis include lidocaine, quinidine, phenytoin, procainamide, aperidine, ajmaline, chloracetylajmaline, and disopyramide [312–316]. The mechanism of the neutropenia for quinidine and procainamide suggests direct drug-induced depression of myelopoisis [315–317]. Marrow epithelioid granulomas concomitant with the development of procainamide-induced neutropenia have been reported [317]. Captopril is an *antihypertensive agent* which has been associated with reversible neutropenia in about 0.2 percent of patients treated. The neutropenia develops during the first 3 to 12 weeks of therapy and is associated with granulo-

TABLE 87-4   Risk of neutropenia with certain common classes of drugs

Drug or type of drug	Frequency of occurrence*	Dose-related	Relative risk*	Reference
Phenothiazines	4	+	4	[283–285]
Phenylbutazone and oxyphenbutazone	4	±	4	[275,294–297]
Sulfonamides	4	±	4	[252,273–280]
Semisynthetic penicillins	3	+	3	[255–258]
Antithyroid drugs	3	+	3	[306–308]
Chloramphenicol	2	±	1	[270,271]
Indomethacin	1	±	2	[294,298]
Aminopyrine and dipyrone	−	0	3	[251,301–304]

*Based on a scale of 1 to 4, with 4 being the greatest.

cytic hypoplasia of the marrow [318]. Methyldopa also may produce mild neutropenia [319].

Little is known concerning the neutropenia-inducing mechanism for the *antimalarial drugs*. Reactions to dapsome [320], amodiaquine [321], quinine [322], and hydroxychloroquine [323] are most consistent with idiosyncratic suppression of myelopoiesis of the phenothiazine type. *Antihistamines* of the H1-receptor type have accounted for relatively little agranulocytosis over the years [324–327]. On the other hand, there has been significant association of cimetidine, a histamine H2-receptor antagonist, on a dose-related basis with moderate leukoneutropenia [328,329]. A small number of cases of agranulocytosis have been attributed to the *sulfonylurea hypoglycemic agents*, particularly chlorpropamide and tolbutamide [330]. Hypersensitivity-type neutropenic reactions have accompanied mercurial *diuretic* therapy [331]. Other diuretics have occasionally been associated with moderate to severe neutropenia [332,333].

A number of *miscellaneous drugs* have been reported to induce neutropenia. Allopurinol has been responsible for several cases of fatal agranulocytosis [334]. The incidence of rapidly reversible, moderate to severe neutropenia in patients with breast cancer and rheumatoid arthritis treated with levamisole approaches that of aminopyrine and antithyroid therapy [335,336]. Increased risk for levamisole-induced agranulocytosis has been noted for persons with HLA-B27–positive rheumatoid arthritis [250,337]. The presence of autoimmune granulocytotoxins [336,338] in these neutropenic patients suggests an immune mechanism, but other clinical features suggest marrow myelotoxicity [335].

The relative frequencies of the classes of drugs that most often cause agranulocytosis have been summarized (Table 87-4).

Evaluation of patients with neutropenia

The objectives of a careful clinical history are to determine (1) frequency and duration of symptoms, (2) possible etiologic factors with particular reference to drugs and toxins, (3) associated illnesses, and (4) family history. The physical examination should focus on the detection of any possible superficial or deep bacterial infections, lymphadenopathy, hepatosplenomegaly, and the signs of underlying chronic illness.

The duration and severity of the neutropenia will greatly influence the extent of laboratory utilization. Patients with chronic neutropenia should have total and differential leukocyte counts performed two or three times a week for 5 or 6 weeks in order to evaluate periodicity. Marrow aspiration and biopsy may be supplemented by cytogenetic studies and special stains in order to rule out leukemia or other hematologic problems. Accurate neutrophil/erythroid ratios may be determined from marrow sections [339]. The presence of neutrophil-specific antibodies may be detected by means of the staphylococcal slide test [340], microleukocyte agglutination [341], antiglobulin consumption [217,342], the alveolar macrophage test [343], tests of granulocyte cytotoxicity [344,345], or inhibition of the hexose monophosphate shunt activity during phagocytosis [310]. Serum folate, vitamin B_{12}, and muramidase levels have limited application in the detection of underlying ineffectual granulopoiesis [126,163]. The Rebuck skin test is useful in an evaluation of neutrophil tissue mobilization [346,347]. Associated autoimmune disease may be detected by means of serum antinuclear antibody or neutrophil cell surface immune complex tests [348].

The serum vitamin B_{12}–binding capacity [349] and prednisolone mobilization studies [350] provide rough indices of pool sizes. More refined studies of neutrophil kinetics involving measurements of mitotic pool size, postmitotic pool turnover, and blood turnover may be measured in suitable patients [31,339]. Indium 111 is a convenient neutrophil label for leukokinetic studies [351]. Colony-forming unit (CFU-c) and colony-stimulating activity (CSA) measurements may be useful in distinguishing between abnormal humoral factors and defective stem cell proliferation [352,353]. Tests have been developed to investigate the possibility of impaired myelopoiesis due to excess suppressor or cytotoxic T cells [145,155,213–215], or serum inhibitory factors [191,211,212].

Therapy of neutropenia

The first important step in reducing the mortality of patients with acute agranulocytosis is the prompt initiation of treatment. All drugs that might possibly be responsible for the neutropenia should be stopped immediately. All neutropenic patients with fever (above 38.0°C) or neutrophil counts less than 500 per microliter should be hospitalized. There is at least a 65 to 70 percent chance that a febrile episode in a severely granulocytopenic patient is due to bacterial infection [354,355]. Unless maximal environmental isolation facilities are available, simple handwashing before and after seeing the patient and possibly the wearing of a mask by the patient are the only protective measures recommended [356,357]. Body temperatures should be recorded every 4 to 6 h. A complete fever evaluation should be followed by the immediate institution of antimicrobial therapy with the occurrence of significant fever (above 38.3°), chills, or other symptoms of infection [354,355]. Patients should be carefully examined for sites of local infection, which frequently are the source of systemic infection. Most infections occur only at a few local sites and by only a narrow spectrum of organisms (i.e., gram-negative bacilli and *Staphylococcus aureus*) [358]. The most common areas of early infection are the lungs, pharynx, anorectal region, skin, and subcutaneous tissues. The fever work-up should include chest x-ray, examination of urinary sediment for bacteria, and cultures of the blood, sputum, urine, and any suspected cutaneous or subcutaneous lesions.

Recommended initial empirical antibiotic therapy is the intravenous administration of ticarcillin disodium (3 g/m²) and gentamicin (45 mg/m²) every 6 h [355,358]. Acceptable alternatives include combinations of carbenicillin or a cephalosporin with an aminoglycoside. These agents are continued until the results of the cultures and sensitivity tests are known, at which time the antimicrobial program may be readjusted. Additional antibiotics may be added to cover organisms isolated from local areas. Antibiotics should be continued for 5 to 7 days after defervescence has occurred. If the fever persists, amphotericin B may be added to the antibiotic regimen [359]. Leukocyte transfusions are of value as additional therapy in the treatment of highly suspected or proven bacteremia which is resistant to appropriate antibiotic therapy (see Chap. 165).

Lithium carbonate is of prophylactic value in the attenuation of chemotherapy-induced neutropenia [360], and may be of value in accelerating recovery from acute agranulocytosis since it directly stimulates stem cells [361]. The effective dose of lithium carbonate is 900 mg per day. Therapy with androgens and glucocorticoids for recovery from agranulocytosis has been disappointing and is not recommended.

General supportive therapy consists of adequate fluid intake and liquid diet if swallowing is painful. Frequent mouth washes will help maintain good oral hygiene. Anesthetic sprays and lozenges may reduce ulcer pain.

Bacterial infections are usually a less serious problem in *chronic neutropenia* than in acute neutropenia, but they may remain a long-term threat to life. Once the chronic pattern is established, efforts are directed toward permanently restoring an adequate level of circulating granulocytes and reducing the risk of infection. Drugs, chemicals, or physical agents possibly harmful to the marrow should be strictly avoided. Patients that have episodes of bacterial infection with chills, fever, and hypotension or any early signs of shock should be treated in the same manner as is any patient with acute agranulocytosis.

No therapy is required for asymptomatic forms of chronic neutropenia. Attempts to achieve higher levels of circulating neutrophils depend on the pathophysiology of the particular disorder (each of which has been discussed separately in previous sections of this chapter).

The critical decision in most patients with significant degrees of chronic neutropenia is whether splenectomy should be performed. Patients with an enlarged spleen, evidence of hypersplenism, or granulocytic hyperplasia of the marrow are most likely to benefit from splenectomy. Primary and secondary forms of hypersplenism respond best, but some improvement has been reported in cyclic neutropenia, various forms of marrow dysplasia, some types of immunoneutropenia, and lymphoma. The overall results achieved in chronically neutropenic patients with glucocorticoids, androgens, splenectomy, and immunosuppressive drugs have been disappointing [362]. The long-term value of lithium carbonate remains to be determined, especially since it is a drug with multiple toxic effects that are dose-related [363].

References

1. Altman, P. L., and Dittmer, D. S.: *Blood and Other Body Fluids*. Federation of American Societies for Experimental Biology, Washington, D.C., 1961.
2. Zacharski, L. R., Elveback, L. R., and Linman, J. W.: Leukocyte counts in healthy adults. *Am. J. Clin. Pathol.* 56:148, 1971.
3. Coulombel, L., Dehan, M., Tchernia, G., Hill, C., and Vial, M.: The number of polymorphonuclear leukocytes in relation to gestational age in the newborn. *Acta. Paediatr. Scand.* 68:709, 1979.
4. Xanthou, M.: Leukocyte blood picture in healthy full-term and premature babies during the neonatal period. *Arch. Dis. Child* 45:242, 1970.
5. Shaper, A. G., and Lewis, P.: Genetic neutropenia in people of African origin. *Lancet* 2:1021, 1971.
6. Ezeilo, G. C.: Non-genetic neutropenia in Africans. *Lancet* 2:1003, 1972.
7. Karayalcin, G., Rosner, F., and Sawitsky, A.: Pseudoneutropenia in Negroes. A normal phenomenon. *N.Y. State J. Med.* 72:1815, 1972.
8. Caramihai, E., Karayalcin, G., Aballi, A. J., and Lanzkowsky, P.: Leukocyte count differences in healthy white and black children 1 to 5 years of age. *J. Pediatr.* 86:252, 1975.

9. Feinaro, M., and Alkan, W. J.: Familial neutropenia in Jews of Yemenite origin, in *Proc. 9th Int. Congr. Life Assurance Medicine, Tel Aviv, 1967.* Karger, Basel, 1968, p. 172.

10. Shoenfeld, Y., et al.: Familial leukopenia among Yemenite Jews. *Isr. J. Med. Sci.* 14:1271, 1978.

11. Weinberger, A., Shoenfeld, Y., Zamir, R., Gazit, E., Joshua, H., and Pinkhas, J.: HLA antigens in genetic neutropenia of Yemenite Jews. *Vox. Sang.* 36:105, 1979.

12. Mason, B. A., Lessin, L., Schechter, G. P.: Marrow granulocyte reserves in black Americans. Hydrocortisone-induced granulocytosis in the ''benign'' neutropenia of the black. *Am. J. Med.* 67:201, 1979.

13. Ezeilo, G. C., and Wacha, D.: Pregnancy-induced leucocytosis in Africans, Asians, and Europeans. *Br. J. Obstet. Gynaecol.* 84:944, 1977.

14. Mintz, U., and Sachs, L.: Normal granulocyte colony-forming cells in the bone marrow of Yemenite Jews with genetic neutropenia. *Blood* 41:745, 1973.

15. Ahmed, P., Minnich, V., and Michael, J. M.: Platelet satellitosis with spurious thrombocytopenia and neutropenia. *Am. J. Clin. Pathol.* 69:473, 1978.

16. Deaton, J. G.: Spuriously low total leukocyte counts in chronic lymphocytic leukemia. *Texas Rep. Biol. Med.* 27:763, 1969.

17. Luke, R. G., Koepke, J. A., and Siegel, R. R.: The effect of immunosuppressive drugs and uremia on automated leukocyte counts. *Am. J. Clin. Pathol.* 56:503, 1971.

18. Kyle, R. A.: Natural history of chronic idiopathic neutropenia. *N. Engl. J. Med.* 302:908, 1980.

19. Dale, D. C., Guerry, D., IV, Wewerka, J. R., Bull, J. M., and Chusid, M. J.: Chronic neutropenia. *Medicine* 58:128, 1979.

20. Pincus, S. H., Boxer, L. A., and Stossel, T. P.: Chronic neutropenia in childhood. Analysis of 16 cases and a review of the literature. *Am. J. Med.* 61:849, 1976.

21. Greenwood, M. F., Jones, E. A., and Holland, P.: Monocyte functional capacity in chronic neutropenia. *Am. J. Dis. Child.* 132:131, 1978.

22. Baehner, R. L., and Johnston, R. B., Jr.: Monocyte function in children with neutropenia and chronic infections. *Blood* 40:31, 1972.

23. Rewald, E., and Moscardi, F.: Chronic granulocytopenia and monocytopenia with apparent good health. *Lancet* 2:935, 1975.

24. Kaufman, D. B.: Granulocytopenia and no infections. *Lancet* 2:1205, 1975 (letter).

25. Howard, M. W., Strauss, R. G., and Johnston, R. B., Jr.: Infections in patients with neutropenia. *Am. J. Dis. Child.* 131:788, 1977.

26. Hopefl, A. W.: Empiric therapy of febrile granulocytopenic patients. *Am. J. Hosp. Pharm.* 36:178, 1979.

27. Sickles, E. A., Greene, W. H., and Wiernik, P. H.: Clinical presentation of infection in granulocytopenic patients. *Arch. Intern. Med.* 135:715, 1975.

28. Kauder, E., and Mauer, A. M.: Neutropenias of childhood. *J. Pediatr.* 69:147, 1966.

29. Cline, M. J., Craddock, C. G., Gale, R. P., Golde, D. W., and Lehrer, R. I.: Granulocytes in human disease. *Ann. Intern. Med.* 81:801, 1974.

30. Price, T. H., and Dale, D. C.: The selective neutropenias. *Clin. Haematol.* 7:501, 1978.

31. Price, T. H., Lee, M. Y., Dale, D. C., and Finch, C. A.: Neutrophil kinetics in chronic neutropenia. *Blood* 54:581, 1979.

32. Weetman, R. M., and Boxer, L. A.: Childhood neutropenia. *Pediatr. Clin. North Am.* 27:361, 1980.

33. de Vaal, O. M., and Seynhaeve, V.: Reticular dysgenesia. *Lancet* 2:1123, 1959.

34. Gitlin, D., Vawter, G., and Craig, J. M.: Thymic alymphoplasia and congenital aleukocytosis. *Pediatrics* 33:184, 1964.

35. Alonso, K., Dew, J. M., and Starke, W. R.: Thymic alymphoplasia and congenital aleukocytosis (reticular dysgenesia). *Arch. Pathol.* 94:179, 1972.

36. Fireman, P., Johnson, H. A., and Gitlin, D.: Presence of plasma cells and gamma 1-M-globulin synthesis in a patient with thymic alymphoplasia. *Pediatrics* 37:485, 1966.

37. Fulginiti, V. A., et al.: Progressive vaccinia in immunologically

38. Nezelof, C.: Thymic dysplasia with normal immunoglobulins and immunologic deficiency: Pure alymphcytosis, in *Immunologic Deficiency Diseases in Man* (Birth defects original article series), edited by D. Bergsma. The National Foundation, New York, 1968, vol. 4, no. 1, p. 104.

39. Lux, S. E., et al.: Neutropenia and abnormal cellular immunity in cartilage-hair hypoplasia. *N. Engl. J. Med.* 282:234, 1970.

40. Leale, M.: Recurrent furunculosis in an infant showing an unusual blood picture. *JAMA* 54:1854, 1910.

41. Ritledge, B. H., Hansen-Prass, O. C., and Thayer, W. S.: Recurrent agranulocytosis. *Bull. Johns Hopkins Hosp.* 46:369, 1930.

42. Morley, A. A., Carew, J. P., and Baikie, A. G.: Familial cyclical neutropenia. *Br. J. Haematol.* 13:719, 1967.

43. Monto, R. W., Shafer, H. C., Brennan, M. J., and Rebuck, J. W.: Periodic neutropenia treated by adrenocorticotrophic hormone and splenectomy. *N. Engl. J. Med.* 246:893, 1952.

44. Page, A. R., and Good, R. A.: Studies on cyclic neutropenia: A clinical and experimental investigation. *Am. J. Dis. Child.* 94:623, 1957.

45. Duane, G. W.: Periodic neutropenia. *Arch. Intern. Med.* 102, 462, 1958.

46. Hahneman, B. M., and Alt, H. L.: Cyclic neutropenia in a father and daughter. *JAMA* 168:270, 1958.

47. Brodsky, L., Reimann, H. A., and Dennis, L. H.: Treatment of cyclic neutropenia with testosterone. *Am. J. Med.* 38:802, 1965.

48. Barkve, H.: Cyclic neutropenia. Report of a case treated with high doses of testosterone. *Acta. Med. Scand.* 182:503, 1967.

49. Evans, D. I., and Holzel, A.: Cyclical neutropenia. *Proc. R. Soc. Med.* 61:302, 1968.

50. Geelhoed, G. W., Kane, M. A., Dale, D. C., and Wells, S. A.: Colon ulceration and perforation in cyclic neutropenia. *J. Pediatr. Surg.* 8:379, 1973.

51. Morley, A. A., Baikie, A. G., and Galton, D. A. G.: Cyclic leucocytosis as evidence for retention of normal homeostatic control in chronic granulocytic leukaemia, *Lancet* 2:1320, 1967.

52. Wright, D. C., Fauci, A. S., Dale, D. C., and Wolff, S. M.: Correction of human cyclic neutropenia with prednisolone. *N. Engl. J. Med.* 298:295, 1978.

53. Dale, D. C., Brown, C. H., Carbone, P., and Wolff, S. M.: Cyclic urinary leukopoietic activity in grey collie dogs. *Science* 173:152, 1971.

54. Dale, D. C., Ward, S. B., Kimball, H. R., and Wolff, S. M.: Studies of neutrophil production and turnover in grey collie dogs with cyclic neutropenia. *J. Clin. Invest.* 51:2190, 1972.

55. Hansen, N. E., Andersen, V., and Karle, H.: Plasma lysozyme in drug induced and spontaneous cyclic neutropenia. *Br. J. Haematol.* 25:485, 1973.

56. Patt, H. M., Lund, J. E., and Maloney, M. A.: Cyclic hematopoiesis in grey collie dogs: A stem cell problem. *Blood* 42:873, 1973.

57. Dale, D. C., and Graw, R. G., Jr.: Transplantation of allogenic bone marrow in canine cyclic neutropenia. *Science* 183:83, 1974.

58. Weiden, P. L., Robinett, B., Graham, T. C., Adamson, J., and Starb, R.: Canine cyclic neutropenia: A stem cell defect. *J. Clin. Invest.* 53:950, 1974.

59. Jones, J. B., Lange, R. D., Yang, T. J., Vodopick, H., and Jones, E. S.: Canine cyclic neutropenia: Erythropoietin and platelet cycles after bone marrow transplantation. *Blood* 45:213, 1975.

60. Hammon, W. P., and Dale, D. C.: Cyclic hematopoiesis: Effects of lithium on colony-forming cells and colony-stimulating activity in grey collie dogs. *Blood* 59:179, 1982.

61. Mangalik, A., and Robinson, W. W.: Cyclic neutropenia: The relationship between urine granulocyte colony stimulating activity and neutrophil count. *Blood* 41:79, 1973.

62. von Schulthess, G. K., and Mazer, N. A.: Cyclic neutropenia (CN): A clue to the control of granulopoiesis. *Blood* 59:27, 1982.

63. Bryan, H. G., and Nixon, R. K.: Dyskeratosis congenita and familial pancytopenia. *JAMA* 192:203, 1965.

64. Good, R. A., and Zak, S. J.: Disturbances in gamma globulin synthesis as ''experiments of nature.'' *Pediatrics* 18:109, 1956.

65. Stiehm, E. R., and Fudenberg, H. H.: Clinical and immunologic fea-

tures of dysgammaglobulinemia Type I. Report of a case diagnosed in the first year of life. *Am. J. Med.* 40:805, 1966.

66. Ackerman, B. D.: Dysgammaglobulinemia: Report of a case with a family history of a congenital gammaglobulin disorder. *Pediatrics* 34:211, 1964.

67. Lonsdale, D., Deodhar, S. D., and Mercer, R. D.: Familial granulocytopenia and associated immunoglobulin abnormality. Report of three cases in young brothers. *J. Pediatr.* 71:790, 1967.

68. Webster, A. D., Slavin, G., Strelling, M. K., Asherson, G. L.: Combined immunodeficiency with hyper-gamma-globulinemia. *Arch. Dis. Child.* 50:486, 1975.

69. Bjorksten, B., and Lundmark, K. M.: Recurrent bacterial infections in four siblings with neutropenia, eosinophilia, hyperimmunoglobulinemia A and defective neutrophil chemotaxis. *J. Infect. Dis.* 133:63, 1976.

70. Mentzer, W. C., Jr., Johnstron, R. B., Jr., Baehner, R. L., and Nathan, D. G.: An unusual form of chronic neutropenia in a father and daughter with hypogammaglobulinemia. *Br. J. Haematol.* 36:313, 1977.

71. Vanderhoof, J. A., Rich, K. C., Stiehm, E. R., and Ament, M. E.: Esophageal ulcers in immunodeficiency with elevated levels of IgM and neutropenia. *Am. J. Dis. Child.* 131:551, 1977.

72. Hitzig, W. H., and Schlapfer, A.: Chronic neutropenia and dysgammaglobulinemia. Possible interrelations. *X Cong. Int. Soc. Hematol. D.*, 1964, p. 23.

73. Dancey, J. T., and Brubaker, L. H.: Neutrophil marrow in chronic benign idiopathic neutropenia. *Am. J. Med.* 68:251, 1980.

74. L'Esperance, P., Brunning, R., Deinard, A. S., Park, B. H., Bigger, W. D., and Good, R. A.: Congenital neutropenia: Impaired maturation with diminished stem-cell input. *Birth Defects* 11:59, 1975.

75. Amato, D., Freedman, M. H., Saunders, E. F.: Granulopoiesis in severe congenital neutropenia. *Blood* 47:531, 1976.

76. Olofosson, T., Ollson, I., Kostmann, R., Malmstom, S., and Thilen, A.: Granulopoiesis in infantile genetic agranulocytosis: In vitro cloning of marrow cells in agar culture. *Scand. J. Haematol.* 16:18, 1976.

77. Greenberg, P. L., Mara, B., Steed, S., and Boxer, L.: The chronic idiopathic neutropenia syndrome: Correlation of clinical features with in vitro parameters of granulocytopoiesis. *Blood* 55:915, 1980.

78. Kostman, R.: Infantile genetic agranulocytosis. *Acta. Paediatr.* 45:105, 1956.

79. Parmley, R. T., Ogawa, M., Darby, C. P., and Spicer, S. S.: Congenital neutropenia: Neutrophil proliferation with abnormal maturation. *Blood* 46:723, 1975.

80. Parmley, R. T., et al.: Congenital dysgranulopoietic neutropenia: Clinical, serologic, ultrastructural, and in vitro proliferative characteristics. *Blood* 56:465, 1980.

81. Chusid, M. J., Pisciotta, A. V., Duquesnoy, R. J., Camitta, B. M., and Tomasulo, P. A.: Congenital neutropenia: Studies of pathogenesis. *Am. J. Hematol.* 8:315, 1980.

82. Chilcote, R. R., Rierden, K. J., Baehner, R. L.: Familial neutropenia, monocytopenia, and nerve deafness with diminished colony stimulating factor activity. *Pediatr. Res.* 9:320, 1975.

83. Rodin, A. E., Haggard, M. E., Nichols, M. M., and Gustavson, L. P.: Infantile genetic agranulocytosis. Two cases occurring in siblings and one in a distant relative. *Am. J. Dis. Child.* 126:818, 1973.

84. Knicker, W. T., and Panos, T. C.: Idiopathic infantile agranulocytosis with hypergammaglobulinemia. *Am. J. Dis. Child.* 94:549, 1957.

85. Miller, D. R., Freed, B. A., and Lapey, J. D.: Congenital neutropenia: Report of a fatal case in a Negro infant with leukocyte function studies. *Am. J. Dis. Child.* 115:337, 1968.

86. Lang, J. E., and Cutting, H. O.: Infantile genetic agranulocytosis. *Pediatrics* 35:596, 1965.

87. Gilman, P. A., Jackson, D. P., and Guild, H. G.: Congenital agranulocytosis: Prolonged survival and terminal acute leukemia. *Blood* 36:576, 1970.

88. Cline, M. J., Golde, D. W., Rich, K., Falk, P., and Feig, S.: Defective granulopiesis in "normal" parents of congenitally neutropenic children. *Clin. Res.* 23:402A, 1975.

89. Matsaniotis, N., Kiossoglou, K. A., Karpouzas, J., and Anastasea-Vlachou, K.: Chromosomes in Kostmann's disease. *Lancet* 2:104, 1966.

90. Pahwa, R. N., et al.: Partial correction of neutrophil deficiency in congenital neutropenia following bone marrow transplantation (BMT). *Exp. Hematol.* 5:45, 1977.

91. Wriedt, K., Kauder, E., and Mauer, A. M.: Defective myelopoiesis in congenital neutropenia. *N. Engl. J. Med.* 283:1072, 1970.

92. Parmley, R. T., Ogawa, M., Darby, C. P., and Spicer, S. S.: Congenital neutropenia: Neutrophil proliferation with abnormal maturation. *Blood* 46:723, 1975.

93. Zucker-Franklin, D., L'Esperance, P., and Good, R. A.: Congenital neutropenia: An intrinsic cell defect demonstration by electron microscopy of soft agar colonies. *Blood* 49:425, 1977.

94. Barak, Y., Paran, M., Levin, S., and Sachs, L.: In vitro induction of myeloid proliferation and maturation in infantile genetic agranulocytosis. *Blood* 38:74, 1971.

95. Lui, V., Ragab, A. H., Findley, H., and Frauen, B.: Infantile genetic agranylocytosis and acute lymphocytic leukemia in two sibs. *J. Pediatr.* 92:1028, 1978.

96. Miller, R. W.: Childhood cancer and congenital defects: A study of U.S. death certificates during the period 1960–1966. *Pediatr. Res.* 3:389, 1969.

97. Rappeport, J. M., Parkman, R., Newburger, P., Camitta, B. M., and Chusid, M. J.: Correction of infantile agranulocytosis (Kostmann's syndrome) by allogeneic bone marrow transplantation. *Am. J. Med.* 68:605, 1980.

98. Levine, S.: Chronic familial neutropenia with marked periodontal lesions: Report of a case. *Oral Surg.* 12:310, 1959.

99. Rossman, P. L., and Hummer, G. J.: Chronic neutropenia in siblings: The effect of steroids. *Ann. Intern. Med.* 52:242, 1960.

100. Bjure, J., Nilsson, L. R., and Plum, C. M.: Familial neutropenia possibly caused by deficiency of a plasma factor. *Acta. Paediatr.* 51:497, 1962.

101. Fanconi, G.: Chronic benign neutropenia of childhood. *Ann. Paediatr. (Basel)* 157:308, 1941.

102. Salomonsen, L: Granulocytopenia in children. *Acta. Paediatr. Scand. (Suppl.)* 35:189, 1948.

103. Dienard, A. S., and Page, A. R.: A study of steroid-induced granulocytosis in a patient with chronic benign neutropenia of childhood. *Br. J. Haematol.* 28:333, 1974.

104. Stahlie, T. O. V.: Chronic benign neutropenia in infancy and early childhood. Report of a case with a review of the literature. *J. Pediatr.* 48:710, 1956.

105. Zuelzer, W. W., and Bajoghli, M.: Chronic granulocytopenia in childhood. *Blood* 23:359, 1964.

106. Kay, A. B., et al.: Leukocyte function in a case of chronic benign neutropenia of infancy associated with circulating leukoagglutinins. *Br. J. Haematol.* 32:451, 1976.

107. Krill, C. E., Jr., Smith, H. D., and Mauer, A. M.: Chronic idiopathic granulocytopenia. *N. Engl. J. Med.* 270:973, 1964.

108. Zuelzer, W. W.: "Myelokathexis"—a new form of chronic granulocytopenia. *N. Engl. J. Med.* 270:699, 1964.

109. O'Regan, S., Newman, A. J., and Graham, R. C.: "Myelokathexis." Neutropenia with marrow hyperplasia. *Am. J. Dis. Child.* 131:655, 1977.

110. Schwachman, H., Diamond, L. K., Oski, F. A., and Khaw, K. T.: The syndrome of pancreatic insufficiency and bone marrow dysfunction. *J. Pediatr.* 65:645, 1964.

111. Bodian, M., Sheldon, W., and Lightwood, R.: Congenital hypoplasia of the exocrine pancreas. *Acta. Paediatr.* 53:282, 1964.

112. Colebatch, J. H., Anderson, C. M., Simons, M. J., and Burke, V.: Neutropenia and pancreatic disorder. *Lancet* 2:496, 1965.

113. Moller, E., Olin, P., and Zetterstrom, R.: Neutropenia and insufficiency of the exocrine pancreas. *Acta. Paediatr. Scand. (Suppl.)* 177:29, 1967.

114. Launiala, K., Furuhjelm, U., Hjelt, L., and Visakorpi, J. K.: A syndrome with pancreatic achylia and granulocytopenia. *Acta Paediatr. Scand. (Suppl.)* 177:28, 1967.

115. Burke, V., Colebatch, J. H., Anderson, C. M., and Simons, M. J.: Association of pancreatic insufficiency and chronic neutropenia in childhood. *Arch. Dis. Child.* 42:147, 1967.

116. Shmerling, D. H., Prader, A., Hitzig, W., Giedion, H., Hadorn, B., and Kuhns, M.: The syndrome of exocrine pancreatic insufficiency, neutropenia, metaphyseal dysostosis, and dwarfism. *Helv. Paediatr. Acta.* 24:547, 1969.

117. Doe, W. F.: Two brothers with congenital pancreatic exocrine insufficiency, neutropenia and dysgammaglobulinanemia. *Proc. R. Soc. Med. 66:*1125, 1973.

118. McCollum, J. P., Muller, D. P., and Harries, J. T.: Congenital pancreatic hypoplasia with neutropenia and skeletal abnormalities. *Proc. R. Soc. Med. 68:*304, 1975.

119. Brueton, M. J., Mavromichalis, J., Goodchild, M. C., and Anderson, C. M.: Hepatic dysfunction in association with pancreatic insufficiency and cyclical neutropenia. Schwachmann-Diamond syndrome. *Arch. Dis. Child. 52:*76, 1977.

120. Aggett, P. J., Harries, J. T., Harvey, B. A. M., and Soothill, J. F.: An inherited defect of neutrophil mobility in Schwachman's syndrome. *J. Pediatr. 94:*391, 1979.

121. Saunders, E. F., Gall, G., and Freedman, M. H.: Granulopoiesis in Schwachman's syndrome (pancreatic insufficiency and bone marrow dysfunction). *Pediatrics 64:*515, 1979.

122. Childs, B., Nyhan, W. L., Borden, M., Bard, L., and Cooke, R. E.: Idiopathic hyperglycinemia and hyperglycinuria: A new disorder of amino acid metabolism. I. *Pediatrics 27:*522, 1961.

123. Soriano, J. R., Taitz, L. S., Finberg, L., and Edelmann, C. W., Jr.: Hyperglycinemia with ketoacidosis and leukopenia. Metabolic studies on the nature of the defect. *Pediatrics 39:*818, 1967.

124. Huguley, C. M., Jr., Bain, J. A., Rivers, S. L., and Scoggins, R. B.: Refractory megaloblastic anemia associated with excretion of orotic acid. *Blood 14:*615, 1959.

125. Rosenberg, L. E., Lilljequist, A., and Hsia, Y. E.: Methylmalonic aciduria: An inborn error leading to metabolic acidosis, long-chain ketonuria, and intermittent hyperglycinemia. *N. Engl. J. Med. 278:*1319, 1968.

126. Blume, R. S., Bennett, J. M., Yankee, R. A., and Wolff, S. M.: Defective granulocyte regulation in the Chediak-Higaski syndrome. *N. Engl. J. Med. 279:*1009, 1968.

127. Boxer, L. A., and Baehner, R. L.: Defects in neutrophil leukocyte function. in *Clinical Immunology Update 1980*, edited by E. E. Franklin, Elsevier North-Holland, Amsterdam, 1981.

128. Huber, H.: Stammbaumuntersuchungen bei Panmyelophthisekranken. *Klin. Wochenschr. 18:*1145, 1939.

129. Gansslen, M.: Konsitutionelle familiare leukopenie (neutropenie) *Klin. Wochenschr. 20:*922, 1941.

130. Bousser, J., and Neyde, R.: La Neutropenie familiale. *Sang 18:*521, 1947.

131. Cutting, H. O., and Lang, J. E.: Familial benign chronic neutropenia. *Ann. Intern. Med. 61:*876, 1964.

132. Burchardt, K., and Zawilska, K.: Benign familial neutropenia with deficiency of alkaline phosphatase in granulocytes. *Pol. Arch. Med. Wewn. 49:*485, 1972.

133. Genz, H.: Klinische beobachtungen und untersuchungen bei einem fall von Fanconi-anamie. *Arch. Kinder 145:*237, 1952.

134. Miller, M. E., Oski, F. A., and Harris, M. B.: Lazy-leukocyte syndrome. A new disorder of neutrophil function. *Lancet 1:*665, 1971.

135. Yoda, S., Morosawa, H., Komiyama, A., and Akabane, T.: Transient "lazy leukocyte" syndrome during infancy. *Am. J. Dis. Child. 134:*467, 1980.

136. Kamada, N., and Uchino, H.: Haematological abnormalities in six cases with the preleukemic stage for 5–13 years. *Acta. Haematol. Jpn. 37:*32, 1974.

137. Pierre, R. V.: Preleukemic states. *Semin. Hematol. 11:*73, 1974.

138. Zak, F. G., and Rubin, E.: Histiocytic medullary reticulosis. *Am. J. Med. 31:*813, 1961.

139. Natelson, E. A., Lynch, E. C., Hettig, R. A., and Alfrey, C. P., Jr.: Histiocytic medullary reticulosis. The role of phagocytosis in pancytopenia. *Arch. Intern. Med. 122:*223, 1968.

140. Pisciotta, A. V.: Clinical and pathological effects of space-occupying lesions of bone marrow. *Am. J. Clin. Pathol. 20:*915, 1950.

141. Pandolfi, F., Strong, D. M., Slease, R. B., Smith, M. L., Ortaldo, J. R., and Herberman, R. B.: Characterization of a suppressor T-cell chronic lymphocytic leukemia with ADCC but not HK activity. *Blood 56:*653, 1980.

142. Brouet, J. C., Flandrin, G., Sasportes, M., Preud'Homme, J. L., and Seligmann, M.: Chronic lymphocytic leukemia of T-cell origin: Immunological and clinical evaluation in 11 patients. *Lancet 2:*890, 1975.

143. McKenna, R. W., Parkin, J., Kersey, J. H., Gajl-Peczalska, K. J., Peterson, L., and Brunning, R. D.: Chronic lymphoproliferative disorder with unusual clinical, morphologic, ultrastructural and membrane surface marker characteristics. *Am. J. Med. 62:*588, 1977.

144. Aisenberg, A. C., Wilkes, B. M., Harris, N. L., Ault, K. A., and Carey, R. W.: Chronic T-cell lymphocytosis with neutropenia: Report of a case studied with monoclonal antibody. *Blood 58:*818, 1981.

145. Bom-Van Noorloos, A. A., et al.: Proliferation of T cells with killer-cell activity in two patients with neutropenia and recurrent infections. *N. Engl. J. Med. 302:*933, 1980.

146. Ringertz, N., and Lindholm, S. O.: Mediastinal tumors and cysts. *J. Thorac. Surg. 31:*458, 1956.

147. Thiele, H. G., and Frenzel, H. I.: Immunoglobulin deficiency syndrome and agranulocytosis in the course of thymoma. *Schwiez. Med. Wochenschr. 97:*1606, 1967.

48. Adams, E. B., and Witts, L. J.: Chronic agranulocytosis. *Q. J. Med. 18:*173, 1949.

149. Spaet, T. H., and Dameshek, W.: Chronic hypoplastic neutropenia. *Am. J. Med. 13:*35, 1952.

150. Murdoch, J. M., and Smith, C. C.: Hematological aspects of systemic disease. *Infection Clin. Haematol. 1:*619, 1972.

151. Cooper, W.: Pancytopenia associated with disseminated tuberculosis. *Ann. Intern. Med. 50:*1497, 1959.

152. Kilbridge, T. M., Gonnella, J. S., and Bolan, J. T.: Pancytopenia and death. Disseminated anonymous mycobacterial infection. *Arch. Intern. Med. 120:*38, 1967.

153. Lakshminarayan, S., and Sahn, S.: Disseminated infection caused by mycobacterium avium: Report of a case with associated leukopenia. *Am. Rev. Respir. Dis. 108:*123, 1973.

154. Cameron, S. J.: Tuberculosis and the blood – A special relationship? *Tubercle 55:*55, 1974.

155. Bagby, G. C., and Gilbert, D. N.: Suppression of granulopoiesis by T-lymphocytes in two patients with disseminated myobacterial infection. *Ann. Intern. Med. 94:*478, 1981.

156. Kies, M. S., Luedke, D. W., Boyd, J. F., and McCue, M. J.: Neutropenic enterocolitis. Two case reports of long-term survival following surgery. *Cancer 43:*730, 1979.

157. Nagaraju, M., Weitzman, S., and Baumann, G.: Viral hepatitis and agranulocytosis. *Am. J. Dig. Dis. 18:*247, 1973.

158. Habib, M. A., Babka, J. C., and Burningham, R. A.: Profound granulocytopenia associated with infectious mononucleosis. *Am. J. Med. Sci. 265:*339, 1973.

159. Koziner, B., Handler, N., Parrillo, J., and Ellman, L.: Agranulocytosis following infectious mononucleosis. *JAMA. 225:*1235, 1973.

160. Stevens, D. L., Everett, E. D., Boxer, L. A., and Landefeld, R. A.: Infectious mononucleosis with severe neutropenia and opsonic antineutrophil activity. *South. Med. J. 72:*519, 1979.

161. Calabro, J. J., Williamson, P., Love, E. S., Kostylo, F., and Jeghers, H.: Kauasaki syndrome. *N. Engl. J. Med. 306:*287, 1982.

162. Rosenthal, N., and Abel, H. A.: The significance of the monocytes in agranulocytosis (leukopenic infectious monocytosis). *Am. J. Clin. Pathol. 6:*205, 1936.

163. Perillie,. P. E., Kaplan, S. S., and Finch, S. C.: Significance of changes in serum muramidose activity in megaloblastic anemia. *N. Engl. J. Med. 277:*10, 1967.

164. Megaloblastic leukopenia. *N. Engl. J. Med. 277:*50, 1967 (editorial).

165. Mauer, A. M., and Krill, C. E.: A study of the mechanisms for granulocytosis. *Ann. N.Y. Acad. Sci. 113:*1003, 1964.

166. Strausz, I., Barcsak, J., Kekes, E., and Szebeni, A.: Prednisolone-induced acute changes in circulating neutrophil granulocytes III in cases of previous anemia. *Haematologia 2:*109, 1968.

167. Cordano, A., Placko, R. P., and Graham, G. G.: Hypocupremia and neutropenia in copper deficiency. *Blood 28:*280, 1966.

168. Cordano, A., Placko, R. P., and Graham, G. G.: Hypocupremia and neutropenia in copper deficiency. *Blood 28:*280, 1966.

169. Al-Rashid, R. A., and Spangler, J.: Neonatal copper deficiency. *N. Engl. J. Med. 285:*841, 1971.

170. Dunlap, W. M., James, G. W., and Hume, D. M.: Anemia and neutropenia caused by copper deficiency. *Ann. Intern. Med. 80:*470, 1974.

171. Zidar, B. L., Shadduck, R. K., Zeigler, Z., and Winkelstein, A.: Observations on the anemia and neutropenia of human copper deficiency. *Am. J. Hematol. 3:*177, 1977.

172. Boxer, L. A., Greenberg, M. S., Boxer, G. J., and Stossel, T. P.: Autoimmune neutropenia. N. Engl. J. Med. 293:748, 1975.

173. Logue, G. L., and Shimm, D. S.: Autoimmune granulocytopenia. Ann. Rev. Med. 31:191, 1980.

174. Lawrence, J. S., Craddock, C. G., Jr., and Campbell, T. N.: Antineutrophilic serum, its use in studies of white blood cell dynamics. J. Lab. Clin. Med. 69:88, 1967.

175. Krantz, S. B.: Pure red-cell aplasia. N. Engl. J. Med. 291:345, 1974.

176. Luhby, A. L., and Slobody, L.: Transient neonatal agranulocytosis in two siblings: Transplacental isoimmunization to a leukocyte factor. Am. J. Dis. Child. 92:496, 1956.

177. Boxer, L. A., Yokoyama, M., and Lalezari, P.: Isoimmune neonatal neutropenia. J. Pediatr. 80:783, 1972.

178. Lalezari, P., and Radel, E.: Neutrophil specific antigens: Immunology and clinical significance. Semin. Haematol. 11:281, 1974.

179. Lalezari, P.: Neutrophil antigens: Immunology and clinical implications. Prog. Clin. Biol. Res. 13:209, 1977.

180. Whang-Peng, J., Leikin, S., Harris, C., Lee, E., and Sites, J.: The transplacental passage of fetal leukocytes into the maternal blood. Proc. Sci. Exp. Biol. Med. 142:50, 1973.

181. Schroder, J.: Passage of leukocytes from mother to fetus. Scand. J. Immunol. 3:369, 1974.

182. Boxer, L. A.: Immune neutropenias: Clinical and biological implications. Am. J. Pediatr. Hematol. Oncol. 3:89, 1981.

183. Lalezari, P., Murphy, G. B., and Allen, F. H., Jr.: NB1, a new neutrophil-specific antigen involved in the pathogenesis of neonatal neutropenia. J. Clin. Invest. 50:1108, 1971.

184. Van Der Weerdt, C. M., and Lalezari, P.: Another example of isoimmune neonatal neutropenia due to anti Na1. Vox. Sang. 22:438, 1972.

185. Christensen, R. D., and Rothstein, G.: Brief clinical and laboratory observations: Exhaustion of mature marrow neutrophils in neonates with sepsis. J. Pediatr. 96:316, 1980.

186. Rossi, J. P., and Brandt, I. K.: Transient granulocytopenia of the newborn associated with sepsis due to Shigella alkalescens and maternal leukocyte agglutinins. J. Pediatr. 56:639, 1960.

187. Payne, R.: Neonatal neutropenia and leukoagglutinins. Pediatrics 33:194, 1964.

188. Abildgaard, H., and Jensen, K. G.: The influence of maternal leucocyte antibodies on infants. Scand. J. Haematol. 1:47, 1964.

189. Moeschlin, S.: Immunological granulocytopenia and agranulocytosis: Clinical aspects. Acta. Med. Scand. (Suppl.) 312:518, 1956.

190. Moeschlin, S.: Leukocyte-autoantibodies. Acta Haematol. 20:167, 1958.

191. Cline, M. J., Opelz, G., Saxon, A., Fahey, J. G., and Golde, D. W.: Autoimmune panleukopenia. N. Engl. J. Med. 295:1489, 1976.

192. Lalezari, P., Jiang, A. F., Yegen, L., and Santorineou, M.: Chronic autoimmune neutropenia due to anti-NA2 antibody. N. Engl. J. Med. 293:744, 1975.

193. Lightsey, A. L., Chapman, R. M., McMillan, R., Mushovic, J., Yelenosky, R., and Longmire, R. L.: Immune neutropenia. Ann. Intern Med. 86:60, 1977.

194. Verheugt, F. W., von dem Borne, A. E., van Noord-Bokhorst, J. C., and Engelfriet, C. P.: Autoimmune granulocytopenia: The detection of granulocyte autoantibodies with the immunofluorescence test. Br. J. Haematol. 39:339, 1978.

195. Verheugt, F. W., von dem Borne, A. E., van Noord-Bokhorst, J. C., van Elven, E. H., and Engelfriet, C. P.: Serological, immunochemical, and immunocytological properties of granulocyte antibodies. Vox Sang., 35:294, 1978.

196. Blaschke, J., Goeken, N. E., Thompson, J. S., Dick, F. R., and Gingrich, R. D.: Acquired agranulocytosis with granulocyte specific cytotoxic autoantibody. Am. J. Med. 66:862, 1979.

197. Ng, R. P., and Prankerd, T. A.: IgA deficiency and neutropenia. Br. Med. J. 1:563, 1976.

198. Linker, C. A., Newcom, S. R., Nilsson, C. M., Wolf, J. L., and Shuman, M. A.: Combined idiopathic neutropenia and thrombocytopenia: Evidence for an immune basis for the syndrome. Ann. Intern. Med. 93:704, 1980.

199. Boxer, L. A., Boxer, G. J., Greenberg, M. S., and Stossel, T. P.: Granulocyte turnover in autoimmune neutropenia. N. Engl. J. Med., 294:165, 1976.

200. Budman, D. R., and Steinberg, A. D.: Hematologic aspects of systemic lupus erythematosus. Current concepts. Ann. Intern. Med. 86:220, 1977.

201. Starkebaum, G., Price, T. H., Lee, M. Y., and Arend, W. P.: Autoimmune neutropenia in systemic lupus erythematosus. Arthritis Rheum. 21:504, 1978.

202. Starkebaum, G., and Arend, W. P.: Neutrophil-binding immunoglobin G in systemic lupus erythematosus. J. Clin. Invest. 64:902, 1979.

203. Cines, D. B., Passero, F., Du Pont, G., IV, Bina, M., Dusak, B., and Schreiber, A. D.: Granulocyte-associated IgG in neutropenic disorders. Blood 59:124, 1982.

204. Rivero, S., Alger, M., and Alarcon-Segovia, D.: Splenectomy for hemocytopenia in systemic lupus erythematosus. Arch. Intern. Med. 139:773, 1979.

205. Spivak, J. L.: Felty's syndrome: An analytical review. Johns Hopkins Med. J. 141:156, 1977.

206. Sienknecht, C. W., Urowitz, M. B., Pruzanski, W., and Stein, H. B.: Felty's syndrome: Clinical and serological analysis of 34 cases. Ann. Rheum, Dis. 36:500, 1977.

207. Cryer, P. E., and Kissane, J. M.: Rheumatoid arthritis with Felty's syndrome, hyperviscosity, and immunologic hyperreactivity. Am. J. Med. 70:89, 1981.

208. Joyce, R. A., Boggs, D. R., Chervenick, P. A., and Lalezari, P.: Neutrophil kinetics in Felty's syndrome. Am. J. Med. 69:695, 1980.

209. Gupta, R. C., Robinson, W. A., and Albrecht, D.: Granulopoietic activity in Felty's syndrome. Ann. Rheum. Dis. 34:156, 1975.

210. Vincent, P. C., Levi, J. A., Mac Queen, A.: The mechanisms of neutropenia in Felty's syndrome. Br. J. Haematol. 27:463, 1974.

211. Duckham, D. J., Rhyne, R. L., Jr., Smith, F. E., and Williams, R. C., Jr.: Retardation of colony growth of in vitro bone marrow culture using sera from patients with Felty's syndrome, disseminated lupus erythematosus (SLE), rheumatoid arthritis, and other disease states. Arthritis Rheum. 18:323, 1975.

212. Goldberg, L. A., Bacon, P. A., Bucknell, P. C., Fitchen, J., and Cline, M. J.: Inhibition of human bone marrow-granulocyte precursors by serum from patients with Felty's syndrome. J. Rheumatol. 7:275, 1980.

213. Bagby, G. C., Jr.: T lymphocytes involved in inhibition of granulopoiesis in two neutrophilic patients are of the cytotoxic/suppressor (T3+ T8+) subset. J. Clin. Invest. 68:1597, 1981.

214. Abdou, N. I., Na Pombejara, C., Balentine, L., and Abdou, N. L.: Suppressor cell-mediated neutropenia in Felty's syndrome. J. Clin. Invest. 61:738, 1978.

215. Bagby, G. C., Jr., and Gabourel, J. D.: Neutropenia in three patients with rheumatic disorders: Suppression of granulopoeisis by cortisol-sensitive thymus-dependent lymphocytes. J. Clin. Invest. 64: 72, 1979.

216. Faber, V., and Elling, P.: Leukocytic-specific anti-nuclear factors in patients with Felty's syndrome, rheumatoid arthritis, systemic lupus erythematosus and other diseases. Acta. Med. Scand. 179:257, 1966.

217. Logue, G.: Felty's syndrome: Granulocyte-bound immunoglobulin G and splenectomy. Ann. Intern. Med. 85:437, 1976.

218. Starkbaum, G., Singer, J. W., and Arend, W. P.: Humoral and cellular immune mechanisms of neutropenia in patients with Felty's syndrome. Clin. Exp. Immunol. 39:307, 1980.

219. Dancey, J. T., and Brubaker, L. H.: Neutrophil marrow profiles in patients with rheumatoid arthritis and neutropenia. Br. J. Haematol. 43:607, 1979.

220. Moore, R. A., Brunner, C. M., Sandusky, W. R., and Leavell, B. S.: Felty's syndrome: Long-term follow-up after splenectomy. Ann. Intern. Med. 75:381, 1971.

221. Laszlo, J., Jones, R., Silberman, H. R., and Banks, P. M.: Splenectomy for Felty's syndrome. Clinicopathological study of 27 patients. Arch. Intern. Med. 138:597, 1978.

222. Blumfelder, T. M., Logue, G. L., and Shimm, D. S.: Felty's syndrome: Effects of splenectomy upon granulocyte count and granulocyte-associated IgG. Ann. Intern. Med. 94:623, 1981.

223. Gowans, J. D. C., and Salami, M.: Response of rheumatoid arthritis with leukopenia in gold salts. N. Engl. J. Med. 288:1007, 1973.

224. Hurd, E. R., and Cheatum, D. E.: Decreased spleen size and in-

creased neutrophils in patients with Felty's syndrome: Effect of gold sodium thiomalate therapy. *JAMA 235:*2215, 1976.

225. Wimer, B. M., and Sloan, M. M.: Remission of Felty's syndrome with long-term testosterone therapy. *JAMA 223:*671, 1973.

226. Hurd, E. R., Andreis, M., and Ziff, M.: Phagocytosis of immune complexes of polymorphonuclear leukocytes in patients with Felty's syndrome. *Clin. Exp. Immunol. 28:*413, 1977.

227. Guptak, R. C., Robinson, W. A., and Kurnick, J. E.: Felty's syndrome. Effect of lithium on granulopoiesis. *Am. J. Med. 61:*29, 1976.

228. Wiseman, B. K., and Doan, C. A.: A newly recognized granulopenic syndrome caused by excessive splenic leukolysis and successfully treated by splenectomy. *Ann. Intern. Med. 16:*1097, 1942.

229. Amorosi, E. L.: Hypersplenism. *Semin. Hematol. 2:*249, 1965.

230. Bishop, C. R., Rothstein, G., Ashenbrucker, H. E., and Athens, J. W.: Leukokinetic studies. XIV. Blood neutrophil kinetics in chronic steady-state neutropenia. *J. Clin. Invest. 50:*1678, 1971.

231. Boxer, L. A., Yokoyama, M., and Wiebe, R. A.: Autoimmune neutropenia associated with chronic active hepatitis. *Am. J. Med. 52:*279, 1972.

232. Horsfall, F. L., and Tamm, L.: *Viral and Rickettsial Infections of Man,* 4th ed. Lippincott, Philadelphia, 1965.

233. Havens, W. P., Jr., and Marck, R. E.: The leukocyte response of patients with experimentally induced infectious hepatitis. *Am. J. Med. Sci. 212:*129, 1946.

234. Cantow, W. F., and Kostinas, J. E.: Studies on infectious mononucleosis. IV. Changes in the granulocyte series. *Am. J. Clin. Pathol. 46:*43, 1966.

235. Downie, A. W.: Pathways of virus infection, in *Mechanisms of Virus Infection,* edited by E. Smith. Academic, New York, 1963.

236. Craddock, P. R., Hammerschmidt, D., White, J. G., Dalmasso, A. P., and Jacob, H. S.: Complement (C5a)-induced granulocyte aggregation in vitro. A possible mechanism of complement-mediated leukostasis and leukopenia. *J. Clin. Invest. 60:*260, 1977.

237. Craddock, P. R., Hammerschmidt, D. E., Moldow, C. E., Yamada, O., and Jacob, H. S.: Granulocyte aggregation as a manifestation of membrane interactions with complement: Possible role in leukocyte margination, microvascular occlusion, and endothelial damage. *Semin. Hematol. 16:*140, 1979.

238. Craddock, P. R., Fehr, J., Brigham, K. L., Kronenberg, R. S., and Jacob, H. S.: Complement and leukocyte-mediated pulmonary dysfunction in hemodialysis. *N. Engl. J. Med. 296:*769, 1977.

239. Craddock, P. R., Fehr, J., Dalmasso, A. P., Brigham, K. L., and Jacob, H. S.: Hemodialysis leukopenia. Pulmonary vascular leukostasis resulting from complement activation by dialyzer cellophane membranes. *J. Clin. Invest. 59:*879, 1977.

240. Schiffer, C. A., Aisner, J., and Wiernik, P. H.: Transient neutropenia induced by tranfusion of blood exposed to nylon fiber filters. *Blood 45:*141, 1975.

241. Chervenick, P. A.: Dialysis, neutropenia, lung dysfunction and complement. *N. Engl. J. Med. 296:*810, 1977.

242. Aster, R. H., and Enright, S. E.: A platelet and granulocyte membrane defect in paroxysmal nocturnal hemoglobinuria: Usefulness for the detection of platelet antibodies. *J. Clin. Invest. 48:*1199, 1969.

243. Drenick, E. J., and Alvarez, L. C.: Neutropenia in prolonged fasting. *Am. J. Clin. Nutr. 24:*859, 1971.

244. Bowers, T. K., and Eckert, E.: Leukopenia in anorexia nervosa. Lack of increased risk of infection. *Arch. Intern. Med. 138:*1520, 1978.

245. Dale, D. C., and Wolff, S. M.: Studies of the neutropenia of acute malaria. *Blood 41:*197, 1973.

246. Brubaker, L. H., and Johnson, C. A.: Correlation of spleen weight and abnormal neutrophil pooling (margination). *Clin. Res. 22:*607A, 1974.

247. Muchmore, H. G., Blackburn, A. B., Shurley, J. T., Pierce, C. M., and McKown, B. A.: Neutropenia in healthy men at the South Polar plateau. *Arch. Intern. Med. (Chicago) 125:*646, 1970.

248. Moltusky, A. G.: Drug reactions, enzymes, and biochemical genetics. *JAMA 165:*835, 1957.

249. Schroder, H., and Evans, D. A.: Acetylator phenotype and adverse effects of sulfasalazine in healthy subjects. *Gut 13:*278, 1972.

250. Symoens, J., Veys, E., Mielants, M., and Pinals, R.: Adverse reactions to levamisole. *Cancer Treatment Rep. 62:*1721, 1978.

251. de Gruchy, C. D. (ed): *Drug-Induced Blood Disorders.* Blackwell, Oxford, chap. v, 1975, p. 76.

252. Arneborn, P., and Palmblad, J.: Drug-induced neutropenia in the Stockholm region 1973–75: Frequency and causes. *Acta Med. Scand. 204:*283, 1978.

253. Arneborn, P., and Palmblad, J.: Drug induced neutropenias in the Stockholm region 1976–77. *Acta Med. Scand. 206:*241, 1979.

254. Levine, P. H., and Weintraub, L. R.: Pseudoleukemia during recovery from Dapsone-induced agranulocytosis. *Ann. Intern. Med. 68:*1060, 1968.

255. Colvin, B., Rogers, M., and Layton, C.: Benzylpenicillin-induced leucopenia. Complication of treatment of bacterial endocarditis. *Br. Heart J. 36:*216, 1974.

256. Kancir, L. M., Tuazon, C. U., Cardella, T. A., and Sheagren, J. N.: Adverse reactions to methicillin and nafcillin during treatment of serious *Staphylococcus aureus* infections. *Arch. Intern. Med. 138:*909, 1978.

257. Westerman, E. L., Bradshaw, M. W., and Williams, T. W., Jr.: Agranulocytosis during therapy with orally administered cloxacillin. *Am. Soc. Clin. Pathol. 69:*559, 1978.

258. Carpenter, J.: Neutropenia induced by semisynthetic penicillin. *South. Med. J. 73:*745, 1980.

259. Weitzman, S. A., and Stossel, T. P.: Drug-induced immunological neutropenia. *Lancet 1:*1068, 1978.

260. Reyes, M. P., Palutke, M., and Lerner, A. M.: Granulocytopenia associated with carbenicillin. Five episodes in two patients. *Am. J. Med. 54:*413, 1973.

261. Borland, C. D., and Farrar, W. E.: Reversible neutropenia from vancomycin. *JAMA 242:*2392, 1979.

262. Spath, P.: The clinical significance of immunohematologic change during therapy with penicillin and cephalosporins. *Wien. Klin. Wochenschr. 85:*1, 1973.

263. Di Cato, M. A., and Ellman, L.: Cephalothin-induced granulocytopenia. *Ann. Intern. Med. 83:*671, 1975.

264. Simon, A. J., and Rogers, D. E.: Agranulocytosis associated with novobiocin administration: Report of a case. *Ann. Intern. Med. 46:*778, 1957.

265. Palva, I. P., and Lehmola, U.: Agranulocytosis caused by nitrofurantoin. *Acta Med. Scand. 194:*575, 1973.

266. Oppenheim, M., and de Meyer, G.: Granulocytopenia and thrombocytopenia from streptomycin treatment. *Schweiz. Med. Wochenschr. 79:*1187, 1949.

267. Graf, M., and Tarlov, A.: Agranulocytosis with monohistiocytosis associated with ampicillin therapy. *Ann. Intern. Med. 69:*91, 1968.

268. Chang, J. C., and Reyes, B.: Agranulocytosis associated with gentamicin. *JAMA 232:*1154, 1975.

269. Fleming, G. F., and Crowe, G. R.: Granulocytopenia due to clindamycin. *Med. J. Aust. 1:*70, 1976.

270. Yuvis, A. A., and Gross, M. A.: Drug-induced inhibition of myeloid colony growth: Modifying effect of colony stimulating factor. *Clin. Res. 23:*49A, 1975.

271. Polak, B. C., Wesseling, H., Schut, D., Herxheimer, A., and Meyler, L.: Blood dyscrasias attributed to chloramphenicol. A review of 576 published and unpublished cases. *Acta Med. Scand. 192:*409, 1972.

272. Moeschlin, S.: Weitere Beobachtungen uber Immunoleukopenien und Agranulocytosen. *Schweiz. Med. Wochenschr. 84:*1110, 1954.

273. Van Hove, W., Hamers, J., and Vermeulen, A.: Hematologische, Bijwerkingen van Trimethoprim-sulfamethoxazole. *Acta Clin. Belg., 28:*176, 1973.

274. Bradley, P. P., Warden, G. D., Maxwell, J. G., and Rothstein, G.: Neutropenia and thrombocytopenia in renal allograft recipients treated with trimethoprimsulfamethoxazole. *Ann. Intern. Med. 93:*560, 1980.

275. Inman, W. H.: Study of fatal bone marrow depression with special reference to phenylbutazone and oxyphenbutazone. *Br. Med. J., 1:*1500, 1977.

276. Fraser, G. L., and Beaulieu, J. T.: Leukopenia secondary to sulfadiazine silver. *JAMA 241:*1928, 1979.

277. Collings, J. R.: Adverse reactions to salicylazolsulfapyridine (azulfidine) in the treatment of ulcerative colitis. *South. Med. J. 61:*354, 1968.

278. Johnson, F. D., and Korst, D. R.: Pancytopenia associated with sulfamethoxy-pyridazine administration. The occurrence of leukopenia suggests an accumulative effect; constant awareness is essential to prevent serious marrow damage. *JAMA* 175:967, 1961.

279. Cochrane, P., Atkins, P., and Ehsanullah, S.: Agranulocytosis associated with sulphasalazine therapy. *Postgrad. Med. J.* 49:669, 1973.

280. Pretty, H. M., Gosselin, G., Colpron, G., and Long, L. A.: Agranulocytosis: A report of 30 cases. *Can. Med. Assoc. J.*, 93:1058, 1965.

281. Ahuja, B. K., and Sabharwal, B. D.: Agranulocytosis due to INH toxicity. A case report. *J. Postgrad. Med.* 16:48, 1970.

282. Jenkins, P. F., Williams, T. D. M., and Campbell, I. A.: Neutropenia with each standard antituberculosis drug in the same patient. *Br. Med. J.* 280:1069, 1980.

283. Pisciotta, A. V.: Immune and toxic mechanisms in drug-induced agranulocytosis. *Semin. Hematol.* 10:279, 1973.

284. Pisciotta, V.: Drug-induced agranulocytosis. *Drugs* 15:132, 1978.

285. Ayd, F. J.: Phenothiazine-induced agranulocytosis: The "at risk patient." *Med. Counterpoint* 2:52, 1970.

286. Albertini, R. S., and Penders, T. M.: Agranulocytosis associated with tricyclics. *J. Clin. Psychiatry* 39:483, 1978.

287. Klerman, G. L., and Cole, J. O.: Clinical pharmacology of imipramine and related antidepressant compounds. *Pharmacol. Rev.* 17:101, 1965.

288. Crammer, J. L., and Elkes, A.: Agranulocytosis after desipramine. *Lancet* 1:105, 1967.

289. Hollis, D. A.: Diazepam: Its scope in anaesthetic practice. *Proc. R. Soc. Med.* 62:806, 1969.

290. Kaelbling, R., and Conrad, F. G.: Agranulocytosis due to chlordiazepoxide hydrochloride. *JAMA* 174:1863, 1960.

291. Greenblatt, D. J., and Shader, R. I.: Meprobamate: A study of irrational drug use. *Am. J. Psychiatry*, 127:1297, 1971.

292. Flexner, J. M., and Hartmann, R. C.: Megaloblastic anemia associated with anticonvulsant drugs. *Am. J. Med.* 28:386, 1960.

293. Tsan, M. F., Mehlman, D. J., Green, R. S., and Bells, W. R.: Dilantin, agranulocytosis, and phagocytic marrow histiocytes. *Ann. Intern. Med.* 84:710, 1976.

294. Cuthbert, M. F.: Adverse reaction to non-steroidal antirheumatic drugs. *Curr. Med. Res. Opinion* 2:600, 1974.

295. McCarthy, D. D., and Chalmers, M. B.: Hematologic complications of phenylbutazone therapy: Review of the literature and report of 2 cases. *Can. Med. Assoc. J.* 90:1061, 1964.

296. Whittaker, J. A., and Evans, D. A. P.: Genetic control of phenylbutazone metabolism in man. *Br. Med. J.* 4:323, 1970.

297. Smith, C. S., Chinn, S., and Watts, R. W. E.: The sensitivity of human bone marrow granulocyte/monocyte precursor cells to phenylbutazone, oxyphenbutazone and gamma-hydroxyphenylbutazone in vitro, with observations on the bone marrow colony formation in phenylbutazone-induced granulocytopenia. *Biochem. Pharmacol.* 26:847, 1977.

298. Thompson, D. M., Pegelow, C. H., Singsen, B. H., Powars, D. R., and Hanson, V.: Neutropenia associated with chrysotherapy for juvenile rheumatoid arthritis. *J. Pediatr.* 93:871, 1978.

299. Kay, A. G. L.: Myelotoxicity of gold. *Br. Med. J.* 1:1266, 1976.

300. Howell, A., Gumpel, J. M., and Watts, R. W. E.: Depression of bone marrow colony formation in gold-induced neutropenia. *Br. Med. J.* 1:432, 1975.

301. Ries, C. A., and Sahud, M. A.: Agranulocytosis caused by Chinese herbal medicines. *JAMA* 231:352, 1975.

302. Rees, J. K. H.: Availability of amidopyrine preparations. *Lancet* 1:581, 1980.

303. Hartl, W.: Drug allergic agranulocytosis (Schultz's disease). *Semin. Hematol.* 2:313, 1965.

304. Moeschlin, S., and Wagner, K.: Agranulocytosis due to occurrence of leukocyte-agglutinins (pyramidon and cold agglutinins). *Acta Haematol.* 8:29, 1952.

305. Barrett, A. J., Weller, B., Rozengurt, H., Longhurst, P., and Humble, J. G.: Amidopyrine agranulocytosis: Drug inhibition of granulocyte colonies in the presence of patient's serum. *Br. Med. J.* 2:850, 1976.

306. Wing, E. S., Jr., and Asper, S. P., Jr.: Observations on the use of propylthiouracil in hyperthyroidism with special reference to long term treatment. *Bull. Johns Hopkins Hosp.* 90:201, 1952.

307. Amrhein, J. A., Kenny, F. M., and Ross, D.: Granulocytopenia, lupus-like syndrome and other complications of propylthiouracil therapy. *J. Pediatr.*, 76:54, 1970.

308. Ahm, Y. S., and Yunis, A. A.: Antithyroid therapy and leukocytes, in *Drugs and Haematologic Reactions*, edited by N. V. Dimitrov and J. H. Nodine. Grune & Stratton, New York, 1973, p. 249.

309. Morton, H.: Agranulocytosis caused by thiouracil: A review of fifty nine cases in the literature and a report of two additional cases. *Am. J. Med.* 2:53, 1947.

310. Tsan, M., and Mc Intyre, P. A.: Stimulation by propylthiourasil of the hexosemonophosphate shunt in human polymorphonuclear leucocytes during phagocytosis. *Br. J. Haematol.* 31:193, 1975.

311. Wiberg, J. J., and Nuttall, F. Q.: Methimazole toxicity from high doses. *Ann. Intern. Med.* 77:414, 1972.

312. Zipes, D. P., and Troup, P. J.: New antiarrhythmic agents: Amiodarone, aprindine, disopyramide, ethmozin, mexiletine, tocainide, verapamil. *Am. J. Cardiol.* 41:1005, 1978.

313. Kohler, G. D.: Antiarrhythmic agents and agranulocytosis. *Lancet* 1:1415, 1980.

314. Opie, L. H.: Aprindine and agranulocytosis. *Lancet* 2:689, 1980.

315. Barzel, U. S.: Quinidine-sulfate-induced hypoplastic anemia and agranulocytosis. *JAMA* 201:325, 1967.

316. Rothman, I. K., and Amorosi, E. L.: Procainamide-induced agranulocytosis and thrombocytopenia. *Arch. Intern. Med.* 139:246, 1979.

317. Riker, J., Baker, J., and Swanson, M.: Bone marrow granulomas and neutropenia associated with procainamide. *Arch. Intern. Med.* 138:1731, 1978.

318. Vidt, D. G., Bravo, E. L., and Fouad, F. M.: Drug therapy: Captopril. *N. Engl. J. Med.* 306:214, 1982.

319. Greene, R., and Spence, A. W.: Neutropenia caused by methyldopa. *Br. Med. J.* 4:618, 1967.

320. Ognibene, A. J.: Agranulocytosis due to dapsone. *Ann. Intern. Med.* 72:52, 1970.

321. Lind, D. E., Levi, J. A., and Vincent, P. C.: Aminodiaquine-induced agranulocytosis: Toxic effects of aminodiaquine in bone marrow cultures *in vitro*. *Br. Med. J.* 1:458, 1973.

322. Sutherland, R., Vincent, P. C., Raik, E., and Burgess, K.: Quinine-induced agranulocytosis: Toxic effect of quinine bisulphate on bone marrow cultures in vitro. *Br. Med. J.* 1:605, 1977.

323. Chernof, D., and Taylor, K. S.: Hydroxychloroquine-induced agranulocytosis. *Arch. Dermatol.* 97:163, 1968.

324. Drake, T. G.: Agranulocytosis during therapy with the anti-histaminic agent methaphenilene (Diatrin). *JAMA* 142:477, 1950.

325. Adams, D. A., and Perry, S.: Agranulocytosis associated with thenalidine (sandostine) tartrate therapy; report of three cases. *JAMA* 167:1207, 1958.

326. Hilker, A. W.: Agranulocytosis from tripelennamine (pyribenzamine) hydrochloride. *JAMA* 143:741, 1950.

327. Hardin, A. C., and Padilla, F.: Agranulocytosis during therapy with a brompheniramine-medication. *J. Arkansas Med. Soc.* 75:206, 1978.

328. Freston, J. W.: Cimetidine and granulocytopenia. *Ann. Intern. Med.* 90:264, 1979.

329. Carloss, H. W., Tavassaloi, M., and MacMillan, R.: Cimetidine-induced granulocytopenia. *Ann. Intern. Med.* 93:57, 1980.

330. Bertoye, A., Garin, J. P., and Monier, P.: À propos d'un cas d'aplasie medullaire après traitment par la carbutamide. *Lyon Med.* 216:1549, 1966.

331. Koszewski, B. J., and Hubbard, T. F.: Immunologic agranulocytosis due to mercurial diuretics. *Am. J. Med.* 20:958, 1956.

332. Havard, C. W. H.: A reappraisal of the thiazide diuretics. *Curr. Med. Drugs* 7:14, 1966.

333. Kim, K. E., Onesti, G., Moyer, J. H., and Swartz, C.: Ethacrynic acid and furosemide. Diuretic and hemodynamic effects and clinical uses. *Am. J. Cardiol.* 27:407, 1971.

334. Scobie, I. N., Maccuish, A. C., Kesson, C. M., and McNeil, I. R.: Neutropenia during allopurinol treatment in total therapeutic starvation. *Br. Med. J.* 280:1163, 1980.

335. Williams, G. T., Johnson, S. A., Dieppe, P. A., and Huskisson, E. C.: Neutropenia during treatment of rheumatoid arthritis with levamisole. *Ann. Rheum. Dis.* 37:366, 1978.

336. Thompson, J. S., et al.: Studies on levamisole-induced agranulocytosis. *Blood* 56:388, 1980.

337. Veys, E. M., Mielants, H., and Verbruggen, G.: Levamisole-in-

duced adverse reactions in HLA B27-positive rheumatoid arthritis. *Lancet* 1:148, 1978.

338. Drew, S. I., Carter, B. M., Nathanson, D. S., and Terasaki, P. I.: Levamisole-associated neutropenia and autoimmune granulocytotoxins. *Ann. Rheum. Dis.* 39:59, 1980.

339. Dancey, J. T., Deubelbeiss, K. A., Harker, L. A., and Finch, C. A.: Neutrophil kinetics in man. *J. Clin. Invest* 58:705, 1976.

340. Harmon, D. C., Weitzman, S. A., and Stossel, T. P.: A staphylococcal slide-test for detection of antineutrophil antibodies. *Blood* 56:64, 1980.

341. Jiang, A. F., and Lalezari, P.: A micro-technique for detection of leukocyte agglutinins. *J. Immunol. Methods.* 7:103, 1975.

342. Logue, G. L., and Silberman, H. R.: Felty's syndrome without splenomegaly. *Am. J. Med.* 66:703, 1979.

343. Boxer, L. A., and Stossel, T. P.: Effects of anti-human neutrophil antibodies *in vitro:* Quantitative studies. *J. Clin. Invest.* 53:1534, 1974.

344. Blaschke, J. W., Severson, C. D., Goeken, N. E., and Thompson, J. S.: Microgranulocytotoxicity. *J. Lab. Clin. Med.* 90:249, 1977.

345. Logue, G. L., Kurlander, R., Pepe, R., Davis, W., and Silberman, H.: Antibody-dependent lymphocyte-mediated granulocyte cytotoxicity in man. *Blood* 51:97, 1978.

346. Rebuck, J. W., and Crowley, J. H.: A method of studying leukocyte functions in vivo. *Ann. N.Y. Acad. Sci.* 59:757, 1955.

347. Senn, H., Holland, J. F., and Banerjee, T.: Kinetic and comparative studies on localized leukocyte mobilization in normal man. *J. Lab. Clin. Med.* 74:742, 1969.

348. Camussi, G., Tetta, C., and Cappio, F. C.: Detection of immune complexes on the surface of polymorphonuclear neutrophils. *Int. Arch. Allergy Appl. Immunol.* 58:135, 1979.

349. Chikkappa, G., Corcino, J., Greenberg, M. L., and Herbert, V.: Correlation between various blood white cell pools and the serum B12-binding capacities. *Blood* 37:142, 1971.

350. Cream, J. J.: Prednisolone-induced granulocytosis. *Br. J. Haematol.* 15:259, 1968.

351. Weiblen, B. J., Forstrom, K., and McCullough, J.: Studies of the kinetics of indium-lll-labeled granulocytes. *J. Lab. Clin. Med.* 94:246, 1979.

352. Senn, J. S., Messner, H. A., and Stanley, E. R.: Analysis of interacting cell populations in cultures of marrow from patients with neutropenia. *Blood* 44:33, 1974.

353. Quesenberry, P., and Levitt, L.: Hematopoietic stem cells. *N. Engl. J. Med.* 301:755, 1979.

354. Gurwith, M. J., Brunton, J. L., Lank, B. A., Ronald, A. R., and Harding, G. K.: Granulocytopenia in hospitalized patients. I. Prognostic factors and etiology of fever. *Am. J. Med.* 64:121, 1978.

355. Wiernik, P. H.: The management of infection in the cancer patient. *JAMA* 244:185, 1980.

356. Nauseef, W. M., and Maki, D. G.: A study of the value of simple protective isolation in patients with granulocytopenia. *N. Eng. J. Med.* 304:448, 1981.

357. Newman, S. B., and Sweet, D. L.: Single protective isolation in patients with granulocytopenia. *N. Engl. J. Med.* 304:1493, 1981.

358. Schimpff, S. C.: Therapy of infection in patients with granulocytopenia. *Med. Clin. North Am.* 61:1101, 1977.

359. Pizzo, P. A., Robichaud, K. J., Gill, F. A., and Witebsky, F. G.: Empiric antibiotic and antifungal therapy for cancer patients with prolonged fever and granulocytopenia. *Am. J. Med.* 72:101, 1982.

360. Lyman, G. H., et al.: Lithium carbonate in patients with small cell lung cancer receiving combination chemotherapy. *Am. J. Med.* 70:1222, 1981.

361. Levitt, L. J., and Quesenberry, P. J.: The effect of lithium on murine hematopoiesis in a liquid culture system. *N. Engl. J. Med.* 302:713, 1980.

362. Crosby, W. H.: How many "polys" are enough? *Arch. Intern. Med.* 123:722, 1969.

363. Hall, R. C., Perl, M., and Pfefferbaum, B.: Lithium therapy and toxicity. *Am. Fam. Physician* 19:133, 1979.

364. Huguley C. M., Jr.: Agranulocytosis induced by dipyrone, a hazardous antipyretic and analgesic. *JAMA* 189:938, 1964.

365. Magis, C. C., Barge, A., and Dausset, J.: Serological study of an allergic agranulocytosis due to naramidopyrine. *Clin. Exp. Immunol.* 3:989, 1968.

366. Forshaw, J.: Penicillin-induced granulopenia. *Br. Med. J.* 3:184, 1968.

367. Elgart, M. L.: Griseofulvin. A review of the literature and summary of present usage. *Med. Ann. D.C.* 36:331, 1967.

368. Rab, S. M., and Alam, M. N.: Severe agranulocytosis during para-aminosalicylic acid therapy. *Br. J. Dis. Chest.* 64:164, 1970.

369. Liederman, E., and Mogabgab, W. J.: Rifampin in beta-hemolytic streptococcal pharyngitis and occurrence of leukopenia. *Clin. Med.* 77:36, 1970.

370. Ahuja, B. K., and Sabharwal, B. D.: Agranulocytosis due to INH toxicity: A case report. *Postgrad. Med. J.* 16:45, 1970.

371. Spittler, J. F.: Agranulocytosis due to ethosuximide with a fatal outcome. *Klin. Paediatr.* 186:364, 1974.

372. Abbott, J. A., and Schwals, R. S.: The serious side effects of the newer antiepileptic drugs: Their control and prevention. *N. Engl. J. Med.* 242:943, 1950.

373. Michelstein, I., and Weiser, N. J.: Fatal agranulocytosis due to trimethadione (Tridione). *Arch. Neurol. Psychiatry* 62:358, 1949.

374. Cahan, A. M., Meilman, E., and Jacobson, B. M.: Agranulocytosis following pyribenzamine. *N. Engl. J. Med.* 241:865, 1949.

375. Sand, B. J., and Shanedling, P. D.: Teratogenesis from Daraprim. *Am. J. Ophthalmol.* 56:1011, 1963.

376. Vanderlaan, W. P., and Storrie, V. M.: A survey of the factors controlling thyroid functions with special reference to newer views on antithyroid substances. *Pharmacol. Rev.* 7:301, 1955.

377. Gavras, H., Brunner, H. R., and Gavras, I.: Captopril in the treatment of hypertension. *Ann. Intern. Med.* 95:505, 1981.

378. Conrad, M. E., Cumbie, W. G., Thrasher, D. R., and Carpenter, J. T.: Agranulocytosis associated with disopyramide therapy. *JAMA* 240:1857, 1978.

379. Nawabi, I. U., and Ritz, N. D.: Agranulocytosis due to propanolol. *JAMA* 223:1376, 1973.

380. Danilo, P., Jr.: Aprindine. *Am. Heart J.* 97:119, 1979.

381. Hoffman, F. G., Zimmerman, S. L., and Reese, J. D.: Fatal agranulocytosis associated with acetazolamide. *N. Engl. J. Med.* 262:242, 1960.

382. Turner, N. A., and Woodliff, H. J.: Neutropenia associated with chlorthalidone therapy. *Med. J. Aust.* 1:361, 1964.

383. Anath, J. V., Valles, J. V., and Whitelaw, J. P.: Usual and unusual agranulocytosis during neurolyptic therapy. *Am. J. Psychiatry* 130:100, 1973.

384. Shabry, F., and Wolk, J. A.: Granulocytopenia in children after phenothiazine therapy. *Am. J. Psychiatry* 137:374, 1980.

385. de la Chapelle, A., Kari, C., Nurminen, M., and Hernberg, S.: Clozapine-induced agranulocytosis. A genetic and epidemiologic study. *Hum. Genet.* 37:183, 1977.

386. Trafton, H. M., and Lind, H. E.: Clinical evaluation of sulfachlorpyridazine in urinary tract infections. *J. Urol.* 90:308, 1963.

387. Jarkowski, T. L., and Martmer, E. E.: Fatal reaction to sulfadimethoxine (Madribon). A case showing toxic epidermal necrolysis and leukopenia. *Am. J. Dis. Child.* 104:669, 1962.

388. Stevens, A. R., Jr.: Agranulocytosis induced by sulfaquanidine. *Arch. Intern. Med.* 123:428, 1969.

389. Kato, K., Sherman, M. S., and Cannon, P. R.: Fatal agranulocytosis following sulfathiazole therapy. *J. Pediatr.* 22:432, 1943.

390. Liu, Y. K.: Leukopenia in alcoholics. *Am. J. Med.* 54:605, 1973.

391. Vigliani, E. C., and Saita, G.: Benzene and leukemia. *N. Engl. J. Med.* 271:872, 1964.

392. Wright, C. S., Doan, C. A., and Haynie, H. C.: Agranulocytosis occurring after exposure to a D.D.T. pyrethrum aerosol bomb. *Am. J. Med.* 2:562, 1946.

393. Goldman, A., and Haber, M.: Acute complete granulopenia with death due to dinitrophenol poisoning. *JAMA* 107:2114, 1936.

394. Parbrook, G. D.: Leucopenic effects of prolonged nitrous oxide treatment. *Br. J. Anaesth.* 39:119, 1967.

395. Corcos, J. M., Soler-Bechara, J., Mayer, K., Freyberg, R. H., Goldstein, R., and Jaffe, I.: Neutrophilic-agranulocytosis during administration of penicillamine (2 cases). *JAMA* 189:265, 1964.

396. Tashjian, A. H., Jr., and Leddy, J. P.: Agranulocytosis associated with phenindione: A case report with review of literature. *Arch. Intern. Med.* 105:121, 1960.

CHAPTER 88

Neutrophilia

STUART C. FINCH

Neutrophilia refers to a concentration of blood neutrophils that is in excess of about 7500 per microliter (total leukocyte count × percent neutrophils) in adults [1]. The definition of neutrophilia varies with age and race. A significant portion of the Negro and Yemenite Jewish populations have low absolute neutrophil counts in comparison to Caucasians [2,3]. During the first few days of life the upper limit of the normal neutrophil counts ranges from about 7000 to 13,000 per microliter for babies born at early and late gestational ages, respectively [4]. Adult levels occur within the first few weeks of life and are maintained thereafter [1]. The term *neutrophilia* is synonymous with the terms *polymorphonuclear leukocytosis* and *neutrophilic leukocytosis*. The term *granulocytosis* refers to an increase in all blood granulocytes (i.e., neutrophils, eosinophils, and basophils), although it has been used often in the past as a synonym for neutrophilia. *Leukemoid reaction* refers to a reactive leukocytosis that resembles the blood picture of leukemia. Moderate to extreme neutrophilic leukocytosis is usually a response to inflammation, infection, tissue damage, tumor, or another marrow stimulus [6–11]. The blood neutrophils can be mature (band and segmented forms) or can include immature cells (promyelocytes and myelocytes). Rarely, it is difficult to differentiate a leukemoid reaction from chronic myelogenous leukemia or another chronic myeloproliferative disorder even with the assistance of a marrow examination [5–9].

Mechanism of neutrophilia

An increase in the concentration of blood neutrophils is the result of a disturbance of the normal equilibrium involving neutrophil marrow production, movement in and out of the marrow storage and blood pools, and neutrophil destruction [10–13]. There are three major mechanisms which alone, or in combination, are responsible for most neutrophilic reactions. Firstly, increased numbers of the preformed neutrophils may be mobilized from either the marrow or marginal storage pools into the circulating pool [13–16]. Secondly, there may be increased blood neutrophil survival due to immaturity or diminished neutrophil outflow into tissue sites [11]. Thirdly, increased effective granulopoiesis can result in expansion of the circulating neutrophil pool [12–13]. This may be due to (1) increased stem cell

differentiation in the direction of the neutrophilic series, (2) stimulation of resting neutrophilic cells in the mitotic pool, or (3) shortening of the cell mitotic cycle of proliferating cells. Models of various acute and chronic forms of neutrophilic leukocytosis and leukemoid reactions are shown in Fig. 88-1.

Acute neutrophilia occurs rapidly and may last for only minutes or hours following stimulation. It is almost always due to the mobilization of neutrophils from one or more of the storage pools. An early type occurs within minutes in response to violent exercise, severe pain, sudden variation in temperature, emotional stress, or the administration of a number of chemical or biological substances [17–22]. This type of rapid neutrophilia has been attributed to mobilization of marginal pool granulocytes in response to accelerated blood flow or stimulation of beta receptors, but the mechanism remains controversial [18–20,22–24]. It sometimes is referred to as *pseudoneutrophilia* since it is due to a shift of neutrophils from one intravascular compartment to another and does not represent any increase in total blood neutrophils.

A more delayed type of acute neutrophilia is recognized with maximal response at 4 to 24 h following stimulation. Inflammation, infection, glucocorticoids, and a wide variety of other organic substances are capable of eliciting this type of neutrophilic reaction [14–17,25–42]. It probably is due to release of marrow storage pool neutrophils into the circulating pool in response to activation of a humoral-releasing factor(s) [25–43]. Neutrophil-releasing activity is probably due to activation of the complement system [34,39,41,43]. Many of the neutrophils released by the marrow during the acute response will marginate before egress to tissue sites or recirculation. This may account for the delayed neutrophilia which occurs in response to many acute stimuli. Glucocorticoids may impede the flow of neutrophils from the circulating pool into the tissues [15]. The magnitude of acute neutrophilia in the circulating pool will depend upon the balance established between neutrophil inflow and outflow rates. The response increment to ordinary stimuli is usually less than twice the baseline for adults, but greater for children.

Chronic neutrophilia frequently is the consequence of a continued neutrophilic stimulus. The resultant shift of marrow neutrophils from the marrow into the circulating pool may increase granulopoiesis through perturbation of a marrow loop feedback mechanism [13]. This may occur by means of direct cell-cell interaction or generation of colony-stimulating activity [12,13,34,36,44,45]. Such a shift of mature cells into the circulating pool occurs in response to prolonged administration of glucocorticoids [15,29,38,40,41], chronic blood loss [46], chronic emotional disturbances [47], or the persistance of inflammation or infection [17]. Most reactions of this type last for days or weeks, but some may persist for many months. Other forms of chronic neutrophilia are due to disturbances in the regulatory mechanisms for

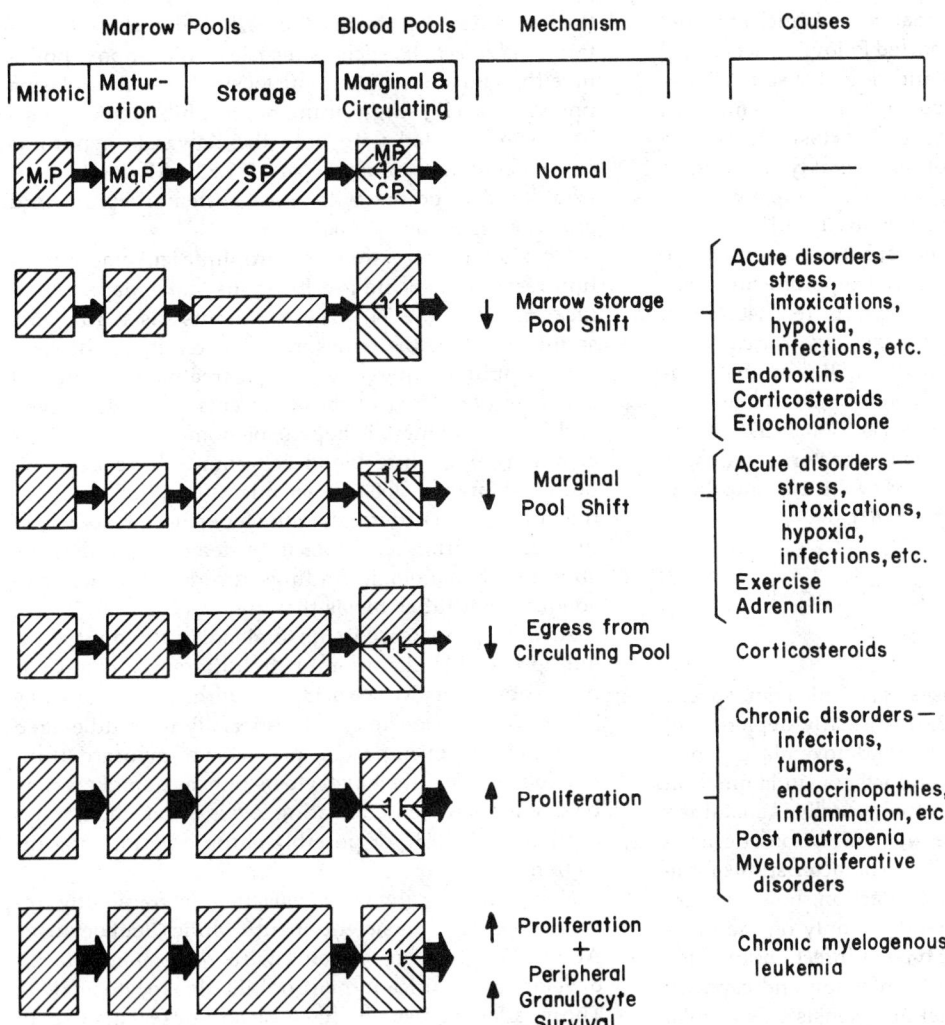

FIGURE 88-1   The mechanisms of producing neutrophilic granulocytosis is represented schematically. The relative size of each neutrophilic granulocyte pool is represented by the size of its corresponding cross-hatched area, and the rate of neutrophilic granulocyte flow through each pool is proportional to the size of each arrow. M.P. = mitotic pool; MaP = maturation pool; SP = marrow neutrophil storage pool; MP = marginal neutrophilic granulocyte pool; CP = circulating neutrophilic granulocyte pool.

granulocyte production such as occur with various myeloproliferative disorders, other forms of primary marrow dysplasia, or chronically increased erythropoiesis [11,13,48–50].

The mechanism for the profound neutrophilic leukemoid reactions that occasionally accompany nonhematologic malignancies remains uncertain. The presence of widespread neoplasm may result in excessive granulopoiesis [51–53], possibly in response to the elaboration of granulopoietic factors [51,52,54–56]. Extensive tissue necrosis or an abnormal host response to tumor breakdown products are other possibilities [52,53]. An alternative explanation is that there is increased accumulation of neutrophils in the blood due to impaired migration of granulocytes from blood into the tissues [57].

Disorders associated with acute neutrophilia

Exercise- and *epinephrine*-induced neutrophilic reactions occur within minutes of the stimulus and are of short duration [19,20,22–24]. A corollary to the exercise-induced neutrophilia of adults is observed in vigorously crying babies who may develop blood neutrophilia with increased numbers of band cells [58]. Acute neutrophilia frequently occurs within minutes of the administration of *cryoprecipitate* [21]. Modest neutrophilic leukocytosis is reported to occur rapidly in response to abrupt changes in *emotion* or *temperature* [17].

There are several types of acute neutrophilia that are probably more delayed in onset, but their precise mechanism is unclear. Profound acute neutrophilic leukocytosis associated with the appearance of nucleated red cells in the blood has been reported following accidental *electric shock* [59]. *Anesthesia* and *surgery* also may precede the development of a neutrophilia which may last for several days [60,61]. The leukocytosis associated with parenteral administration of several types of anesthetic or hypnotic agents may be due to complement activation or immunologic hypersensitivity [61].

The most clearly recognized substances which are known to induce the more delayed type of acute neutrophilia are the *glucocorticoids* [15,16,29,40,42,62], *etiocholanolone* [30,32,39], *hydroxyethyl starch* [37], *typhoid vaccine* [14,25,26], *turpentine* [29], *bacterial endotoxin* [31,32], *antigen-antibody complexes* [34,41], and *activated third component of complement* [30,37,39]. Acute *anoxia*, *inflammation*, and *infection* of bacterial, parasitic and rarely of viral etiologies may evoke a prompt left-shifted neutrophilic response [63–67].

Disorders associated with chronic neutrophilia

One of the most common causes of chronic neutrophilia is *bacterial infection* [7,8,17,63,64,68]. Early depletion of marrow neutrophils as a result of endotoxemia, complement activation, or other products of inflammation results in acute neutrophilia, which usually is sustained in response to continued excessive utilization of granulocytes at sites of infection. The characteristics of the leukocyte responses to chronic infection, however, are extremely variable. They depend not only on the virulence of the organism and the type of infection, but also in the individual's resistance to infection and capacity to react. For example, overwhelming sepsis may invoke rapid depletion of marrow neutrophils and depression of granulopoiesis resulting in neutropenia rather than neutrophilia. The neutrophil response to bacterial infection may be attenuated or absent in debilitated alcoholic patients or persons with chemotherapy-induced granulocytopenia. The magnitude of the neutrophil response in children is usually greater than in adults [69,70]. Absolute neutrophil counts of 12,000 to 14,000 per microliter are common with mild localized infections, and counts in the range of 20,000 to 25,000 per microliter occur with many systemic infections. Counts as high as 50,000 to 70,000 per microliter are occasionally observed with severe infection due to virulent organisms. Total leukocyte counts in the range of 75,000, 104,000, and 112,000 per microliter have been reported with osteomyelitis, empyema, and septicemia, respectively [7,8].

The magnitude of the neutrophilia in most patients with bacterial infections is predictable, but there are exceptions. Moderate to marked leukocytosis occurs in response to pneumonia, endocarditis, meningitis, pyelonephritis, cellulitis, and similar acute bacterial infections. On the other hand, typhoid fever, brucellosis, and whooping cough often are associated with neutropenia rather than neutrophilia. A mild neutrophilic leukocy-

tosis may develop during the early acute phase of certain *viral infections* such as measles, chickenpox, poliomyelitis, infectious mononucleosis, and mycoplasma pneumonia [17]. Significant neutrophilic leukocytosis has been reported with both the Kawasaki syndrome and infectious mononucleosis [71,72]. Moderate neutrophilia also occurs with most systemic *mycotic* and *protozoal* infections [17,66].

Occasionally an extreme neutrophilic leukemoid reaction resembling acute myelogenous leukemia is due to *tuberculosis* [7,8,73,74]. These patients, as a rule, are seriously ill with widespread, necrotizing disease. Death rapidly supervenes unless treatment is prompt and vigorous. Most of these patients have high fever, and frequently there is hepatosplenomegaly. Anemia is common, and white blood cell counts have been reported as high as 200,000 per microliter [8]. Sometimes the only way to differentiate the leukemoid response of tuberculosis from leukemia is to demonstrate that the abnormal hematologic findings revert to normal with adequate antituberculosis therapy.

An average increase in the total leukocyte count without appreciable alteration of the differential count has been observed in association with heavy *smoking* [75,76]. The leukocyte count, especially in middle-aged men, may be an important predictor of myocardial infarction [77,78]. The leukocytosis of heavy smokers may be due to increased circulating levels of catecholamines or nicotine [77,78], or possibly chronic periodontal infection [68].

Nonbacterial *chronic inflammation* is frequently responsible for persistent neutrophilic leukocytosis. About 25 percent of patients with *rheumatoid arthritis* develop a significant neutrophilic leukocytosis [79]. Those affected usually have severe-onset disease of short duration. Disorders that are frequently associated with tissue damage, such as *eclampsia, azotemia, glomerulonephritis, hepatic necrosis, diabetic acidosis, thyroid storm, gout, cutaneous inflammation,* and reactions due to certain *drugs* or *chemicals,* may be accompanied by severe neutrophilia [7,8,80–85]. Secondary amyloidosis in association with leprosy has induced neutrophilic leukocytosis [86].

Chronic stimulation of the marrow due to *hemolysis* or *bleeding* may result in a moderate leukocytosis with significant left shift in the myeloid series [69,87–89]. Transient "rebound" or "overshoot" neutrophilia with total leukocyte counts reaching 20,000 to 30,000 per microliter frequently follows *recovery from acute agranulocytosis* [69,90–92]. These reactions usually last from 1 to 3 weeks, during which time the hematologic picture may resemble that of acute leukemia. The marrow may contain 80 to 90 percent myeloblasts and promyelocytes, and 20 to 30 percent of the blood leukocytes may be immature myeloid forms [92].

About 20 percent of *pregnant women* develop neutrophilic leukocytosis, which almost always occurs during the last trimester [93,94]. About 25 percent of those with neutrophilia will have either myelocytes or metamyelocytes in the peripheral blood. At the onset of labor the total leukocyte count may rise to 25 to 30 per microliter [95].

Neutrophilic leukemoid reactions due to *tumors* are most frequently reported with bronchogenic carcinoma [5–8,52,96,97], but they also occur with gastric carcinoma [8,97,98], renal cancer [99,100], and a wide variety of other tumors [5–9,52,56,97]. Often the tumors are widespread and necrotic [52,53,96,100]. Difficulties in the differentiation from leukemia may be increased in the presence of anemia, thrombocytopenia, or leukoerythroblastic peripheral blood picture [9,70,96,97]. Total leukocyte counts above 50,000 per microliter are unusual, but counts in the range of 100,000 to 200,000 per microliter have been reported [7,8].

Transient neonatal leukemoid reactions which closely resemble congenital leukemia are frequently associated with *Down's syndrome* [101]. Usually these reactions last only for a few weeks or months. Current evidence suggests that in Down's syndrome there is an intrinsic intracellular defect in the regulation of leukocyte multiplication and maturation which is related to chromosome 21 trisomy [102,103]. Relatively minor stimuli may induce exaggerated myeloproliferation which resembles acute leukemia [100]. Newborn infants have also been described with leukemoid reactions in association with *amegakaryocytic thrombocytopenia* and *congenital skeletal defects* [105–107].

A benign form of *idiopathic neutrophil leukocytosis* of unknown cause may persist for many years [108]. Physical findings and all other hematologic values are normal, but the condition may be difficult to differentiate from chronic myelogenous leukemia. Total leukocyte counts average about 15,000 per microliter, but may be as high as 40,000 per microliter.

A benign form of lifelong *hereditary neutrophilia* with autosomal dominant inheritance has been described [109]. Functionally normal granulocytes with total leukocyte counts ranging from 14,000 to 164,000 per microliter are present in the affected persons. Associated findings are hepatosplenomegaly, Gaucher-type histiocytes, thickened calvariae, increased leukocyte alkaline phosphatase, increased serum vitamin B_{12} levels, and heat-labile serum alkaline phosphatase activity.

A peculiar form of *familial myeloproliferative disease* simulating granulocytic leukemia in childhood has also been described [110]. These patients have hepatosplenomegaly, retardation of growth, anemia, leukocytosis, and immature myeloid forms in the peripheral blood [110]. Some of the children die early in life, whereas others remain unchanged or improved. There also is a form of *familial cold urticaria* in which leukocyte counts up to 36,000 per microliter occur following exposure to cold [111]. Injection of gram-negative endotoxin prior to cold exposure prevents the development of leukocytosis, suggesting that the cold urticarial reaction mobilizes the marrow storage pool.

Continued oral or parenteral administration of glucocorticoids in moderate doses results in a significant neutrophilic leukocytosis which tends to peak at 10 to 14 days following the onset of drug therapy [38,42]. The neutrophil count gradually returns to near the normal range in the course of the next few weeks with continuation of the corticosteroids. The most remarkable group of new substances found to produce granulocytosis, however, are the *lithium salts* [112–115]. A dose-related increase in neutrophils, associated with some lymphopenia, is noted several days after the initiation of drug therapy. The average neutrophil response is a rise of 3000 to 5000 per microliter, which persists for the duration of drug administration. The increased granulopoiesis which occurs during therapy [115–116] is associated with increased colony-stimulating activity [117,118], possibly due to direct lithium stimulation of marrow granulocyte precursors [119,120].

Sustained moderate neutrophilia invariably follows the occurrence of either surgical or disease-induced functional *asplenia* [121,122]. This may be due to persistent circulation of those leukocytes which normally are transiently detained in the intact spleen rather than to increased granulopoiesis.

Chronic *emotional disturbances* such as panic, fear, agitation, and anxiety are reported to be associated with moderate leukocytosis [17,47]. Emotional response to sedation is usually accompanied by modification of the leukocytosis.

Erroneously high leukocyte counts that may mimic a neutrophilic leukemoid reaction sometimes are an artifact of *automated blood counting*. Cryoprotein, for instance, may aggregate when blood is cooled, and this may result in the recording of a false leukocytosis due to the counting of protein crystals [123,124]. Some of the various substances and medical conditions associated with chronic neutrophilia are summarized in Table 88-1.

Evaluation of patients with neutrophilia

It is important to differentiate neutrophilic leukocytosis of benign origin from that due to leukemia or other serious underlying disorders as rapidly as possible in order to avoid undue patient apprehension. Each patient will require detailed medical history with emphasis on the family history, environmental exposure, and current medications. The physical examination should include a careful search for evidence of underlying inflammation, infection, metabolic disturbance, trauma, tumor, or hemopoietic disorder.

The total and differential leukocyte count, hematocrit, red cell indices, platelet count, and reticulocyte count are essential for the proper evaluation of most patients. The leukocyte alkaline phosphatase score may provide valuable leads, and marrow examination is often of considerable diagnostic value if the cause of neutrophilia is not obvious from study of the blood. The serum vitamin B_{12} level and B_{12} binding capacity are of little help since they tend to be elevated in virtually all types of neutrophilic leukocytosis [125].

TABLE 88-1   Major causes of neutrophilia

Acute neutrophilia	Chronic neutrophilia
Physical stimuli [17,18,20,58,60, 61,127]: Cold, heat, exercise, convulsions, tachycardia, pain, labor, nausea, vomiting, anesthesia, surgery	Infections [7,8,17,63,64,66–74]: Persistance of many infections that cause acute neutrophilia
Emotional stimuli [17,47,58,127]: Panic, rage, severe stress	Inflammation [8,17,69,75,76,79,81–83]: Continuation of most acute inflammatory reactions, such as rheumatic fever, rheumatoid arthritis, gout, chronic vasculitis, myositis, nephritis, colitis, pancreatitis, dermatitis, thyroiditis, drug-sensitivity reactions, periodontitis, Sweet's syndrome
Infections [17,66,69]: Many localized and systemic acute bacterial, mycotic, rickettsial, spirochetal, and certain viral infections	Emotional stress [17,47,127]: Chronic state of panic, agitation, depression with anxiety, elation, and anger
Inflammation or tissue necrosis [21,27,34,41,43,59,64,65]: Burns, electric shock, trauma, infarction, turpentine reactions, gout, anoxia, ovulation, antigen-antibody complexes, activated complement, acute vasculitis	Tumors [5–9,11,51–57,69,96–100]: Gastric, bronchogenic, breast, renal, hepatic, pancreatic, uterine, and squamous cell cancers. Rarely Hodgkin's disease, other lymphoma, brain tumors, melanoma, and multiple myeloma
Drugs, hormones, and toxins [19,22–26,29–33,37,39,40]: Epinephrine, etiocholanolone, endotoxin, corticosteroids, serotonin, histamine, venoms, typhoid vaccine, casein, peptone, CO, hydroxyethyl starch	Drugs, hormones, and toxins [7,38,42, 62,82,84–86,112–120]: Continued exposure to many substances that produce acute neutrophilia. Chronic exposure to heparin, benzene, lead, mercury, ethylene glycol, cysteine, digitalis, lithium, chlorpropamide, etc.
	Metabolic and endocrinologic disorders [7,17,29,80,93–95]: Eclampsia, azotemia, hepatic necrosis, acidosis, gout, pregnancy, lactation, thyroid storm, overproduction of ACTH or glucocorticoids
	Hematologic disorders [7,46,49,50,69,70,72 87–92,108,121,122]: Rebound from agranulocytosis or therapy of megaloblastic anemia, chronic hemolysis or hemorrhage, asplenia, myeloid leukemia, other myeloproliferative disorders, infectious mononucleosis, continued leukapheresis, chronic idiopathic leukocytosis
	Hereditary and congenital disorders [101–107,109–111]: Down's syndrome, congenital amegakaryocytic thrombocytopenia, hereditary neutrophilia, familial, myeloproliferative disease, familial cold urticaria

The early acute neutrophilic response in the blood is characterized by the appearance of "left-shifted" neutrophils which are identified by their band or monolobed nuclei. Neutrophils containing "toxic" granules or Döhle bodies will appear in the presence of persistent acute or chronic bacterial infections. Neutrophils are the predominant cell type throughout the course of most chronic infections, but a concomitant monocytosis also usually develops.

Marrow aspiration and biopsy in conjunction with

the red cell, reticulocyte, and platelet counts are important in the diagnosis of various underlying erythroid disturbances, most myeloproliferative disorders, and many types of cancer. Marrow cytogenetic studies for trisomy 21 in infants [101–103], or the Philadelphia chromosome at all ages, are of value in the differential diagnosis of chronic myelogenous leukemia.

Appropriate metabolic, bacteriologic, and roentgenologic studies should be obtained for diagnosis of any of the large number of possible underlying causes (Table 88-1).

Anergy occurs in the presence of some benign forms of leukocytosis [126]. This should be considered in the interpretation of negative skin tests to tuberculin or similar antigens.

Therapy

Attention is directed in most neutrophilic states to the treatment of the underlying cause.

References

1. Altman, R. L., and Dittmer, D. S.: *Blood and Other Body Fluids.* Federation of American Societies for Experimental Biology, Washington, D.C. 1961.
2. Karayalcin, G., Rosner, F., and Sawitsky, A.: Pseudoneutropenia in Negroes. A normal phenomenon. *N.Y. State J. Med.* 72:1815, 1972.
3. Shoenfeld, Y., et al.: Familial leukopenia among Yemenite Jews. *Isr. J. Med. Sci.* 14:1271, 1978.
4. Coulombel, L., Dehan, M., Tchernia, G., Hill, C., and Vial, M.: The number of polymorphonuclear leukocytes in relation to gestational age in the newborn. *Acta Paediatr. Scand.* 68:709, 1979.
5. Krumbhaar, E. B.: Leukemoid blood pictures in various clinical conditions. *Am. J. Med. Sci.* 172:519, 1926.
6. Hill, J. M., and Duncan, C. N.: Leukemoid reactions. *Am. J. Med. Sci.* 201:847, 1941.
7. Wintrobe, M. M.: Diagnostic significance of changes in leukocytes. *Bull. N.Y. Acad. Med.* 15:223, 1939.
8. Hilts, S. V., and Shaw, C. C.: Leukemoid blood reactions. *N. Engl. J. Med.* 249:434, 1953.
9. Welsh, J. D., and Denny, W. F.: Diagnostic problems presented by the leukemoid reaction. *Med. Times* 88:16, 1960.
10. Athens, J. W., et al.: Leukokinetic studies. III. The distribution of granulocytes in the blood of normal subjects. *J. Clin. Invest.* 40:159, 1961.
11. Cartwright, G. E., Athens, J. W., Haab, O. P., Raab, S. O., Boggs, D. R., and Wintrobe, M. M.: Blood granulocyte kinetics in conditions associated with granulocytosis. *Ann. N.Y. Acad. Sci.* 113:963, 1964.
12. Cronkite, E. P.: Kinetics of granulopoiesis. *Clin. Haematol.* 8:351, 1979.
13. Von Schulthess, G. K., and Mazer, N. A.: Cyclic neutropenia (CN): A clue to the control of granulopoiesis. *Blood* 59:27, 1982.
14. Perry, S., Weinstein, I. M., Craddock, C. G., Jr., and Lawrence, J. S.: The combined use of typhoid vaccine and P32 labeling to assess myelopoiesis. *Blood* 12:549, 1957.
15. Bishop, C. R., Athens, J. W., Boggs, D. R., Warner, H. R., Cartwright, G. E., and Wintrobe, M. M.: Leukokinetic studies. 13. A non-steady-state kinetic evaluation of the mechanism of cortisone-induced granulocytosis. *J. Clin. Invest.* 47:249, 1968.
16. Dale, D. C., Fauci, A. S., Guerry, D., IV, and Wolff, S. M.: Comparison of agents producing a neutrophilic leukocytosis in man. *J. Clin. Invest.* 56:808, 1975.
17. Murdoch, J. Mc C., and Smith, C. C.: Infection. *Clin. Haematol.* 1:619, 1972.
18. Athens, J. W.: Leukocyte physiology. *JAMA* 198:38, 1966.
19. Athens, J. W., et al.: Leukokinetic studies. IV. The total blood, circulating, and marginal granulocyte pools and the granulocyte turnover rate in normal subjects. *J. Clin. Invest.* 40:989, 1961.
20. Ahlborg, B., and Ahlborg, G.: Exercise leukocytosis with and without beta-adrenergic blockade. *Acta Med. Scand.* 187:241, 1970.
21. Mayne, E. E., Fitzpatrick, J., and Nelson, S. D.: Leukocytosis following administration of cryoprecipitate. *Acta Haematol. (Basel)* 44:155, 1970.
22. Mishler, J. M., and Sharp, A. A.: Adrenaline: Further discussion of its role in the mobilization of neutrophils. *Scand. J. Haematol.* 17:78, 1976.
23. Steel, C. M., French, E. B., and Aitchison, W. R. C.: Studies on adrenaline-induced leukocytosis in normal man. I. The role of the spleen and of the thoracic duct. *Br. J. Haematol.* 21:413, 1971.
24. French, E. B., Steel, C. M., and Aitchison, W. R. C.: Studies on adrenaline-induced leukocytosis in normal man. II. The effects of adrenergic blocking agents. *Br. J. Haematol.* 21:434, 1971.
25. Steinberg, B., and Martin, R. A.: Plasma factor increasing circulating leukocytes. *Am. J. Physiol.* 161:14, 1950.
26. Gordon, A. S., et al.: Evidence for a circulating leukocytosis-inducing factor (LIF). *Acta Haematol. (Basel)* 23:323, 1960.
27. Bierman, H. R., Marshall, G. J., Kelly, K. H., and Byron, R. L., Jr.: Leucopheresis in man. II. Changes in circulating granulocytes, lymphocytes, and platelets in the blood. *Br. J. Haematol.* 8:77, 1962.
28. Gordon, A. S., Handler, E. S., Siegel, C. D., Dornfest, B. S., and Lo Bue, J.: Plasma factors influencing leukocyte release in rats. *Ann. N.Y. Acad. Sci.* 113:766, 1964.
29. Strausz, I., Kekes, E., and Szebeni, A.: Mechanism of prednisolone-induced leukocytosis in man. *Acta Haematol.* 33:40, 1965.
30. Wolff, S. M., Kimball, H. R., Perry, S., Root, R., and Kappas, A.: The biological properties of etiocholanolone. *Ann. Intern. Med.* 67:1268, 1967.
31. Boggs, D. R., Marsh, J. C., Chervenick, P. A., Cartwright, G. E., and Wintrobe, M. M.: Neutrophil releasing activity in plasma of normal human subjects injected with endotoxin. *Proc. Soc. Exp. Biol. Med.* 127:689, 1968.
32. Godwin, H. A., Zimmerman, T. S., Kimball, H. R., Wolff, S. M., and Perry, S.: The effect of etiocholanolone on the entry of granulocytes into the peripheral blood. *Blood* 31:461, 1968.
33. Ostlund, R. E., Bishop, C. R., and Atkins, J. W.: Evaluation of non-steady-state neutrophil kinetics during endoxin-induced granulocytosis. *Proc. Soc. Exp. Biol. Med.* 137:763, 1971.
34. Rother, K.: Leukocyte mobilizing factor: A new biological activity from the third component of complement. *Eur. J. Immunol.* 2:550, 1972.
35. Chervenick, P. A.: Relationships between neutrophil releasing factor (NRF) and colony stimulating factor (CSF). *Blood* 40:949, 1972.
36. Cline, M. J., Craddock, C. G., Gale, R. P., Golde, D. W., and Lehrer, R. I.: Granulocytes in human disease. *Ann. Intern. Med.* 81:801, 1974.
37. Mishler, J. M.: Hydroxyethyl starch as an experimental adjunct to leukocyte separation by centrifugal means: Review of safety and efficacy. *Transfusion* 15:449, 1975.
38. Clemmensen, O., et al.: Sequential studies of lymphocytes, neutrophils, and serum proteins during prednisone treatment. *Acta Med. Scand.* 199:105, 1976.
39. Dale, D. C., Guerry, D., IV, and Wolff, S. M.: Neutrophil-releasing activity in plasma of normal human subjects injected with etiocholanolone. *Proc. Soc. Exp. Biol. Med.* 156:192, 1977.
40. Mishler, J. M., and Emerson, P. M.: Development of neutrophilia by serially increasing doses of dexamethasone. *Br. J. Haematol.* 36:249, 1977.
41. Ghebrehiwet, B., and Müeller-Eberhard, H. J.: C3e: An acidic fragment of human C3 with leukocytosis-inducing activity. *J. Immunol.* 123:616, 1979.
42. Shoenfeld, Y., Gurewich, Y., Gallant, L. A., and Pinkhas, J.: Prednisone-induced leukocytosis. Influence of dosage, method, and duration of administration on the degree of leukocytosis. *Am. J. Med.* 71:773, 1981.

43. Craddock, P. R., Hammerschmidt, D. E., White, J. G., and Jacob, H. S.: Granulocyte (PMN) aggregometry—A new technique for the study of complement (C) and C5a effects upon PMN and their plasma membranes. *Blood* 48:961, 1976.

44. Chikkappa, G., Chanana, A. D., Chandra, P., and Cronkite, E. P.: Kinetics and regulation of granulocyte precursors during a granulopoietic stress. *Blood* 50:1099, 1977.

45. Morra, L., Ponassi, A., Gigli, G., Vercelli, N., and Sacchetti, C.: Blood colony-forming cells (CFU-C) and leukocyte colony-stimulating activity (CSA) in patients with neutrophilic leukocytosis. *Scand. J. Haematol.* 22:311, 1979.

46. Craddock, C. G., Perry, S., and Lawrence, J. S.: Dynamics of leukopoiesis and leukocytosis, as studied by leukopheresis and isotopic techniques. *J. Clin. Invest.* 35:285, 1956.

47. Milhorat, A. T., Small, S. M., and Diethelm, O.: Leukocytosis during various emotional states. *Arch. Neurol. Psychiatr.* 47:779, 1942.

48. Morley, A., King-Smith, E. A., and Stohlman, F., Jr.: The oscillatory nature of hemopoiesis, in *Hemopoietic Cellular Proliferation,* edited by F. Stohlman, Jr. Grune & Stratton, New York, 1970, p. 3.

49. Adamson, J. W., and Fialkow, P. J.: The pathogenesis of myeloproliferative syndromes. *Br. J. Haematol.* 38:229, 1978.

50. Rodriquez, A. R., and Lutcher, C. L.: Marked cyclic leukocytosis-leukopenia in chronic myelogenous leukemia. *Am. J. Med.* 60:1041, 1976.

51. Delmonte, L., and Liebelt, R. A.: Granulocytosis-promoting extract of mouse tumor tissue: Partial purification. *Science* 148:521, 1965.

52. Robinson, W. A.: Granulocytosis in neoplasia. *Ann. N.Y. Acad. Sci.* 230:212, 1974.

53. Lee, M., Durch, S., Dale, D., and Finch, C.: Kinetics of tumor-induced murine neutrophilia. *Blood* 53:619, 1979.

54. Reincke, U., Burlington, H., Carstein, A. L., Cronkite, E. P., and Laissue, J. A.: Hemopoietic effects in mice of a transplanted, granulocytosis-inducing tumor. *Exp. Hematol.* 6:421, 1978.

55. Burlington, H., Cronkite, E. P., Laissue, J. A., Reincke, U., and Shadduck, R. K.: Colony-stimulating activity in cultures of granulocytosis-inducing tumor. *Proc. Soc. Exp. Biol. Med.* 154:86, 1977.

56. Sato, N., et al.: Granulocytosis and colony-stimulating activity (CSA) produced by a human squamous cell carcinoma. *Cancer* 43:605, 1979.

57. Boggs, D. R., Malloy, E., Boggs, S. S., Chervenick, P. A., and Lee, R. E.: Kinetic studies of a tumor-induced leukemoid reaction in mice. *J. Lab. Clin. Med.* 89:80, 1977.

58. Christensen, R. D., and Rothstein, G.: Pitfalls in the interpretation of leukocyte counts of newborn infants. *Am. J. Clin. Path.* 72:608, 1979.

59. Rey, J. J., and Wolf, P. L.: Extreme leukocytosis in accidental electric shock. *Lancet* 1:18, 1968.

60. Ryhanen, P.: Effects of anesthesia and operative surgery on the immune response of patients of different ages. *Ann. Clin. Res. 9* (Suppl.):19, 1977.

61. Watkins, J., Ward, A. M., and Appleyard, T. M.: Changes in peripheral blood leukocytes following I.V. anaesthesia and surgery. *Br. J. Anaesth.* 49:953, 1977.

62. Cream, J. J.: Prednisolone-induced granulocytosis. *Br. J. Haematol.* 15:259, 1968.

63. Stephens, D. J.: The occurrence of myelocytes in the peripheral blood in lobar pneumonia. *Am. J. Med. Sci.* 188:332, 1934.

64. Nettleship, A.: Leukocytosis associated with acute inflammation. *Am. J. Clin. Pathol.* 8:398, 1938.

65. Cress, C. H., Clare, F. B., and Gellhorn, E.: The effect of anoxic and anemic anoxia on the leukocyte count. *Am. J. Physiol.* 140:299, 1943.

66. Brown, H. W.: *Basic Clinical Parasitology.* Appleton-Century-Crofts, New York, 1975.

67. Douglas, R. G., Jr., Alford, R. H., Cate, T. R., and Couch, R. B.: The leukocyte response during viral respiratory illness in man. *Ann. Intern. Med.* 64:521, 1966.

68. Berman, C. L.: Peridontitis and leukocytosis. *N. Engl. J. Med.* 291:366, 1974.

69. Holland, P., and Mauer, A. M.: Myeloid leukemoid reactions in children. *Am. J. Dis. Child.* 105:568, 1963.

70. Chandra, R. K., and Bhakoo, O. N.: Leuco-erythroblastic (leukemoid) reaction in infants and children. *Indian J. Pediatr.* 2:411, 1965.

71. Calabro, J. J., Williamson, P., Love, E. S., Kostylo, F., and Jeghers, H.: Kawasaki syndrome. *N. Engl. Med.* 306:237, 1982.

72. Finch, S. C.: *Laboratory Findings in Infectious Mononucleosis,* edited by R. L. Carter and H. G. Penman. Blackwell, Oxford, 1969, p. 57.

73. Skarberg, K. O., Lagerlof, B., and Reizenstein, P.: Leukaemia, leukaemoid reaction and tuberculosis. *Acta Med. Scan.* 182:427, 1967.

74. Cameron, S. J.: Tuberculosis and the blood—A special relationship? *Tubercle* 55:55, 1974.

75. Corre, F., Lellouch, J., and Schwartz, D.: Smoking and leukocyte-counts. Results of an epidemiological survey. *Lancet* 2:632, 1971.

76. Friedman, G. D., Siegelaub, A. B., and Seltzer, C. C.: Smoking habits and the leukocyte count. *Arch. Environ. Health* 26:137, 1973.

77. Friedman, G. D., Klatsky, A. L., and Siegelaub, A. B.: The leukocyte count as a predictor of myocardial infarction. *N. Engl. J. Med.* 290:1275, 1974.

78. Zalokar, J. B., Richard, J. L., and Claude, J. R.: Leukocyte count, smoking and myocardial infarction. *N. Engl. J. Med.* 304:465, 1981.

79. Short, C. L., Bauer, W., and Reynolds, W. E.: Rheumatoid arthritis: A definition of the disease and a clinical description based on a numerical study of 293 patients and controls. Harvard University Press, Cambridge, Mass., 1957, p. 352.

80. Tullis, J. L.: A cause of leukocytosis in diabetic acidosis: Effects of experimental hypertonia on circulating leukocytes. *J. Clin. Invest.* 26:1098, 1947.

81. Colman, R. W., and Shein, H. M.: Leukemoid reaction, hyperuricemia, and severe hyperpyrexia complicating a fatal case of acute fatty liver of the alcoholic. *Ann. Intern. Med.* 57:110, 1962.

82. Wright, J. S.: Phenindione sensitivity with leukaemoid reaction and hepato-renal damage. *Postgrad. Med. J.* 46:452, 1970.

83. Shapiro, L., Baraf, C. S., and Richheimer, L. L.: Sweet's syndrome (acute febrile neutrophilic dermatosis), report of a case. *Arch. Dermatol.* 103:81, 1971.

84. Terry, S. I.: Transient dysaesthesiae and persistent leukocytosis after clioquinol therapy. *Br. Med. J.* 3:745, 1971.

85. Handelsman, M. B., Levitt, L., and Calabretta, M. F.: A laboratory and clinical study of chlorpropamide in ambulatory diabetics. *Ann. N.Y. Acad. Sci.* 74:632, 1959.

86. Mc Adams, K. P. W. J., Anders, R. F., Smith, S. R., Russell, D. A., and Price, M. A.: Association of amyloidosis with erythema nodosum leprosum reactions and recurrent neutrophil leukocytosis in leprosy. *Lancet* 2:572, 1975.

87. Dacie, J. V.: The haemolytic anaemias: Congenital and acquired, Part II, in *The Auto-immune Haemolytic Anaemias,* 2d ed. Grune & Stratton, New York, 1962, chap. 7, p. 360.

88. Ritchie, G. M.: Extensive myeloid response during folic acid therapy in megaloblastic anaemia of pregnancy. *J. Clin. Pathol.* 5:329, 1952.

89. Sclare, G., and Cragg, J.: A leukaemoid blood picture in megaloblastic anaemia of puerperium. *J. Clin. Pathol.* 11:45, 1958.

90. Michaelson, A. K.: Severe leukemoid reaction after promazine-induced agranulocytosis (1 case). *J. Fl. Med. Assoc.* 45:1418, 1959.

91. Rudivic, R., and Jelic, S.: Haematological aspects of drug-induced agranulocytosis. *Scand. J. Haematol.* 9:18, 1972.

92. Levine, P. H., and Weintraub, L. R.: Pseudoleukemia following recovery from dapsone-induced agranulocytosis. *Ann. Intern. Med.* 68:1060, 1968.

93. Kuvin, S. F., and Brecher, G.: Differential neutrophil counts in pregnancy. *N. Engl. J. Med.* 266:877, 1962.

94. Kinnealey, A. E., and Sweet, D. L., Jr.: Granulocyte in pregnancy. *J. Reprod. Med.* 19:172, 1977.

95. Efrati, P., Presentey, B., Margalith, M., and Rozenszajn, L.: Leukocytes of normal pregnant women. *Obstet. Gynecol.* 23:429, 1964.

96. Fahey, R. J.: Unusual leukocyte responses in primary carcinoma of the lung. *Cancer* 4:930, 1951.

97. Chen, H., and Walz, D. V.: Leukemoid reaction in the bone marrow, associated with malignant neoplasms. *Am. J. Clin. Pathol.* 29:345, 1958.

98. Meyer, L. M., and Rotter, S. D.: Leukemoid reaction (hyperleukocytosis) in malignancy. *Am. J. Clin. Pathol.* 12:218, 1942.

99. Tveter, K. J.: Unusual manifestations of renal carcinoma: A review of the literature. *Acta Chir. Scand.* 139:401, 1973.

100. Rubins, J., and Wakem, C. J.: Hypoglycemia and leukemoid reaction with hypernephroma. *N.Y. State J. Med. 77:*406, 1977.

101. Weinstein, H. J.: Congenital leukemia and the neonatal myeloproliferative disorders associated with Down's syndrome. *Clin. Haematol. 7:*147, 1978.

102. Brodeur, G. M., Dahl, G. V., Williams, D. L., Tipton, R. E., and Kalwinsky, D. K.: Transient leukemoid reaction and trisomy 21 mosaicism in a phenotypically normal newborn. *Blood 55:*691, 1980.

103. Heaton, D. C., Fitzgerald, P. H., Fraser, G. J., and Abbott, G. D.: Transient leukemoid proliferation of cytogenetically unbalanced T 21 cell line of a constitutional mosaic boy. *Blood 57:*883, 1981.

104. Ross, J. D., Maloney, W. C., and Desforges, J. F.: Ineffective regulation of granulopoiesis masquerading as congenital leukemia in a mongoloid child. *J. Pediatr. 63:*1, 1963.

105. Emery, J. L., Gordon, R. R., Rendle-Short, J., Varadi, S., and Warrack, A. J.: Congenital amegakaryocytic thrombocytopenia with congenital deformities and a leukemoid blood picture in the newborn. *Blood 12:*567, 1957.

106. Dignan, P. S., Mauer, A. M., and Frantz, C.: Phocomelia with congenital hypoplastic thrombocytopenia and myeloid leukemoid reactions. *J. Pediatr. 70:*561, 1967.

107. Rubin, S. L.: A case of congenital amegakaryocytic thrombocytopenia with leukemoid blood picture and congenital deformities. *Arch. Pediatr. 76:*251, 1959.

108. Ward, H. N., Reinhard, E. H.: Chronic idiopathic leukocytosis. *Ann. Intern. Med. 75:*193, 1971.

109. Herring, W. B., Smith, L. B., Walker, R. I., and Herion, J. C.: Hereditary neutrophilia. *Am. J. Med. 56:*729, 1974.

110. Randall, D. L., Reiquam, C. N., Githens, J. H., and Robinson, A.: Familial myeloproliferative disease. A new syndrome closely simulating myelogenous leukemia in childhood. *Am. J. Dis. Child. 110:*479, 1965.

111. Tindall, J. P., Beeker, S. K., and Rosse, W. F.: Familial cold urticaria. A generalized reaction involving leukocytosis. *Arch. Intern. Med. 124:*129, 1969.

112. Shopsin, B., Friedman, R., and Gershon, S.: Lithium and leukocytosis. *Clin. Pharmacol. Ther. 12:*923, 1971.

113. Murphy, D. L., Goodwin, F. K., and Bunney, W. E., Jr.: Leukocytosis during lithium treatment. *Am. J. Psychiatry 127:*1559, 1971.

114. Bille, P. E., Jensen, M. K., Jensen, J. P. K., and Poulsen, J. C.: Studies on the haematologic and cytogenetic effect of lithium. *Acta Med. Scand. 198:*281, 1975.

115. Stein, R. S., Hanson, G., Koethe, S., and Hansen, R.: Lithium-induced granulocytosis. *Ann. Intern. Med. 88:*809, 1978.

116. Rothstein, G., Clarkson, D. R., Larsen, W., Grosser, B. I., and Athens, J. W.: Effect of lithium on neutrophil mass and production. *N. Engl. J. Med. 298:*178, 1978.

117. Harker, W. G., Rothstein, G., Clarkson, D., and Athens, J. W.: Enhancement of colony-stimulating activity by lithium. *Blood 49:*263, 1977.

118. Turner, A. R., and Allalunis, M. J.: Mononuclear cell production of colony stimulating activity in humans taking oral lithium carbonate. *Blood 52 (Suppl. 1):*234, 1978.

119. Morley, D. C., and Galbraith, P. R.: Effect of lithium on granulopoiesis in culture. *Can. Med. Assoc. J. 118:*228, 1978.

120. Levitt, J. L., and Quesenberry, P. J.: The effect of lithium on murine hematopoiesis in a liquid culture system. *N. Engl. J. Med. 302:*713, 1980.

121. McBride, J. A., Dacie, J. V., and Shapley, R.: The effect of splenectomy on the leucocyte count. *Br. J. Haematol. 14:*225, 1968.

122. Spencer, R. P., Mc Phedran, P., Finch, S. C., and Morgan, W. S.: Persistent neutrophilic leukocytosis associated with idiopathic functional asplenia. *J. Nucl. Med. 13:*224, 1972.

123. Taft, E., Grossman, J., Abraham, G., Leddy, J., and Lichtman, M.: Pseudoleukocytosis due to cryoprotein crystals. *Am. J. Clin. Pathol. 60:*669, 1973.

124. Shah, P. C., Rao, K., Noble, V., Kumaraiah, V., and Patel, A. R.: Transient pseudoleukocytosis caused by cryocrystalglobinemia. *Arch. Pathol. Lab. Med. 102:*172, 1978.

125. Carmel, R., and Coltman, C. A., Jr.: Nonleukemic elevation of serum Vitamin B12 and B12-binding capacity levels resembling that in chronic myelogenous leukemia. *J. Lab. Clin. Med. 78:*289, 1971.

126. Heiss, L. I., and Palmer, D. L.: Anergy in patients with leukocytosis. *Am. J. Med. 56:*323, 1974.

127. Garrey, W. E., and Bryan, W. R.: Variations in white blood cell counts. *Physiol. Rev. 15:*597, 1935.

Neutrophil disorders—qualitative abnormalities of neutrophils

CHAPTER *89*

Qualitative abnormalities of neutrophils

LAURENCE A. BOXER
THOMAS P. STOSSEL

Chemotaxis and phagocytosis must be intact for neutrophils to function in their key role of protecting the host against infection. A structural or biochemical abnormality of neutrophils that impairs either of these functions places the host at an increased risk to infection. The first disease described which resulted from a neutrophil functional defect was chronic granulomatous disease of childhood (CGD) in which neutrophils are capable of ingesting but not of killing certain microorganisms.

Disorders of neutrophil function may arise from abnormalities of the (1) antibodies required to opsonize microorganisms or the plasma factors which provide chemotactic signals for neutrophils, (2) neutrophil's capability to respond to these proteins, (3) motile responses of the neutrophil, or (4) bactericidal mechanisms of the neutrophil (see Chap. 83). In the present chapter disorders of neutrophils in which the pathogenesis is relatively well understood are reviewed. Other comprehensive reviews of these syndromes are available to the interested reader [1–4].

Abnormalities of the signal mechanism—humoral defects

Table 89-1 provides an outline of the humoral abnormalities associated with neutrophil dysfunction. The references to the original articles describing these disorders are included in the table.

Since a synergistic action of immunoglobulins and complement proteins create the opsonins that coat microorganisms and stimulate the development of chemo-

tactic factors, either deficiency may result in impaired neutrophil function. The most profound disturbances arise from abnormalities of C3, since this protein is the focal point for generation of opsonins and chemotactic factors. Activation of C3 can occur in the absence of antibody or of the classical complement proteins, C1, C4, and C2, and thus disorders of these molecules are of less clinical significance. Patients with C3 deficiency have been described. Total deficiency is associated with recurrent severe pyogenic infections and is inherited in an autosomal recessive pattern. The C3 concentration in the serum of heterozygotes is half the normal level. A second defect in patients which results in pyogenic infections is a deficiency of the C3b inactivator, a protein inhibitor of the alternate complement pathway. Unchecked activation of this pathway leads to hypercatabolism of C3 and factor B.

The large number of chemotactic substances generated during inflammation makes it difficult to establish that a reduction in one compound is important. Furthermore, chemotactic factors and opsonins are involved in the activity of both neutrophils and mononuclear phagocytes. Therefore it may not be clear whether the clinical consequences of disorders involving these substances are unique to one or the other of these phagocytic cells. Patients with antibody- or complement-deficiency syndromes suffer mainly from infections with virulent encapsulated pathogens, such as *Hemophilus influenzae*, pneumococci, streptococci, and meningococci. Splenectomized individuals, deprived of an organ rich in mononuclear phagocytes, which provides intimate contact between these cells and circulating microorganisms, have a small but finite risk of sepsis due to the same microorganisms [20]. These encapsulated pathogens are not the ones characteristically associated with neutropenic states. These observations suggest that the interaction between humoral mediators and phagocytes may be most important to opsonize certain encapsulated microorganisms so as to ensure clearance by mononuclear phagocytes and may be less important for their ingestion by neutrophils.

Abnormalities of the cellular responses—defects in cytoplasmic movement (Table 89-2)

THE CHÉDIAK-HIGASHI SYNDROME
This rare autosomal recessive disease was initially recognized as a disorder in which neutrophils, monocytes, and lymphocytes contained giant cytoplasmic granules [21,22] (Fig. 89-1). The Chédiak-Higashi syndrome is now recognized as a generalized cellular dysfunction characterized by increased fusion of cytoplasmic granules. Albinism, involving the hair, skin, and ocular fundi, results from pathologic aggregation of melanosomes. Increased susceptibility of the patients to infection can be explained, in part, by defective degranulation of abnormal neutrophil granules. Other features

TABLE 89-1   Humoral abnormalities associated with neutrophil dysfunction

Abnormality	Etiology	Effect on neutrophil function	Clinical consequences
Antibody-deficiency syndromes	Early infancy Genetic Acquired idiopathic Secondary to lymphatic neoplasms	Deficiency of serum chemotactic activity and opsonic activity for encapsulated pathogens [5,6]	Recurrent pyogenic infections
Disorders of complement: C1r, C2, C4	Genetic absence	Subtle alterations in serum chemotactic and opsonic activity [7,8]	Possible increase in susceptibility to infection
C3 deficiency	Genetic absence Genetic hypercatabolism	Profoundly deficient serum chemotactic and opsonic activity [9]	Recurrent pyogenic infections
Properdin factor B deficiency	Some neonates	Deficient serum opsonic activity [10]	(?) A cause of susceptibility to infections
C5 deficiency	Genetic absence	Deficient serum chemotactic activity [11,12]	Recurrent pyogenic infections
Activation of C5a	Bacterial sepsis Systemic lupus erythematosus Post-cellophane dialysis	Enhanced neutrophil stickiness [13–15]	Neutropenia and formation of embolic leukoaggregates
Depletion of multiple factors; inhibitors of activation	Rheumatoid arthritis, systemic lupus erythematosus, hepatic cirrhosis, immune complex disease, severe infections, thermal burns, sickle cell anemia, Hodgkin's disease, sarcoidosis, renal disease, other inflammatory states	Deficient serum chemotactic and/or opsonic activity [3,4,16–18]	Recurrent infections
Disorders of other humoral systems: Plasminogen proactivator deficiency	Genetic absence	Deficient serum chemotactic activity [19]	None

of the disease include neutropenia, thrombocytopenia, deficiency of natural-killer-cell activity of lymphocytes, recurrent unexplained fever, and peripheral neuropathy [23,24].

Chédiak-Higashi syndrome patients have prolonged bleeding with normal platelet counts resulting from impaired platelet aggregation associated with a deficiency of the storage pools of ADP and serotonin [25,26]. There is a peculiar propensity for lymphohistiocytic proliferation to occur in the liver, spleen, and marrow, which intensifies the pancytopenia. This proliferation is associated with recurrent bacterial and viral infections, fever, and prostration, and usually results in death. What effect the lack of natural killer cells has in this process is unknown. This constellation has been termed the *accelerated phase* of the Chédiak-Higashi syndrome. Similar genetic syndromes have been discovered in mice, mink, cats, cattle, and killer whales [27,28].

PATHOGENESIS
The basic abnormality underlying the Chédiak-Higashi syndrome is unknown, but altered membrane fusion probably is important [29–33]. Neutrophils behave as if

they were unable to regulate membrane activation. They spontaneously aggregate surface molecules into "caps"; exhibit high resting rates of oxygen consumption and hexose monophosphate shunt activity; and demonstrate impaired adherence to surfaces and reduced chemotactic responses [34–39]. In addition, beginning early in neutrophil development, there is fusion of giant primary granules with each other, with normal-sized primary and secondary granules, and with cytoplasmic membrane components converting the massive primary granules into huge secondary lysosomes, which contain a reduced content of hydrolytic enzymes [31,40–42]. In spite of normal ingestion of particles and active oxygen metabolism, the neutrophils kill microorganisms relatively slowly. This delay reflects a slow and inconsistent delivery of diluted amounts of hydrolytic enzymes from the giant granules into the phagosome [31,36,37,43,44]. The functional derangements of neutrophils in this syndrome have also been found in monocytes [45].

Molecular movements within the membrane are probably critical to cell function. Thus altered membrane structure could lead to defective regulation of

Table 89-2 Neutrophil dysfunction—cellular abnormalities

Abnormality	Etiology	Impaired neutrophil functions	Clinical consequences
Chédiak-Higashi syndrome [21–47]	Unknown; pathologically activated membrane (?)	Neutropenia Decreased chemotactic responsiveness Defective degranulation Delayed microbial killing	Recurrent pyogenic infections
Neutrophil actin dysfunction [48]	Defective polymerization of neutrophil cytoplasmic actin	Impaired chemotactic responsiveness and ingestion, regulation of granule fusion	Frequent bacterial infections without pus
Neutrophil anchoring deficiency [49]	Absence of 180,000-dalton membrane protein	Decreased adherence to surfaces and particles	Recurrent pyogenic infections
Neutrophil ATP deficiency [50,51]	Hyperalimentation without phosphate supplementation	Impaired chemotactic responsiveness and ingestion	Cause of frequent infections (?)
Neutrophil "paralysis" [52–75]	Various inhibitors associated with hepatic cirrhosis, rheumatoid arthritis, immune complex diseases, systemic lupus erythematosus, severe infections, multiple myeloma, thermal burns, graft-vs.-host disease, products of the bacteria *Capnocytophaga*	Impaired chemotactic responsiveness, adhesion, ingestion, microbial killing	
Drug effects [76–87]	Ethanol; corticosteroids, cyclic adenosine monophosphate	Impaired locomotion	Possible cause for frequent infections Neutrophilia seen with epinephrine
Chronic granulomatous disease [88–130]	Absence of neutrophil oxidase function	Absent activation of neutrophil O_2 metabolism	Recurrent pyogenic infections with catalase-positive microorganisms
	Total glucose-6-phosphate-dehydrogenase deficiency	Failure to kill catalase-positive microbes	
	Other	Selective defect in activation of neutrophil O_2	Recurrent pyogenic infections
Myeloperoxidase [131–139]	Genetic Associated with myeloproliferative disorders	Hydrogen peroxide–dependent antimicrobial activity not potentiated by myeloperoxidase	None
Glutathione reductase and glutathione synthetase deficiency [140–144]	Failure to maintain adequate GSH levels	Excessive formation of hydrogen peroxide	Minimal problem with recurrent pyogenic infections
Miscellaneous defects [145–152]	Patients receiving craniospinal irradiation, chronic granulocyte leukemia, other myeloproliferative disorders, malnutrition	Not determined	Unknown

membrane activation by Chédiak-Higashi syndrome neutrophils. Indeed, investigation of human and mouse neutrophil and erythrocyte membranes by spin-labeled electron spin resonance spectrometry indicate that the Chédiak-Higashi syndrome blood cell membranes are more fluid than controls [30,33]. The specific effect on membrane fluidity on cell function is unknown, but surface receptor expression is influenced, which could possibly lead to elevated levels of cyclic adenosine monophosphate, disordered assembly of microtubules, and defective interaction of microtubules with lysosomal membranes, all of which occur in this disorder [32,34,44].

A unifying hypothesis for the aberrations of the Chédiak-Higashi syndrome is that the abnormal membrane leads to uncontrolled granule fusion as well as other defects [31,40,46], including the inability of the cells to move normally, concentrate serotonin into platelets, and express natural killer lymphocyte function. Secretion of pyrogens from fixed monuclear phagocytes could explain the recurrent febrile episodes.

CLINICAL FEATURES

The patient has light skin, silvery hair, and photophobia. Solar sensitivity may be a complaint. Other signs and symptoms vary considerably. These include infections, neuropathy, and concomitants of the accelerated phase (see below). The diagnosis is established by the presence of large inclusions in all nucleated blood cells. These can be seen on Wright's-stained blood films but are accentuated by peroxidase stains.

The infections involve the skin, respiratory tract, and mucous membranes, and are caused by gram-positive and gram-negative bacteria and by fungi. The most common organism is *Staphylococcus aureus*. The neuropathy may be sensory or motor in type. Ataxia may also be a prominent feature. The onset of the accelerated phase may occur at any age. Typically, the patients develop hepatosplenomegaly and high fever in the absence of bacterial sepsis. The pancytopenia becomes worse at this stage, producing hemorrhage and increasing the susceptibility to infection. Overwhelming sepsis resulting in death follows. At autopsy, the lymphohistiocytic infiltrates in the liver, spleen, and lymph nodes are extensive but not clearly neoplastic by histopathologic criteria. Therefore, despite the malignant nature of the accelerated phase, it is not entirely correct to designate it a lymphoma.

TREATMENT

The Chédiak-Higashi syndrome presents a therapeutic dilemma, particularly when the accelerated phase begins. Prophylactic antibiotics do not control infections [46]. Glucocorticoids and vincristine therapy have been used, but their efficacy is not established [23]. Treatment of neutrophils in vitro with ascorbate reduces membrane fluidity to normal values and enhances the bactericidal activity of the cells. When ascorbate was administered to patients in vivo, it resulted in functional and clinical improvements in some patients but not in all [44,47].

NEUTROPHIL ACTIN DYSFUNCTION

Neutrophil actin dysfunction has been observed in a male infant who had repeated infections with grampositive and gram-negative bacteria from birth but failed to produce pus [48]. The infections involved the skin and gastrointestinal tract. The patient's blood contained large numbers of morphologically normal band and segmented neutrophils. Although the patient's serum was active in generating chemotactic factors and opsonins, his neutrophils did not migrate toward inflamed sites in vivo or toward a source of chemotactic factor in vitro. They ingested at a markedly depressed rate. The neutrophils had normal to high ATP levels, rates of lactate production, and rates of reactions associated with oxygen metabolism. Oxygen metabolism of the neutrophils was activated in response to the ingestion of particles, and markedly increased quantities of granule enzymes were extruded into the extracellular medium and into phagosomes. Monocytes of the patient functioned normally. A unifying explanation for the abnormalities of neutrophil function was provided by the finding that monomeric actin in homogenates of the patient's neutrophils did not polymerize into fila

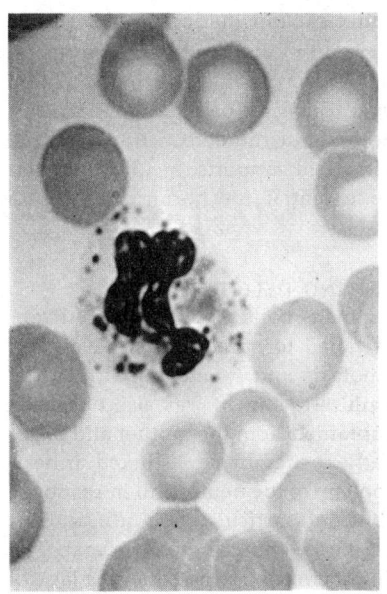

a

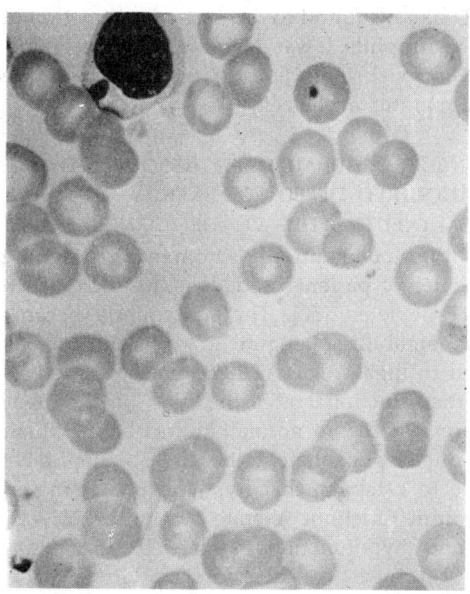

b

FIGURE 89-1 Blood films of patients with the Chédiak-Higashi syndrome. (*a*) The granulocyte contains large amorphic cytoplasmic granulations. (*b*) A large inclusion is easily seen in a lymphocyte.

ments under conditions which polymerized normal neutrophil actin. The basis of the defective polymerization of the actin was not determined, but the fact that a marrow graft resulted in normally functioning neutrophils suggested that the cause might be genetic. The failure of actin to assemble into filaments was consistent with the putative role assigned to reversible polymerization of this protein in the formation of pseudopodia for locomotion and ingestion and as a barrier regulating granule fusion with the membrane. The failure to cre ate pseudopodia would explain the impaired motility, while the failure to produce a barrier to granule fusion would explain the increased granule enzyme secretion in response to a given quantity of ingested particles. The discovery of the basis of the defect in locomotion and ingestion in this patient supports the idea that contractile proteins are essential for normal neutrophil function.

NEUTROPHIL ANCHORING DEFICIENCY

Neutrophils from a male child who had recurrent pyrogenic infections failed to spread on surfaces and had a defect in chemotaxis and a mild impairment in phagocytosis [49]. Failure to spread was also observed in a fraction of cells obtained from the mother and sister but not from the father, suggesting X-linked inheritance. Oxygen metabolism of the neutrophil in response to soluble stimuli (but not particulate stimuli) and release of granule enzyme by the cell were normal. The defects in neutrophil function were not due to a lack of IgG or C3 receptors nor to a defect in actin polymerization but were associated with an absence of a protein of $M_r = 180,000$ daltons found in the particulate fraction of the normal neutrophils. It was suggested that the inability to anchor to surfaces led to impairment in the locomotor apparatus of the cell.

IMPAIRED NEUTROPHIL MOTILITY ASSOCIATED WITH AN ACQUIRED DEFECT OF ENERGY METABOLISM (NEUTROPHIL ATP DEFICIENCY)

In one study the blood neutrophils from hyperalimented hypophosphatemic patients and dogs were found to become ATP-depleted [50]. The neutrophils became deficient in their ability to migrate toward a chemotactic gradient and to ingest. The ATP content of the leukocytes and the functional abnormalities of the neutrophils were restored to normal by incubating them with adenosine or phosphate. Other investigators have been unable to establish that hypophosphatemia impairs neutrophil function. A state of neutrophil ATP deficiency and hypofunction manifested by an impaired ability to ingest can be created in vitro by poisoning the mitochondria of phosphoglycerate kinase–deficient neutrophils with potassium cyanide [51]. Energy in the form of ATP is important for the motile responses of polymorphonuclear leukocytes.

OTHER DISORDERS OF NEUTROPHIL MOTILITY (NEUTROPHIL "PARALYSIS")

Patients with recurrent infections whose neutrophils were believed to have impairments of chemotactic responsiveness, ingestion, or both have been described, although the basis of the abnormalities was not defined [52–54]. In one series of patients with congenital neutropenia it was concluded that blood and marrow neutrophils were defective in locomotion [55]. Toxic products from the microbe *Capnocytophaga* inhibited neutrophil motility and were implicated in the pathogenesis or periodontal disease [56]. Abnormal neutrophil motile responses have been observed in various patients with systemic illnesses. In some patients with bacterial sepsis, Felty's syndrome, systemic lupus erythematosus, and post-cellophane membrane dialysis, neutropenia and enhanced neutrophil adhesiveness have acccompanied the diminished chemotactic responses and ability to ingest [14,15,57–61]. Complement activation leading to the generation of C5a has been observed in some of these disorders, which in turn affects the surface properties of neutrophils, causing the cells to adhere avidly to endothelial surfaces and aggregate with each other [14,15]. After thermal injury, several circulating substances that inhibit neutrophil chemotaxis have been found [17]. In patients with a burn exceeding 40 percent of the total body surface area defective chemotaxis of the neutrophils has been observed. Coincident with the impaired chemotaxis, the thermally injured neutrophils contain diminished specific granule contents. These studies in burned patients suggested that in vivo neutrophil secretion of specific granule contents may result in impaired chemotaxis through release of acidic proteins and lactoferrin, which have been shown to enhance neutrophil "stickiness" [62,63]. In cases of severe eczema associated with eosinophilia, hypergammaglobulinemia E, and recurrent skin infections primarily with *S. aureus*, defective chemotaxis has been observed [17,64,65]. In patients with multiple myeloma, viral infection, IgA paraproteinemia, or those undergoing graft-versus-host reaction following marrow transplantation, chemotaxis has also been depressed [4,66–68]. Although the basis of the chemotactic defect in these diseases is unknown, it is possible that circulating immune complexes, endotoxin, or aggregated IgG could absorb to the neutrophil membranes, causing general activation of the cell, thereby leading to impaired chemotaxis, high resting states of oxygen metabolism, and granule enzyme release [60,69,70]. Little is known about treatment of the chemotactic disorders, although the antihelminthic agent levamisole has improved the chemotactic response of neutrophils from patients with hypergammaglobulinemia E syndrome [71].

Hyperosmolarity impairs neutrophil function, as shown in patients with diabetic ketoacidosis or poorly controlled hyperglycemia whose neutrophils did not perform adequately [72,73]. Decreased neutrophil chemotactic responsiveness has also been reported in leukocytes from patients with diabetes mellitus in experiments which were performed in media of normal osmolarities [74,75]. The reproducibility of the findings and their relevance to the problem of infection in diabetes mellitus requires further study.

DRUGS THAT IMPAIR NEUTROPHIL MOTILITY

Although many pharmacologic agents can influence neutrophil functions (see Chap. 83), few drugs used in clinical medicine have been shown to alter neutrophil activities in vivo. Ethanol, in concentrations that occur in human blood, has been found to inhibit neutrophil locomotion and ingestion [76–78]. Glucocorticoid therapy, especially with high and sustained doses, has been shown to inhibit neutrophil migration, adhesiveness, and ability to ingest [79–85]. Administration of glucocorticoids on alternative days did not interfere with neutrophil movement [82]. If such treatment diminishes functional capabilities of neutrophils, the rise in the total-body granulocyte pool and granulocyte production might constitute a compensatory response. Indeed, a decrease in granulocyte egress from the blood has been observed in kinetic studies of patients receiving glucocorticoids [86]. Cyclic AMP, which is released from endothelial cells following exposure to epinephrine, can also depress neutrophil chemotaxis and adherence [4,87]. Similarly elevated cyclic adenosine monophosphate levels following epinephrine administration in vivo may impair neutrophil adherence leading to diminished neutrophil margination and account for the frequently observed neutrophilia seen with epinephrine [87].

Defects in microbicidal activity

CHRONIC GRANULOMATOUS DISEASE
Chronic granulomatous disease of childhood (CGD) is a genetic disorder in which polymorphonuclear leukocytes and monocytes ingest but do not kill catalase-positive microorganisms because the cells fail to generate oxygen metabolites that normally kill these microbes.

PATHOGENESIS
The metabolism of oxygen to superoxide anion and hydrogen peroxide by neutrophils is described in Chap. 83. The functional defects in CGD neutrophils, which are embedded in the genetic program of neutrophil progenitor cells, could be due to absence of the oxidase enzyme system, which reduces oxygen, or a more generalized abnormality of the membrane leading to a failure of this system to be activated by membrane stimulation [88–92]. It is not possible to choose between these alternatives, because neither the activation mechanism nor the responsible oxygen-metabolizing enzymes have been definitely identified. In fact, CGD, defined as a disorder in which neutrophils do not metabolize oxygen, may be biochemically heterogeneous.

The genetics of CGD support this concept. In some families, CGD is clearly transmitted as an X-linked disorder [93]. In others, it is either sporadic, is autosomally inherited, or represents X-inactivation of normally functioning cells in female carriers [94–98]. Attempts to distinguish biochemically the patients with different patterns of inheritance have been inconclusive. Some investigators reported somewhat diminished hydrogen peroxide–mediated reduced glutathione (GSH)–oxidizing activity in leukocytes of female patients with (presumed) autosomally inherited CGD [99]. However, such changes were not found in other female patients [100]. Although subnormal bactericidal and oxygen-metabolizing activity in leukocytes of putative female carriers of the sex-linked variety of

CGD has been documented, it has not been shown that leukocytes from relatives of other CGD patients have abnormal functional or metabolic capacities. Most patients with CGD have leukocytes with normal glucose-6-phosphatase dehydrogenase activity, but a few individuals have been described with clinical findings of CGD and with neutrophils totally or almost totally lacking in glucose-6-phosphate dehydrogenase activity [101,102]. The erythrocytes of these patients also lacked the enzyme, and the patients had chronic hemolysis. As in other CGD patients, the neutrophils failed to activate their oxygen metabolism in response to membrane stimulation. The observations support the concept that reduced pyridine nucleotides, which are regenerated by activity of glucose-6-phosphate dehydrogenase, are involved in the production of oxygen metabolites by neutrophils. CGD may thus be the final common pathway of a number of different molecular defects.

The manner in which the metabolic deficiency of the CGD neutrophil predisposes the host to infection is shown schematically in Fig. 89-2. Normal neutrophils accumulate hydrogen peroxide (and other oxygen metabolites) in the phagosome containing ingested microorganisms. Hydrogen peroxide plus myeloperoxidase, delivered to the phagosome by degranulation, kills the incorporated microbe. The quantity of hydrogen peroxide produced by the normal neutrophil is sufficient to exceed the capacity of catalase, a hydrogen peroxide–catabolizing enzyme, possessed by many aerobic microorganisms, including *S. aureus*, most gram-negative enteric bacteria, *Candida albicans*, and *Aspergillus* species. However, when these organisms gain entry to CGD neutrophils, they are not exposed to hydrogen peroxide, because the neutrophil does not produce it, and the hydrogen peroxide generated by the microbes themselves is destroyed by the accompanying catalase. The catalase-positive microbes can multiply intracellularly, where they are protected from most circulating antibiotics and can be transported to distant sites and released to establish new foci of infection [103,104]. The granulomatous nature of the lesions of CGD is reminiscent of infections by organisms which survive intracellularly in normal phagocytes, such as mycobacteria. In hema-

FIGURE 89-2 The pathogenesis of chronic granulomatous disease (CGD). (See text for explanation.)

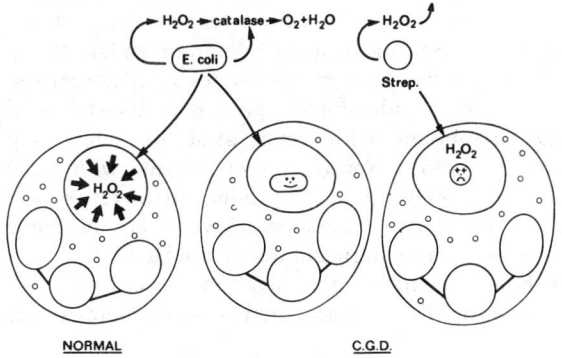

TABLE 89-3   Clinical manifestations of chronic granulomatous disease [104,118–121]

System	Disease
Skin	Eczematous dermatitis
	Granulomas
	Pyoderma
Ear-nose-throat	Otitis
	Rhinitis
	Sinusitis
Cardiopulmonary	Pericarditis
	Mediatinitis
	Pneumonia
	Focal lung abscess
	Diffuse persistent pulmonary infiltrates
Gastrointestinal	Ulcerative stomatitis
	Esophagitis
	Antral granuloma or thickening with obstruction
	Subphrenic abscess
	Focal liver abscess
	Miliary liver abscesses
	Granulomatous ileitis/colitis
	Vitamin B_{12} malabsorption
	Steatorrhea
	Perianal fistulae
Genitourinary	Renal abscess
	Pyelonephritis
	Cystitis
	Dysuria of unknown cause
Endocrine	Septic thyroiditis with thyrotoxicosis
Neurologic	Meningitis
	Epidural abscess
Hematologic	Granulocytosis
	Hypochromic/microcyctic anemia
Immunologic	Diffuse hypergammaglobulinemia
	Lymphadenopathy
	Suppurative lymphadenitis
	Splenomegaly
	Urticaria, arthralgias, costochondritis
Musculoskeletal	Osteomyelitis
	Septic arthritis
	Pyomyositis

toxylin-eosin-stained sections of tissue from patients with CGD, macrophages may contain a golden pigment, which is thought to reflect abnormal accumulation of ingested material [105].

When CGD neutrophils ingest pneumococci or streptococci, they kill them, because these organisms do not contain catalase. These organisms generate hydrogen peroxide which, together with myeloperoxidase delivered to the phagosomes of CGD neutrophils, kills them. The pathogenetic mechanisms just described are consistent with the epidemiologic pattern of infections of CGD patients and with results of studies employing bacterial mutants. Neutrophils of patients with CGD can kill pneumococci which produce hydrogen peroxide, but not mutant pneumococci which are incapable of producing it in sufficient quantities [106].

Although the most impressive functional disorder of CGD neutrophils is their failure to activate their oxygen

metabolism in response to membrane stimulation, other functional abnormalities have been reported. Some [107–109], but not all [37,110–114], investigators have described quantitative deficiencies of degranulation or ingestion by CGD neutrophils. Impaired chemotactic responsiveness has also been noted [115–116]. These findings may reflect the heterogeneity of CGD or may be the consequences of chronic infection itself.

CLINICAL FEATURES

The clinical presentation of CGD is variable, and not all its manifestations, summarized in Table 89-3, are explained by its pathogenesis. The onset of clinical signs and symptoms may occur at any age, ranging from early infancy to adulthood. By analyzing the ability of fetal neutrophils to generate superoxide anion, it is also possible to establish the diagnosis of CGD in utero after obtaining fetal cells by fetoscopy [117]. The attack rate and severity of infections are exceedingly variable.

The most common pathogen is *S. aureus*, although any catalase-positive microorganism may be involved. *Serratia marcescens* and *Salmonella* species appear frequently. Infections are characterized by microabscess and granuloma formation; the presence of pigmented histiocytes [105] is helpful in establishing the diagnosis. Patients may suffer from sequelae of chronic infection, including the anemia of chronic disease, arthralgias, urticaria, and costochondritis possibly related to the presence of circulating immune complexes.

Several mothers of patients in whom X-linked inheritance was established had an illness resembling systemic lupus erythematosus [122]. Most carriers of CGD are clinically well, although in some instances X-inactivation of normally functioning cells can lead to phenotypic CGD in carriers [99].

Another surprising finding in CGD is that some male patients have a rare Kell blood group erythrocyte and neutrophil phenotype, rendering them unusually susceptible to sensitization with Kell antigens [123].

Other patients have been described with recurrent bacterial infection whose neutrophils showed a selective defect in activation of the respiratory burst. In two siblings from one family, ingestion of unopsonized particles, in contrast to IgG-coated particles, failed to result in burst activation [124]. In another family neutrophils from a 2-year-old boy could not be activated with opsonized particles but could be activated with soluble stimuli [125]. These studies suggest that there is more than one pathway leading to activation of the respiratory burst.

TREATMENT

Attempts to correct the defect in bacterial killing by treating neutrophils or patients with agents affecting the redox activities of the cells have not been successful [3]. It has been necessary to focus on prophylaxis or therapy of infections in the management of these patients. Since the early description of this disease, the course and prognosis have improved. The reason for this improvement is unknown but may be due to better medical and surgical therapy or to discovery of milder cases which previously escaped diagnosis. The variable infection rate makes it very difficult to assess the value of prophylactic antibacterial regimens [126,127]. The use of antistaphylococcal antibiotics by these patients carries the risk of an increased incidence of infections with resistant pathogens [1,128].

When the diagnosis of CGD is established, it is advisable to obtain certain studies which aid in the management of septic episodes. These include chest and skeletal roentgenograms and liver and spleen scans. Arrangements should be made for prompt medical attention at the first signs of infection. With early intervention, many lesions can be managed by conservative medical techniques. For example, enlarging lymph nodes often regress when treated with local heat and orally administered antistaphylococcal antibiotics. More serious infections require hospitalization and diagnostic and therapeutic approaches applicable to any patient with severe infection. In general, antibiotic therapy for the offending organism is indicated, and purulent collections should be drained surgically. Unfortunately, the cause of fever and prostration cannot always be established, and empiric treatment with broad-spectrum parenteral antibiotics is required while establishing a specific diagnosis. The use of chloramphenicol has been advocated since it may penetrate more readily into neutrophils than do other antibiotics. Rifampin also has the capacity to diffuse into neutrophils [129], but its usefulness is limited by the rapid emergence of microbial resistance. Granulocyte transfusion therapy has been utilized in a desperately ill CGD patient with aspergillosis [130]. The CGD patient is abnormally susceptible to sensitization by transfusions, and it is difficult to recommend this treatment. CGD patient treated with glucocorticoids have fared poorly, and the use of glucocorticoids is not advocated.

MYELOPEROXIDASE DEFICIENCY
Functional and immunochemical absence of the enzyme myeloperoxidase from granules of neutrophils and monocytes but not from eosinophils is inherited as an autosomal recessive trait [131–135]. The lack of myeloperoxidase, an enzyme that potentiates the microbicidal effectiveness of hydrogen peroxide in the phagosome, causes a microbicidal deficiency of the neutrophils. Although detectable in vitro, the functional impairment is not as severe as that observed in the CGD neutrophil. Myeloperoxidase-deficient neutrophils accummulate more hydrogen peroxide than do normal neutrophils, and this higher peroxide concentration improves the bactericidal activity of the affected neutrophils [135]. Recent surveys suggest that myeloperoxidase deficiency may be common. The patients with this genetic disorder have not been unusually susceptible to pyogenic infections, although two affected patients who also had diabetes mellitus suffered from infection with *C. albicans* [133,136].

Deficiency of neutrophil myeloperoxidase has also been observed as an acquired disorder in patients with hematologic abnormalities such as refractory anemias or myeloproliferative disorders [137–139].

GLUTATHIONE REDUCTASE AND GLUTATHIONE SYNTHETASE DEFICIENCIES
The neutrophil has enzymes to inactivate potentially damaging reduced oxygen by-products. Disposal of superoxide anion is accomplished through dismutase, a soluble enzyme which converts superoxide to hydrogen peroxide. Hydrogen peroxide is detoxified by catalase and by a glutathione peroxidase–glutathione reductase system, which employs reduced glutathione to convert hydrogen peroxide to water and oxygen [3]. In addition to the soluble enzymes, cellular vitamin E serves as an antioxidant to prevent damage to the surface of activated cells while releasing hydrogen peroxide [140]. Inadequate reduced glutathione resulting from deficiencies in glutathione reductase or synthetase, which are inherited as autosomal recessive traits, can lead to bacterial impairment associated with oxidative damage of membranes and microtubules [141,142]. In contrast a congenital deficiency of neutrophil catalase can result in surface damage from external sources of hydrogen peroxide [143]. The glutathione redox cycle not only decomposes hydrogen peroxide as does catalase but is involved in repairing oxidized cell components [144]. Like the patients with myeloperoxidase-deficient neutrophils, the patients with glutathione reductase deficiency, glutathione synthetase deficiency, and catalase deficiency have not usually been susceptible to bacterial infections.

MISCELLANEOUS DISORDERS OF NEUTROPHIL FUNCTION
Tests of neutrophil bactericidal function have been performed in various disease states, and abnormalities have been reported. Abnormalities have been found in patients receiving craniospinal irradiation for acute lymphoblastic leukemia [145], in patients in remission from various leukemias [146], and in patients with protein-calorie malnutrition [147], paraproteinemia [148], rheumatoid arthritis [149], recurrent staphyloccal infections [150,151], and chronic myelogenous leukemia [152]. In most reports it is not possible to determine the cause or the significance of the findings.

Diagnostic approach to the patient with suspected neutrophil dysfunction

Susceptibility to pyogenic infection is determined by the adequacy of host defense and by the microbes to which the host is exposed and the conditions of the exposure. It is not always easy to establish a diagnosis of a specific neutrophil dysfunction on clinical grounds alone. Patients with recurrent pyogenic infections often

TABLE 89-4   Tests of neutrophil function

Test	Basis of test	Diagnoses established	Advantages	Limitations
Neutrophil morphology	Wright's stain	Chédiak-Higashi syndrome	Simple	Most disorders have normal morphology
	Peroxidase stain	Myeloperoxidase deficiency		
	Immunoperoxidase stain with lactoferrin antibody	Specific granule abnormality [153]		
Rebuck window assay	Neutrophils migrate into dermal abrasion and adhere to glass slide [154]	Severe impairment of neutrophil locomotion	An in vivo assay	Semiquantitative. Depends on blood neutrophil count. Not useful in neutropenic states [157]
Levels of serum factors involved in neutrophil functions	Functional or chemical tests of serum proteins	Complement and antibody deficiencies		Not all serum proteins involved have been isolated
Aggregation [57]	Neutrophils stick to each other during activation	Detection of complement activation	Multiple tests can be run	
Boyden chamber assay [155]	Neutrophils migrate through filters toward chemotactic source	Moderate to severe impairment of locomotion. Deficient chemotactic factors. Inhibitors against serum factors or cell movement	Multiple tests can be run	Great variation in results depending on source, handling of sera cells [156, 157]
Ingestion assays: Morphologic	Count "ingested" particles	Severe ingestion abnormality	Historic	Impossible to differentiate "ingested" from adherent particles
Quantitative	Assay initial rate of uptake of labeled particles	Subtle ingestion abnormalities	Precise	
Degranulation assays: Extracellular	Release of β-glucuronidase activity into medium			Most meaningful when corrected for magnitude of eliciting stimulus, e.g., ingestion rate
Intracellular	Release of β-glucuronidase into phagosomes [37]	Granule fusion abnormalities	Precise	
Assays of oxygen metabolism: Oxygen consumption	Assay of primary oxidase activity	Not activated by membrane stimulation in CGD		Most meaningful when corrected for magnitude of eliciting stimuli, e.g., ingestion rate [111]

yield no clues as to why they are afflicted, and patients with established deficiencies of a defense mechanism may have an unimpressive clinical history.

Unfortunately, many of the tests of neutrophil function are bioassays with great variability, and they may be inadequate for establishing mild impairments. For example, the profound failure of CGD neutrophils to active their rates of oxygen metabolism is easily documented; however, the detection of the carrier state in female relatives of male patients is difficult because of the test variability. This variation is intensified by inflammation or infection. Laboratory tests are listed in Table 89-4, along with assessments of their usefulness and limitations.

The interrelationship between the various neutrophil functions, especially those which are elicited by membrane activation is important in evaluating results of assays. For example, the microbicidal activity of neu-

trophils as measured by the bactericidal test in vitro is very dependent on the ingestion rate. It is necessary to perform quantitative measurements of ingestion rates before concluding that deficient bacterial killing is due to this abnormality. Some of the metabolic activities of neutrophils are also complex, and the interpretation of abnormalities is not possible without specific assays for functions which account for this complexity. The results of most of the tests shown in Table 89-4 must be scrutinized with great care. The assays are most rewarding when performed in laboratories which have acquired familiarity with their limitations and the wide variation in "normal" values.

Although specific therapy for the basic defect in neutrophil function is rarely possible, diagnosis of neutrophil disorders aids affected patients by allowing the physician to predict the type of problem likely to be encountered and to plan management.

TABLE 89-4   Tests of neutrophil function *(Continued)*

Test	Basis of test	Diagnoses established	Advantages	Limitations
Nitroblue tetrazolium reduction; redox dye reduced to blue insoluble formazan by superoxide anion [159]	Spectrophotometric assay for superoxide anion production in phagosomes of ingesting cells [95]	Not activated by membrane stimulation in CGD		
	Histochemical assay for determining individual cells that have reduced the dye to formazan	CGD and CGD carrier state		Morphologic findings difficult to interpret
Glucose oxidation Oxidation of [^{14}C]-1-glucose equivalent to hexose monophosphate shunt activity in neutrophils	Assay for hydrogen peroxide detoxification and reduced pyridine nucleotide turnover	Not activated by membrane stimulation in CGD		Dependent on multiple factors that must be recognized: radio-nucleide uptake and distribution, ingestion, rate of various metabolic reactions involved in the final measured value
Hydrogen peroxide formation [160]	Spectrofluorometic assay for hydrogen peroxide in activated cells	CGD		
Iodination: incorporation of radioactive iodide into covalent bond with proteins of phagosome of neutrophils	Assay for activity of myeloperoxidase in the presence of hydrogen peroxide [161]	Not activated by membrane stimulation in CGD or myeloperoxidase deficiency		
Assays of bactericidal activity: Bactericidal assay Diminution in viable microorganisms by colony-forming assay [162]	Assay for overall bactericidal activities of neutrophils	Abnormal in many disease states	Screening procedures	Dependent on multiple factors; not reliable unless abnormalities large Involved and time-consuming
Autoradiography	Tests ability of live bacteria inside neutrophils to incorporate tritiated thymidine [163]		Small samples	Time required for developing autoradiograms
Dye exclusion	Tests ability of live *Candida* inside neutrophils to exclude methylene blue [164]		Small samples	Semiquantitative
Specific bactericidal substances	Chemical and functional analysis of specific antibacterial and antifungal substances in neutrophils [165]			

References

1. Quie, P. G.: Pathology of bactericidal power of neutrophils. *Semin. Hematol. 12:*143, 1975.
2. Vilde, J. L.: Pathologie congénitale du polynucleaire neutrophile. *Nouv. Rev. Fr. Hematol. 14:*274, 1974.
3. Boxer, L. A., and Baehner, R. L.: Defects in neutrophil leukocyte function, in *Clinical Immunology Update,* edited by E. C. Franklin. Elsevier North-Holland, New York, 1981, p. 357.
4. Klebanoff, S. J., and Clark, R. A.: *The Neutrophil: Function and Clinical Disorders.* Elsevier North-Holland, New York, 1978, p. 489.
5. Gewurz, H., Page, A. R., Pickering, R. J., and Good, R. A.: Complement activity and inflammatory neutrophil exudation in man: Studies in patients with glomerulonephritis, essential hypocomplementemia, and agammaglobulinemia. *Int. Arch. Allergy Appl. Immunol. 32:*64, 1967.
6. Johnston, R. B., Jr., Klemperer, M. R., Alper, C. A., and Rosen, F. S.: The enhancement of bacterial phagocytosis by serum: The role of complement components and two cofactors. *J. Exp. Med. 129:*1275, 1969.
7. Gallin, J. I., Clark, R. A., and Frank, M. M.: Kinetic analysis of chemotactic factor generation in human serum via activation of the classical and alternate complement pathways. *Clin. Immunol. Immunopathol. 3:*334, 1975.
8. Root, R. K., Ellman, L., and Frank, M. M.: Bactericidal and opsonic properties of C4-deficient guinea pig serum. *J. Immunol. 109:*477, 1972.
9. Alper, C. A., and Rosen, F. S.: Complement deficiencies in humans, in *Clinical Immunology Update,* edited by E. C. Franklin. Elsevier North-Holland, New York, 1981, p. 59.
10. Stossel, T. P., Alper, C. A., and Rosen, F. S.: Opsonic activity in the newborn: Role of properdin. *Pediatrics 52:*134, 1973.
11. Rosenfeld, S. I., and Leddy, J. P.: Hereditary deficiency of fifth component of complement (C5) in man. *J. Clin. Invest. 53:*67a, 1974.
12. Synderman, R., Durack, D. J., McCarthy, G. A., Ward, F. E., and Meadows, L: Deficiency of the fifth component of complement in human subjects. *Am. J. Med. 67:*638, 1979.

13. O'Flaherty, J. I., and Ward, P. A.: Leukocyte aggregation induced by chemotactic factors: A review. *Inflammation 3*:177, 1978.

14. Craddock P. R., Hammerschmidt, D. E., Moldow, C. F., Yamado, O., and Jacob, H. S.: Granulocyte aggregation as a manifestation of membrane interactions with complement: Possible role in leukocyte margination, microvascular occlusion and endothelial damage. *Semin. Hematol. 16*:140, 1979.

15. Jacob, H. S., Craddock, P. R., Hammerschmidt, D. E., and Moldow, C. F.: Complement-induced granulocyte aggregation: An unsuspected mechanism of disease. *N. Engl. J. Med. 302*:789, 1980.

16. Van Epps, D. E., and Williams, R. C.: Serum inhibitors of leukocyte chemotaxis and their relationship to skin test allergy, in *Leukocyte Chemotaxis: Methods, Physiology, and Clinical Implications*, edited by J. I. Gallin and P. G. Quie. Raven Press, New York, 1978, p. 237.

17. Gallin, J. I., et al.: Disorders of phagocyte chemotaxis. *Ann. Intern. Med. 92*:520, 1980.

18. Johnston, R. B., Jr., Newman, S. L., and Struth, A. G.: An abnormality of the alternate pathway of complement activation in sickle-cell disease. *N. Engl. J. Med 288*:803, 1973.

19. Weiss, A. S., Gallin, J. I., and Kaplan, A. P.: Fletcher factor deficiency: A diminished rate of Hageman factor activation caused by absence of prekallikrein with abnormalities of coagulation, fibrinolysis, chemotactic activity, and kinin generation. *J. Clin. Invest. 53*:622, 1974.

20. Bisno, A. L., and Freeman, J. C.: The syndrome of asplenia, pneumococcal sepsis, and disseminated intravascular coagulation. *Ann. Intern. Med. 72*:389, 1970.

21. Chédiak, M.: Nouvelle anomalie leucocytaire de caractère constitutionnel familial. *Rev. Hematol. 7*:362, 1952.

22. Higashi, O.: Congenital gigantism of peroxidase granules: First case ever reported of qualitive abnormality of peroxidase. *Tohoku J. Exp. Med. 59*:315, 1954.

23. Blume, R. S., and Wolff, S. M.: The Chédiak-Higashi syndrome: Studies in four patients and a review of the literature. *Medicine (Baltimore) 561*:247, 1972.

24. Haliotis, T., et al.: Chédiak-Higashi gene in humans. I. Impairment of natural-killer function. *J. Exp. Med. 151*:1039, 1980.

25. Buchanan, G. R., and Handin, R. I.: Platelet function in the Chédiak-Higashi syndrome. *Blood 47*:941, 1976.

26. Boxer, G. J., et al.: Abnormal platelet function in Chédiak-Higashi syndrome. *Br. J. Haematol. 35*:521, 1977.

27. Prieur, D. J., and Collier, L. L.: Chédiak-Higashi syndrome of animals. *Am. J. Pathol. 90*:533, 1975.

28. Kramer, J. W., Davis, W. C., and Prieur, D. J.: The Chédiak-Higashi syndrome of cats. *Lab. Invest. 36*:554, 1977.

29. Kritzler, R. A., et al.: Chédiak-Higashi syndrome. Cytologic and lipid observations in a case and family. *Am. J. Med. 36*:583, 1964.

30. Haak, R. A., Ingraham, L. M., Baehner, R. L., and Boxer, L. A.: Membrane fluidity in human and mouse Chédiak-Higashi leukocytes. *J. Clin. Invest. 64*:138, 1979.

31. White, J. G., and Clawson, C. C.: The Chédiak-Higashi syndrome: The nature of the giant neutrophil granules and their interactions with cytoplasm and foreign particulates. *Am. J. Pathol. 98*:151, 1980.

32. Ostlund, R. E., Jr., Tucker, R. W., Leung, J. T., Okun, N., and Williamson, J. R.: The cytoskeleton in Chédiak-Higashi syndrome fibroblasts. *Blood 56*:806, 1980.

33. Ingraham, L. M., Burns, C. P., Boxer, L. A., Baehner, R. L., and Haak, R. A.: Fluidity properties and lipid composition of erythrocyte membranes in Chédiak-Higashi syndrome. *J. Cell Biol.* In press.

34. Oliver, J. M., and Zurier, R. B.: Correction of characteristic abnormalities of microtubule function and granule morphology in Chédiak-Higashi syndrome with cholinergic agonists. Studies in vitro in man and in vivo in the beige mouse. *J. Clin. Invest. 57*:1239, 1976.

35. Wolff, S. M., Dale, D. C., Clark, R. A., Root, R. L., and Kimball, H. R.: The Chédiak-Higashi syndrome: Studies of host defenses. *Ann. Intern. Med. 76*:293, 1972.

36. Root, R. K., Rosenthal, A. S., and Balestra, D. K.: Abnormal bactericidal, metabolic, and lysosomal functions of Chédiak-Higashi syndrome leukocytes. *J. Clin. Invest. 51*:649, 1972.

37. Stossel, T. P., Root, R. K., and Vaughan, M.: Phagocytosis in

chronic granulomatous disease and the Chédiak-Higashi syndrome. *N. Engl. J. Med. 286*:120, 1972.

38. Clark, R. A., and Kimball, H. R.: Defective granulocyte chemotaxis in the Chédiak-Higashi syndrome. *J. Clin. Inves. 50*:2645, 1971.

39. Boxer, L. A., Allen, J. M., Watanabe, A. M., Besch, H. R., and Baehner, R. L.: Role of microtubules in granulocyte adherence. *Blood 51*:1045, 1978.

40. Rausch, P. G., Pryzwansky, K. B., and Spitznagel, J. K.: Immunocytochemical identification of azurophilic and specific granulocyte markers in the giant granules of Chédiak-Higashi neutrophil. *N. Engl. J. Med. 298*:693, 1978.

41. Kimball, H. R., Ford, G. H., and Wolff, S. M.: Lysosomal enzymes in normal and Chédiak-Higashi blood leukocytes. *J. Lab. Clin. Med. 86*:616, 1975.

42. Vassalli, J. D., Granelli-Piperno, A., Griscelli, C., and Reich, E.: Specific protease deficiency in polymorphonuclear leukocytes of Chédiak-Higashi syndrome and beige mice. *J. Exp. Med. 147*:1285, 1978.

43. Boxer, L. A., Rister, M., Allen, J. M. and Baehner, R. L.: Improvement of Chédiak-Higashi leukocyte function by cyclic guanosine monophosphate. *Blood 49*:9, 1977.

44. Boxer, L. A., et al.: Correction of leukocyte function in Chédiak-Higashi syndrome by ascorbate. *N. Engl. J. Med. 295*:1041, 1976.

45. Gallin, J. I., Klimerman, J. A., Padgett, G. A., and Wolff, S. M.: Defective mononuclear leukocyte chemotaxis in the Chédiak-Higashi syndrome of humans, mink and cattle. *Blood 45*:863, 1975.

46. Dale, D. C., Alling, D. W., and Wolff, S. M.: Cloxacillin prophylaxis in the Chédiak-Higashi syndrome. *J. Infect. Dis. 125*:393, 1972.

47. Gallin, J. I., et al.: Efficacy of ascorbic acid in Chédiak-Higashi syndrome. Studies in humans and mice. *Blood 53*:226, 1979.

48. Boxer, L. A., Hedley-Whyte, E. T., and Stossel, T. P.: Neutrophil actin dysfunction and abnormal neutrophil behavior. *N. Engl. J. Med. 291*:1093, 1974.

49. Crowley, C. A., et al.: An inherited anomaly of neutrophil adhesion. Its genetic transmission and its association with a missing protein. *N. Engl. J. Med. 302*:1163, 1980.

50. Craddock, P. R., Yawata, Y., Van Santen, L., Giberstadt, S., Silvis, S., and Jacob, H. S.: Acquired phagocytic dysfunction: A complication of parenteral hyperalimentation. *N. Engl. J. Med. 290*:1403, 1974.

51. Baehner, R. L., Feig, S. A., Segel, G. B., Anderson, H. M., and Jaffe, E. R.: Metabolic phagocytic, and bactericidal properties of phosphoglycerate kinase deficient (PGK) polymorphonuclear leukocytes (PMN). *Blood 38*:833, 1971.

52. Steerman, R. L., Synderman, R., Leikin, L., and Colten, H. R.: Intrinsic defect of the polymorphonuclear leukocytes resulting in impaired chemotaxis and phagocytosis. *Clin. Exp. Immunol. 9*:939, 1971.

53. Edelson, P. J., Stites, D. P., Gold, S., and Fudenberg, H. H.: Disorders of neutrophil function: Defects in the early stages of the phagocytic process. *Clin. Exp. Immunol. 13*:21, 1973.

54. Miller, M. E., Norman, M. E., and Koblenzer, P. J.: A new familial defect of neutrophil movement. *J. Lab. Clin. Med. 82*:1, 1973.

55. Miller, M. E., Oski, F. A., and Harris, M. B.: Lazy leukocyte syndrome. *Lancet 1*:665, 1971.

56. Shurin, S. B., Socransky, S. S., Sweeney, E., and Stossel T. P.: A neutrophil disorder induced by Capnocytophaga, a dental microorganism. *N. Engl. J. Med. 301*:849, 1979.

57. Hammerschmidt, D. E., Bowers, T. L., Lammi-Keefe, C. J., Jacob, H. S., and Craddock, P. R.: Granulocyte aggregometry: A sensitive technique for the detection of C5a and complement activation. *Blood 55*:898, 1980.

58. Turner, R. A., Schumacher, H. R., and Myers, A. R.: Phagocytic function of polymorphonuclear leukocytes in rheumatic diseases. *J. Clin. Invest. 52*:1632, 1973.

59. Brandt, L., and Hedberg, H.: Impaired phagocytosis by peripheral blood granulocytes in systemic lupus erythematosus. *Scand. J. Haematol. 6*:548, 1969.

60. McCall, C. E., Caves, J., Cooper, M. R., and DeChatelet, L. R.: Functional characteristics of human toxic neutrophils. *J. Infect. Dis. 124*:68, 1971.

61. Van Epps, D. E., Palmer, D. L., and Williams, R. C., Jr.: Character-

ization of serum inhibitors of neutrophil chemotaxis associated with anergy. *J. Immunol.* 113:189, 1974.

62. Bockenstedt, L. K., and Goetzl, E. J.: Constituents of human neutrophils that mediate enhanced adherence to surfaces. Purification and identification of acidic proteins of the specific granules. *J. Clin. Invest.* 63:1372, 1980.

63. Oseas, R., Yang, H-H., Baehner, R. L., and Boxer, L. A.: Lactoferrin: A promoter of polymorphonuclear leukocytes adhesiveness. *Blood.* In press.

64. Buckley, R. J., Wray, B. B., and Belmaker, E. Z.: Extreme hyperimmunoglobulinemia E and undue susceptibility to infection. *Pediatrics* 49:59, 1972.

65. Schopfer, K. D., Baerlocher, K., Price, P., Krech, U., Quie, P. G., and Douglas, S. D.: Staphylococcal IgE antibodies, hypergammaglobulinemia E and *Staphylococcus aureus* infections. *N. Engl. J. Med.* 300:835, 1979.

66. Spitler, L. E., Spath, P., Petz, L., Cooper, N., and Fudenberg, H. H.: Phagocytes and C4 in paraproteinemia. *Br. J. Haematol.* 29:279, 1975.

67. Van Epps, D. E., and Williams, R. C., Jr.: Suppression of leukocyte chemotaxis by human IgA myeloma components. *J. Exp.Med.* 144:1227, 1976.

68. Clark, R. A., Johnson, F. L., Klebanoff, S. J., and Thomas, E. D.: Defective neutrophil chemotaxis in bone marrow transplant patients. *J. Clin. Invest.* 58:22, 1976.

69. Weissmann, G., Zurier, R. B., and Hoffstein, S.: Leukocyte proteases and the immunologic release of lysosomal enzymes. *Am. J. Pathol.* 68:539, 1972.

70. Strauss, R. G., Mauer, A. M., Asbrock, T., Spitzer, R. E., and Stitzel, A. E.: Stimulation of neutrophil oxidative metabolism by the alternate pathway of complement activation: A mechanism for the spontaneous NBT test. *Blood* 45:843, 1975.

71. Wright, D. G., Kirkpatrick, C. H., and Gallin, J. I.: Effects of levamisole on normal and abnormal leukocyte locomotion. *J. Clin. Invest.* 59:941, 1977.

72. Bybee, J. D., and Rogers, D. E.: The phagocytic activity of polymorphonuclear leukocytes obtained from patients with diabetes mellitus. *J. Lab. Clin. Med.* 64:1, 1964.

73. Drachman, R. H., Root, R. L., and Wood, W. B., Jr.: Studies on the effect of experimental nonketotic diabetes on antibacterial defense. I. Demonstration of a defect in phagocytosis. *J. Exp. Med.* 124:227, 1966.

74. Hill, H. R., Sauls, H. S., Dettloff, J. L., and Quie, P. G.: Impaired leukotactic responsiveness in patients with juvenile diabetes mellitus. *Clin. Immunol. Immunopathol.* 2:395, 1974.

75. Miller, M. E., and Baker, L.: Leukocyte functions in juvenile diabetes mellitus: Humoral and cellular aspects. *J. Pediatr.* 81:980, 1972.

76. Brayton, R. G., Stokes, P. E., Schwartz, M. S., and Louria, D. B.: Effect of alcohol and various diseases on leukocyte mobilization, phagocytosis and intracellular bacterial killing. *N. Engl. J. Med.* 282:123, 1970.

77. Stossel, T. P., Mason, R. J., Hartwig, J., and Vaughan, M.: Quantitative studies of phagocytosis: Use of emulsions to measure the initial rate of phagocytosis. *J. Clin. Invest.* 51:615, 1972.

78. Phelps, P., and Stanislaw, D.: Polymorphonuclear leukocyte motility in vitro. I. Effect of pH, temperature, ethyl alcohol and caffeine, using a modified Boyden chamber technique. *Arthritis Rheum.* 12:181, 1969.

79. Cohen, Z. A.: Determinants of infection in the peritoneal cavity. II. Factors influencing the fate of *Staphylococcus aureus* in the mouse. *Yale J. Biol. Med.* 35:29, 1962.

80. Boggs, D. R., Athens, J. W., Cartwright, G. E., and Wintrobe, M. M.: The effect of adrenal glucocorticosteroids upon the cellular composition of inflammatory exudates. *Am. J. Pathol.* 44:763, 1964.

81. Gallin, J. I., Durocher, J. R., and Kaplan, A. P.: Interaction of leukocyte chemotactic factors with the cell surface. I. Chemotactic factor-induced changes in human granulocyte surface charge. *J. Clin. Invest.* 55:967, 1975.

82. Dale, D. C., Fauci, A. S., and Wolff, S. M.: Alternate-day prednisone: Leukocyte kinetics and susceptibility to infections. *N. Engl. J. Med.* 291:1154, 1974.

83. Handin, R. I., and Stossel, T. P.: Effect of corticosteroid therapy on the phagocytosis of antibody-coated platelets. *Blood* 51:771, 1978.

84. Hammerschmidt, D. E., White, J. G., Craddock, P. R., and Jacob, H. S.: Corticosteroids inhibit complement-induced granulocyte aggregation. A possible mechanism for their efficacy in shock states. *J. Clin. Invest.* 63:798, 1979.

85. MacGregor, R. R., Thorner, R. E., and Wright D. M.: Lidocaine inhibits granulocyte adherence and prevents granulocyte delivery to inflammatory sites. *Blood* 56:203, 1980.

86. Athens, J. W., et al.: Leukokinetic studies. IV. The total blood, circulating and marginal granulocyte pools and the granulocyte turnover rate in normal subjects. *J. Clin. Invest.* 40:989, 1961.

87. Boxer, L. A., Allen, J. M., and Baehner, R. L.: Diminished polymorphonuclear leukocyte adherence. Function dependent on release of cyclic AMP by endothelial cells after stimulation of β-receptors by epinephrine. *J. Clin. Invest.* 66:268, 1980.

88. Newburger, P. E., et al.: Chronic granulomatous disease. Expression of the metabolic defect by in vitro culture of bone marrow progenitors. *J. Clin. Invest.* 66:599, 1980.

89. Karnovsky, M. L.: Chronic granulomatous disease: Pieces of a cellular and molecular puzzle. *Fed. Proc.* 32:1527, 1973.

90. Curnutte, J. T., Whitten, D. M., and Babior, B. M.: Defective superoxide production by granulocytes from patients with chronic granulomatous disease. *N. Engl. J. Med.* 290:593, 1974.

91. Hohn, D. C., and Lehrer, R. I.: NADPH oxidase deficiency in X-linked chronic granulomatous disease. *J. Clin. Invest.* 55:707, 1975.

92. Seligmann, B. E., and Gallin, J. I.: Use of lipophilic probes of membrane potential to assess human neutrophil activation abnormality in chronic granulomatous disease. *J. Clin. Invest.* 66:493, 1980.

93. Whitin, J. C., Chapman, C. E., Simons, E. R., Chovaniec, M., and Cohen, H. J.: Correlation between membrane potential changes and superoxide production in human granulocytes stimulated by phorbol myristate acetate. *J. Biol. Chem.* 255:1874, 1980.

94. Windhorst, D. B., Page, A. R., Holmes, B., Quie, P. G., and Good, R. A.: The pattern of genetic transmission of the leukocyte defect in fatal granulomatous disease of childhood. *J. Clin. Invest.* 47:1026, 1968.

95. Baehner, R. L., and Nathan, D. G.: Quantitative nitroblue tetrazolium test in chronic granulomatous disease. *N. Engl. J. Med.* 278:971, 1968.

96. Quie, P. G., Kaplan, E. L., Page, A. R., Gruskay, F. L., and Malawista, S. E.: Defective polymorphonuclear leukocyte function and chronic granulomatous disease in two female children. *N. Engl. J. Med.* 278:976, 1968.

97. Dupree, E., Smith, C. W., MacDougall, N. L. T., Long, W. K., and Goldman, A. S.: Undetected carrier state in chronic granulomatous disease. *J. Pediatr.* 81:770, 1972.

98. Azimi, P. H., Bodenbender, J. G., Hintz, R. L., and Kontras, S. B.: Chronic granulomatous disease in three female siblings. *JAMA* 206:23, 1968.

99. Mills, E. L., Rholl, K. S., and Quie, P. G.: X-linked inheritance in females with chronic granulomatous disease. *J. Clin. Invest.* 66:332, 1980.

100. Holmes, B., Park, B. H., Malawista, S. E., and Good, R. A.: Chronic granulomatous disease in females: A deficiency of leukocyte glutathione peroxidase. *N. Engl. J. Med.* 283:217, 1970.

101. Nathan, D. G., and Baehner, R. L.: Disorders of phagocytic cell function. *Prog. Hematol.* 7:235, 1971.

102. Cooper, M. R., DeChatelet, L. R., McCall, C. E., LaVia, M. F., Spurr, C. L., and Baehner, R. L.: Complete deficiency of leukocyte glucose-6-phosphate dehydrogenase with defective bactericidal activity. *J. Clin. Invest.* 51:769, 1972.

103. Gray, G. R., et al.: Neutrophil dysfunction, chronic granulomatous disease, and nonspherocytic haemolytic anaemia caused by complete deficiency of glucose-6-phosphate dehydrogenase. *Lancet* 2:530, 1973.

104. Johnston, R. B., Jr., and Baehner, R. L.: Chronic granulomatous disease: Correlation between pathogenesis and clinical findings. *Pediatrics* 48:730, 1971.

105. Landing, B. H., and Shirkey, H. S.: A syndrome of recurrent infec-

tion and infiltration of viscera by pigmented lipid histiocytes. *Pediatrics* 20:431, 1957.

106. Kaplan, E. L., Laxdal, T., and Quie, P. G.: Studies of polymorphonuclear leukocytes from patients with chronic granulomatous disease of childhood: Bactericidal capacity for streptococci. *Pediatrics* 41:591, 1968.

107. Pitt, J., and Bernheimer, H. P.: Role of peroxide in phagocytic killing of pneumococci. *Infect. Immun.* 9:48, 1974.

108. Eschenbach, C.: Zur Atiologie der progressiven Septischen granulomatose. *Pediatr. Res.* 4:493, 1970.

109. Gold, S. B., Hanes, D. M., Stites, D. P., and Fudenberg, H. H.: Abnormal kinetics of degranulation in chronic granulomatous disease. *N. Engl. J. Med.* 291:332, 1974.

110. Stossel, T. P.: Evaluation of opsonic and leukocyte function with a spectrophotometric test in patients with infection and with phagocytic disorders. *Blood* 42:121, 1973.

111. Kauder, E., Kahle, L. L., Moreno, H., and Partin, J. C.: Leukocyte degranulation and vacuole formation in patients with chronic granulomatous disease of childhood. *J. Clin. Invest.* 47:1753, 1968.

112. Baehner, R. L., Karnovsky, M. J., and Karnovsky, M. L.:Degranulation of leukocytes in chronic granulomatous disease. *J. Clin. Invest.* 47:187, 1968.

113. Ulevitch, R. K., Henson, P., Holmes, B., and Good, R. A.: An in vitro study of exocytosis of neutrophil granule enzymes in chronic granulomatous disease neutrophils. *J. Immunol.* 112:1383, 1974.

114. Biggar, W. D.: Phagocytosis in patients and carriers of chronic granulomatous disease. *Lancet* 1:991, 1975.

115. Usui, T., et al.: Studies on the pathogenesis of chronic granulomatous disease. III. Impaired chemotactic response of leukocytes with normal levels of nine components of hemolytic complement in serum of patients with chronic granulomatous disease. *Ann. Paediatr. Jap.* 19:22, 1973.

116. Ward, P. A., and Schlegel, R. A.: Impaired leucotactic responsiveness in a child with recurrent infections. *Lancet* 2:344, 1969.

117. Clark, R. A., and Klebanoff, S. J.: Chronic granulomatous disease. Studies of a family with impaired neutrophil chemotactic, metabolic, and bactericidal function. *Am. J. Med.* 65:941, 1978.

118. Newberger, P., et al.: Prenatal diagnosis of chronic granulomatous disease. *N. Engl. J. Med.* 300:178, 1979.

119. Ament, M. E., and Ochs, H. D.: Gastrointestinal manifestations of chronic granulomatous disease. *N. Engl. J. Med.* 288:382, 1973.

120. Good, R. A., et al.: Fatal (chronic) granulomatous disease of childhood: A hereditary defect of leukocyte function. *Semin. Hematol.* 5:215, 1968.

121. Griscom, N. T., et al.: Gastric antral narrowing in chronic granulomatous disease of childhood. *Pediatrics* 54:456, 1974.

122. Schaller, J.: Illness resembling lupus erythematosus in mothers of boys with chronic granulomatous disease. *Ann. Intern. Med.* 76:747, 1972.

123. March, W. L., Oyen, R., Nichols, M. E., and Allen, F. J., Jr.: Chronic granulomatous disease and the Kell blood group. *Br. J. Haematol.* 29:247, 1975.

124. Weening, R. S., Roos, D., Weemaes, C. M. R., Homan-Muller, J. W. T., and van Schaik, M. K. J.: Defective initiation of the metabolic stimulation in phagocytizing granulocytes. A new congenital defect. *J. Lab. Clin. Med.* 88:757, 1976.

125. Havath, L. and Anderson, B. R.: Defective initiation of polymorphonuclear leukocyte oxidative metabolism. *M. Engl. J. Med.* 300:1130, 1979.

126. Philippart, A. I., Colodny, A. H., and Baehner, R. L.: Continuous antibiotic therapy in chronic granulomatous disease: Preliminary communication. *Pediatrics* 50:923, 1972.

127. Johnston, R. B., Jr., Wilfert, C. M., Buckley, R. H., Webb, L. S., DeChatelet, L. R., and McCall, C. E.: Enhanced bactericidal activity of phagocytes from patients with chronic granulomatous disease in the presence of sulphisoxazole. *Lancet* 1:824, 1975.

128. Lazarus, G. M., and Neu, H. C.: Agents responsible for infection in chronic granulomatous disease of childhood. *Pediatrics* 86:415, 1975.

129. Lobo, M. C., and Mandell, G. L.: Treatment of experimental staphylococcal infection with rifampicin. *Antimicrob. Agents Chemother.* 2:195, 1972.

130. Raubitschek, A. A., Levis, A. S., Stites, D. O., Shaw, E. B., and Fudenberg, H. H.: Normal granulocyte infusion therapy for aspergillosis in chronic granulomatous disease. *Pediatrics* 51:230, 1973.

131. Grignaschi, V. J., Sperperato, A. M., Etcheverry, M. J., and Macario, A. J. L.: Un nuevo cuadro citoquímico: Negatividad spontanea de las reacciones de peroxidasas, oxidasas y lípido en la progenie neutrofila y en los monocitos de dos hermanos. *Rev. Assoc. Med. Argentina* 77:218, 1963.

132. Kithara, M., Simonian, Y., and Eyre, H. J.: Neutrophil myeloperoxidase: A simple, reproducible technique to determine activity. *J. Lab. Clin. Med.* 93:232, 1979.

133. Lehrer, R. I., and Cline, M. J.: Leukocyte myeloperoxidase deficiency and disseminated candidiasis: The role of myeloperoxidase in resistance to Candida infection. *J. Clin. Invest.* 48:1478, 1969.

134. Salmon, S. E., Cline, M. J., Schultz, J., and Lehrer, R. I.: Myeloperoxidase deficiency: Immunologic study of a genetic leukocyte defect. *N. Engl. J. Med.* 282:250, 1970.

135. Klebanoff, S. J., and Pincus, S. H.: Hydrogen peroxide utilization in myeloperoxidase-deficient leukocytes: A possible control mechanism. *J. Clin. Invest.* 50:2226, 1971.

136. Chech, P., Stolder H., Widmann, J. J., Rohner, A., and Miesher, P.: Leukocyte myeloperoxidase deficiency and diabetes mellitus associated with Candida albicans liver abscess. *Am. J. Med.* 66:149, 1979.

137. Lehrer, R. I., Goldbert, L. S., Apple, M. A., and Rosenthal, N. P.: Refractory megaloblastic anemia with myeloperoxidase-deficient neutrophils. *Ann. Intern. Med.* 76:447, 1972.

138. Higashi, O., Katsuyama, N., and Satodate, R.: A case with hematological abnormality characterized by the absence of peroxidase activity in blood polymorphonuclear leukocytes. *Tohoku J. Exp. Med.* 87:77, 1965.

139. Breton-Gorius, J., Houssay, D., Vilde, J. L., and Dreyfus, B: Partial myeloperoxidase deficiency in a case of preleukemia. II. Defects of degranulation and abnormal bacteriocidal activity of blood neutrophils. *Br. J. Haematol.* 30:279, 1975.

140. Boxer, L. A., Harris, R. E., and Baehner, R. L. Regulation of membrane peroxidation in health and disease. *Pediatrics* 64 (Suppl.):713, 1979.

141. Roos, D., et al.: Protection of phagocytic leukocytes by endogenous glutathione: Studies in a family with glutathione reductase deficiency. *Blood* 53:851, 1979.

142. Boxer, L. A., Oliver, J. M., Spielberg, S. P., Allen, J. M., and Schulman, J. D.: Protection of granulocytes by vitamin E in glutathione synthetase deficiency. *N. Engl. J. Med.* 301:901, 1979.

143. Roos, D., Weening, R. S., Wyss, S. R., and Aebi, H. E.: Protection of human neutrophils by endogenous catalase. Studies with cells from catalase-deficient individuals. *J. Clin. Invest.* 65:1515, 1980.

144. Burchill, B. R., Oliver, J. M., Pearson, C. B., Leinbach, E. D., and Berlin, R. B.: Microtubule dynamics and glutathione metabolism in phagocytizing human polymorphonuclear leukocytes. *J. Cell Biol.* 76:439, 1978.

145. Baehner, R. L., Neiburger, R. G., Johnson, D. E., and Murrmann, S. M.: Transient bactericidal defect of peripheral blood phagocytes from children with acute lymphoblastic leukemia receiving craniospinal irradiation. *N. Engl. J. Med.* 289:1209, 1973.

146. Souillet, G. Germain, D., Carraz, M., Veysseyre, C., and Fobert, Y.: Étude de l'activité phagocytaire et bactéricide des polynucleaires de malades atteints de leucémie aiguë lymphoblastique en remission. *Rev. Inst. Pasteur Lyon* 6:87, 1973.

147. Seth, V., and Chandra, R. K.: Opsonic activity, phagocytosis, and bactericidal capacity of polymorphs in under-nutrition. *Arch. Dis. Child.* 47:282, 1972.

148. Douglas, S. D., Lahav, M., and Fudenberg, H. H.: A reversible neutrophil bactericidal defect associated with a mixed cryoglobulin. *Am. J. Med.* 49:274, 1970.

149. Rodey, G. E., Park, B. H., Ford, D. K., Gray, B. H., and Good, R. A.: Defective bactericidal activity of peripheral blood leukocytes in lipochrome histocytosis. *Am. J. Med.* 49:322, 1970.

150. Davis, W. C., Douglas, S. D., and Fudenberg, H. H.: A selective neutrophil dysfunction syndrome: Impaired killing of staphylococci. *Ann. Intern. Med.* 69:1237, 1968.

151. Mandell, G. L.: Staphylococcal infection and leukocyte bactericidal defect in a 22-year-old woman. *Arch. Intern Med. 130*:754, 1972.

152. Odeberg, H., Olofsson, T., and Olsson, I.: Granulocyte function in chronic granulomatous leukaemia. I. Bactericidal and metabolic capabilities during phagocytosis in isolated granulocytes. *Br. J. Haematol. 29*:427, 1975.

153. Breton-Gorius, J., Mason, D. Y., Buriot, D., Vilde, J.-L., and Griscelli, C.: Lactoferrin deficiency as a consequence of a lack of specific granules in neutrophils from a patient with recurrent infections. *Am. J. Pathol. 99*:413, 1980.

154. Rebuck, J. W., and Crowley, J. H.: A method of studying leukocytic functions *in vivo*. *Ann. N.Y. Acad. Sci. 59*:757, 1955.

155. Boyden, S.: The chemotactic effect of mixtures of antibody antigen on polymorphonuclear leukocytes. *J. Exp. Med. 115*:453, 1962.

156. Dale, D. C., and Wolff, S. M.: Skin window studies of the acute inflammatory responses of neutropenic patients. *Blood 38*:138, 1971.

157. Keller, H. U., Hess, M. W., and Cottier, H.: Inhibiting effects of human plasma and serum on neutrophil random migration and chemotaxis. *Blood 44*:843, 1974.

158. Nathan, D. G., Baehner, R. L., and Weaver, D. K.: Failure of nitroblue tetrazolium reduction in the phagocytic vacuoles of leukocytes in chronic granulomatous disease. *J. Clin. Invest. 48*:1895, 1969.

159. Baehner, R. L., Boxer, L. A., and Davis, J., Jr.: The biochemical basis of nitroblue tetrazolium reduction in normal human and chronic granulomatous disease polymorphonuclear leukocytes. *Blood 48*:309, 1976.

160. Root, R. K., Metcalf, J., Oshine, N., and Chance, B.: H_2O_2 release from human granulocytes during phagocytosis. *J. Clin. Invest. 55*:945, 1975.

161. Pincus, S. H., and Klebanoff, S. J.: Quantitative leukocyte iodination. *N. Engl. J. Med. 284*:744, 1971.

162. Hirsh, J. G., and Strauss, B.: Studies on heat-labile opsonin in rabbit serum. *J. Immunol. 92*:145, 1964.

163. Cline, M. J.: A new white cell test which measures individual phagocyte function in a mixed leukocyte population. I. A neutrophil defect in acute myelocytic leukemia. *J. Lab. Clin. Med. 81*:311, 1973.

164. Lehrer, R. I., and Cline, M. J.: Interaction of *Candida albicans* with human leukocyte and serum. *J. Bacteriol. 98*:996, 1969.

165. Lehrer, R. I.: The fungicidal mechanisms of human monocytes. I. Evidence for myeloperoxidase-linked and myeloperoxidase-independent candidacidal mechanisms. *J. Clin. Invest. 55*:338, 1975.

Eosinophils and basophils

CHAPTER 90

Morphology, biochemistry, and function of eosinophils

DOROTHEA ZUCKER-FRANKLIN

The eosinophil was recognized by Paul Ehrlich as a special type of granulocyte in 1879. Its large, refractile granules aroused such interest that by 1914 Schwartz was able to write a review which included more than 2700 references [1]. In recent years, updated comprehensive monographs have become available bearing witness to the fact that interest in this cell has not subsided [2–5].

Morphology

Eosinophils arise in the marrow, where they can be distinguished from neutrophils at the promyelocyte stage of development. The granules of eosinophilic promyelocytes are larger than those of their neutrophilic counterpart. They contain peroxidase, acid phosphatase, arylsulfatase, and a number of other lysosomal enzymes [6]. In addition, eosinophilic promyelocytes contain a few large granules which stain blue with Romanovsky stains. These appear to be lost by attrition as a consequence of subsequent mitotic divisions.

Mature eosinophils have a diameter of 12 to 17 μm on blood films, and because of their large, bright red–staining granules are easily recognized in blood films or sections of tissues [7]. The nucleus usually has two lobes, though further segmentation may occur, especially with folic acid or vitamin B_{12} deficiency. On electron microscopy, the amount of euchromatin, the synthetically active form of chromatin, is more abundant than in mature neutrophils, in keeping with the eosinophil's ability to engage in major biosynthetic processes.

The granules of mature eosinophils are ovoid, membrane-bound organelles, 0.15 to 1.5 μm in length and 0.3 to 1.0 μm in width. Human eosinophil granules have a central, electron-opaque core, or crystalloid, which is surrounded by a less dense matrix (Fig. 90-1). The hydrolytic enzymes as well as peroxidase are located in the matrix. The crystalloid contains basic proteins which are rich in arginine and lysine, phospholipids, and probably melanin [8].

The major basic protein makes up about 50 percent of the core [9]. It consists of a single polypeptide chain with an M_r of 10,800. Either because of its basic nature or its free sulfhydryl groups, this protein adsorbs to membranes, precipitates DNA, and neutralizes heparin. A radioimmunoassay can be used to determine major basic protein levels in the blood and urine of patients with eosinophilia [10]. Other cationic proteins contribute to about 30 percent of the eosinophilic granule core [11]. The relationship between these proteins, if any, is not clear. The Charcot-Leyden crystals, which are found in areas where degeneration of eosinophils and granule release occurs, as in the nasal mucus of patients with allergic asthma, pleural fluid of patients with pulmonary eosinophilic infiltrates, or the stools of patients with parasitic infestation, consist of the fused cores of the eosinophilic granules [12]. The Charcot-Leyden crystals stain red with eosin. The Charcot-Leyden crystals are thought to be conglomerates of basic proteins and other substances present in the core of the granules. The cationic proteins should not be equated with Charcot-Leyden crystals, which differ antigenically. Among granule matrix enzymes, peroxidase and arylsulfatase are of interest.

Among granule matrix enzymes, peroxidase and arylsulfatase are of special interest. Eosinophil peroxidase is found in higher concentration and differs in its physical properties, substrate specificity, and sensitivity to inhibitors from myeloperoxidase in neutrophils [13–15]. Its physiologic substrate has not been defined. Arylsulfatase has an eightfold higher concentration in eosinophils than in other leukocytes [16]. Alkaline phosphatase has not been detected in eosinophils. Other enzymes believed to play a role in eosinophil function, such as phospholipase D, lysophospholipase, and histamine oxidase, have not been localized subcellularly.

The cytoplasm of the cell is rich in vesicles, smooth endoplasmic reticulum, and glycogen (Fig. 90-1). A few profiles of rough endoplasmic reticulum and some single or clustered ribosomes are seen even in mature cells. The size of the Golgi zone varies.

The plasma membrane of the eosinophil is not distinguished structurally from that of other leukocytes. Eosinophils have receptors for the Fc region of particular isotypes of IgG, and the densities of these receptors increase when the cell is activated [17]. There are IgE receptors [18,19] and receptors for complement components C4, C3b, and C3d [20] on the eosinophil, also. Receptors for IgA, IgM, and IgD have not been demonstrated. Eosinophils possess both H1 and H2 histamine receptors, although histamine-induced chemotaxis is probably not mediated by these receptors [21]. The chemotactic tetrapeptides (Val-Gly-Ser-Glu and Ala-Gly-Ser-Glu), which are components of the eosinophil chemotactic factor of anaphylaxis (ECF-A), as well as histamine, have been reported to enhance the number of receptors for C3b and C4 in a dose-dependent fashion [22]. The eosinophil membranes also possess magnesium-dependent ATPase and alkaline phosphodiesterase. 5′-Nucleotidase, an enzyme used as a membrane marker for other cells, has not been detected on eosinophils.

Prostaglandins D_2 and E_2 appear to stimulate the membrane to enhance random motility and chemotaxis. Release of the arachidonic acid derivatives by other cells, such as mast cells,. may attract eosinophils to inflammatory sites. Moreover, the high lysophospholipase activity of the eosinophil membrane may modulate hypersensitivity reactions [23].

Kinetic features

Although the eosinophils constitute a biologically important component of the human granulocyte compartment, relatively little is known about the kinetics of these cells [4,24,25]. Eosinophilic promyelocytes may be identified in the marrow, and together with the eosinophilic myelocytes constitute the mitotic pool. Differentiation proceeds in a manner analogous to that of cells of the neutrophil series, and mature eosinophils are stored in the marrow for several days prior to release [25]. Studies in normal subjects and patients with eosinophilia suggest a mean transit time of about 9 days in the marrow and a postmitotic transit time of 2.5 days [26,27].

An eosinophil-releasing factor has been described [28,29], as has an eosinophilopoietin [28,30,31]. Low-molecular-weight eosinophilopoietin has been identified in mice made eosinophilopenic by injection of antieosinophil antibody [30]. The differentiation of eosinophils can be studied in soft agar cultures where discrete colonies of eosinophils develop from progenitors present in normal marrow and blood [32]. These colonies are composed entirely of eosinophils, indicating that basophils, neutrophils, and monocytes arise from separate progenitors. This implies that commitment into the three different types of granulocytes antedates the myeloblast stage of differentiation.

There seems to be a close relation between the immune system and eosinophil production in that eosinophilopoietic factors can be derived from lymphocytes [4,32,33]. Rats thymectomized at birth or given antilymphocyte serum do not develop eosinophilia when infected with *Trichinella spiralis*. Moreover, thymus grafts from syngeneic mice can reconstitute the ability to develop eosinophilia after *T. spiralis* infection. T lymphocytes appear to play a key role in the induction phase of eosinophilia [34].

Probably less than 1 percent of the total number of eosinophils in the body are found in the blood. Most of these cells are in the marrow and tissues [25]. In dogs, the circulating $T_{1/2}$ of the eosinophil is approximately 30 min, compared with a $T_{1/2}$ of 4 to 6 h for the neutrophil [35]. In humans half of the eosinophils leave the blood during the first circulation after release from the marrow, and most of the cells enter the tissues within 1 h [36]. However, studies in humans using ³H-thymidine

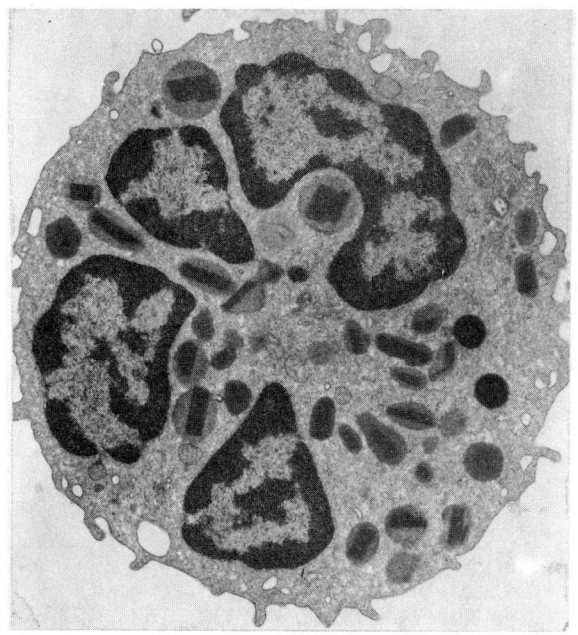

FIGURE 90-1   Electron photomicrograph of a mature eosinophil (for details see text). ×16,500.

indicated a mean $T_{1/2}$ of 8 h [37]. In two patients with eosinophilia the blood $T_{1/2}$ was calculated at 4.5 to 5 h [36]. The eosinophil appears to survive for longer periods than does the neutrophil. In very early studies, eosinophils were reported to survive 8 to 12 days in tissue culture, compared with 2 to 4 days for neutrophils [38]. Eosinophils preferentially reside in the skin, lung, and gastrointestinal tract, and they may enter respiratory or gastrointestinal secretions directly or by way of lymphatic channels. Once eosinophils leave the circulation and enter the tissues, most may not reenter the blood in normal subjects. However, in two patients with eosinophilia, recirculation was demonstrated [26], and similar findings have been reported by others [24].

The normal human circulating eosinophil count averages 150 per microliter [28,39] and roughly parallels the eosinophilopoietic activity of the marrow. Eosinopenia is induced by injections of glucocorticosteroids, ACTH, or epinephrine [40,41], and eosinophilia is produced by the chronic administration of histamine [28].

Glucose provides the main source of energy for eosinophils and inhibition of glycolysis blocks functional responses of these cells. Glucose transport across the membrane is stimulated during chemotaxis induced by C5a or by the synthetic oligopeptide *N*-formyl-methionylleucylphenylalanine (fMLP). Oxidative metabolism in resting eosinophils is greater than in resting neutrophils [42]. When activated, the oxidative burst associated with the production of hydrogen peroxide, superoxide, chemiluminescence, and iodination of protein is much greater in eosinophils than in other leukocytes [43,44]. The function of the oxidative burst in eosinophils is less certain, for despite the availability of all enzymes involved in the hexose monophosphate shunt,

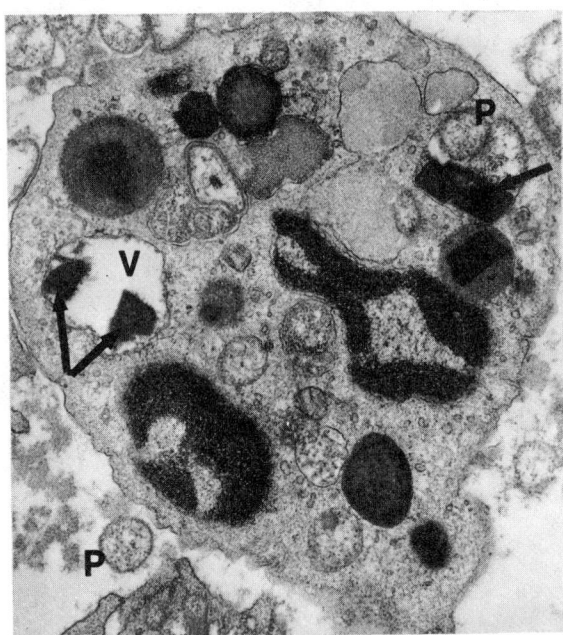

FIGURE 90-2   Blood eosinophil from a buffy coat specimen that had been incubated with *Mycoplasma pneumoniae* (P). The microorganisms are seen attached to the plasma membrane as well as within phagocytic vacuoles. Note that in some vacuoles (V) the core of the granules (*arrows*) has remained intact. ×9500.

secreted to the exterior during "frustrated phagocytosis," when the cells flatten against an object too large to be engulfed. A variety of larval helminths are killed in this manner following attachment of the cells to the parasite which is believed to be mediated by antibody and complement [60,61] (see Fig. 90-3). Release of granule proteins may play a major role in the injury to schistosomula by the attached cells [62,63].

The second important function of eosinophils is their ability to abrogate hypersensitivity reactions as well as nonimmunologic inflammatory responses. These reactions are mediated by an amine oxidase which neutralizes histamine [64,65]. In addition, eosinophils elaborate a substance referred to as *eosinophil-derived inhibitor* likely to consist of prostaglandins [66]. Prostaglandins raise the level of cAMP of mast cells and inhibit their degranulation.

FIGURE 90-3   Detail showing a human eosinophil (E) adhering to a schistosomulum of *Schistosoma mansoni* (S). Note the electron-dense material (*arrows*) between the eosinophil and the schistosomulum. This has been discharged by the cell and resembles the material in the core of the granules (G). ×16,000. (Courtesy of G. Korman, A. Butterworth, and J. Caulfield, Harvard Medical School.)

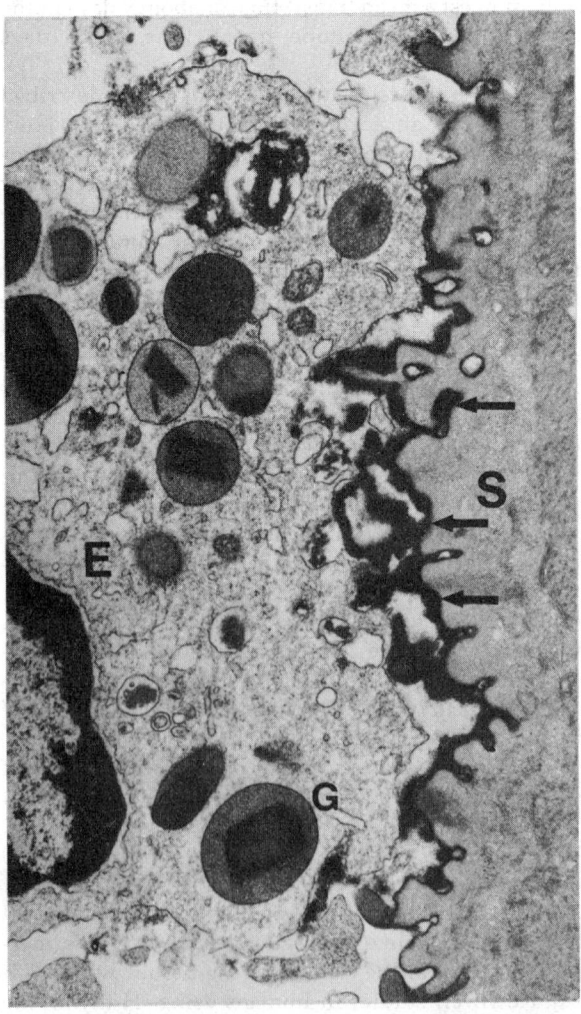

the cells appear to have less intracellular killing ability than neutrophils [45]. Direct toxicity by hydrogen peroxide has been implicated in the killing of *Trichinella* larvae [46]. Unfortunately, most of the metabolic studies have been carried out on eosinophils obtained from patients with eosinophilia. Such eosinophils may be activated, and their surface charge, hexose transport, and lysosomal and hexose monophosphate shunt activities may be different from resting cells [47].

Function

Like neutrophils, eosinophils will undergo chemotaxis in response to bacterial products and components of the complement system [48]. Factors which attract eosinophils preferentially are elaborated by mast cells, e.g., histamine [49] and ECF-A [50], and by sensitized lymphocytes [51,52]. These in vitro observations may explain why eosinophils may accumulate at sites where either degranulating mast cells or activated lymphocytes are found. The role of the eosinophil in host defense is summarized in Table 90-1.

Eosinophils are phagocytic and bactericidal in vitro, but the extent to which eosinophils kill bacteria in vivo is not certain [53–56].

Bacteria, fungi, mycoplasma, or inert particles ingested by eosinophils are taken into phagocytic vacuoles (Fig. 90-2). The granules coalesce with the vacuoles, as a result of membrane fusion, and release of granule content occurs [57–59]. The granule content may also be

TABLE 90-1 Eosinophil in host defense

Role	Special function	Eosinophil constituent or activity	References
Dampening of immediate hypersensitivity reactions	Inhibitor of mediator release by raising intracellular levels of cyclic AMP in basophils	PGE_1/PGE_2	[67,68]
	Removal of secreted mast cell granules	Phagocytosis	[69]
	Enzymatic degradation of:		
	Histamine	Histaminase	[70]
	Platelet lytic factor	Phospholipase D	[71]
	Lysophospholipids	Lysophospholipase	[72]
	Oxidation of mediators	Binding of peroxidase to mast cell granules	[73]
Damage to helminths	Cytotoxicity for opsonized larval and adult forms	C3b and IgG receptors	[2,60,61]
		Superoxide anion	[47]
		Halogenation of the larval surface	[74]
		Major basic protein	

References

1. Schwartz, E.: Das Wesen der Eosinophilie. Jahreskurse fur ärtzliche Fortbildung, in *Zwölf Monatshefte*. München, 1914, vol. 1, p. 5.
2. Zucker-Franklin, D.: Eosinophil function and disorders. *Adv. Intern. Med. 19*:1, 1974.
3. Beeson, P. B., and Bass, D. A.: The eosinophil, in *Major Problems in Internal Medicine*, edited by L. H. Smith. Saunders, Philadelphia, 1977, vol. 14.
4. Mahmoud, A. A. F., and Austen, K. F. (eds.): *The Eosinophil in Health and Disease*. Grune & Stratton, New York, 1980.
5. Zucker-Franklin, D.: Pathophysiology of eosinophilia, in *Clinical Immunology Update*, edited by E. C. Franklin. Elsevier North-Holland, New York, 1979, p. 227.
6. Bainton, D. F., Farquhar, M. G.: Segregation and packaging of granule enzymes in eosinophilic leukocytes. *J. Cell Biol. 45*:54, 1970.
7. Zucker-Franklin, D.: Eosinophils, in *Atlas of Blood Cells: Function and Pathology*. D. Zucker-Franklin, M. F. Greaves, C. E. Grossi, and A. M. Marmont. Edi Ermes, Milano, Lea & Febiger, Philadelphia, 1981, chap. 6, p. 257.
8. Okun, M. R., Donellan, B., Pearson, H., and Edelstein, L. M.: Melanin: A normal component of human eosinophils. *Lab. Invest. 30*:681, 1974.
9. Gleich, G. J., Loegering, D. A., Mann, K. G., and Maldonado, J. E.: Comparative properties of Charcot-Leyden crystal protein and the major basic protein from human eosinophils. *J. Clin. Invest. 57*:633, 1976.
10. Wasson, D. L., et al.: Elevated serum levels of the eosinophil granule major basic protein in patients with eosinophilia. *J. Clin. Invest. 67*:651, 1981.
11. Olsson, I., Venge, P., Spitznagel, J. K., and Lehrer, R. J.: Arginine-rich cationic proteins of human eosinophil granules. Comparison of the constituents of eosinophilic and neutrophilic leukocytes. *Lab. Invest. 36*:493, 1977.
12. Welsh, R. A.: The genesis of the Charcot-Leyden crystal in the eosinophilic leukocyte of man. *Am. J. Pathol. 35*:1091, 1959.
13. Archer, G. T., Air, G., Jackas, J., and Morell, D. B.: Studies on rat eosinophil peroxidase. *Biochim. Biophys. Acta 99*:96, 1965.
14. West, B. C., Gelb, N. A., and Rosenthal, A. S.: Isolation and partial characterization of human eosinophil granules. *Am. J. Pathol. 81*:575, 1975.
15. Zucker-Franklin, D., and Grusky, G.: The identification of eosinophil colonies in soft agar cultures by differential staining for peroxidase. *J. Histochem. Cytochem. 24*:1270, 1976.
16. Tanaka, K. R., Valentine, W. N., and Fredricks, R. E.: Human leukocyte aryl sulfatase activity. *Br. J. Hematol. 8*:86, 1962.
17. Tai, P. C., and Spry, C. J. F.: Studies on blood eosinophils. I. Patients with transient eosinophilia. *Clin. Exp. Immunol. 24*:415, 1976.
18. Hübscher, T.: Role of the eosinophil in the allergic reactions. I.

EDI—An eosinophil-derived inhibitor of histamine release. *J. Immunol. 114*:1379, 1975.
19. Capron, M., and Capron, A.: Schistosomes and eosinophils. *Trans. R. Soc. Trop. Med. Hyg. 74 (Suppl.)*:44, 1980.
20. Anwar, A. R. E., and Kay, A. B.: Membrane receptors for IgG and complement (C_4, C3b and C3d) on human eosinophilis and neutrophils and their relation to eosinophilia. *J. Immunol. 119*:976, 1977.
21. Gallin, J. I., Weinstein, A. M., Cramer, E. B., and Kaplan, A. P.: Histamine modulation of human eosinophil locomotion in vitro and in vivo, in *The Eosinophil in Health and Disease*, edited by A. A. F. Mahmoud and K. F. Austen. Grune & Stratton, New York, 1980, p. 185.
22. Kay, A. B., and Anwar, A. R. E.: Eosinophil surface receptors, in *The Eosinophil in Health and Disease*, edited by A. A. F. Mahmoud and K. F. Austen. Grune & Stratton, New York, 1980, p. 207.
23. Weller, P. F., Wasserman, S. I., and Austen, K. F.: Selected enzymes preferentially present in the eosinophil, in *The Eosinophil in Health and Disease*, edited by A. A. F. Mahmoud and K. F. Austen. Grune & Stratton, New York, 1980, p. 115.
24. Clark, R. A. F., and Kaplan, A. P.: Eosinophil leucocytes: Structure and function. *Clin. Haematol. 4*:635, 1975.
25. Archer, R. K.: *The Eosinophil Leucocytes*. Blackwell Scientific Publications, Oxford, 1963.
26. Herion, J. C., Glasser, R. M., Walker, R. I., and Palmer, J. G.: Eosinophil kinetics in two patients with eosinophilia. *Blood 36*:361, 1970.
27. Stryckmans, P. A., Cronkite, E. P., Greenberg, M. L., and Schiffer, L. M.: Kinetics of eosinophil leukocyte proliferation in man. *Abstr. Simultaneous Sessions XII Cong. Int. Soc. Hematol.*, 1968, p. 41.
28. Archer, R. K.: Regulatory machanisms in eosinophil leukocyte production, release, and distribution, in *Regulation of Hematopoiesis*, edited by A. S. Gordon. Appleton Century Crofts, New York, 1970, vol. II, p. 917.
29. Spry, C. J. F.: Mechanism of eosinophilia. VI. Eosinophil mobilization. *Cell Tissue Kinet. 4*:365, 1971.
30. Mahmoud, A. A. F., Stone, M. K., and Kellermeyer, R. W.: Eosinophilopoietin: A circulating low molecular weight peptide-like substance which stimulates the production of eosinophils in mice. *J. Clin. Invest. 60*:675, 1977.
31. Miller, A. M., and McGarry, M. P. A diffusible stimulator of eosinophilopoiesis produced by lymphoid cells as demonstrated with diffusion chambers. *Blood 48*:293, 1976.
32. Zucker-Franklin, D., Grusky, G., and L'Esperance, P.: Granulocyte colonies derived from lymphocyte fractions of normal human blood. *Proc. Natl. Acad. Sci. 71*:2711, 1974.
33. Greene, B. M., and Colley, D. G. Eosinophils and immune mechanisms. II. Partial characterization of the lymphokine eosinophil stimulation promoter. *J. Immunol. 113*:910, 1974.
34. The mechanism of eosinophilia. *Lancet II*:1187, 1971 (editorial).
35. Carper, H. A., and Hoffman, P. L.: The intravascular survival of

transfused canine Pelger-Huet neutrophils and eosinophils. *Blood* 27:739, 1966.

36. Osgood, E. E.: Number and distribution of human hemic cells. *Blood* 9:1141, 1954.

37. Parwaresch, M. R., Walle, A. J., and Arndt, D.: The peripheral kinetics of human radiolabelled eosinophils. *Virchows Arch. B:* 21:57, 1976.

38. Osgood, E. E.: Culture of human marrow: Length of life of the neutrophils, eosinophils, and basophils of normal blood as determined by comparative cultures of blood and sternal marrow from healthy persons. *JAMA* 109:933, 1937.

39. Uhrbranh, H.: The number of circulating eosinophils. Normal figures and spontaneous variations. *Acta Med. Scand.* 160:99, 1958.

40. Anderson, V., Bro-Rasmussen, F., and Hougaard, K.: Autoradiagraphic studies of eosinophil kinetics: Effects of cortisol. *Cell Tissue Kinet.* 2:139, 1969.

41. Thevathasan, O. I., and Gordon, A. S.: Adrenocortical-medullary interactions on the blood eosinophils. *Acta Haematol.* 19:162, 1958.

42. Bujak, J. S., and Root, R. K.: The role of peroxidase in the bactericidal activity of human blood eosinophils. *Blood* 43:727, 1974.

43. Bass, D. A., Lewis, J. C., and DeChatelet, L. R.: Biochemistry and metabolism of human eosinophils. *Trans. R. Soc. Trop. Med. Hyg.* 74 (Suppl.):11, 1980.

44. DeChatelet, L. R., Shirley, P., Muss, H., McPhail, L., and Bass, D.: Oxidative metabolism of the human eosinophil. *Blood* 50:525, 1977.

45. DeChatelet, L. R., Migler, R., Shirley, P., Muss, H., and Bass, D. A.: Comparison of intracellular bacterial abilities of human neutrophils and eosinophils. *Blood* 52:609, 1978.

46. Bass, D. A. and Szejda, P.: Mechanism of killing of newborn larvae of *Trichinella spiralis* by neutrophil and eosinophil leukocytes: Killing by generators of hydrogen peroxide in vitro. *J. Clin. Invest.* 64:1558, 1979.

47. Bass, D. A., Grover, W. H., Lewis, J. Szejda, P., DeChatelet, L. R., and McCall, C. E.: Comparison of human eosinophils from normals and patients with eosinophilia. *J. Clin. Invest.* 66:1265, 1980.

48. Ward, P. A.: Chemotaxis of human eosinophils. *Am. J. Pathol.* 54:121, 1969.

49. Clark, R. A. F., Gallin, J. I., and Kaplan, A. P.: The selective eosinophil chemotactic activity of histamine. *J. Exp. Med.* 132:1462, 1975.

50. Goetzl, E. J. and Austen, K. F.: Natural eosinophilotactic peptides: Evidence of heterogeneity and studies of structure and function, in *Clinical Immunology Update*, edited by E. C. Franklin. Elsevier North-Holland, New York, 1979, chap. 9, p. 149.

51. Colley, D. G.: Eosinophils and immune mechanisms. I. Eosinophil stimulation promoter (ESP): A lymphokine induced by specific antigen or phytohemagglutin, *J. Immunol.* 110:1419, 1973.

52. Greene, B. M., and Colley, D. G.: Eosinophils and immune mechanisms. II. Partial characterization of the lymphokine eosinophil stimulation promoter. *J. Immunol.* 113:910, 1974.

53. Baehner, R. L., and Johnston, R. B., Jr.: Metabolic and bactericidal activities of human eosinophils. *Br. J. Haematol.* 20:277, 1971.

54. Cline, M. J.: Microbicidal activity of human eosinophils. *J. Reticuloendothel. Soc.* 12:332, 1972.

55. Klebanoff, S. J., Durack, D. T., Rosen, H., and Clark, R. A.: Functional studies on human peritoneal eosinophils. *Infect. Immun.* 17:167, 1977.

56. Mickenberg, I. D., Root, R. K., and Wolff, S. M.: Bactericidal and metabolic properties of human eosinophil. *Blood* 39:67, 1972.

57. Zucker-Franklin, D., and Hirsch, J. G.: Electron microscope studies on degranulation of rabbit peritoneal leukocytes during phagocytosis. *J. Exp. Med.* 120:569, 1964.

58. Zucker-Franklin, D., Davidson, M., and Thomas, L.: The interaction of mycoplasmas with mammalian cells. I. HeLa cells, neutrophils and eosinophils. *J. Exp. Med.* 124:521, 1966.

59. Cotran, R. S., and Litt, M.: The entry of granule-associated peroxidase into the phagocytic vacuoles of eosinophils. *J. Exp. Med.* 129:1291, 1964.

60. Glauert, A. M., Butterworth, A. E., Sturrock, R. F. and Houba, V.: The mechanism of antibody-dependent, eosinophil-mediated damage to schistosomula of *Schistosoma mansoni* in vitro: A study by phase contrast and electron microscopy. *J. Cell Sci.* 34:173, 1978.

61. Butterworth, A. E., et al.: Antibody-dependent eosinophil-mediated damage to ⁵¹Cr-labelled schistosomula of *Schistosoma mansoni:* Damage by purified eosinophils. *J. Exp. Med.* 145:136, 1977.

62. Vadas, M. A., David, J. R., Butterworth, A., Pisani, N. T., and Siongok, T. A.: A new method for the purification of human eosinophils and neutrophils and a comparison of the ability of these cells to damage schistosomula of *Schistosoma mansoni.* *J. Immunol.* 122:1228, 1979.

63. Butterworth, A. E., Wasson, D. L., Gleich, G. J., Loegering, D. A., and David, J. R.: Damage to schistosomula of *Schistosoma mansoni* induced directly by eosinophil major basic protein. *J. Immunol.* 122:221, 1979.

64. Vercauteren, R.: The properties of the isolated granules from blood eosinophils. *Enzymologia* 16:1, 1953.

65. Kovacs, A.: Antihistamine effect of eosinophilic leukocytes. *Experientia* 6:349, 1950.

66. Hubscher, T.: Role of the eosinophil in the allergic reactions. II. Release of prostaglandins from human eosinophil leukocytes. *J. Immunol.* 114:1389, 1975.

67. Weller, P. F., and Goetzl, E. J.: The human eosinophil: Roles in host defense and tissue injury. *Am. J. Pathol.* 100:791, 1980.

68. Hubscher, T.: Role of the eosinophil in the allergic reactions. 1. EDI — An eosinophil-derived inhibitor of histamine release. *J. Immunol.* 114:1379, 1975.

69. Mann, P. R.: An electron-microscopic study of the relations between mast cells and eosinophil leukocytes. *J. Pathol.* 98:182, 1969.

70. Zeiger, R. S., Yurdin, D. L., and Colten, H. R.: Histamine metabolism. II. Cellular and subcellular localization of the catabolic enzymes, histaminase, and histamine methyl transferase in human leukocytes. *J. Allergy Clin. Immunol.* 58:172, 1976.

71. Valone, F. H., Whitmer, D. I., Pukett, W. C., Austen, K. F., and Goetzl, E. J.: The immunological generation of a platelet-activating factor and a platelet-lytic factor in the rat. *Immunology* 37:841, 1979.

72. Strandberg, K., Sydbom, A., and Uvnas, B.: Incorporation of choline serine, ethanolamine and inositol into phospholipids of isolated rat mast cells. *Acta. Physiol. Scand.* 94:54, 1975.

73. Henderson, W. R., Jong, E. C. and Klebanoff, S. J.: Binding of eosinophil peroxidase to mast cell granules with retention of peroxidation activity. *J. Immunol.* 124:1383, 1980.

74. Butterworth, A. E., and David, J. R.: Eosinophil function. *N. Engl. J. Med.* 304:154, 1981.

CHAPTER *91*

Morphology, biochemistry, and function of basophils

STEPHEN J. GALLI
ANN M. DVORAK
HAROLD F. DVORAK

The human basophil is the least common blood granulocyte, with a prevalence of 0.5 percent of total leukocytes and 0.3 percent of nucleated marrow cells [1]. Although the basophil's prominent metachromatic cytoplasmic granules allow unmistakable identification in Wright-Giemsa–stained films of blood or marrow, accurate basophil determinations require absolute counting methods [2]. Differential counts of blood films yield valid results if the percentage of basophils is substantially elevated or if many thousands of leukocytes are counted.

Morphology and kinetics

Ultrastructurally, human basophils contain round or oval cytoplasmic granules surrounded by a membrane and containing a substructure of dense particles, less dense matrix, and, occasionally, membrane whorls [3]. A second minor population of small uniform granules is characteristically located close to the nucleus [4] (Figs. 91-1 to 91-3). The cytoplasm of mature human basophils also contains glycogen particles and small membrane-bound vesicles. Other organelles are inconspicuous.

Despite certain striking similarities in biochemistry and function, mammalian basophils and mast cells are not identical [5], a distinction appreciated by Paul Ehrlich, who described both of these cells in the late nineteenth century. Basophils share a common precursor with other granulocytes and monocytes, have a short life-span similar to that of eosinophils [6,7], and retain granulocytic features even after emigrating into tissues (Fig. 91-2). The precise fate of basophils in the tissues is unknown. The ^{3}H-thymidine-labeling index of basophilic myelocytes is similar to that of neutrophilic myelocytes [7]. Labeled basophils first appear in

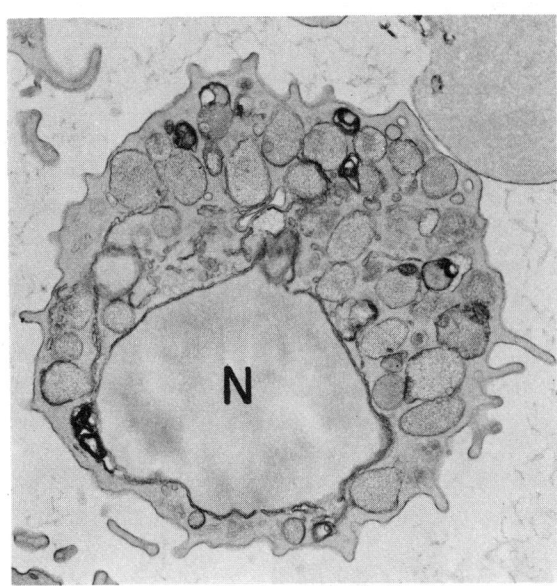

FIGURE 91-1   Normal human blood basophil demonstrating numerous cytoplasmic granules. N = nucleus. Osmium potassium ferrocyanide (OPF) processing, ×12,000.

the blood 2½ days after in vivo administration of ^{3}H-thymidine, and the maximum number of labeled basophils is present in the blood at 7 days [7]. Although the signals controlling human basophil proliferation

FIGURE 91-2   Mast cell (M) and basophil (B) in the ileal submucosa of a patient with Crohn's disease. The mast cell is a larger, mononuclear cell with a more complex plasma membrane surface and cytoplasmic granules that are smaller and more numerous than those of the basophil. In this section plane, the basophil exhibits two nuclear lobes. Several basophil cytoplasmic granules contain whorls of membranes (*arrows*). Osmium collidine uranyl en bloc processing, ×8500. (Dvorak et al. [24], with permission.)

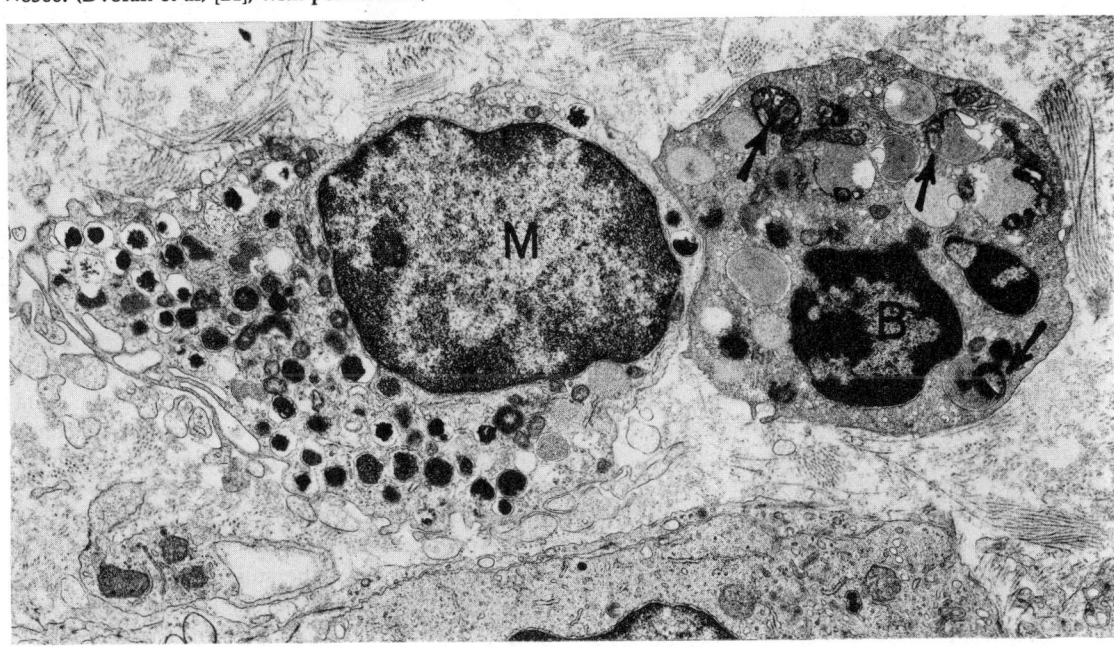

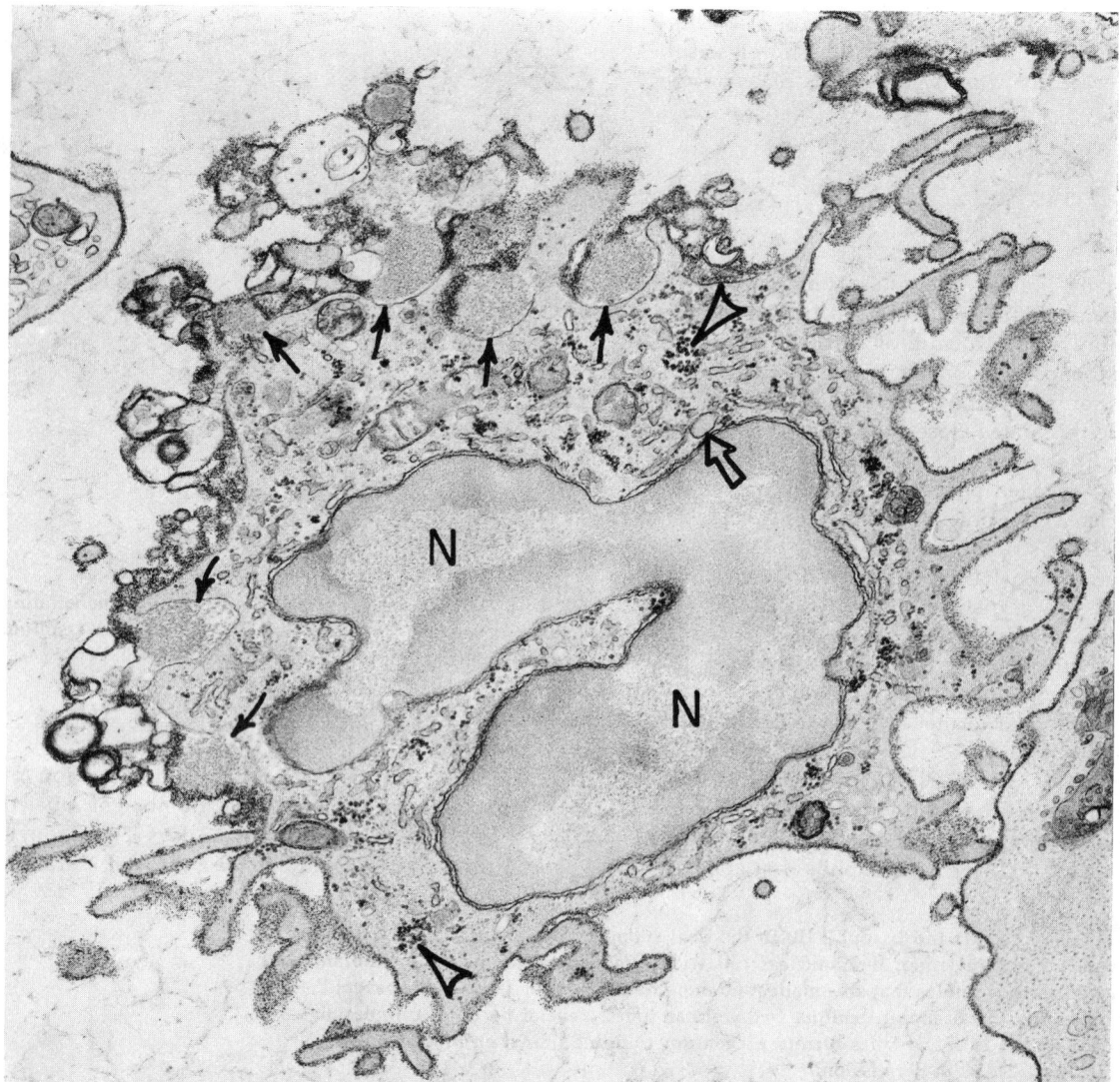

FIGURE 91-3 IgE-mediated degranulation of basophil from ragweed-sensitive patient. Exposure to specific antigen in vitro results in exocytosis of individual cytoplasmic granules from multiple plasma membrane openings (*closed arrows*). The plasma membrane and exteriorized granules are coated with cationic ferritin tracer. Open arrow indicates minor granule type that isn't released during degranulation. Open arrow heads indicate cytoplasmic glycogen. N = nucleus. OPF processing, ×22,000. (Dvorak et al. [17], with permission.)

have not been defined, a T lymphocyte–derived basophilopoietin has been described in the guinea pig [8].

Mast cells normally reside in the connective tissue, particularly beneath epithelial surfaces and around blood vessels, and, in some species, in serous cavities [5]. Although mature mast cells are a normal, if numerically minor, component of human marrow [1], mast cells have not been demonstrated in normal human blood. Unlike basophils, mast cells are very long-lived cells that can proliferate locally in the tissues during a variety of inflammatory and reparative processes. Although the ontogeny of human mast cells is unsettled, in murine species at least some, and perhaps all, mast cells are derived from hemopoietic progenitors [9–12].

Biochemistry and role in immediate hypersensitivity

The cytoplasmic granules of basophils and mast cells contain sulfated glycosaminoglycans that stain metachromatically with basic dyes under appropriate conditions. In the rat mast cell, this substance is predominantly heparin [13]. Human basophils also have been considered to contain heparin, but studies of leukemic basophils have demonstrated little, if any, synthesis of true heparin [5]. Instead, the sulfated glycosaminoglycans of human leukemic basophils, like those of normal guinea pig basophils, consist predominantly of chondroitin sulfates. The functions of these substances are unknown; even the heparin of rat mast cell granules is a poor anticoagulant. Like mast cells, human basophils synthesize and store histamine, and basophils are the source of most, if not all, of the histamine in normal human blood [14].

Basophils also generate many other mediators that can influence the course of inflammatory processes; similar or identical molecules also are elaborated by mast cells [5,15]. These substances are either preformed and granule-associated (glycosaminoglycans, histamine, eosinophil-chemotactic factors) or are produced during activation of the cell (see below), such as leukotrienes (slow-reacting substances of anaphylaxis) and other metabolites of arachidonic acid. Basophils also possess neutral proteases that may have a role in inflammatory processes, such as the granule-associated trypsin- and chymotrypsin-like enzymes and a plasma membrane plasminogen activator in the guinea pig [5] and the basophil kallikrein of anaphylaxis [16] in humans. A variety of other enzymatic activities have been identified by cytochemical approaches [17]. While many of the preformed granule-associated mediators are unique to, or at least highly concentrated in, basophils and mast cells, most of the substances produced during activation are also generated, sometimes in significantly greater amounts, by other leukocytes such as macrophages and neutrophils.

Basophils and mast cells have specific, high-affinity plasma membrane receptors for the Fc region of homocytotropic immunoglobulins; in humans this is largely IgE [18]. When basophil or mast cell surface IgE antibodies are bridged by specific di- or multivalent antigens, anaphylactic degranulation is triggered (Fig. 91-3). The critical signal in this event is probably related to the approximation of IgE receptors on the plasma membrane, and antibodies to the receptors may initiate degranulation in vitro [18]. Antigen binding is independent of divalent cations. However, later steps in degranulation require both Ca^{2+} and physiological temperatures [19]. Morphologically, anaphylactic degranulation involves the fusion of plasma membranes with the membranes delimiting individual cytoplasmic granules, leading to rapid noncytolytic release of granule contents, such as histamine and other preformed mediators. The biochemical and morphological events of anaphylactic degranulation, and the rationale of their pharmacological manipulation, have been reviewed [5,18–23].

The sudden, massive release of mediators from basophils and mast cells is thought to provoke the clinical manifestations of immediate hypersensitivity in such disorders as certain forms of bronchial asthma, urticaria, allergic rhinitis, and anaphylaxis to drugs, insect stings, and other antigens. Other diverse stimuli, including certain complement fragments (anaphylotoxins), neutrophil lysosomal proteins, a variety of basic peptides and peptide hormones, insect venoms, radiocontrast solutions, cold, calcium ionophores, and certain drugs such as narcotics and muscle relaxants, may also initiate rapid release of mediators from basophils and mast cells, independently of IgE [15]. The clinical reactions provoked by these agents closely mimic those of immediate hypersensitivity.

The fate of mature basophils that have undergone anaphylactic degranulation in vivo is unclear. Circulating granulocytes generally have been considered functionally end-stage cells unable to reconstitute their specific cytoplasmic granules; however, mature guinea pig basophils can synthesize additional granules after antigen-induced degranulation in vitro [24].

Cutaneous basophil hypersensitivity

Although a role for basophils in immediate hypersensitivity has been evident for some time, recent studies have established that basophils also participate prominently in reactions of cell-mediated hypersensitivity [5,25]. The identification of basophils in these and other inflammatory processes is critically dependent on proper techniques of fixation, embedding, and staining, since basophils are difficult or impossible to identify in routinely processed tissue sections [5,25].

Guinea pigs and rabbits immunized without mycobacterial adjuvants develop a systemic form of T-lymphocyte–mediated, delayed-onset reactivity termed *cutaneous basophil hypersensitivity* (CBH) [5,25]. In contrast to classic, tuberculin-type delayed hypersensitivity, CBH skin reactions have significant infiltrations of basophils, and, with many antigens, can be elicited only at early intervals after immunization. Reactions having a similar histology are characteristic of the response to important immunogens, including contact allergens, viruses, parasites, tumors, and vascularized allografts. Basophils may account for 60 percent or more of infiltrating cells in these reactions, although blood basophil levels are generally not significantly altered. Basophils are less numerous in human reactions comparable to CBH but may account for 5 to 15 percent of infiltrating cells in allergic contact dermatitis and skin allograft rejection. Basophils in much smaller numbers participate in tuberculin reactions and other classic expressions of delayed hypersensitivity.

Sensitized lymphocytes are essential for the induction and expression of CBH. Also, CBH-like reactions can be elicited in unsensitized animals by skin test with T-cell mitogens. Certain lymphocyte products are chemotactic for basophils and may attract basophils to local skin test sites. Other lymphocytes products may provoke basophil degranulation [26].

Fewer than 5 percent of basophils in CBH reactions bear detectable specific homocytotropic antibody, and an even smaller fraction exhibit evidence of anaphylactic degranulation. However, basophils in cell-mediated reactions may undergo a progressive piecemeal loss of granule matrix over 3 days. Piecemeal degranulation is distinct from anaphylactic degranulation and may involve transport of mediators from granules to the cell surface in vesicles of the type ordinarily associated with pinocytosis [27].

With many soluble protein antigens CBH reactivity may be transient, declining as significant amounts of antibody appear in the circulation. The CBH response persists indefinitely following immunization with antigens which do not generate significant antibody titers (e.g., certain viruses, contact allergens, tumor cells).

CBH may be superseded by "late reactions," i.e., complex lesions comprised of sequential but overlapping phases of cutaneous anaphylaxis and Arthus reactivity in addition to a basophil component. In contrast to CBH, such reactions contain many basophils bearing specific homocytotropic antibody. These late reactions in animals may be analogous to the basophil-containing IgE-mediated "late-phase" reactions that occur in a sizable fraction of atopic patients following an immediate cutaneous hypersensitivity response [5]. Basophil-rich reactions may also develop in animals challenged with antigen after passive transfer of specific antibodies [28].

Participation in other inflammatory processes

Because factors capable of inducing basophil or mast cell degranulation are generated in a wide variety of inflammatory processes, basophils and mast cells may contribute to the pathogenesis of reactions that are neither of immediate nor delayed hypersensitivity type. For example, basophils contribute to the cellular infiltrate in entities as diverse as Crohn's disease [29] and bullous pemphigoid [30].

The basophil's role in inflammatory reactions is obscure, but is presumably related to the mediators expressed on, or released from, these cells upon appropriate stimulation. Such mediators can influence the course of individual reactions in many ways. Histamine, for example, can both promote and dampen inflammation. It augments vascular permeability, resulting in edema formation and egress of antibody, fibrinogen, and other biologically active plasma proteins, but it inhibits MIF production, IgE-mediated histamine release, neutrophil lysosomal enzyme release, and certain T-cell functions [5]. Despite the abundance of theoretical roles for basophils in inflammation and immunity, there is little direct evidence concerning their function in reactions other than those of immediate hypersensitivity. In the guinea pig, basophils appear to be required for the expression of immune resistance to ixodid tick infestation [31]. In the mouse, there are remarkable similarities between basophils and cloned leukocytes that express natural killer cell function in vitro [32]. These cloned cells do not contain histamine, however, and their precise relationship to mouse basophils [33] is not yet clear.

References

1. Juhlin, L.: Basophil leukocyte differential in blood and bone marrow. *Acta Haematol. 29*:89, 1963.
2. Gilbert, H. S., and Ornstein, L.: Basophil counting with a new staining method using alcian blue. *Blood 46*:279, 1975.
3. Zucker-Franklin, D.: Electron microscopic study of human basophils. *Blood 29*:878, 1967.
4. Hastie, R. L.: A study of the ultrastructure of human basophil leukocytes. *Lab. Invest. 31*:223, 1974.
5. Galli, S. J., and Dvorak, H. F.: Basophils and mast cells: Structure, function, and role in hypersensitivity, in *Cellular, Molecular, and Clinical Aspects of Allergic Disorders*, edited by S. Gupta and R. A. Good. Plenum, New York, 1979, p. 1.
6. Osgood, E. E.: Culture of human marrow: Length of life of the neutrophils, eosinophils and basophils of normal blood as determined by comparative cultures of blood and sternal marrow from healthy persons. *JAMA 109*:933, 1937.
7. Murakami, I., Ogawa, M., Amo, H., and Ota, K.: Studies on kinetics of human leukocytes in vivo with ³H-thymidine autoradiography. II. Eosinophils and basophils. *Acta Haematol. Jpn. 32*:384, 1969.
8. Denburg, J. A., Davison, M., and Bienenstock, J.: Basophil production. *J. Clin. Invest. 65*:390, 1980.
9. Kitamura, Y., Shimada, M., Go, S., Matsuda, H., Hatanaka, K., and Seki, M.: Distribution of mast cell precursors in hematopoietic and lymphopoietic tissues of mice. *J. Exp. Med. 150*:482, 1979.
10. Schrader, J. W.: The in vitro production and cloning of the P cell, a bone-marrow derived null cell that expresses H-2 and Ia-antigen, has mast cell-like granules, and is regulated by a factor released by activated T cells. *J. Immunol. 126*:452, 1981.
11. Nabel, G., Galli, S., Dvorak, A. M., Dvorak, H. F., and Cantor, H.: Another inducer T cell function: Synthesis of a factor that stimulates proliferation of cloned mast cells. *Nature 291*:332, 1981.
12. Tertian, G., Yung, Y.-P., Guy-Grand, D., and Moore, M. A. S.: Long-term in vitro culture of murine mast cells. I. Description of a growth-factor dependent culture technique. *J. Immunol. 127*:788, 1981.
13. Yurt, R. W., Leid, R. W., Jr., Austen, K. F., and Silbert, J. E.: Native heparin from rat peritoneal mast cells. *J. Biol. Chem. 252*:518, 1977.
14. Porter, J. F., and Mitchell, R. G. L.: Distribution of histamine in human blood. *Physiol. Rev. 52*:361, 1972.
15. Ho, P. C., Lewis, R. A., Austen, K. F., and Orange, R. P.: Mediators of immediate hypersensitivity, in *Cellular, Molecular, and Clinical Aspects of Allergic Disorders*, edited by S. Gupta and R. A. Good. Plenum, New York, 1979, p. 179.
16. Newball, H. H., Berninger, R. W., Talamo, R. C., and Lichtenstein, L. M.: Anaphylactic release of a basophil kallikrein-like activity. *J. Clin. Invest. 64*:457, 1979.
17. Parwaresch, W. R.: *The Human Basophil*. Springer-Verlag, New York, 1976.
18. Ishizaka, K., and Ishizaka, T.: Immunoglobulin E: Biosynthesis and immunological mechanisms of IgE-mediated hypersensitivity, in *Cellular, Molecular, and Clinical Aspects of Allergic Disorders*, edited by S. Gupta and R. A. Good. Plenum, New York, 1979, p. 153.
19. Plaut, M., and Lichtenstein, L. M.: Pharmacologic control of mediator release. in *Immediate Hypersensitivity: Modern Concepts and Developments*, edited by M. K. Bach. Marcel Dekker, New York, 1978, p. 503.
20. Dvorak, A. M., Newball, H. H., Dvorak, H. F., and Lichtenstein, L. M.: Antigen-induced IgE-mediated degranulation of human basophils. *Lab. Invest. 43*:126, 1980.
21. Dvorak, A. M., Lett-Brown, M., Thueson, D., and Grant, J. A.: Complement-induced degranulation of human basophils. *J. Immunol. 126*:523, 1981.
22. Findlay, S. R., Dvorak, A. M., Kagey-Sobotka, A., and Lichtenstein, L. M.: Hyperosmolar triggering of histamine release from human basophils. *J. Clin. Invest. 67*:1604, 1981.
23. Siraganian, R. P., and Hook, W. A.: Complement-induced histamine release from human basophils. II. Mechanism of the histamine release reaction. *J. Immunol. 116*:639, 1976.
24. Dvorak, A. M., Galli, S. J., Morgan, E., Galli, A. S., Hammond, M. E.,

and Dvorak, H. F.: Anaphylactic degranulation of guinea pig baso-philic leukocytes. II. Evidence for regranulation of mature basophils during recovery from degranulation *in vitro. Lab. Invest.* 46:461, 1982.

25. Dvorak, H. F., Galli, S. J., and Dvorak, A. M.: Expression of cell-mediated immunity in vivo. Recent advances. *Int. Rev. Exp. Pathol.* 21:119, 1980.

26. Thueson, D. O., Speck, L. S., Lett-Brown, M. A., and Grant, J. A.: Histamine-releasing activity (HRA). I. Production by mitogen- or antigen-stimulated human mononuclear cells. *J. Immunol.* 123:626, 1979.

27. Dvorak, A. M. Mihm, M. C., Jr., and Dvorak, H. F.: Degranulation of basophilic leukocytes in allergic contact dermatitis reactions in man. *J. Immunol.* 116:687, 1976.

28. Haynes, J. D., Rosenstein, R. W., and Askenase, P. W.: A newly described activity of guinea pig IgG₁ antibodies: Transfer of cuta-neous basophil reactions. *J. Immunol.* 120:886, 1978.

29. Dvorak, A. M., Monahan, R. A., Osage, J. E., and Dickersin, G. R.: Crohn's disease: Transmission electron microscopic studies. II. Im-munologic inflammatory responses: Alterations of mast cells, baso-phils, eosinophils, and the microvasculature. *Hum. Pathol.* 11:606, 1980.

30. Dvorak, A. M., Mihm, M. C., Jr., Osage, J. E., Kwan, T. H., Austen, K. F., and Wintroub, B. U.: Bullous pemphigoid, an ultrastructural study of the inflammatory response: Eosinophil, basophil, and mast cell granule changes in multiple biopsies from one patient. *J. Invest. Dermatol.* 78:91, 1982.

31. Brown, S. J., Galli, S. J., Gleich, G. J., and Askenase, P. W.: Ablation of immunity to *Amblyomma americanum* by anti-basophil serum: Cooperation between basophils and eosinophils in expression of immunity to ectoparasites (ticks) in guinea pigs. *J. Immunol.* 129:790, 1982.

32. Galli, S. J., et al.: A cloned cell with natural killer function resembles basophils by ultrastructure and expresses IgE receptors. *Nature* 298:288, 1982.

33. Dvorak, A. M., Nabel, G., Pyne, K., Cantor, H., Dvorak, H. E., and Galli, S. J.: Ultrastructural identification of the mouse basophil. *Blood* 59:1279, 1982.

CHAPTER *92*

Eosinopenia and eosinophilia

DOROTHEA ZUCKER-FRANKLIN

The eosinophil count

The normal nonallergic subject has an absolute blood eosinophil count of less than 350 per microliter. Only about 1 percent of eosinophils circulate. There is a marked diurnal variation in the level of circulating eosinophils, with the highest level occurring in the morning and the lowest in the afternoon. This variation should be taken into account when eosinophils are enu-merated, particularly if serial counts are obtained for ex-perimental purposes.

Eosinopenia

Acute infections, glucocorticoids, ACTH, prostaglan-dins, and epinephrine decrease eosinophil levels [1–4], whereas administration of the β-adrenergic blocking agent propranolol prevents the eosinopenia of epineph-rine administration and may induce a rise of 30 per-cent in the blood eosinophil count [5]. Eosinopenia caused by glucocorticoid hormones is attributed to an inhibition of release of mature cells from the marrow and an increased margination of cells in small blood vessels. Splenectomy does not abolish the eosinopenic response to glucocorticoids. Only a few cases of complete aneosinophilia have been reported, and the clinical consequence of an absence of eosinophils is uncertain.

Eosinophilia

BLOOD EOSINOPHILIA

A "physiologic" eosinophilia is seen during the first 3 months of life, when eosinophil counts may be three times as high as in adults [6]. The mechanism underly-ing reactive eosinophilia in most situations has been elucidated by an elegant series of experiments [7,8]. Accelerated marrow proliferation appears to be induced by factors originating from T lymphocytes. Neonatal thymectomy and treatment with antilymphocyte serum deprive most mammals of the ability to raise their eosinophil count above normal levels. Eosinophilia is not necessarily related to the type of antigen but rather to its tissue localization [9]. This observation may ex-plain eosinophilic conditions associated with the cellu-lar immune response elicited by diverse stimuli (Table 92-1). In allergies to drugs, foods, or toxins released by insects or parasites, lymphocytes are sensitized and the degree of sensitization corresponds to the level of eosin-ophilia [9]. Occult tumors, particularly those undergo-ing necrosis, should be considered in cases of unex-plained eosinophilia. Chronic inflammatory reactions are best exemplified by various cutaneous disorders such as mycosis fungoides or Kimura's disease [10] where lymphocytic skin infiltrates devoid of eosino-phils are frequently accompanied by blood eosinophi-lia.

TISSUE EOSINOPHILIA

A different mechanism must be invoked to explain local or generalized eosinophilia of tissues. Chemotaxis plays a role in these conditions. During immediate hypersen-sitivity reactions, mast cells release histamine and eo-sinophil chemotactic factor of anaphylaxis (ECF-A), agents that attract eosinophils preferentially. Therefore, tissues rich in mast cells, such as the respiratory or gas-trointestinal tract, are particularly common sites for eosinophil invasion. In addition, an eosinophilotactic factor, eosinophil stimulation promoter, is elaborated by antigenically or nonspecifically stimulated lympho-

TABLE 92-1   Disorders associated with eosinophilia

PARASITES [31–36]

Protozoan infections:
Pneumonocytis toxoplasmosis, amebiasis, malaria

Metazoan infections:
Nematodes: strongyloidiasis, enterobiasis, ascariasis, toxocariasis (visceral larva migrans), hookworm disease, trichinosis, filariasis; *trematodes:* schistosomiasis, paragonimiasis, clonorchiasis; *cestodes:* cysticercosis, echinococcosis, taeniasis, sparganosis

Arthropods: scabies, *Tunga penetrans*

ALLERGIC DISORDERS [10,36–38]

Hay fever, asthma, hypersensitivity pneumonitides, Heiner's syndrome, angioneurotic edema, urticaria and angioedema, serum sickness, allergic vasculitis, Stevens-Johnson syndrome

DERMATITIS [36–38]

Psoriasis, eczema, dermatitis herpetiformis, dermatitis venenata, pemphigus vulgaris, prurigo, ichthyosis, pityriasis, rubra, facial granulomas

HYPEREOSINOPHILIC SYNDROMES [12–26,30,39–41,53–54,66]

Eosinophilic leukemia, Loeffler's syndrome, Loeffler's endocarditis, disseminated eosinophilic connective tissue disease, polyarteritis nodosa

GASTROINTESTINAL DISORDERS [36,42–44]

Eosinophilic gastroenteritis, milk precipitin disease, ulcerative colitis, protein-losing enteropathy, regional enteritis, allergic granulomatosis

TUMORS [37,45–48,57–59,61–62]

Carcinomatosis, epithelial tumors, brain tumors, melanoma, mycosis fungoides, Hodgkin's and non-Hodgkin's lymphoma, acute lymphocytic leukemia, eosinophilic granuloma, familial histiocytosis, Kimura's disease, myeloproliferative disorders

HEREDITARY (AND FAMILIAL) [49–52]

Familial eosinophilia, hereditary eosinophilia

MISCELLANEOUS [36,55,56,60,63,64,66]

Thymic disorders, hypoxia, peritoneal dialysis, chronic renal disease, Goodpasture's syndrome, sarcoidosis, splenectomy, radiotherapy, febrile illness convalescence, pneumonia, hypoadrenocorticism, pleural effusion, eosinophilic fascitis

cytes [11]. Theoretically, this makes any site of lymphoid proliferation susceptible to eosinophil infiltration.

REACTIVE HYPEREOSINOPHILIC SYNDROMES

The reactive hypereosinophilic syndromes (HES) include a wide spectrum of diseases which may be acute or chronic, fatal, or benign [12,13]. What these conditions have in common is persistent blood eosinophilia of more than 1500 per microliter, eosinophilic infiltration of tissues, and an unknown etiology. Therefore, the category of HES is a catchall from which a syndrome should be removed as the cause of a condition becomes defined. The best example supporting this contention is tropical eosinophilia, a debilitating disease which occurs in India and Southeast Asia. A very high eosinophil count is associated with pulmonary infiltrates; granulomatous changes in liver, spleen, and lymph nodes; an 80 percent male predominance; and unre-

sponsiveness to glucocorticoids [14]. The disease is caused by a filarial organism [15] and can be cured with diethylcarbamazine. Other "pulmonary eosinophilias" include the transient Loeffler's syndrome, described in 1930 [16], in which pulmonary infiltrates may spontaneously subside within a month; the more severe syndrome referred to as *pulmonary infiltrates with eosinophilia* (PIE) [17], which usually responds to glucocorticoids [18]; and a very serious, often fatal, syndrome which consists of asthma, pulmonary infiltrates, central nervous system involvement, or peripheral neuropathy and periarteritis nodosa [19]. These conditions may represent an exogenously or endogenously induced hypersensitivity response with reactive eosinophilia. Tissue damage associated with persistent eosinophilia may be secondary to the effects of substances released by the disintegrating cells.

FATAL HYPEREOSINOPHILIC SYNDROMES

These include the disseminated eosinophilic collagen diseases and eosinophilic leukemia. In addition to persistent eosinophilia and a leukocytosis of more than 15,000 per microliter, there is multiple-organ involvement, hepatosplenomegaly, central nervous system damage, and endomyocardial fibrosis with mural thrombi, fever, weight loss, and anemia. The syndromes have a marked male predominance and affect patients in early middle age. A total leukocyte count over 100,000 per microliter foretells a poor prognosis.

The question of whether some of these cases represent eosinophilic leukemia is addressed in every paper on this subject [20–23]. Chromosome abnormalities in marrow cells are strongly suggestive of leukemia [24–26]. In rare cases, the Ph[1] chromosome has been found, and the disease represents a type of chronic myelogenous leukemia with eosinophil predominance. At this point the disease may follow an acute course. The diagnosis of eosinophilic leukemia is difficult because most of the blood eosinophils are mature, or show morphologic changes also described in severe eosinophilias of a benign nature [27]. Tissue damage may ensue before a blastic crisis or other criteria for the diagnosis of leukemia have developed. The majority of patients succumb to congestive heart failure. Tissue injury caused by persistent hypereosinophilia is attributable to substances released by disintegrating eosinophils. Among these are lysosomal enzymes, peroxidase, and the strongly cationic proteins which react with cell membranes.

MANAGEMENT OF HYPEREOSINOPHILIC SYNDROMES

Although patients have tolerated eosinophilia of unknown etiology for many years without ill effect [28], when eosinophilia exceeds 5000 per microliter, an attempt to suppress this reaction with antihistamines or glucocorticoids is warranted. Chemotherapeutic agents, particularly hydroxyurea [29,30], have been used in patients in whom the height of the eosinophil count and the morbidity warrants such an approach. Leukapheresis therapy has also been beneficial in the management of hypereosinophilic syndromes [65]. If the findings of eosinophilic leukemia are present, the patient can be treated like other patients with acute myelogenous leukemia.

References

1. Anderson, V., Bro-Rasmussen, F., and Hougaard, K.: Autoradiographic studies of eosinophil kinetics: Effects of cortisol. *Cell Tissue Kinet.* 2:139, 1969.
2. Thevathasan, O. J., and Gordon, A. S.: Andrenocortical-medullary interactions on the blood eosinophils. *Acta Haematol.* 19:162, 1958.
3. Kurosawa, M., et al.: Prostaglandin-induced eosinopenia in splenectomized rats. *J. Allergy Clin. Immunol.* 62:33, 1978.
4. Bass, D. A.: Eosinopenia of acute infection. Production of eosinopenia by chemotactic factors of acute inflammation. *J. Clin. Invest.* 65:1265, 1980.
5. Koch-Weser, J.: Beta-adrenergic blockade and circulating eosinophils. *Arch. Intern. Med.* 121:255, 1968.
6. Matheson, A., Rosenblum, A., Glazer, R., and Dacanay, E.: Local tissue and blood eosinophils in newborn infants. *J. Pediatr.* 51:502, 1957.
7. Basten, A., Boyer, M. H., and Beeson, P. B.: Mechanism of eosinophilia. I. Factors affecting the eosinophil response of rats to *Trichinella spiralis*. *J. Exp. Med.* 131:1271, 1970.
8. Basten, A., and Beeson, P. B.: Mechanisms of eosinophilia. II. Role of the lymphocyte. *J. Exp. Med.* 131:1288, 1970.
9. Schriber, R. A., and Zucker-Franklin, D.: Induction of blood eosinophilia by pulmonary embolization of antigen-coated particles. The relationship to cell-mediated immunity. *J. Immunol.* 114:1348, 1975.
10. Zucker-Franklin, D.: Eosinophil function related to cutaneous disorders. *J. Invest. Dermat.* 71:100, 1978.
11. Colley, D. G.:Eosinophils and immune mechanisms. I. Eosinophil stimulation promoter (ESP): A lymphokine induced by specific antigen or phytohemagglutinin. *J. Immunol.* 110:1419, 1973.
12. Hardy, W. R., and Anderson, R. E.: The hypereosinophilic syndromes. *Ann. Intern. Med.* 68:1220, 1968.
13. Chusid, M. F., Dale, D. C., West, B. C. and Wolff, S. M.: The hypereosinophilic syndrome: Analysis of fourteen cases with review of the literature. *Medicine* 54:1, 1975.
14. Donohugh, D. C.: Tropical eosinophilia: An etiologic inquiry. *N. Engl. J. Med.* 269:1357, 1963.
15. Danaray, T. J., Pachecho, G., Shanmugaratnam, K., and Beaver, P. G.: The etiology and pathology of eosinophilic lung (tropical eosinophilia). *Am. J. Trop. Med. Hyg.* 15:183, 1966.
16. Löffler, W.: Die flüchtigen Lungeninfiltrate mit Eosinophilie. *Schweiz. Med. Wochenscher.* 66:1069, 1936.
17. Carrington, C., et al.: Chronic eosinophilic pneumonia. *N. Engl. J. Med.* 280:787, 1969.
18. Liebow, A. A., and Carrington, C. B.: The eosinophilic pneumonias. *Medicine* 48:251, 1969.
19. Churg, J., and Strauss, L.: Allergic granulomatosis, allergic angiitis and periarteritis nodosa. *Am. J. Pathol.* 27:277, 1951.
20. Engfeldt, B., and Zetterstrom, R.: Disseminated eosinophilic "collagen disease." *Acta Med. Scand.* 153:337, 1956.
21. Odeberg, B.: Eosinophilic leukemia and disseminated eosinophilic collagen disease—a disease entity? *Acta Med. Scand.* 177:129, 1965.
22. Benvenisti, D. S., and Ultmann, J. E.: Eosinophilic leukemia. Report of five cases and review of literature. *Ann. Intern. Med.* 71:731, 1969.
23. Bentley, H. P., Reardon, A. E., Knoedler, J. P. and Krivit, W.: Eosinophilic leukemia. *Am. J. Med.* 30:310, 1961.
24. Gruenwald, H., Kiossoglou, K. A., Mitus, W. J., and Dameshek, W.: Philadelphia chromosome in eosinophilic leukemia. *Am. J. Med.* 39:1003, 1965.
25. Goh, K., Swisher, S. N. and Rosenberg, C. A.: Cytogenetic studies of eosinophilic leukemia and chronic myelocytic leukemia. *Ann. Intern Med.* 62:80, 1965.
26. Bitran, J. D., Rowley, J. D., Plapp, F., Golomb, H. M. and Ultmann, J. E.: Chromosomal aneuploidy in a patient with hyperosinophilic syndrome. *Am. J. Med.* 63:1010, 1977.
27. Zucker-Franklin, D.: Eosinophils, in *Atlas of Blood Cells: Function and Pathology*, edited by D. Zucker-Franklin, M. F. Greaves, C. E. Grossi, and A. M. Marmont. Edi Ermes, Milano, Lea & Febiger, Philadelphia, 1981, chap. 6, p. 257.
28. Hildebrand, F. L., Christensen, N. A., and Hanlon, D. G.: Eosinophilia of unknown cause. *Arch. Intern Med.* 113:129, 1964.
29. Kennedy, B. J.: Hydroxyurea therapy in chronic myelogenous leukemia. *Cancer* 29:1052, 1972.
30. Parrillo, J. E., Fauci, A. S. and Wolff, S. M.: Therapy of the hypereosinophilic syndrome. *Ann. Intern. Med.* 89:167, 1978.
31. Brown, H. W.: *Basic Clinical Parasitology*, 3d ed. Appleton-Century-Crofts, New York, 1969.
32. Lenezner, M. M.: Tropical and parasitic diseases: The impact on our civilization. *Mod. Med.* 36:52, 1968.
33. Donohugh, D. L.: Tropical eosinophilia: An etiologic inquiry. *N. Engl. J. Med.* 269:1357, 1963.
34. Beaver, P. D., Snyder, C. H., Carrera, G. M., Dent, J. H., and Lafferty, J. W.: Chronic eosinophilia due to visceral larva migrans. Report of three cases. *Pediatrics* 9:7, 1952.
35. Monshuta, K., Komaya, Y., and Matsubayasha, H. (eds.): *Progress of Medical Parasitology in Japan*, Vols. I and II. Meguro Parasitology Museum, Tokyo, 1964.
36. Lecks, H. I., and Kravis, L.: The allergist and the eosinophil. *Pediatr. Clin. North Am.* 16:125, 1969.
37. Donohugh, D. L.: Eosinophils and eosinophilia. *Calif. Med.* 104:421, 1966.
38. Wolf-Jurgensen, P.: Eosinophil and histamine in Asboe Hansen's disease. *Acta. Derm. Venereol.* 46:500, 1966.
39. Kauer, G. L., and Lugle, R. L., Jr.: Eosinophilic leukemia with Ph^1-positive cells. *Lancet* 2:1340, 1964.
40. Hardy, W. R., and Anderson, R. E.: The hypereosinophilic syndromes. *Ann. Intern. Med.* 68:1220, 1968.
41. Benvenisti, D. S., and Ultmann, J. I.: Eosinophilic leukemia: Report of five cases and review of literature. *Ann. Intern. Med.* 71:731, 1969.
42. Abell, M. R., Limond, R. V., Blamey, W. E., and Martel, W.: Allergic granulomatosis with massive gastric involvement. *N. Engl. J. Med.* 282:665, 1970.
43. Thomas, E., Lev, R., McCahan, J. F., and Pitchumoni, C. S.: Case report: Eosinophilic gastroenteritis with malabsorption, extensive villous atrophy, recurrent hemorrhage and chronic pulmonary fibrosis. *Am. J. Med. Sci.* 46:259, 1975.
44. Haeberle, M. G., and Griffen, W. O., Jr.: Eosinophilia and regional enteritis: A possible diagnostic aid. *Am. J. Dig. Dis.* 17:200, 1972.
45. Fahey, R. J.: Unusual leukocyte responses in primary carcinoma of the lung. *Cancer* 4:930, 1951.
46. Reed, R. J., and Terasaki, N.: Subcutaneous angioblastic lymphoid hyperplasia with eosinophilia (Kimura's disease). *Cancer* 29:489, 1972.
47. Ochs, H. D., Davis, S. D., Mickelson, E., Lerner, K. G., and Wedgewood, R. J.: Combined immunodeficiency and reticuloendotheliosis with eosinophilia. *J. Pediatr.* 85:463, 1974.
48. Barth, R. F., Vergara, G. G., and Khurana, S. K.: Rapidly fatal familial histiocytosis associated with eosinophilia and primary immunological deficiency. *Lancet* 2:503, 1972.
49. Stefanin, M., and Kavara, M.: Familial eosinophilia and splenomegaly. *Am. J. Med. Sci.* 245:125, 1963.
50. Cascone, A.: Su di un caso di leucocitosi eosinofila familiare. *Minerva Med.* 59:2572, 1968.
51. Dalous, A., Rochicciolo, P., and Ghisolfi, I.: Eosinophilic familiale. *Rev. Med. Foulouse.* 4:335, 1968.
52. Nauman, J. I., Oski, F. A., Allen, I. M., Jr., and Diamond, L. K.: Hereditary eosinophilia. Report of a family and review of literature. *Am. J. Hum. Genet.* 16:195, 1971.
53. Zuelzer, W., and Apt, L.: Disseminated visceral lesions associated with extreme eosinophilia. *Am. J. Dis. Child.* 78:153, 1949.
54. Choremis, C., Thomaidis, T., and Kattamis, C.: Hyperleucocytosis and severe eosinophilia in children: A review of nine instances. *Helv. Paediatr. Acta.* 20:628, 1965.
55. Lee, S., and Schoen, L.: Eosinophilia of peritoneal fluid and periph-

eral blood associated with chronic peritoneal dialysis. *Am. J. Clin. Pathol.* 47:638, 1967.

56. Panush, R. S., Franco, A. L., and Schur, P. H.: Rheumatoid arthritis associated with eosinophilia. *Ann. Intern. Med.* 75:199, 1971.

57. Isaacson, N. H., and Rapoport, P.: Eosinophilia in malignant tumors: Its significance. *Ann. Intern. Med.* 25:893, 1946.

58. Banerjee, R. N., and Narang, R. M.: Haematological changes in malignancy. *Br. J. Haematol.* 13:829, 1967.

59. Major, R. M., and Leget, L. H.: Marked eosinophilia in Hodgkin's disease. *JAMA* 112:2601, 1939.

60. Hoy, W. E., and Cestero, R. V. M.: Eosinophilia in maintenance hemodialysis patients. *J. Dialysis* 3:73, 1979.

61. Wasserman, S. I., Goetzl, E. J., Ellman, L., and Austen, K. F.: Tumor-associated eosinophilotactic factor. *N. Engl. J. Med.* 290:420, 1974.

62. Dillon, A. L., Hume, R. B., Chretien, P. B.: Eosinophilia in bronchogenic carcinoma. *N. Engl. J. Med.* 291:207, 1974.

63. Beekman, J. F., Bosniak, S., and Canter, H. G.: Eosinophilia and elevated IgE in a serous pleural effusion following trauma. *Am. Rev. Respir. Dis.* 110:484, 1974.

64. Michet, C. J., Doyle, J. A., and Ginsburg, W. W.: Eosinophilic fasciitis. *Mayo Clin. Proc.* 56:27, 1981.

65. Ellman, L., Miller, L., and Rappeport, J.: Leukapheresis therapy of a hypereosinophilic disorder. *JAMA* 230:1004, 1974.

66. Litt, M.: Eosinophils and antigen antibody reactions. *Ann. N.Y. Acad. Sci.* 116:964, 1964.

CHAPTER 93

Basophilopenia, basophilia, and mastocytosis

DOROTHEA ZUCKER-FRANKLIN

The morphologic and functional similarities of basophils (Fig. 93-1) and of mast cells (Fig. 93-2) are so great that one cell cannot be considered without the other (see Chap. 91). Both appear to be derived from an early hemopoietic progenitor cell in marrow [1–4]. Basophils are circulating leukocytes, whereas mast cells are found in connective tissues. Overlapping morphology between mast cells and basophils is observed in some human pathologic conditions. Transformation of basophils into mast cells or vice versa has never been observed, however, and the granules of these two cells have distinct structural differences (Fig. 93-3).

Blood basophil count

The normal blood basophil count has not been defined precisely. One study reports the normal range to be between 20 and 45 basophils per microliter [5], whereas another study reports it to be 10 to 80 basophils per microliter [6]. The total number of mast cells cannot be assessed because of the wide and variable distribution of these cells in different tissues [7,8]. Therefore, it is difficult to ascertain whether factors which regulate

basophil proliferation affect mast cells equally. Basophils are mature end-stage cells which leave the blood within a few hours, whereas mast cells can undergo mitosis. In the absence of physiologic or pathologic stimuli, the life-span of mast cells has been estimated to be about 2 years. However, when stimulated the mast cell reservoir can be replenished or increased by an influx of morphologically unidentifiable marrow precursors as well as by proliferation of mast cells already residing in tissues [2].

Diurnal variations in basophil levels have been reported in some individuals [9,10], as have alterations related to age [9,11,12]. Sex differences in basophil counts have been found by some authors [12] but not by others [9]. In some individuals, basophil degranulation apparently follows ingestion of large amounts of fat [5,13].

Basophilopenia

Basophilopenia has been recorded in urticaria and immediately after anaphylaxis [9,14], but the extent to which this finding represents a loss of metachromatic

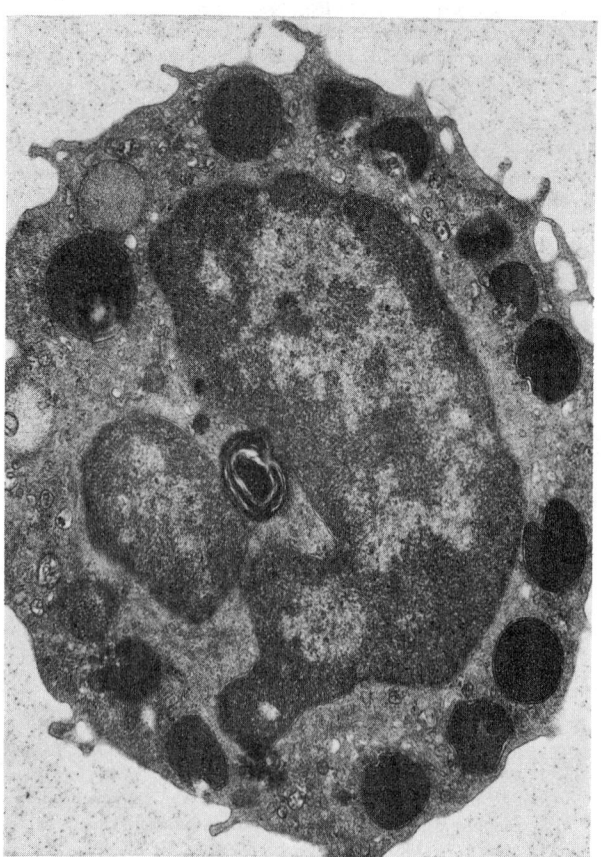

FIGURE 93-1 Ultrastructure of a mature basophil. Note segmented nucleus and abundant electron dense heterochromatin. Higher magnification of typical granules is illustrated in Fig. 93-3*a*. ×18,000 (Reproduced from Zucker-Franklin [4], with permission.)

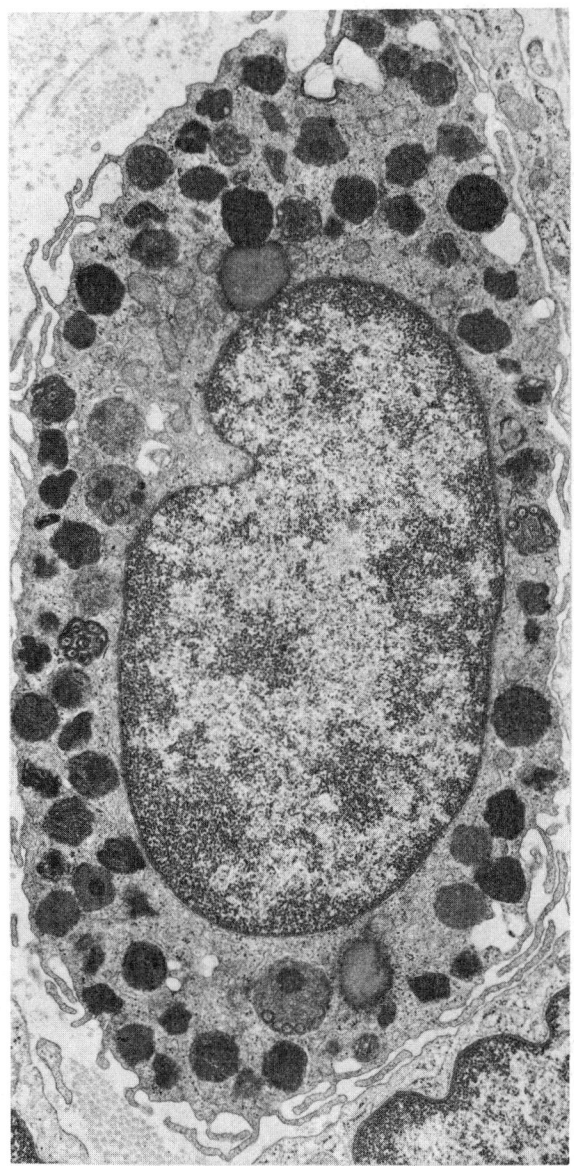

FIGURE 93-2 Ultrastructure of a mast cell. Nucleus is not segmented and has more finely dispersed chromatin than the basophil. Higher magnification of a typical mast cell granule is illustrated in Fig. 93-3*b*. ×14,000. (Reproduced from Zucker-Franklin [4], with permission.)

staining of circulating, degranulated cells is undetermined.

Basophilopenia occurs in conditions that are associated with eosinophilopenia, that is, in situations which stress the pituitary-adrenal axis. Basophil counts may diminish, sometimes markedly, during leukocytosis accompanying infection, inflammatory states, immunologic reactions, neoplasia, or hemorrhage [15,16]. A decrease in basophil count is related to increased levels of glucocorticoids [15,17–19]. Also, basophil counts are diminished in thyrotoxicosis or after treatment with thyroid hormones, and, conversely, they may

be increased in myxedema or after pharmacological ablation of thyroid function [15,18]. A rapid and significant drop of up to 50 percent in blood basophil levels has been documented at ovulation [10,18]. A single patient with an apparent total lack of basophils has been reported [20]. This man also lacked eosinophils, had low levels of IgA and IgE, and appeared to have normal numbers of skin and marrow cells. In addition to clinical problems that could be due to IgA deficiency, he had recurrent warts and persistent scabies, findings consistent with the role basophils have in the expression of cellular immunity [21].

A morphological abnormality expressed in the majority of eosinophils and basophils but not in other leukocytes or mast cells has been described as an autosomal dominant condition affecting four members of a family [22]. Prominent cytoplastic inclusions and crystals of uncertain composition found in basophils resembled those of the May-Hegglin anomaly. The individuals were all clinically healthy, although specific studies of basophil or eosinophil function were not performed. Little has been written about the appearance of basophils in other genetic disorders of granulocyte morphology.

Basophilia

Disorders associated with basophilia are presented in Table 93-1.

INFLAMMATORY REACTIONS
An increase in the number of basophils is commonly associated with hypersensitivity reactions of the immediate type (Table 93-1). This is often accompanied by in-

TABLE 93-1   Disorders associated with basophilia

Allergy or inflammation [9,24–27,46,56–59]:
  Colitis
  Drug, food, inhalant hypersensitivity
  Erythroderma, urticaria
  Hookworm
  Rheumatoid arthritis
Endocrinopathy [18,54,55]:
  Estrogen administration
  Hypothyroidism (myxedema)
  Diabetes mellitus
Infections [56,60,65]:
  Influenza
  Chickenpox
  Smallpox
  Tuberculosis
Neoplasias [29,30,31,35,37–40,47,61–64]:
  Carcinoma
  Myeloproliferative diseases (especially chronic myelogenous leukemia, also polycythemia vera, agnogenic myeloid metaplasia)
  Basophilic leukemia (unrelated to CML)
  Mastocytosis

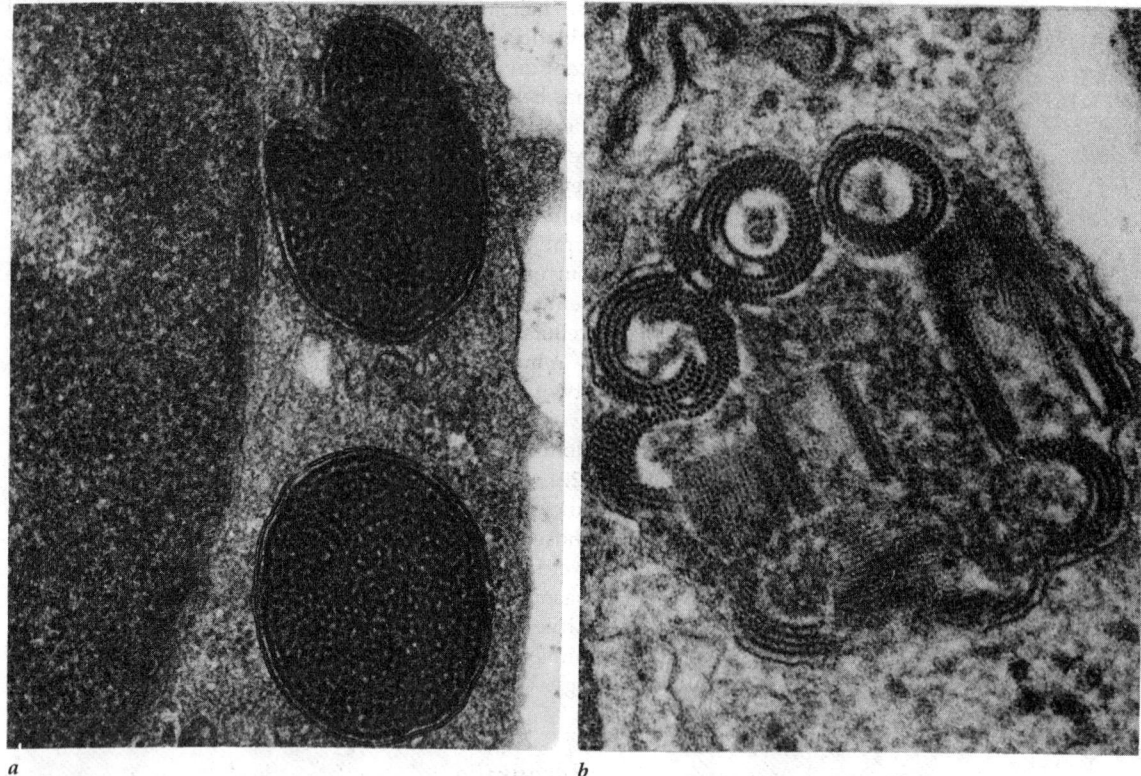

FIGURE 93-3 (*a*) Basophil granules show particles surrounded by unit membrane. ×72,000. (*b*) The ultrastructure of a mast cell granule. ×150,000. (Reproduced from Zucker-Franklin [4], with permission.)

creased levels of IgE. However, parallelism of IgE levels and basophil numbers is neither constant nor causally related [23]. During hypersensitivity reactions, large numbers of basophils move into tissues by diapedesis. They can be distinguished from mast cells by morphological and histochemical methods, e.g., in the lesions caused by allergic contact dermatitis such as poison ivy [24] or in the nasal secretions of patients with allergic rhinitis [25].

Basophil levels may be elevated in ulcerative colitis [26] and juvenile rheumatoid arthritis [27] despite the observation that most inflammatory conditions which cause a leukocytosis are associated with basophilopenia. Basophilia is commonly found in subjects exposed to radiation [28,29].

MYELOPROLIFERATIVE DISEASES

Basophil levels are increased in the chronic myeloproliferative disorders, a finding useful in differentiating these diseases from leukemoid reactions in which low basophil counts are the rule [28]. The basophil count may be moderately elevated in myeloid metaplasia and polycythemia vera, with levels in excess of 1000 per microliter [28]. The highest basophil counts are seen in chronic myelogenous leukemia (CML), where basophils often account for 2 to 20 percent of circulating leukocytes [5,28]. Basophil counts exceeding 30 percent can

occur during the course of CML, particularly late in the disease, and this often heralds its terminal phase [30]. The basophils of CML are neoplastic, not reactive, cells since they possess the Philadelphia chromosome [5,31] and exhibit a variety of morphological and histochemical abnormalities [5,32–36]. Ultrastructurally, overlapping morphology may make the distinction between a typical basophil and a typical mast cell in CML impossible (Fig. 93-4), suggesting that basophils and mast cells arise from the same marrow precursor [4]. Very rarely, cells resembling normal basophils account for over 80 percent of circulating leukocytes early in CML [5,37]. Such cases have been designated *basophilic leukemia*. Occasional patients with basophil-rich myelogenous leukemia, particularly those with extraordinarily elevated basophil counts, may exhibit clinical effects attributable to the liberation of histamine and perhaps other basophil mediators [38].

Basophilic leukemia

Although some observers deny the existence of basophilic leukemia as a disease entity distinct from chronic myelogenous leukemia, the term seems justified when the basophil count is high at the beginning of the disease and remains between 40 and 80 percent of an extremely high white cell count throughout the course, and the Ph[1] chromosome is not present in marrow cells. Acute and chronic forms have been recognized [37]. The clinical and pathologic features are similar to those of myelogenous leukemia, but may occasionally be complicated by symptoms due to potent mediators derived from degranulating cells. The disease is not readily amenable to current modalities of therapy, which, even when effective, may lead to shock due to the massive release of histamine associated with cytolysis [38]. Such individuals may benefit from the administration of antihistamines or, perhaps, inhibitors of arachidonic acid metabolism.

Mastocytosis

REACTIVE MASTOCYTOSIS
An increase in the number of mast cells may be seen in any tissue involved in a hypersensitivity reaction of the immediate or delayed type. Humoral factors released by sensitized T lymphocytes are believed to induce the local response. Allergic rhinitis, allergic asthma, and urticaria are the most common conditions in which increased numbers of mast cells are seen in the affected tissues. Mast cell hyperplasia is also present in the lymph nodes of patients with filariasis and in the nodes draining a large variety of benign and malignant tumors [39,40]. The nodes of patients with lymphoproliferative diseases, particularly Hodgkin's disease, are often replete with mast cells. In all these instances, it is likely that biogenic amines and heparin-like material are secreted in situ. These substances may dilate blood vessels to recruit inflammatory cells or prevent the formation of microthrombi. Mast cell hyperplasia in the marrow of women after the age of 50 has been correlated with an increased incidence of osteoporosis [41].

MAST CELL NEOPLASIA

BENIGN MAST CELL NEOPLASIA
Localized mastocytomas are extremely rare lesions, most often occurring as solitary brown nodules on the ventral aspect of the wrist [42]. Such lesions may resolve spontaneously. The more generalized cutaneous form of mastocytosis, urticaria pigmentosa, makes its appearance before the age of 2 years in 50 percent of cases [43]. The disease is manifested by macules, papules, vesicles, nodules, plaques, or sometimes generalized erythroderma [44,45]. Biopsy of the lesions is diagnostic. Patients may experience intense pruritis and exhibit the Darier's sign, i.e., urticaria as a consequence of mild friction of the skin. Sequential biopsies following mild trauma have confirmed that the skin reaction accompanies local degranulation of mast cells (Fig. 93-5a and b). In the majority of patients, urticaria pigmentosa subsides at puberty. However, a small proportion of cases

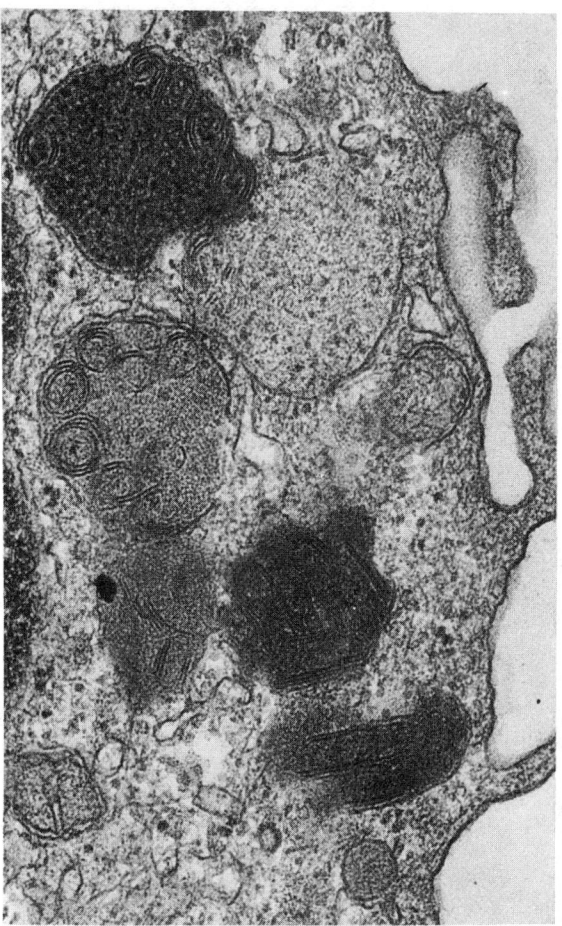

FIGURE 93-4 Detail of a cell from the blood of a patient with CML illustrates the overlap in morphology between basophil and mast cell granules. The granules exhibit particles as well as "scrolls." (Reproduced from Zucker-Franklin [4], with permission.)

continue into adulthood, when the prognosis becomes more guarded. Urticaria pigmentosa in adults rarely remains limited to the skin, but usually develops into systemic mastocytosis. Therefore, adults with urticaria pigmentosa should be examined for systemic spread at regular intervals. Hepatosplenomegaly and enlarged lymph nodes are early signs of systemic involvement.

MALIGNANT MAST CELL NEOPLASIA
The malignant form of systemic mastocytosis may develop as a primary disease. However, one-third of the cases with the benign condition may evolve into the malignant variety. In these instances, cutaneous involvement may be absent. The peak incidence is in the sixth and seventh decade of life. There is a male/female ratio of 2:1. The marrow, spleen, liver, and lymph nodes are almost always infiltrated. Many mitotic mast cells are seen on biopsy. Infiltrated tissues, such as the marrow and liver, may become fibrotic. The prognosis for survival is less than 2 years [39,43,45].

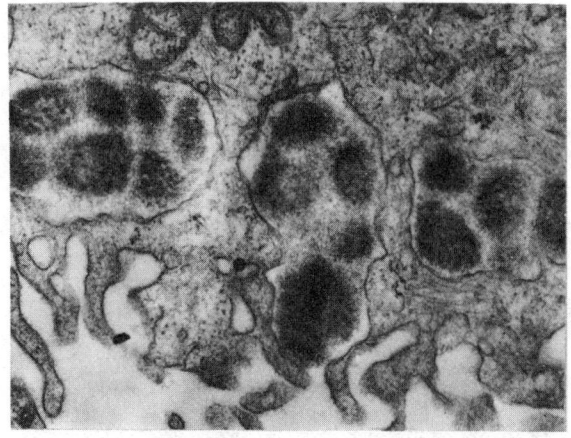

a

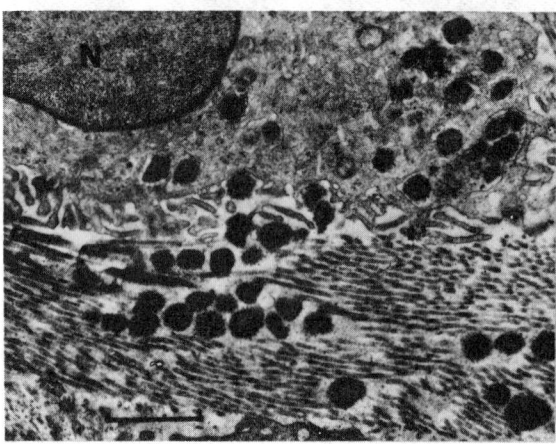

b

FIGURE 93-5   (*a*) Detail of the periphery of a mast cell in the process of discharging its granules. From a biopsy of a patient with urticaria pigmentosa after friction was applied to the skin. ×17,0000. (*b*) Subsequent stage of mast cell degranulation (same patient as in Fig. 93-4*a*). The granules are now seen among collagen fibrils. N = nucleus. ×13,000.

MAST CELL LEUKEMIA

Leukemia develops in about 15 percent of patients with malignant mast cell neoplasia [39]. The morphology of the cells may vary from typical mast cells to monocytoid cells with some metachromatic granules and large nucleoli. Erythrophagocytosis has been reported [44]. The existence of this disease entity has also been adduced in support of the contention that the mast cells belong to the hemopoietic system. Neoplasms of other than lympho- and monocytic leukemias have been observed during the course of malignant mastocytosis more often than would be likely by coincidence.

MAST CELL SARCOMA

Only one well-documented case of mast cell sarcoma has been reported [39]. In this patient, tumor nodules developed initially at various cutaneous and mucosal sites. Subsequently almost every organ became in-

volved. Terminally, the blood showed 95 percent immature mast cells with a monocytoid appearance. This observation is taken as additional evidence for the view that mast cells are marrow-derived.

MANAGEMENT

Since many of the symptoms of benign or malignant mastocytosis are attributable to the release of biogenic amines or heparin-like material from degranulating mast cells, a rational approach to therapy is to block the effects of these agents or to impair degranulation itself. Combined blockade of both H1 and H2 receptors with histamine antagonists such as cimetidine and chlorpheniramine should be attempted [46,47]. In addition, some patients with urticaria pigmentosa appear to have marked overproduction of the arachidonic acid metabolite, prostaglandin D_2 [48]. Therefore, the use of aspirin in addition to histamine antagonists may be of benefit in some cases [49]. Mast cell secretion may be inhibited in vitro with cromoglycate, which blocks the uptake of calcium ions necessary for degranulation [50]. The drug has been used in patients with allergic bronchospasm [51] and in other conditions associated with mast cell hyperplasia, but its efficacy is controversial.

In malignant systemic mastocytosis or mast cell leukemia, a trial of chemotherapeutic protocols used in the treatment of other myeloproliferative diseases is indicated.

References

1. Zucker-Franklin, D.: Basophils, in *Atlas of Blood Cells*, D. Zucker-Franklin, M. F. Greaves, C. E. Grossi, and A. M. Marmont. Lea & Febiger, Philadelphia, 1981, chap. 7.
2. Hatanaka, K., Kitamura, Y., and Nishimune, Y.: Local development of mast cells from bone marrow-derived precursors in the skin of mice. *Blood* 53:142, 1979.
3. Kitamura, Y., Shimada, M., Go, S., Matsuda, H., Hatanaka, K., and Seki, M.: Distribution of mast cell precursors in hematopoietic and lymphopoietic tissues of mice. *J. Exp. Med.* 150:482, 1979.
4. Zucker-Franklin, D.: Ultrastructural evidence for the common origin of human mast cells and basophils. *Blood* 56:534, 1980.
5. Parwaresch, M. R.: *The Human Blood Basophil.* Springer-Verlag, New York, 1976, p. 4.
6. Gilbert, H. S., and Ornstein, L.: Basophil counting with a new staining method using alcian blue. *Blood* 46:279, 1975.
7. Cowen, T., Trigg, P., and Eady, R. A. J.: Distribution of mast cells in human dermis: Development of a mapping technique. *Br. J. Dermatol.* 100:635, 1979.
8. Eady, R. A. J., Cowen, T., Marshall, T. F., Plummer, V., and Greaves, M. W.: Mast cell population density, blood vessel density and histamine content in normal human skin. *Br. J. Dermatol.* 100:623, 1979.
9. Rorsman, H.: Studies on basophil leukocytes with special reference to urticaria and anaphylaxis. *Acta Derm. Venereol.* 42 (Suppl. 48):1, 1962.
10. Osada, Y.: Diurnal rhythms of the numbers in circulating basophils and eosinophils in healthy adults. *Bull. Inst. Public Health* 5:5, 1956.
11. Mitchell, R. G.: Circulating basophilic leukocyte counts in the newborn. *Arch. Dis. Child.* 30:130, 1955.
12. Thonnard-Neumann, E.: Studies of basophils. Variations with age and sex. *Acta Haematol.* 30:221, 1963.
13. Shelley, W. B., and Juhlin, L.: Degranulation of the basophil of man induced by lipemia. *Am. J. Med. Sci.* 242:211, 1961.

14. Shelley, W. B., and Juhlin, L.: New test for detecting anaphylactic sensitivity: Basophil reaction. *Nature* 191:1056, 1961.
15. Juhlin, L.: Basophil and eosinophil leukocytes in various internal disorders. *Acta Med. Scand.* 174:249, 1963.
16. Mitchell, R. G.: Basophilic leukocytes in children in health and disease. *Arch. Dis. Child.* 33:193, 1958.
17. Kelemen, E., and Bikich, G.: Insufficiency of acute response of basophil and eosinophil leukocytes and of blood histamine after the administration of ACTH and cortisone in untreated myelocytic leukemia. *Acta Haematol.* 15:202, 1956.
18. Mettler, L., and Shirwani, D.: Direct basophil count for timing ovulation. *Fertil. Steril.* 25:718, 1974.
19. Juhlin, L.: The effect of corticotropin and corticosteroids on the basophil and eosinophil granulocytes. *Acta Haematol.* 29:157, 1963.
20. Juhlin, L., and Michäelsson, G.: A new syndrome characterized by absence of eosinophils and basophils. *Lancet* i:1233, 1977.
21. Galli, S. J., Colvin, R. B., Orenstein, N. S., Dvorak, A. M., and Dvorak, H. F.: Patients without basophils. *Lancet* ii:409, 1977.
22. Tracey, R., and Smith, H.: An inherited anomaly of human eosinophils and basophils. *Blood Cells* 4:291, 1978.
23. Malveaux, F. J., Conroy, M. C., Adkinson, N. F., and Lichtenstein, L. M.: IgE receptors on human basophils. *J. Clin. Invest.* 62:176, 1978.
24. Dvorak, H. F., and Mihm, M. C.: Basophilic leukocytes in allergic contact dermatitis. *J. Exp. Med.* 135:235, 1972.
25. Levy, D. A., Hastie, R., Chir, B., Heroy, J. H., and Rody, E.: Mast cells and basophils in allergic rhinitis. *Monogr. Allergy* 14:261, 1979.
26. Juhlin, L.: Basophil leukocytes in ulcerative colitis. *Acta Med. Scand.* 173:351, 1963.
27. Athreya, B. H., Moser, G., and Raghavan, T. E. S.: Increased circulating basophils in juvenile rheumatoid arthritis. *Am. J. Dis. Child.* 129:935, 1975.
28. Fredericks, R. E., and Moloney, W. C.: The basophilic granulocyte. *Blood* 14:571, 1959.
29. Moloney, W. C., and Lange, R. D.: Cytologic and biochemical studies on the granulocytes in early leukemia among atom bomb survivors. *Tex. Rep. Biol. Med.* 12:887, 1954.
30. Doan, C. A., and Reinhart, H. L.: The basophil granulocyte, basophilicytosis and myeloid leukemia basophil and mixed granule types; an experimental, clinical and pathological study, with the report of a new syndrome. *Am. J. Clin. Pathol.* 11:1, 1941.
31. Shohet, S. B., and Blum, S. F.: Coincident basophilic chronic myelogenous leukemia and pulmonary tuberculosis. *Cancer* 22:173, 1968.
32. Dvorak, A. M., Dickersin, G. R., Connell, A. B., Carey, R. W., and Dvorak, H. F.: Degranulation mechanisms in human leukemic basophils. *Clin. Immunol. Immunopathol.* 5:235, 1976.
33. Lichtenstein, L. M., Sobotka, A. K., Malveaux, F. J., and Gillespie, E.: IgE-induced changes in human basophil cyclic AMP levels. *Int. Arch. Allergy Appl. Immunol.* 56:473, 1978.
34. Lewis, R. A., Goetzl, E. J., Wasserman, S. I., Valone, F. H., Rubin, R. H., and Austen, K. F.: The release of four mediators of immediate hypersensitivity from human leukemic basophils. *J. Immunol.* 114:87, 1975.
35. Mitrakul, C., Othaganonda, B. O., Manothal, P., Bhanichaya-Bhongsa, S.: Basophilic leukemia. Report of a case. *Clin. Pediatr.* 8:178, 1969.
36. Dvorak, A. M., Monahan, R. A., and Dickersin, G. R.: Diagnostic electron microscopy. I. Hematology: Differential diagnosis of acute lymphoblastic and acute myeloblastic leukemia. Use of ultrastructural peroxidase cytochemistry and routine electron microscopic technology, in *Pathology Annual. Part I*, edited by S. C. Summers and P. P. Rosen. Appleton-Century-Crofts, New York, 1981.
37. Lennert, K., Koster, E., and Martin, H.: Uber die Mastzellen-leukaemie. *Acta Haematol.* 16:255, 1956.
38. Youman, J. D., Taddeini, L., and Cooper, T.: Histamine excess, symptoms in basophilic chronic granulocytic leukemia. *Arch. Intern. Med.* 131, 560, 1973.
39. Lennert, K., and Parwaresch, M. R.: Mast cells and mast cell neoplasia: A review. *Histopathology* 3:349, 1979.
40. Bowers, H. M., Mahapatro, R. C., and Kennedy, J. W.: Numbers of mast cells in the axillary lymph nodes of breast cancer patients. *Cancer* 43:568, 1979.
41. Frame, B., and Nixon, R. K.: Bone marrow mast cells in osteoporosis of aging. *N. Engl. J. Med.* 279:626, 1968.
42. Sagher, F. and Even-Paz, Z.: Mastocytosis and the mast cell. Year Book, Chicago, 1967.
43. Fine, J. D.: Mastocytosis (Review). *Intern. Soc. Trop. Dermatol.* 19:117, 1980.
44. Mutter, R. D., Tannenbaum, M., and Ultmann, J. E.: Splenic mast cell disease. *Ann. Intern. Med.* 59:887, 1963.
45. van Kammen, E.: Generalized mastocytosis. *Acta Haematol.* 52:129, 1974.
46. Gerrard, J. W. and Ko, C.: Urticaria pigmentosa: Treatment with cimetidine and chlorpheniramine. *J. Pediatr.* 94:843, 1979.
47. Hirschowitz, B. I. and Groarke, J. F.: Effect of cimetidine on gastric hypersecretion and diarrhea in systemic mastocytosis. *Ann. Intern. Med.* 90:769, 1979.
48. Lewis, R. A., Roberts, L. J., II, Holgate, S. T., Oates, J. A., and Austen, K. F.: Immunologic generation of mast cell prostaglandins and their effects on mast cell cyclic nucleotides. *J. Allergy Clin. Immunol.* 65:235, 1980.
49. Roberts, L. J., Swetman, B. J., Lewis, R. A., Austen, K. F., and Oates, J. A.: Increased production of prostaglandin D_2 in patients with systemic mastocytosis. *N. Engl. J. Med.* 303:1400, 1980.
50. Mazurek, N., Berger, G., and Pecht, I.: A binding site on mast cells and basophils for the anti-allergic drug cromolyn. *Nature* 286:722, 1980.
51. Hyde, J. S.: Cromolyn prophylaxis for chronic asthma. *Ann. Intern. Med.* 78:966, 1973.
52. Shelley, W. B., and Parnes, H. M.: The absolute basophil count. *JAMA* 192:368, 1965.
53. Nan, R. C., and Hoagland, H. C.: A myeloproliferative disorder manifested by persistent basophilia, granulocytic leukemia and erythroleukemic phases. *Cancer* 28:662, 1971.
54. Hirsch, S. R., Rimm, A. A., and Zastrow, I. E.: The absolute peripheral basophil count: A new and more precise method. *J. Allergy Clin. Immunol.* 53:303, 1974.
55. Boseila, A. W. A.: Hormonal influence on blood and tissue basophilic granulocytes. *Ann. N.Y. Acad. Sci.* 103:394, 1963.
56. Shelley, W. B.: The circulating basophil as an indicator of hypersensitivity in man. *Arch. Dermatol.* 88:759, 1963.
57. Asboe-Hansen, G.: Urticaria pigmentosa with generalized tissue mastocytosis and blood basophils. *Arch. Dermatol.* 31:195, 1960.
58. Rebuck, J. W., Hodson, J. M., Priest, K. J., and Barth, C. I.: Basophilic granulocytes in inflammatory tissues of man. *Ann. N. Y. Acad. Sci.* 103:409, 1963.
59. Michels, N. A. L.: The mast cell. *Ann. N.Y. Acad. Sci.* 103:232, 1963.
60. Paar, J. A., Scheinman, M. M., and Weaver, R. A.: Disseminated nonreactive tuberculosis with basophilia, leukemoid reaction and terminal pancytopenia. *N. Engl. J. Med.* 274:335, 1966.
61. Demis, D. J.: The mastocytosis syndrome. *Ann. Intern. Med.* 59:194, 1963.
62. Mutter, R. D., Tannenbaum, M., and Ultmann, J. E.: Systemic mast cell disease. *Ann. Intern. Med.* 59:887, 1963.
63. Kyle, R. A., and Pease, G. L.: Basophilic leukemia. *Arch. Intern. Med.* 118:205, 1966.
64. Goh, K., and Anderson, F.: Cytogenic studies in basophilic chronic myelocytic leukemia. *Arch. Pathol. Lab. Med.* 103:288, 1979.

PART SIX *Monocytes and macrophages*

Morphology of monocytes and macrophages

CHAPTER 94

Morphology of monocytes and macrophages

SAMUEL K. ACKERMAN
STEVEN D. DOUGLAS

Since modern study of mammalian phagocytes began with Metchnikoff in the nineteenth century, classification of these cells has been controversial. Studies of the ontogeny, kinetics, and function of phagocytic cells in animals has led to the concept of the monocyte-macrophage (mononuclear phagocyte) system [1,2]. The system consists of marrow promonocytes, blood monocytes, and both mobile and fixed tissue macrophages. Vascular endothelium, reticular cells, and dendritic cells of lymphoid germinal centers are not included, although past terms such as the *reticuloendothelial system* [3] denoted these cells and mononuclear phagocytes collectively. The justification for the present classification includes the findings that (1) tissue macrophages share important functional characteristics, particularly, pronounced phagocytic ability in vivo and in vitro and adhesiveness to glass or plastic surfaces in vitro, and (2) kinetic studies identify a marrow cell as the precursor of the blood monocyte, and the monocyte as the precursor of most, though not all, tissue macrophages. The blood monocyte is a medium-to-large motile cell which can marginate along vessel walls and has a propensity for adherence to surfaces. The monocyte responds to inflammation and chemotactic stimuli by active diapedesis across the vessel wall into the inflammatory focus, where it can differentiate into the larger free macrophage, with greater phagocytic capacity and increased content of hydrolytic enzymes. Free macrophages also are present in pleural, peritoneal, and synovial fluid. The functions of mononuclear phagocytes include the following: phagocytosis and digestion of microorganisms, particulate material, or tissue debris; secretion of chemical mediators and regulators of the inflammatory response; interaction with antigen and lymphocytes in the generation of the immune response; cytotoxicity,

such as killing of some tumor cells; and other functions specific for macrophages of particular tissues.

Monocytes and macrophages contain organelle systems which function in phagocytosis and endocytosis. Together with the neutrophil, mononuclear phagocytes constitute the major antimicrobial system of the body, and the cell's structure can be understood from this standpoint.

Macrophages produce and secrete an extraordinary array of chemical mediators and regulators (Table 94-1) which play vital roles in control of inflammation. Mononuclear phagocytes present antigen during specific immune responses by lymphocytes. The immune response, in turn, enhances phagocyte function by production of factors which "activate" the macrophage.

The morphology of the mononuclear phagocyte has been investigated by light microscopy, including histologic and cytochemical stains and phase-contrast, Normarski, and reflection-contrast optics [4]. Scanning and transmission electron microscopy and, more recently, the freeze-fracture and freeze-etch procedures have also been used [5].

Morphology of monoblasts and promonocytes

These cells are the precursors of the monocytes, bearing finely dispersed nuclear chromatin and nucleoli when observed in the stained film of the blood or marrow. Specific means for the recognition of the monoblast are lacking, although this cell is presumed to be a marrow cell, perhaps indistinguishable by light microscopy from the myeloblast.

In animal studies a small percentage of marrow cells are phagocytic, synthesize DNA, adhere to glass surfaces, and contain nonspecific esterases [6]. These have been referred to as *promonocytes* and are considered to be intermediates between monoblasts and the mono-

---

TABLE 94-1 Secretory products of mononuclear phagocytes

Enzymes:
  Lysozyme, lysosomal enzymes (acid phosphatase, glycosidases, other), neutral proteinases (collagenase, elastase, plasminogen activator)
Complement components:
  C1, C2, C3, C4, C5, factor B, factor D, C1INH
Arachidonic acid metabolites:
  Prostaglandins, leukotrienes, platelet-activating factor (1-*O*-alkyl-phosphatides)
Interferon
Fibronectin
Endogenous pyrogen
Lymphocyte-activating factors (interleukins)
α_2-Macroglobulin
Colony-stimulating factor for neutrophil-monocyte eosinophil and erythroid progenitors

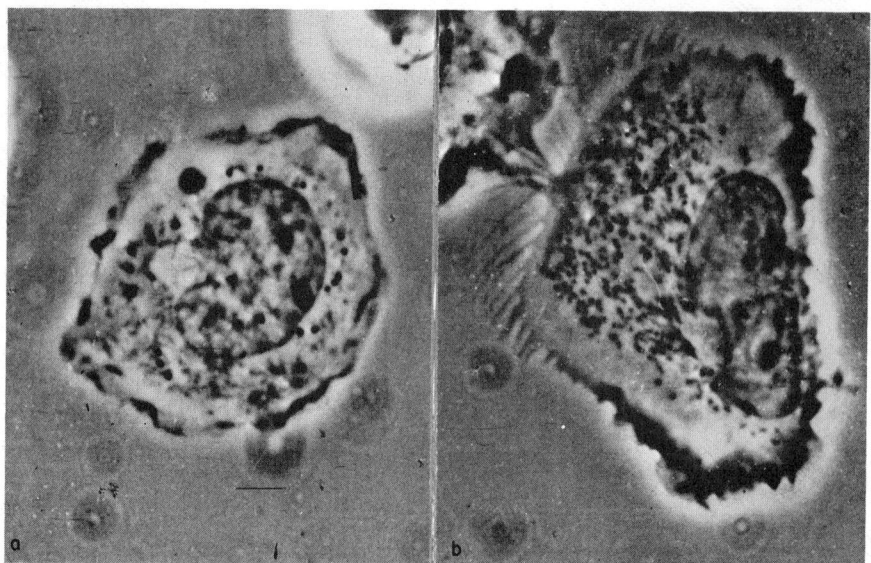

FIGURE 94-1   Phase-contrast micrographs of living monocyte (*a*) and macrophage (*b*). Examination of the living monocyte by phase-contrast microscopy reveals the characteristic reniform nucleus, which is eccentrically placed, surrounded by small phase-dense granulations and a variety of cytoplasmic vacuoles. Adherent to the glass surface, the monocyte is spread and displays irregularly serrated borders. It is a motile cell which displays an undulating centrosomal region located in the juxtanuclear depression. The living macrophage (*b*) as seen in the phase-contrast microscope shows a marked increase in motility. Its fusiform nucleus, in which one or two nucleoli are clearly visible, is eccentrically placed. Phase-dense granulations are markedly increased, and the cell appears to be surrounded by a granule-free hyaloplasm which shows marked ruffling of its active cell margin.

cytes of the blood [6–8]. Cytochemical studies can identify the promonocyte in normal human marrow. These cells have deeply indented and irregularly shaped nuclei, and bundled and scattered single filaments in the cytoplasm; these morphologic features distinguish the promonocyte from the progranulocyte [9,10]. Peroxidase is present throughout the cell secretory apparatus: all cisternae of the rough-surfaced endoplasmic reticulum, the Golgi complex, associated vesicles, and all immature and mature granules. Cytochemical reaction products for acid phosphatase and arylsulfatase are also deposited throughout the secretory apparatus of the promonocyte.

Morphology of monocytes

LIGHT MICROSCOPY
Monocytes are found both in the blood and in tissues and body cavities in which they have morphologic variation.

In the stained blood film, the *monocyte* has a diameter of 12 to 15 μm. (See Plate 1.) Its nucleus occupies about half the area of the cell in a film and is usually eccentrically placed. The nucleus is most often reniform but may be round or irregular. It contains a characteristic chromatin net with fine strands bridging small chroma-

tin clumps. Chromatin aggregates are arranged along the internal aspect of the nuclear membrane. The nuclear chromatin pattern has been called "raked" because of its fine-stranded appearance. The cytoplasm is spread out, stains grayish blue with Wright's stain, and contains a variable number of fine, pink-purple granules which at times are sufficiently numerous to give the entire cytoplasm a pink hue. Clear cytoplasmic vacuoles and a variable number of larger azurophilic granulations are often encountered in these cells.

PHASE MICROSCOPY
Under the phase-contrast microscope (Fig. 94-1) the monocyte nucleus shows a distinct chromatin pattern on a somewhat cloudy background. The cytoplasm is clear and gray. Mitochondria are extremely fine and on occasion form a small, juxtanuclear rosette surrounding the centrosome. The phase-dense cytoplasmic granules, varying in number, are generally at the limit of resolution of light microscopy and appear as fine intracytoplasmic dust. Monocytes contain several types of cytoplasmic vacuoles. Characteristic of the monocyte is its reniform nucleus with a juxtanuclear depression filled by the centrosome, which shows active undulating movement similar to that of other leukocytes [12]. The locomotion of the monocyte exhibits the same pattern of undulating cytoplasmic veils seen in the macrophages. The monocyte generally assumes a triangular

shape as it moves, with one point trailing behind and the other two points advancing before the cell. It adheres and spreads on glass surfaces [8,12,13]. Blood monocytes undergo cytoplasmic spreading following attachment to glass surfaces [84]. The extent of spreading is increased in the presence of antigen-antibody complexes, certain divalent metals, and proteolytic enzymes [14–16]. The spread form of the monocyte is characteristic, with the nucleus and granulations located centrally and the very abundant hyaloplasm about the periphery of the cell, terminating in a fringed border which displays characteristic undulating movement (Fig. 94-1). The small monocyte may be difficult to distinguish from the large lymphocyte when examined by phase-contrast microscopy, although the two cells can be differentiated by the ability of small monocytes to adhere to glass surfaces.

A striking feature on phase-contrast microscopy is the ruffled plasma membrane, which is visible as prominent phase-dense folds at the cell surface and edges (Fig. 94-1). Some cells have a dense thickening at the edge of the cytoplasm with microextensions on the thickened edge.

Heterogeneity of monocyte surfaces

Two techniques used to purify human blood monocytes—adherence to glass and centrifugal elutriation—also purify a smaller cell which is less active than the monocyte (it has fewer Fc receptors, it exhibits weaker phagocytosis, and some of its other functions are less active) [17–19]. This cell has been called a small immature monocyte, but its significance is not clear.

Recently the use of monoclonal antibodies [20] has been introduced for analysis of monocyte surface structures. Several monoclonal antibodies which react with monocytes [21–26] have been developed, although some cross-react with lymphocytes or granulocytes. At least two, MO2 [25] and Mac-120 [26], seem specific for monocytes. The use of fluorescent-labeled monoclonal antibody together with the fluorescence-activated cell sorter permits the identification and separation of human blood cell subpopulations [21–25]. If monoclonal antibodies can be developed that interfere with only a single cellular function (e.g., phagocytosis), it may be possible to use such antibodies to relate specific cell functions to cell surface structures. Also, monoclonal antibodies may be of use therapeutically against neoplasms which bear tumor-specific antigens.

SCANNING ELECTRON MICROSCOPY
Figure 94-2 shows a scanning micrograph of a human monocyte following isolation and 1 h in vitro culture [27,28]. Very prominent ruffles and small surface blebs are apparent. Extensive ruffling of the monocyte plasma membrane is of functional significance. The monocyte is both motile and phagocytic, and these functions require physical contact with fibers or cell surfaces. Reduction in the radius of curvature of the cell surface by formation of ruffles or microvilli may reduce repulsive

FIGURE 94-2   Scanning electron micrograph of human blood monocyte cultured 1 h in vitro. The cell is flattened against the substratum to which it is firmly attached. Note the prominent surface ruffles. ×2750.

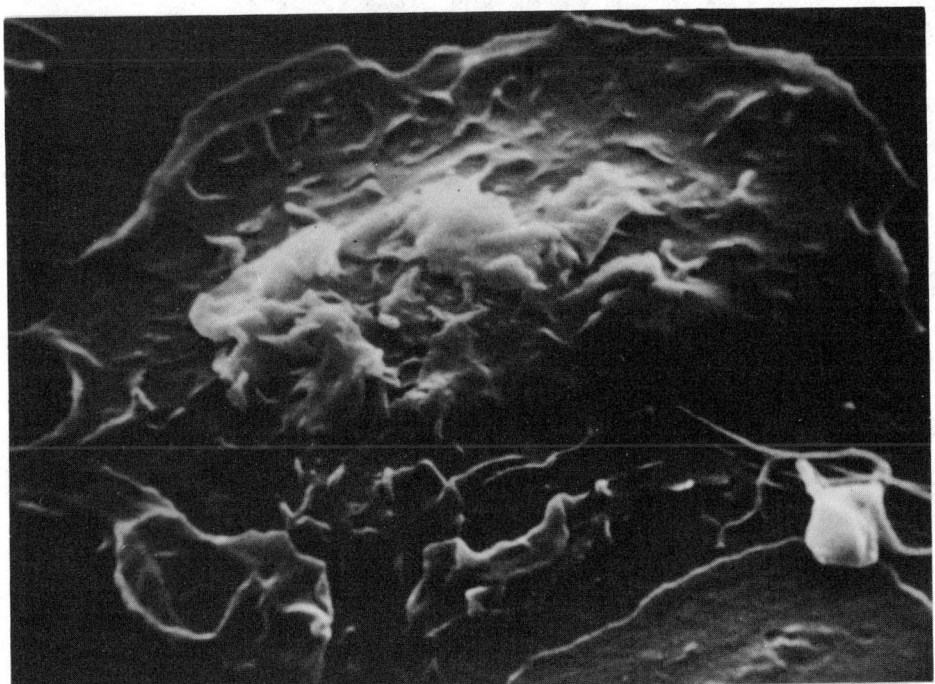

forces when surface negative-charge groups on the cell approach and contact a negatively charged substratum or cell [29]. Also, redundancy of the cell membrane may provide reserve membrane required for locomotion and for phagocytosis.

TRANSMISSION ELECTRON MICROSCOPY

The nucleus of the monocyte contains one or two small nucleoli surrounded by nucleolar-associated chromatin (Fig. 94-3) [30–32]. The cytoplasm contains a relatively small quantity of endoplasmic reticulum and a variable

FIGURE 94-3 Transmission electron micrograph of a large monocyte. The eccentric reniform nucleus has a thinly dispersed chromatin pattern. The centrosome with a centriole (c) and the Golgi complex (G) is in a juxtanuclear position. Small electron-dense granules can be seen evolving in the Golgi complex. A small amount of rough endoplasmic reticulum (er) and polyribosomes (r) are present, particularly about the cell periphery. Mitochondria (m) are concentrated in the region of the Golgi apparatus and are scattered in the cell periphery as well. Lysosomal granulations (L) are composed of small electron-dense granules surrounded by a limiting membrane. The irregular ruffled cell margin is apparent with numerous microprojections and evidence of pinocytosis with vesicle formation (pv).

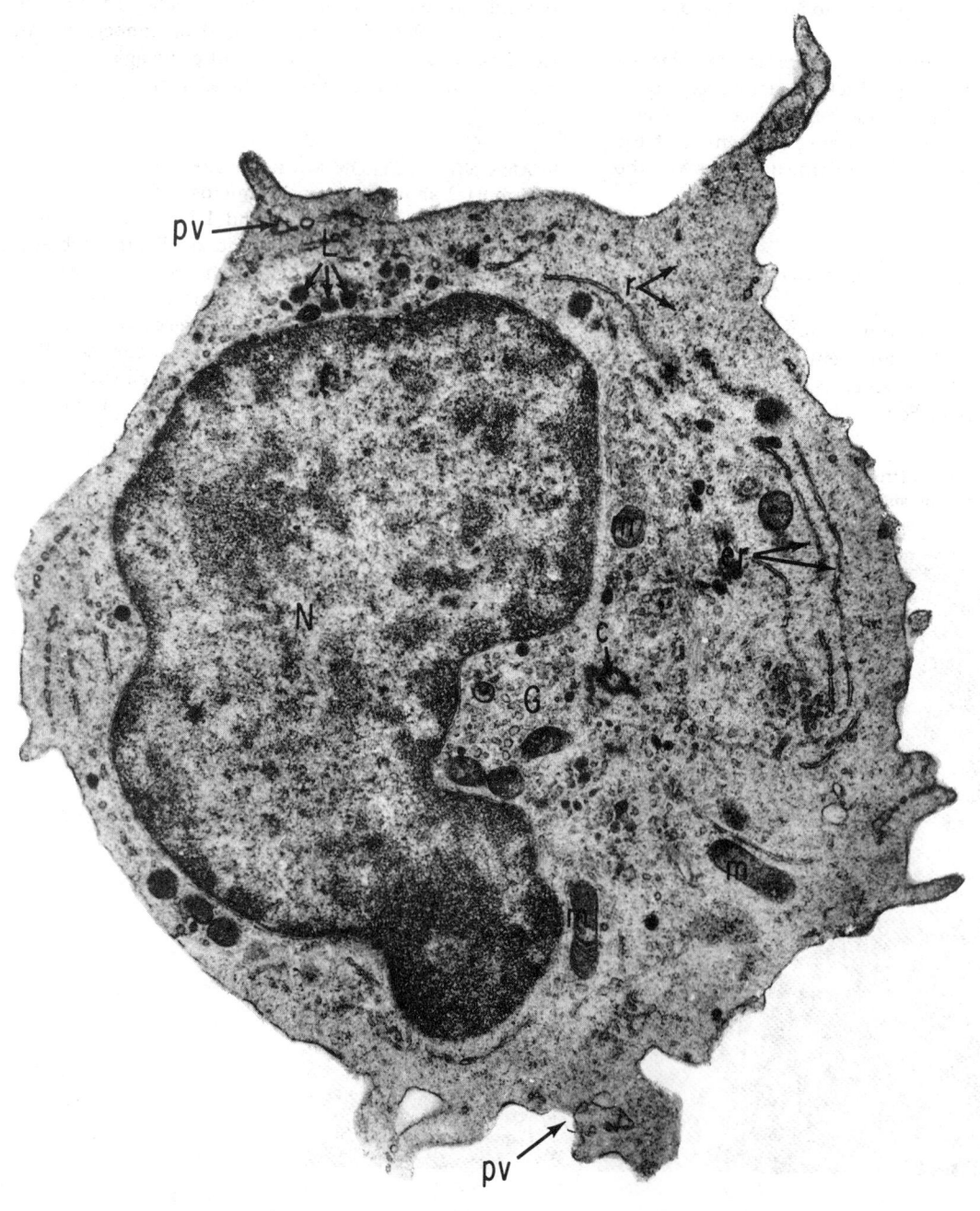

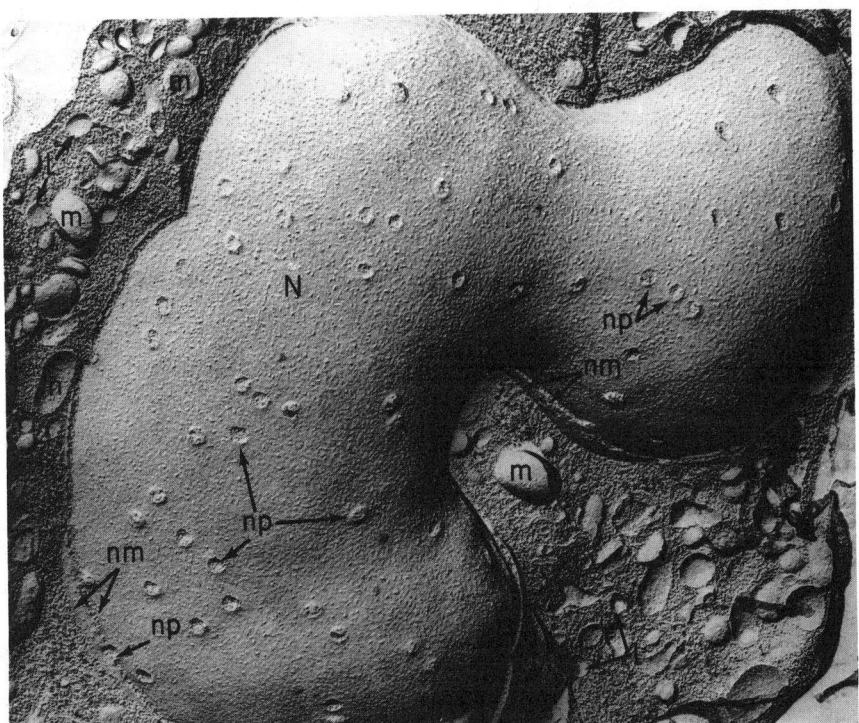

FIGURE 94-4   Freeze-etching electron micrograph of a monocyte. Fracture plane displays the large nucleus (N) with multiple nuclear pores (np) and the two lamellae of the fractured nuclear membrane (nm) evident in some regions. Membrane and cleaved surfaces of mitochondria (m) and lysosomal granules (L) can also be identified in the cytoplasm.

quantity of ribosomes and polysomes. The mitochondria are usually numerous, small, and elongated. The Golgi complex is well developed and is always situated about the centrosome within the nuclear indentation. Centrioles and filamentous centriolar satellites are often visualized in this region. Microtubules are numerous, and microfibrils are found in bundles surrounding the nucleus [31]. In cultured macrophages collections of microfilaments are present underneath the plasma membrane near sites of cell attachment to either a substratum or to phagocytizable particles [33]. Despite biochemical characterization of macrophage contractile proteins [34], the contractile mechanism which powers motility and phagocytosis in intact cells is not understood. The cell surface is characterized by numerous microvilli and vesicles of micropinocytosis. The cytoplasmic granules resemble the small granules found in the granulocytic series, measuring approximately 0.05 to 0.2 μm. They are dense and homogeneous and are surrounded by a limiting membrane. These granules, as with the lysosomal granules of other leukocytes, are packaged by the Golgi apparatus after their enzymatic content has been produced by the ribosomal complex of the cell [9,10,32,35,36]. These cytoplasmic granules contain acid phosphatase and arylsulfatase and are therefore primary lysosomes [37]. After endocytosis, lysosomes fuse with the phagosome, forming secondary lysosomes [13]. Monocyte granules may give a positive

reaction for peroxidase, although a large proportion of monocytes can be found in which this reaction is negative [9,10,38]. Freeze-etch electron micrographs of the monocyte show nuclear pores traversing both lamellae of the nuclear membrane and contours of cytoplasmic lysosomes and mitochondria (Fig. 94-4).

Histochemistry of monocytes

Hydrolytic enzyme content of monocytes, neutrophils, and lymphocytes are compared in Table 94-2 [39–42]. Monocytes also give a weak but positive periodic acid–Schiff (PAS) reaction (for polysaccharides) and Sudan black B reaction (for lipids).

Nonspecific esterase is an enzyme on the external side of the plasma membrane (ectoenzyme) on alveolar macrophages [43] and blood monocytes [44] (Fig. 94-5). Nonspecific esterase [39–42] is frequently used as a marker for monocytes. Monocyte esterases are inhibited by sodium fluoride, whereas the esterases of the granulocytic series are not. The nonspecific esterase reaction is positive in promyelocytes and myelocytes, and therefore analysis of fluoride inhibition is necessary to distinguish marrow monocytes from early myelocytes [40]. Monocyte granules, although heterogeneous in size (0.3 to 0.6 μm), are not separable into populations by routine electron microscopic criteria (except in the rat [46]).

TABLE 94-2   Cytochemical reactions of leukocyte enzymes

Chemical	Monocytes	Neutrophils	Lymphocytes
Acid phosphatase	++	+	+
β-Glucuronidase	++	+	0 to +
Sulfatase	+	+	0
N-Acetylglucosaminidase	++	++	0
Lysozyme*	++	++	0
Naphthylamidase	++	+	0 to +
α-Naphthyl butyrate esterase†	++	0 to +	0
Naphthol AS-D chloroacetate esterase	0 to +	++	0
Peroxidase	+	++	0
Alkaline phosphatase	0	0 to +	0

*Most lysozyme produced by mononuclear phagocytes is secreted rather than stored intracellularly [see also Ref. 82].
†α-Naphthyl acetate and α-naphthyl butyrate esterase activities may appear in human T lymphocytes under certain conditions [85].
SOURCE: Modified from Braunsteiner and Schmalzl [41] and Li et al. [42].

Identification of monocyte granule populations has depended on subcellular localization of monocyte enzymes by electron microscopic cytochemistry [9]. Human marrow promonocytes and blood monocytes contain granules that comprise two functionally distinct populations [9,10]. One population contains the enzymes acid phosphatase, arylsulfatase, and, in the human (but not in the rabbit), also peroxidase; these granules are therefore modified primary lysosomes and are analogous to the azurophil granules of the neutrophil. The monocyte azurophil granule population is heterogeneous with respect to cytochemical reactivity for peroxidase, acid phosphatase, and arylsulfatase [47,83]. Moreover, primary granules which are morphologically identical with other vesicles may be identified as lysosomes cytochemically. The content of the other population of monocyte granules is unknown; however, they lack alkaline phosphatase [47] and hence are not strictly analogous to the specific granules of neutrophils. The function of the lysosomal granule is presumably digestive; that of the second population is not known.

About 10 percent of granules in normal human blood monocytes stain with reagents which identify complex acid carbohydrates, or "acid mucosubstances" [48]. These substances are found in leukemic monocyte granules as well as in granules of normal neutrophils [49], and their function is unknown.

FREEZE-FRACTURE MICROSCOPY
In this technique a cell suspension is first frozen then placed in a high-vacuum chamber and struck with a blunt edge. A fracture is propagated through the frozen specimen. The utility of the procedure comes from the remarkable finding that when the fracture encounters a cell it tends to propagate along the interior of the plasma membrane and thus split the lipid bilayer in half. After fracture, the specimen is coated with platinum, which is electron-dense, and viewed with transmission electron microscopy (TEM). All cell types examined thus far by the freeze-fracture technique have shown intra-membrane particles (IMP) as the predominant feature of the topography of the interior of the bilayer. Studies of the erythrocyte have shown that at least some particles may contain intercalated membrane proteins [50], and this has been assumed to be the case with nucleated cells as well. The distribution of IMP is dramatically altered in a number of cell systems by physiologic stimuli, e.g., hormonal stimulation. The precise role of the IMP remains to be defined, but they may be proved to be of great importance in many membrane-mediated intracellular events.

Profound changes in the distribution of IMP on mononuclear phagocytes occur following binding of antibody-coated erythrocytes [5]. Since redistribution also occurs in some nonphagocyte Fc receptor–bearing cells [5] and after exposure to aggregated IgG [51], this alteration in IMP presumably reflects interaction with the Fc receptor.

Monocyte-macrophage transformation

The classic studies of Lewis and Lewis in 1926 [52], Maximow in 1932 [53], and Ebert and Florey in 1939 [54] have shown that monocytes transform into macrophages and multinucleated giant cells in vitro. These studies have been reproduced utilizing pure populations of monocytes [55], and the alterations of ultrastructure during the transformation into macrophages, epithelioid cells, and giant cells have been described [8,30]. As the monocyte begins its evolution into a macrophage, the cell enlarges in size and the lysosomal content is increased, along with the amount of hydrolytic enzymes within the lysosomes (phosphatases, esterases, β-glucuronidase, lysozyme, arylsulfatase, etc.). At the same time the size and number of mitochondria increase, with a concomitant increase in their energy metabolism and production of lactate. The Golgi complex, which packages lysosomes, increases in size and vesicle complexity. Numerous secondary lysosomes are formed by the fusion of primary lysosomes and phago-

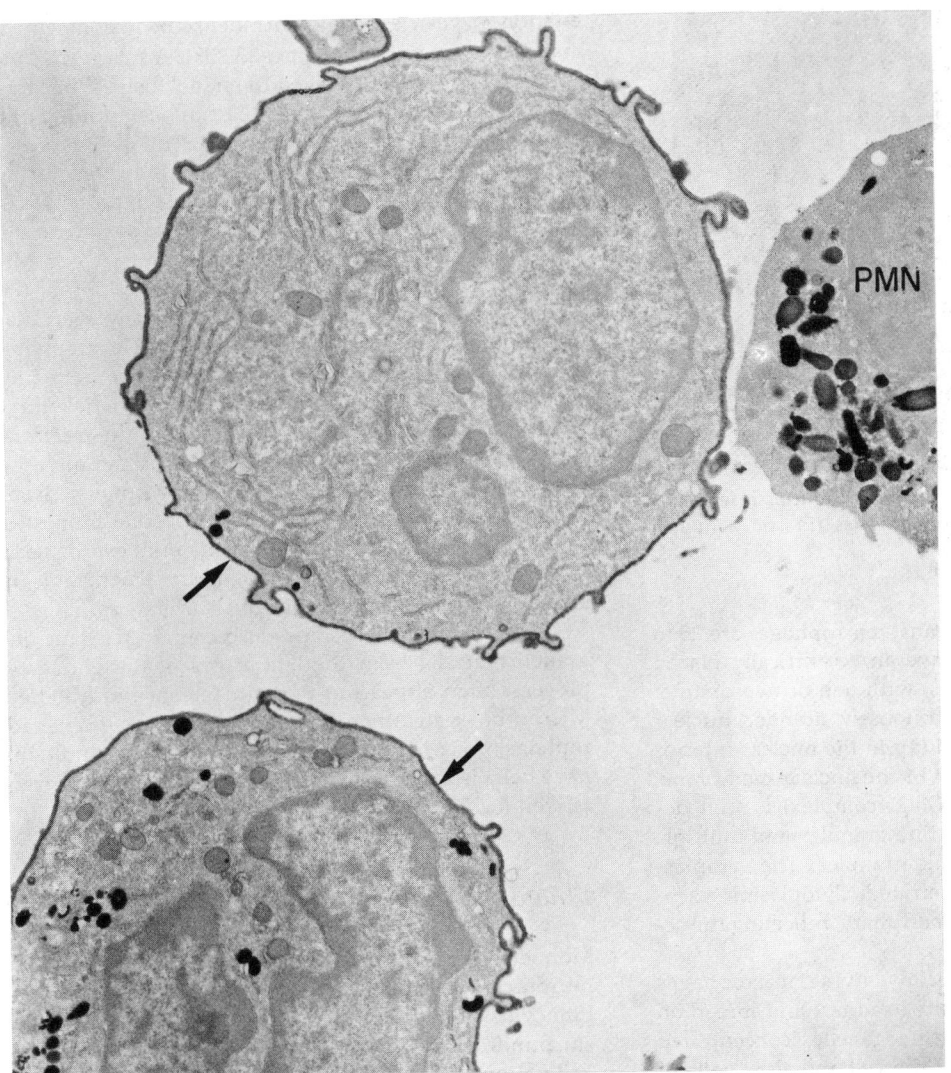

FIGURE 94-5 Electron micrograph of cells inoculated with reagents for simultaneous demonstration of α-naphthyl butyrate (nonspecific) esterase and peroxidase. Note dense esterase reaction product around monocyte plasma membrane (arrows), but the neutrophil (PMN) membrane shows none. Intracellular peroxidase-positive granules are larger and more numerous in PMN than in monocyte. ×12,500. (Bozdech and Bainton [44].)

somes as pinocytosis and phagocytosis increase at the cell margins [55–57].

Morphology of macrophages

LIGHT AND PHASE MICROSCOPY
The macrophages of the pulmonary alveoli, peritoneal and pleural cavities, and inflammatory exudates are hypermature cells, which have undergone in vivo stimulation and maturation. This results in enhanced bactericidal activity [1,2] due to augmentation of the cytoplasmic number of lysosomes and acid hydrolase content.

Macrophages display attributes of morphologic specialization specific to their location and function. The fixed macrophages of the spleen (littoral cells) are involved in the sequestration and destruction of effete or abnormal red cells and display stages of erythrophagocytosis and intracytoplasmic aggregates of ferritin, the storage form of iron. The macrophages of the marrow, the "nurse cells" of the erythroblastic island, play a similar role in erythrophagocytosis and iron storage and transfer (see Chap. 29). Hepatic macrophages (Kupffer cells), found in liver sinusoids, also phagocytize red cells and other cellular elements and are important sites of iron storage. Macrophages of the pulmonary alveoli, the lamina propria of the gastrointestinal tract, and the peritoneal and pleural fluids reflect in their morphology a specific function of phagocytosis of microorganisms, cells, and cellular and noncellular debris, characteristic of the specific organ location.

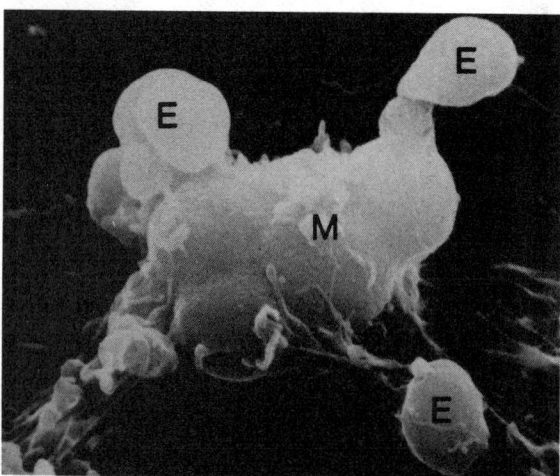

FIGURE 94-6 Scanning electron micrograph of rosette formation between IgG-coated erythrocytes (E) and a human blood monocyte (M). ×6850.

On Wright-stained films, most macrophages are 25 to 50 μm in diameter. They have an eccentrically placed reniform or fusiform nucleus, with one or two distinct nucleoli and finely dispersed, loosely stranded nuclear chromatin which tends to clump in the nuclear interior and along the internal aspect of the nuclear membrane. A juxtanuclear clear zone (Golgi complex) is well defined. The cytoplasm shows fine granules and multiple pink-purple, large azurophilic granules. The cytoplasmic borders are irregularly serrated. Cytoplasmic vacuoles are present near the cell periphery, reflecting the active pinocytosis in these cells.

On phase-contrast microscopy, living macrophages are large cells with a propensity to adhere and spread on glass surfaces, leaving the cell organelles concentrated within the central portion of the cell and clear veils of hyaloplasm spreading about the cell, with intense ruffling of the membrane borders [12] (Fig. 94-1b). Vesicles and contractile vacuoles are seen about the cell periphery and in the cell interior. The juxtanuclear clear zone bearing the centrosome and the Golgi complex is particularly dynamic and displays an undulating motion.

ELECTRON MICROSCOPY
Macrophages show a variable degree of differentiation, nuclear "maturity," ribosomes, mitochondria, and lysosome content [8]. In thin sections, the nucleus varies from horseshoe-shaped to fusiform. The heterochromatin is disposed in fine clumps in the interior of the nucleus and along the internal aspect of the nuclear membrane. Clear spaces between membrane-fixed chromatin aggregates mark the sites of nuclear pores, which are relatively abundant in freeze-etch electron micrographs of macrophages as well as monocytes (Fig. 94-4). Polyribosomes and scant smooth and rough endoplasmic reticulum are seen about the cell periphery. A well-developed Golgi complex is in a juxtanuclear location. It is often multicentric and contains a concat-

enation of vesicles, some with dense inclusions which mark them as early lysosomes [32,58]. A relatively constant feature of cells engaged in endocytosis is the large number of microvilli at the cell surface forming the equivalent of a "brush border" [59]. The degree of development of this surface adaptation is related to the phagocytic activity of the cell and its rate of pinocytosis. The number and size of the mitochondria vary with the phagocytic and hence metabolic activity of the cell. Mitochondria tend to be grouped about the region of the Golgi complex, although several are usually seen dispersed about the cell periphery, presumably supplying energy for the active endocytic processes occurring there. The most constant and characteristic ultrastructural features of the macrophages are the electron-dense membrane-bound lysosomes which can often be seen fusing with phagosomes to form secondary lysosomes [13,58]. Within the secondary lysosomes ingested cellular, bacterial, and noncellular material can be seen in various stages of degradation, often recognizable as degenerating mitochondria or nuclear material.

These secondary lysosomes also contain partially degraded material from the late stages of the endocytic process, often appearing as multilamellar lipid bodies. Microtubules and microfilaments are prominent in macrophages [60,61], and actin and myosin-like proteins have been isolated from monocytes and partially characterized [62,63].

Phagocytosis and pinocytosis

Monocytes display active chemotaxis and particularly necrotaxis, or attraction toward devitalized material. Pinocytosis and micropinocytosis, incorporation of the surrounding medium and soluble molecules by invagination of the cell surface, become increasingly active as the cell differentiates from the monocyte to the macrophage as the metabolic activity increases. As pinocytic vesicles move into the central cytoplasm, they acquire a variety of acid hydrolases by fusion with primary lysosomes [13,64]. After chemotaxis, the mononuclear phagocyte initiates the *attachment phase* of phagocytosis, which appears to require the presence of specific immunoglobulins on the surface of the cell to be phagocytized [54,65–70]. The mononuclear phagocyte has plasma membrane binding sites for the Fc portion of immunoglobulin, for the third component of complement, and for lymphocyte attachment [70–74,86] (Figs. 94-6 and 94-7). The binding site of IgG (IgG$_1$ and IgG$_3$) has been localized to a decapeptide on the Ig molecule [75,76]. These studies indicate that fewer binding sites are required for attachment than for ingestion [77]. They have been interpreted as support for the hypothesis that ingestion requires the sequential, circumferential interaction of particle-bound ligands with specific plasma membrane receptors not involved in the initial attachment. Studies of cytoplasmic spreading of human blood monocytes show that when cells are induced to spread on antigen-antibody complexes, Fc receptor activity disappears, whereas C3 binding is unaltered. These changes in Fc binding do not occur during cytoplasmic spreading on plain glass and are not induced by subtilisin [16]. Following phagocytosis of latex particles, there is disappearance of human monocyte Fc receptor activity but little change in C3 binding [78]. Studies of rabbit and human pulmonary alveolar macrophages also demonstrate differences between Fc and C3 receptors.

The relationships between changes in cell shape, membrane topography, and perhaps receptors may be related to alterations in actin, myosin, and associated binding proteins [63]. During phagocytosis of polystyrene particles, oriented microfilaments have been shown to surround the ingested particles [60,61]. Following attachment, the *ingestion phase* occurs by pseudopodia extension and engulfment to form a phagosome.

Three-dimensional aspects of the attachment and ingestion phases of erythrophagocytosis have recently been visualized by stereoscan electron microscopy [79–81]. Attachment initially takes place over a very small area of the surface of the red blood cell. After the red cell spheres, it is surrounded by a hyaloplasmic veil of the phagocyte, which advances to either envelop or bisect it. *Secondary lysosome formation* then occurs by fusion of the phagosome with primary lysosomes, which inject their acid hydrolases into the secondary lysosome to initiate the *digestion phase*. Partial degradation of lipid components of cell membranes or bacterial cell walls often results in a vesicle which, on electron microscopy, is seen to contain multilaminar "onion skin" bodies. Red cell hemoglobin is broken down to heme degradation products and iron; the latter then complexes with macrophage apoferritin to form ferritin, which is stored in membrane-bound aggregates within the cell, awaiting eventual exit and transport to other storage or erythropoietic sites, bound to transferrin (see Chap. 95). It is probable that indigestible material in secondary lysosomes may leave the cell by *exocytosis*, a process which is the reverse of the ingestion phase.

References

1. van Furth, R. (ed): *Mononuclear Phagocytes in Immunity, Infection and Pathology*. Blackwell, Oxford, 1975.
2. Nelson, D. S. (ed.): *Immunobiology of the Macrophage*. Academic, New York, 1976.
3. Aschoff, L.: Das reticulo-endotheliale System. *Ergeb. Inn. Med. Kinderheilkd*. 26:1, 1924.
4. Ploem, J. S.: Reflection contrast microscopy as a tool in investigations of the attachment of living cells to a glass surface, in *Mononuclear Phagocytes in Immunity, Infection, and Pathology*, edited by R. van Furth. Blackwell, Oxford, 1975, p. 405.
5. Douglas, S. D., Alterations in intramembrane particle distribution during interaction of erythrocyte-bound ligands with immunoprotein receptors. *J. Immunol*. 120:151, 1978.
6. van Furth, R.: Origin and kinetics of monocytes and macrophages. *Semin. Hematol*. 7:125, 1970.
7. van Furth, R., and Cohn, Z. A.: The origin and kinetics of mononuclear phagocytes. *J. Exp. Med*. 128:415, 1968.
8. Fedorko, M., and Hirsch, J. G.: Structure of monocytes and macrophages. *Semin. Hematol*. 7:109, 1970.
9. Nichols, B. A., Bainton, D. F., and Farquhar, M. G.: Differentiation of monocytes: Origin, nature and fate of their azurophil granules. *J. Cell. Biol*. 50:498, 1971.
10. Nichols, B. A., and Bainton, D. F.: Differentiation of human monocytes in bone marrow and blood: Sequential formation of two granule populations. *Lab. Invest*. 29:27, 1973.
11. Kay, N. E., and Douglas, S. D.: Mononuclear phagocytes. *N.Y. State J. Med*. 77:327, 1977.
12. Bessis, M.: Cytologic aspects of immunohematology: A study with phase contrast cinematography. *Ann. N.Y. Acad. Sci*. 59:986, 1955.
13. North, R. J.: Endocytosis. *Semin. Hematol*. 7:161, 1970.
14. Rabinovitch, M., and DeStefano, M. J.: Macrophage spreading *in vitro*. I. Inducers of spreading. *Exp. Cell Res*. 77:323, 1973.
15. Rabinovitch, M., Manejias, R. E., and Nussenzweig. V.: Selective phagocytic paralysis induced by immunobilized immune complexes. *J. Exp. Med*. 142:827, 1975.
16. Douglas, S. D.: Human monocyte spreading *in vitro*: Inducers and effects on Fc and C3 receptors. *Cell Immunol*. 21:344, 1976.
17. Kwan, D., Epstein, M. B., and Norman, A.: Studies on human monocytes with a multiparameter cell sorter. *J. Histochem. Cytochem*. 24:355, 1976.
18. Norris, D. A., Morris, R. M., Sanderson, R. J., and Kohler, P. F.: Isolation of functional subsets of human peripheral blood monocytes. *J. Immunol*. 123:166, 1979.
19. Arensen, E. B., Epstein, M. B., and Seeger, R. C.: Volumetric and functional heterogeneity of human monocytes. *J. Clin. Invest*. 65:613, 1980.
20. Kohler, G., and Milstein, C.: Continuous cultures of fused cells secreting antibody of predefined specificity. *Nature* 256:495, 1975.

FIGURE 94-7 **Monocyte rosette produced by adherence of antibody-coated red cells to a human mononuclear cell. Monocytes and macrophages bear surface receptors which specifically bind a portion of the Fc fragment of immunoglobulin G molecules attached to the surface of sensitized red cells. The sequestered red cells undergo sphering following attachment, but may not undergo phagocytosis.** (LoBuglio, Cotran, and Jandl [41].)

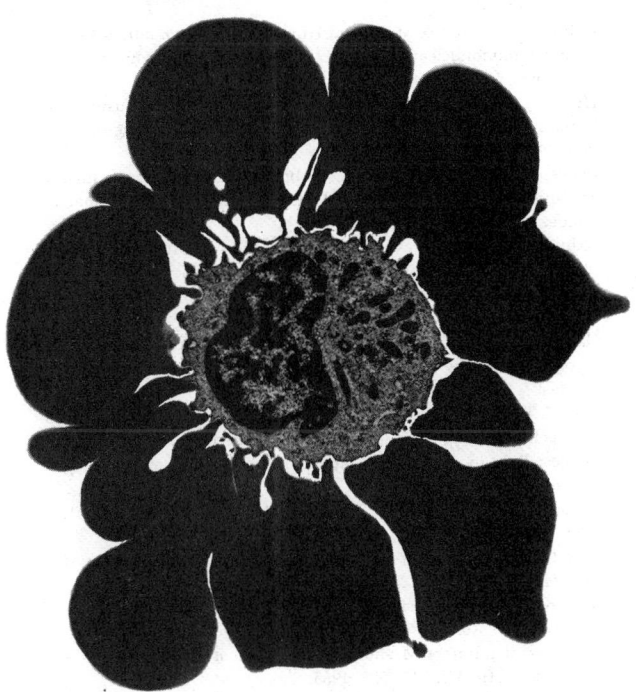

21. Ault, K. A., and Springer, T. A.: Cross-reaction of a rat-anti-mouse phagocyte-specific monoclonal antibody (anti-Mac-1) with human monocytes and natural killer cells. *J. Immunol.* 126:359, 1981.

22. Rosenberg, S. A., Ligler, F. S., Ugolini, V., and Lipsky, P. E.: A monoclonal antibody that identifies human peripheral blood monocytes, recognizes the accessory-cells required for mitogen-induced T lymphocyte proliferation. *J. Immunol.* 126:1473, 1981.

23. Haynes, B. F., et al.: Characterization of a monoclonal antibody (4F2) that binds to human monocytes and to a subset of activated lymphocytes. *J. Immunol.* 126:1409, 1981.

24. Breard, J., Reinherz, E. I., Kung, P. C., Goldstein, G., and Schlossman, S. F.: A monoclonal antibody reactive with human peripheral blood monocytes. *J. Immunol.* 124:1943, 1980.

25. Todd, R. F., III, Nadler, L. M., and Schlossman, S. F.: Antigens on human monocytes identified by monoclonal antibodies. *J. Immunol.* 126:1435, 1981.

26. Hausman, P. B., Raff, H. U., Gilbert, R. C., Picker, L. J., and Stobo, J. D.: T cells and macrophages involved in the autologous mixed lymphocyte reaction are required for the response to conventional antigen. *J. Immunol.* 125:1374, 1980.

27. Ackerman, S. K., and Douglas, S. D.: Purification of human monocytes on microexudate-coated surfaces. *J. Immunol.* 120:1372, 1978.

28. Zuckerman, S. H., Ackerman, S. K., and Douglas, S. D.: Long-term peripheral blood monocyte cultures: Establishment and morphology of primary human monocyte-macrophage cell culture. *Immunology* 38:401, 1979.

29. van Oss, C. J., Gillman, C. F., and Neuman, A. W.: *Phagocytic Engulfment and Adhesiveness as Cellular Surface Phenomena.* Dekker, New York, 1975.

30. Sutton, J. S., and Weiss, L.: Transformation of monocytes in tissue culture into macrophages, epithelioid cells and multinucleated giant cells. *J. Cell Biol.* 28:303, 1966.

31. DePetris, S., Karlsbad, G., and Pernis, B.: Filamentous structures in the cytoplasm of normal mononuclear phagocytes. *J. Ultrastruct. Res.* 7:39, 1962.

32. Cohn, Z. A.: The structure and function of monocytes and macrophages, in *Advances in Immunology,* edited by F. J. Dixon and H. G. Kunkel. Academic, New York, 1968, p. 163.

33. Reaven, E. P., and Axline, S. G.: Subplasmalemmal microfilaments and microtubules in resting and phagocytizing cultivated macrophages. *J. Cell Biol.* 59:12, 1973.

34. Hartwig, J. H., and Stossel, T. P.: Isolation and properties of actin, myosin and a new actin-binding protein in rabbit alveolar macrophages. *J. Biol. Chem.* 250:5696, 1975.

35. Wetzel, B. K., Spicer, S. S., and Horn, R. G.: Fine structural localization of acid and alkaline phosphatases in cells of rabbit blood and bone marrow. *J. Histochem. Cytochem.* 15:311, 1967.

36. Cohn, Z. A., and Benson, B.: The differentiation of mononuclear phagocytes: Morphology, cytochemistry, and biochemistry. *J. Exp. Med.* 121:153, 1965.

37. Axline, S. G.: Functional biochemistry of the macrophage. *Semin. Hematol.* 7:142, 1970.

38. Breton-Corius, J., and Cuichard, J.: Étude au microscope électronique de la localisation des peroxydases dans les cellules de la moelle asseuse humaine. *Nouv. Rev. Fr. Hematol.* 9:678, 1969.

39. Wachstein, M., and Wolf, G.: The histochemical demonstration of esterase activity in human blood and bone marrow smears. *J. Histochem. Cytochem.* 6:457, 1958.

40. Braunsteiner, H., and Schmalzl, F.: Étude cytochemique des monocytes: Mise en évidence d'une esterase caracteristique. *Nouv. Rev. Fr. Hematol.* 8:289, 1968.

41. Braunsteiner, H., and Schmalzl, F.: Cytochemistry of monocytes and macrophages, in *Mononuclear Phagocytes,* edited by R. van Furth. Blackwell, Oxford, 1970, p. 62.

42. Li, C. Y., Lam, K. W., and Yam, L. T.: Esterases in human leukocytes. *J. Histochem. Cytochem.* 21:1, 1973.

43. Jaubert, F., Monnet, J. P., Danel, C., Chretien, J., and Nezelof, C.: The location of non-specific esterase in human lung macrophages. *Histochemistry* 59:141, 1978.

44. Bozdech, M. J., and Bainton, D. F.: Identification of α-naphthyl butyrate esterase as a plasma membrane ectoenzyme of monocytes and as a discrete intracellular membrane bounded organelle in lymphocytes. *J. Exp. Med.* 153:182, 1981.

45. Spitznagel, J. K.: Advances in study of cytoplasmic granules of human polymorphonuclear leukocytes, in *The Phagocytic Cell in Host Resistance,* edited by J. A. Bellanti and D. H. Dayton. Raven Press, New York, 1975.

46. van der Rhee, H. J., de Winter, C. P. M., and Daems, W. T.: Fine structure and peroxidatic activity of rat blood monocytes. *Cell Tissue Res.* 185:1, 1977.

47. Nichols, B. A., and Bainton, D. F.: Ultrastructure and cytochemistry of mononuclear phagocytes, in *Mononuclear Phagocytes in Immunity, Infection, and Pathology,* edited by R. van Furth. Blackwell, Oxford, 1975, p. 17.

48. Parmley, R. T., Spicer, S. S., and O'Dell, R. F.: Ultrastructural identification of acid complex carbohydrate in cytoplasmic granules of normal and leukaemic human monocytes. *Br. J. Haematol.* 39:33, 1978.

49. Horn, R. G., and Spicer, S. S.: Sulfated mucopolysaccharide and basic protein in certain granules of rabbit leukocytes. *J. Lab. Invest.* 13:1, 1964.

50. Weinstein, R. S., Khoudadad, J. K., and Steck, T. L.: Ultrastructural characterization of proteins at the natural surfaces of the red cell membrane, in *The Red Cell,* edited by G. J. Brewer. Alan Liss, New York, 1978, p. 413.

51. Douglas, S. D., Zuckerman, S. H., and Cody, C. S.: Alterations in intramembrane particle distribution during interaction of erythrocyte-bound ligands with immunoprotein receptors. Effect of the membrane mobility agent A_2C on immunologic and non-immunologic ligand binding. *J. Reticuloendothel. Soc.* 28:91, 1980.

52. Lewis, M. R., and Lewis, W. H.: Transformation of mononuclear blood-cells into macrophages, epithelioid cells, and giant cells in hanging-drop blood-cultures from lower vertebrates. Carnegie Institute of Washington, Pub. 96. *Contrib. Embryol.* 18:95, 1926.

53. Maximow, A. A.: The macrophages or histiocytes, in *Special Cytology: The Form and Functions of the Cell in Health and Disease,* 2d ed., edited by E. V. Cowdry. Hoeber-Harper, New York, 1932, vol. II, sec. 19, p. 711.

54. Ebert, R. H., and Florey, H. W.: The extravascular development of the monocyte observed *in vivo. Br. J. Exp. Pathol.* 20:342, 1939.

55. Bennett, W. E., and Cohn, Z. A.: The isolation and selected properties of blood monocytes. *J. Exp. Med.* 123:145, 1966.

56. Cohn, Z. A., and Benson, B.: The in vitro differentiation of mononuclear phagocytes. II. The influences of serum on granule formation, hydrolase production, and pinocytosis. *J. Exp. Med.* 121:835, 1965.

57. Cline, M. J., and Lehrer, R. I.: Phagocytosis by human monocytes. *Blood* 32:423, 1968.

58. Cohn, Z. A., Fedorko, M. E., and Hirsch, J. G.: The in vitro differentiation of mononuclear phagocytes. V. The formation of macrophage lysosomes. *J. Exp. Med.* 123:737, 1966.

59. Hirsch, J. G., Fedorko, M. E., and Cohn, Z. A.: Vesicle fusion and formation at the surface of pinocytic vacuoles in macrophages. *J. Cell Biol.* 38:629, 1968.

60. Reaven, E. P., and Axline, S. G.: Subplasmalemmal microfilaments and microtubules in resting and phagocytizing cultivated macrophages. *J. Cell. Biol.* 59:12, 1973.

61. Axline, S. G., and Reaven, E. P.: Inhibition of phagocytosis and plasma membrane mobility of the cultivated macrophage by cytochalasin B: Role of subplasmalemmal microfilaments. *J. Cell Biol.* 62:647, 1974.

62. Hartwig, J. H., and Stossel, T. P.: Isolation and properties of actin, myosin and a new actin-binding protein in rabbit alveolar macrophages. *J. Biol. Chem.* 250:5696, 1975.

63. Stossel, T. P., and Hartwig, J. H.: Interactions of actin, myosin and a new actin-binding protein of rabbit pulmonary alveolar macrophages: Role in cytoplasmic movement and phagocytosis. *J. Cell. Biol.* 68:602, 1976.

64. Gordon, S., and Cohn, Z. A.: The macrophage. *Int. Rev. Cytol.* 36:171, 1973.

65. Mudd, S., McCutcheon, M., and Lucke, B.: Phagocytosis. *Physiol. Rev.* 14:210, 1934.

66. Rowley, D.: Phagocytosis. *Adv. Immunol.* 2:241, 1962.

67. Robbins, J. B., Kenney, K., and Suter, E.: The isolation and biological activities of rabbit γ M and γ G-anti-*Salmonella typhimurium* antibodies. *J. Exp. Med.* 122:385, 1965.

68. Rabinovitch, M.: Studies on the immunoglobulins which stimulate

the ingestion of glutaraldehyde-treated red cells attached to macrophages. *J. Immunol. 99*:1115, 1967.

69. LoBuglio, A. F., Cotran, R. S., and Jandl, J. H.: Red cells coated with immunoglobulin G: Binding and sphering by mononuclear cells in man. *Science 155*:1582, 1967.

70. Huber, H., Polley, M. J., Linscott, W. D., Fudenberg, H. H., and Muller-Eberhard, H. J.: Human monocytes: Distinct receptor sites for the third component of complement and for immunoglobulin G. *Science 162*:1231, 1968.

71. Huber, H., Douglas, S. D., and Fudenberg, H. H.: The IgG receptor: An immunologic marker for the characterization of mononuclear cells. *Immunology 17*:7, 1969.

72. Rosenthal, A. S., Lipsky, P. E., and Shevach, E. M.: Macrophage-lymphocyte interaction: Morphologic and functional correlates, in *Mononuclear Phagocytes in Immunity, Infection and Pathology*, edited by R. van Furth. Blackwell, Oxford, 1975, p. 813.

73. Rhodes, J.: Macrophage heterogeneity in receptor activity: The activation of macrophage Fc receptor function *in vivo* and *in vitro*. *J. Immunol. 114*:976, 1975.

74. Daughaday, C. C., and Douglas, S. D.: Membrane receptors on rabbit and human pulmonary alveolar macrophages. *J. Reticuloendothel. Soc. 19*:37, 1976.

75. Yasmeen, D., Ellerson, J. R., Dorrington, K. J., and Painter, R. H.: Evidence for the domain hypothesis: Location of the site of cytophilic activity toward guinea pig macrophages in the CH3 homology region of human immunoglobulin G. *J. Immunol. 110*:1706, 1973.

76. Ciccimarra, F., Rosen, F. S., and Merler, E.: Localization of the IgG effector site for monocyte receptors. *Proc. Natl. Acad. Sci. U.S.A. 72*:2081, 1975.

77. Griffin, F. M., Griffin, J. A., Leider, J. E., and Silverstein, S. C.: Studies on the mechanism of phagocytosis. I. Requirements for circumferential attachment of particle-bound ligands to specific receptors on the macrophage plasma membrane. *J. Exp. Med. 142*:1263, 1975.

78. Schmidt, M. E., and Douglas, S. D.: Disappearance and recovery of human monocyte IgG receptor activity following phagocytosis. *J. Immunol. 109*:914, 1972.

79. Rosse, W. S., Bois-Fleury, A., and Bessis, M.: The interaction of phagocytic cells and red cells modified by immune reactions: Comparison of antibody and complement coated red cells. *Blood Cells 1*:345, 1975.

80. Rosse, W. S., and Bois-Fleury, A.: The interaction of phagocytic cells and red cells following alteration of their form or deformability. *Blood Cells 1*:359, 1975.

81. Bessis, M., and de Boisfleury, A.: Étude des différentes étapes de l'erythrophagocytose, par microcinématographie et microscopie électronique a balayage. *Nouv. Rev. Fr. Hematol. 10*:223, 1970.

82. Osserman, E. F., and Lawler, D. P.: Serum and urinary lysozyme (muramidase) in monocytic and monomyelocytic leukemia. *J. Exp. Med. 124*:921, 1966.

83. Bodel, P. T., Nichols, B. A., and Bainton, D. F.: Appearance of peroxidase reactivity within the rough ER of blood monocytes after surface adherence. *J. Exp. Med. 145*:264, 1977.

84. Bumol, T. F., and Douglas, S. D.: Human monocyte cytoplasmic spreading *in vitro* — Early kinetics and scanning electron microscopy. *Cell Immunol. 34*:70, 1977.

85. Totterman, T. H., Ranki, A., and Hayry, P.: Expression of the acid alpha-naphthyl acetate esterase marker by activated and secondary lymphocytes in man. *Scand. J. Immunol. 6*:305, 1977.

86. Zuckerman, S. H., and Douglas, S. D.: Dynamics of the macrophage plasma membrane. *Ann. Rev. Microbiol. 33*:267, 1979.

87. van Furth, R. (ed.): *Mononuclear Phagocytes*, Martinus-Nijhoff, Holland, 1980.

Biochemistry and function of monocytes and macrophages

CHAPTER 95

Biochemistry and function of monocytes and macrophages

JEROME E. GROOPMAN
DAVID W. GOLDE

The mononuclear phagocytes constitute a family of cells that originate in the marrow, circulate in the blood, and form transient and resident populations in various organs and tissues. Although long recognized as phagocytes, monocytes and macrophages are also secretory cells that release a variety of regulatory substances and other bioactive compounds which may act locally or systemically.

The cells of the monocyte-macrophage series and neutrophilic granulocytes are believed to arise from a common progenitor termed the *colony-forming unit, neutrophil-monocyte* (CFU-NM) [1–3]. The CFU-NM gives rise to the first morphologically identifiable cell of the monocyte-macrophage series, the *promonocyte*. The promonocyte matures into the monocyte; the monocyte is released into the blood and then exits into tissue, where it may die or mature into a macrophage [4–6]. Resident tissue macrophages (histiocytes) exist in protean forms, including the hepatic Kupffer cell, alveolar macrophage of the lung, giant cell of granulomas, dermal Langerhans cell, microglial cell of brain, peritoneal and pleural macrophage, and probably the osteoclast [7–9]. Although macrophages, endothelial cells, and fibroblasts are anatomically associated in what has been termed *reticuloendothelial tissue*, these cell types are not developmentally related. Macrophages are derived from marrow hemopoietic progenitors, whereas endothelial cells and fibroblasts are somatic cells derived from the entoderm and mesenchyme, respectively [10].

The concept of a continuum from marrow promono-cyte to circulating monocyte and tissue macrophage is useful in understanding the metabolism and function of these cells, because at different levels of differentiation there are distinctive biochemical, morphologic, and functional characteristics.

Composition and metabolism

The first morphologically identifiable cell of the mono-nuclear phagocyte series, the marrow promonocyte, has a well-developed Golgi complex and contains peroxidase-positive granules. This cell is about 10 to 18 μm in diameter on a blood film, is capable of endocytosis, and shows some adherence to glass, but it is poorly phagocytic. The blood monocyte is smaller than its precursor, has a reniform nucleus with gray-blue cytoplasm and faint azurophilic granules. As the monocyte matures into a macrophage, it increases in size and may eventually reach 5 to 10 times the original cell diameter. There is a concomitant increase in the number of lysosomes. Accompanying these morphologic changes are increases in lysosomal enzymes, including β-glucuronidase, acid phosphatase, cathepsins, lysozyme, sulfatases, glycosidases, lipases, elastases, collagenases, deoxyribonucleases, arginase, and plasminogen activator [6,8,9, 11–13]. This diversity of degradative enzymes is appropriate for a cell whose functions include phagocytosis, microbial killing and digestion, and removal and catabolism of damaged or senescent blood cells.

Concurrent with the transition from monocyte to macrophage, there is an increase in number of mitochondria, activity of mitochondrial enzymes, and rate of cellular respiration [14]. Both glucose oxidation and lactate production increase with cellular maturation. Monocytes have active aerobic glycolysis and, unlike neutrophils, have scant glycogen stores and therefore require externally supplied substrates [15–17]. It appears that glycolysis, not respiration, provides the energy required for the phagocytic activity of mammalian monocytes. As human monocytes differentiate into macrophages in vitro, phagocytosis remains dependent upon glycolytic mechanisms, although the mature macrophage employs both glycolytic and aerobic pathways in the generation of energy [18,19]. Even under anaerobic conditions, most macrophages are effective phagocytes. This anaerobic phagocytic capability is advantageous to cells that often function in granulomata or abscess cavities remote from oxygenated blood. The human pulmonary alveolar macrophage is incapable of phagocytosis under severely anaerobic conditions and requires a partial pressure of oxygen greater than 25 mmHg for phagocytosis and energy production [20–22]. In contrast to other phagocytes, the pulmonary alveolar macrophage depends on both oxidative and glycolytic metabolism during particle ingestion.

The lysosomal enzymes involved in degradation of phagocytosed material are synthesized in the endoplasmic reticulum and packaged by the Golgi apparatus into structures called *primary lysosomes* [11,23]. These primary lysosomes may fuse with phagocytic or pinocytic vacuoles (phagosomes) containing ingested materials. These structures are termed *secondary lysosomes* (phagolysosomes). The mechanism of fusion of the primary lysosome and the phagosome is not known, but it is clear that formation of the secondary lysosome is necessary for degradation and disposal of the ingested material [24].

Activation of macrophages generally refers to a state of enhanced mobility, cellular metabolism, glass adherence, lysosomal enzyme activity, and cytocidal capacity [25–27]. Macrophage activation may be mediated by direct contact with microorganisms or their products, inert agents such as beryllium, or by-products released by sensitized lymphoid cells (lymphokines). The concept of the activated macrophage is important in understanding its participation in defense against infection, removal of cell debris, modulation of immune reactions, and possibly rejection of spontaneously arising tumors. Macrophage activation is usually accompanied by increased elaboration of important products of mononuclear phagocytes. These products include lysosomal neutral proteases and acid hydrolases, complement components, enzyme inhibitors, binding proteins, endogenous pyrogens, prostaglandins, chemotactic factors for neutrophils, interferon, and factors promoting replication of hemopoietic progenitors [13].

Mononuclear phagocytes are able to distinguish among self, senescent self, neoplastic self, and foreign. Insights into such cognitive cell functions can be derived from study of the macrophage surface membrane. Receptors on the monocyte-macrophage surface include those for the Fc fragment of IgG, the third component of complement, and the attachment of lymphocytes [5–9]. In addition, immune complexes may specifically bind to a membrane site other than the Fc receptor. There is a progressive increase in the density of IgG and complement receptors as the promonocyte matures into the circulating monocyte and eventually the tissue macrophage [28]. Activation of both blood monocytes and macrophages also markedly increases surface receptor activity [26,27,29]. Recognition and phagocytosis of foreign particles and microorganisms are greatly facilitated when these targets are coated with IgG or complement (opsonization), allowing their binding to the appropriate receptor [30]. Recognition of nonopsonized antigen by the macrophage is not well understood. Immune-response (Ir) genes may code for surface markers that identify host cells as self [31]. These gene products, like the Ia (Dr) antigens, are also thought to function on the macrophage surface as receptors which bind and present antigen to T lymphocytes [32,33]. The T lymphocyte, in response to presentation of antigen, releases factors that modulate macrophage activity [34] (see Chap. 105).

Phagocytosis

Monocytes, macrophages, and neutrophils provide the phagocytic defense, protecting the host against microbial invasion. The neutrophil, in general, is a more efficient phagocyte, except when the particle is large in relation to the cell or when the particle load is great [14]. Under the latter circumstances, mononuclear phagocytes are more effective than neutrophils. Particle ingestion by monocytes may occur over a broad pH range and is accompanied by enhanced glucose oxidation similar to that which occurs with phagocytosis by neutrophils [17,30]. Phagocytosis by monocytes and macrophages occurs but is less efficient in the presence of inhibitors of oxidative metabolism and of RNA synthesis.

As previously noted, the alveolar macrophage is exceptional in that it requires aerobic energy production for phagocytosis [22,35]. Pinocytosis, a process similar to phagocytosis but differing in that soluble molecules rather than particulate matter are internalized, is also markedly diminished when tissue macrophages are exposed to agents that interfere with aerobic energy production or RNA and protein synthesis [14].

Although many microbes are phagocytized and destroyed with comparable facility by both neutrophils and macrophages, there are certain pathogens that parasitize macrophages and replicate within them. When the macrophage is activated, these intracellular pathogens may be inhibited or destroyed. *Listeria, Salmonella, Brucella, Mycobacteria, Chlamydia, Rickettsia, Leishmania, Toxoplasma, Trypanosoma,* and, recently, the agent of Legionnaires' disease, *Legionella pneumophila,* have been found capable of invading and inhabiting nonactivated macrophages [13,36,37]. The antimicrobial potency of the macrophage is markedly enhanced upon activation. Activated macrophages may kill ingested and extracellular microorganisms by the generation of toxic oxygen metabolites. Monocytes from patients with chronic granulomatous disease manifest a microbial killing defect, suggesting the importance of oxidative metabolites generated by the respiratory burst [38]. Killing or inhibition of intracellular replication of protozoa by murine peritoneal macrophages correlates well with the generation of hydrogen peroxide by these cells [39]. Inhibition of growth of *Toxoplasma gondii* within macrophages appears to require both hydrogen peroxide and superoxide generation [13]. In vitro manipulations that reduce the levels of superoxide, hydrogen peroxide, and oxygen radicals within activated macrophages markedly diminish antiprotozoal activity. In addition, the toxicity of hydrogen peroxide for intracellular microbes can be augmented by the enzyme myeloperoxidase and an oxidizable halide [40,41]. The blood monocyte of most species, like the neutrophil, contains myeloperoxidase, while the tissue macrophage often loses this enzyme during maturation [17,22,42].

Thus, there are differences in the mechanism by which blood monocyte and tissue macrophage kill some microbes. For example, human monocytes kill *Candida albicans* readily, whereas macrophages do not; macrophages, however, kill *C. pseudotropicalis* as well since this organism does not require peroxidase activity in order to be destroyed [41,43].

Certain microorganisms are able to escape the potent microbicidal activity of the mononuclear phagocytes. *Mycobacterium tuberculosis* may release certain substances such as sulfolipids that interfere with fusion of primary lysosomes with phagosomes and thereby avoid exposure to the macrophages' lysosomal enzymes [44]. *Leishmania* and *M. lepraemurium* survive within secondary lysosomes despite exposure to lysosomal enzymes; this may be due to the resistance of the microbial cell wall to the macrophages' degradative enzymes [13,45].

In addition to hydrogen peroxide, superoxide, and possibly myeloperoxidase-mediated microbial killing, mononuclear phagocytes are capable of interferon production, which may aid in protection against viral infection [46]. Monocyte cationic proteins other than myeloperoxidase have been shown to have fungicidal activity [43]. Macrophages activated by lymphokines elaborated by immune lymphocytes have greater microbicidal capacities than nonactivated cells [24–25]. Macrophages from mice immunized with living tubercle bacilli are better equipped to control these organisms than are cells from nonimmunized animals. The resultant enhanced resistance is nonspecific in that it may be directed against intracellular parasites other than the immunizing organism [13,24]. Nonlethal infection with many of the facultative intracellular organisms enumerated above is characterized by development of delayed hypersensitivity and enhanced antibacterial activity of the macrophages of the host. It is likely that the mechanism of enhanced cellular resistance is that of lymphokine-mediated macrophage activation upon rechallenge with the invading organism.

Role of the mononuclear phagocyte in immunity

There is an intimate interplay between the mononuclear phagocyte and the T lymphocyte. The mononuclear phagocyte is essential for the development of cellular and humoral immunocompetence [47,48]. Recognition of protein antigens by the T lymphocyte is usually preceded by phagocytosis and processing of antigen by the macrophage [49,50]. This initial macrophage function is not dependent on or restricted by the previous immune status of the animal. Macrophages and lymphocytes must share genetic identity at some portion of the major histocompatibility complex (MHC) if the T lymphocyte is to recognize the antigenic signal presented by the macrophage [31,47]. These mechanisms have been best studied in the mouse and guinea pig; their applicability to human beings remains uncertain.

Inhibitors of microfilament assembly and function, such as cytochalasin B, apparently do not affect macrophage uptake of immunogenic protein [48]. In addition, antibody directed against antigen does not appear to affect the ability of antigen-exposed macrophages to initiate T-cell proliferation [49,50]. It is still not known precisely how antigen processed by macrophages is presented to lymphocytes. There may be several mechanisms, including secretion of antigen complexed to soluble macrophage products, as well as direct cell-to-cell interaction [48]. Antisera to the major histocompatibility complex antigens block antigen-specific T-cell responses, probably by preventing the physical or functional interaction between macrophage and T cell [57]. Stimulation of B lymphocytes and their subsequent elaboration of antibody requires not only the antigen but also a differentiation signal from the T cell. Thus, the primary interaction in immune recognition is probably that between the macrophages and the T lymphocyte, which then allows effective interactions between T and B lymphocytes with resultant antibody production. Immune-response (Ir) genes are those that control the response to antigenic proteins. The I region of the major histocompatibility locus is the genetic segment that includes the Ir genes, and it is this region that codes for protein molecules termed Ia or Dr antigens that are expressed on the surface membranes of mononuclear phagocytes, B cells, and activated T lymphocytes [33,48]. The Ia molecule of the macrophage is critical for the recognition of macrophage-processed antigen by the T lymphocyte. Although the precise mechanism of this process is not yet known, the Ia antigen may serve as substrate for the attachment of antigen or as a cell-cell interaction site.

Macrophages produce a lymphocyte-activating factor (LAF), also known as interleukin 1, which stimulates the elaboration of a variety of lymphokines by target T lymphocytes including a T-cell growth factor [52,53]. T-cell growth factor may induce proliferation of a clone of specifically immunized T lymphocytes and thereby act in the efferent limb of the immune response. The efferent limb of this same immune response may consist of macrophage activation resulting from T-lymphocyte–derived lymphokines. These lymphokines have not been well characterized but include activities that inhibit macrophage migration, increase macrophage cytocidal capacity, and are chemotactic for macrophages expressing Ia antigen [54–56].

Macrophages and the inflammatory response

The tissue macrophage elaborates a number of secretory products that may modulate the inflammatory response. The physiologic significance of macrophage functions observed in vitro is still to be determined, but it is likely that the tissue macrophage is a pivotal modulator of inflammation. Macrophages secrete proteases active at neutral pH, including plasminogen activator, collagenase, and elastase [13,57,58]. Plasminogen activator catalyzes the cleavage of plasmin from plasminogen. Plasmin is capable of lysing fibrin and thereby degrading clot at sites of inflammation. In addition, plasmin activates complement components C1 and C3, and separates activated Hageman factor into subunits that augment formation of kallikrein from prekallikrein [13]. Breakdown of complement components yields products chemotactic for macrophages and neutrophils [30]. Macrophage collagenase and elastase may act to degrade the structural components of vessel walls, perivascular tissue, and joint surfaces. In this fashion, the macrophage can participate in tissue inflammation and destruction. The macrophage also appears capable of mitigating the inflammatory response. Tissue macrophages secrete plasmin inhibitors as well as α_2-macroglobulin, which inhibits plasmin and many other proteases [59]. The macrophage is then also capable of turning off destructive inflammatory responses.

Mononuclear phagocytes are important cells in the complement system. Macrophages synthesize and secrete numerous complement components, bind activated complement by specific cell surface receptors, and are capable of degrading complement through the action of secreted proteases [13,30,60,61]. Complement components are capable of affecting macrophage migration, endocytosis, and secretion, as well as aiding macrophage ingestion of target antigens via opsonization.

At acid pH at inflammatory sites, macrophage lysosomal acid hydrolases, once regarded solely as intracellular degradative enzymes, are now known to be secreted into the extracellular milieu in response to activation of the macrophage [62]. Acid hydrolases are capable of degrading collagen, basement membrane, and other connective tissue components. In addition, these enzymes can hydrolyze complement, immunoglobin, and kinins and markedly augment the inflammatory response. Likewise, release of superoxide, hydrogen peroxide, and hydroxyradicals by activated macrophages may facilitate the destruction of proteins, lipids, and nucleic acids [13]. Finally, mononuclear phagocytes appear to be the major source of endogenous pyrogen, a factor that causes fever via its effects upon the temperature regulation center of the hypothalamus [63].

Macrophages and tumor cells

Although there are abundant animal data that suggest a role for mononuclear phagocytes as antitumor cells, the participation of the human macrophage in combating neoplasia has not been well defined [56,64]. Macrophage activation in vitro and in certain in vivo situa-

tions is apparently necessary but not sufficient for cytotoxic effects on target tumor cells. Cytolysis may be mediated by secretion of hydrogen peroxide and oxygen radicals after macrophages are stimulated by pharmacologic agents or lymphokines [65]. Macrophages may be capable of recognizing malignant cells as such or may be directed by cytophilic antibody to tumor targets. The mechanism whereby activated macrophages kill tumor cells is incompletely understood.

Control of granulopoiesis and erythropoiesis

The growth of committed hemopoietic progenitor cells in vitro requires factors that may be derived from mononuclear phagocytes and/or T lymphocytes [1,2]. Colony-stimulating factor for human CFU-NM is secreted by normal human monocytes and macrophages [66–68]. Neoplastic monocytes have also been noted to produce colony-stimulating factor [69]. There is evidence that colony-stimulating factor does regulate granulopoiesis in vivo. Cells of the monocyte-macrophage series may also participate in inhibition of CFU-NM development in vitro. Prostaglandins of the E series synthesized by macrophages have been shown to suppress CFU-NM committed to mononuclear phagocyte differentiation in vitro [70]. Colony-stimulating factor seems to act on the macrophage to stimulate prostaglandin secretion, thereby theoretically maintaining monocytopoietic homeostasis. Mononuclear phagocytes may also participate in regulation of early erythroid development as well as secreting a growth factor for fibroblasts [71–74].

Removal of senescent blood cells

Macrophages phagocytose senescent erythrocytes during their circulation through the spleen. The mechanism whereby macrophages recognize senescent cells is unknown. One of several theories of the removal of aged red cells holds that as the normal erythrocyte ages its membrane nonspecifically binds increasing quantities of immunoglobulin until it may be sufficiently coated to be recognized by the macrophage Fc receptor and phagocytosed [75]. In addition, activated macrophages are capable of ingesting cells coated with complement [29]. It is possible that removal of effete leukocytes and platelets is mediated by similar mechanisms.

Macrophages function importantly in hemoglobin degradation and iron transport. Macrophages liberate iron from heme, store iron in protein complexes, and transfer iron to developing erythroblasts [76]. Iron-deficiency anemia has been described in Gaucher's disease despite stainable marrow iron, presumably indicating the failure of the afflicted macrophage to transfer iron efficiently to the developing erythrocyte [77].

References

1. Metcalf, D.: *Hematopoietic Colonies. In Vitro Cloning of Normal and Leukemic Cells.* Springer-Verlag, Berlin, 1977.

2. Golde, D. W., and Cline, M. J.: Regulation of granulopoiesis. *N. Engl. J. Med.* 291:1388, 1974.

3. Metcalf, D.: Transformation of granulocytes to macrophages in bone marrow colonies in vitro. *J. Cell. Physiol.* 77:277, 1971.

4. Van Furth, R.: Origin and kinetics of mononuclear phagocytes. *Ann. N.Y. Acad. Sci.* 278:161, 1976.

5. Territo, M. C., and Cline, M. J.: Mononuclear phagocyte proliferation, maturation and function. *Clin. Haematol.* 4:685, 1975.

6. Nelson, D. S. (ed.): *Immunobiology of the Macrophage.* Academic, New York, 1976.

7. Carr, I.: The biology of macrophages. *Clin. Invest. Med.* 1:59, 1978.

8. Van Furth, R., Langevoort, H. L., and Schaberg, A.: Mononuclear phagocytes in human pathology: Proposal for an approach to improved classification, in *Mononuclear Phagocytes in Immunity, Infection, and Pathology,* edited by R. Van Furth. Blackwell Scientific Publications, Oxford, 1975, p. 1.

9. Carr, I., and Daems, W. T. (eds.): *The Reticuloendothelial System. A Comprehensive Treatise,* vol. 1: *Morphology.* Plenum, New York, 1980.

10. Golde, D. W., Hocking, W. G., Quan, S. G., Sparkes, R. S., and Gale, R. P.: Origin of human bone marrow fibroblasts. *Br. J. Haematol.* 44:183, 1980.

11. Nichols, B. A., Bainton, D. F., and Farquhar, M. G.: Differentiation of monocytes. Origin, nature, and fate of their azurophil granules. *J. Cell Biol.* 50:498, 1971.

12. Cohn, Z. A., and Ehrenreich, B. A.: The uptake, storage, and intracellular hydrolysis of carbohydrates by macrophages. *J. Exp. Med.* 129:201, 1969.

13. Nathan, C. F., Murray, H. W., and Cohn, Z. A.: The macrophage as an effector cell. *N. Engl. J. Med.* 303:622, 1980.

14. Cohn, Z. A.: Structure and function of monocytes and macrophages. *Adv. Immunol.* 9:163, 1968.

15. Frei, J., Borel, Cl., Horvath, G., Cullity, B., and Vannotti, A.: Enzymatic studies in the different types of normal and leukemic human white cells. *Blood* 18:317, 1961.

16. West, J., Morton, D. J., Esmann, V., and Stjernholm, R. L.: Carbohydrate metabolism in leukocytes. VIII. Metabolic activities of the macrophage. *Arch. Biochem. Biophys.* 124:85, 1968.

17. Cline, M. J., Lehrer, R. I., Territo, M. C., and Golde, D. W.: Monocytes and macrophages: Functions and diseases. *Ann. Intern. Med.* 88:78, 1978.

18. Sbarra, A. J., and Karnovsky, M. L.: The biochemical basis of phagocytosis. I. Metabolic changes during the ingestion of particles by polymorphonuclear leukocytes. *J. Biol. Chem.* 234:1355, 1959.

19. Oren, R., et al.: Metabolic patterns in three types of phagocytizing cells. *J. Cell. Biol.* 17:487, 1963.

20. Ouchi, E., Selvaraj, R. J., and Sbarra, A. J.: The biochemical activities of rabbit alveolar macrophages during phagocytosis. *Exp. Cell Res.* 40:456, 1965.

21. Cohen, A. B., and Cline, M. J.: The human alveolar macrophage: Isolation, cultivation in vitro, and studies of morphologic and functional characteristics. *J. Clin. Invest.* 50:1390, 1971.

22. Hocking, W. G., and Golde, D. W.: The pulmonary-alveolar macrophage. *N. Engl. J. Med.* 301:580, 639, 1979.

23. Nichols, B. A., and Bainton, D. F.: Differentiation of human monocytes in bone marrow and blood: Sequential formation of two granule populations. *Lab. Invest.* 29:27, 1973.

24. Dannenberg, A. M., Jr.: Macrophages in inflammation and infection. *N. Engl. J. Med.* 293:489, 1975.

25. Mackaness, G. B.: Cellular immunity, in *Mononuclear Phagocytes,* edited by R. Van Furth. Blackwell Scientific Publications, Oxford, 1970, p. 461.

26. North, R. J.: The concept of the activated macrophage. *J. Immunol.* 121:806, 1978.

27. Karnovsky, M. L., and Lazdins, J. K.: Biochemical criteria for activated macrophages. *J. Immunol.* 121:809, 1978.

28. Van Furth, R., Raeburn, J. A., and van Zwet, T. L.: Characteristics of human mononuclear phagocytes. *Blood* 54:485, 1979.

29. Bianco, C., Griffin, F. M., Jr., and Silverstein, S. C.: Studies of the macrophage complement receptor. Alteration of receptor function upon macrophage activation. *J. Exp. Med.* 141:1278, 1975.

30. Stossel, T. P.: Phagocytosis. *N. Engl. J. Med.* 290:717, 774, 833, 1974.

31. Benacerraf, B.: Role of major histocompatibility complex in genetic regulation of immunologic responsiveness. *Transplant. Proc.* 9:825, 1977.

32. Niederhuber, J. E., and Shreffler, D. C.: Anti-Ia serum blocking of macrophage function in the in vitro humoral response. *Transplant. Proc.* 9:875, 1977.

33. Moraes, M. E., Moraes, J. R., and Stastny, P.: Separate Ia-like determinants in human lymphocytes and macrophages. *Transplant. Proc.* 9:1211, 1977.

34. Wahl, S. M., Wilton, J. M., Rosenstreich, D. L., and Oppenheim, J. J.: The role of macrophages in the production of lymphokines by T and B lymphocytes. *J. Immunol.* 114:1296, 1975.

35. Forman, H. J., Nelson, J., and Fisher, A. B.: Rat alveolar macrophages require NADPH for superoxide production in the respiratory burst: Effect of NADPH depletion by paraquat. *J. Biol. Chem.* 255:9879, 1980.

36. Drutz, D. J., Chen, T. S. N., and Lu, W.-H.: The continuous bacteremia of lepromatous leprosy. *N. Engl. J. Med.* 287:159, 1972.

37. Golde, D. W.: Disorders of mononuclear phagocyte proliferation, maturation and function. *Clin. Haematol.* 4:705, 1975.

38. Babior, B. M.: Oxygen-dependent microbial killing by phagocytes. *N. Engl. J. Med.* 298:659, 721, 1978.

39. Klebanoff, S. J., and Hamon, C. B.: Antimicrobial systems of mononuclear phagocytes, in *Mononuclear Phagocytes in Immunity, Infection, and Pathology,* edited by R. Van Furth. Blackwell Scientific Publications, Oxford, 1973, p. 507.

40. Klebanoff, S. J.: Antimicrobial activity of catalase at acid pH. *Proc. Soc. Exp. Biol. Med.* 132:571, 1969.

41. Lehrer, R. I., and Cline, M. J.: Leukocyte myeloperoxidase deficiency and disseminated candidiasis: The role of myeloperoxidase in resistance to *Candida* infection. *J. Clin. Invest.* 48:1478, 1969.

42. Bainton, D. F., and Golde, D. W.: Differentiation of macrophages from normal human bone marrow in liquid culture: Electron microscopy and cytochemistry. *J. Clin. Invest.* 61:1555, 1978.

43. Lehrer, R. I.: The fungicidal mechanisms of human monocytes. I. Evidence for myeloperoxidase-linked and myeloperoxidase-independent candidacidal mechanisms. *J. Clin. Invest.* 55:338, 1975.

44. Shurin, S. B., and Stossel, T. P.: Complement (C3)-activated phagocytosis by lung macrophages. *J. Immunol.* 120:1305, 1978.

45. Chang, Y. T., and Neikirk, R. L.: *Mycobacterium lepraemurium* and *Mycobacterium leprae* in cultures of mouse peritoneal macrophages (preliminary results). *Int. J. Lepr.* 33:586, 1965.

46. Smith, T. J., and Wagner, R. R.: Rabbit macrophage interferons. I. Conditions for biosynthesis by virus-infected and uninfected cells. *J. Exp. Med.* 125:559, 1967.

47. Unanue, E. R.: The regulation of lymphocyte functions by the macrophage. *Immunol. Rev.* 40:227, 1978.

48. Rosenthal, A. S.: Regulation of the immune response: Role of the macrophage. *N. Engl. J. Med.* 303:1153, 1980.

49. Waldron, J. A., Jr., Horn, R. G., and Rosenthal, A. S.: Antigen-induced proliferation of guinea pig lymphocytes in vitro: Obligatory role of macrophages in the recognition of antigen by immune T-lymphocytes. *J. Immunol.* 111:58, 1973.

50. Rosenthal, A. S., and Shevach, E. M.: Function of macrophages in antigen recognition by guinea pig T lymphocytes. I. Requirement for histocompatible macrophages and lymphocytes. *J. Exp. Med.* 138:1194, 1973.

51. Shevach, E. M., Green, I., and Paul, W. E.: Alloantiserum-induced inhibition of immune response gene product function. I. Genetic analysis of target antigens. *J. Exp. Med.* 139:679, 1974.

52. Rosenstreich, D. L., and Mizel, S. B.: The participation of macrophages and macrophage cell lines in the activation of T lymphocytes by mitogens. *Immunol. Rev.* 40:102, 1978.

53. Ruscetti, F. W., and Gallo, R. C.: Human T-lymphocyte growth factor: Regulation of growth and function of T lymphocytes. *Blood* 57:379, 1981.

54. Ruco, L. P., and Meltzer, M. S.: Macrophage activation for tumor cytotoxicity: Induction of tumoricidal macrophages by supernatants of

PPD-stimulated *Bacillus Calmette-Guérin*-immune spleen cell cultures. *J. Immunol. 119*:889, 1977.

55. Lazdins, J. K., Kühner, A. L., David, J. R., and Karnovsky, M. L.: Alteration of some functional and metabolic characteristics of resident mouse peritoneal macrophages by lymphocyte mediators. *J. Exp. Med. 148*:746, 1978.

56. Fink, M. A. (ed.): *The Macrophage in Neoplasia.* Academic, New York, 1976.

57. Werb, Z., and Gordon, S.: Elastase secretion by stimulated macrophages: Characterization and regulation. *J. Exp. Med. 142*:361, 1975.

58. Wahl, L. M., Wahl, S. M., Mergenhagen, S. E., and Martin, G. R.: Collagenase production by lymphokine-activated macrophages. *Science 187*:261, 1975.

59. Hovi, T., Mosher, D., and Vaheri, A.: Cultured human monocytes synthesize and secrete α_2-macroglobulin. *J. Exp. Med. 145*:1580, 1977.

60. Ehlenberger, A. G., and Nussenzweig, V.: The role of membrane receptors for C3b and C3d in phagocytosis. *J. Exp. Med. 145*:357, 1977.

61. Colten, H. R., Ooi, Y. M., and Edelson, P. J.: Synthesis and secretion of complement proteins by macrophages. *Ann. N.Y. Acad. Sci. 332*:482, 1979.

62. Cardella, C. J., Davies, P., and Allison, A. C.: Immune complexes induce selective release of lysosomal hydrolases from macrophages. *Nature 247*:46, 1974.

63. Bernheim, H. A., Block L. H., and Atkins, E.: Fever: Pathogenesis, pathophysiology, and purpose. *Ann. Intern. Med. 91*:261, 1979.

64. Cameron, D. J., and Churchill, W. H.: Cytotoxicity of human macrophages for tumor cells. Enhancement by human lymphocyte mediators. *J. Clin. Invest. 63*:977, 1979.

65. Nathan, C. F., Brukner, L. H., Silverstein, S. C., and Cohn, Z. A.: Extracellular cytolysis by activated macrophages and granulocytes. I. Pharmacologic triggering of effector cells and the release of hydrogen peroxide. *J. Exp. Med. 149*:84, 1979.

66. Golde, D. W., and Cline, M. J.: Identification of the colony-stimulating cell in human peripheral blood. *J. Clin. Invest. 51*:2981, 1972.

67. Chervenick, P. A., and LoBuglio, A. F.: Human blood monocytes: Stimulators of granulocyte and mononuclear colony formation in vitro. *Science 178*:164, 1972.

68. Golde, D. W., Finley, T. N., and Cline, M. J.: Production of colony-stimulating factor by human macrophages. *Lancet 2*:1397, 1972.

69. Golde, D. W., Rothman, B., and Cline, M. J.: Production of colony-stimulating factor by malignant leukocytes. *Blood 43*:749, 1974.

70. Pelus, L. M., Broxmeyer, H. E., Kurland, J. I., and Moore, M. A. S.: Regulation of macrophage and granulocyte proliferation: Specificities of prostaglandin E and lactoferrin. *J. Exp. Med. 150*:277, 1979.

71. Ascensao, J. L., Kay, N. E., Earenfight-Engler, T., Koren, H. S., and Zanjani, E. D.: Production of erythroid potentiating factor(s) by a human monocytic cell line. *Blood 57*:170, 1981.

72. Zuckerman, K. S.: Human erythroid burst-forming units. Growth in vitro is dependent on monocytes, but not T lymphocytes. *J. Clin. Invest. 67*:702, 1981.

73. Leibovich, S. J., and Ross, R.: A macrophage-dependent factor that stimulates the proliferation of fibroblasts in vitro. *Am. J. Pathol. 84*:501, 1976.

74. Wahl, S. M., Wahl, L. M., and Mergenhagen, S. E.: Lymphokine and monokine regulation of fibroblast function, in *Biochemical Characterization of Lymphokines*, edited by A. de Weck. Academic, New York, 1980, p. 267.

75. Kay, M. M. B.: Mechanism of removal of senescent cells by human macrophages in situ. *Proc. Natl. Acad. Sci. U.S.A. 72*:3521, 1975.

76. Hershko, C.: Storage iron regulation, in *Progress in Hematology*, edited by E. B. Brown. Grune & Stratton, New York, 1977, vol. X, p. 105.

77. Van Slyck, E. J., Waldmann, R., and Rebuck, J. W.: Unavailability of iron in Gaucher's cells. *N. Engl. J. Med. 291*:261, 1974.

Cellular kinetics of monocytes and macrophages

CHAPTER 96

Production, distribution, and fate of monocytes and macrophages

DAVID W. GOLDE
JEROME E. GROOPMAN

The blood monocyte is an intermediate phase in a cell lineage whose youngest morphologically identifiable precursor in the marrow is the promonocyte and whose most mature form in the tissue is the macrophage. The concept of a continuum of cells from the marrow promonocyte through the monocyte to the larger tissue macrophage and multinucleate giant cell is illustrated in Fig. 96-1 and is critical to the understanding of the development and function of these cells. Cells of this line are called *mononuclear phagocytes.*

The *monocyte-macrophage system* or *mononuclear phagocyte system* is now known to serve the functions previously attributed to the reticuloendothelial system [1] and either of the former terms should replace *reticuloendothelial system.* The concept of a system of specialized phagocytic cells widely scattered throughout the body was first evolved by Metchnikoff at the turn of the century. Aschoff [2] further elaborated upon this concept and introduced the term *reticuloendothelial system* (RES). He conceived of a system of widely scattered but embryologically related cells, which together constituted an organization for defense against microorganisms. In this system he included the "reticular cells" of the spleen and lymph nodes, Kupffer cells, monocytes, splenic macrophages, and histiocytes (macrophages) widely scattered in the tissues. Other investigators, however, have reappraised the nomenclature and the fundamental concept of the RES [1]. For example, among this group of cells only those of the monocyte-macrophage system have well-developed phagocytic properties. Thus, although macrophages, endothelial cells, and fibroblasts are structurally associated in what was formerly called the reticuloendothelial system,

these cell types are not developmentally closely related. Macrophages derive from marrow hemopoietic progenitors [1,3,4], whereas endothelial cells and fibroblasts are of entodermal and mesenchymal origin [5,6].

The prefix *reticulo-* is frequently used imprecisely with respect to the mononuclear phagocyte system. Reticulin is a silver-staining, immature collagen produced by fibroblasts. Reticular cells are a subclass of fibroblasts which synthesize reticulin. Cells of the mononuclear phagocyte system are best referred to as monocytes and macrophages or by their special names relating to the tissue of residence (for example, the Kupffer cell of the liver, the Langerhans cell of skin, and the alveolar macrophage).

Proliferation and maturation

ORIGIN
Phylogenetically, the mononuclear phagocyte is a very primitive cell type. Cells related to the mononuclear phagocyte are found in early life forms, and certain single-cell protozoa exhibit features quite similar to the mammalian macrophage. Ontogenically, the macrophage has its origin in the yolk sac [7], but in the adult, monocytes derive from the marrow [8].

All of the circulating cells of blood are ultimately derived from pluripotential stem cells in the marrow. Hierarchies of stem and progenitor cells have been developed with increasing restriction on their capacity to differentiate [9]. Hemopoietic stem cells give rise to committed progenitors that have extensive capacity for replication but are restricted to maturation along one or two cell lineages [10]. There is considerable evidence indicating that monocytes and neutrophils derive from a common bipotential progenitor cell [10,11]. This common progenitor is referred to as the CFU-NM (colony-forming unit, neutrophil-monocyte) because of its ability to give rise to colonies of mononuclear phagocytes and neutrophils in semisolid marrow cultures. Single-cell transfer experiments have shown that such progenitors are capable of differentiation along both pathways [12]; however, it is not known with certainty at what level of differentiation a progenitor cell becomes irrevocably committed to monocytic differentiation. It is likely that a decision is made at a level preceding the promonocyte and promyelocyte stage, although recent evidence with human leukemic cell lines suggests that cells may switch at a later point [13–15]. For example, the human progranulocytic leukemic cell line, HL-60, differentiates to neutrophils in the presence of dimethyl sulfoxide and to monocytes and macrophages in the presence of certain phorbol esters [16].

REGULATION OF MONOCYTE PRODUCTION
The growth of granulocyte and monocyte colonies in semisolid culture requires the presence of a hormone referred to as colony-stimulating factor (CSF) [17,18]. Factors with colony-stimulating activity are active in

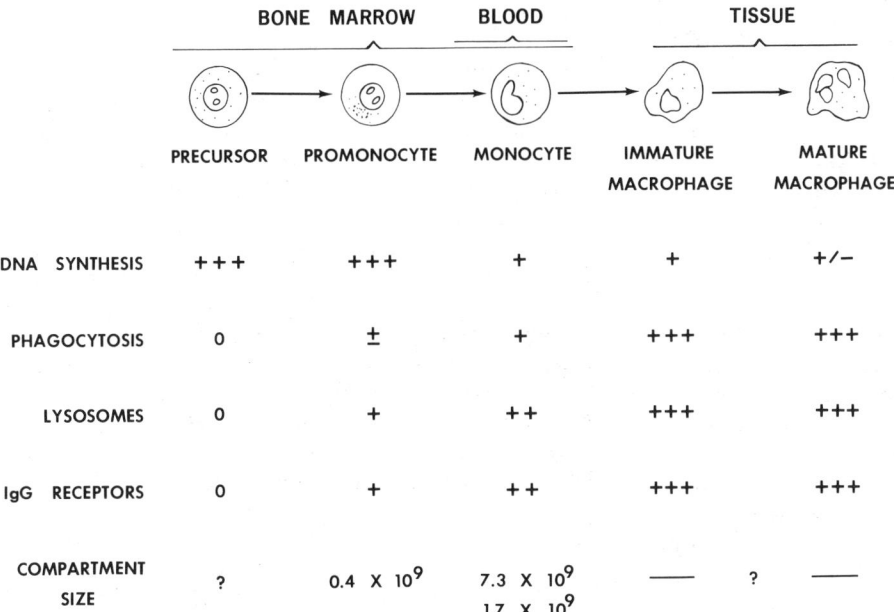

	BONE MARROW		BLOOD	TISSUE	
	PRECURSOR	PROMONOCYTE	MONOCYTE	IMMATURE MACROPHAGE	MATURE MACROPHAGE
DNA SYNTHESIS	+++	+++	+	+	+/−
PHAGOCYTOSIS	0	±	+	+++	+++
LYSOSOMES	0	+	++	+++	+++
IgG RECEPTORS	0	+	++	+++	+++
COMPARTMENT SIZE	?	0.4×10^9	7.3×10^9 1.7×10^9	—— ? ——	

FIGURE 96-1   The mononuclear phagocyte system. Monocytes, promonocytes, and more primitive precursors are found in the marrow. Monocytes circulate in the blood and enter the tissues to differentiate into macrophages. Normally only promonocytes and earlier cells actively proliferate, although cells are capable of division through the immature macrophage stage. The development of phagocytic activity, lysosomes, and IgG receptors is illustrated. Figures for compartment size are estimates for a normal adult. There are approximately 7.3×10^9 monocytes in the marrow compartment and 1.7×10^9 monocytes in the blood.

vitro at extremely low concentrations and are believed to act specifically on CFU-NM in a manner analogous to the action of erythropoietin on committed erythroid precursors. There is mounting evidence that CSF is an important in vivo regulator of neutrophil and monocyte production. Colony-stimulating factors represent a family of glycoprotein hormones with an M_r ranging between 20,000 and 50,000 daltons. The previously described macrophage growth-stimulating factor is identical to CSF [19]. Colony-stimulating factors from murine sources have been purified to homogeneity, and a radioimmunoassay and radioreceptor assay have been developed [17,20,21]. The CSF that has been most highly purified and studied is obtained from murine L cells and stimulates only the growth of mononuclear phagocytes in vitro [20,21]. It has no effect on the growth of granulocytic precursors.

Although CSF is produced by many tissues [10,22], cells of the monocyte-macrophage system are prominent sources of human CSF [17,23–25]. Additionally, T lymphocytes responding to mitogen or antigen release a potent CSF [25]. These observations have suggested that the regulation of monocytopoiesis may be modulated by mononuclear phagocytes themselves, as well as the thymus-dependent lymphoid cells. The release of CSF by mononuclear cells in vitro is augmented by a number of materials that have in common the property of activating macrophages. These compounds include bacteria, endotoxin, polyinosinic-polycytidylic acid, bacillus Calmette-Guèrin (BCG), glucan, etc. [10,25–27]. Neo-

plastic monocytes in monocytic leukemia also have the ability to elaborate CSF [28], and a permanent human monocytic cell line has been developed which produces CSF [29]. The concept has evolved that circulating monocytes and resident macrophages may respond to appropriate stimuli by increasing elaboration of CSF and thereby increasing the proliferation of monocyte precursors. It is also thought that immunologic reactions involving T-cell activation can lead to increased CSF production and the production of increased numbers of mononuclear phagocytes. [25].

In many proliferative systems there is a balance between stimulation and inhibition. It has been postulated that monocyte production is regulated by positive feedback of CSF and also by inhibitory factors elaborated by macrophages [10,18,25]. Prostaglandins of the E series produced by macrophages are potent and specific inhibitors of monocyte generation in vitro [30,31]. It may be that elaboration of prostaglandins or other types of inhibitors by mature macrophages can be modulated by CSF and affect the proliferation of monocyte progenitors. Products released by neutrophils, such as lactoferrin, are said to impair CSF release, although the physiologic importance of lactoferrin as a modulator is uncertain [32–34].

MATURATION OF MONONUCLEAR PHAGOCYTES
With currently available techniques, the youngest monocyte progenitors are not identifiable in normal marrow since they have no unique morphologic features that

allow unequivocal identification. Blast cells presumed to be progenitors of differentiated mononuclear cells can be recognized in monocytic leukemia. These cells show little motility or adhesiveness to glass and are rarely phagocytic. When these undifferentiated blast cells develop a complex Golgi apparatus and a definite granule population, they can be distinguished with certainty and are designated promonocytes—the first clearly identifiable cell of the mononuclear phagocyte system [4,35].

The promonocyte has poorly developed phagocytic capacity and few receptors for the Fc portion of IgG. It is characterized by relatively large size (10 to 15 μm), a high nucleus/cytoplasm ratio, basophilic cytoplasm, peroxidase activity, glass adherence, and the ability to incorporate ^{3}H-thymidine. Monocytes are generally smaller than the antecedent promonocytes, but have a more highly developed lysosomal system and increased phagocytic activity. Under ordinary circumstances they are nondividing, but with appropriate stimulation some may be induced to proliferate.

THE TISSUE MACROPHAGE

Tissue macrophages exist in many forms, including the hepatic Kupffer cell, alveolar macrophage of the lung, giant cell of granuloma, dermal Langerhans cell, microglial cell of brain, peritoneal, pleural, and lymph node macrophages, and the osteoclast. Recent data substantiating the marrow origin of human hepatic and alveolar macrophages have been obtained using sex chromosome markers in patients undergoing allogeneic marrow transplantation [36–38]. Similar investigations have shown that the dermal Langerhans cell is marrow-derived [39,40]. The osteoclast resembles the multinucleated giant cell of granulomata; however, evidence indicating that the osteoclast is developmentally related to the monocyte-macrophage complex has been provided by studies showing that osteopetrosis in mice and humans is cured by marrow transplantation [41,42].

Human macrophages are large cells measuring 20 to 80 μm in diameter when spread on a surface and contain one or more large vesicular nuclei, often with prominent nucleoli. The maturational scheme of human mononuclear phagocytes to mature macrophages can be studied in liquid culture [4]. The mature macrophages usually lose peroxidase activity. Multinucleate giant cells may form by the process of cell fusion or by nuclear endoreduplication. The striking and characteristic ruffled membrane of macrophages and their large processes referred to as lamellipodia can be observed in the scanning electron microscope.

Although tissue macrophages derive from circulating monocytes, which in turn have their origin in the marrow, the resident macrophage population retains the ability to proliferate [36,38]. Thus, resident macrophages in liver and lung are able to divide and may not depend on a constant inflow of monocytes to maintain their population size [43,44]. The proliferation of resident macrophages may be regulated by local factors.

Kinetics

Investigations of monocyte kinetics in rodents and humans have often led to discrepant conclusions [45–52]. There are a minimum of three, and probably more, generations separating the earliest morphologically identifiable precursor and the mature circulating monocyte [46]. In the mouse, the generation time for promonocytes has been estimated at 16 to 19 h [45,48]; in humans it is about 30 to 48 h [45,46,49]. The DNA synthesis time (S phase) usually occupies approximately 70 percent of the cell cycle. DNA synthesis time for human promonocytes is estimated at 34 to 38 h [50]. The ^{3}H-thymidine labeling index (percentage of cells in S phase) for promonocytes is about 80 percent [50], which suggests that at any given time the majority of these cells are in the DNA-synthetic phase of the cycle. In an adult the total number of monocytes in the marrow is estimated at 7.3×10^9 cells [50] (Fig. 96-1). Monocytes leave the marrow spaces shortly after completing their last division. This normally occurs after 2 h in mice, 10 to 18 h in rats, and within 24 h in humans [46,50]. Thus, there is no marrow reserve pool of monocytes analogous to the granulocyte reserve.

Using ^{3}H-thymidine as a marker of newly formed monocytes, kinetic studies in humans have yielded data indicating a mean half-time of disappearance of 71 h (with a range of 36 to 104 h) for monocytes in the circulation [47,50]. Using DF[32]P as a label, a considerably shorter half-life (8.4 h) has been reported [50–52]. The ^{3}H-thymidine data are probably more accurate, and it is possible that the short half-life observed using DF[32]P was due to damaging of the cells during manipulation in vitro.

Although previous studies have suggested that there is a substantial marginated pool of peripheral monocytes, recent kinetic investigations of labeled murine monocytes have not provided evidence for a marginated pool [50]. The total number of circulating monocytes in humans is estimated at 1.7×10^9 cells in the adult [50] (Fig. 96-1). Although circulating mature monocytes have some capacity for proliferation, the ^{3}H-thymidine-labeling index is very low for monocytes both in the marrow and blood, usually averaging less than 1 percent. Circulating blood monocytes leave the blood randomly, and in the normal adult this amounts to 1.6×10^7 monocytes per hour, or 40×10^7 cells per day [50]. Once the monocytes enter the tissues, it is believed that they are not capable of reentering the circulation.

In the normal adult, the relative monocyte count is generally between 1 and 6 percent of the total leukocyte count and rarely exceeds 10 percent. The absolute monocyte count in the adult ranges between 300 and 700 cells per microliter of blood. In children the average count is about 9 percent and the absolute number ranges up to 750 cells per microliter. Monocyte counts of 1000 to 1200 are normal in the first 2 weeks of life. In response to moderate inflammatory stimuli the promonocyte pool size, labeling index, and monocyte birth rate rapidly increase. Also, the promonocyte cell-cycle times shorten. Ultimately, however, increased monocytopoiesis must be sustained by an expansion of precursor cell compartments.

A relatively selective and severe monocytopenia occurs in rodents treated with glucocorticoids [53], and a similar monocytopenia is seen in patients treated with prednisone. When prednisone is given in an alternate-day regimen, monocytopenia and decreased monocyte inflammatory response measured by skin window is observed in both the "on" and "off" days of therapy [54]. In contrast, prednisone causes a neutrophilia and does not impair neutrophil migration to tissues [54].

References

1. Van Furth, R., Cohn, Z. A., Hirsch, J. G., Humphrey, J. H., Spector, W. G., and Langevoort, H. L.: *Bull. WHO* 46:845, 1972.
2. Aschoff, L.: Das retikulo-endotheliale System. *Ergeb. Inn. Med. Kinderheilkd.* 26:1, 1924.
3. Van Furth, R. (ed.): *Mononuclear Phagocytes in Immunity, Infection and Pathology.* Blackwell, Oxford, 1975.
4. Bainton, D. F., and Golde, D. W.: Differentiation of macrophages from normal human bone marrow in liquid culture. *J. Clin. Invest.* 61:1555, 1978.
5. Wilson, F. D., Greenberg, B. R., Konrad, P. N., Klein, A. K., and Walling, P. A.: Cytogenetic studies on bone marrow fibroblasts from a male-female hematopoietic chimera: Evidence that stromal elements in human transplantation recipients are of host type. *Transplantation* 25:87, 1978.
6. Golde, D. W., Hocking, W. G., Quan, S. G., Sparkes, R. S., and Gale, R. P.: Origin of human bone marrow fibroblasts. *Br. J. Haematol.* 44:183, 1980.
7. Moore, M. A. S., and Metcalf, D.: Ontogeny of the haemopoietic system: Yolk sac origin of in vivo and in vitro colony forming cells in the developing mouse embryo. *Br. J. Haematol.* 18:279, 1970.
8. Cline, M. J., Lehrer, R. I., Territo, M. C., and Golde, D. W.: Monocytes and macrophages: Functions and diseases. *Ann. Intern. Med.* 88:78, 1978.
9. Abramson, S., Miller, R. G., and Phillips, R. A.: The identification in adult bone marrow of pluripotent and restricted stem cells of the myeloid and lymphoid systems. *J. Exp. Med.* 145:1567, 1977.
10. Quesenberry, P., and Levitt, L.: Hematopoietic stem cells. *N. Engl. J. Med.* 301:755, 819, 868, 1979.
11. Metcalf, D.: *Hematopoietic Colonies. In Vitro Cloning of Normal and Leukemic Cells.* Springer-Verlag, Berlin, 1977.
12. Metcalf, D.: Transformation of granulocytes to macrophages in bone marrow colonies in vitro. *J. Cell. Physiol.* 77:277, 1971.
13. Rovera, G., Santoli, D., and Damsky, C.: Human promyelocytic leukemia cells in culture differentiate into macrophage-like cells when treated with a phorbol diester. *Proc. Natl. Acad. Sci. U.S.A.* 76:2779, 1979.
14. Rovera, G., Olashaw, N., and Meo, P.: Terminal differentiation in human promyelocytic leukaemic cells in the absence of DNA synthesis. *Nature* 284:69, 1980.
15. Territo, M. C., and Koeffler, H. P.: Induction by phorbol esters of macrophage differentiation in human leukaemia cell lines does not require cell division. *Br. J. Haematol.* 47:479, 1981.
16. Koeffler, H. P., and Golde, D. W.: Human myeloid leukemia cell lines: A review. *Blood* 56:344, 1980.
17. Burgess, A. W., and Metcalf, D.: The nature and action of granulocyte-macrophage colony stimulating factors. *Blood* 56:947, 1980.
18. Brennan, J. K., Lichtman, M. A., DiPersio, J. F., and Abboud, C. N.: Chemical mediators of granulopoiesis: A review. *Exp. Hematol.* 8:441, 1980.
19. Stanley, E. R., Cifone, M., Heard, P. M., and Defendi, V.: Factors regulating macrophage production and growth: Identity of colony-stimulating factor and macrophage growth factor. *J. Exp. Med.* 143:631, 1976.
20. Stanley, E. R.: Colony stimulating factor (CSF) radioimmunoassay: Detection of a CSF subclass stimulating macrophage production. *Proc. Natl. Acad. Sci. U.S.A.* 76:2969, 1979.
21. Guilbert, L. J., and Stanley, E. R.: Specific interaction of murine colony-stimulating factor with mononuclear phagocytic cells. *J. Cell Biol.* 85:153, 1980.
22. Knudtzon, S., and Hertz, W.: Human tissues as source of colony-stimulating factor in human bone marrow cultures. *Scand. J. Haematol.* 19:482, 1977.
23. Golde, D. W., and Cline, M. J.: Identification of the colony-stimulating cell in human peripheral blood. *J. Clin. Invest.* 51:2981, 1972.
24. Chervenick, P. A., and LoBuglio, A. F.: Human blood monocytes: Stimulators of granulocyte and mononuclear colony formation in vitro. *Science* 178:164, 1972.
25. Cline, M. J., and Golde, D. W.: Cellular interactions in haematopoiesis. *Nature* 277:177, 1979.
26. Burgaleta, C., and Golde, D. W.: Effect of glucan on granulopoiesis and macrophage genesis in mice. *Cancer Res.* 37:1739, 1977.
27. Ruscetti, F. W., and Chervenick, P. A.: Release of colony-stimulating factor from monocytes by endotoxin and polyinosinic-polycytidylic acid. *J. Lab. Clin. Med.* 83:64, 1974.
28. Golde, D. W., Rothman, B., and Cline, M. J.: Production of colony-stimulating factor by malignant leukocytes. *Blood* 43:749, 1974.
29. DiPersio, J. F., Brennan, J. K., Lichtman, M. A., Abboud, C. N., and Kirkpatrick, F. H.: The fractionation, characterization, and subcellular localization of colony-stimulating activities released by the human monocyte-like cell line, GCT. *Blood* 56:717, 1980.
30. Pelus, L. M., Broxmeyer, H. E., Kurland, J. I., and Moore, M. A. S.: Regulation of macrophage and granulocyte proliferation: Specificities of prostaglandin E and lactoferrin. *J. Exp. Med.* 150:277, 1979.
31. Kurland, J. I., Bockman, R. S., Broxmeyer, H. E., and Moore, M. A. S.: Limitation of excessive myelopoiesis by the intrinsic modulation of macrophage-derived prostaglandin E. *Science* 199:552, 1978.
32. Broxmeyer, H. E., Smithyman, A., Eger, R. R., Meyers, P. A., and de Sousa, M.: Identification of lactoferrin as the granulocyte-derived inhibitor of colony-stimulating activity production. *J. Exp. Med.* 148:1052, 1978.
33. Winton, E. F., Kinkade, J. M., Jr., Vogler, W. R., Parker, M. B., and Barnes, K. C.: In vitro studies of lactoferrin and murine granulopoiesis. *Blood* 57:574, 1981.
34. Breton-Gorius, J., Mason, D. Y., Buriot, D., Vilde, J.-L., and Griscelli, C.: Lactoferrin deficiency as a consequence of a lack of specific granules in neutrophils from a patient with recurrent infections. *Am. J. Pathol.* 99:413, 1980.
35. Nichols, B. A., and Bainton, D. F.: Differentiation of human monocytes in bone marrow and blood: Sequential formation of two granule populations. *Lab. Invest.* 29:27, 1973.
36. Hocking, W. G., and Golde, D. W.: The pulmonary-alveolar macrophage. *N. Engl. J. Med.* 301:580, 639, 1979.
37. Thomas, E. D., Ramberg, R. E., Sale, G. E., Sparkes, R. S., and Golde, D. W.: Direct evidence for a bone marrow origin of the alveolar macrophage in man. *Science* 192:1016, 1976.
38. Gale, R. P., Sparkes, R. S., and Golde, D. W.: Bone marrow origin of hepatic macrophages (Kupffer cells) in humans. *Science* 201:937, 1978.
39. Katz, S. I., Tamaki, K., and Sachs, D. H.: Epidermal Langerhans cells are derived from cells originating in bone marrow. *Nature* 282:324, 1979.
40. Frelinger, J. G., Hood, L., Hill, S., and Frelinger, J. A.: Mouse epidermal Ia molecules have a bone marrow origin. *Nature* 282:321, 1979.
41. Walker, D. G.: Control of bone resorption by hematopoietic tissue: The induction and reversal of congenital osteopetrosis in mice through use of bone marrow and splenic transplants. *J. Exp. Med.* 142:651, 1975.
42. Coccia, P. F., Krivit, W., Cervenka, J., et al.: Successful bone-marrow transplantation for infantile malignant osteopetrosis. *N. Engl. J. Med.* 302:701, 1980.

43. Kelly, L. S., and Dobson, E. L.: Evidence concerning the origin of liver macrophages. *Br. J. Exp. Pathol.* 52:88, 1971.
44. Golde, D. W., Finley, T. N., Cline, M. J.: The pulmonary macrophage in acute leukemia. *N. Engl. J. Med.* 290:875, 1974.
45. Volkman, A.: Monocyte kinetics and their changes in infection, in *Immunobiology of the Macrophage*, edited by D. S. Nelson. Academic, New York, 1976, p. 291.
46. Whitelaw, D. M., and Batho, H. F.: Kinetics of monocytes, in *Mononuclear Phagocytes in Immunity, Infection, and Pathology*, edited by R. Van Furth. Blackwell, Oxford, 1975, p. 175.
47. Van Furth, R.: Origin and kinetics of monocytes and macrophages. *Semin. Hematol.* 7:125, 1970.
48. Van Furth, R., and Diesselhoff-Den Dulk, M. M. C.: The kinetics of promonocytes and monocytes in the bone marrow. *J. Exp. Med.* 132:813, 1970.

49. Whitelaw, D. M.: Observations on human monocyte kinetics after pulse labeling. *Cell Tissue Kinet.* 5:311, 1972.
50. Van Furth, R., Raeburn, J. A., and van Zwet, T. L.: Characteristics of human mononuclear phagocytes. *Blood* 54:485, 1979.
51. Meuret, G., and Hoffmann, G.: Monocyte kinetic studies in normal and disease states. *Br. J. Haematol.* 24:275, 1973.
52. Meuret, G., Batara, E., and Fürste, H. O.: Monocytopoiesis in normal man: Pool size, proliferation activity and DNA synthesis time of promonocytes. *Acta Haematol.* 54:261, 1975.
53. Thompson, J., and Van Furth, R.: The effect of glucocorticosteriods on the proliferation and kinetics of promonocytes and monocytes of the bone marrow. *J. Exp. Med.* 137:10, 1973.
54. Dale, D. C., Fauci, A. S., and Wolff, S. M.: Alternate-day prednisone: Leukocyte kinetics and susceptibility to infections. *N. Engl. J. Med.* 291:1154, 1974.

Monocyte and macrophage disorders—classification

CHAPTER 97

Classification of disorders of monocytes and macrophages

MARSHALL A. LICHTMAN

Classification of monocytic disorders is difficult because few abnormalities result solely in a disturbance of monocytes or macrophages. For example, two striking examples of monocytopenia are observed in patients with aplastic anemia (a hemopoietic stem cell disorder) and hairy-cell leukemia (a lymphoma). In some severe isolated neutropenias, for example, chronic hypoplastic neutropenia, blood monocyte counts are normal. See Table 97-1 for a list of disorders of monocytes and macrophages.

Monocytosis is often the manifestation of an inflammatory or nonhemopoietic, neoplastic disease (see Chap. 98). Several rare types of blood or tissue monocytosis and histiocytosis may mimic malignant disease and are serious systemic diseases with a high fatality rate; however, the cytopathologic changes in monocytes or macrophages are not indicative of a malignant transformation. Histiocytic medullary reticulosis is such a disorder, and it and others are listed in this classification as systemic histiocytoses.

Certain hemopoietic tumors, especially acute and chronic monocytic leukemia, have as their principal manifestation a predominance of monocytic cells in blood and marrow. Rarely, chronic monocytosis can precede the onset of acute myelogenous leukemia. These abnormalities are also hemopoietic stem cell disorders, not singular abnormalities of a committed monocyte progenitor. Histiocytic lymphoma was so named because it was thought to be a tumor of malignant macrophages. It is now known to be a lymphocytoma usually composed of large B lymphocytes. Occasional cases have the phenotype of a true histiocytic (macrophagic) tumor. This determination is based on cell surface marker studies, which are not conclusive proof of such a

derivation. It, therefore, is still uncertain if macrophages ("tissue monocytes") can undergo malignant transformation or whether all monocytic and macrophagic malignancies originate in the marrow hemopoietic stem cell (monocytic leukemia).

Qualitative abnormalities of macrophages can occur which lead to disorders fundamental to these cells. In these situations, the abnormality is usually shared by other cells also, such as is the case in chronic granulomatous disease and Chédiak-Higashi disease. Also, enzyme deficiencies can result in accumulation of undegraded macromolecules in macrophages leading to various types of storage diseases. A classic example is Gaucher's disease, which results from a deficiency of the enzyme glucocerebrosidase.

It is probable that in complex systems, such as that of

TABLE 97-1 Disorders of monocytes and macrophages

1. Monocytopenia
   a. Aplastic anemia [1]
   b. Hairy cell leukemia [2,3]
   c. Glucocorticoid therapy [4]
2. Macrophage deficiency
   a. Osteopetrosis [5,6]
3. Monocytosis
   a. Benign
      (1) Infectious monocytosis [7]
      (2) Reactive monocytosis [8]
4. Premalignant monocytosis
   a. Chronic idiopathic monocytosis [9]
5. Malignant monocytosis or histiocytosis
   a. Acute monocytic leukemia [10]
   b. Acute myelomonocytic leukemia [11]
   c. Chronic myelomonocytic leukemia [12]
   d. Chronic monocytic leukemia [13]
   e. "True" histiocytic lymphoma [14]
   f. Malignant histiocytosis [15,16]
   g. Malignant (fibrosing) histiocytoma [17]
6. Primary histiocytosis [18–20]
   a. Localized
      (1) Eosinophilic granuloma [21]
      (2) Letterer-Siwe disease [22]
   b. Systemic
      (1) Hand-Schuller-Christian disease [20]
      (2) Sea-blue histiocyte syndrome [23]
      (3) Histiocytic medullary reticulosis [24]
      (4) Sinus histiocytosis [25]
      (5) Histiocytic cytophagic panniculitis [26]
      (6) Multicentric histiocytosis [27]
      (7) Familial erythrophagocytic histiocytosis [28]
7. Secondary histiocytosis [29,30]
   a. Gaucher's disease [31,32]
   b. Niemann-Pick disease [32,33]
   c. Gangliosidosis [34]
   d. Other [32,34,35]
8. Monocyte or macrophage dysfunction [36,37]
   a. Chronic granulomatous disease [38]
   b. Glucocorticoid therapy [39]
   c. Disseminated mucocutaneous candidiasis [40]
   d. Chédiak-Higashi syndrome [41]
   e. Tobacco smoking [42]

antibody production, abnormal monocytes might lead to faulty modulation of normal antibody synthetic rates. The absence of monocytes from the inflammatory response and the failure of monocytes to elaborate chemical mediators (monokines) such as prostaglandins, plasminogen activator, elastase, colony stimulating factors for hemopoiesis, and others, also may contribute to disease causation, although specific disorders of these functions have not been defined.

References

1. Twomey, J. J., Douglass, C. C.,. and Sharkey, O., Jr.: The monocytopenia of aplastic anemia. *Blood* 41:187, 1973.
2. Seshadri, R. S., Brown, E. J., and Zipursky, A.: Leukemic reticuloendotheliosis. A failure of monocyte production. *N. Engl. J. Med.* 295:181, 1976.
3. Turner, A., and Kjeldsberg, C. R.: Hairy cell leukemia. *Medicine* 57:477, 1978.
4. Fauci, A. S., and Dale, D. C.: The effect of *in vivo* hydrocortisone on subpopulations of human lymphocytes. *J. Clin. Invest.* 53:240, 1974.
5. Ash, P., Loutit, J. F., and Townsend, K. M. S.: Osteoclasts derived from haematopoietic stem cells. *Nature* 283:669, 1980.
6. Coccia, P. F., et al.: Successful bone marrow transplantation of infantile malignant osteopetrosis. *N. Engl. J. Med.* 302:701, 1980.
7. Stone, G. E., and Redmond, A. J.: Leukopenic infectious monocytosis. *Am. J. Med.* 34:541, 1963.
8. Maldonado, G. E., and Hanlon, D. G.: Monocytosis. *Proc. Mayo Clin.* 40:248, 1965.
9. Hindle, A. D. F., Garson, O. M., and Buist, D. G. P.: Clinical and cytogenetic studies in chronic myelomonocytic leukaemia. *Br. J. Haematol.* 22:773, 1972.
10. Byrnes, R. K., et al.: Acute monocytic leukemia. *Am. J. Clin. Pathol.* 65:471, 1976.
11. Saarni, M. I., and Linman, J. W.: Myelomonocytic leukemia. *Cancer* 27:1221, 1971.
12. Geary, C. G., et al.: Chronic myelomonocytic leukemia. *Br. J. Haematol.* 30:289, 1975.
13. Bearman, R. M. et al.: Chronic monocytic leukemia in adults. *Cancer* 48:2239, 1981.
14. Berard, C. W., et al.: Immunologic aspects and pathology of the malignant lymphomas. *Cancer* 42:911, 1978.
15. Vardiman, J. W., Byrne, G. E., and Rappaport, H.: Malignant histiocytosis with massive splenomegaly in asymptomatic patients. A possible chronic form of the disease. *Cancer* 36:419, 1975.
16. Lewis, B. A., et al.: Malignant histiocytosis. *Br. J. Haematol.* 41:291, 1979.
17. Fu, Y.-S., et al.: Malignant soft tissue tumors of probable histiocytic origin (malignant fibrous histiocytoma). *Cancer* 35:176, 1975.
18. Sims, D. G., Histiocytosis X. *Arch. Dis. Child.* 52:433, 1977.
19. Vogel, J. M., and Vogel, P.: Idiopathic histiocytosis. *Semin. Hematol.* 9:349, 1972.
20. Greenberger, J. S., et al.: Results of treatment of 127 patients with systemic histiocytosis (Letterer-Siwe syndrome, Schuller-Christian syndrome and multifocal eosinophilic granuloma). *Medicine* 60:311, 1981.
21. Zinkham, W. H.: Multifocal eosinophilic granuloma. *Am. J. Med.* 60:457, 1976.
22. Wolfson, W. L., Gossett, T., and Pagani, J.: Systemic giant-cell histiocytosis. Report of a case and review of the adult form of Letterer-Siwe disease. *Cancer* 38:2529, 1976.
23. Sawitsky, A., Rosner, F., Chodsky, S.: The sea-blue histiocyte syndrome, a review: Genetic and biochemical studies. *Semin. Hematol.* 9:285, 1972.
24. Abele, D. C., and Griffin, T. B.: Histiocytic medullary reticulosis. *Arch. Dermatol.* 106:319, 1972.
25. Sanchez, R., Rosai, J., and Dorfman, R. F.: Sinus histiocytosis with massive lymphadenopathy. *Lab. Invest.* 36:349, 1977.
26. Winkelmann, R. K., and Bowie, E. J. W.: Hemorrhagic diathesis associated with benign histiocytic, cytophagic panniculitis and systemic histiocytosis. *Arch. Intern. Med.* 140:1460, 1980.
27. Barrow, M. V., and Holubar, K.: Multicentric reticulohistiocytosis. *Medicine* 48:287, 1969.
28. Koto, A., Morecki, R., and Santorineou, M.: Congenital hemophagocytic reticulosis. *Am. J. Clin. Pathol.* 65:495, 1976.
29. Brady, R. O.: The lipid storage diseases: New concepts and control. *Ann. Intern. Med.* 82:257, 1975.
30. Groopman, J. E., and Golde, D. W.: The histiocytic disorders: A pathophysiologic analysis. *Ann. Intern. Med.* 94:95, 1981.
31. Peters, S. P., Lee, R. E., and Glew, R. H.: Gaucher's disease. *Medicine* 56:425, 1977.
32. Kolodny, E. H.: Clinical and biochemical genetics of the lipoidosis. *Semin. Hematol.* 9:251, 1972.
33. Long, R. G. et al.: Adult Niemann-Pick disease — Its relationship to the syndrome of sea-blue histiocyte. *Am. J. Med.* 62:627, 1976.
34. Brady, R. O.: Biochemical and metabolic basis of familial sphingolipidoses. *Semin. Hematol.* 9:273, 1972.
35. Part IV. Disorders characterized by evidence of abnormal lipid metabolism, in *The Metabolic Basic of Inherited Disease*, edited by J. B. Stanbury, J. B. Wyngaarden, and D. S. Fredrickson, 3d ed. McGraw-Hill, New York, p. 493, 1972.
36. Territo, M. C., and Cline, M. J.: Monocyte function in man. *J. Immunol.* 118:187, 1977.
37. Cline, M. J., et al.: Monocytes and macrophages: Functions and diseases. *Ann. Intern. Med.* 88:78, 1978.
38. Davis, W. C., Huber, H., Douglas, S. D., and Fudenberg, H. H.: A defect in circulating mononuclear phagocytes in chronic granulomatous disease of childhood. *J. Immunol.* 101:1093, 1968.
39. Rinehart, J. J., et al.: Effects of corticosteroid therapy on human monocyte function. *N. Engl. J. Med.* 292:236, 1975.
40. Snyderman, R., Altman, L. C., Frankel, A., and Blaese, R. M.: Defective mononuclear leukocyte chemotaxis. *Ann. Intern. Med.* 78:509, 1973.
41. White, J. G.: The Chediak-Higashi syndrome: A possible lysosomal disease. *Blood* 28:143, 1966.
42. Green, G. M., and Carolin, D.: The depressant effect of cigarette smoke on the *in vitro* antibacterial activity of alveolar macrophages. *N. Engl. J. Med.* 276:421, 1967.

Monocyte and macrophage disorders— self-limited proliferative responses

CHAPTER 98

Monocytosis

PETER A. CASSILETH

The blood monocyte is derived from the hemopoietic progenitor cell pool, and its differentiation is closely linked to the neutrophil. For example, in viscous culture human marrow progenitors form mixed colonies of neutrophils and monocytes. Mixed colonies containing eosinophils or basophils and either monocytes or neutrophils have not been identified. These findings have indicated that the monocyte and neutrophil are derived from a common progenitor cell.

The regulation of monocyte proliferation and differentiation is not fully understood. The monocyte elaborates a growth factor, colony-stimulating factor, which is a glycoprotein of M_r 25,000 daltons that stimulates the proliferation and differentiation of the common progenitor of neutrophils and monocytes. Neutrophils contain an inhibitor of the neutrophil-monocyte progenitor cell's growth. It is thought that an interplay of these or similar factors, acting locally in marrow, may regulate monocyte production. (See Chap. 18, "Hemopoietic Stem Cells," and Chap. 96, "Production, Distribution, and Fate of Monocytes and Macrophages.") Increases in the concentration of blood monocytes frequently accompany increases in neutrophils. Although this could be a reflection of imperfect regulation of the response to demands for one or the other cell type, it is more likely a reflection of the coordinated role these two cells play in the inflammatory process and other reactions to tissue injury.

The blood monocyte is a cell in transit from marrow to tissues. In tissues it is capable of transformation under the influence of local environmental factors into a macrophage. These cells may be fixed in certain organs. Examples of these are Kupffer cells and splenic, marrow, lymph node, and placental macrophages and microglia. Free macrophages include those in connective tissue, serosal surfaces, inflammatory exudates, and the alveoli

of lung. All the macrophages are derived from blood monocytes. Most evidence indicates that the blood monocyte represents a single pool of cells which mature into different types of macrophages in different sites. This theory is under challenge since monocytes with different physical properties have been identified, raising the possibility that blood monocytes may be subdivided into different classes of cells despite their similarity when examined by light microscopy.

The monocyte plays an important role in several types of inflammatory reactions, especially granulomatous reactions, the reaction to neoplasia, immunologic reactions, and many infections, especially those that involve delayed hypersensitivity, such as tuberculosis. It also is a cell that is involved in repair and reorganization of tissues. Because of its role in a variety of pathological reactions, a modest elevation in blood monocyte concentration occurs in many conditions.

Normal blood monocyte concentration

Monocytes constitute 1 to 9 percent of blood leukocytes [1–3]. The average absolute blood monocyte count is about 1000 per microliter in the first 2 weeks of life [4]. There is a gradual decline in the normal monocyte count to a mean of 400 per microliter in adulthood. Monocytosis is present when the absolute count exceeds 800 per microliter in adults [5,6]. Men tend to have slightly higher monocyte counts than women [6]. Increments in the number of blood monocytes correlate directly with increases in the total blood monocyte pool and the monocyte turnover rate [7].

Disorders associated with monocytosis

Table 98-1 outlines the disease entities reported to be associated with monocytosis. In a review of the subject in 1965 [8], hematologic disorders represented more than 50 percent, collagen vascular diseases about 10 percent, and malignant disease about 8 percent of cases of monocytosis.

HEMATOLOGIC DISORDERS

In patients with preleukemia [see Chap. 22, "Dyshemopoietic (Preleukemic) Disorders"], monocytosis is a common feature [9]. Promonocytes and monocytes may be increased in patients with acute myelogenous leukemia of the myelomonocytic or monocytic types [10]. In some cases the monocytes are immature or have features of monoblasts, but in many cases they are indistinguishable from normal mature monocytes by light microscopy [11,12]. Patients with chronic myelogenous leukemia may have unusual proportions of monocytes, and in variants of chronic myelogenous leukemia the monocytosis may be striking. Such cases have been classified as subacute or chronic myelomonocytic or monocytic leukemia [13–16]. Most of these cases trans-

TABLE 98-1   Disorders associated with monocytosis

Hematologic disorders:
 Hemopoietic stem cell disorders
  Preleukemia
  Acute myelogenous leukemia
   Myelomonocytic type
   Monocytic type
  Chronic myelogenous leukemia
   Myelomonocytic type
   Monocytic type
  Polycythemia vera
 Lymphocytic tumors
  Lymphoma
  Hodgkin's disease
  Multiple myeloma
 Hemolytic anemia
 Idiopathic thrombocytopenic purpura
 Chronic neutropenias
  Familial benign
  Infantile genetic
  Hypoplastic
 Malignant histiocytosis
 Postsplenectomy state
Inflammatory and immune disorders:
 Collagen diseases
  Rheumatoid arthritis
  Systemic lupus erythematosus
  Temporal arteritis
  Myositis
  Polyarteritis nodosa
 Gastrointestinal disorders
  Ulcerative colitis
  Regional enteritis
  Sprue
 Sarcoidosis
 Infections
  Tuberculosis
  Subacute bacterial endocarditis
  Syphilis
 Fever of unknown origin
Nonhemopoietic cancers
Miscellaneous conditions:
 Tetrachloroethane poisoning
 Hand-Schüller-Christian disease

form to acute leukemia after a period measured in months, although a small proportion may have a protracted course [17].

Monocytosis occurs in a number of neutropenic states: cyclic neutropenia [18], chronic granulocytopenia of childhood [19], familial benign chronic neutropenia [20], infantile genetic agranulocytosis [21,22], and chronic hypoplastic neutropenia [23]. Transient elevations of the monocyte count have been reported in the acute phases of drug-induced agranulocytosis [24,25]. This is in contrast to earlier studies in which monocytosis appeared later in the recovery phase of agranulocytosis [26,27]. Although one study [28] found the appearance of monocytes to be of no prognostic value, most reports [24,26,27], but not all [28], have indicated that normal or increased numbers of monocytes is a har-

binger of recovery from agranulocytosis. Agranulocytosis with an accompanying monocytosis has been entitled *leukopenic infectious monocytosis* [29], but it is not a separate entity.

Monocytosis can occur with lymphomas and can vary with disease activity [30]. Monocytosis has been noted in about 25 percent of cases of Hodgkin's disease, although it does not correlate with prognosis [31–33]. Blood monocytosis is likely to occur in diseases associated with histiocytic proliferation, such as malignant histiocytosis (histiocytic medullary reticulosis) [34]. Monocytosis may also occur in individuals who have had splenectomy [35].

INFLAMMATORY AND IMMUNE DISORDERS

COLLAGEN VASCULAR DISEASE
Collagen vascular disease, including rheumatoid arthritis, systemic lupus erythematosus, temporal arteritis, myositis, and periarteritis nodosa may be associated with monocytosis, although monocytosis is not common in these diseases. The usual white cell alterations of systemic lupus erythematosus, for example, are neutropenia and lymphopenia [36], but 10 percent of patients have a mild monocytosis [37].

INFECTIONS
In past years infectious diseases were very common causes of monocytosis. The decreased frequency of chronic infections has accounted for the decreased prevalence of infectious diseases in patients with unexplained monocytosis. Only a few instances of infection were noted in the 1965 series, including tonsillitis, dental infection, recurrent liver abscesses, candidiasis, and one instance of tuberculous peritonitis [8]. Tuberculosis was one of the leading causes of monocytosis, because of the role of monocytes in granuloma (tubercle) formation [38], and monocytic leukemoid reactions have been reported in this disease [39]. The monocyte count and the monocyte/lymphocyte ratio do not correlate with the stage or activity of tuberculosis [40,41] as was once thought.

Monocytosis is found in 15 to 20 percent of patients with subacute bacterial endocarditis [42,43] but is not correlated with the concentration of blood macrophages that appear in this disease [44]. Rarely, in acute bacterial infections, blood monocytes can exceed 20,000 per microliter. Increased monocytes and monocyte precursors may also be present in the marrow, mimicking acute monocytic leukemia.

It has been shown that a number of infections that were formerly thought to be associated with monocytosis are not associated with it, e.g., rickettsial diseases [45–48], brucellosis [49], leishmaniasis [50], typhoid fever [51], malaria [52], and disseminated candidiasis [53]. A monocytosis in the resolution phase of acute infections has been noted [54], and monocytosis appears in neonatal, primary, and secondary syphilis [55]. In addition, fevers of unknown origin have been associated with monocytosis [8].

Gastrointestinal disease and sarcoid

Sprue, ulcerative colitis, and regional enteritis have been associated with monocytosis [8]. Elevation of the blood monocyte count occurs in sarcoid [56] and is inversely related to a reduction in circulating T lymphocytes [57]. A similar correlation has also been noted in patients with malignant disease [58].

MALIGNANT DISEASE

Sixty-two percent of patients with nonhematologic malignancy exhibited a monocytosis, which did not correlate with the presence or absence of metastatic disease [59]. Thus unexplained monocytosis should raise the possibility of a malignancy.

MISCELLANEOUS

Other disorders associated with monocytosis include tetrachloroethane poisoning [60] and Hand-Schüller-Christian disease [61]. Increased monocyte counts do not occur in Niemann-Pick disease [62] and Gaucher's disease [63].

Factitious elevations of the blood monocyte count can occur when blood is obtained from the fingertips of patients who have peripheral vascular disease, such as Raynaud's syndrome [64].

Perspective

Because monocytes play such an important role in inflammation, immune reactions, reactions to neoplasia, and tissue remodeling and repair, they may increase in the blood in many seemingly diverse conditions. In many situations, monocytosis occurs as an expected accompaniment of a clinical disorder such as tuberculosis.

Similarly, in a patient with acute myelomonocytic or monocytic leukemia, monocytosis is an inherent feature of the disease. In some cases monocytosis may be present and the associated disease is not apparent. Such situations can be vexing for the physician. The pathogenetic considerations and specific diseases in Table 98-1 can provide a framework on which to approach the evaluation of the patient with monocytosis.

The blood monocyte concentration can undergo transient fluctuations as a result of minor stresses [65,66]. Thus a single blood count showing monocytosis should be confirmed by further observations. Moreover, reactive lymphocytes and monocytes can be confused by inexperienced observers. Indeed, recent studies of functional properties indicate that cells looking like lymphocytes may be more closely related to monocytes [67]. These complexities need not interfere with the use of the monocyte count as determined by traditional methods. They serve to indicate that mild variations in monocyte counts, especially if transient, reflect the dynamic nature of the cell pool being measured. Only if monocytosis is persistent, and especially if other signs or symptoms are present, should it be considered a harbinger of a more serious disturbance.

References

1. Davidsohn, I., and Henry, J. B.: *Todd-Sanford Clinical Diagnosis*, 15th ed. Saunders, Philadelphia, 1974.
2. deGruchy, G. C.: *Clinical Haematology in Medical Practice*, 4th ed. Blackwell Scientific Publications, Oxford, 1978.
3. Miale, J. B.: *Laboratory Medicine: Hematology*, 5th ed. Mosby, St. Louis, 1977.
4. Albritton, E. C.: *Standard Values in Blood*. Saunders, Philadelphia, 1952.
5. Nathan, D. G. and Oski, F. A.: *Hematology of Infancy and Childhood*, 2d ed. Saunders, Philadelphia, 1981.
6. Munan, L. and Kelly, A.: Age-dependent changes in blood monocyte populations in man. *Clin. Exp. Immunol.* 35:161, 1979.
7. Meuret, G., and Hoffman, G.: Monocyte kinetic studies in normal and disease states. *Br. J. Haematol.* 24:275, 1973.
8. Maldonado, J. E., and Hanlon, D. G.: Monocytosis: A current appraisal. *Mayo Clin. Proc.* 40:248, 1965.
9. Saarni, M. I., and Liman, J. W.: Preleukemia. The hematologic syndrome preceding acute leukemia. *Am. J. Med.* 55:38, 1973.
10. Firkin, B., and Moore, C. V.: Clinical manifestations of leukemia. Recent contributions. *Am. J. Med.* 28:764, 1960.
11. Doan, C. A., and Wiseman, B. K.: The monocyte, monocytosis and monocytic leukosis: A clinical and pathological study. *Ann. Intern. Med.* 8:383, 1934.
12. Shaw, M. T.: The distinctive features of acute monocytic leukemia. *Am. J. Hematol.* 4:97, 1978.
13. Sexauer, J., Kass, L., Schnitzer, B.: Subacute myelomonocytic leukemia. *Am. J. Med.* 57:853., 1974.
14. Geary, C. G., et al.: Chronic myelomonocytic leukemia. *Br. J. Hematol.* 30:289, 1975.
15. Sinn, C. M., and Dick, F. W.: Monocytic leukemia. *Am. J. Med.* 20:588, 1956.
16. Pearson, H. A., and Diamond, L. K.: Chronic monocytic leukemia in childhood. *J. Pediatr.* 53:259, 1958.
17. Knospe, W. H. and Gregory, S. A.: Smoldering acute leukemia. Clinical and cytogenetic studies in six patients. *Arch. Intern. Med.* 127:910, 1971.
18. Brodsky, I., Reimann, H. A., and Dennis, L. H.: Treatment of cyclic neutropenia with testosterone. *Am. J. Med.* 38:802, 1965.
19. Zuelzer, W. W., and Bajoghli, M.: Chronic granulocytopenia in childhood. *Blood* 23:359, 1964.
20. Cutting, H. O., and Lang, J. E.: Familial benign chronic neutropenia. *Ann. Intern. Med.* 61:876, 1964.
21. Krill, C. E., and Mauer, A. M.: Congenital agranulocytosis *J. Pediatr.* 68:361, 1966.
22. Lang, J. E., and Cutting, H. O.: Infantile genetic agranulocytosis. *Pediatrics* 35:596, 1965.
23. Spaet, T. H., and Dameshek, W.: Chronic hypoplastic neutropenia. *Am. J. Med.* 13:35, 1952.
24. Cassileth, P. A.: Monocytosis in chlorpromazine-associated agranulocytosis: Termination in acute leukemia. *Am. J. Med.* 43:471, 1967.
25. 25. Graf, M., and Tarlov, A.: Agranulocytosis with monohistiocytosis associated with ampicillin therapy. *Ann. Intern. Med.* 69:91, 1968.
26. Reznikoff, P.: The etiologic importance of fatigue and the prognostic significance of monocytosis in neutropenia (agranulocytosis). *Am. J. Med. Sci.* 195:627, 1938.
27. Rosenthal, N., and Abel, H. A.: The significance of the monocytes in agranulocytosis (leukopenic infectious agranulocytosis). *Am. J. Clin. Pathol.* 6:205, 1936.

28. Pretty, H. M., Gosselin, G., Colprian, G., and Long, L.-A.: Agranulo-cytosis: A report of 30 cases. *Can. Med. Assoc. J.* 93:1058, 1965.

29. Stone, G. E., and Redmond, A. J.: Leukopenic infectious monocytosis. Report of a case closely simulating acute monocytic leukemia. *Am. J. Med.* 34:541, 1963.

30. Hurst, D. W., and Meyer, O. O.: Giant follicular lymphoblastoma. *Cancer* 14:753, 1961.

31. Wiseman, B. K.: The blood pictures in the primary diseases of the lymphatic system: Their character and significance. *JAMA* 107:2016, 1936.

32. Levinson, B., Walter, B. A., Wintrobe, M. M., and Cartwright, G. E.: A clinical study of Hodgkin's disease. *Arch. Intern. Med.* 99:519, 1957.

33. Ultmann, J. E.: Clinical features and diagnosis of Hodgkin's disease. *Cancer* 9:297, 1966.

34. Warnke, R. A., Kim, H. and Dorfman, R. F.: Malignant histiocytosis (histiocytic medullary reticulosis). Clinicopathologic study of 29 cases. *Cancer* 35:215, 1975.

35. Lipson, R. L., Bayrd, E. D., and Watkins, C. H.: The post splenectomy blood picture. *Am. J. Clin. Pathol.* 32:526, 1959.

36. Budman, D. R., and Steinberg A. D.: Hematologic aspects of systemic lupus erythematosus. Current concepts. *Ann. Intern. Med.* 86:220, 1977.

37. Michael, S. R., Vural, I. L., Bassen, F. A., and Schaefer, L.: The hematologic aspects of disseminated (systemic) lupus erythematosus. *Blood* 6:1059, 1951.

38. Groopman, J. E., and Golde, D. W.: The histiocytic disorders: A pathophysiologic analysis. *Ann. Intern. Med.* 94:95, 1981.

39. Gibson, A.: Monocytic leukemoid reaction associated with tuberculosis and a mediastinal teratoma. *J. Pathol. Bacteriol.* 58:469, 1946.

40. Flinn, J. W.: A study of the differential blood count in 1000 cases of active pulmonary tuberculosis. *Ann. Intern. Med.* 2:622, 1929.

41. Stobie, W., England, N. J., and McMenemy, W. H.: The interpretation of haemograms in pulmonary tuberculosis. *Am. Rev. Tuberc.* 46:1, 1942.

42. Daland, G. A., Gottlieb, L., Wallerstein, R. O., and Castle, W. B.: Hematologic observations in bacterial endocarditis. *J. Lab. Clin. Med.* 48:827, 1956.

43. Hill, R. W., and Bayrd, E. D.: Phagocytic reticuloendothelial cells in subacute bacterial endocarditis with negative cultures. *Ann. Intern. Med.* 52:310, 1960.

44. Dameshek, W.: The appearance of histiocytes in the peripheral blood. *Arch. Intern. Med.* 47:968, 1931.

45. Horsfall, F. L., Jr., and Tamm, I.: *Viral and Rickettsial Diseases of Man,* 4th ed. Lippincott, Philadelphia, 1965.

46. Harrel, G. T., Aikawa, J. K., and Kelsey, W. M.: Rocky Mountain Spotted Fever. *Am. Pract.* 1:425, 1947.

47. Morgan, H. R., Neva, F. A., Fahey, R. J., and Finland, M.: Brill's dis-ease: Report of two serologically proved cases of typhus fever in Irish-born residents of Boston. *N. Engl. J. Med.* 238:87, 1948.

48. Murray, E. S., et al.: Brill's disease. I. Clinical and laboratory diagnosis. *JAMA* 142:1059, 1950.

49. Spink, W. W.: *The Nature of Brucellosis.* University of Minnesota Press, Minneapolis, 1956.

50. Cartwright, G. E., Chung, H.-L., and Chang, A.: Studies on the pancytopenia of kala-azar. *Blood* 3:249, 1948.

51. Dubos, R. J., and Hirsch, J. G.: *Bacterial and Mycotic Infections,* 4th ed. Lippincott, Philadelphia, 1965.

52. Vryonis, G.: Blood studies in malaria. *Am. J. Med. Sci.* 200:809, 1940.

53. Louria, D. B., Stiff, D. P., and Bennett, B.: Disseminated moniliasis in the adult. *Medicine* 41:307, 1962.

54. Hickling, R. A.: The monocytes in pneumonia: A clinical and hematologic study. *Arch. Intern. Med.* 40:594, 1927.

55. Rosahn, P. D., and Pearce, L.: The blood cytology in untreated and treated syphilis. *Am. J. Med. Sci.* 187:88, 1934.

56. Goodwin, J. S., DeHoratius, R., Israel, H., Peake, G. T., and Messner, R. P.: Suppressor cell function in sarcoidosis. *Ann. Intern. Med.* 90:169, 1979.

57. Daniele, R. P., Dauber, J. H., and Rossman, M. D.: Immunologic abnormalities in sarcoidosis. *Ann. Intern. Med.* 92:406, 1980.

58. Wood, G. W., Neff, J. E., and Stephens, R.: Relationship between monocytosis and T-lymphocyte function in human cancer. *J. Natl. Cancer Inst.* 63:587, 1979.

59. Barrett, O'N., Jr.: Monocytosis in malignant disease. *Ann. Intern. Med.* 73:991, 1970.

60. Minot, G. R., and Smith L. W.: The blood in tetrachlorethane poisoning. *Arch. Intern. Med.* 28:687, 1921.

61. Avioli, L. V., Lasersohn, J. T., and Lopresti, J. M.: Histiocytosis X (Schüller-Christian disease): A clinico-pathological survey, review of ten patients and the results of prednisone therapy. *Medicine* 42:119, 1963.

62. Crocker, A. C., and Farber, S.: Niemann-Pick disease: A review of eighteen patients. *Medicine* 37:1, 1958.

63. Reich, C., Seife, M., and Kessler, B. J.: Gaucher's disease: A review and discussion of twenty cases: *Medicine* 30:1, 1951.

64. Czaczkes, J. W., and Dreyfuss, F.: Discrepancy of fingertip and ear lobe leucocyte counts in Raynaud's disease. *Am. J. Med. Sci.* 234:325, 1957.

65. Meuret, G., Detel, U., Kilz, H. P., Senn, H. J., and Van Lessen, H.: Human monocytopoiesis in acute and chronic inflammation. *Acta Haematol.* 54:328, 1975.

66. Meuret, G., Bremer, C., Bammert, J., and Ewen, J.: Oscillation of blood monocyte counts in healthy individuals. *Cell Tissue Kinet.* 7:223, 1974.

67. Horowitz, D. A., and Steagall, R. V., Jr.: The development of macrophages from large mononuclear cells in the blood of patients with inflammatory disease. *J. Clin. Invest.* 51:760, 1972.

Monocyte and macrophage disorders—lipid storage diseases

CHAPTER **99**

Lipid storage diseases

ERNEST BEUTLER

Definitions and history

The lipid storage diseases are hereditary disorders in which one or more tissues become engorged with a lipid. The type of lipid and its distribution have a characteristic pattern in each different disorder; this chapter will deal primarily with those lipid storage disorders in which the monocyte-macrophage system plays a significant role. The most important of these are Gaucher disease, in which glucocerebroside is stored, and Niemann-Pick disease, in which the storage material is sphingomyelin. Related disorders in which monocyte-macrophage storage is less prominent will be discussed briefly.

Gaucher disease was first described by Philippe Gaucher, who thought that the peculiar large cells in the spleen were evidence of a primary neoplasm [1]. Although it was believed at one time that the glycolipid which accumulated in Gaucher disease was a *galacto*cerebroside, it was shown in 1934 that in fact *gluco*cerebroside accumulated [1]. In 1965, the primary defect was recognized as the inability to degrade glucocerebroside [2,3]. Niemann-Pick disease was first described in an infant who died at 18 months of age. Niemann, the Berlin pediatrician who reported the case of this infant, considered the disorder to be unique because of its early onset and rapid course, which seemed atypical for Gaucher disease. The predominant phospholipid accumulating in this disorder is sphingomyelin, and in 1966 a deficiency of sphingomyelinase activity was demonstrated in a patient with Niemann-Pick disease [4].

Etiology

In the course of normal growth, development, and senescence parts of cells or whole cells are continually replaced in all tissues. Breakdown of the complex constituents of cells requires sequential, enzymatic degradation. Such degradation takes place largely in secondary lysosomes, organelles formed by the fusion of primary lysosomes with the phagocytic vacuole containing the ingested material.

Glycolipid storage diseases such as Gaucher disease or Tay-Sachs disease arise as the result of hereditary absence of one of the lysosomal enzymes required for glycolipid degradation. The parent substance is most commonly either a globoside or a ganglioside (Fig. 99-1). In the degradation of globosides and gangliosides it is necessary for the carbohydrate portion to be removed before hydrolysis of the sphingosine–fatty acid complex, ceramide. Removal of carbohydrate always proceeds from the free end of the polysaccharide chain: the distal glycosidic linkage must be cleaved with removal of the terminal sugar before the other glycosidic linkages can be enzymatically hydrolyzed. In the glycolipid storage diseases, the hereditary lack of a lysomal enzyme required for hydrolysis of one of the glycosidic bonds results in the accumulation of the glycolipid which serves as a substrate for the missing enzyme. As shown in Fig. 99-1, the absence of the β-glucosidase which cleaves glucocerebroside (glucocerebrosidase) will result in accumulation of glucocerebroside. Storage of this glycolipid results in Gaucher disease. In Fabry disease, a deficiency of α-galactosidase results in the accumulation of ceramide trihexoside, and in Tay-Sachs and Sandhoff disease a deficiency of β-D-N-acetylgalactosaminidase results in the accumulation of G_{M2} ganglioside. In an analogous fashion, deficiency of the enzyme sphingomyelinase, required to cleave the bond between ceramide and phosphorylcholine, results in Niemann-Pick disease, characterized by accumulation of sphingomyelin (Fig. 99-1). Chronic (type 1) Gaucher disease, typical Niemann-Pick disease, and Tay-Sachs disease all occur with elevated frequencies among Ashkenazic Jews. The explanation for the elevated gene frequencies of these physiologically related diseases is not known. Genetic drift, random shift in gene frequency, is not likely for nonrandomly related disorders. Elevated mutation rates in one ethnic group are also highly improbable. It is more likely to result from some heterozygote advantage such as that found in sickle cell anemia, thalassemia, and glucose-6-phosphate dehydrogenase deficiency among African and Mediterranean peoples (see Chap. 16). The basis for such a possible advantage is unknown [5].

Gaucher disease

GENETICS AND INCIDENCE

Three types of Gaucher disease have been differentiated [1]. The chronic adult type (type 1) and the acute infantile neuronopathic variety (type 2) are both characterized by a deficiency of glucocerebrosidase and accumulation of glucocerebroside, but they are genetically

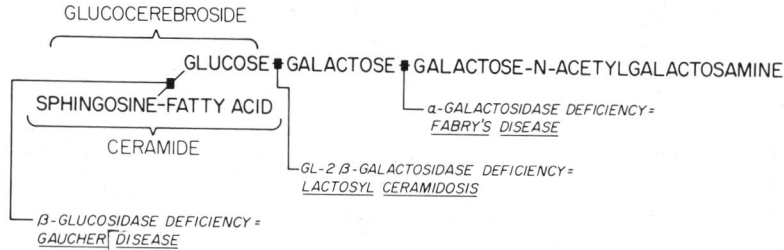

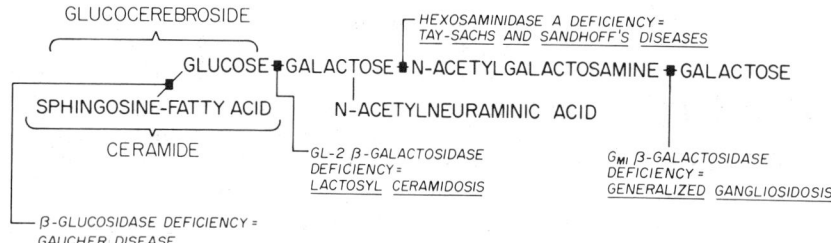

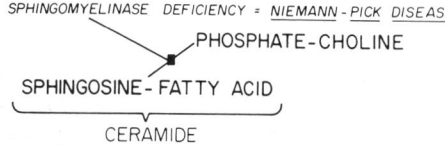

FIGURE 99-1   **The structure of some of the lipids involved in lipid storage diseases. The solid squares indicate the bonds which fail to be cleaved in the diseases specified. The globosides are sometimes designated GL-1, GL-2, etc., the number designating the number of sugar residues attached to ceramide. There are many systems of nomenclature for the gangliosides; the designation G_{M2} is commonly applied to ganglioside which accumulates in Tay-Sachs disease.**

and clinically quite distinct. The infantile disorder is exceedingly rare, does not occur predominantly in Jewish families, and is characterized by rapid neurologic deterioration and early death. The adult type occurs in children as well as in adults, but is clearly differentiated from the infantile variety by the absence of neurologic symptoms. Type 3 is a less well defined subacute neuronopathic disorder with later onset of neurologic symptoms and a somewhat better prognosis than the acute infantile neuronopathic type.

Gaucher disease is inherited as an autosomal recessive disorder. The occurrence of the disease in several successive generations once led to the erroneous conclusion that inheritance followed a dominant pattern [6]. It now seems clear that such pedigrees are best explained by the marriage of a person with Gaucher disease to a carrier [7]. This is not a rare event since estimates of frequency of this disorder in Jewish populations suggest that at least 1 out of 50 persons may be a heterozygote. Among Ashkenazic (European) Jews in Israel, the estimated incidence of the disease is at least 1 in 12,000 [8].

PATHOLOGY AND CLINICAL MANIFESTATIONS

The clinical manifestations of Gaucher disease are produced by the accumulation of glucocerebroside-laden macrophages in spleen, liver, and marrow (Fig. 99-2). These cells have small, usually eccentrically placed nuclei, and cytoplasm with characteristic wrinkles or striations. The cytoplasm is stained by the periodic acid–Schiff (PAS) technique. Electron microscopy reveals that the cytoplasm contains spindle- or rod-shaped, membrane-bound inclusion bodies 0.6 to 4 μm in diameter. These bodies appear to consist of numerous small tubules 130 to 750 Å in diameter [9]. The spleen may become massively enlarged and produce symptoms both as a result of its great bulk and because of sequestration of formed elements. Hemolysis is usually a relatively mild manifestation of splenic sequestration, but moderate leukopenia and severe thrombocytopenia are often present. Hepatic enlargement, like splenic enlargement, may cause mechanical symptoms, and liver fibrosis accompanied by functional abnormalities and varices may develop. Severe pulmonary disease with

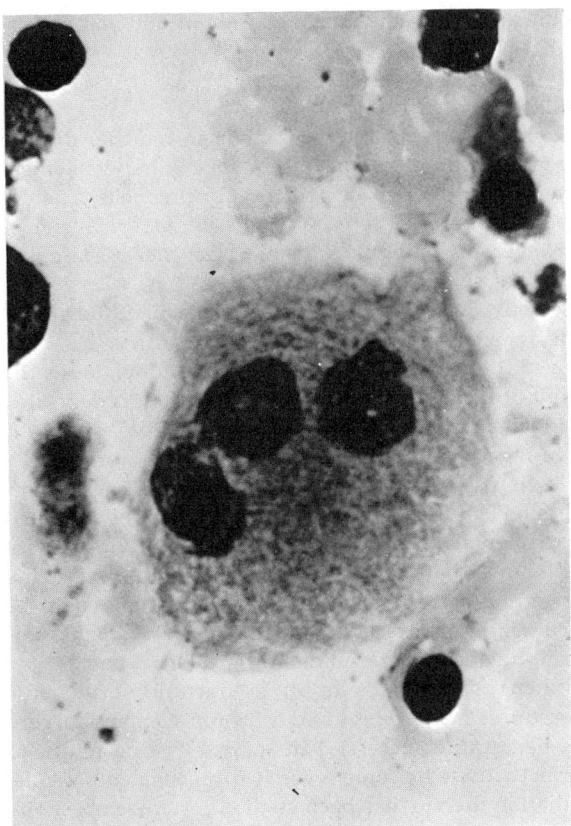

FIGURE 99-2   A Gaucher disease cell from the marrow (×915).

reticulocytosis is often present in anemic patients. The white cell count may be decreased to levels as low as 1000 per microliter, although milder degrees of leukopenia are much more common. The differential count is

FIGURE 99-3   X-rays of distal femora and pelvis of a 27-year-old woman with Gaucher disease. The distal femur shafts are flared with thinning bone trabeculae and scattered sclerotic zones to bone infarcts. The most extensive changes are seen in the left tibia proximally. The pelvis and upper femurs demonstrate extensive cystic and sclerotic changes with collapse of both femoral heads and of the right acetabulum. (X-rays courtesy of Dr. Hyman Gildenhorn, City of Hope Medical Center.)

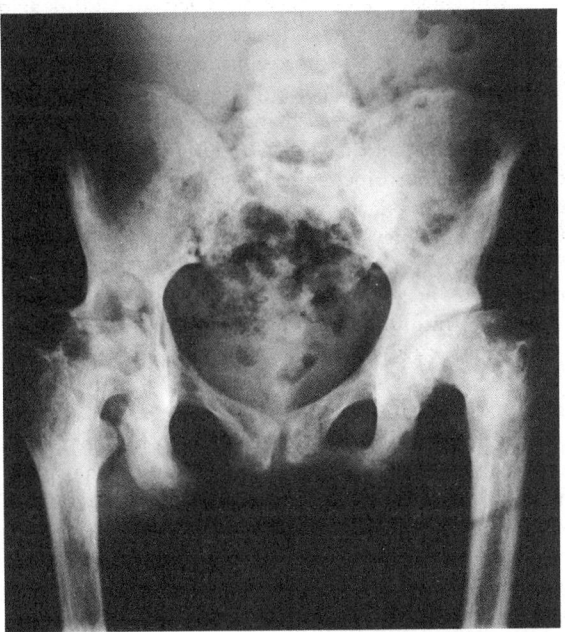

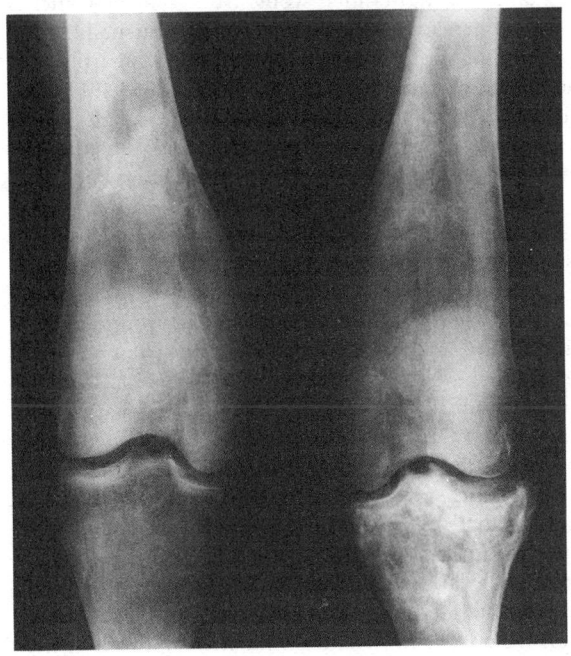

cyanosis and clubbing occurs in some patients with advanced liver involvement. In such individuals, it is probably the consequence of shunting through the lung secondary to the liver disease. In some children, however, direct involvement of the lungs with Gaucher cells has also been observed [10].

Skeletal lesions are often widespread. Patchy areas of bone demineralization are found, and widening of the distal femur gives rise to a typical "Erlenmeyer flask" deformity (Fig. 99-3). Bone pain is probably the most troublesome clinical manifestation of Gaucher disease. Pain may occur anywhere. It generally has a deep, somewhat dull character, and may be very severe. Bone pain may occur in areas with no involvement detectable by x-ray examination. It may last for weeks or months but almost invariably subsides spontaneously, only to reappear later in the same or in another location. Destructive lesions of the hips are a particularly common, crippling complication [11]. Fever may occur in patients in whom a meticulous search fails to reveal evidence of infection [12].

LABORATORY FEATURES

The blood of patients with Gaucher disease may be normal or may manifest effects of hypersplenism. A normocytic, normochromic anemia is frequently present, but hemoglobin levels rarely fall below 8 g/dl. A modest

normal. Thrombocytopenia may become quite severe. If splenectomy has been carried out, severe anisocytosis and poikilocytosis occur, with many target cells, some nucleated red cells, and Howell-Jolly bodies usually present. In splenectomized patients the white cell count and platelet count may be higher than normal. Biochemical examination of leukocytes for β-glucosidase activity shows a severe deficiency of a pH 4 β-glucosidase and a much milder deficiency of pH 5 β-glucosidase activity [13].

A striking, consistent feature of Gaucher disease is increased serum acid phosphatase activity. Since measurement of acid phosphatase activity can be carried out in any clinical laboratory, increased activity of this acid hydrolase is the one most detected. Activities of other hydrolases such as β-hexosaminidase [14] and β-glucuronidase [14], and of angiotensin-converting enzyme [5] are also increased in the serum of most patients with Gaucher disease. When liver involvement is extensive, various biochemical stigmata of liver disease, including clotting-factor abnormalities, may be present. Factor IX deficiency seems to be particularly common, and does not appear to be related to liver disease (see Chap. 156). In older patients with Gaucher disease, monoclonal immunoglobulins are commonly found in the plasma [16,17].

DIFFERENTIAL DIAGNOSIS

The diagnosis of Gaucher disease should be considered in patients with splenomegaly, particularly if the splenomegaly has been present for an extended period of time. Most patients with Gaucher disease have readily demonstrable Gaucher cells in their marrow. The number of these cells may be relatively small, and thorough examination of the marrow film under a low-power objective may be required to find them. Cells indistinguishable by light microscopy from typical Gaucher cells are also found in patients with unusually rapid turnover of granulocytes in the marrow, particularly those with chronic granulocytic leukemia [18,19]. These patients do not lack the capacity to catabolize glucocerebroside [20], but the great inflow of globoside into phagocytic cells exceeds their normal capacity to hydrolyze this glycolipid.

Measurement of serum acid phosphatase activity is useful in confirming the diagnosis of Gaucher disease. When clinical findings strongly suggest the presence of Gaucher disease but Gaucher cells are not found or their authenticity is questionable, a definitive diagnosis can be established by determining leukocyte [13,21] or cultured fibroblast [22] β-glucosidase activity. Prenatal diagnosis of Gaucher disease may be established by examining cultured amniocentesis cells and measuring their β-glucosidase activity [22]. Heterozygotes for Gaucher disease do not have Gaucher cells in their marrow, nor do thay have other stigmata of the disease. Existence of a carrier state can be established in most cases by assaying leukocytes [13,23,24] or fibroblasts [22] for β-glucosidase activity and demonstrating the reduction

in the activity of the enzyme to about one-half of normal.

THERAPY

Thrombocytopenia and leukopenia in Gaucher disease are more frequently the consequence of hypersplenism than of marrow replacement by Gaucher cells. The cytopenias respond very satisfactorily to splenectomy. However, the pathophysiology of Gaucher disease dictates that splenectomy be avoided as long as possible. The body must continue to metabolize all of the globoside which is formed; after the spleen has been removed, the glucocerebroside which accumulates as the result of incomplete globoside metabolism is deposited in the liver and marrow. A number of clinical observers have suggested that bone lesions progress more rapidly following surgical removal of the spleen [25]. This impression is difficult to quantitate and cannot be verified experimentally. While it seems reasonable, in view of the known pathophysiology of Gaucher disease, no worsening of bone lesions after splenectomy could be documented in a recent study [26]. Conservatism is advised, however, in recommending splenectomy.

When bone lesions result in fractures, orthopedic procedures may be required. Hip-replacement surgery has been quite successful in some, allowing return to normal activity by some severely incapacitated patients. Radiation therapy has been credited by some observers with relief of bone pain [11,27], but failure to produce a satisfactory response has also been reported [28,29].

Decreasing globoside inflow by repeated phlebotomy has not yielded clinically significant results [30], probably because most of the glucocerebroside is formed from sequestered white cells. Splenic transplantation was attempted in one patient, without success [31]. Initial reports of marked decrease in liver and erythrocyte glucocerebroside content after infusion of human placental glucocerebrosidase [32] have not been consistently confirmed in later studies [33]. Moreover, only minimal changes, if any, in clinical manifestations of Gaucher disease have been observed following attempts of enzyme-replacement therapy [34]. Accordingly, the effectiveness of this potentially promising therapeutic approach has not been established.

COURSE AND PROGNOSIS

While patients with the neuronopathic forms (type 2 and type 3) of Gaucher disease usually die within a few months to a few years, respectively, the prognosis in the adult type of Gaucher disease is much better. Although in some families early death follows rapid progressive deterioration with extensive involvement of marrow, liver, and spleen, the disease is sometimes not detected until middle age. In one study of 26 patients in whom the disease was diagnosed between the ages of 2 and 50, after at least 10 years only 4 had died, at ages ranging from 22 to 58 years. Several patients have lived beyond the age of 80 [35]. Death may occur as a result of liver disease, bleeding, or sepsis.

Niemann-Pick disease

GENETICS AND INCIDENCE

Niemann-Pick disease is inherited as an autosomal recessive disorder. The disease appears to be quite rare, and although it is more common among Ashkenazic Jews than among other population groups, precise data concerning its incidence are not available. A very similar disorder has been described in mice [36].

PATHOLOGY AND CLINICAL MANIFESTATIONS

The most characteristic histopathologic feature of Niemann-Pick disease is the presence of foam histocytes (Fig. 99-4). These cells are found mainly in lymphoid tissues, but widespread involvement of phagocytes and of some parenchymal cells is present throughout the body [37]. The foam cells contain largely sphingomyelin, but a brown pigment, ceroid, is also present [38].

Typical Niemann-Pick disease is an affliction of infancy. During the first months of life, affected infants gain weight poorly, the abdomen enlarges, and development is delayed. They usually do not learn to sit, and they lose those capabilities already achieved. They may become blind and deaf. Some infants have a protracted course of jaundice of unknown cause. During the second year of life, the child lies still with nearly flaccid hyporeflexic extremities, an abdomen enlarged with enormous spleen and liver, mild lymphadenopathy, and often a fine xanthomatous rash. Bone lesions may be present but are less prominent than in Gaucher disease.

A few cases have been reported of children who have sphingomyelinase deficiency with typical visceral involvement, but with no cerebral manifestations and none of the somatic wasting so characteristic of the infantile form. The typical disease has been designated as type A, and the disease without cerebral manifestations as type B. Other rare variants with late onset and atypical features have also been described and have been designated as types C, D, and E. Although total sphingomyelinase activity of the tissues of patients with such atypical features may be normal, in the case of type C Niemann-Pick disease one of the two major isozymes of sphingomyelinase is missing [39].

LABORATORY FEATURES AND DIFFERENTIAL DIAGNOSIS

The hemoglobin concentration of the blood may be normal, or mild anemia may be present. The lymphocytes may show characteristic vacuolization. Electron microscopy reveals that these vacuoles are lipid-filled lysosomes. The leukocytes of patients with Niemann-Pick disease lack sphingomyelinase activity [40].

The marrow contains typical foam cells, ranging in size from 20 to 100 μm in diameter and containing small droplets throughout the cytoplasm (Fig. 99-4). The cytoplasm of these cells stains only very faintly with the periodic acid–Schiff reagent. Phase microscopy of unstained preparations clearly reveals droplets in the cytoplasm of Niemann-Pick foam cells, which distin-

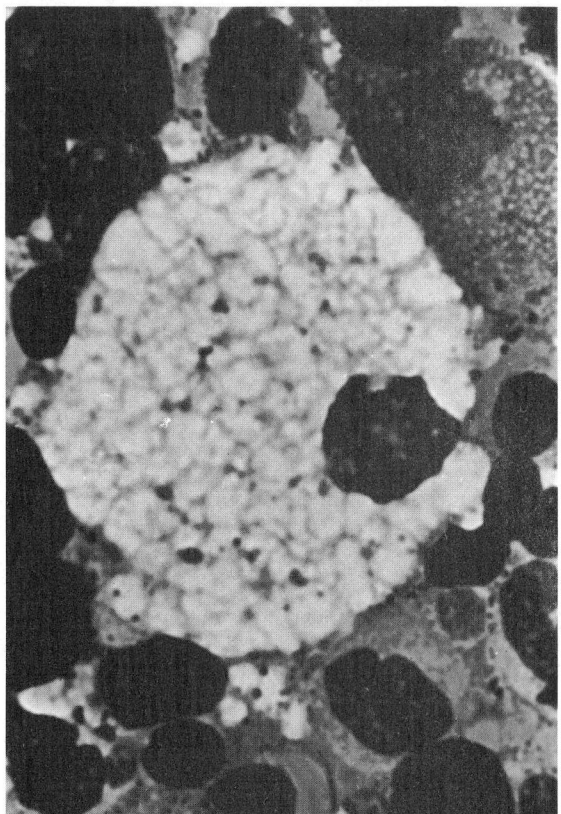

FIGURE 99-4   A foam cell from the marrow of a patient with Niemann-Pick disease (×875).

guishes them from Gaucher cells. In polarized light the droplets may be birefringent, and in ultraviolet light they manifest a greenish-yellow fluorescence [41].

Foam cells resembling those seen in Niemann-Pick disease are also observed in generalized gangliosidosis (see below). Occasionally the storage cells in Gaucher disease may present a somewhat vacuolated appearance and thereby be misinterpreted.

Niemann-Pick disease can be distinguished from other disorders by identification of the lipid as sphingomyelin and by demonstration of sphingomyelinase deficiency in blood leukocytes or in cultured fibroblasts. Heterozygotes may be detected by measurement of sphingomyelinase activity of cultured fibroblasts [38]. Prenatal diagnosis by amniocentesis has been achieved [38,42]. An artificial substrate which is very useful for the measurement of sphingomyelinase activity has been introduced [43].

TREATMENT

There is no effective treatment for Niemann-Pick disease. Splenectomy is only rarely required, because death usually occurs from other manifestations of the disease before hypersplenism becomes clinically important. Liver transplantation was carried out in one case with somewhat encouraging results [44].

COURSE AND PROGNOSIS

The prognosis in typical Niemann-Pick disease is very poor; death nearly always occurs before the third year of life. Some of the rare variants of Niemann-Pick disease carry a better prognosis, with a few patients reaching adult life.

GENERALIZED GANGLIOSIDOSIS
(G_{M1} GANGLIOSIDOSIS TYPE 1)

Generalized gangliosidosis is a rare disease characterized by β-galactosidase deficiency and consequently by greatly increased concentrations of the main (G_{M1}) monosialoganglioside in brain and viscera (Fig. 99-1) [45]. Associated with this ganglioside is its asialo derivative, a tetrasaccharide sphingolipid. At least two mucopolysaccharide compounds are also stored. One is identical with, or closely related to, keratan sulfate, and the other is a sialic acid–containing compound, possibly related to keratan sulfate [46]. The β-galactosidases form a complex system of isozymes differing in pH optimum, molecular weight, charge, and substrate specificity [47]. In generalized gangliosidosis, all forms of the liver enzyme are lacking [48]. The same defect has been described in peripheral blood leukocytes [49]. Reduced activity causes accumulation of the tetrasaccharide sphingolipid and of G_{M1}. Presumably the same enzymes are normally responsible for the hydrolysis of galactose from keratan sulfate and a related sialic acid compound, both of which accumulate when the enzyme is defective.

Clinical manifestations appear in the first year of life and reflect disease in the brain, skeleton, kidney, and monocyte-macrophage system. In typical cases, a peculiar facies, mild hepatosplenomegaly, limitation of motion in the extremities, kyphosis, and mental retardation combine to cause clinical resemblance to the Hurler syndrome. One or more of these features, together with facial edema, may be present even in very early infancy. In a few instances the cherry-red retinal spots typical of Tay-Sachs disease have been noted. Death usually occurs in the first or second year of life. Pathologically, there is generalized ballooning of neurons similar to that seen in Tay-Sachs disease, generalized presence of foam cells as found in Niemann-Pick disease, and cytoplasmic swelling of glomerular epithelial cells as seen in Fabry disease. The stored material stains with the periodic acid–Schiff technique. The presence of foam cells in marrow aspirates is a diagnostic aid. Vacuolation of the peripheral lymphocytes is common [50]. A closely related disorder, juvenile G_{M1} gangliosidosis (G_{M1} gangliosidosis type 2) is a more slowly progressive disorder with onset in late infancy and mild or absent bone involvement. No treatment is known for either form.

Tay-Sachs disease and Sandhoff disease

Tay-Sachs disease and Sandhoff disease are glycolipid storage disorders characterized by a recessively inherited deficiency of β-hexosaminidase. This enzyme cleaves the terminal N-acetylgalactosamine from G_{M2} ganglioside. With deficiency of β-hexosaminidase, large amounts of this ganglioside, and some other glycolipids and mucopolysaccharides, accumulate in the tissues, particularly in the central nervous system. Tay-Sachs disease and Sandhoff disease are clinically very similar. However, infants with Tay-Sachs disease lack only hexosaminidase A, one of the two isozymes of hexosaminidase, while in Sandhoff disease both isozymes are missing. Clinically, these disorders are exclusively an affliction of the nervous system, in which progressive developmental failure begins in the first few months of life. They are associated with blindness and the presence of cherry-red spots in the retinas, and usually terminate in the third or fourth year of life with decerebrate rigidity [51]. The brain becomes larger and heavier than normal, and microscopic examination discloses generalized neuronal ballooning with a PAS-positive material in the cytoplasm. The viscera appear normal microscopically, but chemical analysis reveals an increased concentration of the same glycosphingolipids which accumulate in the brain [52]. The fact that ganglioside accumulation in Tay-Sachs disease does not result in visceral histologic abnormalities whereas mucopolysaccharide accumulation does produce this effect in the Hurler syndrome and other mucopolysaccharidoses suggests that visceral changes in generalized gangliosidosis are attributable to the excess mucopolysaccharide.

Fabry disease

Fabry disease is characterized by the accumulation of ceramide trihexoside in all areas of the body, particularly in endothelial, perithelial, and smooth muscle cells of blood vessels, and to a lesser degree in cells of the macrophage-monocyte line. The glycolipid accumulates because of a deficiency in one of the isozymes of α-galactosidase, α-galactosidase A [53,54].

Clinically, patients suffer from recurrent fever, decreased sweating, burning paresthesias in the extremities, and renal failure. Characteristic cutaneous lesions consisting of small red spots are found primarily on the lower abdomen, thighs, and scrotum. Because of the occurrence of these lesions the disease has been designated as *angiokeratoma corporis diffusum universale*. Fabry disease is sex-linked. The diagnosis is best made by showing the absence or profound deficiency of α-galactosidase A in leukocytes [53], fibroblasts [55], urine, or plasma [56].

The course of Fabry disease is quite variable, but renal failure usually develops in the third or fourth decade of life and is the most common cause of death. Renal transplantation has been attempted as treatment not only for azotemia, but for the disease itself. It does not seem to effect any improvement in the basic disease process [57]. Preliminary studies of the effect of infusion of partially purified enzymes have been mildly encouraging in that a decrease in plasma glycolipid levels has been observed [58]. However, the fact that female heterozygotes for Fabry disease usually manifest stigmata of the disease, and these may be severe, even when plasma levels of α-galactosidase A are relatively high suggests that enzyme replacement therapy will not be helpful in this disorder [59]. The use of diphenylhydantoin [60] and phenoxybenzamine [61] to control symptoms has been suggested.

Wolman's disease

Wolman's disease is a rare disorder characterized by a severe deficiency of acid esterase [62], resulting in accumulation of triglycerides and cholesterol esters in many tissues. The disorder is clinically similar to Niemann-Pick disease. Severe cases manifest vomiting, diarrhea, malabsorption, cachexia, and death in early infancy, with hepatosplenomegaly, and diffuse punctate calcification of the adrenal by x-ray. Foam cells are found in marrow aspirates and in most tissues, including intestine, liver, spleen, adrenals, lymph nodes, thymus, and lungs. Typical ballooning of neurons is found in the retinal ganglion cells and in the myenteric plexus, but is not prominent in the central nervous system, where the major changes are in endothelial cells [63].

A milder type of lipidosis, cholesteryl ester storage disease, has also been described [64,65]. Patients with this disorder also have a defect in acid esterase activity and thus may be considered to have a phenotypically mild variant of Wolman's disease.

Tangier disease

Tangier Island in Chesapeake Bay was the home of the first reported patients with a very rare, recessively inherited disease in which cholesterol esters are stored in foam cells in many tissues, including tonsils, lymph nodes, thymus, spleen, liver, marrow, and rectal mucosa [66]. The underlying defect is a deficiency of one of the high-density lipoproteins (HDL; α-lipoprotein). A unique finding is an orange banding of greatly enlarged tonsils. Splenomegaly, lymphadenopathy, and less frequently hepatomegaly or hypersplenism may occur. Mild weakness and hyporeflexia in older adults suggest the possibility of neurolipidosis as a late complication. The disease is benign in childhood, but it is not clear that it remains so in adulthood, when the arterial deposition of lipid carried risk of pulmonic stenosis or coronary occlusion. Plasma cholesterol levels are subnormal, and electrophoresis and ultracentrifugation reveal a virtual absence of high-density α-lipoproteins. Immunoelectrophoresis further shows that the level of the protein carrier itself is reduced to a small percentage of normal. It is not apparent how this finding, evidently a basic gene-determined protein defect, leads to tissue storage of cholesterol esters. In contrast to abetalipoproteinemia (Chap. 57), Tangier disease does not cause acanthocytosis.

Hyperlipidemia

Tissue foam cells and tissue lipid storage may also be found in various other conditions associated with high plasma cholesterol, triglyceride, and phospholipid concentrations. Disease states in which impressive hyperlipidemia may occur as a secondary phenomenon include diabetes mellitus and type 1 glycogen storage disease.

In one condition the hyperlipidemia and tissue lipidosis are primary expressions of a recessively inherited defect, a deficiency of lipoprotein lipase [67]. The disease becomes apparent in childhood, even in infancy, because of hepatosplenomegaly, recurrent acute episodes of abdominal pain, and eruptive xanthomas of the skin and mucous membranes. Hypersplenism is not a recorded complication. The cause of the abdominal pain is usually unknown, but may sometimes be associated with pancreatitis. Lipemia retinalis is a common feature. Premature atherosclerosis is not ordinarily found, and the life-span may not be compromised. Tissue foam cells occur in lymphoreticular tissues, marrow, and xanthomas. There is nothing distinctive about these foam cells; they resemble those seen in many other conditions, including Niemann-Pick disease, Wolman's disease, and generalized gangliosidosis. The number of foam cells seem to correlate with the degree of hyperlipidemia [68]. Plasma triglycerides, cholesterol esters, and chylomicra attain such high levels that the plasma becomes lactescent. With use of low-fat diets the hyperlipidemia and the clinical manifestations are reduced but not eliminated.

Familial hypercholesterolemia due to a receptor defect is the best-studied form of hyperlipidemia [69]. Although foam cells are not seen in the common heterozygous form of this disorder, they may be present in the homozygous form, in which striking degrees of hypercholesterolemia are apparent even in childhood.

References

1. Fredrickson, D. S., and Sloan, H. R.: Glucosyl ceramide lipidoses: Gaucher's disease, in *The Metabolic Basis of Inherited Disease*, 3d ed., edited by J. B. Stanbury and J. B. Wyngaarden, McGraw-Hill, New York, 1972, p. 730.

2. Brady, R. O., Kanfer, J. N., and Shapiro, D.: Metabolism of glucocerebrosides II: Evidence of an enzymatic deficiency in Gaucher's disease. *Biochem. Biophys. Res. Commun.* 18:221, 1965.

3. Patrick, A. D.: Short Communications: A deficiency of glucocerebrosidase in Gaucher's disease. *Biochem. J.* 97:17C, 1965.

4. Brady, R. O., Kanfer, J. N., Mock, M. B., and Fredrickson, D. S.: The metabolism of sphingomyelin. II: Evidence of an enzymatic deficiency in Niemann-Pick disease. *Proc. Natl. Acad. Sci. U.S.A.* 55:366, 1966.

5. Knudson, A. G., and Kaplan, W. D.: Genetics of the sphingolipidoses, in *Cerebral Sphingolipidoses*, edited by S. M. Aronson and B. W. Volk. Academic, New York, 1962, p. 395.

6. Groen, J. J.: Gaucher's disease: Hereditary transmission and racial distribution. *Arch. Intern. Med. 113*:543, 1964.

7. Ho, M. W., et al.: Adult Gaucher's disease: Kindred studies and demonstration of a deficiency of acid β-glucosidase in cultured fibroblasts. *Am. J. Hum. Genet. 24*:37, 1972.

8. Groen, J. J.: Present status of knowledge of Gaucher's disease. *Isr. J. Med. Sci. 1*:507, 1965.

9. Brady, R. O., and King, F. M.: Gaucher's disease, in *Lysosomes and Storage Diseases*, edited by H. G. Hers and F. Van Hoof. Academic, New York, 1973, p. 381.

10. Schneider, E. L., Epstein, C. J., Kaback, M. J., and Brandes, D.: Severe pulmonary involvement in adult Gaucher's disease. *Am. J. Med. 63*:475, 1977.

11. Amstutz, H. C.: The hip in Gaucher's disease. *Clin. Orthop. 90*:83, 1773.

12. Billings, A. A., Post, M. and Shapiro, C. M.: Febrile reaction of Gaucher's disease. *Ill. Med. J. 145*:222, 1973.

13. Beutler, E., and Kuhl, W.: The diagnosis of the adult type of Gaucher's disease and its carrier state by demonstration of deficieny of β-glucosidase activity in peripheral blood leukocytes. *J. Lab. Clin. Med. 76*:747, 1970.

14. Oeckerman, P. A., and Kohlin, P.: Acid hydrolases in plasma in Gaucher's disease. *Clin. Chem. 15*:61, 1969.

15. Lieberman, J., and Beutler, E.: Elevation of serum angiotensin-converting enzyme in Gaucher's disease. *N. Engl. J. Med. 294*:1442, 1976.

16. Pratt, P. W., Estren, F., and Kochwa, S.: Immunoglobulin abnormalities in Gaucher's disease: Report of 16 cases. *Blood 31*:633, 1968.

17. Shoenfeld, Y., Berliner, S., Pinkhas, J., and Beutler, E.: The association of Gaucher's disease and dysproteinemias. *Acta Haematol. 64*:241, 1980.

18. Rosner, F., Dosik, H., Kaiser, S. S., Lee, S. L., and Morrison, A. N.: Gaucher cell in leukemia. *JAMA 209*:935, 1969.

19. Hopfner, C., Potron, G., Adnet, J. J., Caulet, A. T., and Boy, J.: Histiocytes bleus et "cellules de Gaucher" avec surcharges splenique et ganglionnaire au cours d'une leucémie myeloide chronique. *Nouv. Rev. Fr. Hematol. 14*:607, 1974.

20. Kattlove, H. E., Williams, J. C., Gaynor, E., Spivack, M., Bradley, R. M., and Brady, R. O.: Gaucher cells in chronic myelocytic leukemia: An acquired abnormality. *Blood 33*:379, 1969.

21. Klinbansky, C. H., et al.: Leukocyte glucocerebrosidase deficiency diagnostic in adult Gaucher's disease with negative bone marrow biopsy: Some properties of the enzyme in leukocytes and spleen. *Eur. J. Clin. Invest. 4*:101, 1974.

22. Beutler, E., Kuhl, W., Trinidad, F., Teplitz, R., and Nadler, H.: β-Glucosidase activity in fibroblasts from homozygotes and heterozygotes for Gaucher's disease. *Am. J. Hum Genet. 23*:62, 1971.

23. Beutler, E., Kuhl, W., Matsumoto, F., and Pangalis, G.: Acid hydrolases in leukocytes and platelets of normal subjects and in patients with Gaucher's and Fabry's disease. *J. Exp. Med. 143*:975, 1976.

24. Raghavan, S. S., Topol, J., and Kolodny, E. H.: Leukocyte β-glucosidase in homozygotes and heterozygotes for Gaucher disease. *Am. J. Hum. Genet. 32*:158, 1980.

25. Silverstein, M. N., and Kelley, P. J.: Osteoarticular manifestations of Gaucher's disease. *Am. J. Med. Sci. 253*:569, 1967.

26. Lee, R. E.: The pathology of Gaucher disease, in *Gaucher Disease: A Century of Delineation and Research*, edited by R. J. Desnick, S. Gatt, and G. A. Grabowski. Alan R. Liss, New York, 1982, pp. 177–217.

27. Davies, F. W. T.: Gaucher's disease in bone. *J. Bone Joint Surg. (Br.), 34B*:454, 1952.

28. Schein, A. J., and Arkin, A. M.: The classic: Hip-joint involvement in Gaucher's disease. *Clin. Orthop. 90*:4, 1973.

29. Moore, M., Jr., and Coley, B. L.: Bone lesions in Gaucher's disease. *J. Tenn. Med. Assoc. 40*:101, 1947.

30. Beutler, E., and Southgate, M. T.: Clinical pathological conference: Hepatosplenomegaly, abdominal pain, anemia, and bone lesions. *JAMA 224*:502, 1973.

31. Groth, C. G., et al.: Splenic transplantation in a case of Gaucher's disease. *Lancet 1*:1260, 1971.

32. Brady, R. O., Pentchev, P. G., Gal, A. E., Hibbert, S. R. and Dekaban, A. S.: Replacement therapy for inherited enzyme deficiency: Use of

33. Brady, R. O., Barranger, J. A., Gal, A. E., Pentchev, P. G. and Furbish, F. S.: Status of enzyme replacement therapy for Gaucher's disease, in *Enzyme Therapy in Genetic Diseases*, edited by R. J. Desnick. Alan R. Liss, 1980, vol. II, p. 361.

34. Beutler, E., Dale, G. L., and Kuhl, W.: Replacement therapy in Gaucher's disease, in *Enzyme Therapy in Genetic Diseases*, edited by R. J. Desnick. Alan R. Liss, 1980, vol. II, p. 369.

35. McKelvie, I. J., and Edwards, L. R.: Gaucher's disease: Report of a case. *Med. J. Aust. 2*:297, 1969.

36. Lyon, M. F., Hulse, E. V., and Rowe, C. E.: Foam-cell reticulosis of mice: An inherited condition resembling Gaucher's and Niemann-Pick disease. *J. Med. Genet. 2*:99, 1965.

37. Bloom, W.: The histogenesis of essential lipoid histiocytosis (Niemann-Pick's disease). *Arch. Pathol. 6*:827, 1928.

38. Brady, R. O., and King, F. M.: Niemann Pick disease, in *Lysosomes and Storage Diseases*, edited by H. G. Hers and F. Van Hoof. Academic, New York, 1973, p. 439.

39. Callahan, J. W., Khalil, M., and Gerrie, J.: Isoenzymes of sphingomyelinase and the genetic defect in Niemann-Pick disease, Type C. *Biochem. Biophys. Res. Commun. 58*:384, 1974.

40. Snyder, R. A., and Brady, R. O.: The use of white cells as a source of diagnostic material for lipid storage diseases. *Clin. Chim. Acta 25*:331, 1969.

41. Brady, R. O.: Sphingomyelin lipidosis Niemann-Pick disease, in *The Metabolic Basis of Inherited Disease*, edited by J. B. Stanbury, J. B. Wyngaarden, and D. S. Fredrickson. McGraw-Hill, New York, 1978, p. 718.

42. Epstein, C. J., Brady, R. O., Schneider, E. L., Bradley, R. M., and Shapiro, D.: In utero diagnosis of Niemann-Pick disease. *Am. J. Hum. Genet. 23*:533, 1971.

43. Gal, A. E., Brady, R. O., Hibberg, S. R., and Pentchev, P. G.: A practical chromogenic procedure for the detection of homozygotes and heterozygous carriers of Niemann-Pick disease. *N. Engl. J. Med. 293*:632, 1975.

44. Delvin, E., Glorieux, F., Daloze, P., Gorman, J., and Bloch, P.: Niemann-Pick type A: Enzyme replacement by liver transplantation. *Am. J. Hum. Genet. 26*:25A, 1974 (abstract).

45. O'Brien, J. S., Stern, M. B., Landing, B. H., O'Brien, J. K., and Donnell, G. N.: Generalized gangliosidosis. *Am. J. Dis. Child. 109*:338, 1965.

46. Suzuki, K., Suzuki, K., and Kamoshita, S.: Chemical pathology of GM1-gangliosidosis (generalized gangliosidosis). *J. Neuropathol. Exp. Neurol. 25*:25, 1968.

47. Robinson, D.: Multiple forms of glycosidases in the normal and pathological states. *Enzyme 18*:114, 1974.

48. Okada, S., and O'Brien, J. S.: Generalized gangliosidosis: β-Galactosidase deficiency. *Science 160*:1002, 1968.

49. Crawford, H., and Mollison, P. L.: Reversal of electrolyte changes in stored red cells after transfusion. *J. Physiol. 129*:639, 1955.

50. Derry, D. M., Fawcett, J. S., Andermann, F., and Wolfe, L. S.: Late infantile systemic lipidosis: Major monosialogangliosidosis, delineation of two types. *Neurology 18*:340, 1968.

51. O'Brien, J. S.: The Gangliosidoses, in *The Metabolic Basis of Inherited Disease*, edited by J. B. Stanbury, J. B. Wyngaarden, D. S. Fredrickson. McGraw-Hill, New York, 1978, p. 841.

52. Eeg-Olofsson, O., Kristensson, K., Sourander, P., and Svennerholm, L.: Tay-Sachs disease: A generalized metabolic disorder. *Acta Paediatr. Scand. 55*:546, 1966.

53. Kint, J. A.: Fabry's disease: α-Galactosidase deficiency. *Science 167*:1268, 1970.

54. Beutler, E., and Kuhl, W.: Biochemical and electrophoretic studies of α-galactosidase in normal man, in patients with Fabry's disease, and in equidae. *Am. J. Hum. Genet. 24*:237, 1972.

55. Romeo, G., and Migeon, B. R.: Genetic inactivation of the α-galactosidase locus in carriers of Fabry's disease. *Science 170*:180, 1970.

56. Desnick, R. J., Allen, K. Y., Desnick, S. J., Raman, M. K., Bernlohr, R. W., and Krivit, W.: Fabry's disease: Enzymatic diagnosis of hemizygotes and heterozygotes: α-Galactosidase activities in plasma, serum, urine, and leukocytes. *J. Lab. Clin. Med. 81*:157, 1973.

57. Rietra, P. J. G., Van Den Bergh, F. A. J., and Tager, J. M.: Recent developments in enzyme replacement therapy of lysosomal storage diseases, in *Enzyme Therapy in Lysosomal Storage Diseases*, edited by J. M. Tager, G. J. M. Hooghwinkel, and W. T. H. Daems. North-Holland Publishing, Amsterdam; American Elsevier, New York, 1974, p. 53.

58. Brady, R. O., et al.: Replacement therapy for inherited enzyme deficiency: Use of purified ceramide-trihexosidase in Fabry's disease. *N. Engl. J. Med. 289*:9, 1973.

59. Beutler, E.: Nature's transplant in Fabry's disease. *Lancet 2*:199, 1979.

60. Lockman, L. A., Hunninghake, D. B., Krivit, W., and Desnick, R. J.: Relief of pain of Fabry's disease by diphenylhydantoin. *Neurology 23*:871, 1973.

61. Liston, E. H., Levine, M. D., and Philippart, M.: Psychosis in Fabry disease and treatment with phenoxybenzamine. *Arch. Gen. Psychiatry 29*:402, 1973.

62. Patrick, A. D., and Lake, B. D.: Deficiency of an acid lipase in Wolman's disease. *Nature 222*:1067, 1969.

63. Guazzi, G. C., et al.: Wolman's disease: Distribution and significance of the central nervous system lesions. *Pathol. Eur., 3*:266, 1968.

64. Patrick, A. D., and Lake, B. D.: Wolman's disease, in *Lysosomes and Storage Diseases*, edited by H. G. Hers and F. Van Hoof. Academic, New York, 1973, p. 453.

65. Sloan, H. R., and Fredrickson, D. S.: Enzyme deficiency in cholesteryl ester storage disease. *J. Clin. Invest. 51*:1923, 1972.

66. Herbert, P. N., Gotto, A. M., and Fredrickson, D. S.: Familial lipoprotein deficiency (abetalipoproteinmia, hypobetalipopoteinemia, and Tangier disease), in *The Metabolic Basis of Inherited Disease*, edited by J. B. Stanbury, J. B. Wyngaarden, and D. S. Fredrickson. McGraw-Hill, New York, 1978, p. 544.

67. Fredrickson, D. S., Goldstein, J. L., and Brown, M. S.: The familial hyperlipoproteinemias, in *The Metabolic Basis of Inherited Disease*, edited by J. B. Stanbury, J. B. Wyngaarden, and D. S. Fredrickson. McGraw-Hill, New York, 1978, p. 604.

68. Roberts, W. C., Levy, R. I., and Fredrickson, D. S.: Hyperlipoproteinemia: A review of the five types with first report of necropsy findings in type 3. *Arch. Pathol. 90*:46, 1970.

69. Goldstein, J. L., and Brown, M. S.: Familial Hypercholesterolemia, in *The Metabolic Basis of Inherited Disease*, edited by J. B. Stanbury, J. B. Wyngaarden, D. S. Fredrickson, J. L. Goldstein, and M. S. Brown. McGraw-Hill, New York, 1983, p. 672.

Monocyte and macrophage disorders—conditions with abnormal proliferation, possibly malignant

CHAPTER *100*

Hystiocytosis (histiocytosis X, reticuloendotheliosis)

F. STANLEY PORTER

Definitions and history

Histiocytosis refers to a group of diseases of unknown cause characterized by the abnormal proliferation of histiocytes without association with any known infectious agent or abnormality of lipid metabolism. They have been classically divided into three clinical entities: eosinophilic granuloma, Hand-Schüller-Christian disease, and Letterer-Siwe disease.

The triad of lytic skull lesions, exophthalmos, and diabetes insipidus associated with Hand-Schüller-Christian disease was first described in a case report by Hand in 1893 [1]. The patient also had hepatosplenomegaly and a petechial rash. Christian and others reported patients with the same triad and considered the disease to be the result of abnormal pituitary function [2–4].

In 1924 Letterer described an infant with an eczematous hemorrhagic rash, hepatosplenomegaly, lymphadenopathy, fever, and anemia progressing to a fatal outcome [5]. Siwe then described seven additional cases in 1933, and the eponym *Letterer-Siwe disease* was given to the clinical entity [6,7].

Lichtenstein and Jaffé reported two patients with solitary lytic bone lesions in 1940 and termed this *eosinophilic granuloma* [8]. Others reporting similar conditions used the term *solitary granuloma of bone* [9]. In 1951 Farinacci and coworkers described two adults with isolated diffuse pulmonary disease in whom lung biopsy showed infiltration with histiocytes and eosinophils [10]. They termed this *pulmonary eosinophilic granuloma* and likened it to eosinophilic granuloma of bone.

Following the description of these classic clinical syndromes, case reports appeared describing "atypical" or "transitional" forms of one syndrome or another, and by 1940 the consensus was that they all represented different expressions of the same basic pathologic process [11–13]. Lichtenstein coined the term *histiocytosis X* to encompass all these syndromes to avoid multiple names and to emphasize the common pathologic findings and the idiopathic nature of these diseases [14]. Recent reviews of idiopathic histiocytosis, however, suggest that these diseases should be separated into two categories: (1) eosinophilic granuloma of bone, solitary or multifocal, the latter being synonymous with Hand-Schüller-Christian disease, and (2) diffuse histiocytosis, or Letterer-Siwe syndrome, which may behave like an atypical form of lymphoma [15,16]. Because there is a great difference in clinical manifestations and prognosis, the diseases will be discussed here under two broad headings: (1) localized histiocytosis, representing disease confined to a single organ system, and (2) systemic histiocytosis, representing disease involving more than one organ system.

Etiology and pathogenesis

Hand suggested that the disease in his original patient resulted from an infectious agent, animal in nature [1,3]. An abnormality of lipid metabolism related to that in the xanthomas was postulated later [17] but finally excluded [18–20]. Infection has been suggested as the cause of histiocytosis, but the evidence is tenuous [21–23]. Organisms have been grown from lesions in a few cases [22], but most are sterile [21]. Material from lesions has been injected into animals without ill effect [12]. The apparent response to antibiotics in a few cases, the response to glucocorticoids, and the histologic features of the lesions are given as evidence for the infectious agent hypothesis.

In a study of 270 deaths due to histiocytosis in the United States from 1960 to 1964, five pairs of siblings, including one set of twins, were found [24]. This, together with the high mortality in patients under 1 year of age, led to the conclusion that the disease has a prenatal origin.

Because of similarities between histiocytosis and some of the immunodeficiency syndromes, it has been suggested that histiocytosis is basically an immunologic disorder [25,26]. The results of routine immunologic studies in six infants with disseminated histiocytosis and seven older children with various degrees of involvement were found to be essentially normal [27]. However, 12 of 17 patients with histiocytosis were found to have circulating lymphocytes which were cytotoxic to human fibroblasts or antibody to autologous erythrocytes [27]. In addition, their T lymphocytes did not have histamine H2 surface receptors. Calf thymus gland extract corrected the lymphocyte abnormalities in vitro and 10 of the 17 patients treated with this extract had a complete remission [28].

Although histiocytosis can be suspected clinically, it is necessary to obtain a biopsy to confirm the diagnosis. The site of biopsy is determined by the location of the lesions. Skin is the easiest tissue to obtain, but biopsy of bone, gums, superficial lymph nodes, or liver may be necessary. The basic histology of all lesions is the same. A particularly clear and concise description of the pathology of reticuloendotheliosis has been published [29]. The lesion consists of a proliferation of histiocytes in sheetlike masses with numerous eosinophils interspersed either singly or in clumps. The histiocytes rarely show mitotic figures but do fuse to form multinucleated giant cells. Collections of so-called "foam cells," vacuolated histiocytes with sudanophilic material in the cytoplasm, may also be found. It has been suggested that the histiocytes present in these lesions are derived from Langerhans cells [30]. The amount of lymphocytic and plasmacytic infiltration, the degree of eosinophilia, the number of foam cells, and the amount of necrosis or fibrosis vary considerably from lesion to lesion. It is generally considered that there is no correlation between the histologic findings and the clinical findings or prognosis. All varieties of histologic abnormalities may be seen in all types of histiocytosis, and, at autopsy, there is wide variability in the appearance of lesions taken from different sites in the same patient. However, in a series of 51 patients, two separate histopathologic types have been described, each with a different prognosis [60]. Type I is characterized by a diffuse infiltration of the organs that compose the monocyte-macrophage system by individual histiocytes without giant cells, eosinophils, or necrosis. Type II is characterized by variable focal involvement of the organs which contain the monocyte-macrophage system by syncytial sheets of histiocytes with eosinophils, giant cells, necrosis, and fibrosis. Of the nine patients who died in this series, seven had the type I lesion.

Localized histiocytosis

EOSINOPHILIC GRANULOMA OF BONE
This is a benign disease confined to the skeletal system. It is characterized usually by one, but occasionally by two or more, circumscribed osseous lytic lesions. Since bone lesions are also a characteristic of system histiocytosis, there may be some confusion concerning prognosis. However, if one adheres to the original definition, that of a disease confined to bone, a more meaningful clinical picture emerges.

CLINICAL FEATURES
There is no sex predilection, and the disease is seen primarily in older children and adults. In one series of

TABLE 100-1   Frequency of bones involved by eosinophilic granuloma in 63 cases from the literature

Skull	19	Humerus	3
Femur	10	Clavicle	3
Rib	8	Mastoid	2
Mandible	6	Scapula	2
Vertebra	6	Fibula	1
Pelvis	4	Tibia	1

SOURCE: Oberman [29], McGavran and Spady [31], and Ochsner [32].

28 cases the average age was 13.3 years [31]. The predominant symptoms are pain and swelling over the affected bone. There have been reports of neurologic sequelae from spinal cord compression as a result of vertebral involvement [29]. Fractures of other bones can also occur. The distribution of bone lesions compiled from three clinical studies is shown in Table 100-1 [27,31,32].

LABORATORY FEATURES
The standard clinical tests and hematologic procedures are nondiagnostic.

TREATMENT
Treatment consists of biopsy followed by curettage and irradiation. The results are good, and the prognosis is excellent. Occasionally other lesions will develop, or the bone lesion is the initial manifestation of systemic histiocytosis. The younger the patient, the more likely it is that additional bone lesions or generalized disease will develop; these individuals should be followed closely [21].

PULMONARY EOSINOPHILIC GRANULOMA
Systemic histiocytosis may involve the lungs, but, as with eosinophilic granuloma in bone, local pulmonary involvement may occur.

CLINICAL FEATURES
A review of the natural history of this entity indicates that it is seen primarily in young adult Caucasian males [33,34]. The onset is relatively sudden, and the symptoms mild, usually just a persistent cough. Chest x-rays show a diffuse, interstitial, small-nodular type of infiltrate with small cystic areas giving a honeycomb pattern (Fig. 100-1). Diagnosis requires lung biopsy. The disease has an apparent period of activity lasting a few months and then spontaneously regresses, leaving a variable degrees of fibrosis. Pulmonary function studies on five such patients showed evidence of an alveolocapillary block which varied with the severity of the disease [35].

TREATMENT AND PROGNOSIS
Glucocorticoids and irradiation have been used with some benefit [34,35]. It is difficult to evaluate the effect of treatment, since pulmonary eosinophilic granuloma

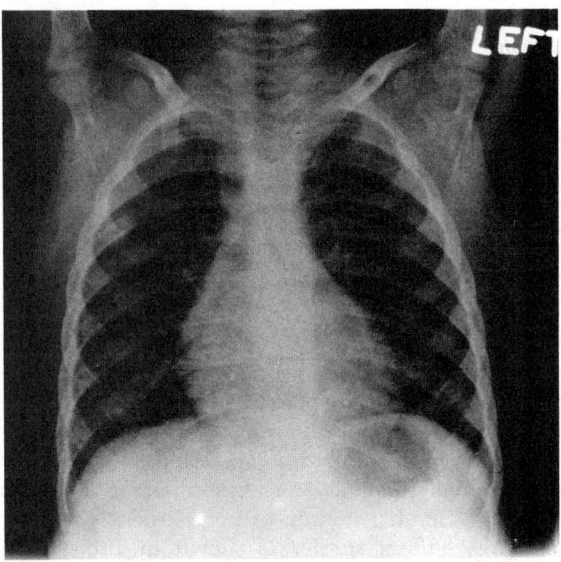

FIGURE 100-1   Chest x-ray showing characteristic pulmonary infiltrates and osteolytic bone lesions in histiocytosis.

has a self-limited course. The prognosis is generally good, and the amount of residual pulmonary fibrosis will vary with the severity of the disease.

LOCALIZED INVOLVEMENT OF OTHER ORGANS
There are numerous reports of so-called eosinophilic granuloma involving other organs, particularly the gastrointestinal tract, but these apparently have no relation to histiocytosis. Isolated involvement of organs other than bone and lung must be very rare. Eosinophilic granuloma of the parotid gland and thymus has been reported, the author citing other examples from the literature [36]. This author has observed a 3-month-old infant with isolated skin involvement, proved by biopsy, which spontaneously resolved. Observation over a 3-year period showed no further disease. Others have reported similar cases [29,37].

LABORATORY FINDINGS
The standard clinical diagnostic procedures and hematologic studies in these instances also are nondiagnostic.

Systemic histiocytosis

An entirely satisfactory, clear-cut distinction between the so-called acute (Letterer-Siwe) and chronic (Hand-Schüller-Christian) forms of systemic histiocytosis cannot be made.

CLINICAL FEATURES
There is a wide spectrum in the clinical expression of systemic histiocytosis, and features frequently overlap. The course varies from an acute fulminating disease to a chronic, relatively benign one, with all variations in between. There may be some predilection of the disease for males [18,21,22]. The disease can occur at any age, but the majority of cases occur in the first 3 years of life, the greatest incidence being in the first year [18,21]. There have been a few instances of the disease in newborn infants [38]. A statistical study indicates that some 270 deaths occurred in the United States from histiocytosis between 1960 and 1964. The probability that a child will develop the disease by the age of 3 years is 3.6 per million [24].

Almost all organ systems can be involved in systemic histiocytosis, some more frequently, however, than others, as is discussed below.

SKELETON
Lytic bone lesions are the most frequent but occur in a somewhat different distribution than in disease localized to bone [21]. The skull is the most frequent site in both, but the sella turcica and sphenoid bone are involved mainly in patients with systemic disease. Involvement of the maxilla, mandible, and bones of the upper extremity likewise seem to be more characteristic of systemic involvement. Examples of extensive bone disease are shown in Fig. 100-2.

The bone lesions themselves are largely asymptomatic. Fractures may occur, of course, but are not as frequent as one would expect. Complications arise from the involvement of adjacent soft tissues, for example, dental problems from disease in the maxilla and mandible, chronically draining ears from destruction of the mastoid and temporal bones, or diabetes insipidus from involvement of the sella turcica.

SKIN
The lesions associated with skin involvement are usually erythematous, papular, and scaly, but are occasionally seborrheic or eczematous as shown in Fig. 100-3. If thrombocytopenia is present, skin lesions may be hemorrhagic or petechial. Xanthomatous-appearing lesions are rare but have been described [39], as have nodular infiltrates [40].

PITUITARY
Diabetes insipidus is a well-known feature of the disease and is due to the involvement of the posterior pituitary. This may be associated with lesions in the sella turcica but can occur without apparent bone disease. In one report of panhypopituitarism associated with histiocytosis, lesions were found at autopsy surrounding the pituitary but not invading it [41]. In another series, growth hormone deficiency was found in seven of eight children with histiocytosis who were of short stature and in three additional patients who had attained adult height before developing the disease [62]. This deficiency was usually found in patients who also had diabetes insipidus, and it was suggested that both abnormalities could be due to a lesion in the hypothalamus. Hyperprolactinemia [42] and hypogonadism [43] have also been reported.

EYES, EARS, MOUTH

Proptosis may be either unilateral or bilateral. The effects are mainly cosmetic since the optic nerve is seldom damaged. Chronically draining ears are characteristic and associated with temporal bone involvement. Granulomatous tissue can be seen in the external auditory canal. The discharge is seldom purulent and is unresponsive to the usual antibiotics. Despite the frequency of temporal bone involvement, facial nerve palsy is extremely rare [44]. Maxillary and mandibular lesions may result in loose or lost teeth. The gums and mucous membranes of the mouth may be directly involved, resulting in ulcerated, hypertrophied, and friable gums as well as mouth ulcers.

FIGURE 100-2 Extensive involvement of skull and long bones in a child with systemic histiocytosis.

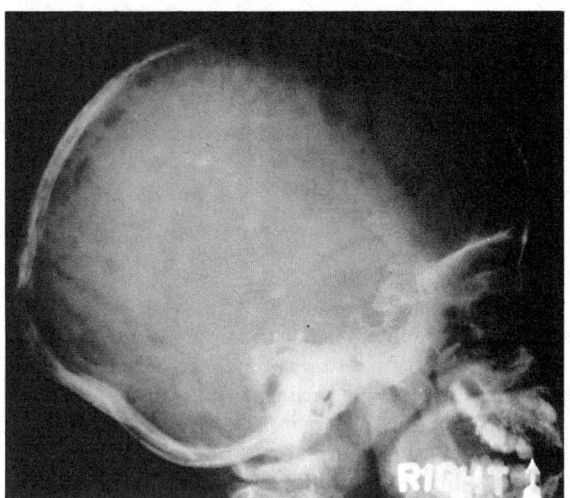

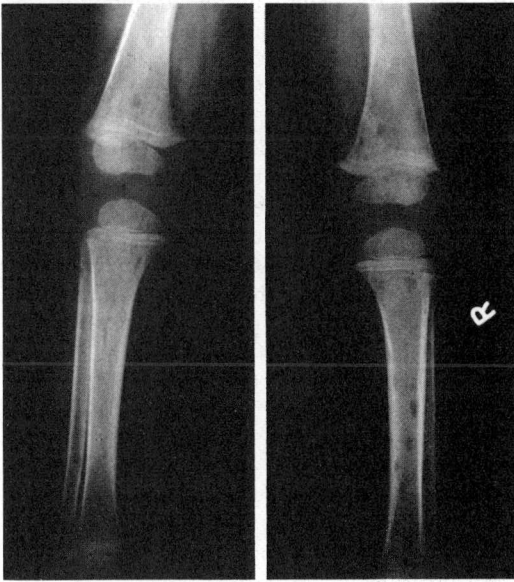

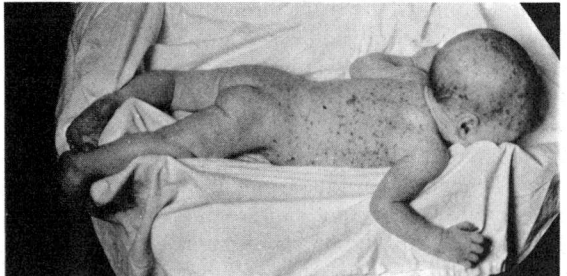

FIGURE 100-3 Eczematous, hemorrhagic rash in an infant with systemic histiocytosis.

LUNGS

The radiographic and clinical findings of lung involvement are essentially the same in systemic histiocytosis as they are in disease localized to the lungs. In fulminant cases the patient may die from cor pulmonale resulting from extensive lung disease. In systemic disease, however, if the patient survives, there are usually no residual fibrotic changes such as develop in patients with localized disease. Spontaneous pneumothorax occurs and may be life-threatening [18]. Recurrent episodes of spontaneous pneumothorax may be the initial manifestation and a clue to the diagnosis in this disease [45].

LYMPH NODES

Lymph node involvement is usually prominent when disease is widespread, but local node enlargement may occur as the initial finding.

LIVER, SPLEEN, AND MARROW

When one of these organs is involved, usually they all are, and this is of grave prognostic significance. Hepatomegaly can occur with or without jaundice or laboratory evidence of hepatocellular damage. Splenomegaly may play a role in the etiology of the thrombocytopenia, anemia, and leukopenia that is sometimes seen, but replacement of marrow tissue by histiocytosis may also produce these findings.

LABORATORY FINDINGS

Standard laboratory procedures show no characteristic deviations from normal. Leukocytosis is frequently seen, but eosinophilia is rare. Nothing diagnostic is ordinarily obtained in aspirated marrow.

TREATMENT

Irradiation, glucocorticoids, antibiotics, and a variety of cytotoxic agents and antimetabolites have been used to treat systemic histiocytosis. Irradiation is effective in arresting the extension of lesions and aids in their resolution. This is particularly true of bone lesions. In systemic disease irradiation is used locally for specific problems such as chronically draining ears, proptosis, or bone lesions where a fracture might occur, particularly in the vertebral bodies. Irradiation of asymptomatic skull lesions is seldom indicated as they often spontaneously resolve, only to recur at another site. Irradiation of the hypophysis for diabetes insipidus, once it is complete, is not effective and is contraindicated. Diabetes insipidus is not always complete, can be of variable severity, and can progress [63,64]. Irradiation of the pituitary-hypothalamic area does not prevent the progression [63]. Diabetes insipidus, when it occurs, can be controlled by the regular administration of Pitressin, which can be given parenterally or inhaled as snuff. Parenteral injection is more satisfactory. A long-acting analog of arginine vasopressin (1-desamino-8-D-arginine vasopressin, DDAVP) given by intranasal spray has been reported to be extremely effective in the management of central diabetes insipidus [46].

There are a number of reports on the efficacy of glucocorticoids used alone [47–49] or in combination with various cytotoxic agents and antimetabolites [22,50]. There is agreement of the value of glucocorticoids in producing symptomatic improvement at least, but whether they alter the outcome is uncertain. Often the fever, constitutional symptoms, skin rash, draining lesions, pulmonary lesions, enlarged lymph nodes, and hemorrhage associated with thrombocytopenia will respond dramatically to glucocorticoid therapy, at least temporarily.

There are reports of some success with almost all antitumor drugs: nitrogen mustard [22], 6-mercaptopurine [22], methotrexate [50], vinblastine sulfate [51–53], cyclophosphamide [53,54], and daunomycin [55], all of which have been used alone and in conjunction with glucocorticoids [56,57]. No agent or combination of agents appears to be most effective.

There are a few case reports that cite long remissions following intensive treatment with antibiotics: streptomycin, penicillin, chloramphenicol, erythromycin, and the tetracyclines, singly and in various combinations [56]. Assessing the value of cytotoxic agents and antibiotics is extremely difficult. Spontaneous long remissions may occur, and the disease has a variable and unpredictable course [58]. In a large study 27 patients had only symptomatic treatment while 64 patients were treated with various combinations of the different agents mentioned above. All the untreated group died within 24 months, and the median survival time was 4 months. In the treated group 70 percent were alive after 24 months, and the median survival time was 18 months. No one therapeutic regimen was found to be most effective [18]. In a study of 17 patients treated with thymus gland extract, 10 patients had remissions [28].

COURSE AND PROGNOSIS
Analysis of 69 patients with systemic histiocytosis collected from three pediatric services showed an overall corrected mortality rate of 34 percent [18]. The factors that correlate with the outcome were age at onset, extent of the disease, and localization of disease. No patient over 3 years of age at onset died. The mortality rate for those under 3 years of age was 50 percent and for those under 6 months of age was 80 percent. Younger patients were more likely to have extensive disease and visceral involvement, and with more extensive disease the prognosis was worse. Involvement of the liver, spleen, marrow, lungs, or skin was an unfavorable prognostic sign, but involvement of the skeleton or pituitary was not necessarily associated with a poor outcome. If a child survived for 3 years, the prognosis was excellent. However, all studies have emphasized the gravity of thrombocytopenia, hemorrhage, splenomegaly, or leukopenia [12,18,21]. A cooperative study of 83 patients [56] showed the same results. An analysis of these patients emphasized the prognostic importance of dysfunction of the liver, lungs, or marrow rather than just histologic evidence of involvement. The greater the number of organs with impaired function as a result of histiocytosis, the worse the prognosis [60]. It should be pointed out that despite the statistics noted above, death from histiocytosis does occur on rare occasions in children over 3 years of age at onset as well as in adults [24]. Although systemic histiocytosis is a serious disease, the majority of children survive, and even in the age group with the greatest mortality, those under 3 years of age, one-half recover.

Familial histiocytosis

Histiocytosis in general is not considered to be a familial disease [7]. In one study, however, 43 cases were cited in 19 sibships [59], including one family in which all 5 siblings had histiocytosis. The cases collected have been variously called familial Letterer-Siwe disease, familial hemophagocytic reticulosis, familial histiocytic reticulosis, familial lymphohistiocytosis, histiocytic medullary reticulosis, familial reticuloendotheliosis with eosinophilia, and familial reticuloendotheliosis. With the exception of one pair of twins, all these children died. Most of them had no skin involvement, and a number had central nervous system infiltration. Erythrophagocytosis was reported in some, and eosinophilia was the prominent feature in one large family in which six siblings were involved.

All instances of familial histiocytosis were characterized by some form of histiocytic proliferation, but whether they are related to each other, to a familial immunologic disorder [25,26], or to histiocytosis proper is not known. The familial cases seem to have enough unique features to indicate that they are a separate category.

Sea-blue histiocyte syndrome

Since the first description in 1950 [65], the concept of a genetic syndrome has evolved, characterized by the presence in the marrow and other tissues of numerous histiocytes filled with sea-blue granules [66,67]. It is thought to be due to an abnormality of lipid metabolism and to be inherited as an autosomal recessive trait. There is no sex predilection. It is most often diagnosed in young adulthood. Almost all patients have hepatosplenomegaly and thrombocytopenia. The skin, lungs, gastrointestinal tract, and nervous system have all been reported to be involved. The course of the disease is usually, but not always, benign. Those diagnosed at an early age may have a less favorable prognosis [68]. The characteristic sea-blue histiocyte can also occur in chronic myelogenous leukemia [69] and adult sphingomyelinase deficiency (Niemann-Pick disease) [70–72].

References

1. Hand, A., Jr.: Polyuria and tuberculosis. *Arch. Pediatr.* 10:673, 1893.
2. Christian, H. A.: Defects in membraneous bones, exophthalmos, and diabetes insipidus, an unusual syndrome of dyspituitarism: A clinical study. *Med. Clin. N. Am.* 3:849, 1920.
3. Kay, T. W., and Hand, A.: Defects of membraneous bones, exophthalmos, and polyuria in childhood: Is it dyspituitarism? *Am. J. Med. Sci.* 162:509, 1921.
4. Schüller, A.: Dysostosis hypophysaria. *Br. J. Radiol.* 31:156, 1926.
5. Letterer, E.: Aleukämische Retikulose (ein Beitrag zu den proliferativen Erkrankungen des Retikuloendothelialapparates). *Frankfurt Z. Pathol.* 30:377, 1924.
6. Siwe, S. A.: Die reticuloendotheliose: Ein neues Krankheitsbild unter den Hepatosplenomegalien. *Z. Kinderheilkd.* 55:212, 1933.
7. Abt, A. F., and Denenholz, E. J.: Letterer-Siwe's disease: Splenohepatomegaly associated with widespread hyperplasia of nonlipid-storing macrophages: Discussion of the so-called reticulo-endothelioses. *Am. J. Dis. Child.* 51:499, 1936.
8. Lichtenstein, L., and Jaffé, H. L.: Eosinophilic granuloma of bone, with a report of a case. *Am. J. Pathol.* 16:596, 1940.
9. Otani, S., and Ehrlich, J. C.: Solitary granuloma of bone stimulating primary neoplasm. *Am. J. Pathol.* 16:479, 1940.
10. Farinacci, C. J., Jeffry, H. C., and Lackey, R. W.: Eosinophilic granuloma of the lung: Report of two cases. *U.S. Armed Forces Med. J.* 2:1085, 1951.
11. Wallgren, A.: Systemic reticuloendothelial granuloma: Nonlipoid reticuloendotheliosis and Schüller-Christian disease. *Am. J. Dis. Child.* 60:471, 1940.
12. Farber, S.: The nature of "solitary or eosinophilic granuloma" of bone. *Am. J. Pathol.* 17:625, 1941.
13. Green, W. T., and Farber, S.: "Eosinophilic or solitary granuloma" of bone. *J. Bone Joint Surg.* 24:499, 1942.
14. Lichtenstein, L.: Histiocytosis X: Integration of eosinophilic granuloma of bone, "Letterer-Siwe disease," and "Schüller-Christian disease" as related manifestations of a single nosologic entity. *Arch. Pathol.* 56:84, 1953.
15. Lieberman, P. H., Jones, C. R., Dargeon, H. W. K., and Begg, C. F.: A reappraisal of eosinophilic granuloma of bone, Hand-Schüller-Christian syndrome and Letterer-Siwe syndrome. *Medicine (Baltimore)* 48:375, 1969.
16. Vogel, J. M., and Vogel, P.: Idiopathic histiocytosis: A discussion of eosinophilic granuloma, the Hand-Schüller-Christian syndrome, and the Letterer-Siwe syndrome. *Semin. Hematol.* 9:349, 1972.
17. Rowland, R. S.: Xanthomatosis and the reticulo-endothelial system: Correlation of an unidentified group of cases described as defects in membranous bones, exophthalmos and diabetes insipidus (Christian's syndrome). *Arch. Intern. Med.* 42:611, 1928.
18. Lahey, M. E.: Prognosis in reticuloendotheliosis in children. *J. Pediatr.* 60:664, 1962.
19. Thannhauser, S. J.: Medical progress: Serum lipids and their value in diagnosis. *N. Engl. J. Med.* 237:515, 1947.
20. Moe, P. J., and Hansen, A. E.: Reticuloendothelial granuloma: Clinical and pathologic observations with lipid analyses of tissues. *Am. J. Dis. Child.* 99:175, 1960.
21. Enriquez, P., Dahlin, D. C., Hayles, A. B., and Henderson, E. D.: Histiocytosis X.: A clinical study. *Mayo Clin. Proc.* 42:88, 1967.
22. Dargeon, H. W.: Considerations in the treatment of reticuloendotheliosis. *Am. J. Roentgenol. Radium Ther. Nucl. Med.* 93:521, 1965.
23. Lichtenstein, L.: Histiocytosis X (eosinophilic granuloma of bone, Letterer-Siwe disease, and Schüller-Christian disease): Further observations of pathological and clinical importance. *J. Bone Joint Surg.* [Am.] 46A:76, 1964.
24. Glass, A. G., and Miller, R. W.: U.S. mortality from Letterer-Siwe disease, 1960–1964. *Pediatrics* 42:364, 1968.
25. Cederbaum, S. D., Niwayama, G., Stiehm, E. R., Neerhout, R. C., Ammann, A. J., and Berman, W., Jr.: Combined immunodeficiency manifested by Letterer-Siwe syndrome. *Lancet* 1:958–63, 1972.
26. Krüger, G. R. F., et al.: Graft versus host disease: Morphologic variation and differential diagnosis in 8 cases of HL-A matched bone marrow transplantation. *Am. J. Pathol.* 63:179, 1971.
27. Leikin, S., Puruganan, G., Frankel, A., Steerman, R., and Chandra, R.: Immunologic parameters in histiocytosis-X. *Cancer* 32:796, 1973.
28. Osband, M. E., et al.: Histiocytosis-X: Demonstration of abnormal immunity, T-cell histamine H2-receptor deficiency, and successful treatment with thymic extract. *N. Engl. J. Med.* 304(3):146, 1981.
29. Oberman, H. A.: Idiopathic histiocytosis: A clinicopathologic study of 40 cases and review of the literature on eosinophilic granuloma of bone, Hand-Schüller-Christian disease and Letterer-Siwe disease. *Pediatrics* 28:307, 1961.
30. Favara, B. E.: The pathology of "histiocytosis". *Am. J. Pediatr. Heme/Onc.* 3:45, 1981.
31. McGavran, M. D., and Spady, H. A.: Eosinophilic granuloma of bone: A study of twenty-eight cases. *J. Bone Joint Surg.* [Am.] 42A:979, 1960.
32. Ochsner, S. R.: Eosinophilic granuloma of bone: Experience with twenty cases. *Am. J. Roentgenol. Radium Ther. Nucl. Med.* 97:719, 1966.
33. Williams, A. W., Dunnington, W. G., and Berte, S. J.: Pulmonary eosinophilic granuloma: A clinical and pathologic discussion. *Ann. Intern. Med.* 54:30, 1961.
34. Bickers, J. N., Buechner, H. A., and Ekman, P. J.: Pulmonary eosinophilic granuloma: Its natural history and prognosis. *Am. Rev. Respir. Dis.* 85:211, 1962.
35. Hoffman, L., Cohn, J. E., and Gaensler, E. A.: Respiratory abnormalities in eosinophilic granuloma of the lung: Long term study of five cases. *N. Engl. J. Med.* 267:577, 1962.
36. Beatty, E. C., Jr.: Eosinophilic granuloma of parotid gland and thymus. *Am. J. Dis. Child* 105:507, 1963.
37. McCraney, H. C., and Falk, A. B.: Eosinophilic granuloma. *Am. J. Dis. Child* 95:214, 1958.
38. Cohen, D. M., Mitchell, G. B., and Alexander, J. W.: Letterer-Siwe disease in a newborn. *Arch. Pathol.* 81:347, 1966.
39. Altman, J., and Winkelmann, R. K.: Xanthomatous cutaneous lesions of histiocytosis X. *Arch. Dermatol.* 87:164, 1963.
40. Ahnquist, G., and Holyoke, J. B.: Congenital Letterer-Siwe disease (reticuloendotheliosis) in a term stillborn infant. *J. Pediatr.* 57:897, 1960.
41. Ezrin, C., Chalkoff, R., and Hoffman, H.: Panhypopituitarism caused by Hand-Schüller-Christian disease. *Can. Med. Assoc. J.* 89:1290, 1963.
42. Braunstein, G. D., Bridson, W. E., and Kohler, P. O.: Acquired hypothalamic growth hormone (GH) deficiency and hyperprolactinemia in Hand-Schüller-Christian disease (HSCD). *Clin. Res.* 20:422, 1972.
43. Sims, D. G.: Histiocytosis X: Follow-up of 43 cases. *Arch. Dis. Child.* 52:433, 1977.
44. Tos, M.: A survey of Hand-Schüller-Christian disease in otolaryngology. *Acta Otolaryngol. (Stockh.)* 62:217, 1966.
45. Roland, A. S., Merdinger, W. F., and Froeb, H. F.: Recurrent spontaneous pneumothorax: A clue to the diagnosis of histiocytosis X. *N. Engl. J. Med.* 270:73, 1964.

46. Robinson, A. G.: DDAVP in the treatment of central diabetes insipidus. *N. Engl. J. Med.* 294:507, 1976.
47. Bass, M. H., Sapin, S. O., and Hodes, H. L.: Use of cortisone and corticotropin (ACTH) in treatment of reticuloendotheliosis in children. *Am. J. Dis. Child.* 85:393, 1953.
48. Avery, M. E., McAfee, J. G., and Guild, H. G.: The course and prognosis of reticuloendotheliosis (eosinophilic granuloma, Schüller-Christian and Letterer-Siwe disease): A study of forty cases. *Am. J. Med.* 22:636, 1957.
49. Avioli, L. V., Lasershon,, J. T., and Lopresti, J. M.: Histiocytosis X (Schüller-Christian disease): A clinico-pathologic survey, review of ten patients and the results of prednisone therapy. *Medicine* 42:119, 1963.
50. Freud, P.: Treatment of reticuloendotheliosis: Use of corticosteroids and antifolic acid compound. *JAMA* 175:82, 1961.
51. Beier, F. R., Thatcher, L. G., and Lahey, M. E.: Treatment of reticuloendotheliosis with vinblastine sulfate: Preliminary report. *J. Pediatr.* 63:1087, 1963.
52. Sharp, H., White, J. G., and Drivit, W.: "Histiocytosis X" treated with vinblastine sulfate (NSC-49842). *Cancer Chemother. Rep.* 39:53, 1964.
53. Siegel, J. S., and Coltman, C. A.: Histiocytosis X: Response to vinblastine sulfate. *JAMA* 197:403, 1966.
54. Starling, K. A., Donaldson, M. H., Haggard, M. E., Viette, T. J., and Sutow, W. W.: Therapy of histiocytosis X with vincristine, vinblastine, and cyclophosphamide. *Am. J. Dis. Child.* 123:Feb. 1972.
55. Segni, G., Mastrangelo, R., and Tortorolo, C.: Daunomycin in Letterer-Siwe's disease. *Lancet* 2:461, 1968.
56. Lahey, M. E.: Histiocytosis X: Comparison of three treatment regimens. *J. Pediatr.* 87 (2):179, Aug. 1975.
57. Komp, D. M., Silva-Sosa, M., Miale, T., Sexauer, C., and Herson, J.: Evaluation of a MOPP-type regimen in histiocytosis-X: A southwest oncology group study. *Cancer Tmt. Rpts.* vol. 61, no. 5, August 1977.
58. Bierman, H. R.: Apparent cure of Letterer-Siwe disease: Seventeen-year survival of identical twins and nonlipoid reticuloendotheliosis. *JAMA* 196:468, 1966.
59. Meenan, F. O., and Cahalane, S. F.: Spontaneous resolution of histiocytosis X: Report of a case. *Arch. Dematol.* 96:532, 1967.
60. Lahey, M. E.: Histiocytosis X: An analysis of prognostic factors. *J. Pediatr.* 87 (2):184, 1975.
61. Miller, D. R.: Familial reticuloendotheliosis: Concurrence of disease in five siblings. *Pediatrics* 38:986, 1966.
62. Newton, W. A., Jr., and Hammondi, A. B.: Histiocytosis: A histiologic classification with clinical correlation. *Perspect. Pediatr. Pathol.* 1:251, 1973.
63. Helbock, H., Krivit, W., and Nesbit, M. E., Jr.: Patterns of anti-diuretic function in diabetes insipidus caused by histiocytosis X. *J. Lab. Clin. Med.* 78:194, 1971.
64. Braunstein, G. D., and Kohler, P. O.: Pituitary function in Hand-Schüller-Christian disease. *N. Engl. J. Med.* 286:1225, 1972.
65. Wewalka, F.: Zur Frage der "blauen pigment Makrophagen un sternal Punktat." *Wien. Klin. Wochenschr.* 62:788, 1950.
66. Sawitsky, A., Rosner, F., and Chodsky, S.: The sea-blue histiocyte syndrome, a review: Genetic and biochemical studies. *Semin. Hematol.* 9:285, 1972.
67. Silverstein, M. N., and Ellefson, R. D.: The syndrome of the sea-blue histiocyte. *Semin. Hematol.* 9:299, 1972.
68. Silverstein, M. N., Ellefson, R. D., and Ahern, E. J.: The syndrome of the sea-blue histiocyte. *N. Engl. J. Med.* 228:1, 1970.
69. Dosik, H., Rosner, F., and Sawitsky, A.: Acquired lipidosis: Gaucher-like cells and "blue cells" in chronic granulocytic leukemia. *Semin. Hematol.* 9:309, 1972.
70. Golde, D. W., et al.: Pathogenesis of one variant of sea-blue histiocytosis. *Lab. Invest.* 33:371, 1975.
71. Briere, J., Calman, F., Lageron, A., Hinglais, N., Emerit, J., and Bernard, J.: Maladie de Niemann-Pick de l'adulte suivie de la naissance a l'age de 26 ans. Forme viscèrale pure avec surcharge en sphingomyeline et déficit en sphingomyelinase. *Nouv. Rev. Fr. Hematol.* 16:185, 1976.
72. Dewhurst, N., Besley, G. T. N., Finlayson, N. D. C., and Parker, A. C.: Sea blue histiocytosis in a patient with chronic non-neuropathic Niemann-Pick disease. *J. Clin. Pathol.* 32:1121, 1979.

PART SEVEN *Lymphocytes and plasma cells*

Morphology of lymphocytes and plasma cells

CHAPTER *101*

Morphology of lymphocytes

STEVEN D. DOUGLAS

The initial descriptions of the lymphocyte were given in the studies of the anatomy of the lymphatics and lymphoid organs by William Hewson in 1774 [1]. In 1879, Paul Ehrlich developed differential staining techniques which led to the delineation of the lymphocyte as an independent cell type [2] (Fig. 101-1). Pfeiffer and Marx (1898) showed that the spleen, lymph nodes, bone marrow, and possibly the lungs were involved in the production of antibody against heat-killed *Vibrio cholerae*, thus implicating lymphocytes in immune phenomena [3]. The demonstration of lymphocyte recirculation by Gowans, namely, that cells traffic from the blood to the lymph via the lymph nodes and back to the blood, indicated a dynamic functional role for the small lymphocyte [4,5]. Using autoradiographic techniques, evidence for short- and long-lived lymphocyte populations was obtained [6–8]. The relationship of lymphocytes and plasma cells to antibody production and cell-mediated immunity has been established by the development of in vitro culture techniques and methodology for the identification of antibody-forming cells [8–11]. Lymphocyte subpopulations are heterogenous and include the T or thymus-derived cells and their functional subsets, e.g., suppressor, helper, or cytotoxic T cells, and B, or marrow-derived, cells of different isotype specificity and stage of maturation. Lymphocytes have been separated using physical properties including size, density, surface negative-charge density, adherence, membrane receptors, and surface antigens [12]. Fluorescence-activated cell sorting, density gradients, discontinuous step gradients, and elutriation have been used in cell separation.

Light microscopy and histochemistry of normal peripheral blood lymphocytes

Classic studies of blood and tissues have demonstrated populations of spherical and/or ovoid cells which are from 8 to 12 μm in diameter when flattened on glass slides [13–17]. In some of these descriptions a distinction has been made between small lymphocytes, which are 6 to 9 μm in diameter, and large lymphocytes, which have a diameter of 9 to 15 μm. Studies of lymphocyte size distribution have been limited, but these findings suggest that there are increased numbers of circulating large lymphocytes in patients with acute viral illnesses and in certain genetic immunologic deficiencies, particularly the Wiskott-Aldrich syndrome [18–20]. Since this morphologic distinction does not appear to relate directly to functional differences, cell age, or distribution, variation in size will not be considered in further detail. Normal Caucasian and Negro adults have a mean absolute number of circulating small lymphocytes of 2.5×10^3 per microliter (with a 95 percent range of 1.5 to 4.0), or 36.1 percent of the total leukocytes (with a 95 percent range of 19.6 to 52.7). Less than 2 percent are large lymphocytes [21].

The typical small lymphocyte as observed with Romanovsky stains (e.g., Giemsa or Wright's) has an ovoid or, at times, kidney-shaped nucleus (Fig. 101-2). The nucleus is dense, stains purple, has densely packed nuclear chromatin, and occupies about 90 percent of the cell area. There is a small rim of cytoplasm which stains

FIGURE 101-1 Blood film from a patient with chronic lymphocytic leukemia. (From P. Ehrlich and A. Lazarus, *Histology of the Blood: Normal and Pathological*, edited and translated by W. Myers, p. 72. Cambridge University Press, 1900.)

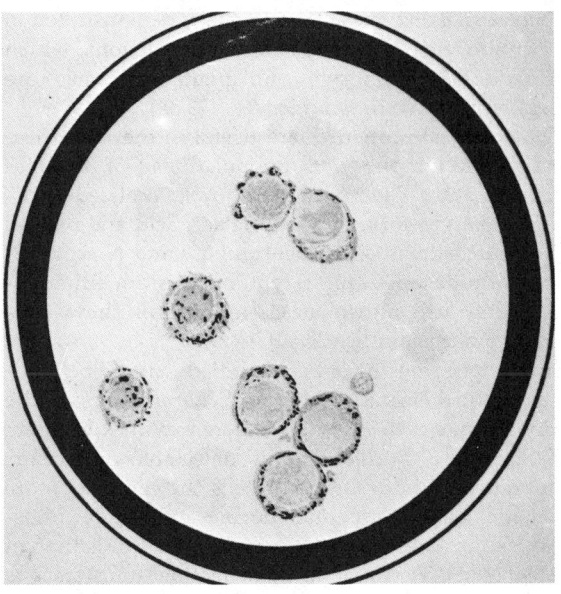

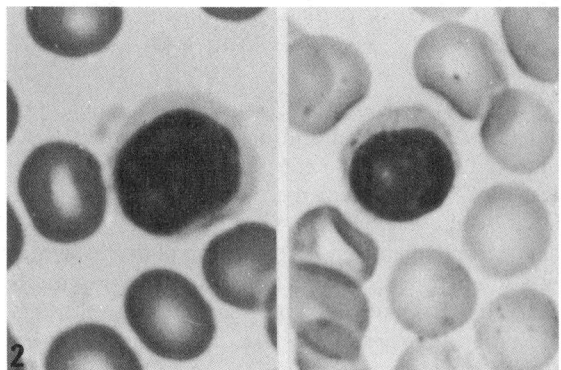

FIGURE 101-2 Photomicrographs of Wright-stained blood films from normal individuals showing typical lymphocytes. (×2000.)

Phase contrast microscopy

By phase contrast, or interference contrast (observation of lymphocytes in the living state), active movement of lymphocytes has been demonstrated. Cytoplasmic spreading which occurs for granulocytes and monocytes does not occur [16]. The moving lymphocyte generally has a "hand mirror" appearance [45–47]. Phase contrast microscopy shows a thickening of the narrow cytoplasmic rim ("Hof" region), and in this area most of the organelles are found corresponding to the Golgi zone. The cells undergo a slow ameboid movement in the hand-mirror contour. Lymphocytes from patients with chronic lymphocytic leukemia have decreased movement [48].

Electron microscopy and cytochemistry of normal peripheral blood lymphocytes

Transmission electron microscopy of fixed, embedded, and sectioned material has made possible the identification and morphologic analysis of various cellular organelles with a limiting biologic resolution of 5 to 10 Å. Several types of artifacts may be introduced by the techniques used for fixation and embedding (e.g., glutaraldehyde, osmium tetroxide, dehydration, embedding media, and an electron beam used during examination). As visualized by electron microscopy [16,49–54] the circulating lymphocyte measures about 5 μm in diameter, presumably its proper size. The nucleus has an abundance of electron-dense condensed heterochromatin, a nuclear feature characteristic of nonproliferating cell systems. The nucleoli are round in section and about 1 to 1.5 μm in diameter. As for other eukaryotic cells, nucleoli are composed of three distinct structural units concentrically arranged (central, middle, and outermost zones) [55,56]. The central region of the nucleolus, the agranular zone, is moderately electron-dense and about 0.5 μm in diameter. The middle, fibrillar region is of greater electron density than the agranular zone and frequently contains intranucleolar chromatin. The outermost zone, or granular zone, of the nucleolus is composed of a moderate electron-dense matrix and granules which are about 150 Å in diameter. The lymphocyte nuclear membrane contains nuclear pores and a perinuclear space.

The cytoplasm of the lymphocyte contains organelle systems which are characteristic of eukaryotic cells [16,49–54]. Some of the organelle systems are poorly developed (e.g., small Golgi zone). The cytoplasm contains many free ribosomes and occasional ribosome clusters and strands of rough-surfaced endoplasmic reticulum (Fig. 101-3). Centrioles are seen in appropriate planes of section. There are frequent, typical mitochondria. In the cytoplasm there are occasional microtubules with a diameter of approximately 250 Å, and adjacent to the cell membrane there are small numbers of 50- to 80-Å diameter microfilaments [57,58]. The cytoplasm contains

light blue. Although nucleoli are rarely observed in Giemsa-stained films, they are always present and can be demonstrated with special stains [22–24]. Furthermore, histochemical studies using methyl green–pyronine have demonstrated nucleolar and cytoplasmic ribonucleoprotein, which is susceptible to ribonuclease [25,26]. Cytoplasmic basophilia is related to RNA content. The lymphocyte cytoplasm contains a number of azurophil granules, usually 5 to 15 per cell, and occasional clear vacuoles. Cytoplasmic glycogen has been demonstrated by a variety of methods, including periodic acid–Schiff and methenamine-silver techniques [27]. The glycogen content among different lymphocytes is variable, and the histochemical distinction between glycogen and glycoproteins may be difficult. Neutral lipids are usually not demonstrable in normal small lymphocytes by means of the Sudan and Nile blue sulfate stains. A number of enzymes, including phosphorylase [28], acid hydrolases [29,30], nucleases [31,32], and mitochondrial enzymes [25], have been demonstrated in the lymphocyte cytoplasm. Peroxidase reactions, which are markers for monocytes and granulocytic cells, are generally negative in lymphocytes [33,34].

Cytochemical properties are useful in the identification of blood lymphocyte subpopulations [35]. The majority of mature T lymphocytes show a localized "dot" staining pattern for acid phosphatase, acid and neutral nonspecific esterases, β-glucuronidase and N-acetyl-β-glucosaminidase [36–40]. B lymphocytes are either esterase- and acid phosphatase–negative or show scattered granular staining [39,40].

Several enzymes have been studied using biochemical and cytochemical techniques. The enzymes in the purine salvage pathway show differences in expression. The enzyme 5'-nucleotidase is detectable on plasma membranes of both B and T cells. In contrast, more adenosine deaminase and purine nucleotide phosphorylase are present in the cytoplasm of T cells than of B cells [41,42]. Terminal deoxynucleotidal transferase is present in cortical thymocytes, undifferentiated stem cells, and many lymphoid leukemias [43,44].

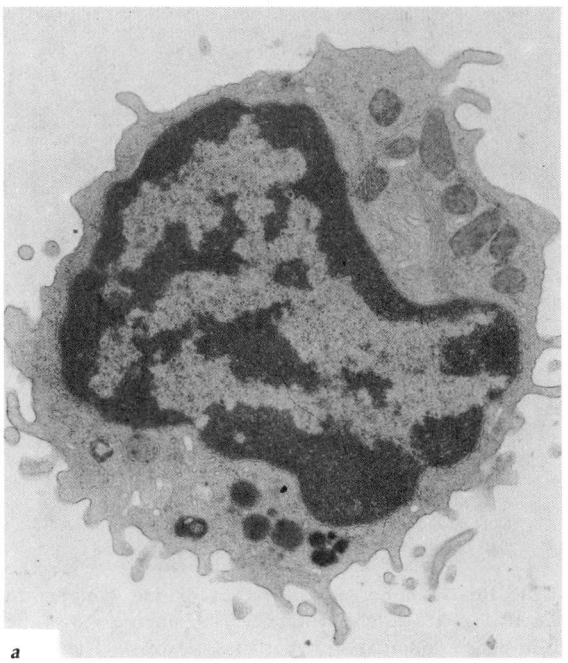

LYMPHOCYTE

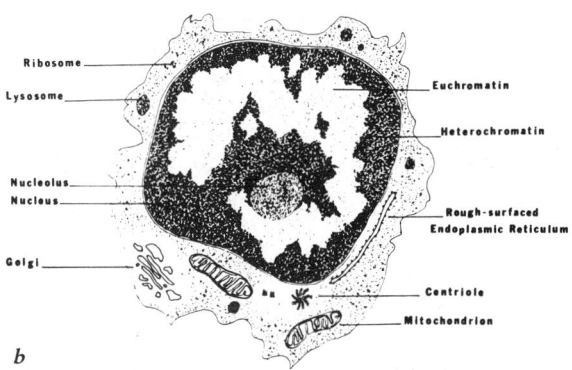

b

FIGURE 101-3 *a.* Electron micrograph of normal human blood lymphocyte. Organelles are labeled in *b.* (×12,000.) *b.* Diagrammatic representation of normal blood lymphocyte.

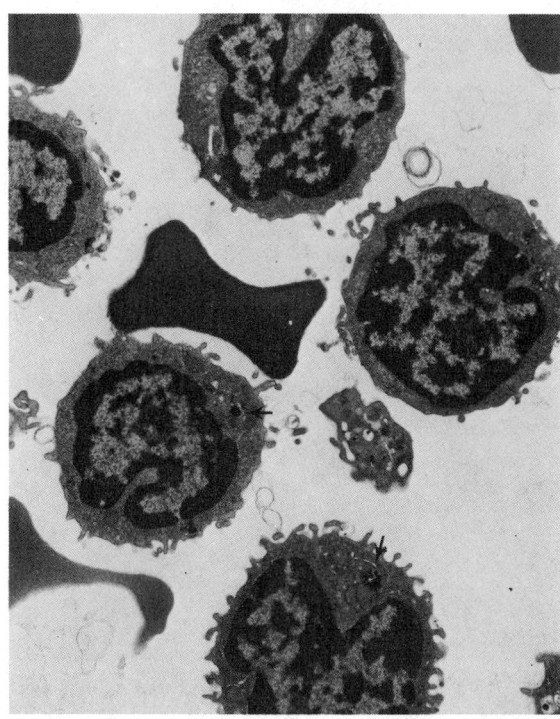

FIGURE 101-4 Normal blood lymphocytes incubated with β-glycerophosphate and lead nitrate to demonstrate acid phosphatase in lysosomes. The lead reaction product is electron-dense (*arrows*). (×5500.)

FIGURE 101-5 Lymphocyte which has been incubated for cytochemical demonstration of acid phosphatase, a lysosomal marker. The electron-dense reaction product in lysosomes is evident (*arrows*). The Golgi zone is indicated (G). (×15,000.)

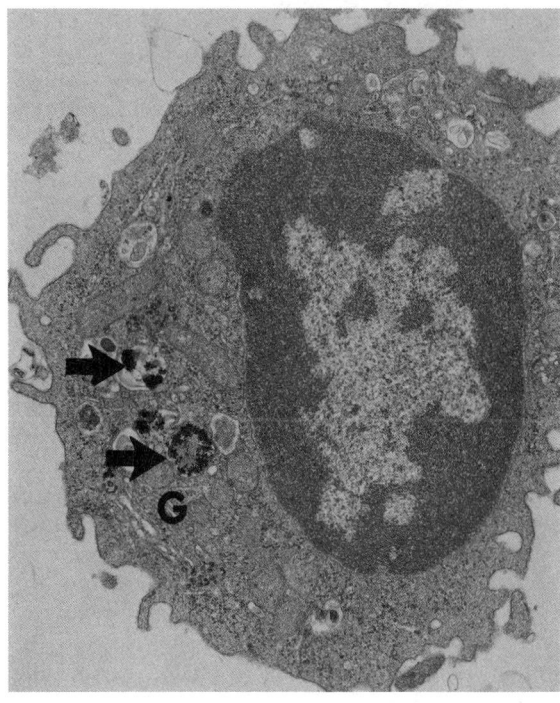

varying numbers of heterogeneous electron-opaque bodies which measure 0.2 to 0.6 μm in diameter; these structures are spherical or ovoid and single-membrane-bound. These organelles have been demonstrated to have acid phosphatase activity and have been isolated in a fraction sedimenting at 20,000 *g* in 0.34 *M* sucrose. They also contain β-glucuronidase and acid ribonuclease and are thus typical lysosomes (Figs. 101-4 and 101-5) [29,59,60]. The lymphocyte plasma membrane frequently shows small projections which are 0.2 to 0.4 μm long. Occasionally broader cytoplasmic projections, or uropods, are observed. The uropod may be significant in attachment between lymphocytes and other cells [61,62]. The lymphocyte plasma membrane has been shown to stain with colloidal iron (Figs. 101-6 and 101-7),

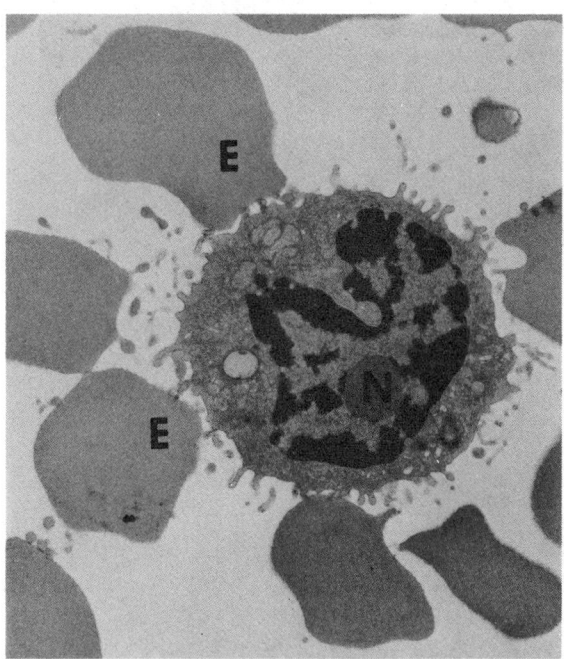

FIGURE 101-6 Normal lymphocyte incubated with sheep erythrocytes (E). Sheep erythrocytes have formed a rosette around the lymphocyte. [This interaction occurs between human thymus–derived (T) lymphocytes and sheep erythrocytes.] The cells were then incubated in colloidal iron, a cytochemical marker for sialic acid, and processed for electron microscopy. The nucleolus is indicated (N). (×7500.)

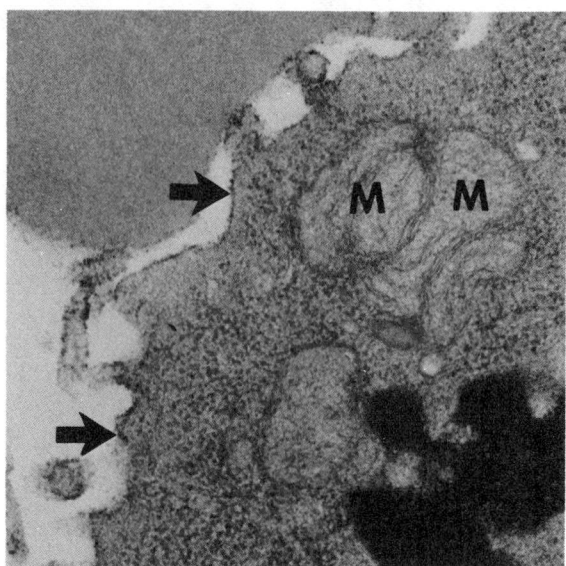

FIGURE 101-7 Higher magnification of the lymphocyte shown in Fig. 101-6. The lymphocyte membrane shows the electron-dense colloidal iron particles (*arrows*). The mitochondria are indicated (M). (×36,000.)

a marker for membrane sialic acid, and there may be differences in staining intensity of different subpopulations using this technique [63–65]. Lymphocyte cell membranes (cell coat glycoproteins) have also been stained with other electron-dense markers including phosphotungstic acid [66], lanthanum colloid [67,68], and ruthenium red [69]. Other aspects of the lymphocyte plasma membrane as they relate to the identification of subpopulations will be considered later in this chapter.

Scanning electron microscopy of normal blood lymphocytes

The technique of scanning electron microscopy (SEM) involves a probing system (where the specimen is located) and a display system which makes possible the visualization of secondary electrons through a time sequence of points. Thus, by this technique, secondary irradiation may be detected using a system which scans the sample. This process, involving a rapid scanning of an electron beam, results in a complete picture which resembles that which occurs in television imaging. These rapidly moving spots are either collected or directly visualized, resulting in an integrated picture of the specimen. In contrast to transmission electron microscopy (TEM), scanning electron microscopy has the

capacity of three-dimensional information transfer [70]. However, the technique is considerably more limited in resolution, about 100 Å, whereas TEM resolution can be 2.0 to 3.0 Å. The development of techniques for cell preparation by freeze-drying or critical point drying has made it possible to analyze the surface topography of a large number of cells using SEM. The analysis and interpretation of SEM data are greatly dependent on the methods used for harvesting cells as well as biologic factors, which include cell cycle, temperature, and cell interaction systems. Although controversial, present evidence suggests that normal lymphocytes, washed and collected onto silver membranes and fixed in glutaraldehyde, have a spherical topography with varying numbers of stubby or fingerlike microvilli (Fig. 101-8) [71–76]. In contrast, monocytes have few microvilli and display ruffled membranes and ridgelike profiles (Fig. 101-9). Studies in several laboratories suggested that it may be possible to recognize lymphocyte subpopulations, namely, marrow-derived (B) and thymus-derived (T) cells on the basis of surface topography. Some investigators have reported that thymus cells and thymus-derived lymphocytes have smaller numbers of microvilli and are smoother than the more villous marrow–derived (B) lymphocytes [72–74]. However, B lymphocytes have a wide spectrum of surface morphology. Many display moderate to markedly villous surfaces, and about 10 to 20 percent of B cells are smooth with few microvilli and thus indistinguishable from most thymus-dependent (T) lymphocytes [76,77]. Furthermore, human lymphocytes fixed in suspension appeared uniformly covered with short microvilli, and no differences between T and B cells were demonstrable

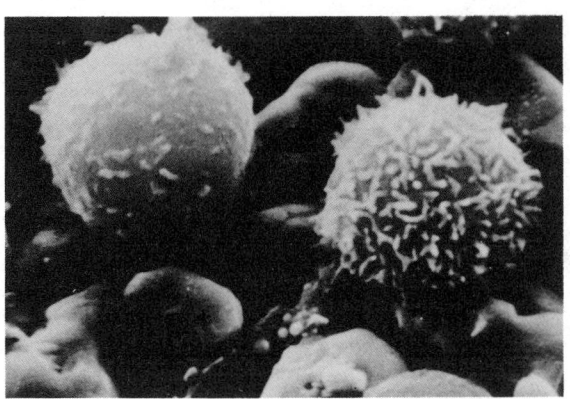

FIGURE 101-8   Scanning electron micrograph (SEM) of normal blood lymphocytes separated by the Ficoll-Hypaque method. Cells show varying numbers of microvilli. (×5000.) (Figs. 101-8 to 101-10 and 101-16 were generously provided by Dr. Aaron Polliack of the Department of Hematology, Hebrew University Hadassah Medical School, Jerusalem, Israel.)

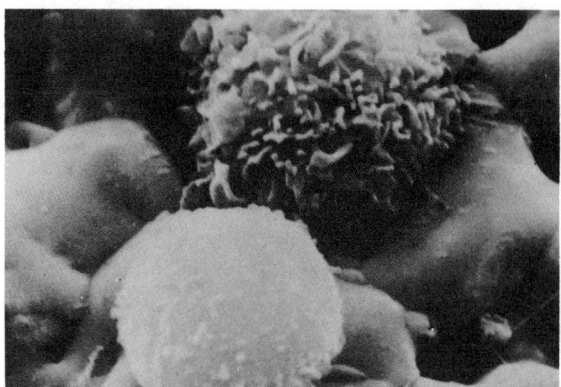

FIGURE 101-9   Scanning electron micrograph of lymphocyte (few microvilli) and monocyte (ruffled membrane). (×5000.) (From Polliack and DeHarven [76], Fig. 2.)

[78]. Thus, careful analysis of the techniques used and extreme caution in interpretation of results are essential.

A number of markers which can be visualized have been utilized in SEM studies. Using cross-linked latex spheres labeled with anti-immunoglobulin it has been possible to label murine B lymphocytes; no differences in microvilli were demonstrable with this technique [79]. It was demonstrated, however, that if the immunolatex reagents were added to unfixed B lymphocytes, a patchy distribution of label was observed. When the cells were prefixed, the label was randomly distributed on the lymphocyte surface [79]. A similar study of rabbit lymphocytes has shown clustering of label on the membrane [80]. Tobacco mosaic virus (TMV), which has a characteristic rodlike shape, has also been used as a label (Fig. 101-10).

Mouse lymphocytes were studied with anti-Ia, anti-Thyl-sera [81,82], and with a rabbit F(ab)'2 antibody using the hybrid antibody technique. This technique involves the preparation of an antibody with dual specificity, one directed against an electron-dense marker which can be visualized (such as ferritin or virus) and the other against the antigen to be studied [83]. Fab fragments are prepared by pepsin treatment of IgG. The univalent Fab fragments of the two antibodies are then reconstituted to form hybrid dimers. In these studies the markers were observed both on microvilli and on the smooth surface of the cell [81,82].

Freeze-fracture of normal circulating lymphocytes

The freeze-fracture and freeze-etching technique has made possible high-resolution studies of large areas of plasma membrane surfaces and the internal structure of membranes. The technique has made possible a detailed analysis of the topography of the plasma membrane and the membranes of intracellular organelles. This method utilizes aldehyde (glutaraldehyde) fixation followed by cryoprotection with glycerol or dimethyl sulfoxide [84]. Cells are frozen in freon cooled over liquid nitrogen, introduced into a vacuum chamber, and maintained at temperatures below −100°C by liquid nitrogen. The specimens are then fractured using a blade microtome. Under these conditions the microtome is used as a mallet and produces symmetrical fracture of the bimolecular leaflets of membranes [85]. The technique thus results in the production of topographical replicas of cell membranes. Etching is performed by warming the stage to sublimate the ice table. Following this, the specimen is shadowed with platinum and carbon. The resultant replicas are then cleared by removing the remaining biologic material. The replicas are examined by conventional electron microscopy. In the freeze-fracture technique membranes are split along their hydrophobic interiors [85]. In order to visualize marker

FIGURE 101-10   Scanning electron micrograph of mouse lymph node cell labeled with the hybrid antibody technique to detect Thy-1 antigen on the lymphocyte [70]. **The presence of the hybrid antibody attached to tobacco mosaic virus (TMV) is recognized on the lymphocyte surface by the erect shape and narrow diameter of the TMV (*arrows*) in comparison with broader microvilli. (×6000.)**

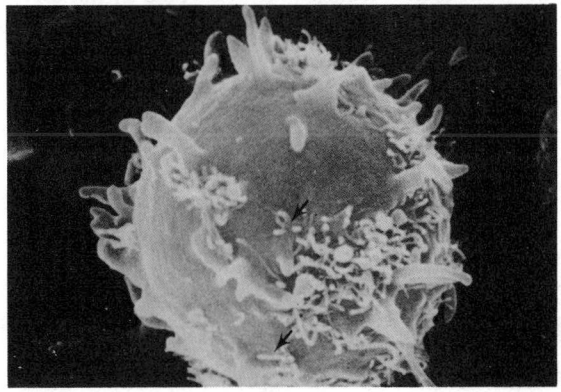

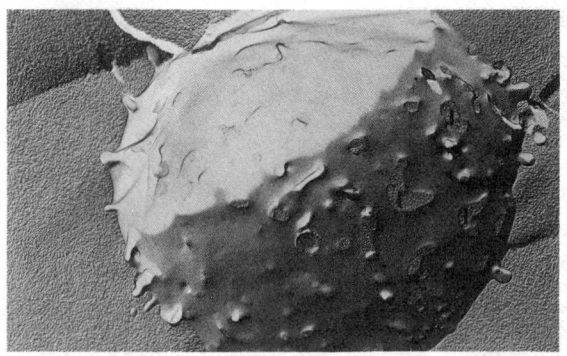

FIGURE 101-11   Normal human peripheral blood lympho-cyte replica. Freeze-fracture at −100°C, followed by platinum-carbon shadowing. Topography of the outer leaflet of the inner half (cytoplasmic portion) of the membrane (A face) is shown. Microvilli are fractured away and ice crystals (I) are present where they were located. (×20,000.)

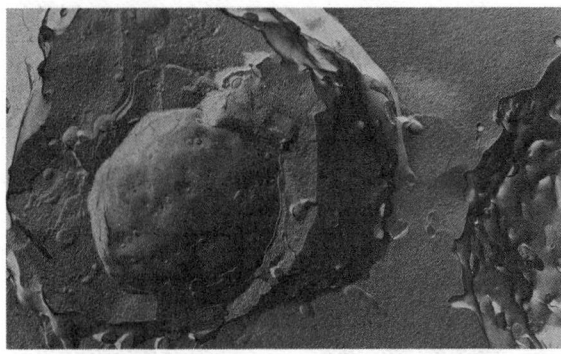

FIGURE 101-13   Freeze-fracture through the cytoplasm of normal lymphocyte. The nucleus, nuclear pores, and cytoplas-mic organelles are revealed in this cell replica. (×16,000.)

macromolecules attached to the surfaces of the mem-brane, etching is performed. This involves sublima-tion of the medium surrounding the membrane expos-ing detail at the surface. By combining freeze-fracture and freeze-etching, simultaneous observation of both the hydrophobic interior and hydrophilic surface of the membrane is possible [86,87]. This technique has re-vealed that membrane structure is characterized by smooth zones and zones containing discrete particles (intramembrane particles). Two faces are exposed: the inner half of the bilayer membrane, or face adjacent to the cytoplasm (A face), and the inner aspect of the outer membrane (B face). Preferential attachment of most in-tramembrane particles with the A face during freeze-fracture suggests that the particles deeply penetrate the inner membrane half (Figs. 101-11 and 101-12). Mem-brane particles have been reported to undergo changes at zones of cell-to-cell contact. The available data in-dicate that the plane of fracture occurs symmetrically between the bimolecular leaflets and that all membranes have intramembrane particles which are about 85 Å in diameter and are present on both the external and inter-

nal faces. Intramembrane particles have been shown to be capable of translational mobility; they can reversibly aggregate [88] and in erythrocyte ghosts have been shown to be the sites of ABO antigens [89]. The particles are distributed differently in relation to cellular metabo-lism and specialized membrane sites (e.g., sites of elec-tronic coupling, gap junctions). Investigations of in-tramembrane particles have been concerned with three major aspects, namely, their size and number, qualita-tive studies of their distribution, and their relation to the structure and fluidity of the cell membrane. Freeze-fracture studies of lymphocytes have thus far been lim-ited (Figs. 101-11 to 101-14). One investigation [90] suggested that the plasma membranes of T lymphocytes contain discrete clusters of intramembrane particles. A subsequent study showed no characteristic differences between B and T lymphocytes using this technique [91]. Mitogen-transformed lymphocytes appear to have an increase in the density of intramembrane particles [92]. An increase in intramembrane particles has been dem-onstrated following incubation of a murine lymphoid cell line with cholera toxin [93]. Intramembrane particles aggregation occurs consequent to interaction of ligands with immunoprotein receptors [94]. In contrast how-ever, the cross-linking of exposed lymphocyte cell-sur-

FIGURE 101-12   Higher magnification of A face. Intramem-branous particles are evident (arrows). Microvilli are fractured, and ice table remains within them (I). (×30,000.)

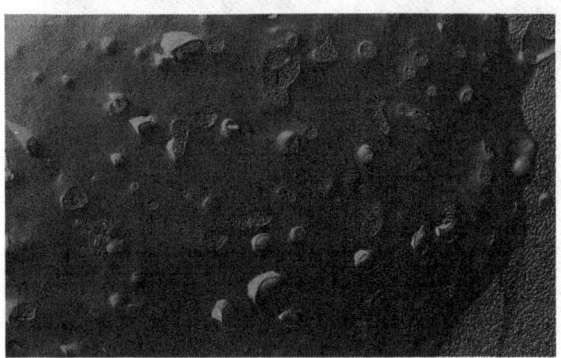

FIGURE 101-14   Higher magnification of replica showing intramembranous particles, replica of normal lymphocyte. (×50,000.)

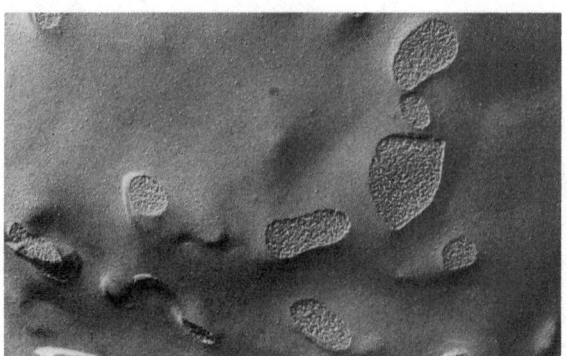

TABLE 101-1 Lymphocyte distribution in various human tissues

| Tissue | Approximate % | |
	T cells	B cells
Blood	55–75	15–30
Marrow	<25	>75
Lymph	>75	<25
Lymph node	75	25
Spleen	50	50
Tonsil	50	50
Thymus	>75	<25

TABLE 101-2 Surface markers on human and murine lymphocytes

Marker	Human	Mouse
Sheep erythrocyte rosette formation	T	
Brain-associated antigen	T	T
Theta (θ)	. .	T
TL, Ly	. .	Thymocytes
Immunoglobulin	B	B
Antigen-antibody complex	B	B
Aggregated Ig (Fc)	B	B
C3	B	B
Antilymphocyte (thymocyte) sera	T	T
Anti-B-cell sera	B	B
Epstein-Barr virus receptors	B	
Anti-T-cell sera	T	T
Helix pomatia hemagglutinin	T	

face proteins did not show obvious redistribution of intramembrane particles, but a decrease in particles [95]. Although it is technically difficult, and there are numerous possible artifacts, the freeze-fracture and freeze-etching technique offers an approach to high-resolution topographical studies of cell membranes and intracellular organelles.

Membrane markers on normal blood lymphocytes

Evidence derived primarily from detailed studies of rodents and avian species has established criteria for the division of lymphocytes into B cells and T cells [for reviews see Refs. 96–100]. Recently, a number of plasma membrane markers have been utilized for the identification and enumeration of B and T lymphocytes from normal and abnormal human blood. A review of the large body of immunologic data which has made possible this tentative classification will not be given here. However, available markers will be briefly reviewed (Tables 101-1 and 101-2). Most studies of human blood have been performed on cells isolated by the Ficoll–sodium metrizoate method [101], which may contain a large percentage of monocytes. The main markers present on B lymphocytes are readily detectable surface immunoglobulin, a receptor for the third component of complement, and receptors for aggregated immunoglobulin [102–105]. There are numerous possible artifacts related to binding of IgG to the B-cell Fc receptor [106]. In order to circumvent some of these difficulties it is necessary to use fluorescein-labeled F(ab)'2 reagents. With this technique, a significant portion of cells with surface staining with IgM and IgD has been observed, but very few cells had surface IgG [106]. A subpopulation of cells has Fc receptors, forms sheep erythrocyte rosettes (a T-cell marker), and lacks membrane immunoglobulin. B cells can also be detected using fluorescein-labeled immunoglobulin aggregates [105,107]. Another marker for B cells is erythrocytes coated with IgM antibody and complement (EAC), which demonstrates a complement receptor (Fig. 101-15) [102]. B cells make up about 10 to 19 percent of the circulating lymphocyte population and bear receptors for C3b, C3d, C1q, and B1H [108,109]. A receptor for Ep-

stein-Barr virus is also present on B lymphocytes or a B-lymphocyte subpopulation [110]. Heteroantisera with specificity for either T or B lymphocytes have been developed [96,97,111,112]. Thymocytes, normal and leukemic T cells, lymphoid cell lines, thymoma cells, and brain have been used as the source of T cells. B-cell heteroantisera have been prepared using lymphoid cell lines and cells from patients with chronic lymphocytic leukemia. For the identification of human T cells, most laboratories have used the capacity of these cells to form rosettes with sheep erythrocytes. Human T lymphocytes also have been reported to bind the hemagglutinin of *Helix pomatia* [116].

A rosette formation assay is also used for the detection of two subpopulations of T cells with receptors for the Fc portions of IgG and IgM, respectively, designated Tγ and Tμ cells [117]. After initial isolation of the T-cell population by erythrocyte rosette formation and dissociation by neuraminidase treatment, the Tγ and Tμ subpopulations are quantitated by rosette formation with ox (or chicken) erythrocytes coated with rabbit IgG or IgM antibodies. The Tγ cells can be identified in freshly

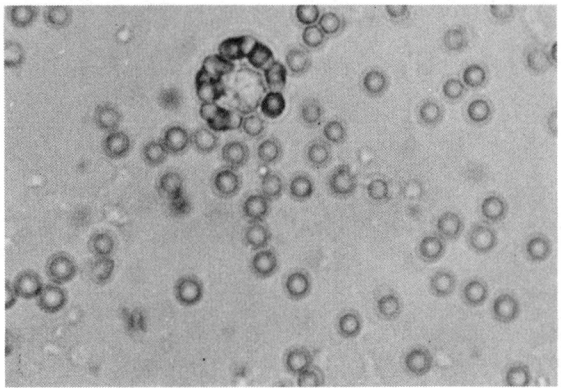

FIGURE 101-15 Photomicrograph of lymphocytes incubated with sheep erythrocytes coated with IgM rabbit antisheep RBC antibody (Forssman) and complement (*EAC*). This type of rosette formation is a marker for bone marrow-dependent (B) lymphocytes. (×400.)

isolated blood, whereas the IgM Fc receptors are saturated with plasma IgM, and thus Tμ cells can be detected only after overnight incubation in culture medium. It was originally thought that Tμ cells were helper and Tγ suppressor cells, but both subpopulations are antigenically and functionally heterogeneous [118]. Imbalances in these two subsets are present in common variable immunodeficiency, selective IgA deficiency, severe combined immunodeficiency following bone marrow transplantation, ataxia telangiectasia, and some lymphoproliferative disorders [119]. Imbalances of circulating Tγ and Tμ subsets have also been correlated with alterations in T-cell subpopulations detected by monoclonal antibodies (see below). Tμ cells can be stimulated in vitro to mature into specific cytotoxic effector cells and to perform helper and suppressor functions for B-cell maturation following pokeweed mitogen stimulation; the γ receptor is expressed on T cells activated in vivo, which are refractory to further in vitro stimulation [120].

The development of the hybridoma technique for the production of monoclonal antibodies and flow microfluorimetry have led to major advances in the analysis of lymphocyte subpopulations. Several monoclonal antibodies react with human T cells and their subsets and can identify helper, suppressor, and cytotoxic T-lymphocyte subpopulations [121].

Monoclonal antibodies to T-cell membrane markers react with human thymocytes at different stages of maturation (Table 101-3). Anti-T1 is a monoclonal antibody reactive with 100 percent of peripheral T cells but only 10 percent of thymocytes. The T1+ thymocytes are the only thymocytes capable of reactivity in mixed lymphocyte culture. Anti-T3 has essentially identical reactivity. Anti-T4 reacts with 75 percent of thymocytes and 60 percent of peripheral T cells; it appears to identify a helper or inducer subset of blood T cells, which also are the only peripheral T cells that show a proliferative response to soluble antigens. This T4+ subset is roughly equivalent to the TH1+ (TH2−) subset defined by heteroantisera. Anti-T5 and anti-T8 react with about 80 percent of thymocytes and 20 to 30 percent of peripheral T cells; anti-T5 appears to identify a subset with both suppressor and cytotoxic capacity, similar to the TH2+ subset. Anti-T6, anti-T9, and anti-T10 react almost exclusively with thymocytes and not with peripheral T cells. The earliest thymocytes appear to bear T9 and T10 markers, or T10 alone; the T10 antigen is apparently lost when the cells leave the thymus for the peripheral compartment. The T5+ subset in human beings is analogous to the murine Ly2,3 subset, which mediates both cytotoxic and suppressor functions, and the human T4+ subset is analogous to the murine Ly1 subset, which has helper function [122]. The T4+ and T5+ subsets make up about 80 to 90 percent of blood T cells; the remainder appear to be equivalent to the JRA+ subset, defined by autoantisera, which probably has feedback regulatory function [123]. Monoclonal antibodies with specificities similar to those of the anti-T reagents are now available commercially from several manufacturers (anti-OKT, anti-Leu).

Functional studies indicate the presence of lymphocyte populations which serve as natural killer cells (NK) and antibody-dependent killer cells (K) in the surveillance of certain tumors and virus-infected cells [124]. The identification and cell lineage of human NK and K cells is controversial, and these cells have been described as bearing T-cell antigens [125], having promonocyte features, and reacting with monoclonal antibodies which bind to macrophages, OKM-1 [126], and MAC-1 [127]. A monoclonal antibody (HNK-1) produced against a membrane antigen from a cultured T-cell line may define a differentiation antigen selectively expressed on human NK and K cells [128].

TABLE 101-3   Stages of human thymocytes as defined by reactivity with monoclonal antibodies*

Cell stage	Cell type	Antibody reactivity
Early thymocyte	Thy1	T10+
	Thy2	T10+,T9+
	(Thy3)†	
Common thymocyte	Thy4	T10+,T6+,T4+,T5+,T8+
	(Thy5)†	
	(Thy6)†	
Mature thymocyte	Thy7	T10+,T1+,T3+,T4+
	Thy8	T10+,T1+,T3+,T5+,T8+

*The cell stage indicates the maturation of the cell in the thymus. The cell type indicates cell populations identified by their reactivity with the antibodies indicated in the right-hand column.
† Hypothetical transition cell between stages.
SOURCE: Adapted from Reinherz and Schlossman [121].

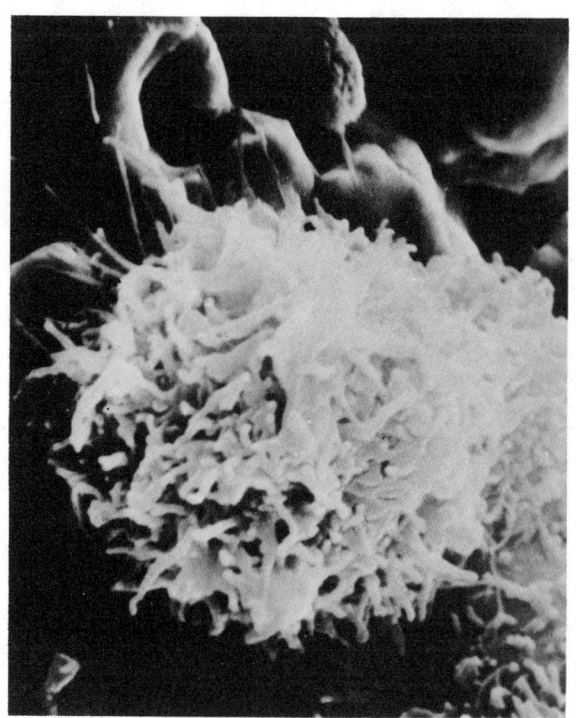

FIGURE 101-16 Scanning electron micrograph of transformed lymphocyte from 3-day culture incubated with phytohemagglutinin (PHA). (×7000.)

Dynamic aspects of lymphocyte morphology and function

The plasma membrane model which best accounts for biochemical and thermodynamic considerations is the "fluid mosaic model" [129]. According to this model, globular amphipathic molecules of the integral proteins are partially embedded in a fluid lipid bilayer matrix. Several experimental results have indicated that membrane components have the capacity for translational motion [130]. The addition of bivalent antibody to lymphocyte membranes results in diffuse membrane fluorescence when the reaction is carried out at 4°C. When the cells are brought to 37°C, the label aggregates into patches of various sizes and then migrates to one pole of the cell, forming a cap ("capping"), which may then be endocytosed [131–133]. The temperature dependence of the phenomenon is probably related to solid-liquid phase transitions in the lipid bilayer of the membrane. When univalent ligands are used, it does not appear possible to induce capping, most likely because of a relationship to the capacity of the antibody to integrate into the membrane. The results of freeze-fracture studies of intramembrane particles during capping have been controversial [133–135], and there is no conclusive information on this important question. Although extensive investigation has been carried out on the possible relation between microtubules and microfilaments and the induction of cap formation, patch formation, and endocytosis, the biologic basis for the in-

teractions involved remains unknown. Agents which are known to alter these organelles appear to impede movement of certain antigenic markers on the membrane [136,137]. It seems reasonable to conclude that these organelles may be important in the dynamics of plasma membrane components. Furthermore, it has been demonstrated that the capping phenomenon and events leading to interiorization of the complex require metabolic energy and are sensitive to diisopropyl fluorophosphate (an inhibitor of serine esterases) [136].

Although not conclusively proved, there appears to be a relation between cap formation and cell locomotion. The addition of a bivalent ligand (e.g., anti-immunoglobulin) leads to an energy-dependent membrane perturbation which can result in capping and cell movement [138,139]. Cell movement requires a bivalent cross-linked antibody; it is inhibited by diisopropyl fluorophosphate and by cytochalasin B. Although capping of θ antigen, H-2, and other lymphocyte determinants is induced by incubation with anti-θ, anti-H-2, and antilymphocyte serum respectively, these antisera do not induce cell movement [138,139].

Morphologic alterations of human lymphocytes during in vitro and in vivo stimulation with mitogens and antigens

A number of reagents including plant lectins [140], bacterial products, polymeric substances, and enzymes have been demonstrated to stimulate lymphocytes in vitro leading to mitosis; these agents have been called *mitogens*. Stimulation leads to a complex sequence of morphologic and biochemical events culminating in transformation of the small lymphocyte into blast or plasmacytoid cells (Figs. 101-16 to 101-19). Some of the mitogens have been demonstrated to have specificity for B or T lymphocytes, whereas others stimulate both (Table 101-4). The analysis of the responses of specific

TABLE 101-4 Selectivity of lymphocyte mitogens for T and B cells

	Human		*Mouse*	
Mitogen	T	B	T	B
Phytomitogens (lectins):				
Phytohemagglutinin (PHA)	+	?	+	−
Concanavalin A (Con A)	+	−	+	−
Wax bean	+	−	ns*	
Pokeweed (PWM)	+	+	+	+
Insoluble PHA, PWM, Con A	+	+	+	+
Bacterial products:				
Salmonella lipopolysaccharide (LPS)	−	−	−	+
Aggregated tuberculin	ns		−	+
Miscellaneous:				
Anti-immunoglobulin sera	−	+	−	+
Dextran PVP	ns		−	+
Trypsin	ns		−	+

*ns = not studied.

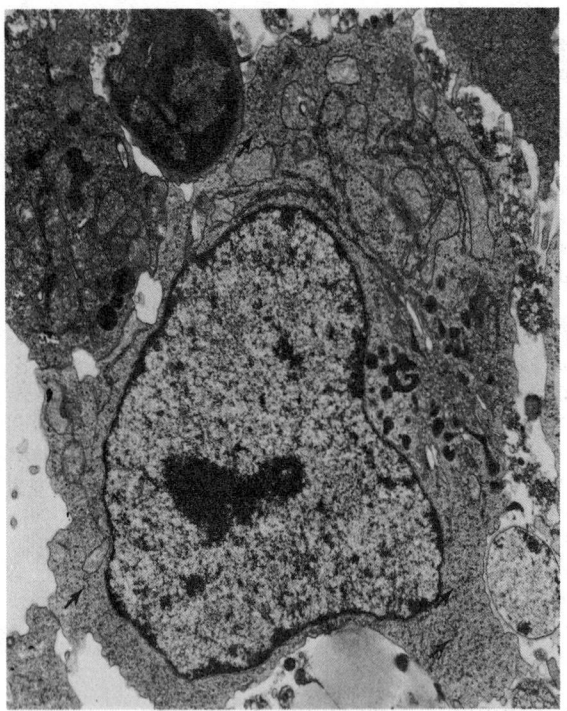

FIGURE 101-17 Transmission electron micrograph (TEM) of lymphocyte from normal individual incubated with PHA for 3 days. The transformed cell has a large Golgi zone (G) and many ribosomal aggregates (*arrows*), and the nucleus is euchromatic. (×7500.)

FIGURE 101-18 Transmission electron micrograph of transformed cell present in lymphocyte culture incubated for 5 days with PHA. This lymphoblast has a prominent uropod (*arrow*). (×7000.) (From Douglas [51], Fig. 2.)

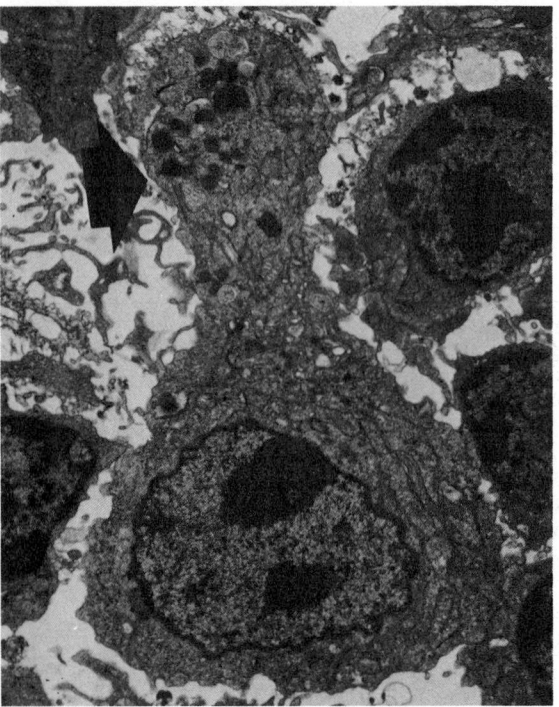

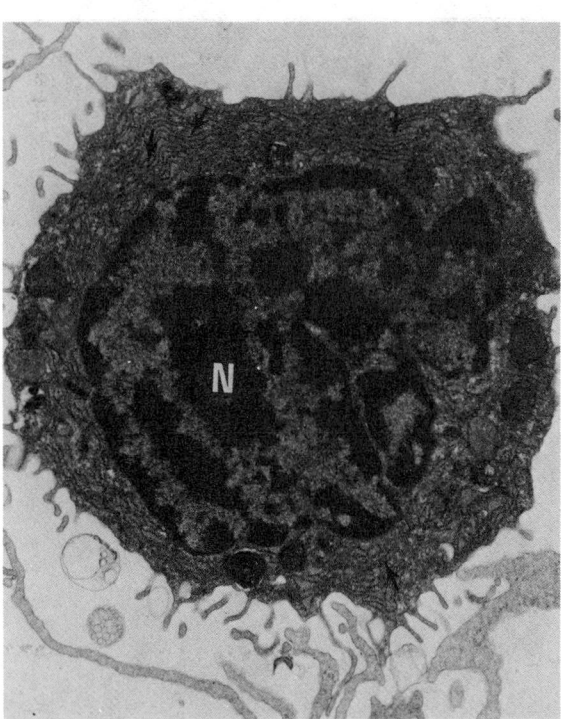

FIGURE 101-19 Transmission electron micrograph of plasmacytoid cell present in culture of lymphocytes from a patient with chronic lymphocytic leukemia incubated with pokeweed mitogen for 7 days. The nucleolus (N) and rough-surfaced endoplasmic reticulum (*arrows*) are evident. (×9000.) (From Cohnen, Douglas, Konig, and Brittinger, *Blood, 42*:591, 1973.)

lymphocyte subpopulations to various mitogens is complex [141]. Nucleolar changes are demonstrated as early as 4 h after exposure to phytohemagglutinin [55]. These morphologic changes consist of an increase in the number and concentration of granules in the granular zone and an increase in nucleolar size. Later in transformation there is an increase in fibrillar zones and increased intranucleolar chromatin. Nucleolar chromatin becomes more electron lucent or dispersed, and electron microscopic autoradiography has shown thymidine grains to be concentrated at the nuclear membrane and throughout the nucleoplasm. Forty-eight to seventy-two hours following the addition of phytomitogens (e.g., phytohemagglutinin) there is an increase in cytoplasmic size. The cytoplasm contains an increase in ribosomal clusters [142], and some increase in rough-surfaced endoplasmic reticulum [143,144]. In the transformed cell (lymphoblast) the Golgi complex is increased in size and in components, and there is an increase in the number of lysosomes [51–55]. Under some circumstances (e.g., cultures of human lymphocytes stimulated with pokeweed mitogen) a subpopulaation of cells characterized by well-developed rough-surfaced endoplasmic reticulum and a well-developed Golgi apparatus appear in 7- and 10-day cultures. This cell type has features of plasmacytoid cells [143,144]. Similar morphologic features (plasmacytoid cells) are observed in antigen-stimulated lymph nodes and during graft rejection in vivo, and in some in vitro systems including the mixed lymphocyte culture.

References

1. Hewson, W., and Johnson, J.: No. 72, Pauls Church Yard, London, 1774, in *Lymphatics, Lymph and Lymphomyeloid Complex*, 3d ed. edited by J. M. Yoffey and F. C. Courtice, Harvard, Cambridge, Mass., 1970, p. 3.
2. Ehrlich, P.: Ueber die specifischen Granulationen des Blutes. *Archiv. Anat. Physiol. (Leipzig)*, vol. 571, 1879.
3. Pfeiffer, R., and Marx, Z.: Untersuchungen uber die Bildungsstatte der Choleraantikorper. *Hyg. Infeckt.* 27:272, 1898.
4. Gowans, J. L.: The recirculation of lymphocytes from blood to lymph in the rat. *J. Physiol.* 146:54, 1959.
5. Gowans, J. L.: Lymphocytes. *Harvey Lect.*, ser. 64, p. 87, 1970.
6. Everett, N. B., Caffey, R. W., and Rieke, W. O.: Recirculation of lymphocytes. *Ann. N.Y. Acad. Sci.* 113:887, 1964.
7. Everett, N. B., and Tyler, R. W.: Lymphopoiesis in the thymus and other tissues: Functional implications. *Int. Rev. Cytol.* 22:205, 1967.
8. Ford, W. L., and Gowans, J. L.: The traffic of lymphocytes. *Semin. Hematol.* 6:67, 1969
9. Coons, A. H., Leduc, E. H., and Connolly, J. M.: Studies on antibody production. I. A method for the histochemical demonstration of specific antibody and its application to a study of the hyperimmune rabbit. *J. Exp. Med.* 102:49, 1955.
10. Nossal, G. J. V., and Makela, O.: Elaboration of antibodies by single cells. *Annu. Rev. Microbiol.* 16:53, 1962.
11. Nossal, G. J. V., and Ada, G. L.: *Antigens, Lymphoid Cells and the Immune Response*. Academic, New York, 1971.
12. Miller, R. G.: Physical separation of lymphocytes in the lymphocyte structure and function. *Immunology Series*, edited by J. J. Marchalonis. Dekker, New York, 1977, vol. 5, p. 205.
13. Rebuck, J. W.: *The Lymphocyte and Lymphatic Tissue*. Hoeber, New York, 1960.
14. Ackerman G. A.: Structural studies of the lymphocyte and lymphocyte development, in *Regulation of Hematopoiesis*, edited by A. S. Gordon. Appleton Century Crofts, New York, 1970, vol. 2, p. 1297.
15. Elves, M. W.: *The Lymphocytes*. Year Book, Chicago, 1972.
16. Bessis, M.: *Living Blood Cells and Their Ultrastructure*. Springer-Verlag, New York, 1973.
17. Yoffey, J. M., and Courtice, F. L.: *Lymphatics, Lymph and the Lympho-Myeloid Complex*. Academic, New York, 1970.
18. Cooper, M. D., Chase, H. P., Lowman, J. T., Krivit, W., and Good. R. A.: Wiskott-Aldrich syndrome: An immunologic deficiency disease involving the afferent limb of immunity. *Am. J. Med.* 44:499, 1968.
19. Wilms-Kretschmer. K., Kretschmer, R. R., and Rosen, F. S.: Ultrastructure of circulating lymphocytes in thymus disorders. *Pediatr. Res.* 5:226, 1971.
20. Heyn, R. M., Tubergen, D. G., and Althouse, N. T.: Lymphocyte size distribution: Determination in normal children and adults and in patients with immunodeficiency states. *Am. J. Dis. Child.* 125:789, 1973.
21. Orfanakis, N., Ostlund. R. E., Bishop, C. R., and Athens, J. W.: Normal blood leukocyte concentration data. *Am. J. Clin. Pathol.* 53:647, 1970.
22. Seman, G.: La Mise en évidence des nucléoles par le bleu de méthylène borate. *Rev. Fr. Clin. Biol.* 5:196, 1960.
23. Smetana, K., Freireich, E. J., and Busch, H.: Chromatin structures in ring-shaped nucleoli of human lymphocytes. *Exp. Cell Res.* 52:112, 1968.
24. Beran, M., and Pospisil, J.: A contribution to the comparative morphology of nucleolar apparatus of lymphocytes in the peripheral blood of man and some mammals. *Folia Haematol. Leipz.* 88:287, 1967.
25. Ackerman, G. A.: Cytochemistry of the lymphocytes: Phase microscopic studies, in *The Lymphocyte and Lymphocytic Tissue*, edited by J. W. Rebuck. Hoeber. New York, 1960. p. 28.
26. Glen. A. C. A.: Measurement of DNA and RNA in human peripheral blood lymphocytes. *Clin. Chem.* 13:299, 1967.
27. Gibb, R. P., and Stowell, R. E.: Glycogen in human blood cells. *Blood* 4:569, 1949.
28. Quaglino, D., and Hayhoe, F. G. J.: Phosphorylase activity in haemic cells. *Nature* 194:929, 1962.
29. Brittinger. G., Hirschhorn, R., Douglas, S. D., and Weissmann, G.: Studies on lysosomes. XI. Characterization of a hydrolase-rich fraction from human lymphocytes. *J. Cell Biol.* 37:394, 1968.
30. Tamaoki. N., and Essner, E.: Distribution of acid phosphatase, β-glucuronidase and N-acetyl-β-glucosaminidase activities in lymphocytes of lymphatic tissues of man and rodents. *J. Histochem. Cytochem.* 17:238, 1969.
31. Atwal, O. S., Enright. J. B., and Frye, F. L.: Acid ribonuclease activity in peripheral leucocytes of mice: A new cytochemical technique. *Proc. Soc. Exp. Biol. Med.* 115:744, 1964.
32. Atwal, O. S., Enright, J. B., and Frye. F. L.: Acid desoxyribonuclease activity in peripheral leucocytes of Swiss mice. *Nature* 205:185, 1965.
33. Yam. L. T., Li. C. Y., and Crosby, W. H.: Cytochemical identification of monocytes and granulocytes. *Am. J. Clin. Pathol.* 55:283, 1971.
34. Li. C. Y., Lam. K. W., and Yam. L. T.: Esterases in human leukocytes. *J. Histochem. Cytochem.* 21:1, 1973.
35. Cawley. J. C., and Burns, G. F.: The cytochemistry of human lymphoreticular subpopulations. *Immunol. Today* 1:85, 1980.
36. Higgy, K. E., Burns, G. F., and Hayhoe. F. G. J.: Discrimination of B, T, and null lymphocytes by esterase cytochemistry. *Scand. J. Haematol.* 18:437, 1977.
37. Knowles, D. M., Hoffman. T., Ferrarini M., and Kunkel, H. G.: The demonstration of acid α-naphthyl acetate esterase activity in human lymphocytes: Usefulness as a T-cell marker. *Cell. Immunol.* 35:112, 1978.
38. Bevan, A., Burns, G. F., Gray, L., and Cawley, J. C.: Cytochemistry of human T-cell subpopulations. *Scand. J. Immunol.* 11:223, 1980.
39. Basso, G., Cocito, M. G., Semenzato, G., Pezzutto, A., and Zanesco, L.: Cytochemical study of thymocytes and T lymphocytes. *Br. J. Haematol.* 44:577, 1980.
40. Machin. G. A., Halper, J. P., and Knowles, D. M.: Cytochemically demonstrable β-glucuronidase activity in normal and neoplastic human lymphoid cells. *Blood* 56:1111, 1980.
41. Tung, R., Silber, R., Quagliata, F., Conklyn, M., Gottesman, J., and Hirschhorn, R.: ADA activity in chronic lymphocytic leukemia—relationship to B- and T-cell subpopulations. *J. Clin. Invest.* 57:756, 1976.
42. Rowe, M., et al.: 5'-Nucleotidase of B and T lymphocytes isolated from human peripheral blood. *Clin. Exp. Immunol.* 36:97, 1979.
43. Greenwood, M. F., et al.: Terminal deoxynucleotidyl transferase distribution in neoplastic and hematopoietic cells. *J. Clin. Invest.* 59:889, 1977.
44. Bollum, F. J.: Terminal deoxynucleotidyl transferase as a hematopoietic cell marker. *Blood* 54:1203, 1979.
45. Rich, A., Wintrobe, M. M., and Lewis, M. R.: The differentiation of myeloblasts from lymphoblasts by their manner of locomotion. *Bull. Johns Hopkins Hosp.* 65:291, 1939.
46. DeBruyn, P. P. H.: The amoeboid movement of the mammalian leukocyte in tissue culture. *Anat. Rec.* 95:177, 1946.
47. Schrek, R.: Motility of normal and leukemic lymphocytes. *J. Lab. Clin. Med.* 61:34, 1963.
48. Cohen, H. J.: Human lymphocyte surface immunoglobulin capping: Normal characteristics and anomalous behavior of chronic lymphocytic leukemic lymphocytes. *J. Clin. Invest.* 55:84, 1975.
49. Zucker-Franklin, D.: The ultrastructure of lymphocytes. *Semin. Hematol.* 6:4, 1969.
50. Huhn, D., and Stich, W.: *Fine Structure of Blood and Bone Marrow.* Lehmanns Verlag, Munich, 1969.
51. Douglas, S. D.: Human lymphocyte growth *in vitro*: Morphologic, biochemical and immunologic significance. *Int. Rev. Exp. Pathol.* 10:42, 1971.
52. Tanaka, Y., and Goodman, J. R.: *Electron Microscopy of Human Blood Cells.* Harper & Row, New York, 1972.
53. Douglas, S. D.: Electron microscopic and functional aspects of human lymphocyte response to mitogens. *Transplant. Rev.* 11:39, 1972.

54. Douglas, S. D., Cohnen, G., and Brittinger, G.: Ultrastructural comparison between phytomitogen transformed normal and chronic lymphocytic leukemic lymphocytes. *J. Ultrastruct. Res.* 44:11, 1973.

55. Tokuyasu, K., Madden, S. C., and Zeldis, L. J.: Fine structural alterations of interphase nuclei of lymphocytes stimulated to growth activity *in vitro*. *J. Cell Biol.* 39:630, 1968.

56. Biberfeld, P.: Morphogenesis in blood lymphocytes stimulated with phytohaemagglutinin (PHA). *Acta Pathol. Microbiol. Scand.* [A] Suppl. 223, 1971.

57. Zucker-Franklin, D., and Berney, S.: Electron microscopic study of surface immunoglobulin-bearing human tonsil cells. *J. Exp. Med.* 135:533, 1972.

58. Yahara, I., and Edelman, G. M.: Electron microscopic analysis of the modulation of lymphocyte receptor mobility. *Exp. Cell Res.* 91:125, 1975.

59. Cohnen, G., Douglas, S. D.: Konig, E., and Brittinger, G.: Acid phosphatase cytochemistry of mitogen-transformed normal and chronic lymphocytic leukemia lymphocytes. *Exp. Cell Res.* 80:297, 1973.

60. Li, C. Y., Yam, L. T., and Lam, K. W.: Studies of acid phosphatase isoenzymes in human leukocytes: Demostration of isoenzyme cell specificity. *J. Histochem. Cytochem.* 18:901, 1970.

61. Biberfeld, P.: Uropod formation in phytohaemagglutinin (PHA) stimulated lymphocytes. *Exp. Cell Res.* 66:433, 1971.

62. Rosenstreich, D. L., Shevach, E., Green, I., and Rosenthal, A. S.: The uropod-bearing lymphocyte of the guinea pig: Evidence for thymic origin. *J. Exp. Med.* 135:1037, 1972.

63. Gasic, G. T., Berwick, L., and Serrentino, M.: Positive and negative colloidal iron as cell surface electron stains. *Lab. Invest.* 18:63, 1968.

64. Giacomelli, F., Wiener, J., Kruskal, J. B., Pomeranz, J. V., and Loud, A. V.: Subpopulations of blood lymphocytes demonstrated by quantitative cytochemistry. *J. Histochem. Cytochem.* 19:426, 1971.

65. Bentwich, Z., Douglas, S. D., Skutelsky, E., and Kunkel, H. G.: Sheep red cell binding to human lymphocytes treated with neuraminidase enhancement of T cell binding and identification of a subpopulation of B cells. *J. Exp. Med.* 137:1532, 1973.

66. Anteunis, A.: Cytochemical and ultrastructural studies concerning the cell coat glycoproteins in normal and transformed human blood lymphocytes. I. Variations of sialic acid containing glycoproteins subsequent to transformation of T and B lymphocytes by various kinds of stimulating agents. *Exp. Cell Res.* 84:31, 1974.

67. Anteunis, A., and Vial, M.: Cytochemical and ultrastructural studies concerning the cell coat glycoproteins in normal and transformed human blood lymphocyes. II. Comparison of lanthanum-retaining cell coat components in T and B lymphocytes transformed by various kinds of stimulating agents. *Exp. Cell Res.* 90:47, 1975.

68. Douglas, S. D., and Huber, H.: Electron microscopic studies of human monocyte and lymphocyte interaction with immunoglobulin-and-complement-coated erythrocytes. *Exp. Cell Res.* 70:161, 1972.

69. Santer, V., Cone, R. E., and Marchalonis, J. J.: The glycoprotein surface coat on different classes of murine lymphocytes. *Exp. Cell Res.* 79:404, 1973.

70. Hayes, T. L.: Scanning electron microscope techniques in biology, in *Advanced Techniques in Biological Electron Microscopy*, edited by J. K. Koehler. Springer-Verlag, New York, 1973, p. 153.

71. Clarke, J. A., and Salsbury, A. J.: Surface ultramicroscopy of human blood cells. *Nature* 215:402, 1967.

72. Polliack, A., et al.: Identification of human B and T lymphocytes by scanning electron microscopy. *J. Exp. Med.* 138:607, 1973.

73. Lin, P. S., Cooper, A. G., and Wortis, H. H.: Scanning electron microscopy of human T cell and B cell rosettes. *N. Engl. J. Med.* 289:548, 1973.

74. Polliack, A., Fu, S. M., Douglas, S. D., Bentwich, Z., Lampen, N., and DeHarven, E.: Scanning electron microscopy of human lymphocyte sheep erythrocyte rosettes. *J. Exp. Med.* 140:146, 1974.

75. Kay, M. M., et al.: Cellular interactions: Scanning electron microscopy of human thymus derived rosette-forming lymphocytes. *Clin. Immunol. Immunopathol.* 2:301, 1974.

76. Polliack, A., and DeHarven, E.: Surface features of normal and leukemic lymphocytes as seen by scanning electron microscopy: An interpretive review. *Clin. Immunol. Immunopathol.* 3:412, 1975.

77. Polliack, A., Hammerling, V., Lampen, N., and DeHarven, E.: Surface morphology of murine B and T lymphocytes: A comparative study by scanning electron microscopy. *Eur. J. Immunol.* 5:32, 1975.

78. Alexander, E. L., and Wetzel, B.: Human lymphocytes: Similarity of B and T cell surface morphology. *Science* 188:732, 1975.

79. Molday, R. S., Dreyer, W. J., Rembaum, A., and Yen, S. P. S.: New immunolatex spheres: Visual markers of antigens on lymphocytes for scanning electron microscopy. *J. Cell. Biol.* 64:75, 1975.

80. Linthicum, D. S., and Sell, S.: Topography of lymphocyte surface immunoglobulin using scanning immunoelectron microscopy. *J. Ultrastruct. Res.* 51:55, 1975.

81. Hammerling, U., Polliack, A., Lampen, N., Sabety, M., and DeHarven, E.: Scanning electron microscopy of tobacco mosaic virus-labeled lymphocyte surface antigens. *J. Exp. Med.* 141:518, 1975.

82. Lipscomb, M. F., Holmes, K. V., Vitetta, E. S., Hammerling, U., and Uhr, J W.: Cell surface immunoglobulin. XII. Localization of immunoglobulin on murine lymphocytes by scanning immunoelectron microscopy. *Eur. J. Immunol.* 5:255, 1975.

83. Andres, G. A., Hsu, K. C., and Seegal, B. C.: Immunologic techniques for the identification of antigens or antibodies by electron microscopy, in *Handbook of Experimental Immunology*, edited by D. M. Weir. Blackwell Scientific Publications, Oxford, 1973.

84. Benedetti, L., and Favard, P.: *Freeze-Etching Techniques and Applications*. Société Francaise de Microscopie Electronique, Paris, 1973.

85. Pinto da Silva, P., and Branton, D.: Membrane splitting in freeze-etching: Covalently bound ferritin as a membrane marker. *J. Cell Biol.* 45:598, 1970.

86. Pinto da Silva, P., and Branton, D.: Membrane intercalated particles: The plasma membrane as a planar fluid domain. *Chem. Phys. Lipids* 8:265, 1972.

87. Pinto da Silva, P., Moss, P. S., and Fudenberg, H. H.: Anionic sites on the membrane intercalated particles of human erythrocyte ghost membranes: Freeze-etch localization. *Exp. Cell Res.* 81:127, 1973.

88. Pinto da Silva, P.: Translational mobility of membrane intercalated particles of human erythrocyte ghosts. *J. Cell Biol.* 53:777, 1972.

89. Pinto da Silva, P., Douglas, S. D., and Branton, D.: Localization of A1 antigen sites on human erythrocyte ghosts. *Nature* 232:194, 1971.

90. Mandel, T. E.: Intramembranous marker in T lymphocytes. *Nature* [New Biol.] 239:112, 1972.

91. McIntyre, J. A., Gilula, N. B., and Karnovsky, M. J.: Cryoprotectant-induced redistribution of intramembranous particles in mouse lymphocytes. *J. Cell Biol.* 60:192, 1974.

92. Scott, R. E., and Marchesi, V. T.: Structural changes in membranes of transformed lymphocytes demonstrated by freeze-etching. *Cell. Immunol.* 3:301, 1972.

93. Zuckerman, S. H., and Douglas, S. D.: Inhibition of Fc receptors on a murine lymphoid cell line by cholera exotoxin. *Nature* 255:410, 1975.

94. Douglas, S. D.: Alterations in intramembrane particle distribution during interaction of erythrocyte-bound ligands with immunoprotein receptors. *J. Immunol.* 120:151, 1978.

95. Kuby, J M., and Wofsy, L.: Intramembrane particles and the organization of lymphocyte membrane proteins. *J. Cell Biol.* 88:591, 1981.

96. Greaves, M. D., Owen, J. J., and Raff, M. C.: *T and B Lymphocytes: Origins, Properties and Roles in Immune Responses*. Elsevier, New York, 1973, pp. 1–315.

97. Moller, G.: T and B lymphocytes. *Transplant. Rev.* 16:3, 1973.

98. Rosenthal, A. S.: *Immune Recognition*. Academic, New York, 1975.

99. Taub, R. N., and Douglas, S. D.: Physiologic and immunologic role of lymphocytes, in *Physiologic Pharmacology*, edited by W. S. Root and N. I. Berlin. Academic, New York, 1974, vol. 5, p. 363.

100. Warner, N. L.: Membrane immunoglobulins and antigen receptors on B and T lymphycytes. *Adv. Immunol.* 19:67, 1974.

101. Boyum, A.: Separation of leucocytes from blood and bone marrow. *Scand. J. Clin. Lab. Invest. Suppl.* 97, 21:9, 1968.

102. Nussenzweig, V.: Receptors for immune complexes on lymphocytes. *Adv. Immunol.* 19:217, 1974.

103. Pernis, B., Forni, L., and Amante, L.: Immunoglobulin spots on the surface or rabbit lymphocytes. *J. Exp. Med.* 132:1001, 1970.

104. Fu, S. M., Winchester, R. J., and Kunkel, H. G.: Occurrence of surface IgM, IgD, and free light chains on human lymphocytes. *J. Exp. Med.* 139:451, 1974.

105. Dickler, H. B., and Kunkel, H. G.: Interaction of aggregated gamma-globulin with B lymphocytes. *J. Exp. Med.* 136:191, 1972.

106. Winchester, R. J., Fu, S. M., Hoffman, T., and Kunkel, H. G.: IgG on lymphocyte surfaces: Technical problems and the significance of a third cell population. *J. Immunol.* 114:1210, 1975.

107. Dickler, H. B.: Studies of the human lymphocyte receptor for heat-aggregated or antigen-complexed immunoglobulin. *J. Exp. Med.* 140:508, 1974.

108. Ross, G. D., Polley, M. J., Rabellino, E. M., and Grey, H. M.: Two different complement receptors on human lymphocytes: One specific for C3$_b$ and one specific for C3$_b$ inactivator cleaved C3$_b$. *J. Exp. Med.* 138:798, 1973.

109. Ross, G. D.: Analysis of the different types of leukocyte membrane complement receptors and their interaction with the complement system. *J. Immunol. Methods* 37:197, 1980.

110. Jondal, M., and Klein, G.: Surface markers on human B and T lymphocytes: Presence of EB virus receptors on B lymphocyte. *J. Exp. Med.* 138:1365, 1973.

111. Identification, enumeration, and isolation of B and T lymphocytes from human peripheral blood: Report of a WHO/IARC–sponsored workshop on human B and T cells. *Scand. J. Immunol.* 3:521, 1974 (special technical report).

112. Brown, G., and Greaves, M. F.: Cell surface markers for human T and B lymphocytes. *Eur. J. Immunol.* 4:302, 1974.

113. Jondal, M., Holm, G., and Wigzell, H.: Surface markers on human T and B lymphocytes. I. A large population of lymphocytes forming non-immune rosettes with sheep red blood cells. *J. Exp. Med.* 136:207, 1972.

114. Wybran, J., Carr, M., and Fudenberg, H. H.: The human rosette forming cell as a marker of a population of thymus-derived cells. *J. Clin. Invest.* 51:2537, 1972.

115. Bentwich, Z., Douglas, S. D., Siegel, F. P., and Kunkel, H. G.: Human lymphocyte–sheep erythrocyte rosette formation. Some characteristics of the interaction. *Clin. Immunol. Immunopathol.* 1:511, 1973.

116. Hammarstrom, S., Hellstrom, V., Perlman, P., and Dillner, M. L.: A new surface marker on T lymphocytes of human peripheral blood. *J. Exp. Med.* 138:1270, 1973.

117. Moretta, L., Moretta, A., Canonica, G. W., Bacigalupo, A., Mingari, M. C., and Cerottini, J. C.: Receptors for immunoglobulins on resting and activated human T cells. *Immunol. Rev.* 56:141, 1981.

118. Reinherz, E. L., et al.: Human T lymphocyte subpopulations defined by Fc receptors and monoclonal antibodies. *J. Exp. Med.* 151:969, 1980.

119. Gupta, S., and Good, R. A.: Subpopulations of human T lymphocytes: Laboratory and clinical studies. *Immunol. Rev.* 56:89, 1981.

120. Pichler, W. J., and Broder, S.: In vitro functions of human T cells expressing Fc-IgG or Fc-IgM receptors. *Immunol. Rev.* 56:163, 1981.

121. Reinherz, E., and Schlossman, S. F.: The differentiation and function of human T lymphocytes. *Cell* 19:821, 1980.

122. Cantor, H., and Boyse, E. A.: Regulation of cellular and humoral immune responses by T cell subclasses. *Cold Spring Harbor Symp. Quant. Biol.* 41:23, 1977.

123. Reinherz, E. L., Rubinstein, A. J., Gela, R. S., Rosen, F. S., and Schlossman, S. F.: Abnormalities of immunoregulatory T cells in disorders of immune function. *N. Engl. J. Med.* 301:1018, 1979.

124. Herberman, R. G., et al.: Natural killer cells: Characteristics and regulation of activity. *Immunol. Rev.* 44:43, 1979.

125. Kaplan, J., and Callewaert, D. M.: Expression of human T-lymphocyte antigens by natural killer cells. *J. Natl. Cancer Inst.* 60:961, 1978.

126. Breard, J., Reinherz, E. L., Kung, P. C., Goldstein, G., and Schlossman, S. F.: A monoclonal antibody reactive with human peripheral blood monocytes. *J. Immunol.* 124:1943, 1980.

127. Ault, K. A., and Springer, T. A.: Cross-reaction of a rat anti-mouse phagocyte-specific monoclonal antibody (anti-Mac-1) with human monocytes and natural killer cells. *J. Immunol.* 126:359, 1981.

128. Abo, T., and Balch, C. M.: A differentiation antigen of human NK and K cells identified by a monoclonal antibody (HNK-1). *J. Immunol.* 127:1024, 1981.

129. Singer, S. J.: Molecular biology of cellular membranes with applications to immunology. *Adv. Immunol.* 19:1, 1974.

130. Edidin, M.: Rotational and translational diffusion in membranes. *Annu. Rev. Biophys. Bioenerget.* 3:179, 1974.

131. Taylor, R. B., Duffus, P. H., Raff, M. C., and dePetris, S.: Redistribution and pinocytosis of lymphocyte surface immunoglobulin molecules induced by anti-immunoglobulin antibody. *Nature [New Biol.]* 233:255, 1971.

132. Loor, F., Forni, L., and Pernis, B.: The dynamics of the lymphocyte membrane: Factors affecting the distribution and turnover of surface immunoglobulin. *Eur. J. Immunol.* 2:203, 1972.

133. Loor, F.: Lymphocyte membrane particle redistribution induced by a mitogen/capping dose of the phytohemagglutinin of *Phaseolus vulgaris*. *Eur. J. Immunol.* 3:112, 1973.

134. Ault, K. A., Karnovsky, M. J., and Unanue, E. R.: Studies on the distribution of surface immunoglobins on human B-lymphocytes. *J. Clin. Invest.* 52:2507, 1973.

135. Matter, A., and Bonnet, C.: Effect of capping on the distribution of membrane particles in thymocyte membranes. *Eur. J. Immunol.* 4:704, 1974.

136. Unanue, E. R., Karnovsky, M. J., and Engers, H. D.: Ligand-induced movement of lymphocyte surface macromolecules. III. Relationship between the formation and fate of anti-Ig-surface Ig complexes and cell metabolism. *J. Exp. Med.* 137:675, 1973.

137. Unanue, E. R., Ault, K. A., and Karnovsky, M. J.: Ligand-induced movement of lymphocyte surface macromolecules. IV. Stimulation of cell motility by anti-Ig and lack of relationship to capping. *J. Exp. Med.* 139:295, 1974.

138. Unanue, E. R., and Karnovsky, M. J.: Ligand-induced movement of lymphocyte membrane macromolecules. V. Capping, cell movement, and microtubular function in normal and lectin-treated lymphocytes. *J. Exp. Med.* 140:1207, 1974.

139. Schreiner, G. F., and Unanue, E. R.: Anti-Ig triggered movements of lymphocytes: Specificity and lack of evidence for directional migration. *J. Immunol.* 114:809, 1975.

140. Nicolson, G. L.: The interactions of lectins with animal cell surfaces. *Int. Rev. Cytol.* 39:89, 1974.

141. Handwerger, B. S., and Douglas, S. D.: The cell biology of blastogenesis, in *Handbook of Inflammation*, edited by G. Weissmann. Elsevier–North Holland, Amsterdam, 1980, vol. 2, pp. 609–706.

142. Soren, L., and Biberfeld, P.: Quantitative studies on RNA accumulation in human PHA–stimulated lymphocytes during blast transformation. *Exp. Cell Res.* 79:359, 1973.

143. Douglas, S. D., Hoffman, P. F., Borjeson, J., and Chessin, L. N.: Studies on human peripheral blood lymphocytes *in vitro*. III. Fine structural features of lymphocyte transformation by pokeweed mitogen. *J. Immunol.* 98:17, 1967.

144. Douglas, S. D., and Fudenberg, H. H.: In vitro development of plasma cells from lymphocytes following pokeweed mitogen stimulation: A fine structural study. *Exp. Cell Res.* 54:277, 1969.

CHAPTER *102*

Morphology of plasma cells

STEVEN D. DOUGLAS

Cells termed *plasma cells* were first reported by Waldeyer in 1875 in descriptions of perivascular connective tissue [1]. Cajal [2] and Unna [3] at about the same time (1890–1891) identified strongly basophilic connective tissue cells which were designated plasma cells. Shortly thereafter, Marschalko (1895) wrote a detailed morphologic characterization of the plasma cell [4]. In 1900 Wright recognized the morphologic similarity between myeloma cells and plasma cells [5]. Bing and Plum [6], in 1937, related plasma cells to antibody production. The relationships, however, between plasma cells and antibody formation, and the differentiation of bone marrow–dependent (B) lymphocytes were not established until the past two decades [for reviews see Refs. 7–10].

Light microscopy, histochemistry, and electron microscopy of plasma cells

By light microscopy, the mature plasma cell is readily identified by its characteristic basophilic cytoplasm and its eccentric nucleus. The nuclear polarity is attributable to a large perinuclear zone which corresponds to the Golgi apparatus. The typical mature plasma cell is usually round or oval and has a diameter from 9 to 20 μm with a mean cell diameter of 14.4 μm and a mean nuclear diameter of 8.5 μm [11]. The nuclear heterochromatin is coarse and distributed in a pattern which appears to resemble the spokes of a wheel (cartwheel nucleus) (Fig. 102-1). The typical small plasma cell with nuclear polarity, radially distributed heterochromatin, prominent Golgi zone, and basophilic cytoplasm has been termed the *Marschalko-type plasma cell*. Plasma cells with several nuclear lobes may occasionally be seen in the bone marrow of normal individuals, but giant plasma cells with tetraploid nuclei are rare. The cytoplasm is characterized by its intense affinity for cationic dyes, the cytoplasmic basophilia is due to ribonucleoprotein. The plasma cell has been shown to stain selectively with methyl green–pyronine; the nucleus stains blue-green with methyl green; and the cytoplasm red with pyronine due to its high content of ribonucleoprotein. This last tinctorial property has led to the designation of plasma cells as *pyroninophilic*. Other cytologic features of the normal plasma cell include cytoplasmic staining with several basic dyes, including toluidine blue and the azures. Plasma cells which occur in pathologic states may have different his-

FIGURE 102-1   Light photomicrograph of marrow aspirate from a patient with multiple myeloma. Typical plasma cells are shown. (×1000.)

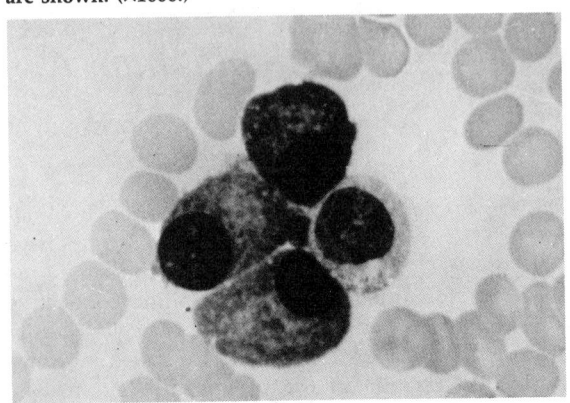

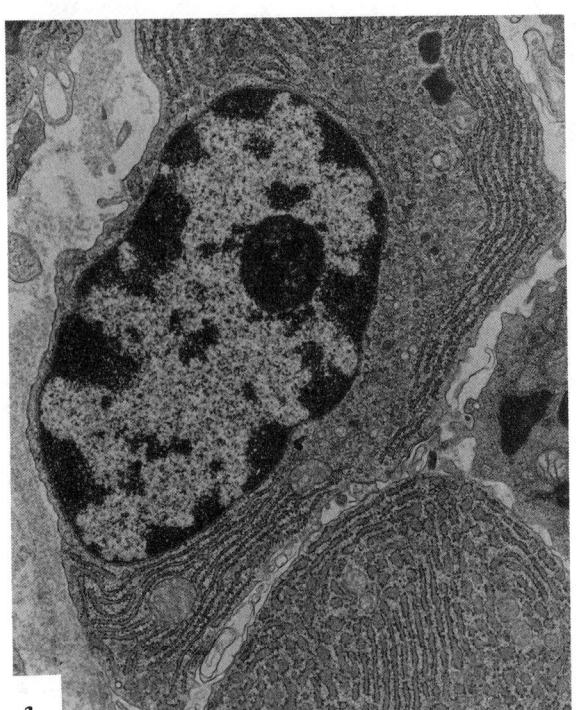

a

PLASMA CELL

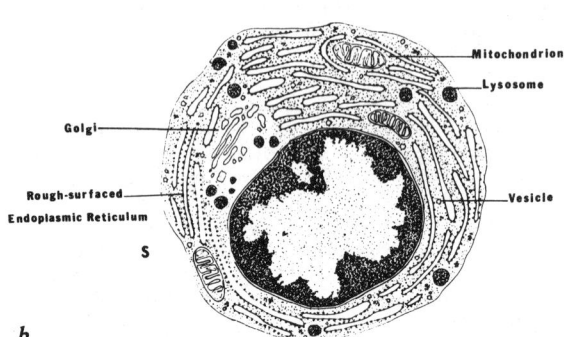

b

FIGURE 102-2   *a.* Electron micrograph of mature plasma cells in normal human lymph node. The organelles are labeled in *b.* (×9000.) *b.* Diagrammatic representation of normal plasma cell.

tochemical properties including alteration in cell size and the presence of inclusions which may be positive with periodic acid–Schiff stains (PAS) [12–15]. In hemochromatosis and hemosiderosis, plasma cells may contain hemosiderin inclusions [16,17]. Other cytochemical features include absence of peroxidase and nonspecific esterase. Plasma cells are strongly positive for β-glucuronidase and for mitochondrial markers [18].

Plasma cell size and morphology may be significantly altered in multiple myeloma and macroglobulinemia [12–15,19–22]. Under some circumstances amyloid inclusions have been described in plasma cells [23].

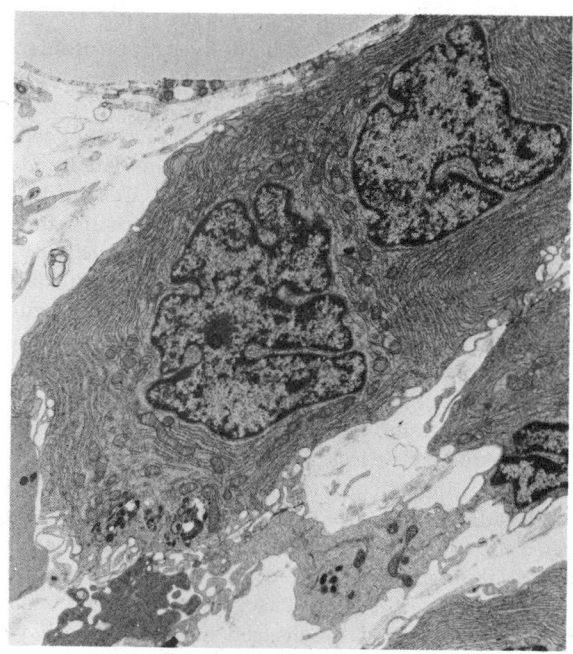

FIGURE 102-3   Electron micrograph of immature plasma cells in marrow of a patient with multiple myeloma. (×4500.)

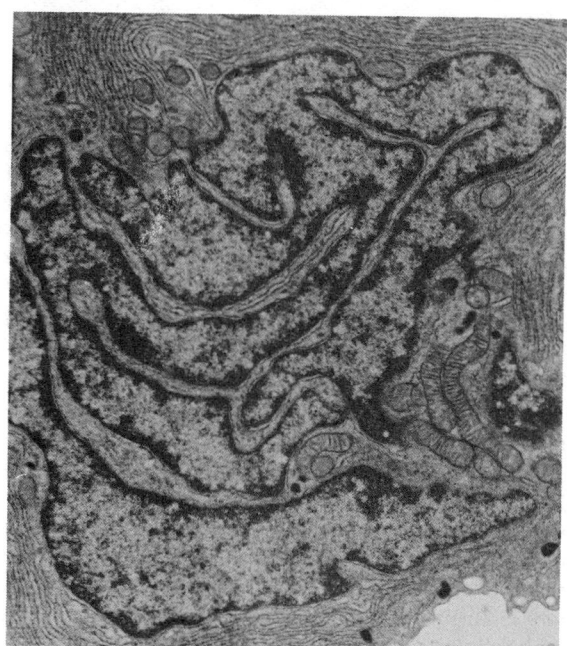

FIGURE 102-5   Marrow plasma cell with extensive nuclear lobulation. Patient with multiple myeloma. (×7500.)

By electron microscopy the plasma cell is packed with rough-surfaced endoplasmic reticulum, which has numerous attached ribosomes. The intracisternal spaces vary in their state of dilatation. There is a large, circumscribed Golgi zone which corresponds to the paranuclear halo present by light microscopy. The nucleus has dense areas of heterochromatin, and nucleoli may be frequently observed. In the Golgi zone there are frequent lamellae, vesicles, and vacuoles, and a number of granules. Between the strands of rough-surfaced endoplasmic reticulum there are frequent mitochondria (Figs. 102-2 to 102-6) [24–26].

FIGURE 102-4   Mature marrow plasma cell. Patient with IgA myeloma. (×12,000.)

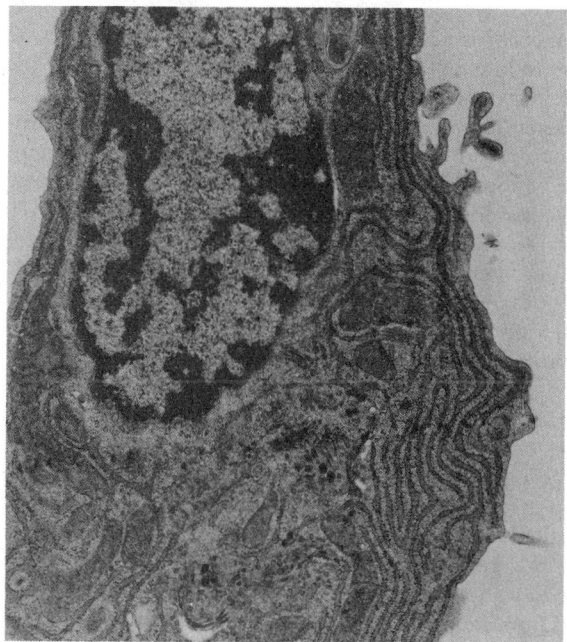

FIGURE 102-6   Higher-magnification micrograph showing plasma cell with dilated rough-surfaced endoplasmic reticulum (E) and attached ribosomes (*arrows*). (×47,000.)

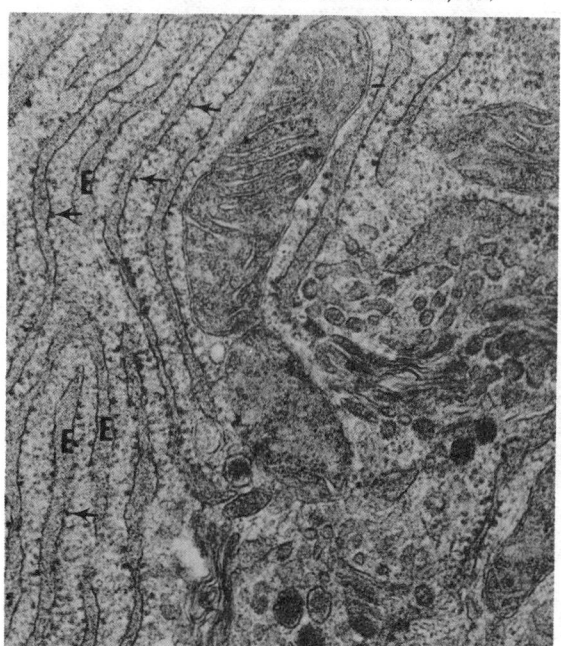

Distribution of plasma cells

Under normal circumstances plasma cells are not seen in the blood. They occur frequently in the lymph nodes, particularly in the medullary cords and germinal centers, and in the white pulp and periarteriolar sheets of the spleen [27]. In the thymus there is a small number of plasma cells [28]. Plasma cells are frequent in the connective tissue, such as in the lamina propria of the intestine. In normal adult bone marrow aspirates, up to 4 percent of nucleated cells may be plasma cells with a mean in one study of 1.3 percent (range, 0.4 to 3.9) [29]. Marrow plasma cells frequently surround reticular cells, an observation which could have immunologic significance. Plasma cells are usually distributed in the region of arteriolar capillaries. Thus, in order to detect plasma cells in marrow films, it is often of value to examine the periphery where capillary fragments are frequently found. Under normal circumstances, plasma cells are rarely present in the thoracic duct or in the lymph. There is an increase in plasma cells in both blood and lymph following antigenic stimulation [30,31].

Blood plasmacytosis

Studies in animal systems following immunization have demonstrated production of large pyroninophilic blast cells in the blood 2 or 3 days after antigenic stimulation. Following this, there is an increase in mature plasma cells which have been demonstrated by autoradiographic techniques to be derived from proliferating blast cells [30,31]. In a study of sheep immunized with human erythrocytes or *Salmonella typhi O* organisms, it was demonstrated that up to 40 percent of cells in the efferent lymph from an antigen-stimulated node were hyperbasophilic lymphoid cells [30]. Cells of this type are discharged into the main lymphatics and then into the circulation. Human responses to *Bordetella pertussis* vaccine, T.A.B. vaccine (*S. typhi* and *S. paratyphi A* and *B*), poliomyelitis vaccine, tetanus vaccine, plague vaccine, and Venezuelan equine encephalitis vaccine have been investigated [32]. In normal control subjects there were never more than 0.5 percent large lymphoid cells (lymphoblasts), and typical plasma cells occurred with a frequency of less than 0.05 percent. Using tritiated thymidine incorporation into DNA as assessed by autoradiography, less than 0.2 percent of cells were labeled [32,33]. Following immunization, there was increased labeling with tritiated thymidine and uridine and an increase in hyperbasophilic lymphoid cells which were observed by electron microscopy to have well-developed endoplasmic reticulum [32].

Circulating plasmacytoid cells also occur in viral infections including mumps and infectious mononucleosis [32,34–37] and in bacterial infections, including endocarditis, typhoid fever, and streptococcal sepsis [34]. Cells of this type have also been observed in patients with serum sickness [38], Waldenström's macroglobulinemia [19], sarcoidosis [39], and kwashiorkor [40], and after severe burns [41] (Fig. 102-7).

FIGURE 102-7 Blood plasma cell from a child with protein-energy malnutrition (kwashiorkor). The rough-surfaced endoplasmic reticulum (RER) is extensively dilated. (×9000.)

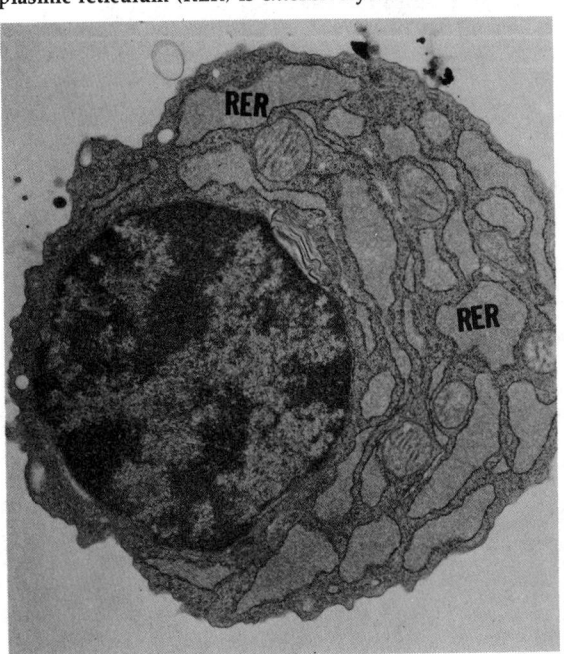

Special techniques for the morphologic and functional investigation of plasma cells

Numerous studies both in vivo and in vitro indicate that following appropriate antigenic stimulation the marrow-dependent (B) lymphocyte has the capacity to differentiate into an antibody-forming plasma cell. Antibody-forming cells have been identified using a number of morphologic and functional techniques. These have included bacterial adherence in microdroplets [7], immunofluorescence [42], light and electron microscopic identification of cells in immune hemolytic plaques using the Jerne technique [43], autoradiography [44], and electron-dense markers which have included ferritin and peroxidase utilized as antigens [45,46], ferritin- or peroxidase-conjugated antibodies [47,48], and modification of these techniques [49,50]. Moreover, it has been possible using electron microscopic autoradiography to observe sequentially some of the events which occur during the formation of immunoglobulin molecules. Studies using tritium-labeled leucine, galactose, and glucosamine have demonstrated the morphologic sequence of events which occurs during immunoglobulin synthesis and assembly [51] in a mouse myeloma. The polypeptide backbone of the immunoglobulin is synthesized in rough-surfaced endoplasmic reticulum (RER) and then probably transported to the Golgi complex. Galactose incorporation occurs primarily at the level of the Golgi complex, whereas glucosamine incorporation occurs both in RER and in the Golgi complex. Although not proved, it is suggested that the completed immunoglobulin reaches the plasma membrane via the Golgi complex and is discharged extracellularly through smooth-surfaced vesicles. This concept of reverse pinocytosis has not yet been conclusively demonstrated. The mechanism whereby immunoglobulin remains bound to the membrane under some circumstances and is secreted in others is unknown but is crucial to an understanding of plasma cell function. Studies of plasma cells from rats immunized with peroxidase and from mouse myeloma cells have shown that there is active membrane traffic between the cell membrane, Golgi cisternae, and lysosomes [72].

In studies utilizing fixation of peroxidase to cells obtained from an animal immunized with peroxidase, it has been demonstrated that antibody first appears in the perinuclear space and in proximity to the RER and then passes through the Golgi apparatus [46]. Reaction product has also been demonstrated on the ribosomes. Early reaction production has been shown in the nucleolus of immature cells [31]. The reactive cells include cells with the morphologic features of transformed lymphocytes, intermediate cells, and cells with the features of plasmablasts and plasma cells [31,46].

Maturation and developmental sequence of plasma cells

The classic studies of Fagraeus [52] suggested that the precursor of the plasma cell was a large transitional cell. Studies using autoradiography showed that the first cell which took up tritiated thymidine during antigenic stimulation was an immature plasma cell of the transitional type [53]. This evidence from animal experiments suggests that there are several sequential mitotic divisions which occur during cellular differentiation from the resting lymphocyte to the plasmablast to the immature plasma cell. Plasma cells were also demonstrated to undergo successive waves of mitosis in the medullary cords of lymph nodes [54]. In cell transfer experiments the differentiation of antibody-forming plasma cells from specific precursors present among transformed cells was demonstrated [55].

Extensive studies of a number of in vitro systems indicate that morphologic and biochemical differentiation of antibody-forming cells can be investigated using these models [56,57]. Studies of human lymphocyte transformation with pokeweed mitogen (PWM) demonstrated the occurrence of cells with electron microscope

features of plasma cells after 7 to 10 days [58]; increased IgM synthesis has also been demonstrated in this system [59].

B cells which have differentiated following pokeweed mitogen treatment show rapid loss of surface IgD. When cytoplasmic immunoglobulin became detectable, the same immunoglobulin isotype was found on the cell membrane [73]. In vitro studies with antibodies to IgG and IgM have demonstrated suppression of pokeweed mitogen—induced antibody synthesis, whereas IgD antibodies resulted in increased Ig synthesis [74]. Studies using *Salmonella* lipopolysaccharide, a known B-cell mitogen for murine cells, have demonstrated in vitro development of plasma cells in these cultures [60]. Moreover, synthesis, assembly, and secretion of immunoglobulins have been demonstrated in vitro. Studies of several murine plasmacytomas in vivo have demonstrated that these represent a sequence in the development and maturation of immunoglobulin-secreting cells [61]. Some murine tumors have primarily membrane-bound immunoglobulin and little intracellular immunoglobulin. Electron microscopic observation reveals that these cells have characteristics of lymphocytes. In contrast, cells which rapidly synthesize and secrete immunoglobulins have these electron microscopic features of mature plasma cells. The murine plasmacytomas are characterized by the presence of A particles in the intracisternal space of the RER; their possible relation, if any, to human disease is unknown (Figs. 102-8 and 102-9) [62]. A number of human plasma cell tumors have been cultured in vitro, and some have

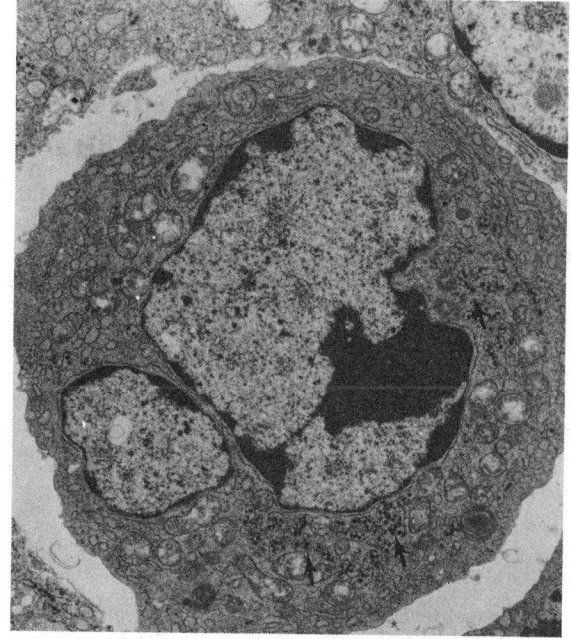

FIGURE 102-8 Plasma cell from IgM producing plasmacytoma (Balb/c mouse). Numerous intracisternal (between RER)–type A particles (*arrows*) are present. (×6000.)

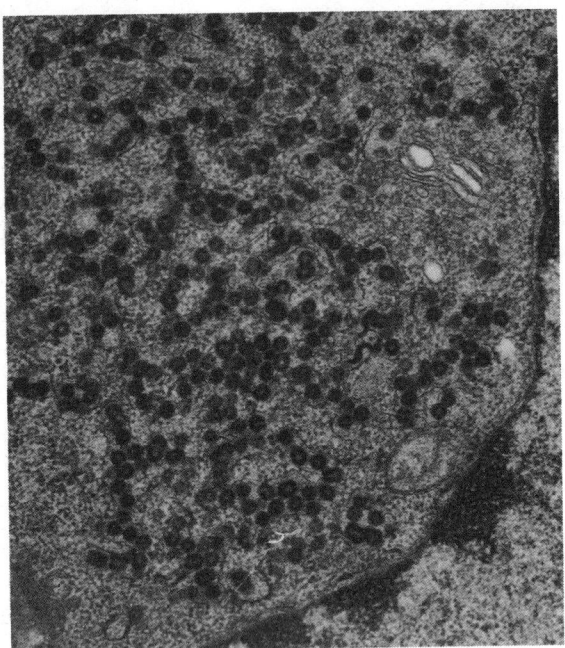

FIGURE 102-9 Higher magnification of plasma cell from mouse plasmacytoma to show morphology of intracisternal A particles. (×30,000.)

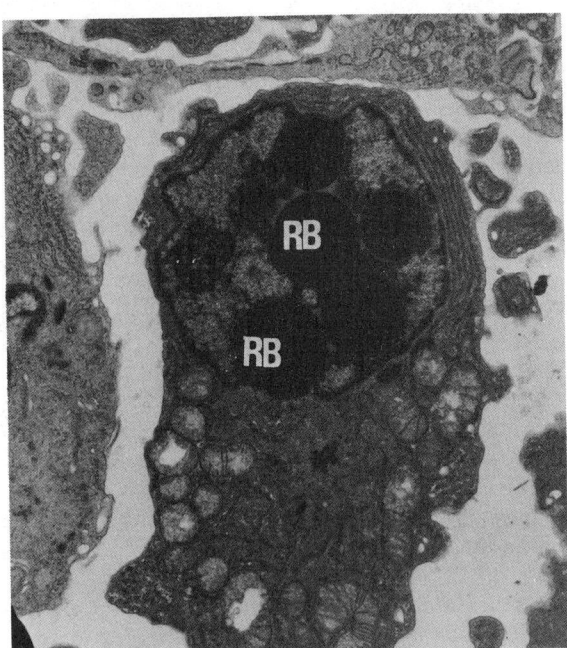

FIGURE 102-10 Intranuclear electron-dense bodies (Russell bodies) (RB) in a plasma cell from the marrow of a patient with multiple myeloma. (×7000.)

been shown to make characteristic myeloma proteins [63].

Application of other morphologic techniques to the investigation of plasma cells

Cytochemistry has yielded no definitive information for either the classification or the identification of plasma cell components. As indicated above, plasma cells infrequently contain large electron-dense inclusions which may measure 2 to 3 μm in diameter (so-called Russell bodies) (Fig. 102-10) [64]. Russell bodies may either stain or be dissolved during the Giemsa staining procedure. They usually occur in pathologic states; however, occasionally they may occur in "normal" situations in lymph nodes. The scanning electron microscope has as yet had little application in the investigation of normal or abnormal plasma cell surface topography. The techniques of freeze-fracture and freeze-etching have been applied to a very limited extent in the investigation of cell membranes of murine plasmacytoma cell lines [65,66,75]; however, thus far it has not been possible to relate intramembrane particles (see Chap. 101) to membrane or secreted immunoglobulin.

Plasma cell membrane markers

In some murine systems an antigen known as PC-1 was reported [67] to be present on most antibody-secreting cells. Although the antigen is present on kidney, liver, and brain cells, it is not present on non-antibody-secreting (resting) B or T lymphocytes, or on leukemic cells. Antibody to PC-1 has been produced by immunization of DBA-2 mice with Balb/c (H-2–compatible) myeloma cells. In addition, a mouse-specific plasma cell antigen (MS-PCA) has been produced in rabbits against mouse myeloma cells and then absorbed with mouse thymocytes; at present the specificity of this marker is still controversial [68–70]. Many of the characteristic B-cell markers (see Chap. 101), which include surface immunoglobulin and the receptor for the third component of complement, appear to be lost during B-cell differentiation toward mature plasma cells [71]. Studies using anti-idiotype antibodies to two human IgA myeloma proteins indicate that the idiotypic markers were present on B lymphocyte precursors (pre-B cells); these findings suggest that the oncogenic event occurs early in B-cell development [76].

Most terminally differentiated Ig-producing plasma cells lack Ia-like antigens. The majority of plasma cells in normal tonsils and blood of patients with Waldenström's macroglobulinemia are negative [77]. Pokeweed mitogen-derived plasma cells are Ia-positive.

References

1. Waldeyer, W: Ueber Bindegewebszellen. *Arch. Mikrobiol. Anat.* 11:176, 1875.
2. Ramon y Cajal, S.: *Manual de anatomia pathologica general*, Intr. de la Casa provincial de Caridad, Barcelona, 1890.

3. Unna, P. G.: Uber Plasmazellen, insbesondere beim Lupus. *Monatsschr. Prakt. Dermatol.* 12:296, 1891.

4. Marschalko, T. von: Über die sogenannten Plasmazellen: Ein Beitrag zur Kenntnis der Herkunft der entzundlichen Infiltrationzellen. *Arch. Dermatol. Syph.* 30:3, 241, 1895.

5. Wright, J. H.: A case of multiple myeloma. *Trans. Assoc. Am. Physicians* 15:137, 1900.

6. Bing, J., and Plum, P.: Serum proteins in leucopenia. *Acta Med. Scand.* 92:415, 1937.

7. Nossal, G. J. V.: Genetic control of lymphopoiesis, plasma cell formation and antibody production. *Int. Rev. Exp. Pathol.* 1:1, 1962.

8. Feldman, J. D.: Ultrastructure of immunologic processes. *Adv. Immunol.* 4:175, 1964.

9. Carr, I.: The fine structure of the mammalian lymphoreticular system. *Int. Rev. Cytol.* 27:283, 1970.

10. Azar, H. A., and Potter, M. (eds.): *Multiple Myeloma and Related Disorders.* Harper & Row, New York, 1973, vol. 1.

11. Sachetti, D.: Le plasmacellule nel midollo osseo delluomo nella norma e nella pathologia: Richerche quantitative citometriche et auxologiche. *Haematologica (Pavia)* 35:13, 1951.

12. White, R. G.: Light and electron microscopic correlations of periodic acid Schiff reaction in the human plasma cell. *Am. J. Pathol.* 40:285, 1962.

13. Quaglino, D., Torelli, V., Sauli, S., and Mauri, C.: Cytochemical and autoradiographic investigations on normal and myelomatous plasma cells. *Acta Haematol. (Basel)* 38:79, 1967.

14. Brecher, G., Tanaka, Y., Malmgren, R. A., and Fahey, J. L.: Morphology and protein synthesis in multiple myeloma and macroglobulinemia. *Ann. N.Y. Acad. Sci.* 113:642, 1964.

15. Brittin, G. M., Tanaka, Y., and Brecher, G.: Intranuclear inclusions in multiple myeloma and macroglobulinemia. *Blood* 21:335, 1963.

16. Goodman, J. R., and Hall, S. G.: Plasma cells containing iron: An electron micrographic study. *Blood* 28:83, 1966.

17. Lerner, R. G., and Parker, J. W.: Dysglobulinemia and iron in plasma cells: Ferrokinetics and electron microscopy. *Arch. Intern. Med.* 121:284, 1968.

18. Suzuki, A., Shibata, A., Onodera, S., Miura, A. B., Sakamoto, S., and Suzuki, C.: Histochemical study on plasma cells. *Tohoku J. Exp. Med.* 97:1, 1969.

19. Zucker-Franklin, D.: Structural features of cells associated with the paraproteinemias. *Semin. Hematol.* 1:165, 1964.

20. Maldonado, J. E., Kyle, R. A., Brown, A. L., Jr., and Bayrd, E. D.: "Intermediate" cell types and mixed cell proliferation in multiple myeloma: Electron microscopic observations. *Blood* 27:212, 1966.

21. Smetana, K., Gyorkey, F., Gyorkey, P., and Busch, H.: Ultrastructural studies on human myeloma plasmacytes. *Cancer Res.* 33:2300, 1973.

22. Zucker-Franklin, D.: Cellular structure and function in normal and neoplastic lymphoid cells. *Arch. Intern. Med.* 135:55, 1975.

23. Franklin, E. C., and Zucker-Franklin, D.: Current concepts of amyloid. *Adv. Immunol.* 15:249, 1972.

24. Braunsteiner, H., Fellinger, K., and Pakesch, F.: Demonstration of a cytoplasmic structure in plasma cells. *Blood* 8:916, 1953.

25. Bessis, M. C.: Ultrastructure of lymphoid and plasma cells in relation to globulin and antibody formation. *Lab. Invest.* 10:1040, 1961.

26. Movat, H. Z., and Fernando, N. V. P.: The fine structure of connective tissue. II. Plasma cell. *Exp. Mol. Pathol.* 1:535, 1962.

27. Weiss, L.: *The Cells and Tissues of the Immune System: Structure, Functions, Interactions,* Foundations of Immunology Series. Prentice-Hall, Englewood Cliffs, N.J., 1972.

28. Sainte-Marie, G.: Plasmocytes in the thymus of the normal rat. *J. Immunol.* 94:172, 1965.

29. Wintrobe, M. M., Lee, G. R., Boggs, D. R., Bithell, T. C., Athens, J. W., and Foerster, J.: *Clinical Hematology,* 7th ed. Lea & Febiger, Philadelphia, 1974, p. 1796.

30. Hall, J. G., Morris, B., Morena, G. D., and Bessis, M. C.: The ultrastructure and function of the cells in lymph following antigenic stimulation. *J. Exp. Med.* 125:91, 1967.

31. Murphy, M. J., Hay, J. B., Morris, B., and Bessis, M. C.: An ultrastructural analysis of antibody synthesis in cells from lymph and lymph nodes. *Am. J. Pathol.* 66:25, 1972.

32. Crowther, D., Fairley, G. H., and Sewell, R. L.: Lymphoid cellular responses in the blood after immunization in man. *J. Exp. Med.* 129:849, 1969.

33. Bond, V. P., Cronkite, E. P., Fliedner, T. M., and Schork, P.: Desoxyribonucleic acid synthesizing cells in peripheral blood of normal human beings. *Science* 128:202, 1958.

34. Turk, W.: *Klinische Untersuchungen uber das Verhalten des Blutes bei akuten: Infektionskrankheiten.* Braumuller, Vienna, 1898.

35. Wood, T. A., and Frenkel, E. P.: The atypical lymphocyte. *Am. J. Med.* 42:923, 1967.

36. Douglas, S. D., Fudenberg, H. H., Glade, P. R., Chessin, L. N., and Moses, H. L.: Fine structure of leukocytes in infectious mononucleosis: In vivo and in vitro studies. *Blood* 34:42, 1969.

37. Farnes, P., and Barker, B. E.: Blood mononuclear cell abnormalities in mumps. *Am. J. Clin. Pathol.* 49:398, 1968.

38. Barnett, E. V., Stone, G., Swisher, S. W., and Vaughan, J. H.: Serum sickness and plasmacytosis: A clinical, immunologic and hematologic analysis. *Am. J. Med.* 35:113, 1963.

39. Biberfeld, P., and Hedfors, E.: Atypical lymphocytes in sarcoidosis: Morphology, cytochemistry and membrane properties. *Scand. J. Immunol.* 3:615, 1974.

40. Schopfer, K., and Douglas, S. D.: In vitro studies of lymphocytes from children with kwashiorkor. *Clin. Immunol. Immunopathol.* 5:21, 1976.

41. Beathard, G. A., Granholm, N. A., Sakai, H. A., and Ritzmann, S. E.: Ultrastructural alterations in peripheral blood lymphocyte profiles following acute thermal burns. *Clin. Immunol. Immunopathol.* 2:488, 1974.

42. Mellors, R. C., and Korngold, L.: The cellular origin of human immunoglobulins: γ2, γ1M, γ1A. *J. Exp. Med.* 118:387, 1963.

43. Hummeler, K., Harris, T. W., and Tomassini, N.: Electron microscopic observations on antibody producing cells in lymph blood. *J. Exp. Med.* 124:255, 1966.

44. Bosman, C., and Feldman, J. D.: Heterogeneity and homogeneity of immunoglobulin-forming cells. *Lab. Invest.* 22:309, 1970.

45. De Petris, S., Karlsbad, G., and Pernis, B.: Localization of antibodies in plasma cells by electron microscopy. *J. Exp. Med.* 117:849, 1963.

46. Avrameas, S., and Leduc, E. H.: Detection of simultaneous antibody synthesis in plasma cells and specialized lymphocytes in rabbit lymph nodes. *J. Exp. Med.* 131:1137, 1970.

47. Zucker-Franklin, D.: Use of tracer techniques in studies on immunoglobulin-producing cells. *J. Histochem. Cytochem.* 21:209, 1973.

48. Taylor, C. R., and Burns, J.: The demonstration of plasma cells and other immunoglobulin-containing cells in formalin-fixed paraffin-embedded tissues using peroxidase-labeled antibody. *J. Clin. Pathol.* 27:14, 1974.

49. Antoine, J. C., Avrameas, S., Gonatas, N. K., Stieber, A., and Gonatas, J. D.: Plasma membrane and internalized immunoglobulins of lymph node cells studies with conjugates of antibody or its Fab fragments with horseradish peroxidase. *J. Cell Biol.* 63:12, 1974.

50. Kuhlmann, W. D., Avrameas, S., and Ternynck, T.: A comparative study for ultrastructural localization of intracellular immunoglobulins using peroxidase conjugates. *J. Immunol. Methods* 5:33, 1974.

51. Zagury, D., Uhr, J. W., Jamieson, J. D., and Palade, G. E.: Immunoglobulin synthesis and secretion. II. Radioautographic studies of sites of addition of carbohydrate moieties and intracellular transport. *J. Cell Biol.* 46:52, 1970.

52. Fagraeus, A.: Antibody production in relation to the development of plasma cells: In vivo and in vitro experiments. *Acta Med. Scand.* 130:1, 1948.

53. Nossal, C. J. V., and Makela, O.: Autoradiographic studies on the immune response. I. The kinetics of plasma cell proliferation. II. DNA synthesis amongst single antibody producing cells. *J. Exp. Med.* 115:209, 1962.

54. Sainte-Marie, G.: Study on plasmocytopoiesis: Description of plasmocytes and of their mitoses in the mediastinal lymph nodes of ten week-old rats. *Am. J. Anat.* 114:207, 1964.

55. Sainte-Marie, G., and Coons, A. H.: Studies on antibody production. X. Mode of formation of plasmocytes in cell transfer experiments. *J. Exp. Med.* 119:743, 1964.

56. Buxbaum, J. N.: The biosynthesis, assembly and secretion of immunoglobulins. *Semin. Hematol.* 10:33, 1973.

57. Scharff, M. D.: The synthesis, assembly and secretion of immunoglobulin: A biochemical and genetic approach. *Harvey Lect.* ser. 69, 1975, p. 125.

58. Douglas, S. D., and Fudenberg, H. H.: In vitro development of plasma cells from lymphocytes following pokeweed mitogen stimulation: A fine structural study. *Exp. Cell. Res. 54:*277, 1969.

59. Parkhouse, R. M. E., Janossy, G., and Greaves, M. F.: Selective stimulation of IgM synthesis in mouse B lymphocytes by pokeweed mitogen. *Nature [New Biol.] 235:*21, 1972.

60. Shands, J. W., Peavy, D. L., and Smith, R. T.: Differential morphology of mouse spleen cells stimulated in vitro by endotoxin, phytohemagglutinin, pokeweed mitogen and staphylococcal entertoxin B. *Am. J. Pathol. 70:*1, 1973.

61. Andersson, J., et al.: IgM-producing tumors in the Balb/c mouse: A model for B-cell maturation. *J. Exp. Med. 140:*742, 1974.

62. Potter, M.: The developmental history of the neoplastic plasma cell in mice: A brief review of recent developments. *Semin. Hematol. 10:*19, 1973.

63. Jobin, M. E., Fahey, J. L., and Price, F.: Long-term establishment of a human plasmacyte cell line derived from a patient with IgD multiple myeloma. *J. Exp. Med. 140:*494, 1974.

64. Welsh, R. A.: Electron microscopic localization of Russell bodies in the human plasma cell. *Blood 16:*1307, 1960.

65. Guerin, C., et al.: Correlation between the mobility of inner plasma membrane structure and agglutination by concanavalin A in two cell lines of MDPC173 plasmocytoma cells. *Proc. Natl. Acad. Sci. U.S.A. 71:*114, 1974.

66. Zuckerman, S. H., and Douglas, S. D.: Inhibition of Fc receptors on a murine lymphoid cell line by cholera exotoxin. *Nature 255:*410, 1975.

67. Takahashi, T., Old, L. J., and Boyse, E. A.: Surface alloantigens of plasma cells. *J. Exp. Med. 131:*1325, 1970.

68. Takahashi, T., Old, L. J., Cheng-Jung, N., and Boyse, E. A.: A new differentiation antigen of plasma cells. *Eur. J. Immunol. 1:*478, 1972.

69. Yutoku, M., Grossberg, A. L., and Pressman, D.: Preparation and properties of rabbit anti-mouse plasmacyte serum purified by in vivo absorption: Further evidence for a new antigenic determinant on plasmacytes. *J. Immunol. 112:*911, 1974.

70. Yutoku, M., Grossberg, A. L. and Pressman, D.: A cell surface antigenic determinant present on mouse plasmacytes and only about one half of mouse thymocytes. *J. Immunol. 112:*1774, 1974.

71. Ramasamy, R., and Munro, A. J.: Surface B and T cell markers on murine lymphomas and plasmacytomas. *Immunology 26:*563, 1974.

72. Ottosen, P. D., Courtoy, P. J., and Farquhar, M. G.: Pathways followed by membrane recovered from the surface of plasma cells and myeloma cells. *J. Exp. Med. 152:*1, 1980.

73. Lucivero, G., Lawton, A., Fuks, A., and Cooper, M. D.: Pokeweed mitogen-induced differentiation of peripheral blood human B lymphocytes (in press).

74. Chiorazzi, N., Fu, S. M., and Kunkel, H. G.: Stimulation of human B lymphocytes by antibodies to IgM and IgG: Functional evidence for the expression of IgG on B-lymphocyte surface membranes. *Clin. Immunol. Immunopathol. 15:*301, 1980.

75. Douglas, S. D., Ooka, M. P., and Zuckerman, S. H.: Effect of cholera toxin on intramembranous particles of a murine lymphoid cell line. *Exp. Cell Res. 101:*111, 1976.

76. Kubagawa, H., Lawton, A. R., and Cooper, M. D.: Studies on the clonal origin of multiple myeloma. *J. Exp. Med. 150:*792, 1979.

77. Halper, J., Fu, S. M., and Kunkel, H. G.: Patterns of expression of human "Ia-like" antigens during the terminal stages of B cell development. *J. Immunol. 120:*1480, 1978.

Biochemistry and function of lymphocytes and plasma cells

CHAPTER *103*

Composition and biochemistry of lymphocytes and plasma cells

DENNIS A. CARSON

Lymphocytes are not a uniform population of cells. Although probably differentiated from a common progenitor, mature lymphocytes can be divided into several types on the basis of cell surface antigens and receptors, most recently defined with monoclonal antibodies [1]. The major classes of lymphocytes are the T, B, and null cells. T lymphocytes can be further subdivided into at least two subsets, helper cells and suppressor/cytotoxic cells. B lymphocytes at various stages of differentiation also differ in cell surface properties [2]. Null lymphocytes have been poorly characterized to date. A detailed account of lymphocyte types and their functions is found in Chap. 105.

T and B lymphocytes have distinguishable metabolic profiles. Unfortunately, most studies of the biochemistry of lymphocytes were performed before methods were available for the separation of lymphocytes from monocytes, or for the clear-cut purification of lymphocyte subpopulations. Since in peripheral blood, helper T cells are the predominant class [1], many reported biochemical parameters are most relevant to this population. In the future, the biochemical characterization of lymphocytes must be performed with highly purified and well-characterized subpopulations.

Wherever possible, this chapter will emphasize those biochemical aspects that distinguish lymphocytes from other nucleated cells, and that differ among lymphocyte subclasses.

Life-span of lymphocytes

The production of lymphocytes is detailed in Chap. 106. From 65 to 85 percent of human peripheral blood lymphocytes are long-lived, with intermitotic periods varying from a few months to up to 5 years [3,4]. The long-lived lymphocytes are predominantly T cells, reversibly arrested in the early G_1 phase of the cell cycle (see Fig. 103-1). This is sometimes termed a G_0 or "resting" state, since the lymphocytes do not progress further through the cycle without an appropriate stimulus [5]. The remaining 15 to 35 percent of peripheral blood lymphocytes are short-lived, with life-spans varying from a few hours to 5 days. Included in this heterogeneous population are T, B, and null cells.

Composition of lymphocytes

In large part the composition and metabolism of long-lived peripheral blood T lymphocytes reflects their resting state. Thus, T cells have a high nuclear-to-cytoplasmic ratio, few ribosomes or mitochondria, and scant endoplasmic reticulum. Glycogen stores are meager. The DNA content of the resting small lymphocyte, 8×10^{-12} g per cell, is the same as in other diploid cells [6]. In contrast, the RNA content averages 2.5×10^{-12} g per cell,

FIGURE 103-1 Approximate sequence of metabolic events during lymphocyte transformation, following the binding of a mitogen to the plasma membrane (time 0).

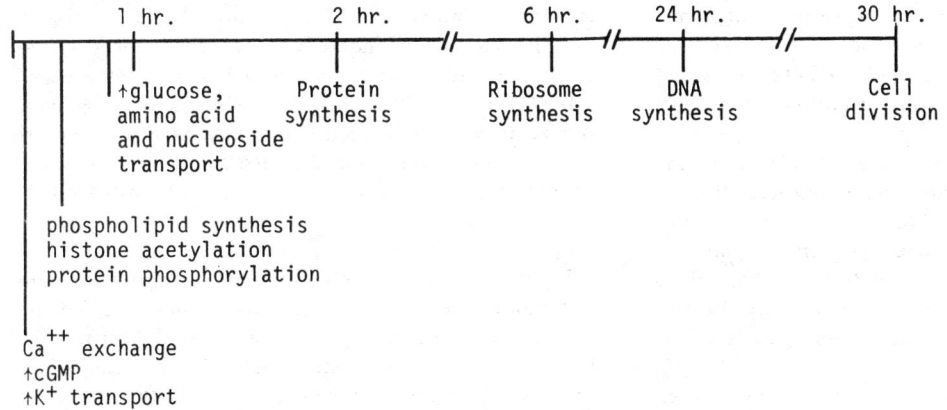

yielding an RNA/DNA ratio of approximately 0.32 [6]. This value is less than in most other human tissues, due to the small amount of ribosomal RNA in lymphocytes.

The resting peripheral blood lymphocyte has a mean cell volume of 200 μm^3, and contains 79 ± 1.2 percent by weight of water [7]. The total lymphocyte cation content is 36×10^{-15} mol per cell, of which 22 to 28×10^{-15} mol per cell is potassium, and $7.9 \pm 3.2 \times 10^{-15}$ mol per cell is sodium [7,8].

The few lysosomes in peripheral blood lymphocytes contain several different acid hydrolases including acid phosphatase, β-glucuronidase, β-galactosidase, β-hexosaminidase, α-arabinosidase, α-galactosidase, α-mannosidase, α-glucosidase, and β-glucosidase [9]. Whether measured cytochemically or in extracts, acid hydrolase activities are generally higher in T than in non-T lymphocytes. Lysosomal acid esterase, assayed histochemically with α-naphthyl acetate as substrate, has a characteristic punctate appearance in mature T lymphocytes [10].

The lymphocyte plasma membrane is composed of equal parts by weight of protein and lipid, and 6 percent by weight of carbohydrate [11]. The molar ratio of cholesterol to phospholipid is approximately 0.5 [12]. The membrane proteins are usually glycosylated.

Enzymes located on the exterior surface of lymphocytes include 5'-nucleotidase, sodium-potassium ATPase, and alkaline phosphatase [13,14]. Levels of 5'-nucleotidase are three- to fourfold higher in B than T lymphocytes, and increase with the maturation of both cell types. The variably low levels of lymphocyte ecto-5'-nucleotidase reported in patients with hypogammaglobulinemia reflect the immature state of the lymphocytes in the peripheral circulation. Levels of ecto-5'-nucleotidase may be useful in distinguishing subclasses of chronic lymphocytic leukemia arising from T or B lymphocytes at various stages of differentiation [15].

It is the specialized membrane proteins of lymphocytes that best distinguish them from other cell types. The immunoglobulin receptors for antigen on B lymphocytes are unique and highly polymorphic recognition molecules that enable the cells to discriminate between self and nonself. The antigen receptors on T lymphocytes have been poorly characterized, and contain polypeptide structures analogous to both immunoglobulin heavy-chain variable regions and Ia antigens. Recently, several additional cell surface components of unknown function have been described that distinguish lymphocyte subpopulations (see Chap. 105).

The various proteins of the lymphocyte plasma membrane have been divided into three types according to their ability to migrate in the fluid mosaic lipid bilayer [16]. Class I components diffuse freely in the plane of the membrane. Class II components are anchored to submembrane microfilaments, while class III components, although attached to microfilaments, have a limited freedom to move.

Beneath the plasma membrane is a fully developed cytoskeleton with several different structural and mechanical proteins, including tubulin, actin, myosin, and α-actinin [16]. The actin myofilaments may play a role in locomotion. Moreover, it may be changes in the reversible interaction of membrane components with microfilamentary structures that trigger the metabolic changes necessary for lymphocyte activation.

Metabolism of the lymphocyte

NUCLEIC ACID SYNTHESIS

Nonreplicating, peripheral blood T lymphocytes are capable of DNA excision/repair and contain exonucleases, endonucleases, and DNA polymerases α and β. Additionally, cortical thymocytes and a small percentage of normal marrow lymphocyte precursors contain a unique terminal deoxynucleotidyl transferase that is template-independent [17]. The latter enzyme is a useful marker in characterizing acute leukemias and chronic myelogenous leukemia in blast crisis [18]. Its physiological function is not known.

Lymphocytes are among the more sensitive cells in the body to the cytotoxic effects of ionizing radiation and ultraviolet light. The reasons for the hypersensitivity are not entirely clear. A contributing factor may be the minute pools of deoxynucleotide triphosphates that limit the rate of DNA repair [19]. Lymphocytes have minimal ribonucleotide reductase activity, and a concomitantly low rate of *de novo* deoxyribonucleotide synthesis.

The DNA sequences coding for the immunoglobulin light and heavy chains undergo several unique physical rearrangements during B-lymphocyte differentiation [20]. These lead to the apposition of DNA segments corresponding to the variable (V), joining (J), and constant (C) regions of immunoglobulin polypeptides, and the deletion of the DNA that separates these genes in embryonic DNA. For uncertain reasons, only one immunoglobulin heavy-chain gene and one light-chain gene is expressed in mature, diploid B lymphocytes, a phenomenon that is known as *allelic exclusion* (see Chap. 104).

The three DNA-dependent RNA polymerases found in other mammalian cell types are also detectable in lymphocyte nuclei. Blood lymphocytes incorporate radioactive uridine into RNA at a slow but measurable rate [21]. The newly synthesized RNA is heterogeneous in size, is largely confined to the nucleus, and turns over rapidly. Blood lymphocytes also synthesize a poorly characterized nonmessenger RNA that has been reported to limit the rate of initiation of protein synthesis [22].

Different species of RNA direct the synthesis of immunoglobin heavy chains that are either inserted into the plasma membrane or secreted. It is the former that predominate in the unstimulated B cell. These RNA species undergo extensive processing in the cytoplasm prior to translation, including the generation of 5'-terminal cap structures, internal methylations, and the selective removal of intervening sequences. The enzymes mediating the RNA rearrangements are under active investigation.

The enzymes for the early pathways of *de novo* purine and pyrimidine synthesis have very low activity in peripheral blood lymphocytes, consistent with the small nucleotide requirements of these nondividing cells [23]. Nevertheless, some *de novo* purine and pyrimidine synthesis probably occurs. In contrast, enzymes of purine and pyrimidine intraconversion are easily detectable, with the exception of xanthine oxidase and guanase which are absent in lymphocytes [23,24]. Patients with a genetic deficiency of the purine salvage enzyme hypoxanthine-guanine phosphoribosyl transferase (the Lesch-Nyhan syndrome) have normal numbers of lymphocytes and adequate immune function. The blood of patients heterozygous for the disorder contains few hypoxanthine-guanine phosphoribosyl transferase-negative lymphocytes, suggesting that the enzyme-deficient cells may have a growth disadvantage [25].

Genetic deficiencies of two enzymes of purine metabolism, adenosine deaminase and purine nucleoside phosphorylase, are associated with a specific impairment of the development and function of the lymphoid system [26,27]. Apparently, the primary function of these enzymes is the catabolism of the potentially toxic nucleosides deoxyadenosine and deoxyguanosine. In adenosine deaminase– and purine nucleoside phosphorylase–deficient patients, phosphorylated derivatives of deoxyadenosine and deoxyguanosine may preferentially accumulate in T lymphocytes. When compared to other cell types, the T lymphocytes have high levels of deoxycytidine kinase, for which the purine deoxyribonucleosides are alternative substrates, and low levels of cytoplasmic deoxynucleotidase [28,29].

FATTY ACID AND LIPID SYNTHESIS
Resting lymphocytes incorporate ^{14}C-acetate into long-chain fatty acids [30]. These are used to replenish unsaturated phospholipids lost during the normal turnover of the lymphocyte plasma membrane [31].

Small lymphocytes, as opposed to monocytes, probably do not synthesize prostaglandins or leukotrienes [32]; however, they do contain prostaglandin receptors. Prostaglandins synthesized by macrophages inhibit lymphocyte function, and may be partially responsible for the impaired immunity associated with chronic inflammatory states such as Hodgkin's disease and systemic fungal infections [33].

CARBOHYDRATE METABOLISM
Blood lymphocytes have few or no insulin receptors [34]. The rate of glucose metabolism is limited by the rate of entry of glucose into the cells [35] as mediated by a facilitated diffusion system. Lymphocytes contain all the enzymes of the glycolytic pathway and tricarboxylic acid cycle. Although resting lymphocytes in vitro consume only small amounts of oxygen, their mitochondria have typically coupled electron transport chains.

The resting lymphocyte requires energy to maintain its ionic milieu via membrane-bound ATPases, to replace degraded proteins and lipids, and for active locomotion [38,39]. The recirculation of long-lived lymphocytes from the vascular space to the interstitial tissues and back into the lymphatic drainage system requires directed cell movement and utilizes considerable amounts of ATP. Lymphocytes treated with nonlethal concentrations of drugs that inhibit mitochondrial respiration, but not with agents that inhibit glycolysis, recirculate sluggishly. This suggests that the energy for lymphocyte locomotion derives largely from oxidative phosphorylation [39].

The enzymes of the hexosemonophosphate shunt account for only a small fraction of energy production in resting lymphocytes [36]. As in other cells types, the pathway provides lymphocytes with high-energy ribose derivatives necessary for purine and pyrimidine synthesis, and with a source of reducing energy in the form of NADPH.

PROTEIN SYNTHESIS AND AMINO ACID METABOLISM
Human peripheral blood lymphocytes actively incorporate radioactive amino acids into protein. The protein synthesis is necessary for survival, and inhibition with cycloheximide or puromycin leads to the rapid death of the lymphocytes.

Among the proteins synthesized uniquely by lymphocytes, immunoglobulin and the interleukin II are of particular interest. The synthesis and assembly of immunoglobulin by activated B lymphocytes and plasma cells is discussed in detail in Chap. 104. Interleukin II (also known as *T-cell growth factor*) is a polypeptide hormone(s) of M_r 15,000 daltons that is synthesized by a subset of activated T cells [40]. It binds to receptors on other dividing T cells, and is necessary for their continued proliferation.

The metabolic pathways for the synthesis of two normally nonessential amino acids, L-cysteine and L-asparagine, are inadequate in thymic lymphocytes, and probably in peripheral blood T cells [41,42]. A similar L-asparagine requirement among certain null and T-cell leukemias is responsible for the L-asparaginase sensitivity of these neoplasms.

HORMONES AND LYMPHOCYTE METABOLISM
Plasma membrane receptors for calcitonin, insulin, and growth hormone have been demonstrated on human B lymphoblastoid cell lines [34]. These receptors are present in much lower density, or absent, on T-cell lines and on resting blood lymphocytes. When T lymphocytes are activated by mitogens, the density of receptors for the growth-related polypeptide hormones increases markedly.

Human T lymphocytes can be fractionated on the basis of the number of histamine receptors on the plasma membrane [43]. T cells of the suppressor/cytotoxic class have greater numbers of histamine receptors than do helper T cells. Lymphocyte membrane receptors for catecholamines and acetylcholine have also been described [43]. When added to in vitro lymphocyte cultures, the latter compounds can alter intracellular levels of cyclic nucleotides, with secondary changes in growth and function.

Glucocorticoids in pharmacologic concentrations have a unique lympholytic effect that is not dependent upon cell division [44]. Among normal lymphocyte subsets, immature T cells in the thymus are most sensitive. The exact mechanism of action of the glucocorticoids on lymphocyte metabolism has eluded definitive investigation. Lymphocytes contain high-affinity receptors for glucocorticoids in the cytoplasm, and perhaps on the cell surface [45,46]. There is evidence that the cytoplasmic glucocorticoid-receptor complexes, after migrating to the nucleus, induce mRNA for specific proteins that inhibit glucose transport and lipid synthesis [47]. Glucocorticoids also profoundly inhibit the synthesis of interleukin II by activated T cells in vitro. The latter effect offer an attractive explanation for some of the immunosuppressive effects of the hormones [47].

LYMPHOCYTE TRANSFORMATION

Both antibody synthesis and the development of cellular immunity require activation and replication of lymphocytes, with subsequent differentiation into plasma cells, or effector T lymphocytes. Lymphocyte activation is a complex and highly regulated process involving the interaction of multiple cell types. Thus, it is now clear that accessory monocyte-macrophages are required for efficient transformation. The macrophages serve both to present mitogenic stimuli in a functional manner, and also to secrete specific hormonelike factors that regulate lymphocyte proliferation and differentiation [48,49]. Once transformation is initiated, soluble factors secreted by helper and suppressor T lymphocytes are important in modulating lymphocyte proliferation [50].

The binding of mitogens, such as phytohemagglutinin or concanavalin A, to the lymphocyte surface membrane leads to the cross-linking of surface membrane receptors, with accompanying changes in microfilamentary organization [14]. Simultaneously there begins a diverse series of metabolic changes, many of which are characteristic of a synchronous cell population moving from the early G_1 phase to the S phase of the cell cycle [51,52]. Within 1 h after mitogen binding, calcium exchange across the plasma membrane accelerates, although total cellular calcium stores remain constant [53–55]. The increased calcium flux may be related to the activity of a specific calcium-ATPase located in the plasma membrane [55]. The binding of phytohemagglutinin or concanavalin A to lymphocytes simultaneously enhances membrane permeability to sodium and potassium by one and one-half– to twofold [56]. The active transport of the two cations, mediated by the specific sodium-potassium ATPase in the plasma mem-

brane, increases proportionately [57]. Transit changes in cyclic nucleotide levels and increases in membrane phospholipid turnover, histone acetylation, and protein phosphorylation also occur soon after mitogen binding to the lymphocyte plasma membrane (see Fig. 103-1) [51,52]. Among the subsequent metabolic events preceeding entry into S phase are increases in RNA, protein, and polyamine synthesis, amino acid, nucleoside, and sugar transport, and hexose monophosphate shunt activity. The energy for these processes is derived initially from glycolysis [58]. Approximately one-third of the total lactate produced early in mitogenesis is used for sodium-potassium transport [59]. By 24 h after the addition of a T-cell mitogen such as phytohemagglutinin, the majority of responsive cells have entered S phase, and within the next 24 h will begin to undergo mitosis.

The exact biochemical control of cellular proliferation in lymphocytes, as in other mammalian cells, is not well understood. The ability of a specific calcium-transporting ionophore to induce lymphocyte proliferation suggest a central role for this cation [60]. However, it must be reiterated that sustained lymphocyte proliferation, and differentiation, is dependent upon specific polypeptide growth factors produced by accessory lymphocytes and monocyte-macrophages.

Plasma cells

Plasma cells are the end product of B-cell differentiation. They are committed to the synthesis, assembly, and secretion of immunoglobulin, and have a well-developed rough endoplasmic reticulum and Golgi apparatus. They lack many of the surface receptors found on B lymphocytes. Mature plasma cells are probably terminally differentiated and have a low rate of DNA synthesis [61]. The detailed biochemical analyses of normal plasma cells have been hindered by the difficulties in obtaining pure, viable populations. Enzymes in the glycolytic and tricarboxylic acid pathways have been demonstrated [62]. The enzymes of the hexose monophosphate shunt are detectable, but of low activity.

References

1. Reinherz, E. L., and Schlossman, S. F.: The differentiation and function of human T lymphocytes. *Cell* 19:821, 1980.
2. Cooper, M. D., Kubagawa, H., Vogler, L. B., Kearney, J. F., and Lawton, A. R.: Generation of clonal and isotype diversity. *Adv. Exp. Med. Biol.* 107:9, 1978.
3. Little, J. R., Brecher, G., Bradley, T. R., and Rose, S.: Determination of lymphocyte turnover by continuous infusion of ³H-thymidine. *Blood* 19:236, 1962.
4. Robinson, S. H., Brecher, G., Lourie, I. S., and Haley, J. E.: Leukocyte labelling in rats during and after continuous infusion with tritiated thymidine. *Blood* 26:281, 1965.
5. Baserga, R.: The cell cycle. *N. Engl. J. Med.* 304:433, 1981.
6. Glen, A. C. A.: Measurement of DNA and RNA in human peripheral blood lymphocytes. *Clin. Chem.* 13:299, 1967.

7. Segal, G. B., Cokelet, G. R., and Lichtman, M. A.: The measurement of lymphocyte volume: Importance of reference particle deformability and counting solution tonicity. *Blood* 57:894, 1981.

8. Segel, G. B., Lichtman, M. A., Hollander, M. M., Gordon, B. R., and Klemperer, M. R.: Human lymphocyte potassium content during the initation of phytohemagglutinin induced mitogenesis. *J. Cell. Physiol.* 86:313, 1975.

9. Pangalis, G. A., Kuhl, W., Waldman, S. R., and Beutler, E.: Acid hydrolases in normal B and T lymphocytes. *Acta Haematol.* 59:285, 1978.

10. Kulenkampff, J., Janossy, G., and Greaves, M. F.: Acid esterase in human lymphoid cells and leukemic blasts: A marker for T lymphocytes. *Br. J. Haematol.* 36:231, 1977.

11. Crumptom, M. J., and Snary, D.: Preparation and properties of lymphocyte plasma membrane. *Contemp. Top. Molec. Immunol.* 3:27, 1974.

12. Johnson, S. M., and Robinson, R.: The composition and fluidity of normal and leukemic or lymphomatous plasma membranes in mouse and man. *Biochim. Biophys. Acta* 558:282, 1979.

13. Muller-Hermelink, H. K.: Characterization of the B-cell and T-cell regions of human lymphatic tissue through enzyme histochemical demonstration of ATPase and 5'-nucleotidase activities. *Virchows Arch. B Cell Pathol.* 16:371, 1974.

14. Rowe, M., De Gost, G. C., Platts-Mills, T. A. E., Asherson, G. L., Webster, A. D. B., and Johnson, S. M.: Lymphocytes 5'-nucleotidase in primary hypogammaglobulinemia and cord blood. *Clin. Exp. Immunol.* 39:337, 1980.

15. Silber, R., Conklyn, M., Grusky, G., and Zucker-Franklin, D.: Human lymphocytes: 5'-Nucleotidase positive and negative subpopulations. *J. Clin. Invest.* 56:1324, 1975.

16. Loor, F.: The lymphocyte membrane and the cytoskeleton, in *Cell Biology and Immunology of Leukocyte Function*, edited by M. R. Quastel. Academic, New York, 1979, p. 1.

17. Beutler, E., and Blume, K. G.: Terminal deoxynucleotidyl transferase: Biochemical properties, cellular distribution, and hematologic significance, in *Progress in Hematology*, vol. XI, 1979, p. 47.

18. McCaffrey, R., Harrison, T. A., Parkman, R., and Baltimore, D.: Terminal deoxynucleotidyl transferase in human leukemic cells and in normal human thymocytes. *N. Engl. J. Med.* 292:775, 1975.

19. Yew, F. H., and Johnson, R. T.: Ultraviolet-induced DNA excision repair in human B and T lymphocytes. III. Repair in lymphocytes from chromic lymphatic leukemia. *J. Cell. Sci.* 39:329, 1979.

20. Battisto, J., and Knight, K. (ed.): *Immunoglobulin Genes and B Cell Differentiation*. Elsevier–North Holland, New York, 1980.

21. Cooper, H. L.: Studies on RNA metabolism during lymphocyte activation. *Transplant. Rev.* 11:3, 1972.

22. Cooper, H. L.: Evidence for a non-messenger RNA which is rate limiting for protein synthesis in resting lymphocytes, in *Cell Biology and Immunology of Leukocyte Function*, edited by M. R. Quastel. Academic, New York, 1979, p. 135.

23. Scholar, E. M., and Calabresi, P.: Identification of the enzymatic pathways of nucleotide metabolism in human lymphocytes and 122B:283, 1980.

24. van Laarhoven, J. P. R. M., Spierenberg, G. T., de Bruyn, C. H. M. M., and Schrellen, E. D. A. M.: Enzymes of purine intraconversions in subfractions of lymphocytes. *Adv. Exp. Biol. Med.* 122B:283, 1980.

25. Albertini, R. J., and DeMars, R.: Mosaicism of peripheral blood lymphocyte population in females heterozygous for the Lesch-Nyhan mutation. *Biochem. Genet.* 11:397, 1971.

26. Giblett, E. R., Anderson, J. E., Cohen, F., Pollara, B., and Meuwissen, H. J.: Adenosine deaminase deficiency in two patients with severely impaired cellular immunity. *Lancet* 2:1067, 1972.

27. Giblett, E. R., Ammann, A. J., Wara, D. W., Sandman, R., and Diamond, L. K.: Nucleoside phosphorylase deficiency in a child with severely defective T-cell immunity and normal B-cell immunity. *Lancet* 1:1010, 1975.

28. Carson D. A., Kaye, J., and Seegmiller, J. E.: Lymphospecific toxicity in adenosine deaminase deficiency and purine nucleoside phosphorylase deficiency: Possible role of nucleoside kinases. *Proc. Natl. Acad. Sci. U.S.A.* 74:5679, 1972.

29. Carson, D. A., Kaye, J., and Wasson, D. B.: The potential importance of soluble deoxynucleotidase activity in mediating deoxyadenosine toxicity in human lymphoblasts. *J. Immunol.* 126:348, 1981.

30. Huber, H., Stueden, N., Winnler, H., Reisen, G., and Koppelstaetler, K.: Studies on the incorporation of ^{14}C-sodium acetate into the phospholipids of phytohemagglutinin stimulated and unstimulated lymphocytes. *Br. J. Haematol.* 15:203, 1968.

31. Morimoto, K., and Kanoke, K.: The role of the *de novo* synthetic pathway in forming molecular species of phospholipids in resting lymphocytes from human tonsils. *Biochim. Biophys. Acta* 617:511, 1980.

32. Kennedy, M. S., Stobo, J. D., and Goldyne, M. E.: In vitro synthesis of prostaglandins and related lipids by populations of human peripheral blood mononuclear cells. *Prostaglandins* 20:135, 1980.

33. Goodwin, J. S., Bankhurst, A. D., and Messner, R. R.: Suppression of human T-cell mitogenesis by prostaglandins: Existence of a prostaglandin-producing suppressor cell. *J. Exp. Med.* 146:1719, 1977.

34. Gavin, J. R., III: Polypeptide hormone receptors on lymphoid cells, in *Comprehensive Immunology*, vol. 3, *Immunopharmacology*, edited by J. W. Hadden, R. G. Coffey, and F. Spreafico. Phenum, New York, 1977, p. 357.

35. Elbrink, J., and Bihler, I.: Membrane transport: Its relation to cellular metabolic rates. *Science* 188:1117, 1975.

36. Hedeskov, C. J.: Early effects of phytohemagglutinin on glucose metabolism of normal human lymphocytes. *Biochem. J.* 110:373, 1968.

37. Pachman, L. M.: The carbohydrate metabolism and respiration of isolated small lymphocytes. *Blood* 30:691, 1967.

38. Segal, G. B., Androphy, E. J., and Lichtman, M. A.: Increased ouabain-sensitive glycolysis of lymphocytes treated with phytohemagglutinin: Relation to potassium transport. *J. Cell. Physiol.* 97:407, 1978.

39. Freitas, A. A., and Bognack, J.: The role of cell locomotion in lymphocyte migration. *Immunology* 34:247, 1979.

40. Ruscetti, F. W., and Gallo, R. C.: Human T lymphocyte growth factor: Regulation of growth and function of T lymphocytes. *Blood* 57:379, 1981.

41. Ohnuma, T., Holland, J. F., Arkin, H., and Minowada, J.: L-Asparaginase requirements of human T-lymphocytes and B-lymphocytes in culture. *J. Natl. Cancer Inst.* 59:1061, 1972.

42. Kamatani, N., and Carson, D.: Differential cysteine requirements of human T and B lymphoblastoid cell lines, submitted for publication.

43. Melmon, K. L., et al.: Receptors for low-molecular-weight hormones on lymphocytes, in *Comprehensive Immunology*, vol. 3, *Immunopharmacology*, edited by J. W. Hadden, R. G. Coffey, and F. Spreafico. Plenum, New York, 1977, p. 33.

44. Claman, H. M.: Corticosteroids and lymphoid cells. *N. Engl. J. Med.* 287:388, 1972.

45. Baxter, J. D., Harris, A. W., Tomkins, G. M., and Cohn, M.: Glucocorticoid receptors in lymphoma cells in culture: Relationship to glucocorticoid killing activity. *Science* 171:189, 1971.

46. Young, D. A., Nicholson, M. L., Voris, B. P., and Lyons, R. T.: Mechanisms involved in the generation of the metabolic and lethal actions of glucorticoid hormones in lymphoid cells, in *Hormones and Cancer*, edited by S. Iacobelli et al. Raven, New York, 1980.

47. Crabtree, G. R., Gillis, S., Smith, K. A., and Munck, A.: Glucocorticoids and immune responses. *Arthritis Rheum.* 22:1246, 1979.

48. Rosenberg, S. A., and Lipsky, P. E.: The role of monocyte factors in the differentiation of immunoglobulin-secreting cells from human peripheral blood cells. *J. Immunol.* 125:232, 1980.

49. Mizel, S. R.: Physiochemical characterization of lymphocyte activating factor. *J. Immunol.* 122:2167, 1979.

50. Cantor, H., and Gershon, R. K.: Generation and analysis of T-cell clones that secrete antigen specific polypeptides mediating different T-cell functions, in *Regulatory T Lymphocytes*, edited by B. Pernis and H. Vogel. Academic, New York, in press.

51. Wedner, H. J., and Parker, C. W.: Lymphocyte activation. *Prog. Allergy* 20:195, 1976.

52. Ling, N. R., and Kay, J. E. (ed.): *Lymphocyte Stimulation*, American Elsevier, New York, 1975.

53. Lichtman, A. H., Segel, S. B., and Lichtman, M. A.: An ultrasensitive method for the measurement of human leukocyte calcium: Lymphocytes. *Clin. Chim. Acta* 97:107, 1979.

54. Lichtman, A. H., Segel, G. B., and Lichtman, M. A.: Total and exchangeable calcium in lymphocytes: Effects of PHA and A23187. *J. Supramol. Structure* 14:65, 1980.

55. Lichtman, A. H., Segel, G. B., and Lichtman, M. A.: Calcium transport and calcium-ATPase activity in human lymphocyte plasma membrane vesicles. *J. Biol. Chem.* 256:6148, 1981.

56. Segel, G. B., Simon, W., and Lichtman, M. A.: Regulation of sodium and potassium transport in phytohemagglutinin-stimulated human blood lymphocytes. *J. Clin. Invest.* 64:834, 1979.

57. Segel, G. B., Kovach, G., and Lichtman, M. A.: Sodium-potassium adenosine triphosphatase activity of human lymphocyte membrane vesicles: Kinetic parameters, substrate specificity, and effects of phytohemagglutinin. *J. Cell. Physiol.* 100:109, 1979.

58. Roos, D., and Loos, J. A.: Changes in the carbohydrate metabolism of mitogenically stimulated human peripheral lymphocytes. I. Stimulation by phytohemagglutinin. *Biochim. Biophys. Acta* 222:565, 1970.

59. Segel, G. B., Androphy, E. J., and Lichtman, M. A.: Increased ouabain-sensitive glycolysis of lymphocytes treated with phytohemagglutinin: Relationship to potassium transport. *J. Cell. Physiol.* 97:407, 1978.

60. Maino, V. C., Green, N. M., and Crumpton, M. J.: The role of calcium ion in initiating transformation of lymphocytes. *Nature* 251:324, 1974.

61. Quagliano, D., Torelli, U., Sauli, S., and Mauri, C.: Cytochemical and autoradiographic investigations on normal and myelomatous plasma cells. *Acta Haematol.* 38:79, 1967.

62. Sternholm, R. L.: Carbohydrate metabolism in leukocytes. VIII. Metabolism of glucose acetate and propionate by human plasma cells. *J. Bacteriol.* 93:1657, 1967.

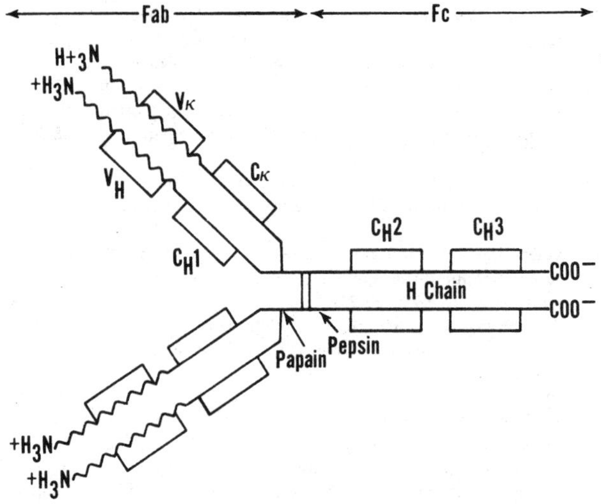

FIGURE 104-1 Schematic model of an IgG molecule of the IgG1 subclass containing kappa (κ) light chains. The sites of proteolytic cleavage by papain and by pepsin are shown. The intrachain disulfide bonds of the variable region domains ($V\kappa$, V_H) and constant region domains ($C\kappa$, C_H, C_H2, C_H3) are shown.

CHAPTER *104*

Functions of lymphocytes and plasma cells— immunoglobulin synthesis

DENNIS A. CARSON

Immunoglobulins are glycoproteins produced by B lymphocytes and plasma cells. Most, if not all, immunoglobulins have antibody activity, and can bind to antigens. A single person can probably synthesize immunoglobulin molecules with more than 1 million distinct amino acid sequences. This great diversity permits the humoral immune system to respond to almost any foreign antigenic challenge by increasing the rate of synthesis of complementary antibody. The binding of antibody to antigen initiates a series of biologically important effector functions, such as complement activation and adherence of the immune complex to receptors on leukocytes. The eventual outcome is the clearance and degradation of the foreign substance.

Immunoglobulin structure and function

All normal immunoglobulin molecules are variants of a 7 S basic unit consisting of two identical heavy (H) chains and two identical light (L) chains (see Fig. 104-1). The four polypeptides are held in a bilaterally symmetrical, Y-shaped structure by disulfide bonds and noncovalent interactions [1,2].

The internal disulfide bonds of the heavy and light chains cause the polypeptides to fold into compact globular shaped regions, called *domains*, each containing about 110 to 120 amino acid residues [3] (see Fig. 104–2). The light chains have two domains; the heavy chains have four or five domains. The amino-terminal domains of the heavy and light chains are designated the variable (V) regions, because their primary structure varies markedly among different immunoglobulin molecules [4]. The carboxy-terminal domains are referred to as constant (C) regions, because their primary structure is the same among immunoglobulins of the same class or subclass.

The amino acids in the light- and heavy-chain variable regions interact to form an antigen-binding site. Each four-chain immunoglobulin basic unit has two identical binding sites. The constant region domains of the heavy and light chains provide stability for the immunoglobulin molecule. The heavy-chain constant regions also mediate the specific effector functions of the different immunoglobulin classes.

Immoglobulin light chains have an approximate M_r of 23,000 daltons. They are divided into two types, kappa (κ) and lambda (λ), based upon multiple amino acid sequence differences in the single constant region domain [4]. The λ chains are divided further into subclasses. The proportion of κ to λ chains in adult human plasma is about 2:1. The constant regions of immunoglobulin light chains have no known effector function.

Immunoglobulin heavy chains have an M_r of 50,000 to 70,000 daltons, depending upon the number and length of the constant region domains. The five major classes of heavy chains, γ, α, μ, δ, and ε, determine the five corresponding classes of immunoglobulin: IgG, IgA, IgM, IgD, and IgE. The individual immunoglobulin molecules of each class may contain either κ or λ light chains, but not both. The distinct physical and functional properties of the human immunoglobulin classes are summarized in Tables 104-1 and 104-2.

Approximately 80 percent of the immunoglobulins in adult plasma are IgG. The IgG molecule is composed of the basic 7 S immunoglobulin four-chain structure, plus about 3 percent carbohydrate. IgG is the predominant antibody produced during the secondary immune response. IgG molecules effectively penetrate extravascular spaces and readily cross the placental barrier to provide passive immunity to the newborn.

Near the junction of the three arms of the Y-shaped immunoglobulin molecule, the two heavy chains interact to form the "hinge" region. Exposed between constant region globular domains, the hinge region is attacked readily by the proteolytic enzymes papain and pepsin. The cleavage sites are shown in Fig. 104-1. The digestion of IgG with papain yields three fragments.

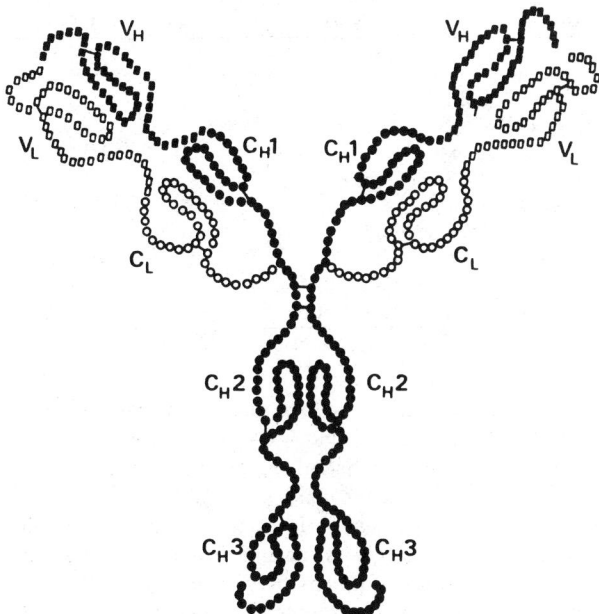

FIGURE 104-2 Folding of IgG. The variable and constant region domains of the heavy chain (V_H, C_H1, C_H2, C_H3) and light chains (V_L, C_L) fold into compact globular structures.

The single Fc piece contains the carboxyterminal region of both heavy chains. The two identical F(ab) pieces contain the entire light chain and the amino-terminal portion of the heavy chain.

TABLE 104-1 Physical properties of human immunoglobulins

WHO designation	IgG (γG)	IgA (γA)	IgM (γM)	IgD (γD)	IgE(γE)
Heavy-chain class	γ	α	μ	δ	ε
Heavy-chain subclass	γ1,γ2,γ3,γ4	α1,α,	μ1,μ2	Ja,La	—
M_r, daltons	150,000	160,000 (monomer) 400,000 (secretory)	900,000	180,000	190,000
Sedimentation coefficient	7 S	7 S, 11 S (secretory)	19 S	7 S	8 S
Antigen-binding valency	2	2	5 or 10	2	2
Concentration in serum, mg/ml	8–16	1.4–4.0	0.5–2.0	0–0.4	17–450 ng/ml
Percent of total immunoglobulin	80	13	6	1	0.002
Electrophoretic mobility	γ	Fast γ to β	Fast γ	Fast γ	Fast γ
Carbohydrate content, %	3	8	12	13	12

TABLE 104-2 Biological properties of human immunoglobulins

	IgG	IgA	IgM	IgD	IgE
Percent of body pool in intravascular space	45	42	76	75	51
Percent of intravascular pool catabolized per day	6.7	25	18	37	89
Normal synthetic rate mg/(kg·day)	33	24	6.7	0.4	0.02
$T_{1/2}$ (half-life in serum in days)	23	5.8	5.1	2.8	2.3
Complement fixation:					
Classical pathway	Yes	No	Yes	No	No
Alternate pathway	No	Yes	No	Weakly	Weakly
Placental transfer	Yes	No	No	No	No
Cytophilic for mast cells and basophils	No	No	No	No	Yes

TABLE 104-3   Characteristics of major subclasses of IgG

	IgG_1	IgG_2	IgG_3	IgG_4
Percent of total IgG	65	23	8	4
Heavy chain	$\gamma 1$	$\gamma 2$	$\gamma 3$	$\gamma 4$
Kappa/lambda ratio	2:1	1:1	1:1	5:1
Metabolism:				
Half-life, days	21	20	7	21
Percent catabolized daily	7	7	17	7
Functional features:				
Complement activation	+	Poor	+	0
Heterologous skin sensitization	+	0	+	+

Within the IgG class are four major subclasses designated IgG1, IgG2, IgG3, and IgG4. Each subclass has a distinct heavy-chain constant region, and mediates different effector functions [5,6] (see Table 104-3). The most abundant subclass is IgG1 which constitutes 65 percent of the total IgG in plasma. The IgG1 and IgG3 subclasses activate complement via the classical pathway; IgG2 proteins fix complement poorly, and IgG4 proteins not at all. IgG3 myeloma proteins may aggregate spontaneously to produce a hyperviscosity syndrome. Either aggregated IgG or antigen-antibody complexes will bind to specific receptors for the Fc fragment on the surface of macrophages and neutrophils. Once attached to the cell surface, the immune complexes are soon phagocytosed and degraded. The average half-life of circulating IgG molecules is approximately 21 days, although the exact value varies among the IgG subclasses (see Table 104-3).

IgA comprises about 13 percent of plasma immunoglobulins [7,8]. Specific IgA antibodies are synthesized during secondary immune responses. IgA circulates as a monomer, dimer, or higher polymer containing approximately 8 percent carbohydrate. The half-life of circulating IgA is 6 days. A modified form of IgA is the principal antibody in saliva, tears, colostrum, and the fluids of the gastrointestinal, respiratory, and urinary tracts. These secretory immunoglobulins consist

of an IgA dimer bound to J (or joining) chain polypeptide [9], and an M_r-70,000-dalton secretory component. The secretory component facilitates the transport of the IgA protein across the epithelial cell, and may protect the secreted IgA molecule from proteolytic digestion by enzymes in the intestinal lumen. IgA antibodies do not cross the placenta, fix complement via the classical pathway, or bind efficiently to cell surfaces. Indeed, their main function may be to prevent foreign substances from adhering to mucosal surfaces and gaining access to the internal immune system.

In normal adults, approximately 6 percent of the total plasma immunoglobulins belong to the IgM class. IgM molecules are 19 S macroglobulins containing 12 percent carbohydrate. The molecules are formed through the linkage of five identical immunoglobulin units by disulfide bonds and by the J chain (see Fig. 104-3) [10]. IgM represents the predominant immunoglobulin class formed during a primary immune response. Along with IgD, IgM is a major immunoglobulin on the surface of B cells [11,12]. IgM macroglobulins do not penetrate easily into extravascular spaces, or readily cross the placenta. Compared to monomeric IgG antibodies, pentavalent IgM antibodies fix complement more efficiently. A single IgM molecule on the surface of a red blood cell can initiate complement-mediated hemolysis. IgM is catabolized rapidly, with a plasma half-life of only 6 days.

IgD is a trace protein, comprising less than 1 percent of total plasma immunoglobulins [13]. The molecule has the basic four-chain immunoglobulin structure. The molecular weight of IgD is slightly higher than IgG, because of a lengthened heavy-chain constant region, and the addition of 11 percent carbohydrate. IgD antibodies do not penetrate extravascular spaces efficiently, cross the placental barrier, or fix complement via the classical pathway. Indeed, the role of soluble IgD in the immune response is not known. Most likely IgD functions primarily as a cell membrane receptor that binds antigen and triggers B-cell proliferation and differentiation.

IgE proteins, also known as reaginic antibodies, normally constitute only 0.004 percent of total plasma immunoglobulins [14,15]. In patients with parasitic infestation, and in some children with atopic diseases, plasma IgE levels may rise to 5 to 20 times normal. The IgE molecule consists of a four-chain basic unit, plus 12 percent carbohydrate. Monomeric IgE binds via the Fc

FIGURE 104-3   Schematic model of an IgM pentamer showing the positions of the heavy (H) chains, light (L) chains, and the single J chain.

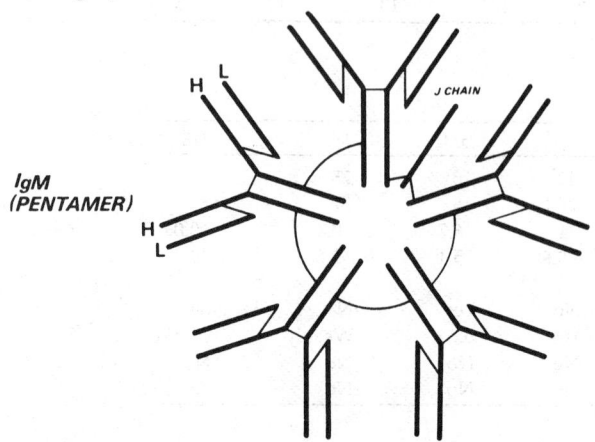

region to high-affinity receptors on the surface membranes of basophils and mast cells. In allergic subjects, the cross-linking of cell-bound IgE antibody by antigen induces the release of histamine, serotonin, slow reactive substance, eosinophilic chemotactic factor, and other vasoactive substances. The physiological functions of IgE antibodies are not known precisely. However, IgE in secretions may facilitate the expulsion of parasites from the gastrointestinal tract.

Genetics of immunoglobulins

Immunoglobulin genes are inherited in three unlinked multigene families, one for κ light chains, one for λ light chains, and one for the heavy-chain classes [16]. The heavy-chain gene family has been mapped to chromosome 14 [17]. Recently, the κ and λ light-chain gene families have been assigned to chromosomes 2 and 22, respectively [18].

As discussed above, each heavy- and light-chain polypeptide has an amino-terminal variable region domain and one to four carboxy-terminal constant region domains. Early sequence studies of myeloma proteins indicated that the variable and constant region domains were coded for by separate genes [19]. For many years, the concept of two genes for one polypeptide chain appeared to violate fundamental genetic precepts. However, it is known that many genes in higher organisms occur in pieces, rather than as continuous stretches of DNA [20]. Indeed, the generation of antibody diversity, the joining of variable and constant regions and the switching of antibody synthesis from one heavy chain class to another, all require DNA rearrangements.

Rearrangement of immunoglobulin variable region genes [20–22]

Two separate DNA segments, V and J, code for the κ light-chain variable region. The V-region segment corresponds to amino acids 1 to 95. The J-region DNA segment (not to be confused with the J polypeptide) codes approximately for amino acids 95 to 110. The human λ light-chain genes have recently been studied, and are organized similarly. Three discontinuous DNA segments, designated V, D, and J, contribute to the variable region domain shared by all the heavy-chain classes.

In embryonic DNA, the different immunoglobulin gene segments are present in multiple copies of closely related sequences arranged linearly along chromosomes 14, 2, and 22. During the differentiation of B lymphocytes, a number of immunoglobulin gene rearrangements occur. A complete light-chain variable region gene is assembled from a randomly chosen V segment, and one of the J segments. In the case of the heavy-chain variable region gene, a D segment is also included (see Fig. 104-4). The process probably is accompanied by the deletion of intervening DNA sequences. The assembled variable region gene is transcribed together with DNA

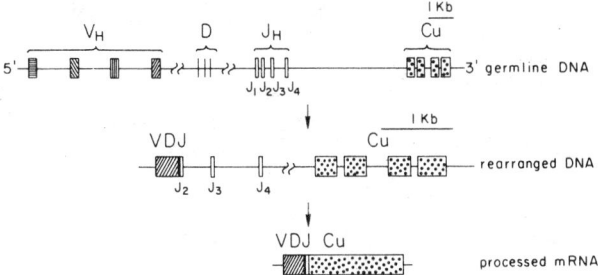

FIGURE 104-4 Rearrangement of heavy-chain gene segments in the mouse. The upper diagram shows the arrangement of gene segments in the germ line. During B-cell differentiation, a V-, D-, and J-gene segment combine to form a complete variable region gene. The process may be accompanied by the deletion of intervening DNA. (From Gearhart [21].)

segments coding for the constant region domains. The splicing of the RNA transcript brings the variable and constant region segments together prior to translation.

Under normal conditions, a B lymphocyte or plasma cell synthesizes only one species of light chain, even though the cell has two different sets of κ-chains genes, and two sets of λ-chain genes. This phenomenon is called *allelic exclusion*. Apparently, when one complete light-chain gene is successfully assembled, all further light-chain gene rearrangements cease. The remaining DNA segments persist in the embryonic configuration, or are improperly rearranged, or deleted. Hence, they are not expressed as immunoglobulin polypeptides. A similar mechanism probably occurs at the level of heavy-chain variable region genes.

Five established mechanisms contribute to the generation of diversity among immunoglobulin polypeptide variable regions [20–23]. They are (1) the presence in the germ line of multiple different V, J, and D gene segments, (2) the random joining together of these DNA segments to produce a complete V gene, (3) uncorrected errors made during the recombination process, (4) somatic mutations within the DNA segments themselves, and (5) the coming together of the heavy- and light-chain polypeptides to produce a complete immunoglobulin monomer capable of binding antigen. Each process works independently and in a different manner. The net result is the enormous diversity of human immunoglobulins.

Heavy-chain class switching

During differentiation, a single B lymphocyte can synthesize heavy chains with different constant regions coupled to the same variable region. Very immature B cells, sometimes called pre-B cells, synthesize cytoplasmic μ chains in the absence of light chains. Subsequently, intact IgM monomers are inserted into the plasma membrane, followed by IgD molecules with the same specificity. The IgM and IgD constant region genes are closely linked in embryonic DNA, and may be

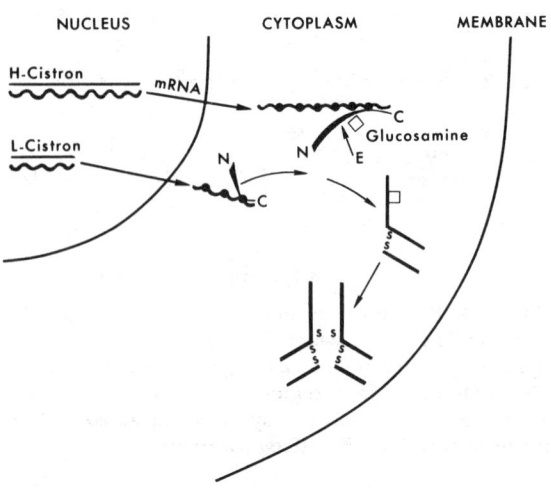

NUCLEUS   CYTOPLASM   MEMBRANE

FIGURE 104-5 Schematic representation of the process of antibody synthesis. The genes for H (heavy) and L (light) polypeptide chains are transcribed, and each mRNA molecule becomes associated with ribosomes in the cytoplasm. Amino acid incorporation into the polypeptide chains is followed by addition of glucosamine (empty box). E designates glycosyltransferase enzymes. The light and heavy chains combine by linkage of SH groups and hydrogen bonding to form half of an immunoglobulin molecule. Two halves are linked by disulfide bonds to form the four-polypeptide-chain immunoglobulin molecule.

transcribed together. The differential splicing of the transcript allows the simultaneous synthesis of the two immunoglobulin heavy chains from a single species of messenger RNA.

The secretion of IgM, and the switch from IgM to IgG or IgA synthesis, probably requires the prior interaction of lymphocytes with antigen or mitogen. Factors produced by antigen-reactive T lymphocytes strongly influence which B cells differentiate into IgM-secreting plasma cells, and which change to the synthesis of another immunoglobulin class. The switch in heavy-chain classes is accompanied by the deletion of intervening DNA segments and the apposition of the previously rearranged variable region gene next to the new constant region gene [22].

Genetic markers on immunoglobulins

Human immunoglobulins have inherited differences in structure, termed *allotypes* [24,25]. These genetic markers usually are detected with agglutinating sera from individuals naturally immunized through transfusion or pregnancy. The antibodies recognize minor amino acid sequence variations in the constant regions of γ, α, and κ chains (see Chap. 163). No definite allotypic differences have been detected on μ, δ, or ϵ chains.

The κ light-chain allotypes are designated Km (formerly called Inv). The Am markers are on the heavy chains of the IgA2 subclass. The G1m, G2m, and G3m allotype markers are on the heavy chains of the IgG1, IgG2, and IgG3 subclasses, respectively. As discussed

earlier, all the heavy-chain constant region genes reside on chromosome 14. Therefore, different combinations of heavy-chain allotype markers are inherited as haplotypic units, in an autosomal codominant manner.

The frequency of the various allelic markers differs among ethnic groups. Immunoglobulin allotyping has been applied clinically in population studies of disease, and in forensic medicine [26].

The Kern, Oz, and Mcg markers reflect minor nonallelic amino acid differences in the constant region of λ-chain [27].

Immunoglobulin synthesis and secretion

The total IgG content of the adult human body is about 75 g, of which 2.2 g is synthesized each day [28]. Most immunoglobulin is produced by mature plasma cells, which have abundant rough endoplasmic reticulum and a well-developed Golgi apparatus [29–31].

The final messenger RNAs for immunoglobulin light and heavy chains are derived from the stepwise cleavage of large nuclear RNA transcripts [22]. In plasma cells, the rearranged and spliced mRNA molecules for the heavy- and light-chain polypeptides are translated on separate ribosomal complexes. An amino-terminal leader peptide approximately 18 to 30 residues long is cleaved prior to the release of the completed light and heavy chains into the cisternae of the endoplasmic reticulum. There the two polypeptides spontaneously combine to form immunoglobulin half-molecules that are stabilized by disulfide bonds. The joining of two identical half-molecules by disulfide bonds yields a basic four-chain immunoglobulin unit (see Fig. 104-5). The entire process usually takes less than 30 min.

Glycosyltransferase enzymes add an orderly sequence of sugars to the assembled immunoglobulin unit to form branched chain oligosaccharides composed of N-acetylglucosamine, mannose, galactose, fucose, and sialic acid. The oligosaccharides are attached covalently to the immunoglobulin heavy chain at several distinct sites. The carbohydrate facilitates the transport of the antibody molecule across the plasma membrane and into the extracellular space [31] (see Fig. 104-6), and increases the solubility of the secreted protein.

Fix 7 S monomeric units of IgM combine to form a pentameric macroglobulin linked by disulfide bonds and a single J-chain polypeptide [9,10]. Usually polymerization immediately precedes or occurs simultaneously with IgM secretion. Similarly, IgA molecules form dimers and polymers linked by the J chain just prior to secretion from the plasma cell [8]. The secretory piece is added to IgA dimers by mucosal epithelial cells.

Regulation of immunoglobulin synthesis

A normal adult has preexisting B lymphocytes that can interact with almost any foreign antigen. In the presence of accessory T lymphocytes and macrophages, an

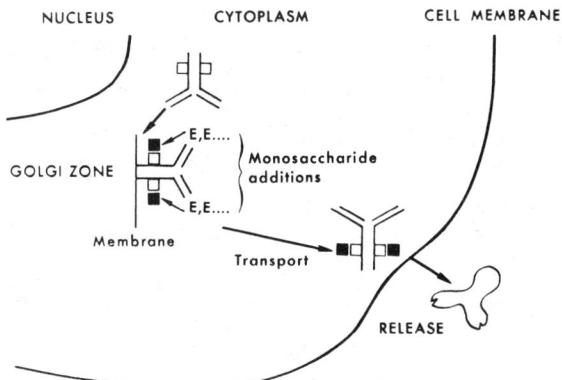

FIGURE 104-6 Schematic representation of carbohydrate addition and antibody secretion. The four-polypeptide-chain molecule becomes attached to membrane in the Golzi zone, where additional carbohydrate (glucosamine, galactosamine) is added. E designates glycosyltransferase enzymes. The completed molecule is transported through the cytoplasm and transferred across the cell membrane into the extracellular milieu. (Adapted from Scherr and Ihr [31].)

antigen-binding clone of B lymphocytes transforms into both memory cells and antibody-secreting plasma cells. Most plasma cells are terminally differentiated and do not divide. Therefore, the continued production of antibody depends upon the rate of plasma cell generation, the functional life-span of the plasma cells, and the half-life of the immunoglobulin protein in the body.

Antibody synthesis is highly regulated by helper and suppressor T lymphocytes. This topic is reviewed in Chaps. 13, 105, and 106. Additionally, secreted immunoglobulin regulates its own production by binding antigen and removing it from the circulation. By preventing the interaction of antigen with immunoglobulin receptors on B lymphocytes, antibody inhibits the generation of more plasma cells.

The body also has an internal, self-contained mechanism for regulating antibody synthesis [32]. Each of the more than 1 million immunoglobulin variants in a single person carries individually specific antigenic determinants, designated *idiotypes*. The idiotypic antigens reflect the unique amino acid sequences of immunoglobulin variable regions, particularly in the area of the antigen binding site. Idiotypes were recognized originally by anti-idiotypic antibodies produced by closely related, genetically nonidentical subjects. However, recent evidence suggests that anti-idiotypic antibodies directed against one's own immunoglobulins are also elicited during a normal immune response [33]. Anti-idiotypic antibodies may bind to complementary idiotypes to form endogenous immune complexes that are removed from the circulation. T lymphocytes may also recognize idiotype antigens. Even in the absence of any external antigenic stimulus, idiotypes and anti-idiotypes probably interact continually. The self-regulating internal network of idiotypes and anti-idiotypes serves to prevent the overproduction of any particular immunoglobulin molecule.

Myelomas and hybridomas

In multiple myeloma, malignant plasma cells or their precursors uncontrollably synthesize large amounts of homogeneous immunoglobulin or immunoglobulin fragments. The excess production of light chains results in the appearance of Bence-Jones proteins ·in the plasma and urine. Patients with heavy-chain disease may produce incompletely or improperly rearranged fragments of one of the heavy chain classes (see Chaps. 121 and 124).

Cell lines capable of continuous growth and tissue culture have been established from mice with transplantable plasmacytomas. These cells retain the plasma cells' capacity to synthesize immunoglobulin. In the presence of polyethylene glycol or inactivated Sendai virus, hypoxanthine phosphoribosyltransferase (HGPRT)–deficient variants of mouse plasma cell lines will fuse successfully with B lymphocytes or plasma cells from an immune mouse to yield somatic cell hybrids, commonly called hybridomas [34–37] (Fig. 104-7).

FIGURE 104-7 Monoclonal antibody production. A mouse plasmacytoma cell line deficient in hypoxanthine phosphoribosyltransferase (HPRT) is fused to spleen cells from an immunized mouse. The hybrid cells are selected in HAT medium (medium containing hypoxanthine, aminopterin, and thymidine) and then are cloned and expanded. (From Diamond et al. [36].)

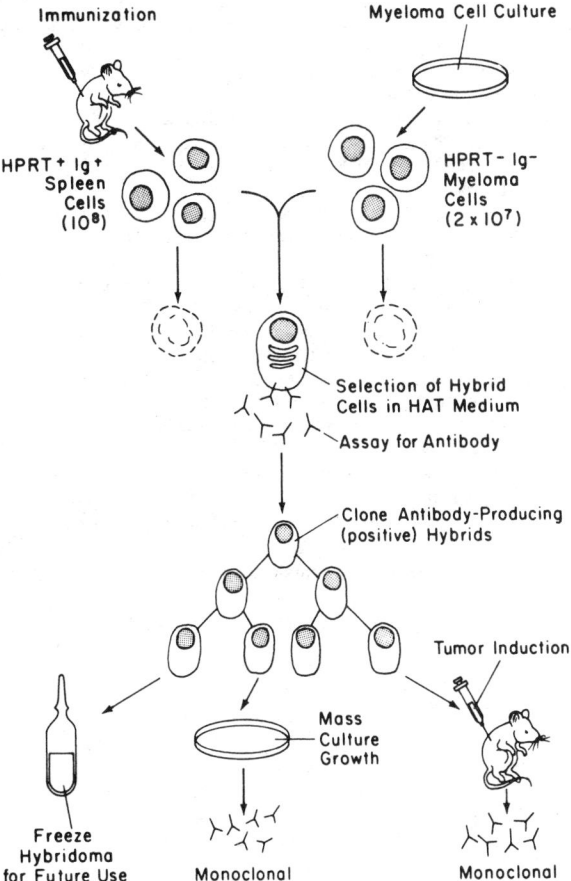

The hybrids, but not the myeloma parental cells, grow in HAT medium (a medium containing hypoxanthine, aminopterin, and thymidine which does not permit growth of HGPRT-deficient cells) in unlimited numbers. They may be further propagated either in tissue culture or in the peritoneal cavity of mice. The hybridomas synthesize massive quantities of monoclonal antibody with the identical antigenic reactivity as the single normal lymphocyte parent which fused with the myeloma cell.

In an intact animal, immunization elicits the synthesis of diverse antibody molecules that recognize antigen with varying degrees of affinity and specificity. In contrast, hybridoma-derived monoclonal antibodies bind antigen with complete uniformity.

The development of hybridoma methodology is the practical outcome of basic experiments concerning immunoglobulin synthesis and assembly. One can now prepare monoclonal antibodies against impure and even uncharacterized substances, such as antigens on cell membranes. Mouse monoclonal antibodies are used in the diagnosis and classification of leukemia and lymphomas [37] (see Chap. 114). Ultimately, the monoclonal proteins may have value as immunotherapeutic agents, replacing conventional antiserums.

References

1. Porter, R. R.: Structural studies of immunoglobulins. *Science 180*:713, 1973.
2. Nisonoff, A., Hopper, J. E., and Spring, S. B.: *The Antibody Molecule.* Academic, New York, 1975.
3. Poljak, R. J., Amzel, L. M., Chen, B. L., Phizackerley, R. P., and Saul, F.: The three-dimensional structure of the Fab' fragment of a human myeloma protein at 2.0A resolution. *Proc. Natl. Acad. Sci. U.S.A. 71*:3440, 1974.
4. Kabat, E. A., Wu, T. T., and Bilofsky, H.: *Sequences of Immunoglobulin Chains.* National Institutes of Health, Washington, D.C., Publication No. 80-2008, 1977.
5. Spiegelberg, H. L.: Biological activities of immunoglobulins of different classes and subclasses. *Adv. Immunol. 19*:259, 1974.
6. Morell, A., Terry, W. D., and Waldmann, T. A.: Metabolic properites of IgG subclasses in man. *J. Clin. Invest. 46*:673, 1970.
7. Tomasi, T. B., and Grey, H. M.: Structure and function of immunoglobulin A. *Progr. Allergy 16*:81, 1982.
8. Mestecky, J., and Lawton, A. R. (eds.): *The Immunoglobulin A System.* Plenum, New York, 1974.
9. Koshland, M. E.: The structure and function of J chains. *Adv. Immunol. 20*:41, 1975.
10. Metzger, H.: Structure and function of γM macroglobulins. *Adv. Immunol. 12*:57, 1970.
11. Warner, N. L.: Membrane immunoglobulins and antigen receptors on B and T lymphocytes. *Adv. Immunol. 19*:67, 1974.
12. Vitetta, E. S., and Uhr, J. W.: Immunoglobulin receptors revisited. *Science 189*:964, 1975.
13. Moller, G. (ed.): Immunoglobulin D: Structure synthesis, membrane representation, and function. *Immunol. Rev. 37*:1, 1977.
14. Ishizaka, K., and Dayton, D. H. (eds): *The Biological Role of the Immunoglobulin E System.* U.S. Department of Health, Education, and Welfare, Washington, D.C., 1973.
15. Bennich, H.: Structure of IgE. *Progr. Immunol. 2*:49, 1974.
16. Fudenberg, H. H. (ed.): *Basic Immunogenetics,* 2d ed. Oxford University Press, New York, 1977.
17. Croce, C. M., et al.: Chromosomal location of the genes for human immunoglobulin heavy chains. *Proc. Natl. Acad. Sci. U.S.A. 76*:3416, 1979.
18. McBride, O. W., Hieter, P. A., Hollis, G. F., Swan, D., Otey, M. C., and Leder, P.: Chromosomal location of human kappa and lambda immunoglobulin light chain constant region genes. *J. Exp. Med. 155*:1480, 1982.
19. Gally, J., and Edelman, G. M.: The genetic control of immunoglobulin synthesis. *Ann. Rev. Genet. 6*:1, 1972.
20. Moller, G. (ed.): Organization of immunoglobulin genes. *Immunol. Rev. 59*:1, 1981.
21. Gearhart, P. J.: Generation of immunoglobulin variable gene diversity. *Immunol. Today 3*:107, 1982.
22. Marx, J. L.: Antibodies: Getting their genes together. *Science 212*:1015, 1981.
23. Baltimore, D.: Somatic mutation gains its place among the generators of diversity. *Cell 26*:295, 1981.
24. Schanfield, M. S.: Immunoglobulins: Genetic markers, in *Basic and Clinical Immunology,* 3d ed., edited by H. H. Fudenberg, D. P. Stites, J. L. Caldwell, and J. V. Wells. Lange Medical, Los Altos, Calif., 1980, pp. 79–83.
25. Natvig, J. R., and Kunkel, H. G.: Human immunoglobulins: Classes, subclasses, genetic variants and idiotypes. *Adv. Immunol. 16*:1, 1973.
26. Sebring, E. S., Polefsky, H. F., and Schonfield, M. S.: Gm and Km allotypes in disputed parentage. *Am. J. Clin. Pathol. 71*:208, 1979.
27. Ein, D.: Nonallelic behavior of the Oz group in human lambda immunoglobulin chains. *Proc. Natl. Acad. Sci. U.S.A. 60*:962, 1968.
28. Waldman, T. A., and Strober, W.: Metabolism of immunoglobulins. *Progr. Allergy 13*:1, 1969.
29. Parkhouse, R. M. E.: Assembly and secretion of immunoglobulin M (IgM) by plasma cells and lymphocytes. *Transplant Rev. 14*:163, 1963.
30. Buxbaum, J. N.: The biosynthesis, assembly, and secretion of immunoglobulin. *Semin. Hematol. 10*:33, 1973.
31. Scherr, C. J., and Ihr, J. W.: Immunoglobulin synthesis and secretion. III. Incorporation of glucosamine into immunoglobulin polyribosomes. *Proc. Natl. Acad. Sci. U.S.A. 64*:381, 1971.
32. Jerne, N. K.: The immune system: A web of V-domain. *Harvey Lectures 70*:93, 1976.
33. Brown, J. C., and Rodkey, L. C.: Autoregulation of an antibody response via network induced auto-anti-idiotype. *J. Exp. Med. 150*:67, 1979.
34. Kohler, G., and Milstein, C.: Continuous cultures of fused cells secreting antibody of a predefined specificity. *Nature 256*:495, 1975.
35. Galfré, G., and Milstien, C.: Preparation of monoclonal antibodies: Strategies and procedures. *Methods Enzymol 73*:1, 1981.
36. Diamond, B. A., Yelton, D. E., and Scharff, M. D.: Monoclonal antibodies. *N. Engl. J. Med. 3(4)*:1344, 1981.
37. Kennett, R. H., McKearn, J. J., and Bechtol, K. B. (eds.): *Monoclonal Antibodies.* Plenum, New York, 1981.

CHAPTER *105*

Function of lymphocytes and plasma cells in immunity

JOHN R. HUDDLESTONE
FRANCIS V. CHISARI

Critical investigations of the structure and function of the cells of the immune system have identified a complex series of interactions by a variety of lymphocytic and nonlymphocytic subpopulations which are necessary for normal immune responses [reviewed in Ref. 1]. Both clinical and experimental studies demonstrate a requirement for three major cellular populations, T lymphocytes, B lymphocytes, and macrophages.

T lymphocytes, whose progenitors are induced to differentiate and express T-lymphocyte phenotypy under the influence of the thymic environment, play both regulatory and effector roles. The effector T lymphocytes are responsible for the phenomena of cell-mediated immunity, including cytolysis of virus-infected cells, defense against fungal or intracellular bacterial infections, graft-versus-host reaction, allograft rejection, and some forms of tumor immunity. Regulatory T lymphocytes control both effector T–lymphocyte and B-lymphocyte functions by either inducing or suppressing their proliferation and differentiation.

B lymphocytes, which derive, postnatally, from bone marrow progenitors, respond to appropriate antigenic stimulation by differentiating into specific antibody–secreting plasma cells, thus providing the major mechanism of defense against pyogenic bacteria and certain viruses.

Macrophages, which derive from marrow stem cells, perform a wide array of functions, including antigen phagocytosis and presentation, secretion of a variety of molecules which modulate lymphocytic function, and cytolysis.

Finally, there is a third class of human lymphoid cell which lacks surface markers characteristic of T or B lymphocytes (*null cell*) and mediates spontaneous killing of tumor cells and antibody-dependent cytolysis.

Surface membrane determinants of human lymphocyte subpopulations and macrophages

B LYMPHOCYTES

B lymphocytes are identified by the presence of surface membrane–bound monomeric immunoglobulin, which functions as an antigen-specific receptor (Table 105-1). Whereas 10 to 16 percent of blood lymphocytes express surface IgM and/or IgD, less than 2 percent of the total blood lymphocytes express IgG, IgA, or IgE [2]. B lymphocytes bear Fc receptors for several immunoglobulin isotypes (IgM, IgG, IgA, and IgE), and these receptors

TABLE 105-1   Characteristics of human lymphocyte/monocyte subpopulations

Cell type	Abbreviation	Function	Markers
Bone marrow–derived lymphocyte	B cell	Antibody synthesis	SmIg, Fc, C, EBV, Ia, Bl, HLA-D
Thymus-derived lymphocyte	T cell	See text	SRBC, HLA-A, HLA-B, HLA-C, OKT1, Leu 1, 17F12
Killer	TK	Antigen-specific HLA-restricted cytolysis	TH2, OKT5, OKT8, Leu 2a, Leu 2b
Helper	TH	Induction and amplification of B- and T-cell responses	Fcγ, OKT4, Leu 3
Suppressor	TS	Suppression of B- and T-cell responses	TH2, OKT5, OKT8, Leu 2a, Leu 2b, Ia, Fcγ, H2
Delayed hypersensitivity	T_{DTH}	Chemotactic lymphokine production (e.g., MIF)	
Null lymphocyte:			
Natural killer	NK	Spontaneous cell-mediated cytotoxicity	Fc, C, Ia, EBV
Killer	K	Antibody-dependent cellular cytotoxicity	Fc, C, Ia, EBV
Monocyte/macrophage	Mφ	Phagocytosis, antigen processing and presentation, suppression of T-cell responses	Ia, OKM1, esterase, peroxidase

NOTE: SmIg = surface membrane immunoglobulin; Fc = Fc receptor; C = complement component receptor; EBV = Epstein-Barr virus receptor; HLA = histocompatibility antigens; Ia = Ia antigens; HTLA = human T-lymphocyte antigen; TH2 = T-cell differentiation; H2 = histamine receptor; B1, OKT4, IKT5, OKT8, Leu 2a, Leu 2b, Leu 3, OKT1, Leu 1, 17F12, OKM1 = differentiation antigens recognized by monoclonal antibodies; SRBC = sheep red blood cell receptor; MIF = migration inhibitory factor.

are spatially associated with Ia-like membrane antigens [3–6]. Ia antigens, products of the immune response (Ir) genes or closely related genes in the major histocompatibility complex, are two-chain glycoproteins which play a critical role in the regulation of the immune response. They are present as surface markers on B lymphocytes, macrophages, null cells, and activated T cells and are also structural components on antigen-specific helper and suppressor factors derived from T cells. Receptors for a variety of complement components, including C3b, C3d, and C4b, exist on the B-lymphocyte membrane [7]. A spatial association also exists between the C3d receptor and the receptor for Epstein-Barr virus which is present on all B lymphocytes [8]. HLA-D coded determinants are present on the B-cell surface and have been designated as B alloantigens or DR antigens analogous to the murine Ia antigens [9].

Heteroantisera recognizing specific B-cell determinants have been produced [10]. With the use of monoclonal hybridoma technology a new antigen, termed B1, has been found on more than 95 percent of peripheral B lymphocytes and is not related to surface immunoglobulin nor to known Ia antigens [11]. Detection of these surface markers may be used both to study cellular collaboration in immune responses and to identify alterations in the qualitative and quantitative composition of B cells in human disease states.

T LYMPHOCYTES

T lymphocytes possess surface receptors for sheep erythrocytes (SRBC) [12] (Table 105-1). Technical factors greatly influence the proportion of SRBC-rosetting lymphocytes. For example, approximately 65 percent of normal blood lymphocytes form rosettes at 4°C, but less than 25 percent form rosettes at 37°C, and neuraminidase treatment of the SRBC increases the rosetting percentage at 4°C to 75 percent [13]. Human T lymphocytes also possess receptors for the Fc portions of IgM (Tμ), IgG (Tγ), IgA (Tα), and IgE (Tϵ). Tγ lymphocytes suppress B-lymphocyte immunoglobulin synthesis, are relatively radiation-sensitive, and contain a subset which mediates spontaneous and antibody-dependent cytotoxicity. In contrast, Tμ lymphocytes induce immunoglobulin synthesis, are insensitive to radiation, and do not mediate cytolysis [14,15].

Differentiation antigens specific for the total T-lymphocyte population and for functionally distinct subpopulations were initially identified using exhaustively absorbed heterologous antisera. Antisera against a human specific T-lymphocyte antigen (HTLA) react with approximately 65 percent of blood lymphocytes and 97 percent of thymocytes [16]. Another heteroantiserum identifies a subpopulation of T lymphocytes, termed TH2, which contains cells that mediate cytolysis in the allogeneic mixed lymphocyte reaction and, presumably, another subset of cells which also suppresses T-cell and B-cell responses [17]. In contrast, TH2-negative cells have markedly less cytotoxic activity but amplify (help) the functions of other cells and proliferate in response to specific antigens [17]. T suppressor lymphocytes also express a histamine–type 2 receptor which may serve to activate the suppressor cells [18].

Application of monoclonal antibody techniques to the identification of T lymphocyte differentiation antigens has resulted in the rapid introduction of a number of markers many of which are still incompletely characterized (Table 105-2). Monoclonal antibodies Leu 1, OKT1, and 17F12 [19–21] bind to more than 95 percent of peripheral T lymphocytes and precipitate a surface molecule of M_r 67,000 daltons. There is recent evidence that the antibodies identify a molecule homologous to murine Ly 1 antigen [21]. Antibody 9.6 is also a pan–T lymphocyte marker and identifies an antigen associated with the SRBC-rosette receptor [22]. Antibody OKT2 [23] precipitates a M_r 20,000-dalton molecule and identifies approximately 90 percent of peripheral T lymphocytes [24].

Monoclonal antibodies which identify the TH2-positive suppressor/cytotoxic population include OKT5, OKT8 [23], and Leu 2a and Leu 2b [21] (Table 105-2). Because Leu 2a and Leu 2b precipitate a macromolecule composed of two subunits with molecular weights of approximately 32,000 and 43,000 daltons, they are hy-

TABLE 105-2   T-lymphocyte differentiation antigens recognized by monoclonal antibodies

Antibody	Molecular weight of target antigen, daltons	Percent positive T lymphocytes	References
9.6	55,000	>99	[22]
Leu 1/17F12	67,000	98	[19]
OKT1	67,000	98	[20]
OKT2	20,000	>90	[23]
Leu 2a*	32,000/43,000	20–40	[21]
Leu 2b*	32,000/43,000	20–40	[21]
Leu 3	55,000	55–65	[21]
OKT4	62,000	55–65	[63]
OKT5	30,000/32,000	20–40	[63]

* Macromolecule composed of dimers of two subunits whose weights are listed.

pothesized to recognize human antigens analogous with murine Ly2 and Ly3 antigens. The TH2-negative, inducer/helper subpopulation is labeled by monoclonal antibodies OKT4 and Leu 3, and the latter antibody precipitates a M_r 55,000-dalton surface protein [21]. Finally activation of T suppressor lymphocytes is associated with the membrane expression of Ia antigens [26].

NULL LYMPHOCYTES

The null lymphocytes representing approximately 15 percent of the peripheral lymphocyte population lack high-affinity SRBC receptors and surface immunoglobulin [27] and therefore cannot be classified with respect to lineage or murine analogue. Null cells express Ia-like antigens and Fc receptors for IgG, but in contrast to B lymphocytes these do not occur in spatial association [28]. Receptors for complement components and Epstein-Barr virus also occur on null cells and have led to the speculation that null cells are of B-lymphocyte lineage. Monoclonal antibody OKM1 labels null cells [29]. Since this antibody also identifies macrophages, it has been suggested that null cells are of monocytic origin, despite the fact that they are not stained by α-naphthyl acetate esterase [30].

MONOCYTES-MACROPHAGES

Macrophages are classically identified by positive α-naphthyl acetate esterase staining, by glass and plastic surface adherence, and by functional tests of phagocytosis. Surface determinants on macrophages include receptors for various complement components and for the Fc region of IgG. The monoclonal antibody OKM1 [29] reacts with all monocyte-macrophages but also cross-reacts with null cells [29] as well as a subpopulation of T lymphocytes which have Fc receptors for IgG [24] and with granulocytes. In contrast, a monoclonal antibody which precipitates a surface protein of M_r 200,000 daltons and only reacts with macrophages and granulocytes has been produced [31].

Functional properties of human lymphocyte subsets

B-LYMPHOCYTE FUNCTION

B-lymphocyte immunoglobulin synthesis in vivo (Table 105-3) is initiated by the binding of macrophage-processed antigen to specific B-lymphocyte surface Ig serving as receptors. Subsequent proliferation and differentiation into specific antibody–producing plasma cells and memory cells (see below) is modulated by interactions with regulatory T lymphocytes. The plasma cells secrete class- and antigen-specific immunoglobulin while the pool of memory cells remains inactive until stimulated to participate in the rapid and abundant production of IgG and IgA following secondary exposure to antigen [1].

In vitro stimulation of human B lymphocytes by a vari-

TABLE 105-3 Functional properties of lymphocyte subsets

Function	B cell	T cell	Null cell	Macrophage
Antibody synthesis	+	−	−	−
Lymphokine synthesis:				
MIF	+	+	+	−
Interferon	−	+	+	−
Lymphotoxin	−	+	−	−
Regulation:				
Induction	−	+	−	+
Suppression	−	+	−	+
Cytolysis:				
HLA-restricted	−	+	−	−
Antibody-dependent	−	+	+	−
Natural killer	−	+	+	−
Proliferation:				
Antigen-specific	+	+	−	−
Allogeneic response	−	+	−	−
EBV-induced	+	−	+	−
Phagocytosis	−	−	−	+

ety of mitogens results in polyclonal, antigen-nonspecific immunoglobulin synthesis. Induction of IgM, IgG, and IgA synthesis by pokeweed mitogen (PWM) requires cellular proliferation and is both monocyte and T-lymphocyte dependent. T-lymphocyte modulation of PWM-stimulated B cells may be provided by either autologous or allogeneic T lymphocytes and exhibits dose-response characteristics [32]. The B-lymphocyte subpopulation which produces IgM and IgG in response to PWM expresses IgG on its surface membrane and therefore represents less than 15 percent of the B-cell population [33]. PWM-stimulated IgM synthesis is accomplished by lymphocytes bearing both surface IgM and IgD, but the IgG-synthesizing subpopulation is heterogeneous with regard to surface IgM expression [34]. There is evidence that other mitogens, such as bacterial lipopolysaccharides (LPS), *Nocardia* water-soluble mitogen, and tuberculin PPD, stimulate subsets of B lymphocytes with different characteristics than those stimulated by PWM [35].

The in vitro synthesis of antigen-specific antibody by human B lymphocytes has been accomplished with a limited number of antigens such as ovalbumin [36] and tetanus toxoid [37]. Although the synthesis is antigen driven and T-lymphocyte dependent, there still exists a separate requirement for mitogen stimulation of the culture. Analogous to nonspecific immunoglobulin synthesis, the subpopulations of B lymphocytes stimulated by different mitogens have widely varying characteristics. Thus, LPS-reactive B lymphocytes are unable to produce tetanus toxoid–specific IgG, while PWM-reactive B cells which produce IgG against tetanus toxoid have surface membrane IgM and IgD, and PPD-reactive B cells making antitetanus IgG lack membrane IgD [38].

The requirement for the presence of mitogen and T helper lymphocytes to induce antigen-specific antibody may be abrogated after in vivo perturbation of the immune system with reimmunization. Commencing 5 to 8 days after booster immunization with tetanus toxoid, lymphoblastoid cells can be isolated which spontaneously secrete antigen-specific IgG in the absence of mitogen or T lymphocytes [39].

T LYMPHOCYTE FUNCTION

T lymphocytes mediate a complex and heterogeneous set of functions in response to antigen- or mitogen-induced activation. The mitogenic responses, triggered by the interaction of a lectin with lymphocyte surface carbohydrates, are polyclonal, and involve 40 to 60 percent of lymphocytes. In contrast, response to a single antigen involves less than 1 percent of the lymphocytes. However, the metabolic and immunologic events triggered by mitogen activation, including proliferation and release of lymphokines, are analogous to those occurring during activation by specific antigens. Of the large number of lectins available, phytohemagglutinin, concanavalin A, and pokeweed mitogen are the best defined. All demonstrate the requirement for a small number of macrophages and all preferentially activate different lymphocyte populations. Phytohemagglutinin and concanavalin A are T-cell mitogens: 90 percent of their activated lymphoblasts derive from T lymphocytes. Moreover helper T lymphocytes are most responsive to phytohemagglutinin while suppressor T lymphocytes are most responsive to concanavalin A [40]. In contrast, 50 percent of pokeweed mitogen—induced blasts are of T-cell and 50 percent of B-cell origin. Immune reactivity to antigenic stimuli depends on the net balance between regulatory influences capable of amplifying or suppressing the effector response, and the T helper and T suppressor subpopulations provide the major cellular basis for this regulation. These T-lymphocyte subpopulations can be distinguished by surface markers. For example, T helper lymphocytes react with OKT4 monoclonal antibody, and T suppressor cells with OKT8. Functional assessment of these regulatory cells may be accomplished in mitogen-activated polyclonal assays as well as in antigen-specific systems. T helper lymphocytes are relatively radioresistant, and soluble T helper lymphocyte products are an absolute requirement for blood lymphocyte proliferation and differentiation in assays as diverse as soluble tetanus toxoid-induced proliferation and pokeweed mitogen–induced B-cell synthesis of immunoglobulin. T helper lymphocyte participation in these assays does not require prior activation [31]. T helper effects, like T suppressor effects, are mediated by lymphokines with varying physicochemical properties. Antigen-specific T helper factors, for example, interact specifically with their stimulating antigen and contain Ia antigen [41], while nonspecific factors exhibit neither of these properties.

T suppressor lymphocytes are only infrequently found activated in blood lymphocytes from normal individuals and therefore usually require activation by interaction with concanavalin A or, in the case of Tγ lymphocytes, with IgG-containing immune complexes. T

suppressor lymphocytes are quite susceptible to radiation, their function being abolished by exposure to as little as 1200 R [42]. Activated T suppressor cells inhibit proliferation of T lymphocytes in specific phytohemagglutinin and antigen-stimulated cultures and probably inhibit pokeweed mitogen—induced B lymphocyte immunoglobulin synthesis by suppression of the necessary T helper lymphocyte induction, as well as by the release of factors which inhibit all lymphocyte proliferation [43].

In addition to specific and nonspecific suppressor and helper factors, activated lymphocytes secrete a large number of lymphokines including migration inhibitory factor and interferon. Migration inhibitory factor (MIF) is a glycoprotein produced by T lymphocytes as a consequence of activation by antigen or lectins. It interacts with macrophage surface receptors and prevents their subsequent migration, thus maintaining a high density of phagocytes at the site of cellular immune reactions. Interferons are produced by lymphocytes as a result of viral infection and immune-specific interactions between virus and sensitized lymphocytes. The latter, termed *immune interferon*, can be distinguished from viral-induced interferon by antigenic and physical properties such as stability at pH 2. Other lymphokines known to be distinct from migration inhibitory factor and interferons include lymphocyte chemotactic factor, osteoclast-activating factor, fibroblast-activating factor, early and late lymphotoxins, and prostaglandin E2. It is presumed, on the basis of animal experiments, that these lymphokines are the in vivo mediators of cellular immune reactions such as delayed hypersensitivity [44].

T-lymphocyte populations which effect cytolysis against allogeneic and virus-infected homologous cells express surface markers homologous to murine Ly 2 and 3 such as OKT5 or Leu 2a and 2b [21]. Normal, asymptomatic subjects do not have detectable levels of circulating antigen-specific cytotoxic T lymphocytes. However, cytotoxic T cells can be generated from blood lymphocytes by in vitro stimulation against the HLA determinants of allogeneic lymphocytes or against the viral antigens of virus-infected autologous cells. In vitro stimulation of blood lymphocytes with allogeneic lymphocytes, as measured in the mixed lymphocytic reaction, requires cellular proliferation by the T-lymphocyte subpopulation expression OKT5 (Leu 2b) and requires the inductive influence of the T helper subpopulation [25]. This stimulation may also be inhibited by T suppressor lymphocytes, either nonspecifically activated or, in rare cases, specifically triggered against a specific allogeneic allele [45]. Cytotoxic T lymphocytes generated in this mixed lymphocytic reaction kill only lymphocytes expressing the same HLA allelic determinant against which they were initially sensitized. In vitro generation of human virus-specific cytotoxic T lymphocytes has been demonstrated with influenza virus [46] and Epstein-Barr virus [47]. The virus-specific cytolysis mediated by these sensitized lymphocytes is

HLA-A and -B restricted, analogous to the H-2 restriction encountered with murine cytotoxic T cells. Thus, the cytotoxic lymphocytes lyse virus-infected cells only if these target cells express HLA-A and HLA-B antigens shared with the cytotoxic cells. Virus-specific cytotoxic lymphocytes are difficult to generate against some viruses. For example, only the blood lymphocytes of a minority of normal subjects generate cytotoxic T-cell responses to measles virus. Nevertheless, cytotoxic T cells have been identified in vivo during acute Epstein-Barr virus and cytomegalovirus infection, suggesting that they may play a significant role in the recovery from these infections [48].

NULL LYMPHOCYTE FUNCTION

Although classification of null cell lineage is poorly understood, at least two null cell functions are well defined: "natural" cytotoxicity (NK) and antibody-dependent cell-mediated cytotoxicity (ADCC). Lysis via ADCC is consequent to attachment of the null cell to the Fc portion of specific IgG antibody bound to target surface antigens. Thus, there is no requirement for prior sensitization of the effector cell, the cytolysis is not HLA-restricted, and specificity of the reaction is conferred by specific antibody [49]. ADCC by human blood lymphocytes in vitro is highly efficient and requires very small concentrations of antibody [48], suggesting that this mechanism of cytotoxicity may be important in vivo in humans.

Natural cytotoxicity (NK) by human blood lymphocytes is mediated primarily by null cells, although some cytolytic activity is found within the T population. Cytotoxicity is directed against various cultured virus-transformed and tumor-derived lines, but the specific surface determinants with which the null cell interacts have not been identified. Also, it is difficult to separate the lymphocytes that have NK activity from those which mediate ADCC, and it may be that the same cell mediates both activities. Interferon is known to regulate NK activity, enhancing cytolysis by human NK cells in vitro and in vivo. Type I interferon (nonimmune, pH stable) is primarily responsible for NK enhancement, but other types may also mediate the effect [50].

MONOCYTE FUNCTION

The role of monocytic phagocytosis and secretion in inflammatory responses and disease pathogenesis is described in Chaps. 95 and 96. Macrophages, however, participate in significant immunoregulatory events which are relevant to the present discussion. Observations of nonspecific suppressive effects which may influence in vivo immunity have been made in two systems. First, in vitro mixed lymphocytic reactions involving irradiated stimulator cells and allogeneic responder lymphocytes may be suppressed by increasing the percentage of phagocytic cells in the irradiated stimulator population [51]. Second, there are patients with neoplastic or inflammatory disorders whose lym-

phocytes manifest a diminished response to mitogenic stimulation. The suppressed response is due to radioresistant adherent monocytes and may be mediated by prostaglandin E [52].

At a more fundamental level macrophages are thought to control immune responses by the presentation of antigen to antigen-specific receptors on T lymphocytes. Hence, for T lymphocytes to be specifically stimulated by antigen and thus provide a helper function for the generation of effector responses, macrophages must first nonspecifically take up the antigen and present it to the T cell. Moreover, the presentation of antigen is believed to occur in the context of gene products of the major histocompatibility complex which are expressed on the macrophage surface and are thought to exert a profound influence on whether the response to specific antigen is induced or suppressed. While these complex interactions have been investigated exclusively in inbred murine models, nevertheless they occur so pervasively that they are thought to be highly conserved and fundamental to the regulation of the human immune response.

Human disease associations

Because of the development of functional assays and surface markers for lymphocyte subsets, considerable information about the mechanisms of several disease states is now available. Since separate chapters are devoted to lymphoproliferative and primary immunodeficiency disorders, we will exclude them from the present discussion.

HEPATITIS B INFECTION

The functional integrity of suppressor cells of both the monocyte-macrophage and the T-cell series has been found to be severely impaired in patients with acute and chronic hepatitis B virus–induced heptocellular injury [53]. When defective, the degree of monocyte suppressor cell deficiency correlated quite well with biochemical parameters of hepatocellular injury. However, in numerous instances hepatocellular injury occurred in the absence of suppressor cell dysfunction suggesting a heterogeneous relationship between suppressor cell dysfunction and liver disease.

In order to determine whether the decreased suppressor cell activities are associated with and perhaps permit the emergence of increased cytotoxic effector cell function, cellular cytotoxicity toward several human liver cell lines has been evaluated. These target cells express host and viral proteins thought to be candidate target antigens in HBV-induced hepatocellular injury. Nevertheless, no evidence of enhanced antigen-specific spontaneous, mitogen-induced, or antibody-dependent cytotoxicity toward any of these target cell lines has been consistently demonstrated [54]. These results suggest either that cellular cytotoxic effector mechanisms are not pathogenetically important in hepatitis B virus infection, or that they are involved but currently available experimental systems are not able to detect them because the appropriate target antigens were not provided or the requirements for genetic restriction were not met.

EPSTEIN-BARR VIRUS INFECTION

Epstein-Barr virus (EBV) causes infectious mononucleosis and has been closely associated with Burkitt's lymphoma and nasopharyngeal carcinoma. EBV infects human B cells in vivo and in vitro and induces polyclonal activation of B cells into immunoglobulin-producing lymphocytes. In vitro, EBV transforms B cells into continuous cell lines that have a number of clearly malignant properties such as the ability to metastasize and to kill immunosuppressed mice following inoculation. Obviously, regulatory mechanisms must be operative in vivo which prevent this outcome in the vast majority of humans infected with EBV.

During the first week of EBV mononucleosis the infected B cells proliferate and become polyclonally activated to produce all classes of immunoglobulin. During the second week of the disease suppressor T cells emerge which inhibit the proliferation and activation of EBV-infected cells in vitro and in vivo [55]. Additionally, cytotoxic T cells specific for EBV appear in the circulation [56]. These cells kill EBV-carrying lymphoid lines without apparent genetic restriction but do not kill EBV-negative cell lines. Each of these processes appears to be critically involved in the termination of a potentially life-threatening lymphoproliferative disease. EBV persists for life, however, in a small number of persistently infected B cells from which continuous cell lines can be regularly generated in vitro. Since neither cytotoxic cells nor suppressor cells can be demonstrated in the blood of seropositive donors convalescent from Epstein-Barr virus infection, it is likely that humoral rather than cellular mechanisms are most important in keeping the latent infection under control.

FUNGAL INFECTION

Thymus-derived immune mechanisms play a crucial role in host defense against fungal infection. Marked, persistent T-cell dysfunction is present in many patients with fungal infection, and the severity of the dysfunction correlates with enhanced risk for dissemination and relapsing infection with the same organism.

Compelling evidence suggests that patients with disseminated fungal infection display suppressor T cells which inhibit the proliferative response of other T cells to antigens and mitogens but have no effect on B-cell responses. Recently, this suppressor T cell has been found to be activated by a soluble product of suppressor macrophages in these patients. Therefore, we are provided with a glimpse of yet another level of complexity in the immunoregulatory network, i.e., the requirement for collaboration between a soluble macrophage product and a population of short-lived, low-density regulatory T cells [57].

SARCOIDOSIS

A defect in cellular immunity in patients with sarcoidosis has long been recognized. Recently a glass-adherent, prostaglandin E₂–producing suppressor cell which inhibits T-cell mitogenesis has been found in the blood of patients with active sarcoidosis [58]. Other, less well defined suppressor cells, perhaps of the monocyte series, also appear to be important in this disease. It is not known whether these abnormalities are primary or secondary to the basic disease process.

GRAFT-VERSUS-HOST DISEASE

Graft-versus-host disease (GVHD) is a major obstacle to the success of allogeneic marrow transplantation. Acute and chronic forms have been defined. It has been postulated that GVHD results from a regulatory imbalance in T suppressor cells permitting development of autocytotoxic cells or of autoantibodies. Patients with acute GVHD have a marked deficiency of T suppressor cells. Patients with chronic GVHD are more heterogeneous. About one-third of patients lack T suppressor cells, have had prior acute GVHD and are hypergammaglobulinemic at the time of study. The remaining patients have increased numbers of T suppressor cells which actively suppress the T-cell response to mitogens and antigens. These patients are hypogammaglobulinemic and very susceptible to infection. The roles played by suppressor cell dysfunction in the induction of GVHD is currently unclear. However, the identification of these abnormalities provides the opportunity to therapeutically modify suppressor cell function in an effort to control the emergence and progression of this devastating disease [59].

SYSTEMIC LUPUS ERYTHEMATOSUS

The mechanisms responsible for autoantibody production in the autoimmune diseases have not yet been conclusively identified. Considerable investigation of systemic lupus erythematosus has been underway for the past several years. The consensus appears to be that this is a multifactorial disease one of the characteristics of which is decreased suppressor cell function [60].

Patients with systemic lupus erythematosus display an assortment of suppressor cell abnormalities. They are relatively deficient in Tγ cells which suppress pokeweed mitogen–induced B-cell immunoglobulin synthesis. They also display a decrease in concanavalin A–inducible T suppressor cells which inhibit T-cell mitogenesis. The latter defect is related to impaired generation of suppressor cells rather than decreased responsiveness to suppressor cell signals. Recent evidence suggests that suppressor cell dysfunction is due to the presence of circulating antibodies to suppressor T precursor cells so that the controversy over the primary importance of intrinsic B-cell hyperactivity versus T suppressor cell deficiency remains unresolved [61,62].

References

1. Katz, D. H.: *Lymphocyte Differentiation, Recognition, and Regulation.* Academic, New York, 1977.
2. Fu, S. M , Winchester, R. J , and Kunkel, H. G.: Occurrence of surface IgM, IgD, and free light chains on human lymphocytes. *J. Exp. Med.* 139:451, 1974.
3. Ferrarini, M., Hoffman, T., Fu, S. M., et al.: Receptors for IgM on certain human B lymphocytes. *J. Immunol.* 119:1525, 1977.
4. Dickler, H. B., and Kunkel, H. G.: Interaction of aggregated gamma immunoglobulin with B lymphocytes. *J. Exp. Med.* 136:191, 1972.
5. Geysta, L., Platsoucas, C. D., and Good, R. A.: Receptors for IgA on subpopulations of human B lymphocytes. *Proc. Natl. Acad. Sci.* 76:4025, 1979.
6. Gonzalez-Molina, A., and Spiegelberg, H. L.: A subpopulation of normal human peripheral blood B lymphocytes that bind IgE. *J. Clin. Invest.* 59:616, 1977.
7. McConnell, I., and Lochmann, P. J.: Complement and cell membranes. *Transplant Rev.* 32:72, 1976.
8. Landal, M., and Klein, G.: Surface markers on human T and B lymphocytes. II. Presence of Epstein-Barr Virus receptors on B lymphocytes. *J. Exp. Med.* 138:1365, 1973.
9. Wernet, P., Winchester, R., and Kunkel, H. G.: Serological detection and partial characterization of human MLC determinants with special reference to B cell specificity. *Transplant. Proc. (Suppl.)* 7:193, 1975.
10. Greaves, M. F., and Brown, G.: A human B lymphocyte specific antigen. *Nature* 246:116, 1973.
11. Stashinko, P., Nadler, L. M., Hardy, R., and Schlossman, S. F.: Characterization of a human B lymphocyte–specific antigen. *J. Immunol.* 125:1678, 1980.
12. Lay, W. H., Mendes, H. F., and Bianco, C.: Binding of sheep red blood cells to a large population of human lymphocytes. *Nature* 230:531, 1971.
13. Bentevich, Z., Douglas, S. D., Skutelsky, E., et al.: Sheep red blood cell binding to human lymphocytes treated with neuraminidase: Enhancement of T cell binding and indentification of a subpopulation of B cells. *J. Exp. Med.* 137:1532, 1973.
14. Moretta, L., Webb, S. K., Grossi, A. E., et al.: Functional analysis of two human T cell subpopulations. Help and suppression of B cell responses by T cells bearing receptors for IgM (TM) or IgG (TG). *J. Exp. Med.* 146:184, 1977.
15. Moretta, L., Ferrarini, M., and Cooper M. D.: Characterizations of human T cell subpopulations as defined by specific receptors for immunoglobulin. *Contemp. Top. Immunobiol.* 8:19, 1978.
16. Ablin, R. L., and Morris, A. J.: Thymus-specific antigens on human thymocytes and on thymus derived lymphocytes. *Transplanatation,* 15:415, 1973.
17. Evans, R. L., Bread, J. M., and Lazarus, J. J., et al.: Detection of two human T cell subclasses bearing unique differentiation antigens. *J. Exp. Med.* 145:221, 1977.
18. Ballet, J. J., and Merler, E.: The separation and reactivity in vitro of a subpopulation of human lymphocytes which bind histamine. Correlation of histamine reactivity with cellular maturation. *Cell Immunol.* 24:250, 1976.
19. Engleman, E. G., and Levy, R.: Immunologic studies of a human T lymphocyte antigen recognized by a monoclonal antibody. *Clin. Res.* 28:511A, 1980.
20. Reinberg, E., Kurg, P., Goldstein, G., and Schlossman, S.: A monoclonal antibody with selective reactivity with functionally mature human thymocytes and all peripheral human T cells. *J. Immunol* 123:1312, 1979.
21. Ledbetter, L. A., Evans R., Lipinski, M., et al.: Evolutionary conservation of surface molecules that distinguish T lymphocyte helper/

inducer and cytotoxic/suppressor subpopulations in mouse and man. *J. Exp. Med.* 153:310, 1981.
22. Hansen, J., Martin, P., Karnour, M., et al.: Monoclonal antibodies recognizing human T-cells. Potential role for preventing graft-versus-host reactions following allogeneic marrow transplantations. *Transplant. Proc.* 13:1133, 1981.
23. Kung, P., Goldstein, G., Reinherz, E., and Schlossman, S.: Monoclonal antibodies defining distinctive human T-cell surface antigens. *Science* 206:347, 1979.
24. Fox, R. I., Thompson, L., and Huddlestone, J. R.: T gamma cells express T-lymphocyte associated antigens. *J. Immunol.* (in press, 1981).
25. Reinherz, E., Kung, P., Goldstein, G., et al.: A monoclonal antibody reactive with human cytotoxic suppressor T cell subset previously defined by a heteroantiserum terminal TH2. *J. Immunol.* 124:1301, 1980.
26. Reinherz, E., Kung, P. Resardo, J., Ritz, J., et al.: Ia determinants on human T cell subsets defined monoclonal antibodies: Activation required for expression. *J. Exp. Med.* 150:1472, 1979.
27. Winchester, R. J., Fu, J. M., Hoffman, T., et al.: IgG on lymphocyte surfaces: technical problems and the significance of the third cell population. *J. Immunol.* 114:1216, 1975.
28. Arebeit, R. D., Henkart, P. O., and Dickler, H. B.: Differences between Fc receptors of two lymphocyte subpopulations of human peripheral blood. *Scand. J. Immunol.* 6:673, 1977.
29. Beard, J., Reinherz, E., Kung, P., et al.: A monoclonal antibody reactive with human blood monocytes. *J. Immunol.* 124:1943, 1980.
30. Knowles, D. M., Hoffman, T., Ferrarini, M., et al.: The demonstration of acid alpha-naphthyl acetate esterase activity in human lymphocytes: Usefulness as a T cell marker. *Cell. Immunol.* 35:112, 1978.
31. Ugolini, V., Nunez, G., and Smith, R. G.: Initial characterization of monoclonal antibodies against human monocytes. *Proc. Natl. Acad. Sci.* 77:6764, 1980.
32. Saxon, A., Stevens, R. H., and Ashman, R. F.: Regulation of immunoglobulin production in human peripheral blood leukocytes: Cellular interactions. *J. Immunol.* 118:1872, 1977.
33. Ault, K., and Towe, M.: Human B lymphocyte subsets. I. IgG-bearing B cell response to pokeweed mitogen. *J. Exp. Med.* 153:339, 1981.
34. Thiele, C. J., and Stevens, R. H.: Antibody potential of human peripheral blood lymphocytes differently expressing surface membrane IgM. *J. Immunol.* 124, 1898.
35. Hammarstrom, L., Bird, A. G., and Smith, C. I. E.: Mitogenic activation of human lymphocytes: A protein A plaque assay evaluation of polyclonal B cell activators. *Scand. J. Immunol.* 11:1, 1980.
36. Ballieux, R. E., Heizner, C. J., and Mytdehaag, F.: Regulation of B cell activity in man: Role of T cells. *Immunol. Res.* 45:1, 1979.
37. Stevens, R. H., and Saxon, G.: Control of antitetanus toxoid antibody after booster immunization. *J. Clin. Invest.* 62:1154, 1978.
38. Thiele, C. J., Morrow, C., and Stevens, R. H.: Multiple subsets of antitetanus toxoid antibody producing cells in human peripheral blood differ by size, expression of membrane receptors, and mitogen reactivity. *J. Immunol.* 126:1146, 1981.
39. Stevens, R. H., Macy, H. E., Morrow, C., and Saxon, A.: Characterization of a circulating subpopulation of spontaneous antitetanus toxoid antibody producing B cell following in vivo booster immunization. *J. Immunol.* 122:2498, 1979.
40. Stobo, J D.: Mitogens. *Clin. Immunobiol.* 4:55, 1980.
41. Mudawarar, F. B., Yunis, E. J., and Geha, R. S.: Antigen-specific helper factor in man. *J. Exp. Med.* 148:1032, 1978.
42. Waldmann, T. A., and Broder, S.: Suppressor cells in the regulation of the immune response, in *Progress in Clinical Immunology,* edited by R. Schwartz. Grune & Stratton, New York, 1977, vol. 3, p. 115.
43. Thomas, Y., Sosman, J., Irigoyen, O., et al.: Functional analysis of human T cell subsets defined by monoclonal antibodies. I. Collaborative T-T interactions in the immunoregulation of B cell differentiation. *J. Immunol.* 125:2402, 1980.
44. Cohen, S.: Lymphokines in delayed hypersivity, in *Progress in Immunology,* edited by M. Fougereau and J. Dausset, Academic, London, New York, 1980, p. 860.
45 Engleman, E. G., McMichael, A. J., Batey, M. C., et al.: A suppressor

T cell of the mixed lymphocyte reaction in man specific for the stimulating alloantigen. Evidence that identity at HLA-D between suppressor and responder is required for suppression. *J. Exp. Med. 147*:137, 1978.

46. McMichael, A., and Askonas, B.: Influenza virus specific cytotoxic T cells in man; induction and properties of the cytotoxic cell. *Eur. J Immunol 8*:705, 1978.

47. Rickinson, A. B., Wallau, L. E., and Epstein, M. A.: HLA-restricted T cell recognition of Epstein-Barr virus-infected B cells. *Nature 283*:865, 1980.

48. Sissons, J. G. P., and Oldstone, M. B. A.: Killing of virus-infected cells by cytotoxic lymphocytes. *J. Infect. Dis. 142*:114, 1980.

49. Perlman, P., and Cerrottini, J. C.: Cytotoxic lymphocytes, in *The Antigens*, edited by M. Lela. Academic, New York, 1979, vol. 5.

50. Santoli, D., and Koprowski, H.: Mechanisms of activation of human natural killer cells against tumor and virus infected cells. *Immunol. Rev. 44*:125, 1979.

51. Laughter, A. H., and Twomey, J. J.: Suppression of lymphoproliferation by high concentrations of normal human mononuclear leukocytes. *J. Immunol. 119*:173, 1977.

52. Sibbitt, W. L., Jr., Bankhurst, A. D., and Williams, R. C., Jr.: Studies of cell subpopulations mediating mitogen hyporesponsiveness in patients with Hodgkin's Disease. *J. Clin. Invest. 61*:55, 1978.

53. Chisari, F. V., Edgington, T. S., Routenberg, J. A., and Anderson, D. S.: Cellular immune reactivity in hepatitis B virus induced liver disease, in *Viral Hepatitis, Proceedings of the UCSF Symposium on Viral Hepatitis*. Franklin Institute, Philadelphia, 1978.

54. Vierling, J. M., Nelson, D. L., Strober, W., Bundy, B. M., and Jones, E. A.: In vitro cell mediated cytotoxicity in primary biliary cirrhosis and chronic hepatitis. *J. Clin. Invest. 60*:1116, 1977.

55. Tosato, G., Magrath, I., Koski, I., Dolley, N., and Blaese, M.: Activation of suppressor T cells during Epstein-Barr-virus–induced infectious mononucleosis. *N. Engl. J. Med. 301*:1133, 1979.

56. Klein, G.: EBV-persistence in human lymphoid and carcinoma cells, in *Persistent Viruses*, edited by J. G. Stevens, G. J. Todaro, and C. F. Fox. Academic, New York, 1978, p. 27.

57. Stobo, J. D., Sigrun, P., Scoy, R. E. V., and Hermans, P. E.: Suppressor thymus-derived lymphocytes in fungal infection. *J. Clin. Invest. 57*:319, 1976.

58. Goodwin, J. S., DeHoratius, R., Israel, H., Peake, G. T., and Messner, R. P.: Suppressor cell function in sarcoidosis. *Ann. Intern. Med. 90*:169, 1979.

59. Reinherz, E. L., Parkman, R., Rappeport, J., Rosen, F. S., and Schlossman, F.: Aberrations of suppressor T cells in human graft-versus-host disease. *N. Engl. J. Med. 300*:1061, 1979.

60. Decker, J. L., et al.: Systemic lupus erythematosus: Evolving concepts. *Ann. Intern. Med. 91*:587, 1979.

61. Bresnihan, B., and Jasin, H. E.: Suppressor function of peripheral blood mononuclear cells in normal individuals and in patients with systemic lupus erythematosus. *J. Clin. Invest. 59*:106, 1977.

62. Sakane, T., Steinberg, A. D., Reeves, J. P., and Green I.: Studies of immune functions of patients with systemic lupus erythematosus. *J. Clin. Invest. 64*:1260, 1979.

63. Terhorst, C., van Agthoven, A., Reinherz, E., and Schlossman, S.: Biochemical analysis of human T lymphocyte differentiation antigens T4 and T5. *Science 209*:520, 1980.

Cellular kinetics of lymphocytes and plasma cells

CHAPTER 106

Production and distribution of lymphocytes and plasma cells

D. ELLIOT PARKS
FRANCIS V. CHISARI

Cellular components

The lymphocytes mediating immune reactivity can be divided into two broad categories based upon both their cellular origin and their ultimate function. The B lymphocytes are derived from stem cells in the bone marrow. No external influence is required for their development. B cells are involved in the synthesis and secretion of humoral antibody which is specific for the stimulating antigen. The T lymphocytes require interaction with the thymus for their differentiation into functionally mature immunocompetent cells. The T-lymphocyte population consists of several subsets, each of which is defined by a distinct effector function:

1. Cytotoxic or killer T cells kill specific cellular targets on contact.
2. Delayed hypersensitivity T cells are involved in antimicrobial and contact sensitivity responses to particulate and soluble antigens.
3. Suppressor T cells inhibit the expression of other lymphocyte functions.
4. Helper T cells induce other T lymphocytes and assist B lymphocytes in the production of antibody.

The T cells in each of the subsets respond to specific antigenic stimulation and accomplish their effector function either by direct interaction with other cells or by synthesizing and secreting soluble mediators termed lymphokines (see Table 105–1).

Cellular networks and interactions

Before an immunocompetent T lymphocyte of any subset can express its effector function, it must first be stimulated by antigen and induced by the inducer-T-cell population. This leads to the establishment of a network of cellular interactions involving at least two cells: the inducer T lymphocyte and the effector T lymphocyte. Furthermore, because suppressor T lymphocytes may inhibit the response of any of the other T lymphocyte subsets, the network of T-lymphocyte interactions becomes increasingly complex. A schematic representation of the interactions in a simplified cellular network is presented in Fig. 106-1. Although the complex network of T-cell interactions serves to enhance or dampen immune reactivity, the presence of foreign antigen is the driving force upon which the interacting T cells depend. The presence or absence of antigen will determine whether or not a cellular immune response is initiated, whereas T cell–T cell interaction will determine the magnitude and duration of that response.

The induction of immune responsiveness in T and B lymphocytes by specific antigen requires another cellular component as well: the phagocytic macrophage, or antigen-presenting cell. This cell is required for the processing and presentation of membrane-bound antigen to T lymphocytes. A requirement for genetic compatibility between the antigen-presenting cell and the T lymphocyte has been demonstrated for most T-cell subsets [1]. The surface structures, called restriction elements, on the antigen-presenting cells and T lymphocytes must be compatible for successful antigen stimulation (genetic restriction). These restriction elements are encoded within the major histocompatibility complex (MHC) of the genome, specifically the H-2 region in mice and the HLA and Dr regions in humans; hence the phenomenon of "genetic restriction" may also be properly termed "MHC restriction" (see Chap. 105). The principles of genetic restriction of T-lymphocyte function extend beyond lymphocyte activation by macrophage-bound antigen to interaction with other genetically compatible cells for the expression of their effector function [12]. Whereas the structure of the restriction element is encoded in the T-lymphocyte genome, the ability to recognize this surface marker is selected for in the thymus, as will be discussed below.

Lymphocytes express immune reactivity by two independent mechanisms. The first involves the synthesis and secretion of specific antibody by B lymphocytes and is commonly termed *humoral immunity*. The second involves the activation of T lymphocytes to express a variety of effector functions and is termed *cell-mediated immunity*. The T-lymphocyte subsets involved in cell-mediated immunity may effect (1) antitissue immunity, such as allograft rejection of antitumor immunity; (2) antimicrobial immunity, such as delayed hypersensitivity, contact sensitivity, and granulomatous reactions; and (3) regulatory functions, such as the induction

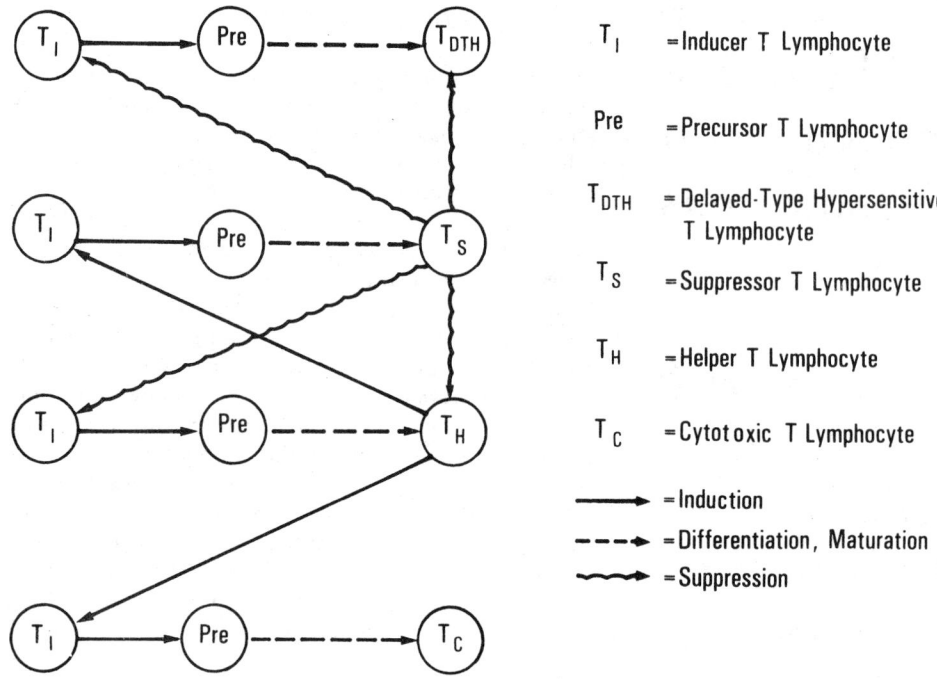

FIGURE 106-1 The network of activation and expression of effector T lymphocytes. The pathway of T-lymphocyte activation following specific antigen exposure includes several functionally different cells and a series of maturational events. The activation of each effector T-cell subset (helper, suppressor, delay-type hypersensitive, cytotoxic) involves the initial triggering of an antigen-specific inducer T cell by the appropriate antigen. This inducer cell acts specifically upon another antigen-specific T cell, the precursor of the effector cell, that matures into the antigen-specific effector. The cells in the pathway of activation of each T-cell subset interact with each other to form a network of T-cell regulation. Mature helper T cells can synergize with inducer cells to enhance the activation of suppressor T cells. Conversely, mature suppressor cells can inhibit the function of inducer cells and thereby suppress the activation of helper T cells. Therefore, each functional subset of T cells may directly or indirectly affect the activation of the other T cell subsets. All possible interactions have not been depicted.

(help) or inhibition (suppression) of T- and B-lymphocyte reactions. The multicellular interactions leading to antigen-specific activation of lymphocytes are known as the *afferent limb* of the immune response. The subsequent antigen-specific immune response by activated T and B lymphocytes is known as the *efferent limb*. Antigen-nonspecific mediator molecules may also be produced by T cells or induced from other cells during the efferent response.

Self-recognition or tolerance

Most tissues with specialized functions develop and differentiate during fetal and neonatal life. Ontogeny within such systems is complete early in life and cellular replication, renewal, or replacement only involves mature cells with fully differentiated characteristics. These systems remain static throughout life with respect to their function. In contrast, ontogeny within the lymphocytic system continues throughout life with exposure to each new foreign antigen requiring the immune system

to discriminate between self and nonself and to produce a new clone of lymphocytes expressing a newly differentiated function. Clonal growth, differentiation, and function are genetically or physiologically determined by the environment at the time of antigenic exposure. Thus, the lymphocytic system has evolved to meet the requirements of antibody diversity, antigenic discrimination, and functional versatility.

Tolerance is the state of specific unresponsiveness established by an initial exposure to antigen. The existence of immunologic tolerance to a particular antigen prevents stimulation of immune reactivity following subsequent challenge with that antigen. Tolerance to self-antigens develops during fetal life. The immature immune system develops in the presence of tissue-specific antigens within the fetus, and the establishment of tolerance to self-constituents during this period precludes subsequent autoimmune reactivity to self.

Several theories have been proposed to explain the mechanism of tolerance to self. They include the blockade of receptors by self-antigens on lymphocytes [3,4]; clonal deletion of cells reacting to self [5]; functional deletion of maturing self-reactive lymphocytes at their earliest stage of immunocompetence, termed *clonal abortion* [6]; the presence of T suppressor cells which inhibit self-reactivity [7]; and more recently the clonal anergy concept, in which a negative signal is provided to immature lymphocytes rendering them immunologically paralyzed [8].

Factors which influence the establishment of immunocompetence or tolerance to both self- and foreign antigens include (1) the amount of antigen present; (2) the number of receptor molecules on potentially responsive lymphocytes; (3) the degree of maturation of lymphocytes at the time of antigen exposure; (4) the mode of antigen presentation; (5) the molecular form of the antigen; (6) the composition of regulatory T lymphocytes present; and (7) the presence of functional antigen-processing cells required for antigen digestion and presentation [9].

IgM and IgG synthesis is detectable as early as 74 and 84 days of gestation, respectively, in the human fetus [10]. Immunoglobulin (Ig) is present on the surface of fetal cells several weeks before it can be found in the serum [11]. A considerable degree of cellular immunocompetence can be detected by mitogen-induced proliferation and antigen-induced cytolysis by 10 to 12 weeks of gestation [12]. Presumably by this early stage in development specific reactivity to antigen has been acquired and therefore tolerance to self must also have been established.

Tolerance can be induced in immature and neonatal lymphocytes more readily than it can be induced in mature adult immunocompetent cells [13,14]. However, a tolerant state can be established in adult animals (and in humans) by certain manipulations which mimic the immune system in the developing fetus. Unresponsiveness to foreign antigens can be established in animals by removing helper T cells [15] or by thymectomy, irradiation, and bone marrow transplantation before exposure to antigen. Immunosuppressive drugs administered to animals or humans prior to engraftment of allogeneic lymphoid tissue facilitates tolerance to the host in the donor tissue. The immunocompetent donor graft will not only restore immune function to the host but will also mount a graft-versus-host reaction unless the donor lymphocytes become tolerant to the recipient tissue during engraftment. The importance of tolerance induction in adult cells is obvious for successful tissue or organ transplantation. The success of these procedures also emphasizes that ontogeny of the lymphocytic system is continuous throughout life.

The ability of the immune system to discriminate between self and nonself is also retained for the lifetime of the individual. Tolerance is an active process, and its maintenance requires the continued presence of antigen. Actively maintained tolerance is also required in the immunologic elimination of somatic cells altered by mutation, trauma, chemicals, or disease while leaving normal host tissue unharmed. Active immune surveillance has been postulated as an important mecha-

nism for the control and rejection of developing tumors. Conversely the breakdown of tolerance to self may result in the activation of self-reactive lymphocytes leading to autoimmune pathology.

Lymphopoietic organs

The marrow and the cortex of the thymus are the primary lymphopoietic organs in adult mammals. These tissues provide a continuous supply of immature differentiating cells through a process of cellular proliferation which is independent of the presence of antigen. The individual cells produced by these tissues are committed to respond to a single antigen but do not become immunocompetent until appropriately stimulated by that antigen. The cells produced by the marrow and thymus migrate to secondary lymphopoietic areas (peripheral lymphatic tissue) where lymphopoiesis continues. The cellular proliferation in peripheral tissue is predominantly a result of antigen-specific stimulation. Although T cells express antigen specificity early in their differentiation, commitment to function may require their interaction with other T cells as well as antigen at the final stage of maturation to immunocompetence.

Cell surface markers

The multiple subpopulations of lymphocytes circulating in blood represent lymphocytes in varying degrees of differentiation and possessing various functional capabilities. Successful identification and separation of each subpopulation requires utilization of cell function, physical properties, and cell surface morphology. Cell separation may be accomplished by exploiting the following: minor differences in cell size and density [16, 17]; adherence to surfaces [18]; antigenic determinants such as surface immunoglobulin molecules on cell membrane [19,20]; and the presence of receptors on the lymphocyte surface, especially those with specificity for red blood cells, the Fc portion of various Ig classes, and complement proteins. In addition, the development of monoclonal antibodies to surface markers on lymphocytes [21,22] has provided a powerful tool for the identification and isolation of physically and functionally distinct subpopulations of lymphocytes (see Chap. 105).

The designation of lymphocytes to a particular functional subpopulation on the basis of surface phenotypes depends on characteristics which are not fully understood at this time. For instance, cell surface or membrane Ig is characteristic of B cells, but is also detectable on granulocytes and monocytes. The binding of cytophilic Ig by Fc receptors on monocytes and macrophages also interferes with characterization of lymphocytes possessing similar Fc receptors. Identification of lymphocyte subpopulations by morphologic characteristics is not possible. Striking surface differences between various lymphocyte populations under scanning electron microscopy have been reported [23] but have not been substantiated [24]. Recent attempts to clone T lymphocytes expressing different functional capabilities have suggested that morphology is not indicative of cellular function. The development of monoclonal antibodies to lymphocyte surface markers appears to provide the greatest promise for separation and identification of the cellular component of the immune response in the near future.

Marrow lymphopoiesis

The marrow stem cell is pluripotential, providing progeny for several differentiated cell lines. Such pluripotential stem cells are also present to a lesser extent in the blood and the spleen of adult mammals. The basic features of stem cell differentiation into lymphocytes are schematically presented in Fig. 106-2. The marrow stem cell with pluripotential capacity provides at least erythrocytic, granulocytic or monocytic, thrombocytic, and lymphocytic cell lines. This pluripotential cell appears first to undergo a fundamental differentiation step into lymphopoietic progenitor cells and hemopoietic progenitor cells. The hemopoietic progenitor cell gives rise to erythrocytes, granulocytes, monocytes, and megakaryocytes. The lymphopoietic progenitor cell results in subsets of T and B lymphocytes. During the differentiation process, a progenitor cell is produced which is restricted to a single functional capacity. Through maturation, effector cells are generated which are capable of immunologic memory upon antigen encounter. The resulting effector cells may themselves become unipotent stem cells, as in the generation of immunologic memory after antigen stimulation.

The primary pluripotential stem cells in the marrow produce secondary progenitor cells which are committed to produce immunocompetent progeny that may enter either the T or B pathway of lymphocyte development. Progeny which migrate to the thymus become any one of a variety of functional T lymphocytes as will be described in more detail below. Functional analysis of human immunodeficiency diseases allows the detection of progenitor cell lines arrested, altered, or deleted at various stages in the development of immunocompetence [see Chap. 112].

The exact stage at which antigen specificity is acquired during lymphopoiesis and the mechanisms that generate antibody diversity have been topics of intense investigation in recent years. Although the genetic information for some antibody specificities is inherited in germ line genes, a large degree of antibody diversity is accomplished by somatic events. Antibody genes are organized in a fashion that allows diversification by combination of various gene segments into new genes during embryonic life [25]. It is unlikely that this rearrangement of genetic information occurs in the bone marrow prior to commitment of stem cells to the

lymphocytic series. However this commitment to a particular amino acid sequence in the variable region of light and heavy chains of the immunoglobulin protein molecule determines the future antigen specificity soon after lymphocytic stem cells enter the T or B pathways if such commitment has not occurred before. Therefore, antigen specificity has been acquired in the T-lymphocyte lineage before these cells acquire functional commitment. RNA splicing prior to translation of immunoglobulin message also plays a role in altering immunoglobulin produced by a single cell [26,27]. These mechanisms account for the differences in membrane and secreted Ig and the switch from production of IgM to production of IgG by a single clone of mature B cells.

B-LYMPHOCYTE MATURATION

In adult mammalian marrow lymphopoiesis the major cellular product is the precursor of B lymphocytes. These cells migrate to peripheral lymphoid tissue where some of them will encounter antigen and be stimulated to differentiate into antibody-secreting plasma cells [28,29]. The maturation of bone marrow lymphocytes to mature B lymphocytes begins in the marrow and continues as these precursor cells leave the marrow, transit to circulation, and "home" to peripheral tissues. Although some of the steps involved in the differentiation from a pre-B lymphocyte in the bone marrow to a mature immunocompetent B cell in the periphery occur in the absence of antigen, the final stage of differentiation requires exposure to specific antigen. Lymphocytes present in the marrow are primarily immunologically immature. When adoptively transferred into immunocompetent irradiated recipients, the marrow cells are unable to replace mature T or B lymphocytes as monitored by a low level of antibody secretion or cellular immune effector reactivity [30]. This indicates that few fully differentiated effector lymphocytes are present in the marrow. In contrast, the marrow is a tissue rich in stem cells which can restore both T- and B-lymphocyte functions in incompetent recipients if given time to mature and differentiate under the influence of peripheral lymphoid tissue of the host [30].

The appearance of cytoplasmic immunoglobulin followed by its subsequent expression on the surface of differentiating B cells can be used to follow the maturation of B cells [31]. Secretion of immunoglobulin by B lymphocytes may precede the maturation of these cells into plasma cells, although differentiated plasma cells synthesize and produce much larger quantities of immunoglobulin than do their B-cell progenitors.

The ontogeny of B lymphocytes in the human fetus has been studied using the appearance of surface markers as indicators of maturation [32]. By 14 weeks of gestation, cells bearing surface immunoglobulin and Fc receptors comprise 9 to 32 percent and 8 to 16 percent of the spleen cells, respectively. In the cord blood of newborn infants, cells expressing surface immunoglobulin are present in numbers equal to or slightly greater than those in adults, confirming that antigen-reactive B cells

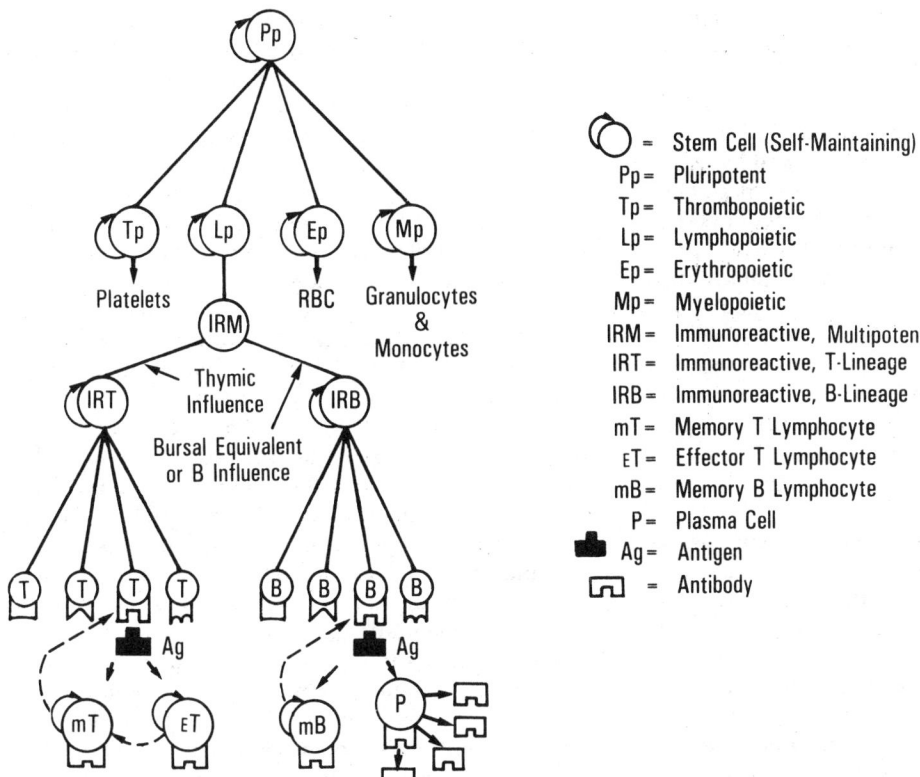

FIGURE 106-2   The production of stem cells for lymphopoiesis. In the context of this chapter, the term *stem cell* means any self-renewing or self-maintaining cell. Stem cells may produce either multiple cell lines, as in the case of the pluripotential stem cell, or single cell lines, as in the case of the lymphopoietic stem cell. The lymphopoietic stem cell is itself pluripotential both with respect to antigen specificity and functional activity of the cells produced. One of the consequences of the clonal production of lymphocytes committed to a single antigenic stimulus may be the development of memory cells, stem cells restricted to a single response. These memory stem cells, exhibiting a long life-span, respond to a subsequent encounter with specific antigen by further clonal proliferation.

The requirements for stimulation of the pluripotential stem cell to produce immunocompetent stem cells is unknown. The multipotential cell capable of supplying either T- or B-lymphocyte precursors resides in the bone marrow. The thymus epithelium produces factors which stimulate stem cells from the marrow to develop into T lymphocytes. Differentiation of stem cells into mature B lymphocytes begins in the marrow in mammals.

The products of extensive thymic and marrow lymphopoiesis are depicted here as possessing receptors of differing antigenic specificity. Cells bearing receptors appropriate for the particular antigen encountered in the periphery are stimulated to proliferate by this encounter. This stimulation results in the clonal selection of responsive cells by proliferation. Interaction with antigen-presenting phagocytic cells, T cells, and antigen is necessary for activation of T or B progenitors and subsequent maturation into effector cells expressing differentiated function. Mature, immunoreactive cells produced by this antigen-specific clonal proliferation mediate the T- and B-lymphocyte responses. Some of these cells persist as fully differentiated memory stem cells.

develop during fetal life [33]. During ontogeny, surface IgM appears first, followed by IgD and then IgG [34].

The cell surface isotypes (immunoglobulin classes) of adult human lymphocytes in peripheral blood have been reported to be approximately 3 percent for IgG, 2 percent for IgA, 9 percent for IgM, 6 percent for IgD, 14 percent for κ chain, and 7 percent for λ chain [35]. These figures would indicate that between 15 and 20 percent of blood lymphocytes are B cells compared with approx-

imately 30 to 40 percent in splenic tissue and slightly less than that in lymph nodes [36,37].

The marrow is the body's major site of production and export of lymphocytes to supply the peripherally distributed immunocompetent tissues. The lymphoid population in the marrow of mice consists of about 20 percent large lymphocytes and 80 percent small lymphocytes. The larger cells are rapidly renewed by local lymphopoiesis in the marrow. The progression in the marrow of large, rapidly dividing lymphocytes expressing no B-cell markers to small lymphocytes bearing multiple B-cell markers [38] is independent of the presence of specific antigen [39].

It appears that B lymphocytes undergo the sequential addition of surface immunoglobulin followed by the C3 receptor as these cells differentiate in the peripheral lymphoid tissues. In human blood only about one-half the immunoglobulin-bearing lymphocytes also express C3 receptors, whereas in the spleen and thoracic duct nearly all of the surface immunoglobulin (sIg)–positive cells do so [40]. The blood contains a higher proportion of cells recently released from the bone marrow than do peripheral tissues. Indeed, the central lymph, fed by the thoracic duct, appears to be made up nearly exclusively of differentiated recirculating cells.

KINETICS AND TURNOVER

The use of radioisotopes to label dividing cells has expanded knowledge of the kinetics of division, fate, and life-span of lymphoid cells. Using this technique it has been demonstrated that the small lymphocyte, the major population in the marrow, consists of two subpopulations. The larger of these two populations represents approximately 93 percent of small lymphocytes in young mice and exhibits a half-life of 14 h. In older mice, this major population of small lymphocytes represents 75 to 80 percent of the small marrow lymphocytes and shows a 50 percent renewal rate of 24 hours [41–43]. In contrast the minor population is made up of long-lived recirculating T and B lymphocytes [44]. It also contains hematopoietic stem cells and other cell types as well.

Rapid advances have occurred in the understanding of B-cell differentiation using cell surface markers as signposts of differentiation [28,29,38]. Random sampling of mouse bone marrow demonstrates that 100 percent of the cells bear H-2 antigens of the major histocompatibility complex, 34 percent bear B-cell–specific antigen, 33 percent bear Fc receptor, 23 percent bear Ig surface immunoglobulin, 8 percent bear T-lymphocyte–specific antigen, and 5 percent bear C3 receptor. The density of surface immunoglobulin displays greater variation on marrow lymphocytes than on lymphocytes in peripheral lymphoid tissue. This variation in surface marker density may reflect the heterogeneity of maturational stages expressed by cells in the bone marrow and a gradual accumulation of B-cell markers with cellular age.

When radioisotopic techniques are employed in conjunction with cell surface studies, the pattern of bone marrow lymphocyte maturation becomes more evident. Only the 'large, rapidly dividing lymphocytes in the bone marrow are radiolabeled with ^{3}H thymidine. Division of these cells results in labeled small lymphocytes [42,43] which are negative for B-lymphocyte surface markers (pre-B cells) and remain so for 30 to 36 h. After this brief lag, detectable cell surface markers are expressed on these small lymphocytes. B-lymphocyte–specific antigen appears first, followed by Fc receptor,

surface immunoglobulin, and C3 receptor. This maturation of small pre-B lymphocytes occurs in the absence of antigen and without further cell division. If these pre-B lymphocytes are injected intravenously, they migrate to the spleen, where maturation continues [28].

B-cell maturation is schematically depicted in Fig. 106-3. The release of pre-B cells into the circulation is one explanation for the presence of small numbers of blood lymphocytes which exhibit neither T- nor B-cell surface markers. Maturation of these virgin pre-B lymphocytes provides the peripheral lymphoid system with a constant source of antigen-specific B cells available for antigen-induced activation, clonal expansion, and maturation [49]. Since the vast majority of virgin B cells do not bear surface immunoglobulin specific for the antigens which they encounter, they are not stimulated to divide and mature into differentiated B cells but rather die after a short interval [45]. The proposed differentiation of small B lymphocytes beginning in the bone marrow and continuing to completion in peripheral tissues can be verified using the C3 receptor as a marker for B-lymphocyte maturation [28,29].

The characteristic high rate of cellular replication in marrow and thymus lymphopoiesis is accompanied by a similar high rate of lymphocyte death and DNA reutilization in these organs [46]. Only a small fraction of the lymphocytes continually produced in these areas survive. This high rate of lymphocyte wastage or ineffective lymphopoiesis may, in part, fill the need for the lymphoid system to supply cells committed to the broad repertoire of antigen specificities required to maintain immunologic integrity. A large proportion of the immunocompetent cells produced by lymphopoiesis are not "selected" by encounter with antigen and therefore die.

The proportion of the two kinetic types of marrow lymphocytes, the large, rapidly dividing pluripotential stem cell and the smaller, long-lived recirculating T lymphocytes, changes with age. The endogenously produced, rapidly renewing cell declines in proportion to the number of recirculating lymphocytes which slowly populate the marrow. In mice the proportion of long-lived cells increases from 7 to 22 percent between 4 and 16 weeks of age [41]. Although the number of small pre-B lymphocytes produced in the marrow declines with age, the production of these cells by lymphopoiesis continues actively throughout life. The character of lymphocyte precursors in marrow also changes with therapeutic or experimental manipulation. Following sublethal whole-body irradiation [47] or endotoxin administration [48], transient marrow depletion is followed by an increase in the numbers of lymphocytes in the marrow. This recovery is due not only to reentry of stem cells from the circulation into the marrow but also to lymphopoiesis in the remaining marrow cells. In patients who are rendered immunoincompetent by whole-body irradiation prior to marrow transplantation, there is a rapid fall in the number of marrow lymphocytes. Following transplantation, donor marrow lymphocytes

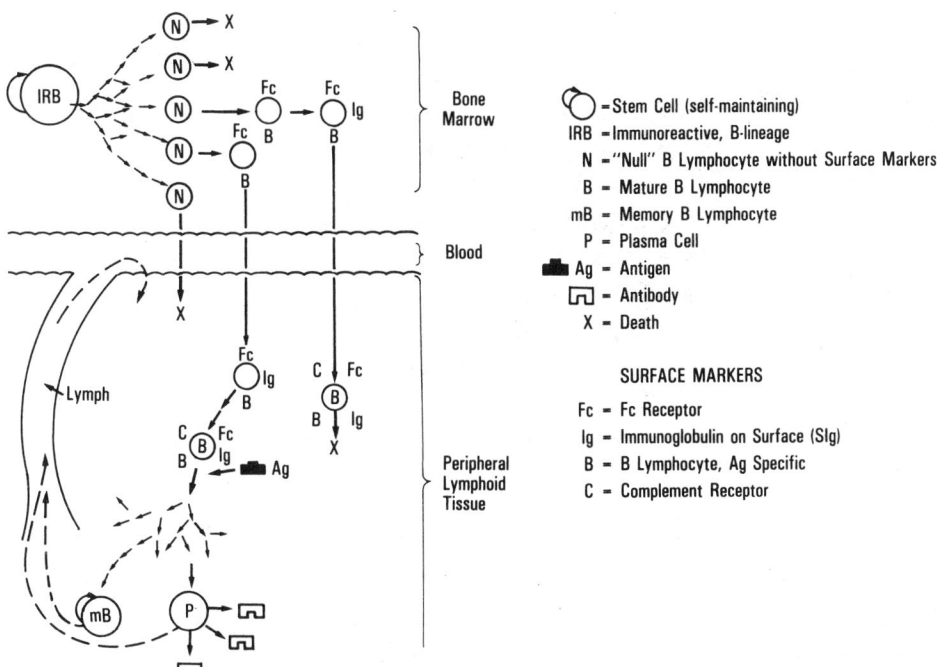

FIGURE 106-3 Differentiation of marrow-derived B lymphocytes. Immature lymphocytes devoid of distinct surface markers are continually produced by the marrow. Many of these cells die in the marrow or in peripheral tissues before further maturation. Maturation can be monitored by the progressive addition of surface markers synthesized by the cell. Differentiation begins in the marrow in the absence of antigen and continues in the periphery. Completion of differentiation, however, does not occur in the absence of antigen. Activation of mature B cells by antigen requires interaction with antigen-presenting cells and T lymphocytes. Some of the fully differentiated B cells resulting from antigen-stimulated, clonal proliferation persist as B memory stem cells. These cells may recirculate in the lymph and blood. A spectrum of B cells with differing membrane markers, representing the varying degrees of maturation, can be found in the circulation having recently left the marrow or reentered the blood from the periphery.

increase as engraftment occurs [49]. From these examples it can be concluded that lymphopoiesis in the marrow can occur at a high rate throughout adult life.

The marrow is the body's largest lymphopoietic mass [50]. Lymphocytes make up more than half of the nucleated cell content of human marrow at birth, but the percentage of lymphocytes in the marrow varies considerably with age. During pubertal growth the percentage decreases [51], and in mature adults only 16 to 21 percent of the nucleated cells in human marrow are lymphocytic (see Chap. 12). Lymphoid follicles, which are characteristic of areas of active antigen responsiveness, are frequent in the marrow of older patients. This may reflect a slow but continued accumulation of recirculating mature T and B lymphocytes in the marrow over time.

Thymus lymphopoiesis

The major function of the normal thymus is to produce and export to peripheral lymphoid tissues T-dependent lymphocytes which recognize antigen and express cell-mediated immune reactivities. This organ is made up of lymphoid cells supported by an epithelial structure in which both medullary and cortical regions can be distinguished morphologically. Lymphopoiesis occurs primarily in the cortical region of the thymus and is dependent on stem cells originating in the marrow [49,52,53]. Cells within the thymus proliferate in an environment which is free of foreign antigen. The genetically determined restriction of thymus-dependent lymphocyte function is established within this organ [2], as is the elimination of clones which react with endogenous self-antigen.

The cortex of the thymus consists predominantly of rapidly dividing immature T lymphocytes. These cortical T lymphocytes, like marrow-derived pre-B lymphocytes, require further maturation before becoming fully immunocompetent. Following migration from the thymus and subsequent maturation in peripheral lymphoid tissues, thymus-dependent cells participate in immunologic reactivity, serving in both afferent and efferent limbs of the immune response. The fully differentiated T lymphocytes consist of several functional cellular subsets which mediate such diverse reactivities as

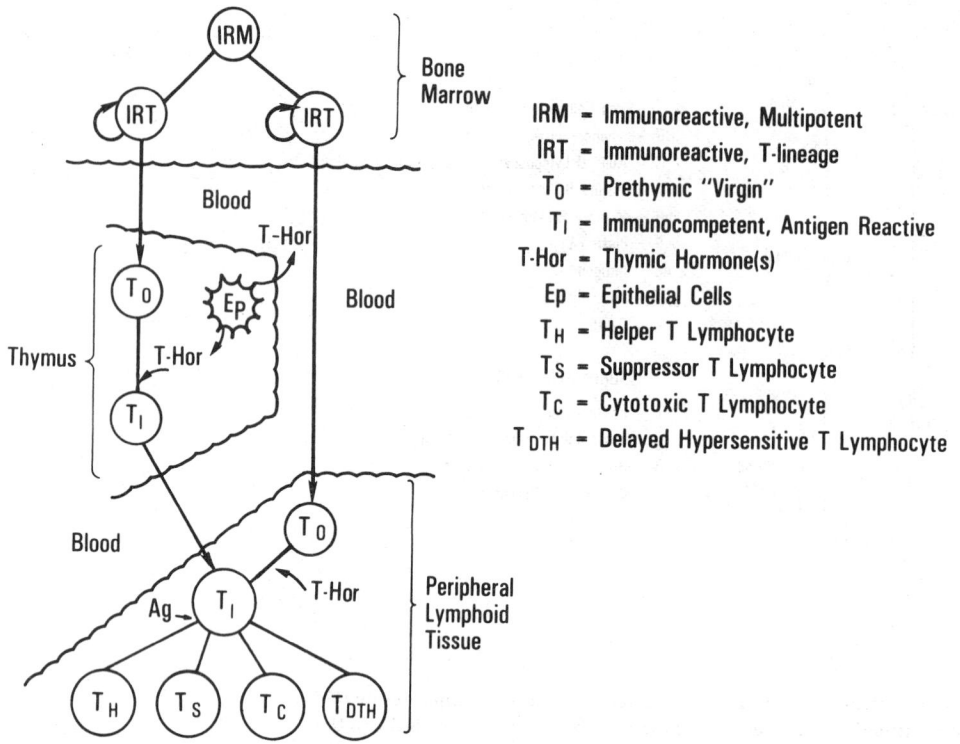

FIGURE 106-4 Production, differentiation, and maturation of T lymphocytes. Immunoreactive stem cells of the T lineage (IRT) are derived from multipotential precursor stem cells (IRM) in the marrow. The IRT stem cells provide prethymic (T_0) precursors to the cortex of the thymus. These cells mature under the influence of thymic hormone(s) secreted by the epithelium of the thymus. As these cells mature into immunocompetent, antigen-reactive (T_1) lymphocytes, they migrate from the cortex to the medulla of the thymus and from there to peripheral lymphoid tissue. However, some prethymic T_0 precursor cells may bypass the thymus to enter peripheral tissue and mature there under the influence of thymic hormones. This T-cell maturation, leading to immunocompetent, antigen-reactive T_1 lymphocytes, occurs in the absence of specific antigen exposure. In the presence of antigen, T_1 lymphocytes proliferate and differentiate into effector T-cell subsets as depicted here and in Fig. 106-1.

(1) cytotoxic or killer T cells, which destroy altered or foreign cells and mediate allograft rejection and antiviral and antitumor responses; (2) delayed hypersensitivity T cells, which mediate antimicrobial and contact sensitivity responses; and (3) regulatory T cells, which can induce or suppress either T- or B-lymphocyte function.

T-LYMPHOCYTE MATURATION

As described in Fig. 106-2, T cells are originally derived from the pluripotential stem cell of the marrow, as are all hemopoietic cells. Stem cells from the marrow seed the thymic cortex to initiate T-cell differentiation (see Fig. 106-4). From 5 to 10 percent of marrow lymphoid cells appear to be the precursors for T lymphocytes, as they can be induced to express T-cell surface markers in vitro [54,55]. Under the influence of the thymus, antigen-specific precursor cells from the marrow differentiate along the pathway toward functional T lymphocytes. The role of the thymus in the maturation of T cells to immunocompetence is well documented by the im-

munodeficiency seen in neonatally thymectomized animals [56–58], by human immune deficiency diseases associated with thymus [59,60], and by the ability of thymic grafts to reverse human thymic deficiencies [61,62].

The thymus may influence precursor cells from the marrow by two major mechanisms: local intrathymic influence and thymic hormonal factors acting distal to the thymus. There is considerable evidence to support the existence of thymic hormones. The epithelial component of the thymus appears to be the source of these secretory products which can induce lymphopoiesis [63]. As with many other biologically active proteins with pharmacologic or hormonal activity, the humoral thymic influence of these thymic hormones is neither species- nor strain-specific [64–66].

Lymphopoiesis occurs predominantly in the thymic cortex. In this region of the thymus the lymphocytes divide rapidly; as many as 95 percent of the cells turn over every 3 days in the rodent thymus [67–69]. After several divisions many of the cells migrate from the thymus to populate peripheral lymphoid tissues, although a significant number of cells remain in the thymus and die there. This thymic lymphopoiesis, which occurs in the cortex, does not require the presence of antigen. Figure 106-4 depicts schematically the maturational sequence of T-dependent lymphocytes and the influence of thymic hormone on this maturation.

Surviving cortical lymphocytes which do not leave the thymus for peripheral lymphoid tissue mature as they migrate into the medulla. These cells differentiate to functional subpopulations of T lymphocytes while acquiring immunocompetence and undergoing changes in cell surface antigens. Whereas some of these immunocompetent T cells remain in the medulla, the majority leave the thymus to seed the thymus-dependent areas of lymph nodes and spleen [67,70] as well as the tonsils and Peyer's patches [69,70]. Migration of T lymphocytes is not limited to the mature medullary cells. Some immature thymic cells leave the thymic cortex to populate the periarteriolar lymphatic sheaths, the deep cortical zones of the lymph nodes, and marginal zones of the spleen [71,72]. These immature T lymphocytes may represent a thymic population available for further extrathymic maturation and may contribute to the development and expansion of immune responses initiated at peripheral sites by mature, effector T lymphocytes.

Recirculating T lymphocytes do not normally migrate into the thymus. A high rate of lymphopoiesis in the cortex of the thymus which produces cells that crowd into the medulla may inhibit the reentry of mature T lymphocytes. This high rate of cellular replication and renewal in the cortex of the thymus may also make entry of new stem cells from the bone marrow unnecessary.

The ability of thymic hormones to influence T-cell maturation in extrathymic locations may explain the continued competence of T lymphocytes in aging individuals many years after the thymus has undergone atrophy. Thymosin is a low-molecular-weight substance isolated from the thymic tissue of several species including humans [66]. A family of thymic hormones containing similar or identical active sites may exist which enhance or restore the development of immune responses in T lymphocytes. These proteins increase DNA synthesis in lymphocytes [66] and restore tumor and skin graft rejection [73] and graft-versus-host reactions [74] in thymectomized mice. Thymosin is also capable of inducing the appearance of T-cell surface markers in precursor cells from the bone marrow and fetal liver [73,75] and of inducing responsiveness to T-cell mitogens [54,55,75], and restoring helper-T-cell function in the spleens of adult thymectomized mice [73]. It would appear that thymic hormones possess the capacity to promote the differentiation of stem cells into immunocompetent T lymphocytes representing a variety of functional subsets [74].

In humans, high levels of thymic hormone are maintained from birth to about 20 to 25 years of age, followed by a gradual decrease in activity to extremely low levels at advanced age [75]. However, even low levels of thymic hormone in aged individuals may play an important role in the maintenance of T-lymphocyte immunocompetence due to the presence of marrow stem cells and immature T cells in the periarteriolar lymphatic sheaths and marginal zones of the spleen. Therefore, functional levels of thymic hormone, produced by the epithelial component of the thymus, may persist long after atrophy of the lymphoid component of the thymus has occurred and this tissue has ceased serving as a primary lymphopoietic organ.

References

1. Rosenthal, A. S.: Determinant selection and macrophage function in genetic control of the immune response. *Immunol. Rev.* 40:136, 1978.
2. Zinkernagel, R. M., et al.: The lymphoreticular system in triggering virus plus self-specific cytotoxic T cells: Evidence for T help. *J. Exp. Med.* 147:897, 1978.
3. Aldo-Benson, M., and Borel, Y.: Direct evidence for receptor blockade by tolerogen. *J. Immunol.* 112:1793, 1974.
4. Schrader, J. W., and Nossal, G. J. V.: Effector cell blockade a new mechanism of immune hyporeactivity induced by multivalent antigens. *J. Exp. Med.* 139:1582, 1974.
5. Burnet, F. M.: *The Clonal Selection Theory of Acquired Immunity.* Cambridge, London, 1959.
6. Nossal, G. J. V., and Pike, B. L.: Evidence for the clonal abortion theory of B lymphocyte tolerance. *J. Exp. Med.* 141:904, 1975.
7. Gershon, R. K.: T cell control of antibody production. *Contemp. Top. Immunobiol.* 3:1, 1974.
8. Nossal, G. J. V., and Pike, B. L.: Clonal anergy: Persistence in tolerant mice of antigen binding B lymphocytes incapable of responding to antigen or mitogen. *Proc. Natl. Acad. Sci. U.S.A.* 77:1602, 1980.
9. Parks, D. E.: Cellular mechanisms of tolerance to self. *Clin. Immunol. Allerg.* 1:3, 1981.
10. Gitlin, D., and Biasucci, A.: Development of γG, γA, γM, β_{1C}/β_{1A}, C'1 esterase inhibitor, ceruloplasmin, transferrin, hemopexin, haptoglobin, fibrinogen, plasminogen, α_1-antitrypsin, orosomucoid, β-lipoprotein, α_2-macroglobulin, and prealbumin in the human conceptus. *J. Clin. Invest.* 48:1433, 1969.
11. Van Furth, R., Schmit, H. R., and Hijmans, W.: The formation of immunoglobulins by human tissues *in vitro*. I. Fetal tissues. *J. Exp. Med.* 122:1173, 1966.
12. Stites, D. P., Carr, M. C., and Fudenberg, H. H.: Segregation of in vitro cellular immune functions in lymphoid organs during early human fetal development, in *Proceedings of the Seventh Leukocyte Culture Conference*, edited by F. Daguillard. Academic, New York, 1973, p. 231.
13. Cambier, J. C., Kettman, J. R., Vitetta, E. S., and Uhr, J. W.: Differential susceptibility of neonatal and adult murine spleen cells to *in vitro* induction of B cell tolerance. *J. Exp. Med.* 144:293, 1976.
14. Metcalf, E. S., and Klinman, N. R.: *In vitro* tolerance induction of neonatal murine B cells. *J. Exp. Med.* 143:1327, 1976.
15. Nelson-Rampy, P. A., Parks, D. E., and Weigle, W. O.: Establishment of unresponsiveness in primed B lymphocytes *in vivo*. *J. Immunol.* 127:1415, 1981.
16. Boyum, A.: Isolation of mononuclear cells and granulocytes from human blood. *Scand. J. Clin. Lab. Invest. (Suppl.)* 97:77, 1968.
17. Wilson, J. D.: The function of immune T and B rosette-forming cells. *Immunology* 24:185, 1973.
18. Shortman, K.: Separation methods for lymphocyte populations. *Contemp. Top. Mol. Immunol.* 2:161, 1974.
19. Wigzell, H., and Andersson, B.: Cell separation of antigen-coated columns: Elimination of high-rate antibody-forming cells and immunological memory cells. *J. Exp. Med.* 129:23, 1969.

20. Schlossman, S. F., and Hudson, L.: Specific purification of lymphocyte populations on a digestible immunoadsorbent. *J. Immunol.* 110:313, 1973.

21. Kung, P. C., Goldstein, G., Reinherz, E. L., and Schlossman, S. F.: Monoclonal antibodies defining distinctive human T cell surface antigens. *Science* 206:347, 1979.

22. Reinherz, E. L., and Schlossman, S. F.: Current concepts in immunology: Regulation of the immune response—Inducer and suppressor T-lymphocyte subsets in human beings. *N. Engl. J. Med.* 303:370, 1980.

23. Lui, P. S., Cooper, A. G., and Wortis, H. H.: Scanning electron microscopy of human T-cell and B-cell rosettes. *N. Engl. J. Med.* 289:548, 1973.

24. Alexander, E. L., and Wetzel, B.: Human lymphocytes: Similarity of B and T surface morphology. *Science* 188:732, 1975.

25. Brack, C., Hirama, M., Lenhard-Schuller, R., and Tonegawa, S.: A complete immunoglobulin gene is created by somatic recombination. *Cell* 15:1, 1978.

26. Alt, F. W., et al.: Synthesis of secreted and membrane-bound immunoglobulin Mu heavy chains is directed by mRNAs that differ in their 3′ ends. *Cell* 20:293, 1980.

27. Rogers, J., et al.: Two mRNAs with different 3′ ends encode membrane-bound and secreted forms of immunoglobulin mu chain. *Cell* 20:303, 1980.

28. Ryser, J., and Vassalli, P.: Mouse bone marrow lymphocytes and their differentiation. *J. Immunol.* 113:719, 1974.

29. Osmond, D. G.: Formation and maturation of bone marrow lymphocytes. *J. Reticuloendothel. Soc.* 17:99, 1975.

30. Miller, J. F. A. P.: Role of the cells which originate from the thymus and bone marrow. *Ann. Immunol. (Paris)* 125:213, 1974.

31. Raff, M. C., Megson, M., Owen, J. J. T., and Cooper, M. D.: Early production of intracellular IgM in B lymphocyte precursors in mouse. *Nature* 259:224, 1976.

32. Lawton, A. R., Self, K. S., Royal, S. A., and Cooper, M. D.: Ontogeny of B-lymphocytes in the human fetus. *Clin. Immunol. Immunopathol.* 1:84, 1972.

33. Froland, S. S., and Natvig, J. B.: Lymphocytes with membrane-bound immunoglobulin (B lymphocytes) in newborn babies. *Clin. Exp. Immunol.* 11:495, 1972.

34. Gathings, W. E., Lawton, A. R., and Cooper, M. D.: Immunofluorescent studies of the development of pre-B cells, B lymphocytes, and immunoglobulin isotype diversity in humans. *Eur. J. Immunol.* 7:804, 1977.

35. Aiuti, J., et al.: International union of immunological societies (IUIS) report, July 1974. *Clin. Immunol. Immunopathol.* 3:584, 1975.

36. Vesakorpe, R., and Repo, H.: T and B lymphocytes in human spleen. *Lancet* 1:740, 1973 (letter).

37. Warner, N. L.: Membrane immunoglobulins and antigen receptors on B and T lymphocytes. *Adv. Immunol.* 19:67, 1974.

38. Osmond, D. G., and Nossal, G. J. V.: Differentiation of lymphocytes in mouse bone marrow. II. Kinetics of maturation and renewal of antiglobulin-binding cells studied by double labeling. *Cell. Immunol.* 13:132, 1974.

39. Shortman, K., Howard, M. C., and Baker, J. A.: Antigen-initiated B lymphocyte differentiation XIV nonspecific effects of antigen stimulation cause proliferation in the "pre-progenator" subset of primary B cells. *J. Immunol.* 121:2060, 1978.

40. Ross, G. D., Rabellino, E. M., Polley, M. J., and Grey, H. M.: Combined studies of complement receptor and surface immunoglobulin-bearing cells and sheet erythrocyte rosette-forming cells in normal and leukemic human lymphocytes. *J. Clin. Invest.* 52:377, 1973.

41. Miller, S. C., and Osmond, D. G.: Lymphocyte subpopulations in mouse bone marrow: Quantitative kinetic studies in young, pubertal and adult C3H mice. *Cell Tissue Kinet.* 8:97, 1975.

42. Everett, N. B., and Tyler (Caffrey), R. W.: Lymphopoiesis in the thymus and other tissues: Functional implications. *Int. Rev. Cytol.* 22:205, 1967.

43. Craddock, C. G.: Bone marrow lymphocytes of the rat as studied by autoradiography. *Acta Haematol. (Basel)* 33:19, 1965.

44. Ropke, C., Hougen, H. P., and Everett, N. B.: Long-lived T and B lymphocytes in the bone marrow and thoracic duct lymph of the mouse. *Cell Immunol.* 15:82, 1975.

45. Strober, S.: Maturation of B lymphocytes in the rat. II. Subpopulations of virgin B lymphocytes in the spleen and thoracic duct lymph. *J. Immunol.* 114:877, 1975.

46. Craddock, C. G., Longmire, R., and McMillan, R.: Lymphocytes and the immune response. *N. Engl. J. Med.* 285:324, 1971.

47. Hulse, E. V.: Lymphocyte recovery after irradiation and its relationship to other aspects of haemopoiesis. *Br. J. Haematol.* 9:376, 1963.

48. Yoffey, J. M.: The lymphocyte. *Ann. Rev. Med.* 15:125, 1964.

49. Thomas, E. D.: Bone marrow transplanatation, in *Clinical Immunology*, edited by F. H. Bach and R. A. Good. Academic, New York, 1974, vol. 2, p. 2.

50. Donahue, D. M., Gabrio, B. W., and Finch, C. A.: Quantitative measurements of hematopoietic cells of the marrow. *J. Clin. Invest.* 37:1564, 1958.

51. Glaser, K., Limarzi, L. R., and Poucher, H. G.: Cellular composition of the bone marrow in normal infants and children. *Pediatrics* 6:789, 1950.

52. Ford, C. E., Micklem, H. S., Evans J. G., Gray J. G., and Ogden, D. A.: The inflow of bone marrow cells to the thymus: Studies with part-body irradiated mice injected with chromosome-marked bone marrow and subjected to antigenic stimulation. *Ann. N.Y. Acad. Sci.* 129:283, 1966.

53. Wu, A. M., Till, J. E., Simmovitch, L., and McCulloch, E. A.: Cytological evidence for a relationship between normal hematopoietic colony-forming cells and cells of the lymphoid system. *J. Exp. Med.* 127:455, 1968.

54. Komuro, K., and Boyse, E. A.: *In vitro* demonstration of thymic hormone in the mouse by conversion of precursor cells into lymphocytes. *Lancet* 1:170, 1973.

55. Touraine, J. L., Incefy, G. S., Touraine, F., Rho, Y. M., and Good, R. A.: Differentiation of human bone marrow cells into T lymphocytes with thymic extracts. *Clin. Exp. Immunol.* 17:151, 1974.

56. Miller, J. F. A. P.: Immunity in the foetus and new born. *Br. Med. Bull.* 22:21, 1966.

57. Aranson, B. G., Jankovic, B. D., and Waksman, B. H.: Effect of thymectomy on delayed hypersensitivity reactions. *Nature* 194:99, 1962.

58. Good, R. A., et al.: The role of the thymus in the development of immunologic capacity in rabbits and mice. *J. Exp. Med.* 116:773, 1962.

59. Nezelof, C., Jammet, M. L., and Lortholary, P.: L'Hypoplasie héréditaire du thymus: Sa place et sa responsabilité dans une observation d'aplasie lymphocytaire, normoplasmocytaire, et normoglobuline que du nourrisson. *Arch. Fre. Pediatr.* 21:897, 1964.

60. Di George, A. M.: Congenital absence of the thymus and its immunological consequences: Concurrence with congenital hypoparathyroidism, in *Immunologic Deficiency Diseases of Man*, edited by D. Bergsma and R. A. Good. National Foundation, New York, 1968, p. 116.

61. August, C. S., et al.: Implantation of a foetal thymus, restoring immunological competence in a patient with thymic aplasia (Di George's syndrome). *Lancet* 2:1210, 1968.

62. Cleveland, W. W., Fogel, B. J., Brown, W. T., and Kay, H. E. M.: Foetal thymic transplant in a case of Di George's syndrome. *Lancet* 2:1211, 1968.

63. Hays, E. F.: The effect of epithelial remnant and whole organ grafts of thymus on the recovery of thymectomized irradiated mice. *J. Exp. Med.* 129:1235, 1969.

64. Roberts, S., and White, A.: Biochemical characterization of lymphoid tissue proteins. *J. Biol. Chem.* 178:151, 1949.

65. Metcalf, D.: The thymic origin of the plasma lymphocytosis stimulating factor. *Br. J. Cancer* 10:442, 1956.

66. Goldstein, A. L., Slater, F. D., and White, A.: Preparations, assay and partial purification of a thymic lymphocytopoietic factor (thymosin). *Proc. Natl. Acad. Sci. U.S.A.* 56:1010, 1966.

67. Craddock, C. G., Nakai, G. S., Fukuta, H., and Vanslager, L. M.: Proliferative activity of the lymphatic tissues of rats as studied with tritium-labeled thymidine. *J. Exp. Med.* 120:389, 1964.

68. Metcalf, D.: The nature and regulation of lymphopoiesis in the normal and neoplastic thymus, in *Ciba Foundation Symposium, Thymus: Experimental Clinical Studies*, edited by G. E. Wolstenholme and R. Porter. Churchill, London, 1966, p. 242.

69. Everett, N. B., and Caffrey, R. W.: Radiographic studies of bone mar-

row small lymphocytes, in *The Lymphocyte in Immunology and Haemopoiesis*, edited by J. M. Yoffey and E. Arnold, London, 1967.

70. Weissman, I. L.: Thymus cell migration. *J. Exp. Med. 126:*291, 1967.

71. Goldschneider, I., and McGregor, D. D.: Anatomical distribution of T and B lymphocytes in the rat: Development of lymphocyte-specific antisera. *J. Exp. Med. 138:*1443, 1973.

72. Waksal, S. D., St. Pierre, R. L., and Hostetler, J. R.: Brain-associated theta antiserum: Differential effects on lymphocyte subpopulations. *Cell Immunol. 12:*66, 1974.

73. Trainin, N., and Linker-Israel, M.: Restoration of immunologic reactivity of thymectomized mice by calf thymus extracts. *Cancer Res. 27:*309, 1967.

74. Hardy, M. A., Quint, J., Goldstein, A. L., State, D., and White, A.: Effect of thymosin and an antithymosin serum on allograft survival in mice. *Proc. Natl. Acad. Sci. U.S.A. 61:*875, 1968.

75. Bach, J. F.: Evaluation of T cells and thymic serum factors in man using the rosette technique. *Transplant. Rev. 16:*196, 1973.

Lymphocytic disorders—classification

CHAPTER *107*

Classification of lymphocyte and plasma cell disorders

MARSHALL A. LICHTMAN

The classification of lymphocyte disorders is complex because the principal manifestation of the diseases can be (1) an altered blood or marrow concentration of lymphocytes or plasma cells, (2) an abnormality of lymphocyte function such as failure of immunoglobulin synthesis or altered T-cell function, or (3) an abnormality of lymph node cells without overt blood or marrow involvement. Many diseases, especially inflammatory states (e.g., rheumatoid arthritis), infection (e.g., tuberculous adenitis) or neoplasia (metastatic carcinoma) can involve lymph nodes or the spleen but are not considered here because the lymph node involvement is a secondary alteration clinically and not in the usual province of hematology.

Three major groups of disease are listed in Table 107-1. First, disorders that are frequently associated with a prominent reactive lymphocytosis. These diseases are the result of infections, especially those caused by viruses, or, less commonly, they are due to drugs.

The second group of diseases result from malignant proliferation of lymphocytes and present a wide array of morphologic and clinical syndromes ranging from a fulminant malignancy such as Burkitt cell leukemia to an indolent disease like chronic lymphocytic leukemia. These lymphocyte tumors have been thought to originate in cells that are at various stages in the pathway of T- or B-lymphocyte differentiation. Thus, acute lymphocytic leukemia is felt to arise from a primitive lymphoid stem cell, chronic lymphocytic leukemia from a more differentiated B-lymphocyte progenitor, and multiple myeloma from a later stage of B-lymphocyte maturation. There is no direct verification of this hypothesis, and it is just as likely that the same stage of differentiation is the site of injury but that the etiologic agent or factor is different or that the type of genetic damage leads to different phenotypic expressions of lesions which occur at the same level of differentiation, for example, at the lymphopoietic stem cell level (see Fig. 20-1). The latter explanation is analogous with the phenotypic variations observed in hemopoietic stem cell diseases, in which injury to the stem cell pool can lead to such widely disparate phenotypes and clinical syndromes as paroxysmal nocturnal hemoglobinuria and chronic myelogenous leukemia. Thus, variability in expression of a lymphopoietic stem cell disorder may result in the spectrum of lymphocytic diseases such as B-lymphocyte or T-lymphocyte neoplasms and different types of B-cell diseases such as hairy cell leukemia, chronic lymphocytic leukemia, or plasma cell myeloma.

The third group of lymphocyte disorders involves those which are expressed as functional abnormalities of marrow derived (B) lymphocytes, thymic derived (T) lymphocytes, or defects involving both systems (impaired humoral and cellular immunity).

Classification of lymphocytic diseases is influenced also by the manifestations of the disease. For example, autoimmune hemolytic disease and autoimmune thrombocytopenia are caused by the inappropriate secretion of autoantibodies by lymphocytes. The blood cell coated with antibody is presumably normal, yet we classify these disorders as an acquired hemolytic anemia or thrombocytopenic purpura because that aspect of the disease is more visible and better understood than is the inappropriate synthesis of anticell antibody by the disturbed lymphocyte population.

References

1. Ryder, R. J. W.: Acute infectious lymphocytosis. *Am. J. Dis. Child.* 110:299, 1965.
2. Lagergren, J.: The white blood cell count and the erythrocyte sedimentation rate of pertussis. *Acta Pediatr.* 52:405, 1963.
3. Wood, T. A., and Frenkel, E. P.: The atypical lymphocyte. *Am. J. Med.* 43:923, 1967.
4. Kantor, G. L., and Goldberg, L. S.: Cytomegalovirus-induced posttransfusion syndrome. *Semin. Hematol.* 8:261, 1971.
5. Theologides, A., and Kennedy, D. K.: Clinical manifestations of toxoplasmosis in the adult. *Arch. Intern. Med.* 117:536, 1966.
6. Horwitz, C. A., et al.: Heterophil-negative infectious mononucleosis and mononucleosis-like illnesses. *Am. J. Med.* 63:947, 1977.
7. Siegel, S., and Berkowitz, J.: Diphenylhydantoin (Dilantin) hypersensitivity with infectious mononucleosis–like syndrome and jaundice. *J. Allergy* 32:447, 1961.
8. Barnett, E. V., Stone, G., Swisher, S. N., and Vaughan, J. H.: Serum sickness and plasmacytosis. *Am. J. Med.* 35:113, 1963.
9. Clark, H., and Muirhead, E. E.: Plasmacytosis of bone marrow. *Arch. Intern. Med.* 94:425, 1954.
10. Ritzman, S. E., et al.: Idiopathic (asymptomatic) monoclonal gammopathies. *Arch. Intern. Med.* 135:95, 1975.
11. Luckes, A. J., and Tindle, B. H.: Immunoblastic lymphadenopathy: A hyperimmune entity resembling Hodgkin's disease. *N. Engl. J. Med.* 292:1, 1975.
12. Thiel, E.: Multimarker classification of acute lymphoblastic leukemia: Evidence for further T-subgroups and evaluation of their clinical significance. *Blood* 56:759, 1980.
13. Bowman, W. P., et al.: A clinical perspective on cell markers in acute lymphocytic leukemia. *Cancer Res.* 91:4794, 1981.

TABLE 107-1   Classification of disorders of lymphocytes and plasma cells

I. Reactive lymphocytosis or plasmacytosis
   A. Viral infectious lymphocytosis [1]
   B. Bordetella pertussis lymphocytosis [2]
   C. Epstein-Barr virus mononucleosis [3]
   D. Cytomegalovirus mononucleosis [4]
   E. Toxoplasma gondii mononucleosis [5]
   F. Other viral mononucleosis [6]
   G. Drug-induced lymphocytosis [7]
   H. Serum sickness [8]
   I. Inflammatory (secondary) plasmacytosis of marrow [9]
II. Premalignant disorders of lymphocytes or plasma cells
   A. Benign monoclonal gammopathy [10]
   B. Angioimmunoblastic lymphadenopathy [11]
III. Malignant disorders of lymphocytes and plasma cells
   A. Acute lymphocytic leukemia
     1. Null type [12]
     2. Common type [13]
     3. B-cell type [14]
     4. Pre-B-cell type [15]
     5. T-cell type [16]
       a. Suppressor type [17]
       b. Helper type [18]
     6. Ph¹+ type [19]
     7. Burkitt type [20]
   B. Chronic lymphocytic leukemia
     1. B-cell type [21]
     2. T-cell type [22]
   C. Cutaneous T-cell lymphomas [23]
     1. Sézary cell
       a. Helper T-cell type [18]
     2. Mycosis fungoides
   D. Prolymphocytic leukemia [24]
   E. Hairy cell leukemia [25]
   F. Lymphoma [26–29]

   G. Hodgkin's disease [30]
   H. Plasma cell myeloma [31]
   I. Macroglobulinemia [32]
   J. The heavy-chain diseases [33]
   K. Primary amyloidosis [34]
IV. B-lymphocyte deficiency or dysfunction
   A. Agammaglobulinemia
     1. Sex-linked of Bruton [35]
     2. Dysgammaglobulinemia with nodular hyperplasia of intestinal lymphoid areas [36]
     3. Acquired agammaglobulinemia [37]
   B. Selective agammaglobulinemia
     1. IgM deficiency (Wiskott-Aldrich syndrome) [38]
     2. IgA deficiency
       a. Isolated asymptomatic [39]
       b. Steatorrheic [40]
     3. IgA and IgM deficiency (type II dysgammaglobulinemia) [41]
V. T-lymphocyte deficiency or dysfunction
   A. Thymic aplasia (DiGeorge's syndrome) [42]
   B. Thymic dysplasia (Nezelof's syndrome) [43]
   C. Hodgkin's disease [44]
   D. Sarcoidosis [45]
   E. Leprosy [46]
   F. Lupus erythematosus [47]
VI. Combined T- and B-cell deficiency or dysfunction
   A. Reticular agenesis (congenital aleukocytosis) [48]
   B. Combined immunodeficiency syndrome
     1. Swiss type—autosomal recessive [49]
     2. Thymic alymphoplasia—sex-linked recessive [50]
   C. Ataxia—telangiectasia [51]
   D. IgG and IgA deficiency and impaired cellular immunity (type I dysgammaglobulinemia) [52]

14. Gajl-Peczalska, K. J., et al.: B-cell markers on lymphoblasts in acute lymphoblastic leukemia. *Clin. Exp. Immunol.* 17:561, 1974.
15. Vogler, L. B., et al.: Pre-B-cell leukemia: A new phenotype of childhood lymphoblastic leukemia. *N. Engl. J. Med.* 298:872, 1978.
16. Lilleyman, J. S., and Sugden, P. J.: T-lymphoblastic leukaemia and the central nervous system. *Br. J. Cancer* 43:320, 1981.
17. Broder, S., et al.: Characterization of a suppressor-cell leukemia. *N. Engl. J. Med.* 298:66, 1978.
18. Broder, S., Uchiyama, T., and Waldmann, T. A.: Neoplasm of immunoregulatory cells. *Am. J. Clin. Pathol.* 72:724, 1979.
19. Bloomfield, C. D., Brunning, R. D., Smith, K. A., and Nesbit, M. E.: Prognostic significance of the Philadelphia chromosome in acute lymphocytic leukemia. *Cancer Gen. Cytogen* 1:229, 1980.
20. Flandrin, G., et al.: Acute leukemia with Burkitt tumor cells. *Blood* 45:183, 1975.
21. Zippin, C., Cutler, J., Reeves, W. J., Jr., and Lum, D.: Survival in chronic lymphocytic leukemia. *Blood* 42:367, 1973.
22. Nair, K. G., Han, T., and Minowada, J.: T-cell chronic lymphocytic leukemia. *Cancer* 44:1652, 1979.
23. Schein, P.: Clinical features. Cutaneous T-cell lymphomas: The Sézary syndrome, mycosis fungoides and related disorders. *Ann. Intern. Med.* 83:542, 1975.
24. Galton, D. A. G., et al.: Prolymphocytic leukemia. *Br. J. Haematol.* 27:7, 1974.
25. Golomb, H. M., Catovsky, D., and Golde, D. W.: Hairy cell leukemia. *Ann. Intern. Med.* 89:677, 1978.
26. Bloomfield, C. D., McKenna, R. W., and Brunning, R. D.: Signifi-

cance of haematological parameters in the non-Hodgkin's malignant lymphomas. *Br. J. Haematol.* 32:41, 1976.
27. Ault, K. A.: Detection of small numbers of monoclonal B-lymphocytes in the blood of patients with lymphoma. *N. Engl. J. Med.* 300:1041, 1979.
28. Gajl-Peczalska, K. J., et al.: B and T cell lymphoma. *Am. J. Med.* 59:674, 1975.
29. Zacharski, L. R., and Linman, J. W.: Chronic lymphocytic leukemia versus chronic lymphosarcoma cell leukemia. *Am. J. Med.* 47:75, 1969.
30. Kaplan, H. S.: *Hodgkin's Disease.* Harvard University Press, Cambridge, Mass., 1972.
31. Mellstedt, H., Hammarström, S., and Holm, G.: Monoclonal lymphocyte population in human plasma cell myeloma. *Clin. Exp. Immunol.* 17:371, 1974.
32. Preud'homme, J. L., and Seligmann, M.: Immunoglobulins on the surface of lymphoid cells in Waldenstrom's macroglobulinemia. *J. Clin. Invest.* 51:701, 1972.
33. Frangione, B., and Franklin, E. C.: Heavy chain diseases. *Semin. Hematol.* 10:53, 1973.
34. Kyle, R. A., and Bayrd, E. D.: Primary systemic amyloidosis and myeloma. *Arch. Intern. Med.* 107:344, 1961.
35. Rosen, F. S., and Janeway, C. A.: The gammaglobulins. *N. Engl. J. Med.* 275:769, 1966.
36. Hermans, P. E., et al.: Dysgammaglobulinemia associated with nodular lymphoid hyperplasia of the small intestines. *Am. J. Med.* 40:78, 1966.

37. Waldmann, T. A., et al.: Role of suppressor T-cells in common variable hypogammaglobulinemia. *Lancet 2*:609, 1974.
38. Cooper, M. D., et al.: Wiskott-Aldrich syndrome. *Am. J. Med. 44*:499, 1968.
39. Ammann, A. J., and Hong, R.: Selective IgA deficiency. *Medicine 50*:223, 1971.
40. Crabbé, P. A., and Heremans, J. F.: Lack of gamma-A-immunoglobulin in serum of patients with steatorrhea. *Gut 7*:119, 1966.
41. Gilbert, C., and Hong, R.: Qualitative and quantitative immunoglobulin deficiency. *Am. J. Med. 37*:602, 1964.
42. DiGeorge, A. M.: Congenital absence of the thymus and its immunologic consequences: Concurrence with congenital hypoparathyroidism, in *Immunologic Deficiency Diseases in Man*. National Foundation, New York, 1968, p. 116.
43. Nezelof, C., et al.: L'Hypoplasie héréditaire des thymus. *Arch. Fr. Pédiatr. 21*:897, 1964.
44. Young, R. C., Corder, M. D., Haynes, H. A., and DeVita, V. T.: Delayed hypersensitivity in Hodgkin's disease. *Am. J. Med. 52*:63, 1972.
45. Tannenbaum, H., Rocklin, R. E., Schur, P. H., and Sheffer, A. L.: Immune function in sarcoidosis. *Clin. Exp. Immunol. 26*:511, 1976.
46. Nath, I., Curtis, J., Bhutani, L. K., and Talwar, G. P.: Reduction of a subpopulation of T-lymphocytes in lepromatous leprosy. *Clin. Exp. Immunol. 18*:81, 1974.
47. Winfield, J. B., Winchester, R. J., and Kunkel, H. G.: Association of cold-reactive antilymphocyte antibodies with lymphopenia in systemic lupus erythematosus. *Arthritis Rheum. 18*:587, 1975.
48. Gitlin, D., Vawter, G., and Craig, J. M.: Thymic alymphoplasia and congenital aleukocytosis. *Pediatrics 33*:184, 1964.
49. Gitlin, D., and Craig, J. M.: The thymus and other lymphoid tissues in congenital agammaglobulinemia. I. Thymic alymphoplasia and lymphatic hypoplasia and their relation to infection. *Pediatrics 32*:517, 1963.
50. Hitzig, W. H., and Willi, H.: Hereditäre lymphoplasmacytäre dysgenesie. *Schweiz. Med. Wochenshr. 52*:1625, 1961.
51. McFarlin, D. E., Strober, W., and Waldmann, T. A.: Ataxia-telangiectasia. *Medicine 51*:281, 1972.
52. Stiehm, E. R., and Fudenberg, H. H.: Clinical and immunological features of dysgammaglobulinemia type I. *Am. J. Med. 40*:805, 1966.

Lymphocytic disorders — self-limited proliferative responses

CHAPTER *108*

Lymph node enlargement and splenomegaly

IRWIN M. WEINSTEIN

The ubiquitous role of the lymphocyte and the lymphoid tissues in reacting to infectious, inflammatory, and immunologic processes is illustrated by the wide variety of diseases in which enlargement of lymph nodes and/or the spleen is a prominent clinical finding. The characteristics of the lymph nodes on palpation, the anatomic distribution of enlargement, and the presence or absence of splenomegaly are often of diagnostic importance. In some instances the physical findings are so typical of a self-limited proliferative response to infection or inflammation that histologic examination of an enlarged lymph node is unnecessary. Benign nodal enlargement results from lymphocytic and/or macrophage hyperplasia. Lymphocytic proliferation is often the result of antigenic stimulation. The lymphocyte is uniquely capable of recognizing foreign antigens by specific surface receptors. Antigen-antibody reactions result in lymphocytic proliferation within the lymph node and clinical enlargement. This is usually transient, but if the antigenic stimulus persists, the lymph node may remain enlarged [1].

Nonmalignant illnesses accompanied by lymph node enlargement and splenomegaly occur most frequently in infancy and childhood. Hyperplasia of lymphoid tissue occurs promptly in response to infection in this age group. The incidence of tonsillitis, adenoiditis, retropharyngeal abscesses, appendicitis, and mesenteric lymphadenitis may be related to the volume of lymphoid tissue in particular areas. For example, appendicitis is rare during infancy, becomes more common after 2 years of age, is most frequent in childhood and adolescence, and becomes quite uncommon in later years. This correlates well with the amount of lymphoid tissue in the appendix, in which the circumferential aggregates of lymph follicles are particularly prone to infection [2].

Occasionally lymphatic hyperplasia is seen in apparently healthy young adults. Approximately 3 percent of college freshmen have palpable spleens not explained by body habitus, recent infections, including infectious mononucleosis, or liver disease. Follow-up evaluation for 10 years reveals no increased incidence of disease [3]. Persistent enlargement of the spleen following infection in younger life may account for half the cases of slight splenomegaly of undetermined cause in adults. Marked asymptomatic splenomegaly is more likely due to portal hypertension, myeloid metaplasia, Gaucher's disease, sarcoidosis, hemangiosarcoma or splenic cysts [4,5].

Benign proliferative reactions producing marked enlargement of lymph nodes may cause striking alterations in the blood, bone marrow, and lymph node morphology. Distinguishing these benign reactions from malignant lymphocyte disorders may be difficult, and may require the most sophisticated histologic interpretation. At times only observation of the patient's clinical course will finally establish whether or not the disorder is benign or malignant [6].

Local infection

Lymph node enlargement may result from either acute or chronic infections. The clinical as well as the histologic appearance of the lymph node depends to a great extent on the nature of the invading organism (bacteria, virus, or parasite), age of the patient, and host resistance.

In many acute infections, particularly with bacteria, such as *Streptococcus* or *Staphylococcus*, the lymph nodes become enlarged, soft, and tender. The overlying skin and surrounding tissues may be reddened and edematous. The histologic reaction is that of acute pyogenic lymphadenitis. Constitutional symptoms are absent or mild unless the infection occurs in a debilitated individual or in the very young. With appropriate antibiotic therapy, spread of the infection to lymph nodes beyond the regional area, with suppuration, abscess, or sinus formation, is now rare.

The persistence of lymph node enlargement in acute infections and the development of severe constitutional symptoms suggest an unusual etiology. Cat-scratch fever can be overlooked if the history of contact with cats is not obtained or the cutaneous lesion has disappeared before the lymph nodes enlarge [7]. Cat-scratch disease usually presents with a single, tender node, but occasionally mesenteric lymph node involvement may mimic appendicitis, or systemic manifestations may resemble lymphoma. Splenomegaly is uncommon [8]. Acute lymphadenitis in an unusual site, such as an epitrochlear lymph node, suggests an uncommon cause, e.g., rat-bite fever or tularemia [9]. Acute cervical lymphadenitis with suppuration (scrofula) is characteristic of tuberculosis [10].

Chronic infections may produce considerable lymph node enlargement without signs of inflammation. The lymph nodes are frequently firmer than in acute infection, and there is a tendency toward fusion and matting. Clinical differentiation from lymphoma may be difficult or impossible. Hard, fixed, and tender nodes are more suggestive of metastatic cancer. Chronic infection produces a granulomatous lymphadenitis in involved lymph nodes. Sinus formation or roentgenographic evidence of calcification suggests tuberculosis. Syphilis, leprosy, many fungal infections, and lymphogranuloma venereum can produce chronic, indolent lymph node enlargement [11]. The anatomic site of lymph node enlargement is sometimes helpful in suggesting the diagnosis, such as the unilateral inguinal lymphadenitis both above and below Poupart's ligament seen in lymphogranuloma venereum [12]. However, excisional biopsy for histologic and bacteriologic evaluation is usualy necessary to establish the precise cause of chronic localized lymph node enlargement.

Enlarged lymph nodes in certain regions take on special clinical significance. The isolated finding of enlarged occipital nodes is often an indication of infection in the scalp, and in children insect bites and ringworm are common causes. Malignant lymphoreticular diseases almost never begin in the occipital lymph nodes, nor are these nodes the site of metastatic disease from carcinomas of the head and neck.

Posterior auricular node enlargement is uncommon in lymphomas but occurs sufficiently often in rubella to be suggestive of this diagnosis [13].

Enlargement of anterior auricular lymph nodes may occur in lymphoma, but these are usually not a primary lesion. Infections of the eyelid and conjunctiva can result in local node enlargement. The intact conjunctiva may be the portal of entry for a number of infectious agents, particularly the viruses producing epidemic keratoconjunctivitis, cat-scratch fever, and adenovirus [14]. Trachoma is the most common cause of oculoglandular fever. The eye infection may be overt, giving the typical oculoglandular syndrome, or, if occult, may produce unilateral anterior auricular lymph node enlargement.

Infections of the head and neck usually do not produce enlargement of the posterior cervical or submental lymph nodes. Exceptions include scalp infections, tuberculosis, and infections of dental origin. Anterior cervical lymph nodes enlarge in response to infections of the oral cavity and pharynx.

Hard and fixed lymph nodes palpable in the supraclavicular fossae are highly suggestive of metastases from intrathoracic or intra-abdominal neoplasia [15]. This type of lymph node enlargement is almost never caused by an inflammatory process.

Enlarged axillary lymph nodes are often produced by infection involving the upper extremity. The cause may be obvious, but unusual infections leading to lymph node enlargement in this site include cat-scratch fever, sporotrichosis, extragenital syphilis, and brucellosis. Axillary lymph nodes may be the primary site in lymphoma, but are much less frequently involved than cervical nodes. In Hodgkin's disease the ratio is approximately 1:3 [16]. Involvement of the axillary nodes is more common in lymphosarcoma than in Hodgkin's disease [17].

Bilateral, painless epitrochlear lymph node enlargement may occur with repeated trivial infections in persons performing manual labor, but may also be a part of the generalized lymphatic reaction typical of many of the childhood viral diseases. Epitrochlear node enlargement is said to be rare in the generalized lymph node enlargement of tuberculosis, but not that of sarcoidosis. Bilateral, painless epitrochlear lymph node enlargement occurs in secondary syphilis, and may persist for life.

Sarcoidosis frequently presents with clinical manifestations suggesting a malignant lymphoreticular disorder. Eighty to ninety percent of patients have generalized lymph node enlargement particularly in the cervical, epitrochlear, and inguinal areas. Symmetrical bilaterally enlarged mediastinal nodes may occur without involvement of superficial lymph nodes and in asymptomatic patients may be virtually diagnostic of sarcoidosis [18]. The reliable differentiation from lymphoma, however, rests on demonstrating the noncaseating epitheloid granulomatous lesions in the lymph node, marrow, or other biopsy sites. Alcohol-induced pain, well recognized in Hodgkin's disease, may also occur in sarcoidosis [19,20]. Syndromes that occur with some regularity in sarcoidosis include the Mikulicz syndrome (enlargement of lacrimal and salivary glands) and uveitis associated with parotid, submaxillary, or submental salivary gland enlargement [21].

Inguinal lymph nodes are easily palpable in almost all adults, possibly due to repeated minor infections and trauma about the lower extremities or perineum. The degree of enlargement is usually modest and roughly symmetrical. Lymphogranuloma venereum in the male may present with unilateral lymph node enlargement, and with advanced disease sinus tracts may develop. In females with lymphogranuloma venereum, lymph node enlargement may be absent. Painless and unilateral enlargement of inguinal lymph nodes may occur in syphilis. Bilateral, tender inguinal lymphadenitis is common in venereal diseases such as gonococcal, mycoplasma, and herpetic urethritis. Progressive enlargement under observation in the absence of overt infection suggests neoplasia. The classic histologic features of malignant disease are often obscured, however, in inguinal lymph nodes by secondary infection and scarring.

Mediastinal or hilar lymph nodes do not become conspicuously enlarged in the ordinary types of pneumonia, but tuberculosis, either primary or hematogenous, can produce unilateral (about 8.5 percent) or bilateral hilar node enlargement. Enlarged nodes can persist after healing of the lung lesion. Coccidioidomycosis and histoplasmosis may also produce symmetrical node enlargement.

Infectious mononucleosis on rare occasions may cause enlargement of the mediastinal lymph nodes, and this may persist for many months [22]. Metastases to hilar lymph nodes are common from carcinoma of the lung but quite rare from distant sites. Mediastinal node enlargement is a frequent feature of malignant reticular disorders, especially Hodgkin's disease of the nodular sclerosing variety. This lymph node enlargement is usually asymmetrical.

Intra-abdominal or retroperitoneal node enlargement is usually not inflammatory in origin, especially when it is gross enough to be palpable or produce radiologically demonstrable displacement of abdominal and/or retroperitoneal structures. Tuberculous mesenteric lymphadenitis is an exception. These affected nodes may grow quite large, calcify, suppurate, and rupture [23].

Systemic infection

Many systemic infections producing regional lymph node enlargement have already been mentioned. A number of these diseases produce a generalized reaction and splenomegaly as well. The most common disorder to do this is infectious mononucleosis, but a number of other viral diseases can produce a very similar syndrome (see Chap. 109). These include viral hepatitis, influenza, cytomegalovirus (CMV), rubella, rubeola, and, less commonly, infectious lymphocytosis, pertussis, roseola infantum, and adenovirus infections [24–26]. Lymph node enlargement is not nearly as prominent in these viral disorders as it is in infectious mononucleosis, and splenomegaly, common in infectious mononucleosis, is unusual except in CMV infections. Atypical lymphocytes are commonly found in the peripheral blood in all the above disorders and are morphologically indistinguishable from those seen in infectious mononucleosis. These lymphocytes are predominantly T (thymus-derived) cells [27].

β-Hemolytic streptococcal pharyngotonsillitis is the bacterial infection most easily confused with infectious mononucleosis [28], and the two infections may coexist. Subacute bacterial endocarditis must be considered in the differential diagnosis of systemic infection versus a malignant lymphoreticular disorder. Lymph node enlargement is usually not impressive in subacute bacterial endocarditis, but the presence of splenomegaly, fever, and often a significant degree of anemia can mimic lymphoma. It is the author's impression that lymphoma is simulated more closely in those patients in whom the valvular infection is caused by an unusual organism [29]. The differential diagnosis between subacute bacterial endocarditis and CMV infection can be vexing, particularly following open heart surgery. The presence of circulating atypical lymphocytes favors a CMV infection, but this diagnosis is usually made by demonstrating a rising titer for CMV complement-fixing antibodies [30,31].

Fever, lymph node enlargement, splenomegaly, and atypical lymphocytes occur occasionally in patients with secondary syphilis and acute brucellosis, and these diseases must be distinguished from both infectious mononucleosis [32] and lymphoma [33]. Occasionally leptospirosis, salmonellosis, typhoid and paratyphoid fevers, tularemia, listeriosis, and diphtheria can present a similar problem in differential diagnosis [22,25,27]. Tuberculous involvement of the spleen resulting from hematogenous spread is not uncommon. Splenomegaly may be the major clinical manifestation of systemic tuberculosis, on occasion, but with diligent search foci of disease can be found elsewhere [34]. Some degree of cytopenia(s) is frequently found in such patients, and the diagnosis may not be established until splenectomy is performed [35].

Toxoplasmosis is another important disorder characterized by lymph node enlargement, atypical circulating lymphocytes and sometimes splenomegaly [36]. The protozoan *Toxoplasma gondii* infects humans and animals throughout the world. This infection may be seen in infants (congenital form) or children and young adults (acquired form). The massive hepatosplenomegaly, anemia, jaundice, skin rash, and fulminating course of congenital toxoplasmosis resembles the acute malignant histiocytosis of infancy and CMV disease [37]. Rapid diagnosis utilizing the toxoplasmosis dye test is essential, as treatment with sulfadiazine and pyrimethamine can be effective in an early infection [38]. The parasite is not ordinarily found in sections of excised lymph node, and histologic criteria do not distinguish toxoplasmosis from viral infections [39]. Acquired toxoplasmosis is usually a mild disorder and may be asymptomatic. Lymph node enlargement is often generalized, but the cervical nodes are the largest. Splenomegaly is less frequent and is usually modest in degree. Splenic enlargement is characteristically transient, but lymph node enlargement may last for months. When constitutional symptoms are present, the illness may closely resemble infectious mononucleosis or occasionally lymphoma. Anemia is rare in the acute, mild variety of acquired toxoplasmosis, but severe hemolytic anemia has been described in the more chronic form [40]. A persistently negative heterophil-antibody test and a rising titer of the toxoplasmosis dye test distinguishes between acquired toxoplasmosis and infectious mononucleosis. Diagnostic titers may not be present, however, until the third week after onset of fever. Because of prior inapparent infection or coexistence of the two disorders [41], a positive dye test without rising titer may be found in patients with malignant reticular disorders.

Up to 10 percent of patients with seronegative infectious mononucleosis may have toxoplasmosis, and this infection may account for some 5 percent of lymph node enlargements of unknown origin [42,43].

Amebiasis is the only other protozoan infection which may produce lymph node enlargement. The histologic picture is that of sclerosing lymphadenitis [44].

Splenomegaly is so common in the tropics that a common saying is, "Most patients have enlarged spleens; some are just larger than others." Malaria is the most important parasite producing splenomegaly [45]. Cytopenias are frequently present, but lymph node enlargement is uncommon. The diagnosis can be difficult at times because the parasite is sequestered in the spleen [46–49]. Malaria must be considered as a possible cause of intermittent fever, splenic enlargement, and anemia in individuals residing in endemic areas. Other important infections causing tropical splenomegaly include schistosomiasis, leishmaniasis, and kala azar [45]. Portal hypertension, hemoglobinopathies, and leukemia may coexist [46]. Chronic worm infestation may cause splenomegaly of considerable magnitude, but conspicuous enlargement of lymph nodes is almost never present in these disorders.

Many fungal infections can produce lymph node enlargement. These include histoplasmosis, coccidioidomycosis, blastomycosis, sporotrichosis, and torulosis. Splenomegaly is uncommon in these infections except in histoplasmosis.

Splenomegaly and lymph node enlargement occur in rickettsial diseases. In the United States the only important disorder is Rocky Mountain spotted fever. Hematologic complications in this disease include disseminated intravascular coagulation [50]. Splenomegaly is present in some 6 to 40 percent of patients. It is usually asymptomatic, but may produce hypersplenism, and rupture after slight trauma.

Splenomegaly and hepatomegaly without nodal enlargement may be found in febrile patients with regional ileitis. The splenomegaly is not due to demonstrable portal hypertension. Histologically the spleen shows atypical histiocytosis [51].

The tropical splenomegaly syndrome has been of recent interest [52,53]. It occurs where malaria is endemic, but its relation to parasite infection is controversial. It is an immune-complex disorder which presents with splenomegaly, often massive, and elevated serum IgM levels. Lymph node enlargement is not a characteristic feature. The disorder may respond to antimalarial therapy. Reticuloendothelial hyperplasia is probably the result of prolonged stimulation by circulating macromolecular immune complexes [53].

A graft-versus-host-like disorder has been described in older patients who present with rapidly enlarging generalized lymph nodes, and often hepatosplenomegaly, with immunologic abnormalities including autoimmune hemolytic anemia and polyclonal dysproteinemia. The lymph node histology shows angiocellular proliferation, considered not to be malignant. The process is often fatal, however, due to infection [54].

Autoimmune hemolytic anemia

Immune hemolytic anemia is frequently associated with lymph node enlargement of a minor degree, but in some children it is accompanied by massive lymph node enlargement which parallels to some extent the severity of the hemolysis [55]. The lymph node enlargement may also be due to episodic CMV infection [1]. In some cases the histologic picture may mimic that of malignant lymphoma.

Collagen-vascular and related disorders

Generalized lymph node enlargement is common in rheumatoid arthritis and systemic lupus erythematosus. Splenomegaly occurs in approximately 5 to 10 percent of patients with the former and in 20 percent of patients with the latter. Splenomegaly may be found in primary amyloidosis, but is considerably less frequent than hepatomegaly. Splenomegaly may also occur in Behçet's disease [56]. The constitutional symptoms of the collagen-vascular disorders, together with lymph node and/or splenic enlargement, and various cytopenias, such as occurs in Felty's syndrome, can make distinction from malignant lymphomas difficult in some cases. The histologic picture of lymph nodes in rheumatoid arthritis is remarkably similar to that seen in nodular lymphoma.

The mucocutaneous lymph node syndrome of infants and young children (Kawasaki's disease) causes nonpurulent cervical lymph node enlargement. Although usually self-limited, it may be fatal due to infantile polyarteritis nodosa [57].

Histiocytic disorders

Certain types of histiocytic disorders can present clinical syndromes indistinguishable from malignant lymphocytic diseases (see Chap. 100).

Massive lymph node enlargement, predominantly in the cervical region but often generalized, has been described in infants, children, and young adults with a unique entity, sinus histiocytosis of the lymph nodes [6]. Splenomegaly is absent but fever and leukocytosis may occur. The disorder is benign, but node enlargement may persist for months to years.

The sea-blue histiocyte syndrome can present as splenomegaly of obscure origin [58,59]. Lymph node enlargement is infrequent.

Gaucher's disease is a frequent cause of asymptomatic splenomegaly in the adult [4,5].

Hypersensitivity reactions

Difficult problems in differentiating benign lymphoreticular disorders from neoplasms are produced by hypersensitivity reactions to anticonvulsant drugs [60]. The clinical findings include fever, lymph node enlargement, splenomegaly, hepatomegaly, arthritis, jaundice, and morbilliform rash. The histologic features mimic those of Hodgkin's disease or "pseudolymphoma." The clinical abnormalities usually disappear rapidly following suspension of drug therapy, but malignant lymphoma has subsequently developed in several instances [61].

Patients with marked splenomegaly, occasionally lymph node enlargement, eosinophilic leukocytosis, and progressive cardiac disease have been described. Diagnostic features of leukemia were not present, and death resulted from cardiac failure [62].

Intensively treated patients with hemophilia may develop splenomegaly from CMV infection or from macrophage hyperplasia as a result of repeated bombardment with foreign antigen [63].

Atypical hyperplasia

Atypical angiofollicular lymph node hyperplasia has been described [64–66]. The clinical presentation is usually an asymptomatic mass in the hilum or mediastinum, but the tumor may obstruct a bronchus. Less commonly, fever, anemia, leukocytosis, elevated sedimentation rate and polyclonal hypergammaglobulinemia may occur. Most patients are young adults. Neither the lymph node tumor nor the systemic manifestations recur after surgical excision. Associated nephrotic syndrome or refractory anemia has also disappeared following removal of the lymph node tumor [67,68]. The solitary, usually asymptomatic thoracic tumor reveals hyaline-vascular changes. Those tumors with systemic manifestations show mature plasma cell infiltration [67]. Amyloid deposits may be found in the involved lymph nodes [69]. The etiology of this unusual benign tumor is unknown. An immunologic pathogenesis seems likely.

A fairly high percentage of patients who present with constitutional symptoms and local, regional, or generalized lymph node enlargement are found to have atypical hyperplasia on initial histological study. Such patients should be followed closely since a "benign" biopsy by no means rules out a collagen-vascular disorder or a malignant lymphoma [70].

Idiopathic splenomegaly is a term used to categorize instances of splenomegaly where clinical and pathological studies are nondiagnostic. The prognosis is usually good, but evolution of frank lymphoma has been described [71,72].

Endocrine diseases

Generalized lymphatic hyperplasia may accompany certain endocrine disorders, particularly hyperthyroidism. Spleen scintiscans reveal splenomegaly in about 50 per-

cent of patients with thyrotoxicosis and 30 percent in Hashimoto's disease [73]. In hyperthyroidism the lymph node and splenic enlargement and symptoms of hypermetabolism can be confused with lymphoma. Enlargement of the spleen in acromegaly has been found to be a manifestation of a second disease, such as cirrhosis of the liver or Gaucher's disease [74].

Dermatopathic lymphadenitis

Patients with exfoliative dermatitis often develop enlarged superficial lymph nodes. On biopsy these nodes show marked reticulum cell hyperplasia associated with melanin pigment and foam cells containing lipoid material. The lymph node enlargement regresses with improvement of the dermatitis [75]. Some patients may subsequently be found to have malignant lymphoma [76].

Gay-related immunodeficiency syndrome

Recent reports have described an outbreak of immunodeficiency diseases among young men belonging to the homosexual community [77]. The illnesses have occasionally been associated with generalized lymphadenopathy, splenomegaly, and atypical lymphocytosis and have ranged from severe opportunistic infection [78] to Kaposi's sarcoma [79]. Although helper T cells have been suppressed in many cases [80], excessive autoantibody response has been found in cases with thrombocytopenic purpura [81]. Infection with immunosuppressive CMV has been invoked as a possible causative mechanism [82], but in most cases, the etiology is unknown.

References

1. Zuelzer, W. W., and Kaplan, J.: The child with lymphadenopathy. *Semin. Hematol. 12*:323, 1975.
2. Solnitzky, O. D., and Jeghas, H.: Lymphadenopathy and disorders of the lymphatic system, in *Signs and Symptoms: Applied Pathologic Physiology and Clinical Interpretation*, 4th ed., edited by C. M. MacBryde. Lippincott, Philadelphia, 1964, p. 469.
3. Ebaugh, F. G. L., and McIntyre, O. R.: Palpable spleens: Ten years follow-up. *Ann. Intern. Med. 90*:130, 1979.
4. Silverstein, M. N., and Maldonado, J. E.: Asymptomatic splenomegaly. *Postgrad. Med. 48(2)*:80, 1970.
5. Goonewardene, A., Bourke, J. B., Ferguson, R., and Toghill, P. J.: Splenectomy for undiagnosed splenomegaly. *Br. J. Surg. 66*:62, 1979.
6. Rosai, J., and Dorfman, R. F.: Sinus histiocytosis with massive lymphadenopathy. *Arch. Pathol. 87*:63, 1969.
7. Spaulding, W. B., and Hennessy, J. N.: Cat-scratch disease: Study of eighty-three cases. *Am. J. Med. 28*:504, 1960.
8. Konbitz, B. C.: Systemic cat scratch disease. *Rocky Mt. Med. J. 70*:23, 1973.
9. Corwin, W. C., and Stubbs, J. P.: Further study on tularemia in the Ozarks. *JAMA 149*:343, 1952.
10. Lincoln, E. M.: Course and prognosis of tuberculosis in children. *Am. J. Med. 9*:623, 1950.

11. Price, L. W.: The pathology of lymph node enlargement. *Postgrad. Med. J.* 23:401, 1947.

12. Shaffar, L. W., and Olansky, S.: Lymphogranuloma venereum, in *Communicable and Infectious Diseases*, 6th ed., edited by F. H. Top, Sr. Mosby, St. Louis, 1968, chap. 34, p. 349.

13. Kalmansohn, R. B.: Rubella: Observations on an epidemic, with particular reference to lymphadenopathy. *N. Engl. J. Med.* 247:428, 1952.

14. Rysor, R., O'Rourke, J. R., and Iser, G.: Conjunctivitis in adenoidal-pharyngeal-conjunctival virus infection. *Arch. Ophthalmol.* 54:211, 1955.

15. Viacasa, E. P., and Pack, G. T.: Significance of supraclavicular signal node in patients with abdominal and thoracic cancer. *Arch. Surg.* 48:109, 1944.

16. Sugarbaker, E. D., and Craver, L. F.: Lymphosarcoma. *JAMA* 115:17, 1940.

17. Goldman, L. B.: Hodgkin's disease: An analysis of 212 cases. *JAMA* 114:1611, 1940.

18. Hodgson, C. H., Olsen, A. M., and Good, C. A.: Bilateral hilar adenopathy: Its significance and management. *Ann. Intern. Med.* 43:83, 1955.

19. Winterbauer, R. H., Belic, N., and Moores, K. D.: A clinical interpretation of bilateral hilar adenopathy. *Ann. Intern. Med.* 78:65, 1973.

20. Sharma, O. P., in *Sarcoidosis: A Clinical Approach*, edited by O. P. Sharma. Charles C Thomas, Springfield, Ill., 1975.

21. Longcope, W. T., and Freidman, D. C.: A study of sarcoidosis. *Medicine (Baltimore)* 31:1, 1952.

22. Finch, S. C.: Clinical symptoms and signs of infectious mononucleosis, in *Infectious Mononucleosis*, edited by R. C. Carter and H. G. Penman. Blackwell Scientific, Oxford, 1969, p. 19.

23. Studley, H. O.: Intra-abdominal rupture of retroperitoneal tuberculous lymph node. *Ann. Surg.* 115:477, 1942.

24. Gardner, H. T., and Paul, J. R.: Infectious mononucelosis at the New Haven Hospital, 1921 to 1946. *Yale J. Biol. Med.* 19:839, 1947.

25. Smith, C. H.: Infectious lymphocytosis. *Am. J. Dis. Child.* 62:221, 1941.

26. Hoagland, R. J.: *Infectious Mononucleosis*. Grune & Stratton, New York, 1967.

27. Virolaine, M., Andersson, L. C., Lalla, M., and Von Essen, R.: T-Lymphocyte proliferation in mononucleosis. *Clin. Immunol. Immunopathol.* 2:114, 1973.

28. Evans, A. S.: Infectious mononucleosis in University of Wisconsin students. *Am. J. Hyg.* 71:342, 1960.

29. Overholt, B. F.: Actinobacillus actinomycetemcomitans endocarditis. *Arch. Intern. Med.* 117:99, 1966.

30. Wheeler, E. O., Turner, J. D., and Scannell, J. G.: Fever, splenomegaly and atypical lymphocytes: A syndrome observed after cardial surgery utilizing a pump oxygenator. *N. Engl. J. Med.* 266:454, 1962.

31. Jordan, M. C., Rousseau, W. E., Stewart, J. A., Noble, G. R., and Chin, T. D.: Spontaneous cytomegalovirus mononucleosis: Clinical and laboratory observations in nine cases. *Ann. Intern. Med.* 79:153, 1973.

32. Rubenstein, A. D., and Shaw, C. I.: Infectious mononucleosis simulating brucellosis. *N. Engl. J. Med.* 231:111, 1944.

33. Goffinet, D. R., Hoyt, C., and Eltringham, J. R.: Secondary syphilis misdiagnosed as lymphoma. *Calif. Med.* 112:22, 1970.

34. Hickling, R. A.: Tuberculous splenomegaly with miliary tuberculosis of the lungs. *Q. J. Med.* 7:263, 1938.

35. Chapman, A. Z., Reader, P. S., and Baker, L. A.: Neutropenia secondary to tuberculous splenomegaly. *Ann. Intern. Med.* 41:1225, 1954.

36. Jones, T. C., Kean, B. H., and Kimball, A. C.: Toxoplasmic lymphadenitis. *JAMA* 192:87, 1965.

37. Krugman, S., and Ward, R.: *Infectious Diseases of Children*, 4th ed. Mosby, St. Louis, 1968, chap. 27, p. 375.

38. Feldman, H. A.: Toxoplasmosis. *Pediatrics* 22:559, 1958.

39. Stansfeld, A. G.: The histological diagnosis of toxoplasmic lymphadenitis. *J. Clin. Pathol.* 14:565, 1961.

40. Kalderon, A. E., Kikkawai, Y., and Berstein, J.: Chronic toxoplasmosis associated with severe hemolytic anemia. *Arch. Intern. Med.* 114:95, 1964.

41. Fleck, D. G., and Ludlam, G. B.: Indications for laboratory tests for toxoplasmosis. *Br. Med. J.* 2:1239, 1965.

42. Beverley, J. K. A., and Beattie, C. P.: Glandular toxoplasmosis: A survey of 30 cases. *Lancet* 2:379, 1958.

43. Penman, H. G.: The problem of seronegative infectious mononucleosis, in *Infectious Mononucleosis*, edited by R. C. Carter and H. G. Penman. Blackwell Scientific, Oxford, 1969, p. 201.

44. Lukes, R. J.: Personal communication, 1970.

45. Balustein, A. U., and Diggs, L. W.: Pathology of the spleen, in *The Spleen*, edited by A. Blaustein. McGraw-Hill, New York, 1963, p. 45.

46. Butler, T., Wilson, M., Sulzer, A. J., and Loan, N. T.: Chronic splenomegaly in Vietnam. I. Evidence for malarial etiology. *Am. J. Trop. Med. Hyg.* 22:1, 1973.

47. Pryor, P. S.: Tropical splenomegaly in New Guinea. *Br. Med. J.* 3:825, 1969.

48. Hermann, R. E.: Splenectomy for the diagnosis of splenomegaly. *Ann. Surg.* 168:895, 1968.

49. Pitney, W. R.: Cold haemagglutinins associated with splenomegaly in New Guinea. *Vox Sang.* 14:438, 1968.

50. Graybill, J. R., Hawiger, J., and Des Prez, R. M.: Complement and coagulation in Rocky Mountain spotted fever. *South. Med. J.* 66:410, 1973.

51. Putnam, M. D., and Hall, D. A.: Asymptomatic regional ileitis manifest as fever, hepatic disease and splenomegaly. *Dis. Colon Rectum* 17:705, 1973.

52. Sagoe, A.: Tropical splenomegaly syndrome: Long term proguanil therapy correlated with spleen size, serum IgM, and lymphocyte transformation. *Br. Med. J.* 3:378, 1970.

53. Ziegler, J. L.: Cryglobulinaemia in tropical splenomegaly syndrome. *Clin. Exp. Immunol.* 15:65, 1973.

54. Frizzera, G., Moran, E. M., and Rappaport, H.: Angioimmunoblastic lymphadenopathy with dysproteinemia. *Lancet* 1:1070, 1974.

55. Zuelzer, W. W., Mastrangelo, R., Stulberg, C. S., Poulik, M. O., Page, R. H., and Thompson, R. I.: Autoimmune hemolytic anemia: Natural history and viral-immunologic interactions in childhood. *Am. J. Med.* 49:80, 1970.

56. Kiernan, T. J., Gillan, J., Murray, J. P., and McCarthy, C. F.: Behçet's disease and splenomegaly. *Br. Med. J.* 2:1340, 1978.

57. Kawasaki, T., Kosaki, F., Okawa, S., Shigematsu, I., and Yanagawa, H.: A new infantile acute febrile mucocutaneous lymph node syndrome (MLNS) prevailing in Japan. *Pediatrics* 54:271, 1974.

58. Silverstein, M. N., and Ellefson, R. D.: The syndrome of the sea-blue histiocyte. *Semin. Hematol.* 9:299, 1972.

59. Vogel, J. M., and Vogel, P.: Idiopathic histiocytosis. *Semin. Hematol.* 9:349, 1972.

60. Siegal, S., and Berkowitz, J.: Diphenyldantoin (Dilantin) hypersensitivity with infectious mononucleosis-like syndrome and jaundice. *J. Allerg.* 32:447, 1961.

61. Hyman, G. A., and Sommers, S. C.: Development of Hodgkin's disease and lymphoma during anticonvulsant therapy. *Blood* 28:416, 1966.

62. Sheperd, A. J. N., Walsh, C. H., Archer, R. K., and Wetherly-Mein, G.: Eosinophilia, splenomegaly and cardiac disease. *Br. J. Haematol.* 20:233, 1971.

63. Levine, P. H., McVerry, B. A., Attock, B., and Dormandy, K. M.: Health of the intensively treated hemophiliac, with special reference to abnormal liver chemistries and splenomegaly. *Blood* 50:1, 1977.

64. Castleman, B., Iverson, L., and Pardo Mendez, V.: Localized mediastinal lymph node hyperplasia resembling thymoma. *Cancer* 9:822, 1956.

65. Tung, K. S. K., and McCormick, L. J.: Mesenteric lymphoid hamartoma: Report of five cases and review of the literature. *Cancer* 20:525, 1967.

66. Keller, A. R., Hochholzer, L., and Castleman, B.: Hyaline-vascular and plasma cell types of giant lymph node hyperplasia of the mediastinum and other locations. *Cancer* 29:670, 1973.

67. Humphreys, S. R., Holley, K. E., Smith, L. H., and McIlrath, D. C.: Mesenteric angiofollicular lymph node hyperplasia (lymphoid hamartoma) with nephrotic syndrome. *Mayo Clin. Proc.* 50:317, 1975.

68. Burgert, E. O., Gilchrist, S. G., and Fairbanks, V. F.: Intraabdominal, angiofollicular lymph node hyperplasia (plasma cell variant) with an antierythropoietic factor. *Mayo Clin. Proc.* 50:542, 1975.

69. Garcia-San Miguel, J., Rozman, C., Palacin, A., and Nomdedu, B.: Mesenteric hyaline plasma cell lymph node hyperplasia with amyloid deposits. *Arch. Intern. Med.* 141:261, 1981.

70. Moore, R. D., Weisberger, A. J., and Bowerfind, E. J., Jr.: An evaluation of lymphadenopathy in systemic disease. *Arch. Intern. Med.* 99:751, 1957.
71. Dacie, J. V., Brain, M. C., Harrison, C. V., Lewis, S. M., and Worlledge, S. M.: Non-tropical idiopathic splenomegaly. *Br. J. Haematol.* 17:317, 1969.
72. Long, J. C., and Aisenberg, A. C.: Malignant lymphoma diagnosed at splenectomy and idiopathic splenomegaly. *Cancer* 33:1054, 1974.
73. Metcalfe-Gibson, C., and Keddie, N.: Spleen size and previous tonsillectomy in autoimmune disease of the thyroid. *Lancet* 1:944, 1978.
74. Sober, A. J., Gorden, P., Roth, J., and AvRuskin, T. W.: Visceromegaly in acromegaly. *Arch. Intern. Med.* 134:415, 1974.
75. Nairn, R. C., and Anderson, T. E.: Erythrodermia with lipomelanotic reticulum-cell hyperplasia of lymph node (dermatopathic lymphadenitis). *Br. Med. J.* 1:820, 1955.
76. Block, J. B., Edgcomb, J., Eisen, A., and Van Scott, E. J.: Mycosis fungoides: Natural history and aspects of its relationship to other malignant lymphomas. *Am. J. Med.* 34:228, 1963.
77. Centers for Disease Control: Epidemiologic aspects of the current outbreak of Kaposi's sarcoma and opportunistic infections. *N. Engl. J. Med.* 306:248, 1982.
78. Mildvan, D., et al.: Opportunistic infections and immune deficiency in homosexual men. *Ann. Intern. Med.* 96:700, 1982.
79. Friedman-Kien, A. E., et al.: Disseminated Kaposi's sarcoma in homosexual men. *Ann. Intern. Med.* 96:693, 1982.
80. Kornfeld, H., et al.: T-lymphocyte subpopulations in homosexual men. *N. Engl. J. Med.* 307:729, 1982.
81. Morris, L., Distenfeld, A., Amorosi, E., and Karpatkin, S.: Autoimmune thrombocytopenic purpura in homosexual men. *Ann. Intern. Med.* 96:714, 1982.
82. Drew, W. L., et al.: Prevalence of cytomegalovirus infection in homosexual men. *J. Infect. Dis.* 143:188, 1981.

CHAPTER *109*

Mononucleosis syndromes

ROBERT F. BETTS

For many years clinicians have recognized a self-limited clinical syndrome known as *infectious mononucleosis* which occurs principally in teenagers and young adults [1–4]. The manifestations include fever, pharyngitis, lassitude, lymphadenopathy, and lymphocytes with atypical morphologic characteristics. An important diagnostic clue is elevated titers of heterophil antibody, an antibody to an antigen occurring on a number of cells including sheep, horse, and beef red blood cells [2,5]. However, not all patients with mononucleosis have elevated heterophil antibody titers, and patients without are designated as having *heterophil-negative mononucleosis* [6]. The chance development of heterophil-positive mononucleosis by a technician infected with a recently discovered herpes virus known as Epstein-Barr virus (EBV) [7] led to further studies which established this virus as the etiologic agent for the heterophil-positive syndrome. Subsequent studies have shown that the heterophil-negative syndrome is caused by other viruses and agents (Table 109-1). Of those the

TABLE 109-1 Etiologic agents associated with mononucleosis syndrome

Heterophil-positive:
  Epstein-Barr virus
Heterophil-negative:
  Cytomegalovirus
  Epstein-Barr virus
  Herpes simplex II
  Rubella
  Toxoplasma gondii
  Adenovirus
  Unknown agents

most important is a closely related herpes virus, cytomegalovirus (CMV), and heterophil-negative mononucleosis is often called *CMV mononucleosis* [6,8–12].

Etiology and pathogenesis

The infectious agents that produce the mononucleosis syndromes have been recognized to cause or be related to other disease states before they were linked to mononucleosis. EBV had been demonstrated in tumor cells from African children with Burkitt's lymphoma [13] and antibody to the antigens of this virus was measurable in sera of the involved children [14]. Although the serum from all other children in the same environment contained antibody, it was present in lower titers than in the sera of children with tumors [15].

After the discovery that EBV also was the cause of mononucleosis, a number of studies of young adults have been conducted prospectively. These studies suggest that there is a steady acquisition of antibody by seronegative subjects eventually yielding an 80 to 90 percent incidence of seropositivity in adults. Such seropositive individuals are immune to heterophil-positive infectious mononucelosis [16–20].

Cytomegalovirus causes intrauterine infection which sometimes results in severe disease of the newborn manifesting as hepatosplenomegaly, thrombocytopenia, hemolytic anemia, and microcephaly [21]. CMV has also been shown to be transmitted by blood and by transplanted allografts. Infection acquired from blood transfusion can produce heterophil-negative mononucleosis syndrome [12]. In the transplant setting primary infection may cause a mild mononucleosis syndrome but all too frequently is followed by severe disease with pneumonitis and death [22–24].

The susceptibility of individuals seropositive for CMV to CMV mononucleosis is not known. However, it is clear from epidemiologic studies that individuals with antibodies to CMV can be superinfected by a second CMV [25]. The clinical consequence of superinfection is not known.

Other herpes viruses can cause a very similar syndrome. Infection with herpes simplex type II and less commonly with varicella-zoster virus can resemble the heterophil-negative syndrome. In addition, rubella virus and adenovirus have occasionally been implicated. Since patients may present with a heterophilnegative mononucleosis syndrome despite absence of all the above-listed agents [6], there are almost certainly unidentified agents that produce this clinical illness.

The only nonviral agent that is regularly associated with the mononucleosis syndrome is *Toxoplasma gondii*. This agent can produce a febrile syndrome with lymph node enlargement, but usually produces asymptomatic infection or isolated lymphadenopathy without fever [26,27].

The pathogenesis of EBV mononucleosis is initiated by the entry of EBV either in epithelial cells in the oropharynx or in B lymphocytes in Waldeyer's ring [28]. Since B lymphocytes possess a specific receptor for EBV, the virus can infect a large number of the B cells, not merely a single clone, and hence a polyclonal B-cell response ensues [29–32]. This probably explains the variety of antibodies which are synthesized. The polyclonal B-cell response in turn elicits a polyclonal T-cell counterresponse. The majority of circulating atypical lymphocytes have T-cell characteristics, but most of them are not functional. A fraction of the T cells function as cytotoxic cells directed at the surface antigens which develop on infected B cells. Furthermore, the cytotoxic T cells may attack the B lymphocytes in the tonsils, which probably explains the severe pharyngitis which ensues. The infection comes under control as a result of a balance between T helper and T suppressor cells that are part of the counterresponse to initial polyclonal B-cell proliferation.

In most instances the disease is self-limited because of the T-B cell interaction. However, occasionally an antibody produced by infected B cells is directed at platelet surface antigens or at i antigen on red blood cells. In such circumstances, thrombocytopenia or hemolytic anemia may result.

In a small number of individuals with a specific type of immune deficiency syndrome, a reciprocal T-cell response may not develop or it may be incomplete. In such instances B-cell proliferation continues and a B-cell lymphoma may develop [33]. Alternatively an excessive T-suppressor-cell response could lead to hypo- or agammaglobulinemia [30,34]. An excessive cytotoxic response if localized to the upper airway may lead to airway obstruction or if more widespread, may lead to graft-versus-host disease [35]. In Africa, EBV has been linked to the development of Burkitt's lymphoma. Some antigens in the tumor cells have the characteristics of EBV and EBV antibodies are found in most affected children. However, the majority of individuals in the United States who have tumors with a similar histologic appearance do not have antibody to EBV and the relationship between the lymphoma and EBV is still poorly understood. Recent epidemiologic studies have also shown an equally unexplained increased incidence of high titer of antibody to EBV antigens in patients with rheumatoid arthritis [36].

The pathogenesis of CMV infection is less well understood. There is no evidence that lymphocytes are lytically infected by this virus and in vitro lytic infection has not been accomplished. Furthermore, the numbers of T cells are not increased and the nature of the atypical cell in CMV is not known. The most recent data suggest that the circulating monocyte may be the infected cell in CMV or at least that there is a defect in monocyte function [34]. This is supported by studies of infected patients and by analysis of in vitro data [37,38].

Epidemiology

The occurrence of the mononucleosis syndrome is uncommon in children under age 10, yet asymptomatic infection with EBV or CMV is quite common. Consequently an understanding of the epidemiology of the etiologic agents is as important as an understanding of the epidemiology of the disease itself [39,40].

The socioeconomic circumstances are an important predictor of the age at which infection with either of these agents first occurs. A large proportion of the population from poor socioeconomic circumstances acquire EBV and CMV infections at an early age [39,40]. Crowding, large families and poor sanitary habits may contribute to this. It has been shown that cytomegalovirus is transmitted from mother to child perinatally either from virus in cervical secretions or in breast milk [41–43]. Since younger women are more likely to have CMV in cervical secretions than older women [44], early marriage contributes to the spread of infection. Where breast-feeding is universal, CMV infection occurs in nearly everyone. EBV on the other hand has not been identified in cervical secretions or breast milk. It is, however, shed for prolonged periods in oral secretions and thereby readily transmitted from mother to child. Thus, by age 5 to 6 nearly all children in poor socioeconomic circumstances have been infected with both of these viral agents without the development of the clinical syndrome of mononucleosis. The epidemiology of infection with *Toxoplasma gondii* in different from either CMV or EBV. Infection is probably acquired from cysts in partially cooked meat or oocysts in cat feces [26,27].

When children do develop primary infection with either CMV or EBV, there may be minor illnesses [16,39,45] resembling those seen is adults [46]. Pneumonitis can occur, but for the most part the infections are inapparent. The incubation period, when apparent, is 20 to 25 days in children.

Young adults who have failed to undergo asymptomatic seroconversion, are very susceptible to EBV and CMV infection and the development of the mononucleosis syndrome [47]. In the teenager, the most common infection is with EBV, and by the age of 30 almost all subjects have had EBV infection. By contrast, in middle class societies, seroconversion to CMV occurs mostly between the ages of 20 and 50. The majority of those who become infected remain free of symptoms, but since so many become infected, these are the years of peak incidence of the mononucleosis syndrome. Consequently, mononucleosis occurring in young adults is almost always due to EBV and is usually heterophil-positive, whereas mononucleosis occurring after the age of 25 or 30 is usually due to CMV and is heterophil-negative.

Because of the high incidence of seropositivity in adults, neither CMV nor EBV causes epidemic outbreaks of mononucleosis. Intrafamilial spread of EBV is infrequent [48], and nurses employed on renal transplant services or on hemodialysis units seldom acquire infection from patients [49,50], in contrast to hepatitis virus, which is spread readily in the dialysis unit. In pediatric neonatal intensive care units the frequency of transmission of CMV from babies to nurses is also very low [51]. This contrasts with the spread of respiratory syncytial virus, which is easily transmitted from babies to nurses in these same nurseries [52]. The reason that EBV and CMV have been maintained in humans is apparently that they persist in saliva and other secretions for prolonged periods of time, affording them ample opportunity to be transmitted during intimate contacts. Since CMV is harbored in cervical secretions and semen [53], its route of transmission in adults is primarily venereal, whereas the transmission of EBV is almost exclusively by salivary contact. Despite these one-to-one modes of transmission, there is a higher incidence of infection with CMV in women than in men [10,54]; however, the sex ratio for EBV infection is equal [55].

Clinical features

The incubation period for EBV and CMV infections is approximately 35 days in adults (range 30 to 55 days). Although there are a number of similarities in the illnesses caused by EBV and CMV, there are two striking differences (see Table 109-2). One is that acute pharyngitis both symptomatically and by physical examination occurs primarily in patients with EBV infection. Pharyngitis may not be obvious initially, but it soon assumes major importance. It may be associated with petechial rash on the palate and interfere with deglutition and breathing, and on rare occasions produce respiratory obstruction [35,56]. In CMV mononucleosis only a small fraction of patients have symptomatic or objective pharyngitis.

The second major difference is that lymphadenopathy usually develops in EBV mononucleosis but is seldom prominent in CMV infection. The adenopathy parallels the pharyngitis both in progression and regression. The nodes are tender and enlarged and can either be confined to the cervical area or found at most peripheral sites.

Aside from these two differences, the clinical features of symptomatic EBV and CMV infections are similar. Both illnesses may begin with lassitude, associated with a sweaty, chilly sensation and weakness. Fever, low-grade at first, soon becomes hectic. Occasionally, illness

TABLE 109-2   Clinical manifestations of mononucleosis syndrome

	Percent of subjects		
	EBV	CMV	Toxoplasma
Fever	90	90	20
Malaise	70	80	80
Pharyngitis	80	10	10
Lymphadenopathy	80	10	60–95
Hepatomegaly	50	40	10
Splenomegaly	40	40	10
Rash	10	5	20
Palatal petechiae	30	5	—

can begin abruptly with shaking chills and fever to 40°C. The symptomatic phase in CMV infection may be much more prolonged, and fever can often persist for 1 to 2 months. Other prominent features of EBV and CMV infection are hepatomegaly and splenomegaly, both of which are more common in EBV infection although in CMV infection the spleen can become markedly enlarged. Rupture of the spleen has been limited to patients with EBV mononucleosis [57]. EBV mononucleosis in older adults is quite uncommon but often more severe than in teenagers [58,59]. CMV mononucleosis, on the other hand, is as common in older adults as in teenagers and equally severe [60].

The major clinical features that are seen in each of these syndromes are outlined above and in Table 109-3. Headache and facial and periorbital swelling are more common in EBV than in CMV infections. In both, a rash can occur, especially if ampicillin is administered [17,61]. Pneumonitis can occur but is unusual in both. Cardiac disease has been observed on rare occasions in EBV mononucleosis. Although not common, acute neurologic syndromes occur in both infections. Guillain-Barré syndrome is most prominent in CMV mononucleosis, whereas transverse myelitis and an acute encephalitis are more common in EBV infection [10,62–64]. Since the other typical features of mononucleosis

TABLE 109-3   Severe disease in normals infected with either EBV or CMV

	EBV	CMV
Hemolytic anemia	++	+
Thrombocytopenia	+	+
Respiratory obstruction	+	—
Splenic rupture	+	—
Jaundice	+	+
Guillain-Barré*	+	++
Encephalitis*	++	+
Transverse myelitis*	+	—
Renal failure	+	—
Pneumonia*	+	+
Myocarditis*	+	—
B-cell lymphoma	+	—
Agammaglobulinemia	+	—

*May occur without other signs of mononucleosis.

NOTES: ++ = common, + = infrequent, − = not reported.

are absent in about half the cases with central nervous system (CNS) syndromes, specific serologic techniques (see below) are necessary to establish the diagnosis. In most instances these neurological syndromes are self-limited and reverse spontaneously, but they may end fatally.

Toxoplasmosis will also produce prominent lymphadenopathy, especially posterior auricular, but it does not produce pharyngitis. Hepatosplenomegaly is less prominent in toxoplasmosis than in either EBV or CMV mononucleosis, but it can occur in some patients. A faint rash occasionally occurs. Fever is usually low-grade or absent. Encephalitis or meningitis can also occur [26,27]. The other agents that produce mononucleosis syndrome may sometimes produce lymphadenopathy. Rubella usually produces a rash, adenovirus usually causes pharyngitis.

Laboratory features

EBV and CMV mononucleosis have many laboratory features in common, the most striking being the presence of atypical lymphocytes [11,65] (see Table 109-4). In each syndrome, over half the white blood cells are lymphocytes and at least 20 percent of these are atypical. The total lymphocyte count may exceed 4500 per microliter, and atypical cells often exceed 1000 per microliter. The cytoplasm/nucleus ratio is much higher than usual, and vacuolization of the cytoplasm is prominent. Cytoplasmic pseudopods and skirting (dark staining of the periphery of the cytoplasm) are prominent. Nuclear chromatin is clumped and may contain inclusions. These lymphocyte abnormalities should not be confused with changes seen in malignancy of the lymphatic system. In the latter instance, the cytoplasm/nucleus ratio is quite low, the peripheral cytoplasmic skirting is lacking, and the nuclei are round and lack clumping of the chromatin [65]. Other hematologic abnormalities include hemolytic anemia due to cold agglutinins usually directed at i antigen [17,66]. Hemolysis is more likely to occur when the thermal activity of the cold agglutinin is broad and is active at temperatures of 30°C or higher. The platelet count is decreased regularly in both EBV and CMV disease and occasionally is suf-

ficiently low to produce petechiae [67,68]. On rare occasions agranulocytosis has developed in association with EBV mononucleosis.

OTHER ABNORMALITIES
Liver function abnormalities, mainly cholestatic in type, occur. Levels of hepatocellular enzymes may be mildly elevated, but jaundice is uncommon [11,69]. Antinuclear factor, rheumatoid factor, cold agglutinins, and cryoglobulins are detected in both diseases. In EBV infection, antibodies to a number of other infectious agents may increase in titer. For this reason, a variety of infectious agents, e.g., Sendai virus, *Listeria monocytogenes*, *Brucella*, and *Streptococcus MG*, were believed at one time or another to be etiologic agents of infectious mononucleosis.

HETEROPHIL ANTIBODY
The one laboratory feature that clearly distinguishes the two syndromes is the heterophil antibody test. This antibody is directed at a heterophil antigen on sheep, horse, and beef red blood cells but not on guinea pig or horse kidney cells. This reactivity is used to establish the diagnosis of EBV mononucleosis in the laboratory. If patients are followed for an adequate period of time, approximately 95 percent of patients with EBV mononucleosis will develop heterophil antibody. If the heterophil antibody develops late, the disease may be more severe [70]. Mild symptoms or even asymptomatic EBV seroconversion can be associated with development of heterophil antibody. The commercial kits used for the demonstration of the diagnosis of heterophil antibody employ horse red blood cells. Because the titer of antibody to these cells in a patient's serum is usually higher than the antibody to either sheep or beef red cells, it is not uncommon for an individual to have heterophil antibody titer to horse red cells for a substantial period of time. Furthermore, after the horse cell–reactive antibody has decreased below diagnostic levels, the titer may increase once again in relationship to another viral infection. Therefore, if a patient has had mononucleosis in the past 12 months and develops another complaint which leads the clinician to perform a test for mononucleosis, an improper diagnosis may be made. Individuals with heterophil-negative mononucleosis but proven Epstein-Barr virus infection have the identical syndrome as individuals who are heterophil-positive [11]. Nevertheless the heterophil antibody is one of the most specific tests available in clinical medicine. Antibody to horse red cells that is not absorbed by guinea pig or horse kidney virtually always indicates EBV infectious mononucleosis. There is not an equivalent serologic test for CMV infectious mononucleosis. CMV-specific serologic evaluation is required to establish this diagnosis.

SPECIFIC VIRAL TESTS
Laboratory tests either measuring specific antiviral antibodies or shedding of virus can be helpful in making a

TABLE 109-4 Laboratory abnormalities in mononucleosis syndrome

	Percent of subjects	
	EBV	*CMV*
Lymphocytosis (4500 per microliter)	90	80
> 20% atypical lymphocytes	90	70
Abnormal liver function	90	70
Cold agglutinins	40	20
Cryoglobulins	40	20
Decreased platelets	50	20
Antinuclear factor	50	20
Heterophil antibody	95	0

specific diagnosis, especially in CMV mononucleosis and EBV heterophil-negative mononucelosis. Tests using immunofluorescent techniques will identify antibodies to specific EBV antigens. There is sequential appearance and disappearance of different antibodies. Almost all infected patients have IgG antibody to the virus capsid antigen (VCA) when first seen. Soon thereafter, IgM antibody develops but only remains for a few months while the IgG anti-VCA persists for life.

Specific antibody to Epstein-Barr nuclear antigen (EBNA) does not develop until after the acute phase of illness but then persists for life. In acute infection, early antigen (EA)–specific antibody, i.e., IgG antibody to nuclear antigens that are synthesized in infected cells before viral directed DNA synthesis commences, appears slightly later in the illness than IgG VCA and persists for only a few months [71–75]. Complement-fixing antibody and neutralizing antibody also develop. Most laboratories that conduct these studies measure VCA and EBNA antibody. The more difficult tests for IgM antibody or antibody to EA are reserved for special cases. A presumptive diagnosis of EBV-induced disease can be reached if VCA antibodies are present and EBNA antibodies are absent.

These antibodies do not cross-react with CMV or react with heterophil antigen. Furthermore EBV antibodies and heterophil antibody occur independently of one another. If techniques are available, EBV can be isolated by inoculating oral secretions into a suspension of umbilical cord lymphocytes [76].

CMV is readily cultured from secretions using human fetal fibroblasts. Virus can be detected in urine, oral and cervical secretions, semen, and in the white blood cells as well as in infected tissue. In addition, most laboratories utilize complement-fixing antibody tests to aid in diagnosis and consider a fourfold rise in antibody titer as diagnostic. Antibodies to different CMV antigens are not as well defined as those to EBV, but IgM and IgG antibody to antigens in CMV infected fibroblasts can be demonstrated by immunofluorescent techniques [77,78]. One major problem is that using these techniques, IgM antibody to CMV infected cells can be detected in serum of patients with EBV mononucleosis [11,79]. A more recent technique which measures cytolytic antibody to CMV-infected cells identifies patients with primary CMV infection [80]. This antibody is an IgM and is not detected in patients with EBV mononucleosis.

HISTOLOGIC FEATURES
Most patients who acquire either EBV mononucleosis or CMV mononucleosis have a self-limited disease. In EBV, scraping of the tonsils yields atypical lymphocytes on smear, and biopsies of lymph nodes reveal a pleomorphic proliferation of lymphatic cells. The few autopsy cases probably represent more extensive disease than usually seen, but tissues from these demonstrate the same pleomorphic proliferation of lymphatic cells in liver, spleen, and most prominently in the tonsils. Atyp-

ical lymphocytes and occasionally granuloma are found within the bone marrow [81]. Granulomatous changes have been detected in the liver in both infections [55,82,83].

Most cases of granulomatous hepatitis due to CMV occur in the setting of CMV mononucleosis syndrome, but occasionally patients have only fever and granuloma.

Differential diagnosis

One disease with which EBV is commonly confused is β-streptococcal pharyngitis. Here, however, the blood count usually shows a predominance of polymorphonuclear leukocytes, and liver function tests are normal. In addition, nearly 100 percent of patients with β-streptococcal pharyngitis have bacteria recoverable from their throat culture. However, one confusing aspect is that between 10 and 25 percent of patients with EBV mononucleosis harbor group A β-streptococci in their throat. Although this organism should be treated, treatment seldom alters the clinical course of the pharyngitis.

The disease with which cytomegalovirus infection is most commonly confused is lymphoma. Since CMV infection can occur in middle-aged subjects and presents with fever and an enlarged spleen without other specific findings, the clinician may suspect that the patient has lymphoma. These patients are often admitted to the hospital and extensively worked up before the diagnosis is reached. By the same token patients with lymphoma can have disease which mimics CMV infection.

The mononucleosis syndrome of toxoplasmosis has features which mimic EBV and CMV mononucleosis, but there are many differences [26,27]. *Toxoplasma gondii* infection tends to involve posterior auricular nodes and is often an afebrile disease. Pharyngitis is uncommon. The liver and spleen are not usually enlarged, and liver function tests are most often normal. Monocytosis occurs rather than atypical lymphocytosis. Of course, a toxoplasma antibody test can quickly differentiate between these possibilities. Both hepatitis A and B viruses can produce a mononucleosis-like syndrome including atypical lymphocytosis and abnormal liver function tests, but the elevated levels of hepatocellular enzymes and the normal heterophil titers usually distinguish these disorders. Furthermore, when liver function becomes abnormal in hepatitis, the fever lyses.

Other infections to be considered include adenovirus infection, which sometimes resembles EBV infection by virtue of pharyngitis and lymphadenopathy. Leptospirosis can cause hepatic abnormalities but usually in conjunction with a polymorphonuclear leukocyte response and is often associated with renal failure. *Listeria monocytogenes* infections may produce disseminated lymphadenopathy fever and mononucleosis. A blood culture positive for *Listeria* will identify these patients.

TABLE 109-5 Special problems in EBV and CMV infection

	EBV	CMV
In utero infection	+	++
Congenital illness	+	++
Neonatal illness	−	++
Transfusion-associated	+	++
Transplant-associated	+	++
Association with rheumatoid arthritis	+	−

NOTES: + = reported, ++ = recognized with significant frequency, − = not reported.

Finally, some patients present with a syndrome which mimics mononucleosis in every respect except that exhaustive evaluation yields no evidence of CMV, EBV, or other recognized etiologic agents. This suggests that there are other causes not yet identified which can produce the mononucleosis syndrome.

Therapy

Since both heterophil-positive and -negative syndromes are self-limited, only symptomatic therapy is usually indicated. If the spleen is large, activity should be temporarily limited to avoid spontaneous rupture. Although aspirin has been recommended to reduce the fever and pharyngeal inflammation, the recent reports of aspirin producing Reye's syndrome in children with varicella [84] suggests that such alternatives such as acetaminophen or gargling with saline be used. Penicillin or erythromycin is indicated if β streptococcus is isolated.

Limited studies carried out with college or military personnel suggest that fever and overall well-being can be improved by glucocorticoids, although the effects on pharyngitis appears to be minimal. Most clinicians, however, are reluctant to use corticosteroids unless there are severe, life-threatening complications such as obstruction of the upper airway, thrombocytopenic purpura, hemolytic anemia, or central nervous system involvement (Table. 109-3). It is advisable to start with the equivalent of 40 to 60 mg per day of prednisone, maintain that dose for 4 days, and then taper over 5 to 7 days. For the patient with life-threatening disease or in the congenital immune deficiency syndrome where EBV has led to B-cell type lymphomas, treatment with a new antiviral agent, acyclovir, is now being considered [85].

There is no definite therapeutic agent available for cytomegalovirus infection. Since the mechanism of disease is not well understood, steroids should not be used unless severe complications such as those listed in Table 109-3 have developed, and no other alternatives seem available.

Patients with the acute infectious mononucleosis syndrome due to *Toxoplasma gondii* usually do not require therapy [26]. If severe complications occur, however, a loading dose of 100 to 200 mg pyrimethamine in two divided doses, followed by 1 mg/kg per day along with sulfadiazine 75 to 100 mg/kg per day in four divided doses should be used. Folinic acid (calcium leucovorin) 2 to 10 mg per day may prevent hematologic toxicity. Total duration of therapy is 2 to 4 weeks. Careful monitoring of the blood count at least once a week is indicated since pyrimethamine can produce leukopenia and thrombocytopenia.

MONONUCLEOSIS IN PREGNANCY

Cytomegalovirus has long been recognized as a cause of cytomegalic inclusion disease of the newborn, but the problem is complex (see Table 109-5). First, there is substantial epidemiologic data to show that the majority of children with in utero infection are born of mothers who were infected many months prior to the onset of their pregnancy and were asymptomatic during pregnancy [86,87]. Second, most babies born with congenital CMV are asymptomatic at birth, and 90 percent of such children will probably develop normally. It is not certain whether the babies who are severely symptomatic at birth are those born of mothers who have had primary infection during the first trimester. However, there is evidence to show that if a mother develops primary CMV infection after the first trimester only a small number of babies will develop congenital infection, usually asymptomatic. The eventual outcome in those babies is not known. Most women in the childbearing age are immune to infection with EBV; hence, congenital infection is rare. Nevertheless, there are rare cases of a severe congenital syndrome including microcephaly, hepatosplenomegaly, cataracts, mental retardation, and/or death following EBV mononucleosis during gestation. Although the data on which to base a therapeutic decision regarding abortion for the mother who does develop either CMV or EBV mononucleosis syndrome during pregnancy are limited, most experts would advise therapeutic abortion if either syndrome develops during the first trimester.

Congenital infection is also a risk in toxoplasmosis. It is clearly established that the mother who has antibody before pregnancy does not transmit the organism to her developing infant. However, infection during the first trimester poses a risk, and most experts suggest therapeutic abortion when toxoplasmosis can be diagnosed during that time. The same is true for rubella.

OTHER SPECIAL PROBLEMS

In the compromised host CMV can cause primary infection if transmitted by blood transfusion or by allografts (see Table 109-5). In some instances the patient with primary infection will develop a heterophil-negative mononucleosis syndrome, whereas in other instances pneumonia will be the major manifestation. The disease may be self-limited, but CMV has been associated with rejection of the allograft and with death.

EBV syndrome also occurs occasionally following renal transplantation either because of development of primary infection, possibly from the donated allograft, or because of reactivation of latent virus.

CMV infection has been observed at an increasing rate in homosexual men, and the CMV has been implicated as a possible etiologic agent for Kaposi's sarcoma, occurring among homosexual men and renal transplant recipients [88,89].

References

1. Sprunt, T. P., and Evans, F. A.: Mononuclear leukocytosis in reaction to acute infections (infectious mononucleosis). *Bull. Johns Hopkins Hosp.* 31:410, 1920.
2. Evans, A. S.: The history of infectious mononucleosis. *Am. J. Med. Sci.* 267:189, 1974.
3. Tidy, H. L., and Daniel, E. C.: Glandular fever and infective mononucleosis with an account of an epidemic. *Lancet* 2:9, 1923.
4. Cabot, R. C.: The lymphocytosis of infection. *Am. J. Med. Sci.* 145:335, 1913.
5. Paul, J. R., and Bunnell, W. W.: The presence of heterophile antibodies in infectious mononucleosis. *Am. J. Med. Sci.* 183:90, 1932.
6. Klemola, E., et al.: Infectious mononucleosis-like disease with negative heterophile agglutination test. Clinical features in relation to Epstein-Barr virus and cytomegalovirus antibodies. *J. Infect. Dis.* 121:608, 1970.
7. Henle, G., Henle, W., and Diehl, V.: Relation of Burkitt's tumor-associated herpes-type virus to infectious mononucleosis. *Proc. Natl. Acad. Sci. U.S.A.* 59:94, 1968.
8. Klemola, E., and Kääriäinen, L.: Cytomegalovirus as a possible cause of a disease resembling infectious mononucleosis. *Br. Med. J.* 2:1099, 1965.
9. Klemola, E., et al.: Cytomegalovirus mononucleosis in previously healthy adults. *Ann. Intern. Med.* 71:11, 1969.
10. Jordan, M. C., et al.: Spontaneous cytomegalovirus mononucleosis. *Ann. Intern. Med.* 79:153, 1973.
11. Horwitz, C. A., et al.: Heterophil-negative infectious mononucleosis and mononucleosis-like illnesses. *Am. J. Med.* 63:947, 1977.
12. Kääriäinen, L., Klemola, E., and Paloheimo, J.: Rise of cytomegalovirus antibodies in an infectious-mononucleosis-like syndrome after transfusion. *Br. Med. J.* 1:1270, 1966.
13. Epstein, M. A., Achong, B. G., and Barr, Y. M.: Virus particles in cultured lymphoblasts from Burkitt's lymphoma. *Lancet* 1:702, 1964.
14. Henle, G., and Henle, W.: Immunofluorescence in cells derived from Burkitt's lymphoma. *J. Bacteriol.* 91:1248, 1966.
15. Gunven, P., Klein, G., Henle, G., Henle, W., and Clifford, P.: Epstein-Barr virus in Burkitt's lymphoma and nasopharyngeal carcinoma. *Nature* 228:1053, 1970.
16. Evans, A. S., Niederman, J. C., and McCollum, R. W.: Seroepidemiologic studies of infectious mononucleosis with EB virus. *N. Engl. J. Med.* 279:1121, 1978.
17. Evans, A. S.: New discoveries in infectious mononucleosis. *Mod. Med.* 42:18, 1974.
18. Niederman, J. C., Evans, A. S., Subrahmanyan, L., and McCollum, R. W.: Prevalence, incidence, and persistence of EB virus antibody in young adults. *N. Engl. J. Med.* 282:361, 1970.
19. Hallee, T. J., Evans, A. S., Niederman, J. C., Brooks, C. M., and Voegtly, J. H.: Infectious mononucleosis at the United States Military Academy: A prospective study of a single class over four years. *Yale J. Biol. Med.* 47:182, 1974.
20. Joint Investigation by University Health Physicians and P.H.I.S. Laboratories: Infectious mononucleosis and its relationship to EB virus antibody. *Br. Med. J.* 4:643, 1971.
21. Weller, T. H., and Hanshaw, J. B.: Virologic and clinical observations on cytomegalic inclusion disease. *N. Engl. J. Med.* 266:1233, 1962.
22. Betts, R. F., et al.: Clinical manifestations of renal allograft–derived primary cytomegalovirus infection. *Am. J. Dis. Child.* 131:759, 1977.
23. Suwansirikul, S., et al.: Primary and secondary cytomegalovirus infection: Clinical manifestations after renal transplantation. *Arch. Intern. Med.* 137:1026, 1977.
24. Pass, R. F., Whitley, R. J., Diethelm, A. G., Whelchel, J. D., Reynolds, D. W., and Alford, C. A.: Cytomegalovirus infection in patients with renal transplants: Potentiation by antithymocyte globulin and an incompatible graft. *J. Infect. Dis.* 142:9, 1980.
25. Huang, E.-S., Alford, C. A., Reynolds, D. N., Stagno, S., and Pass, R. F.: Molecular epidemiology of cytomegalovirus infection in women and their infants. *N. Engl. J. Med.* 303:958, 1980.
26. Kean, B. H.: Clinical toxoplasmosis—50 years. *Trans. R. Soc. Trop. Med. Hyg.* 66:549, 1972.
27. Krick, J. A., and Remington, J. S.: Current concepts in parasitology: Toxoplasmosis in the adult—An overview. *N. Engl. J. Med.* 298:550, 1978.
28. Epstein, M. A., and Adrong, B. G.: Pathogenesis of infectious mononucleosis. *Lancet* 3:1270, 1977.
29. Yefenef, E., et al.: Epstein-Barr virus receptors, complement receptors, and EBV infectibility of different lymphocyte fractions of human peripheral blood. I and II. *Cell. Immunol.* 35:34 and 43, 1978.
30. Tosato, G., et al.: Activation of suppressor T cells during Epstein-Barr virus induced infectious mononucleosis. *N. Engl. J. Med.* 301:1133, 1979.
31. Schwartz, R. S.: Epstein-Barr virus—Oncogen or mitogen? *N. Engl. J. Med.* 302:1307, 1980.
32. DeWaele, M., Thielemans, C., and VanCamp, B. K. G.: Characterization of immunoregulatory T cells in EBV-induced infectious mononucleosis by monoclonal antibodies. *N. Engl. J. Med.* 304:460, 1981.
33. Robinson, J. E., et al.: Diffuse polyclonal B-cell lymphoma during primary infection with Epstein-Barr virus. *N. Engl. J. Med.* 302:1293, 1980.
34. Provisor, A. J., Iacuone, J. J., Chilcotte, R. R., Nieburger, R. G., Crussi, F. G., and Baehner, R. L.: Acquired agammaglobulinemia after a life-threatening illness with clinical and laboratory features of infectious mononucleosis in three related male children. *N. Engl. J. Med.* 293:62, 1975.
35. Britton, S., et al.: Epstein-Barr immunity and tissue distribution in a fatal case. *N. Engl. J. Med.* 298:89, 1978.
36. Ferrell, P. B., Aitcheson, C. T., Pearson, G. R., and Tan, E. M.: Seroepidemiological study of relationship between Epstein-Barr virus and rheumatoid arthritis. *J. Clin. Invest.* 67:681-687, 1981.
37. Rinaldo, C. R., Jr., Carney, W. P., Richter, B. S., Black, P. H., and Hirsch, M. S.: Mechanisms of immunosuppression in cytomegaloviral mononucleosis. *J. Infect. Dis.* 141:448, 1980.
38. Carney, W. P., and Hirsch, M. S.: Mechanism of immunosuppression in cytomegalovirus mononucleosis. *J. Infect. Dis.* 144:47, 1981.
39. Fleisher, G., Henle, G., Henle, W., Sennette, E. T., and Biggar, R. J.: Primary infection with Epstein-Barr virus in infants in the United States. Clinical and serological observations. *J. Infect. Dis.* 139:553, 1979.
40. Li, F., and Hanshaw, J. B.: Cytomegalovirus infection among migrant children. *Am. J. Epidemiol.* 86:137, 1967.
41. Stagno, S., Reynolds, D. W., Pass, R. F., and Alford, C. A.: Breast milk and the risk of cytomegalovirus infection. *N. Engl. J. Med.* 302:1073, 1980.
42. Reynolds, D. W., Stagno, S., Hosty, T. S., Tiller, M., and Alford, C. A., Jr.: Maternal cytomegalovirus and perinatal infection. *N. Engl. J. Med.* 289:1, 1973.
43. Hayes, K., Danks, D. M., Gibas, H., and Jack, I.: Cytomegalovirus in human milk. *N. Engl. J. Med.* 287:177, 1972.
44. Knox, G. E., Pass, R. F., Reynolds, D. W., Stagno, S., and Alford, C. A.: Comparative prevalence of subclinical cytomegalovirus and herpes simplex virus infections in the genital and urinary tracts of low-income, urban women. *J. Infect. Dis.* 140:419, 1979.
45. Hanshaw, J. B., et al.: Acquired cytomegalovirus infection. *N. Engl. J. Med.* 272:602, 1965.
46. Fleisher, G. R., Paradose, J. E., and Lennette, E. T.: Leukocyte response in children with infectious mononucleosis caused by Epstein-Barr virus. *Am. J. Dis. Child.* 135:699, 1981.

47. Sawyer, R. N., Evans, A. S., Niederman, J. C., and McCollum, R. W.: Prospective studies of a group of Yale University freshmen. I. Occurrence of infectious mononucleosis. *J. Infect. Dis.* 123:263, 1971.

48. Pejme, J.: The contagiousness of infectious mononucleosis. *J. Ir. Med. Assoc.* 58:48, 1966.

49. Tolkoff-Rubin, N. E., et al.: Cytomegalovirus infection in dialysis patients and personnel. *Ann. Intern. Med.* 89:625, 1978.

50. Betts, R. F., et al.: Epidemiology of cytomegalovirus infection in end stage renal disease. *J. Med. Virol.* 4:89, 1979.

51. Yeager, A. S.: Longitudinal serologic study of cytomegalovirus infections in nurses and in personnel without patient contact. *J. Clin. Microbiol.* 2:445, 1975.

52. Hall, C. B.: The shedding and spreading of respiratory syncytial virus. *Pediatr. Res.* 11:236-239, 1977.

53. Lang, D. J., and Kummer, J. F.: Demonstration of cytomegalovirus in semen. *N. Engl. J. Med.* 287:756, 1972.

54. Luby, J. P., and Shasby, D. M.: A sex difference in the prevalence of antibodies to cytomegalovirus. *JAMA* 222:1290, 1972.

55. Evans, A. S.: Infectious mononucleosis in University of Wisconsin students. *Am. J. Hyg.* 71:342, 1960.

56. Penman, H. G.: Fatal infectious mononucleosis: A critical review. *J. Clin. Pathol.* 23:765, 1970.

57. Hoagland, R. J., and Henson, H. M.: Splenic rupture in infectious mononucleosis. *Ann. Intern. Med.* 46:1184, 1957.

58. Horwitz, C. A., et al.: Clinical and laboratory evaluation of elderly patients with heterophile antibody positive infectious mononucleosis. *Am. J. Med.* 61:333, 1976.

59. Corey, L., et al.: HB$_s$-Ag-negative hepatitis in a hemodialysis unit —Relation to Epstein-Barr virus. *N. Engl. J. Med.* 293:1273, 1975.

60. Betts, R. F.: Syndromes of cytomegalovirus infection. *Adv. Intern. Med.* 26:447, 1980.

61. Klemola, E.: Hypersensitivity reactions to ampicillin in cytomegalovirus mononucleosis. *Scan. J. Infect. Dis.* 2:29, 1970.

62. Schmitz, H., and Enders, G.: Cytomegalovirus as a frequent cause of Guillain-Barré syndrome. *J. Med. Virol.* 1:21, 1977.

63. Grose, C., Henle, W., Henle, G., and Feorino, P. M.: Primary Epstein-Barr virus infections in acute neurologic diseases. *N. Engl. J. Med.* 292:392, 1975.

64. Phillips, C. A., et al.: Cytomegalovirus encephalitis in immunologically normal adults. Successful treatment with vidarabine. *JAMA* 238:2299, 1977.

65. Downey, H., and McKinlay, C. A.: Acute lymphoadenosis compared with acute lymphatic leukemia. *Arch. Intern. Med.* 32:82, 1923.

66. Coombs, J.: Cytomegalic inclusion disease associated with autoimmune hemolytic anemia. *Br. Med. J.* 2:743, 1968.

67. Harris, A. J., Meyer, F. J., and Brody, E. A.: Cytomegalovirus-induced thrombocytopenia and hemolysis in an adult. *Ann. Intern. Med.* 83:670, 1975.

68. Clark, B. F., and Davies, S. H.: Severe thrombocytopenia in infectious mononucleosis. *Am. J. Med. Sci.* 248:703, 1964.

69. Gelb, D., West, M., and Zimmerman, H. J.: Serum enzymes in disease. IX. Analysis of factors responsible for elevated values in infectious mononucleosis. *Am. J. Med.* 33:249, 1962.

70. Chretien, J. H., et al.: Predictors of duration of infectious mononucleosis. *South. Med. J.* 70:437, 1977.

71. Henle, G., Henle, W., Haltia, K., Klemola, E., and Niederman, J. C.: Antibodies to early antigens induced by Epstein-Barr virus in infectious mononucleosis. *J. Infect. Dis.* 124:58, 1971.

72. Schmitz, H., and Scherer, M.: IgM antibodies to Epstein-Barr virus in infectious mononucleosis. *Arch. Gesamte Virusforsch.* 37:332, 1972.

73. Henle, W., Henle, G., and Horwitz, C. A.: Epstein-Barr–specific diagnostic tests in infectious mononucleosis. *Human Pathol.* 5:552, 1974.

74. Henle, G., Henle, W., and Horwitz, C. A.: Antibodies to Epstein-Barr virus–associated nuclear antigen in infectious mononucleosis. *J. Infect. Dis.* 130:231, 1974.

75. Evans, A. S., Niederman, J. C., Cenabre, L. C., West, B., and Richards, V. A.: Specificity, sensitivity, and persistence of heterophile and EB-virus specific IgM antibodies in clinical and subclinical infectious mononucleosis. *J. Infect. Dis.* 132:546, 1975.

76. Miller, G., Niederman, J. C., Andrews, L.-L.: Prolonged oro-pharyngeal excretion of Epstein-Barr virus after infectious mononucleosis. *N. Engl. J. Med.* 288:229, 1973.

77. Betts, R. F., et al.: Comparative activity of immunofluorescent antibody and complement fixing antibody in cytomegalovirus infection. *J. Clin. Microbiol.* 4:151, 1976.

78. Hanshaw, J. B., Steinfeld, H. J., and White, C. J.: Fluorescent antibody test for cytomegalovirus macroglobulin. *N. Engl. J. Med.* 279:566, 1968.

79. Hanshaw, J. B., Niederman, J. C., and Chessin, L. N.: Cytomegalovirus macroglobulin in cell-associated herpes virus infections. *J. Infect. Dis.* 125:304, 1972.

80. Betts, R. F., and Schmidt, S. G.: Cytolytic IgM antibody to cytomegalovirus in primary cytomegalovirus in humans. *J. Infect. Dis.* 143:821, 1981.

81. Rothwell, D. J.: Bone marrow granulomas and infectious mononucleosis. *Arch. Pathol.* 99:508, 1975.

82. Reller, L. B.: Granulomatous hepatitis associated with acute cytomegalovirus infection. *Lancet* 1:20, 1973.

83. Clark, J.: Cytomegalovirus granulomatous hepatitis. *Am. J. Med.* 66:264, 1979.

84. Starko, K. M., Ray, C. G., Dominguez, L. B., Stromberg, W. L., and Woodal, D. F.: Reye's syndrome and salicylate use. *Pediatrics* 66:859, 1980.

85. King, D. A.: Proceedings of a symposium on acyclovir. *Am. J. Med.* 73:1, 1982.

86. Schopfer, K., Lauber, E., and Krech, U.: Congenital cytomegalovirus infection in newborn infants of mothers infected before pregnancy *Arch. Dis. Child.* 53:536, 1978.

87. Goldburg, G. N., et al.: In utero Epstein-Barr virus (infectious mononucleosis) infection. *JAMA* 246:1579, 1981.

88. Durack, D. T.: Opportunistic infections and Kaposi's sarcoma in homosexual men. *N. Engl. J. Med.* 305:1465, 1981.

89. Fauci, A. S.: The syndrome of Kaposi's sarcoma and opportunistic infections: An epidemiologically restricted disorder of immunoregulation. *Ann. Intern. Med.* 96:777, 1982.

CHAPTER *110*

Lymphocytosis

PETER A. CASSILETH

Lymphocytosis, defined as an absolute increase in the number of circulating lymphocytes, occurs in various disease states but is less common than relative lymphocytosis secondary to granulocytopenia. When an absolute lymphocytosis does develop, the total white blood cell count is rarely elevated above the range of normal. Exceptions to this generalization are the pronounced lymphocytosis and leukocytosis that occur commonly in infectious mononucleosis (and occasionally in the infectious mononucleosis-like syndromes caused by *Toxoplasma gondii* and cytomegalovirus), infectious lymphocytosis, *Bordetella pertussis* infection, and lymphocytic leukemias.

The normal lymphocyte count varies with age [1]. From birth to 6 months the mean absolute lymphocyte count increases from 5500 tp 7300 per microliter then gradually falls during the first 10 years of life to reach the adult level of about 2500 per microliter. Lymphocytosis is defined as an increase in lymphocytes of greater than 9000 per microliter in infants and young children, 7200 per microliter in older children, and 4000 per microliter in adults [1].

As important as determining the absolute or relative number of lymphocytes in the blood is a careful analysis of their morphologic characteristics. In the normal blood film the appearance of the lymphocytes varies considerably. The cell diameter ranges from 7 to 18 μm. The nuclear chromatin may appear densely clumped and "mature" or may have a fine reticular appearance and occasionally a nucleolus. The cytoplasm of normal lymphocytes may be pale blue or slate gray, resembling that of the monocyte, or may have the rich, deep blue color characteristic of plasma cells. Some cells may contain up to six to eight round, azurophilic granules. The nucleus can be round or slightly indented and the cytoplasm abundant or scanty. The term *atypical lymphocyte* has been applied to cells whose appearance deviates to a greater or lesser degree from that of normal lymphocytes. In normal blood as many as 4 to 11 percent of all mononuclear cells (lymphocytes plus monocytes) may be classified as atypical lymphocytes [2]. Studies of DNA synthesis utilizing labeled thymidine in lymphocytes from normal persons and patients with various disease states reveal that atypical lymphocytes actively synthesize DNA. Increase in the number of atypical lymphocytes may represent a response to some antigenic stimulus (see Table 110-1)

Marked increases in atypical lymphocytes occur in infectious mononucleosis, infectious mononucleosis–like syndromes caused by *T. gondii* and cytomegalovirus, infectious hepatitis, and hypersensitivity reactions, especially to such drugs as diphenylhydantoin and *p*-aminosalicylic acid. In *Bordetella pertussis* infections and in infectious lymphocytosis there is characteristically a great increase in normal-appearing small lymphocytes. This phenomenon in whooping cough seems to be caused by a redistribution of these lymphocytes from tissue pools to the peripheral blood.

Acute infectious lymphocytosis

The first reported cases of this entity appeared in 1941 [3], and subsequently epidemic outbreaks in confined populations have been recognized [4–6]. Although most of the epidemics occurred in young children in the first decade of life, teenagers and young adults have been affected [4,7]. Most of the affected individuals were asymptomatic, and the diagnosis was determined only by finding elevated white cell counts in patient contacts [6].

The disease has an incubation period of 12 to 21 days [9] and an infectivity rate of about 50 percent [4]. The heterophil and cold agglutinin titers and the cultures

TABLE 110-1   Causes of absolute lymphocytosis

Infectious mononucleosis
Acute infectious lymphocytosis
Bordetella pertussis infection
Toxoplasma gondii infection
Cytomegalovirus infection
Acute and chronic lymphocytic leukemia
Hypersensitivity reactions (occasionally)

and titers for *B. pertussis* infection are negative [8]. Serial studies of antibody titers to a variety of viruses, including Epstein-Barr (EB) virus, cytomegalovirus, and herpes simplex, were negative [9–11]. In other studies, increased antibody titers to Coxsackie A [6], ECHO 7 [11], and Coxsackie B6 [12] were found, but there has been no evidence to incriminate a single etiologic agent. It has been suggested that different enteric viruses may be responsible for this syndrome [12].

The outstanding feature of this illness is the striking elevation of the lymphocyte count. Although the average is about 20,000 to 30,000 per microliter [3,6], levels to 110,000 per microliter occur [3,9]. The circulating lymphocytes in this disorder are normal-appearing small lymphocytes. Pharyngitis is absent, and less than 50 percent of subjects have a slight elevation in temperature. Symptoms, if present, are mild and usually restricted to diarrhea for 1 to 3 days. Physical examination shows no rash, lymph node enlargement, or splenomegaly [13]. The lymphocyte count is highest during the first week, gradually falls over the next 3 weeks, and may persist at a level of 8000 to 10,000 per microliter for as long as 3 months [5]. The increased lymphocyte count seems to be primarily due to T-lymphocyte proliferation [14]. At the height of the lymphocyte count the number of eosinophils is low [5], but as the lymphocytosis subsides, the eosinophils increase to an average of 2000 to 3000 per microliter [4], then slowly fall to normal in a period of some 4 to 6 weeks. No other blood abnormalities have been found. The few marrow examinations that have been done have been normal or have shown only a minimal increase in the percentage of lymphocytes [4,5,9]. An occasional patient develops evidence of meningoencephalitis [9] or of an acute abdominal condition [15], but the original impression that the illness is uniformly benign has been confirmed by long-term follow-up studies [16].

Bordetella pertussis infection

Substantial elevations of the absolute lymphocyte count occur in *B. pertussis* infections. Counts as high as 50,000 per microliter occur [17] and are said to indicate a poor prognosis, but the usual levels are 15,000 to 25,000 per microliter. The lymphocytes are typical small lymphocytes, and the elevation usually occurs in the first 3 weeks of the illness. The lymphocytosis in this disease seems to be due to a redistribution of lymphocytes [18,19]. A lymphocytosis-promoting factor (LPF) can be obtained from the supernatant of *B. pertussis* cultures [20]. In mice this material causes impaired delayed hypersensitivity and antibody responses [21]. LPF appears to attach directly to lymphocytes and inhibit their migration from the blood to lymph nodes [22]. This leads to a gradual depletion of small lymphocytes in the lymph nodes and expansion of the circulating lymphocyte pool.

Toxoplasmosis

Toxoplasma infection in the neonate [22] is manifested by the neonatal tetrad of chorioretinitis, hydrocephalus or microcephaly, psychomotor retardation, and cerebral calcifications. In the immunosuppressed adult [23] it occurs as a disseminated opportunistic infection with a predilection for the central nervous system, heart, and lung [24]. It may also cause chorioretinitis in the adult. A fourth variety of toxoplasma (lymphadenopathic) infection mimics the features of infectious mononucleosis: the patient presents with fever, enlarged lymph nodes, and atypical lymphocytosis. The possibility of toxoplasmosis should be considered in such patients when the heterophil antibody test is negative [25]. Clinically the disease, unlike infectious mononucleosis, tends to involve the lymphatic tissue generally rather than producing predominant posterior cervical lymph node enlargement. Splenomegaly, a consistent finding in infectious mononucleosis, is less common, and patients ordinarily do not have a sore throat or the abnormal liver function tests found in infectious mononucleosis. *Absolute lymphocytosis is rare,* but a relative lymphocytosis with very atypical cells is common. The atypical cells may resemble lymphoblasts or may show clefts, similar to circulating lymphoma cells. The large lymphocytes with abundant vacuolated cytoplasm seen in large numbers in infectious mononucleosis are rare. Marrow aspiration and biopsies are normal. The diagnosis can be confirmed by demonstrating marked elevations of antibody to toxoplasmosis by the indirect fluorescent antibody or indirect hemagglutination techniques [22].

Cytomegalovirus infection

Like toxoplasmosis, cytomegalovirus may produce a variety of clinical syndromes which vary with the age and the health status of the host [26].

CONGENITAL
Congenital infection can produce a small, microcephalic, icteric newborn infant with hepatosplenomegaly, purpura, and extensive brain damage.

OPPORTUNISTIC
The predilection of the virus for the central nervous system prenatally also appears postnatally in im-

munosuppressed patients [27]. The commonest clinical manifestation in patients with leukemia [28,29] and in patients given immunosuppressants [27] is diffuse pulmonary involvement, which is frequently associated with concomitant *Pneumocystis carinii* infection of the lung [30]. Asymptomatic infections are common in adults with neoplastic disease. One-third of these patients excrete virus in their sputum or urine. The onset of infection seems to coincide with prednisone therapy or the development of hypogammaglobulinemia [31]. The recent reports of cytomegalovirus infection [58], Kaposi's sarcoma [59], and immunosuppression [60] in homosexual men have suggested a relationship and the possibility that immunosuppression may be caused by, rather than be the cause of, cytomegalovirus infection.

POSTPERFUSION SYNDROME
Atypical lymphocytosis appearing in patients after cardiopulmonary bypass was first reported in 1958 [32]. The association of fever and splenomegaly in such patients was noted subsequently [33] and other manifestations documented [34–36]. The illness starts 19 to 48 days after operation, usually with a low-grade fever, and persists for 10 to 21 days. Despite the fever, patients are usually comfortable and have no specific complaints. Enlargement of the spleen is usually recognized 5 to 17 days after the onset of fever. Lymph node enlargement is minimal or absent. Splenomegaly often persists for 2 to 3 months. Atypical lymphocytes resembling those of infectious mononucleosis are present at the onset of fever or appear within a week. The total white cell count is normal or slightly elevated, rarely to more than 12,000 per microliter. Atypical lymphocytes may comprise 15 to 60 percent of the circulating leukocytes and disappear slowly in 1 to 3 months. Other blood abnormalities are unusual, but acute hemolytic anemia has been reported [37]. Mild abnormalities of liver function may be present transiently. The heterophil and toxoplasma antibodies are absent [38]. Occasional patients have been reported with positive tests for antinuclear antibody (ANA), rheumatoid factor, cold agglutinins, and cryoglobulins [39].

Rising titers of complement-fixing antibodies to cytomegalovirus have been demonstrated [39–41], and virus has been recovered from urine and blood [37]. Evidence of clinical infection has been found even in patients with preexisting antibodies to cytomegalovirus [40]. Using a fourfold increase in antibody titer as evidence of infection, the incidence of seroconversion in patients undergoing open heart surgery was 38 percent [41]. Studies of patients given blood during open heart or other surgical procedures showed that the incidence of seroconversion increased with the quantity of blood transfused, from 6 to 10 percent with 1 to 5 units of blood up to 40 to 60 percent when 10 to 15 units of blood were administered [42–44]. The ratio of inapparent to apparent cytomegalovirus infection after blood transfusion is 3:4 to 4:5 [42]. The virus appears to be transmitted in the leukocytes of donor blood [45]. The incidence of infection after transfusion may be reduced by using leucocyte-depleted blood [46].

CYTOMEGALOVIRUS MONONUCLEOSIS

Spontaneous cytomegalovirus infection in the healthy adult leads to an illness that may resemble infectious mononucleosis and generally to more severe clinical symptoms than those which result from blood transfusions. High and irregular fever develops, along with profound malaise that persists for some 3 weeks [47,48]. Pharyngitis is not present. A transient rubelliform rash develops in a few patients [49]. Enlargement of the spleen and lymph nodes is seen only occasionally, and hepatomegaly does not occur. Elevation of the white blood cell count to more than 10,000 per microliter occurs regularly, with an absolute lymphocytosis, and atypical lymphocytes are prominent. Minor abnormalities in liver function tests are common. The Guillain-Barré syndrome, splenic infarction [49], interstitial pneumonia, and myocarditis [49] have been reported as complications, and a variety of serologic abnormalities have been observed, such as cold agglutinins, cryoglobulins, and ANA. In one study, about 20 percent of patients who presented with an infectious mononucleosis–like illness and a negative heterophil test [50]. Of the heterophil-negative patients older than 15 years, 45 percent had cytomegalovirus infections as indicated by rising antibody titers and viruria.

As with infectious mononucleosis most cytomegalovirus infections are subclinical. In one study, 55 percent of adult blood donors had evidence of previous infection [51]. The presence of complement-fixing antibodies does not prevent the carrier state, since cytomegalovirus may be harbored in white blood cells, nor does it protect against reinfection in blood recipients.

Viral-related lymphocytosis

A moderate lymphocytosis, nearly always relative, associated with the appearance of young, atypical lymphocytes, has long been recognized as a characteristic response to viral and other infections, especially in children [2]. In measles, mumps, chickenpox, roseola infantum, infectious hepatitis [52], and some respiratory infections lymphopenia and neutropenia develop soon after the onset of symptoms and are followed in a few days with a relative or absolute lymphocytosis. The magnitude of the blood changes depends partly on the severity of the clinical illness. The cellular reaction is always pleomorphic but usually involves a disproportionate increase in the number of large, atypical cells with deeply basophilic cytoplasm. The reactive lymphocytes occasionally contain a few small vacuoles, and the nucleus ordinarily has a fine chromatin pattern. These cells may be difficult to differentiate from those of infectious mononucleosis, which also stain deep blue with Wright's stain, but generally have a heavily vacuolated cytoplasm, giving them a distinctive foamy appearance. Another differential feature is that the increase in hand-mirror lymphocytes in infectious mononucleosis does not occur in other viral syndromes [53]. As the infection or reaction subsides and the lymphocytosis regresses, the percentage of small lymphocytes increases and some of the large lymphocytes become plasmacytoid. A moderate lymphocytosis may be a diagnostic clue pointing to the viral etiology of some acute infections, but it has to be remembered that the same type of cellular response may occur in bacterial infections (e.g., brucellosis) [54] and rickettsial infections [2]. Moreover, a variety of inflammatory diseases, such as ulcerative colitis, and immune reactions, such as serum sickness, drug hypersensitivity, immune thrombocytopenic purpura, and warm antibody hemolytic anemia, are frequently accompanied by a moderate increase in the number of atypical lymphocytes in the circulating blood.

Endocrine disorders

About 10 percent of patients with thyrotoxicosis have neutropenia and at least a relative increase in the number of circulating lymphocytes [55]. About the same percentage of patients have enlargement of the spleen and lymph nodes. Lymphocytic and some plasma cell infiltration of the hyperplastic thyroid gland in Graves' disease is a well-known histologic feature. The blood aberrations do not occur in patients with acute or chronic thyroiditis and apparently do not have an autoimmune pathogenesis. The lymphocytosis in thyrotoxicosis may relate in part to a disturbance in adrenocortical function [55].

Neutropenia, relative lymphocytosis, and eosinophilia occur in 50 percent of patients with Addison's disease and subside promptly with glucocorticoid therapy [56]. The mean lymphocyte diameter is increased in adrenal insufficiency, and this also corrects with therapy [57].

References

1. Miale, J. B.: *Laboratory Medicine: Hematology*, 5th ed. Mosby, St. Louis, 1977.
2. Wood, T. A., and Frenkel, E. P.: The atypical lymphocyte. *Am. J. Med.* 42:923, 1967.
3. Smith, C. H.: Infectious lymphocytosis. *Am. J. Dis. Child.* 62:231, 1941.
4. Barnes, G. R., Jr., Yannet, H., and Lieberman, R.: A clinical study of an institutional outbreak of acute infectious lymphocytosis. *Am. J. Med. Sci.* 218:646, 1949.
5. Lemon, B. K., and Kaump, D. H.: Infectious lymphocytosis: A report of an epidemic in children. *J. Pediatr.* 36:61, 1950.
6. Horwitz, M. S., and Moore, G. T.: Acute infectious lymphocytosis: An etiologic and epidemiologic study of an outbreak. *N. Engl. J. Med.* 279:399, 1968.

7. Duncan, P. A.: Acute infectious lymphocytosis in young adults. *N. Engl. J. Med.* 233:177, 1945.

8. Olson, L. C., Miller, G., and Hanshaw, J. B.: Acute infectious lymphocytosis presenting as a pertussis-like illness: Its association with adenovirus type 12. *Lancet* 1:200, 1964.

9. Scalletar, H. E., Maisel, J. E., and Bramson, M.: Acute infectious lymphocytosis: Report of an outbreak. *Am. J. Dis. Child.* 88:15, 1954.

10. Blacklow, N. R., and Kapikian, A. Z.: Serological studies with EB virus in infectious lymphocytosis. *Nature* 226:647, 1970.

11. Mandal, B. K., and Stokes, K. J.: Acute infectious lymphocytosis and enteroviruses. *Lancet* 2:1392, 1973.

12. Nkrumah, F. K., and Addy, P. A. K.: Acute infectious lymphocytosis. *Lancet* 1:1257, 1973.

13. Smith, C. H.: Acute infectious lymphocytosis, a specific infection: Report of four cases showing its communicability. *JAMA* 125:342, 1944.

14. Cassuto, J. P., Schneider, M., Bourg, M., Bertrand, A., and Mariani, R.: Acute infectious lymphocytosis as a T-cell lymphoproliferative syndrome. *Br. Med. J.* 2:1331, 1977.

15. Ryder, R. J. W.: Acute infectious lymphocytosis. *Am. J. Dis. Child.* 110:299, 1965.

16. Putnam, S. M., Moore, G. T., and Mitchell, D. W.: Infectious lymphocytosis: Long term follow-up of an epidemic. *Pediatrics* 41:588, 1968.

17. Lagergren, J.: The white blood cell count and the erythrocyte sedimentation rate in pertussis. *Acta Paediatr.* 52:405, 1963.

18. Morse, S. I., and Barron, B. A.: Studies on the leucocytosis and lymphocytosis induced by *Bordetella pertussis*. III. The distribution of transfused lymphocytes in pertussis-treated and normal mice. *J. Exp. Med.* 132:663, 1970.

19. Rai, K. R., Chanana, A. D., and Cronkite, E. P.: Studies on lymphocytes. XVIII. Mechanism of lymphocytosis induced by supernatant fluids of *Bordetella pertussis* cultures. *Blood* 38:49, 1971.

20. Adler, A., and Morse, S. I.: Interaction of lymphoid and nonlymphoid cells with the lymphocytosis-promoting factor of *Bordetella pertussis*. *Infect. Immunol.* 7:461, 1973.

21. Ochiai, T., Okumura, K., and Tada, T.: Effect of lymphocytosis-promoting factor of *Bordetella pertussis* on the immune response. *Int. Arch. Allergy* 43:196, 1972.

22. Feldman, H. A.: Toxoplasmosis. *N. Engl. J. Med.* 279:1370, 1968.

23. Ruskin, J., and Remington, J. S.: Toxoplasmosis in the compromised host. *Ann. Intern. Med.* 84:193, 1976.

24. Remington, J. S.: Toxoplasmosis in the adult. *Bull. N.Y. Acad. Med.* 50:211, 1974.

25. Evans, A. S.: Infectious mononucleosis and related syndromes *Am. J. Med. Sci.* 276:325, 1978.

26. Weller, J. H.: The cytomegaloviruses: Ubiquitous agents with protean clinical manifestations. *N. Engl. J. Med.* 285:203, 267, 1971.

27. Rifkind, D., Goodman, N., and Hill, R. B., Jr.: The clinical significance of cytomegalovirus infection in renal transplant recipients. *Ann. Intern. Med.* 66:1116, 1967.

28. Bodey, G. P., Wertlake, P. T., and Douglas, G.: Cytomegalic inclusion disease in patients with acute leukemia. *Ann. Intern. Med.* 62:899, 1965.

29. Sutton, R. N. P., Darby, C. W., and Gumpel, S. M.: Cytomegalovirus infection in childhood leukemia. *Br. J. Haematol.* 20:437, 1971.

30. Abdallah, P. S., Mark, J. B. D., and Merigan, T. C.: Diagnosis of cytomegalovirus pneumonia in compromised hosts. *Am. J. Med.* 61:326, 1976.

31. Durall, C. P., Casazza, A. R., Grimley, P. M.: Recovery of cytomegalovirus from adults with neoplastic disease. *Ann. Intern. Med.* 64:531, 1966.

32. Battle, J. D., Jr., and Hewlett, J. S.: Hematologic changes observed after extracorporeal circulation during open heart operations. *Cleve. Clin. Q.* 25:112, 1958.

33. Kreel, I., Zaroff, L. I., and Canter, J. W.: A syndrome following total body perfusion. *Surg. Gynecol. Obst.* 111:317, 1960.

34. Seaman, A. J., and Starr, A: Febrile postcardiotomy lymphocytic splenomegaly: A new entity. *Ann. Surg.* 156:956, 1962.

35. Wheeler, E. O., Turner, J. D., and Scannell, J. G.: Fever, splenomegaly, and atypical lymphocytes. A syndrome observed after cardiac surgery utilizing a pump oxygenator. *N. Engl. J. Med.* 266:454, 1962.

36. Smith, D. R.: A syndrome resembling infectious mononucleosis after open-heart surgery *Br. Med. J.* 1:945, 1964.

37. Lang, D. L., and Hanshaw, J. B.: Cytomegalovirus infection and the postperfusion syndrome. *N. Engl. J. Med.* 280:1145, 1969.

38. Kantor, G. L., Goldberg, L. S., and Johnson, B. L., Jr.: Immunologic abnormalities induced by postperfusion cytomegalovirus infection. *Ann. Intern. Med.* 73:553, 1970.

39. Kääriäinen, L., Klemola, E., and Paloheimo, J.: Rise of cytomegalovirus antibodies in an infectious-mononucleosis-like syndrome after transfusion. *Br. Med. J.* 1:1270, 1966.

40. Foster, K. M., and Jack, I.: A prospective study of the role of cytomegalovirus in posttransfusion mononucleosis. *N. Engl. J. Med.* 280:1311, 1969.

41. Caul, E. O., Clarke, S. K. R., and Mott, M. G.: Cytomegalovirus after open heart surgery: A prospective study. *Lancet* 1:777, 1971.

42. Henle, W., Henle, G., and Scriba, M.: Antibody responses to the Epstein-Barr virus and cytomegaloviruses after open-heart and other surgery. *N. Engl. J. Med.* 282:1068, 1970.

43. Stevens, D. P., Barker, L. F., and Ketcham, A. S.: Asymptomatic cytomegalovirus infection following blood transfusion in tumor surgery *JAMA* 211:1341, 1970.

44. Prince, A. M., Szmuness, W., and Millian, S. T.: A serologic study of cytomegalovirus infections associated with blood transfusions. *N. Engl. J. Med.* 284:1125, 1971.

45. Kantor, G., and Johnson, B. L., Jr.: Latent cytomegalovirus and blood transfusion. *Ann. Intern. Med.* 73:333, 1970 (editorial).

46. Benson, J. W. T., Bodden, S. J., and Tobin, J. O'H.: Cytomegalovirus and blood transfusion in neonates. *Arch. Dis. Child.* 54:538, 1979.

47. Klemola, E., and Kääriäinen, L.: Cytomegalovirus as a possible cause of a disease resembling infectious mononucleosis. *Br. Med. J.* 2:1099, 1965.

48. Klemola, E., von Essen, R., and Wagner, O.: Cytomegalovirus mononucleosis in previously healthy individuals. Five new cases and follow-up of 13 previously published cases. *Ann. Intern. Med.* 71:11, 1969.

49. Jordan, M. C., Rousseau, W. E., and Stewart, J. A.: Spontaneous cytomegalovirus mononucleosis: Clinical and laboratory observations in nine cases. *Ann. Intern. Med.* 79:153, 1973.

50. Klemola, E.: Cytomegalovirus infection in previously healthy adults. *Ann. Intern. Med.* 79:267, 1973.

51. Perham, J. G. M., Caul, E. O., and Conway, P. J.: Cytomegalovirus infection in blood donors: A prospective study. *Br. J. Haematol.* 20:307, 1971.

52. Havens, W. P., Jr., and Marck, R. E.: The leucocytic response of patients with experimentally induced infectious hepatitis. *Am. J. Med. Sci.* 212:129, 1946.

53. Thomas, W. J., Yasaka, K., Strong, D. M., Woodruff, C. M., Stass, S. A., and Schumacher, H. R.: Hand-mirror lymphocytes in infectious mononucleosis. *Blood* 55:925, 1980.

54. Castaneda, M. R., and Guerrero, G.: Studies on the leucocytic picture in brucellosis. *J. Infect. Dis.* 78:43, 1946.

55. Herbert, V.: Blood, in *The Thyroid*, edited by S. C. Werner and S. H. Ingbar. Harper & Row, New York, 1978, p. 775.

56. Baez-Villaseñor, J., Rath, C. E., and Finch, C. A.: The blood picture in Addison's disease. *Blood* 3:769, 1948.

57. Hernberg, C. A.: Observations on the size of lymphocytes in the blood in Addison's disease: Panhypopituitarism and Cushing's syndrome during treatment. *Acta Med. Scand.* 144:380, 1953.

58. Drew, W. L., et al.: Prevalence of cytomegalovirus infection in homosexual men. *J. Infect. Dis.* 143:188, 1981.

59. Urmacher, C., et al.: Outbreak of Kaposi's sarcoma with cytomegalovirus in young homosexual men. *Am. J. Med.* 72:569, 1982.

60. Rinaldo, C. R., Jr., et al.: Mechanisms of immunosuppression in cytomegaloviral mononucleosis. *J. Infect. Dis.* 141:488, 1980.

CHAPTER *111*

Lymphocytopenia

PETER A. CASSILETH

An absolute lymphocytopenia is generally defined as a lymphocyte count of less than 1500 per microliter in adults [1,2] and less than 3000 per microliter in children [3], although levels as low as 1400 per microliter in children and 1000 per microliter in adults may be within normal limits [4,5]. Table 111-1 lists the diseases and circumstances associated with lymphocytopenia. The mechanisms resulting in lowered lymphocyte counts are decreased production, increased destruction, or increased loss. Failure of lymphocyte production occurs on a genetic basis (ataxia-telangiectasia) [6,7], in association with thymic abnormalities (thymic dysplasia syndromes) [8], or in aplastic anemia [9]. Increased destruction of lymphocytes may be due to the cytotoxic effects of steroid or ACTH administration [10], irradiation [11–14], cancer chemotherapy [15], or the administration of antilymphocyte globulin [16,17], and may occur in episodic lymphopenia [18]. Even relatively localized radiation treatment fields can cause lymphocytopenia due to destruction of circulating lymphocytes as they pass through the treated area [19]. Increased loss of lymphocytes occurs in thoracic duct drainage [20] and in states of excessive intestinal lymph loss due to congenital lymphatic abnormalities (intestinal lymphangiectasia) [21], acquired intestinal disease (Whipple's disease) [22,23], and increased venous pressure (severe right-sided heart failure) [24].

Patients with acute and chronic renal insufficiency exhibit lymphocytopenia whether or not they are undergoing hemodialysis [25]. Long-term maintenance hemodialysis has been variably reported to worsen [25] or to improve [26] the depressed lymphocyte count. Immunosuppressive therapy in renal allograft recipients is also associated with lymphocytopenia. Such therapy may abrogate the lymphocytosis of supervening cytomegalovirus infections in these patients [27].

Qualitative differences in the lymphopenias also exist. Thus, thoracic duct drainage depletes predominantly the "long-lived," small lymphocyte whereas corticoid administration causes a major decrease in the "short-lived," small lymphocyte [10]. Most of the disorders with lymphocytopenia listed in Table 111-1 are associated with impaired delayed hypersensitivity reactions, but the direct correlation seen in sarcoid [28] between lymphocytopenia and altered immunity is not always found. Patients with early active Hodgkin's disease often show diminished delayed hypersensitivity responses, but lymphocytopenia only occurs late in advanced disease [1].

TABLE 111-1 Causes of lymphocytopenia

1. Decreased lymphocyte production
   a. Immunoglobulin disorders [29]
      (1) Wiskott-Aldrich syndrome [21,30]
      (2) Ataxia telangiectasia [6,7]
      (3) Thymoma-associated syndromes [32,33]
      (4) Di George's syndrome (III–IV pharyngeal cleft pouch)
      (5) Combined immunodeficiency disease [34]
      (6) Sex-linked thymic alymphoplasia [8]
      (7) Lymphopenia with dysgammaglobulinemia [8]
      (8) Thymic alymphoplasia with aleukocytosis [35]
   b. Aplastic anemia [9]
   c. Terminal carcinoma [1]
   d. Advanced Hodgkin's disease [1]
2. Increased lymphocyte destruction
   a. Irradiation [11–14,19]
   b. Chemotherapy of cancer [15]
   c. Antilymphocyte globulin administration [16,17]
   d. Episodic lymphopenia: lymphocytotoxin [18]
   e. Increased plasma corticoids
      (1) ACTH or adrenal steroid administration [10]
      (2) Stress [36]
      (3) Congestive heart failure [37]
      (4) Cushing's syndrome [38]
3. Increased intestinal lymph loss [23]
   a. Thoracic duct drainage [20]
   b. Intestinal lymphectasia [21]
   c. Impaired intestinal lymphatic drainage [21–23]
      (1) Whipple's disease
      (2) Intestinal lymphangitis
      (3) Intestinal lymphatic obstruction due to infiltration, tumor, or fibrosis
   d. Severe right-sided heart failure [24]
      (1) Tricuspid insufficiency
      (2) Constrictive pericarditis
      (3) Cardiomyopathy
4. Various causes
   a. Sarcoid [28]
   b. Myasthenia gravis [39]
   c. Systemic lupus erythematosus [40,41]
   d. Miliary tuberculosis [42,43]
   e. Renal failure [25–27]
      (1) Acute and chronic
      (2) Chronic hemodialysis
      (3) Immunosuppressive therapy

In a review of disease associated with lymphocytopenia [44], the two most frequently noted categories were malignancy (43 percent of cases) and collagen inflammatory disease (14 percent of cases). Further discussion of lymphocytes and lymphocyte function in disease states can be found in other chapters and in the references cited in the table.

References

1. Aisenberg, A.: Lymphocytopenia in Hodgkin's disease. *Blood* 25:1037, 1965.
2. Miale, J. B.: *Laboratory Medicine—Hematology.* Mosby, St. Louis, 1977.

3. Kretschmer, R., Say, B., Brown, D., and Rosen, F.: Congenital aplasia in the thymus gland (Di George's syndrome). *N. Engl. J. Med. 279:*1296, 1968.
4. Albritton, E. C.: *Standard Values in Blood.* Saunders, Philadelphia, 1952.
5. Linman, J. W.: *Principles of Hematology.* Macmillan, New York, 1966.
6. Eisen, A. H., Karpati, G., Laszlo, T., Andermann, F., Robb, J. P., and Bacal, H. L.: Immunologic deficiency in ataxia-telangiectasia. *N. Eng. J. Med. 272:*18, 1965.
7. Peterson, R. D. A., Cooper, M. D., and Good, R. A.: Lymphoid tissue abnormalities associated with ataxia-telangiectasia. *Am. J. Med. 41:*342, 1966.
8. Rosen, F. S.: The lymphocyte and the thymus gland: Congenital and hereditary abnormalities. *N. Engl. J. Med. 279:*643, 1968.
9. Scott, J. L., Cartwright, G. E., and Wintrobe, M. M.: Acquired aplastic anemia: An analysis of thirty-nine cases and review of the pertinent literature. *Medicine (Baltimore) 38:*119, 1959.
10. Esteban, J. N.: The differential effect of hydrocortisone on the short-lived small lymphocyte. *Anat. Rec. 162:*349, 1968.
11. Warren, S., and Bowers, J. Z.: The acute radiation syndrome in man. *Ann. Intern. Med. 32:*207, 1950.
12. Kohn, H. I.: Changes in the human leucocyte count during x-ray therapy for cancer and their dependence upon the integral dose. *Radiology 64:*382, 1955.
13. Osgood, E. E.: Radiobiologic observations on human hemic cells *in vivo* and *in vitro. Ann. N.Y. Acad. Sci. 95:*828, 1961.
14. Stryckmans, P. A., Chanana, A. D., Cronkite, E. P., Greenberg, M. L., and Schiffer, L. M.: Studies on lymphocytes. X. Influence of extracorporeal irradiation of the blood on lymphocytes in chronic lymphocytic leukemia: Apparent correlation with RNA turnover. *Radiat. Res. 37:*118, 1968.
15. Calabresis, P., and Parks, R. E., Jr.: Chemotherapy of neoplastic diseases, in *The Pharmacological Basis of Therapeutics,* 6th ed., edited by L. S. Goodman and A. Gilman. Macmillan, New York, 1980.
16. Russell, P. S.: Antilymphocyte serum as an immunosuppressive agent. *Ann. Intern. Med. 68:*483, 1968 (editorial).
17. Baum, J., Liebermann, G., and Frenkel, E. P.: The effect of immunologically induced lymphopenia on antibody formation. *J. Immunol. 102:*187, 1969.
18. Kretschmer, R., August, C. S., Rosen, F. S., and Janeway, C. A.: Recurrent infections, episodic lymphopenia, and impaired cellular immunity: Further observations on "immunologic amnesia" in two siblings. *N. Engl. J. Med. 281:*285, 1969.
19. Harisiadis, L., Kopelson, G., and Chang, C. H.: Lymphopenia caused by cranial irradiation in children receiving craniospinal radiotherapy. *Cancer 40:*1102, 1977.
20. Ueo, T., Tanaka, S., Tominaga, Y., Ogawa, H., and Sakurami, T.: The effect of thoracic duct drainage on lymphocyte dynamics and clinical symptoms in patients with rheumatoid arthritis. *Arthritis Rheum. 22:*1405, 1979.
21. Strober, W., Wochner, R. D., Carbone, P. P., and Waldmann, T. A.: Intestinal lymphectasia: A protein-losing enteropathy with hypogammaglobulinemia, lymphocytopenia, and impaired homograft rejection. *J. Clin. Invest. 46:*1643, 1967.
22. Waldmann, T. A.: Protein-losing enteropathy. *Gastroenterology 50:*422, 1966.
23. Foldi, M.: *Diseases of Lymphatics and Lymph Circulation.* Charles C Thomas, Springfield, Ill., 1969.
24. Strober, W., Cohen, L. S., Waldman, T. A., and Braunwald, E.: Tricuspid regurgitation: A newly recognized cause of protein-losing enteropathy, lymphocytopenia and immunologic deficiency. *Am. J. Med. 44:*842, 1968.
25. Goldblum, S. E., and Reed, W. P.: Host defenses and immunologic alterations associated with chronic hemodialysis. *Ann. Intern. Med. 93:*597, 1980.
26. Hoy, W. E., Cestero, R. V. M., and Freeman, R. B.: Deficiency of T and B lymphocytes in uremic subjects and partial improvement with maintenance hemodialysis. *Nephron 20:*182, 1978.
27. Peterson, P. K., Balfour, H. H., Jr., Marker, S. C., Fryd, D. S., Howard, R. J., and Simmons, R. L.: Cytomegalovirus disease in renal allograft recipiencts: A prospective study of the clinical features, risk factors, and impact on renal transplantation. *Medicine 59:*283, 1980.
28. Daniele, R. P., Dauber, J. H., and Rossman, M. D.: Immunologic abnormalities in sarcoidosis. *Ann. Intern. Med. 92:*406, 1980.
29. Hoyer, J. R., Cooper, M. D., Gabrielsen, A. E., and Good, R. A.: Lymphopenic forms of congenital immunologic deficiency diseases. *Medicine (Baltimore) 47:*201, 1968.
30. Blaese, R. M., Strober, W., Brown, R. S., and Waldmann, T. A.: The Wiskott-Aldrich syndrome: A disorder with a possible defect in antigen processing or recognition. *Lancet 1:*1056, 1968.
31. Cooper, M. D., Chase, H. P., Lowman, J. T., Krivit, W., and Good, R. A.: Wiskott-Aldrich syndrome: An immunologic deficiency disease involving the afferent limb of immunity. *Am. J. Med. 44:*499, 1968.
32. Korn, D., Gelderman, A., Cage, G., Nathanson, D., and Strauss, A. J. L.: Immune deficiencies, aplastic anemia and abnormalities of lymphoid tissue in thymoma. *N. Engl. J. Med. 276:*1333, 1967.
33. Waldman, T. A., Strober, W., Blaese, R. M., and Strauss, A. J. L.: Thymoma, hypogammaglobulinemia, and absence of eosinophils. *J. Clin. Invest. 46:*1127, 1967.
34. Miller, M. E.: Thymic dysplasia ("Swiss agammaglobulinemia"). I. Graft versus host reaction following bone marrow transfusion. *J. Pediatr. 70:*730, 1967.
35. Gitlin, D., Vawter, G., and Craig, J. M.: Thymic alymphoplasia and congenital aleucocytosis. *Pediatrics 33:*184, 1964.
36. Hoagland, H., Elmadjian, F., and Pincus, G.: Stressful psychomotor performance and adrenal cortical function as indicated by the lymphocyte response. *J. Clin. Endocrinol. 6:*301, 1946.
37. Hurdle, A. D. F., Gyde, O. H. B., and Willoughby, J. M. T.: Occurrence of lymphopenia in heart failure. *J. Clin. Pathol. 19:*60, 1966.
38. DeLaBalze, F. A., Reifenstein, E. C., Jr., and Albright, F.: Differential blood counts in certain adrenal cortical disorders (Cushing's syndrome, Addison's disease, and panhypopituitarism). *J. Clin. Endocrinol. 6:*312, 1946.
39. Adner, M. M., Sherman, J. D., Ise, C., Schwab, R. S., and Dameshek, W.: An immunologic survey of forty-eight patients with myasthenia gravis. *N. Engl. J. Med. 271:*1327, 1964.
40. Budman, D. R., and Steinberg, A. D.: Hematologic aspects of systemic lupus erythematosus: Current concepts. *Ann. Intern. Med. 86:*220, 1977.
41. Rivero, S. J., Diaz-Jouanen, E., and Alarcon-Segovia, D.: Lymphopenia in systemic lupus erythematosus. *Arthritis Rheum. 21:*295, 1978.
42. Fountain, J. R.: Blood changes associated with disseminated tuberculosis: Report of four fatal cases and reviews. *Br. Med. J. 2:*76, 1954.
43. Chapman, C. B., and Whorton, C. M.: Acute generalized miliary tuberculosis in adults: A clinicopathological study based on sixty-three cases diagnosed at autopsy. *N. Engl. J. Med. 235:*239, 1946.
44. Zacharski, L. R., and Linman, J. W.: Lymphocytopenia: Its causes and significance. *Mayo Clin. Proc. 46:*168, 1971.

SECTION SIX

Lymphocytic disorders— benign abnormalities of immunoglobulin synthesis

CHAPTER *112*

Immunodeficiency diseases

FRED S. ROSEN

The immunodeficiency diseases are characterized by a decreased capacity to mount an immune defense against foreign antigens. The specific humoral or cellular defects of these diseases are listed in Table 112-1 and their pathophysiologic and clinical manifestations are detailed below.

X-linked agammaglobulinemia

DEFINITION AND HISTORY
In 1952 Bruton reported the remarkable finding of the absence of γ-globulin from the serum of an 8-year-old boy who had been well up to the age of 4 years, when septic arthritis of the left knee developed. During the next four years, the boy had 19 episodes of pneumococcal sepsis, repeated attacks of otitis media, and two bouts of pneumococcal pneumonia. Although these illnesses were successfully treated with antibiotics, immunization with polyvalent pneumococcal vaccines was not protective and did not lead to the appearance of serum antibodies. Further investigation demonstrated that he was unable to produce antibodies after typhoid vaccination, and a Schick test remained positive after attempted diphtheria immunization. Electrophoresis of the serum revealed normal levels of albumin and α- and β-globulins, but no γ-globulin. When given intramuscular injections of γ-globulin, the patient remained well [1].

ETIOLOGY AND PATHOGENESIS
The study of kindreds with multiple occurrences of agammaglobulinemia has shown that it is inherited as an X-linked recessive trait. In most cases no B cells are present in the blood, marrow, or lymph nodes. In rare instances B cells are present in the blood but are unresponsive to signals from T lymphocytes and will not mature to synthesize and secrete antibody. T-cell function is normal. Blood T lymphocytes of agammaglobulinemic children respond normally to phytohemagglutinin and to antigenic and allogenic stimuli [2]. Homograft rejection is intact in the few agammaglobulinemic patients who have been studied. Delayed hypersensitivity reactions of both the tuberculin and the skin-contact type can be elicited.

CLINICAL FEATURES
Male infants with X-linked agammaglobulinemia usually remain well during the first 9 months of life, probably because of the passive protection afforded by the maternal γ-globulin. Undue susceptibility to infection gradually develops during the second year of life, but the onset of frequent infections may depend on the environment of the child and the presence of older sibs

TABLE 112-1 Immunoglobulin levels and lymphocyte counts in the immunodeficiency diseases

	IgG	IgA	IgM	B cells*	T cells†
X-linked agammaglobulinemia	↓	↓	↓	↓	N
Hyper IgM immunodeficiency	↓	↓	↑	N	N
Selective IgA deficiency	N	↓	N	N	N
Selective IgG subclass deficiency	↓	N	N	N	N
Transient hypogammaglobulinemia	↓	N	N	N	↓
Common varied agammaglobulinemia	↓	↓	↓	N or ↓	N or ↓
Severe combined immunodeficiency	↓	↓	↓	↓	↓
Hereditary ataxia-telangiectasia	N	↓	N	N	↓
Congenital thymic aplasia	↓ or N	N	N	N	↓
Wiskott-Aldrich syndrome	N	↑	↓	N	↓

*As enumerated by surface Ig staining.
†As enumerated by E-rosetting, or by mitogenic response to phytohemagglutinin.
NOTE: ↑ = elevated concentration of immunoglobulin or increased number of cells in the blood;
↓ = decreased concentration of immunoglobulin or decreased number of cells in the blood;
N = normal concentration of immunoglobulin or normal number of cells in the blood.

and social contacts. Almost invariably these children contract infections from the pyogenic organisms, principally staphylococci, pneumococci, streptococci, and *Hemophilus influenzae*. Purulent sinusitis, pneumonia, bacteremia, meningitis, and furunculosis are the most common types of infection. They can usually be readily controlled with antimicrobial chemotherapy, but they recur persistently until proper prophylactic therapy is undertaken.

Agammaglobulinemic children do not have increased susceptibility to the common viral diseases and exanthems of childhood. They usually overcome measles, mumps, varicella, and rubella in an ordinary fashion. When vaccinated with vaccinia virus, they generally exhibit the usual course of a primary take. They have no unusual infections with enterococci or gram-negative bacilli, nor do they have undue susceptibility to mycotic infections. A number of deaths from *Pneumocystis carinii* have been reported in agammaglobulinemic infants and young children.

One-third to one-half of all patients with agammaglobulinemia develop a disease of the large joints which resembles rheumatoid arthritis. The joint disease may develop before susceptibility to infection leads to the establishment of the diagnosis. Joint complications disappear once replacement therapy with γ-globulin is begun.

Other collagen-vascular diseases have been observed in children with agammaglobulinemia. One of the most distressing (and ultimately fatal) is a syndrome resembling dermatomyositis. Edema, ligneous induration of the muscles, weakness, and rash over the extensor surfaces of the joints are the salient features of this complication. Biopsy and autopsy material show lymphorrhages around the small blood vessels. Similar involvement of the central nervous system has been observed, producing a progressive and eventually fatal neurologic disease. Although the distribution of the lymphocytic infiltrates is characteristic of neoplasia, the individual cells in the infiltrate appear to be normal. The disease is uniformly fatal despite the use of glucocorticoids and antimetabolite therapy. Echo virus has been persistently cultured from the cerebrospinal fluid of several of these patients [3].

Hemolytic anemia, drug eruptions, atopic eczema, poison ivy sensitivity, allergic rhinitis, and asthma occur frequently in agammaglobulinemic patients. Wheal and flare reactions cannot be elicited.

LABORATORY FEATURES
The serum contains less than 100 mg/dl of IgG. Other serum immunoglobulins, IgA, IgM, IgD, and IgE are undetectable. Isohemagglutinin is lacking or at a low level. Immunization can be used to demonstrate the basic defect. Stimulation with diphtheria-pertussis-tetanus (DPT) or with any number of other antigens fails to elicit an antibody response. Other serum constituents involved in resistance to infection are normal. Serum complement, lysozyme, and properdin levels, phagocytosis, and interferon synthesis are within normal limits.

The basic deficiency in the disease is an absence of plasma cells from the lymph nodes, spleen, intestine, and marrow. Moreover, plasma cells do not appear in lymph nodes, which are stimulated with antigen. There are no normal lymph node follicles but the thymus is normal.

PROGNOSIS AND THERAPY
The periodic injection of immune serum globulin has proved to be an effective means of preventing the severe recurrent pyogenic infections which affect these patients. Patients with congenital agammaglobulinemia have been given repeated injections at monthly or more frequent intervals for more than 20 years without any ill effect or untoward reaction. Untreated, many of these children develop chronic progressive bronchiectasis and ultimately die of the pulmonary complications if they survive the innumerable infections [4]. The complication resembling dermatomyositis and that involving the central nervous system (see above) are uniformly fatal.

The dose of immune serum globulin that provides effective prophylaxis was determined empirically. If the serum level is raised by approximately 200 mg/dl, invasive bacterial infections can be prevented. To achieve the desired level, a previously untreated patient should be given 1.8 ml, or 300 mg, of immune serum globulin per kilogram of body weight intramuscularly, usually in three divided doses of 0.6 ml (100 mg) per kilogram. This raises the serum concentration by about 300 mg/dl. Since the half-life of the immune serum globulin injected is 30 days or more in these patients, injections must be given at least once a month in a dose of 0.6 ml (100 mg) per kilogram to maintain the desired level of approximately 200 mg/dl. Smaller doses are ineffective. Preparations of immune serum globulin suitable for intravenous administration are still in the investigative phase. The dose of immune serum globulin cited above is applicable to patients with other forms of IgG deficiency, discussed below.

The selective immunoglobulin deficiencies

The advent of immunoelectrophoretic techniques led to a more precise definition of immunoglobulin defects in a number of situations in which the hypogammaglobulinemia involved only one or two of the immunoglobulin classes. Six combinations of deficiency involving the three major immunoglobulins are obviously possible, although only two of these have been extensively reported. It has been estimated that about 1 in 200 random hospital admissions has some form of dysgammaglobulinemia or selective immunoglobulin deficiency [5].

ABSENCE OF IgA AND IgG WITH NORMAL OR ELEVATED IgM

One of the common partial immunoglobulin abnormalities is a deficiency of IgA and IgG with an increased amount of IgM in the serum [6]. IgM levels in this entity range from 150 to 1000 mg/dl, but in spite of the enormous elevation in IgM level, monoclonal components are not present. The IgM appears to contain a normal distribution of molecules with antibody activity, particularly those usually associated with the macroglobulins, and have a normal distribution of κ and λ chains. Some, but not all, of these patients have an elevated level of serum IgD and IgM subunits. Both hereditary and acquired forms of this defect have been observed. In addition to their undue susceptibility to infection, many of these patients develop thrombocytopenia, neutropenia, renal lesions, and aplastic or hemolytic anemia, presumably manifestations of "autoimmune" processes [7]. Optimal treatment includes immune serum globulin replacement as in patients with sex-linked agammaglobulinemia.

ABSENCE OF IgA WITH NORMAL IgG AND IgM

The isolated absence of IgA in the serum occurs in a small but significant proportion of the normal population [8]. IgA deficiency has been associated with steatorrhea and nontropical sprue. These patients lack IgA-producing cells in the lamina propria of the intestinal tract, where for physiologic reasons IgA-producing cells normally occur in greatest abundance. Other patients with connective tissue disease and about 80 percent of patients with ataxia-telangiectasia lack serum and secretory IgA [9].

Although the occurrence of IgA deficiencies in families is well documented, the mode of inheritance is not clear. Several patients with absent IgA have circulating anti-IgA antibodies. This may result in rapid catabolism of IgA, or in plasma transfusion reactions [10]. Some patients with partial deletions of the long arm of chromosome 18 have IgA deficiency, but this is not a consistent finding.

SELECTIVE IgG SUBCLASS DEFICIENCY

A number of patients have been described with recurrent pyogenic infections and selective deficiency of IgG_1, IgG_2, IgG_3, or a combination of these subclasses. Other immunoglobulins are found in normal quantities in the serum. Although the mode of inheritance of these IgG subclass deficiencies is not clear, individuals with deletions of both G1m and G3m markers have been encountered (see Chap. 163). Those heterozygous for such deletions have no immunodeficiency disease but do have decreased serum IgG_1 or IgG_3 levels. The child of parents of whom one was heterozygous for a G1m deletion and the other for a G3m deletion had symptomatic hypogammaglobulinemia. These immunoglobulin gene deletions are rare and account for only a small portion of patients with immunodeficiency disease [11,12].

Transient hypogammaglobulinemia of infancy

The human fetus is capable of forming antibodies in utero when adequately stimulated after the twentieth week of gestation. Intrauterine infection with syphilis, cytomegalovirus, rubella virus, or toxoplasma results in antibody synthesis. The antibodies synthesized by the human fetus are mainly IgM and at times IgA.

In normal circumstances the full-term newborn infant is provided with maternal IgG, so that umbilical cord serum contains as much IgG as the maternal serum. Infants born of agammaglobulinemic mothers have no detectable immunoglobulin in cord serum. Virtually no maternal IgA and very little maternal IgM traverses the placenta into the fetal circulation. The cord blood contains less than 1 percent of maternal serum levels of IgA, IgD, and IgE and about 10 percent of the maternal IgM level.

The transplacental passage of IgG appears to involve an active transport system which recognizes some specific structural attribute of the Fc fragment. Studies with radioactive iodinated proteins injected into pregnant women near term confirm this conclusion [13].

The newborn infant continues to synthesize IgM antibodies, and their level rises rapidly, and by the end of the first year of life it is about 75 percent of the adult level. The newborn infant can synthesize IgA by the third week of life. The level of this globulin tends to rise more slowly and approaches 75 percent of the normal adult concentration by the end of the second year. Thereafter the level rises very slowly throughout childhood. IgA appears in secretions such as tears, however, by the age of 3 weeks. The maternal IgG is slowly catabolized, so that the infant's serum IgG level reaches its low point of approximately 300 mg/ml by the end of the second month of life. With increased synthesis of IgG by the infant, the serum level rises rapidly toward normal adult values by the age of 1 year.

As the infant matures immunologically, there is concomitant maturation of the lymphoid tissue. Follicular organization in lymph nodes, with the appearance of plasma cells, becomes evident during the third month of life. In some infants, the development of immunoglobulin synthesis is abnormally delayed. This unphysiologic event has been designated *transient hypogammaglobulinemia*. It occurs with equal frequency in males and females. These infants usually develop the ability to synthesize immunoglobulin between 18 and 30 months of age. Before they develop the capacity for normal immunoglobulin synthesis, however, infants with transient hypogammaglobulinemia may have undue susceptibility to infections of the skin, meninges, or respiratory tract, usually due to gram-positive organisms. Recurrent otitis media, bronchitis, and bronchiolitis are the most common types of infection in these infants. Multiple cases in a single family have been observed. Despite the presence of a normal number of B cells in the blood, lymph nodes display small or no germinal centers and few, if any, plasma cells. During the period of hypogammaglobulinemia, they require immune serum globulin replacement therapy as described above.

Common varied, unclassifiable immunodeficiency

Most patients with immunodeficiency do not readily fall into any of the aforementioned defined syndromes. Some patients are said to have "acquired" or "late-onset" agammaglobulinemia. Deterioration of T-cell function may also be observed in some instances. The acquisition of agammaglobulinemia has been documented in several cases, but the cause for this depression of immunoglobulin synthesis is unknown.

Primary acquired agammaglobulinemia has been found to occur with equal frequency in males and females. Although there is no clear-cut genetic pattern in its occurrence, multiple cases in a single kindred have been reported. In relatives of patients there has been a high incidence of other immunologic abnormalities, such as lupus erythematosis, immune hemolytic anemia, increased rheumatoid factor titer, and thrombocytopenic purpura.

Undue susceptibility to pyogenic infections, particularly with recurrent sinusitis and pneumonia, is the prominent clinical feature of acquired agammaglobulinemia. Patients with chronic progressive bronchiectasis should as a routine be evaluated for this abnormality.

A prominent and frequent complication of acquired agammaglobulinemia, which is rarely seen in the X-linked disease, is a spruelike syndrome. More than half of all adults with agammaglobulinemia have diarrhea, steatorrhea, protein-losing enteropathy, and a whole range of malabsorption difficulties. Intestinal biopsies usually appear normal, without the characteristic flattening of villi seen in nontropical sprue. In some cases, nodular lymphoid hyperplasia has been reported. *Giardia lamblia* infection is common. Some of these patients have improved when given a gluten-free diet and others after the elimination of milk from the diet. Flagyl (metronidazole) therapy is usually helpful [14].

Another singular feature of the variable form is the frequent occurrence of noncaseating granulomas. The lungs, spleen, skin, and liver are most frequently involved. No microorganisms have been consistently found in these lesions. Steroid therapy has been useful. Several patients have had splenomegaly or hepatosplenomegaly and enlarged lymph nodes, and in some, manifestations of hypersplenism have developed. Pernicious anemia has also been reported in patients with agammaglobulinemia [15].

Quantitation of serum immunoglobulin levels in patients with acquired agammaglobulinemia usually reveals IgG levels under 500 mg/dl—higher than those encountered in the sera of patients with X-linked disease. The IgG, however, may not exhibit normal heterogeneity. Both IgA and IgM may be detected in significant quantity in the sera of these patients.

Lymph nodes lack plasma cells, but in contrast to the absence of follicles noted in X-linked agammaglobulinemia, follicular abiotropy or striking follicular hyperplasia may be evident. Lymph node transplants have survived and functioned for a time in these patients. From in vitro and in vivo studies, it does not appear that an inhibitory factor causes this disease.

B lymphocytes which react with fluorescein-tagged antibody to immunoglobulins are usually, but not always, observed in blood [16]. Thymomas are sometimes associated with common variable immunodeficiency, and these patients may have refractory anemia and declining T-cell function.

Ig replacement therapy, given as outlined above in reference to X-linked agammaglobulinemia, is helpful in the treatment of patients with severe antibody deficiency.

Immunoregulatory defects

The homeostasis of the immune system is carefully regulated by T cells that induce or suppress the immune response. Recently monoclonal antibodies have been developed to the surface antigens of mature T cells and thymocytes [17]. Such an antibody to all mature T cells is designated T3. Another antibody directed against the inducer-helper subset is designated T4, and yet others to the suppressor-cytotoxic subset, T5 and T8. The blood lymphocytes at the helper subset are stated to be $T3^+T4^+$ and the suppressor subset $T3^+T5^+/T8^+$. Mature thymocytes bear another antigen, T6, and such matured thymocytes are $T3^+T6^+T4^+T5^+/T8^+$. Upon exiting from the thymus these cells lose $T6^+$ and diverge into the $T3^+T4^+$ subset and the $T3^+T5^+/T8^+$. Thus, not yet fully matured T cells bear simultaneously the phenotype of helper and suppressor cells; they are not fully functional until they display the divergent markers of the different subsets. Early thymocytes bear another antigen, T10, that is lost during their differentiation [18].

Transient hypogammaglobulinemia of infancy is characterized by a deficiency of $T4^+$ cells. When infants recover from this syndrome their $T4^+$ cells rise to the normal range [19].

Rare cases of common varied immunodeficiency appear to result from immunoregulatory defects rather than from intrinsic defects in B lymphocytes. A patient has been described with no $T4^+$ cells [20]. Another patient had activated $T5^+/T8^+$ cells in his circulation that suppressed Ig production by his own normal B lymphocytes [21]. Yet another patient had $T4^+$ cells that were phenotypically normal but failed to function in helping Ig synthesis [22].

Severe combined immunodeficiency

DEFINITION AND HISTORY

In 1950, Glanzmann and Riniker described two unrelated infants who succumbed to overwhelming infection during the second year of life after a succession of serious infections, including intractable diarrhea, thrush, and persistent morbilliform rash [23]. They noted persistent and profound lymphopenia in these two infants and designated the disease *essential lymphocytophthisis.* Over 200 cases of this disease have by now been described. In 1958, Swiss workers pointed out that agammaglobulinemia is a prominent feature of this disease entity. No antibody synthesis can be detected. These infants lack B and T cells and are prey to all kinds of overwhelming infection. The immunodeficiency is uniformly fatal.

ETIOLOGY AND PATHOGENESIS

Initially, it appeared that the disease was transmitted as an autosomal recessive phenomenon, since consanguinity was demonstrated in approximately one-third of the parents of affected children. Further study of these families in America and Europe strongly suggested an additional X-linked transmission of the defect, on the basis of (1) the documentation of affected males in three generations; (2) the appearance of the disease in sons of identical-twin mothers; and (3) the appearance of the disease in sons of the same mother but different fathers. The two different modes of inheritance, autosomal and X-linked recessive, probably account for the 3:1 ratio of males and females observed in the reported cases.

About half of the infants with the autosomal recessive form have a concomitant deficiency of adenosine deaminase, the aminohydrolase which converts adenosine to inosine [24]. Prenatal diagnosis is possible by finding this enzyme deficiency in cultured amnion cells [25]. Another cause of defective T-cell immunity is nucleoside phosphorylase deficiency [26].

CLINICAL FEATURES

There is no discernible difference in the clinical course of the two genetic types, nor can they be separated on grounds of the morbid anatomy of the disease. Infection starts early, between 3 and 6 months of age, and a rapid succession of debilitating infections brings about early demise. Death within the first 2 years of life is the rule. Almost all infants with this disease have chronic watery diarrhea. Stool cultures frequently reveal strains of *Salmonella* or of enteropathic *Escherichia coli.*

Pulmonary infection is also almost universal. Lung abscesses which contain *Pseudomonas aeruginosa* are a common cause of death, as is pneumonitis due to *Pneumocystis carinii.* Extensive moniliasis of the mouth or diaper area that persists beyond the neonatal period is often the first sign of the disease and is usually present even before any antibiotic therapy is instituted. These infants, furthermore, are incapable of limiting or overcoming the most benign viral infections. Death has resulted from generalized chickenpox, measles with Hecht's giant cell pneumonia, and in a few instances cytomegalovirus and adenovirus infection. Vaccination results in progressive, ultimately fatal vaccinia infection. BCG inoculation has also resulted in progressive BCG infection.

LABORATORY FEATURES

Leukopenia is usually present because the lymphocyte count is usually less than 2000 per microliter. The number of lymphocytes may be variable, declining from initially normal neonatal levels (greater than 3000 per microliter) to profound lymphopenic levels later. A single lymphocyte count is, accordingly, not a reliable index of disease presence. Neutrophils and platelets are normal, although leukocytosis may not occur in the presence of overt infection. Eosinophilia is common, and abnormal granulation of eosinophils has been reported.

Marrow in normal infants contains up to 20 percent lymphocytic elements, but in severe combined immunodeficiency the marrow is uniformly deficient in plasma cells, lymphocytes, and lymphoblasts. Lymph node biopsies, when feasible, show complete lack of germinal elements, plasma cells, and lymphocytes. The stroma of the node may contain an occasional mast cell and eosinophils or, rarely, small collections of lymphoid cells without any apparent organization. The blood contains no mature $T3^+T4^+$ or $T3^+T5^+/T8^+$ cells. When present, they are of maternal origin. The affected infants have $T10^+$ cells or $T3^+T4^+T5^+/T8^+$ cells in their circulation, a highly abnormal finding [20].

None of the indications of delayed sensitivity can be elicited in these infants. The blood lymphocytes are unresponsive to phytohemagglutinin or allogenic stimulation. Skin grafts are accepted without microscopic or macroscopic signs of rejection. At autopsy, no lymphoid tissue is found in the spleen, tonsils, appendix, or intestinal tract. The thymus has usually failed to descend in the normal manner into the anterior mediastinum and is found with difficulty in the neck. It ordinarily weighs less than 1 g and is composed of primordial spindle-shaped cells, occasionally forming swirls or rosettes. No Hassall's corpuscles and few, if any, lymphocytes are present. The embryonal appearance of the thymus is the uniform characteristic of this entity.

PROGNOSIS AND THERAPY

Death within the first 2 years of life, from infection and malnutrition, is almost invariable in this disease. Graft-versus-host disease, however, arising after marrow or whole blood transfusions has resulted in several fatalities. In one case this complication resulted from the persistence of transplacentally acquired maternal lymphoid cells. The onset of graft-versus-host disease in any event is marked by the appearance of a characteristic maculopapular rash, starting on the face about 7 days after the injection of immunocompetent incompatible cells. The rash spreads rapidly to involve all skin surfaces ultimately, including the palms and soles. Thrombocytopenia, leukopenia, jaundice, and anasarca follow in quick succession, and the marrow aplasia leads to death from massive hemorrhage by the twelfth or fourteenth day [27].

On the basis of experimental observations, it has been reasoned that transplants of marrow cells, as a source of immunopotential stem cells, might restore immunologic competence to these infants. It was also apparent from the aforementioned misadventures that it would be necessary to circumvent the difficulties of graft-versus-host disease by administering completely histocompatible marrow cells. This remarkable feat has now been achieved in some infants with severe combined immunodeficiency [29,30].

Transplants of histoidentical marrow from sibling donors equip such infants with T- and B-cell function, and their lymphoid chimerism can be readily demonstrated. Despite HL-A identity between marrow donors and recipients, some degree of graft-versus-host reactivity is almost invariably noted, but its course is less severe and it is not fatal. In one of these cases the donor and recipient were ABO-incompatible, and the recipient had an aplastic crisis, which was treated with a second marrow transplant, which in turn produced complete erythrocyte and leukocyte chimerism in the recipient. Thus far, such transplants have not succeeded in the presence of a positive mixed lymphocyte reaction (MLR). Variable success has been achieved with fetal liver cells or fetal thymus transplants. These therapies are still in an experimental phase [31,32].

Hereditary ataxia-telangiectasia

Hereditary ataxia-telangiectasia is transmitted as an autosomal recessive disease. Affected persons are first noted to be ataxic and to develop choreoathetoid movements and pseudopalsy of eye movements during infancy.

The telangiectasias appear later, at 5 or 6 years, or occasionally not until adolescence. They invariably involve the conjunctivae and other exposed body areas such as the face, ears, eyelids, and arms. Progressive sinopulmonary infection also appears later in the course. Death from chronic respiratory infection or lymphoreticular malignancy is common in the second or third decade of life.

About 80 percent of patients with ataxia-telangiectasia lack both serum and secretory IgA. In some patients, antibody to IgA and rapid catabolism of injected, radioactively labeled IgA have been noted.

All patients with ataxia-telangiectasia have a defect in cellular immunity. The thymus gland is dysplastic or hypoplastic, and there is depletion of thymus-dependent areas in the lymph nodes. Delayed hypersensitivity reactions, in vitro response of blood lymphocytes ot phytohemagglutinin, and allograft rejection are blunted [33]. Immunoglobulin replacement and symptomatic measures have had limited therapeutic success.

Wiskott-Aldrich syndrome

The Wiskott-Aldrich syndrome is characterized by eczema, thrombocytopenia, and recurrent infections. Inheritance of the syndrome is X-linked. Affected boys rarely survive beyond the first decade of life and succumb to overwhelming infection, hemorrhage, or lymphoreticular malignancy. Both gram-positive and gram-negative bacteria, as well as viruses and fungi, produce severe infections. There appears to be a progressive deterioration of thymus-dependent cellular immunity, with concomitant changes in the histopathology of lymph nodes, which show progressive depletion of the paracortical area in the older surviving patients. Serum IgM concentration is usually low, but IgG and IgA levels are normal or elevated. Isohemagglutinins are regularly absent from the serum. This observation suggests a specific inability to respond to polysaccharide antigens. This has now been demonstrated quite conclusively with A and B blood group substances, *Salmonella* Vi lipopolysaccharide, and other similar antigens. T cells of affected infants lack a surface glycoprotein of 115,000 daltons, and platelets have defective glycoprotein Ia and Ib [34]. Many aspects of the syndrome have been ameliorated by the administration of transfer factor obtained from dialysates of normal donor lymphocytes [35], and several cases have been treated successfully with marrow transplants.

Congenital thymic aplasia (DiGeorge's syndrome)

During the sixth week of embryonic life, the thymic primordium arises from the floor of the third pharyngeal pouch and, to a lesser extent, from the fourth pharyngeal pouch. The endodermal epithelial masses rapidly elongate, move down into the neck, and fuse in the midline behind the thyroid primordium in the eighth week of embryonic life. By the twelfth week, the gland comes to occupy its ultimate position in the anterior mediastinum. The epithelial cells form Hassall's corpuscles, and the primordium is invaded by proliferating lymphoblasts.

While the thymus is forming, the parathyroid glands arise simultaneously from the third and fourth pharyngeal pouches and start their downward migration posterior and lateral to the thyroid primordium. During this same period, the nasomedial processes fuse to form the philtrum of the lip, and the ear tubercles around the hyomandibular cleft form into the external ear.

DiGeorge observed that a congenital anomaly may result from the failure of embryogenesis of the endodermal derivatives of the third and fourth pharyngeal pouches—aplasia of the parathyroid and thymus glands. This abnormality has no increased familial incidence and does not appear to be hereditary. All infants with this syndrome thus far studied have manifested neonatal tetany. The hypocalcemia tends to ameliorate with development during the first year of life. Hypertelorism, a shortened lip philtrum, low-set, notched pinnae, and nasal clefts cause these infants to resemble one another. In addition, anomalies of the great blood vessels are almost always present; tetralogy of Fallot and right-sided aortic arch are the most common defects [37].

Infants with thymic aplasia who survive the neonatal period exhibit untoward susceptibility to virus, fungus, and bacterial infections, which may ultimately be overwhelming. At autopsy, some parathyroid tissue and a miniature thymus gland may be found in an ectopic position by carefully sectioning the neck organs. Nephrocalcinosis has been found in over half the infants examined. The lymphoid tissue, marrow, spleen, and gastrointestinal tract contain a normal number of plasma cells, and the cortical germinal centers of the lymph nodes are normal or hyperplastic. The subcortical "thymus-dependent region" shows a moderate to severe depletion of lymphocytes, so that the reticulum cells in this area appear to be unusually prominent. The lymphoid sheaths of the spleen are also depleted of lymphocytes. Blood exhibits profound lymphopenia, and $T5^+/T8^+$ cells are relatively more deficient than $T4^+$ cells [20].

Antibody responses to primary stimuli may be normal. Serum concentrations of immunoglobulins are normal. However, delayed hypersensitivity is not manifested to common antigens such as *Candida* or streptokinase. Sensitization to dinitrofluorobenzene (DNFB) is unsuccessful. Skin allograft rejection has been absent or abnormally delayed. Lymphocyte transfer tests and macrophage-immobilizing factor synthesis are abnormal. The blood lymphocytes respond poorly, if at all, to in vitro stimulation by phytohemagglutinin, allogenic cells, and antilymphocyte serum.

All these deficits in in vitro and in vivo lymphocyte function are dramatically reversed by transplants of fetal thymic tissue into children with this syndrome. Increase in lymphocyte count, population of thymus-dependent areas with lymphocytes, normal skin allograft rejection, and normal responses to intradermal antigens and to DNFB, as well as normalization of phytohemagglutinin response in vitro, have been documented after fetal thymus transplants [38,39].

Hereditary angioneurotic edema (hereditary angioedema)

DEFINITION AND HISTORY

In 1963, the serum of a woman with hereditary angioneurotic edema was found to lack inhibitory activity for a synthetic esterase (*p*-tosyl-L-arginine methyl ester HCl), and it was concluded that a kallikrein inhibitor was absent from the serum [40]. Simultaneously the serum of another affected woman was found to be unable to inhibit the esterolysis of *N*-acetyltyrosine ethyl ester by C1. It was concluded that the defect resulted from the absence of a C1 inhibitor. This was confirmed by im-

munologic studies, which demonstrated the absence or marked reduction of antigenic C1 inhibitor levels in sera from patients with this disease. About 15 percent of patients with low levels of functional C1 inhibitor in their serum have normal or increased amounts of antigenic C1 inhibitor (CRM+) [41] (see below).

ETIOLOGY AND PATHOGENESIS

Attacks of angioedema are associated with the generation of activated C1 (C$\overline{1}$) in the plasma, an event which cannot be measured in normal plasma. C4 and C2, the natural substrates of C$\overline{1}$, are consumed, so that their serum concentration falls precipitously as the attack progresses. The terminal components of the complement system remain unaffected [42]. Highly purified C$\overline{1}$s, when injected intradermally into normal skin or into patients, induces angioedema. This reaction does not occur in people genetically deficient in C2 [43] or in guinea pigs genetically deficient in C4, thus suggesting that the interaction of C$\overline{1}$ with C4 and C2 generates one or more factors which enhance vascular permeability. The effect is on the postcapillary venule. A polypeptide kininlike substance which has vasopermeability-inducing properties has also been generated in the plasma of patients in vitro [44]. The generation of this peptide is inhibited by soybean trypsin inhibitor, purified C1 inhibitor, heparin, and antibody to C4 and C2, but not by antibody to C3. In addition to enhancing vascular permeability, the peptide contracts estrus rat uterus and causes histamine release from mast cells. Patients with angioneurotic edema have massive histaminuria, but antihistaminics or histamine-depleting substances, such as 48/80, do not inhibit the angioedema induced by C$\overline{1}$s or the peptide. Antihistamine drugs are not effective in the therapy of angioedema.

The autosomal dominant inheritance of hereditary angioneurotic edema presents an interesting puzzle. Obviously affected persons are heterozygous for the abnormality. Despite this, their serum contains very little C1 inhibitor (average 17 percent of normal), and liver biopsies can be shown to contain no hepatic parenchymal cells detectably engaged in C1 inhibitor synthesis, whereas 3 to 5 percent of normal hepatic cells will give positive fluorescence with a fluorescein-labeled antibody to C1 inhibitor [45].

The C1 inhibitor, or α_2-neuraminoglycoprotein, is the most highly glycosylated glycoprotein of serum [46–48]. It contains over 40 percent carbohydrate, almost half of which is neuraminic acid. It has a molecular weight of 106,000 but behaves like a 7 S protein on gel filtration. It is a single chain consisting of three identical polypeptide subunits. In addition to its capacity to inactivate C$\overline{1}$s, it also has an inhibitory effect on C$\overline{1}$r, plasmin, kallikrein, factor XIa of the clotting system, and activated Hageman factor (factor XIIa) [49]. The latter activities, however, are also inhibited by α_2-macroglobulin or antithrombin III. C1 inhibitor is the only inhibitor of C1 in the serum. It is inactivated by plasmin, trypsin, and exposure to pH levels below 7.

In 15 percent of affected kindred, sera of patients contain normal or elevated amounts of cross-reacting, immunologically nonfunctional protein (CRM+). The CRM+ nonfunctional C1 inhibitors differ among different kindreds with respect to their electrophoretic mobility, binding affinity to $C\bar{1}s$, and capacity to inhibit the hydrolysis of N-acetyltyrosine ethyl ester by $C\bar{1}s$. All CRM+ C1 inhibitors, however, fail to inhibit the destruction of C4 by C1. The clinical course of the disease is the same in CRM+ and CRM− patients, and the CRM+ proteins are inherited as autosomal dominant traits [50].

CLINICAL FEATURES

Patients with hereditary angioneurotic edema have recurrent episodes of swelling. Edema accumulates rapidly in the affected part, which becomes tense but not discolored. There is no itching, pain, or redness associated with the edema. Laryngeal edema may be fatal because of airway obstruction and consequent pulmonary edema. If the intestine, most often the jejunum, is involved, severe abdominal cramps and bilious vomiting ensue. Clear and watery diarrhea may occur if the colon is affected. The attacks usually last 48 to 72 h. Although they often develop spontaneously and unpredictably, they may occur after trauma or with menses, excessive fatigue, or mental stress. Attacks of angioedema are infrequent in early childhood; the disease exacerbates at adolescence and tends to subside in the sixth decade of life. In children especially, transient mottling of the skin, reminiscent of erythema marginatum may occur frequently but not necessarily in association with attacks of angioedema [41–43].

THERAPY

Approximately 50 percent of patients with hereditary angioneurotic edema have complete relief of symptoms by taking 10 mg methyltestosterone sublingually, 10 mg fluoxymesterone, or 5 to 10 mg oxymetholone daily. The synthetic androgen, danocrine, is also recommended for therapy in doses of 100 to 200 mg every day. ϵ-Aminocaproic acid and its analog, tranexamic acid, are also effective as prophylactic therapy [54–56]. It is well known that plasmin can activate C1, and this may explain the efficacy of inhibitors of plasminogen activators in the therapy of this disease. Although plasma infusions have been given for the therapy of acute attacks of angioedema, this procedure has no merit in the light of present knowledge and may, in fact, be dangerous, since substrate for C1 is being infused along with inhibitor.

COURSE AND PROGNOSIS

As previously indicated, patients with hereditary angioneurotic edema tend to become much wose at pubescence, and in the sixth decade of life the frequency of attacks subsides. The attacks are self-limited, but many patients are subjected to unnecessary abdominal surgery if they and their physicians are unaware that severe cramping abdominal pain is a frequent manifestation of the disease. At one time it was reported that one-third of patients died of the disease by the end of the fourth decade of life, almost invariably from laryngeal edema. These deaths can be eliminated entirely if the patient and attending physicians are aware of the diagnosis and arrange for prompt tracheostomy during episodes of laryngeal obstruction. The long-term prophylactic value of androgen therapy has not been assessed.

Other genetic defects of the complement system

At least five children with a genetically determined deficiency of C3 have been found [57,58]. The defect is transmitted as an autosomal recessive trait, and heterozygous carriers are readily detected by their half-normal levels of C3 [59]. These children are subject to recurrent bouts of pyogenic infection, much like patients with agammaglobulinemia. A similar clinical course has been observed in a single patient with a hereditary deficiency of the C3b inactivator, which resulted in spontaneous consumption of the proteins of the alternative pathway and C3 [60].

The most common complement component deficiency in human beings is that of C2 [61]. At least two dozen C2-deficient subjects are known. This deficiency is also transmitted as an autosomal recessive characteristic, and heterozygous carriers of the defect are easily detected. At least four propositi presented with a disease resembling lupus erythematosus (SLE), three with Henoch-Schönlein purpura, and one with polymyositis. These observations suggest the possibility that C2-deficient persons are especially susceptible also to the development of connective tissue disease. In this regard, a single kindred with C1r deficiency [62], two others with C4 deficiency, and one with C5 deficiency have been identified when they presented with an SLE-like illness [63,64].

Deficiencies of these early-acting components C1r, C4, and C2 are not associated with recurrent pyogenic infections. However, systemic gonococcal infection led to the discovery of patients with deficiencies of C6 and of C8 [65,66]. This finding suggests that the serum bactericidal mechanism may be important in protection against systemic neisserial invasion.

References

1. Bruton, O. C.: Agammaglobulinemia. *Pediatrics* 9:722, 1952.
2. Cooperband, S. R., Rosen, F. S., and Kibrick, S.: Studies on the in vitro behavior of agammaglobulinemic lymphocytes. *J. Clin. Invest.* 47:836, 1968.
3. Ziegler, J. B., and Penny, R.: Fatal Echo 30 virus infection and amyloidosis in X-linked hypogammaglobulinemia. *Clin. Immunol. Immunopathol.* 3:347, 1975.
4. Rosen, F. S., and Janeway, C. A.: The gamma globulins. III. The antibody deficiency syndromes. *N. Engl. J. Med.* 275:709, 1966.

5. Hobbs, J. R.: Immune imbalance in dysgammaglobulinemia type IV. *Lancet* 1:110, 1968.

6. Rosen, F. S., Kevy, S. V., Merler, E., Janeway, C. A., and Gitlin, D.: Recurrent bacterial infections and dysgammaglobulinemia: Deficiency of 7S gamma globulins in the presence of elevated 19S gamma globulins. *Pediatrics* 28:182, 1961.

7. Hinz, C. F., Jr., and Boyer, J. T.: Dysgammaglobulinemia in adult manifested as autoimmune hemolytic anemia. *N. Engl. J. Med.* 269:1329, 1963.

8. Bachmann, R.: Studies on the serum gamma A globulin level: III. The frequency of agamma A globulinemia. *Scand. J. Clin. Lab. Invest.* 17:316, 1965.

9. Ammann, A. J., and Hong, R.: Selective IgA deficiency and autoimmunity. *Clin. Exp. Immunol.* 7:343, 1970.

10. Vyas, G. N., Perkins, H. A., and Fudenberg, H. H.: Anaphylactoid transfusion reactions associated with anti-IgA. *Lancet* 2:312, 1968.

11. Schur, P., Borel, H., Gelfand, E. W., Alper, C. A., and Rosen, F. S.: Selective gamma G globulin deficiencies in patients with recurrent pyogenic infection. *N. Engl. J. Med.* 283:631, 1970.

12. Yount, W. S., Hong, R., Seligmann, M., Good, R., and Kunkel, H. G.: Imbalances of gamma globulin subgroups and gene defects in patients with primary hypogammaglobulinemia. *J. Clin. Invest.* 49:1957, 1970.

13. Gitlin, D., Kumate, J., Urrusti, J., and Morales, C.: Selectivity of human placenta in transfer of plasma proteins from mother to fetus. *J. Clin. Invest.* 43:1938, 1964.

14. Ochs, H. D., Ament, M. E., and Davis, I. D.: Giardiasis with malabsorption in X-linked agammaglobulinemia. *N. Engl. J. Med.* 287:341, 1972.

15. Twomey, J. J., Jordan, P. H., Jarrold, T., Trubowitz, S., Ritz, N. D., and Conn, H. O.: The syndrome of immunoglobulin deficiency and pernicious anemia. *Am. J. Med.* 47:340, 1969.

16. Geha, R. S., Schneeberger, E., Merler, E., and Rosen, F. S.: Heterogeneity of common variable agammaglobulinemia. *N. Engl. J. Med.* 291:1, 1974.

17. Reinherz, E. L., and Schlossman, S. F.: Regulation of the immune response—Inducer and suppressor T lymphocyte subsets in human beings. *N. Engl. J. Med.* 303:370, 1980.

18. Reinherz, E. L., Kung, P. C., Goldstein, G., Levey, R. H., and Schlossman, S. F.: Discrete stages of intrathymic differentiation: Analysis of normal thymocytes and leukemic lymphoblasts of T lineage. *Proc. Natl. Acad. Sci. U.S.A.* 77:1588, 1980.

19. Siegel, R. L., Issekutz, T., Schwaber, J., Rosen, F. S., and Geha, R. S.: Deficiency of T helper cells in transient hypogammaglobulinemia of infancy. *N. Engl. J. Med.* 305:1307, 1981.

20. Reinherz, E. L., Cooper, M. D., Schlossman, S. F., and Rosen, F. S.: Abnormalities of T cell maturation and regulation in human beings with immunodeficiency disorders. *J. Clin. Invest.* 68:699, 1981.

21. Reinherz, E. L., Rubinstein, A., Geha, R. S., Strelkauskas, A. J., Rosen, F. S., and Schlossman, S. F.: Abnormalities of immunoregulatory T cells in disorders of immune function. *N. Engl. J. Med.* 301:1018, 1979.

22. Reinherz, E. L., Geha, R., Wohl, M. E., Morimoto, C., Rosen, F. S., and Schlossman, S. F.: Immunodeficiency associated with loss of T4+ T-cell function. *N. Engl. J. Med.* 304:811, 1981.

23. Glanzmann, E., and Riniker, P.: Essentielle lymphocytophthise. *Ann. Paediatr.* 175:1, 1950.

24. Giblett, E. R., Anderson, J. E., Cohen, F., Pollara, B., and Meuwissen, H. J.: Adenosine-deaminase deficiency in two patients with severely impaired cellular immunity. *Lancet* 2:1067, 1972.

25. Hirschhorn, R., Beratis, N., Rosen, F. S., Parkman, R., Stern, R., and Polmar, S.: Adenosine deaminase deficiency in a child diagnosed prenatally. *Lancet* 1:73, 1975.

26. Giblett, E. R., Ammann, A. J., Wara, D. W., Sandman, R., and Diamond, L. K.: Nucleoside-phosphorylase deficiency in a child with severely defective T-cell immunity and normal B-cell immunity. *Lancet* 1:1010, 1975.

27. Kretschmer, R., Jeannet, M., Mereu, T. R., Kretschmer, K., Winn, H., and Rosen, F. S.: Hereditary thymic dysplasia: A graft-versus-host reaction induced by bone marrow cells with a partial 4A series histo-incompatibility. *Pediatr. Res.* 3:34, 1969.

28. Gatti, R. A., Meuwissen, H. J., Allen, H. D., Hilaire, J., Hong, R., and Good, R.: Immunologic reconstitution of sex-linked lymphopenic immunologic deficiency. *Lancet* 2:1366, 1968.

29. Bortin, M. N., and Rimm, A. A.: Severe combined immunodeficiency disease: Characterization of the disease and results of transplantation. *JAMA* 238:591, 1977.

30. Parkman, R., Gelfand, E. W., Rosen, F. S., Sanderson, A., and Hirschhorn, R.: Severe combined immunodeficiency and adenosine deaminase deficiency. *N. Engl. J. Med.* 292:714, 1975.

31. Buckley, R. H., Whisnant, J. K., Schiff, R. I., Gilbertsen, R. B., Huang, A. T., and Platt, M. S.: Correction of severe combined immunodeficiency by fetal liver cells. *N. Engl. J. Med.* 294:1076, 1976.

32. Githens, J. H.: Immunologic reconstitution with fetal tissue. *N. Engl. J. Med.* 294:116, 1976 (editorial).

33. Petersen, R. D. A., Cooper, M. D., and Good, R. A.: Lymphoid tissue abnormalities associated with ataxia telangiectasia. *Am. J. Med.* 41:342, 1966.

34. Parkman, R., Remold-O'Donnell, E., Kenney, D. M., Perrine, S., and Rosen, F. S.: Surface protein abnormalities in the lymphocytes and platelets from patients with the Wiskott-Aldrich syndrome. *Lancet* 2:1387, 1981.

35. Cooper, M. D., Chase, H. P., Lowman, J. T., Krivit, W., and Good, R. A.: Wiskott-Aldrich syndrome: An immunologic deficiency disease involving the afferent limb of immunity. *Am. J. Med.* 44:499, 1968.

36. Parkman, R., et al.: Complete correction of the Wiskott-Aldrich syndrome by allogeneic bone marrow transplantation. *N. Engl. J. Med.* 298:921, 1978.

37. DiGeorge, A. M.: Congenital absence of thymus and its immunologic consequences: Concurrence with congenital hypoparathyroidism, in *Immunologic Diseases in Man,* edited by D. Bergsma. *Birth Defects* 4:116, 1968.

38. August, C. S., Rosen, F. S., Filler, R. M., Janeway, C. A., Markowski, B., and Kay, H. E. M.: Implantation of a foetal thymus, restoring immunological competence in a patient with thymic aplasia (DiGeorge's syndrome). *Lancet* 2:1210, 1968.

39. Cleveland, W. W., Fogel, B. J., Brown, W. T., and Kay, H. E. M.: Foetal thymic transplant in a case of DiGeorge's syndrome. *Lancet* 2:1211, 1968.

40. Landerman, N. S.: Hereditary angioneurotic edema. *Am. J. Med. Sci.* 33:316, 1962.

41. Donaldson, V. H., and Evans, R. R.: A biochemical abnormality in hereditary angioneurotic edema. *Am. J. Med.* 35:37, 1963.

42. Rosen, F. S., Charache, P., Pensky, J., and Donaldson, V.: Hereditary angioneurotic edema: Two genetic variants. *Science* 148:957, 1962.

43. Donaldson, V. H., and Rosen, F. S.: Action of complement in hereditary angioneurotic edema: The role of C'1-esterase. *J. Clin. Invest.* 43:2204, 1964.

44. Donaldson, V. H., and Rosen, F. S.: Studies on a peptide from hereditary angioneurotic edema plasma with permeability factor and kinin activity. *J. Immunol.* 101:518, 1968 (abstract).

45. Johnson, A. M., et al.: C1 inhibitor: Evidence for decreased hepatic synthesis in hereditary angioneurotic edema. *Science* 123:553, 1971.

46. Levy, L. R., and Lepow, I. H.: Assay and properties of serum inhibitor of C'1-esterase. *Proc. Soc. Exp. Biol. Med.* 101:608, 1959.

47. Pensky, J., Levy, L. R., and Lepow, I. H.: Partial purification of a serum inhibitor of C'-esterase. *J. Biol. Chem.* 236:1674, 1961.

48. Pensky, J., and Schwick, H. G.: Human serum inhibitor of C'1-esterase: Identity with α_2-neuraminoglycoprotein. *Science* 163:695, 1969.

49. Kaplan, A. P.: The Hageman factor dependent pathways of human plasma. *Microvasc. Res.* 8:97, 1974.

50. Rosen, F. S., Alper, C. A., Pensky, J., Klemperer, M. R., and Donaldson, V. H.: Genetically determined heterogeneity of the C1 esterase inhibitor in patients with hereditary angioneurotic edema. *J. Clin. Invest.* 50:2143, 1971.

51. Spaulding, W. B.: Methyltestosterone therapy for hereditary episodic edema (hereditary angioneurotic edema). *Ann. Intern. Med.* 53:739, 1960.

52. Davis, P. J., Davis, F. B., and Charache, P.: Long-term therapy of hereditary angioedema (HAE): Preventive management with fluoxymesterone and oxymetholone in severely affected males and females. *Johns Hopkins Med. J.* 135:391, 1974.

53. Rosse, W. F., Logue, G. L., and Silberman, H. R.: Synthetic androgens in the treatment of hereditary angioneurotic edema (HANE): Effect on levels of the inhibitor of the first component of complement. *Trans. Assoc. Am. Phys.* 89:122, 1976.

54. Nilsson, I. M., Anderson, L., and Björkman, S. E.: Epsilon-aminocaproic acid (E-ACA) as a therapeutic agent based on 5 years' clinical experience. *Acta Med. Scand. (Suppl.)* 448:1, 1966.

55. Frank, M. M., Sergent, J. S., Kane, M. A., and Alling, David W.: Epsilonaminocaproic acid therapy of hereditary angioneurotic edema: A double blind study. *N. Engl. J. Med.* 286:808, 1972.

56. Blohme, G.: Treatment of hereditary angioneurotic oedema with tranexamic acid. *Acta Med. Scand.* 192:293, 1972.

57. Alper, C. A., Colten, H. R., Rosen, F. S., Rabson, A. R., MacNab, G. M., and Gear, J. S. S.: Homozygous deficiency of C3 in a patient with repeated infections. *Lancet* 2:1179, 1972.

58. Ballow, M., Shira, J. E., Harden, L., Yang, S. Y., and Day, N. K.: Complete absence of the third component of complement in man. *J. Clin. Invest.* 56:703, 1975.

59. Alper, C. A., and Rosen, F. S.: Studies of a hypomorphic variant of human C3. *J. Clin. Invest.* 50:324, 1971.

60. Alper, C. A., Abramson, N., Johnston, R. B., Jr., Jandl, J. H., and Rosen, F. S.: Complement defect associated with increased susceptibility to infection. *N. Engl. J. Med.* 392:349, 1970.

61. Klemperer, M. R., Woodworth, H. C., Rosen, F. S., and Austen, K. F.: Hereditary deficiency of the second component of complement (C'2) in man. *J. Clin. Invest.* 45:880, 1966.

62. Pickering, R. J., Naff, G. B., Stroud, R. M., Good, R. A., and Gewurz, H.: Deficiency of C1r in human serum: Effects on the structure and function of macromolecular C1. *J. Exp. Med.* 141:803, 1970.

63. Rosenfield, S. I., Kelly, M. E., and Leddy, J. P.: Hereditary deficiency of the fifth component of complement in man. I. Clinical, immunochemical, and family studies. *J. Clin. Invest.* 57:1626, 1976.

64. Rosenfield, S. I., Baum, J., Steigbigel, R. T., and Leddy, J. P.: Hereditary deficiency of the fifth component of complement in man. II. Biological properties of C5-deficiency human serum. *J. Clin. Invest.* 57:1626, 1976.

65. Leddy, J. P., Frank, M. M., Gaither, T., Baum, J., and Klemperer, M. R.: Hereditary deficiency of the sixth component of complement in man. I. Immunochemical, biologic and family studies. *J. Clin. Invest.* 53:544, 1974.

66. Boyer, J. T., Gall, E. P., Norman, M. E., Nilsson, V. R., and Zimmerman, T. S.: Hereditary deficiency of the seventh component of complement. *J. Clin. Invest.* 56:905, 1975.

CHAPTER *113*

Benign monoclonal gammopathy

MARSHALL A. LICHTMAN

Definition and history

The syndrome of benign monoclonal gammopathy has two important characteristics. The first is a plasma-immunoglobulin or a urinary-immunoglobulin light chain that has the molecular features of the product of a single clone of B lymphocytes or plasma cells: homogeneous electrophoretic migration and a single light-chain type. The second is the absence of evidence for a neoplastic disorder of B lymphocytes or plasma cells such as multiple myeloma.

The observations that Bence Jones proteinuria could precede by many years the clinical signs of multiple myeloma [1] and that hyperglobulinemia without evidence of multiple myeloma occurred in some patients [2] antedated the concept of benign monoclonal gammopathy. With the more frequent application of paper electrophoresis of plasma proteins during the 1950s and 1960s, patients were discovered who had a monoclonal immunoglobulin either without an associated disease or with diseases, such as nonlymphoid cancers, infections, or inflammatory disorders, which are not typically associated with a monoclonal proliferation of B lymphocytes [3–29]. These two circumstances are categorized as benign (asymptomatic) monoclonal gammopathy, if not associated with a disease, or secondary (symptomatic) monoclonal gammopathy, if related to a coincidental disease. Over 30 synonyms for the syndrome have been used, although *benign monoclonal gammopathy* and *secondary monoclonal gammopathy* seem to have gained general favor [17]. A classification of monoclonal gammopathies is presented in Table 113-1.

Occurrence

Benign monoclonal gammopathy is the most common disorder of immunoglobulins. It can occur at any age, but it is unusual before puberty, and its frequency increases with age. The frequency of M components is about 1 percent in those over 25 years of age [6] and is about 3 percent in those over age 70 years [6,7]. Immunoglobulin levels remain stable in such subjects for over 10 years, and less than 5 percent develop myeloma [8,9]. Benign monoclonal gammopathy is present in about 10 percent of persons over 80 years of age [10]. Benign monoclonal gammopathy is much more frequent than myeloma, which has a prevalence of about 1 per 35,000 [10–13].

Etiology and pathogenesis

The etiology of benign monoclonal gammopathy is not known. Monoclonal gammopathy has been compared with a benign tumor [15] such as a colonic polyp which stays the same size for years but then may undergo malignant transformation.

Benign monoclonal gammopathy is viewed as the proliferation of a single B-lymphocyte or plasma cell progenitor leading to a population that reaches a steady state of less than 1×10^{11} total cells. Marrow plasma cell prevalence is similar to normal in benign monoclonal gammopathy, presumably a result of the lower steady-state number of cells in comparison to myeloma. The expanded clone secretes monoclonal immunoglobulin, but neither causes osteolysis, inhibits hemopoietic proliferation and differentiation, nor impairs normal B-lymphocyte to plasma cell differentiation and function sufficiently to lead to a defect in the immune response to antigen and thus to infection. The cells in the benign clone are qualitatively different from myeloma cells (less neoplastic) and do not elaborate osteoclast-activating factor (OAF), which is responsible for bone destruction. These inferences are supported by a type of benign monoclonal gammopathy that exists in the C57BL mouse. The frequency of monoclonal gammopathy increases with mouse age [30]. The disease can be transferred to either irradiated or nonirradiated mice by marrow or spleen cells [31]. Four consecutive transplantations is the maximum observed, and there is no effect on the survival of the recipient when compared to appropriate controls. In contrast, if mouse B-cell lymphoma or myeloma cells are transplanted into normal mice, the engraftment frequency is higher than that of B cells from mice with benign gammopathy; passage from original recipient to a new recipient is unlimited; progressive disease develops; and survival of recipients decreases. Thus, there is an intrinsic difference in the growth potential (degree of malignancy) of these two B-cell clones [31].

Monoclonal gammopathy has been associated with many diseases but especially with carcinoma [10,15,17,32–34]. This relationship could be the result of (1) patients with an M component having an increased risk of developing carcinoma; (2) the M component being an antibody against some antigen in the carcinoma; (3) the globulin being the product of cancer cells; (4) coincidence. The last possibility is favored by one epidemiologic study which found the same frequency of monoclonal gammopathy in a matched control group as in cancer patients [27]. Further, where the monoclonal immunoglobulin is associated with a cancer, it often persists after surgical excision of the tumor.

The possibility that benign monoclonal gammopathy arises from stimulation of one B-lymphocyte clone by an infection or an endogenous antigen has been raised [35]. For example, patients with the cold agglutinin syndrome may have monoclonal macroglobulins for years. A few monoclonal macroglobulins are known to act like rheumatoid factors and also to be involved in formation of cryoglobulins through complex formation with the usual IgG molecules.

Clinical and laboratory features and differential diagnosis

The monoclonal protein is usually IgG; however, IgM, IgA, urinary light chains, biclonal gammopathy involving IgA and IgG or IgM and IgA, and triclonal gammopathy can occur (Table 113-1) [36–38]. Features of a malignant B-lymphocyte or plasma cell disorder are absent, including a lymphocytic or plasmacytic infiltrate in the marrow, enlargement of lymph nodes, liver, or spleen, osteolysis, unifocal infiltrates of lymphoma or

TABLE 113-1   Types of monoclonal gammopathies

BENIGN (ASYMPTOMATIC) MONOCLONAL GAMMOPATHY
Types of Ig synthesized by abnormal cell clones:
  Monoclonal IgG, IgA, or IgM
  Biclonal IgG + IgA, IgG + IgM; triclonal IgG + IgA + IgM
  Monoclonal light chain (Bence Jones proteinuria)

SECONDARY (SYMPTOMATIC) MONOCLONAL GAMMOPATHY
Types of diseases coincident with monoclonal gammopathy:
  Neoplasias of cell types not known to produce immunoglobulins (i.e., carcinoma of colon, other)
  Infectious diseases (i.e., *Mycobacterium tuberculosis*, cytomegalovirus, others)
  Liver disease (e.g., hepatitis, cirrhosis)
  Miscellaneous diseases (e.g., lupus erythematosus, myasthenia gravis, pernicious anemia, Gaucher's disease, others)

MONOCLONAL GAMMOPATHY ASSOCIATED WITH A
B-LYMPHOCYTE MALIGNANCY
Plasma cell myeloma
Waldenström's macroglobulinemia
Lymphoma or lymphocytic leukemia
Heavy-chain diseases

PSEUDOMONOCLONAL GAMMOPATHY
Iron-deficiency anemia with hypertransferrinemia

myeloma cells, or suppression of hemopoiesis (see Table 113-2).

The patient with benign monoclonal gammopathy is usually discovered incidentally. The monoclonal immunoglobulin concentration is usually constant for long periods, unlike that in most patients with untreated multiple myeloma, whose plasma or urinary concentration of immunoglobulin increases within weeks to months (see Fig. 113-1).

In the benign monoclonal gammopathy of the IgG type the concentration of monoclonal immunoglobulin is usually less than 3.0 g/dl, and in the IgA or IgM type

FIGURE 113-1   Serial determinations of γ-globulin concentrations (in grams per deciliter) of monoclonal M proteins in six persons (two females and four males) who have been observed 8 to 15 years without showing signs of myeloma and with no increase in globulin levels. At the time of death of one patient (†), autopsy did not disclose evidence of multiple myeloma. (J. Waldenström, personal observations.)

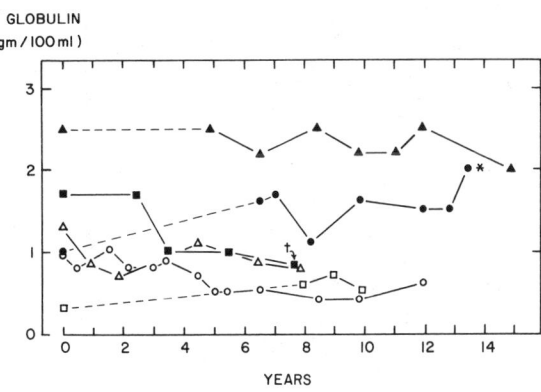

γ GLOBULIN
(gm / 100 ml)

YEARS

* New Technique

TABLE 113-2 Features that can be used to distinguish benign from malignant monoclonal gammopathy

Marrow plasma cell concentration
Plasma cell morphology
Bone integrity
Monoclonal immunoglobulin or light-chain concentration
Stability of monoclonal immunoglobulin concentration over time
Concentration of alternative immunoglobulins
Serum albumin concentration
Blood hemoglobin, neutrophil, or platelet concentration

usually below 1.5 g/dl. However, there are dramatic exceptions to this rule with occasional patients having concentrations as high as 6.0 g/dl. Occasional patients have Bence Jones proteinuria as the manifestation of benign monoclonal gammopathy [1,18,19]. The amount of urinary light chains excreted may occasionally be large (> 1.0 g per day), and renal tubular dysfunction can develop.

Nearly all patients with myeloma or macroglobulinemia have a significant depression in the alternative immunoglobulin levels. For example, the patient with IgG myeloma usually has very low IgA and IgM concentrations. Patients with benign monoclonal gammopathy usually have normal levels, but depression of alternative immunoglobulins occurs in about one-third of cases. If present, the depression of alternative immunoglobulins is usually not as severe as in myeloma.

The nucleolar size of plasma cells is larger [39] and the proportion of blood B lymphocytes lower [40] in myeloma than in benign monoclonal gammopathy. The plasma-cell acid phosphatase is usually markedly elevated in myeloma and is normal in benign monoclonal gammopathy [41].

Secondary monoclonal gammopathy occurs with cancers of the colon, lung, gallbladder, prostate or another site [33,34], pernicious anemia [42], a collagen disease [43], hepatitis [43], myasthenia gravis [44], severe osteoporosis (pseudomyeloma) [45,46], chronic hemolytic anemia [47], or other disorders [10,25,48–50]. The high prevalence of benign, asymptomatic, monoclonal gammopathy dictates that some of these associations are coincidental, as has been suggested in regard to cancers [27].

In patients with severe iron deficiency, the increase in transferrin concentration can be great enough to produce a homogeneous peak on the serum paper electrophoresis that can be mistaken for an immunoglobulin peak.

The major features that can be used to distinguish between benign and malignant monoclonal gammopathies are summarized in Table 113-2.

Course, prognosis, and therapy

Most patients (~75 percent) with benign monoclonal gammopathy will have a stable concentration of their monoclonal immunoglobulin and no signs or symptoms of a plasma cell or lymphocytic neoplasm [23]. In a small proportion of subjects (~ 10 percent) overt myeloma will develop after a short period or as long as 20 years after the diagnosis of benign monoclonal gammopathy (see Fig. 113-2) [18,26,51]. The relationship of benign monoclonal gammopathy to myeloma is strengthened by reports of families with both disorders [21], making it possible that benign monoclonal gammopathy is a premyelomatous lesion with a low likelihood of malignant transformation. In occasional patients (~10 percent) the monoclonal immunoglobulin concentration gradually increases to a new, higher steady-state concentration without other clinical evidence for a transformation to a more malignant state. In rare patients the monoclonal protein has disappeared.

It may not be possible in all cases of suspected benign monoclonal gammopathy to be certain of the correct diagnosis at the time of first evaluation. Therapy should not be administered unless there is a confirmed diagnosis of myeloma, macroglobulinemia, or lymphoma with evidence of progressive disease and significant impairment of bone structure, hemopoiesis, or other vital functions.

FIGURE 113-2 Serial determinations of γ-globulin concentrations in five patients (three females and two males) with multiple myeloma who initially were regarded as having benign nonprogressive gammopathy. It can be seen from the graph that two (△ and □) may have had a steady increase in γ-globulin at an early stage, although the final myeloma phase was accompanied by a much steeper increase. In the other three patients it is possible that there was an early constant level at around 1 g/dl before the rapid increase started. A = Alkeran therapy. (J. Waldenström, personal observations.)

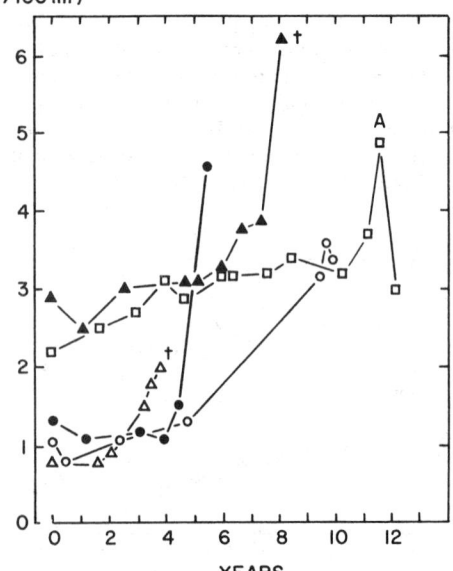

γ GLOBULIN
(gm/100 ml)

YEARS

References

1. Prentiss, R. G., Jr.: Multiple myeloma with diffuse skeletal involvement: Case report. *Milit. Surgeon* 80:294, 1937.

2. Waldenstrom, J. G.: Incipient mye'omatosis or essential hyperglobulinemia with fibrinogenopenia· A new syndrome? *Acta Med. Scand.* 117:216, 1944.

3. Osserman, E. F.: Natural history of multiple myeloma before evidence of radiological disease. *Radiology* 71:157, 1958.

4. Waldenstrom, J. G.: Studies on conditions associated with disturbed gamma globulin formation (gammopathies). *Harvey Lect.* 56:211, 1961.

5. Waldenstrom, J. G.: *Monoclonal and Polyclonal Hypergammaglobulinemia: Clinical and Biological Significance.* Cambridge, London, 1968.

6. Axelsson, U., Bachmann, R., and Hallen, J.: Frequency of pathological proteins (M-components) in 6995 sera from an adult population. *Acta Med. Scand.* 179:235, 1966.

7. Hallen, J.: Discrete gammaglobulin (M-components) in serum. *Acta Med. Scand. (Suppl.)* 462:1966.

8. Axelsson, U., and Hallen J.: Review of fifty-four subjects with monoclonal gammopathy. *Br. J. Haematol.* 15:417, 1968.

9. Axelsson, U.: An eleven-year follow-up on 64 subjects with M-components. *Acta Med. Scand.* 201:173, 1977.

10. Hallen, J.: Frequency of "abnormal serum globulins" (M-components) in the aged. *Acta Med. Scand.* 173:737, 1963.

11. Williams, R. C., Jr., Bailly, R. C., and Howe, R. B.: Studies of "benign" serum M-components. *Am. J. Med. Sci.* 257:275, 1969.

12. Derycke, C., Fine, J. M., and Boffa, G. A.: Dysglobulinémies "essentielles" chez les sujets agés. *Nouv. Rev. Fr. Hematol.* 5:729, 1965.

13. Kyle, R. A., Finkelstein, S., Elveback, L. R., and Kurland, L. T.: Incidence of monoclonal proteins in a Minnesota community with a cluster of multiple myelomas. *Blood* 40:719, 1972.

14. Waldenstrom, J. G.: Benign monoclonal gammopathies, in *Multiple Myeloma and Related Disorders,* edited by H. A. Azar and M. Potter. Harper & Row, New York, 1973, vol. 1 p. 247.

15. Zawadski, Z. A., and Edwards, G. A.: Nonmyelomatous monoclonal immunoglobulinemia. *Prog. Clin. Immunol.* 1:105, 1972.

16. Dammacco, F., and Waldenstrom, J. G.: Bence Jones proteinuria in benign monoclonal gammopathies. *Acta Med. Scand.* 184:403, 1968.

17. Ritzmann, S. E., Loukes, D., Sakai, H., Daniels, J. C., and Levin, W. C.: Idiopathic (asymptomatic) monoclonal gammopathies. *Arch. Intern. Med.* 135:95, 1975.

18. Kyle, R. A.: Monoclonal gammopathy of undetermined significance: Natural history in 241 cases. *Am. J. Med.* 64:814, 1978.

19. Kyle, R. A., Maldonado, J. E., and Bayrd, E. D.: Idiopathic Bence-Jones proteinuria: a distinct entity. *Am. J. Med.* 55:222, 1973.

20. Cronstedt J., Carlong, L., and Ostberg, H.: Idiopathic light chain dyscrasia—a new distinct entity? Report of a case. *Acta Med. Scand.* 196:445, 1974.

21. Meiyers, K. A. E., DeLeeuw, B., and Voormolen-Kalova, M.: The multiple occurrence of mye'oma and asymptomatic paraproteinaemia within one family. *Clin. Exp. Immunol.* 12:185, 1972.

22. Pruzanski, W., Underdoun, B., Silver, E. H., and Katz, A.: Macroglobulinemia-myeloma double gammopathy: A study of four cases and a review of the literature. *Am. J. Med.* 57:259, 1974.

23. Carter, A., and Tatarsky, I.: The physiopathological significance of benign monoclonal gammopathy: A study of 64 cases. *Br. J. Haematol.* 46:565, 1980.

24. Lindstrom, F. D., and Dahlstrom, V.: Multiple myeloma or benign monoclonal gammopathy? A study of differential diagnostic criteria in 44 cases. *Clin. Immunol. Immunopathol.* 10:168, 1978.

25. Zawadzki, Z. A., and Edwards, G. A.: Dysimmunoglobulinemia in the absence of c'inical features of multiple mye'oma and macroglobulinemia. *Am. J. Med.* 42:67, 1967.

26. Nørgaard, O.: Three cases of multiple myeloma in which the preclinical asymptomatic phases persisted throughout 15 to 24 years. *Br. J. Cancer* 25:417, 1971.

27. Migliore, P. J., and Alexanian, R.: Monoclonal gammopathy in human neoplasia. *Cancer* 21:1127, 1968.

28. Michaux, J.-L., and Heremans, J. F.: Thirty cases of monoclonal immunoglobulin disorders other than myeloma or macroglobulinemia. *Am. J. Med.* 46:562, 1969.

29. Amies, A., Ko, H. S., and Pruzanski, W.: M-components—A review of 1242 cases. *Can. Med. Assoc. J.* 114:889, 1976.

30. Radl, J., and Hollander, C. F.: Homogeneous immunoglobulins in sera of mice during aging. *J. Immunol.* 112:2271, 1974.

31. Radl, J., De Glopper, E., Schuit, H. R. E., and Zurcher, C.: Idiopathic paraproteinemia. II. Transplantation of the paraprotein-producing clone from old to young C57Bl/KaLwRij mice. *J. Immunol.* 122:609, 1979.

32. Ky e, R. A., and Bayrd, E. A.: *The Monoclonal Gammopathies.* Charles C Thomas, Springfield, Ill., 1976.

33. Solomon, A.: Homogeneous (monoclonal) immunoglobulins in cancer. *Am. J. Med.* 63:169, 1977.

34. Colls, B. M., and Lorier, M. A.: Immunocytoma, cancer, and other associations of monoclonal gammopathy: A review of 224 cases. *N. Z. Med. J.* 82:221 1975.

35. Osserman, E. F., and Takatsuki, K. Considerations regarding the pathogenesis of the plasmacytic dyscrasias. *Ser. Hematol.* 4:28, 1965.

36. Imhof, J. W., Ballieux, R. E., Mul N. A. J., and Poen, H.: Monoclonal and diclonal gammapathies. *Acta. Med. Scand.* 179 (Suppl. 445):102, 1966.

37. Jensen, K., Jensen, B., and Olesen, H. Three M-components in serum from an apparently healthy person. *Scand. J. Haematol.* 4:485, 1967.

38. Natvig, J. B., and Kunkel, H. G.: Human immunoglobulins: Classes, subclasses, genetic variants, and idiotypes. *Adv. Immunol.* 16:1, 1973.

39. Turesson, I.: Nucleolar size in benign and malignant plasma ce'l proliferation. *Acta Med. Scand.* 197:7, 1975.

40. Lindstrom, F. D., Hardy, W. R., Eberle, B. J., and Williams, R. C., Jr.: Multiple myeloma and benign monoclonal gammopathy: Differentiation by immunofluorescence of lymphocytes. *Ann. Intern. Med.* 78:837, 1973.

41. Cassuto, J. P., Hammore, J. C., Pastorelli, E., Dujardin P., and Masseyeff, R.: Plasma cell acid phosphatase, a discriminative test for benign and malignant monoclonal gammopathies. *Biomed.* 27: 97, 1977.

42. Burner, E., Zwahlen, A., and Cruchaud A.: Nonmalignant monoclonal immunoglobulinemia, pernicious anemia, and gastric carcinoma. A model of immunologic dysfunction. *Am. J. Med.* 60:1019, 1976.

43. Abramson, N., and Shattil, S. J.: M-components. *JAMA* 223:156, 1973.

44. Rowland, L. P., Osserman, E. F., Scharfman, W. B., Balsam, R. F., and Ball, S.: Myasthenia gravis with a myeloma-type gamma-G (IgG) immunoglobulin abnormality. *Am. J. Med.* 46:599, 1969.

45. Buonocore, E., Solomon, A., and Kerley, H. E.: Pseudomyeloma. *Radiology* 95:41, 1970.

46. Maldonado, J. E., Riggs, L., and Bayrd, E. D.: Pseudomyeloma. *Arch. Intern. Med.* 135:267, 1975.

47. Schafer, A. I., Miller, J. B., Lester, E. P., Bowers, T. K., and Jacob, H. S.: Monoclonal gammopathy in hereditary spherocytosis: A possible pathogenetic relation. *Ann. Intern. Med.* 88:45, 1978.

48. Michaux, J.-L., and Heremans, J. F.: Thirty cases of monoclonal immunoglobulin disorders other than myeloma or macroglobulinemia. *Am. J. Med.* 46:562, 1969.

49. Joseph, R. R., Barry, W. E., and Durant, J. R.: Prolonged immunological disorders terminating in hematological malignancy. A human analogue of animal disease? *Ann. Intern. Med.* 72:699, 1970.

50. Shoenfeld, Y., Berliner, S., Pinkhas, J., and Beutler, E.: The association of Gaucher's disease and dysproteinemias. *Acta Haematol* 64:241, 1980.

51. Kyle, R. A., and Bayrd, E. D.: "Benign" monoclonal gammopathy: A potentially malignant condition. *Am. J. Med.* 40:426, 1966.

Lymphocytic disorders—malignant proliferative response—leukemia

CHAPTER *114*

Acute lymphocytic leukemia

EDWARD S. HENDERSON

Definition

Acute lymphocytic leukemia (ALL) is a malignant disease of primitive lymphopoietic progenitors which occurs predominantly in children. The leukemia originates in the marrow, thymus, and lymph nodes. The abnormal cell is a nongranular leukocyte, with little cytoplasm and a round nucleus which resembles that of a normal lymphoblast. Impairment of immunologic response, immunoglobulin deficiencies, and autoimmunity are uncommon features of ALL, suggesting that uninvolved areas containing immunocytes can sustain nearly normal antibody formation and delayed hypersensitivity reactions. Normal marrow hemopoietic cells are markedly suppressed by the leukemic blast cells. There is no evidence that the basic abnormality involves multipotent hemopoietic stem cells which differentiate into erythrocytes, granulocytes, and megakaryocytes; rather these cells fail to proliferate and differentiate as the result of a secondary effect on the lymphoblastic tumor in marrow.

INCIDENCE AND CLASSIFICATION

ALL has a peak incidence between 2 and 10 years of age, and a second rise in frequency from middle age onward [1]. Although its incidence may have declined slightly during the last decade [1–3], it is still the most common malignant disorder in childhood, and the principal cause of death due to disease in the pediatric age group. Data regarding etiology and epidemiology have been reviewed in Chap. 29.

Although the abnormal cells have always been considered to be lymphoid progenitors on morphologic grounds, studies have now shown unequivocally that ALL in its diverse forms is a disease of early lymphoid cells (see Table 114-1). The most frequent and possibly the least differentiated form is the common-type ALL variety which lacks mature B- or T-cell characteristics but can be identified by a distinct membrane glycoprotein known as the *common ALL antigen (cALLa)* [4,5]. This antigen can be detected also in the lymphocytic form of the blastic crisis of chronic myelogenous leukemia, in a pre-B-cell variant of ALL, and in a minority of T-cell and B-cell leukemias. It is found in a very small number of normal marrow cells and essentially never in normal thymus or spleen [6]. The second most frequent form of ALL in both adults and children exhibits T-cell membrane markers: sheep erythrocyte receptors or T cell–specific antigens [7–15]. A few cases have been noted whose blast cells appear to suppress immunoglobulin synthesis and resemble T suppressor cells [16]. Both common ALL and T-cell leukemic lymphoblasts contain terminal deoxynucleotidyl transferase (TdT) [17–30], an enzyme found normally in immature thymocytes [18], in rare marrow lymphocyte precursors [20], in the blasts of about 20 percent of cases with blastic crisis of CML [21–23], and rarely in cases of acute myelogenous leukemia (AML) [19,24,25]. Finally, cell-associated immunoglobulin, a characteristic of B-lymphocyte differentiation, has been found in some cases of ALL. Cytoplasmic immunoglobulin (cIg), a feature of pre-B lymphocytes, is found in one-quarter of otherwise typical common-type ALLs and lymphoid blastic crises of chronic myelogenous leukemia (CML) [26]. Surface immunoglobulin (SmIg), a feature of mature B lymphocytes, is found on the cells of rare patients with acute "lymphoma cell" leukemia and Burkitt cell leukemia [10–13,26]. These distinctive immunological features not only support the lymphocytic origin of these leukemias, but influence to a significant extent the clinical course and the response to treatment of the various forms of ALL (see below).

Certain acute leukemias, while morphologically indistinguishable from ALL, lack the cytochemical and immunological characteristics of T-cell, B-cell, or common ALL. Some of these truly undifferentiated cases may be of early myeloid origin, or may derive from pluripotential stem cells, and exhibit no evidence of differentiation. These cases are rare, more common in adults than children, and respond poorly to therapy [27,28].

Clinical features

The clinical features of ALL resemble those in other varieties of acute leukemia (see Chap. 29).

The onset of ALL is nearly always acute and the course of the disease is steadily progressive. In contrast to acute myelogenous leukemia (AML), ALL is rarely heralded by preleukemic manifestations. Symptoms are usually of short duration and ordinarily have not been present for more than a few weeks before the diagnosis

TABLE 114-1   Immunologic variants of acute lymphocytic leukemia

Type	Features of abnormal cells in bone marrow	Clinical clues
Acute lymphocytic leukemia:		
Common-type ALL	1. Lymphoblasts are usually small, with scant, nongranular cytoplasm. Nuclear chromatin and nucleoli are indistinct. 2. Lymphoblasts are negative for myeloperoxidase, naphthol chloroacetate, nonspecific esterases, and Sudan stains. Acid phosphatase–negative. 3. Lymphoblast cytoplasm usually contains large blocks of PAS-staining material. 4. Contain common ALL antigen (cALLa+); lack sheep RBC receptors and surface Ig. 5. Subsets may have cytoplasmic Ig (pre-B). 6. Philadelphia chromosome present in about 5%.	1. Common in children; rare in adults. 2. Lymphadenopathy common. 3. Gum and skin infiltration uncommon. 4. Muramidase normal or low.
T-cell ALL	1. Indistinguishable morphologically from common-type ALL. 2. Acid phosphatase and nonspecific esterase–staining areas in cytoplasm. May contain PAS blocks. Negative for peroxidase, Sudan stains. 3. Membrane receptors for sheep RBC; T-cell antigens.	1. Most common ages, 10–20 years. 2. Frequent mediastinal lymphadenopathy, CNS infiltration, and high blast cell counts.
B-cell ALL	1. Large blasts with vacuolate, deeply basophilic cytoplasm. 2. Contain surface membrane immunoglobulin.	1. Poor long-term response to treatment. 2. Muramidase low or normal.
Acute undifferentiated leukemia	1. Indistinguishable morphologically from ALL or acute myeloblastic leukemia 2. Peroxidase-, Sudan-, and PAS-negative. 3. Lack common ALL antigen, T- or B-cell determinants.	1. More common in adults. 2. Poor response and survival. 3. Muramidase low or normal.

is established. The most common complaints include malaise, fatigue, weight loss, pallor, ease of bruising, or bleeding. Sweating is relatively common. Chills and fever are usually indicative of infection. Enlargement of superficial lymph nodes, splenomegaly, and hepatomegaly are common in ALL, but the organomegaly is seldom prominent and may be absent. Aching along the spine and hips and tenderness of the superficial bones are common. Gait disturbances may be observed in children, and may be the result of swelling or tenderness about the large joints or epiphyses. In extreme instances, there may be radiologic evidence of joint involvement or areas of bone destruction. In rare instances, cranial nerve paralysis and increased intracranial pressure, or other signs of leukemic meningitis, may be present when the disease is first discovered.

Laboratory features

The leukocyte count is usually increased in ALL, often to 100,000 per microliter or more, but in about one-third of patients the total count is normal or low. The absolute neutrophil and platelet count in the blood is almost always decreased. Anemia is almost always present at the time of diagnosis, but deformed erythrocytes and nucleated red blood cells are usually not present in the blood.

The marrow is almost always hypercellular and heavily infiltrated or replaced by leukemic lymphoblasts which tend to appear less mature than those in the blood. Normal hemopoietic cells are usually reduced in number and frequently appear to be almost totally replaced.

In contrast to myelogenous leukemia, smoldering, or oligoblastic varieties of ALL are very uncommon. Increased reticulin fibers in the marrow are present in 15 percent of all patients with ALL, and are often associated with bone pain [29].

The lymphoblasts in the blood in ALL are usually small cells. They have little cytoplasm and a round or oval nucleus with indistinct chromatin and poorly outlined nucleoli. Auer bodies and primary granules are never present in the leukemic lymphoblasts. In common-type ALL, characteristically seen in children, the leukemic cells have a uniform appearance. They tend to be small and have immature nuclei but with indistinct nucleoli and scant cytoplasm. This corresponds primarily to what has been classified as the L1 morphology and makes up about 85 percent of cases of ALL [30]. Alternative forms of ALL may have larger, more immature-appearing lymphoid cells with prominent nucleoli in marrow and blood, the so-called L2 morphology. They make up about 15 percent of cases of ALL. The rare Burkitt cell ALL, a B-cell variant, presents with larger lymphoblasts, usually with deeply basophilic, heavily vacuolated cytoplasm, and represents the L3 type of morphology.

Histochemical staining of ALL cells typically reveals large PAS-staining aggregates, or "blocks," in the cytoplasm, and an absence of myeloperoxidase, sudanophilic vacuoles, and naphthol-AS-D chloroacetate and α-naphythyl acetate (nonspecific) esterases. Arylsulfatase is frequently identifiable in the blast cells of ALL, but this enzyme is occasionally demonstrable in acute granulocytic leukemia as well [31]. Acid phosphatase and nonspecific esterase are seen in paranuclear collections in T-cell leukemic blasts [32]. Cytogenetic abnormalities, which occur in about 45 percent of patients with ALL, include aneuploidy (usually hyperploidy) and a variety of marker chromosomes usually involving the C and G groups [33–35]. These chromosome anomalies appear to be disease-specific, since they are consistently demonstrable to an extent that parallels the amount of leukemic cell infiltration of all body sites tested (marrow, blood, and cerebrospinal fluid). In about 5 percent of children and 25 percent of adults with ALL, the Ph^1 chromosome is present in the lymphoblasts [35–26].

Biochemical abnormalities in the plasma of patients with ALL are nonspecific. They can reflect organ infiltration and disturbances in function, or release of cell breakdown products (see Chap. 27). Serum lactic acid dehydrogenase (LDH) [37], serum uric acid, and plasma fibrinogen [38] levels are frequently elevated when the disease is in relapse. The absolute levels vary considerably from individual to individual. There are no biochemical "markers" in plasma which can be used with any accuracy for the diagnosis of ALL, or in the measurement of disease activity, although LDH, when present, varies fairly consistently with the extent of leukemic involvement [38,39].

Differential diagnosis

The diagnosis of ALL ordinarily requires little more than the examination of a blood and marrow film. On occasion, however, difficult and critical distinctions must be made between ALL and infectious diseases, any one of which may coexist with leukemia. Those of particular importance include infectious mononucleosis, toxoplasmosis, and cytomegalovirus (CMV) infec-

tions. Numerous benign viral infections may present with fever, enlargement of superficial lymph nodes, splenomegaly, and cytopenias with atypical lymphocytes in the circulating blood. Transient thrombocytopenia and granulocytopenia may occur on occasion and add to the difficulty of differential diagnosis.

ALL can be confused with chronic lymphocytic leukemia, prolymphocytic leukemia, lymphocytic or lymphoblastic lymphomas, or "hairy cell" leukemia. The latter usually presents with progressive pancytopenia, splenomegaly, and the presence of bizarre "lymphoid" cells in the circulating blood. Marrow aspiration in individuals with this disease is usually difficult, and a needle biopsy often is required for adequate morphologic characterization.

In the lymphocytic lymphomas, particularly in children, the lymphoid tissue may appear to be exclusively involved at first. Within a short period of time, however, marrow infiltration characteristically develops, with or without overt leukemia. The differential diagnosis in such instances may be aided by immunologic studies. Lymphoma cells tend to have B-cell characteristics, while the abnormal lymphocytes in most patients with ALL resemble neither T nor B cells. Furthermore, the nuclei of lymphoma cells are frequently cleft and irregular, and occupy less of the cell volume than is the case in ALL. T-cell lymphoblastic lymphomas like T-cell ALL have a tendency to involve the mediastinum, but spare the marrow. Unlike T-cell ALL, T-cell lymphoma may be curable with aggressive drug therapy [40].

Neuroblastomas frequently metastasize to the marrow and may produce clinical and hematologic abnormalities that resemble acute leukemia. The presence of clumps or rosettes of neuroblastoma cells are most helpful in differentiating tumor metastases from leukemic cell infiltrates. If there is doubt regarding the diagnosis in children under 8 years of age, determination of the urinary catecholamine excretion may be of diagnostic assistance.

In older individuals, Ewing's sarcoma and small cell carcinoma of the lung frequently metastasize to the bone marrow. Nucleated red cells and immature granulocytes may be present in the blood (leukoerythroblastic reaction). Micrometastases in the marrow tend to form clusters, which may be more evident in sections of marrow obtained by biopsy. Metastatic tumors usually have a bizarre and pleomorphic nuclear configuration, and more prominent nucleoli than lymphoblasts. In Ewing's sarcoma, the cytoplasmic cell borders tend to be indistinct. Histochemistry is of little value in distinguishing ALL from the above tumors, but on occasion electron microscopic examination may be helpful.

Therapy

GENERAL CONSIDERATIONS

The treatment of ALL has two major components: therapy directed at eliminating the leukemic cells from the

TABLE 114-2 Drugs used in the treatment of acute lymphocytic leukemia

Agent	Class	Mechanism of antitumor action	Usual dose, route, schedule	Pharmacology	Usual limiting toxicities	Other toxicities
Prednisone	Synthetic adrenocortico-steroid	Lymphoblast lysis	40 mg/m² PO bid	Plasma $T_{1/2}$ 1–3 h; metabolized in liver, excreted in urine; enters CNS promptly	Occasional psychosis, hypertension, peptic ulceration	Fluid retention, osteoporosis, immunosuppression
Vincristine	Plant alkaloid	Inhibits RNA synthesis, mitotic spindle assembly	2 mg/m² IV every week initially	Rapid plasma clearance; excreted in bile; (?)CNS entry	CNS and peripheral nerve injury	Alopecia, ileus, inappropriate ADH secretion, locally corrosive
Asparaginase	Enzyme extracted from strain of *Escherichia coli*	Depletion of endogenous asparagine	500 IU/m² per day IV for 10 days	Plasma $T_{1/2}$ 3–30 h (depends on lot and source); metabolized, does not enter CNS but depletes CSF asparagine	Allergic reaction	Hepatotoxicity; inhibition of production of albumin, fibrinogen, insulin; immunosuppression
Daunorubicin	Antibiotic	Binds to DNA; inhibits DNA, RNA synthesis	30–60 mg/m² per day for 3 days IV	Plasma $T_{1/2}$ 45 min; metabolized, excreted through kidneys; excluded from CNS	Acute: myelosuppression Chronic: cumulative cardiac toxicity	Alopecia; locally corrosive
Doxorubicin	Antibiotic	Binds to DNA; inhibits DNA, RNA synthesis	30–45 mg/m² per day for 3 days IV	Plasma $T_{1/2}$ 30 min metabolized, excreted through kidneys; excluded from CNS	Acute: myelosuppression; Chronic: cumulative cardiotoxicity	Alopecia, locally corrosive
Methotrexate	Folic acid antimetabolite	Inhibits formation of folic acid coenzymes; inhibits *de novo* pyrimidine synthesis and, thus, DNA synthesis	25 mg/m² PO every week or twice a week, or 15 mg/m² per day PO, IM or IV for 5 days every 2 weeks or every month	Plasma $T_{1/2}$ 2.5 h; minimal metabolism; excreted by kidney; slow entry into CNS	Myelosuppression, mucositis, gastroenteritis, hepatic toxicity	Immunosuppression, renal toxicity (high dose), pneumonitis; arachnoiditis, and rare leukoencephelopathy with intrathecal injection
6-Mercaptopurine	Purine antimetabolite	Inhibits *de novo* purine synthesis, and thus, DNA synthesis	90 mg/m² PO daily 500 mg/m² per day for 5 days	Plasma $T_{1/2}$ metabolized in liver, etc., excreted by kidney; slow entry into CSF	Myelosuppression	Hepatic injury; mucositis
Cyclophosphamide	Synthetic polyfunctional alkylating agent	Cross-links DNA stands; must be metabolized to be active	100 mg/m² PO daily	Must be metabolized for activity; plasma $T_{1/2}$ 4 h; metabolized in liver; excreted by kidney; minimal entry into CSF	Acute: myelosuppression Chronic: immunosuppression, cystitis	Alopecia: hemorrhagic cystitis; inappropriate antiuresis; cardiac injury at high doses
Cytosine arabinoside	Pyrimidine antimetabolite	Inhibits DNA synthesis; blocks DNA polymerase	100 mg/m² daily IV infusions or q 8 h SC injection	Plasma $T_{1/2}$ < 30 min; deaminated in liver, blood, gut; Excreted in urine; good access into CSF	Myelosuppression	Immunosuppression; hepatotoxicity

marrow and other lymphopoietic tissues and viscera and treatment specifically directed toward eliminating residual foci of disease within the central nervous system. The most successful regimens, judged by the frequency, quality, and duration of the remissions they produce as well as the percentage of apparent cures in children, have included both objectives using multiple therapeutic agents.

The first successful treatment of ALL involved the use of anti-folic acid compounds, and the development of other effective agents soon followed—the antipurines, glucocorticoids, and cyclophosphamide (see Table 114-2) [41]. In the 1960s more drugs effective against ALL were developed, particularly vincristine [42], cytosine arabinoside, and daunorubicin [43]. The important concept of multiagent chemotherapy, giving repeated maximal doses of combinations of active drugs with different toxicities in cycles, led to the design of drug regimens

TABLE 114-3 Acute lymphocytic leukemia—single agent chemotherapy for remission induction

Drug	Usual dose, route, schedule	Complete remission, % Child	Adult
Prednisone	40–80 mg/m², PO daily	51–76	36
Vincristine	2 mg/m², IV each week	55	40
Asparaginase	500–5,000 IU/m², IV daily	67	*
Methotrexate	5 mg, PO daily	22	14
6-Mercaptopurine	90 mg/m², PO daily	27	8–9
Daunorubicin	45–60 mg/m², IV daily 5 times	32–38	*
Cyclophosphamide	100–150 mg/m², PO daily	40	8
Cytosine arabinoside	90–150 mg/m², IV daily	18	22

*Insufficient data.
SOURCE: Goldin et al. [32].

adapted for remission induction and maintenance [44–46]. Subsequent advances can be largely attributed to the effective control of small numbers of leukemic cells remaining within the meninges after successful remission induction [47–51] through the use of drugs [52–54], radiation therapy [51,55,56], or combinations of the two modalities [51,54,56,57]. At the present time unsuccessful treatment is the result either of the failure to eradicate all leukemic cells with currently available agents or the severe toxicity of most effective treatment regimens. The major drugs of value in the treatment of ALL, together with their significant pharmacologic and toxicologic properties, are listed in Table 114-2.

REMISSION INDUCTION

Eliminating visible leukemic marrow and blood cells, followed by restoration of normal hemopoiesis, is relatively simple in most patients. Advanced age, extreme lymphoblastic leukocytosis, and extensive mediastinal or central nervous system involvement are features which imply a poor long-term prognosis [10,58–63]. Complete first remissions, however, can be produced even in the majority of those classified as poor-risk patients.

Successful remission induction can be achieved in a significant number of patients with the use of single agents, particularly the glucocorticoids, vincristine, or L-asparaginase (see Table 114-3). Multiagent chemotherapy should be used since there is no reliable way to predict the response to these agents, and combinations of agents produce a higher proportion of complete remissions and rapid resolution of disease within 3 to 4 weeks.

Virtually all remission induction plans currently involve the use of two or more agents. The most common combination, vincristine plus a glucocorticoid, produced "complete remissions" in 88 percent of children and in 50 percent of adults (see Table 114-4). Often a third drug is added, generally daunorubicin or L-asparaginase [52,64,65]. There is little evidence that daunorubicin or doxorubicin is of special value in childhood ALL, whereas they are particularly beneficial in adults [66–70]. The addition of L-asparaginase to vincristine and prednisone has increased the frequency of complete remission in ALL in adults [66], and has lengthened the duration of remissions in children [64]. The best remission rates achieved in adults have resulted from combinations of vincristine and prednisone with daunorubicin alone or daunorubicin plus asparaginase [66–68]. The best regimens produce 85 to 95 percent complete remissions in children up to 10

TABLE 114-4 Acute lymphocytic leukemia—combination drug therapy for remission induction

Drugs	Complete remission, % Children	Adults	Reference
Prednisone + vincristine	88	50	[46]
Prednisone + daunorubicin	65	*	[46]
Prednisone + mercaptopurine	48–99	*	[46]
Prednisone + methotrexate	57	*	[46]
Prednisone + cyclophosphamide	59	*	[46]
Prednisone + vincristine + asparaginase	87	50–60	[67,68]
Prednisone + vincristine + daunorubicin	89–100	50–88	[53,66]
Prednisone + vincristine + mercaptopurine + methotrexate	50–90	43–60	[44,46]
Prednisone + vincristine + asparaginase + daunorubicin	—	74–80	[67,68]
Prednisone + vincristine + asparaginase + adriamycin	—	71	[69]
Methotrexate + asparaginase	—	69	[128,130]
Cytosine arabinoside + daunorubicin	—	69	[70]

*Insufficient data.

years of age and 75 percent complete remissions in teenagers and adults

REMISSION MAINTENANCE

Suspension of antileukemic treatment after a complete remission is inevitably followed by relapse, usually within 2 to 3 months. Longer remissions may be produced, with some possibility of cure, if therapy is continued. However, patients in whom drug treatment is suspended after 2 to 3 years appear to have a prognosis that is as good as those in whom treatment is maintained longer [51,65,71]. Treatment during the first 2 to 3 years of remission has also been designated *cytoreductive therapy* [72] or *remission consolidation* [73].

Careful studies have been carried out to define the minimum cytoreductive therapy that should be applied and to demonstrate that minor changes in technique have an important influence on the successful outcome of such therapy. As with remission induction, single agents are effective (see Table 114-5) but are less reliable than combinations of drugs (see Table 114-6). The simplest drug regimen with the potential of cure is 6-mercaptopurine (MP) 90 mg/m² orally, daily, plus methotrexate (MTX) 20 mg/m² orally weekly. These drugs are started after a complete remission and continued for 30 months, in conjunction with treatment of the central nervous system early in the period of remission (see below). The evaluation of this treatment program is still incomplete, but the following data support its use:

1. All programs in childhood ALL which have resulted in 50 percent observed or projected 5-year disease-free survival have included MP and MTX [45,51,53,54,57,62,64,65]. Similarly the best reported results in adults have used these two drugs [66–69].

2. The addition of daunorubicin (DNR) or cyclophosphamide (cyclo) to the MP + MTX regimen has not increased its effectiveness [52–74].

TABLE 114-5 Acute lymphocytic leukemia — maintenance with single drugs

Treatment	Median duration of complete remission, days
None	60
Prednisone	79
Vincristine	60
Methotrexate	349
6-Mercaptopurine	147
Daunorubicin	90
Asparaginase	90
Cytosine arabinoside	60
Cyclophosphamide	120

3. The addition of vincristine (V) plus prednisone (P) has been advocated by some [64,74] but not others [51,65,75]. Vincristine and prednisone were shown to improve the effectiveness of either MP or MTX alone [54,74], but this advantage has not been confirmed for MP plux MTX [51,65,75].

4. All the most successful programs have used chemotherapy and/or radiation therapy directed at central nervous system sanctuaries [45,53,56,57,64–69].

5. Continuation of treatment beyond 2.5 to 3 years has not prevented late relapse [59,71], but late relapse is rare following the discontinuance of systemic chemotherapy in patients who have been given adequate central nervous system treatment [56].

Since nearly 50 percent of children and most adults with ALL still die of the disease or the complications of treatment, continued efforts to improve therapy are required.

Many investigators consider immunologic factors to be important for long-term disease control or cure [12,72,73]. Leukemia-associated antigens have been detected in ALL cells [74–77], and some remarkable suc-

TABLE 114-6 Acute lymphocytic leukemia — combination maintenance programs

Induction drugs	Systemic maintenance	CNS treatment	Median duration remission, months		References
			Children	Adults	
POMP*	POMP	None	14	8	[41,44]
V + P	MTX, P + V	None	18	—	[64]
V + P	MP, MTX, cyclo, VCR	None	15	—	[45]
V + P	MP, MTX, cyclo, VCR	1200 rads, craniospinal	14	—	[45]
V + P	MP, MTX, cyclo, V + P	2400 rads, cranial + intrathecal MTX	60	—	[45]
V + P	MP, MTX, V + P	Intrathecal MTX ± RT	60	18	[64]
V + P + DNR	Ara-C, TG, ASN'ase, BCNU, cyclo, MTX, D, HU, P	Intrathecal MTX	60	24–48	[53,66]
V + P + ASN'ase + D	MP, MTX, V + P	Intrathecal MTX + RT	60	18	[67,68]

NOTES: V = vincristine (O = Oncovin); P = prednisone; DNR = daunorubicin, MTX = methotrexate; MP = 6-mercaptopurine; cyclo = cyclophosphamide; TG = 6-thioguanine; ANS'ase = L-asparaginase; BCNU = bis β-chloroethyl nitrosourea; HU = hydroxyurea; RT = radiation therapy; ARA-C = cytosine arabinoside.
*POMP = P + V + MTX + MP.

cess in treating patients with ALL with injections of *bacillus Calmette-Guérin* (BCG) and leukemic cells following extensive cytoreductive therapy has been reported [72]. Others have been less convinced that the immunologic reactions to ALL are significant [78–80], and most attempts at immunotherapy have been disappointing [78–80].

Those patients with ALL whose leukemic cells contain identifiable determinants of T-cell and B-cell differentiation respond poorly to existing chemotherapy [9–12]. The poor response, i.e., early relapse, of T-cell ALL may be related to the extent of extramedullary disease. Patients with T-cell disease who do not have meningeal leukemia, mediastinal widening, and high blood lymphoblast counts have been reported to do as well as those with common-type ALL [63]. There is no explanation for the refractoriness of B-cell ALL to remission induction treatment.

CENTRAL NERVOUS SYSTEM (CNS) LEUKEMIA AND ITS TREATMENT

CNS leukemia with rare exceptions is synonymous with meningeal leukemia (see Chap. 29). Leukemic cells enter the leptomeninges during relapse, either by direct extension from the blood and marrow along meningeal vessels [47] or by intracranial inoculation during petechial bleeding [48,49]. If untreated, these infiltrates extend deep into the cortical sulci and along cranial and spinal nerve sheaths. Cerebrospinal fluid dynamics are altered through mechanical obstruction of normal outflow channels (e.g., arachnoid villi and nerve sheaths) so that meningeal leukemia if untreated will eventually lead to hydrocephaly and death.

CNS leukemia (CNS-L) is one of the most common forms of relapse in children, developing in over 50 percent of those who survive 2 years or longer unless specific treatment to the brain and spinal column is administered early in remission [55,81]. The cumulative incidence of CNS leukemia in adults has been estimated at 40 percent for ALL and 30 percent for acute undifferentiated leukemia [82]. Four factors may account for its high incidence: (1) a selective ability of lymphoblasts as compared to myeloblasts to enter the CNS, (2) the seeding of leukemic cells into the meninges during relapse [48], (3) the fact that most drugs effective against ALL enter the cerebrospinal fluid slowly or in concentrations insufficient to inhibit the replication of leukemic cells, and (4) the slower proliferation of leukemic cells within the spinal fluid, as compared with their counterparts in the marrow, which may require a longer drug exposure than is required for the eradication of leukemic cells elsewhere in the body [83].

The two major modes of CNS leukemia treatment are intrathecal administration of drugs and irradiation of the central nervous system. For either modality to be effective, treatment must encompass the entire brain and spinal axis, and must be given with sufficient intensity and duration for the desired effect to be achieved. Intrathecal administration of aminopterin was the first

successful therapy [84,85]. This drug was later supplanted by methotrexate, despite the demonstration that aminopterin was equally effective in primates at concentrations which caused less neurotoxicity [86]. Intrathecal cytosine arabinoside (ara-C) [87] and glucocorticoids given either systemically or intrathecally [88,90] were subsequently shown to be effective against CNS leukemia. Combination intrathecal chemotherapy for CNS leukemia using two or three of the above agents is effective and may indeed be the optimal drug therapy at present [91].

Craniospinal radiotherapy is also highly effective in the treatment of CNS leukemia. This modality has the advantages of predictable penetration into all leukemic foci, regardless of cerebrospinal fluid dynamics, and the property of killing or sterilizing leukemic cells whether or not they are undergoing cell division. While radiotherapy given in doses of 1000 rads or less is inadequate [56,92], some studies have suggested that doses of 1200 to 1800 rads may be effective particularly in good-risk cases, i.e., those less than 12 years of age and with low blast cell counts [93,94]. The amount most commonly given is 2400 rads administered at the rate of 200 rads daily [56,64]. The most serious disadvantage of radiotherapy is its effect on the marrow of the axial skeleton. Posttreatment myelosuppression is consistently greater after radiation therapy than after intrathecal drug therapy [56,95].

A combination of radiotherapy to the cranium and intrathecal chemotherapy has been recommended in order to combine the advantages of both modalities [55,56,64,96]. In patients without evidence of meningeal leukemia this approach has been as effective as craniospinal radiation [51,56,65] and has been used in a high proportion of the most successful ALL treatment regimens. Prolonged intrathecal MTX also has been successful in one large, but uncontrolled, trial [53,66]. In established CNS leukemia the most effective treatments have used intrathecal MTX to induce CNS remission, followed by either maintenance intrathecal MTX or craniospinal radiation [92,95,97].

Relatively unsuccessful attempts have been made to circumvent the need for repeated intrathecal injections. Glucocorticoids given orally and ara-C given parenterally [88,89] have produced only limited benefit, as have oral bis β-chloroethyl nitrosourea (BCNU) [85,98,99] and oral pyrimethamine (Daraprim) [100,101]. Intravenous infusions of moderately high dose MTX, with or without intrathecal drug therapy, have proved more successful, but are still under evaluation [102,104].

All methods for the treatment of active or potential CNS-L carry a significant risk, and in multimodality regimens the individual contributions of MTX, ara-C, vincristine, cranial radiation, etc., are never clear. MTX has been implicated in the production of somnolence, seizures [105,106], chemical meningitis [107,110], paraparesis [108,111,112], paraplegia [113,116], and gliosis and leukoencephalopathy [112,117–119]. Ara-C given intrathecally can also cause chemical meningitis

[87,122], chronic arachnoiditis, and rarely, more severe neurotoxicity, e.g., paraplegia [87,116] and the Guillain-Barré syndrome. The observation that radiotherapy has been given before intrathecal MTX in most patients who have developed leukoencephalopathy has led to the suggestion that irradiation may increase the diffusion of MTX from the blood into the brain substance. Abnormalities in cerebrospinal fluid drug clearance may also be related to meningeal, arachnoid, or neural sheath leukemic infiltration.

Radiotherapy alone appears to have produced aseptic meningitis, paraplegia, and leukoencephalopathy in a small percentage of children with ALL [56], and an increased frequency of severe systemic infections has been encountered when either craniospinal radiotherapy or combined cranial radiotherapy and intrathecal MTX are given. Of great concern also are the reports of cortical thinning [122], neuropsychiatric abnormalities [123], and impaired intellect [124] in children receiving radiotherapy plus intrathecal drug.

In spite of these hazards most patients with ALL should be given some form of central nervous system antileukemic treatment if they enter a complete remission. If radiotherapy is used, a total of 1200 to 2400 rads should be given to the cranium, including the optic nerves and upper cervical spine, and supplemented by intrathecal MTX with or without the addition of ara-C and hydrocortisone. Chemotherapy given in conjunction with radiotherapy should be administered in a minimum of five installments over a period of at least 3 weeks. If drugs alone are employed, monthly maintenance doses should be continued for at least 1 year. Intrathecal drug(s) should be diluted in 10 ml of spinal fluid or artificial spinal fluids (e.g., Elliot's B solution).

Since the spinal fluid volume is not proportional to body weight or surface area, a maximum of 6 mg of MTX or 25 mg of ara-C per injection should be given to infants, and no more than double that amount to older children and adults. In selected patients, drugs may be given through an intraventricular catheter attached to a semipermanent subcutaneous reservoir (e.g., an Ommaya pump). This is technically easier than repeated lumbar punctures, and provides an opportunity for giving frequent, smaller doses of drug [107,120,121].

The treatment of CNS leukemia is most successful when it is started before there is overt or symptomatic meningeal involvement. The most advantageous time to treat is early remission. If treatment is deferred until clinical signs of CNS-L develop or spinal fluid leukemic cell pleocytosis is detectable, responses are usually temporary and side effects more severe [56]. Effective central nervous system treatment has not only decreased the incidence of central nervous system relapse but in several studies has prolonged the median duration of hematologic remissions and the number of 5-year survivals [53,64].

Extramedullary leukemic infiltrates are not limited to the central nervous system. Control of meningeal leukemia has led to increasingly frequent relapses in other organs, in particular the gonads. Indeed the testes are a most frequent site of relapse in males, and this has been considered to be the reason for the poorer survival of boys than of girls with ALL [125–127]. High-dose MTX may forestall testicular relapse, although this has not been established by a controlled trial. Prophylactic irradiation is unwarranted; it has not prevented systemic relapse and leads to permanent sterility [126,127]. Early diagnosis and treatment of testicular swelling with radiation and repeat induction-consolidation drug regimens will salvage some patients and appears the preferable approach to the problem. Relapses in other organs usually reflect generalized recurrence of leukemia for which a total change of chemotherapy is indicated.

At relapse vincristine and prednisone will be effective in inducing remission in about half the patients, but these remissions will generally be short-lived. Combinations of 1-day MTX or drug combinations followed immediately by asparaginase, which is repeated in 7 to 12 days, appear to be effective in two-thirds or more of relapsed patients [128–130]. The combination of cytosine arabinoside and Adriamycin originally used in AML appears equally active, and equally toxic, in ALL. After relapse, when a second remission is induced, marrow transplantation is the most effective treatment for young patients who have an HLA-matched sibling donor [131].

Course and prognosis

The outlook for children who develop ALL has improved dramatically since 1960. The most striking results have been observed in those between 2 and 10 years of age. Such patients given a combination drug induction and maintenance regimen, which includes early central nervous system prophylactic therapy, have a median survival without evidence of disease of at least 5 years (see Table 114-6).

Despite the response in most patients, about one-half of children and most adults will either relapse or succumb to side effects of therapy [64–67]. Although some patients who relapse can be successfully retreated [65,129,133], most of them will die of the acute leukemia.

High-risk groups have been identified (see Table 114-7). These include patients diagnosed as having ALL in infancy or after puberty, those with extensive mediastinal or central nervous system disease, those whose leukemic cells have B-cell markers [8–11,36] or Ph[1] chromosomes, those with very high blast cell counts [36] and black patients [59]. Patients with T-cell, pre-B-cell, and undifferentiated acute leukemias may not do well, but whether this is due to those cellular features or to associated clinical problems is not yet clear [10,23,25,36,58,59,62,132].

Adults with ALL have a much higher probability of early relapse. The median survival of such patients is about 2 years, and only 10 to 25 percent of patients survive for 5 years.

TABLE 114-7   Features of acute lymphocytic leukemia affecting prognosis

Feature	Probability of survival
Age:	
< 2 years old	Less
2–10 years old	Greater
> 10 years old	Less
Elevated white blood cell count (or blast cell count)	Less
Histology: greater immaturity, greater nuclear atypism, L3, L2(?) cytology	Less
Race:	
Caucasian	Greater
Black	Less
Extramedullary disease:	
Mediastinum, CNS, testes	Less
B-cell characteristics	Less
T-cell characteristics	Less?

References

1. *Third National Cancer Survey: Incidence Data,* edited by S. J. Cutler and J. L. Young, Jr. *Natl. Cancer Inst. Monogr. 41*:102, 1975.
2. Cutler, S. J., Axtell, H., and Heise, H.: Ten thousand cases of leukemia: 1940–1962. *J. Natl. Cancer Inst. 39*:993, 1967.
3. Zippin, C., Cutler, S. J., Reeves, W. J., Jr., and Lum, D.: Variations in survival among patient with acute lymphocytic leukemia. *Blood 37*:59, 1971.
4. Greaves, M. F., Brown, G., Rapson, N., and Lister, T. A.: Antisera to acute lymphoblastic leukaemia cells. *Clin. Immunol. Immunopathol. 4*:67, 1975.
5. Ritz, J., Pesando, J. M., Notis-McConarty, J., Lazarus, H., and Schlossman, S. A.: A monoclonal antibody to human acute lymphoblastic leukemia antigen. *Blood 54 (Suppl. 1)*:204a, 1979 (abstract 545).
6. Janossy, G., Roberts, M., Capellaro, D., Greaves, M. F., and Francis, G.: Use of the fluorescence activated cell sorter in human leukemia, in *Immunofluorescence and Related Staining Techniques,* edited by W. Knapp, K. Holubar, and G. Wick. Elsevier–North Holland, 1978, Amsterdam, p. 111.
7. Sen, L., and Borella, L.: Clinical importance of lymphoblasts with T markers in childhood acute leukemia. *N. Engl. J. Med. 292*:828, 1975.
8. Catovsky, D., Goldman, S. M., Okos, A., Frisch, B., and Galton, D. A. G.: T-lymphoblastic leukaemia: A distinct variant of acute leukemia. *Br. Med. J. 2*:o42, 1974.
9. Kersey, J. H., Sabad, A., Gajl-Peczalska, K., Hallgren, H. M., Yunis, E., and Nesbit, M.: Acute lymphoblastic cells with T (thymus derived) lymphocyte markers. *Science 182*:1355, 1973.
10. Falletta, J. M., Mukhopadhyay, N., Starling, K. A., and Fernbach, D. J.: Leukemic blasts with membrane characteristics of either T or B cells.
11. Belpomme, D., et al.: T and B lymphocyte markers on the neoplastic cells of 20 patients with acute and 10 with chronic lymphocytic leukemia. *Biomedicine 20*:109, 1974.
12. Tsukimoto, I., Wong, K. Y., and Lapkin, B. C.: Surface markers and prognostic factors in acute lymphoblastic leukemia. *N. Engl. J. Med. 294*:245, 1976.
13. Chin, A. H., Saiki, J. H., Trujillo, J. M., and Williams, R. C., Jr.: Peripheral blood T- and B-lymphocytes in patients with lymphoma and acute leukemia. *Clin. Immunol. Immunopathol. 1*:499, 1973.
14. Smith, R. W., Terry, W. D., Buell, D. N., and Sell, K. W.: An antigen marker for human thymic lymphocytes. *J. Immunol. 110*:884, 1973.
15. Seligman, M., Preud'homme, J. L., and Brouet, J. C.: B and T cell markers in human proliferative blood diseases and primary immunodeficiencies. *Transplant. Rev. 16*:83, 1973.
16. Broder, S., et al.: Characterization of a suppressor cell leukemia: Evidence for the requirement of an interaction of two cells in the development of human suppressor effector cells. *N. Engl. J. Med. 298*:66, 1978.
17. Srivastava, B. I. S., and Minowada, J.: Terminal deoxynucleotidyl transferase activity in a cell line (MOLT-4) derived from the peripheral blood of a patient with acute lymphoblastic leukemia. *Biochem. Biophys. Res. Commun. 51*:529, 1973.
18. McCaffrey, R., Harrison, T. A., Parkman, R., and Baltimore, D.: Terminal deoxynecleotidyl transferase in human leukemic cells and in human thymocytes. *N. Engl. J. Med. 292*:775, 1975.
19. Beutler, E., and Blume, K. G.: Terminal deoxynucleotidyl transferase: Biochemical properties, cellular distribution, and hematologic significance. *Prog. Hematol. 11*:47, 1979.
20. Janossy, G., Bollum, F., Bradstock, K., Rapson, N., and Greaves, M. F.: Terminal deoxynucleotidyl transferase positive cells in normal human bone marrow have the antigenic phenotype of acute lymphoblastic leukemia cells. *J. Immunol. 123*:1525, 1979.
21. Sarin, P. S., and Gallo, R. C.: Terminal deoxyribonucleotidyl transferase in chronic myelogenous leukemia. *J. Biol. Chem. 249*:8051, 1974.
22. Marks, J. M., Baltimore, D., and McCaffrey, R.: Terminal transferase as a predictor of initial responsiveness to vincristine and prednisone in blastic crisis myelogenous leukemia. *N. Engl. J. Med. 298*:812, 1978.
23. Srivastava, B. I. S., Khan, S. A., Minowada, J., Gomez, G., and Rakowski, I.: Terminal deoxynucleotidyl transferase ability in the blastic phase of chronic myelogenous leukemia. *Cancer Res. 37*:3612–3618, 1977.
24. Coleman, M. S., Hutton, J. J., De Simone, P., and Bollum, F. J.: Terminal deoxynucleotidyl transferase in human leukemia. *Proc. Natl. Acad. Sci. U.S.A. 71*:4404, 1974.
25. Srivastava, B.I.S., Khan, S. A., and Henderson, E. S.: High terminal transferase in acute myelogenous leukemia. *Cancer Res. 36*:3847, 1976.
26. Volger, L., Crist, W. M., Bockman, D. E., Pearl, E. R., Lawton, A. R., and Cooper, M. D.: Pre-B cell leukemia. A new phenotype of childhood lymphoblastic leukemia. *N. Engl. J. Med. 298*:872, 1978.
27. Gajl-Peczalska, K. J., Bloomfield, C. D., Nesbit, M. E., and Kersey, J. H.: B-cell markers on lymphoblasts in acute lymphoblastic leukemia. *Clin. Exp. Immunol. 17*:561, 1974.
28. Van't Veer, M. B., and Von den Borne, K. V.: Differences in immunological characterization of blast cells in adult and childhood acute lymphoblast leukemia, in *Proceedings of XV Congress International Society of Hematology,* Montreal, 1980 (abstract 1008).
29. Nies, B. A., Kundel, D. W., Thomas, L. B., and Freireich, E. J.: Leukopenia, bone pain, and bone necrosis in patients with acute leukemia. *Ann. Intern. Med. 62*:698, 1965.
30. Gralnick, H. R., Galton, D. A., Catovsky, D., Sultan, C., and Bennett, J. M.: Classification of acute leukemia. *Ann. Intern. Med. 87*:740, 1977.
31. Peterson, H. S.: Nuclear aryl sulfatase activity in leukaemia and some other haematological disorders. *Scand. J. Haematol. 10*:35, 1973.
32. Catovsky, O., Greaves, M. F., Pain, C., Cherchi, M., Janossy, G., and Kay, H. E. M.: Acid-phosphatase reaction in acute lymphoblastic leukaemia. *Lancet 1*:749, 1978.
33. Whang-Peng, J., Freireich, E. J., Oppenheim, J. J., Frei, E., III, and Tjio, J. H.: Acute lymphocytic leukemia. Cytogenetic studies in 45 patients. *J. Natl. Cancer Inst. 42*:881, 1969.
34. Sandberg, A. A., Ishihara, T., Kikuchi, Y., and Crosswhite, L. H.: Chromosome differences among the acute leukemias. *Ann. N.Y. Acad. Sci. 113*:663, 1974.
35. Rowley, J. D.: Chromosome abnormalities in human leukemia. *Ann. Rev. Genet. 14*:17, 1980.
36. Bloomfield, D. C., and Gajl-Peczalska, K. J.: The clinical relevance of lymphocyte surface markers in leukemia and lymphoma. *Curr. Top. Hematol. 3*:175, 1980.
37. Gunz, F., and Baikie, A. G.: *Leukemia,* 3d ed. Grune & Stratton, New York, 1974, p. 524.

38. Brakman, P., Snyder, J., Henderson, E. S., and Astrup, T.: Blood coagulation and fibrinolysis in acute leukemia. *Br. J. Haematol.* 18:135, 1970.
39. Kornberg, A., and Pollack, A.: Serum lactic dehydrogenase (LDH) levels in acute leukemia: Marked elevations in lymphoblastic leukemia. *Blood* 56:351, 1980.
40. Weinstein, H. W., Vance, Z. B., Jaffe, N., Buell, D., Cassady, J. R., and Nathan, D. G.: Improved prognosis for patients with mediastinal lymphoblastic lymphoma. *Blood* 53:687, 1979.
41. Henderson, E. S.: Treatment of acute leukemia. *Semin. Hematol.* 6:271, 1969.
42. Karon, M., et al.: The role of vincristine in the treatment of childhood leukemia. *Clin. Pharmacol. Ther.* 7:332, 1966.
43. Boiron, M., et al.: Daunorubicin in the treatment of acute myelocytic leukaemia. *Lancet* 1:330, 1969.
44. Freireich, E. J., Henderson, E. S., Karon, M. R., and Frei, E., III: The treatment of acute leukemia considered with respect to cell population kinetics, in *The Proliferation and Spread of Neoplastic Cells* (editors anonymous). Williams & Wilkins, Baltimore, 1968, p. 441.
45. Pinkel, D., Simone, J., Hustu, H. O., and Aur, R. J. A.: Nine years experience with "total therapy" of childhood acute lymphocytic leukemia. *Pediatrics* 50:246, 1972.
46. Goldin, A., Sandberg, J. S., Henderson, E. S., Newman, J. W., Frei, E., III, and Holland, J. F.: The therapy of human and animal acute leukemia. *Cancer Chemother. Rep.* 55:309, 1971.
47. Thomas, L. B.: Pathology of leukemia in the brain and meninges: Postmortem studies of patients with acute leukemia and of mice given inoculation of L1210 leukemia. *Cancer Res.* 25:1555, 1965.
48. Price, R. A., and Johnson, W. W.: The central nervous system in childhood leukemia. I. The arachnoid. *Cancer* 31:520, 1973.
49. West, R. J., Graham-Pole, J., Hardisty, R. M., and Pike, M. C.: Factors in pathogenesis of central nervous system leukemia. *Br. Med. J.* 3:311, 1972.
50. Bernard, J., and Boiron, M.: Current status: Treatment of acute leukemia. *Semin. Hematol.* 7:427, 1970.
51. Pinkel, D.: Treatment of childhood acute lymphocytic leukemia, in *Modern Trends in Human Leukemia III*, edited by R. Neth, R. C. Gallo, P. H. Hofschneider, and K. Mannweiler. Springer, Berlin, 1979, p. 31.
52. Sinks, L. F.: Impact of controlled clinical trials in progress toward the cure of leukemia in children, in *Cancer in Childhood*, edited by J. O. Godden. Ontario Cancer Treatment and Research Foundation, Toronto, 1973, p. 216.
53. Hagbin, M., Tan, C. T., Clarkson, B. D., Mikie, V., Burchenal, J. H., and Murphy, M. L.: Treatment of acute lymphoblastic leukemia in children with "prophylactic" intrathecal methotrexate and intensive chemotherapy. *Cancer Res.* 35:807, 1975.
54. Holland, J. F., and Glidewell, O.: An oncologist's reply: Survival expectancy in acute lymphocytic leukemia. *N. Engl. J. Med.* 287:769, 1972.
55. Medical Research Council: Treatment of acute lymphoblastic leukemia: Effect of "prophylactic" therapy against central nervous system leukemia. *Br. Med. J.* 2:381, 1973.
56. Hustu, H. O., Aur, R. J. A., Verzosa, M. S., Simone, J. V., and Pinkel, D.: Prevention of central nervous system leukemia by irradiation. *Cancer* 32:585, 1973.
57. Green, D. M., et al.: A comparison of three methods of central nervous system prophylaxis in childhood acute lymphoblastic leukemia. *Lancet* 1:1398, 1980.
58. Bernard, J., Weil, M., and Jacquillat, C.: Prognostic factors in human acute leukemia. *Adv. Biosci.* 14:97, 1975.
59. Simone, J. V.: Prognostic factors in childhood acute lymphocytic leukemia. *Adv. Biosci.* 14:27, 1975.
60. George, S. L., et al.: Factors influencing survival in pediatric acute leukemia. *Cancer* 32:1542, 1973.
61. Karon, M., Weiner, J. M., and Meshnik, R.: The interaction of disease factors, host variability, and treatment in acute lymphocytic leukemia. *Adv. Biosci.* 14:3, 1975.
62. Miller, D. R.: Acute lymphoblastic leukemia. *Pediatr. Clin. North Am.* 21:269, 1980.
63. Hann, H. W. L., Lustbader, E. D., Evans, A. E., Toledano, S. R., Lillia, P. D., and Jasko, L. D.: Lack of influence of T-cell marker and

64. Holland, J. F., and Glidewell, O.: Chemotherapy of acute lymphocytic leukemia of childhood. *Cancer* 30:1480, 1972.
65. Simone, J., Aur, R. J. A., Hustu, H. O., Verzosa, M. S., and Pinkel, D.: Three to five years after cessation of therapy in children with leukemia. *Cancer* 42:839, 1978.
66. Schauer, P., et al.: The treatment of acute lymphoblastic leukemia in adults: Results of the L-10/L-10M protocol. *Proc. AACR/ASCO* 21:180, 1980 (abstract 719).
67. Henderson, E. S., et al.: Combined chemotherapy and radiotherapy for acute lymphocytic leukemia in adults: Results of CALGB protocol 7113. *Leukemia Res.* 3:395, 1979.
68. Gottlieb, A. J., and Weinberg, V.: Efficacy of daunorubicin induction therapy of adult acute lymphocytic leukemia (ALL). A controlled phase II study. *Blood* 50 (Suppl. 1):188a, 1979 (abstract 496).
69. Lister, T. A., et al.: Combination chemotherapy for acute lymphoblastic leukaemia in adults. *Br. Med. J.* 1:199, 1978.
70. Early, A. P., Preisler, H. D., Gottlieb, A. J., and Lachant, N. A.: Treatment of refractory adult acute lymphocytic leukemia with anthracycline antibiotic and cytosine arabinoside. *Br. J. Haematol.*, 48:369, 1981.
71. Krivit, W., Gilchrist, G., and Beatty, E. C., Jr.: The need for chemotherapy after prolonged complete remission in acute leukemia of childhood. *J. Pediatr.* 76:138, 1970.
72. Mathe, G., et al.: Methods and strategy for the treatment of acute lymphoblastic leukemia. *Recent Results Cancer Res.* 30:109, 1970.
73. Frei, E., III, and Freireich, E. J.: Progress and perspectives in the chemotherapy of acute leukemias. *Adv. Chemother.* 2:269, 1965.
74. Kung, F. H., Nyhan, W. L., and Cuttner, J.: Effect of periodic reinforcement therapy with vincristine or daunorubicin and prednisone on 6-mercaptopurine maintained remission in children with recurrent acute lymphoblastic leukemia. *Cancer*, 1981, in press.
75. Leventhal, B. G.: New looks in leukemia. *Cancer* 35:1015, 1975.
76. Greaves, M. F., Brown, G., Rapson, N. T., and Lister, T. A.: Antisera to acute lymphoblastic leukemia cells. *Clin. Immunol. Immunopathol.* 4:67, 1975.
77. Gutterman, J. V., et al.: Immunoglobulin on tumor cells and tumor-induced lymphocyte blastogenesis in human acute leukemia. *N. Engl. J. Med.* 288:169, 1973.
78. Medical Research Council: Treatment of acute lymphoblastic leukemia: Comparison of immunotherapy (BCG), intermittent methotrexate, and no therapy after a five-month intensive cytotoxic regimen (Concord trial). *Br. Med. J.* 3:189, 1971.
79. Heyn, R., et al.: BCG in the treatment of acute lymphocytic leukemia (ALL). *Proc. AACR/ASCO* 14:45, 1973 (abstract 180).
80. Leventhal, B. G., LePourhiet, A., Halterman, R. H., Henderson, E. S., and Herberman, R. B.: Immunotherapy in previously treated acute lymphocytic leukemia. *Natl. Cancer Inst. Monogr.* 39:177, 1973.
81. Evans, A. E., Gilbert, E. J., and Zandstra, R.: The increasing incidence of central nervous system leukemia in children. *Cancer* 26:404, 1970.
82. Wolk, R. W., Masse, S. R., Conklin, R., and Freireich, E. J.: The incidence of central nervous system leukemia in adults with acute leukemia. *Cancer* 33:863, 1974.
83. Kuo, A. H.-M., Yataganas, X., Galicich, Y. Y., Fried, J., and Clarkson, B. D.: Proliferative kinetics of central nervous system leukemia. *Cancer* 36:232, 1975.
84. Sansone, G.: Pathomorphosis of acute infantile leukemia treated with modern therapeutic agents: "Meningo leukemia" and "Frohlich's obesity," *Ann. Pediatr.* 183:33, 1954.
85. Nies, B. A., Thomas, L. B., and Freireich, E. J.: Meningeal leukemia: A follow-up study. *Cancer* 18:546, 1965.
86. Rieselbach, R. E., Morse, E. E., Rall, D. P., Frei, E., III, and Freireich, E. J.: Treatment of meningeal leukemia with intrathecal Aminopterin. *Cancer Chemother. Rep.* 16:191, 1962.
87. Band, P. R., Holland, J. F., Bernard, J., Weil, M., Walker, M., and Rall, D.: Treatment of central nervous system leukemia with intrathecal cytosine arabinoside. *Cancer* 32:746, 1973.
88. Mitus, A.: Dexamethasone: Its effectiveness in the treatment of

importance of mediastinal mass on the prognosis of acute lymphocytic leukemia of childhood. *J. Natl. Cancer Inst.* 66:285, 1981.

acute symptoms of meningeal leukemia. *Am. J. Dis. Child. 117:*307, 1969.

89. Shaw, R. K., Moore, E. W., Freireich, E. J., and Thomas, L. G.: Meningeal leukemia: A syndrome resulting from increased intracranial pressure in patients with acute leukemia. *Neurology (Minneap.) 10:*823, 1960.

90. Sullivan, M. P.: Intracranial complications of leukemia in children. *Pediatrics 20:*757, 1957.

91. Sullivan, M. P., Moon, T. F., Trueworthy, R., Vietti, T. S., Humphrey, G. B., and Komp, D.: Combination intrathecal (IT) therapy for meningeal leukemia: Two vs. three drugs. *Blood 50:*471, 1977.

92. Sullivan, M. P., Vietti, T. J., Fernbach, D. J., Griffith, K. M., Haddy, T. B., and Watkins, W. L.: Clinical investigations in the treatment of meningeal leukemia: Radiation therapy regimens vs. conventional intrathecal methotrexate. *Blood 34:*301, 1969.

93. Kim, T., Nesbit, M. E., D'Angio, G. D., and Levitt, S.: The role of central nervous system irradiation in children with acute lymphoblastic leukemia. *Radiology 104:*635, 1972.

94. Bleyer, W. A.: Current status of intrathecal chemotherapy for human meningeal neoplasms. *Natl. Cancer Inst. Monogr. 46:*171, 1977.

95. Sullivan, M. P., Humphrey, G. B., Vietti, T. J., Haggard, M. E., and Lee, E.: Superiority of conventional intrathecal methotrexate therapy, unmaintained, or radiotherapy (2000–2500 rads tumor dose) in treatment for meningeal leukemia. *Cancer 35:*1066, 1975.

96. Duttera, M. J., Bleyer, W. A., Pomeroy, T. C., Leventhal, C. M., and Leventhal, B.: Irradiation, methotrexate toxicity, and the treatment of meningeal leukemia. *Lancet 2:*703, 1973.

97. Willoughby, M. L. N.: Treatment of overt leukemia in children: Results of the second MRC meningeal leukemia trial. *Br. Med. J. 1:*864, 1976.

98. Iriarte, P. V., Hananian, J., and Cortner, J. A.: Central nervous system leukemia and solid tumors of childhood: treatment with 1,(2-chloroethyl)-1-nitrosourea (BCNU). *Cancer 19:*1187, 1966.

99. Sullivan, M. P., Vietti, T. J., Haggard, M. E., Donaldson, M. H., Kroll, M. M., and Gehan, E. A.: Remission maintenance therapy for meningeal leukemia: Intrathecal methotrexate vs. intravenous bisnitrosourea. *Blood 38:*680, 1971.

100. Geils, G. P., Scott, C. W., Baugh, C. M., and Butterworth, C. E.: Treatment of meningeal leukemia with pyrimethamine. *Blood 38:*191, 1971.

101. Wiernik, P., and Schimpff, S. C.: Daunorubicin (D) alone vs. daunorubicin, pyrimethamine, cytosine arabinoside, and thioguanine (DDTA) for the treatment of acute non-lymphocytic leukemia (ANLL). *Proc. AACR/ASCO 16:*236, 1975.

102. Wang, J. J., Freeman, A. I., and Sinks, L. F.: Treatment of acute lymphocytic leukemia using high dose methotrexate. *Cancer Res. 36:*1441, 1976.

103. Shapiro, W., Young, D. F., and Mehta, B. M.: Methotrexate: Distribution in cerebrospinal fluid after intravenous, ventricular, and lumbar injections. *N. Engl. J. Med. 293:*161, 1975.

104. Freeman, A. I., Wang, J. J., and Sinks, L. F.: Intermediate dose MTX (IDM) in acute lymphocytic leukemia (ALL), in *Modern Trends in Leukemia III,* edited by R. Neth, R. C. Gallo, P. H. Hofschneider, and K. Mannweiler. Springer, Berlin, 1979, p. 115.

105. Abelson, H. T., Beardsley, G. P., and Henderson, J. C.: Intraventricular methotrexate therapy for central nervous system tumors. *Proc. AACR/ASCO 21:*341, 1980.

106. Yap, H. Y., Blumen, S., Chein, G. R., and Yap, B. S.: High-dose methotrexate for advanced breast cancer. *Cancer Treat. Rep. 63:*757, 1979.

107. Rubin, R. C., Ommaya, A. K., Henderson, E. S., Bering, E. A., and Rall, D. P.: Cerebrospinal fluid perfusion therapy for the treatment of central nervous system neoplasms. *Neurology (Minneap.) 16:*680, 1966.

108. Baum, E. S., Koch, H. F., Corby, D. G., and Plunket, D. C.: Intrathecal methotrexate. *Lancet 1:*649, 1971.

109. Naiman, J. L., Rupprecht, L. M., Tanyeri, G., and Philippedis, P.: Intrathecal methotrexate. *Lancet 1:*571, 1970.

110. Rosner, F., Lee, S. L., Kagen, M., and Morrison, A. N.: Intrathecal methotrexate. *Lancet 1:*249, 1970.

111. Pasquinicci, G., Pardini, R., and Fedi, F.: Intrathecal methotrexate. *Lancet 1:*309, 1970.

112. Hendin, B., DeVino, D. C., Torack, R., Lell, M. E., Ragab, A. H., and Vietti, T. J.: Parenchymatous degeneration of the central nervous system in childhood leukemia. *Cancer 33:*468, 1974.

113. Back, E. H.: Death after intrathecal methotrexate. *Lancet 2:*1005, 1969.

114. Bagshawe, K. D., Magrath, I. T., and Golding, P. R.: Intrathecal methotrexate. *Lancet 2:*1258, 1969.

115. Luddy, R. E., and Gilman, P. A.: Paraplegia following intrathecal methotrexate *J. Pediatr. 83:*988, 1973.

116. Saiki, J. H., Thompson, S., Smith, F., and Atkinson, R.: Paraplegia following intrathecal chemotherapy. *Cancer 29:*370, 1972.

117. Kay, H. E. M., et al.: Severe neurological damage associated with methotrexate therapy. *Lancet 2:*542, 1971.

118. McIntosh, S., and Aspnes, G. T.: Encephalopathy following CNS prophylaxis in childhood lymphoblastic leukemia. *Pediatrics 52:*612, 1973.

119. Shapiro, W. R., Chernik, N. L., and Posner, J. B.: Necrotizing encephalopathy following intraventricular instillation of methotrexate. *Arch. Neurol. 28:*96, 1973.

120. Bleyer, W. A., Drake, J. C., and Chabner, B. A.: Neurotoxicity and elevated cerebrospinal-fluid methotrexate concentration in meningeal leukemia. *N. Engl. J. Med. 289:*770, 1973.

121. Spiers, A. S. D., and Booth, A. E.: Reservoirs for intraventricular chemotherapy. *Lancet 1:*1263, 1973.

122. Peylan-Ramu, N., Poplack, D. G., Pizzo, P. A., Adornato, B. T., and DiChiro, G.: Abnormal CT scans of the brain in asymptomatic children with acute lymphocytic leukemia after prophylactic treatment of the central nervous system with radiation and intrathecal chemotherapy. *N. Engl. J. Med. 298:*815, 1978.

123. Obetz, S. W., et al.: Neuropsychological follow-up study of children with acute lymphocytic leukemia. A preliminary report. *Am. J. Pediat. Hematol. Oncol. 1:*207, 1979.

124. Eiser, C.: Intellectual abilities among survivors of childhood leukemia as a function of CNS irradiation. *Arch. Dis. Childh. 53:*391, 1978.

125. Finkelstein, J. Z., Dyment, P. G., and Hammond, G. D.: Leukemia infiltration of the testes during bone marrow remission. *Pediatrics 43:*1042, 1969.

126. Kay, H. E. M.: Testicular disease in acute lymphoblastic leukemia, in *Proceedings of the XVIIIth Congress of the International Society of Hematology,* Montreal, 1980, p. 32 (abstract 122).

127. Nesbit, M., Ortega, J., Donaldson, M., Hittle, R., Hammond, D., and Weiner, J.: Prevention of testicular relapse by prophylactic irradiation (XRT). *Proc. AACR/ASCO 18:*317, 1977.

128. Capizzi, R. L.: Improvement in the therapeutic index of methotrexate (SC-740) by l-asparaginase (NSC 104229). *Cancer Chemother. Rep. 6:*37, 1975.

129. Reaman, G., Wesley R., Scialla, S., and Poplack, D.: Long-term second remissions in acute lymphoblastic leukemia (ALL) following relapse during initial maintenance therapy. *Proc. AACR/ASCO 21:*435, 1980 (abstract 467).

130. Harris, R. E., McCallister, J. A., Provisor, D. S., Weetman, R. M., and Baechner, R. L.: Methotrexate/asparaginase combination chemotherapy for patients with acute leukemia in relapse: A study of 36 children.

131. Johnson, F. L., et al.: A comparison of marrow transplantation with chemotherapy for children with acute lymphoblastic leukemia in second or subsequent remission. *N. Engl. J. Med. 305:*846, 1981.

132. Keating, M. J., et al.: Factors related to length of complete remission in adult acute leukemia. *Cancer 45:*2017, 1980.

133. Leventhal, B. G., Levine, A. A., Graw, R. G., Jr., Simon, R., Freireich, E. J., and Henderson, E. S.: Long-term second remissions in acute lymphatic leukemia. *Cancer 35:*1136, 1975.

CHAPTER 115

Chronic lymphocytic leukemia

R. WAYNE RUNDLES

Definitions and history

Chronic lymphocytic leukemia (CLL) is the commonest type of leukemia seen in Western countries. It is a generalized malignancy of the lymphoid tissues affecting the small lymphocytes [1]. The life-span of lymphocytes in CLL is long, and their immunologic function is frequently defective; thus, the disorder has been described as an "accumulative disease of immunologically incompetent lymphocytes" [2]. As the disease progresses, lymphocytes accumulate in the marrow, spleen, liver, superficial and deep lymph nodes, and along the walls of the respiratory and gastrointestinal tracts. The major signs of the disease are enlarged lymph nodes, splenomegaly, and abnormal lymphocytes in the blood. Hypogammaglobulinemia usually develops with advanced disease.

The identification of surface membrane immunoglobulin (SmIg) on the abnormal cells or in their cytoplasm (cIg) identifies them as B lymphocytes in about 95 percent of cases. The clonal nature of CLL, and evidence of defective or arrested cell maturation, is shown by the restriction in Ig class, IgG subclass, and light-chain type. The predominant cells ordinarily have only one type of light chain, κ or λ. In most instances, IgM, IgD, IgM combined with IgD, or less frequently IgG and IgA membrane receptors occur with the single κ or λ light chain [3]. The basic defect in CLL apparently develops during a pre-B-cell stage in the differentiation of normal B lymphocytes.

In 2 to 5 percent of patients the cells have characteristics of T lymphocytes. Lymphocyte morphology, T- or B-cell phenotyping, and different clinical expressions permit the identification of subgroups of lymphocytic leukemias, which have B-lymphocyte phenotypes or T-lymphocyte phenotypes (Table 115-1). B-cell and "lymphosarcoma cell" CLL are by far the most common entities. It is important to recognize, however, that most clinical, pathologic, therapeutic, and end-result compilations pertaining to CLL in the past have included variable numbers of the other related diseases.

After leukemia was recognized as a new disease entity in 1845, Virchow soon identified a second type that differed from the original "splenic" leukemia in that lymph nodes were larger, the spleen smaller, and the color of the blood more normal [4]. The latter contained, nevertheless, a large number of small, colorless, nongranular globules similar to those which could be scraped from the lymph nodes. Virchow thought this type of leukemia was primarily a disease related to the lymph nodes rather than to the spleen.

In 1893, Kundrat introduced the term *lymphosarcoma* to describe a chronic disease which affected lymph nodes [5]. The node involvement in lymphosarcoma was often localized and locally invasive, and a leukemic blood picture was often absent. In 1903, Türk reviewed nosologic problems in reference to the *lymphomatoses*, called attention to the similarity of lymphosarcoma and CLL, and thought there might be transitions between the two entities [6]. In the following year Sternberg introduced the term *leukosarcoma*, which was used in confusing ways for more than a generation before it was largely abandoned [7].

The first comprehensive description of CLL was that by Minot and Isaacs in 1924 [8]. The clinical and hematologic features relating to prognosis, overall survival, and the effects of x-ray and radium therapy were documented in detail. The benefits from radiation therapy were far less impressive in CLL than in chronic myelogenous leukemia. Enlargement of the superficial nodes and spleen could be controlled, but anemia, thrombocytopenia, and/or neutropenia resulting from the disease itself or from radiation therapy became the major clinical problems. Later, when marrow examinations became commonplace, observers found that marrow infiltration by abnormal lymphocytes was a frequent occurrence in the course of the disease [9]. Cytopenias associated with marrow replacement continued to be a major complication, difficult to prevent or treat effectively even after ^{32}P was introduced as a therapeutic agent in 1936 [10,11]. Therapeutic prospects improved somewhat with the introduction of the orally administered nitrogen mustard derivatives in 1949 and 1954 [12–15] and with the use of adrenocorticotropic hormone (ACTH) and glucocorticoids after 1950. The development of the Coombs' antiglobulin test in 1945 facilitated the recognition of autoantibodies to red cells in CLL [16] and when isotopic methods for measuring red cell life-span became available, investigators found that erythrocyte survival was reduced in anemic patients with CLL [17–20].

Etiology and pathogenesis

In contrast to the situation in chronic myelogenous leukemia, ionizing radiation plays no part in the etiology of CLL. Genetic and age factors, the male sex predominance, and inherited or acquired immunologic defects, which predispose some individuals to disease produced by leukemogenic agents, appear to be most important.

FAMILIAL PATTERNS
The possibility that genetic factors might play a significant role in the etiology of leukemia in man was suggested over a hundred years ago by Biermer and

TABLE 115-1   Chronic lymphocytic leukemia (CLL), subgroups, and related lymphoproliferative diseases

Disease	Outstanding clinical and hematologic features; cell habitat, origin (?); histopathology	Cell markers	Biochemical features
1. B-cell chronic lymphocytic leukemia (B-CLL)	Lymphocytosis with small cells, uniform in size, condensed nuclei, originating or proliferating in bone marrow, spleen, and medullary cords of lymph nodes. *Node histology:* WDLL-D or WDLL-N.	SIg + EAC (complement, C3d) +, mouse red cell rosettes (MR) ++, sheep red cell rosettes − (E–rosettes), antithymus globulin (ATG) −, Ig "capping" poor, Ia antigen–like ±, Fc portion of IgG ±.	Adenosine deaminase (ADA) + to +++ 5'-Nucleotidase (5'N) 0 to +++ Purine nucleoside phosphorylase (PNP) + to ++ Terminal deoxynucleotidyl transferase (TdT) 0 Hypogammaglobulinemia, occasional monoclonal IgG, IgA, or IgM components
2. T-cell chronic lymphocytic leukemia of adults (T-CLL)	Erythroderma, infiltration of skin and deep paracortex of lymph nodes with large cells having convoluted nuclei; hepatosplenomegaly; early neurologic involvement; commonest type of CLL in Japanese. Poor response to therapy.	SIg −, EAC −, E–rosettes +, ATG + (one subset); Ia antigen–like −; mature T-cell subsets.	TdT 0 Serum Ig normal
3. Cutaneous T-cell lymphomas (Sézary's syndrome)	Lymphocytic skin infiltration, with systemic involvement in late stages. Pleomorphic lymphocytes with lobulated, convoluted nuclei. Poor response to therapy.	SIg −, EAC −, E–rosettes +, ATG + (helper subset). Mature T-cell subset antigens +.	ADA ++ to +++ 5'-N + to ++ PNP + TdT 0 to ±
4. "Lymphosarcoma cell" leukemia (LS-CLL) (see "Clinical Features")	Lymphocytosis, large cells with cleaved or folded nuclei and prominent nucleoli, follicle center origin. *Node histology:* PDLL-N or-D	SIg ++ to +++, EAC + or −, E–rosettes −, MR ±, Fc −, Ig "capping" ++.	Not well differentiated from B–CLL. TdT ± Serum proteins normal
5. Prolymphocytic leukemia	Massive splenomegaly, lymph nodes ± , extreme lymphocytosis with large cells. Poor response to therapy.	SIg +++ to ++++, MR + EAC +. Increased T lymphocytes. Ia antigen–like +, T-cell variants rare.	
6. "Hairy cell" leukemia (HCL)	Pancytopenia, splenomegaly, reticulin-fibrosis of marrow. Hairy cells with actively motile villi, avid phagocytosis.	SIg (monoclonal) +, E–rosettes −, Fc +. (Rare T-cell variants.)	Cytoplasmic acid phosphatase Isoenzyme 5 resistant to tartrate inhibition
7. Macroglobulinemia of Waldenström	Moderate hepatosplenomegaly and lymph node enlargement; hyperviscosity; anemia, marrow replacement with lymphoplasma cells. Variable number of abnormal lymphocytes in circulating blood.	Cytoplasmic and/or surface IgM present, plus SIgG or SIgA receptors.	Homogeneous IgM components present in serum; IgG and IgA normal

NOTES: ADA = adenosine deaminase; ATG = antithymus globulin; EAC = complement, C3d; E-rosettes = sheep red cell rosettes; Fc = receptors for Fc of IgG; Ig = immunoglobulin; MR = mouse red cell rosettes; PNP =purine nucleoside phosphorylase; 5'-N = 5'-nucleotidase; SIg = surface immunoglobulin; TdT = terminal deoxynucleotidyl transferase; WDLL-D or -N = well-differentiated lymphocytic lymphoma (D = diffuse, N = nodular); PDLL-D or -N = poorly differentiated lymphocytic lymphoma (D = diffuse, N = nodular).

others, who reported the occurrence of multiple instances of leukemia in some families. Perennial interest continued but increased sharply in 1929, when Dameshek and collaborators reported twin brothers, 56 years of age, who died within 68 days of each other of CLL. Twenty-five years later a son of one of the twins developed CLL when he was 53 years of age, and, although no consanguinity was involved, it was noted that the husband of an older sister died of CLL, too [21].

Many other families with multiple cases of CLL have been described [22–30]. Videbaek in 1947 [24] reviewed 26 instances of familial leukemia, and added 17 additional cases from 14 families. The incidence of leukemia in this group of relatives was at least 8.1 percent, a striking increase in comparison with that in a control group in whom the incidence was only 0.5 percent. By 1964, over 100 cases of familial leukemia had been reported [1]. Leukemia occurring in close relatives was usually CLL, acute leukemia, or less often other lymphoproliferative diseases [25–29].

An important study of hereditary factors in leukemia in New Zealand focused on CLL [30]. Fifty-four patients were found to have CLL in the South Island of New Zealand between 1962 and 1966. The families of this group of patients included 578 first-degree relatives, children, siblings, parents, and cousins. Among the siblings of the patients with CLL there had been seven deaths from leukemia, six of them in brothers, as compared with an expectation of 0.56. In addition there were two deaths from myelomatosis and one from "lymphosarcoma." Two living sisters had lymphoma, too, and one living son was known to have leukemia. In brothers the familial incidence of lymphocytic leukemia was 8.8 percent. There were no specific abnormalities in lymphocyte morphology, blood counts, distribution of blood groups, and haptoglobin or transferrin types found among the healthy relatives of patients with CLL [30].

These findings were extended in a survey in Australia which included 909 patients with various types of leukemia [31]. Among 41,807 relatives, 72 had leukemia. The incidence of the disease in first-degree relatives was nearly three times that in the general population, and even in distant relatives it was increased by a factor of 2.3. The increased incidence of leukemia in these families was due to CLL and to acute leukemia. There was no definite increase in the familial incidence of chronic myelogenous leukemia [31] or of other malignancies.

In studies of familial leukemia, CLL has been the type most frequently involved. While it tends to occur in closely related individuals, there is no clear-cut pattern of inheritance. Consanguinity does not appear to be a factor.

In a Southern United States family two brothers were found to have hairy cell leukemia and CLL when they were 45 and 48 years old, respectively [32]. Their nephew developed lymphocytic lymphoma at the age of 25 years. The father of the two brothers died of chronic myelogenous leukemia. Several members of the family had a significantly reduced lymphocyte response to phytohemagglutinin and concanavalin A. Antibody titers to eight viral test antigens and delayed cutaneous hypersensitivity reactions were impaired.

CHROMOSOME ABNORMALITIES

Characteristic chromosome abnormalities have not been found in CLL, possibly because of technical difficulties [33–36]. In direct marrow preparations there are very few spontaneously dividing lymphocytes. In blood cultures, B-CLL lymphocytes do not respond well to commonly used mitogens, which stimulate T cells more or less selectively. Dividing cells may, thus, represent nonneoplastic T cells which proliferate better than neoplastic B cells. The 14q+ chromosome translocation, which seems to be the chromosome abnormality most frequently encountered in the lymphoproliferative diseases, has been observed in a few instances [33,35,36]. With the use of polyclonal B-cell mitogen stimulation, e.g., Epstein-Barr virus or lipopolysaccharide from *Escherichia coli*, other nonrandom chromosome abnormalities have been reported as well as trisomy for chromosome 12. The latter was found in 5 of 11 patients [34]. This trisomy may be present in as many as half of all patients with CLL and thus may represent a fundamental abnormality in these patients.

A chromosome anomaly known as the Christchurch chromosome (Ch¹) was found to be present in cultured skin cells and in lymphocytes of several members of a New Zealand family in which lymphoproliferative disease had occurred in two generations. Three siblings developed CLL at ages 56, 67, and 79 years, respectively, but some carriers of the Ch¹ chromosome had no evidence of hematologic disease. The Ch¹ chromosome is an autosome from which the short arm is missing. The Ch¹ chromosome has no general significance in the etiology of CLL.

IMMUNOLOGIC ABNORMALITIES

The progeny of the abnormal stem cells responsible for the genesis of CLL are immunoglobulin-producing B lymphocytes. In CLL these cells appear to have a long life, little proliferative capacity, and tend to be immunologically dysfunctional. The restriction in Ig class and subclass suggests the existence of defective or arrested B-cell maturation, or possibly the existence of lymphocyte subsets which might have an increased vulnerability to some leukemogenic stimuli [40–56].

Hypogammaglobulinemia involving all immunoglobulin classes occurs in 40 to 50 percent of patients with CLL [57]. It may be present in individuals who have early asymptomatic disease or may be observed to develop in patients as disease advances [58–65]. Anomalous monoclonal proteins occur in the sera of 3 to 5 percent of patients with CLL also, particularly in those with subleukemia forms of the disease [58,65–69]. "Mu chain disease" [70–72] and the presence of intracellular crystalline inclusions staining specifically for IgM [73] have been described in a few patients.

In families in which more than one member has had CLL or a related lymphoproliferative disease, some apparently healthy individuals have immunoglobulin abnormalities and/or defective in vitro lymphocyte transformation in response to phytohemagglutinin (PHA) stimulation [28,74]. In the New Zealand families in which there was at least one member with CLL, abnormally high and low concentrations of γ globulin were found sporadically [30]. In a West Virginia family in which 3 of 12 children had CLL, immunoglobulin deficiencies were found in three nonleukemic siblings, and in one of the latter lymphocyte transformation was impaired also [74]. Qualitative and quantitative abnormalities of serum proteins, connective tissue–vascular diseases, and autoimmunity or other abnormal immune responses have been observed in the families of patients with lymphocytic malignancies [28,75–84]. Abnormalities in the regulation of antibody and cellular immune responses thus appear to be an inherited trait in the families that have an increased incidence of lymphocytic malignancies.

An interaction of hereditary and environmental factors may be required to produce leukemia. An example is provided by a family in which six individuals in three generations developed acute myelogenous leukemia and two others hemopoietic malignancies [85]. In a sibship of six children, the oldest two died of acute leukemia before the fourth child developed the disease. The latter patient, a girl 11 years old, three of her siblings, and two of her cousins were found to have low serum IgA levels.

Skin fibroblasts were tested for susceptibility to transformation by the simian virus SV40, an agent known to produce tumors in several animal species and to increase the frequency of fibroblast transformation in cultures from patients with Fanconi's anemia and Down's syndrome [85]. Five to fifty times the expected number of transformed colonies were found in cells cultured from the patient, her mother, and a sister. The transformation frequency of cells obtained from the father and two brothers was normal. Immunoglobulin deficiencies were present in some individuals in the family, but this trait, like that of lymphocyte transformation in response to PHA stimulation, did not parallel the increased susceptibility to oncogenic virus transformation [85].

Susceptibility to infection became the major cause of morbidity and mortality in patients with CLL after the oral mustard compounds and glucocorticoids became available to control the excessive proliferation accumulation of lymphocytes. Some degree of hypogammaglobulinemia and/or neutropenia was present in most patients, but the liability to infection in most instances appeared to be an acquired trait and not congenital.

The mitotic response of CLL lymphocytes to PHA and other antigens in vitro is greatly reduced, absent, or delayed, as is their capacity to synthesize γ globulin [86–95]. The important factor predisposing to infections is the immunologic deficiency characteristic of the disease.

The immunologic abnormalities in CLL resemble in some ways those of immunodeficiency diseases, in which there is also a high incidence of lymphocytic and other malignancies [96–103]. The relationship of the Epstein-Barr virus (EBV) to Burkitt's lymphoma and to the self-limited lymphocytic proliferation in infectious mononucleosis has led to speculation that an immunologic defect might have rendered individuals who develop CLL susceptible to a leukemogenic virus like the EBV, which preferentially infects B lymphocytes. Acute infection by EBV induces a short-lived B-cell proliferative response following which B cells altered in antigenicity appear. The presence of the EBV-infected B cells provokes a massive proliferative response of host T cells, including transformed T cells which are cytoxic for B cells [100]. Normal immune mechanisms are almost effective enough to eliminate the infection, but EBV can produce a chronic or a fulminating, fatal illness in individuals who have an immunologic deficiency. EBV and other virus infections, furthermore, may suppress normal immunologic responses, lead to the appearance of monoclonal "autoantibodies," or

interfere with the proliferation of hemopoietic stem cells and thus produce a variety of other disease manifestations or distinct disease entities. The data which describe these phenomena have been reviewed [100–103].

The immunoglobulin abnormalities and/or the defective immune responses observed in apparently healthy relatives of patients with CLL provide an opportunity to study its etiology and pathogenesis. The autoimmune and hypersensitivity reactions in CLL and the development of antibodies without identified antigens are a late functional aberration in the disease rather than phenomena related to either its etiology or pathogenesis. The immunologic incompetence of lymphocytes may be important in pathogenesis: CLL lymphocytes are relatively unresponsive to antigenic stimuli, and this characteristic may allow them to accumulate in or lie more or less dormant in blood, lymph nodes, marrow, and spleen. T-lymphocyte subsets may interact with each other or with B lymphocytes to produce the immunologic aberrations in CLL or fail to terminate the lymphoproliferation triggered by viral or other antigens.

AGE

Some relationship of aging to CLL has long been apparent, since it occurs predominantly in old persons. Ninety percent of patients with CLL are over 50 years of age, and nearly two-thirds are over 60 [104]. The link may be the reduction in immunologic competence associated with aging, as evidenced by a decrease in immunoglobin concentration, reduced phagocytic efficiency, and impairment of lymphocyte transformation 105–110].

SEX

All varieties of leukemia occur oftener in men than in women, and in CLL the sex disparity is greatest. The overall male/female ratio in CLL is more than 2:1. Both sexes presumably have an equal exposure to leukemogenic hazards, at least in modern times, and there are no known sex differences in lymphocyte physiology, in immune responsiveness, or in the course of the disease once it develops. The precise role of sex hormones in the etiology of CLL has never been defined, but important clues may be provided by recent studies of immune deficiencies which predispose to EBV-induced lymphoproliferative disease [111]. Boys who have the X-linked recessive lymphoproliferative disease are prone to die from overwhelming EBV infection, and approximately 40 percent of them develop lymphocytic malignancies [102]. Other immunodeficiency diseases occur in male children predominantly and predispose them to comparable hazards [103].

Clinical features

The clinical features of B-cell CLL, and "lymphosarcoma cell" leukemia are indistinguishable. The basic abnormality in the common varieties of CLL, the proliferation and accumulation of abnormal lymphocytes in the lymph nodes, marrow, and spleen, varies considerably in severity from patient to patient, and the course of the disease ranges from nearly acute to benign. In its natural evolution, the amount of abnormal lymphatic tissue in a given individual seems to increase at a fairly steady rate [1,112]. The tendency for CLL to undergo progression or acute exacerbation at an early or late stage, with or without treatment, is less than with any other variety of leukemia [113]. The median survival of patients after the disease has been discovered has been reported to be 3 to 4 years [8,114–121]. For patients in collected series and those in cancer registries, about half of whom are never given specific therapy, the median survival is only 2 years [104,122]. Ten to fifteen percent of patients may have good health for 10 to 15 years with little or no treatment, and a somewhat greater percentage who have severe and aggressive disease die within a year [118–122]. The survival curves of adult patients do not suggest the existence of clear-cut subgroups of disease [118,121] (see below).

The earliest clinical manifestations of CLL generally are fatigue and reduced exercise tolerance, sometimes severe enough to suggest myasthenia gravis, enlargement of superficial lymph nodes, or splenomegaly. In most patients, symptoms and signs of disease develop so insidiously that there is no way to date the onset. In a quarter of patients the first evidence of CLL is discovered more or less by accident in routine or other examinations during which enlarged lymph nodes, splenomegaly, or abnormal blood counts are found.

When CLL is discovered at an early or asymptomatic stage and its course followed without treatment, reduced exercise tolerance and chronic fatigue usually develop within a period of 1 to 2 years. Enlarged lymph nodes gradually increase in size, and new regions of node enlargement develop, particularly in the cervical, axillary, brachial, mesenteric, retroperitoneal, and inguinal regions. The spleen ordinarily continues to enlarge, and hepatomegaly develops. Lymph tissue may grow in unusual locations in the scalp, orbit, subconjuctivae, pharynx, pleura, lung parenchyma, walls of the gastrointestinal tract, liver, prostate, and gonads. Periportal infiltration may produce obstructive jaundice, and very rarely myocardial infiltration may cause congestive failure. Symptoms of more advanced or aggressive CLL include severe and more incapacitating fatigue, exceeding that explained by anemia, recurrent or persistent infection, bruising, pallor or jaundice associated with anemia, fever, edema or thrombophlebitis from node obstruction, and increased bone tenderness.

Unusual signs or symptoms such as massive splenomegaly; mediastinal tumor; meningeal or CNS involvement; nodular, diffuse, or pigmented skin infiltration; and the circulatory manifestations of hyperviscosity are suggestive of some of the other lymphoproliferative diseases outlined in Table 115-1 (see "Differential Diagnosis").

Laboratory features

The diagnosis of CLL is ordinarily made by finding a persistently increased number of immature or abnormal lymphocytes in the blood.

In those with mild disease, the microscopic appearance of the lymphocytes may be virtually normal. In the average patient with CLL, however, lymphocytes are somewhat larger than normal and more easily ruptured in making films. Nucleoli tend to be prominent, and the nuclear chromatin is clumped or condensed and apparently increased in amount [123,124]. The abnormal lymphocytes tend to have moderately basophilic, nongranular, and abundant cytoplasm. In patients with more severe or aggressive disease, the lymphocytes may be pleomorphic or very small and have narrow rims of cytoplasm and deeply clefted nuclei suggestive of a follicular cell origin [124–127].

Others have large cells that appear immature and have densely basophilic and somewhat granular cytoplasm. Abnormal lymphocytes with large, reticulated nuclei and prominent, well-delineated nucleoli are sometimes called *lymphosarcoma cells* [121,128]. The lymphocytes in CLL may have a heterogeneous pattern of growth in lymph nodes and tissues, but microscopically they are monotonously similar in the blood of a given patient.

Unique structural, biochemical, or biologic features by which CLL lymphocytes can be differentiated from normal lymphocytes have not been identified [129]. B and T cells and their subsets are morphologically indistinguishable [129–133]. CLL lymphocytes do contain more glycogen, however, than normal lymphocytes (positive periodic acid–Schiff reaction) [124] and have a higher rate of RNA synthesis [130]. There are no distinctive ultrastructural features or surface geographic characteristics demonstrable by scanning electron microscopy [124,131–133].

The abnormal lymphocytes in CLL ordinarily have receptors for a single type of light chain, and for heavy chains of IgM or IgD. The latter may coexist or be present with receptors for IgG or IgA [3]. The type of monoclonal B-cell markers on CLL lymphocytes are identical with those found in lymphocytes obtained from the lymph nodes of patients who have well-differentiated lymphocytic lymphoma [127,134–139]. The type of marker does not change with disease progression. Ia-like antigens may be found in very mature B lymphocytes but are usually not present in B-CLL lymphocytes. The amount of SmIg on the surface membranes of B-CLL lymphocytes demonstrable by immunofluorescence is less than that of normal cells, and the migration of Ig on the cell surface ("capping") is defective, or harder to see [127,140].

All types of plasma immunoglobulins are usually reduced in CLL, either early in the course of the disease or, more regularly, as disease progresses. The γ-globulin level may fall as low as 0.3 to 0.4 g/dl, at which point patients become vulnerable to bacterial, viral, or fungal infections. About 5 percent of patients with CLL have monoclonal Ig "spikes" in their plasma. The majority are IgM components, but anomalous IgG and IgA constituents also occur [58–63]. Clinical manifestations of dysproteinemia usually stem from immunoglobulin deficiency, or rarely from paraprotein-induced hyperviscosity or the effects of a cryoglobulin.

The biochemical characteristics of normal and malignant lymphocytes have been reviewed [141]. In immunodeficiency diseases there is a partial or complete absence of adenosine deaminase and purine nucleotide phosphorylase [142–146]. Neither of these deficiencies has been found in CLL. The serum urate level is usually normal in patients with CLL, and usually neither it nor the amount of urate excreted in the urine increases significantly during treatment. The DNA polymerase, terminal deoxynucleotidyl transferase, increased in thymocytes and in immature lymphocytes, is absent or present in very low concentration in CLL lymphocytes [147,148].

Lactate dehydrogenase (LDH), often used as a measure of disease activity in lymphoproliferative diseases, is a tetramer made up from two polypeptides which can combine to form any of five isoenzymes LDH 1 through 5. The intracellular content of LDH 3 and LDH 5 is higher in B cells than in normal blood T cells, but the latter have relatively more LDH 1. This difference may be a sign of a cell immaturity since thymocytes have a high percentage of LDH-3 activity. Plasma LDH is elevated in many lymphoproliferative diseases, but comparisons of the intracellular enzyme content of cells in parallel with membrane surface markers have not been carried out.

Acid phosphatase is widely distributed in hemopoietic cells, and at least three isoenzymes have been obtained from lymphocytes. Low levels of isoenzyme 3 were found in B-CLL lymphocytes, but considerably more was present in lymphocytes from a patient with T-CLL. Increased isoenzyme 5 was present in three of four patients with hairy cell leukemia. Both isoenzymes 3 and 5 appear to be resistant to tartrate inhibition [149]. 5'-Nucleotidase levels correlate with the degree of lymphocyte maturity, and are elevated in the cells of some patients with CLL [150,151].

The absolute lymphocyte count in CLL ordinarily ranges between 10 and 150 × 10³ per microliter but counts up to 1000 × 10³ per microliter may occur in patients with severe untreated disease. There is relatively little spontaneous fluctuation in total leukocyte count. The abnormal lymphocytes in CLL are smaller than the lymphoblasts and myeloblasts in acute leukemia, and the incidence of thrombotic and embolic complications is low. The percentage of neutrophils in CLL is often reduced, but their absolute number is normal or slightly increased in early stages of the disease [120].

Examination of the marrow is usually not necessary for the diagnosis of CLL, but aspiration and needle biopsies are often performed to confirm the diagnosis or to evaluate the need for therapy. Infiltration of the mar-row usually develops slowly over years in parallel with the advancing stage of the disease. An important degree of involvement may be demonstrable, however, in patients who appear to have early or asymptomatic CLL, and it is sometimes the major site of the disease in individuals who have no enlargement of lymph nodes, splenomegaly, and few or no abnormal cells in the circulating blood (subleukemia or "aleukemic" lymphocytic leukemia). The growth pattern of lymphoid tissue in the marrow may be nodular, interstitial, or paratrabecular, depending somewhat on the stage of the disease, but eventually it becomes diffuse [127,152–156]. When lymphoid tissue comprises 50 percent or more of the marrow, patients tend to develop cytopenias, especially following blood loss, infection, or the aggressive use of antileukemic agents. The plasma cells in the marrow are usually greatly decreased. Mast cells may be increased in number, and at times the erythroid precursors may appear megaloblastic. Spotty or diffuse erythroid hyperplasia is suggestive of hemolytic complications.

As the amount of lymphoid tissue in the marrow increases, fat disappears, and the proportion of normal marrow precursor cells decreases until eventually almost nothing remains but lymphocytes [127,152–156].

When patients with CLL develop anemia, the erythrocytes are ordinarily normochromic and normocytic and the number of reticulocytes normal or reduced. After a great excess of lymphatic tissue has accumulated, in the marrow or elsewhere, the red cell survival is characteristically short even when there is no autoantibody [18–20]. Neutropenia and thrombocytopenia, ranging in severity from mild to severe, are present in patients with marrow replacement in the late stages of CLL. Red cell aplasia and hypogammaglobulinemia have been reported to develop with the proliferation of T lymphocytes which have Fc receptors for IgG [157].

Anemia in chronic leukemia has traditionally been attributed to reduced red cell production associated with leukemic marrow involvement. The rate of red cell production in some anemic patients, however, may be normal or even greater than normal [158,159], and the red cell survival significantly reduced [18–20]. Thus, in some patients with CLL, anemia may be due to hemolysis or sequestration in lymphatic tissues with relative marrow insufficiency. In CLL while anemia is not a feature of early disease, pancytopenia begins to develop when half or more of the marrow is usurped by lymphoid tissue. In patients with gross splenomegaly or bulky accumulation of lymphatic tissue, red cell survival is reduced, and patients with advanced disease are thus subject to double jeopardy—reduced erythrocyte production capacity plus shortened red cell survival.

A third factor responsible for anemia in patients with CLL is immune hemolysis which develops in perhaps 5 to 10 percent of patients who have relatively severe or advanced disease [160]. "Triggering" by therapeutic agents, disease progression, virus infections, and membrane damage by abnormal proteins have been suggested as being responsible [161–166]. Characteristic features of the autoimmune hemolytic anemia in CLL include a shortened red cell survival, mild jaundice, reticulocytosis, often spherocytosis, erythroid hyperplasia in the marrow, and a positive Coombs' test. The latter is due to fixation of IgG and sometimes complement on red cells [166,167].

Differential diagnosis

The diagnosis of CLL is ordinarily not difficult in patients who have an increased number of clearly abnormal lymphocytes in their circulating blood, enlarged lymph nodes, splenomegaly, and no evidence of an acute infection or hypersensitivity reaction. If the lymphocytosis is sustained or increases and if lymphocites in the marrow make up 30 percent or more of the cells present, the diagnosis of CLL is practically certain. If the absolute lymphocyte count is less than 5000×10^9 per microliter, however, and the cells appear relatively normal and mature, or distinctly pleomorphic, then virus or other infections and the other entities outlined in Table 115-1 should be considered. Since the diagnosis of CLL is rarely an emergency, repeated observations made over the course of a few weeks or months are most definitive if the diagnosis is uncertain.

The major problem in differential diagnosis pertains less to disease recognition than to classification difficulties. Lymphocyte surface markers are useful in classification (see Table 115-1). There is a close relationship of lymphoma to lymphocytic leukemia, especially of well-differentiated lymphocytic lymphoma to CLL.

Lymphomas differ from the leukemias primarily in anatomic distribution and in cell type. Lymphomas can originate as localized tumors, whereas leukemias develop as generalized tumors with involvement of the marrow and blood. Some lymphomas are more likely to involve the blood and marrow than are others. Hodgkin's disease is an entity that rarely, if ever, becomes leukemic. Well-differentiated B-cell and T-cell lymphomas in adults frequently involve marrow and blood, whereas the large-cell (formerly histiocytic) lymphomas do so less often.

There is considerable variation among patients in the tendency for lymphocytes either to remain in the tissues—lymph nodes, marrow, or spleen—or to circulate through lymph channels to the blood. These features are not entirely fixed and eternal in a given patient, but are subject to some therapeutic and experimental manipulation. A sharp increase in the number of abnormal lymphocytes in the blood follows splenectomy, and increased lymphocytosis plus a simultaneous reduction in the size of the spleen and lymph nodes may be produced by the administration of glucocorticoids. Subleukemic lymphocytic leukemia may be converted to more typical CLL, for a time at least, by the use of glucocorticoids. Conversely, a change from what appears to be a generalized to a more localized type of lymphocytic proliferation may be produced on occasion by treating patients with CLL for some time with chlorambucil. After therapy is suspended, abnormal lymph nodes may grow again and splenomegaly reappear but without the development of lymphocytosis. CLL may thus be converted to a disease with the features of well-differentiated lymphocytic lymphoma and remain so for months or years.

The pattern of lymph node histopathology tends to be diffuse medullary cord infiltration in B-CLL, nodular or follicular proliferation in "lymphosarcoma cell" leukemia, and deep paracortical involvement in T-CLL [139]. The pattern of involvement, however, is not a reliable clue to blood or marrow involvement, i.e., it does not differentiate lymphocytic leukemia from lymphocytic lymphoma.

A wide variety of dermatologic manifestations or complications occur during the course of CLL, including nodular and diffuse lymphocytic infiltration of the skin, erythroderma, exfoliative dermatitis, and secondary infections. In these instances the possibility of T-cell disease should be considered (see Table 115-1).

Hairy cell leukemia is a rare but important disease that may be difficult to differentiate from CLL. Splenomegaly, severe progressive pancytopenia, atypical mononuclear, lymphocytoid cells in the circulating blood, and marrow that is difficult to aspirate due to reticulin fibrosis or diffuse infiltration with abnormal cells are features that suggest the diagnosis of hairy cell leukemia (see Chap. 116). Although lymphocytosis can occur, most patients have leukopenia. This disease is probably the same as that described as lymphoid myelofibrosis [168]. Waldenström's macroglobulinemia ordinarily appears as a form of subleukemic (lymphocytic) leukemia with an abnormal monoclonal IgM component in the plasma. Large numbers of small lymphocytes, plasmacytoid lymphocytes, and some plasma cells are found in the marrow. The numbers of mast cells in the marrow is often increased (see Chap. 123).

T-lymphocyte leukemia in adults is rare in Western countries. The major clinical features are erythroderma with pruritis, some enlargement of lymph nodes, splenomegaly, and hepatomegaly. The lymphocytes have lobulated, convoluted, or cerebriform nuclei similar to "Sézary/mycosis" cells [169–175]. T-cell malignancies tend to disseminate via the circulation and preferentially involve epidermal sites. There is less marrow infiltration than in chronic B-cell leukemias. Involvement of the central nervous system is common. Japanese patients in one geographic locality have a high frequency of T-cell lymphoma [172] (see Chap. 120).

Treatment

There is no complete and lasting cure for CLL and all forms of therapy involve some cost, risk, and inconvenience to the patient. Once the diagnosis of CLL is

TABLE 115-2 Clinical staging system for chronic lymphocytic leukemia

Stage	Findings at diagnosis
0	Lymphocytes in blood 15,000 × 10⁹ per liter or higher, and 40 percent or more lymphocytes in marrow
I	Above plus enlarged lymph nodes
II	Above plus splenomegaly, hepatomegaly, or both
III	Above plus anemia (Hb less than 11 g/dl)
IV	Above plus thrombocytopenia (platelets less than 100,000 per microliter)

NOTE: In stages II to IV, lymph node enlargement may be present or absent; in stages III and IV, splenomegaly and hepatomegaly are not essential features.
SOURCE: Rai et al. [153].

established, the advisability of treatment, therapeutic options, and logistics should be considered. Decisions require data relating to prognosis, the presence or absence of unrelated disease, and possible complications of therapy. One of the most important prognostic factors is the amount and location of abnormal lymphoid tissue, and particularly the extent to which marrow function is compromised. Other prognostic factors include age; possibly sex; rapidity of disease onset; the presence or absence of systemic symptoms such as impaired muscle strength and endurance, weight loss, and fever; the number and type of lymphocytes in the blood; and the presence of hypogammaglobulinemia.

Pretreatment studies should include a detailed hematologic survey with Coombs' test, marrow aspiration and needle biopsy, and serum electrophoresis. If abnormal protein components are present, they are typed by immunoelectrophoresis. X-rays of the chest and abdominal films are advisable in most patients, as are intravenous pyelograms, abdominal CT scans, lower extremity lymphangiograms, and liver/spleen scans in some instances. Appropriate surveys to rule out the possibility of occult tuberculosis and fungal infections

TABLE 115-3 International clinical staging scheme for chronic lymphocytic leukemia

Stage A	Lymphocytosis in blood, 15,000 × 10⁹ per liter or higher, and 40 percent or more marrow lymphocytes. No anemia or thrombocytopenia, and less than three areas of nodal involvement.*
Stage B	Above with three or more areas of lymphoid involvement, enlarged lymph nodes, spleen, or liver. No anemia or thrombocytopenia.
Stage C	Above with anemia (Hb less than 11 g/dl in men or less than 10 g/dl in women) or thrombocytopenia (less than 100,000 × 10⁹ per liter) regardless of the number of areas of lymphoid involvement.

*Each cervical, axillary and inguinal area, whether unilateral or bilateral, spleen, and liver count as one area. The number of areas of lymphoid involvement, thus, range from one to five [176].

are advisable. Node biopsies may be helpful to exclude the possibility of such entities as Boeck's sarcoid. The presence of latent diabetes mellitus may be important to document if glucocorticoid therapy is contemplated. In CLL the serum urate level and the amount excreted in the urine is usually normal, both in patients with untreated disease and following therapy.

A clinical staging system applicable to the findings at the time of diagnosis has been introduced. It involved the quantitation of the amount, location, and hematologic effects of the abnormal lymphoid tissue (see Table 115-2) [153]. A simpler scheme has now been adopted by an international study group (see Table 115-3) [176,177]. Patients are classified into three groups, in each of which there is a significantly different prognosis making the classification useful in therapeutic decisions. Since the survival of untreated patients in group A approximates that of the general population, they are ordinarily not treated but should be seen periodically to detect disease progression or the development of other complications. Patients in group B tend to have more evidence of disease and their median survival is about 7 years. Many in this group have specific complaints or disabilities that can be controlled with the use of a single agent such as chlorambucil. Patients in group C have more advanced disease and their median survival is less than 2 years. They may require multiagent treatment regimens as outlined below.

A list of the principal agents and procedures used in the treatment of CLL is given in Table 115-4. At one time, irradiation was the standard palliative treatment, and local irradiation therapy is still useful in patients with lymphoid tumors and marked splenomegaly. The systemic benefit from irradiation of the spleen was surprising, in view of the widespread and diffuse nature of the disease, but this can now be explained on the basis of lymphocyte kinetics. Although abnormal lymphocytes grow or accumulate in the nodes, spleen, and marrow, in the hepatic parenchyma and elsewhere, there is brisk interorgan traffic. Circulating lymphocytes move in and out of the spleen, filter out into the marrow, thymus, and lymph nodes and return to the blood. Irradiation of any major site of disease may affect not only lymphocytes *in situ* but also those in transit. This lymphocyte migration has led to the exploratory use of extracorporeal irradiation [193,194] and leukapheresis [226–228] to eliminate the abnormal circulating lymphocytes without damaging the marrow or other organs.

The development of the nitrogen mustard compounds and the glucocorticoids revolutionized the treatment of the lymphoproliferative diseases. The effect of the original very reactive and unstable mustard compound HN₂ in CLL was not particularly encouraging, probably because it was given infrequently, and in large doses, for too short a time. Triethylene melamine (TEM) appeared to be an equally reactive and unstable compound, but since it could be given by mouth in small doses, at optimal intervals, and for prolonged periods of time, a superior degree of disease control was soon demonstrated.

TABLE 115-4   Therapeutic agents and procedures used in the treatment of chronic lymphocytic leukemia

Agent	References
Irradiation:	
Orthovoltage, local and "spray"	[1,8,114–119]
	[178–182]
Phosphorus 32	[10,11,113,117,183–187]
Supervoltage	[188–192]
Extracorporeal	[193,194]
Nitrogen mustard and derivatives, HN_2:	[119,120,195,196]
Triethylene melamine	[1,12,13,120,185–187,197–199]
Chlorambucil	[1,15,120,181,182,185–187,200–207]
Cyclophosphamide	[1,204,209–212]
Sulfonic acid derivatives: Busulfan	[202,213]
Antibiotic derivatives and plant alkaloids:	
Streptonigrin	[207,214,215]
Mitomycin C	[216]
Vinblastine	[217]
ACTH, glucocorticoids	[1,120,121,181,182,218–222]
Splenectomy	[1,167,181,223–226]
Leukapheresis	[227–229]

Extreme sensitivity to the effects of nitrogen mustard compounds proved to be a fundamental biologic property of normal and neoplastic lymphocytes, while antimetabolites and compounds primarily active during some phase of cell division were ineffective. Prolonged treatment with TEM and other nitrogen mustard derivatives, moreover, could be used without producing permanent hypocellularity of the marrow, in contrast to the cumulative effects of ionizing radiation. During the course of therapy, as abnormal lymphocytes were gradually eliminated from the marrow, myeloid and erythroid regeneration occurred with alleviation of anemia, neutropenia, and thrombocytopenia. These effects were aided by the adjuvant use of glucocorticoids and androgens.

With the development of chlorambucil, a stable, well-tolerated, and well-absorbed aromatic mustard derivative, and later cyclophosphamide, practical agents with a somewhat different spectrum of therapeutic activity became available. Extensive clinical studies have now shown that chlorambucil is most effective in suppressing the growth of well-differentiated small lymphocytes, while cyclophosphamide is sometimes superior in suppressing the growth of less mature lymphocytes, with relative sparing of neutrophils and platelets.

The use of standard therapeutic agents in the treatment of CLL and the eventual outcome in a patient with moderately severe (stage C, III) disease are illustrated in Figure 115-1. The length and quality of life is noteworthy. Issues regarding the treatment of CLL, including the comparative merits of different classes of therapeutic agents, evaluation of response, early and late complications associated with the disease and its treatment and survival have been clarified by a large-scale cooperative study [186]. Beginning in 1957, all untreated patients with CLL seen at 10 hospitals were assigned at random to one of three therapeutic agents, ^{32}P, chlorambucil, or TEM, and to one of two regimens, regularly maintained therapy or intermittent treatment given when disease became symptomatic and continued to the point of maximum response. Indications for active therapy included chronic fatigue or lack of exercise tolerance reflected by a significant decline in performance status, enlarged troublesome lymph nodes, progressive enlargement of the spleen, cytopenias due to lymphocytic replacement of the marrow or hemolysis, or other atypical but unequivocal manifestations of disease.

Adjuvant therapeutic measures were used sparingly when needed, but uniformly in all groups of patients. In late stages of the disease, when the degree of therapeutic response to the primary agent was unsatisfactory or hemolytic manifestations appeared, 15 to 20 mg of prednisone was added to the regimen daily and continued more or less indefinitely [187].

One hundred and forty patients were entered into the study, and with one exception all were followed to death or for a period of at least 10 years. After 4 years had elapsed, the use of ^{32}P was suspended when it became apparent that the clinical and hematologic benefit and survival with this agent were clearly inferior to those with chlorambucil and TEM (Fig. 115-2). The effects of chlorambucil and TEM were equal, but chlorambucil was easier and safer to use. The symptomatic group of patients had a shorter survival than the asymptomatic, but even those with mild CLL lived longer when their disease was controlled without allowing morbidity to develop (see Fig. 115-3) [187]. Less therapeutic benefit using the same agents has been reported in previously treated patients with more advanced disease in whom therapy was maintained for a short period of time.

In therapeutic evaluations, it is necessary to grade responses quantitatively. The group cited about used the terms *none, questionable, fair, good,* and *excellent* to

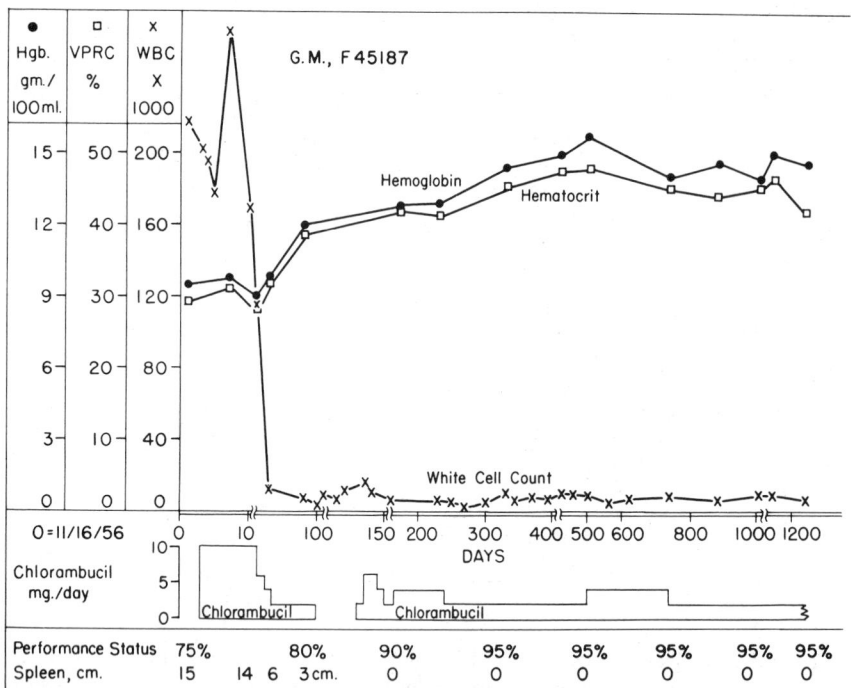

FIGURE 115-1 This 56-year-old woman gradually developed fatigue, lack of exercise tolerance, upper abdominal fullness, and edema over 7 months. She had generalized enlargement of lymph nodes and conspicuous splenomegaly. The lymphocyte count was 200×10^9 per milliliter and the hemoglobin concentration was 9 g/dl. The marrow was heavily infiltrated with lymphocytes.

She was given chlorambucil intermittently. The lymphocytic leukocytosis, splenomegaly, and anemia regressed and after 3 months of treatment she had no major signs or symptoms of disease. Mild neutropenia persisted. With therapy she remained well for over 11 years. Mild anemia, neutropenia, and increasing lymphocytic immaturity then developed. The γ-globulin concentration fell from 0.6 to 0.3 g/dl, and the serum albumin from over 5 to 2.8 g/dl. Prednisone given in a dose of 15 mg daily produced some symptomatic and hematologic benefit. Later a skull tumor developed which on biopsy seemed to originate from the diploic tissues but was too undifferentiated for histologic classification. The tumor regressed following radiation therapy, but the patient's general status worsened, with progressive anemia, lymphocytic immaturity, and recurrent infections. She died 13 years after the appearance of her disease.

specify the degree to which all basic manifestations of disease were controlled in a given set of circumstances [202]. Evidence of disease in CLL rarely disappears completely, and the all-or-none terms *remission* and *relapse* are not useful. Chlorambucil is usually given to adult patients in one oral dose of 6 to 10 mg each day, fasting, for 1 to 2 weeks and then reduced to 2 to 6 mg daily.

Blood counts repeated at intervals of 1 week or so initially are usually sufficient to guard against undue depression of marrow function. Evidence of disease activity begins to subside in 2 or 3 weeks and reaches a maximum in 2 to 4 months. If there is no substantial evidence of disease present at 6 months, therapy can be suspended until signs of relapse develop. This may occur within a period of 1 to 2 months in patients with very aggressive disease, but ordinarily not before 6 to 12 months or longer, at which time another course of therapy may be necessary.

The proliferation or accumulation of abnormal lymphocytes in the blood, marrow, spleen, and lymph nodes may be controlled to a fair or better degree in 70 percent of patients with chlorambucil alone [187,202]. In those whose clinical and hematological response to chlorambucil is less than *good*, the addition of prednisone in a dose of 10 to 20 mg daily, or every other day, improves the degree of disease control. It is advisable to give most of these patients a small dose of an androgen or anabolic steroid with the prednisone to avoid skeletal demineralization and to promote erythropoiesis (see below).

Cyclophosphamide is a useful agent for the treatment of CLL, also. Oral doses of 50 to 100 mg given daily in the fasting state, also are ordinarily well tolerated. Cyclophosphamide metabolites are excreted in the urine, and chronic exposure of the bladder mucosa to these compounds may produce "hemorrhagic cystitis." For this reason, the fluid intake in the early morning should be increased during therapy to enhance urine output.

Patients with CLL who relapse within a few weeks of

suspending treatment may need therapy continuously. Those with milder disease may require a few weeks of chemotherapy once or twice a year to maintain a good status.

The administration of chlorambucil intermittently in doses of 20 to 40 mg at intervals of 2 to 4 weeks produces gastrointestinal side reactions, a slower therapeutic response, more toxicity, and little, if any, increase in therapeutic efficiency [230–232]. Attempts to produce complete remissions are probably not worth the risk [181]. Long remissions without evidence of disease [233,234], like spontaneous remissions and some of the extraordinarily long survivals reported [235,236], probably indicate unusually mild disease or extreme sensitivity to the agents used rather than a superior therapeutic regimen.

Once hypogammaglobulinemia develops in patients with CLL, it ordinarily persists. Little or no improvement occurs even in patients who respond well to treatment and in whom abnormal lymphocytic proliferation is eliminated. Improvement of in vitro lymphocyte transformation by lectins has been reported after effective treatment [206,237], but it may lag several months behind other evidence of clinical and hematologic response.

Prednisone has well-substantiated anti-CLL effects, too, which are useful in patients with severe, or advanced disease. When the response to the oral mustard compound has been inadequate, 10 to 20 mg of prednisone daily or every other day can be given as adjuvant therapy. If immune hemolytic anemia develops, usually in patients with more severe and advanced disease, prednisone becomes a necessary therapeutic adjunct [182]. Satisfactory control of hemolysis is not attained, however, unless the antileukemic regimen otherwise has been effective. In postmenopausal women or others prone to develop skeletal demineralization, an anabolic steroid should be given also. The use of prednisone as a sole or primary agent in CLL results in poor disease control and increases the risk of infection. Large doses, 40 to 60 mg per day, given for any prolonged length of time to patients with CLL are hazardous, since this increases the risk of infections and gastrointestinal hemorrhage [182,218–222,239].

Radiotherapy is used mainly to treat enlarged lymph nodes or massive splenomegaly resistant to alkylating agent–prednisone regimens. A renewed interest in whole-body external irradiation, however, using cobalt teletherapy, has led to some favorable reports [188,189, 240]. Some success with the use of local radiotherapy in the treatment of hypersplenism or splenomegaly with intractable pain has been reported [191], but surgical splenectomy is generally preferred [224–226].

Patients with subleukemic lymphocytic leukemia have disease that varies considerably in severity and in the extent to which marrow function is compromised. The principles of management in these individuals are the same as for CLL [58,203,211,241,242].

Vincristine as a single agent has little effect on lymphocytic proliferation in CLL, but used in combination with cyclophosphamide and prednisone (CVP), moderately good therapeutic effects have been produced in patients with advanced or aggressive disease [127,243–246]. Patients with CLL who develop a rare complication, autoimmune thrombocytopenic purpura [247], may benefit from the administration of vincristine for reasons other than effects on lymphocyte proliferation (see Chap. 145). The addition of doxorubicin and/or bleomycin to the CVP regimen may produce some additional benefit in patients with severe or refractory disease [127,244]. The present consensus regarding the chemotherapy of CLL is that it is best controlled by the

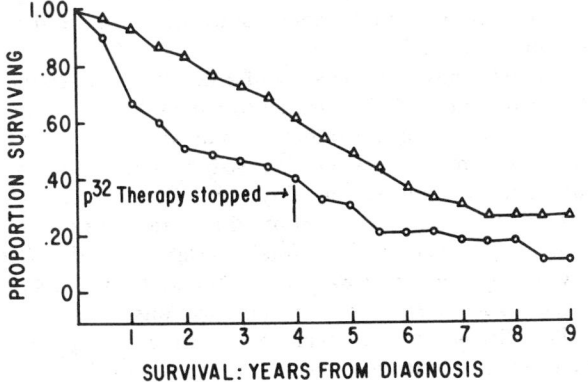

FIGURE 115-2 Southeastern Group comparison of therapeutic agents in patients with previously untreated chronic lymphocytic leukemia. This study was begun on Dec. 1, 1957, and accession stopped on Dec. 1, 1961. The use of ^{32}P was terminated on Dec. 1, 1961. Follow-up status was given as of April 1, 1967. △ = 95 patients treated with chlorambucil or TEM; ○ = 45 patients treated with ^{32}P. (Huguley [295].)

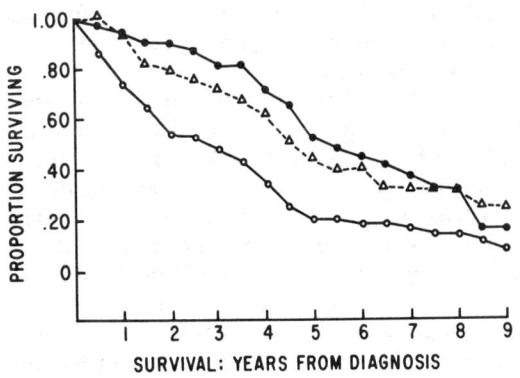

FIGURE 115-3 Southeastern Group comparison of continuous versus intermittent therapy in asymptomatic patients with chronic lymphocytic leukemia. Symptomatic patients required more continuous therapy than asymptomatic, and their survival was poorer. ● = asymptomatic group, continuous therapy (31 patients); △ = asymptomatic group, intermittent therapy (28 patients); ○ = symptomatic group (total) (80 patients).

use of milder regimens, including the use of single agents when feasible, without risking major toxicity.

Leukapheresis is useful in the treatment of CLL particularly when the mass of circulating white cells is great enough to produce vascular thrombosis or embolism in patients with severe cytopenias refractory to alkylating agents, and for the treatment of variants such as prolymphocytic leukemia, T-cell CLL, or the Sézary syndrome, which are comparatively refractory to standard agents [227–229,248–253]. Malignant lymphocytes are more buoyant than granulocytes and can be removed with great efficiency, but removal of the less dense red cells often leads to the development of anemia requiring blood transfusions. Thrombocytopenia has not been a major problem with this procedure.

With repeated leukapheresis the abnormal lymphocytosis, enlargement of lymph nodes, and the hepatosplenomegaly in CLL can all be significantly improved for a few weeks or longer. In some patients, therapeutic failure results from apparent lymphocyte compartmentalization [229].

Interferon(s) produces changes in lymphocyte distribution in CLL but has no established role in standard therapy at this time.

Course and prognosis

The disease develops insidiously and may produce few or no signs or symptoms until it is advanced. Earlier and more accurate recognition of abnormal lymphocyte proliferation is now possible using methods to detect the presence of small numbers of monoclonal B lymphocytes [254,255]. Proliferation of the latter may be induced or allowed to proceed without restraint if there are qualitative or quantitative aberrations in the function of T-lymphocyte subsets [256–261]. Prospective studies of the etiology and pathogenesis of CLL have been carried out using the family members who may have pre-CLL abnormalities, such as splenomegaly of uncertain origin [262], immune Coombs' positive hemolytic anemia [161], Coombs'-positive reactions due to complement-coated red cells [166,167] or hypogammaglobulinemia [69]. Cold hemagglutinin disease may eventuate in CLL or some related lymphoproliferative disorder [262–264]. The cold agglutinin is a monoclonal protein which sometimes is responsive to chlorambucil chemotherapy [264,265].

The course of CLL after discovery or diagnosis varies widely in different patients. Terms used to categorize the disease, such as "benign," asymptomatic, "indolent," or "active," should be replaced by staging designations such as those in Tables 115-2 and 115-3. Clinical staging of the disease at the time of diagnosis by determining the number of major areas of lymph node involvement and the degree to which marrow function has been impaired has a prognostic significance [153,176]. Proper classification is important in making

therapeutic decisions and in comparing different therapeutic programs [153,156,176,177,266–269].

The survival of patients with stage A disease is approximately the same as that of the general population. The median survival of those with stage B disease is about 7 years and those with stage C disease less than 2 years [176]. Staging the disease at the outset as described does not make allowance for other factors that may eventually lead to the identification of patient subgroups. Multivariate statistical analysis of a large number of patients has shown no definite relationship between age, sex, neutrophil count before treatment, cell morphology or hypogammaglobulinemia, and survival [176]. In prospective studies the possible value of determining cell size [270], lymphocyte kinetics [271], immunologic markers, the use of lymphangiographic and CT scanning procedures or identifying T-cell subsets has yet to be determined.

After CLL is diagnosed, serial observations over the course of months or years may show that the disease is stable. The rapidity with which the abnormal lymphocytes accumulate or proliferate, the degree to which the disease responds to therapy with chlorambucil, and the duration of remissions without specific treatment all have prognostic significance. Patients should be restaged whenever there is a material change in disease status. In CLL there is no well-defined group of systemic symptoms (fever, night sweats, weight loss) comparable to those in Hodgkin's disease that reflect effects of the disease on the host.

The 5-year survival of patients registered as having different types of chronic leukemia increased from 15 to 30 percent from 1940 to 1969 [272]. Virtually all of the improvement occurred in patients with CLL. The 5-year survival of patients with CLL increased from 46 percent in 1960–1963 to 59 percent in 1970–1973 [273]. The survival of those with T-cell CLL is about 6 months [274,275].

With well-designed and monitored therapy, the risks of long-term complications are much less than those of the underlying disease [276]. An increased risk of hypersensitivity and infectious phenomena such as autoimmune and hemolytic anemia, hypersensitivity reactions to insect bites [277], and susceptibility to opportunistic infections occur in patients who have immunologic deficiency and disordered immune reactions. These complications contribute to morbidity and mortality [277–279].

CLL becomes more severe and difficult to treat in the course of time [280]. The extent to which this evolution can be retarded by treatment is unknown. The stage is eventually reached when increasing cellular immaturity, fever, neutropenia, thrombocytopenia, and refractory anemia develop, all of which are more or less resistant to therapy. The final phase of the disease develops gradually over a period of 6 months to 2 years when patients succumb to complications of uncontrolled disease, and intercurrent infection complicated by anemia, inanition, or bleeding. About 5 percent of patients with CLL eventually develop what has been called Richter's syndrome (large-cell lymphoma) [281–283]. Involvement of the meninges is an occasional complication, particularly in T-cell malignancies [284,285].

A final acute phase of the disease is seen more frequently now in patients whose survival has been greatly prolonged by therapy [280–286]. During the acute transformation phase the type of heavy- and light-chain markers remain unchanged [287]. A variable number of nonlymphoid neoplasias develop in patients during the course of CLL, but whether the incidence is actually increased or not is uncertain [287]. An unusual late complication in CLL is progressive multifocal demyelinization (leukoencephalopathy) which has been attributed to virus infection [289–294].

References

1. Dameshek, W., and Gunz, F.: *Leukemia*, 2d ed. Grune & Stratton, New York, 1964.
2. Dameshek, W.: Chronic lymphocytic leukemia—an accumulative disease of immunologically incompetent lymphocytes. *Blood* 29:566, 1967.
3. Koziner, B., Kempin, S., Passe, S., Gee, T., Good, R. A., and Clarkson, B. D.: Characterization of B-cell leukemias: A tentative immunomorphological scheme. *Blood* 56:815, 1980.
4. Virchow, R.: Die Leukämie, in *Gesammelte Abhandlungen zur wissenschaftlichen Medizin*. Meidinger, Frankfurt, 1856, p. 190.
5. Kundrat, H.: Ueber Lympho-Sarkomatosis. *Wien. Klin. Wochenschr.* 6:211, 234, 1893.
6. Türk, W.: Ein System der Lymphomatosen. *Wien. Klin. Wochenschr.* 16:1073, 1903.
7. Sternberg, C.: Uber lymphatische Leukämie. *Z. Heilk.* 25:170, 201, 1904.
8. Minot, G. R., and Isaacs, R.: Lymphatic leukemia: Age incidence, duration, and benefit derived from irradiation. *Boston Med. Surg. J.* 191:1, 1924.
9. Leitner, S. J.: *Bone Marrow Biopsy: Haematology in Light of Sternal Puncture*, English translation by C. J. C. Britton and E. Neumark. Grune & Stratton, New York, 1949.
10. Lawrence, J. H., Low-Beer, B. V. A., and Carpenter, J. W. J.: Chronic lymphatic leukemia. *JAMA* 140:585, 1949.
11. Reinhard, E. H., Neely, C. L., and Samples, D. M.: Radioactive phosphorus in the treatment of chronic leukemias: Long-term results over a period of 15 years. *Ann. Intern. Med.* 50:942, 1959.
12. Rundles, R. W., and Barton, W. B.: Triethylene melamine in the treatment of neoplastic disease. *Blood* 7:483, 1952.
13. Rundles, R. W., Coonrad, E. V., and Willard, N. L.: Summary of results obtained with TEM. *Ann. N.Y. Acad. Sci.* 68:926, 1958.
14. Everett, J. L., Roberts, J. R., and Ross, W. C. J.: Aryl-2-halogenoalkylamines. 12. Some carboxylic derivatives of NN-di-2-chloroenphylaniline. *J. Chem. Soc. (London)*, 1953, p. 2386.
15. Galton, D. A. G., Israels, L. G., Nabarro, J. D. N., and Till, M.: Clinical trials of p-(di-2-chloroethylamino)-phenylbutyric acid (CB 1348) in malignant lymphoma. *Br. Med. J.* 2:1172, 1955.
16. Coombs, R. R. A., Maurant, A. E., and Race, R. R.: A new test for the detection of weak and "incomplete" Rh agglutinins. *Br. J. Exp. Pathol.* 26:255, 1945.
17. Berlin, R.: Red cell survival studies in normal and leukaemic subjects. *Acta Med. Scand. [Suppl.]* 252:139, 1951.
18. Brown, G. M., Elliott, S. M., and Young, W. A.: The hemolytic factor in the anemia of lymphatic leukemia. *J. Clin. Invest.* 30:130, 1951.
19. Ross, J. F., Crockett, C. L., and Emerson, C.P.: The mechanism of anemia in leukemia and malignant lymphoma. *J. Clin. Invest.* 30:668, 1951.
20. Berlin, N. I., Lawrence, J. H., and Lee, H. C.: The pathogenesis of the anemia of chronic leukemia: Measurement of the life span of the red blood cell with glycine-2-C^{14}. *J. Lab. Clin. Med.* 44:860, 1954.
21. Gunz, F. W., and Dameshek, W.: Chronic lymphocytic leukemia in a family, including twin brothers and a son. *JAMA* 164:1323, 1957.
22. Decastello, A.: Beitrag zur Kenntnis der familiären Leukämie. *Med. Klin.* 35:1255, 1939.
23. Hornbaker, J. H.: Chronic leukemia in three sisters. *Am. J. Med. Sci.* 203:322, 1942.
24. Videbaek, A.: *Heredity in Human Leukemia and Its Relation to Cancer*. H. R. Lewis, London, 1947.
25. Reilly, E. B., Rappaport, S. I., Karr, N. W., Mills, H., and Carpenter, G. E.: Familial chronic lymphatic leukemia. *Arch. Intern. Med.* 90:87, 1952.
26. Rigby, P. G., Pratt, P. T., Rosenlof, R. C., and Lemon, H. M.: Genetic relationships in familial leukemia and lymphoma. *Arch. Intern. Med.* 121:67, 1968.
27. Anderson, R.C.: Familial leukemia: A report of leukemia in five siblings, with a brief review of the genetic aspects of this disease. *Am. J. Dis. Child.* 81:313, 1951.
28. Fraumeni, J. F., Jr., Wertelecki, W., Blattner, W. A., Jensen, R. D., and Leventhal, B. G.: Varied manifestations of a familial lymphoproliferative disorder. *Am. J. Med.* 59:145, 1975.
29. Gunz, F. W., Fitzgerald, P. H., Crossen, P. E., Mackenzie, I.S., Powles, C. P., and Jensen, G. R.: Multiple cases of leukemia in a sibship. *Blood* 27:482, 1966.
30. Gunz, F. W., and Veale, A. M. O.: Leukemia in close relatives—accident or predisposition? *J. Natl. Cancer Inst.* 42:517, 1969.
31. Gunz, F. W., Gunz, J. P., Veale, A. M. O., Chapman, C. J., and Houston, I. B.: Familial leukaemia: A study of 909 families. *Scand. J. Haematol.* 15:117, 1975.
32. Cohen, H. J., Shimm, D., Paris, S. A., Buckley, C. E., and Dremer, W. B.: Hairy cell leukemia–associated familial lymphoproliferative disorder. *Ann. Intern. Med.* 90:174, 1979.
33. Mitelman, F.: Marker chromosome 14q+ in human cancer and leukemia. *Adv. Cancer Res.* 34:141, 1981.
34. Gahrton, G., Robert, K.-H., Friberg, K., Zech, L., and Bird, A. G.: Nonrandom chromosomal aberrations in chronic lymphocytic leukemia revealed by polyclonal B-cell-mitogen stimulation. *Blood* 56:640, 1980.
35. Whang-Peng, J., and Knutsen, T.: Lymphocytic leukaemias, acute and chronic. *Clin. Haematol.* 9:87, 1980.
36. Atkin, N. B.: Lymphoma and dysproteinaemias. *Clin. Haematol.* 9:175, 1980.
37. Gunz, F. W., Fitzgerald, P. H., and Adams, A.: An abnormal chromosome in chronic lymphocytic leukemia. *Br. Med. J.* 2:1097, 1962.
38. Fitzgerald, P. H., Crossen, P. E., Adams, A. C., Sharman, C. V., and Gunz, F. W.: Chromosome studies in familial leukemia. *J. Med. Genet.* 3:96, 1966.
39. Fitzgerald, P. H., and Hamer, J. W.: Third case of chronic lymphocytic leukemia in a carrier of the inherited Ch^1 chromosome. *Br. Med. J.* 3:752, 1969.
40. Fu, S. M., Winchester, R. J., and Kunkel, H. G.: Occurrence of surface IgM, IgD and free light chains on human lymphocytes. *J. Exp. Med.* 139:409, 1972.
41. Pincus, S., Bianco, C., and Nussenzweig, V.: Increased proportion of complement-receptor lymphocytes in the peripheral blood of patients with chronic lymphocytic leukemia. *Blood* 40:303, 1972.
42. Shevach, E. M., Herberman, R., Frank, M. M., and Green, I.: Receptors for complement and immunoglobulin on human leukemic cells and human lymphoblastoid cell lines. *J. Clin. Invest.* 51:1933, 1972.
43. Lille, I., Desplaces, A., Meeus, L., and Saracino, R. T.: Thymus-derived proliferating lymphocytes in chronic lymphocytic leukemia. *Lancet* 2:263, 1973.
44. Piessens, W. F., Schur, P. H., Maloney, W. C., and Churchill, W. H.: Lymphocyte surface immunoglobulins: Distribution and frequency in lymphoproliferative diseases. *N. Engl. J. Med.* 288:176, 1973.
45. McLaughlin, H., Wetherly-Mein, G., Pitcher, C., and Hobbs, J. R.: Nonimmunoglobulin-bearing "B" lymphocytes in chronic lymphatic leukaemia? *Br. J. Haematol.* 25:7, 1973.

46. Ross, G. D., Polley, M. J., Rabellino, E. M., and Grey, H. M.: Two different complement receptors on human lymphocytes, one specific for C3b and one specific for inactivator cleaved C3b. *J. Exp. Med.* 138:798, 1973.

47. Seligman, M., Preud'Homme, J. L., and Brouet, J. C.: B and T cell markers in human proliferative blood diseases and primary immunodeficiencies, with special reference to membrane bound immunoglobulins. *Transplant. Rev.* 16:85, 1973.

48. Wilson, J. D., and Hurdle, A. D. F.: Surface immunoglobulins on lymphocytes in chronic lymphocytic leukaemia and lymphosarcoma. *Br. J. Haematol.* 24:563, 1973.

49. Catovsky, D., Miliani, E., Okos, A., and Galton, D. A. G.: Clinical significance of T-cells in chronic lymphocytic leukaemia. *Lancet* 2:751, 1974.

50. Seligmann, M.: B-cell and T-cell markers in lymphoid proliferations. *N. Engl. J. Med.* 290:1483, 1974.

51. Brouet, J. C., Sasportes, M., Flandrin, G., Preud'Homme, J. L., and Seligmann, M.: Chronic lymphocytic leukaemia of T-cell origin: Immunological and clinical evaluation in eleven patients. *Lancet* 2:890, 1975.

52. Davis, S.: The variable pattern of circulating lymphocyte subpopulations in chronic lymphocytic leukemia. *N. Engl. J. Med.* 294:1150, 1976.

53. Nowell, P. C., Daniele, R., Winger, L., and Rowlands, D. T., Jr.: T cells in chronic lymphocytic leukaemia. *Lancet* 1:915, 1975.

54. Schiffer, L. M.: Kinetics of chronic lymphocytic leukemia. *Ser. Haematol.* 1:3, 1968.

55. Zimmerman, R. S., Goodwin, H. A., and Perry, S.: Studies of leukocyte kinetics in chronic lymphocytic leukemia. *Blood* 31:277, 1968.

56. Spivak, J. L., and Perry, S.: Lymphocyte kinetics in chronic lymphocytic leukaemia. *Br. J. Haematol.* 18:511, 1970.

57. Slungaard, A., and Smith, M. J.: Serum immunoglobulin levels in chronic lymphatic leukaemia. *Scand. J. Haematol.* 12:112, 1974.

58. Rundles, R. W., Coonrad, E. V., and Arends, T.: Serum proteins in leukemia. *Am. J. Med.* 16:842, 1954.

59. Brem, T. H., and Morton, M. E.: Defective serum gammaglobulin formation. *Ann. Intern. Med.* 43:465, 1955.

60. Jim, R. T. S., and Reinhard, E. H.: Agammaglobulinemia and chronic lymphocytic leukemia. *Ann. Intern. Med.* 44:790, 1956.

61. Jim, R. T. S.: Serum gamma globulin levels in chronic lymphocytic leukemia. *Am. J. Med. Sci.* 234:44, 1957.

62. Prasda, A.: The association of hypogammaglobulinemia and chronic lymphatic leukemia. *Am. J. Med. Sci.* 236:610, 1958.

63. Ultmann, J. E., Fish, W., Osserman, E., and Gellhorn, A.: The clinical implications of hypogammaglobulinemia in patients with chronic lymphocytic leukemia and lymphocytic lymphosarcoma. *Ann. Intern. Med.* 51:501, 1959.

64. Boggs, D. R., and Fahey, J. L.: Serum protein changes in malignant disease. II. The chronic leukemias, Hodgkin's disease, and malignant melanoma. *J. Natl. Cancer Inst.* 25:1381, 1960.

65. Heremans, J. F., et al.: Studies on "abnormal" serum globulins (M-components) in myeloma, macroglobulinemia and related diseases. *Acta Med. Scand.* 170 (Suppl. 367), 1961.

66. Schwartz, T. B., and Jager, B. V.: Cryoglobulinemia and Raynaud's syndrome in a case of chronic lymphocytic leukemia. *Cancer* 2:319, 1949.

67. Azar, H. A., Hill, W. T., and Osserman, E. F.: Malignant lymphoma and lymphatic leukemia associated with myeloma-type serum proteins. *Am. J. Med.* 23:239, 1957.

68. Moore, D. F., Migliore, P. F., Shullenberger, C. C., and Alexanian, R.: Monoclonal macroglobulinemia in malignant lymphoma. *Ann. Intern. Med.* 72:43, 1970.

69. Waldenström, J. G.: *Monoclonal and Polyclonal Hypergammaglobulinemia.* Vanderbilt University Press, Nashville, Tenn., 1968.

70. Lee, S. L., Rosner, F., Ruberman, W., and Glasberg, S.: Mu-chain disease. *Ann. Intern. Med.* 75:407, 1971.

71. Jonsson, V., Videbaek, A., Axelsen, N. H., and Harboe, M.: Mu chain disease in a case of chronic lymphocytic leukaemia and malignant histiocytoma. I. Clinical aspects. *Scand. J. Haematol.* 16:209, 1976.

72. Axelsen, N. H., Harboe, M., Jonsson, V., and Videbaek, A.: Mu chain disease in a case of chronic lymphocytic leukaemia and malignant histiocytoma. II. Immunochemical studies. *Scand. J. Haematol.* 16:218, 1976.

73. Clark, C., Rydell, R. E., and Kaplan, M. E.: Frequent association of IgM with crystalline inclusions in chronic lymphatic leukemic lymphocytes. *N. Engl. J. Med.* 289:113, 1973.

74. Fraumeni, J. F., Vogel, C. L., and De Vita, V. T.: Familial chronic lymphocytic leukemia. *Ann. Intern. Med.* 71:279, 1969.

75. Williams, R. C., Jr., Erickson, J. L., Polesky, H. F., and Swaim, W. R.: Studies of monoclonal immunoglobulins (M-components) in various kindreds. *Ann. Intern. Med.* 67:309, 1967.

76. Seligmann, M.: A genetic predisposition to Waldenström's macroglobulinemia. *Acta Med. Scand.* 179 (Supp. 445):140, 1966.

77. Seligmann, M., Danon, F., Mihaesco, C., and Fudenberg, H. H.: Immunoglobulin abnormalities in families of patients with Waldenström's macroglobulinemia. *Am. J. Med.* 43:66, 1967.

78. Hallen, J.: Frequency of "abnormal" serum globulins (M-compounds) in the aged. *Acta Med. Scand.* 173:737, 1963.

79. Axelsson, U., and Hallen, J.: Familial occurrence of pathological serum proteins of different gammaglobulin groups. *Lancet* 2:369, 1965.

80. Axelsson, U., Bachmann, R., and Hallen, J.: Frequency of pathological proteins (M-components) in 6,995 sera from an adult population. *Acta Med. Scand.* 179:235, 1966.

81. Fudenberg, H., German, J. L., and Kunkel, H. G.: The occurrence of rheumatoid factor and other abnormalities in families of patients with agammaglobulinemia. *Arthritis Rheum.* 5:565, 1962.

82. Wolf, J. K.: Primary acquired agammaglobulinemia with a family history of collagen disease and haematological disorders. *N. Engl. J. Med.* 266:473, 1962.

83. Wollheim, F. A., Belfrage, S., Coster, C., and Lindholm, H.: Primary "acquired" hypogammaglobulinemia: Clinical and genetic aspects of nine cases. *Acta Med. Scand.* 176:1, 1964.

84. Wollheim, F. A., and Williams, R. C., Jr.: Immunoglobulin studies in six kindred of patients with adult hypogammaglobulinemia. *J. Lab. Clin. Med.* 66:433, 1965.

85. Snyder, A. L., Li, F. P., Henderson, E. S., and Todaro, G. J.: Possible inherited leukaemogenic factors in familial acute myelogenous leukaemia. *Lancet* 1:586, 1970.

86. Shaw, R. K., et al.: Infection and immunity in chronic lymphocytic leukemia. *Arch. Intern. Med.* 106:467, 1960.

87. Miller, D. G., and Karnofsky, D. A.: Immunologic factors and resistance to infection in chronic lymphatic leukemia. *Am. J. Med.* 31:748, 1961.

88. Miller, D. G., Budinger, J. M., and Karnofsky, D. A.: A clinical and pathologic study of resistance to infection in chronic lymphatic leukemia. *Cancer* 15:307, 1962.

89. Miller, D. G.: Patterns of immunological deficiency in lymphomas and leukemias. *Ann. Intern. Med.* 57:703, 1962.

90. Fahey, J. L., Scoggins, R., Utz, J. P., and Szwed, C. F.: Infection, antibody response and gamma globulin components in multiple myeloma and macroglobulinemia. *Am. J. Med.* 35:698, 1963.

91. Cone, L., and Uhr, J. W.: Immunological deficiency disorders associated with chronic lymphocytic leukemia and multiple myeloma. *J. Clin. Invest.* 43:2241, 1964.

92. Quaglino, D., and Cowling, D. C.: Cytochemical studies on cells from chronic lymphatic leukemia and lymphosarcoma cultures with phytohemagglutinin. *Br. J. Haematol.* 10:358, 1964.

93. Oppenheim, J. J., Whang, J., and Frei, E., III: Immunologic and cytogenic studies of chronic lymphocytic leukemic cells. *Blood* 26:121, 1965.

94. Rubin, A. D., Havemann, K., and Dameshek, W.: Studies in chronic lymphocytic leukemia: Further studies of the proliferative abnormality of the blood lymphocyte. *Blood* 33:313, 1969.

95. Forbes, I. J., and Henderson, D. W.: Globulin synthesis by human peripheral lymphocytes: *In vitro* measurements using lymphocytes from normals and patients with disease. *Ann. Intern. Med.* 65:69, 1966.

96. Dent, P. B., Peterson, R. D. A., and Good, R. A.: The relationship between immunologic function and oncogenesis. *Birth Defects* 4:443, 1968.

97. Grottum, K. A., Hovig, T., Holmsen, H., Abrahamsen, A. F.,

Jeremic, M., and Seip, M.: Wiskott-Aldrich syndrome: Qualitative platelet defects and short platelet survival. *Br. J. Haematol.* 17:373, 1969.

98. Haerer, A. F., Jackson, J. F., and Evers, C. G.: Ataxia-telangiectasia with gastric adenocarcinoma. *JAMA* 210:1884, 1969.

99. Kersey, J. H., and Spector, B. D.: Immune deficiency diseases, in *Persons at High Risk of Cancer: An Approach to Cancer Etiology and Control*, edited by J. F. Fraumeni, Jr. Academic, New York, 1975, p. 55.

100. Carter, R. L.: Infectious mononucleosis: Model for self-limiting lymphoproliferation. *Lancet* April 12, 1975, p. 846.

101. Klein, G.: The Epstein-Barr virus and neoplasia. *N. Engl. J. Med.* 293:1353, 1975.

102. Purtilo, D. T., Paguin, L., DeFlorio, D., Virzi, F., and Sakhuja, R.: Immunodiagnosis and immunopathogenesis of the X-linked recessive lymphoproliferative syndrome. *Semin. Hematol.* 16:309, 1979.

103. Purtilo, D. T.: Immune deficiency predisposing to Epstein-Barr virus–induced lymphoproliferative diseases: The X-linked lymphoproliferative syndrome as a model. *Adv. Cancer Res.* 34:279, 1981.

104. Cutler, S. J., Axtell, L., and Heise, H.: Ten-thousand cases of leukemia: 1940–62. *J. Natl. Cancer Inst.* 39:993, 1967.

105. Hallen, J.: Frequency of "abnormal" serum globulins (M-components) in the aged. *Acta Med. Scand.* 173:737, 1963.

106. Aoki, T., Teller, M. M., and Robitaille, M.: Aging and cancerigenesis. II. Effect of age on phagocytic activity of the reticuloendothelial system and on tumor growth. *J. Natl. Cancer Inst.* 34:255, 1965.

107. Wigzell, H., and Stjernsward, J.: Age-dependent rise and fall of immunological reactivity in the CBA mouse. *J. Natl. Cancer Inst.* 37:513, 1966.

108. Gross, L.: Immunological defect in aged population and its relationship to cancer. *Cancer* 18:201, 1965.

109. Pisciotta, A. V., Westring, D. W., DePrey, C., and Walsh, B.: Mitogenic effect of phytohaemagglutinin at different ages. *Nature* 215:193, 1967.

110. Wexler, M. D., Hutteroth, T. H.: Impaired lymphocyte function in aged humans. *J. Clin. Invest.* 53:99, 1974.

111. Bar, R. S., DeLor, C. J., Clausen, K. P., Hurtubise, P., Henle, W., and Hewetson, J. F.: Fatal infectious mononucleosis in a family. *N. Engl. J. Med.* 290:363, 1974.

112. Galton, D. A. G.: The pathogenesis of chronic lymphocytic leukemia. *Can. Med. Assoc. J.* 94:1005, 1966.

113. Osgood, E. E.: Contrasting incidence of acute monocytic and granulocytic leukemias in P³²-treated patients with polycythemia vera and chronic lymphocytic leukemia. *J. Lab. Clin. Med.* 64:560, 1964.

114. Panton, P. N., and Valentine, F.: Chronic lymphoid leukaemia. *Lancet* 1:914, 1929.

115. Leavell, B. S.: Chronic leukemia: A study of the incidence and factors influencing the duration of life. *Am. J. Med. Sci.* 196:329, 1938.

116. Bethel, F. H.: Lymphogenous (lymphatic) leukemia. *JAMA* 118:95, 1942.

117. Osgood, E. E.: Titrated, regularly spaced radioactive phosphorus or spray roentgen therapy of leukemias. *Arch. Intern. Med.* 87:329, 1951.

118. Shimkin, M. B., Lucia, E. L., Oppermann, K. C., and Mettier, S. R.: Lymphocytic leukemia: An analysis of frequency, distribution and mortality of the University of California Hospital, 1913–1947. *Ann. Intern. Med.* 39:1254, 1953.

119. Green, R. A., and Dixon, H.: Expectancy for life in chronic lymphatic leukemia. *Blood* 25:23, 1965.

120. Boggs, D. R., Sofferman, S. A., Wintrobe, M. M., and Cartwright, G. E.: Factors influencing the duration of survival of patients with chronic lymphocytic leukemia. *Am. J. Med.* 40:243, 1966.

121. Zacharski, L. R., and Linman, J. W.: Chronic lymphocytic leukemia versus chronic lymphosarcoma cell leukemia. *Am. J. Med.* 47:75, 1969.

122. Lockwood, K., Stancke, B., and Clemmesen, J.: Survival rates for leukemia in various countries. *Natl. Cancer Inst. Monogr.* 15:341, 1964.

123. Schrek, R., Knospe, W. H., and Trobaugh, F. E., Jr.: Chromatin and other cytologic indices in chronic lymphocytic leukemia. *J. Lab. Clin. Med.* 75:217, 1970.

124. Spiro, S., Galton, D. A. G., Wiltshaw, E., and Lohman, R. C.: Follicular lymphoma: A survey of 75 cases with special reference to the syndrome resembling chronic lymphocytic leukaemia. *Br. J. Cancer* 31:60, 1975.

125. Lennert, K., Stein, H., and Kaiserling, E.: Cytological and functional criteria for the classification of malignant lymphomata. *Br. J. Cancer (Suppl. 2)* 31:29, 1975.

126. McKenna, R. W., Bloomfield, C. D., and Brunning, R. D.: Nodular lymphoma: Bone marrow and blood manifestations. *Cancer* 36:428, 1975.

127. Aisenberg, A. C.: Case records of the Massachusetts General Hospital. *N. Engl. J. Med.* 301:1332, 1979.

128. Isaacs, R.: Lymphosarcoma cell leukemia. *Ann. Intern. Med.* 11:657, 1937.

129. Perrera, D. J. B., and Pegrum, G. D.: The lymphocyte in chronic lymphatic leukaemia. *Lancet* 1:1207, 1974.

130. Henry, P., Reich, P., Karon, M., and Weissman, S. M.: Characteristics of RNA synthesized in vitro by lymphocytes of chronic lymphocytic leukemia. *J. Lab. Clin. Med.* 69:47, 1967.

131. Schumacher, H. R., Maugel, T. K., and Davis, K. D.: The lymphocyte of chronic lymphatic leukemia. I. Electron microscopy: Onset. *Cancer* 26:895, 1970.

132. Catovsky, D., Frisch, B., and Van Noorden, S.: B, T and "null" cell leukemias: Electron cytochemistry and surface morphology. *Blood Cells.* 1:115, 1975.

133. Newell, D. G., Roath, S., and Smith, J. L.: The scanning electron microscopy of normal human peripheral blood lymphocytes. *Br. J. Haematol.* 32:309, 1976.

134. Aisenberg, A. C., and Long, J. C.: Lymphocyte surface characteristics in malignant lymphoma. *Am. J. Med.* 58:300, 1975.

135. Braylan, R. C., Jaffe, E. S., and Bernard, C. W.: Malignant lymphomas: Current classification and new observations. *Pathol. Ann.* 10:213, 1975.

136. Braylan, R. C., Jaffe, E. S., Burback, J. W., Frank, M. M., Johnson, R. C., and Berard, C. W.: Similarities of surface characteristics of neoplastic well-differentiated lymphocytes from solid tissues and from peripheral blood. *Cancer Res.* 36:1619, 1976.

137. Leventhal, B. G., Mirro, J., and Yarbro, G. S. K.: Immune reactivity to tumor antigens in leukemia and lymphoma. *Semin. Hematol.* 15:157, 1978.

138. Foon, K. A., Billing, R. J., and Terasaki, P. I.: Dual B and T markers in acute and chronic lymphocytic leukemia. *Blood* 55:16, 1980.

139. Berard, C. W., Jaffe, E. S., Braylan, R. C., Mann, R. B., and Nanba, K.: Immunologic aspects and pathology of the malignant lymphomas. *Cancer* 42:911, 1978.

140. Cohen, H. J.: Human lymphocyte surface immunoglobulin capping: Normal characteristics and anomalous behavior of chronic lymphocytic leukemic lymphocytes. *J. Clin. Invest.* 55:84, 1975.

141. Blatt, J., Reaman, G., and Poplack, D. G.: Biochemical markers in lymphoid malignancy. *N. Engl. J. Med.* 303:918, 1980.

142. Giblett, E. R., and Anderson, J. E., Cohen, F., Pollara, B., and Meuwissen, H. J.: Adenosine deaminase deficiency in two patients with severely impaired cellular immunity. *Lancet* 2:1067, 1972.

143. Giblett, E. R., Ammann, A. J., Wara, D. W., Dandman, R., and Diamond, L. K.: Nucleoside-phosphorylase deficiency in a child with severely defective T-cell immunity and normal B-cell immunity. *Lancet* 1:1010, 1975.

144. Biggar, W. D., Giblett, E. R., Ozere, R. L., Grover, B. D.: A new form of nucleoside phosphorylase deficiency in two brothers with defective T-cell function. *J. Pediatr.* 92:354, 1978.

145. Edwards, N. L., Magilavy, D. B., Cassidy, J. T., and Fox, I. H.: Lymphocyte ecto-5′-nucleotidase deficiency in agammaglobulinemia. *Science* 201:628, 1978.

146. Johnson, S. M., North, M. E., Asherson, G. L., Allsop, J., Watts, R. W. E., and Webster, A. D. B.: Lymphocyte purine 5′-nucleotidase deficiency in primary hypogammaglobulinaemia. *Lancet* 1:168, 1977.

147. McCaffrey, R., Harrison, T. A., Parkman, R., and Baltimore, D.: Terminal deoxynucleotidyl transferase activity in human leukemic

cells and in normal human thymocytes. *N. Engl. J. Med.* 292:775, 1975.

148. Bollum, F. J.: Terminal deoxynucleotidyl transferase as a hematopoietic cell marker. *Blood* 54:1203, 1979.

149. LaFuente, R., Woessner, S., and Sans-Sabrafen, J.: Isoenzymatic study of leucoacid phosphatase in haematologic diagnosis. *Scand. J. Haematol.* 23:146, 1979.

150. Lopes, J., Zucker-Franklin, D., and Silber, R.: Heterogeneity of 5'-nucleotidase activity in lymphocytes in chronic lymphocytic leukemia. *J. Clin. Invest.* 52:1297, 1974.

151. Quagliata, F., Faig, D., Conklyn, M., and Silber, R.: Studies on the lymphocyte 5'-nucleotidase in chronic lymphocytic leukemia, infectious mononucleosis, normal subpopulations, and phytohemagglutinin-stimulated cells. *Cancer Res.* 34:3197, 1974.

152. Gray, J. L., Jacobs, A., and Block, M.: Bone marrow and peripheral blood lymphocytosis in the prognosis of chronic lymphocytic leukemia. *Cancer* 33:1169, 1974.

153. Rai, K. R., Sawitsky, A., Cronkite, E. P., Chanana, A. D., Levy, R. N., and Pasternack, B. S.: Clinical staging of chronic lymphocytic leukemia. *Blood* 46:219, 1975.

154. Carbone, A., Santoro, A., Pilotti, S., and Rilke, F.: Bone marrow patterns and clinical staging in chronic lymphocytic leukemia. *Lancet* 1:606, 1978.

155. Sweet, D. L., Golomb, H. M., and Ultmann, J. E.: Chronic lymphocytic leukaemia and its relationship to other lymphoproliferative disorders. *Clin. Haematol.* 6:141, 1977.

156. Lipshutz, M. D., Mir, R., Rai, K. R., and Sawitsky, A.: Bone marrow biopsy and clinical staging in chronic lymphocytic leukemia. *Cancer* 46:1422, 1980.

157. Nagasawa, T., Abe, T., and Nakagawa, T.: Pure red cell aplasia and hypogammaglobulinemia associated with Tr-cell chronic lymphocytic leukemia. *Blood* 57:1025, 1981.

158. Huff, R. L., Hennessy, T. G., and Lawrence, J. H.: Iron metabolism studies in normal subjects and in patients having blood dyscrasias. *J. Clin. Invest.* 28:790, 1949.

159. Huff, R. L., Hennessy, T. G., Austin, R. E., Garcia, J. F., Roberts, B. M., and Lawrence, J. H.: Plasma and red cell iron turnover in normal subjects and in patients having various hematopoietic disorders. *J. Clin. Invest.* 29:1041, 1950.

160. Young, L. E., Miller, G., and Christian, R. M.: Clinical and laboratory observations on auto-immune hemolytic disease. *Ann. Intern. Med.* 35:507, 1951.

161. Rosenthal, M. C., Pisciotta, A. V., Komninos, Z. D., Goldenberg, H., and Dameshek, W.: The auto-immune hemolytic anemia of malignant lymphocytic disease. *Blood* 10:197, 1955.

162. Lewis, F. B., Schwartz, R. S., and Dameshek, W.: X-radiation and alkylating agents as possible "trigger" mechanisms in the autoimmune complications of malignant lymphoproliferative disease. *Clin. Exp. Immunol.* 1:1, 1966.

163. Schwartz, R. S., and Costea, N.: Autoimmune hemolytic anemia: Clinical correlations and biological implications. *Semin. Haematol.* 3:2, 1966.

164. van Loghem, J. J.: Concepts on the origin of autoimmune diseases: The possible role of viral infection in the aetiology of idiopathic autoimmune diseases, in *Concepts of Autoimmunity and Their Application in Haematology*, edited by S. E. Bjorkman. Williams & Wilkins, Baltimore, 1965, p. 1.

165. Zuelger, W. W., Mastrangelo, R., Stulberg, C. S., Poulik, M. D., Page, R. H., and Thompson, R. I.: Autoimmune hemolytic anemia: Natural history and viral-immunologic interactions in childhood. *Am. J. Med.* 49:80, 1970.

166. Dacie, J. V.: *The Haemolytic Anemias: Congenital and Acquired. Part III. Secondary or Symptomatic Haemolytic Anemias.* Grune & Stratton, New York, 1967.

167. Eyster, M. E., and Jenkins, D. E.: Erythrocyte coating substances in patients with positive direct antiglobulin reactions: Correlation of γG globulin and complement coating with underlying diseases, overt hemolysis and response to therapy. *Am. J. Med.* 46:360, 1969.

168. Duhamel, G.: Lymphoid myelofibrosis. *Acta Haematol.* 45:89, 1971.

169. Brouet, J.-C., Flandrin, G., and Seligmann, M.: Indications of the thymus-derived nature of the proliferative cells in six patients with Sézary's syndrome. *N. Engl. J. Med.* 289:341, 1973.

170. Brouet, J.-C., Flandrin, G., Sasportes, M., Preud'Homme, J. L., and Seligmann, M.: Chronic lymphocytic leukemia of T-cell origin. Immunological and clinical evaluation in eleven patients. *Lancet* 2:890, 1975.

171. Lutzner, M., Edelson, R., Schein, P., Green, I., Kirkpatrick, C., and Aftab, A.: Cutaneous T-cell lymphomas: The Sézary syndrome, mycosis fungoides, and related disorders. *Ann. Intern. Med.* 83:534, 1975.

172. Uchiyama, T., Yodoi, J., Sagawa, K., Takatsuki, K., and Uchino, H. Adult T-cell leukemia: Clinical and hematologic features of 16 cases. *Blood* 50:481, 1977.

173. Reinherz, E. L., Nadler, L. M., Rosenthal, D. S., Moloney, W. C., Schlossman, S. F.: T-cell subset characterization of human T-cell. *Blood* 53:1066, 1979.

174. Nair, K. G., Han, T., and Minowada, J.: T-cell chronic lymphocytic leukemia: Report of a case and review of the literature. *Cancer* 44:1652, 1979.

175. Bunn, P. A.: Prospective staging evaluation of patients with cutaneous T-cell lymphomas. *Ann. Intern. Med.* 93:223, 1980.

176. Binet, J. L., et al.: A new prognostic classification of chronic lymphocytic leukemia derived from multivariate survival analysis. *Cancer* 48:198, 1981.

177. Binet, J. L., Catovsky, D., Chandra, P., Montserrat, E., Rai, K., and Sawitsky, A.: Chronic lymphocytic leukemia: A proposal for a revised prognostic staging system. *Br. J. Haematol.*, to be published.

178. Rosenthal, N., Harris, W.: Leukemia: Its diagnosis and treatment. *JAMA* 104:702, 1935.

179. Medinger, F. G., and Craver, L. F.: Total body irradiation with review of cases. *Am. J. Roentgenol.* 48:651, 1942.

180. Djaldetti, M., de Vries, A., and Levie, B.: Hemolytic anemia in lymphocytic leukemia. *Arch. Intern. Med.* 110:449, 1962.

181. Han, T., Ezdinli, E. Z., and Sokal, J. E.: Complete remission in chronic lymphocytic leukemia and leukolymphosarcoma. *Cancer* 20:243, 1967.

182. Galton, D. A. G., Wiltshaw, E., Szur, L., and Dacie, J. V.: The use of chlorambucil and steroids in the treatment of chronic lymphocytic leukemia. *Br. J. Haematol.* 7:73, 1961.

183. Osgood, E. E.: The threshold dose of P^{32} for leukemia cells of the lymphocytic and granulocytic series. *Blood* 16:1104, 1960.

184. Hill, J. M., Loeb, E., and Speer, R. J.: Colloidal zirconyl phosphate P^{32} in the treatment of chronic leukemias and lymphomas. *JAMA* 187:106, 1964.

185. Miller, D., Diamond, H., and Craver, L.: The clinical use of chlorambucil: A critical study. *N. Engl. J. Med.* 261:525, 1959.

186. Huguley, C. M.: Long-term study of chronic lymphocytic leukemia: Interim report after 45 months. *Cancer Chemother. Rep.* 16:241, 1962.

187. Huguley, C. M.: Survey of current therapy and of problems in chronic leukemia, in *Leukemia-Lymphoma*, edited by R. W. Cumley et al. Year Book, Chicago, 1970, p. 317.

188. Johnson, R. E.: Total body irradiation of chronic lymphocytic leukemia: Incidence and duration of remission. *Cancer* 25:523, 1970.

189. Johnson, R. E.: Treatment of chronic lymphocytic leukemia by total body irradiation alone and combined with chemotherapy. *Natl. J. Rad. Oncol.* 5:159, 1979.

190. Johnson, R. E.: Total body irradiation of chronic lymphocytic leukemia: Relationship between therapeutic response and prognosis. *Cancer* 37:2691, 1976.

191. Byhardt, R. W., Brace, K., and Wiernik, P. H.: Role of splenic irradiation in chronic lymphocytic leukemia. *Cancer* 35:1622, 1975.

192. Richards, F., Spurr, C. L., Pajak, T. F., Blake, D. D., and Raben, M.: Thymic irradiation: An approach to chronic lymphocytic leukemia. *Am. J. Med.* 57:862, 1974.

193. Cronkite, E. P.: Extracorporeal irradiation of the blood. *Hosp. Practice* 81, 1970.

194. Field, E. O., et al.: The response of chronic lymphocytic leukemia to treatment by extracorporeal irradiation of the blood, assessed by isotope-labeling procedures. *Blood* 36:87, 1970.

195. Goodman, L. S., Wintrobe, M. M., Dameshek, W., Goodman, M. J., Gilman, M. A., and McLennan, M. T.: Nitrogen mustard therapy. *JAMA* 132:126, 1946.

196. Jacobson, L. O., Spurr, C. L., Barron, E. S. G., Smith, T., Lushbaugh, C., and Dick, G. F.: Nitrogen mustard therapy. *JAMA* 132:263, 1946.

197. Karnofsky, D. A., et al.: Triethylene melamine in the treatment of neoplastic disease. *Arch. Intern. Med.* 87:477, 1951.

198. Silverberg, J. H., and Dameshek, W.: Use of triethylene melamine in treatment of leukemia and leukosarcoma. *JAMA 148*:1015, 1952.

199. Bond, W. H., Rohn, R. J., Dyke, R. W., and Fouts, P. J.: Clinical use of triethylene melamine: Report of seventy-five cases. *Arch. Intern. Med. 91*:602, 1953.

200. Bouroncle, B., Doan, C., Wiseman, B., and Frajola, W.: Evaluation of CB 1348 in Hodgkin's disease and allied disorders. *Arch. Intern. Med. 97*:703, 1956.

201. Ultmann, J. E., Hyman, G. A., and Gellhorn, A.: Chlorambucil in treatment of chronic lymphocytic leukemia and certain lymphomas. *JAMA 162*:178, 1956.

202. Rundles, R. W., et al.: Comparison of chlorambucil and Myleran in chronic lymphocytic and granulocytic leukemia. *Am. J. Med. 27*:424, 1959.

203. Clatanoff, D. V., and Meher, O. O.: Response to chlorambucil in macroglobulinemia. *JAMA 183*:40, 1963.

204. Kaung, D. T., Whittington, R. M., and Patno, M. E.: Chemotherapy for chronic lymphocytic leukemia. *Arch. Intern. Med. 114*:521, 1964.

205. Ezdinli, E. Z., and Stutzman, L.: Chlorambucil therapy for lymphomas and chronic lymphocytic leukemia. *JAMA 191*:100, 1965.

206. Bouroncle, B. A., Clausen, K. P., and Aschenbrand, J. F.: Studies of the delayed response of phytohemagglutinin (PHA) stimulated lymphocytes in 25 chronic lymphatic leukemia patients before and during therapy. *Blood 34*:166, 1969.

207. Kaung, D. T., Whittington, R. M., Spencer, H. H., and Patno, M. E.: Comparison of chlorambucil and streptonigrin (NSC-45383) in the treatment of chronic lymphocytic leukemia. *Cancer 23*:597, 1969.

208. Knospe, W. H., Loeb, V., and Huguley, C. M.: Bi-weekly chlorambucil treatment of chronic lymphocytic leukemia. *Cancer 33*:555, 1974.

209. Rundles, R. W., Laszlo, J., Garrison, F. E., and Hobson, J. B.: The antitumor spectrum of cyclophosphamide. *Cancer Chemother. Rep. 16*:407, 1962.

210. Solomon, J., Alexander, M. J., and Steinfeld, J. L.: Cyclophosphamide. *JAMA 183*:165, 1963.

211. Bouroncle, B. A., Datta, P., and Frajola, W. J.: Waldenström's macroglobulinemia. *JAMA 189*:729, 1964.

212. Coco, F., and Merritt, J. A.: Cyclophosphamide-induced changes in circulating lymphocytic kinetics in chronic lymphocytic leukemia. *Cancer 25*:721, 1970.

213. Bean, R. H. D.: Myleran in the treatment of chronic lymphatic leukemia. *Isr. J. Med. Sci. 1*:801, 1965.

214. Miller, D. S., Laszlo, J., McCarty, K. S., Guild, W. R., and Hochstein, P.: Mechanism of action of streptonigrin in leukemic cells. *Cancer Res. 27*:632, 1967.

215. Rivers, S. L., Whittington, R. M., and Medrek, T. J.: Methyl ester of streptonigrin (NSC-45384) in treatment of malignant lymphoma. *Cancer Chemother. Rep. 46*:17, 1965.

216. Whittington, R. M.: Clinical experience with mitomycin (NSC 26 980). *Cancer Chemother. Rep. 54*:195, 1970.

217. Hill, J. M., and Loeb, E.: Treatment of leukemia, lymphoma, and other malignant neoplasms with vinblastine. *Cancer Chemother. Rep. 15*:41, 1961.

218. Hill, J. M., Marshall, G. J., and Falco, D. J.: Massive prednisone and prednisolone therapy in leukemia and lymphomas in the adult. *J. Am. Ceriatr. Soc. 4*:627, 1956.

219. Granville, N. B., Rubio, F., Unugur, A., Schulman, E., and Dameshek, W.: The treatment of leukemia in adults with massive doses of prednisone and prednisolone, *N. Engl. J. Med. 259*:207, 1958.

220. Freymann, J. G., Vander, J. B., Marler, E. A., and Meyer, D. G.: Prolonged corticosteroid therapy of chronic lymphocytic leukemia and the closely allied malignant lymphomas. *Br. J. Haematol. 6*:303, 1960.

221. Shaw, R. K., Boggs, D. R., Silberman, H. R., and Frei, E., III: A study of prednisone therapy in chronic lymphocytic leukemia. *Blood 17*:182, 1961.

222. Burningham, R. A., et al.: Weekly high-dosage glucocorticosteroid treatment of lymphocytic leukemias and lymphomas. *N. Engl. J. Med. 270*:1160, 1964.

223. Christensen, B. E., Hanses, L. K., Kristensen, J. K., and Videbaek, A.: Splenectomy in haematology: Indications, results and complications in 41 cases. *Scand. J. Haematol. 7*:247, 1970.

224. Yam, L. T., and Crosby, W. H.: Early splenectomy in lymphoproliferative disorders. *Arch. Intern. Med. 133*:270, 1974.

225. Alder, S., Stutzman, L., Sokal, J. E., and Mittelman, A.: Splenectomy for hematologic depression in lymphocytic lymphoma and leukemia. *Cancer 35*:521, 1975.

226. Christensen, B. E., Hansen, M. M., and Videbaek, A. A.: Splenectomy in chronic lymphocytic leukaemia. *Scand. J. Haematol. 18*:279, 1977.

227. Vallejos, C. S., McCredie, K. B., Britten, G. M., and Freireich, E. J.: Biological effects of repeated leukapheresis of patients with chronic myelogenous leukemia. *Blood 42*:925, 1973.

228. Hadlock, D. C., Fortuny, I. E., McCullough, J., and Kennedy, B. J.: Continuous flow centrifuge leukapheresis in the management of chronic myelogenous leukaemia. *Br. J. Haematol. 29*:443, 1975.

229. Lowenthal, A. M.: Chronic leukaemias: Treatment by leukapheresis. *Exp. Haematol. (Suppl.) 5*:73, 1977.

230. Sprague, C. C.: Evaluation of the effectiveness of radioactive phosphorus and chlorambucil in patients with chronic lymphocytic leukemia. *Cancer Chemother, Rep. 16*:235, 1962 11.

231. Knospe, W. H., Loeb, V., and Huguley, C. M.: Bi-weekly chlorambucil treatment of chronic lymphocytic leukemia. *Cancer 33*:555, 1974.

232. Sawitsky, A., Rai, K. R., Glidewell, O., and Silver, R. T.: Comparison of daily versus intermittent chlorambucil and prednisone therapy in the treatment of patients with chronic lymphocytic leukemia. *Blood 50*:1049, 1977.

233. Lane, S. D., Besa, E. C., Justh, G., et al.: Fatal interstitial pneumonitis following high-dose intermittent chlorambucil therapy for chronic lymphocytic leukemia. *Cancer 47*:32, 1981.

234. Schott, M.: Ten-year recovery from chronic lymphocytic leukaemia. *Br. Med. J. 1*:877, 1955.

235. Walter, L. H., Szur, L., and Lewis, S. M.: Prolonged remission in chronic lymphatic leukaemia. *Br. Med. J. 1*:859, 1958.

236. Durant, J. R., and Finkbeiner, J. A.: "Spontaneous" remission in chronic lymphatic leukaemia? *Cancer 17*:105, 1964.

237. Chervenick, P. A., Boggs, D. R., and Wintrobe, M. M.: Spontaneous remission in chronic lymphocytic leukemia. *Ann. Intern. Med. 67*:1239, 1967.

238. Sharman, D., Crossen, P. E., and Fitzgerald, P. H.: Lymphocyte number and response to phytohaemagglutinin in chronic lymphocytic leukemia. *Scand. J. Haematol. 3*:375, 1966.

239. Murray, J. F., et al.: Opportunistic pulmonary infections. *Ann. Intern. Med. 65*:566, 1966.

240. Editorial: Total lymphoid irradiation. *Lancet 2*:837, 1980.

241. Sanders, J. H., Fahey, J. L., Finegold, I., Ein, D., Reisfeld, R., and Berard, C.: Multiple anomalous immunoglobulins. *Am. J. Med. 47*:43, 1969.

242. Cass, R. M., Anderson, B. R., and Vaughan, J. H.: Waldenström's macroglobulinemia with increased serum IgG levels treated with low doses of cyclophosphamide. *Ann. Intern. Med. 71*:971, 1969.

243. Ezdinli, E., et al.: Comparison of intensive versus moderate chemotherapy of lymphocytic lymphomas: A progress report. *Cancer 28*:1060, 1976.

244. Wiltshaw, E.: Chemotherapy in chronic lymphocytic leukaemia. *Clin. Haematol. 6*:223, 1977.

245. Oken, M. W., and Kaplan, M. E.: Usefulness of cyclophosphamide-vincristine-prednisone (CVP) therapy in refractory chronic lymphocytic leukemia (CLL). *Blood 50*:202, 1977.

246. Liepman, M., and Votaw, M.: The treatment of chronic lymphocytic leukemia with COP chemotherapy. *Cancer 41*:1664, 1978.

247. Carey, R. W., McGinnia, A., Jacobson, B. M., and Carvalho, A.: Idiopathic thrombocytopenic purpura complicating chronic lymphocytic leukemia. *Arch. Intern. Med. 136*:62, 1976.

248. Rosenberg, S. A.: Current concepts in cancer: Non-Hodgkin's lymphoma—Selection of treatment on the basis of histologic type. *N. Engl. J. Med. 301*:924, 1979.

249. Curtis, J. E., Hersh, E. M., and Freireich, E. M.: Leukapheresis therapy of chronic lymphocytic leukemia. *Blood 39*:163, 1972.

250. Galton, D. A. G., Goldman, J. M., Wiltshaw, E., Cataovsky, D., Henry, K., and Goldberg, G. J.: Prolymphocytic leukaemia. *Br. J. Haematol. 27*:7, 1974.

251. Hoecker, P., Pittermann, E., and Gobets, M.: Application of cell separators in leukemia treatment. *Folia Haematol. 102*:283, 1975.

252. Buskard, N. A., Lowenthal, R. M., Goldman, J. M., and Galton, D. A. G.: Treatment of prolymphocytic leukaemia by leucapheresis, in *Leucocytes: Separation, Collection and Transfusion*, edited by J. M. Goldman and R. M. Lowenthal. Academic, London, 1975, pp. 543–547.

253. Edelson, R., Facktor, M., Andrews, A., Lutzner, M., and Schein, P.: Successful management of the Sézary syndrome. *N. Engl. J. Med.* 291:293, 1974.

254. Ault, K. A.: Detection of small numbers of monoclonal B lymphocytes in the blood of patients with lymphoma. *N. Engl. J. Med.* 300:1401, 1979.

255. Ligler, F. S., Smith, R. G., Kettman, J. R., et al.: Detection of tumor cells in the peripheral blood of nonleukemic patients with B-cell lymphoma: Analysis of "clonal excess." *Blood* 55:792, 1980.

256. Fu, S. M., Chiorazzi, N., Kunkel, H. G., Halper, J. P., and Harris, S. R.: Induction of in vitro differentiation and immunoglobulin synthesis of human leukemic B lymphocytes. *J. Exp. Med.* 148:1570, 1978.

257. Leventhal, B. G., Mirro, J., and Yarbro, G. S. K.: Immune reactivity to tumor antigens in leukemia and lymphoma. *Semin. Hematol.* 15:157, 1978.

258. DeWaele, M., Thielemans, C., and Van Camp. B. K. G.: Characterization of immunoregulatory T cells in EBV-induced infectious mononucleosis by monoclonal antibodies. *N. Engl. J. Med.* 304:460, 1981.

259. Haynes, B. F., Metzgar, R. S., Minna, J. D., and Bunn, P. A.: Phenotypic characterization of cutaneous T-cell lymphoma; use of monoclonal antibodies to compare with other malignant T cells. *N. Engl. J. Med.* 304:1319, 1981.

260. Broder, S., et al.: Activation of leukemic pro-suppressor cells to become suppressor-effector cells: Influence of cooperating normal T cells. *N. Engl. J. Med.* 304:1382, 1981.

261. Chiorazzi, N., Fu, S. M., Ghodrat, M., Kunkel, H. G., Rai, K., and Gee, T.: T-cell helper defect in patients with chronic lymphocytic leukemia. *J. Immunol.* 122:1087, 1979.

262. Dacie, J. V., Brain, M. C., Harrison, C. V., Lewis, S. M., and Worlledge, S. M.: "Non-tropical idiopathic splenomegaly" ("primary hypersplenism"): A review of ten cases and their relationship to malignant lymphomas. *Br. J. Haematol.* 17:317, 1969.

263. Schubothe, H.: The cold hemagglutinin disease. *Semin. Hematol.* 3:27, 1966.

264. Harboe, M., van Furth, R., Schubothe, H., Lind, K., and Evans, R. S.: Exclusive occurrence of K chains in isolated cold haemagglutinins. *Scand. J. Haematol.* 2:259, 1965.

265. Macris, N. T., Capra, D., Frankel, G. J., Ioachim, H. L., Satz, H., and Bruno, M. S.: A lambda light chain cold agglutinin cryomacroglobulin occurring in Waldenström's macroglobulinemia. *Am. J. Med.* 48:524, 1970.

266. Phillips, E., Kempin, S., Passe, S., et al.: Prognostic factors in chronic lymphocytic leukemia and their implications for therapy. *Clin. Haematol.* 6:203, 1977.

267. Foa, R., et al.: Clinical staging and immunological findings in chronic lymphocytic leukemia. *Cancer* 44:483, 1979.

268. Peterson, L. C., Bloomfield, C. D., and Brunning, R. D.: Relationship of clinical staging and lymphocyte morphology to survival in chronic lymphocytic leukaemia. *Br. J. Haematol.* 44:563, 1980.

269. Rozman, C., Hernandez-Nieto, L., Montserrat, E., and Brugues, R.: Prognostic significance of bone marrow patterns in chronic lymphocytic leukaemia. *Br. J. Haematol.* 47:529, 1981.

270. Binet, J. L., Vaugier, G., Dighiero, G., D'Athis, P., and Charron, D.: Investigation of a new parameter in chronic lymphocytic leukemia: The percentage of large peripheral lymphocytes determined by the Hemalog D. Prognostic significance. *Am. J. Med.* 63:683, 1977.

271. Moayeri, H., and Sokal, J. E.: In vitro leukocyte thymidine uptake and prognosis in chronic lymphocytic leukemia. *Am. J. Med.* 66:773, 1979.

272. Cutler, S. J., Meyers, M. H., and Green, S. B.: Trends in survival rates of patients with cancer. *N. Engl. J. Med.* 293:122, 1975.

273. Myers, M. H., and Hankey, B. F.: *Cancer Patient Survival Experience.* NIH Publication No. 80-2148, June 1980.

274. Takatsuki, K., Uchiyama, T., Ueshima, Y., and Hattori, T.: Adult T-cell leukemia: Further clinical observations and cytogenetic and functional studies of leukemic cells. *Jpn. J. Clin. Oncol. (Suppl.)* 9:317, 1979.

275. Matsumoto, M., et al.: Adult T-cell leukemia-lymphoma in Kagoshima District, Southwestern Japan: Clinical and hematological characteristics. *Jpn. J. Clin. Oncol. (Suppl.)* 9:325, 1979.

276. Sieber, S. M., and Adamson, R. H.: Toxicity of antineoplastic agents in man: Chromosomal aberrations, antifertility effects, congenital malformations and carcinogenic potential, in *Advances in Cancer Research*, edited by G. Klein, S. Weinhouse, and A. Haddow. Academic, New York, 1975, vol. 22, p. 57.

277. Weed, R. I.: Exaggerated delayed hypersensitivity to mosquito bites in chronic lymphocytic leukemia. *Blood* 26:257, 1965.

278. Pisciotta, A. V., Jermain, J. F., and Hinz, J. E.: Chronic lymphocytic leukemia, hypogammaglobulinemia and autoimmune hemolytic anemia. *Blood* 15:748, 1960.

279. Daily, M. O., Coleman, C. N., and Kaplan, H. S.: Radiation-induced splenic atrophy in patients with Hodgkin's disease and non-Hodgkin's lymphomas. *N. Engl. J. Med.* 302:215, 1980.

280. Zarrabi, M. H., Grunwald., H. W., and Rosner, F.: Chronic lymphocytic leukemia terminating in acute leukemia. *Arch. Intern. Med.* 137:1059, 1977.

281. Trump, D. L., Mann, R. B., Phelps, R., et al.: Richter's syndrome: Diffuse histiocytic lymphoma in patients with chronic lymphocytic leukemia. *Am. J. Med.* 68:539, 1980.

282. Foucar, K., and, Rydell, R. E.: Richter's syndrome in chronic lymphocytic leukemia. *Cancer* 46:118, 1980.

283. Fitzgerald, P. H., McEwan, C. M., Hamer, J. W., and Beard, M. E. J.: Richter's syndrome with identification of marker chromosomes. *Cancer* 46:135, 1980.

284. Goodson, J. D., and Strauss, G. M.: Diagnosis of lymphomatous leptomeningitis by cerebrospinal fluid lymphocyte cell surface markers. *Am. J. Med.* 66:1057, 1979.

285. Liepman, M. K., and Votaw, M. L.: Meningeal leukemia complicating chronic lymphocytic leukemia. *Cancer* 47:2482, 1981.

286. McPhedran, P., and Heath, C. W., Jr.: Acute leukemia occuring during chronic lymphocytic leukemia. *Blood* 35:7, 1970.

287. Enno, A., Catovsky, D., O'Brien, M., et al.: Prolymphocytoid transformation of chronic lymphocytic leukemia. *Br. J. Haematol.* 41:9, 1979.

288. Manusow, D., and Weinerman, B. H.: Subsequent neoplasia in chronic lymphocytic leukemia. *JAMA* 232:267, 1975.

289. Astrom, K. E., Mancall, E. L., and Richardson, E. P., Jr.: Progressive multifocal leuko-encephalopathy: A hitherto unrecognized complication of chronic lymphatic leukaemia and Hodgkin's disease. *Brain* 81:93, 1958.

290. ZuRhein, G. M., and Chou, S. M.: Papova virus in progressive multifocal leukoencephalopathy. *Res. Publ. Assoc. Res. Nerv. Ment. Dis.* 44:307, 1968.

291. Manz, H. J., Dinsdale, H. B., and Morrin, P. A. F.: Progressive multifocal leukoencephalopathy after renal transplantation: Demonstration of papova-like virions. *Ann. Intern. Med.* 75:77, 1971.

292. Weiner, L. P., et al.: Isolation of virus related to SV40 from patients with progressive multifocal leukoencephalopathy. *N. Engl. J. Med.* 286:385, 1972.

293. Bauer, W. R., Turel, A. P., and Jojnson, K. P.: Progressive multifocal leukoencephalopathy and cytarabine. *JAMA* 226:174, 1973.

294. Rubenstein, L., Herman, M. M., Long, T. F., and Wilbur, J. R.: Disseminated necrotizing leukoencephalopathy: A complication of treated central nervous system leukemia and lymphoma. *Cancer* 35:291, 1975.

295. Huguley, C. M.: Survey of current therapy and of problems in chronic leukemia, in *Leukemia-Lymphoma*, edited by R. W. Cumley et al. Year Book, Chicago, 1970, p. 317.

CHAPTER *116*

Hairy cell leukemia

HARVEY M. GOLOMB

Hairy cell leukemia is a malignant lymphoproliferative disease first described in 1958 and referred to originally as leukemic reticuloendotheliosis [1]. By the mid 1970s, it was a clearly recognized disease entity, characterized by pancytopenia and splenomegaly and the presence of abnormal mononuclear cells with irregular, cytoplasmic projections in blood, marrow, and other tissues, especially the spleen [2–8].

Etiology and pathogenesis

The etiology of the disease is unknown, although an association with radiation exposure has been suggested in one study [9]. There is one report of familial involvement [10]. The normal cell pool which is affected, thereby initiating the disease, is uncertain. In most cases, the pathological cells have features of B lymphocytes [11,12] or of B lymphocytes with phagocytic capabilities [13,14]. Occasionally cytological features of monocytes [15] and less often features of T lymphocytes have been identified [16,17]. One explanation for this phenotypic diversity is that the lesion is in a pluripotential stem cell pool and the nature of the genetic injury favors B-lymphocyte maturation and less often that of other lineages [18,19]. The finding of acquired dyserythropoiesis in association with hairy cell leukemia also could be explained by a lesion in a pluripotential cell [20,21].

Clinical features

The median age of onset of hairy cell leukemia is about 50 years. Although the distribution of the age of onset is broad, it is rare in children. Eighty percent of the patients are men [2,3,7,8].

Abdominal fullness or discomfort, associated with splenomegaly, is the principal complaint of about one-fourth of the patients. Fatigue, weight loss, and weakness are reported by another one-fourth, and one-fourth have bruising associated with thrombocytopenia or infections associated with severe granulocytopenia and monocytopenia. The later cell deficiency is a very common feature of the disease. Patients with abnormal blood counts or splenomegaly, detected during a routine checkup or during evaluation for an unrelated disease, account for the remainder of cases.

Splenomegaly is frequently massive and may be the most prominent physical finding. In about one-sixth of the patients, the spleen may not be palpable. Enlargement of lymph nodes is rare and, when present, is minimal and localized. Mild hepatomegaly occurs occasionally.

Laboratory features

BLOOD FINDINGS

Moderate to severe pancytopenia is present in about two-thirds of the patients. The hematocrit is usually between 20 and 35 percent. The white cell count (WBC) is often less than 4000 per microliter, although about 10 percent of patients have a WBC above 10,000 per microliter. The percentage of leukocytes that are hairy cells varies widely. In patients with a low white cell count, usually fewer than 20 percent of the leukocytes are hairy cells, whereas they are the majority of cells in the occasional patient whose white cell count is greater than 10,000 per microliter. Over 80 percent of patients have absolute neutropenia [22] and monocytopenia [23], and thus a relative increase in lymphocytes without cytoplasmic projections is frequent. Mild or moderate thrombocytopenia is common, but platelet counts under 20,000 per microliter are rare at the time of diagnosis.

The diameter of hairy cells varies from 10 to 15 μm in the blood film. The cytoplasm is pale blue to blue-gray, with cytoplasmic projections that may be fine and hair-like or broader, resembling ruffles [24]. The nucleus is sometimes eccentrically placed and may be oval or indented with loose, lacy chromatin and, at times, one or two visible nucleoli. The nucleus may be bilobed infrequently. (See Plate 4.)

MARROW EXAMINATION

The marrow aspirate is unsuccessful in a high proportion of patients with hairy cell leukemia, and a biopsy should be performed in patients in whom the diagnosis is suspected. The marrow biopsy nearly always contains an infiltrate of mononuclear cells, with round or indented nuclei surrounded by a halo of clear or pale cytoplasm. This characteristic appearance is the result of the abundant cytoplasm and some shrinkage during fixation. The "hairy" nature of the cells is not apparent in marrow sections. Mitoses and nuclear pleomorphism are uncommon; bilobed nuclei in the abnormal cells can be found in about 5 percent of patients. The marrow infiltrate is usually diffuse, replacing the normal hemopoietic tissue, but in about one-third of cases it may be patchy with interspersed areas of normal hemopoiesis [25]. The silver stain of the biopsy usually demonstrates increased marrow reticulin, which accounts for the failure to aspirate marrow. The aspirate may reveal that a lymphoproliferative process is present; however, the cytoplasmic projections of the hairy cells are often inconspicuous in such samples. Cells found in the thin area of the aspirate may show the characteristic irregular cytoplasmic margin.

ELECTRON MICROSCOPY OF HAIRY CELLS

The irregular cytoplasmic processes that characterize the cells by light microscopy are particularly well demonstrated by phase or scanning electron microscopy [26]. In about 50 percent of cases, a ribosome-lamella complex can be found in the cytoplasm by transmission electron microscopy. This cytoplasmic inclusion is a cylindrical structure composed of a central hollow space and an outer sheath of multiple parallel lamellae, with ribosomelike granules in the interlamellar space [27]. These structures may also be seen by light microscopy as rod-shaped inclusions which may be helpful in diagnosis [28].

HISTOCHEMISTRY OF HAIRY CELLS

Tartrate-resistant acid phosphatase activity (isoenzyme 5) has been described in the cells of nearly all patients with hairy cell leukemia [29,30]. Although a very useful tool to substantiate the diagnosis, tartrate-resistant acid phosphatase activity is not a prerequisite for the diagnosis of hairy cell leukemia [8,30].

SPLENIC HISTOPATHOLOGY

The spleen is nearly always enlarged in hairy cell leukemia, and tumor cells can be found infiltrating this organ. Lymphoid follicles, periarterial lymphoid sheaths, and follicular arteries are frequently atrophic [31]. Prominent pseudosinuses can often be seen formed either by damage to true sinus walls with engorgement by red cells and hairy cells or by hairy cells arranged to appear like endothelial cells with engorgement of red cells in a false lumen between hairy cells. Expansion of pulp cords is a dramatic finding.

PARAPROTEINEMIA

The serum protein electrophoresis and immunoelectrophoresis are usually normal or nondiagnostic, although several patients with a monoclonal immunoglobulin component have been reported [32,33]. Three patients who had typical features of both hairy cell leukemia and multiple myeloma and a paraprotein have been reported also [34]. These associations have been of particular interest because of the B-lymphocyte nature of most cases of hairy cell leukemia and of multiple myeloma.

Differential diagnosis

The coincidence of pancytopenia and splenomegaly, the most common presentation of hairy cell leukemia, occurs in about 5 percent of patients with malignant lymphoma, 15 percent of patients with agnogenic myeloid metaplasia, and often in patients with Waldenström's macroglobulinemia. The confusion with myeloid metaplasia can be heightened because of the reticulin fibrosis present in marrow biopsies in hairy cell leukemia. Careful histological and cytochemical analysis of blood, marrow, and occasionally splenic tissue as well as other important clinical and laboratory differences among these diseases will usually permit the specific diagnosis to be made.

In the small proportion of patients with hairy cell leukemia and lymphocytosis, distinction from chronic lymphocytic leukemia, lymphoma with marrow and blood involvement, and related diseases need to be considered. The data derived from morphologic and histochemical analysis of blood and marrow are the most important for making a specific diagnosis.

Rare patients may mimic aplastic anemia in that there is severe pancytopenia and hypoplastic marrow [35]. The presence of splenomegaly should always heighten suspicion that true aplastic anemia is not present. Careful analysis of blood and of marrow has shown characteristic hairy cells. Analysis of splenic histopathology following splenectomy also has confirmed the diagnosis in these cases.

Treatment

If a patient has no symptoms associated with the pancytopenia or splenomegaly, no therapy may be necessary. Since hypersplenism contributes to the pancytopenia, the most efficacious therapy in symptomatic patients is removal of the spleen. There is more blood cell sequestration by the spleen in hairy cell leukemia than by spleens of equal size in patients with other lymphoproliferative or myeloproliferative diseases [20]. Splenectomy should be performed in cases of bleeding secondary to thrombocytopenia, repeated or severe infections secondary to granulocytopenia, marked red cell transfusion requirements, splenic infarction, or abdominal discomfort due to massive splenomegaly. Splenectomy may be advised even in the rare patient in whom the spleen cannot be palpated if another indication is present, since the response to splenectomy is not related to spleen size [7]. Splenectomy produces benefit in a large proportion of patients. This improvement can be of long duration. Alternatively, at some time after splenectomy, progressive marrow involvement may result in recurrent pancytopenia and increased concentrations of hairy cells in the blood.

Early studies of the use of alkylating agents suggested that chemotherapy did not benefit patients and possibly even shortened their survival [3,4]. Rare reports of success with intensive chemotherapy have been published [36], but the great proportion of patients do not benefit from this approach. Recently, however, it was found that a single alkylating agent at a low dose may result in long-term benefit [7,8]. Chlorambucil, 4 mg given orally each day, can be used at first, then decreased as necessary for long-term treatment [37]. Aggressive chemotherapy can do more harm than good, at least initially. Patients who have an increasing concentration of abnormal blood mononuclear cells after splenectomy can also be given a low dose of an oral alkylating agent like chlorambucil before symptoms of organ infiltration appear. Multiple-drug combination chemotherapy should be reserved for patients who do not benefit from single-drug therapeutic regimens [8,36]. Recently, beneficial treatment of one patient with intensive leukapheresis has been reported [38].

Glucocorticoids have not been shown to be cytolytic for hairy cells, and may contribute to the infectious complications that are prevalent in this disease [5,39,40].

Course and prognosis

Hairy cell leukemia is a chronic disease. Most patients live for more than 5 years after the diagnosis is made [41]. Some older patients with minimal splenomegaly have been followed without treatment for greater than 10 years, and about 20 percent of patients do not require splenectomy during the course of their disease. About 80 percent of patients will require splenectomy, and benefit ensues in nearly every patient undergoing splenic removal. In one-third of patients the hemoglobin will reach 12 g/dl, the granulocyte count will rise above 1000 per microliter, and the platelet count above 100,000 per microliter. The remaining two-thirds of the patients will have an increase in one or two of the blood cell lines after splenectomy. The patients tolerate splenectomy in nearly all cases if it is performed by an experienced surgeon. Although in one analysis, there was one postoperative death from clostridial sepsis in over 65 splenectomies [40], the benefits of surgery in severely affected patients exceed its risks.

Approximately one-third of patients who have undergone splenectomy relapse with either a progressive leukemic form of the disease or an increasing pancytopenia in association with replacement of the marrow by hairy cells. Relapse can occur within months of splenectomy or as long as after 10 years in some cases.

Infections with gram-negative bacteria occur in a high proportion of patients [38,42]. Fungal infections occur, especially in granulocytopenic patients treated with glucocorticoids. The overwhelming proportion of infections occur prior to splenectomy. Splenectomy reduces the risk of infection by increasing the blood neutrophil count.

Patients rarely die of progressive disease when treated with available methods. Deaths are usually from infection associated with granulocytopenia and monocytopenia. Hairy cell leukemic patients are susceptible to many types of unusual infections such as disseminated atypical mycobacterial disease [26]. Aggressive evaluation of fever in a hairy cell patient will usually uncover an infection and appropriate antibiotic treatment can be instituted. Splenectomy may be required to raise the granulocyte count and permit resolution of the infection.

References

1. Bouroncle, B. A., Wiseman, B. K., and Doan, C. A.: Leukemic reticuloendotheliosis. *Blood 13*:609, 1958.
2. Katayama, I., and Finkel, H. E.: Leukemic reticuloendotheliosis. A clinicopathologic study with review of the literature. *Am. J. Med. 57*:115, 1974.
3. Burke, J. S., Byrne, G. E., Jr., and Rappaport, H.: Hairy cell leukemia (leukemic reticuloendotheliosis). I. A clinical pathologic study of 21 patients. *Cancer 33*:1339, 1974.
4. Catovsky, D., Pettit, J. E., Galton, D. A. G., Spiers, A. J. D., and Harrison, C. V.: Leukaemic reticuloendotheliosis ("hairy" cell leukaemia): A distinct clinicopathological entity. *Br. J. Haematol. 26*:9, 1974.
5. Naeim, F., and Smith, G. S.: Leukemic reticuloendotheliosis. *Cancer 34*:1813, 1974.
6. Turner, A., and Kjeldsberg, C. R.: Hairy cell leukemia: A review. *Medicine 57*:477, 1978.
7. Golomb, H. M.: Hairy cell leukemia: An unusual lymphoproliferative disease: A study of 24 patients. *Cancer 42*:946, 1978.
8. Catovsky, D.: Hairy cell leukemia and prolymphocytic leukemia. *Clin. Haematol. 6*:245, 1977.
9. Stewart, D. J., and Keating, M. J.: Radiation exposure as a possible etiologic factor in hairy cell leukemia (leukemic reticuloendotheliosis). *Cancer 46*:1577, 1980.
10. Ramseur, W. L., Golomb, H. M., Vardiman, J. W., and Collins, J. L.: Hairy cell leukemia in father and son. *Cancer 48*:1825, 1981.
11. Catovsky, D., Pettit J. E., Galetto, J., Okos, A., and Galton, D. A. G.: The B-lymphocyte nature of the hairy cell of leukaemic reticuloendotheliosis. *Br. J. Haematol. 26*:29, 1974.
12. Rieber, E. P., et al.: Hairy cell leukemia: Surface markers and functional capacities of the leukaemic cells analyzed in eight patients. *Br. J. Haematol. 42*:175, 1979.
13. Fu, S. M., Winchester, R. J., Rai, K. R., and Kunkel, H. G.: Hairy cell leukemia: Proliferation of a cell with phagocytic and B-lymphocyte properties. *Scand. J. Immunol. 3*:847, 1974.
14. Utsinger, P. D., Yount, W. J., Fuller, C. R., Logue, M. J., and Orringer, E. P.: Hairy cell leukemia: B-lymphocyte and phagocytic properties. *Blood 49*:19, 1977.
15. Scheinberg, M., Brenner, A. L., Sullivan, A. L., Catheart, E. S., and Katayama, I.: The heterogeneity of leukemic reticuloendotheliosis, "hairy cell leukemia." Evidence for its monocyte origin. *Cancer 37*:1302, 1976.
16. Cawley, J. C., et al.: Hairy-cell leukemia with T-cell features. *Blood 51*:61, 1978.
17. Saxon, A., Stevens, R. H., and Golde, D. W.: T-lymphocyte variant of hairy-cell leukemia. *Ann. Intern. Med. 88*:323, 1978.
18. Golomb, H. M., Vardiman, J., Sweet, D. L., Jr., Simon, D., and Variakojis, D.: Hairy cell leukemia: Evidence for the existence of a spectrum of functional characteristics. *Br. J. Haematol. 38*:161, 1978.
19. Cooper, W. C., Buss, D. H., and Pacher, C. L.: Leukemic reticuloendotheliosis (hairy cell leukemia): A review of the evidence concerning the immunology and origin of the cell. *Leukemic Res. 4*:489, 1980.
20. Berkowitz, L. R., Ross, D. W., and Orringer, E. P.: Hairy cell leukemia with acquired dyserythropoiesis. *Arch. Intern. Med. 140*:554, 1980.
21. Martelli, M. R., Falini, B., Rambotti, P., Tonato, M., and Davis, S.: Sideroblastic anemia associated with hairy cell leukemia. *Cancer 48*:762, 1981.
22. Yam, L. T., Chaudhry, A. A., and Janckila, A. J.: Impaired marrow granulocyte reserve and leucocyte mobilization in leukemic reticuloendotheliosis. *Ann. Intern. Med. 87*:444, 1977.
23. Seshadri, R. S., Brown, E. J., and Zipursky, A.: Leukemic reticuloendotheliosis. A failure of monocyte production. *N. Engl. J. Med. 295*:181, 1976.
24. Shrek, R., and Donnelly, W. G.: "Hairy" cells in blood in *lymphoreticular* neoplastic disease and "flagellated" cells of normal lymph nodes. *Blood 27*:199, 1966.
25. Vykoupil, K. F., Thiele, J., and Georgii, A.: Hairy cell leukemia: Bone

marrow findings in 24 patients. *Virchows Arch. [Pathol. Anat. Histol.] 370:*273, 1976.

26. Golomb, H. M., Braylan, R., and Polliack, A.: "Hairy" cell leukemia (leukemic reticuloendotheliosis): A scanning electron microscopic study of 8 cases. *Br. J. Haematol. 29:*455, 1975.

27. Rosner, M. C., and Golomb, H. M.: Ribosome-lamella complex in hairy cell leukemia: Ultrastructure and distribution. *Lab. Invest. 42:*236, 1980.

28. Katayama, I., Nagy, G. K., and Balogh, K., Jr.: Light microscopic identification of the ribosome-lamella complex in "hairy cells" of leukemic reticuloendotheliosis. *Cancer 32:*843, 1973.

29. Yam, L. T., Li, C. Y., and Lam, K. W.: Tartrate-resistant acid phosphatase isoenzyme in the reticulum cells of leukemic reticuloendotheliosis. *N. Engl. J. Med. 284:*357, 1971.

30. Katayama, I., and Yang, I. P.: Reassessment of a cytochemical test for differential diagnosis of leukemic reticuloendotheliosis. *Am. J. Clin. Pathol. 68:*268, 1977.

31. Nanba, K., Jaffe, E. S., Soban, E. J., Braylan, R. C., and Berard, C. W.: Hairy cell leukemia. *Cancer 39:*2323, 1977.

32. Golde, D. W., Saxon, A., and Stevens, R. H.: Macroglobulinemia and hairy cell leukemia. *N. Engl. J. Med. 296:*92, 1977.

33. Cawley, J. C., et al.: Typical hairy cell leukemia with Ig paraproteinemia. *Br. J. Haematol. 43:*215, 1979.

34. Catovsky, D., et al.: Hairy cell leukemia and myelomatosis: Chance association or clinical manifestations of the same B-cell disease spectrum. *Blood 57:*758, 1981.

35. Brearley, R. L., Chapman, R. M., and Brozovic, B.: Hairy cell leukemia presenting as aplastic anemia. *Ann. Intern. Med. 91:*228, 1979.

36. Davis, T. E., Waterbury, L., Abeloff, M., and Burke, P. J.: Leukemic reticuloendotheliosis: Report of a case with prolonged remission following intensive chemotherapy. *Arch. Intern. Med. 136:*620, 1976.

37. Golomb, H. M.: Progress report on chlorambucil therapy in postsplenectomy patients with progressive hairy cell leukemia. *Blood 57:*464, 1981.

38. Fay, J., Moore, J. O., Logue, G. L., and Huang, A. T.: Leukapheresis therapy of leukemic reticuloendotheliosis (hairy cell leukemia). *Blood 54:*747, 1979.

39. Bouza, E., Burgaleta, C., and Golde, D. W.: Infections in hairy cell leukemia. *Blood 51:*851, 1978.

40. Golomb, H. M., and Hanauer, S. B.: Infectious complications in HCL. *J. Infect. Dis. 143:*639, 1981.

41. Golomb, H. M., Catovsky, D., Golde, D. W.: Hairy cell leukemia: A clinical review based on 71 cases. *Ann. Intern. Med. 89:*677, 1978.

42. Cawley, J. C., Burns, G. F., and Hayhoe, F. G. J.: *Hairy Cell Leukemia. Recent Advances in Cancer Research.* Springer-Verlag, 1980, vol. 72.

Lymphocytic disorders—malignant proliferative response—lymphoma

CHAPTER *117*

Histopathology of malignant lymphomas

TIMOTHY W. MORGAN
PETER M. BANKS

Malignant lymphomas, traditionally considered tumors of the lymphatic system, have more recently been defined as solid neoplasms of the immune system [1–3]. Cells of the lymphatic system are present throughout the body, often in close association with elements of the monocyte-macrophage system (see Chap. 96) and the hemopoietic system (see Chaps. 12 to 14). Not unexpectedly, therefore, malignant lymphoma can arise in virtually any site, although organs with large concentrations of lymphoid tissue, for example, lymph nodes, tonsils, spleen, or marrow, are primarily involved [4]. While some forms of lymphoma tend consistently to retain cohesion and remain as solid tumorous proliferations, others readily disperse into marrow and blood as leukemic progression. The distinction between lymphoma and lymphoid leukemia is purely distributional, so that in many instances a particular lymphoid neoplasm may manifest both lymphomatous and leukemic features during the course of disease (see Chaps. 114 and 115). Certain lymphomas characteristically exhibit selective affinity for specific organs; for example, mycosis fungoides shows strong cutaneous tropism and hairy cell leukemia preferentially involves spleen and marrow (see Chaps. 116 and 120).

In hemopathology, current controversy centers on rival classification systems which are the result of attempts to correlate new data from immune physiology and immunopathology with the histomorphology of malignant lymphomas (see Fig. 117-1). For practical purposes, certain histopathologic features of lymphomas can be recognized as predictive for clinical progression and response to specific therapeutic modalities [5] (see Chaps. 118 and 119). Modern refinement in the recognition of these features is the result of more than a century of progress [6].

FIGURE 117-1 A comparison of the proposed ''Working Formulation'' with classifications for non-Hodgkin's lymphomas.

WORKING FORMULATION (1981)	RAPPAPORT (1966, modified 1976)	KIEL (1978)	LUKES-COLLINS (1974, modified 1979)
Low Grade	A. Well differentiated lymphocytic, with or without plasmacytoid differentiation	**Low Grade**	? U Cell (Undefined)
A. Small lymphocytic, with or without plasmacytoid differentiation		A. Lymphocytic: B-CLL T-CLL T-zone	**B Cell**
B. Follicular, small cleaved	Poorly differentiated lymphocytic	Hairy cell leukemia	A. Small Lymphocytic
C. Follicular, mixed small cleaved and large cell	B. nodular E. diffuse	Cutaneous T-cell group	A. Plasmacytoid Lymphocytic
		A. Immunocytomas:	Follicular Center Cell Types: (follicular or diffuse)
Intermediate Grade	Mixed histiocytic-lymphocytic		
D. Follicular, large cell	C. nodular F. diffuse	Lymphoplasmacytic	(B or E) Small cleaved
E. Diffuse, small cleaved		Lymphoplasmacytoid	(D or G) Large cleaved
F. Diffuse, mixed, small and large cell	Histiocytic	Polymorphous	(D or G) Large noncleaved
	D. nodular	? Plasmacytomas	(J) Small noncleaved
G. Diffuse, large cell	G, H. diffuse	E. Centrocytic	
			H Immunoblastic Sarcoma
High Grade	I. Lymphoblastic	Centrocytic/Centroblastic:	
H. Large cell, immunoblastic			**T Cell**
	Undifferentiated	B,C,D follicular	A. Small lymphocytic
I. Lymphoblastic (convoluted or nonconvoluted)	J. Burkitt's	F. diffuse	I. Convoluted lymphocytic
	J. pleomorphic		? Cerebriform (cutaneous)
J. Small noncleaved cell		**High Grade**	F,G Lymphoepithelioid cell
		G. Centroblastic	H. Immunoblastic sarcoma
Others			
Hairy Cell, Cutaneous T-Cell, etc.		Lymphoblastic:	**Histiocytic** (?G, H)
		J. B - (Burkitt's and others)	
		I. T - (convoluted cell and others)	
		I. Unclassified	
		H. Immunoblastic (B or T)	

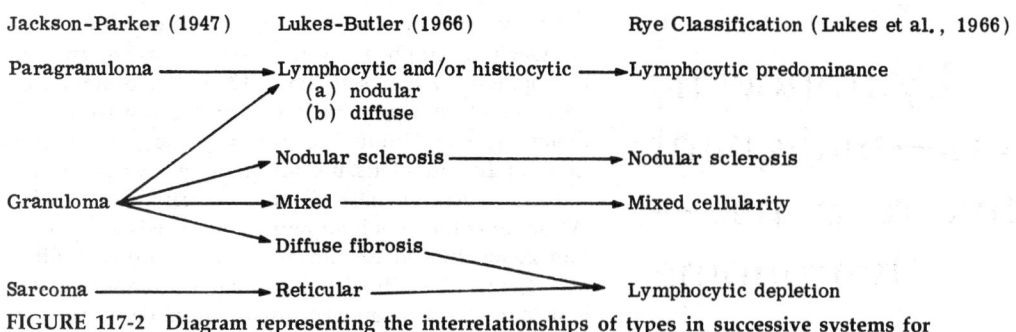

FIGURE 117-2 Diagram representing the interrelationships of types in successive systems for the subclassification of Hodgkin's disease.

Historical background

In 1832, Thomas Hodgkin published the first treatise on primary lymphoid malignancy: tumors of "the absorbent glands" and spleen. His work was derived from clinical and gross autopsy findings in seven cases [7]. Subsequently, Virchow distinguished lymphoma from leukemia in 1846 [8] and coined the terms *lymphoma* [9] and *lymphosarcoma* [10]. Billroth, in 1871, was the first to use the term *malignant lymphoma* [11].

In 1865, Wilks discerned, within a large series of cases, a group of 11 cases with findings that he considered distinctive, and memorialized Hodgkin's original study by applying the eponymic term *Hodgkin's disease* [12]. Retrospective studies indicate that probably only four of Hodgkin's original seven cases were actually examples of the disease that now bears his name. Sternberg, in 1898 [13], and Reed, in 1902 [14], described the histopathologic features of Hodgkin's disease and emphasized the abnormal giant cells characteristic of this disease, which to this day are designated *Reed-Sternberg cells.*

The category of follicular lymphomas was initially recognized in 1916 by Ghon and Roman, who, perhaps ahead of their time, related such neoplasms to normal lymphoid follicles [15]. In subsequent studies, Brill and others, in 1925 [16], and Symmers, in 1927 [17], failed to appreciate the truly neoplastic nature among many of their cases of "giant follicular hyperplasia"; however, this oversight was corrected in 1938 with information gained through long-term follow-up [18]. Thus, the indolent but still malignant nature of this category of lymphomas became recognized.

In addition to perceiving the aggressive nature of lymphomas of large cell composition, Roulet, in 1930, proposed that the origin of such neoplasms was the sinus lining, and he compared their morphology with that of the normal reticulum or syncytial network of nodal sinuses [19]. His term *Retothelsarkom* was subsequently popularized, but mistranslated as *reticulum cell sarcoma,* and the term *reticulum cell* attained an uncontrolled diversity of characterizations [20].

Without the benefit of pathologic studies, Cooke, in 1932, related tumors of older male children, often with anterior mediastinal involvement, to the development of acute lymphoblastic leukemia [21]. Cooke's clinically recognized syndrome remained without pathogenetic explanation until the modern investigations of lymphoblastic disease.

By the middle of the twentieth century clinically applicable systems of classification were being formulated. For Hodgkin's disease, the Jackson and Parker system (1947) separated the unfavorable sarcoma and favorable (but rare) paragranuloma from the large intermediate grouping of granuloma [22]. In 1966, Lukes, Butler, and Hicks, eclectically including the observations of past observers, proffered a six-part pathologic subclassification of Hodgkin's disease that correlated closely with clinical survival [23]. This classification was closely related to the Jackson-Parker system, with subdivision of each of the earlier single categories into two separate types (see Fig. 117-2). Simplified into a four-part classification, the Rye modification [24], this system has proved to be extremely useful clinically (see Chap. 118).

Classification systems for the non-Hodgkin's lymphomas were derived from a few fundamental concepts regarding the association of certain cell types and growth patterns to survival. Neoplasms composed of small, nonreplicating lymphocytes (lymphocytic, well-differentiated lymphocytic) were recognized as a favorable group. Those featuring atypical, mitotically active lymphocytes (lymphoblastic, poorly differentiated lymphocytic) were less favorable. Those made up of large cells were considered as nonlymphoid (stem cell, clasmatocytic, undifferentiated, or histiocytic) in derivation. The presence of a follicular or nodular growth pattern was an important, favorable predictive feature [25,26]. Based upon these simple principles, with ever-increasing detail and precision, sequential classification systems were developed: those of Gall and Mallory (1942), Gall and Rappaport (1958), and Rappaport (1966) [27–29]. During the 1970s, great strides were achieved in the therapy of non-Hodgkin's lymphomas, demonstrating the utility of the Rappaport system (see Chap. 119) [5,30,31]. Nevertheless, during this same decade the validity of this system was questioned by data derived from newly applied methods.

Recent classifications

As early as 1966, Lennert alluded to the potential implications of lymphoid blast transformation for use in classification of lymphomas, noting that such observations in immunology could provide a new, alternative explanation for large cell lymphomas, other than the then-popular "reticulum cell" or histiocytic theories of cytogenesis (see Chap. 106) [32]. Pioneer efforts by Lennert and his coworkers in Kiel, Germany, analyzing immunoglobulin fractions from whole-tumor homogenates, indicated a monoclonal B-cell nature for the majority of non-Hodgkin's lymphomas, including the large cell types—reticulum cell or histiocytic [33,34]. Subsequently, numerous studies using various immunologic cell surface markers, immunofluorescence, and immunohistochemical and cytochemical techniques have characterized these large cell lymphomas as either B- or, less commonly, T-lymphoid-cell proliferations [35–43]. Only rare cases of true histiocytic derivation have been recognized [37,38,44].

Lymphomas with a nodular or follicular growth pattern have been shown conclusively to be the neoplastic counterparts of germinal centers. Ultrastructural examination reveals the presence of desmosomal dendritic reticulum cells in both benign and neoplastic follicles [45,46], and immunologic analyses show that they have common functional properties [47,48].

The category designated *undifferentiated* in the Rappaport system, with Burkitt's and pleomorphic variants, was demonstrated consistently to be a B-cell neoplasm with surface immunoglobulin [49].

Lymphoblastic lymphoma, an important clinicopathologic entity, was distinguished from other lymphomas with which it has been included as "poorly differentiated lymphocytic" in the original Rappaport system [50]. Immunologic, enzymatic, and cytochemical evidence revealed this neoplasm to be of T-cell or precursor T-cell type [51,52], uniformly possessing nuclear terminal deoxynucleotidyl transferase activity [53]. This neoplasm corresponds, and often progresses, to an unfavorable form of acute lymphocytic leukemia (see Chap. 114), thus explaining the clinical observations of Cooke made four decades previously (see "Historical Background").

Some unusual lymphomas composed of "intermediately differentiated lymphocytes" correspond cytochemically to the normal mantle layer of lymphoid cells which normally rims the germinal centers. Both the neoplastic and normal cell types demonstrate alkaline phosphatase activity [54].

T-cell lymphomas, not of the lymphoblastic type, vary greatly in morphologic expression, while in general having an unfavorable prognosis [1,37,38,41–43]. A distinct subtype of T-cell lymphoma with helper T-cell activity was recognized among the cutaneous T-cell processes (mycosis fungoides and the Sézary syndrome) [55,56]. The high proportion of T-cell lymphomas noted in Japan has allowed characterization of subsets [57], although subclassification of these tumors is less developed as compared to B-cell malignancies.

Experimental efforts to define the cytogenesis of Hodgkin's disease have been frustrated because of the intimate association of benign reactive elements with neoplastic cells of this disease process. Direct studies of human tumor tissue consistently failed to demonstrate the hydrolytic enzyme activities of histiocytes in neoplastic cells. Immunohistochemical methods showed immunoglobulin within the cytoplasm of some of the neoplastic cells; however, the polyclonal nature of this immunoglobulin and its distribution within cellular organelles suggest that its presence is on a passive rather than a synthetic basis [58,59]. In vitro short-term cell culture methods have indicated a (latent?) histiocytic nature for the neoplastic cell of Hodgkin's disease [59]. Unexpectedly, the uncommon and clinically most favorable type of Hodgkin's disease, designated as "nodular histiocytic-lymphocytic type" in the original Lukes-Butler-Hicks classification (see Fig. 117-2), has been shown by immunohistochemical methods to involve polyclonal B-cell proliferation emanating from germinal centers [60]. Accordingly, questions have been raised regarding the legitimacy of inclusion of this process within Hodgkin's disease.

Proposed classifications and the "Working Formulation"

With recognition of the scientific inaccuracies of the Rappaport system, a number of new classification systems were proposed as replacements. Several of these, namely those of the World Health Organization, the British Lymphoma Group, and Dorfman of Stanford University, were based entirely on morphologic features without direct implication as to immunologic cell type [61]. Only two systems emphasized immunologic cell type and thereby were capable of assimilating the rapidly amassing data from immune studies.

The so-called Kiel classification of Lennert and coworkers in Kiel, Germany, consists of morphologically and immunologically defined categories which are separated into two major groupings according to clinical behavior (low-grade and high-grade) [1] (see Fig. 117-1). Within each major grouping the categories are further subgrouped by morphologic features; for example, small lymphocytic processes together (B-cell and T-cell chronic lymphocytic leukemia) and immunoblastic lymphomas together (B-cell and T-cell). The Kiel classification recognizes certain lymphomas for their characteristic heterogeneous cellular composition; for example, the mixture of various follicular center cell types in follicular lymphomas (centrocytic-centroblastic type) and the inclusion of the entire range of B-cell types in certain plasmacytoid lymphomas (polymorphic immunocytoma). Reference to the immunologic properties attributable to each cell type of the normal immune system and to each corresponding neoplastic category of the Kiel classification has been exhaustively detailed [1,62]. Lennert's system takes into account all three aspects of non-Hodgkin's lymphomas: morphology, immunology, and prognostic implication.

A rival American system, proposed by Lukes and Collins, emphasizes immunologic cell type primarily [63]. Categories of neoplasia are designated only by a single cell type counterpart of the normal immune system. While the Kiel system recognizes the morphologic similarity of some different immune cell types, implicit in the Lukes-Collins system is the ability to distinguish the many immunologic cell types by cytomorphology alone.

In an effort to resolve the classification controversy, the National Cancer Institute sponsored a large, multi-institutional, international comparison study [64]. Over 1000 cases with long-term clinical follow-up information were reviewed by pathologists representing each respective classification system, as well as by a panel of "referee" pathologists who individually applied the various systems to each case. Computerized analysis of the encoded data revealed a highly significant predictive value for *all* of the systems. As a practical means to allow future interinstitutional and interstudy group comparisons of survival figures, a simple, morphologically based system, or "Working Formulation," was proposed (see Fig. 117-1). This was not intended to be a replacement for the more detailed classification systems. Although this working formulation will be used as a basis for describing the histopathology of the non-Hodgkin's lymphomas in this chapter, the limitations of such a simple schema in certain disease categories also will be addressed. It is anticipated that eventually a much more complex system which recognizes the extreme heterogeneity of the lymphomas will supersede the working formulation. However, much time and effort will be required to achieve a universally agreeable system that can withstand, or absorb, the explosion of new information which has been accruing in recent years.

Lymph node histopathology

Pathologists confronted by sections of a biopsied lymph node face a formidable challenge. On the basis of morphologic findings, they must interpret functional aspects within this sampling of the patient's immune system. Is the process recognizable as an orderly response? Are there features that suggest a specific cause, for example, an infection? Is there evidence of neoplasia, and, if so, is it lymphoid in origin? And what are the implications for the therapist?

Effective study of lymph node biopsy specimens is hindered by inadequacies in tissue sampling or deficiencies in technical processing. The hematologist and surgeon should confer on each case beforehand to assure that the largest, most affected nodes are biopsied. The pathologist must closely monitor the histo-

technology in the laboratory, so that sections of adequate quality are produced [65].

REACTIVE LYMPHOID HYPERPLASIA

Reactive hyperplastic responses of lymph nodes exhibit subtle morphologic features that furnish clues as to the pathogenesis of the lymphadenopathy [66]. Certain infectious agents, such as *Toxoplasma* and the virus of cat-scratch fever, elicit specific patterns of cellular response in lymph nodes. Other well-defined clinicopathologic entities are angiofollicular lymph node hyperplasia (Castleman's disease) and sinus histiocytosis with massive lymphadenopathy (Rosai-Dorfman disease) [67,68]. Actually, the commonest and most important problem for the pathologist is the distinction of benign from malignant proliferations. Benign hyperplasia often demonstrates worrisome features: extreme cellular pleomorphism, abundant mitotic activity, and cellular atypia. Conversely, a lymphoid neoplasm can be difficult to recognize when there is only early, partial nodal involvement or when the neoplasm is composed of small, mitotically inactive cells. In general, the diagnosis of malignancy can be confidently made if the normal functional components of a lymph node are totally replaced by a process of uniform cellular composition (Plate 9-3) or if cytomorphologic study reveals features of atypia beyond the limits of reactive lymphoid or histiocytic response.

There are exceptions to even these cautious generalizations. For example, *angioimmunoblastic lymphadenopathy* has pathologic and clinical features which are both malignant and benign [69]. Pathologically, there is total effacement of lymph node architecture by a polymorphic cell population intimately associated with proliferating venular blood vessels. Clinically, the process is disseminated with multisystem involvement and may be either rapidly or slowly progressive, often fatal in outcome. Nevertheless this entity appears to be a profound immunologic disturbance and not an actual neoplastic proliferation.

Similarly, exceptionally strong immune stimuli, especially in patients with primary or induced immunodeficiency, can elicit cellular responses in nodal or tonsillar tissues so atypical in appearance as to simulate neoplasia [70]. In some cases, such processes actually progress to frank lymphoma [71].

Even when a lymph node biopsy suggests neoplasia, it is sometimes difficult to be certain that it is lymphoid in nature. The morphologic appearance of the large cell lymphomas, in particular, is closely simulated by other neoplasms, such as granulocytic sarcoma (*chloroma*) and anaplastic carcinoma. Special methods, including histochemistry (chloroacetate esterase for granulocytic differentiation) and electron microscopy (for subtle features of epithelial differentiation), may be required to determine cellular origin. The clinical features and further studies on new tissue samples may be needed in order to arrive at a definite diagnosis.

HODGKIN'S DISEASE

The histologic hallmark of Hodgkin's disease, which sets it apart from most non-Hodgkin's lymphomas, is the mixture of benign, reactive cellular elements with the neoplastic cells. This appearance suggests an active host response to the malignancy. Generally, the diagnosis of Hodgkin's disease should not be made unless bizarre, malignant, giant Reed-Sternberg cells are present (Plate 9-5). To qualify, a cell must be large and have two or more nuclei (or nuclear lobes), each containing a large amphophilic or eosinophilic inclusionlike nucleolus. The presence of Reed-Sternberg cells by themselves, however, is not diagnostic, since cells with similar morphology may be present in other benign and malignant diseases [72]. The presence of reactive cells is particularly important for the diagnosis of Hodgkin's disease.

Although the simplified four-part Rye Conference modification may be used in classifying Hodgkin's disease, the pathologist should remain familiar with the original six-part classification of Lukes, Butler, and Hicks. Each of these subcategories has distinctive features and may be of importance in the differential diagnosis [23] (see Fig. 117-2).

Lymphocytic predominance Hodgkin's disease, clinically the most favorable type, exhibits a very low ratio of neoplastic/reactive cellularity, and very few Reed-Sternberg cells. Variant forms of atypical cells, so-called L and H cells, predominate. These have sparse cytoplasm and delicate, multilobated nuclei with small nucleoli. Reactive cells consist of any combination of small lymphocytes, benign histiocytes, and occasional plasma cells. Neutrophils and eosinophils are usually not present, and necrosis is not associated with this type of disease. Two forms of this type are recognized in the original six-part system: the nodular and the diffuse forms of lymphocytic-histiocytic disease. The diffuse type is more common. In this type, although neoplastic cells may show some clustering, the background cellularity has a diffuse pattern, resembling a diffuse non-Hodgkin's lymphoma at low magnification. In the nodular type the reactive cells of the background are massed into nodules and the neoplastic cells are centrally located within these nodules. At low magnification, this process resembles follicular lymphoma. As was mentioned above, the nodular type may be an aberrant form of follicular hyperplasia rather than a true neoplasm [60].

Mixed cellularity–type Hodgkin's disease contains an intermediate ratio of neoplastic/reactive cells. Reed-Sternberg cells are usually but not always easily identified, and mononuclear variant forms of malignant cells are abundant (Plate 9-5). Reactive cells consist of a combination of lymphocytes, histiocytes, plasma cells, neutrophils, and eosinophils. A "mixed" background, however, of all the various reactive cell types need not be present. There may be suppuration or necrosis or both.

Lymphocytic depletion Hodgkin's disease is clinically the least favorable type. The more common reticular form has a high neoplastic/reactive cell ratio, and extremely large, bizarre, malignant giant cells are often present. Without border zones containing more reactive cells, reticular lymphocytic depletion Hodgkin's disease may not be morphologically distinguishable from large cell non-Hodgkin's lymphoma, or even from anaplastic carcinoma. The diffuse fibrosis form is extremely rare and occurs primarily in starved and exhausted patients. Rare neoplastic cells are present among expanses of loose collagenous matrix and scattered lymphocytes.

Nodular sclerosing Hodgkin's disease is distinctive both clinically and pathologically. There is a strong predilection for supradiaphragmatic disease involving the anterior mediastinum, and young adult females are most commonly affected (see Chap. 118). Part of the reactive background includes fibrosis emanating from the capsule and connective tissue trabeculae. This response begins with the formation of cellular granulation tissue and progresses to the formation of dense bands of hyaline fibrosis which encircle remaining nodules of cells (Plate 9-4). Within these nodules are a mixture of reactive and neoplastic cells, and the cellularity may range from "lymphocytic predominance" to "lymphocytic depletion." Although typical Reed-Sternberg cells are sometimes present, there is often only the presence of so-called lacunar cell variants on which to base the diagnosis. These lacunar cells contain abundant clear cytoplasm which, with formalin fixation, retracts from the surrounding lymphocytes, producing a hole, or lacuna. These bizarre cells contain many nuclear lobes, sometimes in circular or semicircular array at the cell margin and sometimes clustered centrally, each containing a small nucleolus (Plate 9-6). Very early involvement of lymph nodes by nodular sclerosing disease does not yet exhibit capsular or trabecular fibrosis but rather shows only nodules with central clusters of lacunar cells. Such a pattern has been described as a *cellular* or *presclerotic phase* of the disease.

NON-HODGKIN'S LYMPHOMAS

Malignant lymphomas other than Hodgkin's disease are generally referred to as *non-Hodgkin's lymphomas,* even though they represent a very diverse group of neoplasms. Their classification is controversial, but categories will be described here in the format of the proposed working formulation. Synonymous or related types from other classification systems are included (see Fig. 117-1). The order of presentation will be from most favorable to most unfavorable prognosis, according to the findings of the Working Formulation Study [64].

SMALL LYMPHOCYTIC (LOW-GRADE) (TYPE A)

Related terms for this lesion are *well-differentiated lymphocytic* (Rappaport); *lymphocytic; chronic lymphocytic leukemia* and *lymphoplasmacytic-lymphoplasmacytoid immunocytoma* (Kiel); and *small lymphocytic* and *plasmacytoid lymphocytic* (Lukes-Collins).

The growth pattern of this lesion is diffuse (Plate 9-3), although there may be *proliferation centers*, zones of larger cells. The predominant cells are small, inactive-appearing lymphocytes with or without some features of plasma cell differentiation (Plate 10-1). Pleomorphic variant forms occur which can be confused with more aggressive forms of lymphoma or with Hodgkin's disease [1]. The mitotic rate is very low, and most nuclei contain peripherally clumped chromatin. Often, this process is an expression of chronic lymphocytic leukemia or an immunosecretory state. Immunologically, this is a rather homogeneous entity, the vast majority of lesions being B-cell counterparts of the small lymphocytes or plasmacytic lymphocytes of the medullary cord region of the lymph node.

FOLLICULAR, PREDOMINANTLY SMALL CLEAVED CELL (LOW-GRADE) (TYPE B)

Related terms for this lesion are *nodular, poorly differentiated lymphocytic* (Rappaport); *centroblastic-centrocytic, follicular* (Kiel); and *small cleaved follicular center cell, follicular* (Lukes-Collins).

A true follicular growth pattern is present—the prime determinant for the very favorable prognosis (Plate 9-2). Various germinal center cell types are usually present; however, small cells (centrocytes) with irregular, angulated nuclei predominate (Plate 9-2). Small nucleoli are present; the mitotic rate is moderately low. As with the other two groups of follicular lymphoma, the follicular growth pattern serves as a dependable immunologic marker. This, then, is an immunologically pure grouping of tumors composed of B cells, with properties similar to those of normal germinal centers [47,48]. The presence of an associated nodular sclerosis has been shown to imply a particularly favorable prognosis [73].

FOLLICULAR, MIXED SMALL CLEAVED AND LARGE CELL (LOW-GRADE) (TYPE C)

Related terms for this lesion are *nodular, mixed lymphocytic-histiocytic* (Rappaport); *centroblastic-centrocytic, follicular* (Kiel); and *small cleaved, follicular center cell, follicular* and *large cleaved follicular center cell, follicular* (Lukes-Collins).

This type is very similar to the previous one; however, a mixture of small and large germinal center cell types (centrocytes and centroblasts) is present without preponderance of either. In lesions with follicular growth pattern of predominantly small cleaved cells or of mixed small cleaved cells and large cells, zones of diffuse growth, if also present, apparently do not confer a less favorable prognosis [74]. The follicular nature of this group reflects its homogeneous B-cell immunology.

FOLLICULAR, PREDOMINANTLY LARGE CELL (INTERMEDIATE) (TYPE D)

Related terms for this lesion are *nodular, histiocytic* (Rappaport); *centroblastic-centrocytic (large), follicular* (Kiel);

and *large cleaved and/or noncleaved follicular center cell, follicular* (Lukes-Collins).

While various germinal center cell types can be identified, the large cells (centroblasts) predominate, and the mitotic rate may be moderately high (Plate 10-3). Fading of the follicular into a diffuse pattern of growth is often present and is indicative of a less favorable prognosis [74]. Immunologically, the follicular pattern marks these neoplasms as of B-cell (germinal center) type.

DIFFUSE, SMALL CLEAVED CELL (INTERMEDIATE) (TYPE E)

Related terms for this lesion are *diffuse, poorly differentiated lymphocytic* (Rappaport); *centrocytic (small)* (Kiel); and *small cleaved follicular center cell, diffuse* (Lukes-Collins).

This tumor is composed of the same small germinal center cell type (centrocytic) as described for the follicular pattern with small cleaved cells; however, the growth pattern is diffuse (Plates 9-3 and 10-2). Without the follicular growth pattern to serve as definite evidence of a B-cell nature, some lesions of T-cell type may fall into this morphologic grouping.

DIFFUSE, MIXED SMALL AND LARGE CELL (INTERMEDIATE) (TYPE F)

Related terms for this lesion are *diffuse, mixed lymphocytic-histiocytic* (Rappaport); *centroblastic-centrocytic, diffuse* (Kiel); *immunocytoma, polymorphic type* (Kiel); and *small cleaved, large cleaved, or large noncleaved follicular center cell, diffuse* (Lukes-Collins).

This grouping undoubtedly includes a number of neoplasms. While many lesions represent a diffuse counterpart of the follicular, mixed small cleaved and large cell, T-cell lymphomas with a morphologically similar mixed cellular composition have been reported [41,43,57]. Non-Hodgkin's lymphomas with a dense interspersion of epithelioid histiocytes, so-called Lennert's lymphomas, are for the most part included in this category [75]. Polymorphic immunocytoma of the Kiel classification, a neoplasm with plasma cellular differentiation, also is placed within this grouping, although its immunosecretory differentiation suggests that it is deserving of separate placement [1].

DIFFUSE, LARGE CELL (INTERMEDIATE) (TYPE G)

Related terms for this lesion are *diffuse, histiocytic* (Rappaport); *centroblastic-centrocytic (large), diffuse* (Kiel); *centrocytic (large)* (Kiel); *centroblastic, diffuse* (Kiel); and *large cleaved or noncleaved, follicular center cell type, diffuse* (Lukes-Collins).

Large cells with round-to-oval or somewhat irregular (cleaved) nuclei predominate in this group. Nuclear membranes are moderately delicate, and two or more small or medium-sized nucleoli are present, often apposed against the nuclear membrane. A modest amount of basophilic cytoplasm is present (Plate 10-3). The mitotic rate is high. There is some question as to how reliably one can recognize the large follicular center cell types in contradistinction to other (T-cell) large cell types [42,43].

LARGE CELL, IMMUNOBLASTIC (HIGH-GRADE) (TYPE H)

Related terms for this lesions are *diffuse, histiocytic* (Rappaport); *immunoblastic* (Kiel); and *immunoblastic sarcoma, T-,* or *B-cell type* (Lukes-Collins).

Most lesions in this category seen in the Western world are composed of B immunoblasts, which are large cells featuring abundant basophilic cytoplasm and vesicular nuclei with one or more central large nucleoli (Plate 10-4). The distinction of this form of lymphoma from anaplastic plasmacytoma may be purely definitional [76].

The features of T-immunoblastic neoplasms can be similar to those of B-immunoblastic composition. For this reason, the Kiel classification separately recognizes those lesions with conspicuous plasmacytoid differentiation (and thereby evidence of B-cell nature) from those without it. In southern Japan, the incidence of T-cell lymphomas is greater than that of B-cell lymphomas, and many cases of T-immunoblastic neoplasia have been described [57]. Features indicative of T-cell nature include hypervascularity, abundant, clear cytoplasm, heterogeneous nuclear size, and irregularity of nuclear contour with delicate nucleoli [41,43,57].

LYMPHOBLASTIC (HIGH-GRADE) (TYPE I)

Related terms for this lesion are *lymphoblastic, convoluted,* and *nonconvoluted* (Rappaport); *lymphoblastic, convoluted,* or *unclassified* (Kiel); and *convoluted T cell* (Lukes-Collins).

These extremely aggressive neoplasms are a tumorous counterpart to the unfavorable form of acute lymphoblastic leukemia. The cells are of uniform, medium size, with delicate nuclei containing dispersed chromatin and small, inapparent nucleoli (Plate 10-5). Only a scant rim of pale-staining cytoplasm is present. Many of these tumors have some nuclei with narrow creasing or convolutions. The mitotic rate is very high. Immunologically, this is a coherent group of neoplasms of T-cell type or, more accurately, precursor T-cell type [52].

SMALL NONCLEAVED CELL (HIGH-GRADE) (TYPE J)

Related terms for this lesion are *undifferentiated, Burkitt's,* and *pleomorphic, non-Burkitt's* (Rappaport); *lymphoblastic, Burkitt's type,* and *other B-lymphoblastic* (Kiel); and *small noncleaved, follicular center cell* (Lukes-Collins).

Two variants within this group are recognized: the Burkitt's type with uniformity of nuclear size and the pleomorphic or non-Burkitt's type with variations in nuclear size. The nuclei are intermediate in size, approximately equivalent to those of phagocytic histiocytes. Many features resemble those of the lympho-

blastic type (type I); however, the nuclear features are coarser, and there is more abundant basophilic cytoplasm. The nuclear membrane is thick and regular without convolutions, and one to four moderate-sized nucleoli are contained within (Plate 10-6). Mitotic figures are abundant, and there is often an interspersion of macrophages, imparting a "starry sky" appearance. Imprint preparations are useful in offering optimal cytomorphologic detail, which aids in the distinction of this type from lymphoblastic types [77]. In imprints, variations in nuclear size are magnified, so that some such variation is detectable in the Burkitt's as well as pleomorphic variant. Lesions studied immunologically have consistently shown properties of a follicular center B-cell type with membrane and cytoplasmic immunoglobulin [49].

UNCLASSIFIABLE

In about 10 percent of non-Hodgkin's lymphomas the morphologic pattern does not fit into any of the above-described groupings. One reason for the inability to classify all lymphomas relates to the phenomenon of so-called composite lymphoma, in which two types occur simultaneously in the same biopsy [78]. Some examples of this phenomenon can be explained by clonal transformation, that is, when both types are of similar lineage, for example, B-cell. However, such an explanation fails to account for many lymphomas that are presumably unrelated in cytogeneology, for example Hodgkin's disease with non-Hodgkin's lymphoma.

OTHER DISTINCT LYMPHOID NEOPLASMS

Several forms of neoplasia not generally included within the non-Hodgkin's lymphomas are recognized as distinct clinicopathologic entities.

HAIRY CELL LEUKEMIA (LEUKEMIC RETICULOENDOTHELIOSIS)

This disease is characterized by pancytopenia, splenomegaly, and myelofibrosis (see Chap. 116). Cells showing pseudopodial "hairs" are present, sometimes only in small numbers, in blood. Because splenectomy often is an effective therapy, this process should not be mistaken for small lymphocytic lymphoma-leukemia. The hairy cells contain a distinctive isoenzyme of acid phosphatase, which is resistant to tartrate inhibition. Exhaustive studies of the cell type remain inconclusive; however, most cases are of B-cell type with a few showing T-cell or monocytic features [79].

CUTANEOUS T-CELL LYMPHOMA

In patients with Sézary's syndrome and mycosis fungoides, the lesions often progress to extracutaneous malignant lymphoma. Most of the lymphomas arising in this disease setting have cells with deep cerebriform nuclear infoldings. However, there is a wide range in nuclear size and shape. Perhaps the early cutaneous manifestations are part of a continuum of neoplastic progression [55]. Immunologic studies have demonstrated these lesions uniformly to be of T-cell type, often made up of helper T cells [56].

MALIGNANT HISTIOCYTOSIS (TRUE HISTIOCYTIC LYMPHOMA)

Malignancies of the fixed phagocytic histiocyte usually have a fulminant clinical course, with systemic distribution of the mononuclear-phagocytic system (see Chap. 96). Patients characteristically suffer pancytopenia due to phagocytic sequestration of the formed elements of the blood. The diagnosis is based on recognition of both the neoplastic and phagocytic features of the process [80,81]. In recent years, with the application of special histochemical, immunohistochemical, and immunologic studies, large cell neoplasia has been described with histiocytic differentiation without evidence of cellular phagocytosis and with localized growth [1,40,44]. Such neoplasms may be equally well considered as lymphadenopathic anaplastic variants of malignant histiocytosis or as true histiocytic lymphoma.

PLASMA CELL NEOPLASMS

With the modern concept of lymphomas as neoplasms of the immune system, their close relationship with plasma cell neoplasia has become implicit. Although most plasma cell neoplasia takes the form of marrow disease with associated serologic abnormalities, lymphomas with plasma cell differentiation often may exhibit overlapping features. Non-Hodgkin's lymphomas at both ends of the clinical spectrum of disease, that is, small lymphocytic type and immunoblastic type, may show plasma cell features. In such cases the distinction from plasmacytoma, that is, well-differentiated and anaplastic, respectively, may be somewhat arbitrary [1,76].

Future developments

The limitations of a morphologically based classification, such as the "Working Formulation," are obvious in view of immunologic and histochemical studies, which have revealed great diversity within some of the major lymphoma groupings. Widespread acceptance of a more complex classification system, however, will depend on the demonstration of significant differences in therapeutic response among the many fine subdivisions of disease. The working formulation should remain satisfactory for those categories in which morphologic structure defines a biologically homogeneous grouping, for example, follicular and lymphoblastic lymphomas. Among heterogeneous categories, separate subsets should be recognized and parenthetically denoted. For example, within the category of diffuse, mixed small and large cell, the plasmacytoid variant or *polymorphic immunocytoma* of the Kiel classification can be distinguished morphologically [1]. By means of immunologic marker studies, a *pleomorphic T-cell* lymphoma [57], included in this same category, could

be detected. The recognition of such subsets will make possible the discernment of any differences in clinical characteristics.

References

1. Lennert, K.: *Malignant Lymphomas: Other Than Hodgkin's Disease; Histology, Cytology, Ultrastructure, Immunology.* Springer-Verlag, New York, 1978.
2. Mann, R. B., Jaffe, E. S., and Berard, C. W.: Malignant lymphomas— A conceptual understanding of morphologic diversity: A review. *Am. J. Pathol.* 94:105, 1979.
3. Lukes, R. J.: The immunologic approach to the pathology of malignant lymphomas. *Am. J. Clin. Pathol.* 72:657, 1979.
4. Freeman, C., Berg, J. W., and Cutler, S. J.: Occurrence and prognosis of extranodal lymphomas. *Cancer* 29:252, 1972.
5. Jones, S. E.: Non-Hodgkin lymphomas. *JAMA* 234:633, 1975.
6. Berard, C. W., and Dorfman, R. F.: Histopathology of malignant lymphomas. *Clin. Haematol.* 3:39, 1974.
7. Hodgkin, T.: On some morbid appearances of the absorbent glands and spleen. *Trans. Med. Chir. Soc. Lond.* 17:68, 1832.
8. Virchow, R.: Weisses Blut and Milztumoren. *Med. Zgt. Berlin* 15:157, 1846.
9. Virchow, R.: *Die Cellularpathologie in ihrer Begründung auf physiologische und pathologische Gewebelehre.* Hirschwald, Berlin, 1858.
10. Virchow, R.: *Die krankhaften Geschwülste.* Hirschwald, Berlin, 1863.
11. Billroth, T.: Multiple lymphome: Erfolgreiche Behandlung mit Arsenik. *Wien. Med. Wochenschr.* 21:1066, 1871.
12. Wilks, S.: Cases of enlargement of the lymphatic glands and spleen (or Hodgkin's disease). *Guys Hosp. Rep.* 11:56, 1865.
13. Sternberg, C.: Ueber eine eigenartige unter dem Bilde der Pseudoleukämie verlaufende Tuberculose des lymphatischen Apparates. *Z. Heilk.* 19:21, 1898.
14. Reed, D. M.: On the pathological changes in Hodgkin's disease, with especial reference to its relation to tuberculosis. *Johns Hopkins Hosp. Rep.* 10:133, 1902.
15. Ghon, A., and Roman, B.: Über das Lymphosarkom. *Frankfurt. Z. Pathol.* 19:1, 1916.
16. Brill, N. E., Baehr, G., and Rosenthal, N.: Generalized giant lymph follicle hyperplasia of lymph nodes and spleen: A hitherto undescribed type. *JAMA* 84:668, 1925.
17. Symmers, D.: Follicular lymphadenopathy with splenomegaly: A newly recognized disease of the lymphatic system. *Arch. Pathol.* 3:816, 1927.
18. Symmers, D.: Giant follicular lymphadenopathy with or without splenomegaly: Its transformation into polymorphous cell sarcoma of the lymph follicles and its association with Hodgkin's disease, lymphatic leukemia and an apparently unique disease of the lymph nodes and spleen—A disease entity believed heretofore undescribed. *Arch. Pathol.* 26:603, 1938.
19. Roulet, F.: Das primäre Retothelsarkom der Lymphknoten. *Virchows Arch [Pathol. Anat.]* 227:15, 1930.
20. Gall, E. A.: Enigmas in lymphoma: Reticulum cell sarcoma and mycosis fungoides. *Minn. Med.* 38:674, 1955.
21. Cooke, J. V.: Mediastinal tumor in acute leukemia: A clinical and roentgenologic study. *Am. J. Dis. Child.* 44:1153, 1932.
22. Jackson, H., Jr., and Parker, F., Jr.: *Hodgkin's Disease and Allied Disorders.* Oxford, New York, 1947, p. 17.
23. Lukes, R. J., Butler, J. J., and Hicks, E. B.: Natural history of Hodgkin's disease as related to its pathologic picture. *Cancer* 19:317, 1966.
24. Lukes, R. J., Craver, L. F., Hall, T. C., Rappaport, H., and Ruben, P.: Report of the nomenclature committee. *Cancer Res.* 26:1311, 1966.
25. Gall, E. A., Morrison, H. R., and Scott, A. T.: The follicular type of malignant lymphoma: A survey of 63 cases. *Ann. Intern. Med.* 14:2073, 1941.
26. Rappaport, H., Winter, W. J., and Hicks, E. B.: Follicular lymphoma: A re-evaluation of its position in the scheme of malignant lymphoma, based on a survey of 253 cases. *Cancer* 9:792, 1956.
27. Gall, E. A., and Mallory, T. B.: Malignant lymphoma: A clinico-pathologic survey of 618 cases. *Am. J. Pathol.* 18:381, 1942.

28. Gall, E. A., and Rappaport, H.: Seminar on diseases on lymph nodes and spleen, in *Proceedings of the 23rd Seminar of the American Society of Clinical Pathologists*, edited by J. R. McDonald. Am. Soc. Clin. Pathol., Chicago, 1958.

29. Rappaport, H.: Tumors of the hematopoietic system, in *Atlas of Tumor Pathology*. Armed Forces Institute of Pathology, Washington, D. C., 1966, sec. III, fasc. 8.

30. Jones, S. E., et al.: Non-Hodgkin's lymphomas. IV. Clinicopathologic correlation in 405 cases. *Cancer* 31:806, 1973.

31. Rosenberg, S. A.: Non-Hodgkin's lymphoma—Selection of treatment on the basis of histologic type. *N. Engl. J. Med.* 301:924, 1979.

32. Lennert, K.: Classification of malignant lymphomas (European concept), in *Progress in Lymphology*, edited by A. Rüttimann. Thieme, Stuttgart, 1967, pp. 103–109.

33. Stein, H., Lennert, K., and Parwaresch, M. R.: Malignant lymphomas of B-cell type. *Lancet* 2:855, 1972.

34. Stein, H., Kaiserling, E., and Lennert, K.: Evidence for B-cell origin of reticulum cell sarcoma. *Virchows Arch.* [*Pathol. Anat.*] 364:51, 1974.

35. Morris, M. W., and Davey, F. R.: Immunologic and cytochemical properties of histiocytic and mixed histiocytic-lymphocytic lymphomas. *Am. J. Clin. Pathol.* 63:403, 1975.

36. Taylor, C. R.: An immunohistological study of follicular lymphoma, reticulum cell sarcoma and Hodgkin's disease. *Eur. J. Cancer* 12:61, 1976.

37. Jaffe, E. S., Braylan, R. C., Nanba, K., Frank, M. M., and Berard, C. W.: Functional markers: A new perspective on malignant lymphomas, *Cancer Treat. Rep.* 61:953, 1977.

38. Lukes, R. J., Taylor, C. R., Parker, J. W., Lincoln, T. L., Pattengale, P. K., and Tindle, B. H.: A morphologic and immunologic surface marker study of 299 cases of non-Hodgkin lymphomas and related leukemias. *Am. J. Pathol.* 90:461, 1978.

39. Van Heerde, P., Feltkamp, C. A., Feltkamp-Vroom, T. M., Koudstaal, J., and van Unnik, J. A. M.: Non-Hodgkin's lymphoma: Immunohistochemical and electron microscopical findings in relation to light-microscopy; a study of 74 cases. *Cancer* 46:2210, 1980.

40. Li, C.-Y., and Harrison, E. G., Jr.: Histochemical and immunohistochemical study of diffuse large-cell lymphomas. *Am. J. Clin. Pathol.* 70:721, 1978.

41. Waldron, J. A., Leech, J. A., Glick, A. D., Flexner, J. M., and Collins, R. D.: Malignant lymphoma of peripheral T-lymphocyte origin: Immunologic, pathologic, and clinical features in six patients. *Cancer* 40:1604, 1977.

42. Pinkus, G. S., Said, J. W., and Hargreaves, H.: Malignant lymphoma, T-cell type: A distinct morphologic variant with large multilobated nuclei, with a report of four cases. *Am. J. Clin. Pathol.* 72:540, 1979.

43. Palutke, M., et al.: T-cell lymphomas of large cell type: A variety of malignant lymphomas; "histiocytic" and mixed lymphocytic-"histiocytic." *Cancer* 46:87, 1980.

44. Koh, S.-J., Vargas, G. F., Caces, J. N., and Johnson, W. W.: Malignant "histiocytic" lymphoma in childhood. *Am. J. Clin. Pathol.* 74:417, 1980.

45. Lennert, K., and Niedorf, H. R.: Nachweis von desmosomal verknüpften Reticulumzellen im follikulären Lymphom (Brill Symmers). *Virchows Arch.* [*Cell Pathol.*] 4:148, 1969.

46. Levine, G. D., and Dorfman, R. F.: Nodular lymphoma: An ultrastructural study of its relationship to germinal centers and a correlation of light and electron microscopic findings. *Cancer* 35:148, 1975.

47. Lennert, K.: Follicular lymphoma: A tumor of the germinal centers. *Gann Monogr. Cancer Res.* 15:217, 1973.

48. Jaffe, E. S., Shevach, E. M. Frank, M. M., Berard, C. W., and Green, I.: Nodular lymphoma—Evidence for origin from follicular B lymphocytes. *N. Engl. J. Med.* 290:813, 1974.

49. Mann, R. B., et al.: Non-endemic Burkitt's lymphoma: A B-cell tumor related to germinal centers. *N. Engl. J. Med.* 295:685, 1976.

50. Nathwani, B. N., Kim, H., and Rappaport, H.: Malignant lymphoma, lymphoblastic. *Cancer* 38:964, 1976.

51. Smith, J. L., Clein, G. P., Barker, C. R., and Collins, R. D.: Characterisation of malignant mediastinal lymphoid neoplasm (Sternberg sarcoma) as thymic in origin. *Lancet* 1:74, 1973.

52. Stein, H., Petersen, N., Gaedicke, G., Lennert, K., and Landbeck, G.: Lymphoblastic lymphoma of convoluted or acid phosphatase type—A tumor of T precursor cells. *Int. J. Cancer* 17:292, 1976.

53. Long, J. C., McCaffrey, R. P., Aisenberg, A. C., Marks, S. M., and Kung, P. C.: Terminal deoxynucleotidyl transferase positive lymphoblastic lymphoma: A study of 15 cases. *Cancer* 44:2127, 1979.

54. Nanba, K., Jaffe, E. S., Braylan, R. C., Soban, E. J., and Berard, C. W.: Alkaline phosphatase–positive malignant lymphoma: A subtype of B-cell lymphomas. *Am. J. Clin. Pathol.* 68:535, 1977.

55. Lutzner, M., Edelson, R., Schein, P., Green, I., Kirkpatrick, C., and Ahmed, A.: Cutaneous T-cell lymphomas: The Sézary syndrome, mycosis fungoides, and related disorders. *Ann. Intern. Med.* 83:534, 1975.

56. Broder, S., et al.: The Sézary syndrome: A malignant proliferation of helper T cells. *J. Clin. Invest.* 58:1297, 1976.

57. Watanabe, S., Nakajima, T., Shimosato, Y., Syimoyama, M., and Minato, K.: T-cell malignancies: Subclassification and interrelationship. *Jpn. J. Clin. Oncol. 9* (Suppl. 1):423, 1979.

58. Kadin, M. E., Stites, D. P., Levy, R., and Warnke, R.: Exogenous immunoglobulin and the macrophage origin of Reed-Sternberg cells in Hodgkin's disease. *N. Engl. J. Med.* 299:1208, 1978.

59. Kaplan, H. S.: Hodgkin's disease: Unfolding concepts concerning its nature, management and prognosis. *Cancer* 45:2439, 1980.

60. Poppema, S., Kaiserling, E., and Lennert, K.: Nodular paragranuloma and progressively transformed germinal centers: Ultrastructural and immunohistologic findings. *Virchows Arch.* [*Cell Pathol.*] 31:211, 1979.

61. Banks, P. M., and Berard, C. W.: Histopathology of the malignant lymphomas, in *Hematology*, 2d ed., edited by W. J. Williams, E. Beutler, A. J. Erslev, and R. W. Rundles. McGraw-Hill, New York, 1977, pp. 1026–1037.

62. Stein, H., Tolksdorf, G., Burkert, M., and Lennert, K.: Cytologic classification of non-Hodgkin's lymphomas based on morphology, cytochemistry, and immunology, in *Advances in Medical Oncology, Research and Education*, edited by D. G. Crowther. Pergamon, New York, 1979, vol. 7, pp. 141–152.

63. Lukes, R. J., and Collins, R. D.: Immunologic characterization of human malignant lymphomas. *Cancer* 34:1488, 1974.

64. The Non-Hodgkin's Lymphoma Pathologic Classification Group: NCI sponsored study of classifications of non-Hodgkin's lymphomas: Summary and description of a working formulation for clinical usage. *Cancer* 49:2112, 1982.

65. Banks, P. M., Long, J. C., and Howard, C. A.: Preparation of lymph node biopsy specimens. *Hum. Pathol.* 10:617, 1979.

66. Dorfman, R. F., and Warnke, R.: Lymphadenopathy simulating the malignant lymphomas. *Hum. Pathol.* 5:519, 1974.

67. Keller, A. R., Hochholzer, L., and Castleman, B.: Hyaline-vascular and plasma-cell types of giant lymph node hyperplasia of the mediastinum and other locations. *Cancer* 29:670, 1972.

68. Rosai, J., and Dorfman, R. F.: Sinus histiocytosis with massive lymphadenopathy: A newly recognized benign clinicopathological entity. *Arch. Pathol.* 87:63, 1969.

69. Frizzera, G., Moran, E. M., and Rappaport, H.: Angio-immunoblastic lymphadenopathy: Diagnosis and clinical course. *Am. J. Med.* 59:803, 1975.

70. Hartsock, R. J.: Postvaccinial lymphadenitis: Hyperplasia of lymphoid tissue that simulates malignant lymphomas. *Cancer* 21:632, 1968.

71. Frizzera, G., et al.: Polymorphic diffuse B-cell hyperplasias and lymphomas in renal transplant recipients. *Cancer Res.* 41:4262, 1981.

72. Strum, S. B., Park, J. K., and Rappaport, H.: Observation of cells resembling Sternberg-Reed cells in conditions other than Hodgkin's disease. *Cancer* 26:176, 1970.

73. Millett, Y. L., Bennett, M. H., Jelliffe, A. M., and Farrer-Brown, G.: Nodular sclerotic lymphosarcoma: A further review. *Br. J. Cancer* 23:683, 1969.

74. Warnke, R. A., Kim, H., Fuks, Z., and Dorfman, R. F.: The coexistence of nodular and diffuse patterns in nodular non-Hodgkin's lymphomas: Significance and clinicopathologic correlation. *Cancer* 40:1229, 1977.

75. Kim, H., Jacobs, C., Warnke, R. A., and Dorfman, R. F.: Malignant lymphoma with a high content of epithelioid histiocytes: A distinct clinicopathologic entity and a form of so-called "Lennert's lymphoma." *Cancer* 41:620, 1978.

76. Banks, P. M., Keller, R. H., Li, C.-Y., and White, W. L.: Malignant

lymphoma of plasmablastic identity: A neoplasm with both "immunoblastic" and plasma cellular features. *Am. J. Med. 64*:906, 1978.

77. Banks, P. M., Arseneau, J. C., Gralnick, H. R., Canellos, G. P., DeVita, V. T., Jr., and Berard, C. W.: American Burkitt's lymphoma: A clinicopathologic study of 30 cases. II. Pathologic correlations. *Am. J. Med. 58*:322, 1975.

78. Kim, H., Hendrickson, M. R., and Dorfman, R. F.: Composite lymphoma. *Cancer 40*:959, 1977.

79. Cawley, J. C., Burns, G. F., and Hayhoe, F. G. J.: Hairy-cell leukaemia. *Recent Results Cancer Res. 72*:1, 1980.

80. Warnke, R. A., Kim, H., and Dorfman, R. F.: Malignant histiocytosis (histiocytic medullary reticulosis). I. Clinicopathologic study of 29 cases. *Cancer 35*:215, 1975.

81. Risdall, R. J., Sibley, R. K., McKenna, R. W., Brunning, R. D., and Dehner, L. P.: Malignant histiocytosis: A light-microscopial and electronmicroscopic and histochemical study. *Am. J. Surg. Pathol. 4*:439, 1980.

CHAPTER *118*

Hodgkin's disease

ERIC P. LESTER
JOHN E. ULTMANN

Definition

Hodgkin's disease (HD) is a neoplastic disorder originating in lymphoid tissue. Usually occurring in adults and initially localized, it subsequently spreads to contiguous lymphoid structures and ultimately disseminates to nonlymphoid tissues with a potentially fatal outcome. It is defined by the presence of the Reed-Sternberg cell. This giant bi- or multinucleated histiocyte-like cell possesses nuclei with large distinctive, acidophilic nucleoli, and occurs in an environment of variable numbers of lymphocytes, plasma cells, eosinophils, granulocytes, and fibroblasts with variable degrees of accompanying fibrosis. Since cells resembling Reed-Sternberg cells may occur in other disorders, both typical Reed-Sternberg cells and an appropriate cellular milieu are required for positive diagnosis. Four main histologic subtypes of HD (lymphocyte predominance, nodular sclerosis, mixed cellularity, and lymphocyte depletion), each associated with characteristic clinical features, are distinguished on the basis of the relative proportions of Reed-Sternberg cells, lymphocytes, and fibrosis. For an individual patient, histologic subtype and anatomic extent of disease are the two primary factors determining prognosis and appropriate therapy.

Over the past 20 years, modern radiotherapy of localized disease and combination chemotherapy for disseminated disease have revolutionized treatment and made HD one of the most curable of major neoplasms. Nonetheless, HD remains for a minority of patients a chronic, relapsing and potentially fatal disease and involves repeated and often unsuccessful courses of therapy. Furthermore, many issues such as the nature of the malignant cell, the role of immunologic defects, proper methods of staging, and optimal treatment strategies remain unresolved.

History

Thomas Hodgkin, of Guy's Hospital, London, was the first to recognize the disease as a distinct entity [1]. In his report to the Medical-Surgical Society in 1832, he described the autopsy findings and brief clinical histories of seven cases, six of whom he had personally examined. While one of these cases had evidence of tuberculosis and another syphilis, be believed that "this enlargement of the glands appeared to be a primitive (i.e., primary) affection of those bodies, rather than the result of an irritation propagated to them from some ulcerated surface or other inflamed texture through the medium of their inferent vessels." He noted that the spleen was involved in six of these cases with "defined bodies of various sizes, in structure resembling that of the diseased glands," and believed that the disease was essentially a "hypertrophy of the lymphatic system" [1]. Subsequent histologic examination of tissues preserved for 97 years in the museum of Guy's Hospital from three of Hodgkin's cases confirmed the diagnosis of HD [2].

In 1856, Sir Samuel Wilks independently described a "peculiar disease of the spleen and an enlargement of the lymphatic glands" [3]. He discovered Hodgkin's earlier report, added six additional cases, and, in 1865, published a subsequent series of 15 cases which definitively established the entity he termed "Hodgkin's disease" [4]. Unaware of the English reports, Wunderlich, in 1858, described two cases of "progressive multiple lymph gland hypertrophy" [5]. Trousseau, in 1865, reported several cases of "l'adénie" [6], adding to the list of synonyms for HD, which has included lymphogranuloma, lymphoadenoma, granuloma malignum, pseudoleukemia, lymphoblastoma, and many others.

Probably because of its similarity to tuberculosis, many physicians believed that HD was reactive or infectious rather than malignant. Wilks, however, lacking all but the crudest histologic information, stated that the disease "must take its place in the rank of malignant diseases, or amongst those afflictions which are characterized by the development of new growths in the system." He believed further that "the lymphatic glands appear to be affected for a considerable period, perhaps many years, before the system suffers, and that next the spleen becomes especially involved and afterwards the other organs; . . . propagation takes place in the course of the lymphatics, and the reason why the corpuscles of the spleen are thus affected arises from the fact of their being intimately connected with the absorbent system" [4].

The works of Virchow [7], Craigie [8], Bennett [9], and many other nineteenth century pathologists gradually established the leukemias and lymphomas as entities related to but distinct from HD. Sternberg [10] in 1898 and Dorothy Reed [11] in 1902 followed these observations with the first definitive descriptions of the histopathology of HD, which Reed characterized as "a peculiar and typical histologic picture, consisting of proliferations of the endothelial and reticular cells, formation of lymphoid cells and characteristic giant cells, and a gradual increase of connective tissue, resulting in fibrosis, and, in most of the specimens, in the presence of great numbers of eosinophiles." These "characteristic giant cells" possess "a nucleus which is always large in proportion to the size of the cell . . . single or multiple . . . often bean-shaped and irregularly indented. . . . The chromatin network is prominent . . . and one or more large nucleoli are always present and have an affinity for acid dyes." Despite the accuracy of these descriptions, Sternberg viewed HD as a form of tuberculosis, and Reed saw it, by virtue of its infrequent invasion through lymph node capsule, as a nonmalignant inflammatory disease distinct from tuberculosis. Controversy over its origin led to investigations of tubercle bacilli [12,13], diphtheroid bacteria [14], *Brucella* [15], *Mycobacterium avium* [16], various fungi, and viruses [17] as possible etiologic agents, but to no avail. Between 1930 and 1950 major advances included the recognition by Rosenthal [18] and Jackson and Parker [19] of histologic subtypes of HD correlating with prognosis, and the development by Peters [20,21] of a clinical staging system to classify the anatomic extent of disease.

Treatment of HD in the nineteenth century consisted of the use of surgery, arsenicals, iodides, serum preparations, and other medications, all ineffective. Pusey in 1902 [22] and Senn in 1903 [23], both working in Chicago, first reported impressive responses of HD to x-ray therapy. Doses of up to 2000 rads, using kilovoltage equipment became standard palliative therapy in the early twentieth century. Gilbert in 1939 proposed the concept of systematically treating both involved and adjacent uninvolved nodal areas [24], and subsequent work [25] demonstrated a modest but significant prolongation of survival in patients thus treated. The development of megavoltage radiotherapy equipment after 1950 permitted Kaplan to explore the relationship between survival and radiation dosage. His evidence indicated that intensive megavoltage doses (>4000 rads) provided far better survival in localized disease than lower orthovoltage doses, and thus it became realistic to speak of the cure of some patients with early HD [26,27]. This potential made accurate estimation of the extent and localization of disease imperative in planning treatment and was responsible for the widespread application of both lymphangiography [28] and staging laparotomy with splenectomy [29] for evaluation of possible intraabdominal sites of disease. Modern concepts of staging were codified at a conference held at Rye, New York, in 1965 [30] and were subsequently refined at the Workshop on the Staging of Hodgkin's Disease held at Ann Arbor, Michigan, in 1971 [31].

Modern, effective chemotherapy was developed concurrently with these advances in staging and radiotherapy. The alkylating agents, created as an outgrowth of studies on nitrogen mustard during World War II by Jacobson et al. [32] and Goodman et al. [33], provided the first agents capable of producing impressive tumor shrinkage and significant palliation of HD. The subsequent development of synthetic adrenal corticosteroids, vinca alkaloids, and procarbazine, agents with differing modes of action and toxicities, made it possible for DeVita and his coworkers to design the first effective combination chemotherapy regimen, MOPP (nitrogen mustard, vincristine, procarbazine, and prednisone) [34].

Etiology and pathogenesis

The etiology of HD remains unknown. The intimate admixture of a wide variety of cellular elements, many having a normal or reactive appearance, initially led to the conclusion that HD was an infectious or inflammatory disease. That it is a true malignancy now seems certain, although controversy remains concerning the origin and behavior of the malignant cell. The characteristic giant cell, either the bi- or multinucleate Reed-Sternberg cell or its uninuclear counterpart the *Hodgkin's cell*, is uniformly present in HD, although its number, and the number of surrounding "reactive" elements, vary. Cases with aggressive clinical behavior often contain large numbers of Hodgkin's or Reed-Sternberg cells, often exhibiting flagrant cytologic features of malignancy (e.g., "Hodgkin's sarcoma," now termed *lymphocyte depletion Hodgkin's disease*). Indolent cases often have only rare Reed-Sternberg cells and an abundance of normal-appearing lymphocytes (e.g., "Hodgkin's paragranuloma" or the modern *lymphocyte predominance HD*). Thus, the malignant cell population appears to be made up of Hodgkin's cells and Reed-Sternberg cells which are capable of eliciting a variety of local responses characterized by a variable infiltration with eosinophils, granulocytes, plasma cells, normal appearing lymphocytes, and fibrosis.

Chromosome analysis of tissue involved with HD has usually revealed a mixture of both normal and abnormal karyotypes. Normal karyotypes are most likely derived from nonmalignant reactive elements, whereas abnormal karyotypes, which are often hypotetraploid in modal chromosome number, are thought to represent the population of Hodgkin's and Reed-Sternberg cells [35]. Many of the abnormal karyotypes contain marker chromosomes and, in some cases, clear-cut evidence of clonal karyotypic abnormalities is found. While no consistent karyotypic abnormality has been found, a number of the relatively small group of cases studied with modern Giemsa banding techniques have shown additional chromatin added to the long arm of chromosome 14 (14q+), an abnormality frequently encountered in the non-Hodgkin's lymphomas [36,37]. Quantitation of the DNA content of individual Reed-Sternberg and Hodgkin's cells in HD tissue has revealed widely ranging DNA contents with many in the diploid or hyperdiploid range and many at hypotetraploid levels [38,39].

Autoradiography of cell suspensions from freshly excised tumor has confirmed that both mononuclear and binuclear Hodgkin's cells are capable of active DNA synthesis as are the surrounding nonmalignant cells [40–43]. Both the malignant and nonmalignant cell populations show very considerable proliferation, and, since the doubling time of such tumors in vivo is of the order of 30 days, substantial cell death must be continuously occurring [44]. Autoradiography indicates that Reed-Sternberg cells originate by a failure of cell division after nuclear replication rather than by cell fusion [42].

The presence of a variety of nonmalignant cell types and the demonstration of DNA synthesis in lymphocytes in Hodgkin's tissue suggests that Hodgkin's disease may represent a "civil war" within the immune system in which the nonmalignant cells are attempting to destroy the Hodgkin's cell population bearing tumor-specific antigens [45–47]. An antiserum initially thought to recognize a Hodgkin's specific tumor antigen was subsequently shown to recognize ferritin which is present in large quantities on the surface of Hodgkin's cells [48,49]. No clear demonstration of a Hodgkin's-specific antigen has been made. The majority of lymphocytes separated from HD biopsies are activated T cells [50]. These T cells respond poorly to the T-cell mitogen phytohemagglutin [51], and may be the source of the ferritin on Hodgkin's cells since peripheral blood lymphocytes from patients with HD show increased synthesis and release of ferritin [52]. A cytotoxic effect of these lymphocytes on Reed-Sternberg cells has been described [53], but recent studies have found no evidence of direct cytotoxicity [54]. Viable, isolated Hodgkin's cells were found to specifically bind T lymphocytes, and clusters of Hodgkin's cells and lymphocytes have persisted in culture for up to 5 weeks with no evidence of cytotoxicity. Nonetheless, other observers have suggested that prognosis is improved in patients who display a high proportion of Hodgkin's cells with attached lymphocytes [55].

Early observers suggested that malignant histiocytes were the neoplastic elements [56]. Furthermore recent ultrastructural examinations of these cells demonstrate numerous cytoplasmic microfibrils and surface processes, indicating that they originate from a macrophage lineage [57]. However, immunoblasts, which are lymphocytes stimulated by an antigen or mitogen, may morphologically resemble Hodgkin's cells, and this led to the proposal that these cells are malignant B lymphocytes [46,47,58]. The finding of surface and cytoplasmic immunoglobulin in these cells lent further support to this hypothesis [59,60]. Subsequent investigation, however, revealed that many Hodgkin's cells in a given preparation may lack immunoglobulin and that κ and λ immunoglobulin light chains are often simultaneously present in a single Hodgkin's cell [61–63]. Since an individual B lymphocyte may synthesize either κ or λ

chains, but never both, this finding strongly suggests that the immunoglobulin in Hodgkin's cells is derived from plasma. T-cell markers, e.g., the capacity to form rosettes with sheep erythrocytes or react with antithymocyte sera, have not been found on these cells. On the other hand, immunofluorescence reactivity with an antiserum raised against malignant B cells, from a patient with chronic lymphocytic leukemia has been reported [64].

The origin of Hodgkin's cells has been most clearly elucidated by studies of these cells in tissue culture. Giant cells with one or more nuclei have been grown for periods of up to a few months in cultures derived from 25 spleens invaded by Hodgkin's disease, but not from 50 control, uninvolved spleens [42]. Many of these cells had the morphologic appearance of Reed-Sternberg cells, possessed aneuploid karyotypes, and grew as tumors when inoculated intracerebrally into nude mice, indicating their neoplastic character. Furthermore, they displayed macrophage characteristics, including cell surface receptors for the Fc portion of immunoglobulin molecules, receptors for the C3b component of complement, phagocytic ability, and lysozyme secretion. They lacked the B-cell characteristics of surface IgG and C3d receptors. Intracellular fibronectin [65], albumin, and α_1 antitrypsin have also been reported in Reed-Sternberg cells [66]. Nonspecific esterase cytochemical activity, a macrophage characteristic, was seen in 30 percent of the cells cultured from one case and has been variably reported in Hodgkin's cells in lymph node biopsies [62,67]. An aneuploid, heterotransplantable cell line from a patient with HD has shown nonspecific esterase activity and phagocytosis, although it does not secrete lysozyme [68]. Thus, present evidence favors a macrophage-histiocyte origin for Hodgkin's cells.

Epidemiology

Hodgkin's disease is an uncommon neoplasm, accounting for about 6900 of all new cases of cancer in the United States and about 1900 deaths per year [69]. In a study of a U.S. metropolitan area, HD had an overall incidence rate of 3.6 per 100,000 person-years for males and 2.6 for females [70]. Unlike most malignancies, which show a steadily increasing incidence with age, the age-distribution of Hodgkin's disease is bimodal for both sexes, with a peak in the late twenties followed by a decline to age 40 to 45, and a subsequent, gradual increase with age [71]. Nodular sclerosis HD and infiltration of involved nodes with eosinophils [72] are more common in younger patients, especially females; infradiaphragmatic presentations and mixed cellularity HD are more frequent in the elderly [73–75]. Some authors have inferred separate etiologies for cases in young adults as opposed to the elderly, but it seems equally likely that tissue responses to HD may differ with age [76].

There is considerable geographic variation in age-incidence pattern for HD, particularly in relation to levels of socioeconomic development. While there appears to be a universal increase with advancing age beyond middle years, the incidence peak in young adults, with low levels in children, is characteristic of developed countries and economically advanced regions within a given country [77]. Underdeveloped countries and less advanced sections of developed countries show a shift of this peak toward childhood, particularly in boys. Countries such as Israel [78] and Yugoslavia and rural regions of developed countries such as Norway [77] and the United States show an intermediate pattern.

Epidemiologic investigations have shown additional associations of HD with higher social and educational levels [70,76,79–82], particularly for nodular sclerosis HD [80] and among females, regardless of the degree of urbanization [79]. Tonsillectomy in childhood, which may be a function of income level, has been reported as a risk factor for HD [83–86]. Some studies using sibling controls have found an association between tonsillectomy and risk of HD [83,86,87], while contrary results have also been found [80,88,89]. Tonsillectomy and higher social class also have been found as risk factors for paralytic poliomyelitis, a rare sequel occurring in older children and adults to infection with a virus commonly associated with a benign, nonparalytic infection in childhood [90]. This evidence has been used to suggest that HD is caused by infection with a widespread virus possessing an oncogenic potential which is low but increases with age at the time of infection [91,92]. In accordance with this hypothesis is the increased risk with decreasing family size and low risk for persons in fifth or subsequent birth-order position. In one study, an only child had an 80 percent greater risk of HD than a child with siblings [83]. Another study using matched controls also documented an inverse association between HD risk and both the number of family units in the childhood dwelling and the number of neighborhood playmates. This study also reported an increased risk in Jews compared to Catholics [70]. Findings in some studies that HD patients were taller than controls may reflect a higher social class and better nutrition [93,94].

A shared environment in childhood may partially explain the up to sevenfold increased risk for the siblings of young adults with HD [95–97]. Additional reports of cases of HD in a parent and child [98,99] and three reports of pairs of HD cases in monozygotic twins [99–101] suggest that genetic factors may also play a role. A family with seven cases of HD, eight other lymphoid malignancies, four embryonic tumors, 13 cases of common variable immunodeficiency, and elevated serum IgD levels has been described in an inbred population in Newfoundland [102,103]. Pooled data from several retrospective studies have suggested a relatively weak association of the A1, B5, and, particularly, B18 antigens with HD [104]. The B18 antigen has been implicated in the Newfoundland population [105]. However, such associations have not been substantiated in prospective studies [106,107].

The possibility of infectious transmission of HD has

been proposed on the basis of evidence suggesting "clustering" of cases within a population. In some familial cases, the dates of onset have been close, suggesting a common exposure to an etiologic environmental agent [108]. In 1971 in Albany, New York, 12 cases, later enlarged to 31, were reported which could be linked by social contact to one high school graduating class [109,110]. A subsequent study of schools in two other New York counties found nearly three times as many HD cases as expected in schools in which an initial case had been present [111]. Similar associations have been observed elsewhere [112–117], but the methodology of such retrospective studies has been criticized, and careful studies of other populations have failed to reveal significant "clustering" [89,118–122]. With one exception [123], no increase in HD in persons occupationally exposed to HD, such as teachers or physicians, has been found [124–126]. Thus, the evidence for the "contagion" hypothesis is unconvincing at present.

Another body of epidemiologic evidence suggests a possible relationship between HD and the Epstein-Barr virus (EBV), the causative agent of infectious mononucleosis. EBV has also been implicated as a cause of Burkitt's lymphoma [127] and is clearly capable of transforming normal B lymphocytes in vitro into cells possessing malignant characteristics [128]. While positive serologic tests indicating prior EBV infection are no more common in HD patients than controls, their antibody titers are generally higher [129–132]. In addition, a number of studies have found an approximately threefold increase in risk of HD in individuals with a clinical history of infectious mononucleosis [70,133–136]. Whether this means that EBV is the cause of at least some cases of HD or simply that clinically apparent infection with EBV may serve as a marker of an individual at greater risk for developing HD is unclear. However, with sensitive nucleic acid hybridization techniques [137], no evidence for the presence of the EBV genome in HD tissue has been found, nor has the EBV-related nuclear antigen been found in Hodgkin's cells [138].

In view of their demonstrated oncogenicity in animal systems [139], type C RNA viruses have also been examined as possible etiologic agents for HD. While no epidemiologic evidence for such a possibility exists, evidence of nucleic acid sequence homology between the RNA of the Rauscher murine leukemia virus and RNA from some tissues involved with HD has been found [140,141]. Furthermore, evidence for the presence of reverse transcriptase, characteristic of type C RNA tumor viruses, has also been found in Hodgkin's tissue [142,143]. However, electron microscopy has generally failed to find in these tissues particles with the characteristic viral morphology seen in animal tumors [144].

Other epidemiologic data suggest that individuals in woodworking occupations have a two- to fourfold increased risk of HD [82,145–147]. The effects of hydantoin drugs such as Dilantin on the immune system have also been used to explain the possible association between their use and HD and non-Hodgkin's lymphoma [148]. In keeping with this concept is the finding of an increased incidence of Hodgkin's and non-Hodgkin's lymphoma in patients with immunodeficiencies [149] and autoimmune diseases [150].

IMMUNOLOGIC ABNORMALITIES

In 1928, Ewing noted that "tuberculosis follows Hodgkin's disease like a shadow" [151]. This clinical association in populations with high endemic rates of tuberculosis, coupled with the lack of cutaneous reactivity to administered tuberculin, even in patients with active tuberculosis, has led to the recognition of serious deficits in the cellular immune system of patients with HD. Systematic studies of skin test reactivity, largely a T-cell function, have revealed a decreased frequency of responsiveness to a variety of ubiquitous natural antigens such as *Candida, Tricophyton,* or mumps [152–159]. Decreased immune reactivity correlates generally with both the advanced stages of HD and the presence of systemic symptoms. Abnormal responses have only occasionally been seen in patients with stage IA disease [154,155,158]. Variations in the responsiveness of an individual patient may correlate with periods of disease activity and remission [160]. Homograft rejection, another function of the cellular immune system, is also delayed in HD patients [161]. More detailed testing using sensitization and subsequent skin testing with suboptimal doses of 2,4-dinitrochlorobenzene (DNCB) has revealed defective responses in the majority of patients, even those with early disease [155–157,160,162].

In contrast, humoral immunity, which is largely a B-cell function, is usually intact in patients with HD until very late in the course of the disease [162–165]. Serum immunoglobulin levels are usually normal or elevated and primary and secondary antibody responses are generally normal [162,166,165]. In spleens from patients with HD, immunoglobulin synthesis may be markedly increased if little or no tumor is present but decreased with heavy tumor involvement [167]. Other studies, however, have noted impaired antibody formation in a proportion of patients, particularly to new antigens [168–170] and in individuals who are post splenectomy and have received combined radiotherapy and chemotherapy [171,172]. Conversely, autoantibodies are sometimes seen; immune thrombocytopenia and Coombs'-positive hemolytic anemia may occur [173]. Elevated serum IgE has been found in about 40 percent of patients [174,175], and rare patients with monoclonal paraproteins have been reported [176]. Antilymphocyte antibodies have been found in HD patients and their relatives, supporting the hypothesis that the immunologic deficit in HD may be an underlying defect predisposing to the development of HD [177,178].

Lymphocytopenia is found in 20 to 50 percent of patients with HD, but is significantly more common in patients with advanced diseased [154–156,179]. A parallel decrease in circulating T and B lymphocytes is seen [180,181] but appears insufficient to explain the in vivo immune deficit since some anergic patients may have normal lymphocyte counts [156,182]. In vitro tests of lymphocyte function have revealed more extensive evidence of deficiencies, particularly in T-cell functions. Morphologic lymphoblastoid transformation and growth stimulation by mitogenic plant lectins such as phytohemagglutinin (PHA) or concanavalin A or by antigens such as PPD are characteristic T-cell responses which are impaired in blood lymphocytes of patients with HD [154,181–185]. However, unstimulated cultures may contain an increased number of large, "transformed" lymphocytes synthesizing DNA. Such in vitro unresponsiveness to antigens is more severe in patients with advanced stages of disease [182,184]. Furthermore, cap formation by concanavalin A bound to the surface of lymphocytes [186,187] and production of cytotoxic T cells [188] and lymphokines [189,190] after mitogen activation are reduced. While the proportion of T lymphocytes in HD patients is usually normal when measured with an assay utilizing cytotoxic anti-human-thymocyte serum, the proportion of these cells capable of binding sheep erythrocytes (E-rosetting cells, another T-cell characteristic) is significantly reduced [181]. Incubation of HD lymphocytes with fetal calf or fetal human serum will restore both their PHA responsiveness and their E-rosetting capacity [181,191] suggesting the prior presence on their surface of a blocking factor which may be present in HD tissue extracts [192] or serum [193]. Evidence that a glycolipid derived from HD tissue [194] or apoferritin [195] may be such a factor has been presented.

The reduced responsiveness of HD lymphocytes to PHA may also be related to the presence of prostaglandin-producing macrophages [196] and to an increased number of supressor T cells [197]. Reduced T-cell colony formation in vitro in soft agar which is not corrected by addition of conditioned medium from normal PHA-stimulated lymphocytes has been reported [198]. An increased proportion of T cells in the spleens of HD patients [199,200] may also play a role in the development of cellular immune defects. Serum complement components are generally normal or elevated [172,201,202], but assays for immune complexes, including the presence of macromolecular C3, C1q binding, and C3d levels have been abnormal in HD patients [202,203].

Radiotherapy and chemotherapy may also decrease cellular immune reactivity in treated HD patients [181,204,205]. Such effects, however, cannot entirely explain the persistence of in vitro immunologic abnormalities seen in long-term survivors of advanced HD after treatment, since patients in remission after similar treatment for advanced histiocytic lymphoma display normal immunologic function [206].

Clinical features

Enlargement of the superficial lymph nodes is the most common presenting complaint and is evident at the time of diagnosis in about 70 percent of patients with

HD; 60 to 80 percent have cervical, 6 to 20 percent axillary, and 6 to 12 percent have inguinal node involvement. Mediastinal nodes are enlarged in up to 60 percent [207] and retroperitoneal nodes in about 25 percent of cases at presentation [208]. Lymphadenopathy is usually "rubbery" and nontender, but may produce pain by compression of adjacent structures. Rarely massive, such nodes have most often been present for weeks to months and may occasionally wax and wane in size. Hepatosplenomegaly, pulmonary signs or symptoms, or other evidence of organ disease is uncommon at presentation, and suggests an advanced stage and adverse histologic subtype such as lymphocyte depletion HD.

Fever, usually low-grade, and night sweats are initially present in about one-quarter to one-third of patients but are more common in later stages of disease [209]. The classic Pel-Epstein fever [210,211], consisting of febrile periods of 1 to 2 weeks alternating with similar afebrile lengths, is rare. Fever, night sweats, and weight loss exceeding 10 percent of baseline body weight during the 6 months preceding diagnosis each denote a poor prognosis and are more common in the prognostically poor histologic subtypes and advanced stages of disease [21,212]. Their presence places a patient for staging purposes in the B category of disease as opposed to the A category of patients who lack such constitutional symptoms (see Table 118-1) [31]. The presence of fever has been related to areas of necrosis within involved nodes, circulating immune complexes [203], and pyrogenic substances in the plasma [213] and spleen [214]. Generalized or, less commonly, localized pruritus occurs in 10 to 15 percent of cases initially [208] and up to 85 percent of cases at later times [13], but lacks prognostic significance [212]. Pain ranging from sharp and severe to a mild, dull ache occurring in involved tissues after ingestion of alcoholic beverages is particularly suggestive of HD, but is uncommon (1 to 10 percent of cases) and of no prognostic import [215]. Cough, chest pain, the superior vena cava syndrome, peripheral edema, ascites, abdominal pain, bone pain, and neurologic symptoms are all uncommon presenting features. Often patients may be entirely asymptomatic and are found to have HD only in the course of a routine physical or radiologic examination.

The clinical pattern at presentation which determines the all-important stage of the disease (see Table 118-1) is strongly influenced by the histologic subtype of HD [216–218]. Lymphocyte predominance HD is a relatively indolent disease, most commonly presenting as stage I (70 percent of patients) or II disease, rarely associated with B symptoms or mediastinal involvement, and without predilection for a specific sex or age range. Nodular sclerosis HD has the next best prognosis, in large part because of an approximately 70 percent likelihood of stage I or II disease. It is distinctive for its pronounced incidence peak in adolescents and young adults, its greater frequency in females, and its high incidence of mediastinal involvement. Mixed cellularity

TABLE 118-1   Ann Arbor staging classification

Stage I	Involvement of a single lymph node region (I) or of a single extralymphatic organ or site (I_E).
Stage II	Involvement of two or more lymph node regions on the same side of the diaphragm (II) or localized involvement of extralymphatic organ or site and of one or more lymph node regions on the same side of the diaphragm (II_E). Optional recommendation: number of node regions involved indicated by subscript (e.g., II_3).
Stage III	Involvement of lymph node regions on both sides of the diaphragm (III), which may also be accompanied by localized involvement of extralymphatic organ or site (III_E), or the spleen (III_S), or both (III_{SE}).
Stage IV	Diffuse or disseminated involvement of one or more extralymphatic organs or tissues with or without associated lymph node enlargement. The reason for classifying the patient as stage IV should be identified further by defining site by symbols.
Systemic symptoms	Each stage is subdivided into A and B categories, B for those with defined symptoms and A for those without. The B classification will be given to those with (1) unexplained weight loss of more than 10 percent of the body weight in the 6 months before admission, (2) unexplained fever with temperatures above 38°C, (3) night sweats.
Staging criteria	Clinical (CS) when based solely on physical examination and laboratory results. Pathologic (PS) when based on biopsies.

SOURCE: Modified from Carbone et al. [31].

HD has an older age incidence peak (30 to 40 years), a higher frequency of both advanced disease at presentation (40 to 50 percent stage III or IV) and B symptoms (40 to 50 percent) and a worse prognosis. The worst prognosis occurs in cases of lymphocyte depletion HD in which 70 percent of patients present with stage III or IV disease and B symptoms, often with a paucity of peripheral or mediastinal adenopathy, but usually with retroperitoneal nodes. Age at onset is usually over 40 and presentation as a fever of unknown origin, or with jaundice, hepatosplenomegaly, or pancytopenia is not uncommon [219]. Lymphocyte predominance HD constitutes about 10 percent, nodular sclerosis 40 to 70 percent, mixed cellularity 30 to 50 percent, and lymphocyte depletion 5 to 10 percent of cases, although nodular sclerosis seems to be less common in underdeveloped countries [220,221]. The histologic subtype is remarkably constant in multiple biopsies within a given patient, whether performed simultaneously during staging [222], or over a period of years during the course of relapsing disease [223]. Alterations in histology are most common in lymphocyte predominance and mixed cellularity HD and almost invariably indicate a progression toward a worse prognostic type [223]. Nodular sclerosis HD rarely progresses to a frankly different type, but may evolve from a cellular phase possessing many "lacunar" Hodgkin's cells (see Chap. 117) to a more fibrotic picture which may show a paucity of normal lymphocytes, a poor prognostic feature in this subgroup either at presentation or on subsequent biopsy [224].

Mode of spread

In most instances, HD appears to begin in an initial focus within the lymphatic system and spreads subsequently via lymphatic channels to contiguous lymphatic structures [225–227]. However, some observers have postulated that various lymph node sites may have intrinsic differences in their susceptibility to HD, accounting for the observed anatomic distributions [228]. Analyses of the location of nodal disease in stage II patients with two or three sites of disease, or of sites of disease extension after radiotherapy for localized disease, are consistent with spread by contiguity in all but a small proportion of patients [227]. The frequency of bilaterally symmetrical noncontiguous involvement is also lower than the "susceptibility" theory would predict [229]. Thus, associations of left supraclavicular and periaortic, mediastinal and supraclavicular, axillary and ipsilateral supraclavicular, and splenic hilar and splenic involvement are frequent. However, when four or more sites of disease are present, noncontiguous locations become more common, and the possibility of spread by hematogenous distribution appears more likely. Noncontiguous spread is also more common in mixed cellularity and lymphocyte depletion HD [227] and may be related to the increased frequency of vascular invasion by HD which has been reported in these subtypes [230]. Such vascular invasion, while controversial [231,232], may be more frequent in the spleen than in nodes involved by HD [233]. Since the spleen is almost invariably involved when HD is present in the liver or marrow [29], vascular invasion in the spleen may lead to hematogenous dissemination. The spleen appears to lack afferent lymphatics [234] and splenic hilar nodes are involved in only about half of the cases with splenic disease [207]. Thus, the spleen may act as a "filter" to which initial hematogenous spread is most likely to occur. Small numbers of Reed-Sternberg cells have been found in the peripheral blood, thoracic duct lymph, and splenic vein blood of HD patients, further supporting these theories [235–237].

Organ involvement

Liver involvement, usually focal, is present in less than 5 percent of patients at diagnosis, but is found in 66 percent of patients at autopsy [238]. The left lobe, to which splenic venous blood predominantly drains, is more frequently involved than the right. Jaundice may result from diffuse involvement of the liver or, rarely, from biliary obstruction by enlarged portal nodes. Noncaseating granulomas and associated lymphoid infiltrates may occur in the liver, marrow, and lymphoid tissues in patients with HD and must be carefully distinguished from true involvement with HD since their presence has no adverse prognostic influence [239].

Marrow involvement, usually asymptomatic, occurs in 5 to 20 percent of new patients [208,240,241] and is almost invariably associated with splenic involvement [242] and usually with clinically advanced disease and an elevated serum alkaline phosphatase level. Since involvement is most often focal and limited, marrow aspiration is rarely diagnostic and one or more marrow biopsies are required to adequately evaluate the possibility of marrow involvement. Localized bony involvement, usually with bone pain, may occur from hematogenous spread in advanced disease (stage IV) or by local extension from adjacent nodal disease (a form of E lesion prognostically much more favorable than stage IV disease [243]). Bone changes on x-ray are usually osteolytic, but osteoblastic lesions are also common [244].

Pulmonary involvement occurs in up to 60 percent of patients at autopsy [245], but in only 10 to 20 percent at presentation. It appears to arise by spread along lymphatics from ipsilateral nodes containing HD, often of the nodular sclerosing type [246]. Pleural effusions, either exudates, transudates, or chylous, may be due to direct pleural spread or central lymphatic obstruction in the mediastinum or thoracic duct. Cytologic examination of the pleural fluid rarely reveals diagnostic Reed-Sternberg cells [247]; culture of the fluid for tuberculosis and other pathogens should always be performed. Myocardial involvement is very rare, but pericardial effusion, occasionally producing tamponade, may occur from direct invasion by adjacent mediastinal HD.

In contrast with other malignant lymphomas, ascites is quite rare, correlating with the low frequency of gastrointestinal tract involvement. When gastrointestinal involvement occurs, it is usually obstructive and related to mesenteric nodal disease, but cases of malabsorption have been seen [248]. Direct renal involvement is rarely clinically significant, but ureteral obstruction and hydronephrosis due to adjacent retroperitoneal lymphadenopathy may require prompt treatment [249]. The nephrotic syndrome, sometimes accompanied by evidence of glomerular immune complex deposition [250] but more commonly presenting as lipoid nephrosis [251], occurs occasionally in association with HD, as does renal amyloidosis [252].

Involvement of the skin by HD by means of retrograde spread along cutaneous lymphatics from adjacent nodal disease [253,254] occurs infrequently, and even more rarely is the skin the initial primary site of disease [255]. A variety of cutaneous manifestations have been associated with HD, including follicular mucinosis [256], erythema nodosum, exfoliative dermatitis, dermatomyositis, urticaria, pemphigus [257], generalized anhydrosis with acquired icthyosis [258], and eczematoid and psoriasiform lesions [259].

The most frequent and potentially devastating neurological manifestation of HD is spinal cord compression, usually due to epidural spread of tumor from paravertebral nodes through intervertebral foramina in the thoracic or lumbar regions [260]. Symptoms of back pain, lower extremity weakness or loss of sensation, or difficulty with bladder or bowel control warrant prompt diagnostic workup including myelography and either surgical decompression or emergency radiotherapy to prevent permanent paraplegia. Parenchymal or meningeal involvement of the central nervous system is quite rare [261], but a variety of paraneoplastic neurological syndromes have been described in HD, including progressive multifocal leukoencephalopathy [262], subacute cerebellar degeneration [263], the Guillain-Barré syndrome [264], and granulomatous angiitis of the central nervous system [265].

Laboratory features

Other than histologic examination of tissues involved by HD, there are no truly diagnostic laboratory tests. Granulocytosis is present initially in about 25 percent of patients and is more frequent in advanced stages [208,266,267]. Eosinophilia, monocytosis, or rarely a leukemoid reaction may also be present. The leukocyte alkaline phosphatase score is often elevated [268], but granulocyte and monocyte function are largely normal [269]. Lymphocytopenia (<1000 per microliter) is an adverse prognostic sign [212] and occurs in about 20 percent of patients at presentation, particularly those with advanced stages of disease or lymphocyte depletion histology.

Anemia is found in about 10 percent of patients at presentation and is more common in advanced disease. It is usually related to impaired iron mobilization and reutilization from macrophage stores (the "anemia of chronic disease") but may be due to concomitant blood loss or nutritional deficiency [208,270]. Low serum iron and elevated ferritin are seen, particularly when constitutional symptoms are present [271]. Hemolytic anemia is found in a few patients, usually in advanced disease, and sometimes in synchrony with episodes of fever [272]. A positive Coombs' test is found in 2 to 10 percent of patients with HD [173,272,273]. The platelet count is usually normal, but thrombocytosis may be present in up to 10 percent of cases at presentation [209]. Thrombocytopenia may occur in advanced disease, either as a result of marrow replacement by HD or treatment with radiation and chemotherapy. It is less commonly due to hypersplenism or an autoimmune mechanism [274–276], although platelet half-lives may be shortened [277].

Elevation of the erythrocyte sedimentation rate is seen in about half of patients at presentation and is particularly associated with B symptoms and advanced disease and may indicate a poor prognosis [279]. While nonspecific, it may provide a useful parameter of disease activity, returning to normal when complete remission is achieved and rising again to herald a relapse [279]. A variety of other nonspecific abnormalities may occur, including elevation of serum levels of copper [280], calcium, uric acid, lactic acid [281], alkaline phosphatase, transaminases, lysozyme, haptoglobin, α, β, and γ globulins, hydroxyproline, C-reactive protein, and other acute phase reactants. Inappropriate antidiuretic hormone secretion may occur. Decreased serum levels of zinc, pyridoxal phosphate, and albumin have been reported [208].

Differential diagnosis

The protean manifestations of Hodgkin's disease lead to an extensive differential diagnosis, but the most common difficulty occurs in distinguishing HD from other malignant lymphomas. Lymphocyte predominance HD may be confused with well-differentiated lymphocytic lymphoma while lymphocyte depletion or mixed cellularity HD may be mistaken for histiocytic or poorly differentiated lymphocytic lymphoma. Since the diagnosis rests upon histopathologic examination, the most abnormal lymph node should be biopsied. While variance in interpretation between pathologists may occur, consultation between experts will usually result in a consensus [282]. Benign diseases producing lymphadenopathy include infectious mononucleosis, in which, unlike HD, nodes are usually in the posterior cervical region. Other viral infections, thyroid and other carcinomas, and autoimmune disorders may also lead to lymphadenopathy. Sarcoidosis often produces mediastinal and hilar nodes visible on chest x-ray. Fever and constitutional symptoms may occur with tuberculosis, fungal or other infections, or other neoplasms such as hypernephroma. Drug reactions, particularly to hydantoin derivatives such as Dilantin, may also produce lymphadenopathy ("pseudolymphoma") [148]. Enlarged lymph nodes must be carefully observed and biopsied if they persist or are atypical, since some benign entities, particularly Sjögren's syndrome, systemic lupus erythematosus, pseudolymphoma, and the recently described entities "immunoblastic" or "angioimmunoblastic lymphadenopathy" [283,284] may be associated with subsequent malignant lymphoma.

Staging

The ability of radiotherapy to cure localized HD, and the need to monitor parameters of disease activity to evaluate the success of treatment, provide the rationale for modern staging practices. If radiotherapy is utilized, sites of disease involvement must be precisely deter-

TABLE 118-2   Recommendations on staging procedures

I. Evaluation procedures
   A. Adequate surgical biopsy, reviewed by a hematopathologist
   B. Detailed history of fever, sweating, pruritus, and weight loss
   C. Complete physical examination with attention to lymphadenopathy, Waldeyer's ring, liver, spleen, and bone tenderness
   D. Laboratory studies
      1. Complete blood count, platelet count, erythrocyte sedimentation rate, serum alkaline phosphatase level
      2. Evaluation of renal function and liver function
   E. Radiologic studies
      1. Chest radiograph (posteroanterior and lateral views)
      2. Computerized tomographic (CT) scan of abdomen
      3. Bilateral lower extremity lymphangiogram
   F. Marrow biopsy, by needle or open surgical technique
II. Evaluation procedures under certain conditions
   A. Whole-chest tomgraphy or CT scan of thorax
   B. IVP, ultrasound, or inferior venacavagram for equivocal lymphangiogram or abdominal CT scan
   C. Skeletal radiographic survey for areas of bone pain or tenderness
   D. Liver biopsy, by percutaneous needle or open surgical technique
   E. Laparoscopy
   F. Exploratory laparotomy and splenectomy, if management decisions will depend on the identification of abdominal disease
III. Useful ancillary procedures
   A. Whole-body gallium-67 tomographic scanning
   B. Liver and spleen scans
   C. Bone scan
   D. Estimate of patient's delayed hypersensitivity

SOURCE: Modified from Carbone et al. [31].

mined to permit treatment with curative intent. If the disease is disseminated beyond the lymphoid system and radiotherapeutic cure is not possible, then chemotherapy may be used as a primary treatment. The goals of staging are (1) to search for evidence of disseminated disease, and, if none is found, (2) to define the location of disease within the lymphoid system, and (3) to find disease manifestations which can be reevaluated during and after treatment to determine the effectiveness of therapy [285,286]. The extent of disease has been classified using a four-stage system (see Table 118-1) [31]. Stage is termed *clinical* (CS) when based solely on physical examination and laboratory results, and *pathological* (PS) when the extent of disease has been proved with appropriate biopsies. The correlation of this staging classification with prognosis has been extensively verified [287–291].

The basic classification is modified by consideration of the poor prognostic implications of constitutional symptoms (B disease) [212] and the realization that localized extranodal extension of disease (E disease) does not carry the same poor prognosis as hematogenous ex-

tranodal dissemination (stage IV disease) [287]. This concept has been challenged for localized extension of HD into the pulmonary parenchyma from hilar nodes [292], but optimal radiotherapy techniques may prevent significant reduction in good prognosis in this situation [293]. The staging and treatment of PS III patients have been controversial [294,295]. Recent results have suggested that PS III disease may be subclassified into a prognostically favorable III$_1$ group, in which abdominal disease is confined to the upper abdomen and radiotherapy is likely to produce cure, and a less favorable III$_2$ group with disease extending to the lower abdomen [296,297].

Recommended staging procedures are outlined in Table 118-2. They should commence promptly after an initial biopsy reveals HD and begin with a complete history and physical examination with attention to lymphadenopathy, hepatosplenomegaly, and constitutional symptoms. Laboratory tests should include a complete blood count, urinalysis, sedimentation rate, renal and liver function tests, including alkaline phosphatase, and a chest x-ray. In an initial attempt to find stage IV disease, bilateral posterior iliac crest marrow biopsies should be performed [298,299]. Marrow aspiration alone is insufficient, but biopsy is omitted in some centers in patients with CS IA or IIA disease without hematologic abnormalities or adverse histologic patterns. A liver scan may provide evidence of hepatomegaly or focal defects and should be performed if liver function tests are abnormal. While percutaneous liver biopsy is rarely diagnostic, if positive it will obviate the necessity for staging laparotomy and should be done if there is strong clinical evidence of hepatic disease [29,300,301]. A bone scan is more sensitive than routine radiographs and should be performed, particularly if the alkaline phosphatase level is elevated or symptoms of localized bone pain are present [302]. Abnormal areas should be biopsied whenever feasible since they often represent areas of early dissemination even in patients with otherwise localized disease. If a pleural effusion is present on chest x-ray, diagnostic thoracentesis, including culture, cytology, and cell block examination, and pleural biopsy should be done. Chest tomography to define precisely the extent of disease, including possible localized E extensions into the pulmonary parenchyma is indicated when hilar or mediastinal disease is present or suspected. Computerized tomography may be particularly valuable both in this regard and to define potential mediastinal or hilar disease.

The most difficult staging questions frequently revolve around the question of intraabdominal disease and the distinction between stage II and III disease. Intravenous pyelography should be performed routinely to rule out hydronephrosis and search for ureteral deviation due to retroperitoneal lymphadenopathy, but is relatively insensitive in detecting nodes [303]. Bipedal lymphangiography is the most sensitive and accurate test for assessing the degree of involvement of retroperitoneal nodes [303,304] and should be done in all cases except those with significant compromise in pulmonary function, large mediastinal mass, or other contraindications. Since the contrast material may remain in nodes for many months, it may be useful for assessing the accuracy of the staging laparotomy and the success of treatment. Alterations in residual contrast may provide an early indication of retroperitoneal relapse. Inferior venacavography is sometimes useful, particularly in assessing high paraaortic nodes which may be poorly visualized on lymphangiography [285,303]. Spleen scans are both insensitive and inaccurate, although usually performed routinely in conjunction with a liver scan [207,305]. Computerized tomography is particularly valuable since it both detects nodal areas poorly visualized on lymphangiography (the celiac, portal, splenic, and mesenteric nodes) and provides a more precise delineation of nodal masses useful in planning radiotherapy [306]. However, it cannot at present replace the lymphangiography since it may be less sensitive in detecting minimal nodal involvement. Ultrasonography is similarly useful in detecting lymphadenopathy and renal obstruction and in delineating masses, but is technically inadequate in 20 percent of patients [307]. Gallium scanning is less sensitive and accurate than lymphangiography in detecting abdominal disease, but may be useful in equivocal situations, particularly in the mediastinum or in areas abnormal on bone scan [308,309]. In view of the low incidence of gastrointestinal involvement in HD, gastrointestinal x-rays are not indicated unless gastrointestinal symptoms are present or occult blood is detected in the stool.

In spite of optimal application of such noninvasive procedures, clinical staging of abdominal disease is inaccurate in 20 to 30 percent of patients, with nearly equal frequencies of over- and underestimation of disease stage [207,285,310]. The spleen is particularly difficult to evaluate clinically and is both a frequent site of early abdominal disease and a harbinger of potential liver involvement. Thus, staging laparotomy with splenectomy is recommended for patients who have neither previous biopsy proof of stage IV disease nor a medical contraindication to laparotomy. Clinical criteria of use to define patients not requiring laparotomy are under evaluation, but are as yet not established [311]. The operation should include splenectomy, a wedge biopsy of the left lobe of the liver and needle biopsies of the right and left lobes, biopsies of the splenic hilar, celiac, portal, mesenteric, right and left paraaortic, and right and left iliac nodes regardless of their clinical appearance at staging, placement of clips at biopsy sites, an open iliac crest marrow biopsy, and midline oophoropexy in females of childbearing age to reduce subsequent radiation to the ovaries [312]. Suspicious inguinal nodes should be biopsied and a blind left scalene biopsy should be done if the patient has no prior evidence of disease above the diaphragm. Such a procedure will advance about one-third of CS I and II patients to PS III or IV and reduce about one-quarter of CS III patients to PS I or II. The surgical mortality rate is about 0.5

percent; the surgical complications less than 9 percent. Careful radiologic evaluation preoperatively is still required both to guide the surgeon and to provide baseline parameters of disease activity to be evaluated during and after treatment. Detailed pathological examination of sites of intraabdominal disease is particularly required to distinguish PS III$_1$ and III$_2$ patients [296,297]. In some cases, staging laparotomy must be deferred until massive mediastinal disease or other threatening complication contraindicating laparotomy has received initial radiotherapy.

Therapy

RADIOTHERAPY

Radiotherapy is generally the treatment of choice for patients with localized HD, PS IA and IIA, since a dose of 4000 to 4400 rads administered to all nodal regions containing known or suspected disease is usually well tolerated and curative. The response of both HD and surrounding normal tissues is dependent upon a number of technical factors. The risk of recurrence of HD within a field of treatment falls from 60 percent with a dose of 1000 rads, to 26 percent at 2500 rads, to 1.3 percent at 4400 rads [313]. Fortunately, many normal tissues may function well after even higher doses, although certain vital organs must be shielded from excessive doses to prevent serious radiation damage (Table 118-3) [314]. Thus, full-dose radiotherapy (4000 rads) can usually be given to a particular field only once, although a subsequent palliative dose (2500 rads) may be given if local relapse occurs. Modern treatment requires the use of a linear accelerator or an appropriate ^{60}Co-teletherapy unit capable of delivering γ rays of sufficient energy to penetrate to deeper nodal regions while sparing the skin and providing treatment fields with sharp margins [26,315–317]. Treatment is usually administered on a schedule of 200 to 250 rads per day, 4 or 5 days per week, over a 3- to 6-week period [318–320]. Depending upon the size and location of the port, acute radiation toxicity including local skin erythema, anorexia sometimes progressing to nausea and vomiting, and hematologic depression (usually leukopenia and thrombocytopenia) may occur and necessitate "rest intervals" of one or more days during therapy. While "split-course" therapy incorporating a 2-week rest period between the first and second halves of treatment has been used with no reported diminution in efficacy [321], more prolonged or frequent intervals during treatment may seriously compromise cure rates. Nodal masses which are either particularly bulky initially (>5 cm) or which respond slowly or only partially to an initial 4000 rads can be given an additional "boost" to provide a total dose of 5000 rads to such areas.

In view of the likelihood of occult spread of HD to adjacent nodal areas and the technical difficulties of aligning adjacent radiation fields without either an untreated gap or a toxic overlap, modern radiotherapists have

TABLE 118-3 Organ tolerance to radiotherapy

Organ	Injury	Rads*	Area radiated
CLASS I: *Organs in which radiation lesions are fatal or result in severe morbidity*			
Marrow	Aplasia, pancytopenia	3,000	Partial
		250	Whole
Liver	Acute and chronic hepatitis	2,500	Whole
Stomach	Perforation, ulcer hemorrhage	4,500	100 cm²
Intestine	Ulcer, perforation, hemorrhage	4,500	400 cm²
Brain and peripheral nerves	Infarction, necrosis, neuritis	6,000	Whole
Spinal cord	Infarction, necrosis	4,500	10 cm
Heart	Pericarditis and pancarditis	4,500	60 percent
		3,000	Partial
Lung	Acute and chronic pneumonitis	1,500	Whole
Kidney	Acute and chronic nephrosclerosis	1,500	Whole
Fetus	Death	200	Whole
CLASS II: *Organs in which radiation lesions result in moderate to mild morbidity and in exceptional circumstances a fatality, but late effects generally are compatible with survival*			
Oral cavity and pharnyx	Ulceration, mucositis	6,000	Partial
Skin	Acute and chronic dermatitis	5,500	Partial
Esophagus	Esophagitis, ulceration	6,000	Partial
Salivary glands	Xerostomia	5,000	Partial
Bladder	Contracture	6,000	Whole
Ureters	Stricture	7,500	Partial
Testes	Sterilization	100	Whole
Ovary	Sterilization	200–300	Whole
Growing cartilage, bone (child)	Growth arrest	1,000	Whole
		1,000	10 cm²
Mature cartilage, bone (adult)	Necrosis, fracture, sclerosis	6,000	Whole
Eye:			
Retina		5,500	Whole
Cornea		5,000	Whole
Lens		500	Whole or partial
Endocrine glands:			
Thyroid	Hypothyroidism	4,500	Whole
Adrenal	Hypoadrenalism	6,000	Whole
Pituitary	Hypopituitarism, neuritis	6,000	Whole
CLASS III: *Organs in which radiation lesions result in mild, transient, reversible effects or in no morbidity*			
Muscle (child)	Atrophy	2,000–3,000	Whole
Muscle (adult)	Fibrosis	6,000	Whole
Lymph nodes and lymphatics	Atrophy, sclerosis	6,000	Whole node
Large arteries and veins	Sclerosis	8,000	10 cm²
Articular cartilage	None	50,000	Joint surface (mm²)
Uterus	Necrosis, perforation	10,000	Whole

* Dose of radiation which produces complication in 5 percent of patients receiving this dose.
SOURCE: Modified from Rubin [314].

treated larger fields which often incorporate adjacent uninvolved nodal regions. While such "extended field" radiotherapy has not been clearly shown to improve survival when compared with treatment of "involved fields" only, the frequency of recurrence at the margin of the initial port is reduced [322,323]. For localized disease above the diaphragm, a *mantle port* covering the cervical, supraclavicular, infraclavicular, axillary, mediastinal, and hilar nodes is usually used [319] (see Fig. 118-1) and is often followed by prophylactic treatment of the paraaortic region and splenic pedicle. Waldeyer's ring is rarely involved by HD but is treated if high cer-

vical or auricular nodes are diseased. Infradiaphragmatic disease is usually treated with an *inverted Y port* [320] (see Fig. 118-1) which included the pelvic, iliac, paraaortic, and splenic pedicle nodes, much of the left lobe of the liver, and a portion of the mesentery. Mesenteric nodes are rarely involved and thus are usually not treated, but, if involved, may be treated with a lateral abdominal port in conjunction with a modified inverted Y [324].

When nodal disease is found on both sides of the diaphragm (PS IIIA), the mantle and inverted Y fields are treated sequentially with initial radiotherapy to the area of predominant involvement, thus comprising *total nodal* or *total lymphoid irradiation* [325–327]. At some institutions PS I or IIB disease or PS I or IIA disease with mixed cellularity or lymphocyte depletion histologies is aggressively treated with total nodal radiotherapy [288,290]. Some centers have combined the mantle port with the paraaortic and splenic pedicle port to make an "extended mantle" which is particularly useful for PS III$_1$ patients in whom abdominal disease is confined to the upper abdomen [328]. Such a port, when followed by a truncated inverted Y, has the added advantage of placing the junction of the two ports (the "splice") below the level of the spinal cord. Another variation on total nodal therapy requires sequential treatment of three ports, mantle, paraaortic, and pelvic, to 2000 rads followed by 1800 rads sequentially to an extended mantle and inverted Y [329,330].

Because of the risk of pulmonary spread from involved hilar nodes, many groups now use a "thin lung block" technique to administer 1500 rads to the entire lung prophylactically when the hilum appears enlarged [331,332]. Similar prophylactic radiation may be given to the right lobe of the liver to a dose of 2500 rads when the spleen is found to be involved and the risk of hepatic dissemination is high [333]. Additional appropriately shaped lead blocks designed to attenuate radiation to vital organs include posterior blocks for the cervical and thoracic spinal cord, a cardiac block used to permit 1500 rads to the pericardium when mediastinal disease is present, a "subcarinal" block to reduce cardiac irradiation during mantle therapy, and blocks to protect the kidneys, larynx, humoral heads, axillary skin folds, and testes.

The radiotherapy of HD is thus a highly complex art requiring port verification films, usually used in conjunction with tatooed position markers on the patient's skin, and careful dosimetry. Even with optimal management significant complications may occur. Radiation pneumonitis develops in 6 to 20 percent of cases receiving mantle radiation and is more common after whole-lung radiation [332,334,335]. Symptoms range from a dry cough to severe and sometimes fatal pneumonitis. Glucocorticoids may provide significant relief, but their rapid withdrawal may itself provoke an episode of pneumonitis in a previously irradiated patient [336]. Radiation pericarditis is also dose-dependent. Asymptomatic pericarditis, most commonly a small effusion seen on echocardiogram, is seen in up to 13 percent of patients receiving mantle radiation [332,337,338]. Myocarditis, constrictive pericarditis, and, rarely, coronary artery disease may ensue [339]. Other complications include hypothyroidism in 20 percent of patients with full-dose radiation to the thyroid [340,341], Lhermitte's sign in 10 percent of patients [332,337], and rare cases of radiation hepatitis, nephritis, transverse myelitis, or peripheral neuropathy. Hemopoietic function is sharply reduced in marrow areas irradiated to full doses, but may partially recover in 1 to 3 years [342].

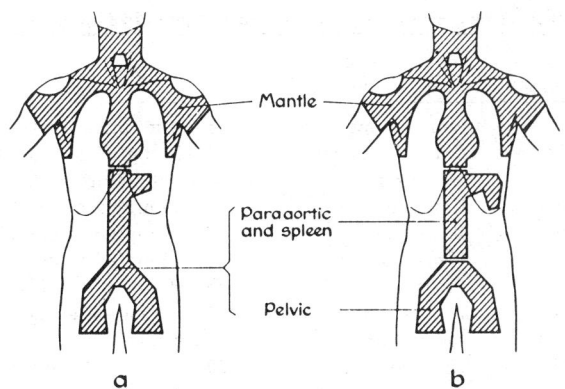

FIGURE 118-1 Diagram of the "mantle" and "inverted-Y" fields used in the radiotherapy of Hodgkin's disease. (*a*) Two-field technique, with small extension to include the splenic pedicle, used in patients who have undergone splenectomy. (*b*) Three-field technique (with full spleen extension) used when the spleen is still present or when hematologic tolerance is poor. Note the gap(s) between adjacent fields. (S. A. Rosenberg and H. S. Kaplan, Hodgkin's disease and other malignant lymphomas, *Calif. Med.* 113:23, 1970, by permission.)

Chemotherapy

A variety of drugs have shown activity when used individually against HD (see Table 118-4) [343–345]. However, significant toxicity may occur with each of these agents (see Table 118-4) and may increase when multiple agents are used [346]. The therapist must be alert for uncommon complications such as Adriamycin-induced cardiomyopathy or bleomycin- or nitrosourea-induced pulmonary fibrosis, both of which may be enhanced by prior or subsequent treatment with radiation or alkylating agents [347]. Unfortunately, the development of tumor resistance to a drug (e.g., an alkylating agent) usually implies cross-resistance to other members of that drug class. By combining agents of known individual efficacy but differing in mechanism of action and toxicity [348–350], a treatment regimen of acceptable toxicity but vastly improved potency became possible. The MOPP regimen [nitrogen mustard, vincristine (Oncovin), procarbazine, prednisone], (see Table 118-5), administered for 6 or more monthly cycles has provided complete remissions in 60 to 80 percent of patients with advanced disease (PS III and IV) [34,351–354]. One-half to two-thirds of these patients have remained in remission, in some cases as long as 15 years. Patients failing to achieve a complete remission have a median duration of survival of about 1 year. In spite of the acute toxicity (nausea, vomiting, alopecia, and marrow suppression) and reduction of drug dose in proportion to myelosuppression, the doses administered should approximate the planned calculated doses.

A variety of clinical variables have been examined as predictors of the occurrence and duration of complete remission [345,351]. The presence of B symptoms re-

TABLE 118-4   Single chemotherapeutic agents in Hodgkin's disease

| Abbreviation | Drug | Dose | Remission rate, % | | | Toxicity |
			Complete	Partial	Total	
HN₂	Nitrogen mustard	15 mg/m² monthly, IV	13	52	65	N, V, A, M
CTX	Cyclophosphamide (Cytoxan)	75–100 mg/m² daily, PO 350–500 mg/m² weekly, IV	12	42	54	N, V, A, M, hemorrhagic cystitis
CLB	Chlorambucil	3.5–7.5 mg/m² daily, PO	16	44	60	M
VLB	Vinblastine	4.5–7.5 mg/m² weekly, IV	30	38	68	N, A, M
VCR	Vincristine	0.7–1.0 mg/m² weekly, IV	36	22	58	A, Neuro, occasionally severe
PCB	Procarbazine	75–150 mg/m² daily, PO	38	31	69	N, M
BCNU	bis-Chlorethyl-nitrosourea	100–200 mg/m² every 6 weeks, IV	4	43	47	Delayed, often severe M, FR
CCNU	cis-Chlorethyl-nitrosourea	100–130 mg/m² every 6 weeks, PO	3	31	34	Delayed, often severe M
PRD	Prednisone	40 mg/m² daily, PO	0	61	61	Cushing's syndrome, infection, psychosis, diabetes
ADM	Adriamycin	25–60 mg/m² every 3 weeks, IV	8	33	41	N, V, A, M, cardiotoxicity, radiation recall reaction
BLM	Bleomycin	5 mg/m² weekly, IV, IM, SC	6	31	37	N, V, FR, pulmonary fibrosis, cutaneous toxicity, radiation recall reaction
STZN	Streptozotocin	500 mg/m² days 1–5, every 2 weeks, IV	6	38	44	Renal tubular injury, tubular acidosis, diabetes
VM26	Epipodophyllotoxin	50 mg/m² twice weekly, IV	12	56	68	N, V, M
DTIC	Dimethyltriazeno imidazole carboxamide	200 mg/m² days 1–5, every 3 weeks, IV	6	50	56	V, occasional M

NOTE: IV = intravenous, PO = orally, IM = intramuscular, SC = subcutaneous, N = nausea, V = vomiting, A = alopecia, M = myelotoxicity, Neuro = neurotoxicity, FR = febrile reactions.
SOURCE: Modified from Kaplan [404].

duces the likelihood of both achieving and maintaining complete remission. Prior chemotherapy greatly reduces response rates, but prior radiotherapy does not inhibit the response to MOPP. Nodular sclerosis histology (especially the subset with lymphocyte depletion), clinical evidence of stage IV disease, lymphocytopenia, age, and poor performance status may all adversely affect prognosis. Continued or "maintenance" chemotherapy after induction of complete remission has been evaluated in an attempt to increase the disease-free duration, but a number of studies have found it to be of no value [355–357]. What is most important is the careful reevaluation of all sites previously involved by HD to provide firm verification that a true *complete* remission has been achieved. Doubtful cases may require rebiopsy or repeat laparotomy. Since a complete remission may occur within the first three cycles of MOPP, it is wise to seek early evidence of improvement in a major disease parameter to ensure that tumor lysis rather than disease progression is occurring and to later undertake a complete reevaluation during the fourth to sixth cycles. An additional two cycles of treatment should be given after verification of complete remission. Some patients may require as many as 12 cycles for induction.

A variety of additional combination chemotherapy regimens have been utilized for HD (see Table 118-5). Vinblastine has been substituted for vincristine [356–

359] and cyclophosphamide [34,356–358], chlorambucil [361], or BCNU [362,363] for nitrogen mustard. In some cases, the substitutions provide a possible amelioration of toxicity in comparison with MOPP. These regimens have generally not resulted in comparable remission duration rates. The addition of bleomycin to MOPP [364] or BCNU to a MOPP-like regimen [365] has not proved superior to MOPP alone. Of particular interest is the ABVD regimen (Adriamycin, bleomycin, Velban, and DTIC [366] which is composed of drugs to which tumor cross-resistance does not develop during MOPP treatment. MOPP and ABVD produced equal remission induction and duration rates in a randomized comparison [366]. Patients resistant to MOPP may respond to ABVD, although the frequency of such responses is controversial [367–370]. Similar regimens useful for the treatment of MOPP failures include B-CAVe [371], B-DOPA [372], SCAB [373], and a combination of CCNU, Velban, and bleomycin [374]. Before these regimens are tried in a patient who relapses after a MOPP-induced complete remission, however, it may be wise to attempt reinduction with MOPP. In one study, patients relapsing after more than 1 year of MOPP-induced complete remission had a 90 percent chance of achieving complete remission with a second trial of MOPP [375]. Recent attempts to improve initial induction rates have employed alternating cycles of MOPP and ABVD for a total of 12 months with promising preliminary results.

TABLE 118-5   Combination chemotherapy in Hodgkin's Disease

Acronym	Drug*	Dose	Remission rates, %			Reference
			Complete	Partial	Total	
MOPP	HN₂	6 mg/m², IV, 1, 8 every 28 days	81	0	81	DeVita et al. [34]
	VCR	1.4 mg/m², IV, 1, 8	83	0	83	Cooper et al. [406]
	PCB	100 mg/m², PO, 1–14	80	0	80	Jacobs et al. [407]
	PRD	40 mg/m², PO, 1–14†	62	17	79	Bonadonna et al. [383]
MVPP	HN₂	6 mg/m², IV, 1, 8, every 42 days	82	0	82	Nicholson et al. [358]
	VLB	6 mg/m², IV, 1, 8				McElwain et al. [408]
	PCB	100 mg/m² PO, 1–14				Sutcliffe et al.[359]
	PRD	40 mg, PO, 1–14				
MVVPP	HN₂	0.4 mg/kg, IV, 1, every 57 days	78	22	100	Levitt et al. [409]
	VCR	1.4 mg/m², IV, 1, 8, 15				
	VLB	6 mg/m², IV, 22, 29, 36				
	PCB	100 mg/day, PO, 22–43				
	PRD	40 mg/m², PO,‡ 2–22				
CVPP	CTX	300 mg/m², IV, 1, 8, every 42 days	74	0	74	Bloomfield et al. [360]
	VLB	10 mg, IV, 1, 8, 15				
	PCB	100 mg/m², PO, 1–15				
	PRD	40 mg/m², PO, 1–15†				
ABVD	ADM	25 mg/m², IV, 1, 15, every 28 days	70	11	81	Bonadonna et al. [383]
	BLM	10 mg/m², IV, 1, 15	22	15	37	Vicente et al. [410]
	VLB	10 mg/m², IV, 1, 15	33	53	86	Krikorian et al. [368]
	DTIC	375 mg/m², IV, 1, 15	0	11	11	Clamon and Corder [411]
CLVPP	CLB	6 mg/m², PO, 1–14, every 28 days	76	17	93	McElwain et al. [361]
	VLB	6 mg/m², IV, 1, 8				
	PCB	100 mg/m², PO, 1–14				
	PRD	40 mg, PO, 1–14				
B-MOPP	MOPP	As above, every 28 days plus	84	14	98	Coltman and Jones [412]
	BLM	2 mg/m², IV, 1, 8				
B-DOPA	BLM	4 mg/m², IM, 2, 5, every 28–35 days	60	20	80	Lokich et al. [372]
	DTIC	150 mg/m², IV, 1–5				
	VCR	1.5/mg/m², PO, 1, 5				
	PRD	40 mg/m², PO, 1–6				
	ADM	60 mg/m², IV, 1				
SCAB	STZN	500 mg/², IV, 1–5, every 42 days	80	10	90	Diggs et al. [413]
	CCNU	100 mg/m², PO, 1	(35)§	(24)	(59)	
	ADM	45 mg/m², IV, 1				
	BLM	15 mg/m², IM, 1, 8				
PAVe	ALK	7.5 mg/m², PO, 1, 2, 8, 9, every 28 days				Rosenberg et al. [377]
	VLB	6 mg/m², IV, 1, 8				
	PCB	100 mg/m², PO, 1–14				
CVB	CCNU	100 mg/m², PO, 1, every 42 days	26	59	85	Goldman and Dawson [374]
	VLB	6 mg/m², IV, 1, 8				
	BLM	15 mg, IM, 1, 8				
B-CAVe	BLM	5 mg/m², IV, 28, 35, every 42 days	50	27	77	Porzig et al. [371]
	CCNU	100 mg/m², PO, 1				
	ADM	60 mg/m², IV, 1				
	VLB	5 mg/m², IV, 1				
ABDV	ADM	25 mg/m², IV, 1, 15 every 28 days	4	57	61	Case et al. [370]
	BLM	2 mg, SC, 4–12, 18–26				
	DTIC	250 mg/m², IV, 1, 15				
	VLB	6 mg/m², IV, 1, 15				

* Abbreviations of drug names are defined in Table 118-4.
† Cycles 1 and 4 only.
‡ Tapered days 23–36, cycle 1 only.
§ Previously treated patients.
SOURCE: Modified from Kaplan [405].

Combined therapy

In view of the curative potentials of both modern radiotherapeutic techniques and combination chemotherapy such as MOPP the possibility that combinations of both treatments might increase remission and survival rates has been tested. A study of PS I and IIA patients has indicated that addition of 6 cycles of "adjuvant" MOPP after involved field radiation provides relapse rates comparable to those achieved by extended field radiation therapy alone [376]. Addition of MOPP to standard extended field or total lymphoid radiation in PS I, II, and IIIA patients may decrease the incidence of relapse, but has had no impact on survival since patients relapsing after radiation therapy alone have a high "salvage" rate with subsequent MOPP [377]. Paradoxically, adjuvant MOPP improved neither relapse rates nor survival in PS I and IIB patients treated with total lymphoid radiation [376]. The results with these patients in other series using less radiation, however, have been sufficiently poor to warrant consideration of combined modality treatment [291,294]. Pathologic stage IIIB patients demonstrated a reduced incidence of relapse with addition of MOPP to total lymphoid radiation although survival was not significantly improved [377]. In view of the increased risk of second neoplasms in patients receiving radiation therapy and chemotherapy it seems clear that combined modality therapy is not indicated in PS I and IIA patients [295]. However, the high incidence of relapse in PS IB and IIB patients and some IIIA patients may warrant the addition of chemotherapy to radiation regimens.

The treatment of PS III patients remains controversial. Both total nodal radiation and combination chemotherapy have produced excellent results in IIIA patients, although one randomized study has reported longer disease-free survival with total lymphoid radiation therapy than with MOPP [378]. No difference in overall survival was noted however. Recent attempts to subclassify such patients have suggested that radiation therapy alone may be adequate for patients with disease limited to the upper abdomen (PS III$_1$A), whereas chemotherapy, with or without supplemental radiation therapy, may be required for more extensive abdominal disease (PS III$_2$A) [296,297,379]. The prognosis of PS IIIB patients and their response to radiation alone in a number of series is so poor as to indicate that chemotherapy should be the primary treatment with possible supplemental radiation [377,380]. Radiation therapy, especially total nodal radiation, may compromise marrow function and severely impair hematologic tolerance to subsequent MOPP in adequate doses. Thus, some institutions give a "sandwich" of MOPP at full dose for 2 to 3 cycles followed by radiation therapy and 3 to 4 further cycles of MOPP when administering combined modality treatment [377,381,382]. Survival appears to be improved in patients receiving alternating therapy as opposed to total lymphoid radiation alone or radiation followed by MOPP.

Relapse in patients with PS IV disease who have achieved complete remission with chemotherapy most commonly occurs in previously involved nodal sites [353]. Thus, radiotherapy to known sites of disease has been added to initial induction chemotherapy in some studies. Two reports of total nodal or extended field radiation following or "sandwiched" within MOPP have failed to show an improvement over MOPP alone [377,382]. Nonetheless, other nonrandomized studies utilizing lower doses of radiation therapy to involved sites in combination with MOPP, ABVD [383], or a five-drug regimen [384] suggest a possible benefit of added radiation.

HD in children may present special problems [385], but localized disease may be effectively treated with standard doses of radiation, although some degree of growth retardation may result. Alternatively, combined modality treatment or MOPP alone have been successfully used [386]. The risk of sepsis after splenectomy in childhood may be significantly higher [387], but staging laparotomy is usually warranted nonetheless. Pregnancy may likewise require modification of treatment plans [388].

Course and prognosis

The 10-year actuarial survival rate of patients with HD has progressively increased from 1 percent with no therapy, to 23 percent with kilovoltage radiation therapy, and now approaches 70 percent at 10 years using modern radiation and/or chemotherapy, with a nearly equal rate of cure [389]. The anatomic extent of disease, histopathologic subtype, and B symptoms remain the most important prognostic factors, but even with initially localized disease a substantial proportion of patients will have one or more relapses. Additional prognostic factors may include anatomic substage III$_2$ [297], five or more sites of involvement, extensive splenic involvement [390], and bulky disease, especially in the mediastinum [292]. When relapse is detected, a complete re-evaluation must be undertaken, often including lymphangiography and occasionally even laparotomy to establish parameters of disease activity and design appropriate treatment. Rather than altering the stage designation established prior to initial therapy, the patient is said to have a "true recurrence" if the relapse is within a previously irradiated area, a "marginal recurrence" if it is confined to nodal areas adjacent to a prior radiation port, a "transdiaphragmatic recurrence" if it is in an untreated transdiaphragmatic area, and "dissemination" if new nonnodal sites of disease are found [391]. For many patients, the course of their disease may thus be subdivided into a series of "therapy courses," each of which consists of initial symptoms or signs, evaluation regarding extent of disease, treatment, and follow-up. True recurrences and dissemination cannot be re-treated with curative intent using radiation and therefore should receive MOPP or a similar combination chemotherapy regimen possibly supplemented by low-dose (2000 rads) radiation to sites of active disease.

Full-dose radiation to marginal recurrences produces a significant relapse-free survival [392], but addition of MOPP is probably wise [393,394].

Complications

The majority of complications arising in the course of HD occur either as a result of direct compromise of vital organs by the growth of tumor or from the toxicities of radiation or chemotherapy. Of particular concern, however, has been the development of second malignancies in patients who have undergone treatment for HD [395]. Acute nonlymphoid leukemia is the most common neoplasm, occurring particularly among patients receiving both radiation therapy and chemotherapy. These leukemias display nonrandom chromosomal abnormalities which differ from those seen in *de novo* leukemias [396] and are usually refractory to treatment. Non-Hodgkin's lymphomas [397] and a variety of other neoplasms have also been reported after HD and total risk of second malignancies may exceed 5 percent, particularly in patients receiving combined modality treatment [395].

Radiation to abdominal ports and chemotherapy share a profound capacity to reduce reproductive fertility in treated patients [398,399]. While both male and female patients have produced normal offspring after treatment, the potential for induction of sterility must be considered, particularly after combined modality therapy. Males may elect to store frozen sperm and females may undergo midline oophoropexy prior to initiation of treatment. Aseptic necrosis of the femoral head has been seen after combination chemotherapy for HD [400].

Herpes zoster occurs in approximately 20 percent of patients with HD [335,401]. Its timing and location may sometimes herald the onset of relapse and in the immunosuppressed host it may become generalized and have a fatal outcome. A variety of infectious complications due to common bacterial pathogens also may be seen, particularly in patients with advanced disease whose defense mechanisms have been further compromised by treatment. Opportunistic infections such as cryptococcosis, local or systemic candidiasis, aspergillosis, or *Pneumocystis carinii* pneumonia are common. Overwhelming sepsis due to encapsulated bacteria has been reported in patients after splenectomy, particularly if they have undergone combined modality treatment [402]. The overall risk may be reduced by the use of pneumococcal vaccine and, at approximately 0.5 percent, is too low to influence decisions regarding staging laparotomy [403].

References

1. Hodgkin, T.: On some morbid appearances of the absorbent glands and spleen. *Med. Chir. Trans.* 17:68, 1832.
2. Fox, H.: Remarks on the presentation of microscopical preparations made from some of the original tissue described by Thomas Hodgkin, 1832. *Ann. Med. History* 8:370, 1926.
3. Wilks, Sir S.: Cases of lardaceous disease and some allied affections, with remarks. *Guys Hosp. Rep. 17* (Ser. II, vol. 2):103, 1856.
4. Wilks, Sir S.: Cases of enlargement of the lymphatic glands and spleen, or Hodgkin's Disease, with remarks. *Guys Hosp. Rep.* 11:56, 1865.
5. Wunderlich, C. A.: Zwei Fälle von progressiven multiplen Lymphdrüsenhypertrophien. *Arch. Physiol. Heilk.* 12:122, 1858.
6. Trousseau, A.: De l'ádenie. *Clin. Med. l'Hôtel-Dieu Paris* 3:555, 1865.
7. Virchow, R.: Weisses blut. *Neue Notizen aus dem Geb. der Natur-und Heilkunde (Frorieps neue Notizen)* 36:151, 1845.
8. Craigie, D.: Case of disease of the spleen, in which death took place in consequence of the presence of purulent matter in the blood. *Edinburgh Med. Surg. J.* 64:400, 1845.
9. Bennett, J. H.: Case of hypertrophy of the spleen and liver, in which death took place from suppuration of the blood. *Edinburgh Med. Surg. J.* 64:413, 1845.
10. Sternberg, C.: Über eine eigenartige unter dem Bilde der Pseudoleukämie verlaufende Tuberculose des lymphatischen Appartes. *Z. Heilk.* 19:21, 1898.
11. Reed, D. M.: On the pathological changes in Hodgkin's disease, with especial reference to its relation to tuberculosis. *Johns Hopkins Hosp. Rep.* 10:133, 1902.
12. Wallhauser, A.: Hodgkin's disease. *Arch. Pathol.* 16:522; 672, 1933.
13. Hoster, H. A., Dratman, M. V., Craver, L.F., and Rolnick, H. A.: Hodgkin's disease—1832–1947. *Cancer Res.* 8:1; 49, 1948.
14. Bunting, C. H., and Yates, J. L.: Bacteriologic results in chronic leukemia and pseudoleukemia. *Bull. Johns Hopkins Hosp.* 26:376, 1915.
15. Wise, N. B., and Poston, M. A.: Coexistence of *Brucella* infection and Hodgkin's disease; clinical bacteriologic and immunologic study. *JAMA* 115:1976, 1940.
16. Branch, A.: Avian tubercle bacillus infection with special reference to mammals and to man; its reported association with Hodgkin's disease. *Am. J. Pathol.* 12:253, 1931.
17. Gordon, M. H.: *Studies on Aetiology of Lymphadenoma. Rose Research on Lymphadenoma.* John Wright, Bristol, England, 1932, pp. 7–76.
18. Rosenthal, S. R.: Significance of tissue lymphocytes in the prognosis of lymphogranulomatosis. *Arch. Pathol.* 21:628, 1936.
19. Jackson, H., Jr., and Parker, F., Jr.: *Hodgkin's Disease and Allied Disorders.* Oxford University Press, New York, 1947.
20. Peters, M. V.: A study of survivals in Hodgkin's disease treated radiologically. *Am. J. Roentgenol.* 63:299, 1950.
21. Peters, M. V., and Middlemiss, K. C. H.: A study of Hodgkin's disease treated by irradiation. *Am. J. Roentgenol.* 79:114, 1958.
22. Pusey, W. A.: Cases of sarcoma and of Hodgkin's disease treated by exposures to x-rays: A preliminary report. *JAMA* 38:166, 1902.
23. Senn, N.: Therapeutical value of röntgen ray in treatment of pseudoleukemia. *New York Med. J.* 77:665, 1903.
24. Gilbert, R.: Radiotherapy in Hodgkin's disease (malignant granulomatosis): Anatomic and clinical foundations; governing principles; results. *Am. J. Roentgenol.* 41:198, 1939.
25. Craft, C. B.: Results with roentgen ray therapy in Hodgkin's disease. *Bul. Staff. Meet. Univ. Minn. Hosp.* 11:391, 1940.
26. Kaplan, H. S.: The radical radiotherapy of regionally localized Hodgkin's disease. *Radiology* 78:553, 1962.
27. Easson, E. C., and Russell, M. H.: The cure of Hodgkin's disease. *Br. Med. J.* 1:1704, 1963.
28. Kinmouth, J. D.: Lymphangiography in man: Method of outlining lymphatic trunks and operation. *Clin. Sci.* 11:13, 1952.
29. Glatstein, E., Guernsey, J. M., Rosenberg, S. A., and Kaplan, H. S.: The value of laparotomy and splenectomy in the staging of Hodgkin's disease. *Cancer* 24:709, 1969.
30. Rosenberg, S. A.: Report of the committee on the staging of Hodgkin's disease. *Cancer Res.* 26:1310, 1966.
31. Carbone, P. P., Kaplan, H. S., Musshoff, K., Smithers, D. W., and Tubiana, M.: Report of the committee on Hodgkin's disease staging. *Cancer Res.* 31:1860, 1971.
32. Jacobson, L. O., Spurr, C. L., Guzman Baron, E. S., Smith, T., Lushbaugh, C., and Dick, G. F.: Nitrogen mustard therapy; studies on the effect of methylbis-(β-chloroethyl)amine hydrochloride on

neoplastic disorders of the hemopoietic system. *JAMA 132*:263, 1946.

33. Goodman, L. S., Wintrobe, M. M., Dameshek, W., Goodman, M. J., Gilman, A. Z., and McLennan, M. T.: Nitrogen mustard therapy: Use of methyl-bis-(β-chloroethyl)amine hydrochloride and tris-(β-chloroethyl)amine hydrochloride for Hodgkin's disease, lympho-sarcoma, leukemia, and certain allied and miscellaneous disorders. *JAMA 132*:126, 1946.

34. DeVita, V. T., Serpick, A. A., and Carbone, P. P.: Combination chemotherapy in the treatment of advanced Hodgkin's disease. *Ann. Intern. Med. 73*:881, 1970.

35. Kaplan, H. S.: *Hodgkin's Disease.* Harvard University Press, Cambridge, Mass., 1980, p. 58.

36. Fukuhara, S., and Rowley, J. D.: Chromosome 14 translocations in non-Burkitt lymphomas. *Int. J. Cancer 22*:14, 1978.

37. Reeves, B. R.: Cytogenetics of malignant lymphomas. *Humangenetik 20*:231–250, 1973.

38. Petrakis, N. L., Bostick, W. L., and Siegel, B. V.: The deoxyribonucleic acid (DNA) content of Sternberg-Reed cells of Hodgkin's disease. *J. Natl. Cancer Inst. 22*:551, 1959.

39. Peckham, M. J., and Cooper, E. H.: Proliferation characteristics of various classes of cells in Hodgkin's disease. *Cancer 24*:135, 1969.

40. Peckham, M. J., and Cooper, E. H.: Cell proliferation in Hodgkin's disease. *Natl. Cancer Inst. Monogr. 36*:179, 1973.

41. Kadin, M. E., and Asbury, A. K.: Long-term cultures of Hodgkin's tissue: A morphologic and radioautographic study. *Lab. Invest. 28*:181, 1973.

42. Kaplan, H. S., and Gartner, S.: "Sternberg-Reed" giant cells of Hodgkin's disease: Cultivation *in vitro*, heterotransplantation, and characterization as neoplastic macrophages. *Int. J. Cancer 19*:511, 1977.

43. Cowley, J. G.: *In vitro* cell proliferation studies in Hodgkin's disease. *Neoplasma 25*:83, 1978.

44. Charbit, A., Galoise, E. P., and Tabiana, M.: Relation between pathological nature growth rate of human tumors. *Eur. J. Cancer 7*:307, 1976.

45. Kaplan, H. S., and Smithers, D. W.: Autoimmunity in man and homologous disease in mice in relation to the malignant lymphomas. *Lancet 2*:1, 1959.

46. Order, S. E., and Hellman, S.: Pathogenesis of Hodgkin's disease. *Lancet 1*:571, 1972.

47. DeVita, V. T.: Lymphocyte reactivity in Hodgkin's disease: A lymphocyte civil war. *N. Engl. J. Med. 289*:801, 1973.

48. Order, S. E.: The history and progress of serologic immunotherapy and radiodiagnosis. *Radiology 118*:219, 1976.

49. Moroz, C., Lahat, N., Biniaminov, M., and Ramot, B.: Ferritin on the surface of lymphocytes in Hodgkin's disease patirents:: A possible blocking substance removed by levamisole. *Clin. Exp. Immunol. 29*:30, 1977.

50. Galili, W., Klein, E., Christensson, B., and Biberfell, P.: Lymphocytes of Hodgkin's disease biopsies exhibit: Stable E-rosette formation, natural attachment, and glucocorticoid sensitivity similar to immunoactivated T cells. *Clin. Immunol. Immunopathol. 16*:173, 1980.

51. William, J. K. L., et al.: Functional characterization of cells separated from suspensions of Hodgkin's disease tumor cells in an isokinetic gradient. *Blood 56*:787, 1977.

52. Sarcione, E. J., et al: Increased ferritin synthesis and release by Hodgkin's disease peripheral blood lymphocytes. *Int. J. Cancer 20*:339, 1977.

53. Kay, M. M. B.: Hodgkin's disease: A war between T-lymphocytes and transformed macrophages?, in *Lymphocytes, Macrophages, and Cancer*, edited by G. Mathé, I. Florentin, and M. C. Simmler. Springer-Verlag. Berlin; *Recent Results Cancer Res. 56*:111, 1976.

54. Payne, S. V., et al.: The Reed-Sternberg cell/lymphocyte interaction. *Am. J. Pathol. 100*:7, 1980.

55. McGuire, R., et al.: Hodgkin's cells and attached lymphocytes. *Cancer 44*:183, 1979.

56. Rappaport, H.: Tumors of the hematopoietic system, in *Atlas of Tumor Pathology*. Armed Forces Institute of Pathology, Washington, D.C., 1966, fasc. 8, sect. 3, p. 156.

57. Carr, I.: The ultrastructure of the abnormal reticulum cells in Hodgkin's disease. *J. Pathol. 115*:45, 1975.

58. Dorfman, R. F., Rice, D. F., Mitchell, A. D., Kempson, R. L., and Levine, G.: Ultrastructural studies of Hodgkin's disease. *Natl. Cancer Inst. Monogr. 36*:221, 1973.

59. Garvin, A. J., Spicer, S. S., Parmley, R. T., and Munster, A. M.: Immunohistochemical demonstration of IgG in Reed-Sternberg and other cells in Hodgkin's disease. *J. Exp. Med. 139*:1077, 1974.

60. Taylor, C. R.: An immunohistochemical study of follicular lymphoma, reticulum cell sarcoma and Hodgkin's disease. *Eur. J. Cancer 12*:61, 1976.

61. Kadin, M. E., Stites, D. P., Levy, R., and Warnke, R.: Exogenous origin of immunoglobulin in Reed-Sternberg cells of Hodgkin's disease. *N. Engl. J. Med. 299*:1208, 1978.

62. Anagnostou, D., Parker, J. W., Taylor, C. R., Tindle, B. H., and Lukes, R. J.: Lacunar cells of nodular sclerosing Hodgkin's disease. *Cancer 39*:1032, 1977.

63. Landaas, T. O., Goodal, T., and Halvorsen, T. B.: Characterization of immunoglobulin in Hodgkin's cells. *Int. J. Cancer 20*:717, 1977.

64. Kadin, M. E., Newcom, S. R., Gold, S. B., and Stites, D. P.: Origin of Hodgkin's cell. *Lancet 2*:167, 1974.

65. Resnick, G. D., and Nachman, R. L.: Reed-Sternberg cells in Hodgkin's disease contain fibronectin. *Blood 57*:339, 1981.

66. Poppema, S., Elema, J. D., and Halie, M. R.: The significance of intracytoplasmic proteins in Reed-Sternberg cells. *Cancer 42*:1973, 1978.

67. Stuart, A. E., Williams, A. R. W., and Habeshaw, J. A.: Rosetting and other reactions of the Reed-Sternberg cell. *J. Pathol. 122*:81, 1977.

68. Roberts, A. N., Smith, K. L., Dowell, B. L., and Hubbard, A. K.: Cultural, morphological, cell membrane, enzymatic, and neoplastic properties of cell lines derived from a Hodgkin's disease lymph node. *Cancer Res. 38*:3033, 1978.

69. American Cancer Society: Cancer statistics, 1979. *CA 29*:15, 1979.

70. Gutensohn, N., and Cole, P.: Childhood social environment and Hodgkin's disease. *N. Engl. J. Med. 304*:135, 1981.

71. Gutensohn, N., and Cole, P.: Epidemiology of Hodgkin's disease. *Semin. Oncol. 7*:92, 1980.

72. Newell, G. R., et al.: Age differences in the histology of Hodgkin's disease. *J. Natl. Cancer Inst. 45*:311, 1970.

73. Stalsberg, H.: Hodgkin's disease in Western Europe: A review. *Natl. Cancer Inst. Monogr. 36*:31, 1973.

74. Silverman, D.T., et al.: A comparison of Hodgkin's disease in Alameda County, California, and Connecticut: Histologic subtype and age distribution. *Cancer 39(4)*:1758, 1977.

75. Li, F. P., et al.: Hodgkin's disease in the elderly. *Lancet 1*:774, 1973.

76. MacMahon, B.: Epidemiology of Hodgkin's disease. *Cancer Res. 26*:1189, 1966.

77. Correa, P., and O'Connor, G. T.: Epidemiological patterns of Hodgkin's disease. *Int. J. Cancer 8*:192, 1971.

78. Sacks, M., Selzer, G., and Steinitz, R.: Hodgkin's disease in Israel. *Natl. Cancer Inst. Monogr. 36*:37, 1973.

79. Hoover, R.: *Persons at High Risk of Cancer: An Approach to Cancer Etiology and Control.* Plenum, New York, 1975, pp. 343–360.

80. Henderson, B. E., et al.: Risk of Hodgkin's disease. *Cancer Res. 39(11)*:4507, 1979.

81. Gutensohn, N., and Cole, P.: Epidemiology of Hodgkin's disease in the young. *Int. J. Cancer 19*:595, 1977.

82. Abramson, J. H., Pridan, H,. Sacks, M. I., Avitzour, M., and Peritzm, E.: A case-control study of Hodgkin's disease in Israel. *J. Natl. Cancer Inst. 61(2)*:307, 1978.

83. Gutensohn, N., Cole, P., and Li, F. P.: Sibship size and Hodgkin's disease. *N. Engl. J. Med. 292*:1025, 1975.

84. Vianna, N. J., Greenwald, P., and Davies, J. N. P.: Tonsillectomy and Hodgkin's disease: The lymphoid tissue barrier. *Lancet 1*:431, 1971.

85. Vianna, N. J., et al.: Tonsillectomy and Hodgkin's disease. *Lancet 2*:131, 1974 (letter).

86. Cole, P., Mack, T., Rothman, K., Henderson, B., and Newell, G.: Tonsillectomy and Hodgkin's disease. *N. Engl. J. Med. 288*:634, 1973.

87. Vianna, N. J., et al.: Tonsillectomy and childhood Hodgkin's disease. *Lancet 1*:338, 1980.

88. Johnson, S. K., and Johnson, R. E.: Tonsillectomy history in Hodgkin's disease. *N. Engl. J. Med. 287*:1122, 1972.

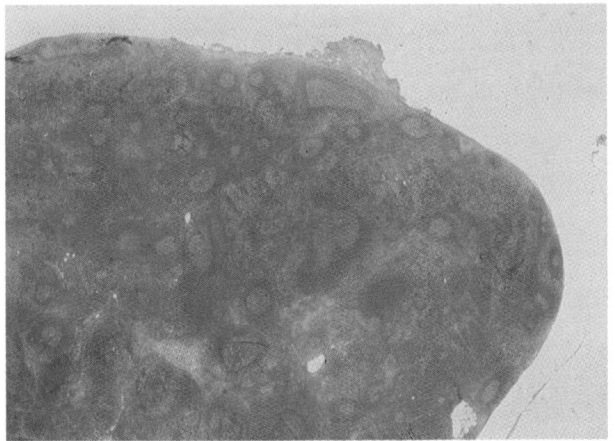

9-1 Orderly hyperplasia of lymph node, with distinct functional components: germinal centers, paracortex, sinuses, and medullary cords. (Original magnification ×4.)

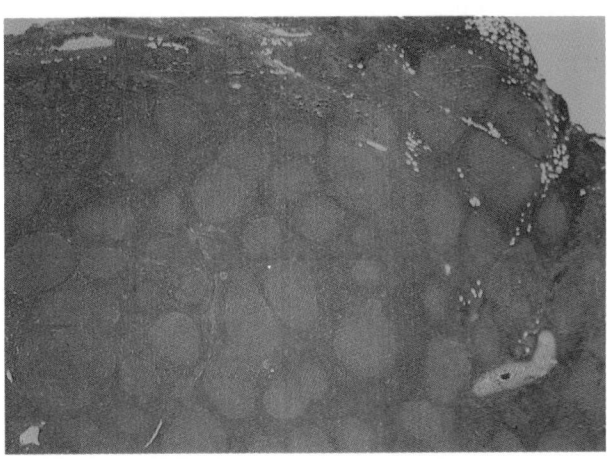

9-2 Follicular lymphoma. Compare with 9-1. Follicles are abnormal and uniformly present without separation throughout node. (Original magnification ×4.)

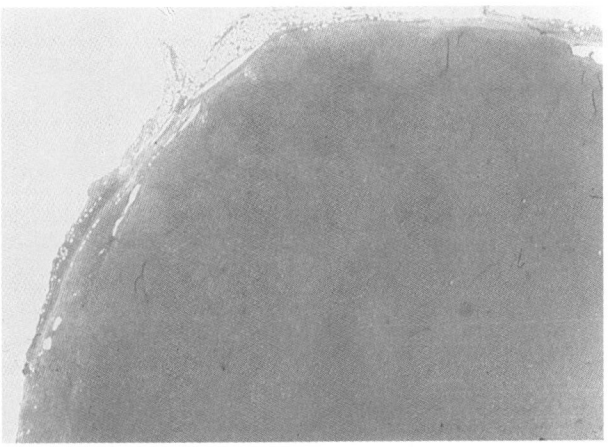

9-3 Diffuse lymphoma. Neoplastic lymphoid cells have grown as a diffuse expanse, totally replacing normal elements. Compare with Plates 9-1 and 9-2. (Original magnification ×4.)

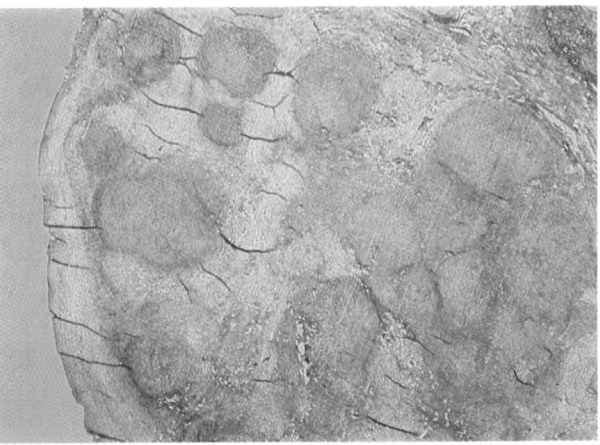

9-4 Nodular sclerosing Hodgkin's disease showing hyaline fibrosis of capsule and trabeculae encircling cellular nodules. (Original magnification ×4.)

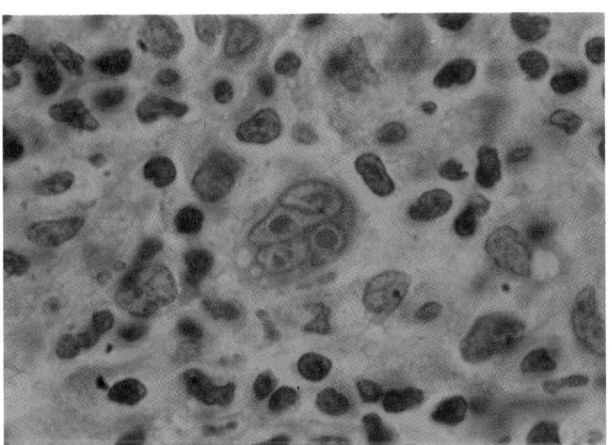

9-5 Reed-Sternberg cell of Hodgkin's disease with multiple nuclear lobes containing large eosinophilic nucleoli. Note surrounding reactive cellularity. (Original magnification ×1000.)

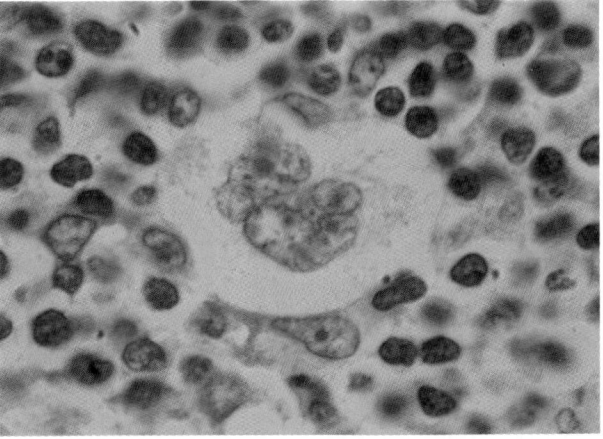

9-6 Lacunar cell variant of nodular sclerosing Hodgkin's disease with abundant clear cytoplasm and multiple nuclear lobes containing small nucleoli. (Original magnification ×1000.)

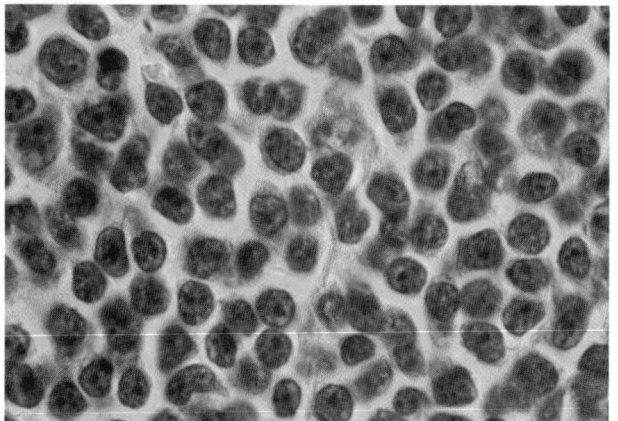

10-1 Small lymphocyte lymphoma (low-grade) composed of small cells with clumped chromatin, some of which show plasmacytoid features with basophilic cytoplasm. (Original magnification ×1000.)

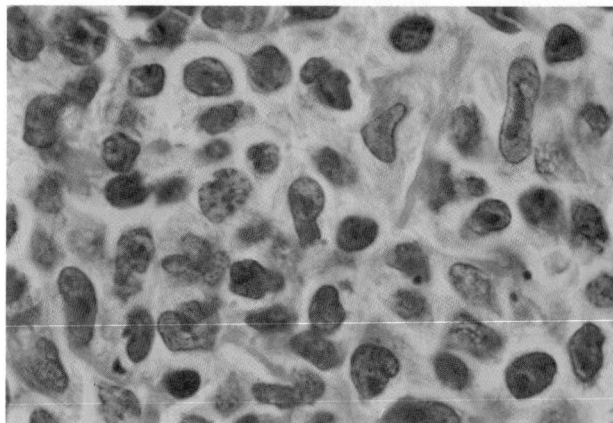

10-2 Small cleaved cell lymphoma with small, irregular nuclei containing nucleoli. If follicular, this is low-grade; if diffuse, intermediate-grade. (Original magnification ×1000.)

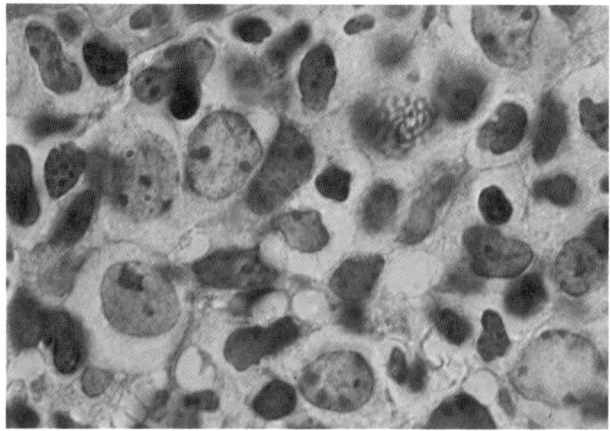

10-3 Large cell lymphoma (intermediate-grade) of large follicular center cell (centroblastic) composition. Nuclear membranes are delicate; nucleoli are small. (Original magnification ×1000.)

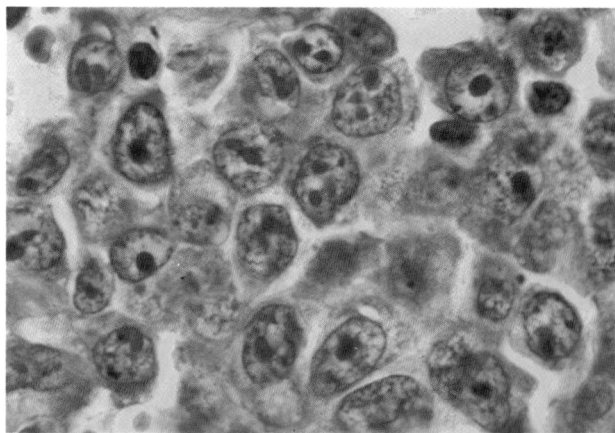

10-4 Large cell, immunoblastic lymphoma (high-grade). Note thick nuclear membranes, large central nucleoli, and abundant basophilic cytoplasm. (Original magnification ×1000.)

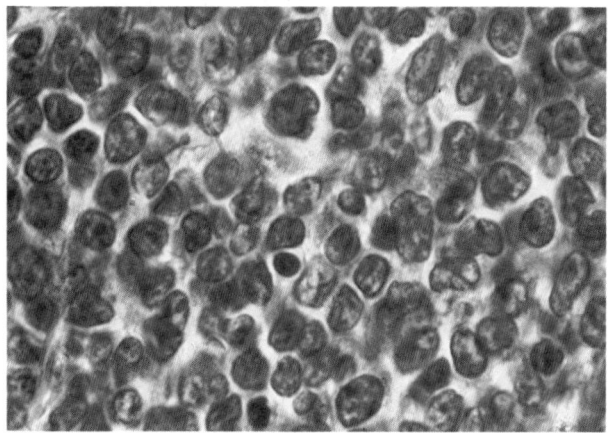

10-5 Lymphoblastic lymphoma (high-grade). There is very little cytoplasm, nuclear membranes are delicate and occasionally convoluted, and nucleoli are small. (Original magnification ×1000.)

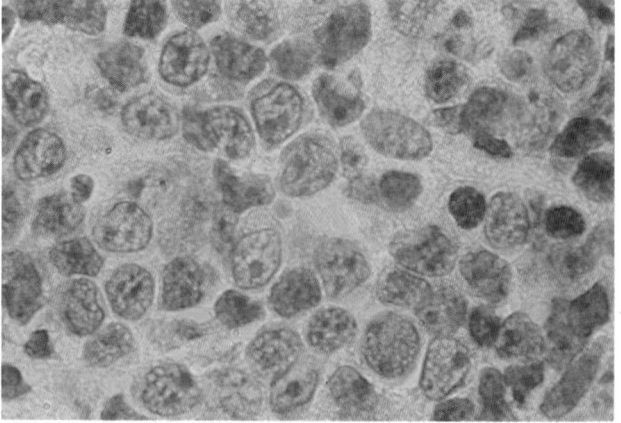

10-6 Small noncleaved cell (Burkitt's) lymphoma (high-grade). Nuclear membranes are thick and smooth, there are large nucleoli, and cytoplasm is basophilic. (Original magnification ×1000.)

PLATE 10   Lymphoma

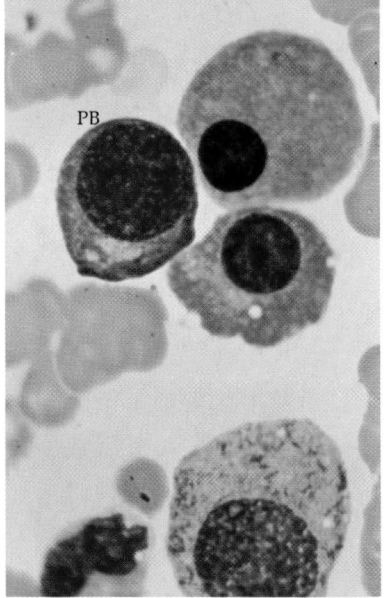

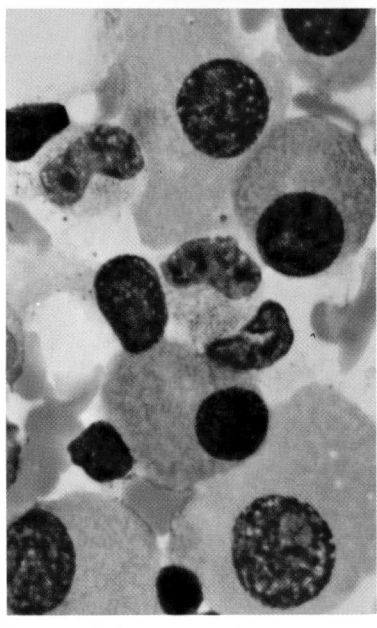

Marrow from patients with multiple myeloma. **11-1** Top, three plasma cells; bottom, reticulum cell. Cell PB, with large nucleus, fine chromatin, and nucleoli, resembles a plasma- blast. These may be hard to distinguish from proerythro- blasts.

11-2,3 Heavy infiltration with abnormal plasma cells, some having immature nuclei with nucleoli.

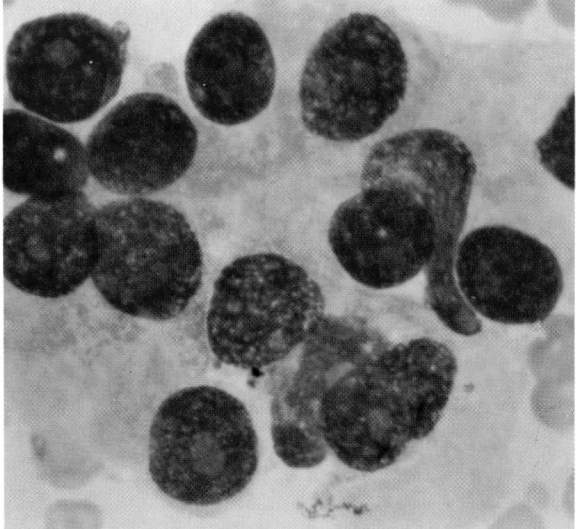

11-4 Marrow from a patient with metastatic carcinoma of the breast. There is a syncytium of carcinoma cells.

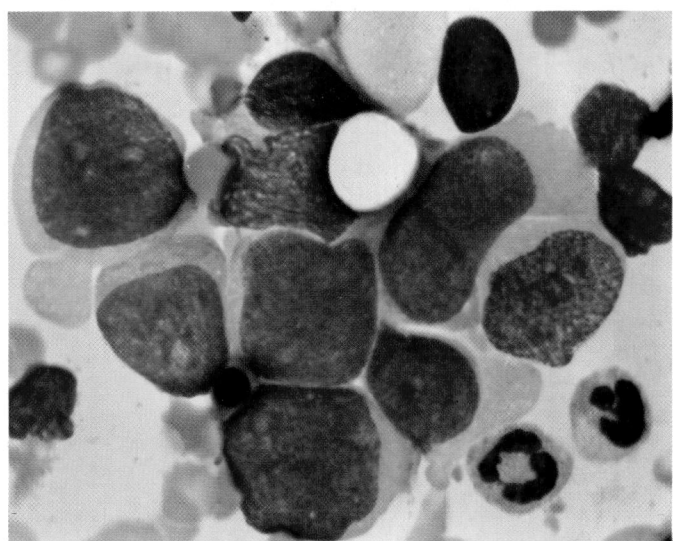

11-5 Marrow from a patient with metastatic carcinoma of the lung, showing a sheet of carcinoma cells.

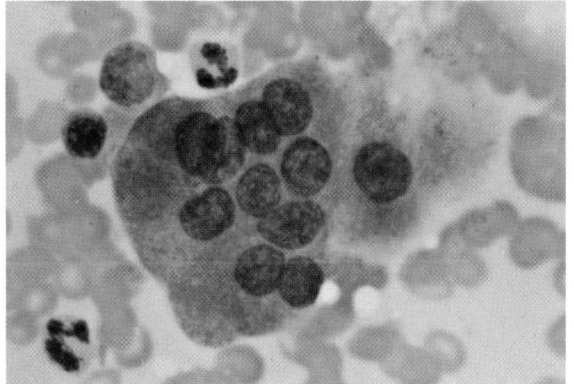

11-6 Osteoclast from marrow.

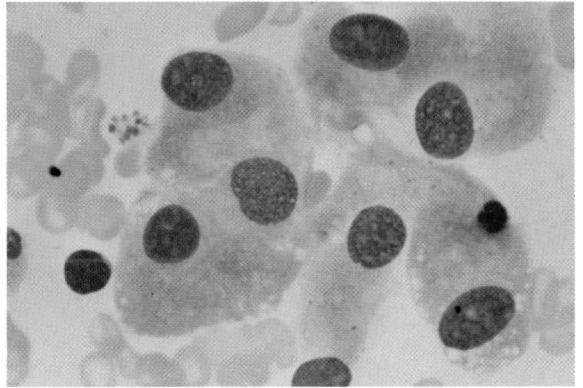

11-7 Osteoblasts from marrow.

Note: All films on this plate, Wright's stain, original magnification ×1000.

Multiple myeloma and metastatic carcinoma **PLATE 11**

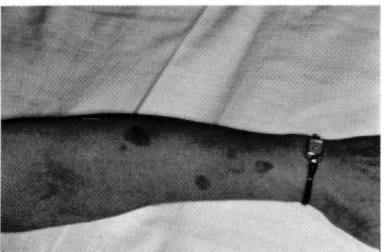

12-1 Steroid purpura.

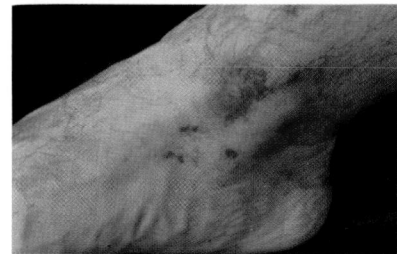

12-2 Schamberg's dermatosis.

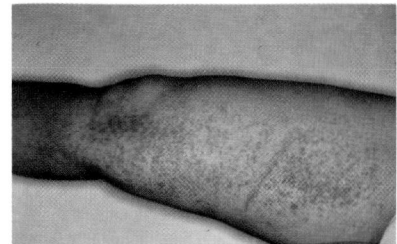

12-3 Macroglobulinemic purpura.

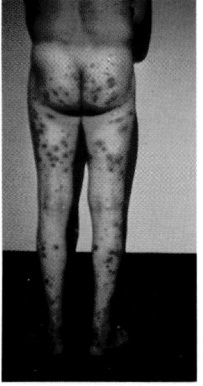

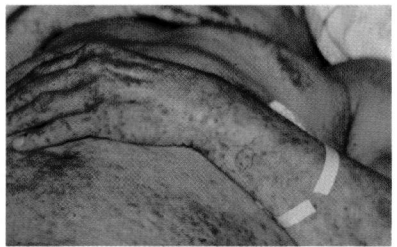

12-4 Henoch-Schönlein purpura.   **12-5** Nonthrombocytopenic purpura due to infection.
12-6 Nonthrombocytopenia drug purpura (mercury).

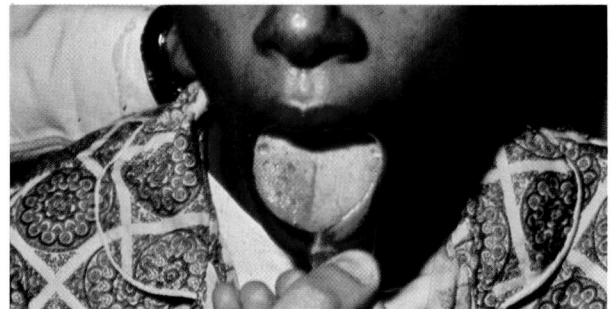

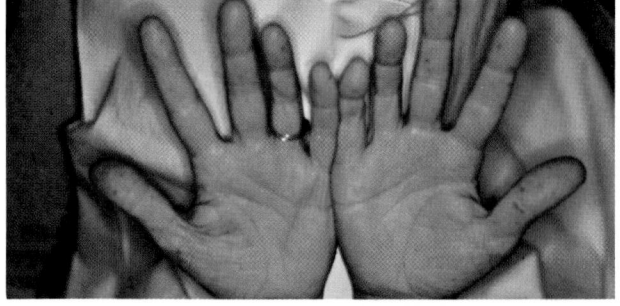

12-7 Hereditary hemorrhagic telangiectasia. Pressing the left side of the tongue with
the glass slide obliterates telangiectases.   **12-8** Hereditary hemorrhagic telangiectasia.
12-1 to 12-8 courtesy of Dr. Steven O. Schwartz.

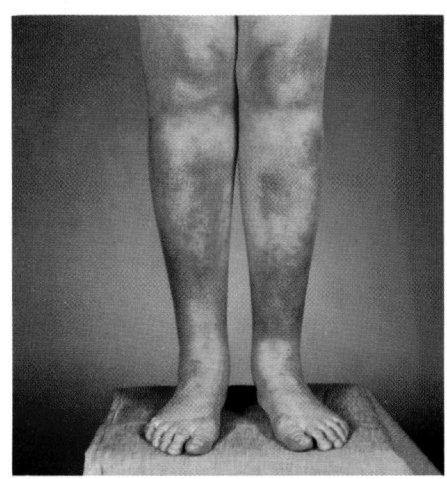

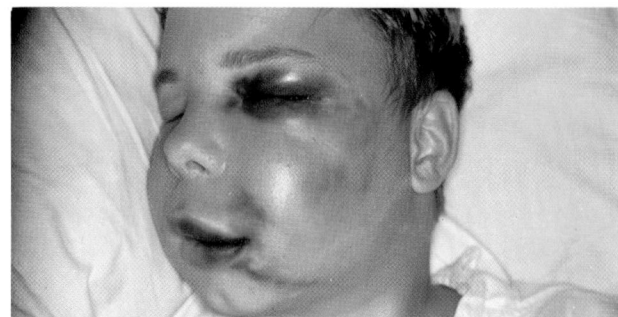

12-9 Purpura due to Cushing's disease. (Courtesy of Dr. William Barry.)   **12-10** Hemophilia-hematoma that developed
after dental treatment. (Courtesy of Dr. E. L. Lozner.)

PLATE 12   Purpura, hereditary hemorrhagic telangiectasia, and hemophilia

89. Paffenberger, R. S., Jr., Wing, A. L., and Hyde, R. T.: Brief communication: Characteristics in youth indicative of adult-onset Hodgkin's disease. *J. Natl. Cancer Inst.* 58:1489, 1977.

90. Paffenberger, R. S.: Previous tonsillectomy and current pregnancy as they affect risk of poliomyelitis attack. *Ann. N.Y. Acad. Sci.* 61:856, 1955.

91. Newell, G. R.: Etiology of multiple sclerosis and Hodgkin's disease. *Am. J. Epidemiol.* 91:119, 1970.

92. Abramson, J. H.: Childhood experience and Hodgkin's disease in adults: An intepretation of incidence data. *Isr. J. Med. Sci.* 10:1365, 1974.

93. Isager, H., and Anderson, E.: Pre-morbid factors in Hodgkin's disease. I. Birth weight and growth patterns from 8 to 14 years of age. *Scand. J. Haematol.* 21(3):250, 1978.

94. Hancock, B. W., Mosley, R., and Coup, A. J.: Height and Hodgkin's disease. *Lancet* 2:1364, 1976.

95. Grufferman, S. G., Cole, P., Smith, P. G., and Lukes, R. J.: Hodgkin's disease in sibs. *N. Engl. J. Med.* 296:248, 1977.

96. Fraumeni, J. F., Jr.: Family studies in Hodgkin's disease. *Cancer Res.* 34:1164, 1974.

97. Rigby, P., Pratt, P., Rosenlof, R., and Lemon, H.: Genetic relationship in familial leukemia and lymphoma. *Arch. Intern. Med.* 121:67, 1968.

98. Vianna, N. J., Davies, J. N. P., Polan, A. K., and Wolfgang, P.: Familial Hodgkin's disease: An environmental and genetic disorder. *Lancet* 2:854, 1974.

99. Razis, D., Diamond, H., and Craver, L.: Familial Hodgkin's disease: Its significance and implications. *Ann. Intern. Med.* 51:933, 1959.

100. Bohunický, L., Poliaková, L., Krizan, Z., Céry, V., and Halko, J.: The incidence of lymphogranulomatosis in single-ovum twins. *Neoplasma* 18:283, 1971.

101. Graza, K., Kofman, S., and Economu, S. G.: Hodgkin's disease in monozygotic twins: A case report. *J. Surg. Oncol.* 12:221, 1979.

102. Beuhler, S. K., Firme, F., Fodor, G., Frase, G. R.: Marshall, W. H., and Vaze, P.: Common variable immunodeficiency, Hodgkin's disease, and other malignancies in a Newfoundland family. *Lancet* 1:195, 1975.

103. Salimonu, L. S., et al.: Immunoglobulins in familial Hodgkin's disease and immunodeficiency in Newfoundland. *Int. Arch. Allergy Appl. Immunol.* 63:52, 1980.

104. Svejgaard, A., Platz, P., Ryder, L. P., Nielsen, L. S., and Thomsen, M.: HL-A and disease association — A survey. *Transplant. Rev.* 22:3, 1975.

105. Marshall, W. H., et al.: HLA in familial Hodgkin's disease: Results and a new hypothesis. *Int. J. Cancer* 19(4):450, 1977.

106. Kissmeyer-Nielsen, F., Kjerbye, K. E., and Lamm, L. U.: HL-A in Hodgkin's disease. III. A prospective study. *Transplant. Rev.* 22:168, 1975.

107. Björkholm, M., Holm, G., Mellstedt, H., and Moller, E.: A prospective study of HL-A antigen phenotypes and lymphocyte abnormalities in Hodgkin's disease. *Tissue Antigens* 6:247, 1975.

108. Kaplan, H. S.: *Hodgkin's Disease.* Harvard University Press, Cambridge, Mass., 1980, pp. 36–37.

109. Vianna, N. J., Greenwald, P., and Davies, J. N. P.: Extended epidemic of Hodgkin's disease in high-school students. *Lancet* 1:1209, 1971.

110. Vianna, N. J., et al.: Hodgkin's disease: Cases with features of a community outbreak. *Ann. Intern. Med.* 77:169, 1972.

111. Vianna, N. J., and Polan, A. K.: Epidemiological evidence for transmission of Hodgkin's disease. *N. Engl. J. Med.* 289:499, 1973.

112. Newell, G. R., et al.: Case-control study of Hodgkin's disease. I. Results of the interview questionnaire. *J. Natl. Cancer Inst.* 51:1437, 1973.

113. Evans, A. R., Hancock, B. W., Brown, M. J., and Richmond, J.: A small cluster of Hodgkin's disease. *Br. Med. J.* 1:1056, 1977.

114. Ramsey, N. M.: Clustering of malignant lymphoma and Hodgkin's disease. *Med. J. Aust.* 2:779, 1975.

115. Klinger, R. J., and Minton, J. P.: Case clustering of Hodgkin's disease in a small rural community, with association among cases. *Lancet* 1:168, 1973.

116. Schimpff, S. C., Schimpff, C. R., Brager, D. M., and Wiernik, P. H.: Leukemia and lymphoma patients linked by prior social contact. *Lancet* 1:124, 1975.

117. Zack, M. M., Jr., Heath, C. W., Jr., Andrews, M. D., Grivas, A. J., Jr., and Christine, B. W.: High school contact among persons with leukemia and lymphoma. *J. Natl. Cancer Inst.* 59:1343, 1977.

118. Smith, P. G., and Pike, M. C.: Case clustering in Hodgkin's disease. A brief review of the present position and report of current work at Oxford. *Cancer Res.* 34:1156, 1974.

119. Smith, P. G., Pike, M. C., Kinlen, L. J., Jones, A., and Harris, R.: Contacts between young patients with Hodgkin's disease: A case control study. *Lancet* 2:59, 1977.

120. Grufferman, S., Cole, P., and Levitan, T. R.: Evidence against transmission of Hodgkin's disease in high schools. *N. Engl. J. Med.* 300:1006, 1979.

121. Abramson, J. H.: Infective agents in the causation of Hodgkin's disease: A review of the epidemiological evidence. *Isr. J. Med. Sci.* 9:932, 1973.

122. Alderson, M. R., and Nayak, R.: Epidemiology of Hodgkin's disease. *J. Chronic Dis.* 25:253, 1972.

123. Vianna, N. J., Keogh, M. D., Polan, A. K., and Greenwald, P.: Hodgkin's disease mortality among physicians. *Lancet* 2:131, 1974.

124. Smith, P. G., Kinlen, L. J., and Doll, R.: Hodgkin's disease mortality among physicians. *Lancet* 2:525, 1974.

125. Matanoski, G. M., Sartwell, P. E., and Elliott, E. A.: Hodgkin's disease mortality among physicians. *Lancet* 1:926, 1975.

126. Hoover, R.: Hodgkin's disease in schoolteachers. *N. Engl. J. Med.* 291:473, 1974.

127. de The, G., et al.: Epidemiological evidence for causal relationship between Epstein-Barr virus and Burkitt's lymphoma from Ugandan prospective study. *Nature* 274:756, 1978.

128. Robinson, J. E., Andiman, W. A., Henderson, E., and Miller, G.: Host-determined differences in expression of surface marker characteristics on human and simian lymphoblastoid cell lines transformed by Epstein-Barr virus. *Proc. Natl. Acad. Sci. U.S.A.* 74:749, 1977.

129. Goldman, J. M., and Aisenberg, A. C.: Incidence of antibody to EB virus, herpes simplex, and cytomegalovirus in Hodgkin's disease. *Cancer* 26:327, 1970.

130. Levine, P. H., Ablashi, D. V., Berard, C. W., Carbone, P. P., Waggoner, D. E., and Malan, L.: Elevated antibody titers to Epstein-Barr virus in Hodgkin's disease. *Cancer* 27:416, 1971.

131. Langenhuysen, M. M. A. C., et al.: Antibodies to Epstein-Barr virus, cytomegalovirus, and Australia antigen in Hodgkin's disease. *Cancer* 34:262, 1974.

132. Henderson, B. E., et al.: Case-control study of Hodgkin's disease. II. Herpesvirus group antibody titers and HL-A type. *J. Natl. Cancer Inst.* 51:1437, 1973.

133. Miller, R. W., and Beebe, G. W.: Infectious mononucleosis and the empirical risk of cancer. *J. Natl. Cancer Inst.* 50:315, 1973.

134. Connelly, R. R., and Christine, B. W.: A cohort study of cancer following infectious mononucleosis. *Cancer Res.* 34:1172, 1974.

135. Rosdahl, N., Larsen, S. O., and Clemmesen, J.: Hodgkin's disease in patients with previous infectious mononucleosis: 30 years' experience. *Br. Med. J.* 2:253, 1974.

136. Carter, C. D., et al.: Cancer incidence following infectious mononucleosis. *Am. J. Epidemiol.* 105:30, 1977.

137. Pagano, J. S., Huang, C. H., and Levine, P.: Absence of Epstein-Barr viral DNA in American Burkitt's lymphoma. *N. Engl. J. Med.* 289:1395, 1973.

138. Lindahl, T., et al.: Relationship between Epstein Barr virus (EBV) DNA and the EBV-determined nuclear antigen (EBNA) in Burkitt lymphoma biopsies and other lymphoproliferative malignancies. *Intl. J. Cancer* 13:764, 1974.

139. Gallo, R. C., Todaro, G. J.: Oncogenic RNA viruses. *Semin. Oncol.* 3:81, 1976.

140. Spiegelman, S., Kufe, D., Hehlman, R., and Peters, W. P.: Evidence for RNA tumor viruses in human lymphomas including Burkitt's disease. *Cancer Res.* 33:1515, 1973.

141. Aulakh, G. S., and Gallo, R. C.: Rauscher-leukemia-virus-related sequences in human DNA: Presence in some tissues of some patients with hematopoietic neoplasias and absence in DNA from other tissues. *Proc. Natl. Acad. Sci. U.S.A.* 74:353, 1977.

142. Schlom, J., and Spiegelman, S.: Simultaneous detection of reverse transcriptase and high-molecular-weight RNA unique to oncogenic RNA viruses. *Science* 174:840, 1971.

143. Chezzi, C., Dettori, G., Manzari, V., Agliano, A. M., and Sanne, A.: Simultaneous detection of reverse transcriptase with high-molecular-weight RNA in tissue of patients with Hodgkin's disease and patients with leukemia. *Proc. Natl. Acad. Sci. U.S.A.* 73:4649, 1976.

144. Hirshaut, Y., Reagan, R. L., Perry, S., DeVita, V., and Barile, M. F.: The search for a viral agent in Hodgkin's disease. *Cancer* 34:1080, 1974.

145. Grufferman, S., Duong, T., and Cole, P.: Occupation and Hodgkin's disease. *J. Natl. Cancer Inst.* 57:1193, 1976.

146. Petersen, G. R., and Milham, S., Jr.: Hodgkin's disease mortality and occupational exposure to wood. *J. Natl. Cancer Inst.* 53:957, 1974.

147. Greene, M. H., Brinton, L. A., Fraumeni, J. F., and D'Amico, R.: Familial and sporadic Hodgkin's disease associated with occupational wood exposure. *Lancet* 2:626, 1978.

148. Li, F. P., Willard, D. R., Goodman, R., and Vowter, G.: Malignant lymphoma after diphenylhydantoin (Dilantin) therapy. *Cancer* 36:1359, 1975.

149. Waldemann, T. P., et al.: Immunodeficiency disease and malignancy. *Ann. Intern. Med.* 77:605, 1972.

150. Miller, D. G.: The association of immune disease and malignant lymphomas. *Ann. Intern. Med.* 66:507, 1967.

151. Ewing, J.: *Neoplastic Diseases*. Saunders, Philadelphia, 1928.

152. Dubin, I. N.: The poverty of the immunological mechanism in patients with Hodgkin's disease. *Ann. Intern. Med* 27:898, 1947.

153. Schier, W. W., Roth, A., Ostroff, G., and Schrift, M. H.: Hodgkin's disease and immunity. *Am. J. Med.* 20:94, 1956.

154. Brown, R. S., Haynes, H. A., Foley, H. T., Godwin, H. A., Berard, C. W., and Carbone, P. P.: Hodgkin's disease: Immunologic, clinical and histologic features of 50 untreated patients. *Ann. Intern. Med.* 67:291, 1967.

155. Young, R. C., Corder, M. P., Berard, C. W., and DeVita, V. T.: Immune alterations in Hodgkin's disease: Effect of delayed hypersensitivity and lymphocyte transformation on course and survival. *Arch. Intern. Med.* 131:446, 1973.

156. Eltringham, J. R., and Kaplan, H. S.: Impaired delayed hypersensitivity responses in 154 patients with untreated Hodgkin's disease. *Natl. Cancer Inst. Monogr.* 36:107, 1973.

157. Case, D. C., Jr., et al.: Comparison of multiple in vivo and in vitro parameters in untreated patients with Hodgkin's disease. *Cancer* 38:1807, 1976.

158. Ziegler, J. B., Hansen, P., and Penny, R.: Intrinsic lymphocyte defect in Hodgkin's disease: Analysis of the phytohemagglutinin dose-response. *Cell Immunol. Immunopathol.* 3:451, 1975.

159. Schulof, R. S., et al.: Multivariate analysis of T-cell functional defects and circulating serum factors in Hodgkin's disease. *Cancer* 48:964, 1981.

160. Aisenberg, A. C.: Studies on delayed sensitivity in Hodgkin's disease. *J. Clin. Invest.* 41:1964, 1962.

161. Miller, D. G., Lizardo, J. G., and Synderman, R. K.: Homologous and heterologous skin transplantation in patients with lymphomatous disease. *J. Natl. Cancer Inst.* 26:569, 1961.

162. DeGast, G. C., Halie, M. R., and Nieweg, H. O.: Immunological responsiveness against two primary antigens in untreated patients with Hodgkin's disease. *Eur. J. Cancer* 11:217, 1975.

163. Aisenberg, A. C.: Immunologic status of Hodgkin's disease. *Cancer* 19:385, 1966.

164. Twomey, J. J., and Rice, L.: Impact of Hodgkin's disease upon the immune system. *Semin. Oncol* 7:114, 1980.

165. Goldman, J. M., and Hobbs, J. R.: The immunoglobulins in Hodgkin's disease. *Immunology* 13:421, 1967.

166. Wagener, D., et al: The immunoglobulins in Hodgkin's disease. *Eur. J. Cancer* 12:683, 1976.

167. Longmire, R. L., McMillan, R., Yelenosky, R., Armstrong, S., Lang, J. E., and Craddock, C. G.: In vitro splenic IgG synthesis in Hodgkin's disease. *N. Engl. J. Med.* 289:763, 1973.

168. Hersh, E. M.: Kinetic approach to the study of cell-mediated immunity in Hodgkin's disease. *Natl. Cancer Inst. Monogr.* 36:123, 1973.

169. Minor, D. R., Schiffman, G., and McIntosh, L. S.: Response of patients with Hodgkin's disease to pneumococcal vaccine. *Ann. Intern. Med.* 90(6):887, 1979.

170. Sybesma, J. P. H. P., Holtzer, J. D., Borst-Eilers, E., Moes, M., and Zegers, B. J. M.: Antibody response in Hodgkin's disease and other lymphomas related to HL-A antigens, immunoglobulin levels, and therapy. *Vox Sang.* 25:254, 1973.

171. Hancock, B. W., Bruce, L., Dunsmore, I. R., Ward, A. M., and Richmond, J.: Follow-up studies on the immune status of patients with Hodgkin's disease after splenectomy and treatment, in relapse and remission. *Br. J. Cancer* 36:347, 1977.

172. Weitzman, S. A., Aisenberg, A. C., Siber, G. R., and Smith, D. H.: Impaired humoral immunity in treated Hodgkin's disease. *N. Engl. J. Med.* 297:245, 1977.

173. Levine, A. M., et al.: Positive Coombs test in Hodgkin's disease: Significance and implications. *Blood* 55:607, 1980.

174. Amlot, P. L., and Green, L. A.: Atopy and immunoglobulin E concentration in Hodgkin's disease and other lymphomas. *Br. Med. J.* 1:327, 1978.

175. Romagnani, S., et al.: Hyperproduction of IgE and T-cell dysfunction in Hodgkin's disease. *Int. Arch. Allergy Appl. Immunol.* 63:64, 1980.

176. Chisesi, T., Capnist, G., and Barbui, T.: Two serum IgG-M components of different light-chain types in a case of Hodgkin's disease. *Acta Haematol.* 55:250, 1976.

177. Grifoni, V.: Recent immunological findings in Hodgkin's disease. *Tumori* 59:363, 1973.

178. Mendius, J. R., et al.: Family distribution of lymphocytotoxins in Hodgkin's disease. *Ann. Intern. Med.* 84(2):151, 1976.

179. Aisenberg, A. C.: Studies of lymphocyte transfer reactions in Hodgkin's disease. *J. Clin. Invest.* 44:555, 1965.

180. Posner, M. R., Reinherz, E. L., Breard, J., Nodler, L. M., Rosenthal, D. S., and Schlossman, S. F.: Lymphoid subpopulations of peripheral blood and spleen in untreated Hodgkin's disease. *Cancer* 48:1170, 1981.

181. Fuks, Z., Strober, S., Bobrove, A.M., Sasazuki, T., McMichael, A., and Kaplan, H. S.: Long-term effects of radiation on T and B lymphocytes in peripheral blood of patients with Hodgkin's disease. *J. Clin. Invest.* 58:803, 1976.

182. Levy, R. A., and Kaplan, H. S.: Impaired lymphocyte function in untreated Hodgkin's disease. *N. Engl. J. Med.* 290:181, 1974.

183. Hersh, E. M., and Oppenheim, J. J.: Impaired in vitro lymphocyte transformation in Hodgkin's disease. *N. Engl. J. Med.* 273:1006, 1965.

184. Matchett, K. M., Huang, A. T., and Kremer, W. B.: Impaired lymphocyte transformation in Hodgkin's disease: Evidence for depletion of circulating T-lymphocytes. *J. Clin. Invest.* 52:1908, 1973.

185. Faguet, G. B.: Quantitation of immunocompetence in Hodgkin's disease. *J. Clin. Invest.* 56:951, 1975.

186. Mintz, U., and Sachs, L.: Membrane differences in peripheral blood lymphocytes from patients with chronic lymphocytic leukemia and Hodgkin's disease. *Proc. Natl. Acad. Sci. U.S.A.* 72:2428, 1975.

187. Ben-Bassat, H., and Goldblum, N.: Concanavalin A receptors on the surface membrane of lymphocytes from patients with Hodgkin's disease and other malignant lymphomas. *Proc. Natl. Acad. Sci. U.S.A.* 72:1046, 1975.

188. Holm, G., Perlmann, and Johansson, B.: Impaired phytohaemagglutinin-induced cytotoxicity in vitro of lymphocytes from patients with Hodgkin's disease or chronic lymphatic leukemia. *Clin. Exp. Immunol.* 2:351, 1967.

189. Churchill, W. H., Rocklin, R. R., Moloney, W. C., and David, J. R.: In vitro evidence of normal lymphocyte function in some patients with Hodgkin's disease and negative delayed cutaneous hypersensitivity. *Natl. Cancer Inst. Mongr.* 36:99, 1973.

190. Rassiga-Pidot, A. L., and McIntyre, O. R.: In vitro leukocyte interferon production in patients with Hodgkin's disease. *Cancer Res.* 34:2995, 1974.

191. Bentwich, Z., Cohen, R., and Brautbar, C.: T and B blocking factors in Hodgkin's disease. *Adv. Exp. Med. Biol.* 66:685, 1976.

192. Bieber, M. M., Fuks, Z., and Kaplan, H. S.: An E-rosette inhibiting substance in Hodgkin's disease spleen extracts. *Clin. Exp. Immunol.* 29:369, 1977.

193. Fuks, Z., Strober, S., and Kaplan, H. S.: Interaction between serum factors and T lymphocytes in Hodgkin's disease. *N. Engl. J. Med.* 295:1273, 1976.

194. Bieber, M. M., King, D. P., Strober, S., and Kaplan, H. S.: Characterization of an E-rossette inhibitor (ERI) in the serum of patients

with Hodgkin's disease as a glycolipid. *Clin. Res.* 27:81A, 1979 (abstract).

195. Moroz, C., Giler, S., Kupfer, B., and Urea, I.: Lymphocytes bearing surface ferritin in patients with Hodgkin's disease and breast cancer. *N. Engl. J. Med.* 296:1172, 1977.

196. Goodwin, J. S., Messner, R. P., Bankhurst, A. D., Peake, G. T., Saiki, J. H., and Williams, R. C., Jr.: Prostaglandin-producing suppressor cells in Hodgkin's disease. *N. Engl. J. Med.* 297:963, 1977.

197. Hillinger, S. M., and Herzig, G. P.: Impaired cell.mediated immunity in Hodgkin's disease mediated by suppressor lymphocytes and monocytes. *J. Clin. Invest.* 61:1620, 1978.

198. Doner, D., and Sachs, L.: Differences in the formation of normal T lymphocyte colonies by peripheral blood cells from patients with chronic lymphocytic leukaemia and Hodgkin's disease. *Clin. Exp. Immunol.* 38:514, 1979.

199. Kaur, J., Spiers, A. S. D., Catovsky, D., and Galton, D. A. G.: Increase of T lymphocytes in the spleen in Hodgkin's disease. *Lancet* 2:800, 1974.

200. Gupta, S., and Tan, C.: Subpopulations of human T lymphocytes. XIV. Abnormality of T-cell locomotion and of distribution of subpopulations of T and B lymphocytes in peripheral blood and spleen from children with untreated Hodgkin's disease. *Clin. Immunol. Immunopathol.* 15:133, 1980.

201. Lichtenfeld, J. L., Wiernik, P. H., Mardiney, M. R., Jr., and Zarco, R. M.: Abnormalities of complement and its components in patients with acute leukemia, Hodgkin's disease, and sarcoma. *Cancer Res.* 36:3678, 1976.

202. Brandeis, W. E., Tan, C., Wang, Y., Good, R. A., and Day, N. K.: Circulating immune complexes, complement, and complement component levels in childhood Hodgkin's disease. *Clin. Exp. Immunol.* 39(3):551, 1980.

203. Amlot, P. L., Russell, B., Slaney, J. M., and Williams, B. D.: Correlation between immune complexes and prognostic factors in Hodgkin's disease. *Clin. Exp. Immunol.* 31:166, 1978.

204. Order, S. E.: The effects of therapeutic irradiation on lymphocytes and immunity. *Cancer* 39 (Suppl. 2):737, 1977.

205. Hancock, B. W., Bruce, L., Ward, A., and Richmond, J.: The immediate effects of splenectomy, radiotherapy, and intensive chemotherapy on the immune status of patients with malignant lymphoma. *Clin. Oncol.* 3:137, 1977.

206. Fisher, P. I., et al.: Persistent immunologic abnormalities in long-term survivors of advanced Hodgkin's disease. *Ann. Intern. Med.* 92(5):595, 1980.

207. Kaplan, H. S., Dorfman, R. F., Nelson, T. S., and Rosenberg, S. A.: Staging laparotomy and splenectomy in Hodgkin's disease: Analysis of indications and patterns of involvement in 285 consecutive, unselected patients. *Natl. Cancer Inst. Monogr.* 36:291, 1973.

208. Ultmann, J. E., and Moran, E. M.: Clinical course and complications in Hodgkin's disease. *Arch. Intern. Med.* 131:332, 1966.

209. Ultmann, J. E., Cunningham, J. K., and Gellhorn, A.: The clinical picture of Hodgkin's disease. *Cancer Res.* 26:1047, 1973.

210. Pel, P. K.: Zur Symptomatologie der sogenannten Pseudoleukämie: II. Pseudoleukämie oder chronisches Rückfallsfieber? *Berlin Klin. Wochenschr.* 24:644, 1887.

211. Ebstein, W. von: Das chronische Rückfallsfiebor eine ne Infectionskrankheit. *Berlin Klin. Wochenschr.* 24:565, 1887.

212. Tubiana, M., Attié, E., Flamont, R., Gérard-Marchant, R., and Hayat, M.: Prognostic factors in 454 cases of Hodgkin's disease. *Cancer Res.* 31:1801, 1971.

213. Young, C. W., and Dowling, M. D., Jr.: Antipyretic effect of cycloheximide, an inhibitor of protein synthesis, in patients with Hodgkin's disease or other malignant neoplasms. *Cancer Res.* 35:1218, 1975.

214. Bodel, P.: Pyrogen release in vitro by lymphoid tissues from patients with Hodgkin's disease. *Yale J. Biol. Med.* 47:101, 1974.

215. Atkinson, M. K., Austin, D. E., McElwain, T. J., and Peckham, M. J.: Alcohol pain in Hodgkin's disease. *Cancer* 37:895, 1976.

216. Lukes, R. J., Butler, J. J., and Hicks, E. B.: Natural history of Hodgkin's disease as related to its pathologic picture. *Cancer* 19:317, 1966.

217. Lukes, R. J., and Butler, J. J.: The pathology and nomenclature of Hodgkin's disease. *Cancer* 26:1063, 1966.

218. Keller, A. R., Kaplan, H. S., Lukes, R. J., and Rappaport, H.: Correlation of histopathology with other prognostic indicators in Hodgkin's disease. *Cancer* 22:487, 1968.

219. Neiman, R. S., Rosen, P. J., and Lukes, R. J.: Lymphocyte-depletion Hodgkin's disease: A clinicopathologic entity. *N. Engl. J. Med.* 288:751, 1973.

220. Dawson, R., and Mangalik, A.: Hodgkin's disease: An analysis of 128 cases. *Am. J. Hematol.* 4:209, 1978.

221. Edington, G. M., and Hendrickse, M.: Incidence and frequency of lymphoreticular tumors in Ibadan and the western state of Nigeria. *J. Natl. Cancer Inst.* 50:1623, 1973.

222. Kadin, M. E., Glatstein, E., and Dorfman, R. F.: Clinical-pathologic studies of 117 untreated patients subjected to laparotomy for staging of Hodgkin's disease. *Cancer* 27:1277, 1971.

223. Strum, S. B., and Rappaport, H.: Interrelations of the histologic types of Hodgkin's disease. *Arch. Pathol.* 91:127, 1971.

224. Coppleson, L. W., Rappaport, H., Strum, S. B., and Rose, J.: Analysis of the Rye classification of Hodgkin's disease: The prognostic significance of cellular composition. *J. Natl. Cancer Inst.* 51:379, 1973.

225. Rosenberg, S. A., and Kaplan, H. S.: Evidence for an orderly progression in the spread of Hodgkin's disease. *Cancer Res.* 26:1225, 1966.

226. Kaplan, H. S.: Contiguity and progression in Hodgkin's disease. *Cancer Res.* 31:1811, 1971.

227. Hutchinson, G. B.: Anatomic patterns by histologic type of localized Hodgkin's disease of the upper torso. *Lymphology* 5:1, 1972.

228. Smithers, D. W.: *Hodgkin's Disease.* Churchill-Livingstone, Edinburgh and London, 1973.

229. Lillicrap, S. C.: Modes of spread of Hodgkin's disease. *Br. J. Radiol.* 46:18, 1973.

230. Strum, S. B.: The natural history, histopathology, staging and mode of spread of Hodgkin's disease. *Ser. Haematol.* 6:20, 1973.

231. Lamoureux, K. B., Jaffe, E. S., Berard, C. W., and Johnson, R. E.: Lack of identifiable vascular invasion in patients with extranodal dissemination of Hodgkin's disease. *Cancer* 31:824, 1973.

232. Naeim, F., Waisman, J., and Coulson, W. F.: Hodgkin's disease: The significance of vascular invasion. *Cancer* 34:655, 1974.

233. Kirschner, R. H., Abt, A. B., O'Connell, M. J., Sklansky, B. D., Greene, W. H., and Wiernik, P. H.: Vascular invasion and hematogenous dissemination of Hodgkin's disease. *Cancer* 34:1159, 1974.

234. Rouviere, H.: Anatomie des lymphatiques de l'homme. Masson, Paris, 1932.

235. Engeset, A., Høeg, K., Høst, H., Liverud, K., and Nesheim, A.: Thoracic duct lymph cytology in Hodgkin's disease. *Int. J. Cancer* 4:735, 1969.

236. Bouroncle, B. A.: Sternberg-Reed cells in the peripheral blood of patients with Hodgkin's disease. *Blood* 27:544, 1966.

237. Schiffer, C. A., Levi, J. A., and Wiernik, P. H.: The significance of abnormal circulating cells in patients with Hodgkin's disease. *Br. J. Haematol.* 31:177, 1975.

238. Levitan, R., Diamond, H. D., and Craver, L. F.: Liver in Hodgkin's disease. *Gut* 2:60, 1961.

239. Sacks, E. L., Donaldson, S. S., Gordon, J., and Dorfman, R. F.: Epithelioid granulomas associated with Hodgkin's disease: Clinical correlations in 55 previously untreated patients. *Cancer* 41:562, 1978.

240. Rosenberg, S. A.: Hodgkin's disease of the bone marrow. *Cancer Res.* 31:1733, 1971.

241. Meyers, L. E., Chabner, B. A., DeVita, V. T., and Gralnick, H. R.: Bone marrow involvement in Hodgkin's disease: Pathology and response to MOPP chemotherapy. *Blood* 44:197, 1974.

242. Kaplan, H. S.: *Hodgkin's Disease.* Harvard University Press, Cambridge, Mass., 1980, p. 284.

243. Musshoff, K., Renemann, H., Boutis, L., and Afkham, J.: Die extranoduläre Lymphogranulomatose: Diagnose, Therapie und Prognose bei zwei unterschiedlichen Formen des Organbefalls: Ein Beitrag zur Stadieneinteilung des Morbus Hodgkin. *Fortschr. Geb. Rontgenstr.* 109:776, 1968.

244. Perttala, Y., and Kijanen, I.: Roentgenologic bone lesions in lymphogranulomatosis maligna. Analysis of 453 cases. *Ann. Chir. Gyn. Fenn.* 54:414, 1965.

245. Stolberg, H. O., Patt, N. L., MacEwen, K. F., Warwick, O. H., and

Brown, T. C.: Hodgkin's disease of the lung: Roentgenologic-pathologic correlation. *Am. J. Roentgenol. 62*:96, 1964.

246. Whitcomb, M. E., Schwartz, M. I., Keller, A. R., Flannery, E. P., and Blom, J.: Hodgkin's disease of the lung. *Am. Rev. Resp. Dis. 106*:79, 1972.

247. Billingham, M. E., Rawlinson, D. G., Berry, P. F., and Kempson, R. L.: The cytodiagnosis of malignant lymphomas and Hodgkin's disease in cerebrospinal, pleural, and ascitic fluids. *Acta. Cytol. 19*:547, 1975.

248. Shreeve, D. R., Horrocks, P., and Mainwaring, A. R.: Steatorrhoea and intra-abdominal lymphoma. *Scand. J. Gastroenterol. 3*:577, 1968.

249. Richmond, J., Sherman, R. S., Diamond, H. D., and Craver, L. F.: Renal lesions associated with malignant lymphomas. *Am. J. Med. 32*:184, 1962.

250. Routledge, R. C., Haun, I. M., and Morris Jones, P. H.: Hodgkin's disease complicated by the nephrotic syndrome. *Cancer 38*:1735, 1976.

251. Moorthy, A. V., Zimmerman, S. W., and Burkholder, P. M.: Nephrotic syndrome in Hodgkin's disease: Evidence for pathogenesis alternative to immune complex deposition. *Am. J. Med. 61*:471, 1976.

252. Yum, M. N., Edwards, J. L., and Kleit, S.: Glomerular lesions in Hodgkin's disease. *Arch. Pathol. 99*:645, 1975.

253. Benninghoff, D. L., Medina, A., Alexander, L. L., and Camiel, M. R.: The mode of spread of Hodgkin's disease to the skin. *Cancer 26*:1135, 1970.

254. Smith, J. L., and Butler, J. J.: Skin involvement in Hodgkin's disease. *Cancer 45*:354, 1980.

255. Szur, L., Levene, G. M., Harrison, C. V., and Samman, P. D.: Primary cutaneous Hodgkin's disease. *Lancet 1*:1016, 1970.

256. Emmerson, R. W.: Follicular mucinosis: A study of 47 patients. *Br. J. Dermatol. 81*:395, 1969.

257. Naysmith, A., and Hancock, B. W.: Hodgkin's disease and pemphigus. *Br. J. Dermatol. 94*:695, 1976.

258. English, R. S., Hurley, H. J., Witkowski, J. A., and Sanders, J.: Generalized anhidrosis associated with Hodgkin's disease and acquired icthyosis. *Ann. Intern. Med. 58*:676, 1963.

259. Bluefarb, S. M.: Cutaneous manifestations of the leukemia-lymphoma group. *Postgrad. Med. 41*:476, 1967.

260. Friedman, M., Kim, T. H., and Panahon, A. M.: Spinal cord compression in malignant lymphoma: Treatment and results. *Cancer 37*:1485, 1976.

261. Cuttner, J., Meyer, R., and Huang, Y. P.: Intracerebral involvement in Hodgkin's disease: A report of 6 cases and review of the literature. *Cancer 43*:1497, 1979.

262. Åström, K.-E., Mancall, E. L., and Richardson, E. P., Jr.: Progressive multifocal leukoencephalopathy: A hitherto unrecognized complication of chronic lymphatic leukemia and Hodgkin's disease. *Brain 81*:93, 1958.

263. Trotter, J. L., Hendin, B. A., and Osterland, C. K.: Cerebellar degeneration with Hodgkin's disease: An immunological study. *Arch. Neurol. 33*:660, 1976.

264. Julien, J., Vital, C., Aupy, G., Laqueny, A., Darriet, D., and Brechenmacher, C.: Guillain-Barré syndrome and Hodgkin's disease — Ultrastructural study of a peripheral nerve. *J. Neurol. Sci. 45(1)*:23, 1980.

265. Rewcastle, N. B., and Tom, M. I.: Non-infectious granulomatous angiitis of the nervous system associated with Hodgkin's disease. *J. Neurol. Neurosurg. Psychiatry 25*:51, 1962.

266. Simmons, A. V., Spiers, A. S. D., and Fayers, P. M.: Haematological and clinical parameters in assessing activity in Hodgkin's disease and other malignant lymphomas. *Q. J. Med. 42*:111, 1973.

267. Tauro, G. P.: Hodgkin's disease associated with raised eosinophil counts. *Med. J. Aust. 2*:604, 1966.

268. Jaffe, N., and Bishop, Y. M. M.: The serum iron level, hematocrit, sedimentation rate, and leukocyte alkaline phosphatase level in pediatric patients with Hodgkin's disease. *Cancer 26*:332, 1970.

269. Steigbigel, R. T., Lambert, L. H., Jr., and Remington, J. S.: Polymorphonuclear leukocyte, monocyte, and macrophage bactericidal function in patients with Hodgkin's disease. *J. Lab. Clin. Med. 88*:54, 1976.

270. Cline, M. J., and Berlin, N. I.: Anemia in Hodgkin's disease. *Cancer 16*:526, 1963.

271. Al-Ismail, S., et al.: Erythropoiesis and iron metabolism in Hodgkin's disease. *Br. J. Cancer 40*:365, 1979.

272. Storgaard, L., and Karle, H.: Fever and haemolysis in Hodgkin's disease. *Acta Med. Scand. 197*:311, 1975.

273. Jones, S. E.: Autoimmune disorders and malignant lymphoma. *Cancer 31*:1092, 1973.

274. Julia, A., and Miller, S. P.: Idiopathic thrombocytopenia purpura in Hodgkin's disease after splenectomy. *Am. J. Hematol. 1*:115, 1976.

275. Cohen, J. R.: Idiopathic thrombocytopenic purpura in Hodgkin's disease: A rare occurrence of no prognostic significance. *Cancer 41(2)*:743, 1978.

276. Kedan, A., et al.: Autoimmune disorders complicating adolescent Hodgkin's disease. *Cancer 44*:112, 1979.

277. Abrahamsen, A. F.: Platelet survival in Hodgkin's disease. *Scand. J. Hematol. 7*:309, 1970.

278. Westling, P.: Studies of the prognosis in Hodgkin's disease. *Acta Radiol. (Suppl.) 245*:5, 1965.

279. Le Bourgeois, J. P., and Tubiana, B.: The erythrocyte sedimentation rate as a monitor for relapse in patients with previously treated Hodgkin's disease. *Int. J. Rad. Oncol. Biol. Phys. 2*:241, 1977.

280. Ray, G. R., Wolf, P. H., and Kaplan, H. S.: Value of laboratory indicators in Hodgkin's disease: Preliminary results. *Natl. Cancer Inst. Monogr. 36*:315, 1973.

281. Nadiminti, Y., et al.: Lactic acidosis associated with Hodgkin's disease. *N. Engl. J. Med. 303*:15, 1980.

282. Coppleson, L. W., Factor, R. M., Strum, S. B., Graff, P. W., and Rappaport, H.: Observer disagreement in the classification and histology in Hodgkin's disease. *J. Natl. Cancer Inst. 45*:731, 1970.

283. Lukes, R. J., and Tindle, B. H.: Immunoblastic lymphadenopathy. A hyperimmune entity resembling Hodgkin's disease. *N. Engl. J. Med. 292*:1, 1975.

284. Frizzera, G., Moran, E. M., and Rappaport, H.: Angio-immunoblastic lymphoadenopathy, diagnosis, and clinical course. *Am. J. Med. 59*:803, 1974.

285. Desser, R. K., Moran, E. M., and Ultmann, J. E.: Staging of Hodgkin's disease and lymphoma: Diagnostic procedures including staging laparotomy and splenectomy. *Med. Clin. North Am. 57*:479, 1973.

286. Sweet, D. L., Jr., Kinnealy, A., and Ultmann, J. E.: Hodgkin's disease: Problems of staging. *Cancer 42 (Suppl. 2)*:957, 1978.

287. Musshoff, K.: Prognostic and therapeutic implications of staging in extranodal Hodgkin's disease. *Cancer Res. 31*:1814, 1971.

288. Kaplan, H. S.: Survival and relapse rates in Hodgkin's disease, Stanford experience, 1961–1971. *Natl. Cancer Inst. Monogr. 36*:487, 1973.

289. Smithers, D. W.: Hodgkin's disease: Survival and relapse free data. *Natl. Cancer Inst. Monogr. 36*:509, 1973.

290. Kaplan, H. S., and Rosenberg, S. A.: The management of Hodgkin's disease. *Cancer 36*:796, 1975.

291. Mintz, U., et al.: Pathologic stage I and II Hodgkin's disease 1968–1975: Relapse and results of treatment. *Cancer 44*:72, 1979.

292. Levi, J. A., Wiernik, P. H.: Limited extranodal Hodgkin's disease: Unfavorable prognosis and therapeutic implications. *Am. J. Med. 63*:365, 1977.

293. Torti, F. M., Portlock, C. S., Rosenberg, S. A., and Kaplan, H. S.: Extranodal (E) lesions in Hodgkin's disease (HD): Prognosis and response to therapy. *Proc. Am. Soc. Clin. Oncol. 19*:367, 1978 (abstract).

294. Aisenberg, P. C.: Current concept in cancer: The staging and treatment of Hodgkin's disease. *N. Engl. J. Med. 299*:1228, 1978.

295. Rosenberg, S. R.: The management of Hodgkin's disease. *N. Engl. J. Med. 288*:1246, 1978.

296. Desser, R. K., et al.: Prognostic classification of Hodgkin disease in pathologic stage III, based on anatomic considerations. *Blood 49(6)*:883, 1977.

297. Golomb, H. M., et al.: Importance of substaging of stage III Hodgkin's disease. *Semin. Oncol. 7*:136, 1980.

298. Menon, N. C., and Buchanan, J. G.: Bilateral trephine bone marrow biopsies in Hodgkin's and non-Hodgkin's lymphoma. *Pathology 11*:53, 1979.

299. Weiss, R. B., Brunning, R. D., and Kennedy, B. J.: Hodgkin's disease in the bone marrow. *Cancer 36*:2077, 1975.

300. Bagley, C. M., Roth, J. A., Thomas, L. B., and DeVita, V. T.: Liver biopsy in Hodgkin's disease: Clinicopathologic correlations in 127 patients. *Ann. Intern. Med.* 76:219, 1972.
301. Lipton, M. J., De Nardo, G. L., Silverman, S., and Glatstein, E.: Evaluation of the liver and spleen in Hodgkin's disease. I. The value of hepatic scintigraphy. *Am. J. Med.* 52:356, 1972.
302. Femant, A., Rodhain, J., Michaux, J. L., Piret, L., Maldague, B., and Sokal, G.: Detection of skeletal involvement in Hodgkin's disease: A comparison of radiography, bone scanning, and bone marrow biopsy in 38 patients. *Cancer* 35:1346, 1975.
303. Lee, B. J., Nelson, J. H., and Schwarz, G.: Evaluation of lymphangiography, inferior venacavography and intravenous pyelography in the clinical staging and management of Hodgkin's disease and lymphosarcoma. *N. Engl. J. Med.* 271:327, 1964.
304. Castellino, R. A., and Blank, N.: Roentgenologic aspects of Hodgkin's disease. I. Current role of lymphangiography. *Natl. Cancer Inst. Monogr.* 36:271, 1973.
305. Silverman, S., DeNardo, G. L., Glatstein, E., and Lipton, M. J.: Evaluation of the liver and spleen in Hodgkin's disease. II. The value of splenic scintigraphy. *Am. J. Med.* 52:362, 1972.
306. Breiman, R. S., Castellino, R. A., Harell, G. S., Marshall, W. H., Glatstein, E., and Kaplan, H. S.: CT-pathologic correlations in Hodgkin's disease and non-Hodgkin's lymphoma. *Radiology* 126:159, 1978.
307. Ferrucci, J. R.: Body ultrasonography. *N. Engl. J. Med.* 300:538, 1977.
308. Hoffer, P. B., Turner, D., Gottschalk, A., Harper, P. V., and Ultmann, J. E.: Whole-body radiogallium scanning for staging of Hodgkin's disease and other lymphomas. *Natl. Cancer Inst. Monogr.* 36:277, 1973.
309. McCaffrey, J. A., et al.: Clinical usefulness of ^{67}gallium scanning in the malignant lymphomas. *Am. J. Med.* 60:523, 1976.
310. Waldor, P. A., and Jaffee, B. E.: Value of preoperative evaluation in patients with lymphoma. *Arch. Surg.* 115:258, 1980.
311. Rutherford, C. J., et al.: The decision to perform staging laparotomy in symptomatic Hodgkin's disease. *Br. J. Haematol.* 44:347, 1980.
312. Ferguson, D. J., Allen, L., Griem, M. L., Moran, M. E., Rappaport, H., and Ultmann, J. E.: Surgical experience with staging laparotomy in 125 patients with lymphoma. *Arch. Intern. Med.* 131:356, 1973.
313. Kaplan, H. S.: *Hodgkin's Disease.* Harvard University Press, Cambridge, Mass., 1980, p. 371.
314. Rubin, P., and Casarett, G.: *Clinical Radiation Pathology.* Saunders, Philadelphia, 1968, p. 34.
315. Anderson, R. E., D'Angio, G. J., and Khan, F. M.: Dosimetry of irregularly shaped radiation therapy fields. II. Isodose contours obtained utilizing a simulated human thorax. *Radiology* 92:1097, 1969.
316. Svahn-Tapper, G., and Landberg, T.: Mantle treatment of Hodgkin's disease with cobalt 60. *Acta Radiol.* 10:33, 1971.
317. Gray, L., and Prosnitz, K. R.: Dosimetry of Hodgkin's disease therapy using a 4 MV linear accelerator. *Radiology* 116:423, 1975.
318. Friedman, M., Pearlman, A. W., and Turgeon, L.: Hodgkin's disease: Tumor lethal dose and iso-effect recovery curve. *Am. J. Roentgenol.* 99:843, 1967.
319. Page, V., Gardner, A., and Karzmark, C. J.: Physical and dosimetric aspects of radiotherapy of malignant lymphomas. I. The mantle technique. *Radiology* 96:609, 1970.
320. Page, V., Gardner, A., and Karzmark, C. J.: Physical and dosimetric aspects of the radiotherapy of malignant lymphomas. II. The inverted-Y technique. *Radiology* 96:619, 1970.
321. Johnson, R. E., Ruhl, R., Johnson, S. K., and Glover, M.: Split-course radiotherapy of Hodgkin's disease. Local tumor control and normal tissue reactions. *Cancer* 37:1713, 1976.
322. Hutchison, G. B., et al.: Survival and complications of radiotherapy following involved and extended field therapy of Hodgkin's disease stages I and II. *Cancer* 38:288, 1976.
323. Staffel, T. J., Maj, M. C., and Cox, J. D.: Hodgkin's disease stage I and II: A comparison between two different treatment strategies. *Cancer* 40:90, 1977.
324. Goffinet, D. R., Glatstein, E., Fuks, Z., and Kaplan, H. S.: Abdominal irradiation in non-Hodgkin's lymphomas. *Cancer* 37:2797, 1976.
325. Kaplan, H. S.: Radiotherapeutic management of the malignant lymphomas. *Med. Rec. Ann.* 58:43, 1965.
326. Kaplan, H. S.: Role of intensive radiotherapy in the management of Hodgkin's disease. *Cancer* 19:356, 1966.
327. Johnson, R. E., Thomas, L. B., Schneiderman, M., Glenn, D. W., Faw, F., and Hafermann, M. D.: Preliminary experience with total nodal irradiation in Hodgkin's disease. *Radiology* 96:603, 1970.
328. Marks, J. E., Moran, E. M., Griem, M. L., and Ultmann, J. E.: Extended mantle radiotherapy in Hodgkin's disease and malignant lymphoma. *Am. J. Roentgenol.* 121:772, 1974.
329. Snyder, E. M.: The 3 and 2 technique for Hodgkin's disease at Memorial Hospital. *Radiol. Technol.* 49:293, 1977.
330. Poussin-Rosillo, H., Nisce, L. Z., and Lee, B. J.: Complications of total nodal irradiation of Hodgkin's disease stages III and IV. *Cancer* 42:437, 1978.
331. Palos, B., Kaplan, H. S., and Karzmark, C. J.: The use of "thin" lead lung shields to deliver limited whole lung irradiation during mantle field treatment of Hodgkin's disease. *Radiology* 101:441, 1971.
332. Carmel, R. J., and Kaplan, H. S.: Mantle irradiation in Hodgkin's disease: An analysis of technique, tumor eradication, and complications. *Cancer* 37:2813, 1976.
333. Schultz, H. P., Glatstein, E., and Kaplan, H. S.: Management of presumptive or proven Hodgkin's disease of the liver: A new radiotherapy technique. *Int. J. Radiat. Oncol. Biol. Phys.* 1:1, 1975.
334. Gross, N. J.: Pulmonary effects of radiation therapy. *Ann. Intern. Med.* 86:81, 1977.
335. Kaplan, H. S., and Stewart, J. R.: Complications of intensive megavoltage radiotherapy for Hodgkin's disease. *Natl. Cancer Inst. Monogr.* 36:439, 1973.
336. Castellino, R. A., Glatstein, E., Turbow, M. M., Rosenberg, S., and Kaplan, H. S.: Latent radiation injury of lungs or heart activated by steroid withdrawal. *Ann. Intern. Med.* 80:593, 1974.
337. Nordman, B.: Complications after megavoltage therapy of Hodgkin's disease. *Ann. Clin. Res.* 9:35, 1977.
338. Markiewicz, W., Glatstein, E., London, E. J., and Popp, R. L.: Echocardiographic detection of pericardial effusion and pericardial thickening in malignant lymphoma. *Radiology* 123:161, 1977.
339. Brosinc, F. C., III, Waller, B. F., and Roberts, W. C.: Radiation heart disease: Analysis of 16 young (aged 15 to 33 years) necropsy patients who received over 3,500 rads to the heart. *Am. J. Med.* 70:519, 1981.
340. Fuks, Z., Glatstein, E., Marsa, G. W., Bagshaw, M. A., and Kaplan, H. S.: Long-term effects of external radiation on the pituitary and thyroid glands. *Cancer* 37:1152, 1976.
341. Schimpff, S. C., Diggs, C. H., Wiswell, J. G., Salvatore, P. C., and Wiernik, P. H.: Radiation-related thyroid dysfunction: Implications for the treatment of Hodgkin's disease. *Ann. Intern. Med.* 92:91, 1980.
342. Sacks, E. L., Goris, M. L., Glatstein, E., Gilbert, E., and Kaplan, H. S.: Bone marrow regeneration following large field radiation: Influence of volume, age, dose, and time. *Cancer* 42:1057, 1978.
343. Desser, R. K., and Ultmann, J. E.: The sensitivity of Hodgkin's disease to chemotherapeutic agents administered singly. *Ser. Haematol.* 6:152, 1973.
344. Carter, S. K., and Livingston, R. B.: Single-agent therapy for Hodgkin's disease. *Arch. Intern. Med.* 131:377, 1973.
345. Coltman, C. A.: Chemotherapy of advanced Hodgkin's disease. *Semin. Oncol.* 7:155, 1980.
346. Gams, R. A.: Complications of chemotherapy in the treatment of Hodgkin's disease. *Semin. Oncol.* 7:184, 1980.
347. Phillips, T. L., and Fu, K. K.: Quantification of combined radiation therapy and chemotherapy effects on critical normal tissues. *Cancer* 37:1186, 1976.
348. Skipper, H. E., Schabel, F. M., Jr., and Wilcox, W. S.: Experimental evaluation of potential anticancer agents. XIII. On the criteria and kinetics associated with "curability" of experimental leukemia. *Cancer Chemotherap. Rep.* 35:3, 1964.
349. Bruce, W. R., Meeker, B. E., and Valeriote, F. A.: Comparison of the sensitivity of normal hematopoietic and transplanted lymphoma colony-forming cells to chemotherapeutic agents administered *in vivo. J. Natl. Cancer Inst.* 37:233, 1966.
350. Capazzi, R. L., Keiser, L. W., and Santorelli, A. C.: Combination chemotherapy: Theory and practice. *Semin. Oncol.* 4:227, 1977.
351. DeVita, V. T., et al.: Curability of advanced Hodgkin's disease with

chemotherapy. Long-term follow-up of MOPP-treated patients at the National Cancer Institute. *Ann. Intern. Med. 92*:587, 1980.

352. DeVita, V. T.: The consequences of the chemotherapy of Hodgkin's disease. *Cancer 47*:1, 1981.

353. Frei, E., et al.: Combination chemotherapy in advanced Hodgkin's disease: Induction and maintenance of remission. *Ann. Intern. Med. 79*:376, 1973.

354. Moore, M. P., Jones, S. E., Bull, J. E., William, L. A., and Rosenberg, S. A.: MOPP chemotherapy for advanced Hodgkin's disease: Prognostic factors in 81 patients. *Cancer 32*:52, 1973.

355. Young, R. C., Canellos, G. P., Chabner, B. A., Schein, P. S., and DeVita, V. T.: Maintenance chemotherapy for advanced Hodgkin's disease in remission. *Lancet 1*:1339, 1973.

356. Diggs, C. H., Wiernik, P. H., Levi, J. A., and Kvols, L. K.: Cyclophosphamide, vinblastine, procarbazine, and prednisone with CCNU and vinblastine maintenance for advanced Hodgkin's disease. *Cancer 39*:1949, 1977.

357. Durant, J. R., Gams, R. A., Velez-Garcia, R., Bantolincci, A., Wirtschafter, D., and Dorfman, R.: BCNU, Velban, cyclophosphamide, procarbazine, and prednisone (BVCPP) in advanced Hodgkin's disease. *Cancer 42*:2101, 1978.

358. Nicholson, W. M., et al.: Combination chemotherapy in generalized Hodgkin's disease. *Br. Med. J. 3*:7, 1970.

359. Sutcliffe, S. B., et al.: MVPP chemotherapy regimen for advanced Hodgkin's disease. *Br. Med. J. 1*:679, 1978.

360. Bloomfield, C. D., Weiss, R. B., Fortuny, I., Vosika, G., and Kennedy, B. J.: Combined chemotherapy with cyclophosphamide, vinblastine, procarbazine, and prednisone (CVPP) for patients with advanced Hodgkin's disease—An alternative program to MOPP. *Cancer 38*:42, 1976.

361. McElwain, T. J., et al.: A combination of chlorambucil, vinblastine, procarbazine, and prednisone for treatment of Hodgkin's disease. *Br. J. Cancer 36*:276, 1977.

362. Harrison, D. T., and Neiman, P. E.: Primary treatment of disseminated Hodgkin's disease with BCNU alone and in combination with vincristine, procarbazine, and prednisone. *Cancer Treat. Rep. 61*:789, 1977.

363. Nissen, N. L., et al.: A comparative study of a BCNU containing 4-drug program versus MOPP versus 3-drug combinations in advanced Hodgkin's disease: A cooperative study by the Cancer and Leukemia Group B. *Cancer 43*:31, 1979.

364. Coltman, C. A., et al.: Bleomycin in combination with MOPP for the measurement of Hodgkin's disease: Southwest Oncology Group experience, in *Bleomycin—Current Status and New Developments*, edited by S. K. Carton, S. T. Crooke, and H. Urmezanva. Academic, New York, 1978.

365. Bennett, J. G., et al.: Clinical trials with BCNU (NSC-409962) in malignant lymphomas by the Eastern Cooperative Oncology Group. *Cancer Treat. Rev. 60*:737, 1976.

366. Bonadonna, G., Zucali, R., Monfardini, S., DeLena, G., and Uslenghi, C.: Combination chemotherapy of Hodgkin's disease with Adriamycin, bleomycin, vinblastine, and imidazole carboxamide versus MOPP. *Cancer 36*:252, 1975.

367. Santoro, A., and Bonadonna, G.: Prolonged disease-free survival in MOPP-resistant Hodgkin's disease after treatment with Adriamycin, bleomycin, vinblastine, and dacarbazine (ABVD). *Cancer Chemother. Pharmacol. 2*:101, 1979.

368. Krikorian, J. G., Portlock, C. S., and Rosenberg, S. A.: Treatment of advanced Hodgkin's disease with Adriamycin, bleomycin, vinblastine, and imidazole carboxamide (ABVD) after failure of MOPP therapy. *Cancer 41*:2107, 1978.

369. Clamon, G. H., and Corder, B. P.: ABVD treatment of MOPP failures in Hodgkin's disease: A re-examination of goals of salvage therapy. *Cancer Treat. Rep. 62*:363, 1978.

370. Case, D. C., Young, C. W., and Lee, B. J.: Combination chemotherapy of MOPP-resistant Hodgkin's disease with Adriamycin, bleomycin, dacarbazine, and vinblastine (ABVD). *Cancer 39*:1382, 1977.

371. Porzig, K. J., Portlock, C. S., Robertson, A., and Rosenberg, S. A.: Treatment of advanced Hodgkin's disease with B-CAVe following MOPP failure. *Cancer 41*:1670, 1978.

372. Lokich, J. J., Frei, E., III, Jaffe, N., and Tullis, J.: New multiple-agent chemotherapy (B-DOPA) for advanced Hodgkin's disease. *Cancer 38*:667, 1976.

373. Levi, J. A., Wiernik, P. H., and Diggs, C. H.: Combination chemotherapy of advanced previously treated Hodgkin's disease with streptozotocin, CCNU, Adriamycin, and bleomycin. *Med. Pediatr. Oncol. 3*:33, 1977.

374. Goldman, J. D., and Dawson, A. A.: Combination therapy for advanced resistant Hodgkin's disease. *Lancet 2*:1224, 1975.

375. Fisher, R. I., et al.: Prolonged disease-free survival in Hodgkin's disease with MOPP reinduction after first relapse. *Ann. Intern. Med. 90*:761, 1979.

376. Rosenberg, S. A., and Kaplan, H. S.: The management of stages I, II, and III Hodgkin's disease with combined radiotherapy and chemotherapy. *Cancer 35*:55, 1975.

377. Rosenberg, S. A., Kaplan, H. S., Glatstein, B. J., and Portlock, C. S.: Combined modality therapy of Hodgkin's disease : A report on the Stanford trials. *Cancer 42*:991, 1978.

378. British National Lymphoma Investigation. *Lancet 2*:991, 1976.

379. Stein, R. S., et al.: Anatomic substages of stage III-A Hodgkin's disease: A collaborative study. *Ann. Intern. Med. 92*:159, 1980.

380. Aisenberg, A. C., Linggood, R. M., and Lew, R. A.: The changing face of Hodgkin's disease. *Am. J. Med. 67*:921, 1979.

381. Hoppe, R. T., Portlock, C. S., Glatstein, E., Rosenberg, S. A., and Kaplan, H. S.: Alternating chemotherapy and irradiation in the treatment of advanced Hodgkin's disease. *Cancer 43*:472, 1979.

382. Kun, L. E., DeVita, V. T., Young, R. C., and Johnson, R. E.: Treatment of Hodgkin's disease using intensive chemotherapy followed by irradiation. *Int. J. Radiat. Oncol. Biol. Phys. 1*:619, 1976.

383. Bonadonna, G., Zucali, R., DeLena, M., and Valagussa, P.: Combined chemotherapy (MOPP or ABVD)–radiotherapy approach in advanced Hodgkin's disease. *Cancer Treat. Rep. 61*:769, 1977.

384. Prosnitz, L. R., Farber, L. R., Fischer, J. J., Bertino, J. R., and Fischer, D. B.: Long-term remissions with combined modality therapy for advanced Hodgkin's disease. *Cancer 37*:2826, 1976.

385. Jenkin, R. D. T., and Berry, G. P.: Hodgkin's disease in children. *Semin. Oncol. 7*:202, 1980.

386. Ziegler, J. L., Blumming, A. Z., Fass, L., Magrath, I. T., and Templeton, A. C.: Chemotherapy of childhood Hodgkin's disease in Uganda. *Lancet 2*:679, 1972.

387. Chilcote, R. R., Baehner, R. L., Hammond, D., and Children's Cancer Study Group: Septicemia and meningitis in children splenectomized for Hodgkin's disease. *N. Engl. J. Med. 295*:798, 1976.

388. Sweet, D. L., Jr., and Golomb H. M. (eds): Hematologic problems during pregnancy and the reproductive years: An invitational symposium. *J. Reprod. Med. 19*:171, 1977.

389. Kaplan, H. S.: *Hodgkin's Disease*. Harvard University Press, Cambridge, Mass., 1980, p. 556.

390. Hoppe, R. T., et al.: Prognostic factors in pathological stage IIIA Hodgkin's disease. *Cancer 46*:1240, 1980.

391. Kaplan, H. S.: Evidence for a tumoricidal dose level in the radiotherapy of Hodgkin's disease. *Cancer Res. 26*:1221, 1966.

392. Musshoff, K., Hartmann, C. H. R., Niklaus, B., and Rössner, R.: The prognostic significance of first and second remission after first and second relapse radiotherapy in Hodgkin's disease. *Z. Krebsforsch. 85*:243, 1976.

393. Weller, S. R., Glatstein, E., Castellino, R. A., Kaplan, H. S., and Rosenberg, S. A.: Initial relapse in previously treated Hodgkin's disease. II. Retrograde transdiaphragmatic extension. *Int. J. Radiat. Oncol. Biol. Phys. 2*:863, 1977.

394. Portlock, C. S., Rosenberg, S. A., Glatstein, E., and Kaplan, H. S.: Impact of salvage treatment on initial relapses in patients with Hodgkin's disease, stages I–III. *Blood 51*:825, 1978.

395. Brody, R. S., and Schottenfeld, D.: Multiple primary cancers in Hodgkin's disease. *Semin. Oncol. 7*:187, 1980.

396. Rowley, J. D., Golomb, H. M., and Vardiman, J.: Nonrandom chromosomal abnormalities in acute nonlymphocytic leukemia in patients treated for Hodgkin's disease and non-Hodgkin's lymphoma. *Blood 50*:759, 1977.

397. Krikorian, J. G., Burke, J. S., Rosenberg, S. A., and Kaplan, H. S.: The occurrence of non-Hodgkin's lymphoma following therapy for Hodgkin's disease. *N. Engl. J. Med. 300*:452, 1979.

398. Chapman, R. M., Satcliffe, S. B., and Gapas, J. S.: Male gonadal dysfunction in Hodgkin's disease. *JAMA 245*:1323, 1981.

399. Horning, S. J., Hoppe, R. T., Kaplan, H. S., and Rosenberg, S. A.:

Female reproductive potential after treatment for Hodgkin's disease. *N. Engl. J. Med. 304:*1377, 1981.

400. Sweet, D. L., Jr., Roth, D. G., Desser, R. K., Miller, J. B., and Ultmann, J. E.: Avascular necrosis of the femoral head with combination therapy. *Ann. Intern. Med. 85:*67, 1976.

401. Ruckdeschel, J. C., Schimpff, S. C., Smyth, A. C., and Harding, M. R.: Herpes zoster and impaired cell-associated immunity to the varicella-zoster virus in patients with Hodgkin's disease. *Am. J. Med. 62:*77, 1977.

402. Weitzman, S., and Aisenberg, A. C.: Fulminant sepsis after the successful treatment of Hodgkin's disease. *Am. J. Med. 62:*47, 1977.

403. Desser, R. K., and Ultmann, J. E.: Risk of severe infection in patients with Hodgkin's disease or lymphoma after diagnostic laparotomy and splenectomy. *Ann. Intern. Med. 77:*143, 1972.

404. Kaplan, H. S.: *Hodgkin's Disease.* Harvard University Press, Cambridge, Mass., 1980, pp. 448–449.

405. Kaplan, H. S.: *Hodgkin's Disease.* Harvard University Press, Cambridge, Mass., 1980, pp. 456–457.

406. Cooper, I. A., Rana, C., Madigan, J. P., Motteram, R., Maritz, J. S., and Turner, C. N.: Combination chemotherapy (MOPP) in the management of advanced Hodgkin's disease: A progress report on 55 patients. *Med. J. Aust. 1:*41, 1972.

407. Jacobs, C., Portlock, C. S., and Rosenberg, S. A.: Prednisone in MOPP chemotherapy for Hodgkin's disease. *Br. Med. J. 2:*146, 1976.

408. McElwain, T. J., et al.: Combination chemotherapy in advanced and recurrent Hodgkin's disease. *Natl. Cancer Inst. Monogr. 36:*395, 1973.

409. Levitt, M., et al.: The Yale combination chemotherapy program for advanced Hodgkin's disease: A preliminary report. *Conn. Med. 34:*862, 1970.

410. Vicente, J., and Cortés Funes, H.: ABVD for the treatment of advanced resistant lymphomas. *Proc. Am. Soc. Clin. Oncol. 17:*189, 1976 (abstract).

411. Clamon, G. H., and Corder, M. P.: ABVD treatment of MOPP failures in Hodgkin's disease. A re-examination of goals of salvage therapy. *Cancer Treat. Rep. 62:*363, 1978.

412. Coltmann, C. A., and Jones, S. E.: MOPP plus low dose bleomycin (MOPP + LDB) for advanced Hodgkin's disease (HD) — A five year follow-up. *Proc. Am. Soc. Clin. Oncol. 19:*329, 1978.

413. Diggs, C. H., Wiernick, P. H., and Aisner, J.: SCAB (streptozotocin, CCNU, Adriamycin, bleomycin) for advanced untreated Hodgkin's disease. *Proc. Am. Soc. Clin. Oncol. 19:*370, 1978.

CHAPTER *119*

Non-Hodgkin's lymphoma

ERIC P. LESTER
JOHN E. ULTMANN

Definition

The non-Hodgkin's lymphomas (NHLs) are a heterogeneous group of neoplastic disorders which originate from cells of the immune system. They are the solid tumor portion of a spectrum of neoplastic diseases which includes chronic lymphocytic leukemia, multiple myeloma, mycosis fungoides, and other related malignancies. Since the cell types making up the immune system are both widely distributed and possess broad functional heterogeneity, it is not surprising that NHL may originate in virtually any organ and show disparate patterns of histology, clinical behavior, and prognosis. The major indicators of both clinical patterns of disease and prognosis are the cell type of origin (state of differentiation of the malignant cell population) and the pattern of growth within involved lymph nodes (follicular or diffuse). Thus, depending upon histology, prognosis even for patients presenting with widespread disease may range from excellent (survival 10 to 20 years) to that of the most malignant neoplasm (survival less than 1 year).

Recent advances in our understanding of the physiology and anatomy of the immune system [1,2] and its division into T cell– and B cell–mediated components have permitted increasingly precise analyses of the state of differentiation of NHL cells and have led to a variety of new schemes for pathologic classification designed to replace the widely accepted Rappaport classification [3] (see Chap. 117). According to the most recent working formulation, three broad groups may be defined: (1) a low-grade or favorable group which has less "aggressive" cell types or possesses a follicular (also called *nodular*) growth pattern; (2) an intermediate-grade group which has either "aggressive" cell types in follicular patterns, or diffuse patterns of cells many or all of which appear aggressive; and (3) a high-grade, unfavorable group in which the pattern of growth is diffuse and the cell type appears highly malignant. Within these general categories an increasing number of entities are being defined on the basis of clinical behavior, histology, and, in some cases, immunologic characteristics (see also Chap. 117).

Most NHLs originate within lymphoid tissue and are widely distributed in nodes, marrow, or blood at the time of clinical presentation. Later dissemination to other organs such as liver, gastrointestinal tract, skin, lungs, or central nervous system is common. Some cases, however, may present with localized disease, often in extranodal sites. Staging, or estimation of the anatomic extent of disease at presentation, is usually expressed using the nomenclature of the Ann Arbor Symposium on the Staging of Hodgkin's Disease (see Table 118-1), but is often less crucial in NHL than in Hodgkin's disease since there is little prognostic difference between stage III and stage IV. It is, however, necessary to distinguish cases of truly localized disease in which radiotherapy to the entire tumor may be curative. If widespread tumor is demonstrated, strict pathologic staging is not necessary and management decisions, ranging from no treatment to aggressive chemotherapy, will depend on the clinical behavior and histology of the tumor. Crucial issues for the clinician caring for a patient with NHL are thus: (1) the histology of the tumor and its prognostic meaning; (2) the distinction of localized disease, potentially curable with radiotherapy, from widespread disease; (3) decisions regarding whether and when to treat if the microscopic examination shows a low-grade malignancy; and (4) choice of an appropriate chemotherapy regimen for intermediate- or high-grade tumors. Low-grade tumors may require no treatment even if widespread and are generally not permanently eradicated by aggressive chemotherapy. Paradoxically, the most malignant tumors may be quite responsive to modern combination chemotherapy so that apparent cure of a significant portion of these patients is now possible.

History

Thomas Hodgkin, in 1832, was the first to clearly recognize a form of malignant lymphoma as a distinct clinical entity originating and spreading primarily within lymphoid tissues [4]. Sir Samuel Wilks, in his extension of these findings in 1865 [5], was able to recognize both the malignant nature of this entity, which he called *Hodgkin's disease*, and to differentiate it from "leucocythemia lymphatica," or leukemia, which had been described earlier by Virchow [6] and others [7,8]. At about the same time, Virchow also distinguished "aleukemic leukemia" (including malignant lymphoma) from leukemia [9], but it was not until the advent of histopathology that such distinctions became routine. Dreschfeld in 1892 [10] and Kundrat in 1893 [11] reported cases of "aleukemic leukemia" in which the disease appeared confined to lymphoid structures. Kundrat applied the term *lymphosarcoma* to these, and this term was accepted by Paltauf who, in 1896 [12], extended the histologic description of these diseases. The recognition by Sternberg in 1898 [13] and Reed in 1902 [14] of the characteristic giant cells found in Hodgkin's disease enabled the separation of Hodgkin's disease from the other lymphomas.

The description of histological subtypes of NHL began with the application of the term *reticulum cell sarcoma* by Oberling in 1928 [15] and Roulet in 1930 [16] to tumors described earlier by Ewing [17] as originating from "reticulum" cells of lymph nodes. Most of these would now be termed *histiocytic* or *large cell* lymphomas. Brill in 1925 [18] and Symmers in 1927 [19] described "giant lymph follicle hyperplasia," now termed *nodular* or *follicular* NHL, composed of smaller cells and following a more benign course although capable of transformation to "lymphosarcoma" with a more malignant behavior and appearance. Many observers remained unconvinced of the existence of histologic subtypes of NHL [20], but ultimately the recognition that cell type and pattern of growth generally allow the prediction of clinical course permitted Rappaport to create a widely accepted classification of NHLs in 1956 [3] (see Chap. 117). While it is not based on current concepts of the immune system, its prognostic utility has made it the standard against which more recent classifications such as the 1981 Working Formulation should be judged. Two additional subtypes with distinct histologic patterns and clinical features have been accepted into the Rappaport classification: Burkitt's

lymphoma, a B-cell neoplasm described in 1958 [21] as "a sarcoma involving the jaws in African children," and "lymphoblastic lymphoma" [22], a T-cell neoplasm closely related to acute lymphocytic leukemia, commonly presenting in children with a mediastinal mass, and corresponding to earlier clinical descriptions by Sternberg [23] and Cooke [24].

No effective therapy was available for NHL until the discovery of x-rays in 1896 and their therapeutic use, initially for the treatment of Hodgkin's disease, by Pusey in 1902 [25] and Senn in 1903 [26]. For the next 50 years their use, usually in doses less than 3000 rads, remained standard treatment for the palliation of symptoms of NHL. In some instances of apparently localized disease, surgical removal was attempted [27,28]. The successful use of intensive radiotherapy for Hodgkin's disease by pioneers such as Gilbert in the 1920s and 1930s [29] and Peters in the 1940s and 1950s [30] led to the development of concepts of clinical staging with emphasis on radiocurable disease which culminated in the Hodgkin's disease staging classification accepted at the Ann Arbor Symposium in 1971 [31]. These concepts have subsequently been applied with variable success to the radiotherapy of NHL [32].

Beginning in 1942 with the development of the alkylating agent nitrogen mustard [33,34], the palliation of advanced disease with single-agent chemotherapy became standard. The subsequent development of additional alkylating agents such as chlorambucil and cyclophosphamide, the antimetabolites such as methotrexate [35] and 5-fluorouracil [36], the vinca alkaloids vincristine and vinblastine [37], synthetic adrenal glucocorticoids such as prednisone [38], and the antitumor antibiotics such as daunorubicin [39] expanded the possibilities for palliation with single agents [40,41]. Experimental work in the 1950s and 1960s in animal systems indicated that combinations of these agents might be more effective than single agents [42,43] and ushered in the modern era of combination chemotherapy. Combinations of an alkylating agent, vincristine, and prednisone were investigated in the treatment of advanced disease in the late 1960s [44–47] and provided the foundations for current research and treatment.

Etiology and pathogenesis

The etiology of NHLs remains unknown. The great heterogeneity in histopathology and clinical behavior of these cancers suggests that a variety of factors including genetic abnormalities, disturbances in the regulation of the immune system, and the ultimate etiologic events may interact in their pathogenesis. Considerable evidence suggests that viruses may act as etiologic agents in at least some cases of NHL. One of the best studied agents is the Epstein-Barr virus (EBV) [48,49] which was first detected in 1964 in cultures of tumor cells taken from African patients with Burkitt's lymphoma [50].

EBV is a DNA virus of the Herpes family, 150 to 200 nm in diameter and surrounded by a lipid containing envelope. While the virus may simply be a "passenger," infecting the tumor cells but not causing their malignant behavior, its capacity to transform and "immortalize" normal B cells suggests an etiologic role. B lymphocytes of humans and primates possess cell surface receptors which specifically bind EBV and permit their infection with the virus [51]. Such infection acts not only as an initial polyclonal mitogenic stimulus to B-cell growth but causes the transformation of some infected B cells into cells possessing properties suggestive of malignancy, particularly the capacity for continuous "immortal" proliferation in culture [52]. The ability of the virus to produce this transformation appears to be modulated by cocultivated normal T cells [53]. The EBV genome may be detected in both a nonintegrated plasmid-like state [54] and in a state in which it is linearly integrated with the human DNA of the infected cells [55]. Such infection often does not result in the production of new virus particles, however, and the EBV remains as a "passenger" in the transformed cells, perhaps accounting for their growth. While the complete viral genome is not often expressed in these cells, the EBV-determined nuclear antigen is usually found. Evidence of EBV infection within the malignant cells in Burkitt's lymphoma, but not other malignant lymphomas, is usually found using both nucleic acid hybridization techniques to detect the viral genome and immunofluorescence techniques to detect the nuclear antigen [56]. Such evidence is more commonly found in African cases of Burkitt's lymphoma, although cases elsewhere have also appeared to possess EBV [57]. Similar evidence of EBV infection has also been found in many cases of nasopharyngeal carcinoma *(lymphoepithelioma)* in China and southeast Asia [58]. Why the virus might cause two such disparate cancers is unclear, but EBV receptors and genomes have been demonstrated in the malignant epithelial cells (not the infiltrating lymphocytes) in these carcinomas [59]. Serologic evidence of antibodies to EBV indicates that infection with EBV occurs at an early age in areas in which Burkitt's lymphoma or nasopharyngeal carcinoma is endemic, and antibody titers are 10 to 15 times higher in tumor-bearing patients [60,61]. Infection early in life, coupled with disordered immune regulation such as that produced by malaria (coendemic with Burkitt's lymphoma), other carcinogens, or genetic susceptibility may act in concert to cause the disease [62].

EBV has been clearly established, using seroepidemiologic [63] and viral culture [64] techniques, as the cause of infectious mononucleosis (see Chap. 109), a disease which bears clinical similarity to an abortive malignant lymphoma. Infectious mononucleosis is characterized by an initial proliferation of EBV-infected B cells followed by a more vigorous proliferation of T cells which are cytotoxic for EBV-infected cells [65]. The *atypical lymphocytes*, which may appear morphologically malignant, come from both cell populations although T cells usually predominate. Infectious mononucleosis may thus represent a "civil war" in which an EBV-induced B-cell proliferation capable of malignant progression is suppressed by a normal T-cell immune response. The B-cell proliferation may be polyclonal and include the recruitment of B-cell clones capable of producing autoantibodies, as is sometimes seen in NHL. In a few patients, often males clustered in particular families, EBV infection may result in either a fatal lymphoproliferative disease [66] or, after a severe illness, agammaglobulinemia [67]. Such patients may have a genetic defect in immunoregulation causing an inability to mount either a humoral or cell-mediated anti-EBV immune response. Inoculation of cotton-top marmosets, a species of primate, with appropriate strains of EBV produces in most animals a spectrum of lymphoproliferative responses ranging from none to frankly malignant lymphomas, usually of the large cell type, from which EBV may be recovered [68].

A variety of DNA and RNA viruses have been identified as etiologic agents for a spectrum of leukemias and solid tumors in rodent, feline, bovine, and primate species [69]. Type C RNA tumor viruses are likely causes of human malignancies; one such virus causes lymphosarcomas in the Gibbon ape and is closely related to a virus causing sarcomas in woolly monkeys [70]. Considerable effort has been spent on isolating similar viruses from human lymphomas and leukemias, and much circumstantial evidence suggests a causative role for them in at least some cases. Permanent cell lines have been established from 20 human lymphoid malignancies including 12 cases of diffuse histiocytic lymphoma, three American Burkitt's lymphomas, two acute lymphocytic leukemias, and three diffuse undifferentiated lymphomas [71]. Seven of these, including two EBV–nuclear antigen-positive Burkitt's cell lines, have spontaneously produced a type C RNA virus which possesses a reverse transcriptase antigenically similar to those of primate, but not feline or murine, leukemia viruses. Infection of normal human blood mononuclear cells with viruses purified from one of these lines produces changes in cell growth and morphology which suggest abortive malignant transformation. Isolation of a similar virus from cultures of malignant cells from patients with cutaneous T-cell lymphomas has also been reported [72] and antibodies to the virus have been found in the serum of both patients and their relatives [73].

While the ultimate etiologic agents of NHL remain unclear, epidemiologic studies have revealed a number of factors which appear to predispose to their development. NHLs make up about 2 percent of all cancers in the United States [74] and have shown a one- to twofold increase in incidence in most Western countries since 1960 [75]. Considerable variation in overall incidence rates is found worldwide; in the United States, age-adjusted incidence rates are somewhat higher in males than females and higher in whites than blacks. Age-specific incidence rates show a preadolescent peak, a late teenage drop, and then a logarithmic rise with increasing age [76]. Higher mortality rates are seen in association with higher socioeconomic status, urban residence, and in the Midwest and coastal California [77,78]. Occupational exposure to a variety of chemicals has also been associated with increases in NHL risk [75,79,80]. The use of hydantoin anticonvulsants may in a few cases be associated with the development of benign "pseudo-lymphomas" which resolve when the drug is discontinued [81]. Hydantoins have also been associated with the development of NHL, although the degree of risk, if any, must be small [82,83]. A small excess of NHL was seen among survivors of the atomic bomb in Japan [84], but lesser doses of radiation do not seem to lead to NHL [85].

The most frequent and significant factor predisposing to NHL appears to be aberration of the immune system [86,87]. Thirty-eight families with multiple cases of NHL, usually in siblings and without predilection for a particular histologic subtype, have been reported and the majority have shown evidence of inherited immune abnormalities [75]. Patients with primary immuno deficiencies have an estimated 10,000-fold increased risk for the development of cancer, the majority of which are malignant lymphomas [88]. Of 267 cases of cancer recorded by the Immunodeficiency Cancer Registry, two-thirds were NHLs and 8 percent were HD [89]. These immunodeficiency diseases include ataxia-telangiectasia, variable immunodeficiency, the Wiskott-Aldrich syndrome, IgA deficiency, severe combined immunodeficiency, immunodeficiency with thymoma, and a variety of other syndromes. Similar phenomena are seen in a number of animal systems, such as the New Zealand black mouse, which displays deficient T-cell functions, autoimmune disorders, and a high frequency of spontaneous malignant lymphomas [90].

Patients suffering from diseases characterized by autoimmune dysfunction likewise have a predisposition to develop NHL. One study has found a threefold increased risk of NHL in rheumatoid arthritis patients [91] and a 44-fold increase in Sjögren's syndrome [92]. Systemic lupus erythematosus also appears to predispose to NHL [93]. Celiac disease, or gluten-sensitive enteropathy, while not a classical autoimmune disease, also shows a marked increase in the incidence of NHL, the "Western" variant of primary intestinal lymphoma, which usually arises in the distal bowel [94]. Another disease of the small intestine, α-heavy-chain disease, is found primarily in lower socioeconomic groups in Mediterranean countries and is characterized by abdominal pain, malabsorption, a plasma cell infiltrate in the bowel producing an α-heavy-chain paraprotein, and a propensity for the development of frank lymphoma [95]. These "Mediterranean" primary intestinal lymphomas usually arise in the proximal small bowel, often display α chains on their surface and are commonly large cell NHLs classified as *immunoblastic sarcomas* [96]. Chronic antigenic stimulation by enteric pathogens may play a role in their development since antibiotic therapy may produce

complete resolution of the premalignant α-heavy-chain disease [96]. *Angioimmunoblastic lymphadenopathy* [97], and the closely related *immunoblastic lymphadenopathy* [98], are disorders in which a morphologically benign proliferation of B-lymphoid immunoblasts is accompanied by polyclonal hyperglobulinemia, and a high incidence of autoimmunity or drug allergy. The disease appears to progress to a frank NHL, usually *immunoblastic sarcoma*, in approximately 35 percent of cases [99]. Other diseases sometimes preceding NHL include dermatitis herpetiformis (related to celiac disease and intestinal lymphoma) [100], sarcoidosis [101], leprosy [102], schistosomiasis [103], and chronic renal failure [104].

Acquired therapeutic immunosuppression, particularly when associated with chronic antigenic stimulation, may likewise predispose to the development of NHL. Patients with renal transplants who are given immunosuppressive agents to prevent graft rejection have a 40- to 100-fold increased risk of NHL, particularly those originating in the central nervous system [105]. A similar risk is seen in cardiac transplant patients [106] and a lesser but still increased risk is found in patients receiving immunosuppressive therapy for non-transplant conditions [105]. The relatively rapid appearance of these tumors, sometimes within 1 year after onset of immunosuppression, has led to the suggestion that activation of oncogenic viruses may play a central role [75]. Graft-versus-host disease in animal models has both been shown to activate type C RNA viruses and to lead to the development of lymphomas [107,108]. Hodgkin's disease, especially when treated with immunosuppressive radiation and chemotherapy, also appears to predispose to NHL [109].

Particularly intriguing evidence for a genetic role in the development of at least some NHL comes from the study of karyotypes in NHL and in ataxia-telangiectasia. Patients with ataxia-telangiectasia have both a high frequency (10 percent of cases) of development of spontaneous NHL, an increase in spontaneous chromosome breakage in cell cultures, and a high incidence of abnormalities in chromosome 14 (usually a translocation of the distal end of one chromosome 14 to the other chromosome 14 or to another chromosome [110]. Nearly all patients with NHL show abnormal karyotypes when carefully studied, the most common abnormality being translocation of genetic material to the long arm of chromosome 14 (14q+) [111]. This appears to be somewhat more common in poorly differentiated lymphocytic lymphoma than in histiocytic lymphoma and is also seen in multiple myeloma, B-cell acute lymphocytic leukemia, and lymphoid malignancies of T-cell origin. A particularly characteristic abnormality is the translocation of material between chromosomes 8 and 14 [t(8;14)] which is seen in over one-half of Burkitt's lymphoma patients and occasionally in other forms of NHL. Infection with EBV of nonmalignant B cells from a patient with ataxia-telangiectasia has resulted in the appearance of an (8;14) translocation in the virally transformed cells [112]. A wide variety of additional chromosome abnormalities are common in NHL cells, particularly those classified as histiocytic or *large cell* lymphomas, although modal chromosome numbers are usually in the diploid range.

Unfortunately, karyotypic data are currently insufficient to provide much diagnostic assistance in distinguishing clinically relevant subtypes of NHL with distinct natural histories. Recent advances in immunology and cell culture techniques, however, are increasingly permitting a precise definition of the state of differentiation (cell of origin) of the malignant cell population [113]. From such studies, particularly immunologic cell surface marker analysis [114], a variety of subtypes of NHL with characteristic clinical features are being distinguished even among histologically similar–appearing diseases. While cellular morphology correlates significantly with immunologic cell type, it is clear that cells of identical appearance may be of types as disparate as T and B cells [115].

The majority of NHLs appear to be of B-cell origin as judged by their possession of surface immunoglobulin (SmIg) and variable expression of surface receptors for complement, surface Ia antigens, and surface receptors for the Fc portion of IgG [113,116–119] (see Chap. 105). This is particularly true of low-grade NHLs, which include well-differentiated lymphocytic, poorly differentiated lymphocytic, and mixed cell nodular lymphomas [120]. While the malignant cells making up the "follicles" in these tumors are of B-cell origin, significant numbers of T cells may also infiltrate involved nodes [117]. These B-cell neoplasms are closely related to chronic lymphocytic leukemia (CLL) in which 98 percent of cases are of B-cell origin but immunofluorescence for SmIg is usually fainter than in NHL [113]. A spectrum of differentiation blending into NHL can be demonstrated [121]. In the intermediate-grade category, diffuse, small cleaved (*poorly differentiated*) or mixed cell lymphoma are of either T, B, or null cell type [116–119]. The T-cell lymphoblastic lymphomas were formerly classified as a subset of diffuse poorly differentiated NHL, but their rapid and distinctive clinical course has led to their inclusion as a separate entity in the high-grade category of NHL [22,116,118]. The diffuse lymphomas composed of large cells (Rappaport's "histiocytic" lymphoma) are of B-cell origin in about one-half of cases, T-cell origin in about one-quarter, and null cell origin in the remaining cases [116–119]. Some of these lymphomas are made up of cells appearing morphologically similar to normal lymphocytes activated by an antigen or mitogen (*immunoblasts*). Many of these immunoblastic sarcomas are of B-cell origin, often occurring as a sequel to a prior immunologic disorder [116,122,123], but some originate from morphologically similar T cells or null cells. A few large cell lymphomas appear to originate from true histiocytes, or tissue macrophages [118]. Another form of aggressive lymphoma, Burkitt's lymphoma, displays surface markers characteristic of B cells at an early stage of differentiation [124]. Lastly, NHL involving the skin, including mycosis fungoides and Sézary's syndrome, is commonly found to originate from T cells [125]. In some cases these neoplastic T cells possess "helper" function immunologically [126]. While many recent classification schemes for NHL are based on immunologic concepts, the simple finding of T- or B-cell markers in a given case of NHL is generally not of great help in diagnosis or prognosis. Clinical features, histologic appearance, and cell surface marker data must be combined to diagnose accurately subtypes of NHL.

A variety of other approaches have recently been utilized to obtain diagnostic and prognostic information. Histochemical analysis of esterases (see Chap. A27) such as α-naphthyl acetate esterase, α-naphthyl butyrate esterase, naphthol ASD chloroacetate esterase, and naphthyl ASD acetate esterase may assist in distinguishing myeloid, monocytoid (histiocytic), and lymphoid cells [118]. Terminal deoxynucleotidyl transferase activity (see Chap. A28) is characteristic of stem cells, and immature lymphoid cells, particularly those of T-cell lineage [118,127]. Acid phosphatase staining (see Chap. A26) appears characteristic of T cells at all stages of differentiation [128], although tartrate-resistant acid phosphatase staining is useful for distinguishing *hairy cell leukemia*, a B-cell–histiocyte malignancy [129]. Alkaline phosphatase reactivity (see Chap. A23) has recently been used to identify a subset of B-cell NHL related to normal follicle cuff cells [117,130–132]. Enzymes of the purine pathway, such as adenosine deaminase and purine nucleoside phosphorylase, lysosomal enzymes, and lactate dehydrogenase are currently under study as markers of lymphoid differentiation [127]. Immunohistochemical staining to detect monoclonal cytoplasmic Ig is also useful in identifying B-cell NHL [133].

Analysis of cell-cycle kinetics and DNA content may provide additional useful information. In one study abnormal DNA content, usually hyperdiploid G_0-G_1 populations, was found in half of the NHLs regardless of histologic type [134]. Most of the low-grade NHLs had < 5 percent of cells in S phase (range 2 to 7 percent), whereas most of the high-grade NHLs had > 5 percent (range 5 to 22 percent). Labeling indices and modal cell volume also correlate independently with histologic subtypes of NHL [135] (see Fig. 119-1). Particularly when used together, they may clearly distinguish favorable histologic types with relatively low cell volumes and labeling indices from unfavorable histologic types which possess higher values reflecting larger and more rapidly growing cells. Another study has shown a median labeling index of 1.5 percent for nodular lymphomas and 6.2 percent for diffuse lymphomas [136]. Patients with tumors with a low labeling index (< 4 percent) were more likely to achieve a complete remission with chemotherapy than those with a higher index even within the nodular and diffuse categories. We must remember, however, that such complete remissions in patients with nodular NHL are usually followed by eventual relapse, whereas chemotherapy may cure some

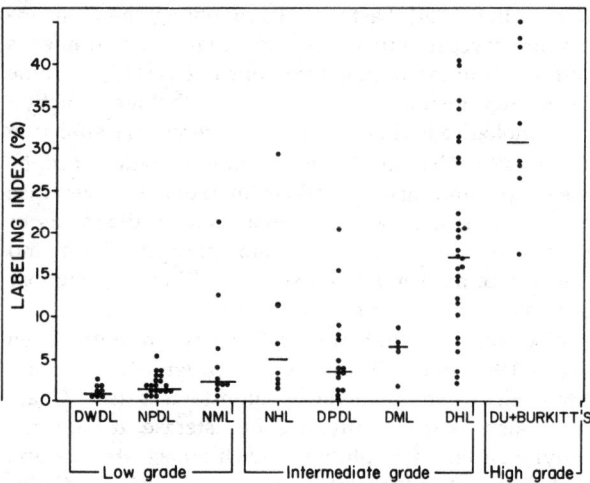

FIGURE 119-1 Labeling index observations in tissues involved by non-Hodgkin's lymphomas. Observations are grouped according to the histopathologic system of Rappaport and the Working Classification. The subclassifications used in the Working Classification are low-grade, intermediate-grade, and high-grade. Horizontal bars represent group medians. The abbreviations used in the Rappaport Classification are as follows: DWDL = diffuse well-differentiated lymphoma; NPDL= nodular poorly differentiated lymphoma; NML = nodular mixed lymphoma; NHL = nodular histiocytic lymphoma; DPDL = diffuse poorly differentiated lymphoma; DML= diffuse mixed lymphoma; DHL = diffuse histiocytic lymphoma; DU = diffuse undifferentiated lymphoma.

patients with diffuse NHL. This may be due to an increased drug sensitivity and an improved killing of tumor cells related to a higher growth rate in some patients with diffuse NHL. Kinetic studies of Burkitt's lymphoma, one of the most malignant NHLs, have shown a growth fraction approaching 100 percent and a potential doubling time of 24 h [137]. In childhood undifferentiated or lymphoblastic NHL, labeling indices have been found highest in B-cell NHL with leukemic involvement, lower in T-cell NHL, and lowest in null cell acute lymphocytic leukemia (ALL) cells [138]. Biochemical measurements of glucocorticoid receptors in NHL cells may also predict responsiveness to therapy with steroids [139]. Physiologic alterations in cell surface events, such as a reduction of "capping" of cell surface receptors for concanavalin A, is also seen in many lymphoproliferative disorders and may be of use in differential diagnosis [140,141].

Clinical features

Lymphadenopathy, usually painless, is the presenting symptom in about two-thirds of patients. The remainder have systemic symptoms (e.g., fever or weight loss) or symptoms related to sites of extranodal involvement [142]. Cervical nodes are most commonly involved, followed by inguinal, axillary, and multiple sites. Up to 10 percent of cases, particularly those with nodular NHL, may show spontaneous regression ranging from minor to complete and lasting a few weeks to years [143]. Presentation in predominantly extranodal sites occurs in about 20 percent of cases, most frequently in diffuse *large cell* ("histiocytic") lymphoma and involving, in order of approximate frequency, Waldeyer's ring, gastrointestinal sites, bone, skin, salivary glands, thyroid, testis, and breast [142,144–147]. Systemic symptoms such as fever, night sweats, or weight loss are found at presentation in 20 to 30 percent of patients and are more common with diffuse NHL and advanced stages of disease [142,147,148]. While they are generally considered not to carry the same prognostic weight as in Hodgkin's disease [147], a correlation between systemic symptoms and survival has been observed [149,150]. Additional presenting symptoms in one large series included abdominal pain (9 percent), fatigue (8 percent), painful adenopathy (8 percent), malaise (7 percent), dysphagia (5 percent), cough (4 percent), bone pain (3 percent), edema (3 percent), and pruritus (2 percent) [142]. However, since NHLs represent a group of widely disparate neoplasms of the immune system, it is best to consider separately the natural history of each of the types of NHL as currently defined by the Working Formulation (see Chap. 117).

Among the *low-grade NHLs* those consisting of a diffuse (rarely follicular) proliferation of *small well-differentiated* lymphocytes represent neoplasms of B cells analogous to the normal B cells of the medullary cords of lymph nodes [118]. Occurring in middle-aged and older patients, they comprise about 10 percent of NHLs [147]. They are, in fact, simply solid tissue forms of chronic lymphocytic leukemia and, as such, the neoplastic cells have a high propensity for entering the blood just as do their nonmalignant counterparts. Thus, widespread, painless adenopathy, advanced anatomic stage of disease, and marrow involvement are common at presentation. The disease often pursues an indolent course for many years regardless of therapy. Subsequent blood invasion occurs frequently and, as with other NHLs, terminal complications are due to marrow replacement, hypersplenism, or involvement of the liver or central nervous system.

A monoclonal Ig is present on the surface of the malignant cells, usually IgM with or without IgD of the same light-chain type and idiotype [151], and usually accompanied by weak cell surface complement receptors. Secretion of the monoclonal Ig, with a serum paraprotein, is found in about 20 percent of cases [152] and hypogammaglobulinemia, as in chronic lymphocytic leukemia, is common, perhaps due to an associated defect in helper-T-cell function [153]. Waldenström's macroglobulinemia represents a closely related disorder in which the neoplastic B cells are more mature and secrete a monoclonal IgM but have a similar tissue distribution (see Chap. 123). A large cell NHL which is clinically and histologically more aggressive may evolve out of any of these well-differentiated lymphoid neoplasms. Such "histiocytic" lymphomas, which occur in the course of chronic lymphocytic leukemia, have been termed *Richter's syndrome* and have been shown to synthesize the same monoclonal Ig as the preceding chronic lymphocytic leukemia, indicating that they represent clonal evolution or *dedifferentiation* of the previously present neoplastic process rather than a new, unrelated NHL [154]. A smaller group of cases of *intermediate differentiation* (between well and poorly differentiated) has recently been described and, while generally similar to diffuse well-differentiated NHL, may have some degree of nodularity and an admixture of cells with cleaved nuclei [117,118,130,131]. Alkaline phosphatase reactivity is often found and the disease usually follows an indolent course in older individuals.

Follicular NHLs, also termed *nodular*, constitute the majority of low-grade lymphomas and about one-half of all NHLs. They occur primarily in the middle-aged and elderly and pursue an indolent course. Three categories may be distinguished on the basis of cytologic composition: poorly differentiated small cleaved cell (20 percent of all NHLs), mixed small cleaved and large cell (20 percent of all NHLs), and large cell (histiocytic) (3 to 10 percent of all NHLs) [147,148]. Each of these is thought to originate from a corresponding type of B cell in normal germinal center follicles, and all are usually characterized, as are their normal counterparts, by brightly staining monoclonal surface IgM, with or without IgD, and strong complement receptors [118]. One study has suggested that patients with small cleaved NHL whose cells lack surface IgD and complement receptor, although possessing surface IgG or IgM, may have a worse prognosis [155]. Like normal germinal center B cells, these neoplastic B cells are capable of circulating throughout blood, marrow, and lymphoid tissue. Disseminated disease with multiple sites of peripheral adenopathy (cervical, retroperitoneal, etc.) is usually present at diagnosis although the mediastinum may not be involved in up to 40 percent of cases [147]. Approximately 60 to 85 percent of patients will have marrow involvement at presentation [156–158], and 90 percent will have involvement of retroperitoneal nodes seen on lymphangiography [158,159]. Even in patients judged to be in clinical stage I and II after lymphangiography, staging laparotomy will demonstrate abdominal disease in up to 60 percent [160]. Positive abdominal nodes usually include the celiac, portal, paraaortic, and mesenteric nodes, unlike Hodgkin's disease, in which mesenteric node involvement is quite uncommon.

Lymph nodes replaced by nodular NHL commonly show variable areas in which the follicular growth pattern has been lost. The significance of these areas of diffuse involvement in follicular NHL has been controversial. In general, significant degrees of nodularity appear to predict a relatively indolent clinical course and good prognosis [148,161]. There generally is a good prognosis with poorly differentiated and mixed cell follicular NHL; prognosis is more guarded for patients with

follicular large cell ("histiocytic") NHL, particularly those in which diffuse areas make up greater than 25 percent of the examined material [161]. When multiple sites are biopsied at the time of diagnosis and staging, a divergence of histologic patterns between sites is found in about one-third of patients [162]. Of these, one-third show different cell types within a uniformly follicular pattern, and two-thirds (18 percent of all NHLs) show a follicular pattern in one site and a diffuse pattern in another. These patients have a prognosis intermediate between those with follicular patterns in all biopsies and those with exclusively diffuse patterns. Divergences in histology both within and between nodes probably reflect the intrinsic tendency of follicular NHL to undergo evolution with the selection and growth of clones of more aggressive behavior. This clonal evolution is reflected in both a tendency to progress from the small cleaved cell type to mixed or large cell types and a progression from follicular to diffuse patterns of growth when multiple biopsies taken over the course of a patient's disease are compared. Up to two-thirds of patients presenting with follicular lymphomas will demonstrate such progression, usually to a diffuse large cell ("histiocytic") lymphoma, at autopsy [163,164]. The term *composite lymphoma* has been applied to cases in which two clearly distinct forms of malignant lymphoma have been found simultaneously within the same tissue; prognosis appears to be determined by the more aggressive of the two forms [165].

The *intermediate-grade NHLs* include the uncommon *follicular large cell NHLs* but consist largely of *diffuse NHLs* with either small cleaved cells or mixed small and large cells, each of which makes up 10 to 15 percent of NHL cases [147,148]. The majority of *diffuse small cleaved cell NHLs* appear to represent B-cell neoplasms closely related to, and often evolving from, the follicular small cleaved cell NHLs. As such, they likewise occur in middle-aged and older patients who most commonly present with generalized adenopathy and, in about two-thirds of cases, with marrow involvement. The disease usually follows a more aggressive course than follicular NHL with involvement and compromise of parenchymal organ function (e.g., liver, lungs, marrow) and a likelihood of refractoriness to therapy or early relapse. A small group of histopathologically distinct cases falling within the group of diffuse small cleaved cell NHL appear to be of T-cell origin and have recently been termed *peripheral T-cell lymphomas*. They usually present in elderly individuals with generalized lymphadenopathy, anorexia, weight loss, and often with pleuropulmonary involvement. They show a pleomorphic nodal infiltrate of malignant T cells associated with prominent capillary proliferation and epithelioid histiocytes [166]. The *diffuse mixed cell NHLs* are a heterogeneous group of lymphomas many of which are B-cell tumors which have evolved from nodular NHL and show clinical features similar to the diffuse small cleaved NHL. A subset of diffuse mixed cell NHLs, however, is characterized by a high content of epithelioid histiocytes and clinical findings of cervical and often generalized adenopathy, a high frequency of splenomegaly, hepatic involvement, B symptoms, and stage III or IV disease in middle-aged or elderly patients [167]. This has been termed *Lennert's lymphoma*, after its discoverer, and may be related to peripheral T-cell lymphomas [168].

The *diffuse large cell NHLs* represent a heterogeneous category of intermediate- or high-grade aggressiveness and constitute about 20 percent of NHLs. Included here are NHLs composed of large cleaved cells probably of follicular center (B-cell) origin which, while still aggressive in behavior, may be somewhat less so than the noncleaved large cell NHLs, many of which may also be of B-cell origin [168-171]. One study, however, reports a good response of the non-cleaved-cell variety to aggressive chemotherapy [172]. Roughly 25 to 30 percent of these patients may present with pathologic stage I, I_E, II, or II_E disease (see Table 118-1). One series found nodal involvement above and below the diaphragm in only 40 percent of cases and determined that patients with this histologic pattern had the lowest incidence of involvement at all nodal sites, the liver, and the marrow [159]. When it occurs, involvement at these sites is more likely to produce bulky masses, in contrast to small cell NHLs which usually enlarge nodes in a discrete fashion and produce small miliary nodules in the liver or spleen [118,163]. Diffuse large cell NHL is the most frequent type for patients with localized NHL, and presentations are common in Waldeyer's ring [173], gastrointestinal sites [174,175], bone, skin, salivary glands, or thyroid [146]. About 10 percent of these NHLs involve the central nervous system, especially if the marrow is concurrently involved [176-178]. They are more likely to present as an intracerebral mass than are other NHLs involving the central nervous system [178]. A subset of diffuse large cell NHL has recently been described with moderate to marked sclerosis within the tumor, a tendency to localized involvement (stage I or II), often in the mediastinum, sometimes causing superior vena-caval obstruction, and in the retroperitoneum, and with resistance to radiotherapy and aggressive chemotherapy [179]. Other studies of sclerosis in NHLs, including follicular types, have also suggested localized presentations and slower rates of progression than in corresponding tumors without sclerosis [180,181].

The *high-grade NHLs* consist of three quite separate diseases which are grouped together in the Working Formulation (see Chap. 117) because of their aggressive clinical behavior and poor prognosis. The first member of this group consists of the *immunoblastic sarcomas*, which may be considered as a subset of the diffuse large cell ("histiocytic") NHL. These usually occur in adults, commonly over age 50, and often in a setting of prior immune or lymphoproliferative disease [123]. Anemia, lymphopenia, diffuse hypergammaglobulinemia, B symptoms, and advanced stage are common at presentation [122]. Poor responses even to aggressive chemotherapy and short survival are characteristic [116,

168,169,182]. The majority of these tumors appear to be of B-cell origin [118,168], although diffuse large cell NHL of T-cell origin have been reported [116,183,184] and may be related to the peripheral T-cell lymphoma discussed above [166,168]. Primary NHLs originating in the central nervous system are most commonly immunoblastic sarcomas in which the frequent finding of intracellular immunoglobulin suggests a B-cell origin [185]. The prognostic significance of B- or T-cell markers is uncertain both within the immunoblastic sarcoma group and the more numerous diffuse large cell category of NHL [116,118]. Immunologic studies have suggested that about half are of B-cell, 5 to 15 percent of T-cell, and 5 percent or less of true histiocytic (monocyte-macrophage) origin, with the remaining one-third of cases lacking markers (so-called null cells). One study has suggested that, for a given histologic subtype of NHL, the simple presence or absence of lymphocyte surface markers may be of more importance than their T- or B-cell classification [186].

Lymphoblastic lymphoma is a high-grade NHL which had previously been included under the terms *diffuse poorly differentiated lymphocytic lymphoma* [3] or *Sternberg leukosarcoma* [23]. It is a T-cell malignancy closely related to T-cell acute lymphocytic leukemia [22,187-190]. Both of these diseases occur primarily in older male children and young male adults. Approximately one-half of patients with lymphoblastic lymphoma present with an anterior mediastinal mass, further suggesting the thymic origin of the tumor, and most show rapid dissemination of disease with early involvement of the marrow, blood, and CNS. While the tumor often responds well to chemotherapy initially, early relapse and a poor prognosis are characteristic. Two histologic variants have been distinguished possessing convoluted or nonconvoluted nuclei [191], but they seem to have similar clinical features and are cytologically indistinguishable from acute lymphocytic leukemia. However, a recent study has shown that tumor cells from most lymphoblastic lymphoma patients possess a surface antigen which is characteristic of the cytotoxic and suppressor cell subpopulation of normal peripheral blood T cells, whereas only 20 percent of T-cell acute lymphocytic leukemia cases display this antigen [192]. Occasionally a "pseudonodular" pattern may be present although prognosis remains poor [193].

Burkitt's lymphoma is the remaining member of the group of high-grade NHLs. It occurs endemically in tropical Africa and New Guinea where it afflicts children, usually in the jaw and retroperitoneum, and commonly with bilateral involvement of the kidneys and ovaries or a paraspinal tumor. Involvement of lymphatic tissue in African cases is uncommon [21,194]. Histologically identical cases occur nonendemically elsewhere, but usually present with lymphatic involvement, most commonly in the ileocecal region of the gastrointestinal tract or in cervical nodes, and more rarely with the tumor distribution seen in Africa [195]. Nonendemic cases show a broader age range (up to 35) and a higher mean age (11 versus 7 in African cases). Males predominate in both endemic and nonendemic areas and other clinical features and prognoses are similar [196]. The tumor is a very aggressive neoplasm of B-cell origin related to the small noncleaved cells of normal lymphoid follicles whose tendency to "home" to germinal centers in mesenteric lymph nodes may account for the tumor distribution seen in nonendemic cases [197]. The explosive growth of which the tumor is capable may account both for the high frequency of central nervous system and marrow involvement, the frequent occurrence of obstructive complications in the gastrointestinal, urinary, and respiratory tracts, and the metabolic abnormalities (hyperuricemia, lactic acidosis). It may also explain its high sensitivity to chemotherapeutic agents such as cyclophosphamide. Rarely, cases may present with leukemic blood involvement [198]. Serum lactic dehydrogenase, uric acid, and antibodies to the early antigen of EBV are often elevated in Burkitt's lymphoma and correlate with both stage and prognosis [199]. Also included in the high-grade category of the Working Formulation is a poorly defined group of neoplasms composed of intermediate to large noncleaved cells differing cytologically from Burkitt's lymphoma cells. Many of these appear to be of B-cell origin [116] and have been termed "undifferentiated, non-Burkitt's" by Rappaport [3] or "blastic" by others [186]. While their prognosis is poor, their natural history is poorly defined because of the confusing and complex nomenclatures used.

Although not included in the Working Formulation of NHL (see Chap. 117), *malignant histocytosis* (histiocytic medullary reticulosis) [200] is a highly aggressive malignancy of histiocytes [201,202]. Occurring at all ages and with a 2:1 male preponderance, it usually presents with the rapid onset of fever, lymphadenopathy (usually localized), hepatosplenomegaly, elevated urinary lysozyme, and pancytopenia [203]. The Coombs' test is negative, but jaundice commonly appears preterminally, and the pancytopenia is thought to be secondary to the phagocytosis of blood elements by malignant histiocytes in the nodes, liver, spleen, and marrow. The disease is rapidly progressive, with a median survival of 6 months. Rare asymptomatic patients have presented with isolated splenomegaly some months before the onset of systemic symptoms [204]. It has been described as a rare terminal finding in patients with acute lymphocytic leukemia [205] and is usually readily distinguished from histiocytosis (see Chap. 100). A *virus-associated hemophagocytic syndrome* has recently been reported to occur commonly in immunosuppressed patients infected with a herpes virus and in some previously healthy individuals [206]. Hepatosplenomegaly, lymphadenopathy, pulmonary infiltrates, pancytopenia, and skin rash were often present, but lymph-node histology, while showing marked benign proliferation of histiocytes with erythrophagocytosis, was clearly distinguishable from malignant histiocytosis, and the marrow was hypocellular, accounting for the pancytopenia.

Organ involvement

Splenic involvement may be proved at staging splenectomy in 30 to 40 percent of patients initially [207,208] and splenomegaly may develop during the course of the disease in a similar proportion of nonsplenectomized patients [142]. Massive involvement of the spleen may lead to pancytopenia due to hypersplenism. At autopsy 40 to 50 percent of patients have splenic involvement [142,163], and the spleen is almost invariably involved when tumor is present in the liver [207,208].

Hepatic involvement can be histologically documented in 20 to 50 percent of patients presenting with NHL and is more common in follicular or diffuse small cleaved cell NHL than in diffuse large cell ("histiocytic") NHL [159,207,208]. Initially, small foci of involvement are found, usually in the portal tracts, but larger masses may be seen, particularly with diffuse large cell lymphomas [163]. At autopsy 50 percent of NHLs of all cell types involve the liver [163]. As in Hodgkin's disease, noncaseating granulomas may be seen in the portal triads and other lymphoid tissue in about 5 percent of cases and must be distinguished from NHL [209]. Liver involvement often occurs without signs or symptoms. Hepatomegaly and jaundice due to intrahepatic or extrahepatic biliary obstruction are uncommon at presentation although they occur in about one-third of patients later in the course of their disease [142].

Marrow involvement may be demonstrated in one-third to one-half of patients presenting with NHL and is more frequent (60 to 80 percent) in the low-grade NHLs, the diffuse small cleaved cell NHLs, and the high-grade lymphoblastic NHLs than in the diffuse large cell ("histiocytic") NHLs (5 to 25 percent) [156–159]. Involvement in the former groups usually consists of diffusely distributed small paratrabecular foci which produce neither symptoms nor hematologic abnormalities. These must be distinguished from normal lymphoid nodules which frequently occur in older persons and are usually not situated in paratrabecular locations. The large cell and mixed cell NHLs are more likely to produce grossly visible nodules and symptomatic lesions. Advanced cases, especially lymphoblastic NHLs, are most likely to show diffuse replacement of the marrow, often associated with peripheral blood involvement or cytopenias. A small proportion of cases (4 percent in one series [142]), usually of diffuse large cell histology may present with isolated bony lesions, with pain as the initial disease manifestation. The lesions are generally lytic but occasionally sclerotic or mixed when examined radiographically. Bones most likely to be involved are the femurs, pelvis, vertebrae, ribs, and skull. Bone scans are usually abnormal at sites of macroscopic disease, but may be normal even with extensive lytic lesions in some cases of B-cell NHL and generally do not reflect microscopic involvement.

Gastrointestinal involvement presents clinically as the initial manifestation of NHL in about 5 percent of cases [142] and may be documented in up to 16 percent of NHL cases at presentation [147,210]. Clinical evidence of gastrointestinal involvement during the course of disease is somewhat less common [158], but it is found at autopsy in about one-half of patients [142,163]. In adults the most frequent sites of primary gastrointestinal NHL are the stomach (50 percent) and small intestine (25 percent) followed by the rectum and colon [174,175,211]. In children small intestinal involvement is much more frequent than gastric involvement [142]. The histologic pattern in adults is most commonly diffuse large cell ("histiocytic"), and localized disease (stage I_E or II_E) is correspondingly more frequent (75 percent) [163,211]. NHL presenting in Waldeyer's ring (up to 7 percent of NHLs [142]) has a particular propensity for associated gastric involvement [173]. Recent studies regarding the pathology of primary gastrointestinal NHL have been controversial, with suggestions of high frequencies of plasmacytoid [212] or histiocytic origin [213] for these tumors. The most common clinical manifestations are pain, abdominal mass, and anorexia and, less commonly, nausea, vomiting, diarrhea, obstruction, or gastrointestinal bleeding [142]. Involvement of adjacent mesenteric nodes (found in about one-half of all NHL cases [160,209]) may also account for many of these symptoms. Ascites is a late and uncommon event and may be due to peritoneal seeding or hepatic involvement. Malabsorption may be seen with extensive gastrointestinal involvement and is particularly common with the so-called Mediterranean lymphoma, or α heavy-chain disease (see Chap. 124).

Central nervous system manifestations are uncommon at presentation but ultimately occur in about 10 percent of patients with NHL [142,177,178,214] and are more frequent in patients with lymphoblastic and diffuse large cell ("histiocytic") NHL [163,177,178]. Clinical evidence of central nervous system spread usually occurs during active, uncontrolled systemic disease and is more frequent in patients with marrow involvement and extranodal sites of disease, particularly the testis [215]. Manifestations include spinal cord compression by an extradural mass often arising by spread through intervertebral foramina from adjacent involved paraspinous nodes and most commonly occurring in the thoracic region. Another common central nervous system manifestation is leptomeningeal spread, often presenting with cranial nerve palsies, signs of meningeal irritation, or increased intracranial pressure. Elevated cerebrospinal fluid protein and low glucose concentrations may suggest meningeal involvement but repeated cytologic examinations of the fluid may be necessary to confirm the diagnosis. Intracerebral mass lesions are less commonly encountered but particularly may be seen with diffuse large cell ("histiocytic") NHL and may present with headache, lethargy, papilledema, focal neurological signs, or seizures. Peripheral nerve involvement, usually by compression or extension from adjacent involved nodes, is not uncommon in advanced disease but does not confer the grave prognosis associated with central nervous system disease. A variety of paraneoplastic neurological syndromes, including progressive multifocal leukoencephalopathy [216], myasthenia gravis, transverse myelopathy, cerebellar degeneration, and peripheral neuropathies have been reported with NHL [217].

Clinical evidence of involvement of the kidneys and urinary tract is uncommon at presentation and is usually related to ureteral obstruction by retroperitoneal nodal disease [218]. However, the kidneys are involved with NHL in about one-half of autopsied cases, usually focally but sometimes with diffuse enlargement [142,163,219]. Renal failure is rare. The nephrotic syndrome occurs rarely and may be due to renal vein occlusion, glomerulonephritis [220], or minimal change glomerulopathy [218], although the latter is more commonly associated with Hodgkin's disease. Hypercalcemia or paraprotein deposition [221] due to NHL are more common, yet still infrequent, causes of renal failure. Involvement of the reproductive tract is uncommon although NHL, usually of the large cell type, may arise in the testis or ovary [222].

Non-Hodgkin's lymphomas occasionally infiltrate the skin as red or purplish nodules, primarily in the head and neck region [223]. While any histologic type of NHL may be found, diffuse large cell is the most common; prognosis is good if the disease remains localized at presentation (see also Chap. 120). Pulmonary involvement with NHL is also uncommon at presentation, although it is found in about one-half of cases at autopsy [142,163,224]. When present, pulmonary parenchymal disease is usually related to lymphatic spread of tumor from hilar and mediastinal nodes, which are involved in about 20 percent of cases at presentation and may sometimes produce superior vena caval obstruction. Pleural effusion occurs during the course of disease in 25 percent of patients either as a result of central lymphatic obstruction or pleural seeding with tumor. Culture and careful cytologic examination should always be performed. While found in about 20 percent of autopsy series, cardiac involvement by NHL is uncommon and is usually related to local growth of tumor from mediastinal nodes to the pericardium [225]. Other sites at which NHL uncommonly presents include the orbit [226,227], salivary glands [228], and thyroid [229], sites which are often previously involved by autoimmune disease and benign lymphoid infiltrates.

Laboratory data

Blood counts are normal in about 90 percent of patients with NHL at the time of presentation [142] in spite of the high frequency of marrow involvement. Anemia ultimately develops in the majority of patients and is related to therapy in most, although anemia may arise from impaired iron reutilization, so-called anemia of chronic disease, extensive replacement of the marrow with NHL, gastrointestinal bleeding, hypersplenism, or hemolysis. A positive Coombs' test is found in a small minority of patients, particularly those with small cell or follicular NHL, and is sometimes associated with a cold agglutinin, but frank autoimmune hemolytic anemia is uncommon. Rarely autoimmune thrombocytopenia is found, sometimes in association with hemolytic anemia. Thrombocytopenia is more commonly due to the effects of radiation or chemotherapy, or occasionally to marrow replacement or hypersplenism. The granulocyte count is normal except when lowered as a side effect of therapy although subtle defects in granulopoiesis [230] and neutrophil function [231] have been found in some patients. Lymphocytopenia is common during the course of disease, particularly in advanced stages [142] and depressed cellular immune responses have been reported [232]. Studies using cytofluorometric detection of lymphocytes with monoclonal surface immunoglobulin have suggested a high incidence (30 to 40 percent) of blood involvement in NHL patients who were thought to have no abnormal blood cells by standard morphologic techniques [233,234]. Frank blood invasion by NHL cells, usually with white blood cell counts in the 15,000 to 40,000 range, occurs in about 10 percent of NHLs, being particularly frequent in diffuse small lymphocytic NHL and lymphoblastic lymphoma. It has been reported in 10 percent of cases of follicular small cleaved NHL and 6 percent of diffuse large cell ("histiocytic") NHL [235]. Its occurrence in diffuse small lymphocytic and most follicular small cleaved cell NHL, either at presentation or during the course of disease, does not connote a poor prognosis. However, a subset of patients with follicular small cleaved NHL with a "blastic" as opposed to the classic "cleaved" nuclear morphology and those with diffuse large-cell or lymphoblastic lymphoma have a very poor prognosis after leukemic invasion [235].

Blood tests are generally normal at the time of presentation. Abnormalities of liver function tests, particularly the alkaline phosphatase, may be seen but are not always indicative of liver involvement. Conversely, these tests are often normal in the face of biopsy proof of NHL in the liver [207]. Likewise, the serum alkaline phosphatase level is an unreliable indicator of marrow involvement [159]. Recent reports have suggested that serum lactate dehydrogenase may be a useful prognostic indicator for patients with aggressive histologic subtypes of NHL [199,236]. The serum uric acid concentration is frequently mildly elevated in NHL and may reach levels capable of producing gout or urate nephropathy when bulky tumors are successfully treated and large amounts of nucleic acid are converted to uric acid after the tumor cells lyse [142]. Hypercalcemia is a rare complication of NHL and usually occurs in patients with advanced bone involvement. In rare cases this is apparently due to secretion of a humoral agent by the tumor [237]. The level of one or more of the serum immunoglobulins may be reduced, most commonly in patients with follicular small cleaved cell NHL (15 to 20 percent), but clinically significant hypogammaglobulinemia is uncommon [232,238]. Polyclonal in-

creases in immunoglobulin concentrations are more common, occurring in up to 40 percent of diffuse intermediate- or high-grade NHL and particularly with the immunoblastic sarcomas (both B- and T-cell type) and lymphoblastic lymphoma [238]. A monoclonal immunoglobulin, most commonly an IgM κ [152], may be found in the serum of about 5 percent of patients with NHLs, particularly of the diffuse small lymphocytic (well-differentiated) types [239].

Differential diagnosis

The diagnosis of NHL rests on the histopathologic examination, and the majority of problems in differential diagnosis lie in distinguishing the various subtypes discussed above and other related lymphoid malignancies. Clinical information is often helpful in distinguishing Hodgkin's disease, hairy cell leukemia (leukemic reticuloendotheliosis), chronic lymphocytic leukemia, Waldenström's macroglobulinemia, plasma cell myeloma, the heavy-chain diseases, mycosis fungoides, and acute lymphocytic leukemia from NHL. It must be recognized, however, that these diseases form a spectrum of lymphoid malignancies and that some cases will display intermediate features between these categories. Certain solid tumors may be confused with NHL. For example, small cell (oat cell) carcinoma of the lung may be mistaken for a small cell NHL, and Ewing's sarcoma or granulocytic sarcoma may be confused with large cell NHL. In difficult cases, biopsy of additional nodal material or other sites of disease may be useful, often in conjunction with specialized procedures such as analysis of cell surface markers [240], histochemistry, or electron microscopy to define better the state of differentiation of the malignant cell population.

Several benign diseases are characterized by lymphoproliferative responses and must be distinguished from NHL [241,242]. Immunoblastic lymphadenopathy [98] and the closely related angioimmunoblastic lymphadenopathy [97] may fall into an intermediate position between benign and malignant diseases. They commonly occur after exposure to a drug, are characterized by systemic symptoms, skin rash, generalized lymphadenopathy, and hepatosplenomegaly and have a histologic appearance which fails to meet the usual criteria for a malignant lymphoma. Nonetheless, the high frequency with which they evolve into an immunoblastic sarcoma, coupled with the finding of abnormal karyotypes in involved nodes [243], suggests that they may be malignant processes from the outset. Localized lymphoid infiltrates which are histologically benign may be termed *pseudolymphomas* [244]. They are sometimes seen in patients with an underlying autoimmune disease such as Sjögren's syndrome [245] and in extranodal sites such as the stomach [246]. *Angiofollicular lymph node hyperplasia*, usually found in the mediastinum, is a similar benign condition [247]. These represent one end of a spectrum of lymphoproliferative lesions and will, in some cases, evolve into a frank malignant lymphoma. *Lymphomatoid granulomatosis* [248] and *lymphocytic interstitial pneumonitis* [249] are related benign pulmonary disorders which may also evolve into malignant lymphoma. *Lymphomatoid papulosis* is a benign lymphoproliferative disorder involving the skin and closely resembling a malignant lymphoma histologically [250]. Viral infections sometimes producing lymphadenopathy include infectious mononucleosis, herpes zoster, postvaccination lymphadenitis, and cat scratch fever [241,242]. Tuberculosis, toxoplasmosis, syphilis, and fungal infections may produce enlarged lymph nodes, and autoimmune disorders such as rheumatoid arthritis or systemic lupus erythematosus likewise frequently produce reactive hyperplasia in nodes. Dermatopathic lymphadenopathy may be seen in nodes draining virtually any type of cutaneous lesion.

Therapy

STAGING

Once a definite histopathologic diagnosis of NHL has been confirmed, and before treatment begins, the patient should undergo a series of procedures designed to estimate the anatomic extent and localization of tumor. The purpose is twofold: first, to define those patients whose disease is of a limited anatomic extent and potentially curable with appropriate radiotherapy; second, to establish parameters of disease activity which may be monitored to determine the progression of disease or the efficiency of therapy. Rarely, a patient may present with a complication such as superior vena cava obstruction or spinal cord compression requiring urgent therapy even before a histologic diagnosis can be obtained. Treatment with local radiotherapy to the tumor mass and systemic glucocorticoids to reduce local edema may be needed to prevent disaster and permit judicious biopsies and staging procedures. While the Ann Arbor staging classification (see Chap. 118, Table 118-1) has been applied to NHL patients for many years, the distinction between stage III and IV disease is rarely relevant since treatment of both is the same and determined on the basis of histology.

Staging procedures begin with a careful and complete history and physical examination with special attention to lymph node–bearing areas, including the epitrochlear, preauricular, femoral, and popliteal areas, which are more frequently involved in NHL than in Hodgkin's disease. Abdominal organomegaly or masses must be carefully sought and the skin, thyroid, salivary glands, Waldeyer's ring, and bones must be examined for extranodal NHL. A complete blood count, including platelet count and examination of the blood film, is required and routine blood examinations must include measures of liver function, calcium, and uric acid. Serum immunoglobulins should be quantitated and immunoelectrophoresis performed to detect potential monoclonal immunoglobulins.

Staging procedures should follow a rational sequence designed to demonstrate, when present, advanced disease early in workup in order to spare the patient more aggressive and invasive procedures [158]. Bilateral posterior iliac crest biopsies should be performed early and on a routine basis since marrow aspirates yield inadequate samples and examination of several sites significantly increases the frequency of a positive biopsy [158,251]. The high frequency of marrow involvement in the favorable NHLs, and its poor prognostic implication in unfavorable NHLs [176], make the early proof of stage IV disease important and will usually obviate the need for additional invasive staging procedures. Similar considerations make it imperative to obtain an early cytologic evaluation of pleural effusions or ascites if they are present. In view of the high frequency of CNS involvement in patients with advanced stages of diffuse lymphoma, especially if the marrow or testicles are involved, such patients should also undergo cytologic examination of the spinal fluid.

Radiologic staging procedures usually begin with a chest radiograph which will reveal lymphomatous nodal involvement in about 25 percent of patients. Chest tomography, either conventional or with computerized axial tomography (CT scan), is usually not needed except in those with significant hilar disease in which it may reveal extension into adjacent pulmonary parenchyma. Radionuclide bone scanning, a more sensitive test than routine radiographs, is often helpful in documenting unsuspected osseous disease, particularly in cases of large cell NHL, and should be routinely performed [252,253]. Gallium 67 scanning may be useful for identifying disease in the chest and bone [254] and in patients with diffuse large cell histologies [255], although its accuracy in the abdomen is less satisfactory. Bipedal lymphangiography has traditionally been the most useful and accurate (80 to 90 percent) noninvasive test for the detection of retroperitoneal nodal disease [159,207,208] although 20 to 30 percent of patients with a negative lymphangiogram may still be found to have abdominal disease at staging laparotomy. Intravenous pyelography, inferior vena cavography [208], and renal or abdominal ultrasound examinations may reveal retroperitoneal disease.

An abdominal CT scan may also provide this information as well as a more detailed view of the retroperitoneal nodes and the mesenteric, portal, and splenic hilar nodes which are not visualized on lymphangiography. Since lymphangiography is unsafe in patients with serious pulmonary or extensive mediastinal or retroperitoneal disease, a CT scan may be preferred. The CT scan has a low false-positive rate but fails to detect many cases of minimally abnormal nodes or involved spleens [256]. Radiologic examination of the stomach and bowel should be performed in patients with involvement of Waldeyer's ring or in those with aggressive disease and evidence of abdominal involvement since therapy may lead to hemorrhage or perforation unless the involved bowel is first resected [257].

About 80 percent of patients undergoing such noninvasive staging procedures will show evidence of advanced (clinical stage III or IV) disease. Those in whom multiple concurrent investigations unequivocally suggest intraabdominal disease require no further staging procedures. Parameters of disease activity will have been established and should be monitored during and after therapy. However, approximately 20 percent of patients will remain in clinical stage I or II in spite of the above tests and require a further sequence of invasive procedures. Percutaneous liver biopsy is positive in 20 percent of such patients, particularly those with follicular or small cell disease [159]. Peritoneoscopy with liver biopsy will yield a positive result in an additional 25 percent of patients [159]. Those patients who remain in clinical stage I or II may be considered for staging laparotomy with splenectomy, as described in Chap. 118. However, laparotomy is indicated only if the demonstration of intraabdominal disease would change the planned therapy. While the mortality of such an operation is very low, the morbidity and expense may be considerable [258]. Laparotomy in two-thirds of patients with low-grade disease who are in clinical stage I or II after lymphangiography will reveal further disease, whereas only 20 percent of those with intermediate-grade [diffuse mixed cell or diffuse large cell ("histiocytic")] disease will be upstaged [159,160]. Since radiation therapy with curative intent is the treatment of choice in most centers for those patients who are confirmed in pathologic stage I or II by laparotomy, the operation is clearly useful for this small group of patients. Patients with high-grade disease (lymphoblastic lymphomas, Burkitt's lymphoma, or immunoblastic sarcoma) are not candidates for staging laparotomy since they will all require aggressive combination chemotherapy.

RADIATION THERAPY

Considerable controversy exists regarding the appropriate role for radiation therapy in the management of NHL. Most cases of NHL are quite sensitive to radiotherapy whether delivered in modest doses (2000 to 2500 rads) for a palliative reduction in a tumor mass or in higher doses to a defined field with curative intent. Patients with low- or intermediate-grade NHL in pathologic stage I, I_E, II, or II_E after complete staging may be considered candidates for curative radiation therapy. However, these tumors have a high propensity for early dissemination, often in quantities below the limits of clinical detection, in blood, marrow, and other organs. This, coupled with their indolent growth, increases the likelihood of eventual relapse in spite of apparent radiotherapeutic eradication of tumor. Furthermore, radiation therapy may also lead to second malignancies, particularly acute nonlymphocytic leukemia, and may at least theoretically accelerate the rate of clonal evolution of the NHL. In the absence of adequate controlled trials addressing these issues, it seems reasonable to attempt to cure low-grade NHL in pathologic stage (PS) I, I_E,

and, in some cases in which total tumor burden appears relatively low, II and II_E. Curative-intent radiotherapy should consist of 4400 rads administered over 4 weeks (or an equivalent dose) to the entire tumor and adjacent nodal areas. While the precise extent of radiation required for cure has not been well defined, extended field radiotherapy is usually given to standard ports such as those used for Hodgkin's disease (see Chap. 118), and the dose response curve for NHL indicates that such treatment will produce a low incidence of relapse within treated areas (6 percent) [259]. Suspected involvement of Waldeyer's ring and distal nodal groups such as preauricular and epitrochlear nodes in NHL sometimes requires extensions of treatment fields. The high frequency of involvement of mesenteric nodes has led to techniques incorporating lateral abdominal radiation therapy when intraabdominal disease is to be treated [260].

In contrast to the low-grade NHL, considerable evidence suggests that patients with PS I and I_E diffuse large cell ("histiocytic") NHLs are cured with radiotherapy alone in over three-quarters of cases, although somewhat higher doses (5000 to 5500 rads) to the tumor mass may be required [261,262]. This represents, at least in part, a reflection of their lower intrinsic potential for early dissemination, the higher accuracy of staging procedures in tumors which are more likely to be characterized by bulky growth as opposed to microscopic foci, and a relative radiosensitivity of these more malignant cells. However, patients with this histology and PS II or II_E disease fare considerably less well (40 percent 5-year disease-free survival) and commonly relapse in the first year after radiation therapy. Current recommendations for these patients include both radiotherapy and aggressive combination chemotherapy [261,263] or chemotherapy [264]. Patients with other intermediate-grade histologies in PS I, I_E, II, or II_E likewise show a high rate of complete remission with radiation therapy but their potential for cure is less certain. The more indolent nature of their disease and its intrinsic biologic tendency to early dissemination may make staging less accurate and may account for the pattern of continued late relapse which has been observed in these patients [32].

Patients with low-grade NHL of stage III or IV extent are not considered curable with either radiation therapy or chemotherapy. Total-body [265,266] or total lymphoid [267,268] irradiation is capable of producing complete remission in 80 to 90 percent of cases, but eventual relapse is the rule. Lacking a realistic strategy for cure, and given the benign clinical course of most such patients, a palliative approach is generally indicated. This may often consist of no therapy at all if disease manifestations are confined to uncomplicated lymphadenopathy [269]. In one such group of untreated patients, therapy was safely deferred for a median of 31 months [270], thus sparing the patient the risk and expense of either radiation or chemotherapy. When disease manifestations become troublesome, palliative radiation therapy to sites of active disease may be sufficient treatment. It may be particularly useful when only a single group of nodes is at fault or when a local problem is acute, such as a ureteral obstruction or spinal cord compression. Alternatively, low-dose whole-body irradiation may provide useful palliation. Palliative radiation therapy may likewise control local problems in patients with advanced stages of intermediate- and high-grade NHL but these patients require aggressive combination chemotherapy which must generally take precedence. The complications of radiation therapy in patients with NHL are similar to those occurring in patients with Hodgkin's disease and are discussed in Chap. 118.

CHEMOTHERAPY

The use of chemotherapy in patients with NHL and the choice of an appropriate regimen depend upon the histologic subtype of the disease. Patients with advanced stages of low-grade NHL may require no therapy at presentation, as discussed above. Some patients, however, will demonstrate more rapidly progressive disease which may be either widespread or accompanied by systemic symptoms. In such instances, palliative chemotherapy is indicated, usually with a single alkylating agent such as chlorambucil (4 to 12 mg, orally, daily) or cyclophosphamide (100 mg, orally, daily) sometimes together with prednisone (1 to 2 mg/kg, orally, daily). Dosage must be regulated by monitoring therapeutic response and blood counts. These or other single agents will produce objective responses in most and complete remissions in approximately 65 percent of previously untreated patients although some months of treatment may be required [271]. Alternatively, a relatively nontoxic combination chemotherapy regimen such as CVP (Table 119-1) [47] may be used. However, a randomized comparison of a single agent versus CVP versus CVP combined with total lymphoid irradiation revealed no difference in therapeutic benefit [272]. Other studies have reached similar conclusions [273–275] and found no difference between CVP and intensive radiation therapy [276]. Some investigators, however, have suggested that patients with follicular mixed cell NHL (the most malignant of the low-grade NHLs) may achieve durable complete remissions with more aggressive combination chemotherapy (C-MOPP, Table 119-1) [277,278]. Other aggressive chemotherapy regimens have failed to prevent relapses in patients with "favorable" disease [279–281], although those who achieve a complete remission may have a better prognosis than those who fail to do so [277].

The biological behavior of the intermediate-grade NHLs is sufficiently aggressive as to require the use of combination chemotherapy promptly after diagnosis and staging in most patients with advanced disease (III and IV). A number of chemotherapy regimens are effective for these NHLs (see Table 119-1). No precise criteria exist for choosing among them except that relatively

mild regimens such as CVP are clearly inappropriate for the more aggressive forms of NHL. A number of studies have shown the superiority of combinations of agents over the use of one or two drugs [282–284]. Cyclophosphamide and doxorubicin are particularly effective agents and are often combined with vincristine, prednisone, and bleomycin (Table 119-1). Such combination chemotherapy regimens are generally administered in a cyclical fashion for 6 to 9 months and produce objective responses in over three-quarters of previously untreated patients with complete remissions in one-half to three-quarters of patients. The dosage and rate of cytotoxic drug administration should generally be at the maximally tolerated level. Such treatments will usually produce significant myelosuppression as well as gastrointestinal and other side effects. Many regimens (e.g., BACOP and COMLA) employ a schedule of administration in which nonmyelotoxic agents are given during periods of myelosuppression to prevent tumor regrowth before the next round of myelotoxic drugs. Paradoxically, such treatment is more beneficial in these more aggressive neoplasms since a substantial proportion of true complete remissions are likely to be of such long duration as to approximate cure, particularly in patients with diffuse large cell ("histiocytic") NHL [285–288]. Thus, it is of great importance to carefully restage patients who are in apparent complete remission after treatment by reexamining those disease parameters which were evident at the time of initial staging even if laparotomy is required [288]. Patients who have only achieved a partial remission should continue chemotherapy, either with additional cycles of the same drugs or with a different regimen. Unfortunately, few controlled studies comparing the efficacy of these regimens exist, although the addition of doxorubicin, which may be synergistic with cyclophosphamide, appears advantageous in two series [280,284]. Likewise the addition of high-dose methotrexate (with leucovorin rescue) or cytosine arabinoside, or both, may be useful in preventing central nervous system spread of lymphoma since both of these agents cross the blood-brain barrier [287]. When these agents are not used, it may be advisable to administer prophylactic central nervous system treatment with cranial irradiation (2400 to 3000 rads) and intrathecal methotrexate (6 mg/m², weekly for 6 doses) with leucovorin rescue in patients at high risk (diffuse large cell NHL with marrow involvement, lymphoblastic lymphoma, or Burkitt's lymphoma [176–178]). Continued maintenance chemotherapy after achievement of a documented complete remission has not been shown to be beneficial although it has been employed in a number of studies. Myelosuppression and subsequent infections are the usual complications of such treatment programs [289]. These are discussed in Chap. 118.

The high-grade forms of NHL are generally also treated with aggressive combination chemotherapy regimens. Patients with an immunoblastic sarcoma usually receive chemotherapy similar to that administered for

TABLE 119-1   Useful drug combinations in the treatment of advanced non-Hodgkin's lymphoma

Regimen	Drug dosage schedule*	Reference
CVP:		[47]
Cyclophosphamide	400 mg/m², PO, days 1–5	
Vincristine	1.4 mg/m², IV, day 1	
Prednisone	100 mg/m², PO, days 1–5	
	(Repeat every 3 weeks)	
C-MOPP:		[286]
Cyclophosphamide	650 mg/m², IV, days 1 & 8	
Oncovin (vincristine)	1.4 mg/m², IV, days 1 & 8	
Procarbazine	100 mg/m², PO, days 1–14	
Prednisone	40 mg/m², PO, days 1–14	
	(Repeat monthly)	
BACOP (NCI):		[288]
Bleomycin	5 mg/m², IV, days 15 & 22	
Adriamycin (doxorubicin)	25 mg/m², IV, days 1 & 8	
Cyclophosphamide	650 mg/m², IV, days 1 & 8	
Oncovin (vincristine)	1.4 mg/m², IV, days 1 & 8	
Prednisone	60 mg/m², PO, days 15–29	
	(Repeat monthly)	
CHOP:		[284]
Cyclophosphamide	750 mg/m², IV, day 1	
Adriamycin (doxorubicin)	50 mg/m², IV, day 1	
Oncovin (vincristine)	1.4 mg/m², IV (max 2 mg), day 1	
Prednisone	100 mg, PO, days 1–5	
	(Repeat every 2–3 weeks)	
HOP:		[284]
Adriamycin (doxorubicin)	80 mg/m², IV, day 1	
Oncovin (vincristine)	1.4 mg/m², IV (max. 2 mg), day 1	
Prednisone	100 mg, PO, days 1–5	
	(Repeat every 2–3 weeks)	
COMLA:		[287]
Cyclophosphamide	1500 mg/m², IV, day 1	
Oncovin (vincristine)	1.4 mg/m², IV (max 2 mg), days 1, 8, 15	
Methotrexate	120 mg/m², IV, days 22, 29, 36, 43, 50, 57, 64, & 71	
Leucovorin	25 mg/m², PO, every 6 hr × 4 doses, 24 h after the methotrexate	
Cytosine arabinoside	300 mg/m², IV, days 22, 29, 36, 43, 50, 57, 64, & 71	
	(Repeat twice after 2-week rest period for total of 3 cycles)	
COP-BLAM:		[285]
Cyclophosphamide	400 mg/m², IV, day 1	
Oncovin (vincristine)	1.0 mg/m², IV, day 1	
Prednisone	40 mg/m², PO, days 1–10	
Bleomycin	15 mg, IV, day 14	
Adriamycin (doxorubicin)	40 mg/m², IV, day 1	
Matulane (procarbazine)	10 mg/m², PO, days 1–10	
	(Repeat every 3 weeks)	
COMP:		[291]
Cyclophosphamide	1000 mg/m², IV, day 1	
Oncovin (vincristine)	1.4 mg/m², IV, day 1	
Methotrexate	12.5 mg/m², IT, days 2 & 5	
Methotrextrate	12.5 mg/m², IV, days 1,3,4	
Prednisolone	1000 mg/m², IV, days 1–5	
	(Repeat every 2 weeks)	

*IT = intrathecal, IV = intravenous, PO = orally.

other diffuse large cell ("histiocytic") NHLs. Burkitt's lymphoma, both endemic and nonendemic, grows with such rapidity as to make extensive staging procedures and local radiotherapy inappropriate. The diagnosis is often made surgically in patients presenting with intraabdominal disease and surgical resection of the tumor ("debulking") appears beneficial when combined with aggressive chemotherapy. The high growth fraction makes it exquisitely sensitive to chemotherapy, which generally consists of a combination of high-dose, intermittent cyclophosphamide combined with vincristine, methotrexate, high-dose glucocorticoids (COMP—see Table 119-1), and central nervous system prophylaxis [290,291]. Modern treatment regimens have resulted in a remarkable improvement in survival (now over 50 percent at 2 years) and the potential for cure in this highly malignant neoplasm.

Lymphoblastic lymphomas are very nearly as aggressive as Burkitt's lymphoma, and staging should be confined to a diagnostic biopsy, examination of bone core biopsies and CSF cytology, and noninvasive radiologic procedures. Chemotherapy should begin promptly. Unfortunately most regimens for lymphoblastic lymphoma have provided only transient responses or brief complete remissions with the rapid emergence of drug-resistant disease and early death for many patients [292]. The most promising approach appears to be the application of intensive chemotherapy regimens designed for the treatment of cases of childhood acute lymphocytic leukemia having poor prognostic features [293,294]. Since the majority of NHLs occurring in children are either Burkitt's or lymphoblastic lymphoma, abbreviated staging, early treatment with aggressive chemotherapy, and central nervous system prophylaxis are generally indicated in children [295]. In addition to the relatively standard combination chemotherapy regimens discussed above, patients with advanced aggressive drug-resistant disease who have failed such treatments may benefit from treatment with newer agents or approaches such as high-dose methotrexate with leucovorin rescue [296], cis-platinum [297], the epipodophyllotoxins VP-16 or VM-26 [298], and streptozotocin [299]. New strategies such as the use of 2-deoxycoformycin, an inhibitor of adenosine deaminase which is cytotoxic to T cells [300], or monoclonal antibodies may also be useful [301,302].

Course, prognosis, and future directions

The underlying biological heterogeneity of the NHLs is reflected in their variable course and prognosis. The indolent behavior of the low-grade NHLs and our inability to eradicate the disease usually leads to a chronic course with multiple episodes of relapse and treatment. Ultimately the disease may evolve into a more aggressive histology or become refractory to treatment and lead to death, although many older patients may die of other causes first. The gradual escalation of treatment leads to progressively increasing toxicity to the marrow and other organs which contribute to the final outcome. Nonetheless, median survivals of 5 to 10 years and even longer for patients with early-stage disease are seen.

Modern chemotherapy programs have revolutionized the prognosis for many of the more aggressive NHLs, particularly the diffuse large cell ("histiocytic") NHLs and Burkitt's lymphoma. For these, median survivals even in advanced stages of disease have increased from a few months to over 2 years [285,287,290,303]. The flattening of the survival curve for these patients after 2 years suggests that cure of a significant proportion of patients is likely. Hopefully, better understanding of the underlying biology of these diseases will in the future lead to new diagnostic approaches capable of identifying patients for whom current methods are unsatisfactory and to new therapies capable of curing them.

References

1. Kay, N. E., Ackerman, S. K., and Douglas, S. D.: Anatomy of the immune system. *Semin. Hematol.* 16:252, 1979.
2. Miller, J. F. A. P.: Cellular interaction in immune response. *Semin. Hematol.* 16:283, 1979.
3. Rappaport, H.: Tumors of the hematopoietic system, in *Atlas of Tumor Pathology.* Armed Forces Institute of Pathology, Washington, D.C., 1966, fasc. 8, sect. 3, p. 91.
4. Hodgkin, T.: On some morbid appearances of the absorbent glands and spleen. *Med. Chir. Trans.* 17:84, 1832.
5. Wilks, S.: Cases of enlargement of the lymphatic glands and spleen. *Guys Hosp. Rep.* 11:56, 1865.
6. Virchow, R.: Weisses blut. *Neue Notizen aus dem Geb. der Natur- und Heilkunde (Froriep's neue Notizen).* 36:151, 1845.
7. Craigie, D.: Case of disease of the spleen, in which death took place in consequence of the presence of purulent matter in the blood. *Edinburgh Med. Surg. J.* 64:400, 1845.
8. Bennett, J. H.: Case of hypertrophy of the spleen and liver, in which death took place from suppuration of the blood. *Edinburgh Med. Surg. J.* 64:413, 1845.
9. Virchow, R.: *Die Krankhoften Geschwulste.* A. Hirschwald, Berlin, vol. I, 1863.
10. Dreschfeld, J.: Clinical lecture on acute Hodgkin's (or pseudoleucocythemia). *Br. Med. J.* 1:893, 1892.
11. Kundrat, H.: Über Lympho-sarkomatosis. *Wien. Klin. Wochenschr.* 6:211, 234, 1893.
12. Paltauf, R.: Lymphosarkom. In Lubarsh and Ostestag, Ergebr. *Allg. Pathol.* 3:652, 1896.
13. Sternberg, C.: Über eine eigenartige unter dem Bilde der pseudoleukämie Verlaufende Tuberculose des Lymphatischen Apparates. *Ztschr. f. Heilk.* 19:21, 1898.
14. Reed, D. M.: On the pathological changes in Hodgkin's disease, with especial reference to its relation to tuberculosis. *Johns Hopkins Hosp. Rep.* 10:133, 1902.
15. Oberling, C.: Les Réticulosarcomes et les réticuloendothéliosarcomes de la moelle ossuese (sarcomes d'Ewing). *Bull. Assoc. Fr. Étude Cancer* 17:259, 1928.
16. Roulet, F.: Das primäre Retothelsarkom der Lymphknoten. *Virchows Arch. [Pathol. Anat.]* 277:15, 1930.
17. Ewing J.: Endothelioma of lymph nodes. *J. Med. Res.* 28:1, 1913.
18. Brill, N. E., Baehr, G., and Rosenthal, N.: Generalized giant lymph follicle hyperplasia of lymph nodes and spleen: A hitherto undescribed type. *JAMA* 84:668, 1925.
19. Symmers, D.: Follicular lymphadenopathy with splenomegaly: A newly recognized disease of the lymphatic system. *Arch. Pathol. Lab. Med.* 3:816, 1927.

20. Mallory, F. B.: *Principles of Pathologic Histology*, 3d ed. Saunders, Philadelphia, 1925.
21. Burkitt, D.: A sarcoma involving the jaws in African children. *Br. J. Surg.* 46:218, 1958.
22. Nathwani, B. N., Kim, H., and Rappaport, H.: Malignant lymphoma, lymphoblastic. *Cancer* 38:964, 1976.
23. Sternberg, C.: Leukosarkomatose und myeloblastic leukämie. *Beitr. Pathol.* 61:75, 1916.
24. Cooke, J. V.: Mediastinal tumor in acute leukemia: A clinical and roentgenologic study. *Am. J. Dis. Child.* 44:1153, 1932.
25. Pusey, W. A.: Cases of sarcoma and of Hodgkin's disease treated by exposures to X-rays: A preliminary report. *JAMA* 38:166, 1902.
26. Senn, N.: Therapeutical value of röntgen ray in treatment of pseudoleukemia. *N.Y. Med. J.* 77:665, 1903.
27. Gall, E. A.: The surgical treatment of malignant lymphoma. *Ann. Surg.* 118:1064, 1943.
28. Craver, L. F.: Lymphomas and leukemias: The value of early diagnosis and treatment. *JAMA* 136:244, 1948.
29. Gilbert, R.: Radiotherapy in Hodgkin's disease (malignant granulomatosis): Anatomic and clinical foundations; governing principles; results. *Am. J. Roentgenol.* 41:198, 1939.
30. Peters, M. V.: A study of survivals in Hodgkin's disease treated radiologically. *Am. J. Roentgenol.* 63:299, 1950.
31. Carbone, P. P., Kaplan, H. S., Musshoff, K., Smithers, D. W., and Tubiana, M.: Report of the committee on Hodgkin's disease staging classification. *Cancer Res.* 31:1860, 1971.
32. Jones, S. E., Fuks, Z., Kaplan, H. S., and Rosenberg, S. A.: Non-Hodgkin's lymphomas. V. Results of radiotherapy. *Cancer* 32:682, 1973.
33. Gilman, A., and Philips, F. S.: The biological actions and therapeutic applications of the β-chlorethylamines and sulfides. *Science* 103:409, 1946.
34. Jacobson, L. O., Spurr, C. L., Guzman-Barron, E. S., Smith, T., Lushbaugh, C., and Dick, G. F.: Nitrogen mustard therapy: Studies on the effect of methylbis (β-chlorethyl) amine hydrochloride on neoplastic disorders and allied disorders of the hematopoietic system. *JAMA* 132:263, 1946.
35. Farber, S., Diamond, L. K., Mercer, R. D., Silvester, R. F., Jr., and Wolfe, J. A.: Temporary remissions in acute leukemia in children produced by folic acid antagonist 4-aminopteroyl glutamic acid (Aminopterin). *N. Engl. J. Med.* 238:787, 1948.
36. Heidelberger, C.: Fluorinated pyrimidines. *Prog. Nucl. Acid. Res. Mol. Biol.* 4:1, 1965.
37. Noble, R. L., Beer, C. T., and Cutts, J. H.: Role of chance observation in chemotherapy: Vinca rosea. *Ann. N.Y. Acad. Sci.* 76:882, 1958.
38. Ezdinli, E. Z., Stutzman, L., Aungst, C. W., and Firat, F.: Corticosteroid therapy for lymphomas and chronic lymphocytic leukemia. *Cancer* 23:900, 1969.
39. Dubost, M., et al.: Un Nouvel Antibiotic a propriétés antitumorales. *C.R. Acad. Sci.* [D](Paris) 257:1813, 1963.
40. Jones, S. E., Rosenberg, S. A., Kaplan, H. S., Kadin, M. E., and Dorfman, R. F.: Non-Hodgkin's lymphomas. II. Single agent chemotherapy. *Cancer* 30:31, 1972.
41. Livingston, D., and Carter, S. K.: In *Single Agents in Cancer Chemotherapy*. IFI/Plenum, New York, 1970, p. 25.
42. Goldin, A., Venditti, J. M., Humphreys, S. R., and Mantel, N.: Quantitative evaluation of chemotherapeutic agents against advanced leukemia in mice. *J. Natl. Cancer Inst.* 21:495, 1958.
43. Skipper, H. E., Schabel, F. M., Jr., and Wilcox, W. S.: Experimental evaluation of potential anticancer agents. XIII. On the criteria and kinetics associated with "curability" of experimental leukemia. *Cancer Chemother. Rep.* 35:3, 1964.
44. Hoogstraten, B., et al.: Combination chemotherapy in lymphosarcoma and reticulum sarcoma. *Blood* 33:370, 1969.
45. Lowenbraun, S., DeVita, V. T., and Serpick, A. A.: Combination chemotherapy with nitrogen mustard, vincristine, procarbazine, and prednisone in lymphosarcoma and reticulum cell sarcoma. *Cancer* 25:1018, 1970.
46. Luce, J. K., et al.: Combined cyclophosphamide, vincristine, and prednisone therapy of malignant lymphoma. *Cancer* 28:306, 1971.
47. Bagley, C. M., DeVita, V. T., Berard, C. W., and Canellos, G. P.: Advanced lymphosarcoma: Intensive cyclical combination chemotherapy with cyclophosphamide, vincristine, and prednisone. *Ann. Intern. Med.* 76:227, 1972.
48. Andiman, W. A.: The Epstein-Barr virus and EB virus infections in childhood. *J. Pediatr.* 95:171, 1979.
49. Zur-Hausen, H., and Fresen, K. D.: Heterogeneity of Epstein-Barr virus. *Biochim. Biophys. Acta* 560:343, 1979.
50. Epstein, M. A., Achang, B. G., and Barr, Y. H.: Virus particles in cultured lymphoblasts from Burkitt's lymphoma. *Lancet* 1:702, 1964.
51. Pattengale, P. K., Smith, R. W., and Gerber, P.: B-cell characteristics of human peripheral and cord blood leukocytes transformed by Epstein-Barr virus. *J. Natl. Cancer Inst.* 52:1081, 1974.
52. Henle, W., Diehl, V., Kohn, G., ZurHausen, H., and Henle, G.: Herpes-type virus and chromosome marker in normal leucocytes after growth with irradiated Burkitt cells. *Science* 157:1064, 1967.
53. Thorley-Larson, D. A.: The suppression of Epstein-Barr virus infection in vitro occurs after infection but before transformation of the cell. *J. Immunol.* 124:745, 1980.
54. Adams, A., and Lindahl, T.: Epstein-Barr virus genomes with properties of circular DNA molecules in carrier cells. *Proc. Natl. Acad. Sci. U.S.A.* 72:1477, 1975.
55. Kaschka-Dierich, C., Falk, L., Bjursell, G., Adams, A., and Lindahl, T.: Human lymphoblastoid cell lines derived from individuals without lymphoproliferative disease contain the same latent forms of Epstein-Barr virus DNA as those found in tumor cells. *Int. J. Cancer* 20:173, 1977.
56. Lindahl, T., Klein, G., Reedman, B. M., Johanssan, B., and Singh, S.: Relationship between Epstein-Barr virus (EBV) DNA and the EBV-determined nuclear antigen (EBNA) in Burkitt lymphoma biopsies and other lymphoproliferative malignancies. *Int. J. Cancer* 13:764, 1974.
57. Anderson, M., Klein, G., Ziegler, J., and Henle, W.: Association of Epstein-Barr viral genomes with American Burkitt lymphoma. *Nature* 260:357, 1976.
58. Nonoyama, M., Huang, C., Pagano, J. S., Klein, G., and Singh, S.: DNA of Epstein-Barr virus detected in tissues of Burkitt's lymphoma and nasopharyngeal carcinoma. *Proc. Natl. Acad. Sci. U.S.A.* 70:3265, 1973.
59. Desgranges, C., et al.: Nasopharyngeal carcinoma. X-Presence of Epstein-Barr genomes in separated epithelial cells of tumours in patients from Singapore, Tunisia and Kenya. *Int. J. Cancer* 16:7, 1975.
60. Henle, G., et al.: Antibodies to Epstein-Barr virus in Burkitt's lymphoma and control groups. *J. Natl. Cancer Inst.* 43:1147, 1969.
61. Henle, W., et al.: Antibodies to Epstein-Barr virus in nasopharyngeal carcinoma, other head and neck neoplasms, and control groups. *J. Natl. Cancer Inst.* 44:225, 1970.
62. de The, G.: The epidemiology of Burkitt's lymphoma. *Epidemiological Rev.* 1:32, 1979.
63. Niederman, J. C., Evans, A. S., McCollum, R. W., and Subrahmanyan, L.: Prevalence, incidence and persistence of EB virus antibody in young adults. *N. Engl. J. Med.* 282:361, 1970. -
64. Gerber, P., Goldstein, L. I., Lucas, S., Nonoyama, B., and Perlin, E.: Oral excretion of Epstein-Barr viruses by healthy subjects and patients with infectious mononucleosis. *Lancet* 2:988, 1972.
65. Royston, I., Sullivan, J. L., Periman, P. O., and Perlin, E.: Cell-mediated immunity to Epstein-Barr-virus-transformed lymphoblastoid cells in acute infectious mononucleosis. *N. Engl. J. Med.* 293:1159, 1975.
66. Robinson, J. E., et al.: Diffuse polyclonal B-cell lymphoma during primary infection with Epstein-Barr virus. *N. Engl. J. Med.* 302:1293, 1980.
67. Purtilo, D. T., Cassel, C. K., Yang, J. P. S., and Harper, R.: X-linked recessive progressive combined variable immunodeficiency (Duncan's disease). *Lancet* 1:935, 1975.
68. Miller, G., et al.: Lymphoma in cotton-top marmosets after inoculation with Epstein-Barr virus: Tumor incidence, histologic spectrum, antibody responses, demonstration of viral DNA and characterization of viruses. *J. Exp. Med.* 145:948, 1977.
69. Rapp, F.: Viruses as an etiologic factor in cancer. *Semin. Oncol.* 3:49, 1976.

70. Gallo, R. C., and Todaro, G. J.: Oncogenic RNA viruses. *Semin. Oncol.* 3:81, 1976.

71. Kaplan, H. S., Goodenow, R. S., Gartner, S., and Bieber, M. M.: Biology and virology of the human malignant lymphomas. *Cancer* 43:1, 1979.

72. Poiesz, B. J., Ruscetti, F. W., Gazdar, A. F., Bunn, P. A., Minna J. D., and Gallo, R. C.: Detection and isolation of type C retrovirus particles from fresh and cultured lymphocytes of a patient with cutaneous T-cell lymphoma. *Proc. Natl. Acad. Sci. U.S.A.* 77:7415, 1980.

73. Robert-Guroff, M., Nakao, Y., Notake, K., Ito, Y., Sliski, A., and Gallo, R. C.: Natural antibodies to human retrovirus HTLV in a cluster of Japanese patients with adult T cell leukemia. *Science* 215:975, 1982.

74. American Cancer Society: Cancer statistics. *CA* 29:6, 1979.

75. Berard, C. W., Greene, M. H., Jaffe, E. S., Magrath, I., and Ziegler, J.: A multidisciplinary approach to non-Hodgkin's lymphomas. *Ann. Intern. Med.* 94:218, 1981.

76. Cutler, S. J., and Young, J. L.: Third national cancer survey: Incidence data. *Natl. Cancer Inst. Monogr.* 41 (Ser. VI), 1975.

77. Hoover, R.: Geographic patterns of cancer mortality in the U.S., in *Persons at High Risk of Cancer*, edited by J. F. Fraumeni, Jr. Academic, New York, 1975, pp. 343–360.

78. Cantor, K. P., and Fraumeni, J. F., Jr.: Distribution of non-Hodgkin's lymphoma in the United States between 1950 and 1975. *Cancer Res.* 40:2645, 1980.

79. Olin, G. R.: The hazards of chemical laboratory environment: A study of the mortality in two cohorts of Swedish chemists. *Am. Ind. Hyg. Assoc. J.* 39:557, 1978.

80. Li, F. P., Fraumeni, J. F., Jr., Mantel, N., and Miller, R. W.: Cancer mortality among chemists. *J. Natl. Cancer Inst.* 43:1159, 1969.

81. Saltzstein, S. L., and Ackerman, L. V.: Lymphadenopathy induced by anticonvulsant drugs and mimicking chemically and pathologically malignant lymphomas. *Cancer* 12:164, 1959.

82. Li, F. P., Willard, D. R., Goodman, R., and Vawter, G.: Malignant lymphoma after diphenylhydantion (Dilantin) therapy. *Cancer* 36:1359, 1975.

83. IARC Working Group on the Evaluation of the Carcinogenic Risk of Chemicals to Man: Phenytoin and phenytoin sodium. IARC World Health Organization, Lyons, France, Monogr. no. 13, 1977.

84. Beebe, G. W., Kato, H., and Land, C.: Studies of the mortality of A-bomb survivors: 6. Mortality and radiation dose, 1950–1974. *Rad. Res.* 75:138, 1978.

85. Advisory Committee on the Biological Effects of Ionizing Radiation, National Academy of Sciences—National Research Council: *The Effects on Populations of Exposure to Low Levels of Ionizing Radiation.* U.S. Government Printing Office, Washington, D.C., 1979.

86. Louie, S., Daoust, P. R., and Schwartz, R. S.: Immunodeficiency and the pathogenesis of non-Hodgkin's lymphoma. *Semin. Oncol.* 7:267, 1980.

87. Miller, D. G.: The association of immune disease and malignant lymphoma. *Ann. Intern. Med.* 66:507, 1967.

88. Gatti, R. A., and Good, R. A.: Occurrence of malignancy in immunodeficiency disease. *Cancer* 28:89, 1971.

89. Spector, B. D., Perry, G. S., III, and Kersey, J. H.: Genetically determined immunodeficiency disease (GDID) and malignancy: A report from the Immunodeficiency Cancer Registry. *Clin. Immunol. Immunopathol.* 11:12, 1978.

90. Talal, N.: Autoimmunity and lymphoid malignancy in New Zealand black mice. *Progr. Clin. Immunol.* 2:101, 1974.

91. Isomaki, H. A., Hakulinen, T., and Joutsenlahti, U.: Excess risk of lymphomas, leukemia, and myeloma in patients with rheumatoid arthritis. *J. Chronic Dis.* 31:691, 1978.

92. Kassan, S. S., et al.: Increased risk of lymphoma in sicca syndrome. *Ann. Intern. Med.* 89:888, 1978.

93. Wyburn-Mason, R.: SLE and lymphoma. *Lancet* 1:156, 1979.

94. Holmes, G. K. T., Stokes, P. L., Sorahan, T. M., Prior, P., Waterhouse, J. A. M., and Cooke, W. T.: Coeliac disease, gluten-free diet, and malignancy. *Gut* 17:612, 1976.

95. Lewin, K. J., Kahn, L. B., and Novis, B. N.: Primary intestinal lymphoma of "Western" and "Mediterranean" type, alpha chain disease and massive plasma cell infiltration: A study of 37 cases. *Cancer* 38:2511, 1976.

96. Alpha-chain disease and related small-intestinal lymphomas: A memo. *Bulletin WHO* 54:615, 1976.

97. Frizzera, G., Moran, E. M., and Rappaport H.: Angio-immunoblastic lymphadenopathy: Diagnosis and clinical course. *Am. J. Med.* 59:803, 1975.

98. Lukes, R. J., and Tindle, B. H.: Immunoblastic lymphadenopathy: A hyperimmune entity resembling Hodgkin's disease. *N. Engl. J. Med.* 292:1, 1975.

99. Nathwani, B. N., Rappaport, H., Moran, E. M., Pangalis, G. A., and Kim, H.: Malignant lymphoma arising in angioimmunoblastic lymphadenopathy. *Cancer* 41:578, 1978.

100. Freeman, H. J., Weinstein, W. M., Shnitka, T. K., Piercey, J. R. A., and Wensel, R. H.: Primary abdominal lymphoma-presenting manifestation of celiac sprue or complicating dermatitis herpetiformis. *Am. J. Med.* 63:585, 1977.

101. Brinker, H., and Wilbek, E.: The incidence of malignant tumors in patients with respiratory sarcoidosis. *Br. J. Cancer* 29:247, 1974.

102. Rodriguez, E., de Bonaparte, Y. P., Morgenfeld, M. C., and Calbrini, R. L.: Malignant lymphomas in leprosy patients: A clinical and histopathologic study. *Int. J. Leprosy* 36:203, 1968.

103. Andrade, Z. A., and Abreu, W. N.: Follicular lymphoma of the spleen in patients with hepatosplenic *Schistosomiasis mansoni. Am. J. Trop. Med. Hyg.* 20:237, 1971.

104. Kinlen, L. J., et al.: Cancer in dialysis patients. *Br. Med. J.* 280:1401, 1980.

105. Kinlen, L. J., Shieil, A. G. R., Peto, J., and Doll, R.: Collaborative United Kingdom–Australasian study of cancer in patients treated with immunosuppresive drugs. *Br. Med. J.* 7:1461, 1979.

106. Anderson, J. L., Bieber, C. P., Fowles, R. E., and Stinson, E. B.: Idiopathic cardiomyopathy, age, and suppressor-cell dysfunction as risk determinants of lymphoma after cardiac transplantation. *Lancet* 2:1174, 1978.

107. Hirsch, M.S., Phillips, S. M., Salnik, C., Black, P. H., Schwartz, R. S., and Carpenter, C. B.: Activation of leukemia viruses by graft-versus-host and mixed lymphocyte reactions in vitro. *Proc. Natl. Acad. Sci. U.S.A.* 69:1069, 1972.

108. Armstrong, M. Y. K., Ruddle, N. H., Lipman, N. B., and Richards, F. F.: Tumor induction by immunologically activated murine leukemic virus. *J. Exp. Med.* 137:1163, 1973.

109. Krikorian, J. H., Burke, J. S., Rosenberg, S. A., and Kaplan, H. S.: Occurrence of non-Hodgkin's lymphoma after therapy for Hodgkin's disease. *N. Engl. J. Med.* 300:452, 1979.

110. Kaiser-McCaw, B., Hecht, F., Harnden, D. G., and Teplitz, R. L.: Somatic rearrangement of chromosome 14 in human lymphocytes. *Proc. Natl. Acad. Sci. U.S.A.* 72:2071, 1975.

111. Rowley, J. D., and Fukuhara, S.: Chromosome studies in non-Hodgkin's lymphomas. *Semin. Oncol.* 7:255, 1980.

112. Jean, P., Richer, C.-L., Murer-Orlando, M., Luu, D. H., and Joncas, J. H.: Translocation 8;14 in ataxia telangiectasia–derived cell line. *Nature* 277:56, 1979.

113. Aisenberg, A. C., Wilkes, B. M., Long, J. C., and Harris, N. L.: Cell surface phenotype in lymphoproliferative disease. *Am. J. Med.* 68:206, 1980.

114. Ross, G. D.: Identification of human lymphocyte subpopulations by surface marker analysis. *Blood* 53:799, 1979.

115. Frizzera, G., Gajl-Peczalska, K. J., Bloomfield, C. D., and Kersey, J. H.: Predicitability of immunologic phenotype of malignant lymphomas by conventional morphology. *Cancer* 43:1216, 1979.

116. Lukes, R. J., Parker, J. W., Taylor, C. R., Tindle, B. H., Cramer, A. D., and Lincoln, T. L.: Immunologic approach to non-Hodgkin lymphomas and related leukemias: Analysis of the results of multiparameter studies of 425 cases. *Semin. Hematol.* 15:322, 1978.

117. Pinkus, G. S., and Said, J. W.: Characterization of non-Hodgkin's lymphomas using multiple cell markers. *Am. J. Pathol.* 94:349, 1979.

118. Mann, R. B., Jaffe, E. S., and Berard, C. W.: Malignant lymphomas—A conceptual understanding of morphologic diversity. *Am. J. Pathol.* 94:105, 1979.

119. Yamanaka, N., Ishii, Y., Koshiba, H., Mikani, C., Ogasawara, M.,

and Kikuchi, K.: A study of surface markers in non-Hodgkin's lymphoma by using anti-T and anti-B lymphocyte sera. *Cancer* 47:311, 1981.

120. Jaffe, E. S., Shevach, E. M., Frank, M. M., Berard, C. W., and Green, I.: Nodular lymphoma-evidence for origin from follicular B lymphocytes. *N. Engl. J. Med.* 290:813, 1974.
121. Koziner, B., Kempin, S., Passe, S., Gee, T., Good, R. A., and Clarkson, B. D.: Characterization of B-cell leukemia: A tentative immunomorphological scheme. *Blood* 56:815, 1980.
122. Lichtenstein, A., et al.: Immunoblastic sarcoma: A clinical description. *Cancer* 43:343, 1979.
123. Michel, R. P., Case, B. W., and Moinuddin, M.: Immunoblastic sarcoma: A light, immunofluorescence, and electron microscopic study. *Cancer* 43:224, 1979.
124. Mann, R. B., et al.: Non-endemic Burkitt's lymphoma: A B-cell tumor related to germinal centers. *N. Engl. J. Med.* 295:685, 1976.
125. Safai, B., and Good, R. A.: Lymphoproliferative disorders of the T-cell series. *Medicine* 59:335, 1980.
126. Broder, S., et al.: The Sézary syndrome: A malignant proliferation of helper T cells. *J. Clin. Invest.* 58:1297, 1976.
127. Blatt, J., Reaman, G., and Poplack, D. G.: Biochemical markers in lymphoid malignancy. *N. Engl. J. Med.* 303:918, 1980.
128. Catovsky, D., Galetto, J., Okos, E., Miliani, E., and Galton, D. A. G.: Cytochemical profile of B and T leukaemic lymphocytes with special reference to acute lymphoblastic leukaemia. *J. Clin. Pathol.* 27:767, 1974.
129. Li, C. Y., Yam, L. T., and Lam, K. W.: Acid phosphatase isoenzyme in human leukocytes in normal and pathologic conditions. *J. Histochem. Cytochem.* 18:473, 1970.
130. Nanba, K., Jaffe, E. S., Braylon, R. C., Soban, E. J., and Berard, C. W.: Alkaline phosphatase-positive malignant lymphoma: A subtype of B-cell lymphomas. *Am. J. Clin. Pathol.* 68:535, 1977.
131. Poppema, S., Elema, J. D., and Halie, M. R.: Alkaline phosphatase positive lymphomas: A morphologic, immunologic, and enzyme-histochemical study. *Cancer* 47:1303, 1981.
132. Van Heerde, P., Feltkamp, C. A., Feltkamp-Vroom, T. M., Koudstaal, J., and Van Unnik, J. A. M.: Non-Hodgkin's lymphoma: Immunohistochemical and electron microscopical findings in relation to light microscopy. *Cancer* 46:2210, 1980.
133. Pangalis, G. A., Nathwani, B. N., and Rappaport, H.: An immunocytochemical study of non-Hodgkin's lymphomas. *Cancer* 48:915, 1981.
134. Diamond, L. W., and Brayland, R. C.: Flow analysis of DNA content and cell size in non-Hodgkin's lymphoma. *Cancer Res.* 40:703, 1980.
135. Hansen, H., Koziner, B., and Clarkson, B.: Kinetic studies in the non-Hodgkin's lymphomas. *Am. J. Med.* 71:107, 1981.
136. Costa, A., Bonnadonna, G., Villa, E., Villegussa, P., and Silvestrini, R.: Labeling index as a prognostic marker in non-Hodgkin's lymphomas. *J. Natl. Cancer Inst.* 66:1, 1981.
137. Iversen, O., et al.: Cell kinetics in Burkitt lymphoma. *Eur. J. Cancer* 10:155, 1974.
138. Murphy, S. B., Melvin, S. L., and Mauer, A. M.: Correlation of tumor cell kinetic studies with surface marker results in childhood non-Hodgkin's lymphoma. *Cancer Res.* 39:1534, 1979.
139. Bloomfield, C. D., et al.: In vitro glucocorticoid studies for predicting response to glucocorticoid therapy in adults with malignant lymphoma. *Lancet* 1:952, 1980.
140. Naeim, F., Bergmann, K., and Gatti, R. A.: Membrane receptors and their redistribution in lymphoproliferative disorders. *Blood* 54:648, 1979.
141. Ben-Bassat, H., et al.:Changes in the Con-A-induced redistribution pattern of lymphocytes: A possible aid in the differential diagnosis between malignant lymphoma and other diseases. *Blood* 55:205, 1980.
142. Rosenberg, S. A., Diamond, H. D., Jaslowitz, B., and Craver, L. F.: Lymphosarcoma: A review of 1269 cases. *Medicine* 40:31, 1961.
143. Gattiker, H. H., Wiltshaw, E., and Galton, D. A. G.: Spontaneous regression in non-Hodgkin's lymphoma. *Cancer* 45:2627, 1980.
144. Rudders, R. A., Ross, M. E., and DeLellis, R. A.: Primary extranodal lymphoma. *Cancer* 42:406, 1978.
145. Lotz, M. J., Chabner, B., DeVita, V. T., Johnson, R. E., and Berard, C. W.: Pathological staging of 100 consecutive untreated patients with non-Hodgkin's lymphomas: Extra-medullary sites of disease. *Cancer* 37:266, 1976.
146. Reddy S., Pellettiere, E., Saxena, V., and Hendrickson, F. R.: Extranodal non-Hodgkin's lymphoma. *Cancer* 46:1925, 1980.
147. Jones, S. E., et al.: Non-Hodgkin's lymphomas. IV. Clinicopathologic correlation in 405 cases. *Cancer* 31:806, 1973.
148. Patchefsky, A. S., Brodovsky, H. S., Menduke, H., Southard, M., Brooks, J., Nicklas, D., and Hoch, W. S.: Non-Hodgkin's lymphomas: A clinicopathologic study of 293 cases. *Cancer* 34:1173, 1974.
149. Bloomfield, C. D., Goldman, A., Dick, F., Brunning, R. D., and Kennedy, B. J.: Multivariate analysis of prognostic factors in the non-Hodgkin's malignant lymphomas. *Cancer* 33:870, 1974.
150. Dewys, W. D., et al.: Prognostic effect of weight loss prior to chemotherapy in cancer patients. *Am. J. Med.* 69:491, 1980.
151. Braylan, R. C., Jaffe, E. S., Burbach, J. W., Frank, M. M., Johnson, R. B., and Berard, C. W.: Similarities of surface characteristics of neoplastic well-differentiated lymphocytes from solid tissues and from peripheral blood. *Cancer Res.* 36:1619, 1976.
152. Pangalis, G. A., Nathwani, B. N., and Rappaport, H.: Malignant lymphoma, well differentiated lymphocytic: Its relationship with chronic lymphocytic leukemia and macroglobulinemia of Waldenström. *Cancer* 39:999, 1977.
153. Fu, S. M., Winchester, R. J., Feizi, T., Walzer, P. D., and Kunkel, H. G.: Idiotypic specificity of surface immunoglobulin and the maturation of leukemic bone-marrow-derived lymphocytes. *Proc. Natl. Acad. Sci. U.S.A.* 71:4487, 1974.
154. Foucar, K., and Rydell, R. E.: Richter's syndrome in chronic lymphocytic leukemia. *Cancer* 46:118, 1980.
155. Rudders, R. A., Ahl, E. T., DeLellis, R. A., Bernstein, S., and Begg, C. B.: Surface marker identification of small cleaved follicular center cell lymphomas with a highly favorable prognosis. *Cancer Res.* 42:349, 1982.
156. Rosenburg, S. A.: Bone marrow involvement in the non-Hodgkin's lymphomata. *Br. J. Cancer* 31 (Suppl. II):261, 1975.
157. Stein, R. S., Ultmann, J. E., Byrne, G. E., Moran, E. M., Golomb, H. M., and Oetzel, N.: Bone marrow involvement in non-Hodgkin's lymphoma. *Cancer* 37:629, 1976.
158. Bitran, J. D., et al.: Non-Hodgkin's lymphoma, poorly differentiated lymphocytic and mixed cell types: Results of sequential staging procedures, response to therapy, and survival of 100 patients. *Cancer* 42:88, 1978.
159. Chabner, B. A., et al.: Sequential nonsurgical and surgical staging of non-Hodgkin's lymphoma. *Ann. Intern. Med.* 85:149, 1976.
160. Heifetz, L. J., et al.: Laparotomy findings in lymphangiogram-staged I and II non-Hodgkin's lymphomas. *Cancer* 45:2778, 1980.
161. Warnke, R. A., Kim, H., Fuks, Z., and Dorfman, R. F.: The coexistence of nodular and diffuse patterns in nodular non-Hodgkin's lymphomas: Significance and clinicopathologic correlation. *Cancer* 40:1229, 1977.
162. Fisher, R. I., et al.: Natural history of malignant lymphomas with divergent histologies at staging evaluation. *Cancer* 47:2022, 1981.
163. Risdall, R., Hoppe, R. T. and Warnke, R.: Non-Hodgkin's lymphoma: A study of the evolution of the disease based upon 92 autopsied cases. *Cancer* 44:529, 1979.
164. Rappaport, H., Winter, W. J., and Hicks, E. B.: Follicular lymphoma: A re-evaluation of its position in the scheme of malignant lymphoma, based on a survey of 253 cases. *Cancer* 9:792, 1956.
165. Kim, H., Hendrickson, M. R., and Dorfman, R. F.: Composite lymphoma. *Cancer* 40:959, 1977.
166. Waldron, J. A., Leech, J. H., Glick, A. D., Flexner, J. M., and Collins, R. D.: Malignant lymphoma of peripheral T-lymphocyte origin. *Cancer* 40:1604, 1977.
167. Kim, H., Jacobs, C., Warnke, R. A., and Dorfman, R. F.: Malignant lymphoma with a high content of epithelioid histiocytes. *Cancer* 41:620, 1978.
168. Nathwani, B. N.: A critical analysis of the classifications of non-Hodgkin's lymphomas. *Cancer* 44:347, 1979.
169. Strauchen, J. A., Young, R. C., DeVita, V. T., Anderson, T., Fantone,

J. C., and Berard, C. W.: Clinical relevance of the histopathological subclassification of diffuse "histiocytic" lymphoma. *N. Engl. J. Med.* 299:1382, 1978.

170. Barcos, M., et al.: The influence of histologic type on survival in non-Hodgkin's lymphoma. *Cancer* 47:2894, 1981.

171. Garvin, A. J., Simon, R., Young, R. C., DeVita, V. T., and Berard, C. W.: The Rappaport classification of non-Hodgkin's lymphomas: A closer look using other proposed classifications. *Semin. Oncol.* 7:234, 1980.

172. Armitage, J. O., Dick, F. R., Platz, C. E., Corder, M. P., and Leimert, J. T.: Clinical usefulness and reproducibility of histologic subclassification of advanced diffuse histiocytic lymphoma. *Am. J. Med.* 67:929, 1979.

173. Banfi, A., et al.: Malignant lymphomas of Waldeyer's ring: Natural history and survival after radiotherapy. *Br. Med. J.* 3:140, 1972.

174. Hermann, R., Panahon, A. M., Barcos, M. P., Walsh, D., and Stutzman, L.: Gastrointestinal involvement in non-Hodgkin's lymphoma. *Cancer* 46:215, 1980.

175. Rosenfeldt, F., and Rosenberg, S. A.: Diffuse histiocytic lymphoma presenting with gastrointestinal tract lesions. *Cancer* 45:2188, 1980.

176. Bunn, P. A., Schein, P. S., Banks, P. M., and DeVita, V. T.: Central nervous system complications in patients with diffuse histiocytic and undifferentiated lymphoma: Leukemia revisited. *Blood* 47:3, 1976.

177. Litam, J. P., Cabanillas, F., Smith, T. L., Bodey, G. P., and Freireich, E. J.: Central nervous system relapse in malignant lymphomas: Risk factors and implications for prophylaxis. *Blood* 54:1249, 1979.

178. Levitt, L. J., Dawson, D. M., Rosenthal, D. J., and Maloney, W. C.: CNS involvement in the non-Hodgkin's lymphomas. *Cancer* 45:545, 1980.

179. Miller, J. B., et al.: Diffuse histiocytic lymphoma with sclerosis: A clinicopathologic entity frequently causing superior venacaval obstruction. *Cancer* 47:748, 1981.

180. Bennett, M. H.: Sclerosis in non-Hodgkin's lymphomata. *Br. J. Cancer* 31 (Suppl. II):44, 1975.

181. Rosas-Uribe, A., and Rappaport, H.: Malignant lymphoma, histiocytic type with sclerosis (sclerosing reticulum cell sarcoma). *Cancer* 29:946, 1972.

182. Rudders, R. A., Ahl, E. T., and DeLellis, R. A.: Surface marker and histopathologic correlation with long-term survival in advanced large-cell non-Hodgkin's lymphoma. *Cancer* 47:1329, 1981.

183. Palutke, M., et al.: T-cell lymphomas of large cell type. *Cancer* 46:87, 1980.

184. Watanabe, S., et al.: Adult T cell lymphoma with hypergammaglobulinemia. *Cancer* 46:2472, 1980.

185. Taylor, C. R., Russell, R., Lukes, R. J., and Davis, R. L.: An immunohistological study of immunoglobulin content of primary central nervous system lymphomas. *Cancer* 41:2197, 1978.

186. Bloomfield, C. D., Gajl-Peczalska, K. J., Frizzera, G., Kersey, J. H., and Goldman A. I.: Clinical utility of lymphocyte surface markers combined with the Lukes-Collins histologic classification in adult lymphoma. *N. Engl. J. Med.* 301:512, 1979.

187. Smith, J. L., Barker, C. R., Clein, G. P., and Collins, R. D.: Characterization of malignant mediastinal lymphoid neoplasm (Sternberg sarcoma) as thymic in orgin. *Lancet* 1:74, 1973.

188. Pinkel, D., Johnson, W., and Aur, R. J. A.: Non-Hodgkin's lymphoma in children. *Br. J. Cancer* 31 (Suppl. II):298, 1975.

189. Williams, A. H., et al.: Childhood lymphoma-leukemia. I. Correlation of morphology and immunological studies. *Cancer* 42:171, 1978.

190. Boucheix, C., et al.: Lymphoblastic lymphoma/leukemia with convoluted nuclei. *Cancer* 45:1569, 1980.

191. Rosen, P. J., et al.: Convoluted lymphocytic lymphoma in adults, a clinicopathologic entity. *Ann. Intern. Med.* 89:319, 1978.

192. Nadler, L. M., Reinherz, E. L., Weinstein, H. J., D'Orsi, C. J., and Schlossman, S. F.: Heterogeneity of T-cell lymphoblastic malignancies. *Blood* 55:806, 1980.

193. Ioachim, H. L., and Finkbeiner, J. A.: Pseudonodular pattern of T-cell lymphoma. *Cancer* 45:1370, 1980.

194. Burkitt, D. P., and O'Conor, G. T.: Malignant lymphoma in African children. I. A clinical syndrome. *Cancer* 14:258, 1961.

195. Arseneau, J. C., Canellos, G. P., Banks, P. M., Berard, C. W., Gral-

nick, H. R., and DeVita, V. T.: American Burkitt's lymphoma: A clinicopathologic study of 30 cases. I. Clinical factors relating to prolonged survival. *Am. J. Med.* 58:314, 1975.

196. Ziegler, J. L.: Treatment results of 54 American patients with Burkitt's lymphoma are similar to the African experience. *N. Engl. J. Med.* 297:75, 1977.

197. Mann, R. B., and Berard, C. W.: Burkitt's tumor: Lessons from mice, monkeys, and man. *Lancet* 2:84, 1977.

198. Prokocimer, M., Matzner, Y., Ben-Bassat, H., and Polliack, A.: Burkitt's lymphoma presenting as acute leukemia (Burkitt's lymphoma cell leukemia). *Cancer* 45:2884, 1980.

199. Magrath, I., et al.: Prognostic factors in Burkitt's lymphoma: Importance of total tumor burden. *Cancer* 45:1507, 1980.

200. Scott, R. B., and Robb-Smith, A. H. T.: Histiocytic medullary reticulosis. *Lancet* 2:194, 1939.

201. Groopman, J. E., and Golde, D. W.: The histiocytic disorders: A pathophysiologic analysis. *Ann. Intern. Med.* 94:95, 1981.

202. Jaffe, E. S., Shevach, E. M., Sussman, E. H., Frank, M., Green, I., and Berard, C. W.: Membrane receptor sites for the identification of lymphoreticular cells in benign and malignant conditions. *Br. J. Cancer* 31 (Suppl. II):107, 1975.

203. Warnke, R. A., Kim, H., and Dortman, R. F.: Malignant histiocytosis (histiocytic medullary reticulosis). I. Clinicopathologic study of 29 cases. *Cancer* 35:215, 1975.

204. Vardiman, J. W., Byrne, G. E., and Rappaport, H.: Malignant histiocytosis with massive splenomegaly in asymptomatic patients. *Cancer* 36:419, 1975.

205. Starkie, C. M., Kenny, M. W., Mann, J. R., Cameron, A. H., and Hill, F. G. H.: Histiocytic medullary reticulosis following acute lymphoblastic leukemia. *Cancer* 47:537, 1981.

206. Risdall, R. J., et al.: Virus-associated hemophagocytic syndrome. *Cancer* 44:993, 1979.

207. Goffinet, D. R., et al.: Staging laparotomies in unselected previously untreated patients with non-Hodgkin's lymphomas. *Cancer* 32:672, 1973.

208. Moran, E. M., Ultmann, J. E., Ferguson, D. J., Hoffer, P. B., Ranniger, K., and Rappaport, H.: Staging laparotomy in non-Hodgkin's lymphoma. *Br. J. Cancer* 31 (Suppl. II):228, 1975.

209. Kim, H., and Dorfman, R. F.: Morphological studies of 84 untreated patients subjected to laparotomy for the staging of non-Hodgkin's lymphomas. *Cancer* 33:657, 1974.

210. Solidoro, A., Salazar, F., Flor, J., Sanchez, J., and Otero, J.: Endoscopic tissue diagnosis of gastric involvement in the staging of non-Hodgkin's lymphoma. *Cancer* 48:1053, 1981.

211. Lewin, K. J., Ranchod, M., and Dorfman, R. F.: Lymphomas of the gastrointestinal tract. *Cancer* 42:693, 1978.

212. Henry, K., and Farrer-Brown, G.: Primary lymphomas of the gastrointestinal tract: I. Plasma cell tumors. *Histopathology* 1:53, 1977.

213. Isaacson, P., Wright, D. H., Judd, M. A., and Mepham, B. L.: Primary gastrointestinal lymphomas. *Cancer* 43:1805, 1979.

214. Herman, T. S., Hammond, N., Jones, S. E., Butler, J. J., Byrne, G. E., and McKelvey, E. M.: Involvement of the central nervous system by non-Hodgkin's lymphoma: The Southwest Oncology Group Experience. *Cancer* 43:390, 1979.

215. Woolley, P. V., Osborne, C. K., Levi, J. A., Wiernik, P. H., and Canellas, G. P.: Extranodal presentation of non-Hodgkin's lymphomas in the testis. *Cancer* 38:1026, 1976.

216. Narayan, O., Penney, J. B., Johnson, R. T., Herndon, R. M., and Weiner, L. P.: Etiology of progressive multifocal leukoencephalopathy. *N. Engl. J. Med.* 289:1278, 1973.

217. Minna, J. D., and Bunn, P. A.: Paraneoplastic syndromes, in *Principles and Practice of Oncology*, edited by V. T. DeVita, S. Hellman, and S. A. Rosenberg. Lippincott, Philadelphia, 1982, pp. 1476–1517.

218. Coggins, C. H.: Renal failure in lymphoma. *Kidney Int.* 17:847, 1980.

219. Richmond, J., Sherman, R. S., Diamond, H. D., and Craver, L. F.: Renal lesions associated with malignant lymphomas. *Am. J. Med.* 32:184, 1962.

220. Petzel, R. A., Brown, D. C., Staley, N. A., McMillen, J. J., Sibley, R. K., and Kjellstrand, C. M.: Cresentic glomerulonephritis and renal failure associated with malignant lymphoma. *Am. J. Clin. Pathol.* 71:728, 1979.

221. Burke, J. F., Flis, R., Lasker, N., and Simenhoff, M.: Malignant

lymphoma with "myeloma kidney" acute renal failure. *Am. J. Med.* 60:1055, 1976.

222. Paladugu, R. R., Bearman, R. M., and Rappaport, H.: Malignant lymphoma with primary manifestation in the gonad. *Cancer* 45:561, 1980.

223. Burke, J. F., Hoppe, R. T., Cibull, M. L., and Dorfman, R. F.: Cutaneous malignant lymphoma: A pathologic study of 50 cases with clinical analysis of 37. *Cancer* 47:300, 1981.

224. Manoharan, A., Pitney, W. R., Schonell, M. E., and Bader, L. V.: Intrathoracic manifestations in non-Hodgkin's lymphoma. *Thorax* 34:29, 1979.

225. Levitt, L. J., Ault, K. A., Pinkus, G. S., Sloss, L. J., and McManus, B. M.: Pericarditis and early cardiac tamponade as a primary manifestation of lymphosarcoma cell leukemia. *Am. J. Med.* 67:719, 1979.

226. Astarita, R. W., Minckler, D., Taylor, C. R., Levine, A., and Lukes, R. J.: Orbital and adnexal lymphomas: A multiparameter approach. *Am. J. Clin. Pathol.* 73:615, 1980.

227. Knowles, D. M., and Jakobiec, F. A.: Orbital lymphoid neoplasms, a clinicopathologic study of 60 patients. *Cancer* 46:576, 1980.

228. Colby, T. V., and Dorfman, R. F.: Malignant lymphomas involving the salivary glands. *Pathol. Ann. 14 (Part 2)*:307, 1979.

229. Burke, J. S., Butler, J. J., and Fuller, L. M.: Malignant lymphomas of the thyroid. *Cancer* 39:1587, 1977.

230. Bull, J. M., DeVita, V. T., and Carbone, P. P.: In vitro granulocyte production in patients with Hodgkin's disease and lymphocytic, histiocytic and mixed lymphomas. *Blood* 45:833, 1975.

231. Fliedner, V. V., Salvatori, V., Higby, D. J., Stuzman, L., and Park, B. H.: Polymorphonuclear neutrophil function in malignant lymphomas and effects of splenectomy. *Cancer* 45:469, 1980.

232. Jones, S. E., Griffin, K., Dombrowski, P., and Gaines, J. A.: Immunodeficiency in patients with non-Hodgkin lymphomas. *Blood* 49:335, 1977.

233. Ault, K. A.: Detection of small numbers of monoclonal B lymphocytes in the blood of patients with lymphoma. *N. Engl. J. Med.* 300:1401, 1979.

234. Ligler, F. S., et al.: Detection of tumor cells in the peripheral blood of nonleukemic patients with B cell lymphoma: Analysis of "clonal excess." *Blood* 55:792, 1980.

235. Come, S. E., et al.: Non-Hodgkin's lymphomas in leukemic phase: Clinicopathologic correlations. *Am. J. Med.* 69:667, 1980.

236. Schneider, R. J., et al.: Prognostic significance of serum lactate dehydrogenase in malignant lymphoma. *Cancer* 46:139, 1980.

237. Greaves, M., and Hancock, B W.: Hypercalcemia in malignant lymphoma. *Postgrad. Med. J.* 56:34, 1980.

238. Lichtenstein, A., and Taylor, C. R.: Serum immunoglobulin levels in patients with non-Hodgkin's lymphoma. *Am. J. Clin. Pathol.* 74:12, 1980.

239. Alexanian, R.: Monoclonal gammopathy in lymphomas. *Arch. Intern. Med.* 135:62, 1975.

240. Pizzolo, G., et al.: Differential diagnosis of malignant lymphoma and nonlymphoid tumor using monoclonal anti-leukocyte antibody. *Cancer* 46:2640, 1980.

241. Dorfman, R. F., and Warnke, R.: Lymphadenopathy simulating the malignant lymphomas. *Human Pathology* 5:519, 1974.

242. Butler, J. J.: Non-neoplastic lesions of lymph nodes of man to be differentiated from lymphomas. *Natl. Cancer Inst. Monogr.* 32:233, 1969.

243. Hossfeld, D. K., Hoffker, K., Schmitt, C. G., and Diedrichs, H.: Chromosome abnormalities in angioimmunoblastic lymphadenopathy. *Lancet* 1:198, 1976.

244. Rosai, J., and Dorfman, R. F.: Sinus histiocytosis with massive lymphadenopathy: A pseudolymphomatus benign disorder. *Cancer* 30:1174, 1972.

245. Anderson, L. G., and Talal, N.: The spectrum of benign to malignant lymphoproliferation in Sjögren's syndrome. *Clin. Exp. Immunol. 9;*199, 1971.

246. Wright, C. J. E.: Pseudolymphoma of the stomach. *Human Pathol.* 4:305, 1973.

247. Keller, A. R., Hochholzer, L., and Castleman, B.: Hyaline-vascular and plasma cell types of giant cell lymph node hyperplasia of the mediastinum and other locations. *Cancer* 29:670, 1972.

248. Liebow, A. A., Carrington, C. R. B., and Friedman, P. J.: Lymphomatoid granulomatosis. *Human Pathol.* 3:457, 1972.

249. Liebow, A. A.: Definition and classification of interstitial pneumonias in human pathology. *Prog. Resp. Res. 8:1*, 1975.

250. Valentino, L. A.: Lymphomatoid papulosis. *Arch. Pathol.* 96:409, 1973.

251. Brunning, R. O., Bloomfield, C. D., McKenna, R. W., and Peterson, L.: Bilateral trephine bone marrow biopsies in lymphoma and other neoplastic diseases. *Ann. Intern. Med.* 82:365, 1975.

252. Schechter, J. P., Jones, S. E., Woolfenden, J. M., Lilien, D. L., and O'Mara, R. E.: Bone scanning in lymphoma. *Cancer* 38:1142, 1976.

253. Chabner, B. A., Fisher, R. I., Young, R. C., and DeVita, V. T.: Staging of non-Hodgkin's lymphoma. *Semin. Oncol.* 7:285, 1980.

254. McCaffrey, J. A., Rudders, R. A., Kahn, P. C., Harvey, H. A., and DeLellis, R. A.: Clinical usefulness of ⁶⁷gallium scanning in the malignant lymphomas. *Am. J. Med.* 60:523, 1976.

255. Longo, D. L., Schilsky, R. L., Blei, L., Cano, R., Johnston, G. S., and Young, R. C.: Gallium⁶⁷ scanning: Limited usefulness in staging patients with non-Hodgkin's lymphoma. *Am. J. Med.* 68:695, 1980.

256. Best, J. J. K., et al.: Computed tomography of abdomen in staging and clinical management of lymphoma. *Br. Med. J. 2:1675*, 1978.

257. Hande, K. R., Fisher, R. I., DeVita, V. T., Chabner, B. A., and Young, R. C.: Diffuse histiocytic lymphoma involving the gastrointestinal tract. *Cancer* 41:1984, 1978.

258. Castellani, R., Bonadonna, G., Spinelli, P., Bajetta, E., Galante, E., and Rilke, F.: Sequential pathologic staging of untreated non-Hodgkin's lymphomas by laparoscopy and laparotomy combined with marrow biopsy. *Cancer* 40:2322, 1977.

259. Fuks, Z., and Kaplan, H. S.: Recurrence rates following radiation therapy of nodular and diffuse malignant lymphomas. *Radiology* 108:675, 1973.

260. Goffinet, D. R., Glatstein, E., Fuks, Z., and Kaplan, H. S.: Abdominal irradiation in non-Hodgkin's lymphoma. *Cancer* 37:2797, 1976.

261. Sweet, D. L., Kinzie, J., Gaeke, M. E., Golomb, H. M., Ferguson, D. L., and Ultmann, J. E.: Survival of patients with localized diffuse histiocytic lymphoma. *Blood* 58:1218, 1981.

262. Bush, R. S., Gospodarowicz, M., Sturgeon, J., and Alison, R.: Radiation therapy of localized non-Hodgkin's lymphoma. *Cancer Treat. Rep.* 61:1129, 1977.

263. Rosenberg, S. A.: Non-Hodgkin's lymphoma-selection of treatment on the basis of histologic type. *N. Engl. J. Med.* 301:924, 1979.

264. Cabanillas, F., Bodey, G. P., and Freireich, E. J.: Management with chemotherapy only of stage I and II malignant lymphoma of aggressive histologic types. *Cancer* 46:2356, 1980.

265. Carabell, S. C., Chaffey, J. T., Rosenthal, D. S., Moloney, W. C., and Hellman, S.: Results of total body irradiation in the treatment of advanced non-Hodgkin's lymphomas. *Cancer* 43:994, 1979.

266. Johnson, R. E.: Management of generalized malignant lymphomata with "systemic" radiotherapy. *Br. J. Cancer 31 (Suppl. II)*:450, 1975.

267. Glatstein, E., Fuks, Z., Goffinet, D. R., and Kaplan H. S.: Non-Hodgkin's lymphomas of stage III extent: Is total lymphoid irradiation appropriate treatment? *Cancer* 37:2806, 1976.

268. Cox, J. D., Komaki, R., Kun, L. E., Wilson, J. F., and Greenberg, M.: Stage III nodular lymphoreticular tumors (non-Hodgkin's lymphoma): Results of central lymphatic irradiation. *Cancer* 47:2247, 1981.

269. Chabner, B. A.: Nodular non-Hodgkin's lymphoma: The case for watchful waiting. *Ann. Intern. Med.* 90:115, 1979.

270. Portlock, C. S., and Rosenberg, S. A.: No initial therapy for stage III and IV non-Hodgkin's lymphomas of favorable histologic types. *Ann. Intern. Med.* 90:10, 1979.

271. Portlock, C. S.: Management of the indolent non-Hodgkin's lymphomas. *Semin. Oncol.* 7:292, 1980.

272. Portlock, C. S., and Rosenberg, S. A.: Chemotherapy of the non-Hodgkin's lymphomas: The Stanford experience. *Cancer Treat. Rep.* 61:1049, 1977.

273. Kennedy, B. J., Bloomfield, C. D., Kiang, D. T., Vosika, G., Peterson, B. A., and Theologides, A.: Combination versus successive single agent chemotherapy in lymphocytic lymphoma. *Cancer* 41:23, 1978.

274. Lister, T. A., et. al.: Comparison of combined and triple-agent che-

motherapy in non-Hodgkin's lymphoma of favorable histological type. *Br. Med. J.* 1:533, 1978.

275. Ezdinli, E. Z., Costello, W. G., Silverstein, M. N., Berard, C., Hartstock, R. J., and Sokal, J. E.: Moderate versus intensive chemotherapy of prognostically favorable non-Hodgkin's lymphoma. *Cancer* 46:29, 1980.

276. Canellos, G. P., DeVita, V. T., Young, R. C., Chabner, B. A., Schein, P. S., and Johnson, R. E.: Therapy of advanced lymphocytic lymphoma: A preliminary report of a randomized trial between combination chemotherapy (CVP) and intensive radiotherapy. *Br. J. Cancer 31 (Suppl. II)*:474, 1975.

277. Anderson, T., et al.: Combination chemotherapy in non-Hodgkin's lymphoma: Results of long-term follow-up. *Cancer Treat. Rep.* 61:1057, 1977.

278. Ezdinli, E. Z., et al.: Nodular mixed lymphocytic-histiocytic lymphoma (NM): Response and survival. *Cancer* 45:261, 1980.

279. Skarin, A. T., Rosenthal, D. S., Moloney, W. C., and Frei, E.: Combination chemotherapy of advanced non-Hodgkin lymphoma with bleomycin, Adriamycin, cyclophosphamide, vincristine, and prednisone (BACOP). *Blood* 49:759, 1977.

280. Jones, S. E., et al.: Superiority of Adriamycin-containing combination chemotherapy in the treatment of diffuse lymphoma. *Cancer* 43:417, 1979.

281. Rodriguez, V., et al.: Combination chemotherapy ("CHOP-BLEO") in advanced (non-Hodgkin) malignant lymphoma. *Blood* 49:325, 1977.

282. Stein, R. S., Moran, E. M., Desser, R. K., Miller, J. B., Golomb, H. M., and Ultmann, J. E.: Combination chemotherapy of lymphomas other than Hodgkin's disease. *Ann. Intern. Med.* 81:601, 1974.

283. Lenhard, R. E., et al.: Treatment of histocytic and mixed lymphomas: A comparison of two, three and four drug chemotherapy. *Cancer* 42:41, 1978.

284. McKelvey, E. M., et al.: Hydroxyldaunomycin (Adriamycin) combination chemotherapy in malignant lymphoma. *Cancer* 38:1484, 1976.

285. Laurence, J., Coleman, M., Allen, S. L., Silver, R. T., and Pasmantier, M.: Combination chemotherapy of advanced diffuse histiocytic lymphoma with the six drug COP-BLAM regimen. *Ann. Intern. Med.* 97:190, 1982.

286. DeVita, V. T., Chabner, B., Hubbard, S. P., Canellos, G. P., Schein, P., and Young, R. C.: Advanced diffuse histiocytic lymphoma, a potentially curable disease. *Lancet* 1:248, 1975.

287. Sweet, D. L., et al.: Cyclophosphamide, vincristine, methotrexate with leucovorin rescue, and Cytarabine (COMLA) combination sequential chemotherapy for advanced diffuse histiocytic lymphoma. *Ann. Intern. Med.* 92:785, 1980.

288. Schein, P. S., et al.: Bleomycin, Adriamycin, cyclophosphamide, vincristine, and prednisone (BACOP) combination chemotherapy in the treatment of advanced diffuse histiocytic lymphoma. *Ann. Intern. Med.* 85:417, 1976.

289. Bishop, J. F., Schimpff, S. C., Diggs, C. H., and Wiernik, P. H.: Infections during intensive chemotherapy for non-Hodgkin's lymphoma. *Ann. Intern. Med.* 95:549, 1981.

290. Ziegler, J. L.: Treatment results of 54 American patients with Burkitt's lymphoma are similar to the African experience. *N. Engl. J. Med.* 297:75, 1977.

291. Ziegler, J. L.: Management of Burkitt's lymphoma: An update. *Cancer Treat. Rev.* 6:95, 1979.

292. Voakes, J. B., Jones, S. E., and McKelvey, E. M.: The chemotherapy of lymphoblastic lymphoma. *Blood* 57:186, 1981.

293. Wollner, N., Wachtel, A. E., Exelby, P. R., and Centore, D.: Improved prognosis in children with intra-abdominal non-Hodgkin's lymphoma following LSA$_2$ L$_2$ protocol chemotherapy. *Cancer* 45:3034, 1980.

294. Weinstein, H. J., Vance, Z. B., Jaffe, N., Buell, D., Cassady, J. R., and Nathan, D. G.: Improved prognosis for patients with mediastinal lymphoblastic lymphoma. *Blood* 53:687, 1979.

295. Murphy, S. B.: Classification, staging and results of treatment of childhood non-Hodgkin's lymphomas: Dissimilarities from lymphomas in adults. *Semin. Oncol.* 7:332, 1980.

296. Skarin, A. T., et al.: High-dose methotrexate with follic acid in the treatment of advanced non-Hodgkin's lymphoma including CNS involvement. *Blood* 50:1039, 1977.

297. Cavalli, F., Jungi, W. F., Sonntag, R. W., Nissen, N. I., and Holland, J. F.: Phase II trial of cis-dichlorodiammineplatinum (II) in advanced malignant lymphoma and small cell lung cancer: Preliminary results. *Cancer Treat. Rep.* 63:1599, 1979.

298. Radice, P. A., Bunn, P. A., and Ihde, D. C.: Therapeutic trials with VP-16-213 and VM-26: Active agents in small cell lung cancer, non-Hodgkin's lymphomas, and other malignancies. *Cancer Treat. Rep.* 63:1231, 1979.

299. Seibert, K., Golub, G., Smiledge, P., and Nystrom, J. S.: Continuous streptozotocin infusion: A phase I study. *Cancer Treat. Rep.* 63:2035, 1979.

300. Grever, M. R., et al.: The biochemical and clinical consequences of 2-deoxycoformycin in refractory lymphoproliferative malignancy. *Blood* 57:406, 1981.

301. Ritz, J., and Schlossman, S. F.: Utilization of monoclonal antibodies in the treatment of leukemia and lymphoma. *Blood* 59:1, 1982.

302. Miller, R. A., Maloney, D. G., Waruke, R., and Levy, R.: Treatment of B-cell lymphoma with monoclonal anti-idiotype antibody. *N. Engl. J. Med.* 306:517, 1982.

303. Armitage, J. O., Corder, M. P., Leimert, J. T., Dick, F. R., and Elliot, T. E.: Advanced diffuse histiocytic lymphoma treated with cyclophosphamide, doxorubicin, vincristine, and prednisone (CHOP) without maintenance therapy. *Cancer Treat. Rep.* 64:649, 1980.

CHAPTER *120*

Cutaneous T-cell lymphomas (mycosis fungoides and Sézary syndrome)

PAUL A. BUNN, Jr.
BERNARD J. POIESZ

Definition and history

Mycosis fungoides and the Sézary syndrome are part of the spectrum of malignant T-cell lymphomas with a predilection for the skin (epidermis and upper dermis) [1–3]. The first case of mycosis fungoides was described by Alibert in 1806 [4], and by 1870 the three classical cutaneous stages were well described including (1) a premycotic, nonspecific erythematous or eczematoid stage; (2) an infiltrated plaque stage; and (3) a cutaneous tumor stage. Characteristically, lesions in individual patients evolved through each of these stages. Two additional cutaneous variants, d'emblée tumors, characterized by the *de novo* appearance of tumors in areas of clinically normal skin, and generalized erythroderma were described in the late 1800s. In 1938, Sézary described a group of patients in whom the generalized erythroderma was accompanied by abnormal mononuclear cells in the blood [5].

The malignant cells in both mycosis fungoides and the Sézary syndrome are mature, thymic-dependent (T) lymphocytes generally with helper-inducer phenotypes [6–12]. The malignant lymphocytes have striking convoluted or cerebriform nuclear contours and almost universally have nonspecific chromosomal abnormalities [13,14]. Recognition of these features led to an appreciation of the frequent and widespread extracutaneous manifestations of these disorders [2,15–18]. Since the malignant cells in mycosis fungoides and the Sézary syndrome have identical cytologic, surface membrane, functional, and cytogenetic characteristics, and the two disorders have overlapping and transitional clinical features, a common nomenclature termed *cutaneous T-cell lymphomas* has been proposed [1,19]. The exact clinical and biologic relationship between these and other T-cell disorders involving the skin, such as T-cell chronic lymphocytic leukemia, non-Hodgkin's T-cell lymphomas involving the skin, "nonepidermotrophic" cutaneous T-cell lymphoma, lymphomatoid granulomatosis, and lymphomatoid papulosis, is unresolved.

Etiology and pathogenesis

The cutaneous T-cell lymphomas are relatively uncommon, the age-adjusted incidence being two to three cases per million individuals in the United States [2]. Current estimates suggest there are 400 to 600 new cases and about 300 deaths per year in this country. Both the incidence and mortality appear to increase with age. The average age at diagnosis is 52 years, and onset before the age of 30 is uncommon. The disorders are more common in males than females and occur in all races.

The etiology is unknown but various environmental, genetic, and infectious factors have been implicated. There is a frequent history of exposure to toxic chemicals, physical agents, and drugs, and a higher-than-expected employment in plants manufacturing textiles, petrochemicals, metals, and machinery [20,21]. These observations are consistent with chronic immunologic stimulation leading to malignant transformation. There are reports of at least four families with more than one member having mycosis fungoides and numerous reports of families with mycosis fungoides in addition to other lymphomas and leukemias [20].

Virus-like particles have been reported in skin biopsies of patients with cutaneous T-cell lymphoma [22]. Further, a new retrovirus, human T-cell lymphoma-leukemia virus has been isolated from the fresh and cultured cells of two patients with cutaneous T-cell lymphoma [23,24]. Studies on the purified reverse transcriptase, core proteins, and nucleic acids indicate that this virus is novel and not endogenous to humans or animals [25,26]. The sera of some, but not all, tested patients with cutaneous T-cell lymphomas have been shown to have high-titer antibody against the structural proteins of this virus, while normals have been consistently negative [27]. A retrovirus capable of lymphocyte transformation has also been isolated from the cultured

lymphocytes of patients with adult T-cell leukemia, a disease of mature T-lymphocytes endemic in southern Japan [28–30]. All comparisons made, to date, suggest that this new isolate is related to human T-cell lymphoma-leukemia virus [31,32]. Close to 100 percent of adult T-cell leukemia patients in Japan have antibodies to human T-cell lymphoma-leukemia virus [33]. While an etiologic role for this virus is not certain, its independently established association with distinct mature T-lymphocyte neoplasias strongly suggests this is the case.

The malignant cells from some patients have been shown to possess (1) functional characteristics of a subset of normal mature lymphocytes including the ability to "help" in vitro immunoglobulin secretion and produce lymphokines, including migration inhibition factor and others, and (2) a characteristic phenotypic expression of membrane antigens similar to normal mature helper-inducer T lymphocytes as defined by monoclonal antibodies [6–12].

As is the case with normal lymphocytes, these neoplastic cells migrate through different body compartments [34]. Although cutaneous T-cell lymphoma cells are epidermotrophic, kinetic and cell-labeling studies indicate that the major region of cell replication is an extracutaneous site (most probably the lymph nodes) with minimal cell turnover occurring in the blood [34,35]. Whether the initial site of oncogenesis in cutaneous T-cell lymphoma is cutaneous or whether the skin acts as a homing organ for these mature neoplastic T-cell remains unresolved.

In culture, activated T lymphoblasts produce a protein of M_r 13,000 daltons termed *T-cell growth factor* or interleukin II which will potentiate the proliferation of mature T lymphocytes which have been stimulated by a mitogen or antigen [36]. Recently, it has been shown that neoplastic cells from some patients with cutaneous T-cell lymphoma will proliferate in response to this growth factor in the absence of prior activation by mitogen, and may become independent of it possibly because of its autonomous production by the tumor cells [37–39]. Unlike normal T lymphocytes, cutaneous T-cell-lymphoma cells subsequently were shown to have exposed T-cell growth factor receptors on their cell surface [39]. It is intriguing to speculate that cutaneous T-cell-lymphoma cells represent an aberrant proliferation secondary to constant stimulation by T-cell growth factor and, perhaps in some cases, by an autostimulatory secretion of it.

Clinical features

CUTANEOUS MANIFESTATIONS
The cutaneous appearance of early skin lesions varies widely, and they are often misdiagnosed as eczema, psoriasis, neurodermatitis, erythema, parapsoriasis-enplaque, poikiloderma, and other such diseases. Typically these early lesions are transitory in nature, and may be associated with or preceded by severe itching. These lesions last for months to years (average 6 years)

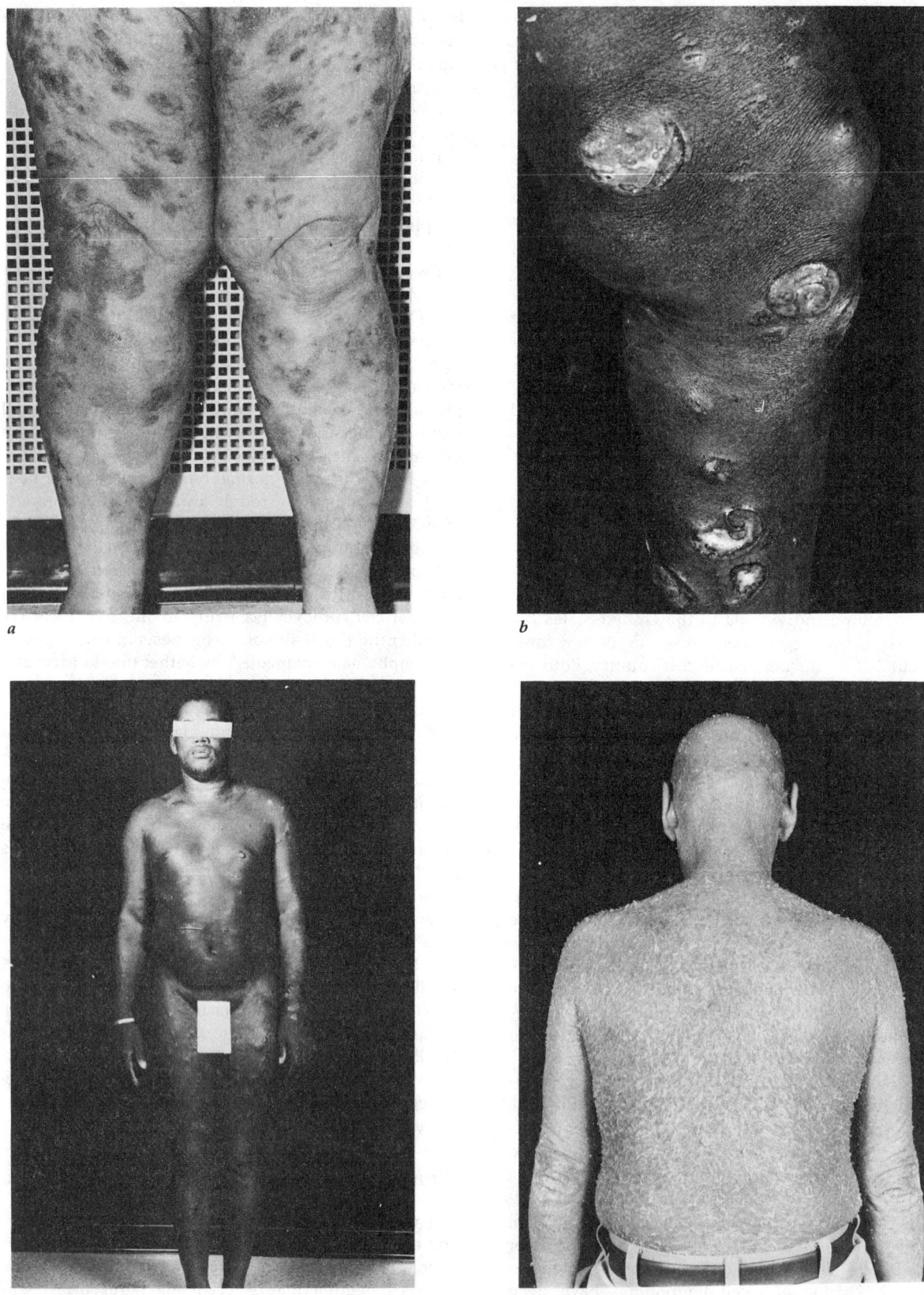

FIGURE 120-1 (*a*) Plaque-stage mycosis fungoides. (*b*) Cutaneous tumor-stage mycosis fungoides. (*c*) Cutaneous tumor d'emblée–stage mycosis fungoides. (*d*) Generalized exfoliative erythroderma (Sézary syndrome).

before becoming indurated plaques which are usually oval or circular with serpiginous, sharply demarcated margins. These plaques are usually more stable than premycotic lesions and gradually may increase in size or coalesce to form extensive lesions. It is useful prognostically to divide these patients into limited plaque stage (<10 percent of the body surface) and generalized plaque state (≥ 10 percent of the body surface) by the extent of skin involvement (see Fig. 120-1a).

Cutaneous tumors usually develop in areas of early skin lesions but may appear in normal skin (d'emblée) (see Fig. 120-1b and c). They occur anywhere but have a predeliction for the face (leonine facies) and body folds. They tend to become generalized and may grow slowly or rapidly. They are usually painless, but often ulcerate and become secondarily infected. Generalized erythroderma involves the majority of the skin surface although areas of seemingly normal skin may persist. It may follow or appear simultaneously with plaque or tumor lesions but most often precedes their development. Exfoliation, hyperkeratosis, alopecia, and ectropions are common (see Fig. 120-1d). Extreme itching is common, often leading to excoriation and exudation.

EXTRACUTANEOUS MANIFESTATIONS

In autopsy series, more than 70 percent of patients with mycosis fungoides have extracutaneous lesions involving nearly every organ system [15–18,40]. The most frequently involved organs in descending order include lymph nodes (61 percent); spleen (52 percent); liver (42 percent); lungs (42 percent); bone marrow (32 percent); gastrointestinal tract (31 percent); kidneys (28 percent); heart (21 percent); and central nervous system (18 percent). In general, patients with more advanced cutaneous disease had more extensive extracutaneous lymphoma, and visceral organs were rarely involved in the absence of lymph node infiltration.

Clinical manifestations of extracutaneous disease are less common than autopsy findings, but reflect widespread organ involvement [13]. Pulmonary lesions including parenchymal nodules, infiltrates, pleural ef-

fusions, and mediastinal and/or hilar adenopathy are reported most frequently. Involvement of the oral cavity and upper respiratory tract, liver, central nervous system, eyes, bones, cardiovascular system, gastrointestinal tract, kidneys, and marrow have been reported.

Extracutaneous disease is most frequently found in lymph nodes and the blood. Lymphadenopathy is present in about 45 percent of all patients with a frequency related to skin stage (17 percent of limited plaque, 44 percent of generalized plaques, 56 percent of cutaneous tumors, and 83 percent of generalized erythroderma) [2,3,15,18,40]. Lymphangiography has not proved to be a useful addition to other staging procedures [2]. Blood involvement is present in 15 to 20 percent of patients with plaque and tumors and over 90 percent of patients with generalized erythroderma by careful review of Wright-Giemsa–stained smears [2,3,15].

A series employing routine pretherapy staging procedures including standard radiographic and biopsy techniques but not laparotomy has demonstrated extracutaneous lymphoma in lymph nodes or blood in 50 percent of patients (100 percent with generalized erythroderma and 23 percent with plaques or tumors [2]). Involvement of viscera was less frequent in this series, with 18 percent of the patients having metastases in the liver and 2 percent in the marrow. When blood and lymph node specimens from the same patients were subjected to cytologic evaluation of T-cell preparations, electron microscopy, and chromosomal analysis, evidence for extracutaneous dissemination was found in 88 percent of patients [2]. These studies suggest that asymptomatic spread to many areas of the monocyte-macrophage system has occurred by the time a biopsy diagnosis is established.

A number of clinical and histologic staging systems have been used to describe the extent of disease. In 1979 the National Workshop on Cutaneous T-Cell Lymphoma adopted a clinical staging system shown in Table 120-1 which is now under study by a number of major institutions [19].

TABLE 120-1   National cutaneous T-Cell Lymphoma Workshop staging classification*

T	Skin	N	Lymph nodes	M	Visceral organs
T_1	Limited plaques (10% BSA)†	N_0	No adenopathy, histology negative	M_0	No involvement
T_2	Generalized plaques	N_1	Adenopathy, histology negative	M_1	Visceral involvement
T_3	Cutaneous tumors	N_2	No adenopathy, histology positive		
T_4	Generalized erythroderma	N_3	Adenopathy, histology positive		

Stage I	Limited (IA) or generalized plaques (IB) without adenopathy or histologic involvement of lymph nodes or viscera (T_1, N_0, M_0, or T_2, N_0, M_0)	
Stage II	Limited or generalized plaques with adenopathy (IIA) or cutaneous tumors with or without adenopathy (IIB); without histologic involvement of lymph nodes or viscera (T_{1-2}, N_1, M_0; T_3, N_{0-1}, M_0)	
Stage III	Generalized erythroderma with or without adenopathy; without histologic involvement of lymph nodes or viscera (T_4, N_{0-1}, M_0)	
Stage IV	Histologic involvement of lymph nodes (IVA) or viscera (IVB) with any skin lesion and with or without adenopathy (T_{1-4}, N_{2-3}, M_0 for IVA; T_{1-4}, N_{0-3}, M_1 for IVB)	

*Blood involvement should be recorded as absent (B_0) or present (B_1) but is not currently used to determine final stage.
†BSA = body surface area.

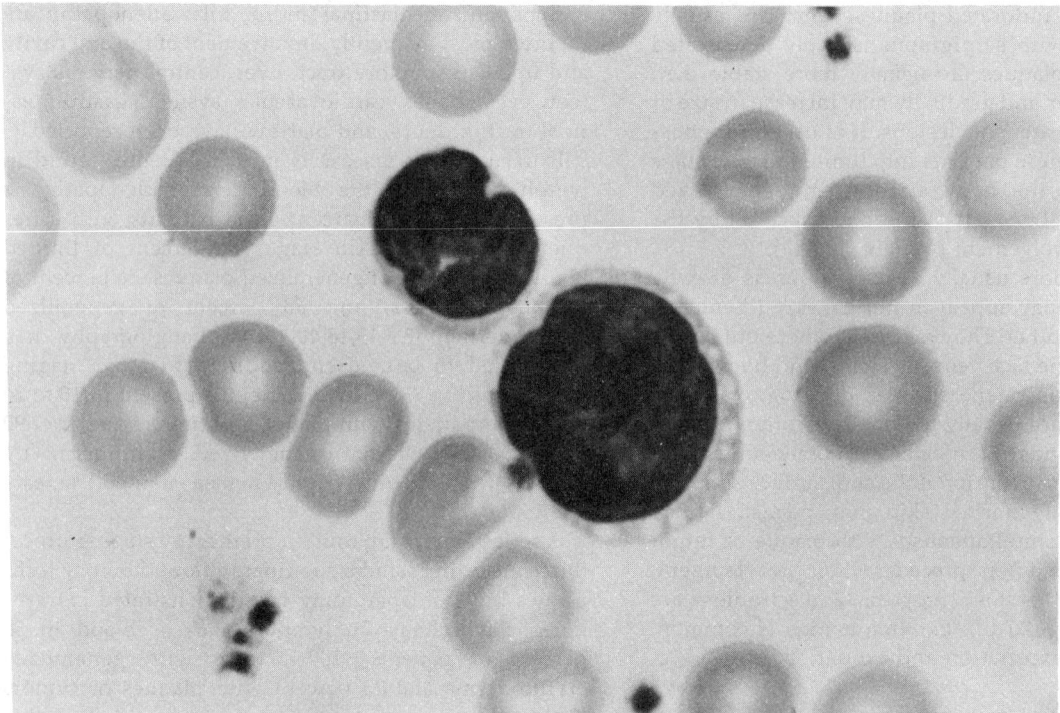

a

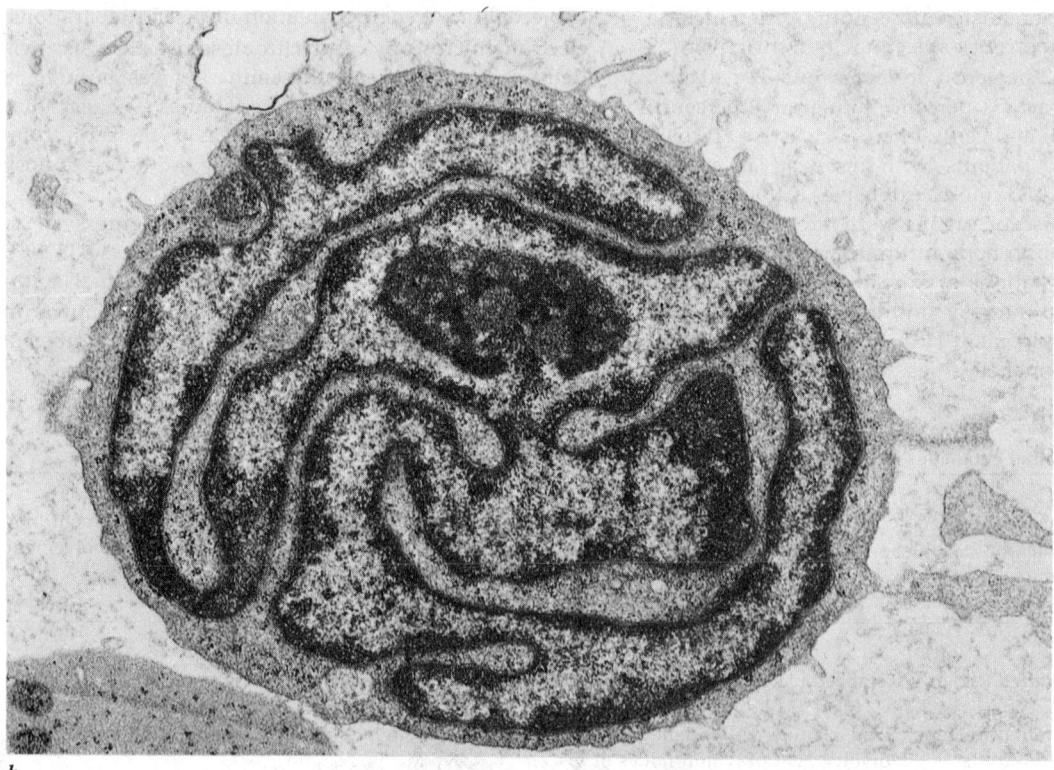

b

FIGURE 120-2   (*a*) Atypical small lymphocyte and atypical large lymphocyte with hyperchromatic, highly convoluted nuclei in the peripheral blood. (Wright-Giemsa, ×1000.) (Courtesy of G. P. Schechter, M.D.) (*b*) Electron micrograph of a markedly convoluted, cerebriform lymphocyte in the peripheral blood. (Uranyl acetate and lead citrate stain, ×6300.) (From Guccion et al. [42], with permission.)

Laboratory features

MYCOSIS/SÉZARY CELL IDENTIFICATION

Cytologic evaluation of blood, lymph nodes, and tumor aspirates The atypical malignant mycosis or Sézary cell varies widely in appearance but can be considered in three categories: (1) Atypical small lymphocyte (see Fig. 120-2): these cells are slightly larger than normal lymphocytes with scant, indistinct cytoplasm and hyperchromatic nuclei with markedly irregular nuclear membranes which may be folded and grooved. (2) Atypical large lymphoblasts (see Fig. 120-2): these cells are considerably larger than normal lymphocytes with scant cytoplasm with large vesicular or hyperchromatic nuclei which are highly convoluted or cerebriform. (3) Atypical blastic lymphocytes: in advanced stages the atypical lymphocytes may have a blastic appearance with large vesicular rounded nuclei and prominent nucleoli.

Ultrastructural appearance Classically Sézary cells have markedly convoluted (cerebriform or ribbonlike) nuclei (see Fig. 120-2*b*) [13]. The nuclear convolutions in the majority of cells are usually less striking and may be described as moderately convoluted. The nuclear contour index (ratio of nuclear perimeter to nuclear area) has been used by several groups to quantitate the degree of nuclear convolutions since convoluted lymphocytes may be seen in other conditions [33]. In general, marked degrees of convolutions with an index of more than 16, or clusters or high percentages (≥ 6 percent) of moderately convoluted cells with an index of more than 8 are highly suggestive of cutaneous T-cell lymphoma [2,41,42].

T-cell membrane properties The mycosis/Sézary cells almost universally have T-cell membrane properties demonstrated by binding polyclonal T-cell antibodies and mature blood T-cell monoclonal antibodies [1,9–12]. In most, but not all, instances the cells will also form spontaneous rosettes with sheep erythrocytes (E rosettes) and have surface antigens characteristic for the helper-inducer subset of T cells. Methods for separation of T cells can be useful in enriching mycosis/Sézary cells for cytologic and other investigations [2].

Other features The finding of aneuploidy by cytogenetic or DNA-content analysis [14,43], abnormal histochemistry (acid phosphatase– and β-glucuronidase–positive; periodic acid–Schiff–positive or –negative; peroxidase and chloracetate esterase–negative), and the absence of Ia antigen and terminal transferase may be useful in distinguishing cutaneous T-cell lymphoma from other conditions [10–12,37,38].

HISTOPATHOLOGY
SKIN BIOPSY
The most important and often most difficult task is to make an early histologic diagnosis of cutaneous T-cell lymphoma on skin biopsy. Since there is often disagreement in early cases, it is important to have skin biopsies reviewed by pathologists familiar with skin histopathology and to obtain multiple biopsies from various sites. Skin biopsies may need to be repeated at later dates in the case of suspicious lesions. Characteristically, the epidermis is infiltrated by mycosis/Sézary cells (exocytosis) either singly or in clusters called Pautrier's microabscesses, and may also show parakeratosis and acanthosis (see Fig. 120-3). The upper dermis contains a variably dense, often bandlike cellular infiltrate in close proximity to the epidermis. In early cases the infiltrate is usually polymorphic, containing lymphocytes, neutrophils, eosinophils, plasma and mast cells, and histiocytes. Atypical convoluted lymphocytes are invariably present in clusters. In more advanced and tumor stages the infiltrate often becomes more monomorphous, and extends deeper into the dermis. The term *nonepidermotrophic cutaneous T-cell lymphoma* has been applied by some investigators to cases with dense cellular infiltrates in the mid and lower dermis with relative sparing of the upper papillary dermis and epidermis [44]. These forms of cutaneous T-cell lymphoma should be distinguished from classic mycosis fungoides and Sézary syndrome until the distinctions between these and other lymphomas involving the skin are resolved.

LYMPH NODES
Histologic interpretation of lymph nodes is controversial. Most often nodal architecture is preserved and "dermatopathic" changes are present as illustrated in Fig. 120-4. The paracortical T-cell zones of these nodes invariably contain atypical convoluted lymphocytes. The density of these cells varies from a few scattered and clustered cells (see Fig. 120-4*a*) to large, dense clusters (Fig. 120-4*b*). Since some atypical convoluted lymphocytes may be seen in other conditions, only nodes with dense clusters are considered positive for cutaneous T-cell lymphoma. In a minority of cases, the nodal architecture is effaced by a relatively monomorphic accumulation of malignant lymphocytes as shown in Fig. 120-4*c*.

OTHER LABORATORY FEATURES
Elevated levels of serum lactic acid dehydrogenase, serum IgE, and eosinophils are frequently found. Delayed hypersensitivity reactions to skin test antigens are usually normal in early stages but become depressed in advanced stages. Mitogenic responses of mycosis/Sézary cells are usually depressed compared to normal lymphocytes [45].

Therapy

There are four well-established therapeutic modalities which will produce at least partial clearing of lesions in the majority of patients. These include (1) topical chemotherapy with mechlorethamine (nitrogen mustard);

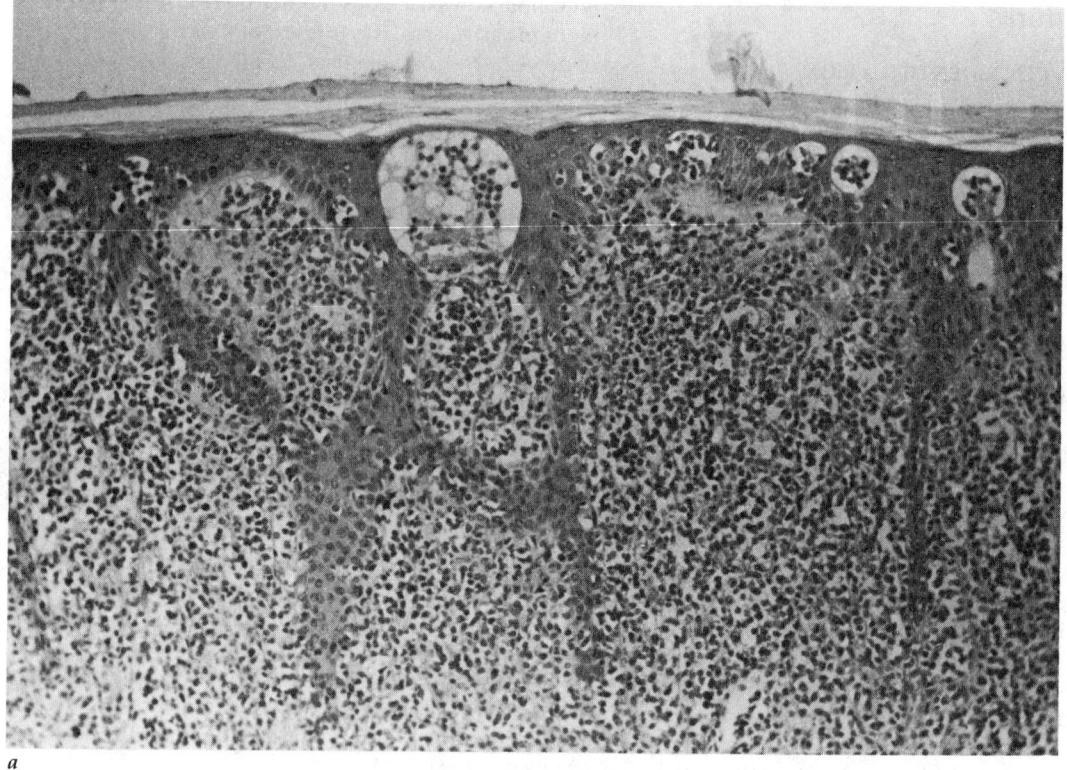

a

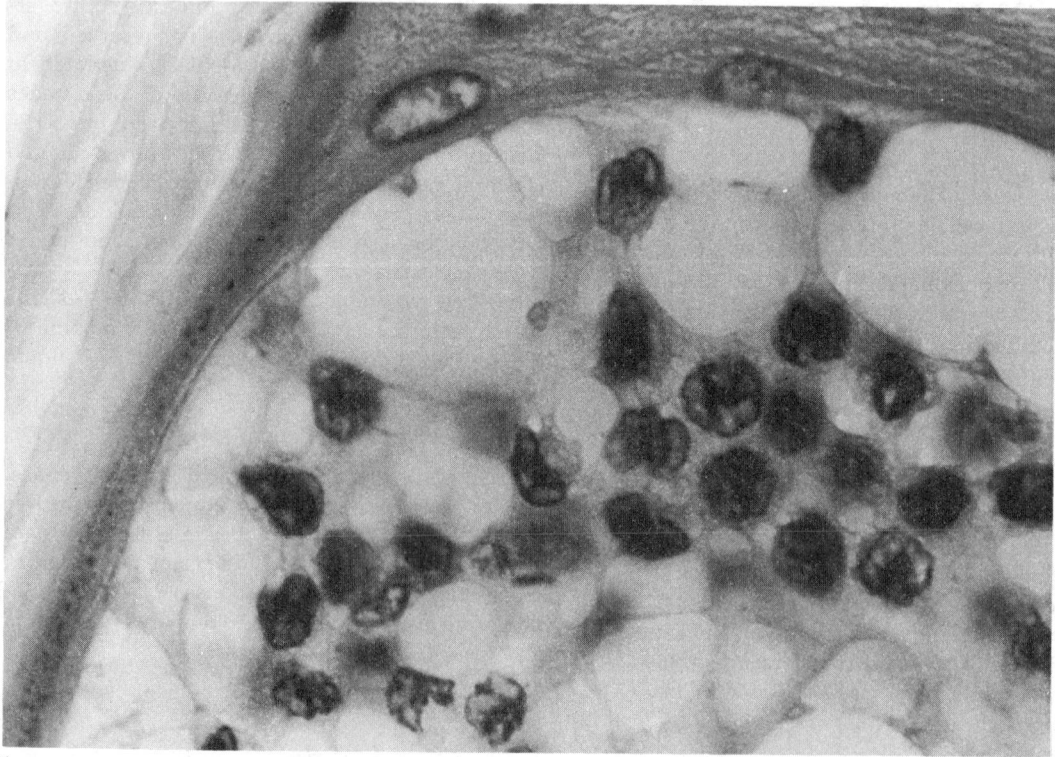

b

FIGURE 120-3   (a and b) Skin biopsy at different powers of magnification showing an infiltrate containing atypical convoluted lymphocytes in the upper dermis and intraepidermal Pautrier abscesses. (Courtesy E. J. Van Scott, M.D.)

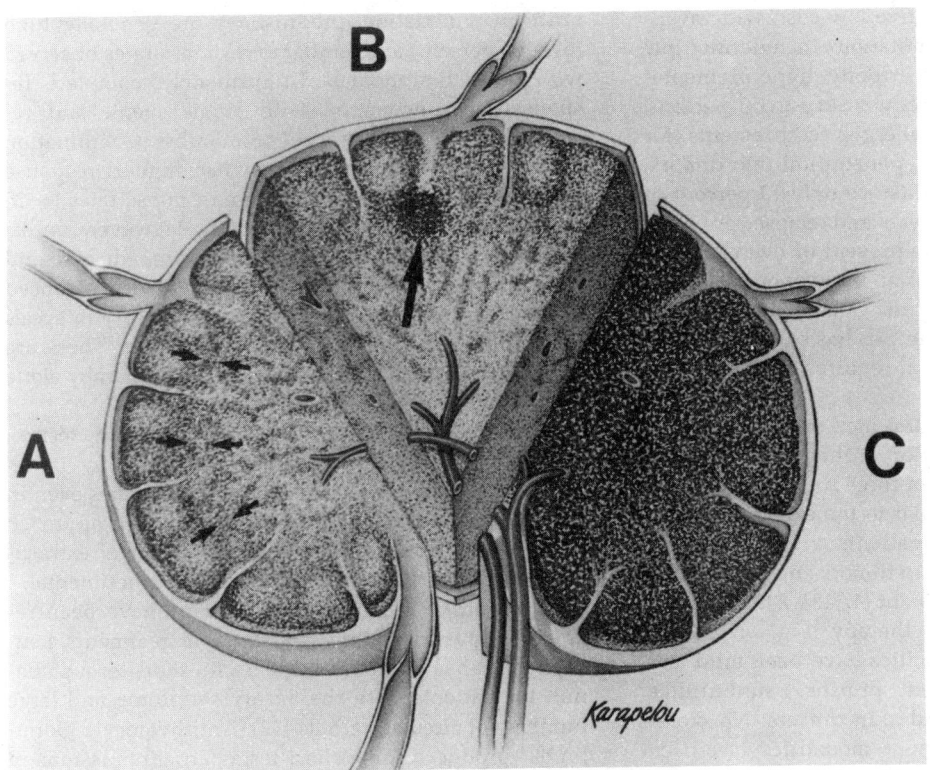

FIGURE 120-4 Schematic of lymph node involvement. In the left third (A) early dermatopathic changes are shown with accumulations of melanin from the inflamed skin, preservation of nodal architecture, and small numbers of atypical convoluted lymphocytes. In the middle third (B) there are focal accumulations of neoplastic atypical convoluted lymphocytes in the paracortical areas (*large arrow*), while nodal architecture is preserved. In the right third (C), a homogeneous accumulation of malignant T cells has replaced the normal lymphoid architecture. (From Edelson [44], with permission.)

(2) photochemotherapy with psoralen and ultraviolet A light; (3) whole-body electron beam irradiation; and (4) systemic chemotherapy. Unfortunately, each of these therapies has major limitations and despite their widespread use nearly all patients still succumb to their underlying lymphoma or its complications. Results reported with these agents alone or in combination are shown in Table 120-2.

Topical mechlorethamine (HN$_2$) applied to the whole body daily for prolonged periods produces complete clearing of skin lesions in the majority of patients with plaque lesions and a minority of patients with tumors or generalized erythroderma (64 percent overall) [46–48]. The therapy consists of 10 mg of HN$_2$ dissolved in 50 ml of water applied daily for 6 to 12 months. Responding patients may be able to reduce the frequency of administration gradually and then discontinue applications after 2 to 3 years [46]. Advantages are the relative

TABLE 120-2 Results of various treatment modalities in cutaneous T-cell lymphoma

Treatment	No. of patients	Percent complete remission	Median response duration, months	Percent 3 year disease free	Estimated median survival, years
Topical HN$_2$	253	64	18†	13	8
EBRT	140	84	16	20	9
PUVA	91	62	Not reported	Too early	Too early
COMB CT	68*	25	8	0	Not reported
EBRT + CT	62†	60	Too early	Too early	Too early

*All with advanced stages.
†Majority with advanced stages.
NOTES: HN$_2$ = mechlorethamine (nitrogen mustard); EBRT = whole-body electron beam irradiation; PUVA = photochemotherapy with psoralen plus ultraviolet A light; CT = chemotherapy; COMB = combination.

lack of systemic toxicity, relative low cost, wide availability, and effectiveness. Limitations include multiple cutaneous toxicities (dryness, atrophy, hyperpigmentation, second skin tumors); frequent (up to 50 percent) development of cutaneous allergy; requirements for daily application; lack of deep penetration into tumors; and lack of curative potential (since only 13 percent of patients are relapse free at 3 years and relapse continues after this period). Attempts to prevent or overcome the allergic reactions with topical or intravenous desensitization have had limited success. Cutaneous hypersensitivity to HN_2 and other chemicals has been associated with an antitumor effect which requires further definition.

Photochemotherapy with oral methoxsalen followed by ultraviolet A light irradiation of the entire skin surface (PUVA) is generally given three times weekly during an induction phase. Similar to the experience with topical HN_2 the majority of patients with plaques are responsive, while patients with tumors and generalized erythroderma tend to be resistant [47,48]. After clearing of skin lesions maintenance therapy is given indefinitely every few weeks. Toxicities have been mild and include nausea, generalized pruritis, sunburnlike changes, atrophy, and second skin cancers. No cross-resistance with other treatment modalities has been reported [47]. Data regarding long-term toxicities are not yet available. However, PUVA dose require prolonged visits to a center having the appropriate facilities, fails to treat deep lesions, and is associated with a high frequency of relapse.

Electron beam irradiation with 3 to 4 MeV electrons can be applied to the entire skin surface since the total depth of penetration will be less than 1 cm [3,48–50]. Responsiveness correlates with the total dose administered and with the type of cutaneous disease. It has been reported that doses in excess of 3000 rads produce complete clearing of skin lesions in 84 percent of patients including nearly all patients with plaques and some patients with tumors or generalized erythroderma (see Table 120-2). In contrast to other modalities, maintenance therapy is not given. The majority of patients relapse within 3 years of treatment but as many as one-third of patients with plaques but without adenopathy will have long, unmaintained disease-free periods [49,50]. Electron beam irradiation is expensive, requires considerable expertise in physics for proper delivery and may cause radiodermatitis, atrophy, alopecia, second skin cancers, edema, loss of sweat glands, and gynecomastia. It should only be undertaken by a facility with the appropriate technical, dosimetric, and physics support and experience. Nonetheless, it is the only single modality reported to produce long-term (>5-year) disease-free remissions.

Systemic chemotherapy has generally been reserved for patients with advanced disease stages [3,18,47,48]. Response rates to single-agent chemotherapy, including standard alkylating agents (cyclophosphamide), antimetabolities (methotrexate), and other agents (dox-

orubicin, vincristine, prednisone), are generally high (over 60 percent) and similar to response rates observed with other lymphomas. Unfortunately, complete responses are uncommon with single agents and responses are generally short (<6 months). Combination chemotherapy produces somewhat higher response rates (~ 80 percent) and complete response rates (~ 25 percent) of slightly longer duration. However, unlike some other lymphomas such as Hodgkin's disease and diffuse histiocytic lymphoma, no patient with advanced disease has had long disease-free (>3-year) intervals following combination chemotherapy alone. There are no reports employing combination chemotherapy alone in early stages.

Combined modality therapy employing both electron beam irradiation and systemic chemotherapy is reported to produce high complete response rates even in patients with advanced disease [3,47,51]. This approach is appealing because of the high frequency of extracutaneous disease but must be regarded as experimental.

Other forms of experimental therapy have been reported for patients failing conventional treatments. Leukapheresis has produced some useful short-term palliation for patients with the Sézary syndrome and large numbers of circulating cells [52]. Antithymocyte globulin has produced some short-term partial remissions in both mycosis fungoides and Sézary syndrome [53]. More recently, responses have been reported from anti-T-cell monoclonal antibodies.

Course and prognosis

The clinical course of individual patients is highly variable but is related to several well-documented prognostic features. Overall survival is shorter than for age-matched controls, and all patients suffer progressive clinical deterioration [18,40]. The interval from first onset of symptoms to biopsy confirmation ranges from several months to two decades or more with an average of 4 to 5 years [18,40]. After the diagnosis is established, median survival is about 8 to 9 years [40,46,50,54]. Infection, particularly with *Staphylococcus aureus* and secondary gram-negative bacteria arising from areas of advanced cutaneous disease occurs frequently, requires prompt antibiotic therapy, and may account for 25 to 50 percent of all deaths [18,40,55]. In recent years, with better therapeutic measures to control skin lesions, progressive lymphoma has become the major cause of death. Since many patients are elderly and long survival is common, deaths due to conditions unrelated to cutaneous T-cell lymphoma (CTCL) are also common.

The most important prognostic factor is the extent or stage of disease, which is determined by evaluation of skin, lymph nodes, blood, and visceral organs. Patients with generalized erythroderma and cutaneous tumors have a worse prognosis than those with plaques; with median survivals of 3 to 4 years compared to more than 8 years [2,3,15,18,46,49,50,54]. Patients with plaques involving less than 10 percent of their body surface (limited plaque stage) respond to therapy more often and live longer than patients with generalized plaques. Patients with blood involvement (median survival 2½ years) have a worse prognosis than those without this finding [2]. Many series have shown that patients with lymphadenopathy have a shorter survival than those without adenopathy irrespective of the type of therapy employed [2,3,15,18,40,46,49,54]. The data on lymph node histology are less certain. Reports from most series suggest that patients with enlarged nodes have a much worse prognosis than patients with lesser or absent lymph node infiltration. Some investigators have found that patients with dermatopathic nodes containing large dense clusters of mycosis/Sézary cells, as in Fig. 120-4b, and nodes with large mycosis/Sézary cells have a worse prognosis than those with lesser degrees of infiltration [2,56].

Clinically apparent visceral organ involvement is associated with a short median survival (6 to 8 months) [18]. If visceral involvement is asymptomatic and discovered during routine pretreatment staging, median survival (1 to 2 years) is somewhat longer, but these patients have a worse prognosis than similarly staged patients with less advanced disease [2].

Age, absolute lymphocyte count, and systemic symptoms (including malaise) have been reported to have prognostic importance, but are not well-established prognostic factors [40,49,54].

References

1. Lutzner, M. A., Edelson, R. L., Schein, P. S., Green, I., Kirkpatrick, C., and Ahmed, A. T.: Cutaneous T-cell lymphomas: The Sézary syndrome, mycosis fungoides, and related disorders. *Ann. Intern. Med.* 83:534, 1975.
2. Bunn, P. A., et al.: Prospective staging evaluation of patients with cutaneous T-cell lymphomas. *Ann. Intern. Med.* 93:223, 1980.
3. Broder, S., and Bunn, P. A.: Cutaneous T-cell lymphomas. *Semin. Oncol.* 7:310, 1980.
4. Ailbert, J. L.: *Déscription des maladies de la peau.* Paris, Barrois, 1806, p. 157.
5. Sézary, A., and Bouvain, Y.: Erythrodermie avec présence de cellules monstreuses dans le derme et dans le sang circulant. *Bull. Soc. Fr. Dermatol. Syph.* 45:254, 1938.
6. Crossen, P. E., Mellor, J. E. L., Finley, A. G., Ravich, R. B. M., Vincent, P. C., and Gunz, F. W.: The Sézary syndrome: Cytogenic studies and identification of the Sézary cell as an abnormal lymphocyte. *Am. J. Med.* 50:24, 1971.
7. Broome, J. D., Zucker-Franklin, D., Weiner, M. S., and Nussenzweig, V.: Leukemic cells with membrane properties of thymus-derived (T) lymphocytes in a case of Sézary's syndrome: Morphologic and immunologic studies. *Clin. Immunol. Immunopathol.* 1:319, 1973.
8. Brouet, J. C., Flandrin, G., and Seligmann, M.: Indications of the thymus-derived nature of the proliferating cells in six patients with Sézary's syndrome. *N. Engl. J. Med.* 289:341, 1973.
9. Broder, S., et al.: The Sézary syndrome: A malignant proliferation of helper T-cells. *J. Clin. Invest.* 58:1297, 1976.
10. Haynes, B. F., Metzgar, R. S., Minna, J. D., and Bunn, P. A.: Clonal origin of cutaneous T-cell lymphomas. Phenotypic comparison with other malignant T-cells using monoclonal antibodies. *N. Engl. J. Med.* 304:1319, 1981.
11. Kung, P. C., Berger, C. L., Goldstein, G., LoGerfo, P., and Edelsen, R. L.: Cutaneous T-cell lymphomas: Characterization by monoclonal antibodies. *Blood* 57:261, 1981.
12. Boumsell, L., et al.: Surface antigens on malignant Sézary and T-CLL cells correspond to those of mature T cells. *Blood* 57:526, 1981.
13. Lutzner, M. A., and Jordan, H. W.: The ultrastructural appearance of an abnormal cell in Sézary's syndrome. *Blood* 31:719, 1968.
14. Whang-Peng, J., et al.: Cytogenic abnormalities in patients with cutaneous T-cell lymphomas. *Cancer Treat. Rep.* 63:575, 1979.
15. Carney, D. N., and Bunn, P. A.: Manifestations of cutaneous T-cell lymphoma. *J. Dermatol. Surg. Oncol.* 6:369, 1980.
16. Long, J. C., and Mihm, M. C.: Mycosis fungoides with extracutaneous T-cell lymphomas. *Cancer Treat. Rep.* 63:575, 1979. 34:1745, 1974.
17. Rappaport, H., and Thomas, L. B.: Mycosis fungoides: The pathology of extracutaneous involvement. *Cancer* 34:1198, 1974.
18. Levi, J. A., and Wiernik, P. H.: Management of mycosis fungoides—Current status and future prospects. *Medicine (Baltimore)* 54:73, 1975.
19. Bunn, P. A., and Lamberg, S. I.: Report of the Committee on Staging and Classification of Cutaneous T-cell Lymphomas. *Cancer Treat. Rep.* 63:725, 1979.
20. Greene, M. H., Dalager, N. A., Lamberg, S. I., Argyropoulos, C., and Fraumeni, J. F.: Mycosis fungoides: Epidemiology observations. *Cancer Treat. Rep.* 62:597, 1979.
21. Fischmann, A. B., Bunn, P. A., Guccion, J. G., Matthews, M. S., and Minna, J. D.: Exposure to chemicals, physical agents, and biologic agents in mycosis fungoides and the Sézary syndrome. *Cancer Treat. Rep.* 63:591, 1979.
22. Van der Loo, E. M., van Muijen, G. N. P., van Vloten, W. A., Beens, W., Scheffer, E., and Meijer, C. L. M.: C-type virus-like particles specifically localized in Langerhans cells and related cells of skin and lymph nodes of patients with mycosis fungoides and Sézary syndrome. *Virchows Arch. B Cell Pathol.* 31:193, 1979.
23. Poiesz, B. J., Ruscetti, F. M., Gazdar, A. F., Bunn, P. A., Minna, J. D., and Gallo, R. C.: Detection and isolation of type c retrovirus particles from fresh and cultured lymphocytes of a patient with cutaneous T-cell lymphoma. *Proc. Natl. Acad. Sci. U.S.A.* 77:7415, 1980.
24. Poiesz, B. J., Ruscetti, F. W., Reitz, M. S., Kalyanaraman, V. S., and Gallo, R. C.: Evidence for nucleic acids and antigens for a new type-C retrovirus (HTLV) in primary uncultured cells of a patient with Sézary T-cell leukemia and isolation of the virus. *Nature* 294:268, 1981.
25. Rho, H., Poiesz, B. J., Ruscetti, F. W., and Gallo, R. C.: Characterization of the reverse transcriptase from a new retrovirus (HTLV) produced by a human cutaneous T-cell lymphoma cell line. *Virology* 112:355, 1981.
26. Reitz, M. S., Poiesz, B. J., Ruscetti, F. W., and Gallo, R. C.: Characterization and distribution of nuclei acid sequences of a novel type-C retrovirus isolated from neoplastic human T-lymphocytes. *Proc. Natl. Acad. Sci. U.S.A.* 78:1887, 1981.
27. Posner, L., et al.: Naturally occurring antibodies against human T-cell lymphoma-leukemia virus (HTLV) in patients with cutaneous T-cell lymphomas. *J. Exp. Med.* 154:333, 1981.
28. Yosida, M., Miyoshi, I., Hinuma, Y.: Isolation and characterization of retrovirus from cell lines of human adult T-cell leukemia and its implication in the disease. *Proc. Natl. Acad. Sci. U.S.A.* 79:2031, 1982.
29. Hinuma, Y., et al.: Adult T-cell leukemia; antigen in an ATL cell line and detection of antibodies to the antigen in human sera. *Proc. Natl. Acad. Sci. U.S.A.* 78:6476, 1981.
30. Miyoshi, I., et al.: Type-C virus particles in a cord T-cell line derived by co-cultivating normal human cord leukocytes and human leukemic T-cells. *Nature* 294:770, 1981.
31. Weiss, R.: A virus associated with human adult T-cell leukemia. *Nature* 294:212, 1981.
32. Lewin, R.: New reports of a human leukemia virus. *Science* 244:530, 1981.
33. Robert-Guroff, M., Nakao, Y., Notake, K., Ito, Y., Slick, A., and Gallo, R.: Natural antibodies to human retrivirus HTLV in a cluster of Japanese patients with adult T-cell leukemia. *Science* 215:975, 1982.
34. Miller, R. A., Coleman, C. N., Fawcett, H. D., Hoppe, R. T., and Mc-

Dougall, I. R.: Sézary syndrome: A model for migration of T-lymphocytes to skin. *N. Engl. J. Med. 303:*89, 1980.

35. Bunn, P. A., Edelson, R., Ford, S. S., and Shackney, S. E.: Patterns of cell proliferation and cell migration in the Sézary syndrome. *Blood 57:*452, 1981.

36. Ruscetti, F. W., and Gallo, R. C.: Human T-lymphocyte growth factor: Regulation of growth and function of T-lymphocytes. *Blood 57:*379, 1981.

37. Gazdar, A. F., et al.: Mitogen requirement for the in vitro propagation of cutaneous T-cell lymphomas. *Blood 55:*409, 1980.

38. Poiesz, B. J., Ruscetti, F. W., Mier, J. W., Woods, A. W., and Gallo, R. C.: T-cell lines established from human T-lymphocytic neoplasias by direct response to T-cell growth factor. *Proc. Natl. Acad. Sci. U.S.A. 77:*6815, 1980.

39. Gootenberg, J. E., Ruscetti, F. W., Mier, J. W., Gazdar, A., and Gallo, R. C.: Human cutaneous T-cell lymphoma and leukemia cell lines produce and respond to T-cell growth factor. *J. Exp. Med. 154:*1403, 1981.

40. Epstein, E. M., Levin, D. L., Croft, J. D., Jr., and Lutzner, M. A.: Mycosis fungoides: Survival, prognostic features, response to therapy, and autopsy findings. *Medicine (Baltimore) 51:*61, 1972.

41. McNutt, N. S., and Crain, W. R.: Quantitative electron microscopic comparison of lymphocyte nuclear contours in mycosis fungoides and in benign infiltrates in skin. *Cancer 47:*698, 1981.

42. Guccion, J. G., Fischmann, A. B., Bunn, P. A., Schechter, G. P., Patterson, R. H., and Matthews, M. J.: Ultrastructural appearance of cutaneous T cell lymphomas in skin, lymph nodes, and peripheral blood. *Cancer Treat. Rep. 63:*565, 1979.

43. Bunn, P. A., Whang-Peng, J., Carney, D. N., Schlam, M. L., Knutsen, T., and Gazdar, A. F.: Correlation of DNA content analysis by flow cytometry and cytogenetic analysis in mycosis fungoides and the Sézary syndrome. *J. Clin. Invest. 65:*1440, 1980.

44. Edelson, R. L.: Cutaneous T-cell lymphoma. *J. Dermatol. Surg. Oncol. 6:*358, 1980.

45. Carney, D. N., Bunn, P. A., Schechter, G. P., and Gazdar, A. F.: Mitogen responses and flow microfluorometry (FMF) of circulating cells in the Sézary syndrome. *Int. J. Cancer 26:*535, 1980.

46. Vonderheid, E. C., Van Scott, E. J., Wallner, P. E., and Johnson, W. C.: A 10-year experience with topical mechlorethamine for mycosis fungoides; comparison with patients treated by total-skin electron-beam radiation therapy. *Cancer Treat. Rep. 63:*691, 1979.

47. Bunn, P. A., and Carney, D. N.: Treatment of cutaneous T-cell lymphoma. *J. Dermatol. Surg. Oncol. 6:*383, 1980.

48. Minna, J. D., Roenigk, H. H., Jr., and Glatstein, E.: Report of the committee on therapy for mycosis fungoides and Sézary syndrome. *Cancer Treat. Rep. 63:*729, 1979.

49. Fuks, Z. Y., Bagshaw, M. A., and Farber, E. M.: Prognostic signs and the management of the mycosis fungoides. *Cancer 32:*1385, 1973.

50. Hoppe, R. T., Cox, R. S., Fuks, Z., Price, N. M., Bagshaw, M. A., and Farber, E. M.: Electronbeam therapy for mycosis fungoides: The Stanford University experience. *Cancer Treat. Rep. 63:*691, 1979.

51. Griem, M. L., Tokars, R. P., Petras, V., Variakojis, D., Baron, J. M., and Griem, S. F.: Combined therapy for patients with mycosis fungoides. *Cancer Treat. Rep. 63:*655, 1979.

52. Edelson, R. L., Rafat, J., Berger, C. L., Grossman, M., Groyer, C., and Hardy, M.: Antithymocyte globulin in the management of cutaneous T-cell lymphoma. *Cancer Treat. Rep. 63:*675, 1979.

53. Edelson, R., Facktor, M., Andrews, A., Lutzner, M., and Schein, P.: Successful management of the Sézary syndrome. Mobilization and removal of extravascular neoplastic cells by leukapheresis. *N. Engl. J. Med. 291:*293, 1974.

54. Lamberg, S. I., et al.: Status report of 376 mycosis fungoides patients at 4 years: Mycosis Fungoides Cooperative Group. *Cancer Treat. Rep. 63:*701, 1979.

55. Posner, L. E., Fossieck, B. E., Eddy, J. L., and Bunn, P. A., Jr.: Septicemic complications of the cutaneous T-cell lymphomas. *Am. J. Med. 71:*210, 1981.

56. Scheffer, G., Meyer, C. J. L., and Van Vloten, W. A.: Dermatopathic lymphadenopathy and lymph node involvement in mycosis fungoides. *Cancer 45:*137, 1980.

Lymphocytic disorders — malignant proliferative response and/or abnormal immunoglobulin synthesis — plasma cell dyscrasias

CHAPTER *121*

Plasma cell neoplasms—general considerations

DANIEL E. BERGSAGEL

Definition

Neoplasms derived from plasma cells or immunoglobulin-producing lymphocytes arise when a cell of the B-lymphocyte lineage undergoes malignant transformation and proliferates to form a clone of abnormal cells. Malignant diseases of this type may be recognized clinically as a lymphocytic or plasma cell tumor, the appearance of circulating lymphoplasmacytic cells in the blood, or a monoclonal immunoglobulin or immunoglobulin fragment in the serum or urine. Two patterns of disease evolution have been recognized: The neoplastic clone may grow in an unrestrained manner to produce systemic disease and often death of the host, as in plasma cell myeloma, Waldenström's macroglobulinemia, and some types of heavy-chain disease. In another entity, benign monoclonal gammopathy, the clone of abnormal cells may expand for a period of time and then become stable or controlled for several years or indefinitely. In rare instances the clone may regress either spontaneously or after treatment with antibiotics, as is the case with α-heavy-chain disease.

Immunoglobulin-producing neoplasms

Many lymphoproliferative diseases are derived from B lymphocytes, and a scheme of B-lymphocyte development is presented in Fig. 121-1 [1]. Lymphocyte progenitors proliferate in their microenvironments and may be exposed to oncogenic factors before or after they develop the capacity to synthesize immunoglobulin. The differentiation of B lymphocytes from lymphoid stem cells is marked by the appearance of membrane-bound immunoglobulin and later by the secretion of immunoglobulin. Cells with membrane-bound IgM and IgD are the least mature, while those with large amounts of surface IgG or IgA are more mature B-lymphocyte derivatives that have been activated by antigen. Plasma cells are the most mature cells in the series and are fully differentiated. As they acquire the ability to produce and secrete immunoglobulin, they lose most of their membrane-bound immunoglobulin.

The immunoproliferative diseases of B-lymphocyte derivation can be classified on the basis of morphology, proliferative activity, and level of differentiation, using such characteristics as C3 receptors, membrane-bound immunoglobulin, and secreted immunoglobulin [1–11] (Table 107-1). In chronic lymphocytic leukemia, for example, the leukemic cells have been identified, in most instances, as B-lymphocyte derivatives [2–7] (see Chap. 115). They are almost always monoclonal in origin, with the membrane immunoglobulin restricted to a single light- and heavy-chain class [3,5,12–14]. IgM has been the most prevalent class of immunoglobulin [6,7], often in association with IgD. In some instances, chronic lymphocytic leukemia lymphocytes secrete monoclonal IgG but have IgA on the cell surface [13]. The same monoclonal immunoglobulin may occasionally be found in the serum and on the cell surface. In several patients, the surface immunoglobulin obtained from leukemic lymphocytes has had antibody activity [13].

CHRONIC LYMPHOCYTIC LEUKEMIA (CLL)
In the usual form of CLL without a serum monoclonal immunoglobulin component, the density of the surface immunoglobulin on the B lymphocyte is much less than on normal B lymphocytes or on the lymphocytes in Waldenström's macroglobulinemia. In a given patient, the fluorescence or radioimmunolabeling pattern is strikingly uniform [4,5,15,16].

BURKITT'S LYMPHOMA
Studies of fresh biopsy specimens of patients with Burkitt's lymphoma have frequently shown several immunoglobulins, usually IgM and IgG, on the cell surfaces [17]. When tissue culture lines of Burkitt's lymphoma were developed, it was found that the membrane-associated IgG gradually disappeared [18] and was predominately antibody to an antigen (probably viral-associated) of the Burkitt lymphoma cell [19]. The membrane IgM persisted for many months in cell cul-

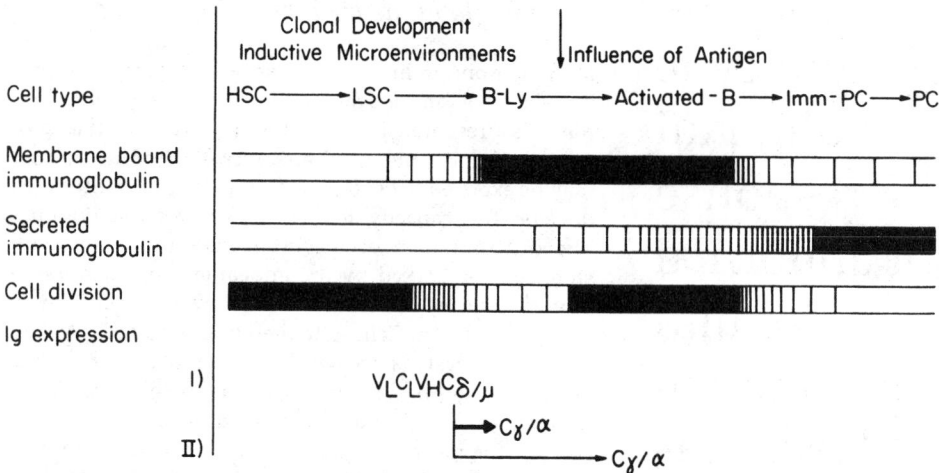

FIGURE 121-1 Scheme of B-cell development. This figure depicts the maturation sequence from pluripotential hemopoietic stem cells (HSC) into a hypothetical lymphoid stem cell (LSC), which is capable of differentiation under thymic influence into T cells or, as depicted above, under the influence of other inductive microenvironments such as the avian bursa of Fabricius or mammalian hemopoietic tissues, into B lymphocytes (B-Ly). During this antigen-independent proliferation, clonal development occurs, with the expression of the variable-region genes of light and heavy chains, the constant light-chain genes, and the μ and (in humans) δ heavy-chain constant-region genes. Some expression of other heavy-chain constant-region genes also occurs in this microenvironment (I), although full clonal expansion and expression of other H-chain genes results from antigen induction (II). The approximate relative concentration of membrane-bound immunoglobulin and secreted immunoglobulin is depicted schematically, with highest activity being fully shaded. Similarly represented is the approximate proportion of cells actively dividing. Antigen-induced differentiation results in initial activation of B cells (activated B) with maturation to immature (imm-PC) and then fully mature plasma cells (PC). (Warner, Potter, and Metcalf [1], with permission.)

tures, however, and soon reappeared if stripped away by trypsin treatment [20], indicating the intrinsic origin of this membrane component. The density of the membrane immunoglobulin in Burkitt's lymphoma is usually high, suggesting that the proliferating cell is an activated B lymphocyte rather than an immature B lymphocyte.

LYMPHOCYTIC AND HISTIOCYTIC LYMPHOMAS

Well-differentiated lymphocytic lymphomas, most nodular lymphomas, and many poorly differentiated lymphocytic lymphomas are monoclonal B-lymphocyte neoplasms, usually with IgM membrane immunoglobulin [14,16,21,22]. The density of membrane immunoglobulin is usually high on the cells of poorly differentiated lymphocytic lymphomas, suggesting that the proliferating cell is an activated B lymphocyte rather than an immature B lymphocyte. The cells of well-differentiated (small cell) lymphocytic lymphomas have a low density of membrane immunoglobulin, comparable to that of CLL lymphocytes [16]. The large cell lymphomas are heterogeneous. While some appear to be B-lymphocyte derivatives, T-lymphocyte markers have been found in others, and in some instances no specific cell markers can be detected (see Chap. 119).

WALDENSTRÖM'S MACROGLOBULINEMIA

The cells in Waldenström's macroglobulinemia have morphologic features which range from lymphoid to plasmacytoid. Immunofluorescence studies of cells obtained from the marrow, lymph nodes, and blood show cytoplasmic IgM only in plasma cells and in some of the large lymphoid cells, whereas membrane immunoglobulin is demonstrated in most lymphocytes and plasma cells [23]. In untreated patients a high proportion of blood lymphocytes carry a monoclonal IgM membrane immunoglobulin [24]. The density of surface immunoglobulin on these lymphocytes is higher than on CLL lymphocytes, more like that of normal lymphocytes [24]. Waldenström's macroglobulinemia is due to the proliferation of a clone of B lymphocytes which, in contrast to those in CLL, maintain a capacity to differentiate and mature into plasma cells (see Table 107-1).

A study of lymphocytes from patients with Waldenström's macroglobulinemia [25] has shown that these cells can carry both IgM and IgD on their membranes and that, as with normal lymphocytes, the IgM and IgD receptors occur independently on the cell surface [26]. The more mature members of the clone, the plasma cells, rarely carry membrane IgD, even when the majority of lymphocytes in the same marrow have these immunoglobulin receptors. These data are consistent with the hypothesis that a switch from the synthesis of δ to μ chains accompanies the maturation of B lymphocytes. In one patient, the IgM and IgD both had anti-γ-globulin activity [25]. This observation suggests that patients with macroglobulinemia may be "double producers," in that the cell is making both IgM and IgD expressing the same variable gene region.

PLASMA CELL MYELOMA

Studies of cellular morphology and immunoglobulin synthesis in patients with myeloma show that this disease involves the growth of plasma cells. The abnormal cells usually contain intracellular immunoglobulin but very little membrane-bound immunoglobulin [18]. In most patients the same monoclonal immunoglobulin is found on the surface and in the cytoplasm of the plasma cells, but in a few instances, IgM molecules are found on the surface of plasma cells which are also producing light chains, IgG or IgA monoclonal protein. In addition, in some patients with myeloma, a high proportion of the circulating lymphocytes carry the same monoclonal immunoglobulin on their surface as that secreted by the marrow plasma cells [27–29]. Plasma cell myeloma may represent a disorder of B lymphocytes in which the majority of cells differentiate into plasma cells. Similar observations have been made in mice with plasma cell tumors [30,31].

HEAVY-CHAIN DISEASES

The heavy chain diseases are immunoproliferative disorders characterized by a serum monoclonal protein consisting of incomplete heavy chains belonging to one γ, α, μ, or δ class and devoid of light chains. The clinical picture varies but often resembles that of a malignant lymphoma with enlarged lymph nodes, liver, and spleen. Biopsies of the marrow and other tissues usually show diffuse pleomorphic infiltration with lymphocytes, plasma cells, eosinophils, and histocytes with variable neoplastic features. Immunoglobulin has not been detected on the surface of the proliferating cells in patients with heavy-chain disease [7]. The cells involved in these disorders are classified as activated lymphocytes and immature plasma cells. By morphologic criteria, both lymphocytes and plasma cells appear to be involved in the secretion of the homogeneous heavy-chain moieties. The neoplastic nature of some of these disorders has not been established: the hyperplastic process has apparently regressed following antibiotic treatment in some patients with α-heavy-chain disease [32].

BENIGN MONOCLONAL GAMMOPATHY

Benign monoclonal gammapathy (BMG) is the most common immunoglobulin disorder [33,34] (see Chap. 113). In some patients a transient immunoglobulin spike appears during acute illness and disappears after recovery [35]. In BMG, the anomalous immunoglobulin component is produced by plasma cells scattered widely throughout the marrow. This disorder cannot be recognized until a single clone of plasma cells becomes sufficiently large to produce enough protein to be detected by serum electrophoresis (approximately 5×10^{11} cells). Once this size has been reached, the clone stops expanding and the amount of monoclonal immunoglobulin in the serum remains constant for years [36].

Pathogenesis

Spontaneous plasma cell tumors or lymphomas producing immunoglobulins have been reported in dogs [37,38], cats [39,40], hamsters [41], rats [42,43], and mice [44–47]. These tumors tend to develop in old animals, but a clearly identifiable etiologic agent has not been found in any species. The plasma cell neoplasms of inbred mouse strains have been investigated most extensively, since they have proved to be useful models for the study of plasma cell neoplasms of humans [48].

MOUSE PLASMA CELL TUMORS

Plasmacytomas can be induced in 70 percent of BALB/c mice by the intraperitoneal implantation of solid plastic materials [49,50] or of mineral oil [51,52]. The subcutaneous injection of oils or adjuvants does not induce plasmacytomas. The possible influence of hormonal factors in the development of plasmacytomas is suggested by the marked reduction in the incidence of tumors produced by cortisol therapy despite continued administration of mineral oil and by the higher incidence in males [53].

The intraperitoneal injection of plastics or oils, including the branched-chain hydrocarbon pristane, induces rapid formation of oil granulomas on the peritoneal and mesenteric surfaces. These granulomas grow progressively if additional injections of oil are given. Plasmacytomas develop within the oil granulomas and remain confined to this tissue except for metastases to regional and superior mediastinal lymph nodes.

The intraperitoneal injection of pristane leads to the appearance of a growth factor which facilitates the sustained proliferation of neoplastic plasma cells [54] and produces local immunosuppression [55]. In cell cultures, the addition of irradiated myeloma-infiltrated spleen cells markedly stimulates colony formation by myeloma stem cells [56]. In this cell culture system, ascorbic acid is required for the progressive growth of myeloma colonies [57]. Phagocytic cells also produce a growth factor for myeloma cells in culture [58], and serum contains a similar factor, the potency of which is markedly increased by the intraperitoneal injection of complete Freund's adjuvant [58]. Whole blood, erythrocytes, marrow or peritoneal cells, and serum from animals injected with endotoxin or bacterial antigens stimulate the growth of myeloma colonies in culture [59]. The active serum factors are nondialysable and heat-labile and migrate electrophoretically like β-globulins [60].

Antigenic stimulation by the normal microbial flora plays an important role in the induction of plasma cell tumors in BALB/c mice, since the incidence of plasmacytomas produced by the intraperitoneal injection of mineral oil is much lower in germfree mice than in others [61].

A long-term cell culture line of plasma cells producing IgD λ derived from a patient with IgD myeloma has been established which requires a growth factor produced by fibroblasts [62].

Genetic factors are important in the induction of plasma cell tumors, for intraperitoneal oil stimulates the formation of these tumors only in inbred mice of the BALB/c or NZB strains. Attempts to induce plasmacytomas by intraperitoneal oil injections in hybrids of BALB/c or NZB mice with mouse strains resistant to plasma cell tumor induction produce very few tumors [48]. BALB/c and NZB mice are unique in having specific genes involved in the pathogenesis of plasma cell tumors and at least one gene is recessive. The findings of the development of plasmacytomas in backcross F2 and intercross combinations involving either BALB/c or NZB parents are also compatible with this interpretation [63].

Although one or more C-type RNA viruses occur endogenously in BALB/c mice or can be activated from cultured BALB/c plasmacytomas, these plasma cell tumors contain intracisternal type-A particles. The etiologic significance of these agents in the induction of plasma cell tumors has not been established [1]. The infectious MLV-A virus accelerates the induction of plasmacytomas in pristane-treated BALB/c mice [64], and the rapidity with which these plasmacytomas develop suggests that they are derived from cells that have been transformed by the MLV-A virus. Since this virus also produces lymphomas derived from B lymphocytes, MLV-A infection may transform B lymphocytes in various stages of development, including some cells that have differentiated to the plasma cell stage [1].

Predisposing factors in humans

There is an increased incidence of myeloma in first-degree relatives. Myeloma has been found in the siblings of 8 among 440 myeloma patients seen over a 6-year period [65], far in excess of the incidence of myeloma in the general population. Familial myeloma has been reported in at least 14 additional families [reviewed in Ref. 65], and there are many reports of benign monoclonal gammopathy occurring in family members of patients with myeloma or macroglobulinemia [reviewed in Ref. 65]. The striking familial association of myeloma, macroglobulinemia, and benign monoclonal gammopathy, the finding that the 4c complex of HLA antigens occurs more frequently in myeloma patients than in the general population, and the increased

incidence of myeloma in blacks, strongly suggest that genetic factors play a role in determining susceptibility to these diseases in humans [65–70]. Although myeloma has been reported in at least five husband and wife pairs in the United States [71,72], the frequency in spouses is less than expected and does not favor the hypothesis of horizontal transmission.

An association between high-dose radiation exposure and plasma cell myeloma has been observed for the period 1950–1976 in a cohort of approximately 100,000 controls and survivors of the atomic bombs in Hiroshima and Nagasaki [73]. The standardized relative risk of developing myeloma was about five times greater than controls for persons with an estimated air-dose exposure of more than 100 rads. The excess risk for myeloma became apparent about 20 years after exposure. An association between low-dose radiation and the development of myeloma has not been established [73].

Chronic antigenic stimulation, for example, in cholecystitis, osteomyelitis, repeated allergen injections, rheumatoid arthritis, hereditary spherocytosis, and Gaucher's disease, has been proposed as a factor predisposing to the development of plasma cell neoplasms in humans [74–87]. The association of a plasma cell neoplasm with these conditions has not been established, however. The incidence of myeloma in Finnish patients with rheumatoid arthritis is about twice the incidence in the general population, and the occurrence of a monoclonal protein in 10 patients with Gaucher's disease and in 2 patients with hereditary spherocytosis may suggest an association between these uncommon disorders [82–87].

The occurrence of 4 patients with myeloma, 1 with macroglobulinemia, and 1 with chronic lymphocytic leukemia in a group of 61 patients with asbestosis raises the question of whether this carcinogen may be involved in the initiation of B-cell neoplasma [88,89].

Aleutian disease of mink is a viral illness characterized by excessive plasmacytosis and hyperglobulinemia. A small proportion of infected mink develop a serum monoclonal protein and light-chain proteinuria [90]. The Aleutian disease virus (ADV) is transmissible to humans, for one-half of the individuals handling high concentrations of ADV developed ADV antibodies, although none became ill [90]. Two cases thought to be Aleutian disease in humans have been described [91,92]. These patients were examined before the ADV antibody assay was developed, so that the diagnosis of ADV infection was not confirmed by demonstrating increased ADV antibodies. A mink handler developed myeloma following exposure to Aleutian disease, but no ADV antibodies could be detected in the patient's serum [93].

Cytogenetic studies have frequently shown chromosome abnormalities in the plasma cells of patients with myeloma, but unique lesions have not been identified [94]. The diversity of the chromosome abnormalities observed suggests that they may be the result rather than the cause of the neoplastic growth.

Clinical evaluation of protein abnormalities

The accurate diagnosis and classification of plasma cell neoplasms requires the identification and measurement of the anomalous proteins produced by the abnormal cell clones. The term *M protein* refers to the electrophoretically homogeneous components in the serum or urine, which may be immunoglobulins, globulin subunits, or fragments containing a single antigenic class of heavy or light chains. The *M* was once used to mean "malignant" or "myeloma," but more recently it has come to signify "monoclonal," in view of the finding that proteins of this type may occur in a variety of diseases, some of which are benign.

Measuring the amount of monoclonal protein in the serum or of light chains excreted in the urine provides an index of tumor activity in a patient, and serial studies are indispensable in evaluating changes in disease status.

Some of the numerous clinical indications for examining serum and urine proteins electrophoretically are outlined in Table 121-1 [95]. If anomalous components are discovered, it is important to recognize that the routine screening of persons 25 years of age or over reveals a monoclonal protein, usually in low concentration, in about 1 percent of all subjects and in about 3 percent of those over 70 years of age. In most instances these protein components, fortunately, represent benign monoclonal gammopathy.

ZONAL ELECTROPHORESIS

Some of the characteristic electrophoretic patterns of serum and urine proteins in patients with various diseases are shown in Fig. 121-2. While it is relatively easy to recognize the presence of anomalous proteins from the densitometer tracing alone or by inspection of the electrophoresis strip, it is essential to quantitate the amount of protein in each band individually, so that changes with time and with treatment can be ascertained.

SERUM

The normal serum electrophoresis pattern (Fig. 121-2a) shows five characteristic bands. Frequently a technical defect, caused by the precipitation of some protein at the site of application, produces a small deflection between the γ and β bands.

Patients with inflammatory or neoplastic disease and those with nephrosis, etc., frequently show a marked elevation of α_2-globulin (Fig. 121-2b). In the nephrotic syndrome hypoalbuminemia may be extreme, since albumin and other normal serum proteins pass through the glomeruli readily and appear in the urine.

Heterogeneous, polyclonal hypergammaglobulinemia (Fig. 121-2c) is a characteristic finding in patients with chronic infection, cirrhosis, chronic active hepatitis, sarcoidosis, the collagen diseases, and "immunoblastic" lymphomas [96]. The serum albumin concentration is

TABLE 121-1 Some clinical indications for the electrophoresis of serum and urine proteins

Clinical indications	Abnormality and interpretation
Unexplained edema or ascites	Hypoalbuminemia
Suspected liver disease	Hypoalbuminemia frequent; hyperglobulinemia suggests cirrhosis or chronic active hepatitis
Collagen diseases, sarcoidosis	Polyclonal hyperglobulinemia
Unusual susceptibility to infections	Hypo- or agammaglobulinemia
CLL, malignant lymphoma	Hypogammaglobulinemia or, rarely, IgG or IgM components
Unexplained proteinuria	Albumin or a mixture of all serum proteins is found with urinary tract infections or the nephrotic syndrome; homogeneous urine proteins that migrate in the globulin region are usually indicative of plasma cell neoplasms secreting free light or heavy chains
Suspected evidence of plasma cell neoplasms, e.g., bone pain, frequent infections, elevated sedimentation rate, rouleaux formation, proteinuria, or osteolytic skeletal lesions.	Serum or urinary monoclonal protein, with reduced normal immunoglobulins and hypoalbuminemia
Amyloidosis	Monoclonal serum or urinary proteins frequent

characteristically reduced in patients with cirrhosis. In patients suspected of havng a lymphocytic or plasma cell malignant disease, immunoelectrophoresis and quantitative immunoglobulin assays are advisable (see below), since a monoclonal IgA or IgM component may be hidden in a broad γ-globulin band [95].

The patterns observed in patients with IgG, IgA, IgM, and IgD plasma cell neoplasms and with those producing only κ and λ light chains are shown in Fig. 121-2d to *h*. IgG components in plasma cell myeloma characteristically appear as tall narrow spikes in the γ-globulin region. Their concentration is usually high (mean 4.3 g/dl), since they are catabolized at a slower rate than most other immunoglobulins [97–100]. The half-life of IgG subclasses 1, 2, and 4 is about 21 days at normal serum concentrations but becomes shorter as the amount in the serum increases. Above a concentration of approximately 3.0 g/dl the half-life stabilizes at about 12.5 days. The half-life of IgG_3 is about 7.1 days and is less affected by the serum concentration [98].

IgA components in plasma cell myeloma usually appear as more broadly based constitutents in the β-globulin region. The peak is broad, because this type of immunoglobulin tends to form polymers of various sizes [99]. The concentration of IgA is usually somewhat

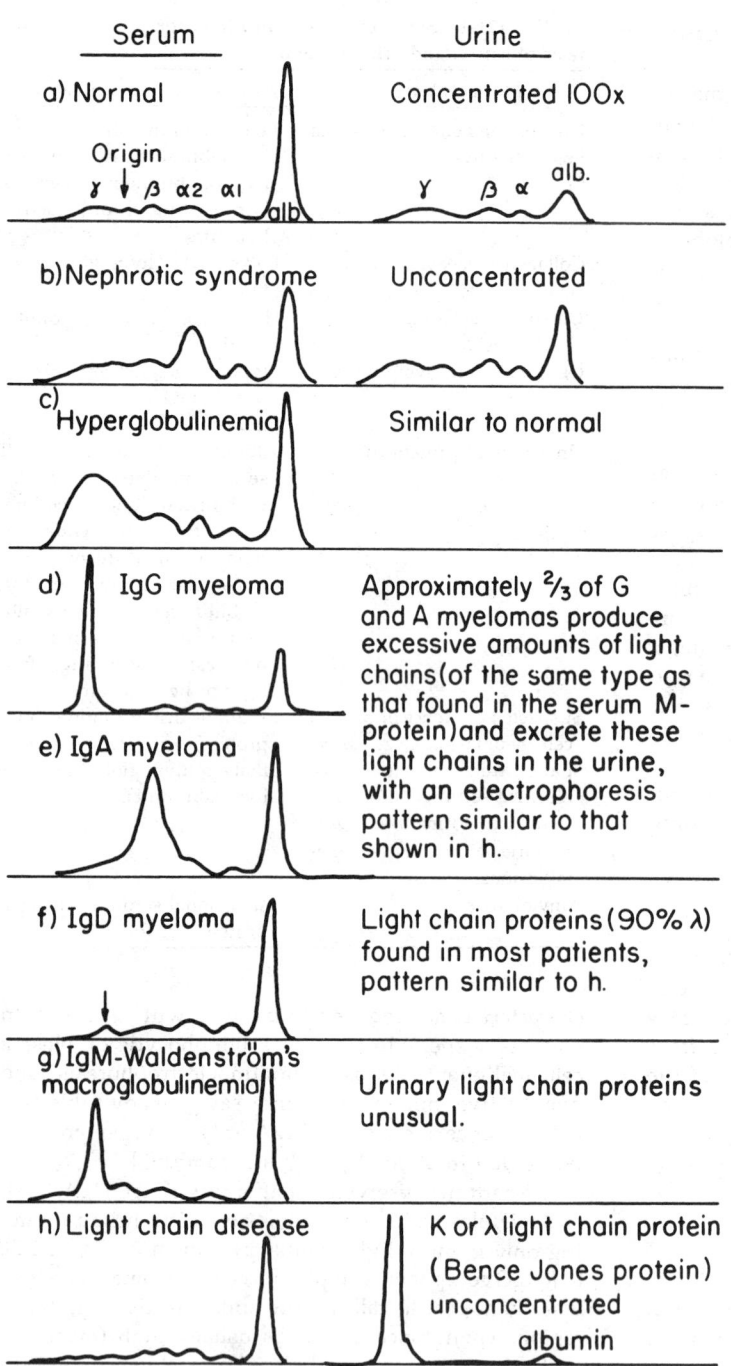

Serum

Urine

a) Normal   Concentrated 100x

Origin

γ   ↓ β α2 α1   γ   β   α   alb.
            alb

b) Nephrotic syndrome   Unconcentrated

c) Hyperglobulinemia   Similar to normal

d)   IgG myeloma   Approximately ⅔ of G and A myelomas produce excessive amounts of light chains (of the same type as that found in the serum M-protein) and excrete these light chains in the urine, with an electrophoresis pattern similar to that shown in h.

e) IgA myeloma

f) IgD myeloma   Light chain proteins (90% λ) found in most patients, pattern similar to h.

g) IgM-Waldenström's macroglobulinemia   Urinary light chain proteins unusual.

h) Light chain disease   K or λ light chain protein (Bence Jones protein) unconcentrated

albumin

FIGURE 121-2 Serum and urinary electrophoresis patterns in various diseases. See text for description.

lower than that of IgG components (mean, 2.8 g/dl). The half-life of IgA proteins is about 5.8 days and is not affected by the serum concentration [97,100].

IgM proteins are large molecules which migrate slowly on the supporting strip and usually appear as narrow bands close to the point of application. The half-life of these proteins is about 5.1 days and is not affected by the serum concentration [97]. In one series of pa-

tients with macroglobulinemia the IgM concentration ranged from 1.2 to 11.1 g/dl, with a mean of 4.4 g [101].

IgD components tend to be present in still lower concentrations and may produce only a small deflection on the densitometer tracing.

IgD protein is catabolized very rapidly, with a half-life of only 2.8 days [97]. The mean serum concentration in patients with IgD myeloma is only 1.7 g/dl [100].

URINE

Patients with light-chain disease, i.e., plasma cell tumors producing only κ or λ light chains, have hypogammaglobulinemia. The small light-chain proteins are so rapidly catabolized by the kidney and excreted in the urine that an abnormal protein component is ordinarily not seen in the serum. Occasionally a small component becomes evident as renal insufficiency progresses, and larger spikes may be detected in the rare patient in whom the light chains form tetramers or polymerize to form large molecules]102].

Anomalies that should not be confused with monoclonal proteins are illustrated in Fig. 121-3.

Patients suspected of having plasma cell neoplasms should have their urine tested for protein, using the sulfosalicylic test or Heller's nitric acid ring test. The Albustix (Ames Company) filter strip does not give a positive reaction with light-chain (Bence Jones) protein [103]. If the urine protein concentration is 0.1 to 0.2 g/dl or more, qualitative tests for Bence Jones protein can be carried out. The pH of the urine should be adjusted to 4.9 with acetate buffer and the urine heated in a waterbath at 58°C. Bence Jones protein almost always precipitates at this temperature or below [104]. The traditional heating and filtration tests for Bence Jones protein are unreliable. Urines that contain protein should be subjected to electrophoresis, since albumin as well as one or more abnormal protein components may be present. If the urine protein concentration is below 0.5 to 1 g/dl, it should be concentrated prior to electrophoresis. Narrow bands in the γ-globulin region usually contain light chains. Determining the percentage of Bence Jones protein in the urine and the total protein excretion per day enables one to calculate the amount of abnormal protein excreted, which is important in evaluating the therapeutic response of patients who excrete light chains. It is usually adequate to measure the total amount of protein excreted, however, with only occasional determination of the electrophoretic pattern once its identity as monoclonal light chains is established.

IMMUNOELECTROPHORESIS

Serum or urine found to contain monoclonal protein components by zonal electrophoresis should be studied by immunoelectrophoresis to identify the class of heavy chain (γ, α, δ, ε, or μ) and the type of light chain (κ or λ) of the protein. In immunoelectrophoresis, the serum or urine sample is first separated by electrophoresis in a supporting gel. Following this, polyvalent antisera to human immunoglobulins or specific antisera for each of the heavy and light chains are allowed to diffuse into the gel from troughs cut laterally parallel to the elongated protein zones separated by electrophoresis. As the antibodies diffuse into the gel and meet their corresponding protein antigens, they produce visible precipitin arcs (Fig. 121-4) [105].

Monoclonal proteins or components that occur in small concentrations, such as IgD, IgE, light chains, and

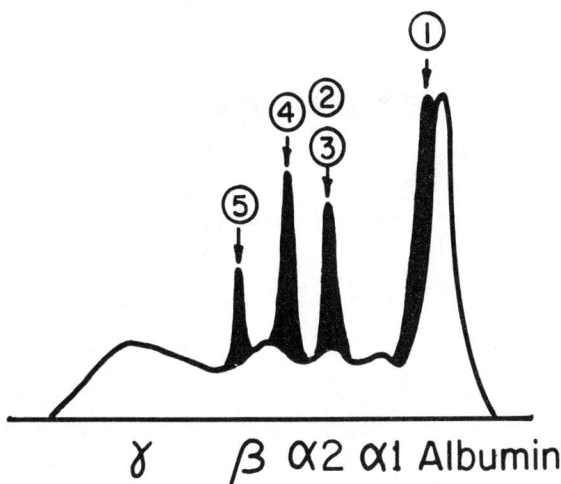

FIGURE 121-3 Some pseudo M components. The non-myelomatous conditions that may cause the abnormalities illustrated here are (1) bisalbuminemia; (2) hyperalpha$_2$-globulinemia associated with chronic inflammatory or neoplastic diseases, or the nephrotic syndrome; (3) hyperlipidemia; (4) presence in the blood of hemoglobin-haptoglobin complexes in association with severe hemolysis; and (5) presence in the blood of fibrinogen, when plasma instead of serum is used for electrophoresis.

some heavy chains, may be difficult to recognize on the electrophoresis strip but can be identified with appropriate antisera. Furthermore, monoclonal protein bands hidden within heterogeneous globulin mixtures, and some in apparently normal sera, can be detected only by immunoelectrophoresis.

QUANTITATIVE IMMUNOGLOBULIN ASSAYS

Immunoglobulin concentrations can be measured by radial immunodiffusion, using gels impregnated with specific antisera. The immunoglobulin assayed precipitates in a ring as it diffuses into the gel (Fig. 121-5). The width of the ring is directly related to the concentration of the immunoglobulin in the sample [106]. These assays are useful for measuring normal or reduced levels of serum immunoglobulin and for detecting some increase in concentration. Radial immunodiffusion, however, is not a reliable method for measuring greatly increased serum immunoglobulin concentrations, since the dilution required leads to inconsistent results. In evaluating the effect of treatment in patients with plasma cell myeloma, it is more reliable to quantitate the anomalous serum proteins by zone electrophoretic methods than by immunodiffusion procedures.

SERUM VISCOSITY

In patients who have visual, central nervous system, or bleeding symptoms which may be due to hyperviscosity (see Chap. 123), it is useful to measure the serum viscosity directly (see Chap. A31). At 24°C, using distilled water as the standard, the relative viscosity of nor-

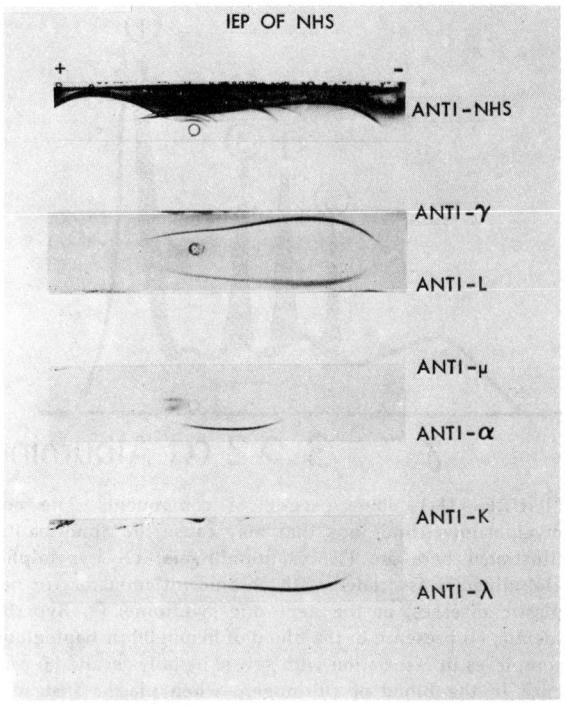

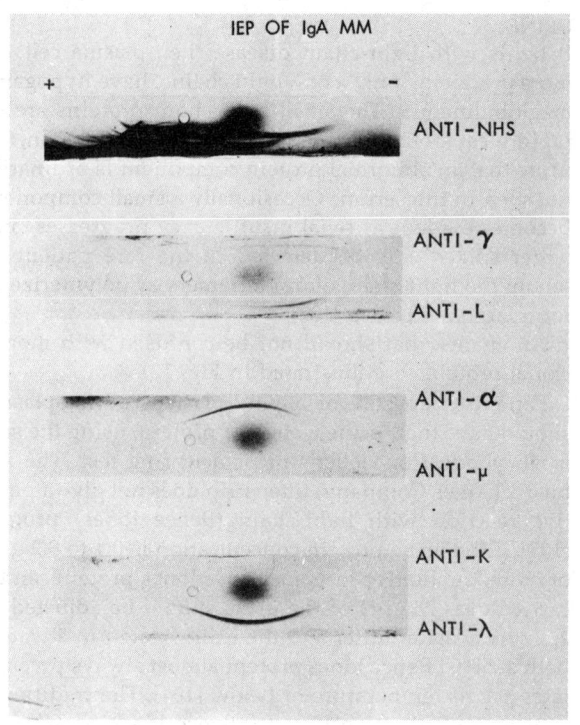

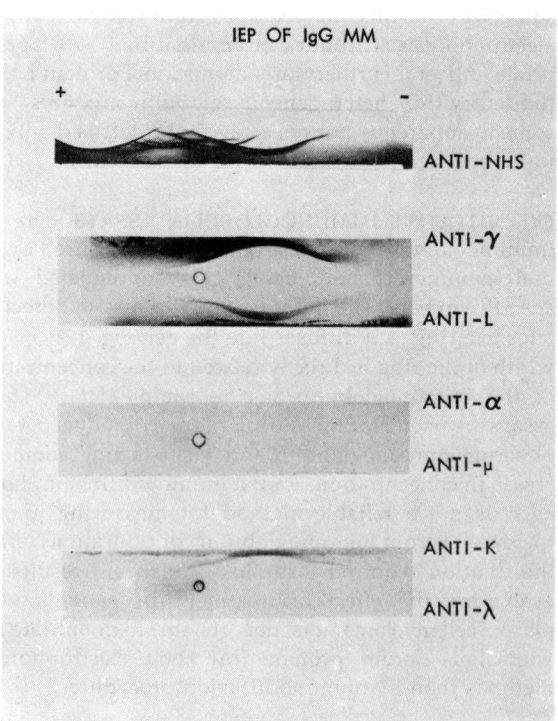

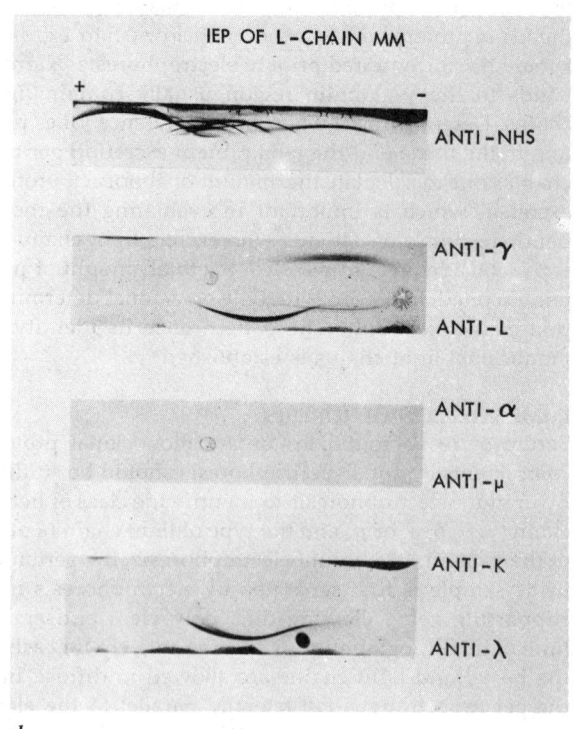

FIGURE 121-4   Representative immunoelectrophoretic (IEP) patterns (2% agar gel, pH 8.6) of normal human serum (NHS) and serum from patients with myeloma (MM). (a) Normal; (b) IgA λ myeloma; (c) IgG κ myeloma; (d) λ light-chain disease. Anti-γ = antibody to the γ heavy chain; anti-L = antibody to κ and λ light chains; anti-μ = antibody to the μ heavy chain; anti-α = antibody to the α heavy chain; anti-κ = antibody to the κ light chain; anti-λ = antibody to the λ light chain. (Courtesy of F. Paraskevas, Department of Medicine, University of Manitoba.)

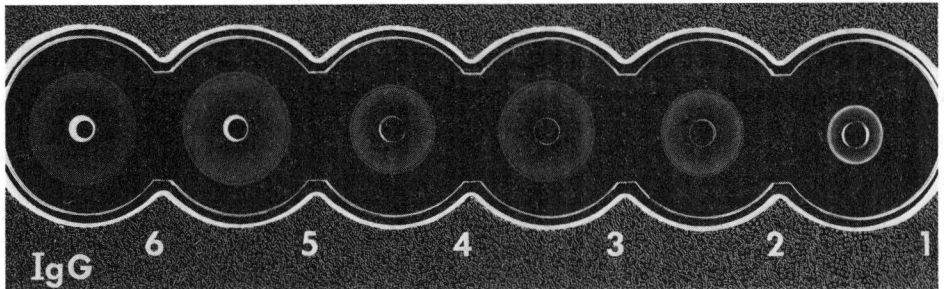

FIGURE 121-5 Assay of IgG by radial immunodiffusion. Serum samples were placed in the central wells of an agar gel impregnated with an antiserum which reacts specifically with IgG (Immunoplate, Hyland, Div. Travenol Laboratories, Inc., Costa Mesa, Calif.) and allowed to diffuse into the gel for 20 h at room temperature. The sera placed in wells 1, 2, and 3 are reference standards, provided by Hyland, containing 285, 782, and 1580 mg/dl of IgG, respectively. The diameter of the precipitate surrounding these wells is measured and plotted against the known IgG concentration on semilogarithmic graph paper. Wells 4, 5, and 6 contain undiluted sera from patients. The diameter of the precipitate surrounding these wells is measured and the IgG concentration read from the standard dilution curve as 860, 2100, and 2100 mg/dl, respectively, for wells 4 to 6.

mal serum may be as high as 1.8. Hyperviscosity symptoms are usually not encountered until the relative serum viscosity is above 4. If the serum contains cryoglobulin, it is important to determine the viscosity at 37°C.

The effect of various proteins on serum viscosity depends on their concentration, size, shape, thermolability, and molecular affinities. Large IgM proteins and some IgA and IgG components which tend to form aggregates are most frequently associated with the hyperviscosity syndrome. In a review of patients with plasma cell myeloma who had hyperviscosity due to IgG serum components, 80 percent of the sera gave a positive Sia test [107]. The Sia water-dilution test is a simple test for recognizing the presence of euglobulins. A drop of serum is added to a cylinder of distilled water, and if a filmy white precipitate appears as the drop settles, the test is read as positive. A positive Sia test in patients with IgG myeloma components thus suggests the possibility of hyperviscosity. Monoclonal IgG_3 proteins tend to form concentration- and temperature-dependent aggregates that are not encountered with other IgG subclasses [108], and to produce hyperviscosity at lower serum concentrations than IgG_1 proteins [107].

ULTRACENTRIFUGATION
Determining the sedimentation velocity of abnormal proteins is useful in estimating their size and tendency to form polymers or aggregates. Ultracentrifugation is especially helpful in separating the usual 19 S pentamer form of IgM (with $M_r = 900,000$ daltons), from the less common 7 S form [109].

OTHER TESTS
The majority of IgM proteins are positive for the Sia water-dilution test [110], and as noted above, 12 percent of one series of patients with myeloma having IgG pro-

teins showed a positive test [107]. A positive Sia test is thus an indication for determining the serum viscosity.

In patients who have Raynaud's phenomenon, purpura, or cold urticaria tests for cryoglobulins may be informative. Blood should be collected with a prewarmed syringe and allowed to clot and retract at 37°C. The serum is cooled at 4 to 10°C for several hours or days. Cryoglobulins settle out as a white precipitate or thick, oily gel on cooling but redissolve completely with warming. Cryoglobulins are usually IgM or IgG proteins [111], but IgA components [112] and light chains [113] have also been reported to form cryoglobulin precipitates.

Monoclonal proteins are occasionally "pyroglobulins," i.e., they precipitate when serum is heated to 50 to 60°C [114,115]. In contrast to the cryoglobulins, the heat precipitation of pyroglobulins is not reversible and represents an unusual susceptibility to heat denaturation.

References

1. Warner, N. L., Potter, M., and Metcalf, D.: *Multiple Myeloma and Related Immunoglobulin-Producing Neoplasms,* UICC Technical Report Series, vol. 13. International Union against Cancer, Geneva, 1974.
2. Klein, E., Eskeland, T., Inoue, M., Strom, R., and Johansson, B.: Surface immunoglobulin moieties on lymphoid cells. *Ann. N.Y. Acad. Sci.* 177:306, 1971.
3. Grey, H. M., Rabellino, E., and Pirofsky, B.: Immunoglobulins on the surface of lymphocytes. IV. Distribution in hypogammaglobulinemia, cellular immune deficiency and chronic lymphatic leukemia. *J. Clin. Invest.* 50:2368, 1971.
4. Pernis, B., Ferrarini, M., Forni, L., and Amante, L.: Immunoglobulins on lymphocyte membranes, in *Progress in Immunology,* First International Congress of Immunology, edited by B. Amos. Academic, New York, 1971, p. 95.
5. Preud'homme, J. L., Klein, M., Verroust, P., and Seligmann, M.: Immunoglobulines monoclonales de membrane dans les leucémies lymphoïdes chroniques. *Rev. Eur. Etud. Clin. Biol.* 16:1025, 1971.

LYMPHOCYTES AND PLASMA CELLS PART SEVEN

6. Warner, N. L.: Membrane immunoglobulins and antigen receptors on B and T lymphocytes. *Adv. Immunol. 19:*67, 1974.

7. Seligmann, M., Preud'homme, J. L., and Brouet, J. C.: B and T cell markers in human proliferative blood diseases and primary immunodeficiencies, with special reference to membrane bound immunoglobulins. *Transplant. Rev. 16:*85, 1973.

8. Shevach, E. M., Herberman, R., Frank, M. M., and Green, I.: Receptors for complement and immunoglobulin on human leukemic cells and human lymphoblastoid cell lines. *J. Clin. Invest. 51:*1933, 1972.

9. Pincus, S., Bianco, C., and Nussenzweig, V.: Increased proportion of complement-receptor lymphocytes in the peripheral blood of patients with chronic lympoycytic leukemia. *Blood 40:*303, 1972.

10. Ross, G. D., Polley, M. J., Rabellino, E. M., and Grey, H. M.: Two different complement receptors on human lymphocytes, one specific for C3b and one specific for C3b inactivator-cleaved C3b. *J. Exp. Med. 138:*798, 1973.

11. Dickler, H. B., Siegal, F. P., Bentwich, Z. H., and Kunkel, H. G.: Lymphocyte binding of aggregated IgG and surface Ig staining in chronic lymphocytic leukemia. *Clin. Exp. Immunol. 14:*97, 1973.

12. Catovsky, D., Galetto, J., Okos, A., Galton, D. A. G., Wiltshaw, E., and Stathopoulos, G.: Prolymphocytic leukaemia of B and T cell type. *Lancet 2:*232, 1973.

13. Preud'homme, J. L., and Seligmann, M.: Surface bound immunoglobulins as a cell marker in human lymphoproliferative diseases. *Blood 40:*777, 1972.

14. Aisenberg, A. C., and Bloch, K. J.: Immunoglobulins on the surface of neoplastic lymphocytes. *N. Engl. J. Med. 287:*272, 1972.

15. Wilson, J. D., and Nossal, G. J.: Identification of human T and B lymphocytes in normal peripheral blood and in chronic lymphocytic leukaemia. *Lancet 2:*788, 1971.

16. Aisenberg, A. C., and Long, J. C.: Lymphocyte surface characteristics in malignant lymphoma. *Am. J. Med. 58:*300, 1975.

17. Klein, G., Clifford, P., Klein, E., and Stjernswärd, J.: Search for tumor-specific immune reactions in Burkitt lymphoma patients by the membrane immunofluorescence reaction. *Proc. Natl. Acad. Sci. U.S.A. 55:*1628, 1966.

18. Klein, E., Klein, G., Nadkarni, J. S., Nadkarni, J. J., Wigzell, H., and Clifford, P.: Surface IgM-kappa specificity on a Burkitt lymphoma cell in vivo and in derived culture lines. *Cancer Res. 28:*1300, 1968.

19. Klein, G., Pearson, G., Henle, G., Henle, W., Goldstein, G., and Clifford, P.: Relation between Epstein-Barr viral and cell membrane immunofluorescence in Burkitt tumor cells. III. Comparison of blocking of direct membrane immunofluorescence and anti-EBV reactivities of different sera. *J. Exp. Med. 129:*697, 1969.

20. Osunkoya, B. O., Mottram, F. C., and Isoun, M. J.: Synthesis and fate of immunological surface receptors on cultured Burkitt lymphoma cells. *Int. J. Cancer 4:*159, 1969.

21. Brouet, J. C., Labaume, S., and Seligmann, M.: Evaluation of T and B lymphocyte membrane markers in human non-Hodgkin's malignant lymphomata. *Br. J. Cancer 31 (Suppl. 2):*121, 1975.

22. Jaffe, E. S., Shevach, E. M., Sussmann, E. H., Frank, M., Green, I., and Berard, C. W.: Membrane receptor sites for the identification of lymphoreticular cells in benign and malignant conditions. *Br. J. Cancer 31 (Suppl. 2):*107, 1975.

23. Preud'homme, J. L., Hurez, D., and Seligmann, M.: Immunofluorescence studies in Waldenström's macroglobulinemia. *Rev. Eur. Etud. Clin. Biol. 15:*1127, 1970.

24. Preud'homme, J. L., and Seligmann, M.: Immunoglobulins on the surface of lymphoid cells in Waldenström's macroglobulinemia. *J. Clin. Invest. 51:*701, 1972.

25. Pernis, B., Brouet, J. C., and Seligmann, M.: IgD and IgM on the membrane of lymphoid cells in macroglobulinemia: Evidence for identity of membrane IgD and IgM antibody activity in a case with anti-IgG receptors. *Eur. J. Immunol. 4:*776, 1974.

26. Rowe, D. S., Hug, K., Forni, L., and Pernis, B.: Immunoglobulin D as a lymphocyte receptor. *J. Exp. Med. 138:*965, 1973.

27. Heller, P., Yakulis, V., Bhoopalam, N., Costea, N., Cabana, V., and Nathan, R. D.: Surface immunoglobulins on circulating lymphocytes in mouse and human plasmacytoma. *Trans. Assoc. Am. Physicians 85:*192, 1972.

28. Lindström, F. D., Hardy, W. R., Eberle, B. J., and Williams, R. C.: Multiple myeloma and benign monoclonal gammapathy: Differentiation by immunofluorescence of lymphocytes. *Ann. Intern. Med. 78:*837, 1973.

29. Preud'homme, J. L., and Seligmann, M.: Surface immunoglobulins on human lymphoid cells, in *Progress in Clinical Immunology,* edited by R. S. Schwartz. Grune & Stratton, New York, 1974, vol. 2, p. 121.

30. Yakulis, V., Bhoopalam, N., Schade, S., and Heller, P.: Surface immunoglobulins of circulating lymphocytes in mouse plasmacytoma. I. Characteristics of lymphocyte surface immunoglobulins. *Blood 39:*453, 1972.

31. Bhoopalam, N., Yakulis, V., Costea, N., and Heller, P.: Surface immunoglobulins of circulating lymphocytes in mouse plasmacytoma. II. The influence of plasmacytoma RNA on surface immunoglobulins of lymphocytes. *Blood 39:*465, 1972.

32. Seligmann, M.: Immunochemical, clinical, and pathological features of α-chain disease. *Arch. Intern. Med. 135:*78, 1975.

33. Axelsson, U., Bachmann, R., and Hällén, J.: Frequency of pathological proteins (M-components) in 6995 sera from an adult population. *Acta Med. Scand. 179:*235, 1966.

34. Axelsson, U.: An eleven-year follow-up on 64 subjects with M-components. *Acta Med. Scand. 201:*173, 1977.

35. Young, V. H.: Transient paraproteins. *Proc. R. Soc. Med. 62:*778, 1969.

36. Kyle, R. A.: Monoclonal gammopathy of undetermined significance. *Am. J. Med. 64:*814, 1978.

37. Hurvitz, A. I.: Animal model for human disease: Canine monoclonal gammopathies/immunoglobulins. *Comp. Pathol. Bull. 3:*4, 1971.

38. Osborne, C. A., Perman, V., Sauttner, J. H., Stevens, J. B., and Hanlon, G. F.: Multiple myeloma in the dog. *J. Am. Vet. Med. Assoc. 153:*1300, 1968.

39. Farrow, B. R., and Penny, R.: Multiple myeloma in a cat. *J. Am. Vet. Med. Assoc. 158:*606, 1971.

40. Kehoe, J. M., Hurvitz, A. I., and Capra, J. D.: Characterization of three feline paraproteins. *J. Immunol. 109:*511, 1972.

41. Cotran, R. S., and Fortner, J. G.: Serum protein abnormality in a transplantable plasmacytoma of the Syrian golden hamster. *J. Natl. Cancer Inst. 28:*1193, 1962.

42. Bazin, H., Deckers, C., Beckers, A., and Heremans, J. F.: Transplantable immunoglobulin-secreting tumours in rats. I. General features of Lou-Wsl strain rat immunocytomas and their monoclonal proteins. *Int. J. Cancer 10:*568, 1972.

43. Bazin, H., Beckers, A., Deckers, C., and Moriamé, M.: Transplantable immunoglobulin secreting tumors in rats. V. Monoclonal immunoglobulins secreted by 250 ileocecal immunocytomas in Lou-Wsl rats. *J. Natl. Cancer Inst. 51:*1359, 1973.

44. Dunn, T. B.: Normal and pathologic anatomy of the reticular tissue in laboratory mice, with a classification and discussion of neoplasms. *J. Natl. Cancer Inst. 14:*1281, 1954.

45. Dunn, T. B.: Plasma-cell neoplasms beginning in the ileocecal area in strain C3H mice. *J. Natl. Cancer Inst. 19:*371, 1957.

46. Pilgrim, H. I.: The relationship of chronic ulceration of the ileocecal junction to the development of reticuloendothelial tumors in C3H mice. *Cancer Res. 25:*53, 1965.

47. Mellors, R. C.: Autoimmune and immunoproliferative diseases of NZB/B1 mice and hybrids. *Int. Rev. Exp. Pathol. 5:*217, 1966.

48. Potter, M.: Immunoglobulin-producing tumors and myeloma proteins of mice. *Physiol. Rev. 52:*631, 1972.

49. Merwin, R. M., and Algire, G. H.: Induction of plasma-cell neoplasms and fibrosarcomas in BALB/c mice carrying diffusion chambers. *Proc. Soc. Exp. Biol. Med. 101:*437, 1959.

50. Merwin, R. M., and Redmon, L. W.: Induction of plasma cell tumors and sarcomas in mice by diffusion chambers placed in the peritoneal cavity. *J. Natl. Cancer Inst. 31:*997, 1963.

51. Anderson, P. N., and Potter, M.: Induction of plasma cell tumours in BALB/c mice with 2,6,10,14-tetramethylpentadecane (pristane). *Nature 222:*994, 1969.

52. Potter, M.: The developmental history of the neoplastic plasma cell in mice: A brief review of recent developments. *Semin. Hematol. 10:*19, 1973.

53. Hollander, V. P., Takakura, K., and Yamada, H.: Endocrine factors in the pathogenesis of plasma cell tumors. *Recent Prog. Horm. Res. 24:*81, 1968.

54. Potter, M., Pumphrey, J. G., and Walters, J. L.: Brief communication: Growth of primary plasmacytomas in the mineral oil-conditioned peritoneal environment. *J. Natl. Cancer Inst.* 49:305, 1972.

55. Potter, M., and Walters, J. L.: Effect of intraperitoneal pristane on established immunity to the Adj-PC-5 plasmacytoma. *J. Natl. Cancer Inst.* 51:875, 1973.

56. Park, C. H., Bergsagel, D. E., and McCulloch, E. A.: Mouse myeloma tumor stem cells: A primary cell culture assay. *J. Natl. Cancer Inst.* 46:411, 1971.

57. Park, C. H., Bergsagel, D. E., and McCulloch, E. A.: Ascorbic acid: A culture requirement for colony formation by mouse plasmacytoma cells. *Science* 174:720, 1971.

58. Namba, Y., and Hanaoka, M.: Immunocytology of cultured IgM-forming cells of mouse. I. Requirement of phagocytic cell factor for the growth of the IgM-forming tumor cells in tissue culture. *J. Immunol.* 109:1193, 1972.

59. Metcalf, D.: Colony formation in agar by murine plasmacytoma cells: Potentiation by hemopoietic cells and serum. *J. Cell Physiol.* 81:397, 1973.

60. Metcalf, D.: The serum factor stimulating colony formation in vitro by murine plasmacytoma cells: Response to antigens and mineral oil. *J. Immunol.* 113:235, 1974.

61. McIntire, K. R., and Princler, G. L.: Prolonged adjuvant stimulation in germ-free BALB/c mice development of plasma cell neoplasia. *Immunology* 17:481, 1969.

62. Jobin, M. E., Fahey, J. L., and Price, Z.: Long-term establishment of a human plasmacyte cell line derived from a patient with IgD myeloma. I. Requirement of a plasmacyte-stimulating factor for the proliferation of myeloma cells in tissue culture. *J. Exp. Med.* 140:494, 1974.

63. Warner, N. L.: Autoimmunity and the pathogenesis of plasma cell tumor induction in NZB inbred and hybrid mice. Quoted in N. L. Warner, M. Potter, and D. Metcalf, *Multiple Myeloma and Related Immunoglobulin-Producing Neoplasms*, UICC Technical Report Series, vol. 13. International Union against Cancer, Geneva, 1974.

64. Potter, M., Sklar, M. D., and Rowe, W. P.: Rapid viral induction of plasmacytomas in pristine-primed BALB/c mice. *Science* 182:592, 1973.

65. Maldonado, J. E., and Kyle, R. A.: Familial myeloma. Report of eight families and a study of serum proteins in their relatives. *Am. J. Med.* 57:875, 1974.

66. MacMahon, B., and Clark, D. W.: Incidence of multiple myeloma. *J. Chronic Dis.* 4:508, 1956.

67. MacFarlane, H.: Multiple myeloma in Jamaica: A study of 40 cases with special reference to the incidence and laboratory diagnosis. *J. Clin. Pathol.* 19:268, 1966.

68. McPhedran, P., Heath, C. W., Jr., and Garcia, J.: Multiple myeloma incidence in metropolitan Atlanta, Georgia: Racial and seasonal variations. *Blood* 39:866, 1972.

69. Bertrams, J., et al.: HL-A antigens in Hodgkin's disease and multiple myeloma. *Tissue Antigens* 2:41, 1972.

70. Smith, G., Walford, R. L., Fishkin, B., Carter, P. K., and Tanaka, K.: HL-A phenotypes, immunoglobulins and K and L chains in multiple myeloma. *Tissue Antigens* 4:374, 1974.

71. Kyle, R. A., Heath, C. W., Jr., and Carbone, P.: Multiple myeloma in spouses. *Arch. Intern. Med.* 127:944, 1971.

72. Peitruszka, M., Rabin, B. S., and Srodes, C.: Multiple myeloma in husband and wife. *Lancet* 1:314, 1976.

73. Ishimaru, M., Ishimaru, T., Mikamin, M., and Matsunaga, M.: *Multiple Myeloma among Atomic Bomb Survivors, Hiroshima and Nagasaki, 1950–1976*, Radiation Effects Research Foundation Technical Report No. 9-79. Radiation Effects Research Foundation, Hiroshima, 1979.

74. Isobe, T., and Osserman, E. F.: Pathologic conditions associated with plasma cell dyscrasias: A study of 806 cases. *Ann. N.Y. Acad. Sci.* 190:507, 1971.

75. Osserman, E. F., and Takatsuki, K.: Considerations regarding the pathogenesis of the plasmacytic dyscrasias. *Ser. Haematol.* 4:28, 1965.

76. Schafer, A. I., and Miller, J. B.: Association of IgA multiple myeloma with pre-existing disease. *Br. J. Haematol.* 41:19, 1979.

77. Wohlenberg, H.: Osteomyelitis and plasmacytoma. *N. Engl. J. Med.* 283:822, 1970.

78. Penny, R., and Hughes, S.: Repeated stimulation of the reticulo-endothelial system and the development of plasma cell dyscrasias. *Lancet* 1:77, 1970.

79. Rosenblatt, J., and Hall, C. A.: Plasma-cell dyscrasia following prolonged stimulation of reticuloendothelial system. *Lancet* 1:301, 1970.

80. Goldenberg, G. J., Paraskevas, F., and Israels, L. G.: The association of rheumatoid arthritis with plasma cell and lymphocytic neoplasms. *Arthritis Rheum.* 12:569, 1969.

81. Wegelius, O., and Skrifvars, B.: Rheumatoid arthritis terminating in plasmacytoma. *Acta Med. Scand.* 187:133, 1970.

82. Isomäki, H. A., Hakulmen, T., and Joutsenlahti, U.: Excess risk of lymphomas, leukemias and myeloma in patients with rheumatoid arthritis. *J. Chron. Dis.* 31:691, 1978.

83. Schafer, A. I., Miller, J. B., Lester, E. P., Bowers, T. K., and Jacob, H. S.: Monoclonal gammopathy in hereditary spherocytosis: A possible pathogenetic relation. *Ann. Intern. Med.* 88:45, 1978.

84. Pratt, P. W., Estren, S., and Kochwa, S.: Immunoglobulin abnormalities in Gaucher's disease: Report of 16 cases. *Blood* 31:633, 1968.

85. Wolf, P.: Monoclonal gammopathy in Gaucher's disease. *Lab. Med.* 4:28, 1973.

86. Turesson, I., and Rausing, A.: Gaucher's disease and benign monoclonal gammopathy. *Acta. Med. Scand.* 197:507, 1975.

87. MacDonald, M., et al.: Gaucher's disease with biclonal gammopathy. *J. Clin. Pathol.* 28:757, 1975.

88. Gerber, M. A.: Asbestosis and neoplastic disorders of the hematopoietic system. *Am. J. Clin. Pathol.* 53:204, 1970.

89. Kagan, E., Jacobson, R. J., Yeung, K.-Y., Haidak, D. J., and Nachnani, G. H.: Asbestosis-associated neoplasms of B cell lineage. *Am. J. Med.* 67:325, 1979.

90. Porter, D. D., Dixon, F. J., and Larsen, A. E.: The development of a myeloma-like condition in mink with Aleutian disease. *Blood* 25:736, 1965.

91. Chapman, I., and Jimenez, F. A.: Aleutian mink disease in man. *N. Engl. J. Med.* 269:1171, 1963.

92. Helmboldt, C. R., Kenyon, A. J., and Dessel, B. H.: *The comparative aspects of Aleutian mink disease*, in *Slow, Latent and Temperate Virus Infections*. National Institutes of Health, Bethesda, Md., NINDB Monograph no. 2, 1964, pp. 315–319.

93. Henry, L. W.: Multiple myeloma in a mink handler following exposure to Aleutian disease. *Cancer* 44:273, 1979.

94. Sandberg, A.: *The Chromosomes in Human Cancer and Leukemia*. Elsevier–North Holland, New York, 1980.

95. Alper, C. A.: Plasma protein measurements as a diagnostic aid. *N. Engl. J. Med.* 291:287, 1974.

96. Lukes, R. J., and Tingle, B. H.: Immunoblastic lymphadenopathy: A hyperimmune entity resembling Hodgkin's disease. *N. Engl. J. Med.* 292:1, 1975.

97. Waldmann, T. A., and Strober, W.: Metabolism of immunoglobulins. *Prog. Allergy* 13:1, 1969.

98. Morell, A., Terry, W. D., and Waldmann, T. A.: Metabolic properties of IgG subclasses in man. *J. Clin. Invest.* 49:673, 1970.

99. Fahey, J. L.: Heterogeneity of myeloma proteins. *J. Clin. Invest.* 42:111, 1963.

100. Jancelwicz, Z., Takatsuki, K., Sugai, S., and Pruzanski, W.: IgG multiple myeloma: Review of 133 cases. *Arch. Intern. Med.* 135:87, 1975.

101. MacKenzie, M. R., and Fudenberg, H. H.: Macroglobulinemia: An analysis of forty patients. *Blood* 39:874, 1972.

102. Parr, D. M., Pruzanski, W., Scott, J. G., and Mills, D. M.: Primary amyloidosis with plasmacytic dyscrasia and a tetramer of Bence-Jones type lambda globulin in the serum and urine. *Blood* 37:473, 1971.

103. Smith, J. K.: The significance of the "protein error" of indicators in the diagnosis of Bence-Jones proteinuria. *Acta Haematol.* 30:144, 1963.

104. Putnam, F. W., Easley, C. W., Lynn, L. T., Ritchie, A. E., and Phelps, R. A.: Heat precipitation of Bence-Jones proteins. I. Optimum conditions. *Arch. Biochem. Biophys.* 83:115, 1959.

105. Grabar, P.: Agar-gel diffusion and immunoelectrophoretic analysis. *Ann. N.Y. Acad. Sci.* 69:591, 1957.

106. Fahey, J. L., and McKelvey, E. M.: Quantitative determination of serum immunoglobulins in antibody-agar plates. *J. Immunol.* 94:84, 1965.

107. Pruzanski, W., and Watt, J. G.: Serum viscosity and hyperviscosity syndrome in IgG multiple myeloma. *Ann. Intern. Med.* 77:853, 1972.

108. Capra, J. D., and Kunkel, H. G.: Aggregation of γG3 proteins: Relevance to the hyperviscosity syndrome. *J. Clin. Invest.* 49:610, 1970.

109. Solomon, A., and Kunkel, H. G.: A "monoclonal" type, low molecular weight protein related to γM-macroglobulin. *Am. J. Med.* 42:958, 1967.

110. MacKay, J. R., Eriksen, N., Motulsky, A. G., and Volwiller, W.: Cryo- and macroglobulinemia: Electrophoretic, ultracentrifugal and clinical studies. *Am. J. Med.* 20:564, 1956.

111. Meltzer, M., and Franklin, E. C.: Cryoglobulinemia: A study of twenty-nine patients. I. IgG and IgM cryoglobulins and factors affecting cryoprecipitability. *Am. J. Med.* 40:828, 1966.

112. Pruzanski, W., Jancelewicz, Z., and Underdown, B.: Immunological and physiochemical studies of IgA1(γ) cryoglobulinaemia. *Clin. Exp. Immunol.* 15:181, 1973.

113. Liss, M., Fudenberg, H. H., and Kritzman, J.: A Bence-Jones cryoglobulin: Chemical, physical and immunological properties. *Clin. Exp. Immunol.* 2:467, 1967.

114. Stefanini, M., McDonnell, E. E., Andracki, E. G., Swansbro, W. J., and Durr, P.: Macropyroglobulinemia: Immunochemical studies in three cases. *Am. J. Clin. Pathol.* 54:94, 1970.

115. Patterson, R., Roberts, M., Rambach, W., and Falleroni, A.: An IgM pyroglobulin associated with lymphosarcoma. *Am. J. Med.* 48:503, 1970.

CHAPTER 122

Plasma cell myeloma

DANIEL E. BERGSAGEL

Plasma cell myeloma (multiple myeloma, PCM) is the most common form of plasma cell neoplasm. The primary abnormality in this disease is an uncontrolled proliferation of malignant plasma cells in the marrow. The clinical manifestations of PCM vary but include tumor formation, osteolysis, hemopoiesis, hypogammaglobulinemia, and renal disease. The neoplastic cells synthesize abnormal amounts of monoclonal immunoglobulin (IgG, IgA, IgD, or IgE) or κ or λ light chains, but rarely there is no detectable secretion of immunoglobulin by the tumor cells.

History

The features of the disease were described in papers published from 1846 through 1850 by John Dalrymple, Henry Bence Jones, and William MacIntyre [1]. Their 46-year-old patient suffered severe bone pain for several months before he died in London on January 1, 1846, from "atrophy from albuminuria." An unusual proteinuria had been recognized during life, and at postmortem examination the bones, particularly the ribs, sternum, and vertebral bones, were extremely soft. The interior of the bones was replaced by a gelatinous blood-red tumor which on microscopic examination was found to be composed of round or oval cells, twice the size of red blood cells. Some of the cells were multinuclear. Rustizky introduced the term *multiple myeloma* in 1873 to emphasize multiple bone tumors as the outstanding feature of the disease [2]. Kahler published a detailed description of multiple myeloma in 1889 [3]. In Europe, plasma cell myeloma is still referred to as *Kahler's disease*. Ellinger [4] called attention to the increased serum protein concentration in the disease and the formation of pathologic erythrocyte rouleaux. The close relationship of myeloma cells to plasma cells was recognized by Wright in 1900 [5], but the clinical diagnosis was difficult and often uncertain until marrow aspiration became a standard procedure in the 1930s. Hyperproteinemia was emphasized as a feature of plasma cell myeloma by Perlzweig in 1929 [6], and with the development of ultracentrifugation and protein electrophoresis in Sweden in the late 1930s, chemical studies of the anomalous serum and urine proteins were undertaken. Magnus-Levy described amyloidosis in about 15 percent of patients with plasma cell myeloma [7]; subsequent evidence indicated that immunoglobulins were involved in the pathogenesis of amyloidosis [8].

The treatment of plasma cell myeloma remained ineffective until 1958. Earlier a few patients had improved with urethane therapy [9,10], but no success was achieved with pentamidine, nitrogen mustard, 6-mercaptopurine, or 5-fluorouracil [10]. In 1958, Blokhin and colleagues reported that DL-phenylalanine mustard (Sarcolysin) produced a significant degree of improvement in three out of six patients, including the healing of skull lesions in one [11]. The value of melphalan (L-phenylalanine mustard) was confirmed by many investigators [12]. Cyclophosphamide was shown to be equally effective [13], and the glucocorticoids were found to have an adjunctive therapeutic usefulness.

Etiology and inheritance

These are discussed in Chap. 121.

Incidence

The annual incidence of plasma cell myeloma is 3.1 per 100,000 people in Olmsted County, Minnesota [14], 2.0 in Atlanta, Georgia [15], 3.0 in Malmo, Sweden [16], and 2.6 in England [17]. The disease occurs more frequently in blacks than whites [15,18,19]. For example, in Atlanta the rates were 4.0 per 100,000 in blacks and 2.1 per 100,000 in whites [15]. The sex incidence is about equal in men and women up to the age of 65 [14,16,20]. The incidence of myeloma increases progressively with age. The mean age at the time of diagnosis is 62 years [20,21].

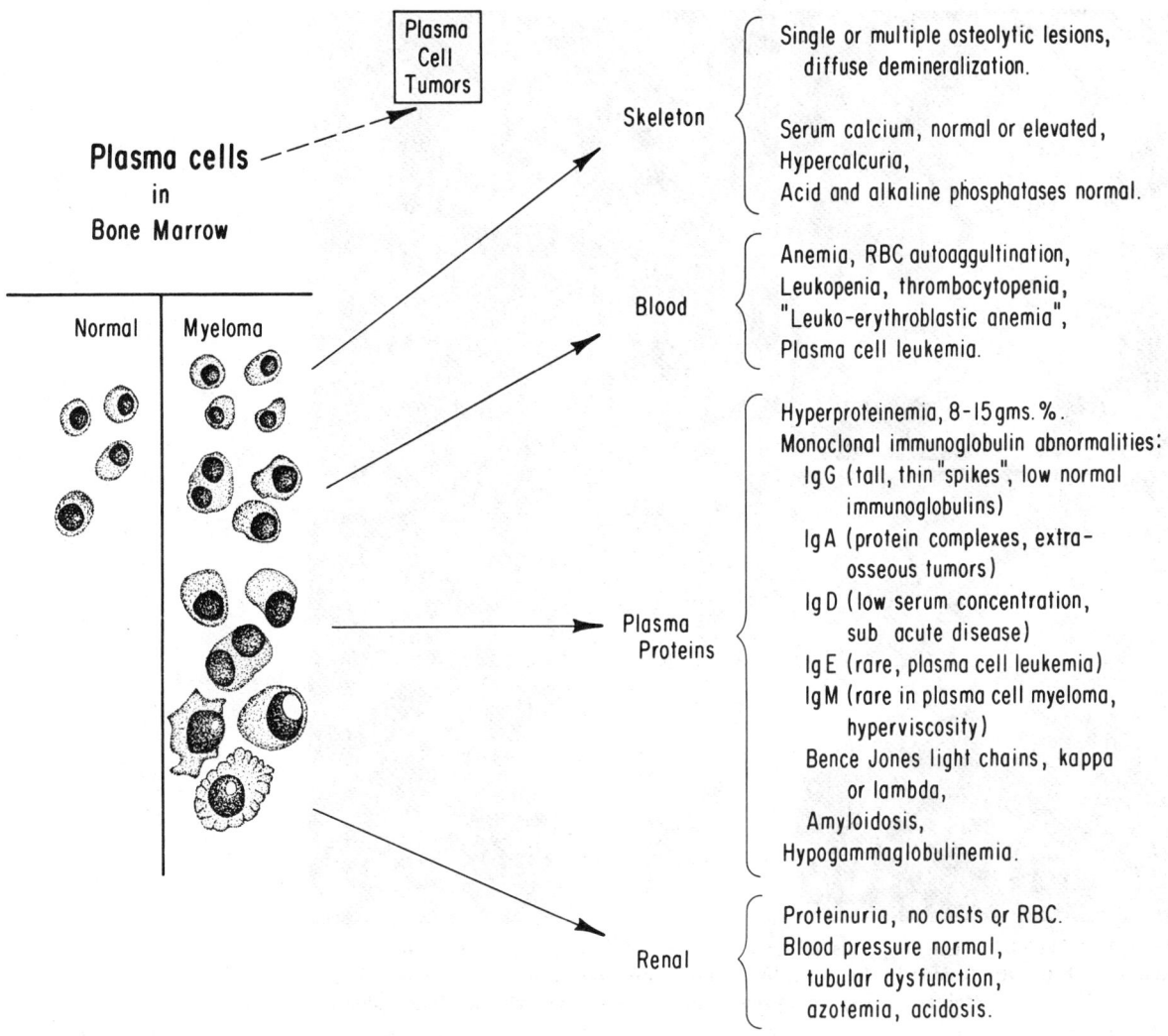

FIGURE 122-1 Pathogenesis of plasma cell myeloma.

Less than 2 percent of patients with PCM are under the age of 40 [22].

Pathogenesis

The pathophysiologic consequences of abnormal plasma cell growth are tumor formation, osteolysis hemopoietic suppression, hypogammaglobulinemia, and paraproteinuria and renal disease (see Fig. 122-1).

PLASMA CELL TUMORS

Plasma cell tumors usually develop in an area of hemopoietically active marrow and grow from a few millimeters to several centimeters in diameter during a period that may range from months to years. These tumors tend to be multiple, firm, fleshy, and pink or reddish in color. They erode adjacent bone and may compress the spinal cord or nerve roots emerging from the spinal canal.

Diffuse infiltration of the marrow by abnormal plasma cells is common also. Plasmacytomas may develop in the jaw, skull, sternum, scapulae, clavicles, ribs, vertebrae, pelvis, or proximal long bones. Occasionally plasma cell tumors develop within the shaft of a long bone—the humerus, femur, or tibia—and on rare occasions they appear to originate in extraskeletal sites such as the nasopharynx, paranasal sinuses, larynx, thorax, paravertebral or epidural tissues, lymph nodes, or gastrointestinal tract. In most instances, plasmacytomas that initially appear to be solitary become generalized [16,23–31].

SKELETAL DISEASE

Symptoms of skeletal disease are prominent initially in 70 percent of patients with PCM [16,20,21]. Diffuse or lo-

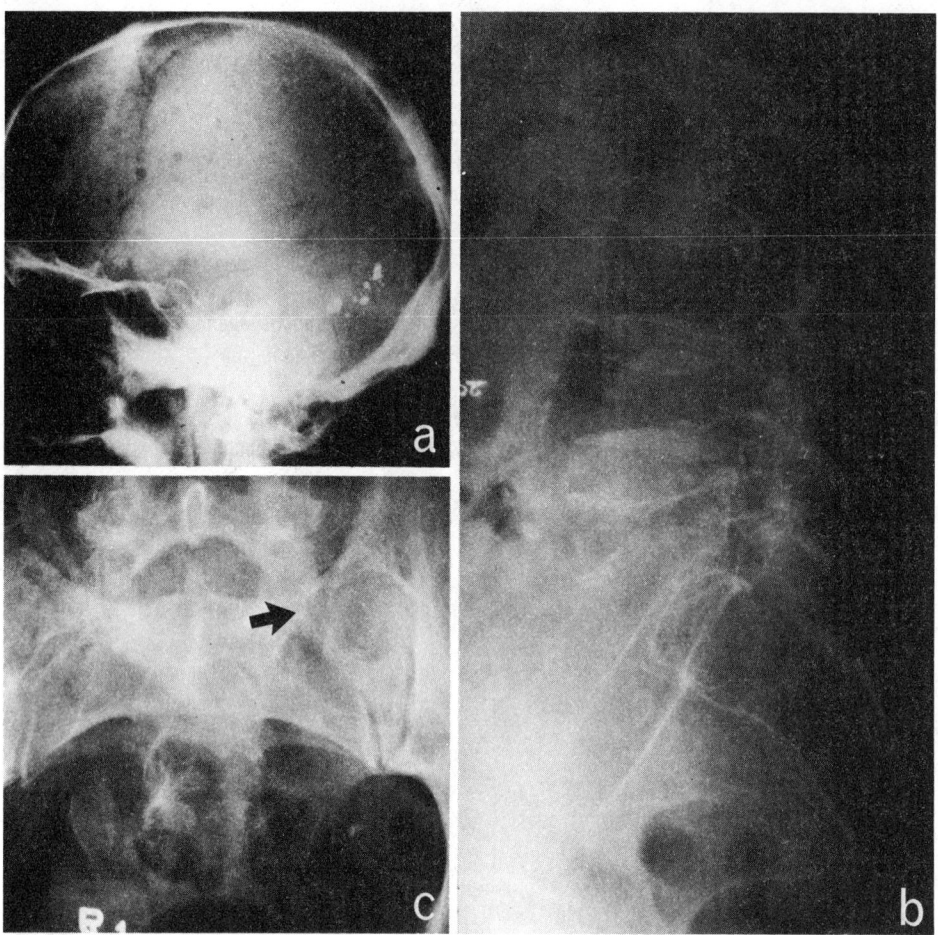

FIGURE 122-2 Skeletal roentgenograms of patients with plasma cell myeloma. (*a*) Small, "punched-out," osteolytic lesions in the skull. (*b*) Severe demineralization of the lumbar spine with partial collapse of vertebral bodies, most pronounced in L4 and L5. (*c*) Osteolytic lesion of the left sacrum.

calized areas of osteolysis develop around foci of abnormal plasma cell growth and produce characteristic symptoms, signs, and radiologic abnormalities (see below). Lesions are most evident in bones that contain hemopoietically active marrow, i.e., the skull, vertebrae, ribs, pelvis, and proximal long bones. The lesions are typically osteolytic (Figs. 122-2 and 122-3). Osteoblastic reaction occurs as a primary process in only 1 to 2 percent of untreated patients, often in association with neuropathy [32–37]. The failure of technetium 99m–labeled phosphate compounds to localize in lesions of PCM is consistent with the purely osteolytic nature of the lesions since the isotope accumulates in areas of new bone formation [38].

The serum calcium and phosphorus levels in untreated patients are usually normal or slightly elevated, although the urinary calcium excretion may be increased. The renal excretion of calcium is impaired by dehydration, and calcium mobilization from the skeleton is promoted by inactivity. Hypercalcemia is commonly observed within the first month after a patient is confined to bed with painful skeletal lesions, and this may lead to the vicious cycle of hypercalciuria → osmotic diuresis and impairment of renal tubular reabsorption → dehydration → reduced renal output → hypercalcemia and azotemia → nausea, vomiting, and further dehydration. The serum acid and alkaline phosphatase activities are usually normal in untreated patients, although some increase in alkaline phosphatase may develop with bone recalcification [37].

The mechanism of bone resorption in patients with PCM has been difficult to ascertain. Plasma cell nodules or infiltrates may not always impinge directly on the bony structures which undergo resorption, but increased osteoclast activity is usually present in these areas. The release of an osteoclast-activating factor into the medium after short-term culture of marrow from patients with PCM has been demonstrated, while in cultures of normal marrow and in those from patients with malignant lymphoma the factor was not present [39]. These observations suggest that the osteolytic lesions and demineralization which occur so frequently in pa-

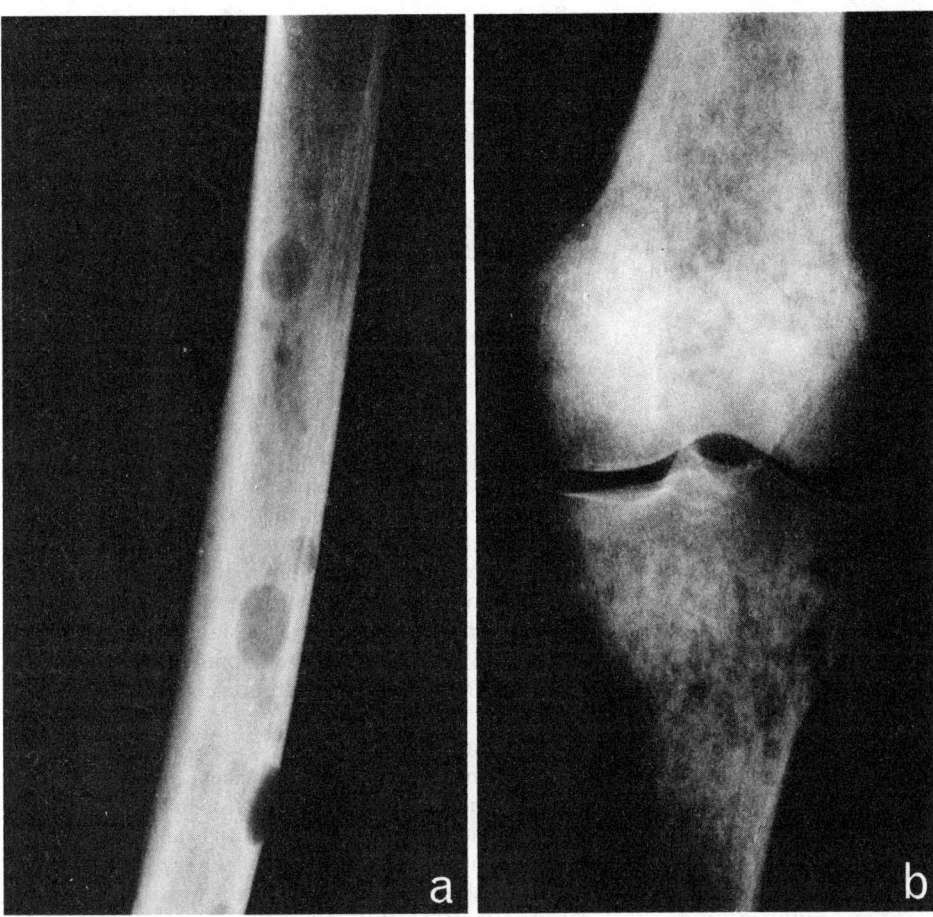

FIGURE 122-3   Bone lesions of plasma cell myeloma compared with those of breast carcinoma. (*a*) Osteolytic lesions in the femur of a patient with plasma cell myeloma. The bone destruction is purely osteolytic. (*b*) Mixed osteolytic-osteoblastic bone destruction in the femur and tibia of a patient with metastatic carcinoma of the breast.

tients with PCM may be produced indirectly by the stimulation of osteoclasts by activating factor released from neoplastic myeloma cells (see Fig. 122-4).

MARROW DYSFUNCTION

Marrow function is often impaired in patients with PCM in proportion to the number of plasma cells in the marrow, but the mechanism responsible for decreased marrow function is not known [40–43]. Anemia is most common, but neutropenia and thrombocytopenia occur also.

MONOCLONAL SERUM AND URINARY PROTEIN

SINGLE MONOCLONAL PLASMA PROTEINS
The normal individual synthesizes several classes of immunoglobulin that differ in chemical structure, metabolism, and biologic function (see Chap. 104). The total-body pool of immunoglobulin is about 1500 mg, and the half-life of different components in the circulation ranges from 2 days to 3 weeks. In plasma cell myeloma, a

FIGURE 122-4   Bone resorption by osteoclasts. Photomicrograph, using polarized light, of a section through an osteolytic lesion of the clavicle from a patient with plasma cell myeloma. The darkly stained cells are plasma cells which are not in contact with bone. The increased numbers of large, multinucleated cells are osteoclasts. (Courtesy of Dr. G. R. Mundy, University of Connecticut Health Center.)

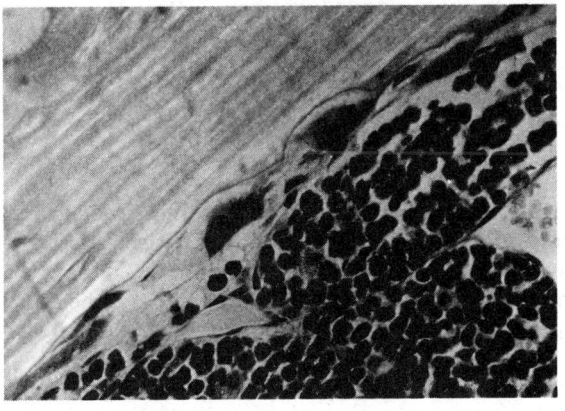

TABLE 122-1 Types of monoclonal protein produced by plasma cell neoplasms

Type of protein	Percent
Monoclonal proteins containing both H and L chains:	
IgG	52
IgA	21
IgM (macroglobulinemia)	12
IgD	2
IgE	<0.01
Monoclonal proteins containing only L chains (κ or λ)	11
Monoclonal proteins containing only H chains (γ, α, or μ)	<1
Two or more monoclonal proteins	0.5
No monoclonal protein in serum or urine	1

SOURCE: Data on 1827 patients compiled by Pruzanski and Ogryzlo [44].

single type of immunoglobulin, or portion of the immunoglobulin molecule, may be produced in excess, and usually there is a concomitant suppression in the synthesis of other classes of immunoglobulin. The anomalous proteins are "homogeneous" by chemical and immunologic criteria and are presumably synthesized by a single species of neoplastic cell.

The frequency with which different types of monoclonal proteins are produced by plasma cell neoplasms is shown in Table 122-1 [44]. The rate at which each immunoglobulin class is synthesized by healthy individuals, expressing the result as a percentage of the total immunoglobulin produced per day, is 52 percent IgG, 37 percent IgA, 10.4 percent IgM, 0.6 percent IgD, and 0.03 percent IgE [45]. Since differentiated plasma cells synthesize immunoglobulin at about the same rate, these percentages reflect the number of cells involved. The close correlation between the number and type of immunoglobulin-producing cells and the incidence of neoplasms derived from them suggests that the malignant transformation process has a random impact on all B-lymphocyte categories [46].

Some plasma cell neoplasms in humans secrete a defective heavy chain, composed primarily of the Fc portion of the molecule (see Chap. 124).

A few human plasma cell tumors produce half-molecules of IgG containing heavy- and light-chain protein [47,48], and some produce a 7 S IgM rather than the usual 19 S pentamer [49].

MULTIPLE MONOCLONAL PROTEINS

Plasma cell tumors producing two or more monoclonal proteins are found in 0.5 percent of patients [44]. The most common combination is IgM with IgG or IgA [50]. The two monoclonal proteins usually have the same type of light chain, but in some cases each type of heavy chain is combined with κ or λ light chains [51–56]. Two separate populations of immunoglobulin-producing cells have sometimes been identified by immunofluorescence studies [52,53,57,58]. Similar studies using anti-idiotypic antisera, however, have shown double staining of individual immunoglobulin-producing cells, implying that a single population of cells was capable of producing two immunoglobulins [59–61]. The structure of heavy and light chains in patients with two monoclonal proteins has been compared.

In several patients, both monoclonal proteins shared idiotypic antigenic determinants [55,56,62–64], while in others, common determinants were not found [64]. In one patient with an IgG-IgM double gammopathy, the amino acid sequence of the variable parts of the light and heavy chains and the constant part of the light chain were very similar, if not identical. In another patient with two monoclonal proteins (IgA and IgM), the light chains had identical variable and constant parts and the variable regions of the heavy chains were very similar [63,65]. These findings suggest that the same gene can code for the variable regions of two different heavy chains and also support the view that in patients with two or more monoclonal proteins, the cells which produce the different immunoglobulins either belong to the same clone or originate from a common ancestor.

LIGHT-CHAIN SECRETION

In approximately 11 percent of plasma cell neoplasms in humans, only light-chain proteins are excreted. It is not known whether the malignant cells fail to synthesize heavy chains, produce abnormal heavy chains which cannot combine with the light chain, or have some other defect in the assembly of light and heavy chains.

The amount of light-chain (Bence Jones) protein excreted in the urine is dependent on a number of factors, such as the rate of unbalanced synthesis of excess light chains, plasma volume, degradation rate, renal catabolism, and urine volume [66]. The renal clearance of light-chain protein is inversely related to the size of the molecule. With a mean molecular radius of 22 to 36 Å, the renal clearance of light-chain protein is between 9 percent and 50 percent of the creatinine clearance [67]. The amount excreted varies from a few milligrams to 25 to 40 g per 24 h. Bence Jones protein was found by the heat coagulation test in 45 percent [68]. With more sensitive techniques, investigators have found light-chain protein to be present in the urine of 70 to 80 percent of patients [21,44].

NONSECRETING MYELOMA

Monoclonal protein cannot be detected in the serum or urine of approximately 1 percent of patients with plasma cell neoplasms. The myeloma cells in some of these patients contain heavy or light chains which they are unable to secrete [69], while others are unable to synthesize either light or heavy chains [70].

NORMAL IMMUNOGLOBULIN SYNTHESIS

The amount of normal immunoglobulin in the plasma of patients with PCM is usually low. It has been suggested that this results from a feedback inhibition of normal immunoglobulin synthesis produced by the myeloma protein, even though the depression in normal immunoglobulin level does not correlate with the increased concentration of anomalous protein. Normal immunoglobulins, furthermore, are very low in patients with PCM who produce only light chains and also in those who do not synthesize detectable myeloma protein [71]. Three hypotheses have been proposed to explain the failure of normal immunoglobulin synthesis in PCM. The first postulates that myeloma cells may release ineffective subunits of RNA that alter the function of normal immunoglobulin receptors on the surface of host B lymphocytes, thereby impairing antigen recognition and antibody formation [72–74]. The second hypothesis suggests that myeloma cells release specific growth inhibitors (chalones) that block the expansion of B-lymphocyte clones in response to antigenic challenge [75,76]; and a third postulates that patients with myeloma develop a population of mononuclear suppressor cells which inhibit the capacity of normal B lymphocytes to secrete immunoglobulin [77]. Whatever mechanism is responsible for the reduced synthesis of normal immunoglobulin in patients with PCM, effective antineoplastic therapy often produces some improvement [78].

EFFECTS OF MONOCLONAL PROTEINS IN BLOOD
The plasma volume often expands as the amount of myeloma protein increases in the serum, and the resulting hemodilution may be great enough to produce a significant reduction in hemoglobin concentration with little or no change in total red cell mass [41].

Pseudohyponatremia may result from the displacement of plasma water by myeloma protein, and patients with cationic monoclonal proteins may have a reduced anion gap [79]. The hyperviscosity syndrome develops in a few patients with PCM who have high concentrations of immunoglobulins with unusual physiochemical properties [80–82], but it occurs more commonly in patients with macroglobulinemia (see below and Chap. 123).

RENAL DISEASE
A unique form of renal disease, not associated with hypertension or notable abnormalities in the urinary sediment, occurs in about 50 percent of patients with PCM. Urinary tract infections and glomerular deposits of amyloid occur in a few cases, but the major cause of renal failure is the tubular damage associated with the excretion of light chains [83,84].

Light chains are filtered and then reabsorbed and catabolized by the renal tubular cells [85–87]. The findings of positive κ and λ immunofluorescent staining within renal tubular cells, and demonstration of protein-like inclusion droplets within tubular cells, are consistent with this observation [88–93]. Renal tubular cells may be damaged during the process of reabsorption or catabolism of light chains, either by the release of lysosomal enzymes or by a direct nephrotoxic effect of the light chain. Renal tubular cell injury is manifested early by defects in the acidification and concentration of urine [84]. Light-chain proteins inhibit a variety of tubular functions in renal cortical slices, including p-aminohippuric acid and organic acid transport, gluconeogenesis, and ammoniagenesis [94,95]. In some patients specific defects in tubular reabsorption result in an increased loss of amino acids, glucose, phosphate, potassium, and other electrolytes in the urine (adult Fanconi syndrome). This syndrome may develop before PCM is recognized, and has been found mainly in patients who excrete κ-type light chains [96,97].

One of the striking features of the "myeloma kidney" is the tubular casts which contain precipitated albumin, other plasma proteins, and complete immunoglobulin molecules, or light chains [44,89]. Cast formation appears to be an end stage of chronic, progressive renal impairment. The glomerular filtration rate decreases progressively if light-chain excretion continues unabated. The load of free light chains must be excreted by fewer nephrons. The resulting increased intratubular light-chain concentration favors their precipitation with resultant cast formation.

Light-chain proteins can be detected in the blood of patients with marked renal impairment [84]. These patients also excrete more than 1.0 g of light-chain protein per 24 h. This high rate of light-chain proteinuria may in part reflect reduced tubular catabolism secondary to progressive renal damage.

Renal tubular acidosis has been reported infrequently in myeloma patients, but in one study acidification defects were found in 14 of 35 patients [84]. This was attributed to light-chain proteinuria in 13, and to hypercalcemia in 1. The renal tubular acidosis of a patient who excreted λ light chains (with a normal serum calcium and normal creatinine clearance) resolved completely as chemotherapy caused the light-chain proteinuria to disappear [75]. These observations suggest that renal tubular acidosis develops in myeloma patients as a result of a specific tubular defect caused by the excretion of light chains.

All light chains, however, are not nephrotoxic. Some patients may excrete large amounts of light chains for many years without developing evidence of renal failure. Patients excreting λ light chains tend to be at greater risk of renal insufficiency than those excreting κ light chains [84]. These findings suggest that the nephrotoxic potential of light chains is variable and related in some way to the structure of the protein. Patients excreting κ light chains survive significantly longer than those producing only λ light chains [98].

When the renal lesion is in the distal and collecting tubules the proteinuria consists primarily of light chains with albumin as a minor component. Glomeruli are not affected in myeloma except in patients who develop glomerular deposits of amyloid or an associated glomerulonephritis [84]. With glomerular lesions the proteinuria is nonselective, large amounts of albumin are excreted, and the electrophoretic pattern of the urinary protein resembles that of the serum.

Other factors which may impair renal function include hyperuricosuria, calciuria, and nephrocalcinosis, each of which occur frequently in myeloma. Dehydration is particularly hazardous in patients with severe disease. Myeloma patients are susceptible to infections, and pyelonephritis may occur. In late stages of the disease, plasma cell infiltration of the kidney may be severe enough to interfere with renal function. Plasma cells may be present in the urinary sediment [99].

Clinical features

ONSET OF MYELOMA

PCM is a progressive disease [16], but rarely the preclinical stage may be years in duration [100]. The doubling time of the abnormal cell population, calculated from the rate of increase in the amount of monoclonal protein in the serum or in the amount of light-chain protein excreted in the urine by untreated patients, has been estimated to be 3 to 10 months [101,102]. Plasmacytomas may remain localized for years before evidence of widespread disease develops. In such patients, careful investigation may lead to the discovery of less advanced multifocal disease permitting earlier treatment.

BONE PAIN

The most frequent symptom of PCM is skeletal pain, which occurs in about 70 percent of patients. Pain in the lower back or ribs aggravated by movement comes on gradually or fluctuates in intensity for weeks or months before it becomes disabling. The sudden onset of severe pain most often signifies the collapse of a vertebra or a spontaneous fracture through a diseased area in a clavicle, a rib, the pelvis, or the shaft of a long bone.

SYSTEMIC SYMPTOMS

Systemic symptoms and signs in patients with PCM include pallor, weakness, fatigue, palpitations, and dyspnea on exertion in part the result of anemia which occurs in about 70 percent of patients at the time of diagnosis. Purpura, epistaxis, or excessive bleeding with injury may result from thrombocytopenia, and signs of infection such as pneumonia, pyoderma, and pyelonephritis may result from immunoglobulin deficiencies and neutropenia. Cold sensitivity and urticaria may result from cryoglobulinemia. Edema may occur and rarely may be associated with the nephrotic syndrome.

HYPERCALCEMIA

In all patients with destructive skeletal lesions, there is an increased resorption of bone salts, which may be well tolerated if hydration is adequate and if the capacity of the kidney to excrete calcium is not exceeded. The serum calcium is elevated about 11.0 mg/dl in about 30 percent of patients at the time of diagnosis, however,

and rises above this level in an additional 30 percent during the course of the disease [10]. Hypercalcemia is most likely to occur in patients with extensive bone disease, azotemia, and hyperuricemia. The deposition of calcium salts in the renal parenchyma may produce or aggravate the kidney damage. The renal excretion of calcium is impaired by dehydration or acidosis, and the amount of calcium to be excreted increases when uncontrolled plasma cell growth produces rapid skeletal demineralization or when painful bone lesions necessitate immobilization. The symptoms of hypercalcemia may develop rapidly, with anorexia, nausea and vomiting, polyuria, polydipsia, constipation, and dehydration. Eventually drowsiness, confusion, and coma develop. The early recognition of incipient hypercalcemia in PCM is important (see below). The occasional M protein can bind calcium firmly [103–105]. These patients do not manifest the symptoms or signs of hypercalcemia, for although the total serum calcium is elevated, there is no increase in free, ionized calcium. An elevated serum calcium in an asymptomatic patient requires measurement of ionized calcium.

SUSCEPTIBILITY TO INFECTION

Patients with PCM have an increased susceptibility to infection and the disease may be discovered during an episode of pneumonia or of infection of the upper respiratory tract, paranasal sinuses, throat, skin, or urinary passages. The absence of leukocytosis in severe infections may be due to the presence of impaired marrow function.

Pneumonia due to pneumococcus infection was once the most common type of infection in patients with PCM [35,106], but recently there has been a predominance of gram-negative organisms [107]. In one study of patients with PCM hospitalized for the treatment of severe infection, 72 percent of the bacterial isolates were gram-negative organisms and none were pneumococci. Gram-negative organisms were isolated from six of the eight patients with pneumonia. The seriousness of these infections in this group of patients is illustrated by the fact that 7 out of the 11 with bacteremia and 6 of the 15 without bacteremia died of infection despite the use of antibiotic regimens [107]. In another study of patients with PCM who developed pneumonia, urinary tract infections, meningitis, and bacteremia, a similar spectrum of organisms was found [108].

Patients with PCM and macroglobulinemia are vulnerable to infection because of neutropenia and hypogammaglobulinemia, but the most important factor in both diseases seems to be deficient antibody response [106,107,109]. Patients may have repeated infections with one type of pneumococcus or may have two or more episodes of herpes zoster infection. Smallpox vaccination is dangerous in these patients because of the risk of producing generalized vaccinia. Impaired granulocyte adhesiveness, defective early granulocyte responsiveness detected by the skin window technique, and reduced levels of the fourth component of complement [110,111] may also contribute to the increased susceptibility to infection. Monoclonal B lymphocytes are increased in PCM, but their immunoglobulin synthetic functions are impaired, especially during periods of disease activity [77,112,113]. Cell-mediated immunity, however, often appears to be preserved [114].

RENAL DISEASE
Impaired renal function is an important clinical feature in 40 to 50 percent of patients.

The nephropathy in PCM may be either chronic or acute [115]. The acute disease is prone to develop in patients who have azotemia, hypercalcemia, hypotension, or infections for which nephrotoxic antibiotics are given and in those who become dehydrated. Dehydration is frequently produced by diagnostic procedures which involve fluid deprivation or the intravenous use of hypertonic contrast media [116]. In patients who may have or are known to have PCM, procedures such as intravenous or retrograde pyelograms or open bone biopsies should not be performed unless there is ample urinary flow, and not until hypercalcemia and hyperuricemia have been corrected. In PCM, as in other diseases with marrow hypercellularity, hyperuricosuria and hyperuricemia are common. The treatment of hyperuricemia and the management of chronic renal insufficiency are discussed below.

HYPERVISCOSITY
The hyperviscosity syndrome refers to a group of circulatory and hemorrhagic disturbances due to increased blood viscosity produced by the monoclonal immunoglobulins [80–82,117–121]. Purpura, ecchymoses, epistaxis, gastrointestinal bleeding, blurred or impaired vision associated with venous congestion, hemorrhages, and exudates, and a variety of ischemic neurologic symptoms are the common manifestations of hyperviscosity. The plasma volume may be greatly expanded and give the appearance of congestive heart failure. The hemodilution, however, may be of some benefit, since it reduces the blood viscosity. Many patients with this syndrome develop renal insufficiency.

The hyperviscosity syndrome occurs most typically in patients with macroglobulinemia, and in this entity its incidence is about 50 percent [120]. In PCM, the syndrome occurs in only 2 percent of patients [120].

The abnormal rheologic properties of the blood depend on the size, shape, and concentration of the anomalous immunoglobulin molecules and on protein-protein and protein-red cell interactions. In some patients, the cryoprecipitation of protein may be an important contributing factor [120,121]. In most instances, the concentration of monoclonal serum protein is at least 3 g/dl, and the plasma viscosity is increased to at least three times above normal before circulatory or hemostatic disturbances become evident. In macroglobulinemia, the increased viscosity is produced by the large, asymmetrical IgM molecules, but in PCM the formation of IgG or IgA aggregates or polymers is responsible [80,81,122,123]. The interference of these proteins with the function of platelets and the activity of coagulation factors is discussed in Chap. 123.

NEUROLOGIC DYSFUNCTION
A variety of neurologic signs and symptoms can develop in patients with plasma cell neoplasms.

MENTAL CONFUSION
Lethargy, mental obtundation, and confusion occur in most patients with hypercalcemia, and hypercalcemia should be suspected whenever these symptoms are associated with polyuria, polydipsia, nausea, vomiting, and constipation. Patients with the hyperviscosity syndrome complain of fatigue, headache, and visual disturbances. These patients often think and respond sluggishly. A history of epistaxis and the finding of cardiomegaly, distended veins, or retinopathy should trigger the measurement of serum viscosity and appropriate treatment. "Coma paraproteinemicum" has become rare now that severe hyperviscosity can be relieved promptly by plasmapheresis.

SPINAL CORD OR NERVE ROOT COMPRESSION
Spinal cord and nerve root compression occurred in about one-third of myeloma patients in the 1960s, but the incidence has decreased to about 10 percent, as a result of increased awareness, earlier diagnosis, and more effective treatment [108,124]. The plasma cell tumor often originates in a rib or vertebra, from which it invades the spinal canal and causes extradural compression. A paraspinal mass is an early warning sign that a patient is at risk of developing cord compression (see Fig. 122-5).

Early recognition of spinal cord compression is the key to successful treatment. Radicular pain, usually well-localized to a dermatome, and aggravated by coughing, sneezing, or straining, is a common early sign. Sensory and motor loss, loss of sphincter control, and paraplegia are late signs. Roentgenograms of the spinal column should be obtained as part of the initial evaluation of all patients with plasma cell neoplasms. If a paraspinal mass or destructive lesions or the vertebrae are seen, a myelogram should be done before neurologic signs become manifest. Radiation therapy can be given before neurologic complications develop.

Patients suspected of having spinal cord compression should have a myelogram, and the radioopaque dye should be left in the subarachnoid space. Follow-up studies can then be done to make sure that the upper margin of the tumor was covered by the radiation field and to check the response to treatment.

MYELOMATOUS MENINGITIS
If the CNS is involved by myeloma, a cytospin preparation of the cerebrospinal fluid (CSF) may contain plasma cells, but the total cell count is usually low. The plasma cells should disappear from the CSF following radiation therapy. The CSF protein concentration may

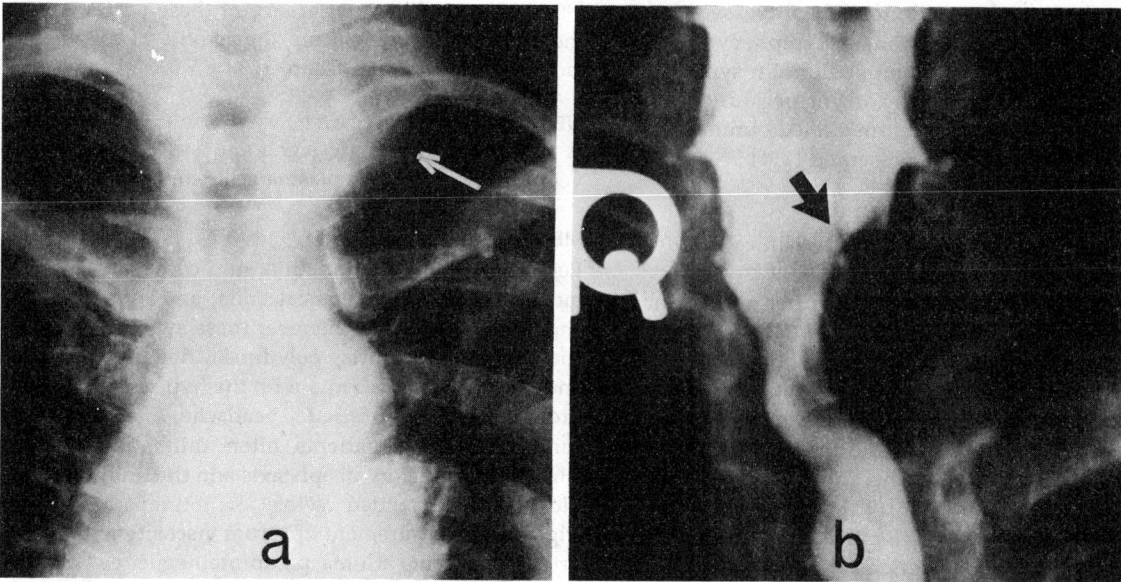

FIGURE 122-5 Chest x-ray and myelogram of a patient with plasma cell myeloma. (*a*) A paraspinal mass is evident along the left border of the upper thoracic vertebra. (*b*) An extradural defect demonstrated by myelography, indicating extension of the plasma cell tumor into the vertebral canal.

be elevated, and the CSF frequently contains the M protein. The presence of M protein in the CSF is difficult to explain when there are no plasma cells in the subarachnoid space.

An M protein was demonstrated by immunoelectrophoresis in the CSF of 16 of 20 unselected myeloma patients with a serum M protein, but no signs of spinal cord or nerve root compression [84]; thus, it is not a sign of significant CSF involvement. Patients with aggressive myeloma may develop myelomatous meningitis with extensive plasma cell infiltration of the meninges and a CSF pleocytosis [86,125].

CARPAL TUNNEL SYNDROME
The deposition of amyloid in the flexor retinaculum of the wrist frequently entraps the medial nerve causing the *carpal tunnel syndrome*. This is the commonest type of neuropathy associated with amyloidosis. The median nerve is not infiltrated with amyloid, and incision of the retinaculum usually gives lasting relief. Other patients with amyloidosis may develop diffuse sensory-motor neuropathy, with involvement of both upper and lower extremities. This neurologic involvement may ascend progressively and eventually lead to the loss of sphincter control. Nerve biopsies have shown infiltration of the nerve fibers by amyloid or amyloid deposited in the perineural vessels without evidence of axonal degeneration [126].

SENSORIMOTOR POLYNEUROPATHY
Somewhat less than 1 percent of patients with plasma cell neoplasms develop a distal sensory motor polyneuropathy that is not caused by infiltration of the nerves with amyloid or plasma cells. This neuropathy appears to occur as a "remote effect" of the plasma cell tumor, because it often improves following irradiation of solitary plasmacytomas, or treatment with melphalan and prednisone for generalized disease [127,128].

The peripheral neurology begins insidiously in the feet, and progresses gradually to involve the legs and hands. Both sensory and motor functions are impaired. In some patients the distal loss of sensation predominates while in others the major effect is loss of motor function. Pain and dysesthesia may be more disabling than the motor or sensory loss. These painful symptoms are uncommon in peripheral neuropathies due to other causes but are found in the majority of patients with plasma cell neoplasms who develop peripheral neuropathies. The CSF protein was found to be elevated above 50 mg/dl in 36 of 40 (90 percent) of myeloma patients with this sensory motor neuropathy [128].

Patients with plasma cell neoplasms who develop a diffuse sensory motor polyneuropathy have several distinctive characteristics that distinguish them from patients without a polyneuropathy [128]. These patients are recognized at a younger age (mean 50.8 years) than those with other plasma cell tumors (mean 64 years). The polyneuropathy is detected before the plasma cell neoplasm in 80 percent, and this may account in part for the earlier age at diagnosis. The polyneuropathy occurs more commonly in males, with a male/female ratio of 4:1. Solitary osseous plasmacytomas account for only 2.8 percent of all plasmacytomas, but 25 percent of those developing polyneuropathy have solitary lesions. The polyneuropathy has been reported most often with tumors producing γ heavy chains, but has also occurred with tumors producing α heavy chains, or only light chains. The light chain was λ in all of the patients tested. The serum M protein is usually low, and rarely exceeds 2.0 g/dl. While osteosclerotic bone lesions occur in much less than 1 percent of patients with plasma cell neoplasms, sclerotic lesions have been found in 22 percent with this type of neuropathy. The fact that the polyneuropathy has improved following treatment of the plasma cell tumor in 20 of the 33 (61 percent) of the reported cases strongly suggests that the neuropathy is a "remote effect" of the tumor. A new syndrome has been reported from Japan of the association of osteosclerotic myeloma, polyneuropathy, certain endocrine disturbances (diabetes, hypertrichosis, and gynecomastia) and skin changes (hyperpigmentation, hyperhidrosis, and skin thickening) [129].

INTRACEREBRAL PLASMACYTOMAS
Plasma cell tumors rarely invade the central nervous system, but examples have been reported, including apparently solitary intracerebral plasma cell tumors [130–132]. Plasma cell tumors in the vault of the skull rarely cause any symptoms, because these tumors tend to grow out rather than in. Tumors involving the base of the skull, however, can compress cranial nerves and cause palsies. Orbital lesions can cause proptosis.

VIRAL INFECTIONS
Herpes zoster was recorded in 2 percent of 169 patients seen at the Mayo Clinic [21], but our own experience suggests a greater prevalance. Repeated infections in the same or in different dermatomes have been reported.

Multifocal leukoencephalopathy is a devastating and currently untreatable, viral infection that may complicate the course of patients with plasma cell neoplasms [132].

Laboratory features

BLOOD
Overgrowth of plasma cells may produce pancytopenia, or may evoke a leukoerythroblastic reaction, with nucleated red cells and immature granulocytes present in the circulating blood (see Chap. 52). In one study the hemoglobin concentration was reduced to less than 12.0 g/dl in 62 percent of the patients, and leukopenia and thrombocytopenia were present in 16 and 13 percent of the patients, respectively [21].

The anemia of patients with PCM is usually normochromic and normocytic, and may be mild to moderately severe. In addition to abnormal marrow function, other contributory factors may include shortened erythrocyte survival, increased blood loss, renal insufficiency, and effects of radiotherapy or chemotherapy. The Coombs' test is almost invariably negative. An increased plasma protein concentration may lead to an ex-

panded plasma volume and a reduction in hemoglobin concentration and in the packed red cell volume disproportionate to the reduction in total red cell mass [41].

The degree of leukopenia and thrombocytopenia in untreated patients with PCM is usually mild. The total leukocyte count is often reduced to 3000 to 4000 per microliter largely because of neutropenia. The failure of some patients to develop a leukocytosis in response to an acute infection such as pneumococcal pneumonia may suggest impaired marrow function. A small number of plasma cells may be found in the circulating blood of many patients, and if the absolute number of plasma cells exceeds 2000 per microliter the diagnosis of plasma cell leukemia may be made. Pathologic rouleaux formation and a rapid red cell sedimentation rate are well-known effects of hyperglobulinemia which occur regardless of etiology and of the presence or relative proportion of monoclonal globulin constituents.

MARROW
In nearly all cases the diagnosis of PCM requires examination of the marrow. Since the distribution of plasma cell foci is often spotty, marrow for aspiration/biopsy is best obtained from areas where there is increased bone tenderness or radiologic evidence of osteolysis. In average patients with moderately advanced disease, 20 to 95 percent of the nucleated cells in the marrow are mature or immature plasma (myeloma) cells. The percent of plasma cells in the marrow varies with the sample and is not a reliable measure of the total amount of disease present.

The neoplastic cells have an abundance of basophilic cytoplasm and eccentric nuclei with a paranuclear clear zone and prominent nucleoli. Multinucleated plasma cells occur frequently, and in some patients, vacuolelike intranuclear inclusions may be present [16]. Various cytoplasmic inclusions, such as multiple grapelike accumulations of immunoglobulin, round bodies which stain cherry-red with Wright's stain, and, rarely, crystalline azurophilic rods, may be present [16].

The plasma cells in patients with chronic disease may appear to be mature and virtually normal in morphology, in contrast to the neoplastic cells in patients with very acute disease, in whom the cells may be small, shaggy, irregular in contour, and even difficult to identify as plasma cells.

Electron microscopic studies of plasma cells in myeloma show a highly developed network of endoplasmic reticulum, in which γ-globulin has been demonstrated with ferritin-labeled antibody [134,135]. The ultrastructure of the abnormal plasma cells is pleomorphic, and in some instances the structural features are intermediate between lymphocytes and plasma cells [136].

The peripheral cytoplasm of the neoplastic plasma cells which produce IgA serum constituents may have a distinctly reddish tinge or even be bright red in areas and may give the appearance of "flaming" plasma cells [137,138]. It is impossible to assess the functional capacity of plasma cells by morphologic criteria, however, or

TABLE 122-2 Clinical features of plasma cell myeloma compared with immunoglobulin status

	IgG	IgA	BJ*
Number of patients	112	54	40
Myeloma protein in serum, mean concentration, g/dl	4.3	2.8	±
Immunoglobulin <20% normal	68	30	19
Hospital admissions, infection, %	60	33	20
Osteolytic bone lesions, %	55	65	78
Hypercalcemia	33	59	62
Azotemia, urea above 79 mg/dl	16	17	33
Detected amyloidosis, %	0.5	7	10
Mean doubling time of myeloma protein, months	10.1	6.3	3.4

*BJ = Bence Jones protein.
SOURCE: Data from Hobbs [100].

sometimes even to distinguish between a benign, reactive plasmacytosis and a neoplastic proliferation when the plasma cells in the bone marrow are few in number or comparatively normal in morphology. The bone marrow of patients with PCM may occasionally contain a greatly increased number of mast cells, but this is more characteristic of macroglobulinemia.

In some patients with PCM the consistency of the marrow makes aspiration difficult, and in others only 5 to 10 percent of the total nucleated cells in the marrow may be plasma cells. In either instance, sections of marrow obtained by needle biopsy may show a heavy focal or diffuse accumulation of abnormal plasma cells. In some patients, myelofibrosis with hypoplasia of the erythroid and granulocytic elements may be present, with only a relative increase in the number of plasma cells. Megaloblastic erythroid maturation may be found in a few patients. When the marrow findings in a given patient suspected of having PCM are equivocal or nondiagnostic, a careful search should be made for the presence of monoclonal immunoglobulin components in the serum or urine and for extraskeletal plasma cell tumors.

BIOCHEMICAL ABNORMALITIES
The serum and urine protein abnormalities are discussed in detail in Chap. 121.

Azotemia is a frequent finding in patients with PCM. Hyperuricemia may accompany renal failure or may occur in the absence of azotemia. Hypercalcemia also occurs frequently. The alkaline phosphatase is normal or slightly elevated, even in patients with extensive bone lesions.

SKELETAL FINDINGS
On x-ray examination the typical bone changes of PCM are multiple, "punched out," purely osteolytic lesions occurring in bones that house hemopoietically active marrow. However, diffuse demineralization or bone lesions in the distal extremities also occur, and rarely the lesions may be osteoblastic [32–37]. Diffuse or spotty osteosclerosis may develop if disorders such as

Paget's disease or metastatic carcinoma are coincidentally present. Localized osteoblastic changes may develop in PCM in regions of the skeleton that have received intensive radiotherapy.

Radioisotope bone scans using technetium 99m–labeled phosphate compounds are rarely helpful in identifying skeletal lesions in patients with PCM since the isotopes used tend to localize in areas of new bone formation and do not concentrate in purely osteolytic lesions [38]. When bone scans do show lesions in PCM it is usually around areas of new bone formation at fracture sites or following radiotherapy.

About 10 to 15 percent of patients with PCM have no demonstrable bone disease, and about 7 percent of patients present with plasmacytomas which appear to be solitary by radiologic criteria [30]. To establish that such lesions are, in fact, "solitary," it is necessary to demonstrate that marrow aspirated from multiple sites is normal and that if an abnormal protein is present in the serum and/or urine, it disappears following excision or radiotherapy. Generalized disease eventually develops in the majority of patients who present with apparently solitary plasmacytomas [30,31].

Relationship between clinical findings and immunoglobulin abnormalities

A possible relationship between specific immunoglobulin abnormalities and particular clinical features is implied by the frequently used cliché describing patients as having "IgG κ" or "IgA λ" myeloma, etc. A tabulation of the findings in a large group of patients with PCM, however, showed that there were only a few general and overlapping correlations (Table 122-2) [139,140]. Patients with IgG components tended to have a more chronic disease, a greater reduction in the amount of normal γ-globulin, and more infections requiring hospitalization than other groups. Patients who excrete Bence Jones light-chain protein in their urine and have no abnormal serum constitutents tend to have more bone and renal disease and amyloidosis. They are likely to have more aggressive disease, as judged by the shorter doubling time of their protein excretion during periods without treatment [139]. These clinical correlations were confirmed later in a study of 97 patients with light-chain disease, in whom the incidence of renal disease was greater than in patients with IgG and IgA serum components [98]. Those with λ light-chain proteinuria had a shorter survival than those with κ light-chain proteinuria [98]. Seven of the 97 patients developed acute plasma cell leukemia during the period of observation (see below).

Patients with IgD serum components have a high incidence of enlarged lymph nodes, hepatosplenomegaly, extramedullary tumors, and amyloidosis. A remarkably high incidence of Bence Jones proteinemia, a preponderance of λ light chain proteinuria, and a short survival due to the tendency of these patients to develop acute terminal exacerbations were observed [141].

Patients with IgE serum components have typical PCM [140,142–144].

Differential diagnosis

The diagnosis of PCM in patients with osteolytic bone lesions, 10 percent or more abnormal plasma cells in the marrow, and monoclonal serum proteins or light-chain proteinuria is not difficult. Each of these manifestations may occur in other diseases: osteolytic bone lesions in metastatic carcinoma or hyperparathyroidism; marrow plasmacytosis in acute serum sickness and in chronic infections or liver disease, which characteristically produce polyclonal hyperglobulinemia; monoclonal globulin components or Bence Jones proteinuria in some benign or hereditary diseases, etc.

In patients with aplastic or hypoplastic anemia, the number of plasma cells in the marrow may be relatively increased. In these instances, it is best to defer interpretation until a meticulous search for other evidences of myeloma has been made and, on occasion, the course of the disease documented. Patients may present with renal failure due to plasma cell myeloma without the basic disease having previously been recognized. An examination of the marrow and search for monoclonal serum and urine proteins ordinarily clarifies the diagnosis. In the chronic cold agglutinin syndrome, the agglutinin is a monoclonal macroglobulin, the level of which, as with benign monoclonal gammopathy, may remain constant for many years [145].

The most common entity in which anomalous serum protein components occur is benign monoclonal gammopathy (see Chap. 113). These patients have no bone disease and only a small percentage of plasma cells in the bone marrow. The monoclonal serum immunoglobulin is usually less than 1 to 1.5 g/dl, and serial measurements over a period of 2 to 3 years show no increase. Progression to myeloma, macroglobulinemia, or amyloidosis has been reported for 11 percent of benign monoclonal gammopathy patients followed for 7 years [146]. Anomalous immunogobulin components occur in 2 to 5 percent of patients with CLL or lymphocytic lymphoma (see Chaps. 115 and 119).

In macroglobulinemia and heavy-chain disease, the abnormal marrow elements are more closely related to lymphocytes than to plasma cells. Skeletal lesions and impairment of renal function are rare. In heavy-chain disease, enlargement of the lymph nodes and splenomegaly are frequent, but the clinical manifestations are variable (see Chap. 124), particularly in those with double gammopathy [50].

Monoclonal proteins have been discovered in association with two dermatologic conditions. Papular mucinosis (lichen myxedematosus) is characterized by the deposition in the skin of mucinous material which forms papules and plaques. Serum electrophoresis shows the presence of a monoclonal protein characteristic of the disease, usually an IgG component with λ-type light chains. The anomalous protein is basic and has a slower mobility than any other γ-globulin constituent. In this entity, marrow plasmacytosis, osteolytic bone lesions, and light-chain proteinuria occur rarely [147–149]. An excellent response to melphalan therapy has been reported [150], which supports the view that papular mucinosis is an unusual variety of plasma cell disease.

Pyoderma gangrenosum is another skin disease in which abnormal monoclonal components have been reported [151]. The proteins may belong to one of the three major classes of immunoglobulin, IgG, IgA, or IgM.

Monoclonal proteins have been reported to occur in association with a variety of neoplasms originating in tissues which normally do not produce immunoglobulins [20]. Some of these tumors have been shown to be infiltrated with plasma cells which can be stained with fluorescent antibodies that react specifically with the class of monoclonal protein in the serum. The anomalous protein is apparently not produced by the neoplasm but may represent an immune response to the tumor or the development of a plasma cell neoplasm as a second malignant disease.

Metastatic carcinomas from the breast, prostate, or lung may produce skeletal lesions which mimic those of PCM, and on occasion more than one malignant growth may be present. When blood-borne tumor metastases infiltrate the bone marrow, tumor cells can usually be demonstrated by aspiration or needle biopsy. Hyperparathyroidism may produce destructive bone lesions, hypercalcemia, and renal dysfunction, but the proteins in this disease are normal, and the alkaline phosphatase level is usually strikingly elevated. Plasma cells in the marrow are not increased, and there is often a great increase in osteoblasts and osteoclasts (see Chap. 52).

Plasmacytosis may occur in the marrow of patients with hepatitis, cirrhosis of the liver, Hodgkin's disease, and occasionally hypernephroma. In these entities, the serum γ-globulin level may be elevated, sometimes to a striking degree, but electrophoresis always shows the presence of a broad-based, heterogeneous, polyclonal hyperglobulinemia.

Several categories of atypical disease are produced by the proliferation of abnormal plasma cells. Many patients who do not have typical myeloma have chronic arthritic symptoms and recurrent evidence of active arthritis or destructive joint disease, which may or may not be associated with amyloidosis (see Chap. 129). Patients who have amyloidosis associated with PCM may present with cutaneous plaques, tumors, hepatosplenomegaly, infiltrative lesions of the gastrointestinal submucosa, or renal infitration producing nephrosis (see Chap. 129) [152,153].

The Fanconi syndrome in adults may be a premyeloma manifestation [96]. Diffuse bone demineralization may be produced by abnormal plasma cell proliferation, as stipulated above, but it may occur as an idiopathic entity associated in retrospect with benign monoclonal gammopathy [154].

The excretion of Bence Jones protein in amounts greater than 60 mg daily usually indicates a plasma cell neoplasm [155], but patients with benign idiopathic Bence Jones proteinuria who excrete a gram or more of light-chain protein daily for several years have been observed [156]. Difficult diagnostic problems may be presented by patients with unusual patterns of disturbed immunoglobulin synthesis. Patients may produce and secrete IgG but produce and retain IgM on the cell membranes [157]; and some patients with nonsecretory myelomatosis, with no monoclonal immunoglobulin in the serum, urine, or inside or outside the neoplastic cell, have been reported [158].

Cervical lymph node metastases may be the first manifestation of extramedullary plasmacytomas, about 75 percent of which arise in the upper respiratory tract and oropharynx [159].

Establishing a diagnosis

The asymptomatic patient who is discovered to have a monoclonal protein should have a marrow aspiration, skeletal roentgenograms, and study of the serum and urinary proteins (see Chap. 125). The occurrence in the marrow of more than 10 percent mature and immature plasma cells, osteolytic skeletal lesions, and a plasma monoclonal protein confirms the diagnosis of PCM. Marrow infiltration with plasma cells is frequently spotty, so that failure to demonstrate marrow plasmacytosis does not rule out PCM. If plasmacytosis is not demonstrated in one site, others should be aspirated, or bone lesions biopsied. The excretion of more than 60 mg per 24 h of a single type of light chain in the urine or a monoclonal serum protein concentration of greater than 2 g/dl is suggestive of a plasma cell tumor. If marrow plasmacytosis is not demonstrated, and if there are no osteolytic skeletal lesions, a search should be made for an extraskeletal plasma cell tumor; possible sites include the nose, paranasal sinuses, oral pharynx, bronchi, skin, lymph nodes, and intestinal mucosa.

If a diagnosis of PCM cannot be made after the above investigation, a search should be made for other malignant diseases (e.g., leukemia, lymphoma, carcinoma) that may be associated with monoclonal serum proteins. A rectal mucosal biopsy may be obtained to search for amyloid deposits. If a diagnosis of PCM cannot be established, the working diagnosis becomes benign monoclonal gammopathy. These patients should be reevaluated periodically. A progressive increase in the concentration of the monoclonal protein is a basic feature of plasma cell neoplasia. Some tumors have such a slow growth rate, however, that it may not be possible to establish the diagnosis until the patient has been observed for 10 years or more.

To establish the diagnosis of a plasma cell neoplasm

one must detect evidence of uncontrolled growth of plasma cells such as invasion and destruction of normal tissues (e.g. osteolytic lesions, or plasma cell tumors in other sites), or a progressive increase in the concentration of serum monoclonal protein or in the amount of Bence Jones protein excreted in the urine.

Treatment

GENERAL PRINCIPLES
The chronic phase of plasma cell neoplasms may last from 1 to more than 10 years after the onset of clinical disease. During this phase most patients respond well to chemotherapy and derive considerable benefit from encouragement and supportive and antineoplastic treatment. The acute terminal phase is usually short and unresponsive to therapy.

An important objective in the management of most patients with plasma cell neoplasms is to relieve pain so that they may remain ambulatory. Skeletal x-rays will serve as a guide to the appropriate form of treatment of the bone pain. Back pain is the most common presenting symptom; and if this is due to localized osteolytic lesions, they may respond well to irradiation. In patients who develop severe demineralization in association with PCM the back pain usually is not relieved by irradiation; for these patients it is better to initiate chemotherapy promptly, and begin to ambulate them cautiously. All patients should be encouraged to be as active as possible in order to avoid further demineralization and weakening of the bone structure. Simple lumbar corsets or a back brace often helps to relieve back pain by stabilizing the spine and preventing rapid rotational movements which may precipitate microfractures and muscle spasms. These supports are usually only required until the back pain is relieved by radiotherapy or chemotherapy. Fractures of the long bones may be fixed with an intramedullary pin and then irradiated. Large osteolytic lesions should be irradiated before a fracture occurs.

Throughout the course of active disease, patients must be reminded to drink 2000 to 3000 ml of fluids daily to maintain the increased urinary output required for the excretion of light chains, calcium, uric acid, and other metabolites. All infections must be investigated and treated promptly.

It is important throughout the course of the disease to record systematically all relevant hematologic and treatment data and indices of the clinical status for each patient. The most useful primary indices of disease activity are measurements of the concentration of monoclonal protein in the serum and determinations of the amount and type of protein excreted in the urine.

ANTINEOPLASTIC THERAPY
Alkylating agents, radiotherapy, and prednisone are the mainstays of treatment. Many other chemotherapeutic agents have been evaluated in the treatment of PCM,

but none have proved to be sufficiently effective to be used regularly (see Table 122-3).

ALKYLATING AGENTS

Many alkylating agents, including melphalan [11,12], cyclophosphamide [13], chlorambucil [160] and carmustine (BCNU) [161], have been reported to produce objective improvement in 30 to 50 percent of patients with plasma cell neoplasms.

Most alkylating agents are equally toxic for resting and proliferating cells. In this respect cyclophosphamide is unique, for regenerating mouse marrow cells are much more sensitive to this agent than are resting marrow cells [162]. Cyclophosphamide has also been shown to be schedule-dependent [163], producing greater antitumor effect when given intermittently than when given daily at doses which produce the same toxicity. This schedule dependency may be partly explained by the fact that the drug becomes increasingly toxic for hematopoietic cells during daily administration as resting stem cells are drawn into cycle to replace injured cells. For these reasons many chemotherapists favor administering cyclophosphamide in large doses intermittently, allowing marrow function to recover before the dose is repeated. However, there has been no clinical trial to determine the superiority of high-dose intermittent cyclophosphamide in the treatment of PCM.

The dose schedules commonly used for these alkylating agents are shown in Table 122-4. Although melphalan and carmustine (BCNU) are not schedule-dependent, the intermittent administration of these agents permits a patient to be seen at 4- to 6-week intervals for blood counts, the measurement of the serum and/or urinary monoclonal proteins and a repeat course of therapy. Alternatively, daily therapy with small dose of

TABLE 122-3 Rationale for using therapeutic agents in plasma cell myeloma

To suppress growth of plasma cells:
  Nitrogen mustard derivatives
    L-Phenylaline mustard (melphalan)
    Cyclophosphamide
  Adrenal corticosteroids, ACTH
  Radiotherapy to local areas, tumors

To promote bone remineralization:
  Activity, physical therapy
  Anabolic steroids
  Androgens
  Fluoride, vitamin D, calcium

To promote erythropoiesis:
  Androgenic steroids
    Testosterone
    Fluoxymesterone

To relieve pain:
  Bed rest (acute), physical therapy,
    orthopedic supports, salicylates,
    analgesics, radiotherapy

alkylating agent may be used [e.g., 164]. Such maintenance therapy may require more frequent visits for blood counts. However, the same proportion of objective responses and the same prolongation of survival is achieved with low-dose continuous melphalan therapy [164] as with the high-dose intermittent regimen.

When intermittent dosage schedules of melphalan or carmustine are used, patients should have blood counts done at weekly intervals after the first course. If the granulocyte count does not fall below 500 per microliter or platelets below 70,000 per microliter and the granulocyte count has increased to more than 1000 per microli-

TABLE 122-4   Dosage schedules for alkylating agents

Drug	Intermittent	Continuous
	The full dose is given for 1 to 4 days and repeated at regular intervals	A *loading dose* is given for a limited period; the drug is stopped until the leukocyte count rises to 4000 per microliter; *daily* therapy is then started and adjusted to maintain the count between 2000 to 3500 per microliter
1. Cyclophosphamide	1000 mg/m² (27 mg/kg) intravenously, or 250 mg/m² per day × 4 days orally; repeat every 3–4 weeks	*Loading:* 10 mg/kg per day for 7 to 10 days orally or intravenously *Daily:* 1–3 mg/kg per day
2. Melphalan	9 mg/m² per day × 4 days (0.25 mg/kg per day × 4) orally; repeat every 4–6 weeks	*Loading:* 10 mg per day for 7 to 10 days orally* *Daily:* 1–3 mg per day
3. BCNU	150 mg/m² intravenously; repeat every 4–6 weeks	
4. Chlorambucil		*Loading:* 0.2 mg/kg per day orally for 3 to 6 weeks *Daily:* 1 to 3 mg per day

* In some successful regimens the loading dose is omitted and therapy started with 2 to 4 mg per day orally, with dosage adjustments according to the blood count [164].

ter, and platelets to more than 100,000 per microliter by the fourth to sixth week, the original dose should be repeated. The dose should be reduced if granulocytopenia or thrombocytopenia is more marked or prolonged. If the counts are too low for therapy to be repeated by the fourth week, the second course of the drug should be delayed for 2 or more weeks, until recovery occurs. The appropriate dose, causing only moderate granulocytopenia or thrombocytopenia with recovery, should be repeated regularly at 4- to 6-week intervals.

The absorption of melphalan from the gastrointestinal tract has been shown to be erratic [166,167]. A dose of 0.25 mg/kg per day for 4 days usually causes some degree of neutropenia and/or thrombocytopenia. However, for occasional patients, the total dose may need to be increased to 1.5 to 2.0 mg/kg, or more, in order to cause marrow toxicity. The dose of melphalan should be increased until there is evidence of a response, or hematologic toxicity. If there is no response, or toxicity, with doses of 0.5 mg/kg per day for 4 days administered orally, consideration should be given to using the intravenous form of melphalan. Intravenous melphalan is more toxic than the oral form. The daily intravenous treatment should be started at a dose of 0.25 mg/kg.

Once the dose which causes moderate toxicity, or a response, has been established, it is usually adequate to check blood counts prior to repeating the drug treatment, to be sure that cumulative toxicity is not developing. Some patients will develop a progressive fall in leukocytes and platelets following repeated courses of melphalan or carmustine. When this happens, treatment should be stopped until the blood counts return to pretreatment levels, and then restarted using longer intervals between courses of treatment.

Following a 1000 mg/m² dose of cyclophosphamide, the leukocyte count falls to a nadir at 10 to 12 days, with recovery by 17 to 21 days [165]. Blood counts should be obtained on days 10, 12, and 21 after a course of cyclophosphamide. If the granulocyte nadir is above 500 per microliter, and the count is near pretreatment levels by day 21, the same dose is repeated. The dose should be reduced if the granulocytopenia is more severe than this. When the appropriate dose is determined, it should be repeated regularly at 3- to 4-week intervals, with blood counts before each treatment. Cumulative toxicity usually does not occur with cyclophosphamide. This drug may be given as a single dose of 1000 mg/m² intravenously, or orally in a dose of 250 mg/m² per day for 4 days. The drug should be given in the morning, and the patients instructed to take 2500 to 3000 ml of fluids to ensure the prompt excretion of the drug and its metabolites to minimize contact with the bladder mucosa. Patients who become so nauseated that they cannot drink adequate amounts of fluid should be hospitalized and given intravenous fluids. These measures are necessary to reduce the chance of the patients' developing cyclophosphamide-induced hemorrhagic cystitis.

The frequency of objective improvement following

the treatment of groups of patients with PCM is probably very similar for melphalan, cyclophosphamide, carmustine, and chlorambucil. Melphalan and cyclophosphamide are the most commonly used drugs, however.

The sensitivity of a plasma cell neoplasm to different alkylating agents may vary considerably. A mouse plasma cell tumor has been described which is highly resistant to carmustine, moderately resistant to melphalan, and very sensitive to cyclophosphamide [168]. It would appear that intrinsic cellular factors determine whether a cell will be sensitive to an alkylating agent, rather than the proliferative state of the cell or the alkylating function of the agent. One-third of a group of patients who were shown to be resistant to melphalan achieved an objective response with high-dose, intermittent cyclophosphamide therapy [169]. An example of a patient who responded well to melphalan, relapsed despite continued treatment, and then achieved another remission with cyclophosphamide is shown in Fig. 122-6. Cyclophosphamide is recommended for the treatment of patients who present with platelet counts of less than 100,000 per microliter, or for those who develop thrombocytopenia during treatment with another alkylating agent. Cyclophosphamide is less toxic to thrombopoiesis than other alkylating agents, and thrombocytopenic patients are usually able to tolerate this drug better than other alkylating agents.

PREDNISONE

Corticosteroid treatment of patients with PCM corrects hypercalcemia by reducing bone resorption [170]; causes a fall in serum protein concentrations, including that of the monoclonal protein; decreases proteinuria; and produces a substantial rise in the hematocrit of some patients [171]. The persistence of marrow plasmacytosis suggests that the fall in the monoclonal protein associated with prednisone therapy may not be due to a direct, injurious effect on myeloma cells, but instead to the induction of hypercatabolism of proteins, resulting in a negative nitrogen balance and lowered serum protein concentrations [172,173]. Prednisone therapy alone, however, has been observed to decrease the size of a plasmacytoma [171], suggesting that this drug may have a direct antineoplastic action in some patients.

OTHER AGENTS

Procarbazine has been shown to lower the serum M-protein concentration, and to lengthen the survival of mice bearing plasma cell tumor LPC-1 [174]. In clinical trials, a lowering of the serum M-protein concentration to less than 50 percent of the pretreatment value was observed in 5 of 36 patients previously treated with melphalan, but this improvement was not associated with a significant change in marrow plasmacytosis [175,176]. This observation suggests that procarbazine may have some activity against plasma cell neoplasms.

Doxorubicin hydrochloride (Adriamycin) produced short objective remissions in 6 of 32 patients who were resistant to other forms of treatment [177,178].

cis-Platinum appears to be an effective agent in the

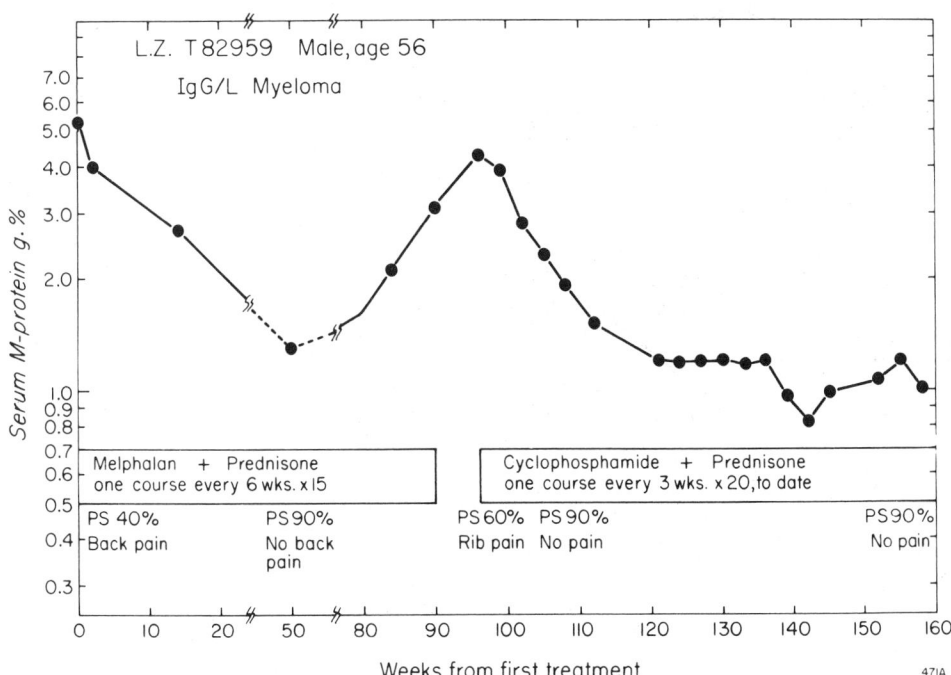

FIGURE 122-6 The effect of the oral administration of melphalan (0.25 mg/kg per day for 4 days) and prednisone (200 mg per day for 4 days), repeated at 6-week intervals, followed by cyclophosphamide (250 mg/m² per day for 4 days) and prednisone (200 mg/day for 4 days), repeated at 3-week intervals, and the monoclonal protein of the patient with plasma cell myeloma. A good initial response to melphalan and prednisone was followed by relapse. A second remission followed treatment with cyclophosphamide and prednisone. PS = performance status, Karnofsky scale. (Bergsagel, Cowan, and Hasselback [169], with permission.)

treatment of mouse myeloma but has not been tested adequately against human myeloma to date [179,180].

INTERFERON

Interferons are potent antiviral glycoproteins which have been shown to inhibit the proliferation of tumor cells in experimental systems. Interferon has been shown to inhibit the growth of neoplastic human cell lines in culture, and has induced objective improvement in at least 11 of 15 myeloma patients [181–183]. Excellent, long-lasting remissions have been achieved, with a fall in serum M protein, improvement in bone pain, and weight gain. The major toxicity is fever, which has been attributed to impurities in the human leukocyte interferon. Other toxic effects, which may be caused by the inhibition of growth and differentiation by interferon, include leukopenia, thrombocytopenia, and hair loss. The biological mechanisms underlying the antitumor properties of interferon are unknown but are of great interest because this substance is produced by normal cells.

DRUG COMBINATIONS

The addition of prednisone to intermittent courses of melphalan doubles the response rate but has little influence on survival [184]. Combining procarbazine with melphalan and prednisone increases the response rate but has little effect on survival [185].

The addition of Adriamycin to melphalan or cyclophosphamide and prednisone did not improve the response rate or survival [186].

The discovery that mouse and human plasma cell tumors that are resistant to one alkylating agent may still respond to another drug of this class, indicated that different alkylating agents are not necessarily cross-resistant [168,169]. Furthermore, combinations of alkylating agents have been shown to be synergistic in the treatment of two murine tumors [187,188]. These observations stimulated clinical trials of combinations of alkylating agents in the treatment of plasma cell myeloma. Combinations containing melphalan and cyclophosphamide with carmustine [186] and with prednisone [189,190] did not significantly change the survival of patients with myeloma, although the response rate of patients may be improved when drugs are given intravenously rather than orally [191,192].

Studies of the labeling index of myeloma marrow plasma cells before and after treatment demonstrated a marked temporary increase in the index after treatment with alkylating agents [193,194].

Trials of cycle-specific agents were initiated in an attempt to destroy the increased fraction of proliferating myeloma cells occurring after treatment with an alkylating agent. In a preliminary trial, vincristine caused a modest additional decrease in myeloma cell number, and was selected for further study in drug combinations

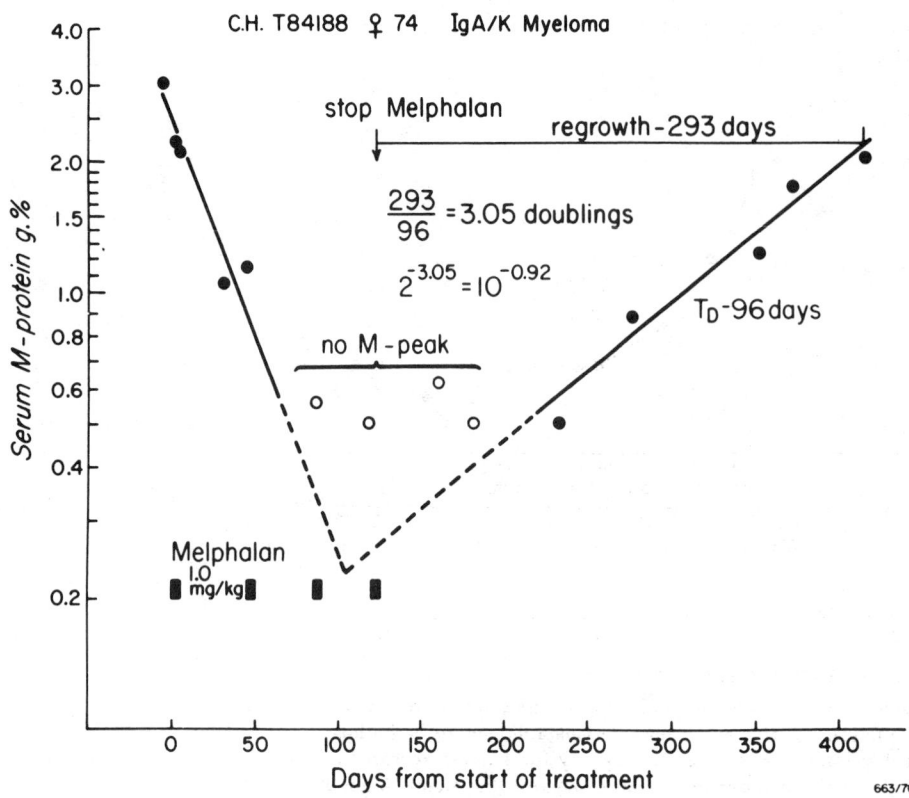

FIGURE 122-7 Estimation of the myeloma cell kill following chemotherapy. A patient with IgA κ myeloma serum component was treated with four courses of melphalan (0.25 mg/kg per day for 4 days). The monoclonal protein disappeared from the serum after the second course of treatment, and melphalan was stopped after the fourth course. The anomalous protein reappeared at 225 days. The amount increased exponentially, with a doubling time (T_D) of 96 days, after 293 days reached the pretreatment value. Dividing the time required for regrowth (293 days) by the T_D (96 days) indicates that the melphalan therapy reduced the tumor mass about tenfold ($10^{-0.92}$).

[195]. Drug combinations of vincristine, Adriamycin, and prednisone plus either melphalan or cyclophosphamide or carmustine appear to improve survival by reducing the number of early deaths [196,197], although longer follow-up will be required to confirm the early results.

TUMOR CELL KILL ACHIEVED BY CHEMOTHERAPY
The amount of monoclonal protein produced by a mouse plasma cell tumor correlates directly with the tumor mass [198]. In humans it is possible to evaluate the effectiveness of chemotherapy by following changes in the concentration of the serum monoclonal protein. One method of estimating tumor cell kill is illustrated in Fig. 122-7. A more sophisticated method for estimating the total myeloma cell number from measurements of the amount of monoclonal protein produced per myeloma cell, the total amount of monoclonal protein in the plasma volume, and the catabolic rate of the monoclonal protein has been developed [101]. Estimates by both of these methods suggest that the maximum tumor cell kill achieved by chemotherapy is between 90 and 99 percent [102], and this is followed by a plateau. In this case the monoclonal protein decreased and then remained con-

stant for many months, despite continued therapy with cyclophosphamide and prednisone.

The results of treating a patient with total-body irradiation are consistent with the view that the duration of response is not determined by the cell kill [199]. The radiation sensitivity of myeloma cells indicates that a dose of 225 rads would reduce the myeloma cell number by 1 log and result in a remission of about 3 years. The administration of this dose to one patient caused the M protein to disappear and lytic skeletal lesions to heal; this excellent remission has now persisted for more than 10 years. It is not possible to explain the duration of this remission on the basis of the myeloma cell kill expected from the dose of irradiation that was used. Prolonged unmaintained remissions following melphalan therapy have been reported [200] and observed in our clinic. It is difficult to attribute these long remissions to the myeloma cell kill achieved with melphalan.

The failure of maintenance therapy to prolong the duration of remission, or survival, provides additional evidence that these response parameters are not determined by the myeloma cell kill [201].

The myeloma growth rate, as reflected by the M-protein doubling time, has been measured repeatedly on myeloma patients in unmaintained remissions [199]. A progressive shortening in the M-protein doubling time was observed. Most of the patients who progressed to an M-protein doubling time of less than 30 days also developed marrow failure [97,202]. This marrow failure did not result from treatment, because the marrow remained cellular and the pancytopenia persisted after all therapy was stopped. About one-third of myeloma patients developed marrow failure and died during the "acute terminal" phase of the disease [189]. The M-protein doubling time during relapse correlates closely with subsequent survival; short M-protein doubling times predict brief survival [199]. The survival of myeloma patients is determined largely by the time required for a progressive loss of myeloma growth control and marrow failure to occur.

RESEMBLANCE OF REMISSIONS TO BENIGN MONOCLONAL GAMMOPATHY (BMG)

In some ways the status of patients during treatment-induced remissions of myeloma resembles that of patients with BMG. In 44 percent of patients the M protein falls progressively during remission-induction to reach a plateau, and then remains stable throughout the remission [203]. The duration of this stable phase is not prolonged by maintenance therapy [201]. Some of these remissions persist for unusually long periods. The persistence of an M protein throughout the remissions, and the demonstration that 12 of 24 remission marrows contained myeloma stem cells capable of forming colonies of plasma cells, indicates that the myeloma clone persists but is controlled during remissions [204].

In both BMG and myeloma remissions there are large monoclonal populations of plasma cells (greater than 10^{10} cells) that remain stable for prolonged periods. Myeloma stem cells capable of forming colonies of plasma cells are present in both conditions. Unmaintained myeloma remissions last for variable periods, from a few months to many years with a median duration of 11 months [205]. A recurrence of progressive, uncontrolled growth of myeloma cells ends the remission of most myeloma patients.

IRRADIATION

Radiotherapy is useful in the palliative treatment of patients with localized lesions, such as fractures, large osteolytic lesions in the long bones which may fracture, extraskeletal plasmacytomas, osteolytic vertebral lesions, and plasma cell tumors causing spinal cord or nerve root compression. Every attempt should be made to avoid neurologic complications by carefully investigating all paraspinal masses to discover plasma cell tumors that are likely to cause spinal cord compression. Surgical laminectomy is indicated when the diagnosis is in doubt or if an acute compression develops.

The field used for irradiating localized lesions must be planned carefully so that all of the lesion is treated. Generous margins should be used in the treatment of osteolytic lesions of the long bones.

Tumor doses of more than 2000 rads in 5 days are rarely required to treat paraspinal masses or large lytic lesions. Smaller lesions in the ribs, vertebrae, or subcutaneous tumors are often effectively treated with a single dose of 800 rads. Solitary plasmacytomas in a bone, or in the naso- or oropharynx should be treated more aggressively with fields and doses designed to be curative; tumor doses of about 4000 rads in 3 to 4 weeks are suggested.

Total-body irradiation has been used successfully in the treatment of at least one patient [199] but is rarely practical. The maximally tolerated dose of total body irradiation (225 to 250 rads) would reduce the tumor cell number by about tenfold. This is justified only if the patient is resistant to all alkylating agents, and has a slowly growing tumor, with a monoclonal protein doubling time of greater than 3 months. If the doubling time is shorter than this, a tumor cell kill of tenfold would produce a remission of less than 9 months.

A TREATMENT PLAN

Patients with generalized PCM who have platelet counts greater than 100,000 per microliter are started on intermittent courses of melphalan (0.25 mg/kg per day for 4 days) and prednisone (100 mg per day for 4 days). Blood counts are done weekly, and therapy is repeated at 4-week intervals. Alternatively the initial loading dose may be followed by daily oral maintenance therapy with 1 to 3 mg of melphalan. Therapy may also be initiated with melphalan given orally in an initial dose of 2 to 4 mg daily. The drug is given continuously, with adjustment of the dose according to changes in the blood count [164] (Table 122-4). Therapy is continued as long as the monoclonal protein continues to decrease. It may be possible to suspend therapy after a satisfactory remission has been induced [201].

If a patient treated with intermittent melphalan therapy has, or develops, thrombocytopenia, or shows no sign of improvement after three courses of treatment, or relapses after demonstrating a response, therapy is changed to intermittent courses of cyclophosphamide and prednisone. Patients who still fail to respond, or who relapse on intermittent or more maintained cyclophosphamide-prednisone regimens, may respond to programs incorporating anabolic steroids (see below) and alkylating agents such as chlorambucil or carmustine.

Painful skeletal lesions and paraspinal masses are irradiated as soon as they are discovered. Patients are permitted to walk as soon as adequate pain relief is achieved and are encouraged to exercise regularly. They are instructed to maintain a good fluid intake, and warned against vaccination.

SPECIAL PROBLEMS

ASYMPTOMATIC PATIENT

Asymptomatic patients with monoclonal proteins should be investigated and followed carefully. No treatment should be given unless progressive disease is confirmed as being responsible for the monoclonal protein.

PLASMACYTOMAS

Solitary plasmacytomas should be treated by irradiation. If the irradiated lesion is truly solitary, the monoclonal protein should disappear from the serum and/or urine, and marrow aspirates should not contain an increased number of plasma cells. The persistence or reappearance of a monoclonal protein in the serum or urine or the development of marrow plasmacytosis following irradiation of an apparently solitary plasmacytoma is an indication that the disease is more extensive and that chemotherapy is required.

HYPERCALCEMIA

Patients with hypercalcemia can be treated with either calcitonin (100 to 200 units subcutaneously every 12 h) or prednisone, 40 to 100 mg per day, or preferably both, until the serum calcium returns to normal, which usually occurs within 1 to 5 days.

Although calcitonin decreases serum calcium, addition of prednisone seems important to maintain a decreased calcium for days to weeks until chemotherapy can reverse the calcium loss from bone [239,240].

Prednisone is known to reduce calcium absorption from the gut, and may exert an antineoplastic effect against myeloma cells. Prednisone has been shown to inhibit the activation of osteoclasts [206], which is probably its most important effect in correcting the hypercalcemia. Improvement is accelerated if therapy with melphalan or cyclophosphamide is started at an early stage. More rapid reduction of hypercalcemia may be accomplished by hydrating the patient with intravenous saline and stimulating urine output with furosemide [207]. If satisfactory lowering of the calcium level is not achieved promptly, mithramycin may be administered in a dose of 25 μg per kilogram of body weight [208]. Mithramycin may worsen thrombocytopenia. These measures are usually successful in correcting hypercalcemia. Oral therapy with 2 g of sodium or potassium phosphate daily may also be useful in controlling hypercalcemia [209].

INFECTION

Infection is the most common cause of death. If patients with PCM become febrile, cultures should be made from the blood, sputum, urine, skin lesions, or other possible sites of infection. Infections with penicillin-resistant staphylococci and gram-negative organisms are frequent, and there is a great danger of septicemia. All infections in patients with plasma cell tumors require immediate attention, and antibiotic therapy is usually administered before the results of cultures and antibiotic sensitivities are available. Treatment of serious infections should be initiated with a combination of antibiotics effective against penicillin-resistant staphylococci and gram-negative organisms (e.g., a cephalosporin and gentamicin), with appropriate attention to nephrotoxicity.

Prophylactic long-acting penicillin (benzathine penicillin G) administration may be useful for patients who have repeated infections with sensitive organisms such as the pneumococcus. Prophylactic γ-globulin administered in conventional doses intramuscular to a random group of patients with PCM produced no reduction in the incidence of severity of infections [210].

Patients with PCM should never be immunized with vaccines containing live organisms (e.g., vaccinia) because of the danger of a generalized viral infection.

HYPERVISCOSITY

Hyperviscosity and hypervolemia are most effectively treated by plasmapheresis. Cryoglobulinemia may also be treated in this way. The aim of this treatment is to remove enough plasma containing the monoclonal protein to reduce the plasma volume towards normal and the relative serum viscosity to less than 4. This procedure will relieve symptoms of bleeding or congestive heart failure temporarily; antineoplastic therapy should be started immediately to inhibit the growth of the PCM and synthesis of the monoclonal protein.

ANEMIA

Anemia may persist in some patients who are otherwise improved by chemotherapy. If the anemia is symptomatic and thought to be due to marrow failure associated with myeloma, rather than to other causes such as blood loss, folic acid deficiency, vitamin B_{12} deficiency or chemotherapy, a trial of androgen therapy is indicated. Treatment with fluoxymesterone, 15 to 30 mg daily by mouth, will raise the hemoglobin level in many of these patients (Fig. 122-8).

HYPERURICEMIA

Hyperuricemia occurs commonly in patients with PCM, but the uric acid level rarely exceeds 9 mg/dl. Marked elevations of serum uric levels are often caused by renal insufficiency, and, in such cases, therapy should be directed primarily toward improving renal function. If hyperuricemia is present, therapy with 300 to 600 mg of allopurinol per day should be instituted in order to avoid the development of uric acid stones or nephropathy.

RENAL FAILURE

When myeloma patients develop acute renal failure as a result of excessive light-chain excretion, there is an urgent need to reduce the load of light chains presented to the kidneys. Plasmapheresis is 10 times more effective than peritoneal dialysis in removing light chains, and appears to be the best method for treating this acute complication [211–213]. Chemotherapy should be started immediately to reduce the production of light chains by myeloma cells. If this treatment is successful, plasmapheresis will be required for a short period and renal function will be improved for as long as the growth of myeloma cells can be controlled. Successful renal transplantation has been reported for a patient with chronic renal failure which did not improve after effective chemotherapy; however, the indications for

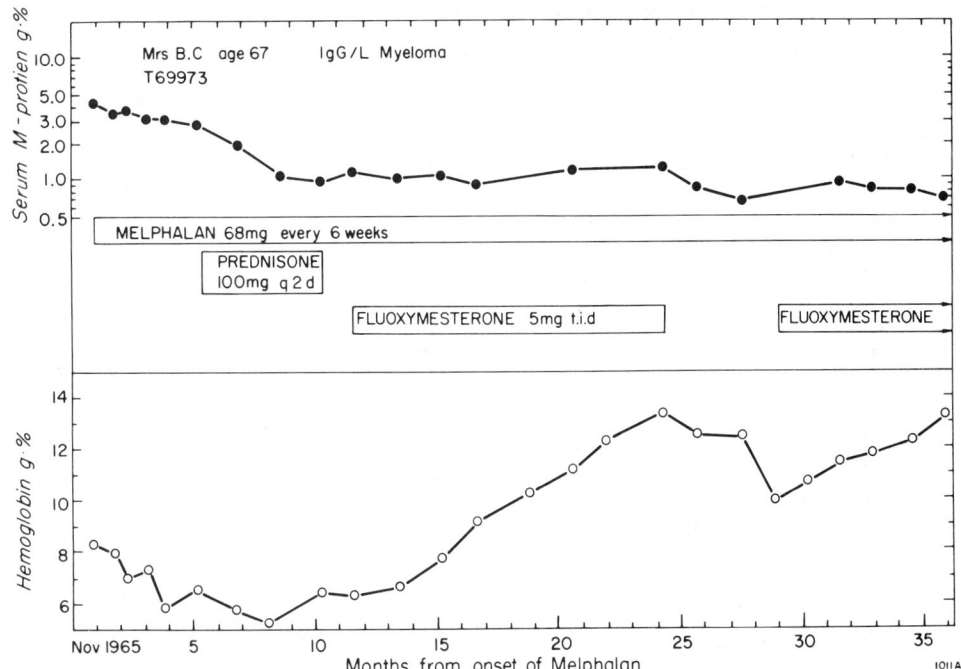

FIGURE 122-8   Treatment of anemia associated with plasma cell myeloma with fluoxymesterone. This patient responded well to melphalan therapy, with a fall in the monoclonal protein and relief of bone pain. The anemia persisted and did not improve with the addition of prednisone. With the administration of fluoxymesterone the hemoglobin rose to normal values but began to fall when fluoxymesterone was suspended. The concentration returned to normal when the hormone was resumed.

renal transplantation in patients with a lethal disease have been questioned [214,215].

The clearance of alkylating agents from the plasma of patients with renal insufficiency has not been examined directly. In practice we have not found that it is necessary to reduce the dose of melphalan administered to myeloma patients with uremia. This alkylating agent is not schedule-dependent, and repeat courses of the drug are given at 4-week intervals. Thus, even if the clearance of melphalan is delayed in patients with renal impairment, excessive toxicity is not observed. Cyclophosphamide, on the other hand, is schedule-dependent, and it has been our practice to reduce the dose of this drug until there is evidence that renal function is adequate to clear the drug and prevent toxic levels of the active form of cyclophosphamide from circulating for prolonged periods.

SKELETAL LESIONS

Demineralization and osteolytic skeletal lesions occur in about two-thirds of patients with PCM, and often lead to incapacitating bone pain and fractures. Therapy with fluorides, calcium, and vitamin D has been considered because of their possible role in strengthening the skeleton. Extensive recalcification of bone has been reported in a patient treated for 22 months with 90 mg of sodium fluoride alone and 3.5 g calcium lactate daily [216]. However, a prospective clinical trial of the effect of sodium fluoride alone on the clinical course of plasma cell myeloma failed to demonstrate any beneficial effect [217].

The administration of fluoride stimulates osteoblasts [218], but the new bone is poorly mineralized, and osteomalacia and secondary hyperparathyroidism occur frequently. The addition of calcium and vitamin D prevents the appearance of poorly mineralized bone in rats. A group of 11 patients with progressive osteoporosis has been treated with fluoride, calcium, and vitamin D. New bone formation was observed in biopsies from all patients receiving more than 45 mg of sodium fluoride per day. Doses of 50 mg of sodium fluoride and at least 900 mg of calcium per day, plus 50,000 units of vitamin D twice weekly, are recommended [218]. It has been suggested [219] that the addition of androgens is required for maximal strengthening of the skeleton.

Course and prognosis

GENERAL

Age and sex have little influence on prognosis. The performance status of the patient reflects the cumulative effects of bony lesions, anemia, renal insufficiency, and other manifestations of the disease. It is not surprising to find that patients with a relatively good performance status have the best prospects for survival [220]. A his-

TABLE 122-5   Immunoglobulin class of monoclonal protein, renal insufficiency, and survival of patients with plasma cell neoplasms.

Monclonal protein	Author	No. patients	Median survival (months from 1st treatment)	Frequency of renal insufficiency (BUN > 30 mg/dl) Affected/evaluated	Percent
IgG/κ	Alexanian et al. [184]	66	35	5/66	8
IgG/λ	Alexanian et al. [184]	37	25	3/37	8
IgG/κ and λ	Acute Leukemia Group B [222]	148	29		
IgA/κ	Alexanian et al. [184]	20	22	3/20	15
IgA/λ	Alexanian et al. [184]	34	19	4/34	11
IgA/κ and λ	Acute Leukemia Group B [222]	67	21		
IgD/κ and λ	Jancelewicz et al. [141]	54*	9†	58/86	67
κ only	Alexanian et al. [184]	23	28	7/23	30
	Shustik, Bergsagel, and Pruzanski [98]	52	30†	32/52	62
λ only	Alexanian et al. [184]	18	11	10/18	58
	Shustik, Bergsagel, and Pruzanski [98]	45	10†	22/45	49
IgM/κ and λ	Krajny and Pruzanski [238]	45	50†	5/38	13

*90% of these patients excreted light chains in the urine.
†Median survival from diagnosis.

tory of a 10 percent or more weight loss is often associated with a high myeloma cell mass, and a poor prognosis [221].

Fever not associated with infection is a bad prognostic factor [97]. In one study all of 17 patients who developed fever without infection died within 1 to 9 months (median 3 months) of the onset of the fever [97].

THE IMMUNOGLOBULIN CLASS OF MONOCLONAL PROTEIN

The malignant transformation which initiates PCM appears to affect a cell that is committed to produce a specific immunoglobulin, subunit, or fragment. Plasma cell tumors producing different classes of immunoglobulins have different clinical manifestations and there is evidence that they grow at different rates [139]. There is considerable difference in the survival prognosis of groups of patients with neoplasms producing different classes of immunoglobulin (Table 122-5) which is confirmation of the view that these neoplasms grow at different rates. The survival prognosis is best for plasma cell neoplasms producing IgM, and decreases progressively for patients with PCM who produce κ light chains only, IgG, IgA, λ light chains only and IgD. Renal insufficiency occurs most often in the two groups of patients with the shortest survival (IgD and λ light chains only).

PROGNOSTIC FACTORS RELATED TO THE TOTAL-BODY MYELOMA CELL MASS

A method for estimating the total-body myeloma cell number has been developed [101,223]. Patients considered to have "early" disease have at least 2×10^{11} myeloma cells, but in most instances well over 1×10^{12} myeloma cells are present at the time of diagnosis. Patients with multiple osteolytic bone lesions have in excess of 2×10^{12} myeloma cells. An increase in the total-body myeloma cell mass to between 5 to 7 percent of

body weight (assuming 10^{12} myeloma cells = 1 kg) almost always causes death (i.e., 3.5 to 5.0×10^{12} cells in a 70-kg patient). In one study the myeloma cell mass was calculated in 50 patients with PCM and evaluated in parallel with conventional clinical and laboratory parameters to determine which most accurately reflected the total myeloma cell number [221]. Multiple lytic bone lesions, a serum calcium of more than 12 mg/dl, hemoglobin levels less than 8.5 g/dl, high serum monoclonal protein concentrations, marked light-chain proteinuria, and low serum albumin levels, were predictive of high myeloma cell numbers. All factors are known to be associated with shorter survival. The percentage of plasma cells in the marrow aspirate also correlated well with cell mass, but was not used as a major criterion because of inherent potential sampling errors. A system has been suggested for classifying the severity of untreated PCM ("clinical staging") based on these variables [224,225].

UREMIA

The occurrence of uremia in patients with PCM is an adverse prognostic factor [189,220–222,226,227]. The median survival of patients who presented with a normal blood urea concentration was 37 months. In others the survival fell progressively as the blood urea rose from 40 to 79 mg/dl. Patients with a blood urea concentration of 80 mg/dl or greater had a median survival of only 2 months. Since the blood urea concentration is approximately twice that of the blood urea nitrogen (BUN), the critical BUN concentration is about 50 mg/dl.

Uremia occurs more frequently in patients who excrete large amounts of light-chain protein in the urine and the adverse effect of light-chain proteinuria appears to be linked with the development of uremia. In one study the correlation of light-chain proteinuria with prognosis disappeared after adjustment for blood urea concentration [226]. However, others have found that the median survival of patients with a blood urea nitrogen of less than 30 mg/dl who have light chain protein in the urine is shorter than for those without such proteinuria [222].

The observation that patients who produce type λ light chains tend to excrete much larger amounts of light-chain protein than those producing type κ light chains, and a higher proportion are therefore uremic [226], may partially explain the poorer survival prognosis that has been reported for patients with PCM producing type λ light chains [97,98,139,222,226,228].

CLINICAL COURSE AND CAUSES OF DEATH

When treatment is started during the symptomatic stage, about 60 percent of patients treated with an alkylating agent and prednisone show objective improvement, marked by a decrease in bone pain and a fall in the serum and/or urine monoclonal protein concentration. These remissions have median durations of 21 months [185]. Eventually the disease progresses and becomes resistant to therapy. Some of the patients who are, or become, resistant to melphalan will respond to treatment with another alkylating agent such as cyclophosphamide, BCNU, or chlorambucil.

About 15 percent of patients die within 3 months after treatment is started with an alkylating agent and prednisone; thereafter, deaths occur at a slower, constant rate, with a median survival of about 30 months [189]. In one large study 46 percent of patients died during the chronic phase of the disease with adequate marrow function and progressive myeloma plus renal failure, sepsis, or both [189]. Another 31 percent died during the acute terminal phase with pancytopenia and a cellular marrow. These patients had evidence of rapidly progressive myeloma with short M-protein doubling times or increasing numbers of plasma cells in the blood. In addition, ring sideroblasts, a presumed preleukemic change [189], were reported in 18 patients. Acute leukemia has developed in 9 of the patients with sideroblasts, and in 6 others. The acute leukemias were classified as myeloblastic in 11, monoblastic in 2, and erythroleukemic in 2 [189,229]. Other serious illnesses, such as myocardial infarctions, chronic obstructive pulmonary disease, and strokes caused deaths in 20 percent, and the cause of death is unknown for 7 percent.

In the management of patients with PCM one should distinguish the chronic phase of the disease, when the growth rate is relatively slow and the majority of patients achieve good objective remissions following treatment with an alkylating agent and prednisone, from the acute terminal phase, when the growth rate is rapid, normal hematopoiesis fails, and the methods of treatment tested to date are usually ineffective.

PLASMA CELL MYELOMA AND ACUTE LEUKEMIA

A high incidence of acute leukemia has been observed in patients with plasma cell myeloma. In one large study the actuarial risk of developing acute leukemia reached 19.6 percent at 50 months after the onset of treatment [189]. It is not possible to decide whether treatment with leukemogenic agents (x-irradiation and alkylating agents) increased the risk of developing acute leukemia, because we do not know what the incidence is in untreated patients. The occurrence of acute leukemia prior to any therapy in at least 17 patients with myeloma, 5 with macroglobulinemia, and 5 with benign monoclonal gammopathy suggests that there is an increased risk of acute leukemia in patients with plasma cell neoplasms in the absence of treatment, and that acute leukemia may occur as part of the natural history of the disease [230–237].

References

1. Clamp, J. R.: Some aspects of the first recorded case of multiple myeloma. *Lancet* 2:1354, 1967.
2. Rustizky, J.: Multiple myeloma. *Dtsch. Z. Chir.* 3:162, 1873.
3. Kahler, O.: Zur Symptomatologie des multiplen Myeloms; Beobachtung von Albumosurie. *Prag. Med. Wochnschr.* 14:33, 1889.
4. Ellinger, A.: Das Vorkommen des Bence Jonesschen Körpers in Harn bei Tumoren des Knochenmarks und seine diagnostische Bedeutung. *Dtsch. Arch. Klin. Med.* 62:255, 1899.
5. Wright, J. H.: A case of multiple myeloma. *Trans. Assoc. Am. Physicians* 15:137, 1900.
6. Perlzweig, W. A., Delrue, G., and Geschickter, C.: Hyperproteinemia associated with multiple myelomas. *JAMA* 90:755, 1929.
7. Magnus-Levy, A.: Multiple myeloma. *Acta. Med. Scand.* 95:217, 1938.
8. Glenner, G. G., Terry, W., Harada, M., Isersky, C., and Page, D.: Amyloid fibril proteins: Proof of homology with immunoglobulin light chains by sequence analyses. *Science* 172:1150, 1971.
9. Alwall, N.: Urethane and stilbamidine in multiple myeloma: Report on 2 cases. *Lancet* 2:388, 1947.
10. Bergsagel, D. E., Griffith, K. M., Haut, A., and Stuckey, W. J., Jr.: The treatment of plasma cell myeloma. *Adv. Cancer Res.* 10:311, 1967.
11. Blokhin, N., Larionov, L., Perevodchikova, N., Chebotareva, L., and Merkulova, N.: Clinical experiences with sarcolysin in neoplastic diseases. *Ann. N.Y. Acad. Sci.* 68:1128, 1958.
12. Bergsagel, D. E., Sprague, C. C., Austin, C., and Griffith, K. M.: Evaluation of new chemotherapeutic agents in the treatment of multiple myeloma. IV. L-Phenylalanine mustard (NSC-8806). *Cancer Chemother. Rep.* 21:87, 1962.
13. Korst, D. R., Clifford, G. O., Fowler, W. M., Louis, J., Will, J., and Wilson, H. E.: Multiple myeloma. II. Analysis of cyclophosphamide therapy in 165 patients. *JAMA* 189:758, 1964.
14. Kyle, R. A., Nobrega, F. T., and Kurland, L. T.: Multiple myeloma in Olmsted County, Minnesota, 1945–1964. *Blood* 33:739, 1969.
15. McPhedran, P., Heath, C. W., Jr., and Garcia, J.: Multiple myeloma incidence in metropolitan Atlanta, Georgia: Racial and seasonal variations. *Blood* 39:866, 1972.
16. Waldenström, J.: *Diagnosis and Treatment of Multiple Myeloma.* Grune & Stratton, New York, 1970.
17. Martin, N. H.: The incidence of myelomatosis. *Lancet* 1:237, 1961.
18. MacMahon, B., and Clark, D. W.: Incidence of multiple myeloma. *J. Chronic Dis.* 4:508, 1956.
19. McFarlane, H.: Multiple myeloma in Jamaica: A study of 40 cases with special reference to the incidence and laboratory diagnosis. *J. Clin. Pathol.* 19:268, 1966.
20. Isobe, T., and Osserman, E. F.: Pathologic conditions associated with plasma cell dyscrasias: A study of 806 cases. *Ann. N. Y. Acad. Sci.* 190:507, 1971.
21. Kyle, R. A.: Multiple myeloma: Review of 869 cases. *Mayo Clin. Proc.* 50:29, 1975.
22. Hewell, G. M., and Alexanian, R.: Multiple myeloma in young persons. *Ann. Intern. Med.* 84:441, 1976.

23. Poole, A. G., and Marchetta, F. C.: Extramedullary plasmacytoma of the head and neck. *Cancer* 22:14, 1968.

24. Kotner, L. M., and Wang, C. C.: Plasmacytoma of the upper air and food passages. *Cancer* 30:414, 1972.

25. Kennedy, J. D., and Kneafsey, D. V.: Two cases of plasmacytoma of the lower respiratory tract. *Thorax* 14:353, 1959.

26. Douglass, H. O., Jr., Sika, J. V., and LeVeen, H. H.: Plasmacytoma: A not so rare tumor of the small intestine. *Cancer* 28:456, 1971.

27. Edwards, G. A., and Zawadzki, Z. A.: Extraosseous lesions in plasma cell myeloma: A report of six cases. *Am. J. Med.* 43:194, 1967.

28. Schweers, C. A., Shaw, M. T., Nordquist, R. E., Rose, D. D., and Kell, T.: Solitary cecal plasmacytoma: Electron microscopic, immunologic and cytochemical studies. *Cancer* 37:2220, 1976.

29. Wile, A., Olinger, G., Peter, J. B., and Dronfeld, L.: Solitary intraparenchymal pulmonary plasmacytoma associated with production of an M-protein: Report of a case. *Cancer* 37:2338, 1976.

30. Cohen, D. M., Svien, H. J., and Dahlin, D. C.: Long-term survival of patients with myeloma of the vertebral column. *JAMA* 187:914, 1964.

31. Meyer, J. E., and Schulz, M. D.: "Solitary" myeloma of bone: A review of 12 cases. *Cancer* 34:438, 1974.

32. Evison, G., and Evans, K. T.: Bone sclerosis in multiple myeloma. *Br. J. Radiol.* 40:81, 1967.

33. Langley, G. R., Sabean, H. B., and Sorger, K.: Sclerotic lesions of bone in myeloma. *Can. Med. Assoc. J.* 94:940, 1966.

34. Morley, J. B., and Schwieger, A. C.: The relation between chronic polyneuropathy and osteosclerotic myeloma. *J. Neurol. Neurosurg. Psychiatry* 30:432, 1967.

35. Snapper, I., and Kahn, A.: *Myelomatosis.* University Park Press, Baltimore, 1971.

36. Case Records of the Massachusetts General Hospital (Case 29-1972). *N. Engl. J. Med.* 287:138, 1972.

37. Rodriguez, A. R., Lutcher, C. L., and Coleman, F. W.: Osteosclerotic myeloma. *JAMA* 236:1872, 1976.

38. Loeffler, R. K., DiSimone, R. N., and Howland, W. J.: Limitations of bone scanning in clinical oncology. *JAMA* 234:1228, 1975.

39. Mundy, G. R., Raisz, L. G., Cooper, R. A., Schechter, G. P., and Salmon, S. E.: Evidence for the secretion of an osteoclast stimulating factor in myeloma. *N. Engl. J. Med.* 291:1041, 1974.

40. Salmon, S. E.: Immunoglobulin synthesis and tumor kinetics of multiple myeloma. *Semin. Hematol.* 10:135, 1973.

41. Kopp, W. L., and MacKinney, A. A., Jr., and Wasson, G.: Blood volume and hematocrit value in macroglobulinemia and myeloma. *Arch. Intern. Med.* 123:394, 1969.

42. Larsson, S. O.: Myeloma and pernicious anemia. *Acta Med. Scand.* 172:195, 1962.

43. Hoffbrand, A. V., Hobbs, J. R., Kremenchuzky, S., and Mollin, D. L.: Incidence and pathogenesis of megaloblastic erythropoiesis in multiple myeloma. *J. Clin. Pathol.* 20:699, 1967.

44. Pruzanski, W., and Ogryzlo, M. A.: Abnormal proteinuria in malignant diseases. *Adv. Clin. Chemo.* 13:355, 1970.

45. Waldmann, T. A., Strober, W.: Metabolism of immunoglobulins. *Prog. Allergy* 13:1, 1969.

46. Schur, P. H., et al.: IgG subclasses: Relationship to clinical aspects of multiple myeloma and frequence distribution among M-components. *Scand. J. Haematol.* 12:60, 1974.

47. Hobbs, J. R., and Jacobs, A.: Case report: A half-molecule GK plasmacytoma. *Clin. Exp. Immunol.* 5:199, 1969.

48. Spiegelberg, H. L., and Fishkin, B. G.: Human myeloma IgA half-molecules. *J. Clin. Invest.* 58:1259, 1976.

49. Solomon, A., and Kunkel, H. G.: A "monoclonal" type, low molecular weight protein related to γM-macroglobulin. *Am. J. Med.* 42:958, 1967.

50. Pruzanski, W., Underdown, B., Silver, E. H., and Katz, A.: Macroglobulinemia-myeloma double gammopathy. *Am. J. Med.* 57:259, 1974.

51. Engle, R. L., Jr., and Nachman, R. L.: Brief report: Two Bence Jones proteins of different immunologic types in the same patient with multiple myeloma. *Blood* 27:74, 1966.

52. Jensen, K., Jensen, K. B., and Olesen, H.: Three M-components in serum from an apparently healthy person. *Scand. J. Haematol.* 4:485, 1967.

53. Bjerrum, O. J., and Weeke, B.: Two M components (gamma-GK and gamma-ML) in different cells of the same patient. *Scand. J. Haematol.* 5:215, 1968.

54. Preud'homme, J. L., and Seligmann, M.: Surface bound immunoglobulins as a cell marker in human lymphoproliferative diseases. *Blood* 40:777, 1972.

55. Hopper, J. E.: Immunofluorescent evidence for a common clonal origin of IgM-λ and IgG-κ paraproteins. *Clin. Res.* 21:557, 1973.

56. Hopper, J. E., Noyes, C., Hendrickson, R. L., and Kingdon, H. S.: Idiotypic antigenic analysis and N-terminal heavy chain sequences of monotypic IgM-λ and IgG-κ from a single patient. *Clin. Res.* 21:581, 1973.

57. Curtain, C. C.: Immuno-cytochemical localization of two abnormal serum globulins in the one bone-marrow smear. *Australia Ann. Med.* 13:136, 1964.

58. Silverman, A. Y., Yagi, Y., Pressman, D., Ellison, R. R., and Tormey, D. C.: Monoclonal IgA and IgM in the serum of a single patient (SC). III. Immunofluorescent identification of cells producing IgA and IgM. *J. Immunol.* 110:350, 1973.

59. Sanders, J. H., Fahey, J. L., Finegold, I., Ein, D., Reisfeld, R., and Berard, C.: Multiple anomalous immunoglobulins: Clinical, structural and cellular studies in three patients. *Am. J. Med.* 47:43, 1969.

60. McNutt, D. R., and Fudenberg, H. H.: IgG myeloma and Waldenström macroglobulinemia: Coexistence and clinical manifestations in one patient. *Arch. Intern. Med.* 131:731, 1973.

61. Fudenberg, H. H., Wang, A. C., Pink, J. R. L., and Levin, A. S.: Studies of an unusual biclonal gammapathy: Implications with regard to genetic control of normal immunoglobulin synthesis. *Ann. N.Y. Acad. Sci.* 190:501, 1971.

62. Penn, G. M., Kunkel, H. G., and Grey, H. M.: Sharing of individual antigenic determinants between a γG and a γM protein in the same myeloma serum. *Proc. Soc. Exp. Biol. Med.* 135:660, 1970.

63. Yagi, Y., and Pressman, D.: Monoclonal IgA and IgM in the serum of a single patient (SC). I. Sharing of individually specific determinants between IgA and IgM. *J. Immunol.* 110:335, 1973.

64. Natvig, J. G., and Kunkel, H. G.: Human immunoglobulins: Classes, subclasses, genetic variants, and idiotypes. *Adv. Immunol.* 16:1, 1973.

65. Seon, B. K., Yagi, Y., and Pressman, D.: Monoclonal IgA and IgM in the serum of a single patient (SC). II. Identity of light chains from IgA (K) and IgM (K). *J. Immunol.* 110:345, 1973.

66. Solomon, A.: Bence Jones proteins and light chains of immunoglobulins. *N. Engl. J. Med.* 294:17, 1976.

67. Harrison, J. F., Blainey, J. D., Hardwiche, J., Rowe, D. S., and Soothill, J. F.: Proteinuria in multiple myeloma. *Clin. Sci.* 31:95, 1966.

68. Carson, C. P., Ackerman, L. V., and Maltby, J. D.: Plasma cell myeloma: Clinical pathologic and roentgenologic review of 90 cases. *Am. J. Clin. Pathol.* 25:849, 1955.

69. Hurez, D., Preud'homme, J.-L., and Seligmann, M.: Intracellular "monoclonal" immunoglobulin in non-secretory human myeloma. *J. Immunol.* 104:263, 1970.

70. River, G. L., Tewksbury, D. A., and Fudenberg, H. H.: "Nonsecretory" multiple myeloma. *Blood* 40:204, 1972.

71. Zolla, S.: The effect of plasmacytomas on the immune response of mice. *J. Immunol.* 180:1039, 1972.

72. Yakulis, V., Bhoopalam, N., Schade, S., and Heller, P.: Surface immunoglobulins of circulating lymphocytes in mouse plasmacytoma. I. Characteristics of lymphocyte surface immunoglobulins. *Blood* 39:453, 1972.

73. Bhoopalam, N., Yakulis, V., Costea, N., and Heller, P.: Surface immunoglobulins of circulating lymphocytes in mouse plasmacytoma. II. The influence of plasmacytoma RNA on surface immunoglobulins of lymphocytes. *Blood* 39:465, 1972.

74. Giacomoni, D., Yakulis, V., Wang, S. R., Cooke, A., Dray, S., and Heller, P.: *In vitro* conversion of normal mouse lymphocytes by plasmacytoma RNA to express idiotypic specificities on their surface characteristic of the plasmacytoma immunoglobulin. *Cell. Immunol.* 11:389, 1974.

75. Salmon, S. E.: "Paraneoplastic" syndromes associated with monoclonal lymphocyte and plasma cell proliferation. *Ann. N.Y. Acad. Sci.* 230:228, 1974.

76. Tanapatchaiyapong, P., and Zolla, S.: Humoral immunosuppressive substance in mice bearing plasmacytomas. *Science 186*:748, 1974.

77. Broder, S., et al.: Impaired synthesis of polyclonal (non-paraprotein) immunoglobulin by lymphocytes from patients with multiple myeloma. *N. Engl. J. Med. 293*:887, 1975.

78. Alexanian, R., and Migliore, P.: Normal immunoglobulins in multiple myeloma: Effect of melphalan chemotherapy. *J. Lab. Clin. Med. 75*:225, 1970.

79. Murray, T., Long, W., and Narins, R. G.: Multiple myeloma and the anion gap. *N. Engl. J. Med. 292*:574, 1975.

80. Pruzanski, W., and Watt, J. G.: Serum viscosity and hyperviscosity syndrome in IgG multiple myeloma. *Ann. Intern. Med. 77*:853, 1972.

81. Capra, J. D., and Kunkel, H. G.: Aggregation of γG3 proteins: Relevance to the hyperviscosity syndrome. *J. Clin. Invest. 49*:610, 1970.

82. Pruzanski, W., Jancelewicz, Z., and Underdown, B.: Immunological and physiochemical studies of IgA1 (γ cryogelglobulinaemia. *Clin. Exp. Immunol. 15*:181, 1973.

83. Zlotnick, A., and Rosenmann, E.: Renal pathologic findings associated with monoclonal gammopathies. *Arch. Intern. Med. 135*:40, 1975.

84. Defronzo, R. A., Cooke, C. R., Wright, J. R., and Humphrey, R. L.: Renal function in patients with multiple myeloma. *Medicine 57*:151, 1978.

85. Solomon, A., Waldmann, T. A., Fahey, J. L., and MacFarlane, A. S.: Metabolism of Bence Jones proteins. *J. Clin. Invest. 43*:103, 1964.

86. Waldmann, T. A., Strober, W., and Mogielnicki, R. P.: The renal handling of low-molecular-weight proteins. II. Disorders of serum protein catabolism in patients with tubular proteinuria, the nephrotic syndrome, or uremia. *J. Clin. Invest. 51*:2162, 1972.

87. Wochner, R. D., Strober, W., Waldmann, T. A.: The role of kidney in the catabolism of Bence Jones proteins and immunoglobulin fragments. *J. Exp. Med. 126*:207, 1967.

88. Clyne, D. H., et al.: Renal effects of intraperitoneal kappa chain infection. Induction of crystals in renal tubular cells. *Lab. Invest. 31*:131, 1974.

89. Levi, D. F., Williams, R. C., Jr., and Lindsrom, F. D.: Immunofluorescent studies of the myeloma kidney with special reference to light chain disease. *Am. J. Med. 44*:922, 1968.

90. Costanza, D. J., and Smoller, M.: Multiple myeloma with the Fanconi syndrome. Study of a case, with electron microscopy of the kidney. *Am. J. Med. 34*:125, 1963.

91. Engle, R. L., Jr., and Wallis, L. A.: Multiple myeloma and the adult Fanconi syndrome. I. Report of a case with crystal-like deposits in the tumor cells and in the epithelial cells of the kidney. *Am. J. Med. 22*:5, 1957.

92. Finkel, P. N., Kronenberg, K., Pesce, A. J., Pollak, V. E., and Pirani, C. L.: Adult Fanconi syndrome, amyloidosis and marked kappa light chain proteinuria. *Nephron. 10*:1, 1973.

93. Sirtoa, J. H., and Hammerman, D.: Renal function studies in an adult subject with the Fanconi syndrome. *Am. J. Med. 16*:138, 1954.

94. Preuss, H. G., Hammack, W. J., and Murdaugh, H. V.: The effect of Bence Jones protein on the *in vitro* function of rabbit renal cortex. *Nephron 5*:210, 1967.

95. Preuss, H. G., Weiss, F. R., Iammarino, R. M., Hammack, W. J., and Murdaugh, H. V., Jr.: Effect on rat kidney slice function *in vitro* of proteins from the urines of patients with myelomatosis and nephrosis. *Clin. Sci. Mol. Med. 46*:283, 1974.

96. Maldonado, J. E., Velosa, J. A., Kyle, R. A., Wagoner, R. D., Holley, K. E., and Salassa, R. M.: Fanconi syndrome in adults: A manifestation of a latent form of myeloma. *Am. J. Med. 58*:354, 1975.

97. Bergsagel, D. E., and Pruzanski, W.: Treatment of plasma cell myeloma with cytotoxic agents. *Arch. Intern. Med. 135*:172, 1975.

98. Shustik, C., Bergsagel, D. E., and Pruzanski, W.: κ and λ light chain disease: Survival rates and clinical manifestations. *Blood 48*:41, 1976.

99. Pringle, J. P., Graham, R. C., and Bernier, G. M.: Detection of myeloma cells in the urine sediment. *Blood 43*:137, 1974.

100. Hobbs, J. R.: Immunochemical classes of myelomatosis, including data from a therapeutic trial conducted by a medical research council working party. *Br. J. Haematol. 16*:599, 1969.

101. Salmon, S. E., and Smith, B. A.: Immunoglobulin synthesis and total body tumor cell number in IgG multiple myeloma. *J. Clin. Invest. 49*:1114, 1970.

102. Sullivan, P. W., and Salmon, S. E.: Kinetics of tumor growth and regression in IgG multiple myeloma. *J. Clin. Invest. 51*:1697, 1972.

103. Lindärde, F., and Zettervall, O.: Hypercalcemia and normal ionized serum calcium in a case of myelomatosis. *Ann. Intern. Med. 78*:396, 1973.

104. Soria, J., Soria, C., and Dao, C.: Immunoglobulin bound calcium and ultrafilterable serum calcium in myeloma. *Br. J. Hematol. 34*:343, 1976.

105. Jaffe, J. P., and Mosher, D. F.: Calcium binding by a myeloma protein. *Am. J. Med. 67*:343, 1979.

106. Fahey, J. L., Scoggins, R., Utz, J. P., and Szwed, C. F.: Infection, antibody response and gamma globulin components in multiple myeloma and macroglobulinemia. *Am. J. Med. 35*:698, 1963.

107. Meyers, B. R., Hirschman, S. Z., and Axelrod, J. A.: Current patterns of infection in multiple myeloma. *Am. J. Med. 52*:87, 1972.

108. Cohen, H. J., and Rundles, R. W.: Managing the complications of plasma cell myeloma. *Arch. Intern. Med. 135*:177, 1975.

109. Harris, J., Alexanian, R., Hersh, E., and Migliore, P.: Immune function in multiple myeloma: Impaired responsiveness to keyhole limpet hemocyanin. *Can. Med. Assoc. J. 104*:389, 1971.

110. Spitler, L. E., Spath, P., Petz, L., Cooper, N., and Fudenberg, H. H.: Phagocytes and C4 in paraproteinaemia. *Br. J. Haematol. 29*:279, 1975.

111. Ziegler, J. B., Hansen, P. J., and Penny, R.: Leukocyte function in paraproteinemia. *Aust. N. Z. J. Med. 5*:39, 1975.

112. Abdou, N. I., and Abdou, N. L.: Monoclonal nature of lymphocytes in multiple myeloma: Effects of therapy. *Ann. Intern. Med. 83*:42, 1975.

113. Mellstedt, H., Pettersson, D., and Holm, G.: Monoclonal B-lymphocytes in peripheral blood of patients with plasma cell myeloma: Relation to activity of the disease. *Scand. J. Haematol. 16*:112, 1976.

114. Linton, A. L., Dunningan, M. G., and Thomson, J. A.: Immune responses in myeloma. *Br. Med. J. 2*:86, 1963.

115. DeFronzo, R. A., Humphrey, R. L., Wright, J. R., and Cooke, C. R.: Acute renal failure in multiple myeloma. *Medicine 54*:209, 1975.

116. Meyers, G. H., and Witten, D. M.: Acute renal failure after excretory urography in multiple myeloma. *Am. J. Roentgenol. 113*:583, 1971.

117. Fahey, J. L.: Serum protein disorders causing clinical symptoms in malignant neoplastic disease. *J. Chron. Dis. 16*:703, 1963.

118. Fahey, J. L., Barth, W. F., and Solomon, A.: Serum hyperviscosity syndrome. *JAMA 192*:464, 1965.

119. Whittaker, J. A., Tuddenham, E. G. D., and Bradley, J.: Hyperviscosity syndrome in IgA multiple myeloma. *Lancet 2*:572, 1973.

120. Somer, T.: Hyperviscosity syndrome in plasma cell dyscrasias. *Adv. Microcirc. 6*:1, 1975.

121. McGrath, M. A., and Penny, R.: Paraproteinemia: Blood hyperviscosity and clinical manifestations. *J. Clin. Invest. 58*:1155, 1976.

122. MacKenzie, M. R., Fudenberg, H. H., and O'Reilly, R. A.: The hyperviscosity syndrome. I. IgG myeloma: The role of protein concentration and shape. *J. Clin. Invest 49*:15, 1970.

123. Bloch, K. J., and Maki, D. G.: Hyperviscosity syndromes associated with immunoglobulin abnormalities. *Semin. Hematol. 10*:113, 1973.

124. Silverstein, A., and Doniger, D. E.: Neurologic complications of myelomatosis. *Arch. Neurol. 9*:534, 1963.

125. Maldonado, J. E., Kyle, R. A., Ludwig, J., and Okazaki, H.: Meningeal myeloma. *Arch. Intern. Med. 126*:660, 1970.

126. Benson, M. D., Cohen, A. S., Brandt, K. D., and Cathcart, E. S.: Neuropathy, M components, and amyloid. *Lancet 1*:10, 1975.

127. Davis, L. E., and Drachman, D. B.: Myeloma neuropathy: Successful treatment of two patients and review of cases. *Arch. Neurol. 27*:507, 1972.

128. Drieger, H., and Pruzanski, W.: Plasma cell neoplasia with peripheral neuropathy. A study of five cases and a review of the literature. *Medicine 59*:301, 1980.

129. Takatsuki, K., Uchiyama, T., Sagawa, K., and Yodi, J.: *Plasma cell dyscrasia with polyneuritis and endocrine disorder: Review of 32 patients.* Excerpta Medica, International Congress Series no. 415, *Topics in Haematology,* Proceedings of the 16th International Congress of Hematology, Kyoto, September 1976, p. 454.

130. Weiner, L. P., Anderson, P. N., and Allen, J. C.: Cerebral plasmacytoma with myeloma protein in the cerebrospinal fluid. *Neurology* 16:615, 1966.

131. Somersen, A., Osgood, C. P., Jr., and Brylski, J.: Solitary posterior fossa plasmacytoma. *J. Neurosurg.* 35:223, 1971.

132. McCarthy, J., and Proctor, S. J.: Cerebral involvement in multiple myeloma: Case report. *J. Clin. Pathol.* 31:259, 1978.

133. Bethlem, J., van Gool, J., and den Hartog Jager, W. A.: Progressive multifocal leucoencephalopathy associated with multiple myeloma. *Acta Neuropathol.* 3:525, 1964.

134. Bessis, M.: Ultrastructure of lymphoid and plasma cells in relation to globulin and antibody formation. *Lab. Invest.* 10:1040, 1961.

135. DePetris, S., Karlsbad, G., and Pernis, B.: Localization of antibodies in plasma cells by electron microscopy. *J. Exp. Med.* 117:849, 1963.

136. Maldonado, J. E., Brown, A. L., Bayrd, E. D., and Pease, G. L.: Ultrastructure of the myeloma cell. *Cancer* 11:1613, 1966.

137. Paraskevas, F., Heremans, J., and Waldenström, J.: Cytology and electrophoretic pattern in γ1A (β2A) myeloma. *Acta Med. Scand.* 170:575, 1961.

138. Maldonado, J. E., Bayrd, E. D., and Brown, A. L., Jr.: The flaming cell in multiple myeloma: A light and electron microscopy study. *Am. J. Clin. Pathol.* 44:605, 1965.

139. Hobbs, J. R.: Growth rates and responses to treatment in human myelomatosis. *Br. J. Haematol.* 16:607, 1969.

140. McIntyre, O. R.: Correlation of abnormal immunoglobulin with clinical features of myeloma. *Arch. Intern. Med.* 135:46, 1975.

141. Jancelewicz, Z., Takatsuki, K., Sugai, S., and Pruzanski, W.: IgD multiple myeloma. *Arch. Intern. Med.* 135:87, 1975.

142. Ogawa, M., Kochwa, S., Smith, C., Ishizaka, K., and McIntyre. O. R.: Clinical aspects of IgE myeloma. *N. Engl. J. Med.* 281:1217, 1969.

143. Johansson, G. O., and Bennich, H.: Immunological studies of an atypical (myeloma) immunoglobulin. *Immunology* 13:381, 1967.

144. Fishkin, B. G., Orloff, N., Scaduto, L. E., Borucki, D. T., and Spiegelberg, H. L.: IgE multiple myeloma: A report of the third case. *Blood* 39:361, 1972.

145. Waldenström, J. G.: Macroglobulinemia. *Adv. Metab. Disord.* 2:115, 1965.

146. Kyle, R. A.: Monoclonal gammopathy of undetermined significance. *Am. J. Med.* 64:814, 1978.

147. Osserman, E. F., and Takatsaki, K.: Role of an abnormal, myeloma-type, serum gamma globulin in the pathogenesis of the skin lesions of papular mucinosis (lichen myxedematosus). *J. Clin. Invest.* 42:962, 1963.

148. James, K., Fudenberg, H., Epstein, W. L., and Shuster, J.: Studies on a unique diagnostic serum globulin in papular mucinosis (lichen myxedematosus). *Clin. Exp. Immunol.* 2:153, 1967.

149. Shapiro, C. M., Fretziu, D., and Norris, S.: Papular mucinosis. *JAMA* 214:2052, 1970.

150. Feldman, P., Shapiro, L., Pick, A. I., and Slatkin, M. H.: Scleromyxedema: A dramatic response to melphalan. *Arch. Dermatol.* 99:51, 1969.

151. Cream, J. J.: Pyoderma gangrenosum with a monoclonal IgM red cell agglomerating factor. *Br. J. Dermatol.* 84:223, 1971.

152. Stone, M. J., and Frenkel, E. P.: Clinical spectrum of light chain myeloma: Study of 35 patients with special reference to occurrence of amyloidosis. *Am. J. Med.* 58:601, 1975.

153. Limas, C., Wright, J. R., Mutsuzaki, M., and Calkins, E.: Amyloidosis and multiple myeloma: A re-evaluation using a control population. *Am. J. Med.* 54:166, 1973.

154. Maldonado, J. E., Riggs, L., and Bayrd, E. D.: Pseudomyeloma: Is association of severe osteoporosis with serum monoclonal gammopathy an entity or a coincidence? *Arch. Intern. Med.* 135:267, 1975.

155. Hobbs, J. R.: Paraproteins, benign or malignant? *Br. Med. J.* 3:699, 1967.

156. Kyle, R. A., Maldonado, J. E., and Bayrd, E. D.: Idiopathic Bence Jones proteinuria: A distinct entity? *Am. J. Med.* 55:222, 1973.

157. Stein, H., and Kaiserling, E.: Myeloma producing nonsecretory IgM and secretory IgG. *Scand. J. Haematol.* 12:274, 1974.

158. Stavem, P., Froland, S. S., Haugen, H. F., and Lislerud, A.: Non-secretory myelomatosis without intracellular immunoglobulin: Immunofluorescent and ultramicroscopic studies. *Scand. J. Haematol.* 17:89, 1976.

159. Fishkin, B. G., and Spiegelberg, H. L.: Cervical lymph node metastasis as the first manifestation of localized extramedullary plasmacytoma. *Cancer* 38:1641, 1976.

160. Southeastern Cancer Study Group: Treatment of myeloma: Comparison of melphalan, chlorambucil, and azathioprine. *Arch. Intern. Med.* 135:157, 1975.

161. Carter, S. K.: Current status of new agents, in *Report of the Chemotherapy Program.* National Cancer Institute, Bethesda, Md., 1972, vol. 2, p. 125.

162. Ogawa, M., Bergsagel, D. E., and McCulloch, E. A.: Chemotherapy of mouse myeloma: Quantitative cell cultures predictive of response *in vivo. Blood* 41:7, 1973.

163. Lane, M.: Preliminary report of animal studies with cytoxan (cyclophosphamide). *Cancer Chemother. Rep.* 3:1, 1959.

164. McArthur, J. R., Athens, J. W., Wintrobe, M. M., and Cartwright, G. E.: Melphalan and myeloma: Experience with a low-dose continuous regimen. *Ann. Intern. Med.* 72:665, 1970.

165. Bergsagel, D. E., Robertson, G. L., and Hasselback, R.: Effect of cyclophosphamide on advanced lung cancer and the hematological toxicity of large intermittent intravenous doses. *Can. Med. Assoc. J.* 98:532, 1968.

166. Tattersall, M. H. N., Jarman, M., Newlands, E. S., Holyhead, I., Milstead, R. A. V., and Weinberg, A.: Pharmacokinetics of melphalan following oral or intravenous administration in patients with malignant disease. *Eur. J. Cancer* 14:507, 1978.

167. Alberts, D. S., et al.: Variability of melphalan absorption in man. *Proc. AACR-ASCO* 19:334, 1978.

168. Bergsagel, D. E., Ogawa, M., and Librach, S. L.: Mouse myeloma as a model for studies of cell kinetics. *Arch. Intern. Med.* 135:109, 1975.

169. Bergsagel, D. E., Cowan, D. H., and Hasselback, R.: Plasma cell myeloma: Response of melphalan-resistant patients to high-dose, intermittent cyclophosphamide. *Can. Med. Assoc. J.* 107:851, 1972.

170. Bentzel, C. J., Carbone, P. P., and Rosenberg, L.: The effect of prednisone on calcium metabolism and Ca⁴⁷ kinetics in patients with multiple myeloma and hypercalcemia. *J. Clin. Invest.* 43:2132, 1964.

171. Salmon, S. E., Shadduck, R. D., and Schilling, A.: Intermittent high-dose prednisone (NSC-10023) therapy for multiple myeloma. *Cancer Chemother. Rep.* 51:179, 1967.

172. Rothschild, M. A., Schreiber, S. S., Oratz, M., and McGee, H. L.: The effects of adrenocortical hormones on albumin metabolism studied with albumin-1¹³¹. *J. Clin. Invest.* 37:1229, 1958.

173. Levy, A. L., and Waldmann, T. A.: The effect of hydrocortisone on immunoglobulin metabolism. *J. Clin. Invest.* 49:1697, 1970.

174. Goldin, A.: Evaluation of chemical agents against the plasma cell tumor LPC-1 in mice. *Biochem. Parmacol.* 16:665, 1967.

175. Moon, J. H., and Edmonson, J. H.: Procarbazine (NSC-77213) and multiple myeloma. *Cancer Chemother. Rep. (Pt. 1)* 54:245, 1970.

176. Samuels, M. L., Leary, W. V., Alexanian, R., Howe, C. D., and Frei, E., III: Clinical trials with N-isopropyl-α-(2-methyl-hydrazino)-p-toluamide hydrochloride in malignant lymphoma and other disseminated neoplasia. *Cancer* 20:1187, 1967.

177. O'Bryan, R. M., Luce, J. K., Talley, R. W., Gottlieb, J. A., Baker, L. H., and Bonadonna, G.: Phase II evaluation of Adriamycin in human neoplasia. *Cancer* 32:1, 1973.

178. Alberts, D. S., Salmon, S. E.: Adriamycin (NSC-123127) in the treatment of alkylator-resistant multiple myeloma: A pilot study. *Cancer Chemother. Rep. (Pt. 1),* 59:345, 1975.

179. Ghanta, V. K., Jones, M. T., Woodard, D. A., Durant, J. R., and Hiramoto, R. N.: cis-Dichlorodiammine platinum (II) chemotherapy in experimental murine myeloma MOPC 104E. *Cancer Res.* 37:771, 1977.

180. Ogawa, M., Gale, G. R., Meischan, S. J., and Cooke, V. A.: Effects of dinitrato (1,2-diaminocyclohexane) platinum (NSC-239851) on murine myeloma and hemopoietic precursor cells. *Cancer Res.* 36:3185, 1976.

181. Mellstedt, H., Björkholm, M, Johansson, B., Ahre, A., Holm, G., and Strander, H.: Interferon therapy in myelomatosis. *Lancet* 1:245, 1979.

182. Ideström, K., Cantell, K., Killander, D., Nilsson, K., Strander, H.,

and Williams, J.: Interferon therapy in multiple myeloma. *Acta Med. Scand.* 205:149, 1979.

183. The big IF in cancer. *Time Magazine,* March 31, 1980.

184. Alexanian, R., et al.: Treatment for multiple myeloma: Combination chemotherapy with different melphalan dose regimens. *JAMA* 208:1680, 1969.

185. Alexanian, R., et al.: Combination chemotherapy for multiple myeloma. *Cancer* 30:382, 1972.

186. Alexanian, R., Salmon, S., Bonnet, J., Gehan, E., Haut, A., and Weich, J.: Combination chemotherapy for multiple myeloma. *Cancer* 40:2765, 1977.

187. Valeriote, F., Bruce, W. R., and Meeker, B. E.: Synergistic action of cyclophosphamide and 1,3 bis (2-chloroethyl)-1-nitrosourea on a transplanted murine lymphoma. *J. Natl. Cancer. Inst.* 40:935, 1968.

188. Lin, H., and Bruce, W. R.: Chemotherapy of the transplanted KHT fibrosarcoma in mice. *Sem. Haematol.* 5:89, 1972.

189. Bergsagel, D. E., Bailey, A. J., Langley, G. R., MacDonald, R. N., White, D. R., and Miller, A. B.: The chemotherapy of plasma-cell myeloma and the incidence of acute leukemia. *N. Engl. J. Med.* 301:743, 1979.

190. Harley, J. P., et al.: Improved survival of increased-risk myeloma patients on combined triple-alkylating agent therapy: A study of the CALGB. *Blood* 54:13, 1979.

191. Tattersall, M. H. N., Jarman, M., Newlands, E. S., Holyhead, I., Milstead, R. A. V., and Weinberg, A.: Pharmacokinetics of melphalan following oral or intravenous administration in patients with malignant disease. *Eur. J. Cancer* 14:507, 1978.

192. Alberts, D. S., et al.: Variability of melphalan absorption in man. *Proc. AACR-ASCO* 19:334, 1978.

193. Alberts, D. S., and Golde, D. W.: Perturbation of DNA synthesis in multiple myeloma cells following cell-cycle–nonspecific chemotherapy. *Cancer Res.* 34:2911, 1974.

194. Drewinko, B., Brown, B. W., Humphrey, R., and Alexanian, R.: Effect of chemotherapy on the labeling index of myeloma cells. *Cancer* 34:526, 1974.

195. Salmon, S. E.: Expansion of the growth fraction in multiple myeloma with alkylating agents. *Blood* 145:119, 1975.

196. Salmon, S. E., Alexanian, R., and Dixon, D.: Non-cross-resistant combination chemotherapy improves survival in multiple myeloma. *Blood* 54 (Suppl. 1):207a, 1979, abstract 552.

197. Case, D. C., Jr., Lee, B. J., III, and Clarkson, B. D.: Improved survival times in multiple myeloma treated with melphalan, prednisone, cyclophosphamide, vincristine, and BCNU: M-2 protocol. *Am. J. Med.* 63:897, 1977.

198. Nathans, D., Fahey, J. L., and Potter, M.: The formation of myeloma protein by a mouse plasma cell tumor. *J. Exp. Med.* 108:121, 1958.

199. Bergsagel, D. E.: Assessment of the response of mouse and human myeloma to chemotherapy and radiotherapy, in *Growth Kinetics and Biochemical Regulation of Normal and Malignant Cells,* edited by B. Drewinko and R. M. Humphreys. University of Texas Cancer Center, M. D., Anderson Hospital and Tumor Institute, 29th Annual Symposium on Fundamental Cancer Research, Williams & Wilkins, Baltimore, 1977, pp. 705–717.

200. Von Schéele, C.: Light chain myeloma with features of adult Fanconi syndrome. Six years remission with one course of melphalan. *Acta. Med. Scand.* 199:533, 1976.

201. Southwest Oncology Group Study: Remission maintenance therapy for multiple myeloma. *Arch. Intern. Med.* 135:147, 1975.

202. Bergsagel, D. E.: Treatment of plasma cell myeloma. *Ann. Rev. Med.* 30:431, 1979.

203. Durie, B. G., Russell, D. H., and Salmon, S. E.: Reappraisal of plateau phase in myeloma. *Lancet* 2:65, 1980.

204. Hamburger, A., and Salmon, S. E.: Primary bioassay of human myeloma stem cells. *J. Clin. Invest.* 60:846, 1977.

205. Alexanian, R., Gehan, E., Haut, A., Saiki, J., and Weick, J.: Unmaintained remissions in multiple myeloma. *Blood* 51:1005, 1978.

206. Raisz, L. G., Luben, R. A., Mundy, G. R., Dietrich, J. W., Horton, J. E., and Trummel, C. L.: Effect of osteoclast activating factor from human leukocytes on bone metabolism. *J. Clin. Invest.* 56:408, 1975.

207. Suki, W. N., Yium, J. J., Von Minden, M., Saller-Herbert, C., Eknoyan, G., and Martinez-Maldonado, M.: Acute treatment of hypercalcemia with furosemide. *N. Engl. J. Med.* 283:836, 1970.

208. Slayton, R. E., Shnider, B. I., Elias, E., Horton, J., and Perila, C. P.: New approach to the treatment of hypercalcemia. The effect of short-term treatment with mithramycin. *Clin. Pharmacol. Ther.* 12:833, 1971.

209. Deftos, L. J., and Neer, R.: Medical management of the hypercalcemia of malignancy. *Ann. Rev. Med.* 24:323, 1974.

210. Salmon, S. E., Samal, B. A., Hayes, D. M., Hosley, H., Miller, S. P., and Schilling, A.: Role of gamma globulin for immunoprophylaxis in multiple myeloma. *N. Engl. J. Med.* 277:1336, 1967.

211. Russell, J. A., Fitzharris, B. M., Corringham, R., Darcy, D. A., and Powles, R.: Plasma exchange *vs.* peritoneal dialysis for removing Bence Jones protein. *Br. Med. J.* 2:1397, 1978.

212. Feest, T. G., Burge, P. S., and Cohen, S. L.: Successful treatment of myeloma kidney by diuresis and plasmapheresis. *Br. Med. J.* 1:503, 1976.

213. Misiani, R., et al.: Plasmapheresis in the treatment of acute renal failure in multiple myeloma. *Am. J. Med.* 66:684, 1979.

214. Humphrey, R. L., Wright, J. R., Zachary, J. B., Sterioff, S., and DeFronzo, R. A.: Renal transplantation in multiple myeloma. A case report. *Ann. Intern. Med.* 83:651, 1975.

215. Trivedi, H., and Kumar, S.: Renal transplantation in lethal disease. *Ann. Intern. Med.* 85:132, 1976 (letter).

216. Cohen, P., and Gardner, F. H.: Induction of subacute skeletal fluorosis in a case of multiple myeloma. *N. Engl. J. Med.* 271:1129, 1964.

217. Harley, J. B., Schilling, A., and Glidewell, O.: Ineffectiveness of fluoride therapy in multiple myeloma. *N. Engl. J. Med.* 286:1283, 1972.

218. Jowsey, J., Riggs, B. L., Kelly, P. J., and Hoffman, D. L.: Effect of combined therapy with sodium fluoride, vitamin D and calcium in osteoporosis. *Am. J. Med.* 53:43, 1972.

219. Gardner, F. H.: Fluorides for multiple myeloma. *N. Engl. J. Med.* 287:1252, 1972.

220. Carbone, P. P., Kellerhouse, L. E., and Gehan, E. A.: Plasmacytic myeloma: A study of the relationship of survival to various clinical manifestations and anomalous protein type in 112 patients. *Am. J. Med.* 42:937, 1967.

221. Salmon, S. E., and Durie, B. G. M.: Cellular kinetics in multiple myeloma. *Arch. Intern. Med.* 135:131, 1975.

222. Acute Leukemia Group B: Correlation of abnormal immunoglobulin with clinical features of myeloma. *Arch. Intern. Med.* 135:46, 1975.

223. Salmon, S. E., and Smith, B. A.: Sandwich solid phase radioimmunoassays for the characterization of human immunoglobulins synthesized *in vitro. J. Immunol.* 104:665, 1970.

224. Durie, B. G. M., and Salmon, S. E.: A clinical staging system for multiple myeloma. Correlation of measured myeloma cell mass with presenting features, response to treatment, and survival. *Cancer* 36:842, 1975.

225. Bergsagel, D. E.: Plasma cell myeloma: Prognostic factors and criteria of response to therapy, in *Cancer Therapy: Prognostic Factors and Criteria of Response,* edited by M. J. Staquet. Raven, New York, 1975, p. 73.

226. Medical Research Council's Working Party for Therapeutic Trials in Leukaemia: Report on the first myelomatosis trial. I. Analysis of presenting features of prognostic importance. *Br. J. Haematol.* 24:123, 1973.

227. Johansson, B.: Prognostic factors in myelomatosis. *Br. Med. J.* 2:327, 1971.

228. Bergsagel, D. E., Migliore, P. J., and Griffith, K. M.: Myeloma proteins and the clinical response to melphalan therapy. *Science* 148:376, 1965.

229. Khaleeli, M., Keane, W. M., and Lee, G. R.: Sideroblastic anemia in multiple myeloma: A preleukemic change. *Blood* 47:17, 1973.

230. Rosner, F., and Grunwald, H.: Multiple myeloma terminating in acute leukemia. Report of 12 cases and review of the literature. *Am. J. Med.* 57:927, 1974.

231. Cleary, B., Binder, R. A., Kales, A. N., and Veltri, B. J.: Simultaneous presentation of acute myelomonocytic leukemia and multiple myeloma. *Cancer* 41:1381, 1978.

232. Tursz, T., Flandrin, G., Brouet, J.-C. Briere, J., and Seligmann, M.: Simultaneous occurrence of acute myeloblastic leukemia and mul-

tiple myeloma without previous chemotherapy. *Br. Med. J.* 1:642, 1974.

233. Salberg, D., Kurtides, E. S., and McKeever, W. P.: Myelomonocytic leukemia in an untreated case of Waldenström's macroglobuline-mia. *Arch. Intern. Med.* 137:514, 1977.

234. Ligorsky, R. D., Axelrod, A. R., Mandell, G. H., Palutke, M., and Prasad, A. S.: Acute myelomonocytic leukemia in a patient with macroglobulinemia and malignant lymphoma. *Cancer* 39:1156, 1977.

235. Osserman, E. F.: The association between plasmacytic and mono-cytic dyscrasias in man. Clinical and biochemical studies, in *Gamma Globulins—Structure and Control Biosynthesis, Third Nobel Symposium held in Stockholm, June 12–17,* edited by J. Killander. In-terscience, New York, 1967, pp. 573–583.

236. Poulik, M. D., Berman, L., and Prasad, A. S.: "Myeloma protein" in a patient with monocytic leukemia. *Blood* 33:746, 1969.

237. Barnard, D. L., et al.: Chronic myelomonocytic leukemia with paraproteinemia but no detectable plasmacytosis. *Cancer* 44:927, 1979.

238. Krajny, M., and Pruzanski, W.: Waldenström's macroglobulinemia: Review of 45 cases. *Can. Med. Assoc. J.* 114:899, 1976.

239. Binstock, M. L., and Mundy, G. R.: Effect of calcitonin and gluco-corticoids in combination on the hypercalcemia of malignancy. *Ann. Intern. Med.* 93:269, 1980.

240. Mazzaferri, E. L., O'Dorisio, T. M., and LoBuglio, A. F.: Treatment of hypercalcemia associated with malignancy. *Semin. Oncol.* 5:141, 1978.

CHAPTER *123*

Macroglobulinemia

DANIEL E. BERGSAGEL

Macroglobulinemia is an increase in the blood concen-tration of IgM. Popular usage of the term *macroglobuline-mia* usually implies that the increase is the result of monoclonal IgM, although polyclonal macroglobuline-mia can occur. The specific disorders listed in Table 123-1 are associated with a monoclonal (M-protein) IgM in the plasma.

The B-lymphocytic and B-lymphoplasmacytic neo-plasms form a spectrum of closely related diseases. In most cases they present in their typical forms and can be distinguished. Waldenström's macroglobulinemia is manifested by a monoclonal IgM in the plasma and very often lymphadenopathy, hepatomegaly, splenomegaly, anemia, and an absence of bone lesions [1].

The other related diseases may occasionally have neoplastic cells that elaborate monoclonal IgM but may not have other features that are typical of Walden-ström's macroglobulinemia [2]. For example, they may have more plasmacytic morphology of tumor cells and osteolytic bone lesions, suggestive of myeloma, or blood counts more in keeping with chronic lympho-cytic leukemia. In these cases classification may be difficult. Fortunately, patient management is dictated by the clinical findings despite the precise classifica-tion, while prognosis is difficult in a single case even if

TABLE 123-1   Diseases associated with monoclonal macro-globulinemia

Diseases	Num-ber of cases	Percent of all cases
B-lymphoplasmacytic neoplasms	133	31
Waldenström's macroglobulinemia (112)*		
IgM myeloma (14)		
Extramedullary plasmacytoma (7)		
B-lymphocytic neoplasms	164	39
Chronic lymphocytic leukemia (31)		
Diffuse lymphomas (133)		
Controlled monoclone	126	30
Cold agglutinin syndrome (9)		
Benign (asymptomatic) monoclonal gammopathy of IgM type (117)		

*The parentheses indicate the number of cases of the specific entity cited. Cases were compiled from Refs. 2 to 4.

it can be easily classified. In general, Waldenström's macroglobulinemia has higher serum IgM levels than other disorders listed in Table 123-1, and hypervis-cosity develops more commonly.

Patients with features of chronic lymphocytic leuke-mia or diffuse lymphocytic lymphomas and a plasma monoclonal macroglobulin rarely have IgM concentra-tions above 2.5 g/dl, and hyperviscosity or cryoglobu-linemia is uncommon. The course of B-lymphocyte neoplasms producing monoclonal IgM is similar to that of those in which the protein is not secreted. The M pro-tein, however, can serve as an index of the response to therapy. The treatment of these patients should be that which is appropriate for chronic lymphocytic leukemia or a diffuse lymphocytic lymphoma.

Cases that resemble Waldenström's macroglobuline-mia but in which monoclonal IgG or IgA proteins are secreted have been described [3], as has the apparent concordance of myeloma and macroglobulinemia with a double gammopathy [4,5].

The IgM level remains constant in patients with the idiopathic cold hemagglutinin syndrome, and the dis-ease behaves like a benign disorder similar to benign monoclonal gammopathy of the IgM type in that the secreting cell population does not grow progressively and invade tissues.

Etiology and pathogenesis

These aspects of the disease are discussed in Chap. 121.

Clinical features

The mean age at diagnosis of patients with macroglobu-linemia associated with a lymphoplasmacytic neoplasm is 64 years [6–10]. In earlier studies 66 percent of the pa-tients were male [8], but in later studies the proportion of males was 50 percent [6,7,9,10].

The common presenting symptoms of macroglobuli-

TABLE 123-2 Presenting symptoms in macroglobulinemia

Symptoms	Percent of 227 cases
Fatigue, weakness	44
Bleeding	44
Weight loss	23
Neurological disturbance	11
Visual disturbance	8
Raynaud's phenomenon	3

SOURCE: McCallister, Bayrd, Harrison, and McGuckin [8].

nemia are listed in Table 123-2, although many patients discovered to have a monoclonal IgM component in their serum are asymptomatic. The most common bleeding manifestation is epistaxis, but bleeding from the gastrointestinal tract and dependent purpura are also frequent. The association of macroglobulinemia with neurologic manifestations has been referred to as the *Bing-Neel syndrome* [11]. Patients may complain of blurred vision or severely reduced visual acuity and other neurologic symptoms described below. Cold hypersensitivity, Raynaud's phenomenon, cold urticaria, or purpura are major symptoms in some patients and may be associated with cryoglobulin in the serum.

The common physical findings are summarized in Table 123-3. The usual constellation of abnormalities which leads to the clinical suspicion of macroglobulinemia are hepatosplenomegaly, enlarged superficial lymph nodes, and retinal abnormalities. The earliest change detectable by funduscopic examination is dilated, tortuous retinal veins. As patients develop more marked hyperviscosity, sausagelike segmentation of distended retinal veins and retinal hemorrhages develop. Clumping of erythrocytes and venocapillary segmentation have also been noted in conjunctival vessels [12]. The most common neurologic presentation is an acute cerebral dysfunction which may resemble either a gross intracerebral or subarachnoid hemorrhage. Confusion, disturbances of consciousness progressing to coma, and a diffuse brain syndrome, sometimes designated *coma paraproteinaemicum* [13], may develop in patients with marked plasma hyperviscosity. The retinal changes and the diffuse brain dysfunction frequently improve following plasmapheresis, which reduces the serum IgM concentration and hyperviscosity.

Polyneuritis or polyradiculitis, with an increase in spinal fluid protein [14–16] and polyneuropathy [16,17],

TABLE 123-3 Physical findings in macroglobulinemia

Finding	Percent in 267 cases
Hepatomegaly	38
Splenomegaly	37
Ocular changes	37
Adenopathy	30
Neurological abnormalities	17
Purpura	15
Congestive heart failure	≈4

SOURCE: Data from McCallister, Bayrd, Harrison, and McGuckin [8], and MacKenzie and Fudenberg [9].

have also been observed in patients with macroglobulinemia. Congestive heart failure may develop as the result of a markedly expanded plasma volume, increased blood viscosity, and anemia. This often becomes an important complication during the course of uncontrolled disease unless it is averted by plasmapheresis and correction of the anemia. Pulmonary findings can be prominent occasionally [18].

Laboratory findings

Some of the common laboratory abnormalities present in patients at the time of diagnosis are shown in Table 123-4. A normochromic, normocytic anemia is usually present. A shortened erythrocyte survival time was found in six of eight patients who had macroglobulinemia, and impairment of erythropoiesis was documented in the other two [19]. Hemodilution by the expanded plasma volume is a factor which also contributes to the low hemoglobulin concentration in macroglobulinemia [9]. The Coombs' test is almost always negative.

Osteolytic lesions were found in only 2 percent of the series of patients shown in Table 123-4. Patients with osteolytic lesions are often classified as having IgM myeloma, and thus it is difficult to determine the frequency of osteolytic lesions in patients with macroglobulinemia.

The marrow findings in monoclonal macroglobulinemia are varied [20]. Typically, a diffuse infiltrate of lymphocytes, plasmacytoid lymphocytes, and a slight increase in plasma cells is associated with Waldenström's macroglobulinemia. Mast cells may also be increased. Periodic acid–Schiff–positive material (Dutcher bodies) can be seen in lymphoid cells and can be seen in blood vessel walls and interstitially. These are not constant features, however. Some patients with benign types of macroglobulinemia may have nodular lymphoid hyperplasia on marrow biopsy. Patients with other types of lymphoma may have pathological lymphoid nodules or infiltrates in the marrow.

The Sia test (Chap. 125) is a simple screening procedure. It was positive in 76 percent of one group of macroglobulinemic sera tested. A negative Sia test does not rule out the diagnosis, and a positive test may also occur in patients with IgG and IgA aggregates or

TABLE 123-4 Abnormal laboratory findings at time of diagnosis

Finding	No. abnormal/ No. tested	Percent abnormal
Hemoglobin <12 g/dl	233/267	88
Osteolytic lesions	5/267	2
Positive Sia test	115/151	76
Relative serum viscosity >4	14/34	41
Cryoglobulinemia	24/65	37
Bence Jones proteinuria	31/126	25

SOURCE: Data from McCallister, Bayrd, Harrison, and McGuckin [8] and MacKenzie and Fudenberg [9].

polymers. Thus, more sensitive and specific measurements of IgM should be used. The relative serum viscosity was elevated above 4 in 41 percent of patients with macroglobulinemia tested in one series, and 36 percent of these patients developed symptoms of hyperviscosity sometime in the course of their disease [9]. Cryoglobulin was demonstrated in the serum of 37 percent of the patients tested. Symptoms of cold hypersensitivity are much more likely to occur if the cryoglobulin begins to precipitate at room temperature or above (20 to 22°C) and if the circulating cryoglobulin is present in a concentration greater than 2 to 3 g/dl.

RENAL FUNCTION AND PROTEINURIA

Bence Jones proteinuria, as detected by the qualitative heat test, has been reported to occur in 25 percent of patients (Table 123-4). A much higher frequency of light-chain proteinuria has been detected in patients with macroglobulinemia when more sensitive and specific tests, such as electrophoresis and immunoelectrophoresis of concentrated urine, are used. In one series urinary light chains were found in 8 of 16 patients, but the heat test for Bence Jones protein was positive in only 1 [21]. Nonselective proteinuria, comparable to that which occurs in the nephrotic syndrome, was present in 2 patients. In two additional series 105 of 157 (67 percent) and 20 of 28 (71 percent) patients were found to be excreting light chains [6,10].

Renal insufficiency occurs in macroglobulinemia [8,22]. In two series the blood urea nitrogen was reported to be greater than 25 mg/dl in 8 of 45 patients [10] and greater than 50 mg/dl in 5 of 16 patients [21].

The renal pathology in patients with myeloma and macroglobulinemia is markedly different. In myeloma, the classic lesions are large casts in the collecting tubules with a surrounding macrophage reaction. Pronounced tubule degeneration has been more strongly emphasized in recent years. The excretion of large amounts of light-chain protein by patients with myeloma and its concentration in the distal tubules are considered to be important in the pathogenesis of renal disease.

Patients with macroglobulinemia excrete much less light-chain protein in the urine, and in one series renal casts were not found [21]. In contrast to myeloma, glomerular lesions appear to be more important features in macroglobulinemia. IgM may be precipitated on the endothelial side of the basement membrane of the tubules, and these deposits may be so voluminous as to occlude capillaries. Deposits of amyloid may be found in the glomeruli, and interstitial infiltrates of lymphocytes and plasma cells, similar to those found in the marrow, are also present [21].

An immunologically mediated glomerulonephritis has been described in a patient with Waldenström's macroglobulinemia who developed the nephrotic syndrome [23]. Deposits of IgG, IgM, and the third component of complement were demonstrated in the glomeruli of this patient by immunofluorescent staining

methods. Improvement in the nephrotic syndrome followed effective treatment with chlorambucil and prednisone.

DISORDERS OF HEMOSTASIS

A bleeding tendency similar to that which may be found in other patients with monoclonal protein abnormalities occurs commonly in patients with macroglobulinemia [24,25]. These patients have bruising, purpura, retinal hemorrhages, epistaxis, and bleeding from mucosal surfaces (see also Chap. 122). The platelet count is usually normal, but abnormalities of platelet function appear to be important causes of bleeding in these patients. Evidence of impaired platelet function includes prolonged bleeding time, positive tourniquet test, impaired clot retraction, defective prothrombin consumption, poor thromboplastin generation with the patient's platelets, defective platelet aggregation in vivo [26], and defective platelet adhesiveness in vitro [27,28]. The impairment of platelet aggregation and the release of platelet factor 3 appears to result from the coating of the platelets by the IgM protein [28–30].

Other abnormalities of the coagulation mechanism can be detected in some patients. It has been postulated that some IgM protein may interact with labile coagulation factors to inhibit coagulation [25]. The coagulation defect detected most frequently is prolongation of the thrombin time. This defect appears to result from the binding of the Fab sites of some immunoglobulins to fibrin during clotting and polymerization, thereby inhibiting fibrin monomer aggregation [31]. This results in a bulky, gelatinous, transparent clot with narrowed fibrin strands and impaired or absent clot retraction. The inhibition of fibrin monomer aggregation does not necessarily produce a bleeding diathesis, however, unless there is a concomitant impairment of platelet function. A variety of monoclonal proteins have been reported to inhibit coagulation factors [25]. These include inhibitors of factor VIII, nonspecific inhibitors usually detected by the thromboplastin generation test, inhibitors of the prothrombin complex, factor V, and factor VII, and factor X deficiency due to in vivo inactivation in patients with primary amyloidosis.

In addition, there are a number of patients who have reduced levels of one or more coagulation factors. Factors II, V, VII, VIII, X, and fibrinogen have all been affected. A clear-cut explanation for the depression of these factors is not apparent. It has been proposed that the anomalous protein complexes with and/or coprecipitates labile coagulation factors [32]. With the exception of fibrinogen [33] the in vitro formation of these complexes has not been confirmed [29,30,34], and their precipitation in cryoglobulinemia could not be demonstrated [24].

THE HYPERVISCOSITY SYNDROME

The hyperviscosity syndrome develops when the size, shape, and concentration of an abnormal plasma protein component or aggregate produces a great increase in blood viscosity. This syndrome is usually associated with macroglobulins, but it has also been reported in patients with IgG and IgA protein aggregates (see Chap. 126). Symptoms usually do not develop unless the serum viscosity (relative to water) rises above 4. Increased whole-blood viscosity measured at low rates of shear correlates well with some vascular complications of hyperviscosity [35]. The clinical syndrome includes (1) a bleeding diathesis, described above; (2) retinopathy with dilatation and segmentation of the retinal and conjunctival veins (link-sausage appearance), retinal hemorrhages, and papilledema; (3) neurologic symptoms, including weakness, fatigability, headache, anorexia, vertigo, nystagmus, transient paresis, and coma; and (4) hypervolemia, distention of peripheral blood vessels, increased vascular resistance, and cardiac failure.

ANTIBODY ACTIVITY OF MONOCLONAL PROTEINS
Although most monoclonal proteins have no demonstrable antibody activity, some have binding specificities for a variety of antigens [36,37]. The antibody activities of monoclonal proteins which may produce clinical manifestations are considered in this section.

Cold agglutinins   Many IgM and a few IgA proteins agglutinate red cells in the cold. Most IgM cold agglutinins have κ light chains and demonstrable anti-I activity. A few IgM λ proteins with cold agglutinin activity have been discovered. They usually have anti-i activity, and many are also cryoglobulins [38]. Normal human serum contains small amounts of cold agglutinin [39], and it is thought that the neoplastic transformation of a normal cell producing a cold agglutinin may be responsible for the development of a neoplastic cell line which continues to produce this type of reactive protein.

Immunoglobulin G   Anti-IgG activity has been found in 5 percent of anomalous IgM proteins [37]. The light chain is usually κ, and the IgM-IgG complex is cryoprecipitable. The patients often have clinical symptoms of cold intolerance, including Raynaud's phenomenon, cold urticaria, and purpura. IgA and IgG components with anti-IgG activity have also been described [37].

Lipoprotein   The unusual association of myeloma, xanthomatosis, and hyperlipidemia prompted a search for antilipoprotein activity among myeloma proteins. Binding activity for lipids was demonstrated in three patients with myeloma and hyperlipidemia (two IgA and one IgG) [40,41]. The interaction of the anomalous protein with serum lipoprotein is thought to produce a complex that is relatively stable and not easily catabolized.

Hemostatic abnormalities   The interaction of monoclonal proteins with coagulation factors is summarized above. There is little evidence that this interference is the result of antibody-binding. The demonstration that Fab fragments of some proteins, however, are effective in binding fibrin monomers suggests that this reaction may be specific [31].

Differential diagnosis

The clinical manifestations of macroglobulinemia may resemble those of chronic lymphocytic leukemia, lymphocytic lymphoma, or a plasma cell neoplasm. The demonstration of a serum component containing μ heavy chains is the feature which distinguishes macroglobulinemia from other entities.

In contrast to plasma cell myeloma, which is relatively easy to differentiate from benign monoclonal gammopathy, the clinical course of macroglobulinemia is not as clearly defined [42]. In general, asymptomatic patients without enlarged lymph nodes, hepatosplenomegaly, lymphocytic and plasmocytic marrow infiltration, or anemia may be considered to have a benign form of the disease and be followed without specific therapy. Even patients with mild anemia, splenic enlargement, or other findings can have a nonprogressive course for years. An increase in the level of the abnormal serum component or the development of clinical manifestations such as worsening anemia, hyperviscosity, or bleeding are manifestations of a more aggressive or progressive form of the disease and constitute an indication for treatment.

Therapy

Waldenström's macroglobulinemia is relatively rare, and patients with this disorder have such variable disease that they are usually excluded from prospective clinical trials of the effectiveness of antineoplastic agents. As a result, recommendations regarding treatment are largely based on the experience of those who have treated only a small number of patients by different regimens over a period of several years.

In one institution, 31 patients with macroglobulinemia were seen between 1955 and 1963 [8]. Five patients were asymptomatic and received no treatment during follow-up periods ranging from 3 to 9 years; 15 were treated with chlorambucil, and 6 of the 9 evaluable patients showed a 50 percent or greater fall in the level of the abnormal serum globulin. The median survival could not be ascertained in this group, since only 12 of the patients had died, but a life table plot suggested that the median survival would be about 6 years from the time of diagnosis.

In another group of 40 patients [9], 8 of 19 (40 percent) treated with chlorambucil, cyclophosphamide, or melphalan for at least 3 months showed a fall in IgM concentration and in serum viscosity. The average survival from the time of diagnosis was 49.2 months for the responding group and 24.1 months for the nonresponders.

The median survival from the time of diagnosis was reported to be 50 months for a group of 45 patients with Waldenström's macroglobulinemia [10]. Treatment with prednisone and an alkylating agent was given to 31 patients; 5 required plasmapheresis, and 14 have not received any therapy.

The median survival from the time of diagnosis in a group of patients with macroglobulinemia associated with chronic lymphocytic leukemia and diffuse lymphoma was 37 months [43]. For the 10 patients who responded to chemotherapy, the median survival was 53 months.

Some patients with macroglobulinemia benefit from treatment with chlorambucil, cyclophosphamide, or melphalan. Patients who have become refractory to alkylating agents but who have responded to doxorubicin have been reported [44]. Prospective, randomized clinical trials will be required to determine when treatment should be instituted, the best agent to use, the optimal dose schedule, and the adjunctive value of prednisone and plasmapheresis.

Since quantitative therapeutic studies have not been carried out, the following approach is suggested. For asymptomatic patients without enlarged superficial lymph nodes, hepatosplenomegaly, bone lesions, anemia, bleeding tendencies, renal insufficiency, hyperviscosity, or neurologic changes, observation without specific treatment is recommended. Patients should be seen regularly, however, and those who have a progressive rise in the IgM concentration or who develop symptoms as enumerated above may require treatment at any time. The disease status may remain stable for many years, and patients may never require treatment.

Patients with symptoms should have treatment as indicated by the type of cellular infiltration in the marrow and other disease features. Those with chronic lymphocytic leukemia, lymphocytic lymphoma, or atypical plasma cell disease should be treated as is appropriate for the cytological diagnosis.

The hyperviscosity syndrome may require special treatment. With the development of fatigue, headache, epistaxis, vertigo, nystagmus, retinopathy, or congestive heart failure, the serum viscosity may be found to have risen to four to eight times that of water. If symptoms are severe, 4 to 6 units of plasma should be removed by plasmapheresis daily until the relative serum viscosity falls to less than 4. Chemotherapy using chlorambucil or cyclophosphamide in combination with prednisone (see Chaps. 119 and 122) controls the underlying disease and should be given in an effort to prevent a recurrence of hyperviscosity.

Course and prognosis

The course of Waldenström's macroglobulinemia is quite variable, but it usually progresses slowly over a period of several years. Hyperviscosity, hemorrhage, thrombosis, hemolytic anemia, and infections are contributory causes of death. Lymphomatous infiltration of lymph nodes, liver, spleen, bone marrow, and gastrointestinal mucosa may occur. In some patients the concentration of IgM may fall as the lymphomatous tumors grow, and this may be associated with rapid clinical deterioration, which suggests that the neoplastic cells can dedifferentiate and grow more rapidly during the terminal phase of the disease. Cases have been reported which have terminated as immunoblastic sarcoma [45] or acute myelogenous leukemia [46].

References

1. Waldenström, J.: Incipient myelomatosis or "essential" hyperglobulinemia with fibrinogenopenia: New syndrome? *Acta Med. Scand.* 117:216, 1944.
2. Ameis, A., Ko, H. S., and Pruzanski, W.: M-components—A review of 1242 cases. *Can. Med. Assoc. J.* 114:889, 1976.
3. Tursz, T., Brouet, J.-C., Flandrin, G., Dannon, F., Clauvel, J.-P., and Seligmann, M.: Clinical and pathologic features of Waldenström's macroglobulinemia in seven patients with serum monoclonal IgG or IgA. *Am. J. Med.* 63:499, 1977.
4. McNutt, D. R., and Fundenberg, H. H.: IgG myeloma and Waldenström's macroglobulinemia. *Arch. Intern. Med.* 131:731, 1973.
5. Pruzanski, W., Underdown, B., Silver, E. H., and Katz, A.: Macroglobulinemia-myeloma double gammopathy. *Am. J. Med.* 57:259, 1974.
6. Carter, P., Koval, J. J., and Jobbs, J. R.: The relation of clinical and laboratory findings to the survival of patients with macroglobulinemia. *Clin. Exp. Immunol.* 28:241, 1977.
7. Stein, R. S., Ellman, L., and Bloch, K. J.: The clinical correlates of IgM M-components: An analysis of thirty-four patients. *Am. J. Med. Sc.* 269:209, 1975.
8. McCallister, B. D., Bayrd, E. D., Harrison, E. G., Jr., and McGuckin, W. F.: Primary macroglobulinemia: Review with a report on thirty-one cases and notes on the value of continuous chlorambucil therapy. *Am. J. Med.* 43:394, 1967.
9. MacKenzie, M. R., and Fudenberg, H. H.: Macroglobulinemia: An analysis of forty patients. *Blood* 39:874, 1972.
10. Krajny, M., and Pruzanski, W.: Waldenström's macroglobulinemia: Review of 45 cases. *Can. Med. Assoc. J.* 114:899, 1976.
11. Bichel, J., Bing, J., and Harboe, N.: Another case of hyperglobulinemia and affection of central nervous system. *Acta Med. Scand.* 138:1, 1950.
12. Ackerman, A. L.: The ocular manifestations of Waldenström's macroglobulinemia and its treatment. *Arch. Ophthalmol.* 67:701, 1962.
13. Wuhrmann, F.: Uber das Coma paraproteinaemicum bei Myelomen and Makroglobulinamien. *Schweiz. Med. Wochenschr.* 86:623, 1956.
14. Logothetis, J., Silverstein, P., and Coe, J.: Neurologic aspects of Waldenström's macroglobulinemia: Report of a case. *Arch. Neurol.* 3:564, 1960.
15. Clinicopathologic Conference, Macroglobulinemia. *Am. J. Med.* 28:951, 1960.
16. Garcin, R., Mallarmé, J., Roudot, P., Endtz, L. J.: Forme névritique de la macroglobulinémie de Waldenström (à propos d'une nouvelle observation). *Sang* 31:441, 1960.
17. Darnely, J. D.: Polyneuropathy in Waldenström's macroglobulinemia: Case report and discussion. *Neurology* 12:617, 1962.
18. Rausch, P. G., and Herion, J. C.: Pulmonary manifestations of Waldenström's macroglobulinemia. *Am. J. Hematol.* 9:201, 1980.
19. Cline, M. J., Solomon, A., Berlin, N. L., and Fahey, J. L.: Anemia in macroglobulinemia. *Am. J. Med.* 34:213, 1963.
20. Rywlin, A. M., Civantos, F., Ortega, R. S., and Dominguez, C. J.: Bone marrow histology in monoclonal macroglobulinemia. *Am. J. Clin. Pathol.* 63:769, 1975.
21. Morel-Maroger, L., Basch, A., Danon, F., Verroust, P., and Richet, G.: Pathology of the kidney in Waldenström's macroglobulinemia: Study of 16 cases. *N. Engl. J. Med.* 283:123, 1970.

22. Waldenstöm, J.: Macroglobulinemia. *Adv. Metab. Disord.* 2:115, 1965.
23. Martelo, O. J., Schultz, D. R., Pardo, V., and Perez-Stable, E.: Immunologically-mediated renal disease in Waldenström's macroglobulinemia. *Am. J. Med.* 58:567, 1975.
24. Perkins, H. A., MacKenzie, M. R., and Fudenberg, H. H.: Hemostatic defects in dysproteinemias. *Blood* 35:695, 1970.
25. Lackner, H.: Hemostatic abnormalities associated with dysproteinemias. *Semin. Hematol.* 10:125, 1973.
26. Godal, H. C., and Borchgrevink, C. F.: The effect of plasmapheresis on the hemostatic function in patients with macroglobulinemia Waldenström and multiple myeloma. *Scand. J. Clin. Lab. Invest.* 17 (Suppl. 84):133, 1965.
27. Doumenc, J., Prost, R. J., Samama, M., and Bousser, J.: Anomalie de l'agrégation plaquettaire au cours de la maladie de Waldenström (à propos de 3 cas). *Nouv. Rev. Fr. Hematol.* 6:734, 1966.
28. Penny, R., Castaldi, P. A., and Whitsed, H. M. Inflammation and haemostasis in paraproteinaemias. *Br. J. Haematol.* 20:35, 1971.
29. Pachter, M. R., Johnson, S. A., Neblett, T. R., and Truant, J. P.: Bleeding, platelets, and macroglobulinemia. *Am. J. Clin Pathol.* 31:467, 1959.
30. Pachter, M. R., Johnson, S. A., and Basinski, D. H.: The effect of macroglobulins and their dissociation units on release of platelet factor 3. *Thromb. Diath. Haemorrh.* 3:501, 1959.
31. Coleman, M., Vigliano, E. M., Weksler, M. E., and Nachman, R. L.: Inhibition of fibrin monomer polymerization by lambda myeloma globulins. *Blood* 39:210, 1972.
32. Henstell, H. H., and Kligerman, M.: A new theory of interference with the clotting mechanism: The complexing of euglobulin with factor V, factor VII and prothrombin. *Ann. Intern. Med.* 49:371, 1958.
33. Brzoza, H., and Lahav, M.: Interaction between macroglobulin and fibrinogen with partial dissociation of macroglobulin after coagulation. *Isr. J. Exp. Med.* 11:165, 1964.
34. Ménaché, D.: Action des macroglobulines de la maladie de Waldenström sur la coagulation étude in vitro. *Ann. Biol. Clin.* 20:170, 1962.
35. McGrath, M. A., and Penny, R.: Paraproteinema: Blood hyperviscosity and clinical manifestations. *J. Clin. Invest.* 58:1155, 1976.
36. Potter, M.: Antigen binding M-components in man and mouse, in *Multiple Myeloma and Related Disorders*, edited by H. A. Azar and M. Potter. Harper & Row, Hagerstown, Md., 1973, vol. 1, p. 195.
37. Seligmann, M., and Brouet, J. C.: Antibody activity of human myeloma globulins. *Semin. Hematol.* 10:163, 1973.
38. Pruzanski, W., Cowan, D. H., and Parr, D. M.: Clinical and immunochemical studies of IgM cold agglutinins and lambda type light chains. *Clin. Immunol. Immunopathol.* 2:234, 1974.
39. Feizi, T., Wernet, P., Kunkel, H. G., and Douglas, S. D.: Lymphocytes forming red cell rosettes in the cold in patients with chronic cold agglutinin disease. *Blood* 42:753, 1973.
40. Beaumont, J. L.: Gamma-globulines et hyperlipidémies: L'hyperlipidémie auto-anticorps. *Ann. Biol. Clin.* 27:611, 1969.
41. Beaumont, J. L., Lorenzelli, L., and Delphanque, B.: Emploi d'un detergent pour la purification d'anticorps antilipoproteins. *Immunochemistry* 7:131, 1970.
42. Seligmann, M., and Basch, A.: The clinical significance of pathological immunoglobulins, in *Plenary Session Papers, XII Congress Int. Soc. Haematol.* New York, 1968, p. 21.
43. Alexanian, R.: Monoclonal gammopathy in lymphomas. *Arch. Intern. Med.* 135:62, 1975.
44. Clamon, G. H., Corder, M. P., and Burns, C. P.: Successful doxorubicin therapy of primary macroglobulinemia resistant to alkylating agents. *Am. J. Hematol.* 9:221, 1980.
45. Leonhard, S. A., Muhleman, A. F., Hurtibise, P. E., and Martello, O. J.: Emergence of immunoblastic sarcoma in Waldenström's macroglobulinemia. *Cancer* 45:3102, 1980.
46. Salberg, D., Kurtides, E. S., and McKeever, W. P.: Monomyelocytic leukemia in an untreated case of Waldenström's macroglobulinemia. *Arch. Intern. Med.* 137:514, 1977.

CHAPTER *124*

The heavy-chain diseases

EDWARD C. FRANKLIN

Heavy-chain diseases represent a special group of plasma cell and lymphocyte neoplasms which produce "immunoglobulin variants," consisting in most instances of separate defective heavy chains with internal deletions. In addition there is usually a failure of light-chain synthesis [1]. The clinical and laboratory features of four types of heavy-chain diseases—gamma (γ), alpha (α), mu (μ), and delta (δ)—have been delineated during the past 20 years [3–7].

Etiology, genetics, and pathogenesis

The anomalous proteins produced by the lymphocytes and plasma cells of patients with heavy-chain disease are of particular interest because they are synthetic rather than degradative products of immunoglobulin molecules, and they represent incomplete molecules; that is, proteins with internal deletions. The largest number of molecules studied, and the most informative, are those of patients with γ heavy-chain disease. Analyses of these proteins have shown that the deletions generally end at the hinge or at the junction of the variable (VH) and constant (CH1) domains and are not randomly distributed (see Chap. 108). The boundaries of these deletions correlate well with the sites where splicing of RNA occurs during RNA processing, a finding which anticipated the concept that the separate domains of the immunoglobulin heavy chain might be coded for by separate genes, recently established by DNA cloning [9]. These RNA splicing errors are probably the result of a genetic event at the DNA level with correction occurring during RNA processing at the sites of splicing of exons. A less likely possibility is an error in transcription or translation [10]. In the case of γ-chain and α-chain disease, there is failure of light-chain synthesis also; in contrast patients with a μ-chain disease usually produce light chains, but they are not assembled into immunoglobulinlike molecules because of the nature of the deletion. Failure of light-chain synthesis is difficult to explain by a second mutation of a gene on another chromosome. Therefore, it is more likely a regulatory defect, perhaps a consequence of the deletion of the CH1 domain of the heavy chain. Structural studies of about 20 heavy-chain-disease proteins have indicated they often represent degradation products which have resulted from cleavage of molecules deleted at the hinge region. Although most patients have pure heavy-chain disease, a few have a heavy-chain-disease fragment in the plasma in addition to an intact myeloma, or more commonly a macroglobulin, molecule.

In one case the original tumor produced a γ_3 myeloma protein and then underwent a further mutation [12]. Although the heavy-chain diseases are uncommon, they usually can be suspected by their characteristic clinical manifestations, which will be described below. As the number of patients has increased, the clinical spectrum has broadened, and some cases of heavy-chain disease have had atypical presentations.

Diagnosis is dependent upon immunochemical investigation of the serum and urine, and can also be supported by immunohistological analysis of lymph node or spleen biopsies.

Gamma heavy-chain disease (γ HCD)

Since its description in 1964 [3], more than 50 patients with γ heavy-chain disease have been described. Most patients have been over 40 years of age, but six have been between 12 and 40 years old. Clinical manifestations consist of lymph node enlargement, anemia, fever, malaise, weakness, and hepatosplenomegaly, symptoms which lead to the suspicion of either a chronic inflammatory disease or a hematological malignancy. Palpable lymph nodes frequently wax and wane in size. A characteristic feature occurring in about one-third the patients is the enlargement of the lymph nodes in Waldeyer's ring, which results in palatal edema [1,3,6]. Unlike myeloma, skeletal lesions are uncommon and have been noted only in two patients. Minimal lymphadenopathy or infiltrates localized in organs like the thyroid, salivary glands, or in the abdomen have been reported. Characteristically patients have mild anemia and leukopenia. Eosinophilia and atypical lymphocytic plasma cell are often seen. A few patients have developed plasma cell leukemia terminally. Thrombocytopenia is not common. The marrow usually has an increase in the number of plasma cells, lymphocytes, lymphocytoid plasma cells, and eosinophils, although the marrow film may be normal. The marrow findings are rarely diagnostic. Spleen and lymph node infiltration with plasma cells or lymphocytes and often eosinophils and macrophages is commonly found. Though in many instances the pathology findings mimic chronic lymphocytic leukemia or multiple myeloma, in about 15 percent of the patients, even after careful study, no evidence of lymphoid malignancy can be detected. Unfortunately, without careful immunohistochemical analysis, the pathologic findings are rarely diagnostic. Two of the patients considered to have heavy-chain disease have been shown to have extensive amyloid infiltration at postmortem examination. Though the amyloid deposits were not examined, in one instance it was possible to make amyloidlike fibrils out of the heavy-chain-disease protein by proteolytic digestion, thus raising the possibility that in these individuals the amyloid may have consisted of the heavy-chain-disease fragment [13].

The diagnosis of γ heavy-chain disease requires a demonstration in the serum, urine, or both of a protein component which reacts with antisera to the γ heavy chain but fails to react with antisera to κ or λ light chains or Fab fragments. Though the first patients to be recognized produced large amounts of the abnormal protein, with the increased awareness of this entity, a number of patients have been diagnosed who have only trace amounts of protein in the serum and virtually none in the urine. Most of the proteins have belonged to the γ_1 subclass. However, proteins belonging to the other subclasses have been recognized, and there appears to be a somewhat higher than expected incidence of γ_3 molecules. On electrophoresis the abnormal protein usually appears as a heterogeneous band and the proteins in the serum and urine are of identical mobility. The concentration of the anomalous component ranges from barely detectable to 3 g/dl with excretion up to 15 g per day in the urine. The course of the disease is variable with survival ranging from a few months to more than 5 years, and in rare instances complete remissions have been noted. Patients usually die of infections or of progression of the disease.

As is true of other types of plasma cell neoplasms, a definitive form of therapy has not been developed. Some of the patients appear to respond to treatment with melphalan or cyclophosphamide and local irradiation applied in a manner similar to that used for multiple myeloma [6].

Alpha heavy-chain disease (α HCD)

α HCD was first described in 1968 [14] and is the most common form of heavy-chain disease. Unlike plasma cell myeloma and macroglobulinemia, the disease usually affects patients under the age of 50 years, with a peak incidence in the second and third decades. There are two clinical forms: the enteric form, which has a high incidence in areas where intestinal infection with parasites, bacteria, and viruses is common (e.g., Mediterranean, Asian, and South American countries), and a respiratory form seen in patients from Europe and the United States [15,16], characterized by a lymphoplasmacytic infiltrate limited to the respiratory tract.

The clinical features of the enteric form, often referred to as "Mediterranean lymphoma," include chronic diarrhea and severe malabsorption with marked weight loss, steatorrhea, hypocalcemia, and excessive fecal losses of water and electrolytes. Abdominal masses are often palpable, and abdominal pain can be a major symptom. Clubbing of the fingers is quite common.

Intestinal mucosal biopsies show diffuse and massive lymphoplasmacytic infiltration of the lamina propria with cells occurring diffusely or in patches. The cells range in appearance from normal plasma cells to those of immunoblastic sarcoma [17]. Villous atrophy and sparsity of crypts have been found in all patients. Mesenteric lymph nodes and rectal biopsies have shown a similar lymphoplasmacytic infiltration. At a late stage tumors may develop and cause intestinal obstruction. Radiologic studies may show bowel wall thickening, villous atrophy, and lymph node enlargement.

Enlarged retroperitoneal nodes have been demonstrated by lymphangiography in a few patients, but involvement of peripheral lymph nodes, the liver, or the spleen usually is not observed. Skeletal lesions have not been reported. Abnormal lymphoid or plasma cells may be found in the blood of patients in the terminal phase of the disease, and abnormal plasma cells have been demonstrated in the marrow by immunofluorescence studies.

The diagnosis of α HCD is dependent on the immunochemical analysis of serum [6,14]. Serum electrophoresis usually reveals a reduced albumin level, a moderate to marked hypogammaglobulinemia, and a broad nonhomogeneous band in the β_2- to α_2-globulin region which can range in concentration from a few hundred milligrams per deciliter to 3 g/dl. The abnormal protein reacts with antisera to α chains but fails to react with antisera to κ or λ light chains. The failure of light-chain antisera to precipitate the abnormal protein is, however, not sufficient evidence to establish a diagnosis, since some IgA paraproteins (usually with λ chains) may have hidden light chains. In doubtful cases immunofixation coupled with immunoelectrophoresis should be employed, and ultimately the abnormal protein should be purified and the absence of light chains demonstrated by polyacrylamide gel electrophoresis. In all the reported cases the abnormal protein has belonged to the α_1 subclass of IgA. Bence Jones proteinuria has not been found, but in many patients the abnormal heavy-chain protein can be demonstrated in concentrated urine. The anomalous protein is usually found in large amounts in the jejunal fluid (as would be expected in view of the intestinal localization of the lymphoplasmacytic infiltrates) and not in the parotid saliva.

Structural and immunochemical studies of several of the abnormal proteins have shown that they contain the Fc and hinge region of the α_1 heavy chain and the J chain (a polypeptide chain found in IgM and polymeric forms of IgA) [2,18]. Most of the Fd protein of the heavy chain is missing, usually as a result of an internal deletion, and there is failure of light-chain production.

The course of the disease is usually progressive and fatal. However, complete clinical remissions have been reported in a number of patients, with disappearance of the abnormal protein from the serum and jejunal fluid and disappearance of the lymphoplasmacytic infiltrate from the intestinal mucosa [6]. In some of the patients remissions were achieved with chemotherapy for a malignant lymphoma, while in others antibiotics alone were employed. The appearance of complete remissions with exclusively antibiotic treatment makes the neoplastic nature of the disease questionable, and raises the possibility that sometimes there is an infectious etiology.

Mu heavy-chain disease (μ HCD)

The 15 known patients with μ HCD have ranged in age from 39 to 79 years, and nearly all have had chronic lymphocytic leukemia (CLL) or some other lymphoid neoplasm [5,20–22]. Yet a survey of more than 300 patients with CLL indicates that this abnormality is rare. The patients differ from the usual patient with CLL in three ways: (1) enlarged peripheral lymph nodes are infrequent while hepatosplenomegaly is common; (2) unusual vacuolated plasma cells are commonly seen in the marrow; similar cells are only rarely encountered in other plasma cell dyscrasias; (3) most of the patients excrete large amounts of κ light chains in the urine.

The diagnosis requires a high index of suspicion. Serum protein electrophoresis is usually normal or shows only hypogammaglobulinemia, but an abnormal protein spike has been demonstrated in some cases [20,21]. The diagnosis usually rests on the demonstration by immunoelectrophoresis of a rapidly migrating component which precipitates with antisera to μ chains but not with antisera to light chains. Often free κ chains having a different mobility can be detected. It is usually necessary to document the diagnosis further by ultracentrifugation or gel filtration, since some intact macroglobulins may not react with κ or λ antisera. A patient with μ-chain fragments and various partially assembled forms of the μ-chain fragments and κ chains has been studied [23]. Treatment for the underlying disease, usually chronic lymphocytic leukemia, should be initiated when the diagnosis is made.

Delta heavy-chain disease (δ HCD)

So far there is only a single case report of patients with δ HCD who presented with renal insufficiency, osteolytic lesions, and a marrow plasmacytosis typical of myeloma [7]. Electrophoresis showed a peak of 700 mg/dl between the γ and β region, reactive in a variety of tests with anti-δ but not anti-κ or anti-λ sera. Molecular weight estimates suggested a tetramer of δ chains with $M_r = 260,000$ daltons, thus explaining its absence from the urine. Unfortunately, careful chemical characterization could not be carried out prior to the patient's death.

References

1. Frangione, B., and Franklin, E. C.: Heavy chain diseases: Clinical features and molecular significance of the disordered immunoglobulin structure. *Semin. Hematol. 10*:53, 1973.
2. Franklin, E. C., and Frangione, B.: Structural variants for human and murine immunoglobulins, in *Contemporary Topics in Molecular Immunology*, edited by F. P. Inman and W. J. Mandy. Plenum, New York, 1975, vol. 4, pp. 89–126.
3. Franklin, E. C., Lowenstein, J., Bigelow, B., and Meltzer, M.: Heavy chain (7S gamma-globulin) disease. A new clinical entity. *Am. J. Med. 37*:332, 1964.

4. Seligmann, M., Mihaesco, E., Hurez, D., Mihaesco, C., Preud'homme, J. L., and Rambaud, J. C.: Immunochemical studies in four cases of alpha chain disease. *J. Clin. Invest.* 48:2374, 1969.
5. Forte, F. A., et al.: Heavy chain disease of the mu type: Report of the first case. *Blood* 36:137, 1970.
6. Seligmann, M., Mihaesco, E., Preud'homme, J. L., Danon, F., and Brouet, J.-C.: Heavy chain diseases: Current findings and concepts. *Immunol. Rev.* 48:145, 1979.
7. Vilpo, J. A., et al.: Delta heavy chain disease: A study of a case. *Clin. Immunol. Immunopathol.* 17:584, 1980.
8. Frangione, B., and Franklin, E. C.: Correlation between fragmented immunoglobulin genes and heavy chain deletion mutants. *Nature* 281:600, 1979.
9. Maki, R., Traunecker, A., Sakano, H., Roeder, W., and Tonegawa, S.: Exon shuffling generates an immunoglobulin heavy chain gene. *Proc. Natl. Acad. Sci. (U.S.A.)* 77:2138, 1980.
10. Early, P., Huang, H., Davis, M., Calame, K., and Hood, L.: An immunoglobulin heavy chain variable region gene is generated from three segments of DNA: V_H, D, and J_H. *Cell* 19:981, 1980.
11. Franklin, E. C.: The structural heterogeneity among degraded gamma heavy chain disease proteins. *J. Immunol.* 121:2582, 1978.
12. Adlersberg, J. B., Grann, V., Zucker-Franklin, D., Frangione, B., and Franklin, E. C.: An unusual case of a plasma cell neoplasm with an IgG3λ myeloma and a γ_3 heavy chain disease protein. *Blood* 51:85, 1978.
13. Pruzanski, W., Katz, A., Nyburg, S. C., and Freedman, M. H.: In vitro production of an amyloid-like substance from γ_3 heavy chain disease protein. *Immunol. Comm.* 3:469, 1974.
14. Seligmann, M., Danon, F., Hurez, D., Mihaesco, E., and Preud'homme, J. L.: Alpha chain disease: A new immunoglobulin abnormality. *Science* 162:1396, 1968.
15. Stoop, J. W., Ballieux, R. E., Higmans, W., and Zegers, B. J. M.: Alpha chain disease with involvement of the respiratory tract in a Dutch child. *Clin. Exp. Immunol* 9:625, 1971.
16. Faux, J. A., Crain, J. D., Rosen, F. S., and Merler, E.: An alpha heavy chain abnormality in a child with hypogammaglobulinemia. *Clin. Immunol. Immunopathol.* 1:282, 1973.
17. Rambaud, J. C., and Seligmann, M.: Alpha chain disease. *Clin. Gastroenterol.* 5:341, 1976.
18. Mestecky, J., Zikan, J., Butler, W. T., and Kulhavy, R.: Studies on human secretory immunoglobulin A—III. J chain. *Immunochem.* 9:883, 1972.
19. Wolfenstein-Todel, C., Mihaesco, E., and Frangione, B.: Variant of a human immunoglobulin: "Alpha chain disease" protein AIT. *Biochem. Biophy. Res. Commun.* 65:47, 1975.
20. Franklin, E. C.: Mu chain disease. *Arch. Intern. Med.* 135:71, 1975.
21. Jonsson, V., Videbaek, A., Axelsen, N. H., and Harboe, M.: Mu chain disease in a case of chronic lymphocytic leukaemia and malignant histiocytoma. *Scand. J. Haematol.* 16:109, 1976.
22. Bonhomme, J., et al.: Mu chain disease in an African patient. *Blood* 43:485, 1974.
23. Kyle, R., and Franklin, E. C.: Unpublished observation.

CHAPTER 125

Amyloidosis

EDWARD C. FRANKLIN

Definition and history

Although amyloid is widely distributed in tissues of human beings and the rest of the animal kingdom, it rarely causes incapacitating disease. On the basis of the color reaction with iodine and sulfuric acid, Virchow designated the substance infiltrating tissues *amyloid* in 1854. Because of its varied manifestations, its association with chronic infection, its subclinical deposition as part of the aging process, and its association with a number of diseases involving the immune system, it has attracted much attention from pathologists and clinicians. Symptoms, and ultimately death, are due to the replacement and destruction of vital organs by the extracellular deposition of proteinaceous amyloid.

This material has been recognized classically by its homogeneous eosinophilic appearance when viewed by light microscopy, and by its staining properties with Congo red and certain metachromatic dyes. Amyloid is a fibrillar substance when viewed in the electron microscope [1–4] and has a characteristic β-pleated sheet appearance by x-ray diffraction [5]. In spite of its rather uniform appearance, the existence of many different types of amyloid has been recognized by clinicians, and this has been documented by biochemical and immunologic studies of the amyloid proteins. Thus, the term *amyloidosis* encompasses a heterogeneous and perhaps unrelated group of disorders whose classification will eventually be based on the nature of the deposits and pathogenetic mechanisms.

Different classification schemes have been presented, based on the clinical features [6–14]. Although some clinical classes of amyloidosis appear to reflect differences in the fibrils or the etiology, they fall short of defining the nature of these disorders. Biochemical studies have led to a classification of these diseases, which includes those in which the infiltrating protein has been characterized and leaves room for those, usually localized, forms that remain to be defined (Table 125-1). This classification, adopted at a symposium on amyloidosis in 1979, bears out the correlation between the old clinical and newer biochemical categories [15]. In this chapter we will use both classifications but anticipate that the newer biochemical one will become predominant in the future. Clinical manifestations and organ distribution are often atypical, and insufficient to categorize a patient. Classification is dependent on the presence or absence of other associated diseases, the tissue distribution of the amyloid deposits, careful immunochemical analyses of the immunoglobulin fractions of serum and urine, and immunohistochemical analysis of tissues [16].

Structure of amyloid proteins

Progress has been hampered by difficulties in isolating the amyloid substance and by the fact that many dissimilar stimuli can induce amyloid deposits. Characterization was advanced when it was discovered that the apparently homogeneous material consists of long fibrils which have a diameter of 100 to 150 Å and are made up of two longitudinal subunits, or filaments, 40 to 60 Å in diameter separated by a clear space of 25 to 50 Å [1–4]. More than 95 percent of the amyloid substance consists of these characteristic fibrils. The fibrils have been isolated, purified, characterized chemically and immunologically, and shown to consist of two major types of amyloid proteins which either singly or in combination form amyloid fibrils [19–21]. One of these proteins is the amyloid A or *AA protein* and the second is the *AL protein*. The latter was formerly classified as the primary and myeloma-associated type and consists of fragments of immunoglobulin light chains [22–28] (see Chap. 104).

AL PROTEINS
This heterogeneous group of proteins now called AL (amyloid L-chain) protein [15] is usually associated with a similar or related L-chain-containing immunoglobulin in the serum [12,20]. The AL proteins have a M_r of 5000 to 25,000 daltons and generally begin at the amino terminal end of the variable region of the light chain. They usually include the variable region in addition to part of the constant region, and may sometimes consist of the entire L chain [20–23]. Proof of their relation to light chains of immunoglobulins is based on three types of studies. The first, and most convincing,

evidence is sequence homologies between the amino terminal region of the amyloid proteins and κ or λ light-chain variable regions [20,22,23]. A new subclass ($V\lambda_6$) has been found in almost a dozen amyloid-related λ-chain proteins [24,25]. Amyloid deposits are usually present when λ_6 proteins are produced [26]. The second line of evidence is the demonstration that fibrils with the appearance of amyloid fibrils can be produced in vitro by proteolytic digestion of some, but not all, Bence Jones proteins, especially those belonging to the $V\lambda_1$ subclass [27,28].

The third is the finding that antisera to amyloid subunits cross-react with κ or λ light chains [29]. While there can be little doubt that these immunoglobulin-related proteins constitute most of the proteins present in primary and myeloma-related amyloid fibrils, it is not known whether the fragments are synthesized as such or whether they are the result of degradation of an intact L chain. While the latter possibility appears more likely, the former can be excluded only by in vitro biosynthetic studies. For unknown reasons, the frequency of λ-related proteins in amyloid fibrils and the sera of patients with amyloidosis is much higher than that of proteins of the κ chain class, although the latter is the predominant L-chain class in all immunoglobulins and myeloma proteins [12,30].

AA PROTEINS
Amyloid fibrils from patients with the *AA* secondary type of amyloidosis, certain familial forms such as familial Mediterranean fever [19,21,31–34], and experimentally induced and naturally occurring amyloid fibrils in all species examined so far [35,36] consist primarily of a protein that is unrelated to any known protein or immunoglobulin. This protein, known as the AA (amyloid A) protein [15], generally has a M_r of 8500 daltons, although a fragment half this size was isolated from the fibrils of one patient with rheumatoid arthritis

TABLE 125-1 Classification of amyloid diseases

Clinical (old)	Chemical (new)	Protein subunit
Primary and myeloma-associated	AL	Amyloid light chain*
Secondary	AA	Amyloid A protein
Familial:		
Portuguese	AF_P	Amyloid prealbumin
Swedish	AF_S	Amyloid prealbumin
Israeli	AF_I	Amyloid prealbumin
Japanese	AF_J	Amyloid prealbumin
Mediterranean fever	FMF	Amyloid A protein
Endocrine:		
Thyroid	AE_T	Amyloid thyrocalcitonin
Pancreas	AE_P	Amyloid–? protein†
Senile:		
Cardiac	AS_C	Amyloid–prealbumin, etc.
Brain	AD_B	Amyloid–? protein
Cutaneous (dermal)	AD	Amyloid–? protein

*Commonly, Amyloid is abbreviated as A.
†Nature of protein remains unknown.
SOURCE: Adapted from Glenner, Costa, and Freites [15].

[34]. Such proteins from humans, baboons, ducks, guinea pigs, mice, and mink have homologies of amino acid sequences [31–36]. The several human proteins that have been sequenced are virtually identical in the amino terminal half but have differences in the carboxy terminal half [32–34]. The human protein can be heterogeneous also at the amino terminus. Several additional residues precede the first residue in duck amyloid. These findings suggest that the AA protein, too, may be derived from a larger precursor by proteolysis perhaps both at the amino and carboxy termini. Further support for its origin from a circulating precursor is provided by the presence in serum of an antigenically related, larger component known as *serum amyloid A–related protein (SAA)* which has a M_r of about 12,000 daltons and on the basis of its amino acid composition and partial sequence appears to be the precursor of the tissue component [37–47]. The two are identical throughout the first 76 residues, but there is a unique 28 residue acidic tail cleaved off during processing [42,43]. This low-molecular-weight protein remains in the circulation complexed to the high-density lipoprotein fraction [44] and to a lesser extent to albumin [45].

The biologic behavior of the serum component has a bearing on the pathogenetic mechanisms in secondary amyloidosis [36–40]. Its concentration is very low (less than 200 μg/ml) during the first five decades of life, and increases in the elderly [39], but the latter point has not been confirmed [46]. Since SAA behaves as an acute phase reactant in many chronic diseases, including all types of amyloidosis, cancer, infections, rheumatoid arthritis, multiple myeloma, macroglobulinemia, lymphomas, and a variety of others, and also in pregnancy, the almost invariable increases noted in the sera of patients with amyloidosis cannot be used as a simple diagnostic test for the disease [38,39]. SAA levels can be used to monitor tumor dissemination, but the complexity of the assay makes this impractical [47].

OTHER AMYLOID PROTEINS
Several other amyloid proteins have been characterized. Three familial forms and the senile cardiac form are related to prealbumin [48–51]. The amyloid in medullary carcinoma of the thyroid is derived from thyrocalcitonin [52]. Furthermore, histochemical studies [53], coupled with the demonstration that β-pleated sheet fibrils can be formed from insulin and glucagon [54], indicate that other peptides may give fibrils with the properties of amyloid [54].

THE P COMPONENT
In addition to the major fibrillar A protein, most amyloid deposits contain a minor component which is known as the P component, or "doughnut," because of its characteristic appearance on electron microscopy [55]. This protein, which may serve as a scaffold for fibril formation [56] has a M_r of 180,000 daltons. It is composed of 5 or 10 identical noncovalently linked subunits, antigenically related to an α_1 serum glycoprotein

[57] and structurally homologous to C-reactive protein [58].

PATHOGENESIS OF AMYLOIDOSIS
In the absence of definitive information, consideration of possible pathogenetic mechanisms must be based on studies of the amyloid substance and the possibility that proteolytic digestion of a variety of proteins and polypeptides can give rise to the characteristic fibrils. Although amyloidosis occurs naturally in many species and can be induced experimentally by a variety of maneuvers, definitive conclusions are difficult to draw, since in many instances apparently contradictory factors appear to be operative [21,59]. In most natural and experimental circumstances, amyloidosis is associated with an exposure to a large antigenic load (case in administration, hyperimmunized horses, and chronic infection in humans) or, alternatively, depression, and, in some instances, neoplastic proliferation of certain components of the immune system. The deposition of amyloid may be accompanied by depressed thymus-derived (T) cell function [60]. It can be accelerated by immunosuppressive agents [59] and often accompanies naturally occurring immunodeficiency states [59]. Thus, in the two common systemic forms amyloid appears to be deposited in situations where the immune system is overwhelmed by an antigenic load or where it has undergone neoplastic transformation [21]. Augmentation of T-cell function with thymic hormone may prevent the development of experimental amyloidosis [61].

Clinical and laboratory features

The clinical and laboratory features associated with this disease are variable and are largely related to the organs involved. Because the clinical patterns associated with the different forms of amyloidosis overlap, it is usually not possible to classify the disease on clinical grounds [8–12]. Nevertheless, the involvement of certain organs gives a clue to the type of amyloid disease in a patient.

AA (SECONDARY) AMYLOIDOSIS
The most common and perhaps the most "typical" form of amyloidosis is that which accompanies chronic illness. While in the past suppurative conditions such as osteomyelitis, tuberculosis, bronchiectasis, and syphilis headed the list of associated diseases, this type of amyloidosis is now more often encountered in illnesses such as paraplegia and other neurological disease, Hodgkin's disease, leprosy, regional ileitis, and rheumatoid arthritis, but only rarely in systemic lupus erythematosus. In patients with long-standing rheumatoid arthritis, the incidence of amyloidosis has been estimated to range between 20 and 60 percent [13,62], although an autopsy study has questioned this frequency [63].

In AA amyloidosis, deposits are most prominent in

the kidneys, spleen, liver, and adrenals, and only rarely involve the heart, musculoskeletal system, or gastrointestinal tract. Renal amyloidosis may be asymptomatic for a time and generally begins with proteinuria, hyposthenuria, and persistent hematuria. It usually progresses to the nephrotic syndrome and may at times produce azotemia. Hypertension is rare in uncomplicated renal amyloidosis. Although renal involvement is considered characteristic of this form, it is frequently encountered in all types of amyloidosis and is the most common cause of death [6–12,64]. Hepatic and splenic enlargement may be asymptomatic or may give rise to abdominal discomfort. Hepatomegaly may be massive, but liver function is relatively unimpaired, and laboratory tests of liver function are normal or minimally altered [6–12,65].

AL (PRIMARY) AMYLOIDOSIS

AL amyloidosis, whether "essential" or associated with an overt lymphocyte or plasma cell neoplasm, is now being recognized with an increased frequency because of the wider use of tissue biopsies and the routine performance of immunochemical analyses of serum and urine. These types of amyloidosis are considered together because the amyloid materials deposited and the organ distribution appear to be identical [12,20–25,30]. An ever-increasing number of patients with AL amyloidosis can be shown to have homogeneous immunoglobulins in the serum and/or urine, and plasmacytosis in the marrow. Ultimately morphologic and clinical evidence of a plasma cell disease may evolve in the majority of individuals with unexplained AL amyloidosis if they are followed long enough [12]. This type of amyloid most often infiltrates the tongue, heart, skeletal muscle, skin, ligaments, and gastrointestinal tract but can involve the same organs as the secondary type [6–12,30]. These patients often come to the attention of a physician because of macroglossia with problems in speaking or swallowing, carpal tunnel syndrome with median nerve compression, articular manifestations due to periarticular or synovial amyloid infiltrates, or peripheral neuropathy with sensory disturbances, weakness, and, on occasion, autonomic nerve dysfunction [65–68]. Amyloid may infiltrate all regions of the gastrointestinal tract and result in obstruction, hemorrhage, diarrhea, malabsorption, protein-losing enteropathy, or disturbances in intestinal motility [69]. Although rare, gastrointestinal involvement can also occur in AA and some of the familial forms. Deposits in the heart may result in cardiomegaly associated with cardiac failure which is often refractory to treatment, conduction disturbances, arrhythmias, and coronary artery insufficiency. The stiff, enlarged, poorly contractile heart often mimics constrictive pericarditis. The ECG usually demonstrates low voltage and disturbances in conduction. Treatment with digitalis may result in serious arrhythmias and is often of little help in improving cardiac contractility [6–12,30,70,71]. On occasion cardiac amyloidosis is seen as an isolated finding in

elderly individuals who present with unexplained congestive heart failure. This form of the disease is commonly called senile cardiac amyloidosis.

The adrenals and other endocrine organs may be involved and lead to hormone insufficiency. All levels of the respiratory tract may be infiltrated and functionally impaired. The larynx and bronchi are often the site of isolated amyloid deposits in the localized form of the disease [6–12,72]. Amyloidosis of the small vessels of the skin and subcutaneous tissues may give rise to purpura and ecchymoses with little or no trauma, especially in the periorbital region and in areas of skin folds [73]. The bleeding tendency may, on occasion, be aggravated by an associated factor X deficiency [74] due to the selective binding of factor X to amyloid [75,76]. In some patients with lichen amyloidosis or the tumefactive form, cutaneous infiltrates of amyloid substances may be the sole clinical manifestation of the disorder, and careful investigation of such patients fails to uncover either a plasma cell infiltrate of the marrow or systemic amyloidosis [77].

AF (FAMILIAL) AMYLOIDOSIS

Familial amyloidosis occurs in a variety of forms, many of which have characteristic geographic and tissue distributions. The most prevalent and best known of these diseases are familial Mediterranean fever (FMF) [78] and the Portuguese type of lower limb neuropathy [79]. The amyloidosis seen in familial Mediterranean fever resembles the secondary type clinically, and at postmortem amyloid deposits are found in virtually every patient with this disease. The predisposition to amyloidosis may be inherited separately, however, since some families develop amyloid deposits in the absence of the febrile disease. The Portuguese type and several other familial forms of the disease are characterized by marked peripheral nerve involvement. The large number and clinical heterogeneity of the familial forms preclude a detailed description of these variants, but they have been carefully reviewed elsewhere [13].

AMYLOID ASSOCIATED WITH AGING (AS)

Though clinically they are often occult, small deposits with many of the histologic and ultrastructural features of amyloid can be found in the senile plaques of the brain and elsewhere such as in the aorta, pancreas, testes, and other endocrine organs in a majority of elderly individuals at autopsy. The incidence of these deposits increases with age. These amyloid deposits may be an invariable accompaniment of aging, and their occurrence may be the best available indicator of the aging process [16,80,81].

AMYLOID OF ENDOCRINE GLANDS (AE)

The amyloid often found in certain endocrine glands in association with diseases such as diabetes and medullary carcinoma of the thyroid is usually localized to a single gland, clinically asymptomatic, and discovered either at autopsy or on pathologic examination of a surgically removed endocrine tumor. On the basis of histopathologic and preliminary chemical studies, it appears wise to consider this as a separate type of amyloidosis [52–54].

Differential Diagnosis

Amyloidosis should be suspected in individuals with unexplained renal disease, especially in those with the nephrotic syndrome, or with hepatosplenomegaly in association with some of the chronic diseases cited above. Amyloidosis should be considered in all patients with a carpal tunnel syndrome, macroglossia, unexplained neuromuscular disease, congestive heart failure, or malabsorption, especially in individuals with plasma cell neoplasms or a homogeneous immunoglobulin in the serum or urine. Clinical studies should include a careful search for homogeneous immunoglobulin components in serum and urine [12,30]. Patients with AL amyloidosis have a high incidence of Bence Jones proteins alone or in association with a myeloma protein. In an extensive study, 92 percent of such patients had a Bence Jones protein [12]. Of interest is the relatively higher frequency of λ-related proteins than is seen in other types of plasma cell or lymphoid neoplasms. In patients suspected of having one of the variants of AL amyloidosis, marrow examination is indicated to document the underlying plasma cell dyscrasia, and to search for amyloid infiltrates which can often be found in the marrow [82]. In contrast, homogeneous immunoglobulin-related proteins are rare in the secondary type of the disease and the familial forms.

In all types of amyloidosis, the diagnosis rests on biopsy of an involved organ. In the event that this is not possible or desirable, as, for example, in hepatic amyloidosis where biopsy is frequently complicated by severe bleeding, a rectal, or a gingival, biopsy can yield the diagnosis in over 90 percent of patients [83,84]. For optimal results, the tissue must be carefully stained with alkaline Congo red or certain metachromatic dyes and studied by polarization microscopy when Congo red is used. Specific fluorescent antisera to the different amyloid proteins are now being used for histochemical studies and will ultimately be employed for the precise antemortem classification of amyloidosis [16,85–88].

Prognosis and treatment

Except for some of the localized forms, amyloidosis tends to be a progressive disease which ultimately leads to death by destruction of the involved tissues. The resistance of amyloid to phagocytosis and proteolysis hampers the removal of the material by normal host defense mechanisms [89–91]. Nevertheless, secondary amyloidosis [92,93] and, in rare instances, primary amyloidosis [94] can be treated with some benefit by controlling the underlying disease or by chemotherapy.

In the case of AL amyloid associated with plasma cell tumors, treatment of the disease with the usual forms of chemotherapy is indicated, but regression of the amyloidosis is usually slow or almost imperceptible. The cause of death in such patients may be either progression of the amyloid infiltrates or of the underlying plasma cell or lymphoid neoplasm. In patients with AL amyloidosis without evidence of abnormal plasma cell proliferation, the rate of regression is variable and spontaneous remissions are occasionally encountered. There is no unanimity on the question of whether to treat amyloidosis without overt myeloma or whether to wait until definite evidence of a plasma cell neoplasm is found, because of possible complications from chemotherapy and a potential of developing drug resistance.

The renal disease of amyloidosis can be treated, in the advanced stages, by hemodialysis or transplantation. Transplantation has been successfully carried out in more than 100 subjects with survival ranging up to 10 years with only few recurrences [95]. Colchicine has been used successfully to abort the febrile episodes of familial Mediterranean fever. Colchicine therapy also can prevent the appearance of amyloidosis in patients with familial Mediterranean fever and cause its regression provided the disease has not progressed too far [96]. Colchicine should be tried in AL, AA, or AF amyloid since it is a relatively innocuous drug. Its effectiveness, appears to be limited, however. Recently dimethylsulfoxide (DMSO) has been reported to be effective in some cases, but it is still too early to judge its therapeutic efficacy [97,98].

References

1. Cohen, A. S., and Calkins, E.: Electron microscopic observations on a fibrous component in amyloid of diverse origin. *Nature* 183:1202, 1959.
2. Spiro, D.: The structural basis of proteinuria in man: Electron microscopic studies of renal biopsy specimens from patients with lipid nephrosis, amyloidosis, and glomerulonephritis. *Am. J. Pathol.* 35:47, 1959.
3. Pras, M., Zucker-Franklin, D., Rimon, A., and Franklin, E. C.: Physical, chemical and ultrastructural studies of human amyloid fibrils. *J. Exp. Med.* 130:777, 1969.
4. Shirahama, T., and Cohen, A. S.: High-resolution electron microscopic analysis of the amyloid fibril. *J. Cell Biol.* 33:679, 1967.
5. Eanes, E. D., and Glenner, G. G.: X-ray diffraction studies of amyloid filaments. *J. Histochem. Cytochem.* 16:673, 1968.
6. Briggs, G. W.: Amyloidosis. *Ann. Intern. Med.* 55:943, 1961.
7. Symmers, W. St. C.: Primary amyloidosis: A review. *J. Clin. Pathol.* 9:187, 1956.
8. Brandt, K., Cathcart, E. S., and Cohen, A. S.: A clinical analysis of the course and prognosis of 42 patients with amyloidosis. *Am. J. Med.* 44:955, 1968.
9. Cohen, A. S.: Amyloidosis. *N. Engl. J. Med.* 277:522, 574, 628, 1967.
10. Barth, W. F., Glenner, G. G., Waldmann, T. A., and Zelis, R. F.: Primary amyloidosis. *Ann. Intern. Med.* 69:787, 1968.
11. Kyle, R. A., and Bayrd, E. D.: Amyloidosis: Review of 236 cases. *Medicine* 54:271, 1975.
12. Isobe, T., and Osserman, E.: Patterns of amyloidosis and their association with plasma cell dyscrasias, monoclonal immunoglobulins and Bence Jones proteins. *N. Engl. J. Med.* 290:473, 1974.
13. Andrade, C., et al.: Hereditary amyloidosis. *Arthritis Rheum.* 13:902, 1970.
14. Wright, J. R., Calkins, E., Breen, W. J., Stolte, G., and Schultz, R. T.: Relationship of amyloid to aging. *Medicine (Baltimore)* 48:39, 1969.

15. Glenner, G. G., Costa, P., and Freitas, A. (eds.): Guidelines for nomenclature, in *Amyloid and Amyloidosis*. Excerpta Medica, Amsterdam, 1980, pp. XI and XII.

16. Cornwell, G. G., III, Husby, G., Westermark, P., Natvig, J. B., Michaelsen, T. E., and Skogen, B.: Identification and characterization of different amyloid fibril proteins in tissue sections. *Scand. J. Immunol.* 6:1071, 1977.

17. Cohen, A. S., and Calkins, E.: The isolation of amyloid fibrils and a study of the effect of collagenase and hyaluronidase. *J. Cell Biol.* 21:481, 1964.

18. Pras, M., Schubert, M., Zucker-Franklin, D., Rimon, A., and Franklin, E. C.: The characterization of soluble amyloid prepared in water. *J. Clin. Invest.* 47:924, 1968.

19. Benditt, E. P., and Eriksen, N.: Amyloid 3: A protein related to the subunit structure of human amyloid fibrils. *Proc. Natl. Acad. Sci. (U.S.A.)* 55:308, 1966.

20. Glenner, G. G.: Amyloid deposits and amyloidosis. *N. Engl. J. Med.* 302:1283, 1333, 1980.

21. Franklin, E. C., and Zucker-Franklin, D.: Current concepts of amyloid. *Adv. Immunol.* 15:249, 1972.

22. Glenner, G. G., Terry, W., Harada, M., Isersky, C., and Page, D.: Amyloid fibril proteins: Proof of homology with immunoglobulin light chains by sequence analysis. *Science* 172:1150, 1971.

23. Terry, W. D., Page, D., Kimura, S., Isobe, T., Osserman, E., and Glenner, G. G.: Structural identity of Bence Jones and amyloid fibril proteins in a patient with plasma cell dyscrasia and amyloidosis. *J. Clin. Invest* 52:1276, 1973.

24. Sletten, K., Husby, G., and Natvig, J. B.: N-terminal amino acid sequence of amyloid fibrillar: Prototypes of a new lambda variable subgroup VλV. *Scand. J. Immunol.* 3:835, 1974.

25. Skinner, M., Benson, M. D., and Cohen, A. S.: Amyloid fibril protein related to immunoglobulin lambda chains. *J. Immunol.* 114:1433, 1973.

26. Solomon, A., Franklin, E. C., and Frangione, B.: Unpublished observation.

27. Glenner, G. G., et al.: The creation of "amyloid" fibrils from Bence Jones proteins in vitro. *Science* 174:712, 1971.

28. Linke, R., Tischendorf, F. W., Zucker-Franklin, D., and Franklin, E. C.: The formation of amyloid-like fibrils in vitro from Bence Jones proteins of the VI subclass. *J. Immunol.* 111:24, 1973.

29. Isersky, C., Ein, D., Page, D. L., Harada, M., and Glenner, G. G.: Immunochemical cross-reaction of human amyloid proteins with immunoglobulin light chains. *J. Immunol.* 108:486, 1972.

30. Cathcart, E. S., Ritchie, R. F., Cohen, A. S., and Brandt, K.: Immunoglobulins and amyloidosis: An immunologic study of 62 patients with biopsy proved disease. *Am. J. Med.* 52:93, 1972.

31. Benditt, E. P., Eriksen, N., Hermodson, M. A., and Ericsson, L. H.: The major proteins of human and monkey amyloid substances: Common properties including N-terminal amino acid sequence. *FEBS Lett.* 19:169, 1971.

32. Levin, M., Franklin, E. C., Frangione, B., and Pras, M.: The amino acid sequence of the major non-immunoglobulin component of amyloid. *J. Clin. Invest.* 51:2773, 1972.

33. Sletten, K., and Husby, G.: The complete amino acid sequence of nonimmunoglobulin amyloid fibril protein AS in rheumatoid arthritis. *Eur. J. Biochem.* 41:117, 1974.

34. Ein, D., Kimura, S., Terry, W. D., Magnotta, J., and Glenner, G. G.: Amino acid sequence of an amyloid fibril protein of unknown origin. *J. Biol. Chem.* 247:5653, 1972.

35. Hermodson, M. A., Kuhn, R. W., Walsh, K. A., Neurath, H., Eriksen, N., and Benditt, E. P.: Amino acid sequence of monkey amyloid protein A. *Biochem.* 11:2934, 1972.

36. Skinner, M., Cathcart, E. S., Cohen, A. S., and Benson, M. D.: Isolation and identification by sequence analysis of experimentally induced guinea pig amyloid fibrils. *J. Exp. Med.* 140:871, 1974.

37. Levin, M., Pras, M., and Franklin, E. C.: Immunologic studies of the major non-immunoglobulin amyloid protein of amyloid. *J. Exp. Med.* 138:373, 1973.

38. Husby, J., and Natvig, J. B.: A serum component related to nonimmunoglobulin amyloid protein AS: A possible precursor of the fibrils. *J. Clin. Invest.* 53:1054, 1974.

39. Rosenthal, C. J., and Franklin, E. C.: Variation with age and disease of an amyloid A protein-related serum component. *J. Clin. Invest.* 55:746, 1975.

40. Gorevic, P. D., Rosenthal, C. J., and Franklin, E. C.: Amyloid-related serum component (SAA)—Studies in acute infections, medullary thyroid carcinoma and postsurgery. Behavior as an acute-phase reactant. *Clin. Immunol. Immunopathol.* 6:83, 1976.

41. Rosenthal, C. J., Franklin, E. C., Frangione, B., and Greenspan, J.: Isolation and partial characterization of SAA: An amyloid-related protein from human serum. *J. Immunol.* 116:1415, 1976.

42. Benditt, E.: Personal communication.

43. Franklin, E. C., and Prelli, F.: The structure of SAA. Manuscript in preparation.

44. Benditt, E. P., and Eriksen, N.: Amyloid protein SAA is associated with high density lipoprotein from human serum. *Proc. Natl. Acad. Sci. (U.S.A.)* 71:4025, 1977.

45. Rosenthal, C. J., and Franklin, E. C.: Serum amyloid A (SAA) protein. Interaction with itself and serum albumin. *J. Immunol.* 119:630, 1977.

46. Hijmans, W., and Sipe, J. P.: Levels of the serum amyloid A protein (SAA) in normal persons of different age groups. *Clin. Exp. Immunol.* 35.96, 1979.

47. Rosenthal, C. J., and Sullivan, L. M.: Serum amyloid A to monitor cancer dissemination. *Ann. Intern. Med.* 91:383, 1979.

48. Costa, P. P., Figueira, A. S., and Bravo, F. R.: Amyloid fibril protein related to prealbumin and familial amyloidotic polyneuropathy. *Proc. Natl. Acad. Sci. (U.S.A.)* 75:4499, 1978.

49. Benson, M. D.: Partial amino acid sequence homology between an heredofamilial amyloid protein and human plasma prealbumin. *J. Clin. Invest.* 67:1035, 1981.

50. Pras, M., Franklin, E. C., Prelli, F., and Frangione, B.: A variant of prealbumin from amyloid fibrils in familial polyneuropathy of Israeli origin. *J. Exp. Med.*, submitted for publication.

51. Sletten, K., Westermark, P., and Natvig, J. B.: Senile cardiac amyloid is related to prealbumin. *Scand. J. Immunol.* 12:503, 1980.

52. Sletten, K., Westermark, P., and Natvig, J. B.: Characterization of amyloid fibrillar proteins from medullary thyroid carcinoma. *J. Exp. Med.* 143:993, 1976.

53. Pearse, A. G. E., Wen, S. W. B., and Polak, J. M.: The genesis of apudamyloid in endocrine polypeptide tumours: Biochemical distinction from immunamyloid. *Virchows Arch. (Zellpathol.)* 10:93, 1972.

54. Glenner, G. G., Eanes, E. D., Bladen, H. A., Linke, R. P., and Turmine, J. D.: Beta-pleated sheet fibrils. A comparison of native amyloid with synthetic protein fibrils. *J. Histochem. Cytochem.* 22:1141, 1974.

55. Bladen, H. A., Nylen, M. U., and Glenner, G. G.: The ultrastructure of human amyloid as revealed by the negative staining technique. *J. Ultrastruct. Res.* 14:449, 1966.

56. Dyck, R. F., et al.: Amyloid P-component is a constituent of normal human glomerular basement membrane. *J. Exp. Med.* 152:1162, 1980.

57. Skinner, M., Cohen, A. S., Shirahama, T., and Cathcart, E. S.: P-component (pentagonal unit) or amyloid: Isolation, characterization and sequence analysis. *J. Lab. Clin. Med.* 84:604, 1974.

58. Levo, Y., Frangione, B., and Franklin, E. C.: Amino acid sequence similarities between amyloid P component Clt and CRP. *Nature* 268:56, 1977.

59. Mandema, E., Ruinen, L., Shulten, J. H., and Cohen, A. S. (eds.): *Amyloidosis*. Excerpta Medica, Amsterdam, 1968.

60. Scheinberg, M. A., and Cathcart, E. S.: Casein-induced experimental amyloidosis. III. Response to mitogens, allogeneic cells and graft versus host reactions in the murine model. *Immunology* 27:953, 1974.

61. Scheinberg, M. A., Goldstein, A. L., and Cathcart, E. S.: Thymosin restores T-cell function and reduces the incidence of amyloid disease in casein-treated mice. *J. Immunol.* 116:156, 1976.

62. Calkins, E., and Cohen, A. S.: Diagnosis of amyloidosis. *Bull. Rheum. Dis.* 10.215, 1960.

63. Ozdemir, A. I., Wright, J. R., and Calkins, E.: Influence of rheumatoid arthritis on amyloid of aging. *N. Engl. J. Med.* 285:534, 1971.

64. Triger, D. R., and Joekes, A. M.: Renal amyloidosis—A fourteen year follow-up. *Q. J. Med.* 42:15, 1973.

65. Levine, R. A.: Amyloid disease of the liver. *Am. J. Med.* 33:349, 1962.

66. Wiernik, P. H.: Amyloid joint disease. *Medicine (Baltimore)* 51:465, 1972.

67. French, J. M., Hall, G., Parish, D. J., and Smith, W. T.: Peripheral and autonomic nerve involvement in primary amyloidosis associated with uncontrollable diarrhoea and steatorrhoea. *Am. J. Med. 39:277*, 1965.

68. Nordborg, C., Kristensson, K., Olsson, Y., and Sourander, P.: Involvement of the autonomic nervous system in primary and secondary amyloidosis. *Acta Neurol. Scand. 49:31*, 1973.

69. Jarnum, S.: Gastrointestinal hemorrhage and protein loss in primary amyloidosis. *Gut 6:14*, 1965.

70. Cassidy, J. T.: Cardiac amyloidosis. Two cases with digitalis sensitivity. *Ann. Intern. Med. 55:989*, 1961.

71. Pomerance, A.: Senile cardiac amyloidosis. *Br. Heart J. 27:711*, 1965.

72. Prowse, C. B.: Amyloidosis of the lower respiratory tract. *Thorax 13:308*, 1958.

73. Brownstein, M. H., and Helwig, E. B.: The cutaneous amyloidoses. *Arch. Dermatol. 102:8*, 1970.

74. Bernhardt, B., Valletta, M., Brooks, J., and Lejnieks, I.: Amyloidosis with factor X deficiency. *Am. J. Med. Sci. 264:411*, 1972.

75. Furie, B., Greene, B., and Furie, B. C.: Syndrome of acquired Factor X deficiency and systemic amyloidosis. *N. Engl. J. Med. 297:81*, 1977.

76. Furie, B., Voo, L., McAdam, K. P. W. J., and Furie, B. C.: Mechanism of factor X deficiency in systemic amyloidosis. *N. Engl. J. Med. 304:827*, 1981.

77. Redleaf, P. D., Davis, R. B., Kucinski, C., Hoilund, L., and Gans, H.: Amyloidosis with an unusual bleeding diathesis: observations on the use of epsilon amino caproic acid. *Ann. Intern. Med. 58:347*, 1963.

78. Sohar, E., Gafni, J., Pras, M., and Heller, H.: Familial Mediterranean fever: A survey of 470 cases and review of the literature. *Am. J. Med. 43:227*, 1967.

79. Andrade, C., Canijo, M., Klein, D., and Kaelin, A.: The genetic aspect of the familial amyloidotic polyneuropathy: Portuguese type of paramyloidosis. *Humangenetik 7:163*, 1969.

80. Terry, R. D.: The fine structure of neurofibrillary tangles in Alzheimer's disease. *J. Neuropathol. Exp. Neurol. 22:629*, 1963.

81. Walford, R. L., and Sjaarda, J. R.: Increase of Thioflavine-T-staining material (amyloid) in human tissues with age. *J. Gerontol. 19:57*, 1964.

82. Kyle, R. A., and Bayrd, E. D.: "Primary" systemic amyloidosis and myeloma. Discussion of relationship and review of 81 cases. *Arch. Intern. Med. 107:344*, 1961.

83. Cohen, A. S.: *Laboratory Diagnostic Procedures in the Rheumatic Diseases.* Little, Brown, Boston, 1967, p. 322.

84. Gafni, J., and Sohar, E.: Rectal biopsy for the diagnosis of amyloidosis. *Am. J. Med. Sci. 240:332*, 1960.

85. Benson, M. D., Skinner, M., and Cohen, A. S.: Amyloid deposition in a renal transplant in familial Mediterranean fever. *Ann. Intern. Med. 87:31*, 1977.

86. Gorevic, P. D., Cleveland, A. B., Wright, J. R., Zucker-Franklin, D., Frangione, B., and Franklin, E. C.: Ultrastructure studies and partial characterization of a low molecular weight component of senile cardiac amyloid fibrils, in *Amyloid and Amyloidosis,* edited by G. G. Glenner, P. P. Costa, and A. Freitas. Excerpta Medica, Amsterdam, 1980, p. 366.

87. Cornwell, G. G., Natvig, J. B., Westermark, P., and Husby, G.: Senile cardiac amyloid: Demonstration of a unique fibril protein in tissue sections. *J. Immunol. 120:385*, 1978.

88. Fujihara, S., and Glenner, G. G.: Primary localized amyloidosis of the genitourinary tract: Immunohistochemical study on eleven cases. *Lab Invest. 44:55*, 1981.

89. Sorenson, G. D., Binington, H. B.: Resistance of murine amyloid fibrils to proteolytic enzymes. *Fed. Proc. 23:550*, 1964.

90. Emeson, E. C., Kikkawa, Y., and Gueft, B.: New features of amyloid found after digestion with trypsin. *J. Cell Biol. 28:570*, 1966.

91. Zucker-Franklin, D.: The submembranous fibrils of human blood platelets. *J. Cell Biol. 47:293*, 1970.

92. Waldenstrom, H.: On formation and disappearance of amyloid in man. *Acta Chir. Scand. 63:479*, 1928.

93. Lowenstein, J., and Gallo, G.: Remission of the nephrotic syndrome in renal amyloidosis. *N. Engl. J. Med. 282:128*, 1970.

94. Cohen, H. J., Lessin, L. S., Hallal, J., and Burkholder, P.: Resolution of primary amyloidosis during chemotherapy: Studies in a patient with nephrotic syndrome. *Ann. Intern. Med. 82:466*, 1975.

95. American College of Surgeons, N. I. H. Organ Transplant Registry, Chicago, May 10, 1974.

96. Zemer, D., Pras, M., Shemer, Y., Sohar, E., and Gafni, J.: Daily prophylactic colchicine in familial Mediterranean fever, in *Amyloid and Amyloidosis,* edited by G. G. Glenner, P. P. Costa, and A. Freitas. Excerpta Medica, Amsterdam, 1980, p. 580.

97. Osserman, E. F., Sherman, W. W., and Kyle, R. A.: Further studies of therapy of amyloidosis with dimethylsulfoxide (DMSO), in *Amyloid and Amyloidosis,* edited by G. G. Glenner, P. P. Costa, and A. Freitas. Excerpta Medica, Amsterdam, 1980, p. 563.

98. van Rijswijk, M. H., et al.: Successful treatment with dimethylsulfoxide of human amyloidosis secondary to rheumatoid arthritis, in *Amyloid and Amyloidosis,* edited by G. G. Glenner, P. P. Costa, and A. Freitas. Excerpta Medica, Amsterdam, 1980, p. 570.

PART EIGHT *Hemostasis*

Morphology of platelets

CHAPTER 126

Platelet morphology and function

JAMES G. WHITE

Since the pioneering efforts of Wolpers and Ruska [1] a large number of studies have been carried out on blood platelets with the aid of the electron microscope. In these studies the emphasis has shifted progressively from pure morphology of platelets to structural physiology. Morphologic studies of blood platelets have been reviewed in detail [2–17]. The morphology of megakaryocytes is reviewed in Chap. 130.

Platelet morphology

Here platelet morphology is considered under functional subdivisions rather than in purely anatomic terms. There are three major structural zones of the platelet, each related to a specific aspect of platelet function. The *peripheral zone* is involved primarily in adhesion, the *sol-gel zone* in contraction, and the *organelle zone* in secretion (Figs. 126-1 and 126-2).

PERIPHERAL ZONE
Adhesion of platelets to sites of vascular injury and to each other is a critical phase in formation of hemostatic plugs. Fundamental steps include conversion of nonsticky platelets to the adhesive state and release of endogenous chemical constituents which promote platelet aggregation [18]. The peripheral zone of the platelet provides the template for chemical interactions generating the platelet response, the physical site for cell-to-cell adhesion, and a trigger mechanism transferring the stimulus from outside the cells to the platelet interior. The peripheral zone of the platelet includes the *exterior coat*, the *unit membrane*, and the *submembrane area*.

EXTERIOR COAT
The component of the peripheral zone in immediate contact with surrounding plasma is the exterior coat (Figs. 126-1 and 126-2). Chemical substances making up

FIGURE 126-1 Platelet from sample of citrated platelet-rich plasma fixed in glutaraldehyde-osmium and embedded in plastic. The cell has been sectioned in the plane of greatest circumference. As a result, the circumferential band of microtubules (MT) is visible inside the cell surface along its entire circumference. The peripheral zone consists of the exterior coat (EC), the lipid bilayer of the cell membrane (CM), and the submembrane area. Channels of the surface-connected open canalicular system (OCS) are continuous with the exposed cell membrane and extend throughout the cytoplasm in a tortuous labyrinth. Elements of the dense tubular system (DTS) are also randomly dispersed. The sol-gel zone forms the dense matrix of the platelet. It contains several filament systems, such as the band of microtubules, and masses of glycogen particles (Gly). The organelle zone comprises many granules (G), a few mitochondria (M), and occasional dense bodies (DB). (×39,000.)

FIGURE 126-2 Cross sections of several platelets prepared from citrated platelet-rich plasma in the same manner as the cell in Fig. 126-1. Groups of microtubules (MT) resembling hollow circular profiles are visible at the polar ends of each cell. Granules (G), dense bodies (DB), and other organelles are randomly dispersed in the cytoplasm of each platelet. Fenestrated channels of the open canalicular system (OCS) are continuous with cell surfaces. (×22,600.)

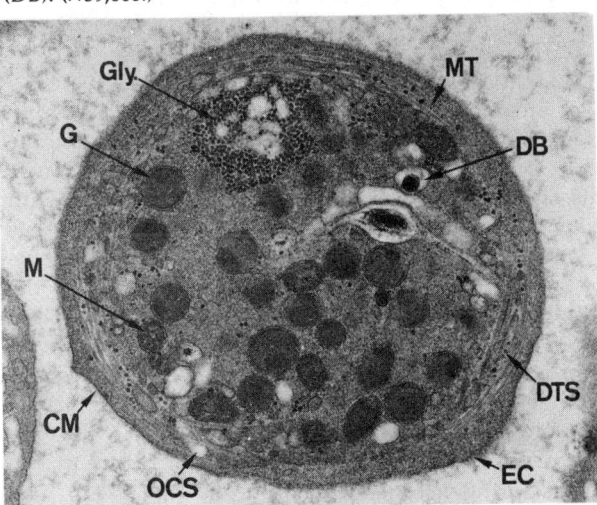

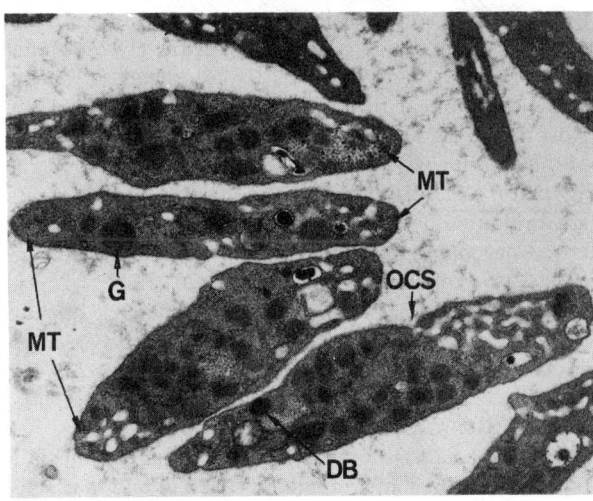

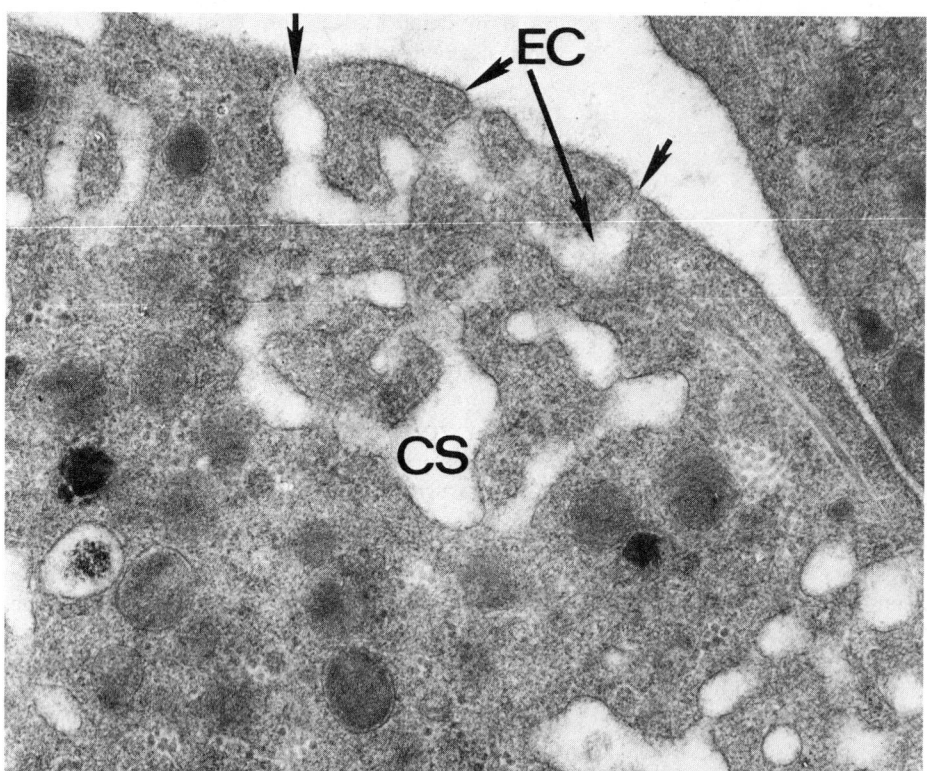

FIGURE 126-3   Higher magnification of the peripheral area of a platelet. The exterior coat (EC) material covers the unit membrane of the cell surface and the linings of the canalicular system (CS). Arrows indicate sites of communication between the canicular system and the outside surface of the platelet. (×41,500.)

the coat were easily extracted by methods formerly used to prepare platelets for study in the electron microscope, but improved fixation and cytochemical techniques have permitted visualization of the platelet exterior coat [12–17,19–23]. Coat material is 150 to 200 Å in thickness and covers the unit membranes of the cell surface and linings of the tortuous canalicular system penetrating the platelet substance (Figs. 126-3 and 126-4). The exterior coat may have structural organization [18], but no firm evidence is available yet as to the precise arrangement of its chemical and physical subunits. Protein antigens, highly specific glycoproteins [23–25], and several enzymes [26] localized in the exterior coat appear to be involved in cell function [27]. Adsorbed plasma proteins are important constituents of the exterior coat where they participate in blood coagulation. Many other intrinsic chemical components are undoubtedly present, but their location is uncertain. Coat material remains on platelets before, during, and after aggregation (Fig. 126-5) [20,23,28]. The exterior coat is the adhesive site of the platelet, but the precise chemical factors and mechanisms involved in stickiness are not clearly defined [29].

UNIT MEMBRANE
The middle layer of the platelet peripheral zone is a typical trilaminar membrane (Fig. 126-6) and is essen-

tial to the integrity of the cell. Surface-active agents, antihistamines, local anesthetics, chelating agents, high and low salt concentrations, and lipid solvents injure the membrane and damage the cells [3]. The changes are characterized by alterations in surface contour or by increased permeability with resultant swelling of the platelet. The unit membrane plays an important role in protecting the integrity of the platelet internal milieu, in platelet adhesion [30], and contraction [31], and in supplying a lipid activator to coagulation [32].

THE SUBMEMBRANE AREA
The area immediately under the unit membrane represents a transition between the peripheral zone and the sol-gel matrix of the hyaloplasm (Fig. 126-6). Because its structural elements appear closely associated with changes in the cell surface, the submembrane area is considered part of the peripheral zone. Fine filaments are evident in the submembrane area peripheral to the circumferential band of microtubules [33–35]. Their close relationship to the cell wall and association with fibrous elements of the hyaloplasm have suggested that submembrane filaments may help to support platelet discoid shape, participate in formation and stabilization of pseudopodia, and aid in retraction of surface projections during viscous metamorphosis.

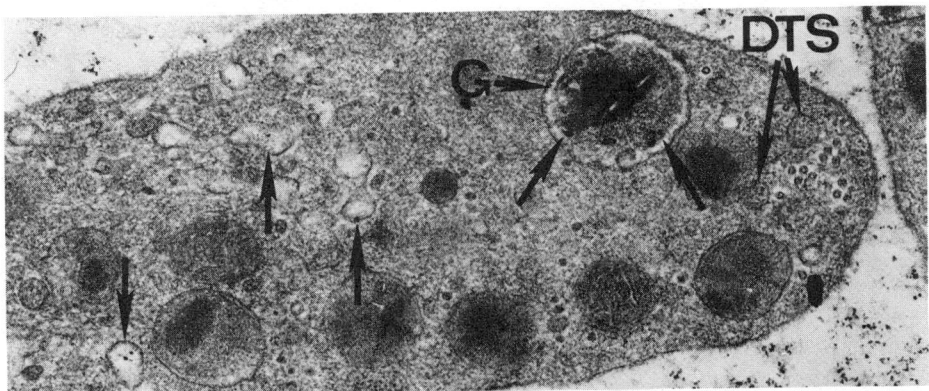

FIGURE 126-4   Discoid platelet from sample of citrated platelet-rich plasma incubated with thorium dioxide. The small electron-dense particles penetrate into open channels (*arrows*) of the canalicular system and are transferred to some platelet granules. The granule containing thorium particles is in an early stage of transformation to a dense body. Elements of the dense tubular system (DTS) associated with the circumferential microtubules are evident in this cell. The sequence of thorium uptake into open channels, transfer to intact granules, and conversion of granules to dense bodies may explain the mechanism of serotonin uptake and storage in platelets. (×33,200.)

FIGURE 126-5   Platelets from sample of citrated platelet-rich plasma aggregated in ADP and stained during fixation with ruthenium red (mucopolysaccharide stain). The agent stains the exterior coat and intracellular material (*arrows*) and enters the platelet canalicular system (CS). The substance of dense bodies (DB) is in close proximity to the stained channels and often mixes with it. Granules also discharge into these channels and are ruthenium red–positive. The channel system and intercellular spaces may serve as the major route for secretion of endogenous platelet constituents. (×38,100.)

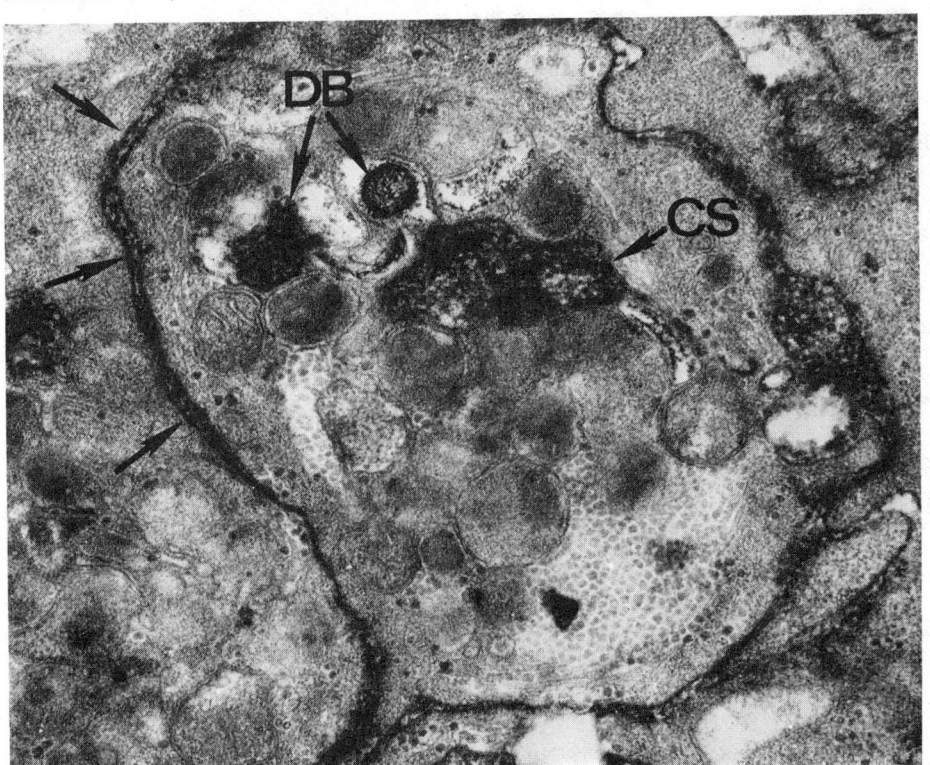

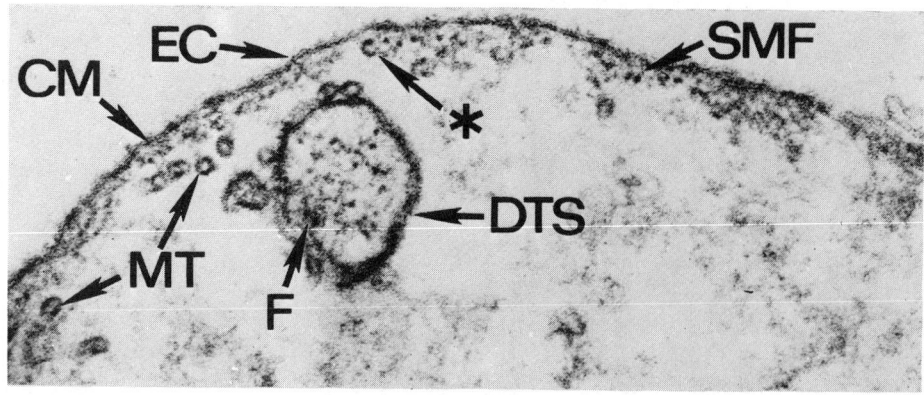

FIGURE 126-6   A portion of a chemically shocked platelet. Mild injury revealed the mat of filaments (SMF) lying just under the unit membrane (CM) of the platelet surface. The submembrane filaments, cell membrane, and exterior coat constitute the platelet peripheral zone. A swollen element of the dense tubular system is filled with filaments (F) similar to SMF and to the subfilaments of microtubules. One microtubule (*arrow with asterisk*) close to the surface is breaking down into component subfilaments. Hyaloplasmic microfilaments not shown in this illustration are identical with SMF and subfilaments of MT. (×116,500.) (Courtesy of the *American Journal of Pathology*.)

FIGURE 126-7   Portion of a platelet swollen by distilled water before whole mounting and negative staining with phosphotungstic acid. The cell membrane (CM) and granule membranes (GM) are relatively electron-transparent. Dense bodies (DB) are inherently electron-opaque. Masses of microfilaments (MF) fill the platelet matrix. The 50-Å fibers are indistinguishable from subfilaments of microtubules (MT) and submembrane filaments. Elements of the channel system (C) also appear electron-transparent in whole-mount preparations. (×71,700.) (Courtesy of *Blood*.)

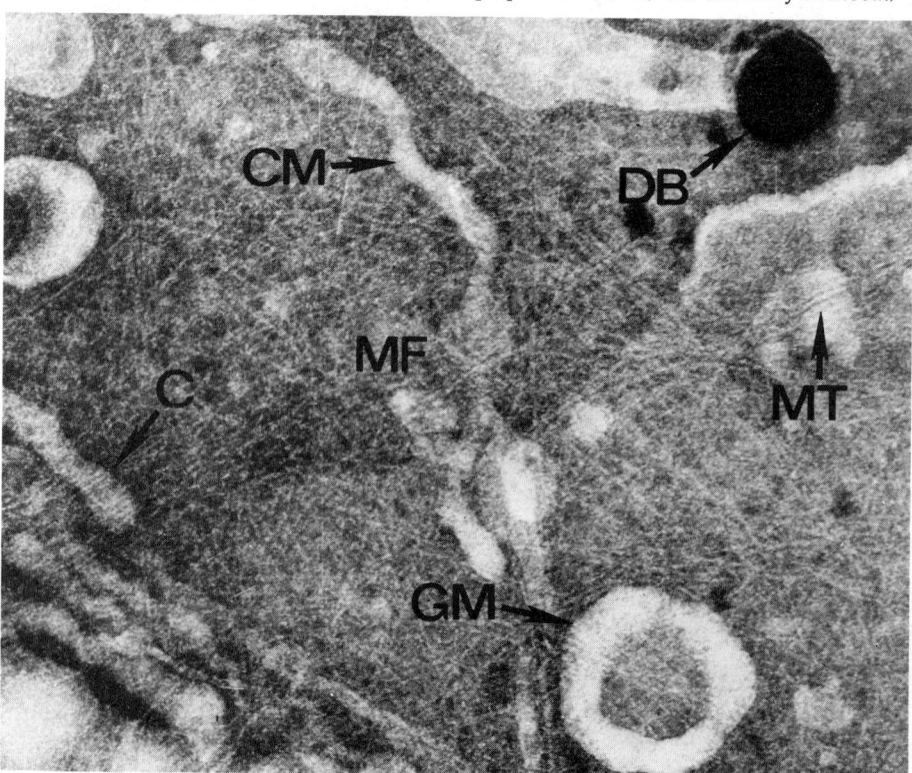

SOL-GEL ZONE

In studies with the light microscope, the interior of platelets appears structureless except for a few granules and is thus called the *hyaloplasm*. However, when examined by electron microscopy, the interior is composed of masses of fibrous elements. An annular bundle of 250-Å microtubules [36] lying under the cell wall along its greatest circumference is the most prominent fibrous system of the hyaloplasm (Figs. 126-1 and 126-2). Microfilaments, 50 Å in diameter, constitute a second system of fibers [37] (Fig. 126-7), and submembrane filaments a third [33–35]. Each microtubule is in itself a fibrous system [38] composed of 12 to 15 subfilaments 50 Å in diameter arranged in parallel association [39] (Fig. 126-8). The subfilaments are more stable than the microtubules [40] and are physically indistinguishable from microfilaments and submembrane filaments. These three fiber systems may differ only in their state of polymerization, aggregation, and location in the cell (Fig. 126-6) [35].

The relative plasticity of the hyaloplasm in unaltered discoid platelets and the rapidity with which the matrix can flow into pseudopodia during platelet shape change suggests characteristics of a sol-gel cytoplasm [41] that exists in nearly every living cell capable of directed self-movement. The highly oriented centripetal movement and subsequent secretion of granules in platelets, contraction of pseudopodia, and clot retraction essential for normal platelet function are dependent upon fibrous elements in the platelet sol-gel zone. For this reason the sol-gel zone is considered as a separate morphologic division of the platelet related to contractile function [42–44].

ORGANELLE ZONE

A variety of formed organelles and particulate elements are embedded in the sol-gel matrix of the platelets (Figs. 126-1 and 126-2). The granules, dense bodies, and mitochondria deserve special comment. In addition, single glycogen particles are evident throughout the matrix, and a compact mass of glycogen not bounded by a membrane is commonly observed (Fig. 126-1). Stacks of flattened saccules resembling a Golgi apparatus are seen in about 3 percent of sectioned platelets (Fig. 126-9*a*). In rare instances bits of endoplasmic reticulum, giant granules, centrioles, and nuclear remnants have been identified in platelets from normal blood.

GRANULES

The granules have been of particular interest because they are so numerous and are believed to be an important source of substances secreted by platelets during viscous metamorphosis [45]. Granules are usually oval or round, but variations in form are common. Each

FIGURE 126-8 Negatively stained whole mount of blood platelet revealing substructure of microtubules (MT). Each tubule is composed of 12 to 15 subfilaments 50 Å in diameter. The subfilaments are in parallel association, but remain individually intact at sites of tubule fracture (X). Subfilaments of microtubules are essentially identical in appearance with microfilaments shown in Fig. 128-7. (×125,400.) (Courtesy of *Blood.*)

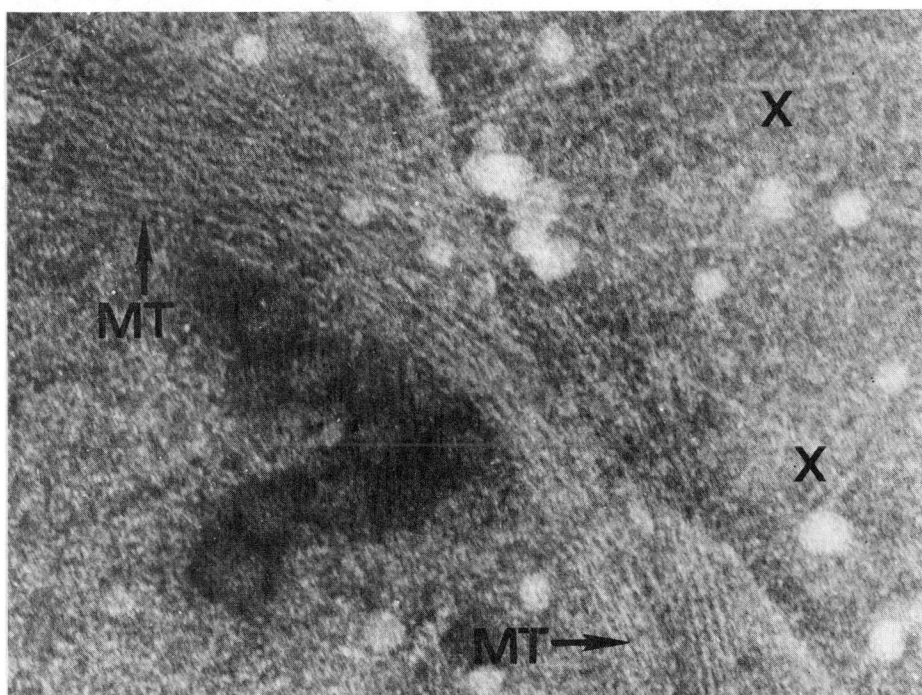

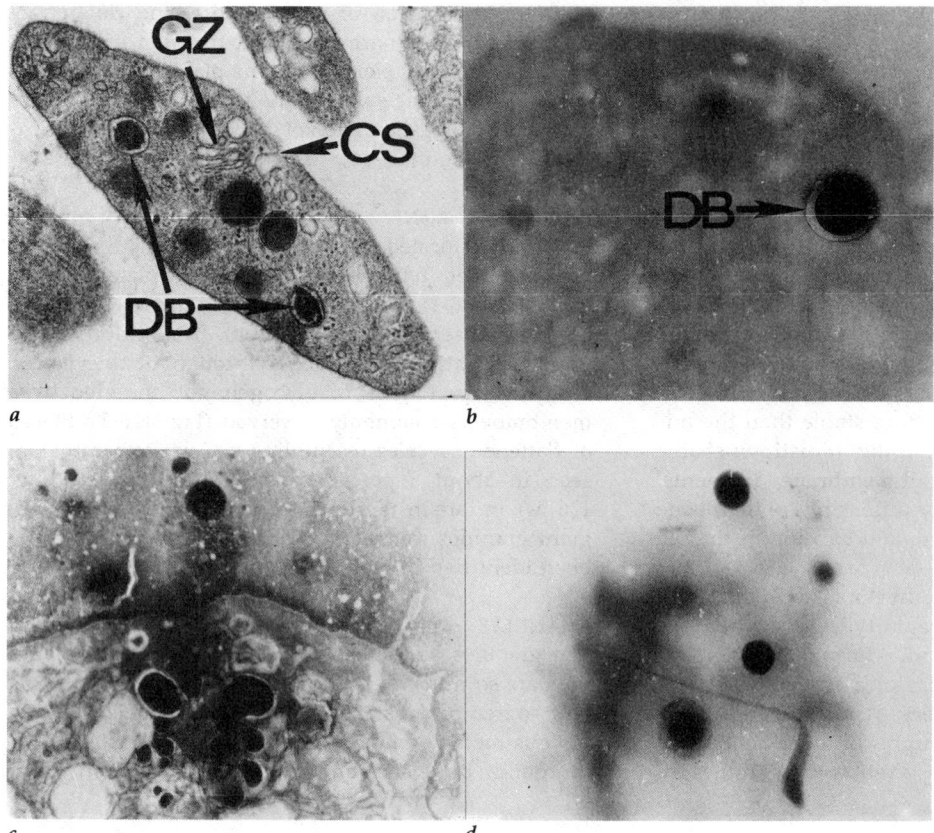

FIGURE 126-9 Platelet dense bodies. Part *a* is a thin section of a platelet from a patient with afibrinogenemia revealing normal dense bodies (DB). Flattened saccules suggestive of a Golgi zone (GZ) are also apparent in this cell. The cell in part *b* was fixed in glutaraldehyde alone. Osmic acid is not essential for the opacity of dense bodies (DB). Part *c* is a negatively stained whole mount revealing dense bodies inside and outside a platelet. Part *d* is an unstained whole mount revealing the inherent electron opacity of dense bodies and their occasional association with long, narrow channels. (Courtesy of *Blood.*)

granule is enclosed by a unit membrane. The internal matrix is usually divided into two zones of differing electron opacity (Figs. 126-1 and 126-4). Tubular elements have been identified in the matrix of granules, but their significance is unknown [46]. One variety of platelet granule, the lysosome, contains hydrolytic enzymes, including acid phosphatase, β glucuronidase, and cathepsin [32,47]. Another, the peroxisome, contains catalase. Platelet factor 4, fibrinogen, β thromboglobulin, thrombin-sensitive protein, growth-promoting factor, and other constituents have been localized in the α-granule fraction [23,26,31,32,48]. Recent cytochemical studies have suggested that the granules contain glycoprotein [25] and mucopolysaccharides [23].

DENSE BODIES

The dense bodies of platelets are relatively few in number but appear to be very important in hemostatic function [49–55] (Fig. 126-9*a* to *d*). Dense bodies are inherently electron-opaque, probably because of a nu-

cleation of calcium within them [56]. Most, if not all, opaque organelles in human platelets may originate from granules [57–58] (Fig. 126-4). The transformation of granules to dense bodies is directly related to the uptake of serotonin [50].

Dense bodies are the primary secretory organelles of the platelets. During the internal transformation following exposure to aggregating agents, dense bodies and granules are shifted to the cell centers [59]. Dense bodies rapidly decrease in number during early viscous metamorphosis and are absent from platelets in late viscous metamorphosis and clot retraction. Serotonin, ADP, catecholamines, calcium, and pyrophosphate have been associated with dense bodies [60].

MITOCHONDRIA

The mitochondria of platelets are simple in structure and few in number (Fig. 126-1). They contribute significantly to the metabolic pool of ATP, for blockade of aerobic glycolysis alone does not affect the level of platelet ATP or energy-requiring functions of the cell. The electron opacity of mitochondria reflects their state of activity. Platelet mitochondria become more opaque to electrons during viscous metamorphosis and often develop precipitates resembling heavy-metal deposits. In addition to their metabolic activity, platelet mitochondria may function as calcium repositories similar to mitochondria of smooth muscle.

ADDITIONAL FEATURES OF PLATELET MORPHOLOGY

The membrane systems constitute a fourth functional zone in blood platelets. Aldehyde fixation techniques markedly improve preservation of platelet ultrastructure and stabilization of associations between the surface membrane and a system of channels which had been regarded as vesicles and vacuoles in early studies [19]. The surface-connected open canalicular system (OCS) consists of tortuous invaginations of the cell wall tunneling throughout the cytoplasm in a serpentine fashion. Studies employing electron-dense tracers reveal that channels of the OCS are patent in activated and aggregated platelets as well as in unaltered cells [12]. Vesicles and vacuoles are virtually absent in doubly fixed platelets, suggesting that these elements are in reality components of the OCS. Canaliculi of the OCS greatly increase the total surface area of the platelet exposed to plasma and provide a route for chemical or particulate substances to reach the deepest recesses of the cell.

The observation that the OCS remains patent throughout the processes of platelet shape change, internal transformation, contraction, adhesion, and aggregation suggests that the channels might serve as conduits for substances extruded by platelets during the release reaction. Experiments employing the cationic polyelectrolytes, polylysine and polybrene, demonstrated that this supposition was correct [61,62]. Both polybrene and polylysine are taken up by platelets during incubation with the agents and deposited in secretory granules. Interaction between polyelectrolytes and the organelles results in polymerization of the matrix and opacification of the granule nucleoids and dense bodies. Polylysine and polybrene stabilize the contents of the organelles so that their egress from activated platelets through channels of the OCS can be followed in the electron microscope. By adding the polyelectrolytes to samples of platelets prior to stirring with specific agents, it is possible to define the sequential extrusion of secretory organelle contents from the cell interior through channels of the OCS to the surrounding plasma.

The second membrane system in platelets, the dense tubular system (DTS), originates from the rough endoplasmic reticulum of the parent megakaryocyte [63,64]. Channels of the dense tubular system (DTS) are distinguished from clear canaliculi of the OCS because of an amorphous material, similar in opacity to surrounding cytoplasm, concentrated within them. Like the OCS, channels of the DTS are randomly dispersed in the platelet cytoplasm. In addition, a channel or two of the OCS can be identified in close association with the circumferential band of microtubules in most thin sections of platelets. Investigations of this relationship suggest that the DTS might have an important role in the elaboration and stabilization of the circumferential microtubules supporting the discoid form of platelets. Although suggested by some workers, there was no evidence of a physical communication between channels of the OCS and DTS. Thus, platelets have two discrete membrane systems not found in other blood cells, the OCS derived from the plasma membrane of the megakaryocyte and the DTS representing residual smooth endoplasmic reticulum of the parent cell.

The OCS and DTS are not completely isolated membrane systems. Canaliculi of the OCS and DTS form intimate physical relationships in nearly every cell. The association of the two channel systems is usually restricted to one or two areas of the cytoplasm and in most examples these are eccentrically located. Elements of the OCS in such areas are gathered in clusters or groups. Even though the open channels are closely approximated, small canaliculi of the DTS can be identified interspersed between them. The relationship is particularly prominent in platelets stained for peroxidase activity in which dense reaction product delineates channels of the DTS and outlines clearly their extremely close relationship to clusters of open canaliculi [64,65]. Examination of the membrane complexes at higher magnification reveals that elements of the DTS are the only structures interspersed between open canaliculi, and that membranes of the two channel systems are practically in apposition. The relationship strongly resembles the association of transverse tubular and sarcotubules in embryonic muscle cells.

The DTS has been shown to be a calcium reservoir similar to muscle sarcotubules [66,67]. Furthermore, the proximity of the dual channel system in platelets to the contractile elements and the demonstration that the DTS selectively binds divalent cations, that platelets do not require exterior calcium for activation, and that vesicles from platelet membranes can sequester calcium as well as sarcotubular vesicles from muscle strongly support the concept that the OCS and DTS in platelets are the equivalent of the sarcoplasmic reticulum of muscle cells [64,67].

Platelets contain a specific peroxidase activity localized to channels of the DTS [64,65]. An inhibitor of platelet peroxidase, 3-amino-1,2,4-triazole, has effects on platelet aggregation similar to those of aspirin [68]. Concentrations of 3-amino-1,2,4-triazole which block cytochemical demonstration of peroxidase inhibit the second wave of aggregation stimulated by release-inducing aggregating agents. 3-Amino-1,2,4-triazole also blocks prostaglandin formation, suggesting that the peroxidase is involved in the synthetic process. Peroxidase activity is contained on prostaglandin endoperoxide synthetase during purification of the enzyme and the heme groups of cyclooxygenase are essential

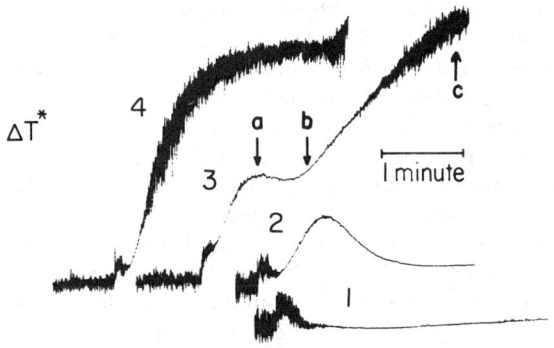

*ΔT - change in light transmission

FIGURE 126-10 The graded response of platelets to thrombin. In tracing 1, citrated platelet-rich plasma was combined with 0.05 unit of thrombin per milliliter. Shape change indicated by narrowing of the baseline took place within a few seconds, but aggregation did not occur. Within 10 min the baseline recovers its normal amplitude as platelet discoid shape is restored. Tracing 2 was from a sample combined with 0.1 unit of thrombin per milliliter of citrated platelet-rich plasma. Upward deflection of the tracing indicates that an increase in light transmission occurred after shape change had developed. The change in light transmission coincides with an initial wave of platelet aggregation. Platelet clumps dispersed completely in this sample as indicated by decrease in light transmission and return of the recording to the base line. The baseline recovers its normal amplitude, and platelet discoid shape is restored within 10 min.

Tracing 3 was recorded where a sample of citrated platelet-rich plasma was exposed to 0.15 unit of thrombin per milliliter. An initial phase of clumping was followed by a brief period in which disaggregation began. This pause was followed by a rapid increase in light transmission as a new wave of aggregation took place. The second phase is entirely dependent for its initiation on endogenous products extruded from platelets during the release reaction. Tracing 4 was obtained when citrated platelet-rich plasma was treated with 0.18 unit of thrombin per milliliter. First and second waves of aggregation are fused together obscuring the biphasic nature of the platelet response. The letters *a, b,* and *c* indicate times during the first and second waves at which samples were fixed for study in the electron microscope.

for its prostaglandin synthetase activity. These findings and studies on platelet subcellular fractions showing that prostaglandin synthetic activity separates with endoplasmic reticulum enzymes and not plasma membrane demonstrate that the DTS is the site of platelet prostaglandin synthesis [15,68].

Structural physiology

Platelets normally circulate as flattened discs. The discoid form can be preserved in vitro by collecting blood in citrate or heparin anticoagulants and separating the platelet-rich plasma at 37°C. Morphologic changes can be induced by adding thrombin directly to small samples of citrated platelet-rich plasma, or spontaneous

evolution of the changes can be secured by recalcification of the platelet-rich plasma. Addition of precise amounts of thrombin provides a better picture of the sequence of events, for the platelet response is proportional to the concentration of the agent. Samples can be fixed for electron microscopic study at selected intervals as the aggregation proceeds. Progress of the reaction is followed by a device (the aggregometer) which records changes in platelet shape and aggregation by measuring changes in light transmission through the reaction mixture [69–71]. Thus, comparisons between morphology, physiology, and biochemistry can be related in time. Figure 126-10 illustrates the effect of thrombin on platelets. If the concentration of thrombin added is 0.1 unit per milliliter of citrated platelet-rich plasma or less, shape change is the only alteration. Discoid shape is lost, and the cells become irregularly spherical with multiple pseudopodia.

Samples prepared for electron microscopy at intervals during this sequence reveal changes entirely consistent with the alterations recorded on the aggregometer. Internal reorganization is a characteristic feature of the platelet response to thrombin (Figs. 126-11 and 126-12). Organelles are moved toward the cell center, and the circumferential bundle of microtubules is shifted internally. The degree of internal reorganization varies from cell to cell, and the number of cells manifesting the change depends on the concentration and nature of the stimulating agent. In platelets exposed to 0.1 unit per milliliter of thrombin, the centrally clumped organelles are loosely arranged, and fusion does not occur. Ten minutes after addition of the small amount of thrombin, the normal appearance of the platelets is restored. The platelets recover their discoid shape, organelles return to their random distribution, and the circumferential band of microtubules is restored to its usual position under the cell wall.

This type of experiment indicates that thrombin can produce effects on platelet form and internal organization at a concentration insufficient to cause platelet adhesiveness (aggregation) or clotting. Shape change precedes adhesiveness (aggregation) but does not cause it, for aggregation does not necessarily follow the shape alterations induced by low concentrations of thrombin. Some other events must occur. Since agents which block the action of adenosine diphosphate (ADP) prevent the aggregating influence of thrombin, the event in question may be related to the appearance of ADP at the platelet surface [71–72].

The capacity of platelets to undergo physical transformation without becoming sticky is perplexing. Yet platelets in circulating blood are constantly exposed to a wide variety of minimal stimuli. If these stimuli were to trigger an all-or-none reaction in each platelet, the host would be in constant danger from thromboembolism. The capacity of the platelet to respond in a manner proportional to the stimulus affords a rapid response to vascular injury as well as protection against overreaction.

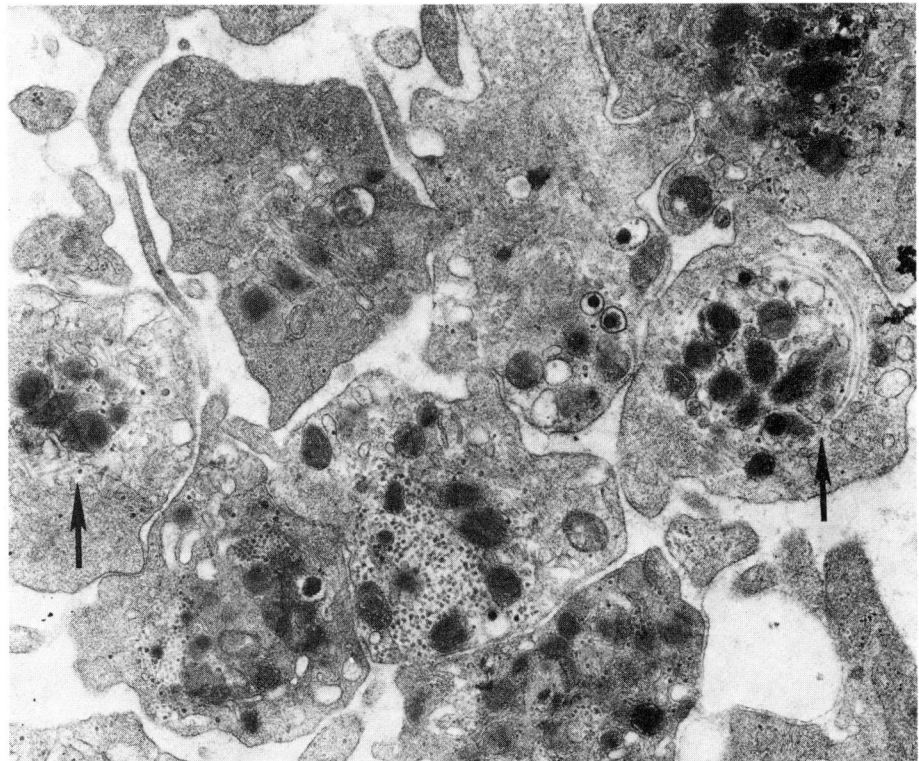

FIGURE 126-11 First wave of aggregation induced in citrated platelet-rich plasma by thrombin. The cells have lost their discoid shape and developed irregular surface projections. Altered surfaces of adjacent platelets are in contact in a few places but are not molded. Organelles in the hyaloplasm are shifted toward the cell centers and encircled by the marginal band of microtubules, which is reduced in circumference. Arrows indicate cells in which the internal reorganization is well demonstrated. (×18,000.)

FIGURE 126-12 Higher magnification of platelet from sample of citrated platelet-rich plasma fixed during first wave after exposure to thrombin. Changes in external contour and attachment of cell surfaces by fuzzy material are evident. Granules are clumped closely together in the cell center, but remain discrete. The band of microtubules (MT) and microfilaments encircles the centrally grouped organelles. (×37,300.)

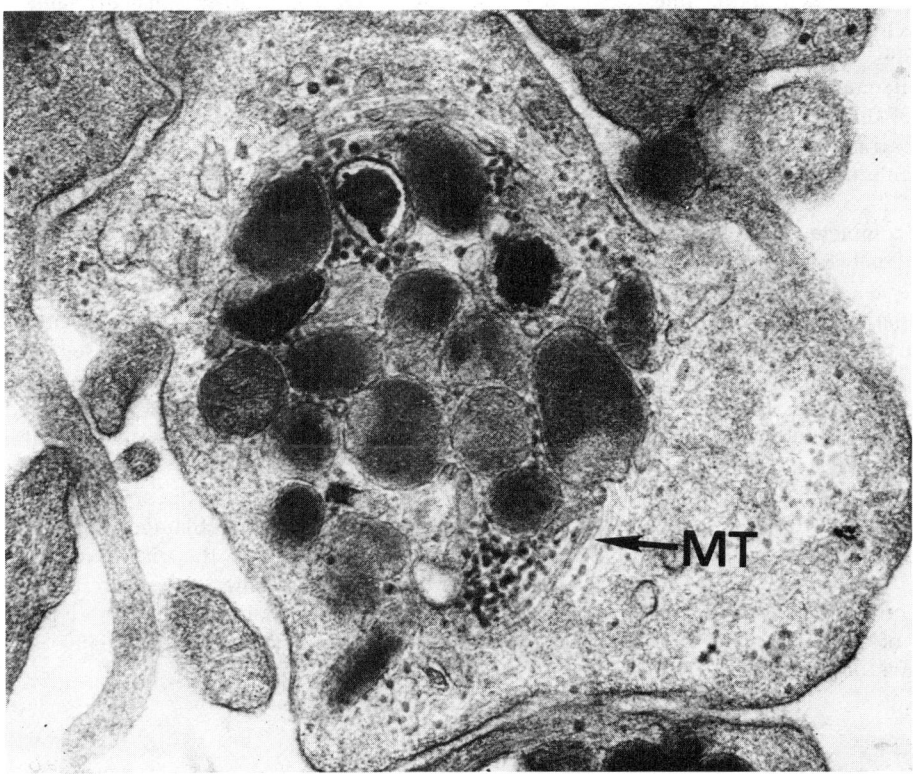

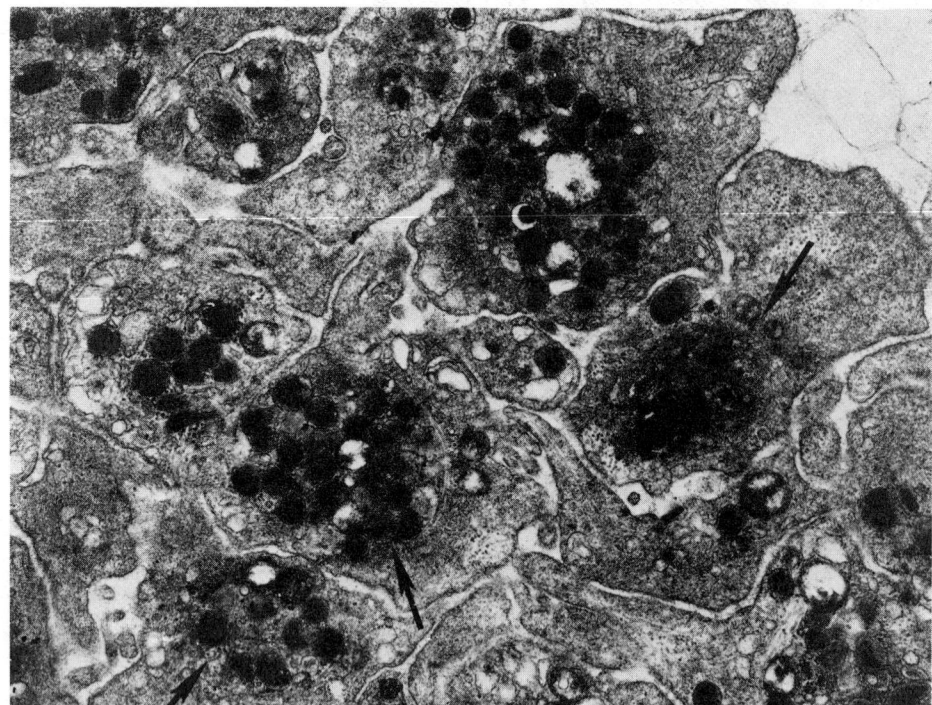

FIGURE 126-13   Early second-wave changes induced in samples of citrated platelet-rich plasma by thrombin. The cells are closely molded to fit each others' contours. Internal changes are similar to first-wave changes, but more advanced. Examples in which granule fusion is in progress are indicated by arrows. This change is not reversible. (×13,900.)

Slightly larger amounts of thrombin, 0.1 to 0.2 units per milliliter of citrated platelet-rich plasma on the aggregometer, cause platelet aggregation as well as the shape change and internal reorganization described above (Fig. 126-10, tracing 2). Samples taken at this time show the cells loosely associated in clumps, but on occasion molded to one another (Figs. 126-11 and 126-12). Internal transformation is similar to that observed in platelets exposed to amounts of thrombin insufficient to cause aggregation, as described above.

The initial wave of aggregation produced by this concentration of thrombin (0.1 to 0.2 unit per milliliter of platelet-rich plasma) reverses completely. Aggregates break up and platelets are gradually restored to their unaltered appearance. A single, completely reversible wave of aggregation is additional evidence for the capacity of platelets to respond in a graded fashion [73–75]. Further, not all platelets undergo shape change or aggregate when exposed to this low concentration of thrombin. The platelet response is individual, and no two cells appear to be at the same stage of transformation at the same time. The degree of internal and external alteration is dependent not only on the nature and concentration of the stimulating agent but on the sensitivity of each cell.

Increasing the concentration of thrombin to approximately 0.2 units per milliliter of citrated platelet-rich plasma results in a double wave of aggregation (Fig. 126-10, tracing 3) [55]. The first phase of clumping reverses partially, and then a new wave of aggregation takes place. Secondary aggregation is usually irreversible and appears to involve most platelets, since light transmission increases nearly to that of platelet-poor plasma. Physical changes observed during the first wave are essentially identical with those observed in samples which undergo complete reversal (Figs. 126-12, sample removed at *a* in tracing 3, and Fig. 126-10). In the trough between the first and second waves two patterns are evident (samples removed at *b* in tracing 3, Fig. 126-10). Some aggregates and platelets appear partially recovered, although it is impossible to determine in which direction they are going. Other cells and clumps appear to have progressed beyond the changes evident in the first wave (Figs. 126-13 to 126-15). Individual cells are more closely molded, and internal changes are more marked. Organelles in many platelets are squeezed tightly together and surrounded by a close-fitting band of microtubules and microfilaments [74,75]. Pseudopodia are both bulbous and filamentous. Microtubules are evident in some pseudopodia, and parallel groups of microfilaments in nearly all. As organelles are crowded to the platelet centers, the peripheral hyaloplasm becomes less electron-dense [76]. Channels of the open canalicular system are more dilated but retain communication with the platelet exterior.

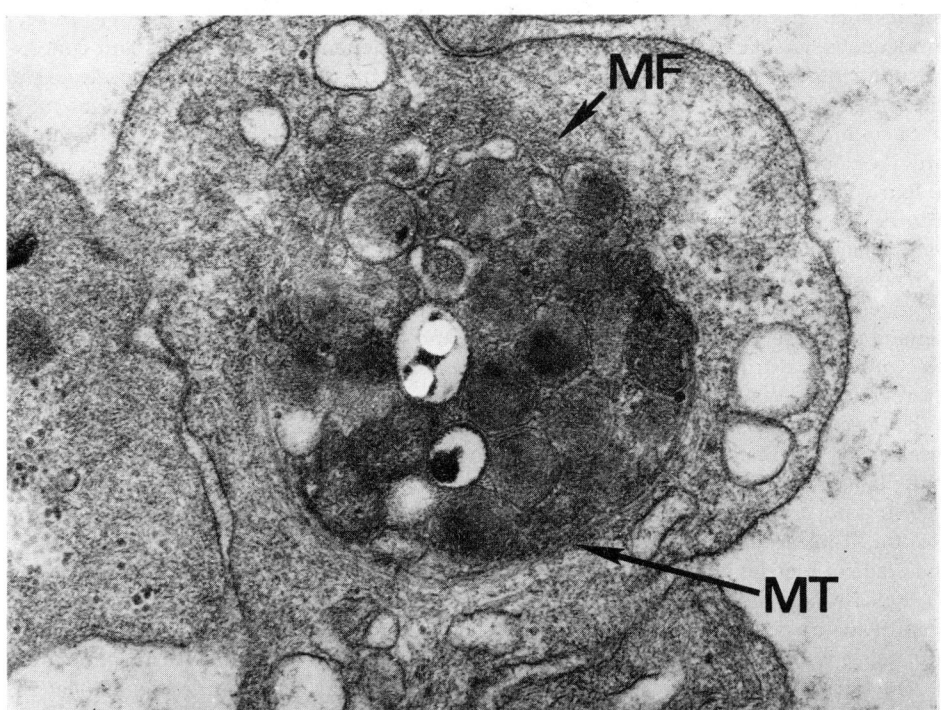

FIGURE 126-14   Second-wave changes due to thrombin at higher magnification. Granules are fused together in some areas. Microfilaments (MF) as well as microtubules (MT) surround the mass of granules. (×41,500.)

FIGURE 126-15   Late second-wave changes due to thrombin. Granule fusion and dissolution are in progress. Peripheral pseudopodia are swollen while those more centrally located are crushed together. Microtubules (MT) fill the pseudopods at this stage. (×17,700.)

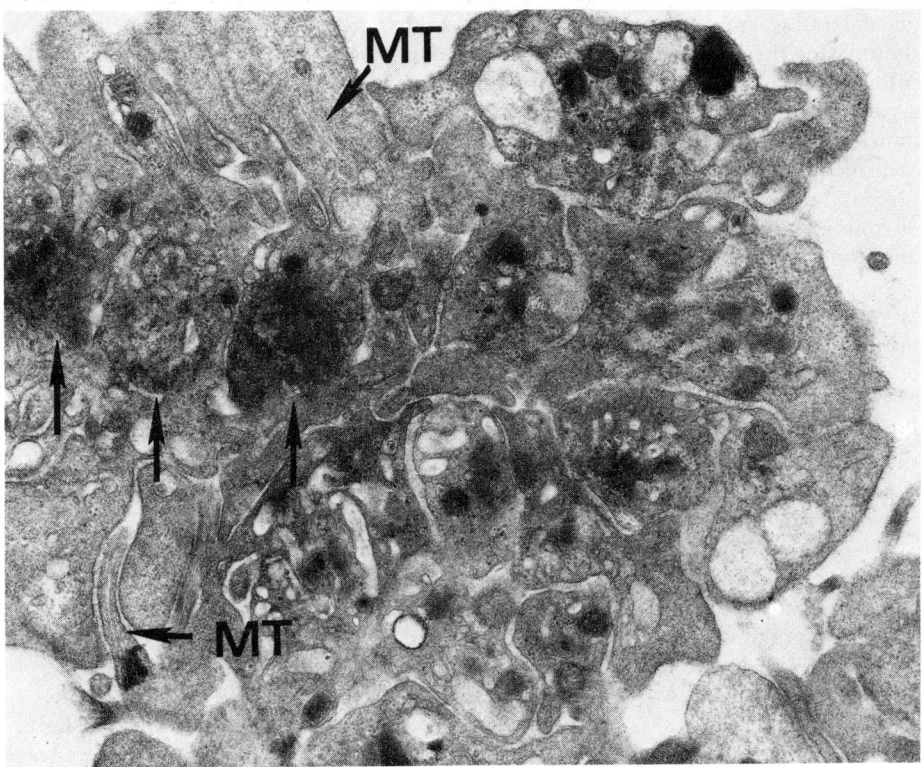

At this point in the biphasic response to thrombin a significant event occurs. Endogenous chemical constituents of the platelets are extruded into the surrounding plasma. The products include ADP, ATP, serotonin, catecholamines, potassium, calcium, lysosomal enzymes, platelet factor 4, β thromboglobulin, and other chemical constituents [47,60]. Extrusion of endogenous chemical components constitutes the *platelet release reaction*. As with other facets of platelet response, the release reaction is not an all-or-none reaction. The process begins after the trough between the first and second waves and builds in intensity as the second wave proceeds. Amounts of platelet products extruded increase with time during the irreversible second wave. The rate and extent to which they become available reflect the nature and concentration of the stimulating agent and the sensitivity of the platelet sample.

The second wave of aggregation is not completely dependent upon the release reaction. If release fails or is artificially blocked, the second stage of platelet clumping can still develop [77–82]. Release does not result from platelet damage, for constituents associated with injury are not extruded from platelets with products of the release reaction [60]. It is clear, therefore, that platelet release is a manifestation of secretory function, resembling the process observed in other cell systems such as the adrenal gland [83].

Platelet secretion is not a passive process [84–86]. It is energy-dependent, is accomplished by the cell's contractile mechanism, and occurs only after internal transformation has developed. The importance of internal transformation has been obscured by the fact that catecholamines, which also trigger the release reaction, cause platelets to aggregate without losing their discoid shape [72–76]. However, sequential studies of epinephrine and norepinephrine aggregates have shown that shape change and internal transformation do occur prior to and during development of the second wave of aggregation [12,81]. Thus, internal transformation is itself a manifestation of platelet contractile activity, for it characteristically precedes the secretion of endogenous chemical constituents. The importance of the centripetally oriented internal wave of contraction which moves platelet organelles to the cell center and surrounds them with a web of tubules and filaments cannot be overemphasized [73,74,79,80]. It is the internal changes which govern the degree of platelet response and the outcome of the aggregation process. This mechanism provides protection against overreaction as well as the dynamic means for extruding the platelet secretory products.

The second wave of thrombin-induced aggregation is characterized by rapid growth of aggregates as shown by increased light transmission and by progression of the physical changes of clumped cells (Figs. 126-13 to 126-16; sampled at *b* and *c* on tracing 3, Fig. 126-10). At this point the aggregometer tracing and physical alterations no longer coincide. Nephelometry indicates only that irreversible aggregation has taken place. The rate

of development and extent of physical changes in secondary aggregates depend on the nature and concentration of the inducing agent and relate closely to the rate and extent of the platelet release reaction.

Individual platelets reveal the physical alterations occurring as this process proceeds. Centrally clumped particles inside the cells are crushed together (Figs. 126-13, 126-14, and 126-16), and the encircling band of microtubules is broken down into its component subfilaments [12–14,74]. As secondary aggregation proceeds, the dense bodies in the clumped cells decrease in number and ultimately disappear. Discharge of dense bodies and granule contents is the physical correlate of the release reaction.

Alterations in the large aggregates during secondary aggregation mimic the transformation observed in the individual platelet (Fig. 126-15). The periphery of the cell clump becomes more electron-transparent and the central area more electron-dense. Swollen pseudopodia, formerly considered to be degranulated platelets, rim the margin of the aggregate. Pseudopodia deeper in the cell mass are interdigitated and appear crushed together. Microtubules are prominent in the pseudopodia of the secondary aggregates. Granules in platelet interiors discharge into the tubular system. Mitochondria remain discrete and are usually more dense than in unaltered cells. Glycogen masses are gone, leaving only a few discrete particles in the cells. The crushing force of contraction inside the aggregates ultimately causes individual platelets to lose their integrity and fuse with each other. This change is late and represents the end stage of platelet viscous metamorphosis, or clot retraction. Thus, a centripetally oriented wave of contraction dominates the physical transformation of large secondary aggregates just as it does individual cells.

The only structural elements which disappear to any significant extent from platelets during early secondary aggregation are the dense bodies [58]. Degranulation in the usual sense is not associated with early release reaction; nor are all the dense bodies lost in the early stages. This is consistent with gradual evolution of the release reaction as physical changes progress during secondary aggregation. The products known to be extruded from platelets early in the release reaction are associated with the dense bodies [60]. A question which has intrigued investigators is how the dense bodies or their products leave platelets, especially after aggregation. The products do not leak through cell walls as a result of increased permeability. The intercellular space between aggregated platelets is not sealed (Fig. 126-5), and it is probable that the open canalicular system and gaps between aggregated platelets serve as the major route of secretion [61,62]. Contraction of individual platelets and the platelet mass facilitate discharge of material into the surrounding plasma. Material from granules is most likely secreted via the same route.

Increasing the concentration of thrombin slightly over the critical amount which produces a double wave pattern results in a single irreversible wave of clumping

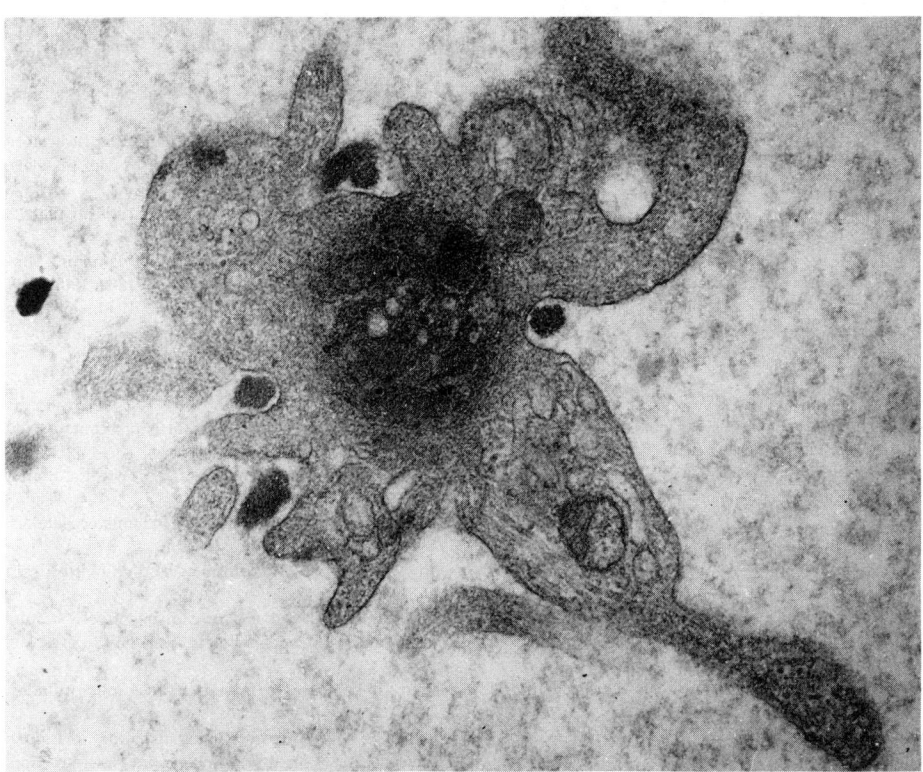

FIGURE 126-16   Platelet from sample of recalcified platelet-rich plasma fixed during clot retraction. The cell reveals completion of internal transformation. Granules are fused into an amorphous mass. Dense bodies are gone. The encircling band of tubules is converted to microfilaments, and other microtubules now appear in the pseudopodia. (×36,400.)

on the aggregometer (Fig. 126-10). This amount is still below that required to clot the sample of citrated platelet-rich plasma. Physical changes throughout the early and late phases of this pattern are identical with those described above, except that they occur more rapidly. The pattern of centripetal contraction in individual cells and in aggregates dominates transformation.

Other chemical agents capable of initiating platelet aggregation and the release reaction produce physical changes essentially identical with those caused by thrombin. Collagen particles, kaolin, adenosine diphosphate, arachidonic acid, the calcium ionophore A23187, and serotonin are typical examples [89]. Collagen produces only a single massive wave of aggregation, whereas ADP causes virtually the same types of single reversible, double, or single irreversible patterns as thrombin (Fig. 126-10) (see Chap. 129). In the case of ADP, however, shape change is virtually simultaneous with development of aggregation. ADP can produce shape change without aggregation, but only if the platelet sample is studied at a pH below 6 [90]. Serotonin is reputed to effectuate only a single, completely reversible wave of clumping [72], but a significant number of normal women manifest a typical double-wave pattern with this agent [91].

Epinephrine and norepinephrine produce unique patterns of platelet response [72]. The cells aggregate without loss of disc shape or increase in volume. Samples observed in the electron microscope reveal only slight alterations in surface contour and formation of a few narrow pseudopodia. The first-wave aggregates gradually transform in appearance until they are indistinguishable from ADP and thrombin aggregates obtained late in the first or between the first and second waves. Alterations during the second wave induced by catecholamines are indistinguishable from those caused by ADP or serotonin, except that they develop more rapidly (Figs. 126-13 to 126-15). In all cases the transformation is virtually identical, differing only in extent and rate at which physical alterations become apparent.

The foregoing description of platelet structural physiology has emphasized the three basic functions of adhesion (aggregation), contraction, and secretion (release reaction). Adhesion (aggregation) and contraction are independent facets of platelet physiology, for adhesion (aggregation) can occur without contraction, and contraction can take place without aggregation. The release reaction is dependent on the contractile system of the platelet, for secretion does not occur without contraction. Yet contraction, as manifested by internal reorganization, can develop up to a point without secretion. Contractile physiology dominates platelet function from the moment that shape change and internal reorganization begin until viscous metamorphosis and clot retraction are complete. Thus, platelets are not merely similar to muscle, or involved in events which resemble contractile processes, but are in fact muscle cells [43,89].

References

1. Wolpers, C., and Ruska, H.: Struktur-untersuchungen zuer Blutgerinnung. *Klin. Wochenschr.* 18:1077, 1939.
2. David-Ferreira, J. F.: The blood platelet: Electron microscopic studies, in *International Review of Cytology*, edited by G. H. Bourne and J. H. Danielli. Academic, New York, 1964, vol. 17, p. 99.
3. Marcus, A. J., and Zucker, M. B.: *The Physiology of Blood Platelets.* Grune & Stratton, New York, 1965, p. 32.
4. Johnson, S. A., and Seegers, W. A. (ed.): *The Physiology of Hemostasis and Thrombosis.* Charles C Thomas, Springfield, Ill., 1967.
5. Johnson, S. A., and Guest, M. M. (eds.): *Dynamics of Thrombus Formation and Dissolution.* Lippincott, Philadelphia, 1969.
6. Brinkhous, K. M. (ed.): Platelets: Their role in hemostasis and thrombosis. *Thromb. Diath. Haemorrh. Suppl.* 26:1967.
7. Haanen, C., and Jurgens, J. (eds.): Platelets in haemostasis, in *Experimental Biology and Medicine*, edited by E. Hagen, W. Wechsler, and F. Zilliken. Karger, Basel, 1968.
8. Kowalski, E., and Niewiarowski, S.: *Biochemistry of Blood Platelets.* Academic, New York, 1967.
9. Schulz, H.: *Thrombocyten und Thrombose im Elektronenmikroskopischen Bild.* Springer-Verlag, New York, 1968.
10. Johnson, S. S., Monto, R. W., Rebuck, F. W., and Horn, R. C. (eds.): *Blood Platelets.* Little, Brown, Boston, 1961.
11. Hovig, T.: The ultrastructure of platelets in normal and abnormal states. *Ser. Haematol.* 1:13, 1968.
12. White, J. G.: Platelet morphology, in *The Circulating Platelet*, edited by S. A. Johnson. Academic, New York, 1971, pp. 45–121.
13. White, J. G.: Physico-chemical dissection of platelet structural physiology, in *Platelets, Production, Function, Transfusion and Storage*, edited by M. G. Baldini and S. Ebbe. Grune & Stratton, New York, 1974, p. 235.
14. White, J. G., and Gerrard, J. M.: Ultrastructural features of abnormal blood platelets. *Am. J. Pathol.* 83:590, 1976.
15. Gerrard, J. M., and White, J. G.: Prostaglandins and thromboxanes: "Middlemen" modulating platelet function in hemostasis and thrombosis. *Prog. Hemostasis Thromb.* 4:87, 1978.
16. White, J. G., and Gerrard, J. M.: The ultrastructure of defective human platelets. *Mol. Cell. Biochem.* 21:109, 1978.
17. White, J. G., and Clawson, C. C.: Biostructure of blood platelets. *Ultrastruct. Pathol.* 1:533, 1980.
18. Grette, K.: Studies on the thrombin catalyzed hemostatic reactions of blood platelets. *Acta Physiol. Scand.* 56 (Suppl. 195):1, 1962.
19. Behnke, O.: Electron microscopic observations on the membrane system of the rat blood platelet. *Anat. Rec.* 158:121, 1967.
20. Behnke, O.: Electron microscopical observations on the surface coating of blood platelets. *J. Ultrastruct. Res.* 24:51, 1968.
21. Behnke, O.: An electron microscope study of the megakaryocyte of the rat bone marrow. I. The development of the demarcation membrane system and the platelet surface coat. *J. Ultrastruct. Res.* 24:412, 1968.
22. Nakao, K., and Angrist, A. A.: Membrane surface specialization of blood platelet and megakaryocyte. *Nature* 217:960, 1968.
23. White, J. G.: Ultrastructural cytochemistry and physiology of blood platelets, in *The Platelet*, edited by K. M. Brinkhous, R. W. Shermer, and F. K. Mastofi. Williams & Wilkins, Baltimore, 1971, pp. 45–121.
24. Bull, B. S.: The ultrastructure of negatively stained platelets: Some physiologic interpretations. *Blood* 28:901, 1966.
25. Rambourg, A., and Leblond, C. P.: Electron microscopic observations on the carbohydrate-rich cell coat present at the surface of cells in the rat. *J. Cell Biol.* 32:27, 1967.
26. White, J. G., and Krivitt, W.: The fine structural localization of adenosine triphosphatase in platelets and other blood cells. *Blood* 26:554, 1965.
27. Cooper, H. A., Mason, R. G., and Brinkhous, K. M.: The platelet surface membrane: Membrane and surface reactions. *Ann. Rev. Physiol.* 38:501, 1976.
28. White, J. G.: Investigation of the exterior coat of platelets during aggregation. *Am. J. Pathol.* 58:19, 1970.
29. Phillips, D. R. Jennings, L. K., and Edwards, H.: Identification of membrane proteins mediating the interactions of human platelets. *J. Cell Biol.* 86:77, 1980.
30. Silver, M. J.: Role of calcium ions and phospholipids in platelet aggregation. *Am. J. Physiol.* 209:1128, 1965.
31. Nachman, R. L., and Marcus, A. J.: Platelet thrombosthenin: Subcellular localization and function. *J. Clin. Invest.* 46:1380, 1967.
32. Marcus, A. J., Zucker-Franklin, D., Safier, L. B., and Ullman, H. L.: Studies on human platelet granules and membranes. *J. Clin. Invest.* 45:14, 1966.
33. White, J. G.: The submembrane filaments of blood platelets. *Am. J. Pathol.* 56:267, 1969.
34. Zucker-Franklin, D.: The submembranous fibrils of human blood platelets. *J. Cell Biol.* 47:293, 1970.
35. Nachmias, V. T.: Cytoskeleton of human platelets at rest and after spreading. *J. Cell Biol.* 86:795, 1980.
36. Haydon, G. B., and Taylor, A. D.: Microtubules in hamster platelets. *J. Cell Biol.* 26:673, 1965.
37. Sixma, J. J., and Molenaar, J.: Microtubules and microfibrils in blood platelets. *Thromb. Diath. Haemorrh.* 16:153, 1966.
38. Behnke, O., and Zelander, T.: Substructure in negatively stained microtubules of mammalian blood platelets. *Exp. Cell Res.* 43:236, 1966.
39. White, J. G.: The substructure of human platelet microtubules. *Blood* 32:638, 1968.
40. White, J. G.: Effects of colchicine and vinca alkaloids on human platelets. I. Influence on platelet microtubules and clot retraction. *Am. J. Pathol.* 53:281, 1968.
41. Allen, R. D., and Kamiya, N.: *Primitive Motile Systems in Cell Biology.* Academic, New York, 1964.
42. Bettex-Galland, M., and Luscher, E.: Extraction of an actomyosin-like protein from human thrombocytes. *Nature* 184:276, 1959.
43. Gerrard, J. M., and White, J. G.: The structure and function of platelets with emphasis on their contractile nature. *Pathobiol. Annu.* 6:31, 1976.
44. Cohen, I., Gerrard, J. M., Bergman, R. N., and White, J. G.: The role of contractile filaments in platelet activation, in *Protides of the Biological Fluids.* Pergamon, Oxford, 1979, p. 55.
45. Fonio, A.: Über das funktionelle Verhalten der isolierten Strukturelements der Thrombocyten, des Hyalomers und des Granulomers. *Acta Haematol. (Basel)* 6:207, 1951.
46. White, J. G.: Tubular elements in platelet granules. *Blood* 32:148, 1968.
47. Kaplan, K. L., Broekman, M. J., Chernoff, A., Lesznik, G. R., and Drillings, M.: Platelet α granule proteins: Studies on release and subcellular organization. *Blood* 53:604, 1979.
48. Baker, R. V., Blaschko, H., and Born, G. V. R.: The isolation from blood platelets of particles containing 5-hydroxytryptamine and adesonine triphosphate. *J. Physiol. (Lond.)* 149:55P, 1959.
49. Solantunturi, E., and Paasonen, M. K.: Intracellular distribution of monamine oxidase, 5-hydroxytryptamine, and histamine in blood platelets of rabbit. *Ann. Med. Exp. Fenn.* 14:427, 1966.
50. Tranzer, J. P., DaPrada, M., and Pletcher, A.: Ultrastructural localization of 5-hydroxytryptamine in blood platelets. *Nature* 212:1574, 1966.
51. Bak, I. J., Hassler, R., May, B., and Westerman, E.: Morphological and biochemical studies on the storage of serotonin and histamine in blood platelets of the rabbit. *Life Sci.* 6:1133, 1967.
52. Etcheverry, G. J., and Zieher, L. M.: Cytochemistry of 5-hydroxytryptamine at the electron microscopic level. I. Study of the specificity of the reaction in isolated blood platelets. *J. Histochem. Cytochem.* 16:162, 1968.
53. Davis, R. B., and White, J. G.: Localization of 5-hydroxytryptamine in blood platelets: A radioautographic and ultrastructural study. *Br. J. Haematol.* 15:93, 1968.
54. DaPrada, M., Pletcher, A., Tranzer, J. P., and Knuchel, H.: Subcel-

lular localization of 5-hydroxytryptamine in blood platelets. *Nature* 216:1315, 1967.

55. Wood, J. G.: Electron microscopic localization of 5-hydroxytryptamine (5-HT). *Tex. Rep. Biol. Med. 23:*838, 1965.
56. White, J. G.: The dense bodies of human platelets: Inherent electron opacity of the serotonin storage particles. *Blood 33:*598, 1969.
57. White, J. G.: The dense bodies of human platelets: Origin of serotonin storage particles from platelet granules. *Am. J. Pathol. 53:*791, 1968.
58. White, J. G.: The origin of dense bodies in the surface coat of negatively stained platelets. *Scand. J. Haematol. 5:*371, 1968.
59. White, J. G.: Fine structural alterations induced in platelets by adenosine diphosphate. *Blood 31:*604, 1968.
60. Holmsen, H., Day, J., and Stormorken, H.: The blood platelet release reaction. *Scand. J. Haematol. (Suppl.) 8:*3, 1969.
61. White, J. G.: Identification of platelet secretion in the electron microscope. *Ser. Haematol. 6:*429, 1973.
62. White, J. G.: Electron microscopic studies of platelet secretion. *Prog. Hemostasis Thromb. 2:*49, 1974.
63. Behnke, O.: The morphology of blood platelet membrane systems. *Ser. Haematol. 3:*3, 1970.
64. White, J. G.: Interaction of membrane systems in blood platelets. *Am. J. Pathol. 66:*295, 1972.
65. Breton-Gorius, J., and Guichard, J.: Ultrastructural localization of peroxidase activity in human platelets and megakaryocytes. *Am. J. Pathol. 66:*277, 1972.
66. Statland, B., Haegan, B., and White, J. G.: The uptake of calcium by platelet relaxing factor. *Nature 223:*521, 1969.
67. White, J. G.: Is the canalicular system the equivalent of the muscle sarcoplasmic reticulum? *Hemostasis 4:*185, 1975.
68. Gerrard, J. M., White, J. G., Rao, G. H. R., and Townsend, D.: Localization of platelet prostaglandin production in the platelet dense tubular system. *Am. J. Pathol. 83:*283, 1976.
69. Born, G. V. R., and Cross, M. J.: The aggregation of blood platelets. *J. Physiol. (Lond.) 168:*178, 1963.
70. O'Brien, J. R.: Platelet aggregation. II. Some results from a new method of study. *J. Clin. Pathol. 15:*452, 1962.
71. Macmillan, D. C.: Secondary clumping effect in human citrated platelet-rich plasma produced by adenosine diphosphate and adrenaline. *Nature 211:*140, 1966.
72. O'Brien, J. R.: Platelet stickiness. *Ann. Rev. Med. 17:*275, 1966.
73. White, J. G.: The muscular system of platelets. *Blood 30:*625, 1967.
74. White, J. G., and Krivit, W.: Changes in platelet granules and microtubules during early clot development. *Thromb. Diath. Haemorrh. (Suppl.) 26:*29, 1967.

75. Thomas, D. P.: Effect of catecholamines on platelet aggregation caused by thrombin. *Nature 215:*298, 1967.
76. Bull, B. S., and Zucker, M. B.: Changes in platelet volume produced by temperature, metabolic inhibitors, and aggregating agents. *Proc. Soc. Exp. Biol. Med. 120:*296, 1965.
77. Mills, D. C. B., and Roberts, G. C. K.: Membrane active drugs and the aggregation of human platelets. *Nature 213:*35, 1967.
78. White, J. G.: Effects of ethylenediamine tetracetic acid (EDTA) on platelet structure. *Scand. J. Haematol. 5:*241, 1968.
79. White, J. G.: A contraction-relaxation cycle in the primary response of platelets to aggregating agents. *Abstracts XII Cong. Int. Soc. of Hematology,* New York, 1968, p. 196.
80. White, J. G.: Effects of colchicine and vinca alkaloids on human platelets. III. Influence on primary internal contraction and secondary aggregation. *Am. J. Pathol. 54:*467, 1969.
81. White, J. G.: Effects of atropine on platelet structure and function. *Scand. J. Haematol. 6:*236, 1969.
82. Rao, G. H. R., Gerrard, J. M., Witkop, C. J., and White, J. G.: Platelet aggregation independent of ADP release or prostaglandin synthesis in patients with Hermansky-Pudlak syndrome. *Prostaglandins Med. 6:*459, 1981.
83. Ruben, R. P., Feinstein, M. B., Joanus, S. D., and Parme, M.: Inhibition of catecholamine secretion and calcium exchange in perfused cat adrenal glands by tetracaine and magnesium. *J. Pharm. Exp. Ther. 155:*463, 1967.
84. Born, G. V. R.: Mechanism of platelet aggregation and of its inhibition by adenosine derivatives. *Fed. Proc. 26:*115, 1967.
85. Karpatkin, S.: Studies on human platelet glycolysis: Effect of glucose, cyanide, citrate, and agglutination on platelet glycolysis. *J. Clin. Invest. 46:*409, 1967.
86. Bettex-Galland, M., and Luscher, E.: Thrombosthenin, the contractile protein from blood platelets, and its relation to other contractile proteins. *Adv. Protein Chem. 20:*1, 1965.
87. Rodman, N. F., Painter, J. C., and McDevitt, N. B.: Platelet disintegration during clotting. *J. Cell Biol. 16:*225, 1963.
88. Behnke, O.: Morphological changes in the hyalomere of rat blood platelets in experimental venous thrombi. *Scand. J. Haematol. 3:*136, 1966.
89. White, J. G., and Gerrard, J. M.: The cell biology of platelets, in *Handbook of Inflammation (The Cell Biology of Inflammation),* edited by G. Weissman. Elsevier–North-Holland, New York, 1980, p. 83.
90. McLean, J. R., and Veloso, H.: Change of shape without aggregation caused by ADP in rabbit platelets at low pH. *Life Sci. 6:*1983, 1967.
91. White, J. G.: A biphasic response of platelets to serotonin. *Scand. J. Haematol. 7:*145, 1970.

Biochemistry and function of platelets

CHAPTER *127*

Composition of platelets

SIMON KARPATKIN
HOLM HOLMSEN

Human platelets contain most of the common cellular constituents except DNA [1–10]. Platelets are a heterogeneous population of megakaryocyte cytoplasmic fragments ranging from <5 to >12 μm^3 in volume [3], with an average volume of 5 to 7.5 μm^3 [3,10]. Glycogen, adenine nucleotides, protein, amino acids, and orthophosphate are all distributed heterogeneously among the platelets [3]. This heterogeneity of volume and composition is probably a reflection of variations in platelet production as well as platelet age. The heavier platelet is a larger and relatively younger platelet, particularly under stress conditions; the lighter platelet is a smaller and probably older platelet [3]. If a total platelet population is employed, there are 119 mg protein or 0.78×10^{11} platelets per gram wet weight or per milliliter packed platelets [3]. (In order to provide uniformity, all data previously published and expressed per number of platelets or per milligram of protein have been converted to gram wet weight.)

Platelets have no nuclei but contain most of the subcellular organelles found in other cells. Thus, mitochondria, microtubules, glycogen granules, occasional Golgi cisternae, and ribosomes are present, although the most conspicuous organelles are the secretory storage granules which account for about 20 percent of the volume of a platelet. These granules are of two main types, the dense granules (also called *dense bodies*) and the α granules. While the dense granules are homogeneous and filled with a strongly osmiophilic material which also is electron-dense without staining or fixation, the α granules are heterogeneous in appearance. They have different sizes and shapes, and appear to contain amorphous material of homogeneous structure or with areas of varying degree of osmiophility. The contents of the two main types of storage granules are shown in Table 127-1, in which the α granules have been subdivided into two types, "true α granules" and acid hydrolase–containing vesicles. Congenital and acquired platelet disorders are known in which the

contents of the dense granules and/or the "true" α granules are absent or present in very small amounts. Patients with these disorders, referred to as *storage pool deficiencies,* have impaired hemostasis. The storage mechanisms and physiological significance of the contents of platelet storage granules have been reviewed [11,12].

Carbohydrates

Carbohydrates represent 1.9 percent of the platelet wet weight, or 8.4 percent of dry weight [5]. No free glucose is detectable in washed platelets [30]. Platelet carbohydrate is composed of poly- and heterosaccharides. Platelet glycogen exists as a particulate form with a sedimentation coefficient of 133 to 155 S [31]. Platelet hexosamine is distributed 75 percent in glycoprotein and 25 percent in mucopolysaccharide. Glucosamine makes up the major hexosamine component of platelet glycoprotein, whereas galactosamine makes up 96 percent of the aminosugar of mucopolysaccharides. Chondroitin 4-sulfate, hyaluronic acid, and/or low-sulfated polysaccharides are probably present [32].

Platelets are rich in acid glycosidases [33–35] and arylsulfatase [34,36], enzymes that are potentially significant for glycoprotein and mucopolysaccharide metabolism. However, since these enzymes are present in subcellular vesicles and in a secretable form, it is uncertain whether they participate in cellular metabolism. Several glycosyltransferases are present in the platelet cytosol [37–40] and probably participate in glycoprotein metabolism.

The sialic acid of platelets consists predominantly of *N*-acetyl neuraminic acid. Treatment of intact platelets with neuraminidase releases 60 percent of total sialic acid, suggesting either that not all sialic acid is available for enzyme action or that not all sialic acid is on the platelet surface. Removal of surface sialic acid by treatment of intact platelets with neuraminidase leads to a reduction in the electrophoretic mobility of the cells at pH 6.4 [41] and to rapid removal of platelets from the circulation [42].

Platelets have an active carbohydrate metabolism (see Chap. 128) and contain enzymes of the Embden-Meyerhof pathway [1,10,43–60], the hexose monophosphate shunt [10,43,56,61–63], the tricarboxylic acid cycle [43–46,60,64], and the glyconeogenic pathway [1,44,55, 64,65], as well as the corresponding intermediates [66,67]. They do not contain a 2,3-diphosphoglycerate shunt [6]. Large, heavy platelets contain approximately twice as much activity of a number of enzymes as do lighter, smaller platelets [10,55,56]. Proteins are the major constituent of platelets, representing 12 percent wet and 52 percent dry weight [3]. Two-dimensional electrophoretic protein separations have revealed between 30 to 50 distinct proteins in total platelet extracts [68–72]. Polyribosomes have been separated on sucrose

TABLE 127-1   Contents of secretory storage granules in human platelets

Dense granules		True α granules		Acid hydrolase–containing vesicles	
Constituent	Source	Constituent	Source	Constituent	Source
Anions:		Platelet-specific		β-N-Hexosaminidase	
ATP	[13,14]	proteins:		β Glucuronidase	
ADP		Platelet factor 4	[17,18]	α and β Galactosidases	[26,27]
GTP		β Thromboglobulin		α and β Fucosidases	[28,29]
GDP	[15]	Coagulation factors:		α Mannosidase	
Pyrophosphate		Fibrinogen	[18]	α Arabinosidase	
Orthophosphate	[16]	Factor V	[19]	β Glycerophosphatase	
Cations:		Factor VIII	[20]	Aryl sulfatase	
Calcium	[12]	Cationic proteins:			
Serotonin		Mitogenic factor			
		Bactericidal factor	[17,18]		
		Permeability factor			
		Chemotactic factor			
		Glycoproteins:			
		Glycoprotein G			
		(thrombospondin)	[21,22]		
		Fibronectin	[23,24]		
		Albumin	[25]		

gradients [73,74] and shown to be increased in heavy platelets [74]

Contractile proteins

Platelets contain a contractile Ca^{2+}-Mg^{2+}–dependent ATPase termed *thrombosthenin,* which is similar in many respects to skeletal muscle actomyosin [75–77]. However, while skeletal muscle has an actin/myosin ratio of about 7, platelets have a ratio of 100 [78]. Platelets do not have the typical organization of myosin (thick filaments) and actin (thin filaments) seen in skeletal muscle, but actin-containing microfilaments appear upon platelet stimulation [79–81]. These observations suggest that actin and myosin are not associated in the resting or activated platelet. However, the ratio of actin to myosin for actomyosin extracted from platelets is the same as that found in skeletal muscle [82]. There is, therefore, a considerable excess of actin within the platelet which does not complex with myosin.

Actin is the most abundant protein in platelets, representing 25 percent of total platelet protein [83,84]. It is a single polypeptide of M_r 43,000 daltons which forms double helical filaments 6 nm thick, with a 39-nm repeat interval [85,86]. Platelet F actin contains 1 mole of ADP per actin monomer. This protein-nucleotide polymer stimulates the ATPase activity of (phosphorylated) myosin [85]. Two different forms of actin have been demonstrated in platelets [87,88], which may correspond to the observation that purified platelet actin consists of β and γ isozymes in a 5:1 proportion typical for nonmuscle actin, despite having the same polymerization-depolymerization properties as skeletal

muscle actin [89]. Actin can exist in several levels of organization. Activated platelets develop microfilaments of F-actin bundles, which are conspicuously absent in resting platelets. The monomer, G actin [90], can polymerize to actin-ADP polymers (F actin). This requires ATP hydrolysis with binding of the liberated ADP to each actin monomer of F actin [90,91]. G actin and F actin coexist in dynamic equilibrium in vitro. F actin depolymerizes at one end and polymerizes at the other at the same velocity. Each molecule of monomer added to the growing end requires one molecule at ATP hydrolysis [91]. Thus, ATP is continuously consumed to maintain F actin; this process, which has been labeled "the actin treadmill" [92], takes place in the platelet [93,94]. It has been estimated that 40 percent of the total ATP consumption of resting platelets is required for the actin treadmill [94,95]. Actin which is insoluble in the nonionic detergent Triton X-100 is thought to be part of the platelet cytoskeleton [96,97]. The content of this insoluble actin increases following stimulation of platelets with thrombin [97]; this is associated with a corresponding conversion of G to F actin [98]. Activation of platelets also leads to exposure of actin on their surface [29,99–101]. In vitro studies have shown that certain cytochalasins depolymerize platelet F actin [102]; a protein has been isolated from platelets that inhibits G-actin polymerization and promotes F-actin depolymerization in a fashion similar to cytochalasin B [103]. A protein of M_r 250,000 to 280,000 daltons that binds actin (actin-binding protein) has also been isolated from platelets and is thought to be involved in actin polymerization [104,105]; it cross-reacts with an antibody to filamin, a protein that is regulated through phosphorylation by a cyclic-AMP (cAMP)–dependent protein kinase [106]. This filamin-like actin-binding protein is present in the platelet cytoskeleton [96] but disappears during platelet storage in parallel to loss of platelet responsiveness [107]. α-Actinin, another protein which binds actin, anchors actin in the Z-band of skeletal muscle cells, is present in platelets [105,108], and is associated with the dense granules [109]. Little is known, however, of how the filamin-like protein and α-actinin control the state of actin polimerization.

A third protein which binds actin in platelets is profilin, a basic protein of M_r 15,000 to 16,000 daltons which is thought to control F-actin polymerization. Profilin is capable of binding at least 55 percent of total platelet actin in an unpolymerizable complex called profilactin [110,111]. The concentration of profilactin decreases sharply during platelet activation; with a concomitant polymerization of F actin. Thus, profilin has been thought to act as a regulator of actin polymerization-depolymerization [112].

Platelet myosin is the best characterized of the contractile proteins [113–121]. It has a M_r of 460,000 daltons and is composed of six polypeptide chains organized in three identical pairs. Two chains have M_r of 200,000 daltons and are referred to as *heavy chains*. Each heavy chain has a globular domain (head) and a stretched domain (rod, tail). The two other pairs are smaller polypeptides, referred to as *light chains*, with molecular weights of 20,000 and 16,000 daltons. Each head of the heavy chain has one binding site for F actin and enzymatic sites for the hydrolysis of ATP to ADP and P_i stimulated by Mg^{2+} or Ca^{2+}. Platelet myosin molecules are different from skeletal muscle myosin in that they form filaments which are 325 nm long and 11 nm thick compared to 1500- by 30-nm filaments for skeletal muscle myosin. Platelet and muscle myosins differ immunologically. The actin-stimulated platelet myosin ATPase [122–129] is in the "on" position when the myosin light chains of M_r 20,000 daltons are phosphorylated and in the "off" position when they are dephosphorylated. The state of phosphorylation is regulated by a Ca^{2+}-myosin light-chain kinase activated by Ca^{2+}-calmodulin; and by a phosphomyosin phosphatase. The myosin light-chain kinase is further regulated by a cAMP–dependent protein kinase which phosphorylates the kinase to an inactive form. There is a linear correlation between the degree of myosin phosphorylation and the tension developed in reconstituted platelet actomyosin fibers [130], suggesting that light-chain phosphorylation regulates contractility in the intact cell. Myosin light chain is present in the dephosphorylated form in the resting platelet [131], and in the phosphorylated form in the stimulated platelet [131–134]. This phosphorylation precedes platelet secretion [133,135,136] and is associated with platelet-supported clot retraction [136]. In contrast to the Ca^{2+}-mediated myosin light-chain phosphorylation that is dominant in platelets, the activation of skeletal muscle myosin ATPase and actomyosin contractility by

Ca^{2+} is transduced through the troponin-tropomyosin complex. Platelets do contain the troponin-tropomyosin complex [137–139], although its physiological significance is obscure.

Microtubules

Platelets contain a marginal bundle of microtubules that are required for platelet structure and platelet secretion [140,141]. Microtubules encompass the periphery of the entire platelet and help maintain its discoid shape [140]. Once platelets are stimulated, this microtubule band appears to move to the center, associated with central movement of platelet granules prior to the release reaction [142]. Once release takes place, microtubules disappear (depolymerize) and then appear in other parts of the platelet, particularly in pseudopodia [143]. Platelet secretion or release does not take place following disruption of microtubule polymerization with nontoxic concentrations of colchicine, which binds to tubulin monomer [141]. The circumferential coil of microtubules in the resting platelet has been isolated from detergent-dissection of the platelet and shown to be a single coil of three turns with clear overlap zones [144]. The microtubules consist of polymerized tubulin made up of monomers with M_r 55,000 daltons, and several different high-molecular-weight proteins, designated *microtubule accessory proteins* [145,146]. Tubulin is composed of two different electrophoretic subunits with identical M_r of 55,000 daltons, termed α and β tubulin [141]. Tubulin represents 2.5 percent of total platelet protein [147]. The tubulin monomer can polymerize in the presence of guanosine triphosphate (GTP) to a polymer or microtubule, containing 1 mole of GDP (guanosine diphosphate) bound per mole of tubulin monomer. The polymerization requires specific free SH groups in the tubulin monomer and presence of the microtubule accessory proteins (MAPs) [148–150]. Both α and β tubulins from platelets are phosphorylated by ATP. The significance of this phosphorylation reaction is not understood [143,151].

Plasma protein analogs

Fibrinogen constitutes 12 percent of total platelet protein [152–154] and is present in α granules (see Table 127-1) as well as on the platelet surface [155–159]. More than 90 percent of total platelet fibrinogen is secreted from intact platelets following platelet activation. The kinetics of release are identical to substances localized in the "true" α granules [157,158]. Significant amounts of externally added fibrinogen bind tightly to specific receptors on the surface of activated platelets in the presence of Ca^{2+} (see below). It is not yet clear whether platelet and plasma fibrinogen are identical gene products [159,160]. Resting platelets do not take up fibrinogen from plasma in vitro [160], and isolated megakaryocytes do not incorporate amino acids into their fibrinogen under conditions where platelet actin is readily synthesized [161]. One is therefore tempted to conclude that neither platelets nor megakaryocytes synthesize fibrinogen and that megakaryocytes or platelets accumulate the fibrinogen by unknown mechanisms [162].

Albumin constitutes 2 percent of all platelet protein [152]. It is present in isolated α granules (see Table 127-1) [163]; more than 9 percent of total platelet albumin is secreted following platelet stimulation with thrombin or collagen [164].

Factor XIII, a transamidase that cross-links fibrin monomers, has been demonstrated in the platelet cytosol [165,166] and purified from these cells [167]. It is not secreted following platelet activation, suggesting that factor XIII is present in the cytoplasm [168]. Cross-linking of platelet actin by factor XIII has been reported [169,285], indicating a potential function for the transamidase in the regulation of actin polymerization.

Platelet factor 4

Two low-molecular-weight proteins with anti-heparin activity are platelet factor 4 (PF4) and low-affinity PF4 (LA-PF4). Platelet factor 4 is a glycoprotein [170] present in the α granules (see Table 127-1) and released from platelets following platelet aggregation by ADP, thrombin, or epinephrine [171–173]. It shortens the thrombin clotting time in the presence of heparin [171–174], potentiates ADP-induced aggregation in vitro, precipitates fibrinogen, nonenzymatically clots soluble fibrin monomer complex [175], and neutralizes certain fibrinogen breakdown products [176]. Large, heavy platelets release 10 times as much PF4 as do small, light platelets. The release of PF4 from small, light platelets is negligible [173]. Platelet factor 4 may be a potent and specific agent triggering platelet aggregation and blood clotting in vivo [175]. The content of PF4 in platelet-poor plasma is 3 to 16 ng/ml [177–180], and in human platelets it is 12 to 18 μg per 10^9 platelets [181,182]. Low-affinity platelet factor 4 (LA-PF4) is immunologically identical with β thromboglobulin (βTG), a specific marker for platelets [181]. LA-PF4 is secreted by platelets and converted to βTG in the circulation by plasmin or neutral proteases which split off a tetrapeptide from the N terminal of LA-PF4 [183]. The content of βTG in plasma is 11 to 39 ng/ml [177,184–187]; and in platelets is 18-24 μg per 10^9 platelets [181,182].

Platelet growth factor

A growth factor capable of stimulating the proliferation of arterial smooth muscle cells has been isolated from platelets. It is a high-molecular-weight compound which is stable at 56°C and labile to pepsin treatment [182,188,189]. A vascular permeability factor has also been isolated from an acid extract of human platelets. It is a heat-stable cationic protein with M_r 30,000 daltons [190].

Acid hydrolases

Acid hydrolases are enzymes which degrade materials in secondary lysosomes where the pH is around 4.5 to 5.0. Platelets are richer in these enzymes compared to other tissues [191]. Many of these enzymes (see Table 127-1) are secreted from platelets by strong (see Chap. 128) stimuli. In contrast to the contents of dense granules and α granules, which are completely secreted, only 25 percent (β glucuronidase) to 60 percent (β-N-hexosaminidase) of the acid hydrolases are secreted [164,192]. Acid hydrolases are also present in membranes of surface and intracellular origin. Platelets are richer than most tissues in the "high uptake" form of some acid hydrolases [194,195], a type that is preferentially taken up by cells through receptor-mediated endocytosis. The role of secreted and retained hydrolase in platelets is not known. However, they are secreted during clotting [196], which greatly increases the levels of acid hydrolases in serum above that of the circulating plasma [196,208]. It has long been known that a significant portion of serum acid *p*-nitrophenylphosphatase (the serum enzyme activity which is elevated in prostatic carcinoma) comes from the platelet [198]. This enzyme activity is not secreted from platelets [192] but is released as a result of lysis of 1 to 2 percent of the platelets during secretion [199].

Amino acids and peptides

The free amino acid pool in platelets has been analyzed and compared with plasma amino acid values [8,9]. The content of taurine [8,9,200] is approximately equivalent to the total content of all other platelet free amino acids (21 μmol/g). Other amino acids present in appreciable concentration are glutamic acid, aspartic acid, serine, and glycine. Cystine, histidine, and methionine are present in trace amounts [8,9]. A comparison of plasma and intracellular platelet amino acid values reveals an appreciable platelet-plasma gradient for all amino acids measured. In this respect the platelet is similar to the leukocyte but different from the red blood cell. The largest gradients obtained were with taurine and aspartic acid [8]. Large heavy platelets contain 2.1 times more total amino acid than small light platelets [3].

Platelets are rich in glutathione [10] which is maintained in the reduced form by a potent hexose monophosphate shunt; one important function of reduced glutathione is to protect platelets from oxidant stress [201].

Lipids

Lipids make up 2.98 percent of the platelet wet weight and 14 percent of the dry weight [3]. Phospholipid makes up 76 percent of the total lipid, neutral lipid 20 percent, and lipoprotein 4 percent [202]. The total phospholipid consists primarily of phosphatidyl choline (lecithin), phosphatidyl ethanolamine, and sphingomyelin. Smaller amounts of phosphatidyl serine, phosphatidyl inositol, lysolecithin, phosphatidic acid, and cardiolipin are also present. The neutral lipid is composed of 85 percent free cholesterol and smaller amounts of tri-, di-, and monoglyceride, free fatty acids, and cholesterol esters. Cerebrosides and gangliosides have also been identified. Details of the fatty acid constituents of the major lipid classes have been published [202,203].

Platelet factor 3 is probably a lipoprotein component of the platelet membrane [60] which becomes available to the coagulant enzymes and cofactors of plasma following platelet aggregation or platelet trauma [204,205]. The active component is the phospholipid moiety, which accelerates plasma clotting, probably by acting as a surface catalyst [205]. The vitamin K–dependent clotting factors, II, VII, IX, and X, each contain γ-carboxyglutamic acid residues which bind to phospholipid via Ca^{2+} bridging [206–209]. Factor Xa also binds to the platelet surface by attaching to Va which, in the presence of Ca^{2+}, attaches to the platelet surface after platelet activation and release of factor V from the α granules [210–213]. The specific phospholipids of the platelet membrane which have been incriminated are phosphatidyl serine and phosphatidyl ethanolamine [214]. These compounds are not chemically altered in this reaction [215]. Lipoprotein (phospholipid) is released during platelet aggregation as a sedimentable fraction [60] and a nonsedimentable fraction [216].

Purines, pyrimidine nucleosides, and nucleotides

Platelets contain nucleotides of the purine bases adenine, guanine, and hypoxanthine and of the pyrimidine bases uracil and cytosine [217–220]. The adenine nucleotides have been studied quantitatively and are present in concentrations similar to those of skeletal muscle as well as other tissues [1,6,217,221–227]. The ATP, ADP, and AMP concentrations reported from one laboratory are 2.52, 1.39, and 0.3 μmol/g, respectively [6]. ATP and ADP are present in two pools: a metabolic pool, which is easily labeled when incubated with radioactive phosphate, adenine, or adenosine; and a storage pool, which is not labeled after 2-h incubation but is labeled in vivo or after prolonged in vitro incubation [228]. The storage pool is present in the dense granules and reflects two-thirds of the total adenine nucleotides [229–231]. The ATP/ADP ratio of the storage pool is 0.8, with 80 percent of total ADP in the storage dense

granules [231]. These dense granules also contain a substantial fraction of platelet guanine nucleotides [15]. The concentration of total nucleotides (anions) and calcium (cation) are extremely high. These components coexist as a complex in the solid state [232] into which serotonin is incorporated after it has entered the dense granule [233].

Mineral and vitamin content

Platelets are capable of maintaining cationic gradients with surrounding plasma [2,234–236]. Thus the intracellular Na^+ and K^+ content of platelets is, respectively, 38.8 and 118 meq/liter of intracellular water [2]. Intracellular K appears to be distributed in two compartments [2,236]. The pumping of this cationic gradient requires energy (ATP), which is probably modulated via a Na^+-K^+–stimulated ATPase on the platelet membrane [2,236]. This ATPase is inhibited by 10^{-4} to 10^{-5} M ouabian as well as by sulfhydryl inhibitors [2,236].

The Ca^{2+}, Mg^{2+}, Zn, and orthophosphate contents are 17 to 32 [237–239], 2.9 [237], 0.36 [240], and 1.2 [6] μmol/g, respectively. Calcium is present in 60 percent of the dense granules [12,241,243]. The phosphorus and sulfate concentrations are 53.3 and 2.9 μmol/g, respectively [4].

Platelets contain 40 to 170 ng of folic acid per gram and 600 to 2100 pg of vitamin B_{12} [244] per gram. They have a high content of ascorbic acid and are capable of reducing dehydroascorbic acid to ascorbic acid [245].

Serotonin (5-hydroxytryptamine)

The smooth muscle vasoconstrictor substance serotonin (5-hydroxytryptamine) is present in platelets and practically absent in plasma or other blood cells. Platelet serotonin is almost exclusively stored in the dense granules [246,247] (see Table 127-1). Platelets possess potent uptake and storage systems for serotonin [248–251].

Platelets do not synthesize serotonin but absorb the amine from the enterochromaffin cells of the intestine [252,253]. Two distinctly different serotonin transport systems are found: a plasma membrane transport system and a granule transport system. The plasma membrane system is inhibited by propranolol, imipramine, and other tricyclic antidepressants and driven by monovalent cation (Na^+, K^+) gradients across this membrane. The ouabain-sensitive, ATP-requiring sodium ATPase pump creates the ion gradients, which in turn makes serotonin transport across the plasma membrane dependent upon cellular energy [254–266]. The serotonin transport mechanism in dense granules is quite different from that found in the plasma membrane [267]. It is inhibited by reserpine, and unaffected by the plasma membrane inhibitors. It is driven by a proton gradient (acid inside) maintained by a membrane ATPase [268–270]. Serotonin is bound to Ca^{2+}-nucleotide aggregates within the dense granules and therefore totally shielded from metabolism [271,272,232,233]. Serotonin is secreted during the platelet release reaction (see Chap. 128). Serotonin can also be released following inhibition of the two transport systems or by exchange with other amines [199]. Platelets have a mitochondrial monamine oxidase [193,273–276] which has been extensively studied in psychiatric disorders, since the platelet has been considered a model for amine-storing neurons. However, little oxidation takes place in normal platelets (in contrast to platelets with absent dense granules [271,278]), since dense-granule serotonin is inaccessible to the mitochondrial monamine oxidase.

Serotonin can also act as a weak agonist of platelets by interaction with receptors on the surface distinctly different from the plasma membrane transport system [279].

Platelet membrane constituents

The platelet membrane consists of two outer electron-dense layers 20 Å thick and an inner, less dense layer. The outer two layers have usually been considered to be protein and the inner one a lipid bimolecular layer.

Preparations of platelet membranes have been shown to contain protein, carbohydrate, neutral lipid, phospholipid, and cholesterol. Biochemical analysis has revealed that the platelet membrane is a lipoglycoprotein. The lipid/protein ratio of platelet membrane is 0.58 compared with a total platelet lipid/protein ratio of 0.28. Phospholipid represents 78 percent of total membrane lipid, with neutral lipid making up the rest. Free cholesterol represents 90 percent of total neutral lipid. The cholesterol/phospholipid ratio is 0.53 [202]. The sugar components are identified as glucose, galactose, mannose, hexosamines (GlcN: GalN = 6:1), sialic acid, and fucose. The chemical composition is protein 36 percent; lipid, 52 percent; carbohydrate, 7.0 percent; RNA, 0.35 percent; DNA, 0.0 percent.

Assymmetry of phospholipids has been reported with respect to their outside-inside orientation [280].

The platelet membrane is composed of over 20 polypeptide chains [281,283], with molecular weights ranging from 13,000 to 200,000 daltons.

Early studies on platelet membranes, employing SDS-polyacrylamide gel electrophoresis and carbohydrate staining revealed three major glycoproteins designated GPI, GPII, and GPIII with apparent molecular weights of 155,000, 135,000, and 103,000 daltons, respectively [283,284,286]. More refined technology [287–291] has revealed, in order of decreasing molecular weight, two glycoproteins and one protein in the GPI region (GPIa, GPIb, and GPIc), two glycoproteins in the GPII region (GPIIa, GPIIb), two in the GPIII region (GPIIIa and GPIIIb, or GPIII and GPIV) and an additional glycoprotein, GPV [292,294] with M_r 82,000 daltons. GPIb, GPIc,

and GPIIb are attached to nonidentical subunits α and β by disulfide bonds. GPIa, GPIIa, GPIII, and the large subunit of GPIIb (GPIIb$_\alpha$) appear to have intramolecular disulfide bonds [290]. GPIb contains the bulk of platelet surface sialic acid [295].

A major antigen noted on crossed immunoelectrophoresis of normal platelet membranes is absent in Glanzmann's thrombasthenia [158,297]. It is composed of a complex of GPIIb and GPIIIa and possibly other glycoproteins which are held together by Ca^{2+} [298,299]. GPIIb and GPIIIa are absent to diminished in Glanzmann's thrombasthenia, suggesting a role in platelet aggregation [286,291]. GPIIIa is probably the carrier for the platelet antigen (PLA) PLA1 since PLA1 antiplatelet antibody does not react with platelets from patients with Glanzmann's thrombasthenia [301]. GPIb (M_r 170,000 daltons) is composed of a "buried" membrane portion and a free portion. The free portion is easily hydrolyzed by a platelet Ca^{2+}-dependent protease during the extraction procedure [302] to a soluble [GPIs] carbohydrate-enriched (60 percent) *glycocalicin* with M_r 148,000 daltons [303]. Glycocalicin probably represents a major part of the platelet membrane carbohydrate [303]. GPIb (and GPIs) is absent to diminished in Bernard-Soulier syndrome [295], a disorder similar to von Willebrand's disease in which platelets do not adhere to basement membrane. Since these patients do have von Willebrand factor, GPIb is thought to have the von Willebrand factor receptor activity [295]. GPIb is also thought to have platelet Fc receptor activity since immune complexes do not bind to platelets from patients with the Bernard-Soulier syndrome [304,305].

The platelet membrane has a negative surface charge which is removed by neuraminidase and is thought to be due to the sialic acid, N-acetylneuraminic acid. There are approximately 1.9×10^6 molecules of sialic acid per square micrometer of platelet surface or approximately 11 times the concentration found in human red blood cells [41].

Specific receptors for binding of various agents to platelet membranes have been reported. Three independent estimations of specific receptors for ADP binding sites have revealed similar values of 0.85, 1.0, and 2×10^5 per platelet [309–311]. The association constant for ADP binding is $6.5 \times 10^6 M$. Binding is temperature-dependent and requires Ca^{2+} or Mg^{2+} as well as intact sulfhydryl groups [311]. The ADP receptor is thought to have a M_r of 100,000 daltons [312].

Receptors for fibrinogen have recently been described which require platelet activation by ADP or other agonists for their exposure and Ca^{2+} for binding [313–317]. ADP stimulation results in the exposure of 1000 to 4000 high-affinity sites per platelet (Kd = $4 \times 10^{-8} M$) and 25,000 to 80,000 low-affinity sites (Kd $\times 10^{-6} M$) [318]. ^{125}I-fibrinogen does not bind to ADP-stimulated thrombasthenic platelets [315–318]. It has been suggested that thrombasthenic platelets contain only high-affinity fibrinogen receptors [318] and that high concentrations of fibrinogen inhibit aggregation of thrombasthenic platelets [318].

Thrombin binding to platelets does not require the presence of its active site [319]. Stimulation of the platelet requires active thrombin and may involve proteolysis of GPV [292–294,308]. GPIb may also have a receptor for thrombin which is not proteolyzed by thrombin because thrombin binds to purified glycocalicin (GPIs). GPIs inhibits thrombin-induced platelet aggregation. Platelets from Bernard-Soulier patients are deficient in GPIs and aggregate poorly with low concentrations of thrombin [306,307]. GPV is the surface protein which is cleaved by thrombin to a fragment of M_r 70,000 daltons [292–294]. Thrombin may bind to GPIb prior to its attack on GPV [308]. Thrombin may aggregate platelets by a two-step reaction which involves binding to a high-affinity receptor, followed by enzymatic modification of this receptor or a nearby receptor, possibly GPV, to yield an activated complex which triggers platelet stimulation [320–322]. One group reported 2×10^4 thrombin-binding sites per platelet, with cooperativity of thrombin binding [320], and concluded that the binding is a reversible catalytic step with no dissociation of enzyme from product [321]. Another group [323] has reported two classes of high-affinity binding sites: at high thrombin concentrations, 4.5×10^4 molecules per platelet, with an apparent dissociation constant of 3 units per milliliter ($30 \times 10^{-9}\ M$); at low thrombin concentrations, 5×10^2 molecules per platelet, with an apparent dissociation constant of 0.02 units per milliliter.

Two types of α-adrenergic receptors have been found in platelets [324]. One type, α-2H, has higher affinity and the other, α-2L, has lower affinity for agonists; both types have similar affinity for antagonists. Norepinephrine has 69 binding sites per platelet with a Kd of $23 \times 10^{-9}\ M$. Platelet receptors for prostaglandins I_2 and D_2 have also been identified [325]. There are two receptors for serotonin: a high-affinity site (Kd = 0.8 nM) concerned with the aggregation response induced by serotonin and a low-affinity site (Kd = 8 nM) involved with transport of serotonin across the plasma membrane [279,296,326].

Also associated with the platelet membrane are surface actin and myosin which are thought to be on the inner surface [327,328], lipoprotein (platelet factor 3), and plasma proteins. The plasma proteins often associated with the platelet membrane and not readily removed by washing include IgG [328], IgM [330], plasminogen [329], factor V (also known as platelet factor 1) [331,332], factor VIII [333], factor XI [332], and factor XII [332,334,335]. Albumin, fibrinogen [158,159], γ globulin, and plasminogen have been identified immunologically and give reactions of identity with plasma proteins. Several enzymes have been localized to the platelet membrane. These include hexokinase, α-glycerol-P-dehydrogenase, glutathione reductase [10], phospholipase A_2 [336], and protease activity [336].

References

1. Luganova, I. S., Seits, I. F., and Teodorovich, V. I.: Metabolism in human thrombocytes. *Biochemistry (U.S.S.R)* 23:379, 1958.
2. Gorstein, F., Carroll, H. J., and Puszkin, E.: Electrolyte concentrations, potassium flux kinetics, and the metabolic dependence of potassium transport in human platelets. *J. Lab. Clin. Med.* 70:938, 1967.
3. Karpatkin, S.: Heterogeneity of human platelets. I. Metabolic and kinetic evidence suggestive of young and old platelets. *J. Clin. Invest.* 47:1073, 1969.
4. Woodside, E. E., and Kocholaty, W.: Carbohydrates of human and bovine platelets. *Blood* 16:1173, 1960.
5. Maupin, B., Saint-Blanchard, J., and Storck, J.: Soufre, taurine, proteins, et ATP plaquettaires. *Rev. Fr. Etud. Clin. Biol.* 7:169, 1962.
6. Karpatkin, S., and Langer, R. M.: Biochemical energetics of simulated platelet plug formation: Effect of thrombin, ADP, and epinephrine on intra- and extracellular adenine nucleotide kinetics. *J. Clin. Invest.* 47:2158, 1968.
7. Soupart, P.: Free amino acids of blood and urine in the human, in *Amino Acid Pools,* edited by J. T. Holden. Elsevier, New York, 1962, p. 220.
8. Gross, R., and Gerok, W.: Quantitative determination of the amino acids and other ninhydrin positive substances in normal human platelets. *Thromb. Diath. Haemorrh.* 6:462, 1961.
9. Karpatkin, S., and Strick, N.: Heterogeneity of human platelets. V. Differences in glycolytic and related enzymes with possible relation to platelet age. *J. Clin. Invest.* 51:1235, 1972.
10. Bull, B. S., and Zucker, M. B.: Changes in platelet volume produced by temperature, metabolic inhibitors, and aggregating agents. *Proc. Soc. Exp. Biol. Med.* 120:296, 1965.
11. Fukami, M. H.: Human platelet storage organelles: A review. *Thromb. Haemost.* 38:963, 1977.
12. Holmsen, H., and Weiss, H. J.: Secretable pools in platelets. *Ann. Rev. Med.* 30:119, 1979.
13. Holmsen, H., Day, H. J., and Storm, E.: Adenine nucleotide metabolism of blood platelets. VI. Subcellular localization of nucleotide pools with different functions in the platelet release reaction. *Biochim. Biophys. Acta* 186:254, 1969.
14. Ugurbil, K., and Holmsen, H.: Nucleotide compartmentation: Radioisotopic and nuclear magnetic resonance studies, in *Platelets in Biology and Pathology,* edited by J. L. Gorden. North Holland, New York, 1981, vol. II, p. 147.
15. Daniel, J. L., Molish, I., and Holmsen, H.: Radiolabeling of purine nucleotide pools as a method to distinguish among subcellular compartments: Studies on platelets. *Biochem. Biophys. Acta* 632:444, 1980.
16. Fukami, M. H., Dangelmaier, C. A., Bauer, J., and Holmsen, H.: Secretion subcellular localization and metabolic status of inorganic pyrophosphate in human platelets: A major constituent of the amine-storing granules. *Biochem. J.* 192:99, 1980.
17. Niewiarowski, S.: Proteins secreted by the platelet. *Thromb. Haemostasis* 38:924, 1977.
18. Kaplan, K. L.: Platelet granule proteins: Localization and secretion, in *Platelets in Biology and Pathology* edited by J. L. Gordon. North Holland, Amsterdam, 1981, vol. 2, p. 77.
19. Vicic, W. J., Lages, B., and Weiss, H. J.: Release of human platelet factor V activity is induced by both collagen and ADP and is inhibited by aspirin. *Blood* 56:448, 1980.
20. Koutts, J., Walsh, P. N., Plow, E. F., Fenton, J. W., Bouma, B. N., and Zimmerman, T. S.: Active release of human platelet factor-VIII–related antigen by adenosine diphosphate, collagen and thrombin. *J. Clin. Invest.* 62:1255, 1978.
21. Hagen, I., Olsen, T., and Solum, N. O.: Studies on subcellular fractions of human platelets by the lactoperoxidase-iodination technique. *Biochim. Biophys. Acta* 455:214, 1976.
22. Lawler, J. H., Slayter, H. S., and Coligan, J. E.: Isolation and characterization of a high molecular weight glycoprotein from human blood platelets, *J. Biol. Chem.* 253:8609, 1978.
23. Zucker, M. B., Mosesson, M. H., Broekman, M. J., and Kaplan, K. L.:

Release of platelet fibronectin (cold-insoluble globulin) from alpha-granules induced by thrombin or collagen: Lack of requirement for plasma fibronectin in ADP-induced platelet aggregation. *Blood* 54:8, 1979.

24. Plow, E. F., Birdwell, C., and Ginsberg, M. H.: Indentification and quantitation of platelet-associated fibronectin antigen. *J. Clin. Invest.* 63:540, 1979.

25. Davey, M. G., and Lüscher, E. F.: Release reactions of human platelets induced by thrombin and other agents. *Biochem. Biophys. Acta* 165:490, 1968.

26. Holmsen, H., and Day, H. J.: The selectivity of the thrombin-induced platelet release reaction: Subcellular localization of released and retained constituents. *J. Lab. Clin. Med.* 75:840, 1970.

27. Schmuckler, M., and Zieve, P. D.: The effect of concanavalin A on human platelets and their response to thrombin. *J. Lab. Clin. Med.* 83:887, 1974.

28. Yatziv, S., White, M., and Eldor, A.: Lysosomal enzyme activities in platelets of normal individuals and of patients with Gaucher's disease. *Thromb. Haemostasis* 32:665, 1974.

29. Bouvier, C. A., Gabbiani, G., Ryan, G. B., Badonnel, M. C., Majno, G., and Lüscher, E. F.: Binding of anti-actin antibodies to platelets. *Thromb. Haemostasis* 37:321, 1977.

30. Karpatkin, S., and Siskind, G. W.: Effect of antibody binding and agglutination on human platelet glycolysis: Comparison with thrombin and epinephrine. *Blood* 30:617, 1967.

31. Scott, R. B., and Still, W. J. S.: Glycogen in human blood platelets: Isolation by ultracentrifugation and characteristics of the isolated particles. *Blood* 35:517, 1970.

32. Olsson, I., and Gardell, S.: Isolation and characterization of glycosaminoglycans from leukocytes and platelets. *Biochim. Biophys. Acta* 141:348, 1967.

33. Bosmann, H. B.: Identification, purification and characteristics of glycosidases of human blood platelets. *Biochim. Biophys. Acta* 258:265, 1972.

34. Dangelmaier, C. A., and Holmsen, H.: Determination of acid hydrolases in human platelets. *Anal. Biochem.* 104:182, 1980.

35. Day, H. J., Holmsen, H., and Hovig, T.: Subcellular particles of human platelets: A biochemical and electronmicroscopic study with particular reference to the influence of fractionation techniques. *Scand. J. Haematol. (Suppl.)* 7:1, 1969.

36. Rotreki, B., and Polasek, J.: Nitrocatechol sulfatase in human blood platelets. *Acta Hematol.* 39:129, 1968.

37. Bosmann, B. B.: Platelet adhesiveness and aggregation: The collagen: glycosyl, polypeptide, N-acetylgalactosamino and glycoprotein galactosyl transferases of human platelet. *Biochim. Biophys. Res. Commun.* 43:1118, 1971.

38. Smith, D. J., Kosow, D. P., Wu, C., and Jameson, G. A.: Characterization of human platelet UDP-glucose-collagen glycosyltransferase using a new rapid assay. *Biochim. Biophys. Acta* 483:263, 1977.

39. Cartron, J. P., and Nurden, A. T.: Galactosyltransferase and membrane glycoprotein abnormality in human platelets from Tn syndrome donors. *Nature* 282:621, 1979.

40. Menashi, S., and Grant, M. E.: Studies on the collagen glucosyltransferase activity present in platelets and plasma. *Biochem. J.* 178:777, 1979.

41. Madoff, M. A., Ebbe, S., and Baldini, M.: Sialic acid of human platelets. *J. Clin. Invest.* 43:870, 1964.

42. Greenberg, J., Packham, M. A., Cazenave, J. P., Reimers, H. J., and Mustard, J. F.: Effects on platelet function of removal of platelet sialic acid by neuraminidase. *Lab. Invest.* 32:476, 1975.

43. Gross, R., Lohr, G. W., and Waller, H. D.: Genetic defects in platelet metabolism as a cause of thrombocytopathia, in *Biochemistry of Blood Platelets*, edited by E. Kowalski and S. Niewiarowski. Academic, New York, 1967, p. 161.

44. Karpatkin, S.: Studies on human platelet glycolysis: Effect of glucose, cyanide, insulin, citrate, and agglutination and contraction on platelet glycolysis. *J. Clin. Invest.* 46:409, 1967.

45. Warshaw, A. L., Laster, L., and Shulman, N. R.: The stimulation by thrombin of glucose oxidation in human platelets. *J. Clin. Invest.* 45:1923, 1966.

46. Chernyak, N. B., and Totskaya, A. A.: Structure and oxidative metabolism of granular fraction isolated from human blood platelets. *Vopr. Med. Khim.* 9:146, 1963.

47. Scott, R. B.: Activation of glycogen phosphorylase in blood platelets. *Blood* 30:321, 1967.

48. Karpatkin, S., and Langer, R. M.: Activation of inactive phosphorylase dimer and monomer from human platelets with magnesium adenosine triphosphate. *J. Biol. Chem.* 244:1953, 1969.

49. Karpatkin, S., and Langer, R. M.: Human platelet phorphorylase. *Biochim. Biophys. Acta* 185:350, 1969.

50. Yunis, A. A., and Arimura, G. K.: Isoenzymes of glycogen phosphorylase in human leukocytes and platelets: Relation to muscle phosphorylase. *Biochem. Biophys. Res. Commun.* 33:119, 1968.

51. Kahn, I., Zucker-Franklin, D., and Karpatkin, S.: Microthrombocytosis and platelet fragmentation associated with idiopathic autoimmune thrombocytopenic purpura. *Br. J. Haematol.* 31:499, 1975.

52. Chaiken, R., Pagano, D., and Detwiler, T. C.: Regulation of phosphorylase. *Biochim. Biophys. Acta* 403:315, 1975.

53. Karpatkin, S., Braun, J., and Charmatz, A.: Requirement of divalent cation for human platelet phosphorylase activity. *Biochim. Biophys. Acta* 220:22, 1970.

54. Gear, A. R. L., and Schneider, W.: Control of platelet glycogenolysis: Activation of phosphorylase kinase by calcium. *Biochim. Biophys. Acta* 392:111, 1975.

55. Karpatkin, S., and Charmatz, A.: Heterogeneity of human platelets. III. Glycogen metabolism in platelets of different sizes. *Br. J. Haematol.* 19:135, 1970.

56. Karpatkin, S., and Strick, N.: Heterogeneity of human platelets. V. *J. Clin. Invest.* 51:1235, 1972.

57. Doery, J. C. G., Hirsh, J., Loder, P. B., and De Gruchy, G. C.: Distribution of platelet hexokinase and the effect of collagen. *Nature* 216:1317, 1967.

58. Akkerman, J. W. N., Gorter, G., Sixma, J., and Staal, G. E. J.: Influence of Mg^{2+}, ITP^{4-}, and ATP^{4-} on human platelet phosphofructokinase. *Biochim. Biophys. Acta* 370:113, 1974.

59. Hule, V.: Isoenzymes of lactic dehydrogenase in human platelets. *Clin. Chim. Acta* 13:431, 1966.

60. Marcus, A. J., Zucker-Franklin, D., Safier, L. B., and Ullman, H. L.: Studies on human platelet granules and membranes. *J. Clin. Invest.* 45:14, 1966.

61. Schettini, F., DiFrancesco, C., Berni Canani, M., and Rea, F.: Study of the enzymatic activity of the blood platelets: 6-Phosphogluconic dehydrogenase and transketolase activities of the platelets of normal children. *Boll. Soc. Ital. Biol. Sper.* 37:797, 1961.

62. Moser, K., Lechner, K., and Vinazzer, H.: A hitherto not described defect in thrombasthenia: Glutathione reductase deficiency. *Thromb. Diath. Haemorrh.* 19:46, 1968.

63. Karpatkin, S., and Weiss, H. J.: Deficiency of glutathione peroxidase associated with high levels of reduced glutathione in Glanzmann's thrombasthenia. *N. Engl. J. Med.* 287:1062, 1972.

64. Karpatkin, S., Charmatz, A., and Langer, R. M.: Glycogenesis and glyconeogenesis in human platelets: Incorporation of glucose, pyruvate and citrate into platelet glycogen: Glycogen synthetase and fructose-1-6-diphosphatase. *J. Clin. Invest.* 49:140, 1970.

65. Negishi, H., Morishita, V., Kodama, S., and Matsuo, T.: Platelet glucose-6-phosphatase activity in patients with von Gierke's Disease. *Clin. Chim. Acta* 53:175, 1974.

66. Kim, B. K., and Baldini, M. G.: Glycolytic intermediates and adenine nucleotides of human platelets. I. The influence of ACD and EDTA-anticoagulants. *Haematologia* 6:437, 1972.

67. Niessner, H., and Beutler, E.: Fluorimetric analysis of intermediates of the glycolytic and citric acid cycle pathway in human platelets. *Am. J. Clin. Pathol.* 62:361, 1974.

68. Phillips, D. R., and Agin, P. P.: Platelet plasma membrane glycoproteins: Evidence for the presence of nonequivalent disulfide bonds using non-reduced–reduced two-dimensional gel electrophoresis. *J. Biol. Chem.* 252:2121, 1977.

69. Clemetson, K. J., Capitanio, A., and Luscher, E. F. L.: High resolution two-dimensional gel electrophoresis of the proteins and glycoproteins of human blood platelets and platelet membranes. *Biochim. Biophys. Acta* 553:11, 1979.

70. McGregor, J. L., Clemetson, K. J., James, E., and Dechavanne, M.: A comparison of techniques used to study externally oriented proteins, proteins and glycoproteins of human blood platelets. *Thromb. Res.* 16:437, 1979.

71. Hagen, J., Bjerrum, O. J., and Solum, N. O.: Characterization of human platelet proteins solubilized with Triton X-100 and examined by crossed immunoelectrophoresis: Reference patterns of extracts from whole platelets and isolated membranes. *Eur. J. Biochem.* 99:9, 1979.

72. McGregor, J. L., Clemetson, K. J., James, E., Lüscher, E. F., and Dechavanne, M.: Characterization of human blood platelet membrane proteins and glycoproteins by their isoelectric point (Pi) and apparent molecular weight using two-dimensional electrophoresis and surface labelling techniques. *Biochim. Biophys. Acta* 59:473, 1980.

73. Steiner, M.: Platelet protein synthesis studied in a cell-free system. *Experientia* 26:786, 1970.

74. Booyse, F. M., Hoveke, T. P., Kisieleski, D., and Rafelson, M. E., Jr.: Studies on human platelets. II. Protein synthetic activity of various platelet populations. *Biochim. Biophys. Acta* 157:660, 1968.

75. Bettex-Galland, M., and Lüscher, E. F.: Thrombosthenin, the contractile protein from blood platelets and its relation to other contractile proteins. *Adv. Protein Chem.* 20:1, 1965.

76. Chambers, D. A., Salzman, E. W., and Neri, L. L.: Characterization of Ecto-ATPase of human platelets. *Arch. Biochem. Biophys.* 119:173, 1967.

77. Nachman, R. L., Marcus, A. J., and Safier, L. B.: Platelet thrombosthenin: Subcellular localization and function. *J. Clin. Invest.* 46:1380, 1967.

78. Pollard, T. D.: Functional implications of the biochemical and structural properties of cytoplasmic contractile protein, in *Molecules and Cell Movement*, edited by S. Inoue and R. E. Stephens. Raven Press, New York, 1976, p. 259.

79. Zucker-Franklin, D., and Grusky, G.: The actin and myosin filaments of human and bovine blood platelets. *J. Clin. Invest.* 51:419, 1972.

80. Behnke, O., Uristenson, B. I., and Engdahl Nielsen, L.: Electron microscopical observations on actinoid and myosinoid filaments in blood platelets. *J. Ultrastruct. Res.* 37:351, 1971.

81. Zucker-Franklin, D.: Microfibrils of blood platelets: Their relationship to microtubules and the contractile protein. *J. Clin. Invest.* 48:165, 1969.

82. Puszkin, S., Kochwa, S., Puszkin, E. G., and Rosenfield, R. E.: A solid-liquid biphasic model for characterization of muscle and platelet contractile proteins. *J. Biol. Chem.* 250:2085, 1975.

83. Lucas, R. C., Gallagher, M., and Stracher, A.: Active and actin-binding protein in platelets, in *Contractile Systems in Non-Muscle Tissues*, edited by S. V. Perry, A. Margreth, and R. S. Adelstein. North Holland, New York, 1976, p. 133.

84. Gordon, D. J., Bayer, J. L., and Korn, E. D.: Comparative biochemistry of non-muscle actins. *J. Biol. Chem.* 252:8300, 1977.

85. Booyse, F. M., Hoveke, T. P., and Rafelson, M. E., Jr.: Human platelet actin. *J. Biol. Chem.* 248:4083, 1973.

86. Probst, E., and Luscher, F.: Studies on thrombosthenin A, the actin-like moiety of the contractile protein from blood platelets. I. Isolation, characterization and evidence for two forms of thrombosthenin A. *Biochim. Biophys. Acta* 278:577, 1972.

87. Abramowitz, J. W. A., Stracher, A., and Detwiler, T. C.: A second form of actin: Platelet microfilaments depolymerized by ATP and divalent cations. *Arch. Biochem. Biophys.* 167:230, 1975.

88. Muszbek, L., Fesus, L., Olveti, E. and Szabo, T.: Cleavage of thrombasthenin A by thrombin: Evidence for the existence of two types of bovine platelet actin. *Biochim. Biophys. Acta* 427:171, 1976.

89. Landau, F., Huc, C., Thome, F., Oriol, C., and Olomucki, A.: Human platelet actin. Evidence of β and γ forms and similarity of properties with sarcomeric actin. *Eur. J. Biochem.* 81:571, 1977.

90. Oosawa, F., and Kasai, M.: Actin, in *Subunits in Biological Systems*, edited by S. N. Timasheff and G. D. Fasman. Dekker, New York, 1971, vol. V, p. 261.

91. Wegner, A.: Head to tail polymerization of actin. *J. Mol. Biol.* 108:139, 1976.

92. Brenner, S. L., and Korn, E. D.: Substoichiometric concentrations of cytochalasin D inhibit actin polymerization: Additional evidence for an F-actin treadmill. *J. Biol. Chem.* 254:9982, 1979.

93. Daniel, J. L., Molish, J. R., and Holmsen, H.: Identification of the precipitable protein–ADP complex in platelets as F-actin–ADP. *Proc. Int. Congress Biochem. XI*, p. 202, 1979.

94. Daniel, J. L., Robkin, L., Salganicoff, L., and Holmsen, H.: Measurement of the nucleotide exchange rate as a possible determination of the cellular state of actin, in *Motility in Cell Function*, edited by F. A. Pepe. Academic, New York, 1979, p. 459.

95. Holmsen, H.: Ethanol-insoluble adenine nucleotides in platelets and their possible role in platelet function. *Ann. N.Y. Acad. Sci.* 201:109, 1972.

96. Muhlrad, A., Eldor, A., and Kahane, J.: Distribution of myosin, actin, and actin-binding proteins in membrane and soluble fraction of human blood platelets. *FEBS Lett.* 92:85, 1978.

97. Jennings, L. K., Fox, J. E. B., Edwards, H. H., and Phillips, D. R.: Changes in the cytoskeletal structure of human platelets following thrombin activation. *J. Biol. Chem.* 256:6927, 1981.

98. Carlsson, L., Markey, F., Blikstad, J., Persson, T., and Lindberg, V.: Reorganization of actin in platelets stimulated by thrombin as measured by the DNase inhibition assay. *Proc. Natl. Acad. Sci. U.S.A.* 76:6376, 1979.

99. Gabbiani, G., et al.: Human smooth muscle auto-antibody. *Am. J. Pathol.* 72:473, 1973.

100. Diggle, T. A., Toh, B. H., Firkin, B. G., and Pfueller, S.: Human platelet actin: Surface expression after platelet activation. *Thromb. Haemostasis* 42:799, 1979.

101. George, J. N., Lyons, R. M., and Morgan, R. K.: Membrane changes associated with platelet activation: Exposure of actin on the platelet surface after thrombin-induced secretion. *J. Clin. Invest.* 66:1, 1980.

102. Howard, T. H., and Lin, S.: Specific interaction of cytochalasins with muscle and platelet actin filaments in vitro. *J. Supramol. Struct.* 11:283, 1979.

103. Grumet, M., and Lin, S.: A platelet inhibitor protein with cytochalasin-like activity against actin polymerization in vitro. *Cell* 21:439, 1980.

104. Lucas, R., Detwiler, T. C., and Stracher, A.: The identification and isolation of a high molecular weight (270,000 daltons) actin-binding protein from human platelets. *J. Cell. Biol.* 70:259A, 1976.

105. Schollmeyer, J. V., Rao, G. H. R., and White, J. G.: An actin-binding protein in human platelets. Interactions with α-actinin on gelation of actin and the influence of cytochalasin B. *Am. J. Pathol.* 93:433, 1978.

106. Wallach, D., Davies, P. J. A., and Pastan, J.: Purification of mammalian filamin: Similarity to high molecular weight actin-binding proteins in macrophages, platelets, fibroblasts, and other tissues. *J. Biol. Chem.* 253:3328, 1978.

107. Robey, F. A., Freitag, C. M., and Jamieson, G. A.: Disappearance of actin-binding protein from human blood platelets during storage. *FEBS Lett.* 102:257, 1979.

108. Gerrard, J. M., Schollmeyer, J. V., Phillips, D. R. and White, J. G.: α-Actinin deficiency in thrombasthenia: Possible identity of α-actinin and glycoprotein III. *Am. J. Pathol.* 94:509, 1979.

109. Jockush, B. M., Burger, M. M., DaPrada, M., Richards, J. G., Chaponnier, C., and Galibianni, G.: α-Actinin attached to membranes of secretory vesicles. *Nature* 270:628, 1977.

110. Markey, F., Lindberg, U., and Eriksson, L.: Human platelets contain profilin, a potential regulator of actin polymerisability. *FEBS Lett.* 88:75, 1978.

111. Harris, H. E., and Weeds, A. G.: Platelet actin: Subcellular distribution and association with profilin. *FEBS Lett.* 90:84, 1978.

112. Markey, F., Persson, T., and Lindberg, U.: Characterization of platelet extracts before and after stimulation with respect to the possible role of profilactin as microfilament precursor. *Cell* 23:145, 1980.

113. Booyse, F. M., Hoveke, T. P., Zschocke, D., and Rafelson, M. E., Jr.: Human platelet myosin. *J. Biol. Chem.* 246:4291, 1971.

114. Adelstein, R. S., Pollard, T. D., and Kuehl, W. M.: Isolation and characterization of myosin and two myosin fragments from human blood platelets. *Proc. Natl. Acad. Sci. U.S.A.* 68:2703, 1971.

115. Adelstein, R. S., and Conti, M. A.: The characterization of contractile proteins from platelets and fibroblasts. *Cold Spring Harbor Symp. Quant. Biol.* 37:599, 1972.

116. Cohen, J., Kaminski, E., and DeVries, A.: Actin-linked regulation of the human platelet contractile system. *FEBS Lett.* 34:315, 1973.

117. Pollard, T. D., Thomas, S. M., and Niewderman, R.: Human platelet myosin. I. Purification by a rapid method applicable to other non-muscle cells. *Anal. Biochem.* 60:258, 1974.

118. Cohen, J., Kaminski, E., Lamed, R., Oplatka, A., and Muhlrad, A.: Characterization of the active site of platelet myosin in comparison to smooth and skeletal muscle myosin. *Arch. Biochem. Biophys.* 175:249, 1976.

119. Niederman, R., and Pollard, T. D.: Human platelet myosin. II. In vitro assembly and structure of myosin filaments. *J. Cell. Biol.* 67:72, 1975.

120. Cove, D. H., and Crawford, N.: Platelet contractile proteins: Separation and characterization of the actin- and myosin-like components. *J. Mechanochem. Cell. Motil.* 3:123, 1975.

121. Pollard, T. D., Fujiwara, K., Handin, R., and Weiss, G.: Contractile proteins in platelet activation and contraction. *Ann. N.Y. Acad. Sci.* 283:218, 1977.

122. Adelstein, R. S., Conti, M. A., Daniel, J. L., and Anderson, W.: The interaction of platelet actin, myosin and myosin light chain kinase, in *Ciba Foundation Symposium on the Biochemistry and Pharmacology of Blood Platelets.* Elsevier–Excerpta Medica–North Holland, Amsterdam, 1975, p. 101.

123. Adelstein, R. S., Conti, M. A., and Anderson, W., Jr.: Phosphorylation of human platelet myosin. *Proc. Natl. Acad. Sci. U.S.A.* 70:3115, 1973.

124. Adelstein, R. S., and Conti, M.A.: Phosphorylation of platelet myosin increases actin-activated myosin ATPase activity. *Nature* 256:597, 1975.

125. Daniel, J. L., and Adelstein, R. S.: Isolation and properties of platelet myosin light chain kinase. *Biochemistry* 15:2370, 1976.

126. Adelstein, B. S., Conti, M. A., and Barylko, B.: The role of myosin phosphorylation in regulation actin-myosin interaction in human blood platelets. *Thromb. Haemostasis* 40:241, 1978.

127. Hathaway, D. R., and Adelstein, R. S.: Human platelet myosin light chain kinase requires the calcium-binding protein calmodulin for activity. *Proc. Natl. Acad. Sci. U.S.A.* 76:1653, 1979.

128. Dabrowski, R., and Hartshorne, D. J.: A Ca^{2+} and modulator-dependent myosin light chain kinase from non-muscle cells. *Biochem. Biophys. Res. Commun.* 85:1352, 1978.

129. Conti, M. A., and Adelstein, R. S.: Phosphorylation by cyclic adenosine 3',5'-monophosphate-dependent protein kinase regulates myosin light chain kinase. *Fed. Proc.* 39:1569, 1980.

130. Lebowitz, E. A., and Cooke R.: Contractile properties of actomyosin from human blood platelets. *J. Biol. Chem.* 253:5443, 1978.

131. Daniel, J. L., Molish, J. R., and Holmsen, H.: Myosin phosphorylation in intact platelets. *J. Biol. Chem.* 256:7510, 1981.

132. Haslam, R. J., and Lynham, J. A.: Relationship between phosphorylation of blood platelet proteins and secretion of platelet granule constituents. I. Effects of different aggregating agents. *Biochem. Biophys. Res. Commun.* 77:71, 1977.

133. Lyons, R. M., and Shaw, J. O.: Interaction of Ca^{2+} and protein phosphorylation in the rabbit platelet release reaction. *J. Clin. Invest.* 65:242, 1980.

134. Haslam, R. J., Lynham, J. A., and Fox, J. E. B.: Effects of collagen, ionophore A23187 and prostaglandin E_1 on the phosphorylation of specific proteins in blood platelets. *Biochem. J.* 178:397, 1979.

135. Daniel, J. L., Holmsen, H., and Adelstein, R. S.: Thrombin-stimulated myosin phosphorylation in intact platelets and its possible involvement in secretion. *Thromb. Haemostasis* 38:984, 1977.

136. Daniel, J. L., Molish, J. R., Holmsen, H., and Salganicoff, L.: *Cold Spring Harbor Conferences on Cell Proliferation,* vol. 8, *Protein Phosphorylation; Phosphorylation of Myosin,* 1981, p. 913.

137. Cohen, I., and Cohen, C.: A tropomyosin-like protein from human platelets. *J. Mol. Biol.* 68:383, 1972.

138. Muszbek, L., Kuznicki, J., Szabo, T., and Drabikowski, W.: Troponin C-like protein of blood platelets. *FEBS Lett.* 80:308, 1977.

139. Cote, G. P., Lewis, W. G., Pato, N. D., and Smillie, L. B.: Platelet tropomyosin: Lack of binding to skeletal muscle troponin and correlation with sequence. *FEBS Lett.* 94:131, 1978.

140. Behnke, O.: Further studies on microtubules: A marginal bundle in human and rat thrombocytes. *J. Ultrastruct. Res.* 13:469, 1965.

141. Menche, D., Israel, A., and Karpatkin, S.: Platelets and microtubules: Effect of colchicine and D_2O on platelet aggregation and release induced by calcium ionophore A23187. *J. Clin. Invest.* 66:284, 1980.

142. White, J. G.: Fine structural changes induced in platelets by adenosine diphosphate. *Blood* 31:604, 1968.

143. Crawford, N., Amos, L. A., and Castle, A. G.: Platelet microtubule subunit proteins: Assembly and disassembly factors, in *Platelets—Cellular Response Mechanisms and Their Biological Significance,* edited by A. Rotman, F. A. Meyer, C. Gitler, and A. Silberberg. Wiley, New York, 1980, p. 171.

144. Nachmias, V., Sullender, J., and Asch, A.: Shape and cytoplasmic filaments in control and lidocaine-treated human platelets. *Blood* 50:39, 1977.

145. Castle, A. G., and Crawford, N.: Isolation of tubulin from pig platelets. *FEBS Lett.* 51:195, 1975.

146. Ikeda, Y., and Steiner, M.: Isolation of platelet microtubule protein by an immunosorptive method. *J. Biol. Chem.* 251:6135, 1976.

147. Steiner, M., and Ikeda, Y.: Quantitative assessment of polymerized and depolymerized platelet microtubules. *J. Clin. Invest.* 63:443, 1979.

148. Castle, A. G., and Crawford, N.: The isolation and characterization of platelet microtubule proteins. *Biochim. Biophys. Acta* 494:76, 1977.

149. Castle, A. G., and Crawford, N.: The [³H]colchicine-binding properties of platelet tubulin. *Int. J. Biochem.* 9:439, 1978.

150. Ikeda, Y., and Steiner, M.: Sulfhydryls of platelets tubulin: Their role in polymerization and colchicine binding. *Biochemistry* 17:3454, 1978.

151. Ikeda, Y., and Steiner, M.: Phosphorylation and protein kinase activity of platelet tubulin. *J. Biol. Chem.* 254:66, 1979.

152. Bezkorovainy, A., and Rafelson, M. E., Jr.: Characterization of some proteins from normal human platelets. *J. Lab. Clin. Med.* 64:212, 1964.

153. Solum, N. O., and Lopaciuk, S.: Bovine platelet proteins. II. Purification of platelet fibrinogen. *Thromb. Diath. Haemorrh.* 21:428, 1969.

154. Keenan, J. P.: Platelet fibrinogen. I. Quantitation using fibrinogen-sensitized tanned red cells. *Med. Lab. Techn.* 29:71, 1972.

155. Nachman, R. L., Marcus, A. J., and Zucker-Franklin, D.: Immunologic studies on proteins associated with subcellular fractions of normal human platelets. *J. Lab. Clin. Med.* 69:651, 1967.

156. Day, H. J., and Solum, N. O.: Fibrinogen associated with subcellular platelet particles. *Scand. J. Haematol.* 11:35, 1973.

157. Kaplan, K. L., Broekman, M. J., Chernoff, A., Lesznik, G. R., and Drillings, M.: Platelet alpha-granule proteins—Studies on release and subcellular localization. *Blood* 53:604, 1979.

158. Shulman, S., and Karpatkin, S.: Crossed immunoelectrophoresis of human platelet membranes: Diminished major antigen in Glanzmann's thrombasthenia and Bernard-Soulier syndrome. *J. Biol. Chem.* 255:4320, 1980.

159. Doolittle, R. F., Takagi, T., and Cottrell, B. A.: Platelet and plasma fibrinogen are identical gene products. *Science* 185:368, 1974.

160. James, H. L., Ganguly, P., and Jackson, C. W.: Characterization and origin of fibrinogen in blood platelets. *Thromb. Haemostasis* 38:939, 1977.

161. Nachman, R. L., Levine, R., and Jaffe, E.: Synthesis of actin by cultured guinea pig megakaryocytes: Complex formation with fibrin. *Biochim. Biophys. Acta* 543:91, 1978.

162. Stahl, P. D., and Schlesinger, P. H.: Receptor-mediated pinocytosis of N-acetylglycosamine-terminated glycoproteins and lysosomal enzymes by macrophages. *Trends Biochemical Sci.* 5:194, 1980.

163. Gogstad, G. O.: A method for the isolation of α-granules from human platelets. *Thromb. Res.* 20:669, 1980.

164. Davey, M. G., and Luscher, E. F.: Release reactions of human platelets induced by thrombin and other agents. *Biochim. Biophys. Acta* 165:490, 1968.

165. Luscher, E. F.: Ein fibrinstabilisierender Faktor aus Thrombozyten. *Schweiz. Med. Wochenschr.* 87:1220, 1957.
166. McDonagh, J., McDonagh, R. P., Sr., Delage, J. M., and Wagner, R. H.: Factor XIII in human plasma and platelets. *J. Clin. Invest.* 48:940, 1969.
167. McDonagh, J., Waggoner, W. G., Hamilton, E. G., Hindenach, B., and McDonagh, R. P.: Affinity chromatography of human plasma and platelet factor XIII on organomercurial agarose. *Biochim. Biophys. Acta* 446:345, 1976.
168. Lopaciuk, S., Lovette, K. M., McDonagh, J., Chuang, H. Y. K., and McDonagh, R. P.: Subcellular distribution of fibrinogen and factor XIII in human blood platelets. *Thromb. Res.* 8:453, 1976.
169. Cohen, J., Blankenberg, T. A., Borden, D., Kahn, D. R., and Veis, A.: Factor XIIIa–catalyzed cross-linking of platelet and muscle actine. *Biochim. Biophys. Acta* 628:365, 1980.
170. Deutsch, E., and Lechner, K.: Platelet clotting factors, in *Biochemistry of Blood Platelets*, edited by E. Kowalski and S. Niewiarowski. Academic, New York, 1967, p. 23.
171. Niewiarowski, S., Lipinski, B., Farbiszewski, R., and Poplawski, A.: The release of platelet factor 4 during platelet aggregation and the possible significance of this reaction in hemostasis. *Experientia* 24:343, 1968.
172. Youssef, A., and Barkhan, P.: Release of platelet factor 4 by adenosine diphosphate and other platelet aggregating agents. *Br. Med. J.* 1:746, 1968.
173. Karpatkin, S.: Heterogeneity of human platelets. II. Functional evidence suggestive of young and old platelets. *J. Clin. Invest.* 48:1083, 1969.
174. Poplawski, A., and Niewiarowski, S.: Method for determining antiheparin activity of platelets and erythrocytes. *Thromb. Diath. Haemorrh.* 13:149, 1965.
175. Farbiszewski, R., Lipinski, B., Niewiarowski, S., and Poplawski, A.: Hypercoagulability and thrombocytopenia after platelet factor 4 infusion into rabbits. *Experientia* 24:578, 1968.
176. Niewiarowski, S., Farbiszewski, R., and Poplawski, A.: Studies on platelet factor 2 (PF2-fibrinogen activating factor) and platelet factor 4 (PF4-antiheparin factor), in *Biochemistry of Blood Platelets*, edited by E. Kowalski and S. Niewiarowski. Academic, New York, 1967, p. 35.
177. Kaplan, K. L., Nossel, H. L., Drillings, M., and Lesznik, G.: Radioimmunoassay of platelet factor 4 and β-thromboglobulin: Development and application to studies of platelet release in relation to fibrin peptide A generation. *Br. J. Haematol.* 39:129, 1978.
178. Botton, A. E., Ludkin, C. A., Pepper, D. S., Moore, S., and Cash, J. D.: A radioimmunoassay for platelet factor 4. *Thromb. Res.* 8:51, 1976.
179. Levine, S. P., and Krentz, L. S.: Development of a radioimmunoassay for human platelet factor 4. *Thromb. Res.* 11:673, 1977.
180. Handin, R. L., McDonough, M., and Leach, M.: Elevation of platelet factor 4 in acute myocardial infarction: Measurement by radioimmunoassay. *J. Lab. Clin. Med.* 91:340, 1978.
181. Rucinski, B., Niewiarowski, S., James, P., Walz, D. A., and Budzynski, A. Z.: Antiheparin proteins secreted by human platelets. Purification, characterization, and radioimmunoassay. *Blood* 53:47, 1979.
182. Weiss, H. J., et al.: Heterogeneity in storage pool deficiency: Studies on granule bound substances in 18 patients including variants deficient in α granules, platelet factor 4, β thromboglobulin, and platelet derived growth factor. *Blood* 54:1296, 1979.
183. Niewiarowski, S., Salz, D. A., James, P., Rucinski, B., and Kueppers, F.: Identification and separation of secreted proteins by isoelectric focusing: Evidence that low affinity platelet factor 4 is converted to β thromboglobulin by limited proteolysis. *Blood* 55:453, 1980.
184. Ludlam, C. A.: Evidence for the platelet specificity of β-thromboglobulin and studies on its plasma concentration in healthy individuals. *Br. J. Haematol.* 41:279, 1979.
185. Ludlam, C. A., Moore, S., Botton, A. E., Pepper, D. S., and Cash, J. D.: The release of a human platelet specific protein measured by a radioimmunoassay. *Thromb. Res.* 6:543, 1975.
186. Han, P., Turpie, A. G. G., and Genton, E.: Plasma β-thromboglobu-

187. Guzzo, J., et al.: Secreted platelet proteins with antiheparin and mitogenic activities in chronic renal failure. *J. Lab. Clin. Med.* 96:102, 1980.
188. Witte, L. D., Kaplan, K. L., Nossel, H. L., Lages, B. A., Weiss, H. J., and Goodman, D. S.: Studies of the release from human platelets of the growth factor for cultured human arterial smooth muscle cells. *Circ. Res.* 42:412, 1978.
189. Ross, R., Glomset, J., Kariya, B., and Harker, L.: A platelet-dependent serum factor that stimulates the proliferation of arterial smooth muscle cells in vitro. *Proc. Natl. Acad. Sci. U.S.A.* 71:1207, 1974.
190. Nachman, R. L., Weksler, B., and Ferris, B.: Characterization of human platelet vascular permeability-enhancing activity. *J. Clin. Invest.* 51:549, 1972.
191. Day, H. J., Holmsen, H., and Hovig, T.: Subcellular particles of human platelets: A biochemical and electron microscopic study with particular reference to the influence of fractionation techniques. *Scand. J. Haematol.* 7:3, 1969.
192. Holmsen, H., and Day, H. J.: The selectivity of the thrombin-induced platelet release reaction: Subcellular localization of released and retained constituents. *J. Lab. Clin. Med.* 75:840, 1970.
193. Holmsen, H., Setkowsky, C. A., Lages, B., Day, H. J., Weiss, H. J., and Scrutton, M. C.: Content and thrombin-induced release of acid hydrolases in gel-filtered platelets from patients with storage pool disease. *Blood* 46:131, 1975.
194. Glaser, J. H., Roozen, K. J., Brot, F. E., and Sly, W. S.: Multiple isoelectric and recognition forms of human beta-glucuronidase activity. *Arch. Biochem. Biophys.* 166:536, 1975.
195. Brot, F. E., Glaser, J. H., Roozen, K. J., and Sly, W. H.: *In vitro* correction of deficient human fibroblasts by β-glucuronidase from different human sources. *Biochem. Biophys. Res. Commun.* 75:1, 1974.
196. Day, H. J., Ang, G., and Holmsen, H.: The release reaction occurring during clotting of platelet-rich plasma. *Proc. Soc. Exp. Med. Biol.* 139:717, 1972.
197. Zucker, M. B., and Borrelli, J.: A survey of some platelet enzymes and functions: The platelets as the source of normal serum acid glycerophosphatase. *Ann. N.Y. Acad. Sci.* 75:203, 1958.
198. Zucker, M. B., and Borrelli, J.: Platelets as a source of serum acid nitrophenylphosphatase. *J. Clin. Invest.* 38:148, 1959.
199. Holmsen, H.: Platelet secretion ("release reaction"), in *Mechanisms of Haemostasis and Thrombosis*, edited by C. H. Mielke and R. Rodevich. Symposia Specialists, Miami, 1978, p. 73.
200. Frendo, J.: Taurine in human blood platelets. *Nature* 183:685, 1959.
201. Koufos, A., and Sagone, A. L., Jr.: Effects of oxidant stress on the hexose monophosphate shunt pathway of platelets. *Blood* 55:835, 1980.
202. Marcus, A. J., Ullman, H. L., and Safier, L. B.: Lipid composition of subcellular particles of human blood platelets. *J. Lipid Res.* 10:108, 1969.
203. Tao, R. V. P., Sweeley, C. C., and Jamieson, G. A.: Sphingolipid composition of human platelets. *J. Lipid Res.* 14:16, 1973.
204. Howell, W. H.: Theories of blood coagulation. *Physiol. Rev.* 15:435, 1935.
205. Surgenor, D. M., and Wallach, D. F. H.: Biophysical aspects of platelet reaction mechanisms of clotting, in *Blood Platelets*, edited by S. A. Johnson, R. W. Monto, J. W. Rebuck, and R. C. Horn, Jr. Little, Brown, Boston, 1961, p. 289.
206. Stenflo, J., Fernlund, P., Egan, W., and Roepstorff, P.: Vitamin K–dependent modifications of glutamic acid residues in prothrombin. *Proc. Natl. Acad. Sci. U.S.A.* 71:2730, 1974.
207. Nelsestuen, G. L., and Zytkovicz, T. H.: The mode of action of vitamin K. *J. Biol. Chem.* 249:6347, 1974.
208. Esmon, C. T., Sadowski, J. A., and Suttie, J. W.: The vitamin K–dependent incorporation of H¹⁴CO₃ into prothrombin. *J. Biol. Chem.* 250:4744, 1974.
209. Stenflo, J., and Suttie, J. W.: Vitamin K–dependent formation of γ-carboxyglutamic acid. *Ann. Rev. Biochem.* 46:157, 1977.

210. Miletich, J. P., Jackson, C. M., and Majerus, P. W.: Properties of the factor Xa binding site on human platelets. *J. Biol. Chem.* 253:6908, 1978.

211. Miletich, J. P., Majerus, D. W., and Majerus, P. W.: Patients with congenital factor V deficiency have decreased factor Xa binding sites on their platelets. *J. Clin. Invest.* 62:824, 1978.

212. Miletich, J. P., Kane, W. H., Hofmann, S. L., Stanford, N., and Majerus, P. W.: Deficiency of factor Xa–factor Va binding sites on the platelets of a patient with a bleeding disorder. *Blood* 54:1015, 1979.

213. Kane, W. H., Lindhout, M. J., Jackson, C. M., and Majerus, P. W.: Factor Va–dependent binding of factor Xa to human platelets. *J. Biol. Chem.* 255:1170, 1980.

214. Marcus, A. J., Ullman, H. L., Safier, L. B., and Ballard, H. S.: Platelet phosphatides: Their fatty acid and aldehyde composition and activity in different clotting systems. *J. Clin. Invest.* 41:2198, 1962.

215. Maurice, P. A., and Wallach, D. F. H.: Étude de l'action thromboplastique de certains phospholipids à l'aide de suspensions de phosphatidyl-éthanolamines radioactives. *Schweiz. Med. Wochenschr.* 90:1259, 1960.

216. Horowitz, H. I.: Non-sedimentable platelet factor 3 during coagulation and after immune platelet injury. *Thromb. Diath. Haemorrh.* [Suppl.] 17:243, 1965.

217. Fantl, P., and Ward, H. A.: Nucleotides of human blood platelets. *Biochem. J.* 64:747, 1956.

218. Mizuno, N. S., Sautter, J. H., and Schultze, M. D.: Acid-soluble nucleotides in bovine thrombocytes. *J. Biol. Chem.* 235:2109, 1960.

219. Da Prada, M., and Pletscher, A.: Identification of guanosine 5'-triphosphate and uridine 5'-triphosphate in subcellular monamine-storage organelles. *Biochem. J.* 119:117, 1970.

220. Rao, G. H. R., White, J. G., Jachinowicz, A. A., and Witkop, C. J.: Nucleotide profiles of normal and abnormal platelets by high-pressure liquid chromatography. *J. Lab. Clin. Med.* 84:839, 1974.

221. Born, G. V. R.: Changes in the distribution of phosphorus in platelet-rich plasma during clotting. *Biochem. J.* 68:695, 1958.

222. Bettex-Galland, M., and Luscher, E. F.: Studies on the metabolism of human blood platelets in relation to clot retraction. *Throm. Diath. Haemorrh.* 4:178, 1960.

223. Zucker, M., and Borrelli, J.: Changes in platelet ATP concentration and phosphate distribution during viscous metamorphosis and clot retraction, in *Blood Platelets*, edited by S. A. Johnson, R. W. Monto, J. W. Rebuck, and R. C. Horn, Jr. Little, Brown, Boston, 1961, p. 383.

224. Holmsen, H., and Rozenberg, M. C.: Adenine nucleotide metabolism of blood platelets. III. Adenine phosphoribosyl transferase and nucleotide formation from exogenous adenine. *Biochim. Biophys. Acta* 157:266, 1968.

225. Haslam, R. J., and Mills, D. C. B.: The adenylate kinase of human plasma, erythrocytes and platelets in relation to the degradation of adenosine diphosphate in plasma. *Biochem. J.* 103:773, 1967.

226. Holmsen, H., and Rozenberg, M. C.: Adenine nucleotide metabolism of blood platelets. I. Adenosine kinase and nucleotide formation from exogenous adenosine and AMP. *Biochim. Biophys. Acta* 155:326, 1968.

227. Ireland, D. M., and Mills, D. C. B.: Detection and determination of adenosine diphosphate and related substances in plasma. *Biochem. J.* 99:283, 1966.

228. Reimers, H. J., Mustard, J. F., and Packham, M. A.: Transfer of adenine nucleotides between the releasable and nonreleasable compartments of rabbit blood platelets. *J. Cell Biol.* 67:61, 1975.

229. Holmsen, H.: Collagen-induced release of adenosine diphosphate from blood platelets incubated with radioactive phosphate in vitro. *Scand. J. Clin. Lab. Invest.* 17:239, 1965.

230. Holmsen, H., and Day, H. J.: Adenine nucleotides and platelet function. *Ser. Haematol.* 4:28, 1971.

231. Ireland, D. M.: Effect of thrombin on the radioactive nucleotides of human washed platelets. *Biochem. J.* 105:857, 1967.

232. Ugurbil, K., Holmsen, H., and Shulman, R. G.: Adenine nucleotide pools and secretion in platelets as studied by ^{31}P nuclear magnetic resonance. *Proc. Nat. Acad. Sci. U.S.A.* 76:2227, 1979.

233. Costa, J. L., Dobson, C. M., Kirk, K. L., Poulsen, F. M., Valeri, C. R.,

and Vecchione, J. J.: Studies of human platelets by ^{19}F and ^{31}P NMR, *FEBS Lett.* 99:141, 1979.

234. Hartman, R. C., Auditore, J. V., and Jackson, D. P.: Studies on thrombocytosis. I. Hyperkalemia due to release of potassium from platelets during coagulation. *J. Clin. Invest.* 37:699, 1958.

235. Zieve, P. H., and Solomon, H. M.: The intracellular pH of the human platelet. *J. Clin. Invest.* 45:125, 1966.

236. Colley, M. H., and Cohen, P.: Potassium transport in human blood platelets. *J. Lab. Clin. Med.* 70:69, 1967.

237. Cousin, C., and Caen, J.: Dosage de magnésium et du calcium dans les plaquettes sanguines humaines. *Rev. Fr. Étud. Clin. Biol.* 9:520, 1974.

238. Wallach, D. F. H., Surgenor, D. M., and Steele, B. B.: Calcium-lipid complexes in human platelets. *Blood* 13:589, 1958.

239. Lages, B., Scrutton, M. C., and Holmsen, H.: Studies on gel-filtered human platelets: Isolation and characterization in a medium containing no added Ca^{2+}, Mg^{2+}, or K^+. *J. Lab. Clin. Med.* 85:811, 1975.

240. Foley, B., Johnson, S. A., Hackley, B., Smith, J. C., Jr., and Halsted, J. A.: Zinc content of human platelets. *Proc. Soc. Exp. Biol. Med.* 128:265, 1968.

241. Salganicoff, L., Hebda, P. A., Yandrasitz, J., and Fukami, M. H.: Subcellular fractionation of pig platelets. *Biochim. Biophys. Acta* 385:394, 1975.

242. Martin, J. H., Carson, F. L., and Race, G. J.: Calcium-containing platelet granules. *J. Cell. Biol.* 60:775, 1974.

243. Skaer, R. J., Peters, P. D., and Emmines, J. P.: The localization of calcium and phosphorus in human platelets. *J. Cell Sci.* 15:679, 1974.

244. Weiss, H. J., Kelly, A., and Herbert, V.: Vitamin B_{12} and folate activity in normal human platelets. *Blood* 31:258, 1968.

245. Sahud, M. A.: Uptake and reduction of dehydroascorbic acid in human platelets. *Clin. Res.* 18:415, 1970.

246. Tranzer, J. P., Da Prada, M., and Pletscher, A.: Ultrastructural localization of 5-hydroxytryptamine in blood platelets. *Nature* 212:1574, 1966.

247. Da Prada, M., Pletscher, A., Tranzer, J. P., and Knuchel, H.: Subcellular localization of 5-hydroxytryptamine and histamine in blood platelets. *Nature* 216:1315, 1967.

248. Zucker, M. B.: Serotonin (5-hydroxytryptamine): Hematologic aspects. *Prog. Hematol.* 2:206, 1959.

249. Zucker, M. B., Lewis, J. H., and Borrelli, J.: Platelet and serum serotonin in normal and hemorrhagic conditions. *Proc. 6th Cong. Int. Soc. Hematol.* Grune & Stratton, New York, 1958, p. 44.

250. Zucker, M. B., and Borelli, J.: Absorption of serotonin (5-hydroxytryptamine) by canine and human platelets. *Am. J. Physiol.* 186:105, 1956.

251. Humphrey, J. H., and Toh, C. C.: Absorption of serotonin (5-hydroxytryptamine) and histamine by dog platelets. *J. Physiol.* 124:300, 1954.

252. Erspamer, V.: *Il sistema cellulare enterocromaffine e l'enteramine (5-idrossitriptamina).* Rendiconti Scientifici Farmitalia, vol. 1, 1954.

253. Sjoerdsma, A., Weissbach, H., and Udenfriend, S.: A clinical, physiologic, and biochemical study of patients with malignant carcinoid (argentaffinoma). *Am. J. Med.* 20:520, 1956.

254. Lingjaerde, O., Jr.: Uptake of serotonin in blood platelets: Dependence on sodium and chloride, and inhibition by choline. *FEBS Lett.* 3:103, 1969.

255. Sneddon, J. M.: Sodium-dependent accumulation of 5-hydroxytryptamine by rat blood platelets. *Br. J. Pharmacol.* 37:680, 1969.

256. Lingjaerde, O., Jr.: Uptake of serotonin in blood platelets in vitro. I. The effects of chloride. *Acta Physiol. Scand.* 81:75, 1971.

257. Barthel, W., and Markwardt, F.: Untersuchungen uber den Einfluss von Herzglykosiden auf die 5-ht-Aufnahme der Blutplattchen. *Biochem. Pharmacol.* 20:2597, 1971.

258. Rudnick, G., and Nelson, P. J.: Platelet 5-hydroxytryptamine transport, an electroneutral mechanism coupled to potassium. *Biochemistry* 17:4739, 1978.

259. Nelson, P. J., and Rudnick, G.: Coupling between platelet 5-hydroxytryptamine and potassium transport. *J. Biol. Chem.* 254:10084, 1979.

260. Ross, S. B., Aperia, B., Beck-Friis, J., Jansa, S., Wetterberg, L., and Aberg, A.: Inhibition of 5-hydroxytriptamine uptake in human

platelets by antidepressant agents in vivo. *Psychopharmacology* 67:1, 1980.

261. Talvenheimo, J., Nelson, P. J., and Rudnick, G.: Mechanism of imipramine inhibition of platelet 5-hydroxytryptamine transport. *J. Biol. Chem.* 254:4631, 1979.

262. Talvenheimo, J., and Rudnick, G.: Solubilization of the platelet plasma membrane transporter in an active form. *J. Biol. Chem.* 255:8606, 1980.

263. Lingjaerde, O.: Inhibitory effect of clomipramine and related drugs on serotonin uptake in platelets: More complicated than previously thought. *Psychopharmacology* 61:245, 1979.

264. Lingjaerde, O.: Inhibition of platelet uptake of serotonin in plasma from patients treated with clomipramine and amitryptaline. *Eur. J. Clin. Pharmacol.* 15:335, 1979.

265. Langer, S. Z., Briley, M. S., Raisman, R., Henry, J. F., and Morselli, P. L.: Specific ³H-imipramine binding in human platelets. *Naunyn Schmiedeberg's Arch. Pharmacol.* 313:189, 1980.

266. Rudnick, G., Bencua, R., Nelson, P. J., and Zito, R. A.: Inhibition of platelet transport by propranolol. *Mol. Pharmacol.* 20:118, 1981.

267. Rudnik, G., Fishkes, H., Nelson, P., and Schuldiner, S.: Evidence for two distinct serotonin transport systems in platelets. *J. Biol. Chem.* 255:3638, 1980.

268. Johnson, R. G., Scarpa, A., and Salganicoff, L.: The internal pH of isolated serotonin containing granules of pig platelets. *J. Biol. Chem.* 253:7061, 1978.

269. Wilkins, J. A., Greenwalt, J. W., and Huang, L.: Transport of 5-hydroxytryptamine by dense granules from porcine platelets. *J. Biol. Chem.* 253:6260, 1978.

270. Wilkins, J. A., and Salganicoff, L.: Participation of a transmembrane proton gradient in 5-hydroxytryptamine transport by platelet dense granules and dense granule ghosts. *Biochem. J.* 198:113, 1981.

271. Berneis, K. H., Da Prada, M., and Pletscher, A.: Metal-dependent aggregation of nucleotides with formation of biphasic liquid systems. *Biochim. Biophys. Acta* 215:547, 1970.

272. Berneis, K. H., Pletscher, A., and Da Prada, M.: Metal-dependent aggregation of biogenic amines: A hypothesis for their storage and release. *Nature* 244:281, 1969.

273. Pletscher, A.: Metabolism transfer and storage of 5-hydroxytryptamine in blood platelets. *Br. J. Pharmacol.* 32:1, 1968.

274. Jain, M.: A rapid, sensitive, radiometric procedure for the determination of human blood platelet monamine oxidase activity. *Clin. Chim. Acta* 47:107, 1973.

275. Fowler, C. J., and Wiberg, A.: Characteristics of human platelet monoamine oxidase. *Arch. Pharmacol.* 313:77, 1980.

276. Friedhoff, A. J., Miller, J. C., and Karpatkin, S.: Heterogeneity of human platelets. VII. Platelet monoamine oxidase activity in normals and patients with autoimmune thrombocytopenic purpura and reactive thrombocytosis: Its relationship to platelet protein density. *Blood* 51:317, 1978.

277. Weiss, H. J., Tschopp, T. B., Rogers, J., and Brand, H.: Studies of platelet 5-hydroxytryptamine (serotonin) in storage pool disease and albinism. *J. Clin. Invest.* 54:421, 1974.

278. Pareti, F. I., Day, H. J., and Mills, D. C. B.: Nucleotide and serotonin metabolism in platelets with defective secondary aggregation. *Blood* 44:789, 1974.

279. Laubscher, A., and Pletscher, A.: Shape change and uptake of 5-hydroxytryptamine in human blood platelets: Action of neuropsychotropic drugs. *Life Sci.* 24:1833, 1979.

280. Schick, P. K., Kurica, K. B., and Chacko, G. K.: Location of phosphatidylethanolamine and phosphatidylserine in the human platelet plasma membrane. *J. Clin. Invest.* 57:1221, 1976.

281. Nachman, R. L., and Ferris, B.: Human platelet membrane protein. *Biochemistry* 9:200, 1970.

282. Barber, A. J., and Jamieson, G. A.: Isolation of glycopeptides from low- and high-density platelet plasma membranes. *Biochemistry* 10:4711, 1971.

283. Phillips, D. R.: Effect of trypsin on the exposed polypeptides and glycoproteins in the human platelet membrane. *Biochemistry* 11:4582, 1972.

284. Nachman, R. L., and Ferris, B.: Studies on the proteins of human platelet membranes. *J. Biol. Chem.* 247:4468, 1972.

285. Cohen, J., Glaser, T., Veis, A., and Bruner-Lorand, J.: Ca²⁺-dependent cross-linking processes in human platelets. *Biochim. Biophys. Acta* 676:137, 1981.

286. Nurden, A. T., and Caen, J. P.: An abnormal platelet glycoprotein pattern in 3 cases of Glanzmann's thromboasthenia. *Br. J. Haematol.* 28:253, 1974.

287. Okumura, T. A., and Jamieson, G. A.: Platelet glycocalicin. I. Orientation of glycoproteins of platelet surface. *J. Biol. Chem.* 251:5944, 1976.

288. Clemetson, K. J., Pfeuller, S. L., Lüscher, E. F., and Jenkins, C. S. P.: Isolation of the membrane glycoproteins of human blood platelets by lectin affinity chromatography. *Biochim. Biophys. Acta* 464:493, 1977.

289. George, J. N., Potterf, R. D., Lewis, P. C., and Sears, D. A.: Studies on platelet plasma membranes. I. Characterization of surface proteins of human platelets labelled with diazotized ¹²⁵I-diiodosulfanilic acid. *J. Lab. Clin. Med.* 88:232, 1976.

290. Phillips, D. R., and Poh Agin, P.: Platelet plasma membrane glycoproteins: Evidence for the presence of nonequivalent disulfide bonds using nonreduced-reduced two-dimensional gel electrophoresis. *J. Biol. Chem.* 252:2121, 1977.

291. Phillips, D. R., and Poh Agin, P.: Platelet membrane defects in Glanzmann's thrombasthenia: Evidence for decreased amounts of two major glycoproteins. *J. Biol. Chem.* 60:535, 1977.

292. Phillips, D. R., and Agin, P. P.: Platelet plasma membrane glycoproteins. *Biochem. Biophys. Res. Commun.* 75:940, 1977.

293. Berndt, M. C., and Phillips, D. R.: Purification and preliminary physiochemical characterization of human platelet membrane glycoprotein V. *J. Biol. Chem.* 256:59, 1981.

294. Mosher, D. F., Vaheri, A., Choate, J. J., and Gahmberg, C. G.: Action of thrombin on surface glycoproteins of human platelets. *Blood* 53:437, 1979.

295. Nurden, A. T., and Caen, J. P.: Specific roles for platelet surface glycoproteins in platelet function. *Nature* 255:720, 1975.

296. Boullin, D. J., Glenton, P. A. M., Molyneux, D., Peters, J. R., and Roach, B.: Binding of 5-hydroxytryptamine to human blood platelets. *Br. J. Pharmacol.* 61:453, 1977.

297. Hagen, I., Bjerrum, O. J., and Solum, N. O.: Characterization of human platelet proteins solubilized with Triton-X-100 and examined by crossed immunoelectrophoresis. *Eur. J. Biochem.* 99:9, 1979.

298. Howard, L., Shulman, S., Sudanandan, S., and Karpatkin, S.: Crossed immunoelectrophoresis of human platelet membranes: The major antigen consists of a complex of glycoproteins held together by Ca²⁺ and is missing in Glanzmann's thrombasthenia. *Clin. Res.* 29:519A, 1981.

299. Kunicki, T. J., Pidard, D., Rosa, J. P., and Nurden, A. T.: The formation of Ca²⁺-dependent complexes of platelet membrane glycoproteins IIb and IIIa in solution as determined by crossed immunoelectrophoresis. *Blood* 58:268, 1981.

300. McEver, R. P., Baenziger, N. L., and Majerus, P. W.: Isolation and quantitation of the platelet membrane glycoprotein deficient in thrombasthenia using a monoclonal hybridoma antibody. *J. Clin. Invest.* 66:1311, 1980.

301. Kunicki, T., and Aster, R. H.: Deletion of the platelet-specific alloantigen PLA1 from platelets in Glanzmann's thrombasthenia. *J. Clin. Invest.* 61:1225, 1978.

302. Solum, N. O., Hagen, I., and Sletbakk, T.: Further evidence for glycocalicin being derived from a large amphiphilic platelet membrane glycoprotein. *Thromb. Res.* 18:773, 1980.

303. Okumura, T., Lombart, C., and Jamieson, G. A.: Platelet glycocalicin. II. Purification and characterization. *J. Biol. Chem.* 251:5950, 1976.

304. Kunicki, T. J., Johnson, M. M., and Aster, R. H.: Absence of the platelet receptor for drug-dependent antibodies in the Bernard-Soulier syndrome. *J. Clin. Invest.* 62:716, 1978.

305. Moore, A., Ross, G. D., and Nachman, R. L.: Interaction of platelet membrane receptors with von Willebrand factor, ristocetin, and the Fc region of immunoglobulin G. *J. Clin. Invest.* 62:1053, 1978.

306. Okamura, T., Hasitz, M., and Jamieson, G. A.: Platelet glycocalicin: Interaction with thrombin and role as thrombin receptor of the platelet surface. *J. Biol. Chem.* 253:3435, 1978.

307. Ganguly, P.: Binding of thrombin to functionally defective platelets: A hypothesis on the nature of the thrombin receptor. *Br. J. Haematol.* 37:47, 1977.

308. Larsen, N. E., and Simons, E. R.: Preparation and application of a photoreactive thrombin analogue: Binding to human platelets. *Biochemistry* 20:4141, 1981.

309. Hampton, J. R., and Mitchell, J. R. A.: An estimate of the number of adenosine diphosphate binding sites on human platelets. *Nature* 211:245, 1966.

310. Born, G. V. R.: Uptake of adenosine and of adenosine diphosphate by human blood platelets. *Nature* 206:1121, 1965.

311. Nachman, R. L., and Ferris, B.: Binding of adenosine diphosphate by isolated membranes from human platelets. *J. Biol. Chem.* 249:704, 1974.

312. Bennett, J. S., Colman, R. F., and Colman, R. W.: Identification of adenine nucleotide binding proteins in human platelet membranes by affinity labeling with 5'-*p*-fluorosulfonylbenzoyl adenosine. *J. Biol. Chem.* 253:7346, 1978.

313. Mustard, J. F., Packham, M. A., Kinlough-Rathbone, R. L., Perry, D. W., and Regoeczi, E.: Fibrinogen-ADP-induced platelet aggregation. *Blood* 52:453, 1978.

314. Marguerie, G. A., Plow, E. F., and Edgington, T. S.: Human platelets possess an inducible and saturable receptor specific for fibrinogen. *J. Biol. Chem.* 24:5357, 1979.

315. Bennett, J. S., and Vilaire, G.: Exposure of platelet fibrinogen receptors by ADP and epinephrine. *J. Clin. Invest.* 64:1393, 1979.

316. Peerschke, E. I., Zucker, M. B., Grant, R. A., Egan, J. J., and Johnson, M. M.: Correlation between fibrinogen binding to human platelets and platelet aggregability. *Blood* 55:841, 1980.

317. Mustard, J. F., Kinlough-Rathbone, R. L., Packham, M. A. Perry, D. W., Harfenist, E. J., and Pai, K. R. M.: Comparison of fibrinogen association with normal and thrombasthenic platelets on exposure to ADP or chymotrypsin. *Blood* 54:987, 1979.

318. Kornecki, E., Niewiarowski, S., Morinelli, T. A., and Kloczewiak, M.: Effects of chymotrypsin and ADP on the exposure of fibrinogen receptors on normal human and Glanzmann's thrombasthenia platelets. *J. Biol. Chem.* 250:5096, 1981.

319. Ganguly, P.: Binding of thrombin to human platelets. *Nature* 247:306, 1974.

320. Detwiler, T. C., and Feinman, R. D.: Kinetics of the thrombin-induced release of Ca(II) by platelets. *Biochemistry* 12:282, 1973.

321. Martin, B. M., Feinman, R. D., and Detwiler, T. C.: Platelet stimulation by thrombin and other proteases. *Biochemistry* 14:1308, 1975.

322. Tam, S. W., Fenton, J. W., and Detwiler, T. L.: Platelet thrombin receptors. *J. Biol. Chem.* 255:6626, 1980.

323. Tollefsen, D., Feagler, J. R., and Majerus, P. W.: The binding of thrombin to the surface of human platelets. *J. Biol. Chem.* 249:2646, 1974.

324. Lynch, C. J., and Steer, M. I.: Evidence for high and low affinity α_2-receptors: Composition of norepinephrine and phentolamine binding to human platelet membranes. *J. Biol. Chem.* 256:3293, 1981.

325. Schaefer, A. I., Cooper, B., O'Hara, D., and Handin, R. I.: Identification of platelet receptors for prostaglandin I_2 and D_2. *J. Biol. Chem.* 254:2914, 1979.

326. Peters, J. R., and Grahame-Smith, D. G.: Human platelet 5HT receptors: Characterization and functional association. *Eur. J. Pharmacol.* 8:243, 1980.

327. Booyse, F. M., and Rafelson, M. E.: Human platelet contractile proteins: Location, properties, and function. *Ser. Haematol.* 4:152, 1971.

328. Bennett, J. S., Vilaire, G., Colman, R. F., and Colman, R. W.: Localization of human platelet membrane-associated actin myosin using the affinity label 5'-*p*-fluorosulfonylbenzoyl adenosine. *J. Biol. Chem.* 256:1185, 1981.

329. Nachman, R. L.: Immunologic studies of platelet protein. *Blood* 25:703, 1965.

330. Salmon, J.: Étude immunoélectrophoretique des antigènes plaquettaires. *Schweiz. Med. Wochenschr.* 88:1047, 1958.

331. Hjort, P. S., Rappoport, S. I., and Owren, P. A.: Evidence that platelet accelerator (platelet factor 1) is adsorbed plasma proaccelerin. *Blood* 10:1139, 1955.

332. Horowitz, H. I., and Fujimoto, M. M.: Association of factors XI and XII with blood platelets. *Proc. Soc. Exp. Biol. Med.* 119:487, 1965.

333. Kao, K-J., Pizzo, S. V., and McKee, P. A.: Demonstration and characterization of specific binding sites for factor VIII/von Willebrand factor on human platelets. *J. Clin. Invest.* 63:656, 1979.

334. Schiffman, S., Rapaport, S. I., and Chong, M. M. T.: Platelets and initiation of intrinsic clotting. *Br. J. Haematol.* 24:633, 1973.

335. Walsh, P. N.: Albumin density gradient separation and washing of platelets and the study of platelet coagulant activities. *Br. J. Haematol.* 22:205, 1972.

336. Aoki, N., Naito, K., and Yoshida, N.: Inhibition of platelet aggregation by protease inhibitors: Possible involvement of proteases. *Blood* 52:1, 1978.

CHAPTER *128*

Metabolism of platelets

HOLM HOLMSEN
SIMON KARPATKIN

Platelets are actively metabolizing cells. Many major metabolic pathways are closely linked to agonist-induced platelet responses. Glyco(geno)lysis and oxidative phosphorylation occur continuously in resting platelets and increase markedly upon stimulation of the cells. Moreover, a number of biochemical processes not occurring in resting platelets are initiated by platelet stimulation, e.g., calcium translocation, protein phosphorylation, phosphatidylinositol breakdown and turnover, phosphatidylcholine breakdown, liberation of arachidonate followed by its oxygenation to prostaglandins and thromboxanes. Inhibition of platelet responses by naturally occurring agents (prostaglandins I_2 and D_2) and drugs is associated with stimulation of other biochemical processes that occur neither in resting nor in stimulated platelets, e.g., cyclic AMP production. This discussion of platelet metabolism is therefore subdivided into that of *resting platelets, stimulated platelets,* and *inhibited platelets.*

Metabolism of resting platelets

Platelets are stimulated or inhibited during handling [1] and therefore studies are performed with platelets that are not representative of resting state. The existence of large, heavy (probably young) and small, light (probably older) platelets further complicates the situation [2], since the relative thrombopoiesis of the platelet donor as well as the manner of platelet isolation (i.e., force of centrifugation, specific gravity of centrifugation media) introduce variables which are functions of the metabolic heterogeneity of platelets [2]. All these variables, in addition to variations in platelet concentration

[3], have significant effects on platelet metabolism and might conceivably explain the great variation in the literature for the flux rates in individual metabolic pathways of "resting" platelets.

CARBOHYDRATE METABOLISM

Glycolysis and glycogenolysis are predominant metabolic pathways of platelets in vitro. The overall glyco-(geno)lytic flux is dependent on, besides the factors described above, the availability of extracellular glucose and oxygen. Addition of glucose to platelets in glucose-free medium containing oxygen increases lactate production and decreases oxygen uptake (Crabtree effect) [4–8]. Conversely, abolition of mitochondrial ATP production in the presence of glucose by anaerobiosis [4,9] or addition of cyanide [10–12], 2,4-dinitrophenol [4], and antimycin A [13] cause a 1.5- to 4-fold increase in lactate production (Pasteur effect). The steady-state level of ATP remains constant during the Crabtree and Pasteur effects; platelets are thus able to maintain ATP homeostasis over large fluctuations in the rate of glycolytic and respiratory flux. The main purpose of carbohydrate catabolism in platelets is to produce ATP, and the capacity of anaerobic glycolysis alone is sufficient to meet the needs for ATP in resting platelets when glucose is available [13]. When glucose is absent, anaerobic glycogenolysis alone is not sufficient to maintain ATP homeostasis, and the ATP level decreases as a result of greater utilization than production of ATP [13]. The failure of glycogenolysis alone to maintain ATP homeostasis supports the contention that glycogen phosphorylase is the rate-limiting step in glycogenolysis [11,14,15].

Anaerobic glycolysis entails the breakdown of glucose 6-phosphate to lactate. Glucose 6-phosphate originates in platelets through two mechanisms: (1) phosphorylation by hexokinase of glucose transported across the platelet membrane, and (2) conversion of glucose 1-phosphate, the phosphorolytic breakdown product of glycogen. Platelets transport glucose by a saturable mechanism which also transports 2-deoxyglucose, fructose, and mannose [16,17], as well as galactose, ribose, xylose, and arabinose [18,19]. Transport of glucose varies between 0.5 [20] and 2.9 [21] μmol/(g·min) at 37°C. All glucose that enters the platelet is phosphorylated to glucose 6-phosphate by ATP and hexokinase, which has maximal activity of 14 μmol/(g·min) in platelet extracts [22]. However, its activity in intact platelets is probably greater, since most of the enzyme is particle-bound [23–25] with a substantial fraction associated with the mitochondria [26]. Hexokinase may be rate-limiting for the glycolytic flux [25]. The conversion of glucose 6-phosphate to lactate in platelets involves 10 reactions catalyzed by enzymes specifically demonstrated in platelets [24,25,27]. Most of these reactions are in equilibrium even during elevated flux rates in intact platelets, and are not believed to regulate glycolytic flux [29,30]. The phosphofructokinase reaction is 10^4 times displaced from equilibrium

[29,30] and is thought to play a central role in flux regulation [11,25,29–31]. Isolated platelet phosphofructokinase is activated by fructose 6-phosphate, ADP, cyclic AMP, and inorganic orthophosphate (P_i) and it is inhibited by ATP, low pH, and citrate; its regulation is conceivably very complex [24]. Another apparent nonequilibrium reaction that may play a role in flux regulation is the pyruvate kinase reaction. In platelets the enzyme is of the M type, with very high affinity for phosphoenolpyruvate [31].

Glucose 6-phosphate is also metabolized in the hexose monophosphate shunt [18,20,21,32]. This pathway produces CO_2 and NADPH. The latter is used for fatty acid synthesis (see below) and to maintain glutathione in the reduced form. Hydroperoxides, hydrogen peroxide in particular, are consumed by platelets [33], and this consumption is associated with a fiftyfold stimulation of the hexose monophosphate shunt [34,35]. This stimulation is probably due to an acute need for NADPH during hydroperoxide reduction by the glutathione peroxidase–glutathione reductase system [24, 34,36]; platelets are rich in the peroxidase and reductase [25,37,38].

Glycogen is a major polysaccharide in platelets (see Chap. 127), which contain the regulatory enzyme for its formation, glycogen synthetase [3,39–43]. This enzyme consists of a glucose 6-phosphate–dependent form (the D form) and a glucose 6-phosphate–independent form (the I form), both of which have maximal activities in platelet extracts of 0.6 to 1.5 μmol/(g·min). Platelets are capable of depositing glucose onto preexistent glycogen primer by 1,4-glucosyl linkages, as well as probably 1,6-glucosyl linkages [3]. The large, heavy platelet population has 5.7 times greater rate of glycogen synthesis than the small, light population [2]. Platelets suspended in glucose-rich media (e.g., plasma) maintain their glycogen stores, and glucose is very slowly incorporated into glycogen (1 percent labeling of glycogen, per hour, at 37°C) [14,32,44,45]. Thus, neither synthesis nor degradation of glycogen appears to take place in resting platelets with adequate supplies of glucose. However, when platelets are transferred to a glucose-free medium, rapid degradation of glycogen takes place [46,179]. This degradation is biphasic, first rapid and then slow, which has been taken as an indication of the presence of two glycogen-degrading enzymes in platelets, glycogen phosphorylase [14,44,47–51] and amylo-1,6-glucosidase (debranching enzyme) [3,42,46]. Glycogen phosphorylase in platelets exists in two active forms, AMP-dependent and AMP-independent phosphorylase a, and one inactive form, phosphorylase b. The latter is converted through ATP-requiring phosphorylation to the active a form by (active) phosphorylase b kinase. In platelets this kinase is activated by Ca^{2+} [14,51] in a calmodulin-dependent manner [47]: elevation of cyclic AMP (cAMP) in platelets does not cause glycogen breakdown, suggesting absence of cAMP-regulated phosphorylase kinase protein kinase in platelets [43]; activation of phosphorylase kinase by a cAMP-activated protein kinase has, however, been demonstrated in platelet extracts [47]. In other tissues phosphorylase a is dephosphorylated by phosphorylase phosphatase, which has not been studied in platelets. The AMP-dependent phosphorylase a is activated by AMP and P_i and inactivated by ATP and glucose 6-phosphate. Therefore, glycogen breakdown by phosphorylase in platelets is controlled by combinations of adenine nucleotides, glucose 6-phosphate, and P_i, and by Ca^{2+}. The maximal rate of glycogen breakdown in platelets is 0.3 to 1.3 μmol glucose residue per gram per minute [24,179].

Aerobic glyco(geno)lysis, i.e., breakdown of glucose 6-phosphate to pyruvate and further oxidation in the mitochondria of the C_2 fragment resulting from decarboxylation of pyruvate, takes place in resting platelets as evidenced by production of $^{14}CO_2$ from 6-^{14}C-labeled glucose [7,18,52] and from the Crabtree and Pasteur effects. Most of the enzymes of the Embden-Meyerhof pathway [25] and Krebs cycle [27] and some mitochondrial cytochromes are present in platelets. ATP synthesis coupled to oxidation of pyruvate and α-glycerophosphate by isolated mitochondria has been reported [53,54]. However, the enzymatic processes that link glycolysis to oxidative phosphorylation, pyruvate dehydrogenase and the α-glycerophosphate shuttle have not yet been elucidated in platelets.

Whether platelets do perform gluconeogenesis and glycogeneogenesis is controversial. Labeled pyruvate can be incorporated into glycogen [3] and glucose [55]. Similarly, platelets can convert labeled citrate to lactate [10], and 2,4-dinitrophenol stimulates incorporation of radioactivity from citrate and pyruvate into glycogen [39,40]. Others have reported exogenous citrate is not metabolized by platelets [56]. In contrast, the key enzymes in gluconeogenesis, phosphoenolpyruvate carboxykinase, pyruvate carboxykinase, and fructose 1,6-phosphatase could not be demonstrated in platelets [31,57], although a fructose 1,6-phosphatase–like enzyme has been described [3].

METABOLISM OF FATTY ACIDS, LIPIDS, AND PHOSPHOLIPIDS

The platelet is the only formed element of the blood which is capable of *de novo* fatty acid synthesis via the malonyl coenzyme A (CoA) (cytoplasmic) pathway [58–66]:

$$Acetyl\ CoA + CO_2 + ATP \rightarrow malonyl\ CoA + P_i$$

Neither mature red blood cells nor leukocytes contain the enzyme acetyl CoA carboxylase which is necessary for malonyl CoA synthesis [58,62,63]. The malonyl CoA that is formed then reacts with acetyl CoA:

$$Acetyl\ CoA + 7\ malonyl\ CoA + 14\ NADPH + 14H^+ \rightarrow$$
$$palmitate + 14\ NADP^+ + 8\ CoA + 7CO_2 + 6HOH$$

This reaction requires the enzyme fatty acid synthetase.

Fatty acid elongation is reduced by inhibition of the hexose monophosphate shunt which provides the NADPH for the elongation process [67]. Platelets also have the capacity for fatty acid chain elongation via the mitochondrial system, where two-carbon fragments of acetyl CoA are added to preexistent long-chain fatty acids [59–61].

Platelets incorporate ^{14}C-acetate into total lipid [59–61,64–66] at a rate of 0.05 to 0.6 μmol/(g·h) at 37°C [61,64]. Platelet lipid synthesis (*de novo* + elongation) represents approximately 30 percent of total lipid synthesis of whole blood [64]. An average platelet incorporates about 1 to 2 percent of the ^{14}C-acetate of an average leukocyte [64,65]. Approximately 40 percent of newly labeled lipid is recovered in plasma [61]. Most of this radioactivity is free fatty acid, particularly myristic and palmitic. Newly labeled fatty acids of platelet phosphatidylcholine exchange with plasma free fatty acids [61]. Some variation has been reported in the distribution of ^{14}C-acetate in platelet lipids. Approximately 75 percent of total platelet-labeled lipid could be accounted for by free fatty acid (37 percent), ceramide (27 percent), and phosphatidylcholine (10 percent) in one study [61], whereas 97 percent of total radioactivity could be accounted for by free fatty acid (47 percent), phospholipid (29 percent), and glyceride (21 percent) in another [66].

Myristic and palmitic acids (14:0 and 16:0) are normally made in platelets by *de novo* synthesis, while fatty acids containing 18 or more carbons are made by chain elongation of a preformed fatty acid [61,65]. Newly synthesized myristic and palmitic acids are found primarily in nonesterified fatty acids [66], while the radioactive fatty acids containing 18 or more carbons are found predominantly in phospholipids [66], glycerides, and ceramides [61,66]. The lipid radioactivity is found primarily in palmitic (16:0), myristic (14:0), and arachidic (20:0) acids [59,61,65].

Long-chain fatty acids in plasma dissociate from albumin, are taken up by platelets, and equilibrate with the nonesterified fatty acid pool [68,69], which also equilibrates with fatty acids synthesized endogenously from acetate [61]. The fatty acids in this pool are incorporated into lipids or phospholipids and undergo oxidative degradation (see below). The mechanism of incorporation of long-chain fatty acids into phospholipids is of particular interest because of the widespread use of platelets labeled in vitro with radioactive arachidonate in order to study arachidonate liberation during stimulation of the cells. Two mechanisms are operative: *de novo* synthesis and remodeling. The *de novo* synthesis pathway [70–80] is shown schematically in Fig. 128-1 (solid lines). All of the enzymes which are involved have been demonstrated in platelets. A fatty acid is esterified, as acyl CoA, with *sn*-glycerol-3-phosphate to yield lysophosphatidic acid. In turn, lysophosphatidic acid is acylated by a second acyl CoA to yield phosphatidic acid (PA), which is dephosphorylated to diglyceride, the common precursor

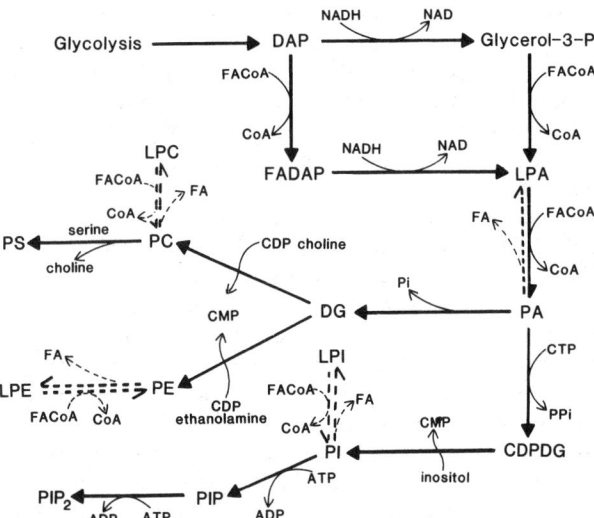

FIGURE 128-1 The *de novo* and remodeling pathways of platelet phospholipid synthesis. The *de novo* pathways are indicated with solid lines and the remodeling pathways are shown with broken lines. Abbreviations used: DAP = dihydroxyacetone phosphate; CoA = coenzyme A (reduced form); FA = fatty acid; FACoA = fatty acid coenzyme A (acyl coenzyme A); NADH and NAD = nicotinamide adenine dinucleotide, reduced and oxidized forms, respectively; FADAP = fatty acid dihydroxyacetone phosphate; LPA = lysophosphatidic acid; PA = phosphatidic acid; CTP = cytidine triphosphate; PP_i = inorganic pyrophosphate; CDPDG = cytidine diphosphate diglyceride; CMP = cytidine monophosphate; PI = phosphatidylinositol; LPI = lysophosphatidylinositol; PIP = phosphatidylinositol 4-phosphate; PIP_2 = phosphatidylinositol 4,5-bisphosphate; DG = diglyceride (diacyl glycerol); PE = phosphatidylethanolamine; LPE = lysophosphatidylethanolamine; CDP = cytidine diphosphate; PC = phosphatidylcholine; LPC = lysophosphatidylcholine; PS = phosphatidylserine.

for the diacylglycerol moiety in phosphatidylcholine (PC), phosphatidylethanolamine (PE), and phosphatidylserine (PS). PA is directly converted (i.e., without dephosphorylation) to the phosphoinositides through activation by cytosine triphosphate, combination with inositol, and successive phosphorylations. For all phospholipids it is evident from Fig. 128-1 that their fatty acid composition obtained by *de novo* synthesis is determined by the two first acylation steps. However, it is not clear whether there exists individual acyltransferases for each acyl CoA species. In the remodeling pathway [75,79–84], preexisting PC, PE, and PA are deacylated by phospholipase A_1 and/or A_2 to the corresponding lysophospholipids, which in turn are reacylated by acyltransferases of varying specificity (Fig. 128-1, broken lines). It is not known how these deacylation and reacylation processes are controlled or how the *de novo* synthesis and remodeling pathways interact in the resting platelet. Strict control of the acyl CoA species entering phosphatidyl inositol (PI) must exist, since this phospholipid contains almost exclusively stearyl

(18:0) in the 1 position and arachidonyl (20:4) in the 2 position [78,85–88]. Another pathway (of uncertain significance) for conversion of PS to PC through decarboxylation to PE followed by three successive methylations has recently been demonstrated in platelets [89, 90]. Besides acyl CoA synthetase(s), platelets also contain acyl CoA hydrolases, both in cytoplasm and mitochondria [91,92]; the latter group of enzymes may also be of importance in selecting the acyl CoA species to be incorporated in platelet phospholipids. There are evidently multiple potential steps in the various routes of phospholipid interconversions at which control of introduction of fatty acids can be exercised.

Fatty acids in the nonesterified pool of platelets are also oxidized to CO_2, in contrast to erythrocytes but similar to leukocytes. The acyl component of acyl CoA is transferred to carnitine by acylcarnitine transferase, and the acylcarnitine complexes can pass into the mitochondria where they undergo classical β oxidation [93–96], at a rate of about 11.9 μmol/(g·min) [94]. Arachidonate, however, is preferentially metabolized along other pathways (see below).

Platelet phospholipid metabolism has also been studied by incorporation into resting cells of various radioactive precursors other than fatty acids. Thus, platelets incorporate ^{32}P-orthophosphate into phospholipid with labeling of PE, PC, PI, and PI-phosphates [97–100]. Incorporation of ^{32}P into platelet phosphatide appears to require a functioning Krebs cycle, since it can be blocked by cyanide, anaerobiosis [97], or malonate and is enhanced four- to fivefold by succinate, citrate, or malate but not by pyruvate [98]. Labeled intermediates of PC synthesis [phosphorylcholine, cytosine diphosphate (CDP)-choline, and cytosine triphosphate (CTP)] have been identified in platelets labeled with [32]P [101]. Platelets can make CDP-diglyceride from CTP and phosphatidic acid [71] and convert CDP-diglyceride to phosphoinositides [72]. Platelets are also capable of incorporating ^{14}C-glycerol into glycerol phosphorylcholine, glycerol phosphorylethanolamine, glycerol phosphorylinositol, and glycerol phosphorylserine [102].

The greater part of albumin-bound arachidonic acid is incorporated into phospholipids as outlined above. However, in the absence of albumin, arachidonate is primarily oxygenated through the cyclooxygenase and lipoxygenase pathways (see below); increasing concentrations of albumin gradually reduces the proportion being oxygenated [103]. The mechanism of the effect of albumin is not clearly understood.

ARACHIDONATE METABOLISM – SYNTHESIS OF PROSTAGLANDINS AND THROMBOXANES

Prostaglandins are a group of complex cyclic fatty acids composed of a cyclopentane ring with two aliphatic side chains. They are present in most tissues and have varied and potent biologic activity. They contain 20 carbon atoms and differ in their degree of unsaturation and/or substitution in the side chain or ring (see Fig.

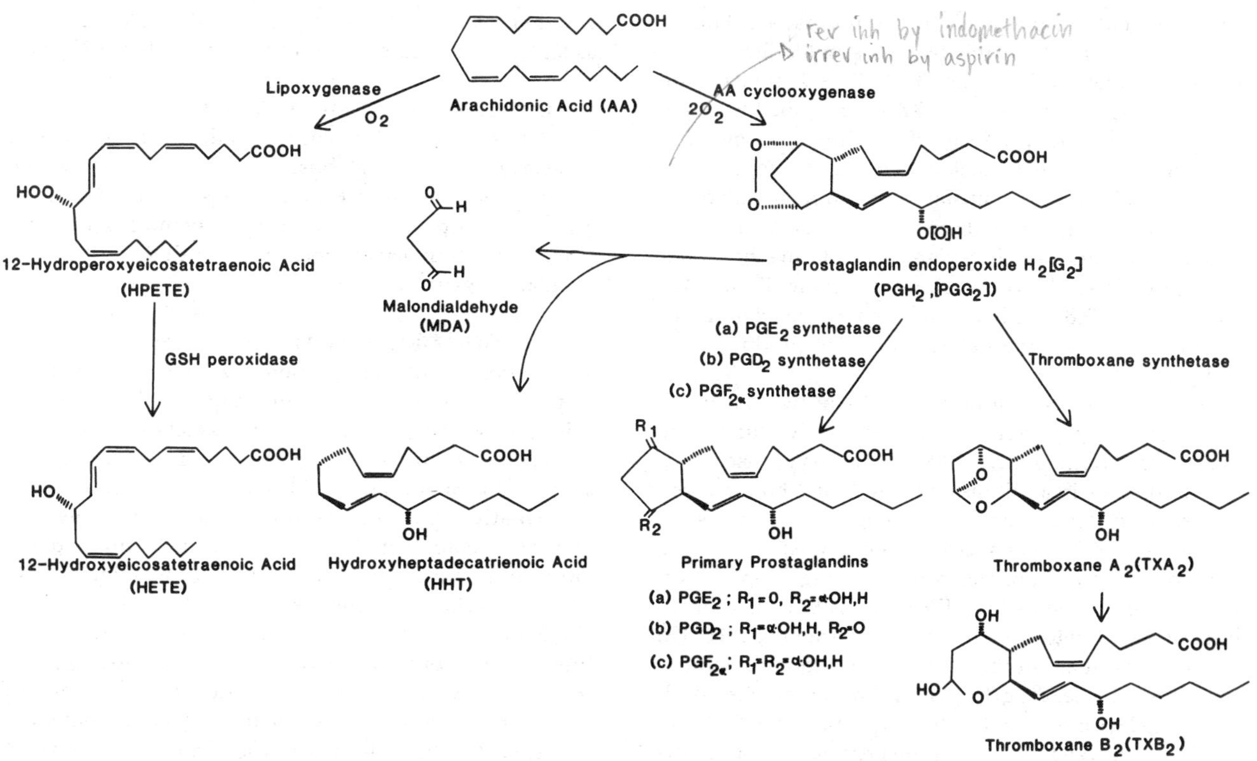

FIGURE 128-2 Pathways of oxygenation of arachidonic acid in platelets: formation of prostaglandins and thromboxanes.

128-2). Platelets synthesize prostaglandins and their derivatives, thromboxanes (Fig. 128-2), from arachidonate, 5,8,11,14-eicosatetraenoate (20:4).

During platelet stimulation arachidonate is liberated from various phospholipids by various pathways (see below) and oxygenated like added arachidonate. Since resting platelets oxygenate arachidonate in the same way as stimulated platelets, we will discuss the oxygenation pathways here (Fig. 128-2). Fatty acid cyclooxygenase (prostaglandin synthetase) may be present in the dense tubular system [104] and catalyzes both cyclooxygenation of arachidonate and peroxidation of the product, prostaglandin G_2 (PGG$_2$, a prostaglandin peroxide) [105–111]. Cyclooxygenation introduces four oxygen atoms into arachidonate together with a concerted cyclization of the molecule, producing PGG$_2$. Hemin is required for this complex reaction. The peroxidase of prostaglandin synthetase reduces the 15-hydroperoxy group of PGG$_2$ to a hydroxyl group, yielding prostaglandin H_2 (PGH$_2$); a suitable donor of reducing equivalents (tryptophan, phenol) is required. It is possible that cytochrome P_{450} also is a functional part of platelet prostaglandin synthetase [112]. Like the enzyme from other sources [113] platelet cyclooxygenase is irreversibly inactivated during catalysis [114]. The cyclooxygenase reaction is inhibited reversibly by indomethacin, and, most importantly, irreversibly by acetylsalicylic acid, *aspirin*; the peroxidase reaction is not inhibited by the drugs. The irreversible inhibition by

aspirin is due to acetylation of the cyclooxygenase moiety [107,115–117]. Salicylate is without effect on platelets but appears to counteract the acetylation by aspirin [118–120]; sulfinpyrazone, an antiplatelet drug, has a similar effect on inhibition by aspirin [120]. Inhibition by aspirin has been used as a nonisotopic method for determination of platelet life-span [121,122].

Prostaglandins G_2 and H_2 undergo a series of enzymatic and nonenzymatic conversions (Fig. 128-2). These endoperoxides are unstable (half-life in aqueous medium = 300 s) and a major proportion is converted into malonyldialdehyde (MDA) and 12-L-hydroxy-5,8,10-heptadecatrienoic acid (HHT) [108,109]. Measurement of MDA is frequently used to determine formation of prostaglandin endoperoxides [123]. A small fraction of PGG$_2$ and PGH$_2$ is converted to other, stable prostaglandins, PGD$_2$, PGE$_2$, and PGF$_{2\alpha}$ [108,109,124–126]. Albumin promotes these conversions, and a PGH$_2$-PGE$_2$ isomerase is present in platelets [127]; it has been suggested that MDA formation is catalyzed by thromboxane synthetase [128]. MDA, HHT, PGE$_2$, and PGF$_{2\alpha}$ have little effect on platelets, while PGD$_2$ is a potent activator of adenylate cyclase (see below). The most important conversion of PGG$_2$ and PGH$_2$ is catalyzed by thromboxane synthetase (Fig. 128-2) and yields the unstable thromboxane A$_2$ [129–134]. This substance is one of the most potent platelet agonists known and is also a powerful vasoconstrictor. Thromboxane synthetase is associated with platelet microsomes, but is not yet well characterized. Several specific inhibitors are known [135–141] which all inhibit platelet stimulation caused by arachidonate or PGG$_2$ and PGH$_2$, thus demonstrating that it is thromboxane A$_2$ (TXA$_2$), and not the many intermediates and products of arachidonate metabolism described above, that is the platelet-active substance. TXA$_2$ is very unstable in aqueous medium ($T_{1/2} = 30$ s), and is hydrated to the stable, platelet-inactive thromboxane B$_2$. Presence of plasma, however, markedly slows the conversion of TXA$_2$ to TXB$_2$ [142]. Antibody to TXB$_2$ has been prepared and used in radioimmunoassays for the determination of production of TXB$_2$ [143].

The lipoxygenase pathway consists of two reactions, catalyzed by lipoxygenase and presumably glutathione peroxidase (Fig. 128-2). Platelet lipoxygenase [105, 144–148] exists in a soluble and membrane-bound form, and requires ferric iron for catalytic activity. It inserts one molecule of oxygen (two linked atoms) at the C-12 position of arachidonate, thus yielding 12-hydroxyperoxyeicosatetraenoate (HPETE). HPETE is subsequently reduced to 12-hydroxyeicosatetraenoate (HETE) in a reaction that is inhibited by exclusion of selenium from the diet leading to glutathione peroxidase deficiency [149]; most likely, the reduction of HPETE to HETE is catalyzed by glutathione peroxidase. HETE, the stable, final product of the lipoxygenase pathway, has been shown to be a chemotactic agent for leukocytes [150]. The two enzymes in the lipoxygenase pathway are not influenced directly by inhibitors of cyclooxygenase (aspirin, indomethacin, nonsteroidal anti-inflammatory drugs) or thromboxane synthetase. Since lipoxygenase and cyclooxygenase have a common substrate, inhibition of one enzyme makes more substrate available for the other. Thus, inactivation of cyclooxygenase in platelets causes a marked increase in the formation of HETE from arachidonate [107]. Direct interactions between the two pathways have also been observed: prostaglandin endoperoxides stimulate lipooxygenase [146], and HPETE has been reported to inhibit cyclooxygenase [151] and thromboxane synthetase [152].

In addition to arachidonate, platelet cyclooxygenase also oxygenates 5,8,11,14,17-eicosapentenoate (20:5) [153,154] and 8,11,14-eicosatrienoic acid (20:3) [155] to the corresponding prostaglandins and thromboxanes. These fatty acids are also metabolized through the lipoxygenase pathway. Both enzymes are inhibited by the acetylenic analog of arachidonate, 5,8,11,14-eicosatetraynoic acid [105] and by 1-phenyl-3-pyrozolidone [156]. Lipoxygenase is selectively inhibited by 5,8,11-eicosatriynoic acid [157].

Endothelial cells have a cyclooxygenase pathway similar to that shown for platelets in Fig. 128-2, except that thromboxane synthetase is substituted by a prostaglandin synthetase that produces prostaglandin I$_2$ (prostacyclin, a powerful inhibitor of platelet stimulation) from PGG$_2$ and PGH$_2$ [158–161]. Prostaglandin I$_2$ is produced from added arachidonate as well as from arachidonate liberated from endothelial phospholipids;

whether platelet-produced PGG$_2$ and PGH$_2$ can serve as substrate appears to be controversial [162,163].

GLYCOSPHINGOLIPID METABOLISM

Platelets also contain glycosphingolipids [164] of which trihexosylceramide, globoside, and hematoside are exposed on the surface of the cells [165]. Glucose is rapidly incorporated into hexosylceramides in vitro [166], indicating active metabolism of this lipid class in circulating platelets.

NUCLEOTIDE METABOLISM

The contents and compartmentalization of nucleotides in platelets were discussed in Chap. 127. Here we will briefly describe the capacity of platelets to synthesize and catabolize nucleotides in the extragranular pool; the control of formation of ATP from ADP in glycolysis and by oxidative phosphorylation is discussed below (see "Energy Metabolism"). The adenine nucleotides are the most abundant in platelets, and their metabolism (Fig. 128-3) has been extensively studied [13,52,167–179]. Circulating platelets do not synthesize adenine nucleotides *de novo* but have a well-developed salvage pathway, i.e., synthesis of nucleotides from preformed bases or ribosides. Thus, platelets take up adenine (reaction 6) through a specific, saturable transport mechanism [180]. Once inside the platelet, adenine reacts with phosphoribosyl pyrophosphate (PRPP) to yield AMP, catalyzed by adenine phosphoribosyltransferase, a cytoplasmic enzyme [25]. PRPP is formed from ATP and ribose 5-phosphate (reaction 10) [174], an intermediate of the hexose monophosphate shunt; stimulation of the shunt elevates the level of ribose 5-phosphate and thereby increases the availability of PRPP which is associated with a 15 to 20 times increase in uptake of adenine [35]. Adenosine is also taken up by a specific transport system (reaction 5) [181] and, at low concentrations, exclusively converted to AMP by the cytoplasmic adenosine kinase and ATP; at high concentrations the kinase reaction is saturated and excess adenosine is deaminated by platelet adenosine deaminase (not shown in Fig. 128-3) [25]. Platelets are rich in adenylate kinase [170,171,175,179] which rapidly equilibrates the newly synthesized AMP among the adenylates (reaction 1). However, platelets contain a powerful AMP deaminase [52,177] which has been purified and characterized [178]. In resting platelets AMP deaminase is practically inactive, but under metabolic stress [13,22,168,169,176] and when platelets are stimulated (see below), the enzyme becomes activated and converts AMP irreversibly to inosine monophosphate (reaction 2). In contrast, when platelets are starved, the ATP level decreases, as during metabolic stress and platelet stimulation, but AMP accumulates [15], indicating that AMP deaminase is not activated. It is presently unclear what controls AMP deaminase; when it is active, the consumption of AMP leads to a decrease in the entire pool of cytoplasmic adenylate because of the rapid equilibration among ATP, ADP, and AMP by adenylate kinase (Fig. 128-3). Thus, AMP deaminase (reaction 2) is essential for controlling the size of the adenylate pool. IMP is dephosphorylated by platelet 5'-nucleotidase to inosine (reaction 3) which is phosphorolyzed to ribose 1-phosphate and hypoxanthine (reaction 4); inosine and hypoxanthine diffuse out of the platelet.

Adenosine is not present in plasma, and adenine is scarce. The formation of adenylates from adenine and adenosine by platelets (above) is therefore probably of minor importance in vivo. The cells have, however, substantial amounts of hypoxanthine-guanine phosphoribosyltransferase (HGPRT) which, in the presence of PRPP, converts hypoxathine to inosine monophosphate (IMP) (reaction 7) and guanine to guanine monophosphate [168]. Hypoxanthine and guanine are taken up very slowly (about 1 percent of uptake of adenine) by resting platelets, but the uptake rate is powerfully stimulated by activation of the hexose monophosphate shunt [35]. The IMP formed is converted to adenylates (and guanylates) in platelets [173,174], demonstrating presence of the anabolic pathway shown in Fig. 128-3 (reactions 9 and 8). Patients with the Lesch-Nyhan syndrome, who lack HGPRT, have reduced levels of total platelet adenine nucleotides [182], suggesting that formation of platelet adenine nucleotides in platelets (or in megakaryocytes) depends partially on HGPRT.

PROTEIN SYNTHESIS

Platelets are capable of incorporating amino acid precursors into platelet protein in an experimental system in which intact platelets [2,18,183,184] or a cell-free system [184–187] is employed. A stable messenger RNA for the synthesis of actomyosin has been reported [186]. The radioactive amino acid precursor has been detected in the peptide map obtained from a proteolytic digest of the isolated platelet protein [183,188]. The incorporation of precursor into protein is inhibited by puromycin [2,18,183,188]. Later studies demonstrated that part of the protein synthesis was inhibited by chloramphenicol and therefore thought to occur in the mitochondria [189]. The degree of total amino acid incorporation, however, is small compared with other tissues and the biological significance uncertain [2]. Actomyosin [190] and fibrinogen [184,185] have both been identified as synthetic products. However, in these studies fibrinogen was isolated as fibrin after clotting with thrombin and the presence of radioactive amino acids was determined in the clot. Using this method in attempts to demonstrate fibrinogen biosynthesis in isolated megakaryocytes, it was found that fibrin formed a tight complex with actin present in the clot and that the radioactivity was only associated with actin and not with fibrin [191]. It is therefore doubtful whether platelets can synthesize fibrinogen. Two types of polyribosomes have been identified, 650 S and 340 S [181]. Human platelet protein synthesis requires iron [192].

Glucose [4] as well as glucosamine and mannose

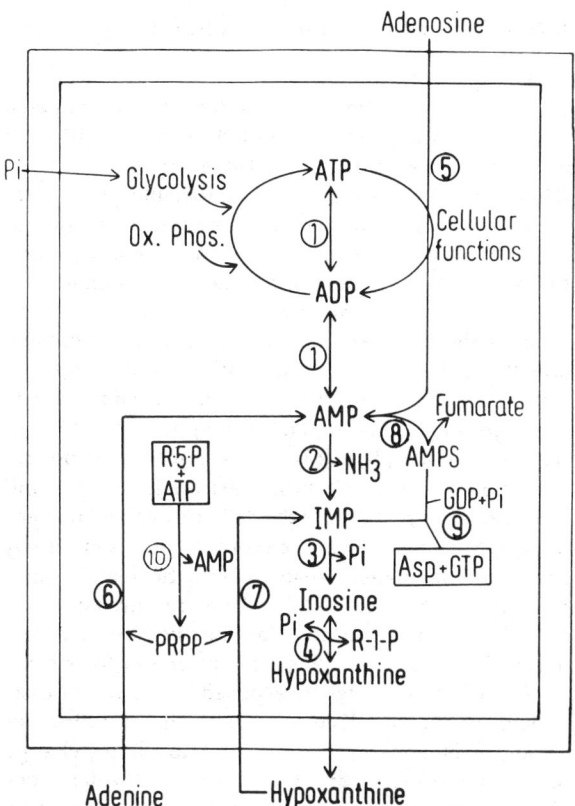

FIGURE 128-3   Adenine nucleotide metabolism in platelets. ATP, ADP, and AMP are kept in equilibrium by adenylate kinase (enzyme 1). AMP is converted irreversibly by adenylate deaminase (enzyme 2) to IMP, which is dephosphorylated to inosine by 5-nucleotidase (enzyme 3). Inosine is converted to hypoxanthine and ribose 1-phosphate (R-1-P) by purine nucleoside phosphorylase (enzyme 4). Adenosine + ATP is converted to AMP via adenosine kinase (enzyme 5). Adenine + phosphoribosyl pyrophosphate (PRPP) is converted to AMP via adenine phosphoribosyltransferase (enzyme 6). In the "salvage pathway," hypoxanthine is converted to IMP by hypoxanthine-guanine phosphoribosyltransferase (enzyme 7). Adenylosuccinate synthetase (enzyme 9) catalyzes the conversion of IMP and asparate (Asp) to adenylosuccinate. This is converted to AMP and fumarate by adenylosuccinate lyase (enzyme 8). PRPP is formed from ribose 5-phosphate and ATP by ribose phosphate pyrophosphokinase (enzyme 10). (From H. Holmsen, L. Salganicoff, and M. H. Fukami, Platelet behaviour and biochemistry, in *Physiology and Biochemistry of Haemostasis*, edited by B. Ogsten and D. Bennet. Wiley, London, 1977. By permission.)

[193,194] are incorporated in an energy-dependent manner [194] into platelet protein in vitro, suggesting the ability of platelets to synthesize the carbohydrate part of glycoproteins; intermediates of the dolichol pathway for this synthesis have been demonstrated [195]. Large, heavy (young) platelets incorporate 2.7 times more leucine into puromycin-inhibitable protein than do light, small platelets [2,196]. It is conceivable that only a relatively young (large, heavy) platelet population is capable of significant protein synthesis [2,197].

Metabolism in stimulated platelets

PLATELET STIMULATION

Platelets have specific receptors for several agonists, and receptor occupancy is coupled to the execution of various platelet responses (see Table 128-1).

There are at least eight distinguishable platelet responses that can be studied in vitro: *adhesion* (to foreign surfaces), *shape change, aggregation, dense granule secretion, α-granule secretion, arachidonate liberation, acid hydrolase secretion,* and *fibrin clot retraction. Shape change* is the first response to stimulation by soluble agonists (epinephrine is an exception), and consists in a rapid transformation of the smooth, discoid platelets (the shape in the resting state) to spherical cells with long pseudopods [279–282]; the response does not require extracellular Ca^{2+}. When extracellular Ca^{2+} and fibrinogen are present, and the cells are allowed to come into close contact with each other (for example by stirring of the platelet suspension), the platelets undergo *aggregation* [283–287]. The requirement for extracellular fibrinogen and Ca^{2+} has been extensively studied. Platelets have "hidden" receptors for fibrinogen (see Chap. 127) that are exposed following agonist-platelet interaction [206,285–291]. The binding of fibrinogen is apparently unrelated to shape change [292], and requires Ca^{2+}. Chymotrypsin, which does not stimulate platelets, exposes fibrinogen binding sites and subsequent addition of fibrinogen (with stirring) causes the platelets to aggregate [291]. Thus, the

active part played by the platelet in agonist-induced aggregation appears to consist in fibrinogen receptor exposure. *Dense granule secretion* and *α-granule secretion,* exocytosis of the contents (Chap. 127) of the dense granules and α-granules, respectively, occur simultaneously and with similar dose-response relationships [293,294]. *Arachidonate liberation,* the hydrolysis of platelet phospholipids by phospholipases and lipases yielding free arachidonate which is oxygenated as outlined above, is a metabolic response which is discussed below. *Acid hydrolase secretion,* the exocytosis of acid hydrolases (see Chap. 127), is a considerably slower process than the two other secretory processes and requires a higher degree of stimulation [294,297].

Intimate interactions exist among the platelet responses and have been extensively studied [198,276, 298–309]. Some responses, or their consequences, promote and others inhibit the propagation of platelet responses. Promotion is caused by (1) secreted substances which are themselves platelet agonists, i.e., ADP and serotonin (see Table 128-1), (2) prostaglandin endoperoxides and thromboxane A_2 synthesized from liberated arachidonate (Fig. 128-2), (3) close cell contact (see Table 128-1) obtained during aggregation, and (4) synergism between applied agonist and agonists secreted or synthesized by the platelets [298,310–314]. Inhibition is caused by (1) tachyphylaxis or "refractoriness" [315–319], (2) substances secreted (ATP antagonizes ADP, see Table 128-1) and their breakdown products in plasma [320], and (3) substances that are

TABLE 128-1 Agonists and platelet receptors

Agonist	Strength	Antagonist	Binding to receptor	References
Vasopressin		Oxytocin	—	[198,199]
Serotonin		Methysergide, metergoline	Yes	[200–202]
ADP	Weak	ATP, 2-methylthio AMP	Yes	[203–212]
Epinephrine		Yohimbine, clonidine	Yes	[210,213–222]
Thromboxane A_2*		13-Azoprostanoate	Yes	[223–226]
Arachidonate†		—	—	[227–228]
Prostaglandin analogs*	Intermediate	9,11-Epoxyethanoprostaglandin H_2	Yes	[229–230]
PAF‡		—	Yes	[231–235]
Collagen		Complement 1q	Yes	[236–244]
Thrombin		Not known	Yes	[245–259]
Proteolytic enzymes	Strong	Not known	—	[260–263]
A23187, free species		(Ca^{2+}, Mg^{2+})	—	[176,264–271]
Close cell contact§	Unknown	—	—	[172,176,271–276]
Foreign surfaces¶		—	—	[277–278]

* Added to platelets. Thromboxane (TXA_2) produced within the platelets may have other characteristics.
† Not an agonist per se; the conversion products prostaglandin endoperoxide and TXA_2 are the active agonists.
‡ Platelet-aggregating factor, 1-alkylether 2-acylglycerol 3-phosphocholine.
§ Platelet-platelet cohesion caused by aggregation; agglutination or physical means.
¶ Nonplatelet surface (subendothelium, glass, gas-liquid interface).
NOTE: The agonists interact with specific receptors on the platelet surface. The specificity of the interaction of a given agonist with its receptor has been demonstrated by use of specific antagonists which inhibit both cellular response and binding of the agonist *without* interfering with response and binding of any other agonists. The strength of an agonist refers to how many responses are triggered when the receptor is saturated with the agonist. Thus, *weak* agonists cause shape change and aggregation; *intermediate* agonists cause shape change, aggregation, and partial secretion-arachidonate liberation; *strong* agonists cause complete activation of all responses.

synthesized from liberated arachidonate, such as HPETE (Fig. 128-2), an inhibitor of thromboxane synthetase [149], and PGD$_2$, which stimulates cyclic AMP production (see below).

There is a striking similarity of the events following stimulation of platelets through interaction between all the different agonists and their receptors. This has led to the belief that they trigger one basic reaction, referred to here as the *basic platelet reaction,* which includes the sequence: shape change → aggregation → dense- and α-granule secretion → arachidonate liberation–acid hydrolase secretion. The agonists are therefore only distinguished qualitatively on the level of agonist-receptor interaction. Close cell contact and cyclooxygenase-dependent secretion is often accompanied by enhanced aggregation, a phenomenon called *secondary aggregation* [209,321–324]; the direct aggregation response to the agonist is called *primary aggregation.* Secondary aggregation is abolished by inhibition of cyclooxygenase (by aspirin), occurs only above 33°C and is inhibited by high calcium levels. Thus, it occurs more promptly with citrate (low Ca^{2+}) than with heparin or hirudin (high Ca^{2+}) [212,325,326] as the anticoagulant. It is usually absent in platelets from patients with storage pool deficiency [327,328] and always absent in cyclooxygenase deficiency [329–332], thromboxane synthetase deficiency [333], and thromboxane receptor anomalies [334,335]. Absence of secondary aggregation is therefore an important diagnostic feature. However, it must be emphasized that vast numbers of drugs, in particular those that contain acetylsalicylate, cause abolition of secondary aggregation [337,338].

Except for the ionophore A23187, prostaglandin analogs, and probably proteolytic enzymes other than thrombin, the platelet agonists listed in Table 128-1 are considered to be of importance in vivo. However, the concentrations of vasopressin and epinephrine obtainable in vivo are too small to stimulate platelets per se, but sufficient to act synergistically with other agonists [312,313]. Platelets become refractory to repeated exposure to epinephrine [315], and the great variation in epinephrine response in vitro, but not to other agonists, indicates that platelets are exposed to epinephrine *in circulation* [339,340]. Platelet-activating factor (PAF) is synthesized in mastocytes, neutrophils, basophils, and macrophages during anaphylactic shock in several animal species [341] and most likely is responsible for the accompanying thrombocytopenia seen [231]. Collagen is an *insoluble* platelet agonist. When a vessel is damaged, platelets adhere first to the collagen-like material of the subendothelium [342]. Platelets are stimulated in vitro by collagen fibers, i.e., polymerized collagen, but not by collagen monomers. The free amino groups and specifically the ε-amino groups of lysine are critical for the platelet-stimulating activity of collagen [238]. An intact tertiary structure [238], an ordered array of polar groups [343,344], hydroxylysine-linked carbohydrate groups [345–347,241–243], and collagen quaternary structure (state of polymerization) [242,243,348] may all be implicated. The degree of polymerization is probably most important, and all other structural collagen requirements are probably related to their ability to enhance or impede collagen polymerization.

Thrombin originates by cleavage of prothrombin in plasma catalyzed by factor Xa, and the reaction is accelerated by factor Va (see Chap. 135). The catalytic activity of the prothrombinase complex, factor Xa–factor Va, is markedly increased in the presence of platelets, and both coagulation factors bind to the platelet surface: factor Va binds to a specific receptor and factor Xa binds to the bound Va [336,349,350]. It is therefore postulated that the first molecules of active thrombin are formed on the platelet surface and will interact with the thrombin receptors [251–259] before thrombin causes fibrin formation in the extracellular system.

CALCIUM METABOLISM (TRANSLOCATION)

About 60 percent of calcium in human platelets is sequestered in the dense granules (see Chap. 127) and secreted when the cells are maximally stimulated [249,351–353]. Platelets possess a nonsecretable pool of 10 μmol calcium per gram that is not present in the dense granules. Some studies seem to indicate that Ca is present in the dense tubular system and the plasma membrane [28,354,355] which is in accordance with the demonstration of Ca-activated ATPases and active Ca accumulation in platelet microsomes [356–362]. The concentration of Ca^{2+} in the cytoplasm of resting platelets is 0.01 to 0.1 μM, corresponding to 0.06 nmol Ca per gram [363–365]. Evidently, all extragranular Ca must be structurally bound in resting platelets. It was suggested earlier that the basic platelet reaction may be mediated by increase in cytosolic calcium [366–368] and a large body of evidence, which has been recently reviewed [369], seems to support this contention. Thus, platelet activation is associated with an increase in cytoplasmic Ca^{2+}, as measured by the techniques mentioned above [363,365], and studies with chlortetracycline suggest rapid loss of structurally bound Ca upon platelet stimulation [370–372]. Some enzymes are stimulated through various mechanisms by minute amounts of Ca, and the formation of their products in intact cells suggests increase of cytoplasmic Ca^{2+}. In platelets three such enzymes are known, glycogen phosphorylase (above), myosin light-chain kinase (see Chap. 127), and phospholipases A$_2$ and C (below); and the immediate formation of glycogen breakdown products [11], phosphorylated myosin light-chain [374–378], and arachidonate [379–383] would suggest increase in cytoplasmic Ca^{2+} during agonist-receptor interaction. The apparent increase in cytoplasmic Ca^{2+} takes place even if EGTA or EDTA are present extracellularly, showing that Ca^{2+} can be exclusively derived from intracellular sites. The time courses for calcium release and performance of responses were, when measured, suggestive of cause-effect relationships, which also is supported by the inhibition of platelet stimulation by *calcium antagonists* [384–385] (although these may have serious side effects [373]) and local anesthetics [386]. Another indication for involvement of intracellular Ca^{2+} in the stimulation of platelets is the inhibition by phenothiazines, known as selective calmodulin inhibitors of every response in the basic platelet reaction [383,387].

The basic platelet reaction is stimulated with the divalent cationophore A23187 [170,264–271]; this ionophore transports magnesium as well as calcium across biological membranes. Ionomycin, an ionophore more specific for calcium than magnesium, also stimulates platelets [392]. All divalent cationophores cause secretion and arachidonate liberation in the absence of extracellular calcium, showing that if calcium mediates these responses, it is derived from intracellular sources, as concluded above. Secretory responses are induced by making the platelet membrane permeable for small molecules with electrical discharge [393] and digitonin [394] when the platelets are suspended in calcium buffers and ATP. Since the degree of stimulation in these experiments was dependent on the extracellular calcium concentration and became saturated at about 1 to 2 μM [Ca^{2+}], these results serve as evidence for stimulation of the platelet response by increases of the cytoplasmic Ca^{2+} concentration.

Thus, platelet responses are apparently triggered concomitantly with increase in cytoplasmic Ca^{2+}. Where does this calcium come from, and what are the mechanisms for release of calcium into cytoplasm? Some evidence suggests that stimulation of platelets with epinephrine, but not ADP, is associated with uptake of cellular calcium prior to aggregation by a process that is inhibited by the Ca^{2+}-channel blocker verapamil [395]; the synergistic interaction of epinephrine and ADP is also accompanied by uptake of extracellular Ca^{2+} [396]. However, the occurrence of the entire basic platelet reaction in the presence of EGTA suggests that calcium can be derived from intracellular sites. The rapid turnover of the phosphoinositides upon platelet stimulation (see below) may be involved in intracellular Ca^{2+} mobilization; the ionophoretic properties of two of the platelet aggregation–promoting substances, prostaglandin endoperoxide [397] and lysophosphatidic acid [398–400], may also be of importance for Ca^{2+} mobilization. Other very early events in platelet stimulation may also be involved, such as membrane depolarization [401–403], change in the microviscosity [404–406] of the plasma membrane, and sodium uptake [402,407,408].

ENERGY METABOLISM
Stimulation of platelets with all agonists listed in Table 128-1 leads to increased production of ATP by glyco(gen)olysis [8,10,11,18,20,24,30,36,179,267,308,409–418] and oxidative phosphorylation [18,308,413,415,418–422]. This increase in ATP production reflects a rapid, extensive demand for ATP. With a novel method which

measures total ATP consumption directly, maximal stimulation by thrombin at 37°C caused an increase in ATP consumption from 5.1 (resting platelets) to 20.5 ATP equivalents (= energy-rich phosphate bonds) per minute per gram [423]. The adenylate energy charge, which is constant when ATP production balances ATP utilization (see above), decreases immediately upon platelet stimulation [424] indicating increased ATP utilization in the very first phase of agonist-platelet interaction. Shape change and aggregation occur without alteration in the ATP level [168,179], but when the basic platelet reaction reaches the secretion phase, the level of ATP decreases with a corresponding accumulation of IMP and hypoxanthine [172,176,179,247,295, 415–417,423,425,426]. This means that although ATP production in glycolysis and by oxidative phosphorylation is markedly stimulated, this production does not balance the consumption during the secretory processes [179]. All evidence quoted above also shows that the further the basic platelet reaction proceeds, the greater is the ATP consumption that accompanies the process, i.e., the stronger the stimulus, the greater is total ATP consumption.

Is ATP consumption coupled to the triggering and performance of the various platelet responses? There is presently no direct answer to this question, although a vast number of observations strongly support (but do not prove directly) coupling between ATP consumption and stimulation-driving of response: Progressive reduction of the availability of ATP by incubation of platelets with inhibitors of glycolysis and oxidative phosphorylation causes progressive inhibition and eventually abolition of shape change [168], aggregation [168,169,427,428], dense granule secretion [297,351,416, 423,425,428], α-granule secretion [423,428], acid hydrolase secretion [297,423,428], and arachidonate liberation [428,429], as well as other platelet responses, e.g., adhesion to glass [427] and collagen [430], clot retraction [427,431], and exposure of fibrinogen receptors [432]. Most importantly, the time course of inhibition of the individual responses are different: at a given reduction in ATP availability the inhibition increases in the order shape change < aggregation < dense granule secretion ≤ α-granule secretion < acid hydrolase secretion = arachidonate liberation [168,297,423,428]. Thus, the responses depend on ATP availability in the same order with which their associated ATP utilization increases. It has also been demonstrated that the degree of dense granule secretion and aggregation is directly proportional to the amount of available ATP when its resynthesis is abolished [433], and that the initial velocity of the three secretory processes are linearly related to the increment in ATP production [423]. These responses also are abolished by starvation but return to normal by refeeding glucose [15,434,435]; a similar glucose dependence has been demonstrated for clot retraction [411,436], which also depends on glycogen stores [44,437]. Another line of evidence for support of this coupling is the activation by platelet stimulation of specific reactions that utilize ATP directly, i.e., the ATP-requiring phosphorylation of myosin light chain [374–378], which in turn activates actomyosin ATPase and contraction (see Chap. 127), of other platelet proteins (see below), and of diglyceride, yielding phosphatidic acid (see below).

CARBOHYDRATE METABOLISM

The increase in ATP production in glyco(gen)olysis [8,10,11,18,20,24,36,179,267,308,409–418] associated with the elevation of ATP consumption in stimulated platelets raises the question of how energy-producing degradation of carbohydrate is controlled by the numerous metabolic changes caused by platelet stimulation.

Glycogen degradation is activated [11,14,30,179] as early as 10 s after addition of strong agonist [11]. Since glycogen phosphorylase is regulated by Ca^{2+}, and there are practically no changes in the other regulators (glucose 6-phosphate, AMP, P_i) at this early stage [11,415,426], phosphorylase is probably solely activated through the increase in cytoplasmic Ca^{2+} accompanying platelet activation. Glucose uptake is also activated during platelet stimulation [18,20,21,179], but its mode of regulation is not known. There is no free glucose within platelets, so that uptake could be controlled through glucose phosphorylation by hexokinase; collagen-platelet interaction has been reported to cause a decrease in structurally bound hexokinase [23], which may be relevant to the activation of glucose uptake. The activity of the nonequilibrium, rate-limiting steps in glycolysis, those catalyzed by phosphofructokinase and pyruvate kinase, is regulated by the levels of ATP, ADP, fructose 6-phosphate and P_i, but there are practically no changes in their levels *before* the increase in glycolytic flux is observed [417]. The subsequent variations in the ATP and P_i levels could explain the sustained increase in the glycolytic flux after the initial increase [30,179, 267,415,417,426]; the massive accumulation of fructose 1,6-diphosphate following platelet stimulation [7,30,179, 417,426] shows that phosphofructokinase is stimulated. The mechanism of the immediate stimulation of glycolysis following platelet stimulation is, however, not yet clear.

The hexose monophosphate shunt is also activated upon platelet stimulation [18,20,21] but the exact time course of this activation and its regulation are not known. The role of the shunt is most likely to maintain glutathione in a reduced form (above), which provides SH groups to a variety of substances. The presence in platelets of intact SH groups is necessary for platelet function: reagents which react specifically with SH groups inhibit clot retraction [438,439] and aggregation [439–441]. By employment of membrane-penetrating as well as nonpenetrating SH-inhibitors, it can be shown that aggregation requires the presence of membrane SH groups, whereas clot retraction requires the presence of intracellular SH groups [439]. Reduction of the level of reduced glutathione with diamide also inhibits aggregation [442]. It is possible, therefore, that the activation of the hexose monophosphate shunt during platelet stimulation reflects consumption of SH groups.

PHOSPHOLIPID METABOLISM

Platelet stimulation causes a marked increase in phospholipid metabolism as outlined in Fig. 128-4. The relative importance of these pathways and their quantitative relationships are obscure, due to the variation in methodologies. The involvement of phospholipid metabolism in agonist-induced signal generation (most likely through calcium mobilization) and in liberation of free arachidonate (Fig. 128-4) are probably interconnected. However, there is no general agreement about exact mechanisms, and the information reviewed below must be taken with reservations.

PHOSPHOLIPID TOPOLOGY

Phospholipids are localized exclusively in the membrane systems of the platelet. Studies with various penetrating and nonpenetrating fluorescent probes and with specific phospholipases have demonstrated an asymmetric arrangement of the phospholipids of the plasma membrane [443,444]. Thus, in the resting platelet practically all sphingomyelin is present on the outside whereas phosphatidylserine (PS) and phosphatidylinositol (PI) are exclusively present on the inside of this membrane; in contrast, phosphatidylethanolamine (PE) and phosphatidylcholine (PC) are unevenly distributed between the inside and outside of the plasma membrane with the larger proportion exposed to the inside. Upon stimulation of platelets, more PE becomes available to the outside, while the distribution of the other phospholipids remains constant [445,446]. Similarly, thrombin causes a reduction in the outside-located trihexosylceramide and globoside and an increase in outside-located hematoside [165].

PHOSPHATIDYLINOSITOL–PHOSPHATIDIC ACID

Minute stimuli, such as ADP in the presence of EDTA (producing shape change, only), cause a rapid incorporation of ^{32}P into phosphatidic acid (PA) in platelets

FIGURE 128-4 Possible mechanisms of liberation of arachidonic acid in stimulated platelets. PLC = phospholipase C; DG lipase = diglyceride lipase; PLA_2 = phospholipase A_2; PG = prostaglandin; TX = thromboxane. For other abbreviations see Fig. 128-1.

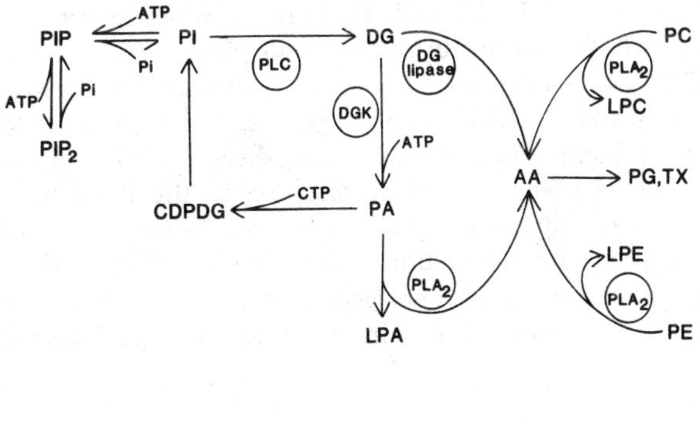

pulse-labeled with $^{32}P_i$; the label appears a few seconds after agonist addition. Other agonists studied (thrombin, epinephrine, collagen) also cause formation of ^{32}P-PA, and the amounts formed are roughly proportional to the strength of the stimulus [447–450]. Immediate formation of PA in platelets in response to stimuli has been shown in many laboratories, using platelets prelabeled with $^{32}P_i$ [260,382,383,447–455], with ^{14}C-arachidonate [260,382,455,456], or by determination of chemical levels of PA [88,457,458]. The three approaches show unequivocally that PA is formed immediately upon addition of agonist. Evidence for coupling between receptor occupancy and PA formation has been found for the thrombin-platelet interaction: formation stops immediately when the agonist is abruptly removed and starts over again when more agonist is added [260], indicating a tight coupling between receptor occupancy and PA formation. Acid hydrolase secretion and arachidonate liberation are immediately stopped by abrupt thrombin removal [260], which suggests a tight coupling between receptor occupancy, and a defined biochemical process and platelet response. This is of special interest, since PA has calcium ionophoretic properties [459,460]. Platelets contain a PA-specific phospholipase A_2 [461], and the product, lyso PA, has calcium ionophoretic activity [398–400] and is formed during thrombin-platelet interaction [451,461]. Thus, early in the platelet-thrombin interaction substances are formed which may liberate calcium from its stores to the cytoplasm. These substances, PA and lyso PA, also stimulate platelets when added in vitro [398–400,460]. PA is formed in response to agonists other than thrombin [447–450], and constitutes a likely candidate for a link between agonist-receptor interaction and calcium mobilization in general.

PA is formed by phosphorylation by ATP of diglyceride (DG) set free from PI by the action of phospholipase C, as shown in Fig. 128-4 [79,88,260,382,383,451–458, 462–464]. Platelet phospholipase C is specific for phosphatidylinositol (PI), is found in the cytosol, and has an absolute requirement for Ca^{2+} at the optimal pH, 6.5 to 7.5 [79,462,463]. The calmodulin inhibitors trifluoperazine and quinacrine do not affect thrombin-induced PI breakdown under conditions where phospholipase A_2 is markedly inhibited [383,455], indicating that phospholipase C activation by calcium may be independent of calmodulin. PA is reconverted to PI in platelets via the reactions shown in Figs. 128-1 and 128-4. With platelets labeled with $^{32}P_i$ (which will be present in ATP), PI will be labeled. There is a marked incorporation of ^{32}P into PI during and after platelet stimulation [79,260,447–450,454,455], demonstrating that PI is resynthesized. Thus, platelets possess a complete cycle for PI degradation and formation, the so-called PI cycle, which is present in all secretory cells; the PI cycle is activated upon receptor-mediated stimulation and thought to be involved in calcium mobilization [465]. In those cells in which it has been studied, the degradation of PI and subsequent phosphorylation of diglyceride

(DG) takes place in the plasma membrane and the formation of cytidine diphosphate diglyceride (CDPDG) and PI takes place in intracellular membrane systems; the transport of PA and PI across the aqueous phase between the two membrane systems is facilitated by specific exchange proteins [466]. Although the entire picture has not been worked out for platelets, there are some important similarities: the first enzyme, phospholipase C, is cytoplasmic [79,462,463]; the second enzyme, DG kinase, is membrane-bound [74]; and an exchange protein for PI is present [467]. In other cells a coupling between receptor occupancy and PI degradation has been suggested, and since phospholipase C is soluble, this degradation has been thought to be brought about by a rearrangement of the membrane-bound PI so it becomes available to phospholipase C [466]; the rearrangement of the phospholipids in the platelet plasma membrane upon stimulation [165,445,446] may be related to this PI exposure. However, no coupling between receptor occupancy and PI breakdown (or resynthesis) could be demonstrated for the platelet-thrombin system [260].

LIBERATION OF ARACHIDONATE

Sufficient platelet stimulation causes liberation of arachidonate esterified in phospholipids, and the free arachidonate is oxygenated as outlined above for resting platelets (Fig. 128-2). However, our understanding of the mechanism for this liberation is controversial, and the four alternate pathways claimed are shown in Fig. 128-4. The controversy is probably due to differences in methodology and a combination of unevenness of arachidonate distribution in the platelet membranes [468] and different phospholipase-susceptible domains in the membrane [469] which makes phospholipid hydrolysis particularly dependent on experimental conditions.

A frequently used approach is to incubate platelets with radioactive arachidonate which becomes esterified in phosphatidylcholine (PC), phosphatidylethanolamine (PE), phosphatidylserine (PS), and PI in a 55:14:14:17 proportion [77,470]. Treatment of such labeled platelets with thrombin causes loss of radioactivity from PI (60 percent decrease) and PC (40 percent decrease) with a corresponding accumulation of radioactive PA and free arachidonate and its oxygenation products [77,79,81,260,451–456,461,463,464,471]. Due to the specificities of platelet phospholipase A_2 (see below) and of phospholipase C (see above) these results suggest that platelet stimulation is associated with activation of phospholipase A_2 which causes liberation of arachidonate from PC and activation of phospholipase C which causes breakdown of PI, but without liberation of arachidonate. This labeling technique has also shown that thrombin causes incorporation of radioactive arachidonate into platelet PE plasmalogen [472], a process that is poorly understood. Labeling with $^{32}P_i$ labels PA and the lyso PA formed during thrombin stimulation [461]; inhibition of phospholipase A_2 with calmodulin inhibitors abolishes both liberation of radioactive arachidonate [383,461] and the formation of lyso PA, suggesting that PA is a source of arachidonate through activation of the PA-specific phospholipase A_2. Free arachidonate may also be produced via a phospholipase C–diglyceride lipase pathway [78,85–88,381,464, 473,474]. Further studies are needed to determine the roles of the remodeling pathway (Fig. 128-1) and the phospholipase C–diglyceride lipase pathway (Fig. 128-4).

Nevertheless, it is clear that phospholipase A_2 is involved in arachidonate liberation and that its regulation is of central importance for the modulation of platelet response through prostaglandins and thromboxanes. The enzyme is membrane-bound, stimulated by Ca^{2+} and detergents [79,474–476]; the calcium activation is enhanced by calmodulin [80], it does not hydrolyse PI, but uses PC, PE, and PS as substrates [79]; hydrolysis depends on the physical state of the substrate [474], and on its conformation in its native milieu, the platelet membrane [469], and is inhibited by certain nonsteroidal anti-inflammatory drugs, i.e., indomethacin, meclofenamate, and flufenamate [476,477].

PROTEIN METABOLISM
Stimulation of platelets is accompanied by phosphorylation, polymerization, depolymerization, and hydrolysis (proteolysis) of various proteins.

PHOSPHORYLATION
Stimulation of platelets with strong agonists leads to rapid phosphorylation of proteins of M_r 20,000, 47,000, and 260,000 daltons [360,374–378,478–481]. The 20,000-dalton protein has been identified as the 20,000-dalton myosin light chain [478]; the 47,000-dalton protein has been purified to homogeneity [482], although its physiological role remains undetermined; and the 260,000-dalton protein may be an actin-binding protein [483]. Myosin light-chain kinase is calcium-calmodulin-activated, and phosphorylation regulates actin-stimulated myosin ATPase and contractile force (see Chap. 127). Thus, the phosphorylation of myosin light chain early in the basic platelet reaction indicates that ATP-consuming contractile processes are initiated. Myosin phosphorylation may be associated with the secretory processes and not with shape change and aggregation [375–377]. However, myosin is phosphorylated up to 60 to 70 percent of maximal phosphorylation during shape change [484,485], and a calmodulin-inhibitor, W-7, inhibits phosphorylation, aggregation, and secretion in parallel [486]. It therefore seems likely that contractile processes are involved in shape change, aggregation, and secretion. Myosin is in the dephosphorylated state in resting platelets [478]; the phosphorylation seen after stimulation usually reverses, probably due to a phosphoprotein phosphatase. A membrane-bound phosphoprotein phosphatase with unknown specificity has been demonstrated in platelets [487].

The apparent close association between platelet response and calcium-dependent myosin phosphorylation strongly supports the view that platelet responses are mediated through increase in cytoplasmic Ca^{2+}. The phosphorylation of the 47,000-dalton protein is dependent on calcium; but also requires phospholipid and diglyceride for activation [488,489].

POLYMERIZATION-DEPOLYMERIZATION
The cytoplasm of resting platelets appears even and granular, while cells which have changed shape have nets of filaments in both cytoplasm and pseudopodia [490,491]; the filamentous material is insoluble in detergents (so-called cytoskeleton) and contains actin, in particular, but also myosin and various actin-binding proteins [492,493]. Actin also is accessible to labeling on the surface of activated, but not resting, platelets [494]. This exposure appears to be restricted to platelets having undergone secretion [495]. The amount of free actin monomer, G actin, decreases rapidly upon platelet stimulation, indicating rapid polymerization (G-F transformation) of this protein [496,497]. The rate of polymerization is slow during shape change, unaffected by aggregation, and rapid and more extensive during secretion [498]. The amounts of profilactin [complex between G actin (60 percent of total) and profilin; see Chap. 127] decreases during actin polymerization and that of free profilin increases, suggesting that the actin in the appearing microfilaments is derived from profilactin [493]. The functional importance of the intracellular actin polymerization following platelet stimulation can be illuminated by experiments with various cytochalasins, which inhibit platelet actin polymerization in vitro [499]. Thus, the polymerization in intact platelets induced by thrombin is inhibited by cytochalasin D [500] in parallel with inhibition of shape change [501]. Platelets that have undergone shape change become discoid in parallel with actin depolymerization when the cells are treated with cytochalasin D [501]. Little is known about the regulation of the state of actin polymerization in platelets. Furthermore, actin undergoes the rapid, endogenous depolymerization upon lysis [493,496]. Nevertheless, induction of the basic platelet reaction is clearly associated with actin polymerization, which probably plays an important role in the mechanism of shape change and secretion.

Ultrastructural alterations during platelet stimulation include disappearance and appearance of microtubules (see Chap. 126), suggesting depolymerization and polymerization of tubulin. Colchicine, an inhibitor of tubulin polymerization which also leads to the depolymerization of polymerized tubulin, inhibits platelet aggregation and secretion, an inhibition that could be counteracted by D_2O, a microtubule-stabilizing agent [502].

Although actin and tubulin polymerization-depolymerization do not involve transamination, binding of microfilaments and microtubules to other proteins may do so. A calcium-dependent transglutaminase has been described in platelets and may be responsible for the cross-linked proteins found in cytoskeleton from stimulated platelets [503].

PROTEOLYSIS

A calcium-dependent protease from platelets has been purified and characterized. It contains free SH groups that are required for its activity and one specific endogenous substrate is the high-molecular-weight actin-binding protein [504]. Proteolysis of membrane glycoprotein V has been observed during the interaction between platelets and thrombin [505–507]. Glycoprotein V has been purified and characterized [508], and thrombin-activated platelets bind isolated membranes from nonactivated platelets [509]. This significance of these findings is not yet clear.

Metabolism in inhibited platelets (the cyclic AMP system)

The complicated mechanism for initiation and performance of the basic platelet reaction can be inhibited in many ways and at various levels of interaction between the pathways involved. In the description above we have mentioned inhibition through interference with agonist binding, arachidonate liberation and oxygenation, energy metabolism, and calcium translocation. However, all platelet responses induced with all agonists listed in Table 128-1 are collectively inhibited by elevation of intracellular cyclic AMP [510–519].

METABOLISM OF CYCLIC AMP

Cyclic AMP is formed from ATP by the membrane-bound enzyme adenylate cyclase and broken down by cyclic AMP phosphodiesterase. Both enzymes are activated and inhibited by agonists that bind to specific membrane receptors or by agents that act directly on the enzymes. Adenylate cyclase has been demonstrated in platelet membranes [520–523], and several forms of platelet phosphodiesterase in both cytoplasm and membranes have been purified and characterized [524,525]. However, since the physiological activity of adenylate cyclase is regulated through agonist-receptor interaction, studies of purified enzyme have not yielded much valuable information. Since it is the intracellular level of cyclic AMP at a given time that is of importance for platelet responsivity, and since it is regulated by adenylate cyclase and phosphodiesterase, most of our knowledge about the cyclic AMP system stems from studies on intact platelets. Table 128-2 shows the agents that stimulate and inhibit adenylate cyclase and phosphodiesterase in platelets; it should be noted that many of these agents are specific for platelet cAMP metabolism, and have no effect on other cell systems.

ADENYLATE CYCLASE (AC)

Formation of cyclic AMP in intact platelets is stimulated through surface receptors by prostaglandins (PG) I_2 (prostacyclin), D_2, and E_1 and by adenosine; fluoride also stimulates cyclic AMP formation presumably by acting directly on adenylase cyclase (see Table 128-2). PGI_2 and PGE_1 share the same receptor, which is distinctly different from the receptor for PGD_2. PGI_2

TABLE 128-2   Agents that influence cyclic AMP formation in platelets

Effect	Agent	Binding to receptor	References
	ADENYLATE CYCLASE		
Promotes cyclic AMP formation	Prostaglandin I_2	Yes	[526–529]
	Prostaglandin D_2	Yes	[528–535]
	Prostaglandin E_1	Yes	[516,530,536–540]
	Adenosine and some derivatives	Yes	[518,521,538,541–543]
	Fluoride	*	[510,520,544]
Counteracts cyclic AMP formation	ADP	Yes	[515,518,530,545–549]
	Epinephrine and norepinephrine	Yes	[510,511,515,518,538, 539,545–548]
	Platelet-stimulating prostaglandins	?	[529,550–554]
	Dideoxyadenosine, SQ 22536	*	[555,562,563]
	Lithium	*	[540,556]
	CYCLIC AMP PHOSPHODIESTERASE		
Inhibits cyclic AMP hydrolysis	Methylxanthines		[516–518,538,541,565]
	Papaverine		[566–568]
	Dipyridamole and other pyrimido-pyrimidines		[517,538,568–570]

* Affects enzyme directly without receptor participation.

(prostacyclin) is produced in the endothelium (see above), and is the most potent stimulator known for platelet cyclic AMP formation, being 10 to 30 times more potent than prostaglandins E_1 and D_2. It has been suggested that PGI_2 is a circulating hormone which regulates the responsivity of circulating platelets [557], which would explain the antithrombotic effect of dipyridamole [558], a phosphodiesterase inhibitor (Table 128-2). However, the measurable levels of circulating PGI_2 are too low to produce enough platelet cyclic AMP to affect platelet responsivity [559,560]. PGD_2 is produced during platelet stimulation (see above) and has been thought to account for the increased levels of cyclic AMP found in thrombin-treated platelets [561]. Prostaglandin E_1 is probably not of importance for control of cyclic AMP in circulating platelets [537]. Adenosine can originate through breakdown of adenine nucleotides (secreted from platelets, released from damaged cells) in plasma [320] or possibly directly from damaged cells; its role for control of platelet reactivity in vivo is not known. Abolition of adenosine uptake has no effect on formation of cyclic AMP [521]. Thus, unlike the three prostaglandins discussed above, adenosine interacts with platelets in two ways: It is transported across the membrane by a specific transport system, and it interacts with the adenosine receptor on the platelet surface that controls adenylate cyclase. Fluoride stimulates cyclic AMP production in platelets as in most other cells, but the concentrations required, 2 to 4 mM, are probably too high for fluoride to be an antiplatelet agent. Optimal concentrations of prostaglandins I_2, D_2, E_1, and adenosine are 10 to 100 nM, 0.1 to 2 μM, 0.5 to 5 μM, and 2 to 10 μM, respectively.

Several platelet-stimulating agents counteract formation of cyclic AMP (Table 128-2). ADP inhibition involves a receptor that appears to be different from the receptor that mediates stimulation of the basic platelet reaction. In contrast, the catecholamine-induced inhibition of adenylate cyclase is abolished by α_2-adrenergic antagonists such as yohimbine, which also antagonizes the catecholamine-induced stimulation of the basic platelet reaction. The inhibition of adenylate cyclase by platelet-stimulating prostaglandins is even more unclear with respect to the question of the existence of specific receptors for adenylate cyclase inhibition and platelet stimulation of the basic platelet reaction. Calcium ions inhibit platelet adenylate cyclase [564], and it is therefore conceivable that platelet-stimulating agents can inhibit adenylate cyclase through their mobilization of intracellular calcium.

It has been claimed that induction of the basic platelet reaction is mediated by inhibition of adenylate cyclase [514], so that resting platelets are kept unresponding because of basal cyclic AMP production, and inhibition of cyclic AMP formation would release this cyclic AMP–induced unresponsiveness. However, specific adenylate cyclase inhibitors such as dideoxyadenosine and SQ 22536 do not stimulate platelets [562,563],

which makes this mechanism unlikely unless compartmentalization plays a significant role. The platelet adenylate cyclase is inhibited by lithium in therapeutic doses.

CYCLIC AMP PHOSPHODIESTERASE

Two forms of phosphodiesterase have been described in platelets, a type I with low affinity to cyclic AMP in the cytoplasm and a type II with high affinity partially associated with membranes [524,525]; the high-affinity enzyme is stimulated by epinephrine and inhibited by prostaglandin E_1, effects that probably are mediated through receptors to the membrane-bound enzyme [524,525]. The low-affinity enzyme is inhibited by dipyridamole, aminophylline, and 6-mercaptopurine [571]. Partially purified phosphodiesterase is also inhibited by adenosine and 2-chloroadenosine [572,573] as well as PGE_1 [525], while it is stimulated by ADP [525]. These substances also influence the formation in intact platelets of cyclic AMP by adenylate cyclase (above); thus, the regulation of intraplatelet cyclic AMP levels by these compounds is apparently very complex.

Some agents that appear to be without effect on adenylate cyclase and that inhibit phosphodiesterase are listed in Table 128-2. They have been widely used in combination with adenylate cyclase stimulators to cause maximal elevation of platelet cyclic AMP. The IC_{50} for some of these substances has been estimated on partially purified phosphodiesterase: papaverine, 5 μM; dipyridamole, 17 μM, theophylline, 0.8 mM, and caffeine, 7 mM [568].

MECHANISM OF INHIBITION OF PLATELET STIMULATION BY INCREASED LEVELS OF CYCLIC AMP

It has been clearly established that the inhibition of the basic platelet reaction by substances that affect formation and destruction of cyclic AMP (Table 128-2) is directly related to the presence of intracellular cyclic AMP at the moment of stimulation. Any direct effect of the substances can be disregarded, since elevation of intracellular cyclic AMP by the penetrable dibutyryl–cyclic AMP causes the same inhibition as when cyclic AMP is formed within the platelets. Furthermore, all responses in the basic platelet reaction are inhibited; inhibition can be overcome by increase of stimulus. It is therefore generally accepted that the major effect of cyclic AMP must be on steps that are common for all responses in the basic platelet reaction.

Elevation of cyclic AMP levels in platelets leads to phosphorylation of distinct proteins which, although different from those phosphorylated during platelet stimulation, have not been clearly identified [360,378, 574]. Proteins that bind cyclic AMP in platelets have been demonstrated [575] and various cyclic AMP-dependent protein kinases have been demonstrated [574, 576–580], although the identification of the kinases or their endogenous substrates is not known.

The uptake of calcium by platelet microsomes is

stimulated by cyclic AMP [581] concomitantly with a cyclic AMP–dependent phosphorylation of a M_r 22,000-dalton protein in the microsomes [582]; this may be the same M_r 22,000-dalton protein that is phosphorylated in intact platelets treated with substances that stimulate adenylate cyclase [360,378,574]. A role of cyclic AMP in stimulating the transport of Ca from cytoplasm to vesicular storage sites, would be in agreement with the inhibition observed: platelet responses are stimulated by increase in cytoplasmic calcium and inhibited by removal of this calcium by a cyclic AMP–dependent uptake system.

Cyclic AMP may also specifically inhibit phosphorylation of myosin light chain, since the corresponding kinase can be regulated by phosphorylation by cyclic AMP–dependent protein kinase [583]. Since myosin phosphorylation appears to be intimately associated with shape change and secretion, cyclic AMP may inhibit these responses by directly interfering with myosin phosphorylation.

References

1. Day, H. J., Holmsen, H., and Zucker, M. B.: International Committee Communication: Report on the working party on platelets. *Thromb. Haemost. 36*:263, 1976.
2. Karpatkin, S.: Heterogeneity of human platelets: Metabolic and kinetic evidence suggestive of young and old platelets. *J. Clin. Invest. 48*:1083, 1969.
3. Karpatkin, S., Charmatz, A. and Langer, R. M.: Glycogenesis and glycogeneogenesis in human platelets: Incorporation of glucose, pyruvate, and citrate into platelet glycogen: Glycogen synthetase and fructose-1-6-diphosphatase activity. *J. Clin. Invest. 49*:140, 1970.
4. Luganova, I. S., Seits, I. F., and Teodorovich, V.: Metabolism in human thrombocytes. *Biochemistry (U.S.S.R.) 23*:379, 1958.
5. Chernyak, N. B.: Process of formation and utilization of energy in human platelets. *Clin. Chim. Acta 12*:244, 1965.
6. Detwiler, T. C., and Zivkovic, R. V.: Control of energy metabolism in platelets: A comparison of aerobic and anaerobic metabolism in washed rat platelets. *Biochim. Biophys. Acta 197*:117, 1970.
7. Doery, J. C. G., Hirsh, J., and Cooper, I.: Energy metabolism in human platelets: Interrelationship between glycolysis and oxidative metabolism. *Blood 36*:159, 1970.
8. Doery, J. C. G., Hirsh, J., and de Gruchy, G. C.: Platelet metabolism and function. *Haematologia 4*:405, 1970.
9. Wu, R., Sessa, G., and Hammerman, D.: P_i transport and glycolysis in leukocytes and platelets. *Biochim. Biophys. Acta 93*:614, 1964.
10. Karpatkin, S.: Studies on human platelet glycolysis: Effect of glucose, cyanide, insulin, citrate and agglutination and contraction on platelet glycolysis. *J. Clin. Invest. 46*:409, 1967.
11. Detwiler, T. C.: Control of energy metabolism in platelets: The effects of thrombin and cyanide on glycolysis. *Biochim. Biophys. Acta 256*:163, 1972.
12. Akkerman, J. W. N., Gorter, G., and Sixma, J. J.: Regulation of glycolytic flux in human platelets: Relation between energy production by glyco(geno)lysis and energy consumption. *Biochim. Biophys. Acta 541*:241, 1981.
13. Holmsen, H., and Robkin, L.: Effects of antimycin A and 2-deoxyglucose on energy metabolism in washed human platelets. *Thromb. Haemost. 42*:1460, 1980.
14. Chaiken, R., Pagano, D., and Detwiler, T. C.: Regulation of platelet phosphorylase. *Biochim. Biophys. Acta 403*:315, 1975.
15. Akkerman, J. W. N., and Gorter, G.: The relation between energy production and adenine nucleotide metabolism in human blood platelets. *Biochim. Biophys. Acta 590*:107, 1980.
16. Solomon, H. M., and Gaut, Z. N.: Accumulation and metabolism of 2-deoxyglucose-1-^{14}C in the human platelet. *Biochem. Pharmacol. 19*:2631, 1970.
17. Detwiler, T. C.: Effects of deoxyglucose on platelet metabolism. *Biochim. Biophys. Acta 244*:303, 1971.
18. Warshaw, A. L., Laster, L., and Shulman, N. R.: The stimulation by thrombin of glucose oxidation in human platelets. *J. Clin. Invest. 45*:1923, 1966.
19. McDonagh, J., Jr., Burns, M. J., Delaimi, K. E., and Faust, R. G.: Sugar penetration into human blood platelets. *J. Cell. Physiol. 72*:77, 1968.
20. Chaudry, A. A., Sagone, A. L., Metz, E. N., and Balcerzak, S. P.: Relationship of glucose oxidation to aggregation of human platelets. *Blood 41*:249, 1973.
21. Cowan, D. H.: Platelet metabolism in acute leukemia. *J. Lab. Clin. Med. 82*:54, 1973.
22. Doery, J. C. G., Hirsch, J., and de Gruchy, G. C.: Platelet glycolytic enzymes: Effects of cellular disruption procedures on activity. *Br. J. Haematol. 19*:145, 1970.
23. Doery, J. C. G., Hirsh, J., Loder, P., and de Gruchy, G. C.: Distribution of platelet hexokinase and the effect of collagen. *Nature 216*:1317, 1967.
24. Akkerman, J. W. N.: Regulation of carbohydrate metabolism in platelets: A review. *Thromb. Haemost. 39*:712, 1978.
25. Karpatkin, S., and Strick, N.: Heterogeneity of human platelets: V. Changes in glycolytic enzymes with possible relation to platelet age. *J. Clin. Invest. 51*:5, 1972.
26. Holmsen, H., Day, H. J., and Pimentel, M. A.: Adenine nucleotide metabolism of blood platelets. V. Subcellular localization and kinetics of some related enzymes. *Biochim. Biophys. Acta 186*:244, 1969.
27. Waller, H. D., Löhr, G. W., Grignani, F., and Gross, R.: Über den Energiestoffwechsel normaler menschlicher Thrombozyten. *Thromb. Diath. Haemorrh. 3*:520, 1959.
28. Howard, L., Shulman, S., Sadanaudan, S., and Karpatkin, S.: Crossed immunoelectrophoresis of human platelet membranes: Presence of a major antigen consisting of glycoproteins IIb, IIIa, and Ca^{++}. *J. Biol. Chem. 257*:8331, 1982.
29. Detwiler, T. C.: Levels of intermediates and cofactors of the glycolytic pathway and the citric acid cycle in rat platelets. *Biochim. Biophys. Acta 177*:161, 1969.
30. Akkerman, J. W. N., Gorter, G., Sixma, J. J., and Staal, G. E. J.: Variations in the levels of glycolytic intermediates in human platelets during platelet-collagen interaction. *Biochim. Biophys. Acta 421*:296, 1976.
31. Schrijver, J., Koster, J. F., and Hulsman, W. C.: Insignificance of gluconeogenesis in human platelets. *Eur. J. Clin. Invest. 5*:7, 1975.
32. Steiner, M., and Kuramoto, A.: Energy metabolism of aggregating platelets. *Ser. Haematol. 4*:98, 1971.
33. Holmsen, H., and Robkin, L.: Hydrogen peroxide lowers ATP levels in platelets without altering adenylate energy charge and platelet function. *J. Biol. Chem. 252*:1752, 1977.
34. Koufos, A., and Sagone, A. L.: Effects of oxidant stress on the hexose monophosphate shunt pathway of platelets. *Blood 55*:835, 1980.
35. Holmsen, H., Robkin, L., and Driver, H. A.: Reduction of the metabolic adenylate pool in platelets by hydroperoxides (HP): Studies on the mechanisms. *Fed. Proc. 38*:826, 1979.
36. Holmsen, H.: Biochemistry of the platelet: Energy metabolism, in *Hemostasis and Thrombosis: Basic Concepts and Clinical Practice*, edited by R. W. Colman, J. Hirsh, V. J. Marder, and E. W. Salzman. Lippincott, Philadelphia, 1982, p. 431.
37. Moser, K., Lechner, K., and Vinazzer, H.: A hitherto not described defect in thrombasthenia: Glutathione reductase deficiency. *Thromb. Diath. Haemorrh. 19*:46, 1968.
38. Karpatkin, S., and Weiss, H. J.: Deficiency of glutathione peroxidase associated with high levels of reduced glutathione in Glanzmann's thrombasthenia. *N. Engl. J. Med. 287*:1062, 1972.
39. Vainer, H., and Wattiaux, R.: Glycogen synthetase activity in blood platelets. *Nature 217*:951, 1968.
40. Karpatkin, S., and Charmatz, A.: Heterogeneity of human platelets. III. Glycogen metabolism in platelets of different sizes. *Br. J. Haematol. 19*:135, 1970.

41. Aguilar, J., and Rosell-Perez, M.: Studies on glycogen metabolism in the human platelet. I. Characteristics and regulation of the glycogen synthetase. *Rev. Esp. Fisiol.* 31:151, 1975.
42. Aguilar, J., and Rosell-Perez, M.: Studies on glycogen metabolism in the human platelet. II. Metabolic levels and enzymes of the glycogen cycle. *Rev. Esp. Fisiol.* 31:163, 1975.
43. Gear, A. R. L., and Schneider, W.: Control of platelet glycogenolysis: Activation of phosphorylase kinase by calcium. *Biochim. Biophys. Acta* 392:111, 1975.
44. Scott, R. B.: Activation of glycogen phosphorylase in blood platelets. *Blood* 30:321, 1967.
45. Scott, R. B., and Still, W. J. S.: Glycogen in human blood platelets: Isolation by ultracentrifugation and characteristics of the isolated particles. *Blood* 35:517, 1970.
46. Fukami, M. H., Salganicoff, L., and Bauer, J.: Pig platelet amylo-1, 6-glucosidase-subcellular localization and possible activation by thrombin. Vth Congr. Int. Soc. Thromb. Haem., Paris, 1975, abstract 438.
47. Gergely, P., Castle, A. G., and Crawford, N.: Platelet phosphorylase kinase activity and its regulation by the calcium-dependent regulatory protein; calmodulin. *Biochim. Biophys. Acta* 612:50, 1980.
48. Karpatkin, S., and Langer, R. M.: Activation of inactive phosphorylase dimer and monomer from human platelets with magnesium ATP. *J. Biol. Chem.* 244:1953, 1969.
49. Karpatkin, S., and Langer, R. M.: Human platelet phosphorylase. *Biochim. Biophys. Acta* 185:350, 1969.
50. Yunis, A. A., and Arimura, G. K.: Isoenzymes of glycogen phosphorylase in human leukocytes and platelets: Relation to muscle phosphorylase. *Biochem. Biophys. Res. Commun.* 33:119, 1968.
51. Karpatkin, S., Braun, J., and Charmatz, A.: Requirement of divalent cation for human platelet phosphorylase activity. *Biochim. Biophys. Acta* 220:22, 1970.
52. Kerby, G. P., and Taylor, S. M.: The effect of added ATP on the pathways of glucose utilization by human washed platelets in vitro. *J. Lab. Clin. Med.* 69:194, 1967.
53. Salganicoff, L., Hebda, P. A., Yandrasitz, J., and Fukami, M. H.: Subcellular fractionation of pig platelets. *Biochim. Biophys. Acta* 385:394, 1975.
54. Fukami, M. H., and Salganicoff, L.: Isolation and properties of human platelet mitochondria. *Blood* 42:913, 1973.
55. Nakamura, N., Zuppinger, K. A., Colombo, J. P., and Walter, P.: Synthesis of glucose in human thrombocytes. *Metabolism* 22:29, 1973.
56. Tegos, C., and Beutler, E.: Platelet glycolysis in platelet storage. III. The inability of platelets to utilize exogenous citrate. *Transfusion* 19:601, 1979.
57. Czapek, E. E., Deykin, D., and Salzman, E. W.: Platelet dysfunction in glycogen storage disease type I. *Blood* 41:235, 1973.
58. Majerus, P. W., Smith, M. B., and Clamos, G. H.: Lipid metabolism in human platelets. I. Evidence for a complete fatty acid synthesizing system. *J. Clin. Invest.* 48:156, 1965.
59. Awai, K., and Hennes, A. R.: Studies of incorporation of radioactivity into lipids by human blood. II. Pattern of incorporation of radioactivity into fatty acids by platelets from normal subjects and patients in diabetic acidosis. *Diabetes* 13:592, 1964.
60. Hennes, A. R., Awai, K., Hammarstrand, K., and Duboff, G.: Carbon-14 in carboxyl carbon of fatty acids formed by platelets from normal and diabetic subjects. *Nature* 210:839, 1966.
61. Deykin, D., and Desser, R. K.: The incorporation of acetate and palmitate into lipids by human platelets. *J. Clin. Invest.* 47:1590, 1968.
62. Pittman, J. G., and Martin, D. B.: Fatty acid biosynthesis in human erythrocytes: Evidence in mature erythrocytes for an incomplete long-chain fatty acid synthesizing system. *J. Clin. Invest.* 45:165, 1966.
63. Majerus, P. W., and Laster, R.: Fatty acid biosynthesis in human leukocytes. *J. Clin. Invest.* 46:1595, 1967.
64. Marks, P. A., Gellhorn, A., and Kidson, C.: Lipid synthesis in human leukocytes, platelets, and erythrocytes. *J. Biol. Chem.* 235:2579, 1960.
65. Hennes, A. R., and Awai, K.: Studies of incorporation of radioactivity into lipids by human blood. IV. Abnormal incorporation

of acetate 1-C-14 into fatty acids by whole blood and platelets from insulin independent diabetics. *Diabetes* 14:709, 1965.
66. Hennes, A. R., Awai, K., and Hammarstrand, K.: Studies of incorporation of radioactivity into lipids by human blood. V. Pattern of fatty acid radioactivity in lipid fractions of platelets. *Biochim. Biophys. Acta* 84:610, 1964.
67. Zieve, P. D., and Schmucler, M.: Stimulation by glucose of fatty acid synthesis in human platelets. *Am. J. Physiol.* 219:1009, 1970.
68. Spector, A. A., Hoak, J. C., Warner, E. D., and Fry, G. L.: Utilization of long-chain free fatty acids by human platelets. *J. Clin. Invest.* 49:1489, 1970.
69. Deykin, D., and Desser, R. K.: The incorporation of acetate and palmitate into lipids by human platelets. *J. Clin. Invest.* 47:1590, 1968.
70. Okuma, M., Yamashita, S., and Numa, S.: Enzymic studies on phosphatidic acid synthesis in human platelets. *Blood* 41:379, 1973.
71. Call, F. L., II, and Williams, W. J.: Biosynthesis of cytidine diphosphate diglyceride by human platelets. *J. Clin. Invest.* 49:392, 1970.
72. Lucas, C. T., Call, F. L., II, and Williams, W. J.: The biosynthesis of phosphatidylinositol by human platelets. *J. Clin. Invest.* 49:1949, 1970.
73. Call, F. L., and Williams, W. J.: Phosphatidate phosphatase in human platelets. *J. Lab. Clin. Med.* 82:663, 1973.
74. Call, F. L., and Rubert, M.: Diglyceride kinase in human platelets. *J. Lipid Res.* 14:466, 1973.
75. Elsbach, P., Pettis, P., and Marcus, A.: Lysolecithin metabolism by human platelets. *Blood* 37:675, 1971.
76. Call, F. L., and Rupert, M.: Synthesis of ethanolamine phosphoglycerides by human platelets. *J. Lipid Res.* 16:352, 1975.
77. Bills, T. K., Smith, J. B., and Silver, M. J.: Metabolism of ^{14}C-arachidonic acid by human platelets. *Biochim. Biophys. Acta* 424:303, 1976.
78. Cohen, P., Broekman, M. J., Verkley, A., Lismann, J. W. W., and Derksen, A. L.: Quantification of human platelet inosities and the influence of ionic environment on their incorporation of orthophosphate-^{32}P. *J. Clin. Invest.* 50:762, 1971.
79. Billah, M. M., Lapetina, E. G., and Cuatrecasas, P.: Phospholipase A_2 and phospholipase C activities of platelets. Differential substrate specificity, Ca^{2+} requirement, pH dependence, and cellular localization. *J. Biol. Chem.* 255:10227, 1980.
80. Wong, P. Y.-K., and Cheung, W. Y.: Calmodulin stimulates human platelet phospholipase A_2. *Biochem. Biophys. Res. Commun.* 90:473, 1979.
81. Rittenhouse-Simmons, S., and Deykin, D.: The activation by Ca^{2+} of platelet phospholipase A_2: Effects of dibutyryl cyclic adenosine monophosphate and 8(N,N-diethyl amino)-octyl-3,4,5-trimethoxybenzoate. *Biochim. Biophys. Acta* 543:409, 1978.
82. Silk, S. T., Wong, K. T., and Marcus, A. J.: Arachidonic acid releasing activity in platelet membranes: Effects of sulfhydryl-modifying agents. *Biochemistry* 20:391, 1981.
83. Lagarde, M., Menashi, S., and Crawford, N.: Localization of phospholipase A_2 and diglyceride lipase activities in human platelet intracellular membranes. *FEBS Lett.* 124:23, 1981.
84. McKean, M. L., Smith, J. B., and Silver, M. J.: Phospholipid biosynthesis in human platelets: Formation of phosphotidylcholine from 1-acyl lysophosphotidylcholine by acyl CoA: 1-acyl-sn-glycerol-3-phosphocholine acyltransferase. *J. Biol. Chem.* 257:11278, 1982.
85. Marcus, A. J., Ullman, H. L., and Safier, L. B.: Lipid composition of subcellular particles of human blood platelets. *J. Lipid Res.* 10:108, 1969.
86. Broekman, M. J., Handin, R. I., Derksen, A., and Cohen, P.: Distribution of phospholipid, fatty acids, and platelet factor 3 activity among subcellular fractions of human platelets. *Blood* 47:963, 1976.
87. Prescott, S. M., and Majerus, P. W.: The fatty acid composition of phosphatidyl inositol from thrombin-stimulated human platelets. *J. Biol. Chem.* 256:579, 1981.
88. Broekman, M. J., Ward, J. W., and Marcus, A. J.: Fatty acid composition of phosphatidyl inositol and phosphatidic acid in stimulated platelets. *J. Biol. Chem.* 256:8271, 1981.
89. Hotchkiss, A., Jordan, J. V., Hirata, F., Shulman, N. R., and Axel-

rod, J.: Phospholipid methylation and human platelet function. *Biochem. Pharmacol. 30*:2089, 1981.

90. Shattil, S. J., McDonough, M., and Burch, J. W.: Inhibition of platelet phospholipid methylation during platelet secretion. *Blood 57*:537, 1981.

91. Berge, R. K., Vollset, S. E., and Farstad, M.: Intracellular localization of palmitoyl CoA hydrolase and synthetase in human blood platelets and liver. *Scand. J. Clin. Lab. Med. 40*:271, 1980.

92. Berge, R. K., Hagen, L. E., and Farstad, M.: Isolation of palmitoyl CoA hydrolase from human blood platelets. *Biochem. J. 199*:639, 1981.

93. Cohen, P., and Wittels, B.: Energy substrate metabolism in fresh and stored human platelets. *J. Clin. Invest. 49*:119, 1970.

94. Donabedian, R., and Nemerson, Y.: Fatty acid oxidation by human platelets and its stimulation by thrombin. *Am. J. Physiol. 221*:1283, 1971.

95. Sander, J., and Farstad, M.: Carnitine palmityltransferase and its relation to palmityl-CoA synthetase in blood platelets from fasting and healthy subjects. *Scand. J. Clin. Lab. Invest. 32*:183, 1973.

96. Giret, M., and Villanueva, V. R.: On the presence of carnitine acetyl transferase in human platelets. *Mol. Cell Biochem. 37*:65, 1981.

97. Grossman, C. M., and Kohn, R.: Enzymatic characteristics in in vitro incorporation of P^{32}-orthophosphate into human platelet phosphatides. *Thromb. Diath. Haemorrh. 13*:126, 1965.

98. Grossman, C. M., and Bartos, F.: Succinate dependence of in vitro incorporation of P^{32}-orthophosphate into human platelet phosphatide. *Arch. Biochem. Biophys. 128*:231, 1968.

99. Firkin, B. G., and Williams, W. J.: The incorporation of radioactive phosphorus into the phospholipids of human leukemic leukocytes and platelets. *J. Clin. Invest. 40*:423, 1961.

100. Westerman, M. P., and Jensen, W. N.: The in vitro incorporation of radiophosphorus into the phosphatides of normal human platelets. *Blood 20*:796, 1962.

101. Holmsen, H.: Incorporation in vitro of P^{32} into blood platelet acid soluble organophosphates and their chromatographic identification. *Scand. J. Clin. Lab. Invest. 17*:230, 1965.

102. Lewis, N., and Majerus, P. W.: Lipid metabolism in human platelets. II. *De novo* phospholipid synthesis and the effect of thrombin on the pattern of synthesis. *J. Clin. Invest. 48*:2114, 1969.

103. Stuart, M. J., Gerrard, J. M., and White, J. G.: The influence of albumin and calcium on human platelet arachidonic acid metabolism. *Blood 55*:418, 1980.

104. Gerrard, J. M., White, J. G., Rao, R. H. R., and Townsend, W.: Localization of platelet prostaglandin production in the dense tubular system. *Am. J. Pathol. 8*:283, 1976.

105. Hamberg, M., and Samuelsson, B.: Prostaglandin endoperoxides: Novel transformations of arachidonic acid in human platelets. *Proc. Natl. Acad. Sci. U.S.A. 71*:3400, 1974.

106. Hamberg, M., Svensson, J., Wakabayashi, T., and Samuelsson, B.: Isolation and structure of two prostaglandin endoperoxides that cause platelet aggregation. *Proc. Natl. Acad. Sci. U.S.A. 71*:345, 1974.

107. Hamberg, M., Svensson, J., and Samuelsson, B.: Prostaglandin endoperoxides: A new concept concerning the mode of action and release of prostaglandins. *Proc. Natl. Acad. Sci. U.S.A. 71*:3824, 1974.

108. Hamberg, M., Svensson, J., Wakabayashi, T., and Samuelsson, B.: Isolation and structure of two prostaglandin endoperoxides that cause platelet aggregation. *Proc. Natl. Acad. Sci. U.S.A. 71*:345, 1974.

109. Nugteren, D. H., and Hazelhof, E.: Isolation and properties of intermediates in prostaglandin synthesis. *Biochem. Biophys. Acta 326*:448, 1973.

110. Miyamoto, T., Yamamoto, S., and Hayishi, O.: Prostaglandin synthetase system—Resolution into oxygenase and isomerase components. *Proc. Natl. Acad. Sci. U.S.A. 71*:3645, 1974.

111. Ho, P. P., Towner, R. D., and Esterman, M. A.: Purification and characterization of fatty acid cyclooxygenase from human platelets. *Prep. Biochem. 10*:597, 1980.

112. Cinti, D. L., and Feinstein, M. B.: Platelet cytochrome P-450: A possible role in arachidonate-induced aggregation. *Biochem. Biophys. Res. Commun. 73*:171, 1976.

113. Egan, R. W., Paxton, J., and Kuchi, F. A., Jr.: Mechanism for irreversible self-deactivation of prostaglandin synthetase. *J. Biol. Chem. 251*:7329, 1976.

114. Lapetina, E. G., and Cuatrecasas, P.: Rapid inactivation of cyclo-

oxygenase activity after stimulation of intact platelets. *Proc. Natl. Acad. Sci. U.S.A. 76*:121, 1979.

115. Smith, J. B., and Willis, A. L.: Aspirin selectively inhibits prostaglandin production in human platelets. *Nature 231*:235, 1971.

116. Roth, G. J., and Majerus, P. W.: The mechanism of the effect of aspirin on human platelets. I. Acetylation of a particulate fraction protein. *J. Clin. Invest. 56*:624, 1975.

117. Roth, G. J., Stanford, N., and Majerus, P. W.: The acetylation of prostaglandin synthetase by aspirin. *Proc. Natl. Acad. Sci. U.S.A. 72*:3073, 1975.

118. Vargaftig, B. B.: The inhibition of cyclooxygenase of rabbit platelets by aspirin is prevented by salicylic acid and by phenanthrolines. *Eur. J. Pharm. 50*:231, 1978.

119. Merino, J., Livio, M., Rajter, G., and DeGaetano, G.: Salicylate reverses in vitro aspirin inhibition of rat platelets and vascular prostaglandin formation. *Biochem. Pharmacol. 29*:1093, 1980.

120. Ali, M., and McDonald, J. W.: Interference by sulfinpyrazone and salicylate of aspirin inhibition of platelet cyclooxygenase activity. *Prostaglandins Med. 3*:327, 1979.

121. Stuart, M. J., Murphy, S., and Oski, F. A.: A simple nonradioisotope technique for the determination of platelet life-span. *N. Engl. J. Med. 292*:1310, 1975.

122. Catalano, P. M., Smith, J. B., and Murphy, S.: Platelet recovery from aspirin inhibition in vivo: Differing patterns under various assay conditions. *Blood 57*:99, 1981.

123. Smith, J. B., Ingerman, C. M., and Silver, M. J.: Malondialdehyde formation as an indicator of prostaglandin production by human platelets. *J. Lab. Clin. Med. 88*:167, 1976.

124. Hamberg, M., and Fredholm, B. B.: Isomerization of prostaglandin H_2 into prostaglandin D_2 in the presence of serum albumin. *Biochim. Biophys. Acta 431*:189, 1976.

125. Christ-Hazelhof, E., Nugteren, D. H., and Van Dorp, D. A.: Conversions of prostaglandin endoperoxides by glutathione-S-transferases and serum albumin. *Biochim. Biophys. Acta 456*:450, 1976.

126. Smith, J. B., Ingerman, C. M., and Silver, M. J.: Formation of prostaglandin D_2 during endoperoxide-induced platelet aggregation. *Thromb. Res. 9*:413, 1976.

127. Raz, A., and Aharony, D.: Prostaglandin biosynthesis in platelets. Demonstration and role of prostaglandin H_2-E_2 isomerase. *Res. Commun. Chem. Pathol. Pharmacol. 21*:507, 1978.

128. McMillan, R. M., MacIntyre, D. E., Booth, A., and Gordon, J. L.: Malondialdehyde formation in intact platelets is catalyzed by thromboxane synthetase. *Biochem. J. 176*:595, 1978.

129. Hamberg, M., Svensson, J., and Samuelsson, B.: Thromboxanes: A new group of biologically active compounds derived from prostaglandin endoperoxides. *Proc. Natl. Acad. Sci. U.S.A. 72*:2994, 1975.

130. Needleman, P., Moncada, S., Bunting, S., Vane, J. R., Hamberg, M., and Samuelsson, B.: Identification of an enzyme in platelet microsomes which generates thromboxane A_2 from prostaglandin endoperoxides. *Nature 261*:558, 1976.

131. Ho, P. P. K., Walters, C. P., and Sullivan, H. R.: Biosynthesis of thromboxane B_2-assay, isolation and properties of the enzyme system in human platelets. *Prostaglandins 12*:951, 1976.

132. Sun, F. F.: Biosynthesis of thromboxanes in human platelets. I. Characterization and assay of thromboxane synthetase. *Biochem. Biophys. Res. Commun. 74*:1432, 1977.

133. Tai, H. H., and Yuan, B.: Studies on the thromboxane synthesizing system in human platelet microsomes. *Biochim. Biophys. Acta 531*:286, 1978.

134. Best, L. C., Jones, P. B. B., and Russell, R. G. G.: Evidence that extracellular calcium ions inhibit thromboxane B_2 biosynthesis by human platelets. *Biochem. Biophys. Res. Commun. 90*:1179, 1979.

135. Needleman, P., Raz, A., Ferrendelli, J. A., and Minkes, M.: Application of imidazole as a selective inhibitor of thromboxane synthetase in human platelets. *Proc. Natl. Acad. Sci. U.S.A. 74*:1716, 1977.

136. Gorman, R. R., Bundy, G. G., Peterson, D. D., Sua, F. F., Miller, D. V., and Fitzpatrick, F. A.: Inhibition of human platelet thromboxane synthetase by 9,11-azoprosta-5,13-dienoic acid. *Proc. Natl. Acad. Sci. U.S.A. 74*:4007, 1977.

137. Needleman, P., et al.: Thromboxane synthetase inhibitors as pharmacological tools—Differential biochemical and biological effects on platelet suspensions. *Prostaglandins 14*:897, 1977.

138. Tai, H. H., Tai, C. L., and Lee, N.: Selective inhibition of thromboxane synthetase by pyridine and its derivatives. *Arch. Biochem. Biophys. 203:758, 1980.*

139. Cross, P. E., Dickinson, R. P., Parry, M. J., and Randall, M. J.: 3-(1-Imidazoylmethyl) indoles: Potent and selective inhibitors of human blood platelet thromboxane synthetase. *Agents Actions 11:274, 1981.*

140. Randall, M. J., Parry, M. J., Hawkeswood, E., Cross, P. E., and Dickinson, R. P.: UK-37,248, a novel, selective thromboxane synthetase inhibitor with platelets anti-aggregatory and anti-thrombotic activity. *Thromb. Res. 23:145, 1981.*

141. Gorman, R. R., Maxey, K. M., and Bundy, G. L.: Inhibition of human platelet thromboxane synthetase by 11A-carbothromboxane A$_2$ analogs. *Biochem. Biophys. Res. Commun. 100:184, 1981.*

142. Smith, J. B., Ingerman, C., and Silver, M. J.: Persistence of thromboxane A$_2$-like material and platelet release-inducing material in plasma. *J. Clin. Invest. 58:1119, 1976.*

143. Kon, H., Inoue, A., Mashimo, N., Numano, F., and Maezawa, H.: A radioimmunoassay of thromboxane B$_2$ with thromboxane B$_2$-^{125}I-1-tyramide and its application for the study of the thromboxane B$_2$ formation during platelet aggregation. *Thromb. Res. 17:403, 1980.*

144. Nugteren, D. H.: Arachidonate lipoxygenase in blood platelets. *Biochim. Biophys. Acta 380:299, 1975.*

145. Ho, P. P. K., Walters, C. P., and Sullivan, H. R.: A particulate arachidonate lipoxygenase in human blood platelets. *Biochem. Biophys. Res. Commun. 76:398, 1977.*

146. Hamberg, M., and Hamberg, G.: On the mechanism of the oxygenation of arachidonic acid by human platelet lipoxygenase. *Biochem. Biophys. Res. Commun. 95:1090, 1980.*

147. Greenwald, J. E., Alexander, M. S., Fertel, R. H., Beach, C. A., Wong, L. K., and Bianchine, J. R.: Role of ferric iron in platelet lipoxygenase activity. *Biochem. Biophys. Res. Commun. 96:817, 1980.*

148. Aharony, D., Smith, J. B., and Silver, M. J.: Inhibition of platelet lipoxygenase by toluene-3,4-dithiol and other ferric iron chelators. *Prostaglandins Med. 6:237, 1981.*

149. Bryant, R. H., and Bailey, J. M.: Altered lipoxygenase metabolism and decreased glutathione peroxidase activity in platelets from selenium-deficient rats. *Biochem. Biophys. Res. Commun. 92:268, 1980.*

150. Turner, S. R., Tainer, J. A., and Lynn, W. S.: Biogenesis of chemotactic molecules by the arachidonate lipoxygenase of platelets. *Nature 257:680, 1975.*

151. Siegel, M. I., McConnell, R. T., Abrahams, S. L., Porter, N. A., and Cuatrecasas, P.: Regulation of arachidonate metabolism via lipoxygenase and cyclooxygenase by 12-HPETE, the product of human platelet lipoxygenase. *Biochem. Biophys. Res. Commun. 89:1273, 1979.*

152. Aharony, D., Smith, J. B., and Silver, M. J.: Inhibition of platelet aggregation, malonyldialdehyde formation and thromboxane function by hydroperoxides of arachidonic acid. *Biochim. Biophys. Acta 718:193, 1982.*

153. Hirai, A., et al.: Eicosapentaenoic acid and platelet function in Japanese. *Lancet 2:1132, 1980.*

154. Hamberg, M.: Transformation of 5,8,11,14,17-eicosapentaenoic acid in human platelets. *Biochim. Biophys. Acta 618:389, 1980.*

155. Falardeau, P., Hamberg, M., and Samuelsson, B.: Metabolism of 8,11,14-eicosatrienoic acid in human platelets. *Biochim. Biophys. Acta 441:193, 1976.*

156. Blackwell, G. J., and Flower, R. J.: 1-Phenyl-3-pyrazolidine-inhibitor of cyclooxygenase and lipoxygenase pathways in lung and platelets. *Prostaglandins 16:417, 1978.*

157. Hammarstrom, S.: Selective inhibition of platelet n-8 lipoxygenase by 5,8,11-eicosatriynoic acid. *Biochim. Biophys. Acta 487:517, 1977.*

158. Bunting, S., Gryglewski, R., Moncada, S., and Vane, J. R.: Arterial walls generate from prostaglandin endoperoxides a substance (prostaglandin X) which relaxes strips of mesenteric and coeliac arteries and inhibits platelet aggregation. *Prostaglandins 12:897, 1976.*

159. Johnson, R. A., et al.: The chemical structure of prostaglandin X (prostacyclin). *Prostaglandins 12:915, 1976.*

160. Weksler, B. B., Marcus, A. J., and Jaffe, E. A.: Synthesis of prostaglandin I$_2$ (prostacyclin) by cultured human and bovine endothelial cells. *Proc. Natl. Acad. Sci. U.S.A. 74:3922, 1977.*

161. MacIntyre, D. E., Pearson, J. D., and Gordon, J. L.: Localization and stimulation of prostacyclin production in vascular cells. *Nature 271:549, 1978.*

162. Hornstra, G., Haddeman, E., and Don, J. A.: Blood platelets do not provide endoperoxides for vascular prostacyclin production. *Nature 279:66, 1979.*

163. Marcus, A. J., Weksler, B. B., Jaffe, E. A., and Broekman, M. J.: Synthesis of prostacyclin from platelet-derived endoperoxides by cultured human endothelial cells. *J. Clin. Invest. 66:979, 1980.*

164. Tao, R. V. P., Sweeley, C. C., and Jamieson, G. A.: Sphingolipid composition of human platelets. *J. Lipid Res. 14:16, 1973.*

165. Wang, C. T., and Schick, P. K.: The effect of thrombin on the organization of human platelet membrane glycosphingolipids. *J. Biol. Chem. 256:752, 1981.*

166. Hughes, H. N., and Liberti, J. P.: In vitro synthesis of glycosyl ceramide in rabbit platelets. *Biochem. Biophys. Res. Commun. 63:555, 1975.*

167. Rozenberg, M. C., and Holmsen, H.: Adenine nucleotide metabolism of blood platelets. II. Uptake of adenosine and inhibition of ADP-induced platelet aggregation. *Biochim. Biophys. Acta 155:342, 1968.*

168. Holmsen, H., Setkowsky, C., and Day, H. J.: Effects of antimycin and 2-deoxyglucose on adenine nucleotides in human platelets. *Biochem. J. 144:385, 1974.*

169. Kattlove, H.: Platelet ATP in ADP-induced aggregation. *Am. J. Physiol. 226:325, 1974.*

170. Holmsen, H., and Rozenberg, M. C.: Adenine nucleotide metabolism of blood platelets. III. Adenine phosphoribosyl transferase and nucleotide formation from exogenous adenine. *Biochim. Biophys. Acta 157:266, 1968.*

171. Holmsen, H., and Rozenberg, M. C.: Adenine nucleotide metabolism of blood platelets. II. Adenosine kinase and nucleotide formation from exogenous adenosine and AMP. *Biochim. Biophys. Acta 155:326, 1968.*

172. Holmsen, H., Day, H. J., and Setkowsky, C. A.: Behaviour of adenine nucleotides during the platelet release reaction induced by adenosine diphosphate and adrenaline. *Biochem. J. 129:67, 1972.*

173. Rivard, G. E., McLaren, J. D., and Brunst, R. F.: Incorporation of hypoxanthine into adenine and guanine nucleotides by human platelets. *Biochim. Biophys. Acta 381:144, 1975.*

174. Jerushalmy, Z., Sperling, O., Pinkhas, J., Kryuska, M., and DeVries, A.: Phosphoribosylpyrophosphate synthetase and purine phosphoribosyltransferase. *Haemostasis 1:279, 1972.*

175. Haslam, R. J., and Mills, D. C. B.: The adenylate kinase of human plasma, erythrocytes, and platelets in relation to the degradation of adenosine diphosphate in plasma. *Biochem. J. 103:773, 1967.*

176. Holmsen, H., and Setkowsky-Dangelmaier, C. A.: Adenine nucleotide metabolism of blood platelets. X. Formaldehyde stops centrifugation-induced secretion after A23187-stimulation and causes breakdown of metabolic ATP. *Biochim. Biophys. Acta 497:46, 1977.*

177. Holmsen, H., Ostvold, A.-C., and Pimentel, M. A.: Properties of platelet 5'-AMP deaminase. *Thromb. Haemost. 37:380, 1977.*

178. Ashby, B., and Holmsen, H.: Platelet AMP deaminase. Purification and kinetic studies. *J. Biol. Chem. 256:10519, 1981.*

179. Karpatkin, S., and Langer, R. M.: Biochemical energetics of simulated platelet plug formation: Effect of thrombin, adenosine diphosphate, and epinephrine on intra- and extracellular adenine nucleotide kinetics. *J. Clin. Invest. 47:2158, 1968.*

180. Sixma, J. J., Trieshnigg, A. M., and Holmsen, H.: Adenine nucleotide metabolism of blood platelets. VIII. Mechanism of adenine uptake by intact cells. *Biochim. Biophys. Acta 298:3, 1973.*

181. Sixma, J. J., Lips, J. P. M., Trieshnigg, A. M., and Holmsen, H.: Transport and metabolism of adenosine in human blood platelets. *Biochim. Biophys. Acta 443:33, 1976.*

182. Rivard, G. E., Izadi, P., Lazerson, J., McLaren, J. D., Parker, C., and Fish, C. H.: Functional and metabolic studies of platelets from patients with Lesch-Nyhan Syndrome. *Br. J. Haematol. 31:245, 1975.*

183. Booyse, F., and Rafelson, M. E.: In vitro incorporation of amino acids into the contractile protein of human blood platelets. *Nature 215:283, 1967.*

184. Rosiek, O., Wegrzynowicz, Z., Sawicki, Z., and Kopec, M.: Fibrinogensynthese in Blutplattchen. *Folia Haematol. (Leipz.)* 92:553, 1970.

185. Cooper, I. A., and Firkin, B. G.: Amino acid transport into human platelets and subsequent incorporation into protein. *Thromb. Diath. Haemorrh.* 23:140, 1970.

186. Booyse, F., and Rafelson, M. E.: Stable messenger RNA in the synthesis of contractile protein in human platelets. *Biochim. Biophys. Acta* 145:188, 1967.

187. Steiner, M.: Platelet protein synthesis studied in a cell-free system. *Experientia* 26:786, 1970.

188. Warshaw, A. L., Laster, L., and Shulman, N. R.: Protein synthesis by human platelets. *J. Biol. Chem.* 242:2094, 1967.

189. Boullin, D. J., Votanova, M., and Green, A. R.: Protein synthesis by human blood platelets after accumulation of leucine and arginine. *Thromb. Diath. Haemorrh.* 28:54, 1972.

190. Booyse, F. M., and Rafelson, M. E.: Human platelet contractile proteins: Location, properties, and function. *Ser. Hematol.* 4:152, 1971.

191. Nachman, R., Levine, R., and Jaffe, E.: Synthesis of actin by cultured guinea pig megakaryocytes—Complex formation with fibrin. *Biochim. Biophys. Acta* 543:91, 1978.

192. Freedman, M. L., and Karpatkin, S.: Requirement of iron for platelet protein synthesis. *Biochem. Biophys. Res. Commun.* 54:475, 1973.

193. Solomon, H. M., and Gaut, Z. N.: Uptake and phosphorylation of D-glucosamine-1-^{14}C in the human platelet. *Biochem. Pharmacol.* 20:2895, 1971.

194. Zieve, P. D., and Schmuckler, M.: Incorporation of carbohydrate into protein of human platelets. *Biochim. Biophys. Acta* 372:225, 1974.

195. DeLuca, S.: Incorporation of mannose and glucose into prenyl-phosphate sugars in isolated human platelet membranes. *Biochim. Biophys. Acta* 498:341, 1977.

196. Booyse, F., Hoveke, T. P., and Rafelson, M. E.: Studies on human platelets. II. Protein synthetic activity of various platelet populations. *Biochim. Biophys. Acta* 157:660, 1968.

197. Karpatkin, S., and Langer, R. M.: Biochemical energetics of simulated platelet plug formation: Effect of thrombin, adenosine diphosphate, and epinephrine on intra- and extracellular adenine nucleotide kinetics. *J. Clin. Invest.* 47:2158, 1968.

198. Haslam, R. J., and Rosson, G. M.: Aggregation of human blood platelets by vasopressin. *Am. J. Physiol.* 223:958, 1972.

199. Holmsen, H.: Classification and possible mechanisms of action of some drugs that inhibit platelet aggregation. *Ser. Haematol.* 8:3, 1976.

200. Drummond, A. H.: Interactions of blood platelets with biogenic amines: Uptake, stimulation and receptor binding, in *Platelets in Biology and Pathology*, edited by J. L. Gordon. North Holland, New York, 1976, vol. I, pp. 203–232.

201. Drummond, A. H., Whigham, K. A. E., and Prentice, C. R. M.: Effects of chlorprothixene isomers on platelet 5-hydroxytryptamine receptors: Evidence for different 5-hydroxytrypamine conformations at uptake and stimulatory sites. *Eur. J. Pharmacol.* 37:385, 1976.

202. Peters, J. R., and Grahame-Smith, D. G.: Human platelet 5HT receptors: Characterization and functional association. *Eur. J. Pharmacol.* 68:243, 1980.

203. Gaarder, A., Jonsen, J., Laland, S., Hellem, A., and Owren, P. A.: Adenosine diphosphate in red cells as a factor in the adhesiveness of human blood platelets. *Nature* 192:531, 1961.

204. Macfarlane, D. E., and Mills, D. C. B.: The effects of ATP on platelets: Evidence against a central role of released ADP in primary aggregation. *Blood* 46:309, 1975.

205. Legrand, C., Dubernard, V., and Caen, J.: Further characterization of human platelet ADP binding sites using 5'-AMP. Demonstration of a highly reactive population of site. *Biochim. Biophys. Res. Commun.* 96:1, 1980.

206. Figures, W. R., Niewiarowski, S., Morinelli, T. A., Colman, R. F., and Colman, R. W.: Affinity labeling of a human platelet protein with 5'-*p*-fluorosulfonbenzoyl adenosine: Concomitant inhibition of ADP-induced platelet aggregation and fibrinogen receptor exposure. *J. Biol. Chem.* 256:7789, 1981.

207. Lips, J. P., Sixma, J. J., and Schiphorst, M. E.: Binding of adenosine diphosphate to human blood platelets and to isolated blood platelet membranes. *Biochim. Biophys. Acta* 628:451, 1980.

208. Legrand, C., and Caen, J.: Binding of ^{14}C-ADP to normal human and thrombasthenic platelet membranes: Study of the dissociation of the nucleotide from its receptors. *Haemostasis* 7:339, 1978.

209. Fantl, P.: Thiol groups of blood platelets in relation to clot retraction. *Nature* 198:95, 1963.

210. Michal, F., Maguire, M. H., and Gough, G.: 2-Methyl-thioadenosine-5'-phosphate: A specific inhibitor of platelet aggregation. *Nature* 222:1073, 1969.

211. Kinlough-Rathbone, R. L., Perry, D. W., and Mustard, J. F.: Factors responsible for ADP-induced release reaction of human platelets. *Am. J. Physiol.* 228:1757, 1975.

212. Macfarlane, D. E., Mills, D. C. B., and Srivistava, P. C.: Binding of 2-azidoadenosine [β-^{32}P] diphosphate to the receptor on intact human blood platelets which inhibits adenylate cyclase. *Biochemistry* 21:544, 1982.

213. Clayton, S., and Cross, M. J.: The aggregation of blood platelets by catecholamines and by thrombin. *J. Physiol.* 169:828, 1963.

214. O'Brien, J. R.: Some effects of adrenaline and anti-adrenaline compounds on platelets in vitro and in vivo. *Nature* 200:763, 1963.

215. Tsai, B. S., and Lefkowitz, R. J.: Agonist-specific effects of guanine nucleotides on α-adrenergic receptors on human platelets. *Mol. Pharmacol.* 16:61, 1979.

216. Rossi, E. C., Louis, G., and Zeller, E. A.: Structure, activity, relationships between catecholamines and the α-adrenergic receptor responsible for the aggregation of human platelets by epinephrine. *J. Lab. Clin. Med.* 93:286, 1979.

217. Scrutton, M. C., and Grant, J. A.: Dihydroergocryptamine is a nonselective antagonist for human platelet α-adrenoreceptors. *Nature* 280:700, 1979.

218. Motulsky, H. J., Shattil, S. J., and Tusel, P. A.: Characterization of α_2-adrenergic receptors on human platelets using ^{3}H-yohimbine. *Biochem. Biophys. Res. Commun.* 97:1562, 1980.

219. Glusa, E., and Markwardt, F.: Influence of clonidine-like hypotensive drugs on adrenergic platelet reactions. *Biochem. Pharmacol.* 30:1359, 1981.

220. Mukherjee, A.: Characterization of a α_2-adrenergic receptors in human platelets by binding of a radioactive ligand ^{3}H-yohimbine. *Biochim. Biophys. Acta* 676:148, 1981.

221. Smith, S. K., and Limbird, L. E.: Solubilization of human platelet α-adrenergic receptors—Evidence that agonist occupancy of the receptor stabilizes receptor effector interactions. *Proc. Natl. Acad. Sci. U.S.A.* 78:4026, 1981.

222. Michel, T., Hoffman, B. B., Lefkowitz, R. J., and Caron, M. G.: Different sedimentation properties of agonist- and antagonist-labelled platelet α_2-adrenergic receptors. *Biochem. Biophys. Res. Commun.* 100:1131, 1981.

223. LeBreton, G. C., Vexton, D. L., Enke, S. E., and Halushka, P. V.: 13-Azoprostanoic acid—Specific antagonist of the human blood platelet thromboxane-endoperoxide receptor. *Proc. Natl. Acad. Sci. U.S.A.* 76:4097, 1979.

224. MacIntyre, D. E., McMillan, R. M., and Gordon, J. L.: Secretion of lysosomal enzymes by platelets. *Biochem. Soc. Trans.* 5:1178, 1977.

225. Bennet, J. S., Vilaire, G., and Burdi, J. W.: A role of prostaglandins and thromboxanes in the exposure of platelet fibrinogen receptors. *J. Clin. Invest.* 68:981, 1981.

226. Huzoor-Akbar, and Ardlie, N. G.: Investigation of the role of arachidonic acid in platelet function and mechanisms for suppression of prostaglandin biosynthesis. *Br. J. Haematol.* 39:71, 1978.

227. Best, L. C., Holland, T. K., Jones, P. B., and Russell, R. G.: The interrelationship between thromboxane biosynthesis, aggregation, and 5-hydroxytryptamine secretion *in vitro*. *Thromb. Haemost.* 43:38, 1980.

228. Vargaftig, B. B., Chignard, M., and Benviste, J.: Present concepts on the mechanisms of platelet aggregation. *Biochem. Pharmacol.* 30:263, 1981.

229. MacIntyre, D. E., Salzman, E. H., and Gordon, J. L.: Prostaglandin receptor on human platelets: Structure-activity relationships of stimulatory prostaglandins. *Biochem. J.* 174:921, 1978.

230. Jones, R. L., Sutherland, R. A., and Wilson, N. H.: Binding of tritium-labelled 9,11-epoxymethano-PGH$_2$ to human platelets. *Br. J. Pharmacol.* 73:304P, 1981.

231. Benviste, J., Camussi, J., and Polonsky, J.: Platelet-activating factor. *Monogr. Allergy* 12:138, 1977.

232. Shaw, J. O., and Henson, P. M.: The binding of rabbit basophil-derived platelet-activating factor to rabbit platelets. *Am. J. Pathol.* 98:791, 1980.

233. Hanahan, D. J., Demopoulos, C. A., Liehr, J., and Pinckard, R. N.: Identification of platelet-activating factor as acetyl glyceryl ether phosphoglycerylcholine. *J. Biol. Chem.* 255:5514, 1980.

234. McManus, L. M., Hanahan, D. J., and Pinckard, R. N.: Human platelet stimulation by acetyl glyceryl ether phosphorylcholine. *J. Clin. Invest.* 67:903, 1981.

235. Marcus, A. J., et al.: Effects of acetyl glyceryl ether phosphorylcholine on human platelet function in vitro. *Blood* 58:1027, 1981.

236. Hovig, T.: Release of platelet aggregating substance (ADP) from rabbit blood platelets induced by saline extract of tendons. *Thromb. Diath. Haemorrh.* 9:264, 1963.

237. Spaet, T. H., and Zucker, M. B.: Mechanism of platelet plug formation and role of adenosine diphosphate. *Am. J. Physiol.* 206:1267, 1964.

238. Wilner, C. D., Noseel, H. L., and LeRoy, E. C.: Aggregation of platelets by collagen. *J. Clin. Invest.* 47:2616, 1968.

239. Cazenave, J. P., Assimeh, S. N., Painter, R. H., Packham, M. A., and Mustard, J. F.: C1q inhibition of the interaction of collagen with human platelets. *J. Immunol.* 116:162, 1976.

240. Suba, E. A., and Csako, G.: C1q (C1) receptor on human platelets: Inhibition of collagen-induced platelet aggregation by C1q (C1) molecules. *J. Immunol.* 117:304, 1976.

241. Kang, A. H., Beachey, E. H., and Katzman, R. L.: Interaction of an active glycopeptide from chick skin collagen (α-1-CB5) with human platelets. *J. Biol. Chem.* 249:1054, 1974.

242. Brass, L. F., and Bensusan, H. B.: The role of collagen quaternary structure in the platelet:collagen interaction. *J. Clin. Invest.* 54:1480, 1974.

243. Muggli, R., and Baugartner, H. R.: Collagen induced platelet aggregation: Requirement for tropocollagen multimers. *Thromb. Res.* 3:775, 1973.

244. Cowan, D.: Platelet adherence to collagen: Role of prostaglandin-thromboxane synthesis. *Br. J. Haematol.* 49:425, 1981.

245. Grette, K.: Studies on the mechanism of thrombin catalyzed hemostatic reactions in blood platelets. *Acta Physiol. Scand. 56 (Suppl. 195)*:9, 1962.

246. Buckingham, S., and Maynert, E. W.: The release of 5-hydroxytryptamine, potassium, and amino acids from platelets. *J. Pharmacol. Exp. Ther.* 143:332, 1964.

247. Holmsen, H., Day, H. J., and Storm, E.: Adenine nucleotide metabolism of blood platelets. VI. Subcellular localization of nucleotide pools with different functions in the platelet release reaction. *Biochim. Biophys. Acta* 186:254, 1969.

248. Davey, M. G., and Luscher, E. F.: Release reactions of human platelets induced by thrombin and other agents. *Biochim. Biophys. Acta* 165:490, 1968.

249. Detwiler, T. C., and Feinman, R. D.: Kinetics of the thrombin-induced release of calcium (II) by platelets. *Biochemistry* 12:282, 1973.

250. Detwiler, T. C., and Feinman, R. D.: Kinetics of the thrombin-induced release of adenosine triphosphate by platelets: Comparison with release of calcium. *Biochemistry* 12:2462, 1973.

251. Martin, B. M., Feinman, R. D., and Detwiler, T. C.: Equilibrium binding of thrombin to platelets. *Biochemistry* 14:1308, 1975.

252. Tollefsen, D. M., Feagler, J. R., and Majerus, P. W.: The binding of thrombin to the surface of human platelets. *J. Biol. Chem.* 249:2646, 1974.

253. Tollefsen, D. M., Jackson, C. M., and Majerus, P. W.: Binding of the products of prothrombin activation to human platelets. *J. Clin. Invest.* 56:241, 1975.

254. Tollefsen, D. M., and Majerus, P. W.: Evidence for a single class of thrombin-binding sites on human platelets. *Biochemistry* 13:2144, 1976.

255. Martin, B. M., Wasiewski, W. W., Fenton, J. W., and Detwiler, T. C.: Equilibrium binding of thrombin to platelets. *Biochemistry* 15:4886, 1976.

256. Workman, E. F., White, G. C., and Lundblad, R. L.: Structure-function relationships in the interaction of α-thrombin with blood platelets. *J. Biol. Chem.* 252:7118, 1977.

257. White, G. C., Lundblad, R. L., and Griffith, M. J.: Structure-function relations in platelet-thrombin reactions: Inhibition of platelet-thrombin interactions by lysine modification. *J. Biol. Chem.* 256:1763, 1981.

258. Larsen, N. E., and Simons, E. R.: Preparation and application of a photoreactive thrombin analogue: Binding to human platelets. *Biochemistry* 20:4141, 1981.

259. Canguli, P., and Fossett, N. G.: Inhibition of thrombin-induced platelet aggregation by a derivative of wheat germ agglutinin: Evidence for a physiologic receptor of thrombin in human platelets. *Blood* 57:343, 1981.

260. Holmsen, H., Dangelmaier, C. A., and Holmsen, H.-K.: Thrombin-induced platelet responses differ in requirement for receptor occupancy: Evidence for tight coupling of occupancy and compartmentalized phosphatidic acid formation. *J. Biol. Chem.* 256:9393, 1981.

261. Davey, M. G., and Luscher, E. F.: Actions of thrombin and other coagulant and proteolytic enzymes on blood platelets. *Nature* 216:857, 1967.

262. Niewiarowski, S., Kirby, E. P., Brudzynski, S., and Stocker, K.: Thrombocytin a serine protease from *Bothrops atrox* venom. 2. Interaction with platelets and plasma clotting factors. *Biochemistry* 18:3570, 1979.

263. Schmaier, A. H., and Colman, R. W.: Crotalocytin: Characterization of the timber rattlesnake platelet-activating protein. *Blood* 56:1020, 1980.

264. Feinman, R. D., and Detwiler, T. C.: Platelet secretion induced by divalent cation ionophores. *Nature* 249:172, 1974.

265. Massini, P., and Luscher, E. F.: Some effects of ionophores for divalent cations on blood platelets: Comparison with the effects of thrombin. *Biochim. Biophys. Acta* 372:109, 1974.

266. White, J. C., Rao, G. F. R., and Gerrard, J. M.: Effects of the ionophore A23187 on blood platelets. I. Influence on aggregation and secretion. *Am. J. Pathol.* 77:135, 1974.

267. Holmsen, H.: Biochemistry of the platelet release reaction. *Ciba Found. Symp. 35 (New Series)*:175, 1975.

268. Kinlough-Rathbone, R. L., Chahil, A., Packham, M. A., Reimers, H.-J., and Mustard, J. F.: Effect of ionophore A23187 on thrombin-degranulated washed rabbit platelets. *Thromb. Res.* 7:435, 1975.

269. Worner, P., and Brossmer, R.: Platelet aggregation and the release reaction induced by ionophores for divalent cations. *Thromb. Res.* 6:295, 1975.

270. Feinstein, M. B., and Fraser, C.: Human platelet secretion and aggregation induced by calcium ionophores: Inhibition by PGE$_1$ and dibutyryl cyclic AMP. *J. Gen. Physiol.* 66:561, 1975.

271. Holmsen, H., and Dangelmaier, C. A.: Evidence that the platelet plasma membrane is impermeable to calcium and magnesium complexes of A23187: A23187-induced secretion is inhibited by Mg^{2+} and Ca^{2+}, and requires aggregation and active cyclooxygenase. *J. Biol. Chem.* 256:10449, 1981.

272. O'Brien, J. R.: Effect of salicylates on human platelets. *Lancet* 1:779, 1968.

273. Massini, P., and Luscher, E. F.: On the mechanism by which cell contact induces the release reaction of blood platelets: The effect of cationic polymers. *Thromb. Diath. Haemorrh.* 27:121, 1972.

274. Zucker, M. B.: Proteolytic inhibitors, contact, and other variables in the release reaction of human platelets. *Thromb. Diath. Haemorrh.* 28:393, 1972.

275. Salzman, E. W. Lindon, J. N., and Rodvien, R.: Cyclic AMP in human blood platelets. Relation to platelet prostaglandin synthesis induced by centrifugation or surface contact. *J. Cyclic Nucl. Res.* 2:25, 1976.

276. Holmsen, H.: Mechanisms of platelet secretion, in *Platelets: Cellular Response Mechanisms and Their Biological Significance,* edited by A. Rotman, F. A. Meyer, C. Gitler, and A. Silberberg. Wiley, New York, 1980, pp. 249–263.

277. Salzman, E. W., Brier-Russell, D., Lindon, J., and Merrill, E. W.:

Platelets and artificial surfaces: The effects of drugs. *Philos. Trans. R. Soc. Lond. (Biol.) 294:389,* 1981.

278. Weiss, H. J., Turitto, V. T., Vicic, W. J., and Baumgartner, H. R.: Effect of aspirin and dipyridamole on the interaction of human platelets with subendothelium: Studies using citrated and native blood. *Thromb. Haemost. 45:136,* 1981.

279. Bull, B. S., and Zucker, M. B.: Changes in platelet volume produced by temperature, metabolic inhibitors, and aggregating agents. *Proc. Soc. Exp. Biol. Med. 120:296,* 1965.

280. Born, G. V. R.: Observations on the changes in shape of blood platelets brought about by adenosine diphosphate. *J. Physiol. (Lond.) 209:487,* 1970.

281. White, J. G.: Shape change. *Thromb. Diath. Haemorrh. Suppl. 60:* 159, 1973.

282. Allen, R. D., Zacharski, L. R., Widirstky, S. T., Rosenstein, R., Zaitler, L. M., and Burgess, D. R.: Transformation and mobility of human platelets. *J. Cell Biol. 83:126,* 1979.

283. Born, G. V. R., and Cross, M. J.: The aggregation of blood platelets. *J. Physiol. 168:178,* 1963.

284. Zucker, M. B., and Peterson, J.: Inhibition of adenosine diphosphate–induced secondary aggregation and other platelet functions by acetyl salicylic acid ingestion. *Proc. Soc. Exp. Biol. Med. 127:* 547, 1968.

285. Bennett, J. S., and Vilaire, G.: Exposure of platelet fibrinogen receptors by ADP and epinephrine. *J. Clin. Invest. 64:1393,* 1979.

286. Peerschke, E. J., Zucker, M. B., Grant, R. A., Egan, J. J., and Johnson, M. M: Correlation between fibrinogen binding to human platelets and platelet aggregability. *Blood 55:841,* 1980.

287. Marguerie, G. A., Edginton, T. S., and Plow, E. F.: Interaction of fibrinogen with its platelet receptor as part of a multistep reaction in ADP-induced platelet aggregation. *J. Biol. Chem. 255:154,* 1980.

288. Marguerie, G. A., Plow, E. F., and Edginton, T. S.: Human platelets possess an inducible and saturable receptor specific for fibrinogen. *J. Biol. Chem. 254:5357,* 1979.

289. Hawiger, J., Parkinson, S., and Timmons, S.: Prostacyclin inhibits mobilization of fibrinogen-binding sites on human ADP- and thrombin-treated platelets. *Nature 283:195,* 1980.

290. Bennett, J. S., Vilaire, G., and Burch, J. W.: A role for prostaglandins and thromboxanes in the exposure of platelet fibrinogen receptors. *J. Clin. Invest. 68:981,* 1981.

291. Niewiarowski, S., Budzynski, A. Z., Morinelli, T. A., Brudzynski, T. M., and Stewart, G. J.: Exposure of fibrinogen receptor on human platelets by proteolytic enzymes. *J. Biol. Chem. 256:917,* 1981.

292. Peerschke, E. I., and Zucker, M. B.: Relationship of ADP-induced fibrinogen binding to platelet shape change and aggregation elucidated by use of colchicine and cytochalasin B. *Thromb. Haemost. 43:58,* 1980.

293. Witte, L. D., Kaplan, H. L., Nossel, H. L., Lages, B. A., Weiss, H. J., and Goodman, D. S.: Studies of the release from human platelets of the growth factor for human arterial smooth muscle cells. *Circ. Res. 42:402,* 1978.

294. Kaplan, K. L., Broekman, M. J., Chernoff, A., Lesznik, G. R., and Drillings, M.: Platelet α-granule proteins: Studies on release and subcellular localization. *Blood 53:604,* 1979.

295. Holmsen, H., and Day, H. J.: The selectivity of the thrombin-induced platelet release reaction: Subcellular localization of released and retained substances. *J. Lab. Clin. Med. 75:840,* 1970.

296. Holmsen, H., Setkowsky, C. A., Lages, B., Day, H. J., Weiss, H. J., and Scrutton, M. C.: Content and thrombin-induced release of acid hydrolases in gel-filtered platelets from patients with storage pool disease. *Blood 46:131,* 1975.

297. Holmsen, H., Robkin, L., and Day, H. J.: Effects of antimycin A and 2-deoxyglucose on secretion in washed human platelets: Differential inhibition of the secretion of acid hydrolases and acid hydrolases. *Biochem. J. 182:413,* 1979.

298. Holmsen, H.: Prostaglandin-thromboxane synthesis and secretion as positive feedback loops in the propagation of platelet responses. *Thromb. Haemost. 38:1042,* 1977.

299. Charo, J. F., Feinman, R. D., Detwiler, T. C., Smith, J. B., Ingerman, C. M., and Silver, M. J.: Prostaglandin endoperoxides and thromboxane A₂ can induce platelet aggregation in the absence of secretion. *Nature 269:66,* 1977.

300. Charo, J. F., Feinman, R. D., and Detwiler, T. C.: Interrelations of platelet aggregation and secretion. *J. Clin. Invest. 60:866,* 1977.

301. Kinlough-Rathbone, R. L., Packham, M. A., Reimers, H.-J., Cazenave, J. P., and Mustard, J. F.: Mechanisms of platelet shape change, aggregation and release induced by collagen, thrombin or A23187. *J. Lab. Clin. Med. 90:707,* 1977.

302. Patscheke, H., and Worner, P.: Common activation of aggregation and release reaction in platelets. *Thromb. Res. 11:391,* 1977.

303. Holmsen, H.: Platelet secretion (release reaction)—Mechanism and pharmacology. *Adv. Pharmacol. Therap. 4:97,* 1978.

304. Bressler, N. M., Broekman, M. J., and Marcus, A. J.: Concurrent studies of oxygen consumption and aggregation in stimulated human platelets. *Blood 53:167,* 1979.

305. Meyers, K. M., Seachord, C. L., Holmsen, H., Smith, J. B., and Prieur, D. J.: A dominant role of thromboxane formation in secondary aggregation of platelets. *Nature 282:331,* 1979.

306. Vargaftig, B. B., Chignard, M., LeCouedic, J. P., and Benviste, J.: One, two, three, or more pathways for platelet activation. *Acta Med. Scand. Suppl. 642:23,* 1980.

307. Best, L. C., Holland, T. K., Jones, P. B. B., and Russell, R. G. G.: The interrelationship between thromboxane biosynthesis, aggregation, and 5-hydroxytryptamine secretion in human platelets in vitro. *Thromb. Haemost. 43:38,* 1980.

308. Akkerman, J. W., and Holmsen, H.: Interrelationships among platelet responses: Studies on the burst in proton liberation, lactate production and oxygen uptake during platelet aggregation and Ca²⁺ secretion. *Blood 57:956,* 1981.

309. Huang, E. M., and Detwiler, T. C.: Reassessment of the evidence for the role of secreted ADP in biphasic platelet aggregation—Mechanism of inhibition by creatine phosphate plus creatine phosphokinase. *J. Lab. Clin. Med. 95:59,* 1980.

310. Kinlough-Rathbone, R. L., Packham, M. A., and Mustard, J. F.: Synergism between platelet aggregating agents. *Biochem. Biophys. Res. Commun. 72:1462,* 1976.

311. Yoshida, N., and Aoki, N.: Potentiation by collagen or epinephrine of platelet responsiveness to aggregation: The possible role of substance(s) released from platelet membranes. *J. Lab. Clin. Med. 89:603,* 1977.

312. Grant, J. A., and Scrutton, M. C.: Positive, interaction between agonists in the aggregation response of human blood platelets: Interaction between ADP and adrenaline and vasopressin. *Br. J. Haematol. 44:109,* 1980.

313. Patscheke, H.: Role of activation in epinephrine-induced aggregation of platelets. *Thromb. Res. 17:133,* 1980.

314. Huang, E. M., and Detwiler, T. C.: Characteristics of the synergistic actions of platelet agonists. *Blood 57:685,* 1981.

315. O'Brien, J. R.: Changes in platelet membranes possibly associated with platelet stickiness. *Nature 212:1057,* 1966.

316. Rozenberg, M. C., and Holmsen, H.: Adenine nucleotide metabolism of blood platelets. IV. Platelet aggregation response to exogenous ATP and ADP. *Biochim. Biophys. Acta 157:280,* 1968.

317. Reimers, H. J., Packham, M. A., Kinlough-Rathbone, R. L., and Mustard, J. F.: Effect of repeated treatment of rabbit platelets with low concentrations of thrombin on their functions, metabolism, and survival. *Br. J. Haematol. 25:675,* 1973.

318. Holme, S., and Holmsen, H.: ADP-induced refractory state in platelets in vitro. I. Methodological studies on aggregation in platelet-rich plasma. *Scand. J. Haematol. 15:96,* 1975.

319. Holme, S., Sixma, J. J., Wester, J., and Holmsen, H.: ADP-induced refractory state of platelets in vitro. II. Functional and ultrastructural studies on gel-filtered platelets. *Scand. J. Haematol. 18:267,* 1977.

320. Holmsen, H., and Day, H. J.: Adenine nucleotides and platelet function. *Ser. Haematol. 4:28,* 1971.

321. O'Brien, J. R.: Some effects of adrenaline and antiadrenaline compounds on platelets in vitro and in vivo. *Nature 200:763,* 1963.

322. Constantine, J. W.: Aggregation of guinea pig platelets by adenosine diphosphate. *Nature 210:162,* 1966.

323. Macmillan, D. C.: Secondary clumping effect in human citrated platelet-rich plasma produced by adenosine diphosphate and adrenaline. *Nature 211:141,* 1966.

324. Hardisty, R. M., Hutton, R. A., Montgomery, D., Richard, S., and

Trebilcock, H.: Secondary platelet aggregation: A quantitative study. *Br. J. Haematol.* 19:307, 1970.

325. Glusa, E., and Markwardt, F.: Adrenaline-induced reactions of human platelets in hirudin plasma. *Haemostasis* 9:188, 1980.

326. Lages, B., and Weiss, H. J.: Dependence of human platelet functional responses on divalent cations: Aggregation and secretion in heparin- and hirudin-anticoagulated platelet-rich plasma and the effects of chelating agents. *Thromb. Haemost.* 45:173, 1981.

327. Weiss, H. J., Chernvenick, P. A., Zalusky, R., and Factor, A.: A familial defect in platelet function associated with impaired release of adenosine diphosphate. *N. Engl. J. Med.* 281:1264, 1969.

328. Pareti, F. I., Day, H. J., and Mills, D. C. B.: Nucleotide and serotonin metabolism in platelets with defective secondary aggregation. *Blood* 44:789, 1974.

329. Malmsten, C., Hamberg, M., Svensson, J., and Samuelsson, B.: Physiological role of an endoperoxide in human platelets: Hemostatic defect due to platelet cyclooxygenase deficiency. *Proc. Natl. Acad. Sci. U.S.A.* 72:1446, 1975.

330. Lagarde, M., Byron, P. A., Vargaftig, B. B., and Dechavanne, M.: Impairment of platelet thromboxane A_2 generation and of the platelet release reaction in two patients with congenital deficiency of platelet cyclooxygenase. *Br. J. Haematol.* 38:251, 1978.

331. Pareti, F. I., Mannucci, P. M., and D'Angelo, A.: Congenital deficiency of thromboxane and prostacyclin. *Lancet* 1:898, 1980.

332. Rak, K., and Boda, Z.: Haemostatic balance in congenital deficiency of platelet cyclooxygenase. *Lancet* 2:44, 1980.

333. Weiss, H. J., and Lages, B.: Possible congenital defect in platelet thromboxane synthetase. *Lancet* 1:760, 1977.

334. Wu, K. K., LeBreton, G. C., Tai, H. H., and Chen, Y.-C.: Abnormal response to thromboxane A_2. *J. Clin Invest.* 67:1801, 1981.

335. Lages, V., Malmsten, C., Weiss, H. J., and Samuelsson, B.: Impaired platelet response to thromboxane A_2 and defective calcium mobilization in a patient with a bleeding disorder. *Blood* 57:545, 1981.

336. Kane, W. H., Lindhout, M. J., Jackson, C. M., and Majerus, P. W.: Factor Va–dependent binding of factor Xa to human platelets. *J. Biol. Chem.* 255:1170, 1980.

337. Buchanan, G. R., Martin, V., Levine, P. H., Scott, K., and Handin, R. D.: The effects of "anti-platelet drugs" on bleeding time and platelet aggregation in normal human subjects. *Am. J. Clin. Pathol.* 68:355, 1977.

338. Amezcua, J. L., O'Grady, J., Salmon, J. A., and Moncada, S.: Prolonged paradoxical effect of aspirin on platelet behavior and bleeding time in man. *Thromb. Res.* 16:69, 1979.

339. O'Brien, J.: Variability in the aggregation of human platelets by adrenaline. *Nature* 202:1188, 1964.

340. Arkel, T. S., Hopt, J. D., Kreutzer, W., Sherwood, J., and Williams, R.: Alteration in second phase platelet associated with an emotionally stressful activity. *Thromb. Haemost.* 38:552, 1977.

341. Vargaftig, B. B., Chignard, M., and Benveniste, J.: Platelet-tissue interaction: Role of platelet-activating factor (PAF-acether). *Agents Actions* 10:502, 1980.

342. Spaet, T., and Erichson, R. B.: The vascular wall in the pathogenesis of thrombosis. *Thromb. Diath. Haemorrh. (Suppl.)* 21:67, 1966.

343. Nossel, H. L., Wilner, G. D., and LeRoy, E. C.: Importance of polar groups for initiating blood coagulation and aggregating platelets. *Nature* 221:75, 1969.

344. Wilner, G. D., Nossel, H. L., and Procupez, T. L.: Aggregation of platelets by collagen: Polar active sites of insoluble collagen. *Am. J. Physiol.* 220:1074, 1971.

345. Katzman, R. L., Kang, A. H., and Beachey, E. H.: Collagen-induced platelet aggregation: Involvement of an active glycopeptide fragment. *Science* 181:670, 1973.

346. Puett, D., Wasserman, B. K., Ford, J. D., and Cunningham, L. W.: Collagen-mediated platelet aggregation: Effects of collagen modification involving the protein and carbohydrate moieties. *J. Clin. Invest.* 52:2495, 1973.

347. Chesney, E. McI., Harper, E., and Colman, R.: Critical role of the carbohydrate side chains of collagen in platelet aggregation. *J. Clin. Invest.* 51:2693, 1972.

348. Meyer, F. A., and Weisman, Z.: Collagen-induced platelet aggregation: Dependence on triple helical structure and fiber diameter. *Thromb. Res.* 22:1, 1981.

349. Miletich, J. P., Kane, W. H., Hofman, S. L., Stanford, N., and Majerus, P. W.: Deficiency of factor X_a–factor V_a binding sites on the platelets of a patient with a bleeding disorder. *Blood* 54:1015, 1979.

350. Tracy, P. B., Nesheim, M. E., and Mann, K. G.: Coordinate binding of Factor Va and Factor Xa to unstimulated platelets. *J. Biol. Chem.* 256:743, 1981.

351. Murer, E. H., and Holme, R.: A study of the release of calcium from human blood platelets and its inhibition by metabolic inhibitors, N-ethyl maleimide and aspirin. *Biochim. Biophys. Acta* 222:197, 1970.

352. Lages, B., Scrutton, M. C., and Holmsen, H.: Secretion in gel-filtered human platelets: Response of platelet Ca^{2+}, Mg^{2+}, and K^+ to secretory agents. *J. Lab. Clin. Med.* 90:873, 1977.

353. Lages, B., Holmsen, H., Weiss, H. J., and Dangelmaier, C. A.: Thrombin- and ionophore A23187–induced dense granule secretion in storage pool deficient platelets: Evidence for impaired nucleotide storage as the primary dense granule defect. *Blood,* 61:154, 1983.

354. Skaer, R. J., Peters, P. D., and Emmines, J. P.: The localization of calcium and phosphorus in human platelets. *J. Cell. Sci.* 15:679, 1974.

355. Daimon, T., Mizuhira, V., and Uchida, K.: Ultrastructural localization of calcium around the membrane of surface-connected system in the human platelet. *Histochemistry* 55:271, 1978.

356. Grette, K.: Relaxing factor in extracts of blood platelets and its function in the cells. *Nature* 198:488, 1963.

357. Statland, B. E., Heagan, B. M., and White, J. G.: Uptake of calcium by platelet relaxing factor. *Nature* 223:521, 1969.

358. Robblee, L. S., Shepro, D., and Belamarich, F. A.: Calcium uptake and associated adenosine triphosphatase activity of isolated platelet membranes. *J. Gen. Physiol.* 61:462, 1973.

359. Kaser-Glanzmann, R., Jakabova, M., George, J. N., and Luscher, E. F.: Further characterization of calcium-accumulating vesicles from human blood platelets. *Biochim. Biophys. Acta* 252:3310, 1979.

360. Fox, J. E. B., Say, A. K., and Haslam, R. J.: Subcellular distribution of the different platelet proteins phosphorylated on exposure of intact platelets to ionophore A23187 or to prostaglandin E_1: Possible role of membrane phosphopolypeptide in the regulation of calcium ion transport. *Biochem. J.* 184:651, 1979.

361. Cutler, L., Rodàn, G., and Feinstein, M. L.: Cytochemical localization of adenylate kinase and of calcium ion, magnesium activated ATPase in the dense tubular system of human blood platelets. *Biochim. Biophys. Acta* 542:357, 1978.

362. Menashi, S., Weintroub, H., and Crawford, N.: Characterization of human platelet surface and intracellular membranes isolated by free flow electrophoresis. *J. Biol. Chem.* 256:4095, 1981.

363. Rink, T. J., Smith, S. W., and Tsieu, R. Y.: Intracellular free calcium in platelet shape change and aggregation. *J. Physiol. (Lond.)* 322:73P, 1981.

364. Murphy, E., Call, K., Rich, T. L., and Williamson, J. R.: Hormonal effects on calcium homeostasis in isolated hepatocytes. *J. Biol. Chem.* 255:6600, 1980.

365. Purdon, D. A., and Holmsen, H.: Determination of the concentration of cytoplasmic calcium in resting and activated platelets by limited digitonin lysis (in preparation).

366. Day, H. J., and Holmsen, H.: Concepts of the blood platelet release reaction. *Ser. Haematol.* 4:3, 1971.

367. Holmsen, H.: Are shape change, aggregation, and release reaction tangible manifestations of one basic cellular process? in *Platelets: Production, Function, Transfusion, and Storage,* edited by M. Baldini and S. Ebbe. Grune & Stratton, New York, 1974, pp. 207–220.

368. Luscher, E. F., and Massini, P.: Common pathways of membrane reactivity after stimulation of platelets with different agents. *Ciba Found. Symp. 135 (New Series)*:5, 1975.

369. Gerrard, J. M., Peterson, D. A. and White, J. G.: Calcium mobilization, in *Platelets in Biology and Pathology,* edited by J. L. Gordon. Elsevier–North Holland, Amsterdam, 1981, vol. 2, p. 407.

370. Feinstein, M. B.: Release of intracellular membrane-bound calcium precedes the onset of stimulus-induced exocytosis in platelets. *Biochim. Biophys. Res. Commun.* 93:593, 1980.

371. Owen, N. E., and LeBreton, G. C.: Ca^{2+} mobilization in blood

platelets as visualized by chlortetra cycline fluorescence. *Am. J. Physiol.* 241:H613, 1981.

372. Murer, E. H., and Siojo, E.: Inhibition of thrombin-induced secretion from platelets with chlortetracycline and its analogs. *Thromb. Haemost.* 47:59, 1982.

373. Murer, E. H., and Siojo, E.: Effects of 8(N,N-diethylamino)octyl 3,4,5-trimethoxybenzoate HCl (TMB-8) on washed blood platelets with special reference to a specific loss of serotonin. *Thromb. Haemost.* 47:62, 1982.

374. Lyons, R. M., Stanford, N., and Majerus, P. W.: Thrombin-induced protein phosphorylation in human platelets. *J. Clin. Invest.* 56:924, 1975.

375. Haslam, R. J., and Lynham, J. A.: Relationship between phosphorylation of blood platelet proteins and secretion of platelet granule constituents. I. Effects of different aggregating agents. *Biochem. Biophys. Res. Commun.* 77:714, 1977.

376. Daniel, J. L., Holmsen, H., and Adelstein, R. S.: Involvement of myosin phosphorylation in platelet secretion. *Thromb. Haemost.* 38:984, 1977.

377. Haslam, R. J., and Lynham, J. A.: Relationships between phosphorylation of blood platelet proteins and secretion of platelet granule constituents. II. Effects of different inhibitors. *Thromb. Res.* 12:619, 1978.

378. Haslam, R. J., Lynham, J. A., and Fox, J. E. B.: Effects of collagen, ionophore A23187, and prostaglandin E₁ on the phosphorylation of specific proteins in blood platelets. *Biochem. J.* 178:397, 1979.

379. Bills, T. K., Smith, J. B., and Silver, M. J.: Selective release of arachidonic acid from phospholipids of human platelets in response to thrombin. *J. Clin. Invest.* 60:1, 1977.

380. Rittenhouse-Simmons, S., Rusell, F. A., and Deykin, D.: Mobilization of arachidonic acid in human platelets. Kinetics and Ca²⁺ dependency. *Biochim. Biophys. Acta* 488:370, 1977.

381. Bell, R. L., Kennerly, D. A., Stanford, N., Majerus, P. W., Costrini, N. V., and Bradshaw, R. A.: Diglyceride lipase pathway for arachidonate release from human platelets. *Proc. Natl. Acad. Sci. U.S.A.* 76:3238, 1979.

382. Lapetina, E. G., and Cuatrecasas, P.: Stimulation of phosphatidic acid production in platelets precedes the formation of arachidonate and parallels the release of serotonin. *Biochim. Biophys. Acta* 573:394, 1979.

383. Walenga, R. W., Opas, E. E., and Feinstein, M. B.: Differential effects of calmodulin antagonists on phospholipases A₂ and C in thrombin-stimulated platelets. *J. Biol. Chem.* 256:12523, 1981.

384. LeBreton, G. C., and Dinerstein, F. J.: Effect of the calcium antagonist TMB-6 on intracellular calcium redistribution associated with shape change. *Thromb. Res.* 10:521, 1971.

385. Charo, I. F., Feinman, R. D., and Detwiler, T. C.: Inhibition of platelet secretion by an antagonist of intracellular calcium. *Biochem. Biophys. Res. Commun.* 72:1462, 1976.

386. Feinstein, M. B., Fiekers, J., and Fraser, C.: An analysis of the mechanism of local anesthetic inhibition of platelet aggregation and secretion. *J. Pharm. Exp. Ther.* 197:217, 1976.

387. Kindness, G., Williamson, F. B., and Long, W. F.: Inhibitory effect of trifluoprazine on aggregation of human platelets. *Thromb. Res.* 17:549, 1980.

388. Rao, G. H., Reddy, K. R., and White, J. G.: Influence of trifluoperazine on platelet aggregation and disaggregation. *Prostagland. Med.* 5:221, 1980.

389. Nishikawa, M., Tanaka, T., and Hidaka, H.: Ca²⁺-calmodulin–dependent phosphorylation and platelet secretion. *Nature* 287:863, 1980.

390. Kao, K.-J., Sommer, J. R., and Pizzo, S. V.: Modulation of platelet shape and membrane receptor binding by Ca²⁺-calmodulin complex. *Nature* 292:82, 1981.

391. Kambayashi, J., Morimoto, K., Hakata, N., Kobayashi, T., and Kosaki, B.: Involvement of calmodulin in platelet reaction. *Thromb. Res.* 22:553, 1981.

392. Massini, P., and Naf, U.: Ca²⁺ ionophores and the activation of human blood platelets: The effects of ionomycin, beceuvericin, lysocellin, virginamycin, lasalocid-derivates, and McN4308. *Biochim. Biophys. Acta* 598:575, 1980.

393. Knight, D. E., and Scrutton, M. C.: Direct evidence for a role for Ca²⁺ in amine storage granule secretion by human platelets. *Thromb. Res.* 20:437, 1980.

394. Holmsen, H.: Unpublished observations.

395. Owen, N. E., Feinberg, H., and LeBreton, G. C.: Epinephrine induces Ca²⁺ uptake in human blood platelets. *Am. J. Physiol.* 239:H483, 1980.

396. Owen, N. E., and LeBreton, G. C.: The involvement of calcium in epinephrine or ADP potentiation of human platelet aggregation. *Thromb. Res.* 17:855, 1980.

397. Gerrard, J. M., Butler, A. M., Graff, G., Stoddard, S. F., and White, J. G.: Prostaglandin endoperoxides promote calcium release from a platelet membrane fraction in vitro. *Prostagland. Med.* 1:373, 1978.

398. Schumacher, K. A., Classen, H. G., and Spath, M.: Platelet aggregation evoked in vitro and in vivo by phosphatidic acids and lysoderivatives: Identity with substances in aged serum (DAS). *Thromb. Haemost.* 42:631, 1979.

399. Gerrard, J. M., Kindom, S. E., Peterson, D. A., Peller, J., Krantz, K. E., and White, J. G.: Lysophosphatidic acids. *Am. J. Pathol.* 96:423, 1979.

400. Tokumurua, A., Fukuzawa, K., Isobe, J., and Tsukatani, H.: Lysophosphatidic-induced aggregation of human and feline platelets: Structure-activity relationship. *Biochem. Biophys. Res. Commun.* 99:391, 1981.

401. Horne, W. C., and Simons, E. R.: Probes of transmembrane potentials in platelets: Changes in cyanine dye fluorescence in response to aggregating stimuli. *Blood* 51:741, 1978.

402. Horne, W. C., and Simons, E. R.: Effects of amiloride on the response of human platelets to bovine α-thrombin. *Thromb. Res.* 13:599, 1978.

403. Friedhoff, L. T., Kim, E., Priddle, M., and Sonenberg, M.: The effect of altered transmembrane ion gradients on membrane potential and aggregation of human platelets in blood plasma. *Biochem. Biophys. Res. Commun.* 102:832, 1981.

404. Nathan, I., Fleischer, G., Livne, A., Dvilansky, A., and Parola, A. H.: Membrane microenvironmental changes during activation of human blood platelets with thrombin. *J. Biol. Chem.* 254:9822, 1979.

405. Nathan, I., Fleischer, G., Dvilansky, A., Livne, A., and Parola, A. H.: Membrane dynamic alterations associated with activation of human platelets by thrombin. *Biochim. Biophys. Acta* 598:417, 1980.

406. Shattil, S. J., and Cooper, R. A.: Membrane viscosity and human platelet function. *Biochemistry* 15:4832, 1976.

407. Feinberg, H., Sandler, W. C., Searer, M., LeBreton, Grossman, B., and Born, G. V. R.: Movement of sodium into platelets induced by ADP. *Biochim. Biophys. Acta* 470:317, 1977.

408. Sandler, W., LeBreton, G. C., and Feinberg, H.: Movement of sodium into human platelets. *Biochim. Biophys. Acta* 600:488, 1980.

409. Corn, M.: Effect of thrombin on glycolysis of fresh and stored platelets. *J. Appl. Physiol.* 21:62, 1966.

410. Bettex-Galland, M., and Luscher, E. F.: Studies on the metabolism of human platelets in relation to clot retraction. *Thromb. Diath. Haemorrh.* 4:178, 1960.

411. Karpatkin, S., and Siskind, G. W.: Effect of antibody binding and agglutination on human platelet glycolysis: Comparison with thrombin and epinephrine. *Blood* 30:617, 1967.

412. Loder, P. B., Hirsch, J., and DeGruchy, G. C.: The effect of collagen on platelet glycolysis and nucleotide metabolism. *Br. J. Haematol.* 14:563, 1968.

413. McElroy, R. A., Kinlough-Rathbone, R. L., Ardlie, N. G., Packham, M. A., and Mustard, J. F.: The effect of aggregating agents on oxidative metabolism of rabbit platelets. *Biochim. Biophys. Acta* 253:64, 1971.

414. Corn, M., Jackson, D. P., and Conley, C. L.: Components of blood necessary for clot retraction. *Bull. Johns Hopkins Hosp.* 107:90, 1960.

415. Fukami, M. H., Holmsen, H., and Salganicoff, L.: Adenine nucleotide metabolism of blood platelets. IX. Time course of secretion and changes in energy metabolism in thrombin-treated platelets. *Biochim. Biophys. Acta* 444:633, 1976.

416. Akkerman, J. W. N., Holmsen, H., and Driver, H. A.: Platelet aggregation and Ca²⁺ secretion are independent on simultaneous ATP production. *FEBS Lett.* 100:286, 1979.

417. Akkerman, J. W. N., Driver, H. A., Dangelmaier, C. A., and Holmsen, H.: Flux control in human platelet glycolysis and glycogenolysis. Unpublished observations.

418. Hussain, Q. Z., and Newcomb, T. F.: Thrombin stimulation of platelet oxygen consumption rate. *J. Appl. Physiol.* 19:297, 1964.

419. Murer, E. H.: Release reaction and energy metabolism in blood platelets with special reference to the burst in oxygen uptake. *Biochim. Biophys. Acta* 162:320, 1968.

420. Muenzer, J., Weinbach, E. C., and Wolfe, S. M.: Oxygen consumption of human platelets. I. Effect of thrombin. *Biochim. Biophys. Acta* 376:237, 1975.

421. Muenzer, J., Weinbach, E. C., and Wolfe, S. M.: Oxygen consumption of human blood platelets. II. Effect of inhibitors of thrombin-induced burst. *Biochim. Biophys. Acta* 376:243, 1975.

422. Bressler, N. M., Broekman, M. J., and Marcus, A. J.: Concurrent studies in oxygen consumption and aggregation in stimulated human platelets. *Blood* 53:167, 1979.

423. Akkerman, J. W., Gorter, G., Schrama, L., and Holmsen, H.: A novel technique for rapid determination of energy consumption in platelets. *Biochem. J.*, 1983, in press.

424. Mills, D. C. B.: Changes in the adenylate energy charge in human blood platelets induced by adenosine diphosphate. *Nature* 243:220, 1973.

425. Ball, G., Fulwood, M., Ireland, D. M., and Yates, P.: Effect of some inhibitors of platelet aggregation on platelet nucleotides. *Biochem. J.* 114:669, 1969.

426. Holmsen, H.: Changes in the radioactivity of P^{32}-labelled acid-soluble organophosphates in blood platelets during collagen and adenosine diphosphate induced platelet aggregation. *Scand. J. Clin. Lab. Invest.* 17:537, 1965.

427. Murer, E. H., Hellem, A. J., and Rozenberg, M. C.: Energy metabolism and platelet function. *Scand. J. Clin. Lab. Invest.* 19:280, 1967.

428. Holmsen, H., Kaplan, K., and Dangelmaier, C. A.: Differential energy requirements for platelet responses. *Biochem. J.* 208:9, 1982.

429. Rittenhouse-Simmons, S., and Deykin, D.: The mobilization of arachidonic acid in platelets exposed to thrombin or ionophore A23187: Effects of adenosine triphosphate deprivation. *J. Clin. Invest.* 60:495, 1977.

430. Mant, M. J.: Platelet adherence to collagen: Metabolic requirements. *Thromb. Res.* 17:729, 1980.

431. Murer, E. H.: Clot retraction and energy metabolism of platelets: Effect and mechanism of inhibitors. *Biochim. Biophys. Acta* 172:266, 1969.

432. Peerschke, E. J., and Zucker, M. B.: Fibrinogen receptor exposure and aggregation of human blood platelets produced by ADP and chilling. *Blood* 57:663, 1981.

433. Holmsen, H., and Akkerman, J. W. N.: On the requirement for ATP availability in platelet responses — A quantitative approach, in *The Regulation of Coagulation* edited by K. G. Mann and F. B. Taylor, Jr. Elsevier–North Holland, New York, 1980, pp. 409–417.

434. Kinlough-Rathbone, R. L., Packham, M. A., and Mustard, J. F.: The effect of glucose on ADP-induced platelet aggregation. *J. Lab. Clin. Med.* 75:780, 1970.

435. Kinlough-Rathbone, R. L., Packham, M. A., and Mustard, J. F.: The effect of glucose on the platelet responses to release-inducing stimuli. *J. Clin. Lab. Med.* 80:247, 1972.

436. Corn, M., Jackson, D. P., and Conley, C. L.: Components of blood necessary for clot retraction. *Bull. Johns Hopkins Hosp.* 107:90, 1960.

437. Weber, E., Littman, W., and Freitag, R.: Über Beziehungen zwischen Glycogengehalt und Retractionsvermogen von Blutplattchen. *Biochem. Pharmacol.* 12:145, 1963.

438. Fantl, P.: Thiol groups of blood platelets in relation to clot retraction. *Nature* 198:95, 1963.

439. Aledort, L. M., Troup, S. B., and Weed, R. I.: Inhibition of sulfhydryl-dependent platelet functions by penetrating and nonpenetrating analogues of parachloromercuribenzene. *Blood* 31:471, 1968.

440. Robinson, C. W., Jr., Mason, R. G., and Wagner, R. H.: Effect of sulfhydryl inhibitors on platelet agglutinability. *Proc. Soc. Exp. Biol. Med.* 113:857, 1963.

441. Harrison, M. J. G., Emmons, P. R., and Mitchell, J. R. A.: The effect of sulfhydryl and enzyme inhibitors on platelet aggregation in vitro. *Thromb. Diath. Haemorrh.* 16:122, 1966.

442. Hofman, J., et al.: Effect of decreased GSH level on human platelet functions. *Artery* 8:431, 1980.

443. Schick, P. K., Kurica, K. B., and Chacko, G. K.: Localization of phosphatidylethanolamine and phosphatidylserine in the human platelet plasma membrane. *J. Clin. Invest.* 57:1221, 1976.

444. Chap, H. J., Zwaal, R. R. A., and Van Deenen, L. L. M.: Action of highly purified phospholipases on blood platelets: Evidence for an asymmetrical distribution of phospholipids in the surface membrane. *Biochim. Biophys. Acta* 467:146, 1977.

445. Schick, P. K.: The organization of aminophospholipids in human platelets: Selective changes induced by thrombin. *J. Lab. Clin. Med.* 91:802, 1978.

446. Schick, P. K.: The role of platelet membrane lipids in platelet hemostatic activities. *Sem. Haematol.* 16:221, 1979.

447. Lloyd, J. V., Nishizawa, E. E., and Mustard, J. F.: Effect of ADP-induced shape change on incorporation of ^{32}P into platelet phosphatidic acid and mono-, di-, and triphosphatidylinositol. *Br. J. Haematol.* 25:77, 1973.

448. Lloyd, J. V., and Mustard, J. F.: Changes in ^{32}P-content of phosphatidic acid and the phosphoinositides of rabbit platelets during aggregation induced by collagen or thrombin. *Br. J. Haematol.* 26:243, 1974.

449. Lloyd, J. V., Nishizawa, E. E., Haldar, J., and Mustard, J. F.: Changes in ^{32}P-labelling of platelet phospholipids in response to ADP. *Br. J. Haematol.* 23:571, 1972.

450. Lloyd, J. V., Nishizawa, E. E., Joist, J. H., and Mustard, J. F.: Effect of ADP-induced aggregation on ^{32}PO$_4$ incorporation into phosphatidic acid and the phosphoinositides of rabbit platelets. *Br. J. Haematol.* 24:589, 1973.

451. Manco, G., Chap, H., Simon, M.-F., and Douste-Blazy, L.: Phosphatidic and lysophosphatidic acid production in phospholipase C- and thrombin-treated platelets: Possible involvement of a platelet lipase. *Biochemistry* 60:653, 1978.

452. Lapetina, E. G., and Cuatrecasas, P.: Ionophore A23187- and thrombin-induced platelet aggregation: Independence from cyclooxygenase products. *Proc. Natl. Acad. Sci. U.S.A.* 75:818, 1979.

453. Walenga, R., Vanderhoek, J. Y., and Feinstein, M. B.: Serine esterase inhibitors block stimulus-induced mobilization of arachidonic acid and phosphatidylinositide-specific phospholipase C activity in platelets. *J. Biol. Chem.* 255:6024, 1980.

454. Lapetina, E. G., Billah, M. M., and Cuatrecasas, P.: The phosphatidylinositol cycle and the regulation of arachidonic acid production. *Nature* 292:367, 1981.

455. Lapetina, E. G., Billah, M. M., and Cuatrecasas, P.: The initial action of thrombin on platelets: Conversion of phosphatidylinositol to phosphatidic acid preceding the production of arachidonic acid. *J. Biol. Chem.* 256:5037, 1981.

456. Lapetina, E. G., Chandrabose, K. A., and Cuatrecasas, P.: Ionophore A23187 and thrombin-induced platelet aggregation: Independence from cyclooxygenase products. *Proc. Natl. Acad. Sci. U.S.A.* 75:818, 1978.

457. Broekman, M. J., Ward, J. W., and Marcus, A. J.: Phospholipid metabolism in stimulated human platelets: Changes in phosphatidylinositol, phosphatidic acid, and lysophospholipids. *J. Clin. Invest.* 66:275, 1980.

458. Bell, R. L., and Majerus, P. W.: Thrombin-induced hydrolysis of phosphatidylinositol in human platelets. *J. Biol. Chem.* 255:1790, 1980.

459. Gerrard, J. M., Butler, A. M., Peterson, D. A., and White J. G.: Phosphatidic acid releases calcium from a platelet membrane fraction in vitro. *Prostaglandins Med.* 1:387, 1978.

460. Ikeda, Y., Kikuchi, M., Toyama, K., Watanabe, K., and Ando, Y.: Ionophoretic activities of phospholipids on human platelets. *Thromb. Haemost.* 41:779, 1979.

461. Billah, M. M., Lapetina, E. G., and Cuatrecasas, P.: Phospholipase A$_2$ activity specific for phosphatidic acid: A possible mechanism for the production of arachidonic acid in platelets. *J. Biol. Chem.* 256:5399, 1981.

462. Mauco, G., Chap, H., and Douste-Blazy, L.: Characterization and properties of a phosphatidylinositol phosphodiesterase (phospholipase C) from platelet cytosol. *FEBS Lett.* 100:367, 1979.

463. Billah, M. M., Lapetina, E. G., and Cuatrecasas, P.: Phosphatidyl-

inosito-specific phospholipase C of platelets: Association with 1,2-diacylglycerol-kinase and inhibition by cyclic-AMP. *Biochem. Biophys. Res. Commun. 90:92, 1979.*

464. Rittenhouse-Simmons, S.: Production of diglyceride from phosphatidylinositol in activated human platelets. *J. Clin. Invest. 63: 580, 1979.*

465. Putney, J. W.: Recent hypotheses regarding the phosphatidylinositol effect. *Life Sci. 29:1183, 1981.*

466. Hawthorne, J. N.: Is phosphatidylinositol now out of the calcium gate? *Nature 295:281, 1982.*

467. Laffont, F., Chap, H., Soula, G., and Douste-Blazy, L.: Phospholipid exchange proteins from platelet cytosol possibly involved in phospholipid effect. *Biochem. Biophys. Res. Commun. 102:1366, 1981.*

468. Perret, B., Chap, J. H., and Dauste-Blazy, L.: Asymmetric distribution of arachidonic acid in the plasma membrane of human platelets. *Biochim. Biophys. Acta 556:434, 1979.*

469. Kannagi, R., Koizumi, K., and Masuda, T.: Limited hydrolysis of platelet membrane phospholipids. *J. Biol. Chem. 256:1177, 1981.*

470. Guichardant, M., and Lagarde, M.: Effects of low doses of thrombin on human platelet phospholipids. *Thromb. Res. 18:285, 1980.*

471. Bills, T. K., Smith, J. B., and Silver, M. J.: Selective release of arachidonic acid from the phospholipids in response to thrombin. *J. Clin. Invest. 60:1, 1977.*

472. Rittenhouse-Simmons, S., Russel, F. A., and Deykin, D.: Transfer of arachidonic acid to human platelet plasmalogen in response to thrombin. *Biochem. Biophys. Res. Commun. 70:295, 1976.*

473. Chan, L. Y., and Tai, H. H.: Release of arachidonate from diglyceride in human platelets requires the sequential action of a diglyceride lipase and a monoglyceride lipase. *Biochem. Biophys. Res. Commun. 100:1688, 1981.*

474. Kannagi, R., and Koizumi, K.: Effect of different physical states of phospholipid substrates on partially purified platelet phospholipase A₂ activity. *Biochim. Biophys. Acta 556:423, 1979.*

475. Apitz-Castro, R. J., Mas, M. A., Cruz, M. R., and Jain, M. K.: Isolation of homogeneous phospholipase A₂ from human platelets. *Biochem. Biophys. Res. Commun. 91:63, 1979.*

476. Jesse, R. L., and Fransson, R. C.: Modulation of purified phospholipase A₂ activity from human platelets by calcium and indomethacin. *Biochim. Biophys. Acta 575:467, 1979.*

477. Franson, R.-C., Eisen, D., Jesse, R., and Lanni, C.: Inhibition of highly purified mammalian phospholipases A₂ by non-steroidal anti-inflammatory agents. *Biochem. J. 186:633, 1980.*

478. Daniel, J. L., Molish, I. R., and Holmsen, H.: Myosin phosphorylation in intact platelets. *J. Biol. Chem. 256:7510, 1981.*

479. Bennet, W. F., Belville, J. S., and Lynch, G.: A study of protein phosphorylation in shape change and Ca²⁺-dependent serotonin release by blood platelets. *Cell 18:1015, 1979.*

480. Lyons, R. M., and Shaw, J. O.: Interaction of Ca²⁺ and protein phosphorylation in the rabbit platelet release reaction. *J. Clin. Invest. 65:242, 1980.*

481. Wallace, W. C., and Bensusan, H. B.: Protein phosphorylation in platelets stimulated by immobilized thrombin at 37°C and 4°C. *J. Biol. Chem. 255:1932, 1980.*

482. Lyons, R. M., and Atherton, R. M.: Characterization of a platelet protein phosphorylated during the thrombin-induced release reaction. *Biochemistry 18:544, 1979.*

483. Gerrard, J. M., and Carroll, R. C.: Stimulation of platelet protein phosphorylation by arachidonic acid and endoperoxide analogs. *Prostaglandins 22:81, 1981.*

484. Gerrard, J. M., and Carroll, R. C.: ADP initiates phosphorylation of platelet myosin light chain (MLC), a 40,000 dalton protein (40P) and actin-binding protein (ABP) independent of secretion. *Thromb. Haemost. 46, 1981 (abstract 282).*

485. Daniel, J. L., and Molish, I. R.: Phosphorylation of myosin light chain during shape change. (In preparation.)

486. Nishikawa, M., Tanaka, T., and Hidaka, H.: Ca²⁺-calmodulin–dependent phosphorylation and platelet secretion. *Nature 287: 863, 1980.*

487. Gergely, P., Castle, A. G., and Crawford, N.: Platelet phosphoprotein phosphatase activity: Its subcellular distribution and regulation. *Biochim. Biophys. Acta 611:384, 1980.*

488. Kawahara, Y., Takai, Y., Minakuchi, R., Sano, K., and Nishizuka, Y.: Possible involvement of Ca²⁺-activated, phospholipid dependent protein kinase in platelet activation. *J. Biochem. 88:913, 1980.*

489. Kawahara, Y., Takai, Y., Minakuchi, R., Sano, K., and Nishizuka, Y.: Phospholipid turnover as a possible transmembrane original for protein phosphorylation during human platelet activation by thrombin. *Biochem. Biophys. Res. Commun. 97:309, 1980.*

490. Nachmias, V. T., Sullender, J., and Asch, A.: Shape and cytoplasmic filaments in control and lidocaine-treated human platelets. *Blood 50:39, 1977.*

491. Nachmias, V. T.: Cytoskeleton of human platelets at rest and after spreading. *J. Cell. Biol. 86:795, 1980.*

492. Gonella, P. A., and Nachmias, V. T.: Platelet activation and microfilament bundling. *J. Cell. Biol. 89:146, 1981.*

493. Markey, F., Persson, T., and Lindberg, V.: Characterization of platelet extracts before and after stimulation with respect to the possible role of profilactin as microfilament precursor. *Cell 23: 145, 1981.*

494. Dingle, T. A., Toh, B. H., Firkin, B. G., and Pfuller, S. L.: Human platelet actin: Surface expression after platelet activation. *Thromb. Haemost. 42:799, 1979.*

495. George, J. N., Lyons, R. M., and Morgan, R. K.: Membrane changes associated with platelet activation: Exposure of actin on the platelet surface after thrombin-induced secretion. *J. Clin. Invest. 66:1, 1979.*

496. Carlsson, L., Markey, F., Blikstad, I., Persson, T., and Lindberg, U.: Reorganization of actin in platelets stimulated by thrombin as measured by the DNase I inhibition assay. *Proc. Natl. Acad. Sci. U.S.A. 76:6376, 1979.*

497. Phillips, D. R., Jennings, L. K., and Edwards, H. H.: Identification of membrane proteins mediating the interaction of human platelets. *J. Cell Biol. 86:77, 1980.*

498. Pribluda, V., Laub, F., and Rotman, A.: The state of actin in activated human platelets. *Eur. J. Biochem. 116:293, 1981.*

499. Howard, T. H., and Lin, S.: Specific interaction of cytochalasins with muscle and platelet actin filaments in vitro. *J. Supramol. Struct. 11:283, 1979.*

500. Fox, J. E. B., and Phillips, D. R.: Inhibition of actin polymerization in blood platelets by cytochalasins. *Nature 292:650, 1981.*

501. Casella, J. F., Flanagan, M. D., and Lin, S.: Cytochalasin D inhibits actin polymerization and induces depolymerization of actin filaments formed during platelet shape change. *Nature 293:302, 1981.*

502. Menche, D., Israel, A., and Karpatkin, S.: Platelets and microtubules: Effect pf colchicine and D₂O on platelet aggregation and release induced by calcium ionophore A23187. *J. Clin. Invest. 66: 284, 1980.*

503. Cohen, I., Glaser, T., Veis, A., and Bruner-Lorand, J.: Ca²⁺-dependent cross-linking processes in human platelets. *Biochim. Biophys. Acta 676:137, 1981.*

504. Truglia, J. A., and Stracher, A.: Purification and characterization of a calcium-dependent sulfhydryl protease from human platelets. *Biochem. Biophys. Res. Commun. 100:814, 1981.*

505. Phillips, D. R., and PohAgin, P.: Thrombin substrates and the proteolytic site of thrombin action on human-platelet plasma membranes. *Biochim. Biophys. Acta 352:218, 1974.*

506. Phillips, D. R., and Agin, P. P.: Platelet plasma membrane glycoproteins: Identification of a proteolytic substrate for thrombin. *Biochem. Biophys. Res. Commun. 75:940, 1977.*

507. Mosher, D. F., Vaheri, A., Choate, J. J., and Gahmberg, C. G.: Action of thrombin on surface glycoproteins of human platelets. *Blood 53:437, 1979.*

508. Berndt, M. C., and Phillips, D. R.: Purification and preliminary physicochemical characterization of human platelet membrane glycoprotein V. *J. Biol. Chem. 256:59, 1981.*

509. Prasanna, J. R., Edwards, H. H., and Phillips, D. R.: Interaction of platelet plasma membranes with thrombin-activated platelets. *Blood 57:305, 1981.*

510. Zieve, P. D., and Greenough, W. B., III: Adenyl cyclase in human platelets: Activity and responsiveness. *Biochem. Biophys. Res. Commun. 35:462, 1969.*

511. Robison, G. A., Cole, B., Arnold, A., and Hartmann, R.: Effects of

prostaglandins on function and cyclic AMP levels of human blood platelets. *Ann. N.Y. Acad. Sci.* 180:324, 1971.

512. Salzman, E. W., and Levin, L.: Cyclic 3',5'-adenosine monophosphate in human blood platelets. II. Effect of N^6-2'-O-dibutyryl cyclic 3',5'-AMP on platelet function. *J. Clin. Invest.* 50:131, 1971.

513. Emmons, P. R., Hampton, J. R., Harrison, M. J. G., Honour, A. J., and Mitchell, J. R. A.: Effect of prostaglandin E₁ on platelet behavior in vitro and in vivo. *Br. Med. J.* 2:468, 1967.

514. Salzman, E. W., and Neri, L. L.: Cyclic 3',5'-adenosine monophosphate in human blood platelets. *Nature* 224:609, 1969.

515. Haslam, R.: Roles of cyclic nucleotides in platelet function, in *Ciba Foundation Symposium on the Biochemistry and Pharmacology of Blood Platelets*, edited by J. Knight. Associated Scientific Publishers, Amsterdam, 1975, p. 21.

516. McDonald, J. W. D., and Stuart, R. K.: Regulation of cyclic AMP levels and aggregation in human platelets by prostaglandin E₁. *J. Lab. Clin. Med.* 81:838, 1973.

517. Robison, G., Arnold, A., Cole, B., and Hartman, R.: Effects of prostaglandins on function and cyclic AMP levels of human blood platelets. *Ann. N.Y. Acad. Sci.* 180:324, 1971.

518. Mills, D. C. B., and Smith, J. B.: The control of platelet responsiveness by agents that influence cyclic AMP levels. *Ann. N.Y. Acad. Sci.* 201:391, 1972.

519. Salzman, E. W., and Weisenberger, H.: Role of cyclic AMP in platelet function. *Adv. Cyclic Nucleotide Res.* 1:231, 1972.

520. Wolfe, S. M., and Shulman, N. R.: Adenyl cyclase in human platelets. *Biochem. Biophys. Res. Commun.* 35:265, 1969.

521. Haslam, R. J., and Rosson, G. M.: Effects of adenosine on levels of adenosine cyclic 3',5'-monophosphate in human platelets in relation to adenosine incorporation and platelet aggregation. *Mol. Pharmacol.* 11:525, 1975.

522. Tsai, B. S., and Lefkowitz, R. J.: Agonist-specific effects of guanine nucleotides on alpha adrenergic receptors in human platelets. *Mol. Pharmacol.* 16:61, 1979.

523. Michel, T., Hoffman, B. B., and Lefkowitz, R. J. Differential regulation of the α-adrenergic receptor by Na and guanine nucleotides. *Nature* 288:709, 1980.

524. Song, S.-Y., and Cheung, W. Y.: Cyclic 3',5'-nucleotide phosphodiesterase: Properties of the enzyme of human platelets. *Biochim. Biophys. Acta* 242:593, 1971.

525. Amer, M., and Maynol, R. F.: Studies with phosphodiesterase. III. Two forms of the enzyme from human platelets. *Biochim. Biophys. Acta* 309:149, 1973.

526. Tateson, J., Moncada, S., and Vane, J. R.: Effects of prostacyclin (PGX) on cyclic AMP concentrations in human platelets. *Prostaglandins* 13:389, 1977.

527. Gorman, R. R., Bunting, S., and Miller, O. V.: Modulation of human platelet adenylate cyclase by prostacyclin (PBX). *Prostaglandins* 13:377, 1977.

528. Schafer, A. I., Cooper, B., O'Hara, D., and Handin, R. I.: Identification of platelet receptors for prostaglandin I₂ and D₂. *J. Biol. Chem.* 254:2914, 1979.

529. Miller, O. V., and Gorman, R. R.: Evidence for distinct prostaglandin I₂ and D₂ receptors in human platelets. *J. Pharmacol. Exp. Ther.* 210:134, 1979.

530. Mills, D. C. B., and Macfarlane, D. E.: Stimulation of human platelet adenylate cyclase by prostaglandin D₂. *Thromb. Res.* 5:401, 1974.

531. Cooper, B.: Agonist regulation of the human platelet prostaglandin D₂ receptor. *Life Sci.* 25:1361, 1979.

532. Siegl, A. M., Smith, J. B., and Silver, M. J.: Specific binding sites for prostaglandin D₂ on human platelets. *Biochem. Biophys. Res. Commun.* 90:291, 1979.

533. Silver, M. J., Smith, J. B., Ingerman, C., and Kocsis, J. J.: Human blood prostaglandins: Formation during clotting. *Prostaglandins* 1:429, 1972.

534. Smith, J. B., Ingerman, C., Kocsis, J. J., and Silver, M. J.: Formation of prostaglandins during the aggregation of human blood platelets. *J. Clin. Invest.* 52:965, 1974.

535. Smith, J. B., Silver, M. J., Ingerman, C. M., and Kocsis, J. J.: Prostaglandin D₂ inhibits the aggregation of human platelets. *Thromb. Res.* 5:291, 1974.

536. Kloeze, J.: Influence of prostaglandins on platelet adhesiveness and platelet aggregation, in *Proceedings of Nobel Symposium II, Stockholm, 1966*. Almquist and Wiksell, Stockholm, 1967, p. 241.

537. Smith, J. B., and Macfarlane, D. E.: Platelets, in *The Prostaglandins*, edited by P. D. Ramwell. Plenum, New York, 1974, vol. 2, pp. 293–343.

538. Mills, D. C. B., and Smith, J. B.: The influence on platelet aggregation of drugs that affect the accumulation of 3',5'-cyclic adenosine monophosphate in platelets. *Biochem. J.* 121, 185, 1971.

539. Steer, M. L., and Wood, A.: Regulation of human platelet adenylate cyclase by epinephrine, prostaglandin E₁, and guanine nucleotides. *J. Biol. Chem.* 254:10791, 1979.

540. Steer, M. L., and Wood, A.: Inhibitory effects of sodium and other monovalent cations on human platelet adenylate cyclase. *J. Biol. Chem.* 256:9990, 1981.

541. Haslam, R. J., and Lynham, J.: Activation and inhibition of blood platelet adenylate cyclase by adenose or by 2-chloroadenosine. *Life Sci.* 11:1143, 1972.

542. Jakobs, K. H., Saur, W., and Johnson, R. A.: Regulation of platelet adenylate cyclase by adenosine. *Biochim. Biophys. Acta* 583:409, 1979.

543. Cusak, N. J., and Hourani, S. M.: 5'-N-Ethyl carboxyamidoadenosine: A potent inhibitor of human platelet aggregation. *Br. J. Pharmacol.* 72:443, 1981.

544. McDonald, J. W.: Lymphocyte and platelet adenylate cyclase. *Can. J. Biochem.* 49:316, 1970.

545. Mills, D. C. B.: Factors influencing the adenylate cyclase system in human blood platelets, in *Platelets and Thrombosis*, edited by S. Sherry and A. Scriabine. University Park, Baltimore, 1974, p. 45.

546. Harwood, J. P., Moskowitz, J., and Krishna, G.: Dynamic interaction of prostaglandin and norepinephrine in the formation of adenosine 3',5'-monophosphate in human and rabbit platelets. *Biochim. Biophys. Acta* 261:444, 1972.

547. Marquis, N. R., Becker, J. A., and Vigdahl, R. L.: Platelet aggregation. III. An epinephrine induced decrease in cyclic AMP synthesis. *Biochem. Biophys. Res. Commun.* 39:783, 1970.

548. Mills, D. C. B.: The regulation of adenylate cyclase activity in human platelets, in *The Regulation of Coagulation*, edited by K. G. Mann and F. B. Taylor. North Holland, New York, 1980, pp. 419–427.

549. Mellwig, K. P., and Jacobs, K. H.: Inhibition of platelet adenylate kinase by ADP. *Thromb. Res.* 18:7, 1980.

550. Salzman, E. W.: Interrelation of prostaglandin endoperoxide PGG₂ and cyclic 3',5' adenosine monophosphate in human blood platelets. *Biochim. Biophys. Acta* 499:48, 1977.

551. Claesson, H.-E., and Malmsten, C.: On the relationship of prostaglandin endoperoxide G₂ and cyclic nucleotides in platelet function. *Eur. J. Biochem.* 76:277, 1977.

552. Miller, O. V., and Gorman, R. R.: Inhibition of PGE₁-stimulated cyclic AMP accumulation by thromboxane A₂. *Prostaglandins* 13:599, 1977.

553. Gorman, R. R.: Modulation of human platelet function by prostacyclin and thromboxane A₂. *Fed. Proc.* 38:83, 1979.

554. Bonne, C., Martin, B., and Regnault, F.: The cyclic-AMP lowering effect of the stable endoperoxide analog U 46619 in human platelets. *Thromb. Res.* 20:701, 1980.

555. Agarwal, K. C., and Parks, R. E., Jr.: 5'-Methylthioadenosine and 2',5'dideoxyadenosine blockage of the inhibitory effects of adenosine-induced platelet aggregation by different mechanisms. *Biochem. Pharmacol.* 29:2529, 1980.

556. Imandt, L., Tijhuis, D., Wessels, H., and Haanen, C.: Lithium inhibits adenylate cyclase of human platelets. *Thromb. Haemost.* 45:142, 1981.

557. Vane, J. R., and Moncada, S.: Prostacyclin. *Ciba Found. Symp.* 71:79, 1980.

558. Moncada, S., and Korbet, R.: Dipyridamole and other phosphodiesterase inhibitors act as antithrombotic agents by potentiating endogenous prostacyclin. *Lancet* 1:1286, 1978.

559. Steer, M. L., MacIntyre, D. E., Levine, L., and Salzman, E. W.: Is prostacyclin a physiologically important circulating antiplatelet agent? *Nature* 283:194, 1980.

560. Haslam, R. J., and McClenagan, M. D.: Measurement of circulating prostacyclin. *Nature* 292:364, 1981.

561. Droller, M. J.: Thrombin-induced platelet production of cyclic AMP and a possible intrinsic modulation of platelet function. *Scand. J. Haematol. 17:167, 1976.*

562. Harris, D. N., Assad, M. M., Phillips, M. B., Goldenberg, H. J., and Antonaccio, M. J.: Inhibition of adenylate cyclase in human blood platelets by 9-substituted adenine derivatives. *J. Cyclic Nucl. 5:125, 1979.*

563. Haslam, R. J., Davidson, M. M. L., and Desjardius, J. V.: Inhibition of adenylate cyclase by adenosine analogues in preparation of broken and intact human platelets. *Biochem. J. 176:83, 1978.*

564. Rodan, G. A., and Feinstein, M. B.: Interrelationships between Ca²⁺ and adenylate and guanylate cyclases in the control of platelet secretion and aggregation. *Proc. Natl. Acad. Sci. U.S.A. 73:1829, 1976.*

565. Ardlie, N. G., Glew, G., Schultz, B. G., and Schwartz, C. J.: Inhibition and reversals of platelet aggregation by methyl xanthines. *Thromb. Diath. Haemorrh. 18:670, 1967.*

566. Markwardt, F., Barthel, W., Glusa, E., and Hoffman, A.: Untersuchungen über den Einfluss von Papaverin auf Reaktionen der Bluttplattchen. *Naunyn Schmiedbergs Arch. Pharmacol. 257:420, 1967.*

567. Markwardt, F., and Hoffman, A.: Effects of papaverine derivatives on cyclic AMP phosphodiesterase of human platelets. *Biochem. Pharmacol. 19:2519, 1970.*

568. Vigdahl, R. M., Mongin, J., Jr., and Marquis, N. R.: Platelet aggregation. 4. Platelet phosphodiesterase and its inhibition by vasodilators. *Biochem. Biophys. Res. Commun. 42:1088, 1971.*

569. Rozenberg, M. C., and Walker, C. M.: The effect of pyrimidine compounds on the potentiation of adenosine inhibition of aggregation, on adenosine phosphorylation and on phosphodiesterase activity of blood platelets. *Br. J. Haematol. 24:409, 1973.*

570. McElroy, F. A., and Philp, R. B.: Relative potencies of dipyridamole and related agents as inhibitors of cyclic nucleotide phosphodiesterases: Possible explanation of mechanism of inhibition of platelet function. *Life Sci. 17:1479, 1976.*

571. Pichard, A. L., Hanoune, J., and Kaplan, J. C.: Multiple forms of cyclic phosphodiesterase from human blood platelets. 1. Kinetic and electrophoretic characterization of two molecular species. *Biochim. Biophys. Acta 315:370, 1973.*

572. Horlington, M., and Watson, P. A.: Inhibition of 3′,5′cyclic AMP phosphodiesterase by some platelet aggregation inhibitors. *Biochem. Pharmacol. 19:955, 1970.*

573. Asano, T., Ochai, Y., and Hidaka, H.: Selective inhibition of separated forms of platelet cyclic phosphodiesterase by platelet aggregation inhibitors. *Mol. Pharmacol. 13:400, 1977.*

574. Haslam, R. J., Salama, S. E., Fox, J. E. B., Lynham, J. A., and Davidson, M. M. L.: Roles of cyclic nucleotides and of protein phosphorylation in the regulation of platelet function, in *Platelets: Cellular Response Mechanisms and Their Biological Significance,* edited by A. Rotman, F. A. Meyer, C. Gitler, and A. Silberberg. Wiley, New York, 1980, pp. 213–231.

575. Lyons, R. M.: Compartmentalization of adenosine 3′5′-monophosphate–binding proteins in human platelets. *Thromb. Res. 19:317, 1980.*

576. Booyse, F. M., Marr, J., Young, D. G., Guiliani, D., and Rafelson, M. E.: Adenosine cyclic 3′,5′-monophosphate–dependent protein kinase from human platelets. *Biochim. Biophys. Acta 422:60, 1977.*

577. Bishop, G. A., and Rozenberg, M. C. The effect of ADP, calcium, and some inhibitors of platelet aggregation on protein phosphokinases from human blood platelets. *Biochim. Biophys. Acta 385:112, 1975.*

578. Steiner, M.: Endogenous phosphorylation of platelet membrane proteins. *Arch. Biochem. Biophys. 171:245, 1975.*

579. Kaulen, H. D., and Gross, R.: Purification and properties of a soluble cyclic AMP–dependent protein kinase of human platelets. *Hoppe Seylers Z. Physiol. Chem. 355:471, 1974.*

580. Assaf, S. F.: Human platelet protein kinases: Reaction with platelet membranes and cytoplasmic enzymes and crystallization of a cyclic AMP-dependent protein kinase. *Ann. N.Y. Acad. Sci. 283:159, 1977.*

581. Kaser-Glanzmann, R., Jakabova, M., George, J. N., and Luscher, E. F.: Stimulation of calcium uptake in platelet membrane vesicles by adenosine 3′,5′-cyclic monophosphate and protein kinase. *Biochim. Biophys. Acta 466:429, 1977.*

582. Kaser-Glanzmann, R.: Regulation of the intracellular calcium level in human blood platelets: Adenosine 3′,5′-monophosphate–dependent phosphorylation of a 22,000 dalton component in isolated Ca²⁺ accumulating vesicles. *Biochim. Biophys. Acta 558:344, 1979.*

583. Hathaway, D. R., Eaton, C. R., and Adelstein, R. S.: Regulation of myosin light-chain kinase by the catalytic subunit of cyclic AMP-dependent protein kinase. *Nature 291:252, 1981.*

CHAPTER *129*

Platelet function

MARJORIE B. ZUCKER

Platelets are important in arresting bleeding from damaged blood vessels, fulfilling their hemostatic function by literally plugging any hole in the vessel wall and providing a surface that promotes blood coagulation. This chapter describes these functions of platelets. The morphologic changes which occur when platelets perform their hemostatic function are presented in Chap. 126, while the biochemical changes are outlined in Chap. 128. A number of books [1–10] and review articles [11–15] may also be consulted for additional details.

The hemostatic plug

The formation of a hemostatic platelet plug can be observed through the light microscope if a small blood vessel in a translucent tissue such as the mesentery is nicked or severed and the blood flowing from the wound is kept from obscuring the field [16,17]. Within 1 or 2 s, a few platelets adhere to the edge of the lesion; over the next few minutes, platelets from the blood flowing out through the wound adhere to those already anchored. The resulting mass fills the gap in the vessel wall (Fig. 129-1) and arrests the bleeding. Although bleeding through the plug is often renewed for brief periods, it is usually permanently arrested within 5 min. Examination of a hemostatic platelet plug with an electron microscope [17–19] (Figs. 129-2 and 129-3) corroborates the impression gained by light microscopy [20] and shows that the plug is composed of platelets which have been altered to varying degrees. Degranulation is especially prominent at the periphery of the plug. Fibrin strands surround the mass of platelets but are rarely seen within it. Erythrocytes and leukocytes are also rarely seen within the plug. If there is a wound tract, it becomes filled with clotted blood—a fibrin meshwork with many entrapped erythrocytes [20]. Within 20 h much more fibrin is evident within the plug; the plate-

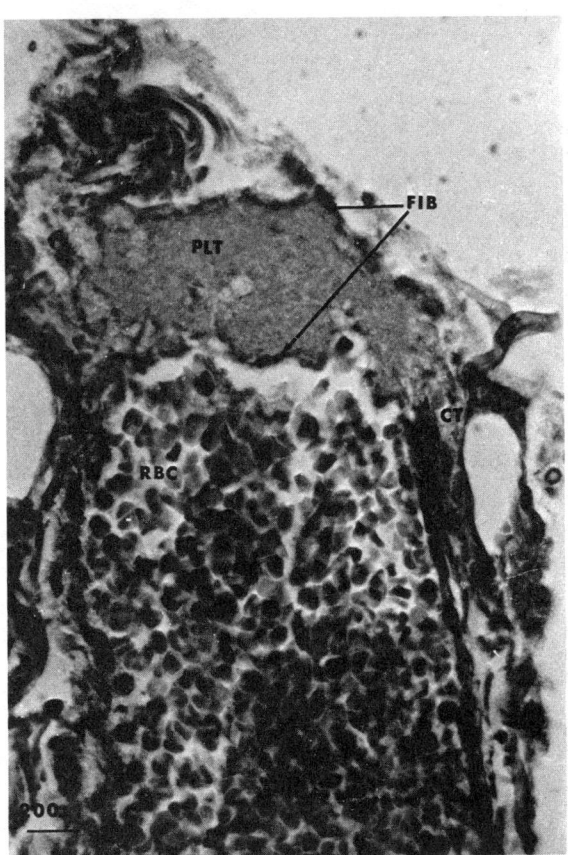

FIGURE 129-1 Hemostatic platelet plug capping blood vessel 10 min after transection. Mass of platelets (PLT) extends across vessel, contacting connective tissue (CT) on either side. Fibrin (FIB) surrounds platelets but is not seen within mass. No fibrin or clotted whole blood is evident within lumen of blood vessel. (Reprinted by permission from Hovig et al. [21].

lets undergo degenerative changes and become more loosely bound [21].

Platelets also interact with the walls of blood vessels which have been denuded of endothelium but not transected (see Chap. 139). Platelets may form a single layer or a *white body* [22] which may become the head of a thrombus as described in Chap. 160.

Platelet function can be conveniently analyzed in terms of the following processes: (1) the interaction of platelets with the blood vessel wall; (2) the interaction of platelets with one another; and (3) the relation of platelets to blood clotting (i.e., thrombin evolution).

The interaction of platelets with the blood vessel wall

When the blood vessel wall is transected, platelets contact and react with subendothelial components and collagen in and around the vessel wall. Only 1 or 2 s elapse between severing of a blood vessel and adhesion of platelets to the cut margin. This interval is too short

for thrombin evolved in the shed blood to be responsible [23], and the observation that platelets adhere to connective tissue strands [24] led to the discovery that they react rapidly with collagen, whether it is purified or present in connective tissue [25–27]. Although formation of a hemostatic platelet plug is triggered by adhesion of platelets to collagen, its major growth depends on cohesive forces between platelets, mediated largely by thrombin and released adenosine diphosphate (ADP) and products of arachidonic acid metabolism (see below).

Vascular trauma which does not breach the vessel wall may detach endothelial cells from either the basement membrane or the less distinct zone that underlies these cells in large vessels [28,29]. The few platelets that may adhere to injured endothelial cells remain normal morphologically. In contrast, the many platelets that adhere to the basement membrane undergo degranulation and may form the nucleus for accumulation of other platelets as well as fibrin [28–30] (Fig. 129-4).

Marked dilation of blood vessels causes adjacent endothelial cells to separate at their junctions exposing the basement membrane. These gaps may then be filled by

FIGURE 129-2 Margin of hemostatic platelet plug, showing degranulated platelets in contact with collagen fibers (COL). Platelets at margin of plug have lost their organelles. No fibrin is seen between platelets. (Courtesy of T. Hovig.)

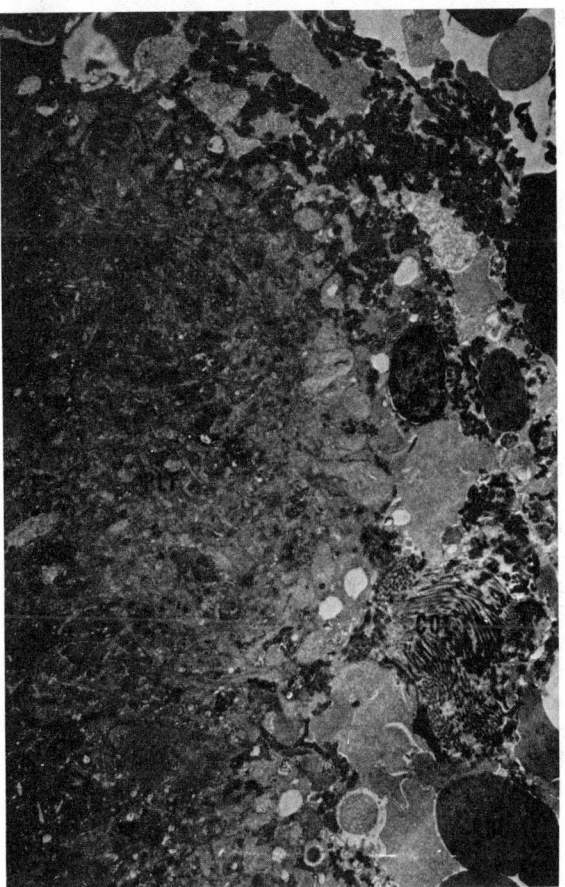

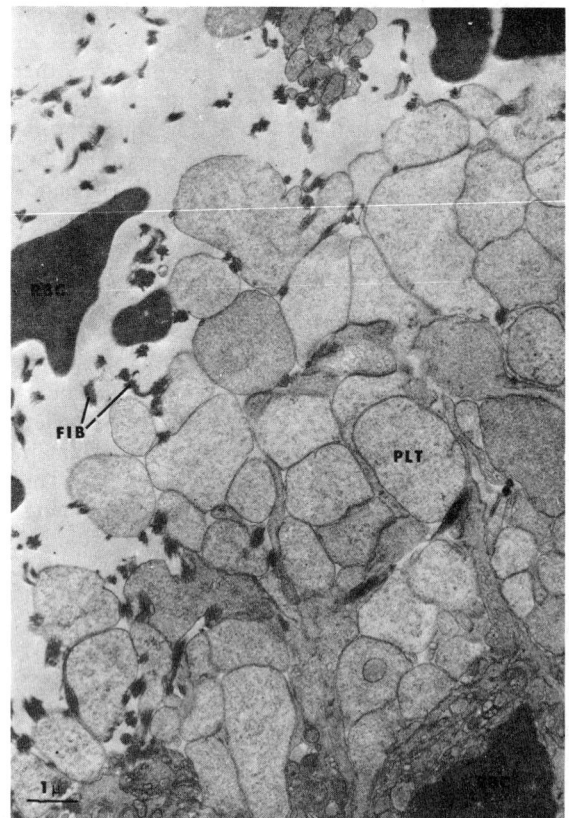

FIGURE 129-3   Higher magnification of degranulated plate-lets and swollen platelet processes at margin of platelet plug. (Courtesy of T. Hovig and J. F. Mustard.)

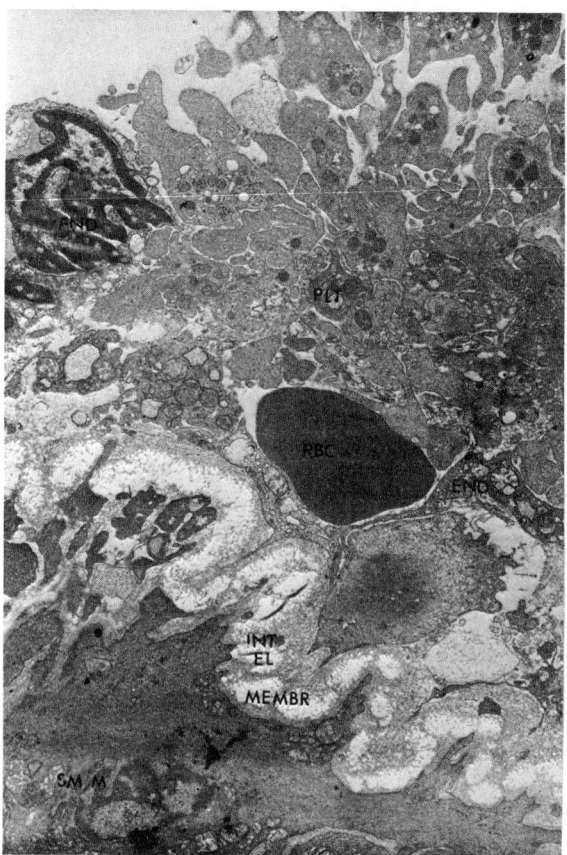

FIGURE 129-4   Platelet aggregate over area of endothelial cell desquamation caused by partial ligation of vein for 2 h. Platelets have not adhered to damaged endothelial cell (END). Note internal elastic membrane (INT EL MEMBR) and under-lying smooth muscle (SM M). (Reprinted by permission from C.-H. Ts'ao and T. H. Spaet, Ultramicroscopic changes in the rabbit inferior vena cava following partial constriction. *Am. J. Pathol.* 51:789, 1967.)

all or part of a platelet [31,32]. When the platelet count is low, red blood cells probably leave the circulation through these gaps. In the skin or mucous membranes these small hemorrhages are recognized as petechiae.

The interaction of platelets with one another (platelet cohesion or aggregation)

ADENOSINE DIPHOSPHATE
The discovery that ADP aggregates platelets was a major advance in understanding platelet function [33]. ADP is effective in low concentrations—less than 1.0 μM—which can readily be derived from endogenous sources in the platelets. The ability of ADP to aggregate platelets is unique—other nucleotides are either in-active or active only at much higher concentrations [34].

Because of the difficulty of examining platelet aggre-gation in vivo, most studies have been carried out in vitro, using platelet-rich plasma prepared by slow centrifugation of citrated blood. Although marked cal-cium depletion inhibits aggregation, citrated plasma

contains enough calcium ions to let it proceed. It is necessary to stir the platelet-rich plasma to provide platelet contact. In vitro studies must be interpreted cautiously because artifacts have been introduced. Thus the low concentration of ionized calcium in citrated plasma facilitates the induction of the release reaction by ADP [35], and the slow centrifugation used in pre-paring platelet-rich plasma alters platelet function [36,37].

Platelets that have been carefully separated from plasma, e.g., by gel filtration [38], will not aggregate with ADP unless fibrinogen is present. The necessary fibrinogen concentration is far below that in normal plasma [39,40].

In vitro platelet aggregation has been studied most extensively by determining changes in the light trans-mission of platelet-rich plasma after addition of an aggregating agent (Fig. 129-5). Platelet-rich plasma is cloudy because the platelets deflect the incident light. As platelets aggregate and form larger masses, the concentration of platelets in the plasma is effectively reduced and light transmission increases. If the aggregates disperse, more particles are present and light transmission decreases.

ADP-induced aggregation may be reversible, biphasic, or irreversible, depending on the concentrations of the reagent used [41] (Fig. 129-5). With low concentrations of ADP (1.0 μM in this experiment), reversible aggregation occurs. The initial platelet aggregation produces an increase in light transmission. This is followed by disaggregation and a decrease in light transmission. With higher concentrations of ADP (e.g., 2.0 μM), a biphasic curve is observed; the initial increase in light transmission is succeeded, after a pause, by a second increase in light transmission indicating further aggregation which proceeds to near completion. The second phase is largely caused by endogenous ADP [41] released from storage granules by the release reaction [42]. With still higher concentrations of ADP (5.0 μM), marked and prolonged aggregation occurs in only one phase.

ADP not only makes platelets sticky but also causes them to lose their characteristic discoid shape and become spiny spheres. This change is evident by phase contrast microscopy [43,44] and also by a loss of the "swirl" noted on agitating a suspension of disc-shaped platelets (or any suspension of asymmetric particles, e.g., erythrocytes or bacteria). The shape change causes a decrease in light transmission (temporary if it is succeeded by aggregation; see Fig. 129-5) and a decrease in the oscillation of the tracing [44,45]. Shape change is not associated with a change in volume [46] and is reversible. Unlike aggregation, ADP-induced shape change is not inhibited by EDTA, does not require fibrinogen [47], is associated with a decrease in energy charge [48], and occurs in platelets of patients with the congenital disorder thrombasthenia [49].

An additional effect of ADP is its ability to promote clot retraction. Reptilase, an enzyme from the venom of the snake *Bothrops atrox*, is capable of clotting fibrinogen, but the clot does not retract because the enzyme does not stimulate platelets as does thrombin. If ADP is added, clot retraction occurs [50].

The mechanisms by which ADP alters platelet shape, induces stickiness, and causes clot retraction are not well understood. Platelets have at least one type of receptor for ADP [51–53], and nucleoside diphosphate kinase may play a part [34]. Stimulation of platelets by ADP causes shape change and induces the appearance of a specific saturable receptor for fibrinogen on the platelet surface [39,40,54,55]. So far, inhibitors which prevent ADP-induced aggregation also prevent fibrinogen binding, and thrombasthenic platelets, which cannot aggregate, fail to bind fibrinogen [15].

OTHER AGGREGATING AGENTS
A number of compounds besides ADP cause platelet aggregation in vitro. These aggregating agents may be divided into four general groups:

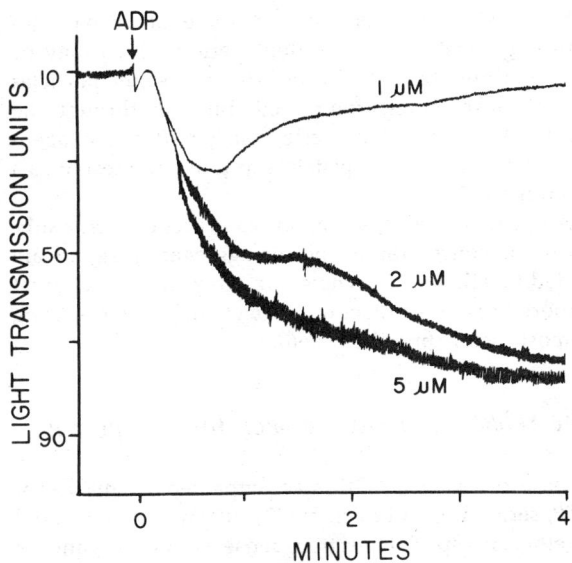

FIGURE 129-5 Aggregometer tracings of effect of ADP on citrated human platelet-rich plasma at 37°C. Note that with the instrument used, increasing light transmission causes a downward deflection.

1. Biogenic amines such as epinephrine [41,56] and serotonin (5-hydroxytryptamine) [56]
2. Certain proteolytic enzymes such as thrombin, trypsin, and those in some snake venoms [57]
3. Particulate materials such as collagen [25–27], aggregated γ-globulin [58], and antigen-antibody complexes [58]
4. Arachidonic acid derivatives [59,60]

When aggregation is studied by recording optical density of citrated platelet-rich plasma, epinephrine at concentrations above about 0.5 μM causes prompt but weak primary aggregation which is not associated with shape change [45]. This is succeeded by marked aggregation associated with ADP liberated during the release reaction [41]. At lower concentrations, epinephrine decreases the threshold for ADP-induced aggregation [61], a property which may be important in human thrombosis. Thrombin induces aggregation at concentrations below those required to clot fibrinogen. At these low concentrations, it causes shape change [62] and often biphasic aggregation [63,64].

ADP is not responsible for primary aggregation caused by epinephrine or thrombin [62]. Thrombasthenic platelets do not aggregate with any of these stimuli [11,49]. It is not yet clear whether primary aggregation induced by amines or thrombin is necessarily associated with fibrinogen binding. Although exogenous fibrinogen need not be added to promote thrombin-induced aggregation, this cofactor is secreted from the platelet α granules, and the inhibition of thrombin-induced aggregation by an antibody to fibrinogen [65] suggests that surface fibrinogen is necessary.

Suspensions of collagen and some other particles cause aggregation after a latent period which may be over a minute [25,26]. This occurs because the particles do not cause aggregation directly but only through the release reaction. Monomeric collagen (tropocollagen) does not interact with platelets; it must be present as a multimer [27].

Aggregation and secretion can occur when subthreshold concentrations of two aggregating agents are added together. This synergistic action may be of great importance in producing platelet aggregates during hemostasis or thrombosis [66].

The release reaction, a secretory response

Release of platelet ADP is accompanied by release of ATP, serotonin, and calcium [42], all of which are stored together in special electron-dense storage organelles (see Chap. 126). The releasable adenine nucleotides are not in equilibrium with metabolically active nucleotides [12]. Release can be monitored in platelets which have taken up radioactive serotonin, since the release of endogenous and newly incorporated serotonin occurs in parallel [67]. The contents of the α granules are also released. These granules contain a variety of proteins. Some, like fibrinogen, factor V, and von Willebrand factor are also present in plasma, whereas others, such as platelet-derived growth factor and the antiheparin compounds platelet factor 4 (PF4) and low-affinity PF4 and its degradation product β-thromboglobulin (βTG), are found only in platelets. In vitro, the contents of both the dense granules and α granules are generally secreted together in response to the same stimuli; the α granules probably require slightly weaker stimuli [68–70].

Thrombin and other strong stimuli also liberate acid hydrolases such as β-glucuronidase from lysosome-like granules which are not easily identified morphologically. Mitochondrial and cytoplasmic enzymes are retained [42]. After secretion has taken place, granules are no longer seen with the electron microscope, i.e., the platelets are degranulated, although the mitochondria remain. The plasma membrane is intact and the platelet aggregates are tightly packed, possibly from activation of the platelet contractile mechanism (see Chap. 128). Thus, the release reaction consists of active secretion from storage granules, not platelet lysis.

Sensitive immunoassays have been developed for PF4 and βTG. Low concentrations of these substances are found in plasma which has been separated from blood with precautions to prevent platelet secretion or lysis. If secretion is induced in vitro by clotting or other stimuli, PF4 and βTG are released in parallel. However, if platelet secretion or lysis occurs in vivo, plasma βTG increases to a greater extent than PF4, probably because the released PF4 binds to endothelial cells [70,71]. Measurement of the concentration of these platelet products in plasma may prove to be clinically valuable.

Platelet secretion can occur by two mechanisms. With ADP, epinephrine, and dilute suspensions of particles such as collagen, it is abolished by aspirin and other nonsteroidal anti-inflammatory agents [72–75] and is therefore due to metabolites of arachidonic acid. This unsaturated 20-carbon fatty acid forms nearly 20 percent of platelet fatty acids, which are largely present in membrane phospholipids. Since prostaglandins are formed only from free fatty acids, the first step in the release reaction must be cleavage of arachidonic acid from phospholipids. The acid is converted enzymatically to endoperoxides and then to thromboxane A_2 [59,60] (see Chap. 128).

Nonsteroidal anti-inflammatory agents inhibit the enzyme cyclooxygenase which converts arachidonic acid to endoperoxides [60,76]. Aspirin differs from other nonsteroidal anti-inflammatory agents in the duration of its effect; ingestion of 650 mg in a single dose may inhibit the release reaction for up to 5 days [73,74]. This drug acetylates platelet cyclooxygenase irreversibly, resulting in inhibition for the life of the platelet [76].

Thromboxane A_2 causes aggregation at a concentration less than 0.1 ng/ml and has a half-life of less than 1 min [59,60]. It causes platelet secretion as well as aggregation, and released ADP is partly but probably not entirely responsible for the associated shape change and aggregation [77,78].

Nonsteroidal anti-inflammatory agents cannot prevent secretion when it is induced by concentrated collagen suspensions or thrombin solutions [64,72–74,79]. Nor do they inhibit lysosomal secretion [80]. Apparently release can be induced by one or more mechanisms that do not involve prostaglandin intermediates.

PROSTAGLANDIN I_2 AND 3',5'-CYCLIC ADENOSINE MONOPHOSPHATE

Another prostaglandin derivative besides thromboxane A_2 exerts a powerful effect on platelets: prostaglandin I_2 (PGI$_2$, prostacyclin) [81]. This compound is synthesized by endothelial and other cells of the blood vessel wall from the endoperoxides derived from arachidonic acid. It is the most powerful known inhibitor of platelet aggregation and secretion, acting at a concentration of less than 1 ng/ml. PGI$_2$ is probably not continuously secreted but is readily formed in response to stimuli including thrombin. Nonsteroidal anti-inflammatory agents prevent its formation [82,83]. Aspirin-induced inhibition of PGI$_2$ production by endothelial cells is reversible and requires a higher drug concentration than thromboxane A_2 production by platelets. Nonetheless, the doses of aspirin in clinical trials of thrombus prevention may have been too high, so that the drug inhibited formation of the inhibitor PGI$_2$ as well as of the aggregator thromboxane A_2 [84].

PGI$_2$ inhibits platelets by stimulating the enzyme adenylate cyclase and thus increasing the platelets' concentration of 3',5'-cyclic adenosine monophosphate (cyclic AMP). Some other inhibitors act by a similar mechanism; among these are PGE₁, PGD₂, and adenosine. Inhibitors of the phosphodiesterase which degrades cyclic AMP (caffeine, for example) also increase the levels of cyclic AMP and inhibit platelet responses. The mechanism of action of cyclic AMP is not clear and is discussed in Chap. 128.

Platelet activation

Platelets exhibit similar responses to a variety of stimuli even though the stimuli or agonists are bound by different receptors in the platelets' plasma membrane. The stimulated or activated platelets change from a discoid shape to spiny spheres, acquire the ability to bind fibrinogen, aggregate when brought into contact with one another in the presence of exogenous or secreted fibrinogen, promote retraction when they are incorporated into fibrin clots, and secrete the contents of their dense granules, α granules, and lysosomes. The stimuli probably cause release of membrane calcium which can directly or indirectly induce actin polymerization and the formation of a larger and more complex cytoskeleton. The mechanisms of these responses have not yet been defined.

Relation of platelets to blood clotting

Platelet activities which contribute to blood coagulation have been designated platelet factors 1 to 4. Platelet factor 1 refers to coagulation factor V in the platelets [85]. Platelet factor 2 accelerates the clotting of fibrinogen by thrombin; it is not released or enhanced by aggregation [85]. These terms are no longer used. Platelet factor 3 (PF3) has a phospholipid-like activity (discussed below), and platelet factor 4 (discussed above) has heparin-neutralizing activity and can be secreted.

In most in vitro studies of blood coagulation, phospholipid suspensions provide the surface on which the complex protein-protein interactions occur. In vivo, platelets presumably carry out this function. The coagulant activity of phospholipid suspensions and PF3 is often assessed by their ability to accelerate clotting induced by the venom from Russell's viper. The venom contains enzymes that activate factors V and X, and the rate of clotting is a function of the concentration of available phospholipid. Using this test or a similar one, PF3 activity is not detectable in circulating platelets, perhaps because the phospholipids active in clotting are negatively charged and are found on the cytoplasmic face of the plasma membrane of platelets and other cells [86,87].

PF3 becomes active when platelets aggregate or are lysed [88]. Activity can develop even when the release reaction does not occur, as after aspirin ingestion or when aggregation is produced by ADP at room temperature [89,90]. Relatively little activity is released into the plasma. The development of PF3 activity as measured with Russell's viper venom may simply be caused by phospholipids exposed by lysis of a few platelets during aggregation [91].

Platelets secrete coagulation factor V. If secretion is stimulated by thrombin, factor V is activated to Va. Factor Va can adhere to the platelet surface and serves there as the receptor for factor Xa; each platelet has only about 200 binding sites for factor Xa [92]. The relationship of the ability of platelets to bind factor Va and their so-called PF3 activity is not clear but platelets probably do not promote clotting more effectively than phospholipids if factor Va is provided [93].

Presumably platelets, like phospholipids, also serve as the surface for the activation of factor X in the intrinsic system, but this has not yet been demonstrated. Platelets can enhance the activation of factors XI and XII [94,95].

The active a chain of factor XIII [96] is present in the platelet cytoplasm and hence cannot be secreted [97].

Clot retraction

The function of platelets in a clot formed in vitro cannot be equated with their function in a physiologic platelet plug. In the body, blood is in motion; this and other factors such as exposed collagen result in a large platelet mass surrounded by a band of fibrin. When blood clots in a test tube, the platelets are well dispersed throughout the fibrin network, and their activation leads to clot retraction. The process is especially obvious in clotted platelet-rich plasma, where the fibrin network and entrapped platelets retract to less than 10 percent of the original volume of the clot. In whole blood, entrapped red cells usually prevent the clot from retracting to less than about 50 percent of its original volume. Since no structure like a blood clot is produced during normal hemostasis, clot retraction is, in a sense, an artifact. However, since clot retraction probably results from contraction of platelet pseudopodia attached to fibrin strands [98], it reflects one of the recognized normal phenomena of platelet function, i.e., platelet contraction, and the same functions required for retraction are probably necessary for the normal formation of a hemostatic platelet plug. The contraction of platelet pseudopodia is due to platelet actomyosin, earlier called thrombosthenin (see Chap. 128).

Role of von Willebrand factor in hemostasis

Patients with von Willebrand's disease have a prolonged bleeding time and a deficiency of factor VIII/von Willebrand factor in their plasma. Thus, plasma of these patients is deficient in coagulant activity, does not support agglutination of platelets by the antibiotic ristocetin, and has reduced levels of factor VIII–related antigen (see Chap. 155).

The prolonged bleeding time and deficiency of von Willebrand factor in von Willebrand's disease, and the normal bleeding time and normal von Willebrand factor in hemophilia, suggest that this factor is necessary for formation of a normal hemostatic platelet plug. This view is strengthened by the fact that both von Willebrand factor levels and the abnormal bleeding time are temporarily improved after transfusion of cryoprecipitate [99]. Histologic studies of bleeding time punctures show that platelet plugs do not adhere to the walls of the cut blood vessels in patients with von Willebrand's disease [100].

The function of von Willebrand factor has been difficult to establish by in vitro tests. In addition to ristocetin-induced agglutination, two tests of platelet function have been abnormal: platelet retention in glass bead columns [101] and adhesion of platelets to perfused aortic subendothelium [102,103]. These tests only require von Willebrand factor when whole blood is used and blood flow is rapid. Although collagen appears to be the substance in the subendothelium to which platelets adhere, platelets in platelet-rich plasma from von Willebrand patients aggregate normally in the usual studies using an aggregometer.

Summary of mechanisms leading to the formation of a hemostatic platelet plug

The development of a hemostatic platelet plug may be somewhat arbitrarily divided into three stages: adhesion, cohesion (aggregation), and consolidation [26]. Platelets adhere to the subendothelium or to more deeply placed collagen fibers (adhesion). Contact of platelets with collagen in vitro releases ADP. Previously this was thought to initiate a chain reaction in which the released ADP caused the recruitment of passing platelets (cohesion), which in turn released their ADP; however, this succession of events now seems unlikely, because ADP does not induce a release reaction in the presence of a normal concentration of ionized calcium [35]. The collagen-induced release reaction presumably plays a role in hemostasis, since aspirin ingestion prolongs the bleeding time [74]. Von Willebrand factor probably takes part in the initial adhesion of platelets to the subendothelium and in subsequent platelet-platelet interactions [104].

Local thrombin evolution is promoted by release of tissue factor from the vessel wall. Thrombin evolution also occurs on the surface of the aggregated platelets. The thrombin, and perhaps ADP as well, causes consolidation and contraction of the platelet plug. Thrombin clots plasma fibrinogen, and the fibrin reinforces the platelet plug, especially at its periphery. Fibrin continues to form during the succeeding hours as the platelets disintegrate. The platelet plug probably fails to develop into a large mixed thrombus because PGI_2 is produced locally, blood flow is not slowed in adjacent branches of the vessels, and the area of vascular injury is not sufficiently extensive.

Correlates outside of hematology

Platelets may play an important role in numerous pathologic situations such as reactions to viruses, antigen-antibody complexes, endotoxin, or prosthetic surfaces [58,105,106].

Clinical tests of platelet function

In contrast to the study of blood coagulation, the number of clinical tests applied to platelet function is small. The screening test for platelet function is the bleeding time (see Chap. A40). The tourniquet test assesses so-called capillary fragility (see Chap. 139). In vitro tests include assessment of platelet aggregation (Chap. A43), secretion, and retention in glass bead columns (Chap. A41), clot retraction (Chaps. A32 and A44), and PF3 activity (Chap. A42).

References

1. Spaet, T. H. (ed.): *Progress in Hemostasis and Thrombosis.* Grune & Stratton, New York, 1972 (vol. I), 1974 (vol. II), 1976 (vol. III), 1978 (vol. IV), and 1980 (vol. V).
2. Mills, D. C. B., and Pareti, F. I. (eds.): *Platelets and Thrombosis.* Academic, New York, 1977.
3. Gordon, J. L. (ed.): *Platelets in Biology and Pathology 2.* Elsevier–North Holland, New York, 1981.
4. Day, H. J., Holmsen, H., and Zucker, M. B. (eds.): *Platelet Function Testing.* DHEW Publication no. (NIH) 78-1087, U.S. Department of Health, Education and Welfare, Washington, D.C., 1978.
5. Schmidt, R. M. (ed.): *Hematology.* CRC Press, Boca Raton, Fla., 1979, vol. I.
6. Mann, K. G., and Taylor, F. B., Jr.: *The Regulation of Coagulation.* Elsevier–North Holland, New York, 1980.
7. Murano, G., and Bick, R. L. (eds.): *Basic Concepts of Hemostasis and Thrombosis.* CRC Press, Boca Raton, Fla., 1980.
8. Rotman, A., Meyer, F. A., Gitler, C., and Silberberg, A.: *Platelets: Cellular Response Mechanisms and Their Biological Significance.* Wiley, New York, 1980.
9. *Biochemistry and Pharmacology of Platelets.* Ciba Foundation Symposium 35 (new series). Elsevier–North Holland, New York, 1975.
10. Weiss, H. J. (ed.): *Platelets and Their Role in Hemostasis. Ann. N.Y. Acad. Sci.* 201, 1972.
11. Weiss, H. J.: Platelet physiology and abnormalities of function. *N. Engl. J. Med.* 293:531,580, 1975.
12. Holmsen, H., Salganicoff, L., and Fukami, M. H.: Platelet behavior and biochemistry in haemostasis, in *Haemostasis: Biochemistry, Physiology, and Pathology,* edited by D. Ogston and B. Bennett. Wiley, New York, 1977, pp. 241–319.
13. Detwiler, T. C., and Charo, I. F.: Research on the biochemical basis of platelet function, in *The Year in Hematology,* edited by A. S. Gordon, R. Silber, and J. LoBue. Plenum, New York, 1977, p. 377.
14. Zucker, M. B.: The functioning of blood platelets. *Sci. Am.* 242:86, 1980.
15. Peerschke, E. I., and Zucker, M. B.: Effects of ADP on blood platelets, in *Contemporary Hematology/Oncology,* edited by A. S. Gordon, R. D. Silber, and J. LoBue. Plenum, New York, 1981, vol. 2, pp. 339–362.

16. Zucker, M. B.: Platelet agglutination and vasoconstriction as factors in spontaneous hemostasis in normal, thrombocytopenic, heparinized and hypoprothrombinemic rats. *Am. J. Physiol.* 148:275, 1947.

17. Hovig, T., Rowsell, H. C., Dodds, W. J., Jørgensen, L., and Mustard, J. F.: Experimental hemostasis in normal dogs and in dogs with congenital disorders of blood coagulation. *Blood* 30:636, 1967.

18. Hovig, T.: The ultrastructure of blood platelets in normal and abnormal states, in *Blood Platelets: Structure, Formation and Function,* edited by K. G. Jensen and S.-A. Killman. *Ser. Haematol.* 1(2):33, 1968.

19. French, J. E., Macfarlane, R. G., and Saunders, A. G.: The structure of hemostatic plugs and experimental thrombi in small arteries. *Br. J. Exp. Pathol.* 45:467, 1964.

20. Zucker, H. D.: Platelet thrombosis in human hemostasis. *Blood* 4:631, 1949.

21. Hovig, T., Dodds, W. J., Rowsell, H. C., and Mustard, J. F.: The transformation of hemostatic platelet plugs in normal and factor IX deficient dogs. *Am. J. Pathol.* 53:355, 1968.

22. Honour, A. J., and Mitchell, J. R. A.: Platelet clumping in injured vessels. *Br. J. Exp. Pathol.* 45:75, 1964.

23. Hugues, J.: Agglutination précoce des plaquettes au cours de la formation du clou hémostatique. *Thromb. Diath. Haemorrh.* 3:177, 1959.

24. Bounameaux, Y.: L'accolement des plaquettes aux fibres sous-endothéliales. *Thromb. Diath. Haemorrh.* 6:504, 1961.

25. Zucker, M. B., and Borrelli, J.: Platelet clumping produced by connective tissue suspensions and by collagen. *Proc. Soc. Exp. Biol. Med.* 109:779, 1962.

26. Spaet, T. H., and Zucker, M. B.: Mechanism of platelet plug formation and role of adenosine diphosphate. *Am. J. Physiol.* 206:1267, 1964.

27. Jaffe, R., and Deykin, D.: Evidence for a structural requirement for the aggregation of platelets by collagen. *J. Clin. Invest* 53:875, 1974.

28. Baumgartner, H. R.: Morphometric quantitation of adherence of platelets to an artificial surface and components of connective tissue. *Thromb. Diath. Haemorrh.* [Suppl.] 60:39, 1974.

29. Stemerman, M. B.: Vascular intimal components: Precursors of thrombosis. *Prog. Hemostasis Thromb.* 2:1, 1974.

30. Ashford, T. P., and Freiman, D. G.: The role of the endothelium in the initial phases of thrombosis: An electron microscope study. *Am. J. Pathol.* 50:257, 1967.

31. Majno, G., and Palade, G. E.: Studies on inflammation. I. The effect of histamine and serotonin on vascular permeability: An electron microscope study. *J. Biophys. Biochem. Cytol.* 11:571, 1961.

32. Tranzer, J. P., and Baumgartner, H. R.: Filling gaps in the vascular endothelium with blood platelets. *Nature* 216:1126, 1967.

33. Gaarder, A., Jonsen, J., Laland, S., Hellem, A., and Owren, P. A.: Adenosine diphosphate in red cells as a factor in the adhesiveness of human blood platelets. *Nature* 192:531, 1961.

34. Mustard, J. F., Packham, M. A., Perry, D. W., Guccione, M. A., and Kinlough-Rathbone, R. L.: Enzyme activities on the platelet surface in relation to the action of adenosine diphosphate, in *Biochemistry and Pharmacology of Platelets.* Ciba Foundation Symposium 35 (new series), Elsevier–North Holland, New York, 1975.

35. Mustard, J. F., Perry, D. W., Kinlough-Rathbone, R. L., and Packham, M. A.: Factors responsible for ADP-induced release reaction of human platelets. *Am. J. Physiol.* 228:1757, 1975.

36. Hampton, J. R., and Mitchell, J. R. A.: Platelet electrophoresis: The present position. *Thromb. Diath. Haemorrh.* 31:204, 1974.

37. Friedberg, N. M., and Zucker, M. B.: ADP as the cause of reversible inhibition of platelet retention in glass bead columns. *J. Lab. Clin. Med.* 80:603, 1972.

38. Day, H. J., Holmsen, H., and Zucker, M. B.: Methods for separating platelets from blood and plasma. *Thromb. Diath. Haemorrh.* 33:648, 1975, and *Thromb. Haemost.* 36:263, 1976.

39. Mustard, J. F., Packham, M. A., Kinlough-Rathbone, R. L., Perry, D. W., and Regoeczi, E.: Fibrinogen and ADP-induced platelet aggregation. *Blood* 52:453, 1978.

40. Marguerie, G. A., Plow, E. F., and Edgington, T. S.: Human platelets possess an inducible and saturable receptor specific for fibrinogen. *J. Biol. Chem.* 254:5357, 1979.

41. Mills, D. C. B., Robb, I. A., and Roberts, G. C. K.: The release of nucleotides, 5-hydroxytryptamine and enzymes from human blood platelets during aggregation. *J. Physiol.* 195:715, 1968.

42. Day, H. J., and Holmsen, H.: Concepts of the blood platelet release reaction. *Ser. Haematol.* 4(1):3, 1971.

43. Zucker, M. B., and Zaccardi, J. B.: Platelet shape change induced by adenosine diphosphate and prevented by adenosine monophosphate. *Fed. Proc.* 23:299, 1964.

44. Macmillan, D. C., and Oliver, M. F.: The initial changes in platelet morphology following the addition of adenosine diphosphate. *J. Atheroscler. Res.* 5:440, 1965.

45. O'Brien, J. R., and Heywood, J. B.: Effect of aggregating agents and their inhibitors on the mean platelet shape. *J. Clin. Pathol.* 19:148, 1966.

46. Feinberg, H., Michel, H., and Born, G. V. R.: Determination of the fluid volume of platelets by their separation through silicone oil. *J. Lab. Clin. Med.* 84:926, 1974.

47. Lloyd, J. V., Nishizawa, E. E., and Mustard, J. F.: Effect of ADP-induced shape change on incorporation of ^{32}P into platelet phosphatidic acid and mono-, di- and triphosphatidyl inositol. *Br. J. Haematol.* 25:77, 1973.

48. Mills, D. C. B.: Changes in the adenylate energy charge in human blood platelets induced by adenosine diphosphate. *Nature (New Biol.)* 243:220, 1973.

49. Zucker, M. B., Pert, J. H., and Hilgartner, M. W.: Platelet function in a patient with thrombasthenia. *Blood* 28:524, 1966.

50. deGaetano, G., Bottecchia, D., and Vermylen, J.: Retraction of Reptilase-clots in the presence of agents inducing or inhibiting the platelet adhesion-aggregation reaction. *Thromb. Res.* 2:71, 1973.

51. Adler, J. R., and Handin, R. I.: Solubilization and characterization of a platelet membrane ADP-binding protein. *J. Biol. Chem.* 254:3866, 1979.

52. Bennett, J. S., Colman, R. F., and Colman, R. W.: Identification of adenosine nucleotide binding proteins in human platelet membrane by affinity labeling with 5'-p-fluorosulfonylbenzoyl adenosine. *J. Biol. Chem.* 253:7346, 1978.

53. Macfarlane, D. E., Srivastava, P. C., and Mills, D. C. B.: 2-Methylthioadenosine-5'-diphosphate (2 MeSADP), a high-affinity probe for ADP receptors on the human platelet. *Thromb. Haemostasis* 42:185, 1979.

54. Bennett, J. S., and Vilaire, G. V.: Exposure of platelet fibrinogen receptors by ADP and epinephrine. *J. Clin. Invest.* 64:1393, 1979.

55. Peerschke, E. I., and Zucker, M. B.: Relationship of ADP-induced fibrinogen binding to platelet shape change and aggregation elucidated by use of colchicine and cytochalasin B. *Thromb. Haemostasis* 43:58, 1980.

56. O'Brien, J. R.: A comparison of platelet aggregation produced by seven compounds and a comparison of their inhibitors. *J. Clin. Pathol.* 17:275, 1964.

57. Davey, M. G., and Luscher, E. F.: Release reactions of human platelets induced by thrombin and other agents. *Biochim. Biophys. Acta* 165:490, 1968.

58. Pfueller, S. L., and Luscher, E. F.: The effects of immune complexes on blood platelets and their relationship to complement activation. *Immunochemistry* 9:1151, 1972.

59. Hamberg, M., Svensson, J., and Samuelsson, B.: Thromboxanes: A new group of biologically active compounds derived from prostaglandin endoperoxides. *Proc. Natl. Acad. Sci. U.S.A.* 72:2994, 1975.

60. Marcus, A. J.: The role of lipids in platelet function: With particular reference to the arachidonic acid pathway. *J. Lipid Res.* 19:793, 1978.

61. Mills, D. C. B., and Roberts, G. C. K.: Effects of adrenaline on human blood platelets. *J. Physiol.* 193:443, 1967.

62. Macfarlane, D. E., and Mills, D. C. B.: The effects of ATP on platelets: Evidence against the role of released ADP in primary aggregation. *Blood* 46:309, 1975.

63. Thomas, D. P.: Effect of catecholamines on platelet aggregation caused by thrombin. *Nature* 215:298, 1967.

64. Charo, I. F., Feinman, R. D., and Detwiler, T. C.: Interrelations of platelet aggregation and secretion. *J. Clin. Invest.* 60:866, 1977.

65. Tollefsen, D. M., and Majerus, P. W.: Inhibition of human platelet aggregation by monovalent antifibrinogen antibody fragments. *J. Clin. Invest.* 55:1259, 1975.

66. Kinlough-Rathbone, R. L., Packham, M. A., and Mustard, J. F.: Synergism between platelet aggregating agents: The role of the arachidonate pathway. *Thromb. Res.* 11:567, 1977.

67. Holmsen, H., Ostvold, A.-C., and Day, H. J.: Behavior of endogenous and newly absorbed serotonin in the platelet release reaction. *Biochem. Pharmacol.* 22:2599, 1973.

68. Broekman, M. J., Handin, R. I., and Cohen, P.: Distribution of fibrinogen, and platelet factors 4 and XIII in subcellular fractions of human platelets. *Br. J. Haematol.* 31:51, 1975.

69. Kaplan, K. L., Broekman, M. J., Chernoff, A., Lesnik, G. R., and Drillings, M.: Platelet α-granule proteins: Studies on release and subcellular localization. *Blood* 53:604, 1979.

70. Kaplan, K. L., and Owen, J.: Plasma levels of β-thromboglobulin and platelet factor 4 as indices of platelet activation in vivo. *Blood* 57:199, 1981.

71. Musial, J., Niewiarowski, S., Edmunds, L. H., Jr., Addonizio, V. P., Nicolaou, K. C., and Colman, R. W.: In vivo release and turnover of secreted platelet antiheparin proteins in Rhesus monkey (*Macaca mulatta*). *Blood* 56:596, 1980.

72. Zucker, M. B., and Peterson, J.: Inhibition of adenosine diphosphate–induced secondary aggregation and other platelet functions by acetylsalicylic acid ingestion. *Proc. Soc. Exp. Biol. Med.* 127:547, 1968.

73. O'Brien, J. R.: Effect of anti-inflammatory agents on platelets. *Lancet* 1:894, 1968.

74. Weiss, H. J., Aledort, L. M., and Kochwa, S.: The effect of salicylates on the hemostatic properties of platelets in man. *J. Clin. Invest.* 47:2169, 1968.

75. Weiss, H. J.: The pharmacology of platelet inhibition, in *Progress in Hemostasis and Thrombosis*, edited by T. H. Spaet. Grune & Stratton, New York, 1972, vol. 1, pp. 199–231.

76. Burch, J. W., Stanford, N., and Majerus, P. W.: Inhibition of platelet prostaglandin synthetase by oral aspirin. *J. Clin. Invest.* 61:314, 1978.

77. Kinlough-Rathbone, R. L., Reimers, H. J., Mustard, J. F., and Packham, M. A.: Sodium arachidonate can induce platelet shape change and aggregation which are independent of the release reaction. *Science* 192:1011, 1976.

78. Meyers, K. M., Seachord, C. L., Holmsen, H., Smith, J. B., and Prieur, D. J.: A dominant role of thromboxane formation in secondary aggregation of platelets. *Nature* 282:331, 1979.

79. Kinlough-Rathbone, R. L., Packham, M. A., Reimers, H.-J., Cazenave, J.-P., and Mustard, J. F.: Mechanisms of platelet shape change, aggregation, and release induced by collagen, thrombin, or A23187. *J. Lab. Clin. Med.* 90:707, 1977.

80. Holmsen, H., Setkowsky, C. A., Lages, B., Day, H. J., Weiss, H. J., and Scrutton, M. C.: Content and thrombin-induced release of acid hydrolases in gel-filtered platelets from patients with storage pool disease. *Blood* 46:131, 1975.

81. Moncada, S., Gryglewski, R., Bunting, S., and Vane, J. R.: An enzyme isolated from arteries transforms prostaglandin endoperoxides to an unstable substance that inhibits platelet aggregation. *Nature* 263:663, 1976.

82. Weksler, B. B., Ley, C. W., and Jaffe, E. A.: Stimulation of endothelial cell prostacyclin production by thrombin, trypsin, and the ionophore A 23187. *J. Clin. Invest.* 63:923, 1978.

83. Czervionke, R. L., Smith, J. B., Fry, G. L., Hoak, J. C., and Haycraft, D. L.: Inhibition of prostacyclin by treatment of endothelium with aspirin: Correlation with platelet adherence. *J. Clin. Invest.* 63:1089, 1979.

84. Harter, H. R., et al.: Prevention of thrombosis in patients on hemodialysis by low-dose aspirin. *N. Engl. J. Med.* 301:577, 1979.

85. Niewiarowski, S., Poplawski, A., Lipinski, B., and Farbieziewski, R.: The release of platelet clotting factors during aggregation and viscous metamorphosis. *Exp. Biol. Med.* 3:121, 1968.

86. Schick, P., Kurica, K. B., and Chacko, G. K.: Localization of phosphatidylethanolamine and phosphatidylserine in the human platelet plasma membrane. *J. Clin. Invest.* 57:1221, 1976.

87. Zwaal, R. F. A., Comfurius, P., and van Deenen, L. E. M.: Membrane asymmetry and blood coagulation. *Nature* 268:358, 1977.

88. Hardisty, R. M., and Hutton, R. A.: Platelet aggregation and the availability of platelet factor 3. *Br. J. Haematol.* 12:764, 1966.

89. Atac, A., Spagnuolo, M., and Zucker, M. B.: Long-term inhibition of platelet functions by aspirin. *Proc. Soc. Exp. Biol. Med.* 133:1331, 1970.

90. Sixma, J. J., and Nijessen, J. B.: Characteristics of platelet factor 3 release during ADP-induced aggregation: Comparison with 5-hydroxytryptamine release. *Thromb. Diath. Haemorrh.* 24:206, 1970.

91. Bevers, E. M., Comfurius, P. C., and Zwaal, R. F. A.: Activation of platelet factor 3. *Thromb. Haemost.* 42:211, 1979.

92. Kane, W. H., Lindhout, M. J., Jackson, C. M., and Majerus, P. W.: Factor Va dependent binding of factor Xa to human platelets. *J. Biol. Chem.* 255:1170, 1980.

93. van Zutphen, H., Bevers, E. M., Hemker, H. C., and Zwaal, R. F. A.: Contribution of the platelet factor V content to platelet factor 3 activity. *Br. J. Haematol.* 45:121, 1980.

94. Walsh, P. N.: Platelet coagulant activities and hemostasis: A hypothesis. *Blood* 43:597, 1974.

95. Walsh, P. N., and Griffin, J. H.: Contributions of human platelets to the proteolytic activation of blood coagulation factors XII and XI. *Blood* 57:106, 1981.

96. Schwartz, M. L., Pizzo, S. V., Hill, R. L., and McKee, P. A.: Human factor XIII from plasma and platelets: Molecular weights, subunit structures, proteolytic activation, and crosslinking of fibrinogen and fibrin. *J. Biol. Chem.* 248:1395, 1973.

97. Joist, J. H., and Niewiarowski, S.: Retention of platelet's fibrin stabilizing factor during the platelet release reaction and clot retraction. *Thromb. Diath. Haemorrh.* 29:679, 1973.

98. DeClerck, D., Borgers, M., deGaetano, G., and Vermylen, J.: Dissociation of clot retraction from platelet granule fusion and degranulation: An ultrastructural study of Reptilase-human platelet-rich plasma clots. *Br. J. Haematol.* 29:341, 1975.

99. Weiss, H. J.: Relationship of von Willebrand factor to bleeding time. *N. Engl. J. Med.* 291:420, 1974.

100. Hovig, T., and Stormorken, H.: Ultrastructural studies on the platelet plug formation bleeding time wounds from normal individuals and patients with von Willebrand's disease. *Acta Pathol. Microbiol. Scand. (Suppl.)* 248:105, 1974.

101. Salzman, E. W.: Measurement of platelet adhesiveness: A simple *in vitro* technique demonstrating an abnormality in von Willebrand's disease. *J. Lab. Clin. Med.* 62:724, 1963.

102. Tschopp, T. B., Weiss, H. J., and Baumgartner, H. R.: Decreased adhesion of platelets to subendothelium in von Willebrand's disease. *J. Lab. Clin. Med.* 83:296, 1974.

103. Sakariassen, K. S., Bolhuis, P. A., and Sixma, J. J.: Human blood platelet adhesion to artery subendothelium is mediated by factor VIII–von Willebrand factor bound to the subendothelium. *Nature* 279:636, 1979.

104. McPherson, J., and Zucker, M. B.: Platelet retention in glass bead columns: Adhesion to glass and subsequent platelet-platelet interactions. *Blood* 47:55, 1976.

105. Zucker, M. B.: Platelets, in *The Inflammatory Process*, edited by B. W. Zweifach, L. Grant, and R. T. McCloskey. Academic, New York, 1974, vol. 1, p. 511.

106. Nachman, R., and Weksler, B.: The platelet as an inflammatory cell, in *Advances in Inflammation Research*, edited by G. Weissman, B. Samuelsson, and R. Paoletti. Raven Press, New York, 1979, vol. 1, p. 169.

SECTION THREE

Platelet kinetics

CHAPTER *130*

Production, distribution, life-span, and fate of platelets

JEAN-MICHEL PAULUS
RICHARD H. ASTER

Production of platelets

Platelets are anucleate fragments of the cytoplasm of the giant, polyploid megakaryocytes. The megakaryocyte-platelet system is unique to mammals, since in lower vertebrates nucleated thrombocytes are derived by multiple division of thromboblasts, in a process similar to erythropoiesis [1]. In the human fetus, megakaryocytes are produced first in the yolk sac and later in the liver and spleen. At 3 months they appear in the marrow [2], where they are found almost exclusively after birth. Megakaryocytes may also be found in the lung in small numbers. Multiple differentiation is a striking feature of the thrombocytic series which integrates the properties of polyploid, secretory, endocytic, and muscular cells as well as those of anucleate elements [3].

CELLULAR COMPARTMENTS

MEGAKARYOCYTE PROGENITORS
Megakaryocytes arise from multipotential stem cells capable of self renewal and of differentiation into the erythrocytic, granulocytic-macrophage, and megakaryocyte series. There may be a close relationship between those cells which generate spleen colonies in lethally irradiated mice, termed colony-forming units—spleen, or CFU-S, and the megakaryocyte progenitors, termed colony-forming units—megakaryocyte, or CFU-Mega, or CFU-M, interposed between the pluripotential cells and the recognizable megakaryocytes [4]. In culture of mouse marrow, megakaryocyte progenitors can form clones [5–7] composed of megakaryocytes [8–13], of megakaryocytes and erythroblasts [6,14], or of several lineages including megakaryocytes [5,7,15,16]. In humans, two culture systems appear to assay distinct progenitor populations [17–19].

Whether progenitors of pure megakaryocyte clones belong to a single homogeneous or to several distinct populations, possibly descending from each other, is debated. In mice, data obtained after 5 days of culture were compatible with the concept of one slowly cycling population of CFU-Mega [12]. The possibility exists, however, that distinct populations peak at different culture times. That this is so was recently shown by establishing cumulative doubling distributions in mega-karyocyte colonies grown from 3 to 14 days [14]. Abrupt shifts of the exponential slopes of these distributions are consistent with the model shown in Fig. 130-1. The two late CFU-Mega (CFU-M) compartments appear to parallel the early erythrocytic progenitors also demonstrated in mice [20].

PROMEGAKARYOBLAST
Staining for acetylcholinesterase in species where this enzyme is specific or quasispecific for the megakaryocyte lineage [21] has delineated a class of probably diploid cells which differ in their physical properties from megakaryocytic colony-forming units (CFU-Mega) [9,22] and which form single megakaryocytes under culture conditions which support the growth of large colonies from CFU-Mega [22]. Such cells appear to be committed to polyploidization and may be termed

FIGURE 130-1 Developmental stages in thrombocytopoiesis (schematic). Megakaryocyte (MKC) progenitors originating from the pluripotential stem cells (S. C.) belong to three consecutive compartments. Bipotent progenitors (BFU-ME) generate mixed erythroblastic-megakaryocytic colonies and are unlikely (probability 0.07) to end multiplication and switch to polyploidization per doubling time. The megakaryocyte precursors CFU-M1 and CFU-M2 are unipotential and have greater probabilities (0.48 and 0.74) to enter the polyploidization phase. The diploid cell committed to polyploidization is termed *promegakaryoblast* (Pro MKB). Polyploidizing blast-like cells are named *megakaryoblasts*. They attain ploidy levels ranging from 4 N to 64 N. They are succeeded by the non-DNA-synthesizing promegakaryocytes (not shown) and megakaryocytes, which liberate platelets. Note that platelets can be released at the 8 N, 16 N, 32 N, or 64 N ploidy level.

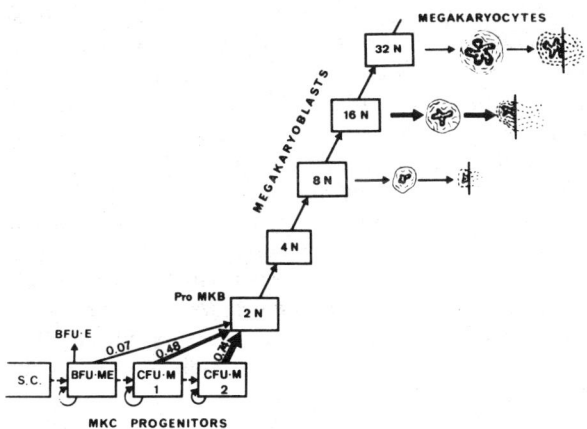

promegakaryoblasts [23]. Similar cells were demonstrated in mice using fluorescent antiplatelet sera [21,24] and in human beings using immunofluorescence [19,25] or the ultrastructural peroxidase reaction which labels the nuclear envelope and endoplasmic reticulum of early and late thrombocytic cells [26].

MEGAKARYOBLAST

Also termed *stage I megakaryocyte,* the megakaryoblast is recognized by its large size, basophilic cytoplasm, and nonlobulated, nonindented nucleus (Plate 2). Polyploidization takes place exclusively in megakaryoblasts [27–30]. Microspectrophotometric studies of the nucleus of megakaryoblasts and megakaryocytes in rats, rabbits, and guinea pigs have demonstrated cells containing 4, 8, 16, 32, or 64 times the haploid DNA complement [28–31], the number most commonly encountered being 16 N. About the same pattern of ploidy distribution appears to hold for human beings [32,33]. Apparently because of differences in megakaryocyte sampling, a somewhat different distribution was obtained on unseparated, suspended marrow using flow cytophotometry, in which the predominant ploidy class was 8 N [34].

Although appearing immature in Wright-stained smears, megakaryoblasts synthesize organelles and other constituents characteristic of mature platelets. The ultrastructure of megakaryoblasts and megakaryocytes has been reviewed [26,35,36]. Cells capable of incorporating tritiated thymidine produce few demarcation membranes and specific granules [30,37]. Megakaryoblasts incorporate sulfates in mucopolysaccharides, and their Golgi complex concentrates these compounds in the α granules [38]. In rodents and cats, megakaryoblasts and megakaryocytes synthesize, transport, and concentrate acetylcholinesterase for later extracellular secretion [39]. Primary lysosomes are formed in the Golgi-endoplasmic reticulum-lysosome (GERL) region [40]. Catalase granules arise by budding of smooth endoplasmic membranes [41] and are not demonstrated in the Golgi apparatus or secreted. Dense storage granules are not produced by megakaryoblasts.

PROMEGAKARYOCYTE AND MEGAKARYOCYTE
Morphology and biochemistry   Also called *stage II* or *basophilic megakaryocyte,* the promegakaryocyte is the intermediate form which develops after the arrest of polyploidization. This event is marked by indentation of the nucleus [28] and by the appearance of recognizable azurophilic granules. The *stage III, mature, acidophilic* or *granular megakaryocyte* is the late giant form. Its nucleus has dense chromatin, no nucleolus, and is irregularly shaped and condensed. The abundant cytoplasm is eosinophilic and packed with fine azurophilic granules, the so-called α granules. Megakaryocytes can be separated from other marrow cells by filtration [42] or, more efficiently, by density gradient and velocity centrifugation [43].

Although synthesis of specialized platelet constituents is initiated at the promegakaryoblast stage, completion of polyploidization is marked by massive synthesis of these products. Factor VIIIR:Ag [25,44], actin [45], fibrinogen, platelet glycoproteins Ib, IIb, and IIIa, platelet myosin, fibronectin, and platelet factor 4 [25] can be demonstrated in more than 85 percent of mature megakaryocytes. Dense granules are rarely recognized [40], but serotonin can be incorporated by isolated megakaryocytes and liberated in a typical release reaction [46]. Microtubules and microfilaments are infrequently seen in developing megakaryocytes, but their constituent proteins have been identified by a variety of techniques [36,47,48].

Delineation of platelet territories   Demarcation membranes, which individualize future platelet territories (Fig. 130-2), develop through a complex fusion-fission process involving fenestrated tubules connected to the plasma membrane [49]. Demarcation membranes and the enclosed open canalicular system serve as an uptake and extrusion route for products absorbed and secreted by megakaryocytes and platelets [50,51]. In some areas of megakaryocyte cytoplasm, demarcation membranes closely associate with the smooth endoplasmic reticulum or dense tubular system [51,52], determining membrane complexes which resemble the association of transverse tubular system (T system) and sarcoplasmic reticulum in muscle and may have a similar function in the control of calcium fluxes [see Fig. 14 in Ref. 53].

Determination of platelet size   Several papers [reviewed in Ref. 54] have established the lognormal distribution of platelet volumes and dry weights, although slight deviations from lognormality can be detected when particle counters using hydrodynamic focusing [55] or computerized analyses [56] are used. Lognormality can be produced by random variations in the percentage changes in volume or weight of platelet territories during successive steps of megakaryocyte cytoplasmic growth and fragmentation [57]. This explanation may account [54] for the correlation between size and platelet functional activity [58], the inverse relationship between size and platelet count [57–61], and the macrothrombocytosis observed in certain clinical conditions [57,59,62]. The kinetics of ^{75}Se-selenomethionine [63,64] or ^{35}S-sulfate [65] incorporation into platelets of different size or density can be interpreted as a function of platelet territory formation [54]. Platelet size may also depend on megakaryocyte ploidy [66], particularly in dysthrombocytopoiesis [67]. The relations between platelet aging, size, and density will be further considered below.

PLATELET-RELEASING MEGAKARYOCYTES
In 1910 Wright showed that mature megakaryocytes extend filaments of cytoplasm into sinusoidal spaces, where they detach and fragment into individual plate-

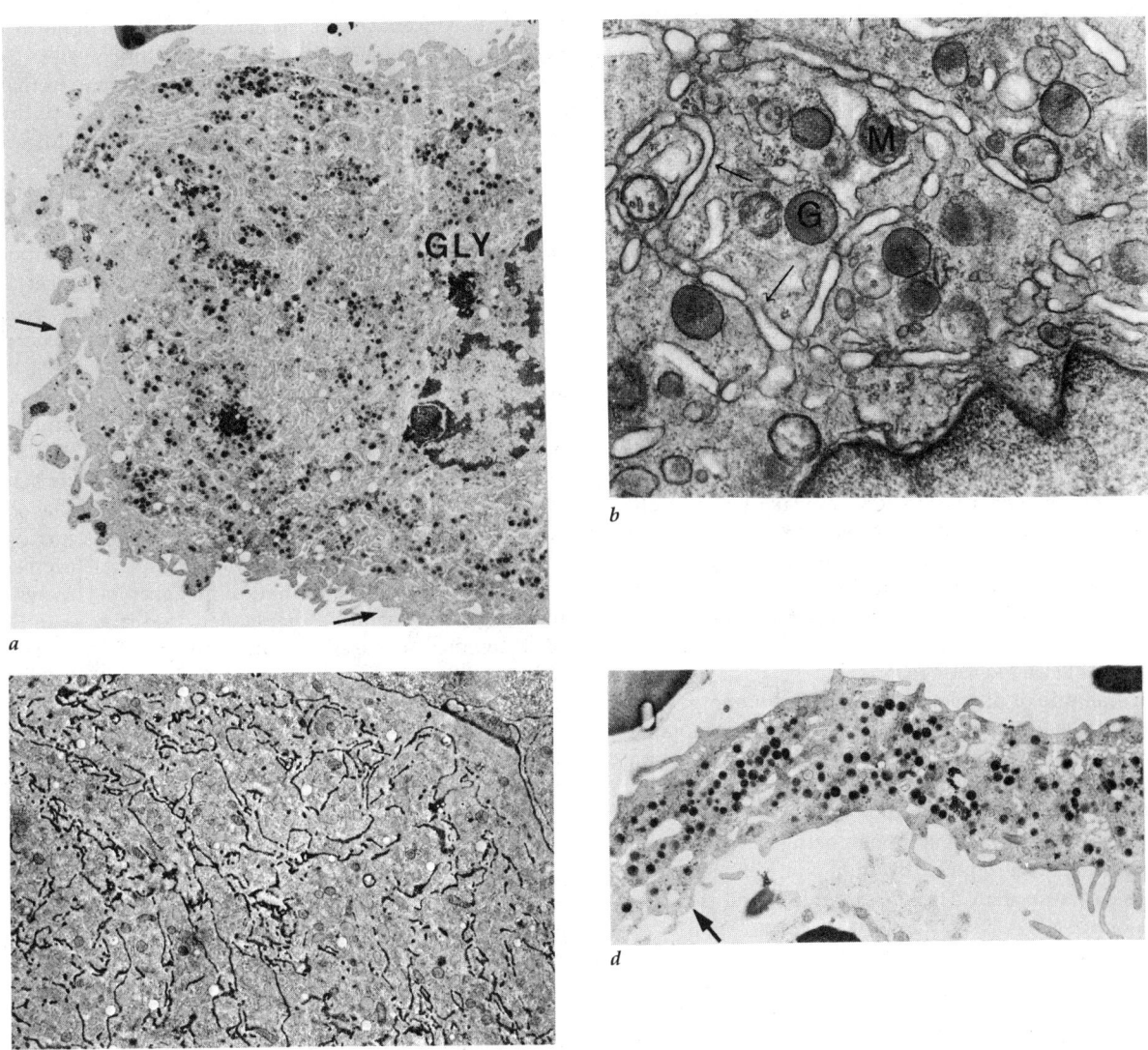

FIGURE 130-2 Electron microscopic studies of megakaryocytes. (*a*) Mature megakaryocyte showing pyknotic nucleus, numerous demarcation membranes, granules, clumps of glycogen (Gly), and the peripheral zone (*arrows*). (×3500.) (*b*) Intermediate zone of rat megakaryocyte showing granules (G), mitochondria (M), and demarcation membranes (*arrows*). (×25,000.) (*c*) Megakaryocyte from rat marrow fixed 30 min after injection of horseradish peroxidase. Reaction product of the peroxidase is electron-dense and may be seen filling the demarcation membrane system. (×2800.) (*d*) Megakaryocyte fragment in a sinusoid of marrow. Arrow indicates possible separation of a small platelet. Note numerous pseudopodia. (×5800.) (Parts *a* and *d* from Breton-Gorius and Reyes [26]; part *b* from J. E. French, *Br. J. Haematol. 13*:595, 1967; part *c* from Behnke [50].)

lets [68]. Later studies utilizing phase contrast microscopy in tissue culture [69] and electron microscopy [70] have confirmed this view (Fig. 130-2). Most megakaryocytes reside less than 1 μm from a marrow sinus, a distribution which is unlikely to be due to chance [71]. Cytoplasmic processes containing longitudinally oriented microtubules, which probably originate from an organizing centriolar center, extend into sinusoids. There they undergo attenuation and develop constric-

tions which rupture to release platelets [72]. This unique process is an example of apocrine secretion [3], a physiological form of metastasis [71], and it shares similarities with the separation of daughter cells in the terminal phase of cytokinesis [72]. It also indicates that platelet size distribution may depend just as much on the manner the released cytoplasmic processes are fragmented as on the arrangement of megakaryocyte demarcation membranes inside megakaryocytes.

KINETICS OF PLATELET PRODUCTION

MATURATION TIME

The time required for the complete sequence of mega-karyocyte maturation is approximately 3 days in the rat [73] and rabbit [74] but, judging from the time required for recovery from acute platelet depletion [75,76], may be 4 to 5 days in human beings.

MEGAKARYOCYTE NUMBER

The iron-normoblast dilution method has shown normal human marrow to contain about 6×10^6 mega-karyocytes per kilogram of body weight [77]. Mega-karyocyte number can also be computed from the amount of injected labeled iron incorporated in a marrow particle and the number of megakaryocytes in that particle [78,79]. Several thousand platelets are probably released per megakaryocyte [69]. Megakaryocyte volume per microliter of marrow was $58 \times 10^5 \pm 30 \times 10^5 \ \mu m^3$ in 25 human controls, and the mean megakaryocyte number per square millimeter of marrow was 19 ± 8, with a mean megakaryocyte area of $296 \pm 60 \ mm^2$ [80].

DAILY PLATELET PRODUCTION

The overall rate of platelet production in human beings can only be estimated indirectly by determining platelet turnover in the blood (see Chap. 131). Estimates of $35,000 \pm 4300$ [77], $44,000 \pm 13,000$ [80], and $66,000 \pm 14,600$ [81] platelets produced per microliter of blood per day have been made in human beings. The fraction of total platelets produced by pulmonary megakaryocytes is no more than 7 to 17 percent [82] and is probably much less.

EXPERIMENTALLY ALTERED THROMBOCYTOPOIESIS

The thrombocytic series reacts specifically to depletion of each of the cellular populations discussed above.

ALTERATIONS IN PLATELET COUNT

Acute thrombocytopenia can be experimentally produced by exchange transfusion [83–86], by plasma-pheresis [87], or by injection of antiplatelet serum [88,89] whereas thrombocytosis has been produced by hypertransfusion of platelets to 4 to 10 times normal level [85]. Evidence for a limited platelet reserve providing immediate compensation for platelet depletion has been obtained in the dog [87] and in humans [90], but this may be derived from platelets pooled in the spleen (see below) rather than from new platelet production. The maximum extent to which platelet production can be increased is disputed. Studies of megakaryocyte mass in thrombocytopenic rats [85] and of platelet turnover in human subjects with chronic idiopathic thrombocytopenic purpura (ITP) [77,80] suggest that platelet synthesis can be increased up to 5- to 8-fold, although the average in ITP was about 2.5-fold [80], and evidence for relatively suppressed platelet production also exists [91]. The remarkable constancy of platelet concentrations for months or years in normal persons [92] suggests that the regulatory system is finely tuned. Only recently has it become apparent that changes in platelet count elicit a direct response at the megakaryoblast-megakaryocyte level and an indirect response at the progenitor level.

The direct response to thrombocytopenia In mice the first recognizable change after induction of thrombocytopenia is an increase within 1 to 2 h in small acetyl-cholinesterase-positive cells [21], nondividing cells which are committed to polyploidization and have been termed *promegakaryoblasts* in Fig. 130-1. Within 24 h, there is an increase in the fraction of recognizable mega-karyoblasts which incorporate tritiated thymidine [86,93,94] and exhibit endomitotic figures [89,94]. By 48 h, there is a marked increase in megakaryocyte size which is due both to a shift to higher ploidy classes [85,89] and to cytoplasmic enlargement [85,93] occurring within each ploidy class [89]. Following platelet depletion, platelet territories in mature megakaryocytes synthesize greater amounts of platelet products, as indicated by the increased specific activity of ^{35}S-sulfate [95] and ^{75}Se-selenomethionine [96] in newly formed platelets. Demarcation membrane formation is not depressed [97–99]. Since platelet volume is a function of both cytoplasmic growth and fragmentation [54,57], acute thrombocytopenia causes only a slight increase in platelet volume. As expected from the increase in small acetylcholinesterase-positive cells, total mega-karyocyte number increases between 24 to 60 h. Whether the overall maturation time of recognizable megakaryocytic cells is reduced by thrombocytopenia is disputed [93,97]. Platelet counts increase initially very slowly [75,76,86,89] but subsequently rise to above normal values [75,76,84,93]. Reciprocal changes occur after platelet hypertransfusion [27,95,100–102].

The indirect response to thrombocytopenia Just as erythroid progenitor cells (BFU-E) are insensitive to the red cell count [103], CFU-Mega are unlikely to be the primary target of the initial reaction to alterations in platelet counts. Support for this view is as follows: (1) CFU-Mega do not increase in number [104,105] until 2 days after platelet depletion, and alterations in the ploidy of the cells they generate [13] is similarly delayed, suggesting that the CFU-Mega respond only indirectly to platelet depletion; (2) in transplanted lethally irradiated mice, platelet hypertransfusion does not affect the number of regenerating CFU-Mega [104]. However, platelet transfusions administered 1 week after transplantation reduce the incidence of splenic mega-karyocyte colonies [106], presumably because the platelet count affects only the immediate precursors of recognizable megakaryocytes.

Thus the thrombocytic response to acute thrombocytopenia appears to consist of an influx of a cohort of promegakaryoblasts and their maturation through all ensuing stages of the series. The latter are programmed for higher ploidy, increased synthesis of platelet constituents, and macrothrombocytosis. Megakaryocyte progenitors are affected secondarily, perhaps by sensing the changes in the size of the more mature compartments.

ALTERATION IN PLATELET FUNCTION

Some of the megakaryocytic responses elicited by thrombocytopenia occur when rats or mice are treated by a single dose of 0.1 mg/kg vincristine [107,108]. Transfusion of platelets from normal donors, but not from vincristine-treated patients, suppresses the megakaryocytopoietic stimulation [108]. These observations suggest that vincristine may inhibit a platelet regulatory function, perhaps the secretion of a substance effecting feedback inhibition of megakaryocytopoiesis.

MEGAKARYOCYTOPENIA

Early studies of the effects of vincristine, hydroxyurea, or total-body irradiation showed that macromegakaryocytosis, a hallmark of megakaryocytopoietic stimulation (see above) can occur when the platelet count is normal or slightly reduced and the megakaryocyte level reduced [109]. Whether megakaryocyte size directly responds to a reduction in megakaryocyte mass or is exquisitely sensitive to thrombocytopenia is unknown.

MEGAKARYOCYTE PROGENITOR AND STEM CELL PERTURBATIONS

Normal platelet counts, megakaryocytopenia, and macrokaryocytosis are associated in the genetically anemic mouse strains W/W^v [110,111] and Sl/Sl^d [112], both of which have reduced numbers of CFU-Mega [113]. These findings illustrate that deficiency in ancestral hemopoietic precursors can be compensated at the level of the circulating cell count. Platelet production depends also on the composition of the stem cell compartment, as evidenced by the greater megakaryocyte repopulating ability of splenic stem cells compared with marrow cells [114] and of stem cells surviving 5-fluorouracil treatment compared with normal cells [115].

THROMBOCYTOPOIESIS-REGULATING FACTORS

There is now evidence for a two-stage regulation of the differentiation of pluripotential stem cells to erythrocytic [103,116], granulocytic [116], and megakaryocytic progeny [104,116,117] as well as modulation by several additional factors.

MEGAKARYOCYTE COLONY–STIMULATING FACTOR(S)

The growth of megakaryocyte colonies from CFU-Mega in semisolid media requires erythropoietin or media conditioned by lectin-treated spleen suspensions [8,18] or by the myelomonocytic leukemic cell line WEHI-3 [10,117]. WEHI-3–conditioned medium stimulated thrombocytopoiesis when injected into irradiated mice reconstituted with marrow cells [118]. A role for erythro-

poietin in platelet production is suggested by the activity of purified preparations of this hormone on megakaryocyte colony formation [119], by the demonstration of thrombopoietic activity in plasma of anemic animals [120], and by the association of renal polycythemia and thrombocytosis [121]. However, injection of purified erythropoietin does not alter platelet levels of monkeys [122], rats [123], or mice [124]. Possibly, a closely related thrombopoietic factor is elevated, together with erythropoietin, in certain pathologic states. Alternatively, erythropoietin at very high concentration may act indiscriminately to increase platelet production [124], particularly when red cell production is ineffective [125].

MEGAKARYOCYTE POTENTIATING ACTIVITY

In vitro growth of megakaryocyte colonies stimulated by WEHI-3–conditioned medium is enhanced if they are supplemented with conditioned medium from various tissues which by themselves do not stimulate colony formation [10,117]. Addition of these conditioned media presumably promotes polyploidization and cytoplasmic maturation of megakaryocyte precursors. The potentiator cell has the physical characteristics of the macrophage [126]. The potentiator has activity in vivo in combination with WEHI-3–conditioned medium [118].

THROMBOPOIETIN

A hormone capable of specifically stimulating platelet production, thrombopoietin, can be demonstrated in the plasma of thrombocytopenic animals [95,127,128], of vincristine-treated mice [107], and of Sl/Sl^d mice (see above) [112]. Administration of thrombopoietin in vivo activates the direct megakaryoblast-megakaryocyte response to thrombocytopenia (see above) while the in vitro activity of the hormone strongly resembles that of the megakaryocyte potentiating activity just discussed [117,129]. Thrombopoietin is best measured by determining the rate of appearance of injected ^{35}S-sulfate or ^{75}Se-selenomethionine in newly formed platelets. Plasma thrombopoietin levels in normal animals can be measured provided endogenous thrombocytopoiesis has been suppressed in assay animals [130]. Stimulation of DNA synthesis in isolated megakaryocytes can also be used as a test for thrombopoietin in vitro [131]. Measurements of platelet count and size are less sensitive than assays of radioisotope incorporation [132] because thrombopoietin probably enhances both the growth and demarcation of platelet territories, thereby causing only moderate macrothrombocytosis. An immunoassay for thrombopoietin has been reported [133].

On the basis of thrombopoietin assays performed on the supernates of cultured human kidney cells, kidney has been considered to be the site of synthesis of thrombopoietin [134]. Since platelet production is fairly well sustained in anephric human beings, it seems unlikely that kidney is solely responsible for thrombopoietin production. However, the thrombopoietic stimulating factor obtained from cultured kidney supernatants shares several physiologic [129] and immunologic [133] properties with thrombopoietin. Partial purification of both thrombopoietin [135] and kidney-derived thrombopoietic stimulating factor have been achieved [136].

In human beings a humoral factor directly affecting megakaryocyte maturation is suggested by studies of a possibly unique child who was severely thrombocytopenic from an early age and whose marrow contained only immature megakaryocytes [137,138]. On repeated occasions, infusion of fresh normal plasma provoked megakaryocyte maturation and an increase in the platelet count to the normal range. Thrombopoietin was generated either by a release mechanism or some other indirect action of the infused plasma [139]. Twenty-two subjects with normal platelet counts had no detectable thrombopoietin in their plasma, while 53 percent of thrombocytotic and 33 percent of thrombocytopenic patients had measurable thrombopoietin in their plasma [140]. Inhibitory activity was also found in some normal and some thrombocytopenic subjects.

ACETYLCHOLINESTERASE
Acetylcholinesterase, an essentially specific and early marker of cells of the rodent thrombocytic series [21], is both a constituent of the cellular membrane and a secretory enzyme. Injection of mice with neostigmine, a cholinesterase inhibitor, caused a significant increase in CFU-Mega per humerus and tripled the fraction of CFU-Mega in DNA synthesis [141]. Cytochemical studies at the ultrastructural level showed that megakaryoblasts and megakaryocytes undergo a typical secretory cycle resulting in the discharge of acetylcholinesterase in the demarcation membrane system and extracellular space [39]. By controlling acetylcholine concentration in hemopoietic tissues, the secretion of acetylcholinesterase by megakaryocytes could conceivably modulate the proliferative activity of megakaryocyte progenitors [39,141].

SPLENIC FACTORS
Thrombocytopenia often accompanies splenic enlargement, and platelet counts can be restored to normal by splenectomy (see Chap. 143). Removal of the spleen in idiopathic thrombocytopenic purpura may also be followed by remission (see Chap. 142). In normal subjects, transient thrombocytosis occurs after splenectomy [142], and the spleen was thought to suppress platelet production through a humoral mechanism [143]. However, the beneficial effect of splenectomy in idiopathic thrombocytopenic purpura is mainly due to removal of a major site of platelet destruction (see Chap. 142), and hypersplenic thrombocytopenia is caused by pooling of platelets in the enlarged spleen rather than by diminished platelet production (see Chap. 143) [144–146].

The spleen may, nonetheless, influence platelet production. In human beings platelet levels increase two- to sixfold after removal of the spleen because of trauma,

reaching a peak level on or about the eleventh postoperative day. This increase is far greater than the 30 to 50 percent rise that normally follows other surgical procedures [147,148] and cannot be accounted for solely by the absence of splenic pooling, which of itself would cause platelets to increase by no more than 50 percent. Since platelet life-span is little changed by splenectomy [146], increased platelet production must play a role in postsplenectomy thrombocytosis. Animal studies suggest this may be due to the absence of a humoral regulator normally produced by the spleen. Reimplantation of a small portion of spleen prevented postsplenectomy thrombocytosis [149,150], even when the implant was encased in a semipermeable chamber [150]. Furthermore, administration of splenic lymphocytes to normal mice caused mild thrombocytopenia and prevented postsplenectomy thrombocytosis in splenectomized animals [151]. As discussed above, activities stimulating megakaryocyte progenitors can be produced from splenic cells conditioned by certain lectins [8,12,16,18].

NONSPECIFIC FACTORS
When given in large doses to dogs and rabbits, estrogenic hormones cause severe thrombocytopenia due to marrow hypoplasia [152]. In the normal human female, a significant reduction of platelet levels often occurs in the course of the menstrual cycle, becoming more pronounced at or just before the onset of menses [153]. A progressive decrease in platelet levels too great to be accounted for by changes in blood volume alone has been noted during normal pregnancy [154]. Contrary findings have also been recorded [155].

Large doses of glucocorticoids given for prolonged periods have been reported to suppress platelet production in some patients with idiopathic thrombocytopenic purpura [156]. Androgenic hormones have not been shown to affect platelet levels.

Egg albumin and ground glass can also increase platelet levels when injected into rats [157] and miscellaneous inflammatory agents have a similar effect [158]. The variability of platelet levels in iron-deficient subjects had led to the suggestion that iron affects platelet production in two ways: (1) a low level of serum iron promotes the action of thrombopoietin by removal of a hypothetical inhibitory factor, and (2) iron is necessary for the synthesis of platelets by megakaryocytes, so that in profound iron deficiency platelet production may be impaired [159].

Distribution of platelets

When platelets labeled with radioactive chromium (^{51}Cr) are transfused to normal persons, only about two-thirds remain in the general circulation [77,146]. In contrast, nearly 100 percent can be recovered in asplenic subjects [77,146], suggesting that the distribution of platelets in the body is affected by the spleen. Intravenous infusion of epinephrine, which reduces blood flow in the spleen and causes the organ to empty passively into the circulation, normally causes platelet levels to increase 30 to 50 percent but does not affect platelet concentrations in asplenic individuals [146]. If ^{51}Cr-labeled platelets are injected prior to administration of epinephrine, the thrombocytosis is accompanied by a decrease in splenic surface radioactivity [146,160]. Large numbers of platelets can be flushed from spleens removed at surgery [146,161]. These observations indicate the existence of a pool of platelets in the spleen constituting about one-third of the total platelet mass and exchanging freely with platelets in the general circulation.

The mechanism of splenic pooling of platelets is unknown. Particles smaller than 2 to 3 μm in diameter tend to pass into the red pulp upon entering the spleen [162] and are, therefore, obliged to follow a tortuous path through the splenic cords rather than the more direct route through the sinusoids. As a result, platelets may traverse the spleen more slowly than larger erythrocytes and leukocytes [146]. An average transit time of about 8 to 10 min must be postulated to account for the known degree of splenic pooling of platelets on this basis alone [146,163]. A scanning electron micrographic study has demonstrated vast numbers of platelets adherent to the surfaces of reticular cells in the splenic cords and endothelial cells of the sinuses, suggesting that the adhesive properties of platelets may delay their passage through the organ [164]. The splenic pool has no apparent physiologic significance, but in diseases characterized by splenic enlargement it may contain 80 to 90 percent of the total platelet mass, causing thrombocytopenia in the peripheral circulation (see Chap. 143). It has been suggested that the spleen contains greater numbers of large platelets [165] and of newly formed platelets than are found in the blood [166].

Platelets can perhaps be released transiently from the lungs by intracardiac injection of epinephrine [167], but they are probably derived from pulmonary megakaryocytes. A nonsplenic platelet pool, making up about 45 percent of the total rapidly mobilizable platelet pool, was inferred from the transient increase in platelet count in splenectomized humans following exercise and in animals treated by epinephrine [168].

Life-span and fate of platelets

PLATELET LIFE-SPAN AND UTILIZATION
Eight to twelve days are required for human platelets labeled with ^{51}Cr-chromate [77,80,81,160,169–171], diisopropylfluorophosphate (DF^{32}P) [90,172], or ^{111}In-indium oxime [173,174] to be cleared from the circulation. The mean life-span in groups of normal humans averaged 6.9 to 9.9 days, and was 8 days in monkeys [175], 5 to 7 days in dogs [176–177], 5 days in rats [144,172], and 3 days in rabbits [179]. In humans, changes in body surface activity following transfusion of ^{111}In-labeled platelets suggest that the marrow plays

a more important part in platelet destruction and liver and spleen a less active one [174,180] than had previously been concluded with ^{51}Cr-labeling [160,181]. Utilization of platelets in the peripheral vessels is not thought to be significant in normal subjects [174].

There is disagreement as to which mathematical model provides the best fit to platelet clearance curves. Even complete accord on this point would not, however, in itself permit firm conclusions to be drawn regarding mechanisms of platelet utilization [182].

Unless they are stabilized by fibrin, many platelet aggregates formed in animals under the action of adenosine diphosphate (ADP), serotonin, epinephrine, thrombin, collagen, antigen-antibody complexes, viruses, and bacteria are unstable and can dissociate. Thrombin, for instance, degranulates and releases platelet constituents [183], causes shedding of unaltered pieces of platelet membrane [184] and reduces platelet density [185], which largely depends on granule concentration [186]. However, thrombin does not affect the residual life-span of subsequently deaggregated platelets [183], indicating that many hemostatic interactions do not inexorably kill platelets and suggesting that normal senescence, if it obeys a multiple hit model [182, 187], is not caused by repeated, thrombin-mediated insults in the circulation. Other experimental insults have been found, however, which drastically reduce platelet survival. Removal of sialoglycoproteins or sialic acid from platelet membrane considerably shortens platelet longevity [188,189]. Thrombin removes little of the sialic acid from platelets, and ADP removes none when tested in the presence of calcium [190].

SENESCENCE AND PLATELET HETEROGENEITY
For reasons given above, the processes of growth and fragmentation within each megakaryocyte induce a marked heterogeneity in platelet properties, including size and synthetic capacities [54]. Recent studies in animals confirm that marrow produces platelets of variable densities, with the most dense platelets originating from platelet territories which incorporates ^{35}S-sulfate at an initially much faster rate than those which produced less dense cells [65]. What additional heterogeneity is mediated by aging is uncertain since in several experimental protocols normal circulating platelets have been compared not to physiological young or old platelets, but rather to young "stress" platelets produced after platelet depletion or to platelets obtained after myelosuppressive treatment. However, density, metabolic, and functional properties are expected to be influenced by the in vivo processes, hemostatic or other, discussed above, as well as by the possible increase in dense granules with aging [191,192]. Decrease in size with aging has been suggested though not definitely established [58,175]. Since newborn platelets are already highly heterogeneous in size [54,57], decrease in platelet size with aging may increase or decrease the overall platelet heterogeneity depending on whether or not it affects platelet fractions uniformly. As an example,

computer simulations showed that even a 30 percent reduction in platelet volume during a normal life-span would cause insignificant alterations in the shape of platelet volume distributions and their coefficient of variation of volumes [193].

References

1. Tavassoli, M.: Megakaryocyte-platelet axis and the process of platelet formation and release. *Blood* 55:537, 1980.
2. Kelemen, E., Calvo, W., and Fliedner, T. M.: *Atlas of Human Hemopoietic Development.* Springer-Verlag, Berlin, 1979.
3. Paulus, J. M.: Multiple differentiation in megakaryocytes and platelets. *Blood* 29:407, 1967.
4. Williams, N.: Megakaryocyte progenitor cells in vitro, in *Megakaryocytes in Vitro,* edited by B. L. Evatt, R. F. Levine, and N. Williams. Elsevier–North Holland, Amsterdam, 1981, pp. 101–108.
5. Metcalf, D., Johnson, G. R., and Mandel, T. E.: Colony formation in agar by multipotential hemopoietic cells. *J. Cell. Physiol.* 98:401, 1979.
6. McLeod, D. L., Shreeve, M. M., and Axelrad, A. A.: Chromosome marker evidence for the bipotentiality of BFU-E. *Blood* 56:318, 1980.
7. Hara, H. V., and Noguchi, K.: Clonal nature of pluripotent hemopoietic precursors in vitro (CFU-mix). *Stem Cells* 1:53, 1981.
8. Metcalf, D., MacDonald, H. R., Odartchenko, N., and Sordat, B.: Growth of mouse megakaryocyte colonies in vitro. *Proc. Natl. Acad. Sci. U.S.A.* 72:1744, 1975.
9. Nakeff, A.: Colony forming unit, megakaryocyte (CFU-M): Its use in elucidating the kinetics and humoral control of the megakaryocytic committed progenitor cell compartment, in *Experimental Hematology Today 1977,* edited by S. J. Baum and G. D. Ledney, Springer-Verlag, Berlin, 1977, pp. 111–123.
10. Williams, N., Jackson, J., Sheridan, A. P. C., Murphy, M. J., Jr., Elste, A., and Moore, M. A. S.: Regulation of megakaryocytopoiesis in long-term murine bone marrow cultures. *Blood* 51:245, 1978.
11. Mizoguchi, H., Kubota, K., Miura, Y., and Takaku, F.: An improved plasma culture system for the production of megakaryocyte colonies in vitro. *Exp. Hematol.* 7:345, 1979.
12. Burstein, S. A., Adamson, J. W., Thorning, D., and Harker, L. A.: Characteristics of murine megakaryocytic colonies in vitro. *Blood* 54:169, 1979.
13. Levin, J., Levin, F. C., Penington, D. G., and Metcalf, D.: Measurement of ploidy distribution in megakaryocyte colonies obtained from cultures: With studies of the effects of thrombocytopenia. *Blood* 57:287, 1981.
14. Paulus, J. M., Prenant, M., Deschamps, J. F., Henry-Amar, M.: Polyploid megakaryocytes develop randomly from a multicompartmental system of committed progenitors. *Proc. Natl. Acad. Sci. U.S.A.* 79:4410, 1982.
15. Humphries, R. K., Eaves, A. C., and Eaves, C. J.: Characterization of a primitive erythropoietic progenitor found in mouse marrow after several weeks in culture. *Blood* 53:746, 1979.
16. Johnson, G. R.: Colony formation in agar by adult bone marrow multipotential hemopoietic cells. *J. Cell. Physiol.* 103:371, 1980.
17. Vainchenker, W., and Breton-Gorius, J.: Induction of human megakaryocyte colonies in vitro and ultrastructural aspects of the maturation, in *Megakaryocytes in Vitro,* edited by B. L. Evatt, R. F. Levine, and N. Williams. Elsevier–North Holland, Amsterdam, 1981, pp. 139–155.
18. Fauser, A. A., and Messner, H. A.: Identification of megakaryocyte, macrophages and eosinophils in colonies of human bone marrow containing neutrophilic granulocytes and erythroblasts. *Blood* 53:1023, 1979.
19. Mazur, M. E., Hoffman, R., Bruno, E., Marchesi, S., and Chasis, J.: Identification of two classes of human megakaryocyte progenitor cells, in *Megakaryocytes in Vitro,* edited by B. L. Evatt, R. F. Levine, and N. Williams. Elsevier–North Holland, Amsterdam, 1981, pp. 281–287.

20. Gregory, C. J.: Erythropoietin sensitivity as a differentiation marker in the hemopoietic system: Studies of three erythropoietic colony responses in culture. *J. Cell. Physiol.* 89:289, 1976.
21. Jackson, C. W.: Some characteristics of rat megakaryocyte precursors identified using cholinesterase as a marker, in *Platelets: Production, Function, Transfusion and Storage,* edited by M. G. Baldini and S. Ebbe. Grune & Stratton, New York, 1974, pp. 33–40.
22. Long, M. W., and Williams, N.: Relationship of small acetylcholinesterase positive cells to megakaryocytes and clonable megakaryocyte progenitor cells, in *Megakaryocytes in Vitro,* edited by B. L. Evatt, R. F. Levine, and N. Williams. Elsevier–North-Holland, Amsterdam, 1981, pp. 293–297.
23. Breton-Gorius, J.: Megakaryoblastic leukemia. *Haematologica* 64:517, 1979.
24. Mayer, M., Schaefer, J., and Queisser, W.: Identification of young megakaryocytes by immunofluorescence and cytophotometry. *Blut* 37:265, 1978.
25. Rabellino, E. M., Levene, R. B., Lawrence, L. K., Leung, and Nachman, R. L.: Human megakaryocytes. II. Expression of platelet proteins in early marrow megakaryocytes. *J. Exp. Med.* 154:88, 1981.
26. Breton-Gorius, J., and Reyes, F.: Ultrastructure of human bone-marrow cell maturation. *Int. Rev. Cytol.* 46:251, 1976.
27. Ebbe, S., and Stohlman, F., Jr.: Megakaryocytopoiesis in the rat. *Blood* 26:20, 1965.
28. de Leval, M.: Contribution à l'étude de la maturation des mégacaryocytes dans la moelle osseuse de cobaye. *Arch. Biol.* 79:597, 1968.
29. Odell, T. T., Jr., and Jackson, C. W.: Polyploidy and maturation of rat megakaryocytes. *Blood* 32:102, 1968.
30. Paulus, J. M.: DNA metabolism and development of organelles in guinea pig megakaryocytes: A combined ultrastructural, autoradiographic, and cytophotometric study. *Blood* 35:298, 1970.
31. Garcia, A. M.: Feulgen-DNA values in megakaryocytes. *J. Cell. Biol.* 20:342, 1964.
32. Kinet-Denoël, C., Bassleer, R., Andrien, J. M., Paulus, J. M., Penington, D. G., and Weste, S. M.: Ploidy histograms in ITP, in *Platelet Kinetics,* edited by J. M. Paulus. North Holland, Amsterdam, 1971, pp. 280–286.
33. Queisser, U., Queisser, W., and Spiertz, B.: Polyploidization in patients with idiopathic thrombocytopenia and with pernicious anemia. *Br. J. Haematol.* 20:489, 1971.
34. Levine, R. F., Bunn, P. A., Jr., Hazzard, K. C., and Schlam, M. L.: Flow cytometric analysis of megakaryocyte ploidy: Comparison with Feulgen microdensitometry and discovery that 8N is the predominant ploidy class in guinea pig and monkey marrow. *Blood* 56:210, 1980.
35. Behnke, O., and Pedersen, T. N.: Ultrastructural aspects of megakaryocyte maturation and platelet release, in *Platelet: Production, Function, Transfusion and Storage,* edited by M. G. Baldini and S. Ebbe, Grune & Stratton, New York, 1974, pp. 21–32.
36. Zucker-Franklin, D.: Megakaryocytes and platelets, in *Atlas of Blood Cells, Function and Pathology,* edited by D. Zucker-Franklin, M. F. Greaves, C. E. Grossi, and A. M. Marmont. Lea & Febiger, Philadelphia, 1981, vol. 2, pp. 557–602.
37. MacPherson, G. G.: Development of megakaryocytes in bone marrow of the rat: An analysis by electron microscopy and high resolution autoradiography. *Proc. R. Soc. Lond. [Biol.]* 177:265, 1971.
38. MacPherson, G. G.: Synthesis and localization of sulfated mucopolysaccharide in megakaryocytes and platelets of the rat: An analysis by electron microscopic autoradiography. *J. Cell. Sci.* 10:705, 1972.
39. Paulus, J. M., Maigne, J., and Keyhani, E.: Mouse megakaryocytes secrete acetylcholinesterase. *Blood* 58:1100, 1981.
40. Bentfeld, M. E., and Bainton, D. F.: Cytochemical localization of lysosomal enzymes in rat megakaryocytes and platelets. *J. Clin. Invest.* 56:1635, 1975.
41. Breton-Gorius, J., and Guichard, J.: Two different types of granules in megakaryocytes and platelets as revealed by the diaminobenzidine method. *J. Microsc. Biol. Cell* 23:197, 1975.
42. Paulus, J. M.: The slit filtration method. Application to megakaryocyte isolation. *Nouv. Rev. Fr. Hematol.* 8:821, 1968.

43. Rabellino, E. M., Nachman, R. L., Williams, N., Winchester, R. J., and Ross, G. D.: Human megakaryocytes. I. Characterization of the membrane and cytoplasmic components of isolated marrow megakaryocytes. *J. Exp. Med. 149:*1273, 1979.

44. Nachman, R., Levine, R., and Jaffe, E. A.: Synthesis of factor VIII antigen by cultured guinea-pig megakaryocytes. *J. Clin. Invest. 60:*914, 1977.

45. Nachman, R., Levine, R., and Jaffe, E. A.: Synthesis of actin by cultured guinea-pig megakaryocytes: Complex formation with fibrin. *Biochim. Biophys. Acta 513:*91, 1978.

46. Fedorko, M. E.: The functional capacity of guinea pig megakaryocytes. I. Uptake of ³H-serotonin by megakaryocytes and their physiologic and morphologic response to stimuli for the platelet release reaction. *Lab. Invest. 36:*310, 1977.

47. Nachman, R. L., Marcus, A. J., and Safier, L. B.: Platelet thrombosthenin: Subcellular localization and function. *J. Clin. Invest. 46:*1380, 1967.

48. Behnke, O., and Emmersen, J.: Structural identification of thrombosthenin in rat megakaryocytes. *Scand. J. Haematol. 9:*130, 1972.

49. Tavassoli, M.: Fusion-fission reorganization of membrane: A developing membrane model for thrombocytogenesis in megakaryocytes. *Blood Cells 5:*89, 1979.

50. Behnke, O.: An electron microscope study of megakaryocytes of rat bone marrow. I. Development of the demarcation membrane system and platelet surface coat. *J. Ultrastruct. Res. 24:*412, 1968.

51. White, J. G.: Interaction of membrane systems in blood platelets. *Am. J. Pathol. 66:*295, 1972.

52. Breton-Gorius, J.: Development of two distinct membrane systems associated in giant complexes in pathological megakaryocytes. *Ser. Haematol. 8:*1, 1975.

53. Gerrard, J. M., and White, J. G.: Prostaglandins and thromboxanes: Middlemen modulating platelet function in hemostasis and thrombosis, in *Progress in Haemostasis and Thrombosis,* edited by T. H. Spaet. Grune & Stratton, New York, 1978, vol. 4, pp. 87–125.

54. Paulus, J. M., Bury, J., and Grosdent, J. C.: Control of platelet territory development in megakaryocytes. *Blood Cells 5:*51, 1979.

55. Paulus, J. M., and Grosdent, J. C.: Platelet size distribution, biological significance and clinical usefulness, in application and interpretation of new electronically derived haematological parameters and techniques. Coulter Electronics, Luton, England, 1982, in press.

56. Dighiero, F., Lesty, C., Leporrier, M., and Couty, M. C.: Computer analysis of platelet volumes. *Blood Cells 6:*365, 1980.

57. Paulus, J. M.: Platelet size in man. *Blood 46:*321, 1975.

58. Karpatkin, S.: Heterogeneity of platelet function: Correlation with platelet volume. *Am. J. Med. 64:*542, 1978.

59. Von Behrens, W. E.: Mediterranean macrothrombocytopenia. *Blood 46:*199, 1975.

60. O'Brien, J. R., and Jamieson, S.: A relationship between platelet volume and platelet number. *Thromb. Diath. Haemorrh. 31:*363, 1974.

61. Zeigler, Z., Murphy, S., and Gardner, F. H.: Microscopic platelet size and morphology in various hematologic disorders. *Blood 51:*479, 1978.

62. Godwin, H. A., and Ginsburg, A. D.: May-Hegglin anomaly: A defect in megakaryocyte fragmentation? *Br. J. Haematol. 26:*117, 1974.

63. Karpatkin, S.: Heterogeneity of rabbit platelets. VI. Further resolution of changes in platelet density volume and radioactivity following cohort labelling with ⁷⁵Se-selenomethionine. *Br. J. Haematol. 39:*459, 1978.

64. Boneu, B., Boneu, A., Raisson, Cl., Guiraud, R., and Biermé, R.: Kinetics of "platelet populations" in the stationary state. *Thromb. Res. 3:*605, 1973.

65. Rand, M. L., Greenberg, J. P., Packham, M. A., and Mustard, J. F.: Density subpopulations of rabbit platelets: Size, proteins and sialic acid content, and specific radioactivity changes following labeling with ³⁵S-sulfate in vivo. *Blood 57:*741, 1981.

66. Penington, D. G., Streatfield, K., and Roxburgh, A. E.: Megakaryocytes and the heterogeneity of circulating platelets. *Br. J. Haematol. 34:*639, 1976.

67. Paulus, J. M., Breton-Gorius, J., Kinet-Denoël, C., and Boniwer, C.: Megakaryocyte ultrastructure and ploidy in human macrothrombocytosis, in *Platelets: Production, Function, Transfusion and Storage,* edited by M. G. Baldini and S. Ebbe. Grüne & Stratton, New York, 1974, pp. 131–142.

68. Wright, J. H.: The histogenesis of the blood platelets. *J. Morphol. 21:*203, 1910.

69. Thiéry, J. P., and Bessis, M.: Mécanisme de la plaquettogenèse: Étude in vivo par la microcinématographie. *Rev. Hematol. 11:*162, 1956.

70. Behnke, O.: An electron microscopic study of the rat megakaryocyte. II. Some aspects of platelet release and microtubules. *J. Ultrastruct. Res. 26:*111, 1969.

71. Lichtman, M. A., Chamberlain, J. K., Simon, W., and Santillo, P. A.: Parasinusoidal location of megakaryocytes in marrow: A determinant of platelet release. *Am. J. Hematol. 4:*303, 1978.

72. Radley, J. M., and Scurfield, G.: The mechanism of platelet release. *Blood 56:*996, 1980.

73. Odell, T. T., Jr.: Megakaryocytopoiesis and its response to stimulation and suppression, in *Platelets: Production, Function, Transfusion and Storage,* edited by M. G. Baldini and S. Ebbe. Grune & Stratton, New York, 1974, pp. 11–20.

74. Cooney, D. P., and Smith, B. A.: Maturation time of rabbit megakaryocytes. *Br. J. Haematol. 11:*484, 1965.

75. Desforges, J. F., Bigelow, F. A., and Chalmers, T. C.: The effects of massive gastrointestinal hemorrhage on hemostasis. I. The blood platelets. *J. Lab. Clin. Med. 43:*501, 1954.

76. Krevans, J. R., and Jackson, D. P.: Hemorrhagic disorder following massive blood transfusion. *JAMA 159:*171, 1955.

77. Harker, L. A., and Finch, C. A.: Thrombokinetics in man. *J. Clin. Invest. 48:*963, 1969.

78. Fillet, G.: The ferrokinetic measurement of marrow cellularity. II. Method using a marrow-cell-erythroid radioiron ratio, in *Platelet Kinetics,* edited by J. M. Paulus. North Holland, Amsterdam, 1971, pp. 166–171.

79. Paulus, J. M., Deschamps, J. F., Prenant, M., and Casals, F. J.: Kinetics of platelets, megakaryocytes and their precursors: What to measure? *Blood Cells 6:*215, 1980.

80. Branehög, I., Kutti, J., Ridell, B., Swolin, B., and Weinfeld, A.: The relation of thrombokinetics to bone marrow megakaryocytes in idiopathic thrombocytopenic purpura (ITP). *Blood 45:*551, 1975.

81. Paulus, J. M.: *Production et destruction des plaquettes sanguines.* Masson, Paris, 1974.

82. Kaufman, R. M., Airo, R., Pollack, S., Crosby, W. H., and Doberneck, R.: Origin of pulmonary megakaryocytes. *Blood 25:*767, 1965.

83. Matter, M., Hartmann, J. R., Kautz, J., DeMarsh, Q. B., and Finch, C. A.: A study of thrombopoiesis in induced acute thrombocytopenia. *Blood 15:*174, 1960.

84. Odell, T. T., Jr., MacDonald, T. P., and Asano, M.: Response of rat megakaryocytes and platelets to bleeding. *Acta Haematol. 27:*171, 1962.

85. Harker, L. A.: Kinetics of thrombopoiesis. *J. Clin. Invest. 47:*458, 1968.

86. Odell, T. T., Jr., and Murphy, J. R.: Effects of degree of thrombocytopenia on thrombocytopoietic response. *Blood 44:*147, 1974.

87. Craddock, C. G., Adams, W. S., Perry, S., and Lawrence, J. S.: The dynamics of platelet production as studied by a depletion technique in normal and irradiated dogs. *J. Lab. Clin. Med. 45:*906, 1955.

88. Ebbe, S., Stohlman, F., Jr., Overcash, J., Donovan, J., and Howard, D.: Megakaryocyte size in thrombocytopenic and normal rats. *Blood 32:*383, 1968.

89. Odell, T. T., Jr., Murphy, J. R., and Jackson, C. W.: Stimulation of megakaryocytopoiesis by acute thrombocytopenia in rats. *Blood 48:*765, 1976.

90. Zucker, M. B., Ley, A. B., and Mayer, K.: Studies on platelet life-span and platelet depots by use of DFP³². *J. Lab. Clin. Med. 58:*405, 1961.

91. Baldini, M. G.: Platelet production and destruction in idiopathic thrombocytopenic purpura: A controversial issue. *JAMA 239:*2477, 1978.

92. Brecher, G., Schneiderman, M., and Cronkite, E. P.: The repro-

ducibility and constancy of the platelet count. *Am. J. Clin. Pathol.* 23:15, 1953.

93. Ebbe, S., Stohlman, F., Jr., Donovan, J., and Overcash, J.: Megakaryocyte maturation rate in thrombocytopenic rats. *Blood* 32:787, 1968.

94. Odell, T. T., Jr., Jackson, C. W., Friday, T. J., and Charsha, D. E.: Effects of thrombocytopenia on megakaryocytopoiesis. *Br. J. Haematol.* 17:91, 1969.

95. Harker, L. A.: Control of platelet production. *Annu. Rev. Med.* 25:383, 1974.

96. Shreiner, D. P., and Levin, J.: The effects of hemorrhage, hypoxia and a preparation of erythropoietin on thrombopoiesis. *J. Lab. Clin. Med.* 88:930, 1976.

97. MacPherson, G. G.: Changes in megakaryocyte development following thrombocytopenia. *Br. J. Haematol.* 26:105, 1974.

98. Bentfeld-Barker, M. E., and Bainton, D. F.: Ultrastructure of rat megakaryocytes after prolonged thrombocytopenia. *J. Ultrastruct. Res.* 61:201, 1977.

99. Penington, D. G., Streatfield, K., and Weste, S. M.: Megakaryocyte ploidy and ultrastructure in stimulated thrombopoiesis, in: *Platelets: Production, Function, Transfusion and Storage*, edited by M. G. Baldini and S. Ebbe. Grune & Stratton, New York, 1974, pp. 115–130.

100. Odell, T. T., Jr., Jackson, C. W., and Reiter, R. S.: Depression of the megakaryocyte platelet system in rats by transfusion of platelets. *Acta Haematol.* 38:34, 1967.

101. Long, M. W., and Henry, K. L.: Thrombocytosis-induced suppression of small acetylcholinesterase positive cells in bone marrow of rats. *Blood* 54:1338, 1979.

102. Evatt, B. L., and Levin, J.: Measurement of thrombopoiesis in rabbits using 75 selenomethionine. *J. Clin. Invest.* 48:1615, 1969.

103. Iscove, N. N.: Erythropoietin-independent stimulation of early erythropoiesis in adult marrow cultures by conditioned media from lectin-stimulated mouse spleen cells, in *Hematopoietic Cell Differentiation*, edited by D. W. Golde, M. J. Cline, D. Metcalf, and C. F. Fox. Academic, New York, 1978, pp. 37–52.

104. Burstein, S. A., Adamson, J. W., Erb, S. K., and Harker, L. A.: Regulation of murine megakaryocytopoiesis, in *Megakaryocytes in Vitro*, edited by B. L. Evatt, R. F. Levine, and N. Williams. Elsevier–North Holland, Amsterdam, 1981, pp. 127–137.

105. Levin, J., Levin, F. C., and Metcalf, D.: The effects of acute thrombocytopenia on megakaryocyte-CFC and granulocyte-macrophage CFC in mice: Studies of bone marrow and spleen. *Blood* 56:274, 1980.

106. Goldberg, J., Phalen, E., Howard, D., Ebbe, S., and Stohlman, F., Jr.: Thrombocytotic suppression of megakaryocyte production from stem cells. *Blood* 49:59, 1977.

107. Mandel, E. M., Bessler, H., and Djaldetti, M: Effect of a low dose of vincristine on platelet production in mice. *Exp. Hematol.* 5:499, 1977.

108. Jackson, C. W., and Edwards, C. C.: Evidence that stimulation of megakaryocytopoiesis by low dose vincristine results from an effect on platelets. *Br. J. Haematol.* 36:97, 1977.

109. Ebbe, S., and Phalen, E.: Does autoregulation of megakaryocytopoiesis occur? *Blood Cells* 5:123, 1979.

110. Ebbe, S., and Phalen, E.: Regulation of megakaryocytes in W/W^v mice. *J. Cell. Physiol.* 96:73, 1978.

111. Petursson, S. R., and Chervenick, P. A.: Abnormalities in megakaryocytopoiesis in W/W^v mice, in *Megakaryocytes in Vitro*, edited by B. L. Evatt, R. F. Levine, and N. Williams. Elsevier–North Holland, Amsterdam, 1981, pp. 323–328.

112. Ebbe, S., Phalen, E., and Howard, D.: Parabiotic demonstration of a humoral factor affecting megakaryocyte size in Sl/Sl^d mice. *Proc. Soc. Exp. Med.* 158:637, 1978.

113. Nakeff, A., and Bryan, J. E.: Megakaryocyte proliferation and its regulation as revealed by CFU-M analysis, in *Haematopoietic Cell Differentiation*, edited by D. W. Golde, M. J. Cline, D. Metcalf, and C. F. Fox. Academic, New York, 1978, pp. 241–259.

114. Bentfeld-Barker, M. E., and Schooley, J. C.: Comparison of the effectiveness of bone marrow and spleen stem cells for platelet repopulation in lethally irradiated mice. *Exp. Hematol.* 9:379, 1981.

115. Jones, B. C., Radley, J. M., Bradley, T. R., and Hodgson, G. S.: En-

hanced megakaryocyte repopulating ability of stem cells surviving 5-fluouracil treatment. *Exp. Hematol.* 8:61, 1980.

116. Metcalf, D., Burgess, A. W., and Johnson, G. R.: Stimulation of multipotential and erythroid precursors cells by GM-CSF, in *Experimental Hematology Today 1980*, edited by S. J. Baum, G. D. Ledney, and D. W. van Bekkum. Karger, Basel, 1980, pp. 3–12.

117. Williams, N., Eger, R. R., Jackson, H. M., and Nelson, D. J.: Two factor requirement for murine megakaryocyte colony formation. *J. Cell Physiol.* 110:101, 1982.

118. Krizsa, F., Dexter, T. M., and Lajtha, L. G.: Stimulation of platelet production in vivo by a factor in cell culture conditioned medium. *Biomedicine* 29:162, 1978.

119. Vainchenker, W., and Breton-Gorius, J.: Differentiation and maturation in vitro of human megakaryocytes from blood and bone marrow precursors, in *Cell Lineage, Stem Cells and Cell Determination*, edited by N. LeDouarin, *Inserm Symposium No. 10.* Elsevier–North Holland, Amsterdam, 1979, pp. 215–226.

120. Linman, J. W.: Factors controlling hemopoiesis: Thrombopoiesis and leukopoietic effects of "anemic" plasma. *J. Lab. Clin. Med.* 59:262, 1962.

121. Brandt, P. W. T., Dacie, J. V., Steiner, R. E., and Szur, L.: Incidence of renal lesions in polycythemia: A survey of 91 patients. *Br. Med. J.* 1:468, 1963.

122. VanDyke, D. C.: Response of monkeys to erythropoietin of rabbit, sheep and human origin. *Proc. Soc. Exper. Biol. Med.* 116:171, 1964.

123. Ebbe, S.: Megakaryocytopoiesis and platelet turnover. *Ser. Haematol.* 1:65, 1968.

124. Evatt, B. L., Spivak, J. L., and Levin, J.: Relationships between thrombopoiesis and erythropoiesis; with studies of the effects of preparations of thrombopoietin and erythropoietin. *Blood* 46:547, 1976.

125. Jackson, C. W., Simone, J. V., and Edwards, C. C.: The relationship of anemia and thrombocytosis. *J. Lab. Clin. Med.* 81:357, 1974.

126. Williams, N., Jackson, H., Ralph, P., and Nakoinz, I.: Cell interactions influencing murine marrow megakaryocytes; nature of the potentiator cell in bone marrow. *Blood* 57:157, 1981.

127. Ebbe, S.: Thrombopoietin. *Blood* 44:605, 1974.

128. Schreiner, D. P., and Levin, J.: Detection of thrombopoietic activity in plasma by stimulation of suppressed thrombopoiesis. *J. Clin. Invest.* 49:1709, 1970.

129. Williams, N., McDonald, T. P., and Rabellino, E. M.: Maturation and regulation of megakaryocytopoiesis. *Blood Cells* 5:43, 1979.

130. McDonald, T. P., Clift, R., Nolan, C., and Tribby, I. I. E.: A comparison of mice in rebound-thrombocytosis with platelet-hypertransfused mice for the assay of thrombopoietin. *Scand. J. Haematol.* 16:326, 1976.

131. Kellar, K. L., Evatt, B. L., McGrath, C. R., and Ramsey, R. B.: Stimulation of DNA synthesis in megakaryocytes by thrombopoietin in vitro, in *Megakaryocytes in Vitro*, edited by B. L. Evatt, R. F. Levine, and N. Williams. Elsevier–North Holland, Amsterdam, 1981, pp. 21–34.

132. McDonald, T. P.: A comparison of platelet size, platelet count and platelet ^{35}S incorporation as assays for thrombopoietin. *Br. J. Haematol.* 34:257, 1976.

133. McDonald, T. P.: Neutralizing antiserum to thrombopoietin. *Proc. Soc. Exp. Biol. Med.* 158:557, 1978.

134. McDonald, T. P., Clift, R., Lange, R. D., Nolan, C., Tribby, I. E., and Barlow, G. H.: Thrombopoietin production by human embryonic culture. *J. Lab. Clin. Med.* 85:59, 1975.

135. Evatt, B. L., Levin, J., and Algazy, K. M.: Partial purification of thrombopoietin from the plasma of thrombocytopenic rabbits. *Blood* 54:377, 1979.

136. McDonald, T. P., Andrews, R. B., Clift, R., and Gottsell, M.: Characterization of a thrombocytopoietic-stimulating factor from kidney cell culture medium. *Exp. Hematol.* 9:288, 1981.

137. Schulman, I., Pierce, M., Lukens, A., and Currimbhoy, Z.: Studies on thrombopoiesis. I. A factor in normal human plasma required for platelet production: Chronic thrombocytopenia due to its deficiency. *Blood* 15:943, 1950.

138. Schulman, I., Abildgaard, C. F., Cornet, J., Simone, J. V., and Currimbhoy, Z.: Studies on thrombopoiesis. II. Assay of human plasma thrombopoietic activity. *J. Pediatr.* 66:604, 1965.

139. McDonald, T. P., and Green, D.: Demonstration of thrombopoietin production after plasma infusion in a patient with congenital thrombopoietin deficiency. *Thromb. Haemostasis* 37:577, 1977 (letter).

140. Schreiner, D. P., Weinberg, J., and Enoch, D.: Plasma thrombopoietic activity in humans with normal and abnormal platelet counts. *Blood* 56:183, 1980.

141. Burstein, S. A., Adamson, J. W., and Harker, L. A.: Megakaryocytopoiesis in culture: Modulation by cholinergic mechanisms. *J. Cell Physiol.* 103:201, 1980.

142. Crosby, W. H.: Hyposplenism: An inquiry into the normal functions of the spleen. *Annu. Rev. Med.* 14:349, 1963.

143. Dameshek, W.: Hypersplenism. *Bull. N.Y. Acad. Med.* 31:133, 1955.

144. Aster, R. H.: Studies of the mechanisms of "hypersplenic" thrombocytopenia in rats. *J. Lab. Clin. Med.* 70:736, 1967.

145. deGabriele, G., and Penington, D. G.: Regulation of platelet production: "Hypersplenism" in the experimental animal. *Br. J. Haematol.* 13:384, 1967.

146. Aster, R. H.: Pooling of platelets in the spleen: Role in the pathogenesis of "hypersplenic" thrombocytopenia. *J. Clin. Invest.* 45:645, 1966.

147. Pepper, H., and Lindsay, S.: Responses of platelets, eosinophiles, and total leukocytes during and following surgical procedures. *Surg. Gynec. Obstet.* 110:319, 1960.

148. Breslow, A., Kaufman, R. M., and Lawsky, A. R.: The effect of surgery on the concentration of circulating megakaryocytes and platelets. *Blood* 32:393, 1968.

149. Jacob, H. S., McDonald, R. A., and Jandl, J. H.: Regulation of spleen growth and sequestering function. *J. Clin. Invest.* 42:1476, 1963.

150. Tarnuzi, A., and Smiley, R. K.: Hematologic effect of splenic implants. *Blood* 29:373, 1967.

151. Bessler, H., Mandel, E. M., and Djaldessi, M.: Role of the spleen and lymphocytes in regulation of the circulating platelet number in mice. *J. Lab. Clin. Med.* 91:760, 1978.

152. Shapter, A. G.: Oestrogens, progesterone, and platelets. *Lancet* 2:569, 1968.

153. Pohle, F. J.: The blood platelet count in relation to the menstrual cycle in normal women. *Am. J. Med. Sci.* 197:40, 1939.

154. Shaper, A. B., Kear, J., MacIntosh, D. M., Kyobe, J., and Njama, D.: The platelet count, platelet adhesiveness and aggregation, and the mechanism of fibrinolytic inhibition in pregnancy and the puerperium. *J. Obstet. Gynaecol. Br. Commonw.* 75:433, 1968.

155. Todd, M. E.: Changes in blood coagulation during pregnancy. *Mayo Clin. Proc.* 40:370, 1965.

156. Cohen, P., and Gardner, F. H.: Thrombocytopenic effect of sustained high dosage prednisone therapy in thrombocytopenic purpura. *N. Engl. J. Med.* 265:611, 1961.

157. Odell, T. T., Jr., MacDonald, T. P., and Howsdan, F. L.: Native and foreign stimulators of platelet production. *J. Lab. Clin. Med.* 64:418, 1964.

158. Abildgaard, C. F., and Simone, J. V.: Thrombopoiesis. *Semin. Haematol.* 4:424, 1967.

159. Karpatkin, S., Garg, S. K., and Freedman, M. E.: Role of iron as a regulator of thrombopoiesis. *Am. J. Med.* 57:521, 1974.

160. Kotilainen, M.: Platelet kinetics in normal subjects and haematological disorders with special reference to thrombocytopenia and to the role of the spleen. *Scand. J. Haematol. (Suppl.)* 5:9, 1969.

161. Penny, R., Rosenberg, M. C., and Firkin, B. G.: The splenic platelet pool. *Blood* 27:1, 1966.

162. Bjorkman, S. E.: The splenic circulation. *Acta Med. Scand. (Suppl.)* 191:7, 1947.

163. Peters, A. M., Klonizakis, I., Lavender, J. P., and Lewis, S. M.: Use of ¹¹¹In-indium–labelled platelets to measure spleen function. *Br. J. Haematol.* 46:587, 1980.

164. Weiss, L.: A scanning electron micrographic study of the spleen. *Blood* 43:665, 1974.

165. Freedman, M. L., and Karpatkin, S.: Heterogeneity of rabbit platelets. V. Preferential splenic sequestration of megathrombocytes. *Br. J. Haematol.* 31:255, 1975.

166. Shulman, N. R., Watkins, S. P., Jr., Itscoitz, S. B., and Students, A. B.: Evidence that the spleen retains the youngest and hemo-

167. Bierman, H. R., Kelly, K. H., Cordes, F. L., Byron, R. L., Jr., Polhemus, J. A., and Rapport, B. S.: The release of leukocytes and platelets from the pulmonary circulation by epinephrine. *Blood* 7:683, 1952.

168. Freedman, M., Altszuler, N., and Karpatkin, S.: Presence of a nonsplenic platelet pool. *Blood* 50:419, 1977.

169. Aster, R. H., and Jandl, J. H.: Platelet sequestration in man: I. Methods. *J. Clin. Invest.* 43:843, 1964.

170. Dassin, E., Balitrand, N., and Najean, Y.: An analysis of the effects of random and ageing mechanisms on the survival of platelets. *Biomedicine* 25:23, 1976.

171. Branehög, I., Ridell, B., and Weinfeld, A.: On the analysis of platelet survival curves and the calculation of platelet production and destruction. *Scand. J. Haematol.* 19:230, 1977.

172. Bithell, J. C., Athens, J. W., Cartwright, G. E., and Wintrobe, M. M.: Radioactive diisopropylfluorophosphate as a platelet label: An evaluation of in vitro and in vivo techniques. *Blood* 29:354, 1967.

173. Hawker, R. J., Hawker, L. M., and Wilkinson, A. R.: Indium (¹¹¹In)-labelled human platelets: Optimal method. *Clin. Sci.* 58:243, 1980.

174. Heyns, du P. A., et al.: Kinetics of distribution and sites of destruction of ¹¹¹Indium-labelled human platelets. *Br. J. Haematol.* 44:269, 1980.

175. Corash, L., Shafer, B., and Porlow, M.: Heterogeneity of human blood platelet subpopulations. II. Use of a subhuman primate model to analyze the relationship between density and platelet age. *Blood* 52:726, 1978.

176. Lötter, M. G., Badenhorst, P. N., Heyns, du P. A., Van Reenen, O. R., Pieters, H., and Minaar, P. C.: Kinetics, distribution and sites of destruction of canine blood platelets with In-111-oxime. *J. Nucl. Med.* 21:36, 1980.

177. Cohen, P., and Gardner, F. H.: Platelet preservation. I. Preservation of canine platelets at 4° C. *J. Clin. Invest.* 41:1, 1962.

178. Hjort, P. F., and Paputchis, H.: Platelet life-span in normal, splenectomized and hypersplenic rats. *Blood* 15:45, 1960.

179. Ebbe, S., Baldini, M., and Donovan, J.: Comparative studies of platelet survival by different methods in the rabbit. *Blood* 25:548, 1965.

180. Klonizakis, I., Peters, A. M., Fitzpatrick, M. L., Kensett, M. J., Lewis, S. M., and Lavender, J. P.: Radionuclide distribution following injection of 111 Indium-labelled platelets. *Br. J. Haematol.* 46:595, 1980.

181. Aster, R. H.: Studies of the fate of platelets in rats and man. *Blood* 34:117, 1969.

182. Mustard, J. F., Rowsell, H. C., and Murphy, E. A.: Platelet economy (platelet survival and turnover). *Br. J. Haematol.* 12:1, 1966.

183. Reimers, H. J., et al.: In vitro and in vivo functions of thrombin-treated platelets. *Thromb. Haemostasis* 35:131, 1976.

184. George, J. N., and Lewis, P. C.: Studies on platelet plasma membranes. III. Membrane glycoprotein loss from circulating platelets in rabbits: Inhibition by aspirin-dipyridamole and acceleration by thrombin. *J. Lab. Clin. Med.* 91:301, 1978.

185. Cieslar, P., Greenberg, J. P., Rand, M. L., Packham, M. A., Kinlough-Rathbone, R. L., and Mustard, J. F.: Separation of thrombin-treated platelets from normal platelets by density-gradient centrifugation. *Blood* 53:867, 1979.

186. Corash, L., Tan, H., and Gralnick, H. R.: Heterogeneity of human whole blood platelet subpopulations. I. Relationship between buoyant density, cell volume and ultrastructure. *Blood* 49:71, 1977.

187. Murphy, E. A.: Models of the destruction of blood platelets, in *Platelet Kinetics*, edited by J. M. Paulus. North Holland, Amsterdam, 1971, pp. 80–91.

188. Greenberg, J. P., Packham, M. A., Guccione, M. A., Rand, M. L., Reimers, H. J., and Mustard, J. F.: Survival of rabbit platelets treated in vitro with chymotrypsin, plasmin, trypsin, or neuraminidase. *Blood* 53:916, 1979.

189. Scott, S., et al.: Effect of viruses on platelet aggregation and platelet survival in rabbits. *Blood* 52:47, 1978.

190. Packham, M. A., Guccione, M. A., Kinlough-Rathbone, R. L., and Mustard, J. F.: Platelet sialic acid and platelet survival after aggregation by ADP. *Blood* 56:876, 1980.

191. Mishory, B., and Danon, D.: Structural aspects of in vivo aging in rabbit blood platelets. *Thromb. Res.* 12:893, 1978.
192. Mezzano, D., Hwang, K. L., Catalano, P., and Aster, R. H.: Evidence that platelet buoyant density, but not size, correlates with platelet age in man. *Am. J. Hematol.* 11:61, 1981.
193. Esch, L., Breny, H., and Paulus, J. M.: A theoretical study of the influence of platelet senescence on platelet size lognormality. *Proc. 5th Cong. Eur. African Div. Int. Soc Haematol,* Hamburg, 1979, vol. 1, p. 29.

CHAPTER *131*

Clinical evaluation of thrombokinetics

JEAN-MICHEL PAULUS
RICHARD H. ASTER

One of the first diagnostic considerations in patients with thrombocytopenia is whether the lowered platelet counts are a consequence of inadequate platelet production, accelerated platelet destruction, pooling of platelets in an enlarged spleen, or loss of platelets from the body (see Chaps. 141 to 144). Often this can be determined on the basis of the clinical findings and a relatively few hematologic measurements. More sophisticated studies of thrombokinetics may be of value in

FIGURE 131-1 **Platelet and erythrocyte log volume distributions from platelet-rich plasma obtained after slow centrifugation of a normal blood sample anticoagulated with EDTA [7]. Discrete points are frequency values while continuous lines are the two lognormal curves fitted to the platelet and erythrocyte histograms. About 1.5 percent of the platelets are not accounted for by the lognormal model, as discussed in Chap. 130. Mean platelet volume was 9.7 fl and the coefficient of variation of volumes, an index of the large platelet heterogeneity, was 73.2 percent.**

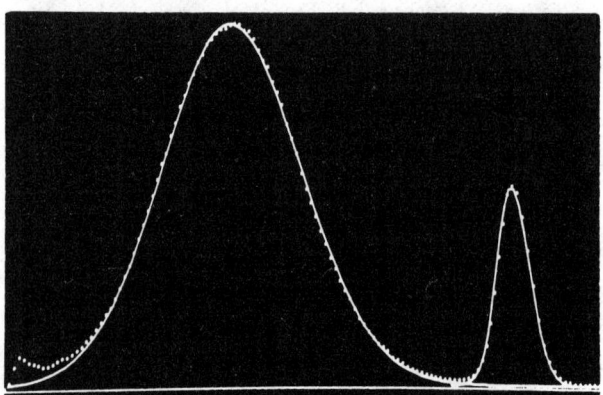

selected cases, e.g., in patients who have compensated for an increased rate of platelet destruction by increasing platelet production to the extent that platelet levels remain normal (compensated thrombocytolysis). The approaches available to the clinician for the evaluation of thrombokinetics are considered here.

Examination of platelets in blood

In addition to fast, accurate, and reproducible platelet enumeration the latest automatic platelet counters can determine platelet volume distributions. However, valuable information can still be obtained from cytological examination of the peripheral blood films.

MORPHOLOGY OF PLATELETS IN BLOOD FILMS
The blood film should be examined to confirm all platelet counts obtained by either manual or automated methods. Spurious thrombocytopenia due to in vitro platelet adherence to neutrophils and/or monocytes ("platelet satellitism") [1] is mediated by IgG platelet agglutinins which react only in ethylenediamine-tetraacetic acid (EDTA)–anticoagulated blood or by IgM antibodies reacting in blood anticoagulated with a variety of chelating agents [2]. Platelet satellitism has been found both in normal individuals and in disease states [2].

Spurious thrombocytosis can also occur, notably when cytoplasmic fragments of leukemic cells artifactually elevate the platelet count. Such fragments can be recognized by careful inspection of the blood film [3] or as a population of small particles distinct from the electronically determined platelet size distributions. Although macrothrombocytosis is most accurately determined by electronic sizing (see below), enumeration of platelets more than 2.5 μm in diameter in Wright-stained blood films (*megathrombocytes*) [4] is a useful diagnostic test. The morphology of megathrombocytes may also be informative. The large platelets found in myeloproliferative diseases or infiltrated marrows are more often hypogranular than are those found in platelet hyperdestruction, and this criterion may be useful in differentiating these causes of macrothrombocytosis [5].

ELECTRONIC PLATELET SIZING
As seen in Chap. 130, the volume distributions of platelets in blood samples anticoagulated with EDTA are lognormal in normal subjects and in most cases of macrothrombocytosis (see Fig. 131-1). Determination of the volume distributions makes it possible to recognize anomalies not only in mean volume but also in coefficient of variation of volumes, an index of platelet heterogeneity [6]. Increased mean platelet volume or macrothrombocytosis is found in cases of (1) platelet hyperdestruction (see Chap. 142) [4,6,7], (2) dysthrombocytopoiesis [5–7], or (3) reduced fragmentation of

platelet territories in megakaryocytes [8–10]. Platelet sizing helps to distinguish thrombocytopenia due to sequestration in the spleen, in which the mean volume is normal, from platelet hyperdestruction, in which the mean platelet volume tends to increase [11], depending on the platelet count [5,7]. Microthrombocytosis has been described in the Wiskott-Aldrich syndrome [12]. An elevated coefficient of variation of volumes, although less completely investigated, appears to have the same clinical significance as macrothrombocytosis but is a more common finding. Particles smaller than platelets can also be detected by electronic counting and have been considered to be red cell and platelet fragments [12–13] or leukemic cell fragments [15]. They are encountered in patients with platelet hyperdestruction [6,13] and in leukemias [6].

Detection of substances released from destroyed platelets

Platelets release certain of their constituents when they participate in hemostasis. Three types of platelet organelles can be distinguished on the basis of the substances they secrete and the patterns of the release reaction [16]. Acid hydrolases are released from lysosomal vesicles while serotonin and adenine nucleotides are liberated from dense granules (see Chap. 127). Alpha granules contain specific platelet proteins which can be measured by sensitive radioimmunoassays. Serum levels of these proteins can be used as indices of platelet activation in vivo. Both platelet factor 4 (PF4) and low-activity platelet factor 4 (LA-PF4) have anti-heparin activity but are structurally and immunologically distinct [17]. LA-PF4 is secreted by platelets and then converted to β-thromboglobulin (βTG) by a platelet protease [18]. Current radioimmunoassays do not differentiate βTG from LA-PF4. While βTG and PF4 are present in similar amounts in platelets and are released in vitro at similar rates, PF4 is cleared from the circulation more rapidly than βTG, due apparently to its immediate binding to endothelial cells. In vivo release is therefore suggested when βTG levels are elevated in the presence of normal or slightly increased levels of PF4. Elevation of the levels of both proteins, however, suggests in vitro release associated with defective sampling [19]. Interpretation of these determinations requires consideration of the increase in βTG levels associated with renal insufficiency [20] and the isolated marked elevation of PF4 levels following heparin infusion [19]. Normal values for plasma βTG (90th percentile) are 6.6 to 47.9 ng/ml and for plasma PF4 1.7 to 20.9 ng/ml [19]. The potential usefulness of measuring these substances is indicated by the inverse correlation between βTG levels and platelet life-span in a study of 91 patients with coronary artery disease [21]. In another study, βTG levels were increased in one patient suffer-

ing from thrombotic thrombocytopenic purpura and in another having disseminated intravascular coagulation but not in cases of immune hyperdestruction of platelets, in which platelets are removed extravascularly by the macrophage system, or in patients with platelet hypoproduction [22].

Evaluation of megakaryocyte number and mass

Estimation of megakaryocyte numbers can be made by assessing total marrow cellularity and comparing the number of megakaryocytic, erythroid, and myeloid elements in a carefully prepared, stained marrow aspirate. Although exceptions are sometimes encountered, thrombocytopenia is nearly always a consequence of accelerated platelet destruction, if megakaryocytes are abundant, their maturation sequence appears normal, and the patient's spleen is not palpable. Evaluation of a marrow biopsy section provides an even better measure of megakaryocyte content. Plastic sections which permit detailed examination of megakaryocytes, use of histochemical procedures, and ultrastructural analysis can now be prepared from human marrow biopsies as rapidly as routine paraffin sections [23]. In a few conditions, such as pernicious anemia, ineffective megakaryopoiesis results in subnormal platelet production despite normal numbers of megakaryocytes. Megakaryocyte morphology may be abnormal in such instances (see Chap 141). In patients with thrombocytopenia due to peripheral destruction of platelets, as in idiopathic thrombocytopenic purpura, megakaryoblasts are usually increased in number and mature megakaryocytes are unusually smooth in contour, with margins free of adherent platelets. It was formerly believed that such megakaryocytes did not produce platelets, i.e., were "nonbudding." As noted in Chap. 130, platelets are released from cytoplasmic processes extending into sinusoids rather than "budding" individually from megakaryocytes. Moreover, measurements of total megakaryocyte mass and platelet turnover in patients with idiopathic thrombocytopenic purpura have shown that the megakaryocytes are effective in platelet production although maximal compensatory hyperproduction of platelets is not the rule in this disorder (see Chap. 130). The absence of platelets adherent to megakaryocytes in the marrow of patients with destructive thrombocytopenias is probably due to the lack of platelets in blood aspirated with the marrow [24]. Total megakaryocyte mass can be measured in human beings [25,27]; but this requires simultaneous evaluation of marrow sections and determination of iron turnover with ^{59}Fe. Other methods yield an estimate of the number of megakaryocytes per cubic millimeter of marrow [28] (see Chap. 130). In most subjects, platelet production appears to be proportional to the total megakaryocyte mass [25].

Platelet survival studies

Although rough estimates of platelet life-span can be inferred from the survival of transfused platelets [29,30], this method is applicable only to thrombocytopenic subjects and necessarily disturbs the stationary state of platelet economy. A steady state is a necessary condition for accurate determination of platelet mean life-span and production from survival curves (see below). Radioisotopic labels provide a more satisfactory means of studying platelet clearance because of the accuracy with which circulating radioactivity can be measured and because small quantities of platelets can be used which do not appreciably alter platelet levels. Two kinds of survival studies have been utilized: (1) *cohort survival curves* derived from the circulating activity of a label which is incorporated by a cell population of uniform age, in practice newly formed cells or their immediate precursors; or (2) *population survival curves* derived from the circulating activity of a random, uniformly labeled sample of the circulating cell population reinfused into an autologous or isologous recipient. Platelet survival studies have been reviewed in detail [31–33].

COHORT SURVIVAL CURVES

LABELING TECHNIQUES
No radioactive label selectively tags newly formed platelets and remains bound to the cells throughout their life-span. ^{35}S-Sulfate appears in circulating platelets only after being incorporated into sulfated mucopolysaccharides by megakaryocytes [34], but its use is limited to animal studies.

In human beings, ^{75}Se-selenomethionine has been used as a platelet cohort label [35,36]. This γ-emitting analog of the amino acid methionine is incorporated into platelets both by adsorption of labeled albumin and fibrinogen and as a component of specific megakaryocyte proteins, mainly thrombosthenin [37]. In rats, measurement of the specific activity of isolated platelet thrombosthenin following ^{75}Se-selenomethionine administration provides an accurate cohort survival curve [37]. This promising but complex method has not been adapted to human studies.

DATA ANALYSIS
Most of the theory of cohort survival curves applies to situations where the radioisotope is taken up only by newly formed cells [38]. In this idealized situation, the mean life-span is equal to the area under the cohort survival curve, expressed as the fraction of injected activity remaining in the circulation at various times. A correction for the artifacts caused by the reutilization of ^{75}Se-selenomethionine by adsorbed platelet proteins has been described [35]. When this correction is made, the time interval between the 50 percent points on the ascending and descending limbs of the circulating

platelet ^{75}Se curve approximates the mean life-span. Normal values of 9.1 days [35] and 7.0 to 11.0 days [36] have thus been obtained in humans. A more sophisticated analysis has been proposed, since platelet cohort curves are determined by the combination of prolonged incorporation of the label into megakaryocytes and of delayed release into circulating platelets [39].

POPULATION SURVIVAL CURVES

LABELING TECHNIQUES
Inhibition of platelet cyclooxygenase This nonradioisotopic technique estimates platelet survival from daily determinations of the fraction of circulating platelets inhibited by a single administration of aspirin [40–44]. It is based on the irreversible acetylation of platelet cyclooxygenase after exposure of platelets in vitro or in vivo to aspirin [45]. Enzyme inhibition persists throughout platelet life-span and can be measured as inhibition of platelet aggregation [40], malondialdehyde (MDA) production [41–49], or thromboxane B_2 (TXB_2) production after N-ethylmaleimide or thrombin stimulation [44]. Under conditions of stationary platelet production, determination of the aspirin-induced inhibition in daily circulating platelet samples provides population survival curves whose special features have recently begun to emerge. First, aspirin inhibition affects not only platelets but also the most mature megakaryocytes, as shown by the persistent inhibition of MDA or TXB_2 production for 24 to 48 h after aspirin administration [44,45]. This feature probably explains the observation that survival times determined from aspirin inhibition studies are longer than those obtained with ^{51}Cr-labeled platelets [44]. Megakaryocyte inhibition also explains the initial upward convexity found in some survival curves [49]. Second, there is evidence that the production of nonacetylated cyclooxygenase does not always occur at a constant rate [32]. The kinetics of platelet recovery differ for low- and high-density platelets [46]. This method has been used to demonstrate normal platelet life-span in pregnant women [47,48] and reduced platelet survival in preeclampsia [48] in patients bearing prosthetic material and in a high proportion of patients with occlusive vascular disease [43].

^{51}Cr-*chromate labeling* This method for the determination of platelet kinetics is discussed in detail in Refs. 49 to 52. Studies comparing the disappearance of the radioisotope with the actual disappearance of transfused platelets, as determined by direct counting of platelets in thrombocytopenic subjects, have shown that disappearance of ^{51}Cr from the circulation is a valid measure of platelet clearance [53,54]. Chromate binds to platelet cytoplasm, and its disappearance can be compared with that of ^{14}C-serotonin–labeled platelets, which estimates dense granule survival [55–57], or with that of ^{125}I-diiodosulfanilic acid–labeled platelets, which may reflect the turnover of platelet membranes [58]. ^{51}Cr-chromate–labeled platelets have been administered to patients with ^{125}I-fibrinogen in order to discriminate between the various types of consumptive hyperdestruction [59,60].

^{111}*In-indium labeling*   The labeled metals ^{99m}Tc-technetium [61], ^{68}Ga-gallium [62], and ^{111}In-indium [63] can be chelated with 8-hydroxyquinoline (oxine) to form lipid-soluble complexes which bind to intracellular components of leukocytes and platelets. Of these compounds, ^{111}In-indium oxine has emerged as a nearly ideal platelet population label [63–73]. While providing platelet survival curves identical with ^{51}Cr-chromate platelets [63–65,69], except for a somewhat higher initial recovery [64,65], ^{111}In-indium has the advantages of a much shorter half-life (2.8 versus 28 days), a higher labeling efficiency (73 to 90 percent versus 6 percent), and a higher yield of γ photons (183 percent versus 9 percent). These features make it possible to label small volumes of platelet suspensions to lessen patient exposure to γ irradiation. Survival studies may be repeated when needed and good imaging of sites of platelet deposition can be obtained. Combined ^{51}Cr-labeling of homologous platelets and ^{111}In-labeling of autologous platelets is also feasible [69].

Diisopropylfluorophosphate (DFP)   Only the ^{32}P-tagged compound has been used to study platelet kinetics in humans, and values for mean life-span of 9 to 11 days have been obtained [74–76].

DATA ANALYSIS
Population survival curves obtained in the steady state after uniform labeling of a circulating cell suspension with a substance that is nontoxic and is not eluted or reutilized permit valid analyses even when the mode of disappearance of cells is unknown. Detailed studies of such curves have been published [38,77]. In practice, platelet survival curves only approximate these ideal conditions [31]. Interpretation of these curves relies on the use of one of several mathematical models, based on linear exponential, mixed linear-exponential [50], or gamma functions [39,50,77]. Estimates of platelet mean life-span, mean age, production, and fraction in the circulation provided by a polynomial model [78] are shown in Fig. 131-2.

Determination of the sites of platelet deposition

The high level of γ emission of ^{111}In-labeled platelets has permitted quantitative imaging of platelet deposition in vivo, using whole-body scanners and scintillation cameras [68–71]. Early and late uptake have been

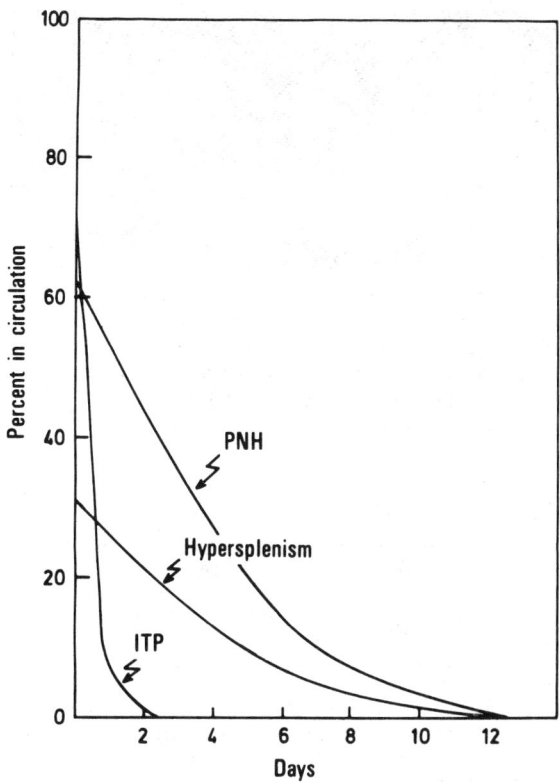

	Plat (/mm³)	μ (j)	a (j)	F (%)	P (/mm³/j)
PNH	120 300	5,4	3,9	62	$\boxed{35\,800}$
HS	86 400	6,0	4,0	$\boxed{31}$	48 000
ITP	90 000	$\boxed{0,83}$	0,58	61	177 800
Norm	144 000	6,1	3,8	49	47 000
	405 000	9,3	4,8	70	90 000

XBL 782- 2828

FIGURE 131-2   Typical platelet survival curves obtained in three patients suffering from platelet hypoproduction due to paroxysmal nocturnal hemoglobinuria (PNH), hypersplenism associated with cirrhosis (HS), and platelet hyperdestruction due to idiopathic thrombocytopenic purpura (ITP). The platelet count (Plat), mean life-span (μ), mean age (a), percent recovered at zero time (F), and production (P) are indicated for each case, and for control subjects (Norm). (With permission from *McGraw-Hill Yearbook of Science and Technology*, McGraw-Hill, New York, 1980.)

measured and visualized for the thorax, head, abdomen, and legs and the activity of the spleen, liver, and heart measured or calculated by use of computer-assisted techniques [68]. Early accumulation in the spleen was described as a single exponential function [68], compatible with a closed compartmental system (see Chap. 130). Physiologic destruction of platelets is also visualized and quantified [68,70] and pathologic deposition of platelets in thrombi can be imaged better than by ^{125}I-fibrinogen counting [72] (see Fig. 131-3).

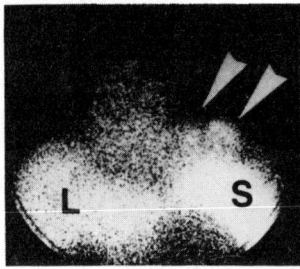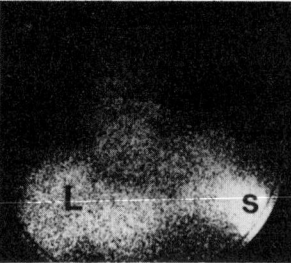

FIGURE 131-3 Left ventricular thrombi (*arrows*) in a patient suffering from heart aneurysm demonstrated by scintigraphy of ^{111}In-labeled platelets. L and S refer to the liver and spleen images. Note lysis of thrombi a few weeks after anticoagulant therapy. (Courtesy of Drs. C. Betz, G. Fillet, and P. Rigo, University of Liege, Belgium; see also Esekowitz et al. [73].)

References

1. Larson, J. H., and Pierre, R. V.: Platelet satellitism as a cause of abnormal Hemalog D differential results. *Am. J. Clin. Pathol. 68*:758, 1977.

2. Onder, O., Weinstein, A., and Hoyer, L. W.: Pseudothrombocytopenia caused by platelet agglutinins that are reactive in blood anticoagulated with chelating agents. *Blood 56*:177, 1980.

3. Armitage, J. O., Goeken, J. A., and Feagler, J. R.: Spurious elevation of the platelet count in acute leukemia. *JAMA 239*:433, 1978.

4. Garg, S. K., Amorosi, E. L., and Karpatkin, S.: The increased percentage of megathrombocytes in various clinical disorders. *Ann. Intern. Med. 77*:361, 1972.

5. Zeigler, Z., Murphy, S., and Gardner, F. H.: Microscopic platelet size and morphology in various hematologic disorders. *Blood 51*:479, 1978.

6. Paulus, J. M., Bury, J., and Grosdent, J. C.: Control of platelet territory development in megakaryocytes. *Blood Cells 5*:59, 1979.

7. Paulus, J. M.: Platelet size in man. *Blood 46*:321, 1975.

8. Godwin, H. A., and Ginsburg, A. D.: May-Hegglin anomaly: A defect in megakaryocyte fragmentation? *Br. J. Haematol. 26*:117, 1974.

9. von Behrens, W.: Mediterranean macrothrombocytopenia. *Blood 46*:199, 1975.

10. Paulus, J. M., and Casals, F. J.: Platelet formation in Mediterranean macrothrombocytosis. *Nouv. Rev. Fr. Hematol. 20*:151, 1978.

11. Karpatkin, S., and Freedman, M. L.: Hypersplenic thrombocytopenia differentiated from increased peripheral destruction by platelet volume. *Ann. Intern. Med. 89*:200, 1978.

12. Murphy, S., Oski, F. A., Naiman, L., Lusch, C. J., Goldberg, S., and Gardner, F. H.: Platelet size and kinetics in hereditary and acquired thrombocytopenia. *N. Engl. J. Med. 286*:499, 1972.

13. Zucker-Franklin, D., and Karpatkin, S.: Red cell and platelet fragmentation in idiopathic autoimmune thrombocytopenic purpura. *N. Engl. J. Med. 297*:517, 1977.

14. Le Tohic, F., Prost-Dvojakovic, R. J., Le Menn, P., and Samama, M.: Problems linked to the estimation of platelet volume in essential thrombocytopenias. *Nouv. Rev. Fr. Hematol. 20*:155, 1978.

15. Roper, P., Johnston, D., Austin, J., Agarwal, S. S., and Drewinko, B.: Profiles of platelet volume distributions in normal individuals and in patients with acute leukemia. *Am. J. Clin. Pathol. 68*:449, 1977.

16. Kaplan, K. L., Broekman, M. J., Chernoff, A., Lesznik, G. R., and Drillings, M.: Platelet alpha-granule proteins: Studies on release and subcellular localization. *Blood 53*:604, 1979.

17. Begg, G. S., Pepper, D. S., Chesterman, C. N., and Morgan, F. J.: Complete covalent structure of human β-thromboglobulin. *Biochemistry 17*:1739, 1978.

18. Niewiarowski, S., Walz, D. A., James, P., Rucinski, B., and Kueppers, F.: Identification and separation of secreted platelet proteins by isoelectric focusing: Evidence that low-affinity platelet factor 4 is converted to β-thromboglobulin by limited proteolysis. *Blood 55*:453, 1980.

19. Kaplan, K. L., and Owen, J.: Plasma levels of β-thromboglobulin and platelet factor 4 as indices of platelet activation in vivo. *Blood 57*:199, 1981.

20. Guzzo, J., et al.: Secreted platelet proteins with antiheparin and mitogenic activities in chronic renal failure. *J. Lab. Clin. Med. 96*:102, 1980.

21. Doyle, D. J., Chesterman, C. N., Cade, J. F., McGready, J. R., Rennie, G. C., and Morgan, F. J.: Plasma concentrations of platelet-specific proteins correlated with platelet survival. *Blood 55*:82, 1980.

22. Han, P., Turpie, A. G. G., and Genton, E.: Plasma β-thromboglobulin: Differentiation between intravascular and extravascular platelet destruction. *Blood 54*:1192, 1979.

23. Beckstead, J. H., Halverson, P. S., Ries, C. A., and Bainton, D. F.: Enzyme histochemistry and immunohistochemistry on biopsy specimens of pathologic human bone marrow. *Blood 57*:1088, 1981.

24. Undritz, V. E., and Rothlin, E.: Zur Frage der Entstehung der geformten Gerinnungselemente und der Entkernung der Erythroblasten. *Helv. Med. Acta 13*:595, 1946.

25. Harker, L. A., and Finch, C. A.: Thrombokinetics in man. *J. Clin. Invest. 48*:963, 1969.

26. Harker, L.: Measurement of total megakaryocyte mass, in *Platelet Kinetics*, edited by J. M. Paulus. North Holland, Amsterdam, 1971, pp. 172–180.

27. Fillet, G.: The ferrokinetic measurement of marrow cellularity. II. Method using a marrow cell–erythroid radioiron ratio, in *Platelet Kinetics*, edited by J. M. Paulus. North Holland, Amsterdam, 1971, pp. 166–174.

28. Branehög, I., Kutti, J., Ridell, B., Swolin, B., and Weinfeld, A.: The relation of thrombokinetics to bone marrow megakaryocytes in idiopathic thrombocytopenic purpura (ITP). *Blood 45*:551, 1975.

29. Hirsh, E. O., and Gardner, F. H.: The life-span of transfused human platelets. *J. Lab. Clin. Med. 39*:556, 1952.

30. Stefanini, M., and Dameshek, W.: Collection, preservation and transfusion of platelets with special reference to factors affecting the "survival rate" and clinical effectiveness of transfused platelets. *N. Engl. J. Med. 248*:797, 1953.

31. Aster, R. H.: Factors affecting the kinetics of isotopically tagged platelets, in *Platelet Kinetics*, edited by J. M. Paulus. North Holland, Amsterdam, 1971, pp. 3–23.

32. Harker, L. A.: Platelet survival time: Its measurement and use. *Prog. Hemost. Thromb. 4*:321, 1978.

33. Mustard, J. F.: Platelet survival. *Thromb. Haemost. 40*:154, 1978.

34. Odell, T. T., Jr.: Use of ^{35}S-sulfate for labeling megakaryocytes and platelets, in *Platelet Kinetics*, edited by J. M. Paulus. North Holland, Amsterdam, 1971, p. 123.

35. Ardaillou, N., Najean, Y., and Eberlin, A.: Study of platelet kinetics using ^{75}Se-selenomethionine, in *Platelet Kinetics*, edited by J. M. Paulus. North Holland, Amsterdam, 1971, pp. 131–142.

36. Brodsky, I., Ross, E. M., Petkov, G., and Kahn, S. B.: Platelet and fibrinogen kinetics with ^{75}Se-selenomethionine in patients with myeloproliferative disorders. *Br. J. Haematol., 22*:179, 1972.

37. Dassin, E., and Najean, Y.: The use of ^{75}Se-methionine as a tracer of thrombocytopoiesis. 1. In vivo incorporation of the tracer into platelet proteins: A biochemical study. *Acta Haematol. 61*:61, 1979.

38. Breny, H.: Fundamental formulae. I. Calculation of mean and distribution of cohort and population survival, in *Platelet Kinetics*, edited by J. M. Paulus. North Holland, Amsterdam, 1971, pp. 38–50.

39. Murphy, E. A.: Models of the destruction of blood platelets, in *Platelet Kinetics*, edited by J. M. Paulus. North Holland, Amsterdam, 1971, pp. 80–91.

40. Schwartz, A. D.: A method for demonstrating shortened platelet survival utilizing recovery from aspirin effect. *J. Pediatr. 84*:350, 1974.

41. Stuart, M. J., Murphy, S., and Oski, F. A.: A simple nonradioisotope technique for the determination of platelet life-span. *N. Engl. J. Med. 292*:1310, 1975.

42. De Haas, H. A., Clark, S. E., Zahavi, J., Kakkar, V. V., and White, A. M.: A modified non-radioisotope method for measurement of platelet production time. *Br. J. Haematol. 43*:137, 1979.

43. Roncucci, R., et al.: Measurement of platelet regeneration time in cardiovascular patients. *Thromb. Res. 14*:3, 1979.

44. Catalano, P. M., Smith, J. B., and Murphy, S.: Platelet recovery from aspirin inhibition in vivo; differing patterns under various assay conditions. *Blood 57*:99, 1981.

45. Burch, J. W., Stanford, N., and Majerus, P. W.: Inhibition of platelet prostaglandin synthetase by oral aspirin. *J. Clin. Invest. 61*:314, 1978.

46. Boneu, B., Sie, P., Caranobe, C., Nouvel, C., and Bierme, R.: Malondialdehyde (MDA) reappearance in human platelet density subpopulations after a single intake of aspirin. *Thrombos. Res. 19*:609, 1980.

47. Wallenburg, H. C. S., and Van-Kessel, P. H.: Platelet life-span in normal pregnancy as determined by a non-radioisotopic technique. *Br. J. Obstet. Gynaecol. 85*:33, 1978.

48. Rakoczi, I., Tallian, F., Bagdany, S., and Gati, I.: Platelet life-span in normal pregnancy and pre-eclampsia as determined by a nonradioisotope technique. *Thromb. Res. 15*:553, 1979.

49. Aster, R. H.: The study of platelet kinetics with ^{51}Cr-labeled platelets, in *Platelet Kinetics*, edited by J. M. Paulus. North Holland, Amsterdam, 1971, pp. 317–323.

50. Panel on Diagnostic Application of Radioisotopes in Hematology, International Committee for Standardization in Hematology: Recommended methods for radioisotope platelet survival studies. *Blood 50*:1137, 1977.

51. Abrahamsen, A. F.: A modification of the technique for ^{51}Cr-labeling of blood platelets giving increased circulating platelet radioactivity. *Scand. J. Haematol. 5*:53, 1968.

52. Tessier, C., Steiner, M., and Baldini, M. G.: Measurement of platelet kinetics using ^{51}Cr, in *Platelets, Production, Function, Transfusion, and Storage*, edited by M. G. Baldini and S. Ebbe. Grune & Stratton, New York, 1974, pp. 327–338.

53. Flatow, F. A., and Freireich, E. J.: Simultaneous determination of platelet disappearance by direct count and by Cr^{51}-labeling. *Clin. Res. 13*:540, 1965.

54. Kummer, H., Von Muhlenen, A., and Laissue, J.: Survival of labeled and non-labeled platelets in the lethally irradiated dog: An evaluation of the ^{51}Cr-chromium method. *Helv. Med. Acta 35*:226, 1969.

55. Zucker, M. B., Hellman, L., and Zumoff, B.: Rapid disappearance of ^{14}C-labeled serotonin from platelets in patients with carcinoid syndrome. *J. Lab. Clin. Med. 63*:137, 1964.

56. Radegran, K.: Double labeling of platelets with 51-chromium and ^{14}C-serotonin. *Thromb. Res. 8*:579, 1976.

57. Hanson, S., and Harker, L. A.: Simultaneous ^{51}Cr- and ^{14}C-serotonin platelet survival measurements. *Thromb. Haemost. 38*:140, 1977 (abstract).

58. George, J. N., Lewis, P. C., and Sears, D. A.: Studies on platelet plasma membranes. II. Characterization of surface proteins of rabbit platelets in vitro and during circulation in vivo using diazotized (^{125}I)-diiodosulfanilic acid as a label. *J. Lab. Clin. Med. 88*:247, 1976.

59. Harker, L. A., and Slichter, S. J.: Platelet and fibrinogen consumption in man. *N. Engl. J. Med. 287*:999, 1972.

60. Harker, L. A., and Hanson, S. R.: Experimental arterial thromboembolism in baboons. Mechanism, quantitation, and pharmacologic prevention. *J. Clin. Invest. 64*:559, 1979.

61. Wistow, B. W., Grossman, Z. D., McAfee, J. G., Subramanian, G., Henderson, R. W., and Roskopf, M. L.: Labeling of platelets with oxine complexes of Tc-99m and In-111. 1. In vitro studies and survival in the rabbit. *J. Nucl. Med. 19*:483, 1978.

62. Welch, M. J., Thakur, M. L., Coleman, R. E., Patel, M., Siegel, B. A., and Ter-Pogossian, M. M.: Gallium-68 labelled red cells and platelets: New agents for position tomography. *J. Nucl. Med. 18*:558, 1977.

63. Thakur, M. L., Welch, M. J., Joist, J. H., and Coleman, R. E.: Indium-111 labeled platelets: Studies on preparation and evaluation of in vitro and in vivo functions. *Thromb. Res. 9*:345, 1976.

64. Scheffel, U., et al.: Evaluation of indium-111 as a new high photon yield gamma-emitting physiological platelet label. *Johns Hopkins Med. J. 140*:285, 1977.

65. Heaton, W. A., et al.: Indium 111: A new radionuclide label for studying human platelet kinetics. *Br. J. Haematol. 42*:613, 1979.

66. Hawker, R. J., Hawker, L. M., and Wilkinson, A. R.: Indium (^{111}In)-labeled human platelets: Optimal method. *Clin. Sci. 58*:243, 1980.

67. Thakur, M. L., Walsh, L., Malech, H. L., and Gottschalk, A.: Indium-111–labeled human platelets: Improved method, efficacy and evaluation. *J. Nucl. Med. 22*:381, 1981.

68. Heyns, du P. A., et al.: Kinetics, distribution and sites of destruction of ^{111}Indium-labelled human platelets. *Br. J. Haematol. 44*:269, 1980.

69. Vigneron, N., Dassin, E., and Najean, Y.: Double marquage des plaquettes par ^{51}Cr et ^{111}In. Application à l'étude simultanée de la durée de vie des plaquettes autologues et homologues. *Nouv. Presse Med. 9*:1835, 1980.

70. Klonizakis, I., Peters, A. M., Fitzpatrick, M. L., Kensett, M. J., Lewis, S. M., and Lavender, J. P.: Radionuclide distribution following injection of ^{111}Indium-labelled platelets. *Br. J. Haematol. 46*:595, 1980.

71. Peters, A. M., Klonizakis, I., Lavender, J. P., and Lewis, S. M.: Use of ^{111}Indium-labelled platelets to measure spleen function. *Br. J. Haematol. 46*:587, 1980.

72. Knight, L. C., Primeau, J. L., Siegel, B. A., and Welch, M. J.: Comparison of ^{111}In-labelled platelets and iodinated fibrinogen for the detection of deep vein thrombosis. *J. Nucl. Med. 19*:891, 1977.

73. Ezekowitz, M.D., Leonard, J. C., Smith, E. O., Allen, E. W., and Taylor, F. B.: Identification of left ventricular thrombi in man using indium-111–labeled autologous platelets. *Circulation 63*:803, 1981.

74. Bithell, T. C., Athens, J. W., Cartwright, G. E., and Wintrobe, M. M.: Radioactive diisopropylfluorophosphate as a platelet label: An evaluation of in vitro and in vivo techniques. *Blood 29*:354, 1967.

75. Zucker, M. B., Ley, A. B., and Mayer, K.: Studies on platelet life-span and platelet depots by use of DFP^{32}. *J. Lab. Clin. Med. 58*:405, 1961.

76. Garg, S. K., Amorosi, E. L., and Karpatkin, S.: Use of the megathrombocyte as an index of megakaryocyte number. *N. Engl. J. Med. 284*:11, 1971.

77. Branehög, I., Ridell, B., and Weinfeld, A.: On the analysis of platelet survival curves and the calculation of platelet production and destruction. *Scand. J. Haematol. 19*:230, 1977.

78. Paulus, J. M.: *Production et destruction des plaquettes sanguines*. Masson, Paris, 1974.

Biochemistry of plasma coagulation factors

CHAPTER *132*

Biochemistry of plasma coagulation factors

WILLIAM J. WILLIAMS

Except for calcium, the plasma coagulation factors are all proteins. The nomenclature used for the plasma coagulation factors has presented many difficulties to nonexperts in the field, and it continues to do so. However, the situation has been simplified by the rather general agreement to utilize the roman numeral system [1] which is presented in Table 132-1, along with synonyms for the factors. The roman numeral system is utilized generally in this book, although usually fibrogen is used for factor I, prothrombin for factor II, tissue factor for factor III, and calcium for factor IV. These terms are well recognized without confusing synonyms and have some value in that they indicate the function or origin of the factors.

TABLE 132-1   International nomenclature for blood coagulation factors

Factor	Synonyms
I	Fibrinogen
II	Prothrombin, prethrombin
III	Tissue factor, tissue thromboplastin
IV	Calcium
V	Proaccelerin, labile factor, Ac globulin
(VI)	Not assigned
VII	Proconvertin, SPCA, stable factor, autoprothrombin I
VIII	Antihemophilic globulin (AHG), antihemophilic factor (AHF), antihemophilic factor A, platelet cofactor I
IX	Plasma thromboplastin component (PTC), Christmas factor, antihemophilic factor B, autoprothrombin II, platelet cofactor II
X	Stuart-Prower factor, Stuart factor, autoprothrombin III
XI	Plasma thromboplastin antecedent (PTA), antihemophilic factor C
XII	Hageman factor
XIII	Fibrin-stabilizing factor, fibrinase, Laki-Lorand factor

NOTE: Activated factors are designated by an "a" after the roman numeral.

The following points should be noted regarding the roman numeral system:

1. The numerals are assigned in the order of discovery and indicating nothing about the sequence of reactions.
2. There is no factor VI.
3. The numerals denote the factors as they exist in plasma [except factor III (tissue factor), which is not normally present in plasma] and do not indicate the active forms. In this book the activated forms are indicated by a lowercase "a" following the roman numeral. Nearly all the activated coagulation factors are enzymes. Exceptions are factors V and VIII, which exist in activated forms not yet shown to function enzymatically. Nevertheless, these are usually designated factor Va and factor VIIIa. In addition, fibrinogen (factor I) is converted to fibrin, which has no activity comparable to any other factor and thus is not called factor Ia. The active form of prothrombin (factor II) is called thrombin rather than factor IIa.
4. Some essential reactants in blood coagulation are *not* represented by a roman numeral. Phospholipid or phospholipoprotein has no assigned numeral, but the phospholipoprotein of platelets is known as platelet factor 3. The most recently described reactants, prekallikrein, its activated form, kallikrein, and high-molecular-weight kininogen have also not been assigned roman numerals.

Modern biochemical techniques have permitted detailed characterization of the plasma coagulation factors in their native and activated forms. Both bovine and human plasma have been used as starting material for studies on the chemistry of the coagulant proteins. The source of the factors discussed below is indicated when it has been made clear in the original report.

Fibrinogen (factor I) and fibrin

Human fibrinogen is a glycoprotein with a molecular weight (M_r) of about 340,000 daltons [2–4]. Human fibrinogen has been extensively purified [5–7]. It is composed of three pairs of peptide chains connected by disulfide bridges to form a molecule composed of symmetrical halves [8–13]. These chains are generally referred to as Aα, Bβ, and γ [14]. Aα designates the chain yielding all types of fibrinopeptide A (see below) when attacked by thrombin, Bβ indicates the chain yielding fibrinopeptide B, and γ is used for the chain which is not attacked by thrombin (Fig. 132-1). In fibrin, where fibrinopeptides A and B have been released, the chains are referred to as α, β, and γ. The molecular weight of the Aα, Bβ, and γ chains are 63,500, 56,000, and 47,000 daltons, respectively [12].

Detailed study of the fibrinopeptides formed when thrombin attacks human fibrinogen has revealed at least three types of fibrinopeptide A, while there is only one type of fibrinopeptide B. Accordingly the chains which yield these subclasses of fibrinopeptide have been named Aα, AYα, and APα [15,16]. The designation "A"α has been used to refer to the sum of Aα, AYα, and APα. About 10 percent of the "A"α chains of human fibrinogen are of the AYα type, and about 20 percent are of the APα type [15].

Fibrinogen and fibrin have six free-amino end groups per mole [5,17–20]. In human fibrinogen there are two residues each of alanine (Aα chain), pyroglutamic acid (Bβ chain), and tyrosine (γ chain) [8,15,17–20]. Aspartic acid is present in small amounts as an N-terminal amino acid in human fibrinogen [17], apparently derived from Aα chains which have lost their N-terminal alanine [5]. These chains are AYα chains [16]. Human fibrin contains four glycine end groups (α and β chains) and two tyrosine end groups (γ chain) per mole [15,18].

Fibrinogen and fibrin both contain carbohydrate in amounts accounting for 3 to 5 percent of the molecule [21–25]. The carbohydrate consists of sialic acid, hexosamines, and hexoses, and is bound by covalent linkages to the Bβ and γ chains [14,26–30]. Fibrin monomer from asialofibrinogen polymerizes more rapidly than normal [31,32]. Asialofibrinogen supports platelet aggregation and adhesion to glass slides [32].

Fibrinogen as isolated from plasma is heterogeneous with regard to solubility, molecular weight, electrophoretic mobility, and chromatographic behavior [5,7,33–38]. Heterogeneity of Aα chains [15,36–40], Bβ chains [26,35], and γ chains [21,26,41–45] has been observed. The former may be due to proteolytic attack (e.g., by plasmin) on the Aα chains in vivo [36,40,46–48]. Heterogeneity of the Bβ and γ chain may be due in part to different contents of sialic acid [26,45] or to other causes [42]. The primary structures of the Aα, Bβ, and γ chains have been established [49–52].

FIBRINOPEPTIDES

Peptides amounting to about 3 percent of the weight of the fibrinogen are released when fibrinogen is converted to fibrin by thrombin [19,53]. Thrombin hydrolyzes four peptide bonds of human fibrinogen, releasing 2 mol each of fibrinopeptides A and B from the Aα and Bβ chains, respectively [15,20] (Fig. 132-1). The fibrinopeptides A are actually heterogeneous, differing by one or more amino acids or substituent groups [16]. Thus, fibrinopeptide AP is identical to fibrinopeptide A except that the serine residue in position 3 is phosphorylated [15]. Fibrinopeptide AY is identical to fibrinopeptide A except that the N-terminal alanine has been removed, leaving aspartic acid as the free-amino end group [15]. There may also be a fibrinopeptide with aspartic acid as the free-amino group and with the serine phosphorylated, an APY fibrinopeptide [16].

The amino acid sequences of fibrinopeptides A, AY, AP, and B have been determined [15] (Fig. 132-1). Thrombin releases fibrinopeptide A from fibrinogen at a more rapid rate than fibrinopeptide B [16,25,54]. Thrombin readily attacks only 4 of about 300 poten-

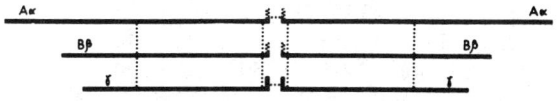

fpp A   ALA.ASP.SER.GLY.GLU.GLY.ASP.PHE.LEU.ALA.GLU.GLY.GLY.GLY.VAL.ARG

fpp B   PYR.GLY.VAL.ASN.ASP.ASN.GLU.GLU.GLY.PHE.PHE.SER.ALA.ARG

FIGURE 132-1 Schematic representation of fibrinogen. The molecule is composed of three pairs of peptide chains (Aα, Bβ, and γ) connected by disulfide bonds to form a symmetrical dimer. The disulfide bonds are indicated by dotted lines. The amino-terminal ends of the half-molecules are connected by disulfide linkages to form the so-called disulfide knot. The fibrinopeptides are indicated by the checked regions at the amino-terminal ends of the Aα and Bβ chains. The structures of the fibrinopeptides (fpp) are illustrated at the bottom of the figure. (From Marder and Budzynski, *Schweiz. Med. Wochenschr. 104*:1338, 1974, by permission.)

tially susceptible arginyl and lysylpeptide bonds in fibrinogen [55], but does attack additional bonds at a slow rate in native fibrinogen or at a more rapid rate in fibrinogen derivatives [16,21,56–58].

An enzyme in the venom of *Bothrops jararaca* or *Bothrops atrox* ("reptilase") [8,9,59,60] and one in venom of the Malayan pit viper ("ancrod") [61] hydrolyze predominantly fibrinopeptide A from intact fibrinogen, and the release of this peptide alone is sufficient to induce clotting. Both reptilase and ancrod can release fibrinopeptide B from N-terminal fragments of fibrinogen [62,63], and ancrod also further digests both the α and the γ chains of fibrin [63,64]. In contrast, the venom of the Southern copperhead snake (*Ancistrodon contortrix contortrix*) contains an enzyme which releases fibrinopeptide B at a much faster rate than fibrinopeptide A [65]. Visible clotting occurs only after appreciable amounts of fibrinopeptide A have been removed [65].

One of the abnormal fibrinogens, fibrinogen Detroit, has serine substituted for arginine in position 19 of the Aα chain. The release of fibrinopeptide A from this fibrinogen by thrombin occurs normally, but fibrinopeptide B is released slowly, and polymerization is grossly impaired [66,67]. Therefore, the primary structural features which determine thrombin action on the Aα chain apparently do not involve the arginine residue in position 19. Fibrin polymer formation after release of fibrinopeptide A by thrombin is followed by enhanced release of fibrinopeptide B and further polymerization [68]. Release of a single fibrinopeptide A may be sufficient to lead to dimer formation [69]. Polymerization is believed to occur by both end-to-end and side-to-side mechanisms [70–73]. It has been suggested that fibrin polymers forming after release of fibrinopeptide A (reptilase fibrin) are formed predominantly end-to-end, while those formed after release of both fibrinopeptides A and B involve both end-to-end and side-to-side mechanisms [74]. The initial polymerization sites may be in the carboxyl-terminal ends of the γ chains [75].

Binding domains [73,76,77] are present in the "N-terminal disulfide knot," representing the amino-terminal portion of the molecule [57], and in "fragment D," a portion of the fibrinogen molecule derived from the carboxyl-terminal portion of the α, β, and γ chains [78]. There is evidence for polymerization sites on both α [79] and γ chains [80]. Grossly deficient polymerization is characteristic of fibrinogen Detroit, one of the inherited fibrinogen abnormalities [66,67]. Since the amino acid substitution in the abnormal fibrinogen is near the amino terminus of the α chain, it seems probable that this region is involved in the polymerization process. Gly-Pro-Arg, a peptide contiguous to fibrinopeptide A in the Aα chain of fibrinogen [16] binds to fibrinogen and interferes with fibrin monomer polymerization, further supporting the concept that a polymerization site is located on the Aα chain near the amino terminal end [81,82].

FIBRIN STABILIZATION

The clot formed from purified fibrinogen and thrombin, in contrast to that formed in plasma, is mechanically weak and is soluble in dilute acid or in concentrated urea solution [83,84]. This difference is due to the presence in plasma of an additional coagulation factor, factor XIII, which is discussed in detail below. Factor XIIIa catalyzes the formation of peptide bonds between the γ-carboxy groups of glutamine and the ϵ-amino groups of lysine in adjacent fibrin molecules and by this mechanism "stabilizes" the fibrin clot [85–87]. Cross-linking occurs between γ chains and between α chains [12,52,88–90].

TERTIARY STRUCTURE

Examinations of fibrinogen by electron microscopy have yielded conflicting results, demonstrating a nodular structure [91–93], perhaps trinodular [72,94,95], or long filaments [96,97]. Physicochemical data have been presented to support both single nodular [98] and trinodular structures [99]. When fibrin molecules combine to form insoluble fibrin, long, thin threads develop [71,72,100]. Fibrin fibers show regular cross-striations with a period of about 230 Å, indicating submolecular structure [101]. Fibrin formed in systems deficient in factor XIII do not show these cross-striations [102]. Immunological evidence substantiates the complexity of the tertiary structure of fibrinogen [103–106].

PLATELET FIBRINOGEN

Platelets contain fibrinogen, which constitutes up to 15 percent of the total platelet protein [107]. Platelet fibrinogen appears to exist both as plasma fibrinogen adsorbed to the platelet surface and as intraplatelet fibrinogen [108–111]. It appears unlikely that megakaryocytes can synthesize fibrinogen [112]. Platelet fibrinogen is not completely coagulated by thrombin, and its carbohydrate content, sedimentation coefficient, and intrinsic viscosity are all different from plasma fibrinogen [111,113–115]. These differences may be due to partial

degradation of the platelet fibrinogen, and it has been concluded that platelet and plasma fibrinogen are products of the same gene [116].

FETAL FIBRINOGEN

The blood of newborn infants contains fetal fibrinogen which can be distinguished from adult fibrinogen by chromatography on DEAE-cellulose [117], tryptic peptide mapping [117,118], phosphorus and carbohydrate content [119,120], and solubility in ethanol solutions [121], but not all of the studies cited have been confirmed [122]. In addition, the clotting time with thrombin is prolonged, especially at high pH [117,120,121], due to slower aggregation of fibrin monomers [122,123], although these changes are slight. Some investigators have denied the existence of fetal fibrinogen [124].

Prothrombin (factor II) and thrombin

Extensive biochemical studies have been carried out on both human and bovine prothrombin [125–127]. Human prothrombin has been highly purified, in some instances to physical homogeneity [128–132]. The M_r of human prothrombin is about 69,000 daltons [129,130]. It is a single polypeptide chain with alanine as the free-amino end group [130,133] (Fig. 132-2). The complete amino acid sequence has been determined [131,134–137]. The molecule contains up to 10 percent of carbohydrate in three chains [129,131,134].

Bovine prothrombin has been highly purified [138–144]. Bovine prothrombin is a single-chain glycoprotein containing 10 to 15 percent carbohydrate [140,143, 145,146–148] localized in three side chains [140,146, 149]. The M_r is about 68,000 to 74,000 daltons [138,143, 146].

The primary structure of prothrombin is characterized by a unique amino acid, γ-carboxyglutamic acid [150–152] (Fig. 132-3). The first 32 amino acids of human prothrombin contain 10 residues of γ-carboxyglutamic acid (Gla) [131–134] (Fig. 132-2). Bovine prothrombin has an almost identical arrangement of Gla residues [153]. The additional carboxyl group of Gla is added by a carboxylation reaction involving CO_2 and requiring vitamin K [154–156]. The Gla residues occur in the region of the molecule essential for calcium-dependent phospholipid binding and for adsorption to inorganic salts such as barium sulfate and are clustered in the end of the molecule which does not yield thrombin [130, 153,157–162].

Thrombin is formed from prothrombin by hydrolysis of peptide bonds by factor Xa and thrombin, as illustrated in Fig. 132-2 [131,141,163,164]. Human and bovine thrombin have been purified [165–168]. The thrombin initially derived from both human and bovine prothrombin has been designated α-thrombin [167,169]. It consists of two polypeptide chains connected by a disulfide bridge [164,169–171]. The M_r of this form of thrombin is 39,000 daltons with the smaller chain, the A

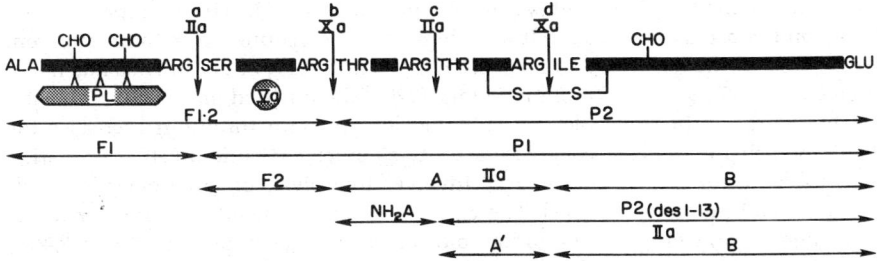

FIGURE 132-2   Human prothrombin. Prothrombin is a single-chain molecule which is converted to thrombin, a two-chain molecule, by the action of factor Xa and thrombin. Prothrombin has three carbohydrate side chains, designated CHO on the figure. The γ-carboxyglutamic acid residues are designated by λ. They are located near the amino-terminal end of the molecule, identified by ALA, and are here shown bound to phospholipid, indicated by the stippled area labeled PL. The factor Va binding site is also indicated by the stippled circle labeled Va. The amino acids at the amino- and carboxyl-terminal ends of the molecule and those surrounding the bonds cleaved by thrombin and factor Xa are designated as follows: ARG for arginine, ALA for alanine, SER for serine, THR for threonine, ILE for isoleucine, and GLU for glutamic acid. The portion of the prothrombin molecule converted to the various intermediates is indicated in the lower half of the figure.

In converting prothrombin to thrombin, factor Xa hydrolyzes the bond labeled *b* to form prothrombin fragment 1·2 (F1·2) and prethrombin 2 (P2), the single-chain precursor of thrombin. Prethrombin 2 is then hydrolyzed at bond *d* to yield thrombin (IIa), a molecule with two chains attached by a disulfide bond. The two chains are designated A and B. The A chain of thrombin may be further attacked by thrombin at bond *c* to release an amino-terminal peptide, designated NH₂A, and produce thrombin (IIa) with a shortened A chain, designated A'.

Thrombin may hydrolyze several other bonds in prothrombin and prothrombin derivatives. For example, thrombin can hydrolyze prothrombin at the bond marked *a* to form prothrombin fragment 1 (F1) and prethrombin 1 (P1), and may attack prothrombin fragment 1·2 to yield prothrombin fragment 1 (F1) and prothrombin fragment 2 (F2). It can also hydrolyze prethrombin 2 to release the amino-terminal peptide NH₂A and produce a shortened form of prethrombin 2, designated P2 (des 1-13). (From Mann and Elion [131], by permission.)

chain, contributing 6000 daltons and the larger chain, the B chain, contributing 33,000 daltons [170]. The active site and the carbohydrate component are located on the B chain [153,169,171]. The amino acid sequence of human and bovine thrombin has been determined [136,153]. α-Thrombin contains about 5 percent carbohydrate [136,170]. β-Thrombin is a two-chain compound of smaller molecular weight than α-thrombin [169], and γ-thrombin is an even smaller three-chain compound [169]. The smaller forms of thrombin appear to be derived from α-thrombin [164,169,172,173]. *Thrombin E* has also been used to designate a degradation product of α-thrombin with smaller molecular weight and with esterase activity but no coagulant activity [164].

Thrombin is one of the family of proteolytic enzymes known as serine proteases [171,174–176] because of the presence of serine in the active site. It is inhibited by reagents which specifically react with serine [177–179] and also by those reacting with histidine [180] and tyrosine [181]. The active center has been mapped as Gly-Asp-Ser-Gly-Gly [136,153]. Its primary structure is homologous with factors IXa and Xa [174–176,182]. The action of thrombin on fibrinogen is discussed above. Thrombin hydrolyzes prothrombin and degradation products of prothrombin [129,146,164], and it also attacks a number of other substrates [183], including amino acid amides and esters [184,185], peptides [186,187], and other proteins [183,188,189]. Thrombin is competitively inhibited by fibrinopeptide A, released from fibrinogen by thrombin action, and by peptides of similar structure [190,191].

Tissue factor (factor III)

Extracts of fresh or acetone-dried tissues accelerate the coagulation of recalcified plasma by two mechanisms. The first is a relatively minor acceleration, caused by the phospholipids or phospholipoproteins in the extracts, e.g., those from erythrocytes [192] and platelets [193,194]. These compounds are involved in the reactions between factor IXa, factor VIII, and calcium and between factor Xa, factor V, and calcium (see Chap. 135).

FIGURE 132-3   Tetrapeptide isolated from normal prothrombin, showing γ-carboxyglutamic acid residues in positions 2 and 3. (From Stenflo et al. [150], by permission.)

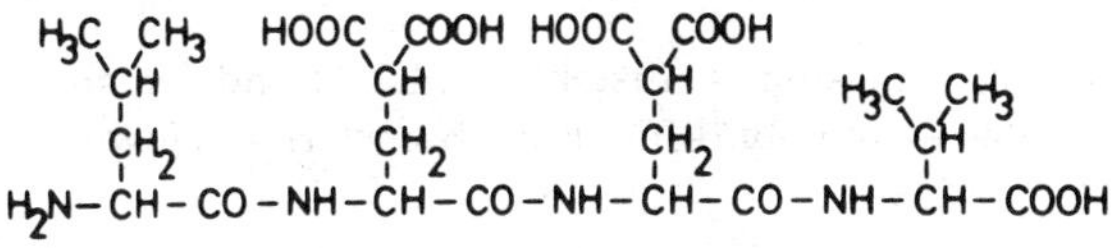

The chemistry of the phospholipids involved in the first mechanism is described below. The second is a major acceleration due to tissue factor (factor III) [195], which reacts with factor VII and calcium (see Chap. 135).

Tissue factor activity is present in many tissues, but lung, brain, and placenta are particularly rich in this material. Lipoprotein complexes with tissue factor activity have been isolated from bovine lung and human placenta as subcellular particles which behave on centrifugation as microsomes [196–199]. These particles are composed of phospholipid, protein, and cholesterol. Tissue factor isolated from acetone-extracted brain is also particulate and is composed of phospholipid and protein [198,200,201].

Both the protein and phospholipid moieties of the tissue factor are required for full activity [200,201]. Heating tissue factor results in loss of activity, which appears to be due to denaturation of the protein moiety, since the heated preparations retain their ability to function as phospholipid in the reactions requiring this cofactor [197,202,203].

The phospholipid and protein components of tissue factor can be separated by treatment with organic solvents, with loss of activity, and then recombined under appropriate conditions with full recovery of activity [200,201,204–206]. The phospholipids extracted from tissue factor preparations are a mixture that contains sphingomyelin, phosphatidylcholine, phosphatidylethanolamine, phosphatidylinositol, and phosphatidylserine [197,198,200,201]. Full tissue factor activity can be restored to the protein moiety with the phospholipid mixture extracted from the tissue factor originally or with purified phospholipids. Recombination experiments with purified phospholipids have indicated no highly specific lipid requirement. The protein fraction separated from tissue factor particles has been solubilized and purified [205,207], and details of the binding of phospholipids to the purified protein component have been studied [206]. Highly purified tissue factor appears to contain carbohydrate [205], and tissue factor activity is inhibited by concanavalin A, a plant lectin known to bind to carbohydrate residues [208,209].

Tissue factor shows species specificity, with preparations from some species having little effect on plasma from others [210]. The species specificity resides in the protein component rather than in the phospholipid moiety [211,212].

Bovine lung tissue factor hydrolyzes a number of peptides, such as leucylglycine, glycylphenylalanine amide, and the oxidized B chain of insulin [213]. This peptidase activity is closely related to the coagulant activity, but its role in blood coagulation, if any, remains undefined.

Factor V

Factor V in plasma is unstable [214,215] and for many years was extremely difficult to characterize. However, highly purified human factor V has been prepared [216–219]. It is a single-chain glycoprotein with an apparent M_r of 330,000 daltons [217–219] or possibly as much as 1 million daltons [220]. The purified material is quite stable [217–219]. Treatment with thrombin increases the coagulant activity as much as 300-fold [219]. Activation of factor V involves hydrolysis of three peptide bonds [219]. The activity appears to reside in some combination of low-molecular-weight components [218,219,466]. The factor V activator from Russell's viper venom yields a similar active product [219].

Bovine factor V has also been purified to homogeneity [221,222]. It is a single-chain glycoprotein of M_r 330,000 daltons [221,222] and is activated by thrombin in a manner similar to human factor V [222,223]. Evidence has been obtained for a bovine factor V of M_r 800,000 to 1,200,000 daltons [220,224,225], but this finding has been questioned [226].

Factor VII

Factor VII has been purified to homogeneity from bovine and human plasma [227–231]. Human factor VII has been purified approximately 140,000-fold [230,231]. It is a single-chain glycoprotein with a M_r of about 50,000 daltons [230,231]. It has alanine as the free-amino end group and contains nine Gla residues per molecule [230,231]. Factor VII is attacked by factor Xa in the presence of phospholipid and calcium to produce a two-chain molecule with enhanced coagulant activity [230,231].

Bovine factor VII has been purified at least 200,000-fold from plasma [227–229]. Bovine plasma factor VII is a single-chain molecule with an apparent M_r of about 53,000 daltons [228,229]. The amino-terminal sequence and the amino acid and carbohydrate composition have been determined [229,232]. The single-chain form of factor VII is rapidly hydrolyzed by factor Xa in the presence of phospholipids and calcium, and by thrombin, to a two-chain molecule of the same molecular weight [228]. The two chains are connected by disulfide bridges [228]. The two-chain form is further hydrolyzed by these enzymes to yield smaller molecules devoid of coagulant activity [228]. The two-chain form of factor VII has at least 85 times the coagulant activity of the single-chain form, but both must be complexed with tissue factor in order to activate factor X at a significant rate [228]. Both the one- and the two-chain forms of bovine factor VII are inactivated by diisopropyl fluorophosphate (DFP) [228,233,234]. Both forms of factor VII have significant esterase activity which is not affected by tissue factor [235]. The two-chain form of factor VII can slowly activate factor X without tissue factor in the system [236]. The enzymatic activity of the tissue factor–factor VII complex appears to reside in factor VII [227,228,237].

The factor VII activity in serum is several times greater than that in plasma [238–241]. Factor VII activity is also increased in plasma which has been exposed to glass or other surfaces [241–245]. In such systems factor VII is activated by factor XIIa and IXa [241,245–247] and by kallikrein [248–251], perhaps indirectly [246].

Factor VIII

Human factor VIII is a complex protein (or a protein complex) which possesses the procoagulant activity deficient in classical hemophilia (hemophilia A) and which maintains a normal bleeding time. Both activities are deficient in classical von Willebrand's disease [252,253]. In this book factor VIII is used to denote the entire protein complex. Factor VIII:C (FVIII:C) refers to the coagulant activity which is deficient in hemophilia, and factor VIII:vWF (FVIII:vWF) refers to the activity which is deficient in patients who have von Willebrand's disease and a prolonged bleeding time. Factor VIII/vWF refers to the protein with FVIII:vWF.

Factor VIII has at least three measurable properties [252,253]: coagulant activity (FVIII:C); antigenic activity, the factor VIII–related antigen usually detected by rabbit antibodies of the precipitating type (FVIIIR:Ag); and the ability to support platelet aggregation initiated by ristocetin, the ristocetin cofactor (FVIIIR:RCo).

Factor VIII has been partially purified from both human [5,254–269] and bovine plasma [270,271]. Nearly all procedures now employ protein inhibitors to limit degradation of the factor VIII during the purification process. Bovine factor VIII has been purified about 300,000-fold from plasma [271]. Factor VIII is a glycoprotein [270,272]. Modification of the carbohydrate component by neuraminidase and galactose oxidase diminishes the von Willebrand factor activity without affecting the coagulant activity [273–275]. Hydrolysis of the carbohydrate moiety has also been reported to reduce the coagulant activity of factor VIII [276].

The molecular structure of factor VIII has not been established. Purified human factor VIII has been reported to have an M_r of 1 to 2 million daltons or more, as determined by gel filtration [272,277,278], and 1.12 million ±98,000 daltons by sedimentation equilibrium [279], but reduction of disulfide bonds reveals subunits of M_r 200,000 to 240,000 daltons, as determined by gel electrophoresis [278–280], or as low as about 105,000 daltons by sedimentation equilibrium [279]. Some studies have supported the concept that FVIII:C, FVIIIR:Ag and FVIIIR:RCo circulate in plasma as separate entities of M_r less than 500,000 daltons, and the high-molecular-weight material is due to artifactual aggregation induced by low-temperature storage [281,282]. Other studies on plasma or purified factor VIII have demonstrated that FVIIIR:Ag exists in multimeric forms derived from a protomer [259,262,283–287].

Treatment of human factor VIII with solvents of high ionic strength (NaCl or CaCl₂) dissociates the complex into high-molecular-weight and low-molecular-weight

components [257,288–295]. The low-molecular-weight component has coagulant activity (FVIII:C), while the high-molecular-weight material has both factor VIII–related antigen (FVIIIR:Ag) and von Willebrand factor activity (FVIII:vWF) [288–290]. The low-molecular-weight component can be activated by thrombin in the same manner as intact factor VIII (see below) [296]. Reassociation of the high- and low-molecular-weight components has been accomplished [294]. Dissociation of FVIII:C from FVIIIR:Ag and FVIIIR:RCo by means of antibodies has also been reported [265–268,297,298]. Dissociation of canine and bovine factor VIII into a small-molecular-weight component with coagulant activity and a large-molecular-weight carrier protein has been noted, using solvents of increased ionic strength or detergents [294,299,300]. Recombination of small-molecular-weight components produced by reduction of disulfide bonds of human and bovine factor VIII has also been reported [295]. Some investigators have been unable to demonstrate dissociation of highly purified factor VIII [301–303], and it has been suggested the apparent dissociation is due to enzymatic proteolysis of the factor VIII [263,302]. However, protease inhibitors have not modified the dissociation [257,304]. A polypeptide fragment with FVIIIR:RCo activity has been isolated from a tryptic digest of factor VIII [264].

Trace amounts of thrombin increase the coagulant activity of factor VIII (FVIII:C) in plasma [305]. With optimal thrombin concentrations the activity of FVIII:C may be increased 63-fold [306]. Thrombin inhibitors such as hirudin and DFP will block activation of FVIII:C but will not deter the deterioration of thrombin-activated FVIII:C [306,307]. Thrombin-activated FVIII:C is stabilized by calcium but eventually the activity decays probably because of inherent instability of the molecule [306,307]. Thrombin-activated FVIII:C appears to be a smaller molecule than unactivated FVIII:C [308]. Thrombin also activates bovine factor VIII by limited proteolysis, and activated bovine factor VIII is inhibited by DFP [271]. Figure 132-4 illustrates a current concept of the structure of factor VIII [309].

Factor IX

Factor IX has been purified to homogeneity from both human [132,310–314] and bovine sources [315,316]. Human factor IX has been purified up to 17,000-fold from plasma [314]. It is a single-chain glycoprotein of M_r about 57,000 daltons [132,310–314]. It contains 17 percent carbohydrate [132,314] and 10 Gla residues per molecule [313,314]. Tyrosine is the free-amino end group [132,314]. Factor IX activated by factor XIa (factor IXaβ) is a two-chain molecule of M_r about 46,000 daltons formed by hydrolysis of two internal peptide bonds with consequent release of a carbohydrate-rich activation peptide of M_r 11,000 daltons [312,313]. The two chains are joined by disulfide bonds. The heavy chain

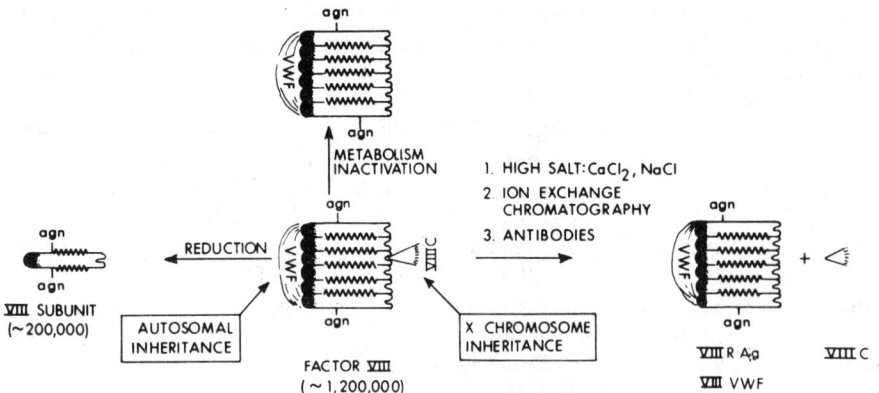

FIGURE 132-4 A concept of factor VIII structure. Factor VIII is here depicted as a complex molecule composed of subunits which can be dissociated by reduction (*left*). The functional properties of the complex are indicated on the figure by VIIIVWF (von Willebrand factor), VIIIC (procoagulant activity), and VIIIRAg (factor VIII-related antigen). Factor VIII:vWF and factor VIIIR:Ag both reside on the high-molecular-weight component of the complex, while factor VIII:C resides on the low-molecular-weight component. Factor VIII:C can be inactivated metabolically (*top*) or dissociated from the complex by various means (*right*). (From Hoyer [309], by permission.)

has an M_r of 28,000 daltons and contains the enzymatically active site [312]. The light chain has an M_r of 18,000 daltons, contains the Gla residues, and represents the original N-terminal sequence of factor IX [312,317]. A protein from Russell's viper venom also activates factor IX but does so by hydrolyzing a single peptide bond yielding an activated factor IX (factor IXaα) with a longer light chain [312]. A partial amino acid sequence has been determined, including the serine active site [312]. There is considerable homology among human and bovine factor IX, factor X, and prothrombin [132,174–176].

Highly purified bovine factor IX is a single-chain molecule of M_r 55,400 daltons, containing approximately 26 percent carbohydrate [315] (Fig. 132-5). The amino acid composition [315] and complete amino acid sequence [182] have been determined.

Bovine factor IXa is composed of two peptide chains ("heavy" and "light"), connected by a disulfide bond(s)

FIGURE 132-5 Structure and activation of factor IX. Factor IX is a single-chain molecule with tyrosine as a free-amino end group and intramolecular disulfide bridge(s). Factor XIa cleaves an internal peptide bond forming a two-chain enzymatically inactive intermediate with free-amino end groups tyrosine and alanine. A second peptide bond is hydrolyzed by factor XIa, releasing an activation peptide from the larger chain and thereby forming a two-chain protein with enzymatic activity. (From Fujikawa et al. [316], by permission of the American Chemical Society.)

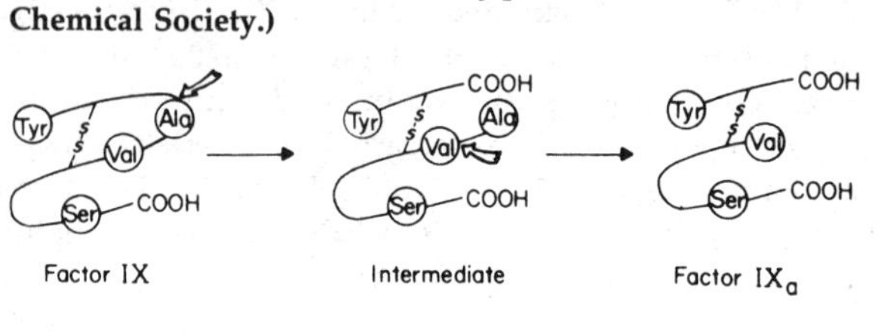

[316] (Fig. 132-5). Activation of factor IX by factor XIa is accompanied by release of an "activation peptide" of M_r 9000 daltons, containing about half of the carbohydrate of the original factor IX molecule [316,318]. The M_r of the heavy chain of factor IXa is 27,000 daltons and of the light chain is 16,000 daltons [316,318]. Thus, the light chain represents the N-terminal portion of factor IX, while the heavy chain originates by hydrolysis of an internal peptide bond [316,318]. Bovine factor IX is also activated by Russell's viper venom by the mechanism employed in activating human factor IX (see above) [318].

Factor X

Human factor X has been purified to homogeneity [132,319,320]. It is a two-chain glycoprotein of M_r approximately 59,000 daltons [132,319]. On SDS-gel electrophoresis the M_r of factor X is 67,000 daltons, the heavy chain M_r is 49,000 daltons, and the light chain 17,000 daltons [132,319]. The free-amino end groups are Ala for the heavy chain and Ser for the light chain [132]. Human factor X contains 15 percent carbohydrate [132]. Human factor Xa has also been highly purified [216].

Bovine factor X [139,142,321–323] and factor Xa [324–326] have been highly purified. Bovine factor X has an M_r of approximately 56,000 daltons [139,142,322,323,326] and is a glycoprotein containing about 10 percent carbohydrate [322,324–326]. Factor X is isolated in two forms (called factor X_1 and factor X_2) by column chromatography on DEAE-Sephadex [142,322,323]. The activation peptides released from factor X_1 and X_2 have different charges but the precise reason for this has not been determined [327]. Factor X consists of two polypeptide chains ("heavy" and "light" chains) connected

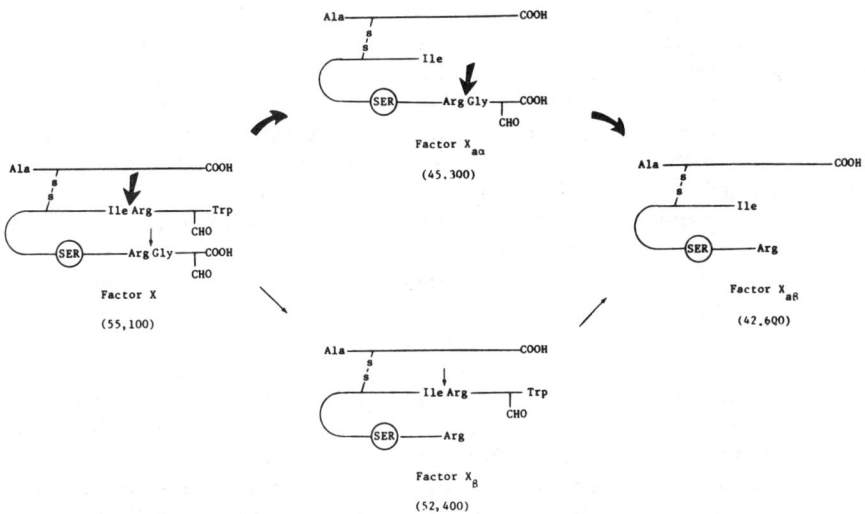

FIGURE 132-6   Structure and activation of factor X. Factor X is composed of a heavy and a light chain connected by disulfide linkage. The serine in the active center of the enzyme is encircled. CHO indicates carbohydrate.

The coagulant protein of Russell's viper venom [329,330] or a complex of tissue factor and factor VII [330] cleave an arginyl-isoleucyl bond in the heavy chain, releasing an activation peptide and forming factor Xaα. Factor Xaα in the presence of phospholipid is then cleaved autocatalytically at an arginyl-glycyl bond to release a second peptide and form factor Xaβ. This activation pathway is depicted by the heavy arrows. Factors Xaα and Xaβ have the same enzymatic activity.

Alternatively the arginyl-glycyl bond is cleaved first to yield an enzymatically inactive intermediate, factor Xβ, which can then be converted to factor Xaβ by hydrolysis of the arginylisoleucyl bond. This minor pathway is depicted by the light arrows. (From Fujikawa et al. [329], by permission.)

by disulfide bridges [139,323,328–330] (Fig. 132-6). The light chain contains 14 Gla residues [331,332]. Evidence has been obtained for a single-chain form of factor X, suggesting the possibility that factor X as usually isolated has already been partially degraded [333]. The primary structure of the heavy and light chains has been reported [331,334,335]. Factor X has two high-affinity metal-binding sites [336].

Activation of factor X by the coagulant protein of Russell's viper venom [324–326] is achieved by hydrolysis of one peptide bond of the heavy chain, releasing a glycopeptide fragment of M_r about 11,000 daltons [329,330,337] (Fig. 132-6). This glycopeptide fragment is firmly but noncovalently bound to the activated factor X [326]. This form of activated factor X is called factor Xaα. It is autocatalytically converted to factor Xaβ by release of a second activation peptide (Fig. 132-6). This modification has no effect on the coagulant activity of the factor Xa [329,330]. Factor X can be activated by several physiologic and nonphysiologic mechanisms [324,325, 329,330]. Factor Xa is a serine protease. It is inhibited by soybean trypsin inhibitor [338]. It is also inhibited by DFP [322,339] and hydrolyzes amino acid esters [322,338]. The active site appears to be on the heavy chain [174,335]. Bovine factor Xa has considerable sequence homology with other mammalian serine proteinases, such as trypsin [174], and with thrombin and factor IXa [175,176,182].

Factor XI

Factor XI has been highly purified from human sources [340–348]. Activated factor XI (factor XIa) has also been purified [349,350]. The M_r of human factor XI is about 180,000 daltons as determined by gel filtration [340,341,344] and 160,000 daltons by disc electrophoresis [345]. The molecule appears to be composed of two subunits of M_r approximately 80,000 daltons [340,345,346]. The amino acid composition has been determined [345]. Human factor XI may circulate in plasma in a complex with high-molecular-weight kininogen [347].

Trypsin and factor XIIa can activate factor XI [340–345,348,351]. Native and activated factor XI behave identically on gel filtration [340,341]. Activation of factor XI by factor XIIa or trypsin is associated with cleavage of the M_r 80,000 daltons subunits to two new components of M_r 35,000 to 50,000 daltons and M_r 25,000 to 33,000 daltons [345,348,351]. Trypsin may yield a third chain of M_r 26,000 daltons [348]. The active center is probably on the M_r 25,000- to 33,000-dalton component [345]. Highly purified human factor XIa has no, or very little, esterase activity [341,342]. The coagulant activity of human factor XIa is inhibited by DFP [343,352,353], as is that of bovine factor XIa [354], suggesting that these enzymes are serine proteases.

Bovine factor XI has been purified to homogeneity

[354–356]. It is a glycoprotein of M_r about 130,000 daltons composed of two similar or identical chains of M_r 55,000 daltons connected by disulfide bonds [355]. It contains 11 percent carbohydrate [345]. The amino acid composition has been determined [345]. It is activated by factor XIIa by hydrolysis of the two chains of the zymogen to yield two heavy chains of M_r 35,000 daltons and two nearly identical light chains of M_r 24,000 and 26,000 daltons [356].

Factor XII

Factor XII has been extensively purified from human [344,357–362] and bovine plasma [363–366]. The M_r of human factor XII is 80,000 daltons as determined by gel electrophoresis [357] and 100,000 to 120,000 daltons as determined by gel filtration [344,359]. It appears to consist of a single polypeptide chain [357] (Fig. 15-3). The amino acid composition has been determined [357,367]. Plasma contains 23 to 47 μg of factor XII per milliliter [357]. Bovine factor XII is a sialoglycoprotein of M_r about 80,000 daltons [364].

Human factor XII is activated by exposure to glass, diatomaceous earth, etc. [368], and by substances such as ellagic acid [369], homocysteine [370], collagen [371], fatty acids [372], and sulfatides [467]. A negatively charged site on the activator appears to be essential for the activation [371,373,374]. The activation of factor XII by ellagic acid or barium carbonate is accompanied by a change in sedimentation properties believed to be the result of a decrease in solubility of the molecule [375]. Factor XII activated on negatively charged surfaces may retain its native molecular weight of about 80,000 daltons [376], but smaller active molecules are also formed (see below). The regions of the molecule responsible for surface binding have been identified [377] (see below).

Factor XII may also be activated in solution by enzymes such as trypsin [357,376,378,379], kallikrein [357, 376], plasmin [357,376,380,381], and factor XIa [376]. Trypsin, plasmin, and kallikrein all attack factor XII at two sites, yielding fragments of apparent M_r of 52,000, 40,000, 28,000, and 12,000 daltons [357], sometimes referred to as factor XIIf. In contact activation of normal plasma the initial split of the factor XII molecule yields fragments of M_r 52,000 and 28,000 daltons [382]. In some molecules the hydrolyzed bond lies within a disulfide bridge and the two-chain product is the same size as the starting material (see Fig. 15-3). In other molecules the fragments are not connected. In either case the M_r 52,000-dalton fragment remains bound to the surface [382]. With prolonged incubation the M_r 52,000-dalton fragment is then split to yield the M_r 40,000- and 12,000-dalton fragments. The M_r 40,000- and 12,000-dalton fragments bind firmly to negatively charged surfaces [377]. The fragment of M_r 28,000 daltons is capable of converting prekallikrein to kallikrein [357,377–379] but has lost as much as 95 to 98 percent of the procoagulant

activity of the parent molecule [357,377–379]. The M_r 28,000-dalton fragment does not bind to negatively charged surfaces [377]. Factor XIIa is also capable of activating prekallikrein [378]. Factor XIIa or the factor XII fragments activate plasminogen proactivator [383]. Thus, the factor XII activation is the initial step of a complex series of reactions involving blood coagulation, kinin formation, and fibrinolysis [384–386]. This is discussed further in Chap. 15.

Factor XIIa appears to function as an enzyme in activating factor XI [345,352] and in the conversion of prekallikrein to kallikrein [387,388]. DFP inhibits this clot-promoting activity [352,389,390]. Factor XIIa possesses esterolytic [391] and amidolytic [392] activities.

Bovine factor XII is a single-chain glycoprotein of M_r 74,000 daltons [365]. Activated bovine factor XII is composed of a light chain (M_r 31,000 daltons) and a heavy chain (M_r 50,000 daltons) attached by disulfide bonds [366,393]. It is a serine protease and is inhibited by DFP and antithrombin III [366]. The active site is on the light chain [366].

Prekallikrein

Prekallikrein has been purified extensively from human plasma [388,394–397]. It is isolated in two functionally equal forms of M_r 88,000 and 85,000 daltons [388]. Factor XIIa converts prekallikrein to kallikrein by hydrolyzing an internal peptide bond, yielding a two-chain enzymatically active product. The heavy chain has an M_r of 52,000 daltons, while the light chain has an M_r of 36,000 or 33,000 daltons. The active site is on the light chain [388,468], and the binding site for high-molecular-weight kininogen is on the heavy chain [468]. Kallikrein attacks prekallikrein with consequent release of a peptide of M_r 10,000 daltons without development of enzymatic activity [388]. Kallikrein also activates plasminogen [388]. Prekallikrein and high-molecular-weight kininogen circulate as a complex in normal plasma [398]. The concentration of prekallikrein in normal plasma is about 15 to 45 μg/ml [399]. Bovine plasma prekallikrein has also been highly purified [400].

High-molecular-weight kininogen

Plasma kininogens exist in several forms which can be separated into two classes: high-molecular-weight kininogen and low-molecular-weight kininogen [401]. High-molecular-weight kininogen has been extensively studied because of its role in blood coagulation. High-molecular-weight kininogen has been highly purified from human plasma [402–405]. It is a single-chain glycoprotein of M_r about 120,000 daltons [402–405]. High-molecular-weight kininogen is digested by kallikrein to release bradykinin. The coagulant activity of the molecule is unaffected by this cleavage [406]. Further attack on high-molecular-weight kininogen by kallikrein yields an intermediate of M_r 102,000 daltons and a final product of M_r 95,000 daltons [404]. The intermediate form is a two-chain compound which yields a single component of M_r 65,000 daltons on reduction, while the final product yields two components of M_r 65,000 and 54,000 daltons [404]. Only the lighter chain of the end product has procoagulant activity [404]. Carbohydrate is attached to the heavier chain but not the lighter [404].

Both prekallikrein [398,407] and factor XI [347] circulate in· biomolecular complexes with high-molecular-weight kininogen. No evidence for complexes involving all three components has been obtained [408].

Bovine high-molecular-weight kininogen has been highly purified and extensively characterized [409–412], and its role in blood coagulation studied in detail [413].

Factor XIII

Factor XIII has been prepared from human plasma and platelets and from bovine plasma [414–421]. Platelet factor XIII has been crystallized [419]. Human factor XIII has an M_r of about 300,000 daltons [419,421–423] and is composed of two pairs of subunits, a and b, of M_r about 75,000 and 80,000 daltons, respectively [417,423,424]. Human platelet factor XIII has an M_r of about 150,000 to 160,000 daltons and consists of two a chains of M_r 75,000 to 80,000 daltons [416,417,419,423,425] each. The b chain of the plasma factor XIII contains carbohydrate, but the a chains of both plasma and platelet factor XIII contain little or none [417,419,423]. The a chains of plasma and platelet factor XIII appear to be identical [189,385, 421,423,425]. The amino acid composition of the plasma and platelet proteins has been determined [417,419,423]. The N-terminal amino acid of the a chain of plasma and platelet factor XIII is blocked by an acetyl group, while that of the b chain is glutamic acid [189]. Sulfhydryl groups are essential for the activity of factor XIIIa, and cysteine stabilizes the purified enzyme [422,426].

Bovine plasma factor XIII has an M_r of about 300,000 daltons [418]. It is probably composed of two pairs of subunits, designated a and b, of M_r 100,000 and 70,000 daltons, respectively [418].

Factor XIII is converted to factor XIIIa by thrombin [423,427–429]. Calcium is not required for this reaction [429]. Factor XIII is also activated by trypsin [423,430,431], reptilase [423,429,430], and papain [423,432]. Thrombin activates plasma and platelet factor XIII by release of a peptide of 36 amino acids from the N-terminal end of the a chains of plasma [189,417, 421,424,425] or platelet factor XIII [189,417,424], or a peptide of 37 amino acids from the a chain of bovine plasma factor XIII [189,433]. The activated a chain has been designated a¹ [421]. The active center of the enzyme is on the a¹ chain [421,434,435].

Calcium is required for the catalytic activity of plasma factor XIIIa [428]. Calcium causes the dissociation of plasma factor XIIIa into a catalytic dimer (a¹₂) and a non-catalytic dimer (b₂) [421,436,437]. Platelet factor XIIIa

exists as a catalytic dimer (a¹₂) with or without calcium in the system [428]. Calcium may thus exert its influence over the activity of plasma factor XIIIa by its effect on dissociation on the subunits of the molecule, thus exposing the active center [421,436,437]. Fibrinogen modulates the reaction of calcium with factor XIIIa, permitting development of full activity with low concentrations of calcium [438].

The cross-linking of fibrin is effected by formation of ϵ-(γ-glutamyl)-lysine bridges [85–87]. Six such bonds are formed for each monomeric fibrin molecule incorporated into the fully cross-linked clot [439]. Two of these are formed intermolecularly between γ chains of adjacent fibrin monomer molecules leading to γ-γ dimers, while the remainder are formed intermolecularly between α chains, leading to α polymers [13,88,89,439–442]. The cross-linking sites are located near the carboxyl-terminals of both the α and γ chains of fibrin [37,52,90,428–432,443–447]. Factor XIIIa catalyzes intermolecular cross-linking of fibrinogen and cross-linking between molecules of fibrinogen and fibrin [423,448]. Fibrinogen may thus act to suppress fibrin stabilization under some circumstances [448]. Other substrates for factor XIIIa include cold insoluble globulin [449], fibronectin [450], platelet myosin [451], platelet actin [452], α_2-macroglobulin [449], and α_2-plasmin inhibitor [453]. The structural features of substrates for factor XIIIa have been studied in detail [454].

Phospholipids

Although not assigned a Roman numeral in the nomenclature system now widely used, phospholipids are essential reactants in blood coagulation. They are effective either as free phospholipids in emulsion or as a component of phospholipoprotein. They accelerate blood coagulation by participating in the reactions involving factor VIII and those involving factor V. The source of phospholipid in in vivo coagulation is either platelets or tissue components. The phospholipid composition of platelets is presented in Chap. 127.

Much research has been done to determine which of the particular phospholipids in a crude mixture is primarily responsible for the coagulant activity. No single phospholipid or combination of phospholipids is uniquely active in coagulation, but the activity depends primarily on the physical properties of the phospholipid in emulsion [455–459]. The degree of unsaturation or oxidaiton of the fatty acids [455,456,458,459] and the size of the phospholipid micelles [456,457] are important parameters. A negative charge on the surface of the phospholipid micelle is essential for coagulant activity [460–463]. A variety of phospholipid mixtures can have the appropriate charge, and even mixtures of phospholipids with synthetic detergents have been found to be active in coagulation [460]. The phospholipids act in coagulation by providing a surface on which the interacting proteins can be localized [464,465].

References

1. Wright, I. S.: The nomenclature of blood clotting factors. *Thromb. Diath. Haemorrh.* 7:381, 1962.

2. Caspary, E. A., and Kekwick, R. A.: Some physiochemical properties of human fibrinogen. *Biochem. J.* 67:41, 1957.

3. Scheraga, H. A., and Laskowski, M., Jr.: The fibrinogen-fibrin conversion. *Adv. Protein Chem.* 12:1, 1957.

4. Blombäck, B., and Laurent, T. C.: N-terminal and light-scattering studies on fibrinogen and its transformation to fibrin. *Arkiv Kemi* 12:137, 1958.

5. Blombäck, B., and Blombäck, M.: Purification of human and bovine fibrinogen. *Arkiv Kemi* 10:415, 1956.

6. Godal, H. C., and Lüscher, E. F.: Chromatography of human fibrinogen. *Scand. J. Clin. Lab. Invest.* 12:47, 1960.

7. Mosesson M. W., and Sherry, S.: The preparation and properties of human fibrinogen of relatively high solubility. *Biochemistry* 5:2829, 1966.

8. Blombäck, B., and Yamashina, I.: On the N-terminal amino acids in fibrinogen and fibrin. *Arkiv Kemi* 12:299, 1958.

9. Clegg, J. B., and Bailey, K.: The separation and isolation of the peptide chains of fibrin. *Biochim. Biophys. Acta* 63:525, 1962.

10. Henschen, A.: S-Sulfo derivatives of fibrinogen and fibrin: Preparation and general properties. *Arkiv Kemi* 22:1, 1963.

11. Henschen, A.: Peptide chains in S-sulfofibrinogen and S-sulfofibrin: Isolation methods and general properties. *Arkiv Kemi* 22:375, 1964.

12. McKee, P. A., Rogers, L. A., Marley, E., and Hill, R. L.: The subunit polypeptides of human fibrinogen. *Arch. Biochem. Biophys.* 116:271, 1966.

13. McKee, P. A., Mattock, P., and Hill, R. L.: Subunit structure of human fibrinogen, soluble fibrin, and cross-linked insoluble fibrin. *Proc. Natl. Acad. Sci. U.S.A.* 66:738, 1970.

14. Blombäck, B., and Johnson, A. J.: Joint report of the subcommittee on nomenclature and on fibrinolysis, thrombolysis, and intravascular coagulation. *Thromb. Diath. Haemorrh.* 51 (Suppl.):251, 1972.

15. Blombäck, B., Blombäck, M., Edman, P., and Heyssel, B.: Human fibrinopeptides: Isolation, characterization, and structure. *Biochim. Biophys. Acta* 115:371, 1966.

16. Blombäck, B., Hessel, B., Iwanaga, S., Reuterby, J., and Blombäck, M.: Primary structure of human fibrinogen and fibrin. I. Cleavage of fibrinogen with cyanogen bromide: Isolation and characterization of NH₂-terminal fragments of the α ("A") chain. *J. Biol. Chem.* 247:1496, 1972.

17. von Korff, R. W., Pollara, B., Coyne, R., Runquist, J., and Kapoor, R.: Application of radioisotopic yield to the quantitation of the N-terminal amino acids of fibrinogen. *Biochim. Biophys. Acta* 74:698, 1963.

18. Abilgaard, U.: N-terminal analysis during coagulation of purified human fibrinogen, fraction I and plasma. *Scand. J. Clin. Lab. Invest.* 17:529, 1965.

19. Lorand, L., and Middlebrook, W. R.: Species specificity of fibrinogen as revealed by end-group studies. *Science* 118:515, 1953.

20. Blombäck, B., Blombäck, M., and Edman, P.: The structure of human fibrinopeptides. *Acta Chem. Scand.* 17:1184, 1963.

21. Henschen, A., and Edman, P.: Large scale preparation of s-carboxymethylated chains of human fibrin and fibrinogen and the occurrence of γ-chain variants. *Biochim. Biophys. Acta* 263:351, 1972.

22. Laki, K.: The transition of fibrinogen to fibrins, in *Blood Clotting and Allied Problems*, edited by J. E. Flynn. Josiah Macy, Jr., Foundation, New York, 1951, p. 217.

23. Szára, S., and Bagdy, D.: On the polysaccharide of fibrinogen and fibrin. *Biochim. Biophys. Acta* 11:313, 1953.

24. Blombäck, B.: On the properties of fibrinogen and fibrin. *Arkiv Kemi* 12:99, 1958.

25. Sherman, L. A., Mosesson, M. W., and Sherry, S.: Isolation and characterization of the clottable low molecular weight fibrinogen derived by limited plasmin hydrolysis of human fraction I-4. *Biochemistry* 8:1515, 1969.

26. Gati, W. P., and Straub, P. W.: Separation of both the Bβ- and the γ-

27. Henschen, A., and Lottspeich, F.: Amino acid sequence of human fibrin. Preliminary note on the completion of the β-chain sequence. *Hoppe Seylers Z. Physiol. Chem.* 358:1643, 1977.

28. Gaffney, P. J.: Localization of carbohydrate in the subunits of human fibrinogen and its plasmin induced fragments. *Biochim. Biophys. Acta* 263:453, 1972.

29. Pizzo, S. U., Schwartz, M. L., Hill, R. L., and McKee, P. A.: The effect of plasmin on the subunit structure of human fibrinogen. *J. Biol. Chem.* 247:636, 1972.

30. Blombäck, B., Gröndahl, N. J., Hessel, B., Iwanaga, S., and Wallén, P.: Primary structure of human fibrinogen and fibrin: II. Structural studies on the NH₂-terminal part of the γ chain. *J. Biol. Chem.* 248:5806, 1973.

31. Martinez, J., Palascak, J., and Peters, C.: Functional and metabolic properties of human asialofibrinogen. *J. Lab. Clin. Med.* 89:367, 1977.

32. Coller, B. S.: Asialofibrinogen supports platelet aggregation and adhesion to glass. *Blood* 53:325, 1979.

33. Finlayson, J. S., and Mosesson, M. W.: Heterogeneity of human fibrinogen. *Biochemistry* 2:42, 1963.

34. Mosesson, M. W., Alkjaersig, N., Sweet, B., and Sherry, S.: Human fibrinogen of relatively high solubility: Comparative biophysical, biochemical, and biological studies with fibrinogen of lower solubility. *Biochemistry* 6:3279, 1967.

35. Gaffney, P. J.: Heterogeneity of human fibrinogen. *Nature [New Biol.]* 230:54, 1971.

36. Mosesson, M. W., Finlayson, J. S., Umfleet, R. A., and Galanaleis, D.: Human fibrinogen heterogeneities. I. Structural and related studies of plasma fibrinogens which are high solubility catabolic intermediates. *J. Biol. Chem.* 247:5210, 1972.

37. Finlayson, J. S., Mosesson, M. W., Bronzert, T. J., and Pisano, J. J.: Human fibrinogen heterogeneities. II. Cross-linking capacity of high solubility catabolic intermediates. *J. Biol. Chem.* 247:5220, 1972.

38. Lipiniska, I., Lipiniski, B., and Gurewich, V.: Fibrinogen heterogeneity in human plasma: Electrophoretic demonstration and characterization of two major fibrinogen components. *J. Lab. Clin. Med.* 84:509, 1974.

39. Murano, G., Wiman, B., Blombäck, M., and Blombäck, B.: Preparation and isolation of the S-carboxymethyl derivative chains of human fibrinogen. *FEBS Lett.* 14:37, 1971.

40. Galanakis, D. K., Mosesson, M. W., and Stathakis, N. E.: Human fibrinogen heterogeneities: Distribution and charge characteristics of chains of Aα origin. *J. Lab. Clin. Med.* 92:376, 1978.

41. Mosesson, M. W., Finlayson, J. S., and Umfleet, R. A.: Human fibrinogen heterogeneities. III. Identification of γ-chain variants. *J. Biol. Chem.* 247:5223, 1972.

42. Martinez, J.: Metabolic studies of human fibrinogen γ/γ' chain heterogeneity. *Blood* 56:417, 1980.

43. Francis, C. W., Marder, V. J., and Martin, S. E.: Demonstration of a large molecular weight variant of the γ chain of normal human plasma fibrinogen. *J. Biol. Chem.* 255:5599, 1980.

44. Wolfenstein-Todel, C., and Mosesson, M. W.: Human plasma fibrinogen heterogeneity: Evidence for an extended carboxyl-terminal sequence in a normal γ chain variant (γ'). *Proc. Natl. Acad. Sci. U.S.A.* 77:5069, 1980.

45. Kuyas, C., Haeberli, A., and Straub, P. W.: A subfraction of human fibrinogen with high sialic acid content and elongated γ chains. *J. Biol. Chem.* 257:1107, 1982.

46. Murano, G., Wiman, B., and Blombäck, B.: Human fibrinogen: Some characteristics of its S-carboxymethyl derivative chains. *Thromb. Res.* 1:161, 1972.

47. Mills, D., and Karpatkin, S.: Heterogeneity of human fibrinogen: Possible relation to proteolysis by thrombin and plasmin as studied by SDS-polyacrylamide gel electrophoresis. *Biochem. Biophys. Res. Commun.* 40:206, 1970.

48. Mills, D., and Karpatkin, S.: The non-plasmin, proteolytic origin of human fibrinogen heterogeneity. *Biochim. Biophys. Acta* 251:121, 1971.

49. Lottspeich, F., and Henschen, A.: Amino acid sequence of human

fibrin. Preliminary note on an internal peptide obtained by cleaving the γ-chain at the arginyl bonds and showing sequence homology with the C-terminus. *Hoppe Seylers Z. Physiol. Chem.* 358:703, 1977.

50. Lottspeich, F., and Henschen, A.: Amino acid sequence of human fibrin. Preliminary note on the completion of the γ-chain sequence. *Hoppe Seylers Z. Physiol. Chem.* 358:935, 1977.

51. Watt, K. W. K., Takagi, T., and Doolittle, R. F.: Amino acid sequence of the β chain of human fibrinogen. *Biochemistry* 18:68, 1979.

52. Doolittle, R. F., Watt, K. W. K., Cottrell, B. A., Strong, D. D., and Riley, M.: The amino acid sequence of the α-chain of human fibrinogen. *Nature* 280:464, 1979.

53. Bailey, K., Bettelheim, F. R., Lorand, L., and Middlebrook, W. R.: Action of thrombin in the clotting of fibrinogen. *Nature (London)* 167:233, 1951.

54. Blombäck, B., Blombäck, M., Hessel, B., and Iwanaga, S.: Structure of N-terminal fragments of fibrinogen and specificity of thrombin. *Nature* 215:1445, 1967.

55. Mihalyi, E., and Godfrey, J. E.: Digestion of fibrinogen by trypsin: I. Kinetic studies of the reaction. *Biochim. Biophys. Acta* 67:73, 1963.

56. Blombäck, B., and Blombäck, M.: The molecular structure of fibrinogen. *Ann. N.Y. Acad. Sci.* 202:77, 1972.

57. Blombäck, B., Blombäck, M., Henschen, A., Hessel, B., Iwanaga, S., and Woods, K. R.: N-terminal disulfide knot of human fibrinogen. *Nature* 218:130, 1968.

58. Iwanaga, S., Wallén, P., Grondahl, N. J., Henschen, A., and Blombäck, B.: Isolation and characterization of N-terminal fragments obtained by plasmin digestion of human fibrinogen. *Biochim. Biophys. Acta* 147:606, 1967.

59. Blombäck, B.: Studies on the action of thrombic enzymes on bovine fibrinogen as measured by N-terminal analysis. *Arkiv Kemi* 12:321, 1959.

60. Holleman, W. H., and Weiss, L. J.: The thrombin-like enzyme from *Bothrops atrox* snake venom. Properties of the enzyme purified by affinity chromatography on p-aminobenzamidine–substituted agarose. *J. Biol. Chem.* 251:663, 1976.

61. Ewart, M. R., Hatton, M. W. C., Basford, J. M., and Dodgson, K. S.: The proteolytic action of Arvin on human fibrinogen. *Biochem. J.* 118:603, 1970.

62. Hessel, B., and Blombäck, M.: The proteolytic action of the snake venom enzymes arvin and reptilase on N-terminal chain-fragments of human fibrinogen. *FEBS Lett.* 18:318, 1971.

63. Pizzo, S. V., Schwartz, M. L., Hill, R. L., and McKee, P. A.: Mechanism of ancrod anticoagulation: A direct proteolytic effect on fibrin. *J. Clin. Invest.* 51:2841, 1972.

64. Edgar, W., and Prentice, C. R. M.: The proteolytic action of ancrod on human fibrinogen and its polypeptide chains. *Thromb. Res.* 2:85, 1973.

65. Herzig, R. H., Ratnoff, O. D., and Shainoff, J. R.: Studies on a procoagulant fraction of southern copperhead snake venom: The preferential release of fibrinopeptide B. *J. Lab. Clin. Med.* 76:451, 1970.

66. Blombäck, B., Blombäck, M., Mammen, E. F., and Prasad, A. S.: Fibrinogen Detroit: A molecular defect in the N-terminal disulphide knot of human fibrinogen? *Nature (London)* 218:134, 1968.

67. Mammen, E. F., Prasad, A. S., Barnhart, M. I., and Au, C. C.: Congenital dysfibrinogenemia: Fibrinogen Detroit. *J. Clin. Invest.* 48:235, 1969.

68. Blombäck, B., Hessel, B., Hogg, D., and Therkildsen, L.: A two-step fibrinogen-fibrin transition in blood coagulation. *Nature* 275:501, 1978.

69. Smith, G. F.: Fibrinogen-fibrin conversion. The mechanism of fibrin-polymer formation in solution. *Biochem. J.* 185:1, 1980.

70. Ferry, J.: The mechanism of polymerization of fibrinogen. *Proc Natl. Acad. Sci. U.S.A.* 38:506, 1952.

71. Siegel, B. M., Mernan J. P., and Scharaga, H. A.: The configuration of native and partially polymerized fibrinogen. *Biochim. Biophys. Acta* 11:329, 1953.

72. Hall, C. E., and Slayter, H. S.: The fibrinogen molecule: Its size, shape and mode of polymerization. *Biophys. Biochem. Cytol.* 5:11, 1959.

73. Blombäck, B., Hessel, B., Okada, M., and Egberg, N.: Mechanism of fibrin formation and its regulation. *Ann. N.Y. Acad. Sci.* 370:536, 1981.

74. Laurent, T. C., and Blombäck, B.: On the significance of the release of two different peptides from fibrinogen during clotting. *Acta Chem. Scand.* 12:1875, 1958.

75. Doolittle, R. F., Cassman, K. G., Chen, R., Sharp, J. J., and Wooding, G. L.: Correlation of the mode of fibrin polymerization with the pattern of cross-linking. *Ann. N.Y. Acad. Sci.* 202:114, 1972.

76. Kudryk, B., Reuterby, J., and Blombäck, B.: Adsorption of plasmin fragment D to thrombin-modified fibrinogen-sepharose. *Thromb. Res.* 2:297, 1973.

77. Kudryk, B. J., Collen, D., Woods, K. R., and Blombäck, B.: Evidence for localization of polymerization sites in fibrinogen. *J. Biol. Chem.* 249:3322, 1974.

78. Budzynski, A. Z., Marder, V. J., and Shainoff, J. R.: Structure of plasmic degradation products of human fibrinogen: Fibrinopeptide and polypeptide chain analysis. *J. Biol. Chem.* 249:2294, 1974.

79. Shen, L. L., McDonagh, R. P., McDonagh, J., and Hermans, J.: Early events in the plasmin digestion of fibrinogen and fibrin. Effects of plasmin on fibrin polymerization. *J. Biol. Chem.* 252:6184, 1977.

80. Olexa, S. A., and Budzynski, A. Z.: Localization of a fibrin polymerization site. *J. Biol. Chem.* 256:3544, 1981.

81. Laudano, A. P., and Doolittle, R. F.: Synthetic peptide derivatives that bind to fibrinogen and prevent the polymerization of fibrin monomers. *Proc. Natl. Acad. Sci. U.S.A.* 75:3085, 1978.

82. Laudano, A. P., and Doolittle, R. F.: Studies on synthetic peptides that bind to fibrinogen and prevent fibrin polymerization. Structural requirements, number of binding sites, and species differences. *Biochemistry* 19:1013, 1980.

83. Laki, K., and Lorand, L.: On the solubility of fibrin clots. *Science* 108:280, 1948.

84. Lorand, L.: Fibrin clots. *Nature (London)* 166:694, 1950.

85. Pisano, J. J., Finlayson, J. S., and Peyton, M. P.: Cross-link in fibrin polymerized by factor XIII: ε-(γ-glytamyl)-lysine. *Science* 160:892, 1968.

86. Matacic, S., and Loewy, A. G.: The identification of isopeptide cross-links in insoluble fibrin. *Biochem. Biophys. Res. Commun.* 30:356, 1968.

87. Lorand, L., Downey, J., Gotoh, T., Jacobsen, A., and Tukura, S.: The transpeptidase system which crosslinks fibrin by γ-glutamyl-ε-lysine bonds. *Biochem. Biophys. Res. Commun.* 31:222, 1968.

88. Chen, R., and Doolittle, R.: Isolation, characterization and location of a donor-acceptor unit from cross-linked fibrin. *Proc. Natl. Acad. Sci. U.S.A.* 66:472, 1970.

89. Lorand, L., Cehnoweth, D., and Domanik, R. A.: Chain pairs in the cross-linking of fibrin. *Biochem. Biophys. Res. Commun.* 37:219, 1969.

90. Fretto, L. J., Ferguson, E. W., Steinman, H. M., and McKee, P. A.: Localization of the α-chain cross-link acceptor sites of human fibrin. *J. Biol. Chem.* 253:2184, 1978.

91. Koppel, G.: Electron microscopic investigation of the shape of fibrinogen molecules: A model for certain proteins. *Nature (London)* 212:1608, 1966.

92. Blakey, P. R., Groom, M. J., and Turner, R. L.: The conformation of fibrinogen and fibrin: An electron microscope study. *Br. J. Haematol.* 35:437, 1977.

93. Mosesson, M. W., Escaig, J., and Feldmann, G.: Electron microscopy of metal-shadowed fibrinogen molecules deposited at different concentrations. *Br J. Haematol.* 43:469, 1979.

94. Fowler, W. E., and Erickson, H. P.: Trinodular structure of fibrinogen. Confirmation by both shadowing and negative stain electron microscopy. *J. Mol. Biol.* 134:241, 1979.

95. Fowler, W. E., Fretto, L. J., Erickson, H. P., and McKee, P. A.: Electron microscopy of plasmic fragments of human fibrinogen as related to trinodular structure of the intact molecule. *J. Clin. Invest.* 66:50, 1980.

96. Hall, C. E.: Electron microscopy of fibrinogen and fibrin. *J. Biol. Chem.* 179:857, 1949.

97. Stewart, G., and Niewiarowski, S.: Non-enzymatic polymerization of fibrinogen by protamine sulfate: An electron microscopic study. *Biochim. Biophys. Acta* 194:462, 1969.

98. Haschemeyer, A. E. V.: A collapsed structure of fibrinogen? New observations of transient electric birefringence. *Thromb. Res.* 7:59, 1975.

99. Doolittle, R. F.: The structures of fibrinogen and fibrin in *The Regulation of Coagulation*, edited by K. G. Mann and F. B. Taylor, Jr. Elsevier–North Holland, New York, 1980, pp. 501–514.

100. Kay, D., and Cuddigan, B. J.: The fine structure of fibrin. *Br. J. Haematol.* 13:341, 1967.

101. Hawn, C. V., and Porter, K. R.: The fine structure of clots formed from purified bovine fibrinogen and thrombin: A study with the electron microscope. *J. Exp. Med.* 86:285, 1947.

102. Duckert, F., Jung, E., and Shmerling, D. H.: Gerinnungsphysiologische Untersuchungen bei einer neuen Gerinnungsstörung. *Schweiz. Med. Wochenschr.* 91:1139, 1961.

103. Plow, E. F., and Edgington, T. S.: A cleavage-associated neoantigenic marker for a γ chain site in the NH$_2$-terminal aspect of the fibrinogen molecule. *J. Biol. Chem.* 250:3386, 1975.

104. Edgington, T. S., and Plow, E. F.: Conformational and structural modulation of the NH$_2$-terminal regions of fibrinogen and fibrin associated with plasmin cleavage. *J. Biol. Chem.* 250:3393, 1975.

105. Cierniewski, C., Plow, E. F., and Edgington, T. S.: An immunochemical homology between the Aα and a D·E complex-dependent site on the γ chains of fibrinogen. *J. Biol. Chem.* 252:8917, 1977.

106. Plow, E. F., and Edgington, J. S.: Localization and characterization of the cleavage-associated neoantigen locus in the E domain of fibrinogen. *J. Biol. Chem.* 254:672, 1979.

107. Slamon, J., and Bounameaux, Y.: Étude des antigènes plaquettes et, en particulier, du fibrinogène. *Thromb. Diath. Haemorrh.* 2:96, 1958.

108. Sokal, G.: Étude morphologique des plaquettes sanguines et de la métamorphose visqueuse au moyen d'anti-sérums fluorescents antifibrinogène et antiplaquettes. *Acta Haematol. (Basel)* 28:313, 1962.

109. Gokcen, M., and Unis, F.: Fibrinogen as a part of platelet structure. *Nature (London)* 200:590, 1963.

110. Nachman, R. L., Mavena, A. J., and Zucker-Franklin, D.: Subcellular localization of platelet fibrinogen. *Blood* 24:853, 1964.

111. Karaca, M., Nilsson, I. M., and Hedner, U.: Quantitative determination of platelet fibrinogen. *J. Lab. Clin. Med.* 77:485, 1971.

112. Nachman, R., Levine, R., and Jaffe, E.: Synthesis of actin by cultured guinea pig megakaryocytes—Complex formation with fibrin. *Biochim. Biophys. Acta* 543:91, 1978.

113. Castaldi, P. A., and Caen, J.: Platelet fibrinogen. *J. Clin. Pathol.* 18:579, 1965.

114. Solum, N. O., and Lopaciuk, S.: Bovine platelet proteins. III. Some properties of platelet fibrinogen. *Thromb. Diath. Haemorrh.* 29:428, 1969.

115. Ganguly, P.: Isolation and some properties of fibrinogen from human blood platelets. *J. Biol. Chem.* 247:1809, 1972.

116. Doolittle, R. F., Takagi, T., and Cottrell, B. A.: Platelet and plasma fibrinogens are identical gene products. *Science* 185:368, 1974.

117. Witt, I., Müller, H., and Künzer, W.: Evidence for the existence of foetal fibrinogen. *Thromb. Diath. Haemorrh.* 22:101, 1969.

118. Witt, I., Karitsky, D., Müller, H., and Künzer, W.: Peptid Muster von hochgereinigtem Fibrinogen aus Neugeborenen und Erwachsenenblut. *Schweiz. Med. Wochenschr.* 98:1648, 1968.

119. Witt, I., and Müller, H.: Phosphorus and hexose content of human foetal fibrinogen. *Biochim. Biophys. Acta* 221:402, 1970.

120. Witt, I., and Hasler, K.: Influence of organically bound phosphorus in foetal and adult fibrinogen on the kinetics of the interaction between thrombin and fibrinogen. *Biochim. Biophys. Acta* 271:357, 1972.

121. Mills, D. A., and Karpatkin, S.: Heterogeneity of human adult and fetal fibrinogen: Detection of derivatives indicative of thrombin proteolysis. *Biochim. Biophys. Acta* 285:398, 1972.

122. Teger-Nilsson, A.-C., and Ekelund, H.: Fibrinogen to fibrin transformation in umbilical cord blood and purified neonatal fibrinogen. *Thromb. Res.* 5:601, 1974.

123. Guillin, M. C., and Menache, D.: Fetal fibrinogen and fibrinogen Paris. I. Comparative fibrin monomers aggregation studies. *Thromb. Res.* 3:117, 1973.

124. Von Felten, A., and Straub, P. W.: Coagulation studies of cord blood, with special reference to "fetal fibrinogen." *Thromb. Diath. Haemorrh.* 22:273, 1972.

125. Mann, K. G.: Prothrombin, in *Methods in Enzymology*, edited by L. Lorand. Academic, New York, 1976, vol. 45, p. 123.

126. Suttie, J. W., and Jackson, C. M.: Prothrombin structure, activation, and biosynthesis. *Physiol. Rev.* 57:1, 1977.

127. Shapiro, S. S., and McCord, S.: Prothrombin, in *Recent Progress in Thrombosis and Hemostasis*, edited by T. H. Spaet. Grune & Stratton, New York, 1978, vol. 4, p. 177.

128. Shapiro, S. S., and Waugh, D. F.: The purification of human prothrombin. *Thromb. Diath. Haemorrh.* 16:468, 1966.

129. Kisiel W., and Hanahan, D. J.: Purification and characterization of human factor II. *Biochim. Biophys. Acta* 304:103, 1973.

130. Downing, M. R., Butkowski, R. J., Clark, M. M., and Mann, K. G.: Human prothrombin activation. *J. Biol. Chem.* 250:8897, 1975.

131. Mann, K. G., and Elion, J.: Prothrombin, in *CRC Handbook Series in Clinical Laboratory Science*, edited by R. M. Schmidt. CRC, Cleveland, 1980, sec. I, p. 15.

132. DiScipio, R. G., Hermodson, M. A., Yates, S. G., and Davie, E. W.: A comparison of human prothrombin, factor IX (Christmas factor), factor X (Stuart factor), and protein S. *Biochemistry* 16:698, 1977.

133. Magnusson, S.: Edman degradation of components of the bovine and human prothrombin-thrombin systems. *Arkiv Kemi* 24:375, 1965.

134. Walz, D. A., Hewett-Emmett, D., and Seegers, W. H.: Amino acid sequence of human prothrombin fragments 1 and 2. *Proc. Natl. Acad. Sci. U.S.A.* 74:1969, 1977.

135. Walz, D. A., Hewett-Emmett, D., and Seegers, W. H.: Primary structure of the amino-terminal (vitamin K–dependent) region of human prothrombin. *Life Sci.* 20:79, 1977.

136. Butkowski, R. J., Elion, J., Downing, M. R., and Mann, K. G.: Primary structure of human prethrombin 2 and α-thrombin. *J. Biol. Chem.* 252:4942, 1977.

137. Thompson, A. R., Enfield, D. L., Ericsson, L. H., Legaz, M. E., and Fenton, J. W., II: Human thrombin: Partial primary structure. *Arch. Biochem. Biophys.* 178:356, 1977.

138. Cox, A. C., and Hanahan, D. J.: The isolation of undegraded bovine prothrombin and its partial characterization. *Biochim. Biophys. Acta* 207:49, 1970.

139. Bajaj, S. P., and Mann, K. G.: Simultaneous purification of bovine prothrombin and factor X: Activation of prothrombin by trypsin-activated factor X. *J. Biol. Chem.* 248:7729, 1973.

140. Nelsestuen, G. L., and Suttie, S. W.: The carbohydrate of bovine prothrombin. Partial structural determination demonstrating the presence of α-galactose residues. *J. Biol. Chem.* 247:6096, 1972.

141. Stenn, K. S., and Blount, E. R.: Mechanism of bovine prothrombin activation by an insoluble preparation of bovine factor Xa (thrombokinase). *Biochemistry* 11:4502, 1972.

142. Esnouf, M. P., Lloyd, P. H., and Jesty, J.: A method for the simultaneous isolation of factor X and prothrombin from bovine plasma. *Biochem. J.* 131:781, 1973.

143. Owen, W. G., Esmon, C. T., and Jackson, C. M.: The conversion of prothrombin to thrombin. I. Characterization of the reaction products formed during the activation of bovine prothrombin. *J. Biol. Chem.* 249:594, 1974.

144. Morita, T., Iwanaga, S., Suzuki, T., and Fujikawa, K.: Characterization of amino-terminal fragment liberated from bovine prothrombin by activated factor X. *FEBS Lett.* 36:313, 1973.

145. Laki, K., Kominz, D. R., Symonds, P., Lorand, L., and Seegers, W. H.: The amino acid composition of bovine prothrombin. *Arch. Biochem.* 49:276, 1954.

146. Heldebrant, C. M., Butkowski, R. J., Bajaj, S. P., and Mann, K. G.: The activation of prothrombin. II. Partial reactions, physical and chemical characterizations of the intermediates of activation. *J. Biol. Chem.* 248:7149, 1973.

147. Magnusson, S.: Structure and function of thrombin and prothrombin. *Thromb. Diath. Haemorrh. (Suppl.)* 38:97, 1970.

148. Thomas, W. R., and Seegers, W. H.: Terminal amino acids of bovine prothrombin and thrombin preparations. *Biochim. Biophys. Acta* 42:556, 1960.

149. Butkowski, R. J., Bajaj, S. P., and Mann, K. G.: The preparation and activation of (sialyl-^{3}H) prothrombin. *J. Biol. Chem.* 249:6562, 1974.

150. Stenflo, J., Fernlund, P., Egan, W., and Rolpstorff, P.: Vitamin K dependent modifications of glutamic acid residues in prothrombin. *Proc. Natl. Acad. Sci. U.S.A.* 71:2730, 1974.

151. Magnusson, S., Sottrup-Jensen, L., Petersen, T. E., Morris, H. R., and Dell, A.: Primary structure of the vitamin K-dependent part of prothrombin. *FEBS Lett.* 44:189, 1974.

152. Nelsestuen, G. L., Zytkovicz, T. H., and Howard, J. B.: The mode of action of vitamin K. Identification of γ-carboxyglutamic acid as a component of prothrombin. *J. Biol. Chem.* 249:6347, 1974.

153. Magnusson, S., Petersen, T. E., Sottrup-Jensen, L., and Clacys, H.: Complete primary structure of prothrombin: Isolation, structure and reactivity of ten carboxylated glutamic acid residues and regulation of prothrombin activation by thrombin, in *Proteases and Biologic Control*, edited by E. Reich, D. B. Rifkin and E. Shaw. Cold Spring Harbor Laboratory, New York, 1975, p. 123.

154. Girardot, J. M., Delaney, R., and Johnson, B. C.: Carboxylation, the completion step in prothrombin biosynthesis. *Biochem. Biophys. Res. Commun.* 59:1197, 1974.

155. Esmon, C. T., and Suttie, J. W.: Vitamin K-dependent carboxylase. Solubilization and properties. *J. Biol. Chem.* 251:6283, 1976.

156. Suttie, J. W., Hageman, J. M., Lehrman, S. R., and Rich, D. H.: Vitamin K-dependent carboxylase. Development of a peptide substrate. *J. Biol. Chem.* 251:5827, 1976.

157. Nelsestuen, G. L., and Suttie, J. W.: The mode of action of vitamin K: Isolation of a peptide containing the vitamin K-dependent portion of prothrombin. *Proc. Natl. Acad. Sci. U.S.A.* 70:5366, 1973.

158. Benson, B. J., Kisiel, W., and Hanahan, D. J.: Calcium binding and other characteristics of bovine factor II and its activation intermediates. *Biochim. Biophys. Acta* 329:81, 1973.

159. Gitel, S. N., Owen, W. G., Esmon, C. T., and Jackson, C. M.: A polypeptide region of bovine prothrombin specific for binding to phospholipids. *Proc. Natl. Acad. Sci. U.S.A.* 70:1344, 1973.

160. Howard, J. B., and Nelsestuen, G. L.: Properties of a Ca^{2+} binding peptide from prothrombin. *Biochem. Biophys. Res. Commun.* 59:757, 1974.

161. Stenflo, J.: Vitamin K and the biosynthesis of prothrombin. IV. Isolation of peptides containing prosthetic groups from normal prothrombin and the corresponding peptides from dicoumarol-induced prothrombin. *J. Biol. Chem.* 249:5527, 1974.

162. Esmon, C. T., Suttie, J. W., and Jackson, C. M.: The functional significance of vitamin K action. Difference in phospholipid binding between normal and abnormal prothrombin. *J. Biol. Chem.* 250:4095, 1975.

163. Esmon, C. T., and Jackson, C. M.: The conversion of prothrombin to thrombin. III. The factor Xa-catalyzed activation of prothrombin. *J. Biol. Chem.* 249:7782, 1974.

164. Seegers, W. H., Walz, D. A., Reuterby, J., and McCoy, L. E.: Isolation and some properties of thrombin-E and other prothrombin derivatives. *Thromb. Res.* 4:829, 1974.

165. Lundblad, R. L., Kingdon, H. S., and Mann, K. G.: Thrombin, in *Methods in Enzymology*, edited by L. Lorand. Academic, New York, 1976, vol. 45, part B, p. 156.

166. Walz, D. A., and Seegers, W. H.: Amino acid sequence of human thrombin A chain. *Biochem. Biophys. Res. Comm.* 60:717, 1974.

167. Fenton, J. W., II, Fasco, M. J., Stackrow, A. B., Aronson, D. L., Young, A. M., and Finlayson, J. S.: Human thrombin. Production, evaluation, and properties of α-thrombin. *J. Biol. Chem.* 252:3587, 1977.

168. Gorman, J. J., Castaldi, P. A., and Shaw, D. C.: The structure of human thrombin in relation to autolytic degradation. *Biochim. Biophys. Acta* 439:1, 1976.

169. Mann, K. G., Yip, R., Heldebrant, C. M., and Fass, D. N.: Multiple active forms of thrombin. III. Polypeptide chain location of the active site serine and carbohydrate. *J. Biol. Chem.* 248:1868, 1973.

170. Magnusson, S.: Thrombin and prothrombin, in *The Enzymes*, edited by P. Boyer. Academic, New York, 1971, vol. III, p. 277.

171. Hartley, B. S.: Homologies in serine proteinases. *Philos. Trans. R. Soc. Lond. [Biol.]* 257:77, 1970.

172. Mann, K. G., Heldebrant, C. M., and Fass, D. N.: Multiple active forms of thrombin. I. Partial resolution, differential activities, and sequential formation. *J. Biol. Chem.* 246:5994, 1971.

173. Mann, K. G., Heldebrant, C. M., and Fass, D. N.: Multiple forms of thrombin. II. Mechanisms of production from prothrombin. *J. Biol. Chem.* 246:6106, 1971.

174. Titani, K., et al.: Bovine factor X_1a (activated Stuart factor): Evidence of homology with mammalian serine proteases. *Biochemistry* 11:4899, 1972.

175. Fujikawa, K., Coan, M. H., Enfield, D. L., Titani, K., Ericsson, L. H., and Davie, E. W.: A comparison of bovine prothrombin, factor IX (Christmas factor), and factor X (Stuart factor). *Proc. Natl. Acad. Sci. U.S.A.* 71:427, 1974.

176. Enfield, D. L., Ericsson, L. H., Fujikawa, K., Titani, K., Walsh, K. A., and Neurath, H.: Bovine factor XI (Christmas factor): Further evidence of homology with factor X (Stuart factor) and prothrombin. *FEBS Lett.* 47:132, 1974.

177. Lundblad, R. L.: A rapid method for the purification of bovine thrombin and the inhibition of the purified enzyme with phenylmethylsulfonyl fluoride. *Biochemistry* 10:2501, 1971.

178. Gladner, J. A., Laki, K., and Stohlman, F.: Labeled DIP-thrombin. *Biochim. Biophys. Acta* 27:218, 1958.

179. Miller, K. D., and van Vunakis, H.: The effect of diisopropyl fluorophosphate on the proteinase and esterase activities of thrombin and on prothrombin and its activators. *J. Biol. Chem.* 223:227, 1956.

180. Glover, G., and Shaw, E.: The purification of thrombin and isolation of a peptide containing the active center histidine. *J. Biol. Chem.* 246:4594, 1971.

181. Lundblad, R. L., Harrison, J. H., and Mann, K. G.: On the reaction of purified bovine thrombin with N-acetylimidazole. *Biochemistry* 12:409, 1973.

182. Katayama, K., et al.: Comparison of amino acid sequence of bovine coagulation factor IX (Christmas factor) with that of other vitamin K-dependent plasma proteins. *Proc. Natl. Acad. Sci. U.S.A.* 76:4990, 1979.

183. Walz, D. A., Seegers, W. H., Reuterby, J., and McCoy, L. E.: Proteolytic specificity of thrombin. *Thromb. Res.* 4:718, 1974.

184. Sherry, S., and Troll, W.: The action of thrombin on synthetic substrates. *J. Biol. Chem.* 208:95, 1954.

185. Sherry, S., Alkjaersig, N., and Fletcher, A. P.: Comparative activity of thrombin on substituted arginine and lysine esters. *Am. J. Physiol.* 209:577, 1965.

186. Mutt, V., Magnusson, S., Jorpes, J. E., and Dahl, E.: Structure of porcine secretin. I. Degradation with trypsin and thrombin: Sequence of the tryptic peptides. The C-terminal residue. *Biochemistry* 4:2358, 1965.

187. Mutt, V., and Jorpes, J. E.: Structure of porcine cholecystokinin pancreozymin. I. Cleavage with thrombin and with trypsin. *Eur. J. Biochem.* 6:156, 1968.

188. Engel, A., and Alexander, B.: Activation of chymotrypsinogen-A by thrombin preparations. *Biochemistry* 5:3590, 1966.

189. Takagi, T., and Doolittle, R. F.: Amino acid sequence studies on factor XIII and the peptide released during its activation by thrombin. *Biochemistry* 13:750, 1974.

190. Bettelheim, F. R.: The clotting of fibrinogen. II. Fractionation of peptide material liberated. *Biochim. Biophys. Acta* 19:121, 1956.

191. Blombäck, B., Blombäck, M., Olsson, P., Svendsen, L., and Aberg, G.: Synthetic peptides with anticoagulant and vasodilating activity. *Scand. J. Clin. Lab. Invest.* 23 (Suppl. 107):59, 1959.

192. Shinowara, G. Y.: Thromboplastic cell component, the lipoprotein of erythrocytes and platelets. *J. Biol. Chem.* 225:63, 1957.

193. Marcus, A. J., and Spaet, T. H.: Platelet phosphatides: Their separation, identification, and clotting activity. *J. Clin. Invest.* 37:1837, 1958.

194. Marcus, A. J., Zucker-Franklin, D., Sofier, L. B., and Ullman, H. L.: Studies on human platelet granules and membranes. *J. Clin. Invest.* 45:14, 1966.

195. Quick, A. J.: The prothrombin in hemophilia and in obstructive jaundice. *J. Biol. Chem.* 109:lxxii, 1935.

196. Chargaff, E., Bendich, A., and Cohen, S. S.: The thromboplastic protein: Structure, properties, disintegration. *J. Biol. Chem.* 156:161, 1944.

197. Williams, W. J.: The activity of lung microsomes in blood coagulation. *J. Biol. Chem.* 239:933, 1964.

198. Williams, W. J.: The activity of human placenta microsomes and brain particles in blood coagulation. *J. Biol. Chem.* 241:1840, 1966.

199. Clarke, N., and O'Meara, R. A. Q.: Intracellular location of thromboplastic activity in the cells of human chorion. *Br. J. Haematol.* 12:536, 1966.

200. Nemerson, Y.: The phospholipid requirement of tissue factor in blood coagulation. *J. Clin. Invest.* 47:72, 1968.

201. Deutsch, E., Irsigler, K., and Lomoschitz, H.: Studien über Gewebethromboplasin. I. Reinigung, chemische Charakaterisierung und Trennung in einen Eiweiss-und Lipoidanteil. *Thromb. Diath. Haemorrh.* 12:12, 1964.

202. Quick, A. J., Stapp, W. F., and Hussey, C. V.: The effect of heating on the thromboplastic activity of rabbit brain extract: A new test for the diagnosis of hemophilia. *J. Lab. Clin. Med.* 39:142, 1952.

203. Jensen, H., Gray, E. J., and Schaffer, E. H., Jr.: Heat stability studies of clotting factors in "thromboplastic" preparations. *Proc. Soc. Exp. Biol. Med.* 86:387, 1954.

204. Hvatum, M., and Prydyz, H.: Studies on tissue thromboplastin: Its splitting into two separable parts. *Thromb. Diath. Haemorrh.* 21:217, 1969.

205. Nemerson, Y., and Pitlick, F. A.: Purification and characterization of the protein component of tissue factor. *Biochemistry* 9:5100, 1970.

206. Pitlick, F. A., and Nemerson, Y.: Binding of the protein component of tissue factor to phospholipids. *Biochemistry* 9:5105, 1970.

207. Nemerson, Y.: Characteristics and lipid requirements of coagulant proteins extracted from lung and brain: The specificity of the protein component of tissue factor. *J. Clin. Invest.* 48:322, 1969.

208. Zacharski, L. R., Rosenstein, R., and Phillips, P. G.: Concanavalin A inhibition of tissue factor (thromboplastin) activity. *Blood* 44:783, 1974.

209. Pitlick, F. A.: Concanavalin A inhibits tissue factor coagulation activity. *J. Clin. Invest.* 55:175, 1975.

210. Mann, F. D., and Hurn, M. M.: Species specificity of thromboplastin. *Proc. Soc. Exp. Biol. Med.* 79:19, 1952.

211. Irsigler, K., Lechner, K., and Deutsch, E.: Studies on tissue thromboplastin. II. Species specificity. *Thromb. Diath. Haemmorrh.* 14:18, 1965.

212. Hecht, E.: Studien über den lipoiden Aktivator der Blutgerinnung. *Thromb. Diath. Haemorrh.* 1:380, 1957.

213. Pitlick, F. A., Nemerson, Y., Gottlieb, A. J., Gordon, R. G., and Williams, W. J.: Peptidase activity associated with the tissue factor of blood coagulation. *Biochemistry* 10:2650, 1971.

214. Quick, A. J.: On the constitution of prothrombin. *Am. J. Physiol.* 140:212, 1943.

215. Owren, P. A.: The coagulation of blood: Investigations on a new clotting factor. *Acta Med. Scand.* 128 (Suppl. 194):1, 1947.

216. Rosenberg, J. S., Becker, D. L., and Rosenberg, R. D.: Activation of human prothrombin by highly purified human factors V and Xa in the presence of human antithrombin. *J. Biol. Chem.* 250:1607, 1975.

217. Bolhuis, P. A., Hakvoort, T. B. M., Breederveld, K., Mochtar, I. A., and Ten Cate, J. W.: Isolation and partial characterization of human factor V. *Biochim. Biophys. Acta* 578:23, 1979.

218. Dahlbäck, B.: Human coagulation factor V purification and thrombin-catalyzed activation. *J. Clin. Invest.* 66:583, 1980.

219. Kane, W. H., and Majerus, P. W.: Purification and characterization of human coagulation factor V. *J. Biol. Chem.* 256:1002, 1981.

220. Bartlett, S., Latson, P., and Hanahan, D. J.: High-molecular-weight factor V of bovine and human plasma. *Biochemistry* 19:273, 1980.

221. Nesheim, M. E., Myrmel, K. H., Hibbard, L., and Mann, K. G.: Isolation and characterization of single chain bovine factor V. *J. Biol. Chem.* 254:508, 1979.

222. Esmon, C. T.: The subunit structure of thrombin-activated factor V. Isolation of activated factor V, separation of subunits, and reconstitution of biological activity. *J. Biol. Chem.* 254:964, 1979.

223. Nesheim, M. E., and Mann, K. G.: Thrombin-catalyzed activation of single chain bovine factor V. *J. Biol. Chem.* 254:1326, 1979.

224. Saraswathi, S., Rawala, R., and Colman, R. W.: Subunit structure of bovine factor V. Influence of proteolysis during blood collection. *J. Biol. Chem.* 253:1024, 1978.

225. Ittyerah, T. R., Rawala, R., and Colman, R. W.: Function of the subunits of factor V, in *The Regulation of Blood Coagulation*, edited by K. G. Mann and F. B. Taylor, Jr. Elsevier–North Holland, New York, 1980, p. 161.

226. Mann, K. G., Nesheim, M. E., and Tracy, P. B.: Molecular weight of undegraded plasma factor V. *Biochemistry* 20:28, 1981.

227. Jesty, J., and Nemerson, Y.: Purification of factor VII from bovine plasma: Reaction with tissue factor and activation of factor X. *J. Biol. Chem.* 249:509, 1974.

228. Radcliffe, R., and Nemerson, Y.: Activation and control of factor VII by activated factor X and thrombin: Isolation and characterization of a single chain form of factor VII. *J. Biol. Chem.* 250:388, 1975.

229. Kisiel, W., and Davie, E. W.: Isolation and characterization of bovine factor VII. *Biochemistry* 14:4928, 1975.

230. Broze, G. J., Jr., and Majerus, P. W.: Purification and properties of human coagulation factor VII. *J. Biol. Chem.* 255:1242, 1980.

231. Bajaj, S. P., Rapaport, S. I., and Brown, S. F.: Isolation and characterization of human factor VII. Activation of factor VII by factor X. *J. Biol. Chem.* 256:253, 1981.

232. Radcliffe, R., and Nemerson, Y.: Mechanism of activation of bovine factor VII. *J. Biol. Chem.* 251:4797, 1976.

233. Nemerson, Y., and Esnouf, M. P.: Activation of a proteolytic system by a membrane lipoprotein: Mechanism of action of tissue factor. *Proc. Natl. Acad. Sci. U.S.A.* 70:310, 1973.

234. Williams, W. J.: The activation of factor X by Russell's viper venom and by the tissue factor system, in *Biophysical Mechanisms in Vascular Homeostasis and Intravascular Coagulation*, edited by P. N. Sawyer. Appleton-Century-Crofts, New York, 1965, pp. 192–203.

235. Zur, M., and Nemerson, Y.: The esterase activity of coagulation factor VII. Evidence for intrinsic activity of the zymogen. *J. Biol. Chem.* 253:2203, 1978.

236. Silverberg, S. A., Nemerson, Y., and Zur, M.: Kinetics of the activation of bovine coagulation factor X by components of the extrinsic pathway. *J. Biol. Chem.* 252:8481, 1977.

237. Williams, W. J., and Norris, D. G.: Purification of a bovine plasma protein (factor VII) which is required for the activity of lung microsomes in blood coagulation. *J. Biol. Chem.* 241:1847, 1966.

238. Johnston, C. L., Jr., Ferguson, J. H., O'Hanlon, F. A., and Black, W. L.: The fate of factor VII and Stuart factor during the clotting of normal and pathological blood. *Thromb. Diath. Haemorrh.* 3:578, 1959.

239. Hougie, C.: Studies on the fate of coagulation factors during the clotting of normal and pathological blood. *Thromb. Diath. Haemorrh.* 3:578, 1959.

240. Johnston, C. L., Jr., and Hjort, P. F.: Development of increased factor VII activity during the spontaneous coagulation of blood. *J. Clin. Invest.* 40:743, 1961.

241. Shanberge, J. W., and Matsuoka, T.: Studies regarding the effect of foreign surface contact on the one-stage prothrombin time determination. *Thromb. Diath. Haemorrh.* 15:442, 1966.

242. Rapaport, S. I., Aas, K., and Owren, P. A.: The effect of glass upon the activity of the various plasma clotting factors. *J. Clin. Invest.* 34:9, 1955.

243. Lewis, J. H., Didisheim, P., Ferguson, J. H., and Hattori, K.: Changes occurring during coagulation in glass. I. Normal human blood. *Thromb. Diath. Haemorrh.* 4:1, 1959.

244. Soulier, J. P., and Prou-Wartelle, O.: New data on Hageman factor and plasma thromboplastin antecedent: The role of "contact" in the initial phases of blood coagulation. *Br. J. Haematol.* 6:88, 1960.

245. Altman, R., and Hemker, H. C.: Contact activation in the extrinsic blood clotting system. *Thromb. Diath. Haemorrh.* 18:525, 1967.

246. Kisiel, W., Fujikawa, K., and Davie, E. W.: Activation of bovine factor VII (proconvertin) by factor XIIa (activated Hageman factor). *Biochemistry* 16:4189, 1977.

247. Seligsohn U., Østerud, B., Brown, S. F., Griffin, J. H., and Rapaport, S. I.: Activation of human factor VII in plasma and in purified systems. Roles of activated factor IX, kallikrein, and activated factor XII. *J. Clin. Invest.* 64:1056, 1979.

248. Gjønnaess, H.: Cold-promoted activation of factor VII. III. Relation to the kallikrein system. *Thromb. Diath. Haemorrh.* 28:182, 1972.

249. Gjønnaess, H.: Cold-promoted activation of factor VII. IV. Relation to the coagulation system. *Thromb. Diath. Haemorrh.* 28:194, 1972.

250. Saito, H., and Ratnoff, O. D.: Alteration of factor VII activity by ac-

tivated Fletcher factor (a plasma kallikrein): A potential link between the intrinsic and extrinsic blood-clotting systems. *J. Lab. Clin. Med.* 85:405, 1975.

251. Laake, K., and Østerud, B.: Activation of purified plasma factor VII by human plasmin, plasma kallikrein, and activated components of the human intrinsic blood coagulation system. *Thromb. Res.* 5:759, 1974.

252. Koutts, J., Howard, M. A., and Firkin, B. G.: Factor VIII physiology and pathology in man, in *Progress in Hematology,* edited by E. B. Brown. Grune & Stratton, New York, 1979, vol. II, p. 115.

253. Hoyer, L.: The factor VIII complex: Structure and function. *Blood* 58:1, 1981.

254. Kekwick, R. A., and Wolf, P.: A concentrate of human antihaemophilic factor: Its use in six cases of haemophilia. *Lancet* 1:647, 1957.

255. Hershgold, E. J., Davidson, A. M., and Janszen, M. E.: Isolation and some chemical properties of human factor VII (antihemophilic factor). *J. Lab. Clin. Med.* 77:185, 1971.

256. Newman, J., Johnson, A. J., Karpatkin, M. H., and Puszkin, S.: Methods for the production of clinically effective intermediate and high-purity factor VIII concentrates. *Br. J. Haematol.* 21:1, 1971.

257. Poon, M.-C., and Ratnoff, O. D.: Evidence that functional subunits of antihemophilic factor (factor VIII) are linked by noncovalent bonds. *Blood* 48:87, 1976.

258. Montgomery, R. R., and Zimmerman, T. S.: Von Willebrand's disease antigen II. A new plasma and platelet antigen deficient in severe von Willebrand's disease. *J. Clin. Invest.* 61:1498, 1978.

259. Counts, R. B., Paskell, S. L., and Elgee, S. K.: Disulfide bonds and the quaternary structure of factor VIII/von Willebrand factor. *J. Clin. Invest.* 62:702, 1978.

260. Hultin, M. B., and Nemerson, Y.: Activation of factor X by factors IXa and VIII; a specific assay for factor IXa in the presence of thrombin-activated factor VIII. *Blood* 52:928, 1978.

261. Kao, K.-J., Pizzo, S. V., and McKee, P. A.: Demonstration and characterization of specific binding sites for factor VIII/von Willebrand factor on human platelets. *J. Clin. Invest.* 63:656, 1979.

262. Weinstein, M., and Deykin, D.: Comparison of factor VIII–related von Willebrand factor proteins prepared from human cryoprecipitate and factor VIII concentrate. *Blood* 53:1095, 1979.

263. Switzer, M. E. P., Pizzo, S. V., and McKee, P. A.: Is there a precursive, relatively procoagulant-inactive form of normal antihemophilic factor (factor VIII)? *Blood* 54:916, 1979.

264. Martin, S. E., Marder, V. J., Francis, C. W., Loftus, L. S., and Barlow, G. H.: Enzymatic degradation of the factor-VIII-von-Willebrand protein: A unique tryptic fragment with ristocetin cofactor activity. *Blood* 55:848, 1980.

265. Koutts, J., Lavergne, J.-M., and Meyer, D.: Immunological evidence that human factor VIII is composed of two linked moieties. *Br. J. Haematol.* 37:415, 1977.

266. Tuddenham, E. G. D., Trabold, N. C., Collins, J. A., and Hoyer, L. W.: The properties of factor VIII coagulant activity prepared by immunoadsorbent chromatography. *J. Lab. Clin. Med.* 93:40, 1979.

267. Barrow, E. S., Reisner, H. M., and Graham, J. B.: The separation of Willebrand factor from factor VIII-related antigen. *Br. J. Haematol.* 42:455, 1979.

268. Cooper, H. A., Lee, D., Lamb, M. A., and Wagner, R. H.: Structure-function of the factor VIII complex studied with an immobilized heteroantisera to VIII:C. *Br. J. Haematol.* 44:149, 1980.

269. Horowitz, B., Lippin, A., and Woods, K. R.: Purification of low molecular weight factor VIII by affinity chromatography using factor VIII-sepharose. *Thromb. Res.* 14:463, 1979.

270. Schmer, G., Kirby, D. E., Teller, D. C., and Davie, E. W.: The isolation and characterization of bovine factor VIII (antihemophilic factor). *J. Biol. Chem.* 247:2512, 1972.

271. Vehar, G. A., and Davie, E. W.: Preparation and properties of bovine factor VIII (antihemophilic factor). *Biochemistry* 19:401, 1980.

272. Hershgold, E. J., Sherman, L., Davison, A. M., and Janszen, M. E.: Native and purified factor VIII: Molecular and electron microscopical properties and a comparison with hemophilic plasma. *Fed. Proc.* 26:488, 1967.

273. Sodetz, J. M., Pizzo, S. V., and McKee, P. A.: Relationship of sialic

acid to function and *in vivo* survival of human factor VIII/von Willebrand factor protein. *J. Biol. Chem.* 252:5538, 1977.

274. Gralnick, H. R.: Factor VIII/von Willebrand factor protein. Galactose, a cryptic determinant of von Willebrand factor activity. *J. Clin. Invest.* 62:496, 1978.

275. Kao, K.-J., Pizzo, S. V., and McKee, P. A.: Factor VIII/von Willebrand protein. Modification of its carbohydrate causes reduced binding to platelets. *J. Biol. Chem.* 255:10134, 1980.

276. Austen, D. E. G., and Bidwell, E.: Carbohydrate structure of factor VIII. *Thromb. Diath. Haemorrh.* 28:464, 1972.

277. Kass, L., Ratnoff, O. D., and Leon, M. A.: Studies on the purification of antihemophilic factor (factor VIII). I. Precipitation of antihemophilic factor by concanavalin A. *J. Clin. Invest.* 48:351, 1969.

278. Marchesi, S. L., Shulman, N. R., and Gralnick, H. R.: Studies on the purification and characterization of human factor VIII. *J. Clin. Invest.* 51:2151, 1972.

279. Legaz, M. E., Schmer, G., Counts, R. B., and Davie, E. W.: Isolation and chemical characterization of human factor VIII. *J. Biol. Chem.* 248:3946, 1973.

280. Shapiro, G. A., Anderson, J. C., Pizzo, S. V., and McKee, P. A.: The subunit structure of normal and hemophilic factor VIII. *J. Clin. Invest.* 52:2198, 1973.

281. Newman, J., Harris, R. B., and Johnson, A. J.: Molecular weights of antihaemophilic factor and von Willebrand factor proteins in human plasma. *Nature* (London) 263:612, 1976.

282. Seghatchian, M. J., Nilsson, I. M., Holmberg, L., and Miller-Andersson, M.: Molecular size distribution of factor VIII in native plasma. *Thromb. Res.* 14:589, 1979.

283. Zimmerman, T. S., Roberts, J., and Edgington, T. S.: Factor-VIII-related antigen: Multiple molecular forms in human plasma. *Proc. Natl. Acad. Sci. U.S.A.* 72:5121, 1975.

284. Perret, B. A., Furlan, M., and Beck, E. A.: Studies on factor VIII-related protein. II. Estimation of molecular size differences between factor VIII oligomers. *Biochim. Biophys. Acta* 578:164, 1979.

285. Meyer, D., et al.: Multimeric structure of factor VIII/von Willebrand factor in von Willebrand's disease. *J. Lab. Clin. Med.* 95:590, 1980.

286. Hoyer, L. W., and Shainoff, J. R.: Factor VIII-related protein circulates in normal human plasma as high molecular weight multimers. *Blood* 55:1056, 1980.

287. Ruggeri, Z. M., and Zimmerman, T. S.: The complex multimeric composition of factor VIII/von Willebrand factor. *Blood* 57:1140, 1981.

288. Weiss, H. J., Hoyer, L. W., Eickles, F. R., Varma, A., and Rogers, J.: Quantitative assay of a plasma factor deficient in von Willebrand's disease that is necessary for platelet aggregation: Relationship of factor VIII procoagulant activity and antigen content. *J. Clin. Invest.* 52:2708, 1973.

289. Weiss, H. J., and Hoyer, L. W.: Von Willebrand factor: Dissociation from antihemophilic factor procoagulant activity. *Science* 182:1149, 1973.

290. Baugh, R., Brown, J., Sargeant, R., and Houghie, C.: Separation of human factor VIII activity from the von Willebrand's antigen and ristocetin platelet aggregating activity. *Biochim. Biophys. Acta* 371:360, 1974.

291. Weiss, H. J., and Kochwa, S.: Molecular forms of antihemophilic globulin in plasma, cryoprecipitate and after thrombin activation. *Br. J. Haematol.* 18:89, 1970.

292. Weiss, H. J., Phillips, L. L., and Rosner, W.: Separation of sub-units of antihemophilic factor (AHF) by agarose gel chromatography. *Thromb. Diath. Haemorrh.* 27:212, 1972.

293. Rick, M. E., and Hoyer, L. W.: Immunologic studies of antihemophilic factor (AHF, factor VIII). V. Immunologic properties of AHF subunits produced by salt dissociation. *Blood* 42:737, 1973.

294. Cooper, H. A., and Wagner, R. H.: The defect in hemophilic and von Willebrand's disease plasmas studied by a recombination technique. *J. Clin. Invest.* 54:1093, 1974.

295. Austen, D. E. G.: Factor VIII of small molecular weight and its aggregation. *Br. J. Haematol.* 27:89, 1974.

296. Rick, M. E., and Hoyer, L. W.: Activation of low molecular weight fragments of antihemophilic factor (factor VIII) by thrombin. *Nature* 252:404, 1974.

297. Zimmerman, T. S., and Edgington, T. S.: Factor VIII coagulant activity and factor VIII-like antigen: Independent molecular entities. *J. Exp. Med.* 138:1015, 1973.

298. Houghie, C., Sargeant, R. B., Brown, J. J., and Baugh, R. F.: Evidence that factor VIII and the ristocetin aggregating factor (VIII Rist) are separate molecular entities. *Proc. Soc. Exp. Biol. Med.* 147:58, 1974.

299. Owen, W. G., and Wagner, R. H.: Antihemophilic factor: Separation of an active fragment following dissociation by salts or detergents. *Thromb. Diath. Haemorrh.* 27:502, 1972.

300. Cooper, H. A., Griggs, T. R., and Wagner, R. H.: Factor VIII recombination after dissociation by CaCl₂. *Proc. Natl. Acad. Sci. U.S.A.* 70:2326, 1973.

301. Beck, E. A., Bachmann, P., and Barbier, P.: Importance of protease inhibition in studies on purified factor VIII (antihaemophilic factor). *Thromb. Haemostasis* 35:186, 1976.

302. Switzer, M. E., and McKee, P. A.: Studies on human antihemophilic factor. Evidence for covalently linked subunit structure. *J. Clin. Invest.* 57:925, 1976.

303. Gralnick, H. R., and Coller, B. S.: Studies of the human factor VIII/von Willebrand's factor protein. II. Identification and characterization of the von Willebrand protein. *Blood* 46:417, 1975.

304. Sussman, I. I., and Weiss, H. J.: Dissociation of factor VIII in the presence of proteolytic inhibitors. *Thromb. Haemostasis* 40:316, 1978.

305. Rapaport, S. I., Schiffman, S., Patch, M. J., and Ames, S. B.: The importance of activation of antihemophilic globulin and proaccelerin by traces of thrombin in the generation of intrinsic prothrombinase activity. *Blood* 21:221, 1963.

306. Switzer, M. E., and McKee, P. A.: Reactions of thrombin with human factor VIII/von Willebrand factor protein. *J. Biol. Chem.* 255:10606, 1980.

307. Rick, M. E., and Hoyer, L. W.: Thrombin activation of factor VIII. II. A comparison of purified factor VIII and the low molecular weight factor VIII procoagulant. *Br. J. Haematol.* 38:107, 1978.

308. Hoyer, L. W., and Trabold, N. C.: The effect of thrombin on human factor VIII. Cleavage of the factor VIII procoagulant protein during activation. *J. Lab. Clin. Med.* 97:50, 1981.

309. Hoyer, L. W.: von Willebrand's disease. *Prog. Hemostasis Thromb.* 3:231, 1976.

310. Rosenberg, J. S., McKenna, P. W., and Rosenberg, R. D.: Inhibition of human factor IXₐ by human antithrombin. *J. Biol. Chem.* 250:8883, 1975.

311. Thompson, A. R.: Factor IX antigen by radioimmunoassay. Abnormal factor IX protein in patients on warfarin therapy and with hemophilia B. *J. Clin. Invest.* 59:900, 1977.

312. DiScipio, R. G., Kurachi, K., and Davie, E. W.: Activation of human factor IX (Christmas factor). *J. Clin. Invest.* 61:1528, 1978.

313. Østerud, B., Bouma, B. N., and Griffin, J. H.: Human blood coagulation factor IX. Purification, properties, and mechanism of activation by activated factor XI. *J. Biol. Chem.* 253:5946, 1978.

314. Chung, K.-S., Madar, D. A., Goldsmith, J. C., Kingdon, H. S., and Roberts, H. R.: Purification and characterization of an abnormal factor IX (Christmas factor) molecule. Factor IX Chapel Hill. *J. Clin. Invest.* 62:1078, 1978.

315. Fujikawa, K., Thompson, A. R., Legaz, M. E., Meyer, R. G., and Davie, E. W.: Isolation and characterization of bovine factor IX (Christmas factor). *Biochemistry* 12:4938, 1973.

316. Fujikawa, K., Legaz, M., Kato, H., and Davie, E. W.: The mechanism of activation of bovine factor IX (Christmas factor) by bovine factor XIa (activated plasma thromboplastin antecedent). *Biochemistry* 13:4508, 1974.

317. Fryklund, L., Borg, H., and Andersson, L.-O.: Amino-terminal sequence of human factor IX: Presence of γ-carboxyl glutamic acid residues. *FEBS Lett.* 65:187, 1976.

318. Lindquist, P. A., Fujikawa, K., and Davie, E. W.: Activation of bovine factor IX (Christmas factor) by factor XIa (activated plasma thromboplastin antecedent) and a protease from Russell's viper venom. *J. Biol. Chem.* 253:1902, 1978.

319. Miletich, J. P., Jackson, C. M., and Majerus, P. W.: Properties of the factor Xa binding site on human platelets. *J. Biol. Chem.* 253:6908, 1978.

320. Kosow, D. P.: Purification and activation of human factor X: Cooperative effect of Ca⁺⁺ on the activation reaction. *Thromb. Res.* 9:565, 1976.

321. Jackson, C. M., Johnson, T. F., and Hanahan, D. J.: Studies on bovine factor X. I. Large-scale purification of the bovine plasma protein possessing factor X activity. *Biochemistry* 7:4492, 1968.

322. Jackson, C. M., and Hanahan, D. J.: Studies on bovine factor X. II. Characterization of purified factor X: Observations on some alterations in zone electrophoretic and chromatographic behavior occurring during purification. *Biochemistry* 7:4506, 1968.

323. Fujikawa, K., Legaz, M. E., and Davie, E. W.: Bovine factors X₁ and X₂ (Stuart factor): Isolation and characterization. *Biochemistry* 11:4882, 1972.

324. Radcliffe, R. D., and Barton, P. G.: Comparisons of the molecular forms of activated bovine factor X. *J. Biol. Chem.* 248:6788, 1973.

325. Dombrose, F. A., and Seegers, W. H.: Evidence for multiple molecular forms of autoprothrombin C (Factor Xa). *Thromb. Res.* 3:737, 1973.

326. Furie, B. C., Furie, B., Gottlieb, A. J., and Williams, W. J.: Activation of bovine factor X by the venom coagulant protein of *Vipera russelli*: Complex formation of the activated fragments. *Biochim. Biophys. Acta* 365:121, 1974.

327. Morita, T., Wilson, E., and Jackson, C. M.: Structural differences between bovine factors X₁ and X₂, in *The Regulation of Coagulation*, edited by K. G. Mann and F. B. Taylor, Jr. Elsevier–North Holland, New York, 1980, p. 189.

328. Jackson, C. M.: Characterization of two glycoprotein variants of bovine factor X and demonstration that the factor X zymogen contains two polypeptide chains. *Biochemistry* 11:4873, 1972.

329. Fujikawa, K., Titani, K., and Davie, E. W.: Activation of bovine factor X (Stuart factor): Conversion of factor Xaα to factor Xaβ. *Proc. Natl. Acad. Sci. U.S.A.* 72:3359, 1975.

330. Jesty, J., Spencer, A. K., Nakashima, Y., Nemerson, Y., and Konigsberg, W.: The activation of coagulation factor X: Identity of cleavage sites in the alternative activation pathways and characterization of the COOH-terminal peptide. *J. Biol. Chem.* 250:4497, 1975.

331. Enfield, D. L., Ericsson, L. H., Walsh, K. A., Neurath, H., and Titani, K.: Bovine factor X₁ (Stuart factor): Primary structure of the light chain. *Proc. Natl. Acad. Sci. U.S.A.* 72:16, 1975.

332. Howard, J. B., and Nelsestuen, G. L.: Isolation and characterization of vitamin K–dependent region of bovine blood clotting factor X. *Proc. Natl. Acad. Sci. U.S.A.* 72:1281, 1975.

333. Mattock, P., and Esnouf, M. P.: A form of bovine factor X with a single polypeptide chain. *Nature [New Biol.]* 242:90, 1973.

334. Enfield, D. L., et al.: Amino acid sequence of the light chain of bovine factor X₁ (Stuart factor). *Biochemistry* 19:659, 1980.

335. Titani, K., Fujikawa, K., Enfield, D. L., Ericsson, L. H., Walsh, K. A., and Neurath, H.: Bovine factor X₁ (Stuart factor): Amino-acid sequence of heavy chain. *Proc. Natl. Acad. Sci. U.S.A.* 72:3082, 1975.

336. Furie, B. C., and Furie, B.: Interaction of lanthamide ions with bovine factor X and their use in the affinity chromatography of the venom coagulant protein of *Vipera russelli*. *J. Biol. Chem.* 250:601, 1975.

337. Fujikawa, K., Legaz, M., and Davie, E. W.: Bovine factor X₁ (Stuart factor): Mechanism of activation by a protein from Russell's viper venom. *Biochemistry* 11:4892, 1972.

338. Esnouf, M. P., and Williams, W. J.: The isolation and purification of a bovine-plasma protein which is a substrate for the coagulant fraction of Russell's viper venom. *Biochem. J.* 84:62, 1962.

339. Leveson, J. E., and Esnouf, M. P.: The inhibition of activated factor X with diisopropyl fluorophosphate. *Br. J. Haematol.* 17:173, 1969.

340. Wuepper, K. D.: Biochemistry and biology of components of the plasma kinin-forming systems, in *Inflammation: Mechanisms and Control*, edited by I. Lepow and P. A. Ward. Academic, New York, 1972, p. 93.

341. Saito, H., Ratnoff, O. D., Marshall, J. S., and Pensky, J.: Partial purification of plasma thromboplastin antecedent (factor XI) and its activation by trypsin. *J. Clin. Invest.* 52:850, 1973.

342. Schiffman, S., and Lee, P.: Preparation, characterization, and activation of a highly purified factor XI: Evidence that a hitherto unrecognized plasma activity participates in the interaction of factors XI and XII. *Br. J. Haematol.* 27:101, 1974.

343. Heck, L. W., and Kaplan, A. P.: Substrates of Hageman factor. I. Isolation and characterization of human factor XI (PTA) and inhibition of the activated enzyme by α_1-antitrypsin. *J. Exp. Med.* 140:1615, 1974.

344. Movat, H. Z., and Ozge-Anwar, A. H.: The contact phase of blood coagulation. Clotting factors XI and XII, their isolation and interaction. *J. Lab. Clin. Med.* 84:861, 1974.

345. Bouma, B. N., and Griffin, J. H.: Human blood coagulation factor XI: Purification, properties, and mechanism of activation by activated factor XII. *J. Biol. Chem.* 252:6432, 1977.

346. Lipscomb, M. S., and Walsh, P. N.: Human platelets and factor XI. Localization in platelet membranes of factor XI-like activity and its functional distinction from plasma factor XI. *J. Clin. Invest.* 63:1006, 1979.

347. Thompson, R. E., Mandle, R., Jr., and Kaplan, A. P.: Association of factor XI and high molecular weight kininogen in human plasma. *J. Clin. Invest.* 60:1376, 1977.

348. Mannhalter, C., Schiffman, S., and Jacobs, A.: Trypsin activation of human factor XI. *J. Biol. Chem.* 255:2667, 1980.

349. Forbes, C. D., and Ratnoff, O. D.: Studies on plasma thromboplastin antecedent (factor XI), PTA deficiency and inhibition of PTA by plasma: Pharmacologic inhibitors and specific antiserum. *J. Lab. Clin. Med.* 79:113, 1972.

350. Özge-Anwar, A. H., Movat, H. Z., and Scott, J. G.: The kinin system of human plasma. IV. The interrelationship between the contact phase of blood coagulation and the plasma kinin system in man. *Thromb. Diath. Haemorrh.* 27:141, 1972.

351. Kurachi, K., and Davie, E. W.: Activation of human factor XI (plasma thromboplastin antecedent) by factor XIIa (activated Hageman factor). *Biochemistry* 16:5831, 1977.

352. Ratnoff, O. D., Davie, E. W., and Mallett, D. L.: Studies on the action of Hageman factor: Evidence that activated Hageman factor in turn activates plasma thromboplastin antecedent. *J. Clin. Invest.* 40:803, 1961.

353. Kingdon, H. S., Davie, E. W., and Ratnoff, O. D.: The reaction between activated plasma thromboplastin antecedent and diisopropylphosphofluoridate. *Biochemistry* 3:166, 1964.

354. Kato, H., Fujikawa, K., and Legaz, M. E.: Isolation and activation of bovine factor XI (plasma thromboplastin antecedent) and its interaction with factor IX (Christmas factor). *Fed. Proc.* 33:1505, 1974.

355. Koide, T., Kato, H., and Davie, E. W.: Bovine factor XI (plasma thromboplastin antecedent), in *Methods in Enzymology*, edited by L. Lorand. Academic, New York, 1976, vol. 45, part B, p. 65.

356. Kurachi, K., Fujikawa, K., and Davie, E. W.: Mechanism of activation of bovine factor XI by factor XII and factor XIIa. *Biochemistry* 19:1330, 1980.

357. Revak, S. D., Cochrane, C. G., Johnston, A. R., and Hugh, T. E.: Structural changes accompanying enzymatic activation of human Hageman factor. *J. Clin. Invest.* 54:619, 1974.

358. Saito, H., Ratnoff, O. D., and Donaldson, V. H.: Defective activation of clotting, fibrinolytic, and permeability-enhancing systems in human Fletcher trait plasma. *Circ. Res.* 34:641, 1974.

359. Griffin, J. H., and Cochrane, C. G.: Human factor XII (Hageman factor), in *Methods in Enzymology*, edited by L. Lorand. Academic, New York, 1976, vol. 45, part 2, p. 56.

360. Chan, J. Y. C., and Movat, H. Z.: Purification of factor XII (Hageman factor) from normal human plasma. *Thromb. Res.* 8:337, 1976.

361. Goldsmith, G. H., Jr., Saito, H., and Ratnoff, O. D.: The activation of plasminogen by Hageman factor (factor XII) and Hageman factor fragments. *J. Clin. Invest.* 62:54, 1978.

362. Silverberg, M., Dunn, J. T., Garen, L., and Kaplan, A. P.: Autoactivation of human Hageman factor. Demonstration utilizing a synthetic substrate. *J. Biol. Chem.* 255:7281, 1980.

363. Schoenmakers, J. G., Kurstjens, R. M., Haanen, C., and Zilliken, F.: Purification of activated bovine Hageman factor. *Thromb. Diath. Haemorrh.* 9:546, 1963.

364. Schoenmakers, J. G., Matze, R., Haanen, C., and Zilliken, F.: Hageman factor: A novel sialoglycoprotein with esterase activity. *Biochim. Biophys. Acta* 101:166, 1965.

365. Fujikawa, K., Walsh, K. A., and Davie, E. W.: Isolation and characterization of bovine factor XII (Hageman factor). *Biochemistry* 16:2270, 1977.

366. Fujikawa, K., Kurachi, K., and Davie, E. W.: Characterization of bovine factor XIIa (activated Hageman factor). *Biochemistry* 16:4182, 1977.

367. McMillin, C. R., Saito, H., Ratnoff, O. D., and Walton, A. G.: The secondary structure of human Hageman factor (factor XII) and its alteration by activating agents. *J. Clin. Invest.* 54:1312, 1974.

368. Ratnoff, O. D.: The biology and pathology of the initial stages of coagulation. *Prog. Hematol.* 5:204, 1966.

369. Ratnoff, O. D., and Crum, J. D.: Activation of Hageman factor by solutions of ellagic acid. *J. Lab. Clin. Med.* 63:359, 1964.

370. Ratnoff, O. D.: Activation of Hageman factor by L-homocystine. *Science* 162:1007, 1968.

371. Wilner, G. D., Nossel, H. L., and LeRoy, E. C.: Activation of Hageman factor by collagen. *J. Clin. Invest.* 12:2608, 1968.

372. Margolis, J.: Activation of Hageman factor by saturated fatty acids. *Aust. J. Exp. Biol. Med. Sci.* 40:505, 1962.

373. Nossel, H., Rubin, H., Drillings, M., and Hsieh, R.: Inhibition of Hageman factor activation. *J. Clin. Invest.* 47:1172, 1968.

374. Margolis, J.: The interrelationship of coagulation of plasma and release of peptides. *Ann. N.Y. Acad. Sci.* 104:133, 1963.

375. Donaldson, V. H., and Ratnoff, O. D.: Hageman factor: Alterations in physical properties during activation. *Science* 150:754, 1965.

376. Cochrane, C. G., Revak, S. D., and Wuepper, K. D.: Activation of Hageman factor in solid and fluid phases: A critical role of kallikrein. *J. Exp. Med.* 138:1564, 1973.

377. Revak, S. D., and Cochrane, C. G.: The relationship of structure and function in human Hageman factor: The association of enzymatic and binding activities with separate regions of the molecule. *J. Clin. Invest.* 57:852, 1976.

378. Cochrane, C. D., and Wuepper, K. D.: The first component of the kinin-forming system in human and rabbit plasma: Its relationship to clotting factor XII (Hageman factor). *J. Exp. Med.* 134:986, 1971.

379. Soltay, M. J., Movat, H. Z., and Ozge-Anwar, A. H.: The kinin system of human plasma. V. The probable derivative of prekallikrein activator from activated Hageman factor (XIIa). *Proc. Soc. Exp. Biol. Med.* 138:952, 1971.

380. Kaplan, A. P., and Austen, K. F.: A prealbumin activator of prekallikrein. II. Derivation of activators of prekallikrein from active Hageman factor by digestion with plasmin. *J. Exp. Med.* 133:696, 1971.

381. Burrowes, C. E., Movat, H. Z., and Soltay, M. J.: The kinin system of human plasma. VI. The action of plasmin. *Proc. Soc. Exp. Biol. Med.* 138:959, 1971.

382. Revak, S. D., Cochrane, C. G., and Griffin, J. H.: The binding and cleavage characteristics of human Hageman factor during contact activation. A comparison of normal plasma with plasmas deficient in factor XI, prekallikrein, or high molecular weight kininogen. *J. Clin. Invest.* 59:1167, 1977.

383. Kaplan, A. P., and Austen, K. F.: The fibrinolytic pathway of human plasma: Isolation and characteristics of the plasminogen proactivator. *J. Exp. Med.* 136:1378, 1972.

384. Schreiberg, A. D., and Austen, K. F.: Interrelationship of the fibrinolytic, coagulation, kinin generating and complement systems. *Ser. Haematol.* 6:4, 1973.

385. Kaplan, A. P.: The Hageman factor dependent pathways of human plasma. *Microvasc. Res.* 8:97, 1974.

386. Cochrane, C. G., Revak, S. D., Wuepper, K. D., Johnston, A., Morrison, D. C., and Ulevich, R.: Soluble mediators of injury of the microvasculature: Hageman factor and the kinin forming, intrinsic clotting and the fibrinolytic systems. *Microvasc. Res.* 8:112, 1974.

387. Wuepper, K. D., and Cochrane, C. G.: Plasma prekallikrein: Isolation, characterization, and mechanism of activation. *J. Exp. Med.* 135:1, 1972.

388. Mandle, R., Jr., and Kaplan, A. P.: Hageman factor substrates. Human plasma prekallikrein: Mechanism of activation by Hageman factor and participation in Hageman factor-dependent fibrinolysis. *J. Biol. Chem.* 252:6097, 1977.

389. Becker, E. L.: Inactivation of Hageman factor by diisopropylfluorophosphate (DFP). *J. Lab. Clin. Med.* 56:136, 1960.

390. Stead, N., Kaplan, A. P., and Rosenberg, R. D.: Inhibition of activated factor XII by antithrombin-heparin cofactor. *J. Biol. Chem.* 251:6481, 1976.

391. Ulevitch, R. J., Letchford, D., and Cochrane, C. G.: A direct enzymatic assay for the esterolytic activity of activated Hageman factor. *Thromb. Diath. Haemorrh. 31:*30, 1974.

392. Ratnoff, O. D., and Saito, H.: Amidolytic properties of single-chain activated Hageman factor. *Proc. Natl. Acad. Sci. U.S.A. 76:*1461, 1979.

393. Fujikawa, K., Heimark, R. L., Kurachi, K., and Davie, E. W.: Activation of bovine factor XII (Hageman factor) by plasma kallikrein. *Biochemistry 19:*1322, 1980.

394. Colman, R. W., and Bagdasarian, A.: Human kallikrein and prekallikrein, in *Methods in Enzymology*, edited by L. Lorand. Academic, New York, 1976, vol. 45, p. 303.

395. Gallimore, M. J., Fareid, E., and Stormorken, H.: The purification of a human plasma prekallikrein with weak plasminogen activator activity. *Thromb. Res. 12:*409, 1978.

396. Bouma, B. N., Miles, L., Beretta, G., and Griffin, J. H.: Human plasma prekallikrein: Studies of its activation by activated factor XII and of its inactivation by diisopropyl phosphofluoridate. *Biochemistry 19:*1151, 1980.

397. Griffin, J. W.: Role of surface-dependent activation of Hageman factor (blood coagulation factor XII). *Proc. Natl. Acad. Sci. U.S.A. 75:*1998, 1978.

398. Mandle, R. J., Colman, R. W., and Kaplan, A. P.: Identification of prekallikrein and high-molecular-weight kininogen as a complex in human plasma. *Proc. Natl. Acad. Sci. U.S.A. 73:*4179, 1976.

399. Bouma, B. N., Kerbiriou, D. M., Vlooswijk, R. A. A., and Griffin, J. H.: Immunological studies of prekallikrein, kallikrein, and high-molecular-weight kininogen in normal and deficient plasma and in normal plasma after cold-dependent activation. *J. Lab. Clin. Med. 96:*693, 1980.

400. Heimark, R. L., and Davie, E. W.: Isolation and characterization of bovine plasma prekallikrein (Fletcher factor). *Biochemistry 18:*5743, 1979.

401. Jacobsen, S., and Kriz, M.: Some data on two purified kininogens from human plasma. *Br. J. Pharmacol. 29:*25, 1967.

402. Saito, H.: Purification of high molecular weight kininogen and the role of this agent in blood coagulation. *J. Clin. Invest. 60:*584, 1977.

403. Thompson, R. E., Mandle, R., Jr., and Kaplan, A. P.: Characterization of human high molecular weight kininogen. Procoagulant activity associated with the light chain of kinin-free high molecular weight kininogen. *J. Exp. Med. 147:*488, 1978.

404. Kerbiriou, D. M., and Griffin, J. H.: Human high molecular weight kininogen. Studies of structure-function relationships and of proteolysis of the molecule occurring during contact activation of plasma. *J. Biol. Chem. 254:*12020, 1979.

405. Schiffman, S., Mannhalter, C., and Tyner, K. D.: Human high molecular weight kininogen. Effects of cleavage by kallikrein on protein structure and procoagulant activity. *J. Biol. Chem. 255:*6433, 1980.

406. Colman, R. W., et al.: Williams trait. Human kininogen deficiency with diminished levels of plasminogen proactivator and prekallikrein associated with abnormalities of the Hageman factor-dependent pathways. *J. Clin. Invest. 56:*1650, 1975.

407. Scott, C. F., and Colman, R. W.: Function and immunochemistry of prekallikrein–high molecular weight kininogen complex in plasma. *J. Clin. Invest. 65:*413, 1980.

408. Kaplan, A. P.: Initiation of the intrinsic coagulation and fibrinolytic pathways of man: The role of surfaces, Hageman factor, prekallikrein, high molecular weight kininogen, and factor XI, in *Progress in Hemostasis and Thrombosis*, edited by T. H. Spaet. Grune & Stratton, New York, 1978, vol. 4, p. 127.

409. Komiya, M., Kato, H., and Suzuki, T.: Bovine plasma kininogens. I. Further purification of high molecular weight kininogen and its physicochemical properties. *J. Biochem. 76:*811, 1974.

410. Komiya, M., Kato, H., and Suzuki, T.: Bovine plasma kininogens. II. Microheterogeneities of high molecular weight kininogens and their structural relationships. *J. Biochem. 76:*823, 1974.

411. Han, Y. N., Komiya, M., Kato, H., Iwanaga, S., and Suzuki, T.: Primary structure of bovine high molecular weight kininogen: Chemical compositions of kinin-free kininogen and peptide fragments released by plasma kallikrein. *FEBS Lett. 57:*254, 1975.

412. Han, Y. N., Kato, H., Iwanaga, S., and Suzuki, T.: Primary structure of bovine plasma high-molecular-weight kininogen. The amino acid sequence of a glycopeptide portion (fragment I) following the C-terminus of the bradykinin moiety. *J. Biochem. 79:*1201, 1976.

413. Sugo, T., et al.: Functional sites of bovine high molecular weight kininogen as a cofactor in kaolin-mediated activation of factor XII (Hageman factor). *Biochemistry 19:*3215, 1980.

414. Loewy, A. G., Dunathan, K., Kriel, R., and Wolfinger, H. L., Jr.: Fibrinase. I. Purification of substrate and enzyme. *J. Biol. Chem. 236:*2625, 1961.

415. Lorand, L., and Gotoh, T.: Fibroligase: The fibrin stabilizing factor system. *Methods Enzymol. 19:*770, 1970.

416. Ganguly, P.: Isolation and properties of a thrombin-sensitive protein from human blood platelets. *J. Biol. Chem. 246:*4286, 1971.

417. Schwartz, M. L., Pizzo, S. V., Hill, R. L., and McKee, P. A.: The subunit structure of human plasma and platelet factor XIII (fibrin-stabilizing factor). *J. Biol. Chem. 246:*5851, 1971.

418. Takagi, T., and Konishi, K.: Purification and some properties of fibrin stabilizing factor. *Biochim. Biophys. Acta 271:*363, 1972.

419. Bohn, H.: Comparative studies on the fibrin-stabilizing factors from human plasma, platelets, and placentas. *Ann. N.Y. Acad. Sci. 202:*256, 1972.

420. Chung, S. I., and Folk, J. E.: Kinetic studies with transglutaminases. The human blood enzymes (activated coagulation factor XIII) and the guinea pig hair follicle enzyme. *J. Biol. Chem. 247:*2798, 1972.

421. Chung, S. I., Lewis, M. S., and Folk, J. E.: Relationships of the catalytic properties of human plasma and platelet transglutaminases (activated blood coagulation factor XIII) to their subunit structures. *J. Biol. Chem. 249:*940, 1974.

422. Loewy, A. G., Dahlberg, A., Dunathan, K., Kriel, R., and Wolfinger, H. H., Jr.: Fibrinase II: Some physical properties. *J. Biol. Chem. 236:*2634, 1964.

423. Schwartz, M. L., Pizzo, S. V., Hill, R. L., and McKee, P. A.: Human factor XIII from plasma and platelets: Molecular weights, subunit structures, proteolytic activation, and cross-linking of fibrinogen and fibrin. *J. Biol. Chem. 248:*1395, 1973.

424. Chung, S. I.: Comparative studies on tissue transglutaminase and factor XIII. *Ann. N.Y. Acad. Sci. 202:*240, 1972.

425. Bohn, H., Haupt, H., and Kranz, T.: Die molekulare Struktur der Fibrinstabilisierenden Faktoren des Menschen. *Blut 25:*235, 1972.

426. Lorand, L., and Jacobsen, A.: Studies on the polymerization of fibrin: The role of the globulin: Fibrin-stabilizing factor. *J. Biol. Chem. 230:*421, 1958.

427. Buluk, K., Januszko, T., Olbromski, J.: Conversion of fibrin to desmofibrin. *Nature 191:*1093, 1961.

428. Lorand, L., and Konishi, K.: Activation of the fibrin stabilizing factor of plasma by thrombin. *Arch Biochem. 105:*58, 1964.

429. Tyler, H. M.: Studies of the activation of purified human factor XIII. *Biochim. Biophys. Acta 222:*396, 1970.

430. Kopeć, M., Latallo, Z. S., Stahl, M., and Wegrzynowicz, Z.: The effect of proteolytic enzymes of fibrin stabilizing factor. *Biochim. Biophys. Acta 181:*437, 1969.

431. Konishi, K., and Takagi, T.: Activation of the fibrin stabilizing factor by trypsin and some of its properties after activation. *J. Biochem. (Tokyo) 65:*281, 1969.

432. Buluk, K., and Zuch, A.: The possibility of proteolytic activation of the fibrin stabilizing factor. *Biochim. Biophys. Acta 147:*593, 1967.

433. Mikuni, Y., Iwanaga, S., and Konishi, K.: A peptide released from plasma fibrin stabilizing factor in the conversion to the active enzyme by thrombin. *Biochim. Biophys. Acta 54:*1393, 1973.

434. Holbrook, J. J., Cooke, R. D., and Kingston, J. B.: The amino acid sequence around the reactive cysteine residue in human plasma factor XIII. *Biochem. J. 135:*901, 1973.

435. Curtis, C. G., Stenberg, P., Chou, C.-H. J., Gray, A., Brown, K. L., and Lorand, L.: Titration and subunit localization of active center cysteine in fibrinoligase (thrombin-activated fibrin stabilizing factor). *Biochem. Biophys. Res. Commun. 52:*51, 1973.

436. Lorand, L., et al.: Dissociation of the subunit structure of fibrin stabilizing factor during activation of the zymogen. *Biochem. Biophys. Res. Commun. 56:*914, 1974.

437. Curtis, C. G., et al.: Calcium-dependent unmasking of active

center cysteine during activation of fibrin stabilizing factor. *Biochemistry* 13:3774, 1974.

438. Credo, R. B., Curtis, C. G., and Lorand, L.: Ca²⁺-related regulatory function of fibrinogen. *Proc. Natl. Acad. Sci. U.S.A.* 75:4234, 1978.

439. Pisano, J. J., Finlayson, J. S., Peyton, M. P., and Nagi, Y.: ε-(γ-Glutamyl) lysine in fibrin: Lack of cross-link formation in factor XIII deficiency. *Proc. Natl. Acad. Sci. U.S.A.* 68:770, 1971.

440. Pisano, J. J., Bronzert, T. J., Peyton, M. P., and Finlayson, J. S.: ε(γ-Glutamyl) lysine cross-links: Determination in fibrin from normal and factor XIII-deficient individuals. *Ann. N.Y. Acad. Sci.* 202:98, 1972.

441. McDonagh, R. P., Jr., McDonagh, J., Blombäck, M., and Blombäck, B.: Cross-linking of human fibrin: Evidence for intermolecular cross-linking involving α-chains. *FEBS Lett.* 14:33, 1971.

442. Doolittle, R. F., Chen, R., and Lau, F.: Hybrid fibrin: Proof of the intramolecular nature of γ-γ cross-linking units. *Biochem. Biophys. Res. Commun.* 44:94, 1971.

443. Chen, R., and Doolittle, R. F.: γ-γ Cross-linking sites in human and bovine fibrin. *Biochemistry* 10:4486, 1971.

444. Doolittle, R. F.: Structural details of fibrin stabilization: Implication for fibrinogen structure and initial fibrin formation. *Thromb. Diath. Haemorrh. (Suppl.)* 54:155, 1973.

445. Sharp, J. J., Cassman, K. G., and Doolittle, R. F.: Amino acid sequence of the carboxy-terminal cyanogen bromide fragment from bovine and human fibrinogen γ-chains. *FEBS Lett.* 25:334, 1972.

446. Finlayson, J. S., and Mosesson, M. W.: Cross-linking of α chain remnants in human fibrin. *Thromb. Res.* 2:467, 1973.

447. Takagi, T., and Doolittle, R. F.: Amino acid sequence studies of the α chain of human fibrinogen: Location of four plasmin attack points and a covalent cross-linking site. *Biochemistry* 14:5149, 1975.

448. Kanaide, H., and Shainoff, J. R.: Cross-linking of fibrinogen and fibrin by fibrin-stabilizing factor (factor XIIIa). *J. Lab. Clin. Med.* 85:574, 1975.

449. Mosher, D. F.: Action of fibrin-stabilizing factor on cold-insoluble globulin and α₂-macroglobulin in clotting plasma. *J. Biol. Chem.* 251:1639, 1976.

450. Keski-Oja, J., Mosher, D. F., and Vaheri, A.: Cross-linking of a major fibroblast surface-associated glycoprotein (fibronectin) catalyzed by blood coagulation factor XIII. *Cell* 9:29, 1976.

451. Cohen, I., et al.: Fibrinoligase-catalyzed cross-linking of myosin from platelet and skeletal muscle. *Arch. Biochem. Biophys.* 192:110, 1979.

452. Cohen, I., et al.: Factor XIIIa catalyzed cross-linking of platelet and muscle actin: Regulation of nucleotides. *Biochim. Biophys. Acta* 628:365, 1980.

453. Sakata, Y., and Aoki, N.: Cross-linking of α₂-plasmin inhibitor to fibrin by fibrin-stabilizing factor. *J. Clin. Invest.* 65:290, 1980.

454. Gorman J. J., and Folk, J. E.: Structural features of glutamine substrates for transglutaminases. *J. Biol. Chem.* 256:2712, 1981.

455. Rouser, G., White, S. G., and Schloredt, D.: Phospholipid structure and thromboplastic activity. I. The phosphatide fraction active in recalcified normal human plasma. *Biochim. Biophys. Acta* 28:71, 1958.

456. Wallach, D. F. H., Maurice, P. A., Steele, B. B., and Surgenor, D. M.: Studies on the relationship between the colloidal state and clot-promoting activity of pure phosphatidylethanolamines. *J. Biol. Chem.* 234:2829, 1959.

457. Turner, D. L., Holburn, R. R., DeSipin, M., Silver, M. J., and Tocantins, L. M.: Thromboplastin activity of phosphatidylethanolamine from natural and synthetic sources. *J. Lipid Res.* 4:52, 1963.

458. Rouser, G., and Schloredt, D.: Phospholipid structure and thromboplastic activity. II. The fatty acid composition of the active phosphatidyl ethanolamines. *Biochim. Biophys. Acta* 28:81, 1958.

459. Grisdale, P. J., and Okany, A.: Phospholipids. II. A correlation of chemical structure with thromboplastic activity. *Can. J. Biochem.* 43:1465, 1965.

460. Bangham, A. D.: A correlation between surface charge and coagulant action of phospholipids. *Nature* 192:1197, 1961.

461. Papahadjopoulos, D., Hougie, C., and Hanahan, D. J.: Influence of surface charge of phospholipids on their clot-promoting activity. *Proc. Soc. Exp. Biol. Med.* 111:412, 1962.

462. Silver, M. J., et al.: Evaluation of activity of phospholipids in blood coagulation *in vitro*. *Thromb. Diath. Haemorrh.* 10:164, 1963.

463. Daemen, F. J., van Arkel, C., Hart, H. C., vander Drift, C., and van Dunen, L. L. M.: Activity of synthetic phospholipids in blood coagulation. *Thromb. Diath. Haemorrh.* 13:194, 1965.

464. Bloom, J. W., Nesheim, M. E., and Mann, K. G.: Phospholipid-binding properties of bovine factor V and factor Va. *Biochemistry* 18:4419, 1979.

465. Zwaal, R. F. A., et al.: Topological and kinetic aspects of phospholipids in blood coagulation, in *The Regulation of Coagulation*, edited by K. G. Mann and F. B. Taylor, Jr. Elsevier–North Holland, New York, 1980, p. 95.

466. Kane, W. H., and Majerus, P. W.: The interaction of human coagulation factor Va with platelets. *J. Biol. Chem.* 257:3963, 1982.

467. Tans, G., and Griffin, J. H.: Properties of sulfatides in factor-XII-dependent contact activation. *Blood* 59:69, 1982.

468. van der Graaf, F., Tans, G., Bouma, B. N., and Griffin, J. H.: Isolation and functional properties of the heavy and light chains of human plasma kallikrein. *J. Biol. Chem.* 257:14300, 1982.

Kinetics of plasma coagulation factors

CHAPTER *133*

Production of plasma coagulation factors

WILLIAM J. WILLIAMS

The liver is the major site of synthesis of fibrinogen (factor I), prothrombin (factor II), and factors V, VII, IX, and X, but the site of synthesis of the remaining plasma coagulation factors has not been determined. The evidence for the site of origin of coagulation factors is derived largely from studies on human subjects with severe liver disease, from experiments on the effect of severe liver damage or hepatectomy in animals on levels of plasma coagulation factors, and from studies on the in vitro synthesis of these factors in tissue preparations.

Fibrinogen (factor I)

The synthesis of fibrinogen in isolated perfused liver, in liver slices, and in isolated hepatocytes has been demonstrated by incorporation of radioactive amino acids or by immunologic methods [1–6]. Studies utilizing immunofluorescence techniques have indicated that the liver parenchymal cell is the site of fibrinogen synthesis [7–9]. Kupffer cells were found to stain for fibrinogen in one study [8]. However, under conditions of increased synthesis, Kupffer cells are generally devoid of fibrinogen [7], while hepatocytes stain intensely for fibrinogen [9]. This raises the possibility that the Kupffer cells are utilized for storage or removal of degradation products. Although fibrinogen is synthesized in the liver, hypofibrinogenemia is rare in patients with liver disease, and when present it may be more a result of fibrinogenolysis [10] or of disseminated intravascular coagulation [11] than of deficient production. Platelets also contain intracellular fibrinogen [12–15] (see Chap. 127). It has been suggested that fibrinogen may be synthesized in the megakaryocyte [15], but in other experiments no evidence for fibrinogen synthesis by megakaryocytes was obtained under conditions which permitted synthesis of actin [16].

Plasma fibrinogen is an "acute phase reactant," and its concentration increases in response to a variety of stimuli [17], including subcutaneous injection of saline [18] or administration of endotoxin [19,20], ACTH [20–22], growth hormone [23], serum [5], or fibrinogen degradation products [9,18,24]. Fibrin degradation products do not increase the rate of fibrinogen synthesis in rabbits [25–28]. ACTH appears to act by some mechanism other than stimulation of the adrenal cortex [21,22], and the effect of fibrinogen degradation products may be nonspecific, since other acute phase reactants are also stimulated by administration of these preparations [24].

Plasma fibrinogen levels in humans are increased in pregnancy [29], postoperatively [30], and in diabetes [31]. Fibrinogen turnover in humans increases with age and is further enhanced in patients with coronary artery disease [32].

Studies utilizing labeled fibrinogen in humans have indicated synthesis of from 1.7 to 5 g per day [4,33] in normal human subjects. Fibrinogen levels can increase from nearly undetectable levels to normal levels in 24 h in individuals receiving effective antiserum therapy following injection of Malayan pit viper venom, a powerful defibrinating agent [34].

Prothrombin (factor II), factor VII, factor IX, and factor X

Prothrombin and factors VII, IX, and X are synthesized in the liver, as indicated by studies on patients with liver disease [10,35] and as demonstrated in experiments on liver slices, isolated perfused liver, suspensions of liver cells, and cell-free liver preparations [36–46]. Studies employing immunofluorescence techniques have supported the concept that the liver is the site of synthesis of prothrombin [9,47,48]. There is evidence that kidney cells can also synthesize factor VII [42,43]. Both cytologic and biochemical studies have indicated that intracellular prothrombin is localized on microsomes [45,47–55].

Vitamin K is required for the maintenance of normal blood levels of these coagulation factors [56,57]. Vitamin K deficiency in vivo has no effect on protein synthesis generally [36,39,52,58]. Vitamin K is a growth factor for some microorganisms [59,60].

The mechanism of action of vitamin K has been studied in animals with dietary deficiency of vitamin K or treated with vitamin K antagonists, such as warfarin or dicumarol. In the normal liver, vitamin K is converted to phylloquinone epoxide by a microsomal epoxidase, and phylloquinone epoxide is converted back to vitamin K by a microsomal reductase [61–67]. Treatment with warfarin leads to accumulation of phylloquinone epoxide [61,62,67], and it has been proposed that the principal mechanism of action of the coumarin drugs is inhibition of regeneration of vitamin K from vitamin K epoxide [68].

Vitamin K acts in the conversion of a polypeptide precursor to the final coagulation factor [38,52,53,69–72]. A polypeptide precursor of prothrombin has been identified in plasma from human beings [73–78] and cows [79–81] with vitamin K deficiency and in the livers of rats with vitamin K deficiency [54,55,82–84]. The prothrombin precursor is found with either drug-induced or dietary vitamin K deficiency. Abnormal forms of factors VII [76,85], IX [76,78,86,87], and X [76,78,88] have also been identified in plasma from anticoagulant-treated human beings. The polypeptide precursor of prothrombin can be detected by reaction with antibodies to normal prothrombin [73,74] and by its ability to be activated by certain enzymes such as staphylocoagulase [75], trypsin [81], or components of the venom of *Echis carinatus* (saw-scaled viper) [81] and *Dispholidus typus* (boomslang snake) [81]. The precursor from human plasma can be activated slowly in a physiologic system [89].

In contrast to normal prothrombin, the precursor does not bind calcium and is not adsorbed to barium sulfate [74,80,81,90,91]. These properties are associated with the presence in prothrombin of a unique amino acid, γ-carboxyglutamic acid (Gla) [92–95]. Vitamin K is essential for the synthesis of this compound, which is formed by addition of CO_2 to the glutamic acid residues in the precursor of prothrombin [96–103]. Factor VII [104,105], factor IX [106,107], factor X [95,108,109] have also been shown to contain γ-carboxyglutamic acid.

Two additional vitamin K–dependent proteins distinct from prothrombin and factors VII, IX, and X have been purified from plasma. One of these proteins, protein C, is a precursor of a serine esterase [110–112], and appears to be autoprothrombin IIA [113], a previously described anticoagulant (see Chap. 136). The other, protein S [114], appears to function as a cofactor of protein C [115,116]. Proteins containing Gla have been detected in bone, nonosseous tissues, and in sites of ectopic calcification [117–121].

The production rate of the vitamin K–dependent factors can be very rapid, with normalization of the blood levels occurring within 10 to 12 h after oral administration of vitamin K to individuals previously treated with vitamin K antagonists [122,123]. The half-time of reappearance of factor VII after administering vitamin K to human subjects treated with vitamin K antagonists was between 250 and 360 min [124,125]. In a quantitative study in humans, the synthetic rate of prothrombin was found to be about 2.5 mg/kg per day [126]. Factor IX production in perfused rabbit liver is inversely proportional to the factor IX concentration in the perfusate, suggesting a feedback control mechanism [127].

There is general agreement that the levels of factors VII and X are increased in pregnancy [128–131]. Prothrombin (factor II) levels are normal [130,132] or slightly increased [129,130], and slight [128–130,132] to marked [123] increases in factor IX levels have been found. Diethylstilbestrol administration leads to a fur-

ther increase in factor IX levels in the puerperium [133]. The low level of factor X in a patient with a congenital deficiency of that factor was found to increase with pregnancy [134].

Estrogen-containing oral contraceptives will increase the levels of plasma factor VII [135], factors VII and X [136], or factors II, VII, and X [137]. Contraceptives containing only progestational hormones do not cause changes in these coagulation factors [128]. Administration of estrogens will also cause an increase in prothrombin levels in vitamin K–deficient male rats [139].

Factor V

The available evidence indicates that factor V is synthesized in the liver. Studies utilizing the immunofluorescence technique have demonstrated factor V in bovine liver cells, although differentiation between synthesis and storage was not possible [140]. Factor V is synthesized in isolated perfused rat liver [46,141], possibly in the Kupffer cells (macrophages) [46]. Animals with experimental liver damage or after hepatectomy have diminished levels of factor V [142,143], and it has been well established clinically that patients with liver disease may be deficient in this factor [10,35,144]. Although factor V is readily destroyed by fibrinolysins [145], activation of the fibrinolytic system appears not to be responsible for the low levels of factor V in liver disease [10,146]. Platelets contain factor V which appears to be intracellular, associated with α granules [147–149]. The site of synthesis of this fraction of factor V has not been determined.

It has been reported that factor V levels in humans increase slightly after the injection of epinephrine [150] but that no change is found after physical exercise [151]. Factor V levels are not changed by pregnancy [128,131,132].

Factor VIII

Most studies on factor VIII synthesis have considered only factor VIII coagulant activity (factor VIII:C or FVIII:C). Liver, spleen, monocyte-macrophage system, and kidney have all been suggested as possible sites of factor VIII synthesis, but none of these has been firmly established. Studies utilizing the immunofluorescence technique have not been conclusive [152]. In an in vivo study, the level of FVIII:C in hepatic venous blood was up to three times higher than that in peripheral venous blood, a result suggesting an abdominal organ as the source but permitting no specific conclusions to be drawn [153]. In experiments with isolated perfused organs it has been demonstrated that FVIII:C appears in perfusion fluid from spleen, liver, kidney, and the hind limb [41,46,127,154–158]. Perfusion of liver or spleen with plasma deficient in FVIII:C increased the yield of this material, suggesting a negative feedback mechanism [127]. In other experiments FVIII:C but not factor VIII–related antigen (FVIIIR:Ag) was released into the perfusate of rat [46,158] or pig [158] livers. FVIII:C release in the perfusate was enhanced by addition of factor VIII–related antigen (FVIIIR:Ag), serum, or cryoprecipitate to the perfusate [158]. Blockade of the monocyte-macrophage system prior to perfusion of rat liver inhibited the synthesis of FVIII:C [46]. Extraction of whole organs has yielded more specific results: of 13 different organs, including liver, spleen, marrow, and kidney, the spleen was the only one from which a large amount of FVIII:C could be extracted with citrate buffer [159].

There is further evidence that the spleen has a definite role in factor VIII homeostasis. In cross-circulation experiments between normal and hemophilic dogs, the FVIII:C level of the normal dog was unchanged, but that of the hemophilic dog increased significantly. If the normal dog was splenectomized, it was still able to contribute FVIII:C to the recipient but was unable to maintain its own FVIII:C level [160]. These results suggest that the spleen may store FVIII:C, and this idea is supported by the finding that FVIII:C levels increase severalfold in normal people after injection of epinephrine [161–165] or after severe exercise [163–171]. The rise in FVIII:C induced by epinephrine is prevented by β-adrenergic blocking agents [172]. It has been reported that splenectomy prevents the postepinephrine rise in FVIII:C levels [162], but contrary results have been obtained by others [165]. Contradictory results have been obtained also regarding the effect of splenectomy on the rise in FVIII:C levels after exercise [165,168,169]. Equivalent amounts of FVIII:C and FVIIIR:Ag are released by exercise and by epinephrine [163,164,169,170]. In some studies postepinephrine or postexercise FVIII:C had a normal half-life when administered to hemophilic patients [162,167], whereas in others, using cryoprecipitate as a source of FVIII:C, the half-life was shorter than expected [171].

Strongly opposed to the concept that the spleen is the primary site of factor VIII synthesis is the fact that splenectomy does not lead to hemophilia. Splenectomy has no effect on the FVIII:C levels of hemophilic dogs [160] and has no clinical effect on human hemophilia [173], further suggesting that the spleen has no regulatory effect on factor VIII.

The liver has not been generally regarded as the source of factor VIII because of the lack of a decrease in the level of this factor in patients with liver disease [10,35] and the absence of a major effect on FVIII:C levels as a result of experimental liver damage [174,175], although both depression and increases have been reported [176,177]. In human beings, marked elevation of FVIII:C levels may occur in association with fatal liver necrosis [178]. Perfusion experiments (see above) and transplant experiments, discussed below, provide evidence in favor of the liver as a major site of synthesis of FVIII:C.

It has been suggested that the monocyte-macrophage system is a source of FVIII:C [157,175]. Cultures of leukocytes [179], fibroblasts [180], and macrophages [181] have been reported to synthesize FVIII:C. However, the coagulant activity in these systems is tissue factor (factor III) rather than FVIII:C [182]. Immunofluorescent staining techniques have demonstrated factor VIII antigens in endothelial cells of blood vessels and in cells lining the splenic and hepatic sinusoids [183–185]. Synthesis of FVIIIR:Ag but not FVIII:C has been demonstrated in cultures of human endothelial cells [186–190] and of human fetal liver and spleen cells [185]. Factor VIIIR:Ag is also synthesized by guinea pig megakaryocytes in culture [191].

The most direct approach to the problem of the origin of factor VIII has been through transplantation of normal organs into hemophilic animals and the reverse. Normal spleen, liver, marrow, and kidney have been transplanted into hemophilic dogs [192–197]. Transplantation of normal spleens into hemophilic dogs has yielded inconclusive results. In one study, splenic transplantation resulted in a somewhat elevated level of FVIII:C for periods of a few weeks [192], but in other studies no significant elevations of FVIII:C levels were found [193,195,196]. Transplantation of normal livers into hemophilic dogs resulted in improved levels of FVIII:C [193–197]. Transplantation of the liver of a hemophilic dog into a normal dog resulted in a fall of factor VIII to 20 to 40 percent of normal, suggesting that other organs may also synthesize some FVIII:C [194, 197]. Transplantation of normal marrow [193] and kidney [196,197] into hemophilic dogs did not improve the FVIII:C level. The site of synthesis of FVIII:C is thus not clearly established. The finding of FVIIIR:Ag in endothelial cells [183–190] is consistent with the widespread distribution of factor VIII in the body and presents an attractive possibility, but one that remains to be proved.

Synthesis of factor VIII appears to involve a substance present in plasma. Patients with von Willebrand's disease frequently have low levels of FVIII:C and respond to the administration of fresh or aged normal plasma, normal serum, or plasma from patients with hemophilia with increased levels of FVIII:C beyond those which would be expected from the FVIII:C content of the administered material [198–202]. The increase in FVIII:C levels appears a few hours after the plasma has been administered, reaches a peak in 24 to 48 h, and then declines slowly over the next few days. The FVIII:C formed appears to be normal as judged by stability and activity in vitro [203]. However, studies of the effects of transfusion on FVIII:C levels in patients with von Willebrand's disease have demonstrated the appearance of procoagulant activity which persists in the circulation much longer than FVIIIR:Ag [204–206]. This finding is consistent with synthesis of a form of factor VIII lacking the antigenic sites characteristic of the normal molecule and therefore of low molecular weight (see Chap. 132). In one study a low-molecular-weight material with procoagulant activity was demonstrated in posttransfusion plasma [205]. However, others could not confirm this finding [206,207], and in one study the factor VIII induced by transfusion had antigenic activity as well as coagulant activity [207]. Normal subjects may also respond to administration of plasma with an elevation of their FVIII:C levels [208].

It is possible that there is a precursor of factor VIII in normal or aged or hemophilic plasma or serum which can be converted to FVIII:C by patients with von Willebrand's disease. A more fundamental mechanism may also be involved, with activation of the gene for FVIII:C synthesis by a substance present in hemophilic plasma but absent from the plasma of patients with von Willebrand's disease [209].

FVIII:C levels in patients with moderately severe von Willebrand's disease increase in response to exercise [201,210], as in normal people [163–171], and may increase in pregnancy [211,212]. FVIII:C increased concomitantly in a pregnant patient with von Willebrand's disease, but the bleeding time remained prolonged [212]. Normal people may show an increase in FVIII:C levels during pregnancy [131,211] and while taking oral contraceptives [133]. Elevated FVIII:C levels also occur in man in a variety of clinical and experimental conditions [210].

Liver transplantation experiments [213] and perfusion experiments [158] employing normal pigs and pigs with von Willebrand's disease have been performed. Livers from normal animals and from animals with von Willebrand's disease appear to be able to synthesize factor VIII:C but not the complete factor VIII complex [158,213].

Factor VIII levels increase in normal individuals or patients with hemophilia or von Willebrand's disease after administration of vasopressin or vasopressin analogs, particularly desamino-8-D-arginine vasopressin (dDAVP) [214–222]. These compounds also cause release of plasminogen activator [214,219]. Plasma levels of factor VIII:C, factor VIIIR:Ag, and the cofactor for ristocetin-induced platelet aggregation, FVIIIR:RCo, all increase promptly after administration of such agents as dDAVP [218–220,222]. The FVIII:C and FVIIIR:Ag produced after administration of dDAVP are apparently normal both in vitro and in vivo [218–220].

The biosynthesis of factor VIII has been reviewed in detail [223].

Factor XI

Little evidence is available to indicate the source of factor XI in the body. Factor XI levels have been reported to be diminished in patients with liver disease [224–226], which suggests that this factor may be produced in the liver. It is not suppressed by treatment with vitamin K antagonists [225–227]. Factor XI appears to be synthesized by isolated perfused rat liver [141]. Factor XI is bound tightly to platelets [228] but does not appear to be synthesized in platelets or megakaryocytes. Factor XI levels fall during pregnancy to about two-thirds of normal [132,229].

Factor XII

The source of factor XII in the body is also obscure. The level of factor XII in liver disease has been reported to be decreased [230], but this has not been confirmed [231]. Factor XII synthesis in isolated perfused rat liver has been reported [141].

Factor XIII

Up to 50 percent of the total factor XIII in the blood is associated with platelets [232,233]. Platelet factor XIII is not derived from plasma factor XIII and therefore may be synthesized by megakaryocytes [233,234]. Immuno-fluorescence studies have demonstrated factor XIII antigen in megakaryocytes but not in liver cells [235]. Factor XIII levels have been found to be decreased in patients with hepatic disease [236–239], and it has been suggested that this is caused by an inhibitor or by failure of the liver to "activate" factor XIII [236]. These studies leave uncertain the role of the liver in factor XIII production.

Prekallikrein (Fletcher factor)

Prekallikrein (Fletcher factor) concentration is reduced in plasma of patients with severe liver disease [240–242], suggesting this coagulation factor is synthesized in the liver. Estrogen administration increases the plasma level of prekallikrein [240].

High-molecular-weight kininogen

The concentration of high-molecular-weight kininogen is reduced in the plasma of patients with severe liver disease [243,244] or of rabbits poisoned with carbon tetrachloride [244], suggesting this factor is also synthesized in the liver.

References

1. Miller, L. L., Bly, C. G., Watson, M. L., and Bale, W. F.: The dominant role of the liver in plasma protein synthesis: A direct study of the isolated perfused rat liver with the aid of lysine-ε-C¹⁴. *J. Exp. Med.* 94:431, 1951.
2. Miller, L. L., and Bale, W. F.: Synthesis of all plasma protein fractions except gamma globulins by the liver. *J. Exp. Med.* 99:125, 1954.
3. John, D. W., and Miller, L. L.: Influence of actinomycin D and puromycin on net synthesis of plasma albumin and fibrinogen by the isolated perfused rat liver. *J. Biol. Chem.* 241:4817, 1966.
4. Straub, P. W.: A study of fibrinogen production by human liver slices *in vitro* by an immunoprecipitin method. *J. Clin. Invest.* 42:130, 1963.
5. Pickart, L. R., and Pilgeram, L. O.: The role of thrombin in fibrinogen biosynthesis. *Thromb. Diath. Haemorrh.* 17:358, 1967.
6. Crane, L. J., and Miller, D. L.: Synthesis and secretion of fibrinogen and albumin by isolated rat hepatocytes. *Biochem. Biophys. Res. Commun.* 60:1269, 1974.

7. Forman, W. B., and Barnhart M. I.: Cellular site for fibrinogen synthesis. *JAMA 187:*128, 1964.

8. Hamashima, Y., Harter, J. G., and Coons, A. H.: The localization of albumin and fibrinogen in human liver cells. *J. Cell Biol. 20:*271, 1964.

9. Barnhart, M. I., and Noonan, S. M.: Cellular control mechanisms for blood clotting proteins. *Thromb. Diath. Haemorrh. (Suppl.) 54:* 59, 1973.

10. Finkbiner, R. B., McGovern, J. J., Goldstein, R., and Bunker, J. P.: Coagulation defects in liver disease, and response to transfusion during surgery. *Am. J. Med. 26:*199, 1959.

11. Tytgat, G. N., Collen, D., and Verstraete, M.: Metabolism of fibrinogen in cirrhosis of the liver. *J. Clin. Invest. 50:*1690, 1971.

12. Sokal, G.: Étude morphologique des plaquettes sanguines et de la métamorphose visqueuse au moyen d'anti-sérums fluorescents antifibrinogène et antiplaquettes. *Acta Haematol. (Basel) 28:*313, 1962.

13. Gokcen, M., and Yunis, E.: Fibrinogen as a part of platelet structure. *Nature 200:*590, 1963.

14. Nachman, R. L., Marcus, A. J., and Zucker-Franklin, D.: Subcellular localization of platelet fibrinogen. *Blood 24:*853, 1964.

15. Cooper, I. A., and Firkin, B. G.: Amino acid transport into human platelets and subsequent incorporation into protein. *Thromb. Diath. Haemorrh. 23:*140, 1970.

16. Nachman, R., Levine, R., and Jaffe, E.: Synthesis of actin by cultured guinea pig megakaryocytes — Complex formation with fibrin. *Biochim. Biophys. Acta 543:*91, 1978.

17. Koj, A., and McFarlane, A. S.: Effect of endotoxin on plasma albumin and fibrinogen synthesis rates in rabbits as measured by the (^{14}C) carbonate method. *Biochem. J. 108:*137, 1968.

18. Bocci, V., and Pacini, A.: Factors regulating plasma protein synthesis. II. Influence of fibrinogenolytic products on plasma fibrinogen concentration. *Thromb. Diath. Haemorrh. 29:*63, 1973.

19. Lerner, R. G., Rapaport, S. I., Siemsen, J. K., and Spitzer, J. M.: Disappearance of fibrinogen-^{131}I after endotoxin: Effects of a first and second injection. *Am. J. Physiol. 214:*532, 1968.

20. Atencio, A. C., and Lorand, L.: Effect of ACTH on biosynthesis of fibrinogen in the rabbit. *Am. J. Physiol. 219:*1161, 1970.

21. Chen, Y., and Reeve, E. B.: ACTH stimulation of fibrinogen biosynthesis. *Am. J. Physiol. 227:*940, 1974.

22. Seligsohn, U., Rapaport, S. I., and Kuefler, P. R.: Extra-adrenal effect of ACTH on fibrinogen synthesis. *Am. J. Physiol. 224:*1172, 1973.

23. Jeejeebhoy, K. N., Bruce-Robertson, A., Sodtke, U., and Foley, M.: The effect of growth hormone on fibrinogen synthesis. *Biochem. J. 119:*243, 1970.

24. Miller, L. L., and John, D. W.: Factors affecting net fibrinogen biosynthesis by the isolated, perfused rat liver. *Thromb. Diath. Haemorrh. (Suppl.) 39:*127, 1970.

25. Kessler, C. M., and Bell, W. R.: Regulation of fibrinogen biosynthesis: Effect of fibrin degradation products, low-molecular-weight peptides of fibrinogenolysis, and fibrinopeptides A and B. *J. Lab. Clin. Med. 93:*758, 1979.

26. Kessler, C. M., and Bell, W. R.: The effect of homologous thrombin and fibrinogen degradation products on fibrinogen synthesis in rabbits. *J. Lab. Clin. Med. 93:*768, 1979.

27. Ittyerah, T. R., Weidner, N., Wochner, R. D., and Sherman, L. A.: Effect of fibrin degradation products and thrombin on fibrinogen biosynthesis. *Br. J. Haematol. 43:*66, 1979.

28. Kessler, C. M., and Bell, W. R.: Stimulation of fibrinogen biosynthesis: A possible functional role of fibrinogen degradation products. *Blood 55:*40, 1980.

29. Plass, E. D., and Matthew, C. W.: Plasma protein fractions in normal pregnancy, labor, and puerperium. *Am. J. Obstet. Gynecol. 12:*346, 1926.

30. Aronsen, K.-F., Ekelund, G., Kindmark, C.-O., and Laurell, C.-B.: Sequential changes of plasma proteins after surgical trauma. *Scand. J. Clin. Lab. Invest. 29 (Suppl. 124):*127, 1972.

31. Jones, R. L., and Peterson, C. M.: Reduced fibrinogen survival in diabetes mellitus: A reversible phenomenon. *J. Clin. Invest. 63:*485, 1979.

32. Pilgeram, L. O.: Turnover rate of autologous plasma fibrinogen-^{14}C

in subjects with coronary thrombosis. *Thromb. Diath. Haemorrh. 20:*31, 1968.

33. Takeda, Y.: Studies of the metabolism and distribution of fibrinogen in healthy men with autologous ^{125}I-labeled fibrinogen. *J. Clin. Invest. 45:*103, 1966.

34. Chan, K. E.: Regeneration of fibrinogen after defibrination with the Malayan pit viper venom. *Thromb. Diath. Haemorrh. (Suppl.) 13:*231, 1964.

35. Rapaport, S. I., Ames, S. B., Mikkelsen, S., and Goodman, J. R.: Plasma clotting factors in chronic hepatocellular disease. *N. Engl. J. Med. 263:*278, 1960.

36. Pool, J. G., and Robinson, J.: In vitro synthesis of coagulation factors by rat liver slices. *Am. J. Physiol. 196:*423, 1959.

37. Pool, J. G., and Borchgrevink, C. F.: Comparison of rat liver response to coumarin administered in vivo versus in vitro. *Am. J. Physiol. 206:*229, 1964.

38. Babior, B. M.: The role of vitamin K in clotting factor synthesis. I. Evidence for the participation of vitamin K in the conversion of a polypeptide precursor to factor VII. *Biochim. Biophys. Acta 123:* 606, 1966.

39. Suttie, J. W.: Control of prothrombin and factor VII biosynthesis by vitamin K. *Arch. Biochem. 118:*116, 1967.

40. Olson, J. P., Miller, L. L., and Troup, S. B.: Synthesis of clotting factors by the isolated perfused rat liver. *J. Clin. Invest. 45:*690, 1966.

41. Dodds, W. J.: Storage, release, and synthesis of coagulation factors in isolated perfused organs. *Am. J. Physiol. 217:*879, 1969.

42. Prydz, H.: Studies on proconvertin (factor VII). V. Biosynthesis in suspension cultures of rat liver cells. *Scand. J. Clin. Lab. Invest. 16:*540, 1964.

43. Prydz, H.: Studies on proconvertin (factor VII). VI. Further studies on the biosynthesis of factor VII in rat cell suspensions. *Scand. J. Clin. Lab. Invest. 17:*143, 1965.

44. Lowenthal, J., and Simmons, E. L.: Failure of actinomycin D to inhibit appearance of clotting factor activity by vitamin K in vitro. *Experientia 23:*421, 1967.

45. Shah, D. V., and Suttie, J. W.: The vitamin K dependent in vitro production of prothrombin. *Biochem. Biophys. Res. Commun. 60:* 1397, 1974.

46. Shaw, E., Giddings, J. C., Peake, I. R., and Bloom, A. L.: Synthesis of procoagulant factor VIII, factor VIII–related antigen, and other coagulation factors by the isolated, perfused rat liver. *Br. J. Haematol. 41:*585, 1979.

47. Anderson, G. F., and Barnhart, M. I.: Prothrombin synthesis in the dog. *Am. J. Physiol. 206:*929, 1964.

48. Barnhart, M. I.: Cellular site for prothrombin synthesis. *Am. J. Physiol. 199:*360, 1960.

49. Gowsami, P., and Munro, H. N.: The role of ribonucleic acid in the formation of prothrombin activity by rat-liver microsomes. *Biochim. Biophys. Acta 55:*410, 1962.

50. Helgeland, L., and Laland, S.: The localization of prothrombin in rat-liver cell fractions. *Biochim. Biophys. Acta 62:*200, 1962.

51. Barnhart, M. J., and Anderson, G. F.: Cellular study of drug alteration of prothrombin synthesis. *Biochem. Pharmacol. 9:*23, 1962.

52. Hill, R. B., et al.: Vitamin K and biosynthesis of protein and prothrombin. *J. Biol. Chem. 243:*3930, 1968.

53. Shah, D. V., and Suttie, J. W.: The effect of vitamin K and warfarin on rat liver prothrombin concentrations. *Arch. Biochem. Biophys. 150:*91, 1972.

54. Morrisey, J. J., Jones, J. P., and Olson, R. E.: Isolation and characterization of isoprothrombin in the rat. *Biochim. Biophys. Res. Commun. 54:*1075, 1973.

55. Carlisle, T. L., Shah, D. V., Schlegel, R., and Suttie, J. W.: Plasma abnormal prothrombin and microsomal prothrombin precursor in various species. *Proc. Soc. Exp. Biol. Med. 148:*140, 1975.

56. Douglas, A. S.: Some observations on the coagulation defect in vitamin K deficiency. *J. Clin. Pathol. 11:*261, 1958.

57. Spaet, T. J., and Kropatkin, M.: Studies on "prothrombin derivatives" in vitamin K deficiency. *Arch. Intern. Med. 102:*558, 1958.

58. Paolucci, A. M., Gaetani, S., and Johnson, B. C.: Vitamin K e sintesi proteica. I. Sintesi indotta de triptofaro pirrolasi in ratti: Caventi di vitamin K. *Quad. Nutr. 24:*275, 1964.

59. Woolley, D. W., and McCarter, J. R.: Antihemorrhagic compounds as growth factors for the Johne's bacillus. *Proc. Soc. Exp. Biol. Med.* 45:357, 1940.

60. Lev, M.: The growth-promoting activity of compounds of the vitamin K group and analogues for a rumen strain of *Fusiformis nigrescens. J. Gen. Microbiol.* 20:697, 1959.

61. Matschiner, J. T., Bell, R. G., Amelotti, J. M., and Knauer, T. E.: Isolation and characterization of a new metabolite of phylloquinone in the rat. *Biochim. Biophys. Acta* 201:309, 1970.

62. Bell, R. G., Sadowski, J. A., and Matschiner, J. T.: Mechanism of action of warfarin: Warfarin and metabolism of vitamin K_1. *Biochemistry* 11:1959, 1972.

63. Bell, R. G., and Matschiner, J. T.: Vitamin K activity of phylloquinone oxide. *Arch. Biochem. Biophys.* 141:473, 1970.

64. Bell, R. G., and Matschiner, J. T.: Warfarin and the inhibition of vitamin K activity by an oxide metabolite. *Nature* 237:32, 1972.

65. Willingham, A. K., and Matschiner, J. T.: Changes in phylloquinone epoxidase activity related to prothrombin synthesis and microsomal clotting activity in the rat. *Biochem. J.* 140:435, 1974.

66. Matschiner, J. T., Zimmerman, A., and Bell, R. G.: The influence of warfarin on vitamin K epoxide reductase. *Thromb. Diath. Haemorrh. (Suppl.)* 57:45, 1974.

67. Zimmerman, A., and Matschiner, J. T.: Biochemical basis of hereditary resistance to warfarin in the rat. *Biochem. Pharmacol.* 23:1033, 1974.

68. Bell, R. G.: Metabolism of vitamin K and prothrombin synthesis: Anticoagulants and the vitamin K–epoxide cycle. *Fed. Proc. 37:* 2599, 1978.

69. Bell, R. G., and Matschiner, J. T.: Synthesis and destruction of prothrombin in the rat. *Arch. Biochem. Biophys.* 135:152, 1969.

70. Suttie, J. W.: The effect of cycloheximide administration on vitamin K-stimulated prothrombin formation. *Arch. Biochem. Biophys.* 141:571, 1970.

71. Prydz, H., and Gaudernack, G.: Studies on the biosynthesis of factor VII (proconvertin): The mode of action of warfarin. *Biochim. Biophys. Acta* 230:373, 1971.

72. Pereira, M., and Couri, D.: Studies on the site of action of dicoumarol on prothrombin synthesis. *Biochim. Biophys. Acta* 237: 348, 1971.

73. Niléhn, J. E., and Ganrot, P. O.: Plasma prothrombin during treatment with dicoumarol. I. Immunochemical determination of its concentration in plasma. *Scand. J. Clin. Lab. Invest.* 22:17, 1968.

74. Ganrot, P. O., and Niléhn, J. E.: Plasma prothrombin during treatment with dicoumarol. II. Demonstration of an abnormal prothrombin fraction. *Scand. J. Clin. Lab. Invest.* 22:23, 1968.

75. Josso, F., Lavergne, J. M., Gouault, M., Prou-Wartelle, O., and Soulier, J. P.: Différents états moléculaires du facteur II (prothrombine): Leur étude à l'aide de la staphylocoagulase et d'anticorps anti-facteur II. *Thromb. Diath. Haemorrh.* 20:88, 1968.

76. Denson, K. W. E.: The levels of factors II, VII, IX and X by antibody neutralization techniques in the plasma of patients receiving phenindione therapy. *Br. J. Haematol.* 20:643, 1971.

77. Ganrot, P. O., and Niléhn, J. E.: Synthesis of an abnormal prothrombin in malnutrition and biliary obstruction and during dicoumarol treatment. *Scand. J. Clin. Lab. Invest.* 28:245, 1971.

78. Reekers, P. P. M., Lindhout, M. J., Kop-Klaassen, B. H. M., and Hemker, H. C.: Demonstration of three anomalous plasma proteins induced by a vitamin K antagonist. *Biochim. Biophys. Acta* 317:559, 1973.

79. Malhotra, O. P., and Carter, J. R.: Isolation and purification of prothrombin from dicoumarolized steers. *J. Biol. Chem.* 246:2665, 1971.

80. Stenflo, J., and Ganrot, P. O.: Vitamin K and the biosynthesis of prothrombin. I. Identification and purification of a dicoumarol-induced abnormal prothrombin from bovine plasma. *J. Biol. Chem.* 247:8160, 1972.

81. Nelsestuen, G. L., and Suttie, J. W.: The purification and properties of an abnormal prothrombin protein produced by dicoumarol-treated cows: A comparison to normal prothrombin. *J. Biol. Chem.* 247:8176, 1972.

82. Suttie, J. W.: Mechanism of action of vitamin K: Demonstration of a liver precursor of prothrombin. *Science* 179:192, 1973.

83. Shah, D. V., Suttie, J. W., and Grant, G. A.: A rat liver protein with potential thrombin activity: Properties and partial purification. *Arch. Biochem. Biophys.* 159:483, 1973.

84. Esmon, C. T., Grant, G. A., and Suttie, J. W.: Purification of an apparent rat liver prothrombin precursor: Characterization and comparison to normal rat prothrombin. *Biochemistry* 14:1595, 1975.

85. Howarth, D. J., Brozović, M., Stirling, Y., and Reed, M.: Factor VII during warfarin treatment. *Scand. J. Haematol.* 12:346, 1974.

86. Larrieu, M. J., and Meyer, D.: Abnormal factor IX during anticoagulant treatment. *Lancet* 2:1085, 1970.

87. Veltkamp, J. J., Muis, H., Muller, A. D., Hemker, H. C., and Loeliger, E. A.: Additional evidence for the existence of a precursor molecule of the prothrombin complex in oral anticoagulation. *Thromb. Diath. Haemorrh.* 25:312, 1971.

88. Prydz, H., and Gladhaug, A.: Factor X: Immunological studies. *Thromb. Diath. Haemorrh.* 25:157, 1971.

89. Hemker, H. C., Muller, A. D., and Loeliger, E. A.: Two types of prothrombin in vitamin K deficiency. *Thromb. Diath. Haemorrh.* 23:633, 1970.

90. Nelsestuen, G. L., and Suttie, J. W.: Mode of action of vitamin K: Calcium binding properties of bovine prothrombin. *Biochemistry* 11:4961, 1972.

91. Stenflo, J., and Ganrot, P. O.: Binding of Ca^{2+} to normal and dicoumarol-induced prothrombin. *Biochem. Biophys. Res. Commun.* 50:98, 1973.

92. Stenflo, J., Fernlund, P., Egan, W., and Rolpstorff, P.: Vitamin K dependent modifications of glutamic acid residues in prothrombin. *Proc. Natl. Acad. Sci. U.S.A.* 71:2730, 1974.

93. Magnusson, S., Sottrup-Jansen, L., Petersen, T. E., Morris, H. R., and Dell, A.: Primary structure of the vitamin K–dependent part of prothrombin. *FEBS Lett.* 44:189, 1974.

94. Nelsestuen, G. L., Zytkovicz, T. H., and Howard, J. B.: The mode of action of vitamin K: Identification of γ-carboxyglutamic acid as a component of prothrombin. *J. Biol. Chem.* 249:6347, 1974.

95. Zytkovicz, T. H., and Nelsestuen, G. L.: [³H] Diborate reduction of vitamin K–dependent calcium-binding proteins: Identification of a unique amino acid. *J. Biol. Chem.* 250:2968, 1975.

96. Girardot, J.-M., Delaney, R., and Johnson, B. C.: Carboxylation, the completion step in prothrombin biosynthesis. *Biochem. Biophys. Res. Commun.* 59:1197, 1974.

97. Esmon, C. T., Sadowski, J. A., and Suttie, J. W.: A new carboxylation reaction: The vitamin K–dependent incorporation of $H^{14}CO_3$ into prothrombin. *J. Biol. Chem.* 250:4744, 1975.

98. Sadowski, J. A., Esmon, D. T., and Suttie, J. W.: Vitamin-K–dependent carboxylase: Requirements of the rat liver microsomal enzyme system. *J. Biol. Chem.* 251:2770, 1976.

99. Mack, D. O., Suen, E. T., Girardot, J. M., Miller, J. A., Delaney, R., and Johnson, B. C.: Soluble enzyme system for vitamin K–dependent carboxylation. *J. Biol. Chem.* 251:3269, 1976.

100. Suttie, J. W., Hageman, J. M., Lehrman, S. R., and Rich, D. H.: Vitamin K–dependent carboxylase: Development of a peptide substrate. *J. Biol. Chem.* 251:5827, 1976.

101. Esmon, C. T., and Suttie, J. W.: Vitamin K–dependent carboxylase: Solubilization and properties. *J. Biol. Chem.* 251:6238, 1976.

102. Jones, J. P., Gardner, E. J., Cooper, T. G., and Olson, R. E.: Vitamin K–dependent carboxylation of peptide-bound glutamate: The active species of "CO_2" utilized by the membrane-bound preprothrombin carboxylase. *J. Biol. Chem.* 252:7738, 1977.

103. Esnouf, M. P., et al.: Evidence for the involvement of superoxide in vitamin K–dependent carboxylation of glutamic acid residues of prothrombin. *Biochem. J.* 174:345, 1978.

104. Broze, G. J., Jr., and Majerus, P. W.: Purification and properties of human coagulation factor VII. *J. Biol. Chem.* 255:1242, 1980.

105. Bajaj, S. P., Rapaport, S. I., and Brown, S. F.: Isolation and characterization of human factor VII: Activation of factor VII by factor Xa. *J. Biol. Chem.* 256:253, 1981.

106. DiScipio, R. G., Kurachi, K., and Davie, E. W.: Activation of human factor IX (Christmas factor). *J. Clin. Invest.* 61:1528, 1978.

107. Fryklund, L., Borg, H., and Anderssen, L.-O.: Amino-terminal sequence of human factor IX: Presence of γ-carboxyl glutamic acid residues. *FEBS Lett.* 65:187, 1976.

108. Enfield, D. L., Ericsson, L. H., Walsh, K. A., Neurath, H., and

Titani, K.: Bovine factor X₁ (Stuart factor): Primary structure of the light chain. *Proc. Natl. Acad. Sci. U.S.A.* 72:16, 1975.

109. Howard, J. B., and Nelsestuen, G. L.: Isolation and characterization of vitamin K–dependent regions of bovine clotting factor X. *Proc. Natl. Acad. Sci. U.S.A.* 72:1281, 1975.

110. Stenflo, J.: A new vitamin K–dependent protein: Purification from bovine plasma and preliminary characterization. *J. Biol. Chem.* 251:355, 1976.

111. Esmon, C. T., Stenflo, J., Suttie, J. W., and Jackson, C. M.: A new vitamin K–dependent protein: A phospholipid binding zymogen of a serine esterase. *J. Biol. Chem.* 251:6238, 1976.

112. Kisiel, W.: Human plasma protein C. Isolation, characterization, and mechanism of activation by α-thrombin. *J. Clin. Invest.* 64: 761, 1979.

113. Seegers, W. H., Novoa, E., Henry, R. L., and Hassouna, H. I.: Relationship of "new" vitamin K–dependent protein C and "old" autoprothrombin II-A. *Thromb. Res.* 8:543, 1976.

114. DiScipio, R. G., Hermodson, M. A., Yates, S. G., and Davie, E. W.: A comparison of human prothrombin, factor IX (Christmas factor), factor X (Stuart factor), and protein S. *Biochemistry* 16:698, 1977.

115. Walker, F. J.: Regulation of activated protein C by a new protein. A possible function for bovine protein S. *J. Biol. Chem.* 255:5521, 1980.

116. Walker, F. J.: Regulation of activated protein C by protein S: The role of phospholipid in factor Va inactivation. *J. Biol. Chem.* 256: 11128, 1981.

117. Hauschka, P. V., Lian, J. B., and Gallop, P. M.: Direct identification of the calcium-binding amino acid, γ-carboxyglutamate, in mineralized tissue. *Proc. Natl. Acad. Sci. U.S.A.* 72:3925, 1975.

118. Lian, J. B., Prien, F. L., Jr., Glimcher, M. J., and Gallop, P. M.: The presence of protein-bound γ-carboxyglutamic acid in calcium-containing renal calculi. *J. Clin. Invest.* 59:1151, 1977.

119. Poser, J. W., Esch, F. S., Ling, N. C., and Price, P. A.: Isolation and sequence of the vitamin K–dependent protein from human bone. *J. Biol. Chem.* 255:8685, 1980.

120. Price, P. A., and Baukol, S. A.: 1,25-Dihydroxyvitamin D₃ increases synthesis of the vitamin K–dependent bone protein by osteosarcoma cells. *J. Biol. Chem.* 255:11660, 1980.

121. Price, P. A., Williamson, M. K., and Lothringer, W.: Origin of the vitamin K–dependent bone protein found in plasma and its clearance by kidney and bone. *J. Biol. Chem.* 256:12760, 1981.

122. Chalmers, J. N. M., Dixon, M. F., and Polack, W.: Antagonistic effect of oral vitamin K₁ on the action of ethyl biscoumacetate and phenylindanedione. *Br. Med. J.* 2:956, 1954.

123. Loeliger, E. A., Hensen, A., Veltkamp, J. J., van der Meer, J., and Hemker, H. C.: On the metabolism of factor IX, in *The Hemophilias,* edited by K. M. Brinkhous. University of North Carolina Press, Chapel Hill, 1964, p. 159.

124. Loeliger, E. A., vanderEsch, B., Cleton, F. J., Booij, H. L., and Mattern, M. J.: On the metabolism of factor VII, in *Proceedings of the 7th Congress of the European Society for Haematology.* London, 1960, part II, p. 764.

125. Marder, V. J., and Shulman, N. R.: Clinical aspects of congenital factor VII deficiency. *Am. J. Med.* 37:182, 1964.

126. Shapiro, S. S., and Martinez, J.: Human prothrombin metabolism in normal man and hypocoagulable subjects. *J. Clin. Invest.* 48: 1292, 1969.

127. Dodds, W. J., and Hoyer, L. W.: Coagulation activities in perfused organs: Regulation by addition of animal plasmas. *Br. J. Haematol.* 26:497, 1974.

128. Fresh, J. W., Ferguson, J. H., and Lewis, J. H.: Blood clotting studies in parturient women and the newborn. *Obstet. Gynec.* 7:117, 1956.

129. Ratnoff, O. D., and Holland, T. R.: Coagulation components in normal and abnormal pregnancies. *Ann. N.Y. Acad. Sci.* 75:626, 1958.

130. Pechet, L., and Alexander, B.: Increased clotting factors in pregnancy. *N. Engl. J. Med.* 265:1093, 1961.

131. Todd, M. E., Thompson, J. H., Jr., Bowie, E. J. W., and Owen, C. A., Jr.: Changes in blood coagulation during pregnancy. *Mayo Clin. Proc.* 40:370, 1965.

132. Nossel, H. L., Lanzkowsky, P., Levy, S., Mibashan, R. S., and Hansen, J. D. L.: A study of coagulation factor levels in women

during labour and in their newborn infants. *Thromb. Diath. Haemorrh.* 16:185, 1966.

133. Daniel, D. G., Bloom, A. L., Giddings, J. C., Campbell, H., and Turnbull, A. C.: Increased factor IX levels in puerperium during administration of diethylstilbestrol. *Br. Med. J.* 1:801, 1968.

134. Brody, J. I., and Finch, S. C.: Improvement of factor X deficiency during pregnancy. *N. Engl. J. Med.* 263:996, 1960.

135. Egeberg, O., and Owren, P. A.: Oral contraception and blood coagulability. *Br. Med. J.* 1:220, 1963.

136. Poller, L., Thomson, J. M., and Thomas, W.: Oestrogen/progestogen oral contraception and blood clotting: A long-term follow-up. *Br. Med. J.* 4:648, 1971.

137. Hougie, C., Rutherford, R. W., Banks, A. L., and Coburn, W. A.: Effect of a progestin-estrogen oral contraceptive on blood coagulation. *Metabolism* 14:411, 1965.

138. Poller, L., Thomson, J. M., Thomas, W., and Wray, C.: Blood clotting and platelet aggregation during oral progestogen contraception: A follow-up study. *Br. Med. J.* 1:705, 1971.

139. Matschiner, J. T., and Bell, R. G.: Effect of sex and sex hormones on plasma prothrombin and vitamin K deficiency. *Proc. Soc. Exp. Biol. Med.* 144:316, 1973.

140. Barnhart, M. I., Ferar, J., and Aoki, N.: Demonstration of Ac-globulin in bovine hepatocytes. *Fed. Proc.* 22:164, 1963.

141. Owen, C. A., and Bowie, E. J. W.: Generation of coagulation factors V, XI, and XII by the isolated rat liver. *Haemostasis* 6:205, 1977.

142. Sykes, E. M., Seegers, W. H., and Ware, A. G.: Effects of acute liver damage on Ac-globulin activity of plasma. *Proc. Soc. Exp. Biol. Med.* 67:506, 1948.

143. Mann, F. D., Shonyo, E. S., and Mann, F. C.: Effect of removal of the liver on blood coagulation. *Am. J. Physiol.* 164:111, 1951.

144. Owren, P. A.: Diagnostic and prognostic significance of plasma prothrombin and factor V levels in parenchymatous hepatitis and obstructive jaundice. *Scand. J. Clin. Lab. Invest.* 1:131, 1949.

145. Lewis, J. H., Howe, A. C., and Ferguson, J. H.: Thrombin formation. II. Effects of lysin (fibrinolysin, plasmin) on prothrombin, Ac-globulin, and tissue thromboplastin. *J. Clin. Invest.* 28:1507, 1949.

146. Ratnoff, O. D., and Donaldson, V. H.: Physiologic and pathologic effects of increased fibrinolytic activity in man. *Am. J. Cardiol.* 6: 378, 1960.

147. Breederveld, K., Giddings, J. C., ten Cate, J. W., and Bloom, A. L.: The localization of factor V within normal human platelets and the demonstration of a platelet-factor V antigen in congenital factor V deficiency. *Br. J. Haematol.* 29:405, 1975.

148. Vicic, W. J., Lages, B., and Weiss, H. J.: Release of human platelet factor V activity is induced by both collagen and ADP and is inhibited by aspirin. *Blood* 56:448, 1980.

149. Tracy, P. B., Eide, L. L., Bowie, E. J. W., and Mann, K. G.: Radioimmunoassay of factor V in human plasma and platelets. *Blood* 60:59, 1982.

150. Forwell, G. D., and Ingram, G. I. C.: The effect of adrenalin infusion on human blood coagulation. *J. Physiol.* 135:371, 1957.

151. Iatridis, S. G., and Ferguson, J. H.: Effect of physical exercise on blood clotting and fibrinolysis. *J. Appl. Physiol.* 18:337, 1963.

152. Barnhart, M. I.: Immunochemistry, in *Blood Clotting Enzymology,* edited by W. H. Seegers. Academic, New York, 1967, p. 217.

153. Gardikas, C., Bakaloudis, P., Hatzioannou, J., and Kokkinos, D.: The factor VIII concentration of the hepatic venous blood. *Br. J. Haematol.* 11:380, 1965.

154. Sise, H. S., Newcombe, J. F., McDermott, W. V., and Norman, J. C.: Inflow-outflow levels of blood coagulation factors in humans during pig liver perfusion for liver failure. *Fed. Proc.* 25:620, 1966.

155. Norman, J. C., Lambilliotte, J., Kojima, Y., and Sise, H. S.: Antihemophilic factor release by perfused liver and spleen: Relationship to hemophilia. *Science* 158:1060, 1967.

156. Norman, J. C., and Sise, H. E.: An auxiliary source of AHF for hemophilia: Experimental studies on isolated spleen perfusions. *J. Natl. Med. Assoc.* 59:330, 1967.

157. Webster, W. P., Reddick, R. L., Roberts, H. R., and Penick, G. D.: Release of factor VIII (antihaemophilic factor) from perfused organs and tissues. *Nature* 213:1146, 1967.

158. Owen, C. A., Jr., Bowie, E. J. W., and Fass, D. N.: Generation of

factor VIII coagulant activity by isolated, perfused neonatal pig livers and adult rat livers. *Br. J. Haematol.* 43:307, 1979.

159. Pool, J. G.: Antihemophilic globulin (AHG, factor VIII) activity in spleen. *Fed. Proc.* 25:317, 1966.

160. Weaver, R. A., Price, R. E., and Langdell, R. D.: Antihemophilic factor in cross-circulated normal and hemophilic dogs. *Am. J. Physiol.* 206:335, 1964.

161. Ingram, G. I. C.: Increase in antihaemophilic globulin activity following infusion by adrenalins. *J. Physiol.* 156:217, 1961.

162. Libre, E. P., Cowan, D. H., Watkins, S. P., Jr., and Shulman, N. R.: Relationships between spleen, platelets and factor VIII levels. *Blood* 31:358, 1969.

163. Prentice, C. R. M., Forbes, C. D., and Smith, S. M.: Rise of factor VIII after exercise and adrenaline infusion, measured by immunologic and biologic techniques. *Thromb. Res.* 1:493, 1972.

164. Denson, K. W. E.: The detection of factor VIII-like antigen in haemophilic carriers and in patients with raised levels of biologically active factor VIII. *Br. J. Haematol.* 24:451, 1973.

165. Goudemand, M., Foucaut, M., Habay, D., and Parquet-Gernez, A.: Les Variations du taux de facteur VIII au cours de l'exercise musculaire: Essai d'interprétation. *Nouv. Rev. Fr. Hematol.* 4:315, 1964.

166. Rizza, C. R.: Effect of exercise on the level of antihaemophilic globulin in human blood. *J. Physiol.* 156:128, 1961.

167. Ikkala, E., Myllylä, G., and Nevanlinna, H. R.: Normal and post-exercise plasma transfusion in patients with haemophilia A and von Willebrand's disease. *Scand. J. Haematol.* 1:300, 1964.

168. Prentice, C. R. M., Hassenein, A. A., McNichol, G. P., and Douglas, A. S.: Studies on the haemostatic mechanism following exercise. *Br. J. Haematol.* 17:611, 1969.

169. Rizza, C. R., and Eipe, J.: Exercise, factor VIII and the spleen. *Br. J. Haematol.* 20:629, 1971.

170. Bennett, B., and Ratnoff, O. D.: Changes in antihemophilic factor (AHF factor VIII) procoagulant activity and AHF-like antigen in normal pregnancy, and following exercise and pneumoencephalography. *J. Lab. Clin. Med.* 80:256, 1972.

171. van Gastel, C., et al.: Preparation and infusion of cryoprecipitate from exercised donors. *Br. J. Haematol.* 25:461, 1973.

172. Ingraham, G. I. C., and Vaughan-Jones, R.: The rise in clotting factor VIII induced in man by adrenaline: Effect of α- and β-blockers. *J. Physiol.* 187:447, 1966.

173. Gross, J. D., Hartmann, R. C., Graham, J. B., and Taylor, C. B.: Splenectomy in hemophilia. *Johns Hopkins Hosp. Bull.* 100:223, 1957.

174. Graham, J. B., Collins, D. L., Jr., Godwin, I. D., and Brinkhous, K. M.: Assay of plasma antihemophilic activity in normal, heterozygous (hemophilia) and prothrombinopenic dogs. *Proc. Soc. Exp. Biol. Med.* 77:294, 1951.

175. Pool, J. G., and Spaet, T. H.: Ethionine-induced depression of plasma antihemophilic globulin in the rat. *Proc. Soc. Exp. Biol. Med.* 87:54, 1954.

176. Penick, G. D., Roberts, H. R., Webster, W. P., and Brinkhous, K. M.: Hemorrhagic states secondary to intravascular clotting. *Arch. Pathol.* 66:708, 1958.

177. Straub, P. S., Riedler, G., and Meili, E. O.: Erhhöhung des antihämophilen Globulins (Faktor 8) bei letaler Lebernekrose. *Schweiz. Med. Wochenschr.* 96:1199, 1966.

178. Meili, E. O., and Straub, P. W.: Elevation of factor VIII in acute fatal liver necrosis. *Thromb. Diath. Haemorrh.* 24:161, 1970.

179. Zacharski, L. R., Bowie, E. J. W., Titus, J. L., and Owen, C. A., Jr.: Synthesis of antihemophilic factor (factor VIII) by leukocytes: Preliminary report. *Mayo Clin. Proc.* 43:617, 1968.

180. Zacharski, L. R., Bowie, E. J. W., Titus, J. L., and Owen, C. A.: Cell-culture synthesis of a factor VIII–like activity. *Mayo Clin. Proc.* 44:784, 1969.

181. Ponn, R. B., Kellog, E. A., Korff, J. M., Pegg, C. A. S., Sise, H. S., and Norman, J. C.: The role of the splenic macrophage in antihemophilic factor (factor VIII) synthesis. *Arch. Surg.* 103:398, 1971.

182. Rickles, F. R., Hardin, J. A., Pitlick, F. A., Hoyer, L. W., and Conrad, M. E.: Tissue factor activity in lymphocyte cultures from normal individuals and patients with hemophilia A. *J. Clin. Invest.* 52:1427, 1973.

183. Bloom, A. L., Giddings, J. C., and Wilkes, C. J.: Factor VIII on the vascular intima: Possible importance in haemostasis and thrombosis. *Nature [New Biol.]* 241:217, 1973.

184. Hoyer, L. W., de los Santos, R. P., and Hoyer, J. R.: Antihemophilic factor antigen: Localization in endothelial cells by immunofluorescent microscopy. *J. Clin. Invest.* 52:2737, 1973.

185. Tuddenham, E. G. D., Shearn, S. A. M., Peake, I. R., Giddings, J. C., and Bloom, A. L.: Tissue localization and synthesis of factor-VIII-related antigen in the human foetus. *Br. J. Haematol.* 26:669, 1974.

186. Jaffe, E. A., Hoyer, L. W., and Nachman, R. L.: Synthesis of antihemophilic factor antigen by cultured human endothelial cells. *J. Clin. Invest.* 52:2757, 1973.

187. Shearn, S. A. M., et al.: The characterization and synthesis of antigens related to factor VIII in vascular endothelium. *Thromb. Res.* 11:43, 1977.

188. Stead, N. W., and McKee, P. A.: The effect of cultured endothelial cells on factor VIII procoagulant activity. *Blood* 54:560, 1979.

189. Wall, R. T., Counts, R. V., Harker, L. A., and Striker, G. E.: Binding and release of factor VIII/von Willebrand's factor by human endothelial cells. *Br. J. Haematol.* 46:287, 1980.

190. Tuddenham, E. G. D., Lazarchick, J., and Hoyer, L. W.: Synthesis and release of factor VIII by cultured human endothelial cells. *Br. J. Haematol.* 47:617, 1981.

191. Nachman, R., Levine, R., and Jaffe, E. A.: Synthesis of factor VIII antigen by cultured guinea pig megakaryocytes. *J. Clin. Invest.* 60:914, 1977.

192. Norman, J. C., Covelli, V. H., and Sise, H. S.: Transplantation of the spleen: Experimental cure of hemophilia. *Surgery* 64:1, 1968.

193. Marchioro, T. L., Hougie, C., Ragde, H., Epstein, R. B., and Thomas, E. D.: Hemophilia: Role of organ homografts. *Science* 163:188, 1969.

194. Marchioro, T. L., Hougie, C., Ragde, H., Epstein, R. B., and Thomas, E. D.: Organ homografts for hemophilia. *Transplant. Proc.* 1:316, 1969.

195. McKee, P. A., Coussons, R. T., Buckner, R. G., Williams, G. R., and Hampton, J. W.: Effects of the spleen on canine factor VIII levels. *J. Lab. Clin. Med.* 75:391, 1970.

196. Penick, G. D., Webster, W. P., Peacock, E. E., Hutchins, P., and Zukoski, C. F.: Organ transplantation in animal hemophilia, in *Hemophilia and New Hemorrhagic States*, edited by K. M. Brinkhous. University of North Carolina Press, Chapel Hill, 1970, p. 97.

197. Webster, W. P., Zukoski, C. F., Hutchin, P., Reddick, R. L., Mandel, S. R., and Penick, G. D.: Plasma factor VIII synthesis and control as revealed by canine organ transplantation. *Am. J. Physiol.* 220:1147, 1971.

198. Nilsson, I. M., Blombäck, M., and Blombäck, B.: Von Willebrand's disease in Sweden. *Acta Med. Scand.* 164:263, 1959.

199. Cornu, P., Larrieu, M. J., Caen, J., and Bernard, J.: Maladie de Willebrand: Étude clinique, génétique and biologique (à propos de 22 observations). *Nouv. Rev. Fr. Hematol.* 1:231, 1961.

200. Cornu, P., Larrieu, M. J., Caen, J., and Bernard, J.: Transfusion studies in von Willebrand's disease: Effect on bleeding time and factor VIII. *Br. J. Haematol.* 9:189, 1963.

201. Biggs, R., and Matthews, J. M.: The treatment of haemorrhage in von Willebrand's disease and the blood level of factor VIII (AHG). *Br. J. Haematol.* 9:203, 1963.

202. Fantl, P., and Sawers, R. J.: Stimulation of factor VIII (antihaemophilic) activity by transfused serum. *Nature* 200:1214, 1963.

203. Barrow, E. M., Roberts, H. R., Pons, H., and Graham, J. B.: Studies on the antihemophilia factor (AHF, factor VIII) produced in von Willebrand's disease. *Proc. Soc. Exp. Biol. Med.* 115:760, 1964.

204. Bennett, B., Ratnoff, O. D., and Levin, J.: Immunologic studies in von Willebrand's disease: Evidence that the antihemophilic factor (AHF) produced after transfusions lacks an antigen associated with normal AHF and the inactive material produced by patients with classic hemophilia. *J. Clin. Invest.* 51:2597, 1972.

205. Bloom, A. L., Peake, I. R., and Giddings, J. C.: The presence and reactions of high and lower-molecular-weight procoagulant factor VIII in the plasma of patients with von Willebrand's disease after treatment: Significance for a structural hypothesis for factor VIII. *Thromb. Res.* 3:389, 1973.

206. Muntz, R. H., Ekert, H., and Helliger, H.: Properties of post-infusion factor VIII in von Willebrand's disease. *Thromb. Res.* 5:111, 1974.
207. Kernoff, P. B. A., Rizza, C. R., and Kaelin, A. C.: Transfusion and gel filtration studies in von Willebrand's disease. *Br. J. Haematol.* 28:357, 1974.
208. Meyer, D., Larrieu, M. J., Maroteaux, P., and Caen, J. P.: Biological findings in von Willebrand's pedigrees: Implications for inheritance. *J. Clin. Pathol.* 20:190, 1967.
209. Graham, J. B., McLester, W. D., Pons, K., Roberts, H. R., and Barrow, E. M.: Genetics of vascular hemophilia and biosynthesis of the plasma antihemophilic factor, in *The Hemophilias*, edited by K. M. Brinkhous. University of North Carolina Press, Chapel Hill, 1964, p. 263.
210. Egeberg, O.: Conditions associated with increased blood factor VIII activity, in *The Hemophilias*, edited by K. M. Brinkhous. University of North Carolina Press, Chapel Hill, 1964, p. 203.
211. Strauss, H. S., and Diamond, L. K.: Elevation of factor VIII (antihemophilic factor) during pregnancy in normal persons and in a patient with von Willebrand's disease. *N. Engl. J. Med.* 269:1251, 1963.
212. Bennett, B., Oxnard, S. C., Douglas, A. S., and Ratnoff, O. D.: Studies on antihemophilic factor (AHF, factor VIII) during labor in normal women in patients with premature separation of the placenta, and in a patient with von Willebrand's disease. *J. Lab. Clin. Med.* 84:851, 1974.
213. Bowie, E. J. W., et al.: Liver transplantation in pigs with von Willebrand's disease. *Br. J. Haematol.* 31:37, 1975.
214. Mannucci, P. M., Aberg, M., Nilsson, I. M., and Robertson, B.: Mechanism of plasminogen activator and factor VIII increase after vasoactive drugs. *Br. J. Haematol.* 30:81, 1975.
215. Mannucci, P. M., et al.: Studies on the prolonged bleeding time in von Willebrand's disease. *J. Lab. Clin. Med.* 88:662, 1976.
216. Mannucci, P. M., Ruggeri, Z. M., Pareti, F. I., and Capitanio, A.: 1-Deamino-8-D-arginine vasopressin: A new pharmacologic approach to the management of haemophilia and von Willebrand's disease. *Lancet* 1:869, 1977.
217. Theiss, W., and Schmidt, G.: DDAVP in von Willebrand's disease: Repeated administration and the behavior of the bleeding time. *Thromb. Res.* 13:119, 1978.
218. Prowse, C. V., Sas, G., Gader, A. M. A., Cort, J. H., and Cash, J. D.: Specificity of the factor VIII response to vasopressin infusion in man. *Br. J. Haematol.* 41:437, 1979.
219. Ludlam, C. A., et al.: Factor VIII and fibrinolytic response to deamino-8-D-arginine vasopressin in normal subjects and dissociated response in some patients with haemophilia and von Willebrand's disease. *Br. J. Haematol.* 45:499, 1980.
220. Nilsson, I. M., Mikaelsson, M., Vilhardt, H., and Walter, H.: DDAVP factor VIII concentrate and its properties in vivo and in vitro. *Thromb. Res.* 15:263, 1979.
221. Ockalford, P. A., Menon, N. C., and Berry, E. W.: Clinical experience with arginine vasopressin (DDAVP) in von Willebrand's disease and mild haemophilia. *N. Z. Med. J.* 92:375, 1980.
222. Mannucci, P. M., Canciani, M. T., Rota, L., and Donovan, B. S.: Response of factor VIII/von Willebrand factor to DDAVP in healthy subjects and patients with haemophilia A and von Willebrand's disease. *Br. J. Haematol.* 47:283, 1981.
223. Bloom, A. L.: The biosynthesis of factor VIII. *Clin. Haematol.* 8:53, 1979.
224. Naeye, R. L.: Hemophilioid factors: Acquired deficiencies in several hemorrhagic states. *Proc. Soc. Exp. Biol. Med.* 94:623, 1957.
225. Rapaport, S. I.: Plasma thromboplastin antecedent levels in patients receiving coumarin anticoagulants and in patients with Laennec's cirrhosis. *Proc. Soc. Exp. Biol. Med.* 108:115, 1961.
226. Horowitz, H. I., Wilcox, W. P., and Fujimoto, M. M.: Assay of plasma thromboplastin antecedent (PTA) with artificially depleted normal plasma. *Blood* 22:35, 1963.
227. Waaler, B. A.: Contact activation in the intrinsic blood clotting system: Studies on a plasma product formed on contact with glass and similar surfaces. *Scand. J. Clin. Lab. Invest.* 11 (Suppl. 37):1, 1959.
228. Horowitz, H. I., and Fujimoto, M. M.: Association of factors XI and XII with blood platelets. *Proc. Soc. Exp. Biol. Med.* 119:487, 1965.

229. Hilgartner, M. W., and Smith, C. H.: Plasma thromboplastin antecedent (factor XI) in the neonate. *J. Pediatr.* 66:747, 1965.
230. Jürgens, J.: The significance of the Hageman factor for the effect of wettable surface on thrombocytes. *Thromb. Diath. Haemorrh.* 7:48, 1962.
231. Ratnoff, O. D.: The biology and pathology of the initial stages of blood coagulation, in *Progress in Hematology*, edited by E. B. Brown and C. V. Moore. Grune & Stratton, New York, 1966, vol. V, p. 204.
232. Kiesselbach, T. H., and Wagner, R. H.: Fibrin-stabilizing factor: A thrombin-labile platelet protein. *Am. J. Physiol.* 211:1472, 1966.
233. McDonagh, J., Kiesselbach, T. H., and Wagner, R. H.: Origin of platelet factor XIII (fibrin stabilizing factor). *Fed. Proc.* 28:745, 1969.
234. McDonagh, J., McDonagh, R. P., Jr., Delage, J.-M., and Wagner, R. H.: Factor XIII in human plasma and platelets. *J. Clin. Invest.* 48:940, 1969.
235. Rookstool, D. J., et al.: Site of synthesis for plasma and platelet transglutaminase by immunofluorescent techniques. *Clin. Res.* 20:742, 1972.
236. Nussbaum, M., and Morse, B.: Plasma fibrin stabilizing factor activity in various diseases. *Blood* 23:669, 1974.
237. Gerhold, W. M., Tiongson, T., and Mandel, E. E.: Studies of fibrin stabilizing factor. *Fed. Proc.* 25:446, 1966.
238. Walls, W. D., and Losowsky, M. S.: Plasma fibrin stabilizing factor (F.S.F.) activity in normal subjects and patients with chronic liver disease. *Thromb. Diath. Haemorrh.* 21:134, 1969.
239. Mandel, E. E., and Gerhold, W. M.: Plasma fibrin stabilizing factor: Acquired deficiency in various diseases. *Am. J. Clin. Pathol.* 52:547, 1969.
240. Colman, R. W., Mason, J. W., and Sherry, S.: The kallikreinogen-kallikrein enzyme system of human plasma. *Ann. Intern. Med.* 71:763, 1969.
241. Bagdasarian, A., et al.: Immunochemical studies of plasma kallikrein. *J. Clin. Invest.* 54:1444, 1974.
242. Saito, H., et al.: Human plasma prekallikrein (Fletcher factor) clotting activity and antigen in health and disease. *J. Lab. Clin. Med.* 92:84, 1978.
243. Saito, H., Goldsmith, G., and Waldmann, R.: Fitzgerald factor (high-molecular-weight kininogen) clotting activity in human plasma in health and disease in various animal plasmas. *Blood* 48:941, 1976.
244. Diniz, C. R., and Carvalho, I. F.: A micromethod for determination of bradykininogen under several conditions. *Ann. N.Y. Acad. Sci.* 104:77, 1963.

CHAPTER *134*

Life-span of plasma coagulation factors

WILLIAM J. WILLIAMS

The life-span of the plasma coagulation factors has been derived from studies of the survival of these substances administered to individuals congenitally deficient in the factor under study, utilizing plasma, serum, or a concentrated preparation of the particular factor. Some studies have been performed by infusing coagulation factors labeled with radioisotopes of iodine, carbon, or sulfur into either normal subjects or factor-deficient patients. Another approach has been to observe the disappearance of factors after their synthesis has been inhibited by a drug.

In the studies measuring the rate of disappearance of a factor after its administration to an appropriate subject, the disappearance curve has the form of either a single or double exponential function [1] (Fig. 134-1). The single exponential curve is assumed to represent disappearance of a factor retained within the vascular compartment. The double exponential curve has an early, rapidly falling portion which is usually interpreted as a result of transfer of the factor to an extravascular compartment. Although coagulation factors have been demonstrated to be present in extracellular spaces, pleural fluid, and lymph [2–6], several alternative explanations are possible for the rapid initial fall in the disappearance curve [1].

The second, more slowly disappearing component is interpreted as representing metabolic destruction of the factor. The double exponential curve has been frequently observed and could be a general property of the coagulation factors. It may be necessary to infuse relatively large quantities of the factors rapidly in order to demonstrate the double exponential curve, and these conditions have not been met for all factors studied.

The biologic half-life of the factor is derived from the second, presumably metabolic, component of the disappearance curve. Because a large proportion of the administered factor may disappear from the circulation rapidly, as occurs, for example, with factor VIII coagulant activity (factor VIII:C or FVIII:C), the half-life may not be a particularly useful parameter in replacement therapy, and a concept of *half-disappearance time* has been developed [1]. This is the time required for one-half of the administered factor to disappear from the circulation, and it is the result of both exponentials, although the initial one may account for most or all of it (Fig. 134-1).

Interpretation of the disappearance curves as indicating normal metabolism requires the assumptions that the administered material has not been altered so as to change its metabolism, that the subject is handling the factor in an entirely normal fashion, and that the presence of the administered factor itself has no effect on the survival or synthesis of the factor in the body. All these assumptions are open to question, but for several of the factors consistent results have been obtained with a variety of preparations administered to both normal subjects and factor-deficient patients, so there is reason to believe the data have validity.

Fibrinogen (factor I)

Fibrinogen metabolism has been studied in human subjects [7–24] and in experimental animals [7,10,13, 25–33], primarily employing radioisotope techniques. Extensive reviews have been published [34,35]. Most

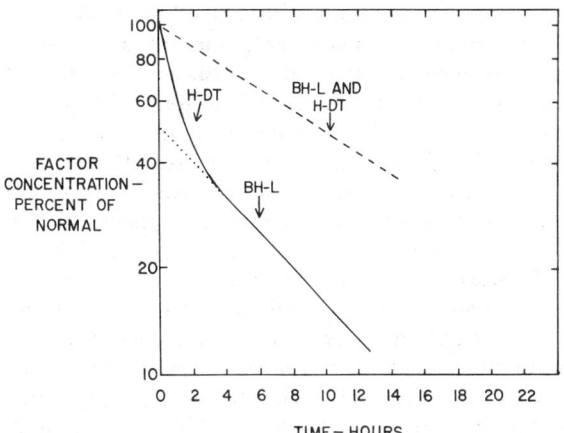

FIGURE 134-1 Single and double exponential disappearance curves for plasma coagulation factors. Time is indicated as hours for this example. The single exponential curve (broken line) describes disappearance of a plasma factor presumably retained within the vascular compartment. The biologic half-life (BH-L) and half-disappearance time (H-DT) are the same. The first component of the double exponential curve (solid line) presumably represents equilibration of the factor with an extravascular compartment, while the second component (continuation of the solid line and dotted extrapolation to zero) represents the biologic degradation of the factor. This is used to calculate the biologic half-life. The H-DT is the time required for one-half of the factor to disappear from the circulation, without regard for the exponential component involved. Thus, in the double exponential systems, the H-DT is shorter than the biologic half-life.

studies have been performed with proteins labeled with radioactive iodine (^{125}I or ^{131}I), which can provide a useful label without causing significant denaturation of the protein [26,30,36] and without the problem of reutilization of the isotope, as may occur with ^{35}S or ^{14}C [7,8,20,25]. Following injection of labeled fibrinogen, about 2 days are required for equilibration to occur, presumably with the extravascular spaces. It has been estimated that from 10 to 25 percent of the total body fibrinogen exists extravascularly [12,15,16,19,20]. Fibrinogen has been demonstrated in the extravascular space by immunofluorescence methods [2], and in a patient with afibrinogenemia no fibrinogen could be demonstrated in the connective tissues of the skin or muscle biopsy specimens until the patient had been transfused with fibrinogen [8]. Fibrinogen is also present in human lymph [3,4].

The biologic half-life of fibrinogen in human beings has been reported to be from 1.5 to 6.3 days [7–24]. The longer half-lives have been obtained in experiments with reutilizable radioisotopes [7–20], and in the studies with radioiodinated fibrinogen the half-lives have ranged between 3 and 4.5 days [15–19,21–24]. The catabolic rate of fibrinogen in normal subjects has been calculated to be from 31 to 46 mg/kg per day [15,16,19, 21,22,36].

The mechanism of fibrinogen catabolism is unknown. Studies utilizing anticoagulants and inhibitors of fibrinolysis have generally demonstrated no effect of these two treatments on the half-life of fibrinogen [13,17,22,24,27–29], but in some patients prolongation of survival of fibrinogen has been noted [17]. Patients with marked impairment of hemostasis because of a congenital disorder of coagulation or a platelet abnormality have had normal fibrinogen survival times [14,17,18,23], but in one report there was a decreased survival time in patients with hemophilia [37]. These results suggest that fibrinogen is not degraded by a continuous coagulation process. However, small amounts of fibrinopeptide A, a fragment of fibrinogen released by thrombin (see Chap. 132), are found in normal human blood, and the quantity of this peptide in blood is reduced, but not eliminated, by heparin therapy [38]. It has been calculated that from 2 to 3 percent of normal fibrinogen catabolism can be accounted for by conversion of fibrinogen to fibrin [38]. It has also been concluded from mathematical analysis of radioisotope data that fibrinogen is catabolized rapidly once it leaves the circulation, and if fibrin formation is involved the fibrin is broken down almost instantaneously [19,30]. Infused fibrin monomer is rapidly removed from the circulation of experimental animals, deposited in various organs, and degraded [39].

Fibrinogen may also be degraded by a pathway involving the plasminogen-plasmin system, the so-called fibrinogenolytic pathway [40,41]. This concept rests on the demonstration that up to 20 percent of circulating fibrinogen in man consists of high-solubility, low-molecular-weight material with properties suggesting partial degradation by plasmin [42–45]. The concentration of this fraction may be increased in patients with advanced liver disease [46]. Studies in experimental animals have indicated that up to 25 percent of fibrinogen may be catabolized via the fibrinogenolytic pathway [32,33]. Objections have been raised to this concept on the basis of the possibility that the high-solubility fibrinogens are artifacts [47,48]. Further work will be necessary to resolve this issue.

Fibrinogen metabolism may be increased in various disease states [11,15–17,20,36,49,50] and in pregnancy [51] and is decreased in hypothyroidism [17]. The fractional catabolic rate tends to remain constant in both health and disease, suggesting that the catabolic mechanisms are not altered by disease and the average lifespan of circulating fibrinogen remains normal [34–36]. In patients with cirrhosis there is increased fibrinogen metabolism, which can be decreased by heparin therapy, suggesting that it is due to disseminated intravascular coagulation [21,52].

Prothrombin (factor II)

The survival of prothrombin (factor II) has been studied by administration of radioiodinated prothrombin [53–55], transfusion of prothrombin-containing materials [56–60], or administration of drugs to block prothrombin synthesis [61–64]. The studies with iodinated human prothrombin have shown a rapid initial fall in plasma radioactivity, with a half-time of about 8 h, probably representing equilibration with extravascular sites. The biologic half-life of prothrombin after equilibration was 2.1 [55], 2.8 [53], and 4.4 [54] days. About 40 percent of the plasma pool was degraded daily. Prothrombin has been demonstrated in lymph [3,4] and in malignant pleural effusions [6]. About 30 to 40 percent of the total body prothrombin is present in the extravascular compartment [53,54]. Plasmapheresis [65] and cross-circulation [66] experiments in dogs suggest that this extravascular prothrombin is not readily available to replenish reduced plasma levels of prothrombin.

Data derived from infusion of prothrombin-containing material into patients with congenital prothrombin deficiency have yielded half-lives of from 2 to 5 days [57–59]. The half-life of prothrombin was estimated to be from 1.25 to 3.5 days in experiments in which prothrombin synthesis was inhibited by vitamin K antagonists [57,61–64].

Prothrombin turnover was normal in patients with hemophilia [53,62], and no products of prothrombin activation could be demonstrated in the circulation of the subjects in one study [53]. Heparin therapy did not alter the turnover of prothrombin in normal subjects [61]. These findings suggest that continuous intravascular coagulation does not play a significant role in the catabolism of prothrombin. Fever and hyperthyroidism probably increase the catabolism of prothrombin, while hypothyroidism decreases it [63].

Factor V

Studies on the half-life of plasma factor V have been limited to patients with a congenital deficiency of this factor who have received transfusions of whole plasma. A decay curve with a single component was detected, although the finding that lymph contains factor V [3,4] suggests an extravascular pool. Values for the half-life have been from 12 to 15 h [67], from 15 to 24 h [68], 20 h [69], and 36 h [70]. The recovery of factor V was between 40 to 65 percent in one study [68] and 100 percent or more in another [70]. Factor V adsorbed to platelets has a survival time of up to 5 days [71].

Factor VII

The survival time of factor VII has been studied after infusion of plasma or serum [64,72–77] or factor VII concentrates [64,72,74,78,79] into patients with congenital or acquired factor VII deficiency, or by studying the disappearance of factor VII from the blood after administration of vitamin K antagonists [62,64,72,75]. In some of the studies with factor VII concentrates [64,78] or with plasma [75], two components of the disappearance curve were detected. The first component of the disappearance curve had a half-time of 18 to 35 min and is thought to be a result of equilibration with extravascular sites. The second component, representing the biologic degradation of factor VII, had a half-time ranging from about 100 to 300 min [64,78]. In all other studies the half-life of factor VII was also short, ranging from 70 to 375 min. The half-life of factor VII derived from serum was shorter than that of factor VII derived from plasma [75,76], but the difference was not considered statistically significant in one study [76]. Recovery of administered factor VII has been 100 percent or more [77,78]. The rate of disappearance of factor VII from the plasma of subjects with hemophilia or from normal subjects treated with coumarin drugs or heparin was the same as in patients congenitally deficient in this factor, suggesting that intravascular coagulation was not involved in the decay of this coagulant protein [61,62]. Factor VII turnover is increased in hypermetabolic states and decreased in myxedema [63].

Factor VIII

The survival of factor VIII in normal human subjects has been studied using plasma labeled in vivo with ^{35}S and an immunologic technique to isolate the factor VIII from samples of circulating plasma [80]. A biphasic survival curve was obtained. The first component, probably a result of equilibration with extravascular sites, had a half-time of 3.8 h, and the second component, representing biologic degradation, had a half-time of 2.9 days. About 25 percent of the administered factor VIII was utilized in the second phase. The size of the extravascular pool was estimated at 1.5 times that of the intravascular pool. Factor VIII coagulant activity (FVIII:C) has been demonstrated in both low and high concentrations in lymph [3,4].

In studies of plasma or factor VIII concentrates administered to patients with factor VIII deficiency [59,81–87], the biologic half-life of FVIII:C was much shorter, varying between 9 and 18 h. FVIII:C and factor VIII–related antigen (FVIIIR:Ag) have been determined after infusion of factor concentrates into patients with hemophilia [88]. The half-life of the FVIII:C was 12 to 14 h, while that of the FVIIIR:Ag was 24 to 40 h [88], approaching the value obtained in the experiments utilizing ^{35}S-labeled factor VIII and an immunologic technique to isolate the labeled factor VIII [80]. Values for the half-life of FVIII:C of 11.5 h and of FVIIIR:Ag of 22 h were found in another study [89].

In the studies with factor VIII concentrates administered to factor VIII–deficient patients, a biphasic disappearance curve for FVIII:C was usually found, with the initial fall of such magnitude that the half-disappearance time was between 3 and 6 h [83], a point of great significance in therapy. The size of the extravascular pool has been estimated at about twice that of the intravascular pool [81]. It has been shown that the initial rapid component of the disappearance curve of FVIII:C may not be observed after very large initial

doses have been given or after prolonged administration of factor VIII, perhaps because of saturation of the extravascular sites [59,84,90]. In some studies a triphasic curve has been observed, with the initial fall in FVIII:C level followed by a plateau or an actual increase before the final phase of exponential decline is observed [82,83]. The duration of the second phase appears to be directly related to the initial level of FVIII:C attained. In these studies on patients with hemophilia, the initial yield of FVIII:C activity has usually ranged from 66 to 100 percent [59,81,87], but with low dosage the yields have been poorer [83]. Factor VIII is bound to platelets and in this form may survive in the circulation for up to 6 days [71].

"Von Willebrand factor" (Factor VIII:vWF)

Administration of plasma or some concentrates of factor VIII (e.g., cryoprecipitate) to patients with von Willebrand's disease results in an increase in FVIII:C and may effect a decrease in the prolonged bleeding time [91–96]. The bleeding time is usually corrected for less than 4 h after administration of normal plasma [91,94], but it has been corrected for up to 24 h after administration of hemophilic plasma to a patient with von Willebrand's disease [97]. The decrease in bleeding time following administration of cryoprecipitate or other concentrates of factor VIII is also short-lived compared to the duration of the elevation of FVIII:C levels [94–96]. The plasma component responsible for stimulation of FVIII:C has not been identified, and its survival time in the circulation is unknown.

FVIII:C and FVIIIR:Ag have been determined after administration of plasma or factor VIII concentrates to patients with von Willebrand's disease [97–102]. In most of the patients the FVIIIR:Ag disappeared from the circulation more rapidly than the FVIII:C [96, 98–102]. For example, in one study FVIIIR:Ag reached pretreatment levels in as little as 24 h, while FVIII:C was at its maximum or still increasing [98]. However, in some patients FVIIIR:Ag and FVIII:C showed similar survival times [99,100], perhaps reflecting the heterogeneity of this disease (see Chap. 155). Data have been reported showing both brief [101] and prolonged [99] correction of ristocetin-induced platelet aggregation following infusion of cryoprecipitate. In one study the following $T_{1/2}$ values were found: FVIII:C, 6 to 12 h; FVIIIR:Ag, 12 to 16 h, and the cofactor for ristocetin-induced platelet aggregation, FVIIIR:RCoF, 12 h [102].

Factor IX

Factor IX survival times have been determined in normal human subjects using ^{35}S-labeled plasma by the techniques used for study of factor VIII (see above) [80]. A biphasic survival curve was obtained, with a half-time for the first phase of 15 h and for the second of 8.4 days. The factor IX was distributed into both intravascular and extravascular pools. The extravascular pool was 2.3 times larger than the intravascular. Factor IX has been demonstrated in lymph [3].

The disappearance of factor IX from the plasma following administration of vitamin K antagonists has also been studied [62,63,104]. Half-times of 20 to 24 h were obtained, values much shorter than those found with labeled factor IX but of the same order as those found with infusion of plasma, serum, or factor IX concentrates into patients with factor IX deficiency. In the studies on deficient patients [59,105–107], the disappearance of factor IX from the circulation followed a biphasic pattern. The first phase had a half-time of from 3 to 8 h [106,107], while the second was from 20 to 52 h, with a mean of about 24 h. It has been observed that after prolonged therapy the initial rapid disappearance phase may no longer be present [59]. Factor IX appears to be distributed in a volume about 2.5 to 3.3 times that of the plasma volume [105,107]. The initial yield of factor IX was less than 50 percent in these studies [59,107,108]. There was no difference in survival between factor IX derived from serum and factor IX derived from plasma [105]. Factor IX catabolism is increased in patients with fever [63,105].

Factor X

The survival of transfused factor X from plasma or concentrates has been studied [5,59,109]. A biphasic curve was obtained, with the first phase showing a half-time of 1.7 to 9 h and the second a half-time of 32 to 48 h [5,59,109]. After multiple transfusions with factor X, the disappearance curve was monophasic [5], a phenomenon observed also in patients deficient in factor IX [59]. Lymph collected from one patient was found to contain factor X after infusion of normal plasma [5], which provides direct evidence for an extravascular component of this factor.

Factor XI

The survival of factor XI has been studied after infusion of plasma into patients congenitally deficient in this procoagulant [110,111]. The initial yield of factor XI activity was about 100 percent [110] and in some cases exceeded 100 percent [111]. Following the initial rise in factor XI, the level sometimes remained constant for 1 to 2 days and then decreased steadily. The biologic half-life was between 40 and 84 h. A half-life of about 30 h has been estimated for factor XI present in commercial prothrombin complex concentrates [112].

Factor XII

Factor XII survival has been studied after plasma infusions in patients with congenital factor XII deficiency

[113,114] and by observing the decrease in factor XII levels in a patient with phosphorus poisoning [114]. The biologic half-lives in the congenitally deficient patients were 48 to 52 h. The half-life in the patient with phosphorus poisoning was about 32 h, but it may have been shortened because of the presence of marked metabolic abnormalities.

Factor XIII

Survival of factor XIII has been studied following administration of plasma or plasma derivatives to patients congenitally deficient in this factor [115–123]. All studies agree that factor XIII survives in the circulation for many days. In some studies a biphasic disappearance curve has been observed [117,118], and the biologic half-life has been estimated as 4.5 to 7 days [117–119]. In another study a biphasic disappearance curve was obtained with a half-life of 11 to 12.5 days [121]. An in vivo yield of 50 to 100 percent of the administered factor has been found [116,117].

Prekallikrein (Fletcher factor)

The half-life of the Fletcher factor determined in one subject after administration of 5 ml of fresh frozen plasma per kilogram of body weight was 35 h [124].

High-molecular-weight kininogen

The half-life of high-molecular-weight kininogen determined in a patient deficient in that substance (Flaujeac factor) was 6.5 days [125].

References

1. Aggeler, P. M.: Physiological basis for transfusion therapy in hemorrhagic disorders: A critical review. *Transfusion* 1:71, 1961.
2. Gitlin, D., Landing, B. H., and Whipple, A.: The localization of homologous plasma proteins in the tissues of young human beings as demonstrated with fluorescent antibodies. *J. Exp. Med.* 97:163, 1953.
3. Blomstrand, R., Nilsson, I. M., and Dahlbäck, O.: Coagulation studies on human thoracic duct lymph. *Scand. J. Clin. Lab. Invest.* 15:248, 1963.
4. Stutman, L. J., Dumont, A. E., and Shinowara, G. Y.: Coagulation factors in human lymph and plasma. *Am. J. Med. Sci.* 250:292, 1965.
5. Roberts, H. R., Lechler, E., Webster, W. P., and Penick, G. D.: Survival of transfused factor X in patients with Stuart disease. *Thromb. Diath. Haemorrh.* 13:305, 1965.
6. Bergsagel, D. E., and Nockolds, E. R.: The activation of proaccelerin. *Br. J. Haematol.* 11:395, 1965.
7. Madden, R. E., and Gould, R. G.: The turnover rate of fibrinogen in the dog. *J. Biol. Chem.* 196:641, 1952.
8. Gitlin, D., and Borges, W. H.: Studies on the metabolism of fibrinogen in two patients with congenital afibrinogenemia. *Blood* 8:679, 1953.
9. Volwiler, W., Goldsworthy, P. D., MacMartin, M. P., Wood, P. A., Mackay, I. R., and Fremont-Smith, K.: Biosynthetic determination

with radioactive sulfur of turnover rates of various plasma proteins in normal and cirrhotic man. *J. Clin. Invest.* 34:1126, 1955.

10. Gerdes, K., and Maurer, W.: Messungen zur Lebensdauer von Fibrinogen beim Menschen und beim Kaninchen. *Biochem. Z.* 328:522, 1957.

11. Christensen, L. K.: The turnover of plasma fibrinogen. *Acta Med. Scand.* 162:407, 1958.

12. Hammond, J. D. S., and Verel, D.: Observations on the distribution and biological half-life of human fibrinogen. *Br. J. Haematol.* 5:431, 1959.

13. Adelson, E., Rheingold, J. J., Parker, O., Buenaventura, A., and Crosby, W. H.: Platelet and fibrinogen survival in normal and abnormal states of coagulation. *Blood* 17:267, 1961.

14. Rausen, A. R., Cruchaud, A., McMillan, C. W., and Gitlin, D.: A study of fibrinogen turnover in classical hemophilia and congenital afibrinogenemia. *Blood* 18:710, 1961.

15. MacFarlane, A. S., Todd, D., and Cromwell, S.: Fibrinogen catabolism in humans. *Clin. Sci.* 26:415, 1964.

16. Amris, A., and Amris, C. J.: Turnover and distribution of ^{131}iodine-labeled human fibrinogen. *Thromb. Diath. Haemorrh.* 11:404, 1964.

17. Hart, H. C.: The biological half-life of I^{131}-fibrinogen. *Thromb. Diath. Haemorrh. Suppl.* 17:121, 1965.

18. Blombäck, B., Carlson, L. A., Franzén, S., and Zetterqvist, E.: Turnover of I^{131}-labeled fibrinogen in man. *Acta Med. Scand.* 179:557, 1966.

19. Takeda, Y.: Studies of the metabolism and distribution of fibrinogen in healthy men with autologous ^{125}I-labeled fibrinogen. *J. Clin. Invest.* 45:103, 1966.

20. Pilgeram, L. O.: Turnover rate of autologous plasma fibrinogen-^{14}C in subjects with coronary thrombosis. *Thromb. Diath. Haemorrh.* 20:31, 1968.

21. Tytgat, G. N., Collen, D., and Verstraete, M.: Metabolism of fibrinogen in cirrhosis of the liver. *J. Clin. Invest.* 50:1690, 1971.

22. Collen, D., Tytgat, G., Claeys, H., and Piessens, R.: Metabolism and distribution of fibrinogen. I. Fibrinogen turnover in physiological conditions in humans. *Br. J. Haematol.* 22:681, 1972.

23. Tytgat, G., Collen, D., and Vermylen, J.: Metabolism and distribution of fibrinogen. II. Fibrinogen turnover studies in polycythemia, thrombocytosis, haemophilia A, congenital afibrinogenaemia, and during streptokinase therapy. *Br. J. Haematol.* 22:701, 1972.

24. Davies, J. W. L., Forsberg, K., Liljedahl, S. O., Martensen, O., and Reizerastein, P.: The effect of anticoagulants on postoperative fibrinogen metabolism. *Acta Med. Scand.* 194:277, 1973.

25. Blombäck, B., Boström, H., and Vestermark, A.: On the (^{35}S) sulphate incorporation in fibrinopeptide B from rabbit fibrinogen. *Biochim. Biophys. Acta* 38:502, 1960.

26. MacFarlane, A. S.: *In vivo* behavior of I^{131}-fibrinogen. *J. Clin. Invest.* 42:346, 1963.

27. Lewis, J. H., Ferguson, E. E., and Schoenfeld, C.: Studies concerning the turnover of fibrinogen I^{131} in the dog. *J. Lab. Clin. Med.* 58:247, 1961.

28. Gajewski, J., and Alexander, B.: Effect of epsilon aminocaproic acid on the turnover of labelled fibrinogen in rabbits. *Circ. Res.* 13:432, 1963.

29. Lewis, J. H.: Effects of epsilon amino caproic acid (EACA) on survival of fibrinogen I^{131} and on fibrinolytic and coagulation factor in dogs. *Proc. Soc. Exp. Biol. Med.* 114:777, 1963.

30. Atencio, A. C., Bailey, H. R., and Reeve, E. B.: Studies on the metabolism and distribution of fibrinogen in young and older rabbits. I. Methods and models. *J. Lab. Clin. Med.* 66:1, 1965.

31. Atencio, A. C., and Reeve, E. B.: Studies on the metabolism and distribution of fibrinogen in young and older rabbits. II. Results. *J. Lab. Clin. Med.* 66:20, 1965.

32. Sherman, L. A., Fletcher, A. P., and Sherry, S.: *In vivo* transformation between fibrinogens of varying ethanol solubilities: A pathway of fibrinogen catabolism. *J. Lab. Clin. Med.* 73:574, 1969.

33. Sherman, L. A.: Fibrinogen turnover: Demonstration of multiple pathways of catabolism. *J. Lab. Clin. Med.* 79:710, 1972.

34. Reeve, E. B., and Franks, J. J.: Fibrinogen synthesis, distribution, and degradation. *Semin. Thromb. Hemost.* 1:129, 1974.

35. Sherman, L. A.: Catabolism of fibrinogen and its derivatives. *Thromb. Haemost.* 38:809, 1977.

36. Regoeczi, E.: Iodine-labelled fibrinogen: A review. *Br. J. Haematol.* 20:649, 1971.

37. Takeda, Y., and Chen, A.: Studies on the metabolism and distribution of fibrinogen in patients with hemophilia A. *J. Clin. Invest.* 46:1979, 1967.

38. Nossell, et al.: Measurement of fibrinopeptide A in human blood. *J. Clin. Invest.* 54:43, 1974.

39. Gurewich, V., Wetmore, R., Nowak, A., and Lipinski, B.: The fate of soluble fibrin monomer, in relation to intravascular fibrin formation and degradation in rabbits. *Blood* 44:723, 1974.

40. Mosesson, M. W.: The fibrinogenolytic pathway of fibrinogen catabolism. *Thromb. Res.* 2:185, 1973.

41. Mosesson, M. W.: Fibrinogen catabolic pathways. *Semin. Thromb. Hemost.* 1:63, 1974.

42. Mosesson, M. W., and Sherry, S.: The preparation and properties of human fibrinogen of relatively low solubility. *Biochemistry* 5:2829, 1966.

43. Mosesson, M. W., Alkjaersig, N., Sweet, B., and Sherry, S.: Human fibrinogen of relatively high solubility: Comparative biophysical, biochemical, and biological studies with fibrinogen of lower solubility. *Biochemistry* 6:3279, 1967.

44. Sherman, L. A., Mosesson, M. W., and Sherry, S.: Isolation and characterization of the clottable, low molecular weight fibrinogen derived by limited plasmin hydrolysis of human fraction I$_4$. *Biochemistry* 8:1515, 1969.

45. Mosesson, M. W., Finlayson, J. S., Umfleet, R. A., and Galanakis, D.: Human fibrinogen heterogeneities. I. Structural and related studies of plasma fibrinogens which are high solubility catabolic intermediates. *J. Biol. Chem.* 247:5210, 1972.

46. Lipinski, B., Lipinska, I., Nowak, A., and Gurewich, V.: Abnormal fibrinogen heterogeneity and fibrinolytic activity in advanced liver disease. *J. Lab. Clin. Med.* 90:187, 1977.

47. Collen, D., Semeraro, N., and Verstraete, M.: The fibrinogenolytic pathway of fibrinogen catabolism: A replay. *Thromb. Res.* 4:491, 1974.

48. Mosesson, M. W., and Finlayson, J. S.: The fibrinogenolytic pathway of fibrinogen catabolism: A rebuttal. *Thromb. Res.* 4:895, 1974.

49. Takeda, Y.: Studies on the metabolism and distribution of fibrinogen in patients with rheumatoid arthritis. *J. Lab. Clin. Med.* 69:624, 1967.

50. Jones, R. L., and Peterson, C. M.: Reduced fibrinogen survival in diabetes mellitus: A reversible phenomenon. *J. Clin. Invest.* 63:485, 1979.

51. Regoeczi, E., and Hobbs, K. R.: Fibrinogen turnover in pregnancy. *Scand. J. Haematol.* 6:175, 1969.

52. Coleman, M., Finlayson, N., Bettigole, R. E., Sadula, D., Cohn, M., and Pasmantier, M.: Fibrinogen survival in cirrhosis: Improvement by 'low-dose' heparin. *Ann. Intern. Med.* 83:79, 1975.

53. Shapiro, S. S., and Martinez, J.: Human prothrombin metabolism in normal man and in hypocoagulable subjects. *J. Clin. Invest.* 48:1292, 1969.

54. Josso, F., Benamon-Dijane, D., and Soulier, J. P.: The biological half-life of ^{131}I-labeled prothrombin in man. *Proc. XIII Cong. Int. Soc. Hematol. New York 1968.* The Society, New York, 1968, p. 176.

55. Bell, W. R., Shapiro, S. R., Martinez, J., and Nossel, H. L.: The effects of ancrod, the coagulating enzyme from the venom of the Malayan pit viper (*A. rhodostoma*) on prothrombin and fibrinogen metabolism and fibrinopeptide A release in man. *J. Lab. Clin Med.* 91:592, 1978.

56. Didisheim, P., Loeb, J., Blatrix, C., and Soulier, J. P.: Preparation of a human plasma fraction rich in prothrombin, proconvertin, Stuart factor, and PTC and a study of its activity and toxicity in rabbits and man. *J. Lab. Clin. Med.* 53:322, 1959.

57. Borchgrevink, C. F., Egeberg, O., Pool, J. G., Skulason, T., Stormorken, H., and Waaler, B.: A study of a case of congenital hypoprothrombinaemia. *Br. J. Haematol.* 5:294, 1959.

58. Soulier, J. P., Prou-Wartelle, O., and Josso, F.: Démie-vie de la prothrombine vraie (fracteur II). *Nouv. Rev. Fr. Hematol.* 2:673, 1963.

59. Biggs, R., and Denson, K. W. E.: The fate of prothrombin and factors VIII, IX, and X transfused to patients deficient in these factors. *Br. J. Haematol.* 9:532, 1963.

60. Tullis, J. L., Melin, M., and Jurigian, P.: Clinical use of human prothrombin complexes. *N. Engl. J. Med.* 273:667, 1965.
61. Hasselback, R., and Hjort, P. F.: Effect of heparin on *in vivo* turnover of clotting factors. *J. Appl. Physiol.* 15:945, 1960.
62. Hjort, P. F., Egeberg, O., and Mikkelsen, S.: Turnover of prothrombin, factor VIII, and factor IX in a patient with hemophilia A. *Scand. J. Clin. Lab. Invest.* 13:668, 1961.
63. Loeliger, E. A., vanderEsch, B., Mattern, M. J., and Hemker, H. C.: The biological disappearance rate of prothrombin, factors VII, IX, and X from plasma in hypothyroidism, hyperthryroidism, and during fever. *Thromb. Diath. Haemorrh.* 10:267, 1964.
64. Marder, V. J., and Shulman, N. R.: Clinical aspects of congenital factor VII deficiency. *Am. J. Med.* 37:182, 1964.
65. Carter, J. R., Chambers, G. H., and Warner, E. D.: Effect on prothrombin of acute massive plasmapheresis with simultaneous chloroform intoxication. *Proc. Soc. Exp. Biol. Med.* 72:52, 1949.
66. Langdell, R. D., Weaver, R. A., and Price, R. E.: Prothrombin homeostasis in cross-circulated normal and dicumarol-treated dogs. *Am. J. Physiol.* 205:803, 1963.
67. Borchgrevink, C. F., and Owren, P. A.: Surgery in a patient with factor V (proaccelerin) deficiency. *Acta Med. Scand.* 170:743, 1961.
68. Rush, B., and Ellis, H.: The treatment of patients with factor-V deficiency. *Thromb. Diath. Haemorrh.* 14:74, 1965.
69. Fantl, P.: Parahemophilia (proaccelerin deficiency): Occurrence and biochemistry, in *Hemophilia and Hemophilioid Diseases*, edited by K. M. Brinkhous. University of North Carolina Press, Chapel Hill, 1957, p. 79.
70. Webster, W. P., Roberts, H. R., and Penick, G. D.: Hemostasis in factor V deficiency. *Am. J. Med. Sci.* 248:194, 1964.
71. Borchgrevink, C. F., and Owren, P. A.: The hemostatic effect of normal platelets in hemophilia and factor V deficiency. *Acta Med. Scand.* 170:375, 1961.
72. Frick, P. G.: Studies on the turnover rate of stable prothrombin conversion factor in man. *Acta Haematol.* 19:20, 1958.
73. Hitzig, W. H., and Zollinger, W.: Kongenitaler, Faktor-VII-Mangel. Familienuntersuchung und physiologische studien über den faktor VII. *Helv. Paediatr. Acta* 13:189, 1958.
74. Caen, J., Yanotti, S., Varangot, J., and Bernard, J.: Étude d'un cas d'hypoproconvertinémie vraie congénitale. *Sang* 30:535, 1959.
75. Loeliger, E. A., vanderEsch, B., Cleton, F. J., Booij, H. L., and Mattern, M. J.: On the metabolism of factor VII. *Proc. 7th Cong. Eur. Soc. Haematol.* London, 1960, part II, p. 764.
76. Roos, J., van Arkel, C., Keuter, E. J. W., and Ballieux, R. E.: Blood coagulation as a continuous process. II. The turnover rate of proconvertin. *Acta Med. Scand.* 168:477, 1960.
77. Hoffman, G. C., and Hewlett, J. S.: Exchange transfusion in hereditary factor VII (proconvertin) deficiency. *Am. J. Clin. Pathol.* 44:198, 1965.
78. Hoag, M. S., Aggeler, P. M., and Fowell, A. H.: Disappearance rate of concentrated proconvertin extracts in congenital and acquired hypoproconvertinemia. *J. Clin. Invest.* 39:554, 1960.
79. Bidwell, E., Booth, J. M., Dike, G. W. R., and Denson, K. W. E.: The preparation for therapeutic use of a concentrate of factor IX containing also factors II, VII, and X. *Br. J. Haematol.* 13:568, 1967.
80. Adelson, E., Rheingold, J. J., Parker, O., Steiner, M., and Kirby, J. C.: The survival of factor VIII (antihemophilic globulin) and factor IX (plasma thromboplastin component) in normal humans. *J. Clin. Invest.* 42:1040, 1963.
81. Shulman, N. R., Marder, V. J., and Hiller, M. C.: A new method for measuring minimum *in vivo* concentrations of factor VIII applied in distribution and survival studies and in detecting factor VIII inhibitors, in *The Hemophilias*, edited by K. M. Brinkhous. University of North Carolina Press, Chapel Hill, 1964, p. 29.
82. Pavlovsky, A., Pavlovsky, A. A., de Tezanos Pinto, M., Canaveri, A. M., and Funes, J. C.: Turnover of factor VIII. *Thromb. Diath. Haemorrh. Suppl.* 13:209, 1964.
83. Abildgaard, C. F., Cornet, J. A., Fort, E., and Schulman, I.: The *in vivo* longevity of antihaemophilic factor (factor VIII). *Br. J. Haematol.* 10:225, 1964.
84. Webster, W. P., Roberts, H. R., Thelin, G. M., Wagner, R. H., and Brinkhous, K. M.: Clinical use of a new glycine precipitated antihemophilic fraction. *Am. J. Med. Sci.* 250:643, 1965.

85. Abildgaard, C. F., et al.: Treatment of hemophilia with glycine-precipitated factor VIII. *N. Engl. J. Med.* 275:471, 1966.
86. Brinkhous, K. M., Shanbron, E., Roberts, H. R., Webster, W. P., Fekete, L., and Wagner, R. H.: A new high-potency glycine-precipitated antihemophilic factor (AHF) concentrate. *JAMA* 205:613, 1968.
87. Johnson, A. J., Karpatkin, M. H., and Newman, J.: Clinical investigation of intermediate- and high-purity antihaemophilic factor (factor VIII) concentrates. *Br. J. Haematol.* 21:21, 1971.
88. Bennett, B., and Ratnoff, O. D.: Studies on the response of patients with classic hemophilia to transfusion with concentrates of antihemophilic factor: A difference in the half-life of antihemophilic factor as measured by procoagulant and immunologic techniques. *J. Clin. Invest.* 51:2593, 1972.
89. Kernoff, P. B. A., Rizza, C. R., and Kaelin, A. C.: Transfusion and gel filtration studies in von Willebrand's disease. *Br. J. Haematol.* 28:357, 1974.
90. Brinkhous, K. M.: Hemophilia: Pathophysiologic studies and the evolution of transfusion therapy. *Am. J. Clin. Pathol.* 41:342, 1964.
91. Weiss, H. J.: The use of plasma and plasma fractions in the treatment of a patient with von Willebrand's disease. *Vox Sang.* 7:267, 1962.
92. Cornu, P., Larrieu, M. J., Caen, J., and Bernard, J.: Transfusion studies in von Willebrand's disease: Effect on bleeding time and factor VIII. *Br. J. Haematol.* 9:189, 1963.
93. Biggs, R., and Matthews, J. M.: The treatment of haemorrhage in von Willebrand's disease and the blood level of factor VIII (AHG). *Br. J. Haematol.* 9:203, 1963.
94. Bennett, E., and Dormandy, K.: Pool's cryoprecipitate and exhausted plasma in the treatment of von Willebrand's disease and factor IX deficiency. *Lancet* 2:731, 1966.
95. Perkins, H. A.: Correction of the hemostatic defects in von Willebrand's disease. *Blood* 30:375, 1967.
96. Holmberg, L., and Nilsson, I. M.: Two genetic variants of von Willebrand's disease. *N. Engl. J. Med.* 288:595, 1973.
97. Larrieu, M. J., Caen, J. P., Meyer, D. O., Vainer, H., Sultan, Y., and Bernard, J.: Congenital bleeding disorders with long bleeding time and normal platelet count. II. von Willebrand's disease (report of thirty-seven patients). *Am. J. Med.* 45:354, 1968.
98. Bennett, B., Ratnoff, O. D., and Levin, J.: Immunological studies in von Willebrand's disease: Evidence that the antihemophilic factor (AHF) produced after transfusion lacks an antigen associated with normal AHF and the inactive material produced by patients with classical hemophilia. *J. Clin. Invest.* 51:2597, 1972.
99. Thomson, C., Forbes, C. D., and Prentice, C. R. M.: Relationship of factor VIII to ristocetin-induced platelet aggregation: Effect of heterologous and acquired factor VIII antibodies. *Thromb. Res.* 3:363, 1973.
100. Bloom, A. L., Peake, I. R., and Giddings, J. C.: The presence and reactions of high and lower-molecular-weight procoagulant factor VIII in the plasma of patients with von Willebrand's disease after treatment: Significance for a structural hypothesis for factor VIII. *Thromb. Res.* 3:389, 1973.
101. Muntz, R. H., Ekert, H., and Helliger, H.: Properties of post-infusion factor VIII in von Willebrand's disease. *Thromb. Res.* 5:111, 1974.
102. Nilsson, I. M., Mikaelsson, M., Vilhardt, H., and Walker, H.: DDAVP factor VIII concentrate and its properties in vivo and in vitro. *Thromb. Res.* 15:263, 1979.
103. Weiss, H. J., and Sussman, I. I.: Synthesis of high-molecular-weight antihaemophilic factor in von Willebrand's disease. *Lancet* 2:402, 1974.
104. Loeliger, E. A., Hensen, A., Veltkamp, J. J., van der Meer, J., and Hemker, H. C.: On the metabolism of factor IX, in *The Hemophilias*, edited by K. M. Brinkhous. University of North Carolina Press, Chapel Hill, 1964, p. 159.
105. Loeliger, E. A., and Hensen, A.: Substitution therapy in haemophilia B. *Thromb. Diath. Haemorrh.* 6:391, 1961.
106. Ménaché, D.: The turnover rate of the coagulation factors II, VII, and IX under normal metabolic conditions. *Thromb. Diath. Haemorrh. Suppl.* 13:187, 1964.

107. Hoag, M. S., Johnson, F. F., Robinson, J. A., and Aggeler, P. M.: Treatment of hemophilia B with a new clotting factor concentrate. *N. Engl. J. Med. 280:*581, 1969.

108. Gilchrist, G. S., Ekert, H., Shanbrom, E., and Hammond, D.: Evaluation of a new concentrate for the treatment of factor IX deficiency. *N. Engl. J. Med. 280:*291, 1969.

109. O'Leary, D. S., Ruymann, F. B., and Conrad, M. E.: Therapeutic approaches to factor X deficiency with emphasis on the use of a new clotting-factor concentrate (Konyne). *J. Lab. Clin. Med. 77:* 23, 1971.

110. Nossel, H. L., Niemetz, J., and Sawitsky, A.: Blood PTA (factor XI) levels following plasma infusion. *Proc. Soc. Exp. Biol. Med. 115:* 896, 1964.

111. Rosenthal, R. L., and Sloan, E.: PTA (factor XI) levels and coagulation studies after plasma infusions in PTA-deficient patients. *J. Lab. Clin. Med. 66:*709, 1965.

112. Beck, R. L., Adams, T., and Radack, K.: Surgical hemostasis with a factor XI-containing concentrate. *JAMA 229:*163, 1974.

113. Fantl, P., Morris, K. N., and Sawers, R. J.: Repair of cardiac defect in patient with Ehlers-Danlos syndrome and deficiency of Hageman factor. *Br. Med. J. 1:*1202, 1961.

114. Veltkamp, J. J., Loeliger, E. A., and Hemker, H. C.: The biological half-time of Hageman factor. *Thromb. Diath. Haemorrh. 13:*1, 1965.

115. Duckert, F., Jung, E., and Schmerling, D. H.: A hitherto undescribed congenital haemorrhagic diathesis probably due to fibrin stabilizing factor deficiency. *Thromb. Diath. Haemorrh. 5:*179, 1960.

116. Ikkala, E., and Nevanlinna, H. R.: Congenital deficiency of fibrin stabilizing factor. *Thromb. Diath. Haemorrh. 7:*567, 1962.

117. Ikkala, E., Myllylä, G., and Nevanlinna, H. R.: Transfusion therapy in factor XIII (F.S.F.) deficiency. *Scand. J. Haematol. 1:*308, 1964.

118. Josso, F., Petrova, M., Ménaché, D., and Sizonenko, P.: Durée de vie du facteur stabilisant de la fibrine (facteur XIII). Incidences thérapeutiques. *Transfusion (Paris) 9:*343, 1966.

119. Britten, A. F. H.: Congenital deficiency of factor XIII (fibrin-stabilizing factor). *Am. J. Med. 43:*751, 1967.

120. Amris, C. J., and Hilden, M.: Treatment of factor XIII deficiency with cryoprecipitate. *Thromb. Diath. Haemorrh. 20:*528, 1968.

121. Miloszewski, K., and Losowsky, M. S.: The half-life of factor XIII in vivo. *Br. J. Haematol. 19:*685, 1970.

122. Ikkala, E.: Transfusion therapy in congenital deficiencies of plasma factor XIII. *Ann. N.Y. Acad. Sci. 202:*200, 1972.

123. Lorand, L., Losowsky, M. S., and Miloszewski, K. J. M.: Human factor XIII: Fibrin-stabilizing factor, in *Progress in Hemostasis and Thrombosis*, edited by T. H. Spaet. Grune & Stratton, New York, 1980, vol. 5, p. 245.

124. Hathaway, W. E., et al.: Clinical and physiological studies of two siblings with prekallikrein (Fletcher factor) deficiency. *Am. J. Med. 60:*654, 1976.

125. Lacombe, M.-J., Varet, B., and Levy, J.-P.: A hitherto undescribed plasma factor acting at the contact phase of blood coagulation (Flaujeac factor): Case report and coagulation studies. *Blood 46:* 761, 1975.

Mechanism of coagulation

CHAPTER *135*

Sequence of coagulation reactions

WILLIAM J. WILLIAMS

Blood coagulation has long been considered to be an enzymatic process. The concept has received its most complete expression in the *cascade* [1] or *waterfall* [2] sequence for blood coagulation (Fig. 135-1). In this conception, most of the coagulation factors circulate as proenzymes which are converted to enzymes during the clotting process. The most obvious exception is fibrinogen, which is converted to insoluble fibrin in the final step. The function of each enzyme formed is to activate the proenzyme which succeeds it in the coagulation sequence. Thus, proenzyme A is converted to enzyme A, which catalyzes the conversion of proenzyme B to enzyme B, which catalyzes the conversion of proenzyme C to enzyme C, and so on, to the formation of the fibrin clot. The cascade concept was developed for the so-called intrinsic system [3], that is, for coagulation occurring as a result of the interaction of substances present in the circulating blood. It also readily accommodates the *extrinsic system* [3], so called because the initial step involves tissue factor (factor III), which is extrinsic to the circulating blood (Fig. 135-1).

Validation of the cascade concept requires demonstration that activated coagulation factors function as enzymes in converting other coagulation factors to enzymatically active forms. Nearly all of the coagulation factors have been highly purified, and application of modern biochemical techniques has demonstrated that most of the reactions follow this mechanism, but at least three involve complex formation rather than enzyme activation. There are the reaction of tissue factor (factor III) with factor VIIa and calcium [4,5]; the reaction involving factor IXa, factor VIIIa, phospholipid or platelets, and calcium [6–11]; and the reaction involving factor Xa, factor Va, phospholipid or platelets, and calcium [12–17].

The conclusions that these reactions involve complex formation have been drawn from their failure to follow classic enzyme kinetics while having properties consis-

FIGURE 135-1 A modified cascade mechanism for blood coagulation. The reactions enclosed by the solid broad lines are those which occur in whole blood exposed to a foreign surface: the *intrinsic system.* **The reactions enclosed in the broken broad lines are those which occur in plasma to which tissue factor and calcium have been added: the** *extrinsic system.* **The solid arrows indicate conversion of a substrate or reactant to a product (e.g., factor X → factor Xa). The narrow solid lines without arrowheads indicate a catalytic function (e.g., thrombin catalyzes the conversion of fibrinogen → fibrin and factor XIII → factor XIIIa). The narrow broken lines with arrows indicate the action of thrombin on factors V and VIII to convert them to a more reactive form designated Va and VIIIa. PL = phospholipid; Ca = calcium.**

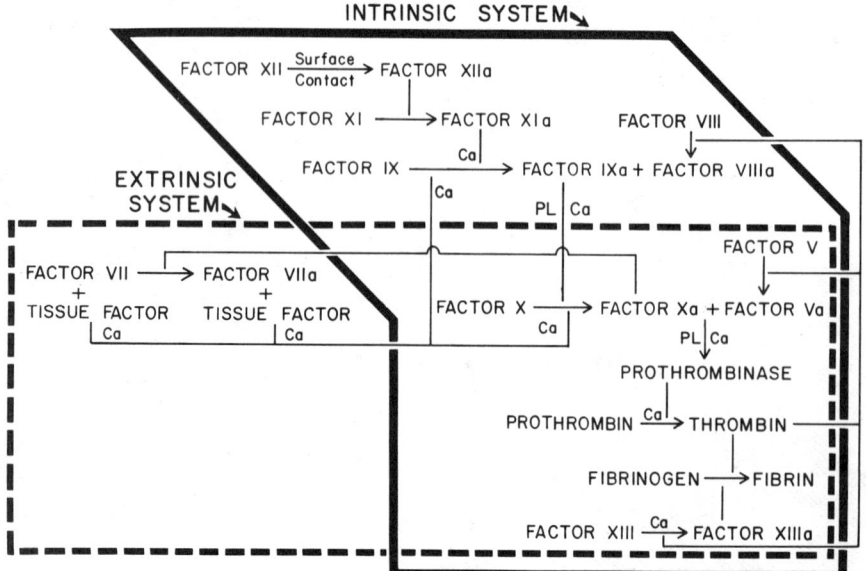

tent with complex formation, from demonstration that the physical and chemical properties of the product can only be accounted for by a substance incorporating more than one component of the reaction mixture, and from recovery of unaltered components following dissociation of the complex [4–17]. Since coagulation in vivo may be initiated by activation of factor XI bound to platelets (see below), all the reactions of the cascade may take place on the platelet surface.

Thus, the present concept of clotting involves both enzymatic conversion of proenzymes to enzymes and the physical combination of reactants. An additional feature of the coagulation mechanism is the influence of activated factors on reactants other than their apparently primary substrates, resulting in feedback effects or autocatalysis (see Chap. 136). Thus, thrombin alters factor V [12,18–27] and factor VIII [20,28–31] to increase their reactivity. Factor Xa can also activate factor VIII [32–34]. The kallikrein formed by factor XIIa–catalyzed activation of prekallikrein in turn activates more factor XII [35,36]. Factor XIIa can also activate factor VII [37,38] and factor IX [39,40]. Plasmin can activate factor XII [35,36,41,42]. Thrombin may play a role in prothrombin activation [43–46], and the activation of factor X may be autocatalytic under some circumstances [47,48]. Finally, the development of coagulant activity is subject to a variety of other control mechanisms, which are reviewed in Chap. 136.

A current version of the cascade concept is presented in Fig. 135-1 and will be discussed in some detail in this chapter. The present scheme represents one interpretation of existing data. It has proved useful in dealing with the phenomena of blood coagulation on both the theoretical and practical levels and is presented in those terms, subject to revision as new data accumulate.

The intrinsic system

Clotting in the intrinsic system in vitro begins with the activation of factor XII by exposure to a foreign surface. Although factor XII is essential for normal clotting in vitro, the function of factor XII in vivo is uncertain, because individuals congenitally deficient in this factor have no significant bleeding disorder [49]. However, factor XII can be activated by substances to which it could be exposed in vivo, such as collagen [50] or fatty acids [51], and this may have pathologic, if not physiologic, significance. A variety of other materials, such as glass, kaolin, Celite, etc., provide surfaces on which factor XII can be activated [52]. Activation of factor XII on a surface may be caused by some alteration in the factor XII itself [53–56], but seems more likely due to increased susceptibility of bound factor XII to enzymatic attack (see below). Calcium is not required for the activation of factor XII [57].

Factor XII has slight enzymatic activity in the zymogen form [58,59], and this low level of intrinsic activity could be responsible for the initiation of the coagulation cascade [58,59]. Factor XII [58,59] or factor XIIa [60,61] can activate factor XII bound to a surface [58–61]. Factor XIIa also activate the conversion of prekallikrein to kallikrein [62,63] and factor XI to factor XIa [64–67] in reactions requiring high-molecular-weight kininogen as a cofactor in addition to an appropriate surface [59,68–71] (Fig. 135-2). High-molecular-weight kinin-

FIGURE 135-2   Reactions of the contact phase of blood coagulation. The solid arrows indicate conversion of a substrate to a product. The narrow solid lines without arrowheads indicate a catalytic function. Factor XIIf denotes the fragments of factor XII produced by the action of kallikrein or plasmin. HMW-kininogen indicates high-molecular-weight kininogen. HMW-kininogen functions both as a cofactor (for the activation of prekallikrein, factor XI, and factor XII) and as a substrate (in the formation of bradykinin). The other reactants subserve a single function, although factor XII yields two products, a high-molecular-weight, surface-bound factor XIIa, and a low-molecular-weight, fluid phase factor XIIf. Kallikrein mediates a positive feedback loop, activating factor XII with HMW-kininogen as a cofactor.

Prekallikrein is also called the Fletcher factor. HMW-kininogen is known variously as the Fitzgerald, Flaujeac, or Williams factor.

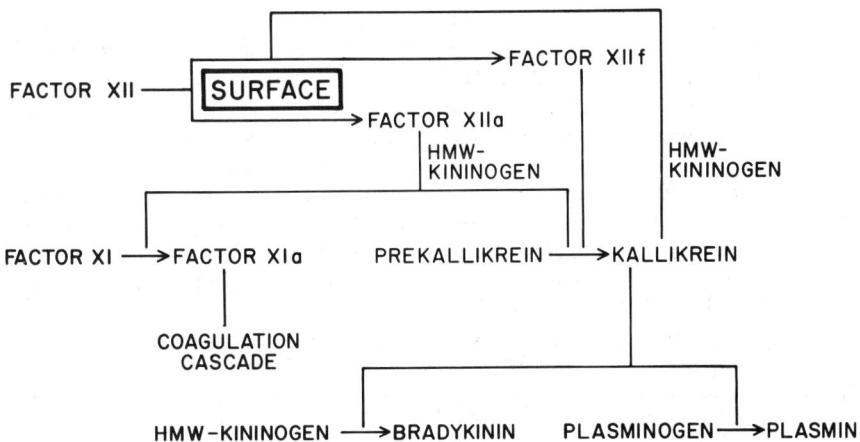

ogen appears to function by binding to the surface and providing a means for orientation of prekallikrein or factor XI [59,68–71]. The prekallikrein and/or factor XI are activated by factor XIIa [59,68–71]. Factor XIa then continues the coagulation cascade sequence.

The kallikrein formed in this reaction remains active at the surface or may be released into the fluid phase [59]. On the surface it attacks factor XII in reactions markedly accelerated by high-molecular-weight kininogen [59,71,72]. Platelets can also promote the proteolytic activation of factor XII by kallikrein [73]. On both the surface and in the fluid phase kallikrein hydrolyzes factor XII at several places, forming activated factor XII, which remains bound to the surface [74], and factor XII fragments [36,59,62,63,71] (Chap. 132). Autodigestion of factor XIIa also produces factor XII fragments [201]. The enzymatically active center of factor XII is located on a small fragment ($M_r = 28,000$ daltons) which is released into the medium, while other enzymatically inactive fragments remain bound to the surface [36,59,71,74]. Factor XII fragments are much more effective in activating prekallikrein and plasminogen proactivator than they are in activating factor XI [75–78]. Activation of factor XII is discussed further in Chap. 15.

Clinical data derived from patients with coagulation abnormalities indicate that maximal rates of activation of factor XII require prekallikrein (Fletcher factor) and high-molecular-weight kininogen as well as adequate concentrations of factor XII and an appropriate surface [79–87]. The abnormality first described as the "Fletcher trait" is characterized by a prolonged activated partial thromboplastin time which progressively shortens as the plasma is incubated with kaolin [88,89] (see also Chap. 152). The defect in Fletcher trait plasma is corrected by addition of normal plasma or small amounts of prekallikrein [79–81]. As noted above, kallikrein appears to function in the early stages of blood coagulation by providing feedback activation of factor XII (Fig. 135-2). Fletcher trait plasma also has defective fibrinolysis, chemotactic activity, kinin generation, and esterase activity [79–82]. All these abnormalities can be explained by the prekallikrein deficiency.

The discovery of prolonged activated partial thromboplastin times in three patients with normal levels of all previously recognized plasma coagulation factors indicated that additional components are involved in the coagulation mechanism. The abnormalities designated Fitzgerald [83,84], Flaujeac [85,86], and Williams [87] traits are due to deficiency of high-molecular-weight kininogen which functions as a cofactor in the activation of factors XII and XI [86,87,90].

Plasmin attacks factor XII in the same manner as kallikrein [36], to yield fragments capable of activating factor XI and prekallikrein [36,62,63,79,91]. The role of this series of reactions in normal blood coagulation is undefined. An additional effect of factor XIIa is the activation of factor VII, which is observed in plasma exposed to a foreign surface [37,38,92,93]. Plasmin may also play a role [94]. Another previously undescribed co-

agulation factor, the Passovoy factor, has been recognized [95], but its function is unknown.

Factor XIIa (activated factor XII) functions as an enzyme in activating factor XI [96–99]. Calcium is not required [64,96], but the reaction is accelerated by high-molecular-weight kininogen [69,70,100,101] and appears to take place on surfaces [56,69,75,102–104]. Optimal activation of factor XI is achieved with stoichiometric rather than catalytic amounts of high-molecular-weight kininogen [68,69]. The consumption of factor XI during clotting is usually minimal, but it becomes complete if the plasma is exposed to a sufficiently large surface [104,105]. The amount of factor XI consumed is in proportion to the amount of factor XIa formed [15,97,104,106]. Factor XI is adsorbed by surfaces but does not appear to be activated in the absence of factor XII [103]. However, factor XI preparations obtained from factor XII-deficient plasma become activated slowly [96]. Long-chain fatty acids may accelerate the activation of factor XI [107].

Because of the absence of a clinical bleeding syndrome in patients with factor XII deficiency [49], it has been suggested that factor XI can be activated by some means other than reaction with factor XIIa. This concept is supported by the observation that factor XI isolated from factor XII–deficient plasma is partially activated, and that purified factor XI undergoes "spontaneous" activation [96]. Platelets may promote activation of factor XI in reactions that are both factor XIIa–dependent and factor XIIa–independent [73,108], and platelets may accelerate the activation of factor IX, possibly by enhancing the effect of traces of factors XI and XII [109].

The product of the reaction of factor XIIa with factor XI has enzymatic activity and is able to activate factor IX [64–67]. Factor XIa appears to be the product [64–67,98], although it has been suggested that the enzyme is actually a complex of factor XIIa with factor XIa [102,104]. Factor XIa is a serine protease [67,110] and is inhibited by heparin–antithrombin III [65,111].

Activation of factor IX by the product of the reaction of factor XIIa with factor XI (assumed here to be factor XIa) requires calcium [65,66]. Factor XIa appears to act as enzyme and factor IX as substrate [65,66,112–114]. Factor VIIa [39,40] and factor Xa [115] also can convert factor IX to its active form. The product, factor IXa, is a serine protease [114,116,117] with powerful coagulant activity which is inhibited by the heparin–antithrombin III complex [118]. Serum contains more factor IX activity than does plasma, probably because of the presence of some factor IXa [112]. The amount of factor IX converted to the active form during clotting is directly proportional to the amount of factor XIa present, and complete consumption of factor IX can be effected [113]. The presence of factor IX in serum may be related to the relatively small amounts of factor XIa generated during normal clotting [113].

Factor IXa next participates in a reaction involving factor VIII, phospholipid or platelets, and calcium [118–120]. This reaction is accelerated by a trace of thrombin

[20,28–31,121–123] or factor Xa [32–34]. The product is a complex of phospholipid, calcium, factor IXa, and factor VIIIa [6–11]. Factor VIII and the platelets must be activated in order to support factor X activation in a purified system [34].

The phospholipid for this reaction is provided by platelets in whole blood. The phospholipids of platelets are bound to both membranes and granules. The membrane lipid is more readily available for participation in clotting [124]. Plasma factors appear generally to be present in excess, and platelet concentration may be the limiting factor in determining the amount of thrombin formed during clotting of blood [125,126].

The product of the reaction involving factors IXa and VIIIa acts as an enzyme to catalyze the activation of factor X, with calcium as cofactor [119,120,127]. Factor Xa is a serine protease [128,129] and is inhibited by the heparin–antithrombin III complex [130–132]. Factor Xa is also capable of inducing platelet aggregation [133]. During normal clotting very little factor X is consumed, but if additional factor VIII is added to plasma, more factor Xa is formed and additional factor X is consumed [127]. These results suggest that factor X remains in serum because insufficient activator of factor X is formed to permit complete conversion of factor X to factor Xa. This may be caused by the marked instability of factor VIII or the factor X activator [28,119,120].

Factor Xa is formed in extrinsic as well as intrinsic clotting and is the product of the action of Russell's viper venom on factor X [134–137]. Factor Xa is the enzyme responsible for the conversion of prothrombin to thrombin; and factor Va, phospholipid or platelets, and calcium serve to accelerate the reaction [14,16,138–151]. Factor Xa can also catalyze the activation of factor IX [98].

The reaction of factor Xa with factor Va, phospholipid or platelets, and calcium yields a complex involving these four components [12–17], referred to in Fig. 135-1 as *prothrombinase*. The complex can be dissociated and the components recovered unchanged [13–16]. The complex acts as an enzyme in catalyzing the conversion of prothrombin to thrombin [14,16]. Factor Xa binds to the surface of thrombin-activated platelets in a calcium-requiring reaction involving factor Va, and prothrombin is converted to thrombin by this complex [139–151]. Factor Va and Xa are bound to the lipid component much more tightly than is prothrombin. The prothrombinase complex is readily formed in the absence of prothrombin [150]. Initiation of blood coagulation and the platelet release reaction may occur simultaneously, and it appears that under some circumstances thrombin formation is associated with the platelet surface [152–155].

Information bearing on the role of the γ-carboxyglutamate residues of prothrombin in its activation has been obtained by comparison of the activation of normal prothrombin with that of the abnormal "prothrombin" formed in animals receiving vitamin K antagonists (dicoumarol prothrombin) (see Chap. 133) [156]. This abnormal "prothrombin" reacts with antibodies to prothrombin [157] but is not activated at a normal rate by systems employing tissue factor [157,158] or by mixtures of factor Xa, phospholipid, and calcium [156]. In contrast, mixtures of factor Xa and calcium and of factor Xa, factor Va, and calcium activate normal prothrombin and dicoumarol prothrombin at identical rates [156].

Normal prothrombin contains several residues of γ-carboxyglutamic acid, but these are missing in the dicoumarol prothrombin [159–161]. The γ-carboxyglutamate residues bind calcium [157,162,163], and calcium is required for binding prothrombin to phospholipid [10–12]. The precise mechanism by which calcium enhances the interaction of prothrombin with phospholipid has not been determined [202]. The phospholipid-binding site(s) are located in the same part of the molecule as the calcium-binding sites and the γ-carboxyglutamic acid residues [164,165]. As would be expected, dicoumarol prothrombin binds to phospholipid much less tightly than does normal prothrombin [156]. The failure of dicoumarol prothrombin to bind to phospholipid may explain why, as noted above, the activation of dicoumarol prothrombin by factor Xa and calcium is not accelerated by the addition of phospholipid to the reaction mixture. Thus, binding of prothrombin to the phospholipid moiety of "prothrombinase" is essential for normal coagulation. Factor X also contains γ-carboxyglutamic acid residues [166,167], which are involved in calcium and phospholipid binding of that molecule as well.

Incubation of factor V with small amounts of thrombin converts factor V to factor Va, a smaller molecule with markedly increased coagulant activity [15,20–22,168,169]. Factor Va binds to platelets in a reaction requiring calcium and stimulated by factor Xa and prothrombin [203]. Factor V is consumed during normal clotting and is absent from serum. Nearly all the prothrombin present in normal plasma is converted to thrombin by prothrombinase, and serum is therefore essentially devoid of this factor. The conversion of prothrombin to thrombin involves a marked change in molecular weight and the appearance of new free-amino end groups and clearly is due to a proteolytic split of the prothrombin molecule. Details of the chemical changes involved are presented in Chap. 132.

Thrombin is a proteolytic enzyme which attacks fibrinogen and converts it to fibrin monomer by hydrolyzing four peptide bonds per mole, releasing 2 mol each of fibrinopeptides A and B (Chap. 132). Sufficient thrombin is formed in normal clotting to convert all the fibrinogen in plasma to fibrin, and normal serum contains no fibrinogen. Although thrombin will clot fibrinogen in the absence of calcium, this reaction is accelerated by calcium [170,171]. The heparin–antithrombin III complex inhibits the proteolytic activity of thrombin [172]. As noted above, thrombin may serve extremely important functions in addition to the conversion of fibrinogen to fibrin by acting on factors V and VIII to increase their reactivity. It also activates factor XIII (see below) and causes platelet aggregation and release of platelet constituents (Chaps. 127–129).

The fibrin monomer formed by the action of thrombin on fibrinogen next polymerizes by hydrogen bonding to form a fibrin clot. The clot formed from purified fibrinogen and thrombin is mechanically unstable and is soluble in concentrated urea solutions, whereas the clot formed in normal plasma is mechanically stronger and is insoluble in concentrated urea solutions [173,174]. These differences are results of the action of factor XIIIa, an enzyme which is formed by the action of thrombin on factor XIII [175,176]. Factor XIII appears to circulate in plasma bound to fibrinogen [177]. Factor XIIIa is a transamidase, catalyzing the formation of peptide bonds between glutamine and lysine groups in adjacent molecules of fibrin monomer in the clot (Chap. 132). It is almost completely absent from serum [178]. The reaction of factor XIIIa with fibrin is the final step in intrinsic clotting and yields a mechanically strong, hemostatically effective clot.

The extrinsic system

The term *extrinsic system* [3] refers to that portion of the coagulation sequence which is activated following addition of tissue extracts and calcium to plasma. The unique step in the extrinsic system is the reaction of tissue factor (factor III) with factor VII. Incubation of tissue factor and calcium with factor VII results in the development of marked coagulant activity, which is sedimentable by high-speed centrifugation [179] and appears to be the result of a complex of these reactants [4,5,180]. Factor VII, a single-chain molecule, is attacked by factor Xa to yield factor VIIa, a two-chain molecule with enhanced coagulant activity [181–183]. The complex of tissue factor and factor VII or VIIa acts enzymatically with calcium as cofactor to convert factor X to factor Xa [4,5,181–183]. The enzymatic activity of the complex appears to be due to the factor VII moiety [4,184–187]. Factor VII is inactivated by diisopropyl fluorophosphate (DFP) in plasma [188] and after purification [185,189], suggesting that it may be circulating in an enzymatically active form, although no coagulant activity can be detected in the absence of tissue factor. The activity of factor VII is increased after exposure of plasma to foreign surfaces [190,191] and during clotting [190,192,193]. This increase in activity appears to be due to the action of factor XIIa [37,38,92,93], kallikrein [92,93,106], thrombin [185], factor Xa [185], and possibly plasmin [94].

One point of apparent difference between the extrinsic and intrinsic systems is the in vitro requirement for added phospholipid in the latter, provided by either platelets or emulsions of extracted phospholipids. This apparent difference can be explained by the observation that tissue factor is composed of phospholipid, protein, and cholesterol and that the phospholipid in this lipoprotein complex is able to function in the formation of prothrombinase [194]. Thus, tissue factor provides its own phospholipid, and the two systems function identically after the activation of factor X, except for the source of the phospholipid: in the extrinsic system from tissue factor and in the intrinsic system from platelets.

The function of the extrinsic system in clotting in vivo is uncertain. The extrinsic system is not required for coagulation to occur, since the intrinsic system functions quite independently of tissue factor or factor VII [195]. However, individuals with congenital deficiencies of factor VII have significant bleeding disorders [196], demonstrating the physiologic importance of the extrinsic system. Congenital deficiencies of tissue factor have not been reported.

The extrinsic system may be important in accelerating coagulation by providing a mechanism for the rapid production of small amounts of thrombin [28]. The thrombin so formed can convert factors V and VIII to more rapidly reactive forms [20,28,29] and initiate or enhance platelet aggregation [197] as well as institute fibrin formation. It may be that tissue factor is released at the site of injury whenever a wound occurs, possibly from the intima of blood vessels [198–200], and then can react rapidly with factor VII in the plasma. Activation of factor VII during clotting [190,192,193] may accelerate this reaction. Since only small amounts of tissue factor and factor VII may initiate rapid thrombin formation, the hypothesis of an acceleratory role for the extrinsic system in vivo seems reasonable. Factor Xa can activate factor IX [115] and may thus provide an additional acceleratory interaction between the extrinsic and intrinsic systems.

Implications of the cascade hypothesis

The essential basis of the cascade concept of blood coagulation is that the active coagulation factors are enzymes, the function of which is to beget other enzymes. The enzymic nature of the products applies even to those steps in which complex formation occurs. Enzymes are catalysts, and a small quantity of enzymes would be expected to convert a large quantity of substrate to product. If the product is also an enzyme, as it is in the cascade concept, a series of such reactions could lead to a rapidly increasing enzymatic activity, with a small amount of enzyme formed initially leading, after several steps, to a relatively enormous quantity of enzyme. Macfarlane [1] originally pointed out the amplification potential of the cascade concept. Whether the amplification possibilities of the cascade are realized in vivo is obviously unknown, as is the more fundamental question of whether or not the cascade concept has any biologic significance at all. In an evaluation of the overall function of the cascade, the concentration of the reactants, their inherent reaction rates, the stability of the enzymes, substrates, and complexes, the activity of inhibitors, effects of competing reactions, etc., must be considered. Precise data on many of these points are slowly accumulating, but a realistic evaluation of the implications of the cascade concept, or of any newer clotting theory, will require much additional research to obtain sufficient information to analyze the system in detail.

References

1. Macfarlane, R. G.: An enzyme cascade in the blood clotting mechanism and its function as a biochemical amplifier. *Nature 202:*498, 1964.

2. Davie, E. W., and Ratnoff, O. D.: Waterfall sequence for intrinsic blood clotting. *Science 145:*1310, 1964.

3. Straub, W., and Duckert, F.: The formation of the extrinsic prothrombin activator. *Thromb. Diath. Haemorrh. 5:*402, 1961.

4. Williams, W. J., and Norris, D. G.: Purification of a bovine plasma protein (factor VII) which is required for the activity of lung microsomes in blood coagulation. *J. Biol. Chem. 241:*1847, 1966.

5. Nemerson, Y.: The reaction between bovine brain tissue factor and factors VII and X. *Biochemistry 5:*601, 1966.

6. Hougie, C., Denson, K. W. E., and Biggs, R.: A study of the reaction product of factor VIII and factor IX by gel filtration. *Thromb. Diath. Haemorrh. 18:*211, 1967.

7. Hemker, H. C., and Kahn, M. J. P.: Reaction sequence of blood coagulation. *Nature 215:*1201, 1967.

8. Barton, P. G.: Sequence theories of blood coagulation reevaluated with reference to lipid-protein interactions. *Nature 215:*1508, 1967.

9. Østerud, B., and Rapaport, S. I.: Synthesis of intrinsic factor X activator: Inhibition of the function of formed activator by antibodies to factor VIII and to factor IX. *Biochemistry 9:*1854, 1970.

10. Hemker, H. C., Kahn, M. J. B., and Devilee, P. P.: The adsorption of coagulant factors onto phospholipids: Its role in the reaction mechanisms of blood coagulation. *Thromb. Diath. Haemorrh. 24:*214, 1970.

11. Chuang, T. F., Sargeant, R. B., and Hougie, C.: The intrinsic activation of factor X in blood coagulation. *Biochim. Biophys. Acta 273:*287, 1972.

12. Papahadjopoulos, D., and Hanahan, D. J.: Observations on the interaction of phospholipids and certain clotting factors in prothrombin activator formation. *Biochim. Biophys. Acta 90:*436, 1964.

13. Cole, E. R., Koppel, J. L., and Olwin, J. H.: Interaction of bovine autoprothrombin C with phospholipids and divalent cation. *Can. J. Biochem. 42:*1595, 1964.

14. Jobin, F., and Esnouf, M. P.: Studies on the formation of the prothrombin converting complex. *Biochem. J. 102:*666, 1967.

15. Barton, P. G., and Hanahan, D. J.: The preparation and properties of a stable factor V from bovine plasma. *Biochim. Biophys. Acta 133:*506, 1967.

16. Barton, P. G., Jackson, C. M., and Hanahan, D. J.: Relationship between factor V and activated factor X in the generation of prothrombinase. *Nature 214:*923, 1967.

17. Hemker, H. C., Esnouf, M. P., Hemker, P. W., Swart, A. C. W., and Macfarlane, R. G.: Formation of prothrombin converting activity. *Nature 215:*248, 1967.

18. Ware, A. G., and Seegers, W. H.: Serum Ac-globulin: Formation from plasma Ac-globulin; role in blood coagulation; partial purification; properties; and quantitative determination. *Am. J. Physiol. 152:*567, 1948.

19. Hjort, P. F.: Intermediate reactions in the coagulation of blood with tissue thromboplastin. *Scand. J. Clin. Lab. Invest. 9 (Suppl. 27):*1, 1957.

20. Rapaport, S. I., Schiffman, S., Patch, M. J., and Ames, S. B.: The importance of activation of antihemophilic globulin and proaccelerin by traces of thrombin in the generation of intrinsic prothrombinase activity. *Blood 21:*221, 1963.

21. Papahadjopoulos, D., Hougie, C., and Hanahan, D. J.: Purification and properties of bovine factor V: A change of molecular size during blood coagulation. *Biochemistry 3:*264, 1964.

22. Hussain, Q. Z., and Newcomb, T. F.: Effects of thrombin on factor V. *Ann. Biochem. Exp. Med. 23:*569, 1963.

23. Bergsagel, D. E., and Nockolds, E. R.: The activation of proaccelerin. *Br. J. Haematol. 11:*395, 1965.

24. Prentice, C. R. M., Ratnoff, O. D., and Breckenridge, R. T.: Experiments on the nature of the prothrombin-converting principle: Alteration of proaccelerin by thrombin. *Br. J. Haematol. 13:*898, 1967.

25. Colman, R. W.: The effects of proteolytic enzymes on bovine factor V. I. Kinetics of activation and inactivation by bovine thrombin. *Biochemistry 8:*1438, 1969.

26. Hanahan, D. J., Rolfs, M. R., and Day, W. C.: Observations on the factor V activator present in Russell's viper venom and its action on factor V. *Biochim. Biophys. Acta 286:*205, 1972.

27. Esmon, C. T., Owen, W. G., Duiguid, D. L., and Jackson, C. M.: Reaction of thrombin on blood clotting factor V: Conversion of factor V to a prothrombin-binding protein. *Biochim. Biophys. Acta 310:*289, 1973.

28. Biggs, R., Macfarlane, R. G., Denson, K. W. E., and Ash, B. J.: Thrombin and the interaction of factor VIII and IX. *Br. J. Haematol. 11:*276, 1965.

29. Özge-Anwar, A. H., Connell, G. E., and Mustard, J. F.: Thrombin and the interaction of factors VIII and IX. *Br. J. Haematol. 11:*276, 1965.

30. Shapiro, G. A., Anderson, J. C., Pizzo, S. V., and McKee, P. A.: The subunit of normal and hemophilic factor VIII. *J. Clin. Invest. 52:*2198, 1973.

31. Legaz, M. E., Schmer, G., Counts, R. B., and Davie, E. W.: Isolation and chemical characterization of human factor VIII. *J. Biol. Chem. 248:*3946, 1973.

32. Vehar, G. A., and Davie, E. W.: Preparation and properties of bovine factor VIII (antihemophilic factor). *Biochemistry 19:*401, 1980.

33. Hultin, M., and Jesty, J.: The activation and inactivation of human factor VIII by thrombin: Effect of inhibitors of thrombin. *Blood 57:*476, 1981.

34. Hultin, M. B.: Role of human factor VIII in factor X activation. *J. Clin. Invest. 69:*950, 1982.

35. Cochrane, C. G., Revak, S. D., and Wuepper, K. D.: Activation of Hageman factors in solid and fluid phases: A critical role of kallikrein. *J. Exp. Med. 138:*1564, 1973.

36. Revak, S. D., Cochrane, C. G., Johnston, A. R., and Hugh, T. E.: Structural changes accompanying enzymatic activation of human Hageman factor. *J. Clin. Invest. 54:*619, 1974.

37. Radcliffe, R., Bagdasarian, A., Colman, R., and Nemerson, Y.: Activation of bovine factor VII by Hageman factor fragments. *Blood 50:*611, 1977.

38. Kisiel, W., Fujikawa, K., and Davie, E. W.: Activation of bovine factor VII (proconvertin) by factor XIIa (activated Hageman factor). *Biochemistry 16:*4189, 1979.

39. Zur, M., and Nemerson, Y.: Kinetics of factor IX activation via the extrinsic pathway. Dependence of Km on tissue factor. *J. Biol. Chem. 255:*5703, 1980.

40. Østerud, B., and Rapaport, S. I.: Activation of factor IX by the reaction product of tissue factor and factor VII: Additional pathway for initiating blood coagulation. *Proc. Natl. Acad. Sci. U.S.A. 74:*5260, 1977.

41. Kaplan, A. P., and Austen, K. F.: A prealbumin activator of prekallikrein. II. Derivation of activators of prekallikrein from active Hageman factor by digestion with plasmin. *J. Exp. Med. 133:*696, 1971.

42. Burrowes, C. E., Morat, H. Z., and Soltay, M. J.: The kinin system of human plasma. VI. The action of plasmin. *Proc. Soc. Exp. Biol. Med. 138:*959, 1971.

43. Stenn, K. S., and Blount, E. R.: Mechanism of bovine prothrombin activation by an insoluble preparation of bovine factor Xa (thrombokinase). *Biochemistry 11:*4502, 1972.

44. Heldebrant, C. M., Butkowski, R. J., Bajaj, S. P., and Mann, K. G.: The activation of prothrombin. II. Partial reactions, physical and chemical characterization of the intermediates of activation. *J. Biol. Chem. 248:*7149, 1973.

45. Owen, W. G., Esmon, C. T., and Jackson, C. M.: The conversion of prothrombin to thrombin. I. Characterization of the reaction prod-

ucts formed during the activation of bovine prothrombin. *J. Biol. Chem.* 249:594, 1974.

46. Esmon, C. T., Owen, W. G., and Jackson, C. M.: The conversion of prothrombin to thrombin. II. Differentiation between thrombin- and factor Xa-catalyzed proteolyses. *J. Biol. Chem.* 249:606, 1974.

47. Jesty, J., Spencer, A. K., and Nemerson, Y.: The mechanism of activation of factor X: Kinetic control of alternative pathways leading to the formation of activated factor X. *J. Biol. Chem.* 249:5614, 1974.

48. Jesty, J., Spencer, A. K., Nakashima, Y., Nemerson, Y., and Konigsberg, W.: The activation of coagulation factor X: Identity of cleavage sites in the alternative pathways and characterization of the COOH terminal peptide. *J. Biol. Chem.* 250:4497, 1975.

49. Ratnoff, O. D., and Steinberg, A. G.: Further studies on the inheritance of Hageman trait. *J. Lab. Clin. Med.* 59:980, 1962.

50. Wilner, G. D., Nossel, H. L., and LeRoy, E. C.: Activation of Hageman factor by collagen. *J. Clin. Invest.* 47:2608, 1968.

51. Margolis, J.: Activation of Hageman factor by saturated fatty acids. *Aust. J. Exp. Biol. Med. Sci.* 40:505, 1962.

52. Ratnoff, O. D.: The biology and pathology of the initial stages of blood coagulation, in *Progress in Hematology*, edited by E. B. Brown and C. V. Moore. Grune & Stratton, New York, 1966, vol. V, p. 204.

53. Donaldson, V. H., and Ratnoff, O. D.: Hageman factor: Alterations in physical properties during activation. *Science* 150:754, 1965.

54. McMillan, C. R., Saito, H., Ratnoff, O. D., and Walton, A. G.: The secondary structure of human Hageman factor (factor XII) and its alteration by activation agents. *J. Clin. Invest.* 54:1312,, 1974.

55. Fair, B. D., Saito, H., Ratnoff, O. D., and Rippon, W. B.: Detection of fluorescence of structural changes accompanying the activation of Hageman factor (factor XII). *Proc. Soc. Exp. Biol. Med.* 155:199, 1977.

56. Hardisty, R. M., and Margolis, J.: The role of Hageman factor in the initiation of blood coagulation. *Br. J. Haematol.* 5:203, 1959.

57. Ratnoff, O. D., and Rosenblum, J. M.: The role of Hageman factor in the initiation of clotting by glass. *J. Lab. Clin. Med.* 50:941, 1957.

58. Wiggins, R. C., and Cochrane, C. G.: The autoactivation of rabbit Hageman factor. *J. Exp. Med.* 150:1122, 1979.

59. Cochrane, C. G., and Griffin, J. H.: Molecular assembly in the contract phase of the Hageman factor system. *Am. J. Med.* 67:657, 1979.

60. Silverberg, M., Thompson, R., Miller, G., and Kaplan, A. P.: Initiation of the intrinsic coagulation pathway: Autoactivatability of human Hageman factor and mechanisms by which the light chain derived from HMW-kininogen functions as a co-factor in the activation of prekallikrenin, factor XI, and Hageman factor, in *The Regulation of Coagulation*, edited by K. G. Mann and F. B. Taylor, Jr. Elsevier–North Holland, New York, 1980, p. 531.

61. Ratnoff, O. D., and Saito, H.: Interactions among Hageman factor, plasma prekallikrein, high molecular weight kininogen, and plasma thromboplastin antecedent. *Proc. Natl. Acad. Sci. U.S.A.* 76:958, 1979.

62. Kaplan, A. P., and Austen, K. F.: A pre-albumin activator of prekallikrein. *J. Immunol.* 105:802, 1970.

63. Cochrane, C. G., and Wuepper, K. D.: The first component of the kinin-forming system in human and rabbit plasma: Its relationship to clotting factor XII (Hageman factor). *J. Exp. Med.* 134:986, 1971.

64. Kingdon, H. S., and Lundblad, R. L.: Factors affecting the evolution of factor XIa during blood coagulation. *J. Lab. Clin. Med.* 85:826, 1975.

65. Ratnoff, O. D., and Davie, E. W.: The activation of Christmas factor (factor IX) by activated plasma thromboplastin antecedent (activated factor XI). *Biochemistry* 1:677, 1962.

66. Schiffman, S., Rapaport, S. I., and Patch, M. J.: The identification and synthesis of activated plasma thromboplastin component (PTC). *Blood* 22:733, 1963.

67. Kingdon, H. S., Davie, E. W., and Ratnoff, O. D.: The reaction between activated plasma thromboplastin antecedent and diisopropylphosphofluoridate. *Biochemistry* 3:166, 1964.

68. Schiffman, S., and Lee, P.: Partial purification and characterization of contact activation cofactor. *J. Clin. Invest.* 56:1082, 1975.

69. Griffin, J. H., and Cochrane, C. G.: Mechanisms for the involvement of high molecular weight kininogen in surface-dependent reactions of Hageman factor. *Proc. Natl. Acad. Sci. U.S.A.* 73:2554, 1976.

70. Meier, H. L., Pierce, J. V., Colman, R. W., and Kaplan, A. P.: Activation and function of human Hageman factor. The role of high molecular weight kininogen and prekallikrein. *J. Clin. Invest.* 60:18, 1977.

71. Kaplan, A. P.: Initiation of the intrinsic coagulation and fibrinolytic pathways of man: The role of surfaces, Hageman factor, prekallikrein, high molecular weight kininogen, and factor XI, in *Progress in Thrombosis and Hemostatis*, edited by T. H. Spaet. Grune & Stratton, New York, 1978, vol. 4, p. 127.

72. Griffin, J. H.: Role of surface in surface-dependent activation of Hageman factor (blood coagulation factor XII). *Proc. Natl. Acad. Sci. U.S.A.* 75:1998, 1978.

73. Walsh, P. N., and Griffin, J. H.: Contributions of human platelets to the proteolytic activation of blood coagulation factors XII and XI. *Blood* 57:106, 1981.

74. Revak, S. D., Cochrane, C. G., and Griffin, J. H.: The binding and cleavage characteristics of human Hageman factor during contact activation. *J. Clin. Invest.* 59:1167, 1977.

75. Cochrane, C. G., and Wuepper, K. D.: The first component of the kinin-forming system in human and rabbit plasma. Its relationship to clotting factor XII (Hageman factor). *J. Exp. Med.* 134:986, 1971.

76. Revak, S. D., Cochrane, C. G., Johnston, A. R., and Hugh, T. E.: Structural changes accompanying enzymatic activation of human Hageman factor. *J. Clin. Invest.* 54:619, 1974.

77. Revak, S. D., and Cochrane, C. G.: The relationship of structure and function in human Hageman factor: The association of enzymatic and binding activities with separate regions of the molecule. *J. Clin. Invest.* 57:852, 1976.

78. Soltay, M. J., Movat, H. Z., and Ozge-Anwar, A. H.: The kinin system of human plasma. V. The probable derivative of prekallikrein activator from activated Hageman factor (XIIa). *Proc. Soc. Exp. Biol. Med.* 138:952, 1971.

79. Wuepper, K. D.: Biochemistry and biology of components of the plasma kinin-forming system, in *Inflammatory: Mechanisms and Control*, edited by I. H. Lepow and P. A. Ward. Academic, New York, 1972, p. 93.

80. Weiss, A. S., Gallin, J. I., and Kaplan, A. P.: Fletcher factor deficiency: A diminished rate of Hageman factor activation caused by absence of prekallikrein with abnormalities of coagulation, fibrinolysis, chemotactic activity, and kinin generation. *J. Clin. Invest.* 53:622, 1974.

81. Saito, H., Ratnoff, O. D., and Donaldson, V. H.: Defective activation of clotting fibrinolytic, and permeability-enhancing systems in human Fletcher trait plasma. *Circ. Res.* 34:641, 1974.

82. Donaldson, V. H., Saito, H., and Ratnoff, O. D.: Defective esterase and kinin-forming activity in human Fletcher trait plasma: A fraction rich in kallikrein-like activity. *Circ. Res.* 34:652, 1974.

83. Waldmann, R., and Abraham, J. P.: Fitzgerald factor: A heretofore unrecognized coagulation factor. *Blood* 44:934, 1974.

84. Saito, H., Ratnoff, O. D., Waldmann, R., and Abraham, J. P.: Fitzgerald trait: Deficiency of a hitherto unrecognized agent, Fitzgerald factor, participating in surface-mediated reactions of clotting, fibrinolysis, generation of kinins, and the property of diluted plasma enhancing vascular permeability (PF/DIL). *J. Clin. Invest.* 55:1082, 1975.

85. Lacombe, M.-J., Varet, B., and Levy, J.-P.: A hitherto undescribed plasma factor acting at the contact phase of blood coagulation (Flaujeac factor): Case report and coagulation studies. *Blood* 46:761, 1975.

86. Wuepper, K. D., Miller, D. R., and Lacombe, M.-J.: Flaujeac trait: Deficiency of human plasma kininogen. *J. Clin. Invest.* 56:1663, 1975.

87. Colman, R. W., et al.: Williams trait: Human kininogen deficiency with diminished levels of plasminogen proactivator and prekallikrein associated with abnormalities of the Hageman factor-dependent pathways. *J. Clin. Invest.* 56:1650, 1975.

88. Hathaway, W. E., Belhasen, L. P., and Hathaway, H. S.: Evidence of a new plasma thromboplastin factor. I. Case report, coagulation studies and physicochemical properties. *Blood* 26:521, 1965.

89. Hattersley, P. G., and Hayse, D.: Fletcher factor deficiency: A report of three unrelated cases. *Br. J. Haematol.* 18:411, 1970.

90. Donaldson, V. H., Glueck, H. I., Miller, M. A., Movat, H. Z., and Habal, F.: Kininogen deficiency in Fitzgerald trait: Role of high

molecular weight kininogen in clotting and fibrinolysis. *J. Lab. Clin. Med.* 87:327, 1976.

91. Soltay, M. J., Movat, H. Z., and Özge-Anwar, A. H.: The kinin system of human plasma. V. The probable derivation of prekallikrein activator from activated Hageman factor (XIIa). *Proc. Soc. Exp. Biol. Med.* 138:952, 1971.

92. Gjønnaess, H.: Cold-promoted activation of factor VII: IV. Relation to the coagulation system. *Thromb. Diath. Haemorrh.* 28:194, 1972.

93. Saito, H., and Ratnoff, O. D.: Alteration of factor VII activity by activated Fletcher factor (a plasma kallikrein): A potential link between the intrinsic and extrinsic blood-clotting systems. *J. Lab. Clin. Med.* 85:405, 1975.

94. Laaki, K., and Østerud, B.: Activation of purified plasma factor VII by human plasmin, plasma kallikrein, and activated components of the human intrinsic blood coagulation system. *Thromb. Res.* 5:759, 1974.

95. Hougie, C., et al.: The Passovoy factor: Further characterization of a hereditary hemorrhagic diathesis. *N. Engl. J. Med.* 298:1045, 1978.

96. Ratnoff, O. D., Davie, E. W., and Mallet, D. L.: Studies on the action of Hageman factor: Evidence that activated Hageman factor in turn activates plasma thromboplastin antecedent. *J. Clin. Invest.* 40:803, 1961.

97. Nossel, H. L.: *The Contact Phase of Blood Coagulation.* Blackwell, Oxford, 1964.

98. Ratnoff, O. D.: Studies on the product of the reaction between activated Hageman factor (factor XII) and plasma thromboplastin antecedent (factor XI). *J. Lab. Clin. Invest.* 80:704, 1972.

99. Movat, H. Z., and Özge-Anwar, A. H.: The contact phase of blood coagulation: Clotting factors XI and XII, their isolation and interaction. *J. Lab. Clin. Med.* 84:861, 1974.

100. Schiffman, S., and Lee, P.: Preparation, characterization and activation of a highly purified factor XI: Evidence that a hitherto unrecognized plasma activity participates in the interaction of factors XI and XII. *Br. J. Haematol.* 27:101, 1974.

101. Schiffman, S., Lee, P., and Waldmann, R.: Identify of contact activation cofactor and Fitzgerald factor. *Thromb. Res.* 6:451, 1975.

102. Vroman, L.: Effects of hydrophobic surfaces on blood coagulation. *Thromb. Diath. Haemorrh.* 10:455, 1964.

103. Soulier, J. P., and Prou-Wartelle, O.: New data on Hageman factor and plasma thromboplastin antecedent: The role of contact in the initial phase of blood coagulation. *Br. J. Haematol.* 6:88, 1960.

104. Haanen, C., Morselt, G., and Schoenmakers, J.: Contact activation of Hageman factor and the interaction of Hageman factor and plasma thromboplastin antecedent. *Thromb. Diath. Haemorrh.* 17:307, 1967.

105. Waaler, B. A.: Contact activation in the intrinsic blood clotting system: Studies on a plasma product formed on contact with glass and similar surfaces. *Scand. J. Clin. Lab. Invest.* 11 (Suppl. 37):1, 1959.

106. Gjønnaess, H.: Cold-promoted activation of factor VII. III. Relation to the coagulation system. *Thromb. Diath. Haemorrh.* 28:182, 1972.

107. Botti, R. E., and Ratnoff, O. D.: The clot-promoting effect of soaps of long-chain saturated fatty acids. *J. Clin. Invest.* 42:1569, 1963.

108. Walsh, P. N., and Biggs, R.: The role of platelets in intrinsic factor Xa formation. *Br. J. Haematol.* 22:743, 1972.

109. Schiffman, S., Rapaport, S. I., and Chong, M. M. Y.: Platelets and initiation of intrinsic clotting. *Br. J. Haematol.* 24:633, 1973.

110. Heck, L. W., and Kaplan, A. P.: Substrates of Hageman factor. I. Isolation and characterization of human factor XI (PTA) and inhibition of the activated enzyme by α_1-antitrypsin. *J. Exp. Med.* 140:1615, 1974.

111. Rosenberg, R. D.: The effects of heparin on factor XIa and plasmin. *Thromb. Diath. Haemorrh.* 33:51, 1974.

112. Cattan, A. D., and Denson, K. W. E.: The interaction of contact product and factor IX. *Thromb. Diath. Haemorrh.* 11:155, 1964.

113. Nossel, H. L.: The activation and consumption of factor IX. *Thromb. Diath. Haemorrh.* 12:505, 1964.

114. Fujikawa, K., Legaz, M., Kato, H., and Davie, E. W.: The mechanism of activation of bovine factor IX (Christmas factor) by bovine factor XIa (activated plasma thromboplastin antecedent). *Biochemistry* 13:4508, 1974.

115. Kalousek, F., Konigsberg, W., and Nemerson, Y.: Activation of fac-

116. Enfield, D. L., Ericsson, L. H., Fujikawa, K., Titani, K., Walsh, K. A., and Neurath, H.: Bovine factor IX (Christmas factor): Further evidence of homology with factor X (Stuart factor) and prothrombin. *FEBS Lett.* 47:132, 1974.

117. Kato, H., Fujikawa, K., and Legaz, M. E.: Isolation and activation of bovine factor XI (plasma thromboplastin antecedent) and its interaction with factor IX (Christmas factor). *Fed. Proc.* 33:1505, 1974.

118. Lundblad, R. L., and Davie, E. W.: The activation of antihemophilic factor (factor VIII) by activated Christmas factor (activated factor IX). *Biochemistry* 3:1720, 1964.

119. Macfarlane, R. G., Biggs, R., Ash, B. J., and Denson, K. W. E.: The interaction of factors VIII and IX. *Br. J. Haematol.* 10:530, 1964.

120. Schiffman, S., Rapaport, S. I., and Chong, M. M. Y.: The mandatory role of lipid in the interaction of factors VIII and IX. *Proc. Soc. Exp. Biol. Med.* 123:736, 1966.

121. Switzer, M. E. P., and McKee, P. A.: Reactions of thrombin with human factor VIII/von Willebrand factor protein. *J. Biol. Chem.* 255:10606, 1980.

122. Rick, M. E., and Hoyer, L. W.: Thrombin activation of factor VIII. II. A comparison of purified factor VIII and the low molecular weight factor VIII procoagulant. *Br. J. Haematol.* 38:107, 1978.

123. Hoyer, L. W., and Trabold, N. C.: The effect of thrombin on human factor VIII. Cleavage of the factor VIII procoagulant protein during activation. *J. Lab. Clin. Med.* 97:50, 1981.

124. Marcus, A. J., Zucker-Franklin, D., Safier, L. B., and Ullman, H. L.: Studies on human platelet granules and membranes. *J. Clin. Invest.* 45:14, 1966.

125. Buckwalter, J. A., Blythe, W. B., and Brinkhous, K. M.: Effect of blood platelets on prothrombin utilization of dog and human plasmas. *Am. J. Physiol.* 159:316, 1949.

126. Penner, J. A.: Prothrombin levels in serum. *Thromb. Diath. Haemorrh.* 10:332, 1964.

127. Macfarlane, R. G., and Ash, B. J.: The activation and consumption of factor X in recalcified plasma: The effect of added factor VIII and Russell's viper venom. *Br. J. Haematol.* 10:217, 1964.

128. Jackson, C. M., and Hanahan, D. J.: Studies on bovine factor X. II. Characterization of purified factor X: Observations on some alterations in zone electrophoretic and chromatographic behavior occurring during purification. *Biochemistry* 7:4506, 1968.

129. Leveson, J. E., and Esnouf, M. P.: The inhibition of activated factor X with diisopropyl fluorophosphate. *Br. J. Haematol.* 17:173, 1969.

130. Seegers, W. F., Cole, E. R., Harmison, C. R., and Monkhouse, F. C.: Neutralization of autoprothrombin C activity with antithrombin. *Can. J. Biochem.* 42:359, 1964.

131. Biggs, R., Denson, K. W. E., Akman, N., Borrett, R., and Hadden, M.: Antithrombin III, antifactor Xa and heparin. *Br. J. Haematol.* 19:293, 1970.

132. Yin, E. T., Wessler, S., and Stoll, P. J.: Biological properties of the naturally occurring plasma inhibitor of activated factor X. *J. Biol. Chem.* 246:3703, 1971.

133. Jerons, S., and Barton, P. G.: Biochemistry of blood platelets: Interaction of activation factor X with platelets. *Biochemistry* 10:428, 1971.

134. Hougie, C.: Reactions of Stuart factor and factor VII with brain and factor V. *Proc. Soc. Exp. Biol. Med.* 101:132, 1959.

135. Esnouf, M. P., and Williams, W. J.: The isolation and purification of a bovine-plasma protein which is a substrate for the coagulant fraction of Russell's viper venom. *Biochem. J.* 84:62, 1962.

136. Marciniak, E., and Seegers, W. H.: Autoprothrombin C: A second enzyme from prothrombin. *Can. J. Biochem. Physiol.* 40:597, 1962.

137. Bergsagel, D. E., and Hougie, C.: Intermediate stages in the formation of blood thromboplastin. *Br. J. Haematol.* 2:113, 1956.

138. Milstone, J. H., Oulianoff, N., and Milstone, V. K.: Outstanding characteristics of thrombokinase isolated from bovine plasma. *J. Gen. Physiol.* 47:315, 1963.

139. Miletich, J. P., Jackson, C. M., and Marjerus, P. W.: Properties of the factor X_a binding site on human platelets. *J. Biol. Chem.* 253:6908, 1978.

140. Walsh, P. N.: Platelets and coagulation proteins. *Fed. Proc.* 40:2086, 1981.

141. Miletich, J. P., Jackson, C. M., and Majerus, P. W.: Interaction of coagulation factor X_a with human platelets. *Proc. Natl. Acad. Sci. U.S.A.* 74:4033, 1977.
142. Kane, W. H., Lindhout, M. J., Jackson, C. M., and Marjerus, P. W.: Factor V_a-dependent binding of factor X_a to human platelets. *J. Biol. Chem.* 255:1170, 1980.
143. Dahlbäck, B., and Stenflo, J.: Binding of bovine coagulation factor X_a to platelets. *Biochemistry* 17:4938, 1978.
144. Østerud, B., Rapaport, S. I., and Lavine, K. K.: Factor V activity of platelets: Evidence for an activated factor V molecule and for a platelet activator. *Blood* 49:819, 1977.
145. White, B. N., Cox, A. C., and Taylor, Jr., F. B.: The procoagulant effect of platelets on conversion of prothrombin to thrombin in nonanticoagulated plasma. *J. Lab. Clin. Med.* 95:827, 1980.
146. Tracy, P. B., Nesheim, M. E., and Mann, K. G.: Coordinate binding of factor V_a and X_a to the unstimulated platelet. *J. Biol. Chem.* 256:743, 1981.
147. Nesheim, M. E., Taswell, J. B., and Mann, K. G.: The contribution of bovine factor V and factor V_a to the activity of prothrombinase. *J. Biol. Chem.* 254:10952, 1979.
148. Nesheim, M. E., Kettner, C., Shaw, E., and Mann, K. G.: Cofactor dependence of X_a incorporation into the prothrombinase complex. *J. Biol. Chem.* 256:6537, 1981.
149. Kane, W. H., and Majerus, P. W.: The interaction of human coagulation factor V_a with platelets. *J. Biol. Chem.* 257:3963, 1982.
150. Nesheim, M. E., Eid, S., and Mann, K. G.: Assembly of the prothrombinase complex in the absence of prothrombin. *J. Biol. Chem.* 256:9874, 1981.
151. Teitel, J. M., Bauer, K. A., Lau, H. K., and Rosenberg, R. D.: Studies of the prothrombin activation pathway utilizing radioimmunoassays for the F_2/F_{1+2} fragment and thrombin-antithrombin complex. *Blood* 59:1086, 1982.
152. Shuman, M. A., and Levine, S. P.: Thrombin generation and secretion of platelet factor 4 during blood clotting. *J. Clin. Invest.* 61:1102, 1978.
153. Prowse, C. V., Vigano, S., Borsey, D. Q., and Dawes, J.: The release of beta-thromboglobulin from platelets during the clotting of whole blood. *Thromb. Res.* 17:433, 1980.
154. Kaplan, K. L., Drillings, M., and Lesznik, G.: Fibrinopeptide A cleavage and platelet release in whole blood in vitro. *J. Clin. Invest.* 67:1561, 1981.
155. Rybak, M. E., Lau, H. K., Tomkins, B., Rosenberg, R. D., and Handin, R. I.: Relationship between platelet secretion and prothrombin cleavage in native whole blood. *J. Clin. Invest.* 68:405, 1981.
156. Esmon, C. T., Suttie, J. W., and Jackson, C. M.: The functional significance of vitamin K action: Difference in phospholipid binding between normal and abnormal prothrombin. *J. Biol. Chem.* 250:4095, 1975.
157. Ganrot, P. O., and Niléhn, J. E.: Plasma prothrombin during treatment with dicoumarol. II. Demonstration of an abnormal prothrombin fraction. *Scand. J. Clin. Lab. Invest.* 22:23, 1968.
158. Nelsestuen, G. L., and Suttie, J. W.: The purification and properties of an abnormal prothrombin protein produced by dicoumarol-treated cows: A comparison to normal prothrombin. *J. Biol. Chem.* 247:8176, 1972.
159. Stenflo, J., Fernlund, P., Egan, W., and Rolpstorff, P.: Vitamin K dependent modifications of glutamic acid residues in prothrombin. *Proc. Natl. Acad. Sci. U.S.A.* 71:2730, 1974.
160. Magnusson, S., Sottrup-Jensen, L., Petersen, T. E., Morris, H. R., and Dell, A.: Primary structure of the vitamin K-dependent part of prothrombin. *FEBS Lett.* 44:189, 1974.
161. Nelsestuen, G. L., Zytkovicz, T. H., and Howard, J. B.: The mode of action of vitamin K: Identification of γ-carboxyglutamic acid as a component of prothrombin. *J. Biol. Chem.* 249:6347, 1974.
162. Nelsestuen, G. L., and Suttie, J. W.: Mode of action of vitamin K: Calcium binding properties of bovine prothrombin. *Biochemistry* 11:4961, 1972.
163. Stenflo, J., and Ganrot, P. O.: Binding of Ca^{2+} to normal and dicoumarol-induced prothrombin. *Biochem. Biophys. Res. Commun.* 50:98, 1973.
164. Gitel, S. N., Owen, W. G., Esmon, C. T., and Jackson, C. M.: A polypeptide region of bovine prothrombin specific for binding to phospholipids. *Proc. Natl. Acad. Sci. U.S.A.* 70:1344, 1973.
165. Benson, B. J., Kisiel, W., and Hanahan, D. J.: Calcium binding and other characteristics of bovine factor II and its activation intermediates. *Biochim. Biophys. Acta* 329:81, 1973.
166. Enfield, D. L., Ericsson, L. H., Walsh, K. A., Neurath, H., and Titani, K.: Bovine factor X_1 (Stuart factor): Primary structure of the light chain. *Proc. Natl. Acad. Sci. U.S.A.* 72:16, 1975.
167. Howard, J. B., and Nelsestuen, G. L.: Isolation and characterization of vitamin K-dependent region of bovine blood clotting factor X. *Proc. Natl. Acad. Sci. U.S.A.* 72:1281, 1975.
168. Dahlbäck, B.: Human coagulation factor V purification and thrombin-catalyzed activation. *J. Clin. Invest.* 66:583, 1980.
169. Kane, W. H., and Majerus, P. W.: Purification and characterization of human coagulation factor V. *J. Biol. Chem.* 256:1002, 1981.
170. Seegers, W. H., and Smith, H. P.: Factors which influence the activity of purified thrombin. *Am. J. Physiol.* 137:348, 1942.
171. Ratnoff, O. D., and Potts, A. M.: The accelerating effect of calcium and other cations on the conversion of fibrinogen to fibrin. *J. Clin. Invest.* 33:206, 1954.
172. Rosenberg, R. D., and Damus, P. S.: The purification and mechanism of action of human antithrombin-heparin cofactor. *J. Biol. Chem.* 248:6490, 1973.
173. Laki, K., and Lorand, L.: On the solubility of fibrin clots. *Science* 108:280, 1948.
174. Lorand, L.: Fibrin clots. *Nature* 166:694, 1950.
175. Tyler, H. M.: Studies on the activation of purified human factor XIII. *Biochim. Biophys. Acta* 222:396, 1970.
176. Schwartz, M. L., Pizzo, S. U., Hill, R. L., and McKee, P. A.: Human factor XIII from plasma and platelets: Molecular weights, subunit structures, proteolytic activation, and cross-linking of fibrinogen and fibrin. *J. Biol. Chem.* 248:1395, 1973.
177. Greenberg, C. S., and Shuman, M. A.: The zymogen forms of blood coagulation factor XIII bind specifically to fibrinogen. *J. Biol. Chem.* 257:6096, 1982.
178. Lorand, L., and Dickenman, R. C.: Assay method for the "fibrin-stabilizing factor." *Proc. Soc. Exp. Biol. Med.* 89:45, 1966.
179. Chargaff, E.: Studies on the mechanism of the thromboplastic effect. *J. Biol. Chem.* 173:253, 1948.
180. Flynn, J. E., and Coon, R. W.: Purification and isolation of certain intermediates formed prior to the activation of prothrombin. *Am. J. Physiol.* 175:289, 1953.
181. Radcliffe, R., and Nemerson, Y.: Activation and control of factor VII by activated factor X and thrombin: Isolation and characterization of a single chain form of factor VII. *J. Biol. Chem.* 250:388, 1975.
182. Broze, G. J., Jr., and Majerus, P. W.: Purification and properties of human coagulation factor VII. *J. Biol. Chem.* 255:1242, 1980.
183. Bajaj, S. P., Rapaport, S. I., and Brown, S. F.: Isolation and characterization of human factor VII. Activation of factor VII by factor X. *J. Biol. Chem.* 256:253, 1981.
184. Jesty, J., and Nemerson, Y.: Purification of factor VII from bovine plasma: Reaction with tissue factor and activation of factor X. *J. Biol. Chem.* 249:509, 1974.
185. Radcliffe, R., and Nemerson, Y.: Activation and control of factor VII by activated factor X and thrombin: Isolation and characterization of a single chain form of factor VII. *J. Biol. Chem.* 250:388, 1975.
186. Zur, M., and Nemerson, Y.: The esterase activity of coagulation factor VII. Evidence for intrinsic activity of the zymogen. *J. Biol. Chem.* 253:2203, 1978.
187. Silverberg, S. A., Nemerson, Y., and Zur, M.: Kinetics of the activation of bovine coagulation factor X by components of the extrinsic pathway. *J. Biol. Chem.* 252:8481, 1977.
188. Nemerson, Y., and Esnouf, M. P.: Activation of a proteolytic system by a membrane lipoprotein: Mechanism of action of tissue factor. *Proc. Natl. Acad. Sci. U.S.A.* 70:310, 1973.
189. Williams, W. J.: The activation of factor X by Russell's viper venom and by the tissue factor system, in *Biophysical Mechanisms in Vascular Homeostasis and Intravascular Thrombosis*, edited by P. N. Sawyer. Appleton-Century-Crofts, New York, 1965, p. 192.
190. Shanberge, J. W., and Matsuoka, T.: Studies regarding the effect of foreign surface contact on the one-state prothrombin time determination. *Thromb. Diath. Haemorrh.* 15:442, 1966.
191. Altman, R., and Hemker, H. C.: Contact activation in the extrinsic blood clotting system. *Thromb. Diath. Haemorrh.* 18:525, 1967.
192. Johnston, C. L., Jr., Ferguson, J. H., O'Hanlon, F. A., and Black,

W. L.: The fate of factor VII and Stuart factor during the clotting of normal and pathological blood. *Thromb. Diath. Haemorrh.* 3:578, 1959.

193. Hougie, C.: Studies on the fate of coagulation factors during the clotting of normal and pathological blood. *Thromb. Diath. Haemorrh.* 3:578, 1959.

194. Williams, W. J.: The activity of lung microsomes in blood coagulation. *J. Biol. Chem.* 239:933, 1964.

195. Ackroyd, J. F.: The function of factor VII. *Br. J. Haematol.* 2:397, 1956.

196. Alexander, B., Goldstein, R., Lendwehr, G., and Cook, C. D.: Congenital SPCA deficiency: A hitherto unrecognized coagulation defect with hemorrhage rectified by serum and serum fractions. *J. Clin. Invest.* 30:596, 1951.

197. Lüscher, E. F.: Viscous metamorphosis of blood platelet and clot retraction. *Vox Sang.* 1:133, 1956.

198. Astrup, T.: Assay and content of tissue thromboplastin in different organs. *Thromb. Diath. Haemorrh.* 14:401, 1965.

199. Kirk, J. E.: Thromboplastin activities of human arterial and venous tissues. *Proc. Soc. Exp. Biol. Med.* 109:890, 1962.

200. Zeldis, S. M., Nemerson, Y., Pitlick, R. A., and Lentz, T. L.: Tissue factor (thromboplastin): Localization to plasma membranes by peroxidase-conjugated antibodies. *Science* 173:766, 1972.

201. Dunn, J. T., Silverberg, M., and Kaplan, A. P.: The cleavage and formation of activated human Hageman factor by autodigestion and kallikrein. *J. Biol. Chem.* 257:1779, 1982.

202. Madar, D. A., et al.: The relationship between protein-protein and protein-lipid interactions and the immunological properties of bovine prothrombin and several of its fragments. *J. Biol. Chem.* 257: 1836, 1982.

203. Kane, W. H., and Majerus, P. W.: The interaction of human coagulation factor Va with platelets. *J. Biol. Chem.* 257:3963, 1982.

CHAPTER *136*

Control of coagulation reactions

WILLIAM J. WILLIAMS

As discussed in the preceding chapters, there have been many efforts to determine the details of the blood coagulation mechanism in vitro and to relate this information to coagulation in vivo. In such work consideration has been given not only to the mechanisms initiating or sustaining coagulation but also to the mechanisms which could prevent coagulation from occurring unnecessarily in localized areas or extending from the physiological response of local hemostasis to generalized intravascular clotting. Blood coagulation appears to be a relentless process once started. The question, then, is not so much why clotting occurs in response to a wound, for example, but why clotting does not occur constantly, with devastating effects. The concept has been advanced that, in fact, intravascular clotting does occur constantly, and maintenance of the fluidity of the blood is the result of a variety of control mechanisms operating continuously [1].

It has been argued that since the plasma coagulation factors have short survival times in the blood relative to proteins such as albumin or γ-globulin [2], they must be utilized continuously in a process of intravascular coagulation, and some evidence suggesting the continuous formation of thrombin intravascularly has been obtained [3]. However, the half-life of fibrinogen is normal or decreased in patients with severe congenital coagulation factor deficiencies [4,5] and in animals or human beings receiving anticoagulants [6,7] or antifibrinolytic therapy [8]. Similar observations have been made with other coagulation factors [9,10]. If intravascular coagulation were occurring normally, one would expect a longer survival time of the coagulation factors in patients with marked impairment of the coagulation mechanism, and this has not been the case.

Anticoagulant therapy appears to prolong platelet survival, suggesting that normal platelet destruction is related to continuous intravascular coagulation [6]. However, platelet survival times have not been changed by some antiplatelet drugs (e.g., aspirin) [11] and have been normal in several diseases characterized by marked impairment of the coagulation mechanism or platelet function [12,13], suggesting that platelet consumption in intravascular coagulation is not a normal mechanism.

Thus, there is no consistent evidence to support the notion of continuous intravascular coagulation. However, a number of control mechanisms exist which could limit continuous intravascular clotting if it should occur either normally or under pathologic conditions (Chap. 158). Except for fibrinolysis, which is reviewed in Chap. 138, these will be discussed in this chapter.

Physiological control mechanisms

BLOOD FLOW

The movement of blood in the vessels may serve to fragment and distribute any small fibrin clots which may have been formed and to dilute any local concentrations of procoagulants. Fibrinogen consumption is not altered in arterial thrombosis, perhaps because the rapid blood flow in arteries causes rapid dilution of coagulants in the vicinity of the thrombogenic focus [11]. This may involve all the coagulation factors, but possibly it has the least influence on tissue factor and factor VII. These two form a complex with marked coagulant activity, and if tissue factor is exposed in situ, e.g., in the endothelium, it may remain there after complexing with factor VII and provide a continuous source of coagulant activity. Factor Xa may also be bound to the tissue factor–factor VII complex, which could enhance this local effect [14–16].

The effect of stasis on intravascular clotting has been studied in experiments dealing with thrombosis following the injection of serum [17,18]. In order to induce thrombus formation, it is essential that a temporary hypercoagulable state be induced by intravenous injection of serum and that blood flow be stopped in a segment of vein during the period of hypercoagulability.

Stasis alone would not induce the thrombus, nor would the hypercoagulable state alone. Damage to the vessel wall was not essential for the clotting to occur, but it could be a factor in other circumstances. Thus, normal blood remains fluid with marked stasis if the coagulation mechanism is normal or in the face of enhanced coagulability if the blood continues to flow freely.

REMOVAL OF ACTIVATED COAGULATION FACTORS FROM THE CIRCULATION

In the experiments on serum-induced thrombosis, it was noted that the hypercoagulable state following serum injection was short-lived, suggesting the existence of some inactivation mechanism. Furthermore, injection of serum into the portal vein rather than into a systemic vein was not followed by development of thrombi in subsequently isolated venous segments [17–19]. These results imply that the liver is able to remove from the circulating plasma the components responsible for the hypercoagulable state. "Blood thromboplastin" (prothrombinase) and factor Xa are rapidly removed from the circulation [20–23], and the liver has been implicated in this phenomenon. The monocyte-macrophage system may be responsible for the removal of particulate procoagulants [20,23,24], while the hepatic cells may remove soluble components [21,22].

Perfusion studies in vitro have confirmed this concept [25]. Components of serum which can induce stasis thrombi have been identified as factor XIa, factor Xa, and factor IX [26,27]. The disappearance of thrombogenicity of serum upon perfusion through rabbit liver in vitro has been associated with a marked decrease in these factors [25]. There was no change in the concentration of factor VII or factor X in these studies, and it was concluded that the liver removes only the activated factors. Similar results have been obtained in a detailed study on factor X [27]. Factor Xa formed by the action of either Russell's viper venom or trypsin on bovine plasma factor X is rapidly cleared by the liver in vitro, but factor X is not. Further, an inhibitor of factor Xa has been isolated from liver, and this material may bind factor Xa in the liver [28]. Thrombin binds rapidly to endothelial cells in culture [29]. This clearance mechanism appears to function in vivo as well [30], and may accelerate inactivation of thrombin by antithrombin III [30,31]. Slow binding of thrombin to endothelium also occurs, but is of uncertain significance [32]. Thrombin binding to endothelium may be mediated by glycosaminoglycans [33]. Particulate fibrin [34,35] and complexes of fibrinogen and fibrin [36] are rapidly removed from the circulating blood, probably by the monocyte-macrophage system [37,38]. Fibrinogen degradation products may also be removed by the monocyte-macrophage system [35,39], but some investigations have found prior reticuloendothelial blockade to have no effect on clearance of these derivatives [40,41]. Fibrinogen fragments D and E are also actively catabolized by the kidney [42].

The effects of intravenously injected tissue factor vary from rapid death of the animal to a mild decrease in some of the coagulation factors, depending on a number of parameters, including dosage [43,44]. Tissue factor particles may be removed in the lung [44].

Biochemical control mechanisms

ANTITHROMBINS

The so-called antithrombins constitute a heterogeneous group of activities having the common attribute of inactivating thrombin. They have been classified in a system employing Roman numerals [45]. Difficulties with definitions of several of the activities has limited the usefulness of this nomenclature. However, the term *antithrombin III* continues to be used [46] (see below).

Thrombin is readily adsorbed to fibrin [47–49]. This has been considered by some to be an inactivation mechanism of major physiologic importance [49–52], but others have questioned its role in vivo [53,54]. The thrombin-adsorbing effect of fibrin has been referred to as *antithrombin I* [45].

ANTITHROMBIN III (FACTOR Xa INHIBITOR, HEPARIN COFACTOR)

Antithrombin III is the principal plasma protein responsible for the progressive inactivation of thrombin. This material is believed to be of major physiological significance [46,55–60]. The phenomenon of progressive inactivation of thrombin is not limited to antithrombin III, however, for thrombin may also be inactivated by two other plasma proteins: the α_2-macroglobulin [56,60–63] and the α_1-proteolytic inhibitor [60,64]. Antithrombin III activity can be separated from the α_2-macroglobulin [65, 66]. The latter accounts for about 25 percent of the total antithrombin activity [65,66]. The α_1-proteolytic inhibitor inactivates thrombin but accounts for a minor fraction of the inhibitory activity of plasma [55,61]. The total progressive antithrombin activity of 1 ml of normal plasma will inactivate about 300 NIH units of thrombin [47], and the reaction rate is such that the half-life of thrombin has been estimated at about 25 [54], 40 [55], and 45 s [48].

Antithrombin III has been purified by a number of procedures [59,67–73], and physically homogeneous preparations have been obtained. Human antithrombin III migrates as an α-globulin on electrophoresis [41] and has a molecular weight of about 62,000 to 67,000 [59,65,71,72]. It contains 9 to 15 percent carbohydrate [69,71,74]. The amino acid sequence has been determined [69,75]. The molecule appears to be a single polypeptide chain with histidine as the free-amino end group [71,73].

Heparin cofactor is the term used for the plasma protein required for the antithrombin activity of heparin. This activity was formerly called "antithrombin II." There is now convincing evidence that heparin cofactor and antithrombin III are the property of a single molecule [58,59,67,71,76]. Evidence has been obtained for other heparin cofactors in human plasma [77–80]. One of these, designated *heparin cofactor II* has been highly purified from human plasma [79,80]. It forms an irreversible, enzymatically inactive complex with thrombin, and heparin accelerates the rate of formation of the complex [79,80]. In comparison with antithrombin III, heparin cofactor II is a relatively ineffective inhibitor of factor Xa [80]. Antithrombin III also inactivates factor Xa [58,81,82], factor IXa [83], factor XIa [84,85], and factor XIIa [86], all serine proteases (see Chap. 132). Antithrombin III also inhibits plasmin [66,85,87] and kallikrein [88]. The inactivation of these enzymes is accelerated by heparin [53,81–85] but in some instances only at high concentrations [257]. Factor VII has been reported to be inactivated slowly by antithrombin III and heparin [89], but others have found no such inhibition [90]. Antithrombin III may also inhibit tissue factor (factor III) [91]. Antithrombin III also inactivates trypsin, chymotrypsin, and plasmin [66]. The inactivation of plasmin is accelerated by heparin [85]. A prothrombin fragment (fragment 2) interferes with the inactivation of thrombin by antithrombin III, apparently by inhibiting binding of thrombin to the antithrombin III molecule [92].

Human antithrombin III appears to inactivate thrombin by forming a complex [56,59,93] in which one molecule of inhibitor and one molecule of thrombin are irreversibly associated [59]. A similar complex is formed between antithrombin III and factor IXa [83,90], Xa [90], or XIIa [86]. When heparin is included in the system, using reagents from human sources, thrombin is not regenerated by neutralization of the heparin with protamine [59] or by platelet antiheparin activity (platelet factor 4) [94]. The active site serine of thrombin (see Chap. 132) and an arginine residue or residues of the inhibitor are involved in the formation of the complex [59]. Acceleration of the rate of formation of the complex by heparin involves lysine residues on the inhibitor [59]. It is believed that the binding of heparin to antithrombin III results in a conformational change which permits more rapid reaction between thrombin and the arginine reactive site of the inhibitor [59].

It appears most likely that heparin assumes a catalytic role in inactivation of thrombin by antithrombin III [95,96]. A heparin–antithrombin III complex initially forms, but is dissociated when the irreversible antithrombin III–coagulation enzyme complex is formed. The released heparin can then bind with another molecule of antithrombin III and enhance its affinity for the coagulation enzyme. Other possible mechanisms of heparin-induced antithrombin III inactivation of coagulation enzymes are neutralization of heparin-enzyme complexes by antithrombin III [97–99] or simultaneous binding of antithrombin III and the coagulation enzyme by heparin with consequent inactivation of the enzyme [100–102]. Heparin is a complex mixture of sulfated glycosaminoglycans which can be separated by several techniques into fractions of different anticoagulant activities [103–107].

Antithrombin III inhibits the action of thrombin in releasing fibrinopeptides from fibrinogen [55] and in hydrolyzing synthetic substrates [59,108]. Heparin accelerates the inhibition of both of these reactions [59,109].

As noted above, factor Xa is inhibited by antithrombin III, and this inhibition is enhanced by heparin. Factor Xa binds readily to phospholipid, and factor Xa mixed with phospholipid is much less readily inactivated by antithrombin III than is factor Xa alone [110]. However, heparin still accelerates the inactivation of factor Xa–phospholipid mixtures [110]. Factor Xa in a complex with factor Va, phospholipid, and calcium (*prothrombinase*, see Chap. 132) is also protected from the action of antithrombin III [111]. Factor Xa bound to platelets is also not inactivated by antithrombin III [112]. Platelet aggregation induced by factor Xa is inhibited by antithrombin III and heparin or by larger amounts of antithrombin III alone [113].

Antithrombin III appears to be synthesized in the liver [114], possibly in endothelial cells [115]. The biologic half-life of antithrombin III was 68 h in normal subjects [116], and 66 h in a patient with antithrombin III deficiency [117], but was 48 h in a patient with fatal phosphorus poisoning [54]. Antithrombin III is distributed widely in body fluids [54], and there apparently is a large extravascular reservoir of this material [118]. Congenital deficiency of antithrombin III has been reported in some families with a tendency to thrombosis [119–126]. In one family the disorder appears to be due to synthesis of an abnormal antithrombin III molecule [121]. Low levels have been found in patients with thrombosis [127], but some investigators have reported normal levels in such patients [85]. Low levels are found in patients with cirrhosis [127–130] and may be found in patients receiving estrogen therapy [131–133]. The effect of heparin therapy on antithrombin III levels is discussed in Chap. 160.

α_2-MACROGLOBULIN INHIBITOR

The α_2-macroglobulin interferes with the clotting activity of thrombin by forming an apparently irreversible complex with the enzyme [56,62]. The rate of inactivation of thrombin is dependent on the concentration of both reactants, although with low concentrations of thrombin this may not be apparent [56,62,63]. The macroglobulin inactivates thrombin in the presence of fibrinogen, but it does not interfere with the polymerization of fibrin [56]. Although the coagulant action of thrombin is inhibited by the macroglobulin, its ability to hydrolyze amino acid esters is retained [62]. The α_2-macroglobulin also forms enzymatically active complexes with trypsin [134,135] and chymotrypsin [135], but it inactivates plasmin [136]. In systems containing both thrombin and plasmin, there appears to be competition between these two enzymes for binding sites on the inhibitor [137].

Thrombin is completely inactivated by incubation for about 20 min with physiological concentrations of the

α_2-macroglobulin [56,62]. The half-life of active thrombin in experiments using α_2-macroglobulin is 2 or more minutes [56], in comparison with the 20 to 45 s obtained in studies on antithrombin III [54,55]. The α_2-macroglobulin may account for about one-fourth of the normal thrombin-inactivating mechanism [65,66].

The concentration of α_2-macroglobulin in plasma is diminished in severe hepatic disease [56] and with fibrinolysis [138] or intravascular coagulation [56]. It is elevated in childhood [139] and in nephrosis [56].

INHIBITORS OF OTHER PROCOAGULANTS

INHIBITORS OF FACTOR Xa
The inhibition of factor Xa by antithrombin III has already been discussed. A second inhibitor of factor Xa is present in the macroglobulin fraction of plasma [140]. The activity of this inhibitor is greatly enhanced by adsorption with $Al(OH)_3$, and therefore its biological significance is uncertain. A competitive inhibitor of factor Xa in prothrombin activation can be derived from prothrombin [141–144]; it is discussed below under "Feedback Controls."

INHIBITORS OF "PLASMA THROMBOPLASTIN" (PROTHROMBINASE)
The activities which interfere with factor Xa would inhibit prothrombinase or plasma thromboplastin as these terms are presently understood (a complex of factor Xa, factor Va, a phospholipid, and calcium). "Plasma thromboplastin" was found to disappear rapidly from reaction mixtures in which it formed [145,146], and this disappearance has been related to inhibitors [147–155]. Two different inhibitors have been identified in serum [150]. They are apparently both proteins, migrating as α_2-globulins on electrophoresis [150]. The relationship of inhibitors of plasma thromboplastin to other better defined inhibitors is unknown.

INHIBITORS OF TISSUE THROMBOPLASTIN (TISSUE FACTOR, FACTOR III) AND FACTOR VII
Inhibitors of tissue thromboplastin have been described [149,155–160], but little is known of their mode of action. Inhibitors of the product of the reaction of tissue factor and factor VII have also been reported [148,149,161–164]. Antithrombin III may be responsible for this latter inhibitory effect [91,165].

INHIBITORS OF FACTORS XIa AND XIIa AND PLASMA KALLIKREIN
The factors activated during the "contact phase" of blood coagulation (factors XI and XII) are inhibited by serum and plasma [166–168]. Factors XIa and XIIa are inhibited by antithrombin III (see above). An inhibitor of factor XIa has been partially purified from human plasma [169]. The preparation inhibited factor Xa as well as XIa but had no effect on factor XIIa. Factor XIa is also inhibited by α_1-antitrypsin [170] and α_1-antiplasmin [258]. α_1-Antitrypsin appears to be responsible for most of the inhibitory activity of plasma [259]. Factor XIa

formed on platelet surfaces is protected from inhibition [171].

An inhibitor of a complement component, $C\bar{1}$ inactivator, has been found to inhibit both factors XIa and XIIa [172,173]. $C\bar{1}$ inactivator also inhibits factor XII fragments [174,175], kallikrein [176], and plasmin [174], all of which appear to play significant roles in the initiation of coagulation, as discussed in Chap. 135. Kallikrein is also inhibited by antithrombin III, with or without heparin [88], and by α_2-macroglobulin [176,177]. Plasminogen activator is inhibited by α_2-macroglobulin [174].

Factor XIIa activity disappears from normal plasma with a half-life of 9 to 15 min [178]. Plasma also contains undefined materials which inhibit the adsorption of factor XII to glass and may also interfere with surface activation of this proenzyme in the initiation of physiological blood coagulation [179]. High concentrations of high-molecular-weight kininogen appear to inhibit factor XII activation [180,181].

INACTIVATION OF FACTOR VIII:C
Factor VIII:C is consumed during clotting [182], and there is evidence that thrombin may be responsible for its destruction [183]. Factor VIII:C is attacked by small amounts of thrombin, with a resulting increase in reactivity (see Chaps. 132 and 135). Factor VIII:C activity disappears in citrated or adsorbed plasma when it is exposed to larger amounts of thrombin [183–186]. This has been interpreted as destruction of factor VIII [183–186].

The activator of factor X derived from the reaction of factor IXa, factor VIIIa, phospholipid, and calcium is unstable [187–189], which may afford an additional mechanism for limiting the action of this complex in coagulation.

The inactivation of factor VIII:C by activated protein C is discussed below.

INACTIVATION OF FACTOR V
Thrombin converts factor V to a more reactive form, factor Va (Chap. 132). As with factor VIII, excess thrombin destroys factor V [190,191]. The reactions of the blood coagulation cascade may occur on the platelet surface [192–194]. In particular, attention has focused on the role of platelet factor V, which after activation to factor Va by thrombin binds factor Xa and prothrombin [112,194–199].

Activated protein C may function as a physiological regulator of coagulation, limiting the activity of factor Va in both plasma and on the platelet surface [86,144,200–209]. Protein C is a vitamin K–dependent plasma protein which circulates as a zymogen and can be converted to an active serine protease by thrombin [200–204] or the coagulant protein of Russell's viper venom [202,203]. Protein C has been highly purified [200,202,207–209] and the primary structure determined [204,210,260,261]. Both plasma and platelet factor Va [204,205,209] and factor VIII:C [206,209] are inactivated by activated protein C. Inactivation of these factors by activated protein C is enhanced by phospholipid and calcium [204–206,209,211,212]. No other coagulation factors are so attacked [204,209]. Both bovine and human activated protein C are highly species-specific. Factor Xa protects factor Va from inactivation by activated protein C [205]. Activation of protein C by thrombin formed from a mixture of platelets, factor Xa, and prothrombin occurs very slowly, suggesting another activation mechanism may be operative if protein C is physiologically important [204]. Endothelial cells may provide a surface on which protein C can be physiologically activated by thrombin [213–216]. Protein S, another vitamin K–dependent plasma protein [200,211, 212,214,217], enhances the activity of activated protein C [211,212]. Activated protein C also induces plasma fibrinolytic activity in vitro and in vivo [218,219]. An inhibitor of activated protein C is present in normal plasma [220].

Protein C levels are low in newborn infants; in patients with chronic liver disease, disseminated intravascular coagulation, and adult respiratory distress syndrome; and after some surgical procedures [262].

INACTIVATION OF FACTOR XIII
Factor XIII is present in only very low concentrations in normal serum [221–223]. The low levels in serum appear to be due to adsorption of both factor XIII and XIIIa to fibrin [223] and to inactivation of factor XIIIa by other plasma factors [223,224].

LIPID INHIBITORS
The anticoagulant effects of various phospholipid preparations have been observed by a number of investigators (Chap. 132). Phosphatidyl serine and phosphatidic acid, alone or in combination, inhibit blood coagulation [225–228] possibly by binding coagulation factors in an inactive complex formed without participation of calcium [226–229]. Factor IX has been reported to be particularly susceptible to this type of inhibition [229]. High concentrations of otherwise active phospholipids can also be inhibiting, probably due to calcium-dependent binding of factor Xa [230].

PLATELETS AND LIPID ACTIVATORS
It has been suggested that platelets may participate in all the reactions of the intrinsic coagulation system [171,192,193,195]. This hypothesis is based on the observation that coagulation may be initiated by reactions involving ADP which lead to activation of factors XII and XI adsorbed to platelet surfaces and/or by the activation of factor XI on platelet surfaces exposed to collagen [231,232]. An alternate possibility is that optimal amounts of phospholipid may markedly enhance the coagulant effect of small amounts of contact product [233]. The reactions of the coagulation cascade following activation of factor XI may also take place on the platelet surface [171].

This concept permits consideration of several control mechanisms, particularly limitation of the reaction sequence to the coagulation factors adsorbed to the platelet surface [171,192,195], protection of the adsorbed activated factors from inhibitors [111,112,171], and modification of the reactions by the participation of components released from the platelet, such as ADP, heparin-neutralizing activity, and platelet factor 3 [192,195] (see Chaps. 127 and 128). Evidence has been obtained for an important role for platelet coagulant activities in physiological hemostasis [194–199,234,235]. The coagulant role of platelet-bound factor V is discussed above.

FEEDBACK MECHANISMS
Both positive and negative feedback controls have been recognized in the coagulation mechanism. Contact activation of factor XII leads to activation of prekallikrein to kallikrein, which is then able to activate further quantities of factor XII [236]. Factor XIIa is also able to activate factor VII [237,238] providing for potential acceleration of the tissue factor pathway in blood coagulation. The obvious function of thrombin in blood coagulation is conversion of fibrinogen to fibrin. However, thrombin also activates factor XIII (see Chaps. 132 and 135), initiates platelet aggregation (see Chaps. 127 to 129), and has profound effects on factors V and VIII, in small amounts enhancing their reactivity but in larger amounts causing their destruction (see Chaps. 132 and 135). Thrombin also has a major effect on prothrombin activation to thrombin [141–144,239–241]. As is shown in Fig. 132-2, prothrombin consists of a single polypeptide chain which is converted to thrombin via a series of intermediates. The intermediate released from the carboxyl-terminal end of the molecule (prethrombin 2) is further attacked by factor Xa to yield thrombin. The free-amino terminal fragment of prothrombin contains the calcium-binding sites of the molecule [242–248] and is not further degraded in the formation of thrombin. This fragment, referred to as fragment 1, is an inhibitor of the activation of prothrombin by factor Xa [243,249–251], probably acting by competing with prothrombin for binding sites on phospholipid. Thrombin can also hydrolyze prothrombin, releasing a carboxyl-terminal fragment referred to as prethrombin 1. Prethrombin 1 can be further hydrolyzed to thrombin but is a poor substrate for prothrombinase [248–250,252]. Thus, thrombin can interfere with prothrombin activation both by creating a competitive inhibitor of prothrombin activation and by converting prothrombin into a poor substrate for prothrombinase. However, the major inhibitory effect of thrombin in the activation of prothrombin appears to be the destruction of factor V [248]. Factor V also appears to exert control over the rate of thrombin formation [3].

Activated factor X also has been shown to influence coagulation by effects on coagulation factors which precede it in the coagulation sequence. Thus, factor Xa converts factor VII from a single-chain molecule to a two-chain form, with an 85-fold increase in coagulant activity [253]. Further digestion of factor VII by factor Xa results in inactivation of the factor VII. Thrombin also converts factor VII to a two-chain form with increased activity and, in larger amounts, inactivates it [253]. This mechanism can thus provide for initial acceleration and rapid dampening of the extrinsic system.

Factor Xa converts factor IX to its active form [254]. Factor VIIa also can activate factor IX [255,256]. These alternate means of activating factor IX may explain the relatively mild hemorrhagic disorder found in patients with factor XI deficiency [254].

Implications of the control mechanisms

The phenomena described in this chapter may readily be assumed to operate in obvious ways in the control of the blood coagulation mechanism, either continuously or intermittently. However, it must be emphasized that such conclusions would be largely conjectural, and it remains for the future to build a realistic concept of the in vivo interaction of these inhibitory or modifying influences on the blood coagulation factors or their derivatives. Such concepts could have major practical importance, and a full understanding of the interactions of this complex system of physiological and biochemical phenomena would not only be intellectually satisfying but would have extensive clinical applications as well.

References

1. Hjort, P. F., and Hasselback, R.: A critical review of the evidence for a continuous hemostasis in vivo. *Thromb. Diath. Haemorrh.* 6:580, 1961.
2. Volwiler, W., Goldsworthy, P. D., MacMartin, M. P., Woods, P. A., Mackay, I. R., and Fremont-Smith, K.: Biosynthetic determination with radioactive sulfur of turnover rates of various plasma proteins in normal and cirrhotic man. *J. Clin. Invest.* 34:1126, 1955.
3. Teitel, J. M., Bauer, K. A., Lau, H. K., and Rosenberg, R. D.: Studies of the prothrombin activation pathway utilizing radioimmunoassays for the F_2/F_{1+2} fragment and thrombin–antithrombin complex. *Blood* 59:1086, 1982.
4. Rausen, A. R., Cruchaud, A., McMillan, C. W., and Gitlin, D.: A study of fibrinogen turnover in classical hemophilia and congenital afibrinogenemia. *Blood* 18:710, 1961.
5. Takeda, Y., and Chen, A. Y.: Studies of the metabolism and distribution of fibrinogen in patients with hemophilia A. *J. Clin. Invest.* 46:1879, 1967.
6. Adelson, E., Rheingold, J. J., Parker, O., Buenaventura, A., and Crosby, W. H.: Platelet and fibrinogen survival in normal and abnormal states of coagulation. *Blood* 17:267, 1961.
7. Lewis, J. H., Ferguson, E. E., and Schoenfeld, C.: Studies concerning the turnover of fibrinogen in the dog. *J. Lab. Clin. Med.* 58:247, 1961.
8. Lewis, J. H.: Effects of epsilon amino caproic acid (EACA) on survival of fibrinogen I^{131} and on fibrinolytic and coagulation factors in dogs. *Proc. Soc. Exp. Biol. Med.* 114:777, 1963.
9. Hjort, P. F., Egeberg, O., and Mikkelsen, S.: Turnover of prothrombin, factor VII and factor IX in a patient with hemophilia A. *Scand. J. Lab. Clin. Invest.* 13:668, 1961.
10. Shapiro, S. S., and Martinez, J.: Human prothrombin metabolism in normal man and in hypocoagulable subjects. *J. Clin. Invest.* 48:1292, 1969.
11. Harker, L. A., and Slichter, S. J.: Platelet and fibrinogen consumption in man. *N. Engl. J. Med.* 287:999, 1972.
12. Raccuglia, G., and Neel, J. V.: Congenital vascular defect associated with platelet abnormality and antihemophilic factor deficiency. *Blood* 15:807, 1960.
13. Mustard, J. F., Rowsell, H. C., and Murphy, E. A.: Platelet economy (platelet survival and turnover). *Br. J. Haematol.* 12:1, 1966.
14. Williams, W. J.: The activity of lung microsomes in blood coagulation. *J. Biol. Chem.* 239:933, 1964.
15. Williams, W. J.: The activity of human placenta microsomes and brain particles in blood coagulation. *J. Biol. Chem.* 241:1840, 1966.
16. Williams, W. J., and Norris, D. G.: Purification of a bovine plasma protein (factor VII) which is required for the activity of lung microsomes in blood coagulation. *J. Biol. Chem.* 241:1847, 1966.
17. Wessler, S.: Studies in intravascular coagulation. III. The pathogenesis of serum-induced venous thrombosis. *J. Clin. Invest.* 34:647, 1955.
18. Wessler, S., Reiner, L., Freiman, D. G., Reiner, S. M., and Lertzman, M.: Serum-induced thrombosis: Studies on its induction and evolution under controlled conditions in vivo. *Circulation* 20:864, 1959.
19. Deykin, D.: The role of the liver in serum-induced hypercoagulability. *J. Clin. Invest.* 45:256, 1966.
20. Spaet, T. H., and Kropatkin, M.: Effect of intravenous soy bean phosphatide on blood coagulation in rabbits. *Proc. Soc. Exp. Biol. Med.* 95:492, 1957.
21. Spaet, T. H., and Cintron, J.: Clearance of blood coagulation product I in rabbits. *Proc. Soc. Exp. Biol. Med.* 104:498, 1960.
22. Spaet, T. H.: Studies on the in vivo behavior of blood coagulation product I in rats. *Thromb. Diath. Haemorrh,* 8:276, 1962.
23. Spaet, T. H., Horowitz, H. I., Zucker-Franklin, D., Cintron, J., and Biezenski, J. J.: Reticuloendothelial clearance of blood thromboplastin by rats. *Blood* 17:196, 1961.
24. Arakawa, T., and Spaet, T. H.: In vitro inactivation of rabbit blood thromboplastin by macrophages. *Proc. Soc. Exp. Biol. Med.* 113:71, 1963.
25. Wessler, S., Yin, E. T., Gaston, L. W., and Nicol, T.: A distinction between the role of precursor and activated forms of clotting factors in the genesis of stasis thrombi. *Thromb. Diath. Haemorrh.* 18:12, 1967.
26. Deykin, D., and Wessler, S.: Activation product, factor IX, serum thrombotic accelerator activity, and serum induced thrombosis. *J. Clin. Invest.* 43:160, 1964.
27. Deykin, D., Cochios, F., DeCamp, G., and Lopez, A.: Hepatic removal of activated factor X by the perfused rabbit liver. *Am. J. Physiol.* 214:414, 1968.
28. Deykin, D., Cochios, F., and Mosher, D.: An hepatic inhibitor of activated clotting factor X (Stuart). *Biochem. Biophys. Res. Commun.* 34:245, 1969.
29. Awbrey, B. J., Hoak, J. C., and Owen, W. G.: Binding of human thrombin to cultured human endothelial cells. *J. Biol. Chem.* 254:4092, 1979.
30. Lollar, P., and Owen, W. G.: Clearance of thrombin from circulation in rabbits by high-affinity binding sites on endothelium. Possible role in the inactivation of thrombin by antithrombin III. *J. Clin. Invest.* 66:1222, 1980.
31. Busch, C., and Owen, W. G.: Identification in vitro of an endothelial cell surface cofactor for antithrombin III. Parallel studies with isolated perfused rat hearts and microcarrier cultures of bovine endothelium. *J. Clin. Invest.* 69:726, 1982.
32. Lollar, P., Hoak, J. C., and Owen, W. G.: Binding of thrombin to cultured human endothelial cells. Nonequilibrium aspects. *J. Biol. Chem.* 255:10279, 1980.
33. Hatton, M. W. C., et al.: Heparin inhibits thrombin binding to rabbit thoracic aorta endothelium. *J. Lab. Clin. Med.* 96:861, 1980.
34. Lewis, J. R., and Szeto, I. L. F.: Clearance of infused fibrin. *Fed. Proc.* 24:840, 1965.
35. Gans, H., and Lowman, J. R.: The uptake of fibrin and fibrin-degradation products by the isolated perfused rat liver. *Blood* 29:526, 1967.
36. Sherman, L. A., Harwig, S., and Lee, J.: In vitro formation and in vivo clearance of fibrinogen:fibrin complexes. *J. Lab. Clin. Med.* 86:100, 1975.
37. Lee, L.: Reticuloendothelial clearance of circulating fibrin in the

pathogenesis of the generalized Schwartzman reaction. *J. Exp. Med.* 115:1065, 1962.

38. Spaet, T. H.: Hemostatic homeostasis. *Blood* 28:112, 1966.

39. Barnhart, M. J., and Cress, D. C.: Plasma clearance of products of fibrinolysis. *Adv. Exp. Med. Biol.* 1:492, 1967.

40. Hayne, O. A., and Sherman, L. A.: In vivo behavior of fibrinogen fragment D in experimental renal, hepatic, and reticuloendothelial dysfunction. *Am. J. Pathol.* 71:219, 1973.

41. Esnouf, M. P., and Marshall, R.: The effect of blockage of the reticuloendothelial system and of hypotension on the response of dogs to *Ancistrodon rhodostoma* venom. *Clin. Sci.* 35:261, 1968.

42. Iio, A., et al.: The roles of renal catabolism and uremia in modifying the clearance of fibrinogen and its degradative fragments D and E. *J. Lab. Clin. Med.* 87:934, 1976.

43. Penick, G. D., Roberts, H. R., Webster, W. P., and Brinkhous, K. M.: Hemorrhagic states secondary to intravascular clotting. *Arch. Pathol.* 66:708, 1958.

44. Astrup, T., and Albrechtsen, O. K.: Serum effects following tissue thromboplastin infusion. *Thromb. Diath. Haemorrh.* 21:117, 1969.

45. Fell, C., Ivanovic, N., Johnson, S. A., and Seegers, W. H.: Differentiation of plasma antithrombin activities, *Proc. Soc. Exp. Biol. Med.* 85:199, 1954.

46. Abildgaard, U.: Antithrombins. *Thromb. Diath. Haemorrh. (Suppl.)* 51:295, 1971.

47. Seegers, W. H.: Multiple protein interactions as exhibited by the blood-clotting mechanism. *J. Phys. Colloid. Chem.* 51:198, 1947.

48. Liu, C. Y., Nossel, H. L., and Kaplan, K. L.: The binding of thrombin by fibrin. *J. Biol. Chem.* 254:10421, 1979.

49. Liu, C. Y., Kaplan, K. L., Markowitz, A. H., and Nossel, H. L.: Thermodynamic characterization of thrombin binding by cross-linked and non-cross-linked fibrin in the presence and absence of Ca^{2+}. *J. Biol. Chem.* 255:7627, 1980.

50. Quick, A. J., and Favre-Gilly, J. E.: Fibrin, a factor influencing the consumption of prothrombin in coagulation. *Am. J. Physiol.* 158:387, 1949.

51. Quick, A. J.: Current blood clotting schemes. *Thromb. Diath. Haemorrh.* 16:318, 1966.

52. Liu, C. Y., Nossel, H. L., and Kaplan, K. L.: Defective thrombin binding by abnormal fibrin associated with recurrent thrombosis. *Thromb. Haemost.* 42:79, 1979.

53. Seegers, W. H., Miller, K. D., Andrews, E. B., and Murphy, R. C.: Fundamental interactions and effect of storage, ether, adsorbants and blood clotting on plasma antithrombin activity. *Am. J. Physiol.* 169:700, 1952.

54. Hensen, A., and Loeliger, E. A.: Antithrombin III: Its metabolism and its function in blood coagulation. *Thromb. Diath. Haemorrh.* 9 (Suppl. 1):1, 1963.

55. Abildgaard, U.: Inhibition of the thrombin-fibrinogen reaction by antithrombin III studied by N-terminal analysis. *Scand. J. Clin. Lab. Invest.* 20:207, 1967.

56. Abildgaard, U.: Inhibition of the thrombin-fibrinogen reaction by α_2-macroglobulin, studied by N-terminal analysis. *Thromb. Diath. Haemorrh.* 21:173, 1969.

57. Monkhouse, F. C., France, E. S., and Seegers, W. H.: Studies on the antithrombin and heparin cofactor activities of a fraction adsorbed from plasma by aluminum hydroxide. *Circ. Res.* 3:397, 1955.

58. Yin, E. T., Wessler, S., and Stoll, P. J.: Identity of plasma-activated factor X inhibitor with antithrombin III and heparin cofactor. *J. Biol. Chem.* 246:3712, 1971.

59. Rosenberg, R. D., and Damus, P. S.: The purification and mechanism of action of human antithrombin-heparin cofactor. *J. Biol. Chem.* 248:6490, 1973.

60. Downing, M. R., Bloom, J. W., and Mann, K. G.: Comparison of the inhibition of thrombin by three plasma protease inhibitors. *Biochemistry* 17:2649, 1978.

61. Steinbuch, M., Blatrix, C., and Josso, F. L.: L'α_2-macroglobuline comme antithrombine progressive. *Proc. XIth Congr. Int. Soc. Haematol., Sydney,* 1966, p. 7.

62. Lanchantin, G. F., Plesset, M. L., Friedmann, J. A., and Hart, D. W.: Dissociation of esterolytic and clotting activities of thrombin by trypsin-binding macroglobulin. *Proc. Soc. Exp. Biol. Med.* 121:444, 1966.

63. Fischer, A. M., Tapon-Bretaudiere, J., Bros, A., and Josso, F.: Respective roles of antithrombin III and alpha 2 macroglobulin in thrombin inactivation. *Thromb. Haemost.* 45:51, 1981.

64. Rimon, A., Shamash, Y., and Shapiro, B.: The plasmin inhibitor of human plasma IV: Its action on plasmin, tryspin, chymotrypsin and thrombin. *J. Biol. Chem.* 241:5102, 1966.

65. Abildgaard, U.: Purification of two progressive antithrombins of human plasma. *Scand. J. Clin. Lab. Invest.* 19:190, 1967.

66. Abildgaard, U., and Egeberg, O.: Thrombin inhibitory activity of fractions obtained by gel filtration of antithrombin III deficient plasma. *Scand. J. Haematol.* 5:155, 1968.

67. Abildgaard, U.: Highly purified antithrombin III with heparin cofactor activity prepared by disc electrophoresis. *Scand. J. Clin. Lab. Invest.* 21:89, 1968.

68. Yin, E. T., Wessler, S., and Stoll, P. J.: Rabbit plasma inhibitor of the activated species of blood coagulation factor X. *J. Biol. Chem.* 246:3694, 1971.

69. Kurachi, K., et al.: Characterization of human, bovine, and horse antithrombin III. *Biochemistry* 15:368, 1976.

70. Yin, E. T., Eisenkramer, L., and Katz, D.: Heparin interaction with activated factor X and its plasma inhibitor. *Adv. Med. Biol.* 52:239, 1974.

71. Miller-Andersson, M., Borg, H., and Andersson, L.-O.: Purification of antithrombin III by affinity chromatography. *Thromb. Res.* 5:439, 1974.

72. Rosenberg, R. D., and Damus, P. S.: Antithrombin-heparin cofactor, in *Methods in Enzymology,* edited by L. Lorand. Academic, New York, 1976, vol. 45, p. 653.

73. Thaler, E., and Schmer, G.: A simple two-step isolation procedure for human and bovine antithrombin II/III (heparin cofactor): A comparison of two methods. *Br. J. Haematol.* 31:233, 1975.

74. Danishefsky, I., Zweben, A., and Slomiany, B. L.: Human antithrombin III. Carbohydrate components and associated glycolipid. *J. Biol. Chem.* 253:32, 1978.

75. Peterson, T. E., Ducek-Wojciechowska, G., Sottrup-Jensen, L., and Magnusson, S.: Antithrombin-III (heparin cofactor) — Human, in *Atlas of Protein Sequence and Structure,* edited by M. O. Dayoff. Natl. Biomed. Res. Foundation, Washington, D.C., 1979, vol. 5, suppl. 3, p. 141.

76. Fagerhol, M. K., and Abildgaard, U.: Immunological studies on antithrombin III. Influence of age, sex and use of oral contraceptives on serum concentration. *Scand. J. Haematol.* 7:10, 1970.

77. Briginshaw, G. F., and Shanberge, J. N.: Identification of two distinct heparin cofactors in human plasma: Separation and partial purification. *Arch. Biochem. Biophys.* 161:683, 1974.

78. Briginshaw, G. F., and Shanberge, J. N.: Identification of two distinct heparin cofactors in human plasma. II. Inhibition of thrombin and activated factor X. *Thromb. Res.* 4:463, 1974.

79. Tollefsen, D. M., and Blank, M. K.: Detection of a new heparin-dependent inhibitor of thrombin in human plasma. *J. Clin. Invest.* 68:589, 1981.

80. Tollefsen, D. M., Majerus, D. W., and Blank, M. K.: Heparin cofactor II. Purification and properties of a heparin-dependent inhibitor of thrombin in human plasma. *J. Biol. Chem.* 257:2162, 1982.

81. Seegers, W. H., Cole, E. R., Harmison, C. R., and Monkhouse, F. C.: Neutralization of autoprothrombin C activity with antithrombin. *Can. J. Biochem.* 42:359, 1967.

82. Biggs, R., Denson, K. W. E., Akman, N., Borrett, R., and Hadden, M.: Antithrombin III, antifactor Xa, and heparin. *Br. J. Haematol.* 19:283, 1970.

83. Rosenberg, J. S., McKenna, P. W., and Rosenberg, R. D.: Inhibition of human factor IXa by human antithrombin. *J. Biol. Chem.* 250:8883, 1975.

84. Damus, P. C., Hicks, M., and Rosenberg, R. D.: Anticoagulant action of heparin. *Nature* 246:356, 1973.

85. Rosenberg, R. D.: The effect of heparin on factor XIa and plasmin. *Thromb. Diath. Haemorrh.* 33:51, 1974.

86. Highsmith, R. F., and Rosenberg, R. D.: Inhibition of human plasmin by human antithrombin-heparin cofactor. *J. Biol. Chem.* 249:4335, 1974.

87. Lahiri, B., et al.: Antithrombin-heparin cofactor: An inhibitor of plasma kallikrein. *Arch. Biochem. Biophys.* 175:737, 1976.

88. Godal, H. C., Rygh, M., and Laake, K.: Progressive inactivation of purified factor VII by heparin and antithrombin III. *Thromb. Res.* 5:773, 1974.

89. Jesty, J.: The inhibition of activated bovine coagulation factors X and VII by antithrombon III. *Arch. Biochem. Biophys.* 185:165, 1978.

90. Egeberg, O.: On the natural blood coagulation inhibitor system: Investigations of inhibitor factors based on antithrombin deficient blood. *Thromb. Diath. Haemorrh.* 14:473, 1965.

91. Walker, F. J., and Esmon, C. T.: The effect of prothrombin fragment 2 on the inhibition of thrombin by antithrombin III. *J. Biol. Chem.* 254:5618, 1979.

92. Abildgaard, U.: Binding of thrombin to antithrombin III. *Scand. J. Clin. Lab. Invest.* 24:23, 1969.

93. Stead, N., Kaplan, A. P., and Rosenberg, R. D.: Inhibition of activated factor XII by antithrombin-heparin cofactor. *J. Biol. Chem.* 251:6481, 1976.

94. Abildgaard, U., Ødegaard, O. R., Kierulf, P., and Pepper, D. S.: Influence of platelet factor 4 on inhibited thrombin substrate reactions. *Thromb. Res.* 5:185, 1974.

95. Jordan, R., Beeler, D., and Rosenberg, R.: Fractionation of low molecular weight heparin species and their interaction with antithrombin. *J. Biol. Chem.* 254:2902, 1979.

96. Jordan, R. E., Oosta, G. M., Gardner, W. J., and Rosenberg, R. D.: The kinetics of hemostatic enzyme–antithrombin interactions in the presence of low molecular weight heparin. *J. Biol. Chem.* 255:10081, 1980.

97. Mackovich, R.: Mechanism of action of heparin through thrombin on blood coagulation. *Biochim. Biophys. Acta* 412:13, 1975.

98. Smith, J. F., and Craft, T. J.: Heparin reacts stoichiometrically with thrombin during thrombin inhibition in human plasma. *Biochem. Biophys. Res. Comm.* 71:738, 1976.

99. Griffith, M. J.: Kinetic analysis of the heparin-enhanced antithrombin III/thrombin reaction. Reaction rate enrichment by heparin-thrombin association. *J. Biol. Chem.* 254:12044, 1979.

100. Gitel, S. N.: Evidence for a catalytic role of heparin in anticoagulation reactions, in *Heparin: Structure and Function and Clinical Implications,* edited by R. A. Bradshaw and S. Wessler. Plenum, New York, 1975, p. 243.

101. Laurent, T. C., et al.: The molecular-weight-dependence of the anticoagulant activity of heparin. *Biochem. J.* 175:691, 1978.

102. Griffith, M. J.: Kinetics of the heparin-enhanced antithrombin III/thrombin reaction. Evidence for a template model for the mechanism of action of heparin. *J. Biol. Chem.* 257:7360, 1982.

103. Lam, L. H., Silbert, J. E., and Rosenberg, R. D.: The separation of active and inactive forms of heparin. *Biochem. Biophys. Res. Commun.* 69:570, 1976.

104. Hook, M., Bjork, I., Hopwood, J., and Lindahl, U.: Anticoagulant activity of heparin. Separation of high-activity and low-activity species by affinity chromatography on immobilized antithrombin. *FEBS Lett.* 66:90, 1976.

105. Andersson, L.-O., Barrowcliffe, T. W., Holmer, E., Johnson, E. A., and Sims, G. E. C.: Anticoagulant properties of heparin fractionated by affinity chromatography on matrix-bound antithrombin III and by gel filtration. *Thromb. Res.* 9:575, 1976.

106. Carter, C. J., Kelton, J. G., Hirsch, J., Cerskus, A., Santos, A. V., and Gent, M.: The relationship between the hemorrhagic and antithrombotic properties of low molecular weight heparin in rabbits. *Blood* 59:1239, 1982.

107. Linhardt, R. J., Grant, A., Cooney, C. L., and Langer, R.: Differential anticoagulant activity of heparin fragments prepared using microbial heparinase. *J. Biol. Chem.* 257:7310, 1982.

108. Blombäck, M., Blombäck, B., Olsson, P., and Svendsen, L.: The assay of antithrombin using a synthetic chromogenic substrate for thrombin. *Thromb. Res.* 5:621, 1974.

109. Blombäck, B.: Studies on the action of thrombic enzymes on bovine fibrinogen as measured by N-terminal analysis. *Arkiv Kemi* 12:321, 1958.

110. Yin, E. T.: Effect of heparin on the neutralization of factor Xa and thrombin by the plasma alpha-2-globulin inhibitor. *Thromb. Diath. Haemorrh.* 33:43, 1974.

111. Marciniak, E.: Factor-Xa inactivation by antithrombin III: Evidence for biological stabilization of factor Xa by factor V-phospholipid complex. *Br. J. Haematol.* 24:391, 1973.

112. Miletich, J. P., Jackson, C. M., and Majerus, P. W.: Properties of the factor Xa binding site on human platelets. *J. Biol. Chem.* 253:6908, 1978.

113. Yin, E. T., Giudice, L. C., and Wessler, S.: Inhibition of activated factor X-induced platelet aggregation: The role of heparin and the plasma inhibitor to activated factor X. *J. Lab. Clin. Med.* 82:390, 1973.

114. Owens, M. R., and Miller, L. L.: Net biosynthesis of antithrombin III by the isolated rat liver perfused for 12–24 hours. Compared with rat fibrinogen and α-2(acute phase) globulin, antithrombin III is not an acute phase protein. *Biochim. Biophys. Acta* 627:30, 1980.

115. Collen, D., et al.: Metabolism of antithrombin III (heparin cofactor) in man: Effect of venous thrombosis and of heparin administration. *Eur. J. Clin. Invest.* 7:27, 1977.

116. Chan, T. K., and Chan, V.: Antithrombin III, the major modulator of intravascular coagulation, is synthesized by human endothelial cells. *Thromb. Haemost.* 46:504, 1981.

117. Mannucci, P. M., Boyer, C., Wolf, M., Tripodi, A., and Larrieu, M. J.: Treatment of congenital antithrombin III deficiency with concentrates. *Br. J. Haematol.* 50:531, 1982.

118. Monkbouse, F. C., and Milojevic, S.: Change in thrombin generation and antithrombin titer following massive bleeding and transfusions in dogs. *Can. J. Biochem. Physiol.* 38:475, 1960.

119. Egeberg, O.: Inherited antithrombin deficiency causing thrombophilia. *Thromb. Diath. Haemorrh.* 13:516, 1965.

120. Marciniak, E., Farley, C. H., and DeSimone, P. A.: Familial thrombosis due to antithrombin III deficiency. *Blood* 43:219, 1974.

121. Sas, G., Blaskó, G., Bánhegyi, D., Jákó, J., and Pálos, L. Á.: Abnormal antithrombin III (antithrombin III Budapest) as a cause of familial thrombophilia. *Thromb. Diath. Haemorrh.* 32:105, 1974.

122. vonKaulla, E., and vonKaulla, K. N.: Deficiency of antithrombin III activity associated with hereditary thrombosis tendency. *J. Med.* 3:349, 1972.

123. Carvalho, A., and Ellman, L.: Hereditary antithrombin III deficiency. Effect of antithrombin III deficiency on platelet function. *Am. J. Med.* 61:179, 1976.

124. Odegard, O. R., and Abildgaard, U.: Anti factor Xa activity in thrombophilia: Studies in a family with AT III deficiency. *Scand. J. Haematol.* 18:86, 1977.

125. Mackie, M., Bennett, B., Ogston, D., and Douglas, A. S.: Familial thrombosis: Inherited deficiency of antithrombin III. *Br. Med. J.* 1:136, 1978.

126. Boyer, C., Wolf, M., Lavergne, J. M., and Larrieu, M. J.: Thrombin generation and formation of thrombin-antithrombin III complexes in congenital antithrombin III deficiency. *Thromb. Res.* 20:207, 1980.

127. vonKaulla, E., and vonKaulla, K. N.: Antithrombin III and diseases. *Am. J. Clin. Pathol.* 48:69, 1967.

128. Hener, U., and Nilsson, I. M.: Antithrombin III in a clinical material. *Thromb. Res.* 3:631, 1973.

129. Abilgaard, U., Fagerhol, M. K., and Egeberg, O.: Comparison of progressive antithrombin activity and the concentrations of three thrombin inhibitors in human plasma. *Scand. J. Clin. Lab. Invest.* 26:349, 1970.

130. Gavrilis, P., Lerner, R. G., and Goldstein, R.: Plasma factor Xa-inhibitory activity in alcoholic liver disease and the effect of heparin. *Thromb. Res.* 4:335, 1974.

131. Fagerhol, M. K., Abilgaard, U., Bergsjö, P., and Jacobsen, J. H.: Oral contraceptives and low antithrombin III concentration. *Lancet* 1:1175, 1970.

132. Bergsjö, P., Fagerhol, M., and Abildgaard, U.: Antithrombin III concentration in women using low-dosage progestin for contraception. *Am. J. Obstetr. Gynecol.* 112:938, 1972.

133. Conrad, J., Samama, M., and Salomon, Y.: Antithrombin III and the oestrogen content of combined oestro-progestagen contraceptives. *Lancet* 2:1148, 1972.

134. Mehl, J. W., O'Connell, W., and DeGrott, J.: Macroglobulin from human plasma which forms an enzymatically active compound with trypsin. *Science* 145:821, 1964.

135. Haverback, B. J., Dyce, B., Bundy, H. F., Wirtschafter, S. K., and Ed-

mondson, H. A.: Protein binding of pancreatic proteolytic enzymes. *J. Clin. Invest.* 41:972, 1962.

136. Steinbuch, M., Quentin, M., and Pejaudier, L.: Technique d'isolement et étude de l'α₂-macroglobuline, in *Protides of the Biological Fluids,* edited by H. Peeters, Elsevier, Amsterdam, 1965, p. 375.

137. Ganrot, P. O., and Niléhn, J.-E.: Competition between plasmin and thrombin for α₂-macroglobulin. *Clin. Chim. Acta* 17:511, 1967.

138. Niléhn, J. E., and Ganrot, P. O.: Plasmin, plasmin inhibitors and degradation products of fibrinogen in human serum during and after intravenous infusion of streptokinase. *Scand. J. Clin. Lab. Invest.* 20:113, 1967.

139. Ganrot, P. O., and Scherstén, B.: Serum α₂-macroglobulin concentration and its variation with age and sex. *Clin. Chim. Acta* 5:113, 1967.

140. Marciniak, E., and Tsukamura, S.: Two progressive inhibitors of factor Xa in human blood. *Br. J. Haematol.* 22:341, 1972.

141. Seegers, W. H., and Marciniak, E.: Some activation characteristics of the prethrombin subunit of prothrombin. *Life Sci.* 4:1721, 1965.

142. Seegers, W. H., Heene, D. L., and Marciniak, E.: Activation of purified prothrombin in ammonium sulfate solutions: Purification of autoprothrombin C. *Thromb. Diath. Haemorrh.* 15:1, 1966.

143. Marciniak, E., Murano, G., and Seegers, W. J.: Inhibitor of blood clotting derived from prothrombin. *Thromb. Diath. Haemorrh.* 18:161, 1967.

144. Murano, G., Seegers, W. H., and Zolton, R. P.: Autoprothrombin II-A: A competitive inhibitor of autoprothrombin C (factor Xa). A review with additions. *Thromb. Diath. Haemorrh. (Suppl.)* 57:305, 1974.

145. Biggs, R., Douglas, A. S., and Macfarlane, R. G.: The formation of thromboplastin in human blood. *J. Physiol.* 119:89, 1953.

146. Spurling, C. L., and King, P. D. W.: Studies on thromboplastin generation. *J. Lab. Clin. Med.* 44:336, 1954.

147. Spaet, T. H., and Garner, E. S.: Inactivation of thromboplastin in human blood. *J. Clin. Invest.* 34:1807, 1955.

148. Egli, H., Kesseler, K., and Klesper, R.: Über die Inaktivierung von Blutthrombokinase: Zugleich ein Beitrag zur Unterscheidung von Blut- und Gewebsthrombokinase. *Acta Haematol. (Basel)* 17:338, 1957.

149. Deutsch, E., and Fuchs, H.: Natürlich vorkommende Koagulationsinhibitoren. *Acta Haematol. (Basel)* 20:97, 1958.

150. Deutsch, E., and Mammen, E. F.: The inactivation of plasma thromboplastin. *Thromb. Diath. Haemorrh.* 2:324, 1958.

151. Berry, C. G.: Antithromboplastin: The degeneration of intrinsic thromboplastin in normal serum. *J. Clin. Pathol.* 11:39, 1958.

152. Soulier, J. P.: Les Inhibiteurs naturels de la coagulation. *Sang* 30: 262, 1959.

153. Israels, L. G., Ferster, J., and Zipursky, A.: A naturally occurring inhibitor of the first stage of blood coagulation. *Br. J. Haematol.* 6:275, 1960.

154. Scott, T. G., Symons, C., and Markham, R. L.: Antithromboplastin in human serum and plasma. *Nature* 186:248, 1960.

155. Schimpf, K., Brieger, G., Mühlhäusler, W., Teupel, R., and Türk, A.: Zur Charakterisierung der Antithrombokinasen. *Acta Haematol. (Basel)* 28:359, 1962.

156. Schneider, C. L.: The active principle of placental toxin: Thromboplastin; its inactivator in blood: Antithromboplastin. *Am. J. Physiol.* 149:123, 1947.

157. Thomas, J.: Studies on the intravascular thromboplastic effect of tissue suspensions in mice. II. A factor in normal rabbit serum which inhibits the thromboplastic effect of the sedementable tissue component. *Bull. Johns Hopkins Hosp.* 81:26, 1947.

158. McClaughery, R. I.: The specificity of antithromboplastic activity. *J. Mich. Med. Soc.* 49:685, 1950.

159. Lanchantin, G. F., and Ware, A. G.: Identification of a thromboplastin inhibitor in serum and in plasma. *J. Clin. Invest.* 32:381, 1953.

160. Berry, C. G.: The degeneration of brain thromboplastin in the presence of normal serum. *J. Clin. Pathol.* 10:342, 1957.

161. Wagner, R. H., Brannan, W. M., Jr., and Brinknous, K. M.: Antiaccelerator (anticonvertin) activity of canine plasma and serum. *Proc. Soc. Exp. Biol. Med.* 89:266, 1955.

162. Jürgens, J.: Factor VII inhibitor: A new physiological serum accelerator inactivation principle. *Acta Haematol. (Basel),* 14:57, 1955.

163. Schaefer, E. H., Jr., Therriault, D. G., and Jensen, H.: Studies on a prothrombin conversion inhibitor fraction from rabbit serum. *J. Appl. Physiol.* 8:300, 1955.

164. Hermansky, F., and Vítek, J.: The role of proconvertin and Stuart factor in the inactivation of tissue thromboplastin by serum. *Experientia* 16:455, 1960.

165. Seegers, W. H., Schröer, H., and Mitsuyasu, K.: Inactivation of purified autoprothrombin I with antithrombin. *Can. J. Biochem.* 42:1425, 1964.

166. Margolis, J.: Initiation of blood coagulation by glass and related surfaces. *J. Physiol.* 137:95, 1957.

167. Waaler, B. A.: Contact activation in the intrinsic blood clotting system: Studies on a plasma product formed on contact with glass and similar surfaces. *Scand. J. Clin. Lab. Invest.* 11 (Suppl. 37):1, 1959.

168. Ratnoff, O. D., and Rosenblum, J. M.: Role of Hageman factor in the initiation of clotting by glass. *Am. J. Med.* 25:160, 1958.

169. Niemetz, J., and Nossel, H. L.: Method of purification and properties of anti-XIa (inhibitor of the contact product). *Thromb. Diath. Haemorrh.* 17:335, 1967.

170. Heck, L. W., and Kaplan, A. P.: Substrates of Hageman factor. I. Isolation and characterization of human factor XI (PTA) and inhibition of the activated enzyme by α₁-antitrypsin. *J. Exp. Med.* 140:1615, 1974.

171. Walsh, P. N., and Biggs, R.: The role of platelets in intrinsic factor-Xa formation. *Br. J. Haematol.* 22:743, 1972.

172. Forbes, C. D., Pensky, J., and Ratnoff, O. D.: Inhibition of activated Hageman factor and activated plasma thromboplastin antecedent by purified serum C̄1 inactivator. *J. Lab. Clin. Med.* 76:809, 1970.

173. Harpel, P. C.: Separation of plasma thromboplastin antecedent from kallikrein by the plasma α₂-macroglobulin, kallikrein inhibitor. *J. Clin. Invest.* 50:2084, 1971.

174. Schreiber, A. D., Kaplan, A. P., and Austen, K. F.: Plasma inhibitors of the components of the fibrinolytic pathway in man. *J. Clin. Invest.* 52:1394, 1973.

175. Schreiber, A. D., Kaplan, A. P., and Austen, K. F.: Inhibition by C̄1 INH of Hageman factor fragment activation of coagulation, fibrinolysis, and kinin generation. *J. Clin. Invest.* 52:1402, 1973.

176. McConnell, D. J.: Inhibitors of kallikrein in human plasma. *J. Clin. Invest.* 51:1611, 1972.

177. Harpel, P. C.: Human plasma alpha-2-macroglobulin. An inhibitor of plasma kallikrein. *J. Exp. Med.* 132:329, 1970.

178. Speer, R. J., and Ridgeway, H.: The formation and "decay" of XIIa. *Thromb. Diath. Haemorrh.* 18:259, 1967.

179. Saito, H., Ratnoff, O. D., Donaldson, V. H., Haney, G., and Pensky, J.: Inhibition of the adsorption of Hageman factor (factor XII) to glass by normal human plasma. *J. Lab. Clin. Med.* 84:62, 1974.

180. Liu, C. Y., et al.: Potentiation of the function of Hageman factor fragments by high molecular weight kininogen. *J. Clin. Invest.* 60:7, 1977.

181. Meier, H. L., Pierce, J. V., Colman, R. W., and Kaplan, A. P.: Activation and function of human Hageman factor. The role of high molecular weight kininogen and prekallikrein. *J. Clin. Invest.* 60:18, 1977.

182. Graham, J. B., Penick, G. D., and Brinkhous, K. M.: Utilization of the antihemophilic factor during clotting of canine blood and plasma. *Am. J. Physiol.* 164:710, 1951.

183. Penick, G. D.: Some factors that influence utilization of antihemophilic activity during clotting. *Proc. Soc. Exp. Biol. Med.* 96:277, 1957.

184. Barrow, E. M., Amos, S. M., Heindel, C., and Graham, J. B.: Separation of the antihemophilic factor (F. VIII) from fibrinogen with thrombin and manganous chloride. *Proc. Soc. Exp. Biol. Med.* 121:1001, 1966.

185. Alexander, B., Goldstein, R., Rich, L., LeBolloc'h, A. G., Diamond, L. K., and Borges, W.: Congenital afibrinogenemia: A study of some basic aspects of coagulation. *Blood* 9:843, 1954.

186. Rizza, C., and Walker, W.: Inactivation of antihaemophilic globulin by thrombin. *Nature* 180:143, 1957.

187. Macfarlane, R. G., Biggs, R., Ash, B. J., and Denson, K. W. E.: The interaction of factors VIII and IX. Br. J. Haematol. 10:530, 1964.

188. Lundblad, R. L., and Davie, E. W.: The activation of antihemophilic factor (factor VIII) by activated Christmas factor (activated factor IX). Biochemistry 3:1720, 1964.

189. Hougie, C., Denson, K. W. E., and Biggs, R.: A study of the reaction product of factor VIII and factor IX by gel filtration. Thromb. Diath. Haemorrh. 18:211, 1967.

190. Ware, A. G., and Seegers, W. H.: Serum Ac-globulin: Formation from plasma Ac-globulin; role in blood coagulation; partial purification; properties; and quantitative determination. Am. J. Physiol. 152:567, 1948.

191. Cox, F. M., Lanchantin, G. F., and Ware, A. G.: Chromatographic purification of human serum accelerator globulin. J. Clin. Invest. 35:106, 1956.

192. Walsh, P. N.: Platelet coagulant activities: Evidence for multiple different functions of platelets in intrinsic coagulation. Ser. Haematol. 6:579, 1973.

193. Walsh, P. N.: Platelet coagulant activities and hemostasis. A hypothesis. Blood 43:597, 1974.

194. Kane, W. H., Lindhout, M. J., Jackson, C. M., and Majerus, P. W.: Factor Va-dependent binding of factor Xa to human platelets. J. Biol. Chem. 255:1170, 1980.

195. Walsh, P. N.: Platelets and coagulation proteins. Fed. Proc. 40:2086, 1981.

196. Miletich, J. P., Jackson, C. M., and Majerus, P. W.: Interaction of coagulation factor Xa with human platelets. Proc. Natl. Acad. Sci. U.S.A. 74:4033, 1977.

197. Dahlbäck, B., and Stenflo, J.: Binding of bovine coagulation factor Xa to platelets. Biochemistry 17:4938, 1978.

198. Østerud, B., Rapaport, S. I., and Lavine, K. K.: Factor V activity of platelets: Evidence for an activated factor V molecule and for a platelet activator. Blood 49:819, 1977.

199. White, B. N., Cox, A. C., and Taylor, F. B., Jr.: The pro-coagulant effect of platelets on conversion of prothrombin to thrombin in nonanticoagulated plasma. J. Lab. Clin. Med. 95:827, 1980.

200. Stenflo, J.: A new vitamin K-dependent protein. Purification from bovine plasma and preliminary characterization. J. Biol. Chem. 251:355, 1976.

201. Esmon, C. T., Stenflo, J., Suttie, J. W., and Jackson, C. M.: A new vitamin K-dependent protein. A phospholipid-binding zymogen of a serine esterase. J. Biol. Chem. 251:3052, 1976.

202. Kisiel, W., Ericsson, L. H., and Davie, E. W.: Proteolytic activation of protein C from bovine plasma. Biochemistry 15:4893, 1976.

203. Amphlett, G. W., Kisiel, W., and Castellino, F. J.: Interaction of calcium with bovine plasma protein C. Biochemistry 20:2156, 1981.

204. Kisiel, W., Canfield, W. M., Ericsson, L. H., and Davie, E. W.: Anticoagulant properties of bovine plasma protein C following activation by thrombin. Biochemistry 16:5824, 1977.

205. Walker, F. J., Sexton, P. W., and Esmon, C. T.: The inhibition of blood coagulation by activated protein C through the selective inactivation of activated factor V. Biochim. Biophys. Acta 571:333, 1979.

206. Vehar, G. A., and Davie, E. W.: Preparation and properties of bovine factor VIII (antihemophilic factor). Biochemistry 19:401, 1980.

207. Comp, P. C., and Esmon, C. T.: Activated protein C inhibits platelet prothrombin-converting activity. Blood 54:1272, 1979.

208. Kisiel, W.: Human plasma protein C. Isolation, characterization, and mechanism of activation by α-thrombin. J. Clin. Invest. 64:761, 1979.

209. Marlar, R. A., Kleiss, A. J., and Griffin, J. H.: Mechanism of action of human activated protein C, a thrombin-dependent anticoagulant enzyme. Blood 59:1067, 1982.

210. Fernlund, P., Stenflo, J., and Tufvesson, A.: Bovine protein C: Amino acid sequence of the light chain. Proc. Natl. Acad. Sci. U.S.A. 75:5889, 1978.

211. Walker, F. J.: Regulation of activated protein C by a new protein: A possible function for bovine protein S. J. Biol. Chem. 255:5521, 1980.

212. Walker, F. J.: Regulation of activated protein C by protein S: The role of phospholipid in factor Va inactivation. J. Biol. Chem. 256:11128, 1981.

213. Esmon, C. T., and Owen, W. G.: Identification of an endothelial cell cofactor for thrombin-catalyzed activation of protein C. Proc. Natl. Acad. Sci. U.S.A. 78:2249, 1981.

214. Owen, W. G., and Esmon, C. T.: Functional properties of an endothelial cell cofactor for thrombin-catalyzed activation of protein C. J. Biol. Chem. 256:5532, 1981.

215. Esmon, N. L., Owen, W. G., and Esmon, C. T.: Isolation of a membrane-bound cofactor for thrombin-catalyzed activation of protein C. J. Biol. Chem. 257:859, 1982.

216. Comp, P. C., Jacocks, R. M., Ferrell, G. L., and Esmon, C. T.: Activation of protein C in vivo. J. Clin. Invest. 70:127, 1982.

217. DiScipio, R. G., and Davie, E. W.: Characterization of protein S, a gamma-carboxyglutamic acid containing protein from bovine and human plasma. Biochemistry 18:899, 1979.

218. Seegers, W. H., McCoy, L. E., Groben, H. D., Sakuragawa, N., and Agrawal, B. L.: Purification and some properties of autoprothrombin II-A; an anticoagulant perhaps also related to fibrinolysis. Thromb. Res. 1:443, 1972.

219. Comp, P. C., and Esmon, C. T.: Generation of fibrinolytic activity by infusion of activated protein C into dogs. J. Clin. Invest. 68:1221, 1981.

220. Marlar, R. A., and Griffin, J. H.: Deficiency of protein C inhibitor in combined factor V/VIII deficiency disease. J. Clin. Invest. 66:1186, 1980.

221. Lorand, L., and Dickenman, R. C.: Assay method for the "fibrin-stabilizing factor." Proc. Soc. Exp. Biol. Med. 89:45, 1955.

222. Dvilansky, A., Britten, A. F. H., and Loewy, A. G.: Factor XIII assay by an isotope method. I. Factor XIII (transamidase) in plasma, serum, leukocytes, erythrocytes and platelets and evaluation of screening tests of clot solubility. Br. J. Haematol. 18:399, 1970.

223. Triantaphyllopoulos, D. C.: The inactivation of factor XIII during blood coagulation. Thromb. Res. 3:241, 1973.

224. Bannerjee, D., Morton, R. O., Delaney, R., and Hampton, J. W.: Inhibitor of fibrin cross-linking transglutaminase (plasma factor XIIIa) in enzyme deficient and normal plasmas, in Abstracts, III Congress of the International Society on Thrombosis and Haemostasis, 1972, p. 67.

225. Silver, M. J., Turner, D. L., and Tocantins, L. M.: Phospholipid antithromboplastin: Assay in vitro and evaluation in vivo of purified fractions. Am. J. Physiol. 190:8, 1957.

226. Bull, R. K., Jevons, S., and Barton, P. G.: Complexes of prothrombin with calcium ions and phospholipids. J. Biol. Chem. 247:2747, 1972.

227. Bajwa, S. S., and Hanahan, D. J.: Interaction of short chain and long chain fatty acid phosphoglycerides and bile salts with prothrombin. Biochem. Biophys. Acta 444:118, 1976.

228. Subbaiah, P. V., Bajwa, S. S., Smith, C. M., and Hanahan, D. J.: Interactions of the components of the prothrombinase complex. Biochim. Biophys. Acta 444:131, 1976.

229. Nelsestuen, G. L., Kisiel, W., and DiScipio, R. G.: Interaction of vitamin K dependent proteins with membranes. Biochemistry 17:2134, 1978.

230. Nelsestuen, G. L.: Interactions of vitamin K-dependent proteins with calcium ions and phospholipid membranes. Fed. Proc. 37:2621, 1978.

231. Walsh, P. N.: The role of platelets in the contact phase of blood coagulation. Br. J. Haematol. 22:237, 1972.

232. Walsh, P. N.: The effects of collagen and kaolin on the intrinsic coagulant activity of platelets: Evidence for an alternative pathway in intrinsic coagulation not requiring factor XII. Br. J. Haematol. 22:393, 1972.

233. Schiffman, S., Rapaport, S. I., and Chong, M. N. Y.: Platelets and initiation of intrinsic clotting. Br. J. Haematol. 24:633, 1973.

234. Walsh, P. N.: Platelet coagulant activities in thrombasthenia. Br. J. Haematol. 23:553, 1972.

235. Walsh, P. N., Rainsford, S. G., and Biggs, R.: Platelet coagulant activities and clinical severity in haemophilia. Thromb. Diath. Haemorrh. 29:722, 1973.

236. Kaplan, A. P.: Initiation of the intrinsic coagulation and fibrinolytic pathways of man: The role of surfaces, Hageman factor, prekal-

likrein, high molecular weight kininogen, and factor XI, in *Progress in Hemostasis and Thrombosis*, edited by T. H. Spaet. Grune & Stratton, New York, 1978, vol. 4, p. 127.

237. Radcliffe, R., Bagdasarian, A., Colman, R., and Nemerson, Y.: Activation of bovine factor VII by Hageman factor fragments. *Blood* 50:611, 1977.

238. Kisiel, W., Fujikawa, K., and Davie, E. W.: Activation of bovine factor VII (proconvertin) by Factor XIIa (activated Hageman factor). *Biochemistry* 16:4189, 1979.

239. Stenn, K. S., and Blout, E. R.: Mechanism of bovine prothrombin activation by an insoluble preparation of bovine factor Xa (thrombokinase). *Biochemistry* 11:4502, 1972.

240. Heldebrant, C. M., Butkowski, R. J., Bajaj, S. P., and Mann, K. G.: The activation of prothrombin. II. Partial reactions, physical and chemical characterization of the intermediates of activation. *J. Biol. Chem.* 248:7149, 1973.

241. Esmon, C. T., Owen, W. G., and Jackson, C. M.: A plausible mechanism for prothrombin activation by factor Xa, factor Va, phospholipid, and calcium ions. *Biol. Chem.* 249:8045, 1974.

242. Nelsestuen, G. L., and Suttie, J. W.: The mode of action of vitamin K. Isolation of a peptide containing the vitamin K-dependent portion of prothrombin. *Proc. Natl. Acad. Sci. U.S.A.* 70:5366, 1973.

243. Benson, B. J., Kisiel, W., and Hanahan, D. J.: Calcium binding and other characteristics of bovine factor II and its activation intermediates. *Biochim. Biophys. Acta* 329:81, 1973.

244. Gitel, S. N., Owen, W. G., Esmon, C. T., and Jackson, C. M.: A polypeptide region of bovine prothrombin specific for binding to phospholipids. *Proc. Natl. Acad. Sci. U.S.A.* 70:1344, 1973.

245. Howard, J. B., and Nelsestuen, G. L.: Properties of a Ca^{2+} binding peptide from prothrombin. *Biochem. Biophys. Res. Commun.* 59:757, 1974.

246. Stenflo, J.: Vitamin K and the biosynthesis of prothrombin. IV. Isolation of peptides containing prosthetic groups from normal prothrombin and the corresponding peptides from dicoumarol-induced prothrombin. *J. Biol. Chem.* 249:5527, 1974.

247. Esmon, C. T., Suttie, J. W., and Jackson, C. M.: The functional significance of vitamin K action: Difference in phospholipid binding between normal and abnormal prothrombin. *J. Biol. Chem.* 250:4095, 1975.

248. Silverberg, S. A., and Nemerson, Y.: The control of prothrombin conversion: Kinetic control by mechanisms inherent in two activation pathways. *Biochemistry* 14:2636, 1975.

249. Mann, K. G., Bajaj, S. P. Heldebrant, C. M., Butkowski, R. J., and Fass, D. N.: Intermediates of prothrombin activation. *Ser. Haematol.* 6:479, 1973.

250. Jackson, C. N., Owen, W. G., Gitel, S. N., and Esmon, C. T.: The chemical role of lipids in prothrombin conversion. *Thromb. Diath. Haemorrh.* 57 (Suppl. 1):273, 1974.

251. Jesty, J., and Esnouf, M. P.: The preparation of activated factor X and its action on prothrombin. *Biochem. J.* 131:791, 1973.

252. Marciniak, E.: Functional and steric characteristics of modified thrombin zymogen. *Throm. Diath. Haemorrh.* 24:361, 1970.

253. Radcliffe, R., and Nemerson, Y.: Activation and control of factor VII by activated factor X and thrombin: Isolation and characterization of a single chain form of factor VII. *J. Biol. Chem.* 250:388, 1975.

254. Kalousek, F., Konigsberg, W., and Nemerson, Y.: Activation of factor IX by activated factor X: A link between the extrinsic and intrinsic coagulation systems. *FEBS Lett.* 50:382, 1975.

255. Østerud, B., and Rapaport, S. I.: Activation of factor IX by the reaction product of tissue factor and factor VII: Additional pathway for initiating blood coagulation. *Proc. Natl. Acad. Sci. U.S.A.* 74:5260, 1977.

256. Zur, M., and Nemerson, Y.: Kinetics of factor IX activation via the extrinsic pathway. Dependence of Km on tissue factor. *J. Biol. Chem.* 255:5703, 1980.

257. Scott, C. F., Schapira, M., and Colman, R. W.: Effect of heparin on the inactivation rate of human factor XIa by antithrombin-III. *Blood* 60:940, 1982.

258. Saito, H., Goldsmith, G. H., Moroi, M., and Aoki, N.: Inhibitory spectrum of α_2-plasmin inhibitor. *Proc. Natl. Acad. Sci. U.S.A.* 76: 2013, 1979.

259. Scott, C. F., Schapira, M., James, H. L., Cohen, A. B., and Colman, R. W.: Inactivation of factor XIa by plasma protease inhibitors. Predominant role of α_1-protease inhibitor and protective effect of high molecular weight kininogen. *J. Clin. Invest.* 69:844, 1982.

260. Fernlund, P., and Stenflo, J.: Amino acid sequence of the light chain of bovine protein C. *J. Biol. Chem.* 257:12170, 1982.

261. Stenflo, J., and Fernlund, P.: Amino acid sequence of the heavy chain of bovine protein C. *J. Biol. Chem.* 257:12180, 1982.

262. Mannucci, P. M., and Vigano, S.: Deficiencies of protein C, an inhibitor of blood coagulation. *Lancet* 2:463, 1982.

CHAPTER *137*

Principles of coagulation tests

WILLIAM J. WILLIAMS

Practical application of the present-day knowledge of the chemistry and the interaction of the coagulation factors occurs most immediately in the coagulation laboratory, where an understanding of the properties of the coagulation factors and their mode of interaction is essential for the proper performance and interpretation of the coagulation tests. In this chapter the properties of the factors and of the tests are considered from a pragmatic viewpoint and with emphasis on the general principles underlying the establishment of these tests.

General considerations

Most of the plasma coagulation factors are measured in terms of their activities, and nearly all the tests use the appearance of a visible fibrin clot as the end point. Conversion of only about 10 percent of the fibrinogen in normal human plasma to fibrin by thrombin is sufficient to lead to a visible clot [1]. Antithrombin activities in plasma also may complicate the use of the fibrin clot as the end point, since larger quantities of thrombin are formed in diluted plasma than appear with undiluted plasma [2–4], and this may change the time required for a clot to form in the test system. These problems have been dealt with empirically, and the fibrin clot remains a useful end point, but caution must be used in interpreting the results.

The relationship of the clotting time in any of the coagulation tests to the activity of a particular factor or factors in the test is complex. In all these tests the clotting time is shortened as the coagulant activity increases. A plot of the clotting time against coagulant activity yields a hyperbola on rectangular coordinates

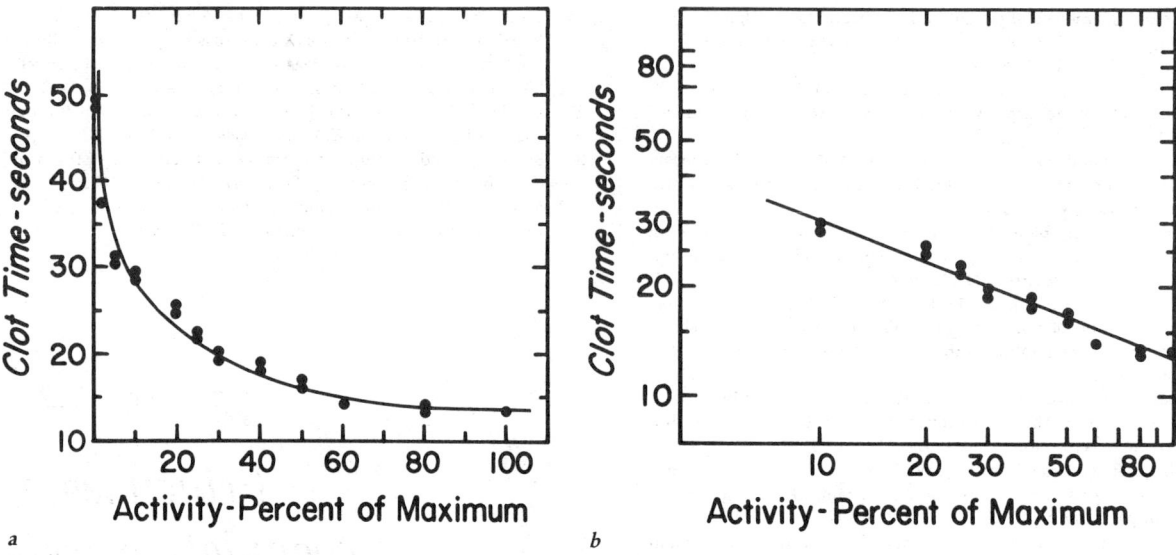

FIGURE 137-1   Plot of coagulant activity against clotting time in a representative assay system. (*a*) Data are plotted on rectangular coordinates. (*b*) Plot is on double logarithmic coordinates. The data were obtained in a study of the coagulation of normal plasma by factor Xa.

[4] and a straight line on double logarithmic coordinates [5,6], as is shown in Fig. 137-1. This relationship is such that small differences in the clotting time represent major differences in activity when the clotting times are short, but they represent minor differences when the clotting times are long. Thus a change in the one-stage prothrombin time [7] from 13 to 15 s may represent a decrease of 40 percent of the coagulant activity, while a change from 23 to 25 s may represent about 3 percent of the coagulant activity. A standard curve must be used with each test to convert the clotting times to units or percentages of maximum activity.

Because it is difficult to isolate the coagulation factors either functionally or chemically, most tests involve the participation of several factors, and there may be serious problems in the interpretation of a single test. Therefore it is essential to perform multiple tests in order to obtain precise information regarding the status of any particular factor or to perform quite complicated and difficult assays for a single factor.

Most of the tests involve the determination of the rate of clotting, and since the coagulation mechanism involves factors which are substrates prior to activation and enzymes afterward, it is well to keep in mind the basically different behavior of these two components of enzymatic systems insofar as the influence of their concentrations on the reaction rate is concerned.

The rate of an enzymatic reaction is directly proportional to the concentration of enzyme present, as is illustrated in Fig. 137-2. The effect of substrate concentration is more complex, and the rate of the reaction may be independent of the amount of substrate present at high concentrations or be nearly directly proportional to the amount of substrate present at low concentrations, as is shown in the substrate concentration curve in Fig.

137-2. Thus, for example, if Russell's viper venom is used to activate factor X [8], the rate of appearance of factor Xa will depend directly on the concentration of Russell's viper venom added. On the other hand, the rate of appearance of factor Xa will be independent of the factor X concentration over a wide range if the concentration of factor X is high, and the test would not measure variations in factor X levels. If the factor X concentration is relatively low, the reaction rate will be nearly directly proportional to the amount of factor X and the test will detect variations in the factor X level. However, in this part of the substrate concentration curve, utilization of the substrate will alter its concentration and hence the reaction rate will decrease, so only brief incubation periods may be employed if accurate data are to be obtained. The same considerations apply to the activation of factor X by the complex of tissue factor, factor VII, and calcium [9], as occurs in the one-stage prothrombin time. Once factor X has been activated, it functions as enzyme [8,10,11], and at this point the reaction rate is directly proportional to the concentration of factor Xa in the system. Thus variations in the concentration of a factor may or may not have major effects on the overall reaction rate in a coagulation system, depending on whether the factor is functioning as an enzyme or as a substrate and whether the substrate concentration is relatively high or low.

These considerations do not apply to those reactions involving complex formation [9,11,12]. Complex formation is generally rapid, and the components react stoichiometrically.

In performing the usual coagulation tests, one generally deals with the concentrations of factors present in plasma at normal or less-than-normal concentrations. Under certain conditions the platelet concentration may be important as well. For example, in studies on the consumpion of prothrombin during clotting, it has been concluded that the plasma factors are present in excess and the platelet concentration is limiting [13–16].

One approach which avoids the issue of the effect of substrate concentration on reaction rate is to permit the reaction to proceed until all the substrate has been activated and then assay the reaction mixture for the product. In this type of study, the yield of activity is measured rather than the rate at which it is formed. This approach may be more complicated, but it can be more accurate and may be conveniently accomplished. The two-stage prothrombin time is an example of a useful application of this approach, in which the amount of thrombin formed during the clotting of whole plasma is measured by its ability to clot exogenous fibrinogen [2,3].

Finally, there are certain points in terminology which deserve comment. The *stages* in coagulation tests indicate how many steps are required to complete the test. Thus a *one-stage test* is completed in one step, while a *two-stage test* requires two steps, etc. *Substrate plasma* must also be defined. This term indicates the plasma which is used in some two-stage tests to determine the clotting time, from which is derived an estimate of the activity of the factor(s) under study. It does not indicate a substrate function in an enzymatic system. Thus the thromboplastin generation test [17] involves two stages (Fig. 139-3). In the first stage, a number of reagents are incubated together to form prothrombinase (plasma thromboplastin). In the second, an aliquot of the first stage is added with calcium to substrate plasma and the clotting time determined. The rate of clotting of the substrate plasma is proportional to the amount of prothrombinase formed in the first stage.

Reagents

The reagents commonly used to provide coagulation factors in clinical tests are plasma, aged plasma, adsorbed plasma, and serum. Platelets are used in some tests. The choice of reagent depends on the combination of factors desired in the particular test. The differences between these reagents are the result of the different properties of the factors.

1. *Plasma* is usually obtained from blood that has been anticoagulated with a decalcifying agent such as oxalate or citrate, and it contains all the factors essential for clotting except calcium. The number of platelets present to provide the phospholipid required for clotting is variable, depending on the centrifugation employed. "Platelet-poor" plasma is an ill-defined reagent, and plasma spun in the ordinary laboratory centrifuge may contain a significant number of platelets [18,19]. Blood is usually exposed to glass during the preparation of plasma, and there is an increase in coagulant activity of plasma after such contact [14–16,20–22]. This is be-

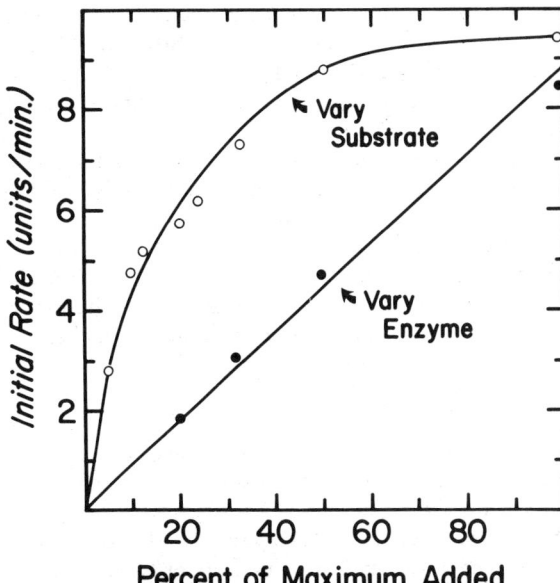

FIGURE 137-2 The effect of enzyme and substrate concentrations on the initial rate of formation of coagulant activity. The curve for the effect of enzyme concentration is given by the solid circles, while that for the effect of substrate concentration is given by the open circles. The rate of formation of coagulant activity is directly proportional to enzyme concentration over the entire range studied, but it is directly proportional to substrate concentration only at low levels. Above approximately 50 percent of maximum substrate concentration, the rate is not significantly affected by substrate concentration. The data were obtained in a study of the activation of factor X by the complex of tissue factor, factor VII, and calcium.

cause of partial activation of factors XII and XI, since these reactions can occur in the absence of calcium [23–25]. There may also be conversion of factors VII and IX to a more reactive form [26–28]. Thus "normal" plasma contains a variable number of platelets and an undefined concentration of activated factors XII and XI, as well as the other coagulation factors in an unactivated state.

2. *Aged plasma* is plasma which has been permitted to stand, usually at 4°C for 1 to 2 weeks. Factor V [29] and VIII [30] activities disappear on aging, particularly in plasma anticoagulated with the more effective decalcifying reagents such as oxalate. Such plasma may be used as a source of factor V–deficient plasma in tests to detect abnormalities in this factor.

3. *Adsorbed plasma* is plasma which has been treated with an insoluble inorganic salt such as barium sulfate or aluminum hydroxide. Barium sulfate is widely used, but it is not effective as an adsorbent if citrate has been used as the anticoagulant. The adsorption removes essentially all prothrombin and factors VII, IX, and X [17,26,31–35], as well as an appreciable amount of factor XI [36]. Thus adsorbed plasma is a source of factors XII, XI, VIII, V, and fibrinogen.

4. *Serum* is obtained from spontaneously clotted

whole blood. Serum must be incubated at 37°C for a few hours to ensure disappearance of thrombin. Serum contains factors VII, IX, X, XI, and XII, but it is essentially devoid of fibrinogen, prothrombin, and factors V and VIII [17,26,28,31–40].

5. *Platelets* are used in some coagulation tests and may be obtained from the patient under study or from a normal donor. Platelets may contribute factor V and VIII to the test system; this can cause confusion in interpreting test results [41,42]. Usually a phospholipid emulsion is used as a platelet substitute [43]. The use of phospholipid emulsions may be responsible for certain abnormalities of coagulation, such as the lupus anticoagulant (see Chap. 157).

The factors adsorbed to barium sulfate are those which are present in serum, except for prothrombin, which is absent from serum as well as being adsorbed to barium sulfate. Factor XI is partially adsorbed and is also present in serum. Thus a mixture of serum and adsorbed plasma provides all the plasma coagulation factors except prothrombin. Further, those factors which are adsorbed to barium sulfate are stable on storage while those which are not adsorbed are unstable, except for factor XII. Factor XI has been reported to increase in activity on storage in deficient plasma, and this must be taken into account in studying stored plasma for this defect.

Principles of selected tests

Figure 137-3 presents the coagulation scheme utilized in the previous discussion of the clotting mechanism (Chap. 135), modified to indicate the factors involved in several of the commonly used tests. Some of the tests involve all the factors in the intrinsic or extrinsic sys-tems, while others involve only a portion of each sequence. It is obvious that none of the tests measures any factor not involved in the reaction sequence included in the test system. Thus the one-stage prothrombin time [7] tells one nothing about factors XII [37], XI [36], IX [32,33], or VIII [44], and the partial thromboplastin time [44] does not measure factor VII [45].

There is wide variation in the rate at which clotting occurs in the various test systems, reflecting a broad difference in inherent reaction rates at the various steps in the coagulation scheme. In general, the earlier reactions are slower, while those from the formation of factor Xa on are extremely rapid. In the thromboplastin generation test [17], for example, a few minutes are required for the appearance of prothrombinase (Fig. 137-3), while only a few seconds are required for prothrombinase to clot normal plasma. Those tests requiring a relatively long time for the clot to occur are generally less sensitive than those in which the clotting time is short.

In those tests employed to study the intrinsic coagulation mechanism (Fig. 137-3), whole plasma is frequently used, but there are uncertainties regarding its composition which require modification of the plasma if discriminating tests are to be performed. The problems are the variable number of platelets and the partial activation of factors XII and XI. The latter depends on the degree of exposure to glass during preparation of the plasma [13–16,20–28]. The recalcification time test and its modification illustrate these difficulties [18,19, 44–47]. The recalcification time test is performed by adding calcium to plasma and determining the time required for clotting to occur at 37°C. After recalcification, normal plasma may clot in from 1 min to over 24 h, depending on the platelet content and extent of surface contact [21]. Under ordinary clinical laboratory conditions, it clots in from 90 to 250 s. In comparison, the

FIGURE 137-3 The clotting scheme modified to show the factors concerned in some of the commonly used coagulation tests. The brackets at the sides indicate the reactions involved in each test. The tests measuring the intrinsic system are indicated on the right of the figure; those involving the extrinsic system are indicated on the left. The indicated times for each test are the approximate normal values.

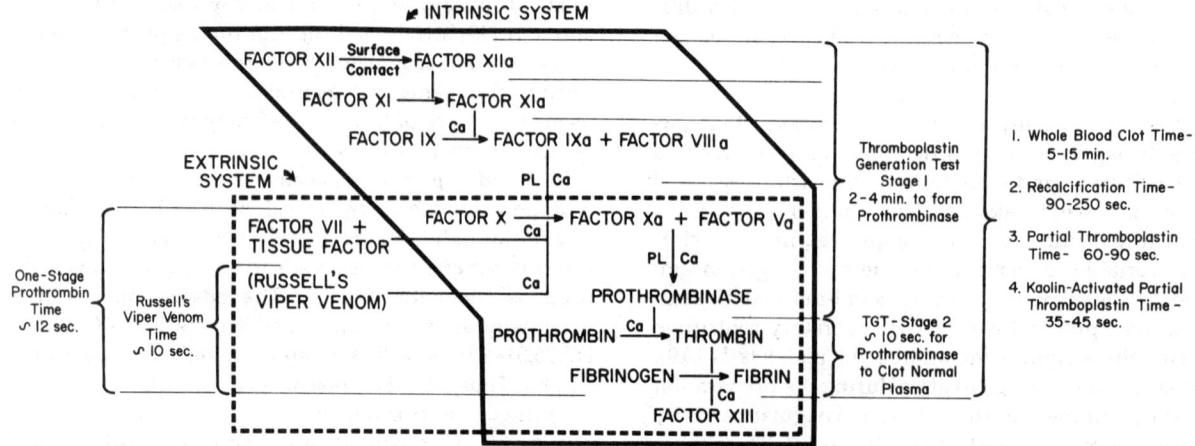

whole-blood clotting time [48] is usually between 5 and 15 min. The shorter recalcification time is a result partly of the difference in technique between the two tests and partly of the activation of coagulation factors during preparation of the plasma for the recalcification time test.

The recalcification time test is not very sensitive, and attempts to improve its utility have been directed toward providing optimal amounts of phospholipid and fully activating factors XII and XI [18,19,44–47]. The phospholipid essential for clotting in the recalcification time test is provided by the platelets remaining in the plasma, and in order to be sure that platelet concentration is not limiting, one may add an emulsion of phospholipid to the plasma prior to recalcification [44,45]. The addition of optimal amounts of phospholipid results in shortening the clotting time to 60 to 90 s in normal plasma [47]. This test is known as the *partial thromboplastin time*, or PTT, so designated because the term *partial thromboplastin* has been used to denote phospholipid emulsions. The PTT is a more useful test than the recalcification time, but it does not eliminate the variable of partial activation of factors XII and XI.

In order to circumvent this problem, a modification of the PTT has been introduced wherein some reagent capable of fully activating factors XII and XI is added to the plasma prior to recalcification [18,19,45–47]. Substances such as kaolin, ellagic acid, Celite, or colloidal silica serve this purpose well [49]. This modification permits optimal phospholipid concentration and full activation of factors XII and XI, and in this system normal plasma will clot in 35 to 45 s after recalcification [19]. This test is more sensitive than its progenitors and has proved useful as a screening test; it has also served as the basis for specific factor assays. It is referred to in Fig. 137-3 as the "kaolin-activated PTT," but it is usually referred to simply as the PTT. The sensitivity of the activated partial thromboplastin time to specific factor deficiencies depends on the reagents used [49,50].

In studies employing tissue factor (the one-stage prothrombin time, for example), the problems of optimal phospholipid concentration and partial activation of factors XII and XI do not occur because tissue factor provides its own phospholipid [9] and the reaction sequence begins at a point in the clotting scheme well beyond the activation of factor XI [36,37]. However, exposure of plasma to glass does increase the reactivity of factor VII and thereby shortens the one-stage prothrombin time [14,22,27,51]. Tests of the extrinsic system may be modified to improve their specificity by adding a reagent known to contain a specific factor or group of factors to a plasma thought to be deficient in that factor or factors in order to determine whether or not correction of the deficiency will occur [45]. Thus an unknown plasma giving a prolonged one-stage prothrombin time might be deficient in factor VII, X, or V, prothrombin, or fibrinogen (Fig. 137-3). Of these factors, normal human serum contains factors VII and X, and if addition of normal serum results in correction of the deficiency,

one could conclude that the problem is with factor VII or X. Similarly, adding adsorbed normal human plasma to the deficient plasma would provide factor V and fibrinogen, and if this addition corrects the defect, the problem would be limited to these two factors. Other additions may be made also, following this general principle.

Normal serum or adsorbed plasma may be added to the patient's plasma and an activated partial thromboplastin time done in order to determine more specifically the factor deficiency responsible for an abnormal result. Thus if substitution of normal serum for that from the patient corrects the abnormal test results, the deficiency must be in factor IX or X. On the other hand, if normal adsorbed plasma corrects the abnormality, the deficiency must be in factor V or VIII. If either normal plasma or serum corrects the abnormality, the deficiency would be in either factor XII or factor XI. Further tests are necessary to differentiate which factor of these pairs is deficient, but these are usually readily done. The activated partial thromboplastin time employing mixing of normal reagents with the patient's plasma is called the *expanded activated partial thromboplastin time.*

Finally, plasma suspected of being deficient in one factor may be mixed with plasma known to be deficient in the same factor in order to ensure that no correction occurs. Thus no improvement in the clotting time of plasma suspected of being deficient in factor XII should result from mixing the plasma with plasma known to be deficient in factor XII. If correction does occur, this is strong evidence against a deficiency of factor XII in the plasma under study. These "mixing" experiments are useful in adding specificity to otherwise nonspecific tests, but they have the disadvantage that plasma known to be deficient in a particular factor may be difficult to obtain.

Factor-deficient plasmas may be employed in the assay of specific factors, using the activated partial thromboplastin time as the test system. Activation of some of the participating factors, as the result of either the patient's illness (e.g., disseminated intravascular coagulation) or improper collection of the blood, can lead to erroneously high values for the factor being assayed. Thus in assays utilizing the activated partial thromboplastin time, activation of prothrombin (factor II) or factor X causes elevated values for factors XI, IX, or VIII [52]. Tissue factor similarly causes elevated values for these factors [52]. It is obviously of extreme importance for any coagulation test to collect the blood with great care to minimize activation of the coagulation mechanism prior to the assay.

Effect of anticoagulant therapy on coagulation tests

Treatment with the coumarin anticoagulants results in a deficiency of prothrombin (factor II) and factors VII, IX, and X and is monitored with the one-stage prothrombin time. Heparin, acting in concert with antithrombin III, inhibits thrombin, factor IXa, factor Xa, factor XIa, factor XIIa, and, possibly, factor VIIa [53–58]. Heparin therapy may be monitored by the whole-blood clotting time, but the activated partial thromboplastin time has been recommended as a convenient and reliable test for the effects of treatment with heparin [59–62]. The activated partial thromboplastin time appears to measure the "antithrombotic" effects of heparin in experimental animals [63]. However, the activated partial thromboplastin time does not always correlate well with the whole-blood clotting time in patients receiving heparin [64], and the sensitivity of the activated partial thromboplastin time to heparin varies with the reagents and techniques used [49,65]. There is also wide variation in the inhibitory effects of heparin on the activated partial thromboplastin times of plasma samples from different patients [66]. It is essential to determine the sensitivity to heparin of any activated partial thromboplastin time system considered for use in monitoring heparin therapy [67]. The prothrombin time may be significantly prolonged in patients receiving intermittent intravenous injections of heparin [68], but this appears not to occur with continuous intravenous heparin therapy [69]. Several techniques are available for neutralization of heparin in plasma [70–73], including methods utilizing ion exchange resins [72,73].

Assays of fibrinogen and factor XIII

Fibrinogen functions in blood coagulation as a substrate and therefore is assayed under conditions different from those used for other coagulation factors. The rate at which a fibrin clot forms when a standard amount of thrombin is added to plasma (thrombin time) is a function of fibrinogen concentration, following the curve described in Fig. 137-2 for "vary substrate." Thus the thrombin time may be abnormal when fibrinogen concentrations are below 100 mg/dl, but the test cannot be used to measure higher fibrinogen levels with any accuracy. Qualitative abnormalities of fibrinogen and inhibitors of fibrin formation also prolong the thrombin time.

The yield of fibrin when thrombin is added to plasma may also be used to estimate fibrinogen concentrations. The fibrin may be measured chemically, or the plasma may be diluted serially before addition of thrombin. The highest dilution yielding a visible clot is taken as the end point. This test is referred to as the fibrinogen titer.

Fibrinogen may also be measured by immunological techniques [74].

The screening tests for factor XIII deficiency depend on the yield of product, since fibrin becomes insoluble in urea, monochloroacetic acid, or acetic acid if it has been sufficiently cross-linked by the action of factor XIIIa [75]. Factor XIIIa can be measured quantitatively by its ability to catalyze the incorporation of fluorescent [76] or radioactive [77] amine compounds into proteins such as casein.

Coagulation factor assays using synthetic substrates

The activated coagulation factors are proteolytic enzymes which attack a specific amino acid sequence or sequences in their substrate proteins (see Chap. 132). Synthetic analogs of the sites of attack are hydrolyzed by the activated coagulation factors at rates proportional to the amount of activated factor (enzyme) in the system [78]. The synthetic substrates contain a chromophore or fluorophore group, and hydrolysis of the peptide is detected by measuring the color or fluorescence which develops when the active group is released [78,79]. For example, a synthetic peptide containing arginine attached by peptide linkage to the chromophore p-nitroaniline releases the p-nitroaniline when attacked by thrombin. p-Nitroaniline is yellow, and the rate of color development is a measure of enzyme activity. This system may also be modified to assay antithrombin III by its ability to inhibit thrombin-catalyzed release of the chromophore [80–82]. Such assays have high specificity and systems satisfactory for clinical use have been developed (e.g., [78]). The general utility of this approach remains to be established.

Practical applications

Specific technical details and the clinical interpretation of platelet studies and coagulation tests are presented in Chaps. A32 to A44. The results one would expect from screening tests in patients with abnormalities of platelets or coagulation factors are presented in Table 137-1. It must be emphasized that the usual coagulation tests are largely empirical, and detailed theoretic understanding of these systems is incomplete at the present time. There are many variables, other than those discussed here, which may influence the coagulation test systems, and occasionally inexplicable, aberrant results are found.

On the practical level, it should be recognized that although experienced coagulation technicians can reproduce clotting times quite precisely with a given set of reagents, there are definite and significant daily variations in reagents, so that it is essential to prepare a standard curve for each set of determinations in order to obtain acceptable accuracy. Coagulation testing must be approached with a highly critical attitude, and workers must be prepared to repeat tests and perform additional tests if a correct conclusion is to be reached.

TABLE 137-1 Reaction to screening tests of patients with abnormalities of platelets or coagulation factors

Abnormality	Bleeding time	Platelet count	Clot retraction	Whole-blood clot time	Activated partial thrombo-plastin time	Prothrombin time	Thrombin time
Thrombocytopenia	A	A	A	N	N	N	N
Qualitative platelet abnormalities	A	N	N[a]	N	N	N	N
Von Willebrand's disease	A	N	N	A–N[b]	A–N[b]	N	N
Deficiency of:							
Fibrinogen	N	N	A	A	A	A	A
Prothrombin	N	N	N	N	A	A	N
Factor V	N	N	N	N–A[c]	A	A	N
Factor VII	N	N	N	N	N	A	N
Factor VIII	N	N	N	N–A[c]	A	N	N
Factor IX	N	N	N	N–A[c]	A	A–B$_M$type[d] N–others	N
Factor X	N	N	N	N–A[c]	A	A	N
Factor XI	N	N	N	N–A[c]	A	N	N
Factor XII	N	N	N	A	A	N	N
Factor XIII[e]	N	N	N	N	N	N	N
Vitamin K deficiency	N	N	N	N–A[f]	A	A	N
Defibrination syndrome	A	A	A	N–A[c]	N–A	A	A

[a] Clot retraction is abnormal in Glantzmann's thrombasthenia.
[b] Abnormal if the deficiency of factor VIII is severe.
[c] Abnormal only if the deficiency is severe.
[d] Hemophilia B$_M$ has abnormal prothrombin times with bovine brain thromboplastin but a normal prothrombin time with human brain thromboplastin (Chap. 152).
[e] Must be detected by special tests (Chap. 154).
[f] Abnormal if marked factor IX deficiency is present.
NOTE: A = abnormal reaction; N = normal reaction.

References

1. Abildgaard, U.: N-terminal analysis during coagulation of purified human fibrinogen, fraction I, and plasma. *Scand. J. Clin. Lab. Invest.* 17:529, 1965.
2. Warner, E. D., Brinkhous, K. M., and Smith, H. P.: A quantitative study on blood clotting: Prothrombin fluctuations under experimental conditions. *Am. J. Physiol.* 114:667, 1936.
3. Ware, A. G., and Seegers, W. H.: Two-stage procedure for the quantitative determination of prothrombin concentration. *Am. J. Clin. Pathol.* 19:471, 1949.
4. Quick, A. J.: On the action of heparin and its relation to thromboplastin. *Am. J. Physiol.* 115:317, 1936.
5. Margolis, J., and Bruce, S.: An experimental approach to the kinetics of blood coagulation. *Br. J. Haematol.* 10:513, 1964.
6. Hemker, H. C., Hemker, P. W., and Loeliger, E. A.: Kinetic aspects of the interaction of blood clotting enzymes. I. Derivation of basic formulas. *Thromb. Diath. Haemorrh.* 13:155, 1965.
7. Quick, A. J.: The prothrombin in hemophilia and obstructive jaundice. *J. Biol. Chem.* 109:LXXIII, 1935.
8. Esnouf, M. P., and Williams, W. J.: The isolation and purification of a bovine plasma protein which is a substrate for the coagulant fraction of Russell's viper venom. *Biochem. J.* 84:62, 1962.
9. Williams, W. J., and Norris, D. G.: Purification of a bovine plasma protein (factor VII) which is required for the activity of lung microsomes in blood coagulation. *J. Biol. Chem.* 241:1847, 1966.
10. Milstone, J. H., Oulianoff, N., and Milstone, V. K.: Outstanding characteristics of thrombokinase isolated from bovine plasma. *J. Gen. Physiol.* 47:315, 1963.
11. Jobin, F., and Esnouf, M. P.: Studies on the formation of the prothrombin-converting complex. *Biochem. J.* 102:666, 1967.
12. Hougie, C., Denson, K. W. E., and Biggs, R.: A study of the reaction product of factor VIII and factor IX by gel filtration. *Thromb. Diath. Haemorrh.* 18:211, 1967.
13. Buckwalter, J. A., Blythe, W. B., and Brinkhous, K. M.: Effect of blood platelets on prothrombin utilization of dog and human plasma. *Am. J. Physiol.* 159:316, 1949.
14. Langdell, R. D., Graham, J. B., and Brinkhous, K. M.: Prothrombin utilization during clotting: Comparison of results with the two-stage and one-stage methods. *Proc. Soc. Exp. Biol. Med.* 74:424, 1950.
15. Dick, F. W., Jackson, D. P., and Conley, C. L.: Surface as a quantitative factor in prothrombin utilization. *J. Clin. Invest.* 33:1423, 1954.
16. Penner, J. A.: Prothrombin levels in serum. *Thromb. Diath. Haemorrh.* 10:332, 1964.
17. Biggs, R., and Douglas, A. S.: The thromboplastin generation test. *J. Clin. Pathol.* 6:23, 1953.
18. Margolis, J.: The kaolin clotting time: A rapid one-stage method for the diagnosis of coagulation defects. *J. Clin. Pathol.* 11:406, 1958.
19. Goulian, M., and Beck, W. S.: The partial thromboplastin time test. *Am. J. Clin. Pathol.* 44:97, 1965.
20. Lozner, E. L., Taylor, F. H. L., and MacDonald, H.: The effect of foreign surfaces on blood coagulation. *J. Clin. Invest.* 21:241, 1942.
21. Margolis, J.: Initiation of blood coagulation by glass and related surfaces. *J. Physiol.* 137:95, 1957.
22. Waaler, B. A.: Contact activation in the intrinsic blood clotting system: Studies on a plasma product formed on contact with glass and similar surfaces. *Scand. J. Clin. Lab. Invest. (Suppl. 37)* 11:1, 1959.
23. Ratnoff, O. D., and Rosenblum, J. M.: Role of Hageman factor in the initiation of clotting by glass. *Am. J. Med.* 25:160, 1958.

24. Rapaport, S. I.: Evidence that glass increases plasma PTA activity. *J. Lab. Clin. Med. 52:*624, 1958.

25. Ratnoff, O. D., Davie, E. W., and Mallett, D. L.: Studies on the action of Hageman factor: Evidence that activated Hageman factor in turn activates plasma thromboplastin antecedent. *J. Clin. Invest. 40:*803, 1961.

26. Biggs, R., Douglas, A. S., and Macfarlane, R. G.: The initial stages of blood coagulation. *J. Physiol. 122:*538, 1953.

27. Rapaport, S. I., Aas, K., and Owren, P. A.: The effect of glass upon the activity of the various plasma clotting factors. *J. Clin. Invest. 34:*9, 1955.

28. Lewis, J. H., Didisheim, P., Ferguson, J. H., and Hattori, K.: Changes occurring during coagulation in vitro. I. Normal human blood. *Thromb. Diath. Haemorrh. 4:*11, 1959.

29. Fahey, J. L., Ware, A. G., and Seegers, W. H.: Stability of prothrombin and ac-globulin in stored human plasma as influenced by conditions of storage. *Am. J. Physiol. 154:*122, 1948.

30. Penick, G. D., and Brinkhous, K. M.: Relative stability of plasma antihemophilic factor (AHF) under different conditions of storage. *Am. J. Med. Sci. 232:*434, 1956.

31. Alexander, B., Goldstein, R., and Landwehr, G.: The prothrombin conversion accelerator of serum (SPCA): Its partial purification and its properties compared with serum ac-globulin. *J. Clin. Invest. 29:*881, 1950.

32. Aggeler, P. M., White, S. G., Glendening, M. B., Page, E. W., Leake, J. B., and Bates, G.: Plasma thromboplastin component (PTC) deficiency: A new disease resembling hemophilia. *Proc. Soc. Exp. Biol. Med. 79:*692, 1952.

33. Biggs, R., et al.: Christmas disease: A condition previously mistaken for haemophilia. *Br. Med. J. 2:*1378, 1952.

34. Duckert, F., Flückiger, P., Isenschmid, H., Matter, M., Vogel-Meng, J., and Killer, F.: A modification of the thromboplastin generation test. *Acta Haematol. (Basel) 12:*197, 1954.

35. Hougie, C., Barrow, E. M., and Graham, J. B.: Stuart clotting defect. I. Segregation of an hereditary hemorrhagic state from the heterogeneous group heretofore called "stable factor" (SPCA, proconvertin, factor VII) deficiency. *J. Clin. Invest. 36:*485, 1957.

36. Rosenthal, R. L., Dreskin, O. H., and Rosenthal, N.: Plasma thromboplastin antecedent (PTA) deficiency: Clinical, coagulation, therapeutic hereditary aspects of a new hemophilia-like disease. *Blood 10:*120, 1955.

37. Ratnoff, O. D., and Colopy, J. E.: A familial hemorrhagic trait associated with a deficiency of a clot-promoting fraction of plasma. *J. Clin. Invest. 34:*602, 1955.

38. Graham, J. B., Penick, G. D., and Brinkhous, K. M.: Utilization of the antihemophilic factor during clotting of canine blood and plasma. *Am. J. Physiol. 164:*710, 1951.

39. Alexander, B., Goldstein, R., Rich, L., LeBolloc'h, A. G., Diamond, L. K., and Borges, W.: Congenital afibrinogenemia: A study of some basic aspects of coagulation. *Blood 9:*843, 1954.

40. Douglas, A. S.: Antihemophilic globulin consumption during blood coagulation. *Blood 11:*423, 1956.

41. Hjort, P. F., Rapaport, S. I., and Owren, P. A.: Evidence that platelet accelerator (platelet factor 1) is adsorbed plasma proaccelerin. *Blood 10:*1139, 1955.

42. Bounameaux, Y.: Dosage des facteurs de coagulation contenus dans l'atmosphère plasmatique des plaquettes humaines. *Rev. Fr. Étud. Clin. Biol. 2:*52, 1957.

43. Bell, W. N., and Alton, H. G.: A brain extract as a substitute for platelet suspensions in the thromboplastin generation test. *Nature 174:*880, 1954.

44. Langdell, R. D., Wagner, R. H., and Brinkhous, K. M.: Effect of antihemophilic factor on one-stage clotting tests: A presumptive test for hemophilia and a simple one-stage antihemophilic factor assay procedure. *J. Lab. Clin. Med. 41:*637, 1953.

45. Rodman, N. F., Jr., Barrow, E. M., and Graham, J. B.: Diagnosis and control of the hemophiloid states with the partial thromboplastin time (PTT) test. *Am. J. Clin. Pathol. 29:*525, 1958.

46. Proctor, R. R., and Rapaport, S. I.: The partial thromboplastin time with kaolin: A simple screening test for first stage plasma clotting factor deficiencies. *Am. Clin. Pathol. 36:*212, 1961.

47. Nye, S. W., Graham, J. B., and Brinkhous, K. M.: The partial thromboplastin time as a screening test for the detection of latent bleeders. *Am. J. Med. Sci. 243:*279, 1962.

48. Lee, R. I., and White, P. D.: A clinical study of the coagulation time of blood. *Am. J. Med. Sci. 145:*495, 1913.

49. Babson, A. L., and Babson, S. R.: Comparative evaluation of a partial thromboplastin reagent containing a non-settling, particulate activator. *Am. J. Clin. Pathol. 62:*856, 1974.

50. Sibley, C., Singer, J. W., and Wood, R. J.: Comparison of activated partial thromboplastin reagents. *Am. J. Clin. Pathol. 59:*581, 1973.

51. Palmer, R. N., and Gralnick, H. R.: Cold-induced contact surface activation of the prothrombin time in whole blood. *Blood 59:*38, 1982.

52. Niemitz, J., and Nossel, H. L.: Activated coagulation factors: In-vivo and in-vitro studies. *Br. J. Haematol. 16:*337, 1969.

53. Rosenberg, R. D., and Damus, P. S.: The purification and mechanism of action of human antithrombin-heparin cofactor. *J. Biol. Chem. 248:*6490, 1973.

54. Yin, E. T., Wessler, S., and Stoll, P. J.: Identity of plasma-activated factor X inhibitor with antithrombin III and heparin cofactor. *J. Biol. Chem. 246:*3712, 1971.

55. Rosenberg, R. D.: The effect of heparin on factor XIa and plasmin. *Thromb. Diath. Haemorrh. 33:*51, 1974.

56. Godal, H. C., Rygh, M., and Laake, K.: Progressive inactivation of purified factor VII by heparin and antithrombin III. *Thromb. Res. 5:*773, 1974.

57. Rosenberg, J. S., McKenna, P. W., and Rosenberg, R. D.: Inhibition of human factor IXa by human antithrombin. *J. Biol. Chem. 250:*8883, 1975.

58. Stead, N., Kaplan, A. P., and Rosenberg, R. D.: Inhibition of activated factor XII by antithrombin-heparin cofactor. *J. Biol. Chem. 251:*6481, 1976.

59. Strüver, G. P., and Bittner, D. L.: The partial thromboplastin time (cephalin time) in anticoagulant therapy. *Am. J. Clin. Pathol. 38:*471, 1962.

60. Spector, J., and Corn, M.: Control of heparin therapy with activated partial thromboplastin times. *JAMA 201:*157, 1967.

61. MacAulay, M. A., Frisch, C. R., and Klionsky, B. L.: Relationship of the partial thromboplastin time to the Lee-White coagulation time. *Am. J. Clin. Pathol. 50:*403, 1968.

62. Basu, D., Gallus, A., Hirsh, J., and Cade, J.: A prospective study of the value of monitoring heparin treatment with the activated partial thromboplastin time. *N. Engl. J. Med. 287:*324, 1972.

63. Zucker, S., and Cathey, M. H.: Control of heparin therapy: Sensitivity of the activated partial thromboplastin time for monitoring the antithrombotic effects of heparin. *J. Lab. Clin. Med. 73:*320, 1969.

64. Pitney, W. R., Pettit, J. E., and Armstrong, L.: Control of heparin therapy. *Br. Med. J. 4:*139, 1970.

65. Soloway, H. B., Cornett, B. M., and Grayson, J. W., Jr.: Comparison of various activated partial thromboplastin reagents on the laboratory control of heparin therapy. *Am. J. Clin. Pathol. 59:*587, 1973.

66. Soloway, H. B., Belliveau, R. R., Grayson, J. W., Jr., and Butler, T. J.: The in vitro effect of heparin on the activated partial thromboplastin time. *Am. J. Clin. Pathol. 58:*405, 1972.

67. Hirsh, J., and Gallus, A. S.: The activated partial thromboplastin time. *N. Engl. J. Med. 288:*1410, 1973.

68. Moser, K. M., and Hajjar, G. C.: Effect of heparin on the one-stage prothrombin time: Source of artifactual "resistance" to prothrombinopenic therapy. *Ann. Intern. Med. 66:*1207, 1967.

69. Salzman, E. W., Deykin, D., Shapiro, R. M., and Rosenberg, R.: Management of heparin therapy. *N. Engl. J. Med. 292:*1046, 1975.

70. LeRoy, B. V., Halpern, B., and Dolkart, R. E.: An indirect, quantitative method for estimation of heparin activity in vitro: The heparin-protamine titration test. *J. Lab. Clin. Med. 35:*446, 1950.

71. Israels, E. D.: Partial thromboplastin time in the presence of heparin. A rapid polybrene neutralization method. *Am. J. Clin. Path. 77:*321, 1982.

72. Thompson, A. R., and Counts, R. B.: Removal of heparin and protamine from plasma. *J. Lab. Clin. Med. 88:*922, 1976.

73. Cowan, J. F., Khan, M. B., Vargo, J., and Joist, J. H.: An improved method for evaluation of blood coagulation in heparinized blood. *Am. J. Clin. Pathol.* 75:60, 1981.

74. Feinberg, J. G.: A new quantitative method for antigen-antibody titration in gels. *Nature* 177:530, 1956.

75. Duckert, F., Jung, E., and Shmerling, D. H.: A hitherto undescribed congenital haemorrhagic diathesis probably due to fibrin stabilizing factor deficiency. *Thromb. Diath. Haemorrh.* 5:179, 1960.

76. Lorand, L., Urayama, T., de Kiewiet, J. W. C., and Nossel, H. L.: Diagnostic and genetic studies on fibrin-stabilizing factor with a new assay based on amine incorporation. *J. Clin. Invest.* 48:1054, 1969.

77. Dvilansky, A., Britten, A. F. H., and Lowey, A. G.: Factor XIII assay by an isotope method. *Br. J. Haematol.* 18:399, 1970.

78. Fareed, J., Messmore, H. L., and Bermes, E. W.: New perspectives in coagulation testing. *Clin. Chem.* 26:1380, 1980.

79. Svendsen, L., Blömback, E., Blömback, M., and Olsson, P.: Synthetic chromogenic substrates for determination of trypsin, thrombin, and thrombin-like enzymes. *Thromb. Res.* 1:267, 1972.

80. Blömback, M. B., Blömback, B., Olsson, P., and Svendsen, L.: The assay of antithrombin using synthetic chromogenic substrate for thrombin. *Thromb. Res.* 5:621, 1974.

81. Abildgaard, U., Lie M., and Ødegard, O. R.: A simple amidolytic method for the determination of functionally active antithrombin III. *Scand. J. Clin. Lab. Invest.* 36:109, 1976.

82. Bartl, K., Dorsch, E., Lill, H. J., and Ziegenhorn, J.: Determination of biological activity of heparin by use of a chromogenic substrate. *Thromb. Haemost.* 42:1446, 1979.

Fibrinolysis

CHAPTER *138*

Mechanisms of fibrinolysis

CHARLES W. FRANCIS
VICTOR J. MARDER

Fibrin formation is a central feature of inflammation, tissue repair, and hemostasis. These reactions are temporary and their effects are curtailed or reversed in order to restore normal tissue structure and function when the inciting stimulus is removed. Thus, a fibrin clot which forms quickly in a torn blood vessel to stem the loss of blood is remodeled and removed to restore blood flow. The principal effector of clot removal is the fibrinolytic system, which controls the enzymatic degradation of fibrin [1–3]. The coordinated action of activators, zymogens, enzymes, and inhibitors provides for local reaction at sites of fibrin accumulation without systemic effects. Fibrinolysis is initiated by enzymes termed *plasminogen activators,* which are present in most body tissues and fluids.

Activators of fibrinolysis

INTRINSIC ACTIVATORS
Activation of the intrinsic coagulation system with kaolin results in plasmin generation as well [4–6], and plasmin in turn can activate Hageman factor (factor XII), leading to amplification of the process. All components of the contact coagulation system are involved in plasminogen activation, but the principal ingredient of the intrinsic system remains controversial. Although little or no plasmin generation occurs in plasma that is deficient in prekallikrein, high-molecular-weight kininogen, or Hageman factor (factor XII) [6], the physiologic importance of the entire Hageman factor (factor XII)–dependent system is uncertain. No clearly identifiable pathologic state referable to impaired fibrinolysis has been identified in patients with profound defects in components of the contact activating system [7–12]. Although, it is of interest that the original factor XII-deficient patient died of a pulmonary embolus which developed after pelvic fracture [13].

EXTRINSIC (TISSUE) ACTIVATORS
The plasminogen activators present in most tissues [14] are serine proteases of M_r 60,000 to 70,000 daltons which share structural and functional properties (Table 138-1). Tissue activators bind avidly to fibrin [15] and express greater enzymatic activity in the presence of fibrin [16],

TABLE 138-1   Molecular components of the plasma fibrinolytic system

Name	Molecular weight, daltons	Baseline plasma concentration	Plasma half-life	Functional properties
Plasminogen	Single chain: M_r 88,000 (Glu₁ form) M_r 80,000 (Lys₇₇ form)	2.4 μM (21 mg/dl)	2.2 days 0.8 days	Zymogen; lysine binding sites to fibrin on "kringle" portions; activator-sensitive site at Arg₅₆₀-Val
Plasmin	Two chains: M_r 85,000 (Glu₁ form) M_r 77,000 (Lys₇₇ form) M_r 38,000 (Val₄₄₂ form)	0	0.1 s	Serine protease; active site on light chain (M_r 26,000); variable size of heavy chain containing "kringle" structures
α_2-Plasmin inhibitor	Single chain: M_r 67,000	1.0 μM (7 mg/dl)	2.6 days	Inhibits fibrinogen lysis by 1:1 complex with plasmin light chain; prevents binding of plasmin to fibrin; is itself bound to fibrin by factor XIIIa
Plasminogen activators:				
Extrinsic (tissue, vascular)	One or two chains: M_r 60,000–70,000	Trace	15 min	Vascular type derived from endothelial cells and secreted into blood; high affinity for fibrin; cleaves Arg₅₆₀-Val site on plasminogen
Exogenous				
Streptokinase	Single chain: M_r 48,000	—		Nonenzymatic, indirect action via 1:1 activator complex with plasminogen
Urokinase	Two chains: M_r 55,000 M_r 32,000	—	10 min	Serine protease; direct action on Arg₅₆₀-Val bond of plasminogen

properties which enhance their fibrinolytic potential at sites of fibrin deposition. Tissue activators have been isolated from human uterus [17], porcine heart [18], and human cadaver limbs [19–21], and they bear striking resemblance to the activator isolated from human blood after strenuous exercise [22,23]. The blood activator is probably identical to the plasminogen activator synthesized and secreted by endothelial cells [24], as well as by some normal, transformed, or malignant cells in culture [25,26]. The common structure and functional properties of all of these extrinsic plasminogen activators and the evidence that the blood activator derives from stimulated endothelial cells supports the concepts of localized extracellular proteolysis as a general defensive reaction to injury [27].

Urokinase is a structurally different type of tissue plasminogen activator which is present in urine [28]. It can be synthesized in vitro by fetal kidney cells [29]. Although urokinase is relatively less efficient in binding to fibrin or activating plasminogen in the presence of fibrin than the other tissue plasminogen activators [2,16,30], it functions to dissolve clots in the extrarenal collecting system and has also been developed as a therapeutic (exogenous) plasminogen activator.

EXOGENOUS (THERAPEUTIC) ACTIVATORS

Urokinase (UK) and streptokinase (SK) are commercially available for the treatment of thrombosis (see Chap. 159). Urokinase is a two-chain serine protease [31] which converts plasminogen to plasmin by hydrolysis of a single peptide bond [32] (see Fig. 138-1). It exists in two molecular weight forms of M_r 55,000 and 32,000 daltons [33], the latter representing a proteolytic derivative of the former. Commercial preparations have been made by affinity chromatography of large volumes of human urine [34] or by chemical purification from the culture medium of human embryonic kidney cells [35]. The two preparations of urokinase produce the same physiologic and therapeutic effect [36].

Streptokinase is a single-chain polypeptide of M_r 48,000 daltons. It is produced by β-hemolytic streptococci and purified for therapeutic use from cultures. Streptokinase alone has no enzymatic or plasminogen activator activity. It acts in a two-step process, the first of which is the formation of an equimolar complex with plasminogen or plasmin. This complex is the plasminogen activator [37,38], which possesses the enzymatic activity required for cleavage of plasminogen. In the second step the streptokinase portion of the complex undergoes molecular degradation, and the attached plasminogen is convered to plasmin with an active serine center. Both streptokinase and urokinase have low affinity for fibrin [39], but the streptokinase-plasmin complex binds to fibrin more avidly [40] and therefore with potentially greater fibrinolytic effect. The advantage of plasminogen activators with high affinity for fibrin is that active protease (plasmin) may be generated primarily in regions of thrombi, with less effect on plasma proteins, especially fibrinogen. The desirability

of fibrin-specific exogenous plasminogen activators for therapy has led to the development of two new agents, acylated streptokinase–plasmin complex [41] and a tissue plasminogen activator derived from a melanoma cell line [42]. Both of these agents at selected doses degrade fibrin and dissolve thrombi with relatively little effect on plasma fibrinogen, especially in comparison with streptokinase or urokinase [43,44].

Conversion of plasminogen to plasmin

All plasminogen activators share the ability to form plasmin from the inactive plasma zymogen plasminogen. The entire sequence of the 790 amino acid residues of plasminogen has been determined [45,46]. It is a single-chain molecule of M_r 88,000 daltons, and exists in plasma at a concentration of 2.4 μM [47] (Table 138-1). Figure 138-1 illustrates the location of disulfide bonds and functional domains for fibrin binding, plasmin activation, and protease activity. The division of the molecule into domains is marked by the cleavage site of plasminogen activators at Arg_{560}-Val. The heavy-chain

FIGURE 138-1 Schematic diagram of human plasminogen, modified from that of Collen [2] and of Sottrup-Jensen [45,46]. The intact form has N-terminal glutamic acid and is called Glu-plasminogen to distinguish it from partially degraded forms with different N-terminal amino acids. Plasminogen activators cleave the Arg_{560}-Val peptide bond which demarcates the heavy (thin line) and light (hatched line) chains of plasmin. Plasmin attacks other plasminogen molecules at several points, most importantly at Lys_{76}-Lys to liberate an "activation peptide" (linked circles) from the amino-terminal portion of the heavy chain, leaving behind Lys_{77}-plasminogen. The heavy chain consists mostly of five repeat "kringle" structures, the first four of which contain a single high-affinity and several low-affinity lysine binding sites for substrate proteins. Plasmin also cleaves plasminogen between the fourth and fifth kringles, producing a smaller plasmin molecule (Val_{442}) (see Table 138-1) that lacks lysine binding sites and therefore is an inefficient protease. The serine active site of plasmin is located on the light chain and represents the major site of interaction with α_2-antiplasmin. This plasma inhibitor is most efficient when the heavy chain of plasmin is also accessible for reaction; for example, when plasmin is in solution rather than bound to fibrin. This indicates that α_2-antiplasmin probably reacts with the heavy-chain kringle portion of plasmin as well, and inhibits binding of the heavy chain to fibrin as well as protease activity of the light chain on protein substrates.

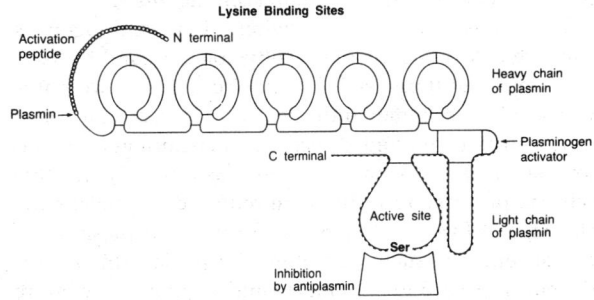

portion on the amino terminal end of the molecule con- tains a five-repeat loop structure, termed "kringles" [46] between amino acids 83 and 560; all but one (442–560) of these loops bind to lysine residues of the fibrin sub- strate (lysine binding sites) [48]. The N-terminal amino acid of intact plasminogen is glutamic acid [49–52] (Glu- plasminogen). The initial amino terminal 76 residues, called the *activation peptide* [53], is readily liberated by plasmin, producing a slightly smaller form of plas- minogen with amino-terminal lysine$_{77}$ (Lys-plas- minogen). The liberation of the amino-terminal acti- vation peptide increases the binding of plasminogen to lysine groups of fibrin [54], perhaps because lysine binding sites are shielded in the Glu-plasminogen form by interaction with part of the activation peptide. The capacity of lysine analogs such as ε-aminocaproic acid (EACA) to compete with fibrin lysine groups and to bind to the lysine binding sites on the heavy chain [55,56] is the basis of their inhibitory potential. After re- action with EACA, neither the precursor plasminogen nor the protease plasmin can effectively reach the fibrin (or other) substrate. The activity of the principal physio- logic inhibitor, α$_2$-plasmin inhibitor, is also mediated in part by its capacity to bind to the lysine binding sites [57,58].

The carboxy-terminal side of the Arg$_{560}$-Val bond is the light chain (561–790), which contains the his- tidine$_{602}$-aspartic acid$_{645}$-serine$_{740}$ active enzyme center [46]. Coincident with cleavage of the Arg$_{560}$-Val bond by any of the plasminogen activators, the plasminogen molecule is converted to a protease [59,60], and the light chain of approximately M_r 26,000 daltons is common to the different molecular weight plasmin molecules (Table 138-1). The latter consist of three major forms, namely, the Glu$_1$ type, which is intact plasminogen with only the Arg$_{560}$-Val bond cleaved, the Lys$_{77}$ form, which is Lys- plasminogen with the Arg$_{560}$-Val bond cleaved, and the Val$_{442}$ form [61], which lacks all but one kringle and all of the lysine binding sites of the heavy chain. All of these plasmin molecules are two-chain endopeptidases which hydrolyze susceptible arginine and lysine bonds in pro- teins at neutral pH and act upon most synthetic sub- strates and proteins susceptible to digestion by trypsin [62]. In addition to fibrinogen and fibrin, plasmin hy- drolyzes plasma proteins such as coagulation factors V and VIII, serum complement components, ACTH, growth hormone, and glucagon [1]. Functional assays for plasmin utilize substrates of protein, synthetic es- ters, and chromogenic or fluorescent agents [3].

The molecular sequence whereby plasminogen is converted to plasmin under physiologic conditions is uncertain, but it proceeds by either or both of two path- ways. One scheme indicates that intact Glu-plas- minogen is converted directly by plasminogen activa- tors such as urokinase to Glu-plasmin [63]. In this scheme protease inhibitors are required to prevent the cleavage of Lys$_{76}$-Lys by newly formed Glu-plasmin. In the absence of such inhibitors, Lys$_{77}$-plasmin is pro- duced. The second scheme would appear to be more

physiologic, and occurs by a two-step sequence. Lys- plasminogen is first produced by release of the activa- tion peptide by trace amounts of Glu-plasmin, followed by rapid cleavage of Arg$_{560}$-Val bond to produce Lys$_{77}$- plasmin [64]. This scheme is supported by the 20 times greater rate of activation of Lys-plasminogen than Glu- plasminogen by urokinase [65], illustrating the self- accelerating feedback mechanism that is characteristic for the fibrinolytic and coagulation enzymatic path- ways.

Inhibition of plasmin by antiplasmin

The physiologic inhibition of plasmin protease activity depends chiefly on the 1:1 irreversible molecular inter- action with α$_2$-antiplasmin [66–68] (Fig. 138-1). This process is central to the physiologic control of fibrinoly- sis, which must provide for its intermittent activation at local sites of fibrin deposition without initiating a sys- temic proteolytic state. In the plasma, α$_2$-antiplasmin reacts exceedingly fast with plasmin [57,58] (Table 138- 1), first binding reversibly, then forming a stable com- plex with the light chain. In the process of complex for- mation, a covalent bond forms between the serine$_{740}$ of plasmin and a leucine residue near the carboxy-ter- minus of α$_2$-antiplasmin, producing a fragment of M_r 8000 daltons from the inhibitor [69] and irreversibly inhibiting the enzyme. Although the primary reaction is with the active center, the rapidity of binding is influenced by availability of lysine binding sites, since prior reaction with lysine analogs such as EACA slows the inhibitory effect considerably [58]. Similarly, plas- min in solution is more readily inactivated than is plas- min that is already bound to a substrate such as fibrin [7,58], since the lysine binding sites are freely accessible to binding by the inhibitor. The functional role of α$_2$-an- tiplasmin is limited to the inhibition of free plasmin in blood, but in this capacity, it represents the major line of defense, while other plasma inhibitors such as α$_2$- macroglobulin [70] serve as backup inhibitors should the capacity of α$_2$-antiplasmin be exceeded [66,68]. Al- though the plasma concentration of α$_2$-macroglobulin is considerable (3 μM), its inhibitory capacity is limited, since the complex formed with plasmin does not com- pletely eliminate protease activity on protein substrates. The other plasma inhibitors such as antithrombin III, α$_1$-antitrypsin, and Cl inactivator have demonstrable antiplasmin activity in purified in vitro systems, but they exert minimal effect in the blood.

Inhibitors of tissue plasminogen activators have been postulated [72] but have been difficult to establish by in vitro techniques, and turnover studies [73] suggest that cellular mechanisms may be more important in clear- ance of intrinsic and extrinsic activators from the blood. Antistreptokinase antibodies are present to varying degree [74] in humans as the result of immunologic response to prior infection with β-hemolytic strepto- cocci. Such antibodies require that streptokinase be administered in sufficient amount to overcome their neutralizing effect. The streptokinase-plasminogen activator complex is resistant to inactivation by α_2-antiplasmin [75] and therefore represents an efficient tool for the activation of plasminogen. However, an anamnestic response is expected to an initial administration of streptokinase, and successful retreatment with this agent is difficult to achieve.

Local augmentation and control of physiologic thrombolysis

The physiologic response to a hemostatic plug or to a thrombus includes localized activation of fibrinolysis. The protein interactions which achieve this are illustrated in Fig. 138-2.

First, approximately 4 percent of the plasminogen in the blood binds to fibrin as it polymerizes [1,76,77]. The zymogen is thus incorporated within the fibrin fibers, attached via the lysine binding sites of the heavy chain (Fig. 138-1). Second, plasminogen activator is released from endothelial cells that are contiguous to the thrombus but not by endothelial cells in vessels that are patent and otherwise unstimulated. This tissue (vascular) plasminogen activator is not only released in the vicinity of the fibrin but also has a high affinity for fibrin or for plasminogen attached to fibrin [16], further localizing the fibrinolytic response. Third, the plasmin that is formed in situ is protected from α_2-antiplasmin, which is an inefficient inhibitor because the lysine binding sites of plasmin are already bound to the fibrin [1,77,78]. The half-life of fibrin-bound plasmin is about 10 s, or two orders of magnitude longer than that of unbound plasmin [78]. Fourth, proteolysis in plasma is limited by the relatively poor affinity of endothelial cell–derived plasminogen activator for plasma proteins and by the efficient inhibition of any liberated plasmin by α_2-antiplasmin.

Plasminogen is very rapidly activated on the fibrin surface, the resulting plasmin rapidly attacks the adjacent fibrin, and the bound plasmin resists inactivation. Such acceleration by complex formation on surfaces has parallels in the coagulation system, in which binding of proteins to platelet surfaces increases their concentration and enhances the velocity of the ensuing reactions. An additional element of local control of fibrinolysis is produced by the covalent binding of α_2-antiplasmin to fibrin through the action of factor XIIIa [79]. Cross-linked fibrin containing bound α_2-antiplasmin is lysed more slowly in vitro than cross-linked fibrin which contains no α_2-antiplasmin. This finding may be related to the relative resistance to plasmin degradation of cross-linked clots compared to non-cross-linked clots [80,81]. In cross-linked clots the fibrin is progressively diminished, presumably by lysis of successive layers of thrombus [82], each of which is in turn exposed to freshly secreted or newly diffused endothelial cell plasminogen activator.

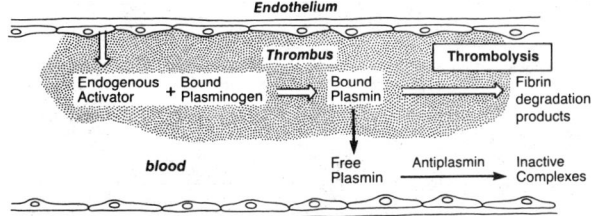

FIGURE 138-2 Molecular interactions of physiologic thrombolysis, in which the process is locally augmented yet systemically inhibited. "Endogenous" activator refers to the tissue plasminogen activator released by endothelial cells, but does not exclude the contribution by intrinsic plasminogen activators generated by the contact coagulation system. The molecular interaction of plasminogen activator, plasminogen, and fibrin takes place on the surface of the particulate fibrin clot, which efficiently directs the protease action onto the desired substrate. The plasma inhibitor, α_2-antiplasmin, rapidly inactivates any plasmin that is released from the thrombus, preventing a systemic proteolytic state that could degrade plasma proteins, especially fibrinogen.

Hyperfibrino(geno)lytic states

Considering that the M_r of α_2-antiplasmin is 67,000 daltons [67,70] and its plasma concentration is 7 mg/dl, the molar concentration in blood is less than half (1.0 versus 2.4 μM) that of plasminogen (Table 138-1). Thus, plasma has a limited capacity to neutralize the maximum potential quantity of plasmin which could result from complete activation of plasminogen. In certain pathological conditions, the backup inhibitory protein, α_2-macroglobulin, also complexes with plasmin, but residual plasmin protease activity still appears in the blood, producing a "plasma proteolytic" or "hyperfibrino(geno)lytic" state [1]. The two major mechanisms whereby this altered state may arise are shown schematically in Fig. 138-3.

In the first instance, excessive amounts of endothelial cell-derived plasminogen activator are released [83] into the blood by a generalized response of the entire vascular system, especially that portion with the highest relative concentration of endothelial cells, the capillaries. This release can be induced by administered vasoactive drugs [84], intrinsic release of catacholamines under severe stress or during exhaustive physical exercise, or by the release of a plasminogen activator releasing hormone from the neurohypophysis [83] that stimulates the endothelial cells directly. Hypotension or surgical trauma may induce a "primary" hyperfibrino(geno)lytic state via these catecholamine-related pathways. However, certain neoplasms secrete a tissue plasminogen activator directly into the blood and produce the same effect. Some patients have a concomitant hypercoagulable state leading to disseminated intravascular coagulation (see Chap. 158) and physiologic (reactive) thrombolysis (see Fig. 138-2).

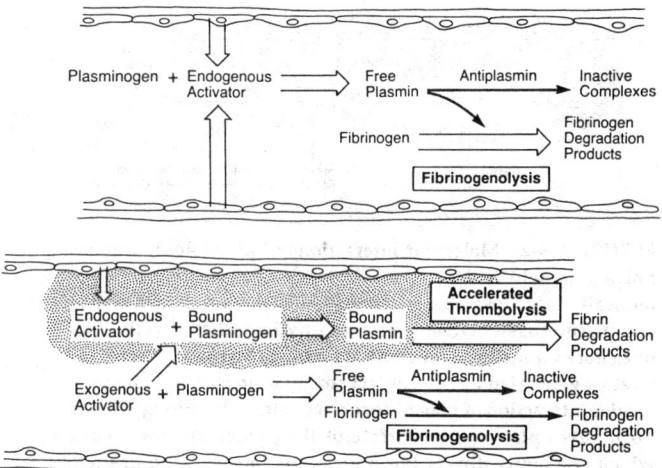

FIGURE 138-3 Molecular interactions in the development of hyperfibrino(geno)lytic state. The top panel illustrates the mechanism whereby excessive vascular plasminogen activator is released from endothelial cells, leading to activation of plasminogen to a degree that α_2-antiplasmin capacity for inhibition is exceeded and fibrinogen is degraded. Usually, only transient or insignificant degrees of hypofibrinogenemia accompany this reaction, which may nevertheless accelerate the lysis of physiologic clots as shown in Fig. 138-2. A similar result could occur in patients with cirrhosis who have decreased cellular clearance of activator or in patients with congenital deficiency of α_2-antiplasmin. The bottom panel shows the mechanism whereby excessive exogenous activator (usually urokinase or streptokinase) is administered, converting both plasma and fibrin-bound plasminogen to plasmin, and producing both the therapeutic effect of rapid thrombolysis and the side effect of fibrino(geno)lysis via the formation of free plasmin in the blood. The "fibrin-specific" plasminogen activator should minimize the blood effect while allowing for preferential fibrin lysis and therapeutic thrombolysis.

A related phenomenon occurs in patients with cirrhosis with a decreased capacity for clearing circulating plasminogen activator, resulting in prolonged elevated levels which are manifest as a shortened clot lysis time or even as a bleeding tendency. Patients have been described with congenitally deficient or congenitally defective α_2-antiplasmin [85,86]. In such cases, even small amounts of plasminogen activator may convert sufficient plasminogen to plasmin to cause clinical manifestations of bleeding. Since the affinity of plasminogen activator for plasminogen is low in the absence of fibrin and since tissue activators and plasminogen or plasmin bind poorly to plasma fibrinogen [16], these hyperfibrino(geno)lytic states rarely cause a significant plasminemia or decrease in plasma fibrinogen concentration [87]. However, bleeding secondary to premature lysis of hemostatic plugs may still occur since the presence of fibrin in local regions of vascular trauma can significantly increase the efficiency of plasmin formation, and accelerate the fibrinolytic response.

This situation is akin to the second example of a lytic state shown in Fig. 138-3 (bottom), namely, that which is induced by exogenous plasminogen activators administered for therapeutic purposes. In this circumstance, urokinase or streptokinase are administered in doses that exceed the inhibitory capacity of the antiactivators, and since urokinase and streptokinase do not have special affinity for fibrin or fibrin-bound plasminogen, an excessive and clinically significant proteolytic state results. The principal deterrent is α_2-antiplasmin, and when this protein is depleted, plasma substrates such as fibrinogen and coagulation factors V and VIII are degraded. The desired therapeutic result of administered exogenous plasminogen activators is the accelerated lysis of thrombi, achieved by the mass action effect of a high concentration of activator on fibrin-bound plasminogen. The potential advantage of fibrin-specific activators can be appreciated from Fig. 138-3 (bottom). Plasma plasminogen would be relatively unaffected by such activators, while plasminogen bound to fibrin would be preferentially activated.

Impairment of the fibrinolytic response can predispose to thrombotic events. Abnormal plasminogen molecules [88,89] are associated with recurrent thromboses. Excessively high levels of plasma fibrinolytic inhibitors can cause similar problems [90–92]. Widespread thrombosis may also occur if a synthetic inhibitor such as EACA were administered to a patient with a predisposition to or an ongoing thrombotic process [93] (see Chap. 158). Some patients may not release vascular plasminogen activator efficiently or appropriately from endothelial cells that are in contact with a growing thrombus [94].

Fibrinogen and fibrin degradation

MOLECULAR CHANGES

The principal substrates of plasmin are fibrinogen and fibrin. Degradation of the former occurs primarily in the blood under circumstances shown in Fig. 138-3 (top) and in clots or thrombi as shown in Figs. 138-2 and 138-3 (bottom). Plasmic degradation of fibrinogen and fibrin is determined primarily by the number and accessibility of critical cleavage sites. Although there are potentially over 300 arginine and lysine bonds susceptible to plasmin hydrolysis [95], only 50 to 60 are cleaved during degradation, and hydrolysis of an even smaller number is responsible for breaking the intact molecule into fragments [96–99]. Fibrinogen has an M_r of 340,000 daltons [100–102] and a plasma concentration of 200 to 300 mg/dl. It consists of three pairs of polypeptide chains, termed Aα, Bβ, and γ, of approximate M_r 67,000, 56,000, and 47,000 daltons, respectively [103]. There are three major domains, a central domain in which the two halves of the molecule are joined by disulfide bonds at their N-terminal region, connected on each side by α helical "coiled coils" [5,104,105] to the terminal domains containing the C-terminal portions of each set of three polypeptide chains [(Fig. 138-4). A long extension of the Aα chain exits from each terminal domain, which consists mostly of β and γ chain components. The major plasmin-susceptible sites which account for the cleavage of fibrinogen into degradation products are located on the Aα chain extension and midway along the coiled coil between central and terminal domains [97,106,107].

Initial plasmic cleavages occur at several points along the exposed carboxy-terminal appendage of the Aα chain [108], liberating a series of peptides and leaving behind a remnant of the chain with M_r 25,000 daltons. This Aα chain cleavage is the principal distinction between intact fibrinogen and the fragment X groups of derivatives, the smallest of which has an M_r of 250,000 daltons [109]. The next cleavages involve all three of the chains in the protease-sensitive portion of the coiled coils (Fig. 138-4). Since one of the coiled coils is usually broken before the other, degradation of fragment X is asymmetric, and it is split into unequal parts, yielding one fragment D and one fragment Y with M_r 100,000 and 150,000 daltons, respectively [110,111]. Fragment Y is a transient intermediate degradation product that is quickly split by plasmin into a second fragment D moiety and fragment E, which represents the central domain standing alone. Fragment E has M_r 50,000 daltons and contains the disulfide-bonded N-terminal part of all six polypeptide chains of the original fibrinogen molecule [112,113].

Degradation products of fibrin differ from those of fibrinogen in having covalent cross-links between fibrin monomers [114–116] and noncovalent attractive forces between central and terminal domain polymerization binding sites [117–119]. Fibrin formation is initiated by thrombin, which liberates fibrinopeptides A and B [120,121] from the central domain. This changes the charge properties of the resultant fibrin monomers and at the same time exposes binding sites on the α and β chains. Both of these effects result in lateral attraction and binding of central and terminal domains (Fig. 138-5), which produces a stepwise longitudinal growth of a fibrin polymer [122–125]. With the end-to-end approximation of terminal domains, portions of the C-terminal region of γ chains interact and are covalently bonded by factor XIIIa [126]. The growing fibrin protofibrils then coalesce by lateral attractive forces into a fibrin fiber, which is further cross-linked by factor XIIIa, producing an α-chain polymer network that effectively stabilizes the clot [80,127]. Plasmic degradation of a crosslinked fibrin clot differs from that of fibrinogen in two ways. First, degradation is slower because the cross-linked bonds join the monomers into a complex, interlacing structure and hold them together in the face of proteolytic cleavage. Second, the degradation products themselves are distinctive because of the covalent and non-covalent bonds that hold the domains together even after solubilization of the clot.

On the other hand, the unique fragments are not the result of any change in the specific cleavages caused by plasmin [128,129]. As with fibrinogen, initial cleavages

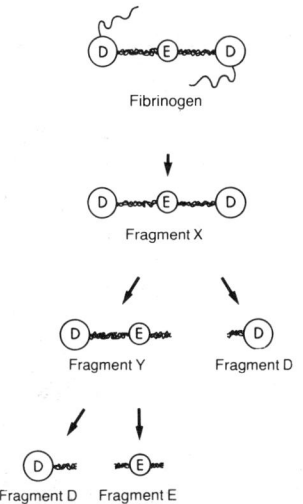

FIGURE 138-4 Asymmetric degradation of fibrinogen by plasmin [110,111]. The principal structures are the three globular domains from which degradation fragments D and E derive, the proposed α-helical coiled coils which connect them, and the long Aα-chain extensions from each of the D domain regions. Intermediate degradation fragment X consists of all three domainal regions, but lacks the Aα-chain extensions. Fragment Y consists of the central E domain with either of the terminal (fragment D) domains connected by the coiled coil. (Figure reproduced with permission from Marder et al. [99].)

degrade the cross-linked α-chain polymer at the same protease-sensitive sites, following which cleavages occur in the connecting coiled coil region between central and terminal domains, again at the same location as in fibrinogen. The "backbone" degradation products consist of domains linked longitudinally by coiled coils or by cross-link bonds, and laterally by noncovalent bonds into complexes that are liberated from fibrin only after the α-chain superstructure has been dismantled (Fig. 138-5). Each complex consists of two fragments, held together by the same forces between central and terminal domains that operated to form the protofibril. The constituent fragments of each complex represent portions of linked fibrin monomers, the terminal domains of which still are joined by cross-linked bonds. The smallest unique degradation product of cross-linked fibrin is fragment DD, which consists of two fragment D moieties joined by cross-linking [130–132]. The smallest complex is a combination of fragment DD with fragment E, joined together by noncovalent bonds [133,134]. The larger complexes are simply combinations of longer portions of each polymer chain of the protofibril [82,99,128,129]. Larger complexes can be progressively degraded by plasmin in vitro to smaller complexes, but it is likely that the larger complexes represent the dominant forms in vivo following clot dissolution [82], since α_2 plasmin inhibitor would limit further plasmic action.

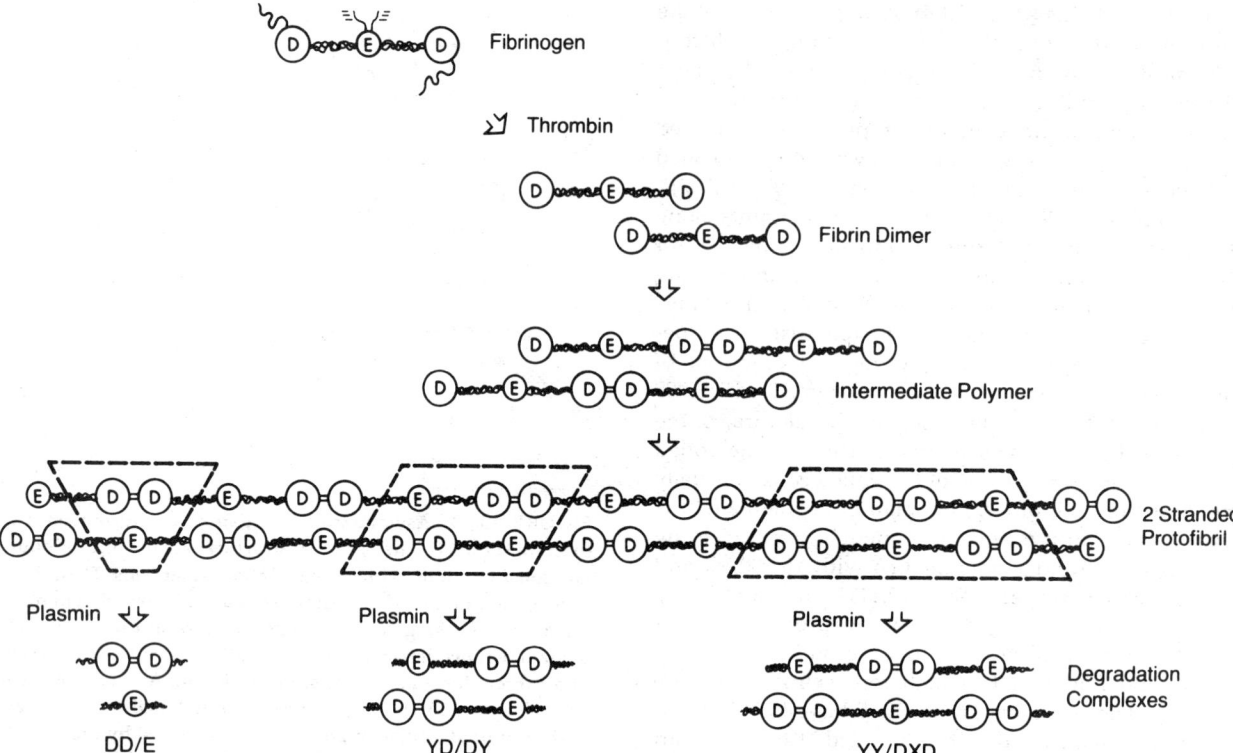

FIGURE 138-5   Fibrin polymerization, cross-linking, and degradation, showing the influence of thrombin, factor XIIIa and plasmin acting in concert on the structure of cross-linked fibrin degradation products [128,129]. After thrombin liberation of the fibrinopeptides, two fibrin monomers form a half-overlap fibrin dimer as the initial step of polymerization. Additional monomers are added to each end by a similar half-overlap process to form an intermediate polymer and then a protofibril. Factor XIIIa catalyzes the formation of crosslinks between γ chains of contiguous terminal domains. Plasmic degradation of a long two-stranded protofibril results in the series of noncovalently bound complexes (*bottom*), the smallest of which is DD/E. The presence of fragments that are larger than DD, such as DY, attached noncovalently to liberated complementary regions of another fibrin strand, provides the basis for this scheme of ever-larger cross-linked fibrin degradation complexes. (Figure reproduced with permission from Marder et al. [99]. For convenience, the α-chain extensions are shown only for the intact fibrinogen molecule.)

TESTS FOR FIBRINOGEN AND FIBRIN DEGRADATION PRODUCTS

Methods to detect these derivatives are based on their functional, immunologic, or structural properties [135,136]. Functional tests for degradation products of fibrinogen or fibrin depend upon their anticoagulant properties or their propensity to form high-molecular-weight complexes with fibrinogen. Tests of clotting function such as thrombin time would assess the anticoagulant effect of degradation products, since the fragments interfere with polymerization of fibrin monomers. Such assays are nonspecific, as other abnormalities such as a decrease in plasma fibrinogen concentration could produce a prolonged clotting time. Complexes of degradation products with fibrinogen or fibrin monomer are larger and less soluble than fibrinogen under certain conditions. The presence of such complexes can be inferred from the formation of precipitates in the presence of ethanol or protamine sulfate [137,138]. Molecular sieve chromatography of plasma samples on calibrated columns [139] separates fibrinogen from its derivatives or complexes by differences in molecular weight, but this method is too cumbersome for routine clinical application.

The most specific and sensitive methods employ immunological techniques. These assays use serum as the test material to avoid interference or cross-reaction with plasma fibrinogen. Unclottable proteolytic derivatives of fibrinogen share antigenic determinants with the undergraded parent molecule and can be quantitatively assayed in serum after removal of fibrinogen by clotting, usually in the presence of excess thrombin to ensure clotting and EACA to prevent in vitro fibrinolysis. Two commonly employed tests are the tanned red cell hemagglutination inhibition immunoassay (TRCHII) [140] and the latex particle flocculation test [141,142]. The TRCHII utilizes fibrinogen-coated tanned erythrocytes that can be agglutinated by antifibrinogen antiserum. Interference with this reaction by prior adsorption of the antiserum with the test serum is evidence that degradation products were present in the sample, and by implication, in the circulation. The test detects as little as 0.5 μg/ml of fibrinogen or degradation product (*fibrinogen-related antigen*). In the latex particle flocculation test, antibody-coated latex particles are clumped by degradation products that react with the antibody (see Chap. A36). The flocculation produced with test serum is compared with the reaction of a standard fibrinogen preparation to quantitate the concentration of degradation products. This assay is exceedingly simple and rapid and may be adjusted for sensitivity that is equivalent to that for the TRCHII. Clinically available tests do not distinguish between degradation products of fibrinogen and cross-linked fibrin, since these derivatives share most immunologic determinants. The distinction would have important physiologic implications [143], since they would arise from either plasminemia or thrombolysis, and the development of specific assays based upon differences such as are shown in Figs. 138-4 and 138-5 would be of major clinical usefulness.

References

1. Sherry, S., Alkjaersig, N., and Fletcher, A. P.: Fibrinolysis and fibrinolytic activity in man. *Physiol. Rev. 39*:343, 1959.
2. Collen, D.: On the regulation and control of fibrinolysis. *Thromb. Haemost. 43*:77, 1980.
3. Robbins, K. C.: The plasminogen-plasmin enzyme system, in *Hemostasis and Thrombosis: Basic Principles and Clinical Practice*, edited by R. W. Colman, J., Hirsh, V. J. Marder, and E. W. Salzman. Lippincott, Philadelphia, 1982 pp. 623–639.
4. Ratnoff, O. D.: The surface-mediated initiation of blood coagulation and related phenomena, in *Haemostasis: Biochemistry, Physiology and Pathology*, edited by D. Ogston, and B. Bennett. Wiley, London, 1977, pp. 25–55.
5. Ogston, D., and Bennett, B.: Surface-mediated reactions in the formation of thrombin, plasmin and kallikrein. *Br. Med. Bull. 34*:107, 1978.
6. Meier, H. L., Pierce, J. V., Colman, R. W., and Kaplan, A. P.: Activation and function of human Hageman factor. The role of high-molecular-weight kininogen and prekallikrein. *J. Clin. Invest. 60*:18, 1977.
7. Ratnoff, O. D., and Colopy, J. E.: A familial hemorrhagic trait associated with a deficiency of a clot-promoting fraction of plasma. *J. Clin. Invest. 34*:601, 1955.
8. Hathaway, W. E., Belhanson, L. P., and Hathaway, H. S.: Evidence for a new thromboplastin factor: Case report, coagulation studies, and physicochemical studies. *Blood 26*:521, 1965.
9. Colman, R. W., et al.: Williams trait. Human kininogen deficiency with diminished levels of plasminogen proactivator and prekallikrein associated with abnormalities of the Hageman factor–dependent pathways. *J. Clin. Invest. 56*:1650, 1975.
10. Saito, H., Ratnoff, O., Waldmann, A., and Abraham, J. P.: Fitzgerald trait. Deficiency of a hitherto unrecognized agent, Fitzgerald factor, participating in surface-mediated reactions of clotting, fibrinolysis, generation of kinins, and the property of diluted plasma enhancing vascular permeability (PF/dil). *J. Clin. Invest. 55*:1082, 1975.
11. Lacombe, N. J.: Déficit constitutionel en un nouveau facteur de la coagulation intervenant au niveau de contact: Le facteur "Flaujeac." *C. R. Acad. Sci. (D) 280*:1039, 1975.
12. Rosenthal, R. H., Dreskin, O. H., and Rosenthal, N.: New hemophilia-like disease caused by deficiency of a third plasma thromboplastin factor. *Proc. Soc. Exp. Biol. Med. 82*:171, 1953.
13. Ratnoff, O. D., Busce, F. J., and Sheon, R. P.: The demise of John Hageman. *N. Engl. J. Med. 279*:760, 1968.
14. Astrup, T.: Tissue activators of plasminogen. *Fed. Proc. 25*:42, 1966.
15. Müllertz, S.: Plasminogen activator in spontaneously active human blood. *Proc. Soc. Exp. Biol. Med. 82*:291, 1953.
16. Wallén, P.: Activation of plasminogen with urokinase and tissue activator, in *Thrombosis and Urokinase*, edited by R. Paoletti and S. Sherry. Academic, London, 1977, pp. 91–102.
17. Rijken, D. C., Wijngaards, G., Zaal-de Jong, M., and Welbergen, J.: Purification and partial characterization of plasminogen activator from human uterine tissue. *Biochim. Biophys. Acta 580*:140, 1979.
18. Cole, E. R., and Bachmann, F. W.: Purification and properties of a plasminogen activator from pig heart. *J. Biol. Chem. 252*:3729, 1977.
19. Aoki, N., and von Kaulla, K. N.: The extraction of vascular plasminogen activator from human cadavers and a description of some of its properties. *Am. J. Clin. Pathol. 55*:171, 1971.
20. Pepper, D. S., and Allen, R.: Isolation and characterization of human cadaver vascular endothelial activator, in *Progress in Chemical Fibrinolysis and Thrombolysis*, edited by J. F. Davidson, R. Rowan, M. Samama, P. C. Desnoyers. Raven Press, New York, 1978, pp. 91–98.
21. Binder, B. R., Spragg, J., and Austen, K. F.: Purification and characterization of human vascular plasminogen activator derived from blood vessel perfusates. *J. Biol. Chem. 244*:1998, 1979.
22. Radcliffe, R., and Heinze, T.: Isolation of plasminogen activator from human plasma by chromatography on lysine-Sepharose. *Arch. Biochem. Biophys. 189*:185, 1978.
23. Rijken, D. C., Wijngaards, G., and Welbergen, J.: Relationship between tissue plasminogen activator and the activator in blood and vascular wall. *Thromb. Res. 18*:815, 1980.
24. Todd, A. S.: The histological localization of fibrinolysin activator. *J. Pathol. 78*:281, 1959.
25. Bernik, M. B., White, W. F., Oller, E. P., and Kwaan, H. C.: Immunologic identity of plasminogen activator in human urine, heart, blood vessels, and tissue culture. *J. Lab. Clin. Med. 84*:546, 1974.
26. Rifkin, D. B., Loeb, J. N., Moore, G., and Reich, E. Properties of plasminogen activators formed by neoplastic human cell cultures. *J. Exp. Med. 139*:1317, 1974.
27. Reich, E.: Activation of plasminogen: A general mechanism for producing localized extracellular proteolysis, in *Molecular Basis of Biological Degradative Processes*, edited by R. D. Berlin, H. Herrmann, I. H. Lepow, and J. M. Tanzer. Academic, New York, 1978, p. 155.
28. Williams, J. R. B.: The fibrinolytic activity of urine. *Br. J. Exp. Pathol. 32*:530, 1951.
29. Bernik, M. B., and Kwaan, H. C.: Origin of fibrinolytic activity in cultures of human kidney. *J. Lab. Clin. Med. 70*:650, 1967.
30. Wallén, P., and Wiman, B.: On the generation of intermediate plasminogen and its significance for activation, in *Proteases and Biological Control*, edited by E. Reich, D. B. Rifkin, and E. Shaw. Cold Spring Harbor Laboratory, 1975, pp. 291–303.
31. Ong, E. B., Soberano, M. E., Johnson, A. J., and Schoellmann, G.: Studies on the biochemistry of urokinase. *Thromb. Haemost. 38*:801, 1977.
32. Summaria, L., Boreisha, I. G., Arzadon, L., and Robbins, K. C.: Activation of human Glu-plasminogen to Glu-plasmin by urokinase in presence of plasmin inhibitors. *Streptomyces leupeptin* and human plasma α_1-antitrypsin and antithrombin III (plus heparin). *J. Biol. Chem. 252*:3945, 1977.
33. Barlow, G. H.: Urinary and kidney cell plasminogen activator. *Methods Enzymol. 45*:239, 1976.
34. Pye, E. K., Maciag, T., Kelly, P., and Ivengar, M. R.: Purification of urokinase by affinity chromatography, in *Thrombosis and Urokinase*, edited by R. Paoletti, and S. Sherry. Academic, London, 1977, p. 43.
35. Barlow, G. H., Lazer, L., Reuter, A., and Tribby, I.: Production of plasminogen activator by tissue culture techniques, in *Thrombosis and Urokinase*, edited by R. Paoletti and S. Sherry. Academic. London, 1977, p. 75.
36. Marder, V. J., et al.: Changes in the plasma fibrinolytic system during urokinase therapy: Comparison of tissue culture urokinase with urinary source urokinase in patients with pulmonary embolism. *J. Lab. Clin. Med. 92*:721, 1978.

37. Robbins, K. C.: Biochemistry of plasminogen and plasmin, in *Haemostasis: Biochemistry, Physiology, and Pathology*, edited by D. Ogsten and B. Bennett. Wiley, London, 1977, p. 208.

38. Castellino, F. J., and Violand, B. N.: The fibrinolytic system — Basic considerations. *Prog. Cardiovasc. Dis.* 21:241, 1979.

39. Camiolo, S. M., Thorsen, S. and Astrup, T.: Fibrinogenolysis and fibrinolysis with tissue plasminogen activator, urokinase, streptokinase-activated human globulin, and plasmin. *Proc. Soc. Exper. Biol. Med.* 138:277, 1971.

40. Cederholm-Williams, S. A.: The effect of streptokinase on the fibrin binding site of plasmin(ogen). *Thromb. Res.* 21:649, 1981.

41. Smith, R. A. G., Dupe, R. G., English, P. D., and Green, J.: Fibrinolysis with acyl-enzymes: A new approach to thrombolytic therapy. *Nature (London)* 290:505, 1981.

42. Rijken, D. C., and Collen, D.: Purification and characterization of the plasminogen activator secreted by human melanoma cells in culture. *J. Biol. Chem.* 256:7035, 1981.

43. Matsuo, O., Collen, D., and Verstraete, M.: On the fibrinolytic and thrombolytic properties of active-site *p*-anisoylated streptokinase-plasminogen complex (BRL 26921). *Thromb. Res.* 24:347, 1981.

44. Matsuo, O., Rijken, D. C., and Collen, D.: Thrombolysis by human tissue plasminogen activator and urokinase in rabbits with experimental pulmonary embolus. *Nature* 291:590, 1981.

45. Sottrup-Jensen, L., Claeys, H., Zajdel, M., Peterson, T. E., and Magnusson, S.: The primary structure of human plasminogen: Isolation of two lysine-binding fragments and one "mini"-plasminogen (M.W. 38,000) by elastase-catalyzed-specific limited proteolysis, in *Progress in Chemical Fibrinolysis and Thrombolysis*, edited by J. F. Davidson, R. M. Rowan, M. M. Samama, and P. C. Desnoyers. Raven Press, New York, 1978, vol. III, pp. 191–209.

46. Sottrup-Jensen, L., Petersen, T. E., and Magnusson, S.: in *Atlas of Protein Sequence and Structure*, vol. 5, suppl. 3, 1978, p. 91.

47. Rabiner, S. F., Goldfine, I. D., Hart, A., Summaria, L., and Robbins, K. C.: Radioimmunoassay of human plasminogen and plasmin. *J. Lab. Clin. Med.* 74:265, 1969.

48. Markus, G., DePasquale, J. L., and Wissler, F. C.: Quantitative determination of the binding of epsilon-aminocaproic acid to native plasminogen. *J. Biol. Chem.* 253:727, 1978.

49. Wallén, P., and Wiman, B.: Characterization of human plasminogen. I. On the relationship between different molecular forms of plasminogen demonstrated in plasma and found in purified preparations. *Biochim. Biophys. Acta* 221:20, 1970.

50. Rickli, E. E., and Cuendet, P. A.: Isolation of plasmin-free human plasminogen with N-terminal glutamic acid. *Biochim. Biophys. Acta* 250:447, 1971.

51. Wallén, P., and Wiman, B.: Characterization of different molecular forms of human plasminogen. *Biochim. Biophys. Acta* 257:122, 1972.

52. Summaria, L., Arzadon, L., Bernabe, P., Robbins, K. C., and Barlow, G. H.: Characterization of the NH_2-terminal glutamic acid and NH_2 terminal lysine forms of human plasminogen isolated by affinity chromatography and isoelectric focusing methods. *J. Biol. Chem.* 248:2984, 1973.

53. Walther, P. J., Steinmann, H. M., Hill, R. L., and McKee, P. A.: Activation of human plasminogen by urokinase. Partial characterization of a preactivation peptide. *J. Biol. Chem.* 249:1173, 1974.

54. Thorsen, S.: Differences in the binding to fibrin of native plasminogen and plasminogen modified by proteolytic degradation. Influence of omega-amino carboxylic acids. *Biochim. Biophys. Acta* 393:55, 1975.

55. Abiko, Y., Iwamoto, M., and Tomikawa, M.: Plasminogen-plasmin system. V. A stoichiometric equilibrium complex of plasminogen and a synthetic inhibitor. *Biochim. Biophys. Acta* 185:424, 1969.

56. Brockway, W. J., and Castellino, F. J.: The mechanism of the inhibition of plasmin activity by ε-aminocaproic acid. *J. Biol. Chem.* 246:4641, 1971.

57. Christensen, U., and Clemmensen, I.: Kinetic properties of the primary inhibitor of plasmin from human plasma. *Biochem. J.* 163:389, 1977.

58. Wiman, B., and Collen, D.: On the kinetics of the reaction between human antiplasmin and plasmin. *Eur. J. Biochem.* 84:573, 1978.

59. Robbins, K. C., Summaria, L., Hsieh, B., and Shah, R. J.: The pep-

60. Summaria, L., Hsieh, B., and Robbins, K. C.: The specific mechanism of activation of human plasminogen to plasmin. *J. Biol. Chem.* 242:4279, 1967.

61. Christensen, U., Sottrup-Jensen, L., Magnusson, S., Petersen, T. E., and Clemmensen, I.: Enzymic properties of the neo-plasmin-val-442 (miniplasmin). *Biochim. Biophys. Acta* 567:472, 1979.

62. Weinstein, M. J., and Doolittle, R. F.: Differential specificities of thrombin, plasmin, trypsin with regard to synthetic and natural substrates and inhibitors. *Biochim. Biophys. Acta* 258:577, 1972.

63. Summaria, L., Arzadon, L., Bernabe, P., and Robbins, K. C.: The activation of plasminogen to plasmin by urokinase in the presence of the plasmin inhibitor trasylol. The preparation of plasmin with the same NH_2-terminal heavy(A) chain sequence as the parent zymogen. *J. Biol. Chem.* 250:3988, 1975.

64. Violand, B. N., and Castellino, F. J.: Mechanism of the urokinase-catalyzed activation of human plasminogen. *J. Biol. Chem.* 251:3906, 1976.

65. Claeys, H., and Vermylen, J.: Physico-chemical and proenzyme properties of NH_2-terminal glutamic acid and NH_2-terminal lysine human plasminogen. Influence of 6-aminohexanoic acid. *Biochim. Biophys. Acta* 342:351, 1974.

66. Collen, D.: Identification and some properties of a new fast-reacting plasmin inhibitor in human plasma. *Eur. J. Biochem.* 69:209, 1976.

67. Moroi, M., and Aoki, N.: Isolation and characterization of alpha 2-plasmin inhibitor from human plasma. A novel proteinase inhibitor which inhibits activator-induced clot lysis. *J. Biol. Chem.* 251:5956, 1976.

68. Mullertz, S., and Clemmensen, I.: The primary inhibitor of plasmin in human plasma. *Biochem. J.* 159:545, 1976.

69. Wiman, B., and Collen, D.: On the mechanism of the reaction between human α_2-antiplasmin and plasmin. *J. Biol. Chem.* 254:9291, 1979.

70. Harpel, P. C.: Human alpha 2-macroglobulin. *Methods Enzymol.* 45:639, 1976.

71. Wiman, B., and Collen D.: Purification and characterization of human antiplasmin, the fast-acting plasmin inhibitor in plasma. *Eur. J. Biochem.* 78:19, 1977.

72. Gurewich, V., Hyde, E., and Lipinski, B.: The resistance of fibrinogen and soluble fibrin monomer in blood to degradation by a potent plasminogen activator from cadaver limbs. *Blood* 46:555, 1975.

73. Fletcher, A. P., Alkjaersig, N., Sherry, S., Genton, E. Hirsh, J., and Bachmann, F.: The development of urokinase as a thrombolytic agent. Maintenance of a sustained thrombolytic state in man by its intravenous infusion. *J. Lab. Clin. Med.* 65:713, 1965.

74. Verstraete, M., Vermylen, J., Amery, A., and Vermylen, C.: Thrombolytic therapy with streptokinase using a standard dosage scheme. *Br. Med. J.* 1:454, 1966.

75. Cederholm-Williams, S. A., De Cock, F., Lijnen, H. R., and Collen, D.: Kinetics of the reactions between streptokinase, plasmin and α_2-antiplasmin. *Eur. J. Biochem.* 100:125, 1979.

76. Rákóczi, I., Wiman, B., and Collen, D.: On the biologic significance of the specific interaction between fibrin, plasminogen and antiplasmin. *Biochim. Biophys. Acta* 540:295, 1978.

77. Alkjaersig, N., Fletcher, A. P., and Sherry, S.: The mechanism of clot dissolution by plasmin. *J. Clin. Invest.* 38:1086, 1959.

78. Wiman, B., and Collen, D.: Molecular mechanisms of physiological fibrinolysis. *Nature* 272:549, 1978.

79. Sakata, Y., and Aoki, N.: Cross-linking of α_2 plasmin inhibitor to fibrin by fibrin-stabilizing factor. *J. Clin. Invest.* 65:290, 1980.

80. McDonagh, R. P., McDonagh, J., and Duckert, F.: The influence of fibrin cross-linking on the kinetics of urokinase-induced clot lysis. *Br. J. Haematol.* 21:323, 1971.

81. Gaffney, P. J., and Whitaker, A. N.: Fibrin crosslinks and lysis rates. *Thromb. Res.* 14:85, 1979.

82. Francis, C. W., Marder, V. J., and Martin, S. E.: Plasmic degradation of cross-linked fibrin. I. Structural analysis of the particulate clot and identification of new macromolecular soluble complexes. *Blood* 56:456, 1980.

83. Cash, J. D.: Control mechanisms of activator release, in *Progress in Chemical Fibrinolysis and Thrombolysis*, edited by J. F. Davidson, R. M. Rowan, M. M. Samama, and P. C. Desnoyers. Raven Press, New York, 1978, vol. III, pp. 65–75.

84. Nilsson, I. M.: Effect of drugs on activator synthesis and release, in *Progress in Chemical Fibrinolysis and Thrombolysis*, edited by J. F. Davidson, R. M. Rowan, M. M. Samama, and P. C. Desnoyers. Raven Press, New York, 1978, vol. III, pp. 77–89.

85. Koie, E., Kamiya, T., Ogata, K., and Takamatsu, J.: α_2-Plasmin-inhibitor deficiency (Miyasato disease). *Lancet* 2:1334, 1978.

86. Aoki, N., Saito, H., Kamiya, T., Koie, K., Sakata, Y., and Kabakura, M.: Congenital deficiency of α_2-plasmin inhibitor associated with severe hemorrhagic tendency. *J. Clin. Invest.* 63:877, 1979.

87. Collen, D., Semeraro, N., Tricot, J. P., and Vermylen, J.: Turnover of fibrinogen, plasminogen, and prothrombin during exercise in man. *J. Appl. Physiol.* 42:865, 1977.

88. Aoki, N., Moroi, M., Sakata, Y., and Yoshida, N.: Abnormal plasminogen. A hereditary molecular abnormality found in a patient with recurrent thrombosis. *J. Clin. Invest.* 61:1186, 1978.

89. Wohl, R. C., Summaria, L., and Robbins, K. C.: Physiological activation of the human fibrinolytic system. Isolation and characterization of human plasminogen variants, Chicago I and Chicago II. *J. Biol. Chem.* 254:9063, 1979.

90. Nilsson, I. M., Krook, H., Sternby, N. H., Soderberg, E., and Soderstrom, N.: Severe thrombotic disease in a young man with bone marrow and skeletal changes and with a high content of inhibitor in the fibrinolytic system. *Acta Med. Scand.* 169:323, 1961.

91. Naeye, R. L.: Thrombotic disorders with increased levels of antiplasmin and antiplasminogen. *N. Engl. J. Med.* 265:867, 1961.

92. Brakman, P., Mohler, E. R., and Astrup, T.: A group of patients with impaired fibrinolytic system and selective inhibition of tissue activator-induced fibrinolysis. *Scand. J. Haematol.* 3:389, 1966.

93. Naeye, R. L.: Thrombotic state after a hemorrhagic diathesis, a possible complication of therapy with epsilon-aminocaproic acid. *Blood* 19:694, 1962.

94. Stead, N., et al.: Familial thrombosis secondary to diminished vascular plasminogen activator release. *Blood* 58:240a, 1981.

95. Doolittle, R. F.: Fibrinogen and fibrin, in *Haemostasis and Thrombosis*, edited by A. Bloom, and D. P. Thomas. Churchill-Livingston, London, 1981, pp. 163–191.

96. Mihalyi, E., Weinberg, R. M., Towne, D. W., and Friedman, M. E.: Proteolytic fragmentation of fibrinogen. I. Comparison of the fragmentation of human and bovine fibrinogen by trypsin or plasmin. *Biochemistry* 15:5372, 1976.

97. Marder, V. J., and Budzynski, A. Z.: The structure of the fibrinogen degradation products, in *Progress in Hemostasis and Thrombosis*, edited by T. Spaet. Grune Stratton, New York, 1974, pp. 141–174.

98. Gaffney, P. J.: The biochemistry of fibrinogen and fibrin degradation products, in *Haemostasis: Biochemistry, Physiology and Pathology*, edited by D. Ogston and B. Bennett. Wiley, London, 1977, pp. 105–168.

99. Marder, V. J., Francis, C. W., and Doolittle, R. F.: Fibrinogen structure and physiology, in *Hemostasis and Thrombosis: Basic Principles and Clinical Practice*, edited by R. W. Colman, J. Hirsh, V. J. Marder, and E. W. Salzman. Lippincott, Philadelphia, 1982, pp. 145–163.

100. Scheraga, H. A., and Laskowski, M., Jr.: The fibrinogen-fibrin conversion. *Adv. Protein Chem.* 12:1, 1957.

101. Doolittle, R. F.: Structural aspects of the fibrinogen-fibrin conversion. *Adv. Protein Chem.* 27:1, 1973.

102. Shulman, S.: The size and shape of bovine fibrinogen studies of sedimentation, diffusion, and viscosity. *J. Am. Chem. Soc.* 75:5846, 1953.

103. McKee, P. A., Rogers, L. A., Marler, E., and Hill, R. L.: The subunit polypeptides of human fibrinogen. *Arch. Biochem. Biophys.* 116:271, 1966.

104. Bouma, H., III., Takagi, T., and Doolittle, R. F.: The arrangement of disulfide bonds in fragment D from human fibrinogen. *Thromb. Res.* 13:557, 1978.

105. Doolittle, R. F., Goldbaum, D. M., and Doolittle, L. R.: Designation of sequences involved in the "coiled coil" interdomainal connector

106. Doolittle, R. F.: Fibrinogen and fibrin, in *The Plasma Proteins: Structure, Function and Genetic Control*, edited by F. W. Putnam. Academic, New York, 1975, vol. 2, p. 109.

107. Doolittle, R. F., Watt, K. W. K., Cottrell, B. A., Strong, D. D., and Riley, M.: The amino acid sequence of the α-chain of human fibrinogen. *Nature* 280:464, 1979.

108. Mills, D., and Karpatkin, S.: Heterogeneity of human fibrinogen: Possible relation to proteolysis by thrombin and plasmin as studied by SDS-polyacrylamide gel electrophoresis. *Biochem. Biophys. Res. Comm.* 40:206, 1970.

109. Budzynski, A. Z., Marder, V. J., and Shainoff, J. R.: Structure of plasmic degradation products of human fibrinogen. Fibrinopeptide and polypeptide chain analysis. *J. Biol. Chem.* 249:2294, 1974.

110. Marder, V. J., Shulman, N. R., and Carroll, W. R.: The importance of intermediate degradation products of fibrinogen in fibrinolytic hemorrhage. *Trans. Assoc. Am. Phys.* 53:156, 1967.

111. Marder, V. J., Shulman, N. R., and Carroll, W. R.: High molecular weight derivatives of human fibrinogen produced by plasmin. I. Physicochemical and immunological characterization. *J. Biol. Chem.* 244:2111, 1969.

112. Marder, V. J.: Identification and purification of fibrinogen degradation products produced by plasmin. Considerations on the structure of fibrinogen, in *Fibrinogen Degradation Products*, edited by M. Verstraete, J. Vermylen, and M. B. Donati. *Scand. J. Haematol. (Suppl.)* 13:21, 1971.

113. Gärdlund, B., Kowalska-Loth, B., Gröndahl, N. J., and Blombäck, B.: Plasmic degradation products of human fibrinogen. I. Isolation and characterization of Fragments E and D and their relation to "disulfide knots." *Thromb. Res.* 1:371, 1972.

114. Loewy, A. G., Dunathan, K., Kriel, R., and Wolfinger, N. L., Jr.: Fibrinase. I. Purification of substrate and enzyme. *J. Biol. Chem.* 236:2625, 1961.

115. Lorand, L., and Konishi, K.: Activation of the fibrin-stabilizing factor of plasma by thrombin. *Arch. Biochem.* 105:58, 1964.

116. Pisano, J. J., Finlayson, J. S., and Peyton, M. P.: Cross-link fibrin polymerized by Factor XIII: ϵ-(γ-glutamyl) lysine. *Science* 160:892, 1968.

117. Laudano, A. P., and Doolittle, R. F.: Studies on synthetic peptides that bind to fibrinogen and prevent fibrin polymerization. Structural requirements, number of binding sites, and species differences. *Biochemistry* 19:1013, 1980.

118. Olexa, S. A., and Budzynski, A. Z.: Evidence for four different polymerization sites involved in human fibrin formation. *Proc. Natl. Acad. Sci. U.S.A.* 77:1374, 1980.

119. Kudryk, B. J., Collen, D., Woods, K. R., and Blombäck, B.: Evidence for localization of polymerization sites in fibrinogen. *J. Biol. Chem.* 249:3322, 1974.

120. Blombäck, B., and Yamashina, I.: On the N-terminal amino acids in fibrinogen and fibrin. *Arkiv Kemi* 12:299, 1958.

121. Lorand, L.: Fibrinopeptide. New aspects of the fibrinogen-fibrin transformation. *Nature* 167:992, 1951.

122. Krakow, W., Endres, G. F., Siegel, B. M., and Scheraga, H. A.: An electron investigation of the polymerization of bovine fibrin monomer. *J. Mol. Microsc. Biol.* 71:95, 1972.

123. Hermans, J., and McDonagh, J.: Fibrin: Structure and interactions. *Semin. Thromb. Haemost.* 8:11, 1982.

124. Ferry, J. D.: The mechanism of polymerization of fibrin. *Proc. Natl. Acad. Sci. U.S.A.* 38:566, 1952.

125. Hermans, J.: Models of fibrin. *Proc. Natl. Acad. Sci. U.S.A.* 76:1189, 1979.

126. Chen, R., and Doolittle, R. F.: γ-γ Cross-linking sites in human and bovine fibrin. *Biochemistry* 10:4486, 1971.

127. Schwartz, M. L., Pizzo, S. V., Hill, R. L., and McKee, P. A.: The effect of fibrin-stabilizing factor on the subunit structure of human fibrin. *J. Clin. Invest.* 50:1506, 1971.

128. Francis, C. W., Marder, V. J., and Barlow, G. H.: Plasmic degradation of crosslinked fibrin. Characterization of new macromolecular soluble complexes and a model of their structure. *J. Clin. Invest.* 66:1033, 1980.

129. Francis, C. W., and Marder, V. J.: A molecular model of plasmic degradation of crosslinked fibrin. *Semin. Thromb. Haemost. 8:*25, 1982.

130. Kopec, M., Teisseyre, E., Dudek-Wojciechowska, G. Kloczewiak, M., Pankiewicz, A., and Latallo, Z. S.: Studies on the "Double D" fragment from stabilized bovine fibrin. *Thromb. Res. 2:*283, 1973.

131. Gaffney, P. J., and Brashner, M.: Subunit structure of the plasmin-induced degradation products of cross-linked fibrin. *Biochim. Biophys. Acta 295:*308, 1973.

132. Pizzo, S. V., Taylor, L. M., Jr., Schwartz, M. L., Hill, R. L., and McKee, P. A.: Subunit structure of Fragment D from fibrinogen and cross-linked fibrin. *J. Biol. Chem. 248:*4584, 1973.

133. Hudry-Clergeon, G., Paturel, L., and Suscillon, M.: Identification d'un complexe (D-D) . . . E dans les produits de degradation de la fibrine bovine stabilisée par la Facteur XIII. *Pathol. Biol. (Suppl.) 22:*47, 1974.

134. Gaffney, P. J., Lane, D. A., Kakkar, V. V., and Brasher, M.: Characterisation of a soluble D dimer-E complex in crosslinked fibrin digests. *Thromb. Res. 7:*89, 1975.

135. Wilner, G. D.: Molecular basis for measurement of circulating fibrinogen derivatives, in *Progress in Hemostasis and Thrombosis,* edited by T. Spaet. Grune & Stratton, New York 1978, vol. 4, pp. 211–248.

136. Marder, V. J., Matchett, M. O., and Sherry, S.: Detection of serum fibrinogen and fibrin degradation products. Comparison of six technics using purified products and application in clinical studies. *Am. J. Med. 51:*71, 1971.

137. Breen, F. A., Jr., and Tullis, J. L.: Ethanol gelation: A rapid screening test for intravascular coagulation. *Ann. Intern. Med. 69:*1197, 1968.

138. Niewiarowski, S., and Gurewich, V.: Laboratory identification of intravascular coagulation. The serial dilution protamine sulfate test for the detection of fibrin monomer and fibrin degradation products. *J. Lab. Clin. Med. 77:*665, 1971.

139. Fletcher, A. P., Alkjaersig, N., O'Brien, J., and Tulevski, V. G.: Blood hypercoagulability and thrombosis. *Trans. Assoc. Am. Phys. 83:*159, 1970.

140. Merskey, C., Lalezari, P., and Johnson, A. J.: A rapid, simple sensitive method for measuring fibrinolytic split products in human serum. *Proc. Soc. Exp. Biol. Med. 131:*871, 1969.

141. Ferreira, H. C., and Murat, L. G.: An immunological method for demonstrating fibrin degradation products in serum and its use in the diagnosis of fibrinolytic states. *Br. J. Haematol. 9:*299, 1963.

142. Marder, V. J., Cruz, G. O., and Schumer, B. R.: Evaluation of a new antifibrinogen-coated latex particle agglutination test in the measurement of serum fibrin degradation products. *Thromb. Haemost. 37:*183, 1977.

143. Marder, V. J., and Budzynski, A. Z.: Degradation products of fibrinogen and crosslinked fibrin. Projected clinical applications. *Thromb. Diath. Haemorrh. 32:*49, 1974.

The role of blood vessels in hemostasis

CHAPTER *139*

Vascular function in hemostasis

ERIC A. JAFFE

Blood vessels form a nonleaking closed circuit which also maintains blood in a fluid state. When a leak does occur, platelets and the coagulation system temporarily close the defect until the cells in the vessel wall permanently repair the leak. If blocked by a thrombus, blood vessels can usually reestablish blood flow by lysing the thrombus. The purpose of this chapter is to discuss the physiological and biochemical mechanisms which give the vasculature these three properties. The participation of the vessel wall in the pathogenesis of thrombosis is discussed in Chap. 160.

The vasculature as a conduit

BLOOD VESSELS AS NONLEAKING CLOSED CIRCUITS
Blood vessels are lined with confluent monolayers of endothelial cells which rest on the subendothelium, an underlying extracellular matrix secreted by the cells. Since each endothelial cell is linked to its adjacent neighbors by continuous and well-organized tight junctions varying in width from 0 to 4 nm [1–4], the endothelial monolayer forms a selectively impermeable membrane which resists the passive transfer of the fluid and cellular phases of blood. While the endothelial monolayer is relatively permeable to gases, the net transendothelial flow of fluid is limited to about 2.5 liters per day, only 0.03 percent of the 7200 liters per day that flows through the vasculature despite the fact that the surface area of the vascular bed is greater than 1000 m² [5]. Transendothelial flow proceeds either by passage of fluid-filled intracellular vesicles from the luminal to abluminal surface of the endothelial cell (endocytosis) [6,7] or by passage between cells [2,8,9]. The normal vessel wall is impermeable to the passive transfer of blood cells since platelets, with a diameter of 2 μm, are far too large to pass through a tight junction. Cells which do migrate through the endothelial monolayer, such as polymorphonuclear leukocytes,

monocytes, and lymphocytes, do so by active processes. Polymorphonuclear leukocytes and monocytes, which adhere to endothelial cells [10–13], probably follow gradients of chemoattractants [14] and migrate out of the circulation by passing between endothelial cells [15,16]. In contrast, lymphocytes migrate out of the circulation mainly in lymph nodes and Peyer's patches by adhering to and then migrating between specialized endothelial cells that are localized to blood vessels in these areas called *high endothelial venules* [17–22].

The subendothelium, which is secreted by the endothelial cell and contains types IV and V (AB₂) collagen [23–27], mucopolysaccharides [28–31], fibronectin [32–36], elastin [25,37,38], microfibrils [25,39,40], and laminin [41–44], anchors endothelial cells to the blood vessel wall. In the absence of endothelial cells, the subendothelium acts as a secondary barrier against the leakage of blood. Endothelial cells and subendothelial extracellular matrix make up the intima. In large vessels, the intima is surrounded by the media, which contains layers of smooth-muscle cells and their extracellular matrix. External to the media is the adventitia, composed mainly of fibroblasts and their extracellular matrix. Both the media and adventitia provide additional mechanical strength and act as barriers against blood loss. Smooth-muscle cells in the media enable blood vessels to constrict or dilate.

NONTHROMBOTIC PROPERTIES
Multiple biochemical mechanisms interact to keep blood fluid and to prevent inappropriate activation of platelets or coagulation proteins.

BLOOD FLOW
The rate of blood flow through a vessel markedly influences the state of activation of platelets and procoagulant factors contained within. During each passage through the capillary bed platelets are exposed to locally high concentrations of prostacyclin and are partially inactivated (see below under "Prostacyclin"). Similarly, the small amounts of activated coagulation factors that form in the circulation are inactivated either by antithrombin III in the presence of its physiological activator, endothelial cell surface mucopolysaccharide (see below under "Antithrombin III"), by activated protein C (see under "Protein C"), or by other circulating protease inhibitors such as α_2-macroglobulin. The first two of these processes occur most effectively in the capillary bed due to its very high endothelial surface/blood volume ratio. Thus low flow or stasis allows the progressive, localized, and unopposed accumulation of activated coagulation factors and platelets which can then lead to thrombosis. As long as thrombosis has not occurred, resumption of flow rapidly disperses the platelets and activated coagulation factors into the circulation, where they are inactivated. While increasing blood flow also increases the delivery of procoagulants, especially platelets, to a site of injury [45], the dispersive effects of blood flow seem much more important since venous thrombosis usually occurs in areas of low flow.

Endothelial cells possess multiple enzyme systems which enable them to influence blood flow, blood pressure, and vascular tone. The cells contain angiotensin-converting enzyme, which converts vasoinactive angiotensin I to the vasoconstrictor angiotensin II and inactivates the vasodilator bradykinin [46–50] and angiotensinases A and C, which inactivate angiotensin II [49,51]. Endothelial cells produce two vasodilators, prostacyclin and adenosine. Endothelial cells inactivate norepinephrine, serotonin, and histamine [52–54].

ANTIPLATELET PROPERTIES

Intrinsic nonthrombogenic properties Unstimulated platelets do not adhere to intact confluent monolayers of endothelial cells in vivo [55–57] and only minimally to intact monolayers in vitro [58–61]. In vitro, platelets that appear to adhere to endothelial cells actually adhere to exposed subendothelium and not to the cells themselves [58]. This nonthrombogenic property seems to be intrinsic to the endothelial cell plasma membrane. It is unrelated to prostacyclin since inhibition of endothelial prostacyclin production does not increase the adhesion of unstimulated platelets [57,59–61]. Prostacyclin does not block the adhesion of unstimulated platelets to fibroblasts or transformed endothelial cells [60–62]. In contrast, the lack of adhesion of stimulated platelets to endothelial cells is highly prostacyclin-dependent [59,61,62].

Prostacyclin Endothelial cells synthesize prostacyclin (PGI_2), a potent vasodilator and inhibitor of platelet function [63–66], from the essential fatty acid arachidonic acid and secrete it into the adjacent fluid [62, 67–70]. Prostacyclin at low nanomolar concentrations binds to a specific receptor on platelet membranes [71,72] and stimulates adenylate cyclase [73–75]. The resulting elevation in intraplatelet cyclic AMP [73–75] inhibits platelet shape change [76], platelet secretion [67], platelet aggregation [63–65], the binding of factor VIII–von Willebrand factor [77] and fibrinogen [78] to specific receptors on the platelet surface membrane, and the development of platelet procoagulant activity [76,79,80]. Higher doses of prostacyclin are required to inhibit platelet adhesion to the subendothelium [81,82]. The inhibition of platelet adhesion by prostacyclin is greatest at high shear rates [81]. Since both shear rates and prostacyclin concentration are highest in the microvasculature [83,84], this may be one of the reasons why the microvasculature is relatively resistant to thrombosis. Prostacyclin has a short half-life (~ 6 min) in whole blood [276] and is not stored by endothelial cells but is synthesized and secreted when the cells are stimulated. Prostacyclin synthesis is markedly stimulated by thrombin and trypsin [62,85,86], histamine [87,277], bradykinin [86,88–90], angiotensin II [90], high-density lipoproteins [91], calcitonin [92], ATP, ADP, and AMP [93], hypoxia [94,95], and platelet-derived growth factor [96]. Synthesis of prostacyclin by endothelial cells is blocked by aspirin [62,84,97,98] and a variety of non-steroidal antiinflammatory agents such as indomethacin

[67,85]; both groups of agents inhibit the enzyme cyclooxygenase. Nicotine also inhibits the release of prostacyclin [99], as does enriching endothelial cells with linoleic acid, the predominant fatty acid in diets high in polyunsaturated fat [100,101].

Under ordinary conditions, the local prostacyclin level in the capillary bed is probably just high enough to mildly inhibit platelet function. When capillary blood is diluted in the general circulation (1:10), the prostacyclin levels become too low to affect platelet function [102–106]. Thus, nonthrombogenicity with respect to platelets is probably a function both of mild platelet inhibition by low levels of prostacyclin in the capillary bed and the innate nonthrombogenicity of the endothelial cell membrane. In contrast, when platelets are activated in areas of stasis or injury in vivo (perhaps due to the generation of low levels of thrombin), both thrombin and components released from platelet granules (such as platelet-derived growth factor) may greatly stimulate local endothelial prostacyclin production, which then locally inhibits platelet function and causes vasodilation [107]. In this situation treatment with aspirin, which blocks prostacyclin synthesis, enhances platelet accumulation at the site of blood vessel wall injury if blood flow is also reduced [57,108]. Prostacyclin also appears to play an important role in compensatory vasodilation [94,95,109,110].

Endothelial cells can also convert prostaglandin endoperoxides secreted by platelets into prostacyclin [68,111]; this mechanism is probably most important in the microvasculature where the endothelial cell/platelet ratio is ≥ 1:1.

Both 6-keto-$PGF_{1\alpha}$, the stable but inactive end product of prostacyclin, and prostacyclin itself can be converted to 6-keto-PGE_1, a stable and active vasodilator and inhibitor of platelet function [112–119]. While measurable levels of 6-keto-PGE_1 are found in normal plasma [120], it is unclear what role, if any, 6-keto-PGE_1 plays in normal human blood vessel wall physiology.

Smooth-muscle cells can also synthesize prostacyclin and are markedly stimulated to do so by platelet-derived growth factor [96] and serotonin [121], singly or in combination [121]. Thus, the pseudointima formed by migration of smooth-muscle cells from the media to an area of denuded endothelium may also be able to release prostacyclin and inhibit platelet function and cause vasodilation [122].

Adenine nucleotides Aggregating platelets release ADP, which recruits nearby platelets into the developing platelet plug and ATP, a vasodilator [123]. Endothelial cells can modulate the effects of the released ADP and ATP because they possess ectoenzymes which rapidly metabolize ADP and ATP to AMP and adenosine, a strong inhibitor of platelet function [124–127]. Endothelial cells can take up exogenous adenosine [128] and convert it to ATP [128]. Endothelial cells can also release ATP [129]. Adenosine is a vasodilator, and is considered to be a local hormone which can regulate blood flow [130].

Serotonin Aggregating platelets also release serotonin from their dense granules [131]. Serotonin is a vasoconstrictor in most vascular beds [132] and by itself is a weak platelet-aggregating agent [131,133] but a potent stimulator of smooth-muscle cell prostacyclin production [121]. Serotonin markedly potentiates the aggregating activity of low doses of other platelet active agents [131] and also markedly potentiates the prostacyclin-stimulating activity of platelet-derived growth factor on smooth-muscle cells [121]. In vivo, pulmonary capillary endothelial cells rapidly remove serotonin from the circulation [134,135] and convert it to vasoinactive products [136–138].

ANTICOAGULANT PROPERTIES

Antithrombin III In vivo, antithrombin III in plasma inactivates thrombin in less than 30 s, forming a covalent thrombin–antithrombin III complex which circulates in plasma until cleared by the liver [139]. The inactivation process is accelerated by heparin or heparan sulfate [140–142] or by endothelial cells [143]. The acceleratory effect of endothelial cells is probably due to heparan sulfate on the cell membrane [28,29, 139,143,144]. Endothelial surface membranes may also support the ability of antithrombin III to inactivate activated factors IX, X, and XII.

During aggregation, platelets release both an endoglycosidase that degrades endothelial cell surface heparan sulfate [144,145] and platelet factor 4, which binds to endothelial cells [146] and blocks the ability of endothelial cells to accelerate the inactivation of thrombin by antithrombin III [143]. Exogenous heparin also binds to endothelial cells [147,148], and appears to promote the inactivation of thrombin by antithrombin III [278]. Antithrombin III is physiologically important since recurrent thrombosis occurs in patients with inherited deficiencies of this protein [149,150].

Protein C Protein C is a vitamin K–dependent protease which circulates in plasma as a zymogen and is rapidly activated in vivo by thrombin [151–155,279]. Activated protein C proteolytically inactivates factors V and VIII and is therefore a powerful anticoagulant [151–155,280]. Endothelial cells markedly accelerate the activation of protein C by thrombin [156,281]. Unlike the antithrombin III–endothelial cell interaction, the acceleration of protein C activation by endothelial cells is not blocked by platelet factor 4 [156]. The activity of protein C is further enhanced by another vitaminK–dependent protein, protein S, which binds protein C to phospholipid [157]. Protein C must play an important role in vivo because heterozygous deficiency of protein C is associated with congenital thrombotic disease [158] and deficiency of an inhibitor of protein C causes combined factor V–factor VIII deficiency [159].

Protease nexin Endothelial cells secrete protease nexin, a protein of M_r 40,000 daltons which inactivates thrombin by forming a covalent complex at its active site [160–165]. The thrombin-protease nexin complex then binds to the endothelial cell, is internalized, and is degraded by lyzosomal enzymes [160,163]. Protease nexin appears to be unrelated to antithrombin III [161,164]. Low doses of thrombin (i.e., 1 to 4 μg/ml) markedly increase protease nexin secretion by endothelial cells [160]. In tissue culture, binding of thrombin–protease nexin complexes to endothelial cells is inversely related to cell density [162]. Mechanically removing part of a monolayer of cultured endothelial cells increases the amount of thrombin–protease nexin complexes that bind per cell [162]. Protease nexin also binds and inactivates trypsin, urokinase, and plasmin [162–164]. Since almost all the thrombin injected into animals rapidly complexes with antithrombin III [139], the role of protease nexin in inhibiting thrombin in vivo is unclear.

Platelets when activated by thrombin or collagen also secrete protease nexin [166]; this may serve to inhibit further platelet activation and/or activation of the coagulation system.

Self-sealing properties of the vasculature

Injuries to blood vessels elicit graded platelet and coagulation system responses which correlate with the degree of injury and tend either to cover the injured area or to seal the leak in the vessel without obstructing the vessel itself. Several mechanisms are involved.

COMPONENTS ACTIVE IN PLATELET AGGREGATION

SUBENDOTHELIUM
Unstimulated platelets do not adhere to intact monolayers of endothelial cells. However, removal or contraction of endothelial cells by injury exposes the subendothelium, which rapidly becomes lined with a monolayer of platelets which subsequently degranulate [55,167]. Subendothelial collagen types IV and V (AB$_2$) and microfibrils cause platelet aggregation and thromboxane A$_2$ release [168–171], whereas laminin [170], elastin [55], and a heparan sulfate proteoglycan [170] do not. Collagen types I and III are found in the media (along with types IV and V), adventitia, and surrounding connective tissue, but not in the subendothelium [23]. Collagen types I and III also induce platelet aggregation and thromboxane A$_2$ release and are, in fact, more potent than types IV and V collagen [169,170,172]. This may partially explain why injuries which penetrate the subendothelium cause a greater hemostatic response [173] than those which do not.

Fibronectin is present in both vascular basement membrane [36,43] and platelet α granules [174–176]. Fibronectin is released from α granules by thrombin treatment [175,176] and then rapidly binds to platelet membrane receptors which are present only after exposure of platelets to thrombin [177]. While fibronectin supports platelet spreading [178,179], its role in other platelet functions remains controversial [177].

FACTOR VIII–VON WILLEBRAND FACTOR

Adhesion of platelets to the subendothelium is dependent on the presence of factor VIII–von Willebrand factor (FVIII/vWF) [180–185]. Endothelial cells synthesize and release FVIII/vWF [186–188], which binds in vitro to collagen types I, II, III, IV, and V [189–193] and human arterial subendothelium [184,185] and is found in vivo in the subendothelium [194]. Since platelets contain a surface receptor for FVIII/vWF [77,195–197], it is likely that platelets adhere to collagen in the subendothelium via FVIII/vWF. This concept is consistent with findings that platelet adhesion to the subendothelium is decreased in von Willebrand disease [180,181] and is corrected by exogenous FVIII/vWF [181] and that antisera to FVIII/vWF block platelet adhesion to the subendothelium [181] and platelet aggregation induced by type III collagen [198]. Platelet aggregation induced by microfibrils is also FVIII/vWF–dependent [171]. The interaction of platelets in flowing blood with the subendothelium is enhanced by increased blood flow [181,183], and whole blood yields greater numbers of adherent platelets than platelet-rich plasma, an effect ascribed to the physical presence of the red cells [199].

COMPONENTS ACTIVE IN COAGULATION

TISSUE FACTOR

Tissue factor reacts with factor VII and calcium and markedly accelerates the ability of factor VII to activate factor X (see Chap. 132). Intact endothelial cells, smooth-muscle cells, and fibroblasts possess little or no tissue factor activity [200]. However, when smooth-muscle cells and fibroblasts are mechanically disrupted and treated with low concentrations of trypsin, their tissue factor activity is markedly increased, whereas that of endothelial cells is enhanced to only 2 to 3 percent of the level seen in smooth-muscle cells or fibroblasts [200]. Exposure of smooth-muscle cells and fibroblasts to platelets also increases their tissue factor activity, whereas endothelial cells are not affected [201]. This suggests that relatively superficial injuries involving only endothelial cells cause either no or only minimal rises in local tissue factor activity. In contrast, deeper injuries involving smooth-muscle cells and fibroblasts in the media, adventitia, or connective tissue probably cause marked rises in local tissue factor activity and thus initiate fluid phase coagulation in a locale beyond the anticoagulant "reach" of endothelial cells. This may partially explain the time-dependent formation of fibrin in hemostatic plugs [173].

HAGEMAN FACTOR (FACTOR XII) ACTIVATOR

Hageman factor (factor XII) circulates in plasma as a single-chain proenzyme which is converted by limited proteolytic cleavage into an active two-chain molecule [202]. Activated Hageman factor (factor XIIa) can activate factors XI and VII and thus initiate coagulation via both the extrinsic and intrinsic pathways [203–208].

Activated Hageman factor (factor XIIa) also may convert prekallikrein to kallikrein leading to plasmin formation [209,210], bradykinin release [211], and activation of the renin-angiotensin [212] and complement systems [213,214]. Homogenates of endothelial cells can activate Hageman factor (factor XII) [215], and activated Hageman factor (factor XIIa), in turn, can activate prekallikrein, high-molecular-weight kininogen, and factor XI. The activator of Hageman factor (factor XII) is a serine protease and is present in the microsomal fraction of endothelial cells [215]. Hageman factor is also activated by a combination of collagen and some other unidentified basement membrane component(s) [216,217]. It is likely that these systems, like the tissue factor system, are activated when endothelial cells are physically disrupted.

VASOCONSTRICTION

Although vasoconstriction alone appears to be inadequate to cause hemostasis without the participation of platelets and the coagulation system, local vasoconstriction contributes to hemostasis in small blood vessels [218]. Vasoconstriction is probably mediated by several systems including the α-adrenergic system and thromboxane A_2 and serotonin secreted by activated platelets.

Maintenance of the integrity of the vessel lumen and vessel wall

FIBRINOLYSIS

During normal hemostasis or the development of a thrombus, endothelial cells may become covered with localized deposits of fibrin. Endothelial cells contain plasminogen activator and therefore can initiate the catabolism of this fibrin [219–224]. Plasminogen activator exists in two forms; the urokinase type activates plasminogen in the fluid phase, whereas the tissue type is active only when bound to fibrin [225–227]. In vivo, endothelial cells apparently make only tissue plasminogen activator [228,229] while in tissue culture both types are made [224,230–232,282]. Endothelial cells also secrete a protein that inhibits urokinase type activators but not tissue-type activators [221,222,230,233]. In tissue cultures with low cell densities endothelial cells secrete small amounts of plasminogen activator and high amounts of plasminogen activator inhibitor, whereas at confluency the secretion of plasminogen activator rises and the inhibitor activity falls [222]. Thrombin and serum both cause a rapid and profound decrease in the secretion of plasminogen activator by the cells [234,235]. Activated protein C, on the other hand, stimulates the generation of fibrinolytic activity probably by stimulating release of endothelial cell plasminogen activator [236,279]. These findings suggest that local conditions can influence the activity of the fibrinolytic system. In turn, the products of the fibrinolytic system affect vascular function since plasmin digestion of fibrinogen produces low-molecular-weight peptides that increase vascular permeability and directly damage endothelial cells [237–239].

REPAIR OF THE VESSEL WALL

Minor injuries to endothelial monolayers heal by migration of adjacent endothelial cells into the wound with subsequent spreading followed by endothelial proliferation which replaces the denuded cells [240–243]. Deeper, penetrating injuries to the vessel wall require migration and proliferation of smooth-muscle cells of the media and fibroblasts of the adventitia. Both cell types are motile and synthesize connective tissue components and secrete elastase and collagenase [23,244–250] and thus have the ability to remodel the components of the vessel wall. Smooth-muscle cells and fibroblasts (but not endothelial cells) have surface-specific receptors for platelet-derived growth factors and proliferate markedly in response to this substance [251–256]. In addition, platelet-derived growth factor is chemotactic for smooth-muscle cells [257]. Thus, exposure to platelets due to vessel wall injury stimulates smooth-muscle cell and fibroblast growth and migration.

ROLE OF PLATELETS IN VESSEL WALL INTEGRITY

Carbon particles [258,259], red cells [259–260], and Thorotrast [259,260] all readily cross the capillary wall into the extravascular space in thrombocytopenic animals but not in normal animals. The ultrastructural and functional changes that develop in the vascular endothelium of thrombocytopenic animals and cause these abnormalities are promptly reversed by elevation of the platelet count [260,261]. Increased capillary resistance after platelet transfusions in thrombocytopenic subjects can be demonstrated in vivo [262]. The vascular integrity of organs perfused in vitro can be better maintained by platelet-rich plasma than by platelet-poor plasma [263]. The molecular basis for these observations is unclear. While intact platelets stimulate the growth of endothelial cells and enhance endothelial integrity [259–264], purified platelet-derived growth factor by itself (see above) does not stimulate endothelial cell proliferation [255,256].

Vascular integrity is influenced by factors other than platelets. Thus, glucocorticoids increase capillary resistance and abate bleeding even when the platelet count does not increase [265,266]. These findings are consistent with the observation that prednisone reverses the endothelial thinning seen in thrombocytopenia [267] and that glucocorticoids cause individual endothelial cells in culture to enlarge 50 percent and also enhance their ability to cover the surface of culture vessels [268]. In nonthrombocytopenic animals, capillary resistance is diminished by stress such as surgery [269] and appears to be influenced by both pituitary and adrenal hormones [270].

Vitamin C deficiency is characterized by petechial bleeding, and in experimental animals made deficient in vitamin C there is breakdown and degeneration of the connective tissue within vessel walls and in the perivascular areas [271]. These observations may be due to defects in basement membrane collagen synthesis since vitamin C is a required cofactor for the lysyl and prolyl hydroxylases involved in collagen synthesis [244], and platelet function is normal in scurvy and experimental vitamin C deficiency [283].

Clinical evaluation of vascular function

The bleeding time (see Chap. A40) is a measure of overall hemostatic function and therefore does not permit evaluation of vascular function. The capillary fragility test has been utilized for this purpose. The test may be performed by applying "negative" pressure to the skin with a suction cup (negative-pressure method) or by increasing intracapillary pressure by occluding venous outflow from the arm (positive-pressure method, Rumpel-Leede test). In the negative-pressure method the least negative pressure maintained for 1 min which elicits one or more petechiae is considered to be the capillary resistance [272]. In one version of the positive-pressure method a blood pressure cuff inflated to a pressure halfway between the systolic and diastolic blood pressure is maintained on the arm of the subject for 5 min. The number of petechiae appearing in a measured area distal to the blood pressure cuff is used to evaluate the capillary fragility. Normally less than five petechiae are encountered in a circle 3 cm in diameter on the volar surface of the forearm [272]. Others prefer to select arbitrarily a fixed pressure which produces few petechiae in normal persons but induces increased numbers of petechiae in individuals with increased capillary fragility. Thus, one may employ a cuff pressure of 80 mmHg for 5 min [273]. The entire arm is examined, and if numerous petechiae appear, the test is considered to be positive. Microscopic observation of the skin vessels during performance of the capillary fragility test has demonstrated that the petechiae result from bleeding at the arteriolar end of the capillary loop [274].

The capillary fragility test is of doubtful value in the clinical evaluation of a patient with a bleeding disorder. At least 8 percent of normal persons have increased capillary fragility [275], and many with significant thrombocytopenias have normal capillary fragility.

References

1. Reese, T. S., and Karnovsky, M. J.: Fine structural localization of a blood-brain barrier to exogenous peroxidase. *J. Cell Biol.* 34:207, 1967.
2. Karnovsky, M. J.: The ultrastructural basis of capillary permeability studied with peroxidase as a tracer. *J. Cell Biol.* 35:213, 1967.
3. Simionescu, M., Simionescu, N., and Palade, G. E.: Segmental dif-

ferentiations of cell junctions in the vascular endothelium: The microvasculature. *J. Cell Biol.* 67:863, 1975.

4. Simionescu, M., Simionescu, N., and Palade, G. E.: Segmental differentiation of cell junctions in the vascular endothelium: Arteries and veins. *J. Cell Biol.* 68:705, 1976.

5. Falkow, B., and Neil, E.: *Circulation.* Oxford University Press, New York, 1971, p. 38.

6. Bruns, R. R., and Palade, G. E.: Studies on blood capillaries. II. Transport of ferritin molecules across the wall of muscle capillaries. *J. Cell Biol.* 37:277, 1968.

7. Bundgaard, M., Frokjaer-Jensen, J., and Crone, C.: Endothelial plasmalemmal vesicles as elements in a system of branching invaginations from the cell surface. *Proc. Natl. Acad. Sci. U.S.A.* 76:6439, 1979.

8. Huttner, I., Boutet, M., and More, R. H.: Studies on protein passage through arterial endothelium. I. Structural correlates of permeability in rat arterial endothelial cells. *Lab. Invest.* 28:672, 1973.

9. Huttner, I., Boutet, M., and More, R. H.: Studies on protein passage through arterial endothelium. II. Regional differences in permeability to fine structural protein tracers in arterial endothelium of normotensive rat. *Lab. Invest.* 28:678, 1973.

10. Lackie, J. M., and DeBono, D.: Interactions of neutrophil granulocytes (PMNs) and endothelium in vitro. *Microvasc. Res.* 13:107, 1977.

11. MacGregor, R. R., Macarak, E. J., and Kefalides, N. A.: Comparative adherence of granulocytes to endothelial monolayers and nylon fiber. *J. Clin. Invest.* 61:697, 1978.

12. Pearson, J. D., Carleton, J. S., Beesley, J. E., Hutchings, A., and Gordon, J. L.: Granulocyte adhesion to endothelium in culture. *J. Cell Sci.* 38:225, 1979.

13. Hoover, R. L., Folger, R., Haering, W. A., Ware, B. R., and Karnovsky, M. J.: Adhesion of leukocytes to endothelium: Roles of divalent cations, surface charge, chemotactic agents, and substrate. *J. Cell Sci.* 45:73, 1980.

14. Snyderman, R., and Goetzl, E. J.: Molecular and cellular mechanisms of leukocyte chemotaxis. *Science* 213:830, 1981.

15. Schoefl, G. I.: The migration of lymphocytes across the vascular endothelium in lymphoid tissue: A reexamination. *J. Exp. Med.* 136:568, 1972.

16. Beesley, J. E., Pearson, J. D., Hutchings, A., Carleton, J. S., and Gordon, J. L.: Granulocyte migration through endothelium in culture. *J. Cell Sci.* 38:237, 1979.

17. Gowans, J. L., and Knight, E. J.: The route of recirculation of lymphocytes in the rat. *Proc. R. Soc. Ser. B* 159:257, 1964.

18. Kuttner, B. J., and Woodruff, J. J.: Adherence of recirculating T and B lymphocytes to high endothelium of lymph nodes in vitro. *J. Immunol.* 123:1421, 1979.

19. Anderson, N. D., Anderson, A. O., and Wyllie, R. G.: Specialized structure and metabolic activities of high endothelial venules in rat lymphatic tissues. *Immunology* 31:455, 1976.

20. Anderson, A. O., and Anderson, N. D.: Lymphocyte emigration from high endothelial venules in rat lymph nodes. *Immunology* 31:731, 1976.

21. Stamper, H. B., and Woodruff, J. J.: Lymphocyte homing into lymph nodes: In vitro demonstration of the selective affinity of recirculating lymphocytes for high-endothelial venules. *J. Exp. Med.* 144:828, 1976.

22. Butcher, E. C., Scollay, R. G., and Weissman, I. L.: Organ specificity of lymphocyte migration: Mediation by highly selective lymphocyte interaction with organ-specific determinants on high endothelial venules. *Eur. J. Immunol.* 10:556, 1980.

23. Madri, J. A., Dreyer, B., Pitlick, F. A., and Furthmayr, H.: The collagenous components of the subendothelium: Correlation of structure and function. *Lab. Invest.* 43:303, 1980.

24. Howard, B. V., Macarak, E. J., Gunson, D., and Kefalides, N. A.: Characterization of the collagen synthesized by endothelial cells in culture. *Proc. Acad. Natl. Sci. U.S.A.* 73:2361, 1976.

25. Jaffe, E. A., Minick, C. R., Adelman, B., Becker, C. G., and Nachman, R.: Synthesis of basement membrane collagen by cultured human endothelial cells. *J. Exp. Med.* 144:209, 1976.

26. Sage, H., Pritzl, P., and Bornstein, P.: Characterization of cell matrix associated collagens synthesized by aortic endothelial cells in culture. *Biochemistry* 20:436, 1981.

27. Sage, H., Crouch, E., and Bornstein, P.: Collagen synthesis by bovine aortic endothelial cells in culture. *Biochemistry* 18:5433, 1979.

28. Buonassisi, V.: Sulfated mucopolysaccharide synthesis and secretion in endothelial cell cultures. *Exp. Cell Res.* 76:363, 1973.

29. Buonassisi, V., and Root, M.: Enzymatic degradation of heparin-related mucopolysaccharides from surface of endothelial cell cultures. *Biochim. Biophys. Acta* 385:1, 1975.

30. Sampson, P., Parshley, M. S., Mandl, I., and Turino, G. M.: Glycosaminoglycans produced in tissue culture by rat lung cells: Isolation from a mixed cell line and a derived endothelial clone. *Connect. Tissue Res.* 4:41, 1975.

31. Kanwar, Y. S., and Farquhar, M. G.: Isolation of glycosaminoglycans (heparan sulfate) from glomerular basement membranes. *Proc. Natl. Acad. Sci. U.S.A.* 76:4493, 1979.

32. Jaffe, E. A., and Mosher, D. F.: Synthesis of fibronectin by cultured human endothelial cells. *J. Exp. Med.* 147:1779, 1978.

33. Macarak, E. J., Kirby, E., Kirk, T., and Kefalides, N. A.: Synthesis of cold-insoluble globulin by cultured calf endothelial cells. *Proc. Natl. Acad. Sci. U.S.A.* 75:2621, 1978.

34. Birdwell, C. R., Gospodarowicz, D., and Nicolson, G. L.: Identification, localization, and role of fibronectin in cultured bovine endothelial cells. *Proc. Natl. Acad. Sci. U.S.A.* 75:3273, 1978.

35. Linder, E., Vaheri, A., Ruoslahti, E., and Wartiovaara, J.: Distribution of fibroblast surface antigen in the developing chick embryo. *J. Exp. Med.* 142:41, 1975.

36. Stenman, S., and Vaheri, A.: Distribution of a major connective tissue protein, fibronectin, in normal human tissues. *J. Exp. Med.* 147:1054, 1978.

37. Carnes, W. H., Abraham, P. A., and Buonassisi, V.: Biosynthesis of elastin by an endothelial cell culture. *Biochem. Biophys. Res. Commun.* 90:1393, 1979.

38. Cantor, J. O., et al.: Synthesis of crosslinked elastin by an endothelial cell culture. *Biochem. Biophys. Res. Commun.* 95:1381, 1980.

39. Majno, G.: Ultrastructure of the vascular membrane, in *Handbook of Physiology,* edited by W. F. Hamilton and H. Dow. American Physiological Society, Washington, 1965, vol. III, p. 2293.

40. Bruns, R. R., and Palade, G. E.: Studies on blood capillaries in muscle. *J. Cell Biol.* 37:244, 1968.

41. Timpl, R., et al.: Laminin—a glycoprotein from basement membrane. *J. Biol. Chem.* 254:9933, 1979.

42. Foidart, J. M., et al.: Distribution and immunoelectron microscopic localization of laminin, a noncollagenous basement membrane glycoprotein. *Lab. Invest.* 42:336, 1980.

43. Madri, J. A., Roll, F. J., Furthmayr, H., and Foidart, J. M.: Ultrastructural localization of fibronectin and laminin in the basement membranes of the murine kidney. *J. Cell Biol.* 86:682, 1980.

44. Gospodarowicz, D., Greenburg, G., Foidart, J. M., and Savion, N.: The production and localization of laminin in cultured vascular and corneal endothelial cells. *J. Cell Physiol.* 107:171, 1981.

45. Turitto, V. T., Weiss, H. J., and Baumgartner, H. R.: The effect of shear rate on platelet interaction with subendothelium exposed to citrated human blood. *Microvasc. Res.* 19:352, 1980.

46. Ryan, J. W., Smith, U., and Niemeyer, R. S.: Angiotensin I: Metabolism by plasma membrane of lung. *Science* 176:64, 1972.

47. Ryan, J. W., et al.: Subcellular localization of pulmonary angiotensin-converting enzyme (kininase II). *Biochem. J.* 146:497, 1975.

48. Caldwell, P. R. B., et al.: Angiotensin-converting enzyme: Vascular endothelial localization. *Science* 191:1050, 1976.

49. Johnson, A. R., and Erdos, E. G.: Metabolism of vasoactive peptides by human endothelial cells in culture. Angiotensin I converting enzyme (kininase II) and angiotensinase. *J. Clin. Invest.* 59:684, 1977.

50. Ody, C., and Junod, A. F.: Converting enzyme activity in endothelial cells isolated from pig pulmonary artery and aorta. *Am. J. Physiol.* 232:C95, 1977.

51. Kumamoto, K., Stewart, T. A., Johnson, A. R., and Erdos, E. G.: Polycarboxypeptidase (angiotensinase C) in human lung and cultured cells. *J. Clin. Invest.* 67:210, 1981.

52. Fishman, A. P., and Pietra, G. G.: Handling of bioactive materials by the lung. *N. Engl. J. Med.* 291:884 and 953, 1974.

53. Junod, A. E.: The metabolic activity of pulmonary endothelial cells. *Pneumonologie* 153:169, 1976.

54. Robinson-White, A., and Beaven, M. A. Presence of histamine and its metabolizing enzymes in rat and guinea pig microvascular endothelial (MVE) cells. *J. Pharmacol. Exp. Ther.*, in press.

55. Stemerman, M.: Vascular intimal components: Precursors of thrombosis, in *Progress in Hemostasis and Thrombosis*, edited by T. H. Spaet. Grune & Stratton, New York, 1974, vol. 2, pp. 1–47.

56. Packham, M. A., Cazenave, J.-P., Kinlough-Rathbone, R. L., and Mustard, J. F.: Drug effects on platelet adherence to collagen and damaged vessel walls. *Adv. Exp. Med. Biol.* 109:253, 1978.

57. Dejana, E., et al.: The effect of aspirin inhibition of PGI_2 production on platelet adherence to normal and damaged aortae. *Thromb. Res.* 17:453, 1980.

58. Booyse, F. M., Bell, S., Sedlak, B., and Rafelson, M. E.: Development of an in vitro vessel wall model for studying certain aspects of platelet-vessel (endothelial) interactions. *Artery* 1:518, 1975.

59. Czervionke, R. L., Hoak, J. C., and Fry, G. L.: Effect of aspirin on thrombin-induced adherence of platelets to cultured cells from the blood vessel wall. *J. Clin. Invest.* 62:847, 1978.

60. Curwen, K. D., Gimbrone, M. A., and Handin, R. I.: In vitro studies of thromboresistance: The role of prostacyclin (PGI_2) in platelet adhesion to cultured normal and virally transformed human vascular endothelial cells. *Lab. Invest.* 42:366, 1980.

61. Fry, G. L., Czervionke, R. L., Hoak, J. C., and Haycraft, D. L.: Platelet adherence to cultured vascular cells: Influence of prostacyclin (PGI_2). *Blood* 55:271, 1980.

62. Czervionke, R., Smith, J. B., Fry, G. L., Hoak, J. C., and Haycraft, D. L.: Inhibition of prostacyclin by treatment of endothelium with aspirin: Correlation with platelet adherence. *J. Clin. Invest.* 63:1089, 1979.

63. Gryglewski, R. J., Bunting, S., Moncada, S., Flower, R. J., and Vane, J. R.: Arterial walls are protected against deposition of platelet thrombi by a substance (prostaglandin X) which they make from postaglandin endoperoxides. *Prostaglandins* 12:685, 1976.

64. Bunting, S., Gryglewski, R., Moncada, S., and Vane, J. R.: Arterial walls generate from prostaglandin endoperoxides a substance (prostaglandin X) which relaxes strips of mesenteric and coeliac arteries and inhibits platelet aggregation. *Prostaglandins* 12:897, 1976.

65. Moncada, S., Gryglewski, R., Bunting, S., and Vane, J. R.: An enzyme from arteries transforms prostaglandin endoperoxides to an unstable substance that inhibits platelet aggregation. *Nature* 263:663, 1976.

66. Weeks, J. R., and Compton, G. D.: The cardiovascular pharmacology of prostacyclin. *Prostaglandins* 17:501, 1979.

67. Weksler, B. B., Marcus, A. J., and Jaffe, E. A.: Synthesis of prostaglandin I_2 (prostacyclin) by cultured human and bovine endothelial cells. *Proc. Natl. Acad. Sci. U.S.A.* 74:3922, 1977.

68. Marcus, A. J., Weksler, B. B., and Jaffe, E. A.: Enzymatic conversion of prostaglandin endoperoxide H_2 (PGH_2) and arachidonic acid to prostacyclin by cultured human endothelial cells. *J. Biol. Chem.* 253:7138, 1978.

69. Moncada, S., Herman, A. G., Higgs, E. A., and Vane, J. R.: Differential formation of prostacyclin (PGX or PGI_2) by layers of the arterial wall: An explanation for the anti-thrombotic properties of vascular endothelium. *Thrombosis Res.* 11:323, 1977.

70. MacIntyre, D. E., Pearson, J. D., and Gordon, J. L.: Localization and stimulation of prostacyclin production in vascular cells. *Nature* 271:549, 1978.

71. Siegl, A. M., Smith, J. B., Silver, M. J., Nicolaou, K. C., and Ahern, D.: Selective binding site for (^{3}H) prostacyclin on platelets. *J. Clin. Invest.* 63:215, 1979.

72. Schafer, A. I., Cooper, B., O'Hara, D., and Handin, R. I.: Identification of platelet receptors for prostaglandin I_2 and D_2. *J. Biol. Chem.* 254:2914, 1979.

73. Gorman, R. R., Bunting, S., and Miller, O.V.: Modulation of human platelet adenylate cyclase by prostacyclin (PGX). *Prostaglandins* 13:377, 1977.

74. Tateson, J. E., Moncada, S., and Vane, J. R.: Effects of prostacyclin (PGX) on cyclic AMP concentrations in human platelets. *Prostaglandins* 13:389, 1977.

75. Best, L. C., Martin, T. J., Russell, R. G. G., and Preston, F. E.: Prostacyclin increases cyclic AMP levels and adenylate cyclase activity in platelets. *Nature* 267:850, 1977.

76. Ehrman, M. L., and Jaffe, E. A.: Prostacyclin (PGI_2) inhibits the development in human platelets of ADP and arachidonic acid–induced shape change and procoagulant activity. *Prostaglandins* 20:1103, 1980.

77. Fujimoto, T., Ohara, S., and Hawiger, J.: Thrombin-induced exposure and prostacyclin inhibition of the receptor for factor VIII/von Willebrand factor on human platelets. *J. Clin. Invest.* 69:1212, 1982.

78. Hawiger, J., Parkinson, S., and Timmons, S.: Prostacyclin inhibits mobilization of fibrinogen-binding sites on human ADP- and thrombin-treated platelets. *Nature* 283:195, 1980.

79. Harsfalvi. J., Muszbek, L., Stadler, I., and Fesus, L.: Inhibition of platelet factor 3 availability by prostacyclin. *Prostaglandins* 20:935, 1980.

80. Bunting, S., Simmons, P. M., and Moncada, S.: Inhibition of platelet activation by prostacyclin: Possible consequences in coagulation and anticoagulation. *Thromb. Res.* 21:89, 1981.

81. Weiss, H. J., and Turitto, V. T.: Prostacyclin inhibits platelet adhesion and thrombus formation on subendothelium. *Blood* 53:244, 1979.

82. Higgs, E. A., Moncada, S., and Vane, J. R.: Effect of prostacyclin on platelet adhesion to rabbit arterial subendothelium. *Prostaglandins* 16:17, 1978.

83. Schmid-Schonbein, G. W., and Zweifach, B. W.: RBC velocity profiles in arterioles and venules in the rabbit omentum. *Microvasc. Res.* 10:153, 1975.

84. Jaffe, E. A., and Weksler, B. B.: Recovery of endothelial cell prostacyclin production after inhibition by low doses of aspirin. *J. Clin. Invest.* 63:532, 1979.

85. Weksler, B. B., Ley, C. W., and Jaffe, E. A.: Stimulation of endothelial cell prostacyclin production by thrombin, trypsin, and the ionophore A23187. *J. Clin. Invest.* 62:923, 1978.

86. Hong, S. L.: Effect of bradykinin and thrombin on prostacyclin synthesis in endothelial cells from calf and pig aorta and human umbilical cord vein. *Thromb. Res.* 18:787, 1980.

87. Baenziger, N. L., Force, L. E., and Becherer, P. R.: Histamine stimulates prostacyclin synthesis in cultured human umbilical vein endothelial cells. *Biochem. Biophys. Res. Commun.* 92:1435, 1980.

88. Needleman, P., Bronson, S. D., Wyche, A., Sivakoff, M., and Nicolaou, K. C.: Cardiac and renal prostaglandin I_2. *J. Clin. Invest.* 61:839, 1978.

89. Mullane, K. M., and Moncada, S.: Prostacyclin mediates the potentiated hypotensive effect of bradykinin following captopril treatment. *Eur. J. Pharmacol.* 66:355, 1980.

90. Lonchampt, M., Ponquin, N., Bonne, C., and Reynault, F.: The effect of angiotensin II on PGI_2 production by endothelial cells in culture. *Thromb. Haemostasis* 46:39, 1981.

91. Fleisher, L. N., et al.: Stimulation of arterial endothelial cell prostacyclin synthesis by high density lipoproteins. *J. Biol. Chem.* 257:6653, 1982.

92. Clopath, P., and Sinzinger, H.: Calcitonin increases porcine vascular prostacyclin formation. *Prostaglandins* 19:1, 1980.

93. Pearson, J. D., Slakey, L. L., and Gordon, J. L.: Stimulation of prostaglandin production through purinergic receptors on endothelial cells and macrophages. *Nature*, in press.

94. Wennmalm, A.: Prostacyclin-dependent coronary vasodilation in rabbits and guinea pig hearts. *Acta Physiol. Scand.* 106:47, 1979.

95. Roberts, A. M., Messina, E. J., and Kaley, G.: Prostacyclin (PGI_2) mediates hypoxic relaxation of bovine coronary arterial strips. *Prostaglandins* 21:555, 1981.

96. Coughlin, S. R., Moskowitz, M. A., Zetter, B. R., Antoniades, H. N., and Levine, L.: Platelet dependent stimulation of prostacyclin synthesis by platelet-derived growth factor. *Nature* 288:600, 1980.

97. Gordon, J. L., and Pearson, J. D.: Effects of sulphinpyrazone and aspirin on prostaglandin I_2 (prostacyclin) synthesis by endothelial cells. *Br. J. Pharmacol.* 64:481, 1978.

98. Preston, F. E., et al.: Inhibition of prostacyclin and platelet thromboxane A_2 after low-dose aspirin. *N. Engl. J. Med.* 304:76, 1981.

99. Wennmalm, A.: Nicotine inhibits hypoxia- and arachidonate-induced release of prostacyclin-like activity in rabbit hearts. *Br. J. Pharmacol.* 69:545, 1980.

100. Spector, A. A., et al.: Effect of fatty acid modification on prosta-

cyclin production by cultured human endothelial cells. *J. Clin. Invest.* 65:1003, 1980.

101. Spector, A. A., Kaduce, T. L., Hoak, J. L., and Fry, G. L.: Utilization of arachidonic and linoleic acids by cultured human endothelial cells. *J. Clin. Invest.* 68:1003, 1981.

102. Smith, J. B., Ogletree, M. L., Lefer, A. M., and Nicolaou, K. C.: Antibodies which antagonize the effects of prostacyclin. *Nature* 274:64, 1978.

103. Steer, M. L., MacIntyre, D. E., Levine, L., and Salzman, E. W.: Is prostacyclin a physiologically important circulating anti-platelet agent? *Nature* 283:194, 1980.

104. Haslam, R. J., and McClenaghan, M. D.: Measurement of circulating prostacyclin. *Nature* 292:364, 1981.

105. Pace-Asciak, C. R., Carrara, M. C., Levine, L., and Nicolaou, K. C.: PGI₂ specific antibodies administered in vivo suggest against a role for endogenous PGI₂ as a circulating vasodepressor hormone in the normotensive and spontaneously hypertensive rat. *Prostaglandins* 20:1053, 1980.

106. FitzGerald, G. A., Brash, A. R., Falardeau, P., and Oates, J. A.: Estimated rate of prostacyclin secretion in the circulation of normal man. *J. Clin. Invest.* 68:1272, 1981.

107. Aiken, J. W., Gorman, R. R., and Shebuski, R. J.: Prevention of blockage of partially obstructed coronary arteries with prostacyclin correlates with inhibition of platelet aggregation. *Prostaglandins* 17:483, 1979.

108. Buchanan, M. R., Dejana, E., Gent, M., Mustard, J. F., and Hirsch, J.: Enhanced platelet accumulation onto injured carotid arteries in rabbits after aspirin treatment. *J. Clin. Invest.* 67:503, 1981.

109. Friedman, P. L., et al.: Coronary vasoconstrictor effect of indomethacin in patients with coronary-artery disease. *N. Engl. J. Med.* 305:1171, 1981.

110. Weiner, E., Messina, E. J., and Kaley, G.: Indomethacin reduces skeletal muscle vasodilation induced by exercise and ischemia. *Artery* 3:52, 1977.

111. Marcus, A. J., Weksler, B. B., Jaffe, E. A., and Broekman, M. J.: Synthesis of prostacyclin from platelet-derived endoperoxides by cultured human endothelial cells. *J. Clin. Invest.* 66:979, 1980.

112. Quilley, C. P., Wong, P. Y. K., and McGiff, J. C.: Hypotensive and renovascular actions of 6-keto-prostaglandin E₁, a metabolite of prostacyclin. *Eur. J. Pharmacol.* 57:273, 1979.

113. Wong, P. Y. K., McGiff, J. C., Sun, F. F., and Lee, W. H.: 6-Keto-prostaglandin E₁ inhibits the aggregation of human platelets. *Eur. J. Pharmacol.* 60:245, 1979.

114. Quilley, C. P., McGiff, J. C., Lee, W. H., Sun, F. F., and Wong, P. Y. K.: 6-Keto-PGE₁: A possible metabolite of prostacyclin having platelet antiaggregatory effects. *Hypertension* 2:524, 1980.

115. Wong, P. Y. K., Malik, K. U., Desiderio, D. M., McGiff, J. C., and Sun, F. F.: Hepatic metabolism of prostacyclin (PGI₂) in the rabbit. Formation of a potent novel inhibitor of platelet aggregation. *Biochem. Biophys. Res. Commun.* 93:486, 1980.

116. Feigen, L. P., et al.: Peripheral vasodilator effects of prostaglandins: Comparison of 6-keto-prostaglandin E₁ with prostacyclin and escape from prostaglandin E₂ in the mesenteric vascular bed. *J. Pharmacol. Exp. Ther.* 214:528, 1980.

117. Miller, O. V., Aiken, J. W., Shebuski, R. J., and Gorman, R. R.: 6-Keto-prostaglandin E₁ is not equipotent to prostacyclin (PGI₂) as an antiaggregatory agent. *Prostaglandins* 20:391, 1980.

118. Wong, P. Y. K., Lee, W. H., Chao, P. H. W., Reiss, R. F., and McGiff, J. C.: Metabolism of prostacyclin by 9-hydroxy-prostaglandin dehydrogenase in human platelets: Formation of a potent inhibitor of platelet aggregation and enzyme purification. *J. Biol. Chem.* 255:9021, 1980.

119. Van Dam, J., et al.: Cardiovascular responses to 6-keto-prostaglandin E₁ in the dog. *Proc. Soc. Exp. Biol. Med.* 166:76, 1981.

120. Jackson, E. K., and Gordon, R. P.: 6-Keto-prostaglandin E₁ and Bartter's syndrome. *N. Engl. J. Med.* 305:287, 1981.

121. Coughlin, S. R., Moskowitz, M. A., Antoniades, H. N., and Levine, L.: Serotonin receptor-mediated stimulation of bovine smooth muscle cell prostacyclin synthesis and its modulation by platelet-derived growth factor. *Proc. Natl. Acad. Sci. U.S.A.* 78:7134, 1981.

122. Eldor, A., Falcone, D. J., Hajjar, D. P., Minick, C. R., and Weksler, B. B.: Recovery of prostacyclin production by de-endothelialized

rabbit aorta. Critical role of neointimal smooth muscle cells. *J. Clin. Invest.* 67:735, 1981.

123. Mills, D. C. B., Robb, I. A., and Roberts, G. C. K.: The release of nucleotides, 5-hydroxytryptamine, and enzymes from human blood platelets during aggregation. *J. Physiol. (Lond.)* 195:715, 1968.

124. Glasgow, J. G., Schade, R., and Pitlick, F. A.: Evidence that ADP hydrolysis by human cells is related to thrombogenic potential. *Thromb. Res.* 13:255, 1978.

125. Dosne, A. M., Legrand, C., Bauvois, B., Bodevin, E., and Caen, J. P.: Comparative degradation of adenylnucleotides by cultured endothelial cells and fibroblasts. *Biochem. Biophys. Res. Commun.* 85:183, 1978.

126. Pearson, J. D., Carleton, J. S., and Gordon, J. L.: Metabolism of adenine nucleotides by ectoenzymes of vascular endothelial and smooth-muscle cells in culture. *Biochem. J.* 190:421, 1980.

127. Crutchley, D. J., Ryan, U. S., and Ryan, J. W.: Effects of aspirin and dipyridamole on the degradation of adenosine diphosphate by cultured cells derived from bovine pulmonary artery. *J. Clin. Invest.* 66:29, 1980.

128. Pearson, J. D., Carleton, J. S., Hutchings, A., and Gordon, J. L.: Uptake and metabolism of adenosine by pig aortic endothelial and smooth muscle cells in culture. *Biochem. J.* 170:265, 1978.

129. Pearson, J. D., and Gordon, J. L.: Vascular endothelial and smooth muscle cells in culture selectively release adenine nucleotides. *Nature* 281:384, 1979.

130. Berne, R. M.: The role of adenosine in the regulation of coronary blood flow. *Circ. Res.* 47:807, 1980.

131. Drummond, A. H.: Interactions of blood platelets with biogenic amines: Uptake, stimulation and receptor binding, in *Platelets in Biology and Pathology*, edited by J. L. Gordon. North Holland, New York, 1976, pp. 203–237.

132. Erspamer, V.: Peripheral physiological and pharmacological actions of indolealkylamines, in *Handbook of Experimental Pharmacology*. Springer, New York, 1966, vol. XIX, pp. 245–359.

133. DeClerck, F., and Van Gorp, L.: Induction of circulating platelet aggregates by release of endogenous 5-hydroxytryptamine in the rat. *Thromb. Haemost.* 46:29, 1981.

134. Alabaster, V. A., and Bakhle, Y. S.: Removal of 5-hydroxytryptamine by rat isolated lung. *Br. J. Pharmacol.* 40:468, 1970.

135. Junod, A. S.: Uptake, metabolism, and efflux of ¹⁴C-5-hydroxytryptamine in isolated perfused lung. *J. Pharmacol. Exp. Ther.* 183:341, 1972.

136. Small, R., Macarak, E., and Fisher, A. B.: Production of 5-hydroxyindoleacetic acid from serotonin by cultured endothelial cells. *J. Cell Physiol.* 90:225, 1977.

137. Roth, J. A., and Venter, J. C.: Predominance of the B form of monoamine oxidase in cultured vascular intimal endothelial cells. *Biochem. Pharmacol.* 27:2371, 1978.

138. Trevethick, M. A., et al.: Monoamine oxidase activities of porcine vascular endothelial and smooth muscle cells. *Biochem. Pharmacol.* 30:2209, 1981.

139. Lollar, P., and Owen, W. G.: Clearance of thrombin from circulation in rabbits by high-affinity binding sites on endothelium. Possible role in the inactivation of thrombin by antithrombin III. *J. Clin. Invest.* 66:1222, 1980.

140. Harpel, P. C., and Rosenberg, R. D.: α₂-Macroglobulin and antithrombin-heparin cofactor: Modulators of hemostatic and inflammatory reactions, in *Progress in Hemostasis and Thrombosis*, edited by T. H. Spaet. Grune & Stratton, New York, 1976, vol. 3, pp. 145–189.

141. Jordan, R. E., Oosta, G. M., Gardner, W. T., and Rosenberg, R. D.: The kinetics of hemostatic enzyme-antithrombin interactions in the presence of low molecular weight heparin. *J. Biol. Chem.* 255:10081, 1980.

142. Hatton, M. W. C., Berry, L. R., and Regoeczi, E.: Inhibition of thrombin by antithrombin III in the presence of certain glycosaminoglycans found in the mammalian aorta. *Thromb. Res.* 13:655, 1978.

143. Busch, P. C., and Owen, W. G.: Identification in vitro of an endothelial cell surface cofactor for antithrombin III. *J. Clin. Invest.* 69:726, 1982.

144. Wasteson, A., et al.: Effect of a platelet endoglycosidase on cell surface associated heparan sulphate of human cultured endothelial and glial cells. *Thromb. Res. 11:*309, 1977.

145. Oldberg, A., Heldin, C. H., Wasteson, A., Busch, C., and Höök, M.: Characterization of a platelet endoglycosidase degrading heparin-like polysaccharides. *Biochemistry 19:*5755, 1980.

146. Busch, C., Dawes, J., Pepper, D. S., and Wasteson, A.: Binding of platelet factor 4 to cultured human umbilical vein endothelial cells. *Thromb. Res. 19:*129, 1980.

147. Hiebert, L. M., and Jaques, L. B.: The observation of heparin on endothelium after injection. *Thromb Res. 8:*195, 1976.

148. Glimelius, B., Busch, C., and Höök, M.: Binding of heparin on the surface of cultured human endothelial cells. *Thromb. Res. 12:*773, 1978.

149. Egeberg, O.: Inherited antithrombin deficiency causing thrombophilia. *Thromb. Diath. Haemorrh. 13:*516, 1965.

150. Marciniak, E., Farley, C. H., and DeSimone, P. A.: Familial thrombosis due to antithrombin III deficiency. *Blood 43:*219, 1974.

151. Kisiel, W., Canfield, W. M., Ericsson, L. H., and Davie, E. W.: Anticoagulant properties of bovine plasma Protein C following activation by thrombin. *Biochemistry 176:*5824, 1977.

152. Walker, F. J., Sexton, P. W., and Esmon, C. T.: The inhibition of blood coagulation by activated Protein C through the selective inactivation of activated factor V. *Biochim. Biophys. Acta 571:*333, 1979.

153. Vehar, G. A., and Davie, E. W.: Preparation and properties of bovine factor VIII (antihemophilic factor). *Biochemistry 19:*401, 1980.

154. Marlar, R. A., Kleiss, A. J., and Griffin, J.: Anticoagulant action of human protein C. *Protides Biol. Fluids Proc. Colloq. 28:*341, 1980.

155. Esmon, C. T., and Owen, W. G.: Identification of an endothelial cell cofactor for thrombin-catalyzed activation of Protein C. *Proc. Natl. Acad. Sci. U.S.A. 78:*2249, 1981.

156. Owen, W. G., and Esmon, C. T.: Functional properties of an endothelial cell cofactor for thrombin-catalyzed activation of Protein C. *J. Biol. Chem. 256:*5532, 1981.

157. Walker, F. J.: Regulation of activated Protein C by Protein S: The role of phospholipid in factor V_a inactivation. *J. Biol. Chem. 256:*11128, 1981.

158. Griffin, J. H., Evatt, B., Zimmerman, T. S., Kleiss, A. J., and Wideman, C.: Deficiency of Protein C in congenital thrombotic disease. *J. Clin. Invest. 68:*1370, 1981.

159. Marlar, R., and Griffin, J. H.: Deficiency of protein C inhibitor in combined factor V/VIII deficiency disease. *J. Clin. Invest. 68:*1186, 1980.

160. Savion, N., Isaacs, J. D., Gospodarowicz, D., and Shuman, M. A.: Internalization and degradation of thrombin and up regulation of thrombin-binding sites in corneal endothelial cells. *J. Biol. Chem. 256:*4514, 1981.

161. Isaacs, J. D., Savion, N., Gospodarowicz, D., Fenton, J. W., and Shuman, M. A.: Covalent binding of thrombin to specific sites on corneal endothelial cells. *Biochemistry 20:*398, 1981.

162. Isaacs, J. D., Savion, N., Gospodarowicz, D., and Shuman, M. A.: Effect of cell density on thrombin binding to a specific site on bovine vascular endothelial cells. *J. Cell Biol. 90:*670, 1981.

163. Low, D. A., Baker, J. B., Koonce, W. C., and Cunningham, D. D.: Released protease-nexin regulates cellular binding, internalization and degradation of serine proteases. *Proc. Natl. Acad. Sci. U.S.A. 78:*2340, 1981.

164. Baker, J. B., Low, D. A., Simmer, R. L., and Cunningham, D. D.: Protease-nexin: A cellular component that links thrombin and plasminogen activator and mediates their binding to cells. *Cell 21:*37, 1980.

165. Perdue, J. F., Lubenskyi, W., Kivity, E., Sonder, S. A., and Fenton, J. W., II: Protease mitogenic response of chick embryo fibroblasts and receptor binding/processing of human α-thrombin. *J. Biol. Chem. 256:*2767, 1981.

166. Maerowitz, T., et al.: A new type of thrombin binding to human platelets. *Clin. Res. 29:*339A, 1981.

167. Warren, B. A., and Vales, O.: The release of vesicles from platelets following adhesion to vessel walls in vitro. *Br. J. Exp. Pathol. 53:*206, 1972.

168. Chiang, T. M., Mainardi, C. L., Seyer, J. M., and Kang, A. H.: Collagen-platelet interaction: Type V (A-B) collagen induces platelet aggregation. *J. Lab. Clin. Med. 95:*99, 1980.

169. Barnes, M. J., Bailey, A. J., Gordon, J. L., and MacIntyre, D. E.: Platelet aggregation by basement-associated collagens. *Thromb. Res. 18:*375, 1980.

170. Tryggvason, K., Oikarinen, J., Viinikka, L., and Ylikorkala, O.: Effects of laminin, proteoglycan, and type IV collagen, components of basement membranes, on platelet aggregation. *Biochem. Biophys. Res. Commun. 100:*233, 1981.

171. Legrand, Y. J., et al.: Microfibrils (MF) platelet interaction: Requirement of von Willebrand factor. *Thromb. Res. 19:*737, 1980.

172. Barnes, M. J., Gordon, J. L., and MacIntyre, D. E.: Platelet-collagen activity of type I and type III collagens from human aorta and chicken skin. *Biochem. J. 160:*647, 1976.

173. Wester, J., Sixma, J. J., Geuze, J. J., and Heijnes, H. F. G.: Morphology of the hemostatic plug in human skin wounds: Transformation of the plug. *Lab. Invest. 41:*182, 1979.

174. Plow, E. F., Birdwell, C., and Ginsberg, M. H.: Identification and quantitation of platelet-associated fibronectin antigen. *J. Clin. Invest. 63:*540, 1979.

175. Zucker, M. B., Mosesson, M. W., Broekman, H. J., and Kaplan, K. L.: Release of platelet fibronectin (cold-insoluble globulin) from alpha granules induced by thrombin or collagen; lack of requirement for plasma fibronectin in ADP-induced platelet aggregation. *Blood 54:*8, 1979.

176. Ginsberg, M. H., Painter, R. G., Birdwell, C., and Plow, E. F.: The detection, immunofluorescent localization, and thrombin induced release of human platelet-aggregation fibronectin antigen. *J. Supramol. Struc. 11:*167,1979.

177. Plow, E. F., and Ginsberg, M. H.: Specific and saturable binding of plasma fibronectin to thrombin-stimulated human platelets. *J. Biol. Chem. 256:*9477, 1981.

178. Hynes, R. O., et al.: A large glycoprotein lost from the surfaces of transformed cells. *Ann. N.Y. Acad. Sci. 312:*317, 1978.

179. Grinell, F., Feld, M., and Snell, W.: The influence of cold insoluble globulin on platelet morphological response to substrate. *Cell Biol. Int. Rep. 3:*585, 1979.

180. Tschopp, T. B., Weiss, H. J., and Baumgartner, H. R.: Decreased adhesion of platelets to subendothelium in von Willebrand's disease. *J. Lab. Clin. Med. 83:*296, 1974.

181. Baumgartner, H. R., Tschopp, T. B., and Meyer, D.: Shear rate dependent inhibition of platelet adhesion and aggregation on collagenous surfaces by antibodies to human factor VIII/von Willebrand factor. *Br. J. Haematol. 44:*127, 1980.

182. Weiss, H. J., Baumgartner, H. R., Tschopp, T. B., Turitto, V. T., and Cohen, D.: Correction by factor VIII of the impaired platelet adhesion to subendothelium in von Willebrand's disease. *Blood 51:*267, 1978.

183. Weiss, H. J., Turitto, V. T., and Baumgartner, H. R.: Effect of shear rate on platelet interaction with subendothelium in citrated and native blood. 1. Shear rate-dependent decrease of adhesion in von Willebrand's disease and the Bernard-Soulier syndrome. *J. Lab. Clin. Med. 92:*750, 1978.

184. Sakariassen, K. S., Bolhius, P. A., and Sixma, J. J.: Human blood platelet adhesion to artery subendothelium is mediated by factor VIII–von Willebrand factor bound to the subendothelium. *Nature 279:*636, 1979.

185. Bolhius, P. A., Sakariassen, K. S., Sander, H. J., Bouma, B. N., and Sixma, J. J.: Binding of factor VIII–von Willebrand factor to human arterial subendothelium precedes increased platelet adhesion and enhances platelet spreading. *J. Lab. Clin. Med. 97:*568, 1981.

186. Jaffe, E. A., Hoyer, L. W., and Nachman, R. L.: Synthesis of antihemophilic factor antigen by cultured human endothelial cells. *J. Clin. Invest. 52:*2757, 1973.

187. Jaffe, E. A., Hoyer, L. W., and Nachman, R. L.: Synthesis of von Willebrand factor by cultured human endothelial cells. *Proc. Natl. Acad. Sci. U.S.A. 71:*1906, 1974.

188. Jaffe, E. A., and Nachman, R L.: Subunit structure of factor VIII antigen synthesized by cultured human endothelial cells. *J. Clin. Invest. 56:*698, 1975.

189. Nyman, D.: Interaction of collagen with the factor VIII antigen–activity–von Willebrand factor complex. *Thromb. Res. 11:*433, 1977.

190. Legrand, Y. J., Rodriguez-Zeballos, A., Kartalis, G., Fauvel, F., and Caen, J. P.: Adsorption of factor VIII antigen-activity complex by collagen. *Thromb. Res. 13:*909, 1978.

191. Nyman, D.: Von Willebrand factor–dependent platelet aggregation and adsorption of factor VIII–related antigen by collagen. *Thromb. Res. 17:*209, 1980.

192. Santoro, S. A.: Adsorption of von Willebrand factor/factor VIII by the genetically distinct interstitial collagens. *Thromb. Res. 21:*689, 1981.

193. Scott, D. M., Griffin, B., Pepper, D. E., and Barnes, M. J.: The binding of purified factor VIII/von Willebrand factor to collagens of differing types and forms. *Thromb Res. 24:*467, 1981.

194. Rand, J. H., Sussman, I. I., Gordon, R. E., Chu, S. V., and Solomon, V.: Localization of factor VIII-related antigen in human vascular subendothelium. *Blood 55:*752, 1980.

195. Kao, K.-J., Pizzo, S. V., and McKee, P. A.: Demonstration and characterization of specific binding sites of factor VIII/von Willebrand factor on human platelets. *J. Clin. Invest. 63:*656, 1979.

196. Kao, K.-J., Pizzo, S. V., and McKee, P. A.: Platelet receptor for human factor VIII/von Willebrand protein: Functional correlation of receptor occupancy and ristocetin-induced platelet aggregation. *Proc. Natl. Acad. Sci. U.S.A. 76:*5317, 1979.

197. Morisato, D. K., and Gralnick, H. R.: Selective binding of the factor VIII/von Willebrand factor protein to human platelets. *Blood 55:*9, 1980.

198. Tschopp, T. B., Baumgartner, H. R., and Meyer, D.: Antibody to human factor VIII (von Willebrand factor) inhibits collagen-induced platelet aggregation and release. *Thromb. Res. 17:*255, 1980.

199. Turitto, V. T., and Weiss, H. J.: Red blood cells: Their dual role in thrombus formation. *Science 207:*541, 1980.

200. Maynard, J. R., Dreyer, B. E., Stemerman, M. B., and Pitlick, F. A.: Tissue-factor coagulant activity of cultured human endothelial and smooth muscle cells and fibroblasts. *Blood 50:*387, 1977.

201. Maynard, J. P.: Tissue factor activity of cultured human vascular cells, in *The Biology of Endothelial Cells,* edited by E. A. Jaffe. Martinus Nijhoff, The Hague, in press.

202. Revak, S. D., Cochrane, C. G., Johnston, A. R., and Hugli, T. E.: Structural changes accompanying enzymatic activation of human Hageman factor. *J. Clin. Invest. 54:*619, 1974.

203. Ratnoff, O. D., Davie, E. W., and Mallet, D. L.: Studies on the action of Hageman factor: Evidence that activated Hageman factor in turn activates plasma thromboplastin antecedent. *J. Clin. Invest. 40:*803, 1961.

204. Bouma, B. N., and Griffin, J. H.: Human blood coagulation factor XI. Purification, properties, and mechanism of activation by activated factor XII. *J. Biol. Chem. 252:*6432, 1977.

205. Koide, T., Kato, H., and Davie, E. W.: Isolation and characterization of bovine factor XI (plasma thromboplastin antecedent). *Biochemistry 16:*2279, 1977.

206. Rapaport, S. I., Aas, K., and Owren, P. A.: The effect of glass upon the activity of the various clotting factors. *J. Clin. Invest. 34:*9, 1955.

207. Laake, K., and Osterud, B.: Activation of purified factor VII by human plasmin, plasma kallikrein, and activated components of the human intrinsic blood coagulation system. *Thromb. Res. 5:*759, 1974.

208. Kisiel, W., Fujikawa, K., and Davie, E. W.: Activation of bovine factor VII (proconvertin) by factor XIIa (activated Hageman factor). *Biochemistry 16:* 4189, 1977.

209. Bouma, B. N., and Griffin, J. H.: Deficiency of factor XII–dependent plasminogen proactivator in prekallikrein-deficient plasma. *J. Lab. Clin. Med. 91:*148, 1978.

210. Mandle, R., Jr., and Kaplan, A. P.: Hageman factor substrates. Human plasma prekallikrein: Mechanism of activation by Hageman factor and participation in Hageman factor–dependent fibrinolysis. *J. Biol. Chem. 252:*6097, 1977.

211. Han, Y. N., Kato, H., Iwanaga, H., and Suzuki, T.: Primary structure of bovine plasma high-molecular-weight kininogen: The amino acid sequence of a glycoprotein portion (Fragment 1) following the C-terminus of the bradykinin moiety. *J. Biochem. (Tokyo) 79:*1201, 1976.

212. Derkx, F. H. M., Bouma, B. N., Schalekamp, M. P. A., and Schalekamp, M. A. D. H.: An intrinsic factor XII-prekallikrein–depen-

dent pathway activates the human plasma renin-angiotensin system. *Nature 280:*315, 1979.

213. Ghebrehiwet, B., Silverberg, M., and Kaplan, A. P.: Activation of the classical pathway of complement by Hageman factor fragment. *J. Exp. Med. 153:*665, 1981.

214. Wiggins, R. C., Giclas, P. C., and Henson, P. M.: Chemotactic activity generated from the fifth component of complement by plasma kallikrein of the rabbit. *J. Exp. Med. 153:*1391, 1981.

215. Wiggins, R. C., Loskutoff, D. J., Cochrane, C. G., Griffin, J. H., and Edgington, T. S.: Activation of rabbit Hageman factor by homogenates of cultured rabbit endothelial cells. *J. Clin. Invest. 65:*197, 1980.

216. Soltay, M. J., Movat, H. Z., and Ozge-Anwar, A. H.: The kinin system of human plasma. V. The probable derivation of prekallikrein activator from the activated Hageman factor (XIIa). *Proc. Soc. Exp. Biol. Med. 138:*952, 1971.

217. Cochrane, C. G., Revak, S. D., Aiken, B. S., and Wuepper, K. D.: The structural characteristic and activation of Hageman factor, in *Inflammation, Mechanisms and Control,* edited by I. M. Lepow and P. A. Ward. Academic, N.Y., 1972, pp. 119–150.

218. Zucker, M. B.: Platelet agglutination and vasoconstriction as factors in spontaneous hemostasis in normal, thrombocytopenic, heparinized, and hypoprothrombinemic rats. *Am. J. Physiol. 148:*275, 1947.

219. Todd, A. S.: Fibrinolysis autographs. *Nature 181:*495, 1958.

220. Todd, A. S.: Localization of fibrinolytic activity in tissue. *Br. Med. Bull. 20:*210, 1964.

221. Loskutoff, D. J., and Edgington, T. S.: Synthesis of a fibrinolytic activator and inhibitor by endothelial cells. *Proc. Natl. Acad. Sci. U.S.A. 74:*3903, 1977.

222. Levin, E. G., and Loskutoff, D. J.: Comparative studies of the fibrinolytic activity of cultured vascular cells. *Thromb. Res. 15:*869, 1979.

223. Laug, W. E., Tokes, Z. A., Benedict, W. F., and Sorgente, N.: Anchorage independent growth and plasminogen activator production by bovine endothelial cells. *J. Cell Biol. 84:*281, 1980.

224. Laug, W. E.: Secretion of plasminogen activators by cultured bovine endothelial cells: Partial purification, characterization and evidence for multiple forms. *Thromb. Haemost. (Stuttgart) 45:*219, 1981.

225. Rijken, D. C., and Collen, D.: Purification and characterization of the plasminogen activator secreted by human melanoma cells in culture. *J. Biol. Chem. 256:*7035, 1981.

226. Matsuo, O., Rijken, D. C., and Collen, D.: Comparison of the relative fibrinogenolytic and thrombolytic properties of tissue plasminogen activator and urokinase in vitro. *Thromb. Haemost. (Stuttgart) 45:*225, 1981.

227. Matsuo, O., Rijken, D. C., and Collen, D. C.: Thrombolysis by human tissue plasminogen activator and urokinase in rabbits with experimental pulmonary embolus. *Nature 291:*590, 1981.

228. Mackie, M., Booth, N. A., and Bennett, B.: Comparative studies on human activators of plasminogen. *Br. J. Haematol. 47:*77, 1981.

229. Binder, B. R., Spragg, J., and Austen, K. F.: Purification and characterization of human vascular plasminogen activator derived from blood vessel perfusates. *J. Biol. Chem. 254:*1998, 1979.

230. Loskutoff, D. J., and Edgington, T. S.: An inhibitor of plasminogen activator in rabbit endothelial cells. *J. Biol. Chem. 256:*4142, 1981.

231. Levin, E., and Loskutoff, D. J.: Cultured bovine endothelial cells produce both urokinase and tissue-type plasminogen activator. *J. Cell Biol. 94:*631, 1982.

232. Luskutoff, D. J., and Mussoni, L.: Interactions between fibrin and the plasminogen activators produced by cultured endothelial cells. *Blood,* in press.

233. Dosne, A. M., Dupuy, E., and Bodevin, E.: Production of a fibrinolytic inhibitor by cultured endothelial cells derived from human umbilical vein. *Thromb. Res. 12:*377, 1978.

234. Loskutoff, D. J.: Effect of thrombin on the fibrinolytic activity of cultured bovine endothelial cells. *J. Clin. Invest. 64:*329, 1979.

235. Levin, E. G., and Loskutoff, D. J.: Serum mediated suppression of cell-associated plasminogen activator activity in cultured endothelial cells. *Cell 22:*701, 1980.

236. Comp, P. C., and Esmon, C. T.: Generation of fibrinolytic activity by infusion of activated protein C into dogs. *J. Clin. Invest.* 68:1221, 1981.

237. Belew, M., Gerdin, B., Porath, J., and Saldeen, T.: Isolation of vasoactive peptides from human fibrin and fibrinogen degraded by plasmin. *Thromb. Res.* 13:983, 1978.

238. Gerdin, B., and Saldeen, T.: Effect of fibrin degradation products on microvascular permeability. *Thromb. Res.* 13:995, 1978.

239. Busch, C., and Gerdin, B.: Effect of low molecular weight fibrin degradation products on endothelial cells in culture. *Thromb. Res.* 22:33, 1981.

240. Sholley, M. M., Gimbrone, Jr., M. A., and Cotran, R. S.: Cellular migration and replication in endothelial regeneration: A study using irradiated endothelial cultures. *Lab. Invest.* 36:18, 1977.

241. Selden, S. C., and Schwartz, S. M.: Cytochalasin B inhibition of endothelial proliferation at wound edges in vitro. *J. Cell Biol.* 81:348, 1979.

242. Reidy, M. A., and Schwartz, S. M.: Endothelial regeneration. III. Time course of intimal changes after small defined injury to rat aortic endothelium. *Lab. Invest.* 44:301, 1981.

243. Schwartz, S. M., Gajdusek, C. M., Reidy, M. A., Selden, S. C., and Haudenschild, C. C.: Maintenance of integrity in aortic endothelium. *Fed. Proc.* 39:2618, 1980.

244. Prockop, D. J., Kivirikko, K. I., Tuderman, L., and Guzman, N. A.: The biosynthesis of collagen and its disorders. *N. Engl. J. Med.* 301:13 and 77, 1979.

245. Layman, D. L., and Titus, J. L.: Synthesis of type I collagen by human smooth muscle cells in vitro. *Lab. Invest.* 33:103, 1975.

246. Rauterberg, J. Allam, S., Brehmer, U., Wirth, W., and Hauss, W.: Characterization of the collagen synthesized by cultured smooth muscle cells from fetal and adult aorta. *Hoppe Seylers Z. Physiol. Chem.* 358:401, 1977.

247. Mayne, R., Vail, M. S., and Miller, E. J.: Characterization of the collagen chains synthesized by cultured smooth muscle cells derived from Rhesus monkey thoracic aorta. *Biochemistry* 17:446, 1978.

248. Nakao, J., Chang, W.-C., Murota, S.-I., and Orimo, H.: Elastinolytic activity in the rat aortic smooth muscle cells in culture. *Atherosclerosis* 36:539, 1980.

249. Valle, K.-J., and Bauer, E. A.: Biosynthesis of collagenase by human skin fibroblasts in monolayer culture. *J. Biol. Chem.* 254:10115, 1979.

250. Bourdillon, M. C., Brechmier, D., Blaes, N., Derouette, J. C. Hornebeck, W., and Robert, L.: Elastase-like enzymes in skin fibroblasts and rat aorta smooth muscle cells. *Cell Biol. Int. Rep.* 4:313, 1980.

251. Ross, R., Gomset, J., Kariya, B., and Harker, L.: A platelet-dependent serum factor that stimulates the proliferation of arterial smooth muscle cells in vitro. *Proc. Natl. Acad. Sci. U.S.A.* 71:1207, 1974.

252. Kohler, N., and Lipton, A.: Platelets as a source of fibroblast growth-promoting activity. *Exp. Cell Res.* 87:297, 1974.

253. Deuel, T. F., et al.: Human platelet-derived growth factor: Purification and resolution into two active protein fractions. *J. Biol. Chem.* 256:8896, 1981.

254. Heldin, C.-H., Westermark, B., and Wasteson, A.: Specific receptors for platelet-derived growth factor on cells derived from connective tissue and glia. *Proc. Natl. Acad. Sci. U.S.A.* 78:3664, 1981.

255. Haudenschild, C. C., Zahniser, D., Folkman, J., and Klagsbrun, M.: Human vascular endothelial cells in culture: Lack of response to serum growth factors. *Exp. Cell Res.* 98:175, 1976.

256. Wall, R. T., Harker, L. A., Quadracci, L. J., and Striker, G. E.: Factors influencing endothelial cell proliferation in vitro. *J. Cell Physiol.* 96:203, 1978.

257. Grotendorst, G. R., Seppa, H. E. J., Kleinman, H. K., and Martin, G. R.: Attachment of smooth muscle cells to collagen and their migration toward platelet-derived growth factor. *Proc. Natl. Acad. Sci. U.S.A.* 78:3669, 1981.

258. Van Horn, D. L., and Johnson, S. A.: The escape of carbon from intact capillaries in experimental thrombocytopenia. *J. Lab. Clin. Med.* 71:301, 1968.

259. Gore, I., Takada, M., and Austin, J.: Ultrastructural basis of experimental thrombocytopenic purpura. *Arch. Pathol.* 90:197, 1970.

260. Roy, A. J., and Djerassi, I.: Effects of platelet transfusions: Plug formation and maintenance of vascular integrity. *Proc. Soc. Exp. Biol. Med.* 139:137, 1972.

261. Kitchens, C. S., and Weiss, L.: Ultrastructural changes of endothelium associated with thrombocytopenia. *Blood* 46:567, 1975.

262. Johnson, S. A., Balboa, R. S., Dessel, B. H., Monto, R. W., Siegesmund, K. A., and Greenwalt, T. J.: The mechanism of the endothelial supporting function of intact platelets. *Exp. Med. Pathol.* 3:115, 1964.

263. Gimbrone, M. A., Jr., et al.: Preservation of vascular integrity in organs perfused in vitro with a platelet-rich medium. *Nature* 222:33, 1969.

264. Maca, R. D., Fry, G. L., Hoak, J. C., and Loh, P.-M.: The effects of intact platelets in cultured human endothelial cells. *Thromb. Res.* 11:715, 1977.

265. Robson, H. N., and Duthie, J. J. R.: Capillary resistance and adrenocortical activity. *Br. Med. J.* 2:971, 1950.

266. Faloon, W. W., Greene, R. W., and Lozner, E. L.: The hemostatic defect in thrombocytopenia as studied by the use of ACTH and cortisone. *Am. J. Med.* 13:12, 1952.

267. Kitchens, C. S.: Amelioration of endothelial abnormalities by prednisone in experimental thrombocytopenia in the rabbit. *J. Clin. Invest.* 60:1129, 1977.

268. Maca, R. D., Fry, G. L., and Hoak, J. C.: The effects of glucocorticoids on cultured human endothelial cells. *Br. J. Haematol.* 38:501, 1978.

269. Kramar, J.: Stress and capillary resistance (capillary fragility). *Am. J. Physiol.* 175:69, 1953.

270. Kramar, J., Meyers, V. W., McCarthy, H. H., and Simay-Kramar, M.: Further studies on the endocrine relations on capillary resistance. *Endocrinology* 60:589, 1957.

271. Stolman, J. M., Goldman, H. M., and Gould, B. S.: Ascorbic acid and blood vessels. *Arch. Pathol.* 72:59, 1961.

272. Kramar, J.: Capillary resistance and its relation to bleeding, in *Blood Platelets*, edited by S. A. Johnson, R. W. Monto, J. W. Rebuck, and R. C. Horn, Jr. Little, Brown, Boston, 1961, p. 41.

273. Conley, C. L.: Unpublished experiments.

274. Humble, J. G.: The mechanism of petechial hemorrhage formation. *Blood* 4:69, 1949.

275. Ashford, T. P., and Freiman, D. G.: The role of the endothelium in the initial phases of thrombosis: An electron microscopic study. *Am. J. Pathol.* 50:257, 1967.

276. Orchard, M. A., and Robinson, C.: Stability of prostacyclin in human plasma and whole blood: Studies on the protective effect of albumin. *Thrombos. Haemostas.* 46:645, 1981.

277. Baenziger, N. L., Fogerty, F. J., Mertz, L. F., and Chernuta, L. F.: Regulation of histamine-mediated prostacyclin synthesis in cultured human vascular endothelial cells. *Cell* 24:915, 1981.

278. Björck, C., Larsson, R., Olsson, P., and Rothman, U.: Uptake and inactivation of thrombin by the fresh, glutardialdehyde or heparin treated human umbilical cord. *Thromb. Res.* 21:603, 1981.

279. Comp, P. C., Jacocks, R. M., Ferrell, G. L., and Esmon, C. T.: Activation of protein C in vivo. *J. Clin. Invest.* 70:127, 1982.

280. Marlar, R. A., Kleiss, A. J., and Griffin, J. H.: Mechanism of action of human activated protein C, a thrombin-dependent anticoagulant enzyme. *Blood* 59:1067, 1982.

281. Esmon, N. L., Owen, W. G., and Esmon, C. T.: Isolation of a membrane-bound cofactor for thrombin-catalyzed activation of protein C. *J. Biol. Chem.* 257:859, 1982.

282. Booyse, F. M., et al.: Immunological identification and comparison of plasminogen activator forms in cultured normal human endothelial cells and smooth muscle cells. *Thromb. Res.* 24:495, 1981.

283. Johnson, G. J., Holloway, D. E., Hutton, S. W., and Duane, W. C.: Platelet function in scurvy and experimental human vitamin C deficiency. *Thromb. Res.* 24:85, 1981.

Disorders of hemostasis—classification

CHAPTER *140*

Classification of disorders of hemostasis

WILLIAM J. WILLIAMS

Disorders of hemostasis may be divided into those caused by abnormalities of platelets, abnormalities of blood vessels, and abnormalities of plasma coagulation factors, or combinations of these. The disorders are best classified in terms of the functional abnormality and the mechanism through which this abnormality is effected. This is generally possible for the quantita-tive and qualitative platelet abnormalities. However, our knowledge of the pathogenesis of the group of diseases referred to as nonthrombocytopenic purpura is limited, and these are classified together as vascular disorders because of clinical similarities and the ap-parent common basis of abnormalities of the small vessels.

The congenital abnormalities of blood coagulation may be classified readily in terms of the deficient activ-ity of a factor. Immunologic studies have demonstrated that some patients with deficiencies of prothrombin (factor II) or of factors VII, VIII, IX, or X have in their blood a substance which reacts with antibodies to the respective normal factor, suggesting the synthesis of an abnormal factor rather than failure of synthesis of the factor. In the case of prothrombin and factors VII, IX, and X, there is evidence of some aberrant function of the abnormal factors. Molecular abnormalities of fibrinogen (dysfibrinogenemias) also occur. Von Wille-brand's disease must be classified as a separate entity and is here considered as a deficiency of a plasma coagulation factor, although it is recognized that the abnormalities in this disease have not been defined precisely. Patients with prekallikrein deficiency (Fletcher trait) and deficiencies of plasma high-molec-ular-weight kininogen (Fitzgerald, Flaujeac, or Williams traits), like those with factor XII deficiency, apparently have no significant hemostatic abnormality, but these conditions are included because they cause abnormal coagulation tests.

TABLE 140-1 Disorders of hemostasis

I. Platelet disorders
  A. Quantitative platelet disorders
    1. Thrombocytopenia
      a. Thrombocytopenia caused by diminished or defective platelet production
        (1) Congenital
          (*a*) Constitutional pancytopenia (Fanconi syn-drome)
          (*b*) Amegakaryocytic thrombocytopenia with congenital malformations
          (*c*) Thrombopoietin deficiency
          (*d*) Hereditary thrombocytopenia (sex-linked, autosomal dominant, autosomal reces-sive)
          (*e*) Marrow infiltration (congenital leukemia, reticuloendotheliosis)
          (*f*) Neonatal rubella
          (*g*) Associated with maternal ingestion of thiazide diuretics
        (2) Acquired
          (*a*) Aplastic anemia
          (*b*) Megakaryocytic aplasia
          (*c*) Marrow infiltration (carcinoma, leukemia, myelofibrosis, tuberculosis, etc.)
          (*d*) Ionizing radiation, myelosuppressive drugs
          (*e*) Drugs which act specifically on platelet production (thiazide diuretics, alcohol, estrogens, interferon)
          (*f*) Cyclic thrombocytopenia
          (*g*) Nutritional deficiency (vitamin B$_{12}$, folic acid, ? iron)
          (*h*) Viral infections (measles, dengue, etc.)
          (*i*) Paroxysmal nocturnal hemoglobinuria
          (*j*) Renal failure
          (*k*) Hyperbaric exposure
      b. Thrombocytopenia caused predominantly by enhanced platelet destruction
        (1) Congenital
          (*a*) Nonimmune
            i. Erythroblastosis fetalis
            ii. Prematurity
            iii. Maternal preeclampsia
            iv. Renal vein thrombosis
            v. Infection
            vi. Indwelling umbilical catheter
            vii. Thrombocytopenia-hemangioma syndrome
          (*b*) Immune
            i. Drug sensitivity
            ii. Isoimmune neonatal thrombocyto-penia
            iii. Maternal idiopathic thrombocytope-nic purpura

TABLE 140-1 Disorders of hemostasis (*Continued*)

    (2) Acquired
        (*a*) Nonimmune
            i. Infection
            ii. Disseminated intravascular coagulation
            iii. Thrombotic thrombocytopenic purpura
            iv. Hemolytic-uremic syndrome
            v. Drug-induced
        (*b*) Immune
            i. Antilymphocyte globulin
            ii. Tn syndrome
            iii. Drug-induced
            iv. Anaphylaxis
            v. Posttransfusion purpura
            vi. Idiopathic thrombocytopenic purpura
                a) Acute
                b) Chronic
    c. Thrombocytopenia caused predominantly by sequestration of platelets
        (1) Hypersplenism
        (2) Hypothermia
    d. Thrombocytopenia caused predominantly by loss of platelets
        (1) Hemorrhage
        (2) Extracorporeal perfusion
  2. Thrombocytosis
    a. Primary (autonomous)
        (1) Essential thrombocythemia
        (2) Other myeloproliferative disorders
    b. Secondary (reactive)
        (1) Chronic inflammatory disorders
        (2) Acute inflammatory disorders
        (3) Acute hemorrhage
        (4) Iron deficiency
        (5) Hemolytic anemia
        (6) Malignant disease
        (7) Postoperative
        (8) Response to drugs
        (9) Response to exercise
 B. Qualitative platelet disorders
  1. Congenital
    a. Defects of adhesion: Bernard-Soulier (giant platelet) syndrome
    b. Defects of primary aggregation: thrombasthenia (Glanzmann's)
    c. Abnormal platelet secretion
        (1) Storage pool disease
        (2) Primary defects in platelet secretion
    d. Abnormal procoagulant activity (platelet factor 3)
    e. Platelet abnormalities associated with other congenital defects
        (1) Thrombocytopenia with absent radius, Wiscott-Aldrich syndrome, Hermansky-Pudlak syndrome (albinism)
        (2) May-Hegglin anomaly
        (3) Connective tissue disorders (Ehlers-Danlos syndrome, etc.)
        (4) Miscellaneous disorders
  2. Acquired
    a. Uremia
    b. Myeloproliferative disorders
    c. Dysproteinemias

    d. Liver disease
    e. Idiopathic thrombocytopenic purpura
    f. Storage pool deficiency
    g. Drug-induced
II. Vascular disorders
 A. Nonthrombocytopenic purpura
  1. Nonallergic, nonthrombocytopenic purpura
    a. Purpura simplex
    b. Mechanical purpura
    c. Orthostatic purpura
    d. Senile purpura
    e. Adrenocortical hyperfunction
    f. Hereditary disorders of connective tissue
    g. Scurvy
    h. Purpura associated with dysproteinemia
    i. Purpura associated with infections
  2. Autoerythrocyte sensitivity
  3. DNA sensitivity
  4. Allergic purpura
 B. Hereditary hemorrhagic telangiectasia
III. Disorders of blood coagulation
 A. Congenital
  1. Caused by abnormalities of plasma factors involved in fibrin formation
    a. Deficient synthesis of specific factors
        (1) Fibrinogen (factor I)
        (2) Prothrombin (factor II)
        (3) Factor V and factors VII to XIII
        (4) Passovoy factor
    b. Synthesis of immunologically reactive but functionally inactive factors
        (1) Prothrombin (factor II)
        (2) Factors VII, VIII, IX, and X
    c. Synthesis of functionally abnormal factors
        (1) Fibrinogen (factor I)
        (2) Prothrombin (factor II)
        (3) Factors VII, IX, or X
        (4) Combined deficiency of prothrombin and factors VII, IX, and X
    d. Deficiency of factors giving abnormal laboratory tests but no clinically significant bleeding
        (1) Factor XII
        (2) Prekallikrein (Fletcher trait)
        (3) High-molecular-weight kininogen (Fitzgerald, Flaujeac, Williams traits)
  2. Caused by abnormalities of plasma factors involved in platelet function and in fibrin formation: von Willebrand's disease
  3. Caused by deficiency of plasma protease inhibitor
    a. Combined deficiency of factors V and VIII
    b. α_2-Antiplasmin deficiency
 B. Acquired
  1. Vitamin K deficiency
  2. Liver disease
  3. Amyloidosis
  4. Nephrotic syndrome
  5. Gaucher's disease
  6. Systemic lupus erythematosus
  7. Circulating anticoagulants
  8. Defibrination syndromes
    a. Disseminated intravascular coagulation
    b. Fibrinolysis
IV. Thrombosis

Disorders of hemostasis—quantitative platelet disorders

CHAPTER 141

Thrombocytopenia due to diminished or defective platelet production

RICHARD H. ASTER

Pseudothrombocytopenia

Artifactual "thrombocytopenia" can be produced by several different mechanisms after blood initially containing a normal number of platelets is collected and anticoagulated; this condition can occur in patients with a wide variety of clinical disorders [1–5]. Platelet autoagglutinins having the characteristics of IgG and IgM immunoglobulins have been described as heterogeneous in their mechanisms of action [1,4,5]. Some cause agglutination only in the presence of EDTA [3–5]; others act independently of the anticoagulant used [1]. In a prospective study, 3 of 1300 blood samples referred for hematologic study manifested autoagglutination [3]. In some patients, pseudothrombocytopenia is associated with the adherence of platelets to neutrophilic granulocytes (rosette formation) in blood anticoagulated with EDTA, a reaction possibly mediated by IgG immunoglobulins [2,6]. In several reported instances, platelet-granulocyte rosetting appears to have been associated with true thrombocytopenia [7]. Pseudothrombocytopenia is particularly prone to confuse the clinician when platelet levels are determined with an automated particle counter. This condition should be ruled out by carefully examining a well-prepared blood film before concluding that a patient is truly thrombocytopenic.

Congenital thrombocytopenia

CONSTITUTIONAL APLASTIC ANEMIA (FANCONI SYNDROME)

Pancytopenia due to aplasia of the marrow can occur with or without other anomalies [8,9]. Hematologic changes usually become prominent at 6 to 8 years of age but may appear as early as 18 months. Thrombocytopenia often precedes granulocytopenia and anemia, and platelets respond less readily to therapy than do other blood elements. For a discussion of treatment and prognosis, see Chap. 20.

AMEGAKARYOCYTIC THROMBOCYTOPENIA WITH CONGENITAL MALFORMATIONS (THROMBOCYTOPENIA WITH ABSENT RADIUS SYNDROME)

Congenital deficiency of megakaryocytes occurring with skeletal, renal, or cardiac malformations is a rare cause of thrombocytopenic purpura in the newborn [10,11]. Bilateral aplasia of the radii is the most commonly associated abnormality. Thrombocytopenia is usually severe, and only occasional megakaryocytes are found in the marrow. A granulocytic leukemoid reaction is sometimes present. As the radii, heart, and megakaryocytes all develop at about 6 to 8 weeks of gestation, the disorder may be a result of an intrauterine disturbance occurring at this stage. Rubella has been implicated in several instances [12]. Siblings and sometimes cousins may be affected [11]. Prenatal radiographic diagnosis is possible at 16 to 20 weeks of gestation [13]. An association with milk allergy has been suggested [14], and in several instances platelets have been shown to be functionally abnormal [15]. In occasional patients, significant bleeding may not occur for the first time until adulthood [16,17].

The prognosis is poor. More than half of the patients die within the first 8 months of life, usually of intracranial hemorrhage. Of the remaining patients, most gradually improve and have less difficulty with bleeding. Those with only moderate thrombocytopenia at birth appear to have a better outlook.

There is no uniformly accepted mode of therapy. Glucocorticoids and splenectomy have generally been found to be without benefit. However, one adult whose marrow contained significant numbers of megakaryocytes responded dramatically to removal of the spleen [16]. Serious hemorrhage can be treated effectively with platelet transfusions. Whether prophylactic platelet transfusions given during the first year of life can reduce overall mortality has not been established.

"THROMBOPOIETIN" DEFICIENCY

As noted in Chap. 130, strong but partially circumstantial evidence suggests that hormonal substances ("thrombopoietins") normally stimulate platelet production. One child who was apparently deficient in thrombopoietin from birth has been studied extensively [18–20]. Bleeding episodes dated from the first year of life. Severe thrombocytopenia was documented at age 8. The hemoglobin level and leukocyte count were normal. Megakaryocytes were present in the marrow, but most were immature or "granular but nonproducing." Treatment with glucocorticoids and splenectomy were ineffective, but after splenectomy transfusions of whole blood or plasma repeatedly caused megakaryocytes to mature and restored platelet levels to normal for approximately 2 weeks. Subsequent studies suggested that the patient lacked an α_2-globulin, which could be recovered from normal plasma and was capable of stimulating thrombopoiesis when injected into rats. The active material was differentiated from erythropoietin [19].

The patient's subsequent course was marked by several remissions lasting for about 1 year and terminated by infections, an episode of hypertension and nephritis at age 13, and a hemolytic process of unknown etiology [20].

It seems probable that this patient lacked a humoral material necessary for normal megakaryocyte development. Whether this substance is a definitive thrombopoietic hormone has not yet been ascertained. A possibly similar disorder involving several members of one family has been described in a brief report [21].

HEREDITARY THROMBOCYTOPENIA

A number of familial forms of thrombocytopenia have been described. In most, the basic abnormality is unknown and data on marrow morphology and platelet kinetics are sketchy. These disorders are therefore best classified by their mode of inheritance. In the interest of covering the hereditary thrombocytopenias together, disorders in which platelet life-span is thought to be shortened because of genetically determined platelet defects will be discussed together with those in which platelet production is thought to be inadequate.

SEX-LINKED THROMBOCYTOPENIA

The Wiskott-Aldrich syndrome is a disorder of males characterized by eczema, thrombocytopenia with microplatelets, and susceptibility to infections associated with defects in cellular and humoral immunity. Death at an early age commonly results from intracranial hemorrhage, infection, or lymphoreticular malignancy [22–24] (see also Chap. 112). Bleeding is common during the first year of life but sometimes becomes less severe thereafter. Both platelets and megakaryocytes show deranged ultrastructure when viewed by electron microscopy [25]. An abnormality of aerobic metabolism of glucose by platelets has been reported [26]. The absolute number of megakaryocytes is normal or increased. Survival of homologous platelets is normal, but autologous platelets have a shortened life-span [23,26]. It is highly probable that thrombocytopenia is caused by an abnormality of megakaryocyte development resulting in both ineffective thrombopoiesis and shortened platelet life-span. Glucocorticoids have little or no effect on platelet levels. In a recently reported series, splenectomy resulted in normalization of platelet size and platelet count in a high percentage of cases [27]. It is essential, however, that patients who undergo splenectomy be maintained on prophylactic antibiotic therapy [27]. Treatment with transfer factor appeared to be beneficial in 14 of 32 cases [28]. In patients for whom a compatible donor is available, marrow transplantation can be curative [29]. An approach to the diagnosis of the heterozygous carrier state based on the effect of glycolytic inhibitors on platelet aggregation has been described [30]. In some cases, selection against cells carrying the Wiskott-Aldrich defect can also be used for this purpose [24].

A number of kindreds are reported in whom sex-linked thrombocytopenia has occurred alone [31], together with partial manifestations of the Wiskott-Aldrich syndrome [32], or in association with other abnormalities [33,34]. Some patients are benefited by glucocorticoid treatment and splenectomy, and most of these disorders appear to be compatible with normal survival [31–34].

AUTOSOMAL DOMINANT THROMBOCYTOPENIA

The May-Hegglin anomaly is a rare disorder inherited as an autosomal dominant trait and characterized by bizarre giant platelets and basophilic inclusions (Döhle bodies) within granulocytes. One-half of the patients have thrombocytopenia, which may be severe on occasion. Megakaryocytes are present in normal numbers, but a defect in their maturation has been suggested on the basis of cytophotometric studies [35]. Platelets are more than twice normal size and contain giant granules, possibly arising by fusion [36]. Survival time of platelets is normal [36,37]. In a minority of cases, platelet functional abnormalities are present [36]. The primary defect may be one of megakaryocyte maturation and fragmentation [35,37].

Thrombocytopenia with giant platelets and a moderately severe bleeding tendency but no associated granulocyte abnormality has been observed in a number of families [38–40]. An association with "variant" von Willebrand's disease has been recorded [41]. Electron microscopic studies have demonstrated decreased numbers of α-granules [38] and normal platelet ultrastructure [41]. In some patients with macrothrombocytopenia, platelet levels fluctuate widely between normal and severely thrombocytopenic values [39]. Both normal and shortened survival of autologous platelets have been reported, indicating that this group of patients is not homogeneous. Glucocorticoids appeared to be of therapeutic value in two instances [38].

Macrothrombocytopenia associated with nerve deafness and nephritis (Alport's syndrome) has been observed in a number of families [42,43]. Platelet ultrastructure is relatively normal [42,43], but abnormal megakaryocytes have been described [44]. Platelet function was found to be normal in some [42] and abnormal in others [43]. Macrothrombocytes and moderate thrombocytopenia and splenomegaly have been described in a high percentage of persons of Mediterranean origin, often in association with stomatocytosis [45]. The mode of inheritance, if any, has not been clearly established. The total circulating platelet mass is almost identical to that of normal subjects, and there is no bleeding tendency. *Mediterranean macrothrombocytopenia* is therefore a benign morphologic variant.

Thrombocytopenia with normal platelet morphology may also be inherited as a dominant trait [46–48]. The bleeding tendency is mild. Platelet function may be impaired [47]. Von Willebrand's disease [49] and factor IX deficiency [50] were found in association with reduced platelet levels in several families. In two well-studied cases from the same family, survival of autologous platelets was much shorter than normal and an intrinsic platelet defect was postulated [47].

AUTOSOMAL RECESSIVE THROMBOCYTOPENIA
Only a few kindreds with thrombocytopenia inherited as an autosomal recessive trait have been reported [51,52]. The number of megakaryocytes was markedly reduced in one instance [51] and increased in another [52]. In the latter family, giant platelets were present which appeared to have a very short life-span. Splenectomy resulted in partial improvement [52]. *The gray platelet syndrome*, characterized by widely fluctuating platelet levels and giant platelets lacking alpha storage granules, is probably an autosomal recessive trait [53]. Two other qualitative platelet disorders, the Bernard-Soulier syndrome and the Montreal platelet syndrome [54], are often associated with thrombocytopenia (see Chap. 146).

INFILTRATIVE DISEASE OF MARROW
Congenital thrombocytopenia caused by marrow infiltration is extremely rare, being limited essentially to cases of disseminated reticuloendotheliosis [55] and congenital leukemia [56].

NEONATAL RUBELLA AND CYTOMEGALOVIRUS INFECTION
Thrombocytopenia, sometimes very severe, is commonly seen in newborn infants infected with rubella [57,58] or cytomegalovirus [59]. Platelet levels were low in 70 of 200 infants with rubella in one series [57]. Megakaryocytes are often diminished in number. A suppressive effect of the virus on platelet production has been postulated but not established [57]. In surviving infants, platelet levels return to normal, but several months may be required [57,58].

MATERNAL INGESTION OF THIAZIDE DIURETICS
Neonatal thrombocytopenic purpura has been reported in seven infants born to mothers being treated with thiazide diuretics during pregnancy [60]. Fatal cerebral hemorrhage occurred in one. Megakaryocytes were diminished in number in three of five marrows examined and were completely absent in a fourth. Recovery occurred 1 to 2 weeks after birth. Platelet antibodies could not be detected in the maternal sera, and a toxic effect of the drug on fetal platelet production was postulated as the cause of thrombocytopenia [60]. In a prospective study, thrombocytopenia was observed in only 1 of 100 infants born to women who had taken thiazide diuretics for at least 3 weeks prepartum [61].

Acquired thrombocytopenia

APLASTIC ANEMIA
Acquired aplastic anemia is fully discussed in Chap. 20. In both the juvenile [8] and the adult [62] forms of the disorder, the platelet response may lag 3 to 9 months behind that of erythrocytes and leukocytes in patients who recover hematologically. Occasionally, thrombocytopenia persists despite restoration of hematocrit and leukocyte levels to normal [8,62].

MEGAKARYOCYTIC APLASIA
Thrombocytopenia due to selective aplasia of megakaryocytes unassociated with other underlying diseases has been reported in a number of patients [63,64]. Maturation of other marrow elements was normal. In one case, thrombopoietic activity was absent from urine and plasma and a defect in megakaryocyte maturation was postulated [63]. Aplastic anemia, systemic lupus erythematosus, and acute leukemia developed later in several instances [64]. By analogy with pure erythroid aplasia, an autoimmune etiology has been suspected but not proved.

MARROW INFILTRATION
Thrombocytopenia may result from marrow replacement by carcinoma, acute and chronic leukemia, lymphoma, and other malignant conditions. Generally, the peripheral blood picture is typical of myelophthisic disease (Chap. 52). When multiple foci of carcinoma are widely disseminated throughout the marrow, however, thrombocytopenia may be the most prominent abnormality [65,66]. Subnormal platelet levels and morphologically abnormal megakaryocytes are typically found in the *preleukemic syndrome* [67]. *Myelofibrosis* often causes thrombocytopenia, although platelet levels may also be elevated. Thrombocytopenia associated with *Gaucher disease* may, in part, be related to marrow infiltration with Gaucher cells, but splenomegaly is usually its major cause (Chap. 99). Thrombocytopenia and anemia are characteristic of the juvenile form of *osteopetrosis* and may be improved by splenectomy [68]. *Miliary tuberculosis* may present as thrombocytopenic purpura, but anemia and leukopenia are usually present as well [69,70]. Other granulomatous disorders in which thrombocytopenia occurs are mentioned in Chap. 142.

IONIZING RADIATION AND MYELOSUPPRESSIVE DRUGS
Platelet precursors may be slightly less sensitive to the effects of *whole-body irradiation* than are lymphocytic, erythroid, and granulocytic precursors [71]. Circulating platelets are unaffected. Following irradiation, platelets do not diminish in number for several days, indicating that committed megakaryocytes are able to mature and release platelets. The hemorrhagic diathesis which follows irradiation is chiefly the result of thrombocytopenia, although other factors, not yet fully understood, may also be operative [72].

All myelosuppressive drugs are capable of causing thrombocytopenia if given in sufficiently large dosage. Cytosine arabinoside is particularly toxic to megakaryocytes, and its use may be followed by sudden, severe thrombocytopenia. Cyclophosphamide, busulfan, methotrexate, and 6-mercaptopurine are intermediate in their toxicity [73]. Vinca alkaloids have relatively little depressant effect on platelet production, although they are effective against erythrocyte precursors [74]. Their use may actually result in elevated platelet levels [75]. Withdrawal of myelosuppressive therapy is often followed by thrombocytosis [76].

SUBSTANCES WHICH ACT SPECIFICALLY ON PLATELET PRODUCTION

The many agents capable of producing generalized marrow aplasia are discussed in Chap. 20. Several substances which appear to have a relatively specific effect on platelet production are considered here.

THIAZIDE DIURETICS

Thrombocytopenia associated with the use of chlorothiazide and other thiazide derivatives has been reported frequently [60,77–79]. In one series, 26 percent of 71 patients receiving these drugs had platelet levels of less than 100,000 per microliter, the lowest being 8000 per microliter [78]. In a few instances, immunologic studies have been interpreted as indicating the presence of drug-dependent antibodies of the type seen in patients with quinidine sensitivity (Chap. 142) [77,79]. Thiazide-induced thrombocytopenia contrasts with the quinidine variety, however, in the following respects: its onset is gradual rather than acute, it is mild rather than severe, megakaryocytes are sometimes diminished rather than increased in number [60], and a longer period, 1 to 4 weeks, of drug administration is required

to reinduce thrombocytopenia in sensitive patients [77,78]. It seems probable, therefore, that in some patients thiazide diuretics cause thrombocytopenia by suppressing platelet production through a toxic effect on the megakaryocytes of sensitive persons. The same drugs sometimes cause an erythematous purpuric rash without inducing thrombocytopenia [80].

ALCOHOL

Thrombocytopenia is commonly seen in patients with chronic alcoholism and may occur without accompanying vitamin deficiency, anemia, or splenomegaly [81,82]. Platelet levels as low as 14,000 per microliter have been recorded [82]. Megakaryocytes are normal [81,82] or diminished [83] in number. Alcohol may also induce platelet dysfunction by several mechanisms [84–86]. Following withdrawal of alcohol, platelet levels usually return to normal within 5 to 21 days and become markedly elevated in some subjects [81–84]. Thrombocytosis may also occur following withdrawal of alcohol from patients who are not thrombocytopenic at the time of hospital admission [81].

The cause of "alcohol thrombocytopenia" has not been definitely established. A transient increase in platelet levels occurred after 4 to 6 hours of alcohol infusion in one patient, suggesting a direct toxic effect on circulating platelets, but a second patient failed to show a similar response [82]. Others have found that ingestion of alcohol for 5 to 10 days is required to produce sustained thrombocytopenia [83,84] (Fig. 141-1) and that this is accomplished by a decrease in the number of

FIGURE 141-1   Effect of alcohol on platelet levels and megakaryocyte levels. On two occasions, a gradual decrease of both platelet and megakaryocyte levels occurred during a 2- to 3-week period of whiskey ingestion regardless of whether or not folic acid was administered simultaneously. (Sullivan [83].)

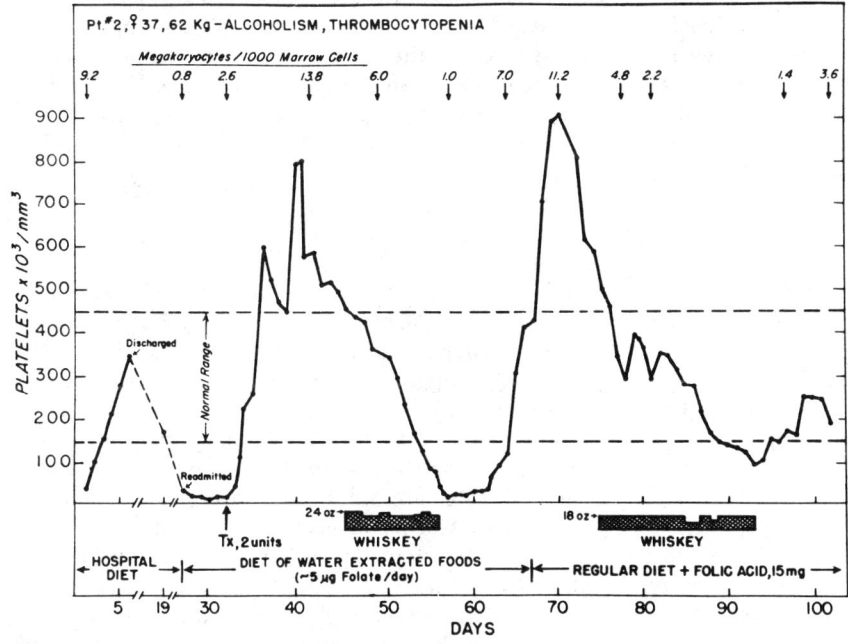

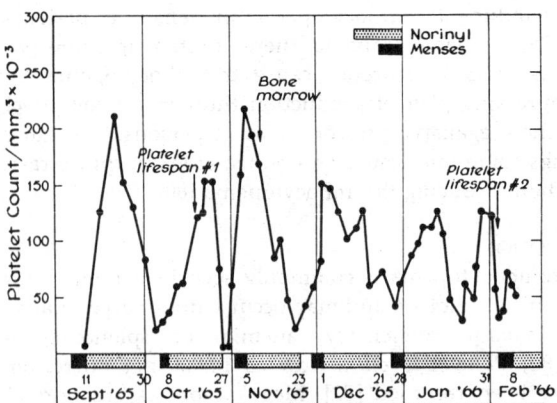

FIGURE 141-2 Cyclic thrombocytopenia in a 28-year-old woman. Cycles were of approximately 28 days. In later studies, they were found to occur out of phase with the menstrual cycle. (Cohen and Cooney [98].)

megakaryocytes [83]. Moreover, ingestion of alcohol inhibited the response to thrombocytopheresis-induced thrombocytopenia in normal men [87]. These observations suggest that alcohol acts to suppress platelet production in some individuals through an as yet unidentified mechanism. Reduction in platelet life-span may also contribute to the lowering of platelet levels [88].

ESTROGENS

Estrogenic hormones have been shown to impair hemopoiesis in animals [89], and numerous reports of thrombocytopenic purpura following prolonged administration of diethylstilbestrol and other estrogenic hormones in human beings have appeared in the literature [90,91]. In most cases, megakaryocytes were normal in number, but occasionally they were "very scanty" [90]. Platelets returned to normal after therapy was withdrawn, but up to 2 months was required. Readministration of diethylstilbestrol caused platelet levels to decrease from normal to less than 100,000 per microliter over a 3- to 5-day period on three occasions [91]. The mechanism of thrombocytopenia was not established, but a "subtle inhibition of platelet production" was postulated [91].

INTERFERON

Moderately severe thrombocytopenia, often associated with leukopenia and apparently due to hematosuppression, is a common side effect of treatment with leukocyte interferon [92,93]. Reduction in platelet levels may occur within 1 week of initial injections and can be reversed by reducing or discontinuing therapy [93].

PLATELETS IN PREGNANCY

A progressive decline in platelet levels during pregnancy to about 80 percent of the initial values, but not to thrombocytopenic levels, has been described [94]. In a second study, a more striking decline was observed [95], but in a third, no consistent change was noted [96].

CYCLIC THROMBOCYTOPENIA

In normal women, platelet levels decrease slightly during the 2 weeks preceding menstruation [97]. Occasionally the reduction is so marked that thrombocytopenic purpura occurs [98,99]. In one case, severe thrombocytopenia developed in midcycle at 28 day intervals over an 8-year-period [100]. Cyclic thrombocytopenia in younger women does not always occur in phase with the menstrual cycle [98] and may be so severe that serious bleeding occurs during the thrombocytopenic interval (Fig. 141-2) It may also affect postmenopausal women and has been reported in several males, each over the age of 50 [101,102]. In both males and females, the period of the thrombocytopenic cycle has averaged about 30 days, with a range of 20 to 40 days. Megakaryocytes have been judged to be diminished in number at the time platelets were lowest [101]. Platelet life-span is normal [98,99,102]. Measurements of plasma thrombopoietin levels in one patient yielded consistently low values [99]. Removal of autologous plasma at a time when platelet levels were falling and its reinfusion when platelets were at their peak was without effect in one case [98], but transfusion of plasma from a normal subject appeared to blunt the decline of platelets in another [99]. No endocrine abnormality has been demonstrated, and the course of this remarkable disorder has been unaffected by oophorectomy [100], splenectomy, and glucocorticoid therapy [98,100]. However, in one instance platelet levels were stabilized following administration of lynestrenol, an inhibitor of ovulation and menstruation [103].

The cause of cyclic thrombocytopenia is presently unknown. A similar disorder can be induced in dogs by infection with a rickettsia-like organism [104], but there is no evidence for an infectious etiology in humans. As noted in Chap. 130, there are feedback mechanisms capable of regulating the production of platelets. The primary defect in this disorder may be abnormal responsiveness of the marrow to either positive or negative feedback stimuli, resulting in regular alternation between excessive and inadequate platelet production, i.e., a state of stable oscillation [105].

NUTRITIONAL DEFICIENCY

MEGALOBLASTIC ANEMIA

In patients with pernicious anemia and folic acid deficiency, platelets are often reduced in number. Occasionally thrombocytopenia is so severe that bleeding is the presenting complaint [106]. Three mechanisms probably account for reduced platelet levels: platelet life-span is shortened by one third to one half [107], ineffective megakaryocytopoeisis occurs [108], and, in severe cases, megakaryocytes are diminished in number or entirely absent [109]. Associated alcoholism may also contribute to the thrombocytopenia (see above). Functional abnormalities of circulating platelets have been described [110,111]. The response of platelets to specific therapy usually parallels that of reticulocytes, but it may occur earlier or later. In one report, it was suggested that red cell transfusions induced lower platelet levels after 2 to 6 days in some patients through an undefined mechanism [112].

IRON DEFICIENCY

Although iron deficiency is commonly associated with thrombocytosis, moderate thrombocytopenia (platelet counts from 50,000 to 100,000 per microliter) is sometimes seen in children and adults with severe iron deficiency anemia [113,114]. The increase in platelet levels which occurs in thrombocytopenic patients after iron therapy has been interpreted as a specific response to iron [113]. It is possible that in some patients the thrombocytopenia is a result of a coexisting folic acid deficiency and that the rise in platelet levels results from correction of that deficiency by a hospital diet and improved gastrointestinal function following iron therapy. However, in several reported instances a rise in platelet levels appeared to result from iron therapy alone [115,116]. Evidence has been presented that iron may be essential for platelet production [117] (see Chap. 130).

VIRAL INFECTIONS

Experimental studies in animals have shown that megakaryocytes provide ideal sites for viral replication both in vitro and in vivo [118,119], suggesting that viruses may interfere with megakaryocyte maturation in infected patients. During the 4 to 5 days following innoculation with live *measles vaccine*, platelet levels became progressively lower in 38 of 44 children, the average reduction being 98,000 per microliter [120] (Fig. 141-3). At the same time, megakaryocytes developed vacuolation and nuclear degeneration and became reduced in number. Up to 2 weeks were required for restoration of platelet levels to normal. Low plasma acid phosphatase values suggested that platelet production was suppressed. In occasional patients, more severe thrombocytopenia with purpura occurs 1 to 2 weeks after measles vaccination [121]. This may, however, be a result of peripheral destruction of platelets by immune mechanisms rather than of suppression of platelet production (Chap. 142).

Thrombocytopenia may occur in the course of many other viral illnesses (Chap. 142). To what extent this is caused by hematosuppression is unclear because few systematic studies of platelet survival have been reported. In congenital *rubella*, discussed earlier, megakaryocytes are sometimes decreased in number, suggesting that platelet production is impaired. In *infectious mononucleosis*, a significant reduction in platelet levels commonly occurs during the incubation period and the acute stage [122]. In *Thai hemorrhagic fever* and the closely related *dengue fever*, thrombocytopenic purpura may be very severe. There are degenerative changes in megakaryocytes [123] similar to those described after administration of live measles vaccine [120]. These changes have been interpreted as indicating that the virus interferes with platelet production

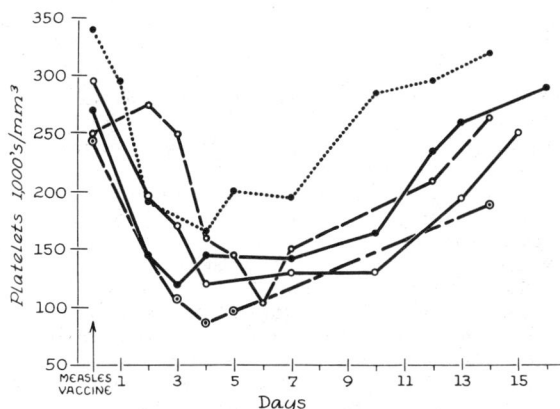

FIGURE 141-3 Effect of live measles vaccine on platelet levels of five normal children. (Oski and Naiman [120].)

[123]. More recent studies indicate that platelet destruction may be a more important cause of reduced platelet levels [124].

PAROXYSMAL NOCTURNAL HEMOGLOBINURIA

Paroxysmal nocturnal hemoglobinuria (PNH) is described in detail in Chap. 21. Platelet levels may be as low as 10,000 per microliter or normal, but are usually in the range of 50,000 to 100,000 per microliter. Although platelets manifest the membrane abnormality characteristic of red blood cells in this disorder [125], platelet lifespan is normal [125,126], indicating that reduced platelet levels are caused primarily by insufficient platelet production. The diagnosis of PNH should be entertained in all patients who have unexplained chronic thrombocytopenia.

RENAL FAILURE

Thrombocytopenia of moderate severity occurs in 15 to 50 percent of patients with renal failure [127–129]. Platelet levels are generally restored to normal after resolution of the primary disorder or effective hemodialysis. In such patients, it is likely that reduction of platelet levels is a consequence of the disorder provoking the renal failure, rather than of the uremic state per se. Platelet dysfunction is more important than thrombocytopenia in the pathogenesis of bleeding [129].

HYPERBARIC EXPOSURE

A progressive reduction in platelet levels to about 75 percent of initial values occurred over a 3-day period in normal persons after exposure to hyperbaric conditions in several simulated diving experiments [130]. Platelet survival remained normal, and it was postulated that platelet production was impaired by an undefined mechanism. In animals subjected to rapid decompression after hyperbaria, severe thrombocytopenia may develop, but this appears to be due to the formation of platelet microaggregates in the lungs and other tissues [131].

References

1. Watkins, S. P., Jr., and Shulman, N. R.: Platelet cold agglutinins. *Blood* 36:153, 1970.
2. Kjeldsberg, C. R., and Hershgold, E. J.: Spurious thrombocytopenia. *JAMA* 227:628, 1974.
3. Mant, M. J., Doery, J. C. G., Gauldie, J., and Sims, H.: Pseudothrombocytopenia due to platelet aggregation and degranulation in blood collected in EDTA. *Scand. J. Haematol.* 15:11, 1975.
4. Veenhoven, W. A., et al.: Pseudothrombocytopenia due to agglutinins. *Am. J. Clin. Pathol.* 72:1005, 1979.
5. Onder, O., Weinstein, A., and Hoyer, L. W.: Pseudothrombocytopenia caused by platelet agglutinins that are reactive in blood anticoagulated with chelating agents. *Blood* 56:177, 1980.
6. Ziegler, Z.: *In vitro* granulocyte-platelet rosette formation mediated by an IgG immunoglobulin. *Haemostasis* 3:282, 1974.
7. White, L. A. Jr., Brubaker, L. H., Aster, R. H., Henry, P. H., and Adelstein, E. H.: Platelet satellitism and phagocytosis by neutrophils: Association with antiplatelet antibodies and lymphoma. *Am. J. Hematol.* 4:313, 1978.
8. Shahidi, N. T., and Diamond, L. K.: Testosterone-induced remission in aplastic anemia in both acquired and congenital types. *N. Engl. J. Med.* 264:953, 1961.
9. Minagi, H. J., and Steinbach, H.: Roentgen appearance of anomalies associated with hypoplastic anemia of childhood: Fanconi's anemia and congenital hypoplastic anemia (erythrogenesis imperfecta). *Am. J. Roentgenol.* 97:100, 1966.
10. Hall, J. G., et al.: Thrombocytopenia with absent radius (TAR). *Medicine* 48:411, 1969.
11. Edelberg, S. B., Cohn, J., and Brandt, N. J., Congenital hypomegakaryocytic thrombocytopenia associated with bilateral absence of the radius—the TAR syndrome: Intra-family variation of the clinical picture. *Hum. Hered.* 27:147, 1977.
12. Berge, T., Brunnhage, F., and Nisson, L. R.: Congenital thrombocytopenia in rubella embryopathy. *Acta Paediatr. Scand.* 52:349, 1963.
13. Luthy, D. A., Hall., J. G., and Graham, C. B.: Prenatal diagnosis of thrombocytopenia with absent radii. *Clin. Genet.* 15:495, 1979.
14. Whitfield, M. F., and Barr, D. G.: Cow's milk allergy in the syndrome of thrombocyotpenia with absent radii. *Arch. Dis. Child.* 51:337, 1976.
15. Day, H. J., and Holmsen, H.: Platelet adenine nucleotide storage pool deficiency in the thrombocytopenic absent radii syndrome. *JAMA* 221:1053, 1972.
16. Armitage, J. O., Hoak, J. C., Elliott, T. E., and Fry, G. L.: Syndrome of thrombocytopenia and absent radii: Qualitatively normal platelets with remission following splenectomy. *Scand. J. Haematol.* 20:25, 1978.
17. Fayen, W. T., and Harris, J. W.: Case report: Thrombocytopenia with absent radii (the TAR syndrome). *Am. J. Med. Sci.* 280:95, 1980.
18. Shulman, I., Pierce, M., Lukens, A., and Currimbhoy, Z.: Studies on thrombopoiesis. I. A factor in normal human plasma required for platelet production: Chronic thrombocytopenia due to its deficiency. *Blood* 16:943, 1960.
19. Schulman, I., Abildgaard, C. F., Cornet, J., Simone, J. V., and Currimbhoy, Z.: Studies on thrombopoiesis. II. Assay of human plasma thrombopoietic activity. *J. Pediatr.* 66:604, 1965.
20. Abildgaard, C. F., and Simone, J. V.: Thrombopoiesis. *Semin. Hematol.* 4:424, 1967.
21. Vildosola, J., and Emparanza, E.: Hereditary familial thrombocytopenia, in *Proceedings of the Xth International Congress on Pediatrics.* Lisbon, 1962, p. 36.
22. Perry, G. S., et al.: The Wiskott-Aldrich syndrome in the United States and Canada (1892–1979). *J. Pediatr.* 97:72, 1980.
23. Ochs, H. D., Slichter, S. J., Harker, L. A., Von Behrens, W. E., Clark, R. A., and Wedgwood, R. J.: The Wiscott-Aldrich syndrome: Studies of lymphocytes, granulocytes, and platelets. *Blood* 55:243, 1980.
24. Prchal, J. T., et al.: Wiskott-Aldrich syndrome: Cellular impairments and their implication for carrier detection. *Blood* 56:1048, 1980.
25. Grottum, K. A., Hovig, T., Holmsen, H., Abrahamsen, A. F., Jeremic, M., and Seip, M.: Wiscott-Aldrich syndrome: Qualitative platelet defects and short platelet survival. *Br. J. Haematol.* 17:373, 1969.
26. Kuramoto, H., Steiner, M., and Baldini, M.: Lack of platelet response to stimulation in the Wiscott-Aldrich syndrome. *N. Engl. J. Med.* 282:475, 1970.
27. Lum, L. G., Tubergen, D. G., Corash, L., and Blaese, R. M.: Splenectomy in the management of the thrombocytopenia of the Wiskott-Aldrich syndrome. *N. Engl. J. Med.* 302:892, 1980.
28. Spitler, L. E.: Transfer factor therapy in the Wiskott-Aldrich syndrome: Results of long-term follow-up in 32 patients. *Am. J. Med.* 67:59, 1979.
29. Parkman, R., et al.: Complete correction of the Wiskott-Aldrich syndrome by allogeneic bone-marrow transplantation. *N. Engl. J. Med.* 298:921, 1978.
30. Shapiro, R. S., Perry, G. S., III, Krivit, W., Gerrard, J. M., White, J. G., and Kersey, J. H.: Wiskott-Aldrich syndrome: Detection of carrier state by metabolic stress of platelets. *Lancet* 1:121, 1978.
31. Moore, G. R.: X-linked thrombocytopenia. *Clin. Genet.* 5:344, 1974.
32. Canales, M. L., and Mauer, A. M.: Sex-linked hereditary thrombocytopenia as a variant of the Wiscott-Aldrich syndrome. *N. Engl. J. Med.* 277:899, 1967.
33. Cohn, J., et al.: Sex-linked hereditary thrombocytopenia with immunological defects. *Hum. Hered.* 25:309, 1975.
34. Thompson, A. R., Wood, W. G., and Stamatoyannopoulos, G.: X-linked syndrome of platelet dysfunction, thrombocytopenia, and imbalanced globin chain synthesis with hemolysis. *Blood* 50:303, 1977.
35. Mayer, M., Sperling, H., Schaefer, J., and Queisser, W.: Megakaryocyte polyploidization in May-Hegglin anomaly. *Acta Haematol.* 60:45, 1978.
36. Hamilton, R. W., Shaikh, B. S., Ottie, J. N., Storch, A. E., Saleem, A., and White, J. G.: Platelet function, ultrastructure, and survival in the May-Hegglin anomaly. *Am. J. Clin. Pathol.* 74:663, 1980.
37. Godwin, H. A., and Ginsburg, A. D.: May-Hegglin anomaly: A defect in megakaryocyte fragmentation? *Br. J. Haematol.* 26:117, 1974.
38. Kurstjens, R., Bolt, C., Vossen, M., and Haanen, C.: Familial thrombopathic thrombocytopenia. *Br. J. Haematol.* 15:305, 1968.
39. Niewiarowski, S., Poplawski, A., Prokopowicz, J., Kansak, B., Lechner, K., and Stockinger, L.: Abnormalities of platelet function and ultrastructure in macrothrombocytic thrombopathia. *Scand. J. Haematol.* 6:377, 1969.
40. Baadenhuijsen, H., and Haanen, C.: Platelet membrane function studies on platelets from patients with hereditary thrombopathic thrombocytopenia. *Haemostasis* 3:98, 1974.
41. Takahashi, H., Nagayama, R., Hattori, A., Ihzumi, T., Tsukada, T., and Shibata, A.: Von Willebrand disease associated with familial thrombocytopenia and increased ristocetin-induced platelet aggregation. *Am. J. Hematol.* 10:89, 1981.
42. Eckstein, J. D., Filip, D. F., and Watts, J. C.: Hereditary thrombocytopenia, deafness, and renal disease. *Ann. Intern. Med.* 82:639, 1975.
43. Clare, N. M., Montiel, M. M., Lifschitz, M. D., and Bannayan, G. A.: Alport's syndrome associated with macrothrombopathic thrombocytopenia. *Am. J. Clin. Pathol.* 72:111, 1979.
44. Parsa, K. P., Lee, D.B.N., Zamboni, L., and Glassock, R. J.: Hereditary nephritis, deafness and abnormal thrombopoiesis: Study of a new kindred. *Am. J. Med.* 60:665, 1976.
45. Von Behrens, W. E.: Mediterranean macrothrombocytopenia. *Blood* 46:199, 1975.
46. Bithell, T. C., Didisheim, P., Cartwright, G. E., and Wintrobe, M. M.: Thrombocytopenia inherited as an autosomal dominant trait. *Blood* 25:231, 1965.
47. Murphy, S., Oski, F. A., and Gardner, F. H.: Hereditary thrombocytopenia with an intrinsic platelet defect. *N. Engl. J. Med.* 281:857, 1969.
48. Law, I. P., Deveny, A., and Meiser, R. J.: Case report: Familial thrombocytopenia in seven members of three generations. *Postgrad. Med.* 63:136, 1978.
49. Rivard, G. E., Daviault, M. B., Brault, N., D'Aragon, L., and

Raymond, R.: Von Willebrand's disease associated with thrombocytopenia and a fast migrating factor VIII related antigen. *Thromb. Res.* 11:507, 1977.

50. Harms, D., and Sachs, V.: Familial chronic thrombocytopenia with platelet autoantibodies. *Acta Haematol.* 34:30, 1965.

51. Myllyla, G., Pelkonen, R., Ikkala, E., and Apajalahti, J.: Hereditary thrombocytopenia: Report of three families. *Scand. J. Haematol.* 4:441, 1967.

52. Cullum, C., Cooney, D. P., and Schrier, S. L.: Familial thrombocytopenic thrombocytopathy. *Br. J. Haematol.* 13:147, 1967.

53. Gerrard, J. M., et al.: Biochemical studies of two patients with the gray platelet syndrome: Selective deficiency of platelet alpha granules. *J. Clin. Invest.* 66:102, 1980.

54. Milton, J. G., and Frojmovic, M. M.: Shape-changing agents produce abnormally large platelets in a hereditary "giant platelets syndrome (MPS)." *J. Lab. Clin. Med.* 93:154, 1979.

55. Hertz, C. G., and Hambrich, G. W.: Congenital Letterer-Siwe disease. *Am. J. Dis. Child.* 116:553, 1968.

56. Wagner, H. P., Tonz, O., and Greyers-Gloor, R. D.: Congenital lymphoid leukemia. *Helv. Paediatr. Acta* 23:591, 1968.

57. Cooper, L. Z., Green, R. H., Krugman, S., Giles, J. P., and Mirick, G. S.: Neonatal thrombocytopenic purpura and other manifestations of rubella contracted in utero. *Am. J. Dis. Child.* 110:416, 1965.

58. Vossaugh, P., Leikin, S., Avery, G., Monif, G., and Sever, T.: Neonatal thrombocytopenia in association with rubella. *Acta Haematol. (Basel)* 35:158, 1966.

59. Hanshaw, H. B.: Congenital and acquired cytomegalovirus infection. *Pediatr. Clin. North Am.* 13:279, 1966.

60. Rodriguez, S. U., Leikin, S., and Hiller, M. C.: Neonatal thrombocytopenia associated with antepartum administration of thiazide drugs. *N. Engl. J. Med.* 270:881, 1964.

61. Jerkner, K., Kutti, J., and Victorin, L.: Platelet counts in mothers and their newborn infants with respect to ante-partum administration of oral diuretics. *Acta Med. Scand.* 194:473, 1973.

62. Scott, J. L., Cartwright, G. E., and Wintrobe, M. M.: Acquired aplastic anemia: An analysis of thirty-nine cases and review of the pertinent literature. *Medicine* 38:119, 1959.

63. Hirsch, E. H., Vogler, W. R., McDonald, T. P., and Stein, S. F.: Acquired hypomegakaryocytic thrombocytopenic purpura: Occurrence in a patient with absent thrombopoietic stimulating factor. *Arch. Intern. Med.* 140:721, 1980.

64. Stoll, D. B., Blum, S., Pasquale, D., and Murphy, S.: Thrombocytopenia with decreased megakaryocytes: Evaluation and prognosis. *Ann. Intern. Med.* 198:170, 1981.

65. Jandl, J. H., and Castleman, B.: Case records of the Massachusetts General Hospital. *N. Engl. J. Med.* 267:452, 1962.

66. Ballas, S. K., and Rubin, R. N.: Microangiopathic hemolytic anemia and thrombocytopenia with disseminated cancer. *Postgrad. Med.* 60:180, 1976.

67. Linman, J. W., and Bagby, G. C.: The preleukemic syndrome (hemopoietic dysplasia). *Cancer* 42:854, 1978.

68. Besselman, D. M.: Splenectomy in the management of the anemia and thrombocytopenia of osteopetrosis (marble bone disease). *J. Pediatr.* 69:455, 1966.

69. Finch, S. C., and Castleman, B.: Case records of the Massachusetts General Hospital. *N. Engl. J. Med.* 268:378, 1963.

70. Cameron, S. J.: Tuberculosis and the blood—A special relationship? *Tubercle* 55:55, 1974.

71. Dameshek, W., and Gunz, F.: *Leukemia*, 2d ed. Grune & Stratton, New York, 1964, p. 451.

72. Jackson, D. P., Cronkite, E. P., LeRoy, G. V., and Halpern, B.: Further studies on the nature of the hemorrhagic state in radiation injury. *J. Lab. Clin. Med.* 39:449, 1952.

73. Karnofsky, D. A.: Cancer chemotherapeutic agents. *CA* 18:80, 1968.

74. Morse, B. S., and Stohlman, F. Jr.: Regulation of erythropoiesis. XVIII. The effect of vincristine and erythropoietin on bone marrow. *J. Clin. Invest.* 45:1241, 1966.

75. Robertson, J. H., and McCarthy, G. M.: Periwinkle alkaloids and the platelet-count. *Lancet* 2:353, 1969.

76. Ogsten, D., Dawson, A. A., and Philip, J. F.: Methotrexate and the platelet count. *Br. J. Cancer* 22:244, 1968.

77. Nordquist, P., Cramer, G., and Bjorntorp, P.: Thrombocytopenia during chlorothiazide treatment. *Lancet* 1:271, 1959.

78. Kutti, J., and Weinfeld, A.: The frequency of thrombocytopenia in patients with heart disease treated with oral diuretics. *Acta Med. Scand.* 183:245, 1968.

79. Eisner, E. V., and Crowell, E. B.: Hydrochlorothiazide-dependent thrombocytopenia due to IgM antibody. *JAMA* 215:480, 1971.

80. Horowitz, H. I., Shapiro, B., and Rubin, J. L.: Athrombocytopenic purpura caused by chlorothiazide. *N.Y. State J. Med.* 59:1117, 1959.

81. Lindenbalm, J.: Thrombocytopenia in alcoholics. *Ann. Intern. Med.* 68:526, 1968.

82. Post, R. M., and Des Forges, J. D.: Thrombocytopenia and alcoholism. *Ann. Intern. Med.* 68:1230, 1968.

83. Sullivan, L. W.: Effect of alcohol on platelet production, in *Platelet Kinetics*, edited by J. M. Paulus. North-Holland, Amsterdam, 1972, p. 247.

84. Cowan, D. H., and Graham, R. C., Jr.: Studies on the platelet defect in alcoholism. *Thromb. Diath. Haemorrh.* 33:310, 1975.

85. Cowan, D. H., Graham, R. C. Jr., and Shook, P.: Hyperosmolality: A factor in ethanol-related platelet dysfunction? *Semin. Hematol.* 13:103, 1976.

86. Pennington, S. N., and Smith, C. P.: The effect of ethanol on thromboxane synthesis by blood platelets. *Prostaglandin in Med.* 2:43, 1979.

87. Sullivan, L. W., Adams, W. H., and Liu, Y. K.: Induction of thrombocytopenia by thrombopheresis in man: Patterns of recovery in normal subjects during ethanol ingestion and abstinence. *Blood* 49:197, 1977.

88. Cowan, D. H.: Thrombokinetic studies in alcohol-related thrombocytopenia. *J. Lab. Clin. Med.* 81:64, 1973.

89. Crandall, T. L., Joyce, R. A., and Boggs, D. R.: Estrogens and hematopoiesis: Characterization and studies on the mechanism of neutropenia. *J. Lab. Clin. Med.* 95:857, 1980.

90. Watson, C. J., Schultz, A. L., and Wikoff, H. M.: Purpura following estrogen therapy with particular reference to hypersensitivity to (diethyl) stilbestrol and with a note on the possible relationship to purpura to endogenous estrogens. *J. Lab. Clin. Med.* 32:606, 1947.

91. Cooper, B. A., and Bigelow, F. S.: Thrombocytopenia associated with the administration of diethylstilbestrol in man. *Ann. Intern. Med.* 52:907, 1960.

92. Merigan, T. C.: Pharmacokinetics and side effects of interferon in man. *Tex. Rep. Biol. Med.* 35:541, 1977.

93. Cheeseman, S. H., et al.: Controlled clinical trial of prophylactic human-leukocyte interferon in renal transplantation: Effects on cytomegalovirus and herpes simplex virus infections. *N. Engl. J. Med.* 300:1346, 1979.

94. Pitkin, R. M., and Witte, D. L.: Platelet and leukocyte counts in pregnancy. *JAMA* 242:2696, 1979.

95. Sejeny, S. A., Eastham, R. D., and Baker, S. A.: Platelet counts during normal pregnancy. *J. Clin. Pathol.* 28:812, 1975.

96. Fenton, V., Saunders, K., and Cavill, I.: The platelet count in pregnancy. *J. Clin. Pathol.* 30:68, 1977.

97. Cederblad, G., Hahn, L., Korsan-Bengtsen, K., Pehrsson, N. G., and Rybo, G.: Variations in blood coagulation, fibrinolysis, platelet function and various plasma proteins during the menstrual cycle. *Haemostasis* 6:294, 1977.

98. Cohen, T., and Cooney, D. P.: Cyclic thrombocytopenia: Case report and review of the literature. *Scand. J. Haematol.* 12:9, 1974.

99. Lewis, M. L.: Cyclic thrombocytopenia: A thrombopoietin deficiency? *J. Clin. Pathol.* 27:242, 1974.

100. Skoog, W. A., Lawrence, J. S., and Adams, W. S.: A metabolic study of a patient with idiopathic cyclical thrombocytopenic purpura. *Blood* 12:844, 1957.

101. Engstrom, K., Linquist, A., and Soderstrom, N.: Periodic thrombocytopenia or platelet dysgenesis occurring in a man. *Scand. J. Haematol.* 3:290, 1966.

102. Wilkinson, T., and Firkin, B.: Idiopathic cyclical acute thrombocytopenic purpura. *Med. J. Aust.* 1:217, 1966.

103. Wahlberg, P., Nyman, D., Ekelund, P., Carlsson, S. A., and Granlund, H.: Cyclical thrombocytopenia with remission during lynestrenol treatment in a woman. *Ann. Clin. Res.* 9:356, 1977.

104. Harvey, J. W., Simpson, C. F., and Gaskin, J. M.: Cyclic thrombocytopenia induced by a Rickettsia-like agent in dogs. *J. Infect. Dis.* 137:182, 1978.

105. Morley, A.: A platelet cycle in normal individuals. *Aust. Ann. Med.* 18:127, 1969.

106. Smith, M. D., Smith, D. A., and Fletcher, M.: Haemorrhage associated with thrombocytopenia in megaloblastic anemia. *Br. Med. J.* 1:982, 1962.

107. Kotilainen, M.: Platelet kinetics in normal subjects in haematological disorders. *Scand. J. Haematol. (Suppl.)*:5, 1969.

108. Harker, L. A., and Finch, C. A.: Thrombokinetics in man. *J. Clin. Invest.* 48:963, 1969.

109. Dameshek, W., and Valentine, E. H.: The sternal marrow in pernicious anemia. *Arch. Pathol.* 23:159, 1937.

110. Levine, P. H.: A qualitative platelet defect in severe vitamin B12 deficiency: Response, hyperresponse, and thrombosis after vitamin-B12 therapy. *Ann. Intern. Med.* 78:533, 1973.

111. Ingeberg, S., and Stoffersen, E.: Platelet dysfunction in patients with vitamin B12 deficiency. *Acta Haematol.* 61:75, 1979.

112. Fillet, G., Andrien, J.-M., and Bury, J.: Effects of transfusion on serum iron, serum lactate dehydrogenase, and platelets in megaloblastic anemia. *Am. J. Clin. Pathol.* 68:458, 1977.

113. Lopas, H., and Rabiner, S. F.: Thrombocytopenia associated with iron deficiency anemia. I. The response to oral and parenteral iron. *Clin. Pediatr.* 5:609, 1966.

114. Dincol, K., and Aksoy, M.: On the platelet levels in chronic iron deficiency anemia. *Acta Haematol.* 41:135, 1969.

115. Scher, H., and Silber, R.: Iron responsive thrombocytopenia. *Ann. Intern. Med.* 84:571, 1976.

116. Beard, M. E. J., and Johnson, S. A. N.: Thrombocytopenia and iron deficiency anaemia in a patient with α_1-thalassaemia trait: Response to iron therapy. *Acta Haematol.* 59:114, 1978.

117. Karpatkin, S., Garg, S. K., and Freedman, M. L.: Role of iron as a regulator of thrombopoiesis. *Am. J. Med.* 57:521, 1974.

118. Osborn, J. E., and Shahidi, N. T.: Thrombocytopenia in murine cytomegalovirus infections. *J. Lab. Med.* 81:53, 1973.

119. Brown, W. M., and Axelrad, A. A.: Effect of Friend leukemia virus on megakaryocytes and platelets in mice. *Int. J. Cancer* 18:764, 1976.

120. Oski, F. A., and Naiman, J. L.: Effect of live measles vaccine on the platelet count. *N. Engl. J. Med.* 275:352, 1966.

121. Alter, H. J., Scanlon, R. T., and Schechter, G. P.: Thrombocytopenic purpura following vaccination with attenuated measles virus. *Am. J. Dis. Child.* 115:111, 1968.

122. Angle, R. M., and Alt, H. L.: Thrombocytopenic purpura complicating infectious mononucleosis. *Blood* 5:499, 1950.

123. Bierman, H. R., and Nelson, E. R.: Hematodepressive virus diseases of Thailand. *Ann. Intern. Med.* 62:867, 1965.

124. Mitrakul, C., Poshyachinda, M., Sangawibha, N., and Ahandrik, S.: Hemostatic and platelet kinetic studies in dengue hemorrhagic fever. *Am. J. Trop. Med.* 26:975, 1977.

125. Aster, R. H., and Enright, S. E.: A platelet and granulocyte membrane defect in paroxysmal nocturnal hemoglobinuria: Usefulness for the detection of platelet antibodies. *J. Clin. Invest.* 48:1199, 1969.

126. Hartmann, R. C., and Jenkins, D. E., Jr.: Paroxysmal nocturnal hemoglobinuria: Current concepts of certain pathophysiologic features. *Blood* 25:850, 1965.

127. Lewis, J. H., Zucker, M. B., and Ferguson, J. H.: Bleeding tendency in uremia. *Blood* 11:1073, 1956.

128. Rath, C. E., Maillard, J. A., and Schreiner, G. E.: Bleeding tendency in uremia. *N. Engl. J. Med.* 257:808, 1957.

129. Rabiner, S. F.: Uremic bleeding, in *Progress in Hemostasis and Thrombosis*, edited by T. H. Spaet. Grune & Stratton, New York, 1972, vol. 1, p. 233.

130. Valeri, C. R., Feingold, H., Zaroulis, C. G., Sphar, R. L., and Adams, G. M.: Effects of hyperbaric exposure on human platelets. *Aerosp. Med.* 45:610, 1974.

131. Philp, R. B., Inwood, M. J., and Warren, B. A.: Interactions between gas bubbles and components of the blood: Implications in decompression sickness. *Aerosp. Med.* 43:946, 1972.

CHAPTER 142

Thrombocytopenia due to enhanced platelet destruction

RICHARD H. ASTER

Congenital thrombocytopenia— nonimmunologic

ERYTHROBLASTOSIS FETALIS

Thrombocytopenia, usually moderate in degree, occurs frequently in infants with erythroblastosis fetalis. Although the red blood cell destruction characteristic of this disorder is antibody-induced, the antigens against which antibodies are directed are not expressed on platelets. Platelets may therefore be destroyed as the result of their interaction with products of red cell breakdown rather than by their direct participation in an immunologic reaction. A further reduction in platelet levels may occur in the course of exchange transfusion, particularly if stored blood containing few viable platelets is used [1]. A modest reduction in platelet levels was observed in a group of infants who received phototherapy for hyperbilirubinemia [2], possibly because of an effect of ultraviolet light on platelets.

THROMBOCYTOPENIA OF PREMATURITY

Thrombocytopenia has been observed in a high percentage of premature infants in several studies [3]. In other studies, however, only 4 of 73 infants weighing less than 2200 g were thrombocytopenic [4] and only 15 percent of 60 low-birth-weight infants had platelet levels of less than 150,000 per microliter [5]. These apparently discrepant observations are perhaps explained by "epidemics" of thrombocytopenia, sometimes associated with gastrointestinal bleeding, which may occur in nurseries for premature infants; possibly these epidemics are caused by some unrecognized toxic or infectious agent [6,7]. A pathologic cause should be sought when significant thrombocytopenia is observed in a premature infant. In one study, an association between maternal smoking and thrombocytopenia in small-for-date infants was observed [8]. Necrotizing enterocolitis in premature infants is sometimes accompanied by severe thrombocytopenia [9].

PREECLAMPSIA

Moderate thrombocytopenia is relatively common in infants born to women with preeclampsia [10,11]. In one study abnormalities consistent with disseminated intravascular coagulation (DIC) were found in cord blood

[10]. In another, the reduction in platelet levels could not be explained on the basis of DIC but was correlated with thrombocytopenia in the mother [11].

RENAL VEIN THROMBOSIS
In a number of reported instances, renal vein thrombosis in the newborn has been complicated by thrombocytopenia [12]. Consumption of circulating platelets in the affected kidney has been suggested as a possible cause [12,13].

INFECTIONS
Thrombocytopenia, usually mild but sometimes very severe occurs frequently in newborn infants suffering from a variety of infections. The acronym *TORCH* has been used in connection with the clinical picture associated with infection by *To*xoplasmosis, *R*ubella, *C*ytomegalic inclusion disease [14], and *H*erpes virus as well as syphilis [15] and other agents. As megakaryocytes are usually present in normal numbers, thrombocytopenia is probably the result of the destruction of circulating platelets by one of several possible mechanisms. Studies to confirm this have not been performed, however. As discussed in Chap. 141, megakaryocyte levels are often diminished in children with neonatal rubella, suggesting that suppression of platelet production may in part be responsible for thrombocytopenia in that disorder.

INDWELLING UMBILICAL ARTERY CATHETER
Moderately severe thrombocytopenia sometimes occurs in association with an indwelling umbilical catheter in a newborn in the absence of disseminated intravascular coagulation and has been ascribed to a "thrombogenic" effect of the catheter [16]. The thrombocytopenia appears to be unrelated to the more severe side effects of catheterization [17].

THROMBOCYTOPENIA WITH GIANT CAVERNOUS HEMANGIOMA (KASABACH-MERRITT SYNDROME)
Thrombocytopenia associated with giant cavernous hemangioma of infancy was first described by Kasabach and Merritt in 1940 [18]. Several hundred cases have since been reported, many of which have been summarized in a review [19]. Although the primary lesion is congenital in the majority of cases, older children and even adults with giant hemangiomas may be similarly affected.

ETIOLOGY AND PATHOGENESIS
Platelets transfused into patients with this disorder are rapidly cleared from the circulation [20,21], and thrombi consisting chiefly of platelets have been found in some biopsy specimens taken from the lesions [20,22]. Data obtained by external scintillation scanning following the injection of radioactively labeled platelets have been interpreted as showing concentration of label within the tumor [20,21,23]. Other studies have suggested that tagged platelets accumulate in the spleen [24]. Since

eradication of the tumor invariably restores platelet levels to normal, it seems probable that thrombocytopenia is mainly a result of platelet destruction induced by the neoplasm itself. The primary mechanism in most instances appears to be intravascular coagulation within the tumor [25] or throughout the entire circulation [26–28]. In an analogous disorder found in the 129/J strain of mice, thrombosis and consumption of platelets occur primarily within the tumors [29].

CLINICAL FEATURES
The hemangioma is usually present at birth but may be internal or so small as to be overlooked. Purpura generally develops within 6 weeks of birth but may appear for the first time later in childhood as the lesion increases in size. Thrombocytopenia may occur neonatally in association with placental chorioangioma [30] or large superficial lesions [31]. Tumors are usually solitary and subcutaneous, involving the extremities, trunk, and neck with approximately equal frequency [19] (Fig. 142-1). Visceral tumors may be located in the tongue, thorax, liver, spleen, gastrointestinal tract, or bones and may be malignant [19]. Subcutaneous and visceral lesions rarely coexist in the same patient. A similar hematologic picture may develop in adults with visceral or, very rarely, cutaneous lesions.

Tumors as small as 6 cm in diameter are capable of causing severe thrombocytopenia [19,23]. For unknown reasons, the lesion sometimes becomes engorged with blood prior to a bleeding episode. Hem-

FIGURE 142-1 Giant cavernous hemangioma of the right upper arm in a 6-month-old child with thrombocytopenia (platelets 7000 per microliter). Platelet levels became normal after successful treatment of the lesion with x-irradiation. (Propp and Scharfman [20].)

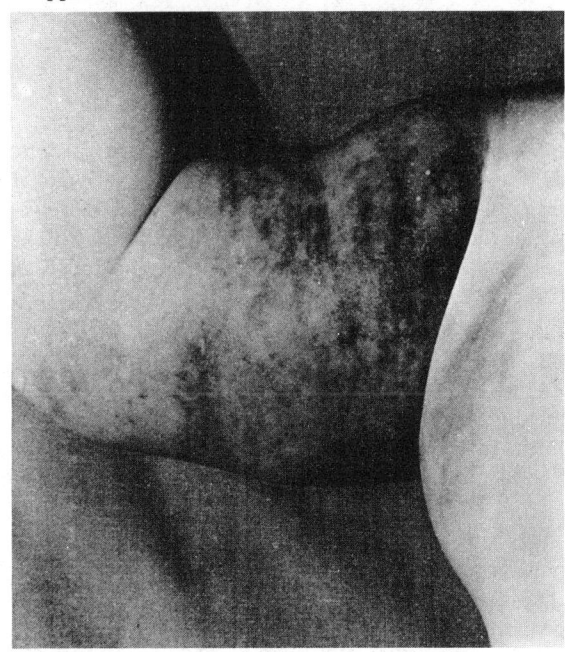

orrhage into subcutaneous tissue may give the primary lesion the appearance of a large hematoma and obscure the diagnosis.

LABORATORY FINDINGS

Platelet levels usually range from 10,000 to 40,000 per microliter. The blood film should be carefully inspected for microangiopathic changes often present in the erythrocytes (Chap. 64). Coagulation abnormalities typical of disseminated intravascular coagulation are often found [24,26–29] but occasionally may be detected only in blood taken directly from the tumor [25]. Rarely, fibrinogen concentration is so low that blood is totally incoagulable [28]. Acquired "storage pool disease" of platelets may aggravate bleeding [32]. Megakaryocyte levels are normal or elevated.

TREATMENT

Although giant hemangiomas sometimes involute spontaneously [33], treatment is often necessitated because of growth of the tumor or the severity of hemorrhagic symptoms. Readily accessible lesions should be excised if disfigurement will not result. Most often, radiation therapy is required. Several courses, with dosage totaling up to 1800 rads, may be necessary to effect regression [28].

Platelet transfusions should be reserved for the treatment of serious hemorrhage. Glucocorticoid therapy is often ineffective [19] but in some instances appears to have been of dramatic benefit [28,34,35]. About 20 percent of reported cases have ended fatally because of hemorrhage, airway obstruction, or infection [19], but mortality among unselected cases is much lower. Surgical excision is invariably followed by rapid correction of the hematologic abnormalities. More than 90 percent of lesions respond to radiation therapy, but a prolonged course of treatment may be needed [19,28].

THROMBOCYTOPENIA DUE TO INHERITED ABNORMALITIES OF PLATELET STRUCTURE OR FUNCTION

In certain of the inherited thrombocytopenic disorders, such as Wiskott-Aldrich syndrome, reduced platelet levels appear to be at least partially the result of accelerated platelet destruction. For the sake of clarity, these are discussed with other inherited thrombocytopenias in Chap. 141.

CONGENITAL CYANOTIC HEART DISEASE

Moderate thrombocytopenia often occurs in children with congenital cyanotic heart disease. This is rarely a problem in the perinatal period and will be discussed under "acquired thrombocytopenias."

PLATELET MICROEMBOLISM

A syndrome associated with platelet microthrombi and vegetative cardiac valve lesions has been described in newborn infants [36]. The etiology of the disorder, which appears to be distinct from thrombotic throm-

bocytopenic purpura and disseminated intravascular coagulation, is unknown.

Congenital thrombocytopenia—immunologic

DRUG SENSITIVITY

Following ingestion of quinine, quinidine, and certain other drugs, antibodies may form which, in the presence of the drug, react with platelets to cause thrombocytopenia (see also pages 1311 to 1316). If the drug is taken by a sensitized pregnant woman shortly before delivery, both she and her offspring may be affected. Quinine, formerly used to facilitate labor, has been implicated as a cause of this type of thrombocytopenia in the newborn [37]. Recovery is usually rapid, but fatal intracranial hemorrhage has been reported [37]. In three reported cases, maternal ingestion of hydralazine was associated with severe neonatal thrombocytopenia [38]. Maternal platelet levels were normal, and no immunologic or marrow findings were reported. Recovery occurred in about 1 week. Maternal ingestion of salicylates sometimes induces perinatal bleeding, but platelet levels are normal [39].

ISOIMMUNE NEONATAL THROMBOCYTOPENIA

Neonatal thrombocytopenia due to immunization of the mother against fetal platelets occurs at least once in 5000 births [40]. If asymptomatic cases were included, the observed frequency might be considerably higher.

ETIOLOGY AND PATHOGENESIS

Destruction of fetal platelets is brought about by their interaction with transplacentally acquired maternal antibodies directed against specific platelet antigens inherited from the father [40,41]. Maternal immunization against the platelet-specific antigen PI^{A1} (Zw^a) (see Chap. 162), found in about 98 percent of the general population, accounts for about two thirds of the cases [42]. A newly defined platelet-specific antigen, Bak^a, provided the apparent immunogenic stimulus in two reported cases [43]. Less well defined platelet antigens have been implicated in other instances [41]. The disorder is similar in pathogenesis to erythroblastosis fetalis except that fetal platelets rather than erythrocytes provide the antigenic challenge.

CLINICAL FEATURES

Firstborn children are often affected, indicating that platelets cross the placenta during gestation. As many as three cases have occurred in the same sibship. Gestation and delivery are generally unremarkable. Affected infants often appear normal at birth but develop scattered petechial and purpuric hemorrhages soon after delivery. Generalized distribution of the petechiae helps to distinguish them from those caused by ordinary birth trauma [44]. Dyspnea or neurologic changes should alert the physician to the possibility of intracranial hemorrhage. Jaundice commonly occurs during the first week, probably because of the limited ability of the newborn infant to metabolize hemoglobin reabsorbed from sites of interstitial hemorrhage [40,45].

LABORATORY FINDINGS
In symptomatic cases, platelet levels are usually lower than 30,000 per microliter and may diminish still further during the first few hours of life. Without treatment, thrombocytopenia persists for an average of about 2 weeks. Occasionally, improvement occurs within 2 to 3 days [46]; rarely, 2 months or more is required. White blood cell counts are normal. Anemia, when present, is due to hemorrhage. The numbers of reticulocytes and erythroblasts are elevated in proportion to blood loss. Megakaryocytes are usually found in normal numbers but occasionally are absent from the marrow, having apparently been destroyed by the same antibody that caused the thrombocytopenia [41,46]. Indirect bilirubin levels may rise sufficiently to threaten kernicterus [40].

In most cases, antibodies reacting with platelets from the infant and the father can be detected in maternal serum when newer methods of antibody detection are used. In a recently reported series, 33 of 38 maternal sera were positive in an indirect immunofluorescence assay [42]. With the use of this technique and others capable of directly measuring platelet-bound immunoglobulin (see Chap. A44), it seems possible that laboratory diagnosis will be feasible in nearly all cases in the future. In one instance, a rising maternal antibody titer was observed before delivery of a thrombocytopenic infant, suggesting that prenatal diagnosis may be possible [47]. Because only 2 percent of the general population lack the Pl^{A1} platelet antigen which provides the immunogenic stimulus in most cases, typing of the mother as Pl^{A1}-negative provides presumptive evidence that the thrombocytopenia is of isoimmune origin.

DIFFERENTIAL DIAGNOSIS
Since definitive serologic tests for detection of platelet antibodies and performance of platelet typing are not yet widely available, the diagnosis of isoimmune neonatal thrombocytopenia is frequently one of exclusion. A normal platelet level in the mother and a history negative for idiopathic (autoimmune) thrombocytopenic purpura help to rule out other types of congenital immune thrombocytopenia. However, isoimmune neonatal thrombocytopenia can occur in infants born to mothers afflicted with autoimmune thrombocytopenia [48,49]. Erythroblastosis fetalis, often characterized by thrombocytopenia, jaundice, anemia, and erythroblastemia, must be excluded by a Coombs' test. Viral or bacterial infection, hemangioma-thrombocytopenia syndrome, congenital absence of megakaryocytes, and thrombocytopenia associated with maternal drug ingestion should also be considered.

TREATMENT
Treatment is difficult to evaluate because the disorder is self-limited.

Glucocorticoids   Use of glucocorticoids was associated with a reduction in the average duration of thrombocytopenia in one retrospective study [40]. In three instances their administration before delivery to a woman who had previously given birth to a thrombocytopenic infant appeared to ameliorate the disease in the next child born to her [40]. In another case, however, a baby born by cesarean section had a platelet level of 4000 per microliter despite administration of prednisone, 60 mg per day, to the mother for 3 days prior to operation [50]. Although the effectiveness of glucocorticoids has not been fully established, it is reasonable to treat severely affected newborn infants with prednisone, 2 mg per kilogram body weight daily, in the immediate postnatal period and to administer dexamethasone prenatally to women carrying an infant at risk to develop the disorder.

Exchange transfusion   This has been used to remove antibody in the hope of shortening the duration of thrombocytopenia [40,41,51,52], but it was apparently ineffective in one infant who remained thrombocytopenic for 42 days [53]. The procedure should be reserved for children with severe thrombocytopenia (platelet levels of less than 20,000 per microliter) or marked hyperbilirubinemia.

Platelet transfusion   This is indicated for the treatment of serious hemorrhage. Even platelets that react with the antibody are of transient benefit and probably without hazard if administered slowly [40,41,51]. Nonreactive platelets are, of course, much more satisfactory and can be obtained by plasmapheresis of the mother since compatibility will be ensured regardless of the antigen-antibody system involved [50–52]. It is essential that maternal platelets be washed so as to avoid administration of additional antibody to the infant [51].

Splenectomy   This has also been advocated [54], but it is generally agreed that the risk of surgery far outweighs its possible usefulness in this self-limited disorder.

Cesarean section   This has been advocated at term in women who have previously given birth to an infant with isoimmune neonatal thrombocytopenia in order to prevent hemorrhage that might occur as a result of trauma in the birth canal [50,55]. Washed maternal platelets can be prepared in advance and transfused immediately if necessary [50]. Performance of platelet counts on fetal scalp blood obtained prior to or early in the course of labor may be helpful in deciding whether to allow a vaginal delivery [56]. Cesarean section may not prevent intracranial hemorrhage in all instances; in at least four reported cases, bleeding was thought to have occurred in utero [57,58].

PROGNOSIS
Approximately 15 percent of cases reported in the literature have ended fatally, chiefly because of intracranial

hemorrhage [40,52]. Infants who survive this complication may suffer severe neurologic damage [55,57,58]. With early diagnosis and therapy, and the use of cesarean section in selected cases, mortality and morbidity should be significantly reduced.

THROMBOCYTOPENIA ASSOCIATED WITH MATERNAL IDIOPATHIC THROMBOCYTOPENIC PURPURA

About 50 percent of children born to women with chronic idiopathic (autoimmune) thrombocytopenic purpura (ITP) are themselves thrombocytopenic at birth, apparently because autoantibody causing the disease in the mother crosses the placenta and binds to fetal platelets [59–64]. In two recently reported cases, binding of maternal antibody to platelets of an affected infant was directly demonstrated by measurement of platelet-associated IgG [47,65]. About 70 percent of children born to mothers with platelet levels of less than 100,000 per microliter are thrombocytopenic at birth, but only 20 to 30 percent are affected if maternal platelet levels are above that [60,63]. If the mother is thrombocytopenic despite having been splenectomized, the probability that her infant will be thrombocytopenic at birth is very high [59,60].

CLINICAL AND LABORATORY FINDINGS
Findings are similar to those in children with isoimmune neonatal thrombocytopenia. Curiously, thrombocytopenia induced by maternal autoantibodies persists for an average of about 1 month and occasionally for as long as 4 to 6 months, whereas the isoimmune disorder usually lasts only 1 to 2 weeks.

THERAPY – PRENATAL
Many cases are so mild as to require no specific treatment.

Glucocorticoids Prenatal administration of glucocorticoids to the mother was associated with a reduction in the severity of thrombocytopenia in the newborn in a recently reported series [66]. In one case treated in this way, the infant had a normal platelet level at birth but became severely thrombocytopenic 1 week later, perhaps because steroids were not continued postnatally [67].

Splenectomy during pregnancy This is associated with increased fetal mortality and should be undertaken only if essential for the well-being of the mother. The operation should preferably be done early in the course of pregnancy but has been successfully performed in the second and third trimesters [62,68].

Cesarean section As with isoimmune neonatal thrombocytopenic purpura, cesarean section has been recommended in ITP to reduce the chances of intracranial hemorrhage [60,62,64]. It has been suggested that this should be routine for all women with a platelet level of less than 100,000 per microliter prenatally [60,64] and for splenectomized women with a history of ITP regardless of platelet count [64]. A contrary view has been expressed [63]. In at least two instances, intracerebral hemorrhage occurred despite delivery by cesarean section [60,62]. Determination of fetal platelet levels in scalp blood obtained before or early in the course of labor has been suggested as a means of determining whether or not cesarean section should be performed [56,69].

THERAPY – POSTNATAL
Treatment of the severely affected newborn is essentially as in isoimmune neonatal thrombocytopenia (see above) except that "incompatible" platelets must necessarily be used for transfusion since the autoantibody of ITP has no known alloantigenic specificity. Many cases are so mild as to require no specific therapy.

Exchange transfusion Experience with exchange transfusion is limited. In one instance the duration of thrombocytopenia appeared to be shortened by exchange [70], but platelet levels remained low for 70 days after exchange in another [71]. As the autoantibody is passively acquired from the mother, exchange transfusion should, in theory, be beneficial and seems advisable in severely thrombocytopenic infants (platelet levels lower than 20,000 per microliter) with severe hemorrhage.

Splenectomy The spleen has been removed in two newborn infants with apparently beneficial results [72], but, as in isoimmune neonatal thrombocytopenic purpura, the operation is difficult to justify in this self-limited disorder.

PROGNOSIS
A fetal mortality rate of 10 to 25 percent was reported in the older literature, but with modern treatment the death rate is very low.

Acquired thrombocytopenia — nonimmunologic

THROMBOCYTOPENIA ASSOCIATED WITH INFECTION
Thrombocytopenia has long been recognized as a complication of various bacterial, viral, and rickettsial infections. Several mechanisms are probably responsible. As summarized in Chap. 141, platelet production may be *suppressed* in certain viral and, possibly, bacterial infections. *Direct interaction* of platelets with viruses [73,74], gram-positive organisms [75–77], lipopolysaccharide from gram-negative bacteria [78–80], and fungi [81] has been demonstrated in vitro and may contribute to the lowering of platelet levels. Complement [82,83], IgG immunoglobulin [78], and fibrinogen [75,77,81] may be in-

volved in such reactions. Of importance in many cases is *disseminated intravascular coagulation* (DIC) (Chap. 158), which can be triggered by either bacterial or viral sepsis. Sensitive techniques for detection of DIC showed that it was present in nearly all septic patients with platelet counts lower than 50,000 per microliter but that moderate thrombocytopenia could occur in its absence [84]. *Circulating immune complexes* are often present in septic patients. Recent studies have shown that platelet-associated IgG is elevated in such patients roughly in proportion to the degree of thrombocytopenia, and it has been suggested that binding of immune complexes to platelets may be important in promoting platelet destruction [85]. However, a cause-and-effect relationship has not been proved. Platelets may also be cleared from the circulation by interaction with endothelial cells damaged by the septic process [86].

Thrombocytopenia in a febrile patient should alert the clinician to the possibility of *septicemia.* More than two-thirds of patients with septicemia have platelet levels of less than 150,000 per microliter; in one-third, levels are below 50,000 per microliter whether or not DIC is present [87–89]. Reduced platelet levels are somewhat more common in patients with gram-negative sepsis than in those with gram-positive sepsis. Thrombocytopenia may provide an important diagnostic clue in patients with undiagnosed gram-negative bacteremia [89–91]. Meningococcemia, in particular, is sometimes confused with idiopathic thrombocytopenia with potentially disastrous consequences [92]. Unexplained thrombocytopenia in a febrile patient should also alert the clinician to the possibility of acute or subacute bacterial endocarditis [93–95]. Other infections often complicated by thrombocytopenia are Rocky Mountain spotted fever [96], typhus [97], typhoid fever [83,98], and diphtheria [99]. Eight of 15 patients with toxic shock syndrome had thrombocytopenia; the lowest platelet level was 14,000 per microliter [100]. Severe, acute thrombocytopenia is occasionally seen in patients with disseminated granulomatous disorders, notably tuberculosis [101], histoplasmosis [81], and brucellosis [102]. Return of platelet levels to normal in patients with bacterial sepsis is a good prognostic sign [89].

Protozoan infections   Thrombocytopenia is often present in patients with malaria [103,104] and trypanosomiasis [105,106]. Chronic thrombocytopenia has been reported in association with toxoplasmosis [107]. Patients with malaria may have disseminated intravascular coagulation [103], but in many of them coagulation parameters are normal [104]. Plasmodia have been found in the platelets of patients with *Plasmodium vivax* infection, and it has been suggested that platelet destruction can be promoted by direct invasion by merozoites [108]. A direct effect of trypanosomes on circulating platelets has also been postulated [105].

Viral infections   Mumps [109,110], varicella [111,112], disseminated herpes simplex [113], cytomegalovirus [114,115], and infectious mononucleosis [116–120] are some of the viral infections associated in their acute stages with severe thrombocytopenia, probably secondary to platelet destruction. In some adults with cytomegalovirus infection, thrombocytopenia appears to have responded to prednisone [114] and splenectomy [115]. In infectious mononucleosis, mild asymptomatic thrombocytopenia lasting 2 to 8 weeks is common [116,117]. In a small percentage of patients, thrombocytopenia is acute, severe, and life-threatening [117–120]. Transfused platelets are rapidly destroyed [118,120]. In one well-studied case, an autoantibody was implicated as the cause of thrombocytopenia [119]. This group of patients should be treated with glucocorticoids [117,118,120] and may require splenectomy [119,120]. As noted elsewhere in this chapter, acute thrombocytopenia that has its onset during convalescence from a viral infection is probably immunologically mediated.

DISSEMINATED INTRAVASCULAR COAGULATION
Disseminated intravascular coagulation (discussed fully in Chap. 158) should always be considered in the differential diagnosis of thrombocytopenia. Occasionally the process is chronic and may be diagnosed as idiopathic thrombocytopenic purpura unless appropriate laboratory studies are performed [121,122].

SNAKE BITES
Bites by certain species of snakes are followed by profound thrombocytopenia [123]. In some cases, the reduction in platelet levels is accounted for by disseminated intravascular coagulation. In several species of snake, however, platelet-activating proteins have been identified which appear to be capable of promoting platelet destruction by mechanisms independent of coagulation [123–125].

HYPOXIC STATES
Moderate thrombocytopenia was observed in about half of 70 patients with cyanotic congenital heart disease, but not in acyanotic patients with cardiac disorders [126]. Platelet survival was shortened in the former group, but not in the latter [127]. Platelet dysfunction, rather than thrombocytopenia, appears to be primarily responsible for bleeding problems encountered at surgery in patients with cyanotic congenital heart disease [128]. About 50 percent of patients with adult respiratory distress syndrome are thrombocytopenic [129,130]. In a group of 15 patients without evidence of disseminated intravascular coagulation, platelet survival was shortened in proportion to the reduction in platelet levels [130]. In a group of patients with chronic obstructive airway disease, platelet survival was shortened in those with hypoxia and was improved during administration of oxygen [131]. The mechanism responsible for platelet destruction was not identified.

BURNS

Moderate thrombocytopenia is frequently present for 2 to 4 days following severe thermal injury to more than 10 percent of the body [132,133]. Reduction in platelet levels is most pronounced in patients with sepsis [133]. The degree of thrombocytopenia does not correlate closely with prognosis, but rising platelet levels are associated with clinical improvement [132]. Studies in rats have shown that platelet life-span is shortened after thermal injury and have suggested that platelets are sequestered in damaged tissue [133]. Functional defects have also been described in platelets of burned patients [134], especially those who are infected [135].

FAT EMBOLISM

Thrombocytopenia, sometimes quite severe, occurs commonly in association with fat embolism in humans [136,137] and in an experimental rat model [136]. Up to 8 days may be required for restoration of platelet levels to normal [137]. The scattered petechiae seen in most patients with fat embolism appear to be caused by microemboli rather than thrombocytopenia [137].

GLOMERULONEPHRITIS

Transient, severe thrombocytopenia has been reported in several patients with poststreptococcal glomerulonephritis [138]. Clinical and laboratory findings suggested that platelet destruction was responsible, but its cause was not determined. Platelet-derived antigens have been detected along the endothelium and as vascular plugs in kidney tissue from patients with membranoproliferative glomerulonephritis [139], and platelet aggregating factors, presumably immune complexes, have been described [140].

RENAL TRANSPLANT REJECTION

Moderately severe thrombocytopenia accompanied by microangiopathic changes in red cells has been reported in patients undergoing rejection of renal transplants [141–143]. Destruction of platelets as a consequence of their interaction with renal vasculature damaged by immune mechanisms has been suggested as the cause. Immediate transplant nephrectomy has been advocated in transplant patients who have the combination of thrombocytopenia and acute renal failure [142]. Intermittent thrombocytopenia associated with megathrombocytes was observed in 20 of 50 patients with well-functioning renal allografts, both in the presence and in the absence of the spleen [144]. This was thought to be unrelated to immunosuppressive therapy.

AORTIC VALVULAR DISEASE

Mild thrombocytopenia was observed in about 20 percent of patients with obstruction to left ventricular outflow secondary to valvular stenosis. Hemolysis was often present as well [145]. In such patients, platelet life-span is probably shortened as a consequence of damage by the deformed valve or by turbulence of blood flow [146].

PRIMARY PULMONARY HYPERTENSION

Severe thrombocytopenia has been reported in at least three patients with "primary" pulmonary hypertension [147,148]. In two, platelets were thought to be sequestered in diffuse pulmonary arterial microthrombi [148]. In a third, whose erythrocytes showed microangiopathic changes, it was suggested that multiple plexiform lesions in the walls of pulmonary arterioles functioned as a massive vascular malformation to induce destruction of platelets and red cells [148].

HEMANGIOMA-THROMBOCYTOPENIA SYNDROME IN ADULTS

Special diagnostic and therapeutic problems may be presented by adults with hemangiomas of the liver [23], spleen [149,150], cerebellum [151], or subcutaneous tissues [152] who have what is essentially a variant of the congenital hemangioma-thrombocytopenia syndrome. The coagulation profile is often characteristic of disseminated intravascular coagulation [23,149,150,152]. A diagnostic clue may be provided by microangiopathic changes in erythrocytes. Heparin may be beneficial [152]. Surgical resection is an effective treatment for accessible lesions [149,150,152].

THROMBOTIC THROMBOCYTOPENIC PURPURA (THROMBOHEMOLYTIC PURPURA, MOSCHCOWITZ'S SYNDROME)

Thrombotic thrombocytopenic purpura (TTP), first described by Moschcowitz in 1925 [153], is characterized by the triad of hemolytic anemia with microangiopathic changes in erythrocytes, thrombocytopenia, and fluctuating, often bizarre, neurologic abnormalities. Fever and renal dysfunction are usually present as well. The typical pathologic lesions—widespread hyaline occlusions in small vessels—were noted by Baehr and coworkers in 1936 [154]. The disorder appears to be increasing in frequency.

ETIOLOGY AND PATHOGENESIS

Despite extensive investigation, the etiology of TTP is presently unknown. Moschcowitz originally postulated the existence of a *circulating "toxin"* that affected red blood cells and platelets, causing microthrombi [153], and much effort has been expended searching for such a factor. Disseminated intravascular coagulation (Chap. 158), can produce microangiopathic changes in red cells and capillary lesions similar to those found in TTP. In TTP, the levels of fibrin split products are often elevated in plasma and urine [155,156], shortened fibrinogen survival has been described in a few cases [157], and occasional patients appear to have responded to heparin [158,159]. However, coagulation changes characteristic of DIC are unusual [160,161], and when they do occur they are probably a secondary rather than a primary phenomenon [160]. One group found a *platelet aggregating factor* in 20 of 30 patients with TTP [162]. This did not appear to be a clotting factor or an immunoglobulin and could be inhibited by prior incubation with normal plasma [162]. Similar activity has been detected in a few patients by some investigators [163,164] but not by others [165,166]. It has been suggested that the basic abnormality in TTP may be a deficiency of a naturally occurring inhibitor of the platelet aggregating factor [162]. *Antibodies* against platelets are rarely detected in TTP, although elevated levels of platelet-associated IgG have been demonstrated in several instances [167]. The specificity of this finding remains to be determined.

An *abnormality of small blood vessels* may be the primary lesion [168]. This concept was supported by the finding of subendothelial, possibly prethrombotic lesions on electron microscopic examination of patent capillaries [169,170] and by studies showing that diffuse disease of the microcirculation can cause hemolysis and microangiopathic changes in red cells [171,172]. TTP has occurred in association with disseminated [173] and discoid [174] lupus erythematosus, rheumatoid arthritis [175], rheumatoid spondylitis [176], polyarteritis [177], and Sjögren's syndrome [178], all of which are characterized by some degree of vasculitis involving small blood vessels. Complement-dependent cytotoxicity against cultured human endothelial cells was detected in serum from seven of nine patients with TTP by one group [179], but this was not confirmed by others [165].

Recognition of the key role played by the vessel wall in regulation of hemostasis led to a search for *abnormalities of endothelial function* in TTP. Plasma from several patients with TTP and the closely related adult hemolytic-uremic syndrome (HUS), in contrast to normal plasma, failed to stimulate prostacyclin synthesis when incubated with exhausted rat aortic rings [180,181] or cultured porcine aortic endothelial cells [182]. These findings were confirmed by others [183,184], who also found that infusion of normal plasma into a patient with TTP appeared to stimulate prostacyclin synthesis in vivo [184]. Abnormal prostacyclin synthesis was observed in two asymptomatic children of one patient with TTP/HUS [180]. On the basis of these findings, it was suggested that some patients with TTP lack a plasma factor required for prostacyclin synthesis by endothelium. Studies in another patient indicated that prostacyclin was destroyed at an excessive rate, and it was proposed that a factor necessary for prostacyclin stabilization might be lacking [185]. These intriguing observations, which have not been confirmed in all instances [186], suggest that in some patients with TTP, platelet aggregation in vivo may result from an abnormality of prostacyclin metabolism, congenital or acquired. The possible association of TTP and adult HUS with oral contraceptives could be related to the action of these drugs on vascular endothelium [187,188]. β-Thromboglobulin released from aggregated platelets might further impair prostacyclin synthesis in patients with TTP [189,190]. An additional abnormality-deficiency of plasminogen activator in the vessel wall adjacent to microthrombi has been described by one group [191].

Etiologic mechanisms in addition to those reviewed above have been implicated in TTP [192]. An *immune etiology* is suggested by the apparent association of TTP with disorders of possible autoimmune origin [173–178,192] and hypersensitivity reactions [193–195], decreased levels of complement [192,196,97], the demonstration of immunoglobulins [170,198] and complement components in the lesions [98,199], and the detection of circulating immune complexes [197,200,201]. In other patients, however, complement levels were normal [192,202,203], immunoglobulins and/or complement components were not found in affected vessels [157,203], and immune complexes were undetectable [165,192,203]. Immune complexes, when present, may be related to associated underlying disease rather than to TTP itself [192,204].

The fulminant, febrile course of TTP in many patients is consistent with *infection*. The disorder is sometimes preceded by a viral infection [157,205], and it has occurred in association with *Mycoplasma pneumoniae* [206], *Bartonella*-like infection [207], vaccination [208], subacute bacterial endocarditis [197,209], and dog bite [210]. Its occasional appearance in families is also consistent with an infectious cause [211].

The occurrence of TTP in siblings [212] and the observation of abnormalities of prostacyclin synthesis in relatives of patients with TTP [180] suggest a genetic predisposition to develop the disorder.

The multitude of etiologies suggested for TTP and the difficulties encountered by clinicians and pathologists in classifying it as a specific disease entity suggests that TTP may occur as a complication of various disorders affecting the microcirculation. It seems possible that both a genetic predisposition and an inciting factor or factors are required to provoke the full-blown syndrome.

CLINICAL FEATURES
Numerous reviews of this subject have been published [155,156,173,213]. TTP has occurred in the newborn [214] and in a 77-year-old man [215], but the majority of patients have been between 20 and 50 years of age. Approximately two-thirds are female. Two forms of TTP are generally recognized: a chronic type, in which symptoms persist for months or sometimes years [216], and a much more common, acute fulminating type, which may be fatal within a few days or weeks. Arthritis, pleuritic pain, Raynaud's phenomenon, and other vague complaints sometimes precede the more severe symptoms and may represent a prodromal phase. The course of the disease is similar in children and adults [217].

Presenting symptoms vary greatly from one patient to another. Hemolysis may cause jaundice or pallor. Generalized purpura is usually present. In women, vaginal bleeding may be the initial complaint [218]. The occlusive lesions of the microcirculation provoke a variety of other symptoms. Neurological abnormalities include seizures, paresthesias, behavioral disorders, and alterations in the state of consciousness. These may fluctuate

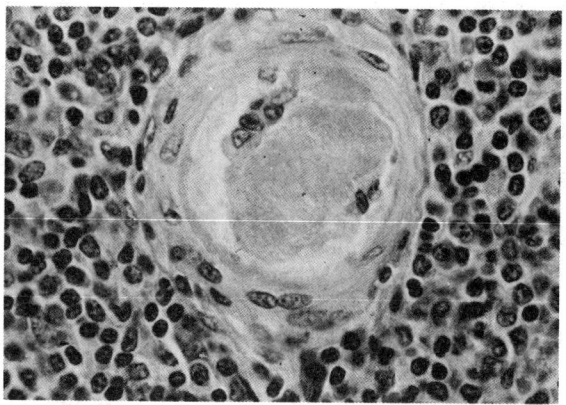

FIGURE 142-2   Cross section of an arteriole in the spleen of a 19-year-old woman with thrombotic thrombocytopenic purpura (surgical specimen; hematoxylin and eosin). The obstructing lesion was PAS-positive and appeared to consist mainly of platelets and fibrin, together with a few leukocytes. (Courtesy of Dr. Anthony V. Pisciotta, Department of Medicine, Medical College of Wisconsin.)

in severity or progress steadily to coma. Cerebral infarction due to embolization from nonbacterial endocarditis has been described [219]. Fever, which occurs in more than 90 percent of patients at some time during their illness, may be the result of lesions in the hypothalamus [173]. Occasional patients present with acute renal failure due to renal cortical necrosis (see also adult hemolytic-uremic syndrome, below). Abdominal pain, due presumably to microinfarctions of abdominal viscera, is often present and on occasion has led to exploratory laparotomy. Heart block due to infarction of the cardiac conduction system [220], sudden cardiac death [221], acute respiratory failure [222,223], and various occular abnormalities [224,225] have been described.

TTP has been reported frequently in pregnancy and in the postpartum period [192,226,227]. Since the disorder occurs most often in women of childbearing age, it is not clear whether the association is significant.

LABORATORY FINDINGS
Anemia is invariably present, and in one-third of these patients the hemoglobin level is less than 6 g/dl. Reticulocytes are nearly always increased in number, sometimes to levels in excess of 30 percent. Nucleated red cells are commonly seen in the peripheral blood. "Helmet" and other fragmented (microangiopathic) red cell forms are invariably present; in fact, the diagnosis of TTP is untenable if they are absent. Spherocytes occasionally dominate the blood picture. The Coombs' test is only rarely positive. Red cell life-span is markedly shortened [228]. Serum biliburbin levels, chiefly unconjugated bilirubin, are elevated in 90 percent of patients. Lactic dehydrogenase levels are elevated in proportion to the severity of the hemolysis.

Platelets are nearly always reduced in number, usu-

ally to the range of 10,000 to 50,000 per microliter. Megakaryocytes are normal or increased in number. Platelet life-span is usually less than 24 h [138,229]. Destruction of platelets in spleen, liver, and marrow was demonstrated in one instance [229].

The white blood cell count is usually elevated with a moderate left shift in the granulocytes. Occasionally a granulocytic leukemoid reaction occurs [173].

Proteinuria and microscopic or gross hematuria are almost invariably present [155,156]. The blood urea nitrogen level is elevated in more than 50 percent of cases initially and in a greater proportion terminally.

Lupus erythematosus preparations were positive in about 15 percent of patients reported prior to 1966 [173]. Lesions typical of lupus erythematosus are occasionally found in biopsy specimens or at autopsy. However, later reports have questioned the relationship between lupus and TTP [192]. Antinuclear antibody levels were elevated in half of 18 patients recently studied [155].

Coagulation tests are usually within normal limits [160,161,173]. In perhaps 25 percent, findings suggestive of DIC are present. Fibrin split product levels are often elevated [155,156]. Fibrinogen turnover is normal or slightly increased [146,157].

MICROSCOPIC PATHOLOGY
The principal histologic abnormality is deposition of hyaline, acidophilic, PAS-positive [230] material within the lumina of arterioles and capillaries [169,170,231] (Fig. 142-2). Endothelial proliferation is often seen in the vicinity of the lesions. Perivascular infiltration with mononuclear cells of the type seen in immune vasculitis is notably lacking. Hyaline material beneath the endothelium of patent vessels has been considered by some to represent a primary, "prethrombotic" process [169,170]. By immunohistochemical methods, both the intraluminal [170,231] and the subendothelial lesions have been shown to contain fibrin. Immunoglobulins and complement components have been demonstrated subendothelially in some cases [170,198,199] but not in others [157,203].

By electron microscopy, the microthrombi have been shown to consist of fibrin-like material, platelet aggregates, and occasional red cells and leukocytes [170,232]. Some lesions consist almost entirely of platelets, which may be loosely or tightly packed together [232]. Possibly, these are newly formed [233].

Microthrombi occur with greatest frequency in the heart, brain, abdominal viscera, and lymph nodes [173,234], but they may be found in any tissue. About 50 percent of gingival biopsies are diagnostic [155, 156,213,235]. A high diagnostic yield has been reported with marrow biopsy [155,156,173,213]. Lymph node biopsy is sometimes helpful [155,156,173], but this tissue is less accessible than gingiva and marrow. Skin and muscle biopsies were usually negative in several series [155,156,173]. In one study, however, each of five biopsies taken at the site of a petechial hemorrhage was interpreted as being diagnostic [191].

DIFFERENTIAL DIAGNOSIS

In typical cases, the triad (thrombocytopenia, microangiopathic hemolytic anemia, and neurologic dysfunction) or often pentad (triad plus fever and renal dysfunction) of clinical findings should suggest the correct diagnosis. Disseminated intravascular coagulation may, as noted above, present with somewhat similar symptoms and laboratory findings, but it is not ordinarily characterized by hemolysis of the severity seen in TTP. Thrombocytopenia together with hemolytic anemia occurs in patients with Evan's syndrome (idiopathic thrombocytopenic purpura with autoimmune hemolytic anemia) and paroxysmal nocturnal hemoglobinuria, but fragmented red cells are not present. HUS occurs chiefly in infancy and may be a variant of TTP. This and other disorders that may be related etiologically to TTP are discussed below.

PROGNOSIS AND THERAPY

Of 271 patients with classic TTP reviewed in 1966 [173], only 17 were alive. More than two-thirds died within 90 days of the onset of symptoms. Mortality was especially high in pregnancy [226,236]. Of the few survivors, most had been treated with glucocorticoids and splenectomy.

In recent years, the use of newer, albeit somewhat empiric, forms of therapy has led to remission in 60 to 80 percent of cases [155,156,205,213,237,238]. Improvement has been achieved most consistently with the combination of glucocorticoids (100 to 1000 mg of prednisone per day), platelet inhibitors (aspirin, dipyridamole, dextran, sulfinpyrazone), and whole-blood or plasma exchange transfusion.

A few patients appear to have responded to glucocorticoids alone [237], but there is no definite evidence to show that this class of drugs is of benefit. Since glucocorticoids have been given to nearly every surviving patient, their use is recommended until a fuller understanding of the etiology of TTP is achieved. Between 200 and 1000 mg of prednisone daily has been given in most instances. A high response rate was achieved by one group with hydrocortisone, 1000 mg per day, in conjunction with other therapy [161].

Agents capable of inhibiting platelet function have been used with the intent of interrupting in vivo platelet aggregation and microthrombus formation [156, 161,205,237–240]. The most frequently used combination has been aspirin, 0.6 to 1.2 g daily, and dipyridamole, 100 mg four times daily. A high rate of remission was achieved in one series of patients treated by infusion of dextran 70. Dipyridamole has been given intravenously to comatose patients [238]. This drug may require prostacyclin for its antiplatelet action [241] and is perhaps most effective when used together with plasma therapy or exchange transfusion (see below). Two patients appear to have responded to treatment with aspirin and dipyridamole alone [242], but there are many documented instances in which platelet inhibitors produced no perceptible improvement. Recently, several patients have been treated by infusion of the most potent known inhibitor of platelet function, prostacyclin. Two failed to respond to infusions lasting 12 h [183] and 8 days [243], respectively, but a third patient, refractory to other therapy, recovered after treatment for 15 days with higher doses [244].

About 25 reported patients have been treated one or more times with *whole-blood exchange transfusion* averaging about one blood volume [237,245]. Some exhibited dramatic improvement while the exchange was still in progress, and more than half recovered completely. One of these received no other therapy [245]. An even higher response rate has been reported in patients treated by machine-assisted *plasmapheresis* [205,237, 238,245,246]. As with whole-blood exchange, improvement was so rapid in some cases as to make a cause-and-effect relationship between treatment and recovery almost certain. In other instances, improvement occurred only after weeks of intensive plasma exchange [246,247].

One well-studied patient with TTP responded repeatedly to *transfusion of normal plasma* but not albumin [248], and, in a larger series, 13 of 18 patients so treated developed a sustained remission [233]. In other cases, infusion of plasma has been without apparent benefit [202,249]. It has been postulated that the beneficial effect of plasma infusion (and exchange transfusion) is related to correction of a deficiency of an inhibitor to a postulated platelet aggregating factor [162,233,248]. Alternatively, plasma may stimulate the production [180–184] or prolong the survival [185] of prostacyclin.

Immunosuppressive therapy in various forms has been used in many patients without apparent effect [reviewed in Ref. 237]. However, improvement occurred after administration of vincristine to six patients [250,251] and cyclophosphamide to one patient [252] refractory to other therapy. The rationale for a possible effect of immunosuppression in TTP is unclear.

Hemodialysis appeared to be of dramatic benefit to one patient who failed to respond to prednisone and splenectomy [253] and may be helpful as adjunctive therapy in patients with severe renal failure [254].

The initial enthusiasm for *splenectomy* in the treatment of TTP [255] has waned because in one series there was little correlation between removal of the spleen and clinical improvement [155,156]. It has been suggested that the apparent benefit of splenectomy may be related to the large quantities of blood and plasma transfused during the operation [237]. However, one of the highest rates of recovery was achieved in a series of patients treated with the combination glucocorticoids, dextran 70, and splenectomy [161].

In a few patients, *heparin* given with glucocorticoids appears to have been effective [158,159]. In the majority of cases, however, heparin has been without benefit and may be dangerous [155].

Platelet *transfusions* are of limited value because platelet life-span is very short. In several instances, rapid clinical deterioration after transfusion of platelet concentrates was attributed to accentuation of microthrombus formation by the transfused cells [233,245]. In view of the role platelets are known to play in microthrombus formation, platelet transfusions are perhaps best avoided. They may be required, however, in patients with life-threatening bleeding [246].

Treatment of TTP is in a state of evolution, and the effectiveness of individual modes of therapy is difficult to evaluate because most patients are treated with multiple agents. On the basis of available information, it seems logical to initiate therapy with high doses of glucocorticoids and platelet inhibitors. In severely affected patients and in those who fail to improve within 24 h on these drugs, exchange plasmapheresis totaling at least one plasma volume daily should be considered. For reasons discussed above, it is probably important to use plasma as the exchange fluid. Sustained reduction of lactic dehydrogenase levels and progressive elevation of the platelet count are perhaps the best indices of improvement [245,246]. In nonresponding patients, remission has been achieved by increasing the frequency and volume of exchange and persisting with this therapy for several weeks where necessary [205,237,238,245,246]. Where plasmapheresis is unavailable, whole-blood exchange transfusion should be instituted. With adequate venous access and capable nursing support, one blood volume can be exchanged in a few hours on an emergency basis in virtually any hospital [245]. Immunosuppressive therapy may be considered in patients who fail to respond to steroids, platelet inhibitors, and plasma exchange. The role of splenectomy in the treatment of TTP is unclear, and heparin should be used only as a treatment of last resort. Further trials to evaluate the possible benefits of dextran 70 and intravenous prostacyclin are clearly warranted.

Recovery from TTP is usually complete and without neurologic deficit even in patients demonstrated to have brain abnormalities suggestive of ischemic infarcts by computerized axial tomography [156]. Blood counts should be followed closely for several months because relapse may occur when the dosage level of glucocorticoids and platelet inhibitors is reduced [205]. Recurrence of the full-blown syndrome has occurred up to 12 years after apparently complete recovery [256] in rare instances.

HEMOLYTIC-UREMIC SYNDROME IN CHILDHOOD

The hemolytic-uremic syndrome (HUS), first described by von Gasser in 1955 [257], is a disease mainly of infancy and early childhood characterized by acute renal failure, fever, hemolytic anemia with microangiopathic changes in the erythrocytes, and thrombocytopenia [258–260]. The disorder is relatively common and appears to be increasing in frequency. A similar disorder of adults with certain distinguishing features is discussed separately below. Thrombotic thrombocytopenic purpura and HUS have many features in common, and the choice between these two diagnoses is sometimes arbitrary, especially in adults.

ETIOLOGY AND PATHOGENESIS

No single etiology has been identified. Many cases are preceded by viral or bacterial infections, especially of the gastrointestinal tract [258–265], and a direct effect of endotoxin [261] and other bacterial toxins on the renal endothelium has been postulated. Disseminated intravascular coagulation may be of importance in some cases [266]. Reduced levels of IgG [267] and complement components [268–270] and evidence of in vivo complement activation [268–270] have been reported, but proof that HUS is immunologically mediated is lacking. Subnormal levels of plasma tocopherol [271], abnormalities of red cell membrane phospholipids [271], and subnormal levels of erythrocyte superoxide-dismutase [272] have been described. A role for dysfunction of the monocyte-macrophage system has been suggested [273]. A deficiency of a plasma factor stimulating prostacyclin production was found in one child [274]. A genetic predisposition is suggested by the occurrence of HUS among members of the same family at different times [275,276]. A relationship to the HLA system has been inferred [212,277]. As with TTP (above), it seems possible that HUS occurs as a consequence of endothelial dysfunction provoked by a variety of causes, perhaps in association with a genetic predisposition to develop the disorder. In HUS, the primary abnormality may be restricted mainly to the kidneys, whereas in TTP it may be more widespread.

CLINICAL FEATURES

Except for the age of onset, HUS closely resembles TTP, the chief differences being that, in HUS, neurologic symptoms are less prominent and renal function is more severely impaired. The peak incidence is between 6 months and 4 years of age [258–260]. Males and females are affected with equal frequency. A febrile illness characterized by diarrhea or respiratory complaints frequently precedes the onset of purpura, hemolysis, and renal failure [258–260,278,279]. Some patients are initially diagnosed as having ulcerative colitis [278,279]. Symptoms suggestive of an acute abdominal emergency are often present and may create diagnostic problems [260,278–280]. In occasional patients, a true surgical emergency is present [280]. In both South Africa [281] and Argentina [266], it has been observed that children of families in the upper socioeconomic brackets are most commonly affected. Neurologic disturbances consisting of seizures and altered states of consciousness occurred in more than one-third of the patients in some series [260,282] and were in part a consequence of renal failure [282]. In other series, neurologic abnormalities have been rare. Hypertension occurs in more than 50 percent of patients and may seriously complicate management [258–260].

LABORATORY FINDINGS

Hemolytic anemia with microangiopathic red cell changes is invariably present. Platelet levels are subnormal in more than 90 percent, but profound thrombocytopenia is less common than in TTP. The urine nearly always contains red cells and protein and, occasionally, red cell casts and platelets. Coagulation tests are usually normal [259,260] except for elevation of fibrin split product levels, but findings typical of DIC are occasionally present [283]. Platelet and red cell survival, but not fibrinogen survival, are shortened [141,284]. Abnormalities in immunoglobulins and complement have been described (see above) [267–270].

On biopsy or at autopsy, fibrin-like material similar to that found in patients with TTP is characteristically present in afferent arterioles and glomerular capillaries of the kidneys [259,260]. Focal abnormalities are found in the glomeruli and arterioles, where the subendothelial space contains granular and fibrillar material that usually stains positively with antifibrin reagents [285]. Abnormalities of the glomerular mesangium are often seen [286]. IgM, occasionally IgG, and C3 have been detected beneath the endothelium in some series [267–270]. In fatal cases, microthrombi may be found in tissues other than the kidney [287].

THERAPY

There is no convincing evidence that glucocorticoids are of general benefit in children with HUS [259]. The same is true of heparin [259,260,288–290], and this agent is perhaps best reserved for children who show definite evidence of DIC. Early fibrinolytic therapy with streptokinase has been advocated [290,291], but its effectiveness has not been fully established. Experience with the platelet inhibitors aspirin and dipyridamole has been generally disappointing [292,293]. Improvement occurred soon after plasma and whole-blood exchange transfusion in three reported cases [246,274]. This form of therapy, the rationale for which would seem to be the same as in TTP (see above), seems deserving of additional trial in severely affected children.

It has become clear that judicious use of peritoneal dialysis and transfusions of red cells as indicated for anemia are of great value [258–260,266,288]. The importance of beginning dialysis early has been stressed [259,260,288]. As in TTP, platelet transfusions are best avoided if possible. Treatment of HUS should be carried out by persons experienced in the management of acute renal failure in childhood.

PROGNOSIS

Formerly, more than one-third of cases ended fatally, due chiefly to renal failure. With dialysis, red cell transfusions, and other supportive care, some groups have reduced mortality to the range of 5 to 15 percent [260,266,294]. The prognosis is worse in children with severe neurologic abnormalities or renal failure of greater than 2 to 3 weeks' duration [260,294].

In some series more than half the survivors had persistent renal dysfunction [260,266], but in others renal function returned to normal in about 90 percent of cases [294]. This difference has been attributed to variability of the populations at risk and of the infectious agents

that may trigger the disease [294]. Occasional patients suffer recurrences of the full-blown syndrome, sometimes on repeated occasions [295]. In one instance, this occurred after renal transplantation [296].

HEMOLYTIC-UREMIC SYNDROME IN ADULTS

A disorder of adulthood similar to TTP but differing from it in that renal failure is more prominent and neurologic abnormalities less so has been termed *adult hemolytic syndrome* [259,297–302]. Prodromal symptoms occur less frequently, and the prognosis is worse than in HUS of childhood. More than two-thirds of patients are women, many of whom develop the disorder in association with preeclampsia, eclampsia, other obstetrical complications, or in the postpartum state [259,299–302]. Although statistical proof is lacking, adult HUS appears to be associated with use of oral contraceptives [298,299,301–303].

Clinical and laboratory findings are similar to those of childhood HUS, but differences in histopathology have been described [301]. Mortality is high. Of 49 cases reported prior to 1979, 61 percent ended fatally [301]. Studies of a plasma prostacyclin-stimulating factor have suggested a genetic predisposition to develop adult HUS [180]. A relationship between adult HUS, TTP, and childhood HUS is inferred from reports in which these disorders have occurred in different members of the same family [207,212,259,300].

Initial treatment is directed toward control of hypertension, anemia, and renal failure, which often requires hemodialysis. Because of the grave prognosis, other, more aggressive forms of therapy have been attempted in recent years. There is evidence that adult HUS, in contrast to the childhood disorder, responds favorably to heparin [259,301,302,304] and to the platelet inhibitors aspirin and dipyridamole [302,305], especially when these are used early. Infusion of a concentrate of antithrombin III was associated with recovery in one instance [306]. Plasma exchange transfusion, which may stabilize or promote synthesis of prostacyclin, has also been utilized with apparent benefit [307]. In at least one case, continuous infusion of prostacyclin for 5 days appeared to be effective [308]. Each of these forms of therapy seems deserving of further trial.

As in childhood HUS, the prognosis is worse if renal failure persists for more than a few weeks [259,302]. However, recovery of renal function has occurred in a few instances after more than 1 year of hemodialysis [302,309]. Renal transplantation has been successful in several cases [685].

INTERMITTENT MICROANGIOPATHIC HEMOLYTIC ANEMIA AND THROMBOCYTOPENIA WITHOUT NEUROLOGIC OR RENAL ABNORMALITIES

In one case, a 29-year-old woman had more than 100 episodes of fever, microangiopathic hemolytic anemia, and thrombocytopenia dating from 6 months of age [310]. There were no associated renal or neurologic abnormalities. She was asymptomatic between the episodes, but red cell and platelet life-span were shortened. Plasma fibronectin was low during an acute episode [311]. On repeated occasions, the hematologic abnormalities were reversed following infusion of plasma [310]. A second patient, at first thought to have a congenital deficiency of thrombopoietic hormones [312], may in fact have had a similar disorder [162,310]. The basis for the response to plasma has not yet been established.

PREECLAMPSIA

A moderate reduction in platelet levels, apparently due to platelet consumption, is commonly seen in women with preeclampsia [686,687]. The mechanism by which platelets are destroyed and the possible relationship between this abnormality and adult HUS is unknown. The occurrence of thrombocytopenia in children born to preeclamptic women was mentioned earlier [10,11].

DRUGS DIRECTLY TOXIC TO CIRCULATING PLATELETS

RISTOCETIN

This antibiotic, no longer in clinical use, is capable of causing thrombocytopenia by a direct action on circulating human platelets [313]. The effect appears to be related to the ability of ristocetin to trigger platelet aggregation by promoting the binding of factor VIII to a platelet receptor [314].

PROTAMINE SULFATE

Following intravenous injection of protamine sulfate, platelet levels were reduced within 5 min by about one-third in patients recovering from surgery on cardiopulmonary bypass and by about one half in normal subjects [315]. The effect was transient, lasting less than 1 h. On the basis of body surface scanning following transfusion of platelets labeled with indium 111, it was concluded that protamine induces temporary sequestration of platelets in the liver.

BLEOMYCIN

Moderately severe, transient thrombocytopenia occurred after bleomycin therapy in five reported cases [316]. It was conjectured that platelets were destroyed upon interacting with pulmonary endothelium damaged by the drug.

HEPARIN

Numerous reports of thrombocytopenia associated with heparin have appeared in the literature and have been reviewed [317,318]. In prospective studies, the frequency of thrombocytopenia in patients receiving heparin has ranged from 1 to 30 percent [317–320]. In one controlled study, heparin from beef lung induced thrombocytopenia significantly more often than did heparin derived from porcine intestinal mucosa [319]. In a second study, fewer than 2 percent of patients receiving either preparation developed thrombocytopenia [318]. The plasma of some patients with heparin-induced thrombocytopenia contains a factor, probably an immunoglobulin, which is capable of inducing platelet aggregation and platelet immunoinjury in the presence of heparin [320–323]. By several criteria, however, this appears not to be a typical drug-induced antibody [324]. In one series, antiplatelet activity could not be detected in plasma from any of eight patients [325]. Since heparin can promote platelet activation in the absence of antibody [326,327], it seems possible that this drug may cause thrombocytopenia by both nonimmunologic and immunologic mechanisms.

In most patients, thrombocytopenia begins after 3 to 10 days of heparin therapy, is relatively mild and of little clinical importance, and resolves after the drug is discontinued. In a minority, however, more severe thrombocytopenia occurs, sometimes in association with disseminated intravascular coagulation and life-threatening thromboembolism [321,322,328,329]. A characteristic radioangiographic picture has been described [330]. The paradoxical association of thromboembolism with heparin administration has not yet been explained, and no in vitro test to predict whether this complication will occur is yet available. Treatment consists of withdrawal of heparin and substitution of an oral anticoagulant. Administration of drugs that inhibit platelet function seems logical, but their effectiveness has not yet been fully established.

PERITONEOVENOUS SHUNTING

Thrombocytopenia, usually associated with disseminated intravascular coagulation, often occurs in patients treated with peritoneovenous shunts for intractable ascites [331,332]. A platelet-aggregating factor, possibly soluble collagen found in ascitic fluid, appears to provoke platelet destruction in such patients [331].

SWAN-GANZ CATHETERIZATION

Prolonged pulmonary artery catheterization following surgery with cardiopulmonary bypass was associated with a significantly greater reduction in platelet levels than in control patients in whom a central venous catheter was used [333]. It was postulated that platelets were destroyed upon interacting with foreign material on the relatively large surface of the indwelling pulmonary catheter.

Acquired thrombocytopenia—immunologic

ANTILYMPHOCYTE GLOBULIN

Thrombocytopenia, sometimes severe enough to cause purpura, is a recognized side effect of using antilymphocyte globulin to prevent or treat allograft rejection [334]. Platelets tagged with chromium 51 are destroyed in the spleen and liver after injection of the antiserum. Only certain batches of antilymphocyte globulin, presumably those that retain specificity for surface antigens of platelets, produce this effect [335]. In a canine model, evidence for non-antigen-specific binding of antilymphocyte globulin to platelets has been obtained [336].

Tn SYNDROME

Moderately severe thrombocytopenia, sometimes accompanied by hemolytic anemia and leukopenia, is commonly seen in patients with Tn syndrome, a chronic disorder associated with polyagglutinable erythrocytes [337,338]. Platelets, like red cells of patients with this disorder, are deficient in T-transferase (UDPGal:GalNAc-β-3-D-galactosyltransferase) and are thus unable to complete the synthesis of oligosaccharide chains of a major membrane glycoprotein, GPIb [338]. This leads to expression of a cryptantigen, Tn, which reacts with naturally occurring antibodies in normal human plasma. Presumably, the thrombocytopenia is a consequence of this reaction.

Another latent antigen, designated "T," is also reactive with naturally occurring antibodies and is expressed on platelets of patients with T activation, an acquired, transient disorder in which red cells are polyagglutinable [339]. This has not been clearly established as a cause of thrombocytopenia.

DRUG-INDUCED IMMUNOLOGIC THROMBOCYTOPENIA

Acute, severe thrombocytopenia purpura following ingestion of quinine was probably first described by Vipan in 1865 [340]. Rosenthal, in 1928, showed that thrombocytopenia could be reinduced in such patients by again administering the drug after their initial recovery [341]. Subsequently, it was found that platelets could be agglutinated or lysed in vitro when mixed with quinine in serum from a thrombocytopenic patient [342] and that sensitivity to quinine could be passively transferred to a normal subject by injecting plasma from a quinine-sensitive patient [343]. These pioneering observations demonstrated that quinine-induced thrombocytopenia is caused by the interaction in vivo of the drug, a plasma factor, and platelets, and they stimulated efforts in many laboratories to determine the pathogenesis of this form of thrombocytopenic purpura.

ETIOLOGY AND PATHOGENESIS

Other drugs have subsequently been observed to cause acute thrombocytopenia in sensitive individuals. Quinine, quinidine, and allylisopropylacetylurea (Sedormid) have been studied most extensively with respect to their mechanism of action.

Ackroyd, in a series of classic papers, showed that the plasma factor present in patients with Sedormid sensitivity has properties of an antibody which reacts with platelets only in the presence of the drug to cause agglutination, lysis, complement fixation, and inhibition of clot retraction[344–346]. Application of Sedormid to the skin caused local purpura in some of his patients. Oral or intravenous administration of the drug caused acute, severe thrombocytopenia.

Using similar techniques, others have demonstrated drug-specific antiplatelet activity in the serum of patients with quinine-induced [342,347,348] and quinidine-induced [349–352] thrombocytopenia. Quinidine-induced antibody, studied more extensively [350–352], is usually an IgG or, rarely, an IgM immunoglobulin which, in the presence of the drug, reacts with platelets from all normal human subjects, weakly with those of the rhesus monkey, and not at all with those of other species [351,353,354]. This antibody reacts with other dextrorotatory cinchona alkaloids, such as cinchonine, but usually not with quinine, the levorotatory isomer of quinidine.

Ackroyd initially postulated from his studies of Sedormid sensitivity that the drug became bound to circulating platelets of patients ingesting it and, acting as a hapten, stimulated antibodies specific for the drug-platelet combination [355]. Such antibodies by themselves would be harmless, but if the patient reingested the drug, platelets would again become coated, combine with antibody, and be destroyed. On the basis of positive patch tests, Ackroyd also hypothesized that antibody could combine with capillary endothelium. Others working with quinidine-dependent antibodies were unable to demonstrate reactivity with vascular tissue [349,351].

An alternative mechanism to explain drug-induced immunologic thrombocytopenia is that the drug may bind initially to a plasma protein or other "carrier" to form the primary antigen [356,357]. Antibodies stimulated by the primary antigen bind to the drug even in the absence of the original carrier protein. Thrombocytopenia is thought to occur when drug-antibody complexes with a peculiar affinity for some component of the platelet membrane are produced. According to this theory, platelets are destroyed as "innocent bystanders" (in the sense that they are unrelated to the primary antigen) upon ingestion of the drug by sensitive persons. Studies using antibodies with quinidine specificity provided important evidence to support this concept by showing that (1) the drug-platelet combination is a very weak one and therefore unlikely to be antigenic; (2) the reaction between antibody and platelets is not inhibited by high concentrations of drug, as would be expected according to classic hapten immunochemistry if platelets were the original carrier; and (3) the affinity of the drug-antibody complex for platelets is very great, with an association constant on the order of 10^7 to 10^8 liters per mole [353,354]. Also supporting this hypothesis are observations that several drugs known to cause immunologic thrombocytopenia—quinine [358], quinidine [359], and stibophen [360]—have on rare occasions stimulated antibodies that bind to an erythrocyte rather than a platelet receptor in the presence of the drug.

The two mechanisms proposed to explain drug-induced thrombocytopenic purpura have been reviewed [353,354,361,362] and are depicted in Fig. 142-3. Evi-

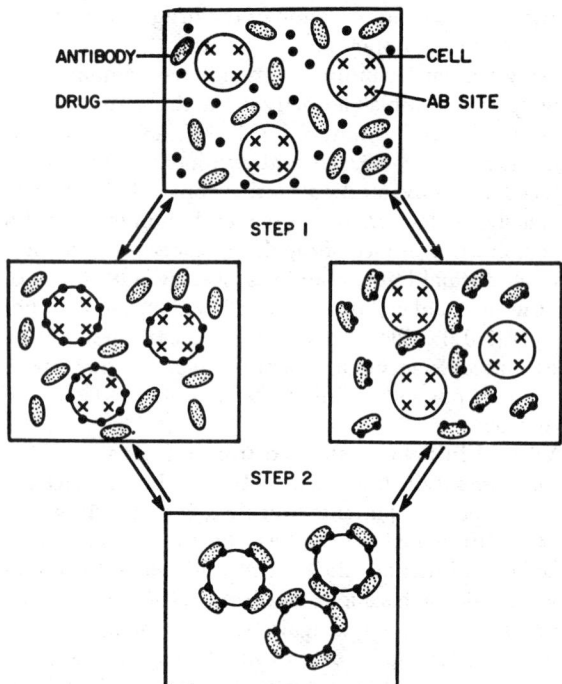

ANTIBODY
DRUG
CELL
AB SITE

STEP I

STEP 2

FIGURE 142-3 Possible mechanisms of drug-induced immunologic thrombocytopenia. Initial mixture consists of platelets, drug, and drug-dependent antibody. (*Left*) The platelets become coated by the drug; the drug-platelet complex then reacts with antibody. (*Right*) The drug combines first with antibody; the drug-antibody complex then coats platelets. (Shulman [353].)

dence cited above suggests that quinidine- and quinine-induced antibodies act by way of the innocent bystander mechanism shown on the right. The binding site for the presumptive drug-antibody complexes appears to be located on a specific platelet membrane glycoprotein, GPIb [363]. Additional complexity has been introduced by findings that platelets coated with quinidine in the presence of plasma and then washed induce proliferation of lymphocytes from quinidine-sensitive subjects [364] and that factor VIII–related antigen may be necessary for quinidine-dependent antibodies to induce platelet immunoinjury [365].

By analogy with the drug-induced hemolytic anemias, it seems possible that some drugs induce thrombocytopenia by other mechanisms, e.g., by binding directly to platelets to form a primary antigen (Fig. 142-3, *left*). It has been suggested that alloantigens may be the platelet receptor in some instances [366]. Other drugs, such as α-methyldopa, may induce true autoantibodies capable of binding to platelets in the absence of the drug.

DRUGS IMPLICATED AS CAUSES OF IMMUNOLOGIC THROMBOCYTOPENIA

A vast number of drugs have been reported to cause immunologic thrombocytopenia (Table 142-1). In many instances the relationship may be coincidental. Numerous

drugs, including Sedormid [344–346], quinidine [349–352,367–369], quinine [347,348,351,367,369], and sulfonamides [367,369–371], have been convincingly shown by both in vitro and in vivo testing to operate through an immunologic mechanism. Quinine and quinidine together account for the largest number of cases. Organic arsenicals [372], sulfisoxazole [371], sodium *p*-aminosalicylic acid [373], α-methyldopa [374], rifampicin [375], oxprenolol [376], and many others have caused a recurrence of acute thrombocytopenia upon being readministered to sensitive patients. Treatment with gold salts [369,377–379] and sulfonamide derivatives has so frequently been followed by thrombocytopenia that a causal relationship of some sort seems nearly certain. More than 10 cases of thrombocytopenia following aspirin ingestion have been reported, and claims have been made for detection of aspirin-dependent antibodies in some of these [367,380,381]. Of 188 patients receiving phenylbutazone, 16 percent were found to have platelet levels of less than 100,000 per microliter [382], but only rare cases of thrombocytopenic purpura have been reported following the use of this drug [383] or its derivative oxyphenbutazone [384]. Similar observations were made with indomethicin in one survey [385]. A history of previous exposure to insecticides is sometimes obtained in patients with "idiopathic" thrombocytopenic purpura [386,387], but there is no definite evidence establishing a cause-and-effect relationship. Occasional cases of thrombocytopenia appear to have been triggered by food [388–393]. In the best-documented example, acute thrombocytopenic purpura occurred on four occasions after ingestion of one variety of bean [392].

Thrombocytopenia is common in patients receiving thiazide diuretics. As noted in Chap. 141, this may sometimes be the result of suppression of platelet production by this class of drugs. The same may be true of thrombocytopenia associated with phenylbutazone [382], trimethoprim-sulfamethoxazole [394], and cimetidine [395]. However, evidence for antibody-mediated platelet destruction has been obtained in patients taking each of these medications.

A summary of drugs and environmental exposures implicated as causes of isolated thrombocytopenia is provided in Table 142-1, together with the approximate number of cases reported and key references. Several recent reviews provide additional information [361, 362,490,491].

CLINICAL FEATURES

Only occasional patients taking quinidine, quinine, and other drugs listed in Table 142-1 develop thrombocytopenia. Those treated with gold salts probably develop purpura most often (about 1 percent of cases). Persons carrying the HLA-DR3 lymphocyte antigen may be at greatest risk when injected with gold [379]. With this possible exception, there is no way at present to predict which patients will develop drug-induced thrombocytopenia. The disorder occurs most commonly in persons

TABLE 142-1   Drugs and other agents implicated as causes of immunologically mediated thrombocytopenia

	Approximate number of cases	Shown to cause platelet destruction by in vitro and/or in vivo criteria	Selected references
Analgesics (nonsteroidal, anti-inflammatory):			
Acetaminophen	6	+	[396–398]
Antipyrine	1	−	[399]
Aspirin	15	+	[380,381]
Clinoril	2	+	[400,401]
Fenoprofen	3	−	[402,403]
Indomethicin	30	−	[385]
Oxyphenbutazone	6	−	[384,404]
Phenylbutazone	6	+	[382,383]
Sodium salicylate	1	−	[405]
Antibacterials:			
Ampicillin	3	+	[367,369,406]
Cephalexin	1	+	[369]
Cephalothin	2	+	[407,408]
Gentamycin	1	+	[409]
Lincomycin	1	−	[410]
Methicillin	1	+	[411]
Novobiocin	1	+	[412]
Oxytetracycline	2	−	[413,414]
p-aminosalicylate	8	+	[373,415]
Penicillin	2	+	[369,416]
Pentamidine	1	−	[417]
Rifampicin	10	+	[375,418]
Streptomycin	1	−	[419]
Sulfonamides	50	+	[367,369–371,420]
Tobramycin	1	−	[421]
Trimethoprim	3	+	[422]
Cinchona alkaloids:			
Quinidine	>100	+	[349,352,367–369]
Quinine	>100	+	[347,348,369]
Foods:			
Beans	1	+	[392]
Citrus fruits	1	−	[389]
Others	10		[388,390,391,393]
Sedatives, hypnotics, anticonvulsants:			
Allylisopropylacetylurea	25	+	[344–346]
Allylisopropylbarbiturate	1	−	[355]
Butabarbitone	1	−	[423]
Carbamazepine	4	+	[367,424]
Centalun	3	+	[425]
Chlordiazepoxide	1	−	[426]
Clonazepam	1	−	[427]
Diazepam	1	+	[370]
Diphenylhydantoin	8	+	[367,370]
Ethylallylacetylurea	1	−	[428]
Ethylchlorvinyl	1	+	[429]
Ethylphenylhydantoin	1	−	[430]
Imprimine	1	+	[367]
Meprobamate	1	−	[367]
Paramethadione	1	−	[431]
Phenytoin	1	−	[432]
Phthalazinol	20	−	[433]
Primidone	1	−	[434]
Valproate Na	10	+	[435,436]
Valproic acid	2	+	[437,438]

TABLE 142-1   Drugs and other agents implicated as causes of immunologically mediated thrombocytopenia (Continued)

	Approximate number of cases	Shown to cause platelet destruction by in vitro and/or in vivo criteria	Selected references
Sulfonamide derivatives:			
Acetazolamide	3	+	[367,439]
Chlorpropamide	6	−	[440,441]
Chlorthalidone	10	+	[367,441]
Clopamide	3	−	[441]
Diazoxide	2	−	[442,443]
Furosemide	10	+	[441,444]
Glymidine	1	−	[441]
Tolbutamide	3	−	[441,445]
Miscellaneous:			
Allopurinol	1	+	[446]
Alphamethyldopa	5	+	[367,374,447]
Amrinone	2	+	[688]
Antazoline	2	+	[355,448]
Arsenical antiluetics	25	+	[372,449]
Bleomycin	5	−	[316]
Chloroquine	10	−	[380]
Chlorothiazide	10	+	[367,441]
Chlorpheniramine	1	+	[450]
Cimetidine	7	+	[369,451–453]
Copper sulfate	1	−	[454]
Desimipramine	2	−	[455]
Digitalis	1	−	[456]
Digitoxin	5	+	[457,458]
Digoxin	1	−	[459]
Disulfiram	1	−	[460]
Gold salts	>100	−	[377–379]
Heparin	>100	+	[320–323]
Heroin	15	−	[461–463]
Hexopropymate	1	−	[464]
Hydrochlorothiazide	4	+	[367,441,465]
Hydroxyquinoline	2	−	[466]
Insect bites	1	−	[467]
Insecticides	7	−	[386,387]
Iopanoic acid	1	−	[468,469]
Isoniazide (INH)	3	−	[470,471]
Levamisole	1	+	[472]
Levodopa	1	−	[473]
Lidocaine	1	+	[474]
Mercurial diuretics	3	−	[475]
Minoxidil	1	+	[476]
Nitrofurantoin	3	−	[441]
Nitroglycerine	1	−	[477]
Oxprenolol	2	+	[376,478]
Penicillamine	1	−	[479]
Pertussis vaccine	3	−	[480]
Procaine amide	2	+	[367,481]
Prochlorperazine	1	−	[482]
Propylthiouracil	1	−	[483]
Spironolactone	1	+	[367]
Stibophen	5	+	[484]
Tetanus toxoid	1	−	[485]
Tetraethylammonium	1	−	[486]
Thioguanine	1	+	[367]
Thiouracil	1	−	[487]
Toluene diisocyanate	2	−	[488]
Turpentine	2	−	[489]
Vinyl chloride	10	−	[689]

over the age of 50, presumably because of greater exposure to drugs [441], but has been described in a child less than 1 year old [373].

A careful history is of the utmost importance in diagnosis. In addition to inquiries about conventional medications, the patient should be asked about ingestion of patent remedies, soft drinks, mixers [348], and aperitifs [492] that may contain quinine. Thrombocytopenia in heroin addicts may be related to adulterants such as quinine injected with the drug [462,463], but this has not been confirmed by in vitro testing. Topical medications may occasionally provide the sensitizing stimulus [466]. In most instances, exposure to the offending drug will have occurred during the 24 h prior to the onset of symptoms. Gold salts, which may be retained for long periods within the body, are an exception to this rule.

Ingestion of a drug to which a patient is specifically sensitive may be followed within minutes by a warm sensation and flushing and later by a chill. Bleeding, characterized first by petechiae, purpura, hemorrhagic bullae of the oral mucosa, and often hemorrhage from the gastrointestinal and urinary tracts, usually appears from 6 to 12 h thereafter in severely affected patients. In some patients, petechial hemorrhages are the only symptom. Bleeding symptoms usually disappear over a period of 3 to 4 days as the offending drug is excreted or metabolized, but thrombocytopenia lasting 10 to 14 days has been observed by the author in a few patients with quinidine sensitivity. In patients with gold sensitivity, platelet levels may remain low for months.

LABORATORY FINDINGS
Thrombocytopenia is often very severe initially, platelet levels being less than 10,000 and sometimes less than 1000 per microliter. The number of megakaryocytes is usually normal or elevated but in a few instances has been reduced despite a suspected immune basis for the thrombocytopenia [409]. Occasionally, red cells [353,493], neutrophils [494], or other tissues [495] are also affected.

Detection of antibodies in vitro   In most but not all cases of thrombocytopenia brought on by quinidine and quinine, drug-dependent antibodies can be detected by a variety of immunologic techniques utilizing mixtures of the patient's serum or plasma, normal platelets, and the offending drug (Chap. A44). Greater sensitivity and specificity have been claimed for the platelet factor 3 release technique in the detection of antibodies stimulated by other drugs [367]. New techniques for directly measuring the deposition of immunoglobulin onto platelets in the presence of drug are likely to facilitate diagnosis in the near future [369]. Transformation of a patient's lymphocytes upon incubation with drug-coated platelets has been described [364], but the general usefulness of this method has not been established. A possible explanation for some negative tests is that drug metabolites formed in vivo, rather than the pharmacologic form of the drug, may provide the antigenic stimulus in some instances [396,415].

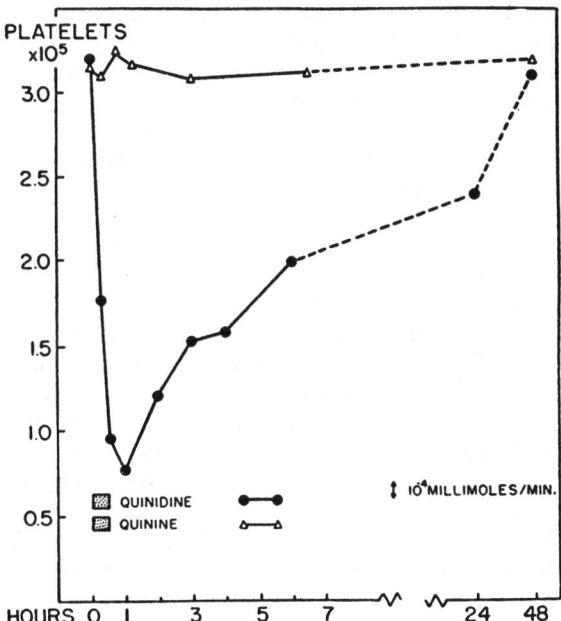

FIGURE 142-4   Induction of thrombocytopenia by infusion of a total of 1.3 mg of quinidine over a 24-min period in a patient with quinidine-dependent antibody. A lower dose of quinidine administered earlier was without effect. (Shulman [352].)

In vivo testing   Sensitivity to quinidine and Sedormid has been demonstrated by patch testing [344,496], but the technique often yields negative results and may carry some risk. Direct challenge of a patient with a drug suspected of causing thrombocytopenia is especially hazardous since as little as 1.3 mg of quinidine [354] and 1.4 μg of Sedormid [344] have been shown to cause severe thrombocytopenia. The nearly disastrous consequence of an in vivo challenge with neoarsphenamine has been graphically described [497]. If in vitro tests for antibody are negative and the drug suspected of causing thrombocytopenia is critical for the patient's welfare, a challenge may be attempted. It is essential, however, that the initial dose be less than 1 μg and that platelet levels be carefully monitored (Fig. 142-4). A single negative challenge in a patient who has not recently taken the suspected drug does not rule out sensitivity, as time may be required for reinduction of antibody.

TREATMENT AND PROGNOSIS
In any patient with thrombocytopenia of unknown etiology, all medications should be stopped until a diagnosis is established. If this is not feasible for medical reasons, other drugs with comparable pharmacologic actions should be substituted. Intracerebral hemorrhage, though fortunately rare, may occur in any patient during the acute stage. Lethal intrapulmonary hemorrhage has also been described [498]. In the author's opinion, hospitalization and observation for at least several days are indicated for patients with severe thrombocytopenia.

Glucocorticoids have not been shown to shorten the duration of thrombocytopenia, but their administration is perhaps advisable because of their possible effect on vascular integrity. Platelet transfusions are usually not helpful, as transfused cells are rapidly destroyed, but they should be given if hemorrhage is life-threatening. As the offending drug is cleared from the circulation, platelet transfusions become more effective [499]. With excretion of the drug to which a patient is sensitive, platelet levels return rapidly to normal, usually within 7 days of the onset of symptoms. As noted above, patients with gold sensitivity may remain thrombocytopenic for many months because of the slow turnover of drug. In such cases, dimercaprol (BAL) may speed recovery by increasing the rate of gold excretion [377,379]. Glucocorticoid therapy and splenectomy have also been used [379], and apparent responses to cyclophosphamide [378] and vincristine [500] have been recorded.

Once induced, sensitivity to drugs causing immunologic thrombocytopenic purpura probably persists indefinitely. Patients should therefore be warned to avoid reexposure. Possible exceptions have been described in patients sensitive to sodium valproate [435,436], valproic acid [438], and levodopa [473] who tolerated readministration of these drugs at lower dosage.

THROMBOCYTOPENIA AS A MANIFESTATION OF ALLERGY

Several authors have commented on a 15 to 50 percent decrease in circulating platelets, lasting several hours, that follows intracutaneous injection of an antigen to which sensitivity has previously been manifested [501,502]. Similar observations have been made following ingestion of foods to which allergy has been suspected [388,691]. One group found that the effect of antigen on platelet levels could be blocked by prior administration of heparin [501]. Platelet dysfunction [503] and activation [504] have been described in association with antigenic challenge in allergic subjects. The usefulness of measurements of platelet levels and platelet function in the evaluation of allergic subjects may deserve further evaluation.

ANAPHYLAXIS

Thrombocytopenia, often very severe, has been observed in laboratory animals subjected to anaphylactic shock [505,506], and it also occurs in humans [507]. Interaction of immune complexes with circulating platelets, together with disseminated intravascular coagulation (Chap. 158), may be responsible for platelet destruction, but the possible role of the recently described platelet-activating factor [508] deserves investigation.

POSTTRANSFUSION PURPURA

Acute thrombocytopenic purpura, comparable in severity to that seen in patients with quinidine sensitivity (see above) but occurring approximately 1 week after transfusion, is a distinct entity. About 30 cases have now been reported [509–520,691].

ETIOLOGY AND PATHOGENESIS

In nearly all cases in which appropriate serologic tests have been performed, an antibody has been detected which is specific for a genetically determined antigen first named Zw [509] and then Pl^{A1} [510]. This antigen is found in 98 percent of the normal population but is lacking from patients who develop posttransfusion purpura (PTP). In a single patient whose platelets were Pl^{A1}-positive, the antibody reacted with another platelet-specific antigen not yet defined [503]. The author has encountered two other cases of PTP in Pl^{A1}-positive patients.

Destruction of autologous platelets in PTP, seemingly mediated by an alloantibody, has thus far defied explanation. The suggestion has been made that a second antibody, arising along with anti-Pl^{A1}, cross-reacts with Pl^{A1}-negative platelets to cause thrombocytopenia. Although no such antibody has yet been demonstrated in humans, a disorder similar to PTP has been induced by injecting one species of marmosets with platelets from another species [521]. A second theory, supported by limited experimental evidence [41,510], is that the antibody stimulated by transfused Pl^{A1} antigen combines with that antigen to form soluble immune complexes having a special affinity for sites on the patient's own Pl^{A1}-negative platelets. The reader will note the similarity between this mechanism and that proposed to explain the destruction of platelets as "innocent bystanders" in drug-induced immunologic thrombocytopenia. Since 1 in 50 recipients is "mismatched" with respect to the Pl^{A1} antigen, while PTP occurs much less frequently, this theory requires one additional postulate: that only certain donor units, possibly those containing the Pl^{A1} antigen in a soluble form, are capable of causing the disorder.

CLINICAL FEATURES

All cases reported thus far except two [513,691] have involved women ranging in age from 39 to 78 years. All but two had previously been pregnant. In each instance the first bleeding symptoms occurred 5 to 8 days after transfusion of one or more units of blood. Hemorrhagic symptoms are usually dramatic at the onset, but a subclinical case has been described [515].

LABORATORY FINDINGS

Platelet levels at the time of the initial bleeding episode are very low, usually less than 10,000 per microliter. Megakaryocytes are usually present in normal or increased numbers but were reduced in one instance [515]. Anti-Pl^{A1} antibody can, in most instances, be detected by a variety of immunologic techniques [515–518]. The antibody inhibited ADP-induced aggregation of normal platelets in two instances [514].

THERAPY AND PROGNOSIS

Thrombocytopenia has persisted for 10 to 48 days in patients untreated or given glucocorticoids [509–518] (Fig.

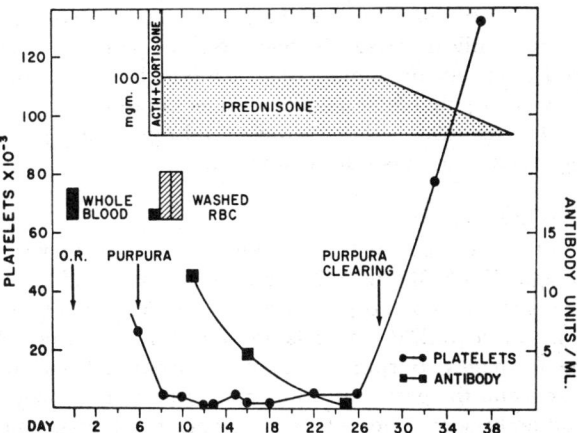

FIGURE 142-5   Clinical course of a 43-year-old woman with posttransfusion purpura. Profound thrombocytopenia occurred 6 days after transfusion of blood during a surgical procedure and persisted for 3 weeks despite treatment with prednisone. Recovery occurred at about the time detectable antibody was cleared from the circulation. (Shulman et al. [510].)

142-5). Two patients treated with whole-blood exchange transfusion recovered completely within 72 h [510,511], presumably because of the removal of antibody and/or immune complexes. Others have recovered rapidly after plasma exchange [512,518,519], but in one instance, plasmapheresis was notably unsuccessful [520]. Because thrombocytopenia is severe and the risk of intracranial hemorrhage is relatively great in the age group affected, whole-blood or plasma exchange therapy early in the course of PTP is deserving of further trial even though the rationale for its effectiveness is still uncertain.

Transfused platelets, even those from a Pl^{A1}-negative donor in one case [516], are usually ineffective in PTP, as they are rapidly destroyed. Moreover, their administration may cause severe, even life-threatening transfusion reactions [510,511]. Accordingly, if exchange transfusion is attempted, the first unit of blood should be given slowly while vital signs are carefully monitored.

Although anti-Pl^{A1} antibody has been shown to persist in some patients following restoration of the platelet level to normal [515,518], PTP does not necessarily recur when patients are later transfused again with Pl^{A1}-positive blood [518]. This appears to have happened in at least one instance, however [515].

IMMUNE COMPLEX–MEDIATED THROMBOCYTOPENIA

Platelets are known to express an Fc receptor capable of binding immune complexes [522,523], and the interaction of platelets with immune complexes has been extensively studied in in vitro systems [524–527]. Studies of patients receiving platelet transfusions suggest that platelets can bind and remove immune complexes from the circulation [528]. Evidence is mentioned elsewhere in this chapter for immune complex–mediated destruction of platelets in drug-induced thrombocytopenia and

posttransfusion purpura and for the association of circulating immune complexes with thrombocytopenia in some patients with infection, thrombotic thrombocytopenic purpura, and the hemolytic-uremic syndrome. Whether immune complexes actually provoke platelet destruction in these or other thrombocytopenic disorders remains to be established.

ACUTE IDIOPATHIC THROMBOCYTOPENIC PURPURA (POSTINFECTIOUS THROMBOCYTOPENIA)

Idiopathic thrombocytopenic purpura (ITP) is a diagnosis usually reached by excluding the other causes of thrombocytopenia discussed in this chapter. Evidence is becoming ever more convincing that platelet destruction in the great majority of patients with ITP is mediated by immune mechanisms. Accordingly, the adjective *idiopathic* may soon be dispensed with.

From its clinical manifestations alone, it is apparent that ITP comprises at least two distinct entities, designated *acute* and *chronic*. Because the two types differ greatly in their clinical course and probably in their pathogenesis, they are discussed separately: acute here and chronic below.

Acute ITP is predominantly a disease of childhood characterized by (1) the abrupt onset of severe thrombocytopenic purpura, (2) a history of infection, usually viral, occurring 2 to 21 days previously in 60 to 80 percent, and (3) spontaneous recovery, usually within 1 to 2 months (Fig. 142-6) [145,146,529–531]. Although its precise frequency has not been calculated, the disorder is quite common, and many large series of cases have been reported [529–533]. An apparently identical disease occasionally occurs in adults of all ages. A form especially prevalent among young adults of central and southern Africa has been designated *onyalai* [534]. Whether the same disorder occurs in American blacks is uncertain [535].

Acute ITP as defined above should be distinguished

FIGURE 142-6   Course of idiopathic thrombocytopenic purpura in an 8-year-old child. Severe thrombocytopenia occurred 1 week after an upper respiratory infection. Remission occurred 4 weeks later.

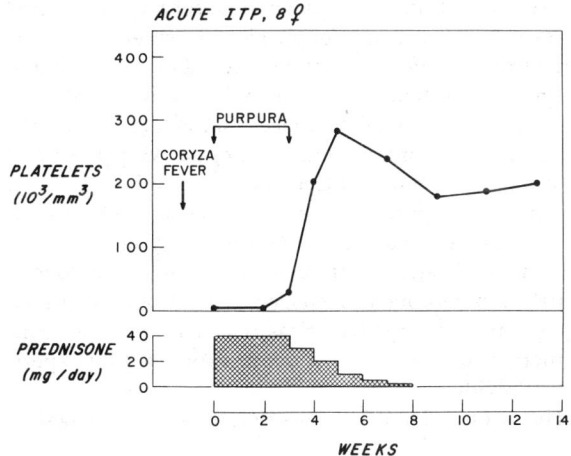

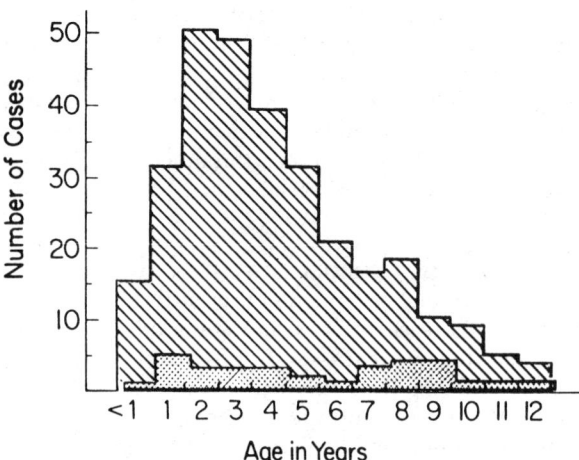

FIGURE 142-7   Age distribution of 305 children with idiopathic thrombocytopenic purpura. (Lusher and Iyer [529].)

from other forms of thrombocytopenia associated with viral infections (Chap. 141 and page 1303). These two forms of thrombocytopenia have been termed *postinfectious* and *infectious,* respectively [536].

ETIOLOGY AND PATHOGENESIS

That acute ITP is often preceded by a viral illness, especially in children, is well established, but the relationship between infection and the subsequent, often fulminating destruction of platelets is not completely understood. The appearance of thrombocytopenia and bleeding at a time when virus is ordinarily cleared from the circulation argues against direct interaction between virus and platelet as the cause of thrombocytopenia and suggests that platelets are somehow affected by the immune response to the primary infection. Immune complexes are known to be capable of binding to human platelets [522–525,537], apparently to an Fc receptor expressed on the platelet membrane. In one study, antibodies in the serum of children with postrubella thrombocytopenia were found to cause platelet aggregation in the presence of rubella antigen, a property that was lacking in the serum of children who experienced rubella without subsequent thrombocytopenia [537]. These clinical and experimental observations suggest that sudden destruction of platelets in patients recuperating from an infection may be a result of the formation of antigen-antibody complexes which have an affinity for sites on the platelet surface; that is, acute ITP, like drug-induced immunologic thrombocytopenia and posttransfusion purpura (see above), may be a form of "immune complex disease." Alternative theories offered to explain acute ITP — that infectious agents somehow alter platelet structure so as to cause autologous platelets to become antigenic or that antibodies formed against an infecting virus cross-react with a surface constituent of platelets — are as yet unsupported by experimental evidence.

That acute ITP rarely occurs in families argues against

a genetic basis. However, the antigen HLA-Aw32 was significantly increased in one group of patients [538], and a variety of immunologic abnormalities was observed in patients and their families in another study [539]. The relationship of these findings to the pathogenesis of the disorder is uncertain.

CLINICAL FEATURES

Acute ITP occurs most frequently in children 2 to 9 years of age [529–533] (Fig. 142-7) but may occur in adults at any age. There is no predilection for either sex. Symptoms of acute ITP are variable, but typically petechial hemorrhages, purpura, and often bleeding from the gums and the gastrointestinal and urinary tracts begin suddenly, sometimes over a period of a few hours. Usually, but not always, the severity of bleeding correlates with the degree of thrombocytopenia. Florid purpura usually persists only for a few days or, at most, 1 to 2 weeks, even though platelet levels may remain depressed for longer periods.

Preceding infections are usually of viral origin. Among these are rubella, rubeola, and chickenpox, but nonspecific respiratory infections are most common [529,531]. Acute ITP may also occur following immunization with live vaccine for measles, chickenpox, mumps, and smallpox [531,540]. In adults, profound but transient thrombocytopenia has occurred following BCG injection for immunotherapy of tumors [541]. The latent period between infection and the onset of purpura is most often 1 to 2 weeks, but it may be as short as 2 days or as long as 6 weeks. Not surprisingly, the disorder is most common during the winter and spring months, when the incidence of infection is high.

Physical examination discloses myriad petechial hemorrhages and often generalized purpura, especially over areas of skin exposed to trauma. Hemorrhagic bullae are often present in the oral mucosa. The liver and spleen are palpable in about 10 percent of cases but are not strikingly enlarged, and shotty lymphadenopathy is common. These findings probably reflect recent viral infection.

LABORATORY FINDINGS

Thrombocytopenia is usually severe at the onset; in most cases platelets are fewer than 20,000 per microliter. Anemia, when present, is related to blood loss. Relative lymphocytosis and slight eosinophilia are common [529]. Normal or increased numbers of megakaryocytes, many of which are "smooth" in contour, are found in the marrow. The latter are probably immature rather than "non-platelet-producing" cells, as discussed below under chronic ITP. The life-span of transfused platelets is extremely short, sometimes only a few hours. Mean IgG levels were subnormal and C3 levels normal in one series [542]. Reduced levels of C3 were observed in another [539].

With a few exceptions [531,543], tests for platelet antibodies in the serum of patients with acute ITP have been negative. However, direct analysis of IgG on autologous platelets has revealed elevated levels of platelet-associated IgG in a high percentage of cases [544–547]. One group has found that platelet IgG is usually higher in children with acute ITP than in adults with chronic ITP [544,545]. Currently available methods do not distinguish between autoantibodies and immune complexes bound to the platelet surface, and the specificity of platelet IgG assays in thrombocytopenic subjects has been questioned [548].

DIFFERENTIAL DIAGNOSIS

The clinical picture presented by a child with acute ITP is usually so typical as to suggest the correct diagnosis immediately. Bacterial sepsis, particularly meningococcemia, which may also be characterized by purpura and thrombocytopenia, must be carefully ruled out, however. Very rarely, acute self-limited thrombocytopenia appears to have been a manifestation of tuberculosis [101] or sarcoidosis. Acute leukemia can readily be excluded by examination of the peripheral blood and marrow. Thrombotic thrombocytopenic purpura and hemolytic-uremic syndrome can be distinguished by the presence of hemolysis and microangiopathic changes in circulating erythrocytes. The latter abnormalities are also found in patients with hemangioma-thrombocytopenia syndrome. Drug-induced immunologic thrombocytopenia must be considered in patients who have been taking medication. Other diagnostic possibilities are discussed under "Chronic Idiopathic Thrombocytopenic Purpura," below.

THERAPY AND PROGNOSIS

Despite the severe thrombocytopenia and hemorrhagic symptoms initially present in patients with acute ITP, more than 80 percent ultimately recover regardless of the treatment administered [529–533]. In half, platelet levels return to normal in less than 6 weeks; 80 to 90 percent are well within 6 months. Recovery is most often permanent, but a few patients have multiple recurrences which sometimes seem to be triggered by infection [529,549] or vaccination [540].

Although acute ITP is usually benign, a mortality of about 1 percent, due chiefly to intracerebral hemorrhage, has been recorded in most series [531,533,550], and higher figures are quoted in the earlier literature. It is generally agreed that the risk of hemorrhage is greatest during the first 1 to 2 weeks. All patients should therefore restrict activity and avoid even minor trauma during the period of severe thrombocytopenia. Those with florid purpura and other bleeding manifestations should be hospitalized and carefully observed. The importance of avoiding aspirin and other drugs that inhibit platelet function has been stressed [550].

Whether *glucocorticoids* should be given to children with acute ITP is still controversial [529,530,551,552]. In several large series the outcome appears to have been unaffected by use or nonuse of these drugs [529,531,553], and in one study they actually seemed to

prolong the time required for recovery [554]. Others have found that platelet levels become elevated more quickly in children given prednisone, 2 to 3 mg per kilogram body weight per day [530,533,555]. Prednisone has also been advocated for its possible effect on vascular resistance [551,556]. Because intracranial hemorrhage is most likely to occur with 2 weeks of the onset of ITP and because the risk of using glucocorticoids for a short period of time is small, it has been suggested that prednisone should be given for several weeks after the onset of symptoms [551,557].

Platelet transfusions may be of transient benefit in treating severe hemorrhage [558,559] but need not be given routinely. Emergency splenectomy combined with high-dose glucocorticoid therapy has been recommended for children with intracranial hemorrhage and should be instituted, where possible, before neurosurgery is undertaken [550,560]. *Therapeutic plasmapheresis* appeared to be of benefit in several severely affected children [558,559]. *Transfusion of fresh normal plasma*, 30 ml per kilogram body weight over a 24-h period, was followed by a dramatic elevation of platelet levels within 72 h in more than half the children so treated in several early studies [561,562]. Recently, each of six children given *intravenous injections of gamma globulin* for 5 successive days responded with an elevation of platelets to normal within 5 to 10 days [563]. Two of these later relapsed, but responded again to additional injections. No explanation for the apparent effectiveness of plasma and gamma globulin is yet available, and this method of treatment, while of great theoretical interest, must be considered experimental.

About 10 percent of children with ITP fail to recover within 6 months. At this point the disorder is generally designated chronic, although, rarely, spontaneous remissions occur after more than 1 year [531]. Among children in whom the disorder is not preceded by infection and who have only moderately severe thrombocytopenia [529], those with lower levels of platelet-associated IgG [544,545], low levels of IgA [529], or an increased basal rate of DNA synthesis in peripheral blood lymphocytes [564] are perhaps more likely to remain thrombocytopenic. Chronicity may be more common among children in Middle East countries [565]. Clinically, children who fail to improve are similar to adults with chronic ITP (below). About one-third of these have mild symptoms which require no specific therapy. In most of the remaining two-thirds, purpura can be controlled with prednisone. Thrombocytopenia almost invariably recurs when the drug is stopped, however, and retardation of growth and other complications may follow its prolonged administration [566]. For these reasons, *splenectomy* is advisable in children who do not recover within 6 to 12 months and require maintenance steroid therapy. Wherever possible, however, the operation should be deferred until 4 or 5 years of age [529]. There is a small but significant risk of serious infection following the procedure [529].

Immunosuppressive therapy has been used in a few

children with chronic ITP. Of 19 children who received azathioprine and glucocorticoids, 7 showed at least temporary improvement [531,566–568]. Vincristine has also been used [569]. In view of the uncertainty about the long-term side effects of such therapy, it should be reserved for the most severe cases.

CHRONIC IDIOPATHIC THROMBOCYTOPENIC PURPURA (WERLHOF'S DISEASE, PURPURA-HEMORRHAGICA, AUTOIMMUNE THROMBOCYTOPENIA)

The first description of idiopathic thrombocytopenic purpura (ITP) is attributed to Werlhof in 1735 [570], but Krauss, in 1883, appears to be the first to associate the hemorrhagic symptoms with thrombocytopenia [571]. Among early descriptions of the disorder are those of Frank [572] and Minot [573]. Many reviews can be found in the more recent literature [574–577].

Chronic ITP, in contrast to the acute disorder (see above), is primarily a disease of adults and rarely resolves spontaneously. It is considerably more common than autoimmune hemolytic anemia (Chap. 67), which, except for the cell type involved, appears to have a similar pathogenesis. Autoimmune thrombocytopenia also occurs in a number of animal species [578].

ETIOLOGY AND PATHOGENESIS

A lively controversy over the pathogenesis of chronic ITP began with the studies of Frank [572], who

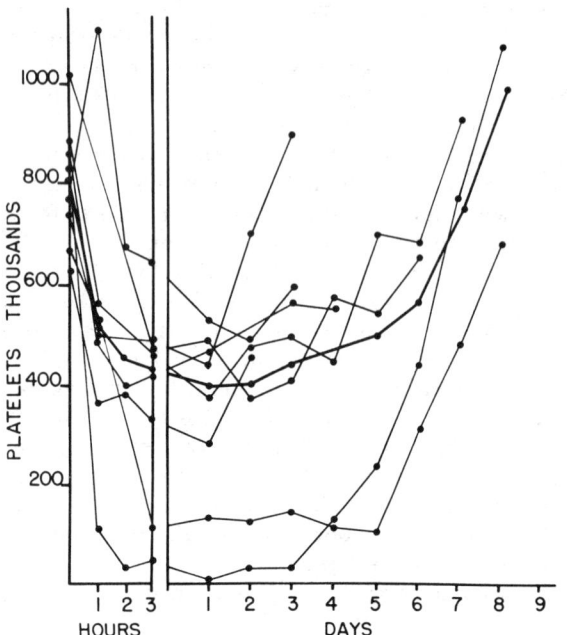

FIGURE 142-8 Effect of infusing 250 ml of plasma from patients with chronic idiopathic thrombocytopenic purpura on platelet levels in normal recipients. On each of eight occasions, a significant decrease in platelet levels was observed. Average change is denoted by the heavy line. High initial platelet concentrations are due to use of an indirect counting technique. (Harrington et al. [585].)

suggested that thrombocytopenia was due to defective megakaryocyte maturation. Minot [573] concluded that platelets were destroyed "as fast as they were formed." Only when platelet transfusions became available was it demonstrated that the life-span of circulating platelets is nearly always shortened [576,577]. Many studies of platelet survival have since been carried out using radioactive labels, and platelet life-span was found to be diminished in nearly every instance [576,577,579–582]. Normal platelet survival has been observed in a few patients who appear to have an as yet unclassified disorder [582,583]. Although the factor responsible for platelet destruction in ITP (see below) may act to some extent on megakaryocytes as well as on platelets [584], platelet production calculated on the basis of platelet turnover is at least normal and usually increased in patients with a shortened platelet life-span [577,581,582].

The observation that women with ITP sometimes give birth to children with thrombocytopenia [61–66] suggested that platelet destruction might be caused by a humoral factor. Confirmation of this was provided by Harrington and coworkers, who found that plasma from about 50 percent of patients with ITP caused thrombocytopenia when transfused to normal persons [585] (Fig. 142-8). Others have demonstrated a comparable effect with plasma from about one-third of patients with ITP [586]. The antiplatelet factor was found to be an immunoglobulin G which can be absorbed by human platelets but does not cause thrombocytopenia in animals. Its reactivity with autologous platelets was demonstrated in one instance by reinduction of thrombocytopenia upon injection of a patient, during a period of remission, with plasma obtained during a previous thrombocytopenic episode [587].

Despite long-standing suspicion that platelet destruction in ITP was immunologically mediated, direct experimental evidence for autoantibodies was difficult to obtain [574]. Technical advances [577] (see also Chap. A43) have led only recently to the consistent demonstration of elevated quantities of platelet-associated IgG in patients with ITP. Of 299 patients studied prior to 1981, platelet-associated IgG was elevated in 278 (93 percent) [577]. Tests for antibody in serum were positive in 169 of 313 (54 percent) [577]. Available methods for measuring platelet-associated IgG do not distinguish between autoantibodies and immune complexes bound to the platelet surface. Moreover, the specificity of platelet-associated IgG measurements in thrombocytopenic patients has been questioned [548,588], and studies of serum antibodies have not always distinguished between allo- and autoreactivity. Nonetheless, observations made to date provide persuasive evidence that platelet destruction is immunologically mediated in nearly all patients with ITP. In most cases, platelet-associated IgG appears to consist of all four subclasses, but mainly IgG1 [589,590]. Complement components have also been detected on autologous platelets [546,591,592]. IgM autoantibodies have been found in a few instances [590]. Circulating immune complexes [593,594], cell-mediated immunity against platelets

[595,596], and a variety of other immunologic abnormalities [597–599] have been demonstrated in some patients. The relationship of the latter findings to platelet destruction is unclear. Diminished suppressor cell activity, implying an abnormality of immunoregulation, was observed in several studies [600,601]. The possibility remains that in some cases of ITP, thrombocytopenia is due to continued exposure to an unrecognized exogenous antigen (see "Drug-Induced Immunologic Thrombocytopenic Purpura," above).

Increased prevalence of the antigens HLA-B8 and HLA-B12 was observed in one series of patients with ITP [602] but not in others [577,603–605]. No association with HLA-DR was found in a large series [606]. Familial occurrence of ITP has been described [607], but this is very unusual. Immunologic abnormalities found in relatives of patients with chronic ITP have been interpreted as evidence of a hereditary tendency to develop the disorder [608].

The effectiveness of splenectomy in the treatment of ITP first drew attention to the spleen as a probable site of platelet destruction and/or autoantibody production [609]. Subsequent studies have demonstrated that in ITP the spleen does remove antibody-coated platelets from the circulation [579,580,587]. The rate at which sensitized platelets are destroyed appears to be directly related to the quantity of platelet-associated IgG [610]. Hepatic destruction of platelets probably occurs only when platelets are very heavily coated with antibody [579,587,610,611] and therefore is seen only in the most severe cases. An added role for the spleen in the pathogenesis of ITP is suggested by studies showing that the organ is a major site of autoantibody synthesis [612,613]. Destruction of platelets in the spleen may therefore be promoted by a high concentration of antibody within the organ [577]. The occurrence of neonatal thrombocytopenia in children born to women previously splenectomized for ITP [61–66] indicates that autoantibody is regularly produced in extrasplenic sites as well. Antibody production by cultured marrow was demonstrated in one instance [614].

That estrogens or other hormones may play a role in the pathogenesis of ITP is suggested by its high frequency in postpubertal, premenopausal women and the relapses that not uncommonly occur during pregnancy [615]. The speculation has been offered that the female preponderance of chronic ITP is related to increased expression of Fc receptors on female platelets [616].

ASSOCIATION WITH OTHER DISORDERS
Thrombocytopenia difficult to distinguish from chronic ITP may be an early manifestation of sarcoidosis [617,618], lymphoma (Hodgkin's disease, chronic lymphocytic leukemia, non-Hodgkin's lymphoma) [619–621], systemic lupus erythematosus [575,622], thyrotoxicosis [623–625], and, possibly, tuberculosis [102], histoplasmosis [626], Hashimoto's thyroiditis [625], scleroderma [627], carcinoma even in the absence of splenic enlargement and/or marrow infiltration [628], and myasthenia gravis [629]. In some of these condi-

tions, the thrombocytopenia is perhaps mediated by immune complexes. The association of chronic ITP and autoimmune hemolytic anemia (Evans' syndrome) in children and adults is well established [575,630]. Concomitant autoimmune abnormalities affecting coagulation [631] and neutrophils [632] have been described in a few patients.

The occurrence of ITP during pregnancy has been mentioned frequently [61–66], but the disease commonly affects women of childbearing age and the association may be coincidental.

CLINICAL FEATURES
Chronic ITP occurs chiefly between the ages of 20 and 50 years but may be seen in the very young and the very old. Women are affected three times as often as men. A history of preceding infection is rarely obtained. The disorder appears to be rare in children [529] and adults [575] among black people.

Presenting symptoms vary greatly from one patient to another, but typically the disease begins somewhat insidiously with scattered petechiae or other minor bleeding manifestations. Occasionally a bruising tendency, menorrhagia, or recurrent epistaxis is present for months or even years before diagnosis. Patients generally feel quite well except for complaints relating to hemorrhage. Petechial and purpuric lesions of a noninflammatory character may occur anywhere on the skin or mucosal surfaces but are most common on the distal upper and lower extremities. Hemorrhagic bullae in the oral mucosa usually indicate that thrombocytopenia is very severe. Deep-lying ecchymoses may be present, especially in regions subjected to trauma, but bleeding into joints or into the retina is unusual as is any type of hemorrhage in the absence of cutaneous lesions [575]. Intracranial hemorrhage, although rare, is a potential hazard in every patient, and neurologic signs should be carefully monitored during the acute stage. The spleen is occasionally palpable on deep inspiration. A greater degree of splenomegaly argues strongly against ITP as the primary diagnosis.

LABORATORY FINDINGS
Platelet levels usually range from 5000 to 75,000 per microliter and are generally somewhat higher than in acute ITP. Bizarre giant platelets and fragmented platelets are commonly seen [633]. Anemia, when present, is usually due to blood loss, but, as noted above, autoimmune hemolytic anemia and ITP occasionally occur together (Evans' syndrome) [575,630], in which case the direct Coombs' test may be positive. Elevated levels of plasma acid phosphatase reflect increased platelet turnover but are not of specific diagnostic value [634]. Adhesion of platelets to leukocytes has been described in a few instances [635]. Perhaps 2 percent of patients with chronic ITP exhibit positive tests for lupus erythematosus and are actually afflicted with this disorder [575,622].

As in any patient with thrombocytopenia, clot retraction is diminished, bleeding time is prolonged, and capillary fragility as measured by the tourniquet test is increased. The active bleeding seen with platelet levels as high as 50,000 per microliter suggests that in some patients the autoantibodies affect platelet function. Recent reports are consistent with this possibility [576,636,637]. In some patients, the autoantibodies may induce platelet dysfunction without causing thrombocytopenia [576,625,638].

As noted above, platelet-associated IgG is almost invariably elevated in severely thrombocytopenic patients [577]. Platelet antibodies have been detected in serum from 20 to 95 percent of patients in different laboratories, the average being about 54 percent [577]. Caveats relating to interpretation of these measurements have already been mentioned. There is a rough, inverse relationship between the quantity of IgG on platelets and the platelet count [544,547,610,639–641] (Fig. 142-9).

In the marrow, megakaryocytes are found in normal or increased numbers but are less granular, more basophilic, and smoother in contour (often described as "nonbudding") than those of normal marrow (Fig. 142-10). These changes have been interpreted as indicating defective maturation or failure of platelet production [576,577]. The demonstration that overall platelet production is usually increased above normal in ITP [577,581,582] suggests, however, that the megakaryocyte population is merely shifted toward immaturity and/or that platelets are released prematurely under the stress of thrombocytopenia. Binding of autoantibodies to megakaryocytes has been demonstrated, however [642],

and the possibility that this affects platelet production adversely has not been totally ruled out [584].

The spleen removed at surgery shows large numbers of lymphatic nodules with highly reactive germinal centers in the white pulp and increased numbers of plasma cells surrounding small vessels of the marginal zone, suggesting active production of antibody [643]. Platelets in various stages of degradation are demonstrable in splenic macrophages by electron microscopy [643,644]. Occasionally the diagnosis of tuberculosis, sarcoidosis, Hodgkin's disease, or lupus erythematosus is established for the first time from splenic histology. Criteria have been suggested by means of which the diagnosis of lupus erythematosus can be made even in the absence of the classic periarterial fibrosis [645]. Lipid-laden macrophages containing phospholipid, cholesterol, and ceroid probably derived from phagocytosed platelets are commonly found in surgical specimens [646–648]. These are manifested as foam cells and sea-blue histiocytes and may be more common in patients treated for prolonged periods with glucocorticoids [647].

DIFFERENTIAL DIAGNOSIS
Until the usefulness of newer diagnostic techniques is fully clarified, each of the disorders discussed in this chapter should be considered before a diagnosis of idiopathic (autoimmune) thrombocytopenia is made. It is essential to exclude drug sensitivity, sepsis, and disseminated intravascular coagulation, as failure to recog-

FIGURE 142-9 Linear (*A*) and double-log (*B*) plots of initial platelet count against platelet-bound antibody in 17 patients with autoimmune thrombocytopenic purpura. (Kernoff, Blake, and Shackleton [610].)

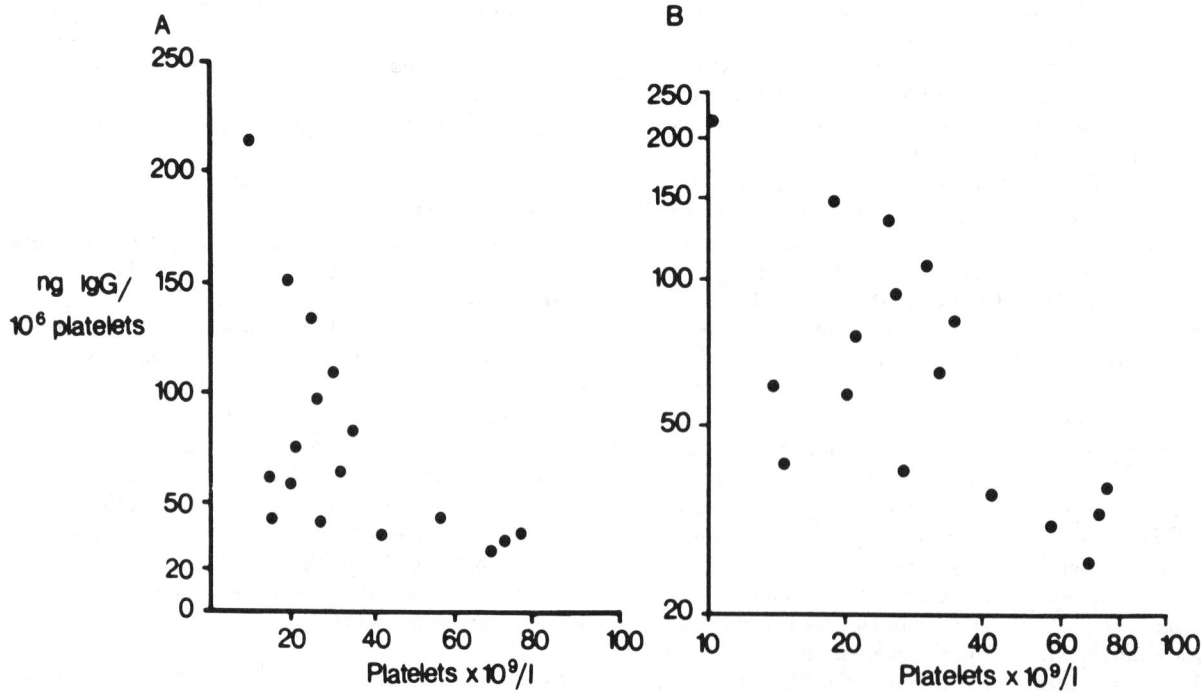

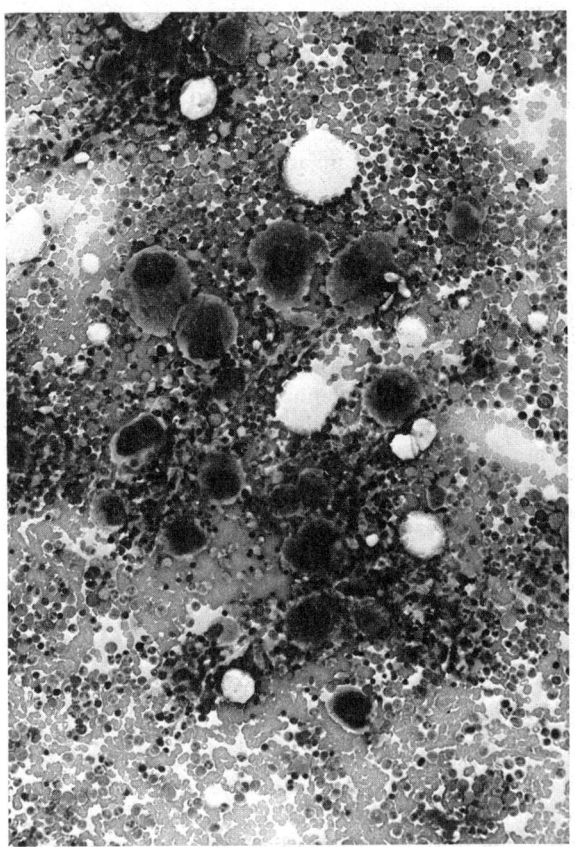

FIGURE 142-10 Cluster of smooth, apparently "nonbudding" megakaryocytes in the marrow of a patient with idiopathic thrombocytopenic purpura. Despite their appearance, platelet production by such cells is probably normal, as noted in the text. (Wright's stain.)

nize these disorders can be disastrous. Thrombotic thrombocytopenic purpura can be ruled out by a careful examination of red cell morphology. Procedures appropriate for the diagnosis of disseminated lupus erythematosus and other connective tissue disorders, tuberculosis, lymphoma, sarcoidosis, and thyrotoxicosis are indicated if there is any suspicion that one of these diseases underlies the thrombocytopenia.

THERAPY AND PROGNOSIS
Numerous reviews of this subject are available [575–577,649–651]. Perhaps 10 to 20 percent of adults with ITP recover spontaneously. Patients in whom thrombocytopenia is very severe and of acute onset may be more apt to do so than those with milder symptoms, but there is no immediate way to differentiate one group from the other with certainty. Patients who recover within a few weeks without splenectomy are perhaps afflicted with acute ITP of the type seen in children or have unsuspected drug sensitivity.

Platelet transfusion   This is effective in treatment of life-threatening hemorrhage [652], but should not be given prophylactically because shortened platelet life-span re-

stricts platelet effectiveness. Moreover, alloantibody formation may limit the usefulness of later transfusions.

Glucocorticoids   The effectiveness of glucocorticoids in the treatment of ITP appears to be due in part to suppression of the phagocytic activity of the monocyte-macrophage system and of the spleen in particular [557,653,654], so that the life-span of antibody-coated platelets is prolonged [579,581]. It is likely that antibody synthesis is inhibited as well, since plasma and platelet-associated autoantibodies usually become undetectable in patients who respond to therapy. Reduction in capillary fragility and shortening of the bleeding time sometimes precede a significant increase in platelet levels in patients treated with glucocorticoids but the mechanism of this effect is uncertain.

The usual starting dose of prednisone is about 1.0 mg/kg. Smaller amounts will elevate platelets in mildly affected patients, but higher doses may be required in others. A minimum of several days and often as long as 2 weeks of treatment may be required before an elevation of platelet levels is observed (Fig. 142-11). Nearly all patients will respond if sufficiently large doses are given, but as many as 250 mg of prednisone per day is sometimes necessary [655]. If improvement does not occur within 2 to 3 weeks or can be maintained only with massive doses of steroids, splenectomy should be considered (see below). In patients who respond to medication, dosage may be reduced gradually over a period of several weeks until platelet levels stabilize at about 50,000 per microliter.

Opinions differ as to how long maintenance therapy with steroids should be continued before performing splenectomy. The prevailing view favors splenectomy in patients who fail to respond spontaneously within 1 to 4 months, who require more than minimal doses of prednisone for maintenance, and who are suitable operative risks [576,656–659].

FIGURE 142-11   Course of chronic idiopathic thrombocytopenic purpura in a 42-year-old woman. Platelets were restored to normal by 3 weeks of prednisone therapy, but thrombocytopenia and purpura recurred after the dosage was reduced. Splenectomy resulted in a sustained remission.

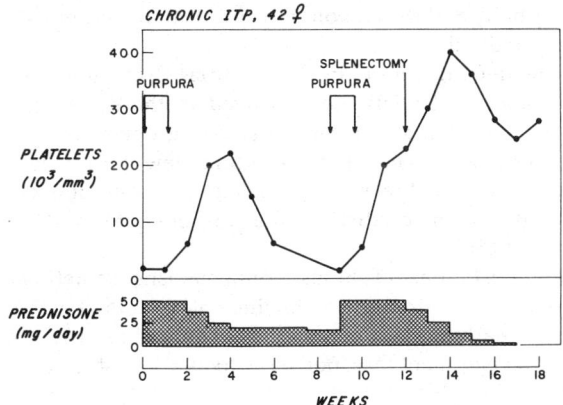

Splenectomy Splenectomy is beneficial primarily because it results in removal of the major site of platelet destruction and an important site of antibody production [577]. In preparation for surgery, the maintenance dose of prednisone may be increased in order to raise the platelet count. In thrombocytopenic patients, platelet transfusions may reduce bleeding if given preoperatively or just after clamping the splenic artery. However, many patients do well without transfusion. At operation, a search should be made for accessory spleens, most often found in or near the base of the splenic pedicle [575].

From 70 to 90 percent of patients improve after splenectomy, and platelet levels are restored permanently to normal in at least two-thirds of them [67,575–577,656–658]. Following splenectomy, platelet levels sometimes increase within 24 h, but more often several days are necessary and occasionally 1 to 2 weeks elapse before there is a response. Patients in whom platelet counts fail to rise may nonetheless be benefited by a reduction in the dosage of glucorcorticoids needed to prevent bleeding.

Plasma- and platelet-associated autoantibody usually becomes undetectable after a response to splenectomy. However, persistent elevation of platelet-associated IgG was found in about one-third of responding patients in several recent studies [544,545]. A modest shortening of platelet life-span observed in some patients who develop a "complete" remission after splenectomy may reflect a compensated thrombocytolytic state [659,660].

There is, unfortunately, no method of predicting with certainty which patients will respond to splenectomy. In several series, the effectiveness of splenectomy correlated reasonably well with the response to glucocorticoid therapy [658,661], but the relationship was by no means absolute. Patients over the age of 50 years have a somewhat lower probability of achieving complete remission than younger patients [575]. Patients in whom platelet levels rise only moderately after splenectomy are less likely to achieve a permanent remission than are those who develop marked thrombocytosis [575,657]. In one series, patients splenectomized early appeared to respond better than those who had their spleen removed late in the course of their disease [662]. The relationship between the level of platelet-associated autoantibody and the response to splenectomy has not yet been defined.

The demonstration by body surface scanning that ^{51}Cr-labeled platelets are destroyed in the spleen has been advocated as a means of selecting operative candidates [660,663,664]. The prevailing view, however, is that studies of the sites of platelet sequestration are not useful in predicting the response to surgery [579,665,666].

Manifestations of lupus erythematosus sometimes appear for the first time following splenectomy for ITP, but the early suggestion that the operation itself triggers this development has not withstood the test of time [667,668].

Following splenectomy, steroids may be withdrawn gradually over a period of 2 to 4 weeks. If platelet levels remain elevated after the drug is stopped, the improvement usually persists indefinitely, but relapses may occur up to 10 years later. In patients who relapse, the question of whether an accessory spleen was overlooked at operation is inevitably raised. It seems clear that accessory splenic tissue has caused recurrences of thrombocytopenia in some patients [575,669,670] even when Howell-Jolly bodies were detectable in the peripheral blood [575], and such tissue should be carefully searched for using modern imaging techniques [670]. However, only about half of these patients respond to removal of accessory splenic tissue [575,670].

The limited but nonetheless significant risks of infection associated with removal of the spleen in adults and precautions that should be taken to minimize these have recently been reviewed [576].

Immunosuppression Immunosuppressive therapy is sometimes effective in ITP. Use of azathioprine with prednisone was associated with a good or excellent response in about 25 percent of 92 patients reported prior to 1981 [577]. About one-half had no response. Several months or longer was usually required for improvement. More than half of 61 patients treated with cyclophosphamide and prednisone obtained good to excellent responses within 1 to 2 months [577,656,671]. About one-third of patients treated with vincristine, 1 mg or 2 mg per week, obtained a good to excellent response in 1 to 2 weeks [577,649,672,673]. However, improvement following the use of vinca alkaloids is sometimes transient [575,577,674]. The effect of vincristine in chronic ITP may in part be a result of direct stimulation of platelet production by the drug [675].

While additional experience in the use of immunosuppressive agents for the treatment of ITP is needed, it seems clear that a trial of immunosuppression should be considered in patients who fail to respond to splenectomy, relapse postoperatively, or are not candidates for operation. The risks of immunosuppressive therapy, including infection and malignancy, should be carefully weighed in considering long-term use of immunosuppressive medications. It should be remembered that some patients do well for long periods of time despite moderately severe thrombocytopenia and that some of these eventually experience a remission without immunosuppressive therapy [651].

Vinblastine-loaded platelets Transfusions of platelets "loaded" with vinblastine, which may act by inhibiting the phagocytic cells that destroy them, seems indicated in occasional patients who remain symptomatic despite the use of other therapeutic measures [676,677]. Because of the dissociation of vinblastine from platelets in vivo, this preparation is likely to be effective only in patients with very short platelet survival times [678].

Therapeutic plasmapheresis Machine-assisted plasma exchange transfusion was followed by significant but transient improvement in several patients refractory to all other forms of therapy [679–681] and deserves consideration in highly selected cases. Dramatic improvement after plasma exchange is distinctly unusual, and this treatment should not be used routinely [682].

Intravenous gamma globulin Infusion of gamma globulin in high doses has been followed by dramatic improvement in patients with ITP [563], including two who had failed splenectomy, but was without benefit in two patients who had not had splenectomy [683]. No explanation for this apparent therapeutic effect is yet available, but this treatment seems worthy of further trial in refractory patients.

Treatment of ITP in pregnancy The course of ITP appears not to be influenced by pregnancy [61–66,684], and treatment is as in nonpregnant women, with appropriate precautions for the welfare of the fetus. Splenectomy should be postponed until after delivery when possible, but the operation has been performed successfully in the second and third trimesters [62,68].

References

1. DeBruijne, J. L., Van Creveld, S. W., and Hoo, U. K.: Clotting factors in hemolytic disease of the newborn. II. Thrombocytopenia after replacement transfusion. *Etud. Neo-natal 5:*109, 1956.
2. Mauer, H. M., et al.: Effects of phototherapy on platelet counts in low-birthweight infants and on platelet production and life span in rabbits. *Pediatrics 57:*506, 1976.
3. Medoff, H. S.: Platelet counts in premature infants. *J. Pediatr. 64:*287, 1964.
4. Fogel, B. J., Arias, D., and Kung, F.: Platelet counts in healthy premature infants. *J. Pediatr. 72:*108, 1968.
5. Appleyard, W. J., and Brinton, A.: Venous platelet counts in low birth weight infants. *Biol. Neonate 17:*30, 1971.
6. Kaplan, E., and Klein, S. W.: Thrombocytopenia and intestinal bleeding in premature infants. *J. Pediatr. 61:*17, 1962.
7. Pearson, H. A.: Thrombocytopenia in premature infants: Pathological or physiological? *J. Pediatr. 73:*60, 1968.
8. Meberg, A., Halvorsen, S., and Orstavik, I. Transitory thrombocytopenia in small-for-date infants, possibly related to maternal smoking. *Lancet 2:*303, 1977.
9. Stein, H., Beck, J., and Solomon, A: Gastroenteritis with necrotizing enterocolitis in premature babies. *Br. Med. J. 2:*616, 1972.
10. Nielson, N.: Influence of pre-eclampsia upon coagulation and fibrinolysis in women and their newborn infants immediately after delivery. *Acta Obstet. Gynecol. Scand. 48:*523, 1969.
11. Kleckner, H. B., Giles, H. R., and Corrigan, J. J., Jr.: The association of maternal and neonatal thrombocytopenia in high-risk pregnancies. *Am. J. Obstet. Gynecol. 128:*235, 1977.
12. Jones, J. E., and Reed, J. F., Jr. Renal vein thrombosis and thrombocytopenia in a newborn infant. *J. Pediatr. 67:*681, 1965.
13. Renfield, M. L., and Kraybill, E. N.: Consumptive coagulopathy and renal-vein thrombosis. *J. Pediatr. 82:*1054, 1973.
14. Hanshaw, J. B.: Congenital and acquired cytomegalovirus infection. *Pediatr. Clin. North Am. 13:*279, 1966.
15. Whitaker, J. A., Sartain, P., and Shaheedy, M.: Hematological aspects of congenital syphilis. *J. Pediatr. 66:*629, 1965.
16. Nachman, R. L., Thomas M., Patel D., and Gottbratten, E.: Thrombocytopenia as evidence of local thrombus in an umbilical artery catheter. *Pediatrics 50:*825, 1972.
17. Mokrohisky, S. T., Levine, R. L., Blumhagen, J. D., Wesenberg, R. L., and Simmons, M. A.: Low positioning of umbilical-artery catheters increases associated complications in newborn infants. *N. Engl. J. Med. 299:*561, 1978.
18. Kasabach, H . H., and Merrit, K. K.: Hemangioma with extensive purpura. *Am. J. Dis. Child. 59:*1063, 1940.
19. Shin, W. K. T.: Hemangiomas of infancy complicated by thrombocytopenia. *Am. J. Surg. 116:*896, 1968.
20. Propp, R. P., and Scharfman, W. B.: Hemangioma-thrombocytopenia syndrome associated with microangiopathic hemolytic anemia. *Blood 28:*623, 1966.
21. Brizel, H. E., and Raccuglia, G.: Giant hemangioma with thrombocytopenia: Radio-isotopic demonstration of platelet sequestration. *Blood 28:*623, 1966.
22. Good, T. A., Carnazzo, S. F., and Good, R. A.: Thrombocytopenia and giant hemangioma in infants. *Am. J. Dis. Child. 90:*260, 1955.
23. Kontras, S. B., Green, O. C., King, L., and Duran, R. J.: Giant hemangioma and thrombocytopenia in a newborn infant treated by irradiation therapy. *Am. J. Dis. Child. 105:*188, 1963.
24. Blix, S., and Aas, K.: Giant hemangioma, thrombocytopenia, fibrinogenopenia, and fibrinolytic activity. *Acta Med. Scand. 169:*63, 1961.
25. Inceman, S., and Tangun, Y.: Chronic defibrination syndrome due to a giant hemangioma associated with micro-angiopathic hemolytic anemia. *Am. J. Med. 46:*997, 1969.
26. Verstraet, M., Amery, A., Vermylen, C., and Robyn, G.: Heparin treatment of bleeding. *Lancet 1:*446, 1963.
27. Hillman, R. S., and Phillips, L. L.: Clotting and fibrinolysis in a cavernous hemangioma. *Am. J. Dis. Child. 113:*1649, 1967.
28. Williams, O. K., Van Buskirk, F. W., Burns, S., and Mellish, R. W. P.: Giant hemangioendothelioma with thrombocytopenia and hypofibrinogenemia. *Am. J. Roentgenol. 106:*204, 1969.
29. Hoak, J. C., Warnee, E. D., Cheng, H. F., Fry, G. L., and Hankenson, E. R.: Hemangioma with thrombocytopenia and microangiopathic anemia (Kasabach-Merritt syndrome): An animal model, *J. Lab. Clin. Med. 77:*941, 1971.
30. Bauer, C. R., Fojaco, R. M., Bancalar, E., and Fernandez, L.: Micro-angiopathic hemolytic-anemia and thrombocytopenia in a neonate associated with a large placental chorioangioma. *Pediatrics 62:*574, 1978.
31. Orenstein, D. M., Yonas, H., Bilenker, R., Rekate, H. L., and White, R. J.: Hemangioma thrombocytopenia syndrome: Case masquerading as an encephalocele. *Am. J. Dis. Child. 131:*680, 1977.
32. Kurana, M. S., Lian, E. C.-Y., and Harkness, D. R.: Storage pool disease of platelets: Association with multiple congenital cavernous hemangiomas. *JAMA 244:*169, 1980.
33. Wallerstein, R. G.: Spontaneous involution of giant hemangioma. *Am. J. Dis. Child. 102:*233, 1961.
34. Fost, N. C., and Esterly, N. B.: Successful treatment of juvenile hemangiomas with prednisone. *J. Pediatr. 72:*351, 1968.
35. Brown, S. H. Jr., Neerhout, R. C., and Fonkalsrud, E. W.: Prednisone therapy in the management of the large hemangiomas in infants and children. *Surgery 71:*168, 1972.
36. Favara, B. E., Franciosi, R. A., and Butterfield, L. J.: Disseminated intravascular and cardiac thrombosis of the neonate. *Am. J. Dis. Child. 127:*197, 1974.
37. Mauer, A. M., DeVaux, L. O., and Lahey, M. D.: Neonatal and maternal thrombocytopenic purpura due to quinine. *Pediatrics 19:*84, 1957.
38. Widerlov, E., Karlman, I., and Storsater, J.: Hydralazine-induced neonatal thrombocytopenia. *N. Engl. J. Med. 303:*1235, 1980 (letter).
39. Haslam, R. H.: Neonatal purpura secondary to maternal salicylism. *J. Pediat. 86:*653, 1975 (letter).
40. Pearson, H. A., Shulman, N. R., Marder, V. J., and Cone, T. E.: Isoimmune neonatal thrombocytopenic purpura: Clinical and therapeutic considerations. *Blood 23:*154, 1964.
41. Shulman, N. R., Marder, V. J., Hiller, M. C., and Collier, E. M.: Platelet and leukocyte isoantigens and their antibodies: Serologic, physiologic and clinical studies. *Prog. Hematol. 4:*222, 1964.
42. Von dem Borne, A. E. G. K., van Leeuwen, E. F., von Riesz, L. E., van Boxtel, C. J., and Engelfriet, C. P.: Neonatal alloimmune throm-

bocytopenia: Detection and characterization of the responsible antibodies by the platelet immunofluorescence test. *Blood* 57:649, 1981.

43. Von dem Borne, A. E. G. K., et al.: Bakᵃ, a new platelet-specific antigen involved in neonatal allo-immune thrombocytopenia. *Vox Sang.* 39:113, 1980.

44. Poley, J. R., and Stickler, G. B.: Petechaie in the newborn infant. *Am. J. Dis. Child.* 102:365, 1961.

45. Rausen, A. R., and Diamond, L. K.: "Enclosed" hemorrhage and neonatal jaundice. *Am. J. Dis. Child.* 101:164, 1961.

46. Shulman, N. R., Aster, R. H., Pearson, H. A., and Hiller, M. C.: Immunoreactions involving platelets. VI. Reactions of maternal isoantibodies responsible for neonatal purpura: Differentiation of a second platelet antigen system. *J. Clin. Invest.* 41:1059, 1962.

47. Kelton, J. G., et al.: Neonatal thrombocytopenia due to passive immunization. *N. Engl. J. Med.* 302:1401, 1980.

48. Mueller-Eckhardt, G., and Mueller-Eckhardt, C.: Die immunhamatologische Diagnostik neonataler Immunthrombozytopenien. *Dtsch. Med. Wochenschr.* 104:1743, 1979.

49. Leeuwen, E. F. V., and von dem Borne, A. E.: Neonatal alloimmune thrombocytopenia complicated by maternal autoimmune thrombocytopenia. *Br. Med. J.* 281:27, 1980 (technical note).

50. Menutti, M., Schwarz, R. H., and Gill, F.: Obstetric management of isoimmune thrombocytopenia. *Am. J. Obstet. Gynecol.* 118:565, 1974.

51. Ander, M. M., Fisch, G. R., Starobin, S. G., and Aster, R. H.: Use of "compatible" platelet transfusions in treatment of congenital isoimmune neonatal thrombocytopenic purpura. *N. Engl. J. Med.* 280:244, 1969.

52. McIntosh, S., Obrien, R. T., Schwarz, A. D., and Pearson, H. A.: Neonatal isoimmune purpura: Response to platelet infusions. *J. Pediatr.* 82:1020, 1973.

53. Colombani, J., Colombani, M., and Dausset, J.: Two cases of neonatal thrombocytopenia due to maternal iso-immunization against leuco-platelet antigens. *Vox Sang.* 14:137, 1968.

54. Bluestone, S. S., and Maslow, H. L.: Essential thrombocytopenic purpura in a newborn infant: Report of first case treated by splenectomy. *Pediatrics* 4:620, 1949.

55. Sitarz, A. L., Driscoll, J. M., and Wolff, J. A.: Management of isoimmune neonatal thrombocytopenia. *Am. J. Obstet. Gynecol.* 124:38, 1976.

56. Scott, J. R., Cruikshank, D. P., Kochenour, N. K., Pitkin, R., M., and Warenski, J. C.: Fetal platelet counts in the obstetric management of immunologic thrombocytopenic purpura. *Am. J. Obstet. Gynecol.* 136:495, 1980.

57. Zalnerai, E. D., Young, R. S. K., and Krishnam, K. S.: Intracranial hemorrhage in utero as a complication of isoimmune thrombocytopenia. *J. Pediat.* 95:611, 1979 (technical note).

58. Jesurun, C. A., Levin, G. S., Sullivan, W. R., and Stevens, D.: Intracranial hemorrhage in utero re thrombocytopenia. *J. Pediat.* 97:695, 1980 (letter).

59. Tancer, M. L.: Idiopathic thrombocytopenic purpura and pregnancy: Report of 5 new cases and review of the literature. *Am. J. Obstet. Gynecol.* 79:148, 1960.

60. Territo, M., Finkelstein, J., Oh, H., Habel, C., and Kattlove, H.: Management of autoimmune thrombocytopenia in pregnancy and in the neonate. *Obstet. Gynecol.* 41:579, 1973.

61. Heys, R. F.: Child bearing and idiopathic thrombocytopenic purpura. *J. Obstet. Gynaecol. Br. Commonw.* 73:205, 1966.

62. Laros, R. K., Jr., and Sweet, R. L.: Management of idiopathic thrombocytopenic purpura during pregnancy. *Am. J. Obstet. Gynecol.* 122:182, 1975.

63. O'Reilly, R. A., and Taber, B.-Z.: Immunologic thrombocytopenic purpura and pregnancy. *Obstet. Gynecol.* 51:509, 1978.

64. Carloss, H. W., McMillan, R., and Crosby, W. H.: Management of pregnancy in women with immune thrombocytopenic purpura. *JAMA* 224:2756, 1980.

65. Kernoff, L. M., Malan, E., and Gunston, K.: Neonatal thrombocytopenia complicating autoimmune thrombocytopenia in pregnancy. *Ann. Intern. Med.* 90:56, 1979.

66. Karpatkin, M., Forges, R. F., and Karpatkin, S.: Platelet counts in infants of women with autoimmune thrombocytopenia: Effect of steroid administration to the mother. *N. Engl. J. Med.* 305:936, 1981.

67. Gardner, F. H.: Idiopathic thrombocytopenic purpura, in *Immunological Diseases*, edited by M. Samter and H. L. Alexander. Little, Brown, Boston, 1965, p. 861.

68. Fitzgerald, G., McCarthy, D., O'Connell, L. G., and McCann, S. R.: Hyperimmune thrombocytopenia and pregnancy treated by splenectomy. *Acta Haematol.* 59:315, 1978.

69. Ayromlooi, J.: A new approach to the management of immunologic thrombocytopenic purpura in pregnancy. *Am. J. Obstet. Gynecol.* 130:235, 1978.

70. Bridges, J. M., and Carre, I. J.: Congenital thrombocytopenic purpura during pregnancy. *Obstet. Gynecol.* 28:532, 1966.

71. Killander, A.: On the use of exchange transfusion in neonatal thrombocytopenic purpura. *Acta Paediatr. Scand. (Suppl.)* 117:29, 1959.

72. Grosfeld, J. L., Naffis, D., and Boles, E. T.: The role of splenectomy in neonatal idiopathic thrombocytopenic purpura. *J. Pediatr. Surg.* 5:166, 1970.

73. Terada, H., Baldini, M., Ebbe, S., and Madoff, M. A.: Interaction of influenza virus with blood platelets. *Blood* 28:231, 1966.

74. Turpie, A. G. G., Chernesky, M. A., Larke, R. P. B., Packham, M. A., and Mustard, J. F.: Effect of Newcastle-disease virus on human and rabbit platelets: Aggregation and loss of constituents. *Lab. Invest.* 28:575, 1973.

75. Clawson, C. C., White, J. G., and Herzberg, M. D.: Platelet interaction with bacteria. 6. The role of contrasting of fibrinogen and fibronectin. *Am. J. Hematol.* 9:43, 1980.

76. Hawiger, J., et al.: Staphylococcal-induced human platelet injury mediated by protein A and immunoglobulin G Fc fragment receptor. *J. Clin. Invest.* 64:913, 1979.

77. Pfueller, S. L., and Costrove, L. J.: Staphylococci-induced human-platelet injury. *Thromb. Res.* 19:733, 1980 (letter).

78. Hawiger, J., Hawiger, A., Steckley, S., Timmons, S., and Cheng, C.: Membrane changes in human platelets induced by lipopolysaccharide endotoxin. *Br. J. Haematol.* 35:285, 1977.

79. Ausprunk, D. H., and Das, J.: Endotoxin-induced changes in human platelet membranes: Morphologic evidence. *Blood* 51:487, 1978.

80. Ginsberg, M. H., and Henson, P. M.: Enhancement of platelet response to immune complexes and IgG aggregates by lipid A-rich bacterial lipopolysaccharides. *J. Exp. Med.* 147:207, 1978.

81. Des Prez, R. M., Steckley, S., Stroud, R. M., and Hawiger, J.: Interaction of histoplasma capsulatum with human platelets. *J. Infect. Dis.* 142:32, 1980.

82. Kane, M. A., May, J. E., and Frank, M. M.: Interactions of the classical and alternate complement pathway with endotoxin lipopolysaccharide. *J. Clin. Invest.* 52:370, 1973.

83. Wautier, J. L.: Mechanism of thrombocytopenia in typhoid: Classical pathway or alternate pathway of complement? *Nouv. Presse Med.* 7:667, 1978.

84. Neame, P. B., Kelton, J. G., Walker, I. R., Stewart, I. O., Nossel, H. L., and Hirsh, J.: Thrombocytopenia in septicemia: The role of disseminated intravascular coagulation. *Blood* 56:88, 1980.

85. Kelton, J. G., Neame, P. B., Gauldie, J., and Hirsh, J.: Elevated platelet-associated IgG in the thrombocytopenia of septicemia. *N. Engl. J. Med.* 300:760, 1979.

86. McGrath, J. M., and Stewart, G. J.: The effects of endotoxin on vascular endothelium. *J. Exp. Med.* 129:833, 1968.

87. Riedler, G. F., Straub, P. W., and Frick, P. G.: Thrombocytopenia in septicemia: A clinical study for the evaluation of its incidence and diagnostic value. *Helv. Med. Acta* 36:23, 1971.

88. Corrigan, J. J.: Thrombocytopenia: Laboratory sign of septicemia in infants and children. *J. Pediatr.* 85:219, 1974.

89. Oppenheimer, L., Hryniuk, W. M., and Bishop, A. J.: Thrombocytopenia in severe bacterial infections. *J. Surg. Res.* 20:211, 1976.

90. Cohen, P., and Gardner, F. H.: Thrombocytopenia as a laboratory sign and complication of gram-negative bacteremic infection. *Arch. Intern. Med.* 117:113, 1966.

91. Beller, F. K., and Douglas, G. W.: Thrombocytopenia indicating gram-negative infection and endotoxemia. *Obstet. Gynecol.* 41:521, 1973.

92. Wilhelm, D. J., and Cherubin, C.: Hypofibrinogenemia and thrombocytopenia with meningococcemia. *Am. J. Dis. Child.* 113:494, 1967.

93. Starobin, O. E., and Castleman, B.: Case records of the Massachusetts General Hospital. *N. Engl. J. Med.* 283:1042, 1970.

94. Murray, H. W., Tuazon, C. U., and Sheagren, J. N.: Staphylococcal septicemia and disseminated intravascular coagulation. *Arch. Intern. Med.* 137:844, 1977.

95. Gould, L., Freisberg, A., Lewnes, G. C., Reddy, R., and Werthamer, S.: Right artrial myxoma associated with thrombocytopenia and bacterial endocarditis. *N.Y. State J. Med.* 78:2081, 1978.

96. Schaffner, W., McLeod, A. C., and Koenig, M. G.: Thrombocytopenia in Rocky Mountain spotted fever: Case study of husband and wife. *Arch. Intern. Med.* 116:857, 1965.

97. Reimann, H. A., Lu, G. Y. C., and Yang, C. S.: The blood platelets in typhus fever. *Arch. Pathol.* 7:640, 1929.

98. Getaz, E. P., and Staples, W. G.: Typhoid fever masquerading as immune thrombocytopenia. *S. Afr. Med. J.* 51:3, 1977 (letter).

99. Karayalcin, G., Saluja, G. S., and Aballi, A. J.: Thrombocytopenia in malignant diphtheria. *N. Engl. J. Med.* 288:914, 1973.

100. Tofte, R. W., and Williams, D. N.: Toxic shock syndrome: Clinical and laboratory features of 15 patients. *Ann. Intern. Med.* 94:1949, 1981.

101. Chia, Y. C., and Machin, S. J.: Tuberculosis and severe thrombocytopenia. *Br. J. Clin. Pract.* 33:55, 1979.

102. Erb, B. D.: Thrombocytopenic purpura accompanying brucellosis: A case report with demonstration of a granuloma in the bone marrow. *J. Tenn. Med. Assoc.* 59:876, 1966.

103. Dennis, L. H., Eichelberger, J. W., Inman, M. M., and Conrad, M. D.: Depletion of coagulation factors in drug resistant plasmodium falciparum malaria. *Blood* 29:713, 1967.

104. Skudowitz, R. B., Katz, J., Lurie, A., Levin, J., and Metz, J.: Mechanisms of thrombocytopenia in malignant tertian malaria. *Br. Med. J.* 2:515, 1973.

105. Davis, C. E., Robbins, R. S., Weller, R. D., and Brande, A. I.: Thrombocytopenia in experimental trypanosomiasis. *J. Clin. Invest.* 53:1359, 1974.

106. Robins-Browne, R. M., Schneider, J., and Metz, J.: Thrombocytopenia in trypanosomiasis. *Am. J. Trop. Med. Hyg.* 24:226, 1975.

107. Diamant, S., and Spirer, Z.: Chronic thrombocytopenic purpura associated with toxoplasmosis. *Br. Med. J.* 280:1505, 1980.

108. Fajardo, L. F., and Tallent, C.: Malarial parasites within human platelets. *JAMA* 229:1205, 1974.

109. Kolars, C. P., and Spink, W. W.: Thrombocytopenic purpura as a complication of mumps. *JAMA* 168:2213, 1958.

110. Graham, D. Y., Brown, C. H., Benry, J., and Butel, J. S.: Thrombocytopenia: A complication of mumps. *JAMA* 227:1162, 1974.

111. Tobin, J. D., and Tenbensen, R. W.: Varicella with thrombocytopenia causing fatal intracerebral hemorrhage. *Am. J. Dis. Child.* 124:577, 1972.

112. Brook, I.: Disseminated varicella with pneumonia, and fatal intracranial hemorrhage. *South. Med. J.* 72:756, 1979.

113. Whitaker, J. A., III, and Hardison, J. E.: Severe thrombocytopenia after generalized herpes simplex virus-2 (HSV-2) infection. *South. Med. J.* 71:864, 1978.

114. Chanarin, I., and Walford, D. M.: Thrombocytopenic purpura in cytomegalovirus mononucleosis. *Lancet* 2:497, 1973.

115. Sahud, M. A., and Bachelor, M. M.: Cytomegalovirus-induced thrombocytopenia: An unusual case report. *Arch. Intern. Med.* 138:1573, 1978.

116. Carter, R. L.: Platelet levels in infectious mononucleosis. *Blood* 24:817, 1965.

117. Sharp, A. A.: Platelets, bleeding, and haemostasis in infectious mononucleosis, in *Infectious Mononucleosis*, edited by R. L. Carter and H. G. Penman. Blackwell, Oxford, 1969, p. 99.

118. Casey, T. P., and Matthews, J.R.D.: Thrombocytopenic purpura in infectious mononucleosis. *N.Z. Med. J.* 77:318, 1973.

119. Ellman, L., Carvallo, A., Jacobson, B. M., and Colman, R. W.: Platelet autoantibody in a case of infectious mononucleosis presenting as thrombocytopenic purpura. *Am. J. Med.* 55:723, 1973.

120. Mazza, J., and Magin, G. E.: Severe thrombocytopenia in infectious mononucleosis. *Wis. Med. J.* 74:124, 1975.

121. Nossel, J. L.: Defibrination syndrome in a patient with chronic thrombocytopenic purpura. *Am. J. Med.* 46:591, 1969.

122. Ginsburg, A. D., Godwin, H. A., and Aster, R. H.: Diagnosis of hemorrhagic illness. *Br. Med. J.* 2:628, 1971.

123. Schmaier, A. H., Claypool, W., and Colman, R. W.: Crotalocytin: Recognition and purification of a timber rattlesnake platelet aggregating protein. *Blood* 56:1013, 1980.

124. Davey, M. G., and Esnouf, M. P.: The isolation of a component of the venom of *Trimeresurus okinavensis* that causes the aggregation of blood platelets. *Biochem. J.* 11:733, 1969.

125. Kirby, E. P., Niewiarowski, S., Stocker, K., Kettner, C., Shaw, E., and Brudzynski, T. M.: Thrombocytin: A serine protease from *Bothrops atrox* venom. *Biochemistry* 18:3564, 1979.

126. Goldschmidt, B.: Platelet functions in children with congenital heart disease. *Acta Paediatr. Scand.* 63:271, 1974.

127. Goldschmidt, B., Sarkadi, B., Gardos, G., and Matlary, A.: Platelet production and survival in cyanotic congenital heart disease. *Scand. J. Haematol.* 13:110, 1974.

128. Mauer, H. M., McCue, C. M., Robertson, L. W., and Haggins, J. C.: Correction of platelet dysfunction and bleeding in cyanotic congenital heart disease by simple red cell volume reduction. *Am. J. Cardiol.* 35:831, 1975.

129. Hill, R. N., Shibel, E. M., Spregg, R. G., and Moser, K. M.: Adult respiratory distress syndrome: Early predictions of mortality. *Trans. Am. Soc. Artif. Intern. Organs* 21:199, 1975.

130. Schneider, R. C., Zapol, W. M., and Carvalho, A. C.: Platelet consumption and sequestration in severe acute respiratory failure. *Am. Rev. Respir. Dis.* 122:445, 1980.

131. Johnson, T. S., Ellis, J. H., and Steele, P. P.: Improvement of platelet survival time with oxygen in patients with chronic obstructive airway disease. *Am. Rev. Respir. Dis.* 117:225, 1978.

132. Hergt, K.: Blood levels of thrombocytes in burned patients: Observations on their behavior in relation to the clinical condition of the patient. *J. Trauma* 12:599, 1972.

133. Eurenius, K., Mortensen, R. F., Meseral, P. M., and Curreri, P. W.: Platelet and megakaryocyte kinetics following thermal injury. *J. Lab. Clin. Med.* 79:247, 1972.

134. Hourdille, P., Bernard, P., Belloc, F., Pradet, A., Sanchez, A., and Boisseau, M. R.: Platelet abnormalities in thermal injury: Study of platelet-dense bodies stained with mepacrine. *Haemostasis* 10:141, 1981.

135. Cowan, D. H., Bowman, L. S., Fratianne, R. B., and Ahmed, F.: Platelet aggregation as a sign of septicemia in thermal injury: A prospective study. *JAMA* 235:1230, 1976.

136. Peltier, L. F.: A few remarks on fat embolism. *J. Trauma* 8:812, 1968.

137. Hoare, E. M.: Platelet response in fat-embolism and its relationship to petechiae. *Br. Med. J.* 2:689, 1971.

138. Kaplan, B. S., and Esseltine, D.: Thrombocytopenia in patients with acute post-streptococcal glomerulonephritis. *J. Pediatr.* 93:974, 1978.

139. Miller, K. M., Gresner, I. G., and Michael, A. F.: Localization of platelet antigens in human kidney disease. *Kidney Int.* 18:472, 1980.

140. Kasai, N., Parbtani, A., Cameron, J. S., Yewdall, V., Shepherd, P., and Verroust, P.: Platelet-aggregating immune complexes and intraplatelet serotonin in idiopathic glomerulonephritis and systemic lupus. *Clin. Exp. Immunol.* 46:64, 1981.

141. Katz, J., Lurie, A., Kaplan, B. S., Krawitz, J., and Metz, J: Coagulation findings in the hemolytic-uremic syndrome of infancy: Similarity to hyperacute renal allograft rejection. *J. Pediatr.* 78:426, 1971.

142. Pillay, V. K. G., Kurtzman, N. A., Manaligod, J. R., and Jonasson, O.: Selective thrombocytopenia due to localized microangiopathy of renal allografts. *Lancet* 2:988, 1973.

143. Bunting, R. W., and Quay, S. C.: Case records of the Massachusetts General Hospital, *N. Engl. J. Med.* 300:1262, 1979.

144. Landis, T. F., von Felten, A., and Berchtold, H.: Thrombocytopenic episodes in patients with well-functioning renal allografts. *Acta Haematol.* 61:2, 1979.

145. Jacobson, R. J., Rath, C. E., and Perloff, J. K.: Intravascular hemolysis and thrombocytopenia in left ventricular outflow obstruction. *Br. Heart J.* 35:849, 1973.

146. Harker, L. A., and Slichter, S. J.: Platelet and fibrinogen consumption in man. *N. Engl. J. Med.* 287:999, 1972.

147. Wang, Y., From, A. H. T., and Krivit, W.: Disseminated pulmonary arterial thrombosis associated with thrombocytopenia: Occurrence in identical twins. *Circulation* 31 (Suppl. 2):215, 1965.

148. Stuard, I. D., Huesinkveld, R. S., and Moss, A. J.: Microangiopathic hemolytic anemia and thrombocytopenia in primary pulmonary hypertension. *N. Engl. J. Med.* 287:869, 1972.

149. Rochmis, P. G.: Splenic angioma with thrombocytopenia. *N.Y. State J. Med. 70:*2133, 1970.

150. Schanberge, J. N., Tanaka, K., and Gruhl, M. C.: Chronic consumption coagulopathy due to hemangiomatous transformation of the spleen. *Am. J. Clin. Pathol. 56:*723, 1971.

151. Scherrer, J. R., Hausser, E., and Berney, J.: Thrombocytopenie associée a un hemangioblastome cérébelleux. *Schweiz. Med. Wochenschr. 95:*456, 1965.

152. Rodriguez-Erdman, F., Button, L., Murray, I. E., and Moloney, W. C.: Kasabach-Merritt syndrome: Coagulo-analytical observations. *Am. J. Med. Sci. 261:*9, 1971.

153. Moschcowitz, E.: An acute febrile pleiochromic anemia with hyaline thrombosis of terminal arterioles and capillaries: An undescribed disease. *Arch. Intern. Med. 36:*89, 1915.

154. Baehr, G., Klemperer, P., and Schifrin, A.: An acute febrile anemia and thrombocytopenic purpura with diffuse platelet thromboses of capillaries and arterioles. *Trans. Assoc. Am. Physicians 51:*43, 1936.

155. Kennedy, S. S., Zacharski, L. R., and Beck, J. R.: Thrombotic thrombocytopenic purpura: Analysis of 48 unselected cases. *Semin. Thromb. Hemostas. 6:*341, 1980.

156. Petitt, R. M.: Thrombotic thrombocytopenic purpura: A thirty year review. *Semin. Thromb. Hemostas. 6:*350, 1980.

157. Berberich, F. R., Cuene, S. A., Chard, R. K., and Hartmann, J. R.: Thrombotic thrombocytopenic purpura: Three cases with platelet and fibrinogen survival studies. *J. Pediatr. 84:*503, 1974.

158. Bernstock, L., and Hirson, C.: Thrombotic thrombocytopenic purpura: Remission on treatment with heparin. *Lancet 1:*28, 1960.

159. Carmichael, D. S., and Medley, D. R. K.: Heparin in thrombotic microangiopathy. *Lancet 1:*1421, 1966.

160. Jaffe, E. A., Nachman, R. L., and Mersky, C.: Thrombotic thrombocytopenic purpura: Coagulation parameters in twelve patients. *Blood 42:*499, 1973.

161. Cuttner, J.: Thrombotic thrombocytopenic purpura: A ten-year experience. *Blood 56:*302, 1980.

162. Lian, E. C. Y.: The role of increased platelet aggregation in TTP. *Semin. Thromb. Hemostas. 6:*401, 1980.

163. Ansell, J. E., Slepchuk, N. I., Jr., and Pechet, L.: Platelet aggregating factor in TTP. *Blood 54:*959, 1979 (letter).

164. Brandt, J. T., Kennedy, M. S., and Senhauser, D. A.: Platelet aggregating factor in thrombocytopenic pupura. *Lancet 2:*463, 1979.

165. Weisenburger, D. D., Fry, G. L., and Hoak, J. C.: Thrombotic thrombocytopenic purpura: Conflicting results of in-vitro studies. *Lancet 1:*99, 1980.

166. Gottschall, J., and Aster, R. H.: Unpublished observations.

167. Morrison, J., McMillan, R., and Newman, D.: Elevated platelet-associated IgG in thrombotic thrombocytopenic purpura. *JAMA 239:*2242, 1978.

168. Altschule, M. D.: A rare type of acute thrombocytopenic purpura: A morphological study of its histogenesis. *Am. J. Pathol. 26:*155, 1950.

169. Gore, I.: Disseminated arteriolar and capillary platelet thrombosis: A morphological study of its histogenesis. *Am. J. Pathol. 26:*155, 1950.

170. Feldman, J. D., Mardiney, M. R., Unanue, E. R., and Cutting, H.: The vascular pathology of thrombotic thrombocytopenic purpura: An immunohistochemical and ultrastructural study. *Lab. Invest. 15:*927, 1966.

171. Brain, M. D., Dacie, J. C., and Hourihane, D. O.: Microangiopathic haemolytic anemia: The possible role of vascular lesions in pathogenesis. *Br. J. Haematol. 8:*358, 1962.

172. Venkatachalam, M. A., Jones, D. B., and Nelson, D. A.: Microangiopathic hemolytic anemia in rats with malignant hypertension. *Blood 32:*278, 1968.

173. Amorosi, E. L., and Ultmann, J. E.: Thrombotic thrombocytopenic purpura: Report of 16 cases and review of the literature. *Medicine (Baltimore) 45:*139, 1966.

174. Meacham, G. C., Orbison, J. L., Heinle, R. W., Steele, H. J., and Schaefer, J. A.: Thrombotic thrombocytopenic purpura: A disseminated disease of arterioles. *Blood 6:*706, 1951.

175. Blackman, N. S., Cohen, B. M., and Watson, J.: Thrombotic thrombocytopenic purpura: Report of a case. *JAMA 148:*546, 1952.

176. Borey, D.A.J., White, J. B., and Daily, W. M.: Thrombotic thrombocytopenic purpura diagnosed by random lymph node biopsy. *Arch. Intern. Med. 98:*821, 1956.

177. Benitz, L., Mathews, M., and Mallory, G. K.: Platelet thrombosis with polyarteritis nodosa: Report of a case. *Arch. Pathol. 77:*116, 1964.

178. Steinberg, A. D., Green, W. T., Jr., and Talal, N.: Thrombotic thrombocytopenic purpura complicating Sjogren's syndrome. *JAMA 215:*757, 1971.

179. Wall, R. T., and Harker, L. A.: The endothelium and thrombosis. *Ann. Rev. Med. 31:*361, 1980.

180. Remuzzi, G., Marchesi, D., Misiani, R., Mecca, G., de Gaetano, G., and Donati, M. B.: Familial deficiency of a plasma factor stimulating vascular prostacyclin activity. *Thromb. Res. 17:*517, 1979.

181. Remuzzi, G., et al.: Prostacyclin and thrombotic microangiopathy. *Semin. Thromb. Hemostas. 6:*391, 1980.

182. Remuzzi, G., et al.: Prostacyclin generation by cultured endothelial cells in haemolytic uraemic syndrome. *Lancet 1:*656, 1980.

183. Jemsbu, C. N., Lewis, P. J., Hilgard, P., Mufti, G. J., Hows, J., and Webster, J.: Prostacyclin deficiency in thrombotic thrombocytopenic purpura. *Lancet 2:*748, 1979.

184. Machin, S. J., Defreyn, G., Chamone, D.A.F., and Vermylen, J.: Plasma 6-keto-PGF$_{1\alpha}$ levels after plasma exchange in thrombotic thrombocytopenic purpura. *Lancet 1:*661, 1980.

185. Chen, Y.-C., Hall, E. R., McLeod, B., and Wu, K. K.: Accelerated prostacyclin degradation in thrombotic thrombocytopenic purpura. *Lancet 2:*267, 1981.

186. Pini, M., Manotti, C., Quintavalla, R., and Dettori, A. G.: Normal prostacyclin-like activity in thrombotic thrombocytopenic purpura. *Thromb. Haemost. 46:*571, 1981.

187. Caggiano, V., Chosney, B., and Way, L. W.: Thrombotic thrombocytopenic purpura, cholangiocarcinoma, and oral contraceptives. *Lancet 1:*365, 1980.

188. Stadel, B. V.: Oral contraceptives and cardiovascular disease. *N. Engl. J. Med. 305:*612, 1981.

189. Hope, W., Martin, T. J., Chesterman, C. N., and Morgan, F. J.: Human β-thromboglobulin inhibits PGI$_2$ production and binds to specific site in bovine aortic endothelial cells. *Nature 282:*210, 1979.

190. Nalbandian, R. M., and Henry, R. L.: A proposed comprehensive pathophysiology and thrombotic thrombocytopenic purpura with implicit novel tests and therapies. *Semin. Thromb. Hemostas. 6:*356, 1980.

191. Kwaan, H. C.: Role of fibrinolysis in thrombotic thrombocytopenic purpura. *Semin. Thromb. Hemostas. 6:*395, 1980.

192. Neame, P. B.: Immunologic and other factors in thrombotic thrombocytopenic purpura (TTP). *Semin. Thromb. Hemostas. 6:*416, 1980.

193. Parker, J. C., and Barrett, D. A.: Microangiopathic hemolysis and thrombocytopenia related to penicillin drugs. *Arch. Intern. Med. 127:*474, 1971.

194. Ahmed, F., Sumalnop, V., Spain, D. M., and Tobin, M. S.: Thrombohemolytic thrombocytopenic purpura during penicillamine therapy. *Arch. Intern. Med. 138:*1292, 1978.

195. Jones, M. B., Armitage, J. O., and Stone, D. B.: Self-limited TTP-like syndrome after bee sting. *JAMA 242:*1121, 1979.

196. Cameron, J. D., and Vick, R.: Plasma C3 in hemolytic-uraemic syndrome and thrombotic thrombocytopenic purpura. *Lancet 2:*975, 1973.

197. Bayer, A. S., Theofilopoulos, A. N., Eisenberg, R., Friedman, S. G., and Guze, L. B.: Thrombotic thrombocytopenic purpura-like syndrome associated with infective endocarditis. *JAMA 238:*408, 1977.

198. Mant, M. J., Cauchi, M. N., and Medley, G.: Thrombotic thrombocytopenic purpura: Report of a case with possible immune etiology. *Blood 40:*416, 1972.

199. Weisenburger, D. D., O'Connor, M. L., and Hart, M. N.: Thrombotic thrombocytopenic purpura with C'3 vascular deposits: Report of a case. *Am. J. Clin. Pathol. 67:*61, 1977.

200. Meister, R. J., Sacher, R. A., and Phillips, T.: Immune complexes in thrombotic thrombocytopenic purpura. *Ann. Int. Med. 90:*717, 1979.

201. Sacher, R. A., Phillips, T. M., Shashaty, G. G., Jacobson, R. J., Rath, C. E., and Lewis, M. G.: Demonstration of immune complexes in thrombotic thrombocytopenic purpura and effect of exchange transfusion. *Scand. J. Haematol. 24:*373, 1980.

202. Ansell, J., Beaser, R. S. and Pechet, L.: Thrombotic thrombocytopenic purpura fails to respond to fresh frozen plasma infusion. *Ann. Intern. Med 89:*647, 1978.

203. Celada, A., and Perrin, L. H.: Circulating immune complexes in thrombotic thrombocytopenic purpura (TTP). *Blood* 52:855, 1978.

204. Cecere, F. A., Yoshinoya, S., and Pope, R. M.: Fatal thrombotic thrombocytopenic purpura in a patient with systemic lupus erythematosus. *Arthritis Rheum.* 24:550, 1981.

205. Myers, T. J.: Treatment of thrombotic thrombocytopenic purpura with combined exchange plasmapheresis and antiplatelet agents. *Semin. Thromb. Hemostas.* 7:37, 1981.

206. Reynolds, P. M., Jackson, J. M., Brine, J. A. S., and Vivian, A. B.: Thrombotic thrombocytopenic purpura: Remission following splenectomy. *Am. J. Med.* 61:439, 1976.

207. Mettler, N. E.: Isolation of a microtatobiote from patients with hemolytic-uremic syndrome and thrombotic thrombocytopenic purpura and from mites in the United States. *N. Engl. J. Med.* 281:1023, 1969.

208. Brown, R. C., Blecher, T. E., French, E. A., and Toghill, P. J.: Thrombotic thrombocytopenic purpura after influenza vaccination. *Br. Med. J.* 2:303, 1973.

209. Moore, M. R., and Poon, M.-C.: Syndrome resembling thrombotic thrombocytopenic purpura associated with bacterial endocarditis. *South. Med. J.* 73:541, 1980.

210. Mars, D. R., Knochel, J. P., Cotton, J. R. and Fuller, T. J.: Thrombotic thrombocytopenic purpura after a dogbite. *South. Med. J.* 73:676, 1980.

211. Watson, C. G., and Cooper, W.: Thrombotic thrombocytopenic purpura: Concomitant occurrence in husband and wife. *JAMA* 215:1821 1971.

212. Hellman, R. M., Jackson, D. V., and Buss, D. H.: Thrombotic thrombocytopenic purpura and hemolytic-uremic syndrome in HLA-identical siblings. *Ann. Intern. Med.* 93:283, 1980.

213. Pisciotta, A. V., and Gottschall, J. L.: Clinical features of thrombotic thrombocytopenic purpura. *Semin. Thromb. Hemostas.* 6:330, 1980.

214. Mounens, L. A. H.: Thrombotic thrombocytopenic purpura in a neonatal infant. *Pediatrics* 7:118, 1967.

215. Tennant, R., and McAdams, G. B.: Thrombotic thrombocytopenic purpura associated with surgery. *Conn. Med.* 22:644, 1958.

216. Cuttner, J.: Chronic thrombotic thrombocytopenic purpura: Report of a case with five relapses and review of the literature. *Mt. Sinai J. Med.* 45:418, 1978.

217. Berman, N., and Finkelstein, J. Z.: Thrombotic thrombocytopenic purpura in childhood: Results of a survey and reexamination of the literature. *Scand. J. Haematol.* 14:286, 1975.

218. Mitch, W. E., Spivak, J. L., Spangler, D. B., and Bell, W. R.: Thrombotic thrombocytopenic purpura presenting with gynaecological manifestations. *Lancet* 1:849, 1973.

219. Vilanova, J. R., Norenberg, M. D., and Stuard, I. D.: Thrombotic thrombocytopenic purpura. *N.Y. State J. Med.* 75:2246, 1975.

220. James, T. N., and Monto, R. W.: Pathology of the cardiac conduction system in thrombotic thrombocytopenic purpura. *Ann. Intern. Med.* 65:37, 1966.

221. Geisinger, K. R., and Solomon, A. R.: Sudden cardiac death in thrombotic thrombocytopenic purpura. *Arch. Pathol. Lab. Med.* 103:599, 1979.

222. Bone, R. C., Henry, J. E., Petterson, J., and Amare, M.: Respiratory dysfunction in thrombotic thrombocytopenic purpura. *Am. J. Med.* 65:262, 1978.

223. Howard, T. P.: Fulminant respiratory failure: A manifestation of thrombotic thrombocytopenic purpura. *JAMA* 242:350, 1979.

224. Benson, D. O., Fitzgibbons, J. F., and Goodnight, S. H.: The visual system in thrombotic thrombocytopenic purpura. *Ann. Ophthalmol.* 12:413, 1980.

225. Lewellen, D. R., Jr., and Singerman, L. J.: Thrombotic thrombocytopenic purpura with optic disk neovascularization, vitreous hemorrhage, retinal detachment, and optic strophy. *Am. J. Opthalmol.* 89:840, 1980.

226. Fitzgibbons, J. F., Goodnight, S. C., Jr., Burkhardt, J. H., and Kirk, P. E.: Survival following thrombotic thrombocytopenic purpura in pregnancy. *Obstet. Gynecol.* 50:66s, 1976.

227. Walker, B. K., Ballas, S. K., and Martinez, J.: Plasma infusion for thrombotic thrombocytopenic purpura during pregnancy. *Arch. Intern. Med.* 149:981, 1980.

228. Swaiman, K., Schaffhausen, M., and Krivit, W.: Thrombotic thrombocytopenic purpura: Report of an unusual clinical case and chromium 51 red cell survival studies. *J. Pediatr.* 60:823, 1962.

229. Heyns, A. Du P., Lotter, M. G., Badenhorst, P. N., Minnaar, P. C., Vorster, B. J., and Retief, F. P.: Thrombotic thrombocytopenic purpura: A case investigated with ¹¹¹In-oxine-labelled platelets. *S. Afr. Med. J.* 56:229, 1979.

230. Moore, R. D., and Schoenberg, M. D.: A polysaccharide component in the vascular lesions of thrombotic thrombocytopenic purpura. *Blood* 15:511, 1960.

231. Craig, J. M., and Gitlin, D.: The nature of the hyaline thrombi in thrombotic thrombocytopenic purpura. *Am. J. Pathol.* 33:251, 1957.

232. Neame, P. B., et al.: Thrombotic thrombocytopenic purpura: A syndrome of intravascular platelet consumption. *Can. Med. Assoc. J.* 114:1108, 1976.

233. Byrnes, J. J.: Plasma infusion in the treatment of thrombotic thrombocytopenic purpura. *Semin. Thromb. Hemostas.* 7:9, 1981.

234. Berkowitz, L. R., Dalldorf, F. G., and Blatt, P. M.: Thrombotic thrombocytopenic purpura: A pathology review. *JAMA* 241:1709, 1979.

235. Goodman, A., Ramos, R., Petrelli, M., Hirsch, S. A., Bukowski, R., and Harris, J. W.: Gingival biopsy in thrombotic thrombocytopenic purpura. *Ann. Intern. Med.* 89:501, 1978.

236. Moon, E. C., and Kitay, D. Z.: Hematologic problems in pregnancy. II. Thrombotic (thrombohemolytic) thrombocytopenic purpura. *J. Reprod. Med.* 9:212, 1972.

237. Bukowski, R. M., Hewlett, J. S., Reimer, R. R., Groppe, C. W., Weick, J. K., and Livingston, R. B.: Therapy of thrombotic thrombocytopenic purpura: An overview. *Semin. Thromb. Hemostas.* 7:1, 1981.

238. Updike, S. J., Bozdech, M. J., Johnson, C. A., and Zimmerman, S. W.: Management of fulminating thrombotic thrombocytopenic purpura. *Semin. Thromb. Hemostas.* 7:33, 1981.

239. Amorosi, E. L., and Karpatkin, S.: Antiplatelet treatment of thrombotic thrombocytopenic purpura. *Ann. Intern. Med.* 86:102, 1977.

240. Cocchetto, D. M., Cook, L., Cato, A. E., and Niedel, J. E.: Rationale and proposal for use of prostacyclin in thrombotic thrombocytopenic purpura therapy. *Semin. Thromb. Hemostas.* 7:43, 1981.

241. Moncada, S., and Korbut, R.: Dipyridamole and other phosphodiesterase inhibitors act as antithrombotic agents by potentiating endogenous prostacyclin. *Lancet* 1:1286, 1978.

242. Gundlach, W. J., and Tarnasky, R.: Thrombotic thrombocytopenic purpura: Remission following treatment with aspirin and dipyridamole. *Minn. Med.* 60:20, 1977.

243. Budd, G. T., Bukowski, R. M., Lucas, F. V., Cato, A. E., and Cocchetto, D. M.: Prostacyclin therapy of thrombotic thrombocytopenic purpura. *Lancet* 2:915, 1980.

244. Fitzgerald, G. A., Maas, R. L., Stein, R., Oates, J. A., and Roberts, J. L.: Intravenous prostacyclin in thrombotic thrombocytopenic purpura. *Ann. Intern. Med.* 95:319, 1981.

245. Gottschall, J. L., Pisciotta, A. V., Darin, J., Hussey, C. V., and Aster, R. H.: Thrombotic thrombocytopenic purpura: Experience with whole blood exchange transfusion. *Semin. Thromb. Hemostas.* 7:25, 1981.

246. Taft, E. G., and Baldwin, S. T.: Plasma exchange transfusion. *Semin. Thromb. Hemostas.* 7:15, 1981.

247. Frankel, A. E., Rubenstein, M. D., and Wall, R. T.: Thrombotic thrombocytopenic purpura: Prolonged coma with recovery of neurologic function with intensive plasma exchange. *Am. J. Hematol.* 10:387, 1981.

248. Byrnes, J. J., and Khurana, M.: Treatment of thrombotic thrombocytopenic purpura with plasma. *N. Engl. J. Med.* 297:1386, 1977.

249. Stern, R., Cornell, C. J., Jr., Beck, R., and Smith, R. E.: Thrombotic thrombocytopenic purpura: Failure of plasma infusion and antiplatelet agents. *Ann. Int. Med.* 90:989, 1979.

250. Abramson, N.: Treatments for thrombotic thrombocytopenic purpura: Plasma, vincristine, hemodialysis and exchange transfusion. *N. Engl. J. Med.* 298:971, 1978 (letter).

251. Gutterman, L., and Stevenson, T. D.: Vincristine in the treatment of thrombotic thrombocytopenic purpura. *Blood* 54:242A, 1979.

252. Wallach, H. W., Oren, M. E., and Herskowitz, A.: Treatment of thrombotic thrombocytopenic purpura with plasma infusions and cyclophosphamide. *South. Med. J.* 72:1345, 1979.

253. Tartaglia, A. P., and Burkhardt, P. T.: Thrombotic thrombocytopenic purpura: Remission following hemodialysis. *JAMA* 281:999, 1971.

254. Rossi, E. C., and Del Greco, F.: The adaptation of hemodialysis to facilitate rapid exchange transfusion in patients with thrombotic thrombocytopenic purpura (TTP). *Semin. Thromb. Hemostas.* 7:22, 1981.

255. Rutkow, I. M.: Thrombotic thrombocytopenic purpura (TTP) and splenectomy: A current appraisal. *Ann. Surg.* 188:701, 1978.

256. Howard, D. J., Roberts, A. B., and Page, F. T.: Late recurrence of thrombotic thrombocytopenic purpura after splenectomy. *Br. Med. J.* 2:317, 1975.

257. Von Gasser, C., Gautier, E., Steck, A., Siebenmann, R. E., and Oechslin, R.: Hamolytisch-Uraemische Syndrome: Bilaterale Nierenrindennekrosen bei akuten Erworbenen hamolytischen Anamien. *Schweiz. Med. Wochenschr.* 85:905, 1955.

258. Musgrave, J. E., Talwalkar, Y. B., Puri, H. C., Campbell, R. A., Loggan, B.: The hemolytic-uremic syndrome. *Clin. Pediatr.* 17:218, 1978.

259. Goldstein, M. H., Churg, J., Strauss, L., and Gribetz, D.: Hemolytic-uremic syndrome. *Nephron* 23:263, 1979.

260. Donckerwolcke, R. A., Kuijten, R. H., Tiddens, H. A., and van Gool, J. D.: Haemolytic uraemic syndrome. *Pediatrician* 8:378, 1979.

261. Koster, F., et al.: Hemolytic-uremic syndrome after shigellosis: Relation to endotoxemia and circulating immune complexes. *N. Engl. J. Med.* 298:927, 1978.

262. Raghupathy, P., Date, A., Shastry, J. C. M., and Sudarsan, A.: Hemolytic-uremic syndrome complicating shigella dysentery in South Indian children. *Br. Med. J.* 1:1518, 1978.

263. Moorthy, B., and Makker, S. P.: Hemolytic-uremic syndrome associated with pneumococcal sepsis. *J. Pediatr.* 95:558, 1979.

264. Sharman, V. L., and Goodwin, F. J.: Hemolytic-uremic syndrome following chicken pox. *Clin. Nephrol.* 14:49, 1980.

265. O'Regan, S., Robitaille, P., Mongeau, J.-G., and McLaughlin, B.: The hemolytic uremic syndrome associated with ECHO 22 infection. *Clin. Pediatr.* 19:125, 1980.

266. Gianantonio, C. A., Vitacco, M., Mendilaharzy, F., and Gallo, G.: The hemolytic-uremic syndrome: Renal status of 76 patients at long-term follow-up. *J. Pediatr.* 72:757, 1968.

267. Monnens, L., Samwell-Mantingh, M., Lestijo, B. J., and van Munster, P.: Serum immunoglobulin levels in the hemolytic-uremic syndrome in children. *Acta Paediatr. Belg.* 33:157, 1980.

268. Kim, Y., Miller, K., and Michael, A. F.: Breakdown products of C3 and Factor B in hemolytic-uremic syndrome. *J. Lab. Clin. Med.* 89:845, 1977.

269. Nolin, L., O'Regan, O., Pelletier, M., Rivard, G. E., Mongeau, J.-G., and Robitaille, P.: Possible C1q bypass loop activation in the haemolytic uraemic syndrome. *Clin. Exp. Immunol.* 35:107, 1979.

270. Monnens, L., Molenaar, J., Lambert, P. H., Proesmans, W., and van Munster, P.: The complement system in hemolytic-uremic syndrome in childhood. *Clin. Nephrol.* 13:168, 1980.

271. O'Regan, S., Chesney, R. W., Kaplan, B. S., and Drummond, K. N.: Red cell membrane phospholipid abnormalities in the hemolytic uremic syndrome. *Clin. Nephrol.* 15:14, 1980.

272. Kobayashi, Y., Okahata, S., Tanabe, K., Tanaka, Y., Ueda, K., and Usui, T.: Erythrocyte superoxide-dismutase activity in hemolytic uremic syndrome. *Hiroshima J. Med. Sci.* 27:181, 1978.

273. Brandslund, I., Petersen, P. H.: Haemolytic uraemic syndrome and reticuloendothelial system. *Lancet* 1:103, 1980.

274. Jørgensen, K. A., and Pedersen, R. S.: Familial deficiency of prostacyclin production stimulating factor in the hemolytic uremic syndrome of childhood. *Thromb. Res.* 21:311, 1981.

275. Kaplan, B. S., Chesney, R. W., and Drummond, K. N.: Hemolytic uremic syndrome in families. *N. Engl. J. Med.* 292:1090, 1975.

276. Hogewind, B. L., Brutel de la Riviere, G., van Es, L. A., and Veltkamp, J. J.: Familial occurrence of the haemolytic uraemic syndrome. *Acta Med. Scand.* 207:73, 1980.

277. Carreras, L., et al.: Familial hypocomplementemic hemolytic uremic syndrome with HLA-A3, B7 haplotype. *JAMA* 245:602, 1981.

278. Whitington, P. F., Friedman, A. L., and Chesney, R. W.: Gastrointestinal disease in the hemolytic-uremic syndrome. *Gastroenterology* 76:728, 1979.

279. Yates, R. S., Osterholm, R. K.: Hemolytic-uremic syndrome colitis. *J. Clin. Gastroenterol.* 2:359, 1980.

280. Schwartz, D. L., Becker, J. M., So, H. B., and Scheider, K. M.: Segmental colonic gangrene: A surgical emergency in the hemolytic-uremic syndrome. *Pediatrics* 62:54, 1978.

281. Kibel, M. A., and Barnard, P. J.: The haemolytic-uraemic syndrome: A survey in southern Africa. *S. Afr. Med. J.* 42:692, 1968.

282. Bale, J. F., Jr., Brasher, C., and Siegler, R. L.: CNS manifestations of the hemolytic-uremic syndrome. *Am. J. Dis. Child.* 134:869, 1980.

283. Avalos, J. S., Vitacco, M., Penalver, J., and Gianantonio, C.: Coagulation studies in the hemolytic-uremic syndrome. *J. Pediatr.* 76:538, 1970.

284. Katz, J., et al.: Platelet erythrocyte and fibrinogen kinetics in hemolytic-uremic syndrome in infancy. *J. Pediatr.* 83:739, 1973.

285. Riella, M. C., et al.: Renal microangiopathy of the hemolytic-uremic syndrome in childhood. *Nephron* 17:188, 1976.

286. Shigematsu, H., Dickman, S. H., Churg, J., Grishman, E., and Duffy, J. L.: Mesangial involvement in hemolytic-uremic syndrome. *Am. J. Pathol.* 85:349, 1976.

287. Upadhyaya, K., Barwick, K., Fishaut, M., Kashgarian, M., and Siegel, N. J.: The importance of nonrenal involvement in hemolytic-uremic syndrome. *Pediatrics* 65:115, 1980.

288. Kaplan, B. S., Katz, J., Krawitz, S., and Lurie, A.: An analysis of the results of therapy in 67 cases of the hemolytic-uremic syndrome. *J. Pediatr.* 78:420, 1971.

289. Vitacco, M., Avalas, J. S., and Gianantonio, C. A.: Heparin therapy in the hemolytic uremic syndrome. *J. Pediatr.* 83:271, 1973.

290. Monnens, L., van Collenburg, J., de Jong, M., Zoethout, H., and van Wieringen, P.: Treatment of the hemolytic-uremic syndrome. *Helv. Paediatr. Acta* 33:321, 1978.

291. Powell, H. R., and Ebert, H.: Streptokinase and anti-thrombotic therapy in the hemolytic-uremic syndrome. *J. Pediatr.* 84:345, 1974.

292. O'Regan, S., Chesney, R. W., Mongeau, J.-G., and Robitaille, P.: Aspirin and dipyridamole therapy in the hemolytic-uremic syndrome. *J. Pediatr.* 97:473, 1980.

293. Gomperts, E. D., and Lieberman, E.: Hemolytic-uremic syndrome. *J. Pediatr.* 97:419, 1980.

294. Dolislager, D., and Tune, B.: The hemolytic-uremic syndrome: Spectrum of severity and significance of prodrome. *Am. J. Dis. Child.* 132:55, 1978.

295. Kaplan, B. S.: Hemolytic uremic syndrome with recurrent episodes: An important subset. *Clin. Nephrol.* 8:495, 1977.

296. Folman, R., Arbus, G. S., Churchill, B., Gaum, L., and Huber, J.: Recurrence of the hemolytic uremic syndrome in a 3½-year-old child, 4 months after second renal transplantation. *Clin. Nephrol.* 10:121, 1978.

297. Clarkson, A. R., Lawrence, J. R., Meadows, R., and Seymour, A. E.: The haemolytic-uraemic syndrome in adults. *Q. J. Med.* 39:227, 1970.

298. Brown, C. B., Robson, J. S., Thomson, D., Clarkson, A. R., Cameron, J. S., and Ogg, C. S.: Haemolytic uraemic syndrome in women taking oral contraceptives. *Lancet* 1:1479, 1973.

299. Schoolwerth, A. C., Sandler, R. S., Klahr, S., and Kissane, J. M.: Nephrosclerosis postpartum and in women taking oral contraceptives: A report of two cases. *Arch. Intern. Med.* 136:178, 1976.

300. Karlsberg, R. P., Lacher, J. W., and Bartecchi, C. E.: Adult hemolytic-uremic syndrome: Familial variant. *Arch. Intern. Med.* 137:1155, 1977.

301. Segonds, A., Louradour, N., Suc, J. M., and Orfila, C.: Postpartum hemolytic uremic syndrome: A study of three cases with a review of the literature. *Clin. Nephrol.* 12:229, 1979.

302. Ponticelli, C., Rivolta, E., Imbasciati, E., Rossi, E., and Mannucci, P. M.: Hemolytic uremic syndrome in adults. *Arch. Intern. Med.* 140:353, 1980.

303. Hauglustaine, D., Van Damme, B., Vanrenteghem, Y., and Michielsen, P.: Recurrent hemolytic uremic syndrome during oral contraception. *Clin. Nephrol.* 15:148, 1981.

304. Khanh, B. T., Bhathena, D., Vasquez, M., and Luke, R. G.: Role of heparin therapy in the outcome of adult hemolytic uremic syndrome. *Nephron* 16:292, 1976.

305. Thorsen, C. A., Rossi, E. C., Green, D., and Carone, F. A.: The treatment of the hemolytic-uremic syndrome with inhibitors of platelet function. *Am. J. Med.* 66:711, 1979.

306. Brandt, P., Jespersen, J., and Gregersen, G.: Postpartum haemolytic-uraemic syndrome successfully treated with antithrombin III. *Br. Med. J. 280:*449, 1980.

307. Remuzzi, G., et al.: Treatment of the hemolytic uremic syndrome with plasma. *Clin. Nephrol. 12:*279, 1979.

308. Webster, J., Rees, A. J., Lewis, P. J., and Hensby, C. N.: Prostacyclin deficiency in haemolytic-uraemic syndrome. *Br. Med. J. 3:*271, 1980.

309. Nissenson, A. R., Krumlovsky, F. A., and del Greco, F.: Postpartum hemolytic uremic syndrome: Late recovery after prolonged maintenance dialysis. *JAMA 242:*173, 1979.

310. Upshaw, J. D., Jr.: Congenital deficiency of a factor in normal plasma that reverses microangiopathic hemolysis and thrombocytopenia. *N. Engl. J. Med. 298:*1350, 1978.

311. Rennard, S., and Abe, S.: Decreased cold-insoluble globulin in congenital thrombocytopenia (Upshaw-Shulman syndrome). *N. Engl. J. Med. 300:*368, 1979.

312. Shulman, I., Pierce, M., Lukens, A., and Currimbhoy, Z.: Studies on thrombopoiesis. I. A factor in normal human plasma required for platelet production: Chronic thrombocytopenia due to its deficiency. *Blood 16:*943, 1960.

313. Gangarosa, E. J., Johnson, T. R., and Ramos, H. S.: Ristocetin-induced thrombocytopenia: Site and mechanism of action. *Arch. Intern. Med. 105:*83, 1960.

314. Howard, M. A., and Firkin, B. G.: Ristocetin: A new tool in the investigation of platelet aggregation. *Thromb. Diath. Haemorrh. 26:*362, 1971.

315. Heyns, A. duP., et al.: Kinetics and in vivo redistribution of ^{111}Indium-labelled human platelets after intravenous protamine sulphate. *Thromb. Haemost. 44:*65, 1980.

316. Hilgard, H., and Hossfeld, D. K.: Transient bleomycin-induced thrombocytopenia: A clinical study. *Eur. J. Cancer 14:*1261, 1978.

317. Godal, H. C.: Thrombocytopenia and heparin. *Thromb. Haemost. 43:*222, 1980.

318. Eika, C., Godal, H. C., Laake, K., and Hamborg, T.: Low incidence of thrombocytopenia during treatment with hog mucosa and beef lung heparin. *Scand. J. Haematol. 25:*19, 1980.

319. Bell, W. R., and Royall, R. M.: Heparin-associated thrombocytopenia: A comparison of three heparin preparations. *N. Engl. J. Med. 303:*902, 1980.

320. Ansell, J., Slepchuk, N., Jr., Kumar, R., Lopez, A., Southard, L., and Deykin, D.: Heparin induced thrombocytopenia: A prospective study. *Thromb. Haemost. 43:*61, 1980.

321. Cimo, P. L., Moake, J. L., Weinger, R. S., Ben-Menachem, Y., and Khalil, K. G.: Heparin-induced thrombocytopenia: Association with a platelet aggregating factor and arterial thromboses. *Am. J. Hematol. 6:*125, 1979.

322. White, P. W., Sadd, J. R., and Nensel, R. E.: Thrombotic complications of heparin therapy. *Ann. Surg. 190:*595, 1979.

323. Cines, D. B., Kaywin, P., Bina, M., Tomaski, A., and Schreiber, A. D.: Heparin-associated thrombocytopenia. *N. Engl. J. Med. 303:*788, 1980.

324. Kelton, J. G., Powers, P. J., Trupie, A. G. G., and Carter, A. J.: Heparin associated thrombocytopenia is not a typical drug induced thrombocytopenia. *Clin. Res. 29:*337A, 1981.

325. Alving, B. M., Shulman, N. R., Bell, W. R., Evatt, B. L., and Tack, K. M.: In vitro studies of heparin-associated thrombocytopenia. *Thromb. Res. 11:*827, 1977.

326. Zucker, M. B.: Biological aspects of heparin action. *Fed. Proc. 36:*47, 1977.

327. Eldor, A., and Weksler, B. B.: Heparin and dextran sulfate antagonize PGI$_2$ inhibition of platelet aggregation. *Thromb. Res. 16:*617, 1979.

328. Ansell, J., and Deykin, D.: Heparin-induced thrombocytopenia and recurrent thromboembolism. *Am. J. Hematol. 8:*325, 1980.

329. Hussey, C. V., Bernhard, V. M., McLean, M. R., and Fobian, J. E.: Heparin induced platelet aggregation: *In vitro* confirmation of thrombotic complications. *Ann. Clin. Lab. Sci. 9:*487, 1979.

330. Lindsey, S. M., Maddison, F. E., and Towne, J. B.: Heparin-induced thromboembolism: Angiographic features. *Radiology 131:*771, 1979.

331. Salem, H. H., Koutts, J., Handley, C., Van Der Weyden, M. B., Dudley, F. J., and Firkin, B. G.: The aggregation of human platelets by ascitic fluid: A possible mechanism for disseminated intravascular coagulation complicating LeVeen shunts. *Am. J. Hematol. 11:*153, 1981.

332. Stein, S. F., et al.: Accelerated fibrinogen and platelet destruction after peritoneovenous shunting. *Arch. Intern. Med. 141:*1149, 1981.

333. Kim, Y. L., Richman, K. A., and Marshall, B. E.: Thrombocytopenia associated with Swan-Ganz catheterization in patients. *Anesthesiology 53:*261, 1980.

334. Anemiya, H., Yokoyama, T., Putnam, C. W., Torisu, M., and Starzl, T. E.: The nature of antiplatelet activity in antilymphoblast ALG with special reference to cross-reacting antibody, immunochemical characterization, and Coombs' positive thrombocytopenia in ALG-treated renal recipients. *J. Exp. Immunol. 10:*417, 1972.

335. Andrassy, K., Ritz, E., Drings, P., and Kommerell, B.: Reversible Thrombopenie bei klinischer Anwendung von Antilymphocytenserum. *Klin. Wochenschr. 49:*47, 1971.

336. Henricsson, A., Husberg, B., and Bergentz, S.-E.: The mechanism behind the effect of ALG on platelets *in vivo. Clin. Exp. Immunol. 29:*515, 1977.

337. Bird, G. W. G., Shinton, N. K., and Wingham, J.: Persistent mixed-field polyagglutination. *Br. J. Haematol. 21:*443, 1971.

338. Cartron, J. P., and Nurden, A. T.: Galactosyltransferase and membrane glycoprotein abnormality in human platelets from Tn-syndrome donors. *Nature 282:*621, 1979.

339. Hysell, J. K., Hysell, J. W., Nichols, M. E., Leonardi, R. G., and Marsh, W. L.: *In vivo* and *in vitro* activation of T-antigen receptors on leukocytes and platelets. *Vox Sang. 31:*9, 1976.

340. Vipan, W. H.: Quinine as a cause of purpura. *Lancet 2:*37, 1865.

341. Rosenthal, N.: The blood picture in purpura. *J. Lab. Clin. Med. 13:*303, 1928.

342. Grandjean, L. C.: A case of purpura haemorrhagica after administration of quinine with specific thrombocytolysis demonstrated *in vitro. Acta Med. Scand. (Suppl. 213) 131:*165, 1948.

343. Steinkamp, R., Moore, C. V., and Doubek, W. G.: Thrombocytopenic purpura caused by hypersensitivity to quinine. *J. Lab. Clin. Med. 45:*18, 1955.

344. Ackroyd, J. F.: The pathogenesis of thrombocytopenic purpura due to hypersensitivity to Sedormid. *Clin. Sci. 7:*249, 1949.

345. Ackroyd, J. F.: The role of complement in Sedormid purpura. *Clin. Sci. 10:*185, 1951.

346. Ackroyd, J. F.: Allergic purpura, including purpura due to food, drugs and infections. *Am. J. Med. 14:*605, 1953.

347. Kissmeyer-Nielsen, F.: Thrombocytopenic purpura following quinine medication: An immunological study. *Acta Med. Scand. 154:*289, 1956.

348. Belkin, G. A.: Cocktail purpura: An unusual case of quinine sensitivity. *Ann. Intern. Med. 66:*583, 1967.

349. Bolton, F. G.: Thrombocytopenic purpura due to quinidine. II. Serologic mechanisms. *Blood 11:*547, 1956.

350. Shulman, N. R.: Immunoreactions involving platelets. I. A steric and kinetic model for formation of a complex from a human antibody, quinidine as a haptene, and platelets, and for fixation of complement by the complex. *J. Exp. Med. 107:*665, 1958.

351. Shulman, N. R.: Immunoreactions involving platelets. III. Quantitative aspects of platelet agglutination, inhibition of clot retraction, and other reactions caused by the antibody of quinidine purpura. *J. Exp. Med. 107:*697, 1958.

352. Shulman, N. R.: Immunoreactions involving platelets. IV. Studies on the pathogenesis of thrombocytopenia in drug purpura using test doses of quinidine in sensitized individuals. Their implications in idiopathic thrombocytopenic purpura. *J. Exp. Med. 107:*711, 1958.

353. Shulman, N. R.: A mechanism of cell destruction in individuals sensitized to foreign antigens and its implications in autoimmunity. *Ann. Intern. Med. 60:*506, 1964.

354. Shulman, N. R.: Immunologic reactions to drugs. *N. Engl. J. Med. 287:*408, 1972.

355. Ackroyd, J. F.: The immunological basis of purpura due to drug hypersensitivity. *Proc. R. Soc. Med. 55:*30, 1962.

356. Miescher, P., and Miescher, R.: Die Sedormid-Anaphlaxie. *Schweiz. Med. Wochenschr. 82:*1279, 1952.

357. Miescher, P., and Straessle, R.: Experimentelle Studien uber den

Mechanismus der Thrombocyten Schadigung durch antigen-antikorper Reactioner. *Vox Sang.* 1:83, 1956.

358. Croft, J. D., Jr., and Weed, R. I.: Coombs'-test positivity induced by drugs: Mechanisms of immunologic reactions, and red cell destruction. *Ann. Intern. Med.* 68:176, 1968.

359. Freedman, A. L., Barr, P. S., and Bordy, E. A.: Hemolytic anemia due to quinidine: Observations on its mechanism. *Am. J. Med.* 20:806, 1956.

360. Harris, J. W.: Studies on the mechanism of a drug-induced hemolytic anemia. *J. Lab. Clin. Med.* 47:760, 1956.

361. Miescher, P. A., and Miescher A.: Immunologic drug-induced blood dyscrasias. *Klin. Wochenschr.* 56:1, 1978.

362. Miescher, P. A., and Graf, J.: Drug-induced thrombocytopenia. *Clin. Haematol.* 9:505, 1980.

363. Kunicki, T. J., Johnson, M. M., and Aster, R. H.: Absence of the platelet receptor for drug-dependent antibodies in the Bernard-Soulier syndrome. *J. Clin. Invest.* 61:716, 1978.

364. Hosseinzadeh, P. K., Firkin, B. G., and Pfueller, S. L.: Study of the factors that cause specific transformation in cultures of lymphocytes from patients with quinine-induced and quinidine-induced immune thrombocytopenia. *J. Clin. Invest.* 66:638, 1980.

365. Pfueller, S. L., Hosseinzadeh, P. K., and Firkin, B. G.: Quinine-dependent and quinidine-dependent antiplatelet antibodies: Requirement of factor VIII-related antigen for platelet damage and for in vitro transformation of lymphocytes from patients with drug-induced thrombocytopenia. *J. Clin. Invest.* 67:907, 1981 (technical note).

366. Claas, F. H. J., Langerak, J., Debeer, L. L., and van Rood, J. J.: Drug-induced antibodies: Interaction of the drug with a polymorphic platelet-antigen. *Tissue Antigens* 17:64, 1981.

367. Karpatkin, M., Siskind, G. W., and Karpatkin, S.: The platelet factor 3 immunoinjury technique re-evaluated: Development of a rapid test for antiplatelet antibody: Detection in various clinical disorders, including immunologic drug-induced and neonatal thrombocytopenias. *J. Lab. Clin. Med.* 82:400, 1977.

368. Kekomaki, R., Rajamaki, A., and Myllyla, G.: Detection of quinidine-specific antibodies with platelet ^{125}I-labeled staphylococcal protein A test. *Vox Sang.* 38:12, 1980.

369. Kelton, J. G., et al.: Drug-induced thrombocytopenia is associated with increased binding of IgG to platelets both in vivo and in vitro. *Blood* 58:524, 1981.

370. Cimo, P. L., Pisciotta, A. V., Desai, R. G., Pino, J. L., and Aster, R. H.: Detection of drug-dependent antibodies by the ^{51}Cr platelet lysis test: Documentation of immune thrombocytopenia induced by diphenylhydantoin, diazepam, and sulfisoxazole. *Am. J. Hematol.* 2:65, 1977.

371. Hamilton, H. E., and Sheets, R. F.: Sulfisoxazole-induced thrombocytopenic purpura. *JAMA* 239:2586, 1978.

372. Schwartz, M., and Vonderheide, E. C.: Thrombocytopenic purpura due to mapharsen. *Am. J. Med. Sci.* 236:475, 1945.

373. Feiging, R. D., Zarkowsky, H. F., Shearer, W., and Anderson, D. C.: Thrombocytopenia following administration of para-aminosalicylic acid. *J. Pediatr.* 83:502, 1973.

374. Manohitharajah, S. M., Jenkins, W. J., Roberts, P. D., and Clark, R. C.: Methyl dopa and associated thrombocytopenia. *Br. Med. J.* 1:494, 1971.

375. Blachman, M. A., Lowry, R. C., Pettit, J. E., and Stradling, P.: Rifampicin-induced immune thrombocytopenia. *Br. Med. J.* 3:24, 1970.

376. Dodds, W. N., and Davidson, R. J. L.: Thrombocytopenia due to slow-release oxprenolol. *Lancet* 2:683, 1978.

377. Stafford, B. T., and Crosby, W. H.: Late onset of gold-induced thrombocytopenia with a practical note on injections of dimercaprol. *JAMA* 239:50, 1978 (technical note).

378. Kozloff, M., Votaw, M., and Penner, J. A.: Gold-induced thrombocytopenia responsive to cyclophosphamide. *South. Med. J.* 72:1490, 1979.

379. Coblyn, J. S., Weinblatt, M., Holdsworth, D., and Glass, D.: Gold-induced thrombocytopenia: A clinical and immunogenetic study of twenty-three patients. *Ann. Intern. Med.* 95:178, 1981.

380. Niewig, H. O., Bouma, H. G., DeVries, K., and Jansz, A.: Haematologic side effects of some anti-rheumatic drugs. *Ann. Rheum. Dis.* 22:240, 1963.

381. Garg, S. K., and Sarker, C. R.: Aspirin-induced thrombocytopenia on an immune basis. *Am. J. Med. Sci.* 267:129, 1974.

382. Stephens, C. A. L., Yoeman, E. E., Holbrook, W. P., Hill, D. F., and Goodin, W. L.: Benefits and toxicity of phenylbutazone (Butazolidin) in rheumatic arthritis. *JAMA* 150:1084, 1952.

383. Davidson, C., and Manohitharajah, S. M.: Drug-induced platelet antibodies. *Br. Med. J.* 3:545, 1973.

384. Handley, A. J.: Thrombocytopenia and LE cells after oxyphenbutazone. *Lancet* 1:245, 1971.

385. Cuthbert, M. D.: Adverse reactions to non-steroidal antirheumatic drugs. *Curr. Med. Res. Opin.* 2:600, 1974.

386. Karpinski, R. E.: Purpura following exposure to DDT. *J. Pediatr.* 37:373, 1950.

387. Kulis, J. C.: Chemically induced selective thrombocytopenic purpura. *Arch. Intern. Med.* 116:559, 1965.

388. Squier, T. L., and Madison, F. W.: Thrombocytopenic purpura due to food allergy. *J. Allergy* 8:143, 1937.

389. Dutton, L. O.: Thrombopenic purpura due to food allergy. *JAMA* 111:1920, 1938.

390. Ancona, G. R., Ellenhorn, M. J., and Falconer, E. H.: Purpura due to food sensitivity: Use of skin testing and etiologic diagnosis. *J. Allergy* 22:487, 1951.

391. Michon, P., and Harmand, J.: Purpura thrombopenique après l'absorption de baies de "viscum albumin." *Sang.* 23:539, 1952.

392. Lavy, R.: Thrombocytopenic purpura due to *Lupinus termis* bean. *J. Allergy* 35:386, 1964.

393. Nagel, H. J.: Verlauf and Therapie einer alimentar-allergischen thrombopenischen Purpura. *Kinderaerztl. Prax.* 35:305, 1967.

394. Bradley, P. P., Warden, G. D., Maxwell, J. G., and Rothstein, G.: Neutropenia and thrombocytopenia in renal allograft recipients treated with trimethoprim-sulfamethoxazole. *Ann. Intern. Med.* 93:560, 1980.

395. Fitchen, J. H., and Koeffler, H. P.: Cimetidine and granulopoiesis: Bone marrow culture studies in normal man and patients with cimetidine-associated neutropenia. *Br. J. Haematol.* 46:361, 1980.

396. Eisner, E. V., and Shaidi, N. T.: Immune thrombocytopenia due to a drug metabolite. *N. Engl. J. Med.* 287:376, 1972.

397. Schieinberg, I. H.: Thrombocytopenic reaction to aspirin and acetaminophen. *N. Engl. J. Med.* 300:678, 1979 (letter).

398. Schoefeld, Y., Shaklai, M., Levni, E., and Pinkhas, J.: Thrombocytopenia from acetaminophen. *N. Engl. J. Med.* 303:47, 1980 (letter).

399. Malinvaud, G., Dausset, J., and Layani, F.: Purpura thrombopenique aigu aux dérives de l'antipyrines. *Sang* 26:130, 1955.

400. Straumbaugh, J. E., Gordon, R. L., and Geller, L.: Leukopenia and thrombocytopenia secondary to clinoril therapy. *Lancet* 2:594, 1980.

401. Rosenbaum, J. T., and O'Connor, M.: Thrombocytopenia associated with sulindac. *Arthritis Rheum.* 24:753, 1981 (letter).

402. Simpson, R. E., Goldstein, D. J., Hjelte, G. S., and Evans, E. R.: Acute thrombocytopenia associated with fenoprofen. *N. Engl. J. Med.* 298:629, 1978 (letter).

403. Katz, M. D., and Wang, P.: Fenoprofen-associated thrombocytopenia. *Ann. Intern. Med.* 92:262, 1980 (letter).

404. Armstrong, F. B., and Scherbel, A.: Review of toxicity of oxyphenbutazone: Reports of a case of thrombocytopenic purpura. *JAMA* 175:614, 1961.

405. Rappoport, A. E., Nixon, C. W., and Barker, W. A.: Fatal secondary toxic thrombocytopenic purpura due to sodium salicylate. *J. Lab. Clin. Med.* 30:916, 1945.

406. Brooks, A. P.: Thrombocytopenia during treatment with ampicillin. *Lancet.* 2:723, 1974.

407. Sheiman, L., Spielvogel, A. R., and Horowitz, H. I.: Thrombocytopenia caused by cephalothin sodium in a penicillin sensitive individual. *JAMA* 203:601, 1968.

408. Gralnick, H. R., McGinniss, M., and Halterman, R.: Thrombocytopenia with sodium cephalothin therapy. *Ann. Intern. Med.* 77:401, 1972.

409. Chen. J.-H., Wiener, L., and Distenfeld, A.: Immunologic thrombocytopenia induced by gentamicin. *N.Y. State J. Med.* 80:1134, 1980.

410. Rolf, M. J.: Lincomycin thrombocytopenia? *Ann. Intern. Med.* 78:799, 1973.

411. Schiffer, C. A., Weinstein, H. J., and Wiernik, P. H.: Methicillin-associated thrombocytopenia. *Ann. Intern. Med.* 85:338, 1967 (letter).

412. Day, H. J., Conrad, F. G., and Moore, J. E.: Immunothrombocytopenia induced by novobiocin. *Am. J. Med. Sci.* 236:475, 1958.

413. Beckett, A. G., and Foxell, A. W. H.: Thrombocytopenic purpura associated with oxytetracycline therapy. *Lancet* 1:1053, 1955.

414. Kounis, N. G.: Oxytetracycline-induced thrombocytopenic purpura. *JAMA* 231:734, 1975.

415. Eisner, E. V., and Kasper, K.: Immune thrombocytopenia due to a metabolite of para-aminosalicylic acid. *Am. J. Med.* 53:709, 1972.

416. Hsi, Y. J., Kuo, H. Y., and Ouyang, A.: Thrombocytopenia following administration of penicillin. *Clin. Med. J.* 85:249, 1966.

417. Levy, M. A., Senior, R. M., and Sneider, R. E.: Severe thrombocytopenic purpura complicating pentamidine therapy for *Pneumocystic carinii* pneumonia. *Cancer* 34:414, 1974.

418. Esposito, R., and Vitali, D.: Rifampicin and thrombocytopenia. *Lancet* 2:491, 1971.

419. Oppenhein, M., and DeMeyer, G.: Granulo- und Thrombocytopenie infolge Streptomycin-Behandlung. *Schweiz. Med. Wochenschr.* 79:1187, 1949.

420. Schwartz, R. H., Rodriguez, W. L., and Luban, N.L.C.: Thrombocytopenia associated with PF3 anti-platelet activity against the sulfa component of trimethoprim-sulfamethoxazole *South. Med. J.* 74:640, 1981 (technical note).

421. Greenlaw, C. W., Stolley, S. N., and Henrietta, G. C.: Tobramycin-induced thrombocytopenia. *Drug Intell. Clin. Pharmacol.* 12:682, 1978 (letter).

422. Claas, F. H., van der Meer, J. W. M., and Langerak, J.: Immunological effect of co-trimoxazole on platelets. *Br. Med. J.* 2:898, 1979.

423. Young, F.: Severe post-operative thrombocytopenic purpura. *Br. Med. J.* 2:919, 1957.

424. Pearce, J.: Thrombocytopenia after carbamazepine. *Lancet* 2:223, 1968.

425. Schmidt, W.: Ein weiterer Fall von allergischer Thrombozytopenie nach Centalun. *Dtsch. Med. Wochenschr.* 93:1152, 1968.

426. Celada, A., Herreros, V., Rudolf, H.: Thrombocytopenic purpura during treatment with librax. *Br. Med. J.* 1:268, 1977 (technical note).

427. Veall, R. M., and Hogarth, H. C.: Thrombocytopenia during treatment with clonazepam. *Br. Med. J.* 4:462, 1975.

428. Graudal, H.: Thrombopenia after Allymid (ethyl-allyl-acetyl-carbamide). *Ugeskr. Laeger* 111:958, 1949.

429. Jacobson, E. S.: Fatal immune thrombocytopenia induced by ethylchlorvinyl. *Ann. Intern. Med.* 77:73, 1972.

430. Jones, D. T., and Jacobs, J. L.: The treatment of obstinate chorea with Nirvanol. *JAMA* 99:18, 1932.

431. Reichelderfer, T. C., Pearson, P. H., and Livingston, S.: Thrombocytopenia occurring in association with Paradione (paramethadione) and Dilantin sodium (phenytoin sodium) therapy. *J. Pediatr.* 43:43, 1953.

432. Fincham, R. W., Hamilton, H. E., and Schottelius, D. D.: Late-onset thrombocytopenia with phenytoin therapy. *Ann. Neurol.* 6:370, 1979.

433. Koller, R. L., and Blank, N. K.: Strawberry picker's palsy. *Arch. Neurol.* 37:320, 1980.

434. Parker, W. A.: Primidone thrombocytopenia. *Ann. Intern. Med.* 81:559, 1974.

435. Cole, A. P.: Transient thrombocytopenia in a child on sodium valproate. *Dev. Med.* 20:487, 1978.

436. Loiseau, P.: Sodium valproate, platelet dysfunction and bleeding. *Epilepsia* 22:141, 1981.

437. Morris, N., Barr, R. D., Pai, K. R. M., and Kelton, J. G.: Valproic acid and thrombocytopenia. *Can. Med. Assoc. J.* 125:63, 1981 (technical note).

438. Barr, B. D., Copeland, S. A., Moore, J. C., Stockwell, M. L., Morris, N., and Kelton, J. C.: Valproic acid and immune thrombocytopenia. *Blood* 58 (Suppl. 1):1889, 1981.

439. Bertino, J. E., Rodman, T., and Myerson, R. M.: Thrombocytopenia and renal lesions associated with acetazolamide (Diamox) therapy. *Arch. Intern. Med.* 99:1006, 1957.

440. Morley, A., and Hirsch, J.: A case of thrombocytopenia associated with chlorpropamide therapy. *Med. J. Aust.* 2:988, 1964.

441. Bottiger, L. E., and Westerholm, B.: Drug-induced thrombocytopenia. *Acta Med. Scand.* 191:541, 1972.

442. Coombs, J. T., Grunt, J. A., and Brant, I. K.: Hematologic reactions to diazoxide. *Pediatrics* 40:90, 1967.

443. Wales, J., and Wolff, F.: Hematologic side effects of diazoxide. *Lancet* 1:53, 1967.

444. Duncan, A., Moore, S. B., and Barker, P.: Thrombocytopenia caused by frusemide-induced platelet antibody. *Lancet* 1:1210, 1981 (letter).

445. Balodimos, M. D., Camerini-Davalos, R. A., and Marble, A.: Nine years' experience with tolbutamide in the treatment of diabetes mellitus. *Metabolism* 15:957, 1966.

446. Rosenbloom, D., and Gilbert, R.: Reversible flu-like syndrome, leukopenia, and thrombocytopenia induced by allopurinol. *Drug Intell. Clin. Pharmacy* 15:286, 1981.

447. Shalev, O., and Brezis, M.: Methyldopa-induced thrombocytopenia in chronic lymphocytic-leukemia. *N. Engl. J. Med.* 297:1471, 1977 (letter).

448. Gassel, W. D., and Schneider, R.: Akute medicamentos-allergische Thrombocytopenie durch antazoline. *Blut.* 29:195, 1974.

449. Falconer, E. H., Epstein, N. N., and Mills, E. S.: Purpura haemorrhagic due to the arsphenamines: Sensitivity in patients as influenced by vitamin C therapy. *Arch. Intern. Med.* 66:319, 1940.

450. Eisner, E. V., LaBocki, N. L., and Pinkney, L.: Chlorpheniramine dependent thrombocytopenia. *JAMA* 231:735, 1975.

451. Yates, V. M., and Kerr, R.E.I.: Cimetidine and thrombocytopenia. *Br. Med. J.* 280:1453, 1980 (letter).

452. Isaacs, A. J.: Cimetidine and thrombocytopenia. *Br. Med. J.* 280:294, 1980 (technical note).

453. McDaniel, J. L., and Stein, J. J.: Thrombocytopenia with cimetitherapy. *N. Engl. J. Med.* 300:864, 1979.

454. Pande, R. S., and Gupta, Y. N.: Thrombocytopenia purpura following copper sulfate therapy. *J. Indian Med. Assoc.* 52:227, 1969.

455. Rachmilewitz, E. A., Dawson, R. B., Jr., and Rachmilewitz, B.: Serum antibodies against Desipramine as a possible cause for thrombocytopenia. *Blood* 32:524, 1968.

456. Perret, J. L., Contasso, J. C., Prost, G., and Tolot, F.: Thrombocytopenia: An unusual complication of digitalis toxicity. *Nouv. Presse Med.* 10:2292, 1981 (letter).

457. Young, R. C., Nachman, R. L., and Horowitz, H. I.: Thrombocytopenia due to digitoxin. *Am. J. Med.* 41:604, 1966.

458. Medecina, R., Hatam, V., Hatam, K., Girard, J. P., and Junet, R.: Mécanisme immunologique de la thrombopenia a la digitoxine: À propos d'un cas. *Helv. Med. Acta* 36:477, 1973.

459. Pirovino, M., Ohnhaus, E. E., and Vonfelte, A.: Digoxin-associated thrombocytopaenia. *Eur. J. Clin. Pharmacol.* 19:205, 1981.

460. Leibetseder, F.: Akute thrombopenische Purpura nach Antabusbehandlung. *Wien. Klin. Wochenschr.* 64:431, 1952.

461. Adams, W. H., Rufo, R. A., Talarico, L., Silverman, S. L., and Brauer, M. J.: Thrombocytopenia and intravenous heroin use. *Ann. Intern. Med.* 89:207, 1978.

462. Moss, R. A.: Heroin-induced thrombocytopenia. *Arch. Intern. Med.* 139:752, 1979.

463. Adams, W. H.: Heroin-associated thrombocytopenia. *Arch. Intern. Med.* 139:740, 1979.

464. Vergoz, D., Vialaltes, T., Perrot, J., and Andre, R.: Thrombocytopenia par sensibilisation à l'hexopropymate. *Nouv. Rev. Fr. Hematol.* 8:408, 1968.

465. Eisner, E. V., and Crowell, E. B.: Hydrochlorothiazide-dependent thrombocytopenia due to IgM antibody. *JAMA* 215:480, 1971.

466. Khaleeli, A. A.: Quinaband-induced thrombocytopenia purpura in a patient with myxoedema coma. *Br. Med. J.* 2:562, 1976.

467. Fatzer, H.: Schwere thrombopenische Purpura nach Insektstich. *Folia Haematol. (Leipz.)* 63:145, 1939.

468. Hysell, J. K., Hysell, J. W., and Gray, J. M.: Thrombocytopenic purpura following iopanoic acid ingestion. *JAMA* 237:361, 1977.

469. Curradi, F., and Abbritti, G.: Acute thrombocytopenia following oral cholecystography with iopanoic acid. *Clin. Toxicol.* 18:221, 1981.

470. Zorab, P. A.: Fulminating purpura during antituberculosis drug treatment. *Tubercle* 41:219, 1960.

471. Hansen, J. E.: Hypersensitivity to isoniazid with neutropenia and thrombocytopenia. *Am. Rev. Respir. Dis.* 83:744, 1961.

472. El-Ghobari, A. F., and Capella, H. A.: Levamisole-induced throm-bocytopenia. *Br. Med. J.* 2:555, 1977.

473. Wanamaker, W. M., Wanamaker, S. J., Celesia, G. G., and Koeller, A. A.: Thrombocytopenia associated with long-term levodopa ther-apy. *JAMA* 235:2217, 1976.

474. Stefanini, M., and Hoffman, M. N.: Case report studies on platelets. XXVIII. Acute thrombocytopenic purpura due to lidocaine (Xylo-caine)-mediated antibody: Report of a case. *Am. J. Med. Sci.* 275:365, 1978.

475. Butt, E. M., and Simonsen, D. G.: Mercury and lead storage in human tissues with special reference to thrombocytopenic pur-pura. *Am. J. Clin. Pathol.* 20:716, 1950.

476. Peitzman, S. J., and Martin, C.: Thrombocytopenia and minoxidil. *Ann. Int. Med.* 92:874, 1980 (letter).

477. Shmuskovich, J., and Davis, E.: Thrombocytopenic skin purpura following treatment with trinitrin. *Br. J. Dermatol.* 67:299, 1955.

478. Hare, D. L., and Hicks, B. H.: Thrombocytopenia due to oxprenolol. *Med. J. Aust.* 2:259, 1979 (letter).

479. Harrison, E. E., and Hickman, J. W.: Hemolytic anemia and throm-bocytopenia associated with penicillamine ingestion. *South. Med. J.* 68:113, 1975.

480. Kugelmass, I. N.: Thrombocytopenic purpura induced by pertussis toxin in allergic children. *JAMA* 107:2120, 1936.

481. Rothman, I. K., and Amorosi, E. L.: Procainamide-induced agranu-locytosis and thrombocytopenia. *Arch. Intern. Med.* 139:246, 1979 (technical note).

482. MacFarland, R. B.: Fatal drug reaction associated with prochlor-perazine (Compazine): Report of a case characterized by jaundice, thrombocytopenia, and agranulocytosis. *Am. J. Clin. Pathol.* 40:284, 1963.

483. Fewell, R. A., Engel, E. F., and Zimmerman, S. L.: Acute throm-bocytopenic purpura associated with propylthiouracil. *JAMA* 143:891, 1950.

484. Kahn, H. R., and Brod, R. C.: Thrombocytopenia due to stibophen. *Arch. Intern. Med.* 108:496, 1961.

485. King, H. E., and Cooper, T.: Thrombocytopenia: A clinical analysis of 500 cases. *Postgrad. Med.* 31:532, 1962.

486. Ham, F. F.: Purpura following treatment with tetraethylammonium chloride. *Calif. Med.* 69:279, 1948.

487. Newcomb, P. B., and Deanne, E. W.: Thiourea causing granulocy-topenia and thrombocytopenia. *Lancet* 1:179, 1944.

488. Jennings, G. H., and Gower, N. D.: Thrombocytopenic purpura in toluene diisocyanate workers. *Lancet* 1:406, 1963.

489. Wahlberg, P., and Nyman, D.: Turpentine and thrombocytopenic purpura. *Lancet* 2:215, 1969.

490. Petz, L. D., and Fudenberg, H. H.: Immunological mechanisms in drug-induced cytopenias. *Prog. Hematol.* 9:185, 1975.

491. Moss, R. A.: Drug-induced immune thrombocytopenia. *Am. J. Hematol.* 9:439, 1980.

492. Siroty, R. R.: Purpura on the rocks—with a twist. *JAMA* 235:2521, 1976.

493. Zeigler, Z., Shadduck, R. K., Winkelstein, A., and Stroupe, T. K.: Immune hemolytic anemia and thrombocytopenia secondary to quinidine: In vitro studies of the quinidine-dependent red cell and platelet antibodies. *Blood* 53:396, 1979.

494. Castro, O., and Nash, I.: Quinidine leukopenia and thrombocy-topenia with a drug-dependent leukoagglutinin. *N. Engl. J. Med.* 296:572, 1977.

495. Alam, M., Duvernoy, W. F. C., Pickard, S. D., and Aronsohn, P. L.: Quinidine-induced hepatitis and thrombocytopenia. *Henry Ford Hosp. Med. J.* 25:53, 1977.

496. Freedman, A. L., Brody, E. A., and Barr, P. S.: Immunothrombocy-topenic purpura due to quinidine: Report of four new cases with special observations on patch testing. *J. Lab. Clin. Med.* 48:205, 1956.

497. Falconer, E. H., Epstein, N. N., and Mills, E. S.: Purpura haemor-rhagica due to the arsphenamines: Sensitivity in patients as in-fluenced by vitamine C therapy. *Arch. Intern. Med.* 66:319, 1940.

498. Fireman, Z., Yust, I., and Abramov, A. L.: Lethal occult pulmonary hemorrhage in drug-induced thrombocytopenia. *Chest* 79:358, 1981 (technical note).

499. Moss, R. A., and Castro, O.: Platelet transfusion for quinidine-in-duced thrombocytopenia. *N. Engl. J. Med.* 288:522, 1973.

500. Ball, G. V.: Gold-induced thrombocytopenia: Response to vincris-tine? *Arthritis Rheum.* 20:1288, 1977 (letter).

501. Johansson, S. A., Lundberg, A., and Sjoberg, H. E.: Influence of heparin on thrombocytopenia in allergic reactions. *Acta Med. Scand.* 168:165, 1960.

502. Storck, H., Hoigne, R., and Koller, F.: Thrombocytes in allergic re-actions. *Int. Arch. Allergy Appl. Immunol.* 6:372, 1955.

503. Gallagher, J. S., Bernstein, I. L., Maccia, C. A., Splansky, G. L., and Glueck, H. I.: Cyclic platelet dysfunction in IgE-mediated allergy. *J. Allergy Clin. Immunol.* 62:229, 1978.

504. Knauer, K. A., Lichtenstein, L. M., Adkinson, N. F., Jr., and Fish, J. E.: Platelet activation during antigen-induced airway reactions in asthmatic subjects. *N. Engl. J. Med.* 304:1404, 1981.

505. Gorog, P., and Kovacs, I. B.: Significance of platelet aggregation in anaphylactic shock in rats. *Int. Arch. Allergy. Appl. Immunol.* 35:411, 1969.

506. Pinckard, R. N., Halonen, M., Palmer, J. D., Butler, C., Shaw, J. O., and Henson, P. M.: Intravascular aggregation and pulmonary sequestration of platelets during IgE-induced systemic anaphylaxis in the rabbit: Abrogation of lethal anaphylactic shock by platelet depletion. *J. Immunol.* 119:2185, 1977.

507. Muller-Eckhardt, C. H.: Immune reactions of platelets and their clinical significance. *Klin. Wochenschr.* 53:889, 1975.

508. Cusack, N. J.: Platelet-activating factor. *Nature* 285:193, 1980.

509. Van Loghem, J. J., Dorfmeijer, H., and Van der Hart, M.: Serological and genetical studies on a platelet antigen (Zw). *Vox Sang.* 4:161, 1959.

510. Shulman, N. R., Aster, R. H., Leitner, A., and Hiller, M. C.: Im-munoreactions involving platelets. V. Post-transfusion purpura due to a complement-fixing antibody against a genetically con-trolled platelet antigen: A proposed mechanism for thrombocy-topenia and its relevance in "autoimmunity." *J. Clin. Invest.* 40:1597, 1961.

511. Cimo, P. L., and Aster, R. H.: Post-transfusion purpura: Successful treatment with exchange transfusion. *N. Engl. J. Med.* 287:290, 1972.

512. Abramson, N., Eisenberg, P. D., and Aster, R. H.: Post-transfusion purpura: Immunologic aspects and therapy. *N. Engl. J. Med.* 291:1163, 1974.

513. Ziegler, Z., Murphy, S., and Gardner, F. H.: Post-transfusion pur-pura: A heterogeneous syndrome. *Blood* 45:529, 1975.

514. Eisenberg, P. D., and Abramson, N.: Post-transfusion purpura revisited. *N. Engl. J. Med.* 296:515, 1977 (letter).

515. Soulier, J.-P., Patereau, C., Gobert, N., Achach, P., and Muller, J.-Y.: Posttransfusional immunologic thrombocytopenia: A case report. *Vox Sang.* 37:21, 1979.

516. Gerstner, J. B., Smith, M. J., Davis, K. D., Cimo, P. L., and Aster, R. H.: Post-transfusion purpura: Therapeutic failure of PI^A1-nega-tive platelet transfusion. *Am. J. Hematol.* 5:71, 1979.

517. Muller-Eckhardt, C., et al.: Post-transfusion thrombocytopenic purpura: Immunological and clinical studies in two cases and review of the literature. *Blut* 40:249, 1980.

518. Lau, P., Sholtis, M., and Aster, R. H.: Post-transfusion purpura: An enigma of alloimmunization. *Am. J. Hematol.* 9:331, 1980.

519. Phadke, K. P., and Isbister, J. P.: Post-transfusion purpura. *Med. J. Aust.* 1:430, 1980.

520. Erichson, R. B., Viles, H., Grann, V., and Ziegler, Z.: Post-trans-fusion purpura: Case report with observation on antibody detec-tion and therapy. *Arch. Intern. Med.* 138:998, 1978.

521. Gengozian, N., and McLaughlin, C. L.: IgG^+ platelets in the mar-moset: Their induction, maintenance, and survival. *Blood* 55:885, 1980.

522. Israels, E. D., Nisli, G., Paraskevas, F., and Israels, L. G.: Platelet Fc receptor as a mechanism for Ag-Ab complex-induced platelet in-jury. *Thromb. Diath. Haemorrh.* 29:434, 1973.

523. Moore, A., Ross, G. D., and Nachman, R. L.: Interaction of platelet membrane receptors with von Willebrand factor, ristocetin and the Fc region of immunoglobulin G. *J. Clin. Invest.* 62:1053, 1978.

524. Pfueller, S. L., and Luscher, E. F.: The effects of immune complexes on blood platelets and their relationship to complement activation. *Immunochemistry* 9:1151, 1972.

525. Kekomaki, R., and Myllyla, G.: Effect of normal human serum on the binding of specific antibodies and platelet-unrelated immune complexes to human platelets. *Scand. J. Immunol.* 9:527, 1979.

526. Fink, P. C., Piening, U., Fricke, M., and Deicher, H.: Platelet aggregation and aggregation inhibition by different antiglobulins and antiglobulin complexes from sera of patients with rheumatoid arthritis. *Arthritis Rheum.* 22:896, 1979.

527. VanZile, J., Kilpatrick, M., Laimins, M., Segal, J., Colwell, J., and Virella, G.: Platelet aggregation and release of ATP after incubation with soluble immune complexes purified from the serum of diabetic patients. *Diabetes* 30:575, 1981.

528. Safai-Kutti, S., Zaroulis, C. G., Day, N. K., Good, R. A., and Kutti, J.: Platelet transfusion therapy and circulating immune complexes. *Vox Sang.* 39:22, 1980.

529. Lusher, J. M., and Iyer, R.: Idiopathic thrombocytopenic purpura in children. *Semin. Thromb. Hemostas.* 3:175, 1977.

530. McWilliams, N. B., and Mauer, H. M.: Acute idiopathic thrombocytopenic purpura in children. *Am. J. Hematol.* 7:87, 1979.

531. McClure, P. D.: Idiopathic thrombocytopenic purpura in children: Diagnosis and management. *Pediatrics* 55:68, 1975.

532. Cohn, J.: Thrombocytopenia in childhood: An evaluation of 433 patients. *Scand. J. Haematol.* 16:226, 1976.

533. Simons, S. M., Main, C. A., Yaish, H. M., and Rutzky, J.: Idiopathic thrombocytopenic purpura in children. *J. Pediatr.* 87:16, 1975.

534. Goldin, R., and Gelfand, M.: Idiopathic thrombocytopaenic purpura and onyalai in Zimbabwean Africans. *Cent. Afr. J. Med.* 26:236, 1980.

535. Harris, M. B., Murphy, S., and Oski, F. A.: Onyalai—a form of idiopathic thrombocytopenic purpura in the United States: Report of 2 patients. *Clin. Pediatr.* 11:705, 1972.

536. Yeager, A. M., and Zinkham, W. H.: Varicella-associated thrombocytopenia: Clues to the etiology of childhood idiopathic thrombocytopenic purpura. *Johns Hopkins Med. J.* 146:270, 1980.

537. Myllyla, G., Vaheri, A., Vesikari, T., and Penttinen, K.: Interaction between human blood platelets, viruses, and antibodies. IV. Post-rubella thrombocytopenic purpura and platelet aggregation by rubella antigen-antibody interaction. *Clin. Exp. Immunol.* 4:323, 1969.

538. Evers, K.-G., Thouet, R., Haase, W., and Kruger, J.: HLA frequencies and haplotypes in children with idiopathic thrombocytopenic purpura (ITP). *Eur. J. Pediatr.* 129:267, 1978.

539. McIntosh, S., Johnson, C., Hartigan, P., Baumgarten, A., and Dwyer, J. M.: Immunoregulatory abnormalities in children with thrombocytopenic purpura. *J. Pediatr.* 99:525, 1981.

540. Carpentieri, U., and Haggard, M. E.: Thrombocytopenia and viral diseases. *Tex. Med.* 71:81, 1975.

541. Norton, J. A., Shulman, N. R., Corash, L., Smith, R. L., Au, F., and Rosenberg, S. A.: Severe thrombocytopenia following intralesional BCG therapy. *Cancer* 41:820, 1977.

542. Khalifa, A. S., Lusher, J. M., Cejka, J., and Zuelzer, W. W.: Immunoglobulins in idiopathic thrombocytopenic purpura in childhood. *Acta Haematol.* 56:205, 1976.

543. Movassaghi, N., Moorhead, J., and Leikin, S.: Antiplatelet antibodies in childhood idiopathic thrombocytopenic purpura. *Am. J. Dis. Child.* 133:257, 1979.

544. Luiken, G. A., et al.: Platelet-associated IgG in immune thrombocytopenic purpura. *Blood* 50:317, 1977.

545. Lightsey, A. L., Koenig, H. M., and McMillan, R.: Platelet-associated immunoglobulin G in childhood idiopathic thrombocytopenic purpura. *J. Pediatr.* 94:201, 1979.

546. Cines, D. B., and Schreiber, A. D.: Immune thrombocytopenia. *N. Engl. J. Med.* 300:106, 1979.

547. Sugiura, K., Steiner, M., and Baldini, M.: Platelet antibody in idiopathic thrombocytopenic purpura and other thrombocytopenias. *J. Lab. Clin. Med.* 96:640, 1980.

548. Mueller-Eckhardt, C., et al.: The clinical significance of platelet-associated IgG: A study of 298 patients with various disorders. *Br. J. Haematol.* 46:123, 1980.

549. Dameshek, W., Ebbe, S., Greenberg, L., and Baldini, M.: Recurrent idiopathic thrombocytopenic purpura. *N. Engl. J. Med.* 269:647, 1963.

550. Woerner, S. J., Abildgaard, C. F., and French, B. N.: Intracranial hemorrhage in children with idiopathic thrombocytopenic purpura. *Pediatrics* 67:453, 1981.

551. McClure, P. D.: Idiopathic thrombocytopenic purpura in children. *Am. J. Dis. Child.* 131:357, 1977.

552. Zuelzer, W. W., and Lusher, J. M.: Childhood idiopathic thrombocytopenic purpura. *Am. J. Dis. Child.* 131:360, 1977.

553. Lammi, A. T., and Lovric, V. A.: Idiopathic thrombocytopenic purpura: Epidemiologic study. *J. Pediatr.* 83:31, 1973.

554. Lusher, J. M., and Zuelzer, W. W.: Idiopathic thrombocytopenic purpura in childhood. *Can. Med. Assoc. J.* 97:562, 1967.

555. Shulman, I.: Diagnosis and treatment: Management of idiopathic thrombocytopenic purpura. *Pediatrics* 33:979, 1964.

556. Alexander, M., VanDenBogart, N., and Fondue, P.: Le Pronostic et le traitement du purpura thrombopenique idiopathique de l'enfant. *Arch. Fr. Pediatr.* 33:829, 1976.

557. McElfresh, A. E.: Idiopathic thrombocytopenic purpura: To treat or not to treat. *J. Pediatr.* 87:160, 1975.

558. Lightsey, A. L., McMillan, R., and Koenig, H. M.: Childhood idiopathic thrombocytopenic purpura: Aggressive management of life-threatening complications. *JAMA* 232:734, 1975.

559. Novak, R., and Wilimas, J.: Plasmapheresis in catastrophic complications of idiopathic thrombocytopenic purpura. *J. Pediatr.* 92:434, 1978.

560. Zerella, J. T., Martin, L. W., and Lampkin, B. C.: Emergency splenectomy for idiopathic thrombocytopenic purpura in children. *J. Pediatr. Surg.* 13:243, 1978.

561. Berglund, G.: Plasma transfusion treatment in six children with idiopathic thrombocytopenic purpura. *Acta Paediatr.* 51:523, 1962.

562. Reiquam, C. W., and Prosper, J. C.: Fresh plasma transfusions in the treatment of acute thrombocytopenic purpura. *J. Pediatr.* 68:880, 1966.

563. Imbach, P., et al.: High-dose intravenous gammaglobulin for idiopathic thrombocytopenic purpura in childhood. *Lancet* 1:1228, 1981.

564. Tomar, R. H., and Stuart, M. J.: Predicting acute vs. chronic childhood idiopathic thrombocytopenic purpura. *Am. J. Dis. Child.* 135:446, 1981.

565. Afifi, A. M., Adnan, M., and Guindi, M. M.: Childhood idiopathic thrombocytopenic purpura in Egypt and the neighboring Arab countries: A regional form with three different patterns of clinical expression. *Acta Haematol.* 65:211, 1981.

566. Lo, S. S., Hitzig, W. H., and Sigg, P.: Management of chronic ITP in children with particular reference to immunosuppressive therapy. *Acta Haematol. (Basel)* 41:1, 1969.

567. Reiquam, C. W., and Prosper, J. C.: Chronic idiopathic thrombocytopenia: Treatment with prednisone, 6-mercaptopurine, vincristine, and fresh plasma transfusions. *J. Pediatr.* 68:885, 1966.

568. Kuzemo, J. A., and Keidan, S. E.: Treatment of chronic idiopathic thrombocytopenic purpura and azathioprine and prednisilone: A clinical trial with three children. *Clin. Pediatr. (Bologna)* 7:216, 1968.

569. Seip, M.: Vincristine in the treatment of post-infectious and neonatal thrombocytopenia. *Acta Paediatr. Scand.* 69:253, 1980 (letter).

570. Paul Gottlieb Werlhof (1699–1767): Thrombocytopenic purpura. *JAMA* 206:2891, 1968 (editorial).

571. Dameshek, W., and Miller, E. B.: The megakaryocytes in idiopathic thrombocytopenic purpura: A form of hypersplenism. *Blood* 1:27, 1946.

572. Frank, E.: Die essentielle Thrombopenie. *Klin. Wochenschr.* 52:454, 1915.

573. Minot, G. R.: Studies on a case of idiopathic purpura hemorrhagica. *Am. J. Med. Sci.* 152:48, 1916.

574. Mueller-Eckhardt, C.: Idiopathic thrombocytopenic purpura (ITP): Clinical and immunologic considerations. *Semin. Thromb. Hemostas.* 3:125, 1977.

575. DiFino, S. M., Lachant, N. A., Kirshner, J. J., and Gottlieb, A. J.: Adult idiopathic thrombocytopenic purpura. Clinical findings and response to therapy. *Am.J. Med.* 69:430, 1980.

576. Karpatkin, S.: Autoimmune thrombocytopenic purpura. *Blood* 56:329, 1980.

577. McMillan, R.: Chronic idiopathic thrombocytopenic purpura. *N. Engl. J. Med.* 304:1135, 1981.

578. Dodds, W. J., Wilkins, R. J.: Animal model: Canine and equine immune-mediated thrombocytopenia and idiopathic thrombocytopenic purpura. *Am. J. Pathol.* 86:489, 1977.

579. Aster, R. H., and Keene, W. R.: Sites of platelet destruction in idiopathic thrombocytopenic purpura. *Br. J. Haematol.* 16:61, 1969.

580. Ries, C. A., and Price, D. C.: Platelet kinetics in thrombocytopenia:

Correlation between splenic sequestration of platelets and response to splenectomy. *Ann. Intern. Med. 80:*702, 1974.

581. Branehog, I., Kutti, J., and Weinfeld, A.: Platelet survival and platelet production in idiopathic thrombocytopenic purpura (ITP). *Br. J. Haematol. 27:*127, 1974.

582. Harker, L. A.: Thrombokinetics in idiopathic thrombocytopenic purpura. *Br. J. Haematol. 19:*95, 1970.

583. Donaldson, G. W. K., Parker, A. C., McArthur, M., and Richmond, J.: Thrombocytopenic purpura with normal platelet survival time. *J. Clin. Pathol. 24:*621, 1971.

584. Baldini, M. G.: Platelet production and destruction in idiopathic thrombocytopenic purpura: A controversial issue. *JAMA 239:*2477, 1978.

585. Harrington, W. J., Minnich, V., Hollingsworth, J. W., and Moore, C. V.: Demonstration of a thrombocytopenic factor in the blood of patients with thrombocytopenic purpura. *J. Lab. Clin. Med. 38:*1, 1951.

586. Watkins, S. P., Jr,. Cowan, D. H., and Shulman, N. R.: Differentiation of immunologic from non-immunologic forms of idiopathic thrombocytopenic purpura. *J. Clin. Invest. 46:*1129, 1967.

587. Shulman, N. R., Marder, V. J., and Weinrach, R. S.: Similarities between known antiplatelet antibodies and the factor responsible for thrombocytopenia in idiopathic purpura: Physiologic, serologic and isotopic studies. *Ann. N.Y. Acad. Sci. 124:*499, 1965.

588. Landolfi, R., Leone, G., Fedeli, G., Storti, S., Laghi, F., and Bizzi, B.: Platelet-associated IgG in acute and chronic hepatic diseases. *Scand. J. Haematol. 25:*417, 1980.

589. Rosse, W. F., Adams, J. P., and Yount, W. J.: Subclasses of IgG antibodies in immune thrombocytopenic purpura (ITP). *Br. J. Haematol. 46:*109, 1980.

590. Von dem Borne, A. E. G. K., Helmerhorst, F. M., van Leeuwen, E. F., Pegels, H. G., von Riesz, E., and Engelfriet, C. P.: Autoimmune thrombocytopenia: Detection of platelet autoantibodies with the suspension immunofluorescence test. *Br. J. Haematol. 45:*319, 1980.

591. Hauch, T. W., and Rosse, W. F.: Platelet-bound complement (C3) in immune thrombocytopenia. *Blood 50:*1129, 1977.

592. McMillan, R., and Martin, M.: Fixation of C3 to platelets in vitro by antiplatelet antibody from patients with immune thrombocytopenic purpura. *Br. J. Haematol. 47:*251, 1981.

593. Lurhuma, A. Z., Riccomi, H., and Masson, P. L.: The occurrence of circulating immune complexes and viral antigens in idiopathic thrombocytopenic purpura. *Clin. Exp. Immunol. 28:*49, 1977.

594. Wautier, J. L., Boizard, B., Wautier, M. P., Kadeva, H., and Caen, J. P.: Platelet-associated IgG and circulating immune complexes in thrombocytopenic purpura. *Nouv. Rev. Fr. Hematol. 22:*29, 1980.

595. Clancy, R.: Cellular immunity to autologous platelets and serum-blocking factors in idiopathic thrombocytopenic purpura. *Lancet 1:*6, 1972.

596. Morimoto, C., Abe, T., Hara, M., and Homma, M.: Cell-mediated immune response in idiopathic thrombocytopenic purpura. *Clin. Immunol. Immunopathol. 8:*181, 1977.

597. Blanchette, V. S., Hallett, J. J., Hemphill, J. M., Winkelstein, J. A., and Zinkham, W. H.: Abnormalities of the peripheral blood as a presenting feature of immunodeficiency. *Am. J. Hematol. 4:*87, 1978.

598. Quagliata, F., and Karpatkin, S.: Impaired lymphocyte transformation and capping in autoimmune thrombocytopenic purpura. *Blood 53:*342, 1979.

599. Gandolfo, G. M., Afeltra, A., Deruggieri, M. A., and Ernandez, M. A.: Determination of serum immunoglobulins in idiopathic thrombocytopenic purpura: IgA reduction in adult patients. *Acta Haematol. 66:*113, 1981.

600. Trent, R., Adams, E., Erhardt, C., and Basten, A.: Alterations in T-gamma-cells in patients with chronic idiopathic thrombocytopenic purpura. *J. Immunol. 127:*621, 1981.

601. Lauria, F., et al.: Tγ cell deficiency in idiopathic thrombocytopenic purpura (ITP). *Scand. J. Haematol. 26:*146, 1981.

602. Goebel, K. M., Hahn, E., and Havemann, K.: HLA matching in autoimmune thrombocytopenic purpura. *Br. J. Haematol. 35:*341, 1977.

603. Mueller-Eckhardt, C., Myr, W., Lechner, K., Muller-Eckhardt, G., Niessner, H., and Pralle, H.: HLA antigens in immunologic thrombocytopenic purpura. *Scand. J. Haematol. 23:*348, 1979.

604. Veenhoven, W. A., Kaars Sijpesteijn, J. A., and van der Schans, G. S.: HLA antigens in idiopathic thrombocytopenic purpura. *Acta Haematol. 62:*153, 1979.

605. Majsky, A., and Fortynova, J.: HLA and idiopathic thrombocytopenic purpura (ITP) *Tissue Antigens 15:*222, 1980.

606. Mayr, W. R., Mueller-Eckhardt, G., Kruger, M., Mueller-Eckhardt, C., Lechner, K., and Niessner, H.: HLA-DR in chronic idiopathic thrombocytopenic purpura (ITP). *Tissue Antigens 18:*56, 1981.

607. Karpatkin, S., Fotino, M., and Winchester, R.: Hereditary autoimmune thrombocytopenic purpura: An immunologic and genetic study. *Ann. Intern. Med. 94:*781, 1981.

608. Stuart, M. J., Tomar, R. H., Miller, M. L., and Davey, F. R.: Chronic idiopathic thrombocytopenic purpura: A familial immunodeficiency syndrome? *JAMA 239:*939, 1978.

609. Kaznelson, P.: Verschwinden die Hamorrhagischen Diathese bei einem Falle von essentielle Thrombopenie (Frank) nach Mil extirpation. *Wien. Klin. Wochenschr. 29:*145, 1919.

610. Kernoff, L. M., Blake, C. H., and Shackleton, D.: Influence of the amount of platelet-bound IgG on platelet survival and site of sequestration in autoimmune thrombocytopenia. *Blood 55:*730, 1980.

611. Aster, R. H., and Jandl, J. H.: Platelet sequestration in man. II. Immunological and clinical studies. *J. Clin. Invest. 43:*856, 1964.

612. McMillan, R., Longmire, R. L., Xelenosky, R., Donnel, R. L., and Armstrong, S.: Quantitation of platelet-binding IgG produced in vitro by spleens from patients with idiopathic thrombocytopenic purpura. *N. Engl. J. Med. 291:*812, 1974.

613. Karpatkin, S., Struck, N., and Siskind, G. W.: Detection of splenic anti-platelet antibody synthesis in idiopathic autoimmune thrombocytopenic purpura (ATP). *Br. J. Haematol. 23:*167, 1972.

614. McMillan, R., Yelenosky, R. J., and Longmire, R. L.: Antiplatelet antibody production by the spleen and bone marrow in immune thrombocytopenic purpura. *Immunoaspects of the Spleen*, edited by J. R. Battisto and J. W. Streilein. North-Holland, Amsterdam, 1976, p. 227.

615. Laros, R. K., and Sweet, R. L.: Management of idiopathic thrombocytopenic purpura during pregnancy. *Am. J. Obstet. Gynecol. 122:*182, 1975.

616. Moore, A., Weksler, B. B., and Nachman, R. L.: Platelet Fc IgG receptor: Increased expression in female patients. *Thromb. Res. 21:*469, 1981.

617. Brent, L. H.: Sarcoidosis with thrombocytopenia. *Del. Med. J. 51:*341, 1979.

618. Knodel, A. R., and Beekman, J. F.: Severe thrombocytopenia and sarcoidosis. *JAMA 243:*258, 1980.

619. Kaden, B. R., Rosse, W. F., and Hauch, T. W.: Immune thrombocytopenia in lymphoproliferative diseases. *Blood 53:*545, 1979.

620. Waddell, C. C., and Cimo, P. L.: Idiopathic thrombocytopenic purpura occurring in Hodgkin disease after splenectomy: Report of two cases and review of the literature. *Am. J. Hematol. 7:*381, 1979.

621. Kirshner, J. J., Zamkoff, K. W., and Gottlieb, A. J.: Idiopathic thrombocytopenic purpura and Hodgkin's disease: Report of two cases and a review of the literature. *Am. J. Med. Sci. 280:*21, 1980.

622. Budman, D. R., and Steinberg, A. D.: Hematologic aspects of systemic lupus erythematosus: Current concepts. *Ann. Intern. Med. 86:*220, 1977.

623. Herman, J., Resnitzky, P., and Fink, A.: Association between thyroxicosis and thrombocytopenia. *Isr. J. Med. Sci. 14:*469, 1978.

624. Kurata, Y., Nishioed, Y., Tsubakio, T., and Kitani, T.: Thrombocytopenia in Graves' disease: Effect of T3 on platelet kinetics. *Acta Haematol. 63:*185, 1980.

625. Hymes, K., Blum, M., Lackner, H., and Karpatkin, S.: Easy bruising, thrombocytopenia, and elevated platelet immunoglobulin G in Graves' disease and Hashimoto's thyroiditis. *Ann. Intern. Med. 94:*27, 1981.

626. Armitage, J. O., and Sheets, R. F.: Idiopathic thrombocytopenic purpura in patients with histoplasmosis. *JAMA 21:*2323, 1977.

627. Neucks, S. H., Moore, T. L., Lichtenstein, J. R., Baldassare, R., Weiss, T. D., and Zuckner, J.: Localized scleroderma and idiopathic thrombocytopenia. *J. Rheumatol. 7:*741, 1980.

628. Kim, H. D., and Boggs, D. R.: A syndrome resembling idiopathic thrombocytopenic purpura in 10 patients with diverse forms of cancer. *Am. J. Med. 67:*371, 1979.

629. Veenhoven, W. A., Oosterhuis, H. J., and van der Schans, G. S.: Myasthenia gravis and Werlhof's disease. *Acta Med. Scand. 206:*131, 1979.

630. Pui, C. H., Wilimas, J., and Wang, W.: Evans syndrome in childhood. *J. Pediatr. 97:*754, 1980.

631. Torres, A., Lucia, J. F., Oliveros, A., and Vazquez, C.: Anti-factor IX circulating anticoagulant and immune thrombocytopenia in a case of Takayasu's arteritis. *Acta Haematol. 64:*338, 1980.

632. Linker, C. A., Newcom, S. R., Nilsson, C. M., Wolf, J. L., and Shuman, M. A.: Combined idiopathic neutropenia and thrombocytopenia: Evidence for an immune basis for the syndrome. *Ann. Intern. Med. 93:*704, 1980.

633. Khan, I., Zucker-Franklin, D., and Karpatkin, S.: Microthrombocytosis and platelet fragmentation associated with idiopathic/autoimmune thrombocytopenic purpura. *Br. J. Haematol. 31:*449, 1975.

634. Oski, F. A., Naiman, J. L., and Diamond, L. K.: Use of the plasma acid phosphatase volume in the differentiation of thrombocytopenic states. *N. Engl. J. Med. 273:*845, 1965.

635. White, L. A., Jr., Brubaker, L. H., Aster, R. H., Henry, P. H., and Adelstein, E. H.: Platelet satellitism and phagocytosis by neutrophils: Association with antiplatelet antibodies and lymphoma. *Am. J. Hematol. 4:*313, 1978.

636. Clancy, R., Jenkins, E., and Firkin, B.: Qualitative platelet abnormalities in idiopathic thrombocytopenic purpura. *N. Engl. J. Med. 286:*622, 1972.

637. Heyns, A. DuP., Fraser, J., and Retief, F. P.: Platelet aggregation in chronic idiopathic thrombocytopenic purpura. *J. Clin. Pathol. 31:*1239, 1978.

638. Weiss, H. J., Rosove, M. H., Lages, B. A., and Kaplan, K. L.: Acquired storage pool deficiency with increased platelet-associated IgG: Report of five cases. *Am. J. Med. 69:*711, 1980.

639. Dixon, R., Rosse, W., and Ebber, L.: Quantitative determination of antibody in idiopathic thrombocytopenic purpura. *N. Engl. J. Med. 292:*230, 1975.

640. Hegde, U. M., Gordon-Smith, E. C., and Worlledge, S.: Platelet antibodies in thrombocytopenic patients. *Br. J. Haematol. 35:*113, 1977.

641. Kelton, J. G., Giles, A. R., Neame, P. B., Powers, P., Hageman, N., and Hirsh, J.: Comparison of two direct assays for platelet-associated IgG (PAIgG) in assessment of immune and nonimmune thrombocytopenia. *Blood 55:*424, 1980.

642. McMillan, R., Luiken, G. A., Levey, R., Yelenosky, R., and Longmire, R. L.: Antibody against megarkaryocytes in idiopathic thrombocytopenic purpura. *JAMA 239:*2460, 1978.

643. Tavassoli, M., and McMillan, R.: Structure of the spleen in idiopathic thrombocytopenic purpura. *Am. J. Clin. Pathol. 64:*180, 1975.

644. Luk, S. C., Musclow, E., and Simon, G. T.: Platelet phagocytosis in the spleen of patients with idiopathic thrombocytopenic purpura (ITP). *Histopathology 4:*127, 1980.

645. Breckenridge, R. T., Moore, R. D., and Ratnoff, O. D.: A study of thrombocytopenia: New histologic criteria for the differentiation of idiopathic thrombocytopenia and thrombocytopenia associated with disseminated lupus erythematosus. *Blood 30:*39, 1967.

646. Salzstein, S. L.: Phospholipid accumulation in histiocytes of splenic pulp associated with thrombocytopenic purpura. *Blood 18:*73, 1961.

647. King, F. M., and Harsock, R. J.: Histochemical identification of lipid in spleens of patients with idiopathic thrombocytopenic purpura. *Am. J. Clin. Pathol. 49:*250, 1968.

648. Takahashi, K., Hakozaki, H., Terashima, K., and Kojima, M.: Two distinctive types of lipid histiocytes appearing in the spleen of idiopathic thrombocytopenic purpura: Sea-blue histiocyte and foam cell. *Acta Pathol. Jpn. 27:*447, 1977.

649. Lacey, J. V., and Penner, J. A.: Management of idiopathic thrombocytopenic purpura in the adult. *Semin. Thromb. Hemostas. 3:*160, 1977.

650. Ikkala, E., Kivilaakso, E., Kotilainen, M., and Hastbacka, J.: Treatment of idiopathic thrombocytopenic purpura in adults: Long-term results in a series of 41 patients. *Ann. Clin. Res. 10:*83, 1978.

651. Picozzi, V. J., Roeske, W. R., and Creger, W. P.: Rate of therapy failures in adult idiopathic thrombocytopenic purpura. *Am. J. Med. 69:*690, 1980.

652. Abraham, J., and Ellman, L.: Platelet transfusion in immune thrombocytopenic purpura. *JAMA 236:*1847, 1976.

653. Shulman, N. R., Weinrach, R. S., Libre, E. P., and Andrews, H. L.: The role of the reticuloendothelial system in the pathogenesis of idiopathic thrombocytopenic purpura. *Trans. Assoc. Am. Physicians 78:*374, 1965.

654. Handin, R. I., and Stossel, T. P.: Effect of corticosteroid therapy on the phagocytosis of antibody-coated platelets by human leukocytes. *Blood 51:*771, 1978.

655. Weisberger, A. S., and Suhrland, L. G.: Massive corticosteroid therapy in the management of resistant thrombocytopenic purpura. *Am. J. Med. Sci. 236:*425, 1958.

656. Finch, S. C., Castro, O., Cooper, M., Covery, W., Erickson, R., and McPhedran, P.: Immunosuppressive therapy of chronic idiopathic thrombocytopenic purpura. *Am. J. Med. 56:*4, 1974.

657. MacPherson, A. I. S., and Richmond, J.: Planned splenectomy in ITP. *Br. Med. J. 1:*64, 1975.

658. Brennan, M. F., Rappeport, J. M., Maloney, W. C., and Wilson, R. E.: Correlation between response to corticosteroids and splenectomy for adult idiopathic thrombocytopenic purpura. *Am. J. Surg. 129:*490, 1975.

659. Branehog, I.: Platelet kinetics in idiopathic thrombocytopenic purpura (ITP) before and at different times after splenectomy. *Br. J. Haematol. 29:*413, 1975.

660. Burger, T., Schmelczer, M., Kett, K., and Kutas, J.: Immune thrombocytolytic purpura (ITP): Diagnosis and therapeutic survey of 86 cases with regard to the results of splenectomy and conservative therapy. *Acta Med. Acad. Sci. Hung. 35:*213, 1978.

661. Thompson, R. L., Moore, R. A., Hess, C. E., Wheby, M. S., and Leavell, B. S.: Idiopathic thrombocytopenic purpura: Long-term results of treatment and the prognostic significance of response to corticosteroids. *Arch. Intern. Med. 130:*730, 1972.

662. Carpenter, A. F., Wintrobe, M. M., Fuller, E. A., Haut, A., and Cartwright, G. E.: Treatment of idiopathic thrombocytopenic purpura. *JAMA 171:*1911, 1959.

663. Nejean, Y., and Ardaillou, N.: The sequestration site of platelets in idiopathic thrombocytopenic purpura: Its correlation with the results of splenectomy. *Br. J. Haematol. 21:*153, 1971.

664. Viala, J. J., Dechevanne, M., and Ville, D.: Les Épreuves radioisotopiques sont les meilleures indications de la splenectomie au cours de purpura thrombopenie idiopathiques chroniques? À propos de 50 observations. *Lyon Med. 234:*419, 1975.

665. Ries, C. A.: Platelet kinetics of autoimmune thrombocytopenia: Relationship between splenic platelet sequestration and response to splenectomy. *Ann. Intern. Med. 86:*194, 1977.

666. Richards, J. D. M., and Thompson, D. S.: Assessment of thrombocytopenic patients for splenectomy. *J. Clin. Pathol. 32:*1248, 1979.

667. Best, W. R., and Darling, D. R.: A critical look at the splenectomy-S.L.E. controversy. *Med. Clin. North. Am. 46:*19, 1962.

668. Homan, W. P., and Dineen, P.: The role of splenectomy in the treatment of thrombocytopenic purpura due to systemic lupus erythematosus. *Ann. Surg. 187:*52, 1978.

669. Verheyden, C. N., Beart, R. W., Jr., Clifton, M. D., and Phyliky, R. L.: Accessory splenectomy in management of recurrent idiopathic thrombocytopenic purpura. *Mayo Clin. Proc. 53:*442, 1978.

670. Davis, H. H., II., Varki, A., Andrew Heaton, A., and Siegel, B. A.: Detection of accessory spleens with indium [111]-labeled autologous platelets. *Am. J. Hematol. 8:*81, 1980.

671. Verlin, M., Laros, R. K., Jr., and Penner, J. A.: Treatment of refractory thrombocytopenic purpura with cyclophosphamide. *Am. J. Hematol. 1:*97, 1976.

672. Ahn, Y. S., Harrington, W. J., Seelman, R. C., and Eytel, C. S.: Vincristine therapy of idiopathic and secondary thrombocytopenias. *N. Engl. J. Med. 291:*376, 1974.

673. Ries, C. A.: Vincristine for treatment of refractory autoimmune thrombocytopenia. *N. Engl. J. Med. 295:*1136, 1976.

674. Ghosh, M. I.: Long-term effect of vincristine in chronic idiopathic thrombocytopenic purpura (ITP). *J. Ir. Med. Assoc. 69:*167, 1976.

675. Robertson, J. F., Crozier, E. F., and Woodend, B. E.: Vincristine therapy of thrombocytopenias. *N. Engl. J. Med. 292:*108, 1975.

676. Ahn, Y. S., et al.: The treatment of idiopathic thrombocytopenia with vinblastine-loaded platelets. *N. Engl. J. Med. 298:*1101, 1978.

677. Nenci, G. G., Agnelli, G., Decunto, M., and Gresele, P.: Infusion of vincristine-loaded platelets in acute ITP refractory to steroids: An alternative to splenectomy. *Acta Haematol.* 66:117, 1981.

678. Kelton, J. G., et al.: The reversible binding of vinblastine to platelets: Implications for therapy. *Blood* 57:431, 1981.

679. Branda, R. F., Tate, D. Y., McCullough, J. J., and Jacob, H. S.: Plasma exchange in the treatment of fulminant idiopathic (autoimmune) thrombocytopenic purpura. *Lancet* 1:688, 1978.

680. Patten, E., and Reuter, F. P.: Evans' syndrome: Possible benefits from plasma exchange. *Transfusion* 20:589, 1980.

681. Marder, V. J., Nusbacher, J., and Anderson, F. W.: One-year follow-up of plasma exchange therapy in 14 patients with idiopathic thrombocytopenic purpura. *Transfusion* 21:291, 1981.

682. Weir, A. B., Poon, M. C., and McGowan, E. I.: Plasma-exchange in idiopathic thrombocytopenic purpura. *Arch. Intern. Med.* 140:1101, 1980 (technical note).

683. Schmidt, R. E., Budde, U., Schafer, G., and Stroehmann, I.: High-dose intravenous gammaglobulin for idiopathic thrombocytopenic purpura. *Lancet* 2:475, 1981.

684. Jones, R. W., Innes Asher, M., Rutherford, C. J., and Munro, H. M.: Autoimmune (idiopathic) thrombocytopenic purpura in pregnancy and the newborn. *Br. J. Obstet. Gynaecol.* 84:679, 1977.

685. Arias-Rodriguez, M., et al.: Renal transplantation and immunological abnormalities in thrombotic microangiopathy of adults. *Transplantation* 23:360, 1977.

686. Redman, C. W. G., Bonnar, J., and Beilin, L.: Early platelet consumption in pre-eclampsia. *Br. Med. J.* 1:467, 1978.

687. Bern, M. M., Driscoll, S. G., and Leavitt, T., Jr.: Thrombocytopenia complicating preeclampsia: Data to support a new model. *Obstet. Gynecol.* 57:28, 1981.

688. Ansell, J., McCue, J., Tiarks, C., Parrilla, N., Rybak, M. E., and Benotti, J.: Amrinone-induced thrombocytopenia. *Blood* 58 (Suppl. 1):187a, 1981.

689. Heuserman, U., and Stutte, H. J.: Zur Atiologie der Thrombozytopenia bei der Vinylchlorid-Krankheit. *Blut* 34:317, 1977.

690. Much, T., and Wuthrich, B.: Erfahrungen mit dem Thrombozytopenietest in der spezifischen Diagnostik der Nahrungsmittel-Allergie. *Schweiz. Med. Wochenschr.* 107:267, 1977.

691. Seidenfeld, A. M., Owen, J., and Glynn, M. F. X.: Posttransfusion purpura cured by steroid therapy in a man. *Can. Med. Assoc. J.* 118:1285, 1978 (technical note).

CHAPTER *143*

Thrombocytopenia due to sequestration of platelets

RICHARD H. ASTER

Thrombocytopenia due to hypersplenism

It has long been known that splenomegaly of diverse etiology may result in pancytopenia. As discussed in Chap. 71, the resulting condition is usually referred to as hypersplenism. While thrombocytopenia due to hypersplenism is rarely severe, its pathogenesis has been of considerable interest because of its relevance to possible control of platelet production by the spleen (Chap. 130).

ETIOLOGY AND PATHOGENESIS

As previously summarized (Chap. 130), controversy raged for years over whether thrombocytopenia of hypersplenism is caused by suppression of the marrow by some humoral factor produced in the spleen or by premature destruction of platelets in the enlarged organ. The finding that the survival time of platelets is normal or only slightly reduced in patients with hypersplenism [1] was consistent with the former view. Studies using ^{51}Cr-labeled platelets, however, strongly support a third alternative: that thrombocytopenia is caused primarily by pooling of a large fraction (up to 90 percent) of the total platelet mass within the spleen itself. This process appears to be an exaggeration of the normal state, in which approximately one-third of the platelet mass is held within the spleen at any given time [2]. Thrombocytopenia resulting from the splenic pooling should not be confused with that which occurs in conditions such as idiopathic thrombocytopenia (Chap. 142), in which platelets are permanently destroyed in the spleen rather than merely being delayed in their transit through the enlarged organ.

Evidence supporting the concept of splenic pooling of platelets is abundant: (1) The percentage of ^{51}Cr-labeled platelets that can be recovered in the peripheral circulation after their transfusion to patients with hypersplenism is very low, ranging from 10 to 30 percent, in contrast to values of 60 to 75 percent and 90 to 100 percent obtained in normal and asplenic subjects, respectively [2,3]. (2) Epinephrine, injected intravenously, causes a pronounced rise in platelet levels in hypersplenic subjects, a moderate increase in normal subjects, and little change in persons who lack a spleen [2,4]. (3) Large quantities of platelets, three to seven times the number present in the general circulation, can be flushed from enlarged spleens removed at operation [2,5]. (4) A comparable disorder in which thrombocytopenia is caused by splenic pooling can be induced in animals by injection of methylcellulose [6]. The rise in platelet levels following injection of epinephrine appears to result from stimulation of α-adrenergic receptors; stimulation of β-receptors causes a reduction in blood platelet counts [7]. Conversely, β-adrenergic blockade causes a significant rise in platelet levels [7]. A small increase in circulating platelets occurs after administration of epinephrine to asplenic subjects, suggesting that there is also a mobilizable platelet pool of nonsplenic origin [8,9].

Splenic pooling of platelets appears to be brought on by the very slow passage of platelets through the spleen [2,10]. Whether this is a result of a "sieving" effect which causes platelets, because of their small size, to take a tortuous course through the sinuous channels of the spleen, of cohesion between platelets and splenic macrophages and endothelial cells, as suggested by electron micrographic studies [11,12], or of some other mechanism has not been determined with certainty. It has been suggested that newly formed platelets [13] and megathrombocytes [14] pool preferentially in the spleen.

CLINICAL AND LABORATORY FEATURES

Clinical findings usually relate to the primary disorder. The most common cause of "hypersplenic" thrombocytopenia is liver disease with portal hypertension and congestive splenomegaly. Thrombocytopenia observed in 5 percent of 395 patients with heart failure was thought to be a consequence of congestive splenomegaly [15]. Gaucher disease [16], lymphomatous disorders [17], sickle cell disease in children, sarcoidosis, kala-azar, myelofibrosis, splenic torsion [18], tuberculosis, and hamartoma [19] of the spleen have also been reported to cause "hypersplenism" [20,21]. In some of these disorders, factors unrelated to the spleen, such as marrow infiltration, should also be considered as possible causes of thrombocytopenia.

In the writer's experience, the spleen must be sufficiently enlarged to be easily palpable in order for pooling to be the cause of thrombocytopenia. Generally speaking, thrombocytopenia is most severe in patients whose spleens are largest [2,22], but there are many exceptions, perhaps related to variations in the ability to compensate for the thrombocytopenia by increasing platelet production. Even in patients with the largest spleens, platelet levels rarely, if ever, fall below 20,000 per microliter on the basis of splenic pooling alone. In most instances, platelet counts range from 50,000 to 100,000 per microliter. Megakaryocytes are usually plentiful but may appear slightly immature.

Occasionally platelet survival studies are helpful in confirming the diagnosis of hypersplenism and ruling out a disorder of platelet destruction such as idiopathic thrombocytopenic purpura (ITP). As shown in Fig.131-2, the curve of platelet survival in patients with "hypersplenic" thrombocytopenia is quite distinctive and contrasts markedly with that obtained in normal subjects and in patients with ITP. The finding of megathrombocytes in ITP and much smaller platelets in hypersplenism may also aid in differential diagnosis [14].

TREATMENT AND PROGNOSIS

As thrombocytopenia from splenic pooling is rarely severe enough to produce a hemorrhagic diathesis in itself, splenectomy is rarely indicated for this cause alone. When the spleen is removed, however, platelet levels are almost invariably restored to normal [23]. Marked thrombocytosis sometimes follows the removal of very large spleens [2,17]. Following portocaval anastomosis, platelet levels increase to normal in more than half the cases, but, curiously, the rise is unrelated to the resulting change in portal pressure [24]. Irradiation of the spleen is occasionally helpful in patients with lymphomatous disorders but not in other conditions [25]. Partial ablation of the spleen by ligation of the splenic artery [26] or induction of splenic artery embolism [27] may ameliorate hematologic abnormalities of hypersplenism. Benefits of the former procedure may be transient, however, [26], and the latter therapy is associated with significant hazard [28].

Thrombocytopenia associated with hypothermia

Thrombocytopenia, usually transient, sometimes very severe, occurs both in animals [29] and in humans [30,31] during induced hypothermia, and it has been implicated as a cause of the hemorrhagic diathesis which sometimes follows restoration of normal body temperature following surgical hypothermia [31]. Body temperatures below 25°C are required to lower platelet levels in both dogs and humans [29–32]. The reduction in platelet levels is much less severe in patients given heparin than in those who receive no anticoagulant [30].

In dogs whose platelets were labeled with ^{32}P before induction of hypothermia, nearly all the tagged platelets returned to the circulation when normal body temperature was restored, demonstrating that thrombocytopenia was a result of temporary sequestration rather than permanent destruction of platelets [29]. Most of the sequestration was thought to occur in the liver and spleen, but a significant amount occurred at other sites [29]. The liver was thought to be the primary site of sequestration in another study [33]. Accumulation of platelets in the splenic cords has been observed in hibernating, hypothermic ground squirrels [34].

Reduction of platelet levels under hypothermic conditions may be caused by increased adhesiveness and a tendency to clump, which can readily be demonstrated when platelets are chilled in vitro [35]. This appears to be harmless in most instances, but in one study platelet aggregates were thought to be a cause of brain damage in children who had been operated on under deep hypothermia (10 to 16°C), even though heparin was given during the procedure [31].

Thrombocytopenia associated with massive trauma and venous stasis

A modest reduction in platelet levels has been observed in dogs subjected to experimental soft-tissue trauma, apparently because of the trapping of platelet aggregates in the lung [36]. This trapping is reduced when the lung is denervated by autotransplantation [37]. The extent to which such trapping occurs in humans is not known. Prolonged occlusion of the venous return of an extremity in humans causes a marked lowering of the platelet level, in the affected limb, which is reversed when the stasis is relieved [38].

References

1. Cohen, P., Gardner, F. H., and Barnett, G. O.: Reclassification of the thrombocytopenias by the ^{51}Cr-labeled method for measuring platelet lifespan. N. Engl. J. Med. 265:1294, 1961.
2. Aster, R. H.: Pooling of platelets in the spleen: Role in the pathogenesis of "hypersplenic" thrombocytopenia. J. Clin. Invest. 45:645, 1964.

3. Toghill, P. J., Green, S., and Ferguson, R.: Platelet dynamics in chronic liver disease with special reference to the role of the spleen. *J. Clin. Pathol.* 30:367, 1977.

4. Libre, E. P., Cowan, D. H., Watkins, S. P., and Shulman, N. R.: Relationships between spleen, platelets, and factor VIII levels. *Blood* 31:358, 1968.

5. Penny, R., Rozenberg, M. C., and Firkin, B. G.: The splenic platelet pool. *Blood* 27:1, 1966.

6. Aster, R. H.: Studies of the mechanism of "hypersplenic" thrombocytopenia in rats. *J. Lab. Clin. Med.* 70:736, 1967.

7. Freden, K., Vilen, L., Lundborg, P., Olsson L.-B., and Kutti, J.: The peripheral platelet count and the isoprenaline-induced splenic platelet pooling in response to beta-adrenoceptor blockade. *Scand. J. Haematol.* 23:245, 1979.

8. Freedman, M., Altszuler, N., and Karpatkin, S.: Presence of a nonsplenic platelet pool. *Blood* 50:419, 1977.

9. Vilen, L., Freden, K., and Kutti, J.: Presence of a nonsplenic platelet pool in man. *Scand. J. Haematol.* 24:137, 1980.

10. Peters, A. M., Klonizakis, I., Lavender, J. P., and Lewis, S. M.: Use of ^{111}Indium-labelled platelets to measure spleen function. *Br. J. Haematol.* 46:587, 1980.

11. Weiss, L.: A scanning electron micrographic study of the spleen. *Blood* 43:665, 1974.

12. Olgjo, R. F.: Platelets, endothelial cells and macrophages in the spleen: An ultrastructural study on perfusion-fixed organs. *Am. J. Anat.* 145:101, 1976.

13. Shulman, N. R., Watkins, S. P. Jr., Iscoitz, S. B., and Students, A. B.: Evidence that the spleen retains the youngest and hemostatically most effective platelets. *Trans. Assoc. Am. Physicians* 81:302, 1968.

14. Karpatkin, S., and Freedman, L.: Hypersplenic thrombocytopenia differentiated from increased peripheral destruction by platelet volume. *Ann. Intern. Med.* 89:200, 1978.

15. Heck, J., Keitel, K., Wusthoff, D., and Gehrmann, G.: Haufigkeit und Pathogenese einer Thrombozytopenie bei Herzinsuffizienz. *Dtsch. Med. Wochenschr.* 101:1381, 1976.

16. Medoff, A. S., and Bayrd, E. D.: Gaucher's disease in 29 cases: Hematologic complications and effect of splenectomy. *Ann. Intern. Med.* 40:481, 1954.

17. Abrahamsen, A. F.: Effects of an enlarged spleen platelet pool in Hodgkin's disease. *Scand. J. Haematol.* 9:153, 1972.

18. Weinreb, N. J., Bauer, J., Dikman, S., and Forte, F. A.: Torsion of the spleen as a cause of hypersplenism. *JAMA* 230:1015, 1974.

19. Ross, C. F., and Schiller, K. F. R.: Hamartoma of spleen associated with thrombocytopenia. *J. Pathol.* 105:62, 1970.

20. Amorosi, E. L.: Hypersplenism. *Semin. Hematol.* 2:249, 1965.

21. Cooney, D. P., and Smith, B. A.: The pathophysiology of hypersplenic thrombocytopenia. *Arch. Inter. Med.* 121:332, 1968.

22. Kutti, J., Weinfeld, W., and Westin, J.: The relationship between splenic platelet pool and spleen size. *Scand. J. Haematol.* 9:351, 1972.

23. Nordoy, A., and Neset, G.: Splenectomy in hematologic diseases. *Acta Med. Scand.* 183:117, 1968.

24. Sullivan, B. H. Jr., and Tumen, H. J.: The effect of portacaval shunt on thrombocytopenia associated with portal hypertension. *Ann. Intern. Med.* 55:598, 1961.

25. Comas, F. V., Andrews, G. A., and Nelson, B.: Splenic irradiation in secondary hypersplenism. *Am. J. Roentgenol.* 104:668, 1968.

26. Witte, C. L., et al.: Circulatory control of splenic hyperfunction in children with peripheral blood dyscrasia. *Surgery* 150:75, 1980.

27. Shaikh, B. S., Nicholas, G. G., and Miller, F. J.: Splenic embolization in hypersplenic thrombocytopenia. *Ann. Intern. Med.* 86:446, 1977.

28. Witte, C. L., et al.: Ischemic therapy in thrombocytopenia from hypersplenism. *Arch. Surg.* 111:1115, 1976.

29. Villalobos, T. J., Adelson, E., Riley, P. A., and Crosby, W. H.: A cause of thrombocytopenia and leukopenia that occurs in dogs during deep hypothermia. *J. Clin. Invest.* 37:1, 1958.

30. Wensel, R. H., and Bigelow, W. G.: The use of heparin to minimize thrombocytopenia and bleeding tendencies during hypothermia. *Surgery* 45:223, 1959.

31. Bjork, V. O., and Hultquist, G.: Brain damage in children after deep hypothermia for open heart surgery. *Thorax* 15:284, 1969.

32. Bunker, J. P., and Goldstein, R.: Coagulation during hypothermia in man. *Proc. Soc. Exp. Biol. Med.* 97:199, 1958.

33. Pina-Cabral, J. M., Amaral, I., Pinto, M. M., and Guerra e Paz, L. H.: Hepatic and splenic platelet sequestration during deep hypothermia in the dog. *Haemostasis* 2:235, 1974.

34. Reddick, R. L., Poole, B. L., and Penick, G. D.: Thrombocytopenia of hibernation: Mechanism of induction and recovery. *Lab. Invest.* 28:270, 1973.

35. Zucker, M. B., and Borrelli, J.: Viscous metamorphosis produced by chilling and by clotting: Failure to find specific defect of viscous metamorphosis in PTA syndrome. *Thromb. Daith. Haemorrh.* 4:424, 1960.

36. Peer, R. M., and Schwartz, S. I.: Development and treatment of post-traumatic pulmonary platelet trapping. *Ann. Surg.* 181:447, 1975.

37. Thorne, L. J., Kuenzig, M., McDonald, H. M., and Schwartz, S. I.: Effect of denervation of a lung on pulmonary platelet trapping associated with traumatic shock. *Surgery* 88:208, 1980.

38. Hladovec, J., Koleilat, Z., and Prebovsky, I: The effect of venous occlusion on the sequestration of blood platelets. *Thromb. Diath. Haemorrh.* 28:383, 1972.

CHAPTER *144*

Thrombocytopenia due to platelet loss

RICHARD H. ASTER

Thrombocytopenia associated with hemorrhage and multiple blood transfusions

Although hemorrhage per se does not cause thrombocytopenia, a reduction in platelet levels may result when the blood lost is replaced by large quantities of stored blood [1–3]. A similar phenomenon may be seen in children who receive exchange transfusions for treatment of erythroblastosis fetalis [4]. The degree of thrombocytopenia is directly related to the number of transfusions given (Fig. 144-1) and occurs regularly in patients who receive 14 or more units of stored bank blood [2,3,5]. It frequently persists for 3 to 5 days.

Thrombocytopenia under these circumstances is caused by replacement of viable platelets lost during hemorrhage with nonviable platelets present in stored blood [5], coupled with the limited ability of the marrow to increase platelet production acutely (Chap. 130). Persistence of thrombocytopenia for several days is presumably a result of "exhaustion" of megakaryocytes.

The development of severe thrombocytopenia in patients receiving massive transfusion therapy can be prevented by administration of an appropriate number of platelet concentrates after each 10 to 12 units of stored blood. However, factors other than thrombocytopenia may be responsible for a bleeding diathesis in patients who receive multiple transfusions [6].

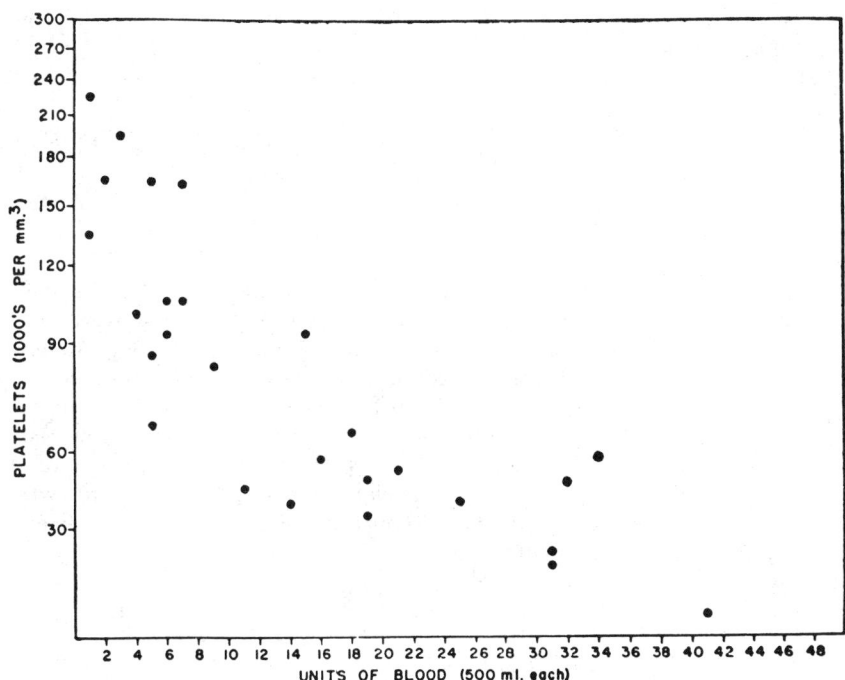

FIGURE 144-1   Platelet levels of 37 patients in whom massive blood loss was treated by infusion of stored blood containing few viable platelets. (Krevans and Jackson [1].)

Thrombocytopenia associated with extracorporeal perfusion

A progressive reduction in platelet levels to about 50 percent of preoperative values occurs in patients who undergo surgery assisted by extracorporeal perfusion [7–12] (Fig. 144-2). The degree of thrombocytopenia is independent of whether "platelet-rich" blood is used in the perfusate [13] or platelet concentrates are transfused during the procedure [14]. Occasionally it is very severe and contributes to the hemorrhagic diathesis which sometimes occurs after perfusion. In such patients, platelet levels usually remain low for 3 to 5 days, and an average of 7 days is required before normal levels are restored.

It is generally assumed that the reduction in platelet levels is caused by damage suffered by platelets in the perfusion apparatus, possibly the result of their attempt to interact with a foreign surface. Adenosine diphosphate released from hemolyzed red blood cells and "consumption" of platelets in coagulation may also be of importance. These effects combine to cause platelets to form microaggregates, which are cleared by the filters of the perfusion apparatus and by the lung [15]. Systems with membrane oxygenators may be less prone than those with bubble oxygenators to provoke microaggregate formation [9,15]. Functional abnormalities characterized by decreased adhesiveness and aggregability may reduce the hemostatic effectiveness of platelets that survive the perfusion procedure [16–18]. This may be related to preferential removal of the youngest, most

active platelets [18]. In some instances, thrombocytopenia may be aggravated by protamine injected postoperatively to neutralize heparin [19].

Platelet levels can readily be elevated by transfusing platelet concentrates to patients who bleed following extracorporeal perfusion. Use of prostaglandin E_1 [20] or prostacyclin [21] in the perfusate may ameliorate or prevent thrombocytopenia altogether. It is important to

FIGURE 144-2   Distribution of platelet counts in patients undergoing open heart surgery with cardiopulmonary bypass. About half the patients were transfused with platelets during the procedure, but their platelet levels did not differ significantly from those of the nontransfused group. (POD = postoperative days.) (Harding, Shakoor, and Grindon [14].)

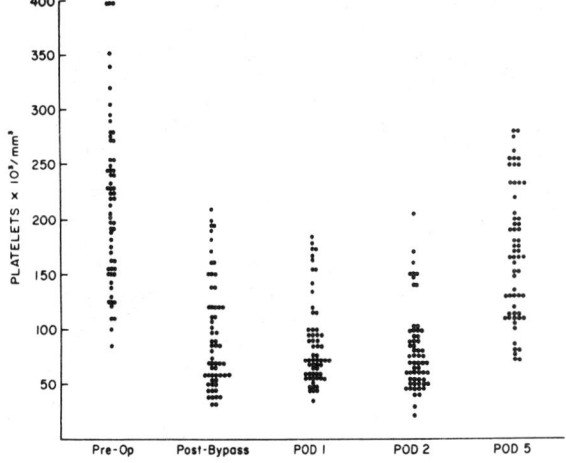

note that many factors other than thrombocytopenia may contribute to the bleeding diathesis which sometimes follows open-heart surgery [8,10,12].

References

1. Krevans, J. R., and Jackson, D. P.: Hemorrhagic disorder following massive whole blood transfusions. *JAMA 159:*171, 1955.
2. Collins, J. A.: Problems associated with the massive transfusion of stored blood. *Surgery 75:*274, 1974.
3. Counts, R. B., et al.: Hemostasis in massively transfused trauma patients. *Ann. Surg. 190:*91, 1979.
4. DesForges, J. F., and O'Connell, L. G.: Hematologic observations of the course of erythroblastosis fetalis. *Blood 10:*302, 1955.
5. Jackson, D. P., Krevans, J. R., and Conley, C. L.: Mechanism of the thrombocytopenia that follows multiple whole blood transfusions. *Trans. Assoc. Am. Physicians 69:*155, 1956.
6. Zucker, M. B., et al.: Generalized excessive oozing in patients undergoing major surgery and receiving multiple blood transfusions. *J. Lab. Clin. Med. 50:*849, 1957.
7. Schmidt, P. J., Peden, J. C. Jr., Brecher, G., and Baranovsky, A.: Thrombocytopenia and bleeding tendency after extracorporeal circulation. *N. Engl. J. Med. 265:*1181, 1961.
8. Pike, O. M., Marquiss, J. E., Weiner, R. S., and Breckenridge, R. T.: A study of platelet counts during cardiopulmonary bypass. *Transfusion 12:*119, 1972.
9. Wandall, H. H., and Silvertson, U.: The puzzle of blood platelets in extracorporeal circulation. *Scand. J. Thorac. Cardiovasc. Surg. 9:*140, 1975.
10. Douglas, A. S., McNicol, G. P., Bain, W. H., and Mackey, W. A.: The haemostatic defect following extracorporeal circulation. *Br. J. Surg. 53:*455, 1966.
11. Bick, R. L.: Alterations of hemostasis associated with cardiopulmonary bypass: Pathophysiology, prevention, diagnosis, and management. *Semin. Thromb. Hemostas. 3:*59, 1976.
12. Harker, L. A., et al.: Mechanism of abnormal bleeding in patients undergoing cardiopulmonary bypass: Acquired transient platelet dysfunction associated with selective α-granule release. *Blood 56:*824, 1980.
13. Grindon, A.J., and Schmidt, P. J.: Platelet-poor blood in open-heart surgery. *N. Engl. J. Med. 280:*1337, 1969.
14. Harding, S. A., Shakoor, M. A., and Grindon, A. J.: Platelet support for cardiopulmonary bypass surgery. *J. Thorac. Cardiovasc. Surg. 70:*350, 1975.
15. Solis, R. T., Kennedy, P. S., Beall, A. C. Jr., Noon, G. P., and DeBakey, M. E.: Cardiopulmonary bypass: Microembolization and platelet aggregation. *Circulation 52:*163, 1975.
16. Salzman, E. W.: Blood platelets and extracorporeal circulation. *Transfusion 3:*274, 1963.
17. McKenna, R., Bachman, F., Wittaker, B., Gilson, J. R., and Weinberg, M., Jr.: The hemostatic mechanism after open-heart surgery. II. Frequency of abnormal platelet functions during and after extracorporeal circulation. *J. Thorac. Cardiovasc. Surg. 70:*298, 1975.
18. Tamari, Y., et al.: Functional changes in platelets during extracorporeal circulation. *Ann. Thorac. Surg. 19:*639, 1975.
19. Heyns, A. duP., et al.: Kinetics and in vivo redistribution of ¹¹¹Indium-labelled human platelets after intravenous protamine sulfate. *Thromb. Haemost. 44:*65, 1980.
20. Addonizio, V. P., Jr., Macarak, E. J., Niewiarowski, S., Colman, R. W., and Edmunds, L. H., Jr.: Preservation of human platelets with prostaglandin E_1 during in vitro simulation of cardiopulmonary bypass. *Circ. Res. 44:*350, 1979.
21. Longmore, D. B., et al.: Prostacyclin: A solution to some problems of extracorporeal circulation. *Lancet 1:*1002, 1979.

CHAPTER 145

Thrombocytosis

WILLIAM J. WILLIAMS

Various physiologic and pathologic states may be associated with elevation of the platelet count above 400,000 per microliter, as listed in Table 145-1 [1–36]. The elevated platelet count in patients with myeloproliferative disorders has been labeled *thrombocythemia* [8] or *autonomous* [7] or *primary thrombocytosis*. The terms *reactive* [7] and *secondary* [4] *thrombocytosis* have been used to describe the platelet count elevation in patients with other diseases. *Thrombocytosis* is used here to denote this latter group.

Pathogenesis

Platelet survival times are normal or somewhat decreased in patients with thrombocytosis resulting from various causes [7,15,37,38]. Platelet production rates are increased, indicating that overproduction is the common mechanism in thrombocytosis [7,15,38]. The thrombocytosis of iron-deficient mice is also due to overproduction [39]. Overproduction may be related to a plasma platelet-stimulating factor (Chap. 130), perhaps produced in response to hemorrhage [40], anemia [19,41], or iron deficiency [42]. Platelet production was stimulated by erythropoietin in some experiments [40,43] but not in others [44,45]. "Rebound" thrombocytosis may also be mediated by a humoral platelet-stimulating factor. Vincristine may cause thrombocytosis by inducing changes in circulating platelets which interfere with their role in regulating thrombopoiesis [46].

Platelet function tests, including aggregation induced by various agents, platelet factor 3 release, and the bleeding time, are usually normal in patients with secondary thrombocytosis but may be abnormal in patients with elevated platelet counts due to myeloproliferative disorders [4,8,20,47].

The thrombotic complications of thrombocytosis appear to arise from increased numbers of platelets, possibly related to marked platelet clumping occurring spontaneously in the blood [48,49] or to increased platelet coagulant activity [50]. If bleeding occurs, it may be due to abnormal platelet coagulant activity [50] or to interference with the coagulation mechanism by the increased number of platelets. It can be shown experimentally that an excessive number of platelets, from either normal or abnormal blood, can interfere with coagulation tests in vitro [51], and this mechanism may operate in vivo as well.

In some cases thrombocytosis may be caused by the release of platelets from storage depots. This appears to be a mechanism of thrombocytosis following administration of epinephrine, where the spleen is probably the source, since the increase in platelet count does not occur in asplenic subjects [27–29]. Others have suggested that the lung is the source of the platelets [52]. Thrombocytosis after exercise is also probably caused by release of platelets, but it appears not to be due to the effect of epinephrine and it does occur in asplenic subjects [31].

Clinical features

Thrombocytosis usually is asymptomatic but may cause thrombosis, usually venous, in a small proportion of cases [e.g., Ref. 19]. There are no data relating the likelihood of complications to the platelet count in patients with thrombocytosis, but levels over 1 million per microliter are generally considered hazardous. Abnormal bleeding is rare in secondary thrombocytosis, in contrast to primary thrombocythemia [8] (see Chap. 26).

Thrombocytosis accompanying the diseases listed in Table 145-1 may persist for prolonged periods of time and disappear with effective therapy of the disease. Thrombocytosis following muscular exercise or epinephrine administration is transient, reaching a peak of up to 50 percent above the baseline in about 15 min and returning to baseline in about 30 min. Thrombocytosis occurring after surgical procedures is preceded by thrombocytopenia at the time of surgery. The platelet count returns to normal in 2 to 6 days and then rises to from 35 to 150 percent above normal. The elevated count slowly returns to normal over a period of 10 to 16 days [22,23]. After splenectomy, the platelet count rises in the first week to levels of up to 1 million or more and then falls slowly to normal over about 2 months [16–19]. Thrombocytosis may persist for prolonged periods after splenectomy [17,19]. In two series, platelet counts between 500,000 and 1,000,000 were found in 40 percent of patients after splenectomy [16,18]. In one of these series, platelet counts exceeding 1 million were found in 13 percent of patients [16].

"Rebound" thrombocytosis usually reaches a peak 10 to 17 days after withdrawal of the offending drug (e.g., alcohol [32] or methotrexate [34,35]) or institution of therapy for thrombocytopenia (e.g., for vitamin B_{12} deficiency [35]). The platelet count may also rise transiently to supernormal levels following prednisone therapy for idiopathic thrombocytopenic purpura [35].

Laboratory features

The platelet count is increased and may reach levels between 1 and 2 million per microliter. Platelet function tests are usually normal [4,8,20,47], as is platelet morphology. Serum obtained from patients with throm-

TABLE 145-1   Conditions in which elevated platelet count may be found

Myeloproliferative disorders:
   Primary thrombocythemia (Chap. 26)
   Polycythemia vera (Chap. 23)
   Chronic myelogenous leukemia (Chap. 24)
   Agnogenic myeloid metaplasia (Chap. 25)
Thrombocytosis:
   Chronic inflammatory disorders
      Rheumatoid arthritis [1–3]
      Acute rheumatic fever [1,2]
      Periarteritis nodosa [4]
      Wegener's granulomatosis [1,2]
      Ulcerative colitis [1,3,5,6]
      Regional enteritis [5]
      Tuberculosis [2,6]
      Hepatic cirrhosis [2,6]
      Sarcoidosis [2,7]
      "Chronic or slowly resolving pneumonitis" [3]
      Osteomyelitis [2,6]
      Gonorrheal arthritis [8]
   Acute inflammatory disease
      Recovery from acute infection [2]
   Acute hemorrhage [2,3,6,9]
   Iron deficiency
      Chronic blood loss or dietary iron deficiency [7,10–12]
Hemolytic anemia [2,3,6,8]
Malignant diseases:
   Carcinoma [2,3,6,7,13–15]
   Hodgkin's disease [3,13]
   "Other lymphomas" [4,9,13]
Postoperative:
   Splenectomy [4,8,16–20]
   Other surgical procedures [21–23]
Response to drugs:
   Vincristine [24–26]
   Epinephrine [27–29]
Response to exercise [30,31]
Recovery from thrombocytopenia ("rebound"):
   Withdrawal of myelosuppressive drugs [32–35], including alcohol [32,33]
   Therapy of vitamin B_{12} deficiency [35]
Miscellaneous:
   Osteoporosis [3]
   Prematurity [36]

bocytosis may contain elevated concentrations of acid phosphatase [53], potassium [54], calcium [55], and phosphorus [55]. In blood samples containing markedly increased numbers of platelets, the Pa_{O_2} may be significantly reduced because of consumption of oxygen by the platelets, particularly if the blood is maintained at room temperature [56]. Elevated levels of plasma β-thromboglobulin also occur [57].

Differential diagnosis

Primary thrombocytosis caused by myeloproliferative disorders can usually be diagnosed from the associated abnormalities of the blood and from the absence of other demonstrable causes. Further, the level of platelets in essential thrombocythemia may be sufficiently high of itself to suggest the diagnosis. In secondary thrombocytosis the diagnosis depends on demonstration of the underlying disorder.

Essential thrombocythemia may be unmasked by splenectomy (Chap. 26) [58]. Usually the thrombocytosis which follows splenectomy develops in the first weeks and subsides spontaneously after about 2 months. However, postsplenectomy thrombocytosis may persist for prolonged periods of time at high levels. Differentiation of these patients from those with myeloproliferative diseases may be difficult. Platelets from patients with myeloproliferative disorders show greater variation in volume and diameter than platelets from patients with reactive thrombocytosis, and this difference may be helpful in differentiating these conditions [59].

Treatment

Treatment of primary thrombocythemia, presented in Chap. 26, involves principally therapy to decrease the autonomous growth of megakaryocytes and resultant excessive platelet production. Patients with thrombocytosis usually do not develop symptoms and therefore do not require treatment. Symptomatic thrombocytosis may be treated by thrombocytapheresis, which can lead to rapid removal of a large number of platelets [60].

Because an increased platelet concentration may interfere with blood coagulation [51], anticoagulant therapy in patients with thrombocytosis may be attended by an increased risk of complicating hemorrhage. On the other hand, heparin therapy in patients with thrombocytosis may require an increased dose because of the antiheparin effect of platelets [61].

Drugs such as aspirin and dipyridamole, which interfere with platelet aggregation, have been advocated for the prevention of thrombosis (see Chap. 160) and could be useful in preventing thrombotic complications in patients with thrombocytosis [48,49,62]. Controlled studies on these agents will be necessary in order to evaluate their effectiveness. Although postoperative patients frequently develop thrombocytosis, patients after splenectomy will occasionally develop thrombocytosis with platelet counts in excess of 1 million. In these patients the increased risk of thrombosis postoperatively is compounded by the markedly elevated platelet count. The question of whether or not these patients should receive heparin to prevent thrombosis is often raised but has not been answered by controlled studies. The risk of thrombosis in patients after splenectomy appears to be low [63,64]. Most physicians do not institute prophylactic therapy with heparin but do treat thrombosis if it develops. Fortunately, thrombocytosis after splenectomy usually does not reach levels greater than 1 million and is usually relatively short-lived.

Prognosis

Most patients with secondary thrombocytosis do not have significant problems caused by thrombocytosis, and the prognosis of the basic disease is not usually significantly affected.

References

1. Bean, R. H. D.: Thrombocytosis in auto-immune disease. *Bibl. Haematol. 23:*43, 1965.
2. Marchasin, S., Wallerstein, R. D., and Aggeler, P. M.: Variation of the platelet count in disease. *Calif. Med. 101:*95, 1964.
3. Levin, J., and Conley, C. L.: Thrombocytosis associated with malignant disease. *Arch. Intern. Med. 114:*497, 1964.
4. Ginsburg, A. D.: Platelet function in patients with high counts. *Ann. Intern. Med. 82:*506, 1975.
5. Morowitz, D. A., Allen, L. W., and Kirsner, J. B.: Thrombocytosis in chronic inflammatory bowel disease. *Ann. Intern. Med. 68:*1013, 1968.
6. Jellett, L. B., and Bonnin, J. A.: Platelet thromboplastic function in polycythaemia and thrombocythaemia. *Aust. Ann. Med. 15:*15, 1966.
7. Harker, L. A., and Finch, C. A.: Thrombokinetics in man. *J. Clin. Invest. 48:*963, 1969.
8. McClure, P. D., Ingram, G. I. C., Stacey, R. S., Glass, U. H., and Matchett, M. D.: Platelet function tests in thrombocythaemia and thrombocytosis. *Br. J. Haematol. 12:*478, 1966.
9. Desforges, J. F., Bigelow, F. S., and Chalmers, T. C.: The effects of massive gastrointestinal hemorrhage on hemostasis. *J. Lab. Clin. Med. 43:*501, 1954.
10. Schlosser, L. L., Kipp, M. A., and Wenzel, F. J.: Thrombocytosis in iron-deficiency anemia. *J. Lab. Clin. Med. 66:*107, 1965.
11. Gross, S., Keefer, V., and Newman, P. J.: The platelets in iron-deficiency anemia. I. The response to oral and parenteral iron. *Pediatrics 34:*315, 1964.
12. Knizley, H., and Noyes, W. D.: Iron deficiency anemia, papilledema, thrombocytosis, and transient hemiparesis. *Arch. Intern. Med. 129:*483, 1972.
13. Davis, R. B., Theologides, A., and Kennedy, B. J.: Comparative studies of blood coagulation and platelet aggregation in patients with cancer and nonmalignant diseases. *Ann. Intern. Med. 71:*67, 1969.
14. Silvis, S. E., Turklas, N., and Duscherholman, A.: Thrombocytosis in patients with lung cancer. *JAMA 211:*1852, 1970.
15. Tranum, B. L., and Haut, A.: Thrombocytosis: Platelet kinetics in neoplasia. *J. Lab. Clin. Med. 64:*615, 1974.
16. Slater, P. P., and Sherlock, E. C.: Splenectomy, thrombocytosis, and venous thrombosis. *Am. Surg. 23:*549, 1957.
17. Lipson, R. L., Bayrd, E. D., and Watkins, C. H.: The postsplenectomy blood picture. *Am. J. Clin. Pathol. 32:*526, 1959.
18. Charlesworth, D., and Torrence, H. B.: Splenectomy in idiopathic thrombocytopenic purpura. *Br. J. Surg. 55:*437, 1968.
19. Hirsh, J., and Dacie, J. V.: Persistent post-splenectomy thrombocytosis and thrombo-embolism: A consequence of continuing anaemia. *Br. J. Haematol. 12:*44, 1966.
20. Zucker, S., and Mielke, C. H.: Classification of thrombocytosis based on platelet function tests: Correlation with hemorrhagic and thrombotic complications. *J. Lab. Clin. Med. 80:*385, 1972.
21. Williams, J. A., and Warren, R.: Endocrine factors in the alterations of the blood coagulation mechanism following surgery. *J. Lab. Clin. Med. 50:*372, 1957.
22. Pepper, H., and Lindsay, S.: Responses of platelets, eosinophils, and total leukocytes during and following surgical procedures. *Surg. Gynecol. Obstet. 110:*319, 1960.
23. Breslow, A., Kaufman, R. M., and Lawsky, A. R.: The effect of surgery on the concentration of circulating megakaryocytes and platelets. *Blood 32:*393, 1968.
24. Carbone, P. P., Bono, V., Frei, E., III, and Brindley, C. O.: Clinical studies with vincristine. *Blood 21:*640, 1963.

25. Robertson, J. H., and McCarthy, G. M.: Periwinkle alkaloids and the platelet count. *Lancet* 2:353, 1969.
26. Robertson, J. H., Crozier, E. H., and Woodend, B. E.: The effect of vincristine on the platelet count in rats. *Br. J. Haematol.* 19:331, 1970.
27. McClure, P. D., Ingram, G. J. C., and Vaughan-Jones, R.: Platelet changes after adrenaline infusions with and without adrenaline blockers. *Thromb. Diath. Haemorrh.* 13:136, 1965.
28. Aster, R. H.: Pooling of platelets in the spleen: Role in the pathogenesis of "hypersplenic" thrombocytopenia. *J. Clin. Invest.* 45:645, 1966.
29. Libre, E. P., Cowan, D. H., Watkins, S. P., Jr., and Shulman, N. R.: Relationships between spleen, platelets and factor VIII levels. *Blood* 31:358, 1968.
30. Biggs, R., Macfarlane, R. G., and Pilling, J.: Observations on fibrinolysis: Experimental production by exercise and adrenaline. *Lancet* 1:402, 1947.
31. Dawson, A. A., and Ogston, D.: Exercise-induced thrombocytosis. *Acta Haematol. (Basel)* 42:241, 1969.
32. Lindenbaum, J., and Hargrove, R. L.: Thrombocytopenia in alcoholics. *Ann. Intern. Med.* 68:526, 1968.
33. Haselager, E. M., and Vreeken, J.: Rebound thrombocytosis after alcohol abuse: A possible factor in the pathogenesis of thromboembolic disease. *Lancet* 1:774, 1977.
34. Ogston, D., Dawson, A. A., and Philip, J. F.: Methotrexate and the platelet count. *Br. J. Cancer* 22:244, 1968.
35. Ogston, D., and Dawson, A. A.: Thrombocytosis following thrombocytopenia in man. *Postgrad. Med. J.* 45:754, 1969.
36. Lundstrom, U.: Thrombocytosis in low birthweight infants: A physiologic phenomenon in infancy. *Arch. Dis. Child.* 54:715, 1979.
37. Najean, Y., Ardaillou, N., and Dresch, C.: Platelet lifespan. *Annu. Rev. Med.* 20:47, 1969.
38. Najean, Y., and Ardaillou, N.: The use of ^{75}Se-methionin for the in vivo study of platelet kinetics. *Scand. J. Haematol.* 6:395, 1969.
39. Choi, S. J., and Simone, J. V.: Platelet production in experimental iron deficiency anemia. *Blood* 42:219, 1973.
40. Shreiner, D. P., and Levin, J.: The effects of hemorrhage, hypoxia, and a preparation of erythropoietin on thrombopoiesis. *J. Lab. Clin. Med.* 88:930, 1976.
41. Jackson, C. W., Simone, J. V., and Edwards, C. C.: The relationship of anemia and thrombocytosis. *J. Lab. Clin. Med.* 84:357, 1974.
42. Karpatkin, S., Garg, S. K., and Freedman, M. L.: Role of iron as a regulator of thrombopoiesis. *Am. J. Med.* 57:521, 1974.
43. McDonald, T. P., and Clift, R.: Effects of thrombopoietin and erythropoietin on platelet production in rebound-thrombocytotic and normal mice. *Am. J. Hematol.* 6:219, 1979.
44. McClure, P. D., and Choi, S. J.: Thrombopoietin and erythropoietin levels in idiopathic thrombocytopenic purpura and iron deficiency anemia. *Br. J. Haematol.* 15:351, 1968.
45. Birks, J. W., Klassen, L. W., and Gurney, C. W.: Hypoxia-induced thrombocytopenia in mice. *J. Lab. Clin. Med.* 86:230, 1975.
46. Jackson, C. W., and Edwards, C. C.: Evidence that stimulation of megakaryopoiesis by low dose vincristine results from an effect on platelets. *Br. J. Haematol.* 36:97, 1977.

47. Neemeh, J. A., Bowie, E. J. W., Thompson, J. H., Jr., Didisheim, P., and Owen, C. A., Jr.: Quantitation of platelet aggregation in myeloproliferative disorders. *Am. J. Clin. Pathol.* 57:336, 1972.
48. Preston, F. E., Emmanuel, I. G., Winfield, D. A., and Malia, R. G.: Essential thrombocythaemia and peripheral gangrene. *Br. Med. J.* 3:548, 1974.
49. Preston, F. E., Martin, J. F., Stewart, R. M., and Davies-Jones, G. A. B.: Thrombocytosis, circulating platelet aggregates, and neurological dysfunction. *Br. Med. J.* 2:1561, 1979.
50. Walsh, P. N., Murphy, S., and Barry, W. E.: The role of platelets in the pathogenesis of thrombosis and hemorrhage in patients with thrombocytosis. *Thromb. Haemost.* 38:1085, 1977.
51. Spaet, T. H., Auer, S., and Melamed, S.: Hemorrhagic thrombocythemia: A blood coagulation disorder. *Arch. Intern. Med.* 98:377, 1956.
52. Bierman, H. R., Kelly, K. H., Cordes, F. L., Byron, R. L., Jr., Polhemus, J. A., and Rappaport, S.: The release of leukocytes and platelets from the pulmonary circulation by epinephrine. *Blood* 7:683, 1952.
53. Zucker, M. B., and Woodward, H. W.: Elevation of serum acid phosphatase activity in thrombocytosis. *J. Lab. Clin. Med.* 59:760, 1962.
54. Hartmann, R. C., Auditore, J. V., and Jackson, D. P.: Studies on thrombocytosis. I. Hyperkalemia due to release of potassium from platelets during coagulation. *J. Clin. Invest.* 37:699, 1958.
55. Rawsley, H. M., and Woodruff, R.: Personal communication, 1970.
56. Hess, C. E., Nichols, A. B., Hunt, W. B., and Suratt, P. M.: Pseudohypoxemia secondary to leukemia and thrombocytosis. *N. Engl. J. Med.* 301:361, 1979.
57. Boughton, B. J., Allington, M. J., and King, A.: Platelet and plasma β-thromboglobulin in myeloproliferative syndromes and secondary thrombocytosis. *Br. J. Haematol.* 40:125, 1978.
58. Bensinger, T. A., Logue, G. L., and Rundles, R. W.: Hemorrhagic thrombocythemia: Control of post-splenectomy thrombocytosis with melphalan. *Blood* 36:61, 1970.
59. Holme, S., Simmonds, M., Ballek, R., and Murphy, S.: Comparative measurements of platelet size by Coulter counter, microscopy of blood smears, and light-transmission studies: Relationship between platelet size and shape. *J. Lab. Clin. Med.* 97:610, 1981.
60. Colman, R. W., Sievers, C. A., and Pugh, R. P.: Thrombocytopheresis: A rapid and effective approach to symptomatic thrombocytosis. *J. Lab. Clin. Med.* 68:389, 1966.
61. Conley, C. L., Hartmann, R. C., and Lalley, J. S.: The relationship of heparin activity to platelet concentration. *Proc. Soc. Exp. Biol. Med.* 69:284, 1948.
62. Rodriquez-Erdmann, F., Goldberg, M. E., Davey, F., and Maloney, W. C.: Treatment of symptomatic thrombocythemia. *N. Engl. J. Med.* 281:854, 1969.
63. Boxer, M. A., Braun, J., and Ellman, L.: Thromboembolic risk of postsplenectomy thrombocytosis. *Arch. Surg.* 113:808, 1978.
64. Coon, W. W., Penner, J., Clagett, P., and Eos, N.: Deep venous thrombosis and postsplenectomy thrombocytosis. *Arch. Surg.* 113:429, 1978.

Disorders of hemostasis—qualitative platelet disorders

CHAPTER *146*

Congenital qualitative platelet disorders

HARVEY J. WEISS

A prolonged bleeding time in a patient whose platelet count is normal suggests an abnormality of platelet function [1]. This may be due either to a qualitative platelet disorder or to a deficiency in a plasma factor necessary for platelet function (see Chap. 155). Tests of platelet aggregation are now widely used to investigate suspected qualitative platelet disorders (see Chap. A43). Aggregation patterns characteristic of various disorders of platelet function are illustrated in Fig. 146-1. Other tests used include the measurement of platelet retention in glass bead filters (see Chap. A41) and studies on the adhesion and aggregation of platelets to the subendothelium of rabbit aorta [2]. Qualitative platelet abnormalities which involve one or more specific platelet functions have been described in a variety of congenital and acquired conditions and are the topics of this chapter and of Chap. 147. Classification of these disorders is based on functional and biochemical defects.

Defects of adhesion

BERNARD-SOULIER (GIANT PLATELET) SYNDROME

DEFINITION AND HISTORY
Bernard and Soulier described a familial bleeding disorder characterized by unusually large platelets with dense condensation of the granules [3,4]. Similar abnormalities have been described by others [5–12]. The characteristic functional abnormalities were a prolonged bleeding time and impaired prothrombin consumption. Thrombocytopenia of varying degrees has been an inconstant feature.

ETIOLOGY AND PATHOGENESIS
Platelet aggregation in response to collagen, ADP, and epinephrine is not impaired [8], but the platelets of these patients, as in von Willebrand's disease, do not aggregate with ristocetin [8,10,12]. However, in contrast to von Willebrand's disease, patients with the Bernard-Soulier syndrome have normal levels of factor VIII/von Willebrand factor and the abnormal ristocetin aggregation is not corrected by this protein [8]. Bernard-Soulier platelets also do not aggregate with either crude [9] or purified [8,10,11] bovine factor VIII. Hence, the platelets of patients with the Bernard-Soulier syndrome are unresponsive to factor VIII/von Willebrand factor in tests of platelet aggregation that require this protein as a cofactor. Impaired adhesion of platelets to the subendothelium probably explains the prolongation of the bleeding time in these patients and in von Willebrand's disease (Chap. 155). Impaired adhesion can be demonstrated in vitro using either directly sampled (native) venous blood [13] or citrated [8] blood. However, unlike von Willebrand's disease, the defect of adhesion in Bernard-Soulier syndrome is intrinsic to the platelet.

A defect in the platelet membrane is probably responsible for the functional defects in the Bernard-Soulier syndrome. The quantity of membrane glycoprotein I (M_r 150,000 daltons) is decreased in platelets from patients with this disorder [14–16]. At least three glyco-

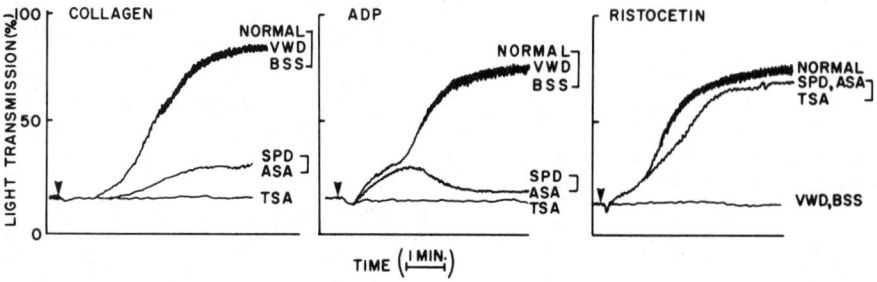

FIGURE 146-1 Platelet aggregation patterns in various disorders. Typical tracings obtained using concentrations of collagen, ADP, and ristocetin that best illustrate the differences between platelet aggregation in normal subjects and in patients with von Willebrand's disease (VWD) (see Chap. 155), Bernard-Soulier syndrome (BSS), thrombasthenia (TSA), storage pool deficiency (SPD), and aspirin ingestion and aspirin-like disorders (ASA). Impaired release of ADP accounts for the SPD and ASA defects. Factor VIII corrects the defective ristocetin aggregation in VWD but not in BSS. (Weiss [1], by permission.)

proteins (GP Is, GP Ib, and GP Ig) contribute to glycoprotein band I [17,18], and both GP Ib [17] and GP Is (glycocalycin) [16,17] are decreased in the Bernard-Soulier syndrome. The deficiencies of the sialic acid–rich GP Ib and GP Is provide a satisfactory explanation for the previously reported reduced sialic acid content and reduced electrophoretic mobility of these platelets [19]. The relationship between the glycoprotein abnormalities and the several defects of platelet function in the Bernard-Soulier syndrome remains to be clarified. Present evidence suggests that factor VIII/von Willebrand factor and the GP I complex are involved both in the aggregation responses of platelets to ristocetin and in the adhesion of platelets to subendothelium. The reported decrease in the uptake of exogenously added factor VIII/von Willebrand factor by Bernard-Soulier platelets [20,21] suggests that some component of the GP I complex could either be a receptor for the factor VIII/von Willebrand factor or, in some other way, be involved in its binding to platelets. Additional defects of Bernard-Soulier platelets, such as impaired binding of thrombin [22], reduced numbers of particles on the external leaflet of freeze-fractured platelets [23], and decrease in some platelet coagulant activities [12], could also be related to the reported abnormalities in membrane glycoproteins. The absence of the platelet receptor for drug-dependent antibodies [24] may be due to additional membrane abnormalities [24].

MODE OF INHERITANCE
The Bernard-Soulier syndrome is inherited as an autosomal recessive disorder. Consanguinity is a common feature, reflecting the rarity of the disorder.

CLINICAL FEATURES
The bleeding diathesis may be severe, and fatal hemorrhage may occur. Cutaneous hemorrhages and muscular and visceral bleeding are common. Hemarthrosis has also been reported. Epistaxis and menorrhagia may be difficult to control.

LABORATORY FEATURES
The bleeding time is usually markedly prolonged (greater than 20 min). The platelet count is highly variable; both normal counts and marked thrombocytopenia can occur, and the count may show considerable fluctuation in the same patient. Over 80 percent of the platelets are usually more than 2.5 μm in diameter on the peripheral blood film. Platelets as large as 15 to 20 μm have been described. Clustering of the granules in the center of the cell sometimes gives the appearance of a pseudonucleus. Marrow megakaryocytes are normal in number. The most consistent laboratory findings are impairment of prothrombin consumption, absence of ristocetin-induced platelet aggregation that is not corrected by addition of plasma or factor VIII, and failure of the platelets to aggregate with bovine factor VIII or crude bovine fibrinogen which contains factor VIII [8–12]. The levels of all plasma clotting factors and compo-

nents of the factor VIII complex (see Chaps. 132 and 155) are normal [8].

DIFFERENTIAL DIAGNOSIS
Differentiation from other congenital platelet disorders is by the laboratory tests described above, for the detection of both functional and morphologic abnormalities. Not all patients with congenital bleeding disorders and giant platelets have the Bernard-Soulier syndrome [8].

THERAPY
Platelet transfusions are the one form of therapy. Neither glucocorticoids nor splenectomy are of any value.

COURSE AND PROGNOSIS
Prognosis must be considered guarded, as fatal hemorrhages may occur. For unknown reasons, the condition tends to improve with age.

Defects of primary aggregation

THROMBASTHENIA

DEFINITION AND HISTORY
Thrombasthenia is the platelet abnormality found in a small group of patients with a congenital bleeding disorder associated with impaired or absent clot retraction and a failure of the platelets to aggregate with most agents. This disorder was described by Glanzmann in 1918 [25] in a heterogenous group of patients with a bleeding disorder characterized by absent or markedly reduced clot retraction. Some of these patients had normal bleeding times and thrombocytopenia and would now be considered atypical. In patients subsequently reported by other authors, the bleeding time was prolonged [26] and the platelets failed to aggregate during coagulation [27] or after addition of ADP [28–30]. These features are now considered to be characteristic of the disorder.

ETIOLOGY AND PATHOGENESIS
The platelets in thrombasthenia adhere normally to collagen [31–33]. They also adhere to the subendothelial surface and undergo degranulation [34]. In addition, they release ADP normally when stimulated by collagen or thrombin [32,35]. Impaired aggregation by ADP (or substances which aggregates platelets through releasing ADP) constitutes the major functional defect, which probably accounts for the prolonged bleeding time.

The impaired aggregation responses of thrombasthenic platelets may be related to an impairment in the binding of fibrinogen to the platelet membrane. The amount of total and surface-associated fibrinogen is reduced in thrombasthenic platelets [29,31,32,35], and these platelets do not bind fibrinogen either in the presence [36–39] or in the absence [40] of ADP. In addition, binding of calcium by thrombasthenic platelets is diminished [37]. Since both fibrinogen and calcium are necessary for platelet aggregation by ADP (see Chap. 129), the defect in ADP-induced aggregation in thrombasthenia may be due to diminished calcium-dependent uptake of fibrinogen by a platelet membrane receptor that is exposed in the presence of ADP. Since fibrinogen uptake is also increased by epinephrine [41] and since thrombin-induced aggregation may also be mediated by fibrinogen [42], a decrease in the binding of fibrinogen to the platelet membrane could explain the various aggregation defects in thrombasthenia.

Glycoprotein I, the membrane glycoprotein which is decreased in the Bernard-Soulier syndrome, is normal in thrombasthenia [15–17,43,44]. However, the concentrations of two other membrane glycoproteins, GP IIb and GP IIIa, are reduced [15,16,43,44]. Glycoproteins IIb and/or IIIa may be involved in platelet aggregation responses [17], and there may be a relationship between the impaired fibrinogen binding and membrane glycoprotein defects. In further support of these possibilities, an IgG antibody obtained from the blood of a transfused thrombasthenic patient specifically interacted with a normal platelet membrane protein of M_r 120,000 daltons, probably GP IIb [45], and inhibited both clot retraction and platelet aggregation responses in normal platelets [46]. Other membrane defects which have been reported in thrombasthenia include decreased amounts of α-actinin [47], actomyosin [48], and the platelet-specific alloantigen PI^{A1} [49,50].

Metabolic abnormalities have also been reported in some patients with this disorder. A decreased platelet content of ATP, associated with decreased activity of the glycolytic enzymes pyruvate kinase and glyceraldehyde-3-phosphate dehydrogenase, was reported in five patients with thrombasthenia [51]. These patients are a minority of those with thrombasthenia and may constitute a subtype of this disorder [52]. Platelet ATP levels were normal in the majority of patients subsequently studied by other investigators [29–31,35]. Other defects in thrombasthenic platelets from some patients include deficiencies of glutathione reductase [53] and glutathione peroxidase [54]. The relationship of these enzyme abnormalities to the defects in platelet function is not clear.

MODE OF INHERITANCE
The disease is one of the rarest of the congenital bleeding disorders [55]. It appears to be transmitted as an autosomal recessive trait [31,55], and consanguinity has been reported in about 10 percent of the cases [55]. In general, no aggregation abnormalities are detected in heterozygotes, but a decreased amount of one of the membrane-specific glycoproteins (see above) has been reported [56].

CLINICAL FEATURES
Bleeding usually begins early in life. Easy bruising and epistaxis, the latter sometimes necessitating blood transfusions, are common. Fatal hemorrhage has been reported [31]. Excessive bleeding may occur during surgical procedures. Joint hemorrhages are rare. There is extreme variability in the clinical symptoms, even among patients with similar degrees of platelet abnormality and prolongation of the bleeding time.

LABORATORY FEATURES
The bleeding time is usually markedly prolonged, although exceptions have been reported [55]. The platelet count and plasma clotting factor levels are normal. In the typical case clot retraction does not occur in 4 h, but some degree of clot retraction may occur [52]. On blood films, the platelets are round and isolated but are otherwise unremarkable. Morphologic abnormalities, detected by electron microscopy, may be nonspecific [31]. Platelets are not retained by glass bead filters [28,30,35], probably owing to the absence of aggregation within the filters. Thrombasthenic platelets do not aggregate with any concentration of ADP or with epinephrine, thrombin, or collagen [29–32,35]. Despite their inability to aggregate, thrombasthenic platelets undergo many of the other changes that are observed in normal platelets after the addition of aggregating agents. Thus, the addition of thrombin to these platelets results in normal ATP consumption, pseudopodium formation, ADP release, degranulation [29,32,52], and prostaglandin synthesis [57–59]. Thrombasthenic platelets also bind ADP [60] and thrombin [61] and respond to these agents by undergoing the change in shape from discs to spiny spheres that is observed with normal platelets [32]. Thrombasthenic platelets also contain fatty acid cyclooxygenase, the enzyme that catalyzes the conversion of arachidonic acid to the cyclic endoperoxide intermediate PGG$_2$ [57–59]. However, when PGG$_2$ is added directly to these platelets, they do not aggregate [62]. Abnormalities in the procoagulant properties of platelets have also been reported [63]. Thrombasthenic platelets are aggregated by ristocetin and by bovine factor VIII, in contrast to the impaired aggregation of platelets from patients with the Bernard-Soulier syndrome [64].

DIFFERENTIAL DIAGNOSIS
The clinical featuers of thrombasthenia do not permit it to be differentiated from other disorders of platelet function of from mild deficiency of one of the plasma coagulation factors or von Willebrand's disease. The differentiation can be made only on the basis of appropriate laboratory studies.

THERAPY
Platelet transfusions are the only therapy available at present. Platelet transfusions may shorten the bleeding time for an unexpectedly brief period, particularly in patients who have been previously treated [55]. Glucocorticoids are of no benefit [31].

COURSE AND PROGNOSIS
The course tends to be highly variable. Fatal hemorrhage has been reported [31].

Abnormalities of platelet secretion

HISTORY

In 1967, several groups independently described patients whose platelets were aggregated by ADP (first-phase aggregation) but not by collagen [65,66]. This impairment of collagen-induced aggregation was associated with, and attributed to, a defect in the secretion of ADP [65,66]. As a result of this abnormality, the second phase of aggregation induced by ADP and epinephrine was also impaired [66,67]. Many other patients with this type of aggregation defect, usually with diminished release of ADP, have been described [68–75], including some patients with oculocutaneous albinism (Hermansky-Pudlak syndrome) [76–80].

Defects in platelet secretion can be broadly classified into two groups. In one group, impaired secretion of ADP is due, in part, to a deficiency of the ADP pool that is stored in dense granules. This type of disorder has been referred to as storage pool disease [81] and, more recently, storage pool deficiency [82]. Initially, storage pool deficiency was defined as a disorder whose characteristic feature was a decreased content of the storage pool ADP (and ATP) in the platelet dense granules [81,83]. Some patients with this disorder also have diminished amounts of secretable substances stored in α granules [82], and some patients may show deficiencies only in α-granule substances [84–86]. It now seems reasonable to enlarge the concept of storage pool deficiency to include all disorders characterized by diminution of secretable substances that are stored in platelet granules. In the second type of platelet secretory defect, the platelets have a normal content of ADP and other granule-bound substances but the platelet secretory mechanism is defective. The patients were initially said to have release [73], or "aspirin-like" [74], defects. As discussed below, the secretory mechanism may also be abnormal in patients with storage pool deficiency.

These two groups of disorders are classified here as *storage pool deficiency* and *primary defects in platelet secretion*.

STORAGE POOL DEFICIENCY

ETIOLOGY AND PATHOGENESIS

Dense granules and substances stored in dense granules
Except for patients with an isolated deficiency of α granules [84–86], a diminution of platelet dense-granule substances is characteristic of storage pool deficiency. The diminished amounts of platelet ATP and ADP [76,79–82] are due specifically to deficiencies of granule-bound nucleotides; the cytosolic nucleotides that participate in platelet metabolism are normal [81,83]. In normal platelets the ATP/ADP ratio in the secretable granule-bound pool of adenine nucleotides is 2:3, whereas the ratio in the cytosolic pool is between 8:1 and 10:1 [87]. Hence, a loss of granule-bound nucleotides has the overall effect of increasing the ATP/ADP ratio in the platelet. This ratio, which in normal platelets

is less than 2.5, is characteristically greater than 3, and frequently 5 to 10, in patients with storage pool deficiency [76,79–82]. The diminished amounts of storage pool ADP can also be demonstrated by incubating platelets with ^{3}H- or ^{14}C-adenine. With normal platelets, radioactivity is incorporated into the ADP and ATP that are actively engaged in metabolism but the storage pool remains unlabeled. The specific radioactivity of ADP and ATP reflects the proportion of nucleotides in these two pools, and normally the unlabeled storage pool reduces the activity of the total pool. When this type of study is done in patients with storage pool deficiency, the uptake of radioactivity into the metabolic pool is normal but the absence of the storage pool, which normally is not labeled, accounts for the very high specific radioactivity of both ADP and ATP [81,83].

The serotonin content of storage pool–deficient platelets is also diminished [76,79–82]. The initial uptake of ^{14}C-serotonin into the platelet reflects membrane transport and is normal. However, the saturation levels are decreased [76,79,80] as a result of the diminished storage capacity of the dense granules. Because of this impaired storage capacity, serotonin that is absorbed into the platelets may be less protected from monoamine oxidases on mitochondrial membranes. This would explain the observation that platelets of patients with storage pool deficiency metabolize ^{14}C-serotonin more rapidly than do normal platelets [79,80].

The concentrations of other dense-granule substances, such as calcium [82,88] and pyrophosphate [89], are also decreased in storage pool deficiency. By contrast, the magnesium and potassium levels are normal, suggesting that the latter cations are not stored in dense granules [88]. The magnitude of the reduction in dense-granule substances varies widely among patients with storage pool deficiency. In a study on 18 patients, the greatest reduction in the content of these substances was observed in 7 patients with the albinism variant (Hermansky-Pudlak syndrome) [82]. Serotonin, in particular, was absent or markedly diminished in these subjects. The decrease in amine-storing organelles, detected by fluorescent microscopy with the dye mepacrine and by electron microscopy with the uranaffin reaction, was also most marked in the albinism variant of storage pool deficiency [90].

Dense granules are generally undetectable in electron micrographs of storage pool-deficient platelets [77,91] (Fig. 146-2). However, dense granules with abnormal ultrastructure have been observed in some patients [92,93], and a normal number of granules has been reported in one patient with Chédiak-Higashi syndrome [94]. A decreased number of dense-body organelles and an increase in atypical organelles have been described in storage pool–deficient platelets [90].

α granules and lysosomal enzymes Deficiencies of α granules have also been described in some patients with storage pool deficiency. Studies on 18 patients demonstrated considerable heterogeneity of the granule

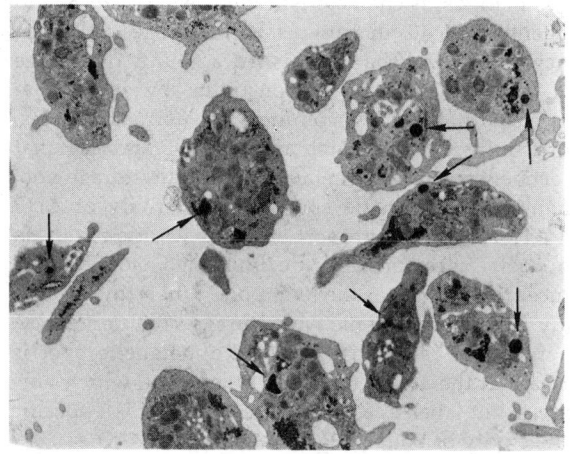

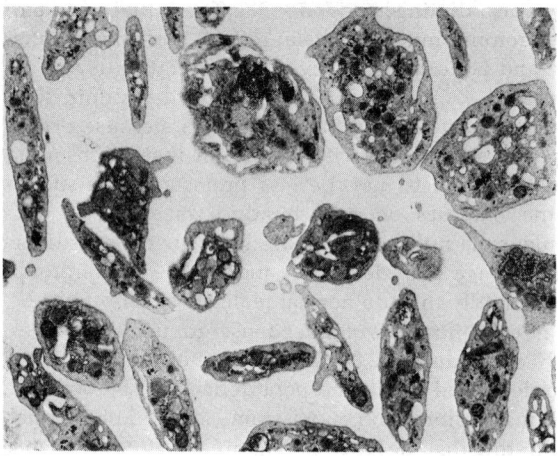

FIGURE 146-2 Platelets in storage pool deficiency. (*a*) Normal platelets, showing the dense bodies (*arrows*) that are the storage sites for serotonin and the releasable pools of ADP and ATP. (*b*) Decreased numbers of dense bodies in a patient with storage pool deficiency, ×12,000. (Weiss [91], by permission.)

defects in this disorder [82]. The number of α granules was normal in patients with the albinism variant (Hermansky-Pudlak syndrome) and in four miscellaneous unrelated patients with storage pool deficiency. A partial deficiency of α granules was observed in members of two unrelated families, and α granules were markedly reduced in one unique patient. In most cases, a reduction in the number of α granules was accompanied by a parallel reduction in substances that were stored in these granules, such as β-thromboglobulin, platelet factor 4, and the platelet-derived growth factor [82]. An isolated deficiency of α granules has recently been reported by two different groups in four patients with gray platelet syndrome [84,86], and the platelets of these patients were also deficient in platelet factor 4, β-thromboglobulin, and platelet-derived growth factor. Both the number and the content of dense granules were normal in these patients.

The platelet content of secretable acid hydrolases (β-glucuronidase, β-galactosidase, and β-N-acetyl-glucosaminidase) and of a membrane-bound acid phosphatase (p-nitrophenylphosphatase) has been consistently normal in patients with storage pool deficiency [82,95], including those with deficiencies of α granules [82]. The normal values obtained for the membrane-bound p-nitrophenylphosphatase in congenital storage pool deficiency are in contrast to the decreased values observed in some patients with an immune-mediated, acquired form of this disorder [96].

Other abnormalities in storage pool deficiency There is evidence that the secretory mechanism is also defective in storage pool deficiency, thereby compounding the functional abnormality of the platelets. For example, although the quantity of platelet factor 4 (heparin-neutralizing activity) is usually normal in this disorder [97], its release by collagen and epinephrine is generally decreased [97]. Release of acid hydrolases by thrombin [95] and release of platelet-bound ^{14}C-serotonin [80] by collagen are also impaired. Abnormalities of the prostaglandin and thromboxane A_2 synthetic pathway have also been described. Although platelets from most storage pool–deficient patients could convert arachidonic acid to prostaglandins PGE_2 and $PGF_2\alpha$ [62] and to thromboxane A_2 [57], impaired synthesis of prostaglandins [58], thromboxane A_2 [57], and malondialdehyde [59] has been observed in response to platelet stimulation by collagen. These findings suggest that the mechanism for activating phospholipase A_2 or C is abnormal in storage pool deficiency [62]. An impaired aggregation response of storage pool-deficient platelets to prostaglandin endoperoxides has been observed in several studies [57,59,98]. Both diminished [57,59,62] and normal [98] aggregation responses to arachidonic acid have been reported, perhaps reflecting the heterogeneity of the defects in storage pool deficiency [59]. Whether these abnormal prostaglandin responses are directly related to the storage pool defect remains to be determined, but they probably contribute to the impairment of platelet aggregation.

Finally, platelets in this disorder do not aggregate normally on the subendothelial surface of rabbit aorta under conditions of arterial flow (Baumgartner technique) [99]. An impairment of platelet aggregation at sites of vascular injury may explain the hemostatic defect in these patients.

Classification and pathogenesis Storage pool deficiency syndromes may be classified in a system that takes into account the results of both morphometric analysis of platelet granules and analysis of granule-bound substances [82]. The term δ-*storage pool deficient* has been assigned to identify patients who show only diminished levels of dense granules and substances stored in dense granules, such as those with the albinism variant (δ-storage pool deficiency:albinism). Patients with both dense-granule defects and either partial or more complete deficiencies in α-granules and granule-bound substances are designated as $\alpha_p\delta$-storage pool deficient and $\alpha\delta$-storage pool deficient. Patients with gray platelet syndrome [84–86], who show normal levels of dense-granule substances but decrease α granule levels, are designated α-storage pool deficient.

The pathogenesis of the various granule defects in patients with storage pool deficiency syndrome remains to be clarified. There is no evidence to suggest that the diminished amounts of granule-bound substances are due to their secretion from platelets in the blood [82]. The defect in these patients, therefore, could arise from an abnormality of granule morphogenesis in the megakaryocyte. In a recent study of two patients with α storage pool deficiency (gray platelet syndrome), a defect in the maturation of α granules in developing megakaryocytes grown in tissue culture was demonstrated [100]. The relationship between platelet granule defects and the defects in melanosome development [101] in the Hermansky-Pudlak and Chédiak-Higashi syndromes remains to be clarified. A variety of defects in platelet granule morphogenesis may be anticipated in the storage pool deficiency syndrome.

MODE OF INHERITANCE
This disorder is heterogeneous, and the term *storage pool deficiency* describes a group of disorders having as their common feature a diminution in secretable substances stored in platelet granules. In one family, the disorder was transmitted as an autosomal dominant trait [67]. The members of that family also showed a specific phospholipid defect, whereas no such defect was observed in other patients in whom the type of inheritance could not be determined [102]. The syndrome may also occur in some patients with oculocutaneous albinism (Hermansky-Pudlak syndrome) [76–80], thrombocytopenia with absent radius (TAR) [103], the Wiskott-Aldrich syndrome [104,105], and the Chédiak-Higashi syndrome [94,106].

CLINICAL FEATURES
Bleeding symptoms are mild, but easy bruising may be troublesome. Excessive bleeding after tooth extraction, tonsillectomy, and other surgical procedures is common. Menorrhagia is frequent; excessive postpartum bleeding may occur but is not the rule. Hemarthrosis has not been reported.

LABORATORY FEATURES
The bleeding time is usually only moderately prolonged. Platelet retention in glass bead filters is decreased [67,73]. The platelet count is normal or slightly decreased. No characteristic morphologic abnormalities are detectable on blood films except in patients deficient in α granules whose platelets appear gray. Platelets are usually of normal size, but somewhat small [67] or large [73] platelets have been observed in some patients. Aggregation by collagen is impaired when tested at the appropriate concentration of collagen (see Chap. A43).

Platelets respond initially to ADP, but no second wave can be demonstrated using ADP concentrations that produce two waves of aggregation in normal subjects (Fig. 146-1). The second wave of epinephrine-induced aggregation is either absent or diminished in most subjects, although exceptions have been reported [107]. The platelets usually respond normally to ristocetin but may show some diminution in the second (ADP-dependent) phase of ristocetin aggregation [64]. Biochemical measurements show a diminution of both platelet ATP and ADP and an increase in the ATP/ADP ratio [67,79–81,83]. Serotonin levels are variably decreased [76,77,80,81,83] but may be only marginally reduced in some cases [80]. Acid hydrolases are present in normal amounts [82,95]. Patients with deficiencies of α granules show variable deficiencies in substances (such as β-thromboglobulin) that are normally stored in these granules. Impaired kaolin-induced platelet factor 3 availability has been observed in patients with well-characterized storage pool deficiency [67,73,74,76]. In patients with abnormalities of second-phase aggregation not clearly identified as storage pool deficiency, normal values have been reported [69,71].

DIFFERENTIAL DIAGNOSIS
The responses of the platelets to aggregating agents are similar to those obtained in normal subjects who ingest drugs such as aspirin and in patients who have primary disorders of platelet secretion (see below). Storage pool deficiency may be differentiated from these defects by biochemical and morphologic analysis of the platelets (increased ATP/ADP ratio; decreased number of these granules). Although both storage pool–deficient and aspirin-treated platelets show diminished aggregation with various agents, significant aggregation is sometimes seen in mixtures containing platelets with both types of defects [62,108,109]. Acquired forms of storage pool deficiency have also been described (Chap. 147).

THERAPY
The administration of platelets, when clinically indicated, may improve hemostasis, although controlled studies have not been done. Glucocorticoids have been reported to shorten the bleeding time in some patients with aggregation defects of the type seen in storage pool deficiency; the aggregation defects were not corrected, however, [72]. Aspirin should be avoided, as in other disorders of platelet function. Finally, in one study, transfusion of cryoprecipitate shortened the bleeding time in patients with the Hermansky-Pudlak variant [110]. The reason for this effect is not clear.

COURSE AND PROGNOSIS
The disease tends to be mild. No fatalities due to hemorrhage have been reported thus far.

PRIMARY DEFECTS IN PLATELET SECRETION
The platelet aggregation tracings in patients with primary defects in platelet secretion are generally similar to

those obtained in patients with storage pool deficiency. However, platelet levels of ATP and ADP are normal. Initially, these patients were said to have a release [73], or "aspirin-like," defect [74], as mentioned above. The true incidence of these disorders is not known, but it may be relatively common [111]. Although more extensive studies on the basic abnormalities in these disorders are needed, several types of defects have recently been described. In several patients, an enzyme defect (cyclooxygenase deficiency) entirely similar to that produced by aspirin has been identified [112]. In others, an impaired platelet response to thromboxane A_2 [113] and defective mobilization of platelet calcium [113,114] have been described. Other types of defects in the platelet secretory process may be anticipated in these patients. The clinical manifestations are the same as described for storage pool deficiencies (see above).

Abnormalities of platelet procoagulant activity

Until 1967, the diagnosis of a qualitative platelet disorder was usually made by demonstrating impairment of platelet factor 3 availability, and patients with these defects were said to have a thrombopathy or a thrombocytopathy [115]. This diagnosis was made by a variety of assays, including the prothrombin consumption test [116], the thromboplastin generation test [117–120], conversion of purified prothrombin [121], and kaolin activation of platelet-rich plasma [65]. Impairment of platelet factor 3 availability may be undetected if the tests are not carried out under optimum conditions [74]. Many of the patients with abnormalities of platelet factor 3 availability had a prolonged bleeding time, a finding that could not be explained by the abnormal platelet coagulant activity per se, since the bleeding time is normal in most coagulation disorders. Subsequently, defects of platelet aggregation and release were found in many of these patients [65,66]. These abnormalities provided a more satisfactory explanation for the prolonged bleeding time, and it was not clear whether the impairment of platelet factor 3 availability, which was probably due to the defects in release and aggregation, was clinically significant. Therefore the distinction that is sometimes made between disorders of platelet aggregation and impairment of platelet factor 3 availability may be more apparent than real.

A patient has been described in whom an isolated deficiency of platelet factor 3 availability was the only abnormality [122]. All studies of platelet aggregation and secretion were normal. Further studies on the platelets of this patient showed impaired binding of factor Xa, due to reduced binding of factor Va [123]. The reduced factor Xa binding to her platelets (approximately 30 percent of that in normal platelets) correlated with the percent reduction in platelet factor 3 availability observed. The studies on this patient suggest that what

has been termed platelet factor 3 availability may, in part, reflect the binding of factor Xa to factor V–associated binding sites that are made available during platelet secretion.

Finally, other procoagulant properties of platelets may be abnormal in thrombasthenia [35,63] and the Bernard-Soulier syndrome [12].

Platelet abnormalities associated with other congenital defects

Reference has been made to the occurrence of storage pool deficiency in association with other congenital defects, such as those occurring with oculocutaneous albinism and increased monocyte-macrophage ceroid [Hermansky-Pudlak syndrome], the Chédiak-Higashi syndrome, and the TAR syndrome. Platelet aggregation defects have been reported in some patients with heritable disorders of connective tissue, such as Ehlers-Danlos syndrome [124] and osteogenesis imperfecta [125]. A storage pool defect has been described in patients with the Wiskott-Aldrich syndrome [104], who may show, in addition, an abnormality in the citric acid cycle [126]. Platelet abnormalities have been described in some [127,128] patients with the May-Hegglin anomaly and in a congenital syndrome characterized by deafness and renal disease (Allport's syndrome) [129]. The platelet aggregation defects in patients with glucose-6-phosphatase deficiency (glycogen storage disease type I) disappear with improvement in their metabolic state [130,131], indicating that such defects are not due to intrinsic platelet abnormalities but rather are secondary to the general metabolic defects in this disorder. Platelet abnormalities occasionally seen in patients with cyanotic congenital heart disease are probably also acquired [132]. Abnormalities of serotonin transport and metabolism have been described in the platelets of patients with Down's syndrome [133].

The bleeding time is often prolonged in patients with congenital afibrinogenemia [134,135], a finding which is difficult to attribute to the clotting abnormalities per se. Although earlier studies suggested that the platelets function normally, more recent reports have described impaired platelet retention in glass bead filters [134,135] and abnormalities in platelet factor 3 activity [134,136] and in ADP-induced aggregation [134–136]. Most of the defects can be corrected in vitro by the addition of fibrinogen [134–136].

Finally, patients with defects in both platelet secretion and the factor VIII complex have been described [64,137–139]. The factor VIII findings may be either those observed in hemophilia (decreased factor VIII coagulant activity; normal levels of factor VIII–related antigen and of von Willebrand's factor) [64,138] or those observed in von Willebrand's disease [64,139]. The relationship between the defects in factor VIII and platelet secretion in these subjects is not clear. Although these findings may be due to a chance association of two inherited diseases, a more fundamental relationship between the two types of defects has not been ruled out.

References

1. Weiss, H. J.: Platelet physiology and abnormalities of platelet function. *N. Engl. J. Med.* 292:531, 1975.
2. Baumgartner, H. R.: Morphometric quantitation of adherence of platelets to an artificial surface and components of connective tissue. *Thromb. Diath. Haemorrh. (Suppl.)* 60:39, 1974.
3. Bernard, J., and Soulier, J. P.: Sur une nouvelle variété de dystrophie thrombocytaire hémorragipare congénitale. *Sem. Hôp. Paris* 24:3217, 1948.
4. Bernard, J., Caen, J., and Maroteau, P.: La Dystrophie thrombocytaire hémorragipare congénitale. *Rev. Hematol.* 12:222, 1957.
5. Alagille, D., Josso, F., Binet, J. L., and Blin, M. L.: La Dystrophie thrombocytaire hémorragipare: Discussion nosologique. *Nouv. Rev. Fr. Hematol.* 4:755, 1964.
6. Kanska, B., Niewiarowski, S., Ostrowski, L., Poplanski, A., and Prokopowicz, J.: Macrothrombocytic thrombopathia: Clinical, coagulation and hereditary aspects. *Thromb. Diath. Haemorrh.* 10:88, 1963.
7. Ulutin, O. N.: Primary thrombocytopathy. *Isr. J. Med. Sci.* 1:857, 1965.
8. Weiss, H. J., Tschopp, T. B., Baumgartner, H. R., Sussman, I. I., Johnson, M. M., and Egan, J. J.: Decreased adhesion of giant (Bernard-Soulier) platelets to subendothelium: Further implications on the role of the von Willebrand factor in hemostasis. *Am. J. Med.* 57:920, 1974.
9. Bithell, T. C., Parekh, S. J., and Strong, R. R.: Platelet function in the Bernard-Soulier syndrome. *Ann. N.Y. Acad. Sci.* 201:145, 1972.
10. Howard, M. A., Hutton, R. A., and Hardisty, R. M.: Hereditary giant platelet syndrome: A disorder of a new aspect of platelet function. *Br. Med. J.* 4:586, 1973.
11. Caen, J. P., Levy-Toledano, S., and Sultan, Y.: La Dystrophie thrombocytaire hémorragipare (interaction des plaquettes et du factor Willebrand). *Nouv. Rev. Fr. Hematol.* 13:593, 1973.
12. Walsh, P., et al.: Hereditary giant platelet syndrome: Absence of collagen-induced coagulant activity and deficiency of factor XI binding to platelets. *Br. J. Haematol.* 29:639, 1975.
13. Weiss, H. J., Turitto, V. T., and Baumgartner, H. R.: Effect of shear rate on platelet interaction with subendothelium in citrated and native blood. I. Shear-dependent decrease of adhesion in von Willebrand's disease and the Bernard-Soulier syndrome. *J. Lab. Clin. Med.* 92:750, 1978.
14. Nurden, A. T., and Caen J. P.: Specific roles for platelet surface glycoproteins in platelet function. *Nature* 255:720, 1975.
15. Hagen I., and Solum, N. O.: Further studies on the protein composition and surface structure of normal platelets and platelets from patients with Glanzmann's thrombasthenia and Bernard-Soulier syndrome. *Thromb. Res.* 13:845, 1978.
16. Jamieson, G. A., Okumura T., Fishback, B., Johnson, M. M., Egan, J. J., and Weiss, H. J.: Platelet membrane glycoproteins in thrombasthenia, Bernard-Soulier syndrome and storage pool disease. *J. Lab. Clin. Med.* 93:652, 1979.
17. Nurden, A. T., and Caen, J. P.: The different glycoprotein abnormalities in thrombasthenic and Bernard-Soulier syndrome and storage pool disease. *J. Lab. Clin. Med.* 93:652, 1979.
18. Solum, N. O., Hagen, I., and Peterka, M.: Human platelet glycoproteins: Further evidence that the GP I band from whole platelets contains three different polypeptides one of which may be involved in the interaction between platelets and factor VIII. *Thromb. Res.* 10:71, 1977.
19. Gröttum, K. A., and Solum, N. O.: Congenital thrombocytopenia with giant platelets: A defect in the platelet membrane. *Br. J. Haematol.* 16:277, 1969.
20. Moake, J., et al.: Defective binding of ¹²⁵I-von Willebrand factor (VWF) to Bernard-Soulier platelets. *Blood* 54:253a, 1979 (abstract).
21. Zucker, M. B., et al.: Binding of factor VIII to platelets in the presence of ristocetin. *Br. J. Haematol.* 35:535, 1977.
22. Jamieson, G. A., and Okumura, T.: Reduced thrombin binding and aggregation in Bernard-Soulier platelets. *J. Clin. Invest.* 61:861, 1978.
23. Chevalier, J., et al.: Freeze-fracture studies on the plasma membranes of normal human thrombasthenic, and Bernard-Soulier platelets. *J. Lab. Clin. Med.* 94;232, 1979.
24. Kunicki, T. J., Johnson, M. M., and Aster, R. H.: Absence of the platelet receptor for drug-dependent antibodies in the Bernard-Soulier syndrome. *J. Clin. Invest.* 62:716, 1978.
25. Glanzmann, E.: Hereditäre haemorrhagische Thrombasthenie, Ein Beitrag zur Pathologie der Blutplättchen. *Jahrb. Kinderheilk.* 88:1, 1918.
26. Naegeli, O.: *Blutkrankheiten und Blutdiagnostik.* Springer-Verlag, Berlin, 1931, vol. 1.
27. Braunsteiner, H., and Pakesch, F.: Thrombocytoasthenia and thrombocytopathia: Old names and new diseases. *Blood* 11:965 1956.
28. Hellem, A. J.: The adhesiveness of human blood platelets in vitro. *Scand. J. Clin. Lab. Invest.* 12 (Suppl. 51), 1960.
29. Jackson, D. P., Morse, E. E., Zieve, P. D., and Conley, C. L.: Thrombocytopathic purpura associated with defective clot retraction and absence of platelet fibrinogen. *Blood* 12:827, 1963.
30. Hardisty, R. M., Dormandy, K. M., and Hutton, R. A.: Thrombasthenia: Studies on 3 cases. *Br. J. Haematol.* 10:371, 1964.
31. Caen, J., et al.: Congenital bleeding time and normal platelet count. I. Glanzmann's thrombasthenia (report of 15 patients). *Am. J. Med.* 41:4, 1966.
32. Zucker, M. B., Pert, J., and Hilgartner, M. W.: Platelet function in a patient with thrombasthenia. *Blood* 28:525, 1966.
33. Huges, J., and Lapiere, C. M.: Nouvelles recherches sur l'accolement des plaquettes aux fibres de collagène. *Thromb. Diath. Haemorrh.* 11:327, 1964.
34. Tschopp, T. B., Weiss, H. J., and Baumgartner, H. R.: Interaction of platelets with subendothelium in thrombasthenia: Normal adhesion, impaired aggregation. *Experientia* 31:113, 1975.
35. Weiss, H. J., and Kochwa, S.: Studies of platelet function and proteins in 3 patients with Glanzmann's thrombasthenia. *J. Lab. Clin. Med.* 71:153, 1968.
36. Bennett, J. S., and Vilaire, G. V.: Exposure of platelet fibrinogen receptors by ADP and epinephrine. *J. Clin. Invest.* 62:1393, 1979.
37. Grant, R. A., Peerschke, E. I., and Zucker, M. B.: Altered surface properties of human blood platelets associated with the loss of aggregability. *J. Cell Biol.* 83:64, 1979.
38. Mustard, J. F., et al.: Comparison of fibrinogen association with normal and thrombasthenic platelets on exposure to ADP or chymotrypsin. *Blood* 54:987, 1979.
39. Peerschke, E. I., et al.: Correlation between fibrinogen binding to human platelets and platelet aggregability. *Blood* 55:841, 1980.
40. Coller, B. S.: Interaction of normal, thrombasthenic, and Bernard-Soulier platelets with immobilized fibrinogen: Defective platelet-fibrinogen interaction in thrombasthenia. *Blood* 55:169, 1980.
41. Plow, E. F., and Marguerie, G. A.: Introduction of the fibrinogen receptor on human platelets by epinephrine and the combination of epinephrine and ADP. *J. Biol. Chem.* 255:10971, 1980.
42. Tollefson, D. M., and Majerus, P. W.: Inhibition of human platelet aggregation by monovalent anti-fibrinogen antibody fragments. *J. Clin. Invest.* 55:1259, 1975.
43. Nurden, A. T., and Caen, J. P.: An abnormal platelet glycoprotein pattern in three cases of Glanzmann's thrombasthenia. *Br. J. Haematol.* 28:253, 1974.
44. Phillips, D. R., and Poh Agin, P.: Platelet membrane defects in Glanzmann's thrombasthenia: Evidence for decreased amounts of two major glycoproteins. *J. Clin. Invest.* 60:535, 1977.
45. Degos, L., et al.: A molecular defect in thrombasthenic platelets. *J. Clin. Invest.* 56:235, 1975.
46. Levy-Toledano, S., et al.: An acquired IgG antibody occurring in a thrombasthenic patient: Its effect on normal human platelet function. *Blood* 51:1065, 1978.
47. Gerrard, J. M., et al.: α-Actinin deficiency in thrombasthenia: Possible identity of α-actinin and glycoprotein III. *Am. J. Pathol.* 94:509, 1979.
48. Booyse, F., et al.: Possible thrombosthenin defect in Glanzmann's thrombasthenia. *Blood* 39:377, 1972.

49. Kunicki, T. J., and Aster, R. H.: Deletion of the platelet-specific alloantigen Pl^A1 from platelets in Glanzmann's thrombasthenia. *J. Clin. Invest.* 61:1225, 1978.

50. Muller, J. Y., Patereau, C., and Soulier, J. P.: Thrombasthenie de Glanzmann antigene Pl^A1 et anticorp anti-Glanzmann. *Rev. Fr. Transfus. Immunohematol.* 21:1069, 1978.

51. Gross, R., Gerok, W., Lohr, G. W., Vogell, W., Waller, H. D., and Theopold, W.: Uber die Natur der Thrombasthenie: Thrombopathie Glanzmann-Naegeli. *Klin. Wochenschr.* 38:193, 1960.

52. Caen, J. P.: Glanzmann thrombasthenia. *Clin. Haemotol.* 1:383, 1972.

53. Moser, K., Lechner, K., and Vinazzer, H.: A hitherto not described enzyme defect in thrombasthenia: Glutathione reductase deficiency. *Thromb. Diath. Haemorrh.* 19:46, 1968.

54. Karpatkin, S., and Weiss, H. J.: Deficiency of glutathione peroxidase associated with raised levels of reduced glutathione in Glanzmann's thrombasthenia. *N. Engl. J. Med.* 287:1062, 1973.

55. Larrieu, M. J., Caen, J., Lelong, J. C., and Bernard, J.: Maladie de Glanzmann: Étude clinique, biologique et pathogenique: À propos de cinq observations. *Nouv. Rev. Fr. Hematol.* 1:662, 1961.

56. Degos, L., et al.: A molecular defect in thrombasthenic platelets. *J. Clin. Invest.* 56:236, 1975.

57. Malmsten, C., et al.: Thromboxane synthesis and the platelet release reaction in Bernard-Soulier syndrome, thrombasthenia Glanzmann and Hermansky-Pudlak syndrome. *Br. J. Haematol* 35:511, 1977.

58. Willis, A. L., and Weiss, H. J.: A congenital defect in platelet prostaglandin production associated with impaired hemostasis in storage pool disease. *Prostaglandins* 4:783, 1972.

59. Weiss, H. J., and Lages, B.: Platelet malondialdehyde production and aggregation responses induced by arachidonate, prostaglandin G$_2$, collagen, and epinephrine in 12 patients with storage pool deficiency. *Blood* 58:27, 1981.

60. Legrand, C., and Caen, J. P.: Binding of ^{14}C-ADP by thrombasthenic platelet membranes. *Haemostasis* 5:231, 1976.

61. White, G. C., Workman, E. F., and Lundblad, R. L.: Thrombin binding to thrombasthenic platelets. *J. Lab. Clin. Med.* 91:76, 1978.

62. Weiss, H. J., et al.: Prostaglandin E$_2$ potential of platelet aggregation by labile aggregation-stimulatory substance (LASS): Abnormal in storage pool disease, normal after aspirin ingestion. *Br. J. Haematol.* 32:257, 1976.

63. Walsh, P. N.: Platelet coagulant activities in thrombasthenia. *Br. J. Haematol.* 23:553, 1972.

64. Weiss, H. J.: Defects of factor VIII and platelet aggregation: Use of ristocetin in diagnosing the von Willebrand syndrome. *Blood* 45:403, 1975.

65. Weiss, H. J.: Platelet aggregation, adhesion and adenosine diphosphate release in thrombopathia (platelet factor 3 deficiency): A comparison with Glanzmann's thrombasthenia and von Willebrand's disease. *Am. J. Med.* 43:570, 1967.

66. Hardisty, R. M., and Hutton, R. A.: Bleeding tendency associated with "new" abnormality of platelet behavior. *Lancet* 1:983, 1967.

67. Weiss, H. J., Chervenick, P. A., Zalusky, R., and Factor, A.: A familial defect in platelet function associated with impaired release of adenosine diphosphate. *N. Engl. J. Med.* 281:1264, 1969.

68. O'Brien, J.: Platelets: Portsmouth syndrome? *Lancet* 2:258, 1967.

69. Sahud, M. A., and Aggeler, P. M.: Platelet dysfunction: Differentiation of a newly recognized primary type from that produced by aspirin. *N. Engl. J. Med.* 280:453, 1969.

70. Caen, J. P., Sultan, Y., and Larrieu, M.: New familial platelet disease. *Lancet* 1:203, 1968.

71. Maurer, H. M., Still, W. J. S., Caul, J., Valdes, O. S., and Laupus, W. E.: Familial bleeding tendency associated with microcytic platelets and impaired release of adenosine diphosphate. *J. Pediatr.* 78:86, 1971.

72. Zucker, S., Meilke, H., Durocher, J. R., and Crosby, W. H.: Oozing and bruising due to abnormal platelet function. *Ann. Intern. Med.* 76:725, 1971.

73. Weiss, H. J., and Rogers, J.: Thrombocytopathia due to abnormalities in the platelet release reaction: Studies on six unrelated patients. *Blood* 39:187, 1972.

74. Weiss, H. J.: Abnormalities in platelet function due to defects in the release reaction. *Ann. N.Y. Acad. Sci.* 201:161, 1972.

75. Ulutin, O. N.: Qualitative platelet disorders: Classification and pathogenesis. *Ann. N.Y. Acad. Sci.* 201:174, 1972.

76. Hardisty, R. M., Mills, D. C. B., and Ketsa-Ard, K.: The platelet defect associated with albinism. *Br. J. Haematol.* 23:679, 1972.

77. White, J. G., Edson, J. R., Desnick, S. J., and Witkop, C. J.: Studies of platelets in a variant of the Hermansky-Pudlak syndrome. *Am. J. Pathol.* 63:319, 1971.

78. Logan, L. J., Rapaport, S. I., and Mather, I.: Albinism and abnormal platelet function. *N. Engl. J. Med.* 284:1340, 1971.

79. Pareti, F. I., Day, H. J., and Mills, D. C. B.: Nucleotide and serotonin metabolism in platelets with defective secondary aggregation. *Blood* 44:789, 1974.

80. Weiss, H. J., Tschopp, T., Brand, H., and Rogers, J.: Studies of platelet 5-hydroxytryptamine (serotonin) in patients with storage-pool disease and albinism. *J. Clin. Invest.* 54:421, 1974.

81. Holmsen, H., and Weiss, H. J.: Further evidence for a deficient storage pool of adenine nucleotides in platelets from some patients with thrombocytopathia—"storage pool disease." *Blood* 39:197, 1972.

82. Weiss, H. J., et al.: Heterogeneity in storage pool deficiency: Studies on granule-bound substances in 18 patients including variants deficient in α-granules, platelet factor-4, β-thromboglobulin and platelet-derived growth factor. *Blood* 54:1296, 1979.

83. Holmsen, H., and Weiss, H. J.: Hereditary defect in the release reaction caused by a deficiency in the storage pool of platelet adenine nucleotides. *Br. J. Haematol.* 19:643, 1970.

84. White, J. G.: Ultrastructural studies of the gray platelet syndrome. *Am. J. Pathol.* 95:445, 1979.

85. Gerrard, J. M., et al.: Biochemical studies of two patients with the gray platelet syndrome. *J. Clin. Invest.* 66:102, 1980.

86. Levy-Toledano, S., et al.: Gray platelet syndrome: α-Granule deficiency. Its influence on platelet function. *J. Lab. Clin. Med.* 98:831, 1981.

87. Holmsen, H., and Weiss, H. J.: Secretable storage pools in platelets. *Ann. Rev. Med.* 30:119, 1979.

88. Lages, B., et al.: Metal ion content of gel-filtered platelets from patients with storage pool disease. *Blood* 46:119, 1975.

89. Silcox, D. C., Jacobelli, S., and McCarty, D. J.: Identification of inorganic pyrophosphate in human platelets and its release on stimulation with thrombin. *J. Clin. Invest.* 52:1595, 1973.

90. Lorez, N. P., et al.: Storage pool disease: Comparative fluorescence microscopical, cytochemical and biochemical studies on amino-storing organelles of human blood platelets. *Br. J. Haematol.* 43:297, 1979.

91. Weiss, H. J., and Ames, R. P.: Ultrastructural findings in storage-pool disease and aspirin-like defects of platelets. *Am. J. Pathol.* 71:447, 1973.

92. Gerritsen, S. M., et al.: The Hermansky-Pudlak syndrome: Evidence for a lowered 5-hydroxytryptamine content in platelets of heterozygotes. *Scand. J. Haematol.* 18:249, 1977.

93. Rendu, F., et al.: Studies on a new variant of the Hermansky-Pudlak syndrome: Qualitative, ultrastructural, and functional abnormalities of the platelet-dense bodies associated with a phospholipase A defect. *Am. J. Haematol.* 4:387, 1978.

94. Boxer, G. J., et al.: Abnormal platelet function in Chediak-Higashi syndrome. *Br. J. Haematol.* 35:521, 1977.

95. Holmsen, H., et al.: Content and thrombin-induced release of acid hydrolase in gel-filtered platelets from patients with storage pool deficiency. *Blood* 46:131, 1975.

96. Weiss, H. J., et al.: Acquired storage pool deficiency associated with increased platelet IgG. *Am. J. Med.* 69:712, 1980.

97. Weiss, H. J., and Rogers, J.: Platelet factor 4 in platelet disorders: Storage location and the requirement of endogenous ADP for its release. *Proc. Soc. Exp. Biol. Med.* 142:30, 1973.

98. Ingerman, C. M., et al.: Hereditary abnormality of platelet aggregation attributable to nucleotide storage pool deficiency. *Blood* 52:332, 1978.

99. Weiss, H. J., Tschopp, T. B., and Baumgartner, H. R.: Impaired interaction (adhesion-aggregation) of platelets with the subendothelium in storage pool disease and after aspirin ingestion: A comparison with von Willebrand's disease. *N. Engl. J. Med.* 293:619, 1975.

100. Breton-Gorius, J., Vainchenker, W., Nurden, A., Levy-Toledano, S., and Caen, J.: Defective α-granule production in megakaryocytes from gray platelet syndrome. *Am. J. Pathol.* 102:10, 1981.

101. Witkop, C. J., Jr., White, J. G., and King, R. A.: Oculocutaneous albinism, in *Heritable Disorders of Amino Acid Metabolism: Patterns of Clinical Expression and Genetic Variation*, edited by W. L. Nylan. Wiley, New York, 1974, p. 177.

102. Safrit, H. F., Weiss, H. J., and Phillips, G. B.: The phospholipid and fatty acid composition of platelets in patients with primary defects of platelet function. *Lipids* 7:60, 1972.

103. Day, H. J., and Holmsen, H.: Platelet adenine nucleotide "storage pool deficiency" thrombocytopenic absent radii syndrome. *JAMA* 221:1053, 1972.

104. Grottum, K. A., Hovig, T., and Holmsen, H.: Wiskott-Aldrich syndrome: Qualitative platelet defects and short platelet survival. *Br. J. Haematol.* 17:373, 1969.

105. Baldini, M. G.: Nature of the platelet defect in the Wiskott-Aldrich syndrome. *Ann. N.Y. Acad. Sci.* 201:437, 1972.

106. Buchanan, G. R., and Handin, R. I.: Platelet function in the Chediak-Higashi syndrome. *Blood* 47:941, 1976.

107. Lages, B., and Weiss, H. J.: Biphasic aggregation responses to ADP and epinephrine in some storage pool deficient platelets: Relationship to the role of endogenous ADP in platelet aggregation and secretion. *Thromb. Haemost.* 43:147, 1980.

108. White, J. G., and Witkop, C. J.: Effects of normal and aspirin platelets on defective secondary aggregation in the Hermansky-Pudlak syndrome: A test for storage pool deficient platelets. *Am. J. Pathol.* 68:57, 1972.

109. Gerrard, J. M., White, J. G., Rao, G.H.R., Krivit, W., and Witkop, C.J., Jr.: Labile aggregation stimulating substance (LASS): The factor from storage pool deficient platelets correcting defective aggregation and release of aspirin treated normal platelets. *Br. J. Haematol.* 29:657, 1975.

110. Gerritsen, S. W., Akkerman, J.-W. N., and Sixma, J. J.: Correction of the bleeding time in patients with storage pool deficiency by infusion of cryoprecipitate. *Br. J. Haematol.* 40:153, 1978.

111. Czapek, E. E., et al.: Intermediate syndrome of platelet dysfunction. *Blood* 52:103, 1978.

112. Malmsten, C., Hamberg, M., Svensson, J., and Samuelsson, B.: Physiological role of an endoperoxide in human platelets: Hemostatic defect due to platelet cyclo-oxygenase deficiency. *Proc. Natl. Acad. Sci. U.S.A.* 72:1446, 1975.

113. Lages, B., Malmsten, C., Weiss, H. J., and Samuelsson, B.: Impaired platelet responses to thromboxane A_2 and defective calcium mobilization in a patient with a bleeding disorder. *Blood* 57:545, 1981.

114. Deykin, D., Rittenhouse-Simmons, S., and Russell, F. A.: Impaired Ca^{2+} mobilization: A possible cause of platelet dysfunction. *Clin. Res.* 21:503A, 1978.

115. Bowie, E. J. W., and Owen, C. A.: Thrombopathy. *Semin. Hematol.* 5:73, 1968.

116. Owen, C. A., and Thompson, J. H.: Soybean phosphatides in prothrombin-consumption and thromboplastin-generation tests: Their use in recognizing "thrombasthenic hemophilia." *Am. J. Clin. Pathol.* 33:197, 1960.

117. Soulier, J. P., and Larrieu, M. J.: Syndrome de Willebrand-Jurgens et thrombopathies. *Rev. Hematol.* 9:77, 1954.

118. Ulutin, O. N., and Karaca, M.: A study on the pathogenesis of thrombopathia using the platelet osmotic-resistance test. *Br. J. Haematol.* 5:302, 1959.

119. Weiss, H. J., and Eichelberger, J. W.: The detection of platelet defects in patients with mild bleeding disorders: Use of a quantitative assay for platelet factor 3. *Am. J. Med.* 32:872, 1962.

120. Bowie, E. J., Thompson, J. H., and Owen, C. A.: A new abnormality of platelet function. *Thromb. Diath. Haemorrh.* 11:195, 1964.

121. Johnson, S. A., Monto, R. W., and Caldwell, M. J.: A new approach to the thrombocytopathies: Thrombocytopathy A. *Thromb. Diath. Haemorrh.* 2:279, 1958.

122. Weiss, H. J., et al.: Isolated deficiency of platelet procoagulant activity. *Am. J. Med.* 67:206, 1979.

123. Miletich, J. P., et al.: Deficiency of factor X_a-factor V_a binding sites on the platelets of a patient with a bleeding disorder. *Blood* 54:1015, 1979.

124. Onel, D., Ulutin, S. B., and Ulutin, O. N.: Platelet defect in a case of Ehlers-Danlos syndrome. *Acta Haematol.* 50:238, 1973.

125. Hathaway, W. E., Solomons, C. C., and Ott, J. E.: Platelet function and pyrophosphates in osteogenesis imperfects. *Blood* 39:500, 1972.

126. Baldini, M. G.: Nature of the platelet defect in the Wiskott-Aldrich syndrome. *Ann. N.Y. Acad. Sci.* 201:437, 1972.

127. Lusher, J. M., et al.: The May-Hegglin anomaly: Platelet function, ultrastructure and chromosome studies. *Blood* 32:950, 1968.

128. Beck, E. S., and Baumgartner, H. R.: Zur Frage der Thrombopathie bei May-Hegglin-Anomalie. *Schweiz. Med. Wochenschr.* 100:330, 1970.

129. Epstein, C. J., et al.: Hereditary macrothrombocytopathia, nephritis and deafness. *Am. J. Med.* 52:299, 1972.

130. Corby, D. G., Putnam, C. W., and Greene, H. L.: Impaired platelet function in glucose-6-phosphatase deficiency. *J. Pediatr.* 85:71, 1974.

131. Czapek, E. E., Deykin, D., and Salzman, E. W.: Platelet dysfunction in glycogen storage disease type I. *Blood* 41:225, 1973.

132. Maurer, H. M., McCue, C. M., Caul, J., and Still, W. J. S.: Impairment in platelet aggregation in congenital heart disease. *Blood* 40:207, 1972.

133. Boullin, D. J., and O'Brien, R. A.: Abnormalities of 5-hydroxytryptamine uptake and binding by blood platelets from children with Down's syndrome. *J. Physiol.* 212:287, 1971.

134. Inceman, S., Caen, J., and Bernard, J.: Aggregation, adhesion, and viscous metamorphosis of platelets in congenital fibrinogen deficiencies. *J. Lab. Clin. Med.* 68:21, 1966.

135. Weiss, H. J., and Rogers, J.: Fibrinogen and platelets in the primary arrest of bleeding: Studies in 2 patients with congenital afibrinogenemia. *N. Eng. J. Med.* 285:369, 1971.

136. Hardisty, R. M., and Hutton, R. A.: Platelet aggregation and the availability of platelet factor 3. *Br. J. Haematol.* 12:764, 1966.

137. Chesney, C., Colman, R. W., and Pechet, L.: A syndrome of platelet-release abnormality and mild hemophilia. *Blood* 43:821, 1974.

138. Crowell, E. B., Jr., and Eisner, E. V.: Familial association of thrombopathia and antihemophilic factor (AHF, factor VIII) deficiency. *Blood* 40:227, 1972.

139. Dowling, S. V., et al.: Platelet release abnormality associated with a variant of von Willebrand's disease. *Blood* 47:265, 1976.

CHAPTER *147*

Acquired qualitative platelet disorders

HARVEY J. WEISS

Qualitative platelet defects have been described in a number of acquired disorders in which abnormal bleeding may be a feature. The nature of the bleeding diathesis in some of these conditions is complex, and the extent to which abnormalities in platelet function contribute to this is not always clear. Some of the defects are similar to those described in congenital disorders of platelet function (see Chap. 146).

Uremia

PLATELET DEFECTS

Abnormal bleeding was formerly a frequent and sometimes fatal complication of uremia, but the incidence of hemorrhagic complications appears to be decreasing [1]. Although decreased plasma coagulation factor levels and thrombocytopenia may occur, these abnormalities are rarely sufficient to account for the hemorrhagic tendency [1]. The bleeding time is often prolonged, suggesting an abnormality in platelet function [2]. The most consistent findings are qualitative platelet defects, demonstrable by a variety of tests. Thus the platelet coagulant activity (platelet factor 3) is abnormal in some patients [3–8]. Decreased platelet retention in glass bead filters has also been repeatedly demonstrated [2,9–11].

Studies of platelet aggregation in uremia have yielded conflicting results. Abnormalities of aggregation induced by collagen and epinephrine have been reported [12]. Abnormalities of ADP-induced aggregation have also been found, including impaired primary aggregation [2,13], rapid disaggregation [13], and an increased ADP requirement for secondary aggregation [14]. In other studies, however, the first and second waves of ADP-induced aggregation [9,15] and the amount of ADP required to induce second-phase aggregation [15] were normal. Enhanced second-phase aggregation has also been observed [16]. These discrepant findings could be related to differences in the calcium concentration used in the tests [15] or to patient selection. There was a high incidence of hemorrhagic manifestations among some patients studied [2], whereas hemorrhage was not a feature of patients studied by other investigators [15].

PATHOGENESIS

The cause of the abnormal platelet function sometimes seen in uremia is not clear. In some studies, normal platelets were made defective by incubating them with uremic plasma [4,6], although negative results in this type of test have also been reported [1]. The defective platelet function and the hemostatic abnormality largely disappear 24 to 48 h after peritoneal dialysis or hemodialysis [1,2,12], suggesting the presence of a low-molecular-weight inhibitor in uremic plasma. However, none has been definitely identified. Addition of urea to normal platelet-rich plasma decreased platelet aggregation [17] and retention in glass bead filters [10], but in other studies urea had no effect on ADP-induced aggregation [2,9], celite-induced platelet factor 3 availability [7], or ADP-induced platelet factor 3 availability [6]. Infusion of urea into normal volunteers increased the bleeding time and decreased platelet retention in glass bead filters [11]. This was observed only after 24 h, suggesting that the platelet and hemostatic defects in uremia may be due to a metabolite of urea, or perhaps to a time-dependent effect of urea on platelets. Defects of ADP-induced aggregation and platelet factor 3 availability have also been observed after the addition to platelet-rich plasma of guanidinosuccinic acid, a metabolite of urea found both in uremic serum and in urine [6,14]. However, guanidinosuccinic acid does not inhibit celite-induced platelet factor 3 availability [7], and its inhibitory effect on platelet function is critically dependent on the concentration of calcium used in the test [14]. The decreased platelet retention in glass bead filters does not appear to be the result of any quantitative or qualitative defect in the factor VIII/von Willebrand factor [18,19]. In uremic patients the plasma concentrations of both factor VIII–related antigen (FVIIIR:Ag) and ristocetin cofactor (FVIIIR:RCo) have been, if anything, increased [18].

The mechanism through which platelet factor 3 activity is decreased and the relationship of this finding to the hemostatic impairment in uremia are not clear. It seems unlikely that abnormalities in platelet factor 3 per se can account for the prolonged bleeding time in these patients (see Chap. 146), which is probably due to abnormalities in adhesion and aggregation.

In uremic patients production of prostacyclin (PGI$_2$, see Chap. 129), a potent inhibitor of platelet aggregation, is increased in vein specimens [20,21], while production of malondialdehyde, which reflects prostaglandin and thromboxane A$_2$ synthesis, was decreased in platelets. Both of these defects could contribute to the impairment of primary hemostasis in these patients.

CLINICAL FEATURES

The in vitro abnormalities in platelet aggregation and retention appear to correlate well with clinical bleeding [2]. The presence or absence of platelet abnormalities in uremia does not appear to be related to the nature of the underlying renal disease. They may be related to the elevation of the blood urea nitrogen [5,11,22], but this has been disputed [7]. In some studies abnormalities appeared to correlate with the duration of uremia [5], while in others this did not appear to be the case [22]. The prolonged bleeding times of uremic patients may be shortened by administration of cryoprecipitate [19]. The reason for this effect, which may be a useful form of therapy in patients with bleeding problems, is not clear at present.

As indicated above, the hemostatic and platelet defects usually disappear after peritoneal dialysis or hemodialysis.

Myeloproliferative disorders

Qualitative platelet defects have been described in all the myeloproliferative disorders (see Chaps. 23 to 28) and may, in some cases, account for the bleeding tendency which is a common feature of these diseases. The basic defect(s) which underlie the abnormalities in platelet function in the myeloproliferative disorders remains to be determined. While these disorders have many features in common, the platelet abnormalities may not be identical in all cases. The clinical significance of the observed platelet defects is not established. In some studies there was a good correlation between platelet abnormalities and clinical bleeding [23], but abnormalities have also been observed in asymptomatic patients [24]. Bleeding or thrombotic complications may correlate with the results of tests measuring various platelet coagulant activities [25].

PRIMARY THROMBOCYTHEMIA
In primary thrombocythemia (see Chap. 26) a variety of qualitative platelet defects have been described. Epinephrine-induced aggregation has been either completely absent [23,24,26,27] or markedly reduced [28], perhaps because of a reduction in the number of α-adrenergic receptors in the platelets of patients with this disorder [29]. ADP-induced aggregation has been either moderately reduced [24,26,28] or normal [27,30]. Collagen-induced aggregation has been reported to be both normal [24] and decreased [26,28,31–33]. Platelet retention in glass bead filters is usually decreased [34,35]. Platelet factor 3 availability was abnormal in some studies, but normal in others [24,26]. Platelet function tests are usually normal in patients with reactive thrombocytosis [23,24,34] (see Chap. 145).

The pathogenesis of the platelet defect in thrombocythemia is not entirely clear. A diminished content [36] and uptake [24,34] of serotonin has suggested a membrane defect [34]. However, these abnormalities are also found in the platelets of patients with storage pool deficiency (see Chap. 146), and decreased levels of both platelet ATP [34] and ADP [28] as well as increased ATP/ADP ratios [32] have been reported in thrombocythemia. It has been suggested that functionally defective platelets may result from platelet damage during disseminated intravascular platelet aggregation [37]. This could account for both the thrombotic and hemorrhagic complications which are characteristic features of this disorder. Response to myelosuppressive therapy has been variable; platelet function often returns to normal but may remain abnormal.

Several patients have been described with a syndrome of repeated attacks of digital ischemia and the isolated finding of an increased platelet count. Their platelets undergo spontaneous aggregation in vitro. Both the latter finding and the clinical symptoms disappeared after treatment with aspirin or with aspirin and dipyridamole [38]. The precise nature of the disorder is not clear, but these patients may have primary thrombocythemia or some variant of that disease.

POLYCYTHEMIA VERA
Abnormalities of platelet factor 3 activity [39], platelet retention, and uptake of serotonin [34] have been reported in polycythemia vera. An unexplained finding is the increased number of free red cells present after the clot has retracted (red cell "fallout" phenomenon). Histologic study of polycythemia clots has demonstrated breaks in the fibrin strands through which red cells could escape [40]. The platelets of some polycythemic

patients have decreased antifibrinolytic activity [41], but normal antifibrinolytic activity has been reported for others [42]. Studies of platelet aggregation have disclosed abnormalities similar to those in primary thrombocythemia [27,32,33,43,44]. The most frequent finding is an impairment of epinephrine-induced aggregation, but aggregation by collagen and ADP are often abnormal as well [32,33,34]. In one study, no relationship was observed between the platelet abnormalities and thrombohemorrhagic episodes [44]. The abnormalities frequently disappear after either myelosuppressive therapy or phlebotomy [44].

MYELOID METAPLASIA
Decreased platelet retention in glass bead filters and abnormal platelet factor 3 activity have also been described in myelofibrosis with myeloid metaplasia [34,45]. Various abnormalities of platelet aggregation, possibly due to a storage pool defect, have also been reported in some patients with this disorder [26,32,33].

CHRONIC MYELOGENOUS LEUKEMIA
Abnormal responses to one or more aggregating agents have been described for platelets from patients with chronic granulocytic leukemia [26,31–33,43,46]. Abnormalities were not found in all patients, and the clinical significance of the findings is not clear. A storage pool type of defect, similar to that described in other myeloproliferative disorders, has been reported [32,47]. Prostaglandin metabolism in response to exogenous arachidonic acid is normal [47]. The plasmas of patients with this disorder have also been reported to show an increased ability to degrade ADP [31,48].

Acute leukemia

Abnormal platelet factor 3 availability has been reported in acute leukemia [49,50]. Defects in collagen-, ADP-, and epinephrine-induced aggregation also occur [51,52] and may be associated with impaired release of ADP [51]. The latter may in some cases be due to both a deficiency of storage pool ADP and a defect in the release mechanism [53]. An abnormal release mechanism has also been indicated by ultrastructural studies [53] and by the finding that thrombin and collagen stimulation fail to elicit either normal consumption of ATP [53] or a net increase in ^{14}C-glucose utilization, lactate production, and $^{14}CO_2$ production [54]. An abnormality in the binding of thrombin to the platelets of patients with acute leukemia has also been reported [55].

Dysproteinemias

Hemorrhagic manifestations frequently occur in dysproteinemias. In one large series, excessive bleeding was observed in 15 percent of patients with IgG myeloma and in over 38 percent with IgA myeloma or macroglobulinemia [56]. The bleeding manifestations have been attributed to abnormalities in the coagulation mechanism, hyperviscosity, quantitative and qualitative platelet defects, and miscellaneous causes [56,57]. In most cases the hemostatic and laboratory abnormalities are related to the concentration of the paraprotein [56,58] and may be corrected by plasmapheresis [57].

Several platelet defects have been described. In macroglobulinemia, abnormalities include decreased platelet retention in glass bead filters [56], impaired platelet aggregation [59,60], decreased adhesiveness of platelets in skin wounds [61], and decreased platelet factor 3 availability [8,56,58]. Impaired factor 3 availability in one patient was attributed to coating of the platelet membrane by the macroglobulin [62]. Inhibition of platelet aggregation by abnormal macroglobulin has also been reported [63,64].

The higher incidence of bleeding in IgA myeloma than in IgG myeloma appears to correlate with the greater frequency of prolonged bleeding times and abnormal platelet retention [56].

Liver disease

The bleeding diathesis in liver disease is complex and has usually been attributed to deficiencies of plasma clotting factors, thrombocytopenia, or enhanced fibrinolysis (see Chap. 156). Qualitative platelet abnormalities, such as decreased platelet factor 3 availability [8,65], impaired adhesiveness in vivo [66], and defective platelet aggregation [67,68], have also been described. In several studies there was a good correlation between impaired platelet aggregation and prolongation of the thrombin time [68,69]. A dialyzable factor present in the plasma of many cirrhotic patients can inhibit the aggregation of normal platelets [67,69]. Fibrinogen degradation products resulting from proteolysis of fibrinogen by plasmin can impair platelet aggregation [70–73] and may be responsible [69] for the abnormal platelet aggregation in liver disease [74,75], but this does not appear to be the complete explanation [68].

Immune thrombocytopenia

Increased platelet destruction in idiopathic thrombocytopenic purpura is usually due to antiplatelet antibodies (see Chap. 142). This mechanism has also been proposed for the thrombocytopenia that occurs in patients with systemic lupus erythematosus [76]. Abnormalities of platelet function, such as decreased platelet factor 3 availability [8,77] or impaired platelet aggregation [79–80], in some patients with these disorders suggests that the platelets might be qualitatively abnormal as well. Abnormalities of both platelet factor 3 availability [77] and aggregation [78,79] can sometimes be induced in normal platelets by incubating them with either serum or serum fractions obtained from some patients with

these disorders. However, the presence of this inhibitor of platelet function does not correlate with the presence of antiplatelet antibody [78,79]. In addition, the relationship of the platelet defects in these disorders to the hemorrhagic manifestation is not clear. Many patients have a shorter bleeding time than would be predicted from their platelet count, possibly due to the presence of younger, more effectively functioning platelets [81]. Finally, an immune mechanism, without thrombocytopenia, has been proposed to explain the abnormal platelet aggregation observed in some patients with "easy bruising" [82].

Acquired storage pool deficiency

The characteristic findings in congenital storage pool deficiency are described in Chap. 146, and acquired types of this disorder, observed in patients with myeloproliferative disorders and acute leukemia, are cited above [32,47,53]. Acquired storage pool deficiency due to depletion of either α granules or dense granules has also been described in other conditions, such as cardiopulmonary bypass surgery [83,84], a collagenvascular disorder associated with a serum factor injurious to platelets [85], alcoholism [86], renal allograft rejection [87], hemolytic uremic syndrome [87], disseminated intravascular coagulation [87,88], and systemic lupus erythematosus [88,89], and in patients with increased platelet-bound IgG but normal platelet counts [89]. In some cases the storage pool defect may be related to the presence in the circulation of "exhausted" platelets following their in vivo exposure to inducers of the release reaction such as damaged endothelium, thrombin, and immune complexes [87].

Other conditions

Impaired platelet aggregation has been described in scurvy [90], pernicious anemia [91], infectious mononucleosis [92], and leukemic reticuloendotheliosis [93]; after transfusion of cryoprecipitate [94]; following major surgery [95]; in some atopic patients [96]; in congenital heart disease [97]; and in patients with Bartter's syndrome [98]. Decreased retention of platelets in glass bead filters has been described in hypothyroidism [99]. In addition, enhanced platelet function has been described in such disorders as ischemic heart disease and diabetes, under conditions of stress, after smoking cigarettes, and in type II hyperlipoproteinemia [100,101].

Drug-induced defects

Impaired hemostasis has been associated with the administration of a number of pharmacologic agents and, in some cases, can be attributed to abnormalities in platelet function. In addition, drugs may inhibit some aspect of platelet reactivity without producing an impairment of hemostasis. Since platelet-induced thrombosis may play a role in a variety of clinical disorders, the possible therapeutic uses of antiplatelet drugs have received attention. Various aspects of platelet pharmacology and its clinical application have been reviewed [100,102,103].

ASPIRIN AND OTHER PROSTAGLANDIN INHIBITORS
Ingestion of aspirin in doses (0.3 to 1.5 g) that do not affect the prothrombin time can prolong the bleeding time in normal subjects [104–107], and its effect on hemostasis may be disproportionately greater in patients with bleeding disorders [104].

Aspirin ingestion impairs the platelet secretory process (release reaction) and thereby results in abnormalities in collagen-induced aggregation and in the second phase of ADP- and epinephrine-induced aggregation [106–110]. In addition, platelet thrombus formation on subendothelium is reduced, although adhesion is unaltered [111]. These defects in platelet-platelet interaction may account for the impairment of hemostasis induced by aspirin ingestion. The effects of aspirin in vitro are achieved with concentrations readily attained in ordinary clinical usage. In adults, oral aspirin doses of 300 to 600 and 2400 to 3600 mg appear to be equally effective in suppressing collagen-induced aggregation [112,113]. The inhibitory effects of a single oral dose of aspirin on both collagen-induced ADP release [107] and epinephrine-induced aggregation [109] may be detected for 4 to 7 days. This period roughly corresponds to the platelet life-span and originally suggested that aspirin produces an irreversible effect on the platelet.

Clinically, the aspirin-induced hemostatic effect must be considered relatively mild. However, aspirin should be avoided when optimum hemostasis is desirable and in patients with bleeding disorders. The analgesic agents acetaminophen, propoxyphene, and codeine do not inhibit platelet function or prolong the bleeding time [114–116].

Aspirin inhibits platelet aggregation and secretion by its effects on arachidonic acid metabolism. Initially, it was found that aspirin prevents the synthesis of platelet prostaglandins [117]. Subsequent studies showed that aspirin irreversibly inactivates a fatty acid cyclooxygenase that converts arachidonic acid to the prostaglandin endoperoxides G_2 and H_2 [118,119], the precursors of various platelet prostaglandins and, more important, of the potent platelet aggregant thromboxane A_2 [120]. Platelet aggregation and secretion in response to a variety of agonists is believed to be due, in part, to the formation of thromboxane A_2. Hence the inhibition of thromboxane A_2 synthesis by aspirin probably accounts for its observed antiplatelet properties. The overall effect of aspirin on hemostasis (and thrombosis as well) is complicated by its ability to inhibit the conversion of arachidonic acid to PGG_2/H_2 in the vessel wall and endothelial cells as well in platelets [121–123]. In endothelial cells, PGG_2/H_2 is converted primarily

to prostaglandin I_2 (prostacyclin), a potent natural *inhibitor* of platelet aggregation [121–123]. Hence, in theory, this might counteract to some extent the effects on platelets.

The effects of other nonsteroidal anti-inflammatory drugs (indomethacin, phenylbutazone, meclofenamic acid, ibuprofen) on platelets appear to be similar to that of aspirin. In comparative in vitro studies, aspirin, indomethacin, and meclofenamic acid at equimolar concentrations were found to be about equally potent inhibitors of platelet function, whereas phenylbutazone was a weaker inhibitor [116,124]. These drugs also inhibit the synthesis of platelet prostaglandins [125]. The prolonged inhibition of platelet function after a single oral dose may be unique for aspirin. For example, the effect of indomethacin is short-lived and after any size dose is no longer detectable after 6 h [126]. The uricosuric agent sulfinpyrazone also inhibits platelet cyclooxygenase activity [127], although in the usual clinical doses its effects on platelet aggregation appear to be less than that of the nonsteroidal anti-inflammatory drugs [128].

PLASMA EXPANDERS
The infusion of plasma expanders, such as dextran and hydroxyethyl starch, is associated with a prolongation of the bleeding time which cannot be explained by the slight decrease in the platelet count which sometimes occurs [129]. The effect is dose-related and is more likely to occur with a dextran of molecular weight greater than 65,000 daltons [130].

Dextran interferes with platelet factor 3 activity, both in vitro and in vivo [131]. Perhaps more relevant to the defect in hemostasis, platelet retention in glass bead filters decreases following the administration of 1 to 2 liters of clinical dextran of M_r 65,000 to 80,000 daltons [130,132]. This defect in retention may be related to adsorption of dextran onto the platelets [133], with consequent alteration of the surface charge, as reflected by measurements of electrophoretic mobility [134]. Since adsorption of dextran onto platelets occurs rapidly, it might be anticipated that its effects would be observed soon after transfusion. However, the maximal prolongation of the bleeding time [129] and the most pronounced decrease in platelet retention [130,132] occur 4 to 8 h after completion of the infusion, suggesting alternative mechanisms. Dextran infusion may produce a time-dependent change in the factor VIII complex identical to that seen in von Willebrand's disease [135].

OTHER DRUGS
Other drugs modify platelet function through several mechanisms [102,103]. Drugs which inhibit platelet function through their effects on membranes include ethanol, local and general anesthetics, phenothiazines, tricyclic antidepressants, and antihistamines. Dipyridamole increases platelet cyclic AMP by inhibiting phosphodiesterase. Other drugs with antiplatelet properties include clofibrate, vitamin E, ticlopidine, furosemide,

and vasodilators, such as hydralazine and nitroprusside. It has not been established that any of these agents seriously impairs hemostasis, although several have been tested for their antithrombotic properties. In contrast, large doses of penicillin and carbenecillin have been shown to prolong the bleeding time and inhibit platelet aggregation [136].

The effects of heparin and coumarin drugs on platelets are controversial. In ordinary clinical doses, coumarin drugs do not inhibit platelet aggregation, as studied in the aggregometer, but defects in platelet function, particularly those influenced by thrombin formation, have been described using other tests [137,138]. Although heparin inhibits platelet aggregation by thrombin [137], very large doses are required in vitro to inhibit aggregation by other agents [139]. Small doses of heparin may actually potentiate platelet aggregation [140], and it has been suggested that this may render the platelet temporarily refractory to other agents [141]. In addition, heparin can sometimes cause thrombocytopenia (see Chap. 142).

References

1. Rabiner, S. F.: Uremic bleeding, in *Progress in Hemostasis and Thrombosis*, edited by T. H. Spaet. Grune & Stratton, New York, 1972, vol. 1, p. 233.
2. Stewart, J. H., and Castaldi, P. A.: Uraemic bleeding: A reversible platelet defect corrected by dialysis. *Q. J. Med.* (new series) 36:409, 1967.
3. Lewis, J. H., Zucker, M. B., and Ferguson, J. H.: Bleeding tendency in uremia. *Blood* 11:1073, 1956.
4. Cahalane, S. F., Johnson, S. A., Monto, R. W., and Caldwell, M. J.: Acquired thrombocytopathy: Observations on the coagulation defect in uremia. *Am. J. Clin. Pathol.* 30:507, 1958.
5. Cheney, K., and Bonnin, J. A.: Haemorrhage, platelet dysfunction and other coagulation defects in uremia. *Br. J. Haematol.* 8:215, 1962.
6. Horowitz, H. I., Cohen, B. D., Martinez, P., and Payayoanou, M. F.: Defective ADP-induced platelet factor 3 activation in uremia. *Blood* 30:331, 1967.
7. Rabiner, S. F., and Hiodek, O.: Platelet factor 3 in normal subjects and patients with renal failure. *J. Clin. Invest.* 47:901, 1968.
8. Weiss, H. J., and Eichelberger, J. W.: Secondary thrombocytopathia: Platelet factor 3 in various disease states. *Arch. Intern. Med.* 112:827, 1963.
9. Salzman, E. W., and Neri, L. J.: Adhesiveness of blood platelets in uremia. *Thromb. Diath. Haemorrh.* 15:84, 1966.
10. Hellem, A. J., Odegaard, A. E., and Skalhegg, B. A.: Platelet adhesiveness in chronic renal failure. *Abstracts, X Congress of the International Society on Haematology*, Stockholm, 1964, p. k:1.
11. Eknoyan, G., Wacksman, S. J., Glueck, H. I., and Will, J. J.: Platelet function in renal failure. *N. Engl. J. Med.* 280:677, 1969.
12. Joist, J. H., Pechan, J., Schikowski, U., Hübner, G., and Gross, R.: Untersuchungen zur Natur und Ätologie der urämischen Thrombocytopathie. *Verh. Dtsch. Ges. Inn. Med.* 75:476, 1969.
13. Holdrinet, A., Ewals, M., Reichert, W. J., and Haanen, C.: Mathematical correlation between ADP-induced aggregation and subsequent disaggregation. *Scand. J. Haematol.* 6:354, 1969.
14. Horowitz, H. I., Stein, I. M., Cohen, B. D., and White, J. G.: Further studies on the platelet inhibitory effect of guanidinosuccinic acid: Its role in uremic bleeding. *Am. J. Med.* 49:336, 1970.
15. Ballard, H. S., and Marcus, A. J.: Primary and secondary platelet aggregation in uraemia. *Scand. J. Haematol.* 9:198, 1972.
16. Hassanein, A. A., McNicol, G. P., and Douglas, A. S.: Relationship between platelet function tests in normal and uraemic subjects. *J. Clin. Pathol.* 23:402, 1970.
17. Davis, J. W., McField, J. R., Phillips, P. L., and Graham, B. A.: Effects of exogenous urea, creatinine, and guanidinosuccinic acid on human platelet aggregation in vitro. *Blood* 39:388, 1972.
18. Warrell, R. P., Hultin, M. B., and Coller, B. S.: Increased factor VIII/von Willebrand factor in renal failure. *Am. J. Med.* 66:226, 1979.
19. Janson, P. A., Jubelirer, S. J., Weinstein, M. J., and Deykin, D.: Treatment of the bleeding tendency in uremia with cryoprecipitate. *N. Eng. J. Med.* 303:1318, 1980.
20. Remuzzi, G., Mecca, G., Cavenaghi, A. E., Donati, M. B., and de Gaetano, G.: Prostacyclin-like activity and bleeding in renal failure. *Lancet* 2:1195, 1977.
21. Remuzzi, G., et al.: Altered platelet function and vascular prostaglandin-generation in patients with renal failure and prolonged bleeding time. *Thromb. Res.* 13:1007, 1978.
22. Castaldi, P. A., Rozenburg, M. C., and Steward, J. H.: The bleeding disorder of uremia. *Lancet* 2:66, 1966.
23. Zucker, S., and Mielke, C. H.: Classification of thrombocytosis based on platelet function tests: Correlation with hemorrhagic and thrombotic complications. *J. Lab. Clin. Med.* 80:385, 1972.
24. Spaet, T. H., Lejnieks, I., Gaynor, I., and Goldstein, M. L.: Defective platelets in essential thrombocythemia. *Arch. Int. Med.* 124:135, 1969.
25. Walsh, P. N., Murphy, S., and Barry, W. E.: The role of platelets in the pathogenesis of thrombosis and hemorrhage in patients with thrombocytosis. *Thromb. Haemost.* 38:1085, 1977.
26. Inceman, S., and Tangun, Y.: Platelet defects in the myeloproliferative disorders. *Ann. N.Y. Acad. Sci.* 201:251, 1972.
27. Neemeh, J. A., Bowie, E. J., Thompson, J. H., Didisheim, P., and Owen, C. A., Jr.: Quantitation of platelet aggregation in myeloproliferative disorders. *Am. J. Clin. Pathol.* 57:336, 1972.
28. Kubisz, P.: Myeloproliferative disorders and platelet functions. *Folia Haematol. (Leipz.)* 99:202, 1973.
29. Kaywin, P., McDonough, M., Insel, P. A., and Shattil, S. J.: Platelet function in essential thrombocythemia: Decreased epinephrine responsiveness associated with deficiency of platelet alpha-adrenergic receptors. *N. Engl. J. Med.* 299:505, 1978.
30. Herrmann, R. P., Gallon, W., Jackson, J. M., and Woodliff, H. J.: Idiopathic thrombocythaemia: A review of seven cases in western Australia. *Aust. N.Z. J. Med.* 3:486, 1973.
31. Caen, J. P., Sultan, Y., and Delobel, J.: Les Thrombopathies acquises. *Nouv. Rev. Fr. Hematol.* 9:553, 1969.
32. Nishimura, J., Okamoto, S., and Ibayashi, H.: Abnormalities of platelet adenine nucleotides in patients with myeloproliferative disorders. *Thromb. Haemost.* 41:787, 1979.
33. Phadke, K., Dean, S., and Pitney, W. R.: Platelet dysfunction in myeloproliferative syndromes. *Am. J. Hematol.* 10:57, 1981.
34. McClure, P. D., Ingram, G. I. G., Stacey, R. S., Glass, T. H., and Matchett, M. O.: Platelet function tests in thrombocythaemia and thrombocytosis. *Br. J. Haematol.* 12:478, 1966.
35. Cronberg, S., Nilsson, I. M., and Gydell, K.: Haemorrhagic thrombocythaemia due to defect in platelet adhesiveness. *Scand. J. Haematol.* 2:208, 1965.
36. Hardisty, R. M., Wolf, H. H.: Haemorrhagic thrombocythemia: A clinical and laboratory study. *Br. J. Haematol.* 1:390, 1955.
37. Boughton, B. J., Corbett, W. E. N., and Ginsberg, A. D.: Myeloproliferative disorders: A paradox of in vivo and in vitro platelet function. *J. Clin. Pathol.* 30:228, 1977.
38. Bierme, R., Boneu, B., Guiraud, B., and Pris, J.: Aspirin and recurrent painful toes and fingers in thrombocythaemia. *Lancet* 1:432, 1972.
39. Abraham, J. P., Johnson, S. A., and Ulutin, O. N.: Platelet function in polycythemia. *J. Lab. Clin. Med.* 54:785, 1959.
40. James, T. N., Johnson, S. A., Diab, G., and Caldwell, J.: Histology of platelet-plasma clots from normal subjects and patients with abnormal coagulation. *Blood* 19:731, 1962.
41. de Vries, S., Braat-van Straaten, M. A. J., Muller, E., and Wettermark, M.: Antiplasmin deficiency in polycythemia vera: A form of thrombopathy. *Thromb. Diath. Haemorrh.* 6:446, 1961.

42. Kwaan, H. C., and Suwanella, N.: Inhibitors of fibrinolysis in platelets in polycythemia vera and thrombocytosis. *Br. J. Haematol.* 21:313, 1971.

43. Tangun, Y.: Platelet aggregation and platelet factor 3 activity in myeloproliferative disorders. *Thromb. Diath. Haemorrh.* 25:241, 1971.

44. Berger, S., Aledort, L. M., Gilbert, H. S., Hanson, J. P., and Wasserman, L. R.: Abnormalities of platelet function in patients with polycythemia vera. *Cancer Res.* 33:2683, 1973.

45. Didisheim, P., and Bunting, K.: Abnormal platelet function in myelofibrosis. *Am. J. Clin. Pathol.* 45:566, 1966.

46. Cardamone, J. M., Edson, J. R., McArthur, J. R., and Jacob, H. S.: Abnormalities of platelet function in the myeloproliferative disorders. *JAMA* 221:270, 1972.

47. Gerrard, J. M., et al.: Platelet storage pool deficiency and prostaglandin synthesis in chronic granulocytic leukaemia. *Br. J. Haematol.* 40:597, 1978.

48. Pinkhas, J., Chivot, J. J., Michel, H., and Caen, J.: Adenosine metabolism in plasma and platelets. IV. Elevated plasmatic adenosine deaminase activity, impaired platelet ^{14}C-adenosine incorporation and hemostatic dysfunction in chronic myeloid leukemia. *Rev. Eur. Etud. Clin. Biol.* 15:1108, 1970.

49. Friedman, I. A., Schwartz, S. O., and Leithold, S. L.: Platelet function defects with bleeding: Early manifestations of acute leukemia. *Arch. Intern. Med.* 113:177, 1964.

50. Bonnin, J. A.: The management of thrombocytopenic states with particular reference to platelet thromboplastic function. II. Acute leukemia and aplastic anaemia. *Br. J. Haematol.* 7:261, 1961.

51. Cowan, D. H., and Haut, M. J.: Platelet function in acute leukemia. *J. Lab. Clin. Med.* 79:893, 1972.

52. Caen, J., et al.: Platelet aggregation and populations in acute leukaemias. *Haemostasis* 1:61, 1972.

53. Cowan, D. H., Graham, R. C., Jr., and Baunach, D.: The platelet defect in leukemia: Platelet ultrastructure, adenine nucleotide metabolism and the release reaction. *J. Clin. Invest.* 56:188, 1975.

54. Cowan, D. H.: Platelet metabolism in acute leukemia. *J. Lab. Clin. Med.* 82:54, 1973.

55. Ganguly, P., Sutherland, S. B., and Bradford, N. R.: Defective binding of thrombin to platelets in myeloid leukemia. *Br. J. Haematol.* 39:599, 1978.

56. Perkins, H. A., MacKenzie, M. R., and Fudenberg, H. H.: Hemostatic defects in dysproteinemias. *Blood* 35:695, 1970.

57. Lackner, H.: Hemostatic abnormalities associated with dysproteinemias. *Semin. Hematol.* 10:125, 1973.

58. Penny, R., Castaldi, P. A., and Whitsed, H. M.: Inflammation and haemostasis in paraproteinemias. *Br. J. Haematol.* 20:35, 1971.

59. Rozenberg, M. C., and Dintenfass, L.: Platelet aggregation in Waldenstrom's macroglobulinaemia. *Thromb. Diath. Haemorrh.* 14:202, 1965.

60. Saraya, A. K., Kasturi, J., and Kishan, R.: A study of haemostasis in macroglobulinaemia. *Acta Haematol.* 47:33, 1972.

61. Borchgrevink, C. F.: Platelet adhesion in vivo in patients with bleeding disorders. *Acta Med. Scand.* 170:245, 1965.

62. Pachter, M. R., Johnson, S. A., and Basinski, D. H.: The effect of macroglobulins and their dissociation units on release of platelet factor 3. *Thromb. Diath. Haemorrh.* 3:501, 1959.

63. Doumenc, J., Prost, J., Samama, M., and Bousser, J.: Anomalie de l'agrégation au cours de la maladie de Waldenstrom (à propos de 3 cas). *Nouv. Rev. Fr. Hematol.* 6:734, 1966.

64. Bang, N. U., Heidenreich, R. O., and Trygstad, C. W.: Plasma protein requirements for human platelet aggregation. *Ann. N.Y. Acad. Sci.* 201:280, 1972.

65. Mandel, E. E., and Lazerson, J.: Thrombasthenia in liver disease. *N. Engl. J. Med.* 265:56, 1961.

66. Cortet, P., Klepping, C., and Devant, J.: Le Facteur plaquettaire au cours des cirrhoses alcooliques: Étude de l'adhésivité in vivo par le test de Borchgrevink. *Arch. Mal. Appar. Digestif* 53:1041, 1964.

67. Thomas, D. P., Ream, V. J., and Stuart, R. K.: Platelet aggregation in patients with Laennec's cirrhosis of the liver. *N. Engl. J. Med.* 276:1344, 1967.

68. Ballard, H. S., and Marcus, A. J.: Platelet aggregation in portal cirrhosis. *Arch. Intern. Med.* 136:316, 1976.

69. Thomas, D. P.: Abnormalities of platelet aggregation in patients with alcoholic cirrhosis. *Ann. N.Y. Acad. Sci.* 201:243, 1972.

70. Kowalski, E., Kopec, M., and Wegrzynowcz, Z.: Influence of fibrinogen degradation products (FDP) on platelet aggregation, adhesiveness and viscous metamophosis. *Thromb. Diath. Haemorrh.* 10:406, 1964.

71. Kowalski, E.: Fibrinogen derivatives and their biologic activities. *Semin. Hematol* 5:45, 1968.

72. Jerushalmy, Z., and Zucker, M. B.: Some effects of fibrinogen degradation products (FDP) on blood platelets. *Thromb. Diath. Haemorrh.* 15:413, 1966.

73. Larrieu, M. J., Inceman, S., and Marder, V.: Action des produits de dégradation du fibrinogène sur les fonctions plaquettaires. *Nouv. Rev. Fr. Hematol.* 7:691, 1967.

74. Stachurska, J., Latallo, Z., and Kopec, M.: Inhibition of platelet aggregation by dialysable fibrinogen degradation products (FDP). *Thromb. Diath. Haemorrh.* 23:91, 1970.

75. Solum, N. O., Rigollot, C., Budzynski, A. Z., and Marder, V. J.: A quantitative evaluation of the inhibition of platelet aggregation by low molecular weight degradation products of fibrinogen. *Br. J. Haematol.* 24:419, 1973.

76. Karpatkin, S., Strick, N., Karpatkin, M. B., and Siskind, G. W.: Cumulative experience in the detection of antiplatelet antibody in 234 patients with idiopathic thrombocytopenic purpura, systemic lupus erythematosus and other clinical disorders. *Am. J. Med.* 52:776, 1972.

77. Bonnin, J. A.: The management of thrombocytopenic states with particular reference to platelet thromboplastic function. I. Idiopathic and secondary thrombocytopenic purpura. *Br. J. Haematol.* 7:250, 1961.

78. Clancy, R., Jenkins, E., and Firkin, B.: Qualitative platelet abnormalities in idiopathic thrombocytopenic purpura. *N. Engl. J. Med.* 286:622, 1972.

79. Regan, M. G., Lackner, H., and Karpatkin, S.: Platelet function and coagulation profile in lupus erythematosus. *Ann. Intern. Med.* 81:462, 1974.

80. Heyns, A. D., Fraser, J., and Retief, F. P.: Platelet aggregation in chronic idiopathic thrombocytopenic purpura. *J. Clin. Pathol.* 31:1239, 1978.

81. Harker, L. A., and Slichter, S. J.: The bleeding time as a screening test for evaluation of platelet function. *N. Engl. J. Med.* 287:155, 1972.

82. Lackner, H., and Karpatkin, S.: On the "easy bruising" syndrome with normal platelet count. *Ann. Intern. Med.* 83:190, 1975.

83. Beurling-Harbury, C., and Galvan, C. A.: Acquired decrease in platelet secretory ADP associated with increased postoperative bleeding in postcardiopulmonary bypass patients and in patients with severe valvular heart disease. *Blood* 52:13, 1978.

84. Harker, L. A., et al.: Acquired transient platelet dysfunction in patients undergoing cardiopulmonary bypass: Association with selective α granule release. *Blood* 56:824, 1980.

85. Zahavi, J., and Marder, V. J.: Acquired "storage pool disease" of platelets associated with circulating antiplatelet antibodies. *Am. J. Med.* 56:884, 1974.

86. Cowan, D. H., and Graham, R. C., Jr.: Studies of the platelet defect in alcoholism. *Thromb. Diath. Haemorrh.* 33:310, 1975.

87. Pareti, F. I., Capitanio, A., Mannucci, L., Ponticelli, C., and Mannucci, P. M.: Acquired dysfunction due to the circulation of "exhausted" platelets. *Am. J. Med.* 69:235, 1980.

88. Pareti, F. I., Capitanio, A., and Mannucci, P. M.: Acquired storage pool disease in platelets during disseminated intravascular coagulation. *Blood* 48:511, 1976.

89. Weiss, H. J., Rosove, M. H., Lages, B. A., and Kaplan, K. K.: Acquired storage pool deficiency with increased platelet-associated IgG: Report of 5 cases. *Am. J. Med.* 69:712, 1980.

90. Wilson, P., McNicol, G. P., and Douglas, A. S.: Platelet abnormality in human scurvy. *Lancet* 1:975, 1967.

91. Levine, P. H.: A qualitative platelet defect in severe vitamin B$_{12}$ deficiency: Response, hyperresponse, and thrombosis after vitamin B$_{12}$ therapy, *Ann. Intern. Med.* 78:533, 1973.

92. Clancy, R., Jenkins, E., and Firkin, B.: Platelet defect of infectious mononucleosis. *Br. Med. J.* 4:646, 1971.

93. Levine, P. H., and Katayama, I.: The platelet in leukemic reticulo-endotheliosis: Functional and morphological evidence of a qualitative disorder. *Cancer* 36:1353, 1975.

94. Hathaway, W. E., Mahasandana, C., Clarke, S., and Humber, J. R.: Paradoxical bleeding in intensively transfused hemophiliacs: Alteration of platelet function. *Transfusion* 13:6, 1973.

95. O'Brien, J. R., Etherington, M., and Jamieson, S.: Refractory state of platelet aggregation with major operations. *Lancet* 2:741, 1971.

96. Solinger, A., Bernstein, I. L., and Glueck, H. I.: The effect of epinephrine on platelet aggregation in normal and atopic subjects. *J. Allergy Clin. Immunol.* 51:29, 1973.

97. Maurer, H. M., McCue, C. M., Caul, J., and Still, W. J. S.: Impairment in platelet aggregation in congenital heart disease. *Blood* 40:207, 1972.

98. Stoff, J. S., Stomerman, M., Steer, M., Salzman, E., and Brown, R. S.: A defect in platelet aggregation in Bartter's syndrome. *Am. J. Med.* 68:171, 1980.

99. Edson, J. R., Fecher, D. R., and Doe, R. P.: Low platelet adhesiveness and other hemostatic abnormalities in hypothyroidism. *Ann. Intern. Med.* 82:342, 1975.

100. Weiss, H. J.: Anti-platelet drugs: A new pharmacologic approach to the prevention of thrombosis. *Am. Heart J.* 92:86, 1976.

101. Cowan, D. H.: Acquired disorders of platelet function, in *Hemostasis and Thrombosis*, edited by R. W. Colman, E. W. Salzman, J. Hirsh, and V. J. Marder, Lippincott, New York, 1982, p. 516.

102. Weiss, H. J.: Antiplatelet therapy. *N. Engl. J. Med.* 298:1344 and 1403, 1978.

103. Packham, M. A., and Mustard, J. F.: Clinical pharmacology of platelets. *Blood* 50:555, 1977.

104. Quick, A. J.: Salicylates and bleeding: The aspirin tolerance test. *Am. J. Med. Sci.* 252:265, 1967.

105. Mielke, C. H., Jr., Kaneshiro, M. M., Maker, I. A., Maher, J. M., Weiner, J. M., and Rapaport, S. I.: The standardized normal Ivy bleeding time and its prolongation by aspirin. *Blood* 34:204, 1969.

106. Weiss, H. J., and Aledort, L. M.: Impaired platelet-connective tissue reaction in man after aspirin ingestion. *Lancet* 2:495, 1967.

107. Weiss, H. J., Aledort, L. M., and Kochwa, S.: The effect of salicylates on the hemostatic properties of platelets in man. *J. Clin. Invest.* 47:2169, 1968.

108. Zucker, M. B., and Peterson, J.: Inhibition of adenosine diphosphate induced secondary aggregation and other platelet functions by acetylsalicylic acid ingestion. *Proc. Soc. Exp. Biol. Med.* 127:547, 1968.

109. O'Brien, J. R.: Effects of salicylates on human platelets. *Lancet* 1:779, 1968.

110. Evans, G., Packham, M. A., Nishizawa, E. E., Mustard, J. F., and Murphy, E. A.: The effect of acetylsalicylic acid on platelet function. *J. Exp. Med.* 128:877, 1968.

111. Weiss, H. J., Tschopp, T. B., and Baumgartner, H. R.: Impaired interaction (adhesion-aggregation) of platelets with the subendothelium in storage pool disease and after aspirin ingestion: A comparison with von Willebrand's disease. *N. Engl. J. Med.* 293:619, 1975.

112. O'Brien, J. R., Tulevski, V., and Etherington, M.: Two in vivo studies comparing high and low aspirin dosage. *Lancet* 1:399, 1971.

113. Stuart, R. K.: Platelet function studies in human beings receiving 300 mg. of aspirin per day. *J. Lab. Clin. Med.* 75:463, 1970.

114. Kasper, C. K., and Rapaport, S. I.: Bleeding time and platelet aggregation after analgesics in hemophilia. *Ann. Intern. Med.* 77:189, 1972.

115. Mielke, C. H., Jr., and Britten, A. F. H.: Use of aspirin or acetaminophen in hemophilia. *N. Engl. J. Med.* 282:1270, 1970.

116. O'Brien, J. R.: Effect of anti-inflammatory agents on platelets. *Lancet* 1:894, 1968.

117. Smith, J. B., and Willis, A. L.: Aspirin selectively inhibits prostaglandin production in human platelets. *Nature (New Biol.)* 231:445, 1972.

118. Hamberg, M., Svensson, J., Wakabayashi, T., and Samuelsson, B.: Isolation and structure of two prostaglandin endoperoxides that cause platelet aggregation. *Proc. Natl. Acad. Sci. U.S.A.* 71:345, 1974.

119. Roth, G., and Majerus, P.: The mechanism of the effect of aspirin on human platelets. I. Acetylation of a particulate fraction protein. *J. Clin. Invest.* 56:624, 1975.

120. Hamberg, M., Svensson, J., Wakabayashi, T., and Samuelsson, B.: Thromboxanes: A new group of biologically active compounds derived from prostaglandin endoperoxides. *Proc. Natl. Acad. Sci. U.S.A.* 72:2994, 1975.

121. Moncada, S., and Vane, J. R.: Prostacyclin platelet aggregation and thrombosis, in *Platelets: A Multidisciplinary Approach*, edited by G. de Gaetano and S. Garattini. Raven Press, New York, 1978, p. 239.

122. Moncada, S., and Vane, J. R.: Prostacyclin in perspective, in *Prostacyclin*, edited by J. R. Vane and S. Bergstrom. Raven Press, New York, 1979, p. 5.

123. Weksler, B. B., Marcus, A. J., and Jaffe, E.: Synthesis of prostaglandin I$_2$ (prostacyclin) by cultured human and bovine endothelial cells. *Proc. Natl. Acad. Sci. U.S.A.* 74:3922, 1977.

124. Zucker, M. B., and Peterson, J.: Effect of acetysalicylic acid, other non-steroidal anti-inflammatory agents, and dipyridamole on human blood platelets. *J. Lab. Clin. Med.* 75:66, 1971.

125. Kocsis, J. J., Hernandovich, J., Silver, M. J., Smith, J. B., and Ingerman, C.: Duration of inhibition of platelet prostaglandin formation and aggregation by ingested aspirin or indomethacin. *Prostaglandins* 3:141, 1973.

126. O'Brien, J. R., Finch, W., and Clark, E.: A comparison of an effect of different anti-inflammatory drugs on human platelets. *J. Clin. Pathol.* 23:522, 1970.

127. Ali, M., and McDonald, J. W. D.: Effects of sulfinpyrazone on platelet release of serotonin. *J. Lab. Clin. Med.* 89:868, 1977.

128. Walz, H. S., and Genton, E.: Altered platelet function in patients with prosthetic heart valves. *Circulation* 42:967, 1970.

129. Langdell, R. D., Adelson, E. A., Furth, F. W., and Crosby, W. H.: Dextran and prolonged bleeding time. *JAMA* 116:346, 1958.

130. Weiss, H. J.: The effect of clinical dextran on platelet aggregation, adhesion and ADP release in man: In vivo and in vitro studies. *J. Lab. Clin. Med.* 69:37, 1967.

131. Ewald, R. A., Eichelberger, J. W., Young, A. A., Weiss, H. J., and Crosby, W. H.: The effect of dextran on platelet factor 3 activity: In vitro and in vivo studies. *Transfusion* 5:109, 1965.

132. Bygdeman, S., Eliasson, R., and Gullbring, B.: Effect of dextran infusion on the adenosine diphosphate induced adhesiveness and the spreading capacity of human blood platelets. *Thromb. Diath. Haemorrh.* 15:451, 1966.

133. Rothman, S., Adelson, E., Schwebel, A., and Langdell, R. D.: Adsorption of carbon-14 dextran to human blood platelets and red blood cells in vitro. *Vox Sang.* 2:104, 1957.

134. Ross, S., and Eber, R.: Microelectrophoresis of blood platelets and the effect of dextran. *J. Clin. Invest.* 38:155, 1959.

135. Aberg, M., Hedner, U., and Bergentz, S. E.: Effect of dextran 70 on factor VIII and platelet function in von Willebrand's disease. *Thromb. Res.* 12:629, 1978.

136. Brown, C. H., Bradshaw, M. W., Natelson, E. A., Alfrey, C. P., and Williams, T. W.: Defective platelet function following the administration of penicillin compounds. *Blood* 47:949, 1976.

137. Weiss, H. J.: The pharmacology of platelet inhibition, in *Progress in Hemostasis and Thrombosis*, edited by T. H. Spaet. Grune & Stratton, New York, 1972, vol. 1, p. 199.

138. Poller, L., Thomason, J. M., and Priest, C. M.: Coumarin therapy and platelet aggregation. *Br. Med. J.* 1:474, 1969.

139. O'Brien, J. R., Shoobridge, S. M., and Finch, W. J.: Comparison of the effect of heparin and citrate on platelet aggregation. *J. Clin. Pathol.* 22:248, 1963.

140. Zucker, M. B.: Proteolytic inhibitors, contact and other variables in the release reaction of human platelets. *Thromb. Diath. Haemorrh.* 28:393, 1972.

141. Gordon, J. L., and Matchinson, M. J.: Coronary artery thrombosis. *Lancet* 1:319, 1974.

Disorders of hemostasis — nonthrombocytopenic purpuras

CHAPTER *148*

Nonallergic purpura

ARLAN J. GOTTLIEB

In the absence of a qualitative or quantitative platelet abnormality or a blood coagulation disorder, the presence of purpura implies an abnormality in one of the vascular factors involved in hemostasis. The diseases associated with vascular purpura are diverse, including the vasculitides, degenerative disorders, avitaminoses (scurvy), heritable disorders of connective tissue (pseudoxanthoma elasticum and the Ehlers-Danlos syndrome), and neoplasia (Kaposi's sarcoma). In this chapter, purpura due to predominantly noninflammatory vascular abnormalities will be discussed. A feature common to all these conditions is the loss of vascular integrity with an increase in both vascular permeability and fragility. The etiology of many of these disorders is incompletely understood. Treatment, therefore, is to a large extent limited to supportive measures. Better definition of the pathogenesis of some of these syndromes will be supplied by application and expansion of our knowledge of vascular integrity and platelet function [1–5]. More specific therapy may then be instituted.

Classically in *purpura simplex* bleeding is mild, taking the form of petechiae or small ecchymoses, and is usually confined to the skin [6]. The majority of patients are women, and exacerbation of the bleeding tendency at the time of menses may be noted. Tourniquet tests are usually negative. Historically, purpura simplex also includes the bruising tendency (devil's nips or pinches) reported in and by women, characterized by small ecchymoses appearing on easily traumatized areas of the body without the inciting incident being recalled. It is probable that many cases previously classed as purpura simplex actually represent mild thrombocytopathies, von Willebrand's disease, or transient allergic or drug-induced vasculitis. In vitro abnormalities of platelet aggregation in response to ADP, epinephrine, and collagen or diminished platelet adhesion to glass beads has been observed in 31 of 75 patients with the "easy bruis-

ing" syndrome [1]. The inhibitory effect of salicylates and other drugs on platelet function may enhance an otherwise mild thrombocytopathy [2,7]. Template bleeding times before and after aspirin has proved valuable as a screening procedure in patients with mild bleeding disorders [3,8].

A *hereditary familial purpura simplex* has been described in several kindreds. The details of hematologic testing are, however, rather scanty [6,9]. The disease is said to occur mainly in females. Positive tourniquet tests are found, although the bleeding times are normal. In one pedigree covering four generations, a dominant transmission was found [10]. Hemorrhagic manifestations are similar to those seen in purpura simplex. In the past, a connection was drawn between both the episodic and familial varieties of purpura simplex and the rheumatic disorders [6,9]. Purpura in the rheumatic disorders is usually related to an underlying vasculitis, to the use of aspirin or other antiplatelet agents, or to steroid administration. The role of anti-IgG factors in the induction of purpura is discussed under hyperglobulinemic purpura.

In *mechanical purpura*, vascular damage results from the marked increase in intraluminal pressure secondary to violent muscular activity. Purpura or ecchymoses may sometimes appear at the site of effort, as over the biceps of a weight lifter, or may be more remote — for example, conjunctival hemorrhage or purpura of the chest wall following strenuous repetitive Valsalva maneuvers or paroxysms of coughing. An increase in intraluminal vascular pressure is also the cause of *stasis*, or *orthostatic purpura*. This condition is usually seen over the lower extremities of the elderly after prolonged periods of standing. Venous insufficiency may also be present. A loss of the supporting framework of the vascular bed, due to atrophy of dermal collagen (senile changes), is probably also important in the pathogenesis of this disorder. When chronic, this condition leads to a dusky, reddish discoloration of the skin of the lower extremities due to the deposition of hemosiderin [11].

Chronic stasis, resulting in a capillaritis, is thought to be the cause of a group of rare pigmented dermatoses. They are *the progressive pigmentary dermatosis of Shamberg* [12–14] (Plate 12), *purpura annularis telangiectodes (Majocchi's disease)* [15], and the *pigmented purpuric lichenoid dermatitis of Gougerot and Blum* [16]. Distinctions among these conditions are probably unwarranted. Each is benign, chronic, unresponsive to therapy, found mainly on dependent areas, and characterized by some degree of capillary proliferation, inflammation, and rupture. Skin pigmentation from hemosiderin deposition is seen as a result of the chronic extravasation of red blood cells. In Majocchi's disease the lesions tend to be confluent and telangiectatic. Pigmented purpuric lichenoid dermatitis is distinguished by the presence of pruritic papules scattered among the larger purpuric lesions [15,17].

In *senile purpura*, purpura or small bluish hematomas appear either spontaneously at sites of pressure from clothing or in response to otherwise trivial trauma [18,19]. The areas of the body usually involved – the face, neck, dorsum of the hands, forearms, and legs – are regions regularly exposed to sunlight. Actinic radiation apparently hastens the degeneration of dermal collagen, which, together with the subcutaneous fat, serves as the supporting framework of the capillary bed. With loss of this latticework of connective tissue, a more friable vascular bed results. A desultory inflammatory response, slow reabsorption of extravasated erythrocytes, and senile degeneration of dermal collagen are found histologically. A loss of the supporting structures of the vascular bed is also thought to cause the purpura seen in severe cachexia. The accentuation of the manifestations of senile purpura seen in liver disease in the absence of thrombocytopenia probably results from the superimposition of acquired deficiencies in circulating procoagulants upon the senile changes in the dermal perivascular bed [20]. Defects in platelet factor 3 release and platelet aggregation have also been described in association with liver disease [21–23] (Chap. 147).

Purpura, in a predominantly dependent distribution, is seen in *Cushing's syndrome* and following the prolonged administration of ACTH or glucocorticoids [24] (Plate 12). Although the exact mechanism by which purpura is produced is unknown, it probably relates to an alteration in the system of dermal vascular support. The purpuric lesions will often disappear, particularly in the young, following withdrawal of the exogenous steroid or treatment of the adrenal hypercorticism.

Hemorrhage into the skin as well as purpura has been reported in *pseudoxanthoma elasticum* [25]. Indeed, spontaneous hemorrhage, primarily from the gastrointestinal tract but also from subarachnoid, retinal, renal, nasal, bladder, and uterine vessels, constitutes the major medical problem in this condition. Surgical intervention may be required for intractable hemorrhage, and in several instances gastrectomy has been lifesaving. A vascular bleeding diathesis ranging from simple easy bruisability to the rupture of major arterial trunks is seen in the *Ehlers-Danlos syndrome* [25]. Most often, however, skin purpura and hematomas bring these patients to the physician. The hyperextensible skin seen in this disorder is slow to heal after trauma. Easy bruisability, frequent epistaxis, and increased bleeding from skin lacerations have been reported in *osteogenesis imperfecta* [26,27], and a mild hemorrhagic tendency has been noted in *Marfan's syndrome* [25,28,29]. Abnormalities in the structure of connective tissue in the vessel wall as well as in the perivascular lattice probably account for the bleeding phenomena and for the increased incidence of disease of the major arterial trunks seen in these mesenchymal dysplasias [25,30]. Deficiencies in circulating coagulation factor appear to be coincidental [25,31,32]. Deficiencies in circulating coagulation factors appear to be coincidental [25,31,32]. Platelet dysfunction, in the form of abnormalities in thromboplastin generation or of reduced platelet aggregation in response to ADP, collagen, or norepinephrine, and giant platelets have been described [26–29,33–35]. These are usually rather mild disturbances found in a minority of patients.

Characteristically, in *scurvy*, perifollicular hemorrhages and edematous, bleeding gums are found. Petechial hemorrhages are among the very first clinical signs to appear [36]. Ecchymoses, particularly over the legs and forearms, and intramuscular hemorrhages are not uncommon. In children, subperiosteal hemorrhages due to the extravasation of blood from the epiphyseal vessels occur. In addition, the skin shows keratotic plugging of the hair follicles and short, broken, "corkscrew" hairs. Capillary fragility is increased. Histologic study has shown the lesions to be noninflammatory [37,38]. In chronic cases, hemosiderin is seen. Ascorbic acid is an obligatory constituent of normal collagen biosynthesis; in its absence there is a decrease in synthesis and accumulation of structurally abnormal collagen [39]. There is edema and degeneration of the connective tissue and nests of detached endothelial cells. The fibroblasts show abnormal morphologic features, and there is a decrease in fibrillogenesis. Synthesis of basement membrane components is also impaired [40]. These changes are most notable in and around vessels and hair follicles and apparently account for the perivascular and perifollicular hemorrhages found in this disorder. Occasionally thrombocytopenia or an intrinsic platelet defect may contribute to the bleeding diathesis [41]. The speed of platelet aggregation in response to ADP appears reduced in experimental scurvy in guinea pigs [42].

The hemorrhagic tendency seen in *Kaposi's hemorrhagic sarcoma* results from proliferation of vascular elements [43]. Males are most frequently involved. The incidence of this malignancy in the United States has been 0.021 to 0.061 per 100,000 population. Those affected have been mainly over 50 years of age [144]. Markedly dilated dermal blood vessels, capillary and endothelial proliferation, local hemorrhage and hemosiderin deposition give the early nodules their violaceous or dark-brown color. Microscopically, the lesions closely resemble granulation tissue. A varying degree of fibroblastic activity is seen. As the lesions mature, an increase in connective tissue elements is often observed. Lesions are most commonly observed on the lower extremities, where they may be associated with lymphedema and tend to ulcerate and bleed. Visceral lesions are present in about 10 percent of sporadic cases [43–45]. Involvement of the gastrointestinal tract, liver, lungs, lymph nodes, and heart is most frequent, and gastrointestinal and pulmonary hemorrhage may pose difficult problems in management. The disease tends to be slowly progressive but is fatal in less than one-fifth of those afflicted [43,44]. An increase in the incidence of second malignancies [140] including lymphoma and multiple myeloma has been reported [43–49]. Kaposi's sarcoma also occurs in patients receiving immunosuppressive therapy [50,51]. The disease is found frequently in various regions of Africa, where it appears to have a greater tendency to widespread visceral dissemination and involves younger patients [52,53]. An aggressive and often fatal variant of the disease has appeared in the United States as part of a syndrome of acquired immunodeficiency [141–143]. Male homosexuals appear at highest risk. The interrelationship of the various clinical aspects of the acquired immunodeficiency and the role of genetic, environmental, and infectious factors in the etiology of these case clusters is under intense investigation. The lesions are extremely radiosensitive, and excellent palliation has been obtained with low-dose radiotherapy [43]. Radionuclide scanning with technetium (^{99m}Tc) has proved a useful means of detecting occult soft tissue disease [54].

A hemorrhagic diathesis in the absence of thrombocytopenia may be encountered in the *malignant dysproteinemic states:* multiple myeloma and the lymphoproliferative disorders. The lymphoproliferative disorder characterized by high levels of circulating macroglobulin, described by Waldenström [55], is particularly noteworthy in this regard [56,57] (see Chap. 123). Epistaxis, the most common hemorrhagic manifestation, occurs in about one-quarter of the patients [57]. Purpura and easy bruisability are seen less frequently (Plate 12). Fibrinogenopenia [55], overt fibrinolysis [58,59], a circulating heparinlike anticoagulant due to mastocytosis [60], acquired deficiencies of coagulation factors [61–65], abnormalities of fibrin formation [66–74], and platelet disorders, including thrombocytopenia and qualitative platelet defects [75–83], have all been implicated in the pathogenesis of the bleeding disorder. Sufficient calcium may be bound to the paraprotein to interfere with coagulation testing in vitro [84,85]. In some instances, purpura may result from an associated cryoglobulinemia or cryofibrinogenemia [84,86,87] or from the intravascular or perivascular deposition of paraprotein.

In one study of multiple myeloma, macroglobulinemia, and cryoglobulinemia [72], overt bleeding was twice as common in IgA myeloma (33 percent) and macroglobulinemia (36 percent) as in IgG myeloma (15 percent). The panorama of previously reported abnormalities in coagulation tests was reproduced in this study. No correlation was found between overt bleeding and the observed abnormalities in platelet count, clot retraction times, platelet function in thromboplastin generation, prothrombin time, thrombin time, partial thromboplastin time, thromboplastin generation time, fibrinolysis, fibrinogen levels, or factor XII levels. A somewhat greater tendency to bleed was found in patients with depressed levels of prothrombin and factors V, VII, X, XI, and XIII. When the levels of these factors were decreased, they did not reach levels usually associated with overt bleeding. Specific factor deficiency was thus thought to be only a contributory factor in the hemorrhagic diathesis. An excellent correlation was obtained between overt hemorrhage and inadequacies of platelet plug formation as evidenced by abnormalities in platelet adhesiveness tests and bleeding times. These

abnormalities were most often seen in association with hyperviscosity [72]. A relationship appears to exist linking platelet membrane-bound immunoglobulin, and serum immunoglobulin or paraprotein level to platelet dysfunction [75].

The most frequently observed inhibitor of coagulation in the dysproteinemic states produces interference in fibrin monomer aggregation, leading to prolonged thrombin and "reptilase" times in association with a structurally abnormal, gelatinous clot [66–74]. These abnormalities appear to arise from the interaction of fibrin monomer with high concentrations of γ-globulin [66–74]. Treatment resulting in a decrease in the level of paraprotein appears to be an effective means of securing hemostasis in these patients. This may most expeditiously be accomplished by plasmapheresis.

Cryoglobulinemic purpura may exist in the absence of hematologic malignancy in essential or primary cryoglobulinemia [86–93]. These cryoglobulins tend to be mixed, or heterogeneous, in type, consisting of a complex of IgG and an immunoglobulin having anti-IgG activity [87,91–93]. The complete complex is necessary for cryoprecipitation. "Mixed" cyroglobulinemia has been associated with a wide variety of disorders, including infectious disease, collagen-vascular disease, and the arthralgia-purpura-weakness syndrome (Peetom-Meltzer syndrome) [87,91–93]. As a consequence of exposure to cold, patients with cryoglobulinemia may experience reactions such as Raynaud's phenomenon, livedo reticularis, skin ulcers, and the hyperviscosity syndrome with central nervous system dysfunction [87]. The syndrome of vasculitis, purpura, arthralgia, and nephritis is far more often observed in patients with mixed cryoglobulinemia and represents a distinct clinical syndrome within the broader group of hypersensitivity vasculitis [87,91–94]. The best management of these disorders is not yet established but probably relates to effective control of the underlying disorder. Plasmapheresis with removal of the cryoglobulin will have short-term benefits.

Purpura often induced by cold, thromboembolic phenomena, and a hemorrhagic diathesis may be seen with high levels of *circulating cryofibrinogen* [95–101]. Retinal hemorrhage and retinal vein thrombosis are also observed. The hemorrhagic manifestations in these disorders are thought to result from tissue anoxia secondary to the "sludging" of blood. Most commonly, an increase in cryofibrinogen is associated with metastatic malignancy [95,97,101]. An intercurrent consumptive coagulopathy should be carefully ruled out in each case. Cryofibrinogens consisting of complexes of fibrin, fibrinogen, and fibronectin have now been identified [102].

In *amyloidosis*, purpura and skin hemorrhage result from an increase in vascular fragility due to the deposition of amyloid in the skin and subcutaneous tissues [103–106]. As a consequence, purpura is found predominantly in areas of the skin which are either dependent or subjected to minor trauma. Purpura may also result from coughing or straining. Intertriginous areas are commonly involved. Of particular note is the occurrence of periorbital purpura. The presence of hemorrhage in an otherwise waxy-appearing cutaneous plaque or papule should suggest the diagnosis of amyloidosis. Induction of skin hemorrhage by gentle stroking with a gauze pad is highly characteristic of dermal amyloidosis [105]. An acquired deficiency of factor X has been reported in amyloidosis [106–114]. Combined factor IX and factor X deficiencies have also been noted [112,113]. In one patient, factor X deficiency proved reversible following removal of an amyloid-laden spleen [113]. Infusion of plasma or of purified factor X has failed to produce the expected rise in factor X level in patients with amyloidosis. It has been suggested that factor X is either selectively destroyed or adsorbed by the amyloid [109–114]. The binding of factor X and, less avidly, of factor IX and prothrombin to isolated, purified amyloid fibrils supports this hypothesis [115].

Chronic, episodic, nonthrombocytopenic purpura of the lower extremities and an electrophoretically diffuse hypergammaglobulinemia are the cardinal features of *benign hyperglobulinemic purpura* [116–139]. Although confusion exists, this syndrome should be distinguished from the bleeding diathesis associated with lymphoproliferative disorders and high circulating levels of predominantly monoclonal macroglobulin [55]. Prodromal symptoms, including local tenderness, burning, or itching, often precede the symmetric appearance, usually in the lower extremities, of a transient petechial, urticarial eruption which may become confluent. As the urticaria subsides, petechial and purpuric areas remain.

Adult females are most frequently involved. A mild anemia may be present, and the erythrocyte sedimentation rate is elevated. Biopsies, when performed, demonstrate a vasculitis in the dermal and subcutaneous tissue [118,119,127,128,130]. The majority of reported cases have had a variety of associated manifestations, including arthritis, hepatosplenomegaly, lymphadenopathy, xerostomia, keratoconjunctivitis sicca, and sialadenitis. In others, a definite diagnosis of Sjögren's syndrome, disseminated lupus erythematosus, rheumatoid arthritis, sarcoidosis, anaphylactoid purpura, lymphoma, or multiple myeloma has been made [119–123,126,128,130]. It would appear that the syndrome of benign hyperglobulinemic purpura actually represents the hemorrhagic cutaneous manifestation of a vasculitis occurring in a number of diseases of diverse etiology [94]. The most common of these disorders appears to be Sjögren's syndrome.

In a study of 24 patients fulfilling the criteria of benign hyperglobulinemic purpura, 22 were female [128]. Half the cases were classed as primary, since no other diagnosis could be established. Sjögren's syndrome, keratoconjunctivitis sicca, lupus erythematosus, chronic lymphocytic leukemia, and undifferentiated collagen vascular disease were diagnosed in the secondary group.

The syndrome was apparent before the age of 40 in the primary group but appeared somewhat later in the secondary group. When performed, biopsies showed vasculitis. Anti-γ-globulin factors were demonstrated in all patients and were IgG, in contrast to rheumatoid arthritis, where they are IgM. Protein complexes having a sedimentation velocity between that of IgG and that of IgM were identified in 19 of the 24 cases by ultracentrifugal analysis. Other studies have served to establish the IgG nature of these anti-γ-globulins and to indicate that the hypergammaglobulinemia characteristic of this syndrome is due in large measure to the presence of these anti-γ-globulins [129,131]. The interaction of these proteins with the native γ-globulins accounts for the intermediate complexes observed in the ultracentrifuge [129,131]. It would thus appear probable that circulating soluble immune complexes are responsible for the characteristic vasculitis observed [94,129,131]. However, cutaneous immunoglobulin deposition has only occasionally been reported [128,132]. Rapid clearance of immunoglobulin complexes from cutaneous sites has been invoked to explain the disparity [132,133].

The purpura that occurs with *infections* is often due to thrombocytopenia, with or without disseminated intravascular coagulation (Chaps. 142 and 158). Nonthrombocytopenic purpura may occur in infections due to bacteria [134–136], viruses [135–137], or rickettsiae [138] (Plate 12). The pathogenesis of the purpura in these diseases is obscure. Petechiae occur commonly in subacute bacterial endocarditis, and purpura may be observed occasionally [139]. These lesions may be due to microemboli or to toxic damage to vascular endothelium. The relationship of infection to allergic purpura is discussed in Chap. 150.

References

1. Lackner, H., and Karpatkin, S.: On the "easy bruising" syndrome with normal platelet count. *Ann. Intern. Med.* 83:190, 1975.
2. Weiss, H. J.: Platelet physiology and abnormalities of platelet function. *N. Engl. J. Med.* 293:580, 1975.
3. Bachmann, F.: Diagnostic approach to mild bleeding disorders. *Semin. Hematol.* 17:292, 1980.
4. Weiss, H. J.: Congenital disorders of platelet functions. *Semin. Hematol.* 17:228, 1980.
5. Malpass, T. W., and Harker, L. A.: Acquired disorders of platelet function. *Semin. Hematol.* 17:242, 1980.
6. Davis, E.: Purpura of the skin: A review of 500 cases. *Lancet* 2:160, 1943.
7. Quick, A. J.: Salicylates and bleeding: The aspirin tolerance test. *Am. J. Med. Sci.* 252:265, 1966.
8. Stuart, M. J., Miller, M. L., Davey, F. R., and Wolk, J. A.: The post-aspirin bleeding time: A screening test for evaluating haemostatic disorders. *Br. J. Haematol.* 43:649, 1980.
9. Davis, E.: Hereditary familial purpura simplex: Review of twenty-seven families. *Lancet* 1:145, 1941.
10. Fisher, B., Zuckerman, G. H., and Douglass, R. C.: Combined inheritance of purpura simplex and ptosis in four generations of one family. *Blood* 9:1199, 1954.
11. Pillsbury, D. M., Shelly, W. B., and Kligman, A. M.: *Dermatology.* Saunders, Philadelphia, 1966, p. 754.
12. Schamberg, J. F.: A peculiar progressive pigmentary disease of the skin. *Br. J. Dermatol.* 13:1, 1901.

13. Templeton, H. J.: Progressive pigmentary dermatosis (Schamberg): With review of literature, report of 2 cases and comparison with angioma serpiginosum and purpura annularis telangiectodes. *Arch. Dermatol. 16:*141, 1927.

14. Randall, S. J., Kierland, R. R., and Montgomery, H.: Pigmented purpuric eruptions. *Arch. Dermatol. 64:*177, 1951.

15. Majocchi, D.: Sopra una dermatosi telangettode non ancora descritta, "purpura annularis." "Telangiectasis follicularis annulata." Studio clinico. *Ital. Mal. Ven. 31:*263, 1896.

16. Gougerot, J., and Blum, P.: Purpura angioscléreux prurigineux avec éléments lichénoides (présentation de malade). *Bull. Soc. Fr. Dermatol. Syphilol. 32:*161, 1925.

17. Nichamin, S. J., and Brough, A. J.: Chronic progressive pigmentary purpura: Purpura annularis telangiectodes of Majocchi-Schamberg. *Am. J. Dis. Child. 116:*429, 1968.

18. Tattersall, R. N., and Seville, R.: Senile purpura. *Q. J. Med. 19:*151, 1950.

19. Shuster, A., and Scarborough, H.: Senile purpura. *Q. J. Med. 30:*33, 1961.

20. Derbes, V. J., and Chernosky, M. E.: Senile purpura and liver disease: A possible relationship. *Arch. Dermatol. 80:*529, 1959.

21. Mandel, E. E., and Lazerson, J.: Thrombasthenia in liver disease. *N. Engl. J. Med. 265:*56, 1961.

22. Weiss, H. J., and Eichelberger, J. W.: Secondary thrombocytopathia: Platelet factor in 3 various disease states. *Arch. Intern. Med. 112:*827, 1963.

23. Thomas, D. P., Ream, V. J., and Stuart, R. K.: Platelet aggregation in patients with Laennec's cirrhosis of the liver. *N. Engl. J. Med. 276:*1344, 1967.

24. Scarborough, H., and Shuster, A.: Corticosteroid purpura. *Lancet 1:*93, 1960.

25. McKusick, V. A.: *Heritable Disorders of Connective Tissue*, 3d ed. Mosby, St. Louis, 1966.

26. Siegal, B. M., Friedman, I. A., and Schwartz, S. O.: Hemorrhagic disease in osteogenesis imperfecta. *Am. J. Med. 22:*315, 1957.

27. Gautier, P., and Guinand-Doniol, J.: Le Cas de maladie de Lobstein associée à une thrombasthénie héréditaire et familiale de Glanzmann. *Bull. Soc. Med. Hôp. Paris 68:*577, 1952.

28. Estes, J. W., Carey, R. J., and Desai, R. G.: Marfans syndrome: Hematological abnormalities in a family. *Arch. Intern. Med. 116:*889, 1965.

29. Estes, J. W.: Platelet size and function in the heritable disorders of connective tissue. *Ann. Intern. Med. 68:*1237, 1968.

30. Kivirkko, K. I., and Risteli, L.: Biosynthesis of collagen and its alterations in pathologic states. *Med. Biol. 54:*159, 1976.

31. Day, H. J., and Zarafonetis, C. J. C.: Coagulation studies in four patients with Ehlers-Danlos syndrome. *Am. J. Med. Sci. 242:*565, 1961.

32. Wigzell, F. W., and Ogston, D.: The bleeding tendency in Ehlers-Danlos syndrome. *Ann. Phys. Med. 7:*55, 1963.

33. Goodman, R. M., Levitsky, J. M., and Friedman, I. A.: The Ehlers-Danlos syndrome and multiple neurofibromatosis in a kindred of mixed derivation, with special emphasis on hemostatis in the Ehlers-Danlos syndrome. *Am. J. Med. 32:*976, 1962.

34. Kashiwagi, H., Riddle, J. M., Abraham, J. P., and Frame, B.: Functional and ultrastructural abnormalities of platelets in Ehlers-Danlos syndrome. *Ann. Intern. Med. 63:*249, 1965.

35. Seibel, B. M., Breidman, I. A., and Schwartz, S. O.: Hemorrhagic disease in osteogenesis imperfecta: Studies of platelet function defect. *Am. J. Med. 22:*315, 1957.

36. Hughes, R. E., Hood, J., Canham, J. E., Sauberlich, H. E., and Baker, E. M.: Clinical manifestations of ascorbic acid deficiency in man. *Am. J. Clin. Nutr. 24:*432, 1971.

37. Stolman, J. M., Goldman, H. M., and Gould, B. S.: Ascorbic acid and blood vessels. *Arch. Pathol. 72:*535, 1961.

38. Ross, R., and Bendett, E. P.: Wound healing and collagen formation. II. Fine structure in experimental scurvy. *J. Cell Biol. 12:*533, 1962.

39. Grant, M. E., and Prockop, D. J.: Biosynthesis of collagen. *N. Engl. J. Med. 286:*194, 242, 291, 1972.

40. Priest, R. E.: Formation of epithelial basement membrane is restricted by scurvy in vitro and is stimulated by vitamin C. *Nature 225:*744, 1970.

41. Centigil, A. I., Ulutin, O.N., and Karaca, M.: A platelet defect in scurvy. *Br. J. Haematol. 4:*350, 1958.

42. Purcell, I. M., and Constantine, J. W.: Platelet and experimental scurvy. *Nature 235:*389, 1972.

43. Bluefarb, S. M.: *Kaposi's Sarcoma: Multiple Idiopathic Hemorrhagic Sarcoma.* Charles C. Thomas, Springfield, Ill., 1959.

44. Reynolds, W. A., Winkelmann, R. K., and Soule, E. H.: Kaposi's sarcoma: A clinicopathologic study with particular reference to its relationship to the reticuloendothelial system. *Medicine 44:*419, 1965.

45. Cox, R. H., and Helwig, E. B.: Kaposi's sarcoma. *Cancer 12:*289, 1959.

46. Anthony, C. W., and Koneman, E. W.: Visceral Kaposi's sarcoma. *Arch. Pathol. 70:*740, 1960.

47. Bluefarb, S. M., and Webster, J. R.: Kaposi's sarcoma associated with lymphosarcoma. *Arch. Intern. Med. 91:*97, 1953.

48. Law, I. P.: Kaposi sarcoma and plasma cell dyscrasia. *JAMA 229:*1329, 1974.

49. Ettinger, D. S., Humphrey, R. L., and Skinner, M. D.: Kaposi sarcoma associated with multiple myeloma. *Johns Hopkins Med. J. 137:*88, 1975.

50. Penn, I., Halgrimson, G. C., and Starzl, T. E.: De novo malignant tumors in organ transplant recipients. *Transplant. Proc. 3:*773, 1971.

51. Myers, B. D., Kessler, E., Levi, J., Pick, A., and Rosenfeld, J. B.: Kaposi sarcoma in kidney transplant recipients. *Arch. Intern. Med. 133:*307, 1974.

52. D'Oliveira, J. J. G., and Torres, F. O.: Kaposi's sarcoma in the Bantu of Mozambique. *Cancer 30:*553, 1972.

53. Templeton, A. C.: Studies in Kaposi's sarcoma: Postmortem findings and disease patterns in women. *Cancer 30:*884, 1972.

54. Rotman, M., Rogow, L., and Roussis, K.: Radioisotope scanning of Kaposi's sarcoma: A modality for treatment planning. *Cancer 33:*58, 1974.

55. Waldenström, J.: Incipient myelomatosis or "essential" hyperglobulinemia with fibrinogenopenia: A new syndrome. *Acta Med. Scand. 117:*216, 1944.

56. Ritzmann, S. E., Thurm, K. H., Truax, W. E., and Levin, W. C.: The syndrome of macroglobulinemia. *Arch. Intern. Med. 105:*939, 1960.

57. McCallister, B. D., Bayrd, E. D., Harrison, E. G., Jr., and McGuckin, W. F.: Primary macroglobulinemia. *Am. J. Med. 43:*394, 1967.

58. Waldenström, J.: Abnormal proteins in myeloma. *Adv. Intern. Med. 5:*398, 1952.

59. Sirridge, M. S., Bowman, K. S., and Garber, P. W.: Fibrinolysis and changes in fibrinogen in multiple myeloma. *Arch. Intern. Med. 101:*630, 1958.

60. Tischendorf, W., and Hartmann, F.: Makroglobulinaemie (Waldenström) mit gleichzeitiger hyperplasie der Gewebsmastzellen. *Acta Haematol. 4:*374, 1950.

61. Perry, S. M., Skoog, W. A., and Adams, W. S.: Clotting defects in the dysproteinemias and paraproteinemias. *Clin. Res. 7:*95, 1959.

62. Long, L. A., et al.: Macroglobulinaemia: Effect of macroglobulins on prothrombin conversion accelerations. *Can. Med. Assoc. J. 73:*726, 1955.

63. Henstell, H. H., and Kligerman, M.: A new theory of interference with the clotting mechanism: The complexing of euglobulin with factor V, factor VII and prothrombin. *Ann. Intern. Med. 49:*371, 1958.

64. Brody, J. I., Haidar, M. E., and Rossman, R. E.: A hemorrhagic syndrome in Waldenström's macroglobulinemia secondary to immunoadsorption of factor VIII: Recovery after splenectomy. *N. Engl. J. Med. 300:*408, 1979.

65. Perry, S.: Coagulation factors in patients with plasma protein disorders. *J. Lab. Clin. Med. 61:*411, 1963.

66. Craddock, C. G., Jr., Adams, W. S., Figueroa, W. G.: Interference with fibrin formation in multiple myeloma by the unusual protein found in blood and urine. *J. Lab. Clin. Med. 42:*847, 1953.

67. Uehlinger, E.: Über eine Blutgerinnungsstörung bei Dysproteinämie (Beitrag zur Kenntnis der körpereigenen Antikoagulantia). *Helv. Med. Acta 16:*508, 1949.

68. Lüscher, E., and Labhart, A.: Blutgerinnungsstörung durch β-Globuline; zur Kenntnis der Gerinnungsstörungen durch körpereigene Antikoagulantien. *Schweiz. Med. Wochenschr. 79:*598, 1949.

69. Friek, P. G.: Inhibition of conversion of fibrinogen to fibrin by abnormal proteins in multiple myeloma. *Am. J. Clin. Pathol. 25*:1263, 1955.

70. Lackner, H., Hunt, V., Zucker, M. B., and Pearson, J.: Abnormal fibrin ultrastructure polymerization, and clot retraction in multiple myeloma. *Br. J. Haematol. 18*:625, 1970.

71. Coleman, M., Vigliano, E. M., Weksler, M. E., and Nachman, R. L.: Inhibition of fibrin monomer aggregation by lambda myeloma globulins. *Blood 39*:210, 1972.

72. Perkins, H. A., MacKenzie, M. R., and Fudenberg, H. H.: Hemostatic defect dysproteinemias. *Blood 35*:695, 1970.

73. Lackner, H.: Hemostatic abnormalities associated with dysproteinemias. *Semin. Hematol. 10*:125, 1973.

74. Davey, F. R., Gordon, G. B., Boral, L. I., and Gottlieb, A. J.: Gamma globulin inhibition of fibrin clot formation. *Ann. Clin. Lab. Sci. 6*:72, 1976.

75. McGrath, K. M., Stuart, J. J., and Richards, F.: Correlation between serum IgG, platelet membrane IgG, and platelet function in hypergammaglobulinemic states. *Br. J. Haematol. 42*:585, 1979.

76. James, T. N., Monto, R. W., and Rebuck, J. W.: Thrombocytopenia and abnormal bleeding in multiple myeloma. *Ann. Intern. Med. 39*:1281, 1953.

77. Godal, H. C., and Borchgrevink, C. F.: The effect of plasmapheresis on the hemostatic function in patients with macroglobulinemia Waldenström and multiple myeloma. *Scand. J. Clin. Lab. Invest. 17 (Suppl. 84)*:133, 1965.

78. Viala, J. J., Thouverez, J. P., Belleville, J., Revol, L., and Croizat, P.: Étude de la coagulation du sang au cours des dysglobulinémies myelomes et maladie de Waldenström: Á propos de 48 observations. *Hemostase 3*:303, 1963.

79. Izarn, P., Paleirac, G., and Robinet, M.: La fonction thromboplastique plaquettaire au cours des dysglobulinémies. *Nouv. Rev. Fr. Hematol. 6*:729, 1966.

80. Pachter, M. R., Johnson, S. A., Neblett, T. R., and Truant, J. P.: Bleeding, platelets, and macroglobulinemia. *Am. J. Clin. Pathol. 31*:467, 1959.

81. Vigliano, E. M., and Horowitz, H. I.: Bleeding syndrome in a patient with IgA myeloma: Interaction of protein and connective tissue. *Blood 29*:823, 1967.

82. Vigliano, E. M., and Horowitz, H. I.: Bleeding syndrome caused by interactions of IgA myeloma protein and connective tissue. *Blood 26*:880, 1965.

83. Pachter, M. R., Johnson, S. A., and Basinski, D. H.: The effect of macroglobulins and their dissociation units on release of platelet factor 3. *Thromb. Diath. Haemorrh. 3*:501, 1959.

84. Kalbfleisch, J. M., and Bird, R. M.: Cryofibrinogenemia. *N. Engl. J. Med. 263*:881, 1960.

85. Glueck, H. I., Wayne, L., and Goldsmith, R.: Abnormal calcium binding associated with hyperglobulinemia clotting defects and osteoporosis: A study of this relationship. *J. Lab. Clin. Med. 59*:40, 1962.

86. Firkin, B. G.: Essential cryoglobulinemia. *Am. J. Med. 24*:974, 1958.

87. Meltzer, M., Franklin, E. C., Elias, K., McCluskey, R. T., and Cooper, N.: Cryoglobulinemia: A clinical and laboratory study. II. Cryoglobulins with rheumatoid factor activity. *Am. J. Med. 40*:837, 1966.

88. Lerner, A. B., and Watson, C. J.: Studies of cryoglobulins: Unusual purpura associated with the presence of a high concentration of cryoglobulin (cold precipitable serum globulin). *Am. J. Med. Sci. 214*:410, 1947.

89. Ritzmann, S. E., and Levin, W. C.: Cryopathies: A review: Classification, diagnostic and therapeutic considerations. *Arch. Intern. Med. 107*:754, 1961.

90. Ellis, F. A.: The cutaneous manifestation of cryoglobulinemia. *Arch. Dermatol. 89*:690, 1964.

91. Brouet, J. C., Clauvel, J. P., Danon, F., Klein, M., and Seligmann, M.: Biologic and clinical significance of cryoglobulinemia: A report of 86 cases. *Am. J. Med. 57*:775, 1974.

92. Lapes, M. J., and Davis, J. S.: Arthralgia-purpura-weakness-cryoglobulinemia. *Arch. Intern. Med. 126*:287, 1970.

93. Grey, H. M., and Kohler, P. F.: Cryoimmunoglobulins. *Semin. Hematol. 10*:87, 1973.

94. Fauci, A. S., Haynes, B. F., and Katz, P.: The spectrum of vasculitis: Clinical, pathologic, immunologic and therapeutic considerations. *Ann. Int. Med. 89*:660, 1978.

95. Korst, D. R., and Kratochvil, C. H.: "Cryofibrinogen" in a case of lung neoplasm associated with thrombophlebitis migrans. *Blood 10*:945, 1955.

96. Jager, B. V.: Cryofibrinogenemia. *N. Engl. J. Med. 266*:579, 1962.

97. McKee, P. A., Kalbfleisch, J. M., and Bird, R. M.: Incidence and significance of cryofibrinogenemia. *J. Lab. Clin. Med. 61*:203, 1963.

98. Glueck, H. I., and Herrmann, L. G.: Cold-precipitable fibrinogen, "cryofibrinogen." *Arch. Intern. Med. 113*:748, 1964.

99. Bell, W., Bahr, R., Waldmann, T. A., and Carbone, P. P.: Cryofibrinogenemia, multiple dysproteinemias, and hypervolemia in a patient with a primary hepatoma. *Ann. Intern. Med. 64*:658, 1966.

100. Waxman, S., and Dove, J. T.: Cryofibrinogenemia aggravated during hypothermia. *N. Engl. J. Med. 281*:1291, 1969.

101. Zlotnick, A., Shahin, W., and Rachmilewitz, E. A.: Studies in cryofibrinogenemia. *Acta Haematol. 42*:8, 1969.

102. Mosseson, M. W., and Amrani, D. L.: The structure and biologic activities of plasma fibronectin. *Blood 56*:145, 1980.

103. Coltz, R.: Systematized amyloidosis: A review of skin and mucous membrane lesions and a report of two cases. *Medicine 31*:381, 1952.

104. Propp, S., Scharfman, W. B., Beebe, R. T., and Wright, A. W.: Atypical amyloidosis associated with nonthrombocytopenic purpura and plasmocytic hyperplasia of the bone marrow. *Blood 9*:397, 1954.

105. Hurley, H. J., and Weinberg, R.: Induced intralesional hemorrhage in primary systemic amyloidosis. *Arch. Dermatol. 89*:678, 1964.

106. Barth, W. F., Willerson, J. T., Waldmann, T. A., and Decker, J. L.: Primary amyloidosis. *Am. J. Med. 47*:259, 1969.

107. Howell, M.: Acquired factor X deficiency associated with systematized amyloidosis: A report of a case. *Blood 21*:739, 1963.

108. Korsan-Bengtsen, K., Kjort, P. F., and Ygge, J.: Acquired factor X deficiency in a patient with amyloidosis. *Thromb. Diath. Haemorrh. 7*:558, 1962.

109. Ménaché, D., and Boivin, P.: Déficit acquis en facteur X chez un malade atteint d'amylose primitive: Injection d'une fraction C.S.B. *Nouv. Rev. Fr. Hematol. 2*:868, 1972.

110. Ottolander, G. J. H., and Perret, L. J.: Verworven hemorragische diathese ten gevolge van geïsoleerde factor-X-deficiëntie. *Ned. Tijdschr. Geneeskd. 109*:852, 1965.

111. Pechet, L., and Kastrul, J. J.: Amyloidosis associated with factor X (Stuart) deficiency. *Ann. Intern. Med. 61*:315, 1964.

112. McPherson, R. A., Onstad, J. W., Ugoretz, R. J., and Wolf, P. L.: Coagulopathyin amyloidosis: Combined deficiency of factor IX and X. *Am. J. Hematol. 3*:225, 1977.

113. Greipp, P. R., Kyle, R. A., and Bowie, E. J. W.: Factor X deficiency in amyloidosis: Resolution after splenectomy. *N. Engl. J. Med. 301*:1050, 1979.

114. Furie, B., Greene, E., and Furie, B. C.: Syndrome of acquired factor X deficiency and systemic amyloidosis: In vivo studies of the metabolic fate of factor X. *N. Engl. J. Med. 297*:81, 1977.

115. Furie, B., Voo, L., McAdam, K. P. W. J., and Furie, B. C.: Mechanism of factor X deficiency in systemic amyloidosis. *N. Engl. J. Med. 304*:827, 1981.

116. Waldenström, J.: Three new cases of purpura hyperglobulinemia: A study in long-lasting benign increase in serum globulin. *Acta Med. Scand. [Suppl. 266] 142*:931, 1952.

117. Lindeboom, G. A.: Purpura hyperglobulinemica. *Dermatologica 96*:337, 1948.

118. Kay, H. E. M., and Robertson, K. M.: Benign hyperglobulinemic purpura. *J. Pathol. Bacteriol. 70*:543, 1955.

119. Seiden, G. E., and Wurzel, H. A.: Idiopathic benign hyperglobulinemic purpura. *N. Engl. J. Med. 255*:170, 1956.

120. Rozengvaig, S., Josephson, A. M., Shapiro, C., and Texidor, T.: Benign purpura hyperglobulinemica. *Arch. Intern. Med. 99*:913, 1957.

121. Symon, W. E., Rohn, R. J., and Bond, W. H.: Some observations on hyperglobulinemic purpura (Waldenström's syndrome). *Am. J. Med. Sci. 234*:160, 1957.

122. Hambrick, G. W., Jr.: Dysproteinemic purpura of hypergammaglobulinemic type: Clinical features and differential diagnosis. *Arch. Dermatol. 77*:23, 1958.

123. Strauss, W. G.: Purpura hyperglobulinemia of Waldenström: Report of a case and review of the literature. *N. Engl. J. Med.* 260:857, 1959.

124. Goltz, R. W., and Good, R. A.: Benign hyperglobulinemic purpura: Relation to Mikulicz's disease, sicca syndrome, and epidermolysis bullosa dystrophica. *Arch. Dermatol.* 83:26, 1961.

125. Waldenström, J.: Studies on conditions associated with disturbed gamma globulin formation (gammapathies). *Harvey Lect.* 56:211, 1961.

126. Birch, C. A., Cooke, K. B., Drew, C. E., London, D. R., Mackenzie, D. H., and Milne, M. D.: Hyperglobulinaemic purpura due to a thymic tumour. *Lancet* 1:693, 1964.

127. Schwartz, H. J., and Fredd, S. B.: The benign purpuric hyperglobulinemia of Waldenström. *JAMA* 187:230, 1964.

128. Kyle, R. A., Bayard, E. D., and Vaughn, J. H.: Benign hyperglobulinemic purpura of Waldenström. *Medicine* 50:113, 1971.

129. Capra, D. J., Winchester, R. J., and Kunkel, H. G.: Hyperglobulinemic purpura: Studies on the unusual anti-γ-globulins characteristic of the sera of these patients. *Medicine* 50:125, 1971.

130. Wilson, S. J., Bolinger, R. E., and Slinker, B. J.: Hyperglobulinemic purpura: Report of 14 cases fulfilling Waldenström's criteria. *J. Kans. Med. Soc.* 58:166, 1957.

131. Clark, R. A., Abraham, G. N., Kyler, R., and Vaughn, J. N.: Gamma globulin complexes in rheumatoid arthritis and hypergammaglobulinemic purpura. *J. Rheum.* 1:54, 1974.

132. Perks, W. H., Green, F., and Gleeson, M. H.: A case of purpura hyperglobulinemica of Waldenström studied by skin immunofluorescence. *Br. J. Dermatol.* 91:563, 1974.

133. Cream, J. J., Bryleson, A. D., and Ryder, G.: Disappearance of immunoglobulin and complement from the Arthus reaction and its relevance to studies of vasculitis in man. *Br. J. Dermatol.* 84:106, 1971.

134. Fox, M. J., and Enzer, N.: A consideration of the phenomenon of purpura following scarlet fever. *Am. J. Med. Sci.* 126:321, 1938.

135. Ackroyd, J. F.: Three cases of thrombocytopenic purpura occurring after rubella with a review of purpura associated with infections. *Q. J. Med.* 18:299, 1949.

136. Ackroyd, J. F.: Allergic purpura, including purpura due to foods, drugs and infections. *Am. J. Med.* 14:605, 1953.

137. Lerner, A. M., Klein, J. O., Cherry, J. D., and Finland, M.: New viral exanthems. *N. Engl. J. Med.* 269:678, 1963.

138. Mengel, C. E., and Trystad, C.: Thrombocytopenia in Rocky Mountain spotted fever. *JAMA* 113:886, 1963.

139. Horwitz, L., and Silber, R.: Subacute bacterial endocarditis presenting as purpura. *Arch. Intern. Med.* 120:483, 1967.

140. Safai, B., Mike, V., Giraldo, G., Beth, E., Good, R. A.: Association of Kaposi's sarcoma with second primary malignancies. Possible etiopathogenic implications. *Cancer* 45:1472, 1980.

141. Hymes, K. B., et al.: Kaposi's sarcoma in homosexual men—A report of eight cases. *Lancet* 2:598, 1981.

142. Urmacher, C., Myskowski, P., Ochoa, M., Jr., Kris, M., Safai, B.: Outbreak of Kaposi's sarcoma with cytomegalovirus infection in young homosexual men. *Am. J. Med.* 72:569, 1982.

143. Durack, D. T.: Opportunistic infections and Kaposi's sarcoma in homosexual men. *N. Engl. J. Med.* 305:1465, 1981.

144. Safai, B., Good, R. A.: Kaposi's sarcoma: A review and recent developments. *Clin. Bull.* 10:62, 1980.

CHAPTER 149

Autoerythrocyte and DNA sensitivity

ARLAN J. GOTTLIEB

Autoerythrocyte sensitivity

Data have been reported on some 170 cases of autoerythrocyte sensitivity since its description in 1955 [1–3]. One report has summarized the findings in 56 patients [3]. Over 95 percent of patients are female [3]. The syndrome is characterized by the spontaneous appearance, either singly or in groups, of painful ecchymoses. The extremities, particularly the hands, are most frequently involved. Usually, local itching, burning, or pain develops before the lesion appears. The presence of erythema helps to differentiate these lesions from "benign" ecchymoses. No distinct histologic picture has emerged. A high percentage of patients have a history of physical or surgical trauma preceding the onset of the disease. Lesions may then appear at the site of trauma or elsewhere. Gastrointestinal bleeding, epistaxis, hematuria, abdominal pain, diarrhea, nausea and vomiting, syncopal attacks, chest pain, headache, and menometrorrhagia have been frequent findings or complaints. Physical examination and laboratory and hematologic examination have failed to reveal a consistent pattern of abnormality. Intradermal injection of autologous erythrocytes or erythrocyte stroma usually results in the rapid appearance of pain, swelling, and induration at the injection site. A positive intradermal test has also been obtained with hemoglobin [4,5]. Intradermal testing with deoxyribonucleic acid (DNA), ribonucleic acid, autologous leukocytes, and plasma has been negative [1–3]. As a result of these studies, the etiology of this condition has been ascribed to an autosensitivity to a component of the erythrocyte membrane [1]. However, attempts to demonstrate this sensitivity by passive cutaneous anaphylaxis or the Prausnitz-Kustner reaction have been unsuccessful [5–7]. Skin tests with phosphatidyl serine, a red cell membrane phospholipid, have been reported to be positive in several patients but negative in others [8]. Similarly, skin tests with erythrocytes have been positive, whereas testing with erythrocyte stroma has been negative [4]. Although the lesions may at times be factitious [9–11], self-infliction has apparently been adequately excluded in a number of reports [2,5,6]. It is extremely important, however, to rule out self-infliction as a cause of the bizarre skin purpura. Extremities temporarily enclosed in plaster casts or inaccessible areas of the back appear to be appropriate locations for skin tests in these patients [6,11].

The relationship between this syndrome and an underlying psychiatric disorder has been emphasized [2,3,7,12–15]. The appearance of new skin lesions was found to correlate with periods of increased psychic stress [1–3,12]. Afflicted individuals were found to have psychosomatic complaints and a rather uniform personality pattern. Typically, they are prone toward hysteria, masochism, depression, and anxiety and have great difficulty expressing hostility. It has been shown, moreover, that both the results of skin tests and the appearance of new lesions may be influenced by hypnotic suggestion [14]. The similarity between the hemorrhagic manifestations of this disorder and religious stigmatization has also been emphasized [2,3,12–14,16]. It has been suggested, therefore, that the condition called autoerythrocyte sensitization is actually psychogenic and should be more appropriately designated *psychogenic purpura* [2,3].

The disease is benign and undergoes periods of exacerbation and sometimes prolonged or lasting remission [1–3]. The administration of antihistamine drugs, glucocorticoids, or chloroquine and splenectomy have had little salutary effect. Supportive psychotherapy has been reported to be of value in some patients [2,3].

A psychiatrically disturbed adolescent female with a disorder characterized by recurrent crops of painful ecchymoses which could be evoked locally by the intradermal or subcutaneous injection of both autologous red cell extract and heterologous DNA has been reported [17]. Consequently it has been suggested that the syndromes of autoerythrocyte sensitivity and DNA sensitivity may be related [17]. Others have suggested that a distinction be made between these two syndromes and a third, autoleukocyte sensitivity [18,19].

Autosensitivity to DNA

Autosensitivity to DNA is a rare and puzzling syndrome. Seven cases have been reported to date, all in women [17,20–25]. Unlike autoerythrocyte sensitization, a consistent history of trauma is lacking. The initial lesion is a painful wheal or nodule, usually on one of the extremities, which rapidly enlarges with accompanying pain and induration. At times localized pruritis may be present before the appearance of the wheal [20]. Within 24 h the lesions are ecchymotic, painful, and sometimes bullous. They vary in size from discrete, coin-sized lesions to large ecchymotic areas almost completely covering the extensor or flexor aspect of a limb. Resolution of lesions usually occurs within 4 to 5 days but may require as long as 2 to 3 weeks. The lesions may occur singly or in groups. Although involvement of the extremities is most common, lesions on the face and trunk have been reported. One case was associated with otherwise inexplicable hematuria [23]. Physical examination reveals only the painful skin lesions. Two of four patients had increased capillary fragility [21,23], but the remainder of the laboratory and hematologic studies,

including serologic and histologic tests for systemic lupus erythematosus, were completely within normal limits.

Characteristically, the lesions may be immediately evoked by the intradermal injection of minute amounts of DNA or a suspension of lysed autologous leukocytes. As little as 0.4 μg of calf thymus DNA has evoked a positive skin test [21]. Negative skin tests have been obtained with deoxyribonuclease or chloroquine-treated DNA or leukocytes, ribonucleic acid, and autologous plasma or erythrocytes. Circulating antibodies to DNA have not been found, nor has it been possible to demonstrate either humoral or cell-bound antibody by passive cutaneous anaphylaxis or the Prausnitz-Kustner reaction. It is intriguing that skin reactivity is confined to localized anatomic locations. For example, the arms may be quite reactive to intradermal tests while the trunk is not. When skin grafts are interchanged between these areas, the site to which the skin has been transplanted rather than the site of origin is the determinant of whether former reactivity is to continue or new sensitivity is to appear [22,23]. Histologically, the induced and spontaneous lesions appear to be identical. Varying degrees of cellular infiltration, edema, and hemorrhage are found. A mild vasculitis has also been noted. The presence of amorphous, basophilic, Feulgen-positive material bearing a close resemblance to hematoxylin bodies, described in the original report of this syndrome [1], has been noted in one subsequent case. In one patient IgM, complement [3], and properdin were demonstrated at the dermal-epidermal junction of a typical lesion [25]. One report [24] has drawn attention to the possible role of leukocyte bradykinin.

While cutaneous hypersensitivity to nuclear antigens has been reported both in patients with disseminated lupus and in normal controls, the reaction is usually of the delayed variety [26]. As yet, there had been little to suggest that patients with autosensitivity to DNA have a collagen-vascular disease.

Treatment with antihistamine drugs and glucocorticoids has been unsuccessful. The administration of chloroquine, however, has induced a prompt, dramatic, and, when continued, apparently lasting response in four of the six patients treated in this manner [20,25]. Chloroquine is administered in a dose of 250 mg four times daily for 1 week and then in a dose of 250 to 500 mg daily. The mechanism of action of chloroquine is unknown but may be related to the high levels attained in the skin as well as to its high affinity for DNA [27–29]. Since the lesions of factitious disease may readily masquerade as those of DNA hypersensitivity [30], diagnostic caution is advisable.

References

1. Gardner, F. H., and Diamond, L. K.: Autoerythrocyte sensitization: A form of purpura producing painful bruising following autosensitization to red blood cells in certain women. *Blood* 10:675, 1955.

2. Ratnoff, O. D., and Agle, D. P.: Psychogenic purpura: A reevaluation of the syndrome of autoerythrocyte sensitization. *Medicine 47:*475, 1968.

3. Ratnoff, O. D.: The psychogenic purpuras: A review of autoerythrocyte sensitization, autosensitization to DNA, "hysterical" and factitial bleeding, and the religious stigmata. *Semin. Hematol. 17:*192, 1980.

4. Ghosh, M. L., and Saudler, G.: Autoerythrocyte sensitization. *Ir. Med. J. 65:*443, 1972.

5. Kremer, W. B., Mengel, C. E., Nowlin, J. B., and Nagaya, H.: Recurrent ecchymoses and cutaneous hyperreactivity to hemoglobulin: A form of autoerythrocyte sensitization. *Blood 30:*62, 1967.

6. Gottlieb, P. M., Stupniker, S., Sandberg, H., and Woldow, I.: Erythrocyte autosensitization. *Am. J. Med. Sci. 233:*196, 1957.

7. McDuffie, F. C., and McGuire, F. L.: Clinical and psychological patterns in auto-erythrocyte sensitivity. *Ann. Intern. Med. 63:*255, 1965.

8. Groch, G. S., Finch, S. C., Rogoway, W., and Fischer, D. S.: Studies in the pathogenesis of autoerythrocyte sensitization syndrome. *Blood 28:*19, 1966.

9. McKeown, K. M.: A case of purpura factitia. *Lancet 2:*555, 1920.

10. Davidson, E.: Factitious purpura presenting as autoerythrocyte sensitization. *Br. Med. J. 1:*104, 1964.

11. Levin, R. M., Chodosh, R., and Sherman, J. D.: Factitious purpura simulating autoerythrocyte sensitization. *Ann. Intern. Med. 70:*1201, 1969.

12. Ratnoff, O. D., and Agle, D. P.: Autoerythrocyte sensitization: Psychiatric patterns in patients with a peculiar protracted purpura. *Trans. Assoc. Am. Physicians 74:*290, 1961.

13. Agle, D. P., and Ratnoff, O. D.: Purpura as a psychosomatic entity: A psychiatric study of autoerythrocyte sensitization. *Arch. Intern. Med. 109:*685, 1962.

14. Agle, D. O., Ratnoff, O. D., and Wasman, M.: Studies in autoerythrocyte sensitization: The induction of purpuric lesions by hypnotic suggestion. *Psychosom. Med. 29:*491, 1967.

15. Hallstrom, T., Hersle, K., and Mobacken, H.: Mental symptoms and personality structure in autoerythrocyte sensitization syndrome. *Br. J. Psychiatry 115:*1269, 1969.

16. Rivas, F. D.: Vicarious bleeding. *Ann. Intern. Med. 50:*811, 1959.

17. Spiera, H., and Schwartz, A. L.: Autoerythrocyte sensitization reproducible by both autologous red cells and heterologous DNA. *Mt. Sinai J. Med. N.Y. 37:*108, 1970.

18. Kahn, S. A., and Cash, J. D.: Autoerythrocyte sensitization syndrome. *Scott. Med. J. 15:*248, 1970.

19. Dilorenzo, P. A., and Peterka, E. S.: Autoleukocyte sensitivity. *Acta Derm.Venereol. (Stockh.) 48:*397, 1968.

20. Levin, M. B., and Pinkus, H.: Autosensitivity to desoxyribonucleic acid (DNA). *N. Engl. J. Med. 264:*533, 1961.

21. Schwartz, R. S., Lewis, B., and Dameshek, W.: Hemorrhagic cutaneous anaphylaxis due to autosensitization to deoxyribonucleic acid. *N. Engl. J. Med. 267:*1105, 1962.

22. Little, A. S., and Bell, H. E.: Painful subcutaneous hemorrhages of the extremities with unusual reaction to injected deoxyribonucleic acid. *Ann. Intern. Med. 60:*886, 1964.

23. Chandler, D., and Nalbandian, R. M.: DNA autosensitivity. *Am. J. Med. Sci. 251:*145, 1966.

24. Leiba, H., Almog, C., Kaufman, S., and Edery, H.: Possible role of bradykinin in a patient with recurrent ecchymoses (DNA sensitization). *Isr. J. Med. Sci. 8:*67, 1972.

25. Pinnas, J. L.: Autosensitization to DNA: Evidence for an immunologic basis. *J. Invest. Dermatol. 72:*157, 1979.

26. Goldman, J. A., Litwin, A., Adams, L. E., Krueger, R. C., and Hess, E. V.: Cellular immunity to nuclear antigens in systemic lupus erythematosus. *J. Clin. Invest. 51:*2669, 1972.

27. Shaffer, B., Cahn, M. M., and Levy, E. J.: Absorption of antimalarial drugs in human skin. *J. Invest. Dermatol. 30:*341, 1958.

28. Parker, F. S., and Irvin, J. L.: The interaction of chloroquine with nucleic acids and nucleoproteins. *J. Biol. Chem. 199:*897, 1952.

29. Cohen, S. N., and Yeilding, K. L.: Stabilization of the structure of native DNA by chloroquine and observations on the nature of the chloroquine-DNA complex. *Arthritis Rheum. 6:*767, 1963.

30. Anderson, P. C., and McCaffree, M. D.: Pseudo DNA autosensitivity: A factitial disease. *JAMA 196:*104, 1966.

CHAPTER 150

Allergic purpura

ARLAN J. GOTTLIEB

The term *allergic purpura* is generally applied to a group of nonthrombocytopenic purpuras characterized by apparently allergic manifestations, including skin rash and edema. Histologically, an aseptic vasculitis of the vessels of the corium is the main finding. Rarely, the inciting agent is presumed to be an allergen in foods, drugs, or insect bites. More commonly, an etiologic agent is not identifiable. When the condition is accompanied by joint pain and gastrointestinal symptoms, the eponym *Henoch-Schönlein purpura* is applied.

HISTORY

In 1808 Willan first described a case of severe purpura associated with polymorphic erythematous cutaneous lesions, abdominal pain, melena, and edema of the extremities [1]. Schönlein in 1837 stressed the concurrent joint symptomatology ("peliosis rheumatica"), while Henoch (1874) called attention to the gastrointestinal symptomatology ("purpura abdominales") [2,3]. Although Johnson in 1852 [4] referred to an association between purpura and nephritis, Henoch [3] and later Osler, at the turn of the century, indicated the frequent and at times serious renal involvement in Henoch-Schönlein purpura [5–8]. Osler first attributed the variable manifestations of the disease to an anaphylactic response to a foreign antigen, a concept developed in greater detail by Glanzmann in 1920 [5–9]. The typical histologic finding of an acute aseptic vasculitis in the skin, noted by Silbermann in 1890 and Osler in 1900, has subsequently been described by others [6,10,11].

ETIOLOGY

The sudden onset, the close resemblance of the symptomatology to that of anaphylaxis, and the lack of an obvious infectious cause led Osler to suggest an immunologic pathogenesis for allergic purpura [5–8]. Cases due to food allergy [12–16], insect bites [12,17–20], and drugs [12,21–25] have been described. Attention has been called to several cases apparently resulting from smallpox vaccination [26–28]. In the majority of these cases, however, reinduction of the disease by reexposure to the presumed offending antigen has not been attempted.

The major impetus to the suggestion that bacteria, particularly the β-hemolytic streptococci, are the offending antigens in a hypersensitivity reaction has been provided by the high incidence of upper respiratory infection prior to the development of allergic purpura, as well as by the striking association between infection and purpura provided by a number of individual cases

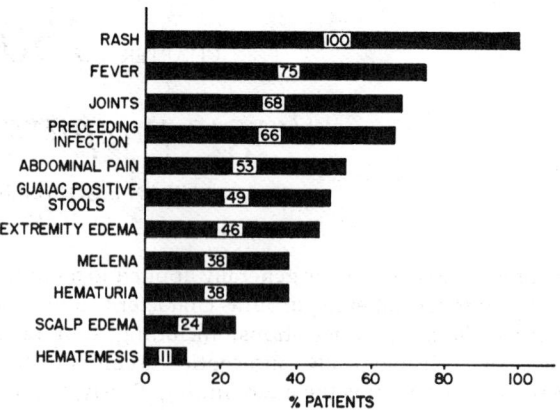

FIGURE 150-1 The occurrence of various signs and symptoms in 131 patients with allergic purpura. (Allen, Diamond, and Howell [34], by permission.)

[5–8,11,12,29–35]. Although the possibility that a specific strain of streptococcus is responsible for allergic purpura cannot be excluded, the evidence that the streptococcus is the sole pathogenic organism is not compelling. Three large series retrospectively examining a total of 40,000 cases of scarlet fever detected only 10 cases of allergic purpura [36–38]. It is possible to culture streptococci in only about a quarter to a third of cases. Similarly, antibody titers to the streptolysin O toxin (ASO) are elevated in only about a third of cases [32–35,39,40]. The incidence of ASO elevation in patients with allergic purpura, moreover, did not differ statistically from a normal control population and was quite distinct from the incidence of over 80 percent found in cases of acute rheumatic fever [32,40]. The frequency of significant antibody elevation to both streptococcal deoxyribonuclease (DNase) and ASO is similar in afflicted and control populations. B_{1C}-globulin levels were also normal [40]. It appears, therefore, that if indeed allergic purpura results from sensitivity to bacterial antigens, in the majority of cases no single type of bacteria can be incriminated.

Skin testing with a variety of bacterial vaccines or filtrates, including *Streptococcus* and *Staphylococcus*, has yielded evidence of hypersensitivity in patients with allergic purpura [41–44]. The hemorrhagic papule and local vasculitis resulting from the intradermal injection of bacteria or their products have also been found in subjects without allergic purpura. The results reported, therefore, serve to distinguish only a state of hypersensitivity. A more convincing argument that bacterial hypersensitivity can be pathogenic can be mustered in those instances in which injection of autogenous or exogenous bacterial filtrates results in local, and occasionally distant, hemorrhagic manifestations in patients with allergic purpura but not in normal controls [45,46]. Bacterial hypersensitivity has also been passively transferred to nonreactors by the transfer of viable leukocytes. Despite the histologic similarities of the induced lesions to those found in the Arthus reaction, the pas-

sively transferred reactivity is of the delayed type [45,46]. Fluorescence microscopy of the lesions indicates the presence of fibrinogen only in the vessel wall, in contrast to the Arthus phenomenon, in which fibrinogen, γ-globulin, and complement are detectable [47].

In accordance with the suggestion that allergic purpura may represent autoimmunity to components of vessel walls [48,49], a generalized nonthrombocytopenic purpura has been produced in experimental animals by the use of antisera to arterial endothelium [50–54]. Preparation of the antigen is, however, extremely difficult, and specific absorption studies of the antibody as well as histologic studies of the induced lesions are limited. The presence and possible role, moreover, of induced anti-γ-globulin factors have not been adequately evaluated [55], and the results of other studies have been negative [56]. Consequently, the significance of this concept of the etiology of allergic purpura is uncertain. It has also been suggested that the syndrome of allergic purpura may be a manifestation of a collagen-vascular disorder akin to rheumatoid arthritis and periarteritis nodosa [11,30,33,49,56,57].

The histopathologic changes observed in allergic purpura may be interpreted as resembling those which have been experimentally induced in "immune-complex" disease [58]. Indeed, the deposition of IgA together with complement components in the inflamed vessel walls and in the glomerular mesangium of patients with Henoch-Schönlein syndrome has suggested that the cutaneous and renal lesions result from the fixation of circulating IgA-containing immune complexes [59–66].

Serum of patients with Henoch-Schönlein purpura frequently contains immune complexes [66–68]. The associated immunoglobulin appears to be IgA more often than is observed in a variety of other disorders [67]. Using one assay, an IgA-immune complex was almost invariably present during the first week of clinical illness. Usually the reactive material disappeared or decreased in titer during the second and third weeks of the disease [67]. Other assays provided evidence for more long-lived circulating IgA-immune complexes [67]. Immune complexes consisting of IgA and of IgG have been observed by others [66]. The IgA complexes occurred more frequently, but the IgG complexes provided better correlation with the existence of nephropathy [66]. Clarification of these data awaits more experience with the technically difficult assays for the detection of IgA-immune complexes. Whether one or the other of the two subclasses of IgA (IgA_1 or IgA_2) occurs more frequently in the renal lesions also requires clarification [68,69]. An increase in serum IgA levels and in polymeric IgA has also been noted in some patients with Henoch-Schönlein purpura [60,68]. The similarity between primary IgA nephropathy (Berger's disease) and the renal lesions of Henoch-Schönlein purpura has also drawn considerable comment [61–64,67–73]. Both syndromes are associated with a nephropathy in which deposition of IgA is prominent, and in both, IgA deposits have been demonstrated in cutaneous biopsies. An increase in serum IgA levels and IgA-bearing and -secreting lymphocytes has also been reported in Berger's disease [74]. These syndromes may represent variants of the same pathogenic mechanism. In IgA nephropathy the extrarenal manifestations are usually absent or, when present, widely separated in time from the development of nephropathy. In contrast, renal disease and systemic illness usually occur concurrently in Henoch-Schönlein syndrome.

PATHOLOGY

Histologic examination shows that the acute skin lesion is an aseptic vasculitis most marked in the vessels of the corium. The cellular perivascular cuff is composed predominantly of polymorphonuclear leukocytes and may contain variable numbers of eosinophils. Fibrinoid necrosis and platelet plugging of vessels may be seen. Interstitial tissue is edematous and contains extravasated erythrocytes [11,35]. Both the venous and the arterial end of the capillary may be involved [75,76]. Since leukocytic nuclear debris is commonly evident in the inflammatory lesions (leukocytoclysis), allergic purpura is considered one of the leukocytoclastic vasculitides [76]. Grossly uninvolved skin is usually histologically normal. When studied by immunofluorescence techniques, the capillary bed in both normal and purpuric skin from patients with allergic purpura has been shown to contain finely granular deposits which are reactive for IgA, C3c, C3d, and C5 [62,69,72]. IgM, C4, and C3b are less frequently identified, and C1q and C3 proactivator have not been found. These findings have been taken to suggest "alternate pathway" activation of complement by IgA [62].

The bowel may be grossly edematous and hemorrhagic. Submucosal hemorrhage is common, and mucosal ulcerations may occur in severe cases. Vascular lesions similar to those seen in the skin are found [11,34,77,78].

Although the renal lesions of allergic purpura have been described as typical of a subacute glomerulonephritis [11,57,78,79], they are probably more focal than diffuse in nature [80–85]. A focal glomerulitis with endothelial proliferation and hypercellularity, and platelet thrombi in capillaries have been most frequently described [35,59,80–85]. As distinct from the findings in glomerulonephritis, mesangial rather than basement membrane localization of fibrinogen, complement, and γ-globulin has been demonstrated by fluorescence microscopy [69,72,81,84]. It has been suggested that the deposition of fibrin in the glomerulus precedes the adhesion of complement and immunoglobulin [82]. In the occasional patient in whom florid, rapidly progressive renal disease is seen, a diffuse glomerulonephritis with epithelial crescent formation, resembling an Ellis type I nephritis, is found [80–85]. Agreement has been reached that the patient with the more diffuse and advanced histopathologic lesion at the time of presentation has the poorer prognosis for recovery of normal renal function [34,83,84]. With chronicity, the pathology is indistinguishable from the end-stage kidney of chronic glomerulonephritis [80–85]. Focal myocarditis [57], hepatic involvement [78], and perivasculitis of the lung [77,85] have also been described.

CLINICAL FEATURES

Allergic purpura is primarily a disease of children. It is relatively uncommon under the age of 2 years and above the age of 20 [11,33,34]. Consequently, while an increasing number of case series in adults are accruing [84–86], our knowledge of the disease stems mainly from the reports of cases in the pediatric age group. The peak incidence is found between the third and seventh year of life, and the mean age of onset given in most series is between 5 and 6 years of age [30,31]. In most reports, males are about twice as frequently afflicted as females [11,29–31,33,34]. A seasonal peak incidence in the early spring, or early spring and autumn, has been suggested [30,33,34]. In adults the disease may not have a predilection for either sex [84,85].

A history of upper respiratory infection within 1 to 3 weeks prior to the onset of symptoms is obtained in a majority of cases. Estimates have ranged from 50 percent to as high as 90 percent or more of pediatric cases [5–8,11,12,29,35] and to as low as 30 percent in the adult age group [85].

The onset of the disease is sudden, but the presenting manifestations are variable [11,34,77]. Malaise, headache, fever, rash, polyarthralgia, or abdominal pain may be the presenting symptoms. The occurrence of various signs and symptoms in 131 patients is presented in Fig. 150-1. The delayed appearance of the skin rash often poses a difficult problem in differential diagnosis, particularly in the patient presenting with colicky abdominal pain. In adults, skin rash is the most common presenting symptom, while joint, renal, and gastrointestinal manifestations are seen in about half the patients [84–86].

The skin lesion of allergic purpura is urticarial at onset [11,34]. As the lesions recede, they gradually become pinkish, then red or at times frankly hemorrhagic (Plate 12); ultimately a brownish-red maculopapular eruption is seen. Petechiae may also be observed. The lesions may occur singly or in clusters, may be confluent or remain discrete, and are painless (Plate 12). Involvement tends to be fairly symmetrical. The extensor surfaces of the lower extremities, particularly the knees and feet, the buttocks, and the extensor surfaces of the arms, particularly the elbows, are commonly involved. Face, trunk, and mucous membrane involvement occurs, but considerably less frequently. Ulceration of the lesions is rare. New crops of lesions may occur throughout the initial 2 to 3 weeks of illness and are the most frequent symptoms during relapse. The hemorrhagic rash has been noted without the preceding urticarial lesion in the adult, and a necrotic, blistered lesion may appear more commonly in the older patient [85].

Nonmigratory polyarthralgias involving, in decreasing frequency, the ankles, knees, hips, wrists, elbows, and fingers are seen. Tenderness and swelling is mainly periarticular. Joint effusion may occur, but the joints themselves are not typically red or warm. Residual joint deformity does not result.

Localized edema, typically of the hands, feet, or scalp, occurs in almost half the patients. Painful swelling of the scalp or face occurs most frequently in children under 3 years of age.

Colicky abdominal pain is the most common gastrointestinal sign or symptom. It is usually associated with frank melena or guaiac-positive stools. Hematemesis may occur. Severe gastrointestinal symptoms are thought to occur with increased frequency in older children [22].

Abdominal tenderness may be elicited on examination, but muscular guarding is usually absent. The increased frequency of intussusception in allergic purpura presumably results from the forward invagination of the relatively rigid edematous or hemorrhagic segment of bowel into a more normally motile segment [87–89]. In this regard, an increase in abdominal pain, melena, the appearance of a palpable mass, or merely the deterioration of the patient may signal the necessity for prompt surgical intervention. The importance of early exploratory laparotomy when doubt exists as to the nature of the intra-abdominal problems has been stressed [90]. Intussusception appears to be less common in adults [84–86]. Intestinal perforation has been reported [91]. Pancreatitis may occur [92]. Transient paresis, convulsions, and cranial nerve palsies, including optic atrophy, have been recorded, due to vasculitis of the nervous system [34,82,93–95].

Renal involvement, as evidenced by either gross or microscopic hematuria, often accompanied by proteinuria, may make its appearance in the second or third week of the disease [34] and is observed in between one-quarter and over one-half of patients [33–35,85]. Males and older children may be at greater risk [11,30,33,34]. Hypertension may develop but is usually easily controlled [34]. Transient renal failure, seen as nitrogen retention or oliguria, occurs in about one-fifth or less of patients with renal involvement. Transient diminution of renal function may accompany exacerbation of the skin lesions [96]. Testicular hemorrhage [34] and torsion [97] have been observed.

LABORATORY FINDINGS

Routine laboratory examinations offer no specific help in the diagnosis of allergic purpura. The platelet count is normal. Anemia is not usually present unless the hemorrhagic manifestations have been severe. The white blood cell count and erythrocyte sedimentation rate are usually elevated. There may be a polymorphonuclear leukocytosis and an increase in eosinophils. Tourniquet tests are, at times, positive. Examination of the urine may show hematuria and proteinuria. Granular and red cell casts may also be seen. The blood urea nitrogen and creatinine are elevated in the presence of renal failure. A protein-losing enteropathy may be a contributing factor when hypoalbuminemia occurs in patients with gastrointestinal involvement [98].

DIFFERENTIAL DIAGNOSIS

As noted, the diagnosis of allergic purpura may require a high index of suspicion and careful examination of the patient presenting without the typical purpuric skin rash. Primarily, it must be distinguished from other forms of nonthrombocytopenic purpura. A number of infectious diseases which may be associated with a purpuric skin lesion must also be considered (see Chap. 148) [12]. The necessary distinctions are usually not difficult to make when the dermatologic and general medical features of each case are reviewed. Drugs such as chlorthiazide and iodides or chemicals such as mercury and bismuth may at times be incriminated [12] (Plate 12). The rash seen in allergic purpura may be differentiated from the purpura that infrequently accompanies acute rheumatic fever and acute glomerulonephritis [99]. Renal involvement, moreover, is not evident early in the course of allergic purpura, nor is it usually associated with carditis [34]. In the adult, only the total clinical and pathologic picture may, at times, serve to distinguish allergic purpura from the cutaneous vasculitides—cutaneous periarteritis nodosa, erythema multiforme, or the vasculitis seen in disseminated lupus erythematosus and Sjögren's syndrome.

THERAPY

Isolated therapeutic successes resulting from the administration of glucocorticoids have been reported [100–103]. No large-scale controlled studies of results of glucocorticoid therapy exist. In general, in children, glucocorticoids have not proved effective in suppressing the appearance of the skin rash or altering either the duration of the illness or its frequency of recurrence [34]. Similarly, glucocorticoid therapy does not appear to alter the course of acute renal involvement, the persistence of hematuria or proteinuria, or the frequency of the development of chronic renal involvement [34,81,82]. Glucocorticoids are apparently effective in controlling edema and joint and abdominal pain during the acute illness and therefore may be of value as supportive measures in the sicker child. Glucocorticoids have been recommended for the child presenting with marked abdominal symptoms [34] as a possible means of preventing intussusception by decreasing bowel edema and hemorrhage.

In chronic renal disease, immunosuppressive therapy with azathioprine has been reported of value in cases with predominantly proliferative glomerular changes [104,105]. Others have been unable to support earlier claims of the efficacy of immunosuppressive and cytotoxic therapy [106,107]. Sufficient data have not yet accrued to support the efficacy of therapy with heparin [108].

COURSE AND PROGNOSIS

In the pediatric age group, the average duration of the initial attack is about 4 weeks. In younger children, the disease runs a somewhat milder and more abbreviated course [34]. One or more recurrences, manifest usually as a reappearance of the skin rash or abdominal pain, occur in almost one-half of patients over the age of 2 years [12,34,83–86]. The initial relapse may be anticipated 6 weeks after the onset of illness, following a period of apparent well-being. The recurrence rate appears highest in the patient with more severe disease during the initial episode. Except for the occasional case in which intussusception or chronic renal disease supervenes, the ultimate prognosis is almost uniformly good. Occasionally death from renal failure has occurred during the acute attack or shorter thereafter. Only 5 such cases, however, were found in three series containing over 440 cases [33,34,83]. A nephritic syndrome may be more frequent in adults [85,86]. In one retrospective series, 38 of 75 cases showed renal involvement. Of these, 19 gave evidence of nephritis, while three others developed progressive renal failure [85].

In the patient with renal involvement, abnormalities of the urinary sediment are slower to subside than the acute illness. Roughly 25 percent of patients with renal disease fall into this group. Morbidity, evidenced mainly by persistent hematuria, is highest among those having severe renal involvement during the initial episode [34,83–86]. Similarly, a renal biopsy indicating diffuse glomerular involvement or crescent formation appears to connote a more prolonged course and less favorable result with regard to renal involvement [83–86]. More usually, an abnormality in the urinary sediment is the sole finding on follow-up examination up to 4 and 5 years after the acute illness. Healing of the lesions has been demonstrated by renal biopsy [35,83–86], and the urinary sediment has been reported to revert to normal in up to 84 percent of patients within 1 year after the initial attack [33]. It would appear, therefore, that in most cases of renal involvement, no permanent renal damage results.

The fate of kidneys transplanted into recipients suffering renal failure in the course of allergic purpura is yet unsettled [84,109]. In one report a graft obtained from an identical twin was surviving normally [84]. A graft from parent to child, however, was rejected [109]. While the immunopathologic findings during rejection in the latter case were similar to those found during active disease, the problems in graft survival may be more related to the difficulties in cross matching than in persistence of the disease.

References

1. Willan, R.: *On Cutaneous Diseases*. Johnson, London, 1808.
2. Schönlein, J.: *Allgemeine und specielle Pathologie und Therapie*, 3d ed. Lit. Compt., Herisau, 1837, vol. 2, p. 48.
3. Henoch, E.: Über eine eigenthümliche Form von Purpura. *Berlin Klin. Wschr.* 11:641, 1874.
4. Johnson, G.: *Diseases of the Kidney*. London, 1852.
5. Osler, W.: On the visceral complications of erythema exudativium multiforme. *Am. J. Med. Sci.* 110:629, 1895.
6. Osler, W.: The visceral lesions of the erythema group. *Br. J. Dermatol.* 12:227, 1900.
7. Osler, W.: On the visceral manifestations of the erythema group of skin diseases. *Am. J. Med. Sci.* 127:1, 1904.
8. Osler, W.: The visceral lesions of purpura and allied conditions. *Br. Med. J.* 1:517, 1914.
9. Glanzmann, E.: Die Konzeption der anaphylaktoiden Purpura. *Jahrb. Kinderh.* 91:391, 1920.
10. Silbermann, O.: *Paediatr. Arb.*, 1890, p. 237.
11. Gairdner, D.: The Schönlein-Henoch syndrome (anaphylactoid purpura). *Q. J. Med.* 17:95, 1948.
12. Ackroyd, J. F.: Allergic purpura, including purpura due to foods, drugs, and infections. *Am. J. Med.* 14:605, 1953.
13. Alexander, H. L., and Eyermann, C. H.: Allergic purpura. *JAMA* 92:2092, 1929.
14. Kahn, I. S.: Henoch's purpura due to food allergy. *J. Lab. Clin. Med.* 14:835, 1929.
15. Ancona, G. R., Ellenhorn, M. J., and Falconer, E. H.: Purpura due to food sensitivity. *J. Allergy* 22:487, 1951.
16. Jensen, B.: Schönlein-Henoch's purpura: Three cases with fish or penicillin as antigen. *Acta Med. Scand.* 152:61, 1955.
17. Siegel, J. M., Brown, H. E., and Dileo, L. W.: Purpura as a result of insect allergy: Treatment with cortisone (adrenocortical preparation). *Postgrad. Med.* 15:46, 1954.
18. Burke, D. M., and Jellinek, H. L.: Nearly fatal case of Schönlein-Henoch syndrome following insect bite. *Am. J. Dis. Child.* 88:772, 1954.
19. Tveteras, E.: Anaphylactoid purpura (Schönlein-Henoch syndrome) complicated by nephritis. *Int. Arch. Allergy* 9:274, 1956.
20. Sharan, G., Anand, R. K., and Sinha, K. P.: Schönlein-Henoch syndrome after insect bite. *Br. Med. J.* 1:656, 1966.
21. Davis, W. C., and Saunders, T. S.: Purpura due to iodides. *Arch. Dermatol.* 53:644, 1946.
22. Spring, M.: Purpura and nephritis after administration of procaine penicillin. *JAMA* 147:1139, 1951.
23. Fitzgerald, E. W., Jr.: Fatal glomerulonephritis complicating allergic purpura due to chlorothiazide. *Arch. Intern. Med.* 105:305, 1960.
24. Carmel, W. J., Jr., and Dannenberg, T.: Nonthrombocytopenic purpura due to Miltown. *N. Engl. J. Med.* 255:770, 1956.
25. Casser, L.: Anaphylactoid purpura following penicillin therapy. *J. Med. Soc. N.J.* 53:133, 1956.
26. Jiménez, E. L., and Dorrington, H. J.: Vaccination and Henoch-Schönlein purpura. *N. Engl. J. Med.* 279:1171, 1968.
27. Castells-Van Dalle, M.: Vaccination and Henoch-Schönlein purpura. *N. Engl. J. Med.* 280:781, 1969.
28. Lane, M. J.: Vaccination and Henoch-Schönlein purpura. *N. Engl. J. Med.* 280:781, 1969.
29. Philpott, M. G.: The Schönlein-Henoch syndrome in childhood with particular reference to the occurrence of nephritis. *Arch. Dis. Child.* 27:480, 1952.
30. Lewis, I. C.: The Schönlein-Henoch syndrome compared with certain features of nephritis and rheumatism. *Arch. Dis. Child.* 30:212, 1955.
31. Wedgewood, R. J. P., and Klaus, M. H.: Anaphylactoid purpura: A long term follow-up study with special reference to renal involvement. *Pediatrics* 16:196, 1955.
32. Bywaters, E. G. L., Isdale, I., and Kempton, J. J.: Schönlein-Henoch purpura. *Q. J. Med.* 26:161, 1957.
33. Sterky, G., and Thilen, A.: A study of the onset of prognosis of acute vascular purpura (the Schönlein-Henoch syndrome) in children. *Acta Paediatr.* 49:217, 1960.
34. Allen, D. M., Diamond, L. K., and Howell, D. A.: Anaphylactoid purpura in children (Schönlein-Henoch syndrome). *Am. J. Dis. Child.* 99:833, 1960.
35. Vernier, R. L., Worthen, H. G., Peterson, R. D., Colle, E., and Good, R. A.: Anaphylactoid purpura. I. Pathology of the skin and kidney and frequency of streptococcal infection. *Pediatrics* 27:181, 1961.

36. Fox, M. J., and Enzer, N.: A consideration of the phenomenon of purpura following scarlet fever. *Am. J. Med. Sci.* 196:321, 1938.
37. Hunt, L. W.: Hemorrhagic purpura in scarlet fever: Report of two cases. *Am. J. Dis. Child.* 56:1086, 1938.
38. Frödin, H.: Purpura fulminans and its relation to scarlatina. *Acta Paediatr.* 34:217, 1947.
39. Gietka, M.: On the aetiology of Schönlein-Henoch syndrome. *Ann. Paediatr.* 203:145, 1964.
40. Ayoub, E. M., and Hoyer, J.: Anaphylactoid purpura: Streptococcal antibody titers and B$_{1C}$-globulin levels. *J. Pediatr.* 75:193, 1969.
41. Coke, H.: Two interesting cases of purpura. *Br. Med. J.* 1:535, 1931.
42. Storck, H.: Purpura rheumatia bei Staphylokokken—enfizierter Monaldi-Höhle. *Dermatologica* 100:387, 1950.
43. Storck, H.: Über hämorrhagische Phänomene en Dermatologie. *Dermatologica* 102:197, 1951.
44. Storck, H.: Hämorrhagische Phänomene en de Dermatologie. *Arch. Dermatol.* 200:257, 1955.
45. Miescher, P., Reymond, A., and Ritter, O.: Le Role de l'allergie bactérienne dans la pathogénèse de certaines vasculites. *Schweiz. Med. Wochenschr.* 86:799, 1956.
46. Miescher, P.: Bakteriell-allergische vasculitiden als Ursache von Organerkrankungen. *Schweiz. Med. Wochenschr.* 87:1339, 1957.
47. Miescher, P. A., Paranetto, F., and Koffler, D.: Immunofluorescence studies in human vasculitis, in *Proceedings of the IVth International Symposium on Immunopathology.* Schwabe, Basel, 1966, p. 446.
48. Dameshek, W.: Acute vascular purpura: An immunovascular disorder. *Blood* 8:382, 1953.
49. Kreidberg, M. B., Dameshek, W., and Latoracca, R.: Acute vascular purpura (Schönlein-Henoch): An immunological disease. *N. Engl. J. Med.* 253:1014, 1955.
50. Katsura, H.: Experimental studies on purpura of guinea pigs: Purpura by the anti-hemangioendothelial cell serum. *J. Osaka Med. Assoc.* 22:373, 717, 816, 1923.
51. Clark, W. G., and Jacobs, E.: Experimental nonthrombocytopenic vascular purpura: A review of the Japanese literature with preliminary confirmatory report. *Blood* 5:32, 1950.
52. Israel, L., Mathe, G., and Bernard, J.: Purpura capillaire provoqué chez le cobaye par un immun-sérum de lapin anti-endothelium de cobaye. *Sang* 26:603, 1955.
53. Israel, L., Mathe, G., and Bernard, J.: Effets des injections dans le derme du cobaye. I. De sérum de lapin anti-endothelium de cobaye. II. De sérum de malades atteints de purpura rhumatoide et glomerulo-néphrite. *Sang* 26:606, 1955.
54. Israel, L., Mathe, G., and Bernard, J.: Sur le syndrome de Schönlein-Henoch. *Rev. Fr. Étude Clin. Biol.* 1:57, 1956.
55. Piomelli, S., Stefanini, M., and Mele, R.: Antigenicity of human vascular endothelium: Lack of relationship to the pathogenesis of vasculitis. *J. Lab. Clin. Med.* 54:241, 1959.
56. Fabuis, A. J. M.: Failure to demonstrate precipitating antibodies against vessel extracts in patients with vascular disorders. *Vox Sang.* 4:247, 1959.
57. Lecutier, M. A.: A case of the Schönlein-Henoch syndrome with myocardial necrosis. *J. Clin. Pathol.* 5:336, 1952.
58. Cochrane, C. G., and Weigle, W. O.: The cutaneous reaction to soluble antigen-antibody complexes: A comparison with the Arthus phenomenon. *J. Exp. Med* 108:591, 1958.
59. Panner, B.: Nephritis of Schönlein-Henoch syndrome. *Arch. Pathol.* 74:230, 1962.
60. Trygstad, C. W., and Stiehm, E. R.: Elevated serum IgA globulin in anaphylactoid purpura. *Pediatrics* 47:1023, 1971.
61. Baart de la Faille-Kupyer, E. H., Kater, L., Dorhut Mees, E. J., and Kooiker, C. J.: Immunohistochemical studies comparing normal skin and kidney tissues in 46 patients with nephropathy. *Neth. J. Med.* 16:60, 1973.
62. Baart de la Faille-Kupyer, E. H., Van der Meer, J. B., Kater, L., and Mul, N.: Alternate pathway complement activation by IgA in Schoenlein-Henoch's syndrome. *Neth. J. Med.* 17:5, 1974.
63. Berger, J.: IgA glomerular deposits in renal disease. *Transplant. Proc.* 1:939, 1969.
64. Tsai, C. C., Giangiacomo, J., and Zuckner, J.: Dermal IgA deposits in Henoch-Schönlein purpura and Berger's nephritis. *Lancet* 1:342, 1975.
65. Giangiacomo, J., and Tsai, C. C.: Dermal and glomerular deposition of IgA in anaphylactoid purpura. *Am. J. Dis. Child.* 131:981, 1977.
66. Levinsky, R. J., and Barratt, T. M.: IgA immune complexes in Henoch-Schönlein purpura. *Lancet* 2:1100, 1979.
67. Kauffmann, R. H., Herrmann, W. A., Meyer, C. J. L. M., Daha, M., and Van Es, L. A.: Circulating IgA-immune complexes in Henoch-Schönlein purpura: A longitudinal study of their relationship to disease activity and vascular deposition of IgA. *Am. J. Med.* 69:859, 1980.
68. André C., Berthoux, F. C., André, F., Gillon, J., Genin, C., and Sabatier, J. C.: Prevalence of IgA$_2$ deposits in IgA nephropathies. *N. Engl. J. Med.* 303:1343, 1980.
69. Conley, M. E., Cooper M. D., and Michael. A. F.: Selective deposition of immunoglobulin A$_1$ in immunoglobulin A nephropathy, anaphylactoid purpura, nephritis, and systemic lupus erythematosus. *J. Clin. Invest.* 66:1432, 1980.
70. McPhane, J. J., Jr.: IgA-associated glomerulonephritis. *Annu. Rev. Med.* 28:37, 1977.
71. Weiss, J. H., Bhathena, D. B., Curtis, J. J., Lucas, B. A., and Luke, R. G.: A possible relationship between Henoch-Schönlein syndrome and IgA nephropathy (Berger's disease): An illustrative case. *Nephron* 22:582, 1978.
72. Nakamoto, Y., et al.: Primary IgA glomerulonephritis and Schönlein-Henoch purpura nephritis: Clinicopathological and immunohistochemical characteristics. *Q. J. Med.* 178:495, 1978.
73. Rifai, A., Small, P. A., Jr., Teaque, P. O., and Ayoub, E. M.: Experimental IgA nephropathy. *J. Exp. Med.* 150:1161, 1979.
74. Nomoto, Y., Sakai, H., and Arimori, S.: Increase of IgA-bearing lymphocytes in peripheral blood from patients with IgA nephropathy. *Am. J. Clin. Pathol.* 71:158, 1979.
75. Humble, J. G.: The mechanism of petechial haemorrhage formation. *Blood* 4:69, 1949.
76. Fauci, A. S., Haynes, B. F., and Katz, P.: The spectrum of vasculitis: Clinical, immunologic and therapeutic considerations. *Ann. Intern. Med.* 89:660, 1978.
77. Norkin, S., and Wiener, J.: Henoch-Schönlein syndrome. *Am. J. Clin. Pathol.* 33:55, 1960.
78. Handel, J., and Schwartz, S.: Gastrointestinal manifestations of the Schönlein-Henoch syndrome. *Am. J. Roentgenol.* 78:643, 1957.
79. Levitt, M. L., and Burbank, B.: Glomerulonephritis as a complication of Schönlein-Henoch syndrome. *N. Engl. J. Med.* 248:530, 1953.
80. Heptinstall, R. H.: *Pathology of the Kidney.* Little, Brown, Boston, 1966, p. 335.
81. Urizar, R. E., Michael, A., Sisson, S., and Vernier, R. L.: Anaphylactoid purpura. II. Immunofluorescent and electronic microscopic studies of the glomerular lesions. *Lab. Invest.* 119:437, 1969.
82. Urizar, R. E., and Herdman, R. C.: Anaphylactoid purpura. III. Early morphologic glomerular changes. *Am. J. Clin. Pathol.* 53:258, 1970.
83. Meadow, S. R., Glasgow, E. F., White, R. H. R., Moncrieff, M. W., Cameron, J. S., and Ogg, L. S.: Schönlein-Henoch nephritis. *Q. J. Med.* 41:241, 1972.
84. Barron, H., and Rosenmann, E.: Schoenlein-Henoch syndrome in adults: A clinical and histologic study of renal involvement. *Isr. J. Med. Sci.* 8:1702, 1972.
85. Cream, J. J., Gumpel, J. M., and Peachey, R. D.: Schönlein-Henoch purpura in the adult: A study of 77 adults with anaphylactoid or Schönlein-Henoch purpura. *Q. J. Med.* 39:461, 1970.
86. Ballard, H. S., Eisenger, R. P., and Gallo, G.: Renal manifestations of the Henoch-Schönlein syndrome in adults. *Am. J. Med.* 49:328, 1970.
87. Balf, C. L.: The alimentary lesion in anaphylactoid purpura. *Arch. Dis. Child.* 26:20, 1951.
88. Wolfsohn, H.: Purpura and intussusception. *Arch. Dis. Child.* 22:242, 1947.
89. Steinhardt, I. D., and Jonas, A. F.: Coexistence of intussusception and Henoch's purpura. *N. Engl. J. Med.* 257:553, 1957.
90. Lindenauer, S. M., and Tank, E. S.: Surgical aspects of Henoch-Schönlein's purpura. *Surgery* 59:982, 1966.
91. DeWolf, W. C.: Anaphylactoid purpura with spontaneous intestinal perforation. *Minn. Med.* 55:1121, 1972.
92. Puppala, A. R., Cheng, J. C., and Steinheber, F. U.: Pancreatitis: A

rare complication of Schönlein-Henoch purpura. *Am. J. Gastroenterol.* 69:101, 1978.

93. Kaplan, J. M., Quintana, P., and Sanson, J.: Facial nerve palsy with anaphylactoid purpura. *Am. J. Dis. Child.* 119:452, 1970.

94. Aita, J. A.: Neurologic manifestations of Henoch-Schöenlein purpura. *Nebr. Med. J.* 58:37, 1973.

95. Lewis, I. C., and Philpott, M. G.: Neurologic complications in the Schöenlein-Henoch syndrome. *Arch. Dis. Child.* 31:369, 1956.

96. Garry, N. E., Mazzara, J. T., and Holfelder, L.: The Schönlein-Henoch syndrome: Report of two patients with recurrent impairment of renal function. *Ann. Intern. Med.* 72:229, 1970.

97. Loh, H. S.: Testicular torsion in Henoch-Schönlein syndrome. *Br. Med. J.* 2:96, 1974.

98. Jones, N. F., Creamer, B., and Gimlette, T. M. D.: Hypoproteinemia in anaphylactoid purpura. *Br. Med. J.* 2:1166, 1966.

99. Jones, R. H., Jr., and Moore, W. W.: Purpuric manifestations of rheumatic fever and acute glomerulonephritis. *Am. Heart J.* 32:529, 1946.

100. Stefanini, M., Roy, C. A., Zannos, L., and Dameshek, W.: The therapeutic effect of pituitary adrenocorticotropic hormones in a case of Henoch-Schönlein vascular (anaphylactoid) purpura. *JAMA* 144:1372, 1950.

101. Levinson, J. E., Horwitz, M., Kulka, J. P., Page, L., and Bauer, W.:

Schönlein-Henoch syndrome response to ACTH: Case with serial skin biopsies. *Ann. Rheum. Dis.* 10:255, 1951.

102. Kuglemass, I. N.: Cortisone in allergic purpura of children. *N.Y. State J. Med.* 51:2504, 1951.

103. Ansell, B. M.: Henoch-Schönlein purpura with particular reference to the prognosis of the renal lesion. *Br. J. Dermatol.* 82:211, 1970.

104. White, R. H. R., Cameron, J. S., and Trounce, J. R.: Immunosuppressive therapy in steroid resistant proliferative glomerulonephritis accompanied by the nephrotic syndrome. *Br. Med. J.* 2:853, 1966.

105. Herdman, R. C., Fish, A. J., and Good, R. A.: Immunosuppressive therapy of chronic renal disease. *N. Engl. J. Med.* 276:817, 1967.

106. Meadow, S. R., Glasgow, E. F., White, R. H. R., Moncrieff, M. W., Cameron, J. S., and Ogg, C. S.: Schönlein-Henoch nephritis. *Perspect. Nephrol. Hypertens.* 5:1089, 1973.

107. Medical Research Council of the Privy Council Working Party: Controlled Study. *Br. Med. J.* 2:239, 1971.

108. Herdman, R. C., Edson, J. R., Pickering, R. J., Fish, A. J., Marker, S., and Good, R. A.: Anticoagulants in renal disease in children. *Am J. Dis. Child.* 119:27, 1970.

109. Baliah, T., Kim, K. H., Anthone, S., Anthone, R., Montes, M., and Andres, G. A.: Recurrence of Henoch-Schönlein purpura glomerulonephritis in transplanted kidneys. *Transplantation* 18:343, 1974.

Disorders of hemostasis—vascular disorders

CHAPTER *151*

Hereditary hemorrhagic telangiectasia

ARLAN J. GOTTLIEB

Hereditary hemorrhagic telangiectasia is an inherited, developmental, structural abnormality of the vasculature characterized by the localized dilatation and convolution of venules and capillaries, giving rise to distinct telangiectases. The hemorrhagic manifestations of the disease result from the friability of the widely disseminated lesions.

HISTORY

The disease was probably first described in 1864 by Sutton, who reported a familial syndrome of epistaxis and gastrointestinal bleeding [1]. No mention of the telangiectases was made either by Sutton or by Babington, who in 1865 described epistaxis in five generations of a family [2]. Legg in 1876 noted developmental vascular nevi in familial epistaxis, as did Chiari in 1887 [3,4]. Both observers, however, discarded a correct notion of the pathogenesis of the disease in favor of a hemophilia-like etiology. The first comprehensive description of the disease as a separate entity was made in 1896 by Rendu, who stressed the widespread nature of the telangiectasia [5]. Osler further provided a view of the visceral distribution of the lesions and clearly distinguished the nature of the diverse hemorrhagic manifestations of the disease [6]. Little has been added to our understanding of the disease that was not noted in the early and excellent reviews of Weber in 1907 [7] and Hanes in 1909 [8]. It was Hanes who first designated the disease *hereditary hemorrhagic telangiectasia* [8].

ETIOLOGY

The basic alteration in hereditary hemorrhagic telangiectasia is a thinning of the vessel walls [8–10]. At times, the walls of venules or capillaries are reduced to a single layer of endothelium. A fragile angiomatous mass of dilated, enlarged vascular elements, the telangiectasis, results. Excellent ultrastructural studies of the

lesions have been published [11,12]. At autopsy, telangiectases have been found in all major organ systems [9,10]. It has been suggested that the lesions are not vascular dilatations but represent new formations of vascular tissue [13], perhaps resulting from embryonal rests [14]. Little specific evidence can be presented to support this contention, however.

MODE OF INHERITANCE

Hereditary hemorrhagic telangiectasia is inherited as an autosomal dominant disorder. The homozygous state may be lethal [15]. The sexes are equally affected [16,17], but it has been suggested that bleeding is less severe in females [17]. Skipping of generations is rare.

CLINICAL FEATURES

The patients' complaints are related to recurrent hemorrhage and anemia. The lesions are usually small (1 to 3 mm), flat, nonpulsatile, and violaceous (Plate 12). Blanching is observed with pressure. Larger aggregates of dilated vascular elements may be raised or at times may resemble spider angiomata. The telangiectases make their appearance throughout life and are usually florid by the fourth or fifth decade [17]. They are found commonly on the nasal mucous membranes; inner surface of the lips; gingiva; buccal mucosa; palate; tongue; skin of the face, trunk, and hands; under the nails; or on the conjunctivae, scalp, or ears. The patients are often unaware of these lesions. Visceral lesions are commonly found in the stomach, respiratory tract, bladder, and liver. Although bleeding may occur wherever the telangiectases are present, recurrent epistaxis is by far the most common symptom [17], occurring in 80 percent or more of those affected. Periodic bleeding from the mouth or from the gastrointestinal or respiratory tract occurs less frequently. Because of the delayed appearance of the lesions, it is not uncommon for a history of recurrent epistaxis during childhood or adolescence to precede overt widespread cutaneous and mucous membrane involvement.

Vascular malformations resulting in pulmonary arteriovenous fistulae are encountered in patients with hereditary telangiectasia. In one study encompassing 231 members of a family, roentgenographic densities suggestive of pulmonary arteriovenous fistulae were found in 15 percent of those with the disease [18]. As might be anticipated, the incidence of pulmonary fistulae was greater in the older patients [18,19]. One-third to almost two-thirds of patients with pulmonary arteriovenous fistulae have hereditary hemorrhagic telangiectasia [18–20]. Occasionally, shunting of blood may be sufficient to cause clubbing of the digits, mild hypoxemia, and even secondary polycythemia when the hemorrhagic manifestations are less severe [18]. A bruit may be heard over the lesion, and a vascular thrill may be palpable [18]. Recurrent cerebral embolism and brain abscess have occurred as a consequence of the pulmonary shunting of blood [18]. The neurologic manifestations of this syndrome are diverse. It is noteworthy that in a significant percentage of patients the neurologic findings may be related to the sequelae of pulmonary arteriovenous shunting (e.g., hypoxemia, paradoxical and septic emboli, brain abscesses) [21].

Arteriovenous fistulae of the cerebral [22] and retinal vessels [23,24] and aneurysms of the hepatic [25] and splenic arteries [9] and of the aorta [26–28] have been reported, as have hemangiomas of the liver [29] and polycystic kidneys [30]. Hepatomegaly and splenomegaly have been noted occasionally [29,31], and cirrhosis and portal hypertension may presumably result from extensive hepatic telangiectasia [32–34].

LABORATORY FEATURES

The laboratory findings relate to the severity of the hemorrhagic manifestations of the disease. Hypochromic, microcytic anemia of varying degree is common. Erythroid hyperplasia of the marrow, reticulocytosis, and depletion of the body iron stores in proportion to the degree of blood loss also should be anticipated. Abnormal platelet function [35,36], factor VIII deficiency [37], and von Willebrand's disease [38,39] have been reported in an occasional patient with hereditary hemorrhagic telangiectasia.

DIFFERENTIAL DIAGNOSIS

The diagnosis of hereditary hemorrhagic telangiectasia is not difficult in patients with characteristic skin or mucous membrane lesions, a history of repeated hemorrhage, and a family history of a similar affliction. Although the history obtained from patients with hemorrhagic telangiectasia is usually quite characteristic for the disease, in some mild cases a congenital platelet or blood coagulation disorder must be considered and appropriate tests performed. The major problem in arriving at the correct diagnosis is in the detection of the telangiectases, which may be hidden in the nasopharynx or an internal organ or which may not be recognized when presenting as slight pink spots on the skin. In the younger patient who presents with recurrent epistaxis but without obvious telangiectases, particular attention should be paid to the family history and to the examination of other family members with histories of repeated hemorrhage. A thorough search should be made for telangiectases. In the absence of detectable skin or mucous membrane lesions, however, the diagnosis should probably be considered uncertain, and other causes of bleeding excluded. Selective angiography and/or endoscopy may prove particularly helpful in patients whose telangiectases are not readily identifiable [40–42]. The skin lesions must be distinguished from purpura, which does not blanch on pressure, and from the pulsatile cutaneous arterial spiders seen in hepatic disease and pregnancy.

THERAPY

Replacement therapy with iron and blood transfusions are the supportive measures to be employed for bleeding. Intramuscular or intravenous iron-dextran complex may be used when adequate iron stores cannot be maintained by the oral route [43,44]. In general, only local therapy for the control of hemorrhage should be employed. Where possible, pressure should be applied to the bleeding point. This may be difficult to accomplish in some cases, as, for example, in the nasopharynx. Such lesions may tax the ingenuity of the otolaryngologist. Control of epistaxis by local tamponade has been accomplished by a lubricated finger cot tied to a catheter and inflated in the nostril. It is of interest that this device was suggested to Osler [6] by a patient with this disease. Absorbable topical hemostatic agents, such as oxidized cellulose, have proved useful. Although temperate use of electrocoagulation may be helpful in less accessible areas, this and techniques such as escharotics, radium, and x-ray therapy are not advised. The use of ε-aminocaproic acid by nasal spray has been advocated for the control of epistaxis [45]. Estrogen therapy has often proved disappointing, but there are also enthusiastic reports of its success, and it may be employed in an attempt to control epistaxis in the difficult case [46–49]. The recommended dose is 0.25 to 1.0 mg of ethinyl estradiol per day in divided doses. Androgens may be administered to male patients to counteract in part the feminizing effect of estrogen. Complaints relating to the dry, crusty nasal mucosa which results from squamous metaplasia of the mucous membrane induced by the estrogen therapy may be treated with petroleum jelly. Considerable debate exists as to whether bleeding is intensified or ameliorated by the low doses of estrogen contained in oral contraceptive agents [50–52].

An obvious approach to the bleeding lesions in this disease is excision. Surgical intervention must be limited by a knowledge of the widespread distribution of the telangiectases and the development of new lesions with time. Septal dermoplasty has been advocated for control of epistaxis [48,53] and has met with some acceptance. Cardiovascular considerations may require excision of pulmonary arteriovenous fistulae. In these circumstances, after the merits of the surgery are carefully weighed in each case, the procedure should be limited to the removal of as little lung tissue as possible and, preferentially, to the larger, more discrete arteriovenous communications [18,19,54]. Similar considerations govern the surgical management of severe gastrointestinal hemorrhage [55].

COURSE AND PROGNOSIS

Patients with hereditary hemorrhagic telangiectasia do surprisingly well despite the lack of specific therapy and the seriousness of their hemorrhagic manifestations. Although they often lead lives restricted by their recurrent hemorrhages, they seldom die from exsanguination. An additional difficulty may be imposed on these patients by the presence of pulmonary arteriovenous fistulae.

References

1. Sutton, H. G.: Epistaxis as an indication of impaired nutrition and of degeneration of the vascular system. *Med. Mirror* 1:769, 1864.

2. Babington, B. G.: Hereditary epistaxis. *Lancet* 2:362, 1865.
3. Legg, W.: A case of haemophilia complicated with multiple naevi. *Lancet* 2:856, 1876.
4. Chiari, O.: *Erfahrungen auf dem Gebiete der Hals und Nasenkrankheiten nach den Ergebnissen des Ambulatoriums.* Toeplitz and Deuticke, Vienna, 1887, p. 60.
5. Rendu, M.: Epistaxis répetées chez un sujet porteur de petits angiomes cutanés et muqueux. *Bull. Soc. Med. Hop. Paris* 13:731, 1896.
6. Osler, W.: On a family form of recurring epistaxis, associated with multiple telangiectases of the skin and mucous membranes. *Bull. Johns Hopkins Hosp.* 12:333, 1901. On multiple hereditary telangiectases with recurring haemorrhages. *Q. J. Med.* 1:53, 1907.
7. Weber, F. P.: Multiple hereditary developmental angiomata (telangiectases) of the skin and mucous membranes associated with recurring haemorrhages. *Lancet* 2:160, 1907.
8. Hanes, F. M.: Multiple hereditary telangiectases causing hemorrhage (hereditary hemorrhagic telangiectasia). *Bull. Johns Hopkins Hosp.* 20:63, 1909.
9. Schuster, N. H.: Familial haemorrhagic telangiectasia associated with multiple aneurysms of the splenic artery. *J. Pathol. Bact.* 44:29, 1937.
10. Bird, R. M., and Jaques, W. E.: Vascular lesion of hereditary hemorrhagic telangiectasia. *N. Engl. J. Med.* 260:597, 1959.
11. Jahnke, V.: Ultrastructure of hereditary telangiectasia. *Arch. Otolaryngol.* 91:262, 1970.
12. Hashimoto, K., and Pritzker, M. S.: Hereditary hemorrhagic telangiectasia: An electron microscopic study. *Oral Surg.* 34:752, 1972.
13. Ravina, A.: Angiomatose héréditaire hémorragique anéurysmes antérioveineux du poumon. *Press Med.* 57:776, 1949.
14. Pierquin, J., Richard, G., and Pierquin, B.: Une Méthode de traitement de la maladie de Rendu-Osler par la radiothérapie. *J. Radiol. Electrol.* 32:787, 1951.
15. Snyder, L. H., and Doan, C. A.: Is the homozygous form of multiple telangiectasia lethal? *J. Lab. Clin. Med.* 29:1211, 1944.
16. Dolowitz, D. A., Rambo, O. N. Jr., and Stephens, F. E.: Hereditary hemorrhagic telangiectasia. *Ann. Otol.* 62:642, 1953.
17. Bird, R. M., Hammarsten, J. F., Marshall, R. A., and Robinson, R. R.: A study of hereditary hemorrhagic telangiectasia. *N. Engl. J. Med.* 257:105, 1957.
18. Hodgson, C. H., Burchell, H. B., Good, C. A., and Clagett, O. T.: Hereditary hemorrhagic telangiectasia and pulmonary arteriovenous fistula. *N. Engl. J. Med.* 261:625, 1959.
19. Hodgson, C. H., and Kaye, R. L.: Pulmonary arteriovenous fistula and hereditary hemorrhagic telangiectasia: A review and report of 35 cases of fistula. *Dis. Chest* 43:449, 1963.
20. Dines, D. E., Arms, R. A., Bernatz, P. E., and Gomes, M. R.: Pulmonary arteriovenous fistulas. *Mayo Clin. Proc.* 49:460, 1974.
21. Roman, G., Fisher, M., Perl, D. P., and Poser, C. M.: Neurologic manifestations of hereditary hemorrhagic telangiectasia (Rendu-Osler-Weber disease): Report of 2 cases and review of the literature. *Ann. Neurol.* 4:130, 1978.
22. Chandler, D.: Pulmonary and cerebral arteriovenous fistula with Osler's disease. *Arch. Intern. Med.* 116:277, 1965.
23. Forker, E. L., and Bean, W. B.: Retinal arteriovenous aneurysm in hereditary hemorrhagic telangiectasia. *Arch. Intern. Med.* 111:778, 1963.
24. Davis, D. G., and Smith, J. L.: Retinal involvement in hereditary hemorrhagic telangiectasia. *Arch. Ophthalmol.* 85:618, 1971.
25. Graham, W. P. III, Eiseman, B., and Pryor, R.: Hepatic artery aneurysm with portal vein fistula in a patient wiht familial hereditary telangiectasia. *Ann. Surg.* 159:362, 1964.
26. Thomas, J. R.: Osler's disease with a dissecting aneurysm of the aorta. *Arch. Intern. Med.* 116:448, 1965.
27. Muggia, F. M.: Osler's disease with aortic aneurysm. *Arch. Intern. Med.* 114:307, 1964.
28. Borman, J. B., and Schiller, M.: Osler's disease with multiple large vessel aneurysms. *Angiology* 20:113, 1969.
29. Smith, J. L., and Lineback, M. I.: Hereditary hemorrhagic telangiectasia. *Am. J. Med.* 17:41, 1954.
30. Solomon, S., and Kleiman, A. H.: Hereditary hemorrhagic telangiectasia associated with polycystic disease of the kidney. *N.Y. State J. Med.* 71:1665, 1971.
31. Fitz-Hugh, T., Jr.: Splenomegaly and hepatic enlargement in hereditary hemorrhagic telangiectasia. *Am. J. Med. Sci.* 181:261, 1931.
32. Feizi, O.: Hereditary hemorrhagic telangiectasia presenting with portal hypertension and cirrhosis of the liver. *Gastroenterology* 63:660, 1972.
33. Daly, J. J., and Schiller, A. L.: The liver in hereditary hemorrhagic telangiectasia (Osler-Weber-Rendu disease). *Am. J. Med.* 60:723, 1976.
34. Martini, G. A.: The liver in hereditary haemorrhagic telangiectasia: An inborn error of vascular structure with multiple manifestations: A reappraisal. *Gut.* 19:531, 1978.
35. Muckle, T. J.: Low in vivo adhesive-platelet count in hereditary haemorrhagic telangiectasia. *Lancet* 2:880, 1964.
36. Larsson, S. O.: Osler's disease with impaired adhesion and aggregation of platelets. *Acta Med. Scand.* 196:133, 1974.
37. Esham, R. H., Skilling, F. C., Jr., Dodson, W. H., and Hammack, W. J.: Hereditary hemorrhagic telangiectasia and factor VIII deficiency. *Arch. Intern. Med.* 134:327, 1974.
38. Ahr, D. J., Rickles, F. R., Hoyer, L. W., O'Leary, D. S., and Conrad, M. E.: Von Willebrand's disease and hemorrhagic telangiectasia: Association of two complex disorders of hemostasis resulting in life-threatening hemorrhage. *Am. J. Med.* 62:452, 1977.
39. Conlon, C. L., Weinger, R. S., Cimo, P. L., Moake, J. L., and Olson, J. D.: Telangiectasia and Von Willebrand's disease in two families. *Ann. Intern. Med.* 89:921, 1978.
40. Campbell, E. W., Jewson, D., and Gilbert, E.: Angiographic identification of enteric lesions: Guide to therapy in hereditary hemorrhagic telangiectasis. *Arch. Intern. Med.* 125:705, 1970.
41. Jacobson, G., and Krause, U.: Hereditary hemorrhagic telangiectasia localized to the gastrointestinal tract. *Scand. J. Gastroenterol.* 5:283, 1970.
42. Sogge, M. R., Dale, J. A., and Butler, M. L.: Detection of typical lesions of hereditary hemorrhagic telangiectasia by colonoscopy. *Gastrointest. Endosc.* 26:52, 1980.
43. Ross, L., and Fremland, H.: Prolonged and massive administration of iron-dextran complex resulting in selective glomerular iron deposition in the kidneys. *Blood* 31:11, 1968.
44. Chernelch, M., Winchell, H. S., Pollycove, M., Sargent, T., and Kusubov, N.: Prolonged intravenous iron-dextran therapy in a patient with multiple hereditary telangiectasia. *Blood* 34:691, 1969.
45. Jash, D. K.: Epistaxis: Topical use of epsilon-aminocaproic acid in its management. *J. Laryngol. Otol.* 87:895, 1973.
46. Koch, H. J., Jr., Escher, G. C., and Lewis, J. S.: Hormonal management of hereditary hemorrhagic telangiectasia. *JAMA* 149:1376, 1952.
47. Harrison, D. F. N.: Familial haemorrhagic telangiectasia: Twenty cases treated with systemic oestrogen. *Q. J. Med.* 33:25, 1964.
48. McCaffrey, T. V., Kern, E. B., and Lake, C. F.: Management of epistaxis in hereditary hemorrhagic telangiectasia: Review of 80 cases. *Arch. Otolaryngol.* 103:627, 1977.
49. Menefee, M. G., Flessa, H. C., and Glueck, H. I.: Hereditary hemorrhagic telangiectasia (Osler-Weber-Rendu disease): An electron microscopic study of the vascular lesions before and after therapy with hormones. *Arch. Otolaryngol.* 101:246, 1975.
50. Rowley, P. T., Kurnich, J., and Cheville, R.: Hereditary hemorrhagic telangiectasia: Aggravation by oral contraceptives. *Lancet* 1:474, 1970.
51. Harris, P. W. R.: Hereditary hemorrhagic telangiectasia and oral contraceptives. *Lancet* 1:615, 1970.
52. Harrison, D. F. N.: Hereditary hemorrhagic telangiectasia and oral contraceptives. *Lancet* 1:721, 1970.
53. Saunders, W. H.: Permanent control of nosebleeds in patients with hereditary hemorrhagic telangiectasia. *Ann. Intern. Med.* 53:147, 1960.
54. Weiss, E., and Gasul, B. M.: Pulmonary arteriovenous fistula and telangiectasia. *Ann. Intern. Med.* 41:989, 1954.
55. Bruusgaard, A., and Juhl, E.: Hereditary hemorrhagic telangiectasis (Render-Weber-Osler's disease) with intestinal involvement successfully treated by surgery. *Gastroenterology* 67:1001, 1974.

Disorders of hemostasis—congenital disorders of blood coagulation factors

Hemophilia and related conditions—congenital deficiencies of prothrombin (factor II), factor V, and factors VII to XII

CECIL HOUGIE

Hemophilia A (factor VIII deficiency)

DEFINITION

Following the classic review of Bulloch and Fildes [1] in 1911, the term *hemophilia* was restricted to a sex-linked disorder of males, characterized by excessive bleeding existing from childhood and a prolongation of the blood clotting time. This definition has had to be modified, however, since the whole-blood clotting time, a very insensitive test, is prolonged only in the more severe hemophilic patients; the test is no longer a *sine qua non* of diagnosis. Furthermore, in unusual cases, manifestations of hemophilia may not be evident in childhood.

Hemophilia can be divided into *hemophilia A* and *hemophilia B*. Hemophilia A, defined as a sex-linked hemorrhagic disease of males characterized by a deficiency of factor VIII:C,* occurs about seven times more fre-

---

* The term *factor VIII*, unmodified, refers to the entire protein complex possessing both the procoagulant activity (factor VIII:C, or FVIII:C) that is deficient in hemophilia and the activity (factor VIII:von Willebrand factor, or FVIII:vWF) whose deficiency accounts for the prolonged bleeding time in von Willebrand's disease. The protein possessing FVIII:vWF activity is referred to as factor VIII/von Willebrand factor (FVIII/vWF). Other properties of this protein are antigenicity, referred to as factor VIII–related antigen (FVIIIR:Ag), and the ability to function as a cofactor for ristocetin-induced platelet aggregation, referred to as factor VIII–related ristocetin cofactor (FVIIIR:RCo). Factor VIII:C may also be detected immunologically; the antigen corresponding to FVIII:C is called factor VIII:CAg or FVIII:CAg.

quently than hemophilia B. The unqualified term *hemophilia* refers to hemophilia A, a terminology used in this book. Hemophilia B, which is clinically indistinguishable from hemophilia A, is also known by its synonym *Christmas disease* and is characterized by a deficiency of factor IX.

HISTORY

The first reference to hemophilia was made in the second century in the Talmud, where the occurrence of fatal bleeding after circumcision in the sons of several sisters is mentioned [2]. The first case of hemophilia recorded in the medical literature was published in 1793 by an anonymous author [3], but the first accurate account was given by Otto, who clearly recognized that the disease was sex-linked, being limited to males and transmitted through apparently normal females married to normal males [4]. Liston, in 1819, had noted the slow coagulation of blood, but it was not until 1893 that Wright developed a technique for measuring the coagulation time. Wright [5] showed that the clotting time was prolonged in hemophilia, and it became accepted that this was the basic abnormality. In 1911, Bulloch and Fildes [1] laid down the criteria for diagnosis which were accepted for over a generation.

Several hypotheses based on Morawitz's concept of coagulation were subsequently put forward to explain the long clotting time. A deficiency of calcium was postulated, but this idea was soon shown to be false. It was suggested that the hemophilic tissues yielded too little thrombokinase, but this was disproved by Lowenburg and Rubenstone [6] in work ignored until relatively recently. In 1911, Addis [7], in a classic experiment, demonstrated that a globulin fraction prepared by dilution and acidification of normal plasma could correct the clotting defect in hemophilia. Since Mellanby [8] had previously shown that this globulin fraction contained prothrombin and fibrinogen and since it was already known that the fibrinogen in hemophilia is normal, Addis assumed a prothrombin abnormality. Later, when it was shown that the prothrombin in hemophilia was normal, Addis's findings were ignored —until 1936. His experiments were then confirmed and repeated by Patek and Taylor [9], who were the first to demonstrate that the defect in hemophilia was due to a deficiency of a globulin fraction subsequently referred to as the antihemophilic globulin or antihemophilic factor. Although the prothrombin content of hemophilic plasma was found to be normal [10,11], Brinkhous showed in 1939 that the prothrombin was converted to thrombin at a relatively slow rate [11]. He also showed that the block in prothrombin conversion could be corrected by blood transfusion and concluded that the basic defect in hemophilia was associated with a lack of blood thromboplastin. In 1947, Quick [12] and Brinkhous [13] independently suggested that the antihemophilic globulin and platelets reacted in some way to generate thromboplastin in the blood. By 1952 hemophilia was defined by these and most other workers as a sex-linked hemorrhagic disease characterized by a normal thrombin time and a defective conversion of prothrombin to thrombin, the abnormality being due to a deficiency of antihemophilic globulin.

In 1947, Pavlovsky [14] showed that mixing the bloods of certain hemophilic patients results in mutual correction of their clotting defects. However, the correct interpretation of this finding was not made until the work of Aggeler and his coworkers [15] in 1952. They studied a male patient who had a severe hemorrhagic diathesis associated with a prolonged clotting time. Although the hemorrhagic features were indistinguishable from those of classic hemophilia, the defect was not corrected either in vivo or in vitro by potent preparations of factor VIII (antihemophilic factor). The patient had normal plasma concentrations of all previously described coagulation factors, namely, fibrinogen, prothrombin, and factors V, VII, and VIII. The clotting abnormality could be corrected by normal serum, but prior treatment of the serum with barium sulfate resulted in a loss of this property. In these respects, the new clotting factor, which Aggeler and coworkers designated plasma thromboplastin component (PTC) and which is now generally known as factor IX, differed from the antihemophilic factor. They suggested that the reported cases of mutual correction of two hemophilic blood specimens occurred because one was deficient in factor VIII and the other deficient in factor IX. Their findings established hemophilia as a heterogeneous disease entity.

The patient of Aggeler and his group had no siblings, living or dead, and there was no family history of a hemorrhagic disorder. Shortly thereafter, Biggs and her associates [16] studied several patients exhibiting a similar defect and showed that the condition was inherited in a manner identical to that of classic hemophilia. They called the factor lacking in their patients *Christmas factor* and the disease *Christmas disease,* after the surname of their first patient.

INCIDENCE
The incidence of hemophilia, including mild cases, in the United States is roughly 1 in 10,000. The disease probably occurs widely in nature and has also been observed in both dogs [17–20] and horses [21].

GENETICS
Hemophilia is the classic example of a sex-linked recessive trait [22]. It is almost exclusively limited to men whose sons are normal but whose daughters are obligatory carriers. The carriers, on a statistical basis, transmit the disorder to half their sons and the carrier state to half their daughters. Hemophilia may occur in homozygous females who are the offspring of a hemophilic father and a carrier mother. The same inheritance pattern occurs in canine hemophilia, a disorder indistinguishable in its clinical and laboratory features from the human disease [17]. A deficiency of factor VIII:C is also

found in von Willebrand's disease, and most of the older reports in the literature of autosomal forms of hemophilia were actually variants of von Willebrand's disease.

A kindred has been reported in whom the mother, daughter, and granddaughter have a mild bleeding disorder associated with a very low FVIII:C level [23]. The laboratory data do not support the diagnosis of von Willebrand's disease, as the FVIIIR:Ag level was normal, the patients' plasma aggregated platelets normally in the presence of ristocetin, and de novo synthesis of FVIII:C did not occur after transfusion. One possibility is that these patients are hemophilia carriers and that the low FVIII:C levels are due to selection of cells in which the X chromosome carrying the mutant gene is active (Chap. 16).

There has been one report of a case of hemophilia in a female who was revealed by chromosomal studies to be genetically a male [24]. In all the other reported cases of female hemophilia, the mother was a carrier and the father had hemophilia. The chances of a homozygous hemophilic female arising from the random or chance mating in the population at large could be theoretically disregarded, as it would be expected to occur in less than 1 out of 100 million matings. However, such a mating may occur more often where members of affected families are brought together socially by a desire to help one another.

A few cases of combined deficiency of factor V and factor VIII affecting both sexes and apparently transmitted as an autosomal recessive trait have been reported [25–27]. A deficiency of a naturally occurring inhibitor of protein C (Chap. 136) has been demonstrated in this disorder [27,28]. It has been proposed that the inhibitor is inherited in an autosomal recessive manner [27]. However, in one of these cases segregation of two separate disorders, parahemophilia (hereditary factor V deficiency) and hemophilia A, appeared likely, as one member of the kindred had an isolated deficiency of factor V [29].

Most hemophilic carriers have FVIII:C levels ranging from 25 to 75 percent, with a mean of approximately half that of the average normal female. Unfortunately, the results of FVIII:C assays have a relatively large standard deviation. Also the FVIII:C level may be markedly increased during pregnancy, following heavy exercise, and in other physiologic states. For these reasons the detection of carriers is usually difficult and often impossible on the basis of a FVIII:C determination. However, under those circumstances in which the FVIII:C level is increased, the FVIIIR:Ag level shows a corresponding increase and the ratio of FVIIIR:Ag to FVIII:C remains unchanged [30–32]. Assuming that the carrier has a normal level of FVIIIR:Ag and only 50 percent FVIII:C the ratio of FVIIIR:Ag to FVIII:C will be twice that of the average female. This ratio is valuable in the recognition of carriers, particularly during late pregnancy and in the differentiation of the carrier state from von Willebrand's disease. When this ratio was used in a study of 54 obligatory carriers, all but one were identified as carriers at the 95 percent confidence level. However at this confidence level 2 of 77 supposedly normal women would have been called carriers [33]. This experience is much better than that in two subsequent studies, in which 4 out of 27 [34] and 4 out of 23 [35] obligatory carriers would have been considered normal on the basis of laboratory tests. That a proportion of carriers can never be detected by a laboratory test might be expected on theoretical grounds. A percentage would be predicted to be phenotypically normal on the basis of random X-chromosomal inactivation and the size of the critical anlage (the number of cells at the early embryo state destined to synthesize factor VIII) [36]. It is difficult and often impossible to detect the carrier state in those very mild forms of hemophilia in which the FVIII:C level is between 20 and 40 percent, as the mean FVIII:C level in the carriers is likely to be borderline or near normal [37]. Carrier detection is performed in only a few specialized centers. Linear discriminant analysis of the ratio of FVIII:C to FVIIIR:Ag or FVIIIR:RCo combined with probability based on pedigree analysis gives the probability of the carrier state [34,35,38]. The importance of carrier testing has increased with the feasibility of diagnosing hemophilia in the fetus (see below).

Hemophilia A results from a mutation of a locus on the X chromosome. The locus lies at one end of a linkage group of approximately 12 units, which also includes the loci for color blindness and glucose-6-phosphate dehydrogenase (G-6-PD) deficiency. The gene for G-6-PD is the middle and that for color blindness the other outside marker. This linkage group is at least 50 map units from both the Xg^a blood group locus and the hemophilia B locus [22,39–41].

PATHOGENESIS

Early studies using antibody neutralization techniques showed that hemophilia is a heterogeneous disorder [42–44]. The plasmas from most patients with the severe form of the disease were found to be incapable of neutralizing naturally occurring antibodies to factor VIII (Chap. 157), and such plasmas are sometimes referred to as being negative for cross-reacting material, or CRM$^-$. However, the plasmas from a small proportion of cases do neutralize human antibodies to factor VIII, and these plasmas are referred to as CRM$^+$. The presence or absence of cross-reacting material is obviously a function of the particular antibody used, and a plasma classified as CRM$^+$ with one antibody might be CRM$^-$ with another.

The procoagulant moiety of factor VIII, FVIII:C, in contrast to FVIII/vWF, is present in plasma in amounts too small to form precipitates with either homologous or heterologous antibodies when most double-diffusion or crossed immunoelectrophoretic methods are used. Moreover, since FVIII:C free of FVIII:vWF is very difficult to prepare, immunologic techniques for the quantitative measurement of FVIII:C are at present restricted to the use of immunoradiometric assays using high-titer homologous factor VIII:C antibodies from patients with hemophilia [45–47] or patients with acquired hemophilia [47,48], or monoclonal antibodies obtained by the hybridoma technique [49]. The results depend on the type of immunoradiometric assay technique (solid versus fluid state) and on the particular antibody used. There is good agreement that most hemophilic patients with less than 1 percent FVIII:C activity have a level of FVIII:CAg below the lower level of discrimination of the immunoradiometric assay (usually 1 percent). However, some hemophilic patients with less than 1 percent of FVIII:C activity have small but significant amounts (1 to 10 percent) of FVIII:CAg [45–47]. In most of the moderate to mild cases the amount of FVIII:CAg closely parallels the coagulant activity, but in some the FVIII:CAg level is within normal limits [46,47]. In one study using an antibody to factor VIII:C derived from a patient with acquired hemophilia, there was no detectable FVIII:CAg in three patients, although their FVIII:C levels ranged from 2 to 6 percent [48]. In another study [47] on plasmas from 43 hemophilic kindred using an antibody to factor VIII:C from a patient with acquired hemophilia and four different hemophilic antibodies, the results obtained with the nonhemophilic antibody corresponded quite closely to the means obtained using the hemophilic antibodies. However, a small but significant amount of antigen was detected in one case with the spontaneous acquired antibody, but none could be detected with any of the four hemophilic antibodies. There is a complex molecular heterogeneity in hemophilia, and a clear understanding of the nature of the disease awaits elucidation of the biochemical nature of the FVIII:C molecule.

The site of synthesis of factor VIII is discussed in Chap. 133.

CLINICAL FEATURES

The clinical severity of the disorder varies markedly from family to family, but among the affected members of a family the baseline level of FVIII:C and the severity of the disease are approximately the same. While it is generally accepted that truly spontaneous bleeding—that is, bleeding unrelated to trauma—does not occur in hemophilia, the trauma may be so slight as to go unnoticed by the patient and therefore the bleeding may appear to be spontaneous.

CLASSIFICATION

The severity of the disease closely parallels the level of FVIII:C, with a continuous spectrum of severity ranging from patients who live completely normal lives to those who are frequently hospitalized. It is, however, convenient and useful to classify cases into three main groups: *severe, moderate,* and *mild.* The severe cases have less than 1 percent FVIII:C, and most, if not all, of these patients suffer from hemarthroses. They give a history of bleeding dating from early infancy, such as following circumcision. The moderate cases have levels of FVIII:C ranging from 1 to 5 percent; most of these patients suffer from occasional hemarthroses but may reach manhood without crippling deformities. The mild cases have levels of FVIII:C ranging from 6 to 40 percent. These patients rarely suffer from hemarthrosis and lead fairly active and normal lives; the diagnosis is often not made until late adolescence, and many of these patients actively participate in sports. Attention is often first drawn to the mild type of hemophilia when bleeding occurs following dental extractions or some other relatively minor surgery. These patients may have periods of complete remission, which may last for many years, especially after the age of puberty.

DENTAL EXTRACTIONS
A symptom common to all forms of hemophilia is excessive bleeding following dental extraction. Normal people may bleed profusely for as long as 12 h following extraction of a molar tooth, especially if there is an associated infection; such bleeding is often from a small blood vessel which has been left exposed. The type of excessive bleeding characteristically encountered in hemophilia occurs during and immediately after the surgery and continues as a very slow ooze. Often the bleeding ceases, only to restart after 1 day, and sometimes as long as after 8 days. If the bleeding persists for 3 days or more, it is almost certain that the patient has a hemorrhagic diathesis. Conversely, the absence of excessive bleeding following dental extractions is a strong point against the diagnosis, provided no prophylactic therapy was given. In the presence of a hemorrhagic diathesis, the suturing of the gum margins without prior replacement therapy sometimes results in blood seeping down into the tissues and accumulating, giving rise to a hematoma which may cause dangerous pharyngeal obstruction (Plate 12-10).

HEMATOMAS
Hematomas are usually subcutaneous or intramuscular (Plate 12-10). The traumatic origin may be so trivial as to go unnoticed, or it may not be recognized because the hemorrhage starts several days later. Such a latent period suggests that the initial trauma may cause mild necrosis and that this breakdown of tissue results in hemorrhage. The hematomas are found mostly on the legs. If they are superficial the ecchymotic area is greater but there is less danger of complications from local pressure. In deep bleeding, discoloration of the skin may be delayed or even absent. Amounts of blood sufficiently large to cause anemia or even severe shock can be lost internally by hemorrhage dissecting along the fascial planes, but such episodes are rarely fatal. A small central nodule surrounded by discoloration due to extravasated blood is helpful in distinguishing this type of bleeding from purpura, which is more superficial and often accompanied by petechiae. Petechiae are not seen in uncomplicated hemophilia. If they are present, some complication such as thrombocytopenia must be considered.

Bleeding may occur in any muscle but is seen most frequently in the calves, thighs, buttocks, and forearms and may be followed by permanent deformity. Thus bleeding into the calf muscle can result in a fixed equinus deformity due to contracture, which in turn leads to abnormal stresses on the ankle joints and results in further hemorrhages and often in permanent joint changes. Volkman's ischemic paralysis occurring in the hand or foot is another grave but fortunately rare complication of intramuscular hematoma.

NEUROLOGIC COMPLICATIONS
Compression of a peripheral nerve may result in peripheral neuropathies, with excruciating pain, paresthesia, and muscle atrophy. This is the most common type of neurologic complication of hemophilia [50]. The compression is usually produced by intramuscular hemorrhage and can produce atrophy of a limb. Loss of deep tendon reflexes may occur, and the majority of patients with peripheral nerve involvement show some evidence of sensory loss in the distribution of the involved nerves. Because of the frequency of hemorrhage within the iliopsoas muscle, the femoral nerve is the most commonly involved; the next most frequently involved nerve is the ulnar. Most peripheral neurologic complications in hemophilia are reversible [50].

One of the major causes of death in hemophilia is hemorrhage within the intracranial cavity. About 10 percent of hemophilic patients develop objective evidence of intracranial hemorrhage [50,51]. A history of trauma can be obtained in almost half these patients. The mortality is high, and survivors may have recurrent episodes. Of the various types of intracranial bleeding, the subarachnoid variety has the best prognosis and intracerebral hemorrhage carries the worst [50]. The differentiation of the various types is often difficult, and hemorrhage may occur in more than one site. Patients with hemophilia who sustain even minor head trauma should be closely observed. As hemophilic patients are subject to the same diseases as the general population, it is important to differentiate intracranial hemorrhage from bacterial meningitis or other conditions that can be treated effectively. Lumbar puncture should be performed only by an experienced physician, following adequate replacement therapy. Hemorrhage in the spinal canal is the least common neurologic complication in hemophilia. It may occur within the cord but more usually is epidural [50].

PRESSURE ON BLOOD VESSELS AND VITAL ORGANS
Deep hemorrhage may produce pressure on blood vessels. This can be severe enough to obstruct the circulation, producing severe ischemia and even gangrene. Occasionally a hemorrhage into the tongue, floor of the mouth, tonsils, or posterior pharyngeal walls will dissect into the neck, producing pharyngeal obstruction. Retroperitoneal bleeding is fairly common; if it occurs in the right iliopsoas region, it may be very difficult to differentiate from acute appendicitis. In some cases bleeding occurs into the abdominal cavity (Fig. 152-1), making the actual site of bleeding difficult if not impos-

sible to determine; an accurate history in such cases, especially with regard to trauma, is of great importance.

HEMARTHROSES

Hemarthroses are the most frequent indication for admission to hospital. Although any joint may be involved, the order of decreasing frequency of involvement is knee, ankle, hip, elbow, wrist, and shoulder (Fig. 152-2). Hemarthroses are unusual in mild cases, and permanent disability is the exception in these patients. In one series, 75 percent of severely affected children were found to have had at least one acute hemarthrosis by the age of 4 years, at 10 years 80 percent had some impairment of function in the knee joint, and by the age of 16, 75 percent had disability associated with bleeding into other joints [52]. There is usually a history of trauma or unusual exertion, although in mild cases a severe degree of trauma is necessary. The affected joints become painful, tender, and later swollen. There is often extreme pain and exquisite tenderness. Usually, the signs and symptoms subside in a few days. In some instances, joints may become painful but there is no swelling and no apparent residual effects. The

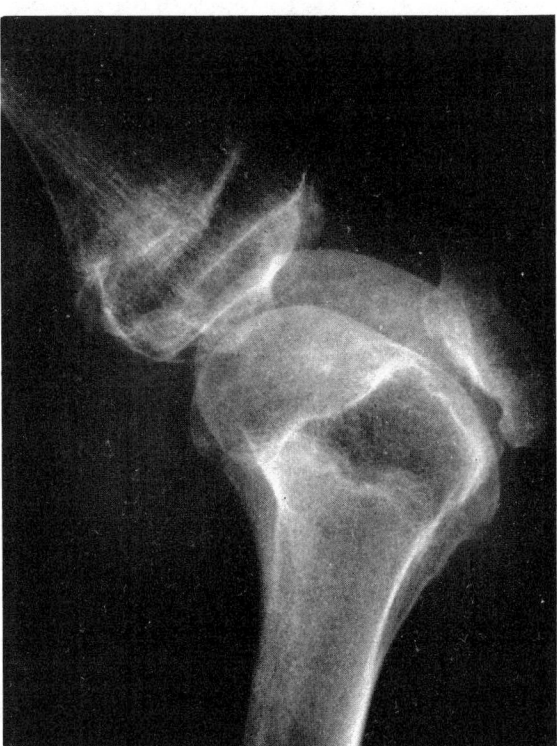

FIGURE 152-2 **Hemarthrosis in a patient with hemophilia.** This x-ray of the knee of a patient with hemophilia shows soft-tissue swelling due to hemorrhage into the joint space. Note also the bone changes characteristic of hemophilic arthropathy: irregularities of the joint surface and cystic areas in the bones. (Courtesy of Dr. F. R. Heitzman.)

pathologic changes involve the joint itself, with extensive destruction and reactive changes in the adjacent bone and tissues. The joint is frequently stiff and occasionally unstable, and movement is greatly restricted. Deformity, muscle wasting, and soft tissue contractures may result. Cystic areas develop in the subchondral bone, and there is narrowing of the joint space. Osteoporosis is common, and in long-standing cases there may be complete loss of articular surfaces and flattening of bone ends. These changes produce a characteristic radiologic picture [53] (Figs. 152-2 and 152-3). All the changes can be minimized or even avoided by good management, which is now available in an increasing number of medical centers [54].

HEMATURIA

Bleeding from the kidneys in hemophilia is often caused by trauma, but usually the cause cannot be determined. It may occasionally be due to infection. Hematuria occurs in approximately 20 percent of the moderate and severe cases and in 5 percent of the mild cases. Blood loss tends to be small, and usually transfusion of whole blood is not required. Intravenous pyelography is safe provided compression of the ureters is not attempted. The ureters may be blocked by blood clots, and painful spasms may occur.

FIGURE 152-1 **Intra-abdominal bleeding in a patient with hemophilia.** The barium enema demonstrates an intraluminal hematoma in the sigmoid colon as an elongated, smooth filling defect, delineated in this illustration by the short arrows. Note also the marked destruction of the hip joint, indicated by the large arrow. (Courtesy of Dr. F. R. Heitzman.)

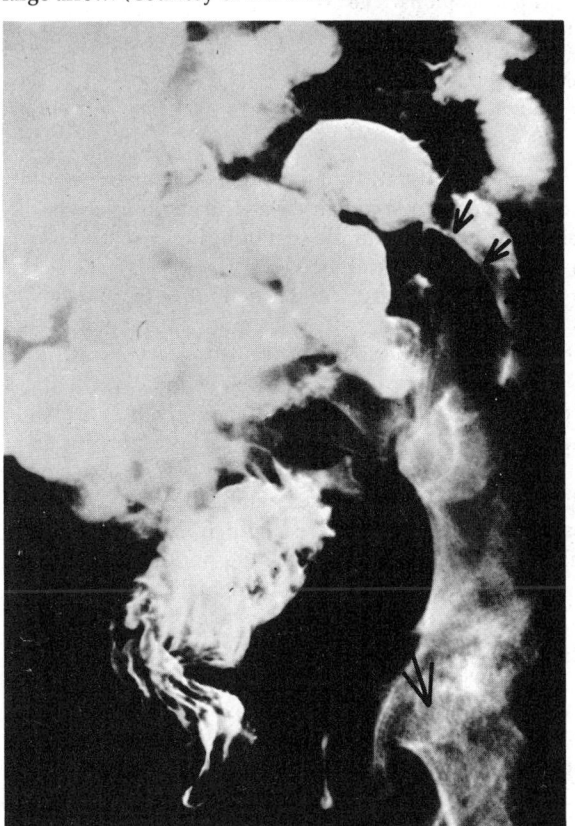

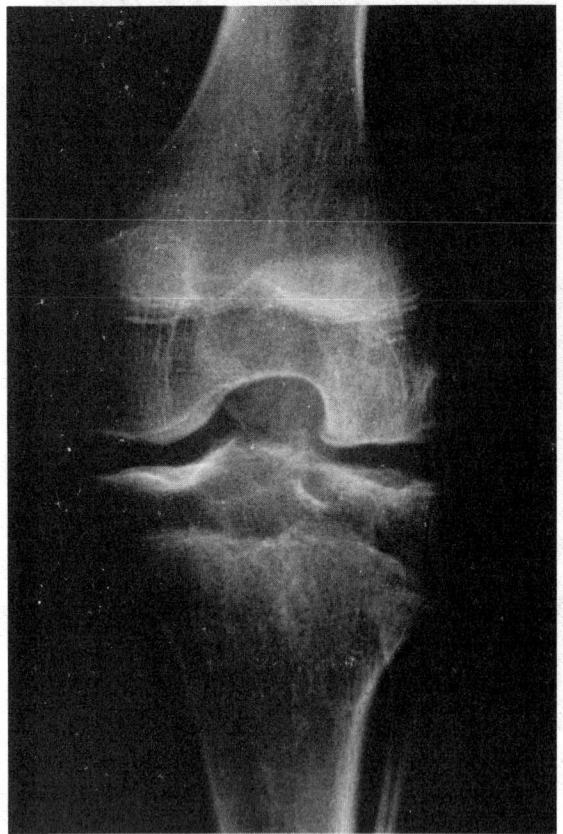 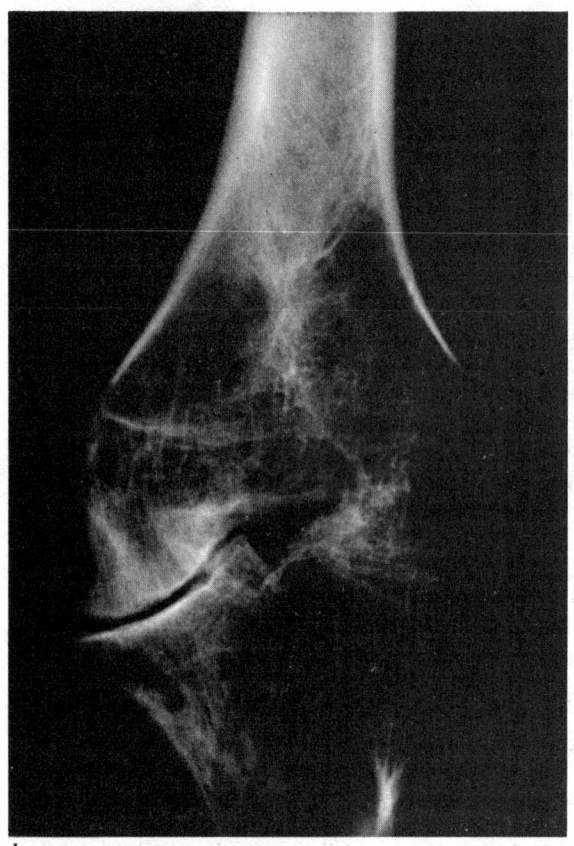

a   b

FIGURE 152-3 (*a*) Early changes in the bones of the knee of a patient with hemophilia. The articular surfaces are irregular, there is widening of the intracondylar notch, and rarefactions are present in the epiphyses. (*b*) Advanced changes in the bones of the knee of a patient with hemophilia. There is marked narrowing of the joint space medially and fusion laterally. Marked rarefaction and cystic changes are also obvious in all the bones. (Courtesy of Dr. F. R. Heitzman.)

EPISTAXES

These are common in hemophilia and in some cases may be the main symptom. However, fewer than 1 in 1000 patients presenting with epistaxes as the only indication of a bleeding tendency prove to have hemophilia or a related condition.

BLEEDING FROM OTHER MUCOUS MEMBRANES

Hematemesis is relatively uncommon and hemoptysis quite unusual. It is important not to overlook the possibility that in known hemophilic patients, a local lesion may be the cause of bleeding rather than the hemophilic state. Thus, tuberculosis or some other lesion of the lung should always be considered in a hemophilic patient who coughs up blood. Bleeding from the mouth, especially the tongue, is common and may be due to trauma associated with eating or to accidental biting of the tongue.

BONE CYSTS AND PSEUDOTUMORS

Hemophilic cysts, also known as *pseudotumors,* are a rare but dangerous complication of hemophilia (Fig. 152-4). There are three main types [55]. The first is a

simple cyst confined by tendinous attachments within the fascial envelope of a muscle. The second variety develops initially as a simple cyst but gives rise to changes in bone due to interference with the periosteal circulation. The third variety, classic pseudotumor, is believed to be caused initially by a subperiosteal hemorrhage which strips the periosteum from the cortex until limited by aponeurotic or tendinous attachments. The mass then compresses and destroys the muscle. It is probable that hemophilic cysts always arise as a result of trauma and usually expand slowly, causing pressure necrosis. They affect chiefly the lower half of the body. They are found in those muscular areas which have profuse vascular connections with underlying periosteum or bone and have extensive ramifications which make them difficult to remove. Unless removed completely, they tend to re-form [56]. These cysts often expand over a period of several years and may become extremely large. The gross appearance of the cyst, together with the radiologic appearance of bone destruction and new bone formation, makes differentiation from a malignant tumor of bone difficult, if not impossible. Infection is prone to occur if needle biopsy is performed. The cysts contain serosanguineous fluid or thick, chocolate-colored material of sticky consistency which is difficult to clear from the surrounding tissue.

LIVER DISORDERS

Most patients with hemophilia who have received transfusions of blood or blood products have a persistent derangement of liver function [57–63], but very few of these patients are symptomatic. Percutaneous liver biopsies have revealed a surprising incidence of structural changes, usually chronic persistent hepatitis, chronic active hepatitis, or fatty infiltration with early cirrhosis, in decreasing order of frequency [62–66]. Acute non-A, non-B hepatitis is relatively common, and acute hepatitis due to hepatitis B virus is still prevalent [67]. The abnormalities of liver function have been reported with greater frequency in hemophiliac patients who have received commercial concentrates than in those who have been transfused only with comparable amounts of cryoprecipitate [61].

SPLENOMEGALY

More than a quarter of hemophilic patients have palpable spleens at some time or another [58]. This may perhaps be related in some way to treatment, as the incidence tends to increase as a function of intensity of therapy [58]. The splenomegaly does not correlate with age, the presence or absence of abnormal liver function tests, or the presence of HBsAg or HBsAb [58]. It may be a monocyte-macrophage response to the continuous bombardment with foreign antigens, including denatured proteins, that these patients often receive. The absence of abdominal symptoms suggests that intrasplenic hemorrhage is not the mechanism of most splenic enlargements [58].

CLINICAL DIAGNOSIS

If a male patient has had repeated joint hemorrhages or a clear-cut sex-linked recessive family history of bleeding of the hemophilic type, the diagnosis of hemophilia A or B can be made with a reasonable degree of confidence. If a sex-linked history and joint hemorrhages are both present, the diagnosis of hemophilia A or B may be considered certain; few exceptions have been reported. If the history is consistent with a sex-linked mode of inheritance but there are only two or three affected males, von Willebrand's disease cannot always be excluded, since such a family history might occur on a chance basis with an autosomal mode of inheritance. Hemarthroses are rare in other hemophilic states and in von Willebrand's disease.

LABORATORY FEATURES

The partial thromboplastin time (PTT), activated or unactivated, is always significantly prolonged in patients with less than 35 percent FVIII:C. Individuals with levels ranging between 35 and 50 percent may have a PTT value either just outside or at the upper end of the normal range. The PTT techniques using activators,

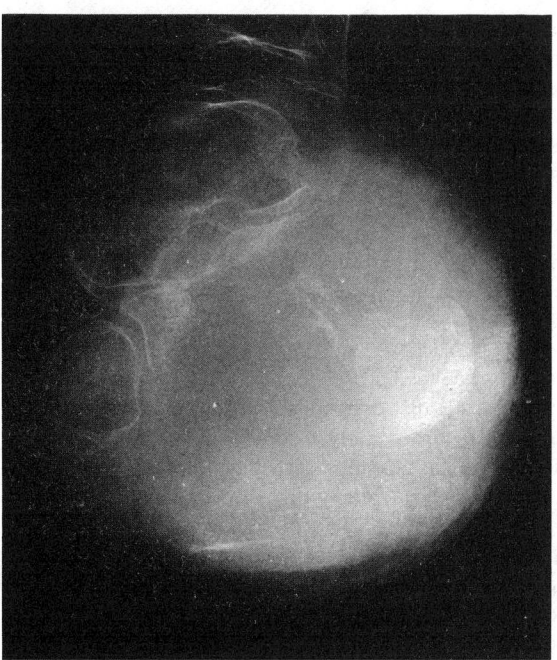

FIGURE 152-4   Hemophilic pseudotumor of the heel. Note extensive destruction of the bones associated with the large soft-tissue mass. (Courtesy of Dr. F. R. Heitzman.)

such as kaolin, celite, or ellagic acid, are more precise than those not using activator. The bleeding time and prothrombin time are not significantly prolonged, and when these tests are normal and the PTT test prolonged, a factor VIII:C assay should be carried out, followed by a factor IX assay if the factor VIII:C is normal.

The diagnosis of hemophilia A can be made with confidence when the patient is a male with a clear-cut sex-linked history of a bleeding disorder and a level of FVIII:C below 40 percent. FVIII:Ag and FVIIIR:RCo levels are usually normal, but since the von Willebrand trait is relatively common and its incidence in hemophilic patients probably the same as in the normal population, about 5 percent of patients may also have the von Willebrand trait with slightly reduced levels of FVIII:vWF (40 to 60 percent). When there is no family history or an unclear inheritance pattern, hemophilia A must be differentiated from von Willebrand's disease. In the latter disease the bleeding time is often increased and the FVIII:C activity is usually the same as or higher than that of FVIIIR:RCo. In hemophilia A, however, the ratio of FVIIIR:RCo to FVIII:C is at least 2. In difficult cases a family study is invaluable, and determination of the FVIII:CAg level is sometimes useful: in hemophilia A the FVIII:CAg level may be higher than the FVIII:C level, although this is not the general rule. In von Willebrand's disease, with the possible exception of the very rare severe case, the FVIII:C and FVIII:CAg levels do not differ significantly. Patients with von Willebrand's disease have a more sustained rise in FVIII:C level following infusion of cryoprecipitate than do patients with hemophilia, but interpretation of results is usually not clear-cut. Factor VIII is an acute-phase protein, and in mild cases of hemophilia A with FVIII:C levels between 15 and 40 percent, normal or even increased levels of FVIII:C may be found following exercise or stress. Accordingly, a normal value found shortly after moderate tissue injury does not exclude a mild form of hemophilia, and the FVIII:C determination should be repeated at a later date. In all patients with hemophilia A, a careful search for a FVIII:C inhibitor should be carried out (Chap. 157).

PRENATAL DIAGNOSIS

Fetal blood collected by fetoscopy may be contaminated by amniotic fluid and thus is often partially clotted, even when immediately mixed with an anticoagulant. This precludes a reliable estimate of FVIII:C activity, which may be spuriously high or low, or even zero, on a normal specimen. The FVIII:CAg activity is more stable, and the lower level of normal is rarely less than 10 percent [68,69] even in serum [45]. Thus a FVIII:CAg value significantly below this in a fetus at risk is good evidence of hemophilia. A normal value excludes the severe to moderate forms of the disease unless the factor is of the relatively rare CRM$^+$ variety, and this must be determined beforehand by performing the assay on an affected family member. Prenatal diagnosis of hemophilia A at mid-trimester has recently been accomplished by two groups [68,69]. One of these [69] used a special small-bore fetoscope to obtain pure fetal blood uncontaminated by amniotic fluid or maternal blood; they performed both FVIII:C and FVIII:CAg determinations and found that either measurement could be used in prediction. The other group [68] used a technique in which there is usually contamination of the fetal blood with amniotic fluid. Using the FVIII:CAg level as their primary indicator, they predicted hemophilia A correctly in three out of six fetuses at risk. Although prenatal diagnosis is claimed to be both reliable and safe [69], it is not without pitfalls [70]. The lower limits of normal for FVIII:CAg levels in these studies were 11 percent [69] and 17 percent [68]. One might therefore expect some mild hemophilic patients to have levels that fall into the normal range. The method should be used only when the hemophilia in the kindred is moderate to severe and it is known that the hemophilia is of the CRM$^-$ type.

GENERAL MANAGEMENT

BETWEEN BLEEDING EPISODES

If the patient is a child or young adult it is essential that the physician gain the confidence of both patient and parents. The physician must keep fully abreast of the current developments in the field and be able to answer the many queries the parents, who are usually already well informed, are likely to direct at him or her. The parents should be encouraged to join a local chapter of the National Hemophilia Society. The patient should know whom to contact in an emergency when the personal physician is not available. The parents should be

carefully instructed concerning when to consult the physician. Indications for hospital attendance are severe pain and swelling of a muscle or joint causing limitation of movement or producing sleeplessness, serious or hard knocks on the head, swelling in the tissues of the neck/or floor of the mouth, severe abdominal pain, hematuria, melena, or skin wounds that would require sutures in a normal person [71]. All deep muscular hematomas should be given careful attention; however, superficial bruises or mild cuts will rarely give rise to serious bleeding. The hospital admission must be managed by a physician who is aware of the special problems involved and is able to give the patient prompt treatment if required.

Psychological support plays an important role in the management of the patient with hemophilia. The patient should be reassured frequently and his morale maintained by emphasizing the achievements of others handicapped in a similar way. The transmission of fears and doubts the physician may have about the outcome of a hemorrhagic episode is likely to have an adverse effect on the patient. An optimistic attitude should be maintained before both patient and parents.

The signs and symptoms of hemophilia are frequently cyclical; the patient has a series of rapidly occurring hemorrhagic episodes followed by a period in which he is asymptomatic. Even in the severe type of hemophilia, remissions lasting months or even years do occur. When the patient reaches adolescence, a significant decrease in the frequency of hemorrhagic episodes is usually seen, and many patients with the moderate or mild types of hemophilia lead almost normal lives. It is possible that the apprehension arising from a first episode after a remission in some way increases the predisposition to bleed and starts a vicious circle. The treatment of every minor hemorrhagic episode with plasma or whole-blood products is to be deprecated, for the patient is likely to become dependent on such treatment. When it is subsequently withheld or delayed he becomes nervous and apprehensive, and an episode which otherwise would almost certainly have resolved spontaneously may continue, confirming the patient's conviction that only with plasma or blood products can his hemorrhagic lesions resolve. There is now general agreement that ε-aminocaproic acid, an inhibitor of plasminogen activation, is a useful agent in the treatment of hemophilic bleeding [72,73], although it has no effect on the level of factor VIII:C.

Patients with hemophilia or any other bleeding disorder should not take aspirin or preparations containing aspirin, since these drugs increase the predisposition to bleed by interfering with platelet function. Acetaminophen or propoxyphene should be used for analgesia; the former is also effective as an antipyretic.

Treatment of a bleeding episode in a hemophilic patient should be initiated as soon as possible. Therefore it is a wise precaution for patients with hemophilia to carry factor VIII concentrate with them when traveling, especially if visiting areas where factor VIII may not be available. Many patients with hemophilia or their parents can be taught to administer the concentrate in an emergency.

There are now home therapy programs in which, with the physician's guidance, the patient (or his family) is taught to administer factor VIII when signs or symptoms of bleeding first appear [74–80]. These programs result in reduced time lost from school and work and a greater sense of security and also prevent the hours spent waiting in emergency rooms, often in considerable pain [81]. A physician's manual of guidelines for home therapy is available from the National Hemophilia Foundation, 25 West 39th Street, New York, NY 10018. Prophylactic therapy in which the patient receives regular doses of factor VIII at short intervals has been used successfully in a few cases [76,81–85]. However, the cost of such therapy is prohibitively high, and the availability of factor VIII is limited.

EDUCATION
Education is of the greatest importance to the hemophilic child, for it is important that he be trained for an occupation not involving physical labor. In general it is best for a hemophilic child to attend a regular school. However, in severe cases the patient may be unable to keep up with his school work because of frequent absences. Also, there is the possibility of accidents during playground periods and sports activities. Schools for the physically handicapped and other types of special schools also present disadvantages, since the treatment of hemophilic children is quite different from that of other physically handicapped children. Special schools for hemophilic children, operated in conjunction with a treatment center, have proved successful in both France and England.

IMMUNIZATION
With the usual type of vaccine, the risk of hemorrhage at the site of injection appears to be relatively low, even in severe cases, perhaps because of the small volume injected [71]. It is recommended, however, that firm pressure be maintained on the puncture with the fingertip for at least 5 full minutes following injection. Subcutaneous and intracutaneous administration carries relatively little risk of bleeding.

TREATMENT OF BLEEDING EPISODES

CUTS AND ABRASIONS
Local measures, such as the application of firm pressure, will usually suffice in the event of a mild cut or abrasion, but if bleeding is persistent, topical administration of thrombin, which is available in most hospital pharmacies, or Russell's viper venom is often helpful. Only rarely is the administration of blood products required for minor injuries. Even if the oozing persists for 1 week or longer, blood products should be withheld unless anemia severe enough to warrant blood

transfusion develops. If the wound is deep and requires sutures, the patient should be hospitalized. It is important not to suture such a wound without raising the factor VIII:C level, for otherwise the patient may continue to bleed into the wound and the blood dissect into the deeper tissues. Injuries to the tongue and small lesions of the mouth may give rise to persistent bleeding. However, it is generally not necessary for the patient to be admitted to the hospital unless the blood loss is unusually rapid or prolonged.

EPISTAXES
Only rarely are these troublesome. More often than not the bleeding will stop without specific therapy, and occasions when blood or blood products will be required are infrequent. A useful device for the application of pressure over the suspected bleeding point is a finger cot tied over the end of a small rubber catheter. This is lubricated and placed well back in the nasal cavity. It is then inflated by the patient so that uniform pressure is applied over the bleeding site.

HEMARTHROSES
In general, the most painful episodes are the most dangerous, and the parents of small children should be instructed to bring them to the hospital if the pain prevents sleep. At the first sign of joint pain, the patient should be told to begin rest without delay and the joint should be immobilized. An elastic bandage, a comfortable plaster of paris back splint, or a complete plaster cast should be applied according to the severity of bleeding. In addition, there is a growing trend, particularly in infants and young children, to raise the plasma factor VIII:C level to 20 to 30 percent. This dose is repeated 24 h later if the swelling does not show evidence of subsiding on immobilization. In most instances pain and swelling are resolved following prompt immobilization alone [86], but sequelae are reduced by administering factor VIII.

If there is evidence of an appreciable amount of fluid in the joint cavity, aspiration may be tried, although in many cases very little blood is removed. All aspirations must be preceded or immediately followed by administration of factor VIII to prevent the accumulation of blood in the joint cavity. It has been customary to give the treatment immediately before aspiration, but it has been pointed out [86] that this treatment might reduce the effect of aspiration by causing the blood in the joint cavity to clot. For this reason, it has been recommended that replacement therapy be given immediately after aspiration [86].

DDAVP IN THE MANAGEMENT OF MILD HEMOPHILIA
Drugs such as catecholamines and insulin may induce a threefold or more increase in FVIII:C and FVIII:vWF levels in normal subjects [87,88]. The same result with fewer side effects can be achieved by intravenous infusion of 1-deamino-8-D-arginine vasopressin (DDAVP),

a synthetic analog of the antidiuretic hormone 8-arginine vasopressin [89]. DDAVP has been used to treat mild to moderate cases of hemophilia and has resulted in a threefold to sixfold increase of factor VIII:C activity [89]. A similar increase in factor VIII:C activity is induced by strenuous exercise or stress.

REPLACEMENT THERAPY
The objective of replacement therapy is to raise the concentration of factor VIII:C to the hemostatic level and maintain this level until healing occurs. The details of the therapeutic regimens available are presented in Chap. 167, including consideration of prophylactic therapy. Acquired immunologic abnormalities in patients receiving replacement therapy for hemophilia A are also discussed in Chap. 167.

SURGERY IN HEMOPHILIA
With the advent of potent concentrates, major surgery in hemophilia has become considerably less dangerous than it was formerly; however, hemostatic failure sometimes occurs for unknown reasons. Surgery still carries a considerable risk in hemophilia [90]. Operations should therefore be avoided unless the indications are compelling. The management of replacement therapy in surgery is discussed in Chap. 167.

A difficult diagnostic problem in hemophilia is the occurrence of right-side abdominal pain and tenderness. In most instances these are due to the formation of a right iliopsoas hematoma rather than to acute appendicitis [91]. In some instances, discoloration of the flank may become apparent several hours after the onset of pain. It is therefore important to examine the flank in a good light. Operation in such a patient is usually contraindicated, for the dangers of surgery may exceed those of conservative therapy [91].

DENTAL EXTRACTION
Prophylactic measures in dental care—including regular visits to the dentist—constitute one of the most important points in the management of hemophilic patients, and no hemophilic patient should be denied the benefits of fluoride [92]. Deciduous teeth, when shed, rarely cause troublesome hemorrhage. If extractions of permanent teeth become inevitable, it is unwise to remove more than two teeth at one time unless factor VIII concentrates are available. When one or two teeth are extracted, a protective acrylic splint should be applied, antibiotic therapy should be given, and the factor VIII:C level should be raised to 50 percent. In addition, ε-aminocaproic acid should be given orally in doses of 24 g per day for 10 days, provided there is no contraindication to its use [72,73]. More extensive dental surgery should be carried out after replacement therapy with factor VIII concentrates [93].

CIRCULATING ANTICOAGULANTS
Approximately 6 percent of hemophilic patients develop specific antibodies against factor VIII, which often present a serious problem in the management of the disease (Chaps. 157 and 167). Every hemophilic patient must therefore be screened for the presence of an antibody directed against factor VIII:C. These anticoagulants are discussed in Chap. 157.

Hemophilia B (factor IX deficiency)

DEFINITION
Hemophilia B (synonyms: *Christmas disease, hereditary PTC deficiency*) is a hemorrhagic disease characterized by a deficiency of factor IX activity. It closely resembles hemophilia A, having a sex-linked, recessive mode of inheritance and practically identical clinical manifestations.

INCIDENCE
The incidence is approximately 1 in 100,000 of the population. There are about seven cases of hemophilia A to every case of hemophilia B. The disease also occurs in dogs [94].

PATHOGENESIS
Several variants of factor IX deficiency have been described. Antibodies against factor IX found in hemophilia B patients can be neutralized by the plasma of some patients with factor IX deficiency, but not by the plasma of others [95–97]. Plasmas from patients with no detectable antibody-neutralizing activity or cross-reacting material are referred to as CRM⁻. Plasmas which neutralize the specific antibody to a degree proportional to the factor IX clotting activity are referred to as CRM reduced or CRMᴿ. Those with normal levels of cross-reacting material are called CRM⁺. In three studies [98–100] involving a total of 352 kindreds, approximately 45 percent had less than 3 percent factor IX with no detectable antigen (CRM⁻), approximately 15 percent had less than 3 percent factor IX with normal levels of antigen (CRM⁺), and the remainder had intermediate amounts of antigen. When a more sensitive radioimmunoassay with a naturally occurring human antibody was used, only 2 of 18 kindreds with less than 3 percent factor IX could be considered CRM⁻ [101]. Clearly, classification based on the ratio of factor IX antigen activity to factor IX coagulant activity is in most cases arbitrary, depending on the antibody and technique used.

All patients with hemophilia B have a prothrombin time which is either normal or 1 or 2 s longer than normal when human brain tissue factor (thromboplastin) is used. However, when bovine brain tissue factor is used, the prothrombin time is markedly prolonged in approximately one-fifth of CRM⁺ patients [98,99,102]. This type of hemophilia B is referred to as hemophilia Bᴹ (M being the first letter of the surname of one of the first patients with this variant) [102–104]. The prolonged bovine brain prothrombin time is due to competitive inhibition of the reaction between factor VII and bovine brain tissue factor by the abnormal factor IX molecule [104–107]. The abnormal factor IX analog has the same physicochemical properties as normal factor IX [104,107], and neutralization of its anticoagulant activity by a specific human factor IX antibody has been demonstrated [105]. Moderate to slight prolongation of the bovine brain thromboplastin times are found in a small percentage of both CRM⁺ and CRM⁻ hemophilia B patients [98,108,109]. Some of these patients appear to have a very mild deficiency of factor VII coagulant activity with a normal amount of the corresponding antigen [108,109]. Levels of factors V and X may be slightly reduced [98]; there is no satisfactory single explanation for these findings.

The degree of clinical severity and factor IX levels do not vary among affected members of the same kindred, but both vary among kindreds [110]. It is probable that a large number of CRM⁺ molecular variants exist, each associated with certain levels of coagulant activity. One such variant is factor IX Chapel Hill [111,112], characterized by mild symptoms and a factor IX molecule which is slowly cleaved at the arginine-alanine bond and yields factor IXa at approximately 60 percent of the rate of normal factor IX [112]. The variant of hemophilia B referred to as hemophilia B Leyden is characterized by an increase in the factor IX level with age [113]. Below the age of 15 years the factor IX level is less than 2 percent, yet after the age of 19 the level may be as high as 58 percent. The clinical manifestations ameliorate with age and may disappear completely. In another variant, the factor IX resembles the factor IX formed in vitamin K deficiency, with low specific coagulant activity, reduced affinity for adsorption to aluminum hydroxide, and increased electrophoretic mobility [114]. The molecular weight of the mutant molecule is higher than that of the normal molecule. It is postulated that the difference is due to an additional polypeptide chain which interferes both with calcium binding and with proteolytic degradation by its physiologic activators [115].

GENETICS
The mode of inheritance of hemophilia B is similar to that of hemophilia A (Fig. 152-5). In one series of 13 obligatory carriers, the range of factor IX levels was 29 to 109 percent, with a mean of 67 percent [110]. In a larger series of 51 obligatory carriers, the range was 12 to 119 percent with a mean of 42 percent [116]. A probability curve derived from these data indicates that a woman who is a daughter of a definite hemophilia B carrier and who has a factor IX activity level of 100 percent still runs a 10 percent risk of being a true carrier of hemophilia B. Conversely, such a woman may have a factor IX activity level of only 60 percent of normal and yet retain approximately a 15 percent chance of not being a carrier [116]. Determinations of factor IX levels permit identification of many carriers. Factor IX antigen determinations are of limited value in improving heterozygote detection in carriers from kindreds in which affected males show no evidence of excess factor

IX antigen relative to activity, but may be useful in kindreds in which the affected males possess an excess of factor IX antigen [98,100,116].

In the detection of the carrier state in kindreds with the relatively rare B^M variant, the bovine brain thromboplastin prothrombin time is a very useful discriminant. A significant prolongation is strong evidence of the carrier state when such prolongation is combined with a reduction in factor IX activity [98,103,104,117]. However, a normal bovine brain thromboplastin prothrombin time with a normal level of factor IX does not exclude the carrier state in B^M kindreds. As is the case in hemophilia A, carriers with any variant of hemophilia B can be phenotypically normal. Roughly 20 percent of obligatory carriers have factor IX levels below 25 percent [98]. Such a marked reduction in factor IX activity is usually associated with abnormal bleeding, and the incidence of bleeding in carriers is significantly higher in hemophilia B than in hemophilia A.

The diagnosis of the carrier state can be made with a reasonable degree of confidence in approximately one-quarter of the cases on the basis of a factor IX assay alone [98,110,118].

In one study [118], two female descendants of carriers were found to have only 5 percent of factor IX; both these women had the B^M variant. There has been a report of hemophilia B in a female with Turner's syndrome [117]. The patient, whose hemorrhagic manifestations included hemarthroses, was also found to have the B^M variant.

CLINICAL FEATURES
Hemophilia B is clinically indistinguishable from hemophilia A.

FIGURE 152-5   Pedigree of a family with hemophilia B. The figures under the symbols representing individual family members give the age of the patient and the level of factor IX. Some of the females not so indicated may be carriers of factor IX deficiency. Males are indicated by the square symbols, females by the circles. (Data contributed by Drs. Eugene L. Lozner and M. Parekh.)

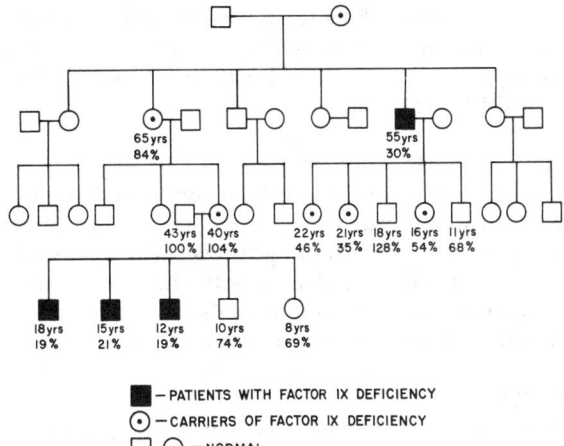

LABORATORY FEATURES

The same tests used for the diagnosis of hemophilia A are also used for the diagnosis of hemophilia B, except, of course, that the definitive diagnosis depends on the assay of factor IX rather than factor VIII. In contrast to hemophilia A, the abnormality in the PTT is corrected by serum but not by adsorbed plasma. The prothrombin time is usually normal but is sometimes prolonged by 1 or 2 s. As mentioned earlier, in approximately 5 percent of cases the prothrombin time is prolonged when bovine brain tissue factor (thromboplastin) is used. With brain extracts of other species, the prolongation is less marked.

The diagnosis of hemophilia B in the fetus has been successfully accomplished using a very-small-bore fetoscope and needle [68]. Contamination with amniotic fluid or partial clotting in the specimen should not affect the factor IX value and factor IX assays can be performed on serum as well as on plasma. In practice this is difficult to accomplish, however, because of the presence of activation products in serum. The normal range in the fetus is wide, and there is uncertainty as to the lower limit of normal, which may be between 10 and 15 percent. Accordingly, carrier detection should be restricted to those forms of hemophilia B in which the factor IX level is less than 3 percent. Factor IX antigen level determinations are of limited value in the detection of hemophilia B in the fetus.

TREATMENT

The general management of patients and the principles of replacement therapy are similar to those in hemophilia A and are discussed in Chap. 167. Prophylactic therapy is considered in that chapter also.

Hereditary deficiency of factor XI

HISTORY

The first case of hereditary deficiency of factor XI was reported in 1953 [119]. Similar cases were soon found in different parts of the world. However, the great majority of recorded cases have been found in New York City and Los Angeles, where the disease is almost as common as classic hemophilia. It has also been called *Rosenthal's syndrome* and *plasma thromboplastin antecedent* (PTA) *deficiency*.

PATHOGENESIS

A relatively large number of kindreds have now been studied using immunologic techniques, and so far in every case the factor XI antigen level was reduced in proportion to the factor XI activity [120,121]. Thus it appears that the defect is due, in the large majority, to reduced or absent synthesis of a normal molecule.

GENETICS

The disease occurs mainly in people of Jewish ancestry. It is transmitted as an autosomal recessive trait. Hetero-

zygotes have 10 to 20 percent of the normal mean level of factor XI [122]. The disease occurs with equal frequency in males and females.

CLINICAL FEATURES

The disorder tends to be exceedingly mild, with bruising, epistaxis, and menorrhagia as the most common clinical manifestations. Hemarthroses are rarely seen, and intramuscular hemorrhages are also unusual. Often the disease presents with persistent bleeding following tooth extraction, tonsillectomy, or some other surgical procedure. A high proportion of patients, including some with no detectable level of factor XI, appear to have completely normal hemostatic mechanisms and do not bleed excessively following major surgery [123]. However, there have been patients who have survived major surgery with no hemostatic problems but on a subsequent occasion have bled excessively [124].

LABORATORY FEATURES

The activated PTT is prolonged and the prothrombin time normal. The bleeding time is normal. Specific assays of factor VIII and factor IX are normal, and in the expanded PTT test normal serum and adsorbed plasma each produce partial correction. Definitive diagnosis is by a factor XI assay using blood from a patient with established factor XI deficiency, but a satisfactory factor XI-deficient plasma can be prepared artificially from normal plasma. Adsorbed normal plasma contains a variable amount of factor XI, and in the expanded PTT test correction with this reagent is slight compared with that produced by normal serum; the results then closely resemble those found in factor IX deficiency, and the two diseases are sometimes confused. All tests to detect factor XI deficiency should be performed on freshly collected plasma, as the PTT of factor XI-deficient plasma may shorten significantly on storage even when the plasma is kept frozen.

TREATMENT

Most patients with severe deficiencies of factor XI respond well to relatively small amounts of plasma (Chap. 167).

Hereditary deficiencies of factor XII and of Fletcher, Fitzgerald, and Passovoy factors

Factor XII (Hageman factor) and Fletcher and Fitzgerald factor deficiencies are not associated with hemorrhagic manifestations. Factor XII deficiency (Hageman trait) was first discovered in 1955 [125] when a long clotting time was found in a patient named Hageman during the course of a preoperative evaluation. Paradoxically, the patient died many years later from pulmonary embolism after a fracture of the pelvis. At least four other patients with this disorder had episodes diagnosed as myocardial infarction or thrombophlebitis [126]. The abnormality is inherited as an autosomal recessive or dominant trait [127]. Approximately 10 percent of the population have persistent mild deficiencies of factor XII with levels of 40 to 60 percent of normal. Orientals have levels of factor XII significantly lower than Caucasians [176]. In a sensitive radioimmunoassay, only 2 out of 49 subjects with factor XII deficiency had antigen levels in excess of procoagulant activity [128].

Fletcher factor deficiency was first described in 1965 [129]. In one family study the deficiency was found to be transmitted as an autosomal recessive trait [130]. The Fletcher factor has been identified as prekallikrein [131,132].

Fitzgerald factor deficiency was first recognized in 1975 [133]. The patient had a prolonged activated PTT and normal levels of all the previously recognized blood clotting factors. Similar cases were independently reported and given the surnames of the patients, Flaujeac [134,135] and Williams [136]. Plasmas from these patients are deficient in high-molecular-weight kininogen. The plasmas from the three patients are not mutually corrective in clotting systems, but there are apparent differences in kininogen levels as determined by immunologic assays [137]. Fitzgerald plasma exhibits impaired surface-mediated fibrinolysis and esterolytic activity, impaired generation of kinins, and the property of enhancing vascular permeability, designated PF/Dil. Both the Flaujeac and Fitzgerald traits appear to be transmitted as autosomal recessive characteristics [133,135].

The Passovoy defect was also described in 1975 [138], and subsequently other cases have been reported [139,177]. The disorder is transmitted as an autosomal dominant trait. Patients with the defect have a mild bleeding diathesis resembling factor XI deficiency.

The laboratory findings are very similar in deficiencies of factor XII and Fletcher, Fitzgerald, and Passovoy factors and closely resemble those found in factor XI deficiency. The activated PTT is prolonged. The most marked prolongation is usually found in the homozygous forms of factor XII deficiency. Only a slight prolongation is usually seen in Fletcher factor deficiency, and this is even less when the incubation period of the reaction mixture is lengthened; the same is true of Passovoy deficiency. However, the Passovoy defect, unlike the other three deficiency states, is associated with a bleeding disorder. The prothrombin and bleeding times are normal in all four disorders. Definitive diagnosis is made by testing against plasma from an established case. As patients with factor XII or Fletcher factor deficiencies do not bleed excessively, there is no need to transfuse these patients preoperatively. Some patients with Passovoy deficiency have bled excessively at surgery and have required plasma transfusions, but on other occasions the same patients have undergone surgery without problems [139]. Thus it seems best not to transfuse preoperatively but to be prepared to trans-

fuse with fresh plasma if significant bleeding occurs in the postoperative period.

Hereditary deficiency of factor V

Hereditary deficiency of factor V was first described in 1944 [140] and is also known as *Owren's disease* or *parahemophilia*. It is transmitted as a highly penetrant, incompletely recessive autosomal characteristic and affects both sexes equally. Three cases, including the original case, have been studied by antibody neutralization techniques, and all appear to be CRM⁻ [141,142].

INCIDENCE
The number of clinically affected patients probably does not exceed 1 per 1 million of the population. However, heterozygotes with factor V levels ranging from 22 to 60 percent of normal are encountered more frequently.

CLINICAL FEATURES
Bruising following trivial injury, epistaxes which may be severe, and bleeding from mucous membranes are the most frequent manifestations. In women, the most troublesome symptom appears to be menorrhagia. Deep intramuscular hematomas or hemarthroses rarely occur. Bleeding frequently follows tonsillectomy or other types of surgery and may be the first sign of the disease. Despite a very long prothrombin time, indicating a very low level of factor V, some patients do not have severe manifestations [143].

LABORATORY FEATURES
The prothrombin time and PTT, activated or unactivated, are all prolonged. The bleeding time is slightly prolonged in approximately one-third of cases. The long prothrombin time is not corrected by Russell's viper venom (RVV) or by aged serum but is shortened by $Al(OH)_3$-treated fresh, normal plasma.

TREATMENT
Replacement therapy is discussed in Chap. 167.

Hereditary factor VII deficiency

DEFINITION AND HISTORY
Hereditary deficiency of factor VII is a hemorrhagic state transmitted as an autosomal recessive trait.

The disease, which is characterized by a prolonged prothrombin time but a normal PTT or whole-blood clotting time, was first described in 1951 [144] under the title of "congenital SPCA deficiency." The term SPCA proved unsatisfactory and has since been abandoned. Evidence of the existence of this factor had been previously obtained indirectly from a study of a patient taking dicumarol [145,146].

PATHOGENESIS

As with hereditary deficiencies of other clotting factors, there is genetic heterogeneity, and factor VII deficiency may be due to decreased or absent synthesis of a normal molecule or to synthesis of an abnormal molecule [147,148]. The latter type can be subclassified on the basis of rabbit and bovine brain prothrombin times. In factor VII Padua the rabbit brain prothrombin time is markedly prolonged, whereas the bovine brain prothrombin time is only slightly prolonged; in factor VII Padua$_2$ the reverse is the case; in factor VII Verona both rabbit and bovine brain times are prolonged [149].

INCIDENCE

The disease is very rare and occurs roughly in 1 out of 500,000 persons. It has been found in beagle dogs [19,20].

CLINICAL FEATURES

The severity of the bleeding depends on the degree of depression of factor VII. Patients who have only a 5- to 7-s prolongation of the one-stage prothrombin time rarely have severe hemorrhagic manifestations and live practically normal lives. However, when the prolongation of the prothrombin time is more marked, significant bleeding manifestations are present. These include bleeding from the mucous membranes and gastrointestinal tract. In women, menorrhagia is often the major problem. Fatal cerebral hemorrhage has been reported, and hemarthroses sometimes occur, although less frequently than in severe hemophilia.

LABORATORY FEATURES

The diagnosis of factor VII deficiency is a relatively simple one. The disease is characterized by a completely normal PTT (activated or unactivated) and a prolonged prothrombin time, which is fully corrected by the addition of Russell's viper venom. All tests which do not use tissue factor (factor III) are normal. Definite diagnosis is made by performing a prothrombin time determination on a mixture of equal parts of the patient's plasma and plasma from a patient with a previously established deficiency. If the prothrombin time of the mixture is significantly shorter than that of one of the plasmas alone, a deficiency of factor VII is excluded.

TREATMENT

Replacement therapy is discussed in Chap. 167. The condition does not respond to vitamin K.

Hereditary deficiency of factor X

DEFINITION AND HISTORY

A hereditary hemorrhagic state due to a deficiency of factor X (Stuart-Prower or Stuart factor) was recognized from investigations of patients with a disorder resembling factor VII deficiency [150–152]. Studies of a female patient who had a prolonged one-stage prothrombin time which was corrected by Russell's viper venom were reported in 1956 [150]. The defect resembled factor VII deficiency in these respects but could be clearly segregated from it on the basis of an abnormality in the serum phase of the thromboplastin generation test. The factor deficient in the patient was called the *Prower factor*, Prower being the patient's surname. Other investigators independently reported on a male patient named Stuart with a similar hemorrhagic condition associated with a prolonged prothrombin time, a serum abnormality in the thromboplastin generation test, and abnormal prothrombin consumption [151,152]. The defect, which was transmitted as an autosomal recessive characteristic [153], was mutually corrected by plasma from the prototype patient with factor VII deficiency. Since the long prothrombin time in the patient Stuart was not corrected by Russell's viper venom, it appeared to differ from the Prower defect. The term *Stuart* was proposed for the clotting activity deficient in Stuart's plasma. It was subsequently shown that the plasmas of the patients Stuart and Prower were not mutually corrective, indicating that both plasmas lacked the same factor [154], and the original observation that the Prower defect was corrected by Russell's viper venom was attributed to a technical error [155]. Further work has demonstrated that the deficiency in both patients is indeed factor X.

INCIDENCE

Fewer than 1 in 500,000 of the population have the disease; however, the heterozygous state occurs in roughly 1 in 500 of the population [153].

PATHOGENESIS

Several types of hereditary factor X deficiency can be distinguished. There may be reduced or absent synthesis of a normal molecule. Stuart, the prototype patient, has this type of abnormality [156]. In these cases the procoagulant activity parallels the level of antigen. There may be a normal amount of antigen but reduced or absent procoagulant activity, or a reduced amount of antigen and a disproportionately greater reduction in procoagulant activity [156,157]. Those cases with relatively more antigen than activity can be further divided according to (1) the degree to which the molecule can be activated by Russell's viper venom, (2) the intrinsic system, and (3) the extrinsic system, as determined by the RVV-cephalin time, the activated PTT, and the prothrombin time, respectively [156].

In factor X Friuli [157,158] the factor X is activated normally by Russell's viper venom but not by the intrinsic or extrinsic systems. Thus, in the standard assay for factor X, in which RVV-cephalin is used [159], the plasma appears to have a normal amount of this factor. When the assay is performed using brain thromboplastin, however, little or no factor X is found [156].

In another variant, the molecule was activated normally by the intrinsic system and RVV-cephalin but not by the extrinsic system [160]. The proband, despite a factor X level of less than 2 percent of normal as measured in an extrinsic system, was completely asymptomatic with respect to excessive bleeding; accordingly, it was suggested that in vivo the extrinsic activation of factor X is only of minor importance. As there were no family studies reported, it is uncertain as to whether the anomaly in this patient was hereditary or acquired.

CLINICAL FEATURES

The manifestations of this deficiency depend on the degree of depression of factor X and may be easy bruising, bleeding from mucous membranes, or menorrhagia. Marked deficiency of factor X may lead to hemarthrosis or serious bleeding after injury.

LABORATORY FEATURES

The prothrombin time is prolonged. As discussed above, the Russell's viper venom time may be normal or prolonged. Prolonged prothrombin time and Russell's viper venom time are both corrected by aged serum but not by $Al(OH)_3$-treated fresh, normal plasma. The PTT is prolonged except in the variant in which the molecule is activated normally by the intrinsic system [160].

TREATMENT

Replacement therapy is discussed in Chap. 167. This disorder does not respond to vitamin K.

Hereditary deficiency of prothrombin

DEFINITION AND INCIDENCE

Most cases of hereditary deficiency of prothrombin reported prior to 1956 have subsequently proved to be due to a deficiency of factor V, factor VII, or factor X. Since then, there have been only a very small number of well-documented case reports, as the condition is very rare. It is divided into two main groups, based on immunologic measurements of prothrombin. Those cases in which the prothrombin antigen level is sig-

nificantly higher than the biologic activity are referred to as the dysprothrombinemias, while those in which the activity and antigen level are reduced proportionately are referred to as true hypoprothrombinemia [161,162]. There are almost as many types of dysprothrombinemias as there are case reports [163–171]. Classification has been based on whether the molecule can be activated by staphylocoagulase, which is a nonenzymatic activator of normal prothrombin, or by certain snake venoms (e.g., Taipan snake, *Echis carinatus*), electrophoretic mobility, and serum immunoelectrophoresis (Table 152-1).

GENETICS

Both true hypoprothrombinemia and the dysprothrombinemias are inherited as recessive autosomal characteristics.

CLINICAL FEATURES

Heterozygotes are either asymptomatic or very mildly affected. Homozygotes have a mild to moderate bleeding tendency with bleeding from mucous membranes, excessive bruising, menorrhagia, etc.

LABORATORY FEATURES

The laboratory findings are a prolonged one-stage prothrombin time test not corrected by adsorbed normal plasma, aged serum, or Russell's viper venom; a prolonged PTT; and normal levels of factors V, VII, and X and fibrinogen. Prothrombin measured by either the one- or two-stage method is significantly decreased. The definitive diagnosis of a case of hereditary prothrombin deficiency is difficult since plasma from an established case is virtually impossible to obtain. The condition must be differentiated from an acquired circulating anticoagulant found in lupus erythematosus, which is associated with an isolated deficiency of prothrombin (Chap. 157).

TREATMENT

The condition does not respond to vitamin K. Replacement therapy is discussed in Chap. 167.

TABLE 152-1   Dysprothrombinemias

	Percent of normal prothrombin activity					
Prothrombin type	Extrinsic system	Staphylo-coagulase	Taipan snake venom	Percent of normal antigen	Electrophoretic mobility	Serum prothrombin fragments on immunoelectrophoresis
Cardeza [163]	30–50	N*		N	N	Abnormal band
Barcelona [164]	12–15	N		75–100	More anodal	
San Juan [165]	15–20	N		N		Abnormal anodal band
Padua [166]	32–52	N	32	N	N	Three abnormal bands
Brussels [167]	27	Decreased		84		Abnormal band
Quick [168,169]	2		Very low	34		
Molise [170]	32–52	50	32	100	N	Two extra bands
Houston [171]	5–10		Markedly reduced	52	N†	

* N = normal.

†The prothrombin antigen from a barium sulfate eluate of patient plasma electrofocused at a more basic isoelectric point than did the prothrombin antigen from an eluate of normal plasma.

Combined deficiency of vitamin K–dependent coagulation factors

Patients with a congenital, combined deficiency of vitamin K–dependent coagulation factors have been described [172–175]. One patient had severe deficiency of all four coagulation factors [172,173], and three others, including two siblings, had mild combined deficiencies of all four factors [174,175]. Evidence of deficient γ-carboxylation of protein precursors of the coagulation factors was obtained in all cases [173–175]. Complete [175], partial [173], and no [174] correction of the abnormalities by administration of vitamin K have been observed. The disorder appears to be due to some abnormality of posttranslational modification of the precursors of the vitamin K–dependent coagulation factors.

References

1. Bulloch, W., and Fildes, P.: *The Treasury of Human Inheritance.* Galton Laboratory for National Eugenics, Cambridge University Press, London, 1911, sec. XIV A, parts V, VI, p. 169.
2. Rosner, F.: Hemophilia in the Talmud and rabbinic writings. *Ann. Intern. Med.* 70:833, 1969.
3. Hynes, H. E., Owen, C. A., Jr., Bowie, E. J. W., and Thompson, J. R., Jr.: Development of the present concept of hemophilia. *Mayo Clin. Proc.* 44:193, 1969.
4. Otto, J. E.: An account of an hemorrhagic disposition existing in certain families. *Med. Repository* 6:1, 1803.
5. Wright, A. E.: On a method of determining the condition of blood coagulability for clinical and experimental purposes, and on the effect of the administration of calcium salts in haemophilia and actual or threatened haemorrhage. *Br. Med. J.* 2:223, 1893.
6. Lowenburg, H., and Rubenstone, A. I.: Hemophilia: Experimental data bearing on the effect of glycerinized extracts of visceral hemophilic tissue on the coagulation time of blood. *JAMA* 71:1196, 1918.
7. Addis, T.: The pathogenesis of hereditary haemophilia. *J. Pathol. Bacteriol.* 15:427, 1911.
8. Mellanby, J.: The coagulation of blood. *J. Physiol.* 38:28, 1909.
9. Patek, A. J., Jr., and Taylor, F. H. L.: Hemophilia. II. Some properties of a substance obtained from normal human plasma effective in accelerating the coagulation defect of hemophilic blood. *J. Clin. Invest.* 16:113, 1937.
10. Quick, A. J., Stanley-Brown, M. A., and Bancroft, F. W.: A study on the coagulation defect in hemophilia and in jaundice. *Am. J. Med. Sci.* 190:501, 1935.
11. Brinkhous, K. M.: A study of the clotting defect in hemophilia: The delayed formation of thrombin. *Am. J. Med. Sci.* 198:509, 1939.
12. Quick, A. J.: Studies on the enigma of the hemostatic dysfunction of hemophilia. *Am. J. Med. Sci.* 214:272, 1947.
13. Brinkhous, K. M.: Clotting defect in hemophilia: Deficiency in a plasma factor required for platelet utilization. *Proc. Soc. Exp. Biol. Med.* 66:117, 1947.
14. Pavlovsky, A.: Contribution to the pathogenesis of hemophilia. *Blood* 2:185, 1947.
15. Aggeler, P. M., White, S. G., Glendenning, M. B., Page, E. W., Leake, T. B., and Bates, G.: Plasma thromboplastin component (PTC) deficiency: A new disease resembling hemophilia. *Proc. Soc. Exp. Biol. Med.* 79:692, 1952.
16. Biggs, R., et al.: Christmas disease: A condition previously mistaken for haemophilia. *Br. Med. J.* 2:1378, 1952.
17. Graham, J. B., Buckwalter, J. A., Harley, L. J., and Brinkhous, K. M.: Canine hemophilia: Observations on the course, the clotting anomaly and the effect of blood transfusions. *J. Exp. Med.* 90:97, 1949.
18. Buckner, R. G., and Hampton, J. W.: Canine hemophilia. *Blood* 27:414, 1966.
19. Hall, D. E.: *Blood Coagulation and Its Disorders in the Dog.* Ballière, London, 1972.
20. Dodds, W. J.: Hereditary and acquired hemorrhagic disorders in animals, in *Progress in Hemostasis and Thrombosis*, edited by T. H. Spaet. Grune & Stratton, New York, 1974, vol. 2, p. 215.
21. Archer, R. K.: Blood coagulation in vertebrate animals other than man, in *Recent Advances in Blood Coagulation*, edited by L. Poller. Churchill, London, 1969, p. 29.
22. Graham, J. B.: Von Willebrand's disease and hemophilia A. *Séminaire sur l'enfance hémophilie* 1:144, 1968.
23. Graham, J. B., et al.: Dominant inheritance of hemophilia A in three generations of women. *Blood* 46:175, 1975.
24. Nilsson, I. M., Bergman, S., Reitalu, J., and Waldenström, J.: Hemophilia A in a "girl" with male sex-chromatin pattern. *Lancet* 2:264, 1959.
25. Jones, J. H., Rizza, C. R., Hardisty, R. M., Dormandy, K. M., and Macpherson, J. C.: Combined deficiency of factor V and factor VIII (antihaemophilic globulin): A report of three cases. *Br. J. Haematol.* 8:120, 1962.
26. Sibinga, C. T. S., Gökemeyer, J. D. M., ten Kate, L. P., and Zwol, F. B.: Combined deficiency of factor V and VIII: Report of a family and genetic analysis. *Br. J. Haematol.* 23:467, 1972.
27. Marlar, R. A., and Griffin, J. H.: Deficiency of protein C inhibitor in combined factor V–VIII deficiency disease. *J. Clin. Invest.* 66:1186, 1980.
28. Giddings, J. C., and Bloom, A. L.: Inhibition of activated protein C in combined factor V/VIII deficiency. *Thromb. Haemost.* 46:61, 1981.
29. Gobbi, F., Ascari, B., and Barbieri, U.: Congenital combined deficiency of factor VIII (antihemophilic globulin) and factor V (proaccelerin) in two siblings: Clinical study and genetic speculations. *Thromb. Diath. Haemorrh.* 17:197, 1967.
30. Bennett, B., and Ratnoff, O. D.: Antihemophilic factor (AHF, factor VIII) procoagulant activity and AHF-like antigen in normal pregnancy and following exercise and pneumoencephalography. *J. Lab. Clin. Med.* 80:251, 1972.
31. Bennett, B., Oxnard, S. C., Douglas, A. S., and Ratnoff, O. D.: Studies on antihemophilic factor (AHF, factor VIII) during labor in normal women, in patients with premature separation of the placenta and in a patient with von Willebrand's disease. *J. Lab. Clin. Med.* 84:851, 1974.
32. Parquet-Gernez, A., Maxurier, U., and Goudemand, D.: Detection of the carrier state for classic hemophilia by comparative assay of factor VIII activity and factor VIII antigen. *Pathol. Biol.* 22:37, 1974.
33. Ratnoff, O. D., and Steinberg, A. G.: Detection of the carrier state of classic hemophilia. *Ann. N.Y. Acad. Sci.* 20:95, 1975.
34. Barrow, E. S., Miller, C. H., Reisner, H. M., and Graham, J. B.: Genetic counselling in haemophilia by discriminant analysis. 1975–1980. *J. Med. Genet.* 19:26, 1982.
35. Peake, I. R., Newcombe, R. G., Davies, B. L., Furlong, R. A., Ludlam, C. A., and Bloom, A. L.: Carrier detection in haemophilia A by measurement of factor VIII clotting antigen (VIIICAg) and factor VIII related antigen (VIIIRAg). *Thromb. Haemost.* 46:187, 1981.
36. Graham, J. B., Barrow, E. S., and Elston, R. C.: Lyonization in hemophilia: A cause of error in direct detection of heterozygous carriers. *Ann. N.Y. Acad. Sci.* 20:141, 1975.
37. Graham, J. B., Barrow, E. S., Glyer, P., Dawson, D. V., and Elston, R. C.: Identifying carriers of mild haemophilia. *Br. J. Haematol.* 44:671, 1980.
38. Graham, J. B.: Genotype assignment (carrier detection) in the haemophilias, in *Clinics in Haematology: Congenital Coagulation Disorders*, edited by C. Rizza. Saunders, London, 1979, p. 115.
39. Whittaker, D. L., Copeland, D. L., and Graham, J. B.: Linkage of color blindness to hemophilias A and B. *Am. J. Hum. Genet.* 14:149, 1962.
40. Davies, S. H., et al.: The linkage relations of hemophilia A and hemophilia B (Christmas disease) to the Xg blood group system. *Am. J. Hum. Genet.* 15:481, 1963.

41. Graham, J. B.: Some genetic aspects of the blood clotting disorders. *Proc. XII Int. Congr. Pediatr. Mexico City* 2:602, 1968.

42. Hoyer, L. W., and Breckenridge, R. T.: Immunologic studies of antihemophilic factor (AHF, factor VIII): Cross-reacting material in a genetic variant of hemophilia A. *Blood* 32:962, 1968.

43. Denson, K. W. E., Biggs, R., Haddon, M. E., Borrett, R., and Cobb, K.: Two types of haemophilia (A+ and A−): A study of 48 cases. *Br. J. Haematol.* 17:163, 1969.

44. Feinstein, D., Chong, M. N. Y., Kasper, C. K., and Rapaport, S. I.: Hemophilia A: Polymorphism detectable by a factor VIII antibody. *Science* 163:1071, 1969.

45. Peake, I. R., Bloom, A. L., Giddings, J. C., and Ludlam, C. A.: An immunoradiometric assay for procoagulant factor VIII antigen: Results in haemophilia, von Willebrand's disease and fetal plasma and serum. *Br. J. Haematol.* 42:269, 1979.

46. Lazarchick, J., and Hoyer, L. W.: Immunoradiometric measurement of the factor VIII procoagulant antigen. *J. Clin. Invest.* 62:1048, 1978.

47. Reisner, H. M., Price, W. A., Blatt, P. M., Barrow, E. S., and Graham, J. B.: Factor VIII coagulant antigen in hemophilic plasma: A comparison of five alloantibodies. *Blood* 56:615, 1980.

48. Holmberg, L., Borge, L., Ljung, R., and Nilsson, I. M.: Measurement of antihaemophilic factor A antigen (VIII:CAg) with a solid phase immunoradiometric method based on homologous non-haemophilic antibodies. *Scand. J. Haematol.* 23:17, 1979.

49. Muller, H. P., van Tilburg, N. H., Bertina, R. M., Derks, J., and Klein-Breteler, E.: A monoclonal antibody to VIII:C produced by a mouse hybridoma. *Thromb. Haemost.* 46:219, 1981.

50. Silverstein, A.: Management of neurologic complications of hemophilia, in *The Hemophilias*, edited by K. M. Brinkhous. University of North Carolina Press, Chapel Hill, 1964, p. 349.

51. Kerr, C. B.: Intracranial hemorrhage in hemophilia. *J. Neurol. Neurosurg. Psychiatry* 27:166, 1964.

52. Kerr, C. B.: *The Management of Hemophilia*. Australian Medical Publishing, Glebe, Australia, 1963.

53. Trueta, J.: The orthopaedic management of patients with haemophilia and Christmas disease, in *Treatment of Hemophilia and Other Coagulation Diseases*, edited by R. Biggs and R. G. Macfarlane. Blackwell, Oxford, 1966, p. 279.

54. Macfarlane, R. G., and Biggs, R.: Haemophilia as a social problem, in *Treatment of Hemophilia and Other Coagulation Diseases*, edited by R. Biggs and R. G. Macfarlane. Blackwell, Oxford, 1966, p. 324.

55. Matthews, J. M., and Valderrama, J. A. F.: The haemophilic pseudo-tumor or haemophilic subperiosteal haematoma. *J. Bone Joint Surg.* 47B:256, 1965.

56. Gunning, A. J.: The surgery of haemophilic cysts, in *Treatment of Hemophilia and Other Coagulation Diseases*, edited by R. Biggs and R. G. Macfarlane. Blackwell, Oxford, 1966, p. 262.

57. Mannucci, P. M., Capitanio, A., del Ninno, E., Colombo, M., Pareti, F., and Ruggeri, Z. M.: Asymptomatic liver disease in haemophilias. *J. Clin. Pathol.* 28:620, 1975.

58. Levine, P. H., McVerry, B. A., Attock, B., and Dormandy, K. M.: Health of the intensively treated hemophilic with special reference to abnormal liver chemistries and splenomegaly. *Blood* 50:1, 1977.

59. Hilgartner, M. W., and Giardina, P.: Liver dysfunction in patients with hemophilia A and B and von Willebrand's disease. *Transfusion* 17:495, 1977.

60. Stirling, M. L., Beckett, G. J., and Percy-Robb, I. W.: Liver function in Edinburgh haemophiliacs: A five-year follow-up. *J. Clin. Pathol.* 34:17, 1981.

61. Hasiba, U., et al.: Liver dysfunction in Pennsylvania's multitransfused hemophiliacs. *Dig. Dis.* 25:776, 1980.

62. Spero, J. H., et al.: Asymptomatic structural liver disease in hemophilia. *N. Engl. J. Med.* 298:1373, 1978.

63. Lesesne, H. R., Morgen, J. E., Blatt, P. M., Webster, W. P., and Roberts, H. R.: Liver biopsy in hemophilia A. *Ann. Int. Med.* 86:703, 1977.

64. Preston, F. E., et al.: Percutaneous liver biopsy and chronic liver disease in hemophilias. *Lancet* 2:592, 1978.

65. Mannucci, P. M., Ronchi, G., Rata, L., and Colombo, M.: A clinico-pathological study of liver disease in hemophiliacs. *J. Clin. Pathol.* 31:779, 1978.

66. McGrath, K. M., Lilleyman, J. S., Triger, D. R., and Underwood, J. C.: Liver disease complicating severe hemophilia in childhood. *Arch. Dis. Child* 7:537, 1980.

67. Kim, H. C., Saidi, P., Ackley, A. M., Bringelsen, K. A., and Gocke, D. J.: Prevalence of type B and non-A, non-B hepatitis in hemophilia: Relationship to chronic liver disease. *Gastroenterology* 79:1159, 1980.

68. Mibashan, R. S., et al.: Plasma assay of fetal factors VIIIC and IX for prenatal diagnosis of haemophilia. *Lancet* 1:1309, 1979.

69. Firshein, S. I., et al.: Prenatal diagnosis of classic hemophilia. *N. Engl. J. Med.* 300:937, 1979.

70. Editorial: Prenatal diagnosis of haemophilia. *Lancet* 13:27, 1979.

71. Matthews, J. M.: The general management of the haemophilic patient at home and in hospital, in *Treatment of Hemophilia and Other Coagulation Diseases*, edited by R. Biggs and R. G. Macfarlane. Blackwell, Oxford, 1966, p. 70.

72. Walsh, P. N., et al.: Epsilon-aminocaproic acid therapy for dental extractions in hemophilia and Christmas disease: A double blind controlled trial. *Br. J. Haematol.* 20:463, 1971.

73. Walsh, P. N., Rizza, C. R., Evans, B. E., and Aledort, L. M.: The therapeutic role of epsilon aminocaproic acid (EACA) for dental extractions in hemophilia. *Ann. N.Y. Acad. Sci.* 20:267, 1975.

74. Abildgaard, C. F.: Current concept in the management of hemophilia. *Semin. Hematol.* 12:223, 1975.

75. Rabiner, S. F., and Telper, M. C.: Home transfusion for patients with hemophilia A. *N. Engl. J. Med.* 283:1011, 1970.

76. Rabiner, S. F., and Lazerson, J.: Home management and prophylaxis of hemophilia. *Prog. Hematol.* 8:223, 1973.

77. Strawczynski, H., Stachewitsch, A., Morgenstern, G., and Shaw, M. E.: Delivery of care to hemophilic children: Home care versus hospitalization. *Pediatrics* 51:986, 1973.

78. Levine, P. H.: Delivery of health care in hemophilia. *Ann. N.Y. Acad. Sci.* 340:201, 1975.

79. LeQuesne, B., Britten, M. I., Maragaki, C., and Dormandy, K. M.: Home treatment for patients with haemophilia. *Lancet* 2:507, 1974.

80. Lazerson, J.: Hemophilic home transfusion program: Effect on school attendance. *J. Pediatr.* 81:330, 1972.

81. Editorial: Hemophilia and home therapy. *Lancet* 2:77, 1979.

82. Lazerson, J.: The prophylactic approach to hemophilia A. *Hosp. Prac.* 6:99, 1971.

83. Ramsay, D. M., and Parker, A. C.: A total of prophylactic replacement therapy in haemophilia and Christmas disease. *J. Clin. Pathol.* 26:243, 1973.

84. Kasper, C. K., Dietrich, S. L., and Rapaport, S. I.: Hemophilia prophylaxis with factor VIII concentrate. *Arch. Intern. Med.* 123:1004, 1970.

85. Aronstam, A., et al.: Twice weekly prophylactic therapy in haemophilia. *Am. J. Clin. Pathol.* 30:65, 1977.

86. Biggs, R., and Matthews, J. M.: The treatment of spontaneous bleeding in haemophilia, in *Treatment of Hemophilia and Other Coagulation Diseases*, edited by R. Biggs, and R. G. Macfarlane. Blackwell, Oxford, 1966, p. 129.

87. Ingram, G. I. C.: Increase in antihemophilic globulin activity following infusion of adrenaline. *J. Physiol.* 156:217, 1961.

88. Mannucci, P. M., Cagnatelli, G., and d'Alonzo, P.: Stress and blood coagulation, in *Thrombosis: Risk Factors and Diagnostic Approaches*, edited by K. M. Brinkhous. Schattauer, Stuttgart, 1972, p. 105.

89. Mannucci, P. M.: Hemophilia diagnosis and management: Progress and problems, in *Recent Advances in Blood Coagulation*, edited by L. Poller. Churchill Livingstone, New York, 1981, p. 193.

90. Biggs, R.: Major surgery in haemophilic patients, in *Treatment of Hemophilia and Other Coagulation Diseases*, edited by R. Biggs and R. G. Macfarlane. Blackwell, Oxford, 1966, p. 166.

91. Macfarlane, R. G., et al.: Surgery in haemophilia: The use of animal antihemophilic globulin and human plasma in thirteen cases. *Lancet* 2:251, 1957.

92. Webster, W. P., Roberts, H. R., and Penick, G. D.: Dental care of patients with hereditary disorders of blood coagulation, in *Treatment of Hemorrhagic Disorders*, edited by O. D. Ratnoff. Harper-Hoeber, New York, 1968, p. 93.

93. Hayton-Williams, D. S.: Dental and oral surgical treatment of pa-

tients with haemophilia and Christmas disease, in *Treatment of Hemophilia*, edited by R. Biggs and R. G. Macfarlane. Blackwell, Oxford, 1966, p. 250.

94. Mustard, J. F., Rowsell, H. C., Robinson, G. A., Hoeksema, T. D., Downie, H. G.: Canine haemophilia B (Christmas disease). *Br. J. Haematol.* 6:259, 1960.

95. Fantl, P., Sawers, R. J., and Marr, A. G.: Investigation of haemorrhagic disease due to beta-prothromboplastin deficiency complicated by a specific inhibitor of thromboplastin formation. *Aust. Ann. Med.* 5:163, 1956.

96. Roberts, H. R., Grizzle, J. E., McLester, W. D., and Penick, G. D.: Genetic variants in hemophilia B: Detection by means of a specific PTC inhibitor. *J. Clin. Invest.* 47:360, 1968.

97. Neal, W. F., Tayloe, D. T., Jr., Cederbaum, A. I., and Roberts, H. R.: Detection of genetic variants of haemophilia B with an immunosorbent technique. *Br. J. Haematol.* 25:63, 1973.

98. Kasper, C. K., Østerud, B., Minami, J. Y., Shonick, W., and Rapaport, S. I.: Hemophilia B: Characterization of genetic variants and detection of carriers. *Blood* 50:351, 1977.

99. Parekh, V. R., Mannucci, P. M., and Ruggeri, Z. M.: Immunological heterogeneity of haemophilia B: A multicentre study of 98 kindreds. *Br. J. Haematol.* 40:643, 1978.

100. Pechet, L., Tiarks, C., Stevens, J., Sudhindra, R. R., and Lipworth, L.: Relationship of factor IX antigen and coagulant in hemophilia B patients and carriers. *Thromb. Haemost.* 40:465, 1978.

101. Thompson, A. R.: Factor IX antigen by radioimmunoassay: Abnormal factor IX protein in patients on warfarin therapy and with hemophilia B. *J. Clin. Invest.* 59:900, 1977.

102. Hougie, C., and Twomey, J. J.: Hemophilia B$_M$: A new type of factor IX deficiency. *Lancet* 1:698, 1967.

103. Gray, G. R., Teasdale, J. M., and Thomas, J. W.: Hemophilia B$_M$. *Can. Med. Assoc. J.* 98:552, 1968.

104. Twomey, J. J., Corless, J., Thornton, L., and Hougie, C.: Studies on the inheritance and nature of hemophilia B$_M$. *Am. J. Med.* 46:372, 1969.

105. Denson, K. W. E., Biggs, R., and Mannucci, P. M.: An investigation of three patients with Christmas disease due to an abnormal type of factor IX. *J. Clin. Pathol.* 21:160, 1968.

106. Østerud, B., Lavine, K., Kasper, C. K., and Rapaport, S. I.: Isolation and properties of the abnormal factor IX molecule of hemophilia B$_M$. *Thromb. Haemost.* 38:514, 1977.

107. Østerud, B., Kasper, C. K., Lavine, K., Prodano, C., and Rapaport, S. I.: Purification and properties of abnormal blood coagulation factor IX (factor IX B$_M$): Kinetics of its inhibition of factor X activation by factor VII and bovine tissue factor. *Thromb. Haemost.* 45:551, 1981.

108. Girolami, A., dal Bo Zanon, R., de Marco, Z., and Cappellato, G.: Hemophilia B with associated factor VII deficiency: A distinct variant of hemophilia B with low factor VII activity and normal factor VII antigen. *Blut* 40:267, 1980.

109. Mazzucconi, M. G., Bertina, R. M., Romoli, D., Orlando, M., Avvisati, G., and Mariani, G.: Factor VII activity and antigen in hemophilia B variants. *Thromb. Haemost.* 43:16, 1980.

110. Barrow, E. M., Bullock, W. R., and Graham, J. B.: A study of the carrier state for plasma thromboplastin component (PTC, Christmas factor) deficiency, utilizing a new assay procedure. *J. Lab. Clin. Med.* 55:936, 1960.

111. Chung, K.-S., Madar, D. A., Goldsmith, J. C., Kingdon, H. S., Brown, H. R., and Roberts, H. R.: Purification and characterization of an abnormal factor IX (Christmas factor) molecule. *J. Clin. Invest.* 62:1078, 1978.

112. Braunstein, K. M., Noyes, C. M., Griffith, M. J., Lundblad, R. L., and Roberts, H. R.: Characterization of the defect in activation of factor IX Chapel Hill by human factor XIa. *J. Clin. Invest.* 68:1420, 1981.

113. Veltkamp, J. J., Meilof, J., Remmelts, H. G., van der Vlerk, D., and Loeliger, E. A.: Another genetic variant of haemophilia B: Haemophilia B Leyden. *Scand. J. Haematol.* 7:82, 1970.

114. Bertina, R. M., and Veltkamp, J. J.: A genetic variant of factor IX with decreased capacity for Ca^{2+} binding. *Br. J. Haematol.* 42:623, 1979.

115. Bertina, R. M., and van der Linden, I. K.: A genetic variant of factor

116. IX with an abnormal high molecular weight. *Thromb. Haemost.* 46:125, 1981 (abstract).

116. Thompson, A. R.: Factor IX antigen by radioimmunoassay in heterozygotes for hemophilia B. *Thromb. Res.* 11:193, 1977.

117. Bithell, T. C., Pizarro, A., and MacDiarmid, W. D.: Variant of factor IX deficiency in female with 45 X Turner's syndrome. *Blood* 36:169, 1970.

118. Kasper, C. K., Minami, J. Y., and Rapaport, S. I.: Detection of the carrier state in hemophilia B. *Clin. Res.* 17:116, 1969.

119. Rosenthal, R. L., Dreskin, R. L., and Rosenthal, N.: New hemophilia-like disease caused by deficiency of a third plasma thromboplastin factor. *Proc. Soc. Exp. Biol. Med.* 82:171, 1953.

120. Forbes, C. D., and Ratnoff, O. D.: Studies on plasma thromboplastin antecedent (factor XI), PTA deficiency and inhibition of PTA by plasma: Pharmacological inhibitors of specific antiserum. *J. Lab. Clin. Med.* 79:113, 1972.

121. Rimon, A., Schiffman, S., Feinstein, D. I., and Rapaport, S. I.: Factor XI activity and factor XI antigen in homozygous and heterozygous factor XI deficiency. *Blood* 48:165, 1976.

122. Rapaport, S. I., Proctor, R. R., Patch, M. J., and Yettra, M.: The mode of inheritance of PTA deficiency: Evidence for the existence of major PTA deficiency and minor PTA deficiency. *Blood* 18:149, 1961.

123. Edson, J. R., White, J. G., and Krivit, W.: The enigma of severe factor XI deficiency without haemorrhagic symptoms: Distinction from Hageman factor and "Fletcher factor" deficiency: Family study and problems of diagnosis. *Thromb. Diath. Haemorrh.* 18:342, 1967.

124. Seligsohn, U.: Personal communication.

125. Ratnoff, O. D., and Colopy, J. E.: A familial hemorrhagic trait associated with a deficiency of a clot-promoting fraction of plasma. *J. Clin. Invest.* 34:602, 1955.

126. Ratnoff, O. D., Busse, R. J., and Sheon, R. P.: The demise of John Hageman. *N. Engl. J. Med.* 279:760, 1968.

127. Bennett, B., Ratnoff, O. D., Holt, J. B., and Roberts, H. R.: Hageman trait (factor XII deficiency): A probable second genotype inherited as an autosomal dominant characteristic. *Blood* 40:412, 1972.

128. Saito, H., Scott, J. G., Movat, H. Z., and Scialla, S. J.: Molecular heterogeneity of Hageman trait (factor XII deficiency): Evidence that two of 49 subjects are cross-reacting material positive (CRM$^+$). *J. Lab. Clin. Med.* 94:256, 1974.

129. Hathaway, W. E., Belhasen, L. P., and Hathaway, H. S.: Evidence for a new plasma thromboplastin factor. I. Case report: Coagulation studies and physiochemical properties. *Blood* 26:521, 1965.

130. Abildgaard, C. F., and Harrison, J.: Fletcher factor deficiency: Family study and detection. *Blood* 43:641, 1974.

131. Wuepper, K. D.: Prekallikrein deficiency in man. *J. Exp. Med* 138:1345, 1973.

132. Donaldson, V. H., Saito, H., and Ratnoff, O. D.: Defective esterase and kinin-forming activity in human Fletcher trait plasma: A fraction rich in kallikreinlike activity. *Circ. Res.* 24:652, 1974.

133. Saito, H., Ratnoff, O. D., Waldmann, R., and Abraham, J. P.: Fitzgerald trait. *J. Clin. Invest.* 55:1082, 1975.

134. Lacombe, M., Varet, B., and Levy, J.: A hitherto undescribed plasma factor acting at the contact phase of blood coagulation (Flaujeac factor): Case report and coagulation studies. *Blood* 46:761, 1975.

135. Wuepper, K. D., Miller, D. R., and Lacombe, M.: Flaujeac trait: Deficiency of human plasma kininogen. *J. Clin. Invest.* 56:1663, 1975.

136. Colman, R. W., et al.: Williams trait: Human kininogen deficiency with diminished levels of plasminogen proactivator and prekallikrein associated with abnormalities of the Hageman factor-dependent pathways. *J. Clin. Invest.* 56:1650, 1975.

137. Wuepper, K.: Personal communication, 1975.

138. Hougie, C., McPherson, R. A., and Aronson, L.: Passovoy factor: A hitherto unrecognized factor necessary for hemostasis. *Lancet* 2:290, 1975.

139. Hougie, C., et al.: The Passovoy factor: Further characterization of a hereditary hemorrhagic diathesis. *N. Engl. J. Med.* 298:1045, 1978.

140. Owren, P. A.: The coagulation of blood: Investigations on a new clotting factor. *Acta Med. Scand.* 128 (Suppl. 194):1, 1947.

141. Feinstein, D. I., Rapaport, S. I., McGehee, W. G., and Patch, M. J.:

Factor V anticoagulants: Clinical, biochemical and immunological observations. *J. Clin. Invest.* 49:1578, 1970.

142. Frantantoni, J. W., Hilgartner, M., and Nachman, R. L.: Nature of the defect in congenital factor V deficiency: Study in a patient with an acquired circulating anticoagulant. *Blood* 39:751, 1972.

143. Friedman, I. A., Quick, A. J., Higgins, F., Hussey, C. V., and Hickey, M. E.: Hereditary labile factor (factor V) deficiency. *JAMA* 175:370, 1961.

144. Alexander, R. B., Goldstein, R., Landwehr, G., and Cook, C. D.: Congenital SPCA deficiency: A hitherto unrecognized coagulation defect with hemorrhage rectified by serum and serum fractions. *J. Clin. Invest.* 30:596, 1951.

145. Owen, C. A., Jr., and Bollman, J. L.: Prothrombin conversion factor of dicumarol plasma. *Proc. Soc. Exp. Biol. Med.* 67:231, 1948.

146. Mann, F. D., and Hurn, M.: Co-thromboplastin, a probable factor in coagulation of blood. *Am. J. Physiol.* 164:105, 1951.

147. Goodnight, S. H., Feinstein, D. I., Østerud, B., and Rapaport, S. I.: Factor VII antibody-neutralizing material in hereditary and acquired factor VII deficiency: *Blood* 38:1, 1971.

148. Mariani, G., et al.: Factor VII deficiency: Immunological characterization of genetic variants and detection of carriers. *Br. J. Haematol.* 48:7, 1981.

149. Girolami, A., Cattarozzi, G., dal Bo Zanon, R., Cella, G., and Toffanin, F.: Factor VII Padua₂: Another factor VII abnormality with defective ox brain thromboplastin activation and a complex hereditary pattern. *Blood* 54:46, 1979.

150. Telfer, T. P., Denson, K. W., and Wright, D. R.: A "new" coagulation defect. *Br. J. Haematol.* 2:308, 1956.

151. Hougie, C., and Graham, J. B.: The blood clotting role and mode of inheritance of the Stuart factor: A new clotting factor distinct from SPCA. *Bibl. Haematol. Fasc. 7,* p. 80, 1956.

152. Hougie, C., Barrow, E. M., and Graham, J. B.: Stuart clotting defect. I. Segregation of an hereditary hemorrhagic state from the heterogeneous group heretofore called "stable factor" (SPCA, proconvertin, factor VII) deficiency. *J. Clin. Invest.* 36:485, 1957.

153. Graham, J. B., Barrow, E. M., and Hougie, C.: Stuart clotting defect. II. Genetic aspects of a new hemorrhagic state. *J. Clin. Invest.* 36:497, 1957.

154. Bachmann, F., Duckert, F., Geiger, M., Baer, P., and Koller, F.: Differentiation of the factor VII complex: Studies on the Stuart-Prower factor. *Thromb. Diath. Haemorrh.* 1:169, 1957.

155. Denson, K. W.: Electrophoretic studies of the Prower factor: A blood coagulation factor which differs from factor VII. *Br. J. Haematol.* 4:313, 1958.

156. Denson, K. W. E., Lurie, A., de Cataldo, P., and Mannucci, P. M.: The factor-X defect: Recognition of abnormal forms of factor X. *Br. J. Haematol.* 18:317, 1970.

157. Fair, D. S., Plow, E. F., and Edgington, T. S.: Combined functional and immunochemical analysis of normal and abnormal human factor X. *J. Clin. Invest.* 64:884, 1979.

158. Girolami, A., Lazzarin, M., Sarpa, R., and Brunetti, A.: Further studies on the abnormal factor X (Factor X Friuli) coagulation disorder: A report on another family. *Blood* 37:534, 1971.

159. Bachmann, F., Duckert, F., Geiger, M., Baer, P., and Koller, F.: Differentiation of the factor VII complex: Studies on the Stuart Prower factor. *Thromb. Diath. Haemorrh.* 1:169, 1957.

160. Bertina, R. M., Alderkamp, G.J.H., and de Nooy, E.: A variant of factor X that is defective only in extrinsic coagulation. *Thromb. Haemost.* 46:88, 1981 (abstract).

161. Kattlove, H. E., Shapiro, S. S., and Spivack, M.: Hereditary prothrombin deficiency. *N. Engl. J. Med.* 282:57, 1970.

162. Girolami, A.: The hereditary transmission of congenital "true" hypoprothrombinaemia. *Br. J. Haematol.* 21:695, 1971.

163. Shapiro, S. S., Martinez, J., and Holborn, R. R.: Congenital dysprothrombinemia: An inherited structural disorder of human prothrombin. *J. Clin. Invest.* 48:2251, 1969.

164. Josso, F., de Sanchez, J. M., Lavergne, J. M., Menache, D., and Soulier, J. P.: Congenital abnormality of the prothrombin molecule (factor II) in four siblings: Prothrombin Barcelona. *Blood* 38:9, 1971.

165. Shapiro, S. S., Maldonada, N. I., Fradera, J., and McCord, S.: Prothrombin San Juan: A complex new dysprothrombinemia. *J. Clin. Invest.* 53:73A, 1974.

166. Girolami, A., Bareggi, G., Brunetti, A., and Sticchi, A.: Prothrombin Padua: A "new" congenital dysprothrombinemia. *J. Lab. Clin. Med.* 84:654, 1974.

167. Kahn, M. J. P., and Govaerto, A.: Prothrombin Brussels: A new congenital defective protein. *Thromb. Res.* 5:141, 1974.

168. Owen, C. A., Henriksen, R. A., McDuffie, F. C., and Mann, K. G.: Prothrombin Quick: A newly identified dysprothrombinemia. *Mayo Clin. Proc.* 53:29, 1978.

169. Henriksen, R. A., Owen, W. G., Nesheim, M. E., and Mann, K. G.: Identification of a congenital dysprothrombin, thrombin Quick. *J. Clin. Invest.* 66:934, 1980.

170. Girolami, A., Coccheri, S., Palareti, G., Poggi, M., Burul, A., and Cappellato, G.: Prothrombin Molise: A "new" congenital dysprothrombinemia, double heterozygosis with an abnormal prothrombin and "true" prothrombin deficiency. *Blood* 52:115, 1978.

171. Weinger, R. S., Rudy, C., Moake, J. L., Olson, J. D., and Cimo, P. L.: Prothrombin Houston: A dysprothrombin identifiable by crossed immunoelectrofocusing and abnormal echis carinatus venom activation. *Blood* 55:811, 1975.

172. McMillan, C. W., and Roberts, H. R.: Congenital combined deficiency of coagulation factors II, VII, IX and X. *N. Engl. J. Med.* 274:1313, 1966.

173. Chung, K.-S., Bezeaud, A., Goldsmith, J. C., McMillan, C. W., Ménaché, D., and Roberts, H. R.: Congenital deficiency of blood clotting factors II, VII, IX, and X. *Blood* 53:776, 1979.

174. Johnson, C. A., Chung, K.-S., McGrath, K. M., Bean, P. E., and Roberts, H. R.: Characterization of a variant prothrombin in a patient congenitally deficient in factors II, VII, IX and X. *Br. J. Haematol.* 44:461, 1980.

175. Goldsmith, G. H., Jr., Pence, R. E., Ratnoff, O. D., Adelstein, D. J., and Furie, B.: Studies on a family with combined functional deficiencies of vitamin K-dependent coagulation factors. *J. Clin. Invest.* 69:1253, 1982.

176. Gordon, E. M., Donaldson, V. H., Saito, H., Su, E., and Ratnoff, O. D.: Reduced titers of Hageman factor (factor XII) in Orientals. *Ann. Int. Med.* 95:697, 1981.

177. Jackson, J. M., Marshall, L. R., and Herrman, R. P.: Passovory factor deficiency in five western Australian kindreds. *Pathology* 13:517, 1981.

CHAPTER *153*

Congenital disorders of fibrinogen

HARVEY R. GRALNICK

Congenital fibrinogen abnormalities can be divided into quantitative defects, termed *hypofibrinogenemia* or *afibrinogenemia,* depending on the severity of the deficiency, and qualitative defects, designated *dysfibrinogenemia.*

Quantitative abnormalities—hypo- and afibrinogenemia

DEFINITION AND PATHOGENESIS

Congenital afibrinogenemia was first described in 1920, and approximately 150 cases have been reported [1–5].

Hypofibrinogenemia, a less clearly defined disorder, was first described in 1935 [6]. Approximately 30 cases have been reported.

The deficiency of fibrinogen in afibrinogenemia appears to be the result of decreased synthesis. The survival of homologous fibrinogen in the circulation of patients is usually normal. Hypofibrinogenemia is probably also due to a synthetic defect, but studies of the half-life of fibrinogen have not been performed. In both conditions the fibrinolytic system is normal and there is no increased utilization or consumption of coagulation factors. Long bleeding times and abnormal platelet aggregation have been reported in afibrinogenemia [3,7,8].

MODE OF INHERITANCE

Afibrinogenemia appears to be transmitted as an autosomal trait. Both sexes are involved, and the ratio of afflicted males to females is approximately 1:1. Consanguinity is present in over half the families [3,7]. Parents of the affected individuals usually have normal fibrinogen concentrations. Affected individuals are homozygous for the deficiency. In a few families presumed heterozygotes exhibit moderately low levels of fibrinogen, and hypofibrinogenemia may represent the heterozygous state of afibrinogenemia.

CLINICAL FEATURES

Patients with congenital afibrinogenemia suffer from a lifelong hemorrhagic diathesis of variable severity. The bleeding may be noted in the first few days of life, with hematomas, hematemesis, melena, or hemorrhage from the umbilical cord [7]. Internal bleeding, particularly gastrointestinal, genitourinary, and central nervous system, and spontaneous splenic rupture are quite common both during and after the newborn period. Severe bleeding may follow minor trauma, and easy bruising and gingival hemorrhages occur frequently. Hemarthroses have been reported in 21 percent of patients with afibrinogenemia [3], and this disorder may be confused with hemophilia. Menstrual bleeding may be severe, but is normal in some cases. The hemorrhagic tendency may be episodic, with troublefree periods which are often preceded or followed by increased spontaneous bleeding. Bleeding after surgery may be severe and protracted.

Most patients with hypofibrinogenemia have no hemorrhagic manifestations, but a few have mild spontaneous bleeding, severe postoperative bleeding, and first-trimester abortions.

LABORATORY FEATURES

In afibrinogenemia the whole-blood clotting time, recalcification time, prothrombin time, partial thromboplastin time, thrombin time, and reptilase time (page 1404) are all prolonged and are all corrected by the addition of normal plasma or normal fibrinogen to the patient's plasma. Plasma fibrinogen is undetectable by almost all physicochemical measurements of functional assays. The most sensitive immunologic techniques usually can demonstrate trace amounts of plasma fibrinogen (usually 5.0 mg/dl) [9–11]. In hypofibrinogenemia, coagulation tests may also be abnormal, depending on the fibrinogen level. There has been one case of hypofibrinogenemia associated with factor VIII deficiency and thrombocytopenia [12], and mild to moderate thrombocytopenia occurs occasionally in patients with afibrinogenemia [3,7,13]. The platelet count is rarely below 100,000 per microliter.

Prolonged bleeding times, unrelated to thrombocytopenia, are found in some patients with either afibrinogenemia [3,7,13,14] or hypofibrinogenemia. Platelet aggregation induced by ADP, collagen, epinephrine, and thrombin is defective in patients with afibrinogenemia [8,15–17], and platelet retention in glass bead columns may also be defective [14]. These abnormalities are totally or partially corrected by the addition of fibrinogen. In afibrinogenemic patients, positive skin tests involving delayed-type hypersensitivity reactions may show only erythema without induration [18].

DIFFERENTIAL DIAGNOSIS

In congenital afibrinogenemia and in some cases of hypofibrinogenemia, all coagulation tests which depend for an end point on the conversion of fibrinogen to fibrin are abnormal. Anticoagulants, such as heparin or fibrinogen degradation products, may also interfere with these coagulation tests. The deficiency of fibrinogen found by physicochemical and thrombin clotting time methods must be confirmed by immunochemical methods. Congenital hypofibrinogenemia may be confused with dysfibrinogenemia [19]. It is imperative to exclude a qualitative defect in addition to a quantitative defect of fibrinogen. Two drugs, sodium valproate and L-asparaginase, can induce moderate to severe hypofibrinogenemia [20,21].

THERAPY

Treatment is given to prevent hemorrhage during surgery or for periods of active bleeding. Long-term prophylaxis has not been attempted for this disease. Fibrinogen levels of 50 to 100 mg/dl are usually adequate to maintain normal hemostasis [11,22,23]. Details of replacement therapy are presented in Chap. 167. Development of antifibrinogen antibodies, associated with severe reactions to infusions and a shortened half-life of administered fibrinogen, has been described [24,25], and major thrombotic episodes have occurred in a few patients after infusions of fibrinogen concentrates [25–27].

COURSE AND PROGNOSIS

Congenital afibrinogenemia has been associated with high mortality in infancy and childhood, primarily due to intracranial hemorrhage. However, with improved replacement therapy the prognosis should be better.

Qualitative abnormalities — congenital dysfibrinogenemia

DEFINITION AND HISTORY
In 1958 a fibrinogen defect was postulated in the plasma of an 8-year-old girl with a severe bleeding disorder and apparent hypofibrinogenemia or afibrinogenemia [28]. Although the concept of dysfibrinogenemia appears to date from this report, the lack of familial coagulation abnormalities and the absence of an immunologically identifiable fibrinogen molecule in the patient's plasma cast doubt on the diagnosis of dysfibrinogenemia. The first well-documented cases of congenital dysfibrinogenemia were described in 1964 [29], in a man and his 14-year-old son. Since then almost 70 abnormal fibrinogens have been described (Table 153-1). The abnormal fibrinogens are named for the locality in which they were first found [30], but since comparative studies between abnormal fibrinogens have not been carried out on a large scale, the present nomenclature is tentative. Fibrinogen Baltimore was described in 1964 and emphasized the familial transmission of the disease [31]. Comparison of the plasma of this family with that of a Canadian family thought to be hypofibrinogenemic [18] established that the latter family also had dysfibrinogenemia [32].

Fibrinogen Zürich was the first fibrinogen demonstrated to have abnormal fibrin monomer aggregation [33], and fibrinogen Bethesda I was the first demonstrated to have defective fibrinopeptide release [34]. Other dysfibrinogenemias have shown abnormal fibrinopeptide release and/or abnormal fibrin monomer aggregation with abnormal cross-linking of the fibrin clot [35–41].

ETIOLOGY AND PATHOGENESIS
Nearly all the congenital dysfibrinogenemias appear to be due to a qualitative defect of the fibrinogen molecule. It is not clear whether the defects result from the synthesis of a mutant protein not present in the plasma of normal individuals or whether one of the subpopulations of fibrinogen found in normal individuals is produced in abnormally high concentration.

In some patients dysfibrinogenemia is accompanied by hypofibrinogenemia without evidence of increased catabolism, suggesting that the abnormal fibrinogen and possibly even normal fibrinogen are synthesized at a reduced rate [42–47]. In two families the disappearance time of the abnormal fibrinogen was shortened in the patient or a normal individual or both, whereas the half-life of normal fibrinogen in the affected individual was normal [48,49]. This group of patients suffers from a combination of hypofibrinogenemia and dysfibrinogenemia.

The conversion of fibrinogen to fibrin may be considered in three steps. Fibrinogen is composed of three pairs of polypeptide chains, designated Aα, Bβ, and γ, joined by disulfide bonds (see Chap. 132). This protein undergoes (1) selective proteolysis by thrombin, which liberates fibrinopeptides A and B from the Aα and Bβ chains, respectively. Under appropriate conditions of pH and ionic strength the resultant molecule, designated *fibrin monomer*, tends to (2) spontaneously aggregate to form a fibrin gel. This step is known as *fibrin monomer aggregation*. The fibrin gel can then (3) be covalently cross-linked to form an insoluble clot in the presence of factor XIIIa. Most of the dysfibrinogenemias exhibit abnormal fibrin monomer aggregation, and fibrinopeptide release is abnormal in 14 [34,38, 40,42,44,50–58]. The defect is solely fibrinopeptide release in 3 families [34,50,51], while in the other 11 families the aggregation and/or fibrin cross-linking are also abnormal. Defective cross-linking of an abnormal fibrinogen was initially suggested as the functional abnormality of fibrinogen Oklahoma [59], but this familial bleeding diathesis may not be related to an abnormal fibrinogen. Fibrin formed from fibrinogen Tokyo is abnormally cross-linked [60]. Analysis of cross-linking of fibrin by polyacrylamide gel electrophoresis revealed a defect in seven other families [35–41].

MODE OF INHERITANCE
In all the families reported to date except three [34,61,62], the dysfibrinogenemia is inherited as an autosomal dominant trait. In fibrinogen Houston, no family member except the propositus was studied [39]. The question of homozygosity for abnormal fibrinogens is frequently raised. In fibrinogen Metz, the propositus, a product of a consanguineous marriage, appears to be homozygous, and both her parents asymptomatic heterozygotes [51]. Homozygotes for fibrinogen Detroit have completely abnormal fibrinogen populations in their plasma, whereas heterozygotes have one-half normal and one-half abnormal molecules [50]. Unfortunately, complete studies on the parents of the Detroit family are not available.

Evidence that most dysfibrinogenemias represent a heterozygous state has come from studies of family members where only one parent is affected and from the separation of abnormal and apparently normal fibrinogens. In fibrinogen Zürich I [63], the enzyme reptilase was used to separate a normal fibrinogen population which appeared to have normal fibrin monomer aggregation from the abnormal fibrinogen, which had a markedly altered aggregation phase. In fibrinogens Cleveland I [35] and Detroit [50], two precipitin bands were present on immunoelectrophoresis against heterologous antihuman fibrinogen. The elution pattern of fibrinogen Baltimore [64] on DEAE-cellulose chromatography suggested that two types of fibrinogen molecules were present. In fibrinogen Bethesda III, ethanol fractionation of plasma separated a population of fibrinogen molecules with a normal monomer aggregation phase from a population which was abnormal [49].

TABLE 153-1   Congenital dysfibrinogenemia*

Designation and reference	Thrombin time, s (patient/control)	Repitilase time, s (patient/control)	Effect on coagulation	IEP compared to normal	Major defect	Site of defect
Asymptomatic:						
Alba/Geneva [72][a]	Abnormal	Abnormal	Inhibitory	Same	A	
Amsterdam [78][b]	32/11	14/2	Inhibitory	Cathodal	A	
Bethesda II [42][b,c,d]	48/30	49/22	Inhibitory	Anodal	A,minor FP	
Bondy [57][e]	Abnormal	Abnormal	None	Same	FP,A	
Buenos Aires II [66][b]	60/24	45/20	None	U	A	
Cleveland I [35][a,f,g,h]	90/26	164/70	Inhibitory	Anodal; 2 components	A,FX	
Copenhagen [38]	30/15	U	None	U	FP,A,FX	
Genova [122]	Abnormal	Abnormal	None	Same	A	
Giessen III [123][b]	40/22	54/23	U	U	A	
Iowa City [117][b]	278/38	173/18	None	Same	U	
Leuven [46][b,d]	43/21	47/20	Inhibitory	Abnormal	A	
Lille [55,100][a]	>24 h/15 s	>24 h/15 s	None	U	FP,A	Aα 7 asp→asn
London [62][a,i]	91/11	215/16	None	Same	A	
Los Angeles [118][b,c]	Abnormal	Abnormal	Inhibitory	Abnormal	A	
Manchester [54][a]	110/24	U	None	Same	FP,A	
Marseille [124][b,g]	73/25	>60/19	U	Same	A	
Montreal I [73][g,j,k]	46/10	80/18	Slightly inhibitory	Same	A	Aα
Nancy [75][f,j]	75/23	67/36	Inhibitory	Anodal	A	
Oslo II [125][b,g]	44/20	U	U	U	A	
Paris I [29,37,65,81,82][a,g,h]	Infinite	Infinite	Inhibitory	Same	A,FX	γ
Paris II [119][b,f]	85/20	60/18	Inhibitory	Same	U	
Paris III [74][a,j]	50/20	45/18	U	Same	A	
Paris IV [66][b]	72/24	46/20	None	U	A	
Quebec I [56][b]	25/17	22/15	U	Same	A	
St. Louis [45][a,d,k]	35/15	40/16	Inhibitory	Same	A	
San Francisco [121,122][c,d,f,g]	Abnormal	U	Inhibitory	Same	A	
Seattle [115][b]	50/17	U	Inhibitory	U	U	
Troyes [51][b]	60/19	98/22	None	Same	A	
Zürich I [33,58,63,101][b,f,g]	38/15	Abnormal	Inhibitory	Same	FP,A	Aα 16 arg→cys
Zürich II [87][b,f]	Abnormal	U	Inhibitory	Same	A	heterozygous
Bleeding:						
Bethesda I [34][b,g]	148/30	106/24	Inhibitory	Anodal	FP	
Bethesda III [49][b,c,d,e]	110/30	100/24	Inhibitory	Anodal	A	
Buenos Aires I [120][a,h,k]	Abnormal	N	U	Anodal	A	
Caracas [36][a]	23/12	25/12	Inhibitory	Anodal	A,FX	? Aα
Chapel Hill [47][d,e,i]	24/17	42/32	U	U	FP,A,FX	? COOH terminus of Aα
Cleveland II [40,121][a,c,f]	68/30	50/21	Inhibitory	Same	FP,A	Aα
Detroit [50,98][b,f,g]	>60/14.5		Inhibitory	Anodal	FP	Aα 19 arg→ser
Geissen I [44,80][b,e,g]	300/20	>1 h/20 s	Inhibitory	Same	FP,A	
Geissen II [68][d,e]	222/18	227/20	U	U	A	
Hanover [69][b,g]	34/20	87/17	U	U	A	
Houston [39][a,e,i]	32/20	21/21	Inhibitory	Same	A,FX	
Metz [51,79][b]	>4 h/19 s	>4 h/22 s	None	Cathodal	FP	Aα 16 arg→cys
Montreal II [67][g,j]	Abnormal	Abnormal	None	U	A	
Philadelphia [48][a,c,d]	84/20	300/39	Inhibitory	Same	A	
Quebec II [56][a,g]	24/17	23/15		Same	FP,A	
Valencia [43][a,d]	>60/11	7 min/15 s	None	U	A	
Vancouver [18,32][a,d]	Abnormal	U	None	Anodal	U	

TABLE 153-1   Congenital dysfibrinogenemia* *(Continued)*

Designation and reference	Thrombin time, s (patient/control)	Repitilase time, s (patient/control)	Effect on coagulation	IEP compared to normal	Major defect	Site of defect
Thrombosis:						
New York [53][a,g]	>300/17	73/33	None	Anodal	FP,A	
Oslo I [77][a]	10–13/15	U	Shortens	U	U	
Bleeding and thrombosis:						
Baltimore [30,31,41,52][b,f]	100/8	No clot formed	None	Anodal	FP,A,FX	? Aα
Marburg [71][b,d]	240/20	>60 min/20 s	Inhibitory	Same	A	
Weisbaden [70][b]	Abnormal	Abnormal	Inhibitory	Same	A	
Uncertain dysfibrinogenemias:						
Oklahoma [59][a]	U	U	U	Same	FX	
Parma [28][a,d]	Infinite	U	None	No arc	U	
Parnham [61][a]	34/11	U	U	Cathodal	U	
Tokyo [60][a]	N	U	U	Anodal	FX	

* The following are several new fibrinogens not included in the table: fibrinogen Charlottesville [146], fibrinogen New Orleans [147], fibrinogen Nagoya [148], fibrinogen Freiburg [149], fibrinogen Frankfurt [150], fibrinogen San Juan [151], and fibrinogen Petoskey [152,153].
[a]Fibrinogen level not determined by thrombin clotting time method.
[b]Fibrinogen level determined by clotting time method lower than level determined by immunologic, chemical, or "total clottable protein" method.
[c]Shortened plasma half-life of abnormal fibrinogen.
[d]Decreased fibrinogen by all methods used.
[e]Abnormal fibrinolysis.
[f]Abnormal carbohydrate composition.
[g]Fibrin(ogen)-related antigen present in serum.
[h] Poor wound healing.
[i]All family members normal.
[j]No difference in fibrinogen level determined by thrombin clotting time or other methods.
[k]Abnormal bleeding time.
NOTE: A = aggregation, arg = arginine, cys = cysteine, ser = serine, FP = fibrinopeptide release, FX = fibrin cross-linking, IEP = immunoelectrophoresis, N = normal, U = unknown.

Fibrinogen Paris I has two populations of fibrinogen molecules, one with a normal γ chain and the other with an abnormal γ chain [37,65]. The mutant γ Paris I chains inhibited the factor XIIIa–catalyzed cross-linking of the normal fibrin α and γ chains.

In fibrinogen St. Louis [47], the propositus had both dysfibrinogenemia and hemophilia A (factor VIII deficiency). These two coagulation defects were transmitted on separate chromosomes, since the son of the propositus inherited the abnormal fibrinogen but not hemophilia A.

CLINICAL FEATURES
Despite the relative uniformity of laboratory and functional abnormalities in patients with congenital dysfibrinogenemia, the symptoms have been varied. The first families with abnormal fibrinogen came to medical attention because of bleeding, thrombosis, or wound dehiscence. Subsequently, the majority of families found to have abnormal fibrinogens have been asymptomatic and have been discovered because of increased use of coagulation tests in a variety of clinical situations. In general, patients who have major defects in fibrinopeptide release have significant clinical bleeding or thrombosis. The majority of individuals who have

major defects in fibrin monomer aggregation and no or minor defects in fibrinopeptide release are usually asymptomatic (27 families), but 13 families are exceptions [36,43,44,47–49,53,66–71]. Those with defects only in the cross-linking of fibrin are symptomatic, but it is not clear whether the defect is specifically related to an abnormal fibrinogen [59,60]. Seven abnormal fibrinogens have a defect in factor XIIIa–catalyzed cross-linking of fibrin and a defect in fibrin monomer aggregation and/or fibrinopeptide release. One of the families is asymptomatic [38], and six families are symptomatic [29,35,36,39–41].

In fibrinogens Paris I and Cleveland I, wound dehiscence was a major complication [29,35]. Recent observations on the abnormal cross-linking of fibrinogens Paris I and Cleveland I suggest that the wound dehiscence may be related to defective tensile strength or increased susceptibility of the fibrin clot to proteolysis.

Sporadic incidents and the presence of other coagulation abnormalities may cloud the clinical symptoms associated with dysfibrinogenemia. In general, symptoms in the symptomatic individuals with dysfibrinogenemia are related to hemorrhage or thrombosis or both. The coagulation abnormalities within a family tend to be similar. Yet, even in symptomatic kindreds, all individuals are not equally affected. In fibrinogen Baltimore, the propositus had thrombosis and bleeding, but others experienced only bleeding [53]; in fibrinogen Bethesda I, the propositus' bleeding was severe enough that he initially was considered to have hemophilia A, yet other affected family members were relatively free of symptoms [34].

Females with one of six different dysfibrinogens have had recurrent abortions, primarily during the first trimester and usually associated with hemorrhage [19,36,49,51,71,72]. In three instances the individual developed thrombophlebitis post partum or post abortion [19,49,71]. Two of these individuals experienced multiple or recurrent episodes of thrombophlebitis.

LABORATORY FEATURES
These congenital variants of fibrinogen are usually suspected from the results of coagulation tests in which plasma fibrinogen is converted to fibrin, e.g., prothrombin time, thrombin time (see Chaps. A33 through A35), and reptilase time.[1] These tests are usually prolonged, but in some cases no clot forms at all (see Table 153-1). In rare instances the Ancrod clotting time is the most abnormal test [47]. The clotting time of whole blood or the recalcification time of platelet-poor plasma has usually been normal, and the partial thromboplastin time has been variable. Even when abnormal, however, the partial thromboplastin time is rarely as prolonged as the prothrombin time or the thrombin time. In some of the dysfibrinogenemias, although the whole-blood clotting time is normal, the clot is small and friable with excessive red cell fallout.

Measurement of plasma fibrinogen has been variable, depending on the technique used. In all but four instances [67,73–75] in which comparisons have been made between the thrombin clotting time (chronometric assay of Clauss [76]) and other techniques for measuring fibrinogen, the results using the thrombin clotting time method have been much lower than those using the other assays. In most cases fibrinogen levels determined by immunologic assays, fibrin tyrosine content [56], or gravimetric methods have been normal. Fibrinogens Vancouver [19], Parma [28], Bethesda II [42], Valencia [43], St. Louis [45], Leuven [46], Chapel Hill [47], Philadelphia [48], and Bethesda III [49] have been designated hypodysfibrinogens since the plasma fibrinogen concentration is decreased when measured by any of these techniques. The fibrinogen levels in fibrinogen Chapel Hill rose 20 to 30 percent when a proteinase inhibitor was added to the incubation mixture. The discordant chronometric fibrinogen values suggest that the normal fibrinogen molecules either inhibit coagulation of the normal fibrinogen or have a markedly delayed clotting time of their own and are present in sufficient concentration to give a falsely low level of fibrinogen in

this assay. Fibrinogen Oslo I was a notable exception, for the plasma and purified fibrinogen have shorter-than-normal thrombin clotting times [77].

Studies of all other coagulation factors have been normal, except in fibrinogens St. Louis (concomitant factor VIII deficiency) and Chapel Hill (slight reduction in factor VIII). When assayed, plasma factor XIII levels and platelet aggregation, including aggregation with thrombin, have been normal. In approximately 20 percent of the patients with abnormal fibrinogen, the euglobulin clot lysis time has been slightly shortened, while plasminogen levels have invariably been normal. In one family, shorter euglobulin clot lysis was a consistent finding [45]. Plasma treated with thrombin and EACA to test for fibrinogen-related antigen or fibrin(ogen) degradation products must be incubated for long periods of time to ensure that the abnormal fibrinogen becomes incorporated into the clot. A false elevation of the level of fibrinogen degradation products was detected in the patient with fibrinogen Bethesda III and led to an initial diagnosis of intravascular coagulation. If serum contains elevated levels of fibrinogen degradation products, it may be important to subject it to immunoelectrophoresis against antifibrinogen antibodies to see if the precipitin arc is characteristic of fibrinogen or of a degradation product. Such studies may differentiate a slowly clottable fibrinogen from true fibrinogen degradation products.

In all instances of congenital dysfibrinogenemia except fibrinogen Caracas [49], double immunodiffusion studies have shown lines of complete identity between the plasma fibrinogen of affected and normal individuals. The same has been true of purified fibrinogen preparations. By immunoelectrophoresis, however, aberrant migrations of several of the abnormal fibrinogens have been noted and are almost invariably an increased anodal migration [51,66,78] (Table 153-1). These migration abnormalities are more marked with plasma than with purified fibrinogen.

Fibrinogen survival times have been determined in a few instances of congenital dysfibrinogenemia. In fibrinogens Bethesda I, Bethesda II, and Chapel Hill [34,38,42], homologous and autologous ^{125}I fibrinogen survival times appear to be normal, with fractional catabolic rates normal or very near normal. In fibrinogen Philadelphia [48], a homologous fibrinogen survival study revealed a normal half-life; the patient's own fibrinogen, however, had a markedly shortened half-life, and the catabolic rate was markedly increased. Similar findings have been observed in fibrinogen Bethesda III [49]. In several other types of dysfibrinogenemia, the half-life of fibrinogen was normal in studies of peak value and disappearance rate after infusion of unlabeled, homologous fibrinogen.

BIOCHEMICAL ABNORMALITIES
Purified preparations of abnormal fibrinogens have migrated normally on electrophoresis on polyacrylamide gel containing sodium dodecyl sulfate. When the

---

[1] The *reptilase time* is similar to the thrombin time except that clotting is initiated with the snake venom enzyme reptilase. Reptilase is discussed in Chap. 132.

disulfide bonds of fibrinogen are disrupted, the migration of the Aα, Bβ, and γ chains is usually indistinguishable from the normal. In fibrinogen Paris I there appear to be two populations of the γ chain with a molecular weight difference of 2500 daltons [37,65]. The population with the higher molecular weight is considered abnormal. In fibrinogens Montreal I [73] and Metz [79], the Aα chain migrates abnormally on polyacrylamide gel electrophoresis. The Aα chains of fibrinogens Baltimore and Caracas also appear to be abnormal [36,41].

Study of the degradation of the abnormal fibrinogens has shown a delay in the evolution of the normal sequence of degradation products [47,49,80] in certain dysfibrinogenemias, and in fibrinogen Geissen and others an aberrant degradation product was present [55,79,81,82]. In these latter instances the aberrant degradation helped localize the specific molecular defect. Fibrinogen Chapel Hill was exquisitely sensitive to Ancrod proteolysis [47]. The increased susceptibility of fibrinogen Houston to fibrinolysis may be related to the defect in α-α polymer formation.

Fibrinogen is a glycoprotein, and the heterogeneity of normal fibrinogen is related, in part, to the presence of different glycosylated Bβ and γ chains [83]. The carbohydrate content of normal and fetal fibrinogen has recently been reported [84]. In general, carbohydrate analysis has revealed no major or constant abnormality in the congenital abnormal fibrinogens. However, individual cases have been reported with an altered sialic acid content or hexosamine/sialic acid ratio (Table 153-1). The significance of these findings is not known, since asialofibrinogen appears to clot either normally or more rapidly than normal [85], although fibrin derived from fibrinogen devoid of sialic acid has increased solubility in urea or acetic acid [86]. The high sialic acid content of fibrinogen Zürich II is related to an increase in the sialic acid–rich variants of the Bβ and γ chains [87]. Multiple studies have elucidated the amino acid sequence of the Aα, Bβ, and γ chains of fibrinogen [87–90] and have provided evidence for heterogeneity of the Aα and γ chains unrelated to the carbohydrate content [91–95]. Polymerization sites involved in fibrin formation [96] and calcium binding sites of fibrinogen [97] have been identified.

Fibrinogen Detroit was the first abnormal fibrinogen in which a molecular defect was elucidated [98]. In position 19 of the Aα chain, arginine has been replaced by a serine residue (see Chap. 132). Fibrinopeptide A is released normally by thrombin, but fibrinopeptide B is not released. It has been suggested that this single amino acid substitution in the Aα chain results in steric hindrance, so that the B peptide of the Bβ chain is inaccessible to the thrombin. In addition, it has been postulated that this amino acid substitution reduces the number of binding sites for carbohydrate on the molecule [50]. The molecular defects in three other dysfibrinogenemias have been identified. In fibrinogen Metz, arginine in position 16 of the Aα chain was replaced by cysteine [99], and in fibrinogen Lille the position 7 of the Aα chain was a mixture of asparagine and aspartic acid rather than solely aspartic acid [100]. Fibrinogen Zürich I has the same substitution as fibrinogen Metz, except in the heterozygous state [101]. Another dysfibrinogen has the same defect as fibrinogen Detroit [101]. When the arginine residue in position 16 is replaced (at the thrombin cleavage site) by a neutral residue, thrombin cleavage is absent. When the arginine residue in position 19 is exchanged, however, the thrombin cleavage occurs but at a reduced rate.

Comparison of the plasma and platelet fibrinogen in Paris I revealed that the platelet fibrinogen was normal [102]. Extrapolation of this result would suggest that platelet aggregation is normal in dysfibrinogenemic individuals because platelet fibrinogen is not altered.

DIFFERENTIAL DIAGNOSIS

It is not clear why there are abnormalities of coagulation tests in certain of the congenital dysfibrinogenemias, since the plasmas or fibrinogens in several instances are not inhibitory in coagulation studies. However, the majority of abnormal fibrinogens do inhibit the conversion of normal fibrinogen to fibrin (Table 153-1). In the differential diagnosis, one must consider all causes of inhibition of the conversion of fibrinogen to fibrin. Acquired dysfibrinogenemia has been reported in association with tumors, particularly hepatoma [103,104], liver disease [105,106], pseudotumor cerebri [107], and cancer metastatic to the liver [108]. The clinical features tend to distinguish the congenital variety from the acquired, and family studies of the acquired states have been normal. Congenital dysfibrinogenemia is differentiated from hypofibrinogenemia by (1) concordant reduction in hypofibrinogenemia of the level of plasma fibrinogen regardless of the technique used, (2) the discrepant result in dysfibrinogenemia between fibrinogen levels determined by physicochemical or immunologic methods and by the thrombin clotting time, and (3) the greater abnormality in the thrombin time in relation to the fibrinogen concentration in dysfibrinogenemia.

Inhibitors of fibrinogen-fibrin conversion which must be considered are heparin, fibrinogen degradation products, and antithrombins. Heparin can be identified simply by a careful history or by the corrective effects of protamine sulfate or toluidine blue on the thrombin time. In addition, the reptilase time is normal in the presence of heparin. The differentiation of congenital dysfibrinogenemia from fibrinolysis or intravascular coagulation with increased fibrinogen degradation products may be difficult at times. In fact, the propositus of fibrinogen Bethesda III was treated with heparin because of an initial diagnosis of intravascular coagulation. Fibrinogen degradation products will not be incorporated into the clot even after prolonged incubation at 37°C. While the abnormal fibrinogens may have residual fibrinogen-related antigen in "serum" after 2 h of incubation, usually after 6 to 12 h all the fibrinogen-related antigen (abnormal fibrinogen) has been incorporated into the clot (Table 153-1). Family studies may be very helpful in differentiating these disorders. Several immunologic and clotting assay techniques are available to measure antithrombin activity.

Another acquired condition which may mimic congenital dysfibrinogenemia is the occurrence in multiple myeloma of abnormal immunoglobulins which interfere with the conversion of fibrinogen to fibrin [109,110]. These paraproteins cause an abnormal fibrin aggregation phase but do not interfere with fibrinopeptide release. Similar abnormalities have been described in systemic lupus erythematosus [111]. Acquired inhibitors of fibrinopeptide release, fibrin polymerization, or fibrin stabilization may mimic dysfibrinogenemia [112–114].

THERAPY

Most patients with congenital dysfibrinogenemia are asymptomatic and require no therapy. In affected individuals, therapy is usually related to acute bleeding disorders and to preoperative procedures in order to maintain fibrinogen levels for hemostasis and adequate wound healing. Whole blood, fresh frozen plasma, fibrinogen concentrates, and cryoprecipitate have been used by various investigators for infusion. Commercial fibrinogen preparations have a high incidence of hepatitis transmission (Chap. 167). Cryoprecipitate infusions have been effective in patients undergoing major surgery [30,34,35,49] and in stopping uterine hemorrhage [49]. Factor VIII concentrates and cryoprecipitate were effective in raising the fibrinogen level and preventing surgical hemorrhage in a patient with dysfibrinogenemia and hemophilia A [69]. The propositus in fibrinogen Seattle underwent open heart surgery without preoperative fibrinogen replacement and did not bleed [115].

In most congenital dysfibrinogenemias that are associated with thrombosis, anticoagulation has proven efficacious. The role of long-term anticoagulation in these patients is unclear at present.

PROGNOSIS

Dysfibrinogenemia does not seem to be associated with an increased mortality. The thromboembolic phenomena which occur in a small group of these patients have not been associated with any deaths. Wound dehiscence was a major complication in patients with fibrinogens Paris I and Cleveland I [29,35] and resulted in the death of one patient. The patient with fibrinogen Zürich I suffered a subarachnoid hemorrhage, and a relative of the propositus of fibrinogen Paris II required surgical removal of an arterial embolus. The high incidence of spontaneous abortions in six dysfibrinogenic patients [19,36,49,51,71,72] is similar to the findings in afibrinogenemia [116]. It is not clear whether this latter complication is related to the abnormal fibrinogens or represent chance association of medical conditions with the qualitative coagulation disorder.

Uncertain dysfibrinogenemias

It is uncertain whether four presumptive dysfibrinogenemias (Parma, Oklahoma, Parnham, and Tokyo) represent true qualitative abnormalities of fibrinogen [28,59–61]. In fibrinogens Parma and Parnham the tested family members were not affected, and in fibrinogen Parma the patient's plasma did not form an immunoprecipitation arc with antihuman fibrinogen. In fibrinogens Oklahoma and Tokyo, abnormalities of clot stabilization have been reported; however, to date this has not been proved to be related to an abnormality of the fibrinogen molecule. In addition, the thrombin clotting time and prothrombin time have been normal. Several dysfibrinogens to date are incompletely described [126–130, 145].

FETAL FIBRINOGEN

Almost 100 years ago [131] it was demonstrated that the rate of clotting of plasma and fibrinogen from normal newborn infants was lower than that of normal adult plasma or fibrinogen. This suggested the existence of a molecular variant of fibrinogen, designated *fetal fibrinogen*. The prolonged thrombin time in newborn plasma may be related to this variant of fibrinogen, but some studies have suggested that heparin-like substances or fibrinogen degradation products are responsible for these abnormalities [132–136]. The prolongation of the umbilical cord blood thrombin time is not related to fibrinogenolysis in vivo [137]. Fetal fibrinogen [138,139] is functionally different from normal fibrinogen in that the thrombin and reptilase times are prolonged in the former, as is the fibrin monomer aggregation phase in the conversion of fibrinogen to fibrin. Fetal and adult fibrinogen are similar in their antigenic determinants, electrophoretic mobility on polyacrylamide gels, molecular weight of the individual fibrinogen chains, and amino acid composition [139–142]. Differences found for fetal fibrinogen are the prolonged coagulation times, different pH-dependent thrombin clotting times, elution on DEAE-cellulose chromatography, fingerprints of tryptic digests [140], and higher phosphorus contents [136]. The sialic acid content of fetal fibrinogen is greater than that of adult fibrinogen, and partial removal of the sialic acid from the fetal fibrinogen corrects the thrombin time [104,143]. There are similarities between fibrinogen Paris I and fetal fibrinogen, and even more striking similarities between fetal fibrinogen and the dysfibrinogenemia found with hepatoma [104] or that found in liver disease [144]. In both instances the sialic acid content of these fibrinogens is increased and the clotting times are corrected by desialation of the abnormal fibrinogens. Like normal fetal fibrinogen, the dysfibrinogens associated with hepatoma and liver disease do not have discrepant results between chronometric and other assay techniques [104], nor are they associated with hemorrhage, thrombosis, or defective wound healing.

References

1. Rabe, F., and Salomon, E.: Über Faserstoffmangel im Blut bei einem Falle von Haemophilie. *Dtsch. Arch. Klin. Med. 132:*240, 1920.

2. Bommer, W., Kunzer, W., and Schroer, H.: Kongenitale Afibrinogenamie, Teil I. *Ann. Paediatr. 200:*46, 1963.

3. Egbring, R., Andrassy, K., Egli, H., and Meyer-Lindenberg, J.: Diagnostische und therapeutische Probleme bei congenitaler Afibrinogenamie. *Blut 22:*175, 1971.

4. Mammen, E. F.: Congenital abnormalities of the fibrinogen molecule. *Semin. Thromb. Hemostas. 1:*184, 1974.

5. Fried, K., and Kaufman, S.: Congenital afibrinogenemia in 10 offspring of uncle-niece marriages. *Clin. Genet. 17:*223, 1980.

6. Risak, E.: Die Fibrinopenie. *Z. Klin. Med. 128:*605, 1935.

7. Bommer, W., Kunzer, W., and Schroer, H.: Kongenitale Afibrinogenamie. Teil II. *Ann. Paediatr. 200:*180, 1963.

8. Solum, N., and Stormorken, H.: Influence of fibrinogen on the aggregation of washed human platelets induced by adenosine diphosphate, thrombin, collagen and adrenalin. *Scand. J. Clin. Lab. Invest. (Suppl.) 84:*170, 1965.

9. Werder, E.: Kongenital Afibrinogenamie. *Helv. Paediatr. Acta 18:*208, 1963.

10. Gross, R., et al.: Untersuchungen an einer angeborenen Afibrinogenamie: Zur Rolle der Blutgerinnung bei der Blutstillung. *Klin. Wochenschr. 41:*695, 1963.

11. Alexander, B., Goldstein, R., Rich, L., Le Balloc'h, A. G., Diamond, L. K., and Borges, W.: Congenital afibrinogenemia: A study of some basic aspects of coagulation. *Blood 9:*843, 1954.

12. Petrescu, C. M., Poppa, C., and Enache, F.: Consideratii asupra unui caz de hemofilie associata cu hipfibrinogenemie si trombocitopatie. *Med. Interna (Bucur.) 20:*613, 1968.

13. Yamagata, S., et al.: A case of congenital afibrinogenemia and review of reported cases in Japan. *Tohoku J. Exp. Med. 96:*15, 1968.

14. Weiss, H., and Rogers, J.: Fibrinogen and platelets in the primary arrest of bleeding: Studies in two patients with congenital afibrinogenemia. *N. Engl. J. Med. 285:*369, 1971.

15. McLean, J. R., Maxwell, R. E., and Hertler, D.: Fibrinogen and adenosine diphosphate–induced aggregation of platelets. *Nature 202:*605, 1964.

16. Gugler, E., and Luscher, E. F.: Platelet function in congenital afibrinogenemia. *Thromb. Diath. Haemorrh. 14:*361, 1965.

17. Bang, N. U., Heidenreich, R. O., and Matsuda, M.: Plasma protein requirement for human platelet aggregation. *Thromb. Diath. Haemorrh. (Suppl.) 42:*37, 1970.

18. Colvin, R. B., Mosesson, M. W., and Dvorak, H. F.: Delayed-type hypersensitivity skin reactions in congenital afibrinogenemia lack fibrin deposition and induration. *J. Clin. Invest. 63:*1302, 1979.

19. Hasselback, R., Marion, R., and Thomas, J.: Congenital hypofibrinogenemia in five members of a family. *Can. Med. Assoc. J. 88:*19, 1963.

20. Dale, B. M., Purdie, G. H., and Rischbieth, R. H.: Fibrinogen depletion with sodium valproate. *Lancet 1:*1316, 1978.

21. Gralnick, H. R., and Henderson, E.: Hypofibrinogenemia and coagulation factor deficiencies with L-asparaginase treatment. *Cancer 27:*1313, 1971.

22. Pinniger, J. L., and Prunty, F. T. G.: Some observations on the blood-clotting mechanism: The role of fibrinogen and platelets with reference to a case of congenital afibrinogenaemia. *Br. J. Exp. Pathol. 27:*200, 1946.

23. Mason, D. Y., and Ingram, G. I. C.: Management of the hereditary coagulation disorders. *Semin. Hematol. 8:*158, 1971.

24. Bronnimann, R.: Kongenitale Afibrinogenamie: Mitteilung eines Falles mit multiplen Knochenzysten und Bildung eines spezifischen Antikorpers (Antifibrinogen) nach Bluttransfusion. *Acta Haemotol. (Basel) 11:*40, 1954.

25. de Vries, A., Rosenberg, S., Kochwa, S., and Boss, J.: Precipitating antifibrinogen antibody appearing after fibrinogen infusions in a patient with congenital afibrinogenemia. *Am. J. Med. 30:*486, 1961.

26. Ingram, D. I. C., McBrien, D. J., and Spencer, H.: Fatal pulmonary embolus in congenital fibrinopenia: Report of two cases. *Acta Haemotol. (Basel) 35:*56, 1966.

27. MacKinnon, H. H., and Fekete, J. F.: Congenital afibrinogenemia: Vascular changes and multiple thromboses induced by fibrinogen infusions and contraceptive medication. *Can. Med. Assoc. J. 140:*597, 1971.

28. di Imperato, C., and Dettori, A. G.: Ipofibrinogenemia congenita con fibrinoastenia. *Helv. Paediatr. Acta 13:*380, 1958.

29. Menache, D.: Constitutional and familial abnormal fibrinogen. *Thromb. Diath. Haemorrh. (Suppl.) 13:*173, 1964.

30. Beck, E. A.: Abnormal fibrinogen (fibrinogen "Baltimore") as a cause of a familial hemorrhagic disorder. *Blood 24:*853, 1964.

31. Beck, E. A., Charache, P., and Jackson, D. P.: A new inherited coagulation disorder caused by an abnormal fibrinogen ("fibrinogen Baltimore"). *Nature 208:*143, 1965.

32. Jackson, D., and Beck, E.: Inherited abnormal fibrinogens, in *Hemophilia and New Hemorrhagic States,* edited by K. M. Brinkhous. University of North Carolina Press, Chapel Hill, 1970, p. 225.

33. von Felten, A., Duckert, F., and Frick, P. G.: Familial disturbance of fibrin monomer aggregation. *Br. J. Haematol. 12:*667, 1966.

34. Gralnick, H. R., Givelber, H. M., Shainoff, J. R. and Finlayson, J. S.: A congenital dysfibrinogenemia with delayed fibrinopeptide release. *J. Clin. Invest. 50:*1819, 1971.

35. Forman, W. B., Ratnoff, O. D., and Boyer, M. H.: An inherited qualitative abnormality in plasma fibrinogen: Fibrinogen Cleveland. *J. Lab. Clin. Med. 72:*455, 1968.

36. Bosch, N., Arocha-Pinnango, C. L., Soria, J., Soria, C., Rodriguez, A., and Rodriguez, S.: An abnormal fibrinogen in a Venezuelan family. *Thromb. Res. 1:*253, 1977.

37. Budzynski, A., Marder, V., Menache, D., and Guillin, M.-C.: Defect in the gamma polypeptide chain of a congenital abnormal fibrinogen. *Nature 252:*66, 1974.

38. Hansen, M. S., Clemmensen, I., and Winther, D.: Fibrinogen Copenhagen: An abnormal fibrinogen with defective polymerization and release of fibrinopeptide A but normal adsorption of plasminogen. *Scand. J. Clin. Lab. Invest. 40:*221, 1980.

39. Weinger, R. S., Rudy, C., Moake, J. L., Conlon, C. L., and Cimo, P. L.: Fibrinogen Houston: A dysfibrinogen exhibiting defective fibrin monomer aggregation and α-chain cross-linkages. *Am. J. Hematol. 9:*237, 1980.

40. Crum, E. D., Shainoff, J. R., Graham, R. C., and Ratnoff, O. D.: Fibrinogen Cleveland II: An abnormal fibrinogen with defective release of fibrinopeptide A. *J. Clin. Invest 53:*1308, 1974.

41. Brown, C., and Crowe, M.: Defective α polymerization in the conversion of fibrinogen Baltimore to fibrin. *J. Clin. Invest. 55:*1190, 1975.

42. Gralnick, H. R., Givelber, H. M., and Finlayson, J. S.: A new congenital abnormality of human fibrinogen: Fibrinogen Bethesda II. *Thromb. Diath. Haemorrh. 29:*562, 1973.

43. Aznar, J., Fernandez-Pavon, A., Reganon, E., Vila, V., and Orellana, F.: Fibrinogen Valencia, a new case of congenital dysfibrinogenemia. *Thromb. Diath. Haemorrh. 32:*564, 1974.

44. Krause, W. H., Heene, D. L., and Lasch, H. G.: Congenital dysfibrinogenemia (fibrinogen Geissen). *Thromb. Diath. Haemorrh. 29:*547, 1973.

45. Sherman, L., Gaston, L., Kaplan, M., and Spivak, A.: Fibrinogen St. Louis: A new inherited fibrinogen variant, coincidentally associated with hemophilia A. *J. Clin. Invest. 51:*590, 1972.

46. Verhaeghe, R., Verstraete, M., Vermylen, J., and Vermylen, C.: Fibrinogen "Leuven": Another genetic variant. *Br. J. Haematol. 26:*421, 1974.

47. McDonagh, R. P., Carrell, N. A., Roberts, H. R., Blatt, P. M., and McDonagh, J.: Fibrinogen Chapel Hill: Hypodysfibrinogenemia with a tertiary polymerization defect. *Am. J. Hematol. 9:*23, 1980.

48. Martinez, J., Holburn, R. R., Shapiro, S. S., and Erslev, A. J.: Fibrinogen Philadelphia: A hereditary hypofibrinogenemia characterized by fibrinogen hypercatabolism. *J. Clin. Invest. 53:*600, 1974.

49. Gralnick, H. R., Coller, B. S., Fratantoni, J. C., and Martinez, J.: Fibrinogen Bethesda III: A hypodysfibrinogenemia. *Blood 53:*28, 1979.

50. Mammen, E. F., Prasad, A. S., Barnhart, M. I., and Au, C. C.: Congenital dysfibrinogenemia: Fibrinogen Detroit. *J. Clin. Invest. 48:*235, 1969.

51. Soria, J., Soria, C., Samama, M., Poirot, E., and Kling, C.: Fibrinogen Troyes-Metz: Two new cases of congenital dysfibrinogenemia. *Thromb. Diath. Haemorrh. 27*:619, 1972.

52. Beck, F. A., Shainoff, J. R., Vogel, A., and Jackson, D. P.: Functional evaluation of an inherited abnormal fibrinogen: Fibrinogen "Baltimore." *J. Clin. Invest. 50*:1974, 1971.

53. Al-Mondhiry, H., Bilezikian, S., and Nossel, H.: Fibrinogen "New York": An abnormal fibrinogen associated with thromboembolism. *Blood 45*:607, 1975.

54. Lane, D. A., et al.: An abnormal fibrinogen with delayed fibrinopeptide A release. *Br. J. Haematol. 46*:89, 1980.

55. Denninger, M.-H., Finlayson, J. S., Reamer, L. A., Parquet-Gernez, A., Goudemand, M., and Menache, D.: Congenital dysfibrinogenemia: Fibrinogen Lille. *Thromb. Res. 13*:453, 1978.

56. Jobin, F., Vu, L., and Delage, J.-M.: Fibrinogenes Quebec I et Quebec II: Deux nouvelles familles de dysfibrinogenemie. *Acta Haematol. 59*:119, 1978.

57. Jandrot-Perrus, M., Aurousseau, M. H., and Josso, F.: A new case of dysfibrinogenemia: Isolation of the abnormal, unclottable fibrinogen population. *Abstracts of the VIII Congress of the International Society for Thrombosis and Haemostasis*, 1981, p. 104.

58. Hofman, V., Gati, W. P., and Straub, P. W.: Fibrinogen Zürich I: Impaired released of fibrinopeptide A. *Thromb. Haemost. 41*:709, 1979.

59. Hampton, J. W.: Qualitative fibrinogen defect associated with abnormal fibrin stabilization. *J. Lab. Clin. Med. 72*:882, 1968.

60. Samori, T., Yatabe, M., Ukita, M., Fujimaki, M., and Fukutabe, K.: A new congenital dysfibrinogenemia (fibrinogen Tokyo) with defective stabilization of fibrin polymer. *Abstracts of the V Congress of the International Society for Thrombosis and Haemostasis*, 1975, p. 64.

61. Fantl, P.: Hypofibrinogenemia with a possibly defective fibrinogen associated with fibrinolysis. *Aust. Ann. Med. 18*:43, 1969.

62. Lane, D. A., Cuddigan, B., VanRoss, M., and Kakkar, V. V.: Dysfibrinogenemia characterized by abnormal fibrin monomer polymerization and normal fibrinopeptide A release. *Br. J. Haematol. 44*:483, 1980.

63. Von Felten, A., Frick, P. G., and Straub, P. W.: Studies on fibrin monomer aggregation in congenital dysfibrinogenemia (fibrinogen "Zürich"): Separation of a pathological from a normal fibrin fraction. *Br. J. Haematol. 16*:353, 1969.

64. Mosesson, M. W., and Beck, E. A.: Chromatographic, ultracentrifugal, and related studies of fibrinogen "Baltimore." *J. Clin. Invest. 48*:1656, 1969.

65. Mosesson, M. W., Amrani, D. L., and Menache, D.: Studies on the structural abnormality of fibrinogen Paris I. *J. Clin. Invest. 57*:782, 1976.

66. Amsellem, M., Samama, M., Conard, J., Levyne, S., and Ohlgiesser, C.: Dysfibrinogenemie congenitale: Deux observations. *Nouv. Presse Med. 7*:3745, 1978.

67. D'Angelo, G., Lacombe, M., Lemay, J., Lavallee, R., Bonney, Y., and Boileau, J.: A new congenital dysfibrinogenemia with hemorrhagic diathesis (fibrinogen Montreal II). *Abstracts of the V Congress of the International Society for Thrombosis and Haemostasis*, 1975, p. 244.

68. Krause, W. H., Huth, K., Heene, D. L., and Lasch, H. G.: Hypodysfibrinogenamie: Fibrinogen Giessen II. *Klin. Wochenschr. 53*:781, 1975.

69. Barthels, M., and Sandvoss, G.: "Fibrinogen Hannover," ein weiteres atypisches Fibrinogen. *Blut 34*:99, 1977.

70. Winkelmann, G., Augustin, R., and Baudilla, K.: Congenital dysfibrinogenemia: Report of a new family (fibrinogen "Weisbaden"). *Abstracts of the II Congress of the International Society for Thrombosis and Haemostasis*, 1971, p. 64.

71. Fuchs, G., Egbring, R., and Havemann, K.: Fibrinogen Marburg: A new genetic variant of fibrinogen. *Blut 34*:107, 1977.

72. Aquercif, M., Soria, J., Soria, C., Ritschard, J., Samama, M., and Bouvier, C.: A new family with dysfibrinogenemia, fibrinogen Alba/Geneva. *Abstracts of the IV Congress of the International Society for Thrombosis and Haemostasis*, 1973, p. 381.

73. Lacombe, M., Soria, J., Soria, C., D'Angelo, G., Lavellee, R., and Bonny, Y.: Fibrinogen Montreal: A new case of congenital dysfibrinogenemia with defective aggregation of monomers. *Thromb. Diath. Haemorrh. 29*:536, 1973.

74. Soria, J., and Soria, C.: Dysfibrinogenemie familiale avec anomalie de l'agrégation des monomeres: Le fibrinogene Paris III. *Pathol. Biol. (Suppl.) 22*:72, 1974.

75. Streiff, F., Alexander, P., Vigneron, C., Soria, J., Soria, C., and Mester, L.: Un Nouveau cas d'anomalie constitutionelle et familiale du fibrinogene sans diatheses hemorragique. *Thromb. Diath. Haemorrh. 26*:565, 1971.

76. Clauss, A.: Gerinnungsphysiologische Schnellmethode zur Bestimmung des Fibrinogens. *Acta Haematol. 17*:237, 1957.

77. Egeberg, O.: Inherited fibrinogen abnormality causing thrombophilia. *Thromb. Diath. Haemorrh. 17*:176, 1967.

78. Janssen, C. L., and Vreeken, J.: Fibrinogen Amsterdam: Another hereditary abnormality of fibrinogen. *Br. J. Haematol. 20*:287, 1971.

79. Soria, J., Soria, C., and Baulard, C.: Anomalie de structure du fibrinogène "Metz," localisée sur la chaine (A) de la molecule. *Biochemie 54*:415, 1972.

80. Bleyl, H., and Krause, W. H.: Studies on the degradation of fibrinogen Geissen I. *Thromb. Res. 9*:329, 1976.

81. Mosesson, M. W., Denninger, M. H., and Menache, D.: Hydrolysis of fibrinogen Paris I by plasmin. *Thromb. Res. 9*:115, 1976.

82. Budzynski, A. Z., and Marder, V. J.: Plasmic degradation of fibrinogen Paris I. *J. Lab. Clin. Med. 88*:817, 1976.

83. Gati, W. P., and Straub, P. W.: Separation of both the Bβ- and the γ-polypeptide chains of human fibrinogen into two main types which differ in sialic acid content. *J. Biol. Chem. 253*:1315, 1978.

84. Lane, D. A., Allen, A. K., Markwick, J., Mackie, I., Thompson, E., and Owen, J.: Carbohydrate composition and catabolism of five abnormal fibrinogens. *Abstracts of the VIII Congress of the International Society for Thrombosis and Haemostasis*, 1981, p. 181.

85. Martinez, J., Palascak, J., and Peters, C.: Functional and metabolic properties of human asialofibrinogen. *J. Lab. Clin. Med. 89*:367, 1977.

86. Laki, K., and Cgabdrasekhar, N.: Sialic acid in fibrinogen and the vulcanization of the fibrin clot. *Nature 197*:1267, 1963.

87. Straub, P. W., and Gati, W. P.: Increase of the sialic acid–rich variants of the Bβ- and γ-chains of fibrinogen Zürich II. *Thromb. Haemostas. 41*:714, 1979.

88. Watt, K. W. K., Cottrell, B. S., Strong, D. C., and Doolittle, R. F.: Amino acid sequence studies on the α chain of human fibrinogen: Overlapping sequences providing the complete sequence. *Biochemistry 18*:5410, 1979.

89. Watt, K. W. K., Takagi, T., and Doolittle, R. F.: Amino acid sequence of the β chain of human fibrinogen. *Biochemistry 18*:68, 1979.

90. Lottspeich, F., and Henschen, A.: Amino acid sequence of human fibrin: Preliminary note on the completion of the γ-chain sequence. *Hoppe Seylers Z. Physiol. Chem. 358*:935, 1977.

91. Galanakis, D. K., Mosesson, M. W., and Stathakis, N. E.: Human fibrinogen heterogeneities: Distribution and charge characteristics of chains of Aα origin. *J. Lab. Clin. Med. 92*:376, 1978.

92. Weinstein, M. J., and Deykin, D.: Low solubility fibrinogen examined by two-dimensional sodium dodecyl sulfate gel electrophoresis and isoelectric focusing. *Thromb. Res. 13*:361, 1978.

93. Stathakis, N. E., Mosesson, M. W., Galanakis, D. K., and Menache, D.: Human fibrinogen heterogeneities: Preparation and characterization of γ and γ' chains. *Thromb. Res. 13*:467, 1978.

94. Francis, C. W., Marder, V. J., and Marin, S. E.: Demonstration of a large molecular weight variant of the γ chain of normal human plasma fibrinogen. *J. Biol. Chem. 255*:5599, 1980.

95. Wolfenstein-Todel, C., and Mosesson, M. W.: Human plasma fibrinogen heterogeneity: Evidence for an extended carboxyl-terminal sequence in a normal γ chain variant (γ). *Proc. Natl. Acad. Sci. U.S.A. 77*:5069, 1980.

96. Olexa, S. A., and Budzynski, A. Z.: Evidence for four different polymerization sites involved in human fibrin formation. *Proc. Natl. Acad. Sci. U.S.A. 77*:1374, 1980.

97. Lindsey, G. G., Brown, G., and Purves, L. R.: Calcium binding to human fibrinogen: Localization of two calcium specific sites. *Thromb. Res. 13*:345, 1976.

98. Blomback, M., Blomback, B., Mammen, E. F., and Prasad, A. S.: Fibrinogen Detroit: A molecular defect in the N-terminal disulphide knot of human fibrinogen? *Nature 218*:134, 1968.

99. Henschen, A., Southan, C., Soria, J., Soria, C., and Samama, M.: Structure abnormality of fibrinogen Metz and its relationship to the clotting defect. *Abstracts of the VIII Congress of the International Society for Thrombosis and Haemostasis,* 1981, p. 103.

100. Morris, S., Denninger, M.-H., Finlayson, J. S., and Menache, D.: Fibrinogen Lille: $A\alpha^{7ASP \rightarrow ASN}$. *Abstracts of the VIII Congress of the International Society for Thrombosis and Haemostasis,* 1981, p. 104.

101. Henschen, A., Southan, C., Kehl, M., and Lottspeich, F.: The structural error and its relation to the malfunction in some abnormal fibrinogens. *Abstracts of the VIII Congress of the International Society for Thrombosis and Haemostasis,* 1981, p. 181.

102. Jandrot-Perrus, M., Mosesson, M. W., Denninger, M.-H., and Menache, D.: Studies of platelet fibrinogen from a subject with a congenital plasma fibrinogen abnormality (fibrinogen Paris I). *Blood* 54:1109, 1979.

103. von Felten, A., Straub, P. W., and Frick, P. G.: Dysfibrinogenemia in a patient with primary hepatoma. *N. Engl. J. Med.* 280:405, 1969.

104. Gralnick, H. R., Givelber, H., and Abrams, E.: Dysfibrinogenemia associated with hepatoma: Increased carbohydrate content of the fibrinogen molecule. *N. Engl. J. Med.* 299:221, 1978.

105. Soria, J., et al.: Dysfibrinogenemies acquises dans les atteintes hepatiques sévères. *Coagulation* 3:37, 1970.

106. Green, G., Thomson, J. M., Dymock, I. W., and Poller, L.: Abnormal fibrin polymerization in liver disease. *Br. J. Haematol.* 34:427, 1976.

107. D'Souza, L., Coots, M. C., and Glueck, H. I.: An acquired abnormal fibrinogen associated with thromboembolic disease and pseudotumor cerebri. *Thromb. Haemost.* 42:994, 1979.

108. Gralnick, H.: Personal observations.

109. Coleman, M., Vigliano, E., Weksler, M., and Nachman, R.: Inhibition of fibrin monomer polymerization by lambda myeloma globulins. *Blood* 39:210, 1972.

110. Lackner, H.: Hemostatic abnormalities associated with dysproteinemias. *Semin. Hematol.* 10:125, 1973.

111. Galahakis, D. K., Ginzler, E. M., and Fikrig, S. M.: Monoclonal IgG anticoagulants delaying fibrin aggregation in two patients with systemic lupus erythematosus (SLE). *Blood* 52:1037, 1978.

112. Marciniak, E., and Greenwood, M. F.: Acquired coagulation inhibitor delaying fibrinopeptid release. *Blood* 53:81, 1979.

113. Hoots, W. K., Carrell, N. A., Wagner, R. H., Cooper, H. A., and McDonagh, J.: A naturally occurring antibody that inhibits fibrin polymerization. *N. Engl. J. Med.* 304:857, 1981.

114. Rosenberg, R. D., Colman, R. W., and Lorand, L.: A new haemorrhagic disorder with defective fibrin stabilization and cryofibrinogenaemia. *Br. J. Haematol.* 26:269, 1974.

115. Branson, H. E., Schmer, G., and Dillard, D. H.: Fibrinogen Seattle: A qualitatively abnormal fibrinogen in a patient with tetralogy of Fallot. *Am. J. Clin. Pathol.* 67:326, 1976.

116. Hahn, L., Lunberg, P. A., and Teger-Nilsson, A. C.: Congenital hypofibrinogenaemia and recurrent abortion. *Br. J. Obstet. Gynecol.* 85:790, 1978.

117. Jacobsen, C. D., and Hoak, J. C.: Fibrinogen Iowa City: An abnormal fibrinogen with no clinical symptoms. *Thromb. Res.* 2:261, 1973.

118. Zietz, B., and Scott, J.: An inherited defect in fibrin polymerization: Fibrinogen Los Angeles. *Clin. Res.* 18:179, 1970.

119. Samama, M., Soria, J., Soria, C., and Bousser, J.: Dysfibrinogenemie congenitale et familiale sans tendance hemorragique. *Nouv. Rev. Fr. Hematol.* 9:817, 1969.

120. Buraschi, J., Sack, E., Quiroga, E., and Hendler, H.: A new fibrinogen anomaly: Fibrinogen Buenos Aires. *Abstracts of the V Congress of the International Society for Thrombosis and Haemostasis,* 1975, p. 244.

121. Ratnoff, O. D., and Forman, W. B.: Criteria for the differentiation of dysfibrinogenemic states. *Semin. Hematol.* 13:141, 1976.

122. Hassan, H. J., et al.: Functional and biochemical studies on a case of dysfibrinogenemia (fibrinogen Genova). *Abstracts of the VIII Congress of the International Society for Thrombosis and Haemostasis,* 1981, p. 360.

123. Matthias, F. R., Krause, W. H., Ganssert, S., Mueller, K., and Lasch, H. G.: Dysfibrinogenamie. Zugleich ein neuer Fall: Dysfibrinogenamie Giessen III. *Klin. Wochenschr.* 55:539, 1977.

124. Soria, J., Soria, C., Juhan, I., Perrimond, H., Haverkate, F., and Orsini, A.: Fibrinogen Marseille: A new case of congenital dysfibrinogenaemia. *Haemostasis* 9:214, 1980.

125. Godal, H. C., Brosstad, F., and Kierulf, P.: Three new cases of an inborn qualitative fibrinogen defect (Fibrinogen Oslo II). *Scand. J. Haematol.* 20:57, 1978.

126. Thaler, E.: Discussion. *XVII Meeting of the German Association of Blood Coagulationists,* Munster, 1973.

127. Papp, A. C., Snopko, R. M., Cole, E. R., Sassetti, R. J., and Wu, K. K.: Recurrent venous thrombosis related to a hereditary dysfibrinogen with abnormal crossed immunoelectrophoretic pattern. *Abstracts of the VIII Congress of the International Society for Thrombosis and Haemostasis,* 1981, p. 360.

128. Pezzoli, A., and Pascali, E.: "Bis"-fibrinogenaemia. *Scand. J. Haematol.* 26:37, 1981.

129. Soria, J., Soria, C., Houbouyan, L., and Goguel, A.: Fibrinogen Boulogue: A congenital abnormality in aggregation of fibrin monomers. *International Society of Haematologists (European-African Division, III Meeting),* London, Abstract 2303.

130. Soria, J., Soria, C., Bezou, M. J., Picot, J., Griffiths-Bernard, J., and Coulet, M.: Dysfibrinogenemie par anomalie de l'agrégation des monomeres. Le fibrinogene Clermont-Ferrand. *Congres Francais d'Hématologie,* Vittel, Abstract 66.

131. Krueger, F.: Ueber das Verhalten des foetalen Blutes in Momente der Geburt. *Arch. Pathol. Anat.* 106:1, 1886.

132. Grossman, B. J., Heyn, R. M., and Rosenfeld, I. H.: Coagulation studies in the newborn infant. *Pediatrics* 9:182, 1952.

133. Aballi, A. J., Lopez-Banus, V., De Lamerens, S., and Rozengvaig, S.: Coagulation studies in the newborn period. I. Alterations of thromboplastin generation and effects of vitamin K on full-term and premature infants. *Am. J. Dis. Child.* 94:954, 1957.

134. Beller, F. J., Douglas, G. W., and Epstein, M. D.: The fibrinolytic enzyme system in the newborn. *Am. J. Obstet. Gynecol.* 96:977, 1966.

135. Bonifaci, E., Baggio, P., and Gravina, E.: Demonstration of split products of fibrinogen in the blood of normal newborns. *Biol. Neonate* 12:29, 1969.

136. von Felten, A., and Straub, P. W.: Coagulation studies of cord blood, with special reference to "fetal fibrinogen." *Thromb. Diath. Haemorrh.* 22:273, 1969.

137. Galanakis, D. K., and Mosesson, M. W.: Evaluation of the role of in vivo proteolysis (fibrinogenolysis) in prolonging the thrombin time of human umbilical cord fibrinogen. *Blood* 48:109, 1976.

138. Guillin, M.-C., and Menache, D.: Fetal fibrinogen and fibrinogen Paris I: Comparative fibrin monomer aggregation studies. *Thromb. Res.* 3:117, 1973.

139. Teger-Nilsson, A.-M., and Ekelund, H.: Fibrinogen to fibrin transformation in umbilical cord blood and purified normal fibrinogen. *Thromb. Res.* 5:601, 1974.

140. Witt, I., Muller, H., and Kunzer, W.: Evidence for the existence of foetal fibrinogen. *Thromb. Diath. Haemorrh.* 22:101, 1969.

141. Witt, I., and Muller, H.: Phosphorus and hexose content of human foetal fibrinogen. *Biochim. Biophys. Acta* 221:402, 1970.

142. Loly, W., Israels, L. G., Bishop, A. J., and Israels, E. D.: A comparative study of adult and fetal sheep fibrinogen: Sulffibrinogen and fibrinogen degradation products. *Thromb. Diath. Haemorrh.* 26:526, 1971.

143. Galanakis, D. K., and Mosesson, M. W.: Correction of the delayed fibrin aggregation of fetal fibrinogen by partial removal of sialic acid. *Abstracts of the VII Congress of the International Society for Thrombosis and Haemostasis,* 1979, p. 79.

144. Martinez, J., Palascak, J., and Kwasniak, D.: Role of sialic acid in the dysfibrinogenemia associated with liver disease. *J. Clin. Invest.* 61:535, 1978.

145. Galanakis, D. K., and Peerschke, E.: Fibrinogen Stony Brook: An Aα chain defect resulting in delayed fibrin assembly and decreased platelet aggregation support. *Blood* 58:216a, 1981.

146. Laugen, R. H., and Bithell, T. C.: Fibrinogen Charlottesville: Hereditary dysfibrinogenemia characterized by slow fibrinopeptide release and competitive inhibition of thrombin. *Blood* 50 (Suppl. I):273, 1977.

147. Andes, W. A., Chavin, S. I., Beltran, G., and Stuckey, W. J.: Fibrinogen New Orleans: Hereditary dysfibrinogenemia with an Aα chain abnormality. *Thromb. Res.* 25:41, 1982.

148. Takamatsu, J., Ogata, K., Kamiya, T., Koie, K., Takagi, T., and Iwanaga, S.: A novel dysfibrinogenemia with abnormal gamma chain (fibrinogen Nagoya). *Thromb. Haemost.* 42:78, 1979.

149. Bottcher, D., Hasler, K., Kottgen, E., and Maurath, J.: Hereditary hypodysfibrinogenemia with defective release of fibrinopeptide A (fibrinogen Freiburg). *Thromb. Haemost.* 42:78, 1979.

150. Scharrer, I., Kirchmaier, C., and Maas, C.: Untersuchungen zur kongenitalen Dysfibrinogenamie ("Fibrinogen Frankfurt"), in *Fibrinogen, Fibrin und Fibrinkleber*, edited by K. I. Schimpf. F. K. Schattauer, Stuttgart, 1980, p. 165.

151. Owen, C. A., Bowie, E. J. W., Fass, D. N., Perez, R. A., Cole, T. L., and Stewart, M.: Hypofibrinogenemia—Dysfibrinogenemia and von Willebrand's disease in the same family. *Mayo Clin. Proc.* 54:375, 1979.

152. Higgins, D. L., Penner, J. A., and Shafer, J. A.: Fibrinogen Petoskey: Identification of a new dysfibrinogenemia characterized by altered release of fibrinopeptide A. *Thromb. Res.* 23:491, 1981.

153. Higgins, D. L., and Shafer, J. A.: Fibrinogen Petoskey, a dysfibrinogenemia characterized by replacement of Arg-Aα16 by a histidyl residue. *J. Biol. Chem.* 256:12013, 1981.

CHAPTER 154

Congenital deficiency of factor XIII (fibrin-stabilizing factor)

WILLIAM J. WILLIAMS

Deficiency of factor XIII (fibrin-stabilizing factor) was described by Duckert, Jung, and Shmerling in 1960, in a boy with a severe hemorrhagic disorder associated with defective wound healing [1]. The fibrin clots formed in this patient's plasma were soluble in 5 M urea, a property shared by clots formed from purified fibrinogen and ascribed to the absence of factor XIII (see Chap. 132).

Etiology and pathogenesis

The disease is due to an inherited deficiency of factor XIII in both plasma and platelets [2]. Both plasma and platelet factor XIII are converted to an enzymatically active form, factor XIIIa, by thrombin, with calcium as cofactor (see Chap. 132). Factor XIIIa catalyzes the formation of peptide bonds between adjacent molecules of fibrin monomer in the fibrin clot and thus imparts chemical and mechanical stability to the clot. Fibrin stabilization is necessary for effective hemostasis.

The poor wound healing observed in some patients [1,3,4] may be related to the structure of the clot. The plasma clot from one patient did not support normal growth of fibroblasts in tissue culture [5]. In affected patients the levels of factor XIII in the plasma are less than 1 percent of normal [6,7]. Plasma from patients with factor XIII deficiency also does not catalyze the incorporation of glycine ethyl ester into casein, a reaction due to factor XIIIa [8].

Factor XIII in plasma is composed of two a chains and two b chains, while platelet factor XIII consists only of two a chains (see Chap. 132). The plasma of most, but not all, patients with congenital factor XIII deficiency contains material which reacts with antibodies to factor XIII [9–12]. The cross-reacting material is the b chain [10,11,13]. No a chain is detectable in plasma from homozygous factor XIII-deficient patients [10,11,13,14], but residual thrombin-activated transamidase activity is 0.5 to 1.7 percent of normal [14].

Mode of inheritance

The disorder appears to be inherited as an autosomal recessive [6,7,15–17], but sex-linked inheritance has been postulated [18]. Family studies utilizing a quantitative assay for factor XIII indicate that inheritance is autosomal recessive, even in a family with only males affected [16]. Consanguineous marriages have been common in the parents of patients with this disorder [6,17,18]. In some families one or both of the parents have been shown to have factor XIII levels less than normal, while the patients have levels near zero [8, 19–23].

Clinical features

Nearly all patients with factor XIII deficiency have bleeding from the umbilical cord during the first few days of life [6,7]. There follows in severely afflicted patients a lifelong bleeding disorder characterized by ecchymoses, hematomas, and prolonged bleeding following trauma. This has been accompanied, in a few instances, by poor wound healing [1,3,4]. Hemarthroses have occurred in several patients [3,6,24–26]. There is a higher incidence of intracranial hemorrhage than in other inherited bleeding disorders [3,17,19,20,26]. Spontaneous abortion has been recurrent in adult female patients [25,27]. In some patients with factor XIII deficiency, the bleeding is delayed for 12 to 36 h following trauma [1,20,24,26], although others have immediate bleeding. In most patients the disorder is manifest in childhood, usually shortly after birth.

Laboratory features

Blood coagulation studies have been normal except for those bearing on fibrin stabilization. Thus the thromboelastogram has been abnormal [1], and the plasma clots are soluble in 5 M urea or dilute monochloroacetic acid or acetic acid [1,28]. The solubility of the patient's plasma clot in 5 *M* urea is a useful screening test (see Chap. A39). Factor XIIIa may be assayed quantitatively by its ability to catalyze the incorporation of fluorescent [29,30] or radioactive [31,32] amines into proteins such as casein. Chemical methods may also be used [33]. Such tests can be used to identify carriers [16]. The bleeding time, platelet counts, and platelet function tests have been normal.

Differential diagnosis

The disorder must be differentiated from other inherited disorders of blood coagulation. It may be sufficiently severe to be confused clinically with classic hemophilia [6]. The diagnosis depends on demonstration of abnormal solubility of the clot or deficient factor XIIIa by quantitative assay. Abnormal clot solubility may also occur as a result of partial proteolysis of the fibrin, interference with fibrin polymerization by fibrin or fibrinogen split products, structurally abnormal fibrinogens, hyperfibrinogenemia, or abnormal plasma protease activity [7,34].

Acquired deficiencies of factor XIII have been demonstrated in some cases of disorders such as liver disease and tumors [35–41]. The significance of this finding is obscure, but in some patients the decrease in factor XIII levels may be due to disseminated intravascular coagulation [37] or fibrinolysis [38]. Deficient factor XIII activity may be due to inhibitors of factor XIII (see Chap. 157).

Therapy

Replacement therapy in factor XIII deficiency is highly satisfactory because of the small quantities needed for effective hemostasis and the long half-life of this material (up to 19 days) [17,42]. Transfusion of only 2 to 3 ml of plasma per kilogram body weight will induce effective hemostasis for periods of up to 4 weeks (see Chap. 167). Prophylactic therapy using infusions of plasma or cryoprecipitate every 3 to 4 weeks has been successful [6,24,27,43]. Placental factor XIII may prove to be useful in prophylaxis [44], but commercial preparations contain several active components [45] some of which have a short half-life [46]. An antibody inhibitory to factor XIII has appeared in a patient following plasma transfusion [29].

Course and prognosis

The disease leads to excessive hemorrhage after trauma or surgery and carries a significant risk of intracranial hemorrhage and spontaneous abortion. Replacement therapy has been successful in preventing hemorrhage in patients undergoing surgery and in terminating hemorrhage occurring spontaneously or after trauma. Abnormal wound healing is also corrected after trans-

fusion of normal plasma. One woman who had had multiple spontaneous abortions completed a pregnancy successfully while receiving prophylactic transfusions [27]. Patients receiving prophylactic transfusion therapy may be able to live a normal life.

References

1. Duckert, F., Jung, E., and Shmerling, D. H.: A hitherto undescribed congenital haemorrhagic diathesis probably due to fibrin stabilizing factor deficiency. *Thromb. Diath. Haemorrh.* 5:179, 1960.
2. McDonagh, J., McDonagh, R. P., Jr., Delâge, J.-M., and Wagner, R. H.: Factor XIII in human plasma and platelets. *J. Clin. Invest.* 48:940, 1969.
3. Amris, C. J., and Raneh, L.: A case of fibrin-stabilizing factor (FSF) deficiency. *Thromb. Diath. Haemorrh.* 14:332, 1965.
4. Tsevrenis, H., Mandalaki, T., Chouliags, C., and Tzimas, S.: Étude d'un cas avec déficit congénital en facteur XIII (FSF). *Thromb. Diath. Haemorrh.* 14:325, 1965.
5. Beck, E., Duckert, F., and Ernst, M.: The influence of fibrin stabilizing factor on the growth of fibroblasts *in vitro* and wound healing. *Thromb. Diath. Haemorrh.* 6:485, 1961.
6. Britten, A. F. H.: Congenital deficiency of factor XIII (fibrin-stabilizing factor): Report of a case and review of the literature. *Am. J. Med.* 43:751, 1967.
7. Duckert, F., and Beck, E. A.: Clinical disorders due to the deficiency of factor XIII (fibrin stabilizing factor, fibrinase). *Semin. Hematol.* 5:83, 1968.
8. Biloszewski, K., Walls, W. D., and Laskowsky, M. D.: Absence of plasma transamidinase activity in congenital deficiency of fibrin stabilizing factor (factor XIII). *Br. J. Haematol.* 17:159, 1969.
9. Duckert, F.: Le Facteur XIII et la protéine XIII. *Nouv. Rev. Fr. Hematol.* 10:685, 1970.
10. Israels, E. D., Paraskevas, F., and Israels, L. G.: Immunological studies of coagulation factor XIII. *J. Clin. Invest.* 52:2398, 1973.
11. Bohn, H., Becker, W., and Trobisch, H.: Die molekulare Struktur der fibrin stabilisierenden Faktoren des Menschen. II. Vergleichende immunologische Untersuchungen von Faktor-XIII-Mangel plasma und Normal plasma. *Blut* 26:303, 1973.
12. Kiesselbach, T. H., and Wagner, R. H.: Fibrin-stabilizing factor: A thrombin-labile platelet protein. *Am. J. Physiol.* 211:1472, 1966.
13. Barbui, T., et al.: Subunits A and S inheritance in four families with congenital factor XIII deficiency. *Br. J. Haematol.* 38:267, 1978.
14. Rodeghiero, F., and Barbui, T.: Fibrin cross-linking in congenital factor XIII deficiency. *J. Clin. Pathol.* 33:434, 1980.
15. Lorand, L., Urayama, T., Atencio, A. C., and Hsia, D. Y.: Inheritance of deficiency of fibrin-stabilizing factor (factor XIII). *Am. J. Hum. Genet.* 22:89, 1970.
16. McDonagh, J., McDonagh, R. P., Jr., Myllylä, G., and Ikkala, E.: Factor XIII deficiency: A genetic study of two affected kindreds in Finland. *Blood* 43:327, 1974.
17. Kitchens, C. S., and Newcomb, T. F.: Factor XIII. *Medicine* 58:413, 1979.
18. Ratnoff, O. D., and Steinberg, A. G.: Fibrin cross-linking and heredity. *Ann. N.Y. Acad. Sci.* 202:186, 1972.
19. Duckert, F.: The fibrin stabilizing factor. *Ser. Haematol.* 5:58, 1965.
20. Josso, F., Prou-Wartelle, D., Alagille, D., and Soulier, J. P.: La Déficit congénital en facteur stabilisant de la fibrine (facteur XIII): Étude de deux cas. *Nouv. Rev. Fr. Hematol.* 4:267, 1974.
21. Losowsky, M. S., and Hall, R.: Estimation of plasma fibrin-stabilizing factor in families showing congenital deficiencies. *Clin. Sci.* 30:171, 1966.
22. Zahir, M.: Congenital deficiency of fibrin-stabilizing factor: Report of a case and family study. *JAMA* 207:751, 1969.
23. Egeberg, O.: New families with hereditary hemorrhage trait due to deficiency of fibrin-stabilizing factor (factor XIII). *Thromb. Diath. Haemorrh.* 20:534, 1968.
24. Greenberg, L. H., Schiffman, S., and Wong, Y. S. S.: Factor XIII deficiency: Treatment with monthly plasma infusions. *JAMA* 209:264, 1969.

25. Ikkala, E., Myllylä, G., and Nevaliuna, H. R.: Transfusion therapy in factor XIII (FSF) deficiency. *Scand. J. Haematol.* 1:308, 1964.

26. Barry, A., and Delage, J.-M.: Congenital deficiency of fibrin-stabilizing factor. *N. Engl. J. Med.* 272:943, 1965.

27. Fisher, S., Rikover, M., and Nady, S.: Factor 13 deficiency with severe hemorrhagic diathesis. *Blood* 28:34, 1966.

28. Tyler, H. M.: A comparative study of the solvents commonly used to detect fibrin stabilization. *Thromb. Diath. Haemorrh.* 16:61, 1966.

29. Lorand, L., Urayama, T., DeKiewiet, W. C., and Nossel, H. L.: Diagnostic and genetic studies on fibrin-stabilizing factor with a new assay based on amine incorporation. *J. Clin. Invest.* 48:1054, 1969.

30. Hendriksson, P., et al.: A specific fluorescent activity staining procedure applied to plasma and red blood cells in congenital factor XIII deficiency. *Br. J. Haematol.* 44:141, 1980.

31. Dvilansky, A., Britten, A. F. H., and Loewy, A. G.: Factor XIII assay by an isotope method. I. Factor XIII (transamidase) in plasma, serum, leucocytes, erythrocytes and platelets and evaluation of screening tests of clot solubility. *Br. J. Haematol.* 18:399, 1970.

32. Schmer, G.: A solid-phase radioassay for factor-XIII activity (fibrin stabilizing factor) in human plasma. *Br. J. Haematol.* 24:735, 1973.

33. Schwartz, M. L., Pizzo, S. V., Hill, R. L., and McKee, P. A.: The effect of fibrin-stabilizing factor on the subunit structure of human fibrin. *J. Clin. Invest.* 50:1506, 1971.

34. Ragaz, S., Kemp, G., Furlan, M., and Beck, E. A.: Bleeding disorder with abnormal wound healing, and soluble clots and normal factor XIII. *Thromb. Haemost.* 36:537, 1976.

35. Nussbaum, M., and Morse, B. S.: Plasma fibrin stabilizing factor activity in various diseases. *Blood* 23:669, 1964.

36. Walls, W. D., and Losowsky, M. S.: Plasma fibrin stabilizing factor (FSF) activity in normal subjects and patients with chronic diseases. *Thromb. Diath. Haemorrh.* 21:134, 1969.

37. Mandel, E. E., and Gerhold, W. M.: Plasma fibrin-stabilizing factor: Acquired deficiency in various disorders. *Am. J. Clin. Pathol.* 52:547, 1969.

38. Baggett, R. T., Hampton, J. W., and Bird, R. M.: Fibrinolytic bleeding complicated by factor XIII defect. *Arch. Intern. Med.* 121:539, 1968.

39. Losowsky, M. S., and Walls, W. D.: Abnormal fibrin stabilization in renal failure. *Thromb. Diath. Haemorrh.* 22:216, 1970.

40. Losowsky, M. S., and Walls, W. D.: Mechanisms of acquired defects of the stabilization of fibrin. *Br. J. Haematol.* 21:377, 1971.

41. Letheby, B. A., Davis, R. B., and Larsen, A. E.: The effect of major surgical procedures on plasma and platelet levels of factor XIII. *Thromb. Diath. Haemorrh.* 31:20, 1974.

42. Ikkala, E.: Transfusion therapy in congenital deficiencies of plasma factor XIII. *Ann. N.Y. Acad. Sci.* 202:200, 1972.

43. Amris, C. J., and Hilden, M.: Treatment of factor XIII deficiency with cryoprecipitate. *Thromb. Diath. Haemorrh.* 20:528, 1968.

44. Miloszewski, K., and Losowsky, M. S.: Factor XIII concentrate in the long term management of congenital factor XIII deficiency. *Thromb. Diath. Haemorrh.* 34:323, 1975.

45. Hendriksson, P., Nilsson, I. M., Ohlsson, K., and Stenberg, P.: Granulocyte elastase activation and degradation of factor XIII. *Thromb. Res.* 18:343, 1980.

46. Stenbjerg, S.: Prophylaxis in factor XIII deficiency. *Lancet* 2:257, 1980.

Disorders of hemostasis — congenital disorders of uncertain pathogenesis

CHAPTER *155*

Von Willebrand's disease

HARVEY J. WEISS

Definition and history

In 1926, and later in 1931, von Willebrand described a bleeding disorder in 23 of 66 members of three branches of a large family living in the Åland Islands, off the coast of Finland [1]. The disease, in these patients, was inherited as an autosomal dominant trait, and the most consistent abnormality was a prolonged bleeding time. In 1957, many members of this family were also found to have a moderate deficiency of factor VIII–coagulant activity [2,3], an abnormality which had been observed in some patients from other countries during the preceding 5 years [4–8].

Von Willebrand's disease is a lifelong bleeding disorder, with either autosomal dominant or recessive inheritance (see below), which is due to an abnormality of the factor VIII complex different from that observed in hemophilia (see Chap. 152). As discussed elsewhere (see Chap. 132), the nomenclature for this complex is still not satisfactory and could be modified in the future. As used in this book, the term *factor VIII* unmodified refers to the entire protein complex (or complex of proteins) possessing both the procoagulant activity (FVIII:C) that is deficient in hemophilia and the activity (FVIII:vWF) whose deficiency accounts for the prolonged bleeding time in von Willebrand's disease. Current evidence strongly suggests that these two activities reside on two distinct proteins, under separate genetic control [9–11]. The protein possessing FVIII:vWF activity is referred to as FVIII/vWF and is synthesized in endothelial cells [9–11]. Other properties of this protein to be discussed here are those related to antigenicity (FVIIIR:Ag) and a property which is related to its function as a cofactor for the aggregation of platelets by ristocetin (FVIIIR:RCo). FVIII/vWF also has other properties, such as those which support platelet-retention in glass bead filters and platelet-adhesion on subendothelium.

A quantitative or qualitative abnormality of FVIII/vWF accounts for the impaired hemostasis that is characteristically observed in patients with von Willebrand's disease. In plasma, FVIII/vWF is complexed to the factor VIII:C protein lacking in hemophilia and is somehow involved in regulating the plasma level of FVIII:C. In addition, FVIII:vWF is necessary for platelets to function normally, and this accounts for the prolonged bleeding time in patients with von Willebrand's disease.

Other terms previously used to describe patients with this disorder, such as *pseudohemophilia, vascular hemophilia,* and *von Willebrand's-Jurgens' thrombopathia,* should probably be discarded, although each name does connote one or more of the types of defects that are characteristic of this complex disorder. Extensive reviews of both von Willebrand's disease and FVIII/vWF have been published [9–14].

Etiology and pathogenesis

VASCULAR ABNORMALITIES

Although capillary abnormalities have been described in patients with von Willebrand's disease [15], similar changes have been reported in normal subjects [16,17]. However, since FVIII/vWF is synthesized in endothelial cells [18], the older concept of von Willebrand's disease as a vascular disorder [15] has some merit. In addition, some patients appear to develop a type of angiodysplasia [19], which may result in protracted bouts of gastrointestinal bleeding, often without an identifiable source.

DEFECTIVE PLATELET FUNCTION

Platelets from patients with von Willebrand's disease do not function normally in several in vitro tests. As early as 1933, von Willebrand and Jurgens reported that the platelets of patients with this disorder did not agglutinate normally in an instrument known as a capillary thrombometer, while platelets from patients with hemophilia did behave normally [20]. In studies on filtration of venous blood through a column of packed glass beads, the platelet count in filtered normal blood was significantly reduced, indicating that platelets had been retained in the column (see Chap. A41). In contrast, platelet retention is decreased in Von Willebrand's disease [21–24], although the abnormality is not specific for this disorder [25].

Another platelet defect in von Willebrand's disease is failure to aggregate with the antibiotic ristocetin [26–28]. Ristocetin causes platelet aggregation when added to the citrated platelet-rich plasma of normal subjects, but no aggregation occurs in the platelet-rich plasma of patients with severe von Willebrand's disease [26–28]. Among congenital bleeding disorders significant impairment of ristocetin-induced aggregation has been observed only in von Willebrand's disease [29] and in the Bernard-Soulier syndrome (see Chap. 146). However, ristocetin aggregation is not decreased in all patients with von Willebrand's disease, and a subtype of the disorder has been described in which ristocetin aggregation is increased (see below).

The conditions used to demonstrate these abnormalities of platelet function are obviously remote from those occurring in and around blood vessels during the primary arrest of bleeding. Nevertheless, the results of these tests suggest that a defect in platelet function at the site of blood vessel injury might account for the prolonged bleeding time in the disorder. Studies on platelet adhesiveness in vivo support this hypothesis [30]. In normal subjects, fewer platelets are found in blood issuing from standardized cuts on the forearm than in venous blood, suggesting that platelets have been "consumed" by adhesion and aggregation at the sites of vascular injury. In contrast, the platelet counts in venous and incisional blood of patients with von Willebrand's disease are the same [30].

It is possible to study and quantify the interaction (adhesion and aggregation) of platelets in either anticoagulated or directly sampled blood with the subendothelial surface of rabbit aorta, under flow conditions similar to those in arteries. With this technique, the adhesion of platelets to the subendothelium is defective in von Willebrand's disease [31–33] and the magnitude of the defect is enhanced with increasing shear rate [33]. This finding, as well as electron microscopic studies of the hemostatic plug in these patients [34,35], suggests that the adhesion of platelets to vascular structures is decreased in von Willebrand's disease. A defect in platelet-to-platelet, as well as platelet-to-surface, interaction in von Willebrand's disease has also been demonstrated [36].

DEFICIENCY OF A PLASMA FACTOR (FVIII/vWF) NECESSARY FOR PLATELET FUNCTION AND PRIMARY HEMOSTASIS

Although the above evidence strongly suggests abnormal platelet function, the abnormality is not intrinsic to the platelet, since the hemostatic and platelet defects in von Willebrand's disease can usually be corrected by plasma or by plasma fractions that contain factor VIII [6,27,28,37–47].

CORRECTION OF ABNORMAL BLEEDING TIME BY PLASMA OR FACTOR VIII

The bleeding time of patients with von Willebrand's disease is transiently shortened after a transfusion of platelet-poor plasma [37]. The factor responsible for this effect is present in the factor VIII–rich fraction (I-O) prepared from normal plasma [2,6]. The "antibleeding" factor (FVIII:vWF) is distinct from factor VIII procoagulant activity (FVIII:C), since a similar effect on the bleeding time can be demonstrated using both plasma and I-O fractions obtained from patients with hemophilia [2, 6,38,39]. Cryoprecipitate also shortens the bleeding time in patients with von Willebrand's disease [40–42]. The antibleeding factor may not be present in all available factor VIII preparations [39,40,48], and when plasma is

used, large amounts may be necessary to demonstrate this effect [34].

CORRECTION OF DEFECTS OF PLATELET FUNCTION BY PLASMA OR FACTOR VIII

Plasma or some purified factor VIII preparations, including cryoprecipitate, can also correct the defective platelet retention [41,43–47], ristocetin aggregation [27,28], and impaired platelet adhesion on subendothelium [49]. The corrective effects on both retention [46] and ristocetin-induced aggregation [27] are inhibited by a rabbit antibody to factor VIII. The property of factor VIII that corrects the platelet defects is distinct from FVIII:C. Thus the platelet defects in von Willebrand's disease are corrected by hemophilic plasma [27,28,45] and by fractions of hemophilic plasma which come off a chromatography column with factor VIII [23, 46,47] but which, of course, lack FVIII:C activity. In addition, human antibodies to factor VIII, such as those which occur in some hemophilic patients following multiple transfusions (see Chap. 157), can neutralize FVIII:C activity without affecting the ability of the preparation to correct the platelet defects in von Willebrand's disease [27].

The above findings suggest that factor VIII, in addition to correcting the coagulation defect in hemophilia (FVIII:C), is also necessary for proper platelet function in certain in vitro tests, such as platelet retention, ristocetin-induced aggregation, and platelet adhesion on subendothelium. Patients with von Willebrand's disease are deficient in this "platelet" property of factor VIII, as well as in FVIII:C. An assay for one of these platelet properties has been developed, based on the observation that ristocetin will aggregate washed normal platelets in proportion to the amount of this factor that is present [28,50]. Plasma levels of this property of factor VIII (FVIIIR:RCo) are 0 to 50 percent of normal in patients with von Willebrand's disease, whereas values are normal in hemophilia [28,50]. The various combinations of defects involving FVIIIR:RCo and other properties of factor VIII are discussed below under "Laboratory Features."

RELATIONSHIP BETWEEN FVIII:vWF AND FVIIIR:RCo

It is tempting to speculate that FVIIIR:RCo and the factor required for a normal bleeding time (FVIII:vWF) are one and the same. In nontransfused patients with von Willebrand's disease, there is a good correlation between the level of FVIIIR:RCo activity and the bleeding time [50,51], although exceptions have been reported [52]. However, increasing the level of FVIIIR:RCo to normal or near-normal levels by transfusing cryoprecipitate does not always ensure a normalization of the bleeding time [51,53]. The reason for this is not clear at present. A deficiency of factor FVIII/vWF in endothelial cells [54,55], uncorrectable by transfusion [56], could be significant. Other nonconcordant changes in the bleeding time and various FVIII/vWF properties have also been observed during stress and pregnancy [57] and after treatment with deamino-D-arginine vasopressin [58]. Whether these results are due to deficiencies of several closely linked proteins or, as seems more likely, are associated with different degrees of multimerization of FVIII/vWF (see below) remains to be determined.

NATURE OF THE FACTOR VIII DEFECT

Any theory of the nature of the factor VIII defect in von Willebrand's disease must explain both the prolonged bleeding time and the decreased levels of FVIII:C that are observed in patients with severe forms of the disease. Current evidence strongly suggests that patients with this disorder have either a quantitative or a qualitative abnormality of a protein, FVIII/vWF, whose synthesis in endothelial cells is controlled by one or more autosomal genes. This protein can bind to both platelets [59,60] and the subendothelium [61] and thereby promotes the accumulation of platelets [31–33] at sites of blood vessel injury and is responsible for the primary arrest of bleeding. In addition, FVIII/vWF somehow regulates the plasma level of another protein with FVIII:C activity, to which it is complexed noncovalently in plasma (see Chap. 132).

FVIII/vWF exists in plasma as a series of multimers with molecular weights extending to 20×10^6 daltons, composed of dimers or tetramers of a basic subunit whose molecular weight is approximately 0.22×10^6 daltons [11] (see Chap. 132). The biologic expression of the protein probably requires the complete multimeric structure, since removal or absence of the higher M_r polymers results in a loss of both FVIIIR:RCo and FVIII:vWF activity [62]. Hence, an abnormality of primary hemostasis might result from diminished production of the FVIII/vWF subunit in the endothelial cell, from an abnormality in the polymerization, from a specific defect in a functional site on the molecule, or from an abnormality of its catabolism. At present, it is difficult to choose among these various possibilities, and it is likely that a variety of heterogenous abnormalities may account for several defects which constitute what may be better termed the *von Willebrand syndrome.* There is a lack of high-molecular-weight multimers in some patients with von Willebrand's disease [63,64], and these types of abnormalities probably account for the disproportionately decreased FVIIIR:RCo activity and increased mobility of FVIIIR:Ag sometimes observed on two-dimensional crossed immunoelectrophoresis [65–68]. Abnormalities of the carbohydrate content of FVIII/vWF have also been reported in some patients [69,70] but not in others [71].

If an abnormality of FVIII/vWF is the primary genetic defect in von Willebrand's disease, the reason for the associated deficiency of FVIII:C is not clear. FVIII/vWF is complexed noncovalently to the protein with FVIII:C activity [11] and may stabilize the coagulant activity of this protein [72]. However, whether FVIII/vWF regulates FVIII:C activity in plasma by stabilizing it or by regulating synthesis, metabolism, or catabolism is not known. The extraordinary response of FVIII:C levels to

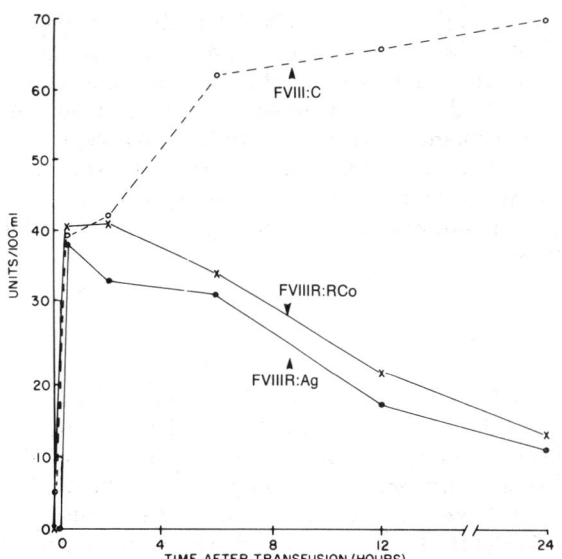

FIGURE 155-1 **Transfusion response in a patient with von Willebrand's disease. Values were obtained after transfusing 10 units of normal cryoprecipitate. Zero-time values are those prior to transfusion.**

transfusion in patients with relatively severe forms of von Willebrand's disease is as yet unexplained. If these patients are transfused with normal plasma, cryoprecipitate, or factor VIII–rich fractions [6,22,73,74] three of the measurable components of factor VIII (VIII:C, VIIIR:Ag, VIIIR:RCo) are increased immediately after transfusion, reflecting their presence in the transfused material (Fig. 155-1). Factor VIII:C often continues to increase while FVIIIR:Ag is decreasing [74] (Fig. 155-1). There is no satisfactory explanation at present for this "new" FVIII:C activity, which is not observed in patients with hemophilia. It could be due to stabilization [72] of normally synthesized FVIII:C by the transfused FVIII/vWF, but other mechanisms are possible.

Mode of inheritance

In contrast to hemophilia, which is sex-linked (see Chap. 152), the inheritance of von Willebrand's disease is autosomal. Although it was previously thought that the disorder was transmitted by a dominant mode of inheritance, a recessive form of the disease, clinically severe and inherited from two clinically normal parents, has been reported [65,75–77]. The dominant form is probably the most commonly encountered type of the disease, and these patients generally are only moderately affected clinically and show variable reductions in components of the factor VIII complex (see below). Patients homozygous for the dominant form of von Willebrand's disease have not been well studied. Patients heterozygous for recessive von Willebrand's disease are generally asymptomatic, but the level of FVIIIR:Ag may sometimes be lower than that of FVIII:C, although the latter finding is inconstant [76–78]. In the homozygous form of recessive von Willebrand's disease, consanguinity is frequent and the clinical symptoms are generally severe. The distinction between recessive and dominant von Willebrand's disease in clinical practice is not always clear-cut, and a more satisfactory description of the genetics of this disorder must await further developments in understanding the molecular biology of factor VIII [14].

Incidence

No racial or ethnic predilection has been reported. The true incidence of the disease has not been clearly established, but the dominant type may be one of the most common congenital bleeding disorders. In Sweden in 1976, there were 785 known cases (240 families) of von Willebrand's disease, which represents a prevalence of 10 cases per 100,000 inhabitants [79]. The corresponding figure for hemophilia in Sweden is 7 per 100,000 [79]. It is likely that very mild cases of von Willebrand's disease remain undiagnosed. The incidence of the severe form has been estimated as 1 per 1 million persons [106].

Clinical features

Symptoms usually appear in early childhood and, for unknown reasons, tend to decrease with age. Fatal bleeding is unusual but does occur [22]. The most common bleeding is mucosal and cutaneous. Epistaxis and easy bruising are among the most frequent symptoms, but petechiae are rare. Gastrointestinal bleeding, often from an undetected site, may be particularly frustrating for both patient and physician. Excessive bleeding associated with surgery often occurs but may be prevented with appropriate therapy (see below). Menorrhagia is common and was present in 15 of 27 women reported in one study [80]. Surprisingly, excessive postpartum bleeding occurred in only 8 of the 22 women who had borne children; this may be related to improvement in the factor VIII:C level and bleeding time abnormalities during pregnancy [80,81]. Hemarthroses are rather infrequent [22] and are usually related to trauma; they are not associated with permanent joint deformity. Some patients with mild laboratory abnormalities may be asymptomatic.

Laboratory features

The laboratory defects are related to the abnormalities of FVIII/vWF and are a reflection of the structural and antigenic properties of this protein and its role in mediating platelet function and the plasma level of FVIII:C.

The bleeding time is prolonged in the majority of patients, but may be at the limit of normal in some pa-

tients having only minimal clinical symptoms or marginally reduced levels of factor VIII–related activities. In general, the incisional (template) Ivy technique for performing the bleeding time is more sensitive than the Duke method in detecting abnormalities [82]. The bleeding time may become excessively prolonged after ingestion of aspirin, even in patients with normal or only slightly prolonged bleeding times [83]. However, an abnormality in this "aspirin-tolerance test" is not specific for von Willebrand's disease and occurs in patients with intrinsic platelet defects as well [83].

The platelet count is usually normal, but thrombocytopenia has been reported in some families [84–87]. Retention of platelets in glass bead filters is usually decreased, provided the test is performed properly [21–24]. However, abnormal platelet retention is not specific for von Willebrand's disease [25]. When abnormal, platelet retention can be corrected by addition of cryoprecipitate or factor VIII [41,45–47]. Aggregation of platelets by collagen and ADP is normal [25]. When the appropriate concentrations of ristocetin are used, ristocetin-induced platelet aggregation in citrated platelet-rich plasma is decreased in most patients with von Willebrand's disease [26–29]. Ristocetin-induced aggregation is almost always decreased in patients with severe clinical symptoms and FVIIIR:RCo levels of 25 percent or less, but may be normal in less severely affected patients [27,29]. In almost all cases, the abnormality of ristocetin-induced aggregation can be corrected by addition of factor VIII or plasma in vitro [27,28], and this correction is probably specific for von Willebrand's disease [29]. Recently, a type of von Willebrand's disease characterized by increased ristocetin aggregation has been described [63,88]. These patients have an abnormal FVIII/vWF that more readily binds to platelets in the presence of ristocetin than does normal FVIII/vWF [88]. In other patients with increased ristocetin-induced aggregation, an enhanced affinity of platelets for FVIII/vWF [89,90,107] and its high-molecular-weight multimers [107] has been demonstrated. This disorder has been termed "pseudo-von Willebrand's disease" [107].

The values of FVIII:C are decreased in the majority of patients with von Willebrand's disease. The lowest values (1 to 5 percent) are found, in general, in patients with the most clinically severe form of the disease who also have very low values for FVIIIR:Ag and FVIIIR:RCo [28,50]. It should be noted that FVIII:C, as well as the bleeding time abnormalities, may show wide fluctuations in the same person on repeated testing. For example, FVIII:C levels and modified Ivy bleeding times were performed simultaneously 100 times on 27 clinically affected members of three families with classic von Willebrand's disease [91]. Both values were abnormal on 53 occasions, only one or the other was abnormal on 36 occasions, and both were normal on 11 occasions. Finally, levels of FVIII:C may be consistently normal in some patients otherwise thought to have von Willebrand's disease by virtue of the FVIII/vWF abnormalities discussed below [65].

The laboratory abnormalities most specific for von Willebrand's disease are those related to the levels and functional properties of the FVIII/vWF, and these are the primary genetic defect in this disorder. The FVIII/vWF, detected by a rabbit antibody to factor VIII, is decreased in von Willebrand's disease but not in hemophilia [92]. Currently, a variety of techniques using specific heterologous antibodies are available for measuring the antigenic properties of FVIII/vWF (FVIIIR:Ag) by electrophoresis and immunoradiometric assays [10–14]. With recent improvements in the assays, detection of FVIIIR:Ag levels as low as 0.01 percent is now possible. The absence of large multimers of FVIIIR:Ag can be detected either by demonstrating a relative lack of slow-moving forms with techniques using two-dimensional crossed electrophoresis or by immunologic analysis of FVIIIR:Ag after separation of the multimers by SDS-agarose gel electrophoresis [11]. Assay of one of the platelet-related properties of FVIII/vWF is based on the observation that ristocetin will aggregate washed normal [50] or formalin-fixed platelets [93] in proportion to the amount of FVIII/vWF present (FVIIIR:RCo activity) [50,93].

The various quantitative and qualitative abnormalities of FVIIIR:Ag, FVIIIR:RCo, and FVIII:C that have been reported in von Willebrand's disease recently emphasize the considerable heterogeneity of the factor VIII–related defects in this disorder. In addition, a tentative classification scheme has been based on the various types of abnormalities found [10,11,64]. There are two main types of the autosomal dominant form of von Willebrand's disease. In type I vWD, levels of FVIIIR:Ag, FVIIIR:RCo, and FVIII:C are usually decreased to about the same extent [10,11,64] and the multimeric structure of FVIII/vWF is normal, as demonstrated by SDS-agarose electrophoresis and by the presence of both fast- and slow-moving forms on crossed immunoelectrophoresis [10,11,64]. In vWD type II, levels of FVIIIR:Ag, FVIIIR:RCo, and FVIII:C are not decreased concordantly; FVIII:C is usually higher than FVIIIR:Ag, and FVIIIR:RCo is even lower or undetectable with current assay techniques [10–14,63–68]. Studies using crossed immunoelectrophoresis and SDS-agarose electrophoresis demonstrate a relative lack of high molecular multimers [63,64], which probably accounts for the disproportionately low FVIIIR:RCo activity. In addition, subtle differences of FVIIIR:Ag may be demonstrated by immunoradiometric assay [94]. Patients with increased ristocetin aggregation (see above) usually show the same general type of plasma abnormalities, although the multimerization defect is somewhat less pronounced than in patients with the typical type II pattern [63,88,107]. Finally, patients with severe recessive von Willebrand's disease usually show an absence of FVIIIR:Ag using sensitive immunoradiometric assays and an absence of FVIIIR:RCo activity [10,14]. FVIII:C activity is usually markedly decreased also, although detectable levels of both FVIII:C and factor VIII coagulant antigen (FVIII:CAg, see Chap. 132) are frequently observed, even when the level of FVIIIR:Ag is less than 0.01 percent [11,14].

Differential diagnosis

Currently, it would seem reasonable to define von Willebrand's disease as a congenital bleeding disorder caused by a quantitative or qualitative defect of FVIII/vWF, assessed by methods described above. The typical patient with this disorder should pose no diagnostic problem, nor should there be any confusion with mild hemophilia, in which FVIIIR:Ag and FVIIIR:RCo are normal. Occasionally, when all values for FVIII/vWF-related properties are borderline, it may be impossible to determine whether the patient has mild von Willebrand's disease or is normal. Patients who show defects of both collagen-induced aggregation and FVIII/vWF (see Chap. 146) have been reported; at present, there is no satisfactory explanation for these findings. Finally, patients have been described who appear to have an acquired form of von Willebrand's disease [95–103]. These have occurred most frequently in patients with autoimmune or lymphoproliferative disorders. Although an immunologic basis for this condition has been suggested, an inhibitor to FVIII/vWF has been detected in only two cases [99,100].

Therapy

Therapy is directed toward increasing the level of FVIII:C and shortening the bleeding time. The FVIII:C level may be increased by the use of cryoprecipitate or fractions that are rich in factor VIII. Correction of the bleeding time is more variable; at present, cryoprecipitate is more predictable than factor VIII–rich preparations, possibly because the latter frequently lack the high-molecular-weight forms of FVIII/vWF [62]. Details of replacement therapy are given in Chap. 167. In patients with clinically mild von Willebrand's disease, the use of ε-aminocaproic acid in association with minor surgical procedures may reduce the amount of perioperative bleeding. In patients with severe and repeated gastrointestinal bleeding in whom no primary site is demonstrable, frequent (weekly to twice weekly) infusions of cryoprecipitate may be necessary.

Intravenously administered deamino-8-D-arginine vasopressin has been used successfully to prevent hemorrhagic complications of surgery in patients with von Willebrand's disease [104,105,108].

Course and prognosis

The prognosis is generally good, although fatal bleeding can occur, particularly in patients with the more severe forms of the disease. For reasons not entirely clear, bleeding episodes may become less frequent with age.

References

1. Von Willebrand, E. A.: Über Hereditäre Pseudohamophilie. *Acta Med. Scand.* 76:521, 1931.
2. Nilsson, I. M., Blomback, M., Jorpes, E., Blomback, B., and Johannsson, S. A.: v. Willebrand's disease and its correction with human plasma fraction I-O. *Acta Med. Scand.* 159:179, 1957.
3. Jürgens, R., Lehmann, W., Wegelius, O., Eriksson, A. W., and Hiepler, E.: Mitteilung uber den Mangel an antihamophilem Globulin (Faktor VIII) bei der Aalandischen Thrombopathie (v. Willebrand-Jurgens). *Thromb. Diath. Haemorrh.* 1:257, 1957.
4. Alexander, B., and Goldstein, B.: Dual hemostatic defect in pseudohemophilia. *J. Clin. Invest.* 32:551, 1953.
5. Nilsson, I. M., Blomback, M., and von Francken, I.: On an inherited autosomal hemorrhagic diathesis with antihemophilic globulin (AHG) deficiency and prolonged bleeding time. *Acta Med. Scand.* 159:35, 1957.
6. Larrieu, M. J., and Soulier, J. P.: Deficit en facteur antihémophilique A chez une fille associée à un trouble saignement. *Rev. Hematol.* 8:61, 1953.
7. Singer, K., and Ramot, B.: Pseudohemophilia type B: Hereditary hemorrhagic diathesis characterized by prolonged bleeding time and decrease in antihemophilic factor. *Arch. Intern. Med.* 97:715, 1956.
8. Bowie, E. J. W., Didisheim, P., and Thompson, J. H.: Von Willebrand's disease: A critical review, in *Hematologic Reviews,* edited by J. L. Ambrus. Dekker, New York, 1968, vol. 1, p. 1.
9. Nilsson, I. M., and Holmberg, L.: Von Willebrand's disease today. *Clin. Haematol.* 8:147, 1979.
10. Meyer, D., and Zimmerman, T. S.: Von Willebrand's disease in *Hemostasis and Thrombosis,* edited by R. Colman, J. Hirsh, V. J. Marder, and E. Salzman. Lippincott, Philadelphia, 1982, p. 64.
11. Zimmerman, T. S., and Meyer, D.: Factor VIII/von Willebrand factor and the molecular basis of von Willebrand's disease, in *Hemostasis and Thrombosis,* edited by R. Colman, J. Hirsh, V. J. Marder, and E. Salzman. Lippincott, Philadelphia, 1982, p. 54.
12. Meyer, D.: Von Willebrand's disease, in *Recent Advances in Blood Coagulation,* 2d ed., edited by L. Poller. Churchill Livingstone, Edinburgh, 1977, p. 183.
13. Hoyer, L. W.: Von Willebrand's disease. *Prog. Hemostasis Thromb.* 3:231, 1976.
14. Bloom, A. L.: The von Willebrand syndrome. *Semin. Hematol.* 17:215, 1980.
15. MacFarlane, R. G.: Critical review: The mechanism of hemostasis. *Q. J. Med.* 10:1, 1941.
16. Jamra, M. M., Lichtenstein, R., Vieira, C. B., and Ribiero-Leite, M. O.: Capilaropatia constitutional: Forma de von Willebrand e forma capilar simples. *Rev. Hosp. Clin. Fac. Med. São Paulo* 7:12, 1952.
17. Buchanan, J. C., and Leavell, B. S.: Pseudohemophilia: Report of 13 new cases and statistical review of previously reported cases. *Ann Intern. Med.* 44:241, 1956.
18. Jaffe, E. A., Hoyer, L. W., and Nachman, R. L.: Synthesis of antihemophilic factor antigen by cultured human endothelial cells. *J. Clin. Invest.* 52:2757, 1973.
19. Ramsay, P. M., et al.: Persistent gastrointestinal bleeding due to angiodysplasia of the gut in von Willebrand's disease. *Lancet* 2:275, 1976.
20. Von Willebrand, E. A., and Jürgens, R.: Über ein neues vererbbates Blutungsübel: Die konstitutionelle Thrombopathie. *Arch. Klin. Med.* 175:453, 1933.
21. Salzman, E. W.: Measurement of platelet adhesiveness: A simple in vitro technique demonstrating an abnormality in von Willebrand's disease. *J. Lab. Clin. Med.* 62:724, 1963.
22. Larrieu, M. J., Caen, J. P., Meyer, D. O., Vainer, H., Sultan, Y., and Bernard, J.: Congenital bleeding disorders with long bleeding time and normal platelet count. II. Von Willebrand's disease (report of 37 patients). *Am. J. Med.* 45:354, 1968.
23. Strauss, H. S., and Bloom, G. E.: Von Willebrand's disease: Use of a platelet adhesiveness test in diagnosis and family investigation. *N. Engl. J. Med.* 273:171, 1965.
24. Weiss, H. J.: Von Willebrand's disease: Diagnostic criteria. *Blood* 32:668, 1968.
25. Weiss, H. J.: Platelet aggregation, adhesion and adenosine diphosphate release in thrombopathia (platelet factor 3 deficiency): A comparison with Glanzmann's thrombasthenia and von Willebrand's disease. *Am. J. Med.* 43:570, 1967.
26. Howard, M. A., and Firkin, B. G.: Ristocetin: A new tool in the investigation of platelet aggregation. *Thromb. Diath. Haemorrh.* 26:362, 1971.
27. Weiss, H. J., Rogers, J., and Brand, H.: Defective ristocetin-induced platelet aggregation in von Willebrand's disease and its correction by factor VIII. *J. Clin. Invest.* 52:2697, 1973.
28. Meyer, D., Jenkins, C. S. P., Dreyfus, D., Fressinaud, E., and Larrieu, M. J.: Willebrand factor and ristocetin-II: Relationship between Willebrand factor, Willebrand antigen and factor VIII activity, *Br. J. Haematol.* 28:579, 1974.
29. Weiss, H. J.: Defects of factor VIII and platelet aggregation: Use of ristocetin in diagnosing the von Willebrand syndrome. *Blood* 45:403, 1975.
30. Borchgrevink, C. F.: Platelet adhesion *in vivo* in patients with bleeding disorders. *Acta Med. Scand.* 170:231, 1961.
31. Tschopp, T., Weiss, H. J., and Baumgartner, H.: Decreased adhesion of platelets to subendothelium in von Willebrand's disease. *J. Lab. Clin. Med.* 83:296, 1974.
32. Weiss, H. J., Tschopp, T. B., and Baumgartner, H. R.: Impaired interaction (adhesion-aggregation) of platelets with the subendothelium in storage pool disease and after aspirin ingestion: A comparison with von Willebrand's disease. *N. Engl. J. Med.* 293:619, 1975.
33. Weiss, H. J., Turitto, V. T., and Baumgartner, H. R.: Effect of shear rate on platelet interaction with subendothelium in citrated and native blood. I. Shear dependent decrease of adhesion in von Willebrand's disease and Bernard-Soulier syndrome. *J. Lab. Clin. Med.* 92:750, 1978.
34. Jorgensen, L., and Borchgrevink, C. F.: The hemostatic mechanism in patients with haemorrhagic disease. *Acta Pathol. Microbiol. Scand.* 60:55, 1964.
35. Hovig, T., and Stormorken, H.: Ultrastructural studies on the platelet plug formation in bleeding time wounds from normal individuals and patients with von Willebrand's disease. *Acta Pathol. Microbiol. Scand. (Suppl. 248)*:105, 1974.
36. Turitto, V. T., Weiss, H. J., and Baumgartner, H. R.: Altered thrombus formation distinct from defective platelet adhesion in von Willebrand's disease (VWD). *Circulation 62 (Suppl. III)*:106, 1980.
37. Schulman, I., Smith, C. H., Erlandson, M., Fort, E., and Lee, R. E.: Vascular hemophilia. *Pediatrics* 18:347, 1956.
38. Cornu, P., Larrieu, M. J., Caen, J., and Bernard, J.: Transfusion studies in von Willebrand's disease: Effect on bleeding time and factor VIII. *Br. J. Haematol.* 9:189, 1963.
39. Weiss, H. J.: The use of plasma and plasma fractions in the treatment of a patient with von Willebrand's disease. *Vox Sang.* 7:267, 1962.
40. Perkins, H. A.: Correction of the hemostatic defects in von Willebrand's disease. *Blood* 30:375, 1967.
41. Weiss, H. J., and Rogers, J.: Correction of the platelet abnormality in von Willebrand's disease by cryoprecipitate. *Am. J. Med.* 53:734, 1972.
42. Hagedorn, B.: Von Willebrand's disease. *JAMA* 216:991, 1971.
43. Salzman, E. W., and Britten, A.: In vitro correction of defective platelet adhesiveness in von Willebrand's disease. *Fed. Proc.* 23:239, 1964.
44. Zucker, M. N.: In vitro abnormality of the blood in von Willebrand's disease correctable by normal plasma. *Nature* 197:601, 1963.
45. Meyer, D., and Larrieu, M. J.: Von Willebrand factor and platelet adhesiveness. *J. Clin. Pathol.* 23:228, 1970.
46. Bouma, B. N., Wiegerinch, Y., Sixma, J. J., von Mourik, J. A., and Mochtar, J. A.: Immunological characterization of purified antihaemophilic factor A (factor VIII) which corrects abnormal platelet retention in von Willebrand's disease. *Nature (New Biol.)* 236:104, 1972.
47. Weiss, H. J., Rogers, J., and Brand, H.: Properties of the platelet re-

tention (von Willebrand) factor and its similarity to the antihemophilic factor (AHF). *Blood 41*:809, 1973.

48. Green, D., and Potter, E. V.: Failure of AHF concentrate to control bleeding in von Willebrand's disease. *Am. J. Med. 60*:357, 1976.

49. Weiss, H. J., Baumgartner, H. R., Tschopp, T. B., Turitto, V. T., and Cohen, D.: Correction by factor VIII of the impaired platelet adhesion to subendothelium in von Willebrand's disease. *Blood 51*:267, 1978.

50. Weiss, H. J., Hoyer, W. W., Rickles, F. R., Varma, A., and Rogers, J.: Quantitative assay of a plasma factor, deficient in von Willebrand's disease, that is necessary for platelet aggregation: Relationship to decreased factor VIII procoagulant activity and antigen content. *J. Clin. Invest. 52*:2708, 1973.

51. Weiss, H. J.: Correlation of the bleeding time with the von Willebrand factor. *N. Engl. J. Med. 291*:420, 1974.

52. Thomson, C., Forbes, C. D., and Prentice, C. R. M.: Evidence for a qualitative defect in factor VIII-related antigen in von Willebrand's disease. *Lancet 1*:594, 1974.

53. Blatt, P. M., Brinkhous, K. M., Culp, H. R., Krauss, J. S., and Roberts, H. R.: Antihemophilic factor concentrate therapy in von Willebrand's disease: Dissociation of bleeding time factor and ristocetin-cofactor activities. *JAMA 236*:2770, 1976.

54. Holmberg, L., Mannucci, P. M., Turesson, I., Ruggeri, A. M., and Nilsson, I. M.: Factor VIII antigen in the vessel walls in von Willebrand's disease and haemophilia A. *Scand. J. Haematol. 13*:33, 1974.

55. Potter, E. V., Chediak, J., and Green, D.: Absence of ristocetin aggregation factor from the skin of a patient with von Willebrand's disease. *Lancet 1*:514, 1976.

56. Mannucci, P. M., Holmberg, L., Ruggeri, Z. M., and Nilsson, I.: Mechanism of the prolonged bleeding time in von Willebrand's disease. *Thromb. Diath. Haemorrh. 34*:607, 1975.

57. Ratnoff, O. D., and Bennett, B.: Clues to pathogenesis of bleeding in Von Willebrand's disease. *N. Engl. J. Med. 289*:1182, 1973.

58. Mannucci, P. M., Pareti, F. I., Holmberg, L., Nilsson, I. M., and Ruggeri, Z. M.: Studies on the prolonged bleeding time in von Willebrand's disease. *J. Lab. Clin. Med. 88*:662, 1976.

59. Doucet-de Bruine, M. H., Sixma, J. J., Over, J., and Beeser-Visser, N. H.: Heterogeneity of human factor VIII. II. Characterization of forms of factor VIII binding to platelets in the presence of ristocetin. *J. Lab. Clin. Med. 92*:96, 1978.

60. Jenkins, C. S. P., Meyer, D., and Larrieu, M. J.: Interaction of ristocetin and von Willebrand factor. *Thromb. Haemost. 35*:752, 1976.

61. Sakariassen, K. S., Bolhuis, P. A., and Sixma, J. J.: Human blood platelet adhesion to artery subendothelium is mediated by factor VIII–von Willebrand factor bound to the subendothelium. *Nature 279*:636, 1979.

62. Weinstein, M., and Deykin, D.: Comparison of factor VIII related von Willebrand factor proteins prepared from human cryoprecipitate and factor VIII concentrate. *Blood 53*:1095, 1979.

63. Ruggeri, Z. M., and Zimmerman, T. S.: Variant von Willebrand's disease: Characterization of two subtypes by analysis of multimeric composition of factor VIII/von Willebrand factor in plasma and platelets. *J. Clin. Invest. 65*:1318, 1980.

64. Meyer, D., Obert, B., Pietu, G., Lavergne, J. M., and Zimmerman, T. S.: Multimeric structure of factor VIII/von Willebrand factor in von Willebrand's disease. *J. Lab. Clin. Med. 95*:590, 1980.

65. Shoai, I., Lavergne, J. M., Ardaillou, N., Obert, B., Ala, F., and Meyer, D.: Heterogeneity of von Willebrand's disease. Study of 40 Iranian cases. *Br. J. Haematol. 37*:67, 1977.

66. Kernoff, P. B. A., Gruson, R., and Rizza, C. R.: A variant of factor VIII related antigen. *Br. J. Haematol. 26*:435, 1974.

67. Peake, I. R., Bloom, A. L., and Giddings, J. C.: Inherited variants of factor VIII-related protein in von Willebrand's disease. *N. Engl. J. Med. 291*:113, 1974.

68. Sultan, Y., Simeon, J., and Caen, J. P.: Electrophoretic heterogeneity of normal factor VIII/von Willebrand protein and abnormal electrophoretic mobility in patients with von Willebrand's disease. *J. Lab. Clin. Med. 87*:185, 1976.

69. Gralnick, H. R.: Factor VIII/von Willebrand factor protein galactose, a cryptic determinant of von Willebrand factor activity. *J. Clin. Invest. 62*:496, 1978.

70. Gralnick, H. R., Coller, B. S., and Sultan, Y.: Carbohydrate deficiency of the factor VIII/von Willebrand factor protein in von Willebrand's disease variants. *Science 192*:56, 1976.

71. Zimmerman, T. S., Wilson, R., and Edgington, T. S.: Carbohydrate of factor VIII/von Willebrand factor in von Willebrand's disease. *J. Clin. Invest. 64*:1298, 1979.

72. Weiss, H. J., Sussman, I. I., and Hoyer, L. W.: Stabilization of factor VIII in plasma by the von Willebrand factor. *J. Clin. Invest. 60*:390, 1977.

73. Biggs, R., and Matthews, J. M.: The treatment of haemorrhage in von Willebrand's disease and the blood level of factor VIII (AHG). *Br. J. Haematol. 9*:203, 1963.

74. Bennett, B., Ratnoff, O. D., and Levin, J.: Immunologic studies in von Willebrand's disease: Evidence that the antihemophilic factor (AHF) produced after transfusion lacks an antigen associated with normal AHF and the inactive material produced by patients with classic hemophilia. *J. Clin. Invest. 51*:2597, 1972.

75. Italian Working Group: Spectrum of von Willebrand's disease: A study of 100 cases. *Br. J. Haematol. 35*:101, 1977.

76. Veltkamp, J. J., and van Tilburg, N. H.: Detection of heterozygotes for recessive von Willebrand's disease by the assay of antihemophilic factor like antigen. *N. Engl. J. Med. 289*:882, 1973.

77. Sultan, Y., Simeon, J., and Caen, J. P.: Detection of heterozygotes in both parents of homozygous patients with von Willebrand's disease. *J. Clin. Pathol. 28*:309, 1975.

78. Zimmerman, T. S., Abildgaard, C., and Meyer, D.: The factor VIII abnormality in severe von Willebrand's disease. *N. Engl. J. Med. 301*:1307, 1979.

79. Silver, J.: Von Willebrand's disease in Sweden. *Acta. Paediatr. Scand. (Suppl.) 238*:5, 1973.

80. Nilsson, I. M., and Blomback, M.: Von Willebrand's disease in Sweden: Occurrence, pathogenesis and treatment. *Thromb. Diath. Haemorrh. 9 (Suppl. 2)*:103, 1963.

81. Strauss, H. S., and Diamond, L. K.: Elevation of factor VIII (antimophilic factor) during pregnancy in normal persons and in a patient with von Willebrand's disease. *N. Engl. J. Med. 269*:1251, 1963.

82. Nilsson, I. M., Magnusson, S., and Borchgrevink, C.: The Duke and Ivy methods for determination of the bleeding time. *Thromb. Diath. Haemorrh. 10*:223, 1963.

83. Bachman, F.: Diagnostic approach to mild bleeding disorders. *Semin. Hematol. 17*:292, 1980.

84. Nielsen, E. G., and Svejaard, A.: Von Willebrand's disease associated with intermittent thrombocytopenia. *Lancet II*:966, 1967.

85. Corder, M. P., Culp, N. W., and O'Neill, B., Jr.: Case report: Familial occurrence of von Willebrand's disease, thrombocytopenia, and severe gastrointestinal bleeding. *Am. J. Med. Sci. 265*:219, 1973.

86. Sultan, Y., Bernal-Hoyos, E. J., Levy-Toledano, S., Jaenneau, C., and Caen, J. P.: Dominant inherited familial factor VIII deficiency (von Willebrand disease) associated with thrombocytopathic thrombocytopaenia. *Pathol. Biol. 22 (Suppl.)*:27, 1974.

87. Rivard, G. E., Daviault, M. B., Brault, N., D'Aragon, L., and Raymond, R.: Von Willebrand's disease associated with thrombocytopenia and a fast migrating factor VIII related antigen. *Thromb. Res. 11*:507, 1977.

88. Ruggeri, Z. M., Pareti, F. I., Mannucci, P. M., Ciavarella, N., and Zimmerman, T. S.: Heightened interaction between platelets and factor VIII/von Willebrand factor in a new subtype of von Willebrand's disease. *N. Engl. J. Med. 302*:1047, 1980.

89. Takahashi, H., Sakuragawa, N., and Shibata, A.: Von Willebrand disease with an increased ristocetin-induced platelet aggregation and a qualitative abnormality of the factor VIII protein. *Am. J. Haematol. 8*:299, 1980.

90. Takashi, H.: Studies on the pathophysiology and treatment of von Willebrand's disease. *Thromb. Res. 19*:857, 1980.

91. Abildgaard, C. F., Simone, J. V., Honig, G. R., Forman, E. N., Johnson, C. A., and Seeler, R. A.: Von Willebrand's disease: A comparative study of diagnostic tests. *J. Pediatr. 73*:355, 1968.

92. Zimmerman, T. S., Ratnoff, O. D., and Powell, A. E.: Immunologic differentiation of classic hemophilia (factor VIII deficiency) and von Willebrand's disease. *J. Clin. Invest. 50*:244, 1971.

93. Allain, J. P., Cooper, H. A., Wagner, R. M., and Brinkhous, K. M.: Platelets fixed with paraformaldehyde: A new reagent for assay of

von Willebrand factor and platelet aggregating factor. *J. Lab. Clin. Med. 85*:318, 1975.

94. Girma, J. P., Ardaillou, N., Meyer, D., Lavergne, J. M., and Larrieu, M. J.: Fluid phase immunoradiometric assay for the detection of qualitative abnormalities of factor VIII/von Willebrand factor in variants of von Willebrand's disease. *J. Lab. Clin. Med. 93*:926, 1979.

95. Simone, J. V., Cornet, J. A., and Abildgaard, C. F.: Acquired von Willebrand's syndrome in systemic lupus erythematosus. *Blood 31*:806, 1968.

96. Ingram, C. I. C., Kingston, P. J., Leslie, J., and Bowie, E. J. W.: Four cases of acquired von Willebrand's syndrome. *Br. J. Haematol. 21*:189, 1971.

97. Mant, M. J., Hirsh, J., Gauldie, J., Bienenstock, J., Pineo, G. F., and Luke, K. H.: Von Willebrand's syndrome presenting as an acquired bleeding disorder in association with a monoclonal gammapathy. *Blood 42*:429, 1973.

98. Ingram, C. I. C., Prentice, C. R. M., Forbes, C. D., and Leslie, J.: Low factor VIII–antigen in acquired von Willebrand's syndrome and response to treatment. *Br. J. Haematol. 25*:137, 1973.

99. Handin, R. I., and Moloney, W. C.: Antibody-induced von Willebrand's disease. *Blood 44*:933, 1974.

100. Wautier, J. L., Levy, S., and Caen, J. P.: Acquired von Willebrand syndrome with inhibitors both to factor VIII clotting activity and ristocetin-induced platelet aggregation. *Br. J. Haematol. 33*:565, 1976.

101. Roseborough, T. K., and Swaim, W. R.: Acquired von Willebrand's

disease, platelet-release defect and angiodysplasia. *Am. J. Med. 65*:96, 1978.

102. Joist, J. H., Cowan, J. F., and Zimmerman, T. S.: Acquired von Willebrand disease: Evidence for a quantitative and qualitative factor VIII disorder. *N. Engl. J. Med. 298*:988, 1978.

103. Meyer, D., Frommel, D., Larrieu, M. J., and Zimmerman, T. S.: Selective absence of large forms of factor VIII–von Willebrand factor in acquired von Willebrand's syndrome: Response to transfusion. *Blood 54*:600, 1979.

104. Mannucci, P. M., Pareti, F. I., Ruggeri, Z. M., and Capitanio, A.: 1-Deamino-8-D-arginine vasopressin: A new pharmacological approach to the management of haemophilia and von Willebrand's disease. *Lancet 1*:869, 1977.

105. Ockelford, P. A., Menon, N. C., and Berry, E. W.: Clinical experience with arginine vasopressin (DDAVP) in von Willebrand's disease and mild haemophilia. *N. Z. Med. J. 92*:375, 1980.

106. Weiss, H. J., Ball, A. P., and Mannucci, P. M.: Incidence of severe von Willebrand's disease. *N. Eng. J. Med. 307*:127, 1982.

107. Weiss, H. J., et al.: Pseudo von Willebrand's disease: An intrinsic platelet defect with aggregation by unmodified human factor VIII/von Willebrand factor and enhanced adsorption of its high molecular weight multimers. *N. Eng. J. Med. 306*:326, 1982.

108. Mannucci, P. M., Canciani, M. T., Rota, L., and Donovan, B. S.: Response of factor VIII/von Willebrand factor to DDAVP in healthy subjects and patients with haemophilia A and von Willebrand's disease. *Brit. J. Haematol. 47*:283, 1981.

Disorders of hemostasis — acquired disorders of blood coagulation

CHAPTER *156*

Disorders of the vitamin K–dependent coagulation factors

BRUCE FURIE

The vitamin K–dependent blood coagulation proteins — factor VII, factor IX, factor X, and prothrombin — are synthesized in the liver. Like other plasma proteins, synthesis requires transcription and translation of nucleic acids and posttranslational modifications including leader sequence cleavage and glycosylation. In a reaction unique to the vitamin K–dependent proteins, certain glutamic acid residues are converted to γ-carboxyglutamic acid by an hepatic carboxylase which requires vitamin K as cofactor (see Chap. 133). Any pathologic process which interferes with the synthetic process in the liver or impairs the availability of vitamin K during protein synthesis can alter the level of activity in plasma of the vitamin K–dependent blood coagulation proteins.

After synthesis, these proteins circulate in the plasma with a characteristic half-life. Deficiency of these factors may also occur by overutilization, as in intravascular coagulation, or by enhanced clearance mechanisms, as has been observed in the factor X deficiency associated with amyloidosis.

Abnormal protein synthesis due to vitamin K deficiency

Factor VII, factor IX, factor X, and prothrombin contain γ-carboxyglutamic acid [1–3]. The complete synthesis of these proteins requires vitamin K as a cofactor for the hepatic vitamin K–dependent carboxylase [4]. In the absence of vitamin K or in the presence of vitamin K

antagonists, these blood clotting proteins contain decreased amounts of γ-carboxyglutamic acid and are functionally inert [5–8]. Clinical manifestations of the deficiency may vary from laboratory evidence of the deficiency state to serious spontaneous hemorrhage.

Ingested food, particularly green leafy vegetables [9], is a primary source of vitamin K in humans. Additionally, intestinal bacteria produce vitamin K_2 which supplements the dietary intake [10]. The daily dietary requirement for vitamin K has been estimated to be less than 1 μg per kilogram body weight [11]. In patients that are severely malnourished and especially those receiving antibiotics, both the dietary source and the bacterial source of vitamin K may be reduced or eliminated [12]. Vitamin K deficiency can develop in an otherwise normal person within 1 to 2 weeks. A common setting of vitamin K deficiency is the postsurgical patient who has developed infectious complications. The absence of dietary intake and the presence of antibiotic therapy often leads to vitamin K deficiency unless vitamin K is administered. Vitamin K deficiency may also be a component of malabsorption syndromes, including sprue, kwashiorkor, or cholestasis.

Vitamin K deficiency is characterized by a prolonged prothombin time and often a prolonged partial thromboplastin time. The diagnosis of vitamin K deficiency is confirmed by the rapid correction by administration of vitamin K of laboratory abnormalities which characterize the deficiency state. By convention, the prothrombin time is used to evaluate and monitor vitamin K deficiency. However, since prolongation of the prothrombin time is not diagnostic of vitamin K deficiency but may be associated with numerous other disorders, the diagnosis of vitamin K deficiency cannot be made unless vitamin K administration completely corrects the prothrombin time. Usually, the prothrombin time becomes normal within 8 to 12 h of administration of vitamin K.

Other laboratory tests which are not now generally available may play an important future role in the diagnosis of vitamin K deficiency. Immunoassay of plasma abnormal prothrombin, the form of prothrombin deficient in γ-carboxyglutamic acid, can be used to diagnose vitamin K deficiency in a single assay [8]. Comparison of thrombin generation by factor Xa and by *Echis carinatus* venom also permits detection of the vitamin K deficiency state and its distinction from other conditions associated with a prolonged prothrombin time, such as liver disease [13].

Vitamin K deficiency should be treated with vitamin K. Since the absorption of oral vitamin K is unreliable, particularly in certain disease states, parenteral vitamin K can be administered. Due to the risks of hematoma formation with intramuscular injection, 10 to 15 mg of vitamin K_1 may be infused intravenously. Because anaphylaxis has been reported, caution must be exercised when one is using this route of administration. Usually, the prothrombin time will approach normal levels within 8 to 12 h. Patients with a significant bleeding disorder who require immediate correction may be treated with fresh frozen plasma as a source of the vitamin K–dependent proteins.

Hemorrhagic disease of the newborn

Hemorrhagic disease of the newborn, first described in 1894 by Townsend [14], is a bleeding disorder in the neonatal period due to vitamin K deficiency [15–17]. Activities of plasma prothrombin, factor VII, factor IX, and factor X are significantly reduced [15,18]. The disorder usually arises between days 2 and 7 after birth, and is manifested by bleeding from mucous membranes, circumcision, and venipuncture sites, and, rarely, internal bleeding and intracranial hemorrhage [19]. Without prophylactic use of vitamin K, about 1 out of 100 children born is afflicted with the syndrome [19] and about 25 percent of those afflicted succumb to serious bleeding. As many as 25 percent of all newborns had laboratory abnormalities consistent with a hemorrhagic potential [20].

The etiology of this disorder is insufficient dietary intake of vitamin K during the newborn period prior to the colonization of the intestine with vitamin K–producing bacteria [21]. Infants that are breast-fed are most susceptible to vitamin K deficiency [19,22], since human milk contains only 15 μg of vitamin K per liter [21,23].

Infants with hemorrhagic disease of the newborn have prolonged prothrombin times and markedly diminished activities of the vitamin K–dependent blood clotting proteins [15,18,19]. The syndrome is rapidly reversed in 4 to 12 h with the administration of vitamin K. A single dose of vitamin K (100 μg) is curative and need not be repeated in the otherwise healthy infant.

In the United States of America all hospital-born infants are now prophylactically treated with vitamin K at birth. Although 25 μg may be an adequate prophylactic dose [24], the usual dosage used is 100 μg to 1 mg [25]. High doses are avoided as vitamin K can interfere with the conjugation of bilirubin in the liver [26] or enhance red cell hemolysis [27].

Deficiency states associated with vitamin K antagonists

Vitamin K, in its reduced form, is required as a cofactor for vitamin K–dependent carboxylation of glutamic acid residues in the precursors of prothrombin, factor VII, factor IX, and factor X. Sodium warfarin, a vitamin K antagonist, inhibits vitamin K–dependent carboxylation, although the mechanism of action of warfarin is not entirely clear [4]. Warfarin may interfere with carboxylation by inhibiting the vitamin K reductase [28].

The vitamin K antagonists, such as sodium warfarin, are widely used as oral anticoagulants. Despite routine monitoring of the prothrombin time, as many as 25 percent of patients treated with warfarin may develop

hemorrhagic complications due to a deficiency of the vitamin K–dependent clotting proteins [29,30]. Occasionally, the accidental use or the surreptitious abuse of these agents can lead to a hemorrhagic disorder [31–33]. Covert anticoagulant ingestion is most likely to be practiced by individuals associated with the medical profession, those with a history of warfarin use, or others with access to these drugs, such as relatives of patients. A behavior disorder often forms the basis for these actions. Treatment of warfarin overdosage varies with the severity of the clinical manifestations and the clinical indication for oral anticoagulation. In the absence of significant bleeding, warfarin may be withheld. Alternatively, the relative vitamin K–deficiency state may be reversed over 6 to 12 h by the administration of vitamin K. Vitamin K (Aquamephyton), 10 to 15 mg, may be infused intravenously. When a bleeding disorder is pronounced and rapid correction is indicated, fresh frozen plasma containing the vitamin K–dependent proteins can be administered.

Liver disease

The liver is the site of synthesis of the vitamin K–dependent blood coagulation proteins [34–36]. Therefore, parenchymal diseases of the liver, including cirrhosis and hepatitis, and infiltrative diseases involving the liver, including metastatic neoplasms, can significantly disrupt the synthesis of the vitamin K–dependent blood coagulation proteins [37–39]. The hemostatic abnormalities of liver disease are often subclinical. Prolongation of the prothrombin time is observed in moderate to severe cases, and is often a poor prognostic sign. The etiology of this laboratory finding may involve multiple abnormalities: (1) decreased synthetic capability of the liver, with a concomitant reduction in the plasma levels of factor V, factor VII, factor X, and prothrombin; the concentrations of all of these proteins influence the prothrombin time; (2) vitamin K deficiency on a dietary basis due to anorexia or improper selection of food; (3) vitamin K deficiency due to malabsorption, based upon intrahepatic or extrahepatic cholestasis or intestinal malabsorption. Fibrinolysis [40] and thrombocytopenia may also contribute to the in vitro laboratory evidence for a potential bleeding disorder. Although des-γ-carboxy forms of prothrombin circulate in the plasma of patients with liver disease, the minor defect in vitamin K–dependent carboxylation does not contribute significantly to the hemostatic disorder [8]. Rather, total synthesis is lowered, as indicated by decreased plasma prothrombin antigen [8,41].

The hemostatic abnormalities often come to clinical attention as a result either of a significant bleeding diathesis associated with liver disease or of a preoperative bleeding evaluation prior to liver biopsy or another surgical procedure. Although a component of the syndrome may be due to vitamin K deficiency, the laboratory disorders are usually not fully corrected by administration of vitamin K. Nonetheless, vitamin K administration assures the clinician that the contribution from cholestasis or malabsorption is corrected. The absence of improvement in the prothrombin time 24 h after administration of vitamin K_1 (10 to 15 mg) intravenously indicates a hemostatic abnormality other than vitamin K deficiency. The administration of fresh frozen plasma in sufficient quantity will partially correct the plasma levels of the vitamin K–dependent proteins and of factor V and may allow surgical intervention [42]. Prothrombin complex concentrates, in the form of factor IX concentrates, have been applied to treatment of the coagulopathy of liver disease [43]. Because numerous cases have been associated with the acute development of thromboembolic disease [44], presumably due to the antithrombin III deficiency which characterizes severe liver disease, these preparations are contraindicated in coagulopathies of hepatic origin.

Enhanced clearance mechanisms

ACQUIRED FACTOR X DEFICIENCY AND AMYLOIDOSIS

Some patients with primary amyloidosis acquire a coagulation disorder characterized by factor X deficiency [45–55] or, occasionally, combined factor IX and factor X deficiency [54,55]. Depending upon the severity of the clotting protein deficiencies, these patients may have hemorrhagic complications superimposed upon the clinical manifestations of amyloidosis.

This disorder is not due to impaired synthesis of factor X. Rather, factor X is rapidly cleared from the blood, and is immobilized along the vasculature and distributed in the monocyte-macrophage system [53]. This is apparently due to the curious affinity of factor X for amyloid fibrils [56].

Therapy of this disorder remains a difficult problem. These patients are refractory to infusion of fresh frozen plasma and to large-volume plasmapheresis and plasma exchange [53]. Transient success with factor IX concentrate, which contains factor X, has been reported [52]. Splenectomy, with concurrent removal of large quantities of amyloid, was associated in a single case with the rapid return of plasma factor X levels to normal [55].

ACQUIRED FACTOR IX DEFICIENCY AND NEPHROTIC SYNDROME

Factor IX deficiency has occasionally been observed in association with the nephrotic syndrome [57,58]. The coincidence of factor IX deficiency and nephrotic syndrome is rare and is usually identified incidentally by a preoperative coagulation test prior to a renal biopsy [59]. The factor IX deficiency is seen in patients with severe proteinuria, with a 24-h urinary protein excretion in excess of 10 g. The etiology of this disorder is not known. The amount of factor IX in the urine protein does not account for the loss of plasma factor IX.

The deficiency state is reversed with remission of the nephrotic syndrome by glucocorticoid therapy.

ACQUIRED FACTOR IX DEFICIENCY AND GAUCHER DISEASE

Acquired factor IX deficiency has also been associated with Gaucher disease [60]. These patients have a shortened plasma factor IX half-life, suggesting that the factor IX is cleared by cerebroside deposits. The factor IX level is not corrected by splenectomy. Despite this and other minor coagulation abnormalities, patients with Gaucher disease have not had hemorrhagic complications due to the factor IX deficiency.

References

1. Nelsestuen, G. L., Zytkowicz, T. H., and Howard, J. B.: The mode of action of vitamin K: Identification of γ-carboxyglutamic acid as a component of prothrombin. *J. Biol. Chem.* 249:6347, 1974.
2. Stenflo, J., Fernlund, P., Egan, W., and Roepstorff, P.: Vitamin K–dependent modifications of glutamic acid residues in prothrombin. *Proc. Natl. Acad. Sci. U.S.A.* 71:2730, 1974.
3. Nemerson, Y., and Furie, B.: Zymogens and cofactors of blood coagulation. *CRC Crit. Rev. Biochem.* 9:45, 1980.
4. Suttie, J. W.: Vitamin K-dependent carboxylation. *CRC Crit. Rev. Biochem.* 8:191, 1980.
5. Ganrot, P. O., and Nilehn, J.-E.: Plasma prothrombin during treatment with dicumarol. *Scand. J. Clin. Lab. Invest.* 22:23, 1968.
6. Friedman, P. A., Rosenberg, R. D., Hauschka, P. V., and Fitz-James, A.: A spectrum of partially carboxylated prothrombins in the plasma of coumarin-treated patients. *Biochim. Biophys. Acta* 494:271, 1977.
7. Esnouf, M. P., and Prowse, C. V.: The gamma-carboxyglutamic acid content of human and bovine prothrombin following warfarin treatment. *Biochim. Biophys. Acta* 490:471, 1977.
8. Blanchard, R. A., Furie, B. C., Jorgensen, M., Kruger, S. F., and Furie, B.: Acquired vitamin K–dependent carboxylation deficiency in liver disease. *New Engl. J. Med.* 305:242, 1981.
9. Almquist, H. J., and Stokstad, E. L. R.: Hemorrhagic chick disease of dietary orign. *J. Biol. Chem.* 111:105, 1935.
10. McKee, R. W., et al.: The isolation of vitamin K_2. *J. Biol. Chem.* 131:327, 1939.
11. Frick, P. G., Riedler, G., and Brogli, H.: Dose response and minimal daily requirement for vitamin K in man. *J. Appl. Physiol.* 23:387, 1967.
12. Ansell, J. E., Kumar, R., and Deykin, D.: The spectrum of vitamin K deficiency. *JAMA* 237:40, 1977.
13. Bertina, R. M., Van der Marel-van Nieuwkoop, W., Dubbeldam, J., Boekhout-Mussert, R. J., and Veltkamp. J. J.: New method for the rapid detection of vitamin K deficiency. *Clin. Chim. Acta* 105:93, 1980.
14. Townsend, C. W.: The hemorrhagic disease of the newborn. *Arch. Pediatr.* 11:559, 1894.
15. Brinkhous, K. M., and Smith, H. P.: Plasma prothrombin level in normal infancy and in hemorrhagic disease of the newborn. *Am. J. Med. Sci.* 193:475, 1937.
16. Dam, H., and Tage-Hansen, E.: Vitamin K lack in normal and sick infants. *Lancet* 2:1157, 1939.
17. Dam, H., and Dyggve, H.: Relation of vitamin K deficiency to hemorrhagic disease of the newborn. *Adv. Pediatr.* 5:129, 1952.
18. Aballi, A. J.: The action of vitamin K in the neonatal period. *South. Med. J.* 58:48, 1965.
19. Sutherland, J. M., Glueck, H. I., and Glesser, G.: Hemorrhagic disease of the newborn. *Am. J. Dis. Child.* 113:524, 1967.
20. Wefring, K. W.: Hemorrhage in the newborn and vitamin K prophylaxis. *J. Pediatr.* 61:686, 1962.
21. Dam, H., et al.: The relation of vitamin K deficiency to hemorrhagic disease of the newborn. *Adv. Pediatr.* 5:129, 1952.

22. Keenan, W. J., Jewett, T., and Glueck, H. I.: Role of feeding and vitamin K in hypoprothrombinemia of the newborn. *Am. J. Dis. Child.* 121:271, 1971.

23. Schneider, D. L., Fluckiger, H. B., and Manes, J. D.: Vitamin K content of infants formula products. *Pediatrics* 53:273, 1974.

24. Aballi, A. J., and de Lamerens, S.: Coagulation changes in the neonatal period and in early infancy. *Pediatr. Clin. North Am.* 9:785, 1962.

25. Committee on Nutrition, American Academy of Pediatrics: Vitamin K supplementation for infants receiving milk substitute infant formulas and for those with fat malabsorption. *Pediatrics* 48:483, 1972.

26. Bound, J. P., and Telfer, J. P.: Effect of vitamin K dosage on plasma bilirubin levels in premature infants. *Lancet* 1:720, 1956.

27. Allison, A. C.: Danger of vitamin K to newborn. *Lancet* 1:669, 1955.

28. Whitlon, R. D. S., Sadowski, J. A., and Suttie, J. W.: Mechanisms of coumarin action: Significance of vitamin K epoxide reductase inhibition. *Biochemistry* 17:1371, 1978.

29. Allen, E. V.: The clinical use of anticoagulants. *JAMA* 134:323, 1947.

30. Wright, I. S., Beck, D. F., and Marple, C. D.: Myocardial infarction and its treatment with anticoagulants. *Lancet* 1:92, 1954.

31. O'Reilly, R. A., and Aggeler, P. M.: Covert anticoagulant ingestion: Study of 25 patients and review of world literature. *Medicine* 55:389, 1976.

32. O'Reilly, R. A., Aggeler, P. M., and Gibbs, J. O.: Hemorrhagic state due to surreptitious ingestion of bishydroxycoumarin. *N. Engl. J. Med.* 267:19, 1962.

33. Bowie, E. J. W., Todd, M., Thompson, J. H., Jr., Owen, C. A., Jr., and Wright, I. S.: Anticoagulant malingerers ("the dicoumarol-eaters"). *Am. J. Med.* 39:855, 1965.

34. Mann, F. D., Shonyo, E. S., and Mann, F. C.: Effect of removal of the liver on blood coagulation. *Am. J. Physiol.* 164:111, 1951.

35. Pool, J., and Robinson, J.: In vitro synthesis of coagulation factors by rat liver slices. *Am. J. Physiol.* 196:423, 1959.

36. Olson, J. P., Miller, L. L., and Troup, S. B.: Synthesis of clotting factors by the isolated perfused rat liver. *J. Clin. Invest.* 45:690, 1966.

37. Ratnoff, O. D.: Hemostatic mechanisms in liver disease. *Med. Clin. North Am.* 47:721, 1963.

38. Rapaport, S. I., Ames, S. B., Mikkelsen, S., and Goodman, J. R.: Plasma clotting factors in chronic hepatocellular disease. *N. Engl. J. Med.* 263:278, 1960.

39. Donaldson, G. W. K., Davies, S. H., Darg, A., and Richmond, J.: Coagulation factors in chronic liver disease. *J. Clin. Pathol.* 22:199, 1969.

40. Pises, P., and Bick, R.: Hyperfibrinolysis in cirrhosis. *Am. J. Gastroenterol.* 60:280, 1973.

41. Corrigan, J. J., and Earnest, D. L.: Factor II antigen in liver disease and warfarin-induced vitamin K deficiency. *Am. J. Hematol.* 8:249, 1980.

42. Spector, I., Corn, M., and Ticktin, H. E.: Effect of plasma transfusions on the prothrombin time and clotting factors in liver disease. *N. Engl. J. Med.* 275:1032, 1966.

43. Green, G., Dymock, I. W., Poller, L., and Thomson, J. M.: Use of factor VII-rich prothrombin complex concentrate in liver disease. *Lancet* 1:1311, 1975.

44. Blatt, P. M., Lundblad, R. L., Kingdon, H. S., McLean, G., and Roberts, H. R.: Thrombogenic materials in prothrombin complex concentrates. *Ann. Intern. Med.* 81:766, 1974.

45. Korsan-Bengsten, K., Hjort, P. F., and Ygge, J.: Acquired factor X deficiency in a patient with amyloidosis. *Thromb. Diath. Haemmorrh.* 7:558, 1962.

46. Howell, M.: Acquired factor X deficiency associated with systematized amyloidosis. *Blood* 21:739, 1963.

47. Pechet, L., and Kastrul, J. J.: Amyloidosis associated with factor X (Stuart) deficiency. *Ann. Intern. Med.* 61:315, 1964.

48. Jacobson, R. J., Sandler, S. G., and Rath, C. E.: Systemic amyloidosis associated with micro-angiopathic haemolytic anaemia and factor X (Stuart factor) deficiency. *S. Afr. Med. J.* 46:1634, 1972.

49. Bernhardt, B., Valletta, M., Brook, J., and Lejnieks, I.: Amyloidosis with factor X deficiency. *Am. J. Med. Sci.* 264:411, 1972.

50. van der Meer, J. W. M., and Mosmans-Smits, A. A. H.: Miltruptuur bij primaire amyloidose. *Ned. T. Geneesk.* 117:1733, 1973.

51. Galbraith, P. A., Sharma, N., Parker, W. L., and Kilgour, J. M.: Acquired factor X deficiency. *JAMA* 230:1658, 1974.

52. Spero, J. A., Lewis, J. H., Hasiba, V., and Ellis, L. D.: Treatment of amyloidosis associated factor X deficiency. *Thromb. Haemostasis* 35:377, 1976.

53. Furie, B., Greene, E., and Furie, B. C.: Syndrome of acquired factor X deficiency and systemic amyloidosis. *N. Engl. J. Med.* 297:81, 1977.

54. McPherson, R. A., Onstad, J. W., Ugoretz, R. J., and Wolf, P. L.: Coagulopathy in amyloidosis: Combined deficiency of factor IX and X. *Am. J. Hematol.* 3:225, 1977.

55. Greipp, P. R., Kyle, R. A., and Bowie, E. J. W.: Factor X deficiency in primary amyloidosis. *N. Engl. J. Med.* 301:1018, 1979.

56. Furie, B., Voo, L., McAdam, K. P. W. J., and Furie, B. C.: Mechanism of factor X deficiency in systemic amyloidosis. *N. Engl. J. Med.* 304:827, 1981.

57. Handley, D. A., and Lawrence, J. R.: Factor IX deficiency in the nephrotic syndrome. *Lancet* 1:1079, 1967.

58. Natelson, E. A., Lynch, E. C., Hettig, R. A., and Alfrey, C. P.: Acquired factor IX deficiency in the nephrotic syndrome. *Ann. Intern. Med.* 73:373, 1970.

59. Vaziri, N. D., Branson, H. E., and Ness, R.: Changes in coagulation factors IX, VIII, VII, X, and V in nephrotic syndrome. *Am. J. Med. Sci.* 280:167, 1980.

60. Boklan, B. F., and Sawitsky, A.: Factor IX deficiency in Gaucher disease. *Arch. Intern. Med.* 136:489, 1976.

CHAPTER *157*

Acquired anticoagulants

BRUCE FURIE

Inhibitors of coagulation factors, also known as acquired or circulating anticoagulants, can cause serious impairment of the hemostatic process. The identification of blood coagulation inhibitors is part of a thorough evaluation of patients with hemorrhagic disorders. Such anticoagulants are usually immunoglobulins. In patients with hemophilia or other hereditary clotting disorders, they are manifestations of an immune response in which antibodies arise by direct stimulation from a "foreign" antigen occurring when the deficient factor is replaced. In patients with systemic lupus erythematosus and other autoimmune diseases, the circulating anticoagulants arise as a result of a disorder of immune regulation. Monoclonal immunoglobulins with inhibitory activity against blood coagulation components can develop in patients with plasma cell or lymphocytic disorders. Acquired anticoagulants may occasionally appear in patients with no evidence of underlying disease and have been the subjects of a number of comprehensive reviews [1–5].

Assay of specificity

Plasma which yields a prolonged partial thromboplastin time (PTT) should be further evaluated to distinguish between a deficiency in a component or components of the intrinsic pathway of blood coagulation and an inhibitor directed at a component of that system. A coagulation inhibitor is assumed to be present if prolongation of the PTT of a mixture of equal parts of the patient's plasma and normal plasma persists after incubation. The specificity of the inhibitor determines the nature of the hemorrhagic disorder. An antibody against one of the contact-phase components, such as factor XII, does not pose a clinical problem. In contrast, antibodies against factor VIII or factor IX can be associated with severe bleeding disorders. Determination of the specificity of an inhibitor may require elaborate laboratory facilities, and often a research coagulation laboratory is needed. Factor-specific assays may be misleading since the inhibitor may interfere with the assay itself (e.g., an anti-factor IX antibody will bind to factor IX in the factor VIII–deficient substrate plasma used to assay factor VIII, suggesting fallaciously that the factor VIII level is low). This problem can be circumvented if the rate of antibody-antigen interaction is slow or if specific factor assays are performed on diluted plasmas [6]. Alternatively, isolated coagulation proteins can be added to test plasma to neutralize the inhibitor [7]. Restoration of the PTT to within the normal range indicates that the added factor is the antigen against which the antibody is directed.

Factor VIII Inhibitors

FACTOR VIII INHIBITORS ASSOCIATED WITH HEMOPHILIA A

Factor VIII inhibitors are most commonly observed in patients with hemophilia A. These antibodies arise in response to factor VIII contained in transfused plasma or plasma products. With one possible exception [8], inhibitors have appeared in patients with factor VIII deficiency only after transfusion therapy [9–13]. Hemophilic patients with the lowest factor VIII levels (less than 1 percent) are most prone to develop circulating factor VIII inhibitors. These patients are also the most severely afflicted and require the most extensive transfusion therapy. However, there appears to be no direct relationship between the transfusion requirement and the development of an inhibitor. Overall, about 6 to 7 percent of patients with hemophilia acquire anti-factor VIII antibodies [9–11]. Such an event represents a turning point in the management of an individual since the therapeutic strategies and problems of the hemophilic patient with an inhibitor are very different from those of patients without anti-factor VIII antibodies. No methods currently exist to predict which patients will develop inhibitors. Although a genetic predisposition must play some role, there are no convincing data to support a familial tendency [11–13].

CHEMISTRY

The circulating anticoagulants directed against factor VIII in patients with hemophilia A are IgG immunoglobulins [14–16]. The inhibitory activity resides in the Fab fragment, presumably in the antibody combining site [16]. These inhibitors are oligoclonal and, as such, are heterogeneous with regard to charge and affinity for factor VIII [17–19]. Although initial studies with anti-κ and anti-λ light-chain antibodies suggested the monoclonality of these inhibitors [20], it is now apparent that they show a restricted heterogeneity but are not monoclonal. Subtyping of antibodies with anti–heavy chain antisera has shown a curious restriction of inhibitors to the following subclasses: IgG$_4$ [21], IgG$_1$ and IgG$_4$ [19], and IgG$_3$ and IgG$_4$ [18]. The dominance of an otherwise minor immunoglobulin subclass, IgG$_4$, is noteworthy. This subclass does not fix complement, which may explain why these patients do not develop serum sickness and immune complex disease. In most cases, the light chain has been of a single class, usually of the κ type. The antibodies form soluble, nonprecipitating complexes with factor VIII and inhibit factor VIII coagulant activity. With rare exception [22], there is no interaction of these antibodies with factor VIII:von Willebrand factor. Comprehensive studies of the inhibitor have been thwarted by the unavailability of purified human factor VIII. However, these inhibitors may be highly potent, based on the low factor VIII concentration in normal plasma and the apparent high affinity of the inhibitor for factor VIII. The kinetics of interaction of the antibody and factor VIII are poorly characterized [23]. Perhaps due to the low concentration of antibody and antigen or to the conformational specificity of the antibody, interaction is often slow and may not be complete even after several hours [15,23]. Some evidence suggests that higher-affinity antibodies are elicited after antigenic stimulation with factor VIII [24].

NATURE OF THE IMMUNE RESPONSE

The immune response in hemophilia A after exposure to factor VIII is variable. Some patients develop low levels of inhibitor despite repeated replacement therapy (low responders), while others develop high levels of inhibitor after any exposure to factor VIII (high responders). Patients who have been low responders to factor VIII administration usually remain low responders. Patients who have been high responders continue to show marked induction of inhibitor after factor VIII exposure. In patients with inducible inhibitors, factor VIII therapy leads to an amnestic rise in the inhibitor which begins 2 to 4 days after the factor VIII is given (Fig. 157-1). The level that the inhibitor reaches is variable, but the peak is usually attained within 1 to 3 weeks [13]. In the absence of further factor VIII therapy, the plasma inhibitor level gradually falls over several months to several years. In some patients, the inhibitor drops to very low titer or may even disappear. In other patients, significant anti-factor VIII antibody titers may circulate years after the last exposure to factor VIII [13]. Several cases have been observed in which the inhibitor disappeared spontaneously despite subsequent factor VIII therapy [13,25]. Because of the varia-

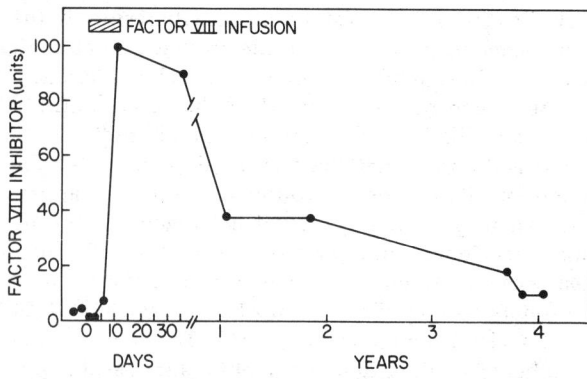

FIGURE 157-1 Immune response of a patient with hemophilia with an inhibitor to factor VIII. A young man with hemophilia A and a factor VIII inhibitor developed a large hematoma in his right quadriceps. Active bleeding persisted despite conservative measures. On day 0, the patient (55 kg) was treated initially with 6000 units of factor VIII followed by 1680 units every 2 h. Levels of plasma FVIII:C between 50 and 100 percent of normal were obtained. Cyclophosphamide, 200 mg per square meter of body area, was given intravenously every day for 3 consecutive days in an attempt to blunt the immune response. The inhibitor was neutralized for 3 days, but the half-life of infused factor VIII was short. The factor VIII infusion dosage was titrated on the basis of the plasma FVIII:C level. Hemostasis was rapidly achieved, and factor VIII treatment was continued on an accelerated schedule as the inhibitor titer rose. On day 11, the inhibitor titer peaked and a factor VIII level above 3 percent could not be maintained. Factor VIII infusions were discontinued on day 12. Clinical rehabilitation continued without complication, and the patient returned to his original status. In the absence of repeated factor VIII exposure, his factor VIII inhibitor titer remains significant 4 years later.

bility of the immune response to factor VIII in patients with hemophilia A, therapies designed to interfere with factor VIII alloantibody production have been difficult to evaluate.

LABORATORY DIAGNOSIS
The presence of a circulating inhibitor may be suspected if, after 2 h of incubation at 37°C, a mixture of the patient's plasma and normal plasma yields a prolonged activated PTT [26]. The loss of factor VIII activity in the mixture can be ascribed to the factor VIII inhibitory activity. Although useful for screening purposes, this test lacks specificity and sensitivity since (1) antibodies against other coagulation proteins can lead to prolongation of the PTT and thus the test is not specific for anti-factor VIII and (2) the PTT precludes measurement of low levels of anti-factor VIII antibody since it is prolonged only if the factor VIII level is below 30 to 40 percent of normal values. Many centers currently use a common protocol for quantitation of factor VIII inhibitors [27]. Citrated test plasma (diluted or undiluted) is incubated at 37°C for 2 h with an equal volume of pooled normal human citrated plasma. Factor VIII coagulant activity (FVIII:C) in this mixture is then assayed

using factor VIII–deficient plasma. A test sample producing a residual factor VIII activity of 50 percent of normal is considered to contain one Bethesda unit of inhibitor per milliliter.

MANAGEMENT OF FACTOR VIII INHIBITORS
Because of the possibility of a factor VIII inhibitor and the induction of an amnestic response to factor VIII, careful evaluation is necessary before factor VIII concentrates or plasma products are administered to a patient with hemophilia. With the possible exception of the most emergent situations, a patient with hemophilia should be questioned as to a past history of an inhibitor. Review of the medical record may also provide valuable information. A positive history should certainly lead to consideration of alternative therapeutic measures. Knowledge of the current titer of the inhibitor, whether or not the inhibitor is inducible, and complete assessment of the severity and implications of the clinical bleeding episode are factors which enable appropriate management of this difficult problem.

Three different approaches are available to treat the bleeding hemophiliac patient with a circulating anticoagulant: (1) conservative management without parenteral therapy, (2) prothrombin complex infusion therapy, and (3) factor VIII concentrate infusion therapy. These therapies should be directed by physicians with experience in the care of patients with hemophilia. The therapeutic goals are to stop bleeding, minimize injury due to inflammation, control pain, and avoid, if possible, induction of anti-factor VIII antibodies.

Simple lacerations, mild hemarthroses, or low-grade mucosal or intramuscular bleeding may be best managed expectantly with direct pressure or cold compresses, judicious use of pain medications, and patience. Aggressive therapy for hemophilic patients with inhibitors should be reserved for serious or life-threatening hemorrhage.

Prothrombin complex concentrates have proved efficacious for the management of hemophilic bleeding complicated by factor VIII inhibitors [28–31]. These concentrates are rich in factor IX, factor X, prothrombin, and, variably, factor VII, and bypass the factor VIII reaction during coagulation by an as yet unknown mechanism. They have been successfully used to treat spontaneous bleeding episodes, traumatic bleeding, and bleeding during surgical procedures in which the operative benefits outweighed the risks. There are no reliable methods to titrate the effect of these agents in vitro, and the major problem is to decide on proper dosage. Administration of too little prothrombin complex concentrate may not alter bleeding in vivo [32]. Too much concentrate is thrombogenic and may lead to venous thrombosis, pulmonary embolization, or death [33,34]. For these reasons, treatment is often empirical and restrained. Although these products often transmit hepatitis, the frequently transfused hemophilic patient is not at risk due to prior exposure. Refinement of the factor IX concentrates have reduced both their thrombogenic potential and their efficacy in the treatment of factor VIII inhibitors. A new product, Autoplex (Hyland Laboratories) has been licensed and demonstrated to be highly effective. One unit of factor VIII correctional activity is that quantity of activated prothrombin complex which will correct the activated PTT of inhibitor plasma. The recommended dosage range is 25 to 100 factor VIII correctional units per kilogram of body weight. The dosage is monitored with the prothrombin time. The postinfusion prothrombin time should be no less than two-thirds of the preinfusion value. As before, this material can induce a hypercoagulable state and may be associated with thromboembolic complications. This material is very expensive and should be reserved for the most serious bleeding episodes. Prothrombin complex concentrates contain small quantities of factor VIII [35] and can lead to an amnestic response, with a rise in the factor VIII inhibitor in about one-third of treated patients [36]. In summary, the activated prothrombin complex concentrate can be very valuable in the treatment of some patients with hemophilia A and factor VIII inhibitors. It should be reserved for patients with high inhibitor levels and serious bleeding episodes. The expense of therapy, the risks of complicating thromboembolic disease, and the inadequacy of dosage monitoring are the major deterrents to its use.

Alternatively, some patients with hemophilia A and factor VIII inhibitors may be successfully treated with factor VIII concentrates. Those patients with low-titer inhibitors which are not inducible (i.e., do not increase upon treatment with factor VIII) can be managed with factor VIII concentrates. Initial doses of factor VIII are used to neutralize the plasma inhibitor. Because the half disappearance time of transfused factor VIII may be shortened, infusions must be given frequently (from every 1 to every 4 h). Because of the neutralization of factor VIII by humoral antibodies and cellular elements, the amount of factor VIII that must be infused is considerably larger than that required to treat hemophilia A without a circulating inhibitor. Factor VIII levels should be assayed regularly to facilitate adjustment of the factor VIII dosage to maintain adequate but not excessive levels.

Hemophilic patients with inducible inhibitors (high responders) may also be treated with factor VIII concentrates if the inhibitor titer is low initially. The quantity of factor VIII needed to neutralize inhibitors in excess of 3 to 6 Bethesda units is large and may not be economically and logistically feasible. If adequate levels of factor VIII can be maintained for 2 to 4 days after the initiation of factor VIII therapy, hemostasis can usually be achieved. As the factor VIII inhibitor level rises during the amnestic response, factor VIII therapy should be continued. If given on a frequent basis (e.g., every hour), a significant factor VIII level may be attained intermittently despite a high inhibitor titer because the rate of neutralization of factor VIII inhibitors is slow [23]. These measures should be reserved for patients

with serious, life-threatening bleeding episodes. Treatment of this type usually precludes use of this same therapeutic strategy for at least several months and maybe several years.

Animal factor VIII, prepared from bovine or porcine plasma, is available in Europe but is restricted to experimental use in the United States. These preparations produce therapeutic levels of factor VIII in treated patients. They carry no hepatitis risk but may lead to the appearance of antibodies to animal factor VIII.

Efforts to reduce inhibitor titers with immunosuppressive agents have not been successful. Regimens including cyclophosphamide [37], cyclophosphamide and prednisone [25], and 6-mercaptopurine [38] have been examined. Although some patients show disappearance of the inhibitor after such treatment, other patients undergo spontaneous remissions without specific therapy. The probability of response to immunosuppressive therapy is not yet known, and this approach should not be considered a standard treatment.

Plasmapheresis can be used as an adjunct to management of the bleeding patient with hemophilia to reduce the concentration of anti-factor VIII in plasma prior to initiation of factor VIII therapy. The reduction in inhibitor levels is transient because the inhibitor is an IgG and rapidly reequilibrates from the extravascular space into the intravascular space.

FACTOR VIII INHIBITORS IN PATIENTS WITHOUT HEMOPHILIA

Factor VIII inhibitors may arise in autoimmune diseases, lymphoproliferative disorders and plasma cell dyscrasias, during and after pregnancy, as an allergic reaction during drug therapy, and, occasionally, spontaneously in otherwise healthy individuals. These inhibitors differ from those which appear in hemophiliacs.

Factor VIII inhibitors may accompany severe allergic reactions to drugs. Multiple cases of hemorrhagic disorders occurring as a complication of penicillin therapy have been due to the development of a circulating inhibitor of factor VIII [21,39–41]. These patients have usually had other major manifestations of penicillin allergy. The factor VIII inhibitors studied have been IgG [21,41,42]. These antibodies do not cross-react with penicillin, nor do antipenicillin antibodies inhibit factor VIII. The etiology of these inhibitors is unknown. Upon discovery of this syndrome, prompt withdrawal of penicillin is indicated. In addition to penicillin, sulfonamides [43] and phenytoin [44] have also been associated with the development of inhibitors to factor VIII.

A rare hemophilia-like disease associated with pregnancy and usually occurring within a year after parturition is caused by an anticoagulant directed against factor VIII [20,45–48]. One patient developed this syndrome prior to delivery [47]. In most cases, affected women have had no underlying disorder and had normal pregnancies and deliveries. The course of the disease is variable but is usually self-limited, lasting for several months.

Factor VIII inhibitors may be associated with collagen-vascular disease [20,40,49,50], including systemic lupus erythematosus, rheumatoid arthritis, and ulcerative colitis [15]. Occasionally, these inhibitors arise spontaneously in apparently well individuals [40]. These patients are often elderly and may have benign monoclonal gammopathies.

Factor VIII inhibitors are occasionally observed in patients with disorders such as multiple myeloma and Waldenstrom's macroglobulinemia [51–54]. In macroglobulinemia, an IgM monoclonal antibody with light chains had anti-factor VIII activity that disappeared with treatment of the macroglobulinemia [52]. A patient with IgA myeloma also manifested factor VIII inhibitor activity [53]. The inhibitor-factor VIII interaction could be eliminated by use of penicillamine to reduce the disulfide bonds in vivo.

An acquired deficiency of factor VIII coagulant activity and factor VIII:von Willebrand factor activity was described in a patient with Waldenstrom's macroglobulinemia and an IgM paraprotein [54]. No circulating plasma inhibitor of blood coagulation was demonstrable [54]. The deficient proteins were adsorbed to peripheral blood lymphocytes, presumably by reacting with IgM on the surface of the cells. This mechanism of factor VIII clearance may be a general phenomenon, as illustrated by the occasional finding of plasma factor VIII deficiency in plasma cell dyscrasias [55,56].

Factor IX inhibitors

With rare exceptions, inhibitors to factor IX develop in patients with hemophilia B, appearing in about 3 percent of patients with hemophilia B who have been transfused with plasma or plasma fractions [11]. As in hemophilia A, patients with the most severe deficiencies of factor IX are most prone to develop inhibitors. One report describes three patients from the same kindred with factor IX deficiency and factor IX inhibitors [57]. Unlike most patients with hemophilia B, these patients lacked factor IX antigen in their plasma. This may make such patients more susceptible to the development of inhibitors.

Factor IX inhibitors are IgG [58]. Two antibodies have been extensively characterized. One of restricted heterogeneity was an IgG$_4$ with λ light chains [59]. The other was a polyclonal IgG, including λ and κ light chains [60]. These antibodies are usually nonprecipitating. In one case, a subpopulation of antibodies was shown to bind to factor IX only in the presence of calcium [61].

Factor IX inhibitors are detected by performing a PTT on a mixture of test plasma and normal plasma. A modified version of the Bethesda assay may be used to quantitate the inhibitor level [27]. A radioimmunoassay has been developed to measure factor IX inhibitors in plasma [61].

Hemophilia B complicated by the presence of factor IX inhibitors can usually be successfully managed with factor IX concentrates, which may neutralize the inhibitor. Alternatively, it is possible that the factor IX concentrates bypass factor IX through a mechanism similar to that in patients with hemophilia A and factor VIII inhibitors.

Factor IX inhibitors have also been observed in patients who do not have hemophilia B. In the cases studied, the inhibitor has been an IgG [62]. The primary diagnoses of these patients have included autoimmune disorders [62] and systemic lupus erythematosus [63].

Factor V inhibitors

The development of a factor V inhibitor is a rare event that is more often associated with plasma transfusion therapy in patients with previously normal hemostasis than in those with congenital factor V deficiency. This inhibitor has been seen in patients who have received a single blood transfusion and in patients who have had multiple transfusions [64]. The inhibitor is usually present for about 2 to 8 weeks [64] but may be more persistent. In the latter event, treatment with cyclophosphamide and prednisone has been used [65]. The factor V inhibitors which have been characterized have been polyclonal IgG [64,66]. A single report has described a patient with congenital factor V deficiency who acquired a factor V inhibitor after multiple transfusions [67]. This inhibitor was also an IgG.

Bleeding patients with factor V inhibitors are usually responsive to large quantities of fresh frozen plasma, but severe hemorrhage leading to death has occurred [68]. In one case involving the spontaneous development of a factor V inhibitor, fresh frozen plasma failed to effect hemostasis [65]. In four separate episodes, platelet transfusions were administered with excellent results. These transfused platelets, with factor V bound to the platelet receptors, may protect factor V from interacting with the plasma inhibitor.

Fibrinogen and fibrin polymerization inhibitors

Although polyclonal immunoglobulins directed against fibrinogen and fibrin have occasionally been described, monoclonal paraproteins associated with multiple myeloma and macroglobulinemia represent the most common inhibitors of fibrin polymerization. About 50 percent of patients with dysproteinemias have abnormalities of the thrombin time [55]. These patients may have purpura, hematuria, gastrointestinal bleeding, or epistaxis. More often, they have no hemostatic disorder despite the laboratory abnormalities.

In vitro, these plasmas form a gelatin-like fibrin clot which is friable and exhibits poor clot retraction. The paraproteins lead to abnormal fibrin monomer polymerization, slowing of the rate of gelation, and reduced opacity of the fibrin clot [69]. Electron microscopy of the clot shows the fibrin strands to be very thin, and aggregates of amorphous material are also observed [70]. The paraprotein binds to certain domains of the fibrin chain during polymerization, interfering with proper development of the clot and precluding normal clot retraction.

Abnormal fibrin polymerization may occur in the presence of IgG, IgA, IgM, or light-chain paraproteins. Bleeding syndromes are more commonly associated with IgA and IgM dysproteinemias, whereas in vitro coagulation tests are more often abnormal in the presence of IgG paraproteins [55]. The inhibitory activity resides on the Fab fragments of the IgG and IgA proteins studied [71]. Isolated heavy chains, light chains, and Fc fragments have no inhibitory activity.

Polyclonal antibodies to fibrinogen have also been observed in patients with hypo- or afibrinogenemia that have been multiply transfused [72,73]. Patients with autoimmune disorders have not developed such antibodies.

Factor XIII inhibitors

Factor XIII inhibitors have been discovered in patients with and without congenital factor XIII deficiency. In those with factor XIII deficiency, the inhibitors arise as apparent complications of plasma transfusion [74–76]. More commonly, factor XIII inhibitors develop after long-term exposure to isoniazid [77,78] or other drugs, such as phenytoin [79,80].

Factor XIII inhibitors which have been characterized have been IgG, with restricted heterogeneity [81]. In one case, antibodies were directed against the α chain of factor XIII [76].

Factor VIII:von Willebrand factor inhibitors

Von Willebrand's disease is a hereditary bleeding disorder characterized in the laboratory by decreased levels of factor VIII:von Willebrand factor (FVIII:vWF) and decreased factor VIII coagulant activity (FVIII:C) (see Chap. 155). A number of patients have been described who have an acquired form of von Willebrand's syndrome. This disorder has appeared in association with systemic lupus erythematosus [82], benign monoclonal gammopathies [83], lymphoma [84,85], and macroglobulinemia [54] and in otherwise normal adults [86]. Two important characteristics of these patients emphasize the acquired nature of the disorder. First, a hemorrhagic disorder is observed in patients who had not had a prior bleeding problem even after trauma or surgical intervention, and, second, family studies show no evidence of a hereditary bleeding disorder.

Two discrete pathogenic mechanisms have been de-

scribed in this disorder. First, a circulating inhibitor directed against FVIII:vWF has been found in the plasma of these patients [84]. This inhibitor, an IgG immunoglobulin, prevents ristocetin-induced aggregation of normal platelets but does not bind to washed platelets and therefore is not an antiplatelet antibody. In the second type of disorder, an inhibitor of FVIII:vWF is not present in the blood. Instead, low levels of FVIII:vWF, factor VIII–related antigen (FVIIIR:Ag), and FVIII:C are found, presumably due to binding of factor VIII to cellular elements in the blood or in tissue. In one patient with a lymphocytic lymphoma, electrophoretic analysis of factor VIII provided evidence for both a quantitative and a qualitative abnormality [85]. Treatment of the lymphocytic lymphoma led to correction of the deficiency state. In a patient with acquired von Willebrand's disease associated with macroglobulinemia, factor VIII was detected on the monoclonal lymphocyte surface [54]. These observations indicate that, in the absence of a circulating antibody in the blood, immunoglobulin on cell surfaces can bind factor VIII, leading to a deficiency state and a bleeding syndrome.

Patients with the inherited form of von Willebrand's disease may develop antibodies to FVIII:vWF as a reaction to infused plasma or plasma products [87–89]. These inhibitors are polyclonal IgG [90,91] and form precipitating complexes with FVIII:vWF. There is a familial tendency to develop these inhibitors [89]. The inhibitors interfere significantly with the treatment of von Willebrand's disease [92]. In addition to poor hemostatic responses, such patients may develop side effects upon infusion of cyroprecipitate, including lumbar and abdominal pain, hypotension, and other early manifestations of immune complex disease [92]. These can be partially reduced with glucocorticoid therapy [92].

Drug-induced inhibitors

Acquired inhibitors which interfere with blood coagulation have been observed in patients in association with the administration of certain medications. The appearance of these inhibitors may be associated with life-threatening hemorrhage or may have no clinically important consequences.

The prevalence of inhibitors in schizophrenic patients treated with chlorpromazine is well documented [93–96]. Patients subjected to long-term chlorpromazine treatment have elevated serum IgM levels and a circulating inhibitor with properties similar to the lupus anticoagulant [96] (see below). A large percentage of these patients also had positive antinuclear antibody tests and antibodies to native DNA.

Procainamide has also been associated with a circulating anticoagulant [7]. This inhibitor, observed in a patient with serologic evidence of drug-induced lupus, was directed at prothrombin and a component of the contact phase of blood coagulation. Isoniazid therapy may lead to the development of antibodies to factor

XIII [77,78], fibrinogen [97], and factor V [68]. In addition, factor V inhibitors have been observed in patients treated with streptomycin [98] and cephalothin [99]. As discussed above, allergic reactions to penicillin, sulfonamides [43], and phenytoin [44] may be associated with development of circulating anticoagulants directed against factor VIII.

Lupus anticoagulants—circulating inhibitors in systemic lupus erythematosus

Circulating anticoagulants are observed in about 5 to 15 percent of patients with systemic lupus erythematosus [100,101]. The lupus anticoagulant was originally described in patients with systemic lupus [102] but has been observed in a variety of clinical conditions, including other autoimmune disorders, drug reactions, neoplastic, neurologic, and gynecologic diseases, and in otherwise healthy individuals [103]. Some patients with systemic lupus erythematosus may have inhibitors other than the lupus anticoagulant, such as those directed against factor VIII.

The PTT is prolonged by the lupus anticoagulant. The prothrombin time is usually slightly prolonged, but may be normal. In a rare patient the prothrombin time is markedly prolonged because of a severe deficiency of prothrombin activity [104]. The anticoagulant reacts rapidly, and the PTTs of mixtures of normal plasma and patient's plasma are prolonged and do not lengthen with further incubation. Owing to the current frequency of ordering of PTTs, an increasing number of patients without hemorrhagic disease have been found to have a prolonged PTT caused by the lupus anticoagulant.

The lupus anticoagulant is not associated with hemostatic defects, but antibodies directed against other hemostatic components may cause abnormal bleeding. Therefore, if the PTT is prolonged due to an inhibitor, efforts must be made to characterize the anticoagulant fully so that the patient may be appropriately managed.

The lupus anticoagulants which have been characterized are immunoglobulins. Both IgG [101,105] and IgM [106,107] have been described. Although most of these inhibitors are polyclonal, occasional patients with monoclonal gammopathies manifest lupus-like inhibitors [107]. There is a correlation between the presence of a lupus anticoagulant and a biologic false-positive serologic test for syphilis [103,108]. The lupus anticoagulant has been thought to be directed against the phospholipids [103] used to accelerate the activation of prothrombin to thrombin by factor Xa in the presence of calcium in in vitro coagulation tests, such as the PTT (see Chap. 135). Evidence for this concept derives from studies of a monoclonal IgMλ, which caused marked prolongation of the PTT of the plasma of a patient with macroglobulinemia [107]. When purified, this immunoglobulin inhibited calcium-dependent binding of pro-

thrombin and factor X to phospholipid micelles. The immunoglobulin also reacted with phosphatidylserine, phosphatidylinositol, and phosphatidic acid, suggesting it was an antibody to phospholipids. In a second study, a monoclonal murine antibody reacting with DNA also reacted with cardiolipin, phosphatidic acid, phosphatidylglycerol, and phosphatidyl serine and had mild anticoagulant activity [109].

Neither the IgM inhibitor nor the hybridoma-derived lupus monoclonal antibody binds to platelets [107,109], and the IgM inhibitor did not interfere with coagulation tests in which platelets were employed instead of phospholipid emulsions [107]. The lack of effect of the inhibitor on coagulation reactions involving platelets may explain the absence of clinical bleeding due to the lupus anticoagulant. Patients with the lupus anticoagulant may actually have a thrombotic tendency [110,111]. The inhibition of the PTT by the lupus anticoagulant may be considered an in vitro laboratory artifact.

Nonimmunoglobulin anticoagulants

In two instances, a circulating proteoglycan with heparin-like anticoagulant properties has been shown to be an inhibitor of blood coagulation and to cause a clinical bleeding disorder [112,113]. One patient had IgA multiple myeloma. The plasma contained a proteoglycan of M_r 116,000 daltons, which bound to platelet factor 4 and functioned similarly to heparin as a cofactor for the inhibition of thrombin by antithrombin III. A second patient, with IgG$_4$ plasma cell leukemia, also had a heparin-like proteoglycan in the plasma.

References

1. Margolius, A., Jackson, D. P., and Ratnoff, O. D.: Circulating anticoagulants: A study of 40 cases and a review of the literature. *Medicine* 40:145, 1961.
2. Bidwell, E.: Acquired inhibitors of coagulants. *Annu. Rev. Med.* 20:63, 1969.
3. Feinstein, D. I., and Rapaport, S. I.: Acquired inhibitors of blood coagulation. *Prog. Hemostasis Thromb.* 1:75, 1972.
4. Shapiro, S. S., and Hultin, M.: Acquired inhibitors to the blood coagulation factors. *Semin. Thromb. Hemostat.* 1:336, 1975.
5. Lewis, R. M., Zeitler, K. D., Blatt, P. M., Reisner, H. M., and Roberts, H. R.: Immunology of inhibitors to clotting proteins, in *Manual of Clinical Immunology*, edited by N. R. Rose and H. Friedman. American Society of Microbiologists, Washington, D.C., 1980, p. 750.
6. Poon, M.-C., Saito, H., Ratnoff, O. D., Forman, W. B., and Wisnieski, J.: Techniques for demonstration of the specificity of circulating anticoagulants against antihemophilic factor (factor VIII), with studies of two cases possibly related to diphenylhydantoin therapy. *Blood* 49:477, 1977.
7. Davis, S., Furie, B. C., Griffin, J. H., and Furie, B.: Circulating inhibitors of blood coagulation associated with procainamide-induced lupus erythematosus. *Am. J. Hematol.* 4:401, 1978.
8. Harmon, M. C., Zipursky, A., and Lahey, M. E.: A study of hemophilia. *Am. J. Dis. Child.* 93:375, 1957.
9. Brinkhous, K. M., Roberts, H. R., and Weiss, A. E.: Prevalence of

inhibitors in hemophilia A and B. *Thromb. Diath. Haemorrh. (Suppl.)* 51:315, 1972.

10. Kasper, C. K.: Incidence and course of inhibitors among patients with classic hemophilia. *Thromb. Diath. Haemorrh.* 30:263, 1973.

11. Biggs, R.: Jaundice and antibodies directed against factor VIII and IX in patients treated for haemophilia or Christmas disease in the United Kingdom. *Br. J. Haematol.* 26:313, 1974.

12. Lusher, J. M., Shuster, J., Evans, R. K., and Poulik, M.D.: Antibody nature of an AHG (factor VIII) inhibitor. *J. Pediatr.* 72:325, 1968.

13. Strauss, H. S.: Acquired circulating anticoagulants in hemophilia A. *N. Engl. J. Med.* 281:866, 1969.

14. Bidwell, E., Denson, K. W. E., Dike, G. W. R., Augustin, R., and Lloyd, G. M.: Antibody nature of the inhibitor to antihaemophilic globulin (factor VIII). *Nature* 210:746, 1966.

15. Shapiro, S.: The immunologic character of acquired inhibitors of antihemophilic globulin (factor VIII) and the kinetics of their interaction with factor VIII. *J. Clin. Invest.* 46:147, 1967.

16. Strauss, H. S., and Merler, E.: Characterization and properties of an inhibitor of factor VIII in the plasma of patients with hemophilia A following repeated transfusions. *Blood* 30:137, 1967.

17. Poon, M.-C., Wine, A. C., Ratnoff, O. D., and Bernier, G. M.: Heterogeneity of human circulating anticoagulants against antihemophilic factor (factor VIII). *Blood* 46:409, 1975.

18. Lavergne, J. M., Meyer, D., and Reisner, H. Characterization of human anti-factor VIII antibodies purified by immune complex formation. *Blood* 48:931, 1976.

19. Hultin, M. B., London, F. S., Shapiro, S. S., and Yount, W. J.: Heterogeneity of factor VIII antibodies: Further immunochemical and biological studies. *Blood* 49:807, 1977.

20. Robboy, S. J., Lewis, E. J., Schur, P. H., and Colman, R. W. Circulating anticoagulants to factor VIII. *Am. J. Med.* 49:742, 1970.

21. Andersen, B. R., and Terry, W. D.: Gamma G$_4$-globulin antibody causing inhibition of clotting factor VIII. *Nature* 217:174, 1968.

22. Koutts, J., Meyer, D., Richard, K., Scott, L., and Firkin, B. G.: Heterogeneity of biological activity of human factor VIII antibodies. *Br. J. Haematol.* 29:99, 1975.

23. Kernoff, P. B. A.: The relevance of factor VIII inactivation characteristics in the treatment of patients with antibodies directed against factor VIII. *Br. J. Haematol.* 22:735, 1972.

24. Allain, J.-P., and Frommel, D. Antibodies to factor VIII: Patterns of immune response to factor VIII in hemophilia A. *Blood* 47:973, 1976.

25. Hultin, M. B., et al.: Immunosuppressive therapy of factor VIII inhibitors. *Blood* 48:95, 1976.

26. Lossing, T. S., Kasper, C. K., and Feinstein, D. I.: Detection of factor VIII inhibitors with the partial thromboplastin time. *Blood* 49:793, 1977.

27. Kasper, C. K., et al.: A more uniform measurement of factor VIII inhibitors. *Thromb. Diath. Haemorrh.* 34:869, 1975.

28. Fekete, L. F., et al.: Auto-factor IX concentrate: A new therapeutic approach to the treatment of hemophilia A patients with inhibitors. *XIV International Congress of Hematology,* 295, 1972.

29. Kurczynski, E. M., and Penner, J. A.: Activated prothrombin concentrate for patients with factor VIII inhibitors. *N. Engl. J. Med.* 291:164, 1974.

30. Kelly, P., and Penner, J. A.: Management of anti-hemophilic inhibitors with prothrombin complex concentrate. *JAMA* 236:2061, 1976.

31. Lusher, J. M., Shapiro, S. S., Palaschak, J. E., Rao, A. V., Levine, P. H., and Blatt, P. M.: Efficacy of prothrombin-complex concentrates in hemophiliacs with antibodies to factor VIII. *N. Engl. J. Med.* 303:421, 1981.

32. Blatt, P. M., Menache, D., and Roberts, H. R.: A survey of effectiveness of prothrombin complex concentrates in controlling hemorrhage in patients with hemophilia and anti-factor VIII antibodies. *Thromb. Haemost.* 44:39, 1980.

33. Kasper, C. K.: Postoperative thrombosis in hemophilia B. *N. Engl. J. Med.* 289:160, 1973 (letter).

34. Blatt, P. M., Lundblad, R. L., Kingdom, H. S., McLean, G., and Roberts, H. R.: Thrombogenic materials in prothrombin complex concentrates. *Ann. Intern. Med.* 81:766, 1974.

35. Onder, O., and Hoyer, L. W.: Factor VIII coagulant antigen in factor IX complex concentrates. *Thromb. Res.* 15:569, 1979.

36. Kasper, C. K.: Effect of prothrombin complex concentrates on factor VIII inhibitor levels. *Blood* 54:1358, 1979.

37. Hruby, M. A., and Schulman, I.: Failure of combined factor VIII and cyclophosphamide to suppress antibody to factor VIII in hemophilia. *Blood* 42:919, 1973.

38. Frenkel, E. P., and Stastny, P.: Use of 6-mercaptopurine in the control of a circulating anticoagulant against antihemophilic globulin. *Clin. Res.* 13:35, 1965.

39. Frick, P. G.: Acquired circulating anticoagulants in systemic "collagen disease." *Blood* 10:691, 1955.

40. Horowitz, H. I., and Fujimoto, M. M.: Acquired hemophilia due to a circulating anticoagulant: Report of two cases with review of the literature. *Am. J. Med.* 33:501, 1962.

41. Green, D.: Spontaneous inhibitors of factor VIII. *Br. J. Haematol.* 15:57, 1968.

42. Klein, K. A., Parkin, J. D., and Madaras, F.: Studies on an acquired inhibitor of factor VIII induced by penicillin allergy. *Clin. Exp. Immunol.* 26:155, 1976.

43. Vera, J. C., Herzig, E. B., Sise, H. S., and Brauer, M. J.: Acquired circulating anticoagulant to factor VIII. *JAMA* 232:1038, 1975.

44. Ratnoff, O. D., and Rabaa, M. S.: Autologous antibodies to AHF and phenytoin. *Blood* 51:768, 1978.

45. Nilsson, I. M., Skanse, B., and Gydell, K.: Circulating anticoagulant after pregnancy and its response to ACTH. *Acta Haematol.* 19:40, 1958.

46. Greenwood, R. J., and Rabin, S. C. Hemophilia-like postpartum bleeding. *Obstet. Gynecol.* 30:362, 1967.

47. Marengo-Rowe, A. J., Murff, G., Levenson, J. E., and Cook, J.: Hemophilia-like disease associated with pregnancy. *Obstet. Gynecol.* 40:56, 1972.

48. Michiels, J. J., Borsch, L. J., Van der Plas, P. M., and Abels, J.: Factor VIII inhibitor postpartum. *Scand. J. Haematol.* 20:97, 1978.

49. Gobbi, F., and Stefanini, M.: Circulating anti-AHF anticoagulant in a patient with lupus erythematosus disseminatus. *Acta Haematol.* 28:155, 1962.

50. Roberts, H. R., Scales, M. B., Madison, J. T., Webster, W. P., and Penick, G. D.: A clinical and experimental study of acquired inhibitors to factor VIII. *Blood* 26:805, 1965.

51. Nilehn, J. E.: On symptomatic anti-haemophilic globulin (AHF) deficiency. *Acta Med. Scand.* 171:491, 1962.

52. Castaldi, P. A., and Penny, R.: A macroglobulin with inhibitory activity against coagulation factor VIII. *Blood* 35:370, 1970.

53. Glueck, H. I., and Hong, R.: A circulating anticoagulant in γ$_1$A-multiple myeloma. *J. Clin. Invest.* 44:1866, 1965.

54. Brody, J. I., Haider, M. E., and Rossman, R. E.: A hemorrhagic syndrome in Waldenstrom's macroglobulinemia secondary to immunoadsorption of factor VIII. *N. Engl. J. Med.* 300:408, 1979.

55. Perkins, H. A., MacKenzie, M. R., and Fudenberg, H. H.: Hemostatic defects in dysproteinemias. *Blood* 35:695, 1970.

56. Lackner, H.: Hemostatic abnormalities associated with dysproteinemias. *Semin. Hematol.* 10:125, 1973.

57. George, J. N., Miller, G. M., and Breckenridge, R. T.: Studies on Christmas disease: Investigation and treatment of a familial acquired inhibitor of factor IX. *Br. J. Haematol.* 21:333, 1971.

58. Colombani, J., and Terrier, E.: Immunochemical investigation of a Christmas factor inhibitor by means of Boyden's technique. *Nature* 196:1111, 1962.

59. Pike, I. M., Yount, W. J., Puritz, E. M., and Roberts, H. R.: Immunochemical characterization of a monoclonal γG$_4$λ human antibody to factor IX. *Blood* 40:1, 1972.

60. Reisner, H. M., Roberts, H. R., Krumholz, S., and Yount, W. J.: Immunochemical characterization of a polyclonal human antibody to factor IX. *Blood* 50:11, 1977.

61. Lewis, R. M., Reisner, H. M., Chung, K.-S., and Roberts, H. R.: Detection of factor IX antibodies by radioimmunoassay: Effect of calcium on antibody–factor IX interaction. *Blood* 56:608, 1980.

62. Largo, R., Sigg, P., von Felton, A., and Straub, P. W.: Acquired factor IX inhibitor in a nonhaemophilic patient with autoimmune disease. *Br. J. Haematol.* 26:129, 1974.

63. Castro, O., Farber, L. R., and Clyne, L. P.: Circulating anticoagulants against factors IX and XI in systemic lupus erythematosus. *Ann. Intern. Med.* 77:543, 1972.

64. Feinstein, D. I., Rapaport, S. I., McGehee, W. G., and Patch, M. J.: Factor V anticoagulants: Clinical, biochemical, and immunochemical observations. *J. Clin. Invest.* 49:1578, 1970.

65. Chediak, J., Ashenhurst, J. B., Garlick, I., and Desser, R. K.: Successful management of bleeding in a patient with factor V inhibitor by platelet transfusions. *Blood* 56:835, 1980.

66. Crowell, E. B., Jr.: Observations on a factor V inhibitor. *Br. J. Haematol.* 29:397, 1975.

67. Fratantoni, J. S., Hilgartner, M., and Nachman, R. L.: Nature of the defect in congenital factor V deficiency. *Blood* 39:751, 1972.

68. Coots, M. C., Muhleman, A. F., and Glueck, H. I.: Hemorrhagic death associated with a high titer factor V inhibitor. *Am. J. Hematol.* 4:193, 1978.

69. Frick, P. G.: Inhibition of conversion of fibrinogen to fibrin by abnormal proteins in multiple myeloma. *Am. J. Clin. Pathol.* 25:1263, 1955.

70. Lackner, H., Hunt, V., Zucker, M. B., and Pearson, J.: Abnormal fibrin ultrastructure, polymerization, and clot retraction in multiple myeloma. *Br. J. Haematol.* 18:625, 1970.

71. Coleman, M., Vigliano, E. M., Weksler, M. E., and Nachman, R. L.: Inhibition of fibrin monomer polymerization by lambda myeloma globulins. *Blood* 39:210, 1972.

72. DeVries, A., Rosenberg, T., Kochwa, S., and Boss, J. H.: Precipitating antifibrinogen antibody appearing after fibrinogen infusions in a patient with congenital afibrinogenemia. *Am. J. Med.* 30:486, 1961.

73. Menache, D.: Abnormal fibrinogens. *Thromb. Diath. Haemorrh.* 29:525, 1973.

74. Lorand, L., Urayama, T., deKiewiet, J. W. C., and Nossel, H. L.: Diagnostic and genetic studies on fibrin stabilizing factor with a new assay based on amine incorporation. *J. Clin. Invest.* 48:1054, 1969.

75. Godal, H. C.: An inhibitor to fibrin stabilizing factor (FSF, factor XIII). *Scand. J. Haematol.* 7:43, 1979.

76. Lopaciuk, S., et al.: Differences between Type I autoimmune inhibitors of fibrin stabilization in two patients with severe hemorrhagic disorder. *J. Clin. Invest.* 64:1196, 1978.

77. Lorand, L., Jacobsen, A., and Bruner-Lorand, J.: A pathological inhibitor of fibrin cross-linking. *J. Clin. Invest.* 47:268, 1968.

78. Otis, P. T., Feinstein, D. I., Rapaport, S. I., and Patch, M. J.: An acquired inhibitor of fibrin stabilization associated with isoniazid therapy: Clinical and biochemical observations. *Blood* 44:771, 1974.

79. Lewis, J. H.: Hemorrhagic disease associated with inhibitors of fibrin cross linkage. *Ann. N.Y. Acad. Sci.* 202:213, 1972.

80. Godal, H. C., and Ly, B.: An inhibitor of factor XIII inhibiting fibrin cross-linking but not incorporation of amine into casein. *Scand. J. Haematol.* 19:443, 1977.

81. Graham, J. E., Yount, W. J., and Roberts, H. R.: Immunochemical characterization of a human antibody to factor XIII. *Blood* 41:661, 1973.

82. Simone, J. V., Cornet, J. A., and Abildgaard, G. F.: Acquired von Willebrand's syndrome in systemic lupus erythematosus. *Blood* 31:806, 1968.

83. Mant, M. J., Hirsh, J., Gauldie, J., Bienenstock, J., Pineo, G. F., and Luke, K. H.: Von Willebrand's syndrome presenting as an acquired disorder in association with a monoclonal gammopathy. *Blood* 42:429, 1973.

84. Handin, R. I., Martin, V., and Moloney, W. C.: Antibody-induced von Willebrand's disease: A newly defined inhibitor syndrome. *Blood* 48:393, 1976.

85. Joist, J. H., Cowan, J. F., and Zimmerman, T. S.: Acquired von Willebrand's disease. *N. Engl. J. Med.* 298:988, 1978.

86. Ingram, G. I. C., Kingston, P. J., Leslie, J., and Bowie, E. J. W.: Four cases of acquired von Willebrand's syndrome. *Br. J. Haematol.* 21:189, 1971.

87. Sarji, K. E., Stratton, R. D., Wagner, R. H., and Brinkhous, K. M.: Nature of von Willebrand's factor: A new assay and a specific inhibitor. *Proc. Natl. Acad. Sci. U.S.A.* 71:2937, 1974.

88. Mannucci, P. M., Meyer, D., Ruggeri, Z. M., Koutts, J., Ciavarella, N., and Lavergne, J. M.: Precipitating antibodies in von Wille-

brand's disease. *Nature* 262:141, 1976.

89. Ruggeri, Z. M., et al.: Familial incidence of precipitating antibodies in von Willebrand's disease: A study of four cases. *J. Lab. Clin. Med.* 94:60, 1979.

90. Stratton, R. D., Wagner, R. H., Webster, W. P., and Brinkhous, K. M.: Antibody nature of circulating inhibitor of plasma von Willebrand factor. *Proc. Natl. Acad. Sci. U.S.A.* 72:4167, 1975.

91. Egberg, N., and Blomback, M.: On the characterization of acquired inhibitors to ristocetin induced platelet aggregation found in patients with von Willebrand's disease. *Thromb. Res.* 9:527, 1976.

92. Mannucci, P. M., Ruggeri, Z. M., Ciavarella, N., Kazatchkine, M.D., and Mowbray, J. F.: Precipitating antibodies to factor VIII/von Willebrand factor in von Willebrand's disease: Effects on replacement therapy. *Blood* 57:25, 1981.

93. Canoso, R. T., Hutton, R. A., and Deykin, D. A.: Chlorpromazine-induced inhibitor of blood coagulation. *Am. J. Hematol.* 2:183, 1977.

94. Glazier, R. L., and Crowell, E. B.: Factor VIII inhibitor associated with chlorpromazine induced hepatic injury. *Thromb. Haemost.* 37:523, 1977.

95. Zucker, S., Zarrabi, M. H., Romano, G. S., and Miller, F.: IgM inhibitor of the contact activation phase of coagulation in chlorpromazine treated patients. *Br. J. Haematol.* 40:447, 1978.

96. Zarrabi, M. H., et al.: Immunologic and coagulation disorders in chlorpromazine-treated patients. *Ann. Intern. Med.* 91:194, 1979.

97. Rosenberg, R. D., Colman, R. W., and Lorand, L.: A new hemorrhagic disorder with defective fibrin stabilization and cryofibrinogenemia. *Br. J. Haematol.* 26:269, 1974.

98. Feinstein, D. I., Rapaport, S. I., and Chong, M. M. Y.: Factor V inhibitor: Report of a case with comments on a possible effect of streptomycin. *Ann. Intern. Med.* 78:385, 1973.

99. Nilsson, I. M., Hedner, U. Ekberg, M., and Denneberg, T.: A circulating anticoagulant against factor V. *Acta Med. Scand.* 195:73, 1974.

100. Meacham, G., and Weisburger, A.: Unusual manifestations of disseminated lupus erythematosus. *Ann. Intern. Med.* 43:143, 1955.

101. Regan, M. G., Lackner, H., and Karpatkin, S.: Platelet function and coagulation profile in lupus erythematosus. *Ann. Intern. Med.* 81:462, 1974.

102. Conley, C. L., and Hartman, R. C.: A hemorrhagic disorder caused by circulating anticoagulant in patients with disseminated lupus erythematosus. *J. Clin. Invest.* 31:621, 1952.

103. Schleider, M. A., Nachman, R. L., Jaffe, E. A., and Coleman, M.: A clinical study of the lupus anticoagulant. *Blood* 48:499, 1976.

104. Rapaport, S. I., Ames, S. B., and Duvall, B. J.: A plasma coagulation defect in systemic lupus erythematosus arising from hypoprothrombinemia combined with antiprothrombinase activity. *Blood* 15:212, 1960.

105. Yin, E. T., and Gaston, L. W.: Purification and kinetic studies on a circulating anticoagulant in a suspected case of lupus erythematosus. *Thromb. Diath. Haemorrh.* 14:88, 1965.

106. Lechner, K.: A new type of coagulation inhibitor. *Thromb. Diath. Haemorrh.* 21:482, 1969.

107. Thiagarajan, P., Shapiro, S. S., and DeMarco, L.: Monoclonal immunoglobulin Mλ coagulation inhibitor with phospholipid specificity. Mechanism of a lupus anticoagulant. *J. Clin. Invest.* 66:397, 1980.

108. Lechner, K.: Acquired inhibitors in non-hemophilic patients. *Haemostasis* 3:65, 1974.

109. Lafer, E. M., et al.: Polyspecific monoclonal lupus autoantibodies against polynucleotides and phospholipids. *J. Exp. Med.* 153:897, 1981.

110. Mueh, J. R., Herbst, K. D., and Rapaport, S. I.: Thrombosis in patients with the lupus anticoagulant. *Ann. Intern. Med.* 92:156, 1980.

111. Bowie, E. J. W., Thompson, J. H., Jr., Pascuzzi, C. A., and Owen, C. A., Jr.: Thrombosis in systemic lupus erythematosus despite circulating anticoagulants. *J. Lab. Clin. Med.* 62:416, 1963.

112. Khorry, M. S., Nesheim, M. E., Bowie, E. J. W., and Mann, K. G.: Circulating heparin sulfate proteoglycan anticoagulant from a patient with a plasma cell disorder. *J. Clin. Invest.* 65:666, 1980.

113. Palmer, R. N., Rick, M. E., and Gralnick, H. R.: Characteristics of a heparin-like inhibitor. *Clin. Res.* 29:343, 1981.

CHAPTER 158

Consumptive thrombohemorrhagic disorders

VICTOR J. MARDER

Known variously as disseminated intravascular coagulation, defibrination, and consumptive coagulopathy, the heterogeneous group of consumptive thrombohemorrhagic disorders can be manifested by the entire range of hemorrhagic and thrombotic phenomena. No single definition covers all varieties, and the term *consumptive thrombohemorrhagic disorders* has a broad interpretation that does not place a limit on clinical manifestations.

These disorders may be either subtle or devastating in clinical presentation and are "intermediary mechanisms of disease" [1] that can complicate a variety of primary conditions. The complexity of the clinical presentation, the variable course, and the multitude of therapies administered to such patients make properly conducted clinical trials difficult. Management therefore must rely on an understanding of the pathologic processes in the patient in question [1–23]. The clinical and laboratory presentations are affected by several parameters (Table 158-1). These variables will determine whether specific therapy of "consumption" is required, beyond that indicated for the underlying disease.

Presented with the patient who may have such a disorder, the physician should judge the *tempo* [17] of the illness, that is, whether the clinical presentation is severe enough to warrant specific therapy and whether the coagulation disorder is likely to be a self-limited problem. The predisposing disorders encompass several pathologic states whose recognition by the physician provides insight for prognosis. Some have been generally accepted as causes for an extreme form of consumptive thrombohemorrhagic disorder, for instance, meningococcal sepsis [24,25] or acute promyelocytic leukemia [26], but variability in the degree of this complication is common [27–29].

Some clinical states may suggest the *location* of consumption, that is, whether it is occurring in a disseminated, or systemic, manner or in an isolated anatomic space. Insults such as sepsis are more likely to have disseminated manifestations. On the other hand, anatomically limited lesions, such as a dissecting aortic aneurysm [30] or giant cavernous hemangioma [31], may consume locally. Other disorders may exceed such anatomic limits. For example, the intrauterine consumption seen in abruptio placentae may liberate thromboplastic material into the circulation and cause disseminated intravascular coagulation [32].

A judgment should be made as to the *pathologic mechanism* involved in the consumption. The elaboration of thrombin leads to the conversion of fibrinogen to fibrin, while the elaboration of plasmin leads to the enzymatic degradation of fibrinogen. Thrombin and other active agents, such as bacterial endotoxin or snake venoms, may consume platelets as well as fibrinogen by their incorporation into clots or aggregates, while other mechanisms may result in isolated thrombocytopenia without hypofibrinogenemia, such as is seen in thrombotic thrombocytopenic purpura [33]. Tempo, location, and pathologic mechanism can all operate as independent variables superimposed on an underlying disorder, and each patient's clinical and laboratory presentation must be individually considered before rational management can be started.

Acute, severe disseminated intravascular coagulation

PATHOGENESIS

INTRAVASCULAR CLOT FORMATION
The extreme end of the spectrum of consumptive thrombohemorrhagic disorders is represented by acute, severe disseminated intravascular coagulation (DIC), defined as a "pathological syndrome resulting from the formation of thrombin, subsequent activation and consumption of certain coagulant proteins, and production of fibrin thrombi" [20]. Several techniques have been used to induce a pathologic state in animals that mimics the clinical condition in humans. One such technique is the injection of such procoagulant materials as thrombin, tissue thromboplastin, and snake venom. Sudden episodes of massive intravascular clotting in patients, e.g., defibrination following abruptio placentae, probably represent clinical examples of this mechanism. A second technique is to inject a weak procoagulant material, such as red cell stroma [34], into an animal whose macrophage function is depressed. This impedes cellular removal mechanisms and allows weaker activated clotting intermediates to remain in the circulation long enough to induce clotting and may be a mechanism in chronic intravascular clotting complicating a malig-

TABLE 158-1 Parameters influencing clinical and laboratory presentation of consumptive thrombohemorrhagic disorders

Parameter	Variation
Tempo	Acute vs. chronic Mild vs. severe
Location	Single site vs. systemic Intravascular vs. extravascular
Pathologic mechanism	Coagulation vs. fibrinolysis Platelets vs. plasma proteins

nancy [35]. In a third method, endotoxin is injected into susceptible animals, resulting in the generalized Schwartzman reaction [36,37], which resembles the ischemic tissue damage following intravascular clotting.

Procoagulant stimuli may act at different steps in the blood coagulation reactions to produce clinical intravascular clotting. For instance, materials directly activating factor X have been identified in mucin [38] and in tumor extracts [39] and may account for the association of thrombosis and intravascular clotting with mucin-secreting adenocarcinomas. Defibrination after certain venomous snake bites is the result of entrance into the circulation of a proteolytic enzyme that directly converts fibrinogen to fibrin [40,41]. Other substances have tissue factor activity which may initiate extrinsic clotting reactions. This can occur with brain tissue after head trauma [42], with uterine contents in patients with obstetrical complications, with granules from promyelocytes in acute leukemia [43–46], and with prostatic tissue after surgery [47].

The blood may come into contact with materials capable of triggering the intrinsic clotting reactions. Extensive injury to small blood vessels—as, for example, in acute allergic [5] or immunologic [48] vasculitis or in the infectious vasculitis of Rocky Mountain spotted fever—presumably exposes the blood to tissue factor activity from damaged endothelial cells and from leukocytes. However, it also exposes the blood to collagen in basement membrane and underlying connective tissue. Collagen activates plasma factor XII (Hageman factor) [49] and, possibly, a factor on the platelet surface that can initiate intrinsic clotting independent of factor XII [50]. Collagen also causes platelets to aggregate and make available platelet factor 3 activity [51]. These combined actions could effectively trigger intrinsic clotting. With extracorporeal circulation, the blood comes into contact with foreign surfaces that can also initiate intrinsic clotting by activating factor XII and by damaging platelets.

Intravascular hemolysis resulting from transfusion of incompatible blood [52–54] or antibody-mediated drug reactions [55] may be associated with extensive intravascular clotting in humans. The clotting probably does not result from the release of large amounts of red cell stroma into the plasma, since massive nonimmune intravascular hemolysis secondary to ingestion of fava beans does not cause hypofibrinogenemia but rather an elevated level of fibrinogen [56].

Gram-negative endotoxinemia may induce clotting in animals by endothelial cell injury, by initiation of intrinsic coagulation by factor XII, or by platelet activation or activation of the extrinsic clotting pathway by tissue factor from leukocytes. Experimental endotoxinemia produces extensive *endothelial cell damage* [57,58], which could lead to both intrinsic and extrinsic clotting. However, endothelial damage is maximal 24 h after the experimental injection of endotoxin, whereas clotting after endotoxin appears to occur primarily during the first few hours [59]. Endotoxin directly activates

purified factor XII [60] and could also activate factor XII in vivo as a consequence of vascular damage [61]. Factor XII levels fall in rabbits given endotoxin [62,63] and in humans with gram-negative septicemia [61], presumably secondary to activation and consumption. Endotoxin damages platelets [64–68] and makes platelet factor 3 available for clotting [66]. Some observers have concluded that platelet injury is the primary mechanism whereby endotoxin induces intravascular clotting [11,67,69].

However, experimentally induced thrombocytopenia does not prevent either endotoxin-induced deposition of fibrin in organs [70–73] or the appearance of soluble fibrin in blood [72]. Moreover, the fall in factor XII levels after injection of endotoxin into rabbits apparently is the result, rather than the cause, of intravascular clotting, since it is prevented by treatment of the animals with warfarin [63,74]. Finally, impeding the activation of factor XII with lysozyme [74] or lowering factor VIII levels with a factor VIII antibody [75] fails to prevent endotoxin-induced clotting.

Leukopenia appears to interfere with the initiation of clotting by endotoxin [63,76–79] but not by thrombin [77] or Ancrod [80]. Leukopenia also prevents the excess consumption of labeled fibrinogen in rabbits given endotoxin [63]. Administration of leukocytes to leukopenic rabbits restores their susceptibility to fibrin deposition in the kidney after endotoxin [78,79]. Granulocytes contain material that can precipitate soluble fibrin monomer in vitro [81] and may be involved in the deposition of fibrin in organs after administration of endotoxin [78,82,83]. Leukopenia prevents factor VIII [63,79], factor V, and factor VII levels from falling and soluble fibrin monomer from forming in the blood after endotoxin [72,80].

Although peritoneal leukocytes from normal rabbits possess only weak tissue factor activity [84], preparations of rabbit or human leukocytes acquire potent tissue factor activity after exposure to endotoxin [85–87], due primarily to the small number of monocytes present in such preparations [88,89]. Intravascular coagulation with deposition of fibrin in the lungs and kidneys was found when normal rabbits were infused with peritoneal leukocytes harvested from rabbits given endotoxin [90]. These data support the hypothesis that endotoxin induces intravascular coagulation primarily through the generation and release of tissue factor activity from leukocytes.

ISCHEMIC TISSUE NECROSIS

In patients with gram-negative endotoxinemia and in experimental animals given thrombin intravenously, fibrin thrombi in small vessels may not be found at autopsy [91–93]. Almost 30 percent of patients with abruptio placentae experience defibrination with a marked fall in fibrinogen level [94], and yet only a rare patient develops renal cortical necrosis as the consequence of fibrin deposition in the kidney [36]. In contrast, ischemic renal necrosis in the hemolytic uremic

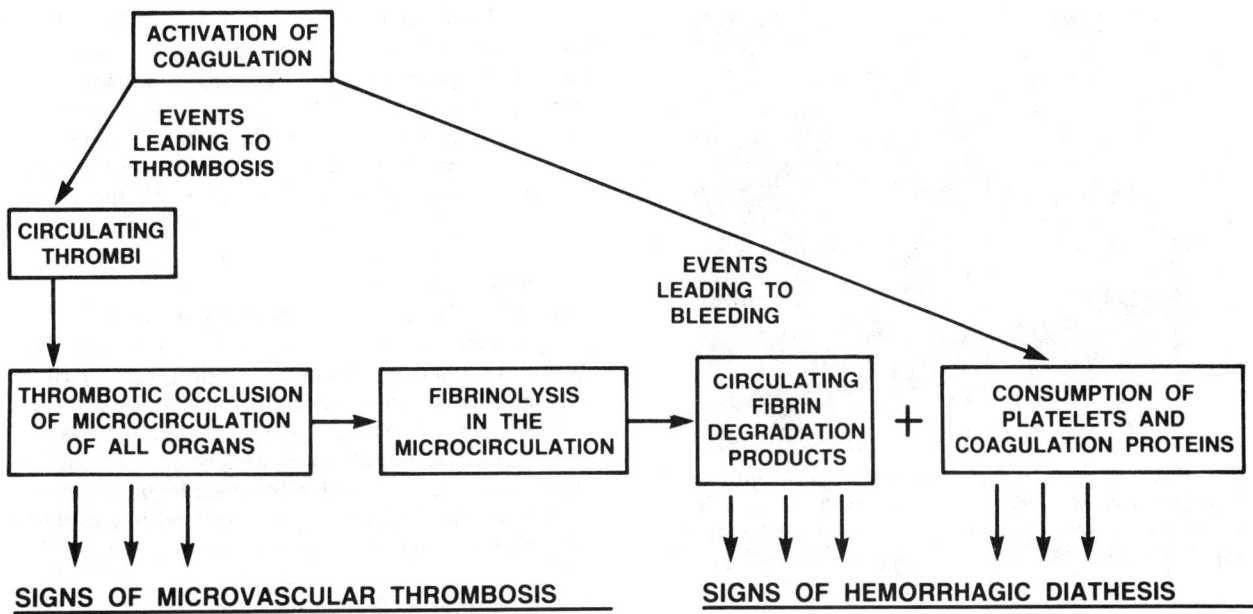

FIGURE 158-1   The sequence of events that occurs during disseminated intravascular coagulation, leading to the clinical appearance of thrombotic and hemorrhagic phenomena. (Marder [110], with permission.)

syndrome may result from gram-negative endotoxinemia with disseminated intravascular clotting insufficient to reduce plasma clotting factor levels [95].

Fibrin deposition in the microcirculation depends on the extent of intravascular clotting and on factors which influence the retention of fibrin in the microcirculation. Animal experiments suggest that impaired clearance of circulating fibrin predisposes to fibrin deposition in the microcirculation. For example, infusing thrombin or homogenized fibrin into rabbits prepared with Thorotrast induces bilateral renal cortical necrosis [91,96–98]. The pattern of blood flow through the microcirculation may critically affect the deposition of fibrin in an organ after intravascular clotting. Sympathetic denervation of the kidney protects rabbits against renal cortical necrosis induced with endotoxin [99], and an α-adrenergic blocking agent prevents the generalized Shwartzman reaction in pregnant rats [100].

Perhaps the most critical determinant is the capacity of the organism to mount a proper local fibrinolytic response to the fibrin deposits. The endothelium of capillaries and veins contains a potent plasminogen activator [101,102]. When fibrin is deposited in small vessels, activator is presumably released from endothelial cells and initiates fibrinolysis locally [103,104]. Inhibition of fibrinolysis by ε-aminocaproic acid enhances deposition of fibrin thrombi in small vessels, such as glomerular capillaries [91,105]. Depletion of renal cortical fibrinolytic activity by the first dose of

endotoxin helps to prepare the rabbit for the generalized Shwartzman reaction after the second dose of endotoxin [106]. Pregnancy enhances the susceptibility of experimental animals and of humans to ischemic tissue necrosis following disseminated intravascular clotting, compatible with the observation that release of activator from blood vessel walls is impaired in pregnancy [107–109].

DEVELOPMENT OF THE CLINICAL DISORDER
The sequence of events that follows the activation of blood coagulation is outlined in Fig. 158-1 [110].

MICROTHROMBOSIS
Thrombotic occlusive events occur first as the result of microthrombi of fibrin and/or platelets that obstruct the microcirculation of organs. These thrombi result from clotting that occurs either in the circulation or from the *in situ* thrombosis of arterioles, capillaries, or venules. Circulatory obstruction produces organ hypoperfusion and even ischemia, infarction, and necrosis. The process is disseminated throughout the microcirculation; therefore all organs are potentially vulnerable. Most obvious to physical examination is involvement of the skin [111], which demonstrates patches of hemorrhagic necrosis sharply separated from intact areas by an irregular border, reflecting the cutaneous distribution of occluded terminal arterioles. These lesions can progress

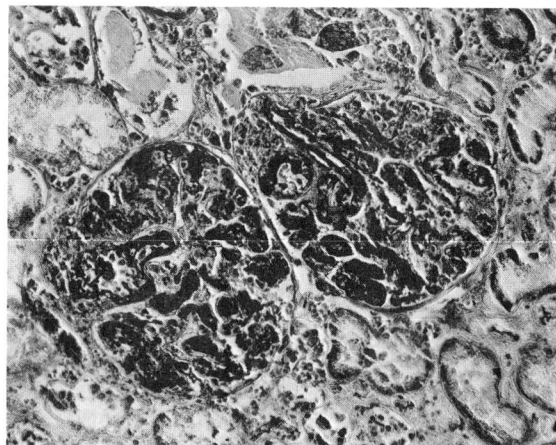

FIGURE 158-2   Section of the kidney (phosphotungstic acid–hematoxylin stain, ×166) from a patient with fulminant meningococcemia. Dark masses of fibrin occlude the glomerular capillaries. (McGehee, Rapaport, and Hjort [112], with permission.)

to hemorrhagic bullae or coalesce as larger vessels are occluded, or they may resolve upon effective treatment of the underlying condition and the thrombotic process. Especially fulminant forms may be manifest as gangrene of the fingers or toes.

Renal involvement affects primarily afferent arterioles or glomerular capillaries. The fibrin clots shown in Fig. 158-2 [112] are often not demonstrable at postmortem examination of patients dying with DIC, presumably because of a local fibrinolytic response within the occluded vessels [5], but they are believed to be the common denominator for the renal and other organ dysfunction. They produce hematuria and acute oliguria or even anuria as the result of ischemic cortical necrosis, and the resultant azotemia represents a serious threat to life, especially when renal function is further compromised by acute tubular necrosis secondary to the hypotension that often accompanies this syndrome.

Cerebral dysfunction most often is manifest as nonspecific changes, such as an altered state of consciousness, convulsions, or coma, rather than as the isolated focal lesions that are characteristic of major vessel occlusive disease. Pulmonary function can likewise be affected as the result of interstitial hemorrhage [113], which produces a clinical picture resembling acute respiratory distress syndrome. If the patient had relatively good pulmonary function prior to the illness, this aspect of DIC is usually not as prominent as that involving the skin, kidneys, and brain, but hypoxemia of some degree occurs in most patients.

Gastrointestinal involvement may produce superficial ulceration in the stomach or duodenum secondary to submucosal necrosis, not infrequently resulting in spontaneous and excessive gastrointestinal bleeding. When complicated by the hemorrhagic diathesis that follows these thrombotic events (Fig. 158-1), gastrointestinal and neurologic pathology are further compli-

cated and even more difficult to manage. The adrenal cortex may be involved in hemorrhagic necrosis (Fig. 158-3) [112], producing the especially fulminant variety of sepsis known as the Waterhouse-Friderichsen syndrome. Thrombotic involvement of organs other than brain, kidneys, lung, skin, and gastrointestinal tract [114,115] usually does not contribute to the clinical picture.

HEMOLYTIC ANEMIA
When fibrin is laid down in loose strands in small blood vessels, blood flow continues but the red cells are damaged as they move through the fibrin [116]. A striking microangiopathic hemolytic anemia may be produced [117–120], with hemoglobinemia, hemoglobinuria, and a characteristic morphologic abnormality of the red blood cells. The red blood cells appear fragmented, with triangular cells, helmet-shaped cells, and microspherocytes on the blood film (Fig. 158-4) (see Chap. 64).

CONSUMPTION AND FIBRINOLYSIS
Formation of microthrombi not only damages organ function but also depletes the supply of platelets and clotting factors in the blood, resulting in serious thrombocytopenia and a dramatic diminution of levels of fibrinogen, prothrombin, and factors V and VIII. This deficiency state is further complicated by the appearance of fibrin degradation products in the blood, resulting from lysis of the thrombi in the microcirculation. The derivatives of fibrin or fibrinogen liberated during clot dissolution have anticoagulant properties and probably contribute to the hemorrhagic state already established by the consumption of platelets and plasma coagulation proteins. Paradoxically, this combination of consumption and anticoagulation predisposes the patient to bleeding manifestations at the same time that thrombotic occlusions are occurring. The bleeding diathesis is manifested by all manner of clinical symptoms. The skin shows ecchymoses, petechiae, and bleeding from venipuncture sites. Hematuria is frequent, as is spontaneous bleeding from the gums and the nose. Gastrointestinal bleeding may be massive, and intracranial hemorrhage may further complicate the thrombotic ischemia of the cerebral circulation. Clearly, any number of possibilities exist for causing the demise of the patient, and an interruption of the underlying cause, inhibition of further thrombosis, and correction of the bleeding state are required in addition to symptomatic treatment of shock, hypovolemia, acidosis, and other secondary effects of tissue ischemia.

Although the initial pathologic events are thrombotic, the patient's clinical problems usually relate to hemorrhagic manifestations, such as mucosal oozing, spontaneous ecchymoses, petechiae, and massive gastrointestinal blood loss. Reflections of the underlying disorder and of concomitant thrombotic vascular occlusions are quickly apparent in such seriously ill patients, and management must consider all of these aspects. Early reports of severe, acute DIC were most often associated with infectious diseases, and purpura fulminans vividly describes the skin manifestations, called spontaneous gangrene by Dick and colleagues in 1934 in their patient with scarlet fever [121].

LABORATORY DIAGNOSIS

In an emergency situation, studies should be simple and specific, in order to determine whether consumption has occurred. To this end, an estimate of platelet number can be quickly accomplished by examination of a Wright-stained blood film or by direct counting. Evaluation of platelet function by the template bleeding time [122] will indicate the degree to which hemostasis is deranged but is not needed if obvious thrombocytopenia is documented. Erythrocyte abnormalities such as schistocytes might be present, but microangiopathic hemolytic anemia [120] alone is a nonspecific finding that is seen in numerous conditions, such as neoplasm, vasculitis, prosthetic valve replacement, or collagen vascular disorder.

Thrombin reacts with fibrinogen, platelets, factor VIII, factor V, and factor XIII. When blood clots in vitro, these factors and prothrombin are consumed and consequently are absent or markedly reduced in serum. In patients with DIC, the concentration of these factors is decreased in vivo. The patient with extensive intravascular clotting may also have reduced levels of clotting factors that are consumed only minimally when blood clots in a glass test tube—factor XI, factor X, factor IX, and factor VII [123]. Possibly these factors undergo more extensive activation during disseminated intravascular clotting.

Activated clotting intermediates are removed from the circulation by cellular clearance and are inactivated by natural inhibitors in the blood [124], particularly antithrombin, whose level falls as the result of the interaction [125,126]. In very ill patients, reduced levels of the vitamin K–dependent clotting factors may also reflect decreased synthesis due to impaired liver function or insufficient vitamin K in patients maintained on intravenous fluids and receiving antibiotics [127,128]. Screening clotting tests, such as activated partial thromboplastin time, prothrombin time, and thrombin time, are prolonged. Quantitative determination of plasmaclottable protein [129] provides relevant information regarding plasma fibrinogen concentration. Care must be taken with inspection of the whole-blood clot to ensure that a small, retracted clot is not overlooked in the mass of loose erythrocytes, since this could be misinterpreted as a systemic fibrinolytic state in which the clot had completely dissolved.

The deposition of fibrin in the microcirculation after disseminated intravascular clotting usually stimulates local secondary fibrinolysis. In this process, plasminogen may be consumed by adsorption onto the extensive fibrin network. In isolated DIC, this local fibrinolysis does not spill over into the systemic circulation to a degree that surpasses the inhibitory ability of plasma antiplasmin, and so the euglobulin lysis time of whole

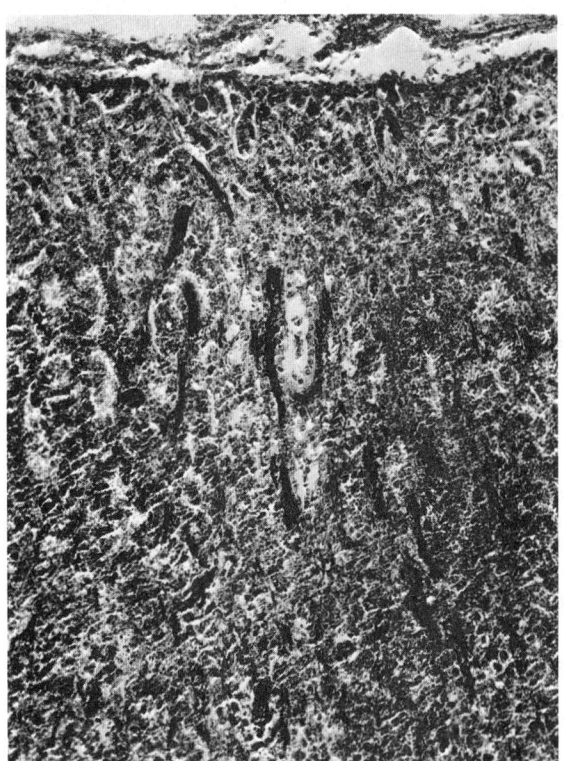

FIGURE 158-3   Section of the adrenal cortex (phosphotungstic acid–hematoxylin stain, ×108) from a patient with fulminant meningococcemia and gross bilateral adrenal hemorrhage at autopsy. Microthrombi in the adrenal sinusoids are seen. (McGehee, Rapaport, and Hjort [112], with permission.)

blood or plasma is not shortened. However, degradation products of fibrin are liberated into the blood, and their presence is important for two reasons. First, one may infer that fibrin has been deposited in vessels and therefore that disseminated intravascular clotting may have occurred. Second, fibrin degradation products interfere with hemostasis, primarily by interfering with

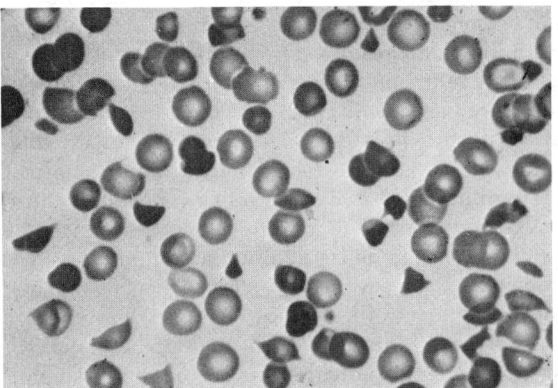

FIGURE 158-4   The appearance of fragmented red blood cells on a peripheral blood film. The deposition of fibrin in small blood vessels after DIC is one mechanism for producing a hemolytic anemia due to red cell fragmentation.

fibrin polymerization, with resultant formation of a defective clot [130–133]. Currently available clinical tests for degradation products do not distinguish between those derived from fibrin and those from fibrinogen (see Chap 138), but the development of such a capacity would be useful for a direct determination that clots were being dissolved.

Clinical tests for fibrin degradation products utilize the unique properties of these derivatives, for instance, their propensity to form soluble complexes with fibrinogen or fibrin that can be precipitated from plasma ("paracoagulation") by low temperature [134], toluidine blue [130], ethanol [135,136], or protamine sulfate [134, 137,138] or demonstrated by gel exclusion chromatography [139,140]. Fibrin degradation products which are unclottable persist in serum and can be detected by their reaction with antisera prepared against native fibrinogen. If blood is clotted by methods assuring full conversion of fibrinogen to fibrin, then the presence in the serum of material immunologically related to fibrinogen must mean that the blood contains nonclottable fibrinogen-fibrin degradation products. Rapid and simple latex-particle agglutination assays [129,141,142], the staphylococcal clumping test [143], or precise hemagglutination tests [144] allow for an estimate of the concentration of serum fibrin degradation products. False-positive results due to incomplete clotting or to in vitro fibrinolysis are avoided by collecting the blood in the presence of excess thrombin and fibrinolytic inhibitor.

The patient with severe DIC may have a normal plasma fibrinogen level if the concentration prior to illness was elevated, as occurs with sepsis and neoplasia. Usually, the blood clot is tiny, the concentration of plasma-clottable protein is less than 100 mg/dl, and serum fibrin degradation product levels are elevated to greater than 40 μg/ml. Although the latter can contribute to bleeding problems, degradation products in the blood reflect the positive feature that the consumed (clotted) fibrinogen is being cleared from the microcirculation by fibrinolysis. Assuming that the factors causing thrombosis can be reversed, this physiologic fibrinolytic response will eventually dissolve all of the offending thrombi and restore normal organ perfusion and function. Evaluation of renal function by monitoring of urine output and blood urea nitrogen or creatinine concentrations provides data for monitoring organ dysfunction that could be due to microthrombi. Normal urine output suggests that excessive consumption has not occurred or that the local fibrinolytic response has kept pace with the deposition of microthrombi.

In patients with severe, acute DIC, virtually all coagulation laboratory studies will be abnormal, and it is not necessary to test further in order to establish the diagnosis. Systemic fibrinolytic states do not cause ischemic skin changes, severe thrombocytopenia, or sudden anuria and azotemia. It is possible that a *systemic* fibrinolytic state may coexist with DIC. In this case, a small, whole-blood clot might dissolve after incubation at 37°C for 1 h or the more sensitive euglobulin lysis time (see Chap. A38) of whole blood or plasma [145] would be shortened from in excess of 4 h to less than 30 min. Even so, treatment should be directed toward the DIC rather than toward the systemic fibrinolytic state.

A minimal laboratory evaluation in the patient who may have DIC would include the following tests:

1. To evaluate platelets and platelet function: bleeding time and platelet count or estimate (blood film)

2. To evaluate plasma clotting reactions: prothrombin time, PTT, thrombin time, fibrinogen concentration, and appearance of whole clot

3. To evaluate fibrinolysis: systemic—clot lysis time of blood or plasma euglobulin; local—fibrin/fibrinogen degradation products

4. To evaluate extent of fibrin deposition in the microcirculation: urine output, blood urea nitrogen, and stained blood film for fragmented red cells

THERAPY

The most important aspects of therapy are those directed toward correction of the underlying disease and general support measures, such as fluid replacement and maintenance of adequate oxygenation and blood pressure. A clinical judgment of whether these therapeutic measures will sustain the patient, curtail the complicating DIC process, and allow for reasonably rapid, spontaneous recovery is the major factor in deciding upon additional, antithrombotic treatments. Thus, life-threatening or progressive, severe microvascular occlusions due to DIC would warrant interruption of thrombosis by heparin anticoagulation, and serious hemorrhagic manifestations would require subsequent aggressive replacement treatment with platelets and plasma clotting factors. This approach has been described and successfully used in acute, severe DIC (purpura fulminans) [146]. There have also been reported the seemingly paradoxical use of an anticoagulant in patients with bleeding manifestations [5,11,147, 148] and benefit both in control of clinical symptoms and in survival [20,21,23]. Others have commented on the limitations, complications, and ineffectiveness of heparin in the treatment of DIC [9,27,149,150] and on the lack of experimental verification of its value to such patients [8,151]. This may be especially confusing when groups of patients with the same underlying condition but with varying degrees of complicating consumptive thrombohemorrhagic disease are subjected to a study of heparin efficacy. Since no prospective, randomized, controlled study on the efficacy of heparin in DIC has been published, the practitioner faces difficult choices in dealing with a case at hand. The approach described below and in Table 158-2 is specifically indicated for the extreme case, according to clinical judgments regarding prognosis, and is not meant to be applied to patients who fall into related but clearly different clinical categories of type or severity of consumptive states.

TABLE 158-2   Treatment of acute, severe disseminated intravascular coagulation

Treatment	Rationale	Details	Expectation
Life-support measures	Self-evident	Fluids, blood, respiratory care, pressors, etc.	Maintain cardiac output, gas exchange, electrolyte balance, etc.
Treatment of underlying disorder	Correct the cause of DIC	Dependent upon primary diagnosis	Inhibit or block complicating pathologic mechanism of DIC, in parallel with response (if any) of disorder
Antithrombotic agents	Block microthrombus formation	Therapeutic doses of heparin by continuous intravenous infusion; monitor by plasma fibrinogen concentration; continue as long as predisposing clinical state persists	Prevent fibrin formation; tip balance within microcirculation toward physiologic fibrinolysis; allow reperfusion of skin, kidneys, brain
Transfusion	Re-establish normal hemostatic potential once thrombosis is blocked by heparin	Infuse platelets and cryoprecipitate for fibrinogen and factors V and VIII; repeat as indicated by laboratory and clinical observation	Increase platelet count and plasma fibrinogen to 50% of normal, if consumption blocked; diminish and stop bleeding during interval of hours to several days
Fibrinolytic inhibitors	Block accumulation of degradation products in blood; protect hemostatic plugs	ϵ-aminocaproic acid, loading dose 4–6 g, then 1 g every 1 or 2 h for limited duration (up to 48 h)	Bleeding ceases rapidly but keeps vascular channels occluded with thrombus; dangerous if thrombotic process not previously treated with heparin

Heparin is administered primarily to inhibit the formation of microthrombi, even though the dominant clinical feature may be hemorrhage. The dose of heparin should be therapeutic (Table 158-2), that is, adequate to overcome the prothrombotic forces, which may have produced a relatively heparin-resistant state in the blood [11]. A bolus intravenous injection of 10,000 units or more could then be followed by intermittent intravenous injections or continuous intravenous administration. The bleeding can be worsened initially by heparin therapy. Therefore, immediately after heparin therapy has been instituted, the bleeding diathesis should be treated by replenishing the depleted (consumed) supply of platelets and clotting factors. For this, platelet concentrates and fresh frozen plasma or cryoprecipitate are used in quantities determined from an expected increase of between 5000 and 10,000 platelets per microliter and 15 mg of fibrinogen per deciliter of plasma for each unit. If consumption is effectively inhibited, the infused material will circulate and the blood concentrations of procoagulants will increase accordingly. From a practical standpoint, *any* increase in platelet count or plasma fibrinogen concentration indicates that the consumption process has been interrupted and that bleeding should be coming under control. Failure to raise the platelet count or plasma fibrinogen level probably means that consumption is continuing. Transfusion without prior administration of heparin only enhances thrombosis and does not effectively correct the plasma deficiency state. Patients with DIC frequently require inordinately large amounts of heparin to overcome intravascular clotting. Such heparin resistance

may be due to increased plasma levels of platelet factor 4 (antiheparin), decreased plasma antithrombin III levels, or other as yet unrecognized influences. Whether antithrombin III infusions will restore responsiveness to heparin awaits evaluation under controlled conditions. With adequate therapy the clinical expectation is for bleeding to decrease, although this may require some hours or even days.

In patients with abruptio placentae [6,152–154] the consumption may be localized in the uterus, but bleeding is severe and laboratory evidence of consumption is striking. Since the primary course of action is to evacuate the uterus, the consumption is effectively terminated; transfused or newly synthesized platelets or fibrinogen will then correct the blood deficiency state. So long as DIC does not coexist, the prior administration of fibrinogen will not produce organ microthrombi. Heparin administration in this circumstance could cause bleeding during the anticipated surgical procedure to relieve the patient of the underlying pathologic process [155]. On the other hand, a patient with septic abortion complicated by DIC may not have a benign course [156,157] even after evacuation of the uterus. In this circumstance, the failure to administer heparin may allow the DIC to progress, given the expected delay before concomitant antibiotic treatment can effectively eliminate the infection.

Fibrinolytic inhibitors should be used with caution in patients with DIC. An excessive concentration of fibrin degradation products in the blood may contribute to the hemorrhagic diathesis. Inhibitors are used to decrease the concentration of degradation products by curtailing the lysis of microthrombi. Fibrinolytic inhibitors may also improve hemostasis by increasing the stability of newly formed hemostatic plugs, but at the same time, the clearance of microthrombi from occluded renal and cerebral vessels will be delayed. The indication for fibrinolytic inhibitors should not be a laboratory value, no matter how abnormal, but rather a clinical state of dangerous, excessive, or extremely bothersome bleeding that has not responded to replacement treatment and is hampering care or threatening life.

In some unfortunate cases, fibrinolytic inhibitors have been administered to patients with severe DIC without prior heparinization, resulting in catastrophic worsening of the thrombotic state [158,159]. Because of this potential problem, fibrinolytic inhibitors are rarely added to the regimen, although their use has been gratifying in selected cases [160]. If DIC is suspected, fibrinolytic inhibitors should not be administered without prior effective antithrombotic treatment with heparin. Antifibrinolytic treatment alone for the relatively unusual case of isolated systemic fibrinolysis should be undertaken only after the diagnosis is clearly established and a concomitant DIC state is excluded. Before deciding on the specifics of therapy in the patient with suspected DIC, it is reasonable to consider the following:

1. Has the mechanism triggering the intravascular clotting been controlled? Has it arrested because of its self-limited nature or is it ongoing and unlikely to respond to treatment for hours or days?

2. Are there clinical effects of tissue ischemia or bleeding or only laboratory changes of the consumption and local fibrinolysis? Stated otherwise, is fibrin in small blood vessels producing harmful effects or does the patient have asymptomatic hypofibrinogenemia and positive tests for serum degradation products?

3. Have all varieties of consumptive thrombohemorrhagic disorder been considered? For instance, is the underlying disorder localized or disseminated and can the laboratory and clinical findings distinguish between a lytic state and thrombosis? These possibilities are discussed below.

Chronic disseminated intravascular coagulation

In contrast to the acutely ill patient with complicating severe DIC, other patients have mild or protracted clinical manifestations of consumption or even subclinical disease manifest only by laboratory abnormalities [20, 161,162]. This clinical picture generally occurs in patients with long-standing illnesses, such as malignancy [35,162–164] or autoimmune disease [165]. A hemorrhagic presentation secondary to thrombocytopenia and hypofibrinogenemia may predominate, but a significant number of patients have deep-vein thrombosis

as the principal manifestation. In a group of patients with malignancy and various manifestations of thrombosis, isolated venous thrombosis occurred in 113 of 182 patients and migratory venous thrombosis (Trousseau syndrome) [166] in 96, while a bleeding state existed in only 75 patients [162]. Signs of microvascular thrombotic occlusive disease are unusual in chronic DIC, even though the patients uniformly have evidence suggestive of intravascular coagulation, namely, positive assays for fibrinopeptide release or circulating fibrin monomers [136,164,167–169]. These may reflect an effective secondary fibrinolytic response that keeps pace with the low-grade intravascular coagulation. The fibrin monomers and polymers that could form obstructive microthrombi are effectively dissolved before tissue ischemia or dysfunction results.

A unique feature of these chronically ill patients, especially those with mucin-producing carcinoma, is nonbacterial thrombotic endocarditis with systemic embolization and infarction [170]. This occurred in 45 of 182 patients in one series [162]. All three clinical reflections of chronic DIC—venous thrombosis, endocarditis, and bleeding—were noted in 12 of this group [162] as well as in single cases reported by others [35, 163].

Patients with no clinical manifestations of DIC but with thrombocytopenia, hypofibrinogenemia, positive serum degradation products, elevated fibrinopeptide A level, or a positive ethanol gelation or protamine sulfate test require only observation and follow-up studies in addition to treatment of the underlying disorder and selective replacement of consumed platelets and/or fibrinogen. In the usual case, the clinical manifestations are controlled and the laboratory evidence of consumption corrected [35,162–165,167]. Attempts at control of the consumption with antiplatelet agents or even with a coumarin agent have proved less effective than heparin treatment in preventing recurrent disease [35]. The treatment of choice remains heparin administered intravenously at first, then chronically by subcutaneous injection. The possibility of an isolated systemic hyperfibrinolytic state should also be evaluated with lysis time assays, but treatment with fibrinolytic inhibitors should be approached with caution in order to avoid their use in patients with a potential for thrombosis.

Systemic fibrino(geno)lysis

Spontaneous systemic hyperfibrinolysis is an unusual occurrence. Its pure form is best illustrated by the changes induced during the therapeutic administration of plasminogen activators, such as streptokinase and urokinase (see Chap. 159). In this circumstance, plasmin is produced and susceptible protein substrates, such as the fibrin in thrombi or hemostatic plugs and plasma fibrinogen, and factors V and VIII are degraded. The clinical manifestations are bleeding, which is a result of both the depletion of clotting factors, especially

TABLE 158-3   Comparison between disseminated intravascular coagulation and primary fibrinogenolysis

	Acute DIC	*Systemic fibrinogenolysis*	*DIC plus systemic fibrinogenolysis*
Incidence	Relatively common	Very rare	Not infrequently
Underlying disease	Present	Often absent, occasionally liver disease	Present
Platelet count	Low	Normal	Low
Euglobulin lysis time	Normal	Rapid	Rapid
Fibrinogen	Low	Low	Low
Serum fibrin/fibrinogen degradation products	Elevated	Elevated	Elevated
Screening coagulation tests	Prolonged	Prolonged	Prolonged

fibrinogen, and the lysis of recently formed hemostatic plugs. The confusing aspects of the fibrinolytic state are (1) that the same clinical states which cause DIC may also predispose to systemic fibrinolysis, (2) that the major presenting symptoms of both DIC and fibrinolysis are usually hemorrhagic, (3) that high concentrations of fibrinogen-fibrin degradation products may circulate in both conditions, and (4) that DIC and fibrinolysis may coexist, both having been induced by the same pathologic insult. Both DIC and hyperfibrinolysis are characterized by a fibrinolytic response, the distinction being primarily one of anatomic location [5]. In DIC, the lysis occurs in, and is typically limited to, the microcirculation; it is a physiologic response to the deposition of thrombi. In systemic hyperfibrinolysis, lysis occurs in the macrocirculation, perhaps as the result of activators released from endothelial cells.

The distinction between DIC and systemic hyperfibrinolysis may be difficult even when abundant laboratory facilities are available since virtually all of the relevant laboratory assays that reflect DIC can be abnormal in systemic fibrinolysis as well (Table 158-3). The simplest laboratory characterization of an isolated fibrinolysis would be a shortened euglobulin lysis time [145] without significant thrombocytopenia. Given this result, along with the absence of any clinical or laboratory indication of concomitant thrombosis and the presence of a serious bleeding disorder, therapy with fibrinolytic inhibitors could be considered. However, if the evaluation of the fibrinolytic state is erroneous and DIC also exists or if subclinical DIC has been masked by an active fibrinolytic response, then treatment with fibrinolytic inhibitors can be dangerous [158,159,171].

Many cases that appear to be systemic fibrinolysis actually are either DIC with secondary fibrinolysis or a combination of DIC and systemic fibrinolysis. For instance, a patient with heat stroke, temperature greater than 108°F, metabolic acidosis, hypotension, gastrointestinal bleeding, and oozing from venipuncture sites was thought to have hypofibrinogenemia secondary to a fibrinolytic state and was treated unsuccessfully with support measures supplemented with ε-aminocaproic acid [172]. The plasma clot lysis time was short, but the platelet count was only 54,000 per microliter, indicating that a fibrinolytic state was not the sole pathologic process producing consumption. Cases such as this are assumed to have coexistent DIC and systemic fibrinolysis. Heparin should be administered first, then platelets and fibrinogen transfused, and fibrinolytic inhibitors should be used only if still indicated for uncontrolled bleeding [173–176].

Fibrinolytic inhibitors have been suggested for routine use in the treatment of systemic fibrinolysis accompanying extracorporeal bypass cardiac surgery, especially that involving cyanotic heart disease and protracted extracorporeal circulation [177–179]. Although the fibrinolytic state can occur during such surgery and excess bleeding may relate to such an abnormality, the use of fibrinolytic inhibitors still represents a potential hazard in the unmasking of a DIC state. Such primary fibrinolytic states are often the result of acute trauma or hypoxic states that are short-lived and self-limited and therefore do not require treatment with fibrinolytic inhibitors; however, those which accompany chronic illness, such as prostatic carcinoma [5], could require long-term therapy.

A rare variant may be localized hyperfibrinolysis, a result of the release of plasminogen activator activity from a tumor, causing persistent local bleeding [180].

Localized consumption

Certain disease states are predictably associated with the consumption of platelets and clotting factors in strictly defined, localized anatomic sites. Laboratory results indicate disseminated intravascular coagulation, inasmuch as the platelet count may be less than 50,000 per microliter and the plasma fibrinogen concentration below 100 mg/dl and significant levels of fibrinogen-fibrin degradation products may be detectable in the serum. The pathologic process may even be manifest clinically as a bleeding disorder if the consumption is excessive and the fibrinolytic response brisk. However, these localized pathologic conditions are typically not associated with thrombosis or consumption anywhere but in the organ or tissue specifically involved.

The risk of not recognizing the limited disorder is twofold: inappropriate therapy may be initiated for a presumed disseminated state, and a potentially reversible underlying disorder may not be recognized. Since management depends more on treatment of the underlying disorder than on correction of the coagulation tests, individual clinical states will be discussed.

AORTIC ANEURYSM

The localized consumption of platelets and fibrinogen which occurs in aortic aneurysms [161] can produce not only striking laboratory abnormalities but even symptomatic bleeding. Although the frequency with which patients with aneurysm demonstrate overt hemorrhagic manifestations is quite low [181], this complication may be particularly associated with acute extensions and enlargements of the aneurysm or false channel [182–187]. In some cases, there is dramatic manifestation of spontaneous bleeding episodes in association with radiographic evidence of an expanding aneurysmal mass or with the sudden onset of severe pain indicative of dissection. Other patients have a chronic hemorrhagic tendency [185,187] with mild bruising and bleeding after minor surgical procedures. Most of the patients respond to treatment with heparin, with increases in platelet count and correction of coagulation tests as well as clinical improvement, reflecting the ability of an otherwise healthy patient to replenish the consumed elements. Definitive treatment depends upon surgical repair, and the best approach to surgery seems to be a prior stabilization of hemostasis with heparin therapy and infusions of platelets and/or fibrinogen, the latter depending upon the urgency of the situation. Symptomatic bleeding signals the need for prompt treatment since significant recent extension had probably occurred. The severity of the underlying condition is reflected in the death of four of the seven cases in two reports [184,186] and the occurrence of dramatic perioperative bleeding during surgical repair [188].

HEMANGIOMAS

The report by Kassabach and Merritt [31] clearly implicated hemangiomas as a cause of hemorrhagic diathesis. Primarily a disorder of infants and children, these hemangiomas are usually benign tumors [189] that may enlarge or otherwise evolve into a convoluted mass of vascular channels that sequester and consume platelets and fibrinogen from the blood. This has been clearly demonstrated by physiologic studies in which the half-life of platelets is shortened [190] and radioactive platelets and fibrinogen accumulate in the tumor

[191]. An animal model has been useful for confirmation of this phenomenon, showing both fibrin deposits and platelet thrombi in transplanted mouse hemangioendotheliomas [192]. The concept of local sequestration [193] is compatible with the demonstration of fibrinolytic activity localized to the tumor [194]. The latter could further explain why fibrin or platelet thrombi are found in some [195] but not all [194] such cases. Although heightened fibrinolytic activity may sometimes be demonstrable in blood, DIC is not a feature of this illness and distant thrombi in organs such as the kidney would not be expected.

Medical treatment of the tumor is often ineffective, and surgery can be dangerous because of problems in achieving hemostasis. Therefore, such patients are usually managed conservatively unless cosmetic corrections are needed or when symptoms of bleeding result from severe thrombocytopenia and hypofibrinogenemia. These symptoms can be persistent and serious, and their control by treatment of the tumor is unpredictable. The mass can occasionally regress spontaneously [189], or it may shrink after radiation therapy. For the remainder of the patients, treatment with either antiplatelet agents [196] or heparin [195,197,198] has been attempted to allow self-correction of the platelet count and fibrinogen concentration and of the bleeding symptoms. This approach is especially recommended when the patient requires surgery, the rationale being first to correct the hemostatic defect by blocking the local consumption and then to remove the tumor. Some patients have had such extensive tumor or involvement of vital organs that postoperative or spontaneous bleeding from the tumor could not be controlled, leading to the patient's demise [194,195].

RENAL DISEASE

The presence in the urine of degradation products of fibrinogen or fibrin at a time when degradation products are absent from the blood or present in only very small amounts indicates that localized consumption has occurred in the kidneys. The most dramatic example of this is in hyperacute renal *allograft rejection*. Destruction of the donor kidney within minutes to hours after transplant is associated with extensive deposition of fibrin in the arterioles and glomeruli [199], probably related to the reaction of humoral antibodies against the mismatched cellular antigens [200]. The vigorous immunologic reaction activates coagulation locally, mimicking the histologic picture of the Shwartzman reaction, and in unusual cases mild systemic consumption occurs as well [201–203].

Fibrin degradation products were first demonstrated in the urine of patients with a slowly evolving homograft rejection [204]. All of the patients excreted fibrin degradation products in the urine in the first 2 weeks after transplantation, whether or not subsequent rejection occurred, but the appearance of urinary degradation products after 2 weeks uniformly heralded rejection. Since serum degradation products were absent, their appearance in the urine was best explained by *in situ* degradation of deposited fibrin by a localized fibrinolytic response, with excretion directly into the draining tubular system. From studies of serial urine samples in patients after renal allotransplantation [205], the initial rise of urinary degradation products after transplant can be attributed to perioperative ischemia and to the onset of spontaneous renal function. These observations explain the occurrence of degradation products in the urine of patients whose transplants were not subsequently rejected. Brief intervals of degradation product excretion were also noted in otherwise asymptomatic patients, possibly representing mild rejection episodes that spontaneously reverse. This measure of localized fibrin dissolution is a convenient tool for monitoring such patients, especially regarding response to changes in treatment with immunosuppressive agents. The addition of heparin anticoagulation may in some cases help to control the local fibrin deposition even though the underlying response may still be active [205], and antiplatelet therapy has also been advocated as a means of limiting the vaso-occlusive phenomena [206].

Other renal disorders may be associated with excretion of fibrin degradation products, reaching concentrations of 2 to 100 μg/ml in patients with *proliferative glomerulonephritis* and glomerulonephritis associated with systemic lupus erythematosus [204,207,208] and 0.25 to 2.5 μg/ml in patients with the nephrotic syndrome of membranous glomerulonephritis [205]. Whereas the amount of urinary degradation product in the proliferative type of glomerulonephritis relates to the amount of deposited intraglomerular fibrin, that which occurs with membranous changes correlates with the degree of proteinuria [205]. In all likelihood, the degradation products in proliferative glomerulonephritis are fibrin-derived, while those in membranous disease result from urokinase degradation of filtered plasma fibrinogen. Patients with autoimmune disorders causing active proliferative glomerulonephritis, such as systemic lupus erythematosus, are likely to have degradation products in the blood as well as in the urine, reflecting some degree of disseminated as well as localized consumption.

Although the etiologic agent or mechanism of the *hemolytic uremic syndrome* is not understood, it is reasonable to consider this entity in the category of localized renal disease. The major pathology is limited to the kidneys, and the underlying process is probably best called a thrombotic angiopathy [209], perhaps of immunologic origin. The initial lesions of afferent arteriolar fibrinoid necrosis and fibrin deposition in glomerular capillaries may be followed in severe cases by major cortical vessel occlusion and renal cortical necrosis [210,211]. The illness most commonly affects infants under 1 year of age and begins with a gastroenteritis which is superseded several days later by oliguria or anuria, by bleeding secondary to thrombocytopenia, and by hemolytic anemia. The course may

proceed rapidly toward recovery or a lethal outcome or may be protracted or even cyclical. The primary determinant of outcome is the degree of renal impairment [212,213]. Mortality has been reported to be as high as 40 percent [214] and as low as 5 percent [215], but the influence of different diagnostic criteria, supportive measures for renal function, and anticoagulant therapy are not the same in all studies [213,216]. The parallels in pathology and laboratory analysis between renal graft rejection and hemolytic uremic syndrome are striking [217,218]. Almost all patients have thrombocytopenia as a result of the localized deposition of thrombi, and microangiopathic hemolytic anemia is a common finding (Fig. 158-4), but levels of serum fibrin degradation products are usually not elevated.

The rationale for heparin therapy is to limit the amount of fibrin deposited in the kidneys and perhaps thereby to limit the amount of renal damage and the duration of thrombocytopenia. Reports of heparin therapy have generally been encouraging [212,219] but are uncontrolled and do not permit firm conclusions. It has been stated that there is compelling evidence against using heparin [216] based upon a controlled study [220] and other observations. Before deciding upon heparin therapy, one must consider the severity of the illness, the extent of ongoing fibrin deposition, and the location of the consumptive process. Heparin and dipyridamole therapy has been successful in three of four patients with hemolytic uremic syndrome [221], and antiplatelet therapy and anticoagulant therapy have been applied together in managing allograft rejections [222]. Fibrinolytic therapy with streptokinase has been used in hemolytic uremic syndrome with inconclusive results in uncontrolled studies [223,224]. The use of any of these agents can be rationalized, but possible benefit must be balanced against the added risk of hemorrhagic complications, especially if the patient already manifests spontaneous bleeding symptoms. Treatment must therefore be directed first toward supportive measures for maintenance of electrolyte balance and vascular volume, especially by hemodialysis and blood and platelet replacement, and then toward possible anticoagulant measures directed at the localized consumption, if individual circumstances suggest their application.

Consumption limited to platelets

A group of disorders which includes thrombotic thrombocytopenic purpura (TTP), hemolytic-uremic syndrome (HUS), systemic lupus erythematosus, diffuse vasculitis, "immune complex" disease, malignant hypertension, and eclampsia is associated with the potential of single or multiple organ ischemic disease as the result of intraluminal platelet thrombus formation. The clinical symptoms and laboratory changes may be remarkably similar among the group, and confusion exists regarding their etiology. The pathologic pictures of HUS and TTP are especially similar, and a strong argument could be made for a common pathogenesis which results in disease localized to the renal circulation in HUS or manifest in multiple organs in TTP [225,226]. TTP in its full-blown clinical presentation would therefore include neurologic symptoms in addition to renal insufficiency and profound thrombocytopenia in addition to microangiopathic hemolytic anemia.

Although untreated TTP carries a higher mortality—up to 80 percent [227]—and appears to affect an older age group than HUS, both disorders may involve platelets exclusively in the intraluminal arteriolar thrombus. The widespread nature of the occlusive disease was initially described by Moschcowitz [33], and soon after it was postulated to result from platelet thrombi [228–230]. Multiple organs have been shown to contain primarily loose platelet aggregates or granular deposits, with minimal regions of interspersed fibrin demonstrable [231]. Thrombocytopenia and microangiopathic hemolytic anemia are striking, but serum fibrin-fibrinogen degradation products are negative and clotting tests and plasma fibrinogen normal, arguing strongly against significant consumption of fibrinogen either locally or systemically. The absence of coagulation factor consumption is also supported by laboratory surveys of patients with TTP [232,233] and by turnover studies indicating the platelets are involved (shorter half-life) to a much greater extent than fibrinogen in HUS, TTP, vasculitis, and malignant hypertension [234,235]. Overlap may occur with syndromes associated with elevated serum fibrin degradation products and significant local or systemic fibrin deposition and may be of special importance in deciding on appropriate therapy. The ischemic symptoms depend almost exclusively on the rapidity of development (acute versus chronic) and location (localized versus disseminated) of platelet thrombi, while the hemorrhagic symptoms depend upon the degree to which the platelets are consumed (mild versus severe) (Table 158-1). Although the hematologic laboratory results may appear similar to those in idiopathic thrombocytopenic purpura, this latter disorder results from direct immune-related platelet destruction and has no thrombotic component.

New approaches to therapy appear to have significantly lessened the mortality rate [236,237]. It is reasonable to consider antiplatelet agents, such as aspirin and persantin [238], as a means of preventing the secondary thrombotic effect following a presumed initial immunologic injury [239]. However, the use of plasma infusion [240] or plasma exchange [241,242], perhaps in combination with antiplatelet agents [243], apparently has been more effective. This approach may remove a noxious agent, such as antibody or immune complex, or may infuse a missing factor [244], perhaps an inhibitor of platelet aggregation [245,246]. Splenectomy has been reported to be effective in some cases [247–250], but concomitant administration of drugs or infusion of plasma during surgery may have contributed to success in these patients [251]. Replacement of consumed platelets, administration of steroids, and general support measures, such as hemodialysis and volume and electrolyte correction, are obviously of importance in the severely affected patient.

Clinical conditions predisposing to consumptive thrombohemorrhagic disorders

Many medical and surgical conditions are associated with consumptive thrombohemorrhagic disorders. Some underlying causes, such as neoplasms, produce highly variable clinical and laboratory manifestations, whereas others, such as the giant cavernous hemangioma, present a uniform pattern of consumption. These associated phenomena are summarized in Table 158-4; some have been described above, and others will be considered individually in the following discussion.

INFECTIONS

Virtually every type of infectious agent has been implicated in the consumptive thrombohemorrhagic disorders. These agents usually produce systemic intravascular coagulation of mild or severe degree, with consumption of both platelets and soluble clotting factors, or isolated thrombocytopenia [252] (Table 158-1). The most flagrant examples are Waterhouse-Friderichsen syndrome [253,254] and purpura fulminans [255], both of which bear pathologic and histologic similarity to the experimental animal model of consumption, the Shwartzman reaction [36,256]. Waterhouse-Friderichsen syndrome is most commonly seen during fulminant meningococcal sepsis [24,25,27,28,113, 257–260], although other organisms, such as Pneumococcus [27,28,261–263], may also precipitate this complication. Widespread intravascular fibrin and platelet thrombi obstruct arterioles, capillaries, and venules of vital organs (as described above), and in addition hemorrhagic necrosis of the adrenal glands leads to profound shock, which is often irreversible and which contributes significantly to the high mortality rate. Purpura fulminans afflicts the young primarily but not exclusively [255] and is characterized by hemorrhagic bullae and hemorrhagic ischemic necrosis of the skin and even gangrene of the extremities. This clinical presentation follows any of a multitude of infections, most commonly streptococcal, which often appears as scarlet fever [27,28,121,146,147,264–267]. Vascular occlusive disease similar to that in the skin occurs in other organs, and thrombosis of larger vessels may occur in severely affected individuals.

Patients with these two clinical entities have the highest mortality risk and the most fulminant clinical course and are the most difficult to treat effectively. Variations in the acuteness of onset and in the degree of consumption, perhaps related to the age and health of the patient and to the type of infectious agent, account for the wide range of clinical manifestations, including

TABLE 158-4   Clinical conditions associated with consumptive thrombohemorrhagic disorders

Underlying disease	Predominant form of consumptive disorder
Sepsis	DIC, variable severity
Neoplasm	DIC, often chronic, but heterogeneous clinical manifestations and rare systemic hyperfibrinolysis
Obstetric	Localized and/or disseminated, wide variation in clinical severity
Hepatic disease	Variable, hyperfibrinolysis more likely than DIC
TTP/HUS	Systemic, predominant platelet involvement
Giant cavernous hemangioma	Localized, intravascular
Arterial aneurysm	Localized, intravascular
Snake bite	DIC, variable thrombocytopenia
Massive hemolysis	DIC
Trauma, surgery, hyperthermia	DIC, occasional fibrinolysis, which may mask an underlying DIC
Streptokinase, urokinase	Systemic fibrinolysis
Menorrhagia, hemorrhagic cystitis	Localized fibrinolysis

some patients with only laboratory abnormalities of consumption. Virtually any gram-negative organism can produce severe DIC [28,268–270], although histopathologic evidence is most often seen in patients with gram-negative shock who died during the first 24 h after presentation [271,272]. Gram-positive bacteria have been less frequently implicated in DIC [28]. A significant number of patients with pneumococcal sepsis and DIC have had functional or anatomic asplenia [261–263], which probably adversely affected the clearance of organisms from the circulation and contributed to the consumptive process. In addition to the association of streptococcal organisms with purpura fulminans, defects of coagulation have been noted during infections with *Staphylococcus* [273] and *Clostridia* organisms have been implicated in the severe DIC of septic abortion [274–276], which has a mortality rate greater than 50 percent when complicated by shock [277].

Viral diseases, such as the exanthems, varicella, variola, rubella, rubeola, and influenza A [278–282], have also led to a consumptive process, and the severity of Dengue hemorrhagic fever has been correlated with shortened fibrinogen survival, thrombocytopenia, prolongation of the PTT, and concentration of fibrin degradation products [283]. The thrombocytopenia that has been reported in about half of the patients with Rocky Mountain spotted fever [284] may reflect intravascular consumption, and, in addition, laboratory evidence of DIC has been associated with a more fulminant clinical course [285–287]. Patients with severe *Plasmodium falciparum* malaria complicated by thrombocytopenia and coagulation abnormalities [288–291] or even by deep-vein thrombosis and tissue necrosis [292] may also have DIC complicating the original infection. Miscellaneous other organisms, such as aspergillus [293], candida [294], trypanosomes [295], and tubercle bacilli [296], have also been implicated as initiators of consumption, suggesting that virtually any infectious agent can be associated with thrombohemorrhagic disorder.

There is much controversy as to whether or not interruption of the hemostatic abnormalities with antithrombotic therapy has a significant influence on the recovery of the patient with severe infection. The rationale for the use of antithrombotic therapy in patients with septic shock derives from experimental data on animal models, in which the Shwartzman reaction in rabbits or the coagulopathy induced by sepsis in primates can be inhibited by heparin [297–301]. The successful use of antithrombotic therapy in purpura fulminans [146,147,255,302], the fall in mortality rate and in renal complications in patients with septic abortion to whom heparin was administered before onset of endotoxic shock [156,303], and the clinical improvement of many acutely ill patients with DIC treated with heparin [11,304] support the role of heparin therapy in DIC, especially in patients who are severely ill and at significant risk of lethal outcome. A statistically significant improvement in survival of heparinized patients (67 percent survival) versus nonheparinized patients (32 percent survival) has been shown among septicemic patients who survive more than 24 h after the start of therapy [20]. On the other hand, analysis of 222 patients with septicemic shock and DIC demonstrated no difference in survival between the group receiving heparin (24 percent) and the group not treated with heparin (21 percent) [305]. It has been suggested that heparinization may have been beneficial in controlling the coagulopathy but that it had no effect on outcome [305]. Treatment of the shock state may be of greater importance than antithrombotic therapy, and reversal of hypotension appears to be the major factor in survival [306]. The possibility that heparin therapy may produce more bleeding complications than would have occurred in the absence of such therapy has been suggested

[307,308], but this has not been demonstrated by controlled studies.

There is no well-controlled, prospective study of heparin therapy in the treatment of DIC associated with sepsis. Therefore it is not possible to substantiate an opinion either in favor of or against the use of heparin in such patients. However, it seems reasonable to use heparin in addition to specific therapy for the underlying disorder in more severely affected patients, that is, those with evolving ischemic skin lesions, renal failure, multifocal neurologic defects or change in the sensorium, or severe bleeding caused by sudden and profound hypofibrinogenemia and thrombocytopenia. In such patients, much higher doses of heparin may be required than those effective in venous thromboembolic disease, and doses adequate to allow transfused platelets and fibrinogen to circulate must be administered. The principles of therapy outlined in Table 158-2—attention to the underlying disease, transfusion of platelets and blood coagulation proteins after administration of heparin, and administration of fibrinolytic inhibitors only after heparin administration and only if hemorrhage is uncontrollable—should be followed.

OBSTETRIC COMPLICATIONS

Since 1901, when DeLee reported a state of "temporary hemophilia" in a patient with premature separation of the placenta and in another with a macerated dead fetus [309], it has become evident that a consumptive thrombohemorrhagic state may be observed in a wide range of obstetric complications, including abruptio placentae, retained dead fetus, amniotic fluid embolism, saline-induced or septic abortion, and toxemia. The manifestations are varied. The site of consumption may be limited to a single, extravascular locus (the uterus), disseminated in the blood, or present in both locations; the pathologic mechanism may involve coagulation, fibrinolysis, or both simultaneously; and the broadest range of tempo may occur, from the fulminant onset of abruptio placentae to the chronic, low-grade effects of retained fetus syndrome. An excellent summary of the clinical, pathologic, diagnostic, and therapeutic aspects of such obstetric complications has been published [310].

A consideration of consumptive disorders before, during, and after delivery must be compared with baseline studies of normal parturition [311,312]. Following uncomplicated single delivery, there is a significant decrease of plasma fibrinogen concentration, a shortening of plasma euglobulin lysis time, and an increase in concentration of fibrinogen degradation products, all occurring 1 to 4 h after delivery. These changes indicate that a minor degree of physiologic defibrination is expected under ordinary circumstances. The changes are similar to, but of lesser magnitude than, those which occur with abruptio placentae or with intrauterine death syndrome.

Abruptio placentae may occur in the absence of clinical symptoms, in which case the diagnosis becomes appar-

ent only upon pathologic examination of the placenta. It may be manifest as a mild-to-moderate episode of vaginal bleeding with excessive contraction of the uterus associated with a significantly increased risk of fetal death, or it may appear with generalized bleeding, hemorrhagic shock, severe abdominal pain and tenderness, and fetal death [12,310]. The incidence of all degrees of abruptio has been variously recorded as somewhat less than 1 percent of all deliveries [313], with the severe form occurring in less than 0.2 percent [152, 153]. Aside from direct trauma [314], the underlying cause of placental separation is not certain [310]. The process that causes consumption in such patients probably represents a combination of localized, intrauterine hemorrhage [314,315] and systemic defibrination caused by release of thromboplastic placental tissue or amniotic fluid constituents [207,316,317]. It is difficult to gauge whether the consumption could result from a localized process alone, since some patients show no preferential accumulation of fibrin in the uterus above that present in a hematoma [152]. On the other hand, the organ effects, such as compromise of renal function, which are presumed to be secondary to DIC, respond dramatically after delivery even with only general support measures and no antithrombotic drugs. This suggests that other factors, such as hypovolemia secondary to the uterine bleeding, may be more important than DIC in the pathogenesis of systemic effects.

Whether consumption is local, disseminated, or a combination of these, the laboratory manifestations include decreases in platelet count and plasma fibrinogen levels and the appearance of fibrin degradation products [152,155,311,312,318,319], the latter resulting principally from physiologic lysis of the intrauterine hematoma. A systemic fibrinolytic state with short euglobulin lysis time is not usually seen [152,311,320].

Although renal cortical necrosis with demonstrable intravascular fibrin occurs in a small proportion of patients with abruptio placentae [321,322], the course of the illness is usually favorable if adequate support measures are taken. Most important, whole blood should be administered to correct hypovolemia and hypotension, improve renal perfusion, and prevent renal cortical necrosis. Using only this therapy, vaginal delivery is usually accomplished without hemorrhagic complication and rapid regeneration of the plasma fibrinogen follows [152,153,311]. If hysterectomy is necessary—for instance, if the fetus is alive and delivery must be performed immediately—or if episiotomy is performed during vaginal delivery, supplementation with fibrinogen (cryoprecipitate) and platelets is reasonable to provide normal hemostasis. Heparin is generally not administered prior to surgery since this could contribute to increased bleeding during vaginal delivery or hysterectomy. Antifibrinolytic agents are contraindicated unless the patient has serious hemorrhagic manifestations that are not corrected by replacement transfusion after delivery.

Amniotic fluid embolism was firmly established as a

syndrome by clinical and histopathologic changes first described in 1941 [323]. Its incidence has been estimated at between 1 in 8000 and 1 in 37,000 live births [324]. Clinically, it is characterized by the sudden onset of severe respiratory distress, cyanosis, and profound circulatory shock in the setting of a multiparous patient during or just after labor. The diagnosis is confirmed antemortem by the demonstration in the buffy coat of fetal debris (scales, lanugo, meconium), which may form a third layer above the leukocytes after centrifugation of blood aspirated from a central venous catheter. Postmortem, patients with amniotic fluid embolism show the same material obstructing the capillaries and arterioles of the lungs. Mortality has been estimated at greater than 80 percent, with 15 percent of these patients dying shortly after the onset of the syndrome [310,324]. In patients who survive the initial episode, excessive bleeding follows in 40 percent of cases, usually after a latent period of 0.5 to 3 h.

The specific pathogenetic mechanism for the clinical manifestations is unclear. An anaphylactoid reaction to the fetal material which enters the maternal circulation has been postulated [323], but a simpler explanation is that the amniotic fluid debris mechanically obstructs the pulmonary circulation, resulting in acute cor pulmonale [310,325,326]. Following the initial pulmonary arterial obstructive phenomena, there can be local activation of the coagulation system and severe consumption with secondary fibrinolysis and a hemorrhagic disorder [310,327–330]. Because of the rarity of this entity and its rapid course, the effectiveness of various treatments has not been fully assessed. Vigorous supportive therapy, including mechanical respiratory assistance for gas exchange and fluid and blood replacement to treat severe hypotension, is essential. In patients in whom continued entry of amniotic fluid debris may be contributing to further intravascular clotting, heparin is a reasonable adjunct to therapy [320,331–335]. When hemorrhage becomes the major manifestation, however, the use of heparin may accentuate the bleeding, especially if adequate replacement of consumed clotting factors has not been achieved [310]. Fibrinolytic inhibitors have been recommended in addition to replacement therapy for treatment of dangerous bleeding, but the precautions regarding its use are the same as those in other settings of DIC and must be considered (Table 158-2).

Dead fetus syndrome exists if the fibrinogen concentration falls below normal in the context of intrauterine fetal death. This syndrome represents a slowly developing, compensated or low-grade form of DIC (Table 158-1). The incidence of DIC increases with longer periods of fetal retention, to as much as 35 percent of patients when retention continues for 5 weeks or longer [336]. Although some patients appear to have an acute primary fibrinolytic response to the dead fetus [155,337], the evidence strongly suggests that intravascular coagulation is the sole mechanism for the defibrination in most patients [155,310,338–340]. As ex-

pected in patients with slowly developing consumption (see above), the secondary fibrinolytic response keeps pace with the formation of fibrin thrombi, and organ obstruction and ischemia are not part of the clinical picture. The low fibrinogen and platelet counts do not usually cause serious spontaneous bleeding, but hemorrhage after delivery is to be expected. Thus, treatment is generally directed at transfusion at the time of delivery since infused plasma fibrinogen will not circulate normally before delivery and since heparin may contribute to bleeding if delivery is traumatic. The use of fibrinolytic inhibitors is not reasonable in the absence of a markedly shortened euglobulin lysis time unless the usual measures for correcting the hemostatic defect fail and bleeding is still intense. As with other obstetric consumptive complications, the essence of treatment is to empty the uterus, and therefore a decision regarding the timing of induced delivery after fetal death should consider the increased potential of this syndrome with delays longer than 2 weeks.

Saline-induced abortion during the second trimester of pregnancy has been documented to cause DIC, based upon demonstration of hypofibrinogenemia, thrombocytopenia, and circulating fibrin degradation products [341–345]. The mechanism for this mild, acute DIC is not certain but presumably is the entry of disintegrated placental tissue into the circulation, resulting in activation of the coagulation system. The laboratory changes are sometimes noted at the time of the abortion but usually follow the procedure after a delay of hours. Systemic manifestations of a bleeding tendency or even problems of excessive bleeding with expulsion of the fetus are unusual. The induced abortion removes the underlying cause of the consumption and is the major consideration in curtailing the consumptive state. Deficiencies of plasma fibrinogen and platelets should be corrected if excessive bleeding is noted at the time of abortion.

In contrast to the relatively mild DIC of saline-induced abortion, *septic abortion* may herald the most fulminant type of severe DIC, similar in all ways to that described above for infections. In a large group of more than 6000 abortion patients treated in one series, 16 percent were infected, of which 40 patients (4 percent) had shock and DIC, leading to death in half of these seriously affected patients [277]. Any of a large number of bacteria, both aerobic and anerobic, may be the inciting agent, and severe hypotension and clinical shock, along with the circulation of endotoxins, contribute to the acute DIC process [310,346,347]. Once DIC is established, the clinical symptoms, laboratory manifestations, and principles of therapy are as noted for the same complication of any severe infection leading to shock, with the added consideration that evacuation of the uterus and sometimes hysterectomy are required in order to neutralize the infection. These patients can be the most refractory to therapy, and vigorous attention must be paid to proper antibiotic choice and to maintenance of blood volume and electrolyte balance. Also, there must be appropriate therapy for the thrombotic process, with consideration of heparin and replacement therapy. As with other circumstances of acute severe DIC, fibrinolytic inhibitors should be withheld unless necessary because of dangerous bleeding, in order not to impair the physiologic fibrinolytic response in the microcirculation of ischemic organs.

A spectrum of renal and neurologic symptoms similar to those seen in thrombotic thrombocytopenic purpura or in hemolytic uremic syndrome has long been recognized in some patients with preeclampsia and especially with eclampsia (*toxemia of pregnancy*) [348,349]. The preeclamptic patients appear to have a chronic DIC process, with levels of fibrinogen, platelets, and other clotting factors no different from those found during normal pregnancy [350–353], but with demonstrable fibrin present in the glomerular capillaries [354,355] and with cyrofibrinogen and soluble fibrin monomer complexes present in the blood [356–358]. Patients with severe eclampsia may develop thrombocytopenia, microangiopathic hemolytic anemia, and moderate hypofibrinogenemia [349,351,352,259–361], and fibrin thrombi have been observed in the kidney, liver, and cerebral vessels of such patients [362–364]. One study reports glomerular capillary thrombosis in all 33 cases of fatal toxemia of pregnancy [365]. The thrombi correspond to the observed clinical manifestations of patients with toxemia of pregnancy, such as convulsions, coma, renal failure, and intracerebral bleeding. It is still uncertain as to whether a low-grade DIC process is the primary event in this syndrome or whether the apparent consumption is secondary to some generalized vascular disorder which causes both the clinical manifestations and the secondary deposition of fibrin. Evidence in favor of a primary consumptive process is based on the finding of cryofibrinogen or soluble fibrin monomer complexes in the blood, and evidence for the consumption as a secondary process is based upon a lack of correlation between thrombocytopenia and the concentration of fibrinogen derivatives in the blood [366]. No significant benefit of heparin therapy in toxemia of pregnancy has been established [360,361, 367–369], and in fact the risk of intracranial bleeding in patients with severe uncontrolled hypertension would make the use of anticoagulants dangerous. Thus, therapy is primarily directed at control of the eclamptic state by the use of antihypertensive agents and by rapid termination of the pregnancy; excellent results with such therapy without the use of heparin have been reported [370].

NEOPLASIA

Although thrombocytopenia in patients with malignancy usually is secondary to decreased marrow production and increased turnover [371], it can also reflect a more generalized consumptive process that leads to low-grade DIC, venous thromboembolic disease, bleeding out of proportion to the thrombocytopenia, microangiopathic hemolytic anemia, or nonthrombotic val-

vular endocarditis. Additionally, a bleeding disorder without thrombocytopenia can occur as the result of pathologic fibrinogenolysis, either systemically or locally in a tumor mass, and all of these various consumptive thrombohemorrhagic disorders can present in any combination of tempo, location, and pathologic mechanism (Table 158-1).

The clinical association between solid tumors of visceral origin and thrombohemorrhagic disorders was described by Trousseau in 1865 [166] and is the topic of an extensive literature, including excellent reviews [162]. Specific features are the following: (1) the high incidence of thrombi in the heart and arterial tree in the absence of underlying inflammation [372]; (2) the migratory nature of venous thrombosis associated with adenocarcinoma [373]; (3) the combination of venous thrombosis, pulmonary emboli, and valvular thrombi with cerebral embolism in patients with tumor [374]; and (4) the association of venous thrombi, nonbacterial thrombotic endocarditis, and mucinous tumors, due to deposition of amorphous fibrin material on valvular surfaces and associated with a hypercoagulable state that could involve veins and arteries simultaneously [170].

Chronic DIC can be considered the basic underlying feature of this group of disorders, which could be manifest by any or all of the thrombotic and hemorrhagic features of DIC or simply by laboratory abnormalities without clinical manifestations. The laboratory alterations include thrombocytopenia and hypofibrinogenemia of variable but usually parallel degree, circulating fibrin-fibrinogen degradation products, and microangiopathic hemolytic anemia. Patients with malignancy may show only the microangiopathic hemolytic anemia, with correction of the abnormality after successful treatment of the tumor [375,376]. A hidden neoplasm may be suggested by unusual clinical thrombotic states—for instance, recurrence of venous thrombi [377], multiple limb thrombosis [378], hemorrhage after reasonable doses of anticoagulation agents [379], myopathy secondary to arterial emboli [380], thrombocytosis [381], cryofibrinogenemia [382–384], phlegmasia cerulea dolens [385], venous gangrene [385,386], combined thrombosis and bleeding, arterial and venous thromboemboli, or all of these in a single patient [162]. Patients with carcinoma of the prostate may have hemorrhagic manifestations that dominate the clinical picture [162,387], and this could reflect the ability of this tumor to produce activators of fibrinolysis [388] as well as activators of intravascular coagulation. The tendency of some tumor cells to produce such clot-dissolving activity has been demonstrated both in vitro and in clinical circumstances following prolonged localized bleeding after biopsy of the tumor [180].

Although patients with such neoplastic disorders require therapy of the underlying malignant process, interruption of clinically evident DIC with anticoagulation agents may provide significant additional benefit. In one study, 29 of 48 such patients had improved hemostatic measurements and 19 had recurrent symptoms after heparin was discontinued [162]. Warfarin therapy is not effective, nor do antiplatelet agents suffice for chronic therapy of the prothrombotic predisposition [35]. For prolonged outpatient therapy, subcutaneous heparin administration is a reasonable alternative to self-administered intravenous heparin given by heparin lock.

Acute promyelocytic leukemia is characterized by leukemic cells containing numerous intracytoplasmic inclusions and granules and is almost uniformly associated with hemostatic abnormalities [26,46,389–391]. Although hemorrhagic phenomena predominate, venous as well as arterial thromboembolic complications may occur in up to 5 percent of such patients, with autopsy evidence of diffuse thrombosis in 15 to 25 percent of the patients [26,46]. The majority of patients show prolongation of the prothrombin time, hypofibrinogenemia, and elevated levels of fibrinogen-fibrin degradation products at the time of admission [391,392]. The half-life of fibrinogen is shortened, even in patients without clinically identifiable disease [390]. Both thromboplastic-type material [393,394] and fibrinolytic proteases [395] are demonstrable in promyelocytic subcellular components, but the former influence predominates in both in vitro analyses and clinical presentation [396].

This clinical disorder may begin abruptly with serious hemorrhagic manifestations due to DIC, further complicated by thrombocytopenia secondary to the effect of tumor on hematopoiesis. The coagulopathy has also been described in patients with chronic myelogenous [167] and monocytic [397] leukemia, acute myelogenous leukemia [29,398,399], and even acute lymphocytic leukemia [400]. The syndrome should be distinguished from thrombotic occlusive disease, which results from excessively high white blood cell counts in acute or chronic leukemia [401]. As with solid tumors, control of the leukemic process will determine the patient's ultimate response. However, the management of acute promyelocytic leukemia may present special problems even if the consumptive disorder is not clinically overt at the time of admission, since the complication may be induced or exacerbated by cell lysis during chemotherapy [392]. Clinical experience suggests that the addition of heparin to platelet transfusion therapy may improve clinical status and laboratory aberrations and contribute to the remission rate and survival of patients with acute promyelocytic leukemia undergoing induction chemotherapy [392,402–404]. A rational approach based on such observations should be individualized for each patient, depending upon the presenting laboratory and clinical features and in anticipation of the release of clot-promoting materials into the circulation during therapy.

LIVER DISEASE

Acute and chronic severe liver disease can be associated with significant hemostatic abnormalities that may lead to or exaggerate a bleeding problem [405]. These hemostatic defects include sequestration of platelets in the spleen and splanchnic vascular bed [406,407], decreased synthesis of vitamin K–dependent clotting factors [408] and antithrombin III [409], and decreased clearance of plasminogen activators from the blood [410]. Additionally, fibrinolytic activity in some tissues may be increased in response to unknown stimuli, such as in the upper gastrointestinal tract [411], further impairing hemostasis in the event of bleeding from trauma or necrosis of mucosa or vessel walls. A consumptive coagulopathy has been postulated as an additional mechanism of deranged hemostasis in patients with liver disease [11,22,61,128], based on the observations that (1) hemorrhagic phenomena and decreased concentrations of plasma clotting factors are not corrected with simple replacement therapy [412,413], (2) infused fibrinogen administered to patients with cirrhosis is rapidly metabolized [414–416], and (3) the shortened fibrinogen half-life is corrected by heparin [415,416] but not by fibrinolytic inhibitors [415].

Despite such evidence, a major role for a consumptive thrombohemorrhagic process in patients with liver disease is still controversial. For example, histopathologic changes compatible with DIC were found in only 4 of 184 cases of acute and chronic liver disease [417]. One must avoid simplistic interpretation of the effects of heparin on the half-life of labeled fibrinogen [418], especially since the changes observed in fibrinogen clearance can be explained by loss of material into extravascular compartments as well as by intravascular coagulation [419]. Laboratory abnormalities similar to those found in clear-cut cases of DIC are not a consistent feature of even severe liver disease, and they can all be explained by other mechanisms, such as, for instance, the synthesis of an abnormal fibrinogen with an inherently prolonged thrombin time [420]. Although correction of the coagulation defect may be facilitated in some cases by adding heparin therapy to treatment with plasma infusions [421], there is no evidence that this treatment improves prognosis [422]. In a controlled trial comparing the use of fresh frozen plasma alone versus fresh frozen plasma with added heparin in the treatment of such coagulation defects in 22 patients with paracetamol-induced heparin necrosis [423], no significant difference was observed either in the rate of correction of the coagulation defect or in the final clinical outcome.

A difficult clinical situation is presented by the patient with liver disease, symptomatic bleeding, thrombocytopenia, hypofibrinogenemia, and increased levels of fibrin degradation products in the plasma who also demonstrates clinical signs suggestive of organ ischemia. Specifically, altered sensorium and decreased urine output may suggest that thrombotic occlusion secondary to DIC has occurred and that heparin treatment is indicated. However, alternative pathologic mechanisms adequately explain the symptoms, namely, shunting of portal blood to produce hepatic precoma and plasma volume shifts leading to decreased renal perfusion and urine volume. The decreased platelet count can be due to splenic sequestration, and the elevated degradation products could be secondary to a shortened euglobulin lysis time caused by inadequate clearance of plasminogen activators. Treatment with heparin under these circumstances will often exaggerate bleeding, even with transfusion therapy with platelets and cryoprecipitate. In fact, patients without evidence of fibrinolysis or vascular obstruction—for instance, if the level of degradation products is not elevated—could benefit by therapy with fibrinolytic inhibitors to stabilize fragile hemostatic plugs in regions of local bleeding, such as a gastric mucosal ulcer or bleeding esophageal varices. As with all instances of possible consumptive thrombohemorrhagic disorders, each patient must be individually considered. Contrary to the situation in which theoretical clot-promoting materials are released into the blood, however, such as with malignancy, infection, or obstetric accidents, there is less evidence that patients with liver disease are predisposed to DIC.

PEDIATRIC DISEASES

DIC may be common in the *seriously ill newborn* [424]. Thrombi without an accompanying cellular infiltrate and resembling the lesions of the generalized Shwartzman reaction were found in the pulmonary arterioles of 15 premature infants dying of infection within the first 2 months of life [425]. Disseminated fibrin thromboemboli were found in 8 of 226 neonates dying of a variety of causes within 48 h of birth [426]. In one survey [424], evidence of disseminated intravascular clotting was found in 11 of 19 sick infants. The newborn may die with bleeding into the brain or lungs, and disseminated intravascular clotting—by giving rise to a hemorrhagic diathesis—may contribute importantly to this bleeding [427–429]. Incipient gangrene that cleared with heparin therapy has been described in a newborn infant with a diarrheal illness [430].

Complications of pregnancy that cause DIC in the mother may also cause the condition in the infant. Thus renal cortical necrosis and cerebral necrosis have been found in newborn infants with a macerated runt twin [431]. Presumably, this results from an intertwin placental shunt that allows thromboplastic material from the dead twin to circulate in the living twin. Defibrination has been observed in the infant of a severely preeclamptic mother [428] and in infants born after abruptio placentae [424,429]. Minor alterations in clotting test results, thought to reflect a lesser degree of intravascular coagulation, were found in a systematic study of infants born to preeclamptic mothers [350].

Intrauterine or neonatal infections, such as disseminated herpes simplex, congenital rubella, and cytomegalic virus infection, may cause DIC with depletion of clotting factors [424]. Infants with severe idiopathic respiratory distress syndrome may also have evidence of DIC, but treating such infants with heparin does not reduce mortality [424].

Purpura fulminans is a rare, catastrophic disorder seen primarily but not exclusively in children (see above, acute DIC). With rare exceptions, it is preceded by an infection that somehow prepares the skin, e.g., scarlet fever, other streptococcal infections, or varicella. After a variable but definite latent period, the patient develops painful, expanding, confluent areas of purpura on the extremities, lower back, buttocks, or face. The affected areas are purplish black, swollen, hard, and tender and are surrounded by a narrow, red border. The more extensive lesions undergo necrosis. Unchecked, the lesion progresses in a wavelike fashion, with the appearance of new areas of involvement and death in many patients. Visceral lesions are uncommon, but instances of associated renal cortical necrosis have been described [432,433].

Coagulation abnormalities characteristic of intravascular clotting—thrombocytopenia, hypofibrinogenemia, and reduced levels of other clotting factors—are found in a high proportion of patients [147,148,205,434–437]. Histologic examination of an affected site reveals widespread thrombosis of capillaries and venules, with a surrounding perivascular inflammatory reaction [147]. The mechanism triggering the intravascular clotting is unknown, but its onset during convalescence from an infection suggests a reaction initiated by an antigen-antibody complex. Heparin has been reported to be an effective means of averting the progress of purpura fulminans [146–148,435–437].

MISCELLANEOUS

Snake bite by certain species, especially the vipers and rattlesnakes (*Vipera, Bothrops, Ankistrodon, Echis, Crotalus*), can produce hypofibrinogenemia with or without accompanying thrombocytopenia, depending upon whether the venom contains enzymes which clot fibrinogen—either directly or via activation of factor X or prothrombin—as well as agents that can aggregate platelets. Most bites cause striking laboratory abnormalities in all victims, but relatively mild clinical disorders in about one-half of the patients [438,439]. The symptoms are characterized by local tenderness and swelling, mild bleeding of the wound or of venipunctures, occasional hypotension without shock, and transient mild oliguria. Although some patients also have shortened euglobulin lysis times [440], the syndrome most closely resembles DIC, but with considerable variation in the rate and degree of consumption and in the chronicity of laboratory changes. Some patients begin to recover spontaneously after 1 to 2 days and are completely normal within 1 week [438], while others demonstrate incoagulable blood without symptoms of hemorrhage for more than 3 weeks [441]. Active secondary fibrinolysis accounts for the rapid recovery of presumed renal microcirculatory obstruction and for the elevated levels of fibrin degradation products in the blood. Patients with combined hypofibrinogenemia and thrombocytopenia [442,443] have been exposed to venoms which contain not only procoagulant enzymes but also a platelet-aggregating factor [444]. Such laboratory changes more closely resemble the DIC induced by infection or malignancy, and these patients have a greater tendency for clinically apparent hemorrhage.

Treatment in most instances has been conservative, concerned primarily with the general principles of neutralizing the venom with antiserum, transfusing with platelets and plasma, and maintaining blood volume, blood pressure, and electrolyte balance. With the exception of one case [442], heparin effect has been unimpressive. In another study, 7 of 14 patients bitten by *Echis carinatus* were treated primarily with antivenom and 7 with antivenom plus heparin [439]. No benefit accrued from the heparin above that obtained with the antivenom alone. The generally benign course in humans and the lack of additive beneficial effect of reasonable doses of heparin suggest that the venom enzymes may not be inhibitable by plasma proteins such as antithrombin III. Defibrinating enzymes, such as Arvin from *Ankistrodon rhodostoma* and Defibrase from *Bothrops atrox,* have been purified for therapeutic defibrination [445,446] as treatment in patients with venous thromboembolic disease [447,448]. The rationale for therapy is that plasma fibrinogen is decreased slowly by conversion to non–cross-linked fibrin, which is in turn quickly lysed without causing any vascular occlusion or organ ischemia. This leaves the patient with sufficient fibrinogen to have normal hemostasis but not enough fibrinogen to allow growth of a thrombus. Repeated injections of the agent keep the fibrinogen level constant. The antithrombotic state that is established and maintained is as safe and effective as that obtained with heparin in preventing thrombus extension or allowing for its recanalization [449]. Some studies have combined therapeutic defibrination with fibrinolytic agents in an attempt to decrease the concentration of degradation products and perhaps to improve efficacy and safety [450,451]. Results are not significantly different from those with fibrinolytic agents alone.

Acute hemolysis, such as that which follows the transfusion of large amounts (500 ml or more) of incompatible blood, can produce a hemorrhagic diathesis characterized by laboratory changes of hypofibrinogenemia and thrombocytopenia [452–454]. The pattern is entirely compatible with acute DIC, with variable effects of intravascular thrombi on renal function (depending on the acuteness and degree of defibrination) and the additional presence of hypovolemia and/or hypotension [453]. Hemolysis of any cause could theoretically produce the same consumptive result, such as was reported for paroxysmal nocturnal hemoglobinuria [455]. However, massive hemolysis does not uniformly produce DIC, as observed in 28 patients with glucose-6-phosphate dehydrogenase deficiency who were exposed to fava beans [56]. Not only was there no DIC, but the hemolysis produced elevated levels of fibrinogen and factors V and VIII, perhaps as a nonspecific reaction to the stress. Tissue macrophages are considered vital in the clearance of the erythrocyte stromal procoagulant

material from the circulation, and possibly some insult which impairs normal monocyte-macrophage function coexists during the hemolytic episode, thereby predisposing the patient to DIC. Hypotension, surgery, anesthesia, and sepsis could qualify as significant additional predisposing factors in the patients who developed DIC after incompatible blood transfusions. This situation should be a self-limited DIC which, in the absence of serious organ damage, such as renal cortical necrosis, will improve rapidly with only supportive measures. Treatment will depend upon maintenance of blood volume and organ perfusion, blood replacement with compatible erythrocytes, and heparin use only if evidence of continued DIC exists.

Prothrombin complex concentrates contain the vitamin K–dependent clotting factors, and efficacy has been established for their use in several conditions including the treatment of patients with congenital or acquired deficiencies of prothrombin or of factor VII, IX, or X or with acquired inhibitors against factor VIII or factor IX [456–458]. However, some of these preparations may contain variable amounts of thrombogenic material in addition to the inactive coagulation factors [459,460]. These include factor IXa, factor Xa [461–463], and material that enhances platelet coagulant activity [464], any or all of which may be implicated in the thrombotic complications attendant the use of such materials [456, 462]. Although administration of these preparations is relatively safe in patients with inhibitors, patients with liver disease may be especially predisposed, perhaps because of impaired clearance of the activated factors or because of a decreased plasma concentration of antithrombin III. Newer concentrates are relatively free of activated coagulation factors, except for those specifically manufactured for treatment of patients with inhibitors, and the latter products are standardized much better than those of a decade ago. Nevertheless, judgment should be exercised for every patient to be certain that simpler materials without thrombogenic potential are considered before resorting to these more potent reagents. For this reason, it has been suggested that factor VIII concentrates be used even for some patients with factor VIII inhibitors, generally those with low-titer antibodies, leaving the use of prothrombin complex concentrates for high-titer inhibitor patients, who are unlikely to respond to factor VIII infusions [457]. An alternative approach is to use the prothrombin complex concentrates for all appropriate deficiency states, including inhibitors of all titers, unless there is a concomitant presence of any disease that may predispose to DIC. Should DIC occur, treatment would follow the principles outlined in Table 158-2.

Reports of *heparin-induced thrombocytopenia* represent a remarkable incongruity, the mechanism and even the incidence of which are still not certain. A few patients have had overt manifestations of DIC [150]. Some have had evidence of heparin-induced platelet aggregation in vitro, arterial occlusions during treatment, and tissue necrosis at sites of subcutaneous injections [465].

Thrombocytopenia (less than 100,000 platelets per microliter) without clinical symptoms has been noted in patients studied prospectively [466], with an observed incidence as low as 0 percent [467] and as high as 30 percent [468], but with most values closer to the lower level. A significant number of patients with thrombocytopenia also had elevated levels of fibrin degradation products (30 percent) and hypofibrinogenemia (60 percent), suggesting that DIC was responsible [468]. However, in another study thrombocytopenia was observed in a high proportion of patients (11.6 percent of 43 patients) but DIC was not detected by either clinical or laboratory evaluation [469]. Most of the patients with thrombocytopenia received bovine lung heparin, although porcine gut heparin is also implicated in some reports [466]. Whatever the real incidence and risk, the mechanism in some cases has been ascribed to the development of platelet agglutinins [469], possibly acting via an immunologic mechanism [470,471].

The reported cases do not represent a homogeneous group, since the delay after the onset of treatment varied from 2 to 11 days [472] or even longer [464,466,469] and since some patients have corrected their thrombocytopenia despite continued heparin administration [469]. Considering the enormous number of patients who receive heparin and the very small number with clinically significant findings, the possibility of heparin-induced thrombocytopenia should not deter one from its use in patients with thrombotic disorders. This association should, however, be a stimulus for developing heparin preparations that are (1) less heterogeneous and (2) free of the tendency to cause platelet aggregation.

Adult respiratory distress syndrome may predispose to local consumption of platelets or even to DIC, and anatomic or functional evidence of thrombotic microvascular organ obstruction in the skin and kidneys as well as in the lungs occurs frequently in such patients [473]. Whatever the initiating stimulus, there is a strong potential for local deposition of platelets and fibrin and even for disseminated consumption, which would in turn further complicate the underlying disorder.

Localized disease in other organs may result in consumption by unique mechanisms, such as the systemic fibrinolytic state associated with *acute pancreatitis*. Although localized consumption in a region of inflammation could contribute to a bleeding diathesis, the proteolytic effect of pancreatic enzymes such as trypsin [474] in blood has been demonstrated [475] in a patient with pancreatitis secondary to L-asparaginase. In such cases, bleeding symptoms depend upon the degree of consumption, and treatment should be directed at the underlying conditions and at replenishment of consumed plasma factors. Heparin would not be indicated without evidence of a coagulation tendency unresponsive to such measures. The indirect association of L-asparaginase with the fibrinolytic state of a patient with pancreatitis [475] points out the possibility of other drug-induced consumptions, such as the report of a hyperfibrinolytic state associated with Adriamycin [476].

Massive trauma that produces irreversible shock unresponsive to multiple transfusions may be associated with evidence of depletion of clotting factors [477]. However, most patients with massive tissue injury do not develop hypofibrinogenemia or other evidence of a consumptive coagulopathy [478–480]. In contrast, patients with head injuries causing brain tissue destruction may undergo striking acute defibrination with severe hypofibrinogenemia, moderate thrombocytopenia, and reduced levels of factor V and factor VIII [42,481–484]. The incidence of serious clotting factor abnormalities after major intracranial injury is not yet known [42,485]. Since a small amount of intracerebral bleeding could precipitate irreversible neurologic damage after intracranial injury, defibrination represents a potentially fatal complication of head trauma.

A special instance of DIC is represented by patients with a *peritoneovenous (LaVeen)* shunt who have evidence of local clotting or systemic consumption, presumably secondary to the procoagulant effect of the ascitis fluid [486]. Heparin may be of use in some of these patients, but the clinical situation is complicated by the multitude of coagulation abnormalities that may be present.

References

1. McKay, D. G.: *Disseminated Intravascular Coagulation: An Intermediary Mechanism of Disease.* Harper-Hoeber, New York, 1965, p. 493.
2. Marder, V. J., Martin, S. E., and Colman, R. W.: Clinical aspects of consumption coagulopathies, in *Hemostasis and Thrombosis: Basic Principles and Clinical Practice,* edited by R. W. Colman, J. Hirsh, V. J. Marder, and E. W. Salzman. Lippincott, Philadelphia, 1982.
3. Rodriguez-Erdmann, F.: Bleeding due to increased intravascular blood coagulation: Hemorrhagic syndromes caused by consumption of blood-clotting factors (consumption-coagulopathies). *N. Engl. J. Med. 273:*1370, 1965.
4. Hardaway, R. M.: *Syndromes of Disseminated Intravascular Coagulation, with Special Reference to Shock and Hemorrhage.* Charles C Thomas, Springfield, Ill., 1966.
5. Merskey, C., et al.: The defibrination syndrome: Clinical features and laboratory diagnosis. *Br. J. Haematol. 13:*528, 1967.
6. Bachmann, F.: Disseminated intravascular coagulation. *Disease of the Month,* December 1969, p. 44.
7. Mammen, E. F., Anderson, G. F., and Barnhard, M. I. (eds.): Disseminated intravascular coagulation. *Thromb. Diath. Haemorrh.* (special issue) *(Suppl.) 36,* 1969.
8. Deykin, D.: The clinical challenge of disseminated intravascular coagulation. *N. Engl. J. Med. 283:*636, 1970.
9. Brodsky, I., and Siegel, N. H.: The diagnosis and treatment of disseminated intravascular coagulation. *Med. Clin. North Am. 54:*555, 1970.
10. Pitney, W. R.: Disseminated intravascular coagulation. *Semin. Hematol. 8:*65, 1971.
11. Colman, R. W., Robboy, S. J., and Minna, J. D.: Disseminated intravascular coagulation (DIC): An approach. *Am. J. Med. 52:*679, 1972.

12. Rapaport, S. I.: Defibrination syndromes, in *Hematology*, 2d ed., edited by W. J. Williams, E. Beutler, A. J. Erslev, and R. W. Rundles. McGraw-Hill, New York, 1977, p. 1454.

13. Verstraete, M., et al.: Excessive consumption of blood coagulation components as cause of hemorrhage diathesis. *Am. J. Med.* 35:899, 1965.

14. Merskey, C.: Defibrination syndrome or . . . ? *Blood* 41:599, 1973.

15. Owen, C. A., Jr., and Bowie, E. J. W.: Chronic intravascular coagulation syndromes: A summary. *Mayo Clin. Proc.* 49:673, 1974.

16. Sharp, A. A.: Diagnosis and management of disseminated intravascular coagulation. *Br. Med. Bull.* 33:265, 1977.

17. Hamilton, P. J., Stalker, A. L., and Douglas, A. S.: Disseminated intravascular coagulation: A review. *J. Clin. Pathol.* 31:609, 1978.

18. Siegel, T., et al.: Clinical and laboratory aspects of disseminated intravascular coagulation (DIC): A study of 118 cases. *Thromb. Haemost.* 39:122, 1978.

19. Bick, R. L.: Disseminated intravascular coagulation and related syndromes: Etiology, pathophysiology, diagnosis and management. *Am. J. Hematol.* 5:265, 1978.

20. Colman, R. W., Robboy, S. J., and Minna, J. D.: Disseminated intravascular coagulation: A reappraisal. *Ann. Rev. Med.* 30:359, 1979.

21. Mant, M. J., and King, E. G.: Severe acute disseminated intravascular coagulation. *Am. J. Med.* 67:557, 1979.

22. Bell, W. R.: Disseminated intravascular coagulation. *Johns Hopkins Med. J.* 146:289, 1980.

23. Spero, J. A., Lewis, J. H., and Hasiba, U.: Disseminated intravascular coagulation: Findings in 346 patients. *Thromb. Haemost.* 43:28, 1980.

24. Dennis, L. H., et al.: Consumptive coagulopathy in fulminant meningococcemia. *JAMA* 205:182, 1968.

25. Winkelstein, A., et al.: Fulminant meningococcemia and disseminated intravascular coagulation. *Arch. Intern. Med.* 124:55, 1969.

26. Albarracin, N. S., and Haust, M. D.: Intravascular coagulation in promyelocytic leukemia: A case study including ultrastructure. *Am. J. Clin. Pathol.* 55:677, 1971.

27. Corrigan, J. J., Jr., Ray, W. L., and May, N.: Changes in the blood coagulation system associated with septicemia. *N. Engl. J. Med.* 279:851, 1968.

28. Yoshikawa, T., Tanaka, K. R., and Guze, L. B.: Infection and disseminated intravascular coagulation. *Medicine (Baltimore)* 50:237, 1971.

29. Gralnick, H. R., Marchesi, S., and Givelber, H.: Intravascular coagulation in acute leukemia: Clinical and subclinical abnormalities. *Blood* 40:709, 1972.

30. Bieger, R., et al.: Arterial aneurysm as a cause of consumption coagulopathy. *N. Engl. J. Med.* 285:152, 1971.

31. Kasabach, H. H., and Merritt, K. K.: Capillary hemangioma with extensive purpura. *Am. J. Dis. Child.* 59:1063, 1940.

32. Sutton, D. M.: Intravascular coagulation in abruptio placentae. *Am. J. Obstet. Gynecol.* 109:604, 1971.

33. Moschcowitz, E.: An acute febrile pleiochromic anemia with hyaline thrombosis of terminal arterioles and capillaries: An undescribed disease. *Arch. Intern. Med.* 36:89, 1925.

34. Rabiner, S. F., and Friedman, L. H.: The role of intravascular haemolysis and the reticulo-endothelial system in the production of hypercoagulable state. *Br. J. Haematol.* 14:105, 1968.

35. Mosesson, M. W., Colman, R. W., and Sherry, S.: Chronic intravascular coagulation syndrome: Report of a case with special studies on an associated plasma cryoprecipitate ("cryofibrinogen"). *N. Engl. J. Med.* 278:815, 1968.

36. Hjort, P. F., and Rapaport, S. I.: The Shwartzman reaction: Pathogenic mechanisms and clinical manifestations. *Annu. Rev. Med.* 16:135, 1965.

37. Josey, W. E., Hoch, W., Moon, E. C., and Thompson, J. D.: Analysis of 21 septic abortion deaths with special reference to the Shwartzman phenomenon. *Obstet. Gynecol.* 28:335, 1966.

38. Pineo, G. F., Regoeczi, E., Hatton, M. W. C., and Brain, M. C.: The activation of coagulation by extracts of mucus: A possible pathway of intravascular coagulation accompanying adenocarcinomas. *J. Lab. Clin. Med.* 82:255, 1973.

39. Gordon, S. G., Franks, J. J., and Lewis, B.: Cancer procoagulant A: A factor X activating procoagulant from malignant tissue. *Thromb. Res.* 6:127, 1975.

40. Regoeczi, E., Gergely, J., and McFarlane, A. S.: In vivo effects of *Agkistrodon rhodostoma* venom: Studies with fibrinogen-^{131}I. *J. Clin. Invest.* 45:1201, 1966.

41. Weiss, H. J., Allan, S., Davidson, E., and Kochwa, S.: Afibrinogenemia in man following the bite of a rattlesnake (*Crotalus adamanteus*). *Am. J. Med.* 47:625, 1969.

42. Goodnight, S. H., Kenoyer, G., Rapaport, S. I., Patch, M. J., Lee, J. A., and Kurze, T.: Defibrination after brain-tissue destruction: A serious complication of head injury. *N. Engl. J. Med.* 290:1043, 1974.

43. Gralnick, H. R., and Abrell, E.: Studies of the procoagulant and fibrinolytic activity of promyelocytes in acute promyelocytic leukaemia. *Br. J. Haematol.* 24:89, 1973.

44. Gouault-Heilmann, M., Chardon, E., Sultan, C., and Josso, F.: The procoagulant factor of leukaemic promyelocytes: Demonstration of immunologic cross reactivity with human brain tissue factor. *Br. J. Haematol.* 30:151, 1975.

45. Didisheim, P., Trombold, J. S., Vandervoort, R. L. E., and Mibasham, R. S.: Acute promyelocytic leukemia with fibrinogen and factor V deficiencies. *Blood* 23:717, 1964.

46. Gralnick, H. R., and Sultan, C.: Acute promyelocytic leukaemia: Haemorrhagic manifestation and morphologic criteria. *Br. J. Haematol.* 29:373, 1975.

47. Friedman, N. J., Hoag, M. S., Robinson, A. J., and Aggeler, P. M.: Hemorrhagic syndrome following transurethral prostatic resection for benign adenoma. *Arch. Intern. Med.* 124:341, 1969.

48. Kazmier, F. J., Didisheim, P., Fairbanks, V. F., Ludwig, J., Payne, W. S., and Bowie, E. J. W.: Intravascular coagulation and arterial disease. *Thromb. Diath. Haemorrh. (Suppl).* 36:295, 1969.

49. Wilner, G. D., Nossel, H. L., and LeRoy, E. C.: Activation of Hageman factor by collagen. *J. Clin. Invest.* 47:2608, 1968.

50. Walsh, P. N.: The effects of collagen and kaolin on the intrinsic coagulant activity of platelets: Evidence for an alternative pathway in intrinsic coagulation not requiring factor XII. *Br. J. Haematol.* 22:393, 1973.

51. Spaet, T. H., and Cintron, J.: Studies on platelet factor 3 availability. *Br. J. Haematol.* 11:269, 1965.

52. Krevans, J. R., Jackson, D. P., Conley, C. L., and Hartmann, R. C.: The nature of the hemorrhagic disorder accompanying hemolytic transfusion reactions in man. *Blood* 12:834, 1957.

53. Rock, R. C., Bove, J. R., and Nemerson, Y.: Heparin treatment of intravascular coagulation accompanying hemolytic transfusion reactions. *Transfusion* 9:57, 1969.

54. Djaldetti, M., Amir, J., Shaklai, M., and Joshua, H.: Haemorrhagic diathesis following transfusion of incompatible blood. *Scand. J. Haematol.* 10:197, 1973.

55. Weiss, H. J., Berger, R. E., Tice, A. D., and Phillips, L. L.: Fatal disseminated intravascular coagulation and hemolytic anemia following stibophen therapy: A study of basic mechanisms. *Am. J. Med. Sci.* 264:375, 1972.

56. Mannucci, P. M., Lobina, G. F., Caocci, L., and Dioguardi, N.: Effect on blood coagulation of massive intravascular haemolysis. *Blood* 33:207, 1969.

57. McGrath, J. M., and Stewart, G. J.: The effects of endotoxin on vascular endothelium. *J. Exp. Med.* 129:833, 1969.

58. Gaynor, E.: The role of granulocytes in endotoxin-induced vascular injury. *Blood* 41:797, 1973.

59. Lerner, R. G., Rapaport, S. I., Siemsen, J. K., and Spitzer, J. M.: Disappearance of fibrinogen-^{131}I after endotoxin: Effects of a first and second injection. *Am. J. Physiol.* 214:532, 1968.

60. Morrison, D. C., and Cochrane, C. G.: Direct evidence for Hageman factor (factor XII) activation by bacterial lipopoylsaccharides (endotoxins). *J. Exp. Med.* 140:797, 1974.

61. Mason, J. W., and Colman, R. W.: The role of Hageman factor in disseminated intravascular coagulation induced by septicemia, neoplasia, or liver disease. *Thromb. Diath. Haemorrh.* 26:327, 1971.

62. Rodriguez-Erdmann, F.: Studies on the pathogenesis of the generalized Shwartzman reaction. III. Trigger mechanism for the activation of the prothrombin molecule. *Thromb. Diath. Haemorrh.* 12:471, 1964.

63. Lerner, R. G., Rapaport, S. I., and Spitzer, J. M.: Endotoxin-induced intravascular clotting: The need for granulocytes. *Thromb. Diath. Haemorrh.* 20:430, 1968.

64. Clark, S. L., and Batchelor, W. H.: The behavior of the formed elements of blood incubated with bacterial endotoxins. *U.S. Naval Med. Res. Inst. Res. Rep.* 15:361, 1957.

65. Davis, R. B., Meeker, W. R., and McQuarrie, D. G.: Immediate effects of intravenous endotoxin on serotonin concentrations and blood platelets. *Circ. Res.* 8:234, 1960.

66. Horowitz, H. I., Des Prez, R. M., and Hook, E. W.: Effects of bacterial endotoxin on rabbit platelets. II. Enhancement of platelet factor 3 activity in vitro and in vivo. *J. Exp. Med.* 116:619, 1962.

67. Fong, J. S. C., and Good, R. A.: Prevention of the localized and generalized Shwartzman reactions by an anticomplementary agent, cobra venom factor. *J. Exp. Med.* 134:642, 1971.

68. Kane, M. A., May, J. E., and Frank, M. M.: Interactions of the classical and alternate complement pathway with endotoxin lipopolysaccharide. *J. Clin. Invest.* 52:370, 1973.

69. Margaretten, W., and McKay, D. G.: The role of the platelet in the generalized Shwartzman reaction. *J. Exp. Med.* 129:585, 1969.

70. Gratia, A., and Linz, R.: Les Phénomènes de Sanarelli et de Shwartzman ou l'allergie hémorragique. *Ann. Inst. Pateur* 49:131, 1932.

71. Levin, J., and Cluff, L. E.: Platelets and the Shwartzman phenomenon. *J. Exp. Med.* 121:235, 1965.

72. Lipinski, B., and Gurewich, V.: The effect of leukopenia versus thrombocytopenia on endotoxin induced intravascular coagulation. *Thromb. Res.* 8:403, 1976.

73. Müller-Berghaus, G., Bohn, E., and Höbel, W.: Activation of intravascular coagulation by endotoxin: The significance of granulocytes and platelets. *Br. J. Haematol.* 33:213, 1976.

74. Müller-Berghaus, G., and Schneberger, R.: Hageman factor activation in the generalized Shwartzman reaction induced by endotoxin. *Br. J. Haematol.* 21:513, 1971.

75. Shen, S. M.-C., Rapaport, S. I., and Feinstein, D. I.: Intravascular clotting after endotoxin in rabbits with impaired intrinsic clotting produced by a factor VIII antibody. *Blood* 42:523, 1973.

76. Thomas, L., and Good, R. A.: Studies on the generalized Shwartzman reaction. I. General observations concerning the phenomenon. *J. Exp. Med.* 96:605, 1952.

77. Hjort, P. F., McGehee, W., and Rapaport, S. I.: Studies on the effect of granulocytes in the generalized Shwartzman reaction. *Abstracts X Congress, Internat. Soc. Haematol.,* Stockholm, 1964, Paper G:1.

78. Horn, H. G., and Collins, R. D.: Studies on the pathogenesis of the generalized Shwartzman reaction: The role of granulocytes. *Lab. Invest.* 18:101, 1968.

79. Forman, E. N., Abildgaard, C. F., Bolger, J. F., Johnson, C. A., and Schulman, I.: Generalized Shwartzman reaction: Role of the granulocyte in intravascular coagulation and renal cortical necrosis. *Br. J. Haematol.* 16:507, 1969.

80. Müller-Berghaus, G., and Eckhardt, T.: The role of granulocytes in the activation of intravascular coagulation and the precipitation of soluble fibrin by endotoxin. *Blood* 45:631, 1975.

81. Hawiger, J., Collins, R. D., and Horn, R. G.: Precipitation of soluble fibrin monomer complexes by lysosomal protein fraction of polymorphonuclear leukocytes. *Proc. Soc. Exp. Biol. Med.* 131:349, 1969.

82. Horn, R. G.: Evidence for participation of granulocytes in the pathogenesis of the generalized Shwartzman reaction: A review. *J. Infect. Dis.* 128:S134, 1973.

83. Lipinski, B., Nowak, A., and Gurewich, V.: The organ distribution of ^{125}I-fibrin in the generalized Shwartzman reaction and its relation to leucocytes. *Br. J. Haematol.* 28:221, 1974.

84. Rapaport, S. I., and Hjort, P. F.: The blood clotting properties of rabbit peritoneal leukocytes in vitro. *Thromb. Diath. Haemorrh.* 17:222, 1967.

85. Lerner, R. G., Goldstein, R., and Cummings, G.: Stimulation of human leukocyte thromboplastic activity by endotoxin. *Proc. Soc. Exp. Biol. Med.* 138:145, 1971.

86. Niemetz, J.: Coagulant activity of leukocytes: Tissue factor activity. *J. Clin. Invest.* 51:307, 1972.

87. Niemetz, J., and Marcus, A. J.: The stimulatory effect of platelets and platelet membranes on the procoagulant activity of leukocytes. *J. Clin. Invest.* 54:1437, 1974.

88. Garg, S. K., and Niemetz, J.: Tissue factor activity of normal and leukemic cells. *Blood* 42:729, 1973.

89. Rivers, R. P. A., Hathaway, W. E., and Weston, W. L.: The endotoxin-induced coagulant activity of human monocytes. *Br. J. Haematol.* 30:311, 1975.

90. Niemetz, J., and Fani, K.: Thrombogenic activity of leukocytes. *Blood* 42:47, 1973.

91. Lee, L.: Reticuloendothelial clearance of circulating fibrin in the pathogenesis of the generalized Shwartzman reaction. *J. Exp. Med.* 115:1065, 1962.

92. Stevens, A. R., Jr., Legg, J. S., Henry, B. S., Dille, J. M., Kirby, W. M. M., and Finch, C. A.: Fatal transfusion reactions from contamination of stored blood by cold growing bacteria. *Ann. Intern. Med.* 39:1228, 1953.

93. Reid, J. D.: Gran-negative bacteraemia. *N.Z. Med. J.* 56:200, 1957.

94. Pritchard, J. A., and Brekken, A. L.: Clinical and laboratory studies on severe abruptio placentae. *Am. J. Obstet. Gynecol.* 97:681, 1967.

95. Ullis, K. C., and Rosenblatt, R. M.: Shiga bacillus dysentery complicated by bacteremia and disseminated intravascular coagulation. *J. Pediatr.* 83:90, 1973.

96. Lee, L., and McCluskey, R. T.: Immunohistochemical demonstration of the reticuloendothelial clearance of circulating fibrin aggregates. *J. Exp. Med.* 116:611, 1962.

97. Gans, H., and Lowman, J. T.: The uptake of fibrin and fibrin-degradation products by the isolated perfused rat liver. *Blood* 29:526, 1967.

98. Rodriguez-Erdmann, F.: Pathogenesis of bilateral renal cortical necrosis: Its production by means of exogenous fibrin. *Arch. Pathol.* 79:615, 1965.

99. Palmerio, C., Ming, S. C., Frank, E., and Fine, J.: The role of the sympathetic nervous system in the generalized Shwartzman reaction. *J. Exp. Med.* 115:609, 1962.

100. Müller-Berghaus, G., and McKay, D. G.: Prevention of the generalized Shwartzman reaction in pregnant rats by α-adrenergic blocking agents. *Lab. Invest.* 17:276, 1967.

101. Todd, A. S.: Localization of fibrinolytic activity in tissues. *Br. Med. Bull.* 20:210, 1964.

102. Warren, B. A.: Fibrinolytic activity of vascular endothelium. *Br. Med. Bull.* 20:213, 1964.

103. Merskey, C., Johnson, A. J., Pert, J. H., and Wohl, H.: Pathogenesis of fibrinolysis in defibration syndrome: Effect of heparin administration. *Blood* 24:701, 1964.

104. Kowalski, E., Budzynski, A. Z., Kopec, M., Latallo, Z. S., Lipinski, B., and Wegrzynowicz, Z.: Circulating fibrinogen degradation products in dog blood after intravenous thrombin infusion. *Thromb. Diath. Haemorrh.* 13:12, 1965.

105. Margaretten, W., Zunker, H. O., and McKay, D. G.: Production of the generalized Shwartzman reaction in pregnant rats by intravenous infusion of thrombin. *Lab. Invest.* 13:552, 1964.

106. Bergstein, J. M., and Michael, A. F., Jr.: Renal cortical fibrinolytic activity in the rabbit following one or two doses of endotoxin. *Thromb. Diath. Haemorrh.* 29:27, 1973.

107. Biezienski, J. J., and Moore, H. C.: Fibrinolysis in normal pregnancy. *J. Clin. Pathol.* 11:306, 1958.

108. Astedt, B.: On fibrinolysis. A. In pregnancy, labour, puerperium and during treatment with sex hormones. B. In human ontogenesis and in human organ culture. *Acta Obstet. Gynecol. Scand.* 51 (Suppl. 18):33, 1972.

109. Bonnar, J.: Blood coagulation and fibrinolysis in obstetrics. *Clin. Haematol.* 2:213, 1973.

110. Marder, V. J.: Microvascular thrombosis, in *The Science and Practice of Clinical Medicine,* edited by J. M. Dietchy. Grune & Stratton, New York, 1980, vol. 6, p. 230.

111. Robboy, S. J., et al.: Skin in disseminated intravascular coagulation: Prospective analysis of thirty-six cases. *Br. J. Dermatol.* 88:221, 1973.

112. McGehee, W. G., Rapaport, S. I., and Hjort, P. F.: Intravascular coagulation in fulminant meningococcemia. *Ann. Intern. Med.* 67:250, 1967.

113. Robboy, S. J., Minna, J. D., and Colman, R. W.: Pulmonary hemor-

rhage syndrome as a manifestation of disseminated intravascular coagulation: Analysis of 10 cases. *Chest* 63:718, 1973.

114. Regoeczi, E., and Brain, M. C.: Organ distribution of fibrin in disseminated intravascular coagulation. *Br. J. Haematol.* 17:73, 1969.
115. Robboy, S. J., Colman, R. W., and Minna, J. D.: Pathology of disseminated intravascular coagulation (DIC): Analysis of twenty-six cases. *Hum. Pathol.* 3:327, 1972.
116. Bull, B. S., Rubenberg, M. L., Dacie, J. V., and Brain, M. C.: Microangiopathic haemolytic anaemia: Mechanisms of red-cell fragmentation: *In vitro* studies. *Br. J. Haematol.* 14:643, 1968.
117. Brain, M. C., Esterly, J. R., and Beck, E. A.: Intravascular haemolysis with experimentally produced vascular thrombi. *Br. J. Haematol.* 13:868, 1967.
118. Brain, M. C., and Hourihane, D. O'B.: Microangiopathic haemolytic anaemia: The occurrence of haemolysis in experimentally produced vascular disease. *Br. J. Haematol.* 13:135, 1967.
119. Rubenberg, M. L., Regoeczi, E., Bull, B. S., David, J. V., and Brain, M. C.: Microangiopathic haemolytic anaemia: The experimental production of haemolysis and red-cell fragmentation by defibrination *in vivo*. *Br. J. Haematol.* 14:617, 1968.
120. Brain, M. C., Dacie, J. V., and Hourihane, D. O'B.: Microangiopathic haemolytic anaemia: The possible role of vascular lesions in pathogenesis. *Br. J. Haematol.* 8:358, 1962.
121. Dick, G., Miller, E. M., and Edmondson, H.: Severe purpura with gangrene of the lower extremity following scarlet fever. *Am. J. Dis. Child.* 47:374, 1934.
122. Mielke, C. H., Jr., et al.: The standardized normal Ivy bleeding time and its prolongation by aspirin. *Blood* 34:204, 1969.
123. Rapaport, S. I., Tatter, D., Coeur-Barron, N., and Hjort, P. F.: Pseudomonas septicemia with intravascular clotting leading to the generalized Shwartzman reaction. *N. Engl. J. Med.* 271:80, 1964.
124. Nossel, H. L.: Differential consumption of coagulation factors resulting from activation of the extrinsic (tissue thromboplastin) or intrinsic (foreign surface contact) pathways. *Blood* 29:331, 1967.
125. Rosenberg, R. D.: Actions and interactions of antithrombin and heparin. *N. Engl. J. Med.* 292:146, 1975.
126. Damus, P. S., and Wallace, G. A.: Immunologic measurement of antithrombin III–heparin cofactor and α2 macroglobulin in disseminated intravascular coagulation and hepatic failure coagulopathy. *Thromb. Res.* 6:27, 1975.
127. Ham, J. M.: Hypoprothrombinaemia in patients undergoing prolonged intensive care. *Med. J. Aust.* 2:716, 1971.
128. Mant, M. J., Hirsh, J., Pineo, G. F., and Luke, K. H.: Prolonged prothrombin time and partial thromboplastin time in disseminated intravascular coagulation not due to deficiency of factors V and VIII. *Br. J. Haematol.* 24:725, 1973.
129. Marder, V. J., Cruz, G. O., and Schumer, B. R.: Evaluation of a new antifibrinogen-coated latex particle agglutination test in the measurement of serum fibrin degradation products. *Thromb. Haemost.* 37:183, 1977.
130. Kowalski, E.: Fibrinogen derivatives and their biologic activities. *Semin. Hematol.* 5:45, 1968.
131. Marder, V. J., and Shulman, N. R.: High molecular weight derivatives of human fibrinogen produced by plasmin. II. Mechanism of their anticoagulant activity. *J. Biol. Chem.* 244:2120, 1969.
132. Fletcher, A. P., Alkjaersig, N., and Sherry, S.: Pathogenesis of the coagulation defect developing during pathological plasma proteolytic ("fibrinolytic") states. I. The significance of fibrinogen proteolysis and circulating fibrinogen breakdown products. *J. Clin. Invest.* 41:896, 1962.
133. Bang, N. U., Fletcher, A. P., Alkjaersig, N., and Sherry, S.: Pathogenesis of the coagulation defect developing during pathological plasma proteolytic ("fibrinolytic") states. III. Demonstration of abnormal clot structure by electron microscopy. *J. Clin. Invest.* 41:935, 1962.
134. Lipinski, B., Wegrzynowicz, Z., Budzynski, A. Z., Kopec, M., Latallo, Z. S., and Kowalski, E.: Soluble unclottable complexes formed in the presence of fibrinogen degradation products (FDP) during the fibrinogen-fibrin conversion and their potential significance in pathology. *Thromb. Diath. Haemorrh.* 17:65, 1967.
135. Godal, H. C., and Abilgaard, U.: Gelatin of soluble fibrin in plasma by ethanol. *Scand. J. Haematol.* 3:342, 1966.

136. Breen, F. A., and Tullis, J. L.: Ethanol gelation: A rapid screening test for intravascular coagulation. *Ann. Intern. Med.* 69:1197, 1968.
137. Seaman, A.: The recognition of intravascular clotting: The 3 P test. *Arch. Intern. Med.* 125:1016, 1970.
138. Niewiarowski, S., and Gurewich, V.: Laboratory identification of intravascular coagulation: The serial dilution protamine sulfate test for the detection of fibrin monomer and fibrin degradation products. *J. Lab. Clin. Med.* 77:665, 1971.
139. Bang, N. U., and Chang, M. L.: Soluble fibrin complexes. *Semin. Thromb. Hemostas.* 1:91, 1974.
140. Alkjaersig, N., Roy, L., and Fletcher, A.: Analysis of gel exclusion chromatography data by chromatographic plate theory analysis: Application to plasma fibrinogen chromatography. *Thromb. Res.* 3:525, 1973.
141. Garvey, M. B., and Black, J. M.: The detection of fibrinogen/fibrin degradation products by means of new antibody-coated latex particle. *J. Clin. Pathol.* 25:680, 1972.
142. Ellman, L., Carvalho, A., and Colman, R. W.: The Thrombo-Wellcotest as a screening test for disseminated intravascular coagulation. *N. Engl. J. Med.* 288:633, 1973.
143. Hawiger, J., et al.: Measurement of fibrinogen and fibrin degradation products in serum by the staphylococcal clumping test. *J. Lab. Clin. Med.* 75:93, 1970.
144. Merskey, C., Lalezari, P., and Johnson, A. J.: A rapid, simple, sensitive method for measuring fibrinolytic split products in human serum. *Proc. Soc. Exp. Biol. Med.* 131:871, 1969.
145. Johnson, A. J., Semar, M., and Newman, J.: Estimation of fibrinolytic activity by whole-blood euglobulin clot lysis, in *Blood Coagulation, Hemorrhage, and Thrombosis*, 2d ed., edited by L. M. Tocantins, and L. A. Kazal. Grune & Stratton, New York, 1964, p. 465.
146. Little, J. R.: Purpura fulminans treated successfully with anticoagulation. *JAMA* 169:36, 1959.
147. Hjort, P. F., Rapaport, S. I., and Jørgensen, L.: Purpura fulminans: Report of a case successfully treated with heparin and hydrocortisone: Review of 50 cases from the literature. *Scand. J. Haematol.* 1:169, 1964.
148. Allen, D. M.: Heparin therapy of purpura fulminans. *Pediatrics* 38:211, 1966.
149. Green, D., et al.: The role of heparin in the management of consumption coagulopathy. *Med. Clin. North Am.* 56:193, 1972.
150. Klein, H. G., and Bell, W. R.: Disseminated intravascular coagulation during heparin therapy. *Ann. Intern. Med.* 80:477, 1974.
151. Straub, P. W.: A case against heparin therapy of intravascular coagulation. *Thromb. Diath. Haemorrh.* 33:107, 1974.
152. Pritchard, J. A., and Brekken, A. L.: Clinical and laboratory studies on severe abruptio placentae. *Am. J. Obstet. Gynecol.* 97:681, 1967.
153. Van der Meer, J., Sluyter, A. M. J., and Vreeken, J.: Early manifestations of clotting in cases of abruptio placentae: Clinical and hematological aspects, in *Coagulation Disorders in Obstetrics*, edited by J. C. de Neef, and G. J. H. den Ottolander. Excerpta Medica Foundation, Amsterdam, 1966, p. 25.
154. Coopland, A. T., et al.: The pathogenesis of defective hemostasis in abruptio placentae. *Am. J. Obstet. Gynecol.* 100:311, 1968.
155. Pritchard, J. A.: Treatment of the defibrination syndromes of pregnancy. *Mod. Treatm.* 5:401, 1968.
156. Heene, D. L.: Disseminated intravascular coagulation: Evaluation of therapeutic approaches. *Semin. Thromb. Haemostas.* 3:291, 1977.
157. Clarkson, A. R., Sage, R. E., and Lawrence, J. R.: Consumption coagulopathy and acute renal failure due to Gram-negative septicemia after abortion: Complete recovery with heparin therapy. *Ann. Intern. Med.* 70:1191, 1969.
158. Naeye, R. L.: Thrombotic state after a hemorrhagic diathesis, a possible complication of therapy with epsilon-aminocaproic acid. *Blood* 19:694, 1962.
159. Gralnick, H. R., and Greipp, P.: Thrombosis with epsilon-aminocaproic acid therapy. *Am. J. Clin. Pathol.* 56:151, 1971.
160. Marder, V. J., Matchett, M. O., and Sherry, S.: Detection of serum fibrinogen and fibrin degradation products. *Am. J. Med.* 51:71, 1971.
161. Straub, P. W.: Chronic intravascular coagulation: Clinical spectrum and diagnostic criteria, with special emphasis on metabolism,

distribution, and localization of I^{131}-fibrinogen. *Acta Med. Scand.* 526 (Suppl.):1, 1971.

162. Sack, G. H., Levin, J., and Bell, W. R.: Trousseau's syndrome and other manifestations of chronic disseminated coagulopathy in patients with neoplasms: Clinical, pathologic, and therapeutic features. *Medicine (Baltimore)* 56:1, 1977.

163. Case records of the Massachusetts General Hospital. *N. Engl. J. Med.* 298:786, 1978.

164. Kierulf, P., and Godal, H. C.: Fibrinaemia and multiple thrombi in pancreatic carcinoma: A case studied with quantitative N-terminal analysis. *Scand. J. Haematol.* 9:370, 1972.

165. Nossel, H. L., et al.: Defibrination syndrome in a patient with chronic thrombocytopenic purpura. *Am. J. Med.* 46:591, 1969.

166. Trousseau, A.: Phlegmasia alba dolens: Clinique Medicale de l'Hotel-Dieu de Paris. *The New Sydenham Society* 3:94, 1865.

167. German, H. J., Smith, J. A., and Lindenbaum, J.: Chronic intravascular coagulation associated with chronic myelocytic leukemia: Use of heparin in connection with a surgical procedure. *Am. J. Med.* 61:547, 1976.

168. Nossel, H. L., et al.: Measurement of fibrinopeptide A in human blood. *J. Clin. Invest.* 54:43, 1974.

169. Lipinski, B., and Worowski, K.: Detection of soluble fibrin monomer complexes in blood by means of protamine sulfate test. *Thromb. Diath. Haemorrh.* 20:44, 1968.

170. Rohner, R. F., Prior, J. T., and Sipple, J. H.: Mucinous malignancies, venous thrombosis and terminal endocarditis with emboli: A syndrome. *Cancer* 19:1805, 1966.

171. Bergin, J. J.: Complications of therapy with epsilon-aminocaproic acid. *Med. Clin. North Am.* 50:1669, 1966.

172. Meikle, A. W., and Graybill, J. R.: Fibrinolysis and hemorrhage in a fatal case of heat stroke. *N. Engl. J. Med.* 276:911, 1967.

173. Bergin, J. J., Crosby, W. H., and Jahnke, E. J.: Massive bleeding with fibrinolysis: Management with heparin and epsilon aminocaproic acid. *Milit. Med.* 131:340, 1966.

174. Shibolet, S., et al.: Heatstroke: Its clinical picture and mechanism in 36 cases. *Q. J. Med.* 36:525, 1967.

175. Weber, M. B., and Blakeley, J. A.: The hemorrhagic diathesis of heatstroke: A consumption coagulopathy successfully treated with heparin. *Lancet* 1:1190, 1969.

176. Stefanini, M., and Spicer, D. D.: Hemostatic breakdown, fibrinolysis, and acquired hemolytic anemia in a patient with fatal heatstroke: Pathogenetic mechanisms. *Am. J. Clin. Pathol.* 55:180, 1971.

177. Kevy, S. V., et al.: The pathogenesis and control of the hemorrhagic defect in open heart surgery. *Surg. Gynecol. Obstet.* 123:313, 1966.

178. McClure, P. D., and Izsak, J.: The use of epsilon-aminocaproic acid to reduce bleeding during cardiac bypass in children with congenital heart disease. *Anesthesiology* 40:604, 1974.

179. Lambert, C. J., et al.: The treatment of postperfusion bleeding using ε-aminocaproic acid, cryoprecipitate, fresh-frozen plasma, and protamine sulfate. *Ann. Thorac. Surg.* 28:440, 1979.

180. Davidson, J. F., et al.: Plasminogen-activator-producing tumour. *Br. Med. J.* 1:88, 1969.

181. Mannick, J. A.: Diagnosis of ruptured aneurysm of the abdominal aorta. *N. Engl. J. Med.* 276:1305, 1967.

182. Fine, N. L., et al.: Multiple coagulation defects in association with dissecting aneurysm. *Arch. Intern. Med.* 119:522, 1967.

183. Kazmier, F. J., et al.: Intravascular coagulation and arterial disease. *Thromb. Diath. Haemorrh.* (Suppl.) 36:295, 1969.

184. Garcia-Zueco, J. C., et al.: Dissecting aneurysm of the aorta and disseminated intravascular coagulation: Report of two cases. *Sangre (Barc.)* 21:839, 1976.

185. Schnetzer, G. W., and Penner, J. A.: Chronic intravascular coagulation syndrome associated with atherosclerotic aortic aneurysm. *South. Med. J.* 66:264, 1973.

186. Ten Cate, J. W., Timmers, H., and Becker, A. E.: Coagulopathy in ruptured or dissecting aortic aneurysms. *Am. J. Med.* 59:171, 1975.

187. Siebert, W. T., and Natelson, E. A.: Chronic consumption coagulopathy accompanying abdominal aortic aneurysm. *Arch. Surg.* 111:539, 1976.

188. Mulcare, R. J., et al.: Disseminated intravascular coagulation as a complication of abdominal aortic aneurysm repair. *Ann. Surg.* 180:343, 1974.

189. Sutherland, D. A., and Clark, H.: Hemangioma associated with thrombocytopenia: Report of a case and review of the literature. *Am. J. Med.* 33:150, 1962.

190. Petit, P., et al.: Les Angiomes géants du nourrisson avec thrombopenie. *Arch. Fr. Pediatr.* 14:789, 1957.

191. Straub, P. W., et al.: Chronic intravascular coagulation in Kasabach-Merritt syndrome: Preferential accumulation of fibrinogen ^{131}I in a giant hemangioma. *Arch. Intern. Med.* 129:475, 1972.

192. Hoak, J. C., et al.: Hemangioma with thrombocytopenia and microangiopathic anemia (Kasabach-Merritt syndrome): An animal model. *J. Lab. Clin. Med.* 77:941, 1971.

193. Good, T. A., Carnazzo, S. F., and Good, R. A.: Thrombocytopenia and giant hemangioma in infants. *Am. J. Dis. Child.* 90:260, 1955.

194. Inceman, S., and Tangrin, Y.: Chronic defibrination syndrome due to a giant hemangioma associated with microangiopathic hemolytic anemia. *Am. J. Med.* 46:997, 1969.

195. Behar, A., Moran, E., and Izak, G.: Acquired hypofibrinogenemia associated with a giant cavernous hemangioma of the liver. *Am. J. Clin. Pathol.* 40:78, 1963.

196. Amir, J., and Krauss, S.: Treatment of thrombotic thrombocytopenic purpura with antiplatelet drugs. *Blood* 42:27, 1973.

197. Rodriguez-Erdmann, F., et al.: Kasabach-Merritt syndrome: Coagulo-analytical observations. *Am. J. Med. Sci.* 261:9, 1971.

198. Hagerman, L. J., Czapek, E. E., and Donnellan, W. L.: Giant hemangioma with consumption coagulopathy. *J. Pediatr.* 87:766, 1975.

199. Starzl, T. E., et al.: Shwartzman reaction after human renal homotransplantation. *N. Engl. J. Med.* 278:642, 1968.

200. Williams, C. M., et al.: "Hyperacute" renal-homograft rejection in man. *N. Engl. J. Med.* 279:611, 1968.

201. Colman, R. W., et al.: Coagulation studies in the hyperacute and other forms of renal-allograft rejection. *N. Engl. J. Med.* 281:685, 1969.

202. Rodriquez-Erdmann, F., and Guttmann, R. D.: Coagulation in renal-allograft rejection. *N. Engl. J. Med.* 281:1428, 1969.

203. Starzl, T. E., et al.: Clotting changes, including disseminated intravascular coagulation, during rapid renal-homograft rejection. *N. Engl. J. Med.* 283:383, 1970.

204. Braun, W. E., and Merrill, J. P.: Urine fibrinogen fragments in human renal allografts: A possible mechanism of renal injury. *N. Engl. J. Med.* 278:1366, 1968.

205. Clarkson, A. R., Morton, J. B., and Cash, J. D.: Urinary fibrin/fibrinogen degradation products after renal homotransplantation. *Lancet* 2:1220, 1970.

206. Sharma, H. M., et al.: Platelets in early hyperacute allograft rejection in kidneys and their modification by sulfinpyrazone (Anturan) therapy. *Am. J. Pathol.* 66:445, 1972.

207. Kanyerezi, B. R., Lwanga, S. K., and Bloch, K. J.: Fibrinogen degradation products in serum and urine of patients with systemic lupus erythematosus: Relation to renal disease and pathogenetic mechanism. *Arthritis Rheum.* 14:267, 1971.

208. Clarkson, A. R., et al.: Serum and urinary fibrin/fibrinogen degradation products in glomerulonephritis. *Br. Med. J.* 3:447, 1971.

209. Habib, R., et al.: Étude anatomopathologique de 35 observations de syndrome hémolytique et uremique de l'enfant. *Arch. Fr. Pediatr.* 26:391, 1969.

210. Lieberman, E., et al.: Hemolytic-uremic syndrome. *N. Engl. J. Med.* 275:227, 1966.

211. Vitsky, B. H., et al.: The hemolytic uremic syndrome: A study of renal pathologic alterations. *Am. J. Pathol.* 57:627, 1969.

212. Lieberman, E.: Hemolytic-uremic syndrome. *J. Pediatr.* 80:1, 1972.

213. Brain, M. C.: The haemolytic-uraemic syndrome. *Semin. Hematol.* 6:162, 1969.

214. Piel, C. F., and Phibbs, R. H.: The hemolytic-uremic syndrome. *Pediatr. Clin. North Am.* 13:295, 1966.

215. Gianantonio, C., et al.: The hemolytic-uremic syndrome. *J. Pediatr.* 64:478, 1964.

216. Kaplan, B. S., Thomson, P. D., and de Chadarévian, J.-P.: The hemolytic uremic syndrome. *Pediatr. Clin. North Am.* 23:761, 1976.

217. Avalos, J. S., et al.: Coagulation studies in the hemolytic-uremic syndrome. *J. Pediatr.* 76:538, 1970.

218. Katz, J., et al.: Coagulation findings in the hemolytic-uremic syndrome of infancy: Similarity to hyperacute renal allograft rejection. *J. Pediatr. 78:*426, 1971.

219. Gilchrist, G. S., et al.: Heparin therapy in the haemolytic-uraemic syndrome. *Lancet 1:*1123, 1969.

220. Vitacco, M., Avalos, J. S., and Gianantonio, C. A.: Heparin therapy in the hemolytic-uremic syndrome. *J. Pediatr. 83:*271, 1973.

221. Thorsen, C. A., et al.: The treatment of the hemolytic-uremic syndrome with inhibitors of platelet function. *Am. J. Med. 66:*711, 1979.

222. Kinkaid-Smith, P.: The modification of the vascular lesions of rejection in cadaveric renal allografts by dipyridamole and anticoagulants. *Lancet 2:*920, 1969.

223. Bergstein, J. M., Edson, J. R., and Michael, A. F.: Fibrinolytic treatment of the haemolytic-uraemic syndrome. *Lancet 1:*448, 1972.

224. Stuart, J., et al.: Thrombolytic therapy in haemolytic-uraemic syndrome. *Br. Med. J. 3:*217, 1974.

225. Ekberg, M., Nilsson, I. M., and Denneberg, T.: Coagulation studies in hemolytic uremic syndrome and thrombotic thrombocytopenic purpura. *Acta Med. Scand. 196:*373, 1974.

226. Umlas, J., and Kaiser, J.: Thrombohemolytic thrombocytopenic purpura (TTP): A disease or a syndrome? *Am. J. Med. 49:*723, 1970.

227. Amorosi, E. L., and Ultmann, J. E.: Thrombotic thrombocytopenic purpura: Report of 16 cases and review of the literature. *Medicine (Baltimore) 45:*139, 1966.

228. Altschule, M. D.: A rare type of acute thrombocytopenic purpura: Widespread formation of platelet thrombi in capillaries. *N. Engl. J. Med. 227:*477, 1942.

229. Baehr, G., Klemperer, P., and Schifrin, A.: An acute febrile anemia and thrombocytopenic purpura with diffuse platelet thrombosis of capillaries and arterioles. *Trans. Assoc. Am. Phys. 51:*43, 1936.

230. Feldman, J. D., Mardiney, M. R., and Unanue, R.: The vascular pathology of thrombotic thrombocytopenic purpura. *Lab. Invest. 15:*927, 1966.

231. Neame, P. B., et al.: Thrombotic thrombocytopenic purpura: Report of a case with disseminated intravascular platelet aggregation. *Blood 42:*805, 1973.

232. Jaffe, E. A., Nachman, R. L., and Merskey, C.: Thrombotic thrombocytopenic purpura: Coagulation parameters in twelve patients. *Blood 42:*499, 1973.

233. Lerner, R. G., Rapaport, S. I., and Meltzer, J.: Thrombotic thrombocytopenic purpura: Serial clotting studies, relation to the generalized Shwartzman reaction, and remission after adrenal steroid and dextran therapy. *Ann. Intern. Med. 66:*1180, 1967.

234. Harker, L. A., and Slichter, S. J.: Platelet and fibrinogen consumption in man. *N. Engl. J. Med. 287:*999, 1972.

235. Berberich, F. R., et al.: Thrombotic thrombocytopenic purpura: Three cases with platelet fibrinogen survival studies. *J. Pediatr. 84:*503, 1974.

236. Thrombotic thrombocytopenic purpura, Part I. *Semin. Thromb. Hemostas. 6:*328, 1980.

237. Management of thrombotic thrombocytopenic purpura. *Semin. Thromb. Hemostas. 7:*1, 1981.

238. Amir, J., and Krauss, S.: Treatment of thrombotic thrombocytopenic purpura with anti-platelet drugs. *Blood 42:*27, 1973.

239. Neame, P. B.: Immunologic and other factors in thrombotic thrombocytopenic purpura (TTP). *Semin. Thromb. Hemostas. 6:*416, 1980.

240. Byrnes, J. J., and Khurana, M.: Treatment of thrombotic thrombocytopenic purpura with plasma. *N. Engl. J. Med. 297:*1386, 1977.

241. Rubinstein, M. A., et al.: Unusual remission in a case of thrombotic thrombocytopenic purpura syndrome following fresh blood exchange transfusions. *Ann. Intern. Med. 51:*1409, 1959.

242. Bukowski, R. M., King, J. W., and Hewlett, J. S.: Plasmapheresis in the treatment of thrombotic thrombocytopenic purpura. *Blood 50:*413, 1977.

243. Myers, T. J., et al.: Thrombotic thrombocytopenic purpura: Combined treatment with plasmapheresis and antiplatelet agents. *Ann. Intern. Med. 92:*149, 1980.

244. Upshaw, J. D., Jr.: Congenital deficiency of a factor in normal plasma that reverses microangiopathic hemolysis and thrombocytopenia. *N. Engl. J. Med. 298:*1350, 1978.

245. Lian, E. C. Y., et al.: The presence of a platelet aggregating factor in the plasma of patients with thrombotic thrombocytopenic purpura and its inhibition by normal plasma. *Blood 53:*333, 1979.

246. Brandt, J. T., Kennedy, M. S., and Senhauser, D. A.: Platelet aggregating factor in thrombotic thrombocytopenic purpura. *Lancet 2:*463, 1979.

247. Rodriguez, H. F., et al.: Thrombotic thrombocytopenic purpura: Remission after splenectomy. *N. Engl. J. Med. 257:*983, 1957.

248. Shapiro, H. D., Doktor, D., and Churg, J.: Thrombotic thrombocytopenic purpura (Moschcowitz's disease): Report of a case with remission after splenectomy and steroid therapy. *Ann. Intern. Med. 47:*582, 1957.

249. Bernard, R. P., Bauman, A. W., and Schwartz, S. I.: Splenectomy for thrombotic thrombocytopenic purpura. *Ann. Surg. 169:*616, 1969.

250. Hill, J. B., and Cooper, W. M.: Thrombotic thrombocytopenic purpura: Treatment with corticosteroids and splenectomy. *Arch. Intern. Med. 122:*353, 1968.

251. Bukowski, R. M., et al.: Therapy of thrombotic thrombocytopenic purpura: An overview. *Semin. Thromb. Hemost. 7:*1, 1981.

252. Neame, P. B., et al.: Thrombocytopenia in septicemia: The role of disseminated intravascular coagulation. *Blood 56:*88, 1980.

253. Rich, A. R.: A peculiar type of adrenal cortical damage associated with acute infections, and its possible relation to circulatory collapse. *Bull. Johns Hopkins Hosp. 74:*1, 1944.

254. Ferguson, J. H., and Chapman, O. D.: Fulminating meningococcic infections and the so-called Waterhouse-Friderichsen syndrome. *Am. J. Pathol. 24:*763, 1948.

255. Spicer, T. E., and Rau, J. M.: Purpura fulminans. *Am. J. Med. 61:*566, 1976.

256. Skjörten, F.: Bilateral renal cortical necrosis and the generalized Shwartzman reaction. I. Review of literature and report of seven cases. *Acta Pathol. Microbiol. Scand. 61:*394, 1964.

257. Evans, R. W., et al.: Fatal intravascular consumption coagulopathy in meningococcal sepsis. *Am. J. Med. 48:*910, 1969.

258. Stiehm, E. R., and Damrosch, D. S.: Factors in the prognosis of meningococcal infection: Review of 63 cases with emphasis on recognition and management of the severely ill patient. *J. Pediatr. 68:*457, 1966.

259. Gerard, P., et al.: Meningococcal purpura: Report of 19 patients treated with heparin. *J. Pediatr. 82:*780, 1973.

260. Hathaway, W. E.: Heparin therapy in acute meningococcemia. *J. Pediatr. 82:*900, 1973.

261. Ratnoff, O. D., and Nebehay, W. G.: Multiple coagulative defects in a patient with the Waterhouse-Friderichsen syndrome. *Ann. Intern. Med. 56:*627, 1962.

262. Whitaker, A. N.: Infection and the spleen: Association between hyposplenism, pneumococcal sepsis and disseminated intravascular coagulation. *Med. J. Aust. 1:*1213, 1969.

263. Bisno, A. L., and Freeman, J. C.: The syndrome of asplenia, pneumococcal sepsis and disseminated intravascular coagulation. *Ann. Intern. Med. 72:*389, 1970.

264. Dyggve, H.: A case of purpura fulminans with fibrinogenopenia in association with scarlatina. *Acta Med. Scand. 127:*382, 1947.

265. Chambers, W. N., Holyoke, J. B., and Wilson, R. F.: Purpura fulminans: Report of two cases following scarlet fever. *N. Engl. J. Med. 247:*933, 1952.

266. Jewett, J. F.: Coagulopathy syndrome due to streptococci. *N. Engl. J. Med. 289:*43, 1973.

267. Hall, W. H.: Purpura fulminans with group B β-hemolytic streptococcal endocarditis. *Arch. Intern. Med. 116:*594, 1965.

268. Beller, F. K.: The role of endotoxin in DIC. *Thromb. Diath. Haemorrh. 36 (Suppl.):*125, 1969.

269. Lipinski, B., and Jeljaszewica, I.: A hypothesis for the pathogenesis of the generalized Shwartzman reaction. *J. Infect. Dis. 120:*160, 1969.

270. Preston, E. F., et al.: Intravascular coagulation and E. coli septicaemia. *J. Clin. Pathol. 26:*120, 1973.

271. McGovern, V. J.: The pathophysiology of gram negative septicaemia. *Pathology 4:*265, 1972.

272. McGovern, V. J.: The pathology of shock, in *Pathology Annual,* edited by S. Somers. Appleton-Century-Crofts, New York, 1971, vol. 6, p. 279.

273. Murray, H. W., Tuazon, C. V., and Sheagren, J. N.: Staphylococcal septicemia and disseminated intravascular coagulation. *Arch. Intern. Med.* 137:844, 1977.

274. Lutz, E. E.: Afibrinogenemia due to postabortal *Clostridium welchii* infection. *Obstet. Gynecol.* 20:270, 1962.

275. Phillips, L. L., Skrodelis, V., and Quigley, H. J.: Intravascular coagulation and fibrinolysis in septic abortion. *Obstet. Gynecol.* 30:350, 1967.

276. Rubenberg, M. L., et al.: Intravascular coagulation in a case of *Clostridium perfringens* septicaemia: Treatment by exchange transfusion and heparin. *Br. Med. J.* 4:271, 1967.

277. Zander, J.: *Septischer Abort und bakterieller Schock.* Springer, Berlin, 1968.

278. McKay, D. G., and Margaretten, W.: Disseminated intravascular coagulation in virus disease. *Arch. Intern. Med.* 120:129, 1967.

279. Talley, N. A., and Assumpcao, C. A. R.: Disseminated intravascular clotting complicating viral pneumonia due to influenza. *Med. J. Aust.* 2:763, 1971.

280. Davison, A. M., Thomson, D., and Robson, J. S.: Intravascular coagulation complicating influenza virus A infection. *Br. Med. J.* 1:654, 1973.

281. Whitaker, A. N., Bunce, I., and Graeme, E. R.: Disseminated intravascular coagulation and acute renal failure in influenza A2 infection. *Med. J. Aust.* 2:196, 1974.

282. Settle, H., and Glueck, H. I.: Disseminated intravascular coagulation associated with influenza. *Ohio State Med. J.* 71:541, 1975.

283. Srichaikul, T., et al.: Fibrinogen metabolism and disseminated intravascular coagulation in Dengue hemorrhagic fever. *Am. J. Trop. Med. Hyg.* 26:525, 1977.

284. Schaffner, W., McLeod, A. C., and Koenig, M. G.: Thrombocytopenic Rocky Mountain spotted fever. *Arch. Intern. Med.* 116:857, 1965.

285. Trigg, J. W., Jr.: Hypofibrinogenemia in Rocky Mountain spotted fever: Report of a case. *N. Engl. J. Med.* 270:1042, 1964.

286. Atkin, M. D., Strauss, H. S., and Fisher, G. U.: A case report of "Cape Cod" Rocky Mountain spotted fever with multiple coagulation disturbances. *Pediatrics* 36:627, 1965.

287. Graybill, J. R., Hawiger, J., and Des Prez, R. M.: Complement and coagulation in Rocky Mountain spotted fever. *South. Med. J.* 66:410, 1973.

288. Dennis, L. H., et al.: Depletion of coagulation factors in drug-resistant *Plasmodium falciparum* malaria. *Blood* 29:713, 1967.

289. Paar, D., et al.: Cerebral malaria and intravascular coagulation. *Br. Med. J.* 4:805, 1970.

290. Butler, T., et al.: Blood coagulation studies in *Plasmodium falciparum* malaria. *Am. J. Med. Sci.* 265:63, 1973.

291. Punyagupta, S., et al.: Acute pulmonary insufficiency in falciparum malaria: Summary of 12 cases with evidence of disseminated intravascular coagulation. *Am. J. Trop. Med. Hyg.* 23:551, 1974.

292. Edwards, I. R.: Malaria with disseminated intravascular coagulation and peripheral tissue necrosis successfully treated with streptokinase. *Br. Med. J.* 280:1252, 1980.

293. Doughten, R. M., and Pearson, H. A.: Disseminated intravascular coagulation associated with *Aspergillus* endocarditis. *J. Pediatr.* 73:576, 1968.

294. Prochazka, J. V., et al.: Systemic candidiasis with disseminated intravascular coagulation. *Am. J. Dis. Child.* 122:255, 1971.

295. Barrett-Connor, E., Ugoretz, R. J., and Braude, A. I.: Disseminated intravascular coagulation in trypanosomiasis. *Arch. Intern. Med.* 131:574, 1973.

296. Kraus, J. S., and Walker, D. H.: Miliary tuberculosis and consumption of clotting factors by multifocal vasculopathic coagulation. *South. Med. J.* 72:1479, 1979.

297. Good, R. A., and Thomas, L.: Studies on the generalized Shwartzman reaction. IV. Prevention of the local and generalized Shwartzman reaction with heparin. *J. Exp. Med.* 97:871, 1953.

298. Corrigan, J. J.: Effect of anticoagulating and non-anticoagulating concentrations of heparin on the generalized Shwartzman reaction. *Thromb. Diath. Haemorrh.* 24:136, 1970.

299. Corrigan, J. J., Jr., and Kiernat, J. F.: Effect of heparin in experimental gram negative septicemia. *J. Infect. Dis.* 131:138, 1975.

300. Gaskins, R. A., Jr., and Palldorf, F. G.: Experimental meningococcal septicemia: Effect of heparin therapy. *Arch. Pathol. Lab. Med.* 100:318, 1976.

301. Horwitz, D. L., Monquin, R. B., and Herman, C. M.: Coagulation changes of septic shock in the subhuman primate and their relationships to hemodynamic changes. *Ann. Surg.* 175:417, 1972.

302. Antley, R. M., and McMillan, C. W.: Sequential coagulation studies in purpura fulminans. *N. Engl. J. Med.* 276:1287, 1967.

303. Kuhn, W., and Graeff, H.: Infizierter Abort und disseminierte intravasculäre Gerinnung (DIG): Heparinprophylaxe und Früh-diagnose der DIG. *Med. Welt* 22:1199, 1971.

304. Colman, R. W., Robboy, S. J., and Minna, J. D.: Therapy of clinically significant disseminated intravascular coagulation, in *Controversy in Internal Medicine II,* edited by F. J. Ingelfinger et al. Saunders, Philadelphia, 1974, p. 633.

305. Corrigan, J. J., Jr.: Heparin therapy in bacterial septicemia. *J. Pediatr.* 91:695, 1977.

306. Corrigan, J. J., Jr., Jordan, C. M., and Bennett, B. B.: Disseminated intravascular coagulation in septic shock: Report of three cases not treated with heparin. *Am. J. Dis. Child.* 126:629, 1973.

307. Niklasson, P. M., et al.: Thrombocytopenia and bleeding complications in severe cases of meningococcemia infection treated with heparin, dextran 70 and chlorpromazine. *Scand. J. Infect. Dis.* 4:183, 1972.

308. Pitney, W. R., Pettit, J. E., and Armstrong, L.: Control of heparin therapy. *Br. Med. J.* 4:139, 1970.

309. DeLee, J. B.: A case of fatal hemorrhagic diathesis, with premature detachment of the placenta. *Am. J. Obstet.* 44:785, 1901.

310. Graeff, H., and Kuhn, W. (eds.): *Coagulation Disorders in Obstetrics: Pathobiochemistry, Pathophysiology, Diagnosis, Treatment.* Georg Thieme, Stuttgard, 1980.

311. Kleiner, G. J., et al.: Defibrination in normal and abnormal parturition. *Br. J. Haematol.* 19:159, 1970.

312. Bonnar, J., et al.: Fibrin degradation products in normal and abnormal pregnancy and parturition. *Br. Med. J.* 3:137, 1969.

313. Bieber, G. F.: Review of three hundred fifty-three cases of premature separation of the placenta. *Am. J. Obstet. Gynecol.* 65:257, 1953.

314. Beller, F. K., and Epstein, M. D.: Traumatic placental abruption. *Obstet. Gynecol.* 27:484, 1966.

315. Nilsen, P. A.: The mechanism of hypofibrinogenemia in premature separation of the normally implanted placenta. *Acta Obstet. Gynecol. Scand.* 42 (Suppl. 2):96, 1963.

316. Page, E. W., Fulton, L. D., and Glendening, M. B.: The cause of the blood coagulation defect following abruptio placentae. *Am. J. Obstet. Gynecol.* 61:1116, 1951.

317. Schneider, C. L.: Rupture of the basal (decidual) plate in abruptio placentae: A pathway of autoextraction from the decidua into the maternal circulation. *Am. J. Obstet. Gynecol.* 63:1078, 1952.

318. Tideman, J. W.: Coagulation disorders in abruptio placentae, in *Coagulation Disorders in Obstetrics,* Proceedings of the Dijkzigt Conference, Rotterdam, February 1966, edited by J. C. de Neef and G. J. H. den Ottolander. Excerpta Medica Foundation, Amsterdam, 1966, p. 13.

319. Graeff, H., and vonHugo, R.: Fibrinogen derivatives in a case of abruptio placentae. *Am. J. Obstet. Gynecol.* 120:335, 1974.

320. Verstraete, M., and Vermylen, J.: Acute and chronic "defibrination" in obstetrical practice. *Thromb. Diath. Haemorrh.* 20:444, 1968.

321. Williams, T. F.: Renal cortical necrosis, renal infarction, and hypertension due to renal vascular disease, in *Diseases of the Kidney,* edited by M. B. Strauss and L. G. Welt. Little, Brown, Boston, 1963, p. 526.

322. Sheehan, H. L., and Moore, H. C.: *Renal Cortical Necrosis and the Kidney of Concealed Accidental Haemorrhage.* Blackwell, Oxford, 1952, p. 186.

323. Steiner, P. E., and Lushbaugh, C. C.: Maternal pulmonary embolism by amniotic fluid. *JAMA* 117:1245, 1941.

324. Russell, W. S., and Jones, W. N.: Amniotic fluid embolism. *Obstet. Gynecol.* 26:476, 1965.

325. Aguillon, A., et al.: Amniotic fluid embolism: A review. *Obstet. Gynecol. Surg.* 17:619, 1962.

326. Liban, E., and Raz, S.: Clinicopathologic study of fourteen cases of amniotic fluid embolism. *Am. J. Clin. Pathol.* 51:477, 1969.

327. Brozman, M. (quoted by O. K. Albrechtsen): Hemorrhagic disorders following amniotic fluid embolism. *Clin. Obstet. Gynecol.* 7:361, 1964.

328. Ratnoff, O. D., and Vosburgh, G. J.: Observations on the clotting defect in amniotic fluid embolism. *N. Engl. J. Med.* 247:970, 1952.

329. Albrechtsen, O. K., Storm, O., and Trolle, D.: Fibrinolytic activity in the circulating blood following amniotic fluid infusion. *Acta Hematol.* 14:309, 1955.

330. Beller, F. K., et al.: The fibrinolytic system in amniotic fluid embolism. *Am. J. Obstet. Gynecol.* 87:48, 1963.

331. Bonnar, J.: Blood coagulation and fibrinolysis in obstetrics. *Clin. Haematol.* 2:213, 1973.

332. Maki, M., et al.: Heparin treatment of amniotic fluid embolism. *Tohoku J. Exp. Med.* 97:155, 1969.

333. Newton, M.: Amniotic fluid embolism: The nonfatal case. *J. Miss. State Med. Assoc.* 7:607, 1966.

334. Owen, C. A., Jr., and Bowie, E. J. W.: *The Intravascular Coagulation-Fibrinolysis Syndromes in Obstetrics and Gynecology,* a Scope Publication, Upjohn, Kalamazoo, Mich., 1976, p. 36.

335. Weiner, A. E., et al.: Coagulation defects with intrauterine death from Rh isosensitization. *Am. J. Obstet. Gynecol.* 60:1015, 1950.

336. Pritchard, J. A., and Ratnoff, O. D.: Studies of fibrinogen and other hemostatic factors in women with intrauterine death and delayed delivery. *Surg. Gynecol. Obstet.* 101:467, 1955.

337. Pfeffer, R. I.: Hypofibrinogenemia in the dead fetus syndrome treated with aminocaproic acid. *Am. J. Obstet. Gynecol.* 95:1095, 1966.

338. Phillips, L. L., and Sciarra, J. J.: Hypofibrinogenemia with a dead fetus treated with intravenous heparin. *Am. J. Obstet. Gynecol.* 92:1161, 1965.

339. Lerner, R., et al.: Heparin in the treatment of hypofibrinogenemia complicating fetal death in utero. *Am. J. Obstet. Gynecol.* 97:373, 1967.

340. Gallup, D. G., and Lucas, W. E.: Heparin treatment of consumption coagulopathy associated with intrauterine fetal death. *Obstet. Gynecol.* 35:690, 1970.

341. Beller, F. K., et al.: Consumptive coagulopathy associated with intra-amniotic infusion of hypertonic salt. *Am. J. Obstet. Gynecol.* 112:534, 1972.

342. Brown, F. D., Davidson, E. C., and Phillips, L. L.: Coagulation studies after hypertonic saline infusion. *Obstet. Gynecol.* 39:538, 1972.

343. Halbert, D. R., et al.: Consumptive coagulopathy with generalized hemorrhage after hypertonic saline-induced abortion. *Obstet. Gynecol.* 39:41, 1972.

344. Schwartz, R., Greston, W., and Kleiner, G. J.: Defibrination in saline abortion. *Obstet. Gynecol.* 40:728, 1972.

345. Talbert, L. M., et al.: Studies on the pathogenesis of clotting defects during salt-reduced abortions. *Am. J. Obstet. Gynecol.* 115:656, 1973.

346. Cavanagh, D., Clark, P. J., and McLeod, A. G. W.: Septic shock of endotoxin type: Some observations based on the management of 50 patients. *Am. J. Obstet. Gynecol.* 102:13, 1968.

347. Valle Ponce, R., Garrido, J., and Bocaz, J. A.: Flora microbiana endouterina en el aborto séptico, con especial referencia a los gérmenes anaerobios. *Rev. Chil. Obstet. Ginecol.* 43:137, 1978.

348. Kistner, R. W., and Assali, N. S.: Acute intravascular hemolysis and lower nephron nephrosis complicating eclampsia. *Ann. Intern. Med.* 33:221, 1950.

349. Pritchard, J. A., et al.: Intravascular hemolysis, thrombocytopenia and other hematologic abnormalities associated with severe toxemia of pregnancy. *N. Engl. J. Med.* 250:87, 1954.

350. Nielsen, N. C.: Influence of pre-eclampsia upon coagulation and fibrinolysis in women and their newborn infants immediately after delivery. *Acta Obstet. Gynecol. Scand.* 48:523, 1969.

351. Bonnar, J., McNicol, G. P., and Douglas, A. S.: Coagulation and fibrinolytic systems in pre-eclampsia and eclampsia. *Br. Med. J.* 2:12, 1971.

352. Galton, M., Merritt, K., and Beller, F. K.: Coagulation studies on the peripheral circulation of patients with toxemia of pregnancy: A study for the evaluation of disseminated intravascular coagulation in toxemia. *J. Reprod. Med.* 6:89, 1971.

353. Sher, G., et al.: Pregnancy, pre-eclampsia, and disseminated intravascular coagulation. *S. Afr. Med. J.* 49:1197, 1975.

354. Morris, R. H., et al.: Immunofluorescent studies on renal biopsies in the diagnosis of toxemia of pregnancy. *Obstet. Gynecol.* 24:32, 1964.

355. Vassalli, P., Morris, R. H., and McCluskey, R. T.: The pathogenic role of fibrin deposition in the glomerular lesions of toxemia of pregnancy. *J. Exp. Med.* 118:467, 1963.

356. McKay, D. G., and Corey, A. E.: Cryofibrinogenemia in toxemia of pregnancy. *Obstet. Gynecol.* 23:508, 1964.

357. Wardle, E. N., and Menon, I. S.: Fibrinolysis in pre-eclamptic toxaemia of pregnancy. *Br. Med. J.* 2:625, 1969.

358. Howie, P. W., Prentice, C. R. M., and Forbes, C. D.: Failure of heparin therapy to affect the clinical course of severe pre-eclampsia. *Br. J. Obstet. Gynecol.* 82:711, 1975.

359. Seftel, H. C., and Metz, J.: Haemolytic anaemia, thrombocytopenia, and uraemia in eclampsia. *S. Afr. Med. J.* 31:1037, 1957.

360. McKay, D. G.: Hematologic evidence of disseminated intravascular coagulation in eclampsia. *Obstet. Gynecol. Surv.* 27:399, 1972.

361. Beecham, J. B., Watson, W. J., and Clapp, J. F., III: Eclampsia, pre-eclampsia, and disseminated intravascular coagulation. *Obstet. Gynecol.* 43:576, 1974.

362. Baker, W. S., et al.: Acute intravascular hemolysis, lower nephron nephrosis, and acute anterior pituitary necrosis complicating a case of severe eclampsia. *Am. J. Obstet. Gynecol.* 66:842, 1953.

363. Counihan, T. B., and Doniach, I.: Malignant hypertension supervening rapidly on pre-eclampsia. *J. Obstet. Gynaecol. Br. Empire* 61:449, 1954.

364. McKay, D. G.: Clinical significance of the pathology of toxemia of pregnancy. *Circulation 29 and 30 (Suppl. II)*:66, 1964.

365. Govan, A. D. T.: Renal changes in eclampsia. *J. Pathol. Bacteriol.* 67:311, 1954.

366. Pritchard, J. A., Cunningham, F. G., and Mason, R. A.: Coagulation changes in eclampsia: Their frequency and pathogenesis. *Am. J. Obstet. Gynecol.* 124:855, 1976.

367. Vardi, J., and Fields, G. A.: Microangiopathic hemolytic anemia in severe pre-eclampsia: A review of the literature and pathophysiology. *Am. J. Obstet. Gynecol.* 119:617, 1974.

368. Brain, M. C., Kuah, K.-B., and Dixon, H. G.: Heparin treatment of haemolysis and thrombocytopenia in pre-eclampsia. *J. Obstet. Gynecol. Br. Commonw.* 74:702, 1967.

369. Butler, B. C., Taylor, H. C., Sr., and Graff, S.: The relationship of disorders of the blood-clotting mechanism to toxemia of pregnancy and the value of heparin in therapy. *Am. J. Obstet. Gynecol.* 60:564, 1950.

370. Pritchard, J. A., and Pritchard, S. A.: Standardized treatment of 154 consecutive cases of eclampsia. *Am. J. Obstet. Gynecol.* 123:543, 1975.

371. Slichter, S. J., and Harker, L. A.: Hemostasis in malignancy. *Ann. N.Y. Acad. Sci.* 230:252, 1974.

372. Sproul, E. E.: Carcinoma and venous thrombosis: The frequency of association of carcinoma in the body or tail of the pancreas with multiple venous thrombosis. *Am. J. Cancer* 34:566, 1938.

373. Edwards, E. A.: Migrating thrombophlebitis associated with carcinoma. *N. Engl. J. Med.* 240:1031, 1949.

374. Barron, K. D., Siqueira, E., and Hirano, A.: Cerebral embolism caused by non-bacterial thrombotic endocarditis. *Neurology* 10:391, 1960.

375. Conley, C. L., Lambird, P. A., and Biesecker, J. L.: Microangiopathic hemolytic anemia with recovery after removal of a huge leiomyoblastoma. *Johns Hopkins Med. J.* 126:51, 1970.

376. Hamm, K., et al.: Microangiopathic hemolytic anemia and cancer: A review. *Medicine* 58:377, 1979.

377. Cooper, T., and Barker, N. W.: Recurrent venous thrombosis: An early complication of obscure visceral cancer. *Minn. Med.* 27:31, 1944.

378. Fountain, J. R., and Taverner, D.: Gangrene of three limbs resulting from venous occlusion. *Ann. Intern. Med.* 44:549, 1956.

379. Goodman, D. H.: Early clue to visceral carcinoma: Hemorrhage after intravenously given warfarin. *JAMA* 166:1037, 1958.

380. Heffner, R. R., Jr.: Myopathy of embolic origin in patients with carcinoma. *Neurology* 21:840, 1971.

381. Levin, J., and Conley, C. L.: Thrombocytosis associated with malignant disease. *Arch. Intern. Med. 114*:497, 1964.

382. McKee, P. A., Kalbfleisch, J. M., and Bird, R. M.: Incidence and significance of cryofibrinogenemia. *J. Lab. Clin. Med. 61*:203, 1963.

383. Ritzmann, S. E., and Levin, W. C.: Cryopathies: A review. *Arch. Intern. Med. 107*:754, 1961.

384. Smith, S. B., and Arkin, C.: Cryofibrinogenemia: Incidence, clinical correlations, and a review of the literature. *Am. J. Clin. Pathol. 58*:524, 1972.

385. Grant, R. N., and Deddish, M. R.: Phlegmasia cerulea dolens and gangrene. *N.Y. State J. Med. 52*:584, 1952.

386. Gaillard, L.: Gangrène humide de pied gauche par thrombose de la veine femorale chez une cancereuse de 27 ans. *Bull. Mém. Soc. Méd. de Hôp. de Paris 11*:315, 1894.

387. Mertens, B. F., et al.: Fibrinolytic split products (FSP) and ethanol gelation test in pre-operative evaluation of patients with prostatic disease. *Mayo Clin. Proc. 49*:642, 1974.

388. Tagnon, H. J., Whitmore, W. F., Jr., and Shulman, N. R.: Fibrinolysis in metastatic cancer of the prostate. *Cancer 5*:9, 1952.

389. Gralnick, H. R., and Tan, H. K.: Acute promyelocytic leukemia: A model for understanding the role of the malignant cell in hemostasis. *Hum. Pathol. 5*:661, 1974.

390. Didisheim, P., et al.: Acute promyelocytic leukemia with fibrinogen and factor V deficiencies. *Blood 23*:717, 1964.

391. Rosenthal, R.: Acute promyelocytic leukemia associated with hypofibrinogenemia. *Blood 21*:495, 1963.

392. Daly, P. A., Schiffer, C. A., and Wiernick, P. H.: Acute promyelocytic leukemia: Clinical management of 15 patients. *Am. J. Hematol. 8*:347, 1980.

393. Kociba, G. J., and Griesemer, R. A.: Disseminated intravascular coagulation induced with leukocyte procoagulant. *Am. J. Pathol. 69*:407, 1972.

394. Gouault-Heilmann, M., et al.: The procoagulant factor of leukaemic promyelocytes: Demonstration of immunologic cross reactivity with human brain tissue factor. *Br. J. Haematol. 30*:151, 1975.

395. Egbring, R., et al.: Demonstration of granulocytic proteases in plasma of patients with acute leukemia and septicemia with coagulation defects. *Blood 49*:219, 1977.

396. Gralnick, H. R., and Abrell, E.: Studies of the procoagulant and fibrinolytic activity of promyelocytes in acute promyelocytic leukaemia. *Br. J. Haematol. 24*:89, 1973.

397. Gingrich, R. D., and Burns, C. P.: Disseminated coagulopathy in chronic myelomonocytic leukemia. *Cancer 44*:2249, 1979.

398. Goodnight, S. H., Jr.: Bleeding and intravascular clotting malignancy: A review. *Ann. N.Y. Acad. Sci. 230*:271, 1974.

399. Baker, W. G., et al.: Hypofibrinogenemic hemorrhage in acute myelogenous leukemia treated with heparin with autopsy findings of widespread intravascular clotting. *Ann. Intern. Med. 61*:116, 1964.

400. Guarini, A., et al.: Defibrination in adult acute lymphoblastic leukaemia: Report of four cases. *Nouv. Rev. Fr. Hematol. 22*:115, 1980.

401. McKee, L. C., Jr., and Collins, R. D.: Intravascular leukocyte thrombi and aggregates as a cause of morbidity and mortality in leukemia. *Medicine 53*:463, 1974.

402. Gralnick, H. R., Bagley, J., and Abrell, E.: Heparin treatment for the hemorrhagic diathesis of acute promyelocytic leukemia. *Am. J. Med. 52*:167, 1972.

403. Drapkin, R. L., et al.: Prophylactic heparin therapy in acute promyelocytic leukemia. *Cancer 41*:2484, 1978.

404. Collins, A. J., et al.: Acute promyelocytic leukemia: Management of the coagulopathy during daunorubicin-prednisone remission induction. *Arch. Intern. Med. 138*:1677, 1978.

405. Lechner, K., Nissner, H., and Thaler, E.: Coagulation abnormalities in liver disease. *Semin. Thromb. Hemostas. 4*:40, 1977.

406. Penny, R., Rozenberg, M. C., and Firkin, B. G.: The splenic platelet pool. *Blood 27*:1, 1966.

407. Aster, R.: Pooling of platelets in the spleen: Role in the pathogenesis of hypersplenic thrombocytopenia. *J. Clin. Invest. 45*:645, 1966.

408. Rapaport, S. I., et al.: Plasma clotting factors in chronic hepatocellular disease. *N. Engl. J. Med. 263*:278, 1960.

409. Braunstein, K. M., and Eurenius, K.: Minimal heparin cofactor activity in disseminated intravascular coagulation and cirrhosis. *Am. J. Clin. Pathol. 66*:488, 1976.

410. Das, P. C., and Cash, J. D.: Fibrinolysis at rest and after exercise in hepatic cirrhosis. *Br. J. Haematol. 17*:431, 1969.

411. Oka, K., and Tanaka, K.: Local fibrinolysis of esophagus and stomach as a cause of hemorrhage in liver cirrhosis. *Thromb. Res. 14*:837, 1979.

412. Zetterqvist, E., and vonFrancken, I.: Coagulation disturbances with manifest bleeding in extrahepatic portal hypertension and in liver cirrhosis. *Acta Med. Scand. 173*:753, 1963.

413. Tytgat, G., et al.: Experience with exchange transfusion in the treatment of hepatic coma. *Digestion 1*:257, 1968.

414. Blombäck, B., et al.: Turnover of ^{131}I-labelled fibrinogen in man: Studies in normal subjects, in congenital coagulation factor deficiency states, in liver cirrhosis, in polycythemia vera, and in epidermolysis bullosa. *Acta Med. Scand. 179*:557, 1966.

415. Tytgat, G. N., Collen, D., and Verstraete, M.: Metabolism of fibrinogen in cirrhosis of the liver. *J. Clin. Invest. 50*:1690, 1971.

416. Coleman, M., et al.: Fibrinogen survival in cirrhosis: Improvement by "low dose" heparin. *Ann. Intern. Med. 83*:79, 1975.

417. Oka, K., and Tanaka, K.: Intravascular coagulation in autopsy cases with liver diseases. *Thromb. Haemost. 42*:564, 1979.

418. Straub, P. W.: Diffuse intravascular coagulation in liver disease *Semin. Thromb. Hemostas. 4*:29, 1977.

419. Rüegg, R., and Straub, P. W.: Exchange between intravascularly and extravascularly injected radioiodinated fibrinogen and its in vivo derivatives. *J. Lab. Clin. Med. 95*:842, 1980.

420. Palascak, J. E., and Martinez, J.: Dysfibrinogenemia associated with liver disease. *J. Clin. Invest. 60*:89, 1977.

421. Rake, M. O., et al.: Early intensive therapy of intravascular coagulation in acute liver failure. *Lancet 2*:1215, 1971.

422. Hillenbrand, P., et al.: Significance of intravascular coagulation and fibrinolysis in acute hepatic failure. *Gut 15*:83, 1974.

423. Gazzard, B. G., et al.: A controlled trial of heparin therapy in the coagulation defect of paracetamol-induced hepatic necrosis. *Gut 15*:89, 1974.

424. Hathaway, W. E., Mull, M. M., and Pechet, G. S.: Disseminated intravascular coagulation in the newborn. *Pediatrics 43*:233, 1969.

425. Groniowski, J.: Thrombotic arteriolar lesions in lungs of newborn. *Arch. Pathol. 75*:144, 1963.

426. Boyd, J. F.: Disseminated fibrin thromboembolism among neonates dying within 48 hours of birth. *Arch. Dis. Child. 42*:401, 1967.

427. Roberts, J. T., Davies, A. J., and Bloom, A. L.: Coagulation studies in massive pulmonary haemorrhage of the newborn. *J. Clin. Pathol. 19*:334, 1966.

428. Leissring, J. C., and Vorlicky, L. N.: Disseminated intravascular coagulation in a neonate. *Am. J. Dis. Child. 115*:100, 1968.

429. Edson, J. R., Blaese, R. M., White, J. G., and Krivit, W.: Defibrination syndrome in an infant born after abruptio placentae. *J. Pediatr. 72*:342, 1968.

430. Manios, S. G., Kanakondi, F., and Miliaras-Vlachakis, M.: Gangrene of lower extremities of a newborn infant associated with intravascular coagulation (recession of gangrene after heparin therapy). *Helv. Paediatr. Acta 27*:193, 1972.

431. Moore, C. M., McAdams, A. J., and Sutherland, J.: Intrauterine disseminated intravascular coagulation: A syndrome of multiple pregnancy with a dead twin fetus. *J. Pediatr. 74*:523, 1969.

432. McGovern, J. P., and Dawson, J. P.: Purpura fulminans: Report of a case coincident with varicella. *Clin. Proc. Children's Hosp. (Wash.) 10*:114, 1954.

433. McKay, G. F., Pisciotta, A. V., and Johnson, S. A.: Hemostatic mechanisms, antithrombin III and purpura fulminans. *Am. J. Clin. Pathol. 38*:357, 1962.

434. Smith, H.: Purpura fulminans complicating varicella: Recovery with low molecular weight dextran and steroids. *Med. J. Aust. 2*:685, 1967.

435. Lo, S. S., Hitzig, W. H., and Frick, P. G.: Clinical experience with

anticoagulant therapy in the management of diffuse intravascular coagulation in children. *Acta Haematol. 45*:1, 1971.

436. De Koning, J., Frederiks, E., and Kerkhoven, P.: Purpura fulminans following varicella: Report of a case with recovery after heparin therapy. *Helv. Paediatr. Acta 27*:127, 1972.

437. Naveh, Y., Tatarsky, I., and Friedman, A.: Disseminated intravascular coagulation complicating chickenpox. *Helv. Paediatr. Acta 27*:193, 1972.

438. Fainaru, M., et al.: The natural course of defibrination syndrome caused by *Echis colorata* venom in man. *Thromb. Diath. Haemorrh. 31*:420, 1974.

439. Warrell, D. A., Pope, H. M., and Prentice, C. R. M.: Disseminated intravascular coagulation caused by the carpet viper *(Echis carinatus)*: Trial of heparin. *Br. J. Haematol. 33*:335, 1976.

440. Reid, H. A.: ∊-Aminocaproic acid and fibrinolysis in viper-bite defibrination. *Lancet 1*:5, 1965.

441. Reid, H. A., Chan, K. E., and Thean, P. C.: Prolonged coagulation defect (defibrination syndrome) in Malayan viper bite. *Lancet 1*:621, 1963.

442. Weiss, H. J., et al.: Heparin therapy in a patient bitten by a saw-scaled viper *(Echis carinatus)*, a snake whose venom activates prothrombin. *Am. J. Med. 54*:653, 1973.

443. Hasiba, U., et al.: DIC-like syndrome after envenomation by the snake *Crotalus horridus horridus*. *N. Engl. J. Med. 292*:505, 1975.

444. Schmaier, A. H., Claypool, W., and Colman, R. W.: Crotalocytin: Recognition and purification of a timber rattlesnake platelet aggregating protein. *Blood 56*:1013, 1980.

445. Sharp, A. A., et al.: Anticoagulant therapy with a purified fraction of Malayan pit viper venom. *Lancet 1*:493, 1968.

446. Reid, H. A.: Therapeutic defibrination by Ancrod (Arvin). *Folia Haematol. (Leipz.) 95*:209, 1971.

447. Davies, J. A., et al.: Controlled trial of Ancrod and heparin in treatment of deep-vein thrombosis of lower limb. *Lancet 1*:113, 1972.

448. Bell, W. R., Pitney, W. R., and Goodwin, J. F.: Therapeutic defibrination in the treatment of thrombotic disease. *Lancet 1*:490, 1968.

449. Kakkar, V. V., et al.: Treatment of deep vein thrombosis: A trial of heparin streptokinase and arvin. *Br. Med. J. 1*:806, 1969.

450. Latallo, Z. S., and Lopaciuk, S.: New approach to thrombolytic therapy: The use of defibrase in connection with streptokinase. *Thromb. Diath. Haemorrh. (Suppl.) 56*:253, 1973.

451. Forbes, C. D., Barbenell, J., and Prentice, C. R. M.: Treatment of thrombosis by sequential therapy with Ancrod followed by streptokinase: Clinical pharmacology and rheology. *Haemostasis 5*:348, 1976.

452. Friesen, S. R., Harsha, W. N., and McCroskey, C. H.: Massive generalized wound bleeding during operation with clinical and experimental evidence of blood transfusion reactions. *Surgery 32*:620, 1952.

453. Hardaway, R. M., McKay, D., and Williams, J. H.: Lower nephron nephrosis (ischemuric nephrosis): With special reference to hemorrhagic diathesis following incompatible blood transfusion reaction. *Am. J. Surg. 87*:41, 1954.

454. Krevans, J. R., et al.: The nature of the hemorrhagic disorder accompanying hemolytic transfusion reactions in man. *Blood 12*:834, 1957.

455. Crosby, W. H., and Stefanini, M.: Pathogenesis of the plasma transfusion reaction with especial reference to the blood coagulation system. *J. Lab. Clin. Med. 40*:374, 1952.

456. White, G. C., II, Lundblad, R. L., and Kingdon, H. S.: Prothrombin complex concentrates: Preparation, properties, and clinical uses. *Curr. Top. Hematol. 2*:203, 1979.

457. Blatt, P. M., et al.: Treatment of anti-factor VIII antibodies. *Thromb. Haemost. 38*:514, 1977.

458. Lusher, J. M., et al.: Efficacy of prothrombin-complex concentrates in hemophiliacs with antibodies to factor VIII. *N. Engl. J. Med. 303*:421, 1980.

459. Kingdon, H. S., et al.: Potentially thrombogenic materials in factor IX concentrates. *Thromb. Diath. Haemorrh. 33*:617, 1975.

460. Pepper, D. S., et al.: In vitro thrombogenicity tests of factor IX concentrates. *Br. J. Haematol. 36*:573, 1977.

461. Hultin, M. B.: Activated clotting factors in factor IX concentrates. *Blood 54*:1028, 1979.

462. Blatt, P. M., et al.: Thrombogenic materials in prothrombin complex concentrates. *Ann. Intern. Med. 81*:766, 1974.

463. White, G. C., II, et al.: Prothrombin complex concentrates: Potentially thrombogenic materials and clues to the mechanism of thrombosis in vivo. *Blood 49*:159, 1977.

464. Vermylen, J., et al.: Evidence that "activated" prothrombin concentrates enhance platelet coagulant activity. *Br. J. Haematol. 38*:235, 1978.

465. White, P. W., Sadd, J. R., and Nensel, R. E.: Thrombotic complications of heparin therapy: Including six cases of heparin-induced skin necrosis. *Ann. Surg. 190*:595, 1979.

466. Godal, H. C.: Report of the International Committee on Thrombosis and Haemostasis: Thrombocytopenia and heparin. *Thromb. Haemost. 43*:222, 1980.

467. Malcolm, I. D., and Wigmore, T. A.: Thrombocytopenia induced by low-dose subcutaneous heparin. *Lancet 1*:444, 1978.

468. Bell, W. R., et al.: Thrombocytopenia during the administration of heparin: A prospective study in 52 patients. *Ann. Intern. Med. 85*:155, 1976.

469. Ansell, J., et al.: Heparin induced thrombocytopenia: A prospective study. *Thromb. Haemost. 43*:61, 1980.

470. Rhodes, G. R., Dixon, R. H., and Silver, D.: Heparin-induced thrombocytopenia with thrombotic and hemorrhagic manifestations. *Surg. Gynecol. Obstet. 136*:409, 1973.

471. Cines, D. B., et al.: Heparin-associated thrombocytopenia. *N. Engl. J. Med. 303*:788, 1980.

472. Alving, B. M., et al.: In vitro studies of heparin-associated thrombocytopenia. *Thromb. Res. 11*:827, 1977.

473. Bone, R. C., Francis, P. B., and Pierce, A. K.: Intravascular coagulation associated with the adult respiratory distress syndrome. *Am. J. Med. 61*:585, 1976.

474. Innerfield, I., and Angrist, A.: Intravenous trypsin: Its anticoagulant fibrinolytic and thrombolytic effects. *J. Clin. Invest. 31*:1049, 1952.

475. Greipp, P. R., Brown, J. A., and Gralnick, H. R.: Defibrination in acute pancreatitis. *Ann. Intern. Med. 76*:73, 1972.

476. Bick, R. L., Fekete, L. F., and Wilson, W. L.: Adriamycin and fibrinolysis. *Thromb. Res. 8*:467, 1976.

477. McGehee, W. G., and Rapaport, S. I.: Systemic hemostatic failure in the severely injured patient. *Surg. Clin. North Am. 48*:1247, 1968.

478. String, T., Robinson, A. J., and Blaisdell, F. W.: Massive trauma: Effect of intravascular coagulation on prognosis. *Arch. Surg. 102*:406, 1971.

479. Innes, D., and Sevitt, S.: Coagulation and fibrinolysis in injured patients. *J. Clin. Pathol. 17*:1, 1964.

480. Simmons, R. L., Collins, J. A., Heisterkamp, C. A., III, Mills, D. E., Andren, R., and Phillips, L. L.: Coagulation disorders in combat casualties. I. Acute changes after wounding. II. Effects of massive transfusion. III. Post-resuscitative changes. *Ann. Surg. 169*:445, 1969.

481. Druskin, M. S., and Drijansky, R.: Afibrinogenemia with severe head trauma. *JAMA 219*:755, 1972.

482. Keimowitz, R. M., and Annis, B. L.: Disseminated intravascular coagulation associated with massive brain injury. *J. Neurosurg. 39*:178, 1973.

483. Drayer, B. P., and Poser, C. M.: Disseminated intravascular coagulation and head trauma: Two case studies. *JAMA 231*:174, 1975.

484. McGauley, J. L., Miller, C. A., and Penner, J. A.: Diagnosis and treatment of diffuse intravascular coagulation following cerebral trauma: Case report. *J. Neurosurg. 43*:374, 1975.

485. Vecht, C. J., Smith-Sibinga, C. T., and Minderhoud, J. M.: Disseminated intravascular coagulation and head injury. *J. Neurol. Neurosurg. Psychiatry 38*:567, 1975.

486. Harmon, D. C., Demirjian, Z., Ellman, L., and Fischer, J. E.: Disseminated intravascular coagulation with the peritoneovenous shunt. *Ann. Intern. Med. 90*:774, 1979.

CHAPTER *159*

Clinical aspects of fibrinolysis

VICTOR J. MARDER
CHARLES W. FRANCIS

Homeostasis of the fibrinolytic system

BALANCE OF OPPOSITE FORCES

Physiologic fibrinolysis is a finely tuned response which leads to the dissolution of hemostatic plugs and thrombi (see Chap. 138). After clot formation, plasminogen activator is released from adjacent endothelial cells by stimuli that may include mechanical injury and thrombin action [1]. Plasminogen and antiplasmin are bound to fibrin [2,3] during clot formation and a balanced process of fibrinolysis is governed by the proportion of these components [4]. During progressive thrombolysis, a systemic fibrinogenolytic state is prevented by the inactivation of free plasmin by antiplasmin in the blood [5]. The process of fibrinolysis, phago-

cytosis, revascularization, and establishment of an intact endothelial lining is completed in about 10 days.

Disruption of the balance or location of fibrinolysis can lead to bleeding, if the balance is shifted toward fibrinolysis, or to thrombosis, if the shift is toward inhibition of lysis. Figure 159-1 shows the complex interaction of fibrinolysis and inhibition, and how disease or pharmacologic intervention can either correct or induce symptoms of bleeding or thrombosis. Bleeding which is caused by an excessive fibrinolytic stimulus can be corrected by administration of a fibrinolytic inhibitor. However, if the patient is predisposed to venous thrombosis or disseminated intravascular coagulation, clinical thrombosis could occur [6]. On the other hand, venous thrombosis may be treated with a fibrinolytic agent. In this case uncomplicated thrombolysis may follow, but bleeding complications may occur in susceptible individuals. Thus, therapy may induce a clinical condition opposite that which existed before treatment.

HYPERFIBRINOLYTIC BLEEDING AND HYPOFIBRINOLYTIC THROMBOSIS

The same clinical manifestation may result from either an excess of fibrinolytic or antifibrinolytic stimuli or a deficiency of opposing stimulus [Table 159-1]. Several hereditary disorders of specific plasma proteins result in hyperfibrinolytic bleeding or hypofibrinolytic throm-

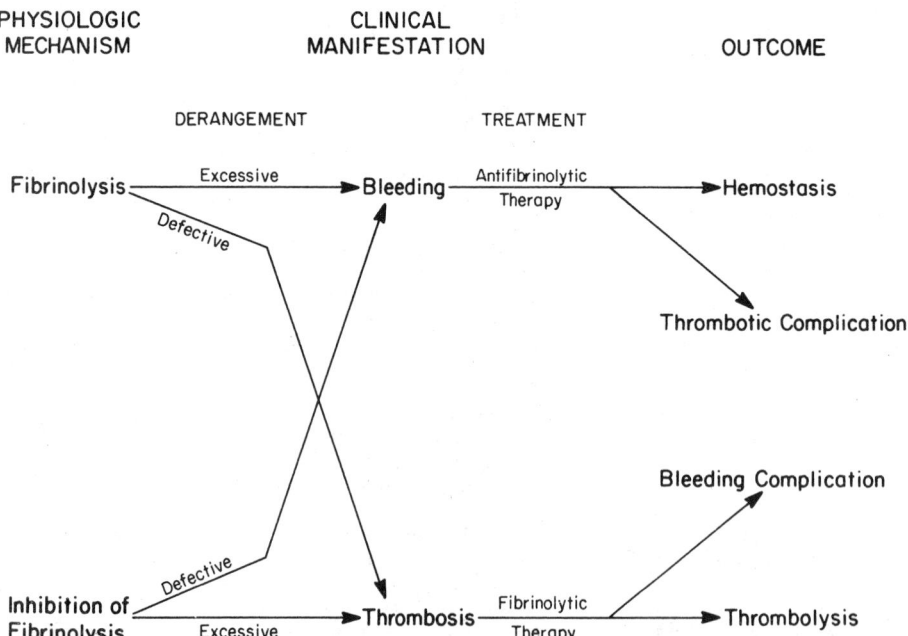

FIGURE 159-1 Disruption of the balance of opposing homeostatic forces of fibrinolysis and antifibrinolysis leading to bleeding or thrombotic manifestations. Therapy with the appropriate pharmacologic agent may correct the clinical disorder, but fibrinolytic therapy may complicate a thrombotic state with a bleeding state and the opposite effect could be produced with antifibrinolytic therapy. Successful therapy, that is, restoration of effective hemostasis or achievement of thrombolysis without complication, depends more on correct selection of the patient to be treated than on variables in dosage.

1462

TABLE 159-1   Pathologic aberrations of the fibrinolytic-antifibrinolytic balance which may cause thrombosis or bleeding

Imbalance	Pathologic cause	Selected clinical disorders
	THROMBOSIS	
Defective fibrinolysis	Inadequate release of vascular plasminogen activator	Endothelial cell defect or injury
	Molecular defect of plasma protein	Hereditary defect or deficiency of plasminogen, fibrinogen, or protein C
Excessive inhibition of fibrinolysis	Iatrogenic	Administration of anti-fibrinolytic agent
	BLEEDING	
Excessive activation of fibrinolysis	Excessive circulating vascular plasminogen activator	Primary hyperfibrinolysis
	Iatrogenic	Administration of exogenous activator
	Defective clearance of activator	Hepatic cirrhosis
	Localized excess activator	Menorrhagia, post-prostatectomy
Defective inhibition of fibrinolysis	Molecular defect of plasma protein	Hereditary deficiency of antiplasmin

bosis. Thus, deficiency of antiplasmin results in unbridled fibrinolysis [7], producing a life-long predisposition to hemorrhage which can be effectively counteracted by chronic administration of synthetic fibrinolytic inhibitors, such as ϵ-aminocaproic acid (EACA) [8]. Inheritance of a form of plasminogen [9,10] which is not converted properly to plasmin by plasminogen activator results in a predisposition to deep-vein thrombosis and pulmonary embolism similar to that of antithrombin III deficiency [11,12]. Patients with abnormal plasminogens may not respond to therapy with fibrinolytic activators since the molecule could resist activation by exogenous as well as endogenous activators.

Two other plasma protein abnormalities may lead to thrombosis. An abnormal fibrinogen with relatively greater reactivity to thrombin than to plasmin [13,14] could predispose to thrombosis. Likewise, a deficiency of protein C [15] (see Chap. 136) may limit the release of plasminogen activator from endothelial cells in response to evolving thrombi [16]. These molecular disorders predispose to thromboembolic disease, although an increase in potential for disseminated intravascular coagulation (DIC) in response to known stimuli (see Chap. 158) would also be theoretically possible.

Bleeding or thrombosis may occur as a complication of therapy with drugs that affect the fibrinolytic system, just as anticoagulant therapy with heparin may result in hemorrhagic complications and infusions of concentrated coagulation factors in patients with deficiency states may result in an excessive procoagulant tendency and laboratory or clinical manifestations of DIC [17,18].

A number of vasoactive hormonal or pharmacologic stimuli may mediate an exaggerated release of endothelial cell fibrinolysis activator [19], leading to a primary fibrinolytic disorder (see Chap. 158), which is a hemorrhagic state that may be acute or chronic, mild or severe. Familial venous thrombosis or thrombosis associated with sepsis or immune complex disorders may be due to defective release of vascular plasminogen activator in response to thrombin [20]. On the other hand, hyperfibrinolytic hemorrhage may be the result of defective clearance of activated plasminogen activator, just as DIC could be precipitated by excessive circulating activated clotting factors. Both could be the result of altered tissue macrophage clearance mechanisms in hepatic cirrhosis.

The site of the hyperfibrinolytic process also influences the type of hemorrhage. For example, excessive circulating fibrinolytic activity due to antiplasmin deficiency [7] presents a threat of bleeding at any injured site, but excessive localized fibrinolytic activity leads to bleeding that is limited to a local site, as, for example, in menorrhagia [21]. Even a physiologic degree of fibrinolysis may contribute to bleeding if there is an accompanying alteration in the hemostatic system, for example, hemophilia or thrombocytopenia.

THERAPEUTIC INTERVENTION

Decisions regarding the use of therapeutic agents which promote or impair fibrinolysis require an understanding of the pathogenesis and natural history of the disorder, of the mode of action of the drug, and of the risks and causes of complications. All of the parameters affecting fibrinolysis must be considered. Thus, a systemic fibrinogenolytic reaction may occur without obvious underlying cause in association with specific disorders of excess production (e.g., malignancy) or decreased clearance (e.g., hepatic cirrhosis) of plasminogen activators. The duration of symptoms may range

TABLE 159-2   Selected characteristics of principal fibrinolytic and antifibrinolytic agents available for use in the United States

	Streptokinase	Urokinase	EACA
Source	Bacterial (streptococcal culture)	Human: urine or kidney cell culture	Synthesized
Desired effect	Accelerate thrombolysis	Accelerate thrombolysis	Inhibit fibrinolysis
Mechanism	Streptokinase-plasminogen complex activates plasminogen	Directly activates plasminogen	Blocks binding of plasmin(ogen) to fibrin(ogen)
Major complication(s)	Bleeding, allergy	Bleeding	Exaggerates existing DIC
Dose	250,000 U IV loading 100,000 U/h IV maintenance Variable duration	4000 U/kg IV loading 4000 U/(kg·h) IV maintenance Variable duration	0.1 g/kg IV or PO loading 0.5–1.0 g/h IV or PO maintenance Variable duration
Laboratory monitoring test	Thrombin time, euglobulin lysis time, fibrinogen level	As with streptokinase	Lysis time or empiric
Available as	Streptase (Hoechst) Kabikinase (KABI/Pharmacia)	Abbokinase (Abbott) Breokinase (Breon)	Amicar (Lederle)

from life-long, as in congenital antiplasmin deficiency [8], to short-lived, as in bleeding due to heat stroke [22].

The basic mechanisms of action of fibrinolytic agents are quite distinct in the plasminogen-to-plasmin cascade which leads to fibrin or fibrinogen degradation (see Chap. 138). Vascular plasminogen activator or the exogenous activators urokinase and streptokinase act primarily to convert the proenzyme plasminogen to the proteolytic enzyme plasmin. The binding of plasminogen to fibrin at its lysine binding sites promotes such activation and protects the plasmin from inhibition by the plasma protein inhibitor, antiplasmin [5,23]. The synthetic analogs of lysine, especially EACA, prevent the binding of plasminogen or plasmin to fibrin or fibrinogen by occupying these lysine binding sites [23–25]. Thus, although the formation of active enzyme

TABLE 159-3   Contraindications to antifibrinolytic and fibrinolytic therapy

Risk	Underlying condition
ANTIFIBRINOLYTIC THERAPY	
DIC or venous thrombosis	Malignancy, especially mucinous visceral adeno-carcinoma
Upper genitourinary bleeding	Hemoglobinopathy, hemophilia
FIBRINOLYTIC THERAPY	
Intracranial hemorrhage	Cerebrovascular accident Neoplasm Injury or surgery (10 days)
Massive localized bleeding	Major thoracic or abdominal surgery or trauma (10 days) Ongoing severe GI bleeding
Generalized bleeding	Severe thrombocytopenia or other hemorrhagic diathesis

may not be prevented and may actually be enhanced [26,27], EACA prevents the alignment of substrate necessary to produce fibrinolysis or fibrinogenolysis.

Antifibrinolytic therapy

PHARMACOLOGY AND COMPLICATIONS

EACA is absorbed rapidly after oral administration (Table 159-2) and is rapidly excreted by the kidneys [28]. It inhibits both fibrin and fibrinogen degradation and may lead indirectly to excessive intravascular thrombosis by unmasking an ongoing DIC process [6,29–32] (Table 159-3). A second complication is the development of clots in the renal pelvis or ureters of patients with upper genitourinary tract bleeding. EACA does not actually cause such clots to form, but rather prevents their dissolution by fibrinolysis mediated by urokinase [33,34]. The patient with upper urinary tract bleeding should be considered for treatment with antifibrinolytic agents only if the symptoms are longstanding, require replacement transfusion, or are being considered for surgical repair. The use of EACA should also be avoided in patients with malignancy, especially of the mucinous adenocarcinoma variety that has been associated with thrombosis [35].

MONITORING OF THERAPY

Laboratory monitoring of antifibrinolytic therapy usually does not require tests. Should a clear-cut plasma hyperfibrinolytic state be the indication for therapy, the shortened euglobulin lysis time, the decrease in plasma fibrinogen concentration, or the increase in fibrinogen degradation product levels can be followed. However, the effect of treatment is best assessed from estimates of the response of the abnormal bleeding, especially since some patients treated with antifibrinolytic agents have normal tests for blood coagulation or fibrinolysis prior to therapy.

CLINICAL FEATURES

The clinical states in which antifibrinolytic therapy has been assessed are considered in Table 159-4 according to pathogenetic mechanism.

SYSTEMIC HYPERFIBRINOLYSIS

Activation of plasma fibrinolysis can occur in acute states, such as heat stroke [22], hypoxia, hypotension, thoracic surgery, or administration of thrombolytic agents, and in chronic states, such as neoplasm or hepatic cirrhosis (see Chap. 158). The hemorrhagic state is accompanied by a shortened euglobulin lysis time, decreased plasma levels of plasminogen and fibrinogen, and elevated levels of fibrinogen degradation products. A short euglobulin lysis time may also be due to DIC, and antifibrinolytic therapy may unmask or accentuate that disorder. Distinguishing systemic hyperfibrinolysis from DIC and other consumption coagulopathies can be difficult. The principal feature of isolated systemic hyperfibrinogenolysis is a hemorrhagic state without thrombotic organ damage, which may disappear spontaneously (e.g., hypotension), persist for months (e.g., neoplasm), or remain as a lifelong state (α_2-antiplasmin deficiency). The unusual congenital absence or reduced levels of α_2-antiplasmin cause a bleeding tendency which can be effectively controlled by therapy with fibrinolytic inhibitors [8,36,37]. Correlation of a shortened euglobulin lysis time with serious bleeding after open heart surgery [38,39] suggests that neutralization of this trauma-associated, systemic hyperfibrinolytic state could be beneficial. A systemic hyperfibrinolytic state is more likely to occur with prolonged procedures and in patients with cyanotic heart disease. One must rule out the possibility of coexisting DIC before instituting therapy with antifibrinolytic agents.

LOCALIZED FIBRINOLYSIS WITH DEFECTIVE CLOT FORMATION

An equilibrium between clot formation and clot dissolution takes place primarily within the smaller vessels serving an injured area, and a hemostatic deficiency of any type may limit the patient's capacity to retain hemostatic plugs until healing has occurred. Replacement therapy is effective in providing normal hemostasis following surgical procedures in patients with hemophilia. Hemarthrosis in patients with hemophilia is easily controlled with small doses of factor VIII, and

TABLE 159-4   Antifibrinolytic therapy with EACA in bleeding states

Pathologic process	Clinical state	Experience	Comment
Systemic hyperfibrinolysis	Spontaneous or iatrogenic	Often self-limited; treatment seldom required	Rule out DIC first
	Extracorporeal bypass surgery	Bleeding reduced, especially with cyanotic heart disease and prolonged pump time	Intrapleural or intrapericardial clots resistant to lysis
	Congenital antiplasmin deficiency	Lifelong bleeding state, controlled with inhibitors	Rare autosomal recessive trait
Excessive localized fibrinolysis	Uterine: spontaneous, intrauterine device, postconization of cervix	Uniformly effective therapy	Evaluate for underlying pathology
	Brain: subarachnoid hemorrhage	Uncertain benefit	No excess risk of thrombosis
	Lower GI tract: ulcerative colitis	Not for routine use	Possible use in unresponsive cases
	Upper GI tract: erosive gastritis, ulcer, varices	Useful adjunctive measure	Carefully evaluate underlying lesion
Normal localized fibrinolysis with defective clot formation	Hemophilia: postsurgical	Proven use for dental extractions, reduces need for factor VIII infusions; not effective as prophylaxis	Reasonable for other surgical procedures
Normal localized fibrinosis with normal clot formation	Lower genitourinary: postprostatectomy	Reduced blood loss, especially in early postoperative period	Indicated primarily in patients with demonstrated excessive bleeding
	Upper genitourinary: spontaneous	Effective in hemophilia and hemoglobinopathies, *but...*	Significant risk of resistant clots in renal collecting system
	Postrenal biopsy	Effective, *but...*	Risk of clots as above; use primarily as alternative to surgery

SOURCE: Modified from Marder, Butler, and Barlow [25], with permission of the publisher.

the addition of EACA has not influenced the frequency or severity of the recurrent bleeding episodes [40,41]. However, antifibrinolytic therapy is highly effective in hemophilic patients who undergo dental extraction, reducing the necessity for factor VIII or IX administration by as much as 80 percent [42,43].

LOCALIZED FIBRINOLYSIS WITH NORMAL CLOT FORMATION

In normal individuals, bleeding can result from localized hyperfibrinolysis. Presumably, organs with higher levels of fibrinolytic activity, such as the uterus and the renal pelvis, would be most severely affected [44]. Any amount of localized fibrinolysis could exaggerate local bleeding and be favorably influenced by fibrinolytic inhibitors [21,45,46]. Excessive bleeding after prostatectomy is reasonably attributed to the presence of urokinase in the urine, which diffuses into the operative site and dissolves newly formed hemostatic plugs [21,46–50]. Several trials of EACA therapy after prostatectomy have demonstrated a significant decrease in blood loss compared to placebo [51–54]. However, postprostatectomy bleeding is usually more bothersome than dangerous, and antifibrinolytic therapy is better reserved for the occasional patient who bleeds excessively [46]. Lower urinary tract bleeding caused by benign prostatic hyperplasia or adenocarcinoma of the prostate may also be ameliorated by antifibrinolytic treatment [55,56]. Caution is required in treating upper urinary tract bleeding, such as that seen in patients with sickle cell disease [57,58] or hemophilia [59,60] or after renal biopsy [61,62], because bleeding from the renal pelvis may be associated with clot formation in the renal collecting system. This complication occurs frequently to a minor degree, but in a significant number of patients the clot is large enough to threaten renal function [52,59,60]. The obstructing clot in the urinary tract may be recognized by a combination of three factors: the disappearance of hematuria, the development of flank pain, and a nephrogram image on intravenous pyelography without dye excretion into the pelvis. EACA therapy produces the additional risk of preventing or retarding the dissolution of such large clots by urokinase. Patients who undergo renal biopsy may have serious and protracted hematuria. Although these patients are at risk of developing urinary tract obstruction, there are reports of cessation of bleeding following treatment with EACA [61,62], even when an arteriovenous fistula was present [63].

Fibrinolysis contributes to menstrual bleeding, and antifibrinolytic therapy has reduced blood loss in *essential menorrhagia* [64,65] as well as in patients with bleeding secondary to the placement of an intrauterine device [66] or after cervical conization [67]. Although one must attempt to document the etiology in patients with fresh or unexplained menorrhagia or postoperative genital tract bleeding, it is reasonable to attempt to control excessive uterine bleeding from any cause with antifibrinolytic therapy.

About 20 percent of patients develop recurrence of *subarachnoid hemorrhage* prior to surgical correction of the underlying lesion [68,69]. Since plasminogen activator is present in the cerebrospinal fluid after subarachnoid hemorrhage, intracranial hemorrhage, or even thrombotic occlusive disease [70,71] and could contribute to lysis of fragile intraaneurysmal thrombi [21], antifibrinolytic therapy has been attempted in patients with subarachnoid hemorrhage. The data from some clinical trials show favorable results [72–74], others show no effect [75,76], and some show a possible detrimental influence [77]. Precise guidelines for treating certain subgroups of patients with subarachnoid hemorrhage have not been defined.

Certain lesions that cause upper or lower *gastrointestinal bleeding* have been associated with increased fibrinolytic activity. For example, increased amounts of plasminogen activator are demonstrable in the rectal mucosa of patients with active ulcerative colitis [78]. Two uncontrolled studies of antifibrinolytic therapy demonstrate a decrease in bleeding in such patients [55,79], but the data are insufficient to conclude that treatment is effective in these conditions. There is also evidence for local fibrinolysis in patients with peptic ulcer [80], erosive hemorrhagic gastritis [81], and cirrhosis of the liver with gastrointestinal hemorrhage [82], and benefit from antifibrinolytic therapy has been observed in patients with bleeding presumably due to diffuse gastritis [83] or esophageal varices [84].

The data for treatment of conditions such as traumatic hyphema [85,86], epistaxis [87], and bleeding after tonsillectomy and adenoidectomy [88,89] are not conclusive.

Fibrinolytic therapy

PHARMACOLOGY AND COMPLICATIONS

The fibrinolytic agents that are currently utilized in the United States are administered by standard dosage schedules (Table 159-2) which uniformly induce a plasma proteolytic state ("lytic state") [5]. Although the desired effect of therapy is the potentiation of fibrin lysis, concomitant degradation of plasma fibrinogen also occurs as a result of the formation of plasmin in amounts exceeding the inhibitory potential of plasma antiplasmin [5,23]. The major complication of fibrinolytic therapy is bleeding, but there is disagreement regarding its pathogenesis. One explanation is that a hypocoagulable state associated with fibrinogenolysis is responsible and the amount of bleeding is related to the degree of hypofibrinogenemia [90]. The alternate explanation is that the fibrin in hemostatic plugs is dissolved along with the fibrin thrombi [91]. This view is supported by the lack of correlation of any laboratory parameter of the lytic state with the occurrence of bleeding [92–94]. The key to avoiding serious bleeding with fibrinolytic agents is a clinical appraisal, especially evaluation for susceptible, recently formed hemostatic

TABLE 159-5   Development of the plasma lytic state

Biochemical alteration	*Laboratory parameter*
Plasminogen converted to plasmin	Decreased plasminogen levels
Antiplasmin inhibits plasmin, to the limit of its concentration	Formation of plasmin-antiplasmin complexes, decreased antiplasmin levels
Free activator and plasmin present	Short lysis time
Fibrinogen degraded	Decreased clottable protein levels; increased levels of fibrin/fibrinogen degradation products
Hypocoagulable state attained	Prolonged thrombin time

plugs. Contraindications to the use of fibrinolytic agents are listed in Table 159-3. The risk of minor bleeding, especially if superficial, or of bleeding from sites not inherently dangerous and manageable by simple measures or transfusion should not preclude continued therapy. If bleeding requires cessation of therapy, normal hemostasis can be achieved within 1 h by clearance of the activator and by infusion of fibrinogen-rich cryoprecipitate. The incidence of hemorrhagic complications with fibrinolytic therapy is higher than with heparin, approximately 9 and 4 percent, respectively [95], but clearly the high incidence of significant complications can be reduced in either case by avoidance of invasive procedures and management of bleeding sites with appropriate local hemostatic measures.

The duration of fibrinolytic treatment will vary according to the clinical condition. Pulmonary embolism is probably adequately treated with only 12 h of infusion [96]. Treatment of deep-vein thrombosis or arterial thrombosis is usually continued for 3 days or more [97–101], but thrombolysis may be accomplished after only 12 h of therapy [97]. From one point of view, fibrinolytic therapy is simply an adjunct to heparin therapy and is initiated approximately 1 h after heparin therapy is discontinued. Similarly, heparin therapy is restarted about 1 h after fibrinolytic therapy is completed. Warfarin is administered for continued prophylactic anticoagulation treatment according to the judgment of the physician.

MONITORING OF THERAPY

There is disagreement regarding the relationship between laboratory abnormalities and the incidence of bleeding in fibrinolytic therapy. In one view, bleeding complications are primarily the result of hemostatic plug dissolution and not of alterations in plasma coagulation proteins [93,97]. For example, plasma plasminogen falls to significantly lower levels after streptokinase treatment than after urokinase treatment but hemorrhagic complications and clinical benefit are equal in both groups [94]. Some patients may have excessive concentrations of antistreptokinase antibodies, or of other inhibitors to fibrinolysis, and monitoring (1) the level of plasma plasminogen, fibrinogen, or fibrinogen degradation products, (2) the thrombin time, or (3) the euglobulin lysis time is useful in determining whether an effective dose of the drug has been

administered. Any degree of derangement of laboratory tests is evidence that a lytic state has been established. However, once a lytic state has been attained (Table 159-5), there is little need to regulate the dose of plasminogen activator during the remainder of the therapeutic infusion, since changes in the laboratory values do not improve the chance of thrombolysis or decrease the risk of hemorrhagic complication [92,93,102].

NEW FIBRINOLYTIC AGENTS

New approaches to plasminogen activator treatment include local rather than systemic infusions, fibrin-specific plasminogen activators, and genetic engineering for more efficient production of fibrinolytic agents. Local installation of plasminogen activators has been suggested for use in pulmonary embolism [103], peripheral arterial occlusion [104], and coronary artery thrombosis [105]. The theoretical basis for this approach is to limit proteolysis to the thrombus itself, thereby avoiding a systemic lytic state and decreasing the risk of hemorrhagic complications. However, even very low doses of streptokinase [104] may result in shortening of euglobulin lysis time, and intracoronary perfusion with fibrinolytic agents may produce hypofibrinogenemia and distant bleeding [106], suggesting that a systemic lytic state is induced. In the case of pulmonary embolism, a systemic lytic state may be desired since it allows for lysis of the source of the embolus as well as of the embolus itself.

Fibrin-specific plasminogen activators represent a biochemical rather than anatomic approach to limiting the fibrinolytic action of the administered agent. Two classes of agent have been prepared: a tissue plasminogen activator from a melanoma cell line [107] and a chemically modified (acylated) streptokinase-plasminogen complex [108]. Both bind preferentially to fibrin rather than to fibrinogen; this is most striking with the tissue plasminogen activator [109,110]. Both agents are effective in dissolving thrombi in animal models [110,111]. They induce less degradation of fibrinogen than urokinase or streptokinase, thereby potentially simplifying therapy. However, the incidence of hemorrhagic complications with the newer drugs is unknown, although bleeding was not a problem in the two patients treated to date with tissue plasminogen activator [112].

Genetic engineering techniques are being applied to

TABLE 159-6   Fibrinolytic therapy with streptokinase or urokinase in thrombotic disorders

Disorder	Experience	Comment
Deep-vein thrombosis	More lysis at 3 to 5 days; fewer patients with postthrombotic symptoms on long-term follow-up	Prompt therapy (7 days after symptoms) yields best response; optimal duration of treatment not established
Pulmonary embolism	More rapid resolution by 24 h; long-term normalization of pulmonary capillary blood volume	Best results with symptoms of less than 48 h, especially in patients with massive PE and shock
Peripheral arterial occlusion	Excellent response in 15%, especially if embolic	Useful if surgery contraindicated or technically not feasible; mural thrombus source could result in further embolic phenomena
Coronary artery thrombosis	Lower mortality in medium-to-high-risk group with systemic administration	Possible advantage of regional perfusion into coronary arteries

studies of synthesis of both tissue plasminogen activator and urokinase, but materials have not yet been produced in sufficient quantity to be tested in clinical trials.

CLINICAL FEATURES

With the exception of patients with a molecular defect of plasminogen [9,10], which theoretically could preclude effective fibrinolysis with activators, all patients with thrombotic occlusion of veins or arteries are potential candidates for fibrinolytic therapy in addition to heparin anticoagulation. Table 159-6 summarizes the clinical status of fibrinolytic therapy.

DEEP-VEIN THROMBOSIS

Most studies of deep-vein thrombosis have utilized 3- to 5-day courses of streptokinase and recorded the effects of treatment soon after the initial course of therapy. The effects of streptokinase therapy have been studied in 297 patients in nine randomized trials that used pretreatment and posttreatment venography as the primary criterion for success [93,97,113–120]. Of those treated with streptokinase, 45 percent showed substantial improvement in the venographic appearance of deep veins after 5 days of treatment. Only 5 percent of heparin- or ancrod-treated patients showed a similar degree of improvement. Although clinical improvement usually paralleled substantial venographic improvement, symptoms such as swelling and discomfort often abated despite persistence of the underlying venous thrombosis. Therapy of venous thrombosis within 5 to 7 days of the onset of symptoms was more likely to result in significant thrombolysis than was treatment of patients with more long-standing symptoms. However, some patients with long-term complaints have responded favorably to fibrinolytic treatment [90]. Thrombi in the popliteal and ileofemoral veins were as likely to dissolve as those in the deep veins of the calf. Except in one study [121], the gender

of the patient did not influence the chance for successful thrombolysis. Patients with pelvic or abdominal carcinoma obstructing venous return from the legs responded to therapy as well as patients without obstructive neoplasms [93].

Most studies had regimens of 3 days or longer, but isolated examples of complete lysis of extensive venous thrombosis have been observed after treatment intervals of only 12 h [97]. Longer intervals of treatment should be avoided if possible since the risk of bleeding continues throughout the course of therapy.

Long-term improvement in venographic appearance after fibrinolytic therapy has been reported in five randomized studies [117,119,120,122–124]. Of the 121 patients, normal venograms were noted in 60 percent of those treated with streptokinase, but in only 11 percent of those treated with anticoagulants alone. Almost all patients (89 percent) treated with anticoagulants had postthrombotic venographic changes or clinical symptoms 3 to 18 months after initial therapy, compared with 45 percent of patients treated with streptokinase [97]. Although one study [125] showed no apparent benefit with fibrinolytic therapy, several studies have demonstrated that fibrinolytic therapy reduced the incidence of postphlebitic symptoms from over 90 percent to less than 10 percent [97].

PULMONARY EMBOLISM

The goal of fibrinolytic therapy in pulmonary embolism is rapid improvement in lung function rather than reduction in mortality, since the latter is highest during the first 10 min [126], often before effective anticoagulant or fibrinolytic therapy can be instituted. In 15 studies, urokinase and streptokinase were evaluated using doses sufficient to activate the blood fibrinolytic system when administered as continuous infusions for intervals of 5 to 72 h. Early studies [127–132] suggested that improved dissolution of pulmonary emboli was possible with either streptokinase or urokinase therapy, but the incidence of hemorrhagic complications was increased. The first controlled clinical trial compared urokinase with heparin and used objective measures of pulmonary perfusion, embolus size, and gas exchange as indicators of the efficacy of therapy [92]. The objective angiographic score was improved by 44 percent over the mean pretreatment value in heparin-treated patients. The patient with pulmonary embolism of acute onset and of massive proportion, especially if associated with clinical shock, benefits most by fibrinolytic therapy. The overall incidence of hemorrhagic complications was 27 and 45 percent in the heparin and urokinase groups, respectively, but the incidence of clinically important hemorrhagic episodes in this [92] and a subsequent study [96] was only approximately 4 and 9 percent. The mortality rate at 14 days was the same, although there was a greater incidence of embolus-related death in the heparin group and a greater incidence of hemorrhage-related death in the urokinase group.

Subsequent trials, such as the urokinase-streptokinase pulmonary embolism trial [96], showed that extending urokinase treatment to 24 h did not increase thrombolysis over that seen with 12 h of treatment. Also, urokinase versus streptokinase therapy for 24 h produced equivalent thrombolytic results. Some patients may have dramatic thrombolysis of a massive pulmonary embolus after only 12 h of fibrinolytic treatment, while others demonstrate progressive lysis with prolonged therapy. The role of fibrinolytic therapy in many patients with pulmonary emboli is not precisely defined, but clinical experience suggests that embolectomy should be reserved for the patient who deteriorates despite medical management with vasopressors, while patients without shock or those who can be maintained with vasopressors should receive thrombolytic therapy [133]. A significant number of patients with pulmonary emboli develop permanent anatomic defects in the pulmonary artery, and only about 20 percent of patients with severe pulmonary embolism have normal pulmonary perfusion scans 4 months after developing the condition [134]. Fibrinolytic treatment resulted in significantly better pulmonary capillary blood volume at 2 weeks and at 1 year than did heparin treatment [135], suggesting that fibrinolytic agents achieve long-term benefits that are not appreciated by pulmonary perfusion scan results.

PERIPHERAL ARTERIAL OCCLUSION
Fibrinolytic therapy provides an alternative to surgical intervention in the treatment of arterial occlusive disease. The results of 11 studies of streptokinase therapy in arterial occlusive disease [136–146] suggest that acute occlusions are more likely to respond dramatically and that occlusions due to embolic phenomena rather than to localized atherosclerosis are more likely to respond to fibrinolytic therapy but that only a minority of patients can be treated successfully with fibrinolytic therapy alone [102,137,147–150]. Occlusions of small

peripheral arteries [97,151,152], such as occur with embolization from proximal sites, are usually not amenable to the surgical approach and therefore represent unique indications for fibrinolytic therapy.

CORONARY ARTERY THROMBOSIS
Early trials suggested that systemic fibrinolytic therapy reduced the immediate mortality rate after myocardial infarction by as much as 40 percent over that expected [153–156]. A number of subsequent trials failed to demonstrate this initial trend, and it appears that the overall short-term mortality rate in unselected patients with myocardial infarction is the same whether or not fibrinolytic agents are administered [97,157–160]. The European Cooperative Study Group compared placebo with systemic streptokinase infusion for 24 h in patients who were stratified to moderate- or high-risk prognosis (approximately 13 percent of the total) [161]. The mortality rate at 6 months was significantly lower (15.6 percent) in the patients receiving streptokinase than in the control group (30.6 percent).

Thrombolytic agents have been perfused directly into thrombosed coronary vessels [105]. The treatment was safe, and benefit was suggested by lower mean values of serum enzymes and by improvement in electrocardiographic changes. All studies of intracoronary artery administration of thrombolytic agents have demonstrated that this therapy can result in recanalization of thrombosed coronary arteries [106,162–166]. However, lysis may also follow nitroglycerine infusion, contrast injection alone, or even guidewire manipulation [164], suggesting that the actual increase in response rate due to the thrombolytic agent is not yet known. The need for prospective, randomized, and controlled studies is further emphasized by the significant proportion of patients with initially thrombosed coronary vessels who spontaneously undergo rapid clearance of the occlusion [167], by the uncertainty over long-term effects [168], and by the occurrence of a significant plasma lytic state in many patients, suggesting that systemic administration of streptokinase may also achieve thrombolysis [162].

MISCELLANEOUS CONDITIONS
Streptokinase has been used successfully for the treatment of thrombosed artificial arteriovenous shunts [169–172]. The fibrinolytic agent is administered locally, and a systemic fibrinolytic effect is not produced. After limited local clot dissolution, which separates the thrombus from the shunt wall, the clot is removed manually. Benefit is often temporary because the clinical condition that predisposed to shunt thrombosis may persist after this therapeutic maneuver is completed.

The data from studies of central retinal vein thrombosis show no clear-cut distinction between fibrinolytic and heparin therapy [173–175]. Local installation of fibrinolytic agents into the vitreous humor or the anterior compartment for the treatment of intraocular hemorrhage is an unproven approach to this refractory clinical problem [176,177].

The possibility that a localized cerebral arterial thrombosis can be lysed has prompted the assessment of thrombolytic agents in patients with cerebral thromboembolic disease or cerebral infarction [178–180], but the risk of intracranial bleeding, even in patients without a clear-cut hemorrhagic stroke, makes this approach unsafe. Intracranial occlusive disease appears to be an absolute contraindication to fibrinolytic therapy.

Successful therapy with fibrinolytic agents has been reported in a variety of unusual or threatening clinical states, including thrombosis of cardiac valves [181], renal artery thrombosis [182], priapism [183], and Budd-Chiari syndrome [184], as well as clots or fibrosis in body cavities, such as occurs after pleural exudates [185].

References

1. Kwaan, H. C., Lo, R., and McFadzean, J. S.: On the production of plasma fibrinolytic activity within veins. *Clin. Sci.* 16:241, 1957.
2. Alkjaersig, N., Fletcher, A. P., and Sherry, S.: The mechanism of clot dissolution by plasmin. *J. Clin. Invest.* 38:1086, 1959.
3. Sakata, Y., and Aoki, N.: Cross-linking of α_2-plasmin inhibitor to fibrin by fibrin-stabilizing factor. *J. Clin. Invest.* 65:290, 1980.
4. Sakata, Y., and Aoki, N.: Significance of cross-linking of α_2 plasmin inhibitor to fibrin in inhibition of fibrinolysis and in hemostasis. *J. Clin. Invest.* 69:536, 1982.
5. Sherry, S., Fletcher, A. P., and Alkjaersig, N.: Fibrinolysis and fibrinolytic activity in man. *Physiol. Rev.* 39:343, 1959.
6. Ratnoff, O. D.: Epsilon aminocaproic acid: A dangerous weapon. *N. Engl. J. Med.* 280:1124, 1969.
7. Aoki, N., et al.: Congenital deficiency of α_2 plasmin inhibitor associated with severe hemorrhagic tendency. *J. Clin. Invest.* 63:877, 1979.
8. Aoki, N., et al.: Fibrinolytic states in a patient with congenital deficiency of α_2 plasmin inhibitor. *Blood* 55:483, 1980.
9. Aoki, N., Moroi, M., Sakara, Y., Yoshida, N., and Matsuda, M.: Abnormal plasminogen: A hereditary molecular abnormality found in a patient with recurrent thrombosis. *J. Clin. Invest.* 61:1186, 1978.
10. Wohl, R. C., Summaria, L., and Robbins, K. C.: Physiological activation of the human fibrinolytic system: Isolation and characterization of human plasminogen variants, Chicago I and Chicago II. *J. Biol. Chem.* 254:9063, 1979.
11. Egberg, O.: Inherited antithrombin deficiency causing thrombophilia. *Thromb. Diath. Haemorrh.* 13:516, 1965.
12. Marciniak, E., Farley, C. H., and DeSimone, P. A.: Familial thrombosis due to antithrombin III deficiency. *Blood* 43:219, 1974.
13. Egberg, O.: Inherited fibrinogen abnormality causing thrombophilia. *Thromb. Diath. Haemorrh.* 17:176, 1967.
14. Al-Mondhiry, H. A. B., Bilezikian, S. B., and Nossel, H. L.: Fibrinogen "New York": An abnormal fibrinogen associated with thromboembolism: Functional evaluation. *Blood* 45:607, 1975.
15. Griffin, J. H., Evatt, B., Zimmerman, T. S., Kleiss, A. J., and Wideman, C.: Deficiency of protein C in congenital thrombotic disease. *J. Clin. Invest.* 68:1370, 1981.
16. Comp, P. C., and Esmon, C. T.: Generation of in vivo fibrinolytic activity by infusion of activated protein C into dogs. *Circulation* 62:3, 1980.
17. Blatt, P. M., et al.: Thrombogenic materials in prothrombin complex concentrates. *Ann. Intern. Med.* 81:766, 1974.
18. White, G. C., II, et al.: Prothrombin complex concentrates: Potentially thrombogenic materials and clues to the mechanism of thrombosis in vivo. *Blood* 49:159, 1977.
19. Kwaan, H. C.: Fibrinolysis: A perspective. *Prog. Cardiovasc. Dis.* 21:397, 1979.
20. Stead, N., et al.: Familial thrombosis secondary to diminished vascular plasminogen activator release. *Blood* 58:240a, 1981.
21. Nilsson, I. M.: Local fibrinolysis as a mechanism for haemorrhage. *Thromb. Diath. Haemorrh.* 34:623, 1975.
22. Meikle, A. W., and Graybill, J. R.: Fibrinolysis and hemorrhage in a fatal case of heat stroke. *N. Engl. J. Med.* 276:911, 1967.
23. Collen, D.: On the regulation and control of fibrinolysis. *Thromb. Haemost.* 43:77, 1980.
24. Markus, G., DePasquale, J. L., and Wissler, F. C.: Quantitative determination of the binding of epsilon-aminocaproic acid to native plasminogen. *J. Biol. Chem.* 253:727, 1978.
25. Marder, V. J., Butler, F. O., and Barlow, G. H.: Antifibrinolytic therapy, in *Hemostasis and Thrombosis: Basic Principles and Clinical Practice*, edited by R. W. Colman, J. Hirsh, V. J. Marder, and E. W. Salzman. Lippincott, Philadelphia, 1982, p. 640.
26. Brockway, W. J., and Castellino, F. J.: Measurement of the binding of antifibrinolytic amino acids to various plasminogens. *Arch. Biochem. Biophys.* 151:194, 1972.
27. Thorsen, S., and Mullertz, S.: Rate of activation and electrophoretic mobility of unmodified and partially degraded plasminogen: Effects of 6-aminohexanoic acid and related compounds. *Scand. J. Clin. Lab. Invest.* 34:167, 1974.
28. McNicol, G. L., et al.: The absorption, distribution, and excretion of ϵ-aminocaproic acid following oral or intravenous administration to man. *J. Lab. Clin. Med.* 59:15, 1962.
29. Clarkson, A. R., Sage, R. E., and Lawrence, J. R.: Consumption coagulopathy and acute renal failure due to gram-negative septicemia after abortion: Complete recovery with heparin therapy. *Ann. Intern. Med.* 70:1191, 1969.
30. Gralnick, H. R., and Greipp, P.: Thrombosis with epsilon aminocaproic acid therapy. *Am. J. Clin. Pathol.* 56:151, 1971.
31. Naeye, R. L.: Thrombotic state after a hemorrhagic diathesis: A possible complication of therapy with epsilon-aminocaproic acid. *Blood* 19:694, 1962.
32. Charytan, C., and Purtilo, D.: Glomerular capillary thrombosis and acute renal failure after epsilon-aminocaproic acid therapy. *N. Engl. J. Med.* 280:1102, 1969.
33. Bergin, J. J.: The complications of therapy with epsilon-aminocaproic acid. *Med. Clin. North Am.* 50:1669, 1966.
34. Gobbi, F.: Use and misuse of aminocaproic acid. *Lancet* 1:472, 1967.
35. Sack, G. H., Levin, J., and Bell, W. R.: Trousseau's syndrome and other manifestations of chronic disseminated coagulopathy in patients with neoplasms: Clinical, pathologic, and therapeutic features. *Medicine (Baltimore)* 56:1, 1977.
36. Kluft, C., Vellenga, E., Brommer, E. J. P., and Wijngaards, G.: A familial hemorrhagic diathesis in a Dutch family: An inherited deficiency of α_2-antiplasmin. *Blood* 59:1169, 1982.
37. Miles, L. A., Plow, E. F., Donnelly, K. J., Hougie, C., and Griffin, J. H.: A bleeding disorder due to deficiency of α_2-antiplasmin. *Blood* 59:1246, 1982.
38. McClure, P. D., and Izsak, J.: The use of epsilon-aminocaproic acid to reduce bleeding during cardiac bypass in children with congenital heart disease. *Anesthesiology* 40:604, 1974.
39. Lambert, C. J., et al.: The treatment of postperfusion bleeding using ϵ-aminocaproic acid, cryoprecipitate, fresh-frozen plasma, and protamine sulfate. *Ann. Thorac. Surg.* 28:440, 1979.
40. Gordon, A. M., et al.: Clinical trial of epsilon-aminocaproic acid in severe haemophilia. *Br. Med. J.* 2:1632, 1965.
41. Bennett, A. E., Ingram, G. I. C., and Inglish, P. J.: Antifibrinolytic treatment in haemophilia: A controlled trial of prophylaxis with tranexamic acid. *Br. J. Haematol.* 24:83, 1973.
42. Walsh, P. N., et al.: Epsilon-aminocaproic acid therapy for dental extractions in haemophilia and Christmas disease: A double-blind controlled trial. *Br. J. Haematol.* 20:463, 1971.
43. Forbes, C. D., et al.: Tranexamic acid in control of haemorrhage after dental extraction in haemophilia and Christmas disease. *Br. Med. J.* 2:311, 1972.
44. Astrup, T.: Tissue activators of plasminogen. *Fed. Proc.* 25:42, 1966.
45. Konttinen, Y. P.: *Fibrinolysis: Chemistry, Physiology, Pathology and Clinics.* Oy Star Ab, Tampere, Finland, 1968.

46. Prentice, C. R. M.: Indications for antifibrinolysis therapy. *Thromb. Diath. Haemorrh.* 34:634, 1975.

47. McNicol, G. P.: Disordered fibrinolytic activity and its control. *Scot. Med. J.* 7:266, 1962.

48. McNicol, G. P., et al.: Impairment of hemostasis in the urinary tract: The role of urokinase. *J. Lab. Clin. Med.* 58:34, 1961.

49. Andersson, L., et al.: Role of urokinase and tissue activator in sustained bleeding and the management thereof with EACA and AMCA. *Ann. N.Y. Acad. Sci.* 146:642, 1968.

50. Andersson, L.: Antifibrinolytic drugs in the treatment of urinary tract haemorrhage. *Prog. Surg.* 10:76, 1972.

51. Andersson, L., and Nilsson, I. M.: Effect of ε-aminocaproic acid (EACA) on fibrinolysis and bleeding conditions in prostatic disease. *Acta Chir. Scand.* 121:291, 1961.

52. McNicol, G. P., et al.: The use of epsilon aminocaproic acid, a potent inhibitor of fibrinolytic activity in the management of postoperative hematuria. *J. Urol.* 86:829, 1961.

53. Sack, E., et al.: Reduction of postprostatectomy bleeding by epsilon-aminocaproic acid. *N. Engl. J. Med.* 266:541, 1962.

54. Vinnicombe, J., and Shuttleworth, K. E. D.: Aminocaproic acid in the control of haemorrhage after prostatectomy: A controlled trial. *Lancet* 1:230, 1966.

55. Nilsson, I. M., Andersson, L., and Björkman, S. E.: Epsilon-aminocaproic acid (E-ACA) as a therapeutic agent: Based on 5 years' clinical experience. *Acta Med. Scand. (Suppl.)* 448:5, 1966.

56. Bennett, B., and Ogston, D.: Natural and drug-induced inhibition of fibrinolysis. *Clin. Haematol.* 2:135, 1973.

57. Immergut, M. A., and Stevenson, T.: The use of epsilon aminocaproic acid in the control of hematuria associated with hemoglobinopathies. *J. Urol.* 93:110, 1965.

58. Vega, R., Shanberg, A. M., and Malloy, T. R.: The use of epsilon aminocaproic acid in sickle cell trait hematuria. *J. Urol.* 105:552, 1971.

59. Hilgartner, M. W.: Intrarenal obstruction in haemophilia. *Lancet* 1:486, 1966.

60. van Itterbeek, H., Vermylen, J., and Verstraete, M.: High obstruction of urine flow as a complication of the treatment with fibrinolysis inhibitors of haematuria in haemophiliacs. *Acta Haematol.* 39:237, 1968.

61. Savdie, E., Mahony, J. F., and Storey, B. G.: Control of bleeding after renal biopsy with epsilon-amino-caproic acid. *Br. J. Urol.* 50:8, 1978.

62. Haygood, T. A., et al.: Aminocaproic acid treatment of prolonged hematuria following renal biopsy. *Arch. Intern. Med.* 127:478, 1971.

63. Silverberg, D. S., et al.: Arteriovenous fistula and prolonged hematuria after renal biopsy: Treatment with epsilon aminocaproic acid. *Can. Med. Assoc. J.* 110:671, 1974.

64. Nilsson, I. M., Björkman, S. K., and Andersson, L.: Clinical experiences with ε-aminocaproic acid (ε-ACA) as an antifibrinolytic agent. *Acta Med. Scand.* 170:487, 1961.

65. Nilsson, L., and Rybo, G.: Treatment of menorrhagia with epsilon aminocaproic acid: A double blind investigation. *Acta Obstet. Gynecol. Scand.* 44:467, 1965.

66. Kasonde, J. M., and Bonnar, J.: Aminocaproic acid and menstrual loss in women using intrauterine devices. *Br. Med. J.* 4:17, 1975.

67. Rybo, G., and Westerberg, H.: The effect of tranexamic acid (AMCA) on postoperative bleeding after conization. *Acta Obstet. Gynecol. Scand.* 51:347, 1972.

68. Sahs, A. L., et al.: *Intracranial Aneurysms and Subarachnoid Hemorrhage: A Cooperative Study.* Lippincott, Philadelphia, 1969, p. 296.

69. Alvord, E. C., Jr., et al.: Subarachnoid hemorrhage due to reptured aneurysms: A simple method of estimating prognosis. *Arch. Neurol.* 27:273, 1972.

70. Smith, R. R., and Upchurch, J. J.: Monitoring antifibrinolytic therapy in subarachnoid hemorrhage. *J. Neurosurg.* 38:339, 1973.

71. Tovi, D., and Nilsson, I. M.: Increased fibrinolytic activity and fibrin degradation products after experimental intracerebral haemorrhage. *Acta Neurol. Scand.* 48:403, 1972.

72. Chowdhary, U. M., Carey, P. C., and Hussein, M. M.: Prevention of early recurrence of spontaneous subarachnoid haemorrhage by ε-aminocaproic acid. *Lancet* 1:741, 1979.

73. Maurice-Williams, R. S.: Prolonged antifibrinolysis: An effective nonsurgical treatment for ruptured intracranial aneurysms? *Br. Med. J.* 1:945, 1978.

74. Nibbelink, D. W., and Sahs, A. L.: Antifibrinolytic therapy and drug-induced hypotension in treatment of ruptured intracranial aneurysms. *Trans. Am. Neurol. Assoc.* 97:145, 1972.

75. Van Rossum, J., et al.: Effect of tranexamic acid on rebleeding after subarachnoid hemorrhage: A double-blind controlled clinical trial. *Ann. Neurol.* 2:242, 1977.

76. Kaste, M., and Ramsay, M.: Tranexamic acid in subarachnoid hemorrhage: A double-blind study. *Stroke* 10:519, 1979.

77. Girvin, J. P.: The use of antifibrinolytic agents in the preoperative treatment of ruptured intracranial aneurysms. *Trans. Am. Neurol. Assoc.* 98:150, 1973.

78. Kwaan, H. C., Cocco, A., and Mendeloff, A. I.: Histologic demonstration of plasminogen activation in rectal biopsies from patients with active ulcerative colitis. *J. Lab. Clin. Med.* 64:877, 1964 (abstract).

79. Salter, R. H., and Read, A. E.: Epsilon-aminocaproic acid therapy in ulcerative colitis. *Gut* 11:585, 1970.

80. Cox, H. T., Poller, L., and Thomson, J. M.: Gastric fibrinolysis: A possible aetiological link with peptic ulcer. *Lancet* 2:1300, 1967.

81. Nilsson, I. M., et al.: Gastric fibrinolysis. *Thromb. Diath. Haemorrh.* 34:409, 1975.

82. Oka, K., and Tanaka, K.: Local fibrinolysis of esophagus and stomach as a cause of hemorrhage in liver cirrhosis. *Thromb. Res.* 14:837, 1979.

83. Cormack, F., et al.: Tranexamic acid in upper gastrointestinal haemorrhage. *Lancet* 2:1207, 1973.

84. Biggs, J. C., Hugh, T. B., and Dobbs, A. J.: Tranexamic acid and upper gastrointestinal haemorrhage: A double-blind trial. *Gut* 17:729, 1976.

85. Jerndal, T., and Frisen, M.: Tranexamic acid (AMCA) and late hyphaema: A double-blind study in cataract surgery. *Acta Ophthalmol.* 54:417, 1976.

86. Mortensen, K. K., and Sjølie, A. K.: Secondary haemorrhage following traumatic hyphaema: A comparative study of conservative and tranexamic acid treatment. *Acta Ophthalmol.* 56:763, 1978.

87. Petruson, B.: Epistaxis: A clinical study with special reference to fibrinolysis. *Acta Otolaryngol. (Suppl.)* 317:1, 1974.

88. Falbe-Hansen, J., Jr., Jacobsen, B., and Lorenzen, E.: Local application of an antifibrinolytic tonsillectomy: A double-blind study. *J. Laryngol. Otol.* 88:565, 1974.

89. Verstraete, M., Vermylen, J., and Tyberghein, J.: Double-blind evaluation of the haemostatic effect of adrenochrome monosemicarbazone, conjugated oestrogens, and epsilon-aminocaproic acid after adenotonsillectomy. *Acta Haematol.* 40:154, 1968.

90. Duckert, F., et al.: Treatment of deep vein thrombosis with streptokinase. *Br. Med. J.* 1:479, 1975.

91. Marder, V. J.: The use of thrombolytic agents: Choice of patient, drug administration, laboratory monitoring. *Ann. Intern. Med.* 90:802, 1979.

92. *The Urokinase Pulmonary Embolism Trial: A National Cooperative Study.* American Heart Association Monograph No. 39, *Circulation* 47 (Suppl. 2):II-1-II-108, 1973.

93. Marder, V. J., et al.: Quantitative venographic assessment of deep vein thrombosis in the evaluation of streptokinase and heparin therapy. *J. Lab. Clin. Med.* 89:1018, 1977.

94. Bell, W. R.: Streptokinase and urokinase in the treatment of pulmonary thromboemboli: From a National Cooperative Study. *Thromb. Haemost.* 35:57, 1976.

95. National Institutes of Health Consensus Panel: Thrombolytic therapy in thrombosis. *Ann. Intern. Med.* 93:141, 1980.

96. Urokinase-streptokinase embolism trial: Phase II results. *JAMA* 229:1606, 1974.

97. Marder, V. J., and Bell, W. R.: Fibrinolytic therapy, in *Hemostasis and Thrombosis: Basic Principles and Clinical Practice,* edited by R. W. Colman, J. Hirsh, V. J. Marder, and E. W. Salzman. Lippincott, Philadelphia, 1982, p. 1037.

98. Fratantoni, J. C., Ness, P., and Simon, T. L.: Thrombolytic therapy: Current status. *N. Engl. J. Med.* 293:1073, 1975.

99. Kakkar, V. V., and Scully, M. F.: Thrombolytic therapy. *Br. Med. Bull.* 34:191, 1978.

100. Verstraete, M.: Biochemical and clinical aspects of thrombolysis. *Semin. Hematol.* 15:35, 1978.

101. Bell, W. R., and Meek, A. G.: Guidelines for the use of thrombolytic agents. *N. Engl. J. Med.* 301:1266, 1979.

102. Samama, M., et al.: La Thrombolyse par la streptokinase. 2. À propos de 66 observations. *Coagulation* 2:221, 1969.

103. Edwards, I. R., MacLean, K. S., and Dow, J. D.: Low-dose urokinase in major pulmonary embolism. *Lancet* 2:409, 1973.

104. Dotter, C. T., Rösch, J., and Seaman, A. J.: Selective clot lysis with low-dose streptokinase. *Radiology* 111:31, 1974.

105. Boucek, R. J., and Murphy, W. P., Jr.: Segmental perfusion of the coronary arteries with fibrinolysin in man following a myocardial infarction. *Am. J. Cardiol.* 6:525, 1960.

106. Rentrop, K. P., et al.: Acute myocardial infarction: Intracoronary application of nitroglycerin and streptokinase. *Clin. Cardiol.* 2:354, 1979.

107. Rijken, D. C., and Collen, D.: Purification and characterization of plasminogen activator secreted by human melanoma cells in culture. *J. Biol. Chem.* 256:7035, 1981.

108. Smith, R. A. G., Dupe, R. J., English, P. D., and Green, J.: Fibrinolysis with acyl-enzymes: A new approach to thrombolytic therapy. *Nature* 290:505, 1981.

109. Matsuo, O., Rijken, D. C., and Collen, D.: Comparison of the relative fibrinogenolytic, fibrinolytic and thrombolytic properties of tissue plasminogen activator and urokinase *in vitro. Thromb. Haemost.* 45:225, 1981.

110. Matsuo, O., Collen, D., and Verstraete, M.: On the fibrinolytic and thrombolytic properties of active-site p-anisoylated streptokinase-plasminogen complex (BRL 26921). *Thromb. Res.* 24:347, 1981.

111. Korninger, C., Matsuo, O., Suy, R., Stassen, J. M., and Collen, D.: Thrombolysis with human extrinsic (tissue-type) plasminogen activator in dogs with femoral vein thrombosis. *J. Clin. Invest.* 69:573, 1982.

112. Weimer, W., Stibbe, J., vanSeyen, A. J., Billiau, A., DeSomer, P., and Collen, D.: Specific lysis of an ileofemoral thrombus by administration of extrinsic (tissue-type) plasminogen activator. *Lancet* 2:1018, 1981.

113. Robertson, B. R., Nilsson, I. M., and Nylander, G.: Thrombolytic effect of streptokinase as evaluated by phlebography of deep venous thrombi of the leg. *Acta Chir. Scand.* 136:173, 1970.

114. Kakkar, V. V.: Treatment of deep vein thrombosis: A comparative study of heparin, streptokinase and Arvin. *Bull. Swiss Acad. Med. Sci.* 29:253, 1973.

115. Tsapogas, M. J., et al.: Controlled study of thrombolytic therapy in deep vein thrombosis. *Surgery* 74:973, 1973.

116. Tibbutt, D. A., et al.: Controlled trial of Ancrod and streptokinase in the treatment of deep vein thrombosis of lower limb. *Br. J. Haematol.* 27:407, 1974.

117. Rösch, J., et al.: Healing of deep venous thrombosis: Venographic findings in a randomized study comparing streptokinase and heparin. *Am. J. Roentgenol.* 127:553, 1976.

118. Arnesen, H., et al.: A prospective study of streptokinase and heparin in the treatment of deep vein thrombosis. *Acta Med. Scand.* 203:457, 1978.

119. Elliot, M. S., et al.: A comparative randomized trial of heparin versus streptokinase in the treatment of acute proximal venous thrombosis: An interim report of a prospective trial. *Br. J. Surg.* 66:838, 1979.

120. Watz, R., and Savidge, G. F.: Rapid thrombolysis and preservation of valvular venous function in high deep vein thrombosis. *Acta Med. Scand.* 205:293, 1979.

121. Seaman, A. J., et al.: Deep vein thrombosis treated with streptokinase or heparin. *Angiology* 27:549, 1976.

122. Kakkar, V. V., Howe, C. T., Laws, J. W., and Flanc, C.: Late results of treatment of deep vein thrombosis. *Br. Med. J.* 1:810, 1969.

123. Common, H. H., et al.: Deep vein thrombosis treated with streptokinase or heparin: Follow-up of a randomized study. *Angiology* 27:645, 1976.

124. Bieger, R., Boekhout-Mussert, R. J., Hohmann, F., and Loeliger, E. A.: Is streptokinase useful in the treatment of deep vein thrombosis? *Acta Med. Scand.* 199:81, 1976.

125. Albrechtsson, U., Anderson, J., Einarsson, E., Eklöf, B., and Norgren, L.: Streptokinase treatment of deep venous thrombosis and the postthrombotic syndrome: Follow-up evaluation of venous function. *Arch. Surg.* 116:33, 1981.

126. Rosenberg, D. M. L., Pearce, C., and McNulty, J.: Surgical treatment of pulmonary embolism. *J. Thorac. Cardiovasc. Surg.* 47:1, 1964.

127. Browse, N. L., and James, D. C. O.: Streptokinase and pulmonary embolism. *Lancet* 1:1039, 1964.

128. Sasahar, A. A., et al.: Urokinase therapy in clinical pulmonary embolism. *N. Engl. J. Med.* 277:1168, 1967.

129. Genton, E., and Wolf, P. S.: Urokinase therapy in pulmonary thromboembolism. *Am. Heart J.* 76:628, 1968.

130. Chesterman, C. N., Biggs, J. C., Morgan, J., and Hickie, J. B.: Streptokinase therapy in acute major pulmonary embolism. *Med. J. Aust.* 2:1096, 1969.

131. Miller, G. A. H., Gibson, R. V., and Sutton, G. C.: Treatment of pulmonary embolism with streptokinase: A preliminary report. *Br. Med. J.* 1:812, 1969.

132. Hirsh, J., McDonald, I. G. M., and Hale, G. S.: Streptokinase in the treatment of major pulmonary embolism: Experience with twenty-five patients. *Aust. Ann. Med. (Suppl.)*19:54, 1970.

133. Miller, G. A. H., Hall, R. J. C., and Paneth, M.: Pulmonary embolectomy, heparin, and streptokinase: Their place in the treatment of acute massive pulmonary embolism. *Am. Heart J.* 93:568, 1977.

134. Tow, D. E., and Wagner, H. N., Jr.: Recovery of pulmonary arterial blood flow in patients with pulmonary embolism. *N. Engl. J. Med.* 276:1053, 1967.

135. Sharma, G. V. R. K., Burleson, V. A., and Sasahara, A. A.: Effect of thrombolytic therapy on pulmonary capillary blood volume in patients with pulmonary embolism. *N. Engl. J. Med.* 303:842, 1980.

136. Hess, H.: Collective Statistics in Thrombolytische Therapie: Symposium der Deutsche Gesselschaft fur Angiologie. Munich, 1966. Shattauer, Stuttgart, 1967.

137. Amery, A., Deloof, W., Vermylen, J., and Verstraete, M.: Outcome of recent thromboembolic occlusions of limb arteries treated with streptokinase. *Br. Med. J.* 4:639, 1970.

138. Salmon, J.: Treatment fibrinolytique: Résultats obtenus au cours d'une expérience intéressant 200 patients, in *International Colloquiam on Streptokinase.* SPEI, Lyon, France, 1970, p. 113.

139. Martin, M., Schoop, W., and Zietler, E.: Streptokinase in chronic arterial occlusive diseases. *JAMA* 211:1169, 1970.

140. Verstraete, M., Vermylen, J., and Donati, M. B.: The effect of streptokinase infusion on chronic arterial occlusions and stenosis. *Ann. Intern. Med.* 74:377, 1971.

141. Deutsch, E., and Ehringer, H.: Thrombolytic therapy in chronic arterial occlusion. *J. Clin. Pathol.* 25:644, 1972.

142. LeVeen, H. H., and Diaz, C. A.: Venous and arterial occlusive disease treated by enzymatic clot lysis. *Arch. Surg.* 105:927, 1972.

143. Poliwoda, H.: Treatment of chronic arterial occlusion with streptokinase. *J. Clin. Pathol.* 25:642, 1972.

144. Heinrich, F.: Ziel und aufbau der studie, in *Streptokinase-therapie bie chronischer arterieller Verschlusskrankheit,* edited by F. Heinrich. Medizinische Verlazsges, Marburg, West Germany, 1975.

145. Fiessinger, J. N., et al.: The indications for streptokinase in arterial occlusions of the limbs. *Coeur Med. Interne* 15:453, 1976.

146. Conard, J., et al.: Complications hémorrhagiques au cours de 98 traitements par la streptokinase: Place de la surveillance biologique. *Nouv. Presse Med.* 8:1319, 1979.

147. Schmutzler, R., and Koller, F.: Thrombolytic therapy, in *Recent Advances in Blood Coagulation,* edited by L. Poller. Churchill, London, 1969, p. 299.

148. Poliwoda, H., et al.: Treatment of chronic arterial occlusions with streptokinase. *N. Engl. J. Med.* 280:689, 1969.

149. Chesterman, C. N., and Briggs, J. C.: Thrombolytic therapy with streptokinase. *Med. J. Aust.* 57:839, 1970.

150. Martin, M.: Thrombolytic therapy in arterial thromboembolism. *Prog. Cardiovasc. Dis.* 21:351, 1979.

151. Kartchner, M. M., and Wilcox, W. C.: Thrombolysis of palmar and digital arterial thrombosis by intra-arterial thrombolysin. *J. Hand Surg.* 1:67, 1976.

152. Cotton, L. T., Flute, P. T., and Tsapogas, M. J. C.: Popliteal artery thrombosis treated with streptokinase. *Lancet* 2:1081, 1962.

153. Schmutzler, R., et al.: On the thrombolytic therapy for recent myocardial infarction. *Dtsch. Med. Wochenschr.* 91:581, 1966.

154. Schmutzler, R., Fritze, E., and Gebauer, D.: Fibrinolytic therapy in acute myocardial infarction, in *Transactions of the 19th Annual Symposium on Blood*, edited by E. F. Mammen, G. F. Anderson, and M. I. Barnhart. Shattauer, Stuttgart, 1971.

155. European Working Party: Streptokinase in recent myocardial infarction: A controlled multicentre trial. *Br. Med. J.* 3:325, 1971.

156. Breddin, K., et al.: Die Kurzzeitfibrinolyse beim akuten Myokardinfarkt. *Dtsch. Med. Wochenschr.* 98:861, 1973.

157. European Collaborative Study: Controlled trial of urokinase in myocardial infarction. *Lancet* 2:624, 1975.

158. Australian multicentre trial of streptokinase in acute myocardial infarction. *Med. J. Aust.* 1:553, 1977.

159. Simon, T. L., Ware, J. H., and Stengle, J. M.: Clinical trials of thrombolytic agents in myocardial infarction. *Ann. Intern. Med.* 79:712, 1973.

160. Duckert, F.: Thrombolytic therapy in myocardial infarction. *Prog. Cardiovasc. Dis.* 21:342, 1979.

161. European Cooperative Study Group for Streptokinase Treatment in Acute Myocardial Infarction: Streptokinase in acute myocardial infarction. *N. Engl. J. Med.* 301:797, 1979.

162. Rentrop, P., et al.: Selective intracoronary thrombolysis in acute myocardial infarction and unstable angina pectoris. *Circulation* 63:307, 1981.

163. Ganz, W., et al.: Intracoronary thrombolysis in evolving myocardial infarction. *Am. Heart. J.* 101:4, 1981.

164. Mathey, D. G., et al.: Nonsurgical coronary artery recanalization in acute transmural myocardial infarction. *Circulation* 63:489, 1981.

165. Reduto, L. W., Smalling, R. W., Freund, G. C., and Gould, K. L.: Intracoronary infusion of streptokinase in patients with acute myocardial infarction: Effects of reperfusion on left ventricular performance. *Am. J. Cardiol.* 48:403, 1981.

166. Gold, H. K., Leinbach, R. C., Buckley, M. J., Akins, C. W., Levine, F. H., and Austen, W. G.: Intracoronary streptokinase in evolving infarction. *Hosp. Pract.* 16:105, 1981.

167. DeWood, M. A., et al.: Prevalence of total coronary occlusion during the early hours of transmural myocardial infarction. *N. Engl. J. Med.* 303:897, 1980.

168. Sobel, B. E., and Bergmann, S. R.: Coronary thrombolysis: Some unresolved issues. *Am. J. Med.* 72:1, 1982.

169. Anderson, D. C., et al.: Eights months' experience in the use of streptokinase for de-clotting arteriovenous cannulae. *Proc. Eur. Dial. Transplant Assoc.* 4:55, 1967.

170. Cocke, T. B., Burgos-Calderon, R. A., and Gonzalez, F.: The use of streptokinase infusions for arteriovenous shunt declotting. *Trans. Am. Soc. Artif. Intern. Organs* 16:292, 1970.

171. Watt, D. A. L., Dunn, B. P., Livingstone, W. R., and MacDougall, A. I.: Declotting of Quinton-Scribner shunts. *Am. Heart J.* 81:292, 1971.

172. Arisz, L., Tegzess, A. M., and Donker, A. J. M.: The use of streptokinase in obstructed arterio-venous shunts. *Postgrad. Med.* 49:99, 1973.

173. Den Ottolander, G. J. H., and Craandijk, A.: Treatment of thrombosis of the central retinal vein with streptokinase. *Thromb. Diath. Haemorrh.* 20:415, 1968.

174. Kohner, E. M., et al.: Streptokinase in central retinal vein occlusion: A controlled clinical trial. *Br. Med. J.* 1:550, 1976.

175. Kwaan, H. C., Dobbie, J. G., and Fetkenhour, C. L.: The use of anticoagulants and thrombolytic agents in occlusive retinal vascular disease, in *Thrombosis and Urokinase*, edited by T. Paoletti and S. Sherry. Academic, New York, 1977, p. 191.

176. Rakusin, W.: Urokinase in the management of traumatic hyphema. *Br. J. Ophthalmol.* 55:826, 1971.

177. Chapman-Smith, J. S., and Crock, G. W.: Urokinase in the management of vitreous hemorrhage. *Br. J. Ophthalmol.* 61:500, 1977.

178. Clarke, R. L., and Cliffton, E. E.: The treatment of cerebrovascular thrombosis and embolism with fibrinolytic agents. *Am. J. Cardiol.* 6:546, 1960.

179. Meyer, J. S., Gilroy, J. Barnhart, M., and Johnson, J. F.: Therapeutic thrombolysis in cerebral thromboembolism: Double-blind evaluation of intravenous plasmin therapy in carotid and middle cerebral arterial occlusion. *Neurology* 13:927, 1963.

180. Fletcher, A. P., et al.: A pilot study of urokinase therapy in cerebral infarction. *Stroke* 7:135, 1976.

181. Luluaga, I. T., et al.: Successful thrombolytic therapy after acute tricuspid-valve obstruction. *Lancet* 1:1067, 1971.

182. Jones, F. E., et al.: Local infusion of urokinase and heparin into renal arteries in impending renal cortical necrosis. *Br. Med. J.* 4:547, 1975.

183. Farrer, J. F., and Goodwin, W. E.: Treatment of priapism: Comparison of methods in 15 cases. *J. Urol.* 86:768, 1961.

184. Warren, R. L., Schlant, R. C., and Wenger, N. K.: Treatment of Budd-Chiari syndrome with streptokinase. *Gastroenterology* 64:200, 1973.

185. Bergh, N. P., Ekroth, R., Larsson, S., and Nagy, I.: Intrapleural streptokinase in the treatment of haemothorax and empyema. *Scand. J. Thorac. Cardiovasc. Surg.* 11:265, 1977.

Disorders of hemostasis—thrombosis

CHAPTER 160

Thrombosis

WILLIAM J. WILLIAMS

The mechanisms by which thrombosis develops have been studied extensively, with attention centering on the role of the blood vessels, blood flow, and blood composition. Emphasis has been placed on the interaction of platelets with the vessel wall, leading to the concept that thrombosis occurs because of an exaggeration or perversion of normal platelet hemostatic reactions. These phenomena are discussed in earlier chapters (Chaps. 126 to 129) but are considered here from the specific vantage point of the pathogenesis of thrombosis. Multiple factors are operative in nearly all experimental and clinical thromboses, and the search for the single determinant which is crucial for effective prevention and treatment has thus far been unsuccessful.

The vessel wall

Damage to the endothelium of blood vessels, with exposure of the subendothelial structures to the blood, results in attachment of platelets to the underlying collagen [1–6], basement membrane [6–9], or microfibrils [6–11] and may be the initiating lesion in thrombosis [2–11]. Factor VIII:von Willebrand factor is required for the initial attachment of platelets to subendothelial structures [6,12]. Subsequent to the attachment of platelets to the vessel wall, additional platelets attach to those already adherent, to form a platelet mass. Extension of this process, coupled with, or resulting from, the initiation of coagulation, may result in formation of a thrombus. Initiation of the coagulation mechanism may be due to activation of factor XII by collagen, activation of factor XI on the platelet surface by exposure to collagen, or release of tissue factor from the endothelium (see below). Blood coagulation is enhanced by release of platelet constituents, such as platelet factor 3 (see Chap. 129). Platelets undergo complex reactions with the vessel wall which may either promote or inhibit thrombosis [13].

Platelets do not attach to undamaged endothelium [3, 5,14,15]. Endothelial damage leading to platelet attachment may be subtle, and sophisticated techniques, including electron microscopy, are necessary to demonstrate some of the minimal lesions of the endothelium [3]. In some instances, endothelial damage can be demonstrated only when fibrinolytic mechanisms are inhibited [15].

Extensive local damage to vascular endothelium may not cause thrombosis [16,17], and in severely damaged arteries maintenance of blood flow usually prevents massive thrombosis [18,19]. However, hypoxia or carbon monoxide may contribute to arterial thrombosis by causing intimal damage [20–22], and in homocysteinuria endothelial damage appears to be responsible for arterial thromboses [23]. Endothelial damage may be more important as a cause of thrombosis in regions of lower blood flow [24]. Tissue injury can induce electric currents of sufficient magnitude to initiate thrombosis [25], perhaps by causing irreversible platelet aggregation [26]. Endothelial cells contain tissue factor, factor VIII–related antigen, and plasminogen activator (see Chap. 139). Possible roles for these substances are discussed below, under "Blood Components."

The nature of the endothelial damage leading to clinical thrombosis has not been defined. Endotoxin [27–30] or mechanical trauma [31,32], perhaps resulting from blood flow [3,33–38], may be causes in some instances. Platelets and leukocytes may initiate or aggravate endothelial injury [39–44]. Carbon monoxide inhalation, as in smoking, causes endothelial changes [21,22,45] and may be of pathogenic significance in atherosclerosis [45,46]. Atherosclerosis may be a major cause of endothelial damage, but it has been suggested that atherosclerosis is the result of thrombosis rather than the cause [13,47–49].

The avidity with which platelets react with components of the vessel wall should influence the development of thrombosis. Thus quantitative increases in platelets predispose to thrombosis [50], and qualitative alterations in platelets which enhance their ability to aggregate may occur in patients with a thrombotic tendency [51,52].

Blood flow

Stasis appears to be an important factor in the induction of thrombosis. Prolonged inactivity may predispose to venous thrombosis [53,54]. Electrical stimulation of leg muscles during surgery decreases the incidence of thrombosis in the leg veins, presumably because of increased blood flow [55]. However, fibrinolytic activity is also increased by this procedure [55]. Experimentally, stasis is necessary to induce thrombosis in animals with increased blood coagulability [56], although marked stasis may occur in normal veins with no apparent predisposition to thrombosis [57,58].

Experimental "stasis" thrombi are "red" and include many erythrocytes in addition to platelets and fibrin in a structure resembling an in vitro clot. Many thrombi formed in veins have a red tail structurally similar to a stasis thrombus. This tail is attached to a "white" head, composed largely of platelets and fibrin. In contrast, arterial thrombi are predominantly white [59]. It has been suggested that the differences between red and white thrombi may not reflect fundamental differences in pathogenesis but rather indicate differences related to factors such as blood flow [60], since red stasis thrombi placed in a rapidly flowing system can assume some of the characteristics of white thrombi [61].

In arteries the rapid blood flow and the pulsatile movement of the vessel wall tend to both dilute and disperse any activated coagulation factor and thereby protect the arterial tree. Although the rapid flow of blood can dilute procoagulants and thus be defensive, it is also possible that rapid blood flow causes endothelial damage and predisposition to thrombosis. Regions of turbulence develop at points of bifurcation or stenosis, and this may be significant in inducing thrombosis [24,60]. The turbulence may cause intimal damage by trauma [33,34], or it may cause deposition of platelets on normal intima [24,35] as the beginning of a thrombus, perhaps predisposing to an atherosclerotic lesion [47].

Polycythemia vera predisposes to thrombosis because of the increased viscosity of blood with an elevated hematocrit [62] as well as the associated thrombocytosis.

Blood components

The role of platelets in thrombosis is discussed above. Platelet adhesion and aggregation can occur without activation of the coagulation mechanism (Chaps. 126 to 129). However, at an early phase of formation of the platelet aggregate in normal hemostasis, the coagulation mechanism is activated. Thrombin is formed and causes further, irreversible platelet aggregation with release of platelet contents, including platelet factor 3 and serotonin. Thrombin, in amounts too small to produce fibrin from fibrinogen, causes platelet aggregation.

The coagulation mechanisms may be initiated by factor XIIa activated by exposure to collagen in the vessel wall [63], by factor XI activated during platelet aggregation induced by collagen [64], or by factor VII reacting with tissue factor in the endothelium of the blood vessels [65–67] or provided by leukocytes [43,44,68,69]. Tissue factor is active in very low concentrations, and the reaction sequence it initiates leads to very rapid thrombin formation. Further, tissue factor and factor VII form an insoluble complex which can bind activated factor X. Thus if tissue factor were exposed in situ, it could form a nidus of coagulant activity in the vessel wall which might lead to thrombosis [70]. A similar nidus may be created by coagulation factors activated on the surface of adherent platelets [64,71]. Factor VIII–related antigen can be demonstrated on vascular endothelium and could also play a role in the pathogenesis of thrombosis [72].

Larger amounts of thrombin cause fibrin formation in addition to platelet aggregation, and platelet aggregates soon become surrounded by fibrin, with extension of the thrombus. Thrombin can also convert factors V and VIII to more reactive forms, thus accelerating the clotting reactions (see Chap. 135), and activate factor XIII, which induces cross-linking of fibrin (see Chap. 132). Cross-linked fibrin is more resistant to the fibrinolytic enzymes, which makes clearance of the thrombus more difficult (see Chap. 138). Some abnormal fibrinogens predispose patients to thrombosis (see Chap. 153).

Hypercoagulability

Systemic hypercoagulability can be operative in the pathogenesis of thrombosis. The term *hypercoagulability* has been used to indicate the presence in plasma of increased activities or concentrations of various procoagulants or the presence in the circulation of activated coagulation factors, either as a result of disease or induced experimentally.

Thromboses occur with increased frequency in patients with elevated levels of coagulation factors, for example, in pregnancy [73,74], in patients taking oral contraceptive drugs [75], and in certain families with supranormal levels of factors V and VIII [76,77]. Clearly, factors such as stasis could be operative in pregnancy, but these are not obvious considerations in thrombosis associated with elevated levels of coagulation factors in nonpregnant women. Thrombosis following the intravenous administration of commercial concentrates of factors VII, IX, and X and prothrombin (prothrombin complex) to patients with liver disease is believed to be due to activated coagulation factors, probably factors Xa and IXa, in the preparation [78], possibly augmented by contaminating phospholipids [335]. In an experimental model of stasis thrombosis, factor IXa, factor Xa, and thrombin can induce thrombosis [79]. Factor IXa is effective in the lowest concentrations [79].

In the hypercoagulable state associated with disseminated intravascular coagulation, there may be thrombotic occlusion of both large and small vessels, although a major effect of this disorder is destruction of the circulating coagulation factors and platelets (see Chap. 158). However, platelets and fibrinogen may be maintained at nearly normal levels by compensatory increases in their production in some patients with disseminated intravascular coagulation and increased platelet and fibrinogen turnover [80]. Experimentally, disseminated intravascular coagulation can be induced by the intravenous administration of a powerful coagulant such as tissue factor (see Chap. 158). Intravenous administration of thrombin or activated factor X causes local coagulation if stasis is induced in some segment of the vascular tree [61], reinforcing the concept that thrombosis is dependent on more than one abnormality.

Phospholipids are known to play a major role in blood coagulation (see Chaps. 132 and 135), and increased concentrations of these substances can lead to enhanced coagulation [81]. Administration of procoagulant phospholipids to animals also receiving activated factor X increases the thrombogenicity of the factor Xa [82]. Sodium salts of long-chain, saturated free fatty acids are also known to enhance coagulability, probably by activation of factor XII and/or XI [83–86]. Both saturated and unsaturated fatty acids cause platelet aggregation and release of platelet constituents [87]. Intravenous administration of fatty acids causes extensive thrombosis [88,89], and the increase in plasma free fatty acids induced by ACTH is associated with thrombosis in animals [90]. Patients with familial hyperbeta-lipoproteinemia (type II hyperlipoproteinemia) have abnormal platelet function characterized by increased sensitivity to aggregating agents (epinephrine, ADP, and collagen) and release increased amounts of nucleotides in response to aggregating agents [52]. These findings suggest the possibility that increased platelet function may be involved in the thrombotic complications of familial hyperbetalipoproteinemia.

Another aspect of hypercoagulability is a decrease in antithrombins or other inhibitors of blood coagulation (see Chap. 136). Decreased antithrombin III activity has been reported as a familial disorder characterized by an increased incidence of thrombosis [91–94] (see Chap. 136).

Defense of the body against thrombosis

Normal endothelium prevents platelet adherence or aggregation and the activation of blood coagulation factors and protects against thrombosis by a variety of mechanisms, including synthesis of prostacyclin (see Chap. 139). The mechanisms available to the body to control the phenomena of coagulation are discussed in Chaps. 136 and 138. The potential of the inhibitors of activated coagulation factor and of the phagocytic clearing mechanisms for preventing or limiting a hypercoagulable state seems clear. The role of antithrombin III in normal defenses is suggested by thrombotic complications attendant on congenital deficiency of this factor [91–94].

The fibrinolytic system also appears to play a major role in defense against thrombosis and may be continuously active under normal conditions. Decreased fibrinolytic activity has been observed in some patients with thrombosis [95–99] (see Chaps. 138 and 159). The endothelium of blood vessels is rich in plasminogen activator [100–102]. This system may protect against thrombosis in the experimental model in which thrombosis is induced by combined intravenous administration of serum and occlusion of blood flow in a segment of a blood vessel [103]. In this model, administration of ε-aminocaproic acid (EACA), an inhibitor of plasminogen activator, along with serum and stasis, enhances thrombus formation [103]. The administration of EACA to patients has occasionally been associated with

widespread thrombosis, supporting the concept of the fibrinolytic system's protective role [104].

Therapy

Therapy in thrombosis has been directed toward interference with the coagulation mechanism, activation of the fibrinolytic system, interference with platelet aggregation, or combinations of these. In addition to these approaches to the therapy of thrombosis, surgical intervention to prevent embolism or to remove thrombi and restore blood flow may be of critical importance in the management of the patient. Immobilization, local heat, etc., are also used. This discussion is limited to those aspects of therapy which are specifically of concern to the hematologist.

ANTICOAGULANT THERAPY

COUMARIN DRUGS
The coumarin drugs (warfarin, or Coumadin, Dicumarol, etc.) act by antagonizing the metabolism of vitamin K [105] and result in depression of the concentration of the procoagulants prothrombin (factor II) and factors VII, IX, and X and also of the anticoagulant proteins C and S (see Chaps. 133 and 136) [106–111]. Details of the action of oral anticoagulants are presented in Chap. 133. The dosage of the drug is regulated by measuring its effect on the coagulation mechanism, utilizing a test which involves the extrinsic system, such as the one-state prothrombin time (see Chap. A34). This test is influenced by the concentration of fibrinogen and factor V, as well as prothrombin and factors VII and X, three of the four factors depressed by the oral anticoagulant. The test does not measure factor IX, which is also depressed by the drug. The concentration of factor VII has the greatest influence on the test. The results of the test are also dependent on which tissue factor preparations are used [112–116] (see Chap. A34). The one-stage prothrombin time has proved invaluable in monitoring therapy with the coumarin drugs, and it, or one of its variants [117], should be utilized systematically to evaluate the degree of anticoagulation achieved. Assay methods using synthetic substrates may prove useful in monitoring anticoagulant therapy [113,118,119]. The details of the use of the one-stage prothrombin time in monitoring anticoagulant therapy are presented in Chap. A34.

Warfarin is the coumarin anticoagulant most widely used in the United States. Warfarin sodium is a racemic mixture of optical isomers with different metabolic characteristics [120]. It is rapidly and completely absorbed [120–122] and is metabolized and excreted with a half-life ranging from 31 to 58 h, with a mean of 44 h [122]. The mean daily dose required for anticoagulation is 6.8 ± 2.8 mg per day [123]. Resistance to warfarin is inherited as an autosomal dominant trait [123–125]. The half-life of warfarin in the plasma of warfarin-resistant patients is normal [123–125], and they respond to very small doses of vitamin K [124,125]. The resistance appears to be due to abnormalities of the receptor site for the drug or vitamin K [125,126]. A similar abnormality has been described in Norway rats resistant to warfarin [127]. There is evidence from these animals that the resistance may be due to lack of inhibition by warfarin of epoxide reductase, an enzyme required for normal vitamin K metabolism [105,128,129] (see Chap. 135). Another type of resistance to warfarin in human beings is due to accelerated disappearance of the drug from the circulation [130].

The rate of development of prolongation of the one-stage prothrombin time following administration of a coumarin drug is a function of the half-life of the vitamin K–dependent plasma coagulation factors. Factor VII levels fall most rapidly ($T_{1/2} \sim 5$ h), while levels of factors IX ($T_{1/2} = 17$ to 40 h), X ($T_{1/2} = 20$ to 48 h), and prothrombin (factor II) ($T_{1/2} = 60$ to 120 h) fall more slowly (see Chap. 134). The initial prolongation of the prothrombin time is primarily due to factor VII deficiency; later the levels of all four factors are decreased equally [131]. The antithrombotic effect of coumarin drug therapy increases over the first several days of drug administration [132,133]. The influence of the vitamin K–dependent anticoagulant proteins, protein C

and protein S [106–111] (see Chap. 136), on the antithrombotic effects of warfarin therapy is not known, but reduction in the levels of these proteins could reduce the therapeutic potential of coumarin drugs.

Warfarin therapy is principally used for the long-term prevention of recurrences of venous thrombosis [e.g., 134–138]. It is also effective for prevention of embolization in patients with mitral valvular diease [139]. The role of oral anticoagulant therapy in patients with myocardial infarction remains controversial [e.g., 140,141].

Initiation of warfarin therapy with a loading dose (50 mg) may lead to a dangerous level of anticoagulation in some patients and does not accelerate the fall of the levels of prothrombin and factors IX and X [142]. With daily administration of smaller doses of warfarin (10 to 15 mg), the rate of decrease in prothrombin and factors IX and X levels is the same as the rate of decrease after a loading dose, and the smaller doses minimize the hazard of over-anticoagulation [142]. This approach yields satisfactory results in practice, and there appears to be no reason for initiating warfarin therapy with doses of more than 10 to 15 mg.

Many drugs interact with warfarin, either increasing or decreasing its activity. Table 160-1 is a partial list of such drugs. The anticoagulant action of warfarin may be modified by several mechanisms, as illustrated in Fig.

TABLE 160-1 Drugs that alter the response to coumarins*

Drug	Mechanism
Drugs that may potentiate the effects of coumarins:	
Phenylbutazone	Displacement [157,158]
	Interference with platelet function [184]
Indomethacin	Displacement [163]
	Interference with platelet function [184]
Clofibrate	Displacement [163]
	Inhibition of coumarin metabolism [174]
	Interference with platelet function [185]
Sulfisoxazole	Displacement [143,164]
Chloramphenicol	Inhibition of coumarin metabolism [170]
Allopurinol	Inhibition of coumarin metabolism [171]
Nortriptyline	Inhibition of coumarin metabolism [171]
Cimetidine	Inhibition of coumarin metabolism [173]
Quinidine	Unknown [180]
Salicylates	Interference with vitamin K metabolism [181]
	Interference with platelet function (aspirin) [184]
Anabolic steroids	Unknown [189]
Trimethoprim-sulfamethoxazole	Unknown [179]
Drugs that may interfere with the effects of coumarins:	
Barbiturates	Acceleration of coumarin metabolism† [165,167]
Glutethimide	Acceleration of coumarin metabolism [165,167]
Griseofulvin	Unknown [168]
Rifampin	Acceleration of coumarin metabolism [169]
Oral contraceptives	Enhancement of synthesis of clotting factors [183]

* Extensive lists of drugs which may interact with coumarin anticoagulants are given in Refs. 149 and 190.
† Heptabarbital also inhibits coumarin absorption [152].

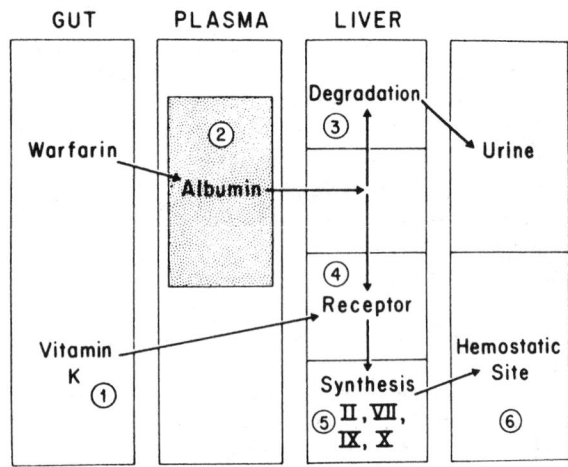

FIGURE 160-1 Sites at which drugs may alter the anticoagulant effects of coumarin drugs. (Reprinted by permission from Deykin [143].)

160-1 [143]. Vitamin K absorption (1 in Fig. 160-1) may be influenced by drugs such as cholestyramine [143,144], which interfere with fat absorption. Cholestyramine may interfere with absorption of warfarin as well (see below).

Vitamin K may be obtained both from the diet and from synthesis by intestinal bacteria, although the relative importance of these two sources is not clear. Excessive dietary intake of vitamin K can significantly reduce the anticoagulant effects of warfarin therapy [145,146]. In human subjects vitamin K appears not to be absorbed from the colon [147]; in experimental animals, vitamin K synthesized by intestinal bacteria is absorbed because of coprophagia [148]. Oral neomycin therapy inconsistently prolonged the prothrombin time in one study of humans anticoagulated with warfarin [147]. However, patients with serious infections treated with various antibiotics may develop vitamin K deficiency [149,150]. It appears that dietary intake is the primary source of vitamin K in human beings, but drug effects on intestinal synthesis may be important if oral intake is low or absent [144,147]. Cholestyramine [151] interferes with the absorption of warfarin, and barbiturates may diminish absorption of dicoumarol [152].

Warfarin is transported in the plasma bound to albumin (2 in Fig. 160-1) [153], and drugs which displace warfarin from albumin transiently increase its effects [154,155]. Normally more than 95 percent of warfarin is protein-bound in plasma [156], and displacement of less than 1 percent of the bound warfarin can cause a significant prolongation of the prothrombin time [154]. The higher concentration of free warfarin increases not only the pharmacologic effects of the drug but also the rate of inactivation, with corresponding decrease in the half-life of the drug [154,155]. Thus this type of drug interaction is characterized by an increased effect of war-

farin with a diminished half-life and a decreased plasma concentration of the drug [144,155]. The interaction of phenylbutazone and warfarin is the prototype of this reaction and has been extensively studied [157,158]. Chloral hydrate is metabolized to trichloroacetic acid, which is able to displace warfarin from albumin and thereby enhance its effects [159]. This interaction may be clinically important during the first few days of combined therapy [159–161] but has been reported not to be significant during chronic combined therapy [161,162].

Drugs may also interact with warfarin by altering its rate of degradation (3 in Fig. 160-1). Warfarin is degraded by hepatic microsomal enzymes [165], and a number of drugs increase the activity of these enzymes [165,166]. This phenomenon of enzyme induction occurs within a few days of administration of the drug, and when the drug is withdrawn the effect disappears in a few days. The increased rate of metabolism of warfarin shortens its plasma half-life, diminishes the serum level of the drug, and decreases its pharmacologic effect [165]. Barbiturates and glutethimide [144,167] appear to interact with warfarin by this mechanism (Table 160-1).

Drugs may also interact with warfarin by decreasing the rate of metabolism, possibly by decreasing the synthesis or activity of the degradative enzymes or by competitively inhibiting the metabolism of warfarin [170,171]. The result is increased anticoagulant effect of the warfarin. Chloramphenicol [170], allopurinol [171], nortriptyline [171], and cimetidine [172,173] interact by this mechanism. Coumarin drugs may cause enhanced effects of other drugs, such as chlorpropamide [175], tolbutamide [176], and dilantin [143,177], presumably by reducing the rate of degradation of the other drug.

Theoretically, drugs could enhance or decrease the effects of warfarin by altering the affinity of the hepatic receptor site for this drug (4 in Fig. 160-1). This mechanism has been suggested for the enhancement of warfarin action by D-thyroxine [178], quinidine [143], and trimethoprim-sulfamethoxazole [179], but no firm evidence has been obtained on this point [144,180].

Drugs which influence the synthesis of prothrombin (factor II) and factors VII, IX, and X may significantly influence the anticoagulant effect of warfarin (5 in Fig. 160-1). Some drugs, such as salicylates, appear to have an anti-vitamin K effect which can be overcome by administration of vitamin K [181].

Known hepatotoxins, such as carbon tetrachloride, in doses which cause no difficulty in normal people, may have profound effects on the levels of coagulation factors in those receiving coumarin drugs [182]. Quinidine may also act in this manner [180]. Oral contraceptives enhance synthesis of several plasma coagulation factors (see Chap. 133) and may thereby diminish the effect of warfarin therapy [183].

Finally, drugs which interfere with other components of the hemostatic system may enhance the effect of warfarin (6 in Fig. 160-1). Examples are drugs which inhibit platelet function, such as aspirin, phenylbutazone, indomethacin, or clofibrate [184,185]. Aspirin, phenylbutazone, and indomethacin and other nonsteroidal anti-inflammatory drugs may also cause gastrointestinal blood loss [186–188] and, as noted, above, can potentiate the anticoagulant effect of coumarin drugs. Administration of any of these drugs to anticoagulated patients is particularly hazardous.

HEPARIN

Heparin is a powerful anticoagulant which acts at several sites in the coagulation sequence: (1) inhibition of factor XIIa [191]; (2) inhibition of factor XIa [192,193]; (3) inhibition of factor IXa [194]; (4) inhibition of factor Xa [195,196]; and (5) inhibition of thrombin [197,198]. The inhibition of thrombin prevents activation of factor XIII [199] as well as other thrombin effects on blood coagulation.

Medicinal heparin is a highly sulfated glycosaminoglycan which is heterogeneous both chemically and physically with multiple bands detected in isoelectric focusing [200]. Its M_r ranges from about 4000 to 30,000 daltons [200–202]. Heparin can be fractionated by several techniques to yield preparations of increased anticoagulant potency [203–213] and differing effects on platelets [208,210,211].

Heparin may be administered intramuscularly, subcutaneously, or intravenously. The intramuscular route carries the risk of development of intramuscular or retroperitoneal hematomas [214], which may be serious complications in patients receiving heparin by injection into the hip or thigh [214]. Furthermore, absorption is unpredictable with both intramuscular and subcutaneous injection of heparin [215]. The intravenous route is therefore preferred and may be employed for continuous or intermittent therapy [216]. Continuous infusion of heparin appears to be safer than intermittent injections [134,216,217]. In most studies both routes of therapy were equally effective [134,216,217]. In one study intermittent heparin was more effective, but the difference might have been due to a higher total daily dose in the group receiving intermittent therapy [218]. If the whole-blood clotting time is used to monitor heparin therapy, it is usually recommended that the heparin dosage be such that the clotting time is maintained at least two to three times normal [117,219,220]. The whole-blood clotting time should be monitored just before each successive dose if intermittent therapy is employed or at any time with continuous intravenous therapy. If the partial thromboplastin time is used to monitor heparin therapy, it is usually recommended that the PTT should be maintained between 1.5 to 2.5 times normal [137,221] or at least twice normal [218] (see below). Effective therapy usually requires a dosage of 5000 to 10,000 units every 3 to 4 h by intermittent intravenous injection, an hourly rate of 1000 to 2000 units by continuous intravenous administration, or 7500 to 15,000 units every 8 to 12 h by subcutaneous injection [117].

Experimental pulmonary emboli develop platelet ac-

cretions on their surfaces [61]. The platelets which attach to the embolus are believed to release serotonin and thus to be responsible for some of the acute physiologic changes accompanying pulmonary embolus, such as airway constriction [222]. The attachment of the platelets to the embolus may be due to thrombin and can be prevented by administration of large doses of heparin [222]. Doses of heparin of 10,000 to 15,000 units intravenously every 4 h have been recommended for therapy of pulmonary emboli, at least initially [223]. Further work is necessary to determine the value of such a treatment program.

Heparin has also been used for the prevention of thrombosis and for the prevention of recurrences of thrombosis [135–138,224–239]. For this purpose, heparin has been given in smaller doses than have been used in therapy. For example, the administration of heparin subcutaneously in doses of 5000 units 2 h preoperatively and every 8 h thereafter for 7 days has been shown to reduce significantly the incidence of thrombophlebitis and pulmonary embolism [228]. Even lower doses of heparin given intravenously have been reported to be effective in preventing venous thrombosis in surgical patients [238]. Heparin administered at a dose of 5000 units every 8 h to a small number of patients with myocardial infarction reduced the incidence of venous thrombosis relative to a control series [226, 230,235,239], but in another study heparin at a dose of 7500 units every 12 h was ineffective [229]. The activated partial thromboplastin time is moderately increased for 5 h after the subcutaneous administration of 5000 units of heparin [226].

Antithrombin III levels are reduced during episodes of active thrombosis and by heparin therapy [240,336]. When heparin therapy is discontinued abruptly, the lowered levels of antithrombin III could increase the risk of thrombosis, although the significance of this possibility is unknown.

The effect of heparin therapy has traditionally been determined by the whole-blood clotting time, but there has been increasing interest in the activated partial thromboplastin time (aPTT) as a means of monitoring heparin therapy [221,241–244]. In the studies cited, prolongation of the aPTT was found to increase with increasing heparin concentrations, and a linear correlation between whole-blood clotting time and aPTT was demonstrated. Prolongation of the aPTT to 1.5 to 2.5 times the control levels has been considered evidence of adequate anticoagulation [216,221,242]. However, the aPTT does not always correlate well with the whole-blood clotting time in patients receiving heparin therapy [245–247], and there are many technical problems in utilizing the aPTT to monitor heparin therapy (see Chap. 137). Careful standardization of the test is required if reliable results are to be obtained. Some clinicians have omitted monitoring the effects of heparin given by intermittent injection and have not encountered an increased incidence of complications [216,218,248].

COMBINED HEPARIN AND ORAL ANTICOAGULANT THERAPY

Therapy is usually initiated with heparin and then switched to oral anticoagulants for long-term treatment. Combined therapy with both heparin and an oral drug should be continued for a few days in order to ensure maximal effect from the oral drug. Heparin can interfere with the one-stage prothrombin time [249], and the oral drugs regularly prolong the partial thromboplastin time [241]. Treatment with the coumarin drugs does not usually alter the whole-blood clotting time in glass but does cause prolongation of the silicone clotting time [250]. If heparin is given by intermittent intravenous injection to patients receiving combined therapy, the prothrombin time should be determined just before an injection of heparin. The prothrombin time appears not to be significantly prolonged when therapeutic doses of heparin are given by continuous intravenous infusion [216], but as the prothrombin time is lengthened by warfarin therapy it may become more sensitive to the inhibitory effects of heparin [249].

COMPLICATIONS OF ANTICOAGULANT THERAPY

Hemorrhage is the principal complication of anticoagulant therapy and occurs in patients in proportion to the intensity of the anticoagulant regimen [114]. Hemorrhage is more likely to occur in the presence of lesions such as peptic ulcers [251]. Women over the age of 60 appear to be particularly likely to develop bleeding complications when treated with heparin [252]. Hemorrhage is a less frequent complication of therapy in patients receiving continuous intravenous infusion of heparin than in those receiving intermittent intravenous therapy [114,216–218]. Heparin can be rapidly neutralized by the intravenous administration of protamine sulfate: 1 mg of protamine sulfate will inactivate about 100 units of heparin. Therapy of overdosage with the coumarin drugs is discussed in Chaps. 156 and 167.

Thrombocytopenia may develop in up to 30 percent of patients receiving heparin therapy [114]. Heparin-associated thrombocytopenia is discussed in Chap. 146.

Uncommon complications of heparin include alopecia [253], osteoporosis [254], and dysesthesia pedis [255]. Both local and systemic hypersensitivity to heparin also occur [256]. A rare complication of therapy with coumarin drugs is necrosis of the skin and subcutaneous tissues [257–259]. Oral anticoagulants cross the placenta and may cause bleeding in the fetus [260], but theoretically heparin does not cross the placenta and may be used in pregnancy [261]. However, complications of pregnancy, including fetal wastage, occur frequently with either warfarin or heparin therapy [262,263].

Thrombosis may occur during anticoagulant therapy, often in patients inadequately treated but also in those whose laboratory tests indicate adequate control. These patients illustrate the limitation of laboratory tests in evaluating antithrombotic effect as opposed to anticoagulant effect. It has been reported that sudden dis-continuation of oral anticoagulant drugs may cause a "rebound" hypercoagulable state, with resulting thrombosis and death [264]. Evidence has been presented that the increased risk of thrombosis upon cessation of oral anticoagulant therapy occurs only when the drugs are discontinued for a hemorrhage complication [265], suggesting that the hypercoagulability is related to the bleeding. However, this conclusion was not confirmed in another study [266]. The possibility that hypercoagulability follows cessation of heparin therapy has also been raised [240].

THROMBOLYTIC AGENTS

Two plasminogen activators, streptokinase and urokinase, have been evaluated in clinical trials and are discussed in Chap. 159.

SNAKE VENOM ENZYMES – ANCROD AND BATROXOBIN

Interest in the venom of the Malayan pit viper as an agent to treat thrombosis arose following reports that the bite of this snake caused prolonged hypofibrinogenemia without significant hemorrhage [267,268]. The disappearance of fibrinogen is due to conversion of fibrinogen to fibrin by the action of a protein in the venom, coupled with fibrinolysis by endogenous fibrinolytic enzymes [269–271]. The coagulant protein has the generic name ancrod. It has no effect on factor VIII [272] or factor XIII [273] and is not inhibited by heparin [270,272]. Clinical investigations of ancrod in the treatment of thrombosis have yielded some encouraging results [e.g., 274–277]. Small doses of ancrod have been administered to surgical patients in attempts to prevent postoperative thromboembolism [278,279]. The pit viper venom enzyme does not appear to be strongly antigenic [276,280] and is not pyrogenic in humans [274–276].

Batroxobin is the generic name for a defibrinating enzyme purified from the venom of *Bothrops atrox moojeni*. It is also known by the trade names Defibrase and Reptilase. Batroxobin, like ancrod, releases fibrinopeptide A from fibrinogen, leading to fibrin formation with subsequent removal from the circulation [271]. Batroxobin has been evaluated clinically both as a single agent and in combination with streptokinase [277,281]. Further studies are necessary to establish the role of these enzymes in clinical medicine.

AGENTS WHICH INTERFERE WITH PLATELET AGGREGATION

Analogs of ADP, such as adenosine and 2-chloroadenosine, are powerful inhibitors of platelet aggregation [282,283] and have been shown to inhibit the formation of platelet aggregates at points of vessel injury in vivo [284]. Unfortunately, these agents have marked side effects, so they cannot be used clinically. A number of drugs, such as aspirin, sulfinpyrazone, phenylbutazone, dipyridamole, clofibrate, and dextran, also interfere with platelet function (see Chap. 147). Aspirin in usual clinical dosage inhibits platelet aggregation and prolongs the bleeding time [285]. Sulfinpyrazone added to blood in vitro inhibits platelet aggregation [184]. However, when administered in vivo it has no effect on platelet aggregation [286], although it does prolong the platelet survival time in normal subjects [287]. Dipyridamole has no effect on platelet aggregation when administered in vivo or in vitro [288,289] but prolongs the platelet survival time in patients with arterial thrombosis or prosthetic heart valves [80]. Clofibrate prolongs platelet survival times and decreases platelet aggregation induced by latex particles [290]. The platelets of patients with familial hyperbetalipoproteinemia (type II hyperlipoproteinemia) are aggregated by abnormally low concentrations of epinephrine, ADP, or collagen and release increased amounts of nucleotide in response to these agents [52]. Administration of clofibrate to these patients diminishes the sensitivity of their platelets to the aggregating agents but does not affect the increased platelet nucleotide release [291]. High-molecular-weight dextran prolongs the bleeding time [292] and interferes with platelet retention on glass bead columns [293,294].

These drugs have been evaluated in clinical trials as antithrombotic agents, with variable results [for reviews see 114,295–297]. Although antiplatelet agents have been studied most extensively in arterial thrombosis, they have also been evaluated in venous thrombosis. Aspirin has been reported to prevent postoperative venous thrombosis [298–300], but other studies have demonstrated no beneficial effect of therapy with this drug [301,302]. Dipyridamole was ineffective in preventing venous thrombosis in two studies [298,303] and did not influence the shortened platelet survival time in patients with venous thrombosis [80]. Dextran was found to be as effective as aspirin or warfarin in the prevention of postoperative venous thrombosis [298]. Sulfinpyrazone therapy reduced the number of episodes of thrombosis in patients with recurrent phlebitis [304, 305]. Platelet survival time was improved by sulfinpyrazone therapy in these patients [304,305].

Antiplatelet drugs have been studied for their antithrombotic effects in patients with prosthetic arteriovenous shunts. Dipyridamole restored to normal the shortened survival time of platelets in patients with arteriovenous shunts [80], and treatment with sulfinpyrazone [306] or small doses of aspirin [307] decreased thrombus formation in such shunts.

Clinical studies have indicated that a combination of dipyridamole and warfarin significantly reduces the incidence of thrombosis in patients with prosthetic heart valves [308]. Dipyridamole, dipyridamole and aspirin in combination, and sulfinpyrazone all increase the shortened platelet survival time in patients with prosthetic heart valves [80,301,309–311].

Antiplatelet drugs correct the shortened platelet survival time in patients with arterial thrombosis [80]. Aspirin has been reported to reduce the number of attacks in patients with amaurosis fugax and transient ischemic attacks [312–318]. Sulfinpyrazone has also been reported to prevent amaurosis fugax [319] but may not prevent transient ischemic attacks [316–318]. Dipyridamole was ineffective in two studies of this disorder [312,320]. The effects of antiplatelet drugs on myocardial infarction have also been evaluated in a number of studies [321–326]. No conclusive benefit has been demonstrated, but a favorable trend has been observed in most series [321,322,324,326]. Sulfinpyrazone may also have a beneficial effect on prevention of death from recurrent myocardial infarction, but the data are not conclusive [327,328]. Treatment with clofibrate was reported to have a favorable effect on both morbidity and mortality from arteriosclerotic heart disease [329–331]. The beneficial effects of clofibrate did not correlate with alterations in the level of blood lipids [329–331], and it is possible that the antiplatelet activity of the drug is responsible. Prostacyclin has been reported to be an effective antithrombotic agent in patients undergoing hemodialysis, with reduced risk of hemorrhage [332,333], and has been evaluated as an antiplatelet aggregating agent in patients maintained on extracorporeal circulation [334].

The concept that platelet aggregation is responsible for the initiation of thrombosis and that interference with platelet aggregation will therefore prevent thrombosis is attractive and is supported by both clinical and experimental evidence. However, much additional work must be done before such therapy can be considered established.

References

1. Zucker, M. B., and Borelli, J.: Platelet-clumping produced by connective tissue suspensions and by collagen. *Proc. Soc. Exp. Biol. Med.* 109:779, 1962.
2. Spaet, T. H., and Erichson, R. B.: The vascular wall in the pathogenesis of thrombosis. *Thromb. Diath. Haemorrh. (Suppl.)* 21:67, 1966.
3. Spaet, T. H., and Ts'ao, C.-H.: Vascular endothelium and thrombogenesis, in *Thrombosis*, edited by S. Sherry, K. M. Brinkhous, E. Genton, and J. M. Stengle, National Academy of Sciences, Washington, D.C., 1969, p. 416.
4. Hugues, J., and Lapiere, C. M.: Nouvelles recherches sur l'accolement des plaquettes aux fibers de collagine. *Thromb. Diath. Haemorrh.* 11:327, 1964.
5. Ashford, T. P., and Freiman, D. G.: The role of the endothelium in the initial phases of thrombosis: An electron microscopic study. *Am. J. Pathol.* 50:257, 1967.
6. Baumgartner, H. R., Muggli, R., Tschopp, T. B., and Turitto, V. T.: Platelet adhesion, release and aggregation in flowing blood: Effects of surface properties and platelet function. *Thromb. Haemost.* 35:124, 1976.
7. Baumgartner, H. R., and Handenschild, C.: Adhesion of platelets to subendothelium. *Ann. N.Y. Acad. Sci.* 201:22, 1972.
8. Baumgartner, H. R.: Platelet interaction with vascular structures. *Thromb. Diath. Haemorrh. (Suppl.)* 51:161, 1972.
9. Baumgartner, H. R.: Morphometric quantitation of adherence of platelets to an artificial surface and components of connective tissue. *Thromb. Diath. Haemorrh.* 60:39, 1974.

10. Baumgartner, H. R., Stemerman, M. B., and Spaet, T. H.: Adhesion of blood platelets to subendothelial surface: Distinct from adhesion to collagen. *Experientia* 27:283, 1971.

11. Stemerman, M. B., Baumgartner, H. R., and Spaet, T. H.: The subendothelial microfibril and platelet adhesion. *Lab. Invest.* 24:179, 1971.

12. Sakariassen, K. S., Bolhuis, P. A., and Sixma, J. J.: Adhesion of human blood platelets to human artery endothelium is mediated by factor VIII:VWF bound to subendothelium. *Nature* 279:636, 1979.

13. Weksler, B. B., and Nachman, R. L.: Platelets and atherosclerosis. *Am. J. Med.* 71:331, 1981.

14. Stebhens, W. E.: Reaction of venous endothelium to injury. *Lab. Invest.* 14:449, 1965.

15. Ashford, T. P., and Freiman, D. G.: Platelet aggregation at sites of minimal endothelial injury: An electron microscopic study. *Am. J. Pathol.* 53:599, 1968.

16. Poole, J. C. F., Sanders, A. G., and Florey, H. W.: The regeneration of aortic endothelium. *J. Pathol. Bacteriol.* 75:133, 1958.

17. Groves, H. M., Kinlough-Rathbone, R. L., Richardson, M., Moore, S., and Mustard, J. F.: Platelet interaction with damaged rabbit aorta. *Lab. Invest.* 40:194, 1979.

18. Williams, A. W., and Montgomery, G. L.: Chemical injury to arteries. *J. Pathol. Bacteriol.* 77:68, 1959.

19. Cotton, R. E., Harwood, T. R., and Wartman, W. B.: Regeneration of aortic endothelium. *J. Pathol. Bacteriol.* 81:175, 1961.

20. Astrup, P.: Carbon monoxide, smoking, and cardiovascular disease. *Circulation* 48:1167, 1973.

21. Morrison, A. D., Orci, I., Berwick, L., Perrelet, A., and Winegrad, A. I.: The effects of anoxia on the morphology and composite metabolism of the intact aortic intima-media preparation. *J. Clin. Invest.* 59:1027, 1977.

22. Asmussen, I., and Kjeldsen, K.: Intimal ultrastructure of human umbilical arteries. Observations on arteries from newborn children of smoking and nonsmoking mothers. *Circ. Res.* 36:579, 1975.

23. Harker, L. A., Ross, R., Slichter, S. J., and Scott, C. R.: Homocystine-induced arteriosclerosis. The role of endothelial cell injury and platelet response in its genesis. *J. Clin. Invest.* 58:731, 1976.

24. Mustard, J. F., Murphy, E. A., Rowsell, H. C., and Downie, H. G.: Factors influencing thrombus formation *in vivo*. *Am. J. Med.* 33:621, 1962.

25. Sawyer, P. N., Suckling, E. E., and Wesolowski, S. A.: Effect of small electric currents on intravascular thrombosis in the visualized rat mesentery. *Am. J. Physiol.* 198:1006, 1960.

26. Sawyer, P. N., Reardon, J. H., and Ogoniak, J. C.: Irreversible electrochemical precipitation of mammalian platelets and intravascular thrombosis. *Proc. Natl. Acad. Sci. U.S.A.* 53:200, 1965.

27. McGrath, J. M., and Stewart, G. J.: The effects of endotoxin on vascular endothelium. *J. Exp. Med.* 129:833, 1969.

28. Gaynor, E., Bouvier, C., and Spaet, T. H.: Vascular lesions: Possible pathogenetic basis of the generalized Shwartzman reaction. *Science* 170:986, 1970.

29. Gaynor, E.: The role of granulocytes in endotoxin-induced vascular injury. *Blood* 41:797, 1973.

30. Gerrity, R. G., Richardson, M., Caplan, B. A., Cade, J. F., Hirsh, J., and Schwartz, C. J.: Endotoxin-induced vascular injury and repair. II. Focal injury, en face morphology, [³H] thymidine uptake and circulating cells in the dog. *Exp. Mol. Pathol.* 24:59, 1976.

31. Robertson, H. R., Moore, J. R., and Mersereau, W. A.: Observations on thrombosis and endothelial repair following application of external pressure to a vein. *Can. J. Surg.* 3:5, 1959.

32. Bedford, R. F., and Wollman, H.: Complications of percutaneous radial-artery cannulation: An objective prospective study in man. *Anesthesiology* 38:228, 1973.

33. Duguid, J. B., and Robertson, W. B.: Mechanical factors in atherosclerosis. *Lancet* 1:1205, 1957.

34. Texon, M., Imparato, A., and Lord, J. W.: Hemodynamic concept of atherosclerosis: The experimental production of hemodynamic arterial disease. *Arch. Surg.* 80:47, 1960.

35. Karino, T., and Goldsmith, H. L.: Adhesion of human platelets to collagen on the walls distal to a tubular expansion. *Microvasc. Res.* 17:238, 1979.

36. Svendsen, E., and Jørgensen, L.: Intimal pits of aorta in rabbits: Imprints of vortices of blood flow? *Acta Pathol. Microbiol. Scand. (Section A)* 85:25, 1977.

37. Gertz, S. D., Uretsky, G., Wajnberg, R. S., Navot, N., and Gotsman, M. S.: Endothelial cell damage and thrombus formation after partial arterial constriction: Relevance to the role of coronary artery spasm in the pathogenesis of myocardial infarction. *Circulation* 63:476, 1981.

38. Turitto, V. T., and Baumgartner, H. R.: Platelet interaction with subendothelium in flowing rabbit blood: Effect of blood shear rate. *Microvasc. Res.* 17:38, 1979.

39. Jorgensen, L., Hovig, T., Korsell, H. C., and Mustard, J. F.: Adenosine diphosphate induced platelet aggregation and vascular injury in swine and rabbits. *Am. J. Pathol.* 61:161, 1970.

40. Mustard, J. F., Jorgensen, L., and Packham, M. A.: Formed elements as a source of vascular injury. *Thromb. Diath. Haemorrh. (Suppl.)* 40:137, 1970.

41. Nachman, R. L., and Weksler, B.: The platelet as an inflammatory cell. *Ann. N.Y. Acad. Sci.* 201:131, 1972.

42. Sacks, T., Moldow, C. F., Craddock, P. R., Bowers, T. K., and Jacob, H. S.: Oxygen radicals mediate endothelial cell damage by complement-stimulated granulocytes. An in vitro model of immune vascular damage. *J. Clin. Invest.* 61:1161, 1978.

43. Stewart, G. J., Ritchie, W. G. M., and Lynch, P. R.: Venous endothelial damage produced by massive sticking and emigration of leukocytes. *Am. J. Pathol.* 74:507, 1974.

44. Lerner, R. G., Goldstein, R., and Nelson, J. C.: Production of thromboplastin (tissue factor) and thrombin by polymorphonuclear leukocytes adhering to vein walls. *Thromb. Res.* 11:11, 1977.

45. Astrup, P., Kjeldsen, K., and Wanstrup, J.: Enhancing influence of carbon monoxide on the development of atheromatosis in cholesterol-fed rabbits. *J. Atheroscler. Res.* 7:343, 1967.

46. Whereat, A. F.: Is atherosclerosis a disorder of intramitochondrial respiration? *Ann. Intern. Med.* 73:125, 1970.

47. Duguid, J. B.: Thrombosis as a factor in the pathogenesis of coronary atherosclerosis. *J. Pathol. Bact.* 58:207, 1946.

48. Hand, R. A., and Chandler, A. B.: Atherosclerotic metamorphosis of autologous pulmonary thromboemboli in the rabbit. *Am. J. Pathol.* 40:469, 1962.

49. Mustard, J. F., Murphy, E. A., Rowsell, H. C., and Downie, H. G.: Platelets and atherosclerosis. *J. Atheroscler. Res.* 4:1, 1964.

50. Hirsh, J., and Dacie, J. V.: Persistent post-splenectomy thrombocytosis and thrombo-embolism. A consequence of continuing anemia. *Br. J. Haematol.* 12:44, 1966.

51. Wu, K. K., and Hoak, J. C.: Increased platelet aggregates in patients with transient ischemic attacks. *Stroke* 6:521, 1975.

52. Carvalho, A. C. A., Colman, R. W., and Lees, R. S.: Platelet function in hyperlipoproteinemia. *N. Engl. J. Med.* 290:434, 1974.

53. Simpson, K.: Shelter deaths from pulmonary embolism. *Lancet* 2:744, 1940.

54. Naide, M.: Prolonged television viewing as cause of venous and arterial thrombosis in legs. *JAMA* 165:681, 1957.

55. Nicolaides, A. N., Kakkar, V. V., Field, E. D., and Fish, P.: Optimal electrical stimulus for prevention of deep vein thrombosis. *Br. Med. J.* 3:756, 1972.

56. Wessler, S.: Studies in intravascular coagulation. III. The pathogenesis of serum-induced venous thrombosis. *J. Clin. Invest.* 34:647, 1955.

57. Stanton, J. R., Freis, E. D., and Wilkins, R. W.: The acceleration of linear flow in the deep veins of the lower extremities by local compression. *J. Clin. Invest.* 28:553, 1949.

58. McLachlin, A. D., McLachlin, J. A., Jory, T. A., and Rawling, E. G.: Venous stasis in the lower extremities. *Ann. Surg.* 152:673, 1960.

59. Poole, J. C. F., and French, J. E.: Thrombosis. *J. Atheroscler. Res.* 1:251, 1961.

60. Leonard, E. F.: The role of flow in thrombogenesis. *Bull. N.Y. Acad. Med.* 48:273, 1972.

61. Wessler, S., Reiner, L., Freiman, D. G., Reimer, S. M., and Lertzman, M.: Serum-induced thrombosis: Studies of its induction and evolution under controlled conditions *in vivo*. *Circulation* 20:864, 1959.

62. Wells, R. E.: Rheologic aspects of stasis in thrombus formation, in *Thrombosis*, edited by S. Sherry, K. M. Brinkhous, E. Genton, and

J. M. Stengle. National Academy of Sciences, Washington, D.C., 1969, p. 469.

63. Wilner, G. D., Nossal, H. L., and LeRoy, R. C.: Activation of Hageman factor by collagen. *J. Clin. Invest.* 47:2608, 1968.

64. Walsh, P. N.: Platelet coagulant activities and hemostasis: An hypothesis. *Blood* 43:597, 1974.

65. Astrup, T., Albrechtsen, O. K., Claassen, M., and Rasmussen, J.: Thromboplastic and fibrinolytic activity of the human aorta. *Circ. Res.* 7:969, 1959.

66. Kirk, J. E.: Thromboplastin activities of human arterial and venous tissues. *Proc. Soc. Exp. Biol. Med.* 109:890, 1962.

67. Zeldis, S. M., Nemerson, Y., Pitlick, F. A., and Lentz, T. L.: Tissue factor (thromboplastin): Localization to plasma membranes by peroxidase-conjugated antibodies. *Science* 175:766, 1972.

68. Niemitz, J.: Coagulant activity of leukocytes: Tissue factor activity. *J. Clin. Invest.* 51:307, 1972.

69. Niemitz, L. P., and Fani, K.: Thrombogenic activity of leukocytes. *Blood* 42:47, 1973.

70. Williams, W. J.: The tissue factor system and its possible role in thrombosis, in *Thrombosis*, edited by S. Sherry, K. M. Brinkhous, E. Genton, and J. M. Stengle. National Academy of Sciences, Washington, D.C., 1969, p. 345.

71. Zwaal, R. F. A.: Membrane and lipid involvement in blood coagulation. *Biochim. Biophys. Acta* 515:163, 1978.

72. Bloom, A. L., Giddings, J. C., and Willes, C. J.: Factor VIII on the vascular intima: Possible importance in haemostasis and thrombosis. *Nature (New Biol.)* 241:217, 1973.

73. Fresh, J. W., Ferguson, J. H., and Lewis, J. H.: Blood clotting studies in parturient women and the newborn. *Obstet. Gynecol.* 7:117, 1956.

74. Strauss, H. S., and Diamond, L. K.: Elevation of factor VIII (antihemophilic factor) during pregnancy in normal persons and in a patient with von Willebrand's disease. *N. Engl. J. Med.* 269:1251, 1963.

75. Egeberg, O., and Owren, P. A.: Oral contraception and blood coagulability. *Br. Med. J.* 1:220, 1963.

76. Gaston, L. W.: Studies on a family with an elevated plasma level of factor V (proaccelerin) and a tendency to thrombosis. *J. Pediatr.* 68:367, 1966.

77. Penick, G. O., Dejanov, I. I., Roberts, H. R., and Webster, W. P.: Elevation of factor VIII in hypercoagulable states. *Thromb. Diath. Haemorrh. (Suppl.)* 20:39, 1966.

78. Blatt, P. M., Lundblad, R. L., Kingdon, H. S., McLean, G., and Roberts, H. R.: Thrombogenic materials in prothrombin complex concentrates. *Ann. Intern. Med.* 81:766, 1974.

79. Gitel, S. N., Stephenson, R. C., and Wessler, S.: In vitro and in vivo correlation of clotting protease activity: Effect of heparin. *Proc. Natl. Acad. Sci. U.S.A.* 74:3028, 1977.

80. Harker, L. A., and Slichter, S. J.: Platelet and fibrinogen consumption in man. *N. Engl. J. Med.* 287:999, 1972.

81. Poole, J. C. F.: Fats and blood coagulation. *Br. Med. Bull.* 14:253, 1958.

82. Barton, P. G., Yin, E. T., and Wessler, S.: Reactions of activated factor X-phosphatide mixtures *in vitro* and *in vivo*. *J. Lipid Res.* 11:87, 1970.

83. Connor, W. E., Hoak, J. C., and Warner, E. D.: The role of lipids in thrombosis. *Thromb. Diath. Haemorrh. (Suppl.)* 21:193, 1966.

84. Connor, W. E.: The acceleration of thrombus formation by certain fatty acids. *J. Clin. Invest.* 41:1199, 1962.

85. Margolis, J.: Activation of Hageman factor by saturated fatty acids. *Aust. J. Exp. Biol. Med. Sci.* 40:505, 1962.

86. Botti, R. E., and Ratnoff, O. D.: The clot-promoting effect of soaps of long-chain saturated fatty acids. *J. Clin. Invest.* 42:1569, 1963.

87. Hoak, J. C., Warner, E. D., and Connor, W. E.: Platelets, fatty acids, and thrombosis. *Circ. Res.* 20:11, 1967.

88. Connor, W. E., Hoak, J. C., and Warner, E. D.: Massive thrombosis produced by fatty acid infusion. *J. Clin. Invest.* 42:860, 1963.

89. Silver, M. J., et al.: Arachidonic acid causes sudden death in rabbits. *Science* 183:1085, 1974.

90. Hoak, J. C., and Robinson, D. S.: Thrombosis associated with mobilization of fatty acids. *Am. J. Pathol.* 43:987, 1963.

91. Koszewski, B. J., and Vahabzadeh, H.: Hypercoagulability syndrome due to heparin co-factor deficiency: A case report and review of the literature. *Thromb. Diath. Haemorrh.* 11:485, 1964.

92. Egeberg, O.: Inherited antithrombin deficiency causing thrombophilia. *Thromb. Diath. Haemorrh.* 13:516, 1965.

93. Marcinick, E., Farley, C. H., and DeSimone, P. A.: Familial thrombosis due to antithrombin III deficiency. *Blood* 43:219, 1974.

94. Sas, G., Blaskó, G., Bánhegyi, P., Jákó, J., and Pálos, L. A.: Abnormal antithrombin III (antithrombin III "Budapest") as a cause of familial thrombophilia. *Thromb. Diath. Haemorrh.* 32:105, 1974.

95. Nilsson, I. M., Krook, H., Sternby, N.-H., Söderberg, E., and Söderström, N.: Severe thrombotic disease in a young man with bone marrow and skeletal changes and with a high content of an inhibitor in the fibrinolytic system. *Acta Med. Scand.* 169:323, 1961.

96. Brakman, P., Mohler, E. R., Jr., and Astrup, T.: A group of patients with impaired plasma fibrinolytic system and selective inhibition of tissue activator-induced fibrinolysis. *Scand. J. Haematol.* 3:389, 1966.

97. Mansfield, A. O.: Alteration in fibrinolysis associated with surgery and venous thrombosis. *Br. J. Surg.* 59:754, 1972.

98. Aoki, N., Moroi, M., Sakara, Y., Yoshida, N., and Matsuda, M.: Abnormal plasminogen. A hereditary molecular abnormality found in a patient with recurrent thrombosis. *J. Clin. Invest.* 61:1186, 1978.

99. Wohl, R. C., Summaria, L., and Robbins, K. C.: Physiological activation of the human fibrinolytic system. Isolation and characterization of human plasminogen variants, Chicago I and Chicago II. *J. Biol. Chem.* 254:9063, 1979.

100. Todd, A. S.: Fibrinolysis autographs. *Nature* 181:495, 1958.

101. Astrup, T.: Tissue activators of plasminogen. *Fed. Proc.* 25:42, 1966.

102. Warren, B. A.: Fibrinolytic activity of vascular endothelium. *Br. Med. Bull.* 25:52, 1966.

103. Ashford, T. P., Freiman, D. G., and Weinstein, M. C.: The role of the intrinsic fibrinolytic system in the prevention of stasis thrombosis in small veins. *Am. J. Pathol.* 52:1117, 1968.

104. Bergin, J. J.: The complications of therapy with epsilonaminocaproic acid. *Med. Clin. North Am.* 50:1669, 1966.

105. Bell, R. G.: Metabolism of vitamin K and prothrombin synthesis: Anticoagulants and the vitamin K-epoxide cycle. *Fed. Proc.* 37:2599, 1978.

106. Stenflo, J.: A new vitamin K–dependent protein. Purification from bovine plasma and preliminary characterization. *J. Biol. Chem.* 251:355, 1976.

107. Esmon, C. T., Stenflo, J., Suttie, J. W., and Jackson, C. M.: A new vitamin K–dependent protein. A phospholipid-binding zymogen of serine esterase. *J. Biol. Chem.* 251:3052, 1976.

108. Kisiel, W.: Human plasma protein C. Isolation, characterization, and mechanism of activation by α-thrombin. *J. Clin. Invest.* 64:761, 1979.

109. Walker, F. J.: Regulation of activated protein C by a new protein. A possible function for bovine protein S. *J. Biol. Chem.* 255:5521, 1980.

110. Walker, F. J.: Regulation of activated protein C by protein S. The role of phospholipid in factor Va inactivation. *J. Biol. Chem.* 256:11128, 1981.

111. Esmon, C. T., and Whyte, G. O.: Identification of an endothelial cell cofactor for thrombin-catalyzed activation of protein C. *Proc. Natl. Acad. Sci. U.S.A.* 78:2249, 1981.

112. Poller, L., Thomson, J. M., Sear, C. H. J., and Thomas, W.: Identification of a congenital defect of factor VII in a colony of beagle dogs: The clinical use of the plasma. *J. Clin. Pathol.* 24:626, 1971.

113. Latallo, Z. S., Thomson, J. M., and Poller, L.: An evaluation of chromogenic substrates in the control of oral anticoagulant therapy. *Br. J. Haematol.* 47:307, 1981.

114. Kelton, J. G., and Hirsh, J.: Bleeding associated with antithrombotic therapy. *Semin. Hematol.* 17:259, 1980.

115. Boekhout-Mussert, M. J., van der Kolk-Schaap. P. J., Hermans, J., and Loeliger, E. A.: Prospective double-blind clinical trial of bovine, human, and rabbit thromboplastins in monitoring long-term oral anticoagulation. *Am. J. Clin. Pathol.* 75:297, 1981.

116. Loeliger, E. A., and Lewis, S. M.: Progress in laboratory control of oral anticoagulants. *Lancet* 2:318, 1982.

117. Aggeler, P. M., and Kosmin, M.: Anticoagulant prophylaxis and treatment of venous embolic disease, in *Thrombosis*, edited by S. Sherry, K. M. Brinkhous, E. Genton, and J. M. Stengle. National Academy of Sciences, Washington, D.C., 1969, p. 639.

118. Italian C.I.S.M.E.L. Study Group: Multicenter evaluation of a new chromogenic factor X assay in plasma of patients on oral anticoagulants. *Thromb. Res.* 19:493, 1980.

119. Avvisati, G., ten Cate, J. W., van Wijk, E. M., Kahlé, L. H., and Mariani, G.: Evaluation of a new chromogenic assay for factor VII and its application in patients on oral anticoagulant treatment. *Br. J. Haematol.* 45:343, 1980.

120. Kelly, J. C., and O'Malley, K. O.: Clinical pharmacokinetics of oral anticoagulants. *Clin. Pharmacokinet.* 4:1, 1979.

121. O'Reilly, R. A., Aggeler, P. M., and Leong, L. S.: Studies on the coumarin anticoagulants: The pharmacodynamics of warfarin in man. *J. Clin. Invest.* 42:1542, 1963.

122. Breckenridge, A., and Orme, M.: Kinetics of warfarin absorption in man. *Clin. Pharmacol. Ther.* 14:955, 1973.

123. O'Reilly, R. A., Pool, J. G., and Aggeler, P. M.: Hereditary resistance to coumarin anticoagulant drugs in man and rat. *Ann. N.Y. Acad. Sci.* 151:913, 1968.

124. O'Reilly, R. A., Aggeler, P. M., Hoag, M. S., Leong, L. S., and Kropatkin, M. L.: Hereditary transmission of exceptional resistance to coumarin anticoagulant drugs: The first reported kindred. *N. Eng. J. Med.* 271:809, 1964.

125. O'Reilly, R. A.: The second reported kindred with hereditary resistance to oral anticoagulant drugs. *N. Engl. J. Med.* 282:1448, 1970.

126. O'Reilly, R. A., and Aggeler, P. M.: Coumarin anticoagulant drugs: Hereditary resistance in man. *Fed. Proc.* 24:1266, 1965.

127. Hermondson, M. A., Suttie, J. W., and Link, K. P.: Warfarin metabolism and vitamin K requirement in the warfarin-resistant rat. *Am. J. Physiol.* 217:1316, 1969.

128. Bell, R. G., and Caldwell, P. T.: Mechanism of warfarin resistance: Warfarin and the metabolism of vitamin K. *Biochemistry* 12:1759, 1973.

129. Zimmerman, A., and Matschiner, J. J.: Biochemical basis of hereditary resistance to warfarin in the rat. *Biochem. Pharmacol.* 23:1033, 1974.

130. Lewis, R. J., Spivack, M., and Spaet, T. H.: Warfarin resistance. *Am. J. Med.* 42:620, 1967.

131. Loeliger, E. A., van der Esch, B., Mattern, M. J., and Brabander, A. S.: Behavior of factors II, VII, IX, and X during long-term treatment with coumarin. *Thromb. Diath. Haemorrh.* 9:74, 1963.

132. Deykin, D., Wessler, S., and Reimer, S. M.: Evidence for an antithrombotic effect of Dicumarol. *Am. J. Physiol.* 199:1161, 1960.

133. Gitel, S. N., and Wessler, S.: The antithrombotic effects of warfarin and heparin following infusions of tissue thromboplastin in rabbits: Clinical implications. *J. Lab. Clin. Med.* 94:481, 1979.

134. Deykin, D.: Current status of anticoagulant therapy. *Am. J. Med.* 72:659, 1982.

135. Bynum, L. J., and Wilson, J. E.: Low-dose heparin therapy in the long-term management of venous thromboembolism. *Am. J. Med.* 67:553, 1979.

136. Coon, W. W., and Willis, P. W.: Recurrence of venous thromboembolism. *Surgery* 73:823, 1973.

137. Hull, R., et al.: Adjusted subcutaneous heparin versus warfarin sodium in the long-term treatment of venous thrombosis. *N. Engl. J. Med.* 306:189, 1982.

138. Hull, R. B., et al.: Warfarin sodium versus-low dose heparin in the long-term treatment of venous thrombosis. *N. Engl. J. Med.* 301:855, 1979.

139. Rogers, P. H., and Sherry, S.: Current status of antithrombotic therapy in cardiovascular disease. *Prog. Cardiovasc. Dis.* 19:235, 1976.

140. The Sixty Plus Reinfarction Study Research Group: A double-blind trial to assess long-term oral anticoagulant therapy in elderly patients after myocardial infarction. *Lancet* 2:989, 1980.

141. Mitchell, J. R. A.: Anticoagulants in coronary heart disease—Retrospect and prospect. *Lancet* 1:257, 1981.

142. O'Reilley, R. A., and Aggeler, P. M.: Studies on coumarin anticoagulant drugs: Initiation of warfarin therapy without a loading dose. *Circulation* 38:169, 1968.

143. Deykin, D.: Warfarin therapy. *N. Engl. J. Med.* 283:691, 801, 1970.

144. Koch-Weser, J., and Sellers, E. M.: Drug interactions with coumarin anticoagulants. *N. Engl. J. Med.* 285:487, 547, 1971.

145. Qureshi, G. D., Reinders, T. P., Swint, J. J., and Slate, M. B.: Ac-

quired warfarin resistance and weight-reducing diet. *Arch. Intern. Med.* 141:507, 1981.

146. Lee, M., and Schwartz, R. N.: Warfarin resistance and vitamin K. *Ann. Intern. Med.* 94:140, 1981.

147. Udall, J. A.: Human sources and absorption of vitamin K in relation to anticoagulant stability. *JAMA* 194:127, 1965.

148. Barnes, R. H., and Fiala, G.: Effects of the prevention of coprophagy in the rat. VI. Vitamin K. *J. Nutr.* 68:603, 1959.

149. Mant, M. J., Hirsch, J., Pineo, G. F., and Luke, K. H.: Prolonged prothrombin time and partial thromboplastin time in disseminated intravascular coagulation not due to deficiency of factors V and VIII. *Br. J. Haematol.* 24:725, 1973.

150. Klissel, A. P., and Pitsinger, B.: Hypoprothrombinemia secondary to antibiotic therapy and manifested by massive gastrointestinal hemorrhage. *Arch. Surg.* 96:266, 1968.

151. Robinson, D., Benjamin, D., and McCormick, J.: Interaction of warfarin and non-systemic gastrointestinal drugs. *Clin. Pharmacol. Ther.* 12:491, 1971.

152. Aggeler, P. M., and O'Reilly, R. A.: Effects of hepatobarbital on the response of bishydroxycoumarin in man. *J. Lab. Clin. Med.* 74:229, 1969.

153. O'Reilly, R. A.: Studies on the coumarin anticoagulant drugs: Interaction of human plasma albumin and warfarin sodium. *J. Clin. Invest.* 46:829, 1967.

154. Sellers, E. M., and Koch-Weser, J.: Kinetics and clinical importance of displacement of warfarin from albumin by acidic drugs. *Ann. N.Y. Acad. Sci.* 179:213, 1971.

155. O'Reilly, R. A.: The binding of sodium warfarin to plasma albumin and its displacement by phenylbutazone. *Ann. N.Y. Acad. Sci.* 226:293, 1973.

156. O'Reilly, R. A., Aggeler, P. M., Hoag, M. S., and Leong, L.: Studies on the coumarin anticoagulant drugs: The assay of warfarin and its biologic application. *Thromb. Diath. Haemorrh.* 8:82, 1962.

157. Aggeler, P. M., O'Reilly, R. A., Leong, L., and Kowitz, P. E.: Potentiation of the anticoagulant effect of warfarin by phenylbutazone. *N. Engl. J. Med.* 276:496, 1967.

158. O'Reilly, R. A., and Aggeler, P. M.: Phenylbutazone potentiation of anticoagulant effect: Fluorimetric assay of warfarin. *Proc. Soc. Exp. Biol. Med.* 128:1080, 1968.

159. Sellers, E. M., and Koch-Weser, J.: Potentiation of warfarin-induced hypoprothrombinemia by chloral hydrate. *N. Engl. J. Med.* 283:827, 1970.

160. Boston Cooperative Drug Surveillance Program: Interaction between chloral hydrate and warfarin. *N. Engl. J. Med.* 286:53, 1972.

161. Udall, J. A.: Warfarin-chloral hydrate interaction: Pharmacological activity and clinical significance. *Ann. Intern. Med.* 81:341, 1974.

162. Kleinman, P. D., and Griner, P. F.: Studies on the epidemiology of anticoagulant drug interactions. *Arch. Intern. Med.* 126:522, 1970.

163. Solomon, H. M., Schrogie, J. J., and Williams, D.: The displacement of phenylbutazone-^{14}C and warfarin-^{14}C from human albumin by various drugs and fatty acids. *Biochem. Pharmacol.* 17:143, 1968.

164. Anton, A.: The effects of disease, drugs, and dilution on the binding of sulfonamide in human plasma. *Clin. Pharmacol. Ther.* 9:561, 1968.

165. Ikeda, M., Conney, A. H., and Burns, J. J.: Stimulatory effect of phenobarbital and insecticides on warfarin metabolism in the rat. *J. Pharmacol. Exp. Ther.* 162:338, 1968.

166. Conney, A. H., and Burns, V.: Metabolic interactions among environmental chemicals and drugs. *Science* 178:576, 1972.

167. MacDonald, M. G., Robinson, D. S., Sylvester, D., and Jaffee, J. J.: The effects of phenobarbital, chloral betaine, and glutethimide administration on warfarin plasma levels and hypoprothrombinemic responses in man. *Clin. Pharmacol. Ther.* 10:80, 1969.

168. Udall, A.: Drug interference with warfarin therapy. *Clin. Med.* 77:20, 1970.

169. O'Reilly, R. A.: Interaction of chronic daily warfarin therapy and rifampin. *Ann. Intern. Med.* 83:506, 1975.

170. Christensen, L. K., and Skousted, L.: Inhibition of drug metabolism by chloramphenicol. *Lancet* 2:1397, 1969.

171. Vissell, E. S., Passananti, G. T., and Greene, F. E.: Impairment of drug metabolism in man by allopurinol and nortiptyline. *N. Engl. J. Med.* 283:1484, 1970.

172. Serlin, M. J., et al.: Cimetidine: interaction with oral anticoagulants in man. *Lancet* 2:317, 1979.

173. Breckenridge, A. M., et al.: Cimetidine increases the action of warfarin in man. *Brit. J. Clin. Pharmacol.* 8:392, 1979.

174. Hunninghake, D. B., and Azarnoff, D. L.: Drug interactions with warfarin. *Arch. Intern. Med.* 121:349, 1968.

175. Kristensen, M., and Hansen, J. M.: Accumulation of chlorpropamide caused by dicoumarol. *Acta Med. Scand.* 183:83, 1968.

176. Kristensen, M., and Hansen, J. M.: Potentiation of the tolbutamide effect by dicoumarol. *Diabetes* 16:211, 1967.

177. Hansen, J. M., Kristensen, M., and Skovsted, L.: Dicumarol-induced diphenylhydantoin intoxication. *Lancet* 2:265, 1966.

178. Solomon, H. M., and Schrogie, J. J.: Change in receptor site affinity: A proposed explanation for the potentiating effect of D-thyroxine on the anticoagulant response to warfarin. *Clin. Pharmacol. Ther.* 8:797, 1967.

179. O'Reilly, R. A., and Motley, C. H.: Racemic warfarin and trimethoprim-sulfamethoxazole interaction in humans. *Ann. Intern. Med.* 91:34, 1979.

180. Koch-Weser, J.: Quinidine-induced hypoprothrombinemic hemorrhage in patients on chronic warfarin therapy. *Ann. Intern. Med.* 68:511, 1968.

181. Shapiro, S.: Studies on prothrombin. VI. The effect of synthetic vitamin K on the prothrombinopenia induced by salicylate in man. *JAMA* 125:546, 1944.

182. Luton, E. F.: Carbon tetrachloride exposure during anticoagulant therapy. *JAMA* 194:1386, 1965.

183. Schrogie, J. J., Solomon, H. M., and Zieve, P. D.: Effect of oral contraceptives on vitamin K-dependent clotting activity. *Clin. Pharmacol. Ther.* 8:670, 1967.

184. Zucker, M. B., and Peterson, J.: Effect of acetylsalicylic acid, other non-steroidal and anti-inflammatory agents, and dipyridamole on human blood platelets. *J. Lab. Clin. Med.* 75:66, 1971.

185. Robinson, R. W., and LeBeau, R. J.: Platelet adhesiveness and aggregation with chlorophenoxyisobutyric ester. *Am. J. Med. Sci.* 253:76, 1967.

186. Scott, J. T., Porter, J. H., Lewis, S. M., and Dixon, A. St. J.: Studies of gastrointestinal bleeding caused by corticosteroids, salicylates, and other analgesics. *Q. J. Med.* 30:167, 1961.

187. Wanka, J., Jones, L. I., Wood, P. H. N., and Dixon, A. St. J.: Indomethacin in rheumatic diseases: A controlled clinical trial. *Ann. Rheum. Dis.* 23:218, 1964.

188. Mauer, F. F.: The toxic effects of phenylbutazone (Butazolidin): Review of the literature and report of the twenty-third death following its use. *N. Engl. J. Med.* 253:404, 1955.

189. Robinson, B. H. B., Hawkins, J. B., Ellis, J. B., and Robinson, M.: Decreased anticoagulant tolerance with oxymethalone. *Lancet* 2:1356, 1971.

190. Bernstein, D.: Drugs known to interact with coumarin-type anticoagulants—revised. *Drug. Intell. Clin. Pharmacol.* 8:172, 1974.

191. Stead, N., Kaplan, A. P., and Rosenberg, R. D.: Inhibition of activated factor XII by antithrombin-heparin cofactor. *J. Biol. Chem.* 251:6481, 1976.

192. Ratnoff, O. D., and Davie, E. W.: The activation of Christmas factor (factor IX) by activated plasma thromboplastin antecedent (activated factor XI). *Biochemistry* 1:677, 1962.

193. Rosenberg, R. D.: The effect of heparin on factor XIa and plasmin. *Thromb. Diath. Haemorrh.* 33:51, 1974.

194. Lundblad, R. L., and Davie, E. W.: The activation of antihemophilic factor (factor VIII) by activated Christmas factor (activated factor IX). *Biochemistry* 3:1720, 1964.

195. Biggs, R., Denson, K. W. E., Akman, N., Borrett, R., and Hadden, M.: Antithrombin III, antifactor Xa and heparin. *Br. J. Haematol.* 19:283, 1970.

196. Yin, E. T., Wessler, S., and Stoll, P. J.: Identity of plasma-activated factor X inhibitor with antithrombin III and heparin cofactor. *J. Biol. Chem.* 246:3712, 1971.

197. Blombäck, B.: Studies on the action of thrombic enzymes on bovine fibrinogen as measured by N-terminal analysis. *Ark. Kemi* 12:321, 1958.

198. Rosenberg, R. D., and Damus, P. S.: The purification and mechanism of action of human antithrombin-heparin cofactor. *J. Biol. Chem.* 248:6490, 1973.

199. Dvilansky, A., Britten, A. F. H., and Loewy, A. G.: Factor XIII assay by an isotope method. II. Heparin inhibition of factor XIII activation. *Thromb. Diath. Haemorrh.* 24:256, 1970.

200. Nader, H. B., McDuffie, N. M., and Dietrich, C. P.: Heparin fractionated by electrofocusing: Presence of 21 components of differing molecular weights. *Biochem. Biophys. Res. Commun.* 57:488, 1974.

201. Rodriguez, H. J., and Vanderwielen, A. J.: Molecular weight determination of commercial heparin sodium USP and its sterile solutions. *J. Pharm. Sci.* 68:588, 1979.

202. Lasker, S. E., and Stivala, S. S.: Physicochemical studies of fractionated bovine heparin. I. Some dilute solution properties. *Arch. Biochem. Biophys.* 115:360, 1966.

203. Lam, L. H., Silbert, J. E., and Rosenberg, R. D.: The separation of active and inactive forms of heparin. *Biochem. Biophys. Res. Commun.* 69:570, 1976.

204. Hook, M., Bjork, I., Hopwood, J., and Lindahl, U.: Anticoagulant activity of heparin. Separation of high-activity and low-activity species by affinity chromatography on immobilized antithrombin. *F.E.B.S. Lett.* 66:90, 1976.

205. Andersson, L.-O., Barrowcliffe, T. W., Holmer, E., Johnson, E. A., and Sims, G. E. C.: Anticoagulant properties of heparin fractionated by affinity chromatography on matrix-bound antithrombin III and by gel filtration. *Thromb. Res.* 9:575, 1976.

206. Barrowcliffe, T. W., Johnson, E. A., Eggleton, C. A., and Thomas, D. P.: Anticoagulant activities of lung and mucous heparins. *Thromb. Res.* 12:27, 1978.

207. Lane, D. A., MacGregor, I. R., Michalski, R., and Kakkar, V. V.: Anticoagulant activities of four unfractionated and fractionated heparins. *Thromb. Res.* 12:257, 1978.

208. Salzman, E. W., et al.: Effect of heparin and heparin fractions on platelet aggregation. *J. Clin. Invest.* 65:64, 1980.

209. Nordenman, B., and Björk, I.: Fractionation of heparin by chromatography on immobilized thrombin. Correlation between the anticoagulant activity of the fractions and their content of heparin with high affinity for antithrombin. *Thromb. Res.* 19:711, 1980.

210. Holmer, E.: Anticoagulant properties of heparin and heparin fractions. *Scand. J. Haematol.* 25 (Suppl. 36):25, 1980.

211. Holmer, E., et al.: Anticoagulant activities and effects on platelets of a heparin fragment with high affinity for antithrombin. *Thromb. Res.* 18:861, 1980.

212. Carter, C. J., Kelton, J. G., Hirsh, J., and Gent, M.: Relationship between the antithrombotic and anticoagulant effects of low molecular weight heparin. *Thromb. Res.* 21:169, 1981.

213. Sache, E., Choay, J., and Fareed, J.: Studies on a highly potent anticoagulant anionic high molecular weight fraction isolated from porcine heparin. *Ann. N.Y. Acad. Sci.* 370:627, 1981.

214. Morrison, F. S., and Wurzel, H. A.: Retroperitoneal hemorrhage during heparin therapy. *Am. J. Cardiol.* 13:329, 1964.

215. Duff, I. F., Linman, J. W., and Birch, R.: The administration of heparin. *Surg. Gynecol. Obstet.* 93:343, 1951.

216. Salzman, E. W., Deykin, D., Shapiro, R. M., and Rosenberg, R.: Management of heparin therapy: Controlled prospective trial. *N. Engl. J. Med.* 292:1046, 1975.

217. Glazier, R. L., and Crowell, E. B.: Randomized prospective trial of continuous vs intermittent heparin therapy. *JAMA* 236:1365, 1976.

218. Wilson, J. E., Bynum, L. J., and Parkey, R. W.: Heparin therapy in venous thromboembolism. *Am. J. Med.* 70:808, 1981.

219. Wessler, S., and Gaston, Q. W.: Anticoagulant therapy in coronary artery disease. *Circulation* 34:856, 1966.

220. Gurewich, V., Thomas, D. P., and Stuart, R. K.: Some guidelines for heparin therapy of venous thromboembolic disease. *JAMA* 199:116, 1967.

221. Basu, D., Gallus, A., Hirsh, J., and Cade, J.: A prospective study of the value of monitoring heparin treatment with the activated partial thromboplastin time. *N. Engl. J. Med.* 287:324, 1972.

222. Thomas, D. P., Gurewich, V., and Ashford, T. P.: Platelet adherence

to thromboemboli in relation to the pathogenesis and treatment of pulmonary embolism. *N. Eng. J. Med.* 274:953, 1966.

223. Thomas, D. P.: The management of pulmonary embolic disease. *Am. J. Med. Sci.* 259:157, 1970.

224. Sharnoff, J. G., and DeBlasio, G.: Prevention of fatal postoperative thromboembolism by heparin prophylaxis. *Lancet* 2:1006, 1970.

225. Kakkar, V. V., et al.: Efficacy of low doses of heparin in the prevention of deep vein thrombosis after major surgery: A double-blind, randomized trial. *Lancet* 2:101, 1072.

226. Gallus, A. S., et al.: Small subcutaneous doses of heparin in prevention of venous thrombosis. *N. Eng. J. Med.* 288:545, 1973.

227. Kakkar, V. V.: Deep vein thrombosis: Detection and prevention. *Circulation* 51:8, 1975.

228. Prevention of fatal postoperative pulmonary embolism by low doses of heparin: An international multicentre trial. *Lancet* 2:45, 1975.

229. Handley, A. J.: Low-dose heparin after myocardial infarction. *Lancet* 2:623, 1972.

230. Thomas, D. P.: Heparin in prophylaxis and treatment of venous thromboembolism. *Semin. Hematol.* 15:1, 1978.

231. Gallus, A. S., et al.: Prevention of venous thrombosis with small, subcutaneous doses of heparin. *JAMA* 235:1980, 1976.

232. Kiil, J., Adelsen, F., Kiil, J., and Andersen, D.: Prophylaxis against postoperative pulmonary embolism and deep-vein thrombosis by low-dose heparin. *Lancet* 1:1115, 1978.

233. Kakkar, V. V.: Low-dose heparin—Present status and future trends. *Scand. J. Haematol.* 25 (Suppl. 36):158, 1980.

234. Mannucci, P. M., Citerio, L. E., and Panajotopoulos, N.: Low-dose heparin and deep-vein thrombosis after total hip replacement. *Thromb. Haemost.* 36:157, 1976.

235. Wessler, S., and Gitel, S. N.: Heparin: New concepts relevant to clinical use. *Blood* 53:525, 1979.

236. Kakkar, V. V., et al.: Prophylaxis for postoperative deep vein thrombosis. *JAMA* 241:39, 1979.

237. Vinazzer, H., Loew, D., Simma, W., and Brücke, P.: Prophylaxis of postoperative thromboembolism by low dose heparin and by acetylsalicylic acid given simultaneously. A double-blind study. *Thromb. Res.* 17:177, 1980.

238. Negus, D., et al.: Ultra-low dose intravenous heparin in the prevention of postoperative deep-vein thrombosis. *Lancet* 1:891, 1980.

239. Wray, R., Maurer, B., and Shillingford, J.: Anticoagulants in myocardial infarction. *N. Engl. J. Med.* 288:815, 1973.

240. Marciniak, E., and Gockerman, J. P.: Heparin-induced decrease in circulating antithrombin III. *Lancet* 2:581, 1977.

241. Struver, G. P., and Bittner, D. L.: The partial thromboplastin time (cephalin time) in anticoagulant therapy. *Am. J. Clin. Pathol.* 38:471, 1962.

242. Spector, J., and Corn, M.: Control of heparin therapy with activated partial thromboplastin times. *JAMA* 201:157, 1967.

243. MacAulay, M. A., Frisch, C. R., and Klionsky, B. L.: Relationship of the partial thromboplastin time to the Lee-White coagulation time. *Am. J. Clin. Pathol.* 50:403, 1968.

244. Blakely, J. A.: A rapid bedside method for the control of heparin therapy. *Can. Med. Assoc. J.* 99:1072, 1968.

245. Pitney, W. R., Pettit, J. C., and Armstrong, L.: Control of heparin therapy. *Br. Med. J.* 4:139, 1970.

246. Hoffmann, J. J. M. L., and Meulendijk, P. N.: Comparison of reagents for determining the activated partial thromboplastin time. *Thromb. Haemost.* 39:640, 1978.

247. Shapiro, G. A., Huntzinger, S. W., and Wilson, J. E., III: Variation among commercial activated partial thromboplastin time reagents in response to heparin. *Am. J. Clin. Pathol.* 67:477, 1977.

248. Bauer, G.: Clinical experience of a surgeon in the use of heparin. *Am. J. Cardiol.* 14:29, 1964.

249. Moser, K. M., and Hajjar, G. C.: Effect of heparin in the one-stage prothrombin time: Souce of artifactual "resistance" to prothrombinopenic therapy. *Ann. Intern. Med.* 66:1207, 1967.

250. Margulies, H., and Baker, N. W.: The coagulation time of blood in silicone tubes in patients receiving dicoumarol. *Am. J. Med. Sci.* 218:52, 1949.

251. Walker, A. M., and Jick, H.: Predictors of bleeding during heparin therapy. *JAMA* 244:1209, 1980.

252. Jick, H., Slone, D., Borda, I. T., and Shapiro, S.: Efficacy and toxicity of heparin in relation to age and sex. *N. Engl. J. Med.* 279:284, 1968.

253. Flesch, P.: Inhibition of keratinizing structures by systemic drugs. *Pharmacol. Rev.* 15:653, 1963.

254. Griffith, G. C., Nichols, G., Jr., Asher, J. D., and Flanagan, B.: Heparin osteoporosis. *JAMA* 193:91, 1965.

255. Robinson, H. J., and VanderVeer, J. B.: Dysesthesia pedis: A heparin reaction. *Arch. Intern. Med.* 111:153, 1963.

256. Turcotte, J. G., Kraft, R. O., and Fry, W. J.: Heparin reaction in patients with vascular disease. *Arch. Surg.* 90:375, 1965.

257. Koch-Weser, J.: Coumarin necrosis. *Ann. Intern. Med.* 68:1365, 1968.

258. Nalbandian, R. M., Beller, F. K., Kamp, A. L., Henry, R. L., and Wolf, P. L.: Coumarin necrosis of skin treated successfully with heparin. *Obstet. Gynecol.* 38:395, 1971.

259. DiCato, M.-A., and Ellman, L.: Coumadin®-induced necrosis of breast, disseminated intravascular coagulation, and hemolytic anemia. *Ann. Intern. Med.* 83:233, 1975.

260. Hirsh, J., Cade, J. F., and Gallus, A. S.: Fetal effects of coumadin administered during pregnancy. *Blood* 36:623, 1970.

261. Flessa, H. C., Kapstrom, A. B., Glueck, H. I., and Will, J. J.: Placental transport of heparin. *Am. J. Obstet. Gynec.* 93:570, 1965.

262. Hall, J. G., Pauli, R. M., and Wilson, K. M.: Maternal and fetal sequelae of anticoagulation during pregnancy. *Am. J. Med.* 68:122, 1980.

263. Stevenson, R. E., et al.: Hazards of oral anticoagulants during pregnancy. *JAMA* 243:1549, 1980.

264. Dinon, L. R., and VanderVeer, J. B.: Recurrent myocardial infarction after cessation of anticoagulant therapy. *Am. Heart J.* 60:6, 1960.

265. Sise, H. S., Moschos, C. B., Gauthier, J., and Becker, R.: The risk of interrupting long-term anticoagulant treatment: A rebound hypercoagulable state following hemorrhage. *Circulation* 24:1137, 1961.

266. Michaels, L.: Incidence of thromboembolism after stopping anticoagulant therapy: Relationship to hemorrhage at the time of termination. *JAMA* 215:595, 1971.

267. Reid, H. A., Thean, P. C., Chan, K. E., and Baharom, A. R.: Clinical effects of bites by Malayan viper (*Ancistrodon rhodostoma*). *Lancet* 1:617, 1963.

268. Reid, H. A., Chan, K. E., and Thean, P. C.: Prolonged coagulation defect (defibrination syndrome) in Malayan viper bite. *Lancet* 1:621, 1963.

269. Regoeczi, E., Gergely, J., and McFarlane, A. S.: *In vivo* effects of *Agkistrodon rhodostoma* venom: Studies with fibrinogen-^{131}I. *J. Clin. Invest.* 45:1202, 1966.

270. Esnouf, M. P., and Tunnah, G. W.: The isolation and properties of the thrombin-like activity from *Ancistrodon rhodostoma* venom. *Br. J. Haematol.* 13:581, 1967.

271. Kwaan, H. C., and Barlow, G. H.: The mechanism of action of Arvin and reptilase. *Thromb. Diath. Haemorrh.* 47 (Suppl.):361, 1971.

272. Chan, K. E., Rizza, C. R., and Henderson, M. P.: A study of the coagulant properties of Malayan pit-viper venom. *Br. J. Haematol.* 11:646, 1965.

273. Schwartz, M. L., Pizzo, S. V., Hill, R. L., and McKee, P. A.: Human factor XIII from plasma and platelets: Molecular weights, subunit structures, proteolytic activation, and cross-linking of fibrinogen and fibrin. *J. Biol. Chem.* 248:1395, 1973.

274. Ashford, A., Ross, J. W., and Southgate, P.: Pharmacology and toxicology of a defibrinating substance from Malayan pit-viper venom. *Lancet* 1:486, 1968.

275. Bell, W. R., Pitney, W. R., and Goodwin, J. F.: Therapeutic defibrination in the treatment of thrombotic disease. *Lancet* 1:490, 1968.

276. Sharp, A. A., Warren, B. A., Paxton, A. M., and Allington, M. J.: Anticoagulant therapy with a purified fraction of Malayan pit-viper venom. *Lancet* 1:493, 1968.

277. Latallo, Z. S.: Report of the task force on clinical use of snake venom enzymes. *Thromb. Haemost.* 39:768, 1978.

278. Barrie, W. W., Wood, E. H., Crumlish, P., Forbes, C. D., and Prentice, C. R. M.: Low-dosage ancrod for prevention of thrombotic complications after surgery for fractured neck of femur. *Br. Med. J.* 4:130, 1974.

279. Lowe, G. D. O., Campbell, A. F., Meek, D. R., Forbes, C. D., Prentice, C. R. M., and Cummings, S. W.: Subcutaneous ancrod in

prevention of deep-vein thrombosis after operation for fractured neck of femur. *Lancet* 2:698, 1978.

280. Lewis, L. J., Martin, D. L., Buckner, S., Finley, R., Lazer, L., and Feder, E. J.: Studies on type specific immunity to the whole venom and a fraction of *Agkistrodon rhodostoma*. *Res. Commun. Chem. Pathol. Pharmacol.* 2:649, 1971.

281. Olsson, P., Blomback, M., Egberg, N., and Ekestrom S.: Experience of extensive vascular surgery on defibrase-defibrinogentated patients. *Thromb. Res.* 9:277, 1976.

282. Born, G. V. R.: Strong inhibition by 2-chloroadenosine of the aggregation of blood platelets by adenosine diphosphate. *Nature* 202:95, 1964.

283. O'Brien, J. R.: A comparison of platelet aggregation produced by seven compounds and a comparison of their inhibitors. *J. Clin. Pathol.* 17:275, 1964.

284. Born, G. V. R., Honour, A. J., and Mitchell, J. R. A.: Inhibition by adenosine and 2-choloradenosine in the formation and embolization of platelet thrombi. *Nature* 202:761, 1964.

285. Weiss, H. J., Aledort, L. M., and Kochwa, S.: The effects of salicylates on the hemostatic properties of platelets in man. *J. Clin. Invest.* 47:2169, 1968.

286. Weily, H. S., and Genton, E.: Altered platelet function in patients with prosthetic mitral valves: Effects of sulfinpyrazone therapy. *Circulation* 42:967, 1970.

287. Smythe, H. A., Ogryzlo, M. A., Murphy, E. A., and Mustard, J. F.: The effect of sulfinpyrazone (Anturane) on platelet economy and blood coagulation in man. *Can. Med. Assoc. J.* 92:818, 1965.

288. Harker, L. A., and Slichter, S. J.: Studies on platelet and fibrinogen kinetics in patients with prosthetic heart valves. *N. Engl. J. Med.* 283:1302, 1970.

289. Rifkin, P. L., and Zucker, M. B.: The effect of dipyridamole and RA 233 on human platelet function in vitro. *Thromb. Diath. Haemorrh.* 29:694, 1973.

290. Glynn, M. F., Murphy, E. A., and Mustard, J. F.: Effect of clofibrate on platelet economy in man. *Lancet* 2:447, 1967.

291. Carvalho, A. C. A., Colman, R. W., and Lees, R. S.: Clofibrate reversal of platelet hypersensitivity in hyperbetalipoproteinemia. *Circulation* 50:570, 1974.

292. Carbone, J. V., Furth, F. W., Scott, R., Jr., and Crosby, W. H.: An hemostatic defect associated with dextran infusion. *Proc. Soc. Exp. Biol. Med.* 85:101, 1954.

293. Bygdemann, S., and Eliasson, R.: Effect of dextrans on platelet adhesiveness and aggregation. *Scand. J. Clin. Lab. Invest.* 20:17, 1967.

294. Weiss, H. J.: The effect of clinical dextran on platelet aggregation, adhesion, and ADP release in man: In vivo and in vitro studies. *J. Lab. Clin. Med.* 69:37, 1967.

295. Wautier, J. L., and Caen, J. P.: Pharmacology of platelet-suppressive agents. *Semin. Thromb. Hemostas.* 5:293, 1979.

296. Fuster, V., and Chesebro, J. H.: Antithrombotic therapy: Role of platelet-inhibitor drugs. II. Pharmacologic effects of platelet-inhibitor drugs. *Mayo Clin. Proc.* 56:185, 1981.

297. Fuster, V., and Chesebro, J. H.: Antithrombotic therapy: Role of platelet-inhibitor drugs. III. Management of arterial thromboembolic and atherosclerotic disease. *Mayo Clin. Proc.* 56:265, 1981.

298. Salzman, E. W., Harris, W. H., and DeSanctis, R. W.: Reduction in venous thromboembolism by agents affecting platelet function. *N. Engl. J. Med.* 284:1287, 1971.

299. Harris, W. H., Salzman, E. W., Athanasoulis, C. A., Waltman, A. C., and DeSanctis, R. W.: Aspirin prophylaxis of venous thromboembolism after total hip replacement. *N. Engl. J. Med.* 297:1246, 1977.

300. McKenna, R., Bachmann, F., Kaushal, S. P., and Galante, J. O.: Thromboembolic disease in patients undergoing total knee replacement. *J. Bone Joint Surg. (AM.)* 58:928, 1976.

301. O'Brien, J. R., Tulevski, V., and Etherington, M.: Two in vivo studies comparing high and low aspirin dosage. *Lancet* 1:399, 1971.

302. Butterfield, W. J. H., and British Medical Research Council: Effect of aspirin on postoperative venous thrombosis. *Lancet* 2:441, 1972.

303. Browse, N. L., and Hall, J. H.: Effect of dipyridamole on the incidence of clinically detectable deep-vein thrombosis. *Lancet* 2:718, 1969.

304. Steele, P., Weily, H. S., and Genton, E.: Platelet survival and adhesiveness in recurrent venous thrombosis. *N. Engl. J. Med.* 288:1148, 1973.

305. Steele, P., Ellis, J., Jr., and Genton, E.: Effects of platelet suppressant, anticoagulant, and fibrinolytic therapy in patients with recurrent venous thrombosis. *Am. J. Med.* 64:441, 1978.

306. Kaeggi, A., Pineo, G. F., Shimizu, A., Trivedi, H., Hirsch, J., and Gent, M.: Arteriovenous-shunt thrombosis: Prevention by sulfinpyrazone. *N. Engl. J. Med.* 290:304, 1974.

307. Harter, H. R., et al.: Prevention of thrombosis in patients on hemodialysis by low-dose aspirin. *N. Engl. J. Med.* 301:577, 1979.

308. Sullivan, J. M., Harken, D. E., and Gorlin, R.: Pharmacological control of thromboembolic complications of cardiac-valve replacement. *N. Engl. J. Med.* 284:1391, 1972.

309. Weily, H. S., Steele, P. P., Davies, H., Pappas, G., and Genton, E.: Platelet survival in patients with substitute heart valves. *N. Engl. J. Med.* 290:534, 1974.

310. Dale, J., Myhre, E., Storstein, O., Stormorken, H., and Efskind, L.: Prevention of arterial thromboembolism with acetylsalicyclic acid: A controlled clinical study in patients with aortic ball valves. *Am. Heart J.* 94:101, 1977.

311. Altman, R., Boullon, F., Rouvier, J., Raca, R., de la Fuente, L., and Favaloro, R.: Aspirin and prophylaxis of thromboembolic complications in patients with substitute heart valves. *J. Thorac. Cardiovasc. Surg.* 72:127, 1976.

312. Harrison, M. J. G., Marshall, J., Meadows, J. C., and Russell, R. W. R.: Effect of aspirin in amaurosis fugax. *Lancet* 2:743, 1971.

313. Mundall, J., Quintero, P., von Kaulla, K. N., Harmon, R., and Austin, J.: Transient monocular blindness and increased platelet aggregability treated with aspirin. *Neurology* 22:280, 1972.

314. Dyken, M. L., Kollar, O. J., and Jones, F. H.: Differences in the occurrence of carotid transient ischemic attacks associated with antiplatelet aggregation therapy. *Stroke* 4:732, 1973.

315. Fields, W. S., Lemak, N. A., Frankowski, R. F., and Hardy, R. J.: Controlled trial of aspirin in cerebral ischemia. *Stroke* 8:301, 1977.

316. The Canadian Cooperative Study Group: A randomized trial of aspirin and sulfinpyrazone in threatened stroke. *N. Engl. J. Med.* 299:53, 1978.

317. Byer, J. A., and Easton, J. D.: Therapy of ischemic cerebrovascular disease. *Ann. Intern. Med.* 93:742, 1980.

318. Barnett, H. J. M.: Prevention of stroke. *Am. J. Med.* 69:803, 1980.

319. Evans, G. E.: Effects of drugs that suppress platelet surface interaction on incidence of amaurosis fugax and transient cerebral ischemia. *Surg. Forum* 23:239, 1972.

320. Acheson, J., Danta, G., and Hutchinson, E. C.: Controlled trial of dipyridamole in cerebral vascular disease. *Br. Med. J.* 1:614, 1969.

321. The Coronary Drug Project Research Group: Aspirin in coronary heart disease. *J. Chronic Dis.* 29:625, 1976.

322. Breddin, K., Loew, D., Lechner, K., Uberla, K., and Walter, E.: Secondary prevention of myocardial infarction: Comparison of acetylsalicyclic acid, phenprocoumon and placebo: A multicenter two-year prospective study. *Thromb. Haemost.* 41:225, 1979.

323. Elwood, P. C., et al.: A randomized controlled trial of acetyl salicylic acid in the secondary prevention of mortality from myocardial infarction. *Br. Med. J.* 1:436, 1974.

324. Elwood, P. C., and Sweetnam, P. M.: Aspirin and secondary mortality after myocardial infarction. *Lancet* 2:1313, 1979.

325. Aspirin Myocardial Infarction Study Research Group: A randomized, controlled trial of aspirin in persons recovered from myocardial infarction. *JAMA* 243:661, 1980.

326. The Persantine-Aspirin Reinfarction Study Research Group: Persantine and aspirin in coronary heart disease. *Circulation* 62:449, 1980.

327. The Anturane Reinfarction Trial Research Group: Sulfinpyrazone in the prevention of cardiac death after myocardial infarction. *N. Engl. J. Med.* 298:289, 1978.

328. The Anturane Reinfarction Trial Research Group: Sulfinpyrazone in the prevention of sudden death after myocardial infarction. *N. Engl. J. Med.* 302:250, 1980.

329. Five-year study by a group of physicians of the Newcastle upon Tyne region: Trial of clofibrate in the treatment of ischaemic heart disease. *Br. Med. J.* 4:767, 1971.

330. Report by a research committee of the Scottish Society of Physicians: Ischaemic heart disease: A secondary prevention trial using clofibrate. *Br. Med. J. 4:*775, 1971.

331. Krasno, L. R., and Kidera, G. J.: Clofibrate in coronary heart disease: Effect on morbidity and mortality. *JAMA 219:*845, 1972.

332. Turney, J. H., et al.: Platelet protection and heparin sparing with prostacyclin during regular dialysis therapy. *Lancet 2:*219, 1980.

333. Zusman, R. M., et al.: Hemodialysis using prostacyclin instead of heparin as the sole antithrombotic agent. *N. Engl. J. Med. 304:*934, 1981.

334. Longmore, D. B.: Experience with prostacyclin in cardiopulmonary bypass in dog and man. *Phil. Trans. Roy. Soc. Lond. 294:*399, 1981.

335. Giles, A. R., Nesheim, M. E., Hoogendoorn, H., Tracy, P. B., and Mann, K. G.: The coagulant-active phospholipid content is a major determinant of in vivo thrombogenicity of prothrombin complex (factor IX) concentrates in rabbits. *Blood 59:*401, 1982.

336. Rao, A. K., Guzzo, J., Niewiarowski, S., and Day, H. J.: Antithrombin III levels during heparin therapy. *Thrombosis Res. 24:*181, 1981.

PART NINE *Replacement therapy and marrow trans-plantation*

Immunologic principles

CHAPTER 161

Erythrocyte antigens and antibodies

ELOISE R. GIBLETT

The red cell alloantigens, representing over 300 serologically determined specificities, belong to a large number of blood group genetic systems with individual chromosomal loci. Only a few of these loci have been determined with near certainty: *Rh* (rhesus) and *Sc* (Sciana) are on the short arm of chromosome 1, and *Fy* (Duffy) is on its long arm. *MN* and *Ss* represent two tandem loci on chromosome 4, *ABO* is on the long arm of chromosome 9, and *Xg* is on the X chromosome, possibly accompanied by *Xk* [see Ref. 1 for a review]. The antigenic determinants called Chᵃ (or Chido) and Rgᵃ (or Rodgers) are located on the C4d fragment of the fourth component of complement, being produced by two tandem loci within the histocompatibility region of chromosome 6. The presence of these C4d antigens on normal red cells probably reflects continuous low-grade complement activation in vivo with subsequent cellular attachment of C4d [2–4].

The medical significance of the blood group antigens is associated mainly with transfusion reactions, tissue graft rejection, and hemolytic disease of the newborn. However, the fact that certain disease states are accompanied by anomalous red cell phenotypes strongly suggests that at least some of the molecules bearing the antigenic determinants are important for structural and physiological functions, including cell differentiation and membrane transport.

Red cell antigens and membrane components

Until recently, most information about red cell antigen biochemistry was obtained by analysis of secreted substances in body fluids. However, modern techniques have permitted studies of antigens extracted from red cells, and these studies, together with the great surge in knowledge about membrane structure (see Chap. 36), have led to the concepts diagrammed in Fig. 161-1.

The integral membrane proteins known as glycophorin A (or α), glycophorin B (or δ), and band 3 glycoprotein have peptides extending beyond the cell surface to which are attached large numbers of carbohydrate chains. Figure 161-1 shows the branched carbohydrate chains on band 3 protein that carry I, i, H, A, and

FIGURE 161-1 Diagram of blood group antigen-bearing molecules on the membrane of red cells, including both glycoproteins and glycosphingolipids. The terminal sugars determining specificities of H, A, and B are not shown; they are discussed in the text. The same is true of adsorbed Leᵃ and Leᵇ. Carbohydrate chains are omitted from the structures of glycophorin molecules (GP-A and GP-B) in order to show the amino acid substitutions associated with M, N, S, and s specificities. (Lux [101]; Blumenfield and Adamany [7]; Dahr et al. [10]; Watkins [19]; Marcus et al. [21]; Anstee [23].)

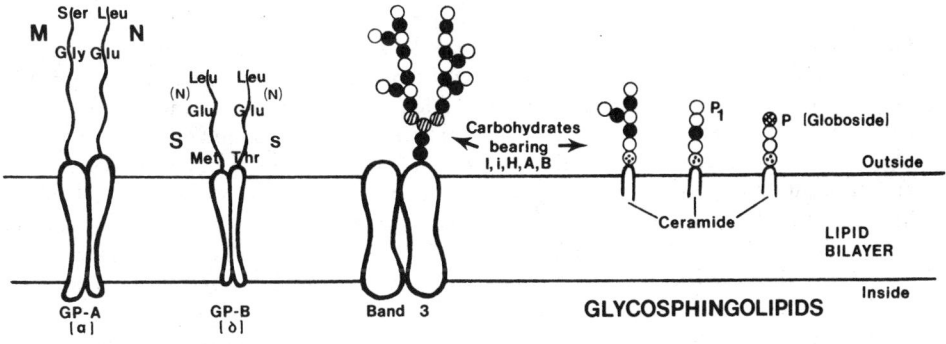

B antigenic specificities. The same specificities are present on glycosphingolipids attached to the lipid membrane by ceramide. In both instances, the carbohydrate chains vary considerably in complexity, the simplest being found on the cells of newborn infants [5]. Band 3 protein possibly also carries the major Rh determinant(s) as a part of the amino acid sequence of its exposed polypeptide chain [6].

Glycophorins A (GP-A) and B (GP-B) have an external sialoglycopeptide moiety. In Fig. 161-1, the large numbers of peptide-linked carbohydrate chains are not shown so that amino acid substitutions can be depicted clearly. In GP-A, the external amino acid sequence of the N terminus varies in two places: the peptides with serine at position 1 and glycine at position 5 carry M specificity, and those with leucine and glutamic acid in corresponding positions carry N specificity [7,8]. In GP-B, the first 25 amino acids are identical to those of GP-A with N specificity [9]. Moreover, in GP-B, residues 26 to 35 differ from those of GP-A and the presence of methionine or threonine at position 29 is said to determine the presence of S or s antigen activity, respectively [10].

In addition, there are glycosphingolipids that carry P system antigens (discussed in the appropriate section). One of these molecular species carries antigens P and P^k, and the other carries P_1. While there is a report that the Fy^a and Fy^b antigens are part of a membrane peptide [11], their protein carrier is unknown.

The serologic detection of blood group antigens

Red cell antigen-antibody interaction is most commonly detected by hemagglutination, using either manual or automated techniques. The most important factors influencing red cell agglutination are the immunoglobulin class of the antibody, the red cell surface, charge, and the distribution and mobility of the antigenic sites. Antibodies of the IgM class often cause agglutination because their pentameric structure provides the length necessary to bridge intercellular gaps. When there are very large numbers of antigen sites on the red cell (e.g., the A and B antigens), specific antibodies of the IgG class can also cause agglutination. However, IgG antibodies with other specificities usually fail to agglutinate red cells unless the negative surface charge is decreased or the antigen sites are brought together in clusters. Treatment of the cells with papain not only removes negatively charged sialopeptides but also causes clustering of antigen sites [12–14], thus facilitating agglutination by IgG antibodies. Addition of albumin may favor agglutination through reduction of the ζ potential [15].

Another way to demonstrate the reactions of IgG antibodies is to treat red cells with antiserum prepared in animals against human IgG. If IgG is present on the cell surface, agglutination occurs. This procedure is known as the antiglobulin (Coombs') test. Since some blood group antibodies fix complement components, antihuman complement can be similarly used to form a lattice of complement-coated cells.

Antibody neutralization tests are used for detecting soluble blood group antigens (such as H, A, B, Le^a, Le^b, Ii, Ch^a, or Rg^a) in body fluids or tissue extracts. Although there are a few exceptions, blood grouping antisera are usually derived from human sources. The antibodies in some blood group systems are characteristically "naturally occurring," i.e., occurring in the absence of exposure to blood from another person. In other systems, antibody formation is usually the result of blood transfusion or pregnancy. In the following discussion, the major blood group systems are divided on that basis into two classes. Fuller accounts of various aspects may be found elsewhere [16–23].

Blood group systems characterized by naturally occurring antibodies

ABO ANTIGENS AND ANTIBODIES

The ABO genetic system was the first to be discovered and remains the most important clinically because nearly all people produce anti-A and/or anti-B antibodies when their red cells lack the corresponding antigens. Absence of the expected antibodies is usually associated with some rare inherited subtype or with an abnormality such as hypogammaglobulinemia.

For routine purposes, red cell ABO typing is performed with two antisera: anti-A and anti-B. In addition, the individual's serum is tested against known A and B red cells, a procedure called *backtyping* or *reverse grouping*, to confirm the presence of the expected agglutinins in this system. Using these tests, the four phenotypes[1] listed in Table 161-1 are found in human populations.

Ideally, patients are transfused with blood of their own ABO type. However, because type AB is relatively rare (occurring in only 2 to 3 percent of many populations), it is not unusual to substitute blood of type A when large amounts of blood are required by AB recipients. The anti-B in type A donors is very rarely capable of destroying the recipient's AB red cells. However, it is preferable in such circumstances to remove most of the plasma and transfuse the packed red cells. Whenever it is necessary to substitute O donor blood for patients of type A, B, or AB, removal of the plasma is much more important because the anti-A and anti-B in the plasma of O donors have a greater potential for destroying the recipient's cells. The difference in reactivity is at least

---

[1] Descriptive characterization of any genetic trait is called a *phenotype* or, more simply, a *type*. However, it is common practice to refer to the ABO phenotype as a *blood group* and the phenotypes in other systems, particularly Rh, as *types*. In this chapter the term *blood group* is reserved for the individual genetic systems, and *type* and *phenotype* are used synonymously to denote serologically detected characteristics of all of the systems, including ABO.

TABLE 161-1   Routine ABO blood typing

Phenotype	Red cell reactions with antisera		Plasma (serum) reactions with red cells of A and B types	
	Anti-A	Anti-B	A	B
O	−	−	+	+
A	+	−	−	+
B	−	+	+	−
AB	+	+	−	−

partly due to the tendency of type O individuals to make IgG, as well as IgM, anti-A and anti-B [24]. Since IgG molecules can cross the placenta during pregnancy, this is also an important consideration in ABO hemolytic disease of the newborn; most cases occur in type A babies of type O mothers [25]. Similarly, most severe transfusion reactions occur in O patients given A, B, or AB blood. However, it is never acceptable medical practice to give A blood to B recipients, or vice versa, since IgM anti-A and anti-B in the recipient's plasma can cause significant red cell destruction.

It is occasionally useful to test red cells with a third antibody, called anti-A_1, to distinguish between A_1 and A_2 types. Cells reacting with both anti-A and anti-A_1 are designated A_1; if they react with anti-A but not anti-A_1, the phenotype is A_2. As shown in Table 161-2, serum of B and O phenotypes contains both anti-A and anti-A_1 antibodies. The "anti-A" used for general typing purposes is actually anti-A + A_1. Anti-A_1 is prepared either by absorbing type B serum with A_2 red cells or by making an extract of certain seeds which contain specific antibody-like substances called *lectins*. Use of anti-A_1 further divides the AB phenotype into A_1B and A_2B. Individuals with A_2 or A_2B types often form weakly reactive cold agglutinins with A_1 specificity, as indicated by the parentheses in Table 161-2. For transfusion, this antibody can generally be ignored.

Table 161-2 also shows the reactions of blood with the very rare O_h (Bombay) phenotype. Its most striking feature is the presence of potent anti-H, as well as anti-A and anti-B, in the plasma. Thus, if a patient of type O_h requires transfusion, the only compatible donors are people of the same rare type. Antibodies with H specifi-

city also occur as weak cold agglutinins, most commonly in people of types A_1 and A_1B, but these are not transfusion hazards.

Two variant phenotypes in the ABO system have special clinical importance. The first is an acquired characteristic found mainly in A_1 patients who develop acute or subacute leukemia [26]. When their red cells are tested with anti-A, only a portion are agglutinated. The unagglutinated cells readily give up anti-A upon elution, indicating a reduced antigen-antibody binding constant. The occurrence of this phenotype in a patient with apparent hypoplastic anemia is a grave prognostic sign. However, it must be differentiated from a similar inherited type, called A_3, which occurs in normal subjects.

The second clinically important variant represents acquisition by A_1 red cells of a weak B antigen not reactive with the anti-B in the patient's own serum. Most individuals with acquired B-like antigen are elderly patients with some form of intestinal malignant disorder. Several explanations have been offered to account for this condition, most of them relating to the action of bacterial enzymes. The phenotype must be distinguished from that of healthy individuals who inherit an unusual gene conferring both A and B specificities on red cells [reviewed in Ref. 27].

INTERACTIONS OF H, ABO, SECRETOR, AND LEWIS SYSTEMS

ABO AND Hh

Two separate genetic loci are involved in determining the presence of H, A, and B antigens on red cells. One

TABLE 161-2   More extensive ABO phenotyping

Phenotype	Red cell reactions with antisera				Plasma (serum) reactions with red cells of A_1, A_2, B, and O types			
	Anti-A	-A_1	-B	-H	A_1	A_2	B	O
O	−	−	−	+	+	+	+	−
A_1	+	+	−	w*	−	−	+	(+)†
A_2	+	−	−	+	(+)	−	+	−
B	−	−	+	w	+	+	−	−
A_1B	+	+	+	w	−	−	−	(+)
A_2B	+	−	+	+	(+)	−	−	−
O_h	−	−	−	−	+	+	+	+

*w = weakly reactive.
†Parentheses indicate the occasional presence in plasma of weakly reactive antibodies with the indicated specificity.

TABLE 161-3   ABO phenotypes and genotypes

Genotype	Phenotype	Phenotype frequencies, %*		
		White	Black	Oriental
A^1O, A^1A^1, A^1A^2	A_1	35	23	35
A^2O, A^2A^2	A_2	10	6	<1
BO, BB	B	8	17	23
A^1B	A_1B	3	3	12
A^2B	A_2B	1	1	<1
OO	O	43	50	30

*These frequencies are representative of U.S. blood donors classified into three quite heterogeneous ethnic groups on the basis of such criteria as color and name.

locus has two allelic genes, H and h; the other locus has four major alleles (disregarding rare variants); these are A^1, A^2, B, and O. The h and O gene products have no detected red cell antigen activity. The H gene has a very high frequency, so that hh homozygotes are extremely rare. These individuals have the O_h type (Bombay) described earlier. Because A and B antigens cannot be expressed when H is missing, type O_h red cells are unreactive with anti-A and anti-B, even when the A and B genes are present [28].

Table 161-3 shows the ABO phenotypes and their respective genotypes. Because the O gene has no active product, usual laboratory tests do not distinguish between the genotypes A^1A^1 and A^1O or between BB and BO. Also, the genotype A^1A^2 cannot be differentiated serologically. Thus, one can infer the genotype from only three phenotypes: A_1B, A_2B, and O. Table 161-3 also presents some typical phenotype frequencies among three ethnic groups living in the United States. Racial differences in gene frequencies are characteristic of nearly all the blood group systems [29].

SECRETOR AND LEWIS SYSTEMS

The ability to secrete water-soluble blood group substances with H, A, and B specificity is determined by a secretor gene called Se; its allele, se, has no known function. Another genetic locus, called Lewis, also affects the antigenic determinants of blood group substances. In this system, there are two major alleles, Le and le, and two major antigens, Le^a and Le^b. Lewis specificity (i.e., Le^a or Le^b) is determined by the Le gene as well as by the presence or absence of H and Se genes (see "Biochemical Explanation of H, A, B, and Lewis Genetics," below). Lewis antigens are not produced by red cells, but are adsorbed onto the cell surface as glycosphingolipids from the surrounding plasma [30]. The three main red cell phenotypes are Le(a+b−), Le(a−b+), and Le(a−b−), the last reflecting the lele genotype.

The plasma of newborn infants contains Lewis substances, but the development of Lewis-specific glycolipids probably lags behind that of Lewis-specific glycoproteins. Thus, the red cells of infants who inherit H, Le, and Se genes are usually Le(a−b−) at birth, becoming Le(a+b−) shortly thereafter. During the next several months of life, the cells react with both anti-Le^a and anti-Le^b, but the eventual phenotype is usually Le(a−b+) [31].

When Le(a+b−) red cells are transfused into an Le(a−b+) recipient, the donor cells take on Le^b specificity over a period of days as a result of the adsorption of glycosphingolipids [32]. These glycosphingolipids also carry A-like determinants, so that O cells transfused to an A recipient gradually become agglutinable by selected type O sera, but not by the usual anti-A typing sera [reviewed in Ref. 33].

The antigenic activity of the secreted blood group substances has been divided into four classes, shown in Table 161-4 [34]. The H activity of plasma glycolipids is not readily detectable, possibly because their chains have type 1 structure [35], as opposed to the type 2 structure on red cells [33]. Secretion of H, A, and/or B substance depends upon the presence of an Se gene (i.e., genotype SeSe or Sese). Nonsecretors of HAB (i.e., those with the sese genotype) who have an Le gene make only Le^a antigen, whereas the Le^b antigen depends upon the presence of H, Se, and Le genes. Homozygotes for the le gene make large amounts of H, A, and B, but no

TABLE 161-4   Gene combinations and their associated H, A, B, and Lewis antigen activities in secreted glycoproteins and in plasma glycosphingolipids

Class	Genes present	Antigenic activities				
		H	A	B	Le^a	Le^b
I	Se, H, AB, Le	++	++	++	+	+++
II.1	sese, H, AB, Le	−	−	−	+++	−
II.2	Se or sese, hh, AB, Le					
III	Se, H, AB, lele	+++	+++	+++	−	−
IV.1	sese, H, AB, lele					
IV.2	Se or sese, hh, AB, lele	−	−	−	−	−

NOTE: In this table, all four classes are shown to have A and B genes. When A and/or B genes are lacking, the respective antigenic activities are not expressed. In Classes I and II, adsorption of plasma glycolipid molecules give red cells the Lewis phenotypes Le(a−b+) and Le(a+b−), depending on the Le, H, and Se genes (see text).

SOURCE: Adapted from Watkins [19].

Le[a] or Le[b]. None of these antigens occur in the secretions of individuals who lack *Se* and *Le* genes or of those who have the rare O_h phenotype (i.e., *hh* homozygotes) and lack of an *Le* gene. These serologic findings combined with biochemical studies led to an understanding of how the gene products interact.

BIOCHEMICAL EXPLANATION OF H, A, B, AND LEWIS GENETICS

The *H, A, B,* and *Le* gene products are not the respective antigenic determinants but, rather, glycosyl transferases which transfer specific monosaccharides from their activating nucleotides (UDP or GDP) to specific acceptor molecules. The latter are short sugar chains (oligosaccharides) occurring independently or as part of glycoprotein or glycolipid molecules. The secreted glycoproteins are macromolecules containing many oligosaccharide chains of varying length with α-N-acetylgalactosamine (Gal-NAc) attached to either serine or threonine in a peptide "backbone" [34]. On red cell membranes, the protein-related carbohydrates with HAB activity are linked through N-acetylglucosamine to asparagine residues on band 3 glycoprotein [22]. The glycosphingolipids, intrinsic to red cells and certain other tissues but also present in the plasma, are composed of ceramide linked to a glucose residue and other sugars in chains varying in structure from simple to very complex [36]. The source of these glycolipids in plasma is unknown, but the liver is a likely candidate [11]. Since the carbohydrate moieties of both molecular classes (i.e., glycoproteins and glycolipids) act as acceptors of sugars from the *H, A, B,* and *Le* gene products, they can have the same H, A, B, and Lewis antigenic determinants. The glycosyl transferases involved in producing blood group substances are active in many tissues. About 20 percent of the *A* transferase in plasma apparently originates in the marrow [37]; the origin of the remainder is unknown [38].

As shown in Table 161-5, the *H* gene product is a fucosyl transferase which produces the H determinant by taking L-fucose (Fuc) from its GDP carrier and attaching it by α-(1→2) linkage to a D-galactose (Gal) residue at the end of a chain of sugars. In the blood group substances of body fluids, the galactose residue is

TABLE 161-5 Glycosyl transferase actions of *H, A, B,* and *Le* gene products and the resultant antigen specificities

Gene	Activated sugar	Acceptor substrate	Resulting structure	Antigen specificity
H	GDP-Fuc*	β-Gal-$\left(\begin{smallmatrix}1\to3\\ \text{or}\\ 1\to4\end{smallmatrix}\right)$-β-GlcNAc—R	β-Gal-$\left(\begin{smallmatrix}1\to3\\ \text{or}\\ 1\to4\end{smallmatrix}\right)$-β-GlcNAc—R ↑2 1 α-Fuc	H
A¹ or *A²*	UDP-GalNAc	β-Gal-$\left(\begin{smallmatrix}1\to3\\ \text{or}\\ 1\to4\end{smallmatrix}\right)$-β-GlcNAc—R ↑2 1 α-Fuc	α-GalNAc-(1→3)-β-Gal-$\left(\begin{smallmatrix}1\to3\\ \text{or}\\ 1\to4\end{smallmatrix}\right)$-β-GlcNAc—R ↑2 1 α-Fuc	A_1 or A_2
B	UDP-Gal	β-Gal-$\left(\begin{smallmatrix}1\to3\\ \text{or}\\ 1\to4\end{smallmatrix}\right)$-β-GlcNAc—R ↑2 1 α-Fuc	α-Gal-(1→3)-β-Gal-$\left(\begin{smallmatrix}1\to3\\ \text{or}\\ 1\to4\end{smallmatrix}\right)$-β-GlcNAc—R ↑2 1 α-Fuc	B
Le	GDP-Fuc	β-Gal-(1→3)-β-GlcNAc—R	β-Gal-(1→3)-β-GlcNAc—R ↑4 1 α-Fuc	Le[a]
Le	GDP-Fuc	β-Gal-(1→3)-β-GlcNAc—R ↑2 1 α-Fuc	β-Gal-(1→3)-β-GlcNAc—R ↑2 ↑4 1 1 α-Fuc α-Fuc	Le[b]

* Abbreviations: Gal = galactose, Glc = glucose, GalNAc = *N*-acetylgalactosamine, GlcNAc = *N*-acetylglucosamine; Fuc = fucose, R = remainder of the molecule, which can vary in the length and branching of the oligosaccharide chains as well as in the peptide or lipid carriers (see text).

joined by either β-$(1{\rightarrow}3)$ or β-$(1{\rightarrow}4)$ linkage to N-acetyl-D-glucosamine (GlcNAc). Chains with $(1{\rightarrow}3)$ linkage are classified as type 1 and those with $(1{\rightarrow}4)$ linkage as type 2. The oligosaccharide chains of glycolipids and glycoproteins intrinsic to the red cell have only type 2 chains [35]. The *O* gene product is a protein molecule which cross-reacts serologically with the *A* and *B* transferases but has little or no enzyme activity [39].

The H-determining fucose provides the conformation required for attachment of the A- and B-determining sugars by their respective gene products, a GalNAc transferase for A and Gal transferase for B [19]. The only difference between these two sugars is the occurrence of either an acetylated amino group (—NHCOCH$_3$) or a hydroxyl group (—OH) on the second carbon atom.

As noted earlier (Table 161-2), A_1 and B cells are poorly agglutinated by anti-H, while O and A_2 cells react strongly. The agglutination of A_2 cells by anti-H is best explained by the fact that the A^1 and A^2 transferases have different kinetic properties [37,40]. Although both enzymes transfer the same sugar (GalNAc) to the same acceptors, the A^1 transferase is much more active than the A^2 transferase. Presumably, the difference between A_1 and A_2 phenotypes is quantitative, the oligosaccharide chains of A_2 subjects having fewer terminal GalNAc residues than those of A_1 subjects [40,41] and thus a larger number of H reactive sites.

The *Le* gene product is also a fucosyl transferase which, like the *H* transferase, takes up Fuc from a GDP carrier, but attaches it by α-$(1{\rightarrow}4)$ linkage to the D-GlcNAc residue in type 1 chains only. Monofucosyl chains of this type have Le^a specificity. Presence of the Le-determining Fuc essentially blocks the *H* gene product from adding its Fuc [42]. However, if the H-determining Fuc is already in place, addition of the Le-determining Fuc creates a difucosyl structure with Le^b specificity.

Nearly all people have an *H* gene, but the presence of its fucosyl transferase in secretions is dependent upon the *Se* gene. The *Se* gene product is unknown; it appears to "switch on" *H* gene activity in secretory cells. About 20 percent of Western Europeans are homozygous for the inactive *se* allele (see Classes II.1 and IV.1 of Table 161-4). Although their red cells accurately express the inheritance of *H, A,* and *B* genes and their plasma contains the appropriate transferase [43], the *H* transferase is absent from their secretions, which also lack A and B as well as H antigens. The *Se* gene is not required for *Le* transferase production, so that in HAB nonsecretors with an *Le* gene (Class II.2), Le^a activity is found both in the secretions and in plasma and the phenotype is Le(a+b−). In *lele* individuals (Classes III and IV of Table 161-4), no Le^a or Le^b antigens are produced.

In HAB secretors with an *Le* gene (Class I in Table 161-4) the secretions and plasma contain Le^a and Le^b activity, but the red cell Lewis phenotype in adults is usually Le(a−b+) and only rarely Le(a+b+), reflecting the predominance of Le^b over Le^a in the plasma of persons with *Le* and *Se* genes. The Le^b difucosyl structure cannot be used as a GalNAc or Gal acceptor by *A* or *B* trans-

ferases [44,45]. The fact that some chains have both A or B and Le^b specificity is due to the ability of the *Le* transferase to attach its Fuc after the *H* and *A* or *B* transferases have added their specific sugars [19].

Absence of all HAB and Lewis antigens from secretions (Class IV of Table 161-4) is associated with lack of either *Se* and *Le* genes or (very rarely) *H* and *Le* genes. In the former case, there is no interference with the activity of *H, A,* and *B* transferases produced by red cell precursors. However, in individuals of Classes II.2 and IV.2 who lack an *H* gene (i.e., with the O$_h$ phenotype), none of the body cells (including erythroblasts) produce the H-determining fucosyl transferase and there is no detectable H antigen. Even though *A* and *B* transferases are produced, there are no H acceptors for their specific sugars [28].

LEWIS ANTIBODIES

Both anti-Le^a and anti-Le^b are naturally occurring antibodies, found most often in Le(a−b−) subjects of types A, B, and AB [46]. When anti-Le^b is found, it usually is accompanied by anti-Le^a or by other less well defined antibodies apparently related to the Lewis system [47]. Lewis antibodies are, with few exceptions, IgM and seem always to fix complement [16,48].

During pregnancy, the red cells tend to lose Lewis antigen reactivity and Lewis antibodies are frequently found in maternal serum [46]. However, there probably has never been a case of hemolytic disease of the newborn due to either anti-Le^a or anti-Le^b, because of their characteristic IgM class and because fetal red cells have very little adsorbed Lewis substance. Anti-Le^a is a potential transfusion hazard, but it is not a common cause of hemolytic reactions, since the plasma of Le(a+b−) donors generally contains sufficient Le^a substance to neutralize the patient's anti-Le^a, unless the latter has unusually high titer and avidity.

Some Lewis antibodies cross-react with antigens of the ABO system. For example, anti-A$_1$Le^b reacts only with cells from persons carrying the A^1, *Le,* and *Se* genes [49]. Such antibodies are IgM molecules and probably have little or no ability to destroy red cells. However, they are of interest because they can be used to detect A$_1$Le^b antigens on the O red cells of A$_1$Le(a−b+) patients who receive a marrow graft from a type O donor [50].

THE P SYSTEM

Naturally occurring antibodies to antigens in the P system occur quite commonly. Several gene loci are involved in determining the various P phenotypes.

Table 161-6 lists the five human P phenotypes, their frequencies, associated antigens, and the antibodies usually found in the plasma. Nearly everyone has either the P_1 or P_2 phenotype. People with p, P_1^k, and P_2^k phenotypes are very rare, but they create serious transfusion problems because their antibodies are usually potent hemolysins.

Table 161-7 shows that the P^k antigen is determined by a ceramide trihexoside, the sugar moiety consisting of Gal attached by α-$(1 \rightarrow 4)$ linkage to a second Gal linked by β-$(1 \rightarrow 4)$ to glucose [51–53]. The P^k antigen is present on all red cells except those of the p phenotype [54], but its detection in individuals of P_1 and P_2 types is more readily accomplished using fibroblasts than red cells [51,101]. The structure of P antigen corresponds to that of globoside, which is simply ceramide trihexoside with a terminal GalNAc attached to Gal by a β-$(1\rightarrow3)$ linkage. Thus, P^k is the precursor of P, in the same way that H is the precursor of A or B. Note that the glycosphingolipid with P_1 specificity does not resemble P^k or P, having a structure similar to that of B in the ABO system [52].

To explain the genetics of these findings, several theories have been proposed. The most likely is that there are three allelic genes: P^k, P^k_1, and p [53]. The first two are α-Gal transferases. Whereas the P^k gene converts ceramide dihexoside (CDH) to ceramide trihexoside (CTH), the P^k_1 gene converts CDH to CTH and also produces P_1 by attaching α-Gal to the paragloboside chain. The p gene is inactive, so that homozygotes have the p phenotype. This theory requires that a second unrelated locus have two allelic genes, one converting CTH to globoside and the other (rare) having no transferase function.

The anti-P_1 frequently found in the serum of people with P_2 phenotype is usually a weak cold agglutinin of no clinical importance. However, obtaining blood for patients of the p and P^k phenotypes usually necessitates calling upon a registry of donors with rare phenotypes.

In the syndrome paroxysmal cold hemoglobinuria, the so-called Donath-Landsteiner autoantibodies often have anti-P (presumably antigloboside) specificity [55]. These antibodies fix complement and cause red cell lysis.

THE MNSs SYSTEM

Of the four common antibodies in the MNSs system, anti-M and anti-N are frequently encountered as naturally occurring antibodies, where as anti-S (often) and anti-s (usually) require the stimulus of transfusion or pregnancy.

TABLE 161-6   Antigens and antibodies in the P system

Phenotype	RBC antigens	Serum antibodies	Phenotype frequency
P_1	P_1, P, P^k	None	About 75%
P_2	P, P^k	Anti-P_1 (often)	About 25%
P^k_1	P_1, P^k	Anti-P	
P^k_2	P^k	Anti-P	Very rare
p	None	Anti-P_1PP^k	

SOURCE: Adapted from Race and Sanger [17] and Naiki and Kato [101].

The antigens in this system are inherited as if they were determined by a single locus. In other words, MS, Ms, NS, and Ns are transmitted as single haplotypes from each parent (Table 161-8). The reason for this phenomenon was mentioned earlier, namely, that the genes for glycophorins A and B, which carry MN and Ss determinants, respectively, are very closely linked on the same chromosome. The amino acid substitutions underlying the antigenic specificities are shown in Fig. 161-1.

The behavior of some rare phenotypes in the MNSs system has recently been explained on the basis of either complete absence or marked changes in the glycophorin molecules. For example, GP-A is missing from the red cells of people with the rare En(a−) phenotype. As would be expected, En(a−) red cells do not react with anti-M, but they do react with anti-N owing to the presence of GP-B, which carries an N-reacting site as well as those for S or s [56,57]. Similarly, the red cells of U-negative subjects (who also lack S and s) have very abnormal GP-B molecules [58]. In another phenotype, called M^k, there is no M, N, S, s, or U activity, probably owing to the absence of both GP-A and GP-B [59]. Finally, in the Class V Miltenberger type, there is a hybrid protein with the amino terminus derived from GP-A and the carboxy terminus from GP-B, consistent with unequal

TABLE 161-7   Structure of human red cell glycosphingolipids with antigens related to the P system compared with structure of paragloboside and B in the ABO system

Name and antigen activity	Structure
Ceramide dihexoside (CDH); present in p phenotype	Gal $(\beta$-$1\rightarrow4)$ Glc-Cer
Ceramide trihexoside (CTH); P^k	Gal $(\alpha$-$1\rightarrow4)$ Gal $(\beta$-$1\rightarrow4)$ Glc-Cer
Globoside; P	GalNAc $(\beta$-$1\rightarrow3)$ Gal $(\alpha$-$1\rightarrow4)$ Gal $(\beta$-$1\rightarrow4)$ Glc-Cer
P_1	Gal $(\alpha$-$1\rightarrow4)$ Gal $(\beta$-$1\rightarrow4)$ GlcNAc $(\beta$-$1\rightarrow3)$ Gal $(\beta$-$1\rightarrow4)$ Glc-Cer
Paragloboside (I, H, A, B precursor)	Gal $(\beta$-$1\rightarrow4)$ GlcNAc $(\beta$-$1\rightarrow3)$ Gal $(\beta$-$1\rightarrow4)$ Glc-Cer
B (type 2 chain)	Gal $(\alpha$-$1\rightarrow3)$ Gal $(\beta$-$1\rightarrow4)$ GlcNAc $(\beta$-$1\rightarrow3)$ Gal $(\beta$-$1\rightarrow4)$ Glc-Cer

$$\uparrow 2$$
$$| 1$$
$$\alpha\text{-Fuc}$$

SOURCE: Adapted from Marcus et al. [21]. See also Fig. 16-1.

TABLE 161-8 Genotypes and phenotypes in the MNSs system

Genotypes	Phenotypes	White	Afro-American*
MS/MS	MS	6	3
MS/Ms	MSs	15	7
Ms/Ms	Ms	9	14
MS/NS	MNS	3	5
MS/Ns Ms/NS	MNSs	23	12
Ms/Ns	MNs	24	33
NS/NS	NS	1	1
NS/Ns	NSs	5	5
Ns/Ns	Ns	14	18

*The frequencies in this column total less than 100% because between 1 and 2% of Afro-Americans lack any of the alleles determining the S or s determinants.
SOURCE: Based on data of Race and Sanger [17].

crossing-over between tandem genes [60]. In all of the above-mentioned rare types, no evidence of hematological abnormality has been found.

In general, anti-M and anti-N antibodies are IgM molecules with little or no red cell destructive capability. A number of patients with renal disease undergoing hemodialysis for prolonged periods form cold agglutinins with anti-N specificity, regardless of the patient's MN phenotype and unrelated to the frequency of blood transfusion. The autoantibody in type N patients is thought to be a cause of graft rejection after renal transplantation when the donor kidney has been chilled [61].

Three antibodies in the MNSs system can cause severe red cell destruction. Anti-S is frequently found as a weak naturally occurring antibody, but many examples are not; anti-s and anti-U rarely occur without previous foreign red cell stimulation. Although anti-s and anti-U are IgG, they are, like anti-M and anti-N, cold-reactive [62]. Anti-U, found only in black people, behaves as if it were anti-Ss in that it reacts with all red cell specimens having S or s specificity; however, it also reacts with some cells which lack S and s [17]. Since nearly all white people are U-positive and only about 1 percent of black people are U-negative, finding compatible blood for patients with anti-U can be very difficult.

THE Ii SYSTEM
The genetics of the Ii system is poorly understood, and the biochemistry also unclear, although carbohydrate structures related to A and B are known to be involved [63,64]. According to current concepts, carbohydrate chain branching is essential for expression of I [22]. Both I and i are detectable on the red cells of nearly all persons, but to a highly variable degree. At birth and up to about 4 months of age, the red cells are strongly agglutinated by anti-i and weakly by anti-I. By age 2 or 3 years, the adult pattern has usually developed, with strong I and weak i expression [65]. Very rarely, normal people are homozygous for a gene associated with absence of I antigen [17]. This failure to switch from a fetal

to an adult characteristic is analogous to the hereditary persistence of fetal hemoglobin, but the mechanism depends on absence of genes which control the branching of carbohydrate chains [22]. In hypoplastic anemia and in certain diseases associated with ineffective erythropoiesis—especially thalassemia and hereditary erythroblastic multinuclearity with positive acidified serum (HEMPAS) [66]—the red cells react much more strongly than usual with anti-i while retaining their I activity [67,68]. Most human plasma contains an i-reactive glycoprotein, but the amount is not correlated with red cell i activity [69].

Both anti-I and anti-i have heterogeneous specificity [70–71]. In patients with autoimmune hemolytic anemia of the "cold" type, the autoagglutinins are usually anti-I or a mixture of anti-I and anti-i. These antibodies react with red cells at body temperature and cause lysis by complement fixation. However, most examples of anti-I and anti-i are clinically harmless, as indicated by their inability to agglutinate red cells in vitro at temperatures about 25 or 30°C.

The formation of anti-i unaccompanied by anti-I is associated with diseases involving lymphoid cells, particularly infectious mononucleosis. In some of these cases, the antibody is apparently IgG attached to red cells with more than the usual amount of i antigen, due to "marrow stress." When the serum also contains IgM anti-IgG molecules, the red cells may be lysed by the IgM-fixed complement [72].

Blood group systems characterized by alloantibody response to immunizing red cells

Many of the naturally occurring antibodies discussed in the previous section are IgM cold agglutinins having little capacity to destroy red cells in vivo. Blood group antibodies formed as the result of transfusion or pregnancy usually belong to the IgG class and react with their antigens at body temperature.

Since alloantibodies can be formed only by individuals who lack the corresponding antigens, a major factor determining alloantibody formation in response to foreign red cell exposure is the population distribution of the antigen. The second major factor is the immunogenicity of the antigen, reflecting such features as the number, conformation, and chemical nature of its determinant as well as the inherited and acquired susceptibility of the exposed individual. Attempts have been made to calculate the approximate risks of sensitization and subsequent transfusion hazards, taking into consideration the individual gene frequencies and observed occurrence of the corresponding antibodies in large populations [73–75] (Table 161-9). A similar assessment can be made for the relative risk of alloimmunization by pregnancy [75]. However, the risk in this situation is altered by the zygosity of the father, the nonrandomness of red cell antigen exposure (except in

TABLE 161-9   Risks of immunization and subsequent transfusion reaction when donors and recipients are matched only for their ABO types

Antigen	Blood group system	Immunogenicity, %*	Rate per 1000 transfusions	
			Immunized by first transfusion†	Reaction to second transfusion‡
D (Rh₀)	Rh	50.00	69.88	58.14
K	Kell	5.00	4.10	0.37
c (hr')	Rh	2.05	3.12	2.54
E (rh'')	Rh	1.69	3.45	0.99
k	Kell	1.50	0.03	0.03
e (hr")	Rh	0.56	0.13	0.13
Fy^a	Duffy	0.23	0.52	0.34
C (rh')	Rh	0.11	0.24	0.16
Jk^a	Kidd	0.07	0.13	0.10
S	MNSs	0.04	0.10	0.05
Jk^b	Kidd	0.03	0.06	0.04
s	MNSs	0.03	0.03	0.03

*Percent of patients lacking the antigen (in column 1) who would be expected to become immunized by a single transfusion of red cells containing that antigen.

†Number per 1000 recipients expected to be immunized by the antigen after a single transfusion of ABO-compatible blood from otherwise random donors. Calculated by multiplying immunogenicity × frequency of antigen-positive × frequency of antigen-negative × 10.

‡Calculated by multiplying the number immunized × the frequency of the antigen. The assumption is made that tests for serologic compatibility are not done.

SOURCE: Data of P. Sturgeon, in *Hematology*, edited by W. J. Williams et al., McGraw-Hill, New York, 1972.

women with many sexual partners), and the protection provided against alloimmunization when the maternal serum is ABO-incompatible with the red cells of the fetus [76].

THE Rh SYSTEM

The Rh system is highly complex, with a very large number of antigenic determinants and many peculiarities of inheritance and serologic behavior. Very little is known about Rh biochemistry, and thus genetic interpretations are based almost entirely on serologic observations. The number of chromosome 1 loci involved is a matter of controversy, and two of the nomenclature systems [17,77] reflect different interpretations of inheritance data. A third system [78] simply lists the antigenic determinants in numerical order (Table 161-10).

One complex genetic model has been proposed which suggests operators of tandem structural genes resembling a lambda phage operon [78]. For practical purposes, a simpler approach is to envision a single Rh region with multiple alleles determining the structure of a peptide component of the red cell membrane, possibly a part of band 3 protein. The multiple antigens determined by each of these alleles may represent amino acid substitutions at particular sites, analogous to those of the Gm and HLA allotypes. There is biochemical evidence for involvement of both protein and phospholipid in Rh antigen expression [6,79,80], and one report indicates that the difference between Rh-positive and Rh-negative red cells depends on the external or internal position of the antigenic determinant [6].

For convenience, this discussion will use the Fisher-Race terminology, the five major Rh determinants being called D, C, E, c, and e (see Table 161-10 for synonyms). The antithetical names Cc and Ee are used because in nearly all populations their genetic determinants behave as alleles, so that C and c or E and e are only very rarely inherited from the same parent. The D determinant has no known antithetical antigen, and so the designation d simply means the absence of D, at least on the red cell surface [6]. Absence of a d-specific antibody

TABLE 161-10   Names given to the antigenic determinants in the RH system in three different nomenclature systems: Ro. (Rosenfield et al.), F.-R. (Fisher-Race), and W. (Wiener)

Ro.	F.-R.	W.	Ro.	F.-R.	W.
Rh1	D	Rh₀	Rh18	....	Hr
Rh2	C	rh'	Rh19	....	hr^s
Rh3	E	rh''	Rh20	VS(e^s)	VS
Rh4	c	hr'	Rh21	C^G	
Rh5	e	hr''	Rh22	CE	
Rh6	f(ce)	hr	Rh23	D^w	
Rh7	Ce	rh$_i$	Rh24	E^T	
Rh8	C^w	rh^{w1}	Rh25	LW	
Rh9	C^x	rh^x	Rh26	....	
Rh10	V(ce^s)	hr^v	Rh27	cE	
Rh11	E^w	rh^{w2}	Rh28	....	hr^H
Rh12	G	rh^G	Rh29	....	
Rh13	....	Rh^A	Rh30	Go^a	
Rh14	....	Rh^B	Rh31	....	hr^B
Rh15	....	Rh^C	Rh32		
Rh16	....	Rh^D	Rh33		
Rh17	....	Hr₀			

SOURCE: Ro. from Rosenfield et al. [78]; F.-R. from Race and Sanger [17]; W. from Wiener [77].

TABLE 161-11 Eight Rh alleles and their major antigenic determinants and approximate frequencies in three ethnic groups

Allele	Antigenic determinants*			Approximate gene frequencies†		
	Ro.	F.-R.	W.	W. European	African	Oriental
R^1	1,2,5	D,C,e	Rh_0,rh′,hr″	0.45	0.10	0.55
r	4,5,6	c,e	hr′,hr″	0.37	0.15	0.10
R^2	1,3,4	D,c,E	Rh_0,hr′,rh″	0.14	0.10	0.35
R^0	1,4,5	D,c,e	Rh_0,hr′,hr″	0.02	0.60	Low
r″	3,4	c,E	hr′,rh″	0.01	Low	Low
r′	2,5	C,e	rh′,hr″	0.01	Low	Low
R^z	1,2,3	D,C,E	Rh_0,rh′,rh″	Low	Low	Low
r^y	2,3	C,E	rh′rh″	Low	Low	Low

*Nomenclature systems as in Table 161-10.
†A low frequency is less than 0.01.

complicates the determination of Rh genotypes: whenever D is inherited, it is difficult to determine whether the individual is homozygous or heterozygous for a D-determining gene. In the absence of family studies, it is necessary to resort to the "most probable" genotype, based on gene frequencies in populations. Depending largely on ethnic origin, the Rh determinants are inherited in certain patterns. For example, the most common Rh gene in most Caucasian populations determines expression of the antigens D, C, and e, and the next in order determines (d), c, and e. However, among most African peoples, the most common Rh gene determines D, c, and e, while the gene associated with D, C, and e is fairly unusual. Table 161-11 lists the best-known Rh genes and their respective antigenic determinants as they are named in the three nomenclature systems. The frequencies are given for the six most common genes in Western European populations. The frequency of any homozygous type is equal to the square of the gene frequency. The frequency of any heterozygous type is determined by doubling the product of the frequencies of the two genes involved. For example, in Western Europeans, the frequency of rr is $(0.37)^2$ and that of R^1r is $2(0.45 \times 0.37)$.

The number of D antigenic sites on red cells varies with the phenotype. According to one estimate [81], the phenotype CcDe (probable genotype R^1r) has only 10,000 to 14,000 D antigen sites per cell, whereas CcDEe (R^1R^2) has 23,000 to 31,000 and cDE (R^2R^2) has 16,000 to 33,000 sites. These sites appear to be dispersed at random on the membrane surface [82].

D (or Rh_0) is by far the most immunogenic of the antigens in this or any other blood group system requiring exposure to blood for antibody formation (Table 161-9). In populations of Western European origin, about 85 percent of people are Rh-positive (i.e., they are either homozygous or heterozygous for an Rh gene determining the D antigen). The 15 percent who do not have this antigen (i.e., those who are Rh-negative) have at least a 50 percent chance of forming anti-D in response to a single transfusion of Rh-positive blood and about an 80 percent chance after repeated stimulation [83]. For this

reason, blood of donors and patients is routinely typed with anti-D. Rh-positive blood should never be given to an Rh-negative premenopausal female, because if she later becomes pregnant with an Rh-positive child, there is a high risk that the infant will develop alloimmune hemolytic disease. In extreme situations, especially when excessive amounts of blood are required, it is sometimes necessary to transfuse unsensitized Rh-negative men or postmenopausal women with Rh-positive blood. However, once this is done, it can rarely be repeated because of the high rate of Rh sensitization. In immunosuppressed patients, the sensitization risk is much lower, but still exists.

The antigens C, c, E, and e are less immunogenic than D, and it is generally impractical to match these antigens in donors with those of blood recipients. However, once formed, all the Rh antibodies are potentially capable of destroying incompatible red cells in vivo and are frequently involved in anamnestic responses causing delayed transfusion reactions.

An Rh-negative person inadvertently transfused with Rh-positive blood can be protected against primary immunization by injection of Rh antibodies [83,84]. However, injections of Rh immune globulin are generally reserved for protecting Rh-negative mothers within 3 days after delivery of an Rh-positive infant [85]. The 3-day limit is based entirely on the experimental model used to prove the value of such treatment. It is quite likely that injection within 5 or even 7 days would also be an effective suppressant. Intramuscular injection of 300 μg of one of the commercial preparations is said to be sufficient to prevent 15 ml of Rh-positive red cells from initiating an immune response [84]. Leakage of as much as 15 ml of red cells during pregnancy and delivery is quite unusual; therefore the standard dose of 300 μg is nearly always enough. However, if the situation involves an Rh-negative patient receiving one or more pints of Rh-positive blood, the required amount of prophylactic anti-D is considerable, being equivalent to about 20 μg for each milliliter of Rh-positive red cells [84].

Some of the "quantitative" Rh variants are of clinical

interest. For example, cells with the D^u phenotype react more weakly than the usual D-positive cells, and their detection requires performance of the indirect antiglobulin test with anti-D selected for broad specificity against a range of D-like antigens. Donors with the D^u phenotype are considered to be Rh-positive because D^u (rarely) can stimulate anti-D formation in D-negative recipients. Patients with the D^u type can (also rarely) be stimulated by D-positive blood to form anti-D antibodies with a narrow specificity range. Thus, they are generally given blood from D-negative donors. Mothers of D^u phenotype are not candidates for prophylactic injection of Rh immune globulin.

Another Rh variant of interest to hematologists is the Rh_{null} phenotype, characterized by failure to react with any of the antibodies specific for Rh antigens or with the autoantibodies produced by many patients with the "warm" type of autoimmune hemolytic anemia. The genetic background of one kind of Rh_{null} is homozygosity for an allele at the Rh locus which has no serologically recognizable product [86]. In another kind of Rh_{null}, the individual inherits and transmits to offspring normally active Rh genes but is homozygous for an unlinked gene which suppresses Rh antigen expression [87]. Rh_{null} red cells have an undefined membrane defect associated with increased i antigen, stomatocytosis, spherocytosis, increased osmotic fragility, and hemolytic anemia [88,89]. The occurrence of this inherited defect provides evidence that the molecule bearing Rh determinants plays an important role in membrane structure [90].

THE KELL SYSTEM

The Kell system resembles the Rh system, having what appear to be four major sets of antithetical antigens: K and k, Kp^a and Kp^b, Js^a and Js^b, and Wk^a and Wk^b, one member of every pair being inherited from each parent. The genes determining k, Kp^b, Js^b, and Wk^b antigens are much more frequent than those determining their antithetical antigens. The Js^a antigen is common in blacks but very rare in other ethnic groups. Additional "para-Kell" antigens are also known to exist [17,91]. About 8 percent of Western Europeans carry the K antigen, which is highly immunogenic in the 92 percent of people who lack the K-determining gene. It is easy to find compatible blood for patients whose serum contains anti-K. However, when k-negative individuals form anti-k, the probability of finding a compatible blood donor among random persons of the same ABO type is about 1 in 500. The probability is even less when a patient has formed anti-Kp^b or anti-Js^b.

Two variant phenotypes of particular interest are K_0 and McLeod. These are characterized by very weak or absent expression of the Kell system antigens and the ability to form antibodies against red cells of all other Kell phenotypes [17]. The McLeod red cell phenotype occurs in a disproportionately large number of boys with the X-linked form of chronic granulomatous disease [92]. The granulocytes of children with this disease are believed to lack Kx, an X-linked Kell precursor which may or may not be missing from their red cells [93]. When these patients are transfused, they are very liable to form antibodies of such wide specificity that further transfusion is virtually impossible. Some people with the McLeod phenotype have normal white cell Kx, but their lack of red cell Kx is associated with acanthocytosis and variable anemia [94].

THE KIDD SYSTEM

There are only two major antigens in the Kidd system: Jk^a and Jk^b. These are determined by allelic genes, each having an average frequency of about 0.50. The major phenotypes are Jk(a+b−), Jk(a−b+), and Jk(a+b+). Nothing is known of their biochemical structure, but these antigens (especially Jk^a) are extremely important in blood transfusion. Their respective antibodies are characteristically transient and difficult to demonstrate serologically, even though they are capable of severe transfusion reactions associated with complement fixation, intravascular hemolysis, and serious renal damage. In some cases, the antibodies react in vitro only with cells from homozygotes, but heterozygote cells are destroyed rapidly after transfusion. There would certainly be some justification for employing Jk^a typing as a routine procedure in blood transfusion laboratories if sufficient antiserum were available. Unfortunately, most examples of anti-Jk^a either react weakly in vitro or lose their potency after relatively brief storage. Whenever a patient has a severe transfusion reaction with intravascular hemolysis not due to anti-A or anti-B, the first suspect should be anti-Jk^a, particularly if the compatibility test is negative or only weakly positive. The Kidd system antibodies are usually IgG, but they are often best detected by using an antiglobulin serum containing anticomplement or by treating the cells with a proteolytic enzyme before performing the anti-human globulin test.

THE DUFFY SYSTEM

The Duffy system is also serologically complex [17]. In white populations, it is nearly always sufficient to consider two major antigens: Fy^a and Fy^b, their respective alleles each having a frequency of about 0.50. The phenotypes are Fy(a+b−), Fy(a−b+), and Fy(a+b+). Among blacks there is a very common phenotype, Fy(a−b−), representing homozygosity for an allele not associated with production of Fy^a or Fy^b. The Fy(a−b−) phenotype protects red cells against parasitism by *Plasmodium vivax* [95]. This important observation provides a good explanation for the prevalence of the phenotype in West Africans, who are unusually resistant to vivax malaria. The possibility that the Duffy antigenic determinants are the red cell receptors for *P. vivax* provides a good clue that blood group antigens are functional. It is possible, for example, that such carbohydrate-determined antigens as H, A, B, I, M, N, and P may act as cell recognition sites, initiating such processes as secretion, cell differentiation, and growth [96].

Anti-Fy^a and anti-Fy^b are usually IgG, and some examples behave as treacherously as anti-Jk^a. However, the strength of their in vitro reactions in the antiglobulin test tends to parallel their in vivo hemolytic capability. Anti-Fy^a, like the antibodies in the Rh system, is known to cause "delayed" transfusion reactions due to an anamnestic rise in antibody titer 1 to 4 weeks after transfusion of cells that were originally compatible.

THE LUTHERAN SYSTEM

This system consists of a large number of antigens, some of which are antithetical [17,97]. The major antigens are Lu^a and Lu^b, with gene frequencies of about 0.02 and 0.98, respectively. In addition to the Lu(a+b−), Lu(a−b+), and Lu(a+b+) phenotypes, there is a very rare Lu(a−b−) type. One form of Lu(a−b−) is associated with dominant inheritance of an unlinked gene which inhibits the expression of Lutheran and certain other blood group antigens [98,99]. Individuals with the other form appear to be homozygous for an inactive allele at the *Lu* locus. Patients whose serum contains anti-Lu^a present no transfusion problems, because most donors are Lu(a−b+). However, finding blood for Lutheran-sensitized Lu(a+b−) or Lu(a−b−) patients necessitates calling upon a rare-blood depository. Most examples of anti-Lu^a are weakly reactive saline agglutinins, whereas anti-Lu^b is usually IgG, best detected by the antiglobulin technique.

THE Xg SYSTEM

The single antigen in this system, Xg^a, is very important to geneticists because the locus of its gene is on the X chromosome. However, it has minimal clinical importance and will not be discussed here. For an excellent summary, see Race and Sanger [17].

Other blood groups systems

Several of the 11 blood group systems described above have one or more rare phenotypes characterized by lack of a very common antigen, e.g., the O$_h$, p, U-negative, Rh$_{null}$, K$_o$, and Lu(a−b−) types. In some of these types, antibodies against the missing antigen regularly occur without exposure to another person's blood, while others require the stimulus of transfusion or pregnancy.

In several other systems, most of them less well defined, one gene has such a high frequency that only a small proportion of people are homozygous for its allelic gene. Some of these high-frequency antigens are Ve^a (Vel), Ge^a (Gerbich), Sd^a (Sid), Yk^a (York), Yt^a (Cartwright), Co^a (Colton), Ch^a (Chido), and Rg^a (Rodgers). Antibodies with corresponding specificities often show a wide range of activity when tested against a panel of red cell specimens, and selection of the most weakly reactive donor blood may be acceptable for transfusion, especially in emergencies.

Ch^a and Rg^a resemble A, B, Le^a, Le^b, and i in that they are detectable as soluble antigens in plasma. The identity of these two antigens as part of the C4d fragment of complement was noted earlier [2–4]. Red cells react variably with anti-Ch^a and anti-Rg^a, but the phenotype can be reliably determined by testing the plasma for hemagglutination inhibition. With this technique, about 2 percent of people lack one or the other of these antigens. Although such people are quite likely to be stimulated by transfusion to form anti-Ch^a or anti-Rg^a of the IgG class, these antibodies have not been found to cause significant red cell destruction. In transfusing subjects who have antibodies against these and several other high-frequency antigens, the major hazard lies in increasing their titer, thus masking the development of more dangerous antibodies with other specificities.

So-called private blood group antigens occur so rarely that they may be found in only one or two families when thousands are tested. An antigen of this kind can cause a laboratory problem when a newborn infant who has inherited the antigen from its father has a positive direct antiglobulin test and the mother's serum fails to react with the red cells used for screening purposes. In these cases, the father's cells must be used to detect the mother's antibody.

Risk of incompatibility in transfusion

Over 300 different antigens have been detected on human red cells, and a large proportion of them have been placed in the 21 blood group genetic systems currently considered to be established [17]. The frequencies of their corresponding alleles vary greatly, but there are several million possible phenotypes. Thus, when a patient is transfused with serologically compatible blood selected only on the basis of ABO and Rh(D) phenotype, the probability that the blood contains one or more antigens foreign to the patient is very high indeed. Fortunately, most red cell antigens are not very immunogenic, and the 12 antigens listed in Table 161-9 are responsible for stimulating most of the clinically significant antibodies which are not naturally occurring. Among the naturally occurring antibodies, anti-A and anti-B present a very serious transfusion hazard, but most of the others have little capability of destroying red cells [100].

There remains a "gray area" of antibodies which, in spite of being IgG, usually do not cause significant red cell destruction, perhaps because their corresponding antigens have fewer active sites or are "buried" by other membrane components. Although such antibodies are, in general, less dangerous than those discussed in the preceding paragraph, it is unsafe to make a blanket statement recommending that they be ignored. Caution, judgment, and experience are clearly necessary in making decisions about transfusing serologically incompatible blood. But, of course, the same prerequisites apply to *all* transfusions, compatible or otherwise.

References

1. Tippett, P.: Chromosomal mapping of the blood group genes. *Semin. Hematol.* 18:4, 1981.

2. O'Neill, G. J., Yang, S. Y., Tegoli, J., Berger, R., and DuPont, B.: Chido and Rodgers blood groups are distinct antigenic components of human complement C4. *Nature* 273:668, 1978.

3. Tilley, C. A., Romans, D. G., and Crookston, M. C.: Localization of Chido and Rodgers determinants to the C4d fragment of human C4. *Nature* 276:713, 1978.

4. Awdeh, Z. L., and Alper, C. A.: Inherited structural polymorphism of the fourth component of human complement. *Proc. Natl. Acad. Sci. U.S.A.* 77:3576, 1980.

5. Watanabe, K., and Hakomori, S.: Status of blood group carbohydrate chains in ontogenesis and in oncogenesis. *J. Exp. Med.* 144:644, 1976.

6. Plapp, F. V., Kowalski, M. M., Tilzer, L., Brown, P. J., Evans, J., and Chiga, M.: Partial purification of $Rh_o(D)$ from Rh positive and Rh negative erythrocytes. *Proc. Natl. Acad. Sci. U.S.A.* 76:2964, 1979.

7. Blumenfield, O. O., and Adamany, A. M.: Structural polymorphism within the amino-terminal region of MM, NN and MN glycoproteins (glycophorins) of the human erythrocyte membrane. *Proc. Natl. Acad. Sci. U.S.A.* 75:2727, 1978.

8. Lisowska, E., and Wasniowska, J.: Immunochemical characterization of cyanogen bromide degradation products of M and N blood group glycopeptides. *Eur. J. Biochem.* 88:247, 1978.

9. Furthmayr, H.: Structural comparison of glycophorins and immunochemical analysis of genetic variants. *Nature* 271:519, 1978.

10. Dahr, W., Beyreuther, K., Steinbach, H., Gielen, W., and Kruger, J.: Structure of the Ss blood group antigens. II. A methionine/threonine polymorphism within the N-terminal sequence of the Ss glycoprotein. *Z. Physiol. Chem.* 361:895, 1980.

11. Davies, D. M., Hall, S. J., Graham, H. A., and Chachowski, R.: The isolation and partial characterization of Duffy antigens from human red cells. *Transfusion* 19:638, 1979 (abstract).

12. Nicolson, G. L.: Anionic sites of human erythrocyte membranes. I. Effects of trypsin, phospholipase C and pH on the topography of bound positively charged colloidal particles. *J. Cell Biol.* 57:373, 1973.

13. Romano, E. L., Stolinski, C., and Hughes-Jones, N. C.: Distribution and mobility of the A, D and c antigens on human red cell membranes: Studies with a gold-labelled antiglobulin reagent. *Br. J. Haematol.* 30:507, 1975.

14. Victoria, E. J., Muchmore, E. A., Sudora, E. J., and Masouredis, S. P.: The role of antigen mobility in anti-$Rh_o(D)$-induced agglutination. *J. Clin. Invest.* 56:292, 1975.

15. Pollack, W., and Reckel, R.: The zeta potential and hemagglutination with Rh antibodies: A physiochemical explanation. *Int. Arch. Allergy Appl. Immunol.* 38:482, 1970.

16. Mollison, P. L.: *Blood Transfusion in Clinical Medicine,* 6th ed. Blackwell, Oxford, 1975.

17. Race, R. R., and Sanger, R.: *Blood Groups in Man,* 6th ed. Blackwell, Oxford, 1975.

18. Issitt, P. D., and Issitt, C. H.: *Applied Blood Group Serology,* 2d ed. Spectra Biologicals, Oxnard, Calif., 1975.

19. Watkins, W. M.: Biochemistry and genetics of the ABO, Lewis and P blood group systems, in *Advances in Human Genetics,* edited by H. Harris and K. Hirschhorn. Plenum, New York, 1980, vol. 10, p. 1.

20. Marcus, D. M.: The ABO and Lewis blood group systems. *N. Engl. J. Med.* 280:994, 1969.

21. Marcus, D. M., Kundu, S. K., and Suzuki, A.: The P blood group system: Recent progress in immunochemistry and genetics. *Semin. Hematol.* 18:63, 1981.

22. Hakomori, S.: Blood group ABH and Ii antigens of human erythrocytes: Chemistry, polymorphism, and their developmental changes. *Semin. Hematol.* 18:39, 1981.

23. Anstee, D. J.: The blood group MNSs-active sialoglycoproteins. *Semin. Hematol.* 18:13, 1981.

24. Kochwa, S., Rosenfield, R. E., Tallal, L., and Wasserman, L. R.: Isoagglutinins associated with erythroblastosis. *J. Clin. Invest.* 40:874, 1961.

25. Rosenfield, R. E.: A-B hemolytic disease of the newborn: Analysis of 1480 cord blood specimens, with special reference to the direct antiglobulin test and to the group O mother. *Blood* 10:17, 1955.

26. Salmon, C., André, R., and Dreyfus, B.: Existe-t-il des mutations somatiques du gène de groupe sanguin A au cours de certaines leucémies aiguës? *Rev. Fr. Etudes Clin. Biol.* 4:468, 1959.

27. Beattie, K. M.: Perspectives on some usual and unusual ABO phenotypes, in *A Seminar on Antigens on Blood Cells and Body Fluids,* edited by C. A. Bell. American Association of Blood Banks, Washington, D.C., 1980, p. 97.

28. Race, C., and Watkins, W. M.: The enzyme products of the human A and B blood group genes in the serum of "Bombay" O_h donors. *F.E.B.S. Lett.* 27:125, 1972.

29. Mourant, A. E., Kopec, A. C., and Domaniewska-Sobczak, K.: *The Distribution of the Human Blood Groups and Other Biochemical Polymorphisms,* 2d ed. Oxford University Press, New York, 1975.

30. Marcus, D. M., and Cass, L. E.: Glycosphingolipids with Lewis blood group activity: Uptake by human erythrocytes. *Science* 164:553, 1969.

31. Cutbush, M., Giblett, E. R., and Mollison, P. L.: Demonstration of the phenotype Le(a+b+) in infants and in adults. *Br. J. Haematol.* 2:210, 1956.

32. Mollison, P. L., Polley, M. J., and Crome, P.: Temporary suppression of Lewis blood group antibodies to permit incompatible transfusion. *Lancet* 1:909, 1963.

33. Crookston, M. C.: Blood group antigens acquired from the plasma, in *Immunobiology of the Erythrocyte,* edited by S. G. Sandler, J. Nusbacher, and M. S. Schanfield. Liss, New York, 1980, vol. 40, p. 99.

34. Watkins, W. M.: Blood-group substances. *Science* 152:172, 1966.

35. Hanfland, P., Egge, H., Dabrowski, J., and Graham, H. A.: Purification and characterization of the Le^{dH} blood group antigens from human plasma. *Abstract 1129,* 16th Congress Int. Soc. Blood Transfusion, 1980.

36. Watanabe, K., Laine, R. A., and Hakomori, S.: On neutral fucoglycolipids having long, branched carbohydrate chains: H-active and I-active glycosphingolipids of human erythrocyte membranes. *Biochemistry* 14:2725, 1975.

37. Schachter, H., Michaels, M. A., Crookston, M. C., Tilley, C. A., and Crookston, J. H.: A qualitative difference in the activity of blood group A-specific N-acetylgalactosaminyltransferase in serum from A_1 and A_2 human subjects. *Biochem. Biophys. Res. Commun.* 45:1011, 1971.

38. Yoshida, A., Schmidt, G. M., Blume, K. G., and Beutler, E.: Plasma blood group glycosyltransferase activities after bone marrow transplantation. *Blood* 55:699, 1980.

39. Yoshida, A., Yamaguchi, Y. F., and Dave, V.: Immunologic homology of human blood group glycosyltransferases and genetic background of blood group ABO determination. *Blood* 54:344, 1979.

40. Schachter, H., Michaels, M. A., Tilley, C. A., Crookston, M. C., and Crookston, J. H.: Qualitative differences in the N-acetyl-D-galactosaminyltransferases produced by human A^1 and A^2 genes. *Proc. Natl. Acad. Sci. USA* 70:220, 1973.

41. Schenkel-Brunner, H., and Tuppy, H.: Enzymatic conversion of human blood group 0 erythrocytes into A_2 and A_1 cells by α-N-acetyl-galactosaminyltransferases of blood group A individuals. *Eur. J. Biochem.* 34:125, 1973.

42. Shen, L., Grollman, E. F., and Ginsburg, V.: Enzymatic basis for secretor status and blood group specificity in humans. *Proc. Natl. Acad. Sci. U.S.A.* 59:224, 1968.

43. Schenkel-Brunner, H., Chester, M. A., and Watkins, W. M.: α-L-Fucosyltransferases in human serum from donors of different ABO, secretor and Lewis blood group phenotypes. *Eur. J. Biochem.* 30:269, 1972.

44. Lloyd, K. O., Kabat, E. A., and Rosenfield, R. E.: Immunochemical studies on blood groups. XXXV. Activity of fucose-containing oligosaccharides isolated from blood group A, B and H substances by alkaline degradation. *Biochemistry* 5:1502, 1966.

45. Hearn, V., Smith, Z. G., and Watkins, W.: An α-N-acetylgalactosaminyltransferase associated with the human blood A character. *Biochem. J.* 109:315, 1968.

46. Kissmeyer-Nielsen, F.: Irregular blood group antibodies in 200,000 individuals. *Scand. J. Haematol.* 2:331, 1965.

47. Arcilla, M. B., and Sturgeon, P.: Le^x, the spurned antigen of the Lewis blood group system. *Vox Sang.* 26:425, 1974.

48. Holburn, A. M.: Quantitative studies with ^{125}IgM anti-Le^a. Immunology 24:1019, 1973.

49. Crookston, M. C., Tilley, C. A., and Crookston, J. H.: Human blood chimaera with seeming breakdown of immune tolerance. Lancet 2:1110, 1970.

50. Swanson, J., Crookston, M. C., Yunis, E., Azar, M., Gatti, R. A., and Good, R. A.: Lewis substances in a human marrow-transplantation chimaera. Lancet 1:396, 1971.

51. Fellous, M., Gerbal, A., Nobillot, G., and Weils, J.: Studies on the biosynthetic pathway of human P erythrocyte antigen using genetic complementation tests between fibroblasts from rare p and P^k phenotype donors. Vox Sang. 32:262, 1977.

52. Naiki, M., Fong, J., Ledeen, R., and Marcus, D. M.: Structure of the human erythrocyte blood group P$_1$ glycosphingolipid. Biochemistry 14:4831, 1975.

53. Graham, H. A., and Williams, A. N.: A genetic model for the inheritance of the P, P$_1$ and P^k antigens. Immunol. Commun. 9:191, 1980.

54. Naiki, M., and Marcus, D. M.: Human erythrocyte P and P^k blood group antigens: Identification as glycosphingolipids. Biochem. Biophys. Res. Commun. 60:1105, 1974.

55. Levine, P., Celano, M. J., and Falkowski, F.: The specificity of the antibody in paroxysmal cold hemoglobinuria. Transfusion 3:278, 1963.

56. Dahr, W., Uhlenbruck, G., Leikola, J., Wagstaff, W., and Lanfrest, K.: Studies on the membrane glycoprotein defect of En(a−) erythrocytes. I. Biochemical aspects. J. Immunogenet. 3:329, 1976.

57. Tanner, M.J.A., and Anstee, D. J.: The membrane change in En(a−) human erythrocytes: Absence of the major erythrocyte sialoglycoprotein. Biochem. J. 153:271, 1976.

58. Tanner, M.J.A., Anstee, D. J., and Judson, P. A.: A carbohydrate deficient membrane glycoprotein in human erythrocytes of phenotype S−s−. Biochem. J. 165:157, 1977.

59. Tokunaga, E., et al.: Two apparently healthy Japanese individuals of type M^{k}M^k have erythrocytes which lack both the blood group MN and Ss-active sialoproteins. J. Immunogenet. 6:383, 1979.

60. Anstee, D. J., Mawby, W. J., and Tanner, M.J.A.: Abnormal blood group Ss-active sialoglycoproteins in the membrane of Miltenberger class III, IV and V human erythrocytes. Biochem. J. 183:193, 1979.

61. Howell, E. D., and Perkins, H. A.: Anti-N-like antibodies in the sera of patients undergoing chronic hemodialysis. Vox Sang. 23:291, 1972.

62. Lalezari, P., Malamut, D. C., Dreisiger, M. E., and Sandra, C.: Anti-s and anti-U cold-reacting antibodies. Vox Sang. 25:390, 1973.

63. Feizi, T., and Kabat, E. A.: Immunochemical studies on blood groups. LIV. Classification of anti-I sera into groups based on their reactivity patterns with various blood group A, B, H, Le^a, Le^b, and precursor substances. J. Exp. Med. 135:1247, 1972.

64. Feizi, T., Childs, R. A., Watanabe, K., and Hakomori, S.: Three types of blood group I specificity among monoclonal anti-I autoantibodies revealed by analogues of a branched erythrocyte glycolipid. J. Exp. Med. 149:975, 1979.

65. Marsh, W. L.: Anti-i: A cold antibody defining the iI relationship in human red cells. Br. J. Haematol. 7:200, 1961.

66. Crookston, J. H., et al.: Hereditary erythroblastic multinuclearity associated with a positive acidified-serum test: A type of congenital dyserythropoietic anaemia. Br. J. Haematol. 17:11, 1969.

67. Giblett, E. R., and Crookston, M. C.: Agglutinability of red cells by anti-i in patients with thalassaemia major and other haematological disorders. Nature (New Biol.) 201:1138, 1964.

68. Hillman, R. S., and Giblett, E. R.: Red cell membrane alteration associated with "marrow stress." J. Clin. Invest. 44:1730, 1965.

69. Cooper, A. G., and Brown, M. C.: Serum i antigen: A new human blood-group glycoprotein. Biochem. Biophys. Res. Commun. 55:297, 1973.

70. Feizi, T., Kabat, E. A., Vicari, G., Anderson, B., and Marsh, W. L.: Immunochemical studies on blood groups. XLIX. The I antigen complex: Specificity differences among anti-I sera revealed by quantitative precipitin studies: Partial structure of the I determinant specific for one anti-I serum. J. Immunol. 106:1578, 1971.

71. Dzierzkowa-Borodej, W., Seyfried, H., and Lisowska, E.: Serological classification of anti-I sera. Vox Sang. 28:110, 1975.

72. Capra, J. D., Dowling, P., Cook, S., and Kunkel, H. G.: An incomplete cold-reactive γG antibody with i specificity in infectious mononucleosis. Vox Sang. 18:10, 1969.

73. Giblett, E. R.: A critique of the theoretical hazard of inter- vs. intraracial transfusion. Transfusion. 1:233, 1961.

74. Sturgeon, P.: Red cells and the hazards of isoimmunization. Ann. Intern. Med. 74:114, 1971.

75. Spielmann, W., and Seidl, S.: Prevalence of irregular red cell antibodies and their significance in blood transfusion and antenatal care. Vox Sang. 26:551, 1974.

76. Giblett, E. R.: Blood group antibodies causing hemolytic disease of the newborn. Clin. Obstet. Gynecol. 7:1044, 1964.

77. Wiener, A. S.: The blood group: Three functional problems—serology, genetics and nomenclature. Blood 27:110, 1966.

78. Rosenfield, R. E., Allen, F. H., and Rubenstein, P.: Genetic model for the Rh blood group system. Proc. Natl. Acad. Sci. U.S.A. 70:1303, 1973.

79. Green, F. A.: Erythrocyte membrane lipids and Rh antigen activity. J. Biol. Chem. 247:881, 1972.

80. Hughes-Jones, N. C., Green, E. J., and Hunt, V.A.M.: Loss of Rh antigen activity following the action of phospholipase A$_2$ on red cell stroma. Vox Sang. 29:184, 1975.

81. Rochna, E., and Hughes-Jones, N. C.: The use of purified ^{125}I-labelled anti-γ globulin in the determination of the number of D antigen sites on red cells of different phenotypes. Vox Sang. 10:675, 1965.

82. Nicolson, G. L., Masouredis, S. P., and Singer, S. J.: Quantitative two-dimensional ultrastructural distribution of Rh$_o$(D) antigenic sites on human erythrocyte membranes. Proc. Natl. Acad. Sci. U.S.A. 68:1416, 1971.

83. Pollack, W., Ascari, W. Q., Kochesky, R. J., O'Connor, R. R., Ho, T. Y., and Tripodi, D.: Studies on Rh prophylaxis. I. Relationship between doses of anti-Rh and size of antigenic stimulus. Transfusion 11:333, 1971.

84. Pollack, W., Ascari, W. Q., Crispen, J. R., O'Connor, R. R., and Ho, T. Y.: Studies on Rh prophylaxis. II. Rh immune prophylaxis after transfusion with Rh-positive blood. Transfusion 11:340, 1971.

85. Pollack, W., Gorman, J. G., and Freda, V. J.: Prevention of Rh hemolytic disease, in Progress in Hematology, edited by E. B. Brown and C. V. Moore. Grune & Stratton, New York, 1969, vol. 6, p. 121.

86. Ishimori, T., and Hasekura, H.: A Japanese with no detectable Rh blood group antigens due to silent Rh alleles or deleted chromosomes. Transfusion 7:84, 1967.

87. Levine, P., Celano, M. J., Falkowski, F., Chambers, J., Hunter, O. B., and English, C. T.: A second example of ---/--- or Rh$_{null}$ blood. Transfusion 5:492, 1965.

88. Schmidt, R. J., Lostumbo, M. M., English, C. T., and Hunter, O. B.: Aberrant U blood group accompanies Rh$_{null}$. Transfusion 7:33, 1967.

89. Sturgeon, P.: Hematological observations on the anemia associated with blood type Rh$_{null}$. Blood 36:310, 1970.

90. Levine, P., Tripodi, D., Struck, J., Zmijewski, C. M., and Pollack, W.: Hemolytic anemia associated with Rh$_{null}$ but not with Bombay blood. Vox Sang. 24:417, 1973.

91. Barrasso, C., Eska, P., Grindon, A. J., Oyen, R., and Marsh, W. L.: Anti-K18: An antibody defining another high-frequency antigen related to the Kell blood group system. Vox Sang. 29:124, 1975.

92. Giblett, E. R., Klebanoff, S. J., Pincus, S. H., Swanson, J., Park, B. H., and McCullough, J.: Kell phenotypes in chronic granulomatous disease: A potential transfusion hazard. Lancet 1:1235, 1971.

93. Marsh, W. L., Oyen, R., Nichols, M. E., and Allen, F. H.: Chronic granulomatous disease and Kell blood groups. Br. J. Haematol. 29:247, 1975.

94. Marsh, W. L.: Molecular defects associated with the McLeod blood group phenotype, in Blood Groups and Other Red Cell Surface Markers in Health and Disease, edited by C. Salmon. Masson, New York, 1982, in press.

95. Miller, L. H., Mason, S. J., Clyde, D. F., and McGinniss, H.: The resistance factor to Plasmodium vivax in blacks. N. Engl. J. Med. 295:302, 1976.

96. Giblett, E. R., and Crookston, M. C.: A, B, or O: What's the difference? N. Engl. J. Med. 288:907, 1973 (editorial).

97. Gralnick, M. A., Goldfinger, D., Hatfield, P. A., Reid, M. E., and Marsh, W. L.: Anti-Lu 11: Another antibody defining a high-

frequency antigen related to the Lutheran blood group system. *Vox Sang.* 27:52, 1974.

98. Taliano, V., Guevin, R.-M., and Tippett, P.: The genetics of a dominant inhibitor of the Lutheran antigens. *Vox Sang.* 24:42, 1973.

99. Crawford, M. N., Tippett, P., and Sanger, R.: Antigens Au^n, i and P$_1$ of cells of the dominant type of Lu(a–b–). *Vox Sang.* 26:283, 1974.

100. Giblett, E. R.: Blood group alloantibodies: An assessment of some laboratory practices. *Transfusion* 17:299, 1977.

101. Lux, S. E.: Spectrin-actin membrane skeleton of normal and abnormal red blood cells. *Semin. Hematol.* 16:21, 1979.

102. Naiki, M., and Kato, M.: Immunological identification of blood group P^k antigen on normal erythrocytes and isolation of anti-P^k with different affinity. *Vox Sang.* 37:30, 1979.

CHAPTER *162*

Human leukocyte and platelet antigens and antibodies

DONNA D. KOSTYU
EMILY G. REISNER

Leukocyte antigens and antibodies are important in the selection of tissues, organs, and endocrine and exocrine glands for transplantation; in the selection of cells for transfusion; and in paternity testing. Also leukocyte and platelet antigens are associated with afebrile transfusion reactions and with the accelerated destruction of transfused platelets and leukocytes by an immunized recipient.

Several independent systems of antigens restricted to platelets and neutrophils have been described. The information that has accumulated about leukocyte antigens over the last several years relates almost exclusively to the human leukocyte antigen (HLA) system.

HLA—the human major histocompatibility complex

The HLA region is a remarkable cluster of genes, including those for histocompatibility antigens, those for complement components, those for immune responses, and those involved in the susceptibility to disease [1,2]. The cluster of genes comprising the HLA system is on the short arm of chromosome 6 (Fig. 162-1) [3]. There are five recognized loci—HLA-A, HLA-B, HLA-C, HLA-D, and HLA-DR [4]. The antigens determined by these five loci are listed in Table 162-1. The markers most easily distinguished by serologic techniques are the HLA-A, HLA-B, and HLA-C antigens. At least 20 distinct specificities have been identified at HLA-A, and over 40 at HLA-B; only a few alleles have been identified at HLA-C. The HLA-A, B, and C antigens are found on most nucleated cells. Because of their similar tissue distribution and biochemistry and because of the occurrence of homologous loci in other species, these antigens are often referred to as class I antigens.

HLA-D, DR, SB, and probably also MB and MT represent a second type, or class, of major histocompatibility complex (MHC) antigens, namely, those that are ex-

FIGURE 162-1   A simplified schematic of the HLA region. Three general types of loci exist. Class I loci code for glycoproteins ($M_r = 44,000$ daltons) associated with β_2-microglobulin. These antigens are found on nearly all nucleated cells. In contrast, class II loci code for B-cell antigens which are defined by antibody-mediated assays or by stimulation in mixed lymphocyte culture. These loci include HLA-D, DR, and SB. The newly described MB and MT loci (not indicated in this figure) also determine B-cell antigens which are probably within the D/DR region. Class III loci determine various complement components, namely the second (C2) and fourth (C4A, C4B) complement components of Bf of the alternative pathway. The exact sequence of HLA-D and DR, and of the complement genes, is unknown. GLO, which determines the red cell enzyme glyoxalase, is the only other known polymorphic locus near HLA. The linkage distances in centimorgans (cM) are given where known. The GLO-to-HLA-B distance has been variably estimated at from 3 to 10 cM.

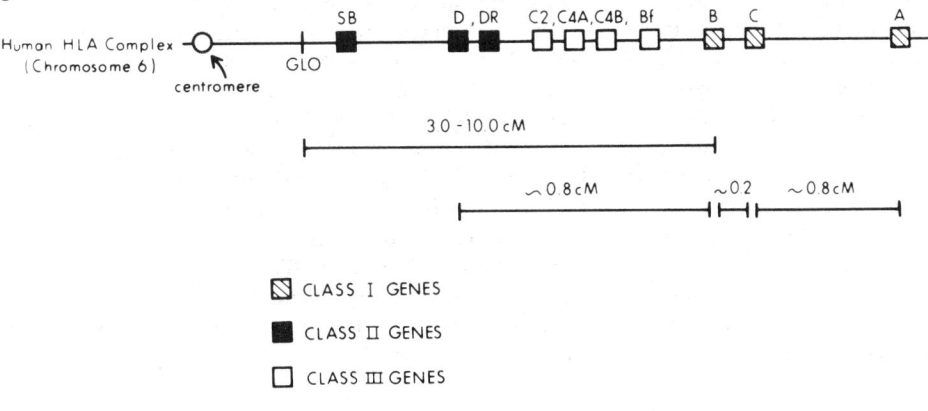

TABLE 162-1 Current HLA antigens

HLA-A locus	HLA-B locus	HLA-C locus	HLA-D locus	HLA-DR locus
A1	B5	Cw1	Dw1	DR1
A2	Bw51	Cw2	Dw2	DR2
A3	Bw52	Cw3	Dw3	DR3
A9	B7	Cw4	Dw4	DR4
Aw23*	B8	Cw5	Dw5	DR5
Aw24	Bw59	Cw6	Dw6	DRw6
A10	B12	Cw7	Dw7	DR7
A25	Bw44	Cw8	Dw8	DRw8
A26	Bw45		Dw9	DRw9
A11	B13		Dw10	DRw10
A28	B14		Dw11	
Aw19	B15		Dw12	
A29	Bw62			
Aw30	Bw63			
Aw31	Bw16			
Aw32	Bw38			
Aw33	Bw39			
Aw34	B17			
Aw36	Bw57			
Aw43	Bw58			
	B18			
	Bw21			
	Bw49			
	Bw50			
	Bw22			
	Bw54			
	Bw55			
	Bw56			
	B27			
	Bw35			
	B37			
	B40			
	Bw60			
	Bw61			
	Bw41			
	Bw42			
	Bw46			
	Bw47			
	Bw48			
	Bw53			
	Bw4			
	Bw6			

*Splits or variants of an antigen.

pressed only on B lymphocytes, macrophages, monocytes, and endothelial cells. The HLA-D antigens are defined by stimulation in mixed lymphocyte culture (MLC), a complex in vitro proliferative T-cell response. At least part of the response is directed to B-cell-specific antigens which can be serologically defined and which have been designated HLA-DR (D-related). Only recently have loci been found which determine other B-cell antigens. Two of these loci, designated MB and MT, are associated with HLA-DR and can be serologically defined as HLA-DR can. A third locus, SB, is closer to GLO, which determines the red cell enzyme glyoxalase. The SB antigens are defined by stimulation in a secondary (primed) MLC. Little is known of the biochemistry of these new antigens. It seems likely that HLA-D is not the functional equivalent of HLA-DR as first thought, but encompasses a response in MLC to many B-cell antigens, including DR, SB, and others.

The HLA-determinant genes are linked to other important loci. Some are responsible for an individual's response to immunogens (IR, or immune response, loci). Also linked to the HLA complex are at least four structural genes involved in the complement system. Genes for C2, C4a, and C4b of the classical complement pathway and Bf of the alternative pathway are located between HLA-B and HLA-D/DR [5]. These are sometimes referred to as class III loci. Other genes within or closely linked to HLA include a locus determining congenital adrenal hyperplasia (21-hydroxylase deficiency) [6] and a locus for olivopontocerebellar ataxia (DPCA-1 or SCA) [7]. T-cell-specific antigens are also reported to be determined by genes in the HLA region.

HLA TERMINOLOGY
HLA terminology is regulated by the World Health Organization and the International Union of Immunologic Societies. HLA designations (e.g., A1, A2, B8) are reserved for the best-established specificities. The letter *w* placed before a number (e.g., Bw16) indicates that a specificity has been identified during one of the periodic workshops on HLA but is not yet fully established. New specificities are given a temporary designation by the individual laboratory. For example, the specificity HLA-A28 was first identified as Ba*; later this was changed to HLA-Aw28 and finally to HLA-A28. Specificities are published in World Health Organization bulletins and in the Joint Reports of the International Histocompatibility Testing Workshops [4,8–12].

INHERITANCE OF HLA
Since each chromosome carries one HLA-A, one HLA-B, one HLA-C, one HLA-D, and one HLA-DR determinant and since each individual has two homologous chromosomes, the maternal and paternal haplotypes can be readily identified in family studies. For example, in the family diagrammed in Fig. 162-2, and Tables 162-2 and 162-3, the father types as HLA-A1, A2, B8, B12, Cw1, Cw2, Dw3, Dw5, DR3, DR5 and the mother as A3, A11, B5, B7, Cw3, Cw4, Dw2, Dw6, DR2, DRw6. These are phenotypes. From the children's types, it can be deduced that A1, B8, Cw1, Dw3, DR3 and A2, B12, Cw2, Dw5, DR5 are the paternal gametic units, or haplotypes. The maternal haplotypes would be A3, B7, Cw3, Dw2, DR2 and A11, B5, Cw4, Dw6, DRw6.

It is often convenient to use a code notation for the HLA haplotypes. The father's two haplotypes are frequently termed A and B, the mother's haplotypes C and D. In most (over 99 percent) families, the children can be only AC, AD, BC, or BD. Two children of identical genotype (e.g., AD and AD) are designated HLA-identical, two children who share only one haplotype (e.g., AC and AD) are termed haploidentical, and those who share neither (e.g., AC and BD) are haplodistinct. In the illustration shown in Fig. 162-2, recombination could occur between the mother's two haplotypes to generate a new A3-B5-Cw4-Dw6-DRw6 haplotype. Crossing-over also occurs between HLA-B and HLA-D, and, very rarely, between HLA-B and HLA-C (see also Chap. 16).

HLA-A, B, AND C

TISSUE DISTRIBUTION
HLA-A, B, and C antigens are found on a wide variety of tissues and organs, on tumors, and on white blood cells and platelets [1,2]. They are reported to be on spermatozoa but are probably not on unfertilized or fertilized eggs, nor on the trophoblast. They are present,

however, on the placenta at term. HLA antigens have been detected in fetal tissue at 6 weeks, on many types of cultured cells, and possibly at low concentration on erythrocytes. There is an association of red cell antigens Bg^a with HLA-B7, Bg^b with B17, and Bg^c with A28 [13].

Certain exceptions should be noted. Platelets often lack some HLA-B antigens [14] and most HLA-C antigens [15], thus facilitating platelet therapy. Fibroblast and cultured amniotic cells may lack HLA-B [16]. Early lymphoid cells reportedly lack HLA-A, B, and C antigens [17]. An absence of HLA-A, B, and C has also been described for circulating lymphocytes and fibroblasts in several cases of immunodeficiency [18,19].

TYPING
The HLA microcytotoxicity test is the fundamental tissue-typing procedure used for defining the HLA-A, B, and C antigens [20]. In this reaction, a suspension of lymphocytes (blood lymphocytes or purified T cells) is incubated with antibody in a specially designed tray. Rabbit serum is added to the mixture to serve as a source of complement, and cell damage is determined, e.g., by the release of radioactive chromium (^{51}Cr) if the cells were labeled or by the uptake of vital stains. For special purposes, other tests are available. These include complement fixation, an antiglobulin cytotoxicity test, and fluorochromasia.

Antisera are usually obtained from multiparous women, and sometimes from multitransfused patients. A number of excellent human sera have also been produced following planned immunization with lymphocytes or, less frequently, with skin grafts. Monoclonal HLA antibodies, now becoming available, will be an important supplement to human alloantisera.

DEFINITION
The definition of the A, B, and C antigens is complicated by the continuing discovery of new antigens and variants and by the extensive cross-reactivity between specific groups of antigens. Such cross-reactive groups (or CREGS) include A1, A10, A11, A3 or Bw51, Bw52, Bw35, B18, Bw49, Bw50. This greatly complicates the procurement of typing sera, since a serum may react with many antigens even though the original immunizing stimulus was a single HLA specificity.

Further complicating analysis of antigens is the occurrence of "splits," or variants. For example, the A9 antigen is now known to be split, that is, to exist in two forms, designated Aw23 and Aw24. Some sera will react with all A9+ cells, i.e., both Aw23+ and Aw24+ cells; some will react only with Aw23+ cells; and others only with Aw24+ cells. As many as three variants of Bw22 have been described. Many variants are extremely rare and thus far have been found only in non-Caucasian populations.

The HLA-B molecule appears to carry two antigenic sites. One is the highly polymorphic site, and the other is a diallelic system, Bw4 and Bw6 [21]. Many HLA-B splits, such as the division of Bw16 into Bw38 and Bw39

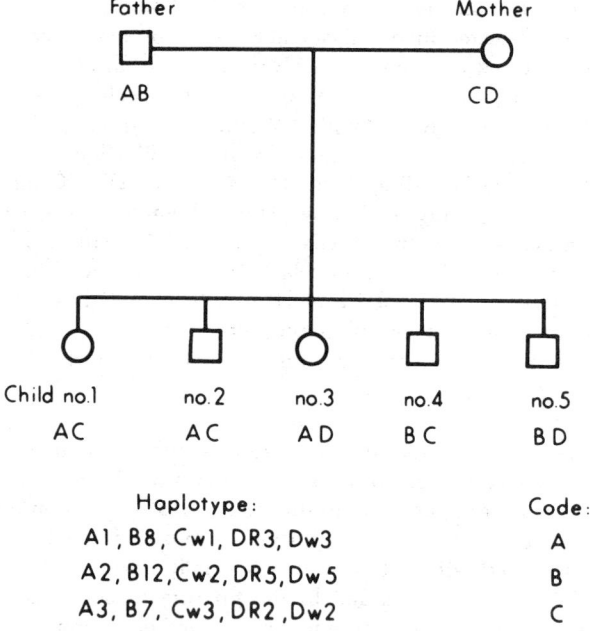

Haplotype:

Haplotype:	Code:
A1, B8, Cw1, DR3, Dw3	A
A2, B12, Cw2, DR5, Dw5	B
A3, B7, Cw3, DR2, Dw2	C
A11, B5, Cw4, DRw6, Dw6	D

FIGURE 162-2 Inheritance of HLA haplotypes. The HLA-A, B, C, and DR antigens are determined by microcytotoxicity and the D types by MLC (Table 162-4).

or Bw21 into Bw49 and Bw50, fall along Bw4 and Bw6 lines. Thus, individuals who are Bw38 or Bw49 invariably are Bw4+, while Bw39+ or Bw50+ cells are Bw6+. Such peculiar associations have been attributed to linkage disequilibrium between closely linked genes or to a complex antigenic site.

BIOCHEMISTRY

The HLA-A, B, and C antigens are transmembrane glycoproteins [22] with an M_r of 56,000 daltons. They are composed of a heavy chain (M_r=45,000 daltons) and a light chain (M_r=11,000 daltons) (Fig. 162-3). The light chain is β_2-microglobulin, a globular protein which can be isolated from serum or urine and which is determined by a gene on chromosome 15. Antigenic specificity resides in the amino acid sequence of the heavy chain. The 45,000-dalton glycoprotein can be divided into multiple domains determined by intrachain disulfide bonds. The amino terminal $\alpha1$ domain consists of 110 amino acids. Two loops ($\alpha2$ and $\alpha3$) of 63 and 36 amino acids, respectively, are followed by a short portion responsible for membrane insertion. The carboxy terminal end projecting into the cytoplasm consists of approximately 30 amino acids and has two half cystines and a serine which can be phosphorylated.

FUNCTION

The physiological function of the HLA-A, B, and C antigens is not known, but recent speculation has centered on an important role in "self" recognition [23]. Much of this evidence comes from studies of the lysis of virally modified cells by cytolytic T cells.

In the mouse, cytolytic T cells are both MHC-specific and virus-specific, i.e., they lyse only infected cells which carry the specific viral antigen and a specific class I antigen. Viruses include the lymphochoriomeningitis virus, vaccinia, Sendai, and influenza. This has led to the hypothesis that the class I antigens are physically modified by viral products or that the cytolytic T lymphocytes must interact with a viral target antigen and a class I molecule in order to be functionally lytic. Similar effects have been seen in humans, using influenza-infected cells [24].

HLA-DR

TISSUE DISTRIBUTION

The HLA-DR antigens are equivalent to the Ia antigens of the mouse. Expression of HLA-DR (and HLA-D) is limited to B lymphocytes, B lymphoblastoid cell lines, monocytes, macrophages, Langerhans cells, and endothelial cells [1]. They may also be present on some mitogen-activated T cells, on early (but not late) cells of the myeloid series, and on some malignant melanoma cells. Although the characterization of three newly discovered loci determining B-cell-specific antigens—the serologically defined MB and MT antigens, and the primed lymphocyte-defined SB antigens—is still incomplete, evidence to date supports a tissue distribution similar to that found with HLA-DR.

TABLE 162-2 Determination of HLA haplotypes within a family: HLA-A and HLA-B antigens determined by microcytotoxicity

	HLA typing sera detecting							
	HLA-A antigens				*HLA-B antigens*			
	A1	A2	A3	A11	B8	B12	B7	B5
Father (AB)*	+	+	−	−	+	+	−	−
Mother (CD)	−	−	+	+	−	−	+	+
Child 1 (AC)	+	−	+	−	+	−	+	−
Child 2 (AC)	+	−	+	−	+	−	+	−
Child 3 (AD)	+	−	−	+	+	−	−	+
Child 4 (BC)	−	+	+	−	−	+	+	−
Child 5 (BD)	−	+	−	+	−	+	−	+

*Haplotype (see Fig. 162-2).

TYPING

DR typing is accomplished by the antibody complement-dependent cytotoxicity assay described earlier, with several modifications. As B cells constitute only 10 to 15 percent of the blood lymphocytes, removal of T cells and macrophages (which may carry monocyte-specific antigens) is a prerequisite. The isolation of an enriched B-cell population from blood cells can be accomplished by several techniques—through depletion of T cells by rosetting with sheep erythrocytes [25] or through positive selection of B cells by their Fc receptor [26], surface immunoglobulin [27], or adherence to nylon [28]. As B cells are HLA-A+B+C+DR+, all DR typing sera that contain HLA-A, B, or C antibodies must be absorbed with platelets and/or T cells before use. Eleven HLA-DR antigens are currently recognized. However, there is support for new variants and new antigens, and so the number of alleles will grow.

BIOCHEMISTRY

Little is known of the biochemistry of HLA-DR. The HLA-DR antigens reside on a molecule formed by two noncovalently associated glycoproteins [22]. The larger α chain ($M_r = 34,000$ daltons) and a smaller β chain ($M_r = 29,000$ daltons) both appear to be determined by genes within the HLA region. The newly identified MB and MT antigens are thought to represent separate antigenic sites on the DR molecule or on other molecules with a similar structure. In the mouse, each chromosome carries genes for several α and β chains [29].

MB AND MT ANTIGENS

Current interest centers on the improved definition of the MB and MT antigens [4]. Typing for these antigens is dependent upon sera that give strong cytolytic patterns, which are inherited with the HLA haplotype in families but which do not conform to known DR antigens. They are less polymorphic than DR, with three MB and three MT alleles identified. Further alleles are likely to be found in the future, as some cells fail to type for MB1, 2, or 3 and presumably carry a new MB antigen.

The association between MB, MT, and DR is remarkably strong. For example, in Caucasians, individuals who

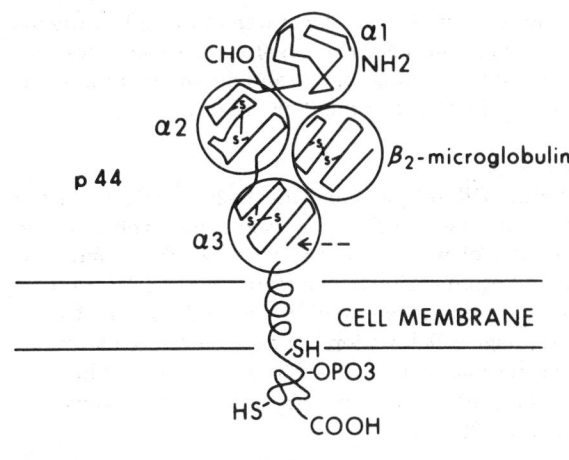

FIGURE 162-3   Schematic of the HLA-A, B, and C molecules. The heavy chain (p44), determined by a structural gene in the HLA region, carries the HLA antigen. It is a transmembrane glycoprotein consisting of three functional sections: an extracellular segment, a hydrophobic portion which spans the membrane, and an intracellular segment. The extracellular segment consists of several domains, designated $\alpha 1$, or $\alpha 2$, and $\alpha 3$ (circled), similar to immunoglobulins. A papain cleavage site close to the membrane is denoted by an arrow. The smaller chain, β_2-microglobulin, is determined by a gene on chromosome 15. It has significant homology with immunoglobulin constant-region domains.

type for DR1 almost invariably type for MB1 and MT1. Those that type for DR3 also type for MB2 and MT2. While it has been proposed that MB and MT represent cross-reactive groups of antigens, three lines of evidence would argue against this. Biochemical data, including sequential binding [30], immunoprecipitation [31], two-dimensional gel analysis [32], and differential susceptibility to papain cleavage [33], suggest that DR, MB, and MT all represent separate antigenic sites. Secondly, serologic data and segregation of MB and MT antigens in families yield unusual DR-MB-MT correlations, e.g., some DR7+ cells are not MB2+ as expected. The third type of evidence is indirect and comes from

TABLE 162-3   Determination of HLA haplotypes within a family: MLC stimulation and identification of HLA-D antigens by use of homozygous typing cells

Responding cell	Stimulating cells								
	Father$_M$*	Mother$_M$	Child 1$_M$	Child 2$_M$	Child 5$_M$	Dw3 HTC$_M$	Dw5 HTC$_M$	Dw2 HTC$_M$	Dw6 HTC$_M$
Father (AB)†	810‡	18,450	5,140	5,400	6,800	930	750	16,700	17,750
Mother (CD)	9,250	520	3,210	2,900	3,500	8,600	9,740	640	550
Child 1 (AC)	3,400	4,600	440	640	9,980	650	9,345	375	10,650
Child 2 (AC)	4,100	4,800	550	550	8,760	675	8,600	460	11,120
Child 5 (BD)	2,350	2,300	8,260	7,550	345	8,840	320	11,550	575

* The subscript M indicates mitomycin-treated stimulating cell.
† Haplotype (see Fig. 162-2).
‡ Counts per minute.

the mouse, where several loci determining Ia antigens have been found [29]. Human studies are now concentrating on the number of loci and on whether these antigens are localized to the β or the α chains.

FUNCTION

The HLA-DR antigens and the H-2 Ia antigens of the mouse (all class II antigens) appear to be involved in the generation of an immune response [34]. The differentiation and proliferation of cytotoxic T cells and antibody-secreting plasma cells require not only T cell–B cell–macrophage collaboration but also class II compatibility between collaborating cells. Moreover, soluble "helper" and "suppressor" factors carry I-A or I-J antigens, respectively [35].

HLA-D

In contrast to the serologically defined antigens just described, HLA-D is determined by a functional test called the mixed lymphocyte culture (MLC) [36]. Fundamentally, it is thought to be an in vitro representation of the primary recognition response of lymphocytes. An MLC consists of the culturing of responding and stimulating lymphocytes together for several days. The stimulating cell itself is prevented from responding by irradiation or by exposure to mitomycin C. A sequence of reactions involving the responding cells leads to DNA synthesis and cell replication. A radioactive label, usually ^{3}H-thymidine, is added, and the amount of thymidine incorporated is proportional to the amount of proliferation. The degree of cellular activation is a measure of HLA-D disparity. Background counts per minute range from 100 to 500 cpm in ideal cases, and the responding cultures often incorporate 20,000 cpm or higher. The average degree of stimulation between family members sharing one haplotype is about one half that found between family members differing in both haplotypes. HLA-identical siblings should not stimulate each other's cells.

The results of an MLC are shown in Table 162-2. Data can be expressed as (1) gross counts per minute; (2) a stimulation index, the ratio of $A + Bx/A + Ax$, where A is the responding cell and Ax and Bx are irradiated stimulating cells; or (3) a relative response, a percentage of the maximum stimulation observed when a cell is tested against a nonrelated panel.

Controls include cultures of cell A, Ax, B, Bx, each alone, etc., and exposure to at least one mitogen to show that the cultured cell in question is capable of responding. Two unrelated individuals should be included as a gauge of the capacity to respond to allogeneic cells.

HLA-D alleles are identified through the use of MLR homozygous typing cells (e.g., Dw1/Dw1) [37]. These cells are most frequently obtained from children of first-cousin marriages who have inherited the same HLA chromosomal segment or genetic complex (haplotype) from one of the great-grandparents. Cells from such an individual do not stimulate cells from other family members carrying the same haplotype. They also do not stimulate unrelated individuals who by chance carry the same HLA-D allele.

RELATIONSHIP BETWEEN HLA-D AND HLA-DR

In an MLC, the predominant responding cell population consists of helper T cells which proliferate in response to disparate antigens found on B lymphocytes. In addition, cytotoxic T cells and suppressor cells are generated which can be measured in alternative assays. The "B-cell antigens" which are recognized include DR, and probably also MB and MT. It was therefore hoped that DR typing would be quicker and less expensive than D typing by MLC. This has not been the case. The MLC is a complex response and appears to include recognition of cell-surface antigens other than HLA-DR, some of which may not be detectable by antibody-mediated assays. For instance, the SB antigens which are determined by a locus separate from DR [24] can be identified only by primed lymphocyte typing [38]. Further complexity is implicated by some rare individuals who type as DR2 but not Dw2, or who carry Dw2 and DR7 on haplotype.

RACIAL DISTRIBUTION OF HLA ANTIGENS

Different races differ markedly in the frequency of HLA antigens (Table 162-4). Examples of divergent frequency distribution would be the comparative rarity of HLA-A1 and A3 in Orientals, the high frequency of the HLA-B5 and Bw35 antigens in American Indians, and the restriction of Bw46 to Orientals. Besides frequency differences of well-defined specificities, two other distinctions can be noted. An HLA specificity is usually allocated on the basis of concordant reactions of a number of antisera. A typical typing panel includes at least two sera reacting with each specificity and often three or four similar sera for detecting more difficult antigens. Sera that are concordant in their reactions with cells from Caucasians may give discordant reactions in non-Caucasians. Sometimes the anomalous reactions are due to unsuspected reactions against HLA-C antigens, while some reactions are against antigens absent from, or rare in, Caucasians. While these new specificities will be of great value in anthropologic and other racial studies, variant alleles greatly complicate tissue typing in many populations, including North American Negroes.

APPLICATIONS OF HLA

HLA TESTING IN PARENTAGE DETERMINATION

HLA-A, B, and C antigen testing is important for parentage determination. The HLA system is an excellent one for this purpose since the large number of antigens makes each HLA-A and B combination rare. Fifteen A and twenty B antigens could produce 20,246 phenotypes (or 45,245 genotypes) [39].

The rarity of any HLA haplotype invests the system with a very high prior probability of exclusion. This

TABLE 162-4 Antigen frequencies in North American Caucasians (NAC), North American Negroes (NAN), and American Indians (AMI)*

	NAC	NAN	AMI		NAC	NAN	AMI
A1	25.7	6.5	2.9	Bw56	1.1	0.0	0.0
A2	46.6	27.3	60.3	Bw57	7.2	7.7	0.0
A3	26.0	14.2	2.9	Bw58	2.2	20.3	0.0
A11	12.5	1.1	1.5	Bw59	0.8	1.6	0.0
Aw23	5.0	20.4	1.5	Bw60	11.0	2.7	18.8
Aw24	12.8	5.7	41.9	Bw61	2.0	0.8	10.1
A25	4.2	0.8	0.0	Bw62	9.5	1.9	40.6
A26	7.2	7.4	0.0	Bw63	1.9	0.6	2.9
A28	9.9	16.6	13.0	N	1029	365	69
A29	8.1	12.3	4.4				
Aw30	5.1	28.3	0.0	Bw4	66.4	65.3	51.6
Aw31	6.2	4.4	39.0	Bw6	82.3	83.1	90.7
Aw32	7.1	3.0	4.4	N	1013	359	69
Aw33	3.4	9.0	0.0				
Aw34	0.5	12.5	0.0	Cw1	6.0	0.1	20.3
Aw36	0.7	3.3	0.0	Cw2	9.1	22.5	1.5
Aw43	0.2	1.9	0.0	Cw3	22.6	17.5	62.3
N†	1029	367	69	Cw4	20.7	29.3	14.5
				Cw5	11.9	5.8	2.9
B7	18.7	17.0	1.5	Cw6	14.9	17.3	2.9
B8	17.1	5.8	2.9	Cw7	6.0	4.8	0.0
B13	5.3	1.4	0.0	Cw8	5.1	0.8	0.0
B14	9.5	8.0	1.5	N	1028	365	69
B18	9.7	7.7	2.9				
B27	7.5	3.0	1.5	DR1	22.0	9.6	3.0
Bw35	15.6	12.1	20.3	DR2	25.3	28.5	46.3
B37	3.2	0.8	0.0	DR3	22.2	31.6	6.0
Bw38	6.2	0.0	1.5	DR4	27.3	9.6	47.8
Bw39	3.6	3.6	21.7	DR5	19.4	24.8	3.0
Bw41	3.9	2.5	0.0	DRw6	7.2	10.2	7.5
Bw42	0.6	14.8	0.0	DR7	23.6	18.6	4.5
Bw44	26.1	13.7	5.8	DRw8	5.3	10.8	37.3
Bw45	1.4	7.7	1.5	DRw9	3.0	5.3	1.5
Bw47	0.4	0.3	0.0	DRw10	1.2	3.7	7.5
Bw48	1.3	2.2	4.4	N	1145	323	67
Bw49	4.7	4.9	1.5				
Bw50	2.6	1.4	0.0	MT1	54.9	62.9	52.2
Bw51	9.3	2.7	43.5	MT2	57.6	75.9	49.3
Bw52	2.8	1.9	4.4	MT3	18.8	13.0	7.5
Bw53	0.9	12.6	1.5	N	1145	323	67
Bw54	0.0	0.0	0.0				
Bw55	4.3	1.6	0.0				

* Data from Terasaki [4].

† N = number tested.

probability is a measure of the power of an antigen system to exclude a falsely accused man of paternity and is derived from the number of antigens and their gene frequencies. The prior probability of exclusion of any system is derived by defining all possible mother–child–alleged father trios which demonstrate an exclusion and determining their frequency in a population. (Several excellent reviews are available [40,41].) The prior probability of exclusion of the ABO system is usually quoted as 17 percent, that of HLA at 90 percent. The prior probability of exclusion is dependent on the number of antigens detected and will change slightly depending on the completeness of a laboratory's reagent panel.

The power of the HLA system to exclude paternity now permits calculation of the statistical likelihood of paternity using a modification of Bayes' theorem. Using population data, one may estimate the chance of the alleged father's producing a single sperm containing the relevant genetic information and compare his chance to that of an unrelated man of the same race. The chance of the unrelated man is derived from population gene frequencies. The comparison of these two figures can be expressed as an odds ratio or as a percentage [41]. The percentage of men not excluded may be calculated in a similar manner using phenotype data. HLA may not exclude in cases where the alleged and natural fathers are close relatives, where the mother and child share three or more HLA antigens, or where unknown antigens are suspected. If an exclusion is not observed, testing with additional systems is imperative. Additional systems may include red cell antigens, red cell enzymes, or serum proteins. A number of cases have been observed [42] in which HLA did not exclude and some other system did.

HLA AND TRANSPLANTATION

HLA functions as the major human histocompatibility system and is implicated in organ and tissue graft rejection and in graft-versus-host reactions following marrow transplantation. The HLA-A and B antigens are the most easily detected marker for the inheritance of the MHC in families. Because the HLA haplotype is inherited as a tightly linked group of loci, with rare exceptions (recombinants), siblings who genotype HLA-A–identical and HLA-B–identical are also identical with respect to HLA-D and HLA-DR. HLA-A and HLA-B identity therefore allows a favorable prognosis for graft survival between HLA-identical siblings. Unfortunately, because many of the other products of the HLA region involved in graft rejection (e.g., HLA-D, HLA-DR) are not easily identified and differ from one individual to another, HLA matching gives incomplete in-

formation about the potential strength of the immune response between haploidentical siblings, between parent and child, or between unrelated individuals.

Moreover, even kidneys transplanted from HLA-identical, ABO-compatible siblings are rejected unless some immunosuppressive agents are given, and HLA-identical marrow not infrequently induces severe graft-versus-host disease. Thus, antigenic systems of white cells and tissues not linked to HLA are manifested in the reactions against transplants. Fortunately, immunity to these other antigenic factors is more readily controlled by immunosuppressive agents, and rejection of HLA genotypically identical kidneys is rare, even with low doses of immunosuppressive agents [43].

Marrow transplantation is useful in patients with immunodeficiency states, marrow aplasia, or leukemia in remission (Chap. 168). When engraftment does take place, there is a significant danger from graft-versus-host reactions [44]. The greatest chances for success come from transplanting HLA- and MLR-identical siblings. Rare successes have been achieved with non-HLA-matched donor-recipient pairs.

HLA ANTIGENS AND DISEASE

One of the most intriguing discoveries has been the association of HLA and susceptibility to disease. A variety of disease associations have been found with, for example, diabetes, gluten-sensitive enteropathy, and multiple sclerosis (Table 162-5). To date, the strongest asso-

TABLE 162-5   Some positive correlations between HLA and disease

HLA	Disease	Frequency, % Patients	Frequency, % Controls	Average relative risk*
A3	Hemochromatosis	72	21	9.7
B27	Ankylosing spondylitis	90	8	103.5
	Reiter's disease	80	9	40.4
	Yersinia arthritis	69	11	18.0
	Acute anterior uveitis	48	9	9.3
	Juvenile rheumatoid arthritis	35	11	4.4
Cw6	Psoriasis:			
	Caucasian	50	23	3.3
	Japanese	53	7	15.0
DR2 (B7)	Multiple sclerosis	55	23	4.1
DR3 (B8)	Gluten-sensitive enteropathy	96	27	64.5
	Dermatitis herpetiformis	77	20	13.4
	Sjögren's disease	75	21	11.3
	Idiopathic Addison's disease	70	21	8.8
	Chronic active hepatitis	68	24	6.7
	Graves' disease	53	18	5.1
	SLE	70	28	5.8
	Myasthenia gravis	30	17	2.1
DR4	Rheumatoid arthritis	56	15	7.2
DR3	Insulin-dependent diabetes	50	21	3.8
DR4	Insulin-dependent diabetes	38	13	4.1

*Woolf's relative risk $= Pd(1 - Pc)/Pc(1 - Pd)$, where Pd = frequency in patients and Pc = frequency in controls.
SOURCE: Modified from Hildeman et al. [67].

TABLE 162-6   Platelet-specific antigens

Antigen	Antibody source	Methods used to detect antigen*	Subjects tested		Approx. gene frequency	Approx. genotype frequency	
			Number	% positive		Homozygous	Heterozygous
Pl^A1 or Zw^a†	17 Maternal 4 Posttransfusion	1, 2, 4, 5	452	97	0.83	0.69	0.28
Pl^A2 or Zw^b†	1 Posttransfusion	1	435	26.5	0.17	0.03	0.28
Pl^E1†	1 Posttransfusion	3	945	>99.9	0.975	0.95	0.049
Pl^E2†	1 Maternal	3	147	5.0	0.025	0.0006	0.049
Ko^a†	4 Posttransfusion	1	435	17	0.08	0.006	0.147
Ko^b‡	1 Posttransfusion	1, 3	1,080	99.4	0.92	0.85	0.147
DUZO^a†	1 Maternal	2	82	22	0.12	0.014	0.21

*Methods used to determine antigens:
1. Agglutination
2. Antiglobulin consumption test
3. Complement fixation
4. Inhibition of clot retraction
5. Inhibition of complement fixation
†Summarized from Shulman et al. [48].
‡Summarized from Svejgaard [68].

ciation of an HLA specificity with disease is HLA-B27 and ankylosing spondylitis and related arthropathies. Other diseases originally associated with particular HLA-B antigens have, in fact, been more strongly associated with the HLA-D and DR antigens. This is due to the strong linkage disequilibrium characteristic of the genes making up the HLA haplotype. Linkage disequilibrium refers to the association of antigens on a haplotype more frequently than would be expected by chance, e.g., the frequent association of B8 and DR3 or of B7 and DR2. This phenomenon may result from population expansion, migration and admixture, or selective pressure, or as a by-product of selection at, or recombination suppression by, some other closely linked locus.

It is important to distinguish between association and linkage. Association implies a concordant observation of a disease and a particular antigen in population studies, e.g., an analysis in which 95 percent of unrelated patients with ankylosing spondylitis are B27 positive, compared with a normal B27 frequency of under 10 percent. Linkage with HLA is determined only by family studies. It allows placement of a disease gene close to or within the HLA region. A primary example is hemochromatosis, where the original findings of an association with HLA-A3 was later followed by linkage studies on multigeneration families. A major gene could be identified. It was recessive, highly penetrant in the homozygous state, near HLA-A, and often, but not always, found with HLA-A3 (see also Chap. 79). A complete summary of HLA and disease associations, the methods of analysis, and some statistical approaches and theories behind these associations are given in detail elsewhere [45].

Platelet antigens

HLA antigens have been demonstrated on platelets by absorption, fluorescence, and complement fixation.

However, the expression of certain antigens may vary considerably [46]. For example, 20 percent of individuals typed as HLA-B12 by lymphocytotoxicity do not appear to have this antigen on their platelets, and an intermediate group expresses the antigen only weakly. Some HLA antigens on transfused platelets seem more immunogenic than others. For example, matching for C-locus antigens is probably not necessary [47].

Platelets also possess platelet-specific antigens unrelated to erythrocyte or leukocyte isoantigens. These include Pl^A1, Pl^A2, Pl^E1, Pl^E2, Ko^a, Ko^b, and DUZO, as described in Table 162-6 [48,49]. Most of these antibodies were discovered in the sera of mothers of infants with neonatal thrombocytopenia or of persons receiving transfusions. The antigen Pl^A1, which is present on 97 percent of the population, is absent from persons with Glansmann's thrombasthenia. These persons cannot synthesize the antigen because of a genetic defect [50].

The major problem when working with platelets, either for antigen detection or for cross-matching for transfusions, is to develop a suitable typing method. Platelets adsorb blood constituents and aggregate easily in a nonspecific fashion. Tests for platelet antigens therefore fall into two groups: direct detection of antigens by agglutination [51] or immunofluorescence [52] and indirect methods, such as complement fixation [53] and antiglobulin consumption [54]. A third group of tests involve some biological function of the platelet, such as platelet factor 3 release [55] or serotonin release [56]. The disadvantage of these latter tests is that the platelets must be physiologically active.

Neutrophil antigens

Neutrophil antigens were first identified in studies of isoimmune neonatal neutropenia due to fetal-maternal incompatibility. Characterization of these antigens has

TABLE 162-7   Neutrophil-specific antigens

System	Gene	Frequency
NA	NA1	0.337
	NA2	0.663
NB	NB1	0.830

SOURCE: Modified from *Semin. Hematol.* 11:281, 1974.

been slow, however, because of technical difficulties. Neutrophil antibodies are detected only by agglutination. This method is slow, requires intact cells, and is extremely sensitive to temperature, method of cell preparation, physiological state of the donor cell, and medium used.

Neutrophil-specific antigens have been described at two independent loci, NA and NB [57]. The NA1 antigen is present on neutrophils but not on eosinophils, monocytes, lymphocytes, and platelets. The NB1 antibody is not absorbable by red blood cells, platelets, lymphocytes, placenta, kidney, liver, lung, or lymph node cells. The frequencies of the antigens determined by genes at the NA and NB loci are given in Table 162-7. Other neutrophil-specific antigens have been defined, including NC, ND [58], and NE [59].

The role of neutrophil antigens in the survival of transplanted neutrophilic cells has not been evaluated. Such an assessment could be relevant to marrow transplantation and transfusion of granulocytes and platelets [60].

Platelet and leukocyte antigens in transfusion

Antibodies to platelet and leukocyte antigens cause problems in transfusion on three levels: masking the presence of specific anti-red cell antibodies, a febrile transfusion reaction, and/or a shortened in vivo survival of transfused cells. Anti-white cell antibodies in the patient's serum may mask specific anti-red cell antibodies by acting as weak panagglutinins of red cells. This problem may be caused by antibodies against Bg antigens. For example, if the patient has an antibody to HLA-A2, it may react with all BgC red cells. This effect can be reduced or eliminated by absorbing the serum sample with pooled or specific platelets before testing with red cells. The second problem, that of the unexplained febrile nonhemolytic transfusion reaction following a transfusion of red cells, may often be explained by the presence of an antibody against white cells. This problem may be eliminated by using washed or frozen red cells for transfusion.

The third and by far the major problem associated with antibodies against white cells or platelets is a markedly reduced in vivo survival of the transfused cells. Unmatched platelets can be given to patients without adverse effects. With repeated administrations, however, the patient may become sensitized, develop-

ing antibodies which shorten the life of the transfused cells. This problem may be minimized or eliminated by the use of matched platelets. How to type and crossmatch is the subject of debate [61]. HLA matching within a family often alleviates the problem of limited platelet survival [62]. However, problems are encountered when this idea is extended to HLA matching among unrelated persons. Such matching (made possible by the testing of many donors and the use of a computer) is often but not always helpful. Persons carrying HLA-A2 need more careful matching than those lacking A2, and matching within a cross-reactive group rather than a specific antigen is often helpful [63]. About 30 percent of sensitized patients are not helped by these methods. Apparently their refractory state is not caused by sensitization to HLA antigens. Such persons are often helped by preparing white cell–poor or white cell–free platelets. Improved cross-matching techniques to identify good matches for these cases has been hampered by difficulties in typing platelets. Promising crossmatching tests are the indirect immunofluorescence test [52] or platelet aggregometry [64]. The latter technique has the disadvantage of needing fresh platelets for testing.

Platelet and leukocyte antibodies and pregnancy

The antibody response to allogenic leukocyte and platelet antigens is unpredictable. It depends on the route of administration, the type and amount of antigenic tissue, the interval between exposures, and the presence of preformed antibody. Antibodies to platelet and leukocyte antigens are ordinarily produced by prior sensitization, usually through exposure to allogeneic tissues, skin grafts, blood transfusions, or pregnancy.

Development of antibodies to platelets and neutrophils are most often associated with transplacental sensitization. Maternal antibodies specific to fetal neutrophils can readily cross the placenta. The resulting neonatal neutropenia, which is occasionally found even in first-born infants, will persist as long as maternal antibody exists in the newborn.

Isoimmunization to HLA antigens is much more frequent than immunization to neutrophil antigens, probably because mothers can become sensitized by fetal granulocytes, lymphocytes, platelets, and placental tissues. Once in the maternal circulation, fetal lymphocytes also persist longer than do granulocytes. At least a third of all multiparous women produce detectable anti-HLA antibodies, and an equal number form anti-B-cell antibodies. Furthermore, mothers who have once been sensitized will often form antibodies to blood transfusions more readily than unsensitized men or women [65]. Even though maternal antibodies to HLA antigens develop, there is little evidence that they reach the fetus. This is most likely due to the adsorption of maternal antibodies onto the trophoblast [66].

References

1. Albert, E. D., and Götze, D.: The major histocompatibility system in man, in *The Major Histocompatibility System in Man and Animals*, edited by D. Götze. Springer-Verlag, New York, 1977, p. 7.
2. Amos, D. B., and Kostyu, D. D.: HLA—A central immunological agency of man. *Adv. Hum. Genet.* 10:137, 1980.
3. Breuning, M. H., et al.: Localization of HLA on the short arm of chromosome 6. *Hum. Genet.* 37:131, 1977.
4. Terasaki, P. I. (ed.): *Histocompatibility Testing 1980.* UCLA Tissue Typing Laboratory, Los Angeles, 1980.
5. Lachmann, P. J., and Hobart, M. J.: Complement genetics in relation to HLA. *Br. Med. Bull.* 34:247, 1978.
6. Dupont, B., Oberfield, S. E., Smithwick, E. M., Lee, T. D., and Levine, L. S.: Close genetic linkage between HLA and congenital adrenal hyperplasia (21-hydroxylase deficiency). *Lancet* ii:1309, 1977.
7. Jackson, J. F., Currier, R. D., Terasaki, P. I., and Morton, N. E.: Spino-cerebellar ataxia and HLA linkage. *N. Engl. J. Med.* 296:1138, 1977.
8. Russell, P. S., and Winn, H. J. (eds.): *Histocompatibility Testing.* Natl. Acad. Sci. Publ. 1229, Washington, D. C., 1965.
9. Curtoni, E. S., Mattiuz, P. L., and Tosi, R. M. (eds.): *Histocompatibility Testing 1967.* Munksgaard, Copenhagen, 1967.
10. Allen, F., et al.: Joint report of the Fourth International Histocompatibility Testing Workshop, in *Histocompatibility Testing 1970*, edited by P. I. Terasaki. Munksgaard, Copenhagen, 1970, p. 17.
11. Bodmer, J. G., Colombani, J., Rocques, P., Degos, L., Bodmer, W. F., and Dausset, J.: Joint report of the Fifth International Histocompatibility Testing Workshop, in *Histocompatibility Testing 1972*, edited by J. Dausset and J. Colombani. Munksgaard, Copenhagen, 1973, p. 619.
12. Bodmer, J.: Joint report of the Sixth International Histocompatibility Testing Workshop, in *Histocompatibility Testing 1975*, edited by F. Kissmeyer-Nielson. Munksgaard, Copenhagen, 1975, p. 21.
13. Morton, J. A., Pickles, M. M., Sutton, L., and Skov, F.: Identification of further antigens on red cells and lymphocytes: Association of Bg^b with w17 (Te57) and Bg^c with w28 (Da15, Ba*). *Vox Sang.* 21:141, 1971.
14. Duquesnoy, R. J., Testin, J., and Aster, R. H.: Variable expression of w4 and w6 on platelets: Possible relevance to platelet transfusion therapy of alloimmunized thrombocytopenic patients. *Transplant Proc.* 9:1829, 1977.
15. Mueller-Eckhardt, G., Hauck, M., Kayser, W., and Mueller-Eckhardt, C.: HLA-C antigens on platelets. *Tissue Antigens* 16:91, 1980.
16. Pollack, M. S., et al.: HLA typing of amniotic cells: The prenatal diagnosis of congenital adrenal hyperplasia (21-OH-deficiency type). *Transplant. Proc.* 11:1726, 1979.
17. Brown, G., Biberfeld, P., Christensson, B., and Mason, D. Y.: The distribution of HLA on human lymphoid, bone marrow and peripheral blood cells. *Eur. J. Immunol.* 9:272, 1979.
18. Schurmann, R.K.B., et al.: Failure of lymphocyte-membrane HLA-A and B expression in two siblings with combined immunodeficiency. *Clin. Immunol. Immunopathol.* 14:418, 1979.
19. Betuel, H., Touraine, J. L., Souillet, G., and Jeune, M.: Absence of cell membrane HLA antigens in an immunodeficient child. *Tissue Antigens* 11:68, 1978.
20. Amos, D. B., Pool, P., and Grier, J.: HLA-A, HLA-B, HLA-C, and HLA-DR, in *Manual of Clinical Immunology*, edited by N. R. Rose and H. Friedmans. American Society for Microbiology, Washington, D.C., 1980, p. 978.
21. Cresswell, P., and Ayres, J. L.: HLA antigens: Rabbit antisera reacting with all A series or B series specificities. *Eur. J. Immunol.* 6:82, 1976.
22. Strominger, J. L., et al.: The biochemical analysis of products of the major histocompatibility complex, in *The Role of the Major Histocompatibility Complex in Immunobiology*, edited by M. Dorf. Garland, New York, 1981, p. 115.
23. Zinkernagel, R. M., and Doherty, P. C.: MHC-restricted cytotoxic T cells: Studies on the biological role of polymorphic major transplantation antigens determining T cell restriction-specificity, function, and responsiveness. *Adv. Immunol.* 27:52, 1979.
24. Shaw, S., Kavathas, P., Pollack, M. S., Charmot, D., and Mawas, C.: Family studies define a new histocompatibility locus, SB, between HLA-DR and GLO. *Nature* 293:745, 1981.
25. Mendes, N. F., Toinai, M.E.A., Silveira, N.P.A., Gilbertsen, R. B., and Metzgar, R. S.: Technical aspects of the rosette tests used to detect human complement receptor (B) and sheep erythrocyte-binding (T) lymphocytes. *J. Immunol.* 111:860, 1973.
26. Mann, D. L., Abelson, L., Harris, S., and Amos, D. B.: Detection of antigens specific for B-lymphoid cultured cell lines with human alloantisera. *J. Exp. Med.* 142:84, 1975.
27. Grier, J. O., Abelson, L. A., Mann, D. L., Amos, D. B., and Johnson, A. H.: Enrichment of B lymphocytes using goat anti-human F(ab')₂. *Tissue Antigens* 10:236, 1977.
28. Lowry, R., Goguen, J., Carpenter, C. B., Strom, T. B., and Garovoy, M. R.: Improved B cell typing for HLA-DR using nylon wool column enriched B lymphocyte preparations. *Tissue Antigens* 14:325, 1979.
29. Silver, J., and Russell, W. A.: Genetic mapping of the component chains of Ia antigens. *Immunogenetics* 8:339, 1979.
30. Tanigaki, N., Tosi, R., Pressman, D., and Ferrara, G. B.: Molecular identification of human Ia antigens coded for by a gene locus closely linked to HLA-DR locus. *Immunogenetics* 10:151, 1980.
31. Tosi, R., Tanigaki, N., Centis, D., Ferrara, G. B., and Pressman, D.: Immunological dissection of human Ia molecules. *J. Exp. Med.* 148:1592, 1980.
32. Markert, M. L., and Cresswell, P.: Polymorphism of human B-cell alloantigens: Evidence for three loci within the HLA system. *Proc. Natl. Acad. Sci. U.S.A.* 77:6101, 1980.
33. Tanigaki, N., Tosi, R., Koyama, K., and Pressman, D.: Purification and separation of subsets of human Ia molecules by papain digestion. *Immunology* 39:615, 1980.
34. Schroer, J., and Rosenthal, A. S.: Function of macrophages as antigen presenting cells. *Springer Semin. Immunopathol.* 3:247, 1980.
35. Germain, R. N., and Banacerraf, B.: Helper and suppressor T cell factors. *Springer Semin. Immunopathol.* 3:93, 1980.
36. Dupont, B., Hansen, J. A., and Yunis, E. J.: Human mixed lymphocyte culture reaction: Genetics, specificity and biological implications. *Adv. Immunol.* 23:108, 1976.
37. Jorgensen, F., Lamm, L. U., and Kissmeyer-Nielsen, F.: Mixed lymphocyte cultures with inbred individuals: An approach to MLC typing. *Tissue Antigens* 3:323, 1973.
38. Sheehy, M. J., and Bach, F. H.: Primed LD typing (PLT): Technical considerations. *Tissue Antigens* 8:157, 1976.
39. Snell, G. D., Dausset, J., and Nathenson, S.: *Histocompatibility.* Academic Press, New York, 1976, p. 210.
40. Silver, H. (ed.): *Paternity Testing.* American Association of Blood Banks, Washington, D.C., 1978.
41. Lee, C. L., and Henry, J. B.: Laboratory evaluation of disputed parentage, in *Clinical Diagnosis and Management by Laboratory Methods*, edited by J. B. Henry, Saunders, Philadelphia, 1979, chap. 44.
42. Reisner, E. G., and MacQueen, M. M.: Problems arising from the use of the HLA system in paternity testing. *Clin. Lab. Haematol.* 3:113, 1981.
43. Seigler, H. F., et al.: Renal transplantation between HL-A identical donor-recipient pairs: Functional and morphological evaluation. *J. Clin. Invest.* 51:3200, 1972.
44. Hansen, J. A., Clift, R. A.,Thomas, E. D., Buchner, C. D., Michaelsen, E. M., and Storb, R.: Histocompatibility and marrow transplantation. *Transplant. Proc.* 11:1924, 1979.
45. Dausset, J., and Svejgaard, A. (eds.): *HLA and Disease.* Munksgaard, Copenhagen, 1977.
46. Aster, R. H., Szatkowski, Liebert, M., and Duquesnoy, R. J.: Expression of HLA-B12, HLA-B8, w4 and w6 in platelets. *Transplant. Proc.* 9:1695, 1977.
47. Duquesnoy, R. J., Filip, D. J., Tomasulo, P. A., and Aster, R. H.: Role of HLA-C matching in histocompatible platelet transfusion therapy of alloimmunized thrombocytopenic patients. *Transplant. Proc.* 9:1827, 1977.
48. Shulman, N. R., Marder, V. J., Hiller, M. C., and Collier, E. M.: Platelet and leukocyte isoantigens and their antibodies: Serologic, physiologic, and clinical studies. *Prog. Hematol.* 4:223, 1964.

49. Perkins, H. A., Payne, R., Vyas, G., and Fudenberg, H. H.: Nonhemolytic reactions to blood transfusion and organ transplantation. *Bibl. Haematol. 38:315, 1971.*

50. Van Leeuwen, E. F., von dem Borne, A.E.G., von Riesz, L. E., Nijenhuis, L. E., and Engelfriet, C. P.: Absence of platelet-specific alloantigens in Glanzmann's thrombasthenia. *Blood 57:49, 1981.*

51. Harrington, W. J., Sprague, C. C., Minnich, V., Moore, C. V., Aulvin, R. C., and Dubach, R.: Immunologic mechanisms in idiopathic and neo-natal thrombocytopenic purpura. *Ann. Intern. Med. 38:433, 1953.*

52. Brand, A., van Leeuwen, A., and Eernesse, J. G.: Platelet transfusion therapy: Optimal donor selection with a combination of lymphocytotoxicity and platelet fluorescence tests. *Blood 51:781, 1978.*

53. Aster, R. H., Cooper, H. E., and Singer, D. L.: Simplified complement fixation test for the detection of platelet antibodies in human serum. *J. Lab. Clin. Med. 53:161, 1964.*

54. Steffen, C.: Results obtained with the antiglobulin consumption test and investigations of autoantibody eluates in immunohematology. *J. Lab. Clin. Med. 55:9, 1980.*

55. Horowitz, H. L., Rapaport, H. I., Young, R. C., and Fujimoto, M. M.: Change in platelet factor 3 as a means of demonstrating immuno reactions involving platelets: Its use as a test for quinidine-induced thrombocytopenia. *Transfusion 5:336, 1965.*

56. Bridges, J. M., Fichera, C., and Baldini, M.: The serotonin test for the detection of antiplatelet antibodies. *Blood 20:797, 1962.*

57. Lalezari, P., and Radel, E.: Neutrophil specific antigens: Immunology and clinical significance. *Semin. Hematol. 11:281, 1974.*

58. Verheught, F. W. A., Borne, A. E. G. Kr. von dem, van Noorde-Bokhorst, J. C., Nijenhuis, L. E., and Engelfriet, C. P.: ND, a new neutrophil granulocyte antigen. *Vox Sang. 35:13, 1978.*

59. Claas, F. J. H., Langerak, J., Sabbe, L. J. M., and van Rood, J. J.: Ne₁, a new neutrophil specific antigen. *Tissue Antigens 13:129, 1979.*

60. Lalezari, P.: Histocompatibility requirements for bone marrow transplantation and transfusion of granulocytes and platelets, in *Immunology of the Major Histocompatibility Complex* (7th Int. Covoc. Immunol.). Karger, Basel, 1981, p. 286.

61. Slichter, S. J.: Controversies in platelet transfusion therapy. *Ann. Rev. Med. 31:509, 1980.*

62. Yankee, R. A.: HL-A antigens and platelet therapy, in *Platelets: Production, Function, Transfusion and Storage,* edited by M. G. Baldini and S. Ebbe. Grune & Stratton, New York, 1974, p. 313.

63. Duquesnoy, R. J., Filip, D. J., and Rodey, G. E.: Successful transfusion of platelets "mismatched" for HLA antigens to alloimmunized thrombocytopenic patients. *Am. J. Hematol. 2:219, 1977.*

64. Wu. K. K., Hoak, J. C., and Thompson, J. S.: Use of platelet aggregometry in selection of compatible platelet donors. *N. Engl. J. Med. 292:130, 1975.*

65. Hattler, B. G., Jr., Young, W. G., Amos, D. B., Hutchen, P., and MacQueen, M.: White blood cell antibodies: Occurrence in patients undergoing open heart surgery. *Arch. Surg. 91:451, 1966.*

66. Amos, D. B.: HL-A fertility and natural selection in *Immunological Approaches to Fertility Control* (Karolinska Symposia on Research Methods in Reproductive Endocrinology, VII Symposium). Karger, Basel, 1973, p. 318.

67. Hildemann, W. H., Clark, E. A., and Raison, R. L.: *Comprehensive Immunogenetics.* Elsevier, New York, 1981, p. 292.

68. Svejgaard, A.: Iso-antigenic systems of human blood platelets: A survey. *Ser. Haematol. 2:3, 1969.*

CHAPTER *163*

The plasma proteins

CHESTER A. ALPER

The plasma is a highly complex mixture of over 100 proteins [1]. In almost every plasma protein that has been intensively investigated, inherited structural variation, or genetic polymorphism, has been found. In most instances, this genetic polymorphism has resulted from point mutation and amino acid substitution. Genetic variation has been detected by protein separation methods sensitive to the net surface charge changes that result from such substitutions. Remarkably, even those substitutions involving amino acids of similar charge may be detected by such sensitive techniques as isolectric focusing. In general, whole serum or plasma can be examined without prior purification or other treatment provided the protein in question can be distinctly seen without interference from or confusion with other plasma proteins. For a few proteins occurring in high concentration, such as albumin, transferrin, C3, and α_1-antitrypsin, interference is minimal and simple protein staining after electrophoresis or isoelectric focusing suffices. For most plasma proteins, however, specific staining methods dependent upon unique functional or physicochemical characteristics or upon reaction with specific antibody (immunofixation) are required.

Although theoretically genetic variation in plasma proteins can lead to alloimmunization following exposure during transfusion or pregnancy, in fact such alloimmunization occurs with only a few of the plasma proteins: certain immunoglobulins, lipoproteins, and the fourth component of complement. Moreover, alloantibodies to plasma proteins, when present, seem rarely, if ever, to cause major transfusion reactions. The one situation where transfusion can result in symptoms is in IgA-deficient subjects who have anti-IgA and receive normal plasma (see Chap. 164). Such patients may have severe reactions with chills, fever, and even hypotension. This antibody is not a true alloantibody, being presumably directed against many antigenic determinants on a molecule completely absent in its producer.

Inherited deficiency states of individual plasma proteins are rare. Those affecting proteins of the coagulation and fibrinolytic systems, considered elsewhere in this book, are associated with dramatic symptoms such as excessive bleeding or clotting in vivo. Deficiencies of immunoglobulins and certain complement proteins are associated with increased susceptibility to bacterial infection, whereas deficiency of α_1-antitrypsin may result in neonatal hepatitis, juvenile cirrhosis, and severe adult chronic obstructive pulmonary disease. Inherited deficiency of α_1-antitrypsin usually involves genetic variants of this protein. Abnormalities in the genetic control of plasma lipoproteins will be touched on only briefly here because this area is a specialty unto itself. However, both deficiency states and inherited tendencies to increased levels of lipoproteins are recognized, with attendant disease susceptibilities and symptoms. Deficiencies of some complement proteins predispose to systemic lupus erythematosus and, in other instances, to angioedema (see Chap. 112). Deficiency of albumin suprisingly produces only mild and intermittent edema. On the other hand, inherited deficiency of transferrin is associated with severe hypochromic microcytic anemia and death in childhood (see Chap. 49).

With the development of methods for direct analysis of mRNA and genomic DNA has come the opportunity to examine inherited variation in the plasma protein genes themselves. Progress in this area is rapid, and broad outlines of the gene structure of several plasma proteins are already known. Just as was first shown for globin, genes for plasma proteins may contain intervening nucleotide sequences (introns) not expressed in their protein products. Rapid methods for the detection of genetic polymorphisms in introns and other nonexpressed DNA using restriction endonucleases promise a wealth of new information on inherited variation in plasma protein genes, including their evolution, chromosomal localization, function, and relation to other genes.

Almost all plasma proteins, with the major exception of the immunoglobulins, are produced by hepatocytes. Plasma cells and B lymphocytes synthesize immunoglobins. Plasma proteins are, in general, synthesized on the polyribosomes and discharged into the rough endoplasmic reticulum. If carbohydrate is part of the circulating protein, it is added during passage through the cisternae of the endoplasmic reticulum and the Golgi apparatus. As it is synthesized, each polypeptide chain may have extra peptides at the amino terminus called pre and pro fragments. Release from the ribosomes of newly synthesized polypeptide chains involves cleavage between the pre fragment and the amino acid which becomes the N-terminal amino acid of the appropriate chain in the circulating protein. A second proteolytic cleavage during processing removes the pro fragment. The latter may serve as a signal for passage through the endoplasmic reticulum. Some proteins are synthesized as single polypeptide chains but then cleaved intracellularly by a plasmin-like enzyme(s) to produce multichain structures which circulate as the major "natural" protein.

Nomenclature

The nomenclature used in this chapter is that endorsed by the International Society for Human Genetics [2] and is meant, by eliminating subscripts and superscripts and by using only capital letters and arabic numerals, to be easily used in computer storage and analysis. Gene loci are designated by two or more italicized letters and/or numbers (preferably four characters or fewer). Alleles are designated by the locus name, an asterisk, and one or more italicized letters and/or numbers (preferably four characters or fewer). All characters are on the same line. Gene products, genetic variants, and phenotypes are noted as alleles are except that the asterisk is replaced by a space and characters are not italicized. Null alleles or variants are designated "Q0" for "quantity zero" and "QL" for "quantity lowered." Table 163-1 lists this new nomenclature for the genetic loci and alleles discussed in this chapter and shows equivalents appearing in the literature.

Albumin

Albumin is the most abundant of the plasma proteins. Because of this and its relatively low M_r of 69,000 daltons, it is the major contributor to colloid osmotic pressure. Its primary structure consists of 585 amino acids cross-linked by 17 disulfide bridges. The arrangement of these bridges is such that they form helical, rodlike structures with tight hairpin loops at their ends [3]. Three such structures in parallel constitute a troughlike subdomain, and a pair of subdomains forms a domain. There are three domains in the whole albumin molecule, each forming a cylinder produced by six parallel rods and having hydrophobic walls. Fatty acids, bilirubin, and other hydrophobic substances are bound to these domains as albumin performs its transport functions. From extensive sequence homology it is postulated that albumin evolved by a series of tandem gene triplications from a 77-residue protein some 700 million years ago.

There are at least two dozen structural variants of albumin. The variants are detected by electrophoretic methods applied to whole serum or, in a few instances, to fragments of the purified proteins [4]. In most populations, the common form, albumin A, is found in well over 99 percent of individuals. In a few American Indian and Turkish populations, variants are found with allele frequencies in excess of 1 percent. Examples are albumin Naskapi (in Indian groups from Quebec) and albumin Mexico (in Indians of the American Southwest and of Mexico). A variant found in Turkey (albumin Mersin) appears identical to albumin Naskapi.

It is likely that albumin B, a rare variant found largely in Caucasians, differs from albumin A in that a lysine is substituted for a glutamate residue at position 570. Similarly, albumin Mexico-2 has glycine at position 550, where albumin A has aspartate. An interesting variant, albumin Christchurch [5], is larger than albumin A by six amino acids. There is a substitution of glutamate for arginine at the point of proteolytic cleavage between the pro fragment and albumin. The substitution prevents

TABLE 163-1   Gene locus and allele designation equivalences

Designation in this chapter		Alternative and prior designations	
Locus	Alleles	Locus	Alleles
PI	M1, M2, M3, M4, Z, S, Q0, M MALTON	Pi	M₁, M₂, M₃, M₄, Z, S, null or −, M^Malton
OR	F, S	Or	F, S
HPA	1F, 1S, 2	Hp	1αF, 1αS, 2α
GC	1F, 1S, 2, 1A1, 2A3	Gc	1F, 1S, 2, Ab, Japan
CP	A, B, C, NH	Cp	A, B, C, B^NH
E1	U, A, J, F, S, K	El	u, a, j, f, s, k
TF	C1, C2, C3, C4, C5, B2, D1	Tf	C₁, C₂, C₃, C₄, C₅, B₂, D₁
AG	X, Y, A1, D, C, G, T, Z, H, I	Ag	x, y, a1, d, c, g, t, z, h, i
LP	A	Lp	a
G1M	A, Z, X, F, NONA	G1m	a or 1, z or 17, x or 2, f or 3, non-a
G2M	N	G2m	n or 23
G3M	B0, B1, B3, B4, B5, C3, C5, S, T, G	G3m	b⁰ or 11, b¹ or 5, b³ or 12, b⁴ or 14, b⁵ or 10, c³ or 6, c⁵ or 24, s or 15, t or 16, g or 21
A2M	1, 2	A2m	1, 2
HV	1	Hv	1
KM	1, 2, 3	Km, InV	1, a, b
PLGN	A, B	Plg	1, 2
F13A	1, 2	FXIIIA	1, 2
F13B	1, 2, 3	FXIIIB	1, 2, 3, (S, F)
BG	N, Q0	Bg	N, D
C3	F, S, Q0	C3	F, S, null or −
BF	F, S, F1, S1	Bf, Gb	F, S, F1, S 0.7, F₁, S₁
C2	C, B, A1, A2	C2	1, 2, (3), (4)

the proteolytic processing, explaining the slightly larger size of this variant.

α₁-Antitrypsin

α₁-Antitrypsin inhibits a number of serine proteases, including pancreatic elastase, trypsin, chymotrypsin, plasmin, and granulocyte proteases. It does so by forming stable equimolar complexes. The M_r of α₁-antitrypsin is 52,000 daltons, and it contains 12.5 percent carbohydrate [6]. There are 30 or more genetic variants of α₁-antitrypsin, of which six occur in European populations with allele frequencies in excess of 1 percent [7]. The variants are detected most definitively by starch gel electrophoresis and by isoelectric focusing in polyacrylamide gel, but agarose gel electrophoresis with immunofixation is adequate for clinical screening. Figure

163-1 shows the variants as detected by starch gel electrophoresis and isoelectric focusing [7].

Table 163-2 lists the frequencies of common alleles for α₁-antitrypsin at its structural locus, designated PI (for protease inhibitor). Of clinical interest are the alleles PI*Z and PI*S, which are associated with markedly and moderately reduced serum concentrations of α₁-antitrypsin. There are several other alleles, rare in all populations, associated with markedly reduced (PI*M MALTON, PI*M NICKINAN) or nondetectable (PI*Q0) serum levels of α₁-antitrypsin. Individuals doubly heterozygous or homozygous for these deficient alleles have an increased risk of severe, early-onset chronic obstructive pulmonary disease (panlobular emphysema). Those homozygous for PI*Z or heterozygous for this allele and another moderately or severely deficient PI allele are susceptible to neonatal hepatitis, juvenile cirrhosis, and primary cancer of the liver. All subjects who

TABLE 163-2   Protease inhibitor (PI) allele frequencies in several populations

Country	M1	M2	M3	M4	S	Z	F	I	V	W
France	0.626	0.092	0.104	0.037	0.141					
China	0.765	0.173	0.051				0.011			*
Australia (Aborigines)	0.280	0.680	0.040							
Sweden	0.946			†		0.024	0.003			
Spain	0.866			†	0.112	0.012	0.003	0.001	0.0026	0.0026
Norway (Lapps)	0.992			†		0.008				
Norway	0.946			†	0.023	0.016	0.013	0.001	0.0004	

*Unspecified "rare" variants.
†PI*M not further subdivided.

ANODAL VARIANTS
α- ANTITRYPSIN (Pi)

CATHODAL VARIANTS
α-ANTITRYPSIN (Pi)

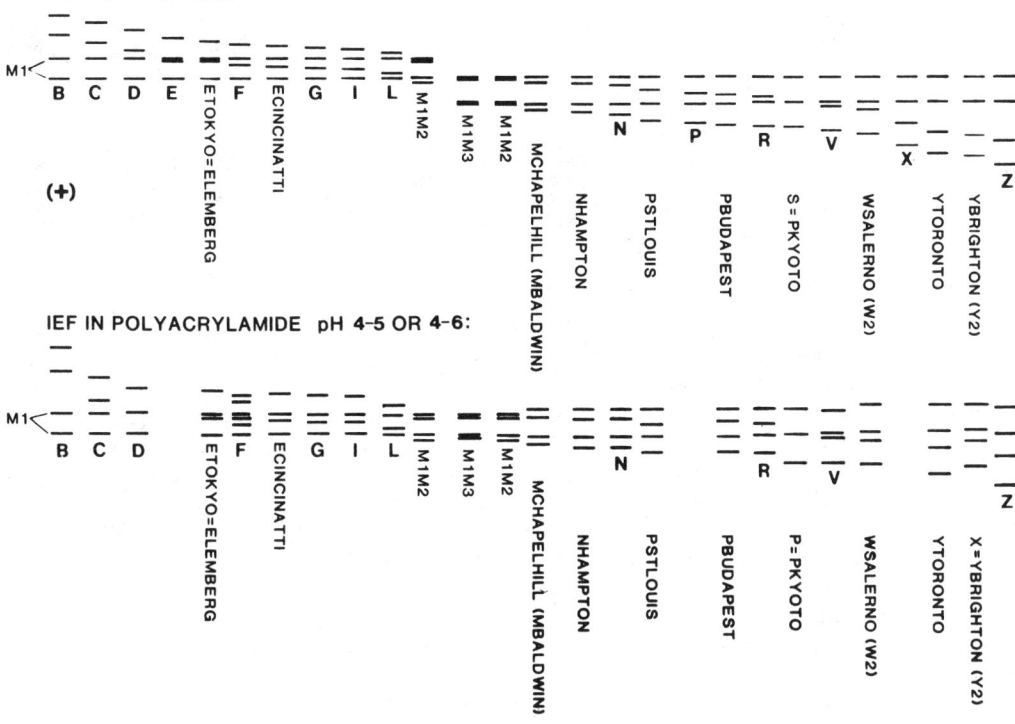

FIGURE 163-1 Diagrammatic representation of genetic variants of α_1-antitrypsin as they appear on acid starch gel electrophoresis and isoelectric focusing. Only the two most prominent bands of each variant are shown. (Adapted from Cox et al. [7].)

have the *PI**Z allele have characteristic inclusion bodies in their hepatocytes. These represent accumulated α_1-antitrypsin in the endoplasmic reticulum. The inclusion bodies appear to contain incompletely glycosylated PI Z protein that is in other ways indentical to the circulating protein.

α_1-Antitrypsin displays considerable microheterogeneity, even in homozygotes, and each allele product consists of five major bands. The basis of this microheterogeneity resides in the carbohydrate portion of the molecule and reflects different numbers of sialic acid residues per protein molecule.

The structural differences between a number of PI variants involve single amino acid substitutions for Glu in PI M1. In P1 M2 it is Asp [8], in PI S it is Val [9], and in PI Z it is Lys [10]; the substitutions are not all at the same Glu residue. There has been identified at least one PI M variant that occurs in normal concentration but is both acid- and heat-labile and therefore "disappears" on either acid gel electrophoresis or isoelectric focusing [11,12].

A cDNA insert of 1352 base pairs coding for baboon α_1-antitrypsin has been cloned [13]. It (and the amino acid sequence it encodes) show 96 percent homology with the human homolog. The cDNA codes for a 15–

amino acid N-terminal signal sequence and 394 amino acids of the mature protein, and has a stop codon and 76 noncoding nucleotides.

The C-terminal 8– to 10–amino acid sequence of human α_1-antitrypsin is virtually identical to that of human and porcine antithrombin III. This suggests a common evolutionary origin for the genes for both proteinase inhibitors.

α_1-Acid glycoprotein

α_1-Acid glycoprotein (orosomucoid, OR) contains 37 percent carbohydrate and transports a number of basic drugs, including local anesthetics and propranolol. On electrophoresis near its isoelectric point or on isoelectric focusing, the protein exhibits marked microheterogeneity, largely ascribable to differences in sialic acid content [14]. Treatment of whole serum with neuraminidase (to remove sialic acid from all serum proteins) followed by analysis by agarose gel electrophoresis at pH 8.6 and immunofixation with antiserum to α_1-acid glycoprotein [15] reveals a simple genetic polymorphism. Two alleles of nearly equal frequency are found in almost all populations studied, as seen in Table 163-3.

TABLE 163-3 α_1-Acid glycoprotein (orosomucoid, *OR*) allele frequencies in some populations

Country	S	F
Botswana	0.62	0.38
Nigeria	0.41	0.59
Zaire	0.47	0.53
United States (Chinese)	0.47	0.53
United States (Amerind)	0.54	0.46
Japan	0.27	0.73
United States (whites)	0.36	0.64
France	0.49	0.51
Sweden	0.67	0.33

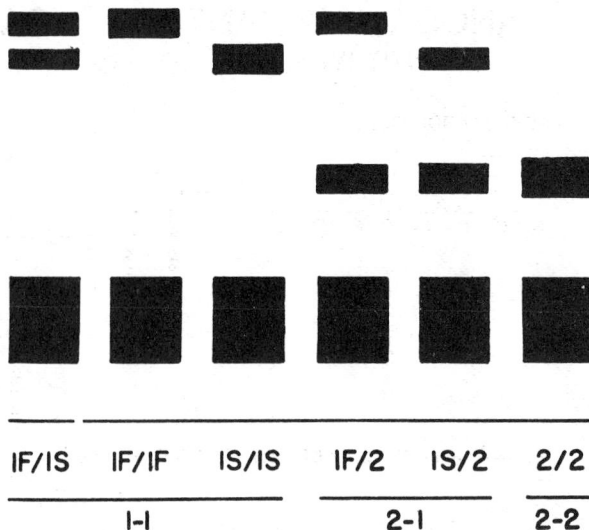

FIGURE 163-2 Electrophoretic patterns produced by purified haptoglobin of different genetic types, shown schematically. Electrophoresis is run in starch or polyacrylamide gel at acidic pH, in the presence of 6 *M* urea and reducing agent, so that the molecules are resolved into subunits: invariant β chains at bottom and polymorphic α chains at top.

Haptoglobin

Haptoglobin is an axially symmetrical molecule consisting of two β chains and two α chains [16]. The protein binds hemoglobin and thereby conserves iron released from red cell destruction [17]. Each β chain of one molecule of haptoglobin binds one half molecule of hemoglobin. The covalent structure of haptoglobin is known. The β chain has 245 amino acids and an M_r of 33,820 daltons, including about 6560 daltons for carbohydrate [18]. The α chain contains either 83 amino acids ($M_r = $ 9189 daltons) or nearly twice this number, depending upon genetic type. The β chain shows about 30 percent homology with serine proteases, suggesting its evolutionary origin from a primordial protease gene. It is not clear whether there is one cistron for each haptoglobin subunit or whether there is a single cistron producing a prohaptoglobin molecule which is then cleaved to form the two-chain half (α-β) molecule.

There are three common variants of human haptoglobin reflecting differences in the α chains (HPA) [19]. The difference between HPA 1F and HPA 1S is determined by the presence of Lys or Glu at position 53. HPA 2 consists of an apparent fusion of HPA 1F and HPA 1S to produce a chain nearly twice the length of either HPA 1 product. It is most likely that an unequal crossover in an individual heterozygous for *HPA*1F/ HPA*1S* with fusion of the two nearly complete genes led to the *HPA*2* gene [20]. Rare examples of *HPA*2* genes consisting of *HPA*1F/1F* or *HPA*1S/1S* have been found and strengthen the argument for unequal crossing over and fusion as the origin of *HPA*2* genes. Patterns given by the different *HPA* phenotypes produced

by these alleles in starch or polyacrylamide gel electrophoresis under acidic, reducing, and dissociating conditions are shown in Fig. 163-2.

Table 163-4 lists *HPA* allele frequencies in a number of populations. In addition to the common alleles, a number of rare *HPA* variants have been described. A few β-chain genetic variants have also been found. It is of interest that some have altered hemoglobin binding. Linkage studies in families with both α- and β-chain variation suggest that there are separate and unlinked loci for the haptoglobin α and β subunits. In addition to direct structural variation, there may be inherited underproduction of one or another *HPA* gene, producing unusual and recognizable electrophoretic patterns.

Gc-Globulin (vitamin D–binding globulin)

There are three common alleles of Gc-globulin [21,22] — *GC*1F, GC*1S,* and *GC*2* — detected by isoelectric focusing of whole serum and immunofixation with specific

TABLE 163-4 Frequencies of major haptoglobin α-chain (HPA) alleles

Country	1F	1S	2
Nigeria	0.473	0.258	0.269
China		0.341	0.659
Korea		0.321	0.679
Japan	0.003	0.227	0.770
Baffin Island (Eskimo)		0.239	0.761
United States (Amerind)		0.374	0.626
Chile (Amerind)		0.774	0.226
Italy	0.118	0.252	0.630
India	0.046	0.104	0.850

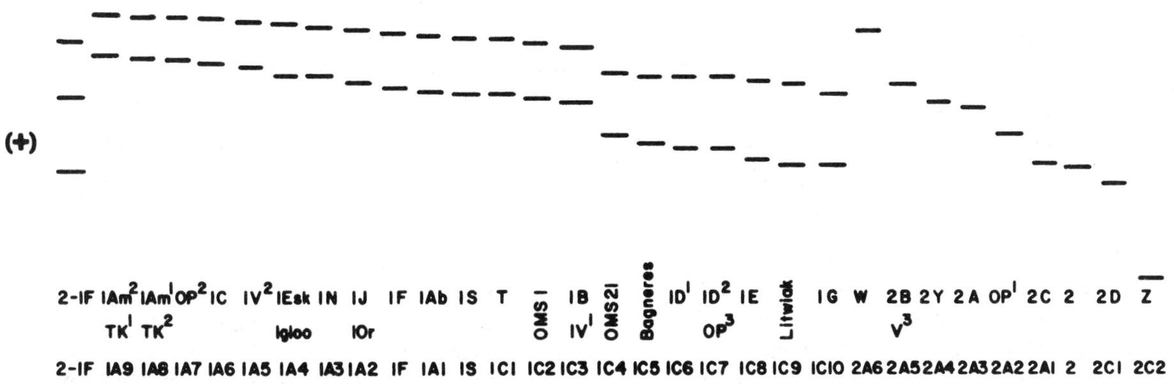

FIGURE 163-3   Diagrammatic representation of variants of Gc-globulin (vitamin D–binding globulin) made visible by isoelectric focusing and immunofixation with specific antiserum. (Adapted from Constans and Cleve [23].)

antiserum. Electrophoresis at alkaline pH, whether in agarose, starch, or polyacrylamide gels or on cellulose acetate, fails to detect the GC 1F-1S difference. Patterns produced by the common alleles and some of the nearly three dozen additional (rare) variants of this protein [23] are shown in Fig. 163-3. Table 163-5 gives the GC allele frequencies in some populations. Two alleles, GC*1A1 and GC*2A3, rare in other populations, are found in high frequencies in African populations.

Gc-globulin is the transport protein for vitamin D [24]. All variants bind this vitamin, although there is evidence that the affinity for GC 1 is greater than that for GC 2. Charge microheterogeneity in the GC system has been shown to reflect sialic acid content (GC 1) and whether or not vitamin D is bound [25].

Ceruloplasmin

The copper-containing blue protein ceruloplasmin has an M_r of approximately 160,000 daltons [26,27]. It is not a copper-transport protein (that function is carried out by albumin), but it has amine oxidase activity and probably detoxifies superoxide and other reactive oxygen-containing species released during phagocytosis.

Ceruloplasmin concentration is usually markedly decreased in the serum of patients with Wilson's disease and with an inherited disorder called kinky hair disease. The latter is a rare autosomal disorder characterized by copper malabsorption and resulting copper

deficiency, mental retardation, and microscopically kinky hair.

Inherited structural variants of ceruloplasmin are detected by electrophoresis in either starch or agarose gel at alkaline pH followed by either amine oxidase staining [28] or immunofixation. CP*B is the most common allele in all populations, and only blacks have other variants in appreciable frequency.

Pseudocholinesterase

The known genetic variation in pseudocholinesterase largely concerns inherited functional deficiency. This is of major clinical importance because deficient patients are subject to prolonged apnea when given the muscle relaxant succinylcholine. Normally, pseudocholinesterase (acylcholine acylhydrolase) rapidly hydrolyzes this drug, which is essentially a dimer of acetyl choline. A number of different mutant genes are responsible for deficiency of the enzyme as defined by kinetics of inhibition with a variety of substrates and inhibitors, including dibucaine and fluoride [29]. The genetic locus has been designated E1. Recognized variants are designated E1 A (atypical); E1 S (silent), with little or no immunoreactive enzyme; E1 J, with 30 to 35 percent activity; E1 K with 65 to 70 percent activity; and E1 F, with nearly normal dibucaine number and markedly reduced fluoride number [30].

The E1*A allele has a frequency of between 0.01 and

TABLE 163-5   Gc-Globulin *(GC)* allele frequencies in several populations

Country	1F	1S	2	1A1	1A9	2A3	1A2
France	0.077	0.512	0.410				
Germany	0.125	0.603	0.272				
Central African Republic	0.584	0.191	0.064	0.054		0.107	
Bolivia (Amerind)	0.231	0.636	0.122		0.009		
Japan	0.466	0.259	0.257				0.018

TABLE 163-6   Transferrin (TF) allele frequencies in several populations

Country	C1	C2	C3	C4	C5	B2	D1
Germany	0.795	0.155	0.042	0.01–0.02		0.008	
United States (whites)	0.787	0.165	0.049				
United States (blacks)	0.840	0.121	0.008		0.03		0.003
Pyrenees	0.788	0.132	0.053			0.027	
Bolivia (Amerinds)				0.03–0.04			

0.02 in most white populations studied, but frequencies as high as 0.05 have been observed in non-Ashkenazi Jews. E1*S and E1*F may also have frequencies in the 0.01 to 0.05 range, but other alleles appear to be rarer.

Transferrin

The protein responsible for iron transport in the blood is the β-globulin transferrin [31]. The molecule is a single chain of M_r 75,000 daltons with two similar domains, each with an iron-binding site, suggesting evolution via gene duplication.

Although a large number of relatively rare alleles at TF, the structural locus for transferrin, have been known for years [32], it is only recently that the true extent of genetic polymorphism has been appreciated. This came about because, on alkaline electrophoresis, the transferrin of most populations appeared the same in most individuals, TF C. With the introduction of isoelectric focusing, it has become possible to detect not only the differences in charge between the molecules with no iron and those with one and two iron atoms but also the extensive polymorphism in TF C [33,34]. There are three common alleles in Caucasians, designated TF*C1, TF*C2, and TF*C3; one variant common in Amerind populations, TF*C4; and another, TF*C5, common in blacks. Table 163-6 gives allele frequencies for TF in a number of populations.

Lipoproteins

A full treatment of the complex subject of genetic control of serum lipoproteins will not be attempted here. For our purposes, it is sufficient to recognize that there are seven well-characterized, distinct apolipoproteins, each almost certainly under separate genetic control, and that almost all "classical" lipoprotein classes (high density, very low density, etc.) consist of components that differ from one another in both lipid and apolipoprotein composition. Finally, individual apoproteins are found in more than one "classical" lipoprotein class.

Three genetic systems have been reasonably well characterized: AG and LP serological variants of Apo B and the electrophoretic variants of Apo E. The AG (antigen) system [35,36] consists of 10 specificities, designated X, Y, A1, D, C, G, T, Z, H, and I. They are detected by precipitin formation in agar gels with antisera obtained mostly from multitransfused patients. The typing antisera are thus alloantisera. The AG markers have been observed to occur as antithetical pairs, and it has therefore been postulated that there are five closely linked tandem genetic loci for Apo B and that specific haplotypes occur more commonly in some populations than in others. Fourteen AG haplotypes have been identified, and some appear to be population-specific [36].

LP A is an antigenic determinant recognized by an antiserum produced in rabbits immunized with β-lipoprotein [37]. It is found in the serum of about 35 percent of Caucasians. It may be that the LP locus controls two overlapping distributions of LP A concentration, as determined from family studies [38]. LP A is carried on electrophoretically pre-β-lipoproteins with physiochemical characteristics different from both low-density and very-low-density lipoproteins (VLDL) [39].

The genetic polymorphism in Apo E, a protein intimately involved with cholesterol metabolism, is detected by isoelectric focusing of the purified apoproteins or VLDL [40,41]. There are three alleles, E*2, E*3, and E*4, for specific proteins that are acidic, medium, and basic with respect to each other. The E 4 protein has Arg at both position 74 and position 158, and the E 3 has Cys at 74 and Arg at 158. The E 2 protein in some individuals has Cys at both 74 and 158 or Cys at 74, Arg at 158, and a Cys for Arg substitution a number of residues toward the C terminus. The frequencies of the alleles are $E*2 = 0.15$, $E*3 = 0.74$, and $E*4 = 0.11$ among Bostonian Caucasians. Individuals with type III hyperlipoproteinemia are homozygous E*2/2. The E 2 protein is cleared slowly in vivo and in a perfused rat liver preparation and binds poorly (when purified from the plasma of some individuals) or not at all (from others) in a fibroblast LDL receptor assay in vitro. Thus, type III hyperlipoproteinemia can be traced to an amino acid substitution in Apo E that abrogates or severely interferes with receptor binding and hence uptake, utilization, and clearance. The situation is in contrast to type II hyperlipoproteinemia, in which an Apo B receptor deficiency or dysfunction has been demonstrated.

Immunoglobulins

The immunoglobulins carry serum antibody activity. The structure of the immunoglobulins and organization of immunoglobulin genes are described in detail in Chap. 104, and the reader is referred to that section as the basis for the present discussion of genetic polymorphisms.

TABLE 163-7 Structural differences related to GM specificities

Specificity	Polypeptide chain	Papain fragment	Sequence number	Amino acid residues
G1M A	γ1	Fc	356–358	Asp-Glu-Leu
GM NONA	γ1, γ2, γ3	Fc	356–358	Glu-Glu-Met
G1M F	γ1	Fd	214	Arg
G1M Z	γ1	Fd	214	Lys
G3M G	γ3	Fc	296	Tyr
GM NONG	γ2, γ3	Fc	296	Phe
G3M BO	γ3	Fc	436	Phe
GM NONBO	γ1, γ2, γ3	Fc	436	Tyr
KM 1	κ	Fab	191	Leu
KM 2	κ	Fab	191	Val

The GM system was discovered over 25 years ago by Grubb and Laurell [42], working with serum from patients with rheumatoid arthritis. They noted that if Rh (D)–positive red cells were coated with incomplete anti-D from single individuals, the agglutination of these red cells produced by the rheumatoid agglutinins (RAgg) could be inhibited by some but not other random normal sera. It was shown that this ability to inhibit resided on IgG molecules and was under genetic control. Subsequently, it was discovered that serum from some normal individuals (SNAgg) was more specific than the RAgg as a reagent for this genetic system, called GM. An additional source of such reagents is rabbits immunized with purified myeloma proteins or M components.

There are a large number of GM specificities [43–45]. They reflect one or more amino acid differences in the constant regions of the heavy chains of IgG molecules of specific subclasses. For example, the specificity G1M 1 or A occurs on IgG1 molecules and is determined by the sequence Asp-Glu-Leu at positions 356 to 358 on the γ_1 chain. The allelic corresponding sequence in IgG1 is Glu-Glu-Met and is called GlM NON1 or NONA. However, this same sequence occurs on all IgG2 and IgG3 molecules at corresponding positions in all individuals and is therefore not allotypic on those molecules. Other markers on IgG1 include G1M Z, X, and F (G1M 17, 2, and 3); those on Ig G3 include G3M B0, B3, B4 (G3M 11, 13, 14); a single marker, G2M N (or G2M 23) is known for IgG2. Some of the known amino acid differences related to the genetic markers on immunoglobulins are given in Table 163-7. There are two genetic markers on the IgA2 minor subclass of IgA: A2M 1 and A2M 2.

There is now considerable indirect and direct evidence that the genetic loci for the heavy chains of the four subclasses of IgG and for those of IgA are adjacent to one another. This and their extensive structural homology strongly suggest a common evolutionary origin and production by repeated tandem gene duplication. Furthermore, groups of specific alleles at each of the loci occur in individuals and in populations as single genetic units or haplotypes. Some of the common haplotypes are given in Table 163-8.

There is a group of serological markers on κ chains that reflect amino acid differences in their constant regions. The system is KM, and the structural differences are given in Table 163-7. As pointed out elsewhere, the genetic loci controlling light-chain synthesis are not linked to those for heavy chains of immunoglobulins. There is evidence for a genetic marker in one of the framework regions of the variable portion of IgG, IgA, and IgM heavy chains [46]. The postulated gene (and locus) *HV*1* are not linked to *GM*.

Plasminogen

There is a common genetic polymorphism in plasminogen, most easily detected by isoelectric focusing of neuraminidase-treated serum or plasma [47]. Two common alleles, *PLGN*A* and *PLGN*B*, are found, as well as a number of rare alleles, and are detected by an overlay containing casein or fibrin (proteolysis) or by immunofixation. Frequencies for the common alleles are given in Table 163-9.

TABLE 163-8 Some common *GM-A2M* haplotypes

Population	G1M	G3M	G2M	A2M
Caucasoid	NONA, F	B0, B1, B3, B4, B5	N	1
Caucasoid	NONA, F	B0, B1, B3, B4, B5	—	1
Caucasoid, Mongoloid	A, Z, X	G	—	1
Caucasoid, Mongoloid, Negroid	A, Z	G	—	1
Mongoloid	A, F	B0, B1, B3, B4, B5	N	1
Mongoloid, Negroid	A, Z	B0, B1, B3, B4, B5	—	2
Negroid	A, Z	B0, B1, B4, B5	—	2
Negroid	A, Z	B0, B1, C3, C5		

TABLE 163-9 Plasminogen *(PLGN)* allele frequencies

Population	A	B	Rare
U.S. blacks	0.795	0.193	0.012
U.S. orientals	0.964	0.029	0.007
U.S. whites	0.686	0.299	0.015

Factor XIII

Using immunofixation with antisera specific for the two separate subunits of coagulation factor XIII, two distinct unlinked genetic polymorphisms have been detected [48,49]. There are two alleles for the A subunit with frequencies of 0.80 *(F13A*1)* and 0.20 *(F13A*2)* in random, unrelated Australian Caucasians. In this same population, allele frequencies for the B subunit were *F13B*1* = 0.747, *F13B*2* = 0.084, and *F13B*3* = 0.169 [49]. In a different genetic interpretation of similar electrophoretic typing patterns, two alleles were postulated for Japanese with frequencies of 0.664 for *F13B*S* and 0.336 for *F13B*F*.

Transcobalamin II

Charge variants of transcobalamin II are detected by the addition of radioisotopically labeled vitamin B_{12} to serum, isoelectric focusing or gel electrophoresis, and autoradiography [50,51]. Four common variants and one rare variant are detected in whites. The allele frequencies are presented in Table 163-10.

β_2-Glycoprotein I

Although no structural variation has been detected, deficiency of β_2-glycoprotein I is sufficiently common to produce a polymorphism [52]. The protein is measured immunochemically by radial immunodiffusion, electroimmunoassay, or any other appropriate means. In sera from random, unrelated persons, the concentration of this protein falls into one of three virtually completely nonoverlapping groups: none detectable, intermediate, and normal, these three corresponding to the genotypes $BG*Q0/BG*Q0$, $BG*Q0/BG*N$, and $BG*N/BG*N$. $BG*Q0$, the deficiency allele, has a frequency of around 0.03 among randomly selected Europeans. Individuals homozygous for deficiency of β_2-glycoprotein I are entirely healthy. The protein appears to be the same as apolipoprotein H.

Complement C3

Genetic polymorphism in the third component of complement is most easily detected by high-voltage electrophoresis of fresh serum in agarose or starch gel [53,54] in the presence of Ca^{2+} or Mg^{2+}. Under these conditions, the C3 can be seen on simple protein staining. There are two common alleles of *C3* in whites and, to a lesser extent, blacks, as seen in Table 163-11. There are a large number of structural variants of C3, as well as a rare deficiency allele, *C3*Q0*. Deficiency states for almost all complement proteins have been described. Almost all are rare, and a description of most of them is beyond the scope of this chapter. They are reviewed elsewhere [55,56].

Complement C6

The sixth component of human complement shows considerable genetic polymorphism [57]. Variants of C6 are most clearly detected by isoelectric focusing in gel of

TABLE 163-10 Transcobalamin II *(TC2)* allele* frequencies in some populations

Country	1	2	3	4	5
United States (whites)	0.450		0.531	0.015	0.004
United States (blacks)	0.178		0.635	0.187	
Guatemala (Amerind)	0.236		0.764		
United States (orientals)	0.486		0.514		
Switzerland	0.406	0.010	0.578	0.004	0.002

*The allele nomenclature is that proposed in Ref. 51, in which variants (and alleles) are named in order of electrophoretic mobility in alkaline gel electrophoresis from cathode to anode. It differs from that in Ref. 50.

TABLE 163-11 *C3* allele frequencies in various populations

Country	S	F	S0.4	Other
United States (whites)	0.77	0.22	0.003	
Norway	0.80	0.19	0.003	
Germany	0.78	0.21	0.003	
United States (blacks)	0.92	0.07		
Angola	0.95	0.05	0.001	
United States (orientals)	0.99			0.001
Tibet	1.00			

whole serum, with development of patterns in an overlay agarose gel containing antibody-sensitized sheep cells and early complement components and C6-deficient rabbit serum.

Complement C7

About 2 percent of the British population carry a variant of the seventh complement component and have the gene C7*2 [58]. Most individuals are homozygous C7*1/C7*1. The gene for C7 is closely linked to that for C6.

Complement C8

The eighth component of human complement consists of three subunits, of which only two are covalently linked (via disulfide bonds). There is now evidence that there are two separate and unlinked loci for C8, one (C81) coding for the α-γ chains and the other (C82) for the β chain of the complete molecule [59]. The C81 locus [60] has three common alleles in blacks and two in whites and orientals. There is also inherited structural variation at the C82 locus, but it is much less extensive than at C81 [59]. Both sets of variants are most easily and clearly detected by isoelectric focusing in 3.1 M urea (to dissociate α-γ from β chains most completely), removal of the urea, and detection in an overlay gel containing antibody-sensitized sheep erythrocytes and serum from humans with homozygous deficiencies in either α-γ or β chains.

Factor B (BF)

Variants of B of the alternative complement pathway are most easily detected by agarose gel electrophoresis and immunofixation [61]. An overlay gel in MgEGTA containing unsensitized guinea pig red cells and serum heated at 52°C for 15 min can also be used to produce bands of B-induced hemolysis. The two most common variants are BF F and BF S (for fast and slow), and two less common variants are BF F1 and BF S1 (Fig. 163-4). Each BF allele produces a protein that forms multiple bands, the most prominent of which is the second from the origin toward the anode. The variants are distinguished by the displacement of all bands toward the anode or cathode.

Complement C2

On isoelectric focusing in polyacrylamide gel [62], the second component of human complement can be detected by hemolysis of antibody-sensitized sheep erythrocytes in an agarose gel overlay containing dilute normal human serum (under these conditions, C2 is the limiting component). Bands of lysis consist of one main and two fainter flanking bands (C2 C). A relatively small

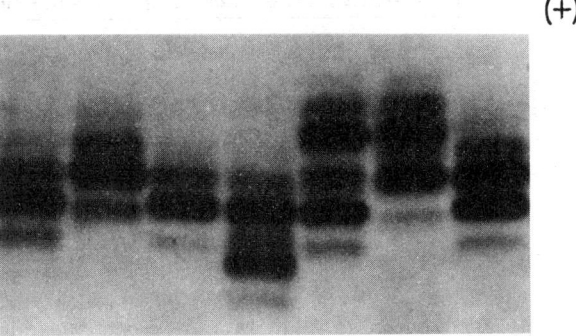

(+)

S   F   S   SSI FIS FIF FS

FIGURE 163-4 Electrophoretic patterns produced by variants of factor B of the alternative complement pathway. Electrophoresis was carried out at pH 8.6, and patterns were developed by immunofixation.

number of serum samples show cathodal duplication (C2 B), and rarely other variants are found.

Complement C4

Definition of genetic polymorphism in human C4 was difficult for many years until it was realized that there were two closely linked loci [63] producing this protein (C4A and C4B) and that there were common C4 haplotypes in which one or the other of these loci was null (Q0). By treating whole serum with neuraminidase to remove sialic acid from C4, the half-null haplotypes could be detected by crossed immunoelectrophoresis [64] and the many structural variants by immunofixation after agarose gel electrophoresis [65]. By the latter technique, each allele produces three equally spaced bands (Fig. 163-5). Usually, the most anodal band is most intense. Our laboratory has detected eight structural variants at each C4 locus, and other laboratories have found other rare variants. Several C4A and C4B variants have identical electrophoretic mobilities, in which case

FIGURE 163-5 Genetic variants of C4 produced by electrophoresis of desialated plasma at alkaline pH followed by immunofixation with anti-C4. (Awdeh and Alper [65].)

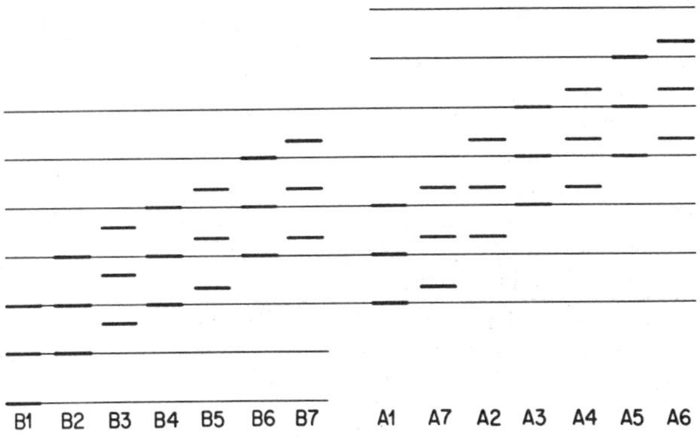

B1 B2 B3 B4 B5 B6 B7   A1 A7 A2 A3 A4 A5 A6

TABLE 163-12 Frequencies of common complotypes in Caucasians

BF	C2	C4A	C4B	Frequency	BF	C2	C4A	C4B	Frequency
S	C	3	1	0.403	F	C	0	1	0.029
S	C	0	1	0.127	S	C	0	2	0.029
F	C	3	1	0.096	S	C	2	1	0.022
S	C	3	0	0.053	S	B	4	2	0.019
S	C	4	2	0.040	S	C	3	3	0.014
S	C	6	1	0.034	S	C	2	2	0.013
F	C	3	0	0.031	S	C	3	2	0.011

other properties of C4A and C4B molecules are used to help decide by which locus the variant is synthesized. Functional overlay using either C4-deficient guinea pig serum or hydrazine-treated normal human serum and antibody-sensitized sheep red cells reveals that almost all hemolytic activity is exhibited by C4B products. Sometimes the different serological properties of C4A and C4B molecules can be used. Anti-Chido and anti-Rodgers are occasionally found in the serum of people who have received blood. The Chido (Ch) [66] and Rodgers (Rg) [67] "blood group" genetic systems were noted to be closely linked to HLA but were not antithetical, and no individual negative for both was initially found. It was recognized that the Ch and Rg antigens were plasma components and were deposited on red cells as an in vitro phenomenon. The solution to the entire puzzle came from noting that individuals homozygous for C4A*Q0 were negative for Rg and those homozygous for C4B*Q0 were negative for Ch [68]. It was also shown that purified C4 from pooled plasma carried Ch and Rg determinants and that the rare individuals homozygous for C4 deficiency were negative for both antigens. As an aid in typing rare C4 structural variants, serological reactions are useful only when family members are available who have C4A*Q0 or C4B*Q0 on the *other* chromosome.

Complotypes

The four genes for complement proteins coded for within the major histocompatibility complex are closely linked to one another, and no crossover among them has been noted in thousands of informative matings [69]. They therefore are regarded as genetic units at both the population and the family level. This is entirely analogous to the Rh and a number of other blood group systems (see Chap. 161) and to the immunoglobulin heavy-chain system described above. Complotypes are given as BF, C2, C4A, and C4B types in shortened form (the order of genes is arbitrary). For example, BF*S, C2*C,C4A*3,C4B*1 is SC31 and BF*F,C2*C,C4A*3,C4B*Q0 is FC30. The complotype loci are very close to HLA-D/DR, perhaps between HLA-D/DR and HLA-B [70].

Over 40 complotypes have been found in family studies of Caucasians. Of these, 14 occur with a frequency of 0.01 or more (Table 163-12) [69]. More important, studies of the relationship of these to HLA have shown that certain major histocompatibility haplotypes occur as extended units held in linkage disequilibrium over 5 to 7 centimorgans (recombination units) [71]. In other words, the whole haplotypes function as gametic units. The mechanisms which maintain such haplotypes are

TABLE 163-13 Chromosomal localization and linkage groups of plasma proteins other than the coagulation system

Protein	Chromosome	Linkage shown with
Antithrombin III	1	Fy
κ chains, C and V	2	
Albumin	4	
Gc globulin	4	ALB–GC–DG1-1–MNSs
Plasminogen	4	
Factor B	6	
C2	6	HLA-A, C, B, D, DR, BF, C2, C4A, C4B, GLO
C4	6	
Ig H chains	14	
α_1-Antitrypsin	14	G1M, G2M, G3M, G4M, A2M, PI
β_2-Microglobulin	15	
α-Haptoglobin	16	
C3	19	C3-Le-Se-Lu-Dm
λ chains, C	22	
Thyroxine-binding globulin	X	

NOTE: DG1-1 = dentiogenesis imperfecta; Dm = myotonic dystrophy.
SOURCE: The author is indebted to C. W. Partridge and F. H. Ruddle, Yale University, for providing the information on which this table is based.

not known, but it appears likely that the main ones are selection and perhaps crossover suppression in meioses with "wild" chromosomes [72] in analogy to mouse *t* variants [73]. It appears certain that it is these extended haplotypes that provide both the observed linkage disequilibrium sets that vary so strikingly from population to population [74] and most major histocompatibility markers for disease.

Chromosomal localization of serum protein genes

A number of serum protein genetic loci have been assigned to specific chromosomes by somatic cell hybridization techniques, by family linkage studies, and, most recently, by recombinant DNA methods. Table 163-13 lists those loci for which such information is available.

References

1. Putnam, F. W.: Alpha, beta, gamma, omega—The roster of the plasma proteins, in *The Plasma Proteins*, edited by F. W. Putnam. Academic, New York, 1977, vol. 1, p. 57.
2. Shows, T. B. et al.: International system for human gene nomenclature (1979). *Cytogenet. Cell Genet.* 25:96, 1979.
3. Brown, J. R., Shockley, P., and Behrens, P. Q.: Albumin: Sequence, evolution and structural models, in *The Chemistry and Physiology of the Human Plasma Proteins*, edited by D. H. Bing. Pergamon, New York, 1979, pp. 23–40.
4. Franklin, S. G., Wolf, S. I., Zweidler, A., and Blumberg, B. S.: Localization of the amino acid substitution site in a new variant of human serum albumin, albumin Mexico-2. *Proc. Natl. Acad. Sci. U.S.A.* 77:2505, 1980.
5. Brennan, S. O., and Carrell, R. W.: A circulating variant of human proalbumin. *Nature* 274:908, 1978.
6. Laurell, C.-B.: Aspects on biochemistry and pathophysiology of α₁-antitrypsin, in *The Chemistry and Physiology of the Human Plasma Proteins*, edited by D. H. Bing. Pergamon, New York, 1979, pp. 329–341.
7. Cox, D. W., Johnson, A. M., and Fagerhol, M. K.: Report of nomenclature meeting for α₁-antitrypsin: INSERM, Rouen/Bois Guillaume-1978. *Hum. Genet.* 53:429, 1980.
8. Yoshida, A., Taylor, J. C., and van den Brock, W. G. M.: Structural difference between the normal PiM₁ and the common PiM₂ variant of human α₁-antitrypsin. *Am. J. Hum. Genet.* 31:564, 1979.
9. Owen, M. C., and Carrell, R. W.: Alpha₁-antitrypsin: Molecular abnormality of S variant. *Br. Med. J.* 1:130, 1976.
10. Jeppsson, J.-O.: Amino acid substitution—Glu Lys in α-1-antitrypsin PiZ. *F.E.B.S. Lett.* 65:195, 1976.
11. Lie-injo, L. E.: α₁-Antitrypsin with unusual behaviour. *Clin. Chim. Acta* 72:83, 1976.
12. Taylor, J. C., Colin, M., Inamizu, T., and Mittman, C.: Familial temperature sensitive alpha 1 protease inhibitor (M1-ANAHEIM). *Clin. Chim. Acta* 104:301, 1980.
13. Kurachi, K., et al.: Cloning and sequence of cDNA coding for α₁-antitrypsin. *Proc. Natl. Acad. Sci. U.S.A.* 78:6826, 1981.
14. Schmid, K.: α₁-Acid glycoprotein, in *The Plasma Proteins*, edited by F. W. Putnam. Academic, New York, 1977, vol. 1, pp. 183–228.
15. Johnson, A. M., Schmid, K., and Alper, C. A.: Inheritance of human α₁-acid glycoprotein (orosomucoid) variants. *J. Clin. Invest.* 48:2293, 1969.
16. Smithies, O., Connell, G. E., and Dixon, G. H.: Gene action in the human haptoglobins. I. Dissociation into constituent polypeptide chains. *J. Mol. Biol.* 21:213, 1966.
17. Laurell, C.-B., and Nyman, M.: Studies on the serum haptoglobin level in hemoglobinemia and its influence on renal excretion of hemoglobin. *Blood* 12:493, 1957.
18. Kurosky, A., et al.: Covalent structure of human haptoglobin: A serine protease homolog. *Proc. Natl. Acad. Sci. U.S.A.* 77:3388, 1980.
19. Connell, G. E., Dixon, G. H., and Smithies, O.: Subdivision of the three common haptoglobin types based on "hidden" differences. *Nature* 193:505, 1962.
20. Smithies, O., Connell, G. E., and Dixon, G. H.: Chromosomal rearrangements and evolution of haptoglobin genes. *Nature* 196:232, 1962.
21. Hirschfeld, J.: Immunoelectrophoretic demonstration of qualitative differences in normal human sera and their relation to the haptoglobins. *Acta Pathol. Microbiol. Scand.* 47:160, 1959.
22. Constans, J., and Viau, M.: Group specific component: Evidence for two subtypes of the Gc¹ gene. *Science* 198:1070, 1977.
23. Constans, J., and Cleve, H.: Group specific component: Report on the first international workshop. *Hum. Genet.* 48:143, 1979.
24. Daiger, S. P., Schanfield, M. S., and Cavalli-Sforza, L. L.: Human group-specific component (Gc) proteins bind vitamin D and 25-hydroxy-vitamin D. *Proc. Natl. Acad. Sci. U.S.A.* 72:2076, 1975.
25. Svasti, J., and Bowman, B. H.: Human group-specific component. Changes in electrophoretic mobility resulting from vitamin D binding and from neuraminidase digestion. *J. Biol. Chem.* 253:4188, 1978.
26. Shreffler, D. C., Brewer, G. J., Gall, J. C., and Honeyman, M. S.: Electrophoretic variation in human serum ceruloplasmin: A new genetic polymorphism. *Biochem. Genet.* 1:101, 1967.
27. Alper, C. A., and Johnson, A. M.: Immunofixation electrophoresis: A technique for the study of protein polymorphism. *Vox Sang.* 17:445, 1969.
28. Holmberg, C. G., and Laurell, C.-B.: Oxidase reactions in human plasma caused by ceruloplasmin. *Scand. J. Clin. Lab. Invest.* 31:103, 1951.
29. Bamford, K. F., and Harris, H.: Studies on "usual" and "atypical" serum cholinesterase using α-naphthyl acetate as substrate. *Ann. Hum. Genet.* 27:417, 1964.
30. Evans, R. T., Iqbal, J., Dietz, A. A., Lubrano, T., and Rubinstein, H. M.: A family segregating for E₁ʲ and E₁ᵏ at cholinesterase locus 1. *J. Med. Genet.* 17:464, 1980.
31. Putnam, F. W.: Transferrin, in *The Plasma Proteins*, edited by F. W. Putnam. Academic, New York, 1977, vol. 1, pp. 265–316.
32. Giblett, E. R.: *Genetic Markers in Human Blood*. Blackwell Scientific, Oxford, 1969, p. 126.
33. Kühnl, P., and Spielmann, W.: Transferrin: Evidence for two common subtypes of the Tfᶜ allele. *Hum. Genet.* 43:91, 1978.
34. Thymann, M.: Identification of a new serum protein polymorphism as transferrin. *Hum. Genet.* 43:225, 1978.
35. Allison, A. C., and Blumberg, B. S.: An isoprecipitation reaction distinguishing human serum protein types. *Lancet* 1:634, 1961.
36. Bütler, R., Brunner, E., and Morganti, G.: Contribution to the inheritance of the Ag groups: A population genetic study. *Vox Sang.* 26:485, 1974.
37. Berg, K.: A new serum type system in man: The Lp system. *Acta Pathol. Microbiol. Scand.* 59:369, 1963.
38. Sing, C. F., Schultz, J. S., and Shreffler, D. C.: The genetics of the Lp antigen. II. A family study and proposed models of genetic control. *Ann. Hum. Genet.* 38:47, 1974.
39. Dahlén, G., Ericson, C., and Berg, K.: In vitro studies of the interaction of calcium ions and other divalent cations with the Lp(a) lipoprotein and other isolated serum lipoproteins. *Clin. Genet.* 14:115, 1978.
40. Utermann, G., Hees, M., and Steinmetz, A.: Polymorphism of apolipoprotein E and occurrence of dysbetalipoproteinemia in man. *Nature* 269:604, 1977.
41. Zannis, V. I., Just, P. W., and Breslow, J. L.: Human apolipoprotein E isoprotein subclasses are genetically determined. *Am. J. Hum. Genet.* 33:11, 1981.
42. Grubb, R., and Laurell, A. B.: Hereditary serological human serum groups. *Acta Pathol. Microbiol. Scand.* 39:390, 1956.
43. Steinberg, A. G.: Globulin polymorphisms in man. *Annu. Rev. Genet.* 3:25, 1969.

44. Van Loghem, E.: Polymorphism of immunoglobulins, in *Transfusion and Immunology* (Plenary Session Lectures of the XIV Congress, International Society for Blood Transfusion), Vammala, Helsinki, 1975, p. 13.

45. Natvig, J. B., and Kunkel, H. G.: Human immunoglobulins: Classes, subclasses, genetic variants, and idiotypes. *Adv. Immunol. 16*:1, 1973.

46. Pandey J. P., et al.: Linkage relationship between variable and constant region allotypic determinants of human immunoglobulin heavy chains. *Nature 286*:406, 1980.

47. Raum, D., Marcus, D., and Alper, C. A.: Genetic polymorphism of human plasminogen. *Am. J. Hum. Genet. 32*:681, 1980.

48. Board, P. G.: Genetic polymorphism of the A subunit of human coagulation factor XIII. *Am. J. Hum. Genet. 31*:116, 1979.

49. Board, P. G.: Genetic polymorphism of the B subunit of human coagulation factor XIII. *Am. J. Hum. Genet. 32*:348, 1980.

50. Daiger, S. P., Labowe, M. L., Parsons, M., Wang, L., and Cavalli-Sforza, L. L.: Detection of genetic variation with radioactive ligands. III. Genetic polymorphism of transcobalamin II in human plasma. *Am. J. Hum. Genet. 30*:202, 1978.

51. Fráter-Schröder, M., Hitzig, W. H., and Bütler, R.: Studies on transcobalamin. I. Detection of transcobalamin II isoproteins in human serum. *Blood 53*:193, 1979.

52. Cleve, H.: Genetic studies on the deficiency of β_2-glycoprotein I of human serum. *Humangenet. 5*:294, 1968.

53. Alper, C. A., and Propp, R. P.: Genetic polymorphism of the third component of human complement (C'3). *J. Clin. Invest. 47*:2181, 1968.

54. Alper, C. A., et al.: Statement on the polymorphism of the third component of complement in man (C3). *Vox Sang. 25*:18, 1973.

55. Alper, C. A., and Rosen, F. S.: Human complement deficiencies, in *Mechanisms of Immunopathology*, edited by S. Cohen, P. A. Ward, and R. T. McCluskey. Wiley, New York, 1979, pp. 289–305.

56. Agnello, V.: Complement deficiency states. *Medicine (Baltimore) 57*:1, 1978.

57. Hobart, M. J., Lachmann, P. J., and Alper, C. A.: Polymorphism of human C6. *Protides Biol. Fl. 22*:575, 1975.

58. Hobart, M. J., Joysey, V., and Lachmann, P. J.: Inherited structural variation and linkage relationships of C7. *J. Immunogenet. 5*:157, 1978.

59. Marcus, D., Spira, T. J., Petersen, B. H., Raum, D., and Alper, C. A.: There are two unlinked genetic loci for human C8. *Mol. Immunol.* (abstract). *19*:1385, 1982.

60. Raum, D., et al.: Genetic control of the eighth component of complement. *J. Clin. Invest. 64*:858, 1979.

61. Alper, C. A., Boenisch, T., and Watson, L.: Genetic polymorphism in human glycine-rich beta-glycoprotein. *J. Exp. Med. 135*:68, 1972.

62. Alper, C. A.: Inherited structural polymorphism in human C2: Evidence for genetic linkage between C2 and Bf. *J. Exp. Med. 144*:1111, 1976.

63. O'Neill, G. J., Yang, S. Y., and Dupont, B.: Two HLA-linked loci controlling the fourth component of human complement. *Proc. Natl. Acad. Sci. U.S.A. 75*:5165, 1978.

64. Awdeh, Z. L., Raum, D., and Alper, C. A.: Genetic polymorphism of C4 and detection of heterozygotes. *Nature 282*:205, 1979.

65. Awdeh, Z. L., and Alper, C. A.: Inherited structural polymorphism of the fourth component of human complement. *Proc. Natl. Acad. Sci. U.S.A. 77*:3576, 1980.

66. Middleton, J., et al.: Linkage of Chido and HL-A. *Tissue Antigens 4*:366, 1974.

67. Giles, C. M., et al.: Rg^a (Rodgers) and the HLA region: Linkage and associations. *Tissue Antigens 8*:143, 1976.

68. O'Neill, G. J., Yang, S. Y., Tegoli, J., Berger, R., and Dupont, B.: Chido and Rodgers are distinct antigenic components of human complement C4. *Nature 273*:668, 1968.

69. Alper, C. A., Raum, D., Karp, S., Awdeh, Z. L., and Yunis, E. J.: Serum complement "supergenes" of the major histocompatibility complex in man (complotypes). *Vox Sang.*, in press.

70. Raum, D. D., Awdeh, Z. L., Glass, D., Yunis, E., and Alper, C. A.: The location of C2, C4, and BF relative to HLA-B and HLA-D. *Immunogenetics 12*:473, 1981.

71. Awdeh, Z. L., Raum, D., Yunis, E. J., and Alper, C. A.: Extended haplotypes involving HLA and complement genes. *Mol. Immunol.* (abstract). *19*:1358, 1982.

72. Alper, C. A., Awdeh, Z. L., Raum, D. D., and Yunis, E. J.: Extended major histocompatibility complex haplotypes in man: Role of alleles analogous to murine t mutants. *Clin. Immunol. Immunopathol. 24*:276, 1982.

73. Bennett, D.: The T-locus of the mouse. *Cell 6*:441, 1975.

74. Bodmer, W. F., and Bodmer, J. G.: Evolution and function of the HLA system. *Br. Med. Bull. 34*:309, 1978.

Preservation and clinical use of blood and blood components

CHAPTER *164*

Preservation and clinical use of erythrocytes and whole blood

S. P. MASOUREDIS

Although the association of blood with life and vitality was recognized by primitive peoples [1,2], the transfusion of blood was not thought possible until Harvey described the circulation in 1628. During the following 40 years, animal blood was transfused directly into animals and humans. In Paris, Denis transfused lamb's blood into three paid volunteers. Unfortunately, the third volunteer died as a consequence of the transfusion, and Denis suffered for years because of litigation with the ungrateful widow. Interest in blood transfusion waned, and it was not until 1828 that Blundell [3] successfully treated postpartum hemorrhage by direct transfusion.

Safe and effective transfusion therapy had to await the discovery of red cell blood group antigens by Landsteiner [4] and the development of nontoxic anticoagulants so that blood could be stored and used for indirect transfusions. During World War I, Rous and Turner [5,6] found that hemolysis developing in blood collected in sodium citrate could be retarded by the addition of sugars. Sterile blood collected in citrate and glucose and refrigerated for up to 26 days was used by Robertson, then a young physician in the U.S. Army, to treat casualties during World War I [7]. In 1937 Fantus [8] described the establishment at Cook County Hospital in Chicago of a blood bank for the collection, storage, and compatibility testing of blood for transfusion therapy.

Blood transfusion therapy played a major role in treating casualties during World War II. The Americans relied unduly on the use of plasma, for reasons that are not clear but possibly related to logistics, supply considerations, and the interest in plasma fractionation by the Harvard group under Cohn. Retrospectively, it is difficult to understand why the successful experience with whole blood, documented during the Spanish Civil War and by the British civilian experience early in World War II, was not fully exploited by American military forces [2]. It was not until the invasion of Italy that the superiority of whole blood over plasma was officially recognized [9].

Since World War II there has been a tremendous increase in the need for whole blood and blood components, brought about by developments in cardiovascular surgery, extensive cancer surgery, renal dialysis, and exchange transfusions. Blood and blood components have also played an increasingly vital role in the therapy and management of cancer patients who sustain marrow depression following intensive irradiation and chemotherapy. Better understanding of the properties and function of blood, as well as advances in technology, has facilitated and promoted its increased use. Major technical developments include the introduction of plastic equipment consisting of a closed system of tubing and bags, which minimizes the risk of contamination, the availability of a practical refrigerated centrifuge, which facilitates separation of components, and the introduction of automated equipment for continuous-flow cell separations [10,11].

Principles of storage and preservation of blood

Before the introduction of component therapy, efforts to preserve whole blood in the liquid state were concerned only with the erythrocytes. Conditions designed for preserving erythrocytes are not optimal for maintenance of the viability of other important components of blood. Storage requirements for maintaining blood platelets, white blood cells, and plasma fractions are described in Chaps. 165 to 167. A fundamental contribution of component preparation is that freshly drawn blood can be fractionated into components and each component stored under those conditions that will maximize its survival (freezing for labile coagulation factors, room temperature storage for platelets, etc.).

Two well-established methods are used for preservation of erythrocytes: liquid storage at 4°C and frozen storage with various cryoprotective agents at either −80 or −150°C. When stored red cells are reinfused into the circulation, some perish within a few hours but the remainder appear to return to an entirely normal state. The survival of those cells not removed within the first 24 h is normal [12]. Many attempts have been made to devise a means of predicting the number of viable erythrocytes in a unit of stored blood. The ATP level of the erythrocytes enjoys a poorly deserved reputation as a predictor of viability of red cells after reinfusion [13,14]. The osmotic fragility and plasma hemoglobin levels are of little value in predicting the viability of stored red cells. Measurements of the plastic properties of red cells and microscopic observation of the ratio of

TABLE 164-1 Preservation of ATP and 2,3-DPG red cell concentrations during storage in different preservative solutions

| | Storage period, weeks | | | | | | | |
| | 1 | | 2 | | 3 | | 4 | |
	ATP	2,3-DPG	ATP	2,3-DPG	ATP	2,3-DPG	ATP	2,3-DPG
ACD	90	60	80	10	60	5	40	5
CPD	75	120	70	85	65	40	40	10
ACD−0.5 mM adenine	85	110	85	70	80	30	65	10
CPD−0.5 mM adenine	95	100	90	40	85	10	70	5
CPD + PIP (10 mM phosphate, 5 mM inosine, 5 mM pyruvate)	70	150	60	150	55	105	45	35
Addition PIP at 14 days					80	120	70	100

NOTE: Whole blood stored at 4°C. Values are in percent of initial values and are approximate since there is considerable variation from donor to donor.
SOURCE: Modified from de Verdier et al. [17].

sphered to biconcave cells may provide some information [15], but in the final analysis preservative solutions have to be evaluated by red cell survival studies in volunteers. Licensure of preservative solutions in the United States requires that more than 70 percent of the transfused red cells remain in the circulation 24 h after administration.

Attention has been focused on the effect of different preservative solutions on red cell oxygen delivery [16,17]. The loss of 2,3-diphosphoglycerate (2,3-DPG) (Chaps. 35 and 37) during storage results in an increase in oxygen affinity that may compromise the ability of the stored erythrocytes to deliver oxygen to the tissues. After reinfusion, the red cell 2,3-DPG level returns to half-normal in 4 h and to normal in 24 h [18,19]. Although the clinical significance of 2,3-DPG loss in stored blood is difficult to assess [16], there is general agreement that blood with nearly normal oxygen affinity should be used for massive transfusions, particularly in infants, older patients, and patients with cardiovascular and pulmonary disease.

Ideally, preservative solutions for erythrocytes should ensure maximum viability for the maximum possible storage time, as measured by survival of the reinfused cells, and should allow optimum oxygen delivery. Unfortunately, with commonly used preservative solutions, optimal storage conditions for either of two critical components, ATP and 2,3-DPG, usually produce adverse effects on the other. The effect of various storage conditions on maintenance of ATP and 2,3-DPG levels during liquid storage is summarized in Table 164-1.

TABLE 164-2 Effect of storage in ACD on erythrocyte properties

Alteration	ATP	2,3-DPG	Viability
↑ pH	↓	↑	↓
↓ pH	↓	↓	↓
↑ P$_i$*	↑		↔
+Adenine	↑	↓	↑
+Inosine	↑	↑	↑

*Inorganic phosphate.

LIQUID PRESERVATION OF ERYTHROCYTES

The preservative solutions used in the past for the storage of whole blood or red cells contain glucose and a citrate buffer at a pH of either 5.0 or 5.6. The function of the citrate ion is to chelate calcium and thus prevent coagulation of the blood. Glucose sustains the metabolism of red cells during storage, and the acid pH counteracts the marked rise of pH that occurs when blood is cooled to 4°C [20]. The two preservative solutions of this type in use until CPD-adenine was introduced in 1978 were acid-citrate-dextrose (ACD) and citrate-phosphate-dextrose (CPD) (page 1532).

When whole blood or packed red cells are stored in either ACD or CPD, a series of well-defined biochemical changes, designated the *storage lesion,* take place in the erythrocytes (Table 164-2). The concentration of red cell ATP falls gradually during storage [19–21]. As ATP is dephosphorylated, the levels of ADP and AMP rise at first but diminish with time as AMP is irreversibly deaminated to inosine monophosphate (IMP), which is ultimately broken down to hypoxanthine [22]. When the ATP level declines to 0.4 mM or less, the capacity of red cells to phosphorylate glucose is impaired and their viability is lost. Hemoglobin oxygen affinity and 2,3-DPG levels change rapidly in ACD blood. Some 40 percent of the 2,3-DPG is lost in the first week of storage, resulting in a significant increase in oxygen affinity. After 2 weeks of storage, virtually all of the 2,3-DPG has disappeared from blood stored in ACD solution. The loss of 2,3-DPG occurs more slowly in blood stored in CPD solution because of its higher pH [21,23]. The oxygen affinity and 2,3-DPG levels remain nearly normal during the first week of storage and then fall rapidly. Potassium rapidly leaks from the stored cells, and sodium seeps in [24] because the sodium-potassium ATPase is exquisitely sensitive to changes in temperature. The osmotic fragility of the red cells gradually increases [25]. This change is largely an artifact produced by the intracellular accumulation of lactate [229]. Some erythrocytes undergo spontaneous lysis, causing a rise of plasma hemoglobin levels. Erythrocytes stored at 4°C show a progressive increase in rigidity as measured by their rate of flow through filters. Their loss of deformability correlates to some extent with the loss of ATP [15,26,27]. Blood stored in ACD or CPD will yield a 70 percent 24-h survival of transfused red cells for up to 21 days of storage.

Major efforts have been directed toward development of preservative solutions which will maintain adequate erythrocyte levels of ATP and 2,3-DPG. Adenine and inosine are two additives that have been extensively studied. Addition of adenine to give a final concentration of 0.25 to 0.75 mM at the beginning of storage helps to prevent the loss of ATP, since it can serve as a substrate for synthesis of adenine nucleotides (Chap. 35). Unfortunately, the addition of adenine does not correct the loss of 2,3-DPG and may slightly hasten its depletion. CPD-containing adenine, a preservative that allows a 35-day shelf life, was approved for use in the United States by the FDA in August 1978.

The addition of adenine alone at the end of storage is not helpful if red cells have lost a substantial portion of their ATP. Under these circumstances, they are unable to phosphorylate glucose and thus are unable to synthesize adenine nucleotides or to phosphorylate ADP and AMP to ATP. If inosine is supplied, ATP formation can occur even when red cell ATP levels are very low. The phosphorolysis of inosine yields ribose 1-phosphate, which can be metabolized to yield high-energy phosphates and maintain 2,3-DPG levels (Chap. 35). The addition of inosine, either at the beginning of storage or before infusion of ATP-depleted blood, markedly improves the storage viability of red cells [28], but a concentration of inosine of the order of 10 mM is required. Infusion of inosine or of the hypoxanthine formed by its catabolism may result in dangerous hyperuricemia.

A number of other additives have been used experimentally to maintain or restore 2,3-DPG levels of stored red cells. The 2,3-DPG content of stored blood can be restored to normal or supranormal levels [29] by incubating the erythrocytes with phosphate, inosine, and pyruvate (PIP). Both 2,3-DPG and ATP levels in outdated blood can be restored by incubation with PIP and adenine. The rejuvenated erythrocytes can be recovered by centrifugation and washing and then either used for transfusion or frozen for future use [30]. Ascorbic acid helps to maintain 2,3-DPG levels even in low-pH media such as ACD-adenine or CPD-adenine [31]. Dihydroxyacetone is metabolized by erythrocytes and helps to maintain 2,3-DPG levels during storage [31,32–34]. Its effect is additive to that of ascorbate [31]. Periodic agitation of blood during storage improves the maintenance of 2,3-DPG levels in some preservatives, probably by preventing a localized decrease in pH in the gravity-sedimented red cells [35], but has little effect on red cells in blood collected in CPD solution [36].

FROZEN STORAGE OF ERYTHROCYTES

Uncontrolled freezing and thawing of erythrocytes results in hemolysis and is a common method for preparing red cell hemolysates. Freeze-thaw injury is dependent on the rate of freezing, the physical structure of ice, and the properties of water, cell membranes, and solutions at various temperatures. A current theory of freeze-thaw hemolysis suggests that slowly cooled red cells are damaged by osmotic dehydration as they are exposed to increasing extracellular electrolyte concentration and osmolality as water is removed by freezing [37]. Damage may result either because of the prolonged exposure of the dehydrated, hypertonic red cell to temperatures insufficiently low to prevent irreversible biochemical changes in the membrane [38] or, if these changes are prevented in lysis of the red cells on return to isotonicity, because of the excess solute content acquired during the hypertonic phase of freezing [39]. Although the precise biochemical and biophysical changes leading to hemolysis are not fully understood, methods have been developed empirically for the practical freeze-preservation of red cells.

Glycerol is the most commonly used cryoprotective agent for freeze-preservation of erythrocytes. Two general techniques using glycerol are in current use: a slow freezing method in which the red cells have been equilibrated with 40 to 50% glycerol and cooled to −80 to −120°C using mechanical refrigeration [40,41] and a rapid freezing technique in which cells equilibrated with 14 to 20% glycerol are cooled in liquid nitrogen (−196°C) within 2 to 3 min [42–44].

All methods of freeze-preservation of erythrocytes involving the use of cryoprotective agents require a technical capability for introducing and removing high concentrations of the agent (glycerol) under sterile conditions. Frozen red cells must be thawed and the glycerol removed gradually by washing in glycerol solutions of decreasing concentration to prevent osmotic hemolysis. Washing is carried out by centrifugation using either a continuous-flow centrifugal device with a specially designed disposable plastic bowl [45] or manual batch centrifugation. An alternative method which does not require centrifugation relies on the agglomeration of erythrocytes as the thawed red cells are serially diluted with sugar solutions of low ionic strength [46]. The clumped red cells settle rapidly by gravity, and the glycerol-containing supernatant is readily decanted.

Equipment for automatic or semiautomatic processing and thawing of frozen blood is commercially available (Elutramatic System of Fenwal, Cytoglomerator, Haemonetics with ADL-Latham bowl, IBM Blood Cell Processor). With automated equipment the total time required for cell washing (deglycerolizing) is about 30 to 45 min. Under optimum conditions of processing, storage, and cell washing, over 80 percent of the freeze-preserved red cells from a unit of blood will survive and function normally after transfusion. Such thawed and washed red cells must be used within 24 h.

Whole blood preparations

Most clinical situations require the use of specific blood components, and the use of whole blood is limited to correction or prevention of hypovolemia in patients who are sustaining or have recently sustained an acutely developing severe blood loss.

ACD (ACID-CITRATE-DEXTROSE) AND CPD (CITRATE-PHOSPHATE-DEXTROSE) WHOLE BLOOD

ACD and CPD are the two preservative-anticoagulant solutions used exclusively in the past in the United States. They are gradually being superseded by the introduction of adenine-containing solutions. Blood is currently collected and stored in plastic bags, although glass bottles were formerly used.

For each 100 ml of whole blood there should be 15 ml of ACD solution or 14 ml of CPD. The ACD solution (formula A) contains 8.0 g of citric acid ($C_6H_8O_7 \cdot H_2O$), 22 g of sodium citrate ($Na_2C_6H_5O_7 \cdot 2H_2O$), and 24.5 g of glucose ($C_6H_{12}O_6 \cdot H_2O$) per liter. CPD is a modified ACD solution which is slightly less acid and which therefore improves the preservation of 2,3-DPG (Table 164-1). It contains 3.27 g of citric acid, 23.6 g of sodium citrate, 25.5 g of glucose, and 2.22 g of $NaH_2PO_4 \cdot H_2O$ per liter.

A unit of whole blood may contain from 435 to 500 ml of blood. The volume of each anticoagulant solution used for 450 ml of whole blood is 67.5 ml of ACD or 63 ml of CPD solution. The total fluid volume actually administered in transfusing 450 ml of whole blood is 517.5 ml for ACD and 513 ml for CPD collected blood.

Whole blood can be divided into partial units; that is, 450 ml of blood can be split into fractions using a double (225 ml), triple (150 ml), or quadruple pack (112.5 ml). These subdivided units of whole blood are especially useful for pediatric transfusions.

With proper collection and storage at 2 to 6°C, ACD whole blood and CPD whole blood can be used up to 21 days after collection. The 21-day storage limit has been established on the basis of 70 percent survival of the transfused erythrocytes (see page 1530). Red cells appear to fare approximately equally well in these preservatives whether stored as whole blood or as packed cells [47] unless the erythrocytes are packed to a hematocrit reading of over 80 percent [48]. There are currently no regulations governing oxygen affinity or red cell 2,3-DPG concentration of stored blood.

On rare occasions whole blood may be available as leukocyte-poor whole blood or as whole blood with cryoprecipitate and/or platelets removed. These products are not available when component utilization is ideal, however. The appropriate products should be leukocyte-poor red blood cells or red blood cells (see below).

CPD WHOLE BLOOD WITH ADENINE

The addition of adenine improves the maintenance of ATP levels in blood collected in ACD or CPD and thereby prolongs the storage life of red blood cells to 35 to 42 days [49–51]. In the various preservative preparations which have been used, the amount of adenine present is sufficient to provide a concentration of from 0.25 to 0.75 mM in the blood-preservative mixture. Preservatives containing adenine are used routinely in Sweden and in some other European countries. CPD with

adenine (CPDA-1) was licensed for use in the United States in 1978. It contains CPD modified to contain 125 percent of the usual concentration of glucose and adenine to provide a final concentration of 0.25 mM. Although still suboptimal, the higher glucose concentration provides an additional supply for cells packed immediately after collection so that the blood may be fractionated into components [52,53]. Currently under development, CPDA-2 provides 0.50 mM adenine and 1.75 times the glucose provided by CPD. Blood collected in CPDA-1 has a 35-day shelf life, and CPDA-2 appears to be adequate for at least 42 days of storage.

HEPARINIZED WHOLE BLOOD

Heparinized whole blood was used primarily for large-volume transfusions in cardiac surgery to avoid cardiac arrythmias resulting from the severe depression of ionized calcium levels by the citrate in ACD and CPD. Blood collected in a heparin anticoagulant solution has relatively poor erythrocyte preservation since it lacks added glucose and tends to clot as the anticoagulant effect of heparin is neutralized during storage. Neutralization of the heparin effect is a result of the release of thromboplastic and antiheparin in materials from the cellular elements of the blood [54]. As a result, such blood must be used within 48 h of collection. Because of these limitations, recalcified heparinized ACD or CPD blood has been adopted as a substitute for blood collected in heparin [55].

FRESH BLOOD

Requests for "fresh" blood are based on the recognition that during liquid storage there is a relatively rapid loss of some blood components and a progressive increase in the levels of such undesirable products as potassium, ammonium, and hydrogen ions [56,57]. Components that deteriorate rapidly include leukocytes, platelets, and some of the coagulation factors. Erythrocytes also undergo undesirable changes, such as loss of ATP and 2,3-DPG but at significantly slower rates. Platelet viability in ACD or CPD blood declines so rapidly in 24 h that such blood can barely provide hemostasis. For all practical purposes, blood stored over 48 h should be considered to be depleted of viable platelets [58]. Factor V remains at adequate levels (greater than 80 percent) for at least 5 days [59], factor VIII remains above 80 percent of its original level for 1 to 2 days [59], and factor XI rapidly drops to about 20 percent of its original level within the first week of storage [60]. All other clotting factors appear to be stable during liquid storage [61,62].

Blood "freshness" cannot be arbitrarily defined, since it depends upon the storage stability of the component needed. A unit of blood is "fresh" after 21 days of storage with respect to its fibrinogen content but not with respect to factor VIII. In general, blood less than 24 h old is used to replace coagulation factors, particularly factor VIII, factor V, and platelets. Whole blood less than 5 to 7 days old is given when such changes as increase in plasma potassium and ammonium, decrease in pH, and decrease in labile plasma coagulation factors must be avoided. These alterations may be harmful to patients with advanced renal or liver disease or to newborn infants who are given exchange transfusions for hemolytic disease due to blood incompatibilities. It is useful to provide patients with refractory anemias red cells that are less than 10 days old so as to avoid the infusion of nonviable cells which add unnecessarily to the patient's iron burden.

There are probably only a few rare clinical situations in which blood should be transfused before it has been stored for more than a few hours. Too frequently, "fresh" blood is requested for situations for which stored blood is equally satisfactory. Indiscriminate use of "fresh" blood may seriously jeopardize the supply of blood by producing increased outdating. The use of specific components, in most situations, will be more effective than the use of fresh whole blood. Severe deficiencies of platelets and coagulation factors should be corrected by the use of specific components.

A relative indication for "fresh" blood is massive transfusion following trauma or surgery in which more than the patient's blood volume (12 to 14 units) is replaced by banked blood within a 24-h period. Thrombocytopenia and decreased levels of labile coagulation factors with oozing of blood may occur [63]. Such patients can be managed if a third of the units of blood subsequently transfused are less than 24 h old [56]. However, in most cases, packed red blood cells, fresh-frozen plasma, and platelet concentrates are superior to "fresh" whole blood. In the seriously ill patient massively transfused with 2- or 3-week-old banked blood, the low levels of 2,3-DPG may compromise tissue oxygenation. Although the 2,3-DPG levels are regenerated within a day or so [18,19], it is probably prudent to administer a significant proportion of CPD blood less than 5 days old or ACD blood less than 2 days old [16,64].

Erythrocyte preparations

There are three types of erythrocyte preparations in common use: packed or sedimented red blood cells, leukocyte-poor red blood cells, and frozen red blood cells. Washed red blood cells can be obtained from liquid stored blood by saline washing using a continuous-flow cell separator or from frozen erythrocytes which have been extensively washed to remove the cryoprotective agent (glycerol).

RED BLOOD CELLS
Erythrocytes can be separated and recovered from whole blood either by centrifugation (packed red cells) or by gravity sedimentation (sedimented red cells) at any time before the expiration date of the blood. The red cells from either ACD, CPD, or CPDA-1 whole blood can be administered after removing 80 percent of the plasma. Packed or sedimented red cells have a hematocrit of 60 to 90 percent. If the hermetic seal has not been broken and the blood has not been exposed to the external environment, red cells packed to a hema-

tocrit of less than 80 percent or sedimented red cells stored at 1 to 6°C are suitable for transfusion for the full shelf life of the preservative-anticoagulant solution (21 or 35 days). "Tightly" packed red cells do not survive as well, chiefly because they exhaust available glucose [48]. If the blood is exposed to the external environment during preparation, the packed or sedimented red cells must be transfused within 24 h [65].

Red blood cells rather than whole blood should be used for the treatment of all patients who require transfusion because of a red cell mass deficit, as in chronic anemia. An absolute requirement for red blood cells exists when transfusing anemia patients with acutal or incipient congestive heart failure. Surgical patients, both before and after operation, should receive red blood cells rather than whole blood. Packed red cells and balanced salt solutions appear to be as effective as whole blood in correcting the blood loss that occurs at surgery [66].

Red blood cells are administered in the same fashion as in whole blood. The rate of administration may be slower with packed red cells but approaches that of whole blood if a 17-gauge or larger needle is used or if a diluting solution such as saline is used [67].

RED BLOOD CELLS—LEUKOCYTE POOR
A variety of methods have been developed for the preparation of leukocyte-poor or HLA antigen–poor blood [68]. These include sedimentation, inverted centrifugation, filtration through nylon or cotton, saline batch washing using an automatic cell processor, and freeze-thawing.

Whole blood which is stored less than 24 h can be separated by centrifugation into a leukocyte-poor red cell layer, a buffy coat layer containing red cells and white cells, and an upper plasma layer. Red cells in the buffy coat layer are removed with the buffy coat so that each unit of leukocyte-poor red cells contains only about two thirds of the red cells present in the unit of whole blood. Removal of white cells by centrifugation is relatively inefficient. If the method of preparation does not involve entering the container, the expiration date is that of the whole blood from which the leukocyte-poor cells are prepared [65].

Passing heparinized blood, warmed to 37°C, through a nylon filter removes nearly all the granulocytes and monocytes and a significant number of platelets. Lymphocytes are not adsorbed on the nylon fibers, so that nylon-filtered blood contains about 98 to 100 percent of the lymphocytes present in the blood. Leukocyte-poor red blood cells prepared in this way have a storage survival of only 24 h because of the poor preservative properties of the heparin anticoagulant and the risk of bacterial contamination during the filtration process.

Filtration through cotton was introduced over 50 years ago by Sir Alexander Fleming [69] as a method of removing leukocytes from blood. Although this technique has been commonly employed to render small volumes of blood leukocyte-free for laboratory purposes, it has only recently been introduced as a means for preparing leukocyte-free erythrocytes for transfusion. It is probably the most efficient means for the preparation of leukocyte-poor red cells [70,71], but apparatus for cotton filtration of blood is not yet commercially available in the United States.

Leukocyte-poor red cells can be prepared by saline washing (see below under "Washed Red Cells"). Frozen red blood cells (see below) are a relatively satisfactory, but expensive, source of leukocyte-poor erythrocytes. It is not the freezing but the extensive washing to remove cryoprotective agents that effectively removes the leukocytes and platelets.

There are two major indications for the use of leukocyte-poor red blood cells: (1) to prevent or avoid febrile reactions due to antibodies to white cells and platelets, which develop in response to previous transfusions or pregnancies (see page 1540), and (2) to avoid immunization against leukocyte and platelet antigens in a recipient who may be a candidate for an organ transplant. There are conflicting views concerning the use of blood and blood products in patients awaiting a kidney transplant (see below).

FROZEN RED CELLS
Red blood cells may be stored continuously at below-freezing temperatures in the presence of a cryoprotective agent [72,73].

The cost of processing and storing frozen red cells is severalfold higher than the cost of liquid storage. However, preservation of erythrocytes by freezing retards or arrests the deleterious biochemical changes that occur during liquid storage. Frozen red cells have a shelf life measured in years rather than weeks, which facilitates the efficient management of blood inventories. They are relatively leukocyte-poor. Initially it was suggested that frozen-thawed red cells did not transmit hepatitis, but more recent reports indicate that this is not true (see below under "Hazards"). These potential advantages of frozen red cells have stimulated intensive efforts to develop more practical procedures for preserving erythrocytes and other cellular blood components by freezing.

Arguments have been presented for and against the large-scale (over 80 percent of all donated blood) use of frozen blood [74]. There is general agreement that frozen red cells play an important role in transfusion therapy. They are admirably suited to autotransfusion, especially for patients with rare blood types or unidentifiable blood group antibodies. Other advantages of frozen blood include availability of an inventory of rare blood [75,76]; promotion of component therapy; reduction in the incidence of nonhemolytic transfusion reaction; a ready supply of metabolically superior red cells (2,3-DPG and ATP); reduction in sensitization to histocompatibility antigens for potential transplant recipients; possibly a reduced incidence of transfusion hepatitis; and more efficient inventory control. Experience from a blood bank that uses only frozen red cells has been reported [77]. The arguments against large-scale conversion to frozen blood include increased costs, increased processing time, and logistic limitations imposed by the short postthaw storage time. With the technology available at this time, a unit of frozen blood costs two or three times as much as a unit stored in the liquid state. On balance it would appear that, while frozen blood plays an important role on a selective basis, large-scale conversion from liquid-stored to frozen blood cannot be justified.

WASHED RED CELLS
Washed red blood cells are usually obtained from whole blood. Packed red blood cells collected by centrifugation can be washed either by batch centrifugation using saline or by continuous-flow cell separators initially designed for removing cryoprotective agents from frozen red cells [78]. Washed red blood cells must be used within a few hours of processing because of the risk of bacterial contamination during preparation. Frozen red blood cells are an excellent albeit expensive source of washed red cells.

Washed red blood cells are indicated in the rare patient who is hypersensitive to plasma. Such patients develop an allergic or febrile reaction following whole blood transfusion; the reaction can be reproduced with the injection of even a small quantity of plasma [79]. Some of these patients have a deficiency of immunoglobulin A (IgA) and have formed antibodies to IgA from a previous transfusion or pregnancy [80–84]. Washing the red cells removes the donor's plasma, which contains the IgA, and prevents the anaphylactoid reaction. Washed red blood cells may also be useful in transfusing patients who have paroxysmal nocturnal hemoglobinuria (Chap. 21).

ARTIFICIAL BLOOD SUBSTITUTES
A number of functions supported by blood, such as maintenance of circulating volume and oncotic pressure, can be replaced with various crystalloids or with colloid macromolecules such as dextran and hydroxyethyl starch. These blood substitutes, however, do not provide for oxygen transport. A variety of materials with the potential of supporting oxygen transport, such as stroma-free hemoglobin solutions, cobalt chelates, and perfluorocarbons, have been under investigation. In 1968 it was demonstrated that rats survived up to 8 h following complete replacement of their blood with liquid fluorocarbon [85]. More recently a perfluorocarbon-hydroxyethyl starch preparation developed in Japan—designated Fluosol-DA, 20 percent—has become available for experimental use. It has been used in clinical trials in Japan and in a few cases in this country involving patients whose religious beliefs prohibit blood transfusions. Numerous reports have appeared on the use of stroma-free hemoglobin in experimental animals [86].

The safety and efficacy of these artificial blood substitutes for oxygen transport is not established, and it remains to be determined what role if any they will play in clinical medicine.

Transfusion therapy

Transfusion therapy is the replacement of blood or one of its components. Safe and effective transfusion therapy requires a basic understanding of the pathophysiology of the disorder under treatment in order to identify the deficiency, recognition of the storage stability and in vivo survival of the deficient component, and an understanding of the hydrodynamic aspects of the circulation. The purpuric patient may have a deficiency of platelets; the patient with hemophilia, a deficiency of factor VIII (antihemophilic globulin) or factor IX (plasma thromboplastin component); the severely burned patient, a deficiency of plasma; and the patient with chronic anemia, diminished blood oxygen-carrying capacity due to decreased hemoglobin concentration.

The decisions to use transfusion therapy also requires an accurate assessment of the possible hazards associated with its use. Not only must an untoward reaction to the transfusion be avoided, but it is equally important that the component transfused has been properly collected and stored so as to ensure its survival and effective function in the recipient. A patient should be transfused only when specific, clearly established indications are present. Most patients require blood components rather than whole blood.

COMPONENT THERAPY

The most important advance in transfusion therapy during the last 25 years has been the introduction and implementation of component therapy. The rationale for component therapy stems from the recognition that blood is a complex tissue with numerous constituents, or components, both cellular and noncellular, which serve diverse functions. Except for conditions which result in acute hemorrhage, transfusion therapy is occasioned by the need to correct a deficiency in a component of whole blood. Component therapy permits the physician to deliver an effective therapeutic dose of the deficient component with minimum risk of circulatory overload or of adverse reaction to the unnecessary blood components. Each component can be collected, processed, and stored under conditions that maximize its storage stability [87]. It is possible to meet the needs of more than one patient from a single blood donation. This more efficient use of the available blood supply should help to keep pace with increasing demands for blood.

Probably fewer than 20 percent of all transfusions require whole blood [88–92]. The indiscriminate use of whole blood denies the patient safe and effective therapy.

INDICATIONS FOR TRANSFUSION THERAPY

One clinical indication for transfusion therapy is the need to restore and maintain the volume of circulating blood to prevent or treat shock, as in hemorrhage or trauma. Another is the need for specific cellular or protein components, such as erythrocytes, specific coagulation factors, or platelets. Exchange transfusions may be required to remove deleterious materials from the blood, usually in infants, but on an experimental basis in adults as well. Both plasma and cell exchange transfusions in adults are now clinically feasible with the introduction of automated equipment for continuous-flow blood cell separation [10,11]. Blood is also used to maintain the circulation in extracorporeal or cardiac bypass shunts [93,94].

HEMORRHAGE AND SHOCK

A major indication for whole blood transfusion is existing or anticipated hemorrhage (Chap. 72). Accurate estimation of blood loss is difficult [95]. An indication of the severity of a hemorrhage may be obtained from changes in blood pressure, pulse rate, and hemoglobin level. Symptoms of severe blood loss include pallor, sweating, thirst, light-headedness, air-hunger, and restlessness.

A helpful guide to blood loss in acute hemorrhage is the systolic blood pressure. If this is below 100 mmHg, the blood volume is probably less than 70 percent of normal [96]. The average patient may compensate for a blood loss of up to 1000 to 1500 ml by vasoconstriction and may appear normal if lying flat [97]. Such a patient may be in latent shock and will become hypotensive and faint if placed in the upright position. The loss of 2000 ml of blood produces clinical shock in most patients.

The pulse rate is not a reliable guide to blood loss, but a persistent pulse rate of 100 or more per minute in a patient with hemorrhage probably indicates a blood volume less than 80 percent of normal.

Measurement of the hemoglobin level may be misleading. Reduced levels of hemoglobin 3 and 6 h after hemorrhage suggest significant blood loss. A normal hemoglobin level 6 h after hemorrhage suggests that the loss has not been large.

Treatment of acute blood loss should be devoted to volume support and only secondarily concerned with loss of red cell mass. A loss of approximately 1 liter of blood in a patient without cardiovascular disease can be treated with electrolyte solutions. Colloids for volume support and possible red cells may be needed with losses of 1 to 2 liters. Acute blood loss in excess of 2 to 3 liters requires correction of both volume deficiency and red cell mass loss [98].

If the history and the clinical picture suggest that the patient has sustained a significant loss of blood, replacement therapy with whole blood or red blood cells is indicated. Clinical [99] and experimental [66] observations in hypovolemic (hemorrhagic) shock suggest that the combination of packed red cells with crystalloids or albumin is as effective as whole blood in correcting volume deficit. Blood of any age within the usual storage limits is suitable. It is essential, however, that primary attention be given to identifying the site of bleeding and instituting the appropriate medical and surgical means to stop the flow of blood. Many patients who have sustained blood loss do not need a whole blood transfusion and should not be exposed to the associated risks (see below under "Hazards").

SURGERY

The loss of 500 ml of blood during a surgical procedure is well tolerated by the average patient. Even patients undergoing open heart surgery have been managed successfully without transfusions [100] despite a severe, acute decrease in red blood cell mass. Blood volume was supported with crystalloid solutions, and maintaining normovolemia appears to be a significant factor in preventing morbidity and mortality. Another report [101] describes 100 patients undergoing major surgery with blood losses greater than 1000 ml who were managed without blood transfusions. They were treated, instead, with Hartmann's solution (lactated Ringer's solution: NaCl, 102 meq/liter; KCl, 4 meq/liter; CaCl₂, 3.5 meq/liter; sodium lactate, 27 meq/liter), using two to three times the volume of blood lost. Postoperative mortality and morbidity were not affected by the lack of blood, and there were no unexpected complications.

Dogs with hemorrhagic shock appear to respond as well to simple saline solutions administered in volumes three times that of the lost blood as to transfusions of autologous blood [102]. More recent experimental studies indicate that the crystalloid requirements for resuscitation in hemorrhagic shock may require a ratio of crystalloid to shed plasma volume in excess of 8:1 [103]. These findings suggest that transfusion requirements in surgical hemorrhage may be relative rather than absolute. Furthermore, if transfusions are indicated, red blood cells may be preferable to whole blood. If transfusion therapy is indicated during surgery, the amount given is based upon the quantity of blood lost, the nature of the operation, the surgeon's skill, and the condition of the patient. Massive transfusions of stored blood given in less than 24 h are associated with problems in hemostasis (p. 1542), oxygen transport, and electrolyte and metabolic abnormalities [104].

The transfusion requirements for elective surgery have been analyzed. A maximum surgical blood order schedule based on this experience has been used in a number of institutions to define preoperative blood orders [105–107]. This practice has been effective in reducing unnecessary cross matches and has reduced blood outdating.

BURNS

The pathophysiology of burn shock is complex, and resuscitation is difficult [108]. Patients with a burn injury of more than 25 percent of body surface area require large volumes of balanced salt solutions during the initial 24 h [109,110]. Plasma loss that ensues during the next 5 days can be corrected with plasma and colloids. The progressive development of anemia during the early postburn period is best treated with packed red cells. Large quantities of whole blood may also be needed to correct blood loss following extensive debridement.

ANEMIA

The necessity for transfusing blood to patients with chronic stable anemia is rare. Blood transfusion of such patients is probably unjustifiable if the hemoglobin is above 7 g per 100 ml, unless severe cardiac or pulmonary disease is present. A recent report, unfortunately, indicates that there is significant misuse of blood transfusion. Among nonoperated patients drawn from 300 hospitals across the country, 401 were transfused for anemia even though they had a hemoglobin concentration greater than 10 g per 100 ml [111].

In most cases, anemia, even when developing quite rapidly, will not cause symptoms sufficiently serious to justify urgent blood transfusion unless the hemoglobin level is below 4 to 5 g per 100 ml [112,113]. When transfusion is indicated, red blood cells should be administered.

Multiple, repeated transfusions of whole blood or packed red cells have been used to suppress erythropoiesis in patients with sickle cell anemia [114] or thalassemia [115,116] (Chaps. 50 and 60). The complication of transfusional hemochromatosis (Chap. 79) may limit the usefulness of this method of managing the hemoglobinopathies.

A recent approach to the control of iron accumulation in patients with thalassemia who require repeated transfusions is the use of red cells enriched in their content of young red cells, "neocytes." Young red cells were obtained on the basis of size and density using a continuous-flow cell separator [117]. A typical neocyte unit had a calculated red cell age of 12.3 days, as compared with 60 days for the unfractionated red cells. The use of neocytes appeared to decrease the transfusion requirements, with the interval between transfusions going from 30 to 43 days.

OTHER INDICATIONS

The clinical uses of other types of blood components are presented in Chaps. 165 (leukocytes), 166 (platelets), and 167 (plasma and plasma fractions).

ADMINISTRATION

The most important action the clinician can take before administering blood or a blood product is to read the label to verify that the unit to be used is the one selected by the laboratory for the patient (see below under "Hazards").

Blood need not be warmed before use unless unusually large amounts must be given (more than 3 liters) at a rapid rate (greater than 100 ml per minute) [112]. With the usual rate of administration [500 ml per 1 to 2 h], the agglutination that may occur in patients with high-titer cold agglutinins is usually dissociated as the transfused blood equilibrates to body temperature.

Blood should be administered slowly during the first 30 min so that, if an untoward reaction occurs, the transfusion can be discontinued before too much blood is given. It is perfectly safe to transfuse 1000 ml of citrated blood within a period of 2 to 3 h in the average patient without cardiovascular disease [112].

A number of intravenous solutions are incompatible with banked blood and should not be administered through the blood lines. Aqueous dextrose solutions cause agglomeration (clumping) of red cells, and calcium-containing solutions, such as Ringer's lactate, may exceed the calcium-binding capacity of the citrate in the anticoagulated blood, with formation of clots [118,119]. Physiological saline is compatible with all blood components.

Most transfusion therapy is administered intravenously. A vein in the forearm or antecubital fossa is ordinarily used, although any accessible vein may be employed. Other routes available for the administration of blood and components are intraarterial, intraperitoneal, and intraosseous. These routes are used infrequently and only for special reasons. The value of intraarterial transfusion for moribund patients has not been clearly established. Because of the hazards, transfusion into an artery should be reserved for patients who have failed to respond to rapid, large-volume intravenous transfusion. Intraperitoneal transfusions may be indicated for children in whom suitable veins are difficult to find or for the fetus in utero [120]. Intraosseous transfusions are generally not used because they are slow, painful, and capable of producing serious complications, such as osteomyelitis, mediastinitis, and injury to the epiphysis [112].

SINGLE-UNIT TRANSFUSION

Although single-unit transfusions cannot be condemned outright, they often represent an unwarranted use of blood. It has been suggested that the patient who needs only one unit of blood is no more in need of the transfusion than the donor. This is certainly the case in "elective" transfusions, such as administration of a unit of blood to correct a preoperative hemoglobin or blood volume deficit which could be corrected by other means or to hasten recovery of convalescing patients. Single-unit transfusion is justifiable in elderly surgical patients with coronary disease; in patients who have sustained an acute loss of two or three units, who may achieve circulatory stability with one unit; and in patients whose bleeding during surgery or from the gastrointestinal tract is controlled after transfusion of the first unit. The administration of single-unit transfusions in such cases represents good judgment and therapeutic skill [121]. An empirical guide for evaluating the appropriateness of single-unit transfusions is that they should represent not more than 10 percent of total hospital blood usage.

AUTOTRANSFUSION

Autotransfusion is a procedure in which blood removed from a patient is returned to the patient's circulation after storage [122]. Autotransfusion averts some of the problems associated with the use of (banked) donor blood, such as febrile and allergic reactions, immunologic incompatibilities which may lead to hemolysis, and the transmission of disease, particularly posttransfusion hepatitis. Isoimmunization, which has been estimated to have an incidence of 3 to 5 percent among hospitalized patients receiving transfusions, can be avoided by use of autologous blood. Three variations of autotransfusion have been used: preoperative blood collection, storage for variable periods of time, and retransfusion during surgery; immediate preoperative phlebotomy, artificial hemodilution, and postoperative return of the phlebotomized blood; and intraoperative collection of shed blood with reinfusion during surgery [123]. Equipment designed for intraoperative autotransfusion is commercially available. In many situations the recipient is able to predeposit up to four units of blood within 10 days before elective surgery [124]. Frozen autologous blood is the ideal component for patients with rare blood types (e.g., Rh_{null}) or for patients with antibodies in numbers and combinations that make it nearly impossible to find compatible units of blood.

SPECIAL TRANSFUSION REQUIREMENTS

There are a number of clinical situations in which the immunologic consequences of transfusion therapy requires special consideration.

BLOOD FOR EXCHANGE TRANSFUSIONS

Exchange transfusions are used to treat the newborn who has severe hemolytic disease due to a fetomaternal blood group incompatibility, a G-6-P deficiency, or an unknown cause (Chaps. 70 and 58). Every effort should be made to minimize factors contributing to the accumulation of bilirubin in the infant. Blood less than 5 days old should be given in order to provide red cells with a maximum survival potential and in order to avoid infusing excess extracellular potassium. The donor blood should be free of the antigen to which the mother has developed an antibody and compatible with the maternal serum [112,125]. Calcium gluconate may be indicated to compensate for excess citrate ion in ACD blood. Exchange transfusions in adults for hepatic coma, renal failure, and other conditions are still considered experimental [126,127].

BLOOD FOR THE PATIENTS WITH AUTOIMMUNE HEMOLYTIC DISEASE

Donor blood selected for the patient with autoimmune hemolytic disease should lack those antigens corresponding to the antibodies in the recipient, whether autoimmune or alloimmune. Patients with autoimmune hemolytic anemia are serologically incompatible with their own red cells and with those of most if not all donors. Sometimes no specificity can be proved, and it may be impossible to find serologically compatible blood. However, some cells may react more weakly than others. Many of these patients will tolerate a hemoglobin level of 5 to 7 g per 100 ml and should not be transfused. In life-threatening situations a transfusion may be required even in the face of serological incompatibility. In such cases, the red cells selected should be at least as compatible as the cells in the patient's own serum. Packed red cells rather than whole blood should be used, and in some cases packed red cells less than 10 days old may be indicated in order to minimize the number and frequency of transfusions required. The decision to use blood in patients with autoimmune hemolytic anemia should be made only by mutual agreement between the clinician and the blood bank director. Transfusion should be avoided in these patients whenever possible [112,128].

BLOOD FOR EMERGENCIES

Emergencies in which no time is available to type, select, and cross-match compatible blood should be a rare occurrence. The hazards of using blood that has not been cross-matched should be weighed against the alternative of no blood. In a civilian population such emergencies may arise because of trauma, unexpected intraoperative hemorrhage, or ruptured aneurysm [129].

If the urgency of the patient's need justifies the administration of unmatched blood, type O, Rh-negative blood with low plasma anti-A and anti-B titers can be used. Unfortunately, tests for donor anti-A and anti-B levels are not done routinely, and it is preferable to use ABO-specific blood if time is available (5 to 15 min) to group and type the patient. Administration of un-cross-matched group-specific blood will prevent hemolysis that may occur if a high-titer anti-A or anti-B group O blood is given to a non-O recipient. If 15 to 30 min is available, an abbreviated antibody screen can be carried out using low-ionic-strength conditions. Group- and type-specific unmatched blood with a negative antibody screen in the recipient provides, in essentially all cases, compatibility equivalent to that of cross-matched blood. The routine cross match should be carried out retrospectively if un-cross-matched or partially cross-matched blood is administered.

BLOOD FOR TRANSPLANT RECIPIENTS

The effect of previous transfusions, both the number of transfusions and the type of component used, on graft survival is complex and not well understood. Until definitive studies become available, the transfusion management of potential graft recipients remains empirical and is based predominantly on retrospective analysis of graft survival.

Kidney grafts   Until 1973, transfusions were avoided in recipients awaiting cadaveric kidney transplants. However, since 1973 numerous reports [130–132] indicate that transfused patients have better cadaver graft survival than those not transfused. Higher graft survival rates have been reported for recipients who have two to five transfusions before grafting and for those in whom the last transfusion is within 3 months of grafting [131]. The effect appears to be related to the type of

product used, frozen red cells being less effective than other blood products [132].

In kidney transplants from a living related donor, there is a beneficial effect of blood transfusion when there is a disparity in one HLA haplotype but no detectable effect in HLA-identical transplants [133]. Studies are under way on the use of systemic transfusions to maximize kidney graft survival [134].

It is clear that the effect of blood transfusion in kidney grafting is complex, and its therapeutic potential will not be resolved until further studies are carried out.

Marrow grafts   Previous blood transfusions, especially from the intended donor, are associated with a high rate of marrow graft rejection in patients with aplastic anemia but do not appear to be a problem in marrow transplantation of leukemic patients [135]. ABO incompatibility in otherwise histocompatible donors does not appear to affect the marrow transplant outcome [136]. There is a need to avoid an immediate transfusion reaction caused by the red cells in the marrow inoculum when an ABO-incompatible engraftment is carried out. Such a complication may be averted either by removing anti-A or -B from the recipient by plasma exchange, by neutralizing in vivo, or by removing mature red cells from the inoculum [136].

Hazards of transfusion therapy

The possibility of a transfusion-induced reaction and consequent morbidity and the possibility of a fatal outcome for the recipient must be taken into account whenever transfusion therapy is contemplated. Federal regulations instituted in December 1975 require the reporting of all transfusion-associated fatalities. Of the 70 fatalities reported for the 3-year period between 1976 and 1978, 44, or 56 percent, were due to acute hemolytic reactions. Of these, 22 were preventable since they involved an ABO mismatch due to a human error in identification. Most of these fatalities (77 percent) were due to administration of the correctly cross-matched blood to the wrong patient, usually in a surgical or intensive care facility [137,138]. These figures dramatically illustrate the importance of specimen and patient identification in blood transfusion. They also significantly underestimate the incidence of transfusion mortality, since the 10 reported posttransfusion hepatitis deaths for the 3-year period are less than the 16 reported to the Center for Disease Control for only the year 1976 [139].

Even under ideal circumstances, transfusion therapy carries a significant risk for the recipient. Untoward reactions to transfusions appear to occur in about 5 percent of cases. Clinical recognition of a transfusion reaction requires an awareness of the possibility of such a reaction and the ability to exclude causes more likely related to the patient's primary clinical condition. An additional complication is that a large proportion of transfusions (about one-third) are given to anesthetized patients [140]. If a reaction is suspected, the transfusion should be immediately discontinued and appropriate laboratory determinations and clinical investigations undertaken to establish the diagnosis and institute appropriate therapy (see below).

The incidence of transfusion reactions can be significantly reduced by using components rather than whole blood. For example, the use of red blood cell preparations rather than whole blood will significantly reduce the frequency of circulatory overload, citrate and ammonia intoxication, and some forms of febrile or allergic reactions.

Transfusion reactions may be categorized as either immediate or delayed.

IMMEDIATE TRANSFUSION REACTIONS
Symptoms of an immediate transfusion reaction begin within minutes to hours and are nonspecific with respect to etiology. They may include chills, fever, urticaria, tachycardia, dyspnea, nausea and vomiting, tightness in the chest, chest and back pain, hypotension, bronchospasm, angioneurotic edema, anaphylaxis, shock, pulmonary edema, and congestive failure. In the anesthetized patient undergoing surgery, an immediate transfusion reaction may manifest itself as generalized oozing and by shock which is not corrected by the administration of blood.

Immediate transfusion reactions may be hemolytic, febrile, allergic, or due to contaminated blood. These reactions are all associated with nonspecific symtomatology which is not necessarily related to the severity of the reaction. A severe hemolytic reaction may not differ in its presentation from that of a self-limiting febrile reaction. An etiologic diagnosis in most cases requires additional laboratory studies.

HEMOLYTIC TRANSFUSION REACTIONS
Hemolytic transfusion reactions may be associated with a variety of signs and symptoms, such as fever, lower-back pain, sensations of chest compression, hypotension, nausea, and vomiting—none of which are pathognomonic of hemolysis. Two mechanisms may account for hemolysis of transfused red cells: (1) intravascular breakdown, most commonly due to an incompatibility in the ABO system, or (2) destruction in the extravascular space, i.e., the macrophage system of the spleen, liver, and marrow.

The primary pathogenetic mechanisms in intravascular hemolysis appear to be disseminated intravascular coagulation (DIC) and a series of hemodynamic alterations leading to ischemic necrosis of tissues, notably the kidneys [141,142]. Abnormal bleeding due to a consumptive coagulopathy may develop in one-half to one-third of patients who develop major intravascular hemolysis following an incompatible transfusion [143,144].

The clinical management of a hemolytic transfusion reaction should include prompt termination of the transfusion and immediate efforts to correct shock, maintain renal circulation, and correct the bleeding diathesis. The risk of serious sequelae appears to be proportional to the volume of incompatible blood transfused, and so it is imperative that the transfusion be stopped immediately. Severe complications rarely follow the transfusion of under 200 ml of red blood cells [141]. If a hemolytic reaction is suspected, therapy designed to correct bleeding and to protect the kidneys (see below) should be instituted promptly without waiting for the laboratory studies to confirm its presence.

The laboratory diagnosis of a hemolytic reaction is based on evidence of hemolysis (hemoglobinemia and/or hemoglobinuria) and of a blood group incompatibility (antibodies in the recipient reacting with blood group antigens or transfused red cells). A sample of blood carefully drawn to avoid artifactual hemolysis is centrifuged for cell separation. The plasma is examined for hemoglobin (pink) ore methemalbumin (brown) and is compared with the pretransfusion specimen. The urine should be examined for hemoglobin (Chap. A15) and urinary output monitored. The entire typing and cross-match procedure should be repeated to identify the blood group incompatibility. The patient and the blood transfused should be retyped, the cross-match reconfirmed, the patient's red cells examined for the presence of bound immunoglobulins and/or complement (antiglobulin or Coombs' test), and the patient's serum tested for the presence of blood group antibodies. The donor's plasma should be examined for the presence of antibodies which may react with the patient's red cells.

The major effort in a hemolytic reaction should be directed toward control of bleeding, if it is present, and prevention of acute tubular necrosis. If bleeding is due to DIC (Chap. 158), heparin may be helpful, particularly in pregnant women [144,145]. Heparin therapy is not without potential risk, and its use should be restricted to cases in which a severe reaction has been confirmed. To be effective, heparin should be used early in the course of DIC [144]. When intravascular coagulation is controlled, the depleted coagulation factors can be restored by transfusing fibrinogen-rich cryoprecipitate, platelet concentrates, and fresh frozen plasma [146].

The prevention of renal complications depends on maintaining renal blood flow. Systolic blood pressure should be sustained above 100 mmHg, if necessary by administration of intravenous fluids and transfusion. Mannitol has been used to protect against renal failure [147,148], but there is a growing consensus that it has no value in preventing renal failure in acute hemolytic transfusion reactions [141]. If mannitol is used, it should be given in quantities sufficient to maintain a urine flow of 100 ml per hour [147]. Initially, 20 g of mannitol (100 ml of a 20% solution) are infused intravenously in 5 min. This dose can be repeated if diuresis does not occur, but not more than 100 g of mannitol should be used in a 24-h period. Diuretics, such as furosemide and ethacrynic acid, may be more effective in maintaining renal blood flow.

Should these measures fail to prevent anuria, the standard measures for an anuric patient should be instituted: (1) restrict fluid intake so as not to exceed fluid requirements for insensible loss by more than 500 ml; (2) administer 100 g of carbohydrate per day to avoid ketosis and decrease the catabolic rate; and (3) control hyperkalemia. Such patients should be evaluated by a nephrologist and considered candidates for dialysis.

FEBRILE REACTIONS

A febrile response associated with the administration of blood may be due to a hemolytic reaction, to sensitivity to leukocytes or platelets, to bacterial pyrogens, and frequently to unidentifiable causes. Febrile reactions due to bacterial pyrogens have become uncommon with the introduction of commercially manufactured disposable transfusion equipment.

The decision to stop the administration of blood in a febrile reaction is a difficult one. Many but not all febrile reactions can be tolerated by the patient with supportive care, e.g., antipyretics, antihistamines. A chill, however, may herald a more serious reaction, such as a hemolytic reaction, or may be due to grossly contaminated blood. Unfortunately, good guidelines are not available to help with this decision. The clinician should exercise judgment but should not hesitate to discontinue the transfusion if there is any doubt about the underlying cause of the reaction.

Sensitivity to leukocytes and platelets A frequent cause of a nonhemolytic febrile reaction is sensitization to white cell or platelet antigens [149–152]. Febrile reactions to buffy coat are predominantly due to leukocyte antigens [153]. Clinically there is a temperature rise during the administration of blood or shortly thereafter. The temperature continues to rise for 2 to 6 h after cessation of transfusion, and this fever may persist for 12 h. Occasionally there may be more severe manifestations and, rarely, a drop in blood pressure with nausea, vomiting, and chest and back pains. Although a reaction due to leukocyte antigens has a good prognosis, it may be confused with a hemolytic transfusion reaction. Nonhemolytic febrile reactions are relatively frequent and are estimated to cause up to 30 percent of all reactions. At least seven transfusions are usually required to induce sensitization to leukocyte antigens in men, nonparous women, or children. In gravid or parous women reactions may occur with the first or second transfusion. Diagnosis depends on laboratory demonstration of antibodies to white cell antigens, usually leukoagglutinins or lymphocytotoxins. Most reactions of this type are associated with sensitivity to granulocytes, but sensitivity to lymphocytes or to platelets can also cause the reaction. Treatment is supportive, with antipyretics such as aspirin, and preventive, with subsequent transfusions utilizing leukocyte-poor or HLA-poor blood or frozen blood. HLA matching of donor and recipient is rarely justified for prevention of this reaction.

PULMONARY HYPERSENSITIVITY REACTION

Incompatibility to leukocyte antigens, both HLA and non-HLA, usually results in a febrile reaction as described above. On occasion it may produce pulmonary edema of noncardiac origin with dyspnea, chills, fever, and tachycardia. Chest x-rays show a diffuse, patchy, bilateral pattern of pulmonary densities without cardiac enlargement [154]. Leukocyte incompatibility can be demonstrated in most cases. Either antibodies of the recipient are reacting with donor leukocytes [155], or passively transferred antibodies are reacting with recipient leukocytes or with recently transfused (interdonor) leukocytes [156]. It is unclear why only a relatively few individuals respond to leukocyte incompatibility with the pulmonary hypersensitivity reaction instead of with the usual febrile response. The reaction can occur with platelet concentrates, fresh frozen plasma, whole blood, and packed red cells. Almost 25 percent of multiparous women donors have leukoagglutinins and lymphocytotoxins which have been shown to be the cause of these reactions in many of the published reports. Some of these reactions can be prevented if blood from multiparous donors is used for packed red cells instead of whole blood [156]. Therapy is supportive, and in a healthy recipient the symptoms are self-limiting and subside in less than 24 h. The reaction in a compromised recipient, however, can be fatal [155].

Severe pulmonary toxicity characterized by respiratory deterioration and alveolar hemorrhage has been reported in neutropenic patients receiving granulocyte transfusions and amphotericin B simultaneously. A recent retrospective study, however, indicates that in most cases causes other than the concomitant administration of granulocytes and amphotericin B could account for the fatal pulmonary toxicity [157]. However, it may be prudent to separate infusions of granulocytes and of amphotericin by as many hours as is practical.

ALLERGIC REACTIONS

Transfusion of blood or blood products in some patients may result in generalized pruritus and urticaria. Occasionally there may be bronchospasm, angioneurotic edema, or anaphylaxis. The underlying cause of allergic reactions is poorly understood. It has been suggested that it is due to a sensitivity to plasma proteins or other agents passively transferred from donor to recipient. Subsequent exposure to the antigen through medication or food precipitates the reaction. Antibodies to leukocytes or platelets do not appear to be causally related to urticarial reactions [158]. These reactions are usually mild and respond readily to parenteral antihistamines. Serious reactions require the prompt parenteral administration of epinephrine.

ANTI-IgA IN IgA-DEFICIENT RECIPIENT

Severe anaphylactoid transfusion reactions can occur in IgA-deficient patients who have formed anti-IgA [80–

84,159–161]. Such patients either lack or have a marked deficiency of IgA and have developed an IgG or occasionally an IgM type of anti-IgA which may be either class-specific (IgA) or allotype-specific (Am) [159]. Deficiency or absence of IgA occurs infrequently; about 1 in 650 donors lacks IgA by immunodiffusion, and about 1 in 886 donors has no demonstrable IgA [160]. The IgA present in the plasma of the transfused blood probably reacts with the anti-IgA to produce the anaphylactoid reaction. Small amounts of plasma (less than 10 ml) can produce the reaction. The reaction usually is not associated with fever but may produce dyspnea, nausea, chills, abdominal cramps, emesis, diarrhea, and profound hypotension. A fatal reaction due to anti-IgA occurring 45 min after administration of about 50 ml of blood has been reported [161]. The diagnosis of this type of transfusion reaction requires laboratory demonstration of the absence of IgA in the recipient and of the presence of anti-IgA in the recipient's circulation. It can usually be prevented by the use of washed red cells or, preferably, frozen blood, procedures effective in removing IgA. Plasma protein components, such as albumin or plasma protein fraction, may contain sufficient IgA to produce a reaction. If platelet or granulocyte transfusions are required for IgA-deficient patients, they should be obtained from donors who lack IgA (Rare Donor File, American Association of Blood Banks).

BACTERIAL CONTAMINATION

Blood may be contaminated by cold-growing organisms (*Pseudomonas* or colon-aerogenes group), by the entrance of contaminated air into the blood-collecting equipment, or by bacteria on the skin of the phlebotomized donor. These microorganisms are ubiquitous, have the ability to grow at 4°C, and are able to utilize citrate as the primary source of carbon. Overgrowth of blood by these microorganisms may deplete its citrate concentration sufficiently to result in clotting. The infusion of large numbers of gram-negative microorganisms results in a serious reaction accompanied by fever, marked hypotension, pain, vomiting, diarrhea, and the development of profound shock [162]. The reaction may start with shaking chills following a latent period of 30 min or more. As little as 50 ml of blood may contain sufficient microorganisms to produce the reaction. Rapid diagnosis is essential and can be made by drawing a small sample of residual donor blood from the container or administration tubing. The plasma obtained by slow centrifugation is transferred to a slide, fixed by heating, and Gram-stained. If the blood is heavily contaminated, several organisms can be clearly identified in most oil-immersion fields.

Septic shock is a complex disorder involving abnormalities of oxygen transport, peripheral perfusion, myocardial function, and metabolism, as well as activation of blood coagulation, complement, kallikrein, kinins, and fibrinolysis [163–167]. The transfusion must be stopped immediately, and comprehensive supportive therapy is essential once the diagnosis is made. Treatment is often ineffective, and heroic measures are required. The fatality rate with this type of overwhelming shock is estimated to be 50 to 80 percent.

Bacterial contamination of blood is an uncommon complication since the introduction of disposable plastic blood bags. This transfusion hazard, however, is significant with platelet concentrates stored at room temperature. Transfusion-induced enterobacterial sepsis has been reported in two patients following platelet transfusion [168].

CIRCULATORY OVERLOAD

Hypervolemia produced by administration of excess blood in patients with a compromised cardiovascular system may provoke the development of congestive heart failure and pulmonary edema. Patients in congestive failure or with an impaired cardiovascular status should be treated with packed red blood cells rather than whole blood to reduce the quantity of sodium and fluid administered. Treatment of this reaction requires rapid digitalization, diuretics, and, if necessary, repeated phlebotomies with reinfusion of the erythrocytes as packed red cells.

Patients with severe chronic anemia (hemoglobin less than 4 g per 100 ml), such as those with pernicious anemia, who are rapidly transfused with whole blood or packed red blood cells may develop congestive heart failure and pulmonary edema. The slow administration of packed red blood cells appears to be well tolerated by the patient in a semiupright position. Venous pressure should be monitored in such patients and the transfusion given at a rate of 1 ml per pound of body weight per hour. It is unlikely that a transfusion will precipitate congestive heart failure if the venous pressure is normal before transfusion [169].

AIR EMBOLISM

Air embolism is now a rare complication of transfusion therapy because of the introduction of plastic equipment, which provides a closed system. In the past, transfusion for massive exsanguination was administered rapidly from glass bottles with the help of air pressure from above. With this procedure, the infusion of significant quantities of air into the circulation was a possibility. Only the infusion of large volumes of air and not the entry of a few bubbles results in clinically significant air embolism. Symptoms associated with air embolism include pain, cough, and sudden onset of dyspnea. Treatment consists of clamping off administration tubing and placing the patient on her or his left side in the head-down position so that air in the right ventricle flows away from the pulmonary outflow tract.

REACTIONS DUE TO EXCESSIVE OR MASSIVE TRANSFUSIONS

The use of large quantities of banked blood for massive transfusions may lead to a number of complications. Among these are circulatory overload, air embolism, citrate intoxication, and a bleeding syndrome.

MICROAGGREGATES IN BLOOD
Particles consisting largely of platelets and fibrin [170] form in blood stored in ACD or CPD solution. Such debris, collectively designated *microaggregates* and ranging in diameter from 13 to 100 μm, is not removed by an ordinary blood filter, which has a pore size of about 170 μm. Microaggregates have been shown to produce pulmonary insufficiency in clinical situations involving massive transfusions of banked blood. Pulmonary complications and histologic changes in the lungs have been observed in Korean and Vietnam combat casualties receiving massive transfusions [171,172]. Comparison of the pulmonary vascular pressures of dogs given filtered blood and dogs given unfiltered blood showed that the infusion of nonfiltered blood resulted in a consistent increase in pulmonary vascular resistance [173]. Patients transfused with more than 20 percent of their blood volume have increased pulmonary arteriovenous shunting when the blood is filtered with standard blood filters, but this can be prevented if microaggregate filters are used [174].

The clinical importance of microaggregates in routine transfusions is unclear. A number of investigators, however, believe that microaggregate filters should be used in cardiac surgery and in critically ill patients with pulmonary insufficiency who will receive more than three to five units of banked blood in less than 12 h. Microemboli filters should not be used with fresh blood or platelet concentrates, since they will substantially reduce the platelet yield. These filters retard the flow of blood and should be avoided if they will compromise the rapid administration of blood into the hemorrhaging patient [88].

BLEEDING SYNDROMES
Bleeding may be a complication of transfusion either because an antigen-antibody reaction involving a red cell antigen initiates DIC or because coagulation factors are diluted following large-volume compatible transfusions of banked blood [143]. *It should always be kept in mind that the most common cause of bleeding in surgical patients is a severed vessel.*

Unexplained bleeding may be the first sign of incompatibility in the anesthetized patient and may follow the administration of 200 to 500 ml of incompatible blood. Local bleeding at the surgical site of generalized bleeding such as epistaxis, bruising, or purpura due to disseminated intravascular coagulation may occur following an acute hemolytic transfusion reaction. The diagnosis and management of this complication are outlined above under hemolytic transfusion reactions.

Bleeding associated with the transfusion of large amounts of compatible stored blood is due largely to the dilution of the intravascular volume with blood lacking in both cellular and plasma coagulation components. Since platelets do not survive in stored blood, transfusion of a volume of blood equal to that of the recipient will produce thrombocytopenia through a dilutional effect. Stored blood is also deficient in factors V, VIII, and

XI, so that these clotting factors may be depleted when a large exchange-type transfusion is performed.

DELAYED TRANSFUSION REACTIONS
A delayed reaction occurs days or weeks following transfusion and may result in jaundice and anemia due to hemolysis, transmission of infectious disease such as hepatitis or malaria, alloimmunization to cellular and plasma antigens, hemosiderosis, and, in certain circumstances, graft-versus-host disease.

DELAYED HEMOLYTIC REACTION
In the delayed hemolytic reaction, development of previously undetected alloantibodies occurs 4 to 14 days after transfusion of apparently compatible blood. In such cases the patient usually has been alloimmunized by a previous pregnancy or transfusion and the concentration of antibody was below the level of serological detection at the time of transfusion. If the transfused blood contains the corresponding antigen, an anamnestic response ensues with formation of detectable amounts of the antibody, which coats the transfused red cells and leads to their hemolysis. The principal clinical signs are onset of jaundice and progressive development of anemia. These reactions occur a few days after transfusion and are associated with a positive direct antiglobulin reaction (Coombs' test) [175,176]. The development of a positive direct antiglobulin reaction in such patients may be confused with an autoimmune hemolytic anemia [177]. Generally, these reactions are clinically less severe than the acute hemolytic reaction and frequently are not detected until more blood is ordered for a transfusion-unresponsive anemia. The frequency of delayed hemolytic anemia was 1 in 4000 in a recent report [176], with no deaths in 37 cases. The incidence of delayed hemolytic anemia is related to the sensitivity of pretransfusion tests and to the clinical awareness that it may occur as a transfusion complication [176,178]. As a result, delayed hemolytic reactions are frequently undetected.

A rare complication of transfusion therapy is post-transfusion purpura, which occurs approximately 1 week after transfusion and is associated with the development of an antibody to the platelet-specific antigen Pl^{A1} [179–183]. In such cases it appears that alloantibodies to the transfused platelets not only decrease their survival time but also lead to the destruction of the patient's autologous platelets, presumably by the adsorption of antigen-antibody complexes (Chap. 142).

TRANSMISSION OF DISEASE
Hepatitis Hepatitis continues to be a major risk of transfusion therapy. Three or more viruses have been associated with hepatitis: type A (infectious), type B (serum), and the non-A, non-B type. Serological markers are available for types A and B so that it is possible to identify the virus causing the disease. The existence of non-A, non-B hepatitis became evident both from epidemiological studies and from the recognition

of a subset of patients with hepatitis that did not have serological markers for either A or B [184,185]. Although all three types are capable of transmitting posttransfusion hepatitis, type A is rarely transmitted by transfusion [186]. In addition, posttransfusion hepatitis may result from the transfusion transmission of the Epstein-Barr virus or the cytomegalovirus.

Screening donors by sensitive radioimmunoassay tests for the hepatitis B surface antigen (HBsAg), mandated by the FDA for licensed blood banks since 1972 and for all blood banks since 1975, has resulted in a reduction in transfusion-associated hepatitis [187]. About 20 to 40 percent of donors whose blood will transmit viral hepatitis have in their serum the HBsAg [188,189], originally described as Australia (Au) antigen [190]. The infective hepatitis B virion is a 42-nm, double-shelled, round particle also known as the Dane particle. The 28-nm inner core contains DNA, DNA polymerase and an antigenic determinant, the hepatitis B core antigen (HBcAg) [191], and the e antigen (HBeAg), which appears to be a structural component of the core of the virus. The core is surrounded by a 7-nm lipoprotein shell which contains the HBsAg. The HBsAg also occurs on noninfective spherical particles as well as on filaments of variable length. Sensitive radioimmunoassay procedures are available for five serological markers of hepatitis B virus: HBsAg, anti-HBs, anti-HBc, HBeAg, and anti-HBe.

In hepatitis B virus (HBV) infection, the virus, DNA polymerase, HBcAg, HBeAg, and HBsAg appear in the blood during the incubation period [192]. In the usual case, HBsAg is first detected 4 to 12 weeks after exposure to HBV and persists in the circulation for less than 3 months. HBeAg appears shortly after HBsAg and persists for varying lengths of time, but usually disappears prior to the clearance of HBsAg. Antibody to HBcAg appears soon after the appearance of e antigen, and high titers of anticore are an excellent index of active viral replication. Antibody to HBsAg usually appears during convalescence and is associated with immunity to HBV infection. Both antibodies may persist for several years, although levels of one or the other may fall to subdetectable quantities with the passage of time. There is a serological gap in the late acute stage and in early convalescence during which neither HBsAg nor antibody to HBsAg is detectable and only antibody to HBcAg is present. Despite the absence of detectable levels of HBsAG, donors in this phase are capable of transmitting HBV infection even though they may be missed when being screened for HBsAg. Anti-HBc will usually be present during this period and serves as a reliable indicator of HBV replication and infectivity under these circumstances [193,194]. Passive immunization to HBV with hyperimmune γ-globulin is available [195], and a vaccine for active immunization will shortly be available for clinical use [196].

Of some 19 million donors processed by the American Red Cross, 2.08 per 1000 first-time donors and 0.77 per 1000 repeat donors were positive for HBsAg [197]. Similar values have been reported for Canadian donors, 2.42 per 1000 first-time donors, except for the province of Quebec, where the rate was 4.05 per 1000 donors [198]. It is well known that the infectivity rate in different populations varies widely [199].

Despite measures taken to control transmission of HBV infection by screening donors for HBsAg, transfusion-associated hepatitis continues to be a significant problem. The incidence of posttransfusion icteric and anicteric (changes in liver enzymes) is still from 5.4 to 18.5 percent of recipients receiving five or fewer units of blood [200]. A lower incidence, 3.4 percent has been reported from the Netherlands [201]. About 90 percent of transfusion-associated hepatitis is now due to an agent or agents of non-A, non-B hepatitis [184]. The remaining 10 percent include some cases of hepatitis B which may be undetectable when donors are screened only for HBsAg [193,194].

The non-A, non-B agent is unrelated to hepatitis A virus, HBV, cytomegalovirus, or Epstein-Barr virus. Non-A, non-B hepatitis differs clinically from HBV. There is a shorter incubation period, the acute phase is less severe than in B disease, and it is more variable in severity so that only elevated enzymes are present in some cases. Two thirds of the cases of HBV infection are icteric, whereas about one third with non-A, non-B are so [202,203]. Chronic infection (chronic hepatitis) appears to occur more frequently with non-A, non-B. For these reasons control of non-A, non-B is a major concern [202,203].

Chimpanzees have been experimentally infected with non-A, non-B [204], and a number of serological tests for detecting antigens and antibodies associated with the virus [205] are under study. Such tests may soon be available for donor screening, and their application should lead to better control of transfusion-associated hepatitis.

The ultimate control of posttransfusion hepatitis depends on screening donors for serological markers of HBV infection and, in the near future, on tests that will identify donors capable of transmitting non-A, non-B. An additional important measure is the use of only voluntary, unpaid blood donors, since the risk of infection for both HBV and non-A, non-B is 3 to 10 times greater when paid donors are used (prisoners, derelicts, etc.).

The effectiveness of controlling posttransfusion hepatitis by identifying and excluding donors with hepatitic dysfunction using alanine aminotransferase (ALT, GPT) levels has been reexamined [206]. There was a significant association between the level of donor ALT and the occurrence of non-A, non-B hepatitis in recipients. Multiunit recipients receiving blood with donor ALT levels below 29 IU per liter had an attack rate of 6 percent or higher; at higher donor ALT levels, the attack rate increased progressively, reaching a level of 45 percent for recipients of a unit with an ALT of 60 IU or higher. ALT screening, however, is a nonspecific index of infectivity, and it lacks both the sensitivity to detect all infectious donors and the specificity to detect only infectious units. In view of these limitations, it is unclear if the added costs of ALT donor screening and the impact of excluding noninfectious donors on the chronically limited supply of blood can be justified.

All blood products with the exception of albumin (because of pasteurization) [207] and immune serum globulin [208] can transmit hepatitis. The risk is directly related to the number of units either transfused or pooled for preparation of a product. Coagulation factor concentrates are known to carry a high risk of non-A, non-B hepatitis presumably because products are now prepared from pools screened for HBsAg [209].

Earlier reports indicated that no recipients of frozen red cells developed hepatitis [210], suggesting that the washing procedure in reconstituting cryopreserved red cells eliminated the hepatitis virus. However, 16 cases of hepatitis resulting from the transfusion of 76 units of frozen, washed cells have been reported [211]; of these frozen cells, 93 percent were obtained from commercial donors. Frozen and thawed blood prepared from units intentionally inoculated with HBV also transmitted hepatitis to chimpanzees [212], indicating that the washing procedure was ineffective in removing the virus.

Malaria The risk of transmitting malaria by transfusion has significantly increased in the United States because of the increasing number of donors who have been tourists or have served in the military in areas endemic for malaria. The transmission of malaria should be considered in patients who develop an unexplained febrile illness many weeks or months following a transfusion. In the past decade there have been at least 20 documented cases of transfusion malaria in the United States [213–216].

Cytomegalovirus Transfusion transmission of cytomegalovirus (CMV) may occur in compromised recipients, such as premature infants, open heart surgery patients, and immunosuppressed transplant recipients. A heterophil-negative, mononucleosis-like syndrome has been described [217] following extracorporeal perfusion associated with the development of serological and/or virological evidence of CMV infection. In most patients CMV seroconversion following transfusion is clinically benign, but in some patient populations, such as neonates, it may cause pneumonia, hepatitis, thrombocytopenia, and neurologic sequelae [218].

Granulocyte transfusions carry a high risk of transmitting CMV infection [219], and the use of leukocyte depleted blood results in a reduction of CMV infection [220], suggesting that seropositive donor leukocytes contain latent CMV that is activated following transfusion. Ideally, susceptible recipients (neonates, immunosuppressed patients, etc.) should receive donor blood free of infectious CMV. Unfortunately, it is difficult to identify donors capable of transmitting CMV since 51 to 72 percent have antibodies to CMV but only 5 percent are capable of transmitting CMV infection [218].

GRAFT-VERSUS-HOST DISEASE

Graft-versus-host (GVH) disease occurs commonly in recipients of marrow transplants [221]. It also may be a complication of transfusion. Some 10 well-documented cases of GVH disease have been reported in patients receiving blood transfusions. It may occur in children with various primary immunodeficiency diseases, after intrauterine or exchange transfusions of neonates with hemolytic disease of the newborn, and after granulocyte transfusions to myelosuppressed and immunodeficient patients with hematological malignancies [222–224]. GVH disease can be prevented by irradiating blood when it is to be given to immunocompromised recipients. With doses of 1500 to 3000 rads there is no gross impairment of red cell, granulocyte, or platelet function [225]. Equipment designed for irradiating blood products is commercially available, or irradiation can be carried out by the hospital radiation therapy unit.

OTHER TYPES OF DELAYED REACTIONS

Other complications of transfusion therapy are iron overload with hemosiderosis or hemochromatosis (Chap. 79), which occurs in patients who receive many transfusions, and alloimmunizations to red cell and histocompatibility antigens.

Blood is matched routinely only with respect to ABO antigens and to one of the Rh antigens, $Rh_0(D)$. There is a high probability that the donor has red cell antigens not present in the recipient. The clinical relevance of this transfusion complication is illustrated by a study of 50 patients with sickle cell disease [226]. Of this group 36 percent developed one or more red cell alloantibodies over a period of 33 months following transfusion with a mean of 9.5 units.

More extensive pretransfusion typing to include matching for additional antigens in recipients who will require frequent transfusions may reduce the risk of alloimmunization. This measure alone may not be cost-effective since not all individuals are capable of mounting an immune response to blood group antigens. Some 30 percent of $Rh_0(D)$-negative individuals fail to produce anti-$Rh_0(D)$ in spite of intentional immunization with the antigen [227]. Recent studies, however, indicate that up to 95 percent of Rh-negative individuals will produce antibodies when large quantities (average 19.4 units) of incompatible blood are administered [228]. More extensive pretransfusion matching would be justifiable if a marker could be found which unequivocally identifies the responder population of recipients.

Transfusion-produced alloimmunization may also play a significant role in some types of organ transplants, as discussed above for marrow transplants.

References

1. Blum, L., and Nelson, W. M.: The antecedents of blood transfer. *Bull. N.Y. Acad. Med.* 31:671, 1955.
2. Schmidt, P. J.: Transfusion in historical perspective: The Emily

Cooley Lecture, in *Seminar on Current Technical Topics*. American Association of Blood Banks, Washington, D.C., 1974, p. 49.

3. Blundell, J.: The after-management of floodings, and on transfusion. *Lancet 13:*673, 1828.

4. Landsteiner, K.: Über Agglutinationser scheinungen normalen menschlichen Blutes. *Wien. Klin. Wochenschr. 14:*1132, 1901.

5. Rous, P., and Turner, J. R.: The preservation of living red blood cells in vitro. I. Methods of preservation. *J. Exp. Med. 23:*219, 1916.

6. Rous, P., and Turner, J. R.: The preservation of living red blood cells in vitro. II. The transfusion of kept cells. *J. Exp. Med. 23:*239, 1916.

7. Robertson, O. H.: Transfusion with preserved red blood cells. *Br. Med. J. 1:*691, 1918.

8. Fantus, B.: Therapy of Cook County Hospital: Blood preservation. *JAMA 109:*128, 1937.

9. Churchill, E. D.: *Surgeon to Soldiers.* Lippincott, Philadelphia, 1972.

10. Jones, A. L.: Continuous-flow blood cell separation. *Transfusion 8:*94, 1968.

11. Hester, J. P., Kellogg, R. M., Mulzet, A. P., Kruger, V. R., McCredie, K. B., and Freireich, E. J.: Principles of blood separation and component extraction in a disposable continuous-flow single-stage channel. *Blood 45:*254, 1979.

12. Gabrio, B. W., Stevens, A. R. Jr., and Finch, C. A.: Erythrocyte preservation. III. The reversibility of the storage lesion. *J. Clin. Invest. 33:*252, 1954.

13. Dern, R. J., Brewer, G. J., and Wiorkowski, J. J.: Studies on the preservation of human blood. II. The relationship of erythrocyte adenosine triphosphate levels and other in vitro measures to red cell storageability. *J. Lab. Clin. Med. 69:*968, 1967.

14. Wood, L., and Beutler, E.: The viability of human blood stored in phosphate adenine media. *Transfusion 7:*401, 1967.

15. Haradin, A. R., Weed, R. I., and Reed, C. F.: Changes in physical properties of stored erythrocytes: Relation to *in vivo* survival. *Blood 30:*876, 1967.

16. Chaplin, H., Beutler, E., Collins, J. A., Giblett, E. R., and Polesky, H. F.: Current status of red-cell preservation and availability in relation to the developing National Blood Policy. *N. Engl. J. Med. 291:*6, 1974.

17. De Verdier, C. H., et al.: Maintenance of oxygen transport function of stored blood, in *Progress in Transfusion and Transplantation*, Proc. AABB-ISBT Transfusion Congress, Washington, D.C., August 1972.

18. Beutler, E., and Wood, L.: The in vivo regeneration of red cell 2,3-diphosphoglyceric acid (DPG) after transfusion of stored blood. *J. Lab. Clin. Med. 74:*300, 1969.

19. Valeri, C. R., and Hirsch, N. M.: Restoration in vivo of erythrocyte adenosine triphosphate, 2,3-diphosphoglycerate, potassium ion, and sodium ion concentrations following the transfusion of acid-citrate-dextrose-stored human red cells. *J. Lab. Clin. Med. 73:*722, 1969.

20. Beutler, E., and Duron, O.: Effect of pH on preservation of red cell ATP. *Transfusion 5:*17, 1965.

21. Beutler, E., Meul, A., and Wood, L. A.: Depletion and regeneration of 2,3-diphosphoglyceric acid in stored red blood cells. *Transfusion 9:*109, 1969.

22. Bishop, C.: Changes in the nucleotides of stored or incubated human blood. *Transfusion 1:*349, 1961.

23. Shafer, A. W., Tague, L. L., and Guenter, C. A.: 2,3-Diphosphoglycerate in red cells stored in acid-citrate-dextrose and citrate-phosphate-dextrose: Implication regarding delivery of oxygen. *J. Lab. Clin. Med. 77:*430, 1971.

24. Wood, L., and Beutler, E.: Temperature dependence of sodium-potassium activated erythrocyte adenosine triphosphatase. *J. Lab. Clin. Med. 70:*287, 1967.

25. Rapoport, S.: Dimensional, osmotic, and chemical changes of erythrocytes in stored blood. I. Blood preserved in sodium-citrate, neutral, and acid-citrate-glucose (ACD) mixtures. *J. Clin. Invest. 26:*591, 1947.

26. La Celle, P. L.: Alteration of deformability of the erythrocyte membrane in stored blood. *Transfusion 9:*238, 1969.

27. La Celle, P. L., and Weed, R. I.: The contribution of normal and pathologic erythrocytes to blood rheology. *Prog. Hematol. 7:*1, 1971.

28. Simon, E. R.: Adenine and purine nucleosides in human red cell preservation: A review. *Transfusion 7:*395, 1967.

29. Duhm, J., Deutich, B., and Gerlach, E.: Complete restoration of oxygen transport function and 2,3-diphosphoglycerate concentration in stored blood. *Transfusion 11:*147, 1971.

30. Valeri, C. R., et al.: Therapeutic effectiveness and safety of outdated human red blood cells rejuvanated to restore oxygen transport function to normal, frozen for 3 to 4 years at −80°C, washed, and stored at 4°C for 24 hours prior to rapid infusion. *Transfusion 20:*159, 1980.

31. Wood, L., and Beutler, E.: The effect of ascorbate and dihydroxyacetone on the 2,3-diphosphoglycerate and ATP levels of stored human red cells. *Transfusion 14:*272, 1974.

32. Brake, J. M., and Deindoerfer, F. H.: Preservation of red blood cell 2,3-diphosphoglycerate in stored blood containing dihydroxyacetone. *Transfusion 13:*84, 1973.

33. Beutler, E., and Guinto, E.: The metabolism of dihydroxyacetone by intact erythrocytes. *J. Lab. Clin. Med. 82:*534, 1973.

34. Beutler, E., and Guinto, E.: Dihydroxyacetone metabolism by human erythrocytes: Demonstration of triokinase activity and its characterization. *Blood 41:*559, 1973.

35. Dern, R. J., Wiorkowski, J. J., and Matsuda, T.: Studies on the preservation of human blood. V. The effect of mixing anticoagulated blood during storage on the poststorage erythrocyte survival. *J. Lab. Clin. Med. 75:*37, 1970.

36. Bensinger, T. A., Metro, J., and Beutler, E.: The effect of agitation on *in vitro* metabolism of erythrocytes stored in CPD-adenine. *Transfusion 25:*140, 1975.

37. Merryman, H. T.: Freezing injury and its prevention in living cells, in *Annual Review of Biophysics and Bioengineering*. Annual Review, Palo Alto, 1974, vol. 3, p. 341.

38. Lovelock, J. E.: Denaturation of lipid protein complexes as a cause of damage by freezing. *Proc. R. Soc. Lond. [Biol.] 147:*427, 1957.

39. Lovelock, J. E.: The haemolysis of human red blood cells by freezing and thawing. *Biochim. Biophys. Acta 10:*414, 1953.

40. Tullis, J. L., et al.: Clinical use of frozen red cells. *Arch. Surg. 81:*169, 1960.

41. Merryman, H. T., and Hornblower, M.: A method for freezing and washing red blood cells using a high glycerol concentration. *Transfusion 12:*145, 1972.

42. Pert, J. H., Schork, P. K., and Moore, R.: A new method of low temperature blood preservation using liquid nitrogen and a glycerol-sucrose additive. *Clin. Res. 11:*197, 1963.

43. Krijnen, H. W., de Wit, J. J., Kuivenhoven, A. C. J., Loos, J. A., and Prins, H. K.: Glycerol treated human red cells frozen with liquid nitrogen. *Vox Sang. 9:*599, 1964.

44. Rowe, A. W., Eyster, E., and Kellner, A.: Liquid nitrogen preservation of red blood cells for transfusion: A low glycerol–rapid freeze procedure. *Cryobiology 5:*119, 1968.

45. Tullis, J. L., Tinch, R. J., Gibson, J. G. III, and Baudanza, P.: A simplified centrifuge for the separation and processing of blood cells. *Transfusion 7:*232, 1967.

46. Huggins, C. E.: Frozen blood: Clinical experience. *Surgery 60:*81, 1966.

47. Szymanski, I. O., and Valeri, C. R.: Clinical evaluation of concentrated red cells. *N. Engl. J. Med. 280:*281, 1969.

48. Beutler, E., and West, C.: The storage of hard-packed red blood cells in citrate-phosphate-dextrose (CPD) and CPD-adenine (CPDA-1). *Blood 54:*280, 1979.

49. De Verdier, C. H., Garby, L., Hjelm, M., and Hogman, C.: Adenine in blood preservation: Posttransfusion viability and biochemical changes. *Transfusion 4:*331, 1964.

50. Akerblom, O., De Verdier, C. H., Finnson, M., Garby, L., Hogman, C. F., and Johansson, S. G. O.: Further studies on the effect of adenine in blood preservation. *Transfusion 7:*1, 1967.

51. Messeter, L., Ugander, L., Monti, M., Lundh, B., and Low, B.: CPD-adenine as a blood preservative: Studies *in vitro* and *in vivo*. *Transfusion 17:*210, 1977.

52. Bensinger, T. A., Metro, J., and Beutler, E.: In vitro metabolism of packed erythrocytes stored in CPD-adenine. *Transfusion 15:*135, 1975.

53. Valeri, C. R., Valeri, D. A., Gray, A., Melaragno, A., Dennis, R. C., and Emerson, C. P.: Viability and function of red blood cell concentrates stored at 4 degrees C for 35 days in CPDA-1, CPDA-2, or CPDA-3. *Transfusion* 22:210, 1982.

54. Perkins, H. A., Rolfs, M. R., and Acra, D. J.: Studies on bank blood collected and stored under various conditions with particular reference to its use in open heart surgery. *Transfusion* 1:151, 1961.

55. Britten, A., Salzman, E. W., Grove-Rasmussen, M., and Shaw, R. S.: The use of ACD bank blood and fresh heparinized blood in open-heart surgery. *Transfusion* 3:368, 1963.

56. Oberman, H. A.: The indications for transfusion of freshly drawn blood. *JAMA* 199:96, 167.

57. Heustis, D. W.: Fresh blood: Fact and fancy, in *Seminar on Current Technical Topics*. American Association of Blood Banks, Washington, D.C., 1974, p. 117.

58. Baldini, M., Costea, N., and Dameshek, W.: The viability of stored human platelets. *Blood* 16:1669, 1960.

59. Bowie, E. J. W., Thompson, J. H., and Owen, C. A., Jr.: The stability of antihemophilic globulin and labile factor in human blood. *Mayo Clin. Proc.* 39:144, 1964.

60. Horowitz, H. I., and Fujimoto, M. M.: Survival of factor XI in vitro and in vivo. *Transfusion* 6:539, 1965.

61. Aggeler, P. M.: Physiological basis for transfusion therapy in hemorrhagic disorders. *Transfusion* 1:71, 1961.

62. Mooreside, D. E., Graybeal, F. Q., Jr., and Langdell, R. D.: Effects of adenine on clotting factors in fresh blood, stored blood, and stored fresh frozen plasma. *Transfusion* 9:191, 1969.

63. Krevans, J. R., and Jackson, D. P.: Hemorrhagic disorder following massive whole blood transfusions. *JAMA* 159:171, 1955.

64. Bunn, H. F., May, M. H., Kocholaty, W. F., and Shields, C. E.: Hemoglobin function in stored blood. *J. Clin. Invest.* 48:311, 1969.

65. *Standards for a Blood Transfusion Service*, 9th ed. American Association of Blood Banks, Washington, D.C., 1978.

66. Moss, G. S., Proctor, H. J., Homer, L. D., Herman, C. M., and Litt, B. D.: Comparison of asanguinous fluids and whole blood in treatment of hemorrhagic shock. *Surg. Gynecol. Obstet.* 129:1247, 1969.

67. Kahn, R. A., Staggs, S. D., Miller, W. V., and Ellis, F. R.: Use of plasma products with whole blood and packed RBCS. *JAMA* 242:2087, 1979.

68. Miller, W. V., Wilson, M. J., and Kalb, H. J.: Simple methods for production of HL-A antigen poor red blood cells. *Transfusion* 13:189, 1973.

69. Fleming, A.: A simple method of removing leucocytes from blood. *Br. J. Exp. Pathol.* 7:281, 1926.

70. Englefriet, C. P., Diepenhorst, P., Gissen, M. V. D., and von Riesz, E.: Removal of leucocytes from whole blood and erythrocyte suspensions by filtration through cotton wool. IV. Immunization studies in rabbits. *Vox Sang.* 28:81, 1975.

71. Diepenhorst, P., and Englefriet, C. P.: Removal of leukocytes from whole blood and erythrocyte suspensions by filtration through cotton wool. V. Results after transfusion of 1,820 units of filtered erythrocytes. *Vox Sang.* 29:15, 1975.

72. Valeri, C. R., Runck, A. H., and Brodine, C. E.: Recent advances in freeze-preservation of red blood cells. *JAMA* 208:489, 1969.

73. Valeri, C. R.: Factors influencing the 24-hour post-transfusion survival and oxygen transport function of previously frozen red cells preserved with 40% (w/v) glycerol and frozen at −80°C. *Transfusion* 14:1, 1974.

74. Chaplin, H., Jr.: Frozen red cell storage: Perspectives and potentials, in *Progress in Transfusion and Transplantation*, AABB-ISBT Transfusion Congress, Washington, D.C., August 1972, p. 329.

75. Grove-Rasmussen, M.: Selection of donors for frozen blood based on specific blood group combinations. *JAMA* 193:48, 1965.

76. Grove-Rasmussen, M., and Huggins, C. E.: Selected types of frozen blood for patients with multiple blood group antibodies. *Transfusion* 13:124, 1973.

77. Tellichi, M., Holberg, R., Rao, K. R. P., and Patel, A. R.: The use of frozen, thawed erythrocytes in blood banking: A report of 28 months' experience in a large transfusion service. *Am. J. Clin. Path.* 68:250, 1977.

78. Contreras, T. J., and Valeri, C. R.: A comparison of methods to wash liquid-stored red blood cells and red blood cells frozen with high or low concentrations of glycerol. *Transfusion* 16:539, 1976.

79. Dameshek, W., and Neber, J.: Transfusion reactions to a plasma constituent of whole blood. *Blood* 5:129, 1950.

80. Vyas, G. N., Perkins, H. A., and Fudenberg, H. H.: Anaphylactoid transfusion reactions associated with anti-IgA. *Lancet* 2:312, 1968.

81. Schmidt, A. P., Taswell, H. F., and Gleich, G. J.: Anaphylactic transfusion reactions associated with anti-IgA antibody. *N. Engl. J. Med.* 280:188, 1969.

82. Vyas, G. N., and Fudenberg, H. H.: Isoimmune anti-IgA causing anaphylactoid transfusion reactions. *N. Engl. J. Med.* 280:1073, 1969.

83. Miller, W. V., Holland, P. V., and Sugarbaker, E.: Anaphylactic reaction to IgA: A difficult transfusion problem. *Transfusion* 54:618, 1970.

84. Leikola, J., Koistinen, M., Lehtinen, M., and Virolainen, M.: IgA-induced anaphylactic transfusion reaction: A report of four cases. *Blood* 42:111, 1973.

85. Geyer, R. P.: Fluorocarbon-polyol artificial blood substitutes. *N. Engl. J. Med.* 289:1077, 1970.

86. Tam, S. C., Blumenstein, J., and Wong, J. T. F.: Blood replacement in dogs by dextran-hemoglobin. *Can. J. Biochem.* 56:981, 1978.

87. Myhre, B. A. (ed.): *A Seminar on Blood Components*. American Association of Blood Banks, Washington, D.C., 1977.

88. Greenwalt, T. J. (ed.): *General Principles of Blood Transfusion* American Medical Association, Chicago, 1977.

89. Myhre, B. A. (ed.): *Blood Component Therapy*, 2d ed. American Association of Blood Banks, Washington, D.C., 1975.

90. McCurdy, P. R.: Blood component therapy, giving what the patient needs. *Postgrad. Med.* 62:143, 1977.

91. Westphal, R. G.: Rational alternatives to the use of whole blood. *Ann. Intern. Med.* 76:987, 1972.

92. Sturgeon, P., Adashek, E. P., Self, J. L., Stiehm, E. R., and Tishkoff, G. H.: Recent developments in blood component therapy. *Ann. Intern. Med.* 74:113, 1971.

93. Roche, J. K., and Stengle, J. M.: Open-heart surgery and the demand for blood. *JAMA* 225:1516, 1973.

94. Plzak, L. F., Jr.: Blood requirements in cardiac surgery, in *Preservation of Red Blood Cells: Proceedings of a Conference*, June 5–6, 1972, edited by H. Chaplin, Jr., et al. National Academy of Sciences, Washington, D.C., 1973, p. 35.

95. Irvin, T. T., Modgill, V. K., Hayter, C. J., and Goligher, J. C.: Clinical assessment of postoperative blood volume. *Lancet* 2:446, 1972.

96. Blackburn, E. K.: Indications for blood transfusion, *Practitioner* 15:14, 1965.

97. Metheny, D.: Clinical estimation of acute blood loss by the tilt test. *Am. Surg.* 33:573, 1967.

98. Hillman, R. S.: Blood-loss anemia. *Postgrad. Med.* 64:88, 1978.

99. Greenwalt, T. J., and Perry, S.: Preservation and utilization of the components of human blood, in *Progress in Hematology*. Grune & Stratton, New York, 1969, vol. 6, p. 157.

100. Golub, S., and Baily, C. P.: Management of major surgical blood loss without transfusion. *JAMA* 198:1171, 1966.

101. Rigor, B., Bosomworth, P., and Rush, B. J., Jr.: Replacement of operative blood loss of more than 1 liter with Hartmann's solution. *JAMA* 203:339, 1968.

102. Moyer, C.: Blood adjuncts in the treatment of hemorrhagic hypovolemias or shock: Conference on blood groups and blood transfusions, in *Blood Transfusion*. Better Bellevue Association, New York, 1967, vol. 2.

103. Cervera, A. L., and Moss, G.: Crystalloid requirements and distribution when resuscitating with RBC's and noncolloid solutions during hemorrhage. *Cir. Shock* 5:357, 1978.

104. Collins, J. A.: Problems associated with the massive transfusion of stored blood. *Surgery* 75:274, 1974.

105. Boral, L. I., and Henry, J. B.: The type and screen: A safe alternative and supplement in selected surgical procedures. *Transfusion* 17:163, 177.

106. Mintz, P. D., Nordine, R. B., Henry, J. B., and Webb, W. R.: Expected hemotherapy in elective surgery. *N.Y. State J. Med.* 76:532, 1976.

107. Friedman, B. A., Oberman, H. A., Chadwick, A. R., and Kingdon, K. I.: The maximum surgical blood order schedule and surgical blood use in the United States. *Transfusion* 16:380, 1976.

108. Moncrief, J. A.: Burns, medical progress. *N. Engl. J. Med.* 288:444, 1973.

109. Baxter, C. R.: Problems and complications of burn shock resuscitation. *Surg. Clin. North Am. 58*:1313, 1978.

110. Pruitt, B. A., Jr.: Fluid and electrolyte replacement in the burned patient. *Surg. Clin. North Am. 58*:1291, 1978.

111. Friedman, B. A.: Patterns of blood utilization by physicians: Transfusion of nonoperated anemic patients. *Transfusion 18*:193, 1978.

112. Mollison, P. L.: *Transfusions in Clinical Medicine*, 6th ed. Blackwell Scientific, Oxford, 1979.

113. Chaplin, H., Jr.: Packed red blood cells. *N. Engl. J. Med. 281*:364, 1969.

114. Status van Eps, L. W., Schouten, H., La Porte-Wijlsman, L., and Struyker-Boudier, A. M.: The influence of red blood cell transfusions on the hyposthenuria and renal hemodynamics of sickle cell anemia. *Clin. Chim. Acta 17*:449, 1967.

115. Necheles, T. F., Chung, S., Sabbah, R., and Whitten, D.: Intensive transfusion therapy in thalassemia major: An eight-year follow-up. *Ann. N.Y. Acad. Sci. 232*:179, 1974.

116. Cavill, I., Ricketts, C., Jacobs, A., and Letsky, E.: Erythropoiesis and the effect of transfusion in homozygous B-thalassemia. *N. Engl. J. Med. 298*:776, 1978.

117. Propper, R. D., Button, L. N., and Nathan, D. G.: New approaches to the transfusion management of thalassemia. *Blood 55*:55, 1980.

118. Ryden, S. E., and Oberman, H. A.: Compatibility of common intravenous solutions with CPD blood. *Transfusion 15*:250, 1975.

119. Dickson, D. N., and Gregory, M. A.: Compatibility of blood with solutions containing calcium. *S. Afr. Med. J. 57*:785, 1980.

120. Liley, A. W.: Intrauterine transfusion of foetus in hemolytic disease. *Br. Med. J. 2*:1107, 1963.

121. Reece, R. L., and Beckett, R. S.: Epidemiology of single-unit transfusion: A one-year experience in a community hospital. *JAMA 195*:801, 1966.

122. Brzica, S. M., Pineda, A. A., and Taswell, H. F.: Autologous blood transfusion. *Mayo Clin. Proc. 51*:723, 1976.

123. Schaff, H. V., Hauer, J. M., and Brawley, R. K.: Autotransfusion in cardiac surgical patients after operation. *Surgery 84*:713, 1978.

124. Newman, M. M., Hamstra, R., and Block, M.: Use of banked autologous blood in elective surgery. *JAMA 218*:861, 1971.

125. Levine, P., and Pollack, W.: Hemolytic disease of the fetus and newborn. *Med. Clin. North. Am. 49*:1647, 1965.

126. McLeod, B. C., Wu, K. K., and Knospe, W. H.: Plasmapheresis in thrombotic thrombocytopenic purpura. *Arch. Int. Med. 140*:1059, 1980.

127. Flaum, M. A., Cuneo, R. A., Appelbaum, F. R., Deisseroth, A. B., Engel, W. K., and Gralnick, H. R.: The hemostatic imbalance of plasma-exchange transfusion. *Blood 54*:694, 1979.

128. Rosenfield, R. E., and Jagathambal: Transfusion therapy for autoimmune hemolytic anemia. *Semin. Hematol. 13*:311, 1976.

129. Blumberg, N., and Bove, J. R.: Uncrossmatched blood for emergency transfusion: One year's experience in a civilian setting. *JAMA 240*:2057, 1978.

130. Opelz, G., Sengan, D. P. S., Mickey, M. R., and Terasaki, P. I.: Effect of blood transfusions on subsequent kidney transplants. *Transplant. Proc. 5*:253, 1973.

131. Hourmant, M., Soulillou, J. P., and Bui-quang, D.: Beneficial effect of blood transfusion: Role of the time interval between the last transfusion and transplantation. *Transplantation 28*:40, 1979.

132. Spees, E. K., et al.: Effects of blood transfusion on cadaver renal transplantation: The Southeastern Organ Procurement Foundation Prospective Study (1977 to 1979). *Transplantation 30*:455, 1980.

133. Solheim, B. G., Flatmark, A., Halvorsen, S., Jervel, J., Pape, J., and Thorsby, E.: Effect of blood transfusions on renal transplantation: Study of 191 consecutive first transplants from living related donors. *Transplantation 30*:281, 1980.

134. Soulillou, J. P., Bignon, J. D., Peyrat, M. A., Guimbretiere, J., and Guenel, J.: Systematic transfusion in hemodialyzed patients awaiting grafts: Kinetics of anti-T and B lymphocyte, immunization and its incidence on graft function. *Transplantation 30*:285, 1980.

135. Thomas, E. D.: Current status of marrow transplantation for aplastic anemia and acute leukemia. The Philip Levine Award Lecture. *Am. J. Clin. Pathol. 72*:887, 1979.

136. Gale, R. P., Feig, S., Ho, W., Falk, P., Rippee, C., and Sparkes, R.: ABO blood group system and bone marrow transplantation. *Blood 5*:185, 1977.

137. Schmidt, P. J.: Transfusion mortality, with special reference to surgical and intensive care facilities. *J. Fl. Med. Assoc. 67*:151, 1980.

138. Honig, C. L., and Bove, J. R.: Transfusion-associated fatalities: Review of Bureau of Biologics Reports, 1976–1978. *Transfusion 20*:653, 1980.

139. Center for Disease Control Hepatitis Surveillance Report No. 42. CDC, Atlanta, June 1978.

140. Van Dijk, P. M., and Kleine, J. W.: The transfusion reaction in anaesthesiological practice. *Acta Anaesthesiol. Belg. 4*:274, 1976.

141. Goldfinger, D.: Acute hemolytic transfusion reactions: A fresh look at pathogenesis and considerations regarding therapy. *Transfusion 17*:85, 1977.

142. Pineda, A. A., Brzica, S. M., and Taswell, H. F.: Hemolytic transfusion reaction: Recent experience in a large blood bank. *Mayo Clin. Proc. 53*:378, 1978.

143. Ingram, G. I. C.: The bleeding complications of blood transfusion. *Transfusion 5*:1, 1965 (editorial review).

144. Rock, R. C., Bove, J. R., and Nemerson, Y.: Heparin treatment of intravascular coagulation accompanying hemolytic transfusion reactions. *Transfusion 9*:57, 1969.

145. Sack, E. S., and Nefa, O. M.: Fibrinogen and fibrin degradation products in hemolytic transfusion reactions. *Transfusion 10*:317, 1970.

146. Bick, R. L., Schmalhorst, W. R., and Fekete, L.: Disseminated intravascular coagulation and blood component therapy. *Transfusion 16*:361, 1976.

147. Barry, K. G., and Crosby, W. H.: The prevention and treatment of renal failure following transfusion reaction. *Transfusion 3*:34, 1963.

148. Luke, R. G., Linton, A. L., Briggs, J. D., and Kennedy, A. C.: Mannitol therapy in acute renal failure. *Lancet 1*:980, 1965.

149. Brittingham, T. E., and Chaplin, H., Jr.: Febrile transfusion reactions caused by sensitivity to donor leukocytes and platelets. *JAMA 165*:819, 1957.

150. Payne, R.: The association of febrile transfusion reactions with leukoagglutinins. *Vox Sang. 2*:233, 1957.

151. Jensen, K. G.: The significance of leuco-agglutinins for development of transfusion reactions. *Dan. Med. Bull. 9*:198, 1962.

152. Perkins, H. A., Payne, R., Ferguson, J., and Wood, M.: Nonhemolytic febrile transfusion reactions: Quantitative effects of blood components with emphasis on isoantigenic incompatibility of leucocytes. *Vox Sang. 11*:578, 1966.

153. Thulstrup, H.: The influence of leukocyte and thrombocyte incompatibility on non-haemolytic transfusion reactions. II. A prospective study. *Vox Sang. 21*:434, 1971.

154. Thompson, J. S., Severson, C. D., Parmely, M. J., Marmorstein, B. L., and Simmons, A.: Pulmonary "hypersensitivity" reactions induced by transfusion of non-HL-A leukoagglutinins. *N. Engl. J. Med. 284*:1120, 1971.

155. Wolf, C. F. W., and Conale, V. C.: Fatal pulmonary hypersensitivity reaction to HL-A incompatible blood transfusion: Report of a case and review of the literature. *Transfusion 16*:135, 1976.

156. Andrews, A. T., Zmijewski, C. M., Bowman, H. S., and Reihart, J. K.: Transfusion reaction with pulmonary infiltration associated with HL-A specific leukocyte antibodies. *Am. J. Clin. Pathol. 66*:483, 1976.

157. Dana, B. W., Durie, B.G.M., White, R. F., and Huestis, D. W.: Concomitant administration of granulocyte transfusions and amphotericin B in neutropenic patients: Absence of significant pulmonary toxicity. *Blood 57*:90, 1981.

158. Thulstrup, H.: The influence of leukocyte and thrombocyte incompatibility on non-haemolytic transfusion reactions. I. A retrospective study. *Vox Sang. 21*:233, 1971.

159. Nadorp, J. H. S., et al.: The significance of the presence of anti-IgA antibodies in individuals with an IgA deficiency. *Eur. J. Clin. Invest. 3*:317, 1973.

160. Vyas, G. N., Perkins, H. A., Yang, Y.-M., and Basantani, G. K.: Healthy blood donors with selective absence of immunoglobulin A: Prevention of anaphylactic transfusion reactions caused by antibodies to IgA. *J. Lab. Clin. Med. 85*:838, 1975.

161. Pineda, A. A., and Taswell, H. F.: Transfusion reactions associated with anti-IgA antibodies: Report of four cases and review of the literature. *Transfusion 15*:10, 1975.

162. Braude, A. I.: Transfusion reactions from contaminated blood: Their recognition and treatment. *N. Engl. J. Med.* 258:1289, 1958.

163. Fine, J.: Septic shock. *JAMA* 188:127, 1965.

164. Vdhoji, V. N., and Weil, M. H.: Hemodynamic and metabolic studies on shock associated with bacteremia. *Ann. Intern. Med.* 62:966, 1965.

165. Cherry, J. W.: Endotoxin shock. *Surg. Clin. North Am.* 50:403, 1970.

166. Siegel, J. H., Glodwyn, R. M., and Friedman, H. P.: Pattern and process in the evolution of human septic shock. *Surgery* 70:232, 1971.

167. Ratnoff, O. D.: Some relationships among hemostasis, fibrinolytic phenomena, immunity and the inflammatory response. *Adv. Immunol.* 10:145, 1969.

168. Buchholz, D. H., Young, V. M., Friedman, N. R., Reilly, J. A., and Mardiney, M. R., Jr.: Bacterial proliferation in platelet products stored at room temperature: Transfusion-induced enterobacter sepsis. *N. Engl. J. Med* 285:429, 1971.

169. Duke, M., Herbert, V. D., and Abelmann, W. H.: Hemodynamic effects of blood transfusion in chronic anemia. *N. Engl. J. Med.* 271:975, 1964.

170. Arrington, P., and McNamara, J. J.: Mechanism of microaggregate formation in stored blood. *Ann. Surg.* 179:146, 1974.

171. Martin, A. M., Simmons, R. L., and Heisterkamp, C. A.: Respiratory insufficiency in combat casualties: Pathologic changes in the lungs of patients dying of wounds. *Ann. Surg.* 170:30, 1969.

172. Moseley, R. V., and Doty, D. B.: Death associated with multiple pulmonary emboli soon after battle injury. *Ann. Surg.* 171:336, 1970.

173. McNamara, J. J., Burran, E. S., Larson, E., Omiya, G., Suchiro, G., and Yamase, H.: Effect of debris in stored blood on pulmonary microvasculature. *Ann. Thorac. Surg.* 14:113, 1972.

174. Barrett, J., Tahir, A. H., and Litwin, M. S.: Increased pulmonary arteriovenous shunting in humans following blood transfusion. *Arch. Surg.* 113:947, 1978.

175. Pineda, A. A., Taswell, H. F., and Brzica, S. M., Jr.: Delayed hemolytic transfusion reaction: An immunologic hazard of blood transfusion. *Transfusion* 18:1, 1978.

176. Moore, S. B., Taswell, H. F., Pineda, A. A., and Sonnenberg, C. L.: Delayed hemolytic transfusion reactions: Evidence of the need for an improved pretransfusion compatibility test. *Am. J. Clin. Pathol.* 74:94, 1980.

177. Croucher, B. E. E., Crookston, M. C., and Crookston, J. H.: Delayed haemolytic transfusion reaction stimulating autoimmune haemolytic anemia. *Vox Sang.* 12:32, 1967.

178. Diamond, W. J., Brown, F. L., Bitterman, P., Klein, H. G., Davey, R. J., and Winslow, R. M.: Delayed hemolytic transfusion reaction presenting as sickle-cell crises. *Ann. Int. Med.* 93:231, 1980.

179. Shulman, N. R., Aster, R. H., Leitner, A., and Hiller, M. C.: Immunoreactions involving platelets. V. Posttransfusion purpura due to a complement-fixing antibody against a genetically controlled platelet antigen: A proposed mechanism for thrombocytopenia and its relevance in "autoimmunity." *J. Clin. Invest.* 40:1597, 1961.

180. Abramson, N., Eisenberg, P. D., and Aster, R. H.: Post-transfusion purpura: Immunologic aspects and therapy. *N. Engl. J. Med.* 291:1163, 1974.

181. Zeigler, Z., Murphy, S., and Gardner, F. H.: Post-transfusion purpura: A heterogenous syndrome. *Blood* 45:529, 1975.

182. Phadke, K. P., and Isbister, J. P.: Post-transfusion purpura. *Med. J. Aust.* 1:430, 1980.

183. Lau, P., Sholtis, C. M., and Aster, R. H.: Post-transfusion purpura: An enigma of alloimmunization. *Am. J. Hematol.* 9:331, 1980.

184. Alter, H. J., Purcell, R. H., Holland, P. V., Feinstone, S. M., Morrow, A. G., and Moritsugu, Y.: Clinical and serological analysis of transfusion-associated hepatitis. *Lancet* 2:838, 1975.

185. Prince, A. M., et al.: Long incubation post transfusion hepatitis without serological evidence of exposure to hepatitis B virus. *Lancet* 2:2441, 1974.

186. Dienstag, J. L., Purcell, R. H., Alter, H. J., Feinstone, S. M., Wong, D. C., and Holland, P. V.: Non-A, non-B post-transfusion hepatitis. *Lancet* 1:560, 1977.

187. Goldfield, M., Black, H. C., Bill, J., Srihongse, S., and Pizzuti, W.: The consequences of administering blood pretested for HBsAg by third generation techniques: A progress report. *Am. J. Med. Sci.* 270:335, 1975.

188. Prince, A. M.: An antigen detected in the blood during the incubation period of serum hepatitis. *Proc. Natl. Acad. Sci. U.S.A.* 60:814, 1968.

189. Gocke, D. J., and Kavey, N. B.: Hepatitis antigen: Correlation with disease and infectivity of blood donors. *Lancet* 1:1055, 1969.

190. Blumberg, B. S., Alter, H. J., and Visnich, S.: A new antigen in leukemia sera. *JAMA* 191:541, 1965.

191. Hirschman, S. Z.: The hepatitis B virus and its DNA polymerase: The prototype three-D virus. *Mol. Cell. Biochem.* 26:47, 1979.

192. Krugman, S., Overby, L. R., Mushahwar, I. K., Ling, C.-M., Frosner, G. G., and Deinhardt, F.: Viral hepatitis, type B: Studies on the natural history and prevention re-examined. *N. Engl. J. Med.* 300:101, 1979.

193. Hoofnagle, J. H., Seeff, L. B., Bales, Z. B., and Zimmerman, H. J.: Type B hepatitis after transfusion with blood containing antibody to hepatitis B core antigen. *N. Engl. J. Med.* 298:1379, 1978.

194. Katchaki, J. N., Siem, T. H., and Brouwer, R.: Serological evidence of the presence of HBsAg undetected by conventional radioimmunoassay in anti-HBc positive blood donors. *J. Clin. Pathol.* 31:837, 1978.

195. Seeff, L. B., et al.: Type B hepatitis after needle-stick exposure: Prevention with hepatitis B immunoglobulin. Final report of the Veterans Administration Cooperative Study. *Ann. Intern. Med.* 88:285, 1978.

196. Szmuness, W., et al.: Hepatitis B vaccine: Demonstration of efficacy in a controlled clinical trial in a high-risk population in the United States. *N. Engl. J. Med.* 303:833, 1980.

197. Bastiaans, M. J. S., Dodd, R. Y., Nath, N., Pineda-Tamondong, G., Sandler, S. G., and Barkee, L. F.: Hepatitis-associated markers in American Red Cross volunteer blood donor population. I. Trends in HBsAg detection, 1975–1978. *Vox Sang.* 39:1, 1980.

198. Moore, B. P. L., and Perrault, R. A.: Hepatitis B antigenemia among blood donors: The changing scene. *Can. Med. Assoc. J.* 112:53, 1975.

199. Cossart, Y. E.: Epidemiology of serum hepatitis. *Br. Med. J.* 28:156, 1972.

200. Aach, R. D., et al.: Transfusion-transmitted viruses: Interim analysis of hepatitis among transfused and non-transfused patients, in *Viral Hepatitis*, edited by G. N. Vyas, S. N. Cohen, and R. Schmid. Franklin Institute Press, Philadelphia, 1978, p. 383.

201. Katchaki, J. N., Siem, T. H., and Brouwer, R.: Post-transfusion non A, non B hepatitis in the Netherlands. *Br. Med. J.* 282:107, 1981.

202. Feinstone, S. M., and Purcell, R. H.: Non-A, non-B hepatitis. *Annu. Rev. Med.* 29:359, 1978.

203. Tabor, E., and Gerety, R. J.: Non-A, non-B hepatitis: New findings and prospects for prevention. *Transfusion* 19:669, 1979.

204. Alter, H. J., Purcell, R. H., Holland, P. V., and Popper, H.: Transmissible agent in non-A, non-B hepatitis. *Lancet* 1:459, 1978.

205. Kabiri, M., Tabor, E., and Gerety, R. J.: Antigen-antibody system associated with non-A, non-B hepatitis detected by indirect immunofluorescence. *Lancet* 2:221, 1979.

206. Aach, R. D., et al.: The transfusion-transmitted viruses study: Serum alanine aminotransferase of donors in relation to the risk of non-A, non-B hepatitis in recipients. *N. Engl. J. Med.* 304:989, 1981.

207. Hoofnagle, J. H., Barker, L. F., Thiel, J., and Gerety, R. J.: Hepatitis B virus and hepatitis B surface antigen in human albumin products. *Transfusion* 16:141, 1976.

208. Schroeder, D. D., and Mozen, M. M.: Australia antigen: Distribution during Cohn ethanol fractionation of human plasma. *Science* 168:1462, 1970.

209. Hoofnagle, J. H., Gerety, R. J., Thiel, J., and Barker, L. F.: The prevalence of hepatitis B surface antigen in commercially prepared plasma products. *J. Lab. Clin. Med.* 88:102, 1976.

210. Tullis, J. L., Hinman, J., Sproul, M. T., and Nickerson, R. J.: Incidence of post transfusion hepatitis in previously frozen blood. *JAMA* 214:719, 1970.

211. Hangen, R. K.: Hepatitis after the transfusion of frozen red cells and washed red cells. *N. Engl. J. Med.* 301:393, 1979.

212. Alter, H. J., et al.: Transmission of hepatitis B virus infection by transfusion of frozen deglycerolized red blood cells. *N. Engl. J. Med.* 298:637, 1978.

213. Black, R. H.: Investigation of blood donors in accidental transfusion malaria: *Plasmodium vivax, falciparum,* and *malariae* infections. *Med. J. Aust.* 2:446, 1960.

214. Chojnacki, R. E., Branzinsky, J. H., and Barrett, O.: Transfusion introduced *falciparum* malaria. *N. Engl. J. Med. 279:*984, 1968.
215. Dover, A. S., and Schultz, M. G.: Transfusion-induced malaria. *Transfusion 11:*353, 1971.
216. Joishy, S., and Lopez, C. G.: Transfusion-induced malaria in a splenectomized β-thalassemia major patient and review of blood donor screening methods. *Am. J. Hematol. 8:*221, 1980.
217. Kaariainen, L., Klemola, E., and Paloheimo, J.: Rise of cytomegalovirus antibodies in an infectious-mononucleosis-like syndrome after transfusion. *Br. Med. J. 1:*1270, 1966.
218. Yeager, A. S.: Transfusion acquired cytomegalovirus infection in newborn infants. *Am. J. Dis. Child. 128:*478, 1974.
219. Winston, D. J., et al.: Cytomegalovirus infections associated with leukocyte transfusions. *Ann. Intern. Med. 93:*671, 1980.
220. Lang, D. J., Ebert, P. A., Rodgers, B. M., Boggess, H. P., and Rixse, R. S.: Reduction of postperfusion cytomegalovirus-infections following the use of leukocyte depleted blood. *Transfusion 17:*391, 1977.
221. Thomas, E. D., Fefer, A., Buckner, C. D., and Storb, R.: Current status of bone marrow transplantation for aplastic anemia and acute leukemia. *Blood 49:*671, 1977.
222. Ford, J. M., Lucey, J. J., Cullen, M. H., Tobias, J. S., and Lister, T. A. Fatal graft-versus-host disease following transfusion of granulocytes from normal donors. *Lancet 2:*1167, 1976.
223. Cohen, D., Weinstein, H., Mihm, M., and Yankee, R.: Non-fatal graft-versus-host disease occurring after transfusion with leukocytes and platelets obtained from normal donors. *Blood 53:*1053, 1979.
224. Lowenthal, R. M., et al.: Granulocyte transfusions in treatment of infections in patients with acute leukemia and aplastic anemia. *Lancet 1:*353, 1975.
225. Dinsmore, R. E., et al.: Fatal graft-versus-host disease following blood transfusion in Hodgkin's disease documented by HLA typing. *Blood 55:*831, 1980.
226. Orlina, A. R., Unger, P. J., and Koshy, M.: Post-transfusion alloimmunization in patients with sickle cell disease. *Am. J. Hematol. 5:*101, 1978.
227. Mollison, P. L., Frame, M., and Ross, M. E.: Differences between Rh(D) negative subjects in response to Rh(D) antigen. *Br. J. Haematol. 19:*257, 1970.
228. Cook, K., and Rush, B.: Rh(D) immunization after massive transfusion of Rh(D)-positive blood. *Med. J. Aust. 1:*166, 1974.
229. Beutler, E., Kuhl, W., and West, C.: The osmotic fragility of erythrocytes after prolonged liquid storage and after reinfusion. *Blood 59:*1141, 1982.

CHAPTER *165*

Preservation and clinical use of leukocytes

JACOB NUSBACHER

History of leukocyte transfusion

The feasibility of leukocyte transfusions in the treatment of marrow failure and granulocytopenia was first explored in 1934, but with little success [1]. Some years later benefit from the use of leukocytes in the supportive therapy of irradiated dogs was demonstrated [2]. In these studies, donor leukocytes were shown to migrate to sites of infection and to be capable of normal phagocytic activity. Practical clinical methods for transfusing granulocytes were slow to develop, possibly because the urgency for granulocyte replacement became less acute with the development of antibiotics and because technical problems made it difficult to procure adequate quantities of normal granulocytes.

In the early studies, granulocytes for transfusion were obtained from normal donors. The lack of clinical benefit and the failure of the number of white cells in the blood to increase were the result of an insufficient number of cells being infused [3]. Subsequently, patients with chronic myelogenous leukemia (CML) were used as donors [4]. CML granulocytes, when given to patients with acute leukemia who had severe granulocytopenia and life-threatening infection, led to improvement in blood counts and appeared to help some patients overcome the infection. These observations led to the development of the continuous-flow centrifuge apparatus [5] and to other methods for collecting large quantities of granulocytes from normal individuals.

Granulocyte collection

Granulocytes are found primarily in the marrow and tissues. Less than 5 percent of the total body granulocyte pool is in the intravascular space [6,7]. Granulocytes use the bloodstream primarily as a mode of transport from the marrow to sites of inflammation and have a half-life of 4 to 10 h in the intravascular compartment [8,9]. Therefore, whole-blood donors are an inadequate source of granulocyte concentrates, as the number of cells that can be collected from each donor is small. The collection of large numbers of granulocytes requires the processing of between 5 to 10 liters per donation. This can be accomplished within 3 h with the leukapheresis devices that are now available.

CENTRIFUGATION LEUKAPHERESIS

Most leukapheresis procedures are done with a centrifuge [10–15]. Modeled after the original continuous-flow cell separator [5], these machines exploit the different densities of red cells, plasma, and the interposed leukocytes and platelets (buffy coat). Donor blood is pumped through the centrifuge, wherein the separation into the three layers occurs. The buffy coat is harvested to form the granulocyte concentrate, and the red cells and plasma are returned to the donor.

Granulocyte collections from healthy donors by centrifugal leukapheresis do not yield adequate quantities of phagocytic cells. Yields of 0.05 to 0.1×10^{10} granulocytes per liter of donor blood processed have been reported [14,16]. This is due to two factors: (1) the difficulty of separating granulocytes from lighter red cells and lymphocytes because of the similarity in their densities and (2) the low number of granulocytes in the circulation. However, the addition of a rouleaux-inducing agent to the blood before it enters the centrifuge enhances cell separation and increases yields by as much as twofold. The most common rouleaux-inducing agent is hydroxyethyl starch [17–20], which is ordinarily used as a volume expander in surgery. Dextran has also been used [21]. Virtually all centrifugal cell separators require the use of cell sedimenting agents to achieve adequate yields of granulocytes.

Donor granulocyte count can also be increased prior to donation by the administration of drugs that either mobilize granulocytes from the marrow or cause a shift of granulocytes from the marginal to the circulating pool [22,23]. Etiocholanolone [17], which raises the donor granulocyte count and improves leukapheresis yields considerably, is associated with donor discomfort. At present, prednisone or another glucocorticoid is administered [14,16,19,23–25], either orally or by intravenous infusion, prior to leukapheresis in order to raise the donor granulocyte count. Various dose schedules have been used, but the usual total dose is the equivalent of 40 to 60 mg of prednisone. Leukapheresis yields have increased by 50 to 100 percent after glucocorticoid administration, and their use is routine in most leukapheresis facilities. The effects of hydroxyethyl starch and steroid administration are additive, and yields of 1.5 to 3.0×10^{10} granulocytes per 10-liter leukapheresis procedure are possible. Hydroxyethyl starch and glucocorticoid treatments have no significant adverse effects on the function of collected granulocytes [23,26–28].

Although centrifugation leukapheresis procedures are safe, some hazards have been identified [14,29–37]. The most common donor reaction is circumoral or digital tingling resulting from mild hypocalcemia from the reinfusion of citrate solution, the anticoagulant used in leukapheresis procedures. This reaction is alleviated by slowing the reinfusion rate. Hypovolemic or vasovagal hypotension, donor chilling, and allergic reactions due to hydroxyethyl starch also occur occasionally. Fluid retention occurs often when hydroxyethyl starch is used.

Other potential adverse effects have been identified. These include the hazards of glucocorticoid administration, retention in the donor of small amounts of hydroxyethyl starch [35,36], and lymphocyte depletion (about 2 to 4×10^9 are removed per procedure) [14,37,38]. At present, none of these have been shown to be deleterious if the frequency and total number of leukapheresis donations are limited.

Decreased granulocyte counts are not a significant problem with centrifugal leukapheresis despite the removal of as many as 2.5×10^{10} granulocytes, the number usually present in the circulating granulocyte pool [14,16]. There is mobilization of granulocytes from the marginal and marrow pools during the leukapheresis procedure, although an increase in "band" or other immature granulocyte forms is not usually seen. The platelet count may fall, usually by less than 30 percent, because these cells are also removed during granulocyte collection. Donor hemoglobin concentration usually also falls. This is due in part to red cell removal but more to hemodilution, especially when hydroxyethyl starch is used. Donor platelet count and hemoglobin concentration return to predonation levels in a few days.

GRANULOCYTE CONCENTRATES FROM CML DONORS
Originally, cell separator collections were performed on donors with CML. High yields, up to 10×10^{10} phagocytic cells, are possible with these donors, depending on the patient-donor white blood cell count [39]. Transfusion of concentrates obtained from CML donors has been shown to increase recipient white cell count and cause lysis of fever in septic neutropenic recipients [4,40]. However, there are few untreated CML patients available, and they are rarely used as leukapheresis donors.

FILTRATION LEUKAPHERESIS
An alternative, noncentrifugal method of granulocyte collection exploits the ability of granulocytes to adhere to nylon in the presence of divalent cations [41]. Thus, heparin replaces citrate as the anticoagulation agent. Donor blood is passed continuously through nylon-filled cylinders, which trap granulocytes and monocytes but permit the passage of other blood cells. After the donation is completed, the phagocytes are retrieved from the filters in vitro by perfusing the cylinders with a calcium chelating solution.

Filtration leukapheresis is simple, requires little equipment, and yields 1.5 to 3.0×10^{10} granulocytes per procedure if glucocorticoid pretreatment is used [14,16,41–43]. The necessity to heparinize the donor has been a major factor in limiting its widespread use, although serious hemorrhage has not been reported. Other donor problems observed include complement activation [44–49], abdominal pain reactions [50], and priapism [51]. Furthermore, some of the granulocytes collected by filtration leukapheresis are damaged [27,42,52–56], as evidenced by the frequent development of shaking chills in the recipient, and the abnormal morphology, poor survival in vivo, and poor chemotaxis in vivo and in vitro of such granulocytes (although their bactericidal capacity is normal or only slightly diminished [28,57]). The quality of filtration-collected granulocytes can be improved by glucocorticoid [43,52] or colchicine [58] pretreatment of the donor or by modification in the formulation of the solution used to elute the cells from the nylon fibers [59].

Despite these problems, there is considerable evidence in both animal models and humans that granulocyte concentrates collected by filtration leukapheresis are efficacious in the treatment of septic neutropenic subjects [53,60–64]. However, the drawbacks and hazards seem to have diminished enthusiasm for this technique in recent years.

Granulocyte transfusion

There is considerable disparity in the composition of granulocyte concentrates collected by different facilities and by different collection devices. Most collection facilities strive for a minimum of 1.0×10^{10} granulocytes per concentrate, but this number is often not achieved. Among the variables that determine the yield of granulocytes are the following: the cell separator used, donor granulocyte count, glucocorticoid pretreatment and donor response, the use of hydroxyethyl starch, the volume of donor blood processed, and the skill of the collection team. The volume of the granulocyte concentrate and the number of contaminating red cells and lymphocytes are also variable. Questions of clinical efficacy, function in vitro and in vivo, immunological considerations, and recipient hazards have been difficult to answer because of this product variability. It is also likely that the lack of efficacy of granulocyte transfusions may result from an inadequate dose of granulocytes being transfused [60].

As with all blood transfusion therapy, granulocyte transfusions are temporizing procedures. Even when transfusion is successful, the patient will continue to be at risk of fatal infection unless marrow recovery occurs. The patient's underlying disease determines the ultimate prognosis.

The setting in which granulocyte concentrates are used often contributes to the poor results. Most granulocyte transfusions are given to patients with acute myelogenous leukemia. Thrombocytopenic bleeding is often present. The patient may have splenomegaly, may have received previous blood transfusions, and may have an infection, all circumstances associated with shortened survival of transfused cells.

Many of the principles that guide granulocyte transfusions were elucidated by studies done with granulocyte concentrates collected from patients with CML using bag leukapheresis methods [4]. A total of 40 granulocytopenic recipients, most of whom had acute leukemia, were given 118 transfusions. The median dose of mature granulocytes and band forms was 5.8×10^{10}, a dose rarely achieved with concentrates obtained from normal donors. The studies showed the following: (1) Only a small portion of all granulocytes transfused are recovered in the circulation 1 h after transfusion (median, 5 percent; range, 0 to 36 percent); most transfused granulocytes enter the marginal or tissue pools immediately. (2) The median increment in circulating granulocytes measured 1 h after transfusion was 1000 per microliter. (3) The posttransfusion increment in recipient granulocyte count was inversely related to the pretransfusion granulocyte count: the more severely granulocytopenic the patient, the smaller the increment. (4) No recipient increments were observed if the number of granulocytes transfused was fewer than 1×10^{10}. (5) The response to granulocyte transfusions, as measured by lysis of fever, was related to the dose of granulocytes given: doses lower than 1×10^{10} were rarely effective, and doses 10 times greater usually were.

Two general principles guiding granulocyte transfusions are derived from these data: (1) The minimum dose of granulocytes transfused should be 1.0×10^{10}.

This points out the need for better granulocyte collection methods and the inadequacy of granulocyte concentrates now being used. (2) Posttransfusion increments in recipient granulocyte count are unlikely to occur with the number of cells usually collected. Furthermore, such increments are generally inadequate in assessing efficacy or in evaluating other factors related to granulocyte transfusion, such as immunological incompatibility.

Despite these difficulties, there is evidence of the clinical efficacy of granulocyte concentrates. Dogs made neutropenic by cyclophosphamide provide the clearest demonstration of the effectiveness of granulocyte transfusions in treating both gram-negative septicemia [53,61] and systemic candidiasis [65]. In humans, probable efficacy of granulocyte transfusion was shown with cells obtained by bag collection methods from patients with CML [4]. Granulocyte concentrates obtained from normal donors were thought to be of value in treating gram-negative septicemia, but the study was not controlled prospectively [66] and daily granulocyte transfusions were required to achieve a good result.

In a randomized prospective study, better survival and more frequent lysis of fever occurred in infected granulocytopenic patients treated with granulocyte transfusion and antibiotics than in a group of patients receiving antibiotics alone [62]. The majority of other controlled studies support these observations [63,64, 67–72]. The clearest demonstration of efficacy has been with granulocyte transfusions given for septicemia, especially with gram-negative organisms [60]. Efficacy in treating nonbacterial infections has not been clearly demonstrated in humans.

INDICATIONS
The indications for granulocyte transfusion are not easy to define. In general, the patient should have (1) an absolute granulocyte count of less than 500 per microliter, (2) fever, (3) preferably a documented infection, and (4) no response of the infection after 48 h of appropriate antibiotic treatment. Also, the patient's underlying condition should not be so severe or so far advanced that a remission is no longer possible.

The risk of infection in granulocytopenic patients is related to the severity and duration of the cytopenia [73]. The risk of infection increases dramatically when the granulocyte count is below 500 per microliter. Perhaps a more important consideration than absolute number in determining the need for granulocyte transfusion is the status of the patient's marrow. If early marrow recovery is expected, granulocyte concentrates are probably superfluous. Conversely, if the neutropenia is expected to last for a time, the patient may benefit from granulocyte transfusions when infection is present.

It may not always be possible to document infection in severely neutropenic patients for whom granulocyte transfusions are contemplated. Further, the sepsis may be so severe that there may not be time for a trial of antibiotic therapy alone.

PROPHYLACTIC TRANSFUSION

A number of studies have evaluated the usefulness of giving prophylactic granulocyte transfusions to neutropenic patients without evidence of infection [74–78]. In the largest randomized study, neutropenic leukemia patients receiving prophylactic granulocyte transfusions did not have an overall reduced incidence of infections when compared with controls, although the proportion of transfused patients with bacterial septicemia was reduced [70]. Also, prophylactic granulocyte transfusions did not improve the rates of remission, survival, or occurrence of marrow recovery. Most other studies agree with these findings.

Two randomized studies have evaluated the use of prophylactic granulocyte transfusions in patients receiving marrow transplants. One study found fewer infections in transfused patients than in controls [76]. In contrast, the other study found a decrease in bacterial septicemia in transfused patients but did not observe a reduction in overall infection; nor was survival improved. Furthermore, 13 of the 18 patients receiving transfusion developed cytomegalovirus (CMV) infections (as compared with only 6 of 17 controls), a significant additional hazard in the severely immunosuppressed patient population.

One major drawback to prophylactic granulocyte transfusion is the increased likelihood of leukocyte and platelet alloimmunization. Patients who receive such treatment have a high incidence of transfusion reactions, alloimmunization, lymphocytotoxic antibodies, repeated fevers, and refractoriness. Refractoriness to platelet transfusion occurs frequently in the transfused group and complicates platelet transfusion therapy [75]. Although there is some reduction in the incidence of infection, the occurrence of alloimmunization is a major deterrent to the successful use of prophylactic granulocyte transfusions. Development of a leukocyte compatibility test could make prophylactic granulocyte transfusions more useful.

HAZARDS

The general hazards of blood transfusion also apply to granulocyte transfusions. Hemolytic reactions may occur because there are red cells in granulocyte concentrates. ABO-compatible concentrates should be given. Recovery of granulocytes in the recipient 1 h after transfusion is adversely affected by ABO incompatibility [66]. The presence of non-ABO erythrocyte antibodies in the recipient should also be ascertained prior to transfusion, but transfusion is often given in the presence of such erythrocyte incompatibilities because of the severity of the patient's infection. This decision is based on weighing the risk of hemolysis against the benefit of transfusion in each situation. If possible, most of the erythrocytes in the concentrate should be re-

moved by differential centrifugation prior to transfusion in these cases.

Febrile transfusion reactions occur frequently with granulocyte transfusions [60]; about 10 percent of recipients have chills and fever after transfusion of cells collected by a centrifugation method. Granulocytes procured by filtration, when transfused, induce febrile reactions in about 30 percent of recipients, probably because some of the cells are damaged by this collection method and pyrogenic substances are released. The presence in the recipient of leukocyte antibodies also can provoke febrile reactions. Glucocorticoids, antihistamines, and meperidine can be given either prophylactically or therapeutically to reduce the frequency or severity of these reactions.

Acute pulmonary insufficiency has been reported with granulocyte transfusions [79]. A number of different mechanisms have been proposed. In neutropenic patients with pneumonia, it has been postulated that the rapid migration of transfused granulocytes to the infected lung may induce such a reaction [79]. Leukoagglutinins in the recipient may also cause pulmonary problems by causing leukocyte aggregates which embolize to the lung [80]. Other mechanisms, involving complement activation with the generation of C5a, which results in granulocyte aggregation or adhesion to endothelial cells, have also been postulated [81]. Finally, severe, even lethal, pulmonary reactions may be associated with the concomitant use of amphotericin B and granulocyte transfusions [82]. These observations are supported by other studies demonstrating that amphotericin B promotes the aggregation of leukocytes exposed to nylon fibers [83]. Therefore, amphotericin B and leukocyte transfusion should be separated in time each day they are coadministered.

Severely immunosuppressed patients are particularly at risk for other serious complications of granulocyte transfusion. Graft-versus-host disease, sometimes fatal, has occurred [84–88]. In those patients receiving intensive chemotherapy, the concentrate should be irradiated with 1500 rads prior to administration to prevent this problem. Severely immunosuppressed patients, especially those undergoing marrow transplantation, may also develop CMV infection, particularly CMV pneumonia, which may be fatal [77]. While it is difficult to ascertain from current studies whether these cases are examples of activation of the recipient's latent virus or result from CMV-infected transfused leukocyte concentrates, it is likely that both mechanisms play a role. Toxoplasmosis associated with transfusion of granulocytes obtained from donors with CML has also been observed in four patients [89].

IMMUNOLOGICAL FACTORS

Prior transfusion and/or immunization to leukocyte antigens adversely affect the outcome of granulocyte transfusion. In dogs, prior whole-blood transfusion decreases the efficacy of granulocyte transfusions given to the same recipient animals made cytopenic with cyclophosphamide [90]. Dogs that had been previously transfused had poorer increments after granulocyte transfusion and a higher mortality rate than dogs who did not have prior transfusion. In this study, lymphocytotoxic cross matching was not useful in ascertaining alloimmunization.

Studies in humans have shown that prior granulocyte transfusion or lymphocytotoxic or leukoagglutinating antibodies in the recipient adversely affect the postransfusion granulocyte increment and recovery [40,66,75, 91]. HLA matching between donor and recipient improves posttransfusion granulocyte increments [66,92, 93]. Febrile reactions or severe pulmonary insufficiency after granulocyte transfusion are more frequent when leukocyte antibodies are present in the recipient [40,75]. Also, noncytotoxic HLA antibodies inhibit granulocyte phagocytosis [94].

It would be desirable to transfuse "compatible" granulocytes. Unfortunately, there are no good methods for performing granulocyte compatibility testing in a timely manner. A study of 50 patients using ^{111}In-labeled granulocytes showed that shortened posttransfusion survival time and failure to localize at sites of infection were predicted by the presence of granulocyte agglutinating antibodies in the recipient, but not by granulocytotoxic or lymphotoxic antibodies [91].

Storage of granulocyte concentrates

It is best to transfuse granulocytes as soon as possible after collection [60,95]. Granulocyte concentrates are collected in an open system and should not be stored for more than 24 h to avoid bacterial contamination.

Granulocyte chemotaxis is the biological function altered first during storage [25,28,95–98]. Changes in phagocytic function, bactericidal capacity, and biochemical functions such as hexose monophosphate shunt activity and oxygen consumption are generally less sensitive indicators of cell damage during storage.

Room temperature storage (about 22°C) and refrigerator storage (about 5°C) of granulocyte concentrates have been evaluated [95–100]. Cell viability and bactericidal capacity seem to be well maintained at either temperature for at least 24 h [100], but chemotaxis and cell ATP are better preserved at 20 to 24°C [96,97,100].

After transfusion, about 15 percent of radioisotope-labeled granulocytes stored at either room temperature or at 1 to 6°C for 24 h can be recovered in the circulation [95,101]. The intravascular half-life is about 4 h. Studies in rabbits have shown that migration of ^{3}H-thymidine–labeled granulocytes to subcutaneous sponges is better when granulocytes are stored at 5°C than when they are stored at room temperature [102]. Stored granulocytes collected by filtration leukapheresis have poor intravascular recovery relative to those collected by centrifugation [28,100,103].

The pH of the suspending medium should probably be over 6.5 [28], since preservation of chemotaxis requires a pH nearer the physiological range of 7.0 to 7.5 [95,100]. Granulocyte concentrates are better stored in plasma than in other suspension fluids [100], especially if collected by filtration leukapheresis. As with platelets, there is evidence that the kind of plastic used in the storate bag is another important storage variable [104].

Cryopreservation of granulocytes would be an ideal method of storage because it would permit the "banking" of large quantities of cells, which would be available when needed. Dimethyl sulfoxide is the best cryoprotective agent, but there are no satisfactory methods for freezing granulocytes. Postthaw recovery of viable cells, as measured by phagocytosis, rarely exceeds 25 percent [105]. A few reports [106,107] suggest better cryopreservation of granulocytes, but further studies are required.

References

1. Strumia, M. M.: Effect of leukocyte cream injection in treatment of neutropenias. *Am. J. Med. Sci.* 187:527, 1934.
2. Brecher, G., Wilbur, K. M., and Cronkite, E. P.: Transfusion of separated leukocytes into irradiated dogs with aplastic marrows. *Proc. Soc. Exp. Biol. Med.* 84:54, 1953.
3. Hirsch, E. O., and Gardner, F. H.: The transfusion of human blood platelets with a note on the transfusion of granulocytes. *J. Lab. Clin. Med.* 39:556, 1952.
4. Freireich, E. J., Levin, R. H., Whang, J., Carbone, P. P., Bronson, J., and Morse, E. E.: The functions and fate of transfused leukocytes from donors with chronic myelocytic leukemia in leukopenic recipients. *Ann. N.Y. Acad. Sci.* 113:1081, 1964.
5. Freireich, E. J., Judson, G., and Levin, R. H.: Separation and collection of leukocytes. *Cancer Res.* 25:1516, 1965.
6. Donohue, D. M., Grabrio, B. W., and Finch, C. A.: Quantitative measurements of hematopoietic cells of the marrow. *J. Clin. Invest.* 37:1564, 1958.
7. Donahue, D. M., Reiff, R. H., Henson, M. L., Betson, Y., and Finch, C. A.: Quantitative measurements of the erythrocytic and granulocytic cells of the marrow and blood *J. Clin. Invest.* 37:1571, 1958.
8. Athens, J. W., Haab, O. P., Mauer, A. M., Ashenbrucker, H., Cartwright, G. E., and Wintrobe, M. M.: Leukokinetic studies. IV. The total blood circulating and marginal granulocyte pools and the granulocyte turnover rate in normal subjects. *J. Clin. Invest.* 40:989, 1961.
9. Cartwright, G. E., Athens, J. W., and Wintrobe, M. M.: The kinetics of granulopoiesis in normal man. *Blood* 24:780, 1969.
10. Graw, R. G., Herzig, G. P., Eisel, R. J., and Perry, S.: Leukocyte and platelet collection from normal donors with the continuous flow blood cell separator. *Transfusion* 11:94, 1971.
11. Mishler, J. M., Higby, D. J., Rhomberg, W., Cohen, E., Nicora, R. W., and Holland, J. F.: Hydroxyethyl starch and dexamethasone as an adjunct to leukocyte separation with the IBM blood cell separator. *Transfusion* 14:352, 1974.
12. Buchholtz, D. H., Schiffer, C. A., Wiernik, P. H., Betts, S. W., and Reilly, J. A.: Granulocyte harvest for transfusion: Donor response to repeated leukapheresis. *Transfusion* 15:96, 1975.
13. Huestis, D. W., White, R. F., Price, M. J., and Inman, M.: Use of hydroxyethyl starch to improve granulocyte collection on the Lathan blood processor. *Transfusion* 15:559, 1975.
14. MacPherson, J. L., Nusbacher, J., and Bennett, J. M.: The acquisition of granulocytes by leukapheresis: A comparison of continuous flow centrifugation and filtration leukapheresis in normal and corticosteroid-stimulated donors. *Transfusion* 16:221, 1976.

15. Hester, J. P., Kellogg, R. M., Mulzet, A. P., Kruger, V. R., McCredie, K. B., and Freireich, E. J.: Principles of blood separation and component extraction in a disposable continuous-flow single-stage channel. *Blood* 54:254, 1979.

16. Nusbacher, J., McCullough, J., and Huestis, D. W.: Granulocyte collection and processing, in *The Granulocyte: Function and Clinical Utilization*, edited by T. J. Greenwalt and G. A. Jamieson. Liss, New York, 1977, p. 175.

17. McCredie, K. B., Freireich, E. J., Hester, J. P., and Vallejos, C.: Increased granulocyte collection with the blood cell separator and the addition of etiocholanolone and hydroxyethyl starch. *Transfusion* 14:357, 1974.

18. Mishler, J. M., Hadlock, D. E., Fortuny, I. E., Nicora, R. W., and McCullough, J.: Increased efficiency of leukocyte separation by the addition of hydroxyethyl starch to the continuous flow centrifuge. *Blood* 44:571, 1974.

19. Mishler, J. M., Higby, D. J., and Rhomberg, W.: Hydroxyethyl starch and dexamethasone as an adjunct to leukocyte separation with the IBM blood cell separator. *Transfusion* 14:352, 1974.

20. Mishler, J. M.: Hydroxyethyl starch as an experimental adjunct to leukocyte separation by centrifugal means: Review of safety and efficacy. *Transfusion* 15:449, 1975.

21. Lowenthal, R. M., and Park, D. S.: The use of dextran as an adjunct to granulocyte collection on the continuous-flow blood cell separator. *Transfusion* 15:23, 1975.

22. Athens, J. W., Heab, O. P., Raab, S. O., Boggs, D. R., Cartwright, G. E., and Wintrobe, M. M.: The mechanism of steroid granulocytosis. *J. Clin. Invest.* 41:1342, 1962.

23. Mischler, J. M.: The effects of corticosteroids on mobilization and function of ventrophils. *Exp. Hematol.* 5 (Suppl.):15, 1977.

24. Higby, D. J., Mishler, J. M., Rhomberg, W., Nicora, R. W., and Holland, J. F.: The effect of a single or double dose of dexamethasone on granulocyte collection with a continuous flow centrifuge. *Vox Sang.* 28:243, 1975.

25. Winton, E. F., and Vogler, W. R.: Development of a practical oral dexamethasone premedication schedule leading to improved granulocyte yields with the continuous-flow centrifugal blood cell separator. *Blood* 52:249, 1978.

26. Glasser, L., Huestis, D. W., and Jones, J. F.: Functional capabilities of steroid-recruited neutrophils harvested for clinical transfusion. *N. Engl. J. Med.* 297:1037, 1977.

27. McCullough, J., Weiblin, B. J., Deinard, A. R., Boen, J., Fortuny, I. E., and Quie, P. G.: In vitro function and post-transfusion survival of granulocytes collected by continuous-flow centrifugation and by filtration leukapheresis. *Blood* 48:315, 1976.

28. Steigbigel, R. T., Baum, J., MacPherson, J. L., and Nusbacher, J.: Granulocyte bactericidal capacity and chemotaxis as affected by continuous-flow centrifugation and filtration leukapheresis, steroid administration, and storage. *Blood* 52:197, 1978.

29. McCullough, J., and Fortuny, I. E.: Laboratory evaluation of normal donors undergoing leukapheresis on the continuous flow centrifuge. *Transfusion* 13:394, 1973.

30. Fraser, I. D.: Which are the principal established or potential risks for donors undergoing cytapheresis procedures and how can they be prevented? *Vox Sang.* 39:173, 1980.

31. Strauss, R. G., Koepke, J. A., Maguire, L. C., and Thompson, J. S.: Clinical and laboratory effects on donors of intermittent-flow centrifugation platelet-leukapheresis performed with hydroxyethyl starch and citrate. *Clin. Lab. Haematol.* 2:11, 1980.

32. Rock, G., and Wise, P.: Plasma expansion during granulocyte procurement: Cumulative effects of hydroxethyl starch. *Blood* 53:1156, 1979.

33. Drescher, W. P., Shih, N., Hess, K., and Tishkoff, G. H.: Massive extracorporeal blood clotting during discontinuous flow leukapheresis. *Transfusion* 18:89, 1978.

34. Kosmin, M.: Bacteremia during leukapheresis. *Transfusion* 20:115, 1980.

35. Maguire, L. C., et al.: The elimination of hydroxyethyl starch from the blood of donors experiencing single or multiple intermittent-flow centrifugation leukapheresis. *Transfusion* 21:347, 1981.

36. Ring, J., Sherkoff, D., and Richter, W.: Intravascular persistence of hydroxyethyl starch (HES) after serial granulocyte collections using HES in man. *Vox Sang.* 34:181, 1980.

37. Sandler, S. G., and Nusbacher, J.: Health risks of leukapheresis donors. *Haematologia* 15:57, 1982.

38. Wright, D. G., Karsh, J., Fauci, A. S., Klippel, H., Deisseroth, A. B., and Decker, J. L.: Lymphocytapheresis, in *The Lymphocyte*, edited by K. W. Sell and W. V. Miller. Liss, New York, 1981, p. 217.

39. Buckner, D., Graw, R. G., Eisel, R. J., Henderson, E. S., and Perry, S.: Luekapheresis by continuous flow centrifugation (CFC) in patients with chronic myelocytic leukemia (CML). *Blood* 33:353, 1969.

40. Eyre, H. J., Goldstein, I. M., Perry, S., and Graw, R. G.: Leukocyte transfusions: Function of transfused granulocytes from donors with chronic myelocytic leukemia. *Blood* 36:432, 1970.

41. Djerassi, I., Kim, J. S., Suvansri, U., Mitrakul, C., and Ciesielka, W.: Continuous flow filtration leukapheresis. *Transfusion* 12:75, 1972.

42. Herzig, G. P., Root, R. K., and Graw, R. G.: Granulocyte collection by continuous-flow filtration leukapheresis. *Blood* 39:554, 1972.

43. Higby, D. J., Henderson, E. S., Burnett, D., and Cohen, E.: Filtration leukapheresis: Effects of donor stimulation with dexamethasone. *Blood* 50:953, 1977.

44. Rubins, J. M., MacPherson, J. L., Nusbacher, J., and Wiltbank, T.: Granulocyte kinetics in donors undergoing filtration leukapheresis. *Transfusion* 16:56, 1976.

45. Schiffer, C. A., Aisner, A. J., and Wiernik, P. H.: Transient neutropenia induced by transfusion of blood exposed to nylon fiber filters. *Blood* 45:141, 1975.

46. Hammerschmidt, D. E., Craddock, P. R., McCullough, J., Kronenberg, R. S., Dalmasso, A. P., and Jacob, H. S.: Complement activation and pulmonary leukastasis during nylon fiber filtration leukapheresis. *Blood* 51:721, 1978.

47. Nusbacher, J., Rosenfeld, S. I., MacPherson, J. L., Thiem, P. A., and Leddy, J. P.: Nylon fiber leukapheresis: Associated complement changes and granulocytopenia. *Blood* 51:359, 1978.

48. Craddock, P. R., Hammerschmidt, D. E., White J. G., and Jacob, H. S.: Complement (C5a)-induced granulocyte aggregation in vitro: A possible mechanism of complement-mediated leukostasis and leukopenia. *J. Clin. Invest.* 60:261, 1977.

49. Nusbacher, J., Rosenfeld, S. I., Leddy, J. P., Klemperer, M. R., and MacPherson, J. L.: The leukokinetic changes and complement activation associated with filtration leukapheresis. *Exp. Hematol.* 7 (Suppl. 4):24, 1979.

50. Wiltbank, T. B., Nusbacher, J., Higby, D. J., and MacPherson, J. L.: Abdominal pain in donors during filtration leukapheresis. *Transfusion* 17:159, 1977.

51. Dahlke, M. B., Shah, S. L., Sherwood, W. C., Shafer, A. W., and Brownstein, P. K.: Priapism during filtration leukapheresis. *Transfusion* 19:482, 1979.

52. Wright, D. G., Kauffman, J. C., Chusid, M. J., Herzig, G. P., and Gallin, J. I.: Functional abnormalities of human neutrophils collected by continuous flow filtration leukapheresis. *Blood* 46:901, 1975.

53. Debalak, K. M., Epstein, R. B., and Anderson, B. R.: Granulocyte transfusions in leukopenic dogs: In vivo and in vitro function of granulocytes obtained by continuous-flow filtration leukapheresis. *Blood* 43:757, 1974.

54. Applebaum, F. R., Norton, L., and Graw, R. G.: Migration of transfused granulocytes in leukopenic dogs. *Blood* 49:483, 1977.

55. McCullough, J., Weiblin, B. J., Peterson, P. K., and Quie, P. G.: Effects of temperature on granulocyte preservation. *Blood* 52:301, 1978.

56. Price, T. H., and Dale, D. C.: Neutrophil transfusion: Effect of storage and of collection method on neutrophil blood kinetics. *Blood* 51:789, 1978.

57. Harris, M., Djerassi, I., and Schwartz, E.: Polymorphonuclear leukocytes prepared by continuous flow filtration leukapheresis: Viability and function. *Blood* 44:707, 1974.

58. Wright, D. G., Ungerleider, R. S., Gallin, J. I., and Deisseroth, A. B.: Pretreatment of filtration leukapheresis donors with colchicine. *Blood* 52:783, 1978.

59. Higby, D. J., Salvatori, V., Burnett, D., and Park, B. H.: Improvement in the quality of granulocytes obtained by filtration leukapheresis. *Exp. Hematol.* 7 (Suppl. 4):36, 1979.

60. Higby, D. H., and Burnett, D.: Granulocyte transfusions: Current status. *Blood* 55:2, 1980.

61. Epstein, R. B., Waxman, F. J., Bennet, B. T., and Anderson, B. R.: Pseudomonas septicemia in neutropenic dogs. I. Treatment with granulocyte transfusions. *Transfusion* 14:51, 1974.

62. Higby, D. J., Yates, J., Henderson, E. S., and Holland, J. F.: Filtration leukapheresis for granulocyte transfusion therapy. *N. Engl. J. Med.* 292:761, 1975.

63. Schiffer, C. A., Buchholz, D. H., Aisner, J., Betts, S. W., and Wiernick, P. H.: Clinical experience with transfusion of granulocytes obtained by continuous flow filtration leukapheresis. *Am. J. Med.* 58:373, 1975.

64. Alavi, J. B., et al.: A randomized clinical trial of granulocyte transfusions for infection in acute leukemia. *N. Engl. J. Med.* 296:706, 1977.

65. Chow, H.-S., Sarpel, S. C., and Epstein, R. B.: Pathophysiology of *Candida albicans* meningitis in normal, neutropenic, and granulocyte transfused dogs. *Blood* 55:546, 1980.

66. Graw, R. G., Herzig, G., Perry, S., and Henderson, E. S.: Normal granulocyte transfusion therapy: Treatment of septicemia due to gram-negative bacteria. *N. Engl. J. Med.* 287:367, 1972.

67. Herzig, R. H., Herzig, G. P., Graw, R. G., Bull, M. I., and Ray, K. K.: Successful granulocyte transfusion therapy for gram-negative septicemia: A prospectively randomized controlled study. *N. Engl. J. Med.* 296:701, 1977.

68. Schwarzenberg, L., et al.: White blood cell transfusions. *Isr. J. Med. Sci.* 1:925, 1965.

69. Lowenthal, R. M., et al.: Granulocyte transfusions in treatment of infections in patients with acute leukaemia and aplastic anaemia. *Lancet* 1:353, 1975.

70. Vallejos, C., McCredie, K. B., Bodey, G. P., Hester, J. P., and Freireich, E. J.: White blood cell transfusions for control of infections in neutropenic patients. *Transfusion* 15:28, 1975.

71. Strauss, R. G., Goedken, M. M., Maguire, L. C., Koepke, J. A., and Thompson, J. S.: Gram-negative sepsis treated with neutrophils collected exclusively by intermittent flow centrifugation leukapheresis. *Transfusion* 20:79, 1980.

72. Ambinder, E. P., Button, G. R., Cheung, T., Goldberg, J. D., and Holland, J. F.: Filtration versus gravity leukapheresis in febrile granulocytopenic patients: A randomized prospective trial. *Blood* 57:836, 1981.

73. Bodey, G. P., Buckley, M., Sathe, Y. S., and Freireich, E. J.: Quantitative relationships between circulating leukocytes and infection in patients with acute leukemia. *Ann. Intern. Med.* 64:328, 1966.

74. Ford, J. M., and Cullen, M. H.: Prophylactic granulocyte transfusions. *Exp. Hematol.* 5 (Suppl. 1):65, 1977.

75. Schiffer, C. A., Aisner, J., Daly, P. A., Schimpff, S. C., and Wiernik, P. H.: Alloimmunization following prophylactic granulocyte transfusion. *Blood* 54:766, 1979.

76. Clift, R. A., Sanders, J. E., Thomas, E. D., Williams, B., and Buckner, C. D.: Granulocyte transfusions for the prevention of infection in patients receiving bone-marrow transplants. *N. Engl. J. Med.* 298:1052, 1978.

77. Winston, D. J., Ho, W. G., Young, L. S., and Gale, R. P.: Prophylactic granulocyte transfusions during human bone marrow transplantation. *Am. J. Med.* 68:893, 1980.

78. Strauss, R. G., et al.: A controlled trial of prophylactic granulocyte transfusions during initial induction chemotherapy for acute myelogenous leukemia. *N. Engl. J. Med.* 305:597, 1981.

79. Higby, D. J., Freeman, A. I., Henderson, E. S., Sinks, L., and Cohen, E.: Granulocyte transfusions in children using filter-collected cells. *Cancer* 38:1407, 1976.

80. Ward, H. N.: Pulmonary infiltrates associated with leukoagglutinin transfusion reaction. *Ann. Intern. Med.* 73:689, 1970.

81. Jacob, H. S.: Granulocyte-complement interaction. *Arch. Intern. Med.* 138:461, 1978.

82. Wright, D. G., Robichaud, K. J., Pizzo, P. A., and Deiseroth, A. B.: Lethal pulmonary reactions associated with the combined use of amphotericin B and leukocyte transfusions. *N. Engl. J. Med.* 304:1185, 1981.

83. Boxer, L. A., Ingraham, L. A., Allen, J., Oseas, R. S., and Baehner, R. L.: Ampotericin-B promotes leukocyte aggregation of nylon-wool-fiber-treated polymorphonuclear leukocytes. *Blood* 58:518, 1981.

84. Ford, J. M., Lucey, J. J., Cullen, M. H., Tobias, J. S., and Lister, T. A.: Fatal graft-versus-host disease following transfusion of granulocytes from normal donors. *Lancet* 2:1167, 1976.

85. Rosen, R. S., Huestis, D. W., and Corrigan, J. J.: Acute leukemia and granulocyte transfusion: Fatal graft-versus-host reaction following transfusion of cells obtained from normal donors. *J. Pediatr.* 93:268, 1978.

86. Cohen, D., Weinstein, H., Mihm, M., and Yankee, R.: Nonfatal graft-versus-host disease occurring after transfusion with leukocytes and platelets obtained from normal donors. *Blood* 53:1053, 1979.

87. Graw, R. G., et al.: Complication of bone-marrow transplantation. Graft-versus-host disease resulting from chronic-myelogenous-leukaemia leucocyte transfusions. *Lancet* 2:338, 1970.

88. Weiden, P. L., et al.: Fatal graft-versus-host disease in a patient with lymphoblastic leukemia following normal granulocytic transfusions. *Blood* 57:328, 1981.

89. Siegel, S. E., et al.: Transmission of toxoplasmosis by leukocyte transfusion. *Blood* 37:388, 1971.

90. Westrik, M. A., Debalak-Fehir, K. M., and Epstein, R. B.: The effect of prior whole blood transfusion on subsequent granulocyte support in leukopenic dogs. *Transfusion* 17:611, 1977.

91. McCullough, J., Weiblin, B. J., Clay, M. E., and Forstrom, L.: Effect of leukocyte antibodies on the fate in vivo of Indium-111-labeled granulocytes. *Blood* 58:164, 1981.

92. Graw, R. G., Goldstein, I., Eyre, H., and Terasaki, I.: Histocompatibility testing for leukocyte transfusions. *Lancet* 2:77, 1970.

93. Higby, D. J., Mishler, J. M., Cohen, E., Rhomberg, W., Nicora, R. W., and Holland, J. F.: Increased elevation of peripheral leukocyte counts by infusion of histocompatible granulocytes. *Vox Sang.* 27:186, 1974.

94. Nusbacher, J., MacPherson, J. L., Gore, I., and Grinberg, R.: Inhibition of granulocyte erythrophagocytosis by HLA antisera. *Blood* 53:350, 1979.

95. McCullough, J.: Liquid preservation of granulocytes. *Transfusion* 20:129, 1980.

96. McCullough, J., Weiblin, B. J., and Quie, P. G.: Chemotatic activity of human granulocytes preserved in various anticoagulants. *J. Lab. Clin. Med.* 84:902, 1974.

97. McCullough, J., and Weiblin, B. J.: Relationship of granulocyte ATP to chemotactic response during storage. *Transfusion* 19:764, 1979.

98. Lane, T. A.: Granulocyte concentrate preservation: 6C versus room temperature. *Transfusion* 18:394, 1978.

99. Lane, T. A.: Storage of granulocyte concentrates (GC): Bacterial killing and chemotaxis. *Transfusion* 18:650, 1978.

100. McCullough, J., Weiblin, B. J., Peterson, P. K., and Quie, P. G.: Effects of temperature on granulocyte preservation. *Blood* 53:301, 1978.

101. McCullough, J.: Liquid preservation of granulocytes for transfusion. *Prog. Clin. Biol. Res.* 13:185, 1977.

102. Price, T. H., and Dale, D. C.: Neutrophil preservation: The effect of short-term storage on in vivo kinetics. *J. Clin. Invest.* 59:475, 1977.

103. Price, T. H., and Dale, D. C.: Neutrophil transfusion: Effect of storage and of collection method on neutrophil blood kinetics. *Blood* 51:789, 1978.

104. Contreras, T. J., Jemionek, J. F., French, J. E., and Shields, L. J.: Effects of plastic polymer surfaces on the liquid preservation of human granulocytes. *Transfusion* 18:650, 1978.

105. Meryman, H. T., and Howard, J.: Cryopreservation of granulocytes, in *The Granulocyte: Function and Clinical Utilization*, edited by T. J. Greenwalt and G. A. Jamieson, Liss, New York, 1977, p. 193.

106. Hill, R. S., and MacKinder, C. A.: Freeze preservation of human granulocytes. *Lancet* 1:878, 1980.

107. Lionetti, F. J., Hunt, S. M., Gore, J. M., and Curby, W. A.: Cryopreservation of human granulocytes. *Cryobiology* 12:181, 1975.

CHAPTER *166*

Preservation and clinical use of platelets

FRANK H. GARDNER

Platelet transfusion therapy is used to improve or correct hemostasis in patients with thrombocytopenia associated with acute leukemia, marrow aplasia, chemotherapy, or cardiac surgery. Initially platelet transfusions were administered directly by using whole blood from donors with thrombocytosis due to polycythemia vera. Blood was withdrawn into siliconized syringes and transfused immediately, without anticoagulant, into the thrombocytopenic recipient. Approximately 70 percent of the transfused platelets remained in the recipient's circulation to provide hemostasis [1], with the remainder sequestered in the spleen. In splenectomized patients the platelet yield was 80 to 90 percent. Similar platelet yields have been obtained with platelet-rich plasma or platelet concentrates prepared with plastic bags or automated centrifugal cell separators.

The initial procedure was to store platelets at 4°C to inhibit metabolic activity, following the earlier concepts of red blood cell preservation. Platelets stored as platelet-rich plasma for 24 h at 4°C survive poorly in the circulation of recipients, and for approximately the last 15 years the use of 4°C-stored platelets has been discouraged. At 4°C, platelets rapidly lose their normal discoid shape and become spherical, with disappearance of circumferential microtubules and loss of viability [2]. These changes are irreversible after several hours. In contrast, if platelet-rich plasma is maintained at 22°C, platelet morphology is preserved. The in vivo life-span of platelets maintained at 22°C is greater than that of those stored at 4°C [3]. Studies on platelets stored at temperatures from 4 to 37°C indicate that 22°C provides maximum viability (Fig. 166-1).

Techniques of platelet preparation

Initially, platelet-rich plasma was used because platelets, less dense than other blood elements, could be separated by low-speed centrifugation. However, the large volume of plasma limited the number of platelets that could be infused unless donors with thrombocytosis were used. Therefore most of the plasma was removed after the platelets were collected by centrifugation, leaving 50 to 60 ml to resuspend the platelets to a concentration of 2 to 3 million per microliter. Platelet concentrates are now prepared by serial centrifugation using individual plastic bags to separate plasma sterilely or by semicontinuous-flow centrifugation using plastic bags that limit the amount of plasma removed.

SERIAL CENTRIFUGATION
In most instances blood from random donors is used to prepare platelet concentrates as a by-product of the donation for other uses. The plastic bag of blood anticoagulated with CPDA (citrate-phosphate-dextrose-adenine) is centrifuged under conditions which achieve maximum retention of platelets in the plasma. The platelet-rich plasma is transferred to a satellite bag, with care to minimize contamination by white and red cells from the buffy coat. The satellite bag is centrifuged again at higher speed, and the platelets collect as a button at the bottom of the bag. A large portion of the supernatant plasma is transferred to another plastic bag to be used for plasma components, and the platelet button is left behind with 50 to 60 ml of plasma. The preparation is then maintained at 22°C for 1 to 2 h to decrease platelet aggregation, possibly by enzymatic degradation of platelet ADP. The platelet button may then be resuspended evenly in the residual plasma [4].

CONTINUOUS-FLOW CENTRIFUGATION
Continuous-flow centrifugation of CPDA-anticoagulated blood may be accomplished in the Latham blood processor [5] or the Aminco Celltrifuge [6]. The platelets and buffy coat leave the spinning bowl and are collected in a satellite bag, and the plasma and red cells are returned to the donor. Six to eight units of blood

FIGURE 166-1 Relationship between storage temperature and platelet survival after transfusion in days ($T_{1/2}$). Platelet-rich plasma was obtained from normal volunteers and stored overnight at the indicated temperatures. Thereafter the platelets were labeled with radioactive chromium and reinfused. In vivo survival is optimal at 22°C and declines abruptly at lower temperatures. Although the platelets stored at 30 and 37°C have a survival equal to that of the samples stored at 22°C, the yield of circulating platelets is less.

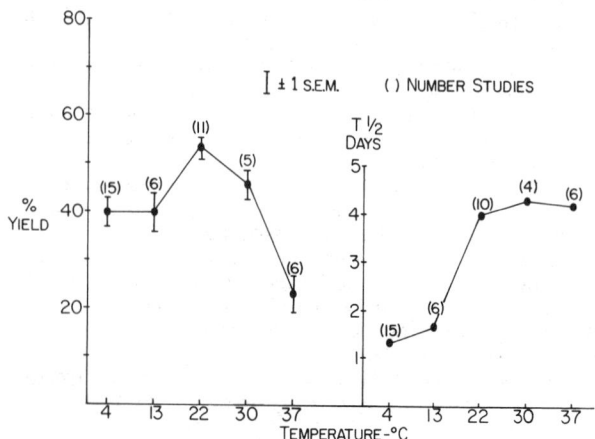

may be processed from a single donor two to three times weekly. With this method the yield of platelets from whole blood is 60 percent and there is significant leukocyte contamination. Indeed, the lymphocyte contamination may be in range of 3 to 4×10^9 cells per unit collected and may induce graft-versus-host disease in an immune-suppressed recipient. These platelets survive normally in vivo and are clinically effective, as demonstrated by shortened bleeding times of thrombocytopenic recipients [7]. The addition of hydroxyethyl starch to the blood bag improves the platelet yield but does not decrease leukocyte contamination [8]. Platelets collected in plastic bags by serial or continuous-flow centrifugation can be preserved by the techniques listed below.

Platelet preservation techniques

Earlier techniques to prolong platelet utilization by suspension in gelatin solution, direct freezing in plasma, or lyophilization did not yield platelets with satisfactory hemostatic capacity after reconstitution.

LIQUID STORAGE

The ability of platelets to control hemostasis after storage as platelet concentrates for 72 h at 22°C has expanded the use of this simple technique for platelet preparation. In contrast, platelets stored at 4°C for 24 to 48 h are only transiently effective in the control of bleeding. In treating patients with chronic thrombocytopenia, better hemostasis can be expected from platelets stored at 22°C because of the increased life-span of the platelets in the recipient. Platelet concentrates can currently be stored for 72 h at 22°C with a loss of only 30 percent of the in vivo recovery. Recently, platelets have been stored for 5 days at 22°C in polyolefin plastic containers. The viability and in vivo recovery of these 5-day samples are comparable to the viability and in vivo recovery of samples stored for only 3 days in the standard polyvinyl chloride plastic bag [9,57]. This additional 2 days will be of great value to hospitals in providing platelets on weekends and holidays and will decrease excessive outdating of platelet concentrates. Also, the use of polyolefin plastic bags can eliminate the questionable toxicity related to di-2-ethylhexylphthalate, the plasticizer used in the current polyvinyl plastic bag, which migrates into the plasma and binds selectively to the platelet [10].

FROZEN STORAGE

GLYCEROL

The prolonged storage of red cells frozen in glycerol encouraged the use of this agent for platelet preservation. Despite the initial encouraging data, the large loss of platelets during freezing and thawing has made this type of preservation not acceptable [11]. However, the nontoxic nature of glycerol as a cryopreservative continues to suggest that different techniques should be tried.

DMSO

Dimethyl sulfoxide (DMSO) is an excellent cryopreservative for long-term tissue freezing and storage [12]. Platelet concentrates may be suspended in a 5% solution of DMSO with or without 5% glucose and frozen successfully at a rate of 3°C per minute [13]. After thawing, the platelets may be washed to remove the DMSO and then infused. In vivo recovery is usually about 45 percent (two-thirds the recovery rate of platelets stored fresh). The recovered platelets have a normal life-span and are hemostatically effective [14]. Further techniques and refinements are needed if frozen platelets are to be available for emergency use. In one clinic, platelets have been collected from patients with acute leukemia during remission, frozen with DMSO, stored, and readministered during relapse of the disease [15]. Certain patients with platelet histocompatibility locus antigen (HLA) antibodies could be supported during transplantation procedures or chemotherapy by collection from compatible donors and preservation by this freezing technique.

During the past 15 years only pilot clinical investigations of frozen platelets have been carried out. The toxicity of prolonged DMSO exposure has been eliminated by washing the drug out of the platelet button prior to infusion. The greater availability of platelet concentrates and the usefulness of platelets stored in liquid phase at 22°C for 3 and probably 5 days have diminished the need for frozen platelets, especially in view of the complex technology involved.

Clinical use of platelets

Platelet transfusions have been used in clinical medicine for over 70 years, beginning with the observation of Duke that thrombocytopenic bleeding could be corrected with fresh blood transfusions that elevated the circulating platelet count [16]. For many years, direct transfusions of whole blood without anticoagulants were used, but in the past 20 years platelet concentrates have been preferred. Early studies of platelet transfusions to control thrombocytopenic bleeding demonstrated that recipients become immunized to the administered platelets, resulting in a decreased yield and shortened life-span of the platelets (Fig. 166-2) [1]. There is great variability among patients as to the number of transfusions required for immunization; usually platelets from 20 donors can be used before immunization develops, but some patients are immunized after a single transfusion, with rapid destruction of all subsequently administered platelets [17]. As a general rule the period of immunization varies from 2 weeks to 6 months with a median of 6 weeks. Previous transfusion of whole blood or packed red cells can produce a refractory state since nonviable platelets remaining in such products can also immunize patients. Rh factor incom-

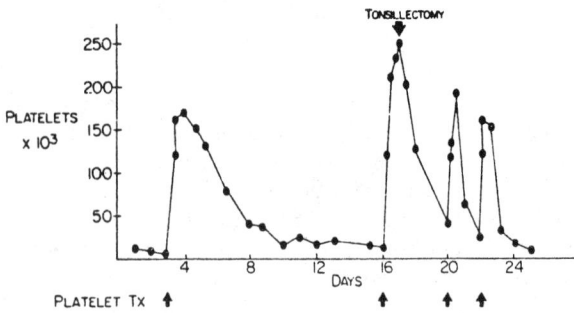

FIGURE 166-2 Platelet response in patient with amegakaryocytic thrombocytopenia receiving transfusions of platelet-rich plasma. One platelet transfusion immunized the patient so that the platelet life-span was shortened progressively during surgery and convalescence. (Data supplied by L. K. Diamond.)

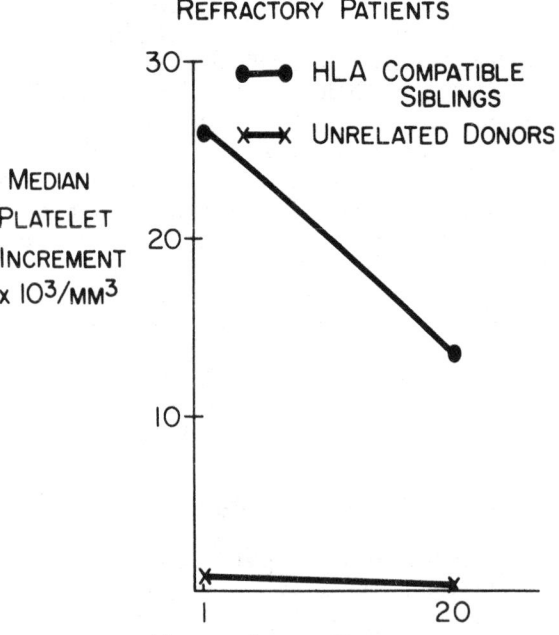

FIGURE 166-3 Effect of HLA-compatible platelets. Five thrombocytopenic patients who were refractory to platelets from random donors had an excellent response when they received platelets from HLA-compatible siblings. The platelet increment charted represents the rise in platelet count per platelet unit infused multiplied by the body surface area (in square meters). A similar curve may be expected in recipients who are not refractory. (Graph drawn from data presented by R. A. Yankee et al. [21].)

patibility does not influence the platelet yield, and usually there are not enough contaminating red cells in the platelet concentrates to produce significant anti-D titers in the recipient [18]. There is some decrease in the in vivo yield if ABO-incompatible platelets are used [19]. However, in many blood banks this loss is considered acceptable and pooled concentrates containing ABO-incompatible units are used.

Platelets have most of the same HLAs as the circulating lymphocytes. Hence platelet types usually can be inferred from some lymphocytotoxicity testing of donors and recipient. It is difficult to find identical (A) matches in the general population because of the highly polymorphic nature of the HLA genetic system. In the past few years it has been observed that certain cross-reactive antigens may not be recognized as foreign by the immunized patient and that some antigens, such as HLA-B12, may have weak reactivity on the platelet and be tolerated [20]. These weak expressions have allowed more flexibility and latitude in donor selection. If patients who have become refractory to transfusion of platelets from random donors are given HLA-compatible platelets, a satisfactory yield can be obtained (Fig. 166-3). In most instances this good response will persist for months. Siblings are likely to have the most complete HLA compatibility. With the ease of collecting multiple platelet concentrates from a single donor by repeated plateletpheresis techniques (described above), an HLA-compatible donor can be used indefinitely. Unrelated donors can be used if they are HLA-compatible, and it is estimated that 1 of 1000 members of a random population will be suitable [22]. Sufficient donors should be available in urban centers, and platelets can be shipped to remote geographic areas as needed.

Some patients receiving multiple blood transfusions develop leukoagglutinins that may cause febrile transfusion reactions [23]. Many patients receiving platelet transfusions also have febrile reactions from contaminating leukocytes, especially if the platelets are obtained by continuous-flow centrifugation techniques. Such reactions to leukocytes may reduce the platelet yield in the recipient [24], possibly by involving the platelets as "in-

nocent bystanders" in the leukoagglutinin reaction. If the platelet preparations are centrifuged carefully to reduce the contaminating leukocytes to less than 3000 per microliter, the circulating platelet yield is restored in such recipients. These observations suggest that a recipient may develop antibodies to leukocytes without developing antibodies to platelets. It is obviously necessary to prepare platelets with minimal leukocyte contamination for the chronically thrombocytopenic recipient. Platelet antibodies also may bind to granulocytes [25], and after transfusions of incompatible platelets there may be a marked decline in the peripheral granulocyte count. With marrow failure and inadequate marrow reserve, this granulocytopenia may expose the patient to an increased risk of infection.

General concepts for platelet transfusion

Platelet transfusions are given to prevent or stop bleeding associated with thrombocytopenia or a qualitative platelet disorder. Usually no serious bleeding problems are encountered until the circulating platelet level falls below 20,000 per microliter. With the platelet count in this range or higher, there is no need for platelet transfusions. Platelet transfusions are indicated if bleeding occurs in a patient with a platelet count below 20,000 per microliter when the thrombocytopenia is due to inadequate platelet production. Platelet transfusions may be considered for patients with higher platelet counts and prolonged bleeding times due to functionally inadequate platelets. Some patients with aplastic anemia may have platelet counts of 5000 per microliter for months without bleeding. In such patients the onset of infection or fever may induce a critical hemorrhage. A possible mechanism for thrombocytopenia associated with fever is the adherence of platelets to foreign particles (bacteria) and their subsequent rapid removal by the monocyte-macrophage system [26]. Indeed, this mechanism may be responsible for the thrombocytopenia seen in some patients assumed to have disseminated intravascular coagulation [27,28]. The yield of transfused platelets is low in all febrile thrombocytopenic patients, and it may be necessary to triple the estimated platelet requirement. Often, following treatment of the infection with proper antibiotics, the platelet count will return to a range that does not require platelet transfusions, or bleeding may cease despite no apparent change in the platelet count.

Menorrhagia can be a distressing problem with thrombocytopenia. Such bleeding may be controlled by adequate platelet transfusions, but the risk of immunization is such that induction of amenorrhea by progestational preparations may be desirable. An initial parenteral dose of 300 mg of medroxyprogesterone followed by a daily oral dose of 20 mg of medroxyprogesterone acetate is usually satisfactory. If the bleeding is brisk in the initial few days after hormone injection, platelet transfusions should be used. Hormonal therapy should be continued until the platelet count is above 60,000 per microliter since the platelet count may decline at the time of menstruation, increasing the risk of recurrent menorrhagia. If there is any indication of vaginal bleeding ("breakthrough bleeding"), the daily oral dose of medroxyprogesterone acetate should be increased by 10 mg at weekly intervals.

Table 166-1 presents the clinical disorders for which platelets transfusion should be considered. Platelet transfusion therapy is largely empirical and has often developed without controlled clinical trials. Hypoproliferative (amegakaryocytic) thrombocytopenia is associated with more severe and frequent bleedings than hyperdestructive (megakaryocytic) thrombocytopenia with similar low platelet counts. This difference may be due to the larger platelets found in the hyperdestructive states [29]. In most instances the hyperdestructive states will destroy transfused as well as autologous platelets on an immune basis. Platelet transfusions therefore are rarely useful, and if used to control serious bleeding, the benefit should be expected only for minutes or a few hours. In the hypoproliferative states, thrombocytopenia is more prolonged, not quickly reversed by therapy, and associated with smaller, less effective platelets. Transfusion will provide hemostasis for several days in the absence of immunization. Currently the physicians's decision to transfuse platelets is based on the bleeding episode correlated with the platelet count.

TABLE 166-1   Indications for platelet transfusion

I. Thrombocytopenia with decreased platelet production (amegakaryocytic thrombocytopenia).
  A. Leukemia.
  B. Aplastic anemia.
  With either A or B, transfuse only for control of bleeding when platelet count is below 20,000 per microliter; consider either prophylactic or therapeutic transfusion program with severe and chronic thrombocytopenia.

II. Thrombocytopenia due to loss, destruction, or sequestration of platelets (megakaryocytic thrombocytopenia).
  A. Platelet loss.
    1. Multiple transfusions: transfuse platelet concentrates when platelet count declines to 40,000 per microliter.
    2. Use of stored blood (washout thrombocytopenia).
    3. Extracorporeal pumps.
  B. Platelet sequestration.
    1. Splenomegaly: triple platelet transfusion units suggested because of sequestration of platelets in splenic pool.
  C. Platelet destruction.
    1. Acute idiopathic thrombocytopenic purpura (postinfectious thrombocytopenia): rarely need platelet transfusions, but they should be used to control severe bleeding.
    2. Chronic idiopathic thrombocytopenic purpura: avoid platelet transfusions since megathrombocytes usually prevent excessive hemorrhage.
    3. Posttransfusion purpura: do not use platelet transfusion; plan to remove antibody by plasmapheresis.
    4. Neonatal isoimmune thrombocytopenia: transfuse with maternal platelets suspended in ABO-compatible plasma.
    5. Drug purpura: platelet transfusion rarely needed if offending drug is removed.
    6. Hereditary defects: use platelet transfusions for acute bleeding and surgery.
    7. Infection: platelet transfusions usually are not helpful until the infection is controlled.

III. Qualitative platelet disorders.
  A. Congenital (usually ADP aggregation defect): use platelet transfusions for acute bleeding and surgery.
  B. Acquired (uremia, PNH, myeloproliferative diseases): dialysis more effective to control uremic bleeding; severe bleeding with PNH may require platelet transfusions.

Platelet counts by automated instruments may be erroneous, particularly if very large or very small platelets, red cell fragments, or cytoplasmic fragments of leukemic blast cells are present [30]. The morphologic appearance of a blood film should be correlated with the automated or manual platelet count.

Amegakaryocytic thrombocytopenia

LEUKEMIA

Although recent chemotherapy programs have improved survival in acute leukemia, hemorrhage associated with thrombocytopenia remains a major cause of death. Even if severe thrombocytopenia is not present at the time of diagnosis, the current intensive therapy programs will induce it quickly. The decline in the proportion of deaths attributed to hemorrhagic complications from 63 percent to 20 percent in the past 20 years has been attributed in part to the vigorous use of platelet transfusions [31]. Hemorrhage-free intervals are prolonged if the platelet count can be maintained at about 20,000 per microliter, and in a controlled study less hemorrhage was observed in those patients who received infusions of platelet concentrates thrice weekly [32]. There is a risk of hepatitis with the prophylactic use of platelets to maintain such a platelet count. In other studies, patients had no more bleeding complications when platelets were used therapeutically to control hemorrhage rather than prophylactically to maintain a desired platelet level [33,34]. In patients achieving a chemotherapy-induced remission from acute leukemia within 10 to 12 weeks, and particularly children, random pooled donors will be sufficient [35]. With intensive therapy for acute nonlymphoid leukemia, many platelet transfusions will probably be needed because the induced thrombocytopenia may be aggravated by sepsis with accentuated bleeding. Currently two treatment approaches are being used, prophylactic and therapeutic. For the prophylactic program transfusions are given three times weekly, usually at a dose of 6 units per square meter of body surface. If the patient is febrile, the dose should be tripled and given daily because the in vivo yield of platelets is poor. In therapeutic management, platelets in the same dosage are used when there is a bleeding episode. Currently there is no significant difference in survival with the two approaches [22]. With the therapeutic approach, fewer platelet transfusions have been used with a lower risk of immunization. Our clinic has used a therapeutic plan with good results.

If the patient has become immunized to platelet antigens, adequate increments of circulating platelets cannot be achieved with random donors. With a prophylactic platelet therapy program, 50 to 60 percent of patients will become immunized in 3 to 6 weeks. It is therefore necessary to match the patient with siblings or with panels of donors with known platelet HLA types. Prolonged repeated plasmapheresis from such donors may allow 4 units of platelet concentrate to be obtained two or three times weekly [7]. If the patients achieve a hematologic remission, the platelets can be collected from the patient and preserved in DMSO. The use of autologous platelets has provided 40 percent of the platelets needed in a maintenance program and allowed random donor platelets to be used effectively after several months of therapy with autologous platelets [15].

APLASTIC ANEMIA
Platelet transfusions are used in aplastic anemia only during intervals of hemorrhage. With continued marrow failure, thrombocytopenia may persist not only before a hematologic remission occurs but also for months or years after, even if the patient has an erythropoietic response from therapy [36]. With platelet counts above 20,000 to 30,000 per microliter, no therapy need

be planned. Patients with more profound thrombocytopenia (5000 to 20,000 per microliter) have been watched expectantly. Nasopharyngeal bleeding, especially continuous oozing epistaxis, has responded well to oral ε-aminocaproic acid in a dosage range of 3 to 5 g every 6 h [37]. In 1 year the use of this fibrinolytic inhibitor decreased our use of platelet concentrates by 35 percent. Patients may use ε-aminocaproic acid for weeks or months to control mucous membrane bleeding. If this agent is not helpful and there is associated gastrointestinal or urinary tract bleeding, platelet transfusions from random donors should be used initially. Siblings are HLA-typed for potential marrow transplantation but may be used as repetitive donors two to three times weekly if transplantation is not done. In a few patients splenectomy has been performed to remove this site of platelet sequestration and thereby obtain better survival of platelets and red cells [38]. However, this operation has been used less and less in the past decade, and the availability of compatible platelets by air transportation would suggest that the procedure should not be done. Drug-induced transient aplastic anemia may lead to such severe thrombocytopenia that prophylactic platelet transfusions are necessary.

Megakaryocytic thrombocytopenia

ACUTE THROMBOCYTOPENIA WITH INCREASED PLATELET LOSS
Massive transfusions of banked whole blood or packed red cells for hemorrhage will deplete the patient's platelets [39]. Usually one can expect the platelet count to fall below 100,000 per microliter after 15 to 20 units of stored red cells. With such bleeding the platelet count and fibrinogen level are most useful to guide subsequent blood replacement. If the platelet count falls to about 20,000 per microliter, 48 h may be required for adequate replacement of platelets by the marrow. If such severe thrombocytopenia develops, further bleeding should be treated with packed red cells and platelet concentrates. Usually 6 units of random platelet concentrates can be given at hourly intervals for intense bleeding, and cryoprecipitate rather than frozen plasma should be used (6 to 8 units) for fibrinogen and coagulation factor replacement.

Extracorporeal pumps may cause a 30 to 50 percent decline in the platelet count during cardiac surgery [40]. This decline usually is not associated with bleeding, and the residual platelets appear to function normally. While prophylactic platelet transfusions may be considered, bleeding episodes have decreased markedly in the past decade as a result of improved operative techniques and smaller volumes of blood in the pump system. With prolonged thoracic surgery and use of the bubble oxygenator bypass, platelet function is altered without marked decline in platelet count. These changes can be improved by use of 6 to 8 units of random donor platelets to correct this transient platelet defect [41]. Recently, prostacyclin has been used in cardiac surgery and hemodialysis to decrease the use of heparin and to maintain a higher platelet count [42]. The use of prostacylin appears to reduce platelet activation and aggregation caused by contact with the artificial membranes of the hemoperfusion pumps and dialyzers [43].

THROMBOCYTOPENIA DUE TO PLATELET SEQUESTRATION
Patients with liver disease and congestive splenomegaly will usually have platelet levels of 50,000 to 80,000 per microliter but rarely have hemorrhagic complications. With severe bleeding, e.g., from varices, these patients do not develop a compensating thrombocytosis because of the large percentage of the total body mass of platelets sequestered in the enlarged spleen [44]. The platelet lifespan is normal, and platelet transfusions should be used to control bleeding during surgical procedures if the platelet count declines. To compensate for the platelets that will remain in the enlarged spleen, the average dose of 3 to 6 units of platelet concentrates per square meter of body surface should be increased threefold to ensure an adequate circulating platelet level.

DESTRUCTION OF PLATELETS

ACUTE IDIOPATHIC THROMBOCYTOPENIC PURPURA
In this condition, also called *postinfectious thrombocytopenia,* serious bleeding is rarely observed, and the thrombocytopenia will usually improve in 10 to 15 days. Glucocorticoid therapy should not be used since it can inhibit the platelet recovery interval [45]. Platelet lifespan is shortened markedly, due to the presence of a platelet antibody. If surgical procedures are needed, platelet transfusions are sometimes used at the time of surgery, recognizing that a protective platelet level can be achieved for only minutes to a few hours because the existing antibody will cause rapid destruction of all transfused platelets.

CHRONIC IDIOPATHIC THROMBOCYTOPENIC PURPURA
With persistent and rapid platelet destruction, the young platelets (megathrombocytes) formed are more protective than normal platelets [46]. With platelet counts in the range of 20,000 per microliter, the bleeding diathesis is minimal. Transfused platelets are short-lived and should be used sparingly. In rare instances of severe menorrhagia, platelet transfusions may be useful until hormonal therapy can be started. While some surgeons have used platelet transfusions during surgery just prior to splenectomy, no adequate evaluation is available to demonstrate that the precaution is helpful. If platelets are used, the transfusion should be withheld until immediately before the operation.

POSTTRANSFUSION PURPURA
This rare clinical syndrome results from the formation of an antibody directed against the platelet antigen Pl^{A1} [47]. Ninety-seven percent of the population is Pl^{A1}-positive, and unless Pl^{A1}-negative platelets are available, transfused platelets will be rapidly destroyed.

Plasma exchange to decrease the circulating antibody has been more successful and is the procedure of choice [48].

NEONATAL ISOIMMUNE THROMBOCYTOPENIA
In 50 percent of these patients, the maternal isoantibody is anti-Pl^{A1}; the other antibodies are not well defined [49]. Maternal platelets are compatible, and after plasmapheresis and concentration by centrifugation they should be resuspended in compatible ABO plasma to eliminate the maternal antibody. Usually the infant requires transfusion of platelets from only 1 unit of blood.

DRUG-INDUCED THROMBOCYTOPENIA (DRUG PURPURA)
A variety of drug-immune thrombocytopenias have been well documented. Quinidine is a common cause. After withdrawal of the drug, the rapid platelet destruction disappears. Prednisone may improve the thrombocytopenia by decreasing sequestration of the platelet-immune complex by the monocyte-macrophage system and is especially useful with drugs that are slowly excreted, such as gold salts. Platelet transfusions should not be used for these patients. Although thrombocytopenia with purpura has been observed frequently in patients receiving chlorothiazide diuretics, bleeding has not been severe enough to warrant transfusions of platelets.

HEREDITARY THROMBOCYTOPENIA
The majority of these patients do not have serious bleeding problems [50], but platelet transfusions are useful for bleeding episodes or to prepare patients for surgery. Patients with the Bernard-Soulier syndrome (Chap. 146) or the Wiskott-Aldrich syndrome (Chap. 141) may need platelet transfusions more frequently to control hemorrhage. Donors should be selected carefully for patients with the Wiskott-Aldrich syndrome if marrow transplantation is considered.

Qualitative platelet disorders

Patients with qualitative platelet disorders have normal platelet counts, but an intrinsic platelet defect causes prolonged bleeding times, impaired adhesion to glass, and altered platelet aggregation [51] (see Chap. 146). For major surgical procedures they may require platelet transfusions, but their bleeding otherwise does not need such treatment. Intrinsic platelet defects also occur in the myeloproliferative syndromes [52] and leukemia [53]. Despite adequate or increased numbers of platelets, these patients may require platelet transfusions for complete hemostasis during surgery or to control bleeding. Finally, platelet transfusions are frequently required for control of bleeding in hereditary thrombasthenia or Glanzmann's disease [54] (see Chap. 146). Because these patients usually have had multiple platelet transfusions, efforts should be made to obtain HLA-type-specific platelets.

Altered platelet membrane function because of drugs or plasmatic factors does not warrant platelet transfusions. One should avoid drugs that can affect platelet aggregation and the bleeding time, such as aspirin, indomethacin, and phenylbutazone (see Chap. 147). Hemodialysis is effective in improving platelet function in the uremic patient. The prolonged bleeding time in uremia can be normalized by large infusions (10 units) of cryoprecipitate to allow surgical procedures. Platelet aggregation is not improved by the cryoprecipitate, and the mechanism has not been defined [55]. Plasmapheresis is helpful in the hemorrhagic diathesis of hypergammaglobulinemia by decreasing protein coating of the platelet [56].

References

1. Hirsch, E. O., and Gardner, F. H.: The transfusion of human blood platelets. *J. Lab. Clin. Med.* 39:556, 1952.
2. Behnke, O.: Some possible practical implications of the lability of blood platelet microtubules. *Vox Sang.* 13:502, 1967.
3. Murphy, S., and Gardner, F. H.: Platelet preservation: Effect of storage temperature on maintenance of platelet viability: Deleterious effect of refrigerated storage. *N. Engl. J. Med.* 280:1094, 1969.
4. Mourad, N.: A simple method for obtaining platelet concentrates free of aggregates. *Transfusion* 8:48, 1968.
5. Tullis, J. L., Eberle, W. G., II, Baudanza, P., and Tinch, R.: Plateletpheresis: Description of a new technic. *Transfusion* 8:154, 1968.
6. McCredie, K. B., et al.: Platelet and leukocyte transfusions in acute leukemia. *Hum. Pathol.* 5:699, 1974.
7. Duquesnoy, R. I., et al.: Histocompatible platelet transfusion service in regional blood center. *Transfusion* 14:503, 1974.
8. Roy, A., Simmons, W. B., Franklin, A., and Djerassi, I.: Hydroxyethyl starch for separation of normal granulocytes. *Fed. Proc.* 29:424, 1970.
9. Murphy, S., et al.: Improved storage of platelets for transfusion in a new container. *Blood* 60:194, 1982.
10. Valeri, C. R., Contreras, T. J., Feingold, H., Sheibley, R. H., and Jaeger, R. J.: Accumulation of di-2-ethylhexyl phthalate (DEHP) in whole blood, platelet concentrates and platelet poor plasma. 1. Effect of DEHP on platelet survival and function. *Environmental Health Perspectives*, January 1973, p. 103.
11. Cohen, P., and Gardner, F. H.: Platelet preservation. IV. Preservation of human platelet concentrates by controlled slow freezing in a glycerol medium. *N. Engl. J. Med.* 274:1400, 1966.
12. Djerassi, I., Farber, S., Roy, A., and Cavins, J.: Preparation and in vivo circulation of human platelets preserved with combined dimethylsulfoxide and dextrose. *Transfusion* 6:572, 1966.
13. Murphy, S., Sayor, S. N., Abdou, N. L., and Gardner, F. H.: Platelet preservation by freezing: Use of dimethylsulfoxide as cryoprotective agent. *Transfusion* 14:139, 1974.
14. Kim, B. K., and Baldini, M. G.: Biochemistry, function, and hemostatic effectiveness of frozen human platelets. *Proc. Soc. Exp. Biol. Med.* 145:830, 1974.
15. Lazarus, H. M., Kaniecki-Green, E. A., Warm, S. E., Masamichi, A., and Herzig, R. H.: Therapeutic effectiveness of frozen platelet concentrates for transfusions. *Blood* 57:243, 1981.
16. Duke, W. W.: The relation of blood platelets to hemorrhagic disease: Description of a method for determining the bleeding time and coagulation time and report of 3 cases of hemorrhagic disease relieved by transfusion. *JAMA* 55:1185, 1910.
17. Sintnicolaas, K., et al.: Delayed alloimmunisation by random single donor platelet transfusions. *Lancet* 1:750, 1981.
18. Pfisterer, H., Thierfelder, S., and Stich, W.: ABO Rh blood groups and platelet transfusion. *Blut* 17:1, 1968.
19. Aster, R.: Effect of anticoagulant and ABO incompatibility on recovery of transfused human platelets. *Blood* 26:732, 1965.
20. Duquesnoy, R. J., Filip, D. H., and Aster, R. H.: Influence of HLA-A2 on the effectiveness of platelet transfusions in alloimmunized thrombocytopenic patients. *Blood* 50:407, 1977.
21. Yankee, R. A., Grumet, F. C., and Rogentine, G. N.: Platelet transfusion therapy: The selection of compatible platelet donors for refractory patients by lymphocyte HL-A typing. *N. Engl. J. Med.* 281:1208, 1969.
22. Slichter, S. J.: Controversies in platelet transfusion therapy. *Ann. Rev. Med.* 31:509, 1980.
23. Dausset, J.: Iso-leuco-anticorps. *Acta Haematol.* 20:156, 1958.
24. Herzig, R. H., et al.: Correction of pooled platelet transfusion responses with leukocyte poor HL-A matched platelet concentrates. *Blood* 46:743, 1975.
25. Herzig, R. H., Poplack, D. G., and Yankee, R. A.: Prolonged granulocytopenia from incompatible platelet transfusions. *N. Engl. J. Med.* 290:1220, 1974.
26. Cohen, P., Brunwald, J., and Gardner, F. H.: Destruction of canine and rabbit platelets following intravenous administration of carbon particles or endotoxin. *J. Lab. Clin. Med.* 66:263, 1965.
27. Cohen, P., and Gardner, F. H.: Thrombocytopenia as a laboratory sign and complication of gram-negative bacteremic infection. *Arch. Intern. Med.* 117:113, 1966.
28. Reedler, G. F., Straub, P. W., and Frick, P. G.: Thrombocytopenia in septicemia. *Helv. Med. Acta* 36:23, 1972.
29. Karpatkin, S., and Freedman, M. D.: Hypersplenic thrombocytopenia differentiated from increased peripheral destruction by platelet volume. *Ann. Int. Med.* 89:200, 1978.
30. Bessman, J. D., Williams, L. J., and Gilmer, P. R. J.: Mean platelet volume: The inverse relation of platelet size and count in normal subjects and an artifact of other particles. *Am. J. Clin. Pathol.* 76:289, 1981.
31. Graw, R. G., Jr., Herzig, G., Perry, S., and Henderson, E. S.: Normal granulocyte transfusion therapy: Treatment of septicemia due to gram-negative bacteria. *N. Eng. J. Med.* 287:367, 1972.
32. Higby, D. J., Cohen, E., Holland, J. F., and Sinks, L.: The prophylactic treatment of thrombocytopenic leukemic patients with platelets: A double blind study. *Transfusion* 14:440, 1974.
33. Murphy, S., et al.: The indications for platelet transfusions in children with acute leukemia. *Am. J. Hematol.* 12:347, 1982.
34. Solomon, J., Bofenkamp, T., Fahey, J. L., Chillar, R. K., and Beutler, E.: Platelet prophylaxis in acute non-lymphoblastic leukemia. *Lancet* 1:267, 1978.
35. Simone, J. V.: Use of fresh blood components during intensive combination therapy of childhood leukemia. *Cancer* 28:562, 1971.
36. Bernard, J., and Najean, Y.: Evolution and prognosis of the idiopathic pancytopenias. *Proceedings of the X Congress of the International Society of Hematologists*, 1965, p. 1.
37. Gardner, F. H., and Helmer, R. E.: Aminocaproic acid: Use in control of hemorrhage in patients with amegakaryocytic thrombocytopenia. *JAMA* 243:35, 1980.
38. Flatlow, F. A., and Freireich, E. J.: Effect of splenectomy on the response to platelet transfusion in three patients with aplastic anemia. *N. Engl. J. Med.* 274:242, 1966.
39. Counts, R. B., Haisch, C., Simon, T. L., Maxwell, N. G., Heimbach, D. M., and Carrico, C. J.: Hemostasis in massively transfused trauma patients. *Ann. Surg.* 190:91, 1979.
40. Kevy, S. V., Glickman, R. M., Bernhard, W. F., Diamond, L. K., and Gross, R. E.: Pathogenesis and control of the hemorrhagic defect in open heart surgery. *Surg. Gynecol. Obstet.* 123:313, 1966.
41. Harker, L. A., Malpass, T. W., Branson, H. E., Hessel, E. A., and Slichter, S. J.: Mechanism of abnormal bleeding in patients undergoing cardiopulmonary bypass: Acquired transient platelet dysfunction associated with selective alpha granule release. *Blood* 56:824, 1980.
42. Zusman, R. M., Rubin, R. H., Cato, A. E., Cocchetto, D. M., Crow, J. W., and Tokloff-Rubin, N.: Hemodialysis using prostacylin instead of heparin as the sole antithrombotic agent. *N. Engl. J. Med.* 304:934, 1981.
43. Coppe, D., Sobel, M., Seamans, L., Levine, F., and Salzman, E.: Preservation of platelet function and number by prostacyclin during cardiopulmonary bypass. *J. Thorac. Cardiovasc. Surg.* 81:274, 1981.
44. Jandl, J. H., and Aster, R. H.: Increased splenic pooling and the pathogenesis of hypersplenism. *Am. J. Med. Sci.* 253:383, 1967.

45. Cohen, P., and Gardner, F. H.: The thrombocytopenic effect of sustained high dosage prednisone therapy in thrombocytopenic purpura. *N. Engl. J. Med.* 265:611, 1961.
46. Karpatkin, S.: Heterogeneity of human platelets. I. Metabolic and kinetic evidence suggestive of young and old platelets. *J. Clin. Invest.* 48:1073, 1969.
47. Shulman, N. R., Aster, R. H., Leitner, A., and Hiller, M. C.: Immunoreactions involving platelets. V. Post-transfusion purpura due to a complement-fixing antibody against a genetically controlled platelet antigen: A proposed mechanism for thrombocytopenia and its relevance in "autoimmunity." *J. Clin. Invest.* 40:1597, 1961.
48. Lau, P., Sholtis, C. M., and Aster, R. H.: Post-transfusion purpura: An enigma of alloimmunization. *Am. J. Hematol.* 9:331, 1980.
49. McIntosh, S., O'Brien, R. T., Schwartz, A. D., and Pearson, H. A.: Neonatal isoimmune purpura: Response to platelet infusions. *J. Pediatr.* 82:1020, 1973.
50. Murphy, S.: Platelet transfusion. *Prog. Hemostasis Thromb.* 3:289, 1976.
51. Weiss, H. J.: Thrombocytopathia, in *Clinics in Haematology*, edited by J. R. O'Brien. Saunders, London, 1972, vol. 1, p. 369.
52. Cardamone, J. M., Edson, J. R., McArthur, J. R., and Jacob, H. S.: Abnormalities of platelet function in the myeloproliferative disorders. *JAMA* 221:268, 1972.
53. Cowan, D. H., and Haut, M. J.: Platelet function in acute leukemia. *J. Lab. Clin. Med.* 79:893, 1970.
54. Brown, C. H., III, Weisberg, R. J., Natelson, E. A., and Alfrey, C. P., Jr.: Glanzmann's thrombasthenia: Assessment of the response to platelet transfusions. *Transfusion* 15:124, 1975.
55. Janson, P. A., Jubelirer, S. J., Weinstein, M. J., and Deykin, D.: Treatment of the bleeding tendency in uremia with cryoprecipitate. *N. Engl. J. Med.* 303:1318, 1980.
56. Perkins, H. A., Mackenzie, M. R., and Fudenberg, H. H.: Hemostatic defects in dysproteinemias. *Blood* 35:695, 1970.
57. Murphy, S., and Holme, S.: Storage of platelets for five days—Value of paired studies. *Transfusion* 21:637, 1981.

CHAPTER *167*

Preparation and clinical use of plasma and plasma fractions

ALAN J. JOHNSON
DAVID L. ARONSON
WILLIAM J. WILLIAMS

Plasma

Technological advances in the collection, storage, and fractionation of plasma permit a single unit to supply concentrated, purified components for different therapeutic uses, while whole plasma has been relegated to a secondary and controversial therapeutic role.

PREPARATION OF PLASMA

Plasma for clinical use can be obtained from whole blood or by plasmapheresis [1]. It is possible to repeat plasmapheresis every 2 to 3 days, with removal of up to 800 ml of plasma weekly from a healthy person [2], but donors participating in these programs must be kept under medical and laboratory surveillance. Plasmapheresis permits collection of both normal plasma, for large-scale fractionation, and special plasma, e.g., plasma with high-titer antibodies [3]. Placentas are also a source of plasma proteins, particularly immunoglobulins and albumin.

Citrate formulas without dextrose may be employed as anticoagulant if the blood is collected for plasma fractionation only; plasma for fractionation is also derived from blood drawn into any of the standard anticoagulants (see Chap. 164). Treatment with EDTA or with an ion exchange resin has been used for special purposes. Heparin is not a satisfactory anticoagulant for plasma that is to be stored longer than 48 h.

Recommended storage temperatures for plasma range from $-20°C$ to as high as $30°C$. The elevated temperature was recommended to inactivate hepatitis virus. Plasma should be maintained at $-20°C$, if possible, to preserve the coagulation factors.

CLINICAL USE OF PLASMA

Plasma has been widely used for a variety of clinical states, including shock, hemorrhage, infection, and bleeding associated with massive trauma. However, few data support the view that it provides the best treatment for these states.

The use of plasma as a plasma expander originated during World War II in the absence of adequate supplies of whole blood and albumin. Several clinical studies and some animal experiments show that fresh plasma may be less effective as an intravascular volume expander than plasma stored at room temperature [4–7]. The difference may be due to changes in vascular permeability when fresh homologous plasma is infused. It would seem that hypovolemia is better treated by infusion of either crystalloid or albumin solutions. In case of hemorrhage, replacement with whole blood is obviously superior to reconstitution of red cell concentrates with albumin or plasma.

While newer fractions have superseded plasma for the treatment of hemophilia A and B, plasma is still the most reasonable therapeutic choice for some congenital and acquired bleeding states. Deficiencies of factor V, XI, or XIII are best treated by plasma infusion. The diffuse bleeding state accompanying massive trauma or extensive transfusion is poorly understood. If in these situations platelet function is not compromised [8], hemorrhage may be due to a deficiency of one or more procoagulant factors and may be alleviated by the infusion of frozen plasma.

Plasma infusion is also useful in several uncommon diseases. While immunoglobulin preparations are, in general, effective in the treatment of hypogammaglobulinemia (see Chap. 112), some patients have an unsatisfactory response even at the maximum tolerated intramuscular dose and can be successfully treated with intravenous infusions of plasma (10 ml/kg every 4 weeks) [9]. Thrombotic thrombocytopenic purpura has been treated by infusions of plasma or by plasma exchange [10,11] (Chap. 142).

UNFAVORABLE EFFECTS OF PLASMA THERAPY
Fever, urticaria, and erythema may occur after plasma therapy. Some reactions are due to infusion of leukocyte and platelet antigens into a patient with high antibody titer; others are reactions to such plasma proteins as the Gm factors [12] (see Chap. 163). These reactions may be prevented by giving antihistamines prior to plasma infusion or by Gm-typing the donor and recipient plasmas.

Pharmacologically active substances, such as vasoactive polypeptides [13], may form in blood after it is drawn, causing reactions when infused into patients. The rapid administration (e.g., 100 ml per minute) of large volumes of plasma may also cause symptoms of citrate toxicity.

Bacterial contamination of plasma may occur during removal of the cells from whole blood and pooling of the plasma. When plasma from many donors is pooled, up to 20 percent of the pools may be contaminated [14]. If the contamination is slight, the organism does not usually multiply; however, residual endotoxins may induce pyrogenic reactions in the recipient.

The most common serious hazard of plasma therapy is hepatitis—with an incidence of at least 10 percent when pooled plasma that has been stored at room temperature or higher (30 to 32°C) for 6 months is used [15,16]. Single-donor plasma, particularly if obtained from volunteers screened for hepatitis B surface antigen (HbsAg, see Chap. 164), diminishes the risk of hepatitis B although the incidence of non-A, non-B hepatitis is still high [17].

Plasma fractionation

With current technology [17–20], at least four clinically useful fractions can be obtained from the same plasma: antihemophilic factor (factor VIII), prothrombin complex (prothrombin and factors VII, IX, and X), γ-globulin, and albumin. Large-scale plasma fractionation permits the final product to be sampled and tested for safety, sterility, pyrogenicity, and potency prior to use.

The single greatest hazard is contamination of the plasma pool with hepatitis virus [7]. Screening donors with a sensitive radioimmunoassay (RIA) has reduced the incidence of hepatitis from blood transfusion by about 50 percent [21]; the remaining cases may be due to other infectious agents [22] or to an insufficiently sensitive hepatitis B assay. Screening plasma prior to fractionation has reduced but not eliminated hepatitis B. However, the incidence of non-A, non-B hepatitis is substantial in patients treated with plasma and plasma derivatives [17,21,22]. If the carrier rate is between 0.1 and 1 percent, a pool of 1000 donors has a 63 to 99 percent chance of being contaminated. Diminishing the pool size is theoretically possible but impractical. Properly prepared γ-globulin and plasma products such as albumin and plasma proteins which have been heat-treated to inactivate the viruses of hepatitis A, hepatitis B, and non-A, non-B hepatitis are no longer associated with hepatitis. A considerable effort is being made to heat-treat other, more labile fractions, such as antihemophilic factor and the prothrombin complex, to prevent transmission of hepatitis by these fractions (see below).

Protein denatured during ethanol fractionation may have toxic effects or may produce new antigens which sensitize the recipient [23–25]. Allergic reactions to plasma fractions are less frequent and less severe than reactions to whole plasma. Enzyme activation during production, e.g., Hageman factor (factor XII), may cause transient adverse reactions [26,27].

PRINCIPLES OF PLASMA FRACTIONATION
Plasma protein fractionation by selective precipitation depends on reducing the interaction of a protein with its solvent by alterations in either one. Methods which depend on changes in pH, alcohol concentration, and ionic strength are widely employed [28–31]. Adsorbents are also used, such as calcium phosphate or diethylaminoethyl (DEAE) cellulose, agarose gels for gel permeation and affinity chromatography, and solid-phase polyelectrolytes [31].

ALBUMIN AND ALBUMIN-RICH FRACTIONS
Albumin-rich solutions for clinical use are generally produced by ethanol fractionation [29,30]. Albumin produced by the Cohn cold ethanol method [29,30] is more than 95 percent pure by electrophoresis. A variation of the Cohn fractionation method yields a product, plasma protein fraction (PPF), which is more than 83 percent albumin. Pasteurization of PPF and albumin at 60°C for 10 h prevents transmission of hepatitis [32]. Albumin is available in 5 and 25% solutions containing 100 to 160 meq/liter of sodium ion. PPF is packaged as a 5% solution.

CLINICAL USE AND ABUSE OF ALBUMIN
Albumin and PPF are widely used in the United States [33]. Indeed, albumin is the major budgetary item for many hospital blood banks. It is used mainly for hypovolemia in surgery or trauma and for chronic hypoalbuminemia in nephrosis, cirrhosis, and the malabsorption syndrome [34] and may be used to maintain the obligatory extracellular space, as in severe burns.

Specific indications for the use of albumin are still unclear, however. Studies on hemorrhagic shock in animals have shown no significant advantage in colloid replacement if sufficient fluid is given to restore arterial pressure [35]. Renal shutdown is prevented in healthy young people with acute trauma by treatment with crystalloids and whole blood [36], although there is a high incidence of pulmonary edema (wet lung, shock lung, respiratory distress). In abdominal surgery these complications have been prevented by infusing albumin during the operation in an amount equal to the total normal circulating albumin [35,36].

Traditionally, large amounts of albumin have been administered to maintain the blood volume in cases of severe burns; during the first 24 h, however, albumin may cause little increase in the plasma volume [37]. After this period, albumin levels in excess of 2 g/dl may help minimize edema formation.

While albumin is considered useful in acute conditions such as hypovolemic shock and burns [38], replacement of albumin in chronic hypoalbuminemic states is usually unnecessary [39] and is generally futile as a supplement in chronic nutritional hypoproteinemia. In adult patients with nephrosis, the loss of albumin is partially offset by a decrease in the rate of degradation and an increase in the rate of synthesis [39]. In cirrhosis, if the patient's diet is adequate, the liver can usually synthesize sufficient albumin [40].

Albumin carries a definite risk of pyrogenic reactions [41] and microbial contamination [42]. One epidemic of hepatitis B from albumin has been documented [43]. Hypotensive reactions following the infusion of al-

bumin and PPF are due to contamination by prekallikrein activator [27]. Albumin prepared after the prekallikrein activator was recognized has a substantially lower content of this activator than do lots produced before it was identified.

General principles of replacement therapy in coagulation disorders

Therapy of coagulation factor deficiencies is based on replacement of the factor, alone or in combination, by administering whole blood, plasma, or purified plasma fractions or concentrates. The optimal dose of the particular factor for each patient is determined by certain general principles, such as the severity of the bleeding episode, the possible danger to the patient, the time interval between doses, and the duration of therapy [44–50] (Table 167-1).

DOSAGE

The deficient coagulation factor should be given in sufficient amounts to ensure adequate hemostasis. The

TABLE 167-1 Recommended factor VIII:C dosage in hemophilic patients with severe factor VIII:C deficiency and various types of hemorrhage

Type of bleeding	Initial dose	Maintenance dosage
Surgically induced		
Orthopedic surgery (joint replacement)	1 PV* 1–2 h preoperatively	1 PV every 8 h for 24 h, then 1 PV every 12 h for 14 days, then 0.25 PV every 12 h for 14–28 days
Other major surgery, including comprehensive dental surgery	1 PV 1–2 h preoperatively	0.5 PV every 8 h for 24 h, then 0.5 PV every 12 h for 7 to 10 days, then 0.25 PV every 12 h for 3–7 days
Major hemorrhage Retroperitoneal hematoma Hemophilic pseudocyst Bleeding in mouth Gastrointestinal bleeding Intra-abdominal bleeding Head injury†	1 PV	0.5 PV every 8 h for 24 h, then 0.5 PV every 12 h until 3–5 days after cessation of bleeding
Minor hemorrhage Hemarthrosis Simple hematoma of muscle Hematuria	0.25–0.5 PV	0.25–0.5 PV, depending on severity, usually in a single dose; if bleeding resumes, 0.5 PV may be given every 12 h for at least 48 h

*PV = plasma volume (about 41 ml per kilogram of body weight); the number of milliliters in the PV fraction corresponds to the number of factor VIII:C units to be administered.

†Even if bleeding is not apparent in head injuries, the indicated dosage should be given prophylactically.

dose is usually calculated in units; one unit is generally defined as the activity present in 1 ml of normal human male plasma. A relatively high dose is usually required to control major hemorrhage; hemorrhage in a potentially dangerous area, such as the head, throat, or abdomen; and hemorrhage during and immediately after surgery or trauma. As healing progresses, smaller doses will suffice. Minor hemorrhage into a joint or muscle may be treated with about half the amount used for major hemorrhage. Typical doses for factor VIII:C[1] are given in Table 167-1.

HEMOSTATIC LEVEL IN VIVO

The hemostatically effective blood level is different for each coagulation factor.

METABOLIC HALF-LIFE

Each factor must be given in sufficiently high doses and often enough to compensate for a decline in the plasma level as it is metabolized. The metabolic half-life varies for each factor. The concentrates are infused rapidly so that the maximal plasma level is reached before metabolic changes or degradation take place.

VOLUME OF DISTRIBUTION

Each coagulation factor has a different apparent volume of distribution, depending on the amount retained intravascularly, the amount diffusing into the extravascular space, and many other factors not yet understood.

PLASMA DILUTION FACTOR

The volume in which the factor is administered influences the plasma levels achieved. A large volume of whole plasma containing a given amount of the deficient factor causes greater expansion of the plasma volume, and thus a lower apparent recovery in vivo, than a highly purified concentrate containing the same amount of the factor.

DIFFERENCES IN PREPARATION METHOD OR STARTING MATERIAL

Small differences in the in vivo recovery may be found following infusion of concentrates of the same factor prepared by different methods [47]. This may be due in part to differences in the degree of denaturation and in the volume of distribution and, in the case of bovine and porcine factor VIII:C, to species differences.

[1] The following nomenclature is used for factor VIII:

Factor VIII:C—procoagulant activity of factor VIII, i.e., antihemophilic factor activity
Factor VIII:CAg—immunologic activity of factor VIII:C
Factor VIII/vWF—protein responsible for von Willebrand factor activity
Factor VIII:vWF—von Willebrand factor activity
Factor VIIIR:RCo—activity which supports platelet aggregation with ristocetin
Factor VIIIR:Ag—factor VIII-related antigen

Factor VIII:C fractionation methods

COHN FRACTION I

One of the first clinically useful factor VIII:C concentrates [51] was a fibrinogen-rich fraction (fraction I). The preparation contained about 70 percent fibrinogen and was only 4 to 6× purified [46].

FRACTION I-0

Further purification of fraction I in small batches by extraction with 1 M glycine-ethanol-citrate solution yields a concentrate that is about 10 to 20× purified and contains 40 to 90 percent of the factor VIII:C activity of the starting plasma [52]. Widely used with good clinical results, it may also contain hemostatically active factor VIIIR:RCo [53–59].

CRYOPRECIPITATE

The development of cryoprecipitate [60] was probably the most important advance in factor VIII:C therapy. In this method, fresh-frozen plasma in bags, each bag from a single donor, is thawed at 2 to 4°C [61,62]. In a process that uses a closed system, undissolved cryoprecipitate is collected by centrifugation and the precipitate and supernatant plasma are placed in separate plastic bags. The precipitate can be redissolved in plasma or saline for use in patients deficient in fibrinogen, factor VIII:C, or factor XIII or in those with von Willebrand's disease. Cryoprecipitate is about one-third fibrinogen and contains small amounts of all the plasma proteins [61]. The supernatant plasma may provide prothrombin and factor V, VII, IX, X, or XI for patients who are deficient in one or more of these factors; it may also be used as a plasma expander in surgical patients or for fractionation of the residual proteins.

Factor VIII:C in cryoprecipitate is 10 to 30× purified. The yield, depending on the factor VIII:C content of the starting plasma, its cryoprecipitability, and losses that occur during processing, averages about 80 to 100 units from 200 ml of plasma [62–66]. The content of factor VIII:C varies from bag to bag and the fibrinogen level is high, preventing over 10-units-per-milliliter concentration. Single units cannot be assayed prior to use without risk of bacterial contamination, therefore the effectiveness of each unit is unpredictable. It must be stored in the frozen state, and residual contaminating white blood cells lead to a moderately high incidence of reactions unless the cells or cell fragments are partially removed by further centrifugation or Millipore filtration. However, because of the inherent nature of the collection method, the incidence of hepatitis in recipients may be lower than that which occurs with concentrates made from large plasma pools and similar to what occurs with single-unit fresh-frozen plasma.

Most commercially available concentrates today are prepared using cryoprecipitation as the initial step followed by tris extraction, cold precipitation, and aluminum hydroxide adsorption [67–70]. The pooled material can be assayed and labeled before use; it is stable in the lyophilized state for long periods. When properly prepared, it causes very few reactions, but the hepatitis risk remains high.

GLYCINE PRECIPITATION
Factor VIII:C (about 20× purified) can be prepared from plasma by glycine precipitation [71]. With cryoprecipitate as the starting material, the yield is lower but the plasma supernatant is much more useful.

POLYETHELENE GLYCOL (PEG) FRACTIONATION, PEG PRECIPITATION
High-purity factor VIII:C (100 to 200× purified) is produced by the further fractionation of intermediate-purity factor VIII:C with PEG-4000 [48,67,68]. The material is readily soluble, is stable for long periods at 4°C, and can be administered to adults by syringe. When preparations containing 500 units per milliliter were injected intramuscularly, they failed to raise the plasma factor VIII:C levels perceptibly. This finding has also been reported for other factor VIII:C preparations [72,73].

PEG FRACTIONATION, GLYCINE PRECIPITATION
A similar type of high-purity factor VIII:C made by glycine precipitation of cryoprecipitated, PEG-fractionated factor VIII:C is approximately 100× purified [74,75]. It is widely available commercially. Use of heparin in the preparation is claimed to increase the yield [76].

PEG fractionation is now the basic method for most commercial preparations of factor VIII:C. Its advantages are high concentration, moderately high purity, low type-specific antibody, moderately reduced hepatitis contamination, and ease of storage and administration. However, the moderate yield is a commercial disadvantage.

HEAT-TREATED FACTOR VIII:C FOR THE ELIMINATION OF HEPATITIS
Liver function tests and liver biopsy samples indicate definite chronic liver disease in about 50 percent of patients treated with plasma concentrates [77–86]. While the exact pathogenesis of the hepatitis is not clear, a high incidence of hepatitis B antibody (up to 90 percent) suggests that this virus may be implicated [77–79]. The use of multiple-donor, pooled products rather than single-donor materials and the higher incidence in patients who have had fewer transfusions supports this theory. However, the apparently benign course of the disease and the high incidence of non-A, non-B hepatitis in sero-negative individuals points to this as a possible cause. At least one manufacturer has initiated heat treatment (60°C for 10 h) of glycine-protected cryoprecipitate to inactivate all the hepatitis viruses [87]. The resulting preparation is freely soluble, and more than 218 infusions were administered to 12 patients for 6 to 12 months without evidence of hepatitis.

POLYELECTROLYTE-PURIFIED FACTOR VIII:C
Highly purified plasma proteins have long been sought for infusion into patients. The higher the purity of factor VIII:C, the more soluble and concentrated it can be and the fewer potentially toxic contaminants are present, such as hepatitis viruses, red cell antibodies [88,89], possible immunogens, fibrinogen, and other proteins.

Polyelectrolyte purification [90] presents the possibility of purifying human factor VIII:C up to 10,000× in a high yield from plasma in only two steps. While initial clinical testing has demonstrated therapeutic effectiveness and lack of toxicity [91], considerable clinical investigation will be necessary before this product becomes commercially available.

ANIMAL FACTOR VIII:C
Concentrates of factor VIII:C and factor VIIIR:RCo with about 100 times the activity of normal human plasma have been prepared from bovine and porcine plasma [92,93]. When infused in humans, the porcine and bovine factor VIII preparations were antigenic and caused pyrogenic reactions as well as a decrease in platelets [44]. The pyrogenicity, decrease in platelets, and antigenicity have diminished with new polyelectrolyte fractionation techniques [94–96].

Hemophilia A—factor VIII:C deficiency

FACTOR VIII

DOSAGE AND DURATION OF THERAPY
Raising the plasma level of factor VIII:C above 25 percent in patients with hemophilia A results in predictably normal hemostasis even during and after major surgery [48–50]. Their factor VIII:C level should be maintained at a minimum of 25 to 30 percent for 8 to 10 days and at 10 to 15 percent for the next 3 to 7 days. However, in patients undergoing orthopedic reconstruction or extensive surgery, plasma levels of about 50 percent should be maintained for 2 weeks and levels of 10 to 15 percent for up to 4 weeks [97,98].

In patients with major spontaneous hemorrhage, levels of 25 to 30 percent should be maintained for 3 to 7 days or until a hemostatically effective thrombus has formed. Under life-threatening circumstances—such as bleeding intracranially, in the throat or floor of the mouth, or intraabdominally—replacement therapy must be continued for 5 to 7 days after bleeding ceases [49,50]. In patients with minor hemorrhage, about half as much factor VIII:C is required as for major hemorrhage and therapy is often continued for only 24 to 48 h (Table 167-1).

The dose should be adjusted according to daily assays of the patient's factor VIII:C levels. When such assays are not available, an empirical dosage schedule may be followed (Table 167-1).

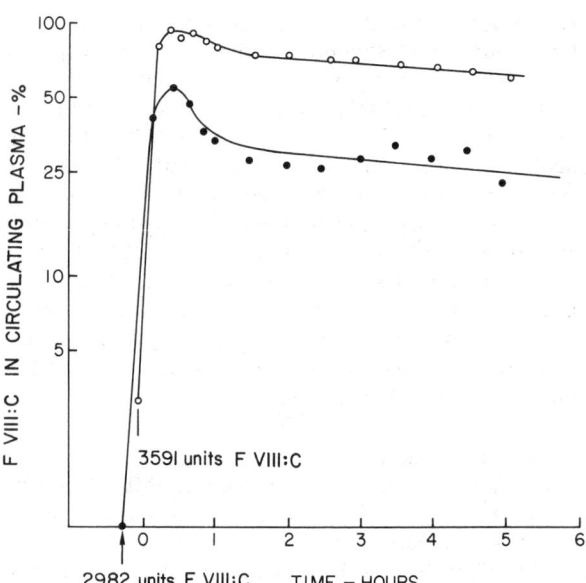

FIGURE 167-1   Plasma levels of factor VIII:C following intravenous infusion of PEG concentrates in 15 untreated patients with severe hemophilia (< 1 percent factor VIII:C) (solid circles) and in 5 of the 15 given an additional intravenous dose 1 day after the first infusion (open circles) (mean of data).

RECOVERY OF FACTOR VIII:C IN VIVO

When an untreated patient with severe factor VIII:C deficiency (less than 1 percent) is given an injection of concentrate intravenously, a semilog plot of the plasma concentration of factor VIII:C against time generally shows three phases (Fig. 167-1) [48,49,57,99–101]: (1) dilution of the infused material in the intravascular space; (2) dilution in the extravascular space [58,59,102] and adsorption onto platelets, red blood cells, and endothelial surfaces [103,104]; and (3) a steady decrease which appears to represent the true metabolic half-life. The second phase disappears after several days of intravenous factor VIII:C administration (Fig. 167-1) and is consequently of less practical concern during prolonged therapy.

CALCULATION OF DOSAGE

The dose of factor VIII:C to be administered is calculated as follows:

Units to be administered
$$= \text{(desired factor VIII:C concentration} \\ - \text{initial factor VIII concentration)} \\ \times \text{plasma volume}$$

where 1 unit is defined as the amount of factor VIII:C in 1 ml of pooled, normal, human male plasma and factor concentrates are in units per milliliter.

The plasma volume may be calculated from an assumed plasma volume of 41 ml per kilogram body weight if the hematocrit reading is nearly normal [105]. Two doses must be infused daily for several days with

peak concentrations of at least 50 to 60 percent and a metabolic half-life of approximately 12 h to ensure a minimum level of 25 to 30 percent factor VIII:C (0.25 to 0.30 unit per milliliter of plasma). However, the extravascular distribution of factor VIII:C must also be considered for the first few days of therapy. Since at least one-fifth of the amount infused during acute therapy probably goes into the extravascular space, it is necessary to allow for this during the early stages of treatment (Fig. 167-1).

Because only 80 percent of each unit (0.80 unit) of infused factor VIII:C remains in the plasma, 1 unit brings about a 1 percent rise in the level of circulating factor VIII:C when diluted in 80 ml of plasma (and 20 ml of extravascular pool). If there is approximately 80 ml of plasma per 2 kilograms of body weight, each unit of infused factor VIII:C causes a 1 percent rise in the plasma level per 2 kilograms of body weight, or a 2 percent rise per kilogram. That is, 1 unit of concentrate per kilogram of body weight causes a 2 percent rise in the plasma factor VIII:C levels.

Factor VIII:C fractions from different species yield different levels of factor VIII:C after infusion of the same size doses [47]. Thus, if the increment in factor VIII:C is taken as 1 for fresh plasma, it is about 0.6 for animal factor VIII:C. Of greater importance is the fact that with most commercially available VIII:C the response to transfusion may vary considerably from patient to patient and must be assessed by the attending physician for each case.

FACTOR VIII:C CONTENT OF PLASMA AND CRYOPRECIPITATE

Although the factor VIII:C content of fresh plasma is normally considered to be 1 unit per milliliter of plasma, in practice it may vary from 0.5 to 2.0 units per milliliter (50 to 200 percent of normal) [106]. In fresh-frozen plasma, the activity after thawing is usually below 80 percent (0.8 unit per milliliter). The yield of factor VIII:C activity in cryoprecipitate prepared from 200 ml of fresh-frozen plasma averages between 80 and 100 units, but may vary from 50 to 120 units. The dosage schedule should be based on a conservative estimate of about 0.8 unit per milliliter for fresh plasma, 0.7 unit per milliliter for fresh-frozen plasma, and 80 units per bag for cryoprecipitate. The factor VIII:C content of commercial concentrates is determined for each batch and given on the label.

PATIENTS WITH FACTOR VIII:C INHIBITOR (ANTIBODY)

INHIBITOR ASSAYS AND ESTIMATION OF DOSAGE

It is estimated that more than 10 percent of patients with severe classic hemophilia A will develop an inhibitor (IgG) to factor VIII:C [49,107–109]. In most instances, inhibitors have formed in individuals who had at least 50 to 100 or more infusions (exposure-days) of factor VIII:C [110], many of them during postoperative treatment. While these patients usually have severe hemophilia, bleeding episodes do not increase appreciably in number. Major bleeding episodes may be effectively treated if factor VIII:C is infused in massive amounts or if the inhibitor level in the plasma is decreased beforehand by plasmapheresis or exchange transfusion [111]. Immunosuppressive drugs have also been used in a variety of protocols [112,113] but with only occasional success. The amount of factor VIII:C neutralized by the inhibitor may be determined by several methods [49, 110,114,115]. It is highly desirable to determine an adequate hemostatic dosage for each patient by assaying the actual level of inhibitor in the plasma, the factor VIII:C level before and after factor VIII:C concentrate is administered, and the therapeutic response. The antigen-antibody complex which develops in most patients with inhibitor is dissociable, is not stoichiometric, and combines very slowly in a time-dependent reaction. Rarely, the inhibitor combines tightly and relatively stoichiometrically with the antigen [107].

The treatment of patients with inhibitor is based on several considerations:

1. The level of inhibitor in the plasma (less than 5 units per milliliter, 5 to 100 units per milliliter, more than 100 units per milliliter)

2. The patient's immunologic response to infused factor VIII:C (patients who form factor VIII:C antibody following infusion of factor VIII:C are called responders, and those who do not form antibody are called nonresponders)

3. The severity of the hemorrhage and/or potential danger to the patient (major or minor hemorrhage)

4. The expected duration of therapy (1 to 2 days for most minor hemorrhages, 1 to 2 weeks following severe trauma or operative intervention)

In patients with inhibitor levels of 5 Bethesda units or less [116–118], hemostasis is usually achieved by continuous infusion of concentrated factor VIII:C with or without a demonstrable increase in the plasma factor VIII:C level. It is believed that hemostasis is effected in these patients prior to complete neutralization of the factor VIII:C because the antigen and antibody may form a dissociable complex [49,107,108].

If the inhibitor level is less than 5 units per milliliter, the patient is a nonresponder, and hemostasis has not been achieved with "normal" doses of factor VIII:C, moderate to large amounts of factor VIII:C may be administered to neutralize most of the intravascular and extravascular inhibitor and provide sufficient amounts of free factor VIII:C for hemostasis.

In some patients with bleeding which is not life-threatening but with moderate or high inhibitor levels that have caused the antigen-antibody complex to form rapidly, it may be necessary to devise an effective factor VIII:C dosage based on therapeutic results, bearing in mind that high doses of factor VIII:C may stimulate antibody production if the patient is a responder.

If a patient with a non-life-threatening hemorrhage is known to be a responder or to have had an anamnestic response, it may be necessary to try sequentially (1) an ordinary, clinical preparation of factor IX; (2) if this does not control bleeding, an "activated" factor IX preparation (Autoplex-Hyland or FEIBA-Immuno); and (3) if this is not effective, porcine VIII:C preparation (Hyate:C-Speywood). However, if a life-threatening hemorrhage has occurred and the patient is an adult with a high factor VIII:C antibody, plasmapheresis and human factor VIII:C may be tried. In the event of an anamnestic response, a clinical-grade factor IX preparation may be tried; if there is little therapeutic response, this should be followed by activated factor IX. If this is not effective, porcine VIII:C may be employed. If prior to therapy there was no cross-reactivity on testing the patient's antibody against porcine VIII:C and if the patient has no clinical evidence of porcine hypersensitivity, therapy may be initiated with the porcine VIII:C.

Similarly, if the patient is a small child difficult to treat by exchange transfusion, it would probably be sensible to use the following therapeutic agents in sequence, as necessary: (1) factor IX, (2) "activated" factor IX, and (3) porcine VIII:C.

USE OF FACTOR VIII:C OF ANIMAL ORIGIN IN PATIENTS WITH INHIBITOR

Animal factor VIII:C has been investigated very nearly as long as human factor VIII:C [119]. In early studies it was demonstrated that infusion of animal factor VIII:C was followed by sustained blood levels of factor VIII:C similar to those achieved by infusion of human factor VIII:C [92,93,120,121]. Animal factor VIII:C was also effective in patients with a high level of factor VIII:C antibody because there was little antigenic cross-reactivity between the human antibody and the porcine procoagulant molecules. However, the concentrate was very impure. Patients infused with large amounts of it formed antibody to it in 5 to 10 days, contraindicating subsequent infusions.

As noted above, individuals with little or no cross-reactivity required about twice as much animal factor VIII:C to reach a specified blood level as did normal hemophiliac patients given human factor VIII:C. There was also a thrombocytopenic effect due to platelet aggregation factor [122] which was much stronger with bovine than with porcine preparations. Early experience with the animal concentrate has been reviewed extensively [44,47].

Polyelectrolyte fractionation methods [90] have been employed in the purification of porcine factor VIII:C [94,123,124]. The clinically effective material is about 1000× purified and contains little measurable platelet aggregation factor, and there is little cross-reactivity with human antibody. It seems to have lower immunogenicity than the above-cited less pure materials [96,125,126]. This porcine material seems to provide a good alternative treatment method for patients with inhibitor; it has no thrombocytopenic effect, it cannot transmit hepatitis, and when given 30 to 40 times to the same patient during 20 to 30 days there was little evidence of immunogenicity [127]. However, porcine concentrate is ultimately immunogenic, and the possible presence of specific porcine antibodies or even anaphylaxis must be considered. Preliminary testing should be carried out with small intravenous doses on each therapeutic occasion, followed by a slow infusion [95].

In general, minor spontaneous bleeding episodes in patients with inhibitor should be treated conservatively or with factor IX. Human or possibly animal factor VIII:C, or "activated" factor IX should be reserved for patients undergoing necessary major surgery or after hemorrhage into a critical region such as the head, neck, or abdomen. Elective surgery for such patients should be planned with great caution since the inhibitor level may rise postoperatively, reaching potentially dangerous levels which could require the use of factor IX, "activated" factor IX, or porcine factor VIII:C.

PROPHYLACTIC AND INTERMITTENT TREATMENT
Patients with hemophilia who have plasma factor VIII:C levels of 2 to 4 percent have mild disease with little spontaneous bleeding. Thus, it would appear that spontaneous bleeding could be avoided by injecting factor VIII:C three times a week in amounts sufficient to give postinfusion plasma levels of 30 percent and minimum plasma levels of 2 to 5 percent [128]. Such therapy for all patients would probably require the fractionation of about 9 to 12 million liters of plasma annually for factor VIII:C in the United States rather than the approximately 3 to 4 million liters of plasma that are now fractionated annually [129] for intermittent therapy of hemophilia A (including home care) [128,130–132].

In view of limited blood supplies and the high cost, about three times as much as for intermittent care [128], the case for prophylaxis must be assessed critically. It is certainly useful and probably necessary as an interim measure in 5 to 10 percent of all hemophilic patients, especially those who are chronically ill and debilitated by their disease. Furthermore, if the patients are carefully selected, it may be less expensive in the long run than intermittent therapy, considering the ultimate cost to the patient and to society [133].

HOME CARE
Home transfusion programs in which factor VIII:C concentrates are administered by the patient or by someone else in the home environment were initiated in 1961 [132] and soon adopted by many of the major clinics [128,131–138]. They have been enthusiastically received, literally changing the quality of life for many patients. At present, about 60 percent of patients with hemophilia in the United States are participating in such programs, and the majority of these administer replacement therapy to themselves as soon as possible after the onset of symptoms. Early treatment substantially decreases the extent of damage which results from spontaneous hemorrhage when therapy is delayed. About 10 percent of the patients on home care are receiving prophylactic therapy.

Patients considered ineligible for home care are those who are reluctant or unable to undergo the necessary training, those whose families do not cooperate, and very young children [137,138]. Psychological factors may be important for individual patients [139]. Home care programs require adequate training opportunities and close supervision and followup of the patients and others responsible for the actual home care. Among the hazards are possible transmission of hepatitis to others through handling of the materials and serious transfusion reactions in the absence of informed supervision.

In one representative study [140] the estimated annual cost of home care (self-care) for each patient, exclusive of surgery, was $5932, only one-third the annual cost ($15,800) for similar patients hospitalized for treatment during the same period or for the same patient prior to admission to the home-care program. There was also a threefold decrease in the number of work or school days lost because of disease-related illness, and only 12.5 percent of the group continued to have long-term clinical problems such as hemarthroses although 90 percent of the patients had previously been affected by them [131,132]. A major increase in use of factor VIII:C or factor IX concentrates was expected, but this has not been the case [132].

SIDE EFFECTS OF THERAPY
The adverse reactions which may occur are qualitatively similar to those discussed above under "Unfavorable Effects of Plasma Therapy." The incidence of allergic reactions is much lower with factor VIII:C concentrates than with whole plasma. The risk of hepatitis seems to be only partially related to the purification of the factor VIII:C. The use of volunteer donors and the testing of starting plasma for hepatitis B surface antigen by third-generation test methods have markedly reduced the incidence of hepatitis in recipients [21,141–143]. The incidence of hepatitis in recipients of different factor VIII:C preparations is unknown. In one series, 31 percent of older children and adults who had little prior exposure to blood products acquired the disease within 6 months of their first infusion [144]. Subsequently, it was recommended that such patients be treated with nonpooled or small-pool plasma components. Overt hepatitis developed in (1) less than 3.5 percent of 1837 patients treated in England [145], (2) 2 percent of multiply transfused patients treated with high-purity PEG-precipitated concentrate fractionated from approximately 50,000 units of plasma from volunteer donors [48], and (3) 5 percent of patients with hemophilia who had been treated previously with cryoprecipitate and then received concentrates prepared from large pools of plasma from professional donors [144]. Up to 90 percent of patients with hemophilia have antibody to hepatitis antigen, probably indicating recent exposure to the antigen [71–81,144,146].

About 72 percent of 1300 patients frequently treated with factor VIII:C had occasional abnormal liver function tests, including elevated transaminase levels [77,79–81]. About 95 percent of patients with persistent abnormal liver function tests showed biopsy evidence of some type of chronic liver disease, including cirrhosis [82–86], although hypersensitivity has also been suggested as a possible mechanism [147].

A few patients with hemophilia have developed *Pneumocystis carinii* pneumonia and have been found to have abnormalities of cellular immunity similar to those of the acquired immunodeficiency syndrome (AIDS) [257]. Further studies on hemophilia patients who appear to be well otherwise have demonstrated reduced ratios of OKT4 cells to OKT8 cells due to a relative decrease in OKT4 (helper) cells and a relative or absolute increase in OKT8 (suppressor) cells (see Chap. 105) [258,259]. The abnormal ratios are associated with functional abnormalities of T cells and elevated levels of serum IgG, and, although the numbers are small, appear to be more frequent in patients who have received commercial factor VIII concentrates than in patients receiving cryoprecipitate [258,259].

Von Willebrand's disease

REPLACEMENT THERAPY: BLEEDING TIME, PLATELET RETENTION, AND PLATELET AGGREGATION

Infusion of plasma, cryoprecipitate, or various plasma fractions into patients with von Willebrand's disease may raise the level of factor VIII:C or decrease the bleeding time or both (Fig. 167-2). The increase in factor VIII:C levels lasts 12 to 40 h [148–150]. Patients with mild disease tend to respond more readily to plasma and plasma fractions than severely affected patients, and with longer-lasting effects, although there is great individual variation. The response also varies with the amount and type of material infused [151–157]. Still to be determined are the specific factors that may be necessary to correct the hemostatic abnormality in von Willebrand's disease and increase the metabolic half-life of the specific plasma component(s) in therapy.

Perhaps the greatest handicap is our difficulty in testing by in vitro assays the hemostatic abnormality in von Willebrand's disease. While most investigators estimate factor VIII:vWF activity by the level of ristocetin cofactor FVIIIR:RCo, high levels of the cofactor have been found in some factor VIII:C preparations that had little hemostatic effect when infused in vivo [158,159]. Thus, the hemostatic effectiveness of factor VIII:vWF in vivo may correlate better with the results of test systems devised to measure (1) the adhesion and subsequent spreading of the platelets on human arterial subendothelium [160,161], (2) the retention of platelets in glass bead columns [162], and/or (3) the size of the factor VIIIR:RCo oligomers in the concentrates [163,164]. However, these tests have not yet been used for the purpose and are complicated to perform and difficult to quantitate.

Replacement therapy in von Willebrand's disease is particularly successful with cryoprecipitate, which con-

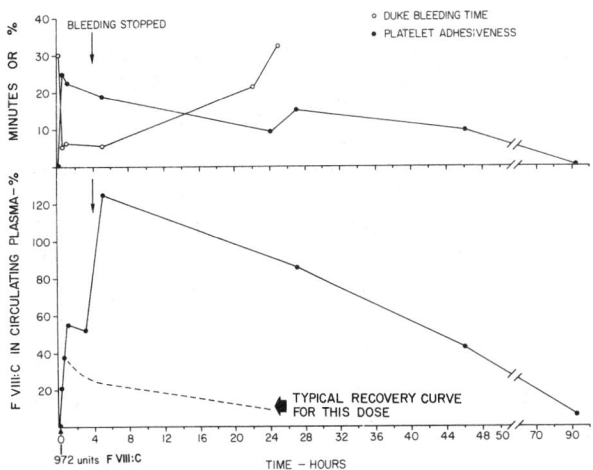

FIGURE 167-2   Effect of intravenous injection of **972 units of intermediate-purity factor VIII:C (extracted from cryoprecipitate with tris-buffer) in a 50-kg patient with severe von Willebrand's disease and intractable rectal hemorrhage.**

tains large amounts of factors VIII:C and VIIIR:RCo, VIII:C-stimulating factor, and the factor(s) which cause shortened bleeding time, increased platelet retention, and increased adhesion and spreading of platelets on arterial subendothelium. Since cryoprecipitate contains a relatively high concentration of these factors and a reduced protein content as compared to plasma, it is the treatment of choice. Fraction I-0 and intermediate-purity fractions usually contain large amounts of factor VIII:C and varying amounts of the other factors. The PEG high-purity factor VIII:C fractions contain large amounts of factor VIII:C and small amounts of the other factors. Most commercially available factor VIII:C concentrates probably should not be used to treat von Willebrand's disease, with the possible exception of Blombäck's fraction I-0 [55]. Factor VIII:C concentrates prepared by different methods usually have similar effects in increasing the level of factor VIII:C but very different effects on the levels of factor VIII:vWF and factor VIIIR:Ag and on platelet retention, bleeding time, and hemostasis [48,154–159].

The quality of cryoprecipitate varies from unit to unit, both when prepared in different laboratories and when prepared at different times in the same laboratory. In one series the content of factor VIIIR:RCo ranged from 10 to nearly 60 percent, with an average of about 30 percent [165]. Storage of cryoprecipitate at −50 to −80°C may preserve "antibleeding" activity for as long as 6 months.

The hemostatic effectiveness of cryoprecipitate or other fractions is usually gauged by the clinical response, and the Duke bleeding time is often shortened [99,166]. While the minimum factor VIII:C level for normal hemostasis in von Willebrand's disease, as in hemophilia A, is about 25 percent, bleeding can occur in patients with much higher plasma factor VIII:C levels [48,159] because of the variable factor VIII:vWF content of the infused materials.

DOSAGE

Although it has been common practice, therapy should not be based on the plasma factor VIII:C levels [44,46] or the levels of factor VIIIR:RCo. Adequate levels of factor VIII:C are usually achieved without difficulty because of the secondary rise in factor VIII:C levels. A dosage schedule of 10 to 15 ml of plasma per kilogram per day or 1 to 1.5 units of cryoprecipitate per 10 kilograms per day [167] has successfully maintained a minimum factor VIII:C level of 25 percent (Table 167-2). With this regimen, platelet retention and factor VIIIR:RCo level are often increased and the bleeding time (Duke method) decreased, although these effects are more variable [47,154,167–169]. The Duke bleeding time has also been used as the principal index of effective treatment [55,166]. In preparing patients for surgery, it is often useful to administer full doses of cryoprecipitate a full day prior to operation as well as 2 to 4 h before.

No large-scale commercially produced plasma fraction except fresh or fresh-frozen cryoprecipitate is now available that will consistently correct the abnormalities in von Willebrand's disease and produce hemostasis when infused in vivo. It is obvious that much more information is needed regarding the clinical significance of the secondary rise in factor VIII:C levels and the methods for quantitating the deficient factor(s) in vitro before optimal criteria and methods can be developed for the treatment of von Willebrand's disease.

Prothrombin and factors VII, IX, and X (prothrombin complex)

FRACTIONATION METHODS

Fractions of proven value in the treatment of a congenital deficiency of one or more of the vitamin K–dependent factors (prothrombin and factors VII, IX, and X)[2] are being produced by several methods which depend on adsorption to either tricalcium phosphate or diethylaminoethyl (DEAE) cellulose [170–173]. The preparations made by calcium phosphate adsorption contain approximately equal amounts of factors II, VII, IX, and X, whereas the DEAE preparations of prothrombin complex contain less factor VII. Heparin (1 to 4 units per milliliter) may be added to some preparations to prevent activation of the concentrated factors. The calcium-binding ions phosphate and citrate are also usually present.

CLINICAL USE OF PROTHROMBIN COMPLEX

Preparations of prothrombin complex have been used to treat both congenital and acquired hemorrhagic disorders. Their efficacy in congenital deficiency states, particularly factor IX deficiency, is well established. However, their usefulness in a variety of acquired hem-

[2] The terms *prothrombin complex* and *factor IX complex* are used interchangeably for the type of preparation containing these four factors.

orrhagic disorders, such as liver disease and coumarin anticoagulant overdosage, is limited by the high risk of transmitting hepatitis.

FACTOR IX

When patients with factor IX deficiency are infused with either plasma or factor IX complex, the in vivo recovery of factor IX activity in the plasma ranges from 30 to 50 percent [174,175]. Intravenously infused factor IX has an initial rapid die-away with a half-life of about 5 h; this is assumed to represent diffusion into the extravascular space. This is followed by a slower phase with a half-life of 24 h, attributed to metabolism of the complex [174,175].

The actual amount administered is based primarily on the patient's weight and on the severity of bleeding. For treatment of patients undergoing surgery, bleeding into the central nervous system, or bleeding after major trauma, the factor IX level should be at least 25 percent of normal [176] (Table 167-2). An initial dose of 50 units per kilogram of body weight is recommended, followed by 20 units per kilogram every 12 to 24 h. In the case of extensive hematomas and trachael, laryngeal, or arterial compression, the patient should be treated according to the same schedule. Patients with hemarthrosis or hematuria can be managed with smaller doses [176].

Therapy should be continued as long as needed. A single dose may suffice for treatment of a minor hemorrhage, but surgical patients should receive replacement therapy for 10 to 14 days or until healing is complete. Where possible, the factor IX levels should be monitored before each infusion.

PROPHYLACTIC THERAPY

The prophylactic management of factor IX deficiency with a single weekly infusion of 10 units per kilogram helps to reduce the frequency and severity of hemorrhagic episodes [176]. Since the metabolic half-life of factor IX is about 24 h, the plasma level is extremely low at the end of 1 week.

PROTHROMBIN AND FACTORS VII AND X

Therapeutic regimens for patients deficient in prothrombin, factor VII, and factor X are not well established (Table 167-2).

FACTOR VII

The clinical severity of factor VII deficiency varies so greatly that therapeutic generalizations are difficult [177]. The half-life is only about 5 h [178]. Administration of the therapeutic material three times daily to maintain a level of 25 percent for several days can ensure adequate hemostasis for surgery in patients with congenital factor VII deficiency or anticoagulated with coumarin drugs. A level as low as 5 percent may be sufficient in such cases.

Therapeutic factor IX concentrates are standardized by their factor IX content, and the content of factor VII varies widely from preparation to preparation. Tricalcium phosphate preparations tend to contain at least as many units of factor VII as factor IX, whereas DEAE preparations may have little factor VII.

FACTOR X

Too few data are available to establish the best method of treating factor X deficiency. Adequate hemostasis during and following dental extraction has been reported with a plasma level of 15 percent [179]. Surgical patients have been effectively treated by infusing an initial dose of 15 units per kilogram, with a maintenance dose of 10 units per kilogram per day postoperatively [101]. The metabolic half-life of infused factor X is variously reported as 30 to 50 h [179,180]. The extravascular distribution volume is about twice the plasma volume.

PROTHROMBIN (FACTOR II)

Effective control of spontaneous hemorrhage in patients with prothrombin deficiency or dysprothrombinemia is achieved at prothrombin levels of 5 to 10 percent of normal. The metabolic half-life of infused prothrombin is 50 to 70 h [101,181], with an apparent volume of distribution about twice the plasma volume. Surgical patients have been effectively treated by infusing an initial dose of 15 units per kilogram with a maintenance dose of 10 units per kilogram per day postoperatively [46].

ACQUIRED DEFICIENCY STATES (REVERSAL OF COUMARIN ANTICOAGULANTS)

The prothrombin complex has proved useful in the treatment of bleeding associated with coumarin drug therapy or when rapid reversal of these anticoagulants is indicated. A level of 30 percent of normal is appropriate for all the vitamin K–dependent factors in the complex. However, the possibility of transmitting hepatitis must be considered, and the complex should be used only for life-threatening emergencies.

POSSIBLE INDICATIONS

Liver disease is associated with a hemorrhagic diathesis and low plasma levels of the vitamin K–dependent factors. Although the prothrombin complex has been administered to patients with liver disease, its therapeutic effectiveness has not yet been established. The prothrombin complex has been given to shorten a prolonged prothrombin time prior to needle biopsy of the liver [182,183], but the necessity for this therapy, or its efficiency, has not been established. In severe liver disease, factor V may be depressed as well as factors II, VII, IX, and X, and for this reason administration of the prothrombin complex may not correct the prothrombin time abnormality [183].

ANTI-INHIBITOR COAGULANT COMPLEX

In 1967 a hemostatic effect was noted when a factor IX complex preparation was infused into a hemophilia A patient undergoing surgery [176]. In a controlled clinical study, this therapeutic effect in hemophilia A patients

with inhibitors was noted when factor IX complex was infused in a dosage of 75 units per kilogram [184].

It has been proposed that an "activated" factor IX (defined as a product capable of in vitro correction of the clotting of hemophilia A plasma) might prove useful in treating patients with antibodies directed against factor VIII [185].

Two such activated products are currently in use clinically, FEIBA (Immuno, Vienna) and Autoplex (Hyland Laboratories, Glendale, California). Both have a pronounced effect in vitro on the clotting of hemophilic plasma and have a hemostatic effect in hemophilic dogs [186]. Both have high levels of activated factors VII, IX, and X [187,188]. However, they differ in content of factor VIII coagulant antigen (FVIII:CAg), with FEIBA containing substantially more than Autoplex. Furthermore, a significant amount of the in vitro activity of FEIBA is inhibited by an antibody against factor VIII [189]. It must be emphasized that there is no evidence for any significance in the measurement of in vitro activity. If either activated factor VII or IX were the effective component, it would have a minimal effect on the in vitro potency measurement. According to several studies, activated factor X is responsible for a large amount of in vitro activity [190] but has little in vivo effect.

While the activated factor IX preparations are usually effective hemostatically in hemophilia A patients with factor VIII antibodies, it is not clear whether they are more effective than nonactivated factor IX complex. In a blind, controlled trial comparing FEIBA and a nonactivated product, FEIBA was shown to be slightly more effective in the treatment of hemarthroses [191].

In light of the ambiguities of the clinical data and the expense of the activated product, strategies have been suggested for use of the nonactivated and activated factor IX products in hemophilia A patients with inhibitor to factor VIII:C [116–118]. For minor bleeding, factor VIII:C should be used. If this is not possible because of high inhibitor levels or an anamnestic response, a standard factor IX concentrate should be the choice. If this fails, one of the activated concentrates should be tried. In the case of a major hemorrhage, factor VIII:C should be tried if possible; if this is ineffective activated factor IX concentrate should be used next, and if this fails, porcine factor VIII:C concentrates should be given.

HAZARDS AND SIDE EFFECTS ASSOCIATED WITH FACTOR IX COMPLEX

The incidence of icteric hepatitis with most factor IX concentrates is higher than reported for any other blood product. Over 60 percent of the recipients of factor IX concentrates with little prior exposure to blood products developed hepatitis [183,192,193]. The incidence of overt hepatitis in frequently transfused patients is lower [145,194]. More than 80 percent of hemophilia B patients have antibody to hepatitis B and possibly a high degree of immunity [195]. With the advent of HBsAg screening of donors, the incidence of hepatitis B has decreased,

TABLE 167-2   Summary of data on replacement therapy of blood coagulation factors

| Deficiency in plasma | Effective plasma level, for hemostasis* | | Plasma or concentrate |
	Minor spontaneous hemorrhage, % of normal	Major trauma or surgery, % of normal	
Factor I (fibrinogen)	50–100 mg/dl	100 mg/dl	Plasma 1,2,3‡
			Cryoprecipitate§
			Fraction 1, any intermediate-purity factor VIII
Factor II (prothrombin)	10–15	20–40	Plasma 1,2‡ Prothrombin complex
Factor V (proaccelerin)	5–15	25	Plasma 1,2,‡ and cryoprecipitate supernatant
Factor VII (proconvertin)	5–10	10–20	Plasma 1,2‡ Prothrombin complex
Factor VIII (antihemophilic factor, AHF)			Plasma 1,2‡ (0.8 U/ml)
Hemophilia A	15–20	25	Fraction I-0 (Blombäck)
(The use of factor IX concentrates to treat patients with hemophilia A and inhibitors of factor VIII:C is discussed on page 1573, and in Refs. 184–191.)			Cryoprecipitate§
			Partially purified AHF
			Bovine and porcine AHF¶
Von Willebrand factor	25	25	Plasma 1,2‡ Cryoprecipitate§
			Factor VIII: Fraction I-0
Factor IX (Christmas factor)	10–15	20–25	Plasma 1,2‡ Prothrombin complex (also used to treat inhibitors of factor VIII:C) DEAE eluate Calcium phosphate eluate "Activated" complex (used only to treat inhibitors of factor VIII:C)
Factor X (Stuart-Power factor)	5–10	15–20	Plasma 1,2‡ Prothrombin complex
Factor XI (plasma thromboplastin antecedent, PTA)	5–15	15–25	Plasma 1,2,3‡ Cryoprecipitate supernate
Factor XII (Hageman factor)	<10	<10	Plasma 1,2,3‡
Factor XIII (fibrin stabilizing factor)	1	5	Plasma 1,2,3‡ Cryoprecipitate§

*Twenty-five percent is now generally considered the *minimal* effective level for patients with most coagulation disorders while undergoing surgery or severe accidental trauma. Furthermore, the range of values encountered under normal clinical conditions is likely to be much wider than depicted here. The disparities are due primarily to differences in patients, in the particular clinical state being treated, and in the assay employed. When therapy is initiated in a particular patient, the dosage employed should maintain plasma levels above the recommended minimum to allow for these variables.

Dosage/kg body weight†		Recovery, %	Metabolic half-life, h	References
Initial	Maintenance per day			
25 U	5–10 U	50	96–144	[44]
2–4 bags/10 kg	1 bag/15 kg	50 (from cryoprecipitate)		[45,46,60,61]
60–100 mg	15–30 mg	50		[29,48,57,200–203]
20 U	15–20 U bid	50–100	50–80	[44,46,101]
40 U	15–20 U	50–100	50–80	[170–178,181]
15–25 U	15–20 U	50	24	[44–46,60–62,204–207]
5–10 U	5 U qid	100	5	[44–46]
5–10 U	5 U qid	100	5	[170,176–178,182]
30 U (Dose limited by volume of plasma administered)	15 U bid	70–80	12	[44–46,106]
40 U	20 U bid	70–80	12	[52–59]
1 bag/2 kg	1 bag/4 kg bid	70–80	12	[47,60–66]
40 U	20 U bid	80	12	[44–59,67–77,81–83,87,90,91,97, 107–118,128,130–140,144–147]
80 U	40 U bid	~40	12	[47,92–96,107–111,114–118, 123–127]
10 U (factor VIII)	10 U (factor VIII)	100		[44,47,148–151,166]
1–2 bags/10 kg	1 bag/10 kg/ 1–2 days	100	~24	[60–64,167–169]
20 U	20 U	100		[44,46,47,55, 150–159,167–169]
40–60 U	5–10 U bid	30–50	20–30	[44,47]
40–60 U	5–10 U bid	30–50	20–30	[170–176,183–199]
100–150 U	100 U bid			[184–191]
10–15 U	10 U	75–100	25–60	[44,46,101,179,180]
10–15 U	10 U	75–100	25–60	[101,170–173,179,180]
10–20 U	5 U	90		[44–46]
10 U	5–10 U	90	40–84	[44–46,208–212]
10 U	5 U	?		[44–46]
2–3 U	Unnecessary	50–100	150	[60–66,213]
1 bag/10 kg	Unnecessary			

† Units of activity are expressed in terms of plasma equivalents: 1 unit is the amount present in 1.0 ml of fresh normal plasma.
‡ 1 = fresh plasma; 2 = fresh frozen plasma; 3 = outdated plasma, approximately 21 days old.
§ 1 bag cryoprecipitate contains 80–100 units factor VIII:C.
¶ Antigenic; reserved for patients with factor VIII:C inhibitor.

but the majority of susceptible recipients acquire non-A, non-B hepatitis [196]. Because of the high risk of infection and mortality in patients who have not received multiple transfusions, prothrombin complex seems to be contraindicated in the absence of compelling reasons.

Another serious and sometimes fatal complication following the infusion of factor IX complex is venous thrombosis or disseminated intravascular coagulation [197,198]. Either or both have been reported in patients with congenital as well as acquired deficiencies. Preformed coagulant activity is present in varying amounts in most factor IX preparations. The phospholipid content is also reported to be an important element in thrombogenicity [199].

Deficiencies in other factors

FIBRINOGEN (FACTOR I) DEFICIENCY

Bleeding problems are infrequent in patients with congenital afibrinogenemia or dysfibrinogenemia and seldom require treatment with fibrinogen (see Chap. 153). Patients with disseminated intravascular coagulation do not usually bleed from this syndrome. If the patient has a very low level of fibrinogen and fails to respond to treatment of the primary disorder or to heparin therapy, and if there is evidence of serious bleeding, it may be necessary to give fibrinogen.

The normal hemostatic level of fibrinogen is above 50 mg/dl, and the infused material has a biologic half-life of about 4 days [200] (Table 167-2). In patients with disseminated intravascular coagulation or primary fibrinolysis, this turnover is markedly increased due to the production of fibrinogen degradation products [201, 202].

Sources of fibrinogen for clinical use include fresh plasma (300 mg/dl) and single-donor cryoprecipitate. Fibrinogen prepared from plasma from a large number of donors is never indicated because of the high risk of hepatitis [203]. Repeated treatment with whole plasma may lead to circulatory overload. Single-donor cryoprecipitate contains 30 to 50 percent of the plasma fibrinogen, or 200 to 300 mg from 220 ml of plasma. Approximately two bags of cryoprecipitate per 10 kilograms of body weight will achieve more than adequate fibrinogen levels for hemostasis. Thrombosis has been reported as a possible complication associated with fibrinogen therapy.

FACTOR V (PROACCELERIN) DEFICIENCY

Factor V plasma levels of 5 to 20 percent seem to prevent hemorrhage after abdominal surgery [204], but levels of 25 percent may be necessary after orthopedic surgery [205] or dental procedures [206] (Table 167-2). The percentage of administered factor V entering both the intravascular and extravascular spaces is probably similar to that found with factor IX [204–206]. The metabolic

half-life is estimated to be 14 to 36 h [207], or approximately 24 h on average.

Since factor V in plasma is labile, fresh-frozen plasma or the supernatant from cryoprecipitate has higher levels of factor V than older plasmas. Plasma levels of 15 to 30 percent may be achieved with an initial dose of 15 to 25 ml/kg; the level should be monitored by a factor V assay or the one-stage prothrombin time. For surgical patients, daily injections of 15 to 20 ml/kg should be continued for about 10 days.

FACTOR XI (PLASMA THROMBOPLASTIN ANTECEDENT, OR PTA) DEFICIENCY

In the treatment of patients with factor XI deficiency, very little of the material administered enters the extravascular space immediately and the initial rise closely approximates the expected rise [208–210] (Table 167-2). Factor XI activity may be monitored by direct assay [211] or by the partial thromboplastin time. The half-life usually ranges from 40 to 84 h [208–210], although in an occasional patient it may be only 10 h [210–212]. Peak plasma factor XI levels of 25 to 50 percent may be achieved after a single injection of 7 to 20 ml of plasma per kilogram [209,210]. Cryoprecipitate supernatant contains approximately 1 unit of factor XI per milliliter and, when administered in daily doses of 10 ml per kilogram of body weight, can maintain plasma levels of 30 to 50 percent in surgical patients. A preoperative dose of approximately 30 ml plasma per kilogram and a maintenance dose of approximately 5 ml per kilogram daily, or 10 ml/kg every 2 days, have been found effective for the treatment of patients undergoing surgery [46]. This dosage might have to be given two or three times a day to those patients in whom the factor XI has a 10-h half-life.

FACTOR XII (HAGEMAN FACTOR) DEFICIENCY

Deficiency of factor XII is not known to be associated with bleeding episodes, and affected persons have undergone major surgery without untoward hemorrhage.

FACTOR XIII (FIBRIN-STABILIZING FACTOR, OR FSF) DEFICIENCY

Factor XIII deficiency is readily treated by replacement therapy with plasma (or cryoprecipitate). The long half-life, about 2 weeks, and the low level needed for normal hemostasis allow for convenient and effective prophylaxis. This is important since the factor XIII–deficient patient may not have frequent hemorrhages, but when hemorrhage occurs or wound healing is delayed in a postoperative patient, it can be catastrophic. Effective prophylaxis can be achieved by the infusion of 500 ml of plasma or 4 to 6 bags of cryoprecipitate [213].

C1 INACTIVATOR DEFICIENCY (HEREDITARY ANGIOEDEMA)

The demonstration that hereditary angioedema is associated with and is probably due to a deficiency of the C1 inactivator level raises the possibility of treating acute episodes by replacement therapy. Both plasma and partially purified C1 inactivator have been used successfully during acute episodes. Dosages of about 1000 units of purified C1 inactivator usually give a favorable clinical response within 6 h [214]. Long-term control of the disease is best accomplished with androgen derivatives [215].

FIBRONECTIN (COLD INSOLUBLE GLOBULIN)

The infusion of fibronectin (purified or as cryoprecipitates) may ameliorate the depression of opsonization following surgical or traumatic shock in patients whose fibronectin levels are also abnormally decreased [216]. The available data must be confirmed by controlled studies, and the risk of hepatitis is real.

Human immunoglobulins (immune globulin, immune serum globulin)

Human immunoglobulins (Ig) [217] are almost always prepared by cold alcohol precipitation, starting with either human plasma or human placenta. The cold alcohol method yields a product which when properly prepared is free of hepatitis virus contamination [218], but rarely hepatitis B is transmitted by such preparations [219, 220]. In the United States, Ig is now prepared from serum free of hepatitis B surface antigen [221]. The product is about 99 percent IgG, with little IgA or IgM [217]. The heavy-chain subtype distribution is similar to that found in plasma. There is some aggregation of the IgG prepared by cold ethanol fractionation.

Ig is marketed as a 16.5 ± 1.5 percent solution for intramuscular use. Ig may be administered by slow, continuous subcutaneous infusion using a portable, battery-powered pump [222,223]. The presently available material is unsatisfactory for intravenous use because of adverse reactions (see below) caused by mechanisms that are poorly understood. Complement activation due to IgG aggregates, contaminating kinin-producing enzymes, or pharmacologic effects such as release of prostaglandins have all been proposed [224–226].

In an early approach to reducing the toxicity of intravenously administered Ig, an attempt was made to reduce its capacity to bind complement in vitro. As a result, the Ig was modified chemically or proteolytically to suppress the Fc binding to C1q.

In a more recent approach, native IgG has been further purified to reduce the content of both aggregates and contaminating trace proteins, yielding products which seem as safe as the modified products but with their Fc functions intact [227,228]. It is still common to have acute reactions if the infusion rate of the 5% solutions is greater than 3 ml/min.

VARIETIES

Ig from normal sources is assumed to contain a normal spectrum of antibodies such as those present in the general population, and in order to ensure this, starting material from pools of 1000 or more donors is required.

Human Ig rich in a particular type of antibody may also be prepared from plasma obtained from patients convalescing from the disease in question or from subjects actively immunized against the appropriate antigen. Those of established efficacy are tetanus immune globulin, hepatitis B immune globulin, rabies immune globulin, measles immune globulin, vaccinia immune globulin, and $Rh_0(D)$ immune globulin.

SIDE EFFECTS OF IMMUNOGLOBULIN THERAPY

The intramuscular administration of Ig is often accompanied by local pain and tenderness; the degree and duration of these symptoms depend on the dosage given. Fever, chills, nausea, vomiting, and headache have also been observed after intramuscular administration of Ig [229]; they are thought to be due to aggregated γ-globulin. Intravenous administration of Ig is accompanied by symptoms of anxiety, flushing of the face, a feeling of constriction in the chest, muscle pain in the legs and thighs, nausea, vomiting, and, in rare instances, circulatory collapse [224,229–231]. These reactions are more common and severe in patients with Ig deficiencies.

Allotypic antibodies may develop to Ig antigens such as Gm (see Chap. 163) [232–235], and apparent hypersensitivity to Ig has also been reported [233].

As noted above, serum hepatitis is not transmitted by properly made human Ig prepared by the cold ethanol procedure but may be transmitted by preparations made from plasma from inadequately screened donors or from very small donor pools.

USE IN HEMATOLOGIC PATIENTS

REPLACEMENT IN PATIENTS WITH IMMUNOGLOBULIN DEFICIENCY

Prophylaxis In certain patients with Ig deficiencies, Ig is effective in preventing serious infections if a circulating IgG level of about 200 mg/dl is maintained, although chronic infections of the respiratory and gastrointestinal tracts may not be prevented [235]. The recommended dosage has ranged from 0.6 to 1.8 ml per kilogram body weight (100 to 300 mg/kg) administered every 3 to 4 weeks. This dosage has been limited by the quantity of Ig than can be administered intramuscularly. It may be that the higher levels achievable with an intravenous preparation will be even more effective. The biologic half-life of IgG is between 3 and 4 weeks, and the suggested interval between doses is based on this value. Clinical trials of intravenously administered modified Ig have yielded encouraging results [236–239]. The usual dose has been 100 to 150 mg per kilogram of body weight per month. In some cases much higher doses have been used [239].

Such prophylactic therapy is effective in the Bruton-type, sex-linked, congenital agammaglobulinemia, in some selective Ig deficiencies, in transient hypogammaglobulinemia of infancy, and in common varied unclassifiable immunodeficiency states (see Chap. 112).

Ig should not be given to patients with Ig deficiencies who have developed antibodies to the Ig missing from their serum [240].

Treatment When patients with Ig deficiency develop infection, they should receive Ig therapy in a dosage of 1 to 2 ml per kilogram body weight or comparable quantities of intravenous Ig.

IDIOPATHIC THROMBOCYTOPENIC PURPURA

The intravenous infusion of large amounts of Ig has been found to give an impressive and prolonged rise in the platelet count of patients with idiopathic thrombocytopenic purpura (ITP) [241–243]. After the infusion of 400 mg/kg of Ig on several successive days, many such patients respond with a platelet count greater than 100,000 per microliter. This increased platelet count can last for weeks or longer [241]. The mechanism may be interference with phagocyte Fc-receptor-mediated immune clearance [243].

PROPHYLAXIS AGAINST HEPATITIS B

Hepatitis B Ig (HBIg) provides significant protection for persons at high risk from multiple or intense exposure [244,245]. After an acute exposure, it is recommended that 0.06 ml/kg of HBIg be given within 24 h of exposure; this dose is repeated 1 month later [221,241]. With the availability of a hepatitis B vaccine, the need for repeat administration of HBIg to chronically exposed individuals may be obviated.

A special group who should receive HBIg are newborn children of antigen-positive mothers. Prompt administration of 0.5 ml of HBIg as soon after birth as possible may prevent development of the carrier state [246].

PROPHYLAXIS AGAINST HEPATITIS A

One of the clearest indications for the use of Ig is for the prevention of hepatitis A either after known exposure or during travel to an area where it is endemic. For postexposure prophylaxis, a dose of 0.02 ml/kg is recommended as soon as possible. For travel of 3 months' duration in an endemic area, 0.02 ml/kg is satisfactory, but for more prolonged exposure, up to 0.06 ml/kg is recommended. This should be repeated every 5 to 6 months as long as necessary [221].

PREVENTION OF HEMOLYTIC DISEASE OF THE NEWBORN

When administered in the postpartum period, human specific Ig anti-Rh(D) has been shown to diminish the formation of anti-Rh(D) antibodies in Rh-negative mothers of Rh-positive babies [247–250]. When administered within 72 h of delivery, doses of 300 μg or more of human specific Ig anti-Rh(D) have proved effective [251–253]. If delivery is complicated by transplacental hemorrhage of more than 30 ml of fetal blood, larger amounts of specific Ig are indicated. A dose of 10 to 25 μg of antibody per milliliter of fetal blood in the maternal circulation has been suggested as sufficient [254,255]. The amount of fetal blood in the maternal circulation can be estimated by differential staining of the red cells [248–250]. Fetal blood may also enter the maternal circulation after abortion [255,256]. Prophylaxis with anti-Rh(D) Ig is therefore recommended for Rh-negative women undergoing abortion. The incidence of sensitization of Rh-negative mothers has been reduced from 14 to 1 percent [253] using anti-$Rh_0(D)$.

The mechanisms responsible for protection following immunization are not clearly established. The principal theories are (1) the antibody blocks the D antigenic sites on the fetal cells and thereby inhibits antibody formation and (2) the administered antibody inhibits new antibody synthesis by a feedback mechanism.

References

1. Kliman, A. J., and Schwab, P. J.: Plasmapheresis with simple equipment. *Am. J. Clin. Pathol.* 36:379, 1961.
2. Simson, L. R., Lien, D. M., Warner, C. L., and Oberman, H. A.: The long-term effects of repeated plasmapheresis. *Am. J. Clin. Pathol.* 45:367, 1966.
3. Smolens, J., Stokes, J., Jr., and Vogt, A. B.: Human plasmapheresis and its effects on antibodies. *J. Immunol.* 79:434, 1957.
4. Pareira, M. D., Serkes, K. D., and Lang, S.: Enhanced efficacy of plasma after aging in treatment of tourniquet shock. *Proc. Soc. Exp. Biol. Med.* 115:660, 1964.
5. Hutchison, J. L., and Burgen, A. S. V.: Infusion of non-autologous plasma: Effects of chlorpheniramine, prednisolone, and adrenaline. *Br. Med. J.* 2:904, 1963.
6. Hutchison, J. L., Freedman, S. O., Richards, B. A., and Burgen, A. S. V.: Plasma volume expansion and reactions after infusion of autologous and non-autologous plasma in man. *J. Lab. Clin. Med.* 56:734, 1960.
7. Hillman, R. S.: Pooled human plasma as a volume expander. *N. Engl. J. Med.* 271:1027, 1964.
8. Harker, L. A., Malpass, T. W., Bronson, H. E., Hessel, E. A., and Slichter, S. J.: Mechanism of abnormal bleeding in patients undergoing cardiopulmonary bypass: Acquired transient platelet dysfunction associated with selective α-granule release. *Blood* 56:824, 1980.
9. Kirkpatrick, C. H.: Treatment of hypogammaglobulinemia with plasma transfusions, in *Immunoglobulins: Characteristics and Uses of Intravenous Preparations,* edited by B. M. Alving and J. S. Finlayson. DHHS Publication No. (FDA)-80-9005.
10. Byrnes, J. J.: Plasma infusion in the treatment of thrombotic thrombocytopenic-purpura. *Semin. Thromb. Hemostas.* 7:9, 1981.
11. Taft, E. G., and Baldwin, S. T.: Plasma exchange transfusion. *Semin. Thromb. Hemostas.* 7:15, 1981.
12. Fedenberg, H. F., Stiehm, E. R., Franklin, E. C., Meltzer, M., and Frangione, B.: Antigenicity of hereditary human gamma globulin (Gm factors): Biological and chemical aspects. *Cold Spring Harbor Sympos. Quant. Biol.* 29:463, 1964.
13. Shimizu, I., Takayame, R., Tohyama, H., and Hoshikowa, M.: Vasoconstrictor substance in preserved blood. *Commun. 8th Congr. Intl. Soc. Blood Transf.,* Tokyo, 1960.
14. Allen, J. G., Sayman, W. A., Humphreys, E. M., Benham. R. S., and Hovens, I.: Blood transfusion and hepatitis: Use of monochloracetate as an antibacterial agent in plasma. *Ann. Surg.* 150:455, 1959.
15. Redeker, A. G., Hopkins, C. E., Jackson, B., and Peck, P.: A controlled study of the safety of pooled plasma stored in the liquid state at 30–32°C for six months. *Transfusion* 8:60, 1968.

16. Murray, R., Ratner, F., Diefenbach, W. E. L., and Geller, H.: Effect of storage at room temperature on the infectivity of icterogenic plasma. *JAMA* 155:13, 1954.

17. *Proceedings of the National Red Cross Symposium on the Development of Plasma Derivatives for Clinical Use,* edited by G. A. Jamieson. *Vox Sang. (Suppl.)* 23:1, 1972.

18. Ness, P. M.: Plasma fractionation in the United States: A review for clinicians. *JAMA* 230:247, 1974.

19. Schwick, H. G.: A survey of the production of plasma derivatives for clinical use. *Vox Sang.* 23:82, 1972.

20. Sgouris, J. T.: The current status of blood fractionation in the United States. *Vox Sang.* 23:45, 1972.

21. Goldfield, M., Black, H. C., Bill, J., Srihongse, S., and Pizzuti, W.: The consequences of administering blood pretested for HBsAg by third generation techniques: A progress report. *Am. J. Med. Sci.* 270:335, 1975.

22. Maynard, J. E., and Bradley, D. W.: Transmission of non-A, non-B hepatitis by blood products and plasma derivatives, in *Non-A, Non-B Hepatitis,* edited by R. J. Gerety. Academic, New York, 1981, p. 71.

23. Richerson, H. B., and Seebohm, P. M.: Anaphylactoid reaction to human gamma globulin. *Arch. Intern. Med.* 117:568, 1966.

24. Henney, C. S., and Ellis, E. F.: Antibody production to aggregated human γ-globulin in acquired hypogammaglobulinemia. *N. Engl. J. Med.* 278:1144, 1968.

25. Ellis, E. F., and Henney, C. S.: Adverse reactions following administration of human gamma globulin. *J. Allergy* 43:45, 1969.

26. Alving, B. M., et al.: Hypotension associated with prekallikrein activator (Hageman-factor fragments) in plasma protein fractions. *N. Engl. J. Med.* 299:66, 1978.

27. Alving, B. M., Tankersley, D. L., Mason, B. L., Rossi, F., Aronson, D. L., and Finlayson, J. S.: Contact-activated factors: Contaminants of immunoglobulin preparations with coagulant and vasoactive peptides. *J. Lab. Clin. Med.* 96:334, 1980.

28. Cohn, E. J., et al.: A system in the separation of the components of human plasma. *J. Am. Chem. Soc.* 72:465, 1950.

29. Cohn, E. J., et al.: Preparation and properties of serum and plasma proteins. IV. A system for the separation into fractions of the protein and lipoprotein components of biological tissues and fluids. *J. Am. Chem. Soc.* 68:459, 1946.

30. Oncley, J. L., Melin, M., Richart, D. A., Cameron, J. W., and Gross, P. M.: The separation of the antibodies, isoagglutinins, prothrombin, plasminogen, and B₁ lipoproteins into subfractions of human plasma. *J. Am. Chem. Soc.* 71:541, 1949.

31. Curling, J. M. (ed.): *Methods of Plasma Protein Fractionation.* Academic, New York, 1980.

32. Gellis, S. S., Neefe, J. R., Stokes, J., Jr., Strong, L. E., Janeway, C. A., and Scatchard, G.: Chemical, clinical, and immunological studies on the products of human plasma fractionation. XXXVI. Inactivation of the virus of homologous serum hepatitis in solutions of normal serum albumin by means of heat. *J. Clin. Invest.* 27:239, 1948.

33. Tullis, J. H.: Albumin. I. Background and use. *JAMA* 237:355, 1977.

34. Moss, G. S.: Malabsorption associated with extreme malnutrition: Importance of replacing plasma albumin. *J. Am. Col. Nutrition* 1:89, 1982.

35. Moss, G. S., Proctor, H. J., Homer, L. D., Herman, C. M., and Litt, B. D.: A comparison of asanguineous fluids and whole blood in the treatment of hemorrhagic shock. *Surg. Gynecol. Obstet.* 129:1247, 1969.

36. Proctor, H. J., Ballantine, T. V. N., and Broussard, N. D.: An analysis of pulmonary function following non-thoracic trauma with recommendations for therapy. *Ann. Surg.* 172:180, 1970.

37. Baxter, C. R.: Crystalloid resuscitation of burn shock, in *Contemporary Burn Management,* edited by H. C. Polk. Little, Brown, Boston, 1971, p. 1.

38. Tullis, J. H.: Albumin. 2. Guidelines for clinical use. *JAMA* 237:460, 1977.

39. Jensen, H.: Plasma protein metabolism in the nephrotic syndrome in adults, in *Physiology and Pathology of Plasma Protein Metabolism,* edited by G. Birke, R. Norberg, and L. O. Plantin. Pergamon, London, 1969, p. 213.

40. Rothschild, M. A., Oratz, M., Zimmon, D., Schreiber, S. S., Weiner,

I., and Van Caneghem, A.: Albumin synthesis in cirrhotic subjects with ascites studied with carbonate-¹⁴C. *J. Clin. Invest.* 48:344, 1969.

41. Pennell, R. B.: Assessment of suitability of normal human serum albumin and of plasma protein fraction for clinical use, in *Proc. Workshop on Albumin,* edited by J. T. Sgouris and A. Rene. DHEW Publication No. (NIH) 76–925, 1975, p. 270.

42. Steere, A. C.: Adverse reactions to albumin caused by bacterial contamination, in *Proc. Workshop on Albumin,* edited by J. T. Sgouris and A. Rene. DHEW Publication No. (NIH) 76–925, 1975, p. 278.

43. Hoofnagle, J. H., and Barker, L. F.: Hepatitis B virus and albumin products, in *Proc. Workshop on Albumin,* edited by J. T. Sgouris and A. Rene. DHEW Publication No. (NIH) 76–925, 1975, p. 305.

44. Biggs, R., and Macfarlane, R. G. (eds.): *Treatment of Haemophilia and Other Coagulation Disorders.* Davis, Philadelphia, 1966.

45. Breckenridge, R. T., and Ratnoff, O. D.: Therapy of hereditary disorders of blood coagulation, in *Modern Treatment,* edited by O. D. Ratnoff. Hoeber-Harper, New York, 1968, vol. 1, p. 39.

46. Shulman, N. R.: Surgical care of patients with hereditary disorders of blood coagulation, in *Modern Treatment,* edited by O. D. Ratnoff. Hoeber-Harper, New York, 1968, vol. 5, p. 61.

47. Rizza, C. R., and Biggs, R.: The use of plasma fractions in the treatment of haemophilia and von Willebrand's disease, in *Progress in Hematology,* edited by E. B. Brown and C. V. Moore. Grune & Stratton, New York, 1969, vol. VI, p. 181.

48. Johnson, A. J., Karpatkin, M. H., and Newman, J.: Clinical investigation of intermediate- and high-purity factor VIII concentrates. *Br. J. Haematol.* 21:21, 1971.

49. Biggs, R. (ed.): *The Treatment of Haemophilia A and B and von Willebrand's disease.* Blackwell, Oxford, 1978.

50. Factor replacement therapy, in *Hemophilia in the Child and Adult,* edited by M. W. Hilgartner. Masson, Plainview, N.Y., 1982.

51. Minot, G. R., Davidson, C. S., Lewis, J. H., Tagnon, H. J., and Taylor, F. H. L.: The coagulation defect in hemophilia: The effect, in hemophilia, of parenteral administration of a fraction of the plasma globulins rich in fibrinogen. *J. Clin. Invest.* 24:704, 1945.

52. Blomback, B., and Blomback, M.: Purification of human and bovine fibrinogen. *Arkiv. Kemi* 10:415, 1956.

53. Blomback, M., and Nilsson, I. M.: Treatment of hemophilia A with human and antihemophilic globulin. *Acta Med. Scand.* 161:301, 1958.

54. Nilsson, I. M., Blomback, M., and Ramgren, O.: Haemophilia in Sweden. VI. Treatment of haemophilia A with the human antihaemophilic factor preparation (fraction 1-0). *Acta Med. Scand.* 171 *(Suppl. 379)*:61, 1962.

55. Nilsson, I. M., Blomback, M., Jorpes, E., Blomback, B., and Johannson, S.: Von Willebrand's disease and its correction with human plasma fraction 1-0. *Acta Med. Scand.* 159:179, 1957.

56. Nilsson, I. M., and Hedner, U.: Characteristics of various factor VIII concentrates used in treatment of haemophilia A. *Br. J. Haematol.* 37:543, 1977.

57. Surgenor, D. M., McMillan, C. W., Diamond, L. K., and Steel, B. B.: Studies with AHF-rich fibrinogen in classical hemophilia. *Vox Sang.* 5:80, 1960.

58. Abildgaard, C. F., Cornet, J. A., Fort, E., and Schulman, I.: The in vivo longevity of antihaemophilic factor (factor VIII). *Br. J. Haematol.* 10:225, 1964.

59. Marder, V. J., and Shulman, N. R.: Major surgery in classic hemophilia using fraction 1: Experience in twelve operations and review of the literature. *Am. J. Med.* 41:56, 1966.

60. Pool, J. G., Hershgold, E. J., and Pappenhagen, A. R.: High-potency antihemophilic factor concentrate prepared from cryoglobulin precipitate. *Nature* 203:312, 1964.

61. Pool, J. G., and Shannon, A. E.: Production of high-potency concentrates of antihemophilic globulin in a closed-bag system: Assay in vitro and in vivo. *N. Engl. J. Med.* 273:1443, 1965.

62. Kasper, C. K., Myre, B. A., McDonald, J. D., Nakasako, Y., and Feinstein, D. I.: Determinants of factor VIII recovery in cryoprecipitate. *Transfusion* 15:312, 1975.

63. Waumans, P., van Itterbeek, R., and Verstraete, M.: The preparation of a human plasma fraction by cryoprecipitation and its use in hemophilia. *Acta Clin. Belg.* 23:139, 1968.

64. Pool, J. G.: Cryoprecipitate quality and supply. *Transfusion* 15:305, 1975.

65. Burka, E. R., Harker, L. A., Kasper, C. K., Levy, S. V., and Ness, P. M.: A protocol for cryoprecipitate production. *Transfusion* 15:307, 1975.

66. Burka, E. R., Puffer, T., and Martinez, J.: The influence of donor characteristics and preparation methods on the potency of human cryoprecipitate. *Transfusion* 15:323, 1975.

67. Johnson, A. J., Newman, J., Howell, M. B., and Puszkin, S.: Purification of antihemophilic factor (AHF) for clinical and experimental use. *Thromb. Diath. Haemorrh. (Suppl.)* 26:377, 1967.

68. Newman, J., Johnson, A. J., Karpatkin, M. H., and Puszkin, S.: Methods for the production of clinically effective intermediate- and high-purity factor VIII concentrates. *Br. J. Haematol.* 21:1, 1971.

69. James, H. L., and Wickerhauser, M.: Development of large-scale fractionation methods. III. Preparation of a factor VIII concentrate of intermediate purity. *Vox Sang.* 23:402, 1972.

70. Hagan, J. J., and Glaser, C.: Antihemophilic factor. U.S. patent 3,973,002, 1976, assigned to E. R. Squibb and Sons, Inc., Princeton, N.J.

71. Webster, W. P., Roberts, H. R., Thelin, G. M., Wagner, R. H., and Brinkhous, K. M.: Clinical use of a new glycine-precipitated antihemophilic fraction. *Am. J. Med. Sci.* 250:643, 1965.

72. Wagner, R. H., Langdell, R. D., Richardson, B. A., Farrell, R. A., and Brinkhous, K. M.: Antihemophilic factor (AHF): Plasma levels after administration of AHF preparations to hemophilic dogs. *Proc. Soc. Exp. Biol. Med.* 96:152, 1957.

73. Pool, J. G., Welton, J., and Creger, W. P.: Ineffectiveness of intramuscularly injected factor VIII concentrate in two hemophilic patients. *N. Engl. J. Med.* 275:547, 1966.

74. Brinkhous, K. M., Shanbrom, E., Webster, W. P., Roberts, H. R., Fekete, L., and Wagner, R. H.: A high-potency glycine-precipitated antihemophilic factor concentrate: Use in hemophilia and hemophilia with inhibitors. *Blood* 30:855, 1967 (abstract).

75. Brinkhous, K. M., Shanbrom, E., Roberts, H. R., Webster, W. P., Fekete, L., and Wagner, R. H.: A new high-potency glycine-precipitated antihemophilic factor (AHF) concentrate: Treatment of classical hemophilia and hemophilia with inhibitors. *JAMA* 205:613, 1968.

76. Fekete, L. F., and Holst, L.: Stabilization of AHF using heparin. U.S. patent No. 3,803,115, April 9, 1974, assigned to Baxter Laboratories, Inc., Morton Grove, Ill.

77. Levine, P. H., McVerry, B. A., Attock, B., and Dormandy, K. M.: Health of the intensively treated hemophiliac, with special reference to abnormal liver chemistries and splenomegaly. *Blood* 50:1, 1977.

78. Lewis, J. H., Maxwell, N. G., and Brandon, J. M.: Jaundice and hepatitis B antigen antibody in hemophilia. *Transfusion* 14:203, 1974.

79. Hilgartner, H. W., and Giardina, P.: Liver dysfunction in patients with hemophilia A, B and von Willebrand's disease. *Transfusion* 17:495, 1977.

80. Hasibu, U., Spero, J. A., and Lewis, J. H.: Chronic liver dysfunction in multi-transfused hemophiliacs. *Transfusion* 17:490, 1977.

81. Cederbaum, A. I., Blatt, P. M., and Levine, P. H.: Abnormal serum transaminase levels in patients with hemophilia A. *Arch. Intern. Med.* 142:481, 1982.

82. Lesene, H. R., Morgan, J. E., Blatt, P. M., Webster, W. P., and Roberts, H. R.: Liver biopsy in hemophilia A. *Ann. Intern. Med.* 86:703, 1977.

83. Mannucci, P. M., Ronchi, G., Rota, L., and Colombo, M.: Liver biopsy in hemophilia. *Ann. Intern. Med.* 88:429, 1978.

84. Spero, J. A., Lewis, J. H., Van Thiel, D. H., Hasibu, U., and Rabin, B. S.: Asymptomatic structural liver disease in hemophilia. *N. Engl. J. Med.* 298:1373, 1978.

85. Schimpf, K. L., et al.: Hepatitis histology and serological findings in 22 patients with severe hemophilia A, hemophilia B and factor VII deficiency: Results of 25 biopsies. *XVII Congress of the International Society of Hematology,* 1978, p. 212 (abstract).

86. Preston, E. E., et al.: Percutaneous liver biopsy and chronic liver disease in haemophiliacs. *Lancet* 2:592, 1978.

87. Heimburger, N., Schwinn, H., and Mouler, R.: Factor VIII-Konzentrat, hepatitissicher: Fortschritte in der behandlung der hamophilie A. *Die Gelben Hefte* 4:165, 1980.

88. Seeler, R. A.: Hemolysis due to anti-A and anti-B with intensive therapy in hemophilia, in *Proceedings of a Workshop on Unsolved Therapeutic Problems in Hemophilia,* edited by J. Fratantoni and D. Aronson. U.S. Government Printing Office, Bethesda, 1976, p. 113.

89. Aledort, L. M., Taub, S., and Diaz, M.: Problems of anti-A and anti-B in concentrates, in *Hemophilia in the Child and Adult,* edited by M. W. Hilgartner. Masson, Plainview, N.Y., 1982, p. 181.

90. Johnson, A. J., et al.: Preparation of the major plasma fractions by solid-phase polyelectrolytes. *J. Lab. Clin. Med.* 92:194, 1978.

91. Tuddenham, E. D. G., et al.: Response to infusions of polyelectrolyte fractionated human factor VIII concentrate in human haemophilia A and von Willebrand's disease. *Brit. J. Haematol.* 52:259, 1982.

92. Bidwell, E.: The purification of bovine antihaemophilic globulin. *Br. J. Haematol.* 1:35, 1955.

93. Bidwell, E.: The purification of antihaemophilic globulin from animal plasma. *Br. J. Haematol.* 1:386, 1955.

94. Middleton, S. M., Fulton, A. J., Costello, W. P., Watson, C. N., and Johnson, A. J.: Preparation of a therapeutic porcine factor VIII concentrate using solid phase polyelectrolyte. Abstract 808, Joint Meeting of the XVIII Congress of the International Society of Hemophilia and XVI Congress of the International Society of Blood Transfusion, Montreal, 1980.

95. Heath, D.: Highly purified porcine factor VIII in hemophilia A with inhibitors to factor VIII. *Br. Med. J.* 282:654, 1981 (letter).

96. Kernoff, P. B. A., Thomas, N. D., Lilley, P. A., and Tuddenham, E. G. D.: Polyelectrolyte fractionated porcine factor VIII concentrate in the treatment of haemophiliacs with antibodies to factor VIII:C. VIII Internat. Congress on Thrombosis and Haemostasis, Toronto, 1981 (abstract).

97. Biggs, R. (ed.): *Human Blood Coagulation, Haemostasis and Thrombosis.* Blackwell, Oxford, 1976.

98. Hilgartner, M.: Hemophilic arthropathy. *Adv. Pediatr.* 21:139, 1974.

99. Biggs, R.: Assay of antihaemophilic globulin in treatment of haemophilic patients. *Lancet* 2:311, 1957.

100. Douglas, A. S.: Antihemophilic globulin assay following plasma infusions in hemophilia. *J. Lab. Clin. Med.* 51:850, 1958.

101. Biggs, R., and Denson, K. W.: The fate of prothrombin and factors VIII, IX and X transfused to patients deficient in these factors. *Br. J. Haematol.* 9:532, 1963.

102. Shulman, N. R., Marder, V. J., and Hiller, M. C.: A new method for measuring minimum in vivo concentrationis of factor VIII applied in distribution and survival studies and in detecting factor VIII inhibitors, in *The Hemophilias,* edited by K. M. Brinkhous. University of North Carolina Press, Chapel Hill, 1964, p. 29.

103. Karpatkin, M. H., and Karpatkin, S.: In vivo and in vitro binding of factor VIII to human platelets. *Thromb. Diath. Haemorrh.* 21:130, 1969.

104. Webster, W. P., Reddick, R. L., Roberts, H. R., and Penick, G. D.: Release of factor VIII (antihaemophilic factor) from perfused organs and tissues. *Nature* 213:1146, 1967.

105. Gray, S. J., and Frank H.: The simultaneous determination of red cell mass and plasma volume in man with radioactive sodium chromate and chromic chloride. *J. Clin. Invest.* 32:1000, 1953.

106. Biggs, R., and Macfarlane, R. G.: *Human Blood Coagulation and Its Disorders,* 3d ed. Davis, Philadelphia, 1962, p. 73.

107. Shapiro, S. S., and Hultin, M.: Acquired inhibitors to the blood coagulation factors. *Semin. Thromb. Hemostas.* 1:336, 1975.

108. Allain, M. P., and Frommel, D.: Antibodies to factor VIII: Specificity and kinetics of iso- and hetero-antibodies in hemophilia A. *Blood* 44:313, 1974.

109. Kasper, C. K.: Incidence and course of inhibitors among patients with classic hemophilia. *Thromb. Diath. Haemorrh.* 30:263, 1973.

110. Strauss, H. S.: Acquired circulating anticoagulants in hemophilia A. *N. Engl. J. Med.* 281:866, 1969.

111. Blatt, P. M., White, G. C., McMillan, C. W., and Roberts, H. R.: Treatment of anti-factor VIII antibodies. *Thromb. Haemost.* 38:514, 1977.

112. Nilsson, I. M., Hedner, U., and Holmberg, L.: Suppression of factor VIII antibody by combined factor VIII and cyclophosphamide. *Acta Med. Scand.* 195:75, 1975.

113. Dormandy, K. M., and Sultan, Y.: Suppression of factor VIII antibodies in haemophilia. *Pathol. Biol.* 23:17, 1975.

114. Kasper, C. K., et al.: A more uniform measurement of factor VIII inhibitors. *Thromb. Diath. Haemorrh.* 34:869, 1975.

115. Pool, J. G., and Miller, R. G.: Assay of the immune inhibitor in classic haemophilia: Application of virus-antibody kinetics. *Br. J. Haematol.* 22:517, 1972.

116. Roberts, H. R.: Hemophiliacs with inhibitors: Therapeutic options. *N. Engl. J. Med.* 305:757, 1981.

117. Shapiro, S. S.: Antibodies to blood coagulations factors. *Clinics in Hematology* 8:207, 1979.

118. Abildgaard, C. F.: Management of inhibitors in hemophilia, in *Hemophilia in the Child and Adult*, edited by M. W. Hilgartner. Masson, Plainview, N.Y., 1982.

119. Patek, A. J., and Taylor, F. H. L.: Hemophilia: Some properties of a substance obtained from normal human plasma effective in accelerating the coagulation of hemophilic blood. *J. Clin. Invest.* 16:113, 1937.

120. Macfarlane, R. G., Biggs, R., and Bidwell, E.: Bovine antihaemophilic globulin in the treatment of haemophilia. *Lancet* 1:1316, 1954.

121. Macfarlane, R. G., et al.: Surgery in hemophilia: The use of animal AHG and human plasma in 13 cases. *Lancet* 2:251, 1957.

122. Forbes, C. D., Barr, R. D., McNicol, G. P., and Douglas, A. S.: Aggregation of human platelets by commercial preparations of bovine and porcine AHF. *J. Clin. Path.* 25:210, 1972.

123. Lee, H. H., Macdonald, V. E., Semar, M., Brind, J., and Johnson, A. J.: The use of solid-phase polyelectrolyte (PE) for the preparation of a porcine factor VIII concentrate. XVIIth Congress International. Society of Hematology, Paris, 1978 (abstract).

124. Heath, D., Middleton, S. M., Williams, D. R., and Costello, W. P.: A new generation of factor VIII:C concentrates. XIVth Congress of the World Federation of Hemophilia, Costa Rica, 1981 (abstract).

125. Mayne, E. E., Madden, M., Crothers, I. S., and Ingles, T.: Highly purified porcine factor VIII in hemophilia A with inhibitors to factor VIII. *Br. Med. J.* 282:318, 1981 (letter).

126. Kernoff, P. B. A., Thomas, N. D., Mathews, K. B., and Tuddenham, E. G. D.: Dose response relationships and the immunogenicity of porcine factor VIII. Proceedings of the British Society of Haematology, London, 1982 (abstract).

127. Kernoff, P. B. A., Thomas, N. D., Lilley, P. A., and Tuddenham, E. G. D.: Clinical experience with polyelectrolyte-fractionated porcine factor VIII concentrate in the treatment of hemophiliacs with antibodies to factor VIII. Proceedings of the 22nd Annual General Meeting of the British Society of Haematology, Sheffield, 1981 (abstract).

128. Levine, P. H.: Delivery of health care in hemophilia. *Ann. N.Y. Acad. Sci.* 240:201, 1975.

129. Fahle, V.: Source Plasma Industry Statistical Report 1979. *Plasma Quarterly* 3:68, 1981.

130. Eyster, M. E., and Haverstick, J.: Annual report of Harrisburg-Hershey Hemophilia Center of the Commonwealth of Pennsylvania Hemophilia Program, 1975.

131. Levine, P. H.: Efficacy of self-therapy in hemophilia: A study of 72 patients with hemophilia A and B. *N. Engl. J. Med.* 291:1381, 1974.

132. Eyster, M. E.: Home therapy programs, in *Hemophilia in the Child and Adult*, edited by M. W. Hilgartner. Masson, Plainview, N.Y., 1982.

133. Kasper, C. K., Dietrich, S. L., and Rapaport, S. I.: Hemophilia prophylaxis with factor VIII concentrates. *Arch. Intern. Med.* 125:1004, 1970.

134. Lazerson, J.: Hemophilia home transfusion programs: Effect of cryoprecipitate utilization. *J. Pediatr.* 82:857, 1973.

135. Rabiner, S. F., and Telfer, M. C.: Home transfusion for patients with hemophilia A. *N. Engl. J. Med.* 283:1011, 1970.

136. Rabiner, S. F., and Lazerson, J.: Home management and prophylaxis of hemophilia. *Prog. Hematol.* 8:223, 1973.

137. Van Eys, J., Agle, D. P., Hilgartner, M., and Lazerson, J.: *Home Therapy for Hemophilia.* National Hemophilia Foundation Medical and Scientific Advisory Council, 1974.

138. Hilgartner, M. W., and Sergis, R. N.: Current therapy for hemophiliacs: Home care and therapeutic complications. *Mt. Sinai J. Med.* 44:316, 1977.

139. Fajardo, R. A.: Psychosocial aspects of hemophilia, in *Symposium on Hemophilia*, edited by D. Green. Charles C Thomas, Springfield, Ill., 1973, p. 62.

140. Levine, P. H.: Personal communication, 1982.

141. Alter, H. J., Barker, L. F., and Holland, P. V.: Hepatitis B immune globulin: Evaluation of clinical trials and rationale for usage. *N. Engl. J. Med.* 293:1093, 1975.

142. Hoofnagle, J. H., Gerety, R. J., Thiel, J., and Barker, L.: The prevalence of hepatitis B surface antigen in commercially prepared plasma products. *J. Lab. Clin. Med.* 88:102, 1976.

143. Koretz, and Gitnick, G.: Prevention of post-transfusion hepatitis: Role of sensitive hepatitis B antigen screening tests, source of blood and volume of transfusion. *Am. J. Med.* 59:754, 1975.

144. Kasper, C. K., and Kipnis, S. A.: Hepatitis and clotting factor concentrates. *JAMA* 221:510, 1972.

145. Biggs, R.: Jaundice and antibodies directed against factors VIII and IX treated for haemophilia or Christmas disease in the United Kingdom. *Br. J. Haematol.* 26:313, 1974.

146. Craske, J., Dilling, N., and Stern, D.: An out break of hepatitis associated with intravenous injection of factor VIII concentrate. *Lancet* 2:221, 1975.

147. Myers, T. J., Tembrevilla-Zubin, C. L., Klatsky, A. U., and Rickles, F. R.: Recurrent acute hepatitis following the use of factor VIII concentrates. *Blood* 55:748, 1980.

148. Nilsson, I. M., Blomback, M., and von Francken, I.: On an inherited autosomal hemorrhagic diathesis with antihemophilia globulin (AHG) deficiency and prolonged bleeding time. *Acta Med. Scand.* 159:35, 1957.

149. Cornu, P., Larrieu, M.-J., Caen, J., and Bernard, J.: Transfusion studies in von Willebrand's disease: Effect on bleeding time and factor VIII. *Br. J. Haematol.* 9:189, 1963.

150. Larrieu, M.-J., Caen, J. P., Meyer, D. O., Vainer, H., Sultan, Y., and Bernard, J.: Congenital bleeding disorders with long bleeding time and normal platelet count. II. Von Willebrand's disease (report of thirty-seven patients). *Am. J. Med.* 43:354, 1968.

151. Bowie, E. J. W., Didisheim, P., Thompson, J. H., Jr., and Owen, C. A.: Von Willebrand's disease: A critical review. *Hematol. Rev.* 1:1, 1968.

152. Muntz, R. H., Ekert, H., and Helliger, H.: Properties of post-infusion factor VIII in von Willebrand's disease. *Thromb. Res.* 5:111, 1974.

153. Weiss, H. J., Hoyer, L. W., Rickles, F. R., Varma, A., and Rogers, J.: Quantitative assay of a plasma factor, deficient in von Willebrand's disease, that is necessary for platelet aggregation: Relationship to factor VIII procoagulant activity and antigen content. *J. Clin. Invest.* 52:2708, 1973.

154. Nilsson, I. M., and Hedner, U.: Characteristics of various factor VIII concentrates used in treatment of haemophilia A. *Br. J. Haematol.* 37:543, 1977.

155. Nilsson, I. M., Holmberg, L., Stenberg, P., and Henriksson, P.: Characteristics of the factor VIII protein and factor XIII in various factor VIII concentrates. *Scand. J. Haematol.* 24:340, 1980.

156. Holmberg, L., Borge, L., and Nilsson, I. M.: Factor VIII:C and VIII:CAg response in patients with haemophilia A and von Willebrand's disease after administration of different factor VIII concentrates or plasma. *Br. J. Haematol.* 47:587, 1981.

157. Perkins, H. A.: Correction of the hemostatic defect in von Willebrand's disease. *Blood* 30:375, 1967.

158. Green, D., and Potter, E. V.: Failure of AHF concentrate to control bleeding in von Willebrand's disease. *Am. J. Med.* 60:357, 1976.

159. Blatt, P. M., Brinkhous, K. M., Culp, H. R., Krauss, J. S., and Roberts, H. R.: Antihemophilic factor concentrate therapy in von Willebrand disease: Dissociation of bleeding time factor and ristocetin-cofactor activities. *JAMA* 236:2770, 1976.

160. Sakariassen, K. S., Bolhuis, P. A., and Sixma, J. J.: Human blood platelet adhesion to artery subendothelium is mediated by factor

VIII-von Willebrand factor bound to subendothelium. *Nature* 279:636, 1979.

161. Bolhuis, P. A., Sakariassen, K. S., Sander, H. J., Bouma, B. N., and Sixma, J. J.: Binding of factor VIII-von Willebrand factor to human arterial subendothelium precedes increased platelet adhesion and enhances platelet spreading. *J. Lab. Clin. Med.* 97:568, 1981.

162. Zucker, M. B.: In vitro abnormality of the blood in von Willebrand's disease correctable by normal plasma. *Nature* 197:601, 1963.

163. Ruggeri, Z. M., Mannucci, P. M., Lombardi, R., Federici, A. B., and Zimmerman, T. S.: Multimeric composition of factor VIII/von Willebrand factor following administration of DDAVP: Implications for pathophysiology and therapy of von Willebrand's disease subtypes. *Blood* 59:1272 1982.

164. Martin, S. E., Marder, V. J., Francis, C. W., and Barlow, G. H.: Structural studies on the functional heterogeneity of von Willebrand protein polymers. *Blood* 57:313, 1981.

165. Johnson, A. J.: Unpublished observations, 1976.

166. Nilsson, I. M., Blomback, M., and Blomback, B.: Von Willebrand's disease with special reference to a plasmatic factor necessary for hemostasis. Proceedings of the 8th Congress of the European Society of Haematology, 1961, p. 354.

167. Bennett, E., and Dormandy, K.: Pool's cryoprecipitate and exhausted plasma in the treatment of von Willebrand's disease and factor XI-deficiency. *Lancet* 2:731, 1966.

168. Meili, E. O., Straub, P. W., and Frick, P. G.: Zur Pathogenese und Behandlung der von Willebrandschen Krankheit. *Schweiz. Med. Wochenschr.* 99:1805, 1969.

169. Weiss, H. J., and Rogers, J.: Correction of the platelet abnormality in von Willebrand's disease by cryoprecipitate. *Am. J. Med.* 53:734, 1972.

170. Dike, G. W. R., Bidwell, E., and Rizza, C. R.: The preparation and clinical use of a new concentrate containing factor IX, prothrombin and factor X and of a separate concentrate containing factor VII. *Br. J. Haematol.* 22:469, 1972.

171. Tullis, J. L., Melin, M., and Jurigian, P.: Clinical use of prothrombin complexes. *N. Engl. J. Med.* 273:667, 1965.

172. Middleton, S. M., Bennett, I. H., and Smith, J. K.: A therapeutic concentrate of coagulation factors II, IX and X from citrated factor VIII-depleted plasma. *Vox Sang.* 24:441, 1973.

173. Heystek, J., Brummelhuis, H. G. J., and Krijnan, H. W.: Contributions to the optimal use of blood. II. The large scale preparation of prothrombin complex: A comparison between two methods using the anion exchangers DEAE-cellulose DE-52 and DEAE Sephadex A-50. *Vox Sang.* 25:113, 1973.

174. Zauber, N. P., and Levin, J.: Factor IX levels in patients with hemophilia B (Christmas disease) following transfusion with concentrates of factor IX or fresh frozen plasma (FFP). *Medicine (Baltimore)* 56:213, 1977.

175. Smith, K. J., and Thompson, A. R.: Labeled factor IX kinetics in patients with hemophilia B. *Blood* 58:625, 1981.

176. Hoag, M. S., Johnson, F. F., Robinson, J. A., and Aggeler, P. M.: Treatment of hemophilia B with a new clotting factor concentrate. *N. Engl. J. Med.* 280:581, 1969.

177. Marder, V. J., and Shulman, R. R.: Clinical aspects of congenital factor VII deficiency. *Am. J. Med.* 37:182, 1964.

178. Menache, D.: The turnover rate of coagulation factors II, VII and IX under normal metabolic conditions. *Thromb. Diath. Haemorrh. (Suppl.)* 13:187, 1963.

179. Graham, J. B.: Stuart clotting defect and Stuart factor. *Thromb. Diath. Haemorrh. (Suppl.)* 1:22, 1960.

180. Roberts, H. R., Lechler, E., Webster, W. P., and Penick, G. D.: Survival of transfused factor X in patients with Stuart disease. *Thromb. Diath. Haemorrh.* 13:305, 1965.

181. Shapiro, S. S., and Martinez, J.: Human prothrombin metabolism in normal men and in hypocoagulable subjects. *J. Clin. Invest.* 48:1292, 1969.

182. Green, G., Bymock, I. W., Poller, L., and Thompson, J.: Use of factor VII–rich prothrombin complex concentrate in liver disease. *Lancet* 1:1311, 1975.

183. Sandler, S. G., Rath, C. E., and Ruder, A.: Prothrombin complex concentrate in acquired hypoprothrombinemia. *Ann. Intern. Med.* 79:485, 1973.

184. Lusher, J. M., Shapiro, S. S., Palascak, J. E., Rao, A. V., Levine, P. H., and Blatt, P. M.: Efficacy of prothrombin-complex concentrates in hemophiliacs with antibodies to factor VIII. *N. Engl. J. Med.* 303:421, 1980.

185. Fekete, L., Holst, S. L., Petoom, F., and de Veber, L. L.: Autofactor IX concentrate: A new approach to treatment of hemophilia A patients with inhibitor. XIV Congress of the International Society of Haematology, São Paulo, 1972 (abstract).

186. Kingdon, H. S., and Hassell, T. M.: Hemophilic dog model for evaluating therapeutic effectiveness of plasma protein fractions. *Blood* 58:868, 1981.

187. Hultin, M. B.: Activated clotting factors in factor IX concentrates. *Blood* 54:1028, 1979.

188. Seligsohn, U., Kasper, C. K., Østerud, B., and Rapaport, S. I.: Activated factor VII: Presence in factor IX concentrates and persistence in the circulation after infusion. *Blood* 53:828, 1979.

189. Barrowcliffe, T. W., Kemball-Cook, G., and Gray, E.: Factor VIII inhibitor bypassing activity: A suggested mechanism of action. *Thromb. Res.* 21:181, 1981.

190. Aronson, D. L., and Bagley, J.: Characterization of the in vivo factor VIII bypassing activity. *Thromb. Haemost.* 46:687, 1981 (abstract).

191. Sjamsoedin, L. J. M., et al.: The effect of activated prothrombin complex on joint and muscle bleeding in patients with hemophilia A and antibodies to factor VIII. *N. Engl. J. Med.* 305:717, 1981.

192. Faria, R., and Fiamara, N. J.: Hepatitis associated with Konyne. *N. Engl. J. Med.* 287:358, 1972.

193. Boklan, B. F.: Factor IX concentrate and viral hepatitis. *Ann. Intern. Med.* 74:298, 1971.

194. Roberts, H. R., and Blatt, P. M.: Post transfusion hepatitis following the use of prothrombin complex concentrates. *Thromb. Diath. Haemorrh.* 33:610, 1975.

195. Hoofnagle, J. H., Aronson, D. L., and Roberts, H. R.: Serologic evidence for hepatitis B virus infection in patients with hemophilia B. *Thromb. Diath. Haemorrh.* 33:606, 1975.

196. Wyke, R. J., et al.: Transmission of non-A, non-B hepatitis to chimpanzees by factor IX concentrates after fatal complications in patients with chronic liver disease. *Lancet* 1:520, 1979.

197. Kasper, C. K.: Post-operative thrombosis in hemophilia B. *N. Engl. J. Med.* 289:610, 1973.

198. Kingdon, H. S., Lundblad, R. L., Veltkamp, J. J., and Aronson, D. L.: Potentially thrombogenic material in prothrombin complex concentrates. *Thromb. Diath. Haemorrh.* 33:617, 1975.

199. Giles, A. R., Nesheim, N. E., Hoogendorn, H., Tracy, P. B., and Mann, K. G.: The coagulant-active phospholipid content is a major determinant of in vivo thrombogenicity of prothrombin complex (factor IX) concentrates in rabbits. *Blood* 59:401, 1982.

200. Hammond, J. D. S., and Verel, D.: Observations on the distribution and biological half-life of human fibrinogen. *Br. J. Haematol.* 5:431, 1959.

201. Al-Mondhiry, H.: Disseminated intravascular coagulation: Experience in a major cancer center. *Thromb. Diath. Haemorrh.* 34:181, 1975.

202. Tytgat, G. N., Collen, D., and Vermylen, J.: Metabolism and distribution of fibrinogen. II. Fibrinogen turnover in polycythemia, thrombocytosis, haemophilia A, congenital afibrinogenaemia and during streptokinase therapy. *Br. J. Haematol.* 22:701, 1972.

203. Bove, J. R.: Fibrinogen: Is the benefit worth the risk? *Transfusion* 18:129, 1978.

204. Borchgrevink, C. F., and Owren, P. A.: Surgery in a patient with factor V (proaccelerin) deficiency. *Acta Med. Scand.* 170:743, 1961.

205. Rush, B., and Ellis, H.: The treatment of patients with factor-V deficiency. *Thromb. Diath. Haemorrh.* 14:74, 1965.

206. Webster, W. P., Roberts, H. R., and Penick, G. D.: Hemostasis in factor V deficiency. *Am. J. Med. Sci.* 248:194, 1964.

207. Prentice, C. R. M., and Ratnoff, O. D.: Genetic disorders of blood coagulation. *Semin. Hematol.* 4:93, 1967.

208. Rosenthal, R. L., and Sloan, E.: PTA (factor XI) levels and coagulation studies after plasma infusions in PTA-deficient patients. *J. Lab. Clin. Med.* 66:709, 1965.

209. Rosenthal, R. L.: Plasma therapy in factor XI (PTA) deficient patients undergoing surgery. *Transfusion* 7:383, 1967 (abstract).

210. Nossel, H. L., Niemetz, J., Mibashan, R. S., and Schulze, W. G.: The measurement of factor XI (plasma thromboplastic antecedent): Diagnosis and therapy of the congenital deficiency state. *Br. J. Haematol.* 12:133, 1966.

211. Rapaport, S. I., Schiffman, S., Patch, M. J., and Ware, A. G.: A simple, specific one-stage assay for plasma thromboplastin antecedent: Diagnosis and therapy of the congenital deficiency state. *Br. J. Haematol.* 12:133, 1966.

212. Horowitz, H. I., and Fujimoto, M. M.: Survival of factor XI in vitro and in vivo. *Transfusion* 5:539, 1965.

213. Kitchens, C. S., and Newcomb, T. F.: Factor XIII. *Medicine* 58:413, 1979.

214. Gadek, J. E., et al.: Replacement therapy in hereditary angioedema. *N. Engl. J. Med.* 302:542, 1980.

215. Gelfand, J. A., Sherins, R. J., Alling, D. W., and Frank, M. M.: Treatment of hereditary angioedema with danazol: Reversal of clinical and biochemical abnormalities. *N. Engl. J. Med.* 295:1444, 1976.

216. Robbins, A. B., Doran, J. E., Reese, A. C., and Mansberger, A. R., Jr.: Cold insoluble globulin levels in operative trauma: Serum depletion, wound sequestration, and biological activity: An experimental and clinical study. *Am. Surgeon* 46:663, 1981.

217. Finlayson, J. S.: Immune globulins. *Semin. Thromb. Hemostas.* 6:44, 1979.

218. Murray, R., and Ratner, F.: Safety of immune serum globulin with respect to homologous serum hepatitis. *Proc. Soc. Exp. Biol. Med.* 83:554, 1953.

219. John, T. J., et al.: Epidemic hepatitis B caused by commercial human immunoglobulin. *Lancet* 1:1074, 1979.

220. Patrilli, F. O., Crovari, P., and de Flora, S.: Hepatitis B in subjects treated with a drug containing immunoglobulins. *J. Infect. Dis.* 135:252, 1977.

221. Immune globulins for protection against viral hepatitis. *MMWR* 30:423, 1981.

222. Berger, M., Cupps, T. R., and Fauci, A. S.: Immunoglobulin replacement therapy by slow subcutaneous infusion. *Ann. Intern. Med.* 93:55, 1980.

223. Berger, M., Cupps, T. R., and Fauci, A. S.: High-dose immunoglobulin replacement therapy by slow subcutaneous infusion during pregnancy. *JAMA* 247:2824, 1982.

224. Barandun, S., Kistler, P., Jeunet, F., and Isliker, H.: Intravenous administration of human γ-globulin. *Vox Sang.* 7:157, 1962.

225. Alving, B. M., Tankersley, D. L., Mason, B. L., Rossi, F., Aronson, D. L., and Finlayson, J. S.: Contact-activated factors: Contaminants of immunoglobulin preparations with coagulant and vasoactive properties. *J. Lab. Clin. Med.* 96:334, 1980.

226. Passwell, J., Rosen, F. S., and Merler, E.: The effect of Fc fragments of IgG on human mononuclear cell responses, in *Immunoglobulins: Characteristics and Uses of Intravenous Preparations,* edited by B. M. Alving and J. S. Finlayson. DHHS Publication No. (FDA)-80-9005, p. 139.

227. Romer, J., Morgenthaler, J. J., Scherz, R., and Skvaril, F.: Characterization of various immunoglobulin preparations for intravenous application. I. Protein composition and antibody content. *Vox Sang.* 42:62, 1982.

228. Romer, J., Spath, P. J., Skvaril, F., and Nydegger, U. E.: Characterization of various immunoglobulin preparations for intravenous application. II. Complement activation and binding to Staphylococcus protein A. *Vox Sang.* 42:74, 1982.

229. Kleinman, P. K., and Weksler, M. E.: Repeated reactions following intramuscular injection of gamma globulin. *J. Pediatr.* 83:827, 1973.

230. Moore, G. E., Sandberg, A., and Amos, D. B.: Experimental and clinical adventures with large doses of gamma and other globulins as anticancer agents. *Surgery* 41:972, 1957.

231. Coon, W. W., Iob, V., Wolfman, E. F., Jr., Hodgson, P. E., and McMath, M.: Experiences with large infusions of γ-globulin. *Am. J. Surg.* 102:548, 1961.

232. Allen, J. C., and Kunkel. H. G.: Antibodies to genetic types of gamma globulin after multiple transfusions. *Science* 139:419, 1963.

233. Stiehm, E. R., and Fudenberg, H. H. S.: Antibodies to gamma globulin in infants and children exposed to isologous gamma globulin. *Pediatrics* 35:229, 1965.

234. Fudenberg, H. H.: Sensitization to immunoglobulins and hazards of immunoglobulin therapy, in *Immunoglobulins,* edited by E. Merley. National Academy of Sciences, Washington, D.C., 1970, p. 211.

235. Janeway, C. A., and Rosen, F. S.: The gamma globulins. IV. Therapeutic uses of gamma globulin. *N. Engl. J. Med.* 275:826, 1966.

236. Nolte, M. T., Pirofsky, B., Gerritz, G. A., and Golding, B.: Intravenous immunoglobulin therapy for antibody deficiency. *Clin. Exp. Immunol.* 36:237, 1979.

237. Ochs, H. D., et al.: Safety and patient acceptability of intravenous immune globulin in 10% maltose. *Lancet* 2:1158, 1980.

238. Yamanaka, T., et al.: Clinical effect and metabolism of S-sulfonated immunoglobulin in 7 patients with congenital humoral immunodeficiency. *Vox Sang.* 37:14, 1979.

239. Barandun, S., Morell, A., and Skvaril, F.: Clinical experiences with immunoglobulin for intravenous use, in *Immunoglobulins: Characteristics and Uses of Intravenous Preparations,* edited by B. M. Alving, and J. S. Finlayson. U.S. Department of Health and Human Services, 1980, p. 31.

240. Immunodeficiency. Report of a WHO Scientific Group. *Clin. Immunol. Immunopath.* 13:296, 1979.

241. Imbach, P., et al.: High-dose intravenous gammaglobulin for idiopathic thrombocytopenic purpura in childhood. *Lancet* 1:1228, 1981.

242. Schmidt, R. E., Budde, U., Schafer, G., and Stroehmann, I.: High-dose intravenous gammaglobulin for idiopathic thrombocytopenic purpura. *Lancet* 2:475, 1981 (letter).

243. Fehr, J., Hofmann, V., and Kappeler, U.: Transient reversal of thrombocytopenia in idiopathic thrombocytopenic purpura by high-dose intravenous gamma globulin. *N. Engl. J. Med.* 306:1254, 1982.

244. Maynard, J. E.: Passive immunization against hepatitis B.: A review of recent studies and comment on current aspects of control. *Am. J. Epidemiol.* 107:77, 1978.

245. Seeff, L. B., and Hoofnagle, J. H.: Immunoprophylaxis of viral hepatitis. *Gastroenterology* 77:161, 1979.

246. Stevens, C. E., et al.: Perinatal hepatitis B virus infection: Use of hepatitis B immune globulin, in *Viral Hepatitis,* edited by W. Szmuness, H. Alter, and J. E. Maynard. Franklin Institute Press, Philadelphia, 1982, p. 527.

247. Freda, V. J., Gorman, J. G., and Pollack, W.: Rh factor: Prevention of isoimmunization and clinical trial on mothers. *Science* 151:828, 1966.

248. Clarke, C. A.: Prevention of Rhesus iso-immunization. *Semin. Hematol.* 6:201, 1969.

249. Woodrow, J. C.: Rh immunization and its prevention. *Ser. Haematol.* 3(3):1, 1970.

250. Zipursky, A.: The universal prevention of Rh immunization. *Clin. Obstet. Gynecol.* 14:869, 1971.

251. Finn, R.: Liverpool experience with Rh immunoglobulin. *Transfusion* 8:148, 1968.

252. Pollack, W., Gorman, J. G., Freda, V. J., Ascari, W. Q., Allen, A. E., and Baker, W. J.: Results of clinical trials with RhoGAM in women. *Transfusion* 8:151, 1968.

253. Freda, V. J., Gorman, J. G., and Pollack, W.: Prevention of Rh-hemolytic disease with Rh-immune globulin. *Am. J. Obstet. Gynecol.* 128:456, 1977.

254. Bowman, J. M., and Chown, B.: Prevention of Rh immunization after massive transfusion. *Can. Med. Assoc. J.* 99:385, 1968.

255. Bowman, J. M.: Prevention of haemolytic disease of the newborn. *Br. J. Haematol.* 19:653, 1970.

256. Freda, V. J., Gorman, J. G., Galen, R. S., and Treacy, N.: The threat of Rh immunization from abortion. *Lancet* 2:147, 1970.

257. *Pneumocystis carinii* pneumonia among persons with hemophilia A. *Morbid. Mortal. Weekly Rep.* 31:365, 1982

258. Lederman, M. M., Ratnoff, O. D., Scillian, J. J., Jones, P. K., and Schacter, B.: Impaired cell-mediated immunity in patients with classic hemophilia. *N. Engl. J. Med.* 308:79, 1983.

259. Menitove, J. E., et al.: T-lymphocyte subpopulations in patients with classic hemophilia treated with cryoprecipitate and lyophilized concentrates. *N. Engl. J. Med.* 308:83, 1983.

Marrow transplantation

CHAPTER 168

Marrow transplantation

KARL G. BLUME

History

The transplantation of marrow to rescue patients from lethal radiation or chemotherapy or to replace malfunctioning marrow has been of interest to hematologists for decades. The first documented attempt was made in 1939, when a woman with gold-induced aplasia was given marrow intravenously from a brother with identical blood group antigens; engraftment did not take place and the patient died 5 days later [1]. The observation that intravenous administration of marrow cells protected animals against lethal radiation reawakened interest in marrow transplantation for patients with fatal marrow disorders [2]. Starting in 1955, patients with hematologic malignancies were treated with ablative radiation and chemotherapy followed by marrow infusion [3–5]. A variety of cell markers were used to demonstrate the persistence of marrow cells in the immunosuppressed host. Radiation accident victims were also given allogeneic marrow infusion, but permanent engraftment was not established and no graft-versus-host disease was observed [6]. The transplantation experience during the following 10 years led to a better appreciation of the clinical problems related to marrow transplantation. Most patients died before engraftment could be evaluated, and those who lived for several weeks succumbed to graft-versus-host disease or recurrent malignancy. The lack of encouraging results dampened the enthusiasm for the procedure, and the number of transplants performed plummeted [7].

Animal research led to a new phase of marrow transplantation in 1970. By that time, histocompatibility typing had been devised, stem cell proliferation was more thoroughly understood, more effective antibiotics had been developed, and improved supportive care, such as platelet and granulocyte transfusions, had become available. As before, transplant recipients generally were patients with acute leukemia who had failed conventional therapy or patients with aplastic anemia who had been multiply transfused and had been treated with androgens and glucocorticoids [8,9]. For the first time, a significant percentage of patients became disease-free, long-term survivors [10].

Since 1975, patients who are early in the course of their respective diseases have been considered suitable candidates for marrow transplantation. The number of marrow transplant centers throughout the world has increased, and by the end of 1980, more than 1000 patients had been treated with marrow transplantation.

General aspects

DONOR SELECTION, RECIPIENT TREATMENT, AND PROCEDURES

At the current time most transplantations are performed with donor-recipient pairs fully compatible for the major histocompatibility complex. Donors are usually siblings of the recipient (allogeneic pair = genetically nonidentical, e.g., brother-sister; syngeneic pair = genetically identical, i.e., monozygotic siblings), and marrow grafting is preceded by heavy, immunosuppressive, marrow ablative treatment of the recipient. Such treatment consists of high-dose chemotherapy and, in cases of hematologic malignancies, total body irradiation also. The marrow graft is obtained from the donor's iliac crests under spinal or general anesthesia. Particles from the aspirate are made into a single-cell suspension by filtration through metal screens [11]. The marrow is then infused intravenously into the recipient. The problem of a mismatching major blood group can be dealt with by total plasma exchange [12], by immunoabsorption of blood group antibodies [13], or by removal of red cells from the marrow inoculum by differential centrifugation [14]. The actual grafting procedure, usually well tolerated, is followed by a phase of extensive aplasia. After about 2 weeks, discrete aggregates of hemopoietic cells are detectable in the marrow. Most of these consist of single cell types; erythroid, granulocytic, and undifferentiated hemopoietic colonies are approximately equal in frequency [15]. During subsequent days, if the transplant is successful, marrow cellularity increases rapidly and a rise in the number of normal blood cells signals graft productivity.

Engraftment can be confirmed by the use of chromosomes [8,16], red cell antigens [8,17], red cell and white cell isozymes [17,18], and immunoglobulin allotypes [19]. Whereas all marrow cells including the cells forming the hemopoietic environment [137] originating from transplanted stem cells are genetically of donor type, cytogenetic studies demonstrate that marrow fibroblasts of host type remain [20]. Additionally, alveolar macrophages and Kupffer cells change to donor type, which indicates that these human lung and hepatic cellular elements originate from donor marrow [21,22].

During the aplastic phase, which lasts approximately 4 weeks, patients frequently become infected with bacteria or fungi, a condition that necessitates therapy with broad-spectrum antibiotics and antifungal agents [23,24]. Granulocyte transfusions decrease the incidence of local and systemic infectious complications of transplanted recipients [25]. However, the benefits of granulocyte transfusions may be offset by a higher incidence later of interstitial pneumonia associated with cytomegalovirus [26]. Most marrow graft recipients require red cell transfusions and intermittent platelet support [27]. Studies of laminar airflow isolation provide no convincing evidence that a protected environment is mandatory for patient management during the aplastic phase [28]. Parenteral nutrition has frequently been utilized, since most patients, especially those who have been treated with total-body irradiation, experience severe mucositis. This occurs mainly in the oral cavity, with variable involvement of other portions of the gastrointestinal tract. Parenteral nutrition can meet the caloric needs of transplant patients during a period when the nutritional requirements are increased [29]. Veno-occlusive disease, another complication of the first posttransplant month, is a consequence of pretransplant radiochemotherapy. Although veno-occlusive disease was thought to be related to graft-versus-host disease [30], studies have shown that a relationship does not exist [31].

During the second and subsequent months varicellazoster virus may be reactivated but most often resolves spontaneously [32,33]. Patients may also develop interstitial pneumonia, which is usually associated with cytomegalovirus infections but may also be idiopathic in nature [34]. In general, patients who can respond to viral infections with adequate antibody production have a much better chance for survival than those who are not able to do so. Bacterial infections are generally caused by gram-positive bacteria and are particularly frequent in patients who have chronic graft-versus-host disease [35,36].

GRAFT-VERSUS-HOST DISEASE

Graft-versus-host reaction, a frequent complication of allogeneic marrow transplantation, is caused by a reaction of immunocompetent lymphoid donor cells against the immunocompromised host. This phenomenon frequently occurs in the face of complete HLA identity and represents an immunologic process due to as yet undefined tissue antigen differences. During the first 3 months after grafting, this disorder may manifest itself as *acute* graft-versus-host disease, principally involving the skin, gastrointestinal tract, and liver [37]. It may vary from a benign syndrome presenting with a mild skin rash, liver function abnormalities, and abdominal discomfort to an extremely severe, frequently fatal form with extensive epidermolysis, massive diarrhea, nausea, abdominal pain, and liver failure. Patients surviving graft-versus-host disease have delayed immunologic recovery, which in turn reduces the patient's ability to cope with later infectious complications [38]. Histopathologic studies on biopsies from involved organs show characteristic changes, especially in cases with severe manifestations [39–41]. Attempts have been made to prevent acute graft-versus-host disease by manipulation of the marrow inoculum through density

gradient centrifugation [42] or by incubation of the marrow concentrate with anti-T-cell antibody [43]. Although such attempts are still experimental, the results with in vitro anti-T-cell antibody incubation appear to be promising. Currently the most widely used regimen for the prevention or amelioration of acute graft-versus-host disease is the administration of methotrexate with or without glucocorticoids [10,33]. Attempts to prevent or treat acute graft-versus-host disease with antithymocyte globulin in vivo have not been successful [44,45]. However, a combination of antithymocyte globulin with methotrexate and glucocorticoids appears to be an effective approach [138]. Cyclosporin A has most recently been added to the list of drugs which have been used for prophylaxis or therapy [46–48]. Very promising observations have been reported [139], and further studies are required to define the role of this drug in the prevention of graft-versus-host disease.

As more patients have become long-term survivors, *chronic* graft-versus-host disease has been recognized as a clinical entity [49–52]. This syndrome involves the same organs as acute graft-versus-host disease and may also include the eyes, mouth, lungs, and musculoskeletal system. The course may be variable, ranging from mild dryness of the conjunctiva and clinically inapparent liver function abnormalities to a very severe, debilitating form with bacterial infections as frequently fatal complications [35]. In many respects chronic graft-versus-host disease resembles autoimmune disorders, such as lupus erythematosus and scleroderma. Pathologic studies reveal characteristic abnormalities of the organ systems [50,53,54]. Patients with chronic graft-versus-host disease have been treated with antithymocyte globulin, glucocorticoids, procarbazine, cyclophosphamide, and azothioprine, as single drugs or in combination [33,52]. The combination of glucocorticoids with azothioprine is an appropriate regimen for severe chronic graft-versus-host disease [52], although further studies are required to evaluate this and other combinations of drugs.

Marrow transplantation for hematologic malignancies

For patients with hematologic malignancies, total-body irradiation (750 to 1200 rads) and high-dose chemotherapy (cyclophosphamide and sometimes other agents) are used as antileukemic combinations in preparation for marrow transplantation [8,33,55–61,140,141].

Of patients with *acute myelogenous* or *lymphoid leukemia* in florid relapse who are transplanted from HLA-identical sibling donors, only about 10 percent become disease-free, long-term survivors, i.e., survive 2 to 10 years after transplantation without any further antileukemic therapy [8,33,58,60]. Although successful marrow engraftment is the rule, severe infections and leukemic recurrence represent the major obstacles to success.

From studies on patients who were in advanced relapse at the time of marrow grafting, it has become apparent that more aggressive pretransplant regimens leads to excessive, often intolerable toxicity without increasing long-term survival [58]. About 20 to 35 percent of patients who undergo marrow transplantation during partial remission, i.e., with less than 25 percent leukemic cells in the marrow and almost normal blood counts, have a long-term, disease-free survival without any further therapy [8,62]. Patients who have a history of extramedullary leukemia, or disease outside the marrow, at the time of transplantation have a higher incidence of leukemic recurrence after transplantation [62,63]. Leukemic relapse after transplantation is projected to reach approximately 70 percent in patients considered to be refractory to conventional combination chemotherapy. Most of the relapses occur during the first 2 years after transplantation; only rarely is a later relapse seen [64]. In most cases the relapse is due to the persistence of leukemic cells in the host. In a few cases cytogenetic markers have indicated that relapse occurs in donor cells [65–69]. This rare but highly interesting phenomenon has stimulated discussion about the nature of leukemic transformation and its transmissibility. Attempts to transplant patients a second time have been generally unsuccessful; resistance of leukemic cells to treatment or overwhelming infections were the major causes for failure [70].

In some patients, a graft-versus-leukemia effect has been observed [71]. One retrospective study indicated that patients who have moderate to severe acute graft-versus-host disease have a significantly lower relapse rate than transplant recipients without manifestation of graft-versus-host disease [72]. Similarly, chronic graft-versus-host disease appears to significantly reduce the risk of leukemic recurrence [73].

Patients who undergo marrow transplantation during complete remission have an excellent chance of benefiting from the procedure. In marrow transplantation done during the first complete remission of acute myelogenous leukemia, 50 to 80 percent of patients under 40 years of age remain free of disease for up to 5 years and are probably cured [33,74–76,142,143]. The causes for failure are principally related to graft-versus-host disease and interstitial pneumonia associated with cytomegalovirus.

Marrow transplantation in patients with acute lymphoid leukemia is frequently performed during second or subsequent remission [77]. Because of a 40 percent incidence of leukemic recurrence after marrow transplantation, disease-free survival for those patients is of the order of 30 to 45 percent [144]. Not enough data have accumulated for patients with acute lymphoid leukemia transplanted during their first complete remission to allow a meaningful evaluation of the clinical results. The influence of the hematologic pretransplant condition on the outcome of marrow transplantation in patients with acute leukemia is demonstrated in Fig. 168-1.

Marrow transplantation for acute myelogenous or lymphoid leukemia with identical twin donors has been carried out in patients who had end-stage disease [78,79]. Of 34 such patients, 70 percent achieved complete remission following marrow grafting and 24 percent were alive and well 2 to 9 years after the transplant [79].

Attempts have been made to use partly HLA-matched family members as marrow donors for patients with acute leukemia [80]. Although the follow-up period of the surviving patients is only about 2 years, the preliminary results indicate that it might be possible to transplant across the histocompatibility barrier. Only rarely are completely HLA-matched unrelated donors found

FIGURE 168-1 Survival of 61 patients with acute leukemia who underwent marrow transplantation during complete remission (CR), partial remission (PR), or advanced relapse (AR). (Blume et al. [33].)

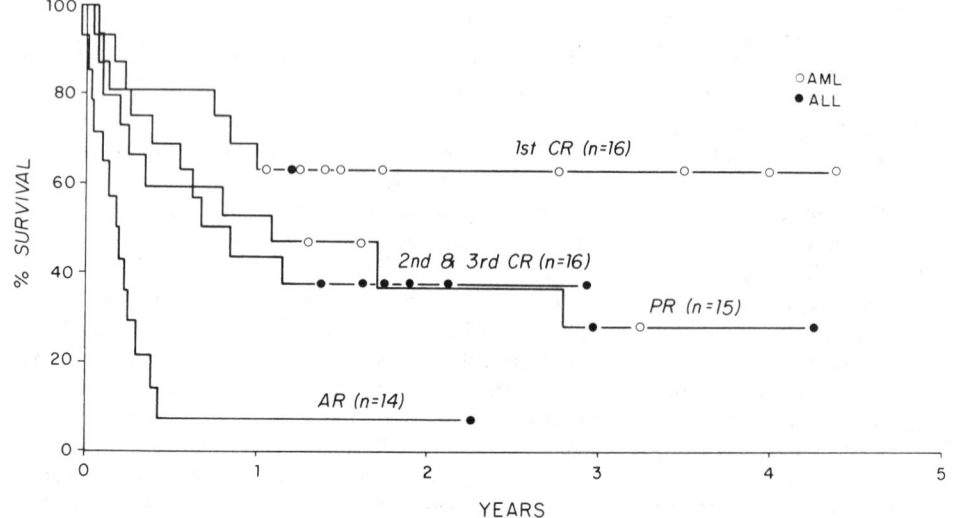

and used as marrow donors for patients who are suffering from acute leukemia. One such successful transplantation has been documented, but the recipient suffered leukemic recurrence 1 year after transplantation [81].

Long-term complications for patients with acute leukemia prepared with total-body irradiation for marrow grafting are permanent sterility and cataract formation [82]. Rarely, solid tumors have been detected in long-term survivors [83]. However, it may be that acute leukemia per se predisposes patients to second malignancies.

Allogeneic marrow transplantation has also been employed in patients with *chronic myelogenous leukemia*. The results were not encouraging when transplantation was done during blast crisis, since most patients succumbed to infections or relapsed within 6 months after transplantation [84]. Conversely, the results of transplantation during the chronic phase for patients who had identical twin donors are very promising; it has been possible to abrogate the Philadelphia chromosome–positive clone and to achieve disease-free, long-term survival [85,145]. The clinical posttransplant courses for such patients have been benign and hospitalizations short. Currently, studies are underway to evaluate allogeneic marrow transplantation during the chronic phase of chronic myelogenous leukemia. Because of the poor short-term prognosis of juvenile chronic myelogenous leukemia, allogeneic marrow transplantation has been performed early during the clinical course and has been successful [86].

Recently, marrow ablation followed by allogeneic marrow grafting has been utilized for patients with *acute myelofibrosis*. Marrow fibrosis and sclerosis were reversible after transplantation, and a disease-free survival of transplanted patients exceeding 1 year has been reported [87,88].

Syngeneic marrow transplantation has also been employed successfully in patients with end-stage lymphoma [89] and hairy cell leukemia [146]. The role of marrow transplantation in the future management of lymphomas remains to be determined.

Autologous marrow "transplantation" (or, better, "rescue") after marrow ablation as a treatment of hematologic malignancies is a very attractive concept since it obviates the need for a suitable donor or the risk of graft-versus-host disease. Attempts have been made to purify the marrow suspension of leukemic cells by discontinuous albumin gradient centrifugation [90] or by incubation with antileukemic antisera [91]. Marrows are collected during complete first remission of acute leukemia, treated, and cryopreserved until the patients' relapses. After high-dose total-body irradiation and chemotherapy, the cell concentrate is reinfused. Hematologic recovery is attained in most patients. However, leukemic recurrence remains a major obstacle in patients who live long enough to be evaluated. It is difficult to determine whether the relapse originates from residual leukemic cells in the marrow inoculum or is caused by cells which survived the antileukemic ther-

apy rendered to the patient. More potent measures to eliminate leukemic cells from the marrow samples and performance of the procedure earlier during the course of the disease are required to determine whether autologous marrow rescue will become a useful form of therapy. A recent study indicates that it may be possible to successfully purge marrow from contaminating leukemic cells by the use of leukemia-specific monoclonal antibodies [147].

Marrow transplantation for nonmalignant disorders

Severe aplastic anemia responds unsatisfactorily to various forms of drug therapy. Therefore, marrow transplantation has been utilized more frequently in this disorder [9,92–94,148]. Certain diagnostic criteria are required for marrow grafting to be indicated [95,96]: (1) a marrow of less than 25 percent of the normal cellularity or a marrow of less than 50 percent of the normal cellularity with less than 30 percent hemopoietic cells and (2) at least two of the following three blood values: granulocytes less than 500 per microliter; platelets less than 20,000 per microliter; anemia with reticulocytes less than 1 percent (corrected for hematocrit reading).

In contrast to transplantation for leukemia, graft rejection is a more frequent complication in marrow transplantation for aplastic anemia, occurring in 10 to 40 percent of all cases. Either a positive relative response index in mixed leukocyte cultures or a low number of nucleated marrow cells used for transplantation strongly correlates with graft rejection [97]. Sensitization by previous blood transfusions is a major factor determining the fate of a marrow graft. Various conditioning regimens have been used to prepare for transplantation. In one regimen, transplant recipients receive high-dose cyclophosphamide followed by infusion of the marrow. Patients who are probably sensitized by previous transfusions or who have positive in vitro tests also should receive unirradiated donor buffy coat to enhance the growth of the graft with circulating stem cells and lymphoid cells [98]. This step, however, may carry a risk for more extensive chronic graft-versus-host disease later. In other attempts to overcome rejection, total-body irradiation [94,99], total lymphoid irradiation [100], or antihuman thymocyte serum [101] has been used with cyclophosphamide. It is difficult to compare the various methods; however, the irradiation should be minimal because of its oncogenic potential.

Currently, about 80 percent of nonsensitized, untransfused patients with an allogeneic donor have been successfully transplanted [102]. Survival falls to 65 percent in transfusion-sensitized patients who receive unirradiated donor buffy coat and is about 45 percent in multiply transfused patients who receive allogeneic marrow without buffy coat cells [98,102,149]. Figure 168-2 illustrates the survival of untransfused and transfused patients with aplastic anemia who underwent

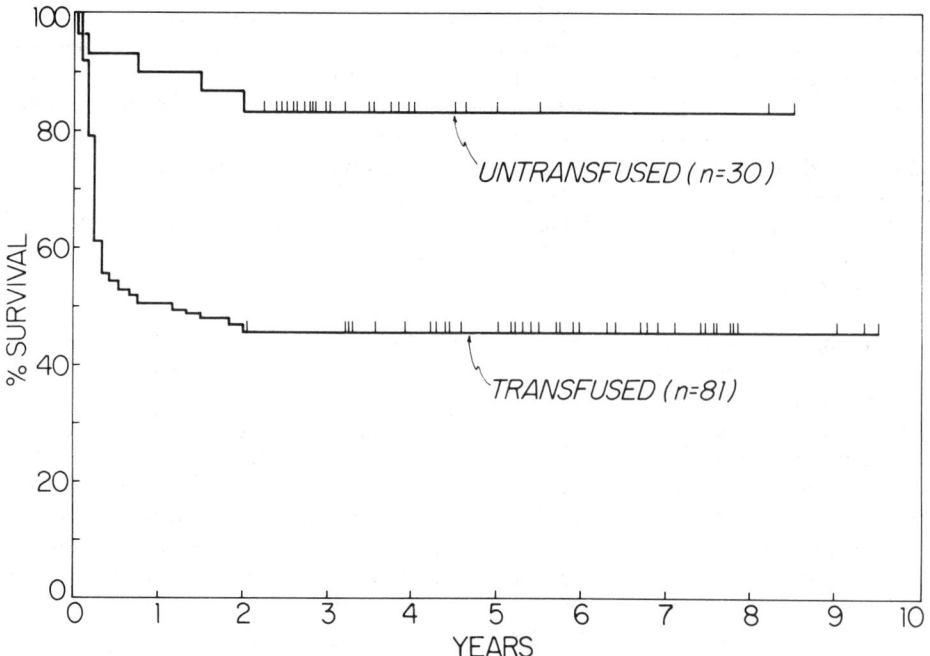

FIGURE 168-2 Survival of 30 untransfused and 81 transfused patients with aplastic anemia who underwent allogeneic marrow grafting after conditioning with cyclophosphamide. (Storb et al. [102].)

allogeneic marrow transplantation after cyclophosphamide conditioning.

In a small number of patients, autologous recovery after rejection of the marrow graft has been documented [103–107]. In those cases, the pretransplant immunosuppression may have influenced the pathogenic mechanism which led to aplastic anemia without totally eliminating donor stem cells. This view is supported by observations in aplastic anemia patients who received marrow grafts from identical twins: whereas most recipients recovered marrow function after infusion of twin donor marrow without prior immunosuppression, some engrafted only after they were conditioned with high-dose cyclophosphamide followed by twin marrow transplantation [108].

Attempts also have been made to prepare aplastic anemia patients with antilymphocyte globulin for marrow infusion from partly histocompatible donors [109]. In one series androgens were administered concomitantly. Permanent engraftment was not achieved, but about 70 percent of the patients survived with return of autologous marrow function [110,150]. The mechanism for this intriguing observation is poorly understood, and further studies are required.

In a limited number of patients with aplastic anemia, partly or fully HLA-identical family members other than siblings have been used as donors. Except for two successfully transplanted recipients who were fully histocompatible with their parental donors, all other patients died with either graft rejection, graft-versus-host disease, or supervening infections [111,112].

A small number of patients with *paroxysmal nocturnal hemoglobinuria* and refractory marrow failure have been treated successfully with allogeneic and syngeneic marrow transplantation [113,114].

With the recognition that lymphatic cells and the immune function are derived in part from marrow stem cells, the concept of marrow transplantation as a means of immunoreconstitution in *severe combined immunodeficiency disease* has been developed. In 1968 a child with this disorder was successfully transplanted with marrow from a histocompatible sibling [115], and soon many additional patients were transplanted [116]. Whereas complete reconstitution after engraftment was achieved in some patients, partial persistence of host marrow function was observed in others [117–119]. Most patients were treated with infusion of marrow without prior immunosuppression, but in some instances cyclophosphamide was administered prior to marrow infusion. The major risk for such patients after transplantation lies in the development of extensive graft-versus-host disease and severe infections. In 24 patients who have received marrow from HLA-identical sibling donors, the survival rate is approximately 50 percent [120]. In a small number of patients who lacked HLA-identical siblings, other family members who were fully histocompatible were used as marrow donors, and three of seven recipients have become long-term survivors [120]. Family donors who were only HLA-D–compatible have also been used with children with severe combined immunodeficiency, and two of nine such patients have become long-term survivors

[120–123]. Marrow from HLA-D–compatible unrelated donors has led to immunologic reconstitution in one child, whereas six others were not transplanted successfully [120,124,125]. Finally, at least 30 children were transplanted with marrow from family members despite clear HLA-D incompatibility since no other donors were available; none of these patients became long-term survivors [120]. The results of marrow transplantation in severe combined immunodeficiency with various types of donors have been reviewed in detail [120,126,127].

Marrow transplantation has also been utilized for some rare congenital disorders with life-threatening immunologic or hematologic abnormalities. Patients with marrow disorders such as *Wiskott-Aldrich syndrome, Kostmann's syndrome, chronic granulomatous disease, primary granulocyte dysfunction, Diamond-Blackfan syndrome, Fanconi anemia, osteopetrosis,* storage disorders such as *Hurler's disease,* and most recently *thalassemia major* have been treated with immunosuppression and marrow grafting [128–136,151–153]. Correction of the underlying disease was achieved in some of those patients. However, in the case of Fanconi anemia, most patients died with severe graft-versus-host disease and toxicity related to cyclophosphamide.

References

1. Osgood, E. E., Riddle, M. C., and Mathews, T. J.: Aplastic anemia treated with daily transfusions and intravenous marrow: Case report. *Ann. Intern. Med.* 13:357, 1939.
2. Lorenz, E., Uphoff, D., Reid, T. R., and Shelton, E.: Modification of irradiation injury in mice and guinea pigs by bone marrow injections. *J. Natl. Cancer Inst.* 12:197, 1951.
3. Thomas, E. D., Lochte, H. L., Jr., Lu, W. C., and Ferrebee, J. W.: Intravenous infusion of bone marrow in patients receiving radiation and chemotherapy. *N. Engl. J. Med.* 257:491, 1957.
4. Thomas, E. D., Lochte, H. L., Jr., Cannon, J. H., Sahler, O. D., and Ferrebee, J. W.: Supralethal whole body irradiation and isologous marrow transplantation in man. *J. Clin. Invest.* 38:1709, 1959.
5. Mathé, G., et al.: Essai de traitement de sujets atteints de leucémie aiguë en rémission par irradiation totale suivie de transfusion de moelle osseuse homologue. *Rev. Fr. Etudes Clin. Biol.* 4:675, 1959.
6. Mathé, G., et al.: Transfusions et greffes de moelle osseuse homologue chez des humains irradiés a haute dose accidentellement. *Rev. Fr. Études Clin. Biol.* 4:226, 1959.
7. Bortin, M. M.: A compendium of reported human bone marrow transplants. *Transplantation* 9:571, 1970.
8. Thomas, E. D., et al: One hundred patients with acute leukemia treated by chemotherapy, total body irradiation, and allogeneic marrow transplantation. *Blood* 49:511, 1977.
9. Storb, R., et al.: Allogeneic marrow grafting for treatment of aplastic anemia. *Blood* 43:157, 1974.
10. Thomas, E. D., et al.: Bone-marrow transplantation. *N. Engl. J. Med.* 292:832, 1975.
11. Thomas, E. D., and Storb, R.: Technique for human marrow grafting. *Blood* 36:507, 1970.
12. Gale, R. P., Feig, S., Ho, W., Falk, P., Rippee, C., and Sparkes, R.: ABO blood group system and bone marrow transplantation. *Blood* 50:185, 1977.
13. Bensinger, W. I., Baker, D. A., Buckner, C. D., Clift, R. A., and Thomas, E. D.: Immunoadsorption for removal of A and B blood-group antibodies. *N. Engl. J. Med.* 304:160, 1981.
14. Braine, H. G., et al.: Bone marrow transplantation with major ABO blood group incompatibility using erythrocyte depletion of marrow prior to infusion. *Blood* 60:420, 1982.
15. Cline, M. J., Gale, R. P., and Golde, D. W.: Discrete clusters of hematopoietic cells in the marrow cavity of man after bone marrow transplantation. *Blood* 50:709, 1977.
16. Borgaonkar, D. S., Bias, W. B., Sroka, B. M., Hutchinson, J. R., and Santos, G. W.: Identification of graft and host cells in bone marrow transplants by the quinacrine banding technique of chromosome identification. *Acta Cytol.* 18:263, 1974.
17. Sparkes, M. C., Crist, M. L., Sparkes, R. S., Gale, R. P., and Feig, S. A.: Gene markers in human bone marrow transplantation. *Vox Sang.* 33:202, 1977.
18. Blume, K. G., Beutler, E., Bross, K. J., Schmidt, G. M., Spruce, W. E., and Teplitz, R. L.: Genetic markers in human bone marrow transplantation. *Am. J. Hum. Genet.* 32:414, 1980.
19. Witherspoon, R. P., Schanfield, M. S., Storb, R., Thomas, E. D., and Giblett, E. R.: Immunoglobulin production of donor origin after marrow transplantation for acute leukemia or aplastic anemia. *Transplantation* 26:407, 1978.
20. Wilson, F. D., Greenberg, B. R., Konrad, P. N., Klein, A. K., and Walling, P. A.: Cytogenetic studies on bone marrow fibroblasts from a male-female hematopoietic chimera: Evidence that stromal elements in human transplantation recipients are of host type. *Transplantation* 25:87, 1978.
21. Thomas, E. D., Ramberg, R. E., Sale, G. E., Sparkes, R. S., and Golde, D. W.: Direct evidence for a bone marrow origin of the alveolar macrophage in man. *Science* 192:1016, 1976.
22. Gale, R. P., Sparkes, R. S., and Golde, D. W.: Bone marrow origin of hepatic macrophages (Kupffer cells) in humans. *Science* 201:937, 1978.
23. Clift, R. A., et al.: Infectious complications of marrow transplantation. *Transplant. Proc.* 6:389, 1974.
24. Winston, D. J., Gale, R. P., Meyer, D. V., and Young, L. S.: Infectious complications of human bone marrow transplantation. *Medicine* 58:1, 1979.
25. Clift, R. A., Sanders, J. E., Thomas, E. D., Williams, B., and Buckner, C. D.: Granulocyte transfusions for the prevention of infection in patients receiving bone-marrow transplants. *N. Engl. J. Med.* 298:1052, 1978.
26. Winston, D. J., Ho, W. G., Young, L. S., and Gale, R. P.: Prophylactic granulocyte transfusions during human bone marrow transplantation. *Am. J. Med.* 68:893, 1980.
27. Storb, R., and Weiden, P. L.: Transfusion problems associated with transplantation. *Semin. Hematol.* 18:163, 1981.
28. Buckner, C. D., et al.: Protective environment for marrow transplant recipients: A prospective study. *Ann. Intern Med.* 89:893, 1978.
29. Schmidt, G. M., Blume, K. G., Bross, K. J., Spruce, W. E., Waldron, J. C., and Levine, R.: Parenteral nutrition in bone marrow transplant recipients. *Exp. Hematol.* 8:506, 1980.
30. Berk, P. D., Popper, H., Krueger, G.R.F., Decter, J., Herzig, G., and Graw, R. G., Jr.,: Veno-occlusive disease of the liver after allogeneic bone marrow transplantation: Possible association with graft-versus-host disease. *Ann. Intern. Med.* 90:158, 1979.
31. Shulman, H. M., et al.: An analysis of hepatic venocclusive disease and centrilobular hepatic degeneration following bone marrow transplantation. *Gastroenterology* 79:1178, 1980.
32. Atkinson, K., Meyers, J. D., Storb, R., Prentice, R. L., and Thomas, E. D.: Varicella-zoster virus infection after marrow transplantation for aplastic anemia or leukemia. *Transplantation* 29:47, 1980.
33. Blume, K. G., et al.: Bone-marrow ablation and allogeneic marrow transplantation in acute leukemia. *N. Engl. J. Med.* 302:1041, 1980.
34. Neiman, P. E., et al.: A prospective analysis of interstitial pneumonia and opportunistic viral infection among recipients of allogeneic bone marrow grafts. *J. Infect. Dis.* 136:754, 1977.
35. Atkinson, K., et al.: Analysis of late infections in 89 long-term survivors of bone marrow transplantation. *Blood* 53:720, 1979.
36. Winston, D. J., et al.: Pneumococcal infections after human bone-marrow transplantation. *Ann. Intern. Med.* 91:835, 1979.
37. Glucksberg, H., et al.: Clinical manifestations of graft-versus-host disease in human recipients of marrow from HL-A-matched sibling donors. *Transplantation.* 18:295, 1974.
38. Noel, D. R., et al.: Does graft-versus-host disease influence the

tempo of immunologic recovery after allogeneic human marrow transplantation? An observation on 56 long-term survivors. *Blood* 51:1087, 1978.

39. Lerner, K. G., Kao, G. F., Storb, R., Buckner, C. D., Clift, R. A., and Thomas, E. D.: Histopathology of graft-vs.-host reaction (GvHR) in human recipients of marrow from HL-A-matched sibling donors. *Transplant. Proc.* 6:367, 1974.

40. Woodruff, J. M., Hansen, J. A., Good, R. A., Santos, G. W., and Slavin, R. E.: The pathology of the graft-versus-host reaction (GVHR) in adults receiving bone marrow transplants. *Transplant. Proc.* 8:675, 1976.

41. Epstein, R. J., McDonald, G. B., Sale, G. E., Shulman, H. M., and Thomas, E. D.: The diagnostic accuracy of the rectal biopsy in acute graft-versus-host disease: A prospective study of thirteen patients. *Gastroenterology* 78:764, 1980.

42. Dicke, K. A., and van Bekkum, D. W.: Allogeneic bone marrow transplantation after elimination of immunocompetent cells by means of density gradient centrifugation. *Transplant. Proc.* 3:666, 1971.

43. Rodt, H., et al.: Effect of anti-T-cell globulin on GVHD in leukemic patients treated with BMT. *Transplant. Proc.* 13:257, 1981.

44. Weiden, P. L., Doney, K., Storb, R., and Thomas, E. D.: Antihuman thymocyte globulin for prophylaxis of graft-versus-host disease. *Transplantation* 27:227, 1979.

45. Doney, K. C., and Weiden, P. L.: Failure of early administration of antithymocyte globulin to lessen graft-versus-host disease in human allogeneic marrow transplant recipients. *Transplantation* 31:141, 1981.

46. Powles, R. L., Clink, H., Sloane, J., Barrett, A. J., Kay, H. E. M., and McElwain, T. J.: Cyclosporin A for the treatment of graft-versus-host disease in man. *Lancet* 2:1327, 1978.

47. Powles, R. L., et al.: Cyclosporin A to prevent graft-versus-host disease in man after allogeneic bone-marrow transplantation. *Lancet* 1:327, 1980.

48. Gluckman, E., Arcese, W., Devergie, A., and Boiron, M.: Cyclosporin-A prophylactic treatment of graft-versus-host disease in human allogeneic bone marrow transplantation: Preliminary results. *Transplant. Proc.* 13:368, 1981.

49. Lawley, T. J., Peck, G. L., Moutsopoulos, H. M., Gratwohl, A. A., and Deisseroth, A. B.: Scleroderma, Sjögren-like syndrome, and chronic graft-versus-host disease. *Ann. Intern. Med.* 87:707, 1977.

50. Shulman, H. M., et al.: Chronic cutaneous graft-versus-host disease in man. *Am. J. Pathol.* 92:545, 1978.

51. Shulman, H. M., et al.: Chronic graft-versus-host syndrome in man: A long-term clinicopathologic study of 20 Seattle patients. *Am. J. Med.* 69:204, 1980.

52. Sullivan, K. M., et al.: Chronic graft-versus-host disease in 52 patients: Adverse natural course and successful treatment with combination immunosuppression. *Blood* 57:267, 1981.

53. Bearman, M. D., et al.: The liver in long-term survivors of marrow transplant—Chronic graft-versus-host disease. *J. Clin. Gastroenterol.* 2:53, 1980.

54. Bernuau, D., et al.: Histological and ultrastructural appearance of the liver during graft-versus-host disease complicating bone marrow transplantation. *Transplantation* 29:236, 1980.

55. Mathé, G., et al.: Successful allogeneic bone marrow transplantation in man: Chimerism, induced specific tolerance and possible antileukemic effects. *Blood* 25:179, 1965.

56. Graw, R. G., Jr., et al.: Bone marrow transplantation from HL-A-matched donors to patients with acute leukemia. *Transplantation* 14:79, 1972.

57. Santos, G. W., et al.: Allogeneic marrow grafts in man using cyclophosphamide. *Transplant. Proc.* 6:345, 1974.

58. UCLA Bone Marrow Transplantation Team: Bone-marrow transplantation in acute leukemia. *Lancet* 2:1197, 1977.

59. Thomas, E. D., Storb, R., and Buckner, C. D.: Total-body irradiation in preparation for marrow engraftment. *Transplant. Proc.* 8:591, 1976.

60. Kim, T. H., Kersey, J., Sewchand, W., Nesbit, M. E., Krivit, W., and Levitt, S. H.: Total-body irradiation with a high-dose-rate linear accelerator for bone-marrow transplantation in aplastic anemia and neoplastic disease. *Radiology* 122:523, 1977.

61. Findley, D. O., Skov, D. D., and Blume, K. G.: Total body irradiation with a 10 MV linear accelerator in conjunction with bone marrow transplantation. *Int. J. Radiat. Oncol. Biol. Phys.* 6:695, 1980.

62. Blume, K. G., et al.: Bone marrow ablation and marrow transplantation in acute leukemia: Influence of clinical pretransplant condition. *Transplant. Proc.* 13:252, 1981.

63. Harrison, D. T., et al.: Relapse, following marrow transplantation for acute leukemia. *Am. J. Hematol.* 5:191, 1978.

64. Oliff, A., Ramu, N.-P., and Poplack, D.: Leukemic relapse 5½ years after allogeneic bone marrow transplantation. *Blood* 52:281, 1978.

65. Fialkow, P. J., Thomas, E. D., Bryant, J. I., and Neiman, P. E.: Leukaemic transformation of engrafted human marrow cells in vivo. *Lancet* 1:251, 1971.

66. Thomas, E. D., et al.: Leukaemic transformation of engrafted human marrow cells in vivo. *Lancet* 1:1310, 1972.

67. Goh, K., and Klemperer, M. R.: In vivo leukemic transformation: Cytogenetic evidence of in vivo leukemic transformation of engrafted marrow cells. *Am. J. Hematol.* 2:283, 1977.

68. Elfenbein, G. J., et al.: Cytogenetic evidence for recurrence of acute myelogenous leukemia after allogeneic bone marrow transplantation in donor hematopoietic cells. *Blood* 52:627, 1978.

69. Newburger, P. E., et al.: Leukemia relapse in donor cells after allogeneic bone-marrow transplantation. *N. Engl. J. Med.* 304:712, 1981.

70. Wright, S. E., et al.: Experience with second marrow transplants. *Exp. Hematol.* 4:221, 1976.

71. Odom, L. F., et al.: Remission of relapsed leukaemia during a graft-versus-host reaction: A "graft-versus-leukaemia reaction" in man? *Lancet* 2:537, 1978.

72. Weiden, P. L., et al.: Antileukemic effect of graft-versus-host disease in human recipients of allogeneic-marrow grafts. *N. Engl. J. Med.* 300:1068, 1979.

73. Weiden, P. L., Sullivan, K. M., Flournoy, N., Storb, R., Thomas, E. D., and the Seattle Marrow Transplant Team: Antileukemic effect of chronic graft-versus-host disease contributes to improved survival after allogeneic marrow transplantation. *N. Engl. J. Med.* 304:1529, 1981.

74. Thomas, E. D., et al.: Marrow transplantation for acute nonlymphoblastic leukemia in first remission. *N. Engl. J. Med.* 301:597, 1979.

75. Powles, R. L., et al.: The place of bone-marrow transplantation in acute myelogenous leukemia. *Lancet* 1:1047, 1980.

76. Mannoni, P., et al.: Marrow transplantation for acute nonlymphoblastic leukemia in first remission. *Blut* 41:220, 1980.

77. Thomas, E. D., et al.: Marrow transplantation for patients with acute lymphoblastic leukemia in remission. *Blood* 54:468, 1979.

78. Fefer, A., et al.: Cure of hematologic neoplasia with transplantation of marrow from identical twins. *N. Engl. J. Med.* 297:146, 1977.

79. Fefer, A., et al.: Bone marrow transplantation for refractory acute leukemia in 34 patients with identical twins. *Blood* 57:421, 1981.

80. Clift, R. A., Hansen, J. A., and Thomas, E. D.: The role of HLA in marrow transplantation. *Transplant. Proc.* 13:234, 1981.

81. Hansen, J. A., Clift, R. A., Thomas, E. D., Buckner, C. D., Storb, R., and Giblett, E. R.: Transplantation of marrow from an unrelated donor to a patient with acute leukemia. *N. Engl. J. Med.* 303:565, 1980.

82. Stewart, P. S., et al.: Allogeneic marrow grafting for acute leukemia: A follow-up of long-term survivors. *Exp. Hematol.* 7:509, 1979.

83. Deeg, H. J., et al.: Increased cancer risk in canine radiation chimeras. *Blood* 55:233, 1980.

84. Doney, K., Buckner, C. D., Sale, G. E., Ramberg, R., Boyd, C., and Thomas, E. D.: Treatment of chronic granulocytic leukemia by chemotherapy, total body irradiation and allogeneic bone marrow transplantation. *Exp. Hematol.* 6:738, 1978.

85. Fefer, A., et al.: Disappearance of Ph¹-positive cells in four patients with chronic granulocytic leukemia after chemotherapy, irradiation and marrow transplantation from an identical twin. *N. Engl. J. Med.* 300:333, 1979.

86. Sanders, J. E., Buckner, C. D., Stewart, P., and Thomas, E. D.: Successful treatment of juvenile chronic granulocytic leukemia with marrow transplantation. *Pediatrics* 63:44, 1979.

87. Smith, J. W., Shulman, H. M., Thomas, E. D., Fefer, A., and Buckner, C. D.: Bone marrow transplantation for acute myelosclerosis. *Cancer* 48:2198, 1981.

88. Wolf, J., et al.: Reversal of acute malignant myelosclerosis by allogeneic bone marrow transplantation. *Blood* 59:191, 1982.

89. Appelbaum, F. R., et al.: Treatment of non-Hodgkin's lymphoma with marrow transplantation in identical twins. *Blood* 58:509, 1981.

90. Dicke, K. A., et al.: Autologous bone marrow transplantation in patients with adult acute leukemia in relapse. *Transplantation* 26:169, 1978.

91. Netzel, B., Haas, R. J., Rodt, H., Kolb, H. J., Belohradsky, B., and Thierfelder, S.: Antileukemic, autologous bone marrow transplantation in childhood acute lymphoblastic leukemia. *Transplant. Proc.* 13:254, 1981.

92. UCLA Bone Marrow Transplant Team: Bone-marrow transplantation in severe aplastic anaemia. *Lancet* 2:921, 1976.

93. Storb, R., et al.: One-hundred-ten patients with aplastic anemia (AA) treated by marrow transplantation in Seattle. *Transplant. Proc.* 10:135, 1978.

94. Gluckman, E., et al.: Bone marrow transplantation in 65 patients with severe aplastic anemia. *Blut* 41:157, 1980.

95. Camitta, B. M., Rappeport, J. M., Parkman, R., and Nathan, D. G.: Selection of patients for bone marrow transplantation in severe aplastic anemia. *Blood* 45:355, 1975.

96. Camitta, B. M., et al.: A prospective study of androgens and bone marrow transplantation for treatment of severe aplastic anemia. *Blood* 53:504, 1979.

97. Storb, R., Prentice, R. L., and Thomas, E. D.: Marrow transplantation for treatment of aplastic anemia: An analysis of factors associated with graft rejection. *N. Engl. J. Med.* 296:61, 1977.

98. Storb, R.: Decrease in the graft rejection rate and improvement in survival after marrow transplantation for severe aplastic anemia. *Transplant. Proc.* 11:196, 1979.

99. Gale, R. P., et al.: Prevention of graft rejection following bone marrow transplantation. *Blood* 57:9, 1981.

100. Ramsay, N. K. C., et al.: Total lymphoid irradiation and cyclophosphamide as preparation for bone marrow transplantation in severe aplastic anemia. *Blood* 55:344, 1980.

101. Parkman, R., Rappeport, J., Camitta, B., Levey, R. H., and Nathan, D. G.: Successful use of multiagent immunosuppression in the bone marrow transplantation of sensitized patients. *Blood* 52:1163, 1978.

102. Storb, R., et al.: Marrow transplantation in thirty "untransfused" patients with severe aplastic anemia. *Ann. Intern. Med.* 92:30, 1980.

103. Thomas, E. D., et al.: Recovery from aplastic anemia following attempted marrow transplantation. *Exp. Hematol.* 4:97, 1976.

104. Speck, B., et al.: Autologous marrow recovery following allogeneic marrow transplantation in a patient with severe aplastic anemia. *Exp. Hematol.* 4:131, 1976.

105. Sensenbrenner, L. L., Steele, A. A., and Santos, G. W.: Recovery of hematologic competence without engraftment following attempted bone marrow transplantation for aplastic anemia: Report of a case with diffusion chamber studies. *Exp. Hematol.* 5:51, 1977.

106. Territo, M. C.: Autologous bone marrow repopulation following high dose cyclophosphamide and allogeneic marrow transplantation in aplastic anaemia. *Br. J. Haematol.* 36:305, 1977.

107. Gmür, J., von Felten, A., Rhyner, K., and Frick, P. G.: Autologous hematologic recovery from aplastic anemia following high dose cyclophosphamide and HLA-matched allogeneic bone marrow transplantation. *Acta Haematol.* 62:20, 1979.

108. Appelbaum, F. R., et al.: Treatment of aplastic anemia by bone marrow transplantation in identical twins. *Blood* 55:1033, 1980.

109. Mathé, G., and Schwarzenberg, L.: Treatment of bone marrow aplasia by bone marrow graft after conditioning with antilymphocyte globulin: Long term results. *Exp. Hematol.* 4:256, 1976.

110. Speck, B., et al.: Severe aplastic anemia: A prospective study on the value of different therapeutic approaches in 37 successive patients. *Blut* 41:160, 1980.

111. Clift, R. A., et al.: Marrow transplantation from donors other than HLA-identical siblings. *Transplantation* 28:235, 1979.

112. Tricot, G. J. K., Jansen, J., Zwaan, F. E., Eernisse, J. G., Sabbe, L., and van Rood, J. J.: Successful bone marrow transplantation for aplastic anemia using an HLA phenotypically identical parent. *Transplantation* 31:86, 1981.

113. Storb, R., et al.: Paroxysmal nocturnal haemoglobinuria and refractory marrow failure treated by marrow transplantation. *Br. J. Haematol.* 24:743, 1973.

114. Fefer, A., et al.: Paroxysmal nocturnal hemoglobinuria and marrow failure treated by infusion of marrow from an identical twin. *Ann. Intern. Med.* 84:692, 1976.

115. Gatti, R. A., Meuwissen, H. J., Allen, H. D., Hong, R., and Good, R. A.: Immunological reconstitution of sex-linked lymphopenic immunological deficiency. *Lancet* 2:1366, 1968.

116. Meuwissen, H. J., Gatti, R. A., Terasaki, P. I., Hong, R., and Good, R. A.: Treatment of lymphopenic hypogammaglobulinemia and bone marrow aplasia by transplantation of allogeneic marrow: Crucial role of histocompatibility matching. *N. Engl. J. Med.* 281:691, 1969.

117. Buckley, R. H., Amos, D. B., Kremer, W. B., and Stickel, D. L.: Incompatible bone-marrow transplantation in lymphopenic immunologic deficiency. *N. Engl. J. Med.* 285:1035, 1971.

118. Stiehm, E. R., et al.: Immunologic reconstitution in severe combined immunodeficiency without bone-marrow chromosomal chimerism. *N. Engl. J. Med.* 286:797, 1972.

119. Goldmann, S. F., et al.: Hemopoietic and lymphopoietic split chimerism in severe combined immunodeficiency disease (SCID). *Transplant. Proc.* 11:225, 1979.

120. Niethammer, D.: Treatment of severe combined immunodeficiency by transplantation. *Blut* 42:137, 1981.

121. Copenhagen Study Group of Immunodeficiencies: Bone-marrow transplantation from an HL-A non-identical but mixed-lymphocyte-culture identical donor. *Lancet* 1:1146, 1973.

122. Niethammer, D., et al.: Bone marrow transplantation for severe combined immunodeficiency with the HL-A-A-incompatible but MLC-identical mother as a donor. *Transplant. Proc.* 8:623, 1976.

123. O'Reilly, R. J., Pahwa, R., Dupont, B., and Good, R. A.: Severe combined immunodeficiency: Transplantation approaches for patients lacking an HLA genotypically identical sibling. *Transplant. Proc.* 10:187, 1978.

124. Horowitz, S. D., Groshong, T., Bach, F. H., Hong, R., and Yunis, E. J.: Treatment of severe combined immunodeficiency with bone-marrow from an unrelated, mixed-leucocyte-culture–non-reactive donor. *Lancet* 2:431, 1975.

125. O'Reilly, R. J., et al.: Reconstitution in severe combined immunodeficiency by transplantation of marrow from an unrelated donor. *N. Engl. J. Med.* 297:1311, 1977.

126. Bortin, M. M., and Rimm, A. A.: Severe combined immunodeficiency disease: Characterization of the disease and results of transplantation. *JAMA* 238:591, 1977.

127. Kenny, A. B., and Hitzig, W. H.: Bone marrow transplantation for severe combined immunodeficiency disease. *Eur. J. Pediatr.* 131:155, 1979.

128. Bach, F. H., Albertini, R. J., Joo, P., Anderson, J. L., and Bortin, M. M.: Bone-marrow transplantation in a patient with the Wiskott-Aldrich syndrome. *Lancet* 2:1364, 1968.

129. Parkman, R., et al.: Complete correction of the Wiskott-Aldrich syndrome by allogeneic bone-marrow transplantation. *N. Engl. J. Med.* 298:921, 1978.

130. Kapoor, N., et al.: Reconstitution of normal megakaryocytopoiesis and immunologic functions in Wiskott-Aldrich syndrome by marrow transplantation following myeloablation and immunosuppression with busulfan and cyclophosphamide. *Blood* 57:692, 1981.

131. Rappeport, J. M., Parkman, R., Newburger, P., Camitta, B. M., and Chusid, M. J.: Correction of infantile agranulocytosis (Kostmann's syndrome) by allogeneic bone marrow transplantation. *Am. J. Med.* 68:605, 1980.

132. Rappeport, J. M., Parkman, R., Belli, J. A., Cassidy, J. R., and Levey, R.: Correction of congenital bone marrow disorders by allogeneic bone marrow transplantation following preparation with anti-human thymocyte serum and total body irradiation. *Transplant. Proc.* 13:241, 1981.

133. August, C. S., et al.: Establishment of erythropoiesis following bone marrow transplantation in a patient with congenital hypoplastic anemia (Diamond-Blackfan syndrome). *Blood* 48:491, 1976.

134. Gluckman, E., et al.: Bone marrow transplantation in Fanconi anaemia. *Br. J. Haematol. 45*:557, 1980.

135. Ballet, J. J., Griscelli, C., Coutris, C., Milhaud, G., and Maroteaux, P.: Bone-marrow transplantation in osteopetrosis. *Lancet 2*:1137, 1977.

136. Coccia, P. F., et al.: Successful bone-marrow transplantation for infantile malignant osteopetrosis. *N. Engl. J. Med. 302*:701, 1980.

137. Keating, A., et al.: Donor origin of the in vitro hematopoietic microenvironment following marrow transplantation in man. *Nature 298*:280, 1982.

138. Ramsay, N. K. C., et al.: A randomized study of the prevention of acute graft-versus-host disease. *N. Engl. J. Med. 306*:392, 1982.

139. Speck, B., et al.: Neue Entwicklung in der Klinischen Knochenmarktransplantation bei Leukämie. *Schweiz. Med. Wschr. 111*:1975, 1981.

140. Shank, B., et al.: Hyperfractionated total body irradiation for bone marrow transplantation: Early results in leukemia patients. *Int. J. Radiat. Oncol. Biol. Phys. 7*:1109, 1981.

141. Thomas, E. D., et al.: Marrow transplantation for acute nonlymphoblastic leukemia in first remission using fractionated or single dose irradiation. *Int. J. Radiat. Oncol. Biol. Phys. 8*:817, 1982.

142. Sanders, J. E., et al.: Marrow transplantation for children with acute nonlymphoblastic leukemia in first remission. *Med. Pediatr. Oncol. 9*:423, 1981.

143. Kersey, J. H., et al.: Allogeneic bone marrow transplantation in acute nonlymphocytic leukemia: A pilot study. *Blood 60*:400, 1982.

144. Johnson, F. L., et al.: A comparison of marrow transplantation with chemotherapy for children with acute lymphoblastic leukemia in second or subsequent remission. *N. Engl. J. Med. 305*:846, 1981.

145. Fefer, A., et al.: Treatment of chronic granulocytic leukemia with chemoradiotherapy and transplantation of marrow from identical twins. *N. Engl. J. Med. 306*:63, 1982.

146. Chever, M. A., et al.: Treatment of hairy-cell leukemia with chemoradiotherapy and identical twin bone marrow transplantation. *N. Engl. J. Med. 307*:479, 1982.

147. Ritz, J., et al.: Autologous bone marrow transplantation in CALLA-positive acute lymphoblastic leukemia after in vitro treatment with J5 monoclonal antibody and complement. *Lancet 2*:60, 1982.

148. Camitta, B. M., Storb, R., and Thomas, E. D.: Aplastic anemia. *N. Engl. J. Med. 306*:645, 1982.

149. Storb, R., et al.: Marrow transplantation with or without donor buffy coat cells for 65 transfused aplastic anemia patients. *Blood 59*:236, 1982.

150. Gratwohl, A., et al.: Behandlung der schweren aplastischen anämie. *Schweiz. Med. Wschr. 111*:1520, 1981.

151. Sorell, M., et al.: Marrow transplantation for juvenile osteopetrosis. *Am. J. Med. 70*:1280, 1981.

152. Hobbs, J. R.: Reversal of clinical features of Hurler's disease and biochemical improvement after treatment by bone-marrow transplantation. *Lancet 2*:709, 1981.

153. Thomas, E. D., et al.: Marrow transplantation for thalassemia. *Lancet 2*:227, 1982.

Hemapheresis procedures

CHAPTER 169

Therapeutic hemapheresis—indications, efficacy, complications

JACOB NUSBACHER

Cell separators were introduced in the late 1960s for the collection of granulocytes for transfusion [1]. These centrifuge machines could remove the major blood cell constituents or plasma rapidly, thereby "processing" large volumes of patient blood efficiently. The earliest procedures were performed on patients with chronic myelogenous leukemia (CML) [2,3]. In these instances, white cell collection for transfusion into neutropenic patients was the goal, but the procedures also served to lower the patient-donor's white cell count. More recently, therapeutic hemapheresis procedures have been used to treat a large number of hematological conditions, including hyperleukocytic leukemias and lymphomas, thrombocythemia, thrombotic thrombocytopenic purpura, sickle cell anemia, and disorders associated with pathological proteins in plasma. Unfortunately, evidence demonstrating efficacy has not been gathered in a rigorous manner in controlled studies.

The generic term best applied to therapeutic cell separator techniques is *therapeutic hemapheresis*. The specific procedure may be described by the blood element being removed: cytapheresis (for any blood cell removed), leukapheresis, lymphapheresis, erythrapheresis (or red cell exchange), plateletpheresis (or, more accurately, thrombocytapheresis), and plasma exchange. This last procedure has also been termed *therapeutic plasmapheresis*, but *plasma exchange* better describes the process.

Rationale for therapeutic hemapheresis

Therapeutic hemapheresis can remove abnormal blood cells or plasma constituents. This procedure often does not alter the underlying abnormality, and more definitive therapy is usually needed. Hemapheresis is best performed when an acute effect is desired, when conventional therapy is ineffective or contraindicated, or as an adjunctive measure to accelerate recovery.

Leukapheresis

Leukapheresis has been performed as therapy in both acute and chronic leukemia and lymphoma [2–10]. The degree of cytoreduction achieved depends on the technique used. Usually a reduction in cell count of 25 to 50 percent occurs after a 3-h therapeutic leukapheresis procedure. Often leukapheresis results in a smaller decrement in the patient's white count than would be expected from the number of cells in the collection bag. This result is due to a reduction in blood volume and to mobilization of leukocytes into the bloodstream during and after the procedure. The rate of mobilization and the rate of cell proliferation dictate the frequency of leukapheresis procedures necessary to achieve a sustained reduction in the leukocyte count. This can usually be achieved in acute leukemia or in CML only if the procedure is performed at least three times per week. Once significant cytoreduction is achieved, however, less frequent procedures may suffice. The frequency and intensity of leukapheresis can be adjusted to meet the needs of each patient.

ACUTE LEUKEMIA

Patients with acute myelogenous leukemia (AML) with high cell counts are prone to vaso-occlusive problems secondary to leukostasis [11,12], pulmonary or cerebral insufficiency, and intracerebral hemorrhage. Early death, within the first week after diagnosis, is much more common when the white cell count is greater than 100,000 per microliter [13]. Similar problems occur in patients with CML, but usually at white cell counts of about 300,000 per microliter [12].

Rapid cytoreduction is indicated in patients with AML or acute lymphocytic leukemia (ALL) with white cell counts of greater than 100,000 per microliter. Leukapheresis, either alone or combined with appropriate chemotherapy, results in a rapid reduction in white cell count and a reversal of symptoms [9,14]. Severe hyperuricemia and renal insufficiency from rapid, chemotherapy-induced cytoreduction may be minimized by decreasing the tumor burden by leukapheresis just prior to cytotoxic drug administration. Also, after leukapheresis, red cell transfusion can be given with less increase in blood viscosity [13,15].

CHRONIC LEUKEMIA

Repeated leukapheresis has been used in the treatment of CML prior to chemotherapy or as chronic treatment in lieu of chemotherapy [2,3,6–8]. In the usual case, leukapheresis procedures are required two to three times per week in order for the cell removal rate to exceed the rate of leukocyte mobilization and new cell production. After a number of weeks of frequent leukapheresis procedures, during which an 80 percent reduction of the initial leukocyte count can be achieved [3], less frequent procedures usually suffice to maintain the count at that level.

In patients with CML treated by leukapheresis, there has been a reduction in organomegaly and remission of symptoms such as sweating, malaise, and pain secondary to splenomegaly [3,6,7]. Leukapheresis is valuable in treating CML during pregnancy because it permits a delay in the use of chemotherapy [10], or when extreme leukocytosis and leukostasis are present and rapid cytoreduction is desired. Leukapheresis has not prolonged longevity or delayed the onset of blastic transformation [3]. Leukapheresis procedures are also expensive and time-consuming, often interfering with the patient's usual activities. Therefore, chemotherapy is preferable to leukapheresis in the usual patient with CML.

Leukapheresis has also been used to treat patients with chronic lymphocytic leukemia (CLL) [4,5]. With frequent treatment, the blood leukocyte count, organomegaly, and the degree of marrow lymphocyte infiltration have been decreased in most patients. Anemia and thrombocytopenia have also been ameliorated. However, leukapheresis for CLL has the same drawbacks as for CML and is indicated only when conventional therapy is ineffective or contraindicated.

There have been a few reports of striking clinical improvement after a course of leukapheresis for both Sézary syndrome [16–18] and hairy cell leukemia [19]. Despite the removal of only a modest number of cells in some cases, hemapheresis therapy resulted in marked reduction in leukocyte counts and complete resolution of skin lesions. In one instance, remission lasted for at least 2 years without additional therapy.

Plateletpheresis

Plateletpheresis is useful as acute therapy in patients with severe thrombocythemia [17,20–22]. A reduction in the platelet count of about 50 percent can be achieved with each procedure [20]. The size of the spleen plays an important role in determining efficacy since mobilization of platelets from the spleen occurs during plateletpheresis [23]. The patient's platelet count returns to pretreatment levels within a few days, and repeated plateletpheresis procedures are often necessary.

It is not known whether the very rapid cytoreduction achieved by plateletpheresis reduces the frequency of thrombotic and/or hemorrhagic complications associated with thrombocythemia compared with that achieved by chemotherapy or radioisotopic therapy. In the symptomatic thrombocythemic patient, however, plateletpheresis may be the treatment of choice because it may dramatically reverse signs and symptoms related to cerebral and myocardial ischemia, gastrointestinal bleeding, and pulmonary embolism. To achieve a lasting effect, more definitive cytotoxic therapy, which may

not take effect for days or weeks, should be started at the same time as hemapheresis.

Chronic plateletpheresis is not the treatment of choice for thrombocythemia [24]. Although platelet count reduction and stabilization can be achieved by hemapheresis, as many as five procedures per week may be required to achieve this effect [21,24]. In one study [21], fewer plateletpheresis procedures were found to be necessary after a more intensive initial therapeutic period, but in another study [24], sustained intensive therapy was needed. Chronic plateletpheresis is a costly therapeutic regimen which interferes with the patient's lifestyle and should be reserved for those cases where conventional therapy is ineffective or contraindicated.

Erythrapheresis

The complications of sickle cell disease have been treated by erythrapheresis, or red cell exchange [25–28]. The rationale for this treatment is to break the cycle of sickling, vascular stasis, and hypoxia by exchanging the patient's red cells for erythrocytes containing hemoglobin A. The degree of exchange required to achieve a therapeutic effect is not known, however. Favorable results have been reported following erythrapheresis for priapism [28] and unremitting painful crises [26]. Red cell exchange has also been used in patients with hemoglobin S disease during pregnancy [25] and preparatory to major surgery [27].

Red cell exchange has been used preoperatively in a patient with paroxysmal nocturnal hemoglobinuria [29] and in a comatose patient with posttransfusion falciparum malaria [30].

Unlike other types of cytapheresis procedures, where the volume of blood removed is small, erythrapheresis requires equivalent red cell replacement. This treatment, analogous to a massive blood transfusion, is associated with hazards, especially hypovolemia, hepatitis, and red cell alloimmunization. The specific red cell exchange kinetics and the distribution of red cell subpopulations within various cell separators require further study [31,32].

Cell separators have been used to collect young erythrocytes, referred to as *neocytes*, from normal donors for transfusions into thalassemic patients or others who need chronic transfusion and in whom iron-overload is inevitable. The transfusion of younger red cells with a longer survival reduces the number of transfusions needed. When combined with "supertransfusion" to maintain the hematocrit reading at over 35 percent and with iron chelation therapy, such transfusions could delay or eliminate the onset of iron-overload [33].

Neocyte units having a mean cell age of 12 to 30 days have been collected [31,32] (mean cell age for regular red cell units is 60 days). The radioactive chromium (^{51}Cr) red cell half-life of transfused neocytes is about 45 days (normal survival is 28 days).

Partial exchange transfusion can be accomplished in thalassemic patients by removing old red cells (*gerocytes*), which are dense and settle to the bottom of the separation module, and replacing them with neocytes [33]. This procedure, repeated at appropriate intervals, could result in little net accumulation of iron in the patient. These cell separator applications may become a useful therapeutic adjunct for this group of patients.

Plasma exchange

Definitive studies of therapeutic plasma exchange are virtually nonexistent. Numerous case reports, or studies on a small series of patients, describe clinical improvement after one or more plasma exchanges. Only tentative conclusions can be reached about the usefulness of plasma exchange in the treatment of certain disorders.

PHYSIOLOGY OF PLASMA EXCHANGE

Therapeutic plasma exchange removes the putative pathological material in the patient's plasma continuously and replaces the plasma with fluid devoid of the material in question. The reduction in concentration of the material being removed can be calculated by the formula

$$X_t = X_o e^{-\frac{b}{v} t}$$

where X_t = the concentration in the patient after time t, X_o = the concentration of the pathological material in the patient's blood before exchange, b = the volume of blood exchanged, t = the duration of the exchange, and v = the patient's blood volume [34,35]. According to this formula, an exchange of one plasma volume would reduce the starting concentration of the patient's pathological material by about 65 percent; a two-volume exchange would achieve only an additional 23 percent reduction. In general, exchanges of smaller amounts of plasma are more efficient than large-volume exchanges.

It is useful to measure the reduction in the concentration of pathological materials achieved with plasma exchange to determine the effectiveness of the therapy. Often, one finds that the decrement in plasma concentration after exchange differs from the expected value [36]. This finding is related to a change in the patient's blood volume, mobilization of plasma constituents from the extravascular space, and new synthesis of plasma constituents [36].

The choice of replacement fluids for plasma exchange varies among different investigators. Crystalloid solutions may suffice when the volume exchanged is small or when the patient is hyperproteinemic, such as in cases of macroglobulinemia. More frequently, albumin solutions are used either alone or in combination with crystalloid. Albumin solutions are accessible, do not require immunological compatibility, and do not transmit hepatitis. Temporary reductions in plasma constituents, including coagulation factors, occur after large-volume plasma exchanges with purified protein fraction (PPF), albumin, or crystalloid [37–39]. Factor IX activity, ristocetin cofactor activity, and factor VIII procoagulant activity return to normal within 4 h; other coagulation abnormalities are corrected within 24 h. Fibrinogen and C3 levels may still be depressed at 72 h [38]. Bleeding resulting from removal of coagulation factors has not been reported. The other alterations in the concentration of plasma constituents are inconsequential but illustrate the complexity of the procedure.

Fresh frozen plasma (FFP) has also been used as an exchange fluid. FFP has the virtue of replacing coagulation factors but requires immunological compatibility, may cause immunological reactions, and can transmit hepatitis. FFP is rarely used as the main replacement fluid, although a few units may be infused to replenish coagulation factors at the end of a large-volume exchange. In thrombotic thrombocytopenic purpura and perhaps idiopathic thrombocytopenic purpura, there is evidence that FFP may have a special effect by supplying a factor required for the therapeutic benefit. Hypocalcemia occurs when FFP is used as the replacement fluid [39,40]. The hypocalcemia has been associated with only minor symptoms which are reversed when the infusion rate is decreased. Calcium supplementation is not the usual practice in most hemapheresis programs [40].

AUTOIMMUNE DISORDERS

Autoimmune hemolytic anemias (AIHA) due to both the warm- and cold-reactive antibodies have been treated by plasma exchange. No definite benefit has been achieved in the warm-antibody type of AIHA [41–44].

Hemapheresis procedures on patients with cold-agglutinin disease are difficult to perform because cooling of the patient's blood in the extracorporeal circuit often results in red cell agglutination, which may lead to hemolysis [44,45,46]. The use of a blood warmer prior to the return of blood to the patient is usually necessary. In most cases, a temporary reduction in cold-agglutinin titer was achieved, but return to pretreatment antibody levels usually occurred within a few days. Clinical improvement was either not apparent or could not be sustained.

The treatment of idiopathic thrombocytopenic purpura (ITP) by plasma exchange may result in long-lasting benefit in some patients with acute ITP [47], but not in patients with chronic ITP [47,48]. The patient's platelet counts increased when FFP was used as the replacement fluid but not when albumin solution was used. This observation is consistent with earlier observations in some patients with ITP [49] and with the observation that intravenous gamma globulin raise the platelet count in ITP patients [50]. In the absence of controlled studies, it is difficult to evaluate the role of plasma exchange in ITP treatment, given the responsiveness of patients to glucocorticoids and splenectomy.

ALLOIMMUNE DISORDERS

Alloantibodies are not harmful to the patient, as they are directed against "foreign" antigens. However, they may seriously constrain transfusion of blood components, and their removal is often desirable. Plasma exchange has been used to remove leukocyte antibodies from a patient receiving granulocyte transfusions [41], factor VIII antibodies from a patient requiring factor VIII infusion [17,51], and factor IX antibodies from a patient requiring surgery [52]. Plasma exchange should be used only rarely for these applications, as other approaches are simpler and more effective.

In patients receiving ABO-incompatible marrow transplants, plasma exchange is necessary to remove anti-A and/or anti-B alloantibody [53–56]. In some instances other techniques of antibody removal are combined with plasma exchange [54].

Plasma exchange has been used to remove (maternal) alloantibody in severe Rh immunization [57–60], but carefully controlled studies are needed to evaluate the utility of this procedure.

Posttransfusion purpura is another alloantibody-mediated condition in which plasma or whole blood exchange has been used [61,62]. Exchange therapy seems to be the treatment of choice for this condition [61,62].

PARAPROTEINEMIA

Plasma exchange is useful for the amelioration of hyperviscosity in patients with macroglobulinemia and, occasionally, in patients in other paraproteinemic states [63]. Signs and symptoms attributable to hyperviscosity, including both vaso-occlusive and hemorrhagic phenomena, have been reversed by exchange techniques that use either traditional bag plasmapheresis or cell separators [36,63–69]. Little difference was found in the efficiency of plasma exchange when performed for IgG or IgA multiple myeloma as compared with those performed for macroglobulinemia. While plasma exchange is effective in reducing hyperviscosity acutely, the paraprotein usually reaccumulates in the patient's blood within a few days, and frequent exchanges are often required. Therefore, this approach must be considered a temporizing strategy until more definitive therapy directed at the protein-producing cells can take effect.

Plasma exchange has also been used successfully in the treatment of the symptoms of cryoglobulinemia [70,71]. Raynaud's disease, a condition that may result from an abnormal plasma factor, has also been treated by plasma exchange [72].

THROMBOTIC THROMBOCYTOPENIC PURPURA

The treatment of thrombotic thrombocytopenia purpura (TTP) by plasma exchange illustrates the complexities in assessing this form of therapy. TTP has been treated in a variety of ways, including splenectomy, glucocorticoids, antiplatelet agents, and heparin, with good results in some instances [73]. The mortality rate has been estimated as high as 80 percent [74]. A large number of

studies have reported considerable improvement in mortality rate by the use of plasma exchange [75–82] or exchange transfusion [83], but no controlled studies have been performed.

In most cases, frequent large-volume plasma exchanges were necessary before a sustained remission was achieved. Most investigators agree that FFP is the exchange fluid of choice in TTP, but the administration of antiplatelet agents—aspirin and dipyridamole—was thought to be an important ancillary therapeutic factor in one study [79]. It is not clear whether plasma exchange produces remission in TTP by the removal of an as yet undefined pathogenic plasma factor, by the action of plasma as the replacement fluid, or by both mechanisms.

References

1. Freireich, E. J., Judson, G., and Levin, R. H.: Separation and collection of leukocytes. *Cancer Res.* 24:1516, 1965.
2. Morse, E. E., Carbone, P. P., Freireich, E. J., Bronson, W., and Kliman, A.: Repeated leukapheresis of patients with chronic myelocytic leukemia. *Transfusion* 6:175, 1966.
3. Vallejos, G. S., McCredie, K. B., Britten, G. M., and Freireich, E. J.: Biological effects of repeated leukapheresis of patients with chronic myelogenous leukemia. *Blood* 49:925, 1973.
4. Curtis, J. E., Hersh, E. M., and Freireich, E. J.: Leukapheresis therapy of chronic lymphocytic leukemia. *Blood* 39:163, 1972.
5. Hocker, P., Pitterman, E., Gobets, M., and Stacher, A.: Treatment of patients with chronic myeloid leukemia (CML) and chronic lymphocytic leukemia (CLL) by leukapheresis with a continuous flow blood cell separator, in *Leukocytes: Separation, Collection and Transfusion*, edited by J. M. Goldman and R. M. Lowenthal. Academic, London, 1975, p. 510.
6. Huestis, D. S., Corrigan, J. J., and Johnson, H. V.: Leukapheresis of a five-year-old girl with chronic granulocytic leukemia. *Transfusion* 15:489, 1975.
7. Lowenthal, R. M., et al.: Intensive leukapheresis as initial therapy for chronic granulocytic leukemia. *Blood* 46:835, 1975.
8. Huestis, D. W., Price, M. J., White, R. F., and Inman, M.: Leukapheresis of patients with chronic granulocytic leukemia (CGL), using the Haemonetics Blood Processor. *Transfusion* 16:255, 1976.
9. Stirling, M. L., Parker, A. C., Keller, A. J., and Urbaniak, S. J.: Leukapheresis for papilloedema in chronic granulocytic leukaemia. *Br. Med. J.* 2:676, 1977.
10. Caplan, S. M., Coco, F. V., and Berkman, E. M.: Management of chronic myelocytic leukemia in pregnancy by cell pheresis. *Transfusion* 18:120, 1978.
11. Fritz, R. D., Forkner, G. E., Freireich, E. J., Frei, E., and Thomas, L. B.: The association of fatal intracranial hemorrhage and "blastic crisis" in patients with acute leukemia. *N. Engl. J. Med.* 261:59, 1959.
12. McKee, L. C., and Collins, R. D.: Intravascular leukocyte thrombi and aggregates as a cause of morbidity and mortality in leukemia. *Medicine* 53:463, 1974.
13. Harris, A. L.: Leukostasis associated with blood transfusion in acute myeloid leukaemia. *Br. Med. J.* 1:1169, 1978.
14. Eisenstadt, R. S., and Berkman, E. M.: Rapid cytoreduction in acute leukemia: Management of cerebral leukostasis by cell pheresis. *Transfusion* 18:113, 1978.
15. Lichtman, M. A.: Rheology of leukocytes, leukocyte suspensions, and blood in leukemia. *J. Clin. Invest.* 52:350, 1973.
16. Edelson, R., Facktor, M., Andrews, A., Lutzner, M. A., and Schien, P.: Successful management of the Sezary syndrome. *N. Engl. J. Med.* 291:293, 1974.
17. Pineda, A. A., Brzica, S. M., and Taswell, H. F.: Continuous-and semicontinuous-flow blood centrifugation systems: Therapeutic

applications, with plasma-, platelet-, lympha-, and eosinapheresis. *Transfusion* 17:407, 1977.

18. Bongiovanni, M. B., Katz, R. S., Tomaszewski, J. E., Ziselman, E. M., Goldwein, M. I., and Wurzel, H. A.: Cytapheresis in a patient with Sezary syndrome. *Transfusion* 21:332, 1981.

19. Fay, J. W., Moore, J. O., Logue, G. L., and Huang, A. T.: Leukopheresis therapy of leukemic reticuloendotheliosis (hairy cell leukemia). *Blood* 54:747, 1979.

20. Taft, E. G., Babcock, R. B., Scharfman, W. B., and Tartaglia, A. P.: Plateletpheresis in the management of thrombocytosis. *Blood* 50:927, 1977.

21. Panlilio, A. L., and Reiss, R. F.: Therapeutic plateletpheresis in thrombocythemia. *Transfusion* 19:147, 1979.

22. Greenberg, B. R., and Watson-Williams, E. J.: Successful control of life-threatening thrombocytosis with a blood processor. *Transfusion* 15:620, 1975.

23. Nusbacher, J., Scher, M. L., and MacPherson, J. L.: Plateletpheresis using the Haemonetics Model 30 cell separator. *Vox Sang.* 33:9, 1977.

24. Goldfinger, D., Thompson, R., Lowe, C., Kurz, L., and Belkin, G.: Long-term plateletpheresis in the management of primary thrombocytosis. *Transfusion* 19:336, 1979.

25. Ricks, P.: Further experience with exchange transfusion in sickle cell anemia and pregnancy. *Am. J. Obstet. Gynecol.* 100:1087, 1968.

26. Brody, J. I., Goldsmith, M. H., Park, S. K., and Sotys, H. D.: Symptomatic crisis of sickle cell anemia treated by limited exchange transfusion. *Ann. Intern. Med.* 72:327, 1970.

27. Kernoff, L. M., Botha, M. B., and Jacobs, P.: Exchange transfusions in sickle cell disease using a continuous-flow blood separator. *Transfusion* 17:269, 1977.

28. Lanzowsky, P., Shende, A., Karayalcin, G., Kim, Y. J., and Abelli, A. M.: Partial exchange transfusion in sickle cell anemia. *Am. J. Dis. Child.* 132:1206, 1978.

29. Cundall, J. R., Moore, W. H., and Jenkins, D. E.: Erythrocyte exchange in paroxysmal nocturnal hemoglobinuria prior to cardiac surgery. *Transfusion* 18:626, 1978 (abstract).

30. Yarrish, R. L., Janas, J. S., Nosanchuk, J. S., Steigbigel, R. T., and Nusbacher, J.: Transfusion-acquired falciparum malaria: Treatment with exchange transfusion following delayed diagnosis. *Arch. Intern. Med.* 142:187, 1982.

31. Propper, R. D., Button, L. M., and Nathan, D. G.: New approaches to the transfusion management of thalassemia. *Blood* 55:55, 1980.

32. Corash, L., et al.: Selective isolation of young erythrocytes for transfusion support of thalassemia major patients. *Blood* 57:599, 1981.

33. Propper, R. D.: Current concepts in the overall management of thalassemia. *Ann. N.Y. Acad. Sci.* 344:375, 1980.

34. Collins, J. A.: Problems associated with the massive transfusion of stored blood. *Surgery* 75:274, 1974.

35. Marsaglia, G., and Thomas, E. D.: Mathematical consideration of cross circulation and exchange transfusion. *Transfusion* 11:216, 1971.

36. Russell, J. A., Toy, J. L., and Powles, R. L.: Plasma exchange in malignant paraproteinemias. *Exp. Hematol. (Suppl.)* 5:105, 1977.

37. Flaum, M. A., Cuneo, R. A., Applebaum, F. R., Deisseroth, A. B., Engle, K. W., and Gralnick, H. R.: The hemostatic imbalance of plasma-exchange transfusion. *Blood* 54:694, 1979.

38. Orlin, J. B., and Berkman, E. M.: Partial plasma exchange using albumin replacement: Removal and recovery of normal plasma constituents. *Blood* 56:1055, 1980.

39. McCullough, J., Fortuny, I. E., Kennedy, B. J., Edson, J. R., Branda, R. F., and Jacob, H. S.: Rapid exchange with the continuous-flow centrifuge. *Transfusion* 13:94, 1973.

40. Watson, D. K., Penny, A. F., Marshall, R. W., and Robinson, E. A. E.: Citrate induced hypocalcemia during cell separation. *Br. J. Haematol.* 44:503, 1980.

41. Branda, R. F., Moldow, G. F., McCullough, J. J., and Jacob, H. S.: Plasma exchange in the treatment of immune disease. *Transfusion* 15:570, 1975.

42. Patten, E., Reuter, F. P., Castle, R., and Mercer, C.: Evans' syndrome: Benefit from plasma exchange. *Transfusion* 18:383, 1978.

43. Petz, L. D., and Garratty, G.: *Acquired Immune Hemolytic Anemias.* Churchill Livingstone, New York, 1980, chap. 11, p. 418.

44. Rosenfield, R. E., and Jagathambal: Transfusion therapy for autoimmune hemolytic anemia. *Semin. Hematol.* 13:311, 1976.

45. Logue, G. L., Rosse, W. F., and Gockerman, J. P.: Measurement of the third component of complement bound to red blood cells in patients with cold agglutinin syndrome. *J. Clin. Invest.* 52:493, 1973.

46. Taft, E. G., Propp, R. P., and Sullivan, S. A.: Plasma exchange for cold agglutinin hemolytic anemia. *Transfusion* 17:173, 1977.

47. Branda, R. F., Tate, D. Y., McCullough, J. J., and Jacob, H. S.: Plasma exchange in the treatment of fulminant idiopathic (autoimmune) thrombocytopenic purpura. *Lancet* 1:688, 1978.

48. Marder, V. J., Nusbacher, J., and Anderson, F. W.: One-year follow-up of plasma exchange therapy in 14 patients with idiopathic thrombocytopenic purpura. *Transfusion* 21:291, 1981.

49. Schulman, I., Pierce, M., Lukens, A., and Currimbhoy, Z.: Studies in thrombopoiesis. I. A factor in normal human plasma required for platelet production; chronic thrombocytopenia due to its deficiency. *Blood* 16:943, 1960.

50. Imbach, P., Barandun, S., Baumgartner, C., Hirt, A., Hofer, F., and Wagner, H. P.: High-dose intravenous gamma globulin therapy of refractory, in particular idiopathic thrombocytopenia in childhood. *Helv. Paediatr. Acta* 46:81, 1981.

51. Pintado, T., Taswell, H. F., and Bowie, E. J. W.: Treatment of life-threatening hemorrhage due to acquired factor VIII inhibitor. *Blood* 46:535, 1975.

52. Nillson, I. M., Jonsson, S., Sundqvist, S. B., Ahlber, A., and Bergentz, S. E.: A procedure for removing high titer antibodies by extracorporeal protein-A-Sepharose adsorption in hemophilia: Substitution therapy and surgery in a patient with hemophilia B and antibodies. *Blood* 58:38, 1981.

53. Berkman, E. M., Caplan, S., and Kim, G. S.: ABO-incompatible bone marrow transplantation: Preparation of plasma exchange and in vivo antibody absorption. *Transfusion* 18:504, 1978.

54. Bensinger, W. I., Baker, D. A., Buckner, C. D., Clift, R. A., and Thomas, E. D.: Immunoadsorption for removal of A and B blood group antibodies. *N. Engl. J. Med.* 304:160, 1981.

55. Bensinger, W. I., Baker, D. A., Buckner, C. D., Clift, R. A., and Thomas, E. D.: In vitro and in vivo removal of anti-A erythrocyte antibody by adsorption to a synthetic immunoadsorbant. *Transfusion* 21:335, 1981.

56. Buckner, C. D., et al.: ABO-incompatible marrow transplants. *Transfusion* 26:233, 1978.

57. Graham-Pole, J., Barr, W., and Willoughby, M. L. N.: Continuous-flow plasmapheresis in management of severe rhesus disease. *Br. Med. J.* 1:1185, 1977.

58. Fraser, I. D., et al.: Intensive antenatal plasmapheresis in severe rhesus immunization. *Lancet* 1:6, 1976.

59. Robinson, E. A. E., and Tovey, L. A. D.: Intensive plasma exchange in the management of severe Rh disease. *Br. J. Haematol.* 45:621, 1980.

60. Tilz, G. P., Weiss, P. A. M., Teubl, I., Lanzer, G., and Vollmann, H.: Successful plasma exchange in rhesus incompatibility. *Lancet* 2:203, 1977.

61. Cimo, P. L., and Aster, R. H.: Post-transfusion purpura: Successful treatment by exchange transfusion. *N. Engl. J. Med.* 287:290, 1972.

62. Abramson, N., Eisenberg, P. D., and Aster, R. H.: Post-transfusion purpura: Immunologic aspects and therapy. *N. Engl. J. Med.* 291:1163, 1974.

63. Solomon, A., and Fahey, J. L.: Plasmapheresis therapy in macroglobulinemia. *Ann. Intern. Med.* 58:789, 1963.

64. Skoog, W. A., Adams, W. S., and Coburn, J. W.: Metabolic balance study of plasmapheresis in a case of Waldenstrom's macroglobulinemia. *Blood* 19:425, 1962.

65. Lawson, N. S., Nosanchuk, J. S., Oberman, H. A., and Myers, M. C.: Therapeutic plasmapheresis in treatment of patients with Waldenstrom's macroglobulinemia. *Transfusion* 8:174, 1968.

66. Luxemberg, M. N., and Mausolf, F. A.: Retinal circulation in the hyperviscosity syndrome. *Am. J. Ophthalmol.* 70:588, 1970.

67. Lindsely, H., Teller, D., Noonan, B., Peterson, M., and Mannik, M.: Hyperviscosity syndrome in multiple myeloma: A reversible, concentration-dependent aggregation of the myeloma protein. *Am. J. Med.* 54:682, 1973.

68. Powles, R., Smith, C. R., and Hamilton Fairley, G.: Method of removing abnormal protein rapidly from patients with malignant paraproteinemias. *Br. Med. J.* 2:664, 1971.

69. Buskard, N. A., et al.: Plasma exchange in the long-term management of Waldenstrom's macroglobulinemia. *Can. Med. Assoc. J.* 117:135, 1977.

70. Berkman, E. M., and Orlin, J. B.: Use of plasmapheresis and partial plasma exchange in the management of patients with cryoglobulinemia. *Transfusion* 20:171, 1980.

71. McLeod, B. C., and Sassetti, R. J.: Plasmapheresis with return of cryoglobulin-depleted autologous plasma (cryoglobulinpheresis) in cryoglobulinemia. *Blood* 55:866, 1980.

72. Talpos, G., Horrocks, M., White, J. M., and Cotton, L. T.: Plasmapheresis in Raynaud's disease. *Lancet* 1:416, 1978.

73. Cuttner, J.: Thrombotic thrombocytopenic purpura: A ten-year experience. *Blood* 56:302, 1980.

74. Amorosi, E. L., and Ultmann, J. E.: Thrombotic thrombocytopenic purpura: Report of 16 cases and review of the literature. *Medicine* 45:139, 1966.

75. Bukowski, R. M., King, J. W., and Hewlett, J. S.: Plasmapheresis in the treatment of thrombotic thrombocytopenic purpura. *Blood* 50:413, 1977.

76. Byrnes, J. J., and Khurana, M.: Treatment of thrombotic thrombocytopenic purpura with plasma. *N. Engl. J. Med.* 297:1386, 1977.

77. Pisciotta, A. V., Garthwaite, T., Darin, J., and Aster, R. H.: Treatment of thrombotic thrombocytopenic purpura by exchange transfusion. *Am. J. Hematol.* 3:73, 1977.

78. Taft, E. G.: Thrombotic thrombocytopenic purpura and dose of plasma exchange. *Blood* 54:842, 1979.

79. Myers, T. J., Wakem, C. J., Ball, E. D., and Tremont, S. G.: Thrombotic thrombocytopenic purpura: Combined treatment with plasmapheresis and antiplatelet agents. *Ann. Intern. Med.* 92:149, 1980.

80. Byrnes, J. J., and Lian, E. C. Y.: Recent therapeutic advances in thrombotic thrombocytopenic purpura. *Semin. Thromb. Hemostas.* 5:199, 1979.

81. Rossi, E. C., DelGreco, F., Kwaan, H. C., and Lerman, B. B.: Hemodialysis-exchange transfusion for treatment of thrombotic thrombocytopenic purpura. *JAMA* 244:1466, 1980.

82. Lian, E. C. Y., Harkness, D. R., Byrnes, J. J., Harkness, H., and Nunez, R.: Presence of a platelet aggregating factor in the plasma of patients with thrombotic thrombocytopenic purpura (TTP) and its inhibition by normal plasma. *Blood* 53:333, 1979.

83. Rubenstein, M. A., Kagan, E. M., MacGillviray, M. H., Reuben, M., and Sachs, H.: Unusual remission in a case of thrombotic thrombocytopenic purpura syndrome following fresh blood exchange transfusions. *Ann. Intern. Med.* 51:1409, 1959.

APPENDIX *Laboratory techniques*

SECTION ONE

Erythrocyte studies

CHAPTER *A1*

Polychrome staining

WILLIAM J. WILLIAMS

PURPOSE OF THE TEST
Staining of blood films with polychrome stains permits identification of the various cell types in the peripheral blood and
marrow.

PRINCIPLE OF THE TEST
The polychrome stains are mixtures of methylene blue altered
by heating in $NaHCO_3$ solution or in acid bichromate (methylene azure) and eosin [1]. Methylene azure is blue-violet and
stains acidic cell components, such as nuclei and cytoplasmic
RNA. Eosin is red and stains more basic components, such as
hemoglobin. Some structures stain with both components. The
stains are methanolic solutions of the precipitate which forms
on mixing the two dyes. Because the dyes are dissolved in
methanol, the solution can be used to fix the blood or marrow
film as well as to stain it.

REAGENTS
1. Wright's stain. Many satisfactory solutions are available
commercially, or the dry stain can be purchased as a powder.
To prepare a solution from the dry stain, 0.1 g is ground in a
mortar with sequential addition of small amounts of absolute
methanol to a final volume of 60 ml. The mixture is allowed to
stand at room temperature for 1 to 2 days. It is then filtered
before use. Wright's stain must be kept in a tightly stoppered
bottle to prevent entry of water vapor and should not be
opened when acidic or basic solutions are being used, e.g.,
while staining for iron.
2. Giemsa stain. Satisfactory solutions are available commercially. They are diluted in distilled water prior to use.
3. Microscopic slides and cover slips. These are available
commercially. Cover slips 22 mm square of thickness No. 2
are convenient if the working distance of the oil immersion
objectives of the microscope is sufficiently great to permit
their use. Otherwise thinner cover slips must be used. Slides
and cover slips must be thoroughly clean.

TECHNIQUE
1. Preparation of films of peripheral blood:
   a. Cover slip method (see Fig. A1-1). After thorough
   cleaning with alcohol, the skin of the fingertip is pierced
   with a disposable lancet. The first drop of blood is wiped off
   with a piece of dry gauze, and a drop of blood about 2 mm in
   diameter is allowed to accumulate at the site of the wound.
   The drop is touched quickly with a cover slip held horizon-
   tally by the thumb and index finger placed on the edges near
   one end. A spot of about 2 or 3 mm in diameter should be
   transferred to the cover slip. A second cover slip is immediately placed over the first, in a position rotated 90° so that the
   corners can be readily grasped between the thumb and index
   finger of the free hand. The blood is allowed to spread be-

FIGURE A1-1 Techniques of preparing blood films on cover slips and slides. [R. O. Greep (ed.),
Histology, 2d ed., McGraw-Hill, New York, 1966.]

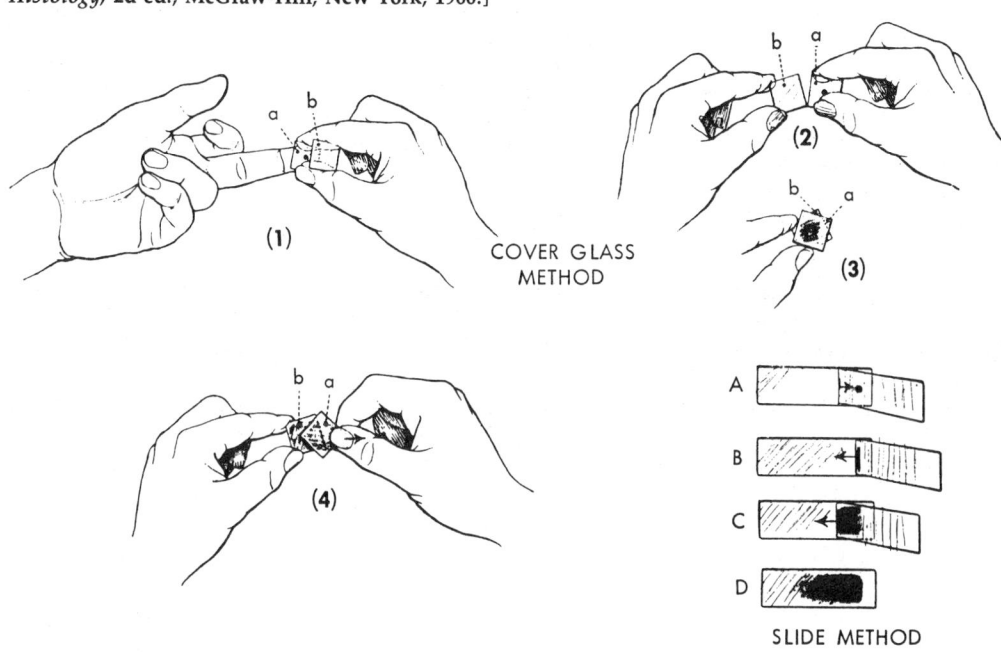

COVER GLASS
METHOD

SLIDE METHOD

tween the cover slips. As soon as the blood stops spreading, the cover slips are separated in a sliding motion so that they remain in the same plane. If there is no lifting motion, there will be an even, thin film of blood on each cover slip.

b. Slide method (see Fig. A1-1). The fingertip is pierced as described above. The slide is touched to the drop of blood so that a spot of blood somewhat larger than that used for the cover slip method is transferred to the slide near one end. The slide is then placed on a flat surface or held in a horizontal position by placing the thumb and index finger on opposite ends. A second slide is held at an angle of about 30° from the horizontal, with its long axis parallel to that of the slide with the blood on its upper surface. The lower edge of the second slide is placed firmly on the surface of the first so that the drop of blood is beneath the second slide. The second slide is then moved slowly toward the blood until contact is made, whereupon the blood will flow evenly along the area of contact between the two slides. The second slide is then pushed rapidly and smoothly in the opposite direction, maintaining contact between the two slides. If the drop of blood appears to be too large, the spreader slide may be lifted, moved a few millimeters from the drop of blood, and the film prepared as described. The film formed should be even and about one-third to one-half the length of the slide. The thickness of the film depends on the rate of movement of the spreader slide and the angle at which the spreader is held; a larger angle makes a thicker slide. Slide films are useful for examining erythrocytes but are less satisfactory for leukocytes because the larger cells (polymorphonuclear leukocytes and monocytes) tend to accumulate near the edge of the slide.

c. Spinner method [2,3]. Blood films with even distribution of cells can be prepared on glass slides using a special centrifuge which provides rapid rotation of the slide in a horizontal plane. A measured aliquot of anticoagulated blood is placed on the center of the slide, and the rate and duration of centrifugation are adjusted to permit even spreading of the blood over the glass surface.

2. Preparation of marrow films: this is described in Chap. 3 in conjunction with the techniques of aspiration and biopsy of marrow.

3. Staining of the films:

a. The films must be supported in a horizontal position. With cover slips this may be accomplished by placing the cover slip atop a small rubber stopper standing on its end in a metal tray. With slides a small rack can be constructed consisting of two parallel glass or metal rods about 2 in. apart. This rack may be placed across a metal tray and the slides placed on it.

b. Wright's stain is placed on the film from a dropper pipette in sufficient quantity to cover the entire surface of the slide or cover slip evenly. The stain is left for 1 to 2 min to fix the film. Optimal times for this step should be determined for each batch of stain.

c. Distilled water, tap water, or buffer from a dropper pipette is then added to dilute the stain. The amount of water

should be enough to cover the slide completely, but none should run off. Because the surface tension of water is much greater than that of alcohol, about 2.5 ml of water can be added to a slide and 0.5 ml to a cover slip without difficulty. A thin film, metallic in appearance, forms on the stain when it is diluted. The water and stain can be mixed by blowing gently on the preparation so that a circular motion is imparted to the liquid. The choice as to tap water, distilled water, or buffer is made empirically. Usually tap or distilled water is satisfactory, but it may be necessary to use 0.05 M sodium phosphate buffer at pH 6.4 to obtain good results (see below). The diluted stain is left on the slide for 3 to 6 min. The optimal time for this step must also be determined for each batch of stain.

d. The stain is washed off the slide or cover slip with running water. The preparation should be kept horizontal and the stain washed off quickly to avoid precipitation of stain on the surface of the film.

e. The staining may be improved by covering the slides with a 1:10 dilution of Giemsa stain for 5 min after the Wright staining is completed. The Giemsa stain is rinsed off with water by the technique that was used for the Wright stain.

f. The film is allowed to dry in air. The preparation may be blotted gently to hasten drying. Cover slips may be mounted temporarily by placing them over a drop of immersion oil on a slide. Permanent mounts can be made with mounting medium.

INTERPRETATION

The details of the appearance of cells stained with Wright's stain are presented in Chaps. 2 and 3. Properly stained films appear pink grossly; microscopically the red cell are pink. In some films the red cells may be blue and the nuclei deeply stained. This may be due to too prolonged staining, inadequate washing, or excessively alkaline stain or diluting fluid. Other films show excessive redness of the red cells and poor staining of the nuclei, which is due to inadequate staining, excessive washing, or excessively acid stain or diluting fluid. Exposure of the stain or diluent to HCl fumes during staining for iron is a common cause of the latter problem.

The procedure is deceptively simple, and films may be improperly stained even when one apparently has followed the procedure carefully. Occasionally it is necessary to obtain all fresh reagents in order to achieve proper results.

References

1. Lillie, R. D.: Factors influencing the Romanowsky staining of blood films and the role of methylene violet. *J. Lab. Clin. Med.* 29:1181, 1944.
2. Ingram, M., and Minter, F. M.: Semiautomatic preparation of coverglass blood smears using a centrifugal device. *Am. J. Clin. Pathol.* 51:214, 1969.
3. Rogers, C. H.: Blood sample preparation for automated differential systems. *Am. J. Med. Technol.* 39:435, 1973.

Heinz body staining

ERNEST BEUTLER

PURPOSE OF THE TEST
Heinz bodies are particles of denatured hemoglobin which are generally attached to the cell membrane. They are found after the administration of chemicals or drugs such as chlorates, phenylhydrazine, or, in sensitive individuals, primaquine [1]; such drugs result in the oxidative denaturation of hemoglobin. Similar inclusion bodies are found when an unstable hemoglobin, such as hemoglobin Zürich, is present.

PRINCIPLE OF THE TEST
Heinz bodies assume a purple color when exposed to certain basic dyes. They are most easily seen when the red cells are slightly distended by suspension in a hypotonic solution.

REAGENTS AND EQUIPMENT
1. Crystal violet solution. Approximately 2 g of crystal violet (C.I. 681) is added to 100 ml of 0.73% sodium chloride solution at room temperature. The mixture is shaken for 5 min and filtered. It is mixed with an equal volume of 0.73% sodium chloride solution.
2. An ordinary light microscope with oil immersion lens and clean slides and cover glasses are needed.

TECHNIQUE
A drop of approximately 0.025 ml of the crystal violet staining solution is placed on a slide. A small droplet of blood (approximately 0.01 ml) is placed on a cover slip using a wooden or glass applicator stick. The cover slip is put on the slide so that the droplet of blood will come in contact with the drop of staining solution. The slide is ready for examination after approximately 5 min.

INTERPRETATION
Heinz bodies appear as small purplish inclusions, usually seen at the margin of the cell. Reticulocytes are not stained by this technique.

SOURCE OF REAGENTS
Crystal Violet (Sigma Chemical Co., St. Louis, Mo.).

References

1. Beutler, E., Dern, R. J., and Alving, A. S.: The hemolytic effect of primaquine. VI. An *in vitro* test for sensitivity of erythrocytes to primaquine. *J. Lab. Clin. Med.* 45:40, 1955.

Blood, marrow, and urine iron stains

ERNEST BEUTLER

PURPOSE OF THE TEST
Iron stains of the marrow are very useful in the diagnosis of iron deficiency anemia (see Chap. 48). Macrophages generally contain no iron in this disorder [1]. Developing erythroblasts which contain stainable iron granules are known as *sideroblasts.* These cells are found normally, but they are absent or their number is greatly diminished in patients with iron deficiency anemia [1–3]. In sideroblastic anemia, on the other hand (see Chap. 54), the number of iron granules in the developing erythroblasts is greatly increased. Iron-containing inclusions in red blood cells are generally seen only in splenectomized individuals and may be observed in such patients with a variety of disturbances in erythropoiesis. Hemosiderin is present in the urinary sediment of patients with intravascular hemolysis and may be demonstrated as free granules or as granules within epithelial cells. It may also sometimes be present in patients with hemochromatosis.

PRINCIPLE OF THE TEST
The stain is based on the well-known Prussian-blue reaction. Ionic iron reacts with an acid ferrocyanide solution to give a blue color.

REAGENTS AND EQUIPMENT
1. 4% hydrochloric acid in water. Carefully pour 40 ml of concentrated (38%) HCl solution into 340 ml of cold distilled water, stirring constantly. This solution is stable for many months at room temperature.
2. 4% potassium ferrocyanide in distilled water. This solution is stable for many months at room temperature.
3. Basic fuchsin stock solution. Dissolve 1 g of basic fuchsin in 10 ml of absolute alcohol and add 90 ml of 5% aqueous phenol solution. Filter. Stable for many months at room temperature.
4. Dilute counterstaining solution. Add 3 ml of basic fuchsin stock solution to 100 ml of distilled water. Stable for several days at room temperature.
5. Formaldehyde solution. Formalin (37% formaldehyde gas in H_2O).

TECHNIQUE

BLOOD AND MARROW
Films of blood or marrow are made in the usual manner. They are air-dried, and immediate fixation is not necessary. Prior to staining, the slides are fixed in formalin vapor by placing them in a staining jar containing a sponge or a piece of filter paper slightly moistened with formalin. The staining jar is closed and permitted to stand for approximately 2 or 3 min. Equal volumes of 4% hydrochloric acid and 4% potassium ferrocyanide solutions are mixed in a staining jar. The fresh mixture is heated to approximately 56°C, and the slides immersed in the solution.

After 30 min they are removed from the staining solution and are rinsed in tap water. They are counterstained for 5 min with dilute basic fuchsin solution. They are again rinsed with water, then with absolute ethyl alcohol, and again with water. After drying they are ready for examination.

URINE SEDIMENT

The sediment from a random specimen of urine is collected by centrifugation. Most of the supernate is decanted, leaving a small volume in which the sediment is resuspended. An equal volume of a mixture of equal parts of 4% HCl and 4% potassium ferrocyanide is added and the mixture incubated at room temperature for 10 min, with frequent agitation. A drop of the suspended sediment is placed on a glass slide, covered with a cover slip, and examined microscopically. Alternatively, a film of the urine sediment may be prepared as a glass slide and stained by the technique used for blood or marrow.

INTERPRETATION

A portion of the film in which marrow cells are well separated is most suitable for the identification of sideroblasts. Sideroblasts appear as nucleated red cells, the pink cytoplasm of which contains one or more small blue granules, usually less than 1 μm in diameter (see Fig. 54-1 and Plate 3). Normally 20 to 50 percent of the erythroblasts contain such inclusions. When these granules surround the nucleus, the cell is known as a *ringed sideroblast*. Sideroblasts are pink-staining, non-nucleated erythrocytes which contain one or more small bluish granules. Macrophage iron is most readily seen in particles on the marrow film. Macrophages which have become separated from marrow particles are much less suitable because the cell membranes of such cells have been torn and the iron particles will be dispersed. Iron particles in macrophages may be spherical, irregularly shaped, finely granular particles, or the cells may be diffusely stained. Although often the macrophage nucleus may not be visible, the intracellular location of the iron may be surmised from the aggregation of the iron particles in small areas, suggesting that they are, indeed, enclosed within the membrane of a single cell.

Occasional contamination with exogenous iron appears to be difficult to avoid, and it is therefore necessary for the individual examining the iron-stained material to learn to distinguish artifacts from iron which is present in the cells. Artifacts may often be recognized by the fact that they are found above or below the plane of the material being studied. Highly refractile particles usually represent artifacts.

Hemosiderin in urine may be seen as free blue granules or as blue granules contained within epithelial cells of the urine sediment. The intracellular hemosiderin is less likely to be artifactual than are the free granules and therefore has greater significance. In conditions such as paroxysmal nocturnal hemoglobinuria, urine hemosiderin is nearly always present and may be a valuable aid in making the diagnosis.

References

1. Beutler, E., Robson, M. J., and Buttenwieser, E.: A comparison of the plasma iron, iron-binding capacity, sternal marrow iron and other methods in the clinical evaluation of iron stores. *Ann. Intern. Med.* 48:60, 1958.
2. Kaplan, E., Zuelzer, W. W., and Mouriquand, C.: Sideroblasts: A study of stainable nonhemoglobin iron in marrow normoblasts. *Blood* 9:203, 1954.
3. Weinfeld, A., and Hansen, H. A.: Further studies on the interrelationship between hemosiderin and sideroblasts in bone marrow smears. *Acta Med. Scand.* 171:23, 1962.

CHAPTER *A4*

Reticulocyte staining

JEAN ATWATER
ALLAN J. ERSLEV

PURPOSE OF THE TEST

The enumeration of immature red cells (reticulocytes) is a simple and direct way in which to assess the effective rate of red cell production. Because of premature or delayed release from the marrow and different rates of maturation, the reticulocyte counts do not always reflect absolute erythroid activity. However, the ease by which reticulocytes can be counted serially in the same individual makes the reticulocyte count an excellent method for estimating changes in the rate of red cell production.

PRINCIPLE OF THE TEST

Residual RNA in immature red blood cells is precipitated and stained with a supravital dye, such as new methylene blue [1] or brilliant cresyl blue. Films are prepared, and the cells containing stained precipitates (reticulum) are counted. The results are reported as a percentage of the red cells examined or as an absolute number per microliter.

REAGENTS AND EQUIPMENT

1. New methylene blue N (C.I. 52030). Dissolve 0.5 g of the dye in 100 ml of distilled water containing 1.6 g of potassium oxalate.

2. Brilliant cresyl blue. Dissolve 1 g of the dye in 100 ml of 0.9% saline solution containing 0.4 g of sodium citrate ($Na_3C_6H_5O_7 \cdot 2\ H_2O$).

3. Microhematocrit tubes.

4. Microscope slides and cover slips.

5. Parafilm squares, 2×2 in.

TECHNIQUE

Place 2 drops of blood on a Parafilm square (or glass slide). Add 2 drops of either of the dye solutions and mix with a microhematocrit tube. Half-fill two or three hematocrit tubes with the mixture. After 10 or 15 min make thin films and air-dry. Using an oil emersion objective and examining areas of the blood film where cells do not overlap, count the number of cells containing any blue granules or reticulum occurring among 1000 red blood cells. For an accurate count, the red cells should not be overlapping, in clumps, or in rouleaux.

CALCULATION OF RESULTS

Report the number of reticulocytes per 100 red blood cells, or convert the percentage to absolute value as follows:

$$\frac{\% \text{ reticulocytes} \times \text{RBC}/\mu l}{100} = \text{reticulocytes}/\mu l$$

The presence of basophilic stippling may introduce an error in the enumeration of reticulocytes on a film stained with new methylene blue. This error can be eliminated by first enumerating stippled cells on a film stained with Wright's stain and then subtracting this number from the number of stippled cells enumerated on a film stained with new methylene blue [2].

INTERPRETATION

Absolute reticulocyte counts average about 60,000 per microliter. The mean percentage for normal adult males is 1.6 ± 0.5 and for females is 1.4 ± 0.5 [3]. Newborn infants have levels of 2.5 to 6.5 percent, but this drops to normal adult levels in 2 weeks [4].

References

1. Brecher, G.: New methylene blue as a reticulocyte stain. *Am. J. Clin. Pathol. 19:895,* 1949.
2. Jensen, W. N., Moreno, G. D., and Bessis, M. C.: An electron microscopic description of basophilic stippling in red cells. *Blood 25:933,* 1965.
3. Atwater, J., and Erslev, A. J.: Unpublished data.
4. Miale, J. B.: *Laboratory Medicine: Hematology,* 4th ed. Mosby, St. Louis, 1972, p. 655.

CHAPTER *A5*

Examination of blood for malaria and other parasites

ALLAN J. ERSLEV
RICHARD A. BURNINGHAM

Purpose of the test

The parasites that inhabit human blood, tissues, and viscera can in general be diagnosed on careful microscopic examination of stained blood films, stained smears of tissue aspirates, histologic sections, or stained touch preparations from infected organs. Serologic and immunologic methods for parasitic detection have been developed [1–5], but the blood film remains the most definitive method. Parasites that infect the blood may be intracellular or extracellular. Extracellular organisms such as the trypanosomes and microfilariae can be observed microscopically in unstained preparations. However, the stained blood film must be examined in order to see smaller forms and to identify the parasitic species. In malaria the diagnosis of the specific species causing the infection can be accomplished only by careful microscopic examination of the stained blood film.

Principle of the test

The demonstration of parasites in blood is accomplished by examination of blood films stained with Giemsa's or Wright's solution. In most circumstances the blood sample to be studied should be obtained during the acute phase of the disease.

Reagents and equipment

1. Standard blood collecting and staining equipment
2. Cleaned, grease-free microscopic slides
3. Wright's stain solution
4. Giemsa's stain solution
5. Absolute methanol
6. 1% saponin solution in 0.9% NaCl
7. 2% formalin solution
8. Distilled water, pH 7.2
9. 10- by 75-mm serologic test tubes
10. Standard laboratory centrifuge
11. Pipettes

Techniques for the detection of intracellular organisms

MALARIA

THIN FILM METHOD

A film of blood from a fingerstick or a tube of anticoagulated blood is prepared in the usual manner, using cleaned, grease-free, properly labeled slides. The film is fixed in methanol for 2 min and stained with Giemsa's solution diluted 1:20 with distilled water at pH 7.2 for 15 min. The slides are washed in running water and allowed to dry at room temperature. When using Wright's stain, no preliminary fixation is required.

THICK PREPARATION OR DROP METHOD

The thick preparation is especially useful in clinically mild malarial infections in which the organisms could easily be missed in the thin film. Two to three drops of blood are placed on a slide to cover an area approximately 15 mm in diameter and allowed to dry completely. Giemsa's solution diluted 1:20 with distilled water at pH 7.2 is carefully poured over the slide, and the blood is stained for 15 min *without* prior fixation. During staining the red blood cells are lysed. The slide is then tilted carefully and the stain allowed to run off. A few drops of distilled water are then placed on the edge of the slide and allowed to wash over the residue gently without detaching it from the slide. The slide is dried at room temperature. Since the red blood cells have been lysed, the intracellular location of the parasites will not be evident. Thick preparations which are 2 to 3 days old should be dehemoglobinized prior to staining with Giemsa's solution. This is accomplished by carefully pouring distilled water on the slide. After 2 min the hemoglobin-containing water is allowed to run off by tilting the slide. Giemsa's solution is then applied as previously de-

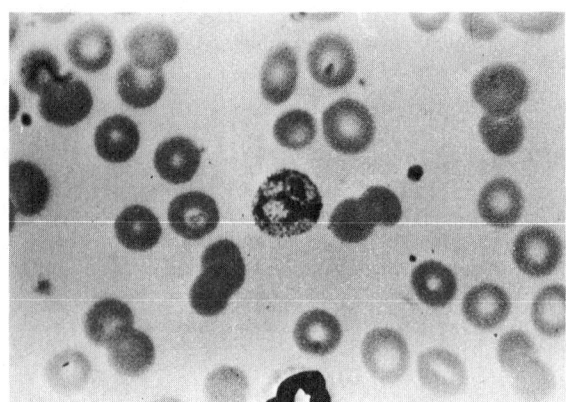

FIGURE A5-1   *Plasmodium vivax*, schizont. (Courtesy of Dr. M. Yoeli.)

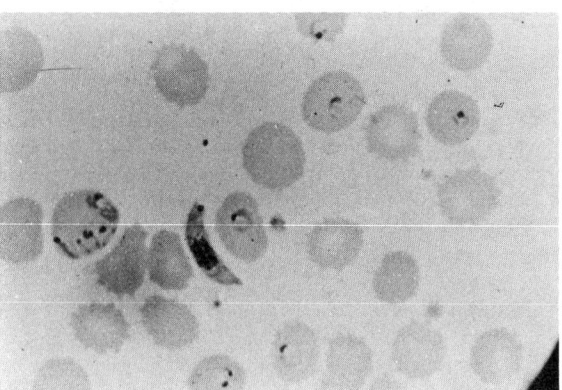

FIGURE A5-3   *Plasmodium falciparum*, gametocyte and ring forms. (Courtesy of Dr. M. Yoeli.)

scribed. Wright's stain should not be used for thick preparations.

CONCENTRATION BY SAPONIN HEMOLYSIS

This method can be used instead of the thick preparation but is not as practical. To 2 ml of whole blood anticoagulated with ethylenediaminetetracetate (1 mg EDTA to 1 ml whole blood) is added 1.5 ml of 1% saponin solution in 0.9% saline solution, using 75-mm serologic test tubes. Lysis of red cells is generally completed in 30 to 60 s. The mixture is centrifuged at 2000 to $2300 \times g$ for 1 min. The supernatant fluid is decanted into a second tube and centrifuged at the same speed for 10 min. The sediments from the first and second centrifugations are then smeared, dried, and stained as described for the thin film. A high concentration of malarial parasites is obtained with well-preserved morphology. Ring forms are found in the first sediment.

Interpretation

When examining a blood film for plasmodia, the observer must be able to distinguish plasmodial forms from other blood elements or artifacts. This can be especially difficult for a thick

film with crowded, lysed red cells. Unless the examiner has considerable experience, prolonged scrutiny of several thin, regularly prepared films may be preferable. Intraerythrocytic inclusions, such as Howell-Jolly bodies, Cabot rings, superimposed platelets, crenated or distorted cells, and precipitated stain, can simulate malaria parasites. The diagnosis of malaria in a properly stained film is not difficult [6]. *Plasmodium vivax* develops in large, pale erythrocytes and imparts a stippled appearance to the red cell—Schüffner's dots (Fig. A5-1). The following forms are visible in the peripheral blood: ring forms, ameboid stage, 14 to 16 merozoites in the mature schizont and gametocyte. *P. malariae* grows in nonenlarged red blood cells and shows no stippling. A characteristic feature of the parasite is a tendency to spread across the cell to form a bandlike structure. Also, the 8 to 10 merozoites of the mature schizont tend to form a rosette (Fig. A5-2). *P. falciparum*, the most dangerous of the malaria parasites, inhabits nonenlarged red cells. Except on rare occasions, only the young trophozoites and gametocytes are present in the blood. The gametocyte tends to form a banana, or sickled, shape (Figs. A5-3 and A5-4). In *P. falciparum* it is important to remember that the development of these parasites takes place extravascularly in internal organs. Therefore the intensity of the parasitemia in the peripheral blood does not always mirror the intensity of the infection. Thus it is essential, especially with suspected *P. falciparum*, to examine

FIGURE A5-2   *Plasmodium malariae*, schizont, rosette formation of merozoites. (Courtesy of Dr. M. Yoeli.)

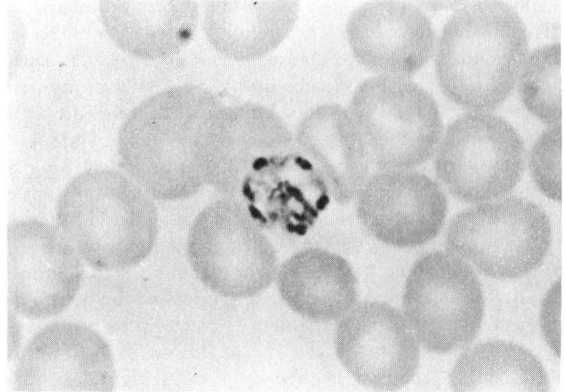

FIGURE A5-4   *Plasmodium falciparum*, ring forms. (Courtesy of Dr. M. Yoeli.)

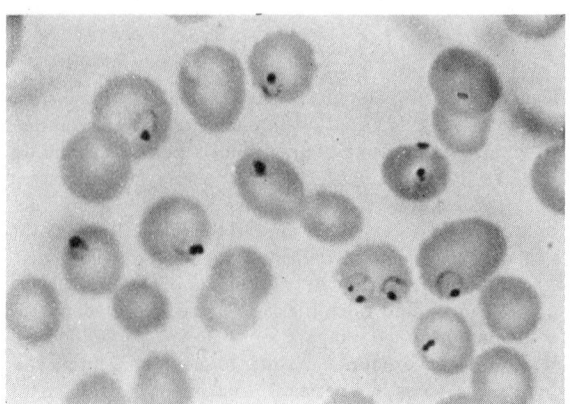

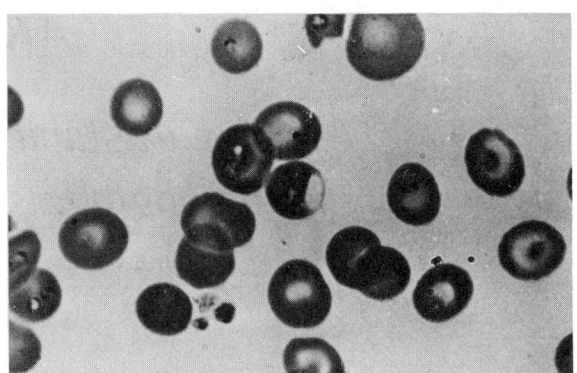

FIGURE A5-5   *Babesia microti,* **transmitted by transfusion of blood from infected individual. (Courtesy of Dr. M. Lichtman.)**

both thin and thick preparations and not to accept the first negative report as final.

OTHER PARASITES

Other blood parasites of humans can be seen with these techniques [7]. *Bartonella baccilliformis,* a parasite confined to certain areas of Central and South America, causing Oroya fever (Carrion's disease), is diagnosed by finding small, elongated, bacillary forms intimately associated with the erythrocyte [8]. *Babesia microti,* a protozoan parasite which infests domestic and wild animals, is endemic to the northeastern coastal region of the United States [9]. It is transmitted to humans by the bite of the deer tick and by transfusion of blood from asymptomatic carriers. Like Bartonella infection, *B. microti* is particularly dangerous for asplenic individuals. The parasite can be demonstrated in red cells as ring-shaped organisms similar to *P. falciparum* (Fig. A5-5). However, the finding of budding and cross-shaped forms facilitates the correct diagnosis. Quinine and Clindamycin are effective chemotherapeutic agents [10]. *Leishmania* organisms are pathogenic protozoa that develop in the macrophages of different organs and in the blood [11]. In the visceral form, kala-azar, *L. donovani* organisms can be seen by examining stained films made from aspirates of the marrow, liver, or spleen (Fig. A5-6). In rare cases the organisms may be seen in the granulocytes of the blood.

Techniques for the detection of extracellular parasites

The diagnoses of filariasis and trypanosomiasis depend on detection of characteristic parasitic forms in peripheral blood films prepared as for the diagnosis of malaria. In those patients who have been treated or are not heavily infected, the microfilariae or trypanosomes can be detected best by the following concentration method: Add 2 ml whole blood to 10 ml 2% formalin solution and mix well. The mixture is centrifuged at $1500 \times g$ for 5 min, and the supernatant is discarded. The sediment is smeared, allowed to dry, fixed, and stained with Giemsa's solution as previously described.

FILARIASIS

The most important filarial infections of humans are those caused by *Wuchereria bancrofti, Brugia malayi, Loa loa,* and *Onchocerca volvulus* [12]. Each species is transmitted by a particular type of blood-sucking insect. The adult worm of *W. bancrofti* lives in lymph nodes and lymphatic channels and produces live embryos—microfilariae (Fig. A5-7). The biologic adaptation to the mosquito vector has resulted in the nocturnal appearance of the microfilariae of *W. bancrofti* in the blood. Therefore the diagnosis can best be made by examining blood obtained between 8 P.M. and 4 A.M. Two methods can be used. A fresh drop of blood is placed on a clean glass slide. A cover slip is carefully placed over the drop, and the blood is examined microscopically under low power. The moving microfilariae, over 200 μm in length, can be seen displacing erythrocytes. Permanent preparations can be made by using the thick preparation method described previously. However, fixation after dehemoglobinization of the specimen is recommended. The same methods are used for diagnosing other forms of filariasis. In *L. loa* the parasites have a diurnal rhythm, and so blood for examination should be taken during the daylight hours. In *O. volvulus* the diagnosis is made by demonstrating microfilariae from skin scrapings or adult worms from subcutaneous nodules.

TRYPANOSOMIASIS

When present in large numbers, trypanosomal parasites, such as *Trypanosoma brucei,* one of the causative agents of African trypanosomiasis, may be seen microscopically in unstained

FIGURE A5-6 *Leishmania donovani,* **touch prep. Hamster. (Courtesy of Dr. M. Yoeli.)**

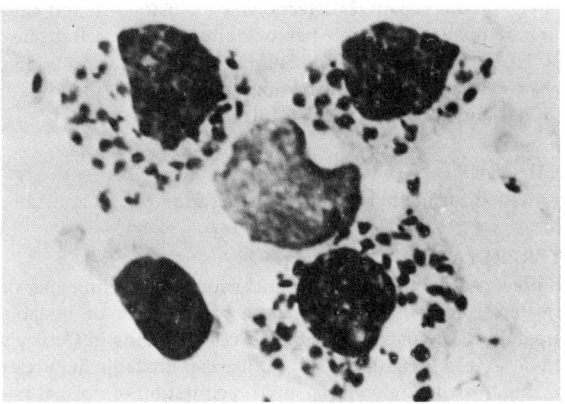

FIGURE A5-7 *Wuchereria bancrofti,* **microfilaria in blood. (Courtesy of Dr. M. Yoeli.)**

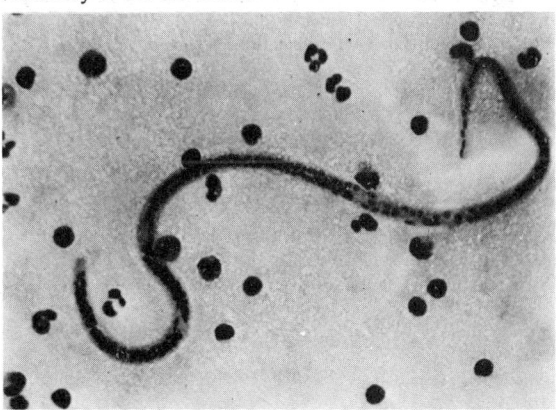

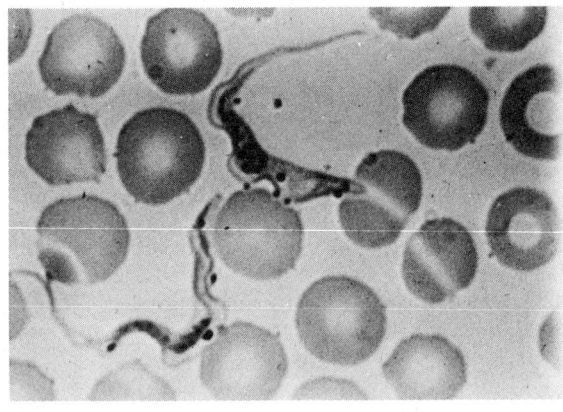

FIGURE A5-8 *Trypanosoma brucei,* **African trypanosomiasis. (Courtesy of Dr. M. Yoeli.)**

wet preparations of human blood. [3]. Here they appear as slender, colorless, tapered forms undulating amid the erythrocytes (Fig. A5-8). The morphology is best seen in thick and/or thin preparations stained with Giemsa's solution. The organisms measure about 14 to 33 μm in length, have a prominent, centrally located nucleus which stains red, and posteriorly have a smaller red dot, the kinetoplast. The cytoplasm may contain irregular-sized bluish granules. *T. cruzi* organisms occur in two forms: the leishmanial form exists in macrophage, or tissue cells, especially in the heart and intestines, and the trypanosomal form circulates in the blood [14]. In the blood the trypanosomal organisms are about 20 μm long and tend to curl into C-shaped forms with a large kinetoplast. Their cellular structure is similar to that of other trypanosomal species.

References

1. Hunter, G. W., Swartzwelder, J. C., and Clyde, D. F.: *Tropical Medicine,* 5th ed. Saunders, Philadelphia, 1976.
2. Voller, A.: The detection and measurement of malarial antibodies. *Trans. R. Soc. Trop. Med. Hyg.* 65:111, 1971.
3. Joshua, R. A., Herbert, W. J., and White, R. J.: Diagnosis of African Trypanosomiasis. *Trans. R. Soc. Trop. Med. Hyg.* 73:602, 1979.
4. Ranque, J., and Guilici, M.: Recent advances in immunodiagnosis of Leishmaniasis. *J. Parasitol.* 56:227, 1970.
5. Smithers, S. R., and Terry, R. J.: Immunology of schistosomiasis. *Adv. Parasitol.* 14:399, 1976.
6. Perrin, L. H., Mackey, L. J., and Miescher, P. A.: The hematology of malaria in man. *Sem. Hematol.* 19:70, 1982.
7. Ristic, M., and Kreier, J. P.: Hemotrophic bacteria, *N. Engl. J. Med.* 301:937, 1979.
8. Reynafarje, C., and Ramos, J.: The hemolytic anemia of human bartonellosis. *Blood* 17:562, 1961.
9. Jacoby, G. A., et al.: Treatment of transfusion-transmitted babesiosis by exchange transfusion. *N. Engl. J. Med.* 303:1098, 1980.
10. Wittner, M., et al.: Successful chemotherapy of transfusion babesiosis. *Ann. Int. Med.* 96:601, 1982.
11. Miescher, P. A., and Belehu, A.: Leishmaniasis: Hematologic aspects. *Sem. Hematol.* 19:93, 1982.
12. Sasa, M.: *Human Filariasis.* University Press, Baltimore, 1976.
13. Wéry, M., et al.: Hematologic manifestations, diagnosis and immunopathology of African trypanosomiasis. *Sem. Hematol.* 19:83, 1982.
14. *American Trypanosomias Research,* PAHO, Scientific Publications 318, 1975.

Tests for unstable hemoglobins

HAEWON C. KIM
JEAN ATWATER
ELIAS SCHWARTZ

Some hemolytic anemias are due to unstable hemoglobins. Many unstable hemoglobins are electrophoretically silent, and some may constitute only a small percentage of the total hemoglobin. If special care is not given to blood samples during preparation, storage, and analysis, these hemoglobins precipitate, resulting in a concentration too low to demonstrate by routine hemoglobin electrophoresis. Toluene or chloroform should not be used to prepare hemolysates when searching for unstable hemoglobins [1]. Unstable hemoglobins already precipitated can be demonstrated by methylviolet staining. If still in solution, they can be detected by exposing red cells or hemolysate to oxidants, heat, isopropanol, or mechanical shaking.

Methyl violet test

PURPOSE OF THE TEST
This supravital stain detects preformed inclusions of precipitated hemoglobin (Heinz bodies) in erythrocytes and erythroblasts.

PRINCIPLE OF THE TEST
Unstable hemoglobins denature, precipitate, and produce Heinz bodies in vivo. Methyl violet stains preformed Heinz bodies but does not induce precipitation of unstable hemoglobin. Since inclusion bodies are selectively removed by the spleen, Heinz bodies are usually not seen in blood in the presence of a functioning spleen but may be present after splenectomy or in erythroblasts of marrow samples. This latter is most common in thalassemia syndromes where excess α or β chains precipitate [2–6]. An alternate method for evaluation of Heinz bodies is the acid elution technique which is primarily used to detect F cells (Chap. A9). However, this technique has been applied for the sensitive detection of inclusions in red cells from patients with unstable hemoglobins or sickle cell disease [7,8]. Heinz bodies are seen as compact, pink inclusion bodies in ghost cells after all soluble hemoglobin with the exception of Hb F has eluted at the proper acidic pH.

TECHNIQUE
The method for methyl violet test is described in Chap. A2.

INTERPRETATION
The presence of violet-stained inclusions in erythrocytes or nucleated red cells indicates previous precipitation of unstable hemoglobin. The usual causes are excess α chains in Cooley's anemia, excess β chains in Hb H disease, unstable hemoglobins due to structural defects, and precipitation of normal he-

moglobin following an oxidative insult in G-6-PD deficiency [9].

Brilliant cresyl blue test

PURPOSE OF THE TEST
This test detects Hb H (β_4) and other unstable hemoglobins by simple microscopic evaluation.

PRINCIPLE OF THE TEST
Incubation of whole blood with brilliant cresyl blue (BCB) causes oxidative denaturation and precipitation of unstable hemoglobins and staining of the precipitates, resulting in diffuse stippling of the red blood cells [6]. This contrasts with the methyl violet and acid elution methods, where precipitation of hemoglobin is not induced during the procedure.

REAGENTS AND EQUIPMENT
1. Fresh blood collected with an anticoagulant
2. Brilliant cresyl blue, 1% in citrate saline (0.4 g of $Na_3C_6H_5O_7 \cdot 2H_2O$ in 100 ml of 0.9% saline)
3. 37°C water bath
4. Whatman #42 filter paper

TECHNIQUE
1. Mix stain and filter the amount to be used through filter paper before use.
2. Incubate equal volumes of whole blood (3 to 4 drops) and the BCB solution at 37°C. Keep tube covered to minimize evaporation.
3. Make and air-dry a blood film at 10 min, 1 h, and 4 h.
4. Remove tubes from water bath and keep at room temperature. Make film again at 24 h.
5. Examine under oil immersion. A sample from a normal control should be included with every run.

INTERPRETATION
The 10-min slide is a control indicating the number of reticulocytes present, since reticulum is stained by BCB. If there is an increase in the number of stained particles on the later slides, it is most probably due to precipitated denatured hemoglobin. The positive pattern is characterized by particles distributed evenly throughout the cell and is quite different from the stained reticulum of reticulocytes. It has been aptly described as resembling the even pattern on a golf ball. The color of the precipitate, pale blue, is also different from the bluish-black particles in reticulocytes.

The even distribution of pale blue inclusions on films indicates the presence of an unstable hemoglobin [10–12]. When the 1-h slide shows numerous cells with inclusions, the presence of Hb H should be strongly suspected since other unstable hemoglobins usually require a longer period of incubation in order to be denatured and precipitated to the same degree. With increases in the time of incubation, the individual precipitates become larger.

Heat stability test

PURPOSE OF THE TEST
Unstable hemoglobins precipitate upon exposure to heat, a property which can be used for in vitro identification [13].

PRINCIPLE OF THE TEST
Heating of the hemolysate enhances dissociation of hemeglobin or alterations in subunit contacts in hemoglobins which are unstable due to structural abnormalities. Unstable hemoglobin can usually be detected by turbidity when a fresh hemolysate in an appropriate buffer is heated at 50°C for 1 to 2 h. Comparison of the optical density of the supernate before and after heating allows detection and estimation of the percentage of unstable hemoglobin.

REAGENTS AND EQUIPMENT
1. Whole blood (drawn within 24 h, using any anticoagulant)
2. Tris buffer, 0.1 M, pH 7.4. Dissolve 12.1 g tris-[2-amino-2-(hydroxymethyl)-1,3-propandiol] in 800 ml distilled water at room temperature. Add HCl (0.1 N) with constant mixing until the pH is 7.4 and then bring the volume to 1 liter with water.
3. Cyanmethemoglobin diluent, 1 liter containing:

Sodium bicarbonate	1.0 g
Potassium cyanide	50 mg
Potassium ferricyanide	200 mg

4. Centrifuge
5. Spectrophotometer (visible light)
6. Water bath, 50°C

TECHNIQUE
1. Wash red cells from 3 to 4 ml of blood with 0.85% NaCl solution three times.
2. Lyse the washed red cells with five volumes of buffer containing 0.5 mM EDTA and 5 mM phosphate at pH 7.4. Mix gently, allow to stand for 5 min, add 0.1 volume of 9.0% saline, and centrifuge at 15,000 × g for 20 min at 4°C. Draw off the clear hemolysate at the top of the tube with a Pasteur pipette.
3. Add 3 ml of the hemolysate to 3 ml of tris buffer.
4. Pipette 2 ml of this solution into each of two tubes. Place one tube in the refrigerator and the other, after covering to prevent evaporation, in a water bath at 50°C.
5. At the end of 2 h, centrifuge both tubes at 2000 × g for 10 min.
6. From each tube remove 0.1 ml of the clear supernate and dilute with 5 ml cyanmethemoglobin solution. (These tubes may be refrigerated overnight if necessary.)
7. Centrifuge at 20,000 × g for 20 min.
8. Remove clear supernate and read optical densities at 540 nm against a blank made by adding 0.1 ml tris buffer to 5 ml of the cyanmethemoglobin solution. A sample known to be normal should be used with every run.

CALCULATION OF RESULTS
Quantitation of the precipitated hemoglobin is calculated by the formula

$$\frac{OD_R - OD_{50°}}{OD_R} \times 100 = \% \text{ precipitated hemoglobin}$$

where OD_R is the optical density of the refrigerated solution at 540 nm and $OD_{50°}$ is the optical density of the incubated sample at 540 nm.

INTERPRETATION
Less than 5 percent of normal hemoglobin will precipitate at 50°C. Phosphate buffers retard precipitation of hemoglobin at 50°C and should not be used for the test [13], but can be used at higher temperatures [14].

The use of 5 mM phosphate buffer containing 0.5 mM EDTA in the preparation of hemolysate does not retard precipitation of hemoglobin because the phosphate concentration is so low. Instead, this buffer promotes the maximum hemolysis of red cells.

Isopropanol stability test

PURPOSE OF THE TEST
This is a simple test to detect unstable hemoglobins and to provide purified fractions for further studies.

PRINCIPLE OF THE TEST
Normal hemoglobin is somewhat unstable at 37°C in a 17% isopropanol solution and will begin to precipitate after 40 min. Unstable hemoglobins will start to precipitate in 5 min under the same conditions and will become flocculent by 20 min [15]. The isopropanol solution is relatively nonpolar and tends to weaken the internal bonding of hemoglobin, thereby decreasing stability of the molecule.

REAGENTS AND EQUIPMENT
1. Fresh hemolysate prepared as for the heat stability test described above. Whole blood may be stored for several days at 4°C before lysis, but precipitation of some unstable hemoglobins may occur during storage.
2. Isopropanol-tris buffer. Tris buffer, 0.1 M pH 7.4, is described above in the heat stability test. Add 170 ml of isopropanol to about 700 ml of tris buffer and adjust the pH again to 7.4. Dilute to 1 liter with tris buffer. Keep in a tightly stoppered bottle at room temperature.
3. Waterbath, 37°C.

TECHNIQUE
1. Heat two small stoppered test tubes containing 2 ml of the isopropanol-tris buffer to 37°C in water bath.
2. Add 0.2 ml of a fresh control hemolysate to one tube and 0.2 ml of the test hemolysate to the other. Restopper and mix by inverting. Return the tubes to the water bath. Check for precipitation at 5 min, 20 min, and 40 min.

INTERPRETATION
Normal hemoglobin does not begin to precipitate until about 30 to 40 min. Unstable hemoglobin shows signs of precipitation by 5 min and flocculation by 20 min.

Shaking test

PURPOSE OF THE TEST
This test provides an alternate method of detecting heat-unstable hemoglobins and sickle hemoglobin by a rapid and simple procedure[16]. A modification of the test allows accurate quantitation of these hemoglobins [17].

PRINCIPLE OF THE TEST
The oxy form of sickle hemoglobin is unstable when subjected to mechanical shaking, either by hand or by machine [18]. This instability is influenced by conformation of the molecule, type of buffer salt, pH, temperature, and rate of shaking. Some hemoglobins, both traditionally unstable ones (e.g., $Hb_{Köln}$ [17],

$Hb_{Gun\ Hill}$ [19], and Hb_{Leiden} [19]) and traditionally stable ones (e.g., Hb C$_{Harlem}$ [14]), precipitate much more quickly than Hb S, whereas others (e.g., Hb H and Hb_{Philly} [20]) need special conditions to demonstrate this abnormality.

REAGENTS AND EQUIPMENT
1. Blood sample collected in a heparinized microhematocrit tube
2. 10 mM sodium phosphate solution, pH 8.0
3. Vials 15 mm by 45 mm, with caps
4. TCS shaker, Model 150 (Southampton, PA 18966)

TECHNIQUE
1. Centrifuge the microhematocrit tubes and break just below the interface between red cell and plasma. Add the red cells in a fragment of the capillary tube to 2 ml of phosphate buffer in the vial.
2. Shake the vial for 2 min in the TCS shaker. The red cells (or hemolysate) may alternatively be added to 2 ml buffer in a test tube, covered, and shaken by hand with a rapid wrist motion for 2 min. This latter method is effective but tiring.
3. A kinetic analysis of the rate of precipitation may be performed easily by determining the absorbency at 542 or 577 nm of the original hemolysate and of the solutions after shaking for several time intervals and centrifuging to remove the precipitate [17].

INTERPRETATION
The presence of turbidity after shaking indicates Hb S or a heat-unstable hemoglobin in the solution.

In a kinetic analysis, the rate of precipitation of the abnormal hemoglobin may be determined from a graph of percent hemoglobin remaining versus time. The percent hemoglobin remaining is calculated as (A_{542} after shaking) $\times$ 100/(A_{542} of original hemolysate). $Hb_{Köln}$ may be easily distinguished from Hb S by this method, since it precipitates at a rate five times as fast. In addition, the percentage of abnormal hemoglobin may be accurately calculated from this type of graph by extrapolation of the portion of the curve representing Hb A (the slow portion) to zero. The percentage of abnormal hemoglobin is equal to 100 minus the value of the intercept of this extrapolated line representing Hb A.

References

1. Asakura, T., Adachi, K., and Schwartz, E.: Stabilizing effect of various organic solvents on proteins. *J. Biol. Chem. 253*:6423, 1978.
2. Fessas, P.: Inclusions of hemoglobin in erythroblasts and erythrocytes of thalassemia. *Blood 21*:21, 1963.
3. Yataganas, X., and Fessas, P.: The pattern of hemoglobin precipitation in thalassemia and its significance. *Ann. N.Y. Acad. Sci. 165*:270, 1969.
4. Friedman, S., Ozsoylu, S., Luddy, R., and Schwartz, E.: Heterozygous beta thalassaemia of unusual severity. *Br. J. Haematol. 32*:65, 1976.
5. Adams, J. G., III, Boxer, L. A., Baehner, R. L., Forget, B. G., Tsistrakis, G. A., and Steinberg, M. H.: Hemoglobin Indianapolis (β112[G14] Arginine), an unstable β-chain variant producing the phenotype of severe β-thalassemia. *J. Clin. Invest. 63*:931, 1979.
6. Rigas, D. A., and Koler, R. D.: Decreased erythrocyte survival in hemoglobin H disease as a result of the abnormal properties of hemoglobin H: The benefit of splenectomy. *Blood 18*:1, 1961.
7. Kleihauer, E., and Kohne, E.: Application of the acid elution technique for the detection of inclusion bodies: Abnormal haemoglo-

bins and thalassaemia, in *Diagnostic Aspects,* edited by R. M. Schmidt. Academic, New York, 1975, p. 149.

8. Kim, H. C., Friedman, S., Asakura, T., and Schwartz, E.: Inclusions in red blood cells containing Hb S or Hb C. *Br. J. Haematol.* 44:547, 1980.

9. Beutler, E.: The hemolytic effect of primaquine and related compounds: A review. *Blood* 14:103, 1959.

10. Gabuzda, T. G.: Hemoglobin H and the red cell. *Blood* 27:568, 1966.

11. Rieder, R. F., Zinkham, W. H., and Holtzman, N. A.: Hemoglobin Zürich. *Am. J. Med.* 39:4, 1965.

12. Rieder, R. F., Oski, F. A., and Clegg, J. B.: Hemoglobin Philly (β 35 tyrosine $\rightarrow$ phenylalanine): Studies in the molecular pathology of hemoglobin. *J. Clin. Invest.* 48:1627, 1969.

13. Schneiderman, L. J., Junga, I. G., and Fawley, D. E.: Effect of phosphate and nonphosphate buffers on thermolability of unstable haemoglobins. *Nature* 225:1041, 1970.

14. Adachi, K., Kinney, T. R., Schwartz, E., and Asakura T.: Molecular stability and function of Hb C-Harlem. *Hemoglobin* 4:1, 1980.

15. Carrell, R. W., and Kay, R.: A simple method for the detection of unstable haemoglobins. *Br. J. Haematol.* 23:615, 1972.

16. Asakura, T., Segal, M. E., Friedman, S., and Schwartz, E.: A rapid test for sickle hemoglobin. *JAMA* 233:156, 1975.

17. Asakura, T., Adachi, K., Shapiro, M., Friedman, S., and Schwartz, E.: Mechanical precipitation of hemoglobin Köln. *Biochim. Biophys. Acta* 412:197, 1975.

18. Asakura, T., Ohnishi, T., Friedman, S., and Schwartz, E.: Abnormal precipitation of oxyhemoglobin S by mechanical shaking. *Proc. Natl. Acad. Sci. U.S.A.* 71:1594, 1974.

19. Roth, E. F., Elbaum, D., and Nagel, R. L.: Observations on the mechanical precipitation of oxy Hb S and other mutants. *Blood* 45:377, 1975.

20. Asakura, T., Adachi, K., Schwartz, E., and Wiley, J.: Molecular stability of Hb Philly (α $\beta^{35(C1) \ Tyr \rightarrow Phe}$): The relationship of hemoglobin stability to ligand state as defined by heat and mechanical shaking tests. *Hemoglobin* 5:177, 1981.

CHAPTER *A7*

Separation of hemoglobins

HAEWON C. KIM
JEAN ATWATER
ELIAS SCHWARTZ

Hemoglobins may be separated by various methods, including electrophoresis and chromatography. An evaluation of a patient suspected of having a hemoglobin variant or one of the thalassemia syndromes should include hemoglobin electrophoresis to detect abnormal hemoglobins and to quantitate Hb A_2 and Hb F. Some abnormal hemoglobins are electrophoretically silent but are unstable or have abnormal oxygen affinity; special tests are used for their detection.

The methods described here combine reliability, accuracy, and relative ease of performance in a clinical laboratory. Readers may refer to specialized texts [1–3] for alternative methods and for those used mainly in the research laboratory.

Hemoglobin electrophoresis

PURPOSE OF THE TEST
Hemoglobin electrophoresis can detect and differentiate hemoglobin variants and allows a presumptive identification of the hemoglobin phenotype.

PRINCIPLE OF THE TEST
Human hemoglobins are made up of two separate pairs of globin chains. Each chain consists of amino acids in linear sequence. Some of these amino acids have hydrophilic side chains and thus can be negatively or positively charged depending upon the pH of the medium. Hemoglobin electrophoresis is based on the different rates of migration of charged hemoglobin molecules in an electric field. Many factors can influence the migration pattern of the various hemoglobins, including pH, temperature, voltage, ionic strength of the buffer, and nature of the supporting medium. Normal adult hemoglobin (Hb A) has an isoelectric point at pH 6.8. It therefore has a negative charge in alkaline buffers and a positive charge in acidic buffers. In an alkaline buffer, hemoglobins with a net charge more positive than Hb A migrate more slowly and those with a more negative charge migrate faster than Hb A toward the positively charged electrode.

Electrophoresis in an alkaline buffer (pH 8.6 to 8.8) is the principal method of differentiating hemoglobins. The supporting medium may be cellulose acetate, starch gel, paper, starch block, agarose, or polyacrylamide gel. Electrophoresis on cellulose acetate is the method of choice for the general clinical laboratory because of commercial availability of equipment, ease of preparation, and rapidity of analysis. Electrophoresis on starch gel provides better resolution of hemoglobins and is presently the most widely used method in specialized hematology laboratories. Electrophoresis in acidic buffer can be helpful in identifying certain abnormal hemoglobins. Electrophoresis in agar gel at pH 6.2 is useful in differentiating Hb S from Hb D, and Hb C from Hb O and Hb E. Electrophoresis in starch gel at pH 6.8 to 7.0 will clearly separate Hb H and Hb Bart's from all other hemoglobins.

Globin-chain electrophoresis can be utilized for further differentiation of hemoglobins with similar mobilities (e.g., Hb E and Hb O) on both alkaline and acidic electrophoreses.

The relative mobilities of several abnormal hemoglobins in various media and buffers are summarized in Table A7-1.

Cellulose acetate electrophoresis

PURPOSE OF THE TEST
Cellulose acetate electrophoresis [4,5] should be the initial procedure in screening for abnormal hemoglobins, including sickle hemoglobin, in anyone over 3 months old. The equipment is commercially available, the procedure can be completed within 1 h, and only a drop of blood is needed. The dried cellulose acetate strips may be saved for permanent storage and for rapid quantitation of major bands of hemoglobin by scanning with a densitometer. This scanning method is not accurate for Hb A_2 quantitation.

PRINCIPLE OF THE TEST
The distance between Hb A and its variants depends on the net charge of the molecules. For example, on cellulose acetate electrophoresis, at pH 8.6, Hb S and Hb C migrate more slowly

TABLE A7-1 Electrophoretic relative mobilities of hemoglobin variants under different conditions

Supporting medium, buffer, and pH	Relative migration rates of various hemoglobins*						
Starch gel, paper, starch block, agarose; barbital, pH 8.6; tris-EDTA-borate buffer, pH 8.8	C E O A₂ 1	S DL 5G P	A FMK	J 4 6N3 2	H I		+
Cellulose acetate; tris-EDTA borate buffer, pH 8.6†	C A₂ 7	S D	A	J	H		+
Starch gel, paper, starch block; phosphate buffer, pH 6.8	C O A₂	L	S DGPF 5 E	A JN K	I 2	H	+
Agar gel; phosphate or citrate buffer, pH 6.2	F	A D E A₂ G ‡	S O 7 HL Q	C			+

*Dotted lines indicate origin.

† With a discontinuous buffer system, migration is to the cathodal side, possibly because of a greater electroendosmotic flow.

‡ Also I, J, P, 1, 2, 3, 4, 5.

1, Alexandra	3, Hopkins I	5, Lepore	7, C$_{Harlem}$
2, Bart's	4, Hopkins II	6, Norfolk	

toward the anode than does Hb A because they are more positively charged. Hbs H, I, and J migrate more rapidly toward the anode than does Hb A because they are more negatively charged. Electroendosmotic flow also influences movement, retarding flow toward the anode.

REAGENTS AND EQUIPMENT

1. Sample:

Crude hemolysate: Crude hemolysate can be prepared by mixing one drop of whole, anticoagulated blood with four drops of distilled water.

Purified hemolysate: Collect the red blood cells by centrifugation in a graduated centrifuge tube of anticoagulated blood and wash three times with NaCl solution, 0.85 g/dl. Add 1.5 volumes of 5 mM phosphate and 0.5 mM EDTA solution. Allow the samples to stand for 5 min. Add 0.1 volume of 9.0% saline and centrifuge the samples at 15,000 $\times$ g for 20 min at 4°C. Remove the clear hemolysate with a Pasteur pipette. It may occasionally be necessary to centrifuge this hemolysate again under the same conditions or to filter it in order to clear the solution of debris. Organic solvents should not be used for the preparation of the hemolysate because they tend to precipitate unstable hemoglobin and free α chains. The hemolysate is used for various electrophoretic procedures as well as for quantitation of Hb A₂ and Hb F and may be stored in the refrigerator for 2 to 4 weeks, although some degeneration of hemoglobin will take place. It is best to use the hemolysate within 1 week after preparation, if possible. Hemolysate can be stored at −70°C indefinitely for future use.

2. Tris-EDTA-borate (TEB) buffer, pH 8.6 [5]:

Tris(hydroxymethyl)aminomethane	12.0 g
Ethylenediaminetetraacetic acid	1.22 g
Boric acid	1.5 g
Distilled water	to 1000 ml

Adjust the pH to 8.6 with boric acid. TEB buffer is commercially available and can be prepared from premixed reagents by adding distilled water according to the manufacturer's directions.

3. Ponceau S stain:

Ponceau S	0.5 g
Trichloroacetic acid	5 g
Distilled water	to 100 ml

4. Destaining solution:

Acetic acid, glacial	50 ml
Distilled water	to 111 ml

5. Clearing solution:

Absolute methanol	80 ml
Acetic acid, glacial	20 ml

6. Power supply.
7. Electrophoresis chamber, aligning base, sample well, and sample applicator.
8. Cellulose acetate plates.
9. Staining containers.
10. Paper wicks.
11. Blotters.
12. Hot tray or oven.
13. Plastic envelopes for permanent mounting.

TECHNIQUE
The appropriate methods differ with the type of equipment used and are described in the technical literature included with each apparatus.

CALCULATIONS
The hemoglobins are reported in the order of decreasing concentration, as estimated visually, with comments about the quantities of Hb A$_2$ and Hb F and the presence of any trace components (e.g., Hb$_{Constant Spring}$, Hb$_{Bart's}$ in the newborn). For example, if Hb A is present in a greater amount than Hb S, the report is Hb AS (sickle cell trait likely) but if the amount of Hb S is greater than Hb A, the report reads Hb SA (sickle-β^+ thalassemia likely).

Hb A$_2$ is usually seen on cellulose acetate, except with newborns, in whom only trace amounts of Hb A$_2$ are present. The thin band cathodal to Hb A$_2$ is carbonic anhydrase stained with Ponceau S. In persons over 2 to 3 years of age, Hb F is present in such small amounts that it may be evident only on citrate agar gel electrophoresis.

INTERPRETATION OF RESULTS
Table A7-1 shows migration patterns of normal and the common abnormal hemoglobins on cellulose acetate. Hb S migrates cathodally to Hb A. Hb C migrates cathodally to Hb S at a distance from Hb A twice that between Hb A and Hb S. Hb C and Hb A$_2$ migrate to the same position on cellulose acetate, but they can usually be distinguished by quantitative differences because the Hb C band is more prominent than the Hb A$_2$ band. To detect an increased amount of Hb A$_2$, the density of the band is best compared with that from a normal subject on the same plate, although confirmation by quantitation of Hb A$_2$ is necessary. Hb F separates from Hb A in this system and migrates slightly closer to the origin. However, cellulose acetate electrophoresis is not recommended as an initial screening test during the neonatal period because large amounts of Hb F form a heavy band overlapping the adjacent bands of Hb A or Hb S. For this reason, the presence of small amounts of Hb A or Hb S may not be detected, resulting in an inaccurate diagnosis. Citrate agar gel electrophoresis is preferable for blood from newborns because of the different relative migration of Hb F.

Certain hemoglobins migrate to similar positions on cellulose acetate and must be differentiated by other means, such as citrate agar gel electrophoresis. For instance, Hbs G, D, and Lepore migrate to the position of Hb S, and Hbs E, O, and C Harlem migrate to that of Hb C (Fig. A7-1). Confirmatory testing should be done to determine the presence of Hb S (Chap. A5) or Hb C (electrophoresis on citrate agar gel).

SOURCE OF REAGENTS AND EQUIPMENT
TEB buffer is available as Super-Heme buffer from Helena Laboratories, P.O. Box 752, Beaumont, TX 77704.

Ponceau S stain is available in ready-to-use form from Helena or in concentrated solution from Beckman, Fullerton, Calif. Ponceau S is available from MCB Manufacturing Chemists, 480 Democrat Rd., Gibbstown, NJ 08029.

A suitable power supply is the SP-2717 model from Heath Company, Benton Harbor, MI 49022.

All electrophoresis equipment and cellulose acetate plates are available from Helena, Beckman, or Isolab, Drawer 4350, Akron, OH 44321.

Starch gel electrophoresis

PURPOSE OF THE TEST
Starch gel [6] provides better resolution of hemoglobin than cellulose acetate and is more sensitive in detecting small amounts of hemoglobin. Elevations of Hb A$_2$ and Hb F may be detected by comparison with a normal sample.

Hb H and Hb Bart's may be differentiated from other hemoglobins in starch gel at pH 6.8 to 7.0.

FIGURE A7-1 Differentiation of hemoglobins by cellulose acetate and citrate–agar gel electrophoresis. Origin is at the left border of the photograph of the cellulose acetate strip. (Kim [41], with permission.)

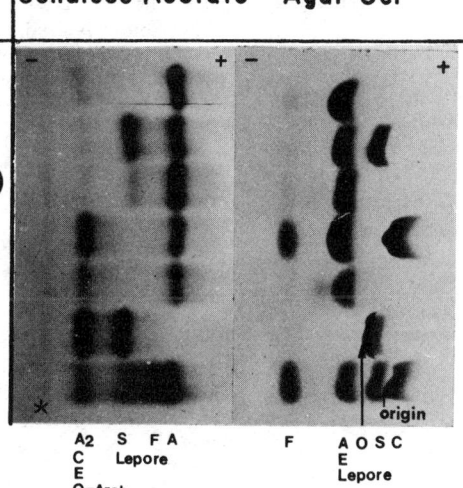

PRINCIPLE OF THE TEST

The principle of starch gel electrophoresis at pH 8.8 is the same as that for cellulose acetate electrophoresis.

Hb A is neutral at pH 6.8, and it will move slightly toward the negative electrode in starch gel at pH 8.8 because of electroendosmotic flow. At this pH, Hb H and Hb Bart's remain negatively charged and move away from the origin toward the positive electrode.

REAGENTS AND EQUIPMENT

1. Hemolysate, as prepared from washed red blood cells for cellulose acetate electrophoresis.
2. Hydrolyzed starch, 50 g.
3. Stock buffers:

Tris-EDTA-borate buffer, pH 8.8

Tris(hydroxymethyl)aminomethane	109.0 g
Sodium diethylenediaminetetraacetate	7.44 g
Boric acid	30.9 g

Dissolve these reagents in distilled water sufficient to make 1000 ml.

Phosphate buffer, pH 6.8

Electrode vessels (0.075 M)		
Na$_2$HPO$_4$ (anhydrous)		10.7 g
Distilled water		1000 ml
Gel (0.011 M)		
Na$_2$HPO$_4$ (anhydrous)		0.81 g
Distilled water		500 ml

Adjust the pH of both of the above solutions to 6.8 with H$_3$PO$_4$.
4. Stains:

> *Benzidine stain.* Stock solution: Dissolve 1 g of *N,N,N',N'*-tetramethylbenzidine in 100 ml of 25% acetic acid. Mild heat may be used. Label and store at room temperature. Working solution: Immediately before use, dilute 1 volume of the stock solution with 2 volumes of distilled water. Add 1 drop of 30% hydrogen peroxide for each 10 ml of the stain and mix. Stain until Hb A$_2$ spots are clearly visible. The staining reaction may be stopped by washing the gel three times in distilled water and then immersing it in 5% acetic acid. Tetramethylbenzidine has not yet been reported as carcinogenic (National Institute for Occupational Safety and Health, December 31, 1981).

Amido black stain

Amido black	1 g
Methanol	100 ml
Acetic acid, glacial	10 ml
Distilled water	100 ml

> Cover gel with this stain and allow to stand for 5 min. Acetic acid (5%) will decolorize a gel stained with amido black.

5. White petrolatum.
6. Starch gel tray with one or two slot formers (10 positions each).
7. Stand for vertical electrophoresis.
8. Buffer vessels fitted with wire electrodes, preferably platinum (two are required, each of 500 ml capacity).
9. Gel slicer.
10. Sheet of soft, clear plastic.
11. Plexiglass sheet slightly larger than the gel mold.
12. Power supply.
13. Flask, 2000-ml, thick-walled, heat-resistant.
14. Bunsen burner.
15. Lead weights.
16. Asbestos gloves.

TECHNIQUE

The separation in TEB buffer, pH 8.8, depends on a discontinuous buffer system [6]; three dilutions of buffer must be prepared:

	Stock buffer		Distilled water
Gel	34 ml	diluted to	500 ml
Cathode tray	71 ml		500 ml
Anode tray	100 ml		500 ml

1. Prepare the gel mold with the ends attached and the slot former in place near one side of the mold. If more than 10 samples are to be run, a second slot former may be placed in the center of the gel mold (in the apparatus from MRA).
2. Pour the diluted buffer for the gel (500 ml) into the 2000-ml, thick-walled, heat-resistant flask, and add the starch (50 g). Swirl to mix. Heat over a flame with constant swirling. The mixture will gradually change consistency and become translucent. The mixture should not boil. Attach the flask to a vacuum source and degas carefully until the gel is clear. Pour immediately into the mold. Cover with the sheet of soft plastic without trapping bubbles. Place the glass sheet over the plastic and apply the lead weights. Allow to stand for 3 to 5 h at room temperature.
3. Dilute the prepared hemolysate by adding 1 to 7 drops of distilled water. The best hemoglobin concentration for the usual analytical purposes is about 1.0 to 1.2 g/dl. The solutions to be analyzed may be adjusted by eye with distilled water so that the hemoglobin concentrations are similar.
4. Remove the lead weights and invert the gel mold. Gently lift the slot former from its position. Apply the samples to the slots with glass capillary tubing. Heat the white petrolatum until it melts and pour into the large depression to cover completely the small slots containing the samples. Allow to cool for a few minutes. Remove the end pieces and stand the mold vertically on a piece of cloth or sponge in the anode tray, using the support to maintain the gel in a vertical position. Cover the exposed top of the gel with a cloth wick that dips in the cathode tray. The electrophoresis should take place in the cold (4 to 8°C) in a refrigerator or a cold room. Run for 15 to 20 h at 20 mA, 250 V. The current will drop somewhat overnight if a constant voltage source is used.
5. After completion of electrophoresis, remove the petrolatum and slice the gel with the gel slicer supplied with the apparatus. One half may be stained with benzidine stain for heme-containing substances and the other half with amido black for proteins. The benzidine stain is usually sufficient and is fully developed in 10 to 20 min.

The gel at neutral pH is prepared and run in the same fashion, except for the different buffers and the placement of the slot former in the center of the mold.

CALCULATIONS

The hemoglobins are reported in order of decreasing concentrations (estimated visually), with comments about the quantities of Hb A$_2$ and Hb F and the presence of any trace components.

INTERPRETATION OF RESULTS

Table A7-1 indicates the relative mobilities of hemoglobins in starch gel at pH 8.8 and pH 6.8. Hb F separates from Hb A and remains slightly closer to the origin. Amounts of Hb F above 2.5 to 3.0 percent can usually be detected by starch gel electrophoresis. Confirmation by quantitation of Hb A_2 and Hb F is advisable.

Certain hemoglobins migrate together and must be tested by other means to ascertain their identity.

The same equipment and buffers may be used for urea–starch gel electrophoresis for separating the globin chains of hemoglobin [7].

SOURCE OF REAGENTS AND EQUIPMENT
Hydrolyzed starch is available from Electrostarch, P.O. Box 1294, Madison, WI 43701, and from Connaught Medical Research Laboratories, University of Toronto, Toronto, Canada (distributed by Fisher Scientific, 191 South Gulph Rd., King of Prussia, PA 19406).

N,N,N',N'-tetramethylbenzidine is available from Aldrich Chemical.

White petrolatum is available from Fisher.

The various pieces of electrophoresis equipment are available from Metaloglass, 466 Blue Hill Ave., Boston, MA 02121; Buchler Instruments, Fort Lee, N.J.; or Otto Hiller, P.O. Box 1294, Madison, WI 53711. A suitable power supply is the SP-2717 model from Heath, Benton Harbor, MI 49022.

Citrate–agar gel electrophoresis

PURPOSE OF THE TEST
Agar gel electrophoresis in an acid buffer system [8,9] is useful for differentiating between several groups of hemoglobins that have similar migration rates in alkaline electrophoresis. In infants less than 3 months old citrate–agar gel electrophoresis is the method of choice as an initial screening procedure because Hb F distinctly separates from Hb A and Hb S, thus allowing small amounts of these hemoglobins to be seen easily.

PRINCIPLE OF THE TEST
The acidic pH and electrical properties of agar provide a separation of normal and abnormal hemoglobins different from those described above. Agar gel electrophoresis in a citrate buffer at pH 6.2 can differentiate Hb C from Hbs O, E, C_{Harlem}, and A_2; Hb S from Hbs D, G, and Lepore; and Hb O from Hbs C, E, and A_2.

REAGENTS AND EQUIPMENT
1. Hemolysate, as prepared for cellulose acetate electrophoresis
2. Citrate buffer, 0.05 M, pH 6.0 to 6.2 [3]:

Stock citrate buffer, 0.5 M

Trisodium citrate ($Na_3C_6H_5O_7 \cdot 2H_2O$)	147.0 g
Citric acid ($H_3C_6H_5O_7 \cdot H_2O$)	4.3 g
Distilled water	to 1000 ml

Working citrate buffer, 0.05 M, pH 6.0 to 6.2

Dilute the stock citrate buffer 1:10 with deionized distilled water. Adjust the pH to between 6.0 and 6.2 with 30% citric acid and store at 4°C. Citrate buffer is commercially available and prepared by diluting premixed reagents in distilled water. Helena citrate buffer, pH 6.0, is found to be satisfactory for routine laboratory use.

3. Agar plates: Precoated agar plates are available. Alternatively, plates can be prepared from agar [2,3,5]. Helena agar plates provide satisfactory resolution of various hemoglobins.

4. Stains:

Bromphenol blue stain

Bromphenol blue	0.1 g
Distilled water	1000 ml
Acetic acid, glacial	10 ml

o-Dianisidine (dimethoxybenzidine) stain

Acetic acid, 5%	10 ml
o-Dianisidine, 0.2% in methanol	5 ml
Sodium nitroferricyanide, 1%	1 ml
Hydrogen peroxide, 3%	1 ml

It is advisable to handle o-dianisidine with maximum care since the question of its carcinogenicity has not been fully resolved. Alternatively, benzidine stain (tetramethylbenzidine), described in the section on starch gel electrophoresis, can be used as a specific heme protein stain.

5. The same equipment required for cellulose acetate electrophoresis.

TECHNIQUE
Satisfactory results can be obtained with commercial kits, but these are costly relative to preparation of agar gel plates and citrate buffers in the laboratory. Below is a brief summary of a technique which is more thoroughly described in the technical literature accompanying the kit from Helena Laboratories.

1. Hemolysate, as prepared for cellulose acetate electrophoresis.
2. Pour 100 ml of citrate buffer, 0.05 M, pH 6.0 to 6.2, into each of the outer compartments of the chamber.
3. Apply hemolysate, including control samples, to the agar plate with sample applicator.
4. Place agar plate, gel side down, in the chamber. Electrophorese at approximately 50 V and 50 mA for 60 min in a cold room or refrigerator at 4 to 6°C.
5. Remove and stain by pouring staining solution over plate. With bromphenol blue, pour off stain after 20 to 30 min and wash agar plate with distilled water. With o-dianisidine, stain for 5 to 10 min and rinse with 5% acetic acid for 10 min.
6. For storage, cover with another gel tray and reseal with tape. Store in cold room or refrigerator.

CALCULATIONS
Hemoglobins are reported in order of decreasing concentration, after estimating the concentrations visually.

INTERPRETATION
Table A7-1 shows migration patterns of hemoglobin variants on agar gel at pH 6.2. This method allows clear separation of Hb F from Hb A and Hb S, and thus it is recommended as an initial screening procedure in infants less than 3 months old. This procedure is also used as a confirmatory test for Hb S and Hb C.

Figure A7-1 shows differentiation by citrate agar gel electrophoresis of hemoglobins that migrate with Hb S and Hb C on cellulose acetate.

SOURCE OF REAGENTS AND EQUIPMENT
Premixed reagents for citrate buffer are available from Helena Laboratories, Box 752, Beaumont, TX 77704, and from Isolab, Drawer 4350, Akron, OH 44321.

Preformed agar plates are also available from Helena, as are o-dianisidine (cat. no. 5032) and sodium nitroferricyanide (cat. no. 5111).

Urea Cellulose Acetate, pH 8.7

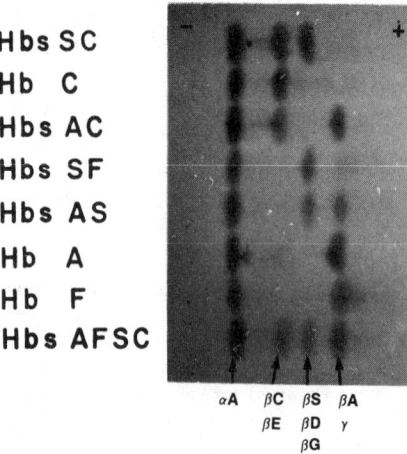

Hbs SC
Hb C
Hbs AC
Hbs SF
Hbs AS
Hb A
Hb F
Hbs AFSC

αA βC βS βA
    βE βD γ
        βG

FIGURE A7-2 Alkaline urea–cellulose acetate electrophoresis pattern (alkaline globin electrophoresis). (Kim [41], with permission.)

Electrophoresis kits may be purchased from Helena (Super Z and Zip Zone Hemo-Citrate Kit) and from Isolab.

Globin chain electrophoresis

PURPOSE OF THE TEST
Separation of globin chains by urea–cellulose acetate or urea–starch-gel electrophoresis provides useful information for further identification when hemoglobins have similar mobility on both cellulose acetate and citrate agar gel (e.g., Hb E and Hb O) [10]. Further characterization of abnormal hemoglobins can be made by comparing mobilities of the mutant globin chains to the mobilities of normal α (α^A) and β chains (β^A) at pH 6.0 and 8.8 [11].

An alternative method of globin chain electrophoresis allows determination of $G\gamma/A\gamma$ ratios for further analysis of high Hb F syndromes, as well as biosynthetic ratios of globin chains [12].

PRINCIPLE OF THE TEST
The use of 2-mercaptoethanol and urea allows the dissociation of heme from globin and the separation of α from non-α chains. Different globin chains have different charges and migrate at a different rate in acidic and alkaline buffers. A variety of supporting media can be used. A method with cellulose acetate is described below.

REAGENTS AND EQUIPMENT
1. The same reagents and equipment required for cellulose acetate electrophoresis
2. Citric acid, 30% (300 g/liter)
3. Urea (purified)
4. 2-Mercaptoethanol
5. Fume hood

TECHNIQUE
1. On the day of the study prepare TEB-urea buffer by adding 54 g of urea to 105 ml of TEB buffer and adjust pH to be-

tween 8.7 and 8.9 for alkaline electrophoresis and to between 6.0 and 6.2 with 30% citric acid for acidic electrophoresis.

2. Set aside 2 ml of TEB-urea buffer for dilution of hemolysate.

3. Add 2 drops of the above buffer, 1 drop of hemolysate, and 1 drop of 2-mercaptoethanol to the test tube. Mix, cover the tube, and incubate at 4 to 6°C for 1 to 2 h. All procedures with 2-mercaptoethanol should be done in a hood because the fumes are irritating.

4. Add 2 ml of 2-mercaptoethanol to the remaining buffer. Mix.

5. Soak the cellulose acetate strip in this buffer for 1 to 2 h.

6. Pour 50 ml of the buffer used to soak the strips into each of the outer compartments of an electrophoresis chamber. Moisten wicks and position in the chamber.

7. Fill the sample well with samples and control.

8. Blot excess buffer from strip.

9. Position strip on the aligning base.

10. Apply the sample using an applicator from sample well. Always run with a control.

11. Apply current for 2.5 to 3 h at 200 V.

12. Remove strip from chamber and stain, rinse, and dry in the same way as for cellulose acetate electrophoresis.

INTERPRETATION OF RESULTS
In both alkaline and acidic globin chain electrophoreses, normal α (α^A) chains move cathodally, remaining close to the origin, and normal β (β^A) chains as well as other globin chains move anodally. Normal γ (γ^F) chains migrate similarly to β^A chains in alkaline globin chain electrophoresis, but γ^F migrates farther toward the anode in acidic globin chain electrophoresis. Figures A7-2 and A7-3 show migration patterns of normal and some abnormal globin chains in alkaline and acidic urea–cellulose acetate electrophoreses. More detailed examples are shown in papers by Schneider et al [10,11,13].

FIGURE A7-3 Acidic urea–cellulose acetate electrophoresis pattern (acidic globin electrophoresis). (Kim [41], with permission.)

Urea Cellulose Acetate, pH 6.0

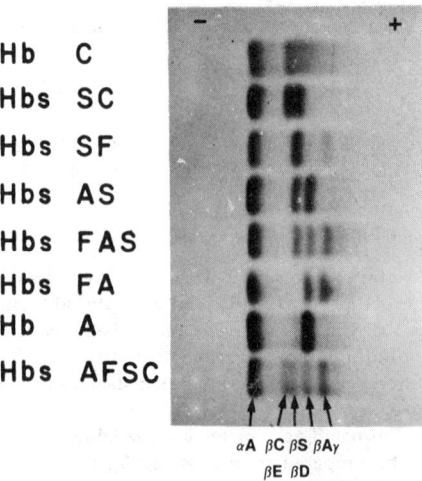

Hb C
Hbs SC
Hbs SF
Hbs AS
Hbs FAS
Hbs FA
Hb A
Hbs AFSC

αA βC βS βAγ
    βE βD
        βO-Arab

Quantitation of Hb A₂

PURPOSE OF THE TEST

There are variations in the level of the minor hemoglobin component Hb A_2 which are of use in the diagnosis of thalassemia.

PRINCIPLE OF THE TEST

Hb A_2 is generally quantitated by any one of three methods: densitometry, elution, or microcolumn chromatography. Scanning a cellulose acetate plate with a densitometer after electrophoresis and staining is not recommended for Hb A_2 analysis and has been shown to be unsatisfactory for detecting β-thalassemia trait [14]. Quantitation of Hb A_2 eluted from cellulose acetate membrane following electrophoresis is a fast and simple procedure and generally gives satisfactory results [15]. However, results of Hb A_2 measurements in the presence of Hb S tend to be higher because Hb A_2 is often not completely separated from Hb S.

The most accurate, simple, and rapid method available at present for measuring Hb A_2 is separation of hemoglobins by DEAE cellulose chromatography [16]. This method is described below. At pH 8.3, a 0.05 M tris-HCl buffer is used to elute Hb A_2 from a column. At this pH and ionic strength, Hb A adheres more strongly to DE52 cellulose than does Hb A_2, resulting in rapid separation and elution of Hb A_2. The optical density of the Hb A_2 eluted from the column is compared to the optical density of the total hemoglobin solution and the percent of Hb A_2 is calculated.

Commercial microcolumns are available for Hb A_2 quantitation, but careful quality control surveillance is necessary to ensure consistent results.

REAGENTS AND EQUIPMENT

1. Anticoagulated whole blood (2 ml).
2. DE52 (diethylaminoethyl cellulose) anion exchanger.
3. Stock buffer, 1.0 M tris buffer:

Tris(hydroxymethyl)aminomethane	60.57 g
Distilled water	to 500 ml

4. Working buffers, 0.05 M tris-HCl, pH 8.5, 8.3, and 7.0:

1.0 M tris buffer	200 ml
KCN	400 mg
Distilled water	to 4000 ml

Pour 2000 ml of buffer into a 2-liter flask and then divide the remaining 2000 ml of buffer equally into two 1-liter flasks. Adjust pH to 8.5, 8.3, and 7.0, respectively, with concentrated HCl and label as buffers 1, 2, and 3, respectively.

5. Cotton.
6. Disposable Pasteur pipettes (14.5 cm length).
7. Volumetric flasks (10 ml, 25 ml).
8. Tygon tubing (1.25 by 0.16).

TECHNIQUE

1. Prepare hemolysate as desribed in the section on cellulose acetate electrophoresis. Dilute 2 drops of this hemolysate with 7 drops of buffer 1.
2. Process 500 g of DE52 cellulose at one time and store for future use. Suspend the DE52 in 2 liters of buffer 1 and allow to settle. Then slowly decant off the supernatant fluid containing the particles which have failed to settle. Repeat this treatment at least four times or until the supernatant fluid has the same pH and conductivity as the buffer. Store the DE52 as a slurry in a covered container with a volume of the supernatant equal to

about 0.7 that of the settled anion exchanger at room temperature.

3. Chromatography is carried out at room temperature. Disposable Pasteur pipettes serve admirably as chromatography columns (0.5 by 6 or 7 cm). Pack a small plug of cotton loosely in the tapered part of the pipette and place the pipette vertically inside a test tube (16 by 100 mm). Moisten the column and the cotton plug with buffer 1. Pack the column to a height of 6 or 7 cm with the DE52 slurry.

4. Remove excess buffer from the top of the column with a Pasteur pipette.

5. Carefully apply 3 drops of the diluted hemolysate to the top of the column. After the sample has entered the column, rinse the walls of the column with 0.5 ml of buffer 2 and allow this to flow into the adsorbent.

6. Make a reservoir by placing a 1-in. piece of Tygon tubing on the stem of a funnel and attach it to the top of the pipette.

7. Discard all the effluent that has been collected in the test tube thus far. Fill the reservoir with 10 ml of buffer 2 and allow buffer to flow into the column from the reservoir. Collect the first 6 to 8 ml of effluent in a 10-ml volumetric flask and adjust volume to 10 ml with distilled water. This effluent contains the Hb A_2.

8. When all the Hb A_2 has been eluted, change the buffer in the reservoir to buffer 3. Collect the first 5 to 10 ml of effluent, which contains the remaining hemoglobins, in a 25-ml volumetric flask. Dilute this effluent with distilled water to 25 ml. The optical density (OD) of Hb A_2 solution and that of the remaining hemoglobin solution collected from the column are read at 415 nm in a spectrophotometer, using distilled water as a blank.

At the completion of the chromatographic separation, discard the pipette and DE52.

CALCULATIONS

$$\frac{\text{OD Hb } A_2}{(\text{OD remaining Hb} \times 2.5) + \text{OD Hb } A_2} \times 100 = \% \text{ Hb } A_2$$

The mean values for normal and for β-thalassemia trait are 2.5 ± 0.15 percent (1 standard deviation) and 4.8 ± 0.27 percent (1 standard deviation), respectively [17]. The upper limit for a normal subject is 3.6 percent.

All determinations should be performed in duplicate and the figures averaged. Always run a known normal and an elevated control with each batch of tests. The normal mean and standard deviation should be established in each laboratory using this procedure. Hbs C, E, and O are eluted with Hb A_2 in this procedure. Using a longer column (0.5 by 15 cm), this procedure is also suitable for the quantitation of Hb A_2 in hemolysates containing Hb S.

INTERPRETATION OF RESULTS

Hb A_2 ($\alpha_2\delta_2$) is a minor component of normal adult hemoglobin. Trace amounts of Hb A_2 are present at birth and rapidly increase to reach near-adult levels by the age of about 6 months [18], with only insignificant increases thereafter. Although the function of Hb A_2 is not known, determination of its level has important diagnostic value because an elevated level indicates the presence of the most common variety of heterozygous β thalassemia. Some persons with homozygous β thalassemia will have elevated levels of Hb A_2, but others will have normal levels. Decreased Hb A_2 levels can be seen in iron deficiency anemia, sideroblastic anemia, or thalassemia syndromes such as Hb H disease, carrier states of α thalassemia, $\delta\beta$ thalassemia,

Hb$_{Lepore}$ syndromes, or hereditary persistence of fetal hemoglobin.

SOURCE OF REAGENTS

Microcolumns may be purchased from Helena Laboratories or Isolab.

DE52 is available from Whatman, 9 Bridewell Pl., Clifton, NJ 07014.

Quantitation of Hb A$_{Ic}$

PURPOSE OF THE TEST

The measurement of Hb A$_{Ic}$ is of use in monitoring the effectiveness of diabetic management [19–21].

PRINCIPLE OF THE TEST

Hb A$_{Ic}$ is the most abundant minor hemoglobin component in human erythrocytes. The structure of Hb A$_{Ic}$ is the same as that of Hb A except for the addition of glucose to the N terminus of the β chain by a Schiff base linkage [22,23]. The formation of Hb A$_{Ic}$ takes place slowly and irreversibly throughout the life span of the red cells by a nonenzymatic process [24]. Therefore, the level of Hb A$_{Ic}$ can be used to assess control of blood glucose levels over the previous several months.

Hb A$_{Ic}$ can be measured by various methods [25], such as chromatography [26], electrophoresis [27], colorimetry [28], and radioimmune assay [29]. Although all of these methods provide good results, some are time-consuming, laborious, or difficult to standardize in clinical laboratories.

To meet the popular need of clinicians for a routine laboratory test in the management of diabetic patients, the simple, rapid, and inexpensive microcolumn chromatographic technique has been shown to be satisfactory. The disposable microcolumns are available commercially [30] and as homemade columns [31,32]. The methods for the three commercially available kits are similar, and the procedures can be finished within 1.5 h. Every kit comes with a hemolysis reagent, disposable microcolumns, and elution buffers. The assay involves the direct application of hemolysates to the column; hemoglobin is adsorbed onto a weakly acidic cation exchange resin, and total Hb A$_I$ is eluted with a low-molarity buffer as a fast hemoglobin component. The OD (415 nm) of the fast-moving hemoglobin is compared with the OD of the total hemoglobin solution, and the percentage of glycosylated hemoglobins (Hb A$_{Ia,b,e}$) is calculated. Special care should be taken with each method since several problems, such as incomplete hemolysis, leakage of fine resin particles from the column, and retention of hemoglobin by the column, are encountered and can cause a significant error in the results [33]. When such care is taken, and when the first eluate is centrifuged prior to measuring absorbance, the Bio-Rad kit provides very satisfactory results.

REAGENTS AND EQUIPMENT

1. Sample: 1 ml of anticoagulated (EDTA) whole blood
2. Microcolumn chromatography kit
3. Spectrophotometer

TECHNIQUE

The methods differ slightly according to the kit used and are described in the technical literature included with each kit. However, errors can be minimized by centrifuging the hemo-lysate before applying it to the column with the Helena kit and centrifuging the first eluate before reading the OD with all three kits [33].

INTERPRETATION OF RESULTS

The normal value of Hb A$_{Ic}$ is 6.5 ± 1.5 percent [26]. Hb A$_{Ic}$ is elevated in the red cells of diabetic patients, as high as three times the normal level. The level of Hb A$_{Ic}$ is relatively stable and usually changes very slowly. However, there have been recent reports of rapid changes in the level of Hb A$_{Ic}$ [34,35], as well as wide variations for normal levels of Hb A$_{Ic}$. Variation of the Hb A$_{Ic}$ level depends in part upon the column procedure. With the rapid microchromatographic method, Hb A$_{Ic}$ cannot be separated from other minor components, such as Hb A$_{Ia}$ and Hb A$_{Ib}$, and the sum of the three components (total Hb A$_I$) will be measured as glycosylated hemoglobin. The total Hb A$_I$ level is an unreliable index in unstable diabetic patients [36]. In fact, the specific measurement of Hb A$_{Ic}$ is recommended in patients with fluctuating blood glucose levels.

Results obtained by the chromatographic method should be interpreted carefully since Hb A$_{Ic}$ is falsely elevated in the presence of increased Hb F levels, abnormal hemoglobins (e.g., Hb S, Hb C), uremia, lead intoxication, aspirin ingestion, etc. [37–40]. Conversely, Hb A$_{Ic}$ levels are falsely reduced in the presence of red cells with a shortened life span.

SOURCE OF EQUIPMENT

Microcolumn chromatography kits are sold by Helena Laboratories, Box 752, Beaumont, TX 77704; Isolab, Drawer 4350, Akron, OH 44321; and Bio-Rad Laboratories, 2200 Wright Ave., Richmond, CA 94804.

References

1. Huisman, T. H. J., and Jonxis, J. H. P.: *The Hemoglobinopathies: Techniques of Identification.* Marcel Dekker, New York, 1977.
2. Weatherall, D. J., and Clegg, J. B.: *The Thalassemia Syndromes,* 2d ed. Blackwell Scientific, Oxford, 1972.
3. Schmidt, R. M., and Brosious, E. M.: *Basic Laboratory Methods of Hemoglobinopathy Detection,* 7th ed. CDC, Atlanta, 1978.
4. Schmidt, R. M., and Holland, S.: Standardization in abnormal hemoglobin detection: An evaluation of hemoglobin electrophoresis kits. *Clin. Chem.* 20:591, 1974.
5. Fairbanks, V. F.: *Hemoglobinopathies and Thalassemias: Laboratory Methods and Case Studies.* Brian C. Decker, New York, 1980, p. 85.
6. Smithies, O.: An improved procedure for starch-gel electrophoresis: Further variations in the serum protein of normal individuals. *Biochem. J.* 71:585, 1959.
7. Garrick, M. G., Balzer, R. H., Jr., and Carlton, J. P.: An improved method for electrophoretic characterization of globin chains from hemolysates, purified hemoglobins, and fractions selected from chromatographic separations of chains. *Anal. Biochem.* 34:312, 1970.
8. Milner, P. F., and Gooden, H.: Rapid citrate-agar electrophoresis in routine screening for hemoglobinopathies using a simple hemolysate. *Am. J. Clin. Pathol.* 64:58, 1975.
9. Hicks, E. J., and Hughes, B. J.: Comparison of electrophoresis on citrate agar, cellulose acetate, and starch for hemoglobin identification. *Clin. Chem.* 21:1072, 1975.
10. Schneider, R. G.: Differentiation of electrophoretically similar hemoglobins—such as S, D, G, and P; or A$_2$, C, E, and O—by electrophoresis of the globin chains. *Clin. Chem.* 20:1111, 1974.
11. Schneider, R. G., and Barwick, R. C.: Measuring relative electrophoretic mobilities of mutant hemoglobins and globin chains. *Hemoglobin* 2(5):417, 1978.

12. Alter, B. P., Goff, S. C., Efremov, G. D., Gravely, M. E., and Huisman, T. H. J.: Globin chain electrophoresis: A new approach to the determination of the G_γ/A_γ ratio in fetal haemoglobin and to studies of globin synthesis. *Br. J. Haematol.* 44:527, 1980.

13. Schneider, R. G., et al.: Abnormal hemoglobins in a quarter million people. *Blood* 48:629, 1976.

14. Schmidt, R. M., Rucknagel, D. L., and Necheles, T. F.: Comparison of methodologies for thalassemia screening by Hb A_2 quantitation. *J. Lab. Clin. Med.* 86:873, 1975.

15. Marengo-Rowe, A. J.: Rapid electrophoresis and quantitation of hemoglobins on cellulose acetate. *J. Clin. Pathol.* 18:790, 1965.

16. Efremov, G. D., Huisman, T. H. J., Bowman, K., Wrightstone, R. N., and Shroeder, W. A.: Microchromatography of hemoglobins. II. A rapid method for the determination of hemoglobin A_2. *J. Lab. Clin. Med.* 83:657, 1974.

17. Efremov, G. D.: An evaluation of the methods for quantitation of hemoglobin A_2: Results from a survey of 10,663 cases. *Hemoglobin* 1(8):845, 1977.

18. Serjeant, B. E., Mason, K. P., and Serjeant, G. R.: The development of haemoglobin A_2 in normal Negro infants and in sickle cell disease. *Br. J. Haematol.* 39:259, 1978.

19. Koenig, R. J., Peterson, C. M., Jones, R. L., Saudek, C., Lehrman, M., and Cerami, A.: Correlation of glucose regulation and hemoglobin A_{1c} in diabetes mellitus. *N. Engl. J. Med.* 295:417, 1976.

20. Gabbay, K. H., Hasty, K., Breslow, J. L., Ellison, R. C., Bunn, H. F., and Gallop, P. M.: Glycosylated hemoglobins and long-term blood glucose control in diabetes mellitus. *J. Clin. Endocrinol. Metab.* 44:859, 1977.

21. Graf, R. J., Halter, J. B., and Porte, D.: Glycosylated hemoglobin in normal subjects and subjects with maturity-onset diabetes. *Diabetes* 27:834, 1978.

22. Bunn, H. F., Haney, D. N., Gabbay, K. H., and Gallop, P. M.: Further identification of the nature and linkage of the carbohydrate in hemoglobin A_{1c}. *Biochem. Biophys. Res. Commun.* 67:103, 1975.

23. Koenig, R. J., Biobstein, S. H., and Cerami, A.: The structure of carbohydrate of hemoglobin A_{1c}. *J. Biol. Chem.* 252:2992, 1977.

24. Bunn, H. F., Haney, D. N., Kamin, S., Gabbay, K. H., and Gallop, P. M.: The biosynthesis of human hemoglobin in vivo. *J. Clin. Invest.* 57:1652, 1976.

25. Bunn, H. F.: Evaluation of glycosylated hemoglobin in diabetic patients. *Diabetes* 30:613, 1981.

26. Trivelli, L. A., Ranney, H. M., and Lai, H. T.: Hemoglobin components in patients with diabetes mellitus. *N. Engl. J. Med.* 284:353, 1971.

27. Menard, L., Dempsey, M. E., Blankstein, L. A., Aleyassine, H., Wacks, M., and Soeldner, J. S.: Quantitative determination of glycosylated hemoglobin A_1 by agar gel electrophoresis. *Clin. Chem.* 26:1598, 1980.

28. Flückiger, R., and Winterhalter, K. H.: In vitro synthesis of hemoglobin A_{1c}. *F.E.B.S. Lett.* 71:356, 1976.

29. Javid, J., Pettis, P. K., Keonig, R. J., and Cerami, A.: Immunologic characterization and quantitation of haemoglobin A_{1c}. *Br. J. Haematol.* 38:329, 1978.

30. Kynoch, P. A. M., and Lehmann, H.: Rapid estimation (2½ hours) of glycosylated haemoglobin for routine purposes. *Lancet* 2:16, 1977.

31. Jones, M. B., Koler, R. D., and Jones, R. T.: Microcolumn method for the determination of hemoglobin minor fractions A_{1a+b} and A_{1c}. *Hemoglobin* 2:53, 1978.

32. Friedman, S., and Humbert, J. R.: A simple microchromatographic column for determination of hemoglobins A_{1a+b} and A_{1c}. *Hemoglobin* 3:411, 1979.

33. Reilly, M. P., Mochan, B., and Asakura, T.: Comparison of microcolumn methods for determination of glycosylated hemoglobin. Submitted for publication, 1982.

34. Widness, J. S., et al.: Rapid fluctuations in glycohemoglobin (Hb A_{1c}) related to acute changes in glucose. *J. Lab. Clin. Med.* 95:386, 1980.

35. Boden, G., Master, R. W., Gordon, S. S., Shuman, C. R., and Owen, O. E.: Monitoring metabolic control in diabetic outpatients with glycosylated hemoglobin. *Ann. Intern. Med.* 92:357, 1980.

36. Compagnucci, P., Cartechini, M. G., Bolli, G., Feo, P. D., San-teusanio, F., and Brunetti, P.: The importance of determining irreversibly glycosylated hemoglobin in diabetics. *Diabetes* 30:607, 1981.

37. Sosenko, J. M., Flückiger, R., Platt, O. S., and Gabbay, K. H.: Glycosylation of variant hemoglobins in normal and diabetic subjects. *Diabetes Care* 3:590, 1980.

38. Flückiger, R., Harmon, W., Meier, W., Loo, S., and Gabbay, K. H.: Hemoglobin carbamylation in uremia. *N. Engl. J. Med.* 304:823, 1981.

39. Charache, S., and Weatherall, D. J.: Fast hemoglobin in lead poisoning. *Blood* 28:377, 1966.

40. Spicer, K. M., Allen, R. C., and Buse, M. G.: A simplified assay of hemoglobin A_{1c} in diabetic patients by use of isoelectric focusing and quantitative microdensitometry. *Diabetes* 27:384, 1978.

41. Kim, H. C.: Inherited hemoglobinopathies in children. *Clin. Pediatr.* 20:161, 1981.

CHAPTER *A8*

Fetal hemoglobin—alkali denaturation test

HAEWON C. KIM
ELIAS SCHWARTZ

PURPOSE OF THE TEST

Hb F, the main hemoglobin component in the fetus, is present at levels of 65 to 90 percent at birth and usually drops to less than 2 percent by 6 to 12 months of age. Hb F levels may be elevated as a result of genetic abnormalities of hemoglobin production or because of hemopoietic stress. The accurate quantitation of Hb F is important for the precise differentiation of hemoglobinopathies or for the evaluation of conditions with marrow stress. The Betke method of Hb F quantitation in hemolysate is described here [1,2]. This method permits accurate quantitation of fetal hemoglobin at levels of less than 10 to 15 percent even in the presence of carboxyhemoglobin. Other methods for measuring Hb F have been described [3–7].

PRINCIPLE OF THE TEST

Most human hemoglobins denature upon exposure to a strong alkali. With this test, denaturation is stopped by the introduction of saturated ammonium sulfate, which precipitates the denatured hemoglobin. However, the fetal hemoglobin is not denatured and remains soluble; thus, the hemoglobin remaining in solution can be filtered, measured, and expressed as the percent of alkali-resistant hemoglobin.

REAGENTS AND EQUIPMENT

1. Hemolysate is prepared from anticoagulated blood, as described in Chap. A7. Three milliliters of blood usually provides sufficient hemolysate for quantitative determination of Hb F and Hb A_2 and for hemoglobin electrophoresis.

2. 1.2 N sodium hydroxide. Dissolve 48 g of NaOH in distilled water to make 1000 ml. Store at 5°C in a polyethylene bottle.

3. Saturated ammonium sulfate. Dissolve 500 g of $(NH_4)_2SO_4$ in distilled water to make 1000 ml of solution.

4. Drabkin's solution. Dissolve 0.05 g of potassium cyanide and 0.20 g of potassium ferricyanide in distilled water to make 1000 ml. Store in dark bottles.

5. Stopwatch.

6. Test tubes, 16 × 100 mm.

7. Funnels, 2-in. diameter.

8. Filter paper, Whatman No. 42, 11-cm diameter.

9. Spectrophotometer.

TECHNIQUE

1. Make a 450 to 600 mg/dl solution of diluted hemolysate by adding 0.6 ml of hemolysate (approximately 8 to 12 g of hemoglobin per deciliter) to 10.0 ml of Drabkin's solution.

2. Add 0.2 ml of 1.2 N NaOH to a test tube containing 2.8 ml of the diluted hemolysate and simultaneously start the stopwatch. Mix the solution gently.

3. At exactly 2 min, add 2.0 ml of saturated ammonium sulfate solution at room temperature and shake the mixture vigorously.

4. Allow to stand for at least 5 min.

5. Filter through a double layer of filter paper into another tube, referred to as the *fetal hemoglobin tube*.

6. While the alkali-resistant hemoglobin is filtering, prepare a control, or *total hemoglobin tube*, by mixing 1.4 ml of the diluted hemolysate, 1.6 ml of distilled water, and 2.0 ml of saturated ammonium sulfate. Using another tube, dilute this control sample 1:10 with Drabkin's solution by mixing 0.5 ml of the control sample and 4.5 ml of Drabkin's solution (total hemoglobin tube).

7. Read the optical density (OD) of the fetal hemoglobin tube and total hemoglobin tube at 415 nm against a blank consisting of 1.4 ml of Drabkin's solution, 0.2 ml of 1.2 N NaOH, and 2 ml of saturated ammonium sulfate solution. All determinations should be performed in duplicate and the figures averaged.

CALCULATION

$$\% \text{ of Hb F} = \frac{\text{OD fetal hemoglobin tube}}{\text{OD total hemoglobin tube}} \times 5$$

INTERPRETATION

In the normal person, less than 1 percent fetal hemoglobin remains after 2 years of age.

In cord blood, Hb F levels are between 65 and 90 percent, but these decrease with time, so that by the age of 4 months Hb F makes up less than 10 percent of the total hemoglobin.

Elevated levels of Hb F, usually between 2 and 5 percent, have been reported in some cases of hereditary spherocytosis, hypoplastic anemia, acute and chronic leukemia, myelophthisic anemia, untreated pernicious anemia, and carcinoma with metastases to the marrow.

Children with hereditary or acquired aplastic anemia may have levels of Hb F in excess of 10 percent.

Approximately 50 percent of patients with β-thalassemia trait will have Hb F levels of 2 to 5 percent. In patients with homozygous β thalassemia the fetal hemoglobin is almost always markedly increased, usually reaching levels of 15 to 100 percent.

Patients who are homozygous for Hb S (sickle cell anemia) may have normal levels of fetal hemoglobin or levels as high as 20 percent. Persons who are heterozygous for the gene for sickle hemoglobin usually have normal levels of Hb F.

When fetal hemoglobin reaches a level of 15 percent in patients with no other apparent hematologic disorder, the presence of the gene for hereditary persistence of fetal hemoglobin should be suspected.

Hb F can be quantitated accurately by this technique at levels of less than 10 to 15 percent, but is usually underestimated at levels higher than 15 to 20 percent. For specimens containing more than 10 percent fetal hemoglobin, more accurate values will be achieved by using column chromatographic techniques [4–7].

References

1. Betke, K., Marti, H. R., and Schlicht, I.: Estimation of small percentages of foetal haemoglobin. *Nature* 184:1877, 1959.

2. Pembrey, M. E., McWade, P., and Weatherall, D. J.: Reliable routine estimation of small amounts of foetal haemoglobin by alkali denaturation. *J. Clin. Pathol.* 25:738, 1972.

3. Singer, K., Chernoff, A. I., and Singer, L.: Studies on abnormal hemoglobins. I. Their demonstration in sickle cell anemia and other hematologic disorders by means of alkali denaturation. *Blood* 6:413, 1951.

4. Armstrong, D. H., Schroeder, W. A., and Fenninger, W. D.: A comparison of the percentage of fetal hemoglobin in human umbilical cord blood as determined by chromatography and by alkali denaturation. *Blood* 22:554, 1963.

5. Schroeder, W. A., Huisman, T. H. J., Shelton, J. R., and Wilson, J. B.: An improved method for quantitative determination of human fetal hemoglobin. *Anal. Biochem.* 35:235, 1970.

6. Abraham, E. C., Reese, A., Stallings, M., and Huisman, T. H. J.: Separation of human hemoglobins by DEAE-cellulose chromatography using glycine-KCN-NaCl developers. *Hemoglobin* 1(1):27, 1976–77.

7. Abraham, E. C., Carver, J., Döbler, J., Milner, P. F., and Huisman, T. H. J.: Microchromatographic quantitation of fetal hemoglobin in patients with sickle cell disease. *Hemoglobin* 3(5):341, 1979.

CHAPTER *A9*

Fetal hemoglobin— differential staining

HAEWON C. KIM
JEAN ATWATER
ELIAS SCHWARTZ

PURPOSE OF THE TEST

The cytologic detection of red blood cells containing fetal hemoglobin is of importance in determining the distribution of fetal hemoglobin in red cells. This technique allows the differentiation of most types of hereditary persistence of fetal hemoglobin from other hemoglobinopathies with elevated Hb F levels and is also useful in determining the presence of fetal red blood cells in the maternal circulation.

PRINCIPLE OF THE TEST

In addition to being alkali-resistant, fetal hemoglobin is also more acid-resistant than other hemoglobins. Hb A and its variants are soluble in an acid citrate-phosphate buffer and thus elute rapidly, whereas Hb F is not soluble under the same conditions [1,2]. After staining with eosin, the percentage of F cells (red cells containing Hb F) can be determined microscopically. Cells containing fetal hemoglobin appear pink, and other cells appear as colorless ghosts.

REAGENTS AND EQUIPMENT

1. Freshly drawn anticoagulated blood (less than 6 h old for best results) and positive and negative controls, as indicated below
2. Ethanol, 80%
3. Citric acid–phosphate buffer, pH 3.3, made fresh from 0.1 M citric acid (store at 4°C) and 0.2 M disodium phosphate
4. Ehrlich's acid hematoxylin
5. Eosin, 0.1% aqueous
6. Coplin staining jar
7. Microscope slides (2.5 by 7.5 cm)
8. Water bath, 37°C

TECHNIQUE

1. Prepare two thin blood films (dilute blood specimen 1:1 with 0.85% saline, if necessary) from each blood sample. A normal, or negative, control can be obtained from a healthy adult and an abnormal, or positive, control from a person with known hereditary persistence of fetal hemoglobin or from cord blood. Allow films to dry for 20 min.
2. Within 2 h of preparation, fix blood film in 80% ethanol for 5 min. Rinse with tap water and dry. Control slides may be saved after this step for use in future tests.
3. Place the Coplin jar in the water bath at 37°C
4. Mix 37.7 ml of 0.1 M citric acid with 12.3 ml of 0.2 M Na_2HPO_4. Check pH and adjust to 3.3, if necessary, by adding additional citric acid or Na_2HPO_4. Pour into the Coplin jar.
5. When the solution has reached 37°C, place the fixed slides in the jar. Incubate for 5 min with gentle agitation.
6. Remove slides, rinse with tap water, and shake dry.
7. Stain with hematoxylin for 2 min and rinse with tap water. Stain with eosin for 2 min, rinse with tap water, and dry.
8. Examine films with the microscope under low power first to scan and then under oil immersion.

INTERPRETATION OF RESULTS

Cells staining pink with eosin contain Hb F since other hemoglobins are not acid-resistant. Hematoxylin stains the white blood cell nuclei and prevents misinterpretation as eosin-positive cells.

On slides made from cord blood, almost all cells have a bright red color, indicating the presence of Hb F. In infants 1 month of age, only about two-thirds of the cells stain bright red while the rest appear as ghosts because they do not contain Hb F. By 4 to 6 months of age only an occasional bright red cell is seen.

Films from adults typically have only ghost cells, but occasionally fewer than 1 percent of cells containing Hb F may be found in persons who are presumably normal.

In the carrier of the gene for hereditary persistence of fetal hemoglobin 99 to 100 percent of red cells show a variable pink color that is less intense than that seen in cord blood. In homozygous hereditary persistence of fetal hemoglobin there is an evenly distributed bright red staining reaction similar to that of the most deeply stained cells of cord blood.

Samples from some patients heterozygous for β thalassemia with elevated Hb F levels and from patients heterozygous for $\delta\beta$ thalassemia have heterogeneous distribution, with some cells being brightly stained, some pink, and other ghosts. It is sometimes difficult to differentiate Hb S-$\delta\beta$ thalassemia from heterozygous HPFH because almost all red cells can be stained to various intensities of pink in S-$\delta\beta$ thalassemia; however, at least 2 percent of the red cells remain unstained as ghosts in Hb S-$\delta\beta$ thalassemia [3].

Other conditions which have been associated with increased fetal hemoglobin-containing cells by the acid elution technique [4–6] or by a fluorescent antibody technique [6–8] are described below. With the acid elution technique, red cells are stained various degrees of pink.

1. Hemopoietic stress: leukemia, pernicious anemia, aplastic anemia, hypoplastic anemia, sideroblastic anemia, polycythemia vera, transient erythroblastopenia of childhood, and congenital hemolytic anemia
2. Chromosomal abnormalities: D-trisomy syndrome, Down's syndrome, and congenital dystrophies associated with cleft palate
3. Complications of pregnancy: molar pregnancy and fetal-maternal transfusions

SOURCE OF REAGENTS AND EQUIPMENT

A commercial kit for this procedure called "Reagent Set — Fetal Hemoglobin" is available through Bio-Dynamics/Boehringer Mannheim, 9115 Hague Rd., Indianapolis, IN 46250.

Ehrlich's acid hematoxylin may be purchased from Harleco Laboratories, 480 Democrat Rd., Gibbstown, NJ 08027 (no. 636X).

References

1. Kleihauer, E., Braun, H., and Betke, K.: Demonstration von fetalem Haemoglobin in die Erythrozyten eines Blutausstrichs. *Klin. Wochenschr.* 35:627, 1957.
2. Betke, K., and Kleihauer, E.: Fetaler und bleibender Blut-farbstoff in Erythrozyten und Erythroblasten von menschlichen Feten und Neugeborenen. *Blut* 4:421, 1958.
3. Kim, H. C.: Variants of sickle cell disease, in *Hemoglobinopathies in Children*, edited by E. Schwartz. PSG Publishing, Littleton, Mass., 1980, p. 238.
4. Lie, J. T., Balazs, N. D. H., Ungar, B., and Cowling, D. W.: Anaemias associated with increased foetal haemoglobin content: A study of the acid elution technique. *Med. J. Austral.* 1:43, 1968.
5. Link, M. P., and Alter, B. P.: Fetal-like erythropoiesis during recovery from transient erythroblastopenia of childhood (TEC). *Pediatr. Res.* 15:1036, 1981.
6. Wood, W. G., Stamatoyannopoulos, G., Lim, G., and Nute, P. E.: F-cells in the adult: Normal values and levels in individuals with hereditary and acquired elevations of Hb F. *Blood* 46:671, 1975.
7. Hoffman, R., et al.: Fetal hemoglobin in polycythemia vera: Cellular distribution in 50 unselected patients. *Blood* 53:1148, 1979.
8. Papayannopoulou, T., Vichinsky, E., and Stamatoyannopoulos, G.: Fetal Hb production during acute erythroid expansion. *Br. J. Haematol.* 44:535, 1980.

Tests for sickle hemoglobin

HAEWON C. KIM
ELIAS SCHWARTZ

Sickling test

PURPOSE OF THE TEST

The sickling of red blood cells, originally described in 1917 by Emmel [1], reflects their content of sickle hemoglobin; its presence is used to identify individuals with sickle cell trait and sickle cell anemia and its variants.

PRINCIPLE OF THE TEST

The sickling phenomenon can be demonstrated by depriving the red blood cells of oxygen by sealing a cover slip over a drop of fresh blood on a slide. The rapidity with which the reaction occurs will vary with the amount of Hb S present in the cells. To expedite the reaction, a number of reducing substances, such as sodium metabisulfite ($Na_2S_2O_5$), have been used successfully [2].

REAGENT

Aqueous sodium metabisulfite, 2%. Capsules containing 200 mg of sodium metabisulfite are available commercially (Curtin Matheson Scientific Co., Houston, Tex.). One capsule is dissolved in 10 ml of distilled water on the day of use. Care must be taken to avoid too much agitation in dissolving the powder. Reagent-grade sodium metabisulfite that has been kept in a firmly closed container when not in use is also an entirely suitable reagent.

TECHNIQUE

On a slide mix 1 or 2 drops of the 2% solution of metabisulfite with a drop of venous or capillary blood. Place a cover slip over the drops and use finger pressure to form a thin layer. Wipe off the excess with gauze or filter paper. A control should be set up with isotonic saline solution instead of reducing agent. The preparations are observed at 15 and 30 min by means of the high dry power objective of a microscope.

INTERPRETATION

The presence of sickled cells is reported as a positive test. All the cells may assume a sickled shape within a short time. The control preparation is helpful when elliptocytosis or poikilocytosis is present, especially in cases of thalassemia. Crenated, or burr, cells are distinguished by their short spikes and their rounded rather than elongated forms.

Cells with mean corpuscular sickle hemoglobin concentration in any proportion over 7 percent will sickle under these conditions. This test, however, will not differentiate the person as being homozygous or heterozygous for sickle hemoglobin. It must also be borne in mind that rare abnormal hemoglobins have been associated with sickling of the red blood cells in the absence of any Hb S [3–7]. In infants with Hb S disorders, the test may not become positive until 1 or 2 months of age.

Solubility test

PURPOSE OF THE TEST

The solubility test [8] is quick and easy to perform as a rapid screening test for Hb S. It can be used as a confirmatory test for sickle hemoglobin after cellulose acetate electrophoresis, in an emergency, or in instances when the only information needed is the presence or absence of Hb S. It is not satisfactory as a primary test for genetic screening.

PRINCIPLE OF THE TEST

The test is based on the insolubility of deoxy-Hb S in concentrated phosphate buffer. One drop of blood is placed in a test tube and mixed with 2 ml of solubility test reagent, which includes saponin to hemolyze red blood cells; dithionite to deoxygenate oxy-Hb S; and phosphate buffer solution, in which deoxy-Hb S is insoluble and forms water crystals (tactoids), producing turbidity [9].

REAGENTS AND EQUIPMENT

1. Potassium phosphate, dibasic anhydrous	216 g
Potassium phosphate, monobasic crystals	169 g
Sodium hydrosulfite (dithionite)	10 g
Saponin (Fisher Scientific Co.)	1 g
Distilled water, to make	1000 ml

Dissolve the dibasic potassium phosphate (K_2HPO_4) in 800 ml of distilled water. Then add the monobasic potassium phosphate (KH_2PO_4) and dissolve. Add the sodium hydrosulfite ($Na_2S_2O_4$) and the saponin. Dilute to 1000 ml with distilled water. Transfer to a labeled, dated, well-stoppered bottle. Store in the refrigerator. Shelf life varies from 2 to 4 weeks.

2. Whole blood (at least 20 μl collected in sodium heparin or disodium EDTA).
3. Glass test tubes (12 × 75 mm).
4. White card with black lines.

TECHNIQUE

1. Include a positive and a negative control with each group.
2. Pipette 2 ml of reagent into each tube. Allow to warm to room temperature.
3. Add 20 μl (0.02 ml) of blood to each tube. Mix and let stand for 5 min.
4. Hold tubes 1 in. in front of white card with black lines and read for turbidity.

INTERPRETATION

Negative: lines are visible; solution may be slightly cloudy. Positive: solution is turbid; lines are not clearly visible.

Hemoglobins S, C_{Harlem}, $C_{Ziguinchor}$, and S_{Travis} give positive results. Hemoglobins A, C, D, E, F, $G_{Philadelphia}$, I, J, and O_{Arab} are negative. The mixture should be pink to red. Light orange may be an indication that the reagent has deteriorated. Blood hemolysates can also be tested by this method if sufficient hemoglobin solution is added to provide a hemoglobin concentration comparable to that of about 40 μl of whole blood. Commercial kits are available from many laboratory supply houses.

Shaking test

PURPOSE OF THE TEST

This test is simple, fast, and reliable and may be used for the same purposes as the solubility test. With modification, this test can be used for the accurate quantitation of sickle hemoglobin.

PRINCIPLE OF THE TEST

The shaking test is based on the fact that oxy-Hb S denatures and precipitates easily upon mechanical shaking [10]. If a mixture of blood and sodium phosphate buffer solution becomes cloudy upon shaking, the presence of Hb S or another unstable hemoglobin is suspected. This unusual property of Hb S is not shared by other relatively common hemoglobins, including hemoglobins A, C, D, E, F, G$_{Philadelphia}$, and O$_{Arab}$. This technique can also be used to distinguish Hb C$_{Harlem}$ from Hb C since Hb C$_{Harlem}$ is unstable.

Technique and interpretation are described in Chap. A6.

References

1. Emmel, V. E.: A study of the erythrocytes in a case of severe anemia with elongated and sickle-shaped red blood corpuscles. *Arch. Intern. Med.* 20:586, 1917.
2. Daland, G. A., and Castle, W. B.: A simple and rapid method for demonstrating sickling of the red blood cells: The use of reducing agents. *J. Lab. Clin. Med.* 33:1085, 1948.
3. Atwater, J., Schwartz, I. R., Erslev, A. J., Montgomery, T. L., and Tocantins, L. M.: Sickling of erythrocytes in a patient with thalassemia—hemoglobin I disease. *N. Engl. J. Med.* 263:1215, 1960.
4. Lie-Injo Luan Eng: Haemoglobin "Bart's" and the sickling phenomenon. *Nature* [New Biol.] 191:1314, 1961.
5. Pierce, L. E., Roth, C. E., and McCoy, K.: A new hemoglobin variant with sickling properties. *N. Engl. J. Med.* 268:862, 1963.
6. Bookchin, R. M., Nagel, R. L., Ranney, H. M., and Jacobs, A. S.: Hemoglobin C$_{Harlem}$: A sickling variant containing amino acid substitutions in two residues of the β-polypeptide chain. *Biochem. Biophys. Res. Commun.* 23:122, 1966.
7. Thompson, R. B., and Holloway, C. H.: Observations on the sickling phenomenon. *Am. J. Med. Technol.* 29:379, 1963.
8. Greenberg, M. S., Harvey, H. A., and Morgan, C.: A simple and inexpensive screening test for sickle hemoglobin. *N. Engl. J. Med.* 286:1143, 1972.
9. Itano, H. A.: Solubilities of naturally occurring mixtures of human hemoglobins. *Arch. Biochem. Biophys.* 47:148, 1953.
10. Asakura, T., Ohnishi, T., Friedman, S., and Schwartz, E.: Abnormal precipitation of oxyhemoglobin S by mechanical shaking. *Proc. Natl. Acad. Sci. U.S.A.* 71:1594, 1974.

Erythrocyte enzyme assays

ERNEST BEUTLER

Quantitative assays

PURPOSE OF THE TEST

Quantitative erythrocyte enzyme assays are useful in the differential diagnosis of nonspherocytic congenital hemolytic anemia (Chap. 59) and drug-induced hemolytic anemia (Chap. 58). In the case of glucose-6-phosphate dehydrogenase deficiency (G-6-PD) and pyruvate kinase deficiency, screening tests are usually adequate (see pages 1625 and 1626).

PRINCIPLE OF THE TEST

Hemolysate is added to a mixture of reagents which have been constituted in such a way that the amount of enzyme being measured represents the limiting step in a series of reactions eventuating in the reduction of an oxidized pyridine nucleotide or the oxidation of a reduced pyridine nucleotide. The optical density of the mixture is followed at 340 nm, since reduced pyridine nucleotides absorb strongly in this region of the spectrum and oxidized pyridine nucleotides do not.

REAGENTS AND EQUIPMENT [1,2]

1. Tris HCl-EDTA buffer, pH 8. Dissolve 12.1 g of tris and 168 mg of disodium EDTA in approximately 80 ml of distilled water at room temperature. The dropwise addition of concentrated hydrochloric acid is carried out while the solution is stirred, and the pH is monitored with a pH meter until it reaches 8. The total volume is then brought to 100 ml. Stable for at least 3 months frozen or at 4°C unless mold forms.

2. 0.1 M magnesium chloride solution. Dissolve 2 g of MgCl$_2$·6H$_2$O in water and bring to a volume of 100 ml. Stable indefinitely at room temperature unless mold forms.

3. 6 mM glucose 6-phosphate solution. A sufficient quantity of dipotassium or disodium glucose 6-phosphate to make a 6 mM solution is brought to 10 ml with distilled water. The exact quantity will depend on hydration, purity, and which salt is used, as stated on the label, but 21.7 mg of the pure disodium salt·3H$_2$O will be required. Stable for at least 6 months frozen or at 4° unless mold forms.

4. 0.02 M glucose solution. Dissolve 36 mg of D-glucose in 10 ml of distilled water. Stable indefinitely when frozen.

5. 0.02 M ATP solution. Dissolve 200 μmoles of ATP in approximately 8 ml of distilled water. The pH is adjusted to approximately 7 with 0.5% NaOH solution, using pH paper or a pH meter. The volume is adjusted to 10 ml with distilled water. The exact quantity will depend on hydration, purity, and on which salt is used, but 101 mg of the pure anhydrous free acid is required. Stable for at least 3 months frozen.

6. 0.27 M EDTA. Add 10 g of disodium EDTA to 80 ml of distilled water and stir constantly. Add 10% NaOH solution in a dropwise manner until the precipitate is all dissolved and the pH is approximately 7, as measured with pH paper or a pH meter. Then adjust the volume to 100 ml. Stable indefinitely at room temperature unless mold forms.

7. 10 μM FAD solution. Approximately 1 mg of flavin aden-

ine dinucleotide is weighed out and dissolved in a sufficient quantity of distilled water to give a concentration of 0.79 mg per 100 ml. Should be prepared fresh each working day, but is stable for at least 8 h at 4° in a dark bottle.

8. 0.033 M GSSG solution. Dissolve 200 mg of oxidized glutathione (GSSG) in 8 ml distilled water. Adjust the pH to approximately 7 with 0.5% NaOH solution using a pH meter or paper. Bring the volume to 10 ml. Stable for at least 3 months frozen or at 4° unless mold forms.

9. 1 M KCl solution. Weigh out 7.5 g of potassium chloride and bring to 100 ml with distilled water. Stable indefinitely at room temperature unless mold forms.

10. 2 mM NADPH solution. Weigh out sufficient NADPH to make a solution of approximately 2 mg per milliliter of distilled water. Place 0.85 ml of distilled water into a 1-ml spectrophotometer cuvette with a 1-cm light path. Add 0.1 ml of 1 M tris HCl-EDTA buffer, pH 8 (see above). Read the optical density at 340 nm (reading R_1), add 0.050 ml of the NADPH solution, and take a second reading (R_2). These volumes may all be doubled or tripled if only spectrophotometer cuvettes with a critical volume of greater than 1 ml are available. The volume of the remaining NADPH solution (V_1) should be adjusted, by the addition of water, to a greater volume (V_2) according to the equation

$$V_2 = \frac{R_2 - R_1}{0.622} \times V_1$$

This solution should be prepared daily, but is stable for at least 8 h at 4°.

11. 2 mM NADH solution. Prepare in exactly the same manner as the 2 mM NADPH solution.

12. 0.030 M ADP. Weigh out 0.30 mmoles of ADP. The exact quantity used will vary with hydration, purity, and which salt is used, but 128 mg of the pure, anhydrous free acid will be required. Proceed exactly as in preparing 0.02 M ATP (see above).

13. Lactic dehydrogenase solution. Dilute commercially available lactic dehydrogenase solution in distilled water so that it contains approximately 60 units per milliliter. This is the amount of enzyme which reduces 60 μmoles of NAD⁺ (or oxidizes 60 μmoles of NADH) per minute. It should be freshly diluted each working day, but is stable for at least 8 h at 4°.

14. α-Glycerophosphate dehydrogenase, 2 units per ml. Dilute α-glycerophosphate dehydrogenase to give approximately 2 units per milliliter of distilled water. It should be freshly diluted each working day, but is stable for at least 8 h at 4° in a dark bottle.

15. DL-Glyceraldehyde 3-phosphate. Dilute the commercially available 50-mg/ml solution 1:5 in distilled water. The diluted material is stable for at least 1 month at 4°.

16. Stabilizing solution. Bring 0.05 ml of β-mercaptoethanol and 10 ml of 0.27 M EDTA to 1 liter with water. Stable for 1 week at 4°.

17. G-6-PD, 10 units per ml. Hexokinase-free yeast G-6-PD is diluted in stabilizing solution at an approximate concentration of 10 units per ml. The exact concentration is not critical. A fresh solution should be prepared for each working day.

18. 0.050 M phosphoenolpyruvate. Weigh out sufficient cyclohexylammonium phosphoenolpyruvate to make a 0.050 M solution. Bring to final with distilled water. Stable indefinitely when frozen.

19. 2 mM NADP solution. Weigh out sufficient NADP to make a 2 mM solution and bring to volume with distilled water. The exact quantity required will depend upon purity,

hydration, and which salt is used. It is 1.7 mg/ml if the tetrahydrate of the monosodium salt is used. Stable several months at 4°.

TECHNIQUE

PREPARATION OF HEMOLYSATES [1,2]

Blood may be drawn into heparin, EDTA, or ACD solution. All enzymes described below are stable for at least 1 week in blood collected in these anticoagulants and stored at 4°. One milliliter of blood is allowed to flow through a small column prepared from equal parts of microcrystallin cellulose (Sigma, 50-μm mean size) and α-cellulose (Sigma). The red cells are washed through the column with 3 ml of isotonic sodium chloride solution and then washed twice using at least 5 volumes of cold isotonic sodium chloride solution for each wash.

One part of packed washed red cells is added to 19 parts of cold stabilizing solution and frozen by immersion of the centrifuge tube in a dry ice-acetone mixture.

After thawing, the hemolysate is kept in the cold. Although several of the enzymes are quite stable even in dilute hemolysates, it is best to carry out all assays on the day on which the hemolysate is prepared. Hemoglobin determinations are carried out on the hemolysates, using the cyanmethemoglobin technique. Ten times the volume of blood which is used for hemoglobin determinations will be required to obtain readings in an acceptable range.

GENERAL CONDITIONS OF ASSAY

All assays are carried out at 340 nm with the cuvette chamber thermostated at 37°. Cuvettes with a critical volume of less than 1 ml are most convenient, and the volumes given below are intended for such a system. When only larger cuvettes are available, the volumes given may be adjusted with a suitable multiplier. The reagents are added to the cuvette in the order given. The symbol * indicates that water is substituted for the reagent in the blank system. The symbol ¶ indicates that the contents of the cuvette are incubated at 37° for 10 min. This may be done in the cuvette compartment of the spectrophotometer or in a specially constructed temperature block. It is also possible to carry out assays at room temperature. Since the activity of various enzymes will increase by approximately 2 to 7 percent per degree, good reproducibility cannot be obtained without thermostatically controlled equipment. In the case of enzyme assays in which a decreasing optical density is observed (glutathione reductase, pyruvate kinase, and triosephosphate isomerase), the blank should be set to an arbitrary optical density reading of 0.6 or 0.7 OD units unless a spectrophotometer with an auxiliary offset control device is available.

SPECIFIC ENZYME ASSAY SYSTEMS

1. Hexokinase. Tris HCl-EDTA buffer 100 μl; MgCl₂, 100 μl; glucose, 100 μl; ATP*, 500 μl; NADP, 100 μl; hemolysate, 50 μl; G-6-PD, 10 μl; water, 40 μl; ¶.

Comment: To make certain that the G-6-PD is hexokinase-free, a system in which hemolyzing solution is substituted for hemolysate should be set up. There should be no change in optical density at 340 nm. A gradually increasing rate is observed in this assay system, and measurements should be continued until the rate becomes constant. This will generally require 30 to 45 min.

2. Glutathione reductase. Water, 690 μl; tris HCl-EDTA buffer, 50 μl; hemolysate, 10 μl; FAD, 100 μl; ¶; GSSG*, 100 μl; ¶; NADPH, 50 μl.

Comment: This assay may also be performed without the addition of FAD. The difference between enzyme activity without and with FAD addition appears largely to be an index of the state of riboflavin nutrition of the subject [3].

3. Pyruvate kinase. Tris HCl-EDTA buffer, 100 μl; KCl, 100 μl; MgCl$_2$, 100 μl; NADH, 100 μl; ADP*, 50 μl; water, 330 μl; hemolysate, 20 μl; lactic dehydrogenase, 100 μl; ¶; phosphoenolypyruvate, 100 μl.

Comment: Pyruvate kinase is an allosteric enzyme. Its activity at low PEP concentrations is strongly dependent upon the presence of traces of fructose diphosphate. The procedure given above will detect most patients with pyruvate kinase deficiency. However, more complex techniques [4] may be required to detect some pyruvate kinase mutants.

4. G-6-PD. Tris HCl-EDTA buffer, 100 μl; MgCl$_2$, 100 μl; NADP, 100 μl; water, 580 μl; hemolysate, 20 μl; ¶; glucose 6-phosphate,* 100 μl.

Comment: This procedure is similar to that proposed by the WHO [5]. The rate measured represents results of the combined activities of G-6-PD and phosphogluconic dehydrogenase. Individual enzyme activities may be measured by preparing one cuvette in which both 6 mmoles of glucose 6-phosphate and 6 mmoles of 6-phosphogluconic acid are supplied as substrate and a second cuvette in which only phosphogluconic acid is present. The rate in the second cuvette represents the phosphogluconic dehydrogenase activity; the difference between the first and the second represents the activity contributed by G-6-PD alone.

5. Triosephosphate isomerase. Tris HCl-EDTA buffer, 100 μl; NADH, 100 μl; hemolysate (1:100 further dilution), 10 μl; water, 640 μl; α-glycerophosphate dehydrogenase, 50 μl; ¶; DL-glyceraldehyde phosphate,* 100 μl.

Comment: The rate depends strongly on the concentration of glyceraldehyde phosphate, and abnormally low results will be obtained if this preparation has lost activity. The reaction often occurs in two components, a rapid first component and a slower second component. The rate of the first component should be measured.

CALCULATION OF RESULTS

Activity is most conveniently expressed as international units (μmoles of substrate metabolized per minute) per gram of hemoglobin:

$$\text{IU per gram Hb} = \frac{\Delta\text{OD} \times 10^5}{6.22 \times \text{Hb} \times V}$$

where ΔOD is the change of optical density per minute, 6.22 represents the millimolar extinction coefficient of NADPH or NADPH, Hb equals the hemoglobin concentration of the hemolysate in grams per 100 ml, and V equals the volume of hemolysate, in microliters, which has been added to the 1-ml assay system. In making these calculations it is assumed that only 1 mole of pyridine nucleotide is oxidized or reduced per mole of substrate metabolized. In the case of G-6-PD, this assumption is clearly incorrect (see above), since nearly 2 moles of NADP are reduced to NADPH for each mole of glucose 6-phosphate oxidized. However, the method of calculation for this enzyme is based by convention upon the reduction of a single mole of NADP for each mole of glucose 6-phosphate oxidized. In the case of hexokinase, the potential for the reduction of 2 moles of NADP to NADPH also exists, but for reasons that are not entirely clear, only a small portion of the 6-phosphogluconate formed in the G-6-PD reaction undergoes

further oxidation, so that the assumption that a single mole of NADPH is formed per mole of glucose phosphorylated is a reasonably accurate one.

INTERPRETATION

Normal values using these techniques are given in Chap. 19. As indicated in this chapter, patients with reticulocytosis may be expected to have increased activities of some of the glycolytic enzymes. Thus, normal G-6-PD or hexokinase activity in a patient with marked reticulocytosis must be regarded with considerable suspicion. Since the hemoglobin concentration is used as a basis for expression of results, patients with hypochromic anemias will appear to have increased enzyme activities.

SOURCE OF REAGENTS

Reliable reagents may be obtained from several commercial suppliers, including Sigma Chemical Corporation, 3500 De-Kalb St., St. Louis, Mo.; Calbiochem, 10933 N. Torrey Pines Rd., La Jolla, CA 92037; and Boehringer-Mannheim Corporation, 20 Vesey St., New York, NY 10007.

Screening procedures [1,6]

PURPOSE OF TESTS

The purpose of these screening procedures is to detect G-6-PD deficiency and pyruvate kinase deficiency (see Chaps. 58 and 59).

PRINCIPLE OF THE TEST

The principles of these procedures are the same as those outlined under "Quantitative Assays." Instead of measuring the absorption of light by reduced pyridine nucleotides, however, the fluorescence of reduced nucleotides when activated with long-wave ultraviolet light is employed for visual evaluation of whether pyridine nucleotide has been reduced (in the case of G-6-PD screening) or whether pyridine nucleotide has been oxidized (in the case of pyruvate kinase screening).

REAGENTS AND EQUIPMENT

1. Long-wave ultraviolet light. Lamps which emit at 366 nm are very satisfactory, e.g., Blak-Ray, Ultraviolet Products, Inc., San Gabriel, Calif.

2. 6 mM glucose 6-phosphate solution. See under "Quantitative Assays" in this chapter.

3. 1% saponin solution. 100 mg of saponin (Sigma) is brought to 10 ml with distilled water.

4. Tris hydrochloride buffer, pH 7.8. Prepared in the same way as tris HCl buffer, pH 8.0, except that the pH is brought to 7.8 (see under "Quantitative Assays").

5. 0.033 M GSSG solution. See under "Quantitative Assays."

6. 7.5 mM NADP solution. Prepare as for 2 mM NADP solution (see under "Quantitative Assays").

7. G-6-PD screening solution. Mix the following quantities, or multiples thereof: 6 mM glucose 6-phosphate, 1.6 ml; 7.5 mM NADP, 1.0 ml; 1% saponin solution, 2.0 ml; tris hydrochloride buffer, pH 7.8, 3.0 ml; 0.033 M GSSG, 0.25 ml; water, 2.15 ml. Dispense 0.1 ml aliquots into tubes, seal with Parafilm, and store in the freezer. Stable for at least 4 months.

8. 0.15 M phosphoenolpyruvate. See under "Quantitative Assays."

9. 3 mM NADH solution. Dissolve 1 mg of NADH in 0.5 ml of distilled water; this solution is stable for only 1 day, and

preweighed vials such as those available from Sigma Chemical Corporation are particularly convenient.

10. 0.08 M magnesium chloride. 0.163 g of $MgCl_2 \cdot 6H_2O$ is brought to a volume of 10 ml. Stable indefinitely at room temperature unless mold forms.

11. 0.25 M potassium phosphate buffer, pH 7.4. Prepare 0.25 M K_2KPO_4 and 0.25 M KH_2PO_4 solutions. Adjust the pH of the K_2HPO_4 solution to 7.4 using the KH_2PO_4 solution.

12. 0.03 M ADP solution. Prepare as described for ATP solution, but weigh out 300 μmoles of ADP.

13. Pyruvate kinase reaction mixture. The following reagents may be premixed and kept frozen in aliquots: phosphoenolpyruvate, 0.3 ml; ADP solution, 1.0 ml; magnesium chloride, 1.0 ml; potassium phosphate buffer, 0.5 ml; water, 2.2 ml. Aliquots (0.5 ml) of this mixture may be placed in the freezer. Prior to use, an aliquot should be thawed and added to 0.5 ml of freshly prepared NADH solution.

14. Whatman No. 1 filter paper. This may be obtained from various commercial suppliers in either discs or sheets.

TECHNIQUE

Blood collected into ACD, heparin, or EDTA is suitable for the screening tests, even after several weeks of storage at 4°.

1. G-6-PD screening procedure. 10 μl of whole blood is mixed with 100 μl of G-6-PD screening solution. After 10 min at room temperature, the mixture is spotted onto Whatman No. 1 filter paper and allowed to dry completely. The paper is then examined under illumination with long-wave ultraviolet light.

2. Pyruvate kinase screening procedure. The blood sample is centrifuged, the plasma and buffy coat are aspirated, and the red cells are resuspended in four volumes of 0.9% sodium chloride solution. 10 μl of the cell suspension is mixed with 100 μl of screening solution, and the mixture is incubated at 37°. It is spotted on Whatman No. 1 paper immediately after mixing, and every 15 min thereafter for 1 h. The paper is examined under illumination with long-wave ultraviolet light after the spots are dry.

INTERPRETATION OF RESULTS

It is well to perform the screening procedure side-by-side with one or two normal samples. When the screening procedure for G-6-PD deficiency is carried out on a normal sample, the dried spot fluoresces brightly when illuminated with long-wave ultraviolet light. Enzyme-deficient samples either fail to fluoresce or show only very dull fluorescence. When normal samples are tested with the pyruvate kinase screening procedure, fluorescence has disappeared at the end of 15 min of incubation. In the case of pyruvate kinase–deficient samples, in contrast, loss of fluorescence fails to occur even at the end of 45 or 60 min.

False-negative results may be observed with either test if the patient has been transfused sufficiently recently so that substantial numbers of transfused cells are still circulating.

SOURCE OF REAGENTS

Reagents may be obtained from the same sources listed for the quantitative assay procedures.

References

1. Beutler, E.: *Red Cell Metabolism: A Manual of Biochemical Methods*, 2d ed. Grune & Stratton, New York, 1975.

2. Beutler, E., Blume, K. G., Kaplan, J. C., Loehr, G. W., Ramot, B,. and Valentine, W. N.: International Committee for Standardization in Haematology: Recommended methods for red-cell enzyme analysis. *Br. J. Haematol.* 35:331, 1977.

3. Beutler, E.: Effect of flavin compounds on glutathione reductase activity: *in vivo* and *in vitro* studies. *J. Clin. Invest.* 48:1957, 1969.

4. Blume, K. G., Arnold, H., Löhr, G. W., and Beutler, E.: Additional diagnostic procedures for the detection of abnormal red cell pyruvate kinase. *Clin. Chim. Acta* 43:443, 1973.

5. WHO: Standardization of procedures for the study of glucose-6-phosphate dehydrogenase. *WHO Tech. Rep. Ser.*, no. 366, 1967.

6. Beutler, E., and Mitchell, M.: Special modifications of the fluorescent screening method for glucose-6-phosphate dehydrogenase deficiency. *Blood* 32:816, 1968.

CHAPTER *A12*

Osmotic fragility

ERNEST BEUTLER

PURPOSE OF THE TEST

The osmotic fragility test is a simplified means of estimating the surface area/volume ratio of erythrocytes. Its greatest usefulness is in the diagnosis of hereditary spherocytosis, but it has also been used in screening for thalassemia.

PRINCIPLE OF THE TEST

When red cells are placed in a hypotonic solution, water is drawn into the erythrocyte osmotically. This results in swelling of the cell, which approaches a spherical shape. After the critical volume of the cell is reached, the membrane at first leaks and then bursts, releasing large molecules, such as hemoglobin. The amount of hemoglobin in the supernatant is measured colorimetrically and compared with a sample of completely lysed cells.

REAGENTS AND EQUIPMENT

1. Stock solution. A stock solution osmotically equivalent to 10% sodium chloride solution and at a pH of 7.4 is prepared as follows: sodium chloride 18.0 g, Na_2HPO_4 (M.W. 142) 2.73 g, and NaH_2PO_4 (M.W. 120) 0.374 g are dissolved in sufficient distilled water to make 200 ml [1]. For the most precise results the sodium chloride should be dried in an oven and be permitted to cool in a desiccator prior to weighing. If the sodium phosphate salts are not anhydrous, a correction for water must be made. This is done by multiplying the weight given (e.g., 2.73 for Na_2HPO_4) by the ratio of the molecular weight of the hydrated salt to that of the anhydrous salt.

2. A photoelectric colorimeter or spectrophotometer is needed.

TECHNIQUE

Either heparinized or defibrinated blood is suitable for osmotic fragility studies. It is usually desirable to determine the osmotic fragility both of the freshly drawn blood and of the autoincubated blood. In this case it is necessary for the blood sample

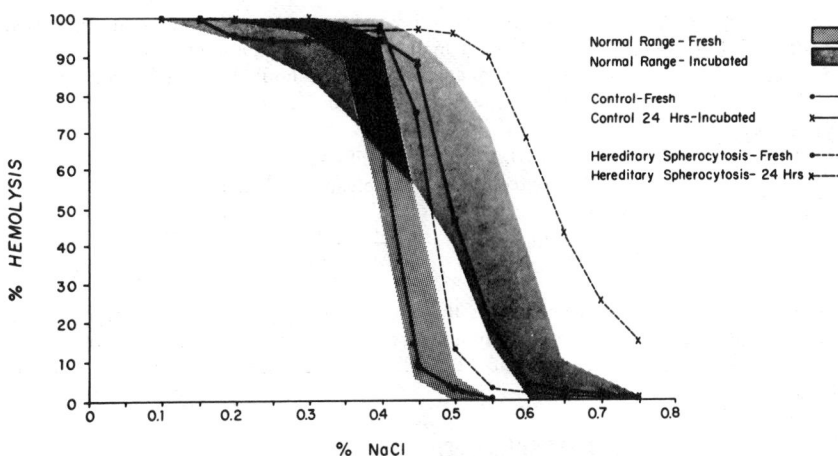

FIGURE A12-1 Osmotic fragility of normal erythrocytes and those from a patient with hereditary spherocytosis. The osmotic fragility is normal in fresh cells from some patients with hereditary spherocytosis, although it is usually increased. The osmotic fragility of normal cells is increased by autoincubation, but that of cells from patients with hereditary spherocytosis is increased to a greater extent than normal.

which is to be autoincubated to be sterile. 2 ml of the sterile blood is placed in a sterile 5-ml screw-cap vial and incubated for 24 h at 37°.

Thirteen 100-ml volumetric flasks are labeled 0.15, 0.20, 0.25, 0.30, 0.35, 0.40, 0.45, 0.50, 0.55, 0.60, 0.65, 0.75, and 0.90. The volume of the stock solution in milliliters equal to 10 times the number on the container is pipetted into each flask, and the total volume is brought to the mark with distilled water. Thus the flask labeled 0.15 contains 1.5 ml of stock solution and 98.5 ml of distilled water and is osmotically equivalent to 0.15% saline solution. Ten milliliters of each solution is placed in a centrifuge tube. An additional tube containing 10 ml of distilled water is labeled 0. Next, 0.1 ml of freshly drawn or autoincubated heparinized or defibrinated whole blood is added to each tube. Each tube is capped with Parafilm and is inverted several times; the suspensions are allowed to stand at room temperature for 60 min. Tubes are then centrifuged to sediment unlysed cells and stroma, and the supernatant solution is removed. Lysis in the tube marked 0 should be complete; only a white or slightly pinkish sediment should be present at the bottom of the tube. If intact red cells are present, the contents of the tube should be resuspended; a small amount of digitonin or saponin should be added to the tube to complete lysis of the erythrocytes, and it should be recentrifuged.

Optical density readings are made at 540 or 545 nm or with a suitable green filter. The cuvette chosen must have a light path sufficiently short (approximately 1.0 cm) so that, when the colorimeter is blanked against the 0.90 sample, the reading of the 0 sample is between 0.4 and 0.8 optical density (OD) units. If such readings cannot be achieved with the cuvettes that are available, all the supernatants should be diluted equally, so that the reading of the 0 tube falls into the acceptable range. Optical density readings are now taken on all the supernatant solutions, using the tube marked 0.9 as a blank.

CALCULATION OF RESULTS
The percent hemolysis in each tube is calculated as follows:

$$\% \text{ hemolysis} = \frac{\text{OD sample}}{\text{OD tube 0}} \times 100$$

TABLE A12-1

NaCl, %	Lysis, %	
	Fresh	Incubated
0.20		95–100
0.30	97–100	85–100
0.35	90–99	75–100
0.40	50–95	65–100
0.45	5–45	55–95
0.50	0–6	40–85
0.55	0	15–70
0.60		0–40
0.65		0–10
0.70		0–5
0.75		0

INTERPRETATION
The normal range of values is presented in Table A12-1 and Fig. A12-1 [2]. Increased osmotic fragility occurs in hereditary spherocytosis and is consistently present in this disorder after autoincubation of the sample (Fig. A12-1). Increased osmotic fragility is also seen, however, in autoimmune hemolytic disease. Increased resistance to hemolysis is characteristic of thalassemia, in both the homozygous and heterozygous forms, in iron deficiency, and in any other condition in which an increase of the surface area/volume ratio of the red cell is present (for example, in some forms of liver disease).

References

1. Dacie, J.: *The Hemolytic Anemias,* 1st ed. Grune & Stratton, New York, 1954, p. 476.
2. Dacie, J.: *The Hemolytic Anemias,* 2d ed. Grune & Stratton, New York, 1960, part I, pp. 37 and 42.

Autohemolysis

ERNEST BEUTLER

PURPOSE OF THE TEST

The autohemolysis test is primarily useful in the diagnosis of hereditary spherocytosis. While it has also been used in the differential diagnosis of hereditary nonspherocytic hemolytic anemia, the availability of specific enzymatic assays has made the autohemolysis test obsolete for this purpose.

PRINCIPLE OF THE TEST

When red cells are incubated in their own plasma or serum, hemolysis occurs gradually. Although the exact mechanism of lysis is probably quite complex, it seems likely that loss of membrane and inability to maintain cation gradients plays an important role, especially in hereditary spherocytosis (see Chap. 55).

REAGENTS AND EQUIPMENT

1. Sterile 125-ml Erlenmeyer flasks with 10 to 20 glass beads, 2 to 4 mm in diameter, or sterile tube with 150 units of sterile heparin or 15 mg of sterile disodium EDTA.
2. Sterile 5-ml screw-cap vials.
3. Sterile pipettes.
4. Photoelectric colorimeter or spectrophotometer with cuvettes with 2.0- to 2.5-cm light path.
5. Sterile 10% glucose in 0.85% NaCl solution.
6. Sterile 0.85% NaCl solution.
7. Ferricyanide-cyanide solution (100 mg of NaCN and 300 mg of $K_3Fe(CN)_6$ per liter).

TECHNIQUE

Approximately 15 ml of blood is drawn into a sterile syringe and defibrinated by swirling it in the sterile flask containing glass beads or anticoagulated with heparin or EDTA. Two 2-ml aliquots of blood are pipetted into two 5-ml sterile screw-cap vials which contain 0.1 ml of 0.85% sodium chloride solution, and another two 2-ml aliquots are pipetted into two vials which contain 0.1 ml of sterile 10% glucose in 0.85% sodium chloride solution. An aliquot of the blood sample is centrifuged, and the serum or plasma is saved. The four tubes (two with glucose and two without) are incubated at 37°C. After 24 and 48 h of incubation each sample is mixed well by swirling. The vials containing one sample with and one sample without glucose are opened, and 0.02 ml of blood is added to 10 ml of ferricyanide-cyanide solution for subsequent determination of the hemoglobin concentration. A hematocrit determination is also carried out on each blood sample.

The remaining two samples are centrifuged, and 0.2 ml of the serum or plasma is added to 10 ml of ferricyanide-cyanide solution. Optical density is measured at 540 or 545 nm, or with an appropriate green filter. Readings on the diluted whole-blood sample are blanked against ferricyanide-cyanide solution, and the diluted serum or plasma samples are blanked against a cuvette containing 10 ml of ferricyanide-cyanide solution to which 0.2 ml of preincubation serum or plasma has been added. If colorimeter cuvettes with a shorter light path must be used, a smaller volume of ferricyanide-cyanide solution is used as diluent. A method designed for the estimation of plasma hemoglobin, e.g., as in Ref. 1, should be used if quantitation of hemolysis levels of less than 2 percent is desired.

CALCULATION OF RESULTS

The percentage of hemolysis is calculated as follows:

$$\% \text{ hemolysis} = \frac{AS_T (100 - Hct_T)}{AB_T \times 10}$$

where AS_T is the optical density given by a serum or plasma sample at time T (24 or 48 h), Hct_T is the hematocrit reading at time T, and AB_T is the optical density given by a blood sample at time T.

INTERPRETATION

Autohemolysis in normal samples is generally less than 3.5 percent at the end of 48 h without added glucose and less than 0.6 percent with added glucose. Autohemolysis in the absence of added glucose is generally greatly increased in hereditary spherocytosis, but the defect is largely corrected by the addition of glucose. Patients with hereditary nonspherocytic hemolytic anemia whose red cells show only moderate autohemolysis (3 to 6 percent), corrected by glucose, have been said to have "type 1" hereditary nonspherocytic hemolytic anemia. Patients in whom autohemolysis is considerable without glucose (7 to 15 percent) and in which correction with glucose does not take place are said to have "type 2" hereditary nonspherocytic hemolytic anemia [2,3]. The effect of other additives, such as ATP and inosine, have also been investigated. However, many of the earlier results are suspect because of failure to neutralize ATP solutions. Furthermore, the effect of some metabolites to which the cell is impermeable may be osmotic.

References

1. Elson, E. C., Ivor, L., and Gochman, N.: Substitution of a nonhazardous chromogen for benzidine in the measurement of plasma hemoglobin. *Am. J. Clin. Pathol.* 69:354, 1978.
2. Selwyn, J. G., and Dacie, J. V.: Autohemolysis and other changes resulting from the incubation in vitro of red cells from patients with congenital hemolytic anemia. *Blood* 9:414, 1954.
3. Young, L. E., Izzo, M. J., Altman, K. I., and Swisher, S. N.: Studies on spontaneous in vitro autohemolysis in hemolytic disorders. *Blood* 11:977, 1956.

CHAPTER *A14*

Studies for paroxysmal nocturnal hemoglobinuria

WENDELL F. ROSSE

Sucrose hemolysis test [1]

PURPOSE OF THE TEST

This test is carried out to screen patients suspected of suffering from paroxysmal nocturnal hemoglobinuria (PNH). It should be performed on patients with hemoglobinuria, marrow aplasia or hypoplasia, or an undiagnosed hemolytic anemia. If the diagnosis is suspected only when a history of nocturnal hemoglobinuria is obtained, less than 25 percent of all patients with PNH will be identified.

PRINCIPLE OF THE TEST

The laboratory diagnosis of PNH is based upon the demonstration of complement-sensitive red cells.

When red blood cells are suspended in an isotonic sucrose solution, osmotic lysis does not occur since sucrose does not penetrate the red cell membrane. In the presence of a small amount of serum, PNH cells undergo lysis in a sucrose solution. The low ionic strength of the sucrose solution used probably enhances the binding of complement components to the red cell membrane. The complement-sensitive cells of PNH develop membrane defects through which sucrose can pass, producing osmotic lysis. Alternatively, it is possible that defects sufficiently large to permit loss of the red cell contents are formed by the action of complement.

MATERIALS

CELLS

The cells to be tested are obtained from defibrinated blood or blood collected in EDTA or acid citrate dextrose solution. The plasma and white blood cells are removed by centrifugation, and the cells are washed three times in $0.15\ M$ NaCl solution. After the last washing, a 50% suspension is made by the addition of approximately an equal volume of $0.15\ M$ NaCl to the packed cells. The ABO blood group of the cells should be determined.

SERUM

Type-compatible fresh or properly stored normal serum is used. Complement activity is rapidly diminished unless the serum is stored at $-90°C$. Serum can be stored for 1 to 2 weeks at $-20°C$. Since normal serum varies considerably in its ability to induce lysis of PNH cells, it is best to have available a known potent serum from an unsensitized AB donor. Serum from the patient or from other patients (especially those with liver disease) should not be used.

STOCK SUCROSE SOLUTION

A stock solution is made up of 486 g of sucrose and 5.1 g of sodium barbital dissolved in 500 ml of distilled water. The pH is adjusted to 7.3 to 7.4 with HCl and distilled water added to make 1 liter. This solution is stable for several months at 4°C.

WORKING SUCROSE SOLUTION

20-ml of stock solution is mixed with 80 ml of distilled water.

TECHNIQUE

The following test mixtures are prepared in small test tubes:

	Tube			
	1	*2*	*3*	*4*
Sucrose, ml	0.90	0.95	0.95	
Cells, ml	0.05	0.05		0.05
Serum, ml	0.05		0.05	
$0.01\ M$ NH$_4$OH, ml				0.95

The mixtures are incubated for 60 min at room temperature. Four milliliters of $0.15\ M$ NaCl is then added, and the cells remaining are removed by centrifugation. The optical density (OD) of the supernatant fluid is read against an H$_2$O blank at 540 nm.

CALCULATION OF RESULTS

The percentage of lysis is calculated as follows:

$$\text{Percent lysis} = \frac{\text{OD}_{\text{tube 1}} - (\text{OD}_{\text{tube 2}} + \text{OD}_{\text{tube 3}})}{(\text{OD}_{\text{tube 4}} - \text{OD}_{\text{tube 2}})} \times 100$$

INTERPRETATION

If more than 5 percent lysis is obtained, the diagnosis of PNH is almost certain. The test does not, however, always accurately reflect the percentage of complement-sensitive cells, and false-positive and false-negative results may be expected under some circumstances.

FALSE-POSITIVE RESULTS

Up to 5 percent of the red cells may be lysed in the absence of a complement-sensitive PNH population as demonstrated by the complement lysis sensitivity test. This is frequently seen in patients with other hematologic diseases, especially megaloblastic anemia and autoimmune hemolytic anemia. Thus, small amounts of lysis must be interpreted with caution since they may or may not represent the lysis of PNH cells. The number of false-positive tests increases as the concentration of serum is increased.

Type-compatible serum must be selected with the same care used in the acidified-serum lysis test. The use of the patient's own serum may give false-positive results, especially in patients with autoimmune hemolytic anemia.

FALSE-NEGATIVE RESULTS

The sucrose lysis test hemolyzes nearly all the complement-sensitive cells (and some of the complement-insensitive cells as well) in the blood of patients with PNH. To date, we have not seen a negative result in a patient with PNH, even with the very small sensitive population, when proper materials are used. Nearly all sera are potent in lysing the complement-sensitive cells in this test; the exceptions include the sera from patients with abnormalities of the complement system.

Acidified-serum lysis test (Ham test) [2]

PURPOSE OF THE TEST
This test is carried out to establish a definitive diagnosis of PNH.

PRINCIPLE OF THE TEST
In his original observations on PNH, Ham remarked that the red cells of patients with PNH appeared to be lysed by fresh normal serum, especially when that serum was acidified, and that this lysis depended on the presence of complement but not antibody. In the acidified-serum lysis test, complement is destroyed by heating, and this leads to loss of hemolytic activity of serum with respect to PNH cells.

MATERIALS

CELLS
Cells are prepared as for the sucrose hemolysis test (above).

SERUM
Serum is prepared as for the sucrose hemolysis test. The pH of the serum is lowered to prepare "acidified serum" by titration to a pH of 6.4 to 6.6 with 0.15 N HCl, using a pH meter to determine the end point. "Heated serum" is prepared by incubation at 56°C for 30 min. To increase the sensitivity of the test, the magnesium content of the serum may be increased by the addition of one-tenth volume of 0.05 M Mg Cl$_2$ (e.g., 5 ml of serum + 0.5 ml of 0.05 M MgCl$_2$).

TECHNIQUE
Reagents are added to six small test tubes as follows:

	Tube					
	1	2	3	4	5	6
Acidified serum, ml	0.5			0.5		
Unacidified serum, ml		0.5				
Heated acidified serum, ml			0.5			
Cells, ml	0.05	0.05	0.05		0.05	0.05
0.15 M NaCl, ml				0.05	0.5	
0.01 M NH$_4$OH, ml						0.5

The tubes are incubated for 60 min at 37°C.

READING THE SAMPLES
After the incubation, 4 ml of 0.15 M NaCl is added to each tube, the tubes are centrifuged, and the optical density of the supernatant fluid is read at 540 nm.

CALCULATION OF RESULTS
The percent lysis (H) in tubes 1, 2, and 3 is calculated as follows:

$$H = \frac{OD_i - (OD_5 + OD_4)}{OD_6 - OD_5} \times 100$$

where OD_i represents the optical density of tubes 1, 2, or 3, and OD_4, OD_5, and OD_6 represent the optical densities of tubes 4, 5, and 6, respectively.

INTERPRETATION
If significant lysis occurs (greater than 1 percent) in tube 1 and *no* lysis occurs in tube 2, the diagnosis of PNH is probable. The percent lysis is roughly commensurate with, but usually less than, the percentage of complement-sensitive cells.

FALSE-POSITIVE RESULTS
Noncompatible serum   The use of serum containing isoantibodies capable of reacting with the test cells may render the test positive when the cells are normal. This is circumvented by using serum from an AB donor or by careful typing of the cells to be tested and of the donor whose serum is to be used.

Overacidification   If the pH of the serum is rendered too low, lysis may occur. With overacidification, lysis usually also occurs in the tube containing heated serum.

Congenital dyserythropoietic anemia   The cells of certain patients with congenital dyserythropoietic anemia, sometimes designated by the acronym *HEMPAS* (hereditary erythrocytic multinuclearity with positive acidified-serum test), will be lysed by the serum of many normal donors [3]. Since this lysis is antibody-mediated, absorption of the serum at 0°C with washed packed red cells from the patient markedly reduces the amount of lysis. No reduction in lysis of PNH cells is seen if serum is absorbed similarly by PNH, normal, or HEMPAS cells.

FALSE-NEGATIVE RESULTS
"Impotent" serum   Serum from some individuals may not readily lyse PNH cells. If serum from a donor is used for the first time, known PNH cells should be run in parallel to be certain that the serum is able to lyse PNH cells. Great care must be used in storing the serum at proper temperatures if fresh serum is not used.

Small complement-sensitive population   Occasionally, the population of complement-sensitive cells may be so small as to make detection of lysis difficult. The amount of lysis may be increased by centrifuging the cells in a hematocrit tube and analyzing the lighter cells (reticulocyte-rich layer), since the proportion of complement-sensitive cells is higher in this fraction.

EVALUATION
The Ham, or acidified-serum, test appears deceptively easy. Great care must be taken to avoid the pitfalls outlined. It is almost never positive in any other disease and is seldom negative in patients with PNH. However, it does not accurately assess the percentage of complement-sensitive cells.

References

1. Hartman, R. C., and Jenkins, D. E.: The "sugar-water" test for paroxysmal nocturnal hemoglobinuria. *N. Engl. J. Med.* 275:155, 1966.
2. Ham, T. H.: Studies on destruction of red blood cells. I. Chronic hemolytic anemia with paroxysmal nocturnal hemoglobinuria: An investigation of the mechanism of hemolysis, with observations on five cases. *Arch. Intern. Med.* 64:1271, 1939.
3. Crookston, J. H., et al.: Hereditary erythroblastic multinuclearity associated with a positive acidified-serum test: A type of congenital dyserythropoietic anaemia. *Br. J. Haematol.* 17:11, 1969.

CHAPTER *A15*

Differentiation of hemoglobin and myoglobin in urine

WENDELL F. ROSSE

PURPOSE OF THE TEST

The correct interpretation of dark, or "Coca-Cola" colored, urine is often important in the diagnosis of hemolytic or myolytic disease. The first steps are excluding the presence of red blood cells by microscopic examination and establishing the presence of heme-containing pigments. If the latter are present, the differentiation between hemoglobin and myoglobin is essential if the clinical course is not clearly indicative of one or the other.

PRINCIPLE OF THE TEST

Both hemoglobin and myoglobin may be detected in a reaction involving hydrogen peroxide and an indicator, such as orthotolidine. Myoglobin is soluble in 80% saturated ammonium sulfate solution, whereas hemoglobin is not. Further, each has particular electrophoretic and spectrophotometric characteristics which can be used in its identification.

REAGENTS AND EQUIPMENT

1. Orthotolidine solution: A 1% solution is prepared by dissolving 1 g in 100 ml of methanol; the reagent is difficult to dissolve but stable.

2. Acid peroxide: 50 ml of glacial acetic acid is carefully mixed with 100 ml of 3% hydrogen peroxide.

3. Sulfosalicylic acid (3% w/v) in distilled water.

4. Ammonium sulfate, reagent grade.

5. Veronal buffer, pH 8.6, ionic strength 0.05: 409 ml of 0.025 M barbital and 100 ml of 0.5 M sodium barbital diluted to 1 liter with water.

6. Red cell hemolysate: This is made exactly as for hemoglobin electrophoresis (see Chap. A7). The concentration should be 10 g/dl. A hemolysate should be made from the patient's own cells, especially if the hemoglobin type of the patient is not known. Hemolysate standards from patients known to have hemoglobin A and hemoglobin C should also be used.

7. Acetate buffer, pH 4.7: Sodium acetate ($Na_2C_2H_3O_2 \cdot 3H_2O$) 27.22 g is dissolved in 1 liter of distilled water. 11.3 ml of glacial acetic acid is brought up to 1 liter with distilled water. Then 535 ml of the sodium acetate solution is mixed with 465 ml of the acetic acid solution.

8. *o*-Dianisidine (3,3-dimethoxybenzidine) stain (should be prepared just before use): 100 mg of 3,3-dimethoxybenzidine is dissolved in 70 ml of 95% ethanol. To this is added 10 ml of acetate buffer, 18 ml of distilled water, and 2 ml of 30% hydrogen peroxide.

9. Commercially available electrophoresis apparatus for cellulose acetate strips is suitable.

10. Applicator for electrophoresis.

11. A power supply capable of providing 200 volts dc.

TECHNIQUE

DEMONSTRATION OF HEME PIGMENTS

1. Add two drops of orthotolidine solution to four drops of urine and then add three drops of acid peroxide solution (in that order). If either hemoglobin or myoglobin in significant amount is present, a blue color will appear.

2. The same reagents are used in Hemastix (see below). These may be used according to the manufacturer's directions.

DIFFERENTIAL SOLUBILITY IN AMMONIUM SULFATE (PRESUMPTIVE DIFFERENTIATION) [1]

1. The urine is clarified by filtration or centrifugation; then 2.8 g of $(NH_4)_2SO_4$ is added to 5 ml of urine, making an 80% saturated solution of $(NH_4)_2SO_4$. The solution is allowed to stand for 5 min.

2. The urine is again filtered and the filtrate examined for heme pigments as noted above.

DIFFERENTIATION BY ELECTROPHORESIS

1. The urine is centrifuged. If the amount of heme-containing pigment is small, the urine may be concentrated by pressure dialysis using a vacuum system and dialysis tubing, or by dialysis against solid Carbowax or concentrated polyvinylpyrrolidone (PVP) solution.

2. Control solutions are prepared by adding one drop of each hemolysate (patient, known hemoglobin A, known hemoglobin C) to 2-ml aliquots of control urine.

3. The cellulose acetate strip is moistened with veronal buffer as for hemoglobin electrophoresis (Chap. A7). The samples (three controls plus patient's urine) are placed on the strip with the applicator. Two applications may be necessary if the sample has little heme pigment.

4. The sample is electrophoresed for 120 min at 150 to 200 volts.

5. The cellulose acetate strip is removed and dried on a glass plate in an oven set lower than 90°C.

6. The strip is then stained by being floated on the freshly prepared *o*-dianisidine stain until soaked through from the bottom, after which it is immersed for 3 to 5 min.

7. The excess stain is then thoroughly rinsed in distilled water, and the strip is dried again in the oven.

INTERPRETATION

DIFFERENTIAL SOLUBILITY

If heme-containing protein is present and is soluble in the presence of 80% ammonium sulfate, myoglobin is presumed to be present. However, the concomitant presence of hemoglobin is not ruled out. Denatured myoglobin may be precipitated in 80% ammonium sulfate. For that reason, freshly voided urine should be used. If the urine is to be stored, the pH should be adjusted to 7.0 and the urine frozen until analysis.

ELECTROPHORESIS

The heme-containing pigments stain blue. Hemoglobin in the urine will have the same electrophoretic mobility as the patient's hemoglobin, whereas myoglobin in the urine will have slower mobility, approximately that of hemoglobin C (or E). Thus, if the patient has hemoglobin C in the red cells, hemoglobinuria cannot be distinguished from myoglobinuria by this method. (*Note:* This method cannot be used to distinguish hemoglobinemia from myoglobinemia, since hemoglobin attached to haptoglobin has the same electrophoretic mobility as free myoglobin.)

SOURCES OF REAGENTS

1. *Hemastix:* Ames Corp., Div. of Miles Laboratories, Inc., Elkhart, IN 46514.

2. *Veronal buffer:* This may be prepared according to directions or purchased from Beckman Instruments, Houston, Tex.

3. *3,3-Dimethoxybenzidine:* Eastman Chemicals, Rochester, N.Y.

4. *Electrophoresis apparatus and sample applicator:* Beckman Instruments, Fullerton, Calif.

5. *Power supply* (see Chap. A7, under "Starch Gel Electrophoresis").

References

1. Blondheim, S. H., Margoliash, E., and Shafrir, E.: A simple test for myohemoglobinuria (myoglobinuria). *JAMA* 167:453, 1958.
2. Brodine, C. E., and Vertrees, K. M.: Differentiation of myoglobinuria from hemoglobinuria, in *Hemoglobin: Its Precursors and Metabolites,* edited by F. W. Sunderman and F. W. Sunderman, Jr. Lippincott, Philadelphia, 1964, p. 90.
3. Wishnant, C. L., Owings, R. H., Cantrell, C. G., and Cooper, G. R.: Primary idiopathic myoglobinuria in a Negro female: Its implications and a new method of laboratory diagnosis. *Ann. Intern. Med.* 51:140, 1959.

CHAPTER *A16*

Carboxyhemoglobin, methemoglobin, and sulfhemoglobin determinations

ERNEST BEUTLER

PURPOSE OF THE TEST

Carboxyhemoglobin is a complex of hemoglobin and carbon monoxide which may be found in increased concentration in the blood as a result of smoking or other toxic exposure. Chronic carboxyhemoglobinemia is a cause of secondary polycythemia; acute intoxication may produce severe brain damage and death.

Methemoglobinemia may occur because of hereditary deficiency in NADH diaphorase (Chap. 77), inheritance of the hemoglobin M's (Chap. 78), or exposure to toxic drugs or chemicals (Chap. 77). Sulfhemoglobinemia also occurs chiefly as a result of toxic exposure, although some cases have been reported in the absence of drug administration or exposure to toxins.

PRINCIPLE OF THE TEST

The estimation of carboxyhemoglobin, methemoglobin, and sulfhemoglobin depends upon the differences in their spectra and those of their derivatives from the spectra of oxyhemoglobin and reduced hemoglobin [1–3]. Quantitation of a mixture of two pigments can be accomplished by measuring the optical density at two wavelengths and solving simultaneous equations. In measuring methemoglobin, advantage is taken of the fact that this pigment has an absorption band in the 630-nm range which disappears upon the addition of cyanide. A band in the 620-nm region is present when hemoglobin degradation products, categorized as sulfhemoglobins, are present. This band does not disappear upon the addition of cyanide.

The measurement of methemoglobin and of carboxyhemoglobin may be achieved by the use of a microprocessor-controlled, fixed-wavelength, dedicated instrument, such as the Co-oximeter (Instrumentation Laboratories, Menlo Park, CA 94025). Such instruments are designed to measure these pigments as well as the percentage of hemoglobin oxygenation. They should be used according to the instructions provided by the manufacturer. Unless measurement of these pigments is to be performed very frequently, it is difficult to justify the cost of such dedicated devices, and they will not be discussed here.

REAGENTS AND EQUIPMENT

1. 1 M K_2HPO_4. Dissolve 17.42 g of K_2HPO_4 (anhydrous) and bring to a final volume of 100 ml with distilled water.

2. 1 M KH_2PO_4. Dissolve 13.61 g of KH_2PO_4 (anhydrous) and bring to a final volume of 100 ml with distilled water.

3. 0.066 M phosphate buffer. Mix 23 ml of 1 M K_2HPO_4 and 43 ml of 1 M KH_2PO_4 and dilute to 1 liter with distilled water to give a buffer with a pH of 6.6

4. 0.0166 M phosphate buffer. Dilute 250 ml of the 0.066 M phosphate buffer to 1 liter with distilled water. Add approximately 0.2 g of saponin.

5. 20% potassium ferricyanide. Dissolve 2 g of potassium ferricyanide in 10 ml of distilled water. This solution may be stored in a dark bottle at room temperature.

6. Sodium cyanide solution. Dissolve 1 g of sodium cyanide in 10 ml of distilled water. This solution may be stored at room temperature. A "poison" label should be affixed.

7. Acetic acid solution. Dilute 12 ml of glacial acetic acid to 100 ml with distilled water.

8. Concentrated ammonium hydroxide. Used as purchased.

9. Neutralized cyanide. Dispense 4 drops of sodium cyanide solution into a small test tube. While agitating the tube, preferably in a vented hood, add 4 drops of acetic acid solution. Stopper the tube or cover with Parafilm because the solution gives off toxic HCN fumes. This solution may be kept at room temperature but must be used within 1 h.

10. 0.1 M phosphate buffer. Dilute 52.7 ml of 1 M K_2HPO_4 and 47.3 ml of 1 M KH_2PO_4 to 1 liter with distilled water to give a buffer with a pH of about 6.85.

11. Lysing solution. Dilute 10 ml of 0.1 M phosphate buffer to 100 ml with distilled water.

12. CO-Hb diluting solution. Immediately before use, add 25 mg of $Na_2S_2O_4$ to 20 ml of the 0.1 M phosphate buffer.

13. Photoelectric colorimeters are suitable for methemoglobin and sulfhemoglobin estimations. A narrow-bandpass spectrophotometer is needed for carboxyhemoglobin measurements.

TECHNIQUE

CARBOXYHEMOGLOBIN

1. Add 0.025 ml of blood to 3 ml of lysing solution in a small test tube. Mix by inverting two or three times.

2. After 5 min, pipette 0.1 ml of the mixture into a cuvette that has a critical volume of less than 1 ml and already contains 1.15 ml of the fresh CO-Hb diluting solution. Alternatively, 0.2 ml of the mixture may be added to 2.3 ml of the CO-Hb diluting solution in a larger cuvette (with a critical volume of less than 2.5 ml).

3. Cover the cuvette with Parafilm, mix by inverting gently several times, and allow to stand at room temperature for 10 min.

4. Using an optically matched cuvette containing CO-Hb diluting solution as the blank, read the optical density at 420 and 432 nm to obtain readings A_{420} and A_{432}, respectively.

METHEMOGLOBIN AND SULFHEMOGLOBIN

1. Pipette 0.1 ml of fresh whole blood into 10 ml of the 0.0166 M phosphate buffer solution. Mix well and read the optical density at 630 nm against a water or buffer blank. This reading is OD_A.

2. Add 1 drop of neutralized cyanide to the cuvette, swirl, and take a second reading at 630 nm after 1 or 2 min. The exact time of reading is not critical, but the reading should be constant. This reading is OD_B.

3. If *sulfhemoglobin* is to be measured, add 1 drop of 20% potassium ferricyanide and 1 drop of concentrated ammonia to the cuvette and mix. Read the optical density at 620 nm and record as OD_C. This step may be omitted if only methemoglobin measurements are to be made.

4. Pipette 2 ml of the cuvette contents into 8 ml of 0.066 M phosphate buffer. If step 3 was omitted, add 1 drop of 20% potassium ferricyanide. Add 1 drop of neutralized cyanide solution. Wait at least 2 min and then read the optical density at 540 nm against a blank containing 10 ml of 0.066 M phosphate buffer. This reading is OD_D.

CALCULATION OF RESULTS

The calibration factors for determining carboxyhemoglobin are

$$F_1 = \frac{\epsilon_{432}^{Hb}}{\epsilon_{420}^{Hb}} \qquad F_2 = \frac{\epsilon_{432}^{CO\text{-}Hb}}{\epsilon_{420}^{CO\text{-}Hb}} \qquad F_3 = \frac{\epsilon_{420}^{CO\text{-}Hb}}{\epsilon_{420}^{Hb}}$$

where ϵ is the molar extinction coefficient of carboxyhemoglobin (CO-Hb) or reduced hemoglobin (Hb) at wavelengths of 420 or 432 nm. These factors may be computed from published molar extinction coefficients [3], giving values of $F_1 = 1.3330$, $F_2 = 0.4787$, and $F_3 = 1.9939$. Because photometer response and accuracy of wavelength calibration may vary with different spectrophotometers, it is probably prudent to determine these factors for the instrument being used. By using the same hemoglobin solution, it is sufficient to measure and substitute the absorbance values $A_{420}^{CO\text{-}Hb}$, $A_{432}^{CO\text{-}Hb}$, A_{420}^{Hb}, and A_{432}^{Hb} for their corresponding extinction coefficients used in computing F_1, F_2, and F_3. The calibration is performed using a hemolysate made from a normal blood sample. Aliquots are converted to 100 percent CO-Hb by gassing with carbon monoxide and to 100 percent Hb by gassing with air while removing traces of CO-Hb by photolysis. To accomplish this, 0.25 ml of blood is added to 30 ml of lysing solution and 2 ml of the hemolysate is added to each of two 25-ml volumetric flasks. One

aliquot is gassed with carbon monoxide for 30 min with frequent swirling of the solution. The other flask is swirled while being gassed with air for 45 min and is exposed to a bright light such as that produced by an ordinary high-intensity desk lamp to aid the dissociation of traces of carbon monoxide. After equilibration with carbon monoxide or air, the contents of each flask are brought to volume with the fresh CO-Hb diluting solution, stoppered, and mixed by inverting several times. After 10 min the optical density of the diluted hemolysates (A_w) is determined at wavelengths (ω) of 420 and 432 nm by reading against matched cuvettes containing CO-Hb diluting solution. These absorbance values are used to calculate F_1, F_2, and F_3.

The carboxyhemoglobin content of blood is calculated from the equation

$$\% \text{ CO-Hb} = \frac{(1 - A_R \times F_1) \times 100}{A_R \times (F_2 - F_1) - F_3 + 1}$$

where A_R is the ratio of the absorbance of the sample in CO-Hb diluting solution at 420 to that at 432 nm:

$$A_R = \frac{A_{420}}{A_{432}}$$

The calibration factors for methemoglobin are derived as follows: A blood sample is lysed by freezing and thawing, and its hemoglobin content is determined accurately using the cyanmethemoglobin technique, measuring against a commercially available cyanmethemoglobin standard. Then 0.1 ml of the sample is added to 10 ml of the 0.0166 M phosphate buffer. One drop of freshly prepared potassium ferricyanide solution is added to the hemolysate, and the remainder of the procedure as listed under "Technique" is carried out.

$$F_D = \frac{\text{hemoglobin (g/dl)}}{OD_D}$$

$$F_A = \frac{\text{hemoglobin (g/dl)}}{OD_A - OD_B}$$

$$F_B = 100 \times \frac{OD_D}{OD_A - OD_B}$$

With a Coleman Junior Spectrophotometer Model 1A with a 25-mm cuvette, the following factors are approximately correct:

$$F_A = 35 \qquad F_B = 84 \qquad F_D = 41$$

The calculation of F_C and F_E, needed for sulfhemoglobin determinations, is based on the published data concerning the theoretical spectrum of pure sulfhemoglobin [2]. These data give an F_C of 15.3/L, where L is the light path of the cuvette in centimeters, and a value of 0.153 for F_E.

The use of such factors is not appropriate with colorimeters such as the Coleman Junior, however, because of the relatively wide spectral bandwidth. Values of $F_C = 9.4$ and $F_E = 0.17$ give fairly satisfactory results with 25-mm cuvettes in the Coleman Junior Spectrophotometer Model 1A.

The concentration of total hemoglobin, methemoglobin, and sulfhemoglobin in grams per deciliter may be calculated as follows:

Total hemoglobin $= F_D \times OD_D$

Methemoglobin (g/dl) $= (OD_A - OD_B) \times F_A$

Percent of pigment which is methemoglobin
$$= \frac{(OD_A - OD_B) \times F_B}{OD_D}$$

Sulfhemoglobin (g/dl) $= F_C \times OD_C - F_E \times F_B \times OD_D$

References

1. Evelyn, K. A., and Malloy, H. T.: Micro determination of oxyhemoglobin, methemoglobin and sulfhemoglobin in a single sample of blood. *J. Biol. Chem.* 126:655, 1938.
2. Drabkin, D. L., and Austin, J. H.: Spectrophotometric studies. II. Preparations from washed blood cells: Nitric oxide hemoglobin and sulfhemoglobin. *J. Biol. Chem.* 112:51, 1935–1936.
3. Rodkey, F. L., Hill, T. A., Pitts, L. L., and Robertson, R. F.: Spectrophotometric measurement of carboxyhemoglobin and methemoglobin in blood. *Clin. Chem.* 25:1388, 1979.

CHAPTER *A17*

Erythropoietin assay

ALLAN J. ERSLEV

PURPOSE OF THE TEST

Determination of the concentration of erythropoietin in plasma or of the 24-h excretion of erythropoietin in urine may add important information in the diagnostic evaluation of patients with erythrocytosis or anemia [1]. Patients with secondary polycythemia may have elevated erythropoietin levels, while patients with polycythemia vera characteristically have no erythropoietin in plasma or urine. This difference becomes more pronounced after phlebotomies have decreased the hematocrit reading to about 50 percent. Patients with anemias caused by marrow dysfunction have high erythropoietin concentration and excretion, while patients with anemia caused by renal disease have only normal or low levels in plasma or urine.

PRINCIPLE OF THE TEST

Erythropoietin levels can be determined and standardized by in vivo bioassays in small laboratory animals in which endogenous erythropoietin production has been reduced by transfusion [2] or starvation [3]. The effect of the test material on the rate of red cell production, reticulocyte count, or ^{59}Fe incorporation is used as a measure of its erythropoietin content. In vitro bioassays use suspensions of erythroid cells obtained from marrow [4] or from fetal liver [5] and measure the erythropoietin content of the test sample by its effect on cellular incorporation of ^{59}Fe or on erythroid colony formation [6]. Immunologic assays measure the competitive effect of the test material on the agglutination of erythropoietin-coated red blood cells by an erythropoietin antibody [7] or on the formation of radioactive antigen-antibody complexes [8].

These tests all provide reasonable estimates of the erythropoietin content of unknown samples. The agglutination inhibition assay is the least reliable and the radioimmune assay the most convenient. This latter test is unfortunately still not generally available. The in vivo biologic assay measures most directly the physiologic effect of erythropoietin on stem cells, and since it serves as a standard for all other tests, it will be described here.

REAGENTS AND EQUIPMENT

1. Adult female mice are used as recipients. They should weigh between 20 and 30 g and be either from an inbred strain or, what is less expensive, from a random-bred Swiss-Webster colony. Whole blood for transfusion is obtained by bleeding normal, large donor mice. The mice are lightly anesthetized in an ether jar. The carotid arteries are severed with a scalpel, and the blood, about 1 ml per mouse, is collected in a beaker containing heparin, penicillin, and streptomycin (125 ml of whole blood to 5 ml of saline, with 1000 units of heparin, 20,000 units of penicillin, and 20 mg of streptomycin). The blood is centrifuged and the plasma removed. The packed cells are washed twice with saline. The hematocrit is adjusted to 85 percent, and the cells are transfused into recipient mice on the schedule presented below. The cells can be stored at 4°C for about 24 h.

2. Polycythemia can also be induced by exposure to 0.4 atmospheric pressure in a hypobaric chamber for 16 h per day for 2 weeks [2].

3. If high titers are expected, plasma or serum is assayed directly. If low titers are expected, it is necessary to concentrate the samples. The most practical method is to take 200 ml of plasma obtained from a phlebotomy, adjust the pH to 5.5 in hydrochloric acid, place it in a boiling water bath for 5 min, cool rapidly, and centrifuge for 30 min at 3000 rpm. This procedure will precipitate almost all protein and leave about 50 percent of the heat-resistant erythropoietin in the supernatant. The supernatant is removed and concentrated fortyfold in a cellophane dialysis bag against Carbowax 6000 (Union Carbide Co.). The resulting concentrate is assayed directly [9].

4. Urine concentrate for assay is prepared by placing 300 ml of urine in a dialysis bag and concentrating it fiftyfold against Carbowax 6000 [10].

5. Radioactive iron (^{59}Fe) may be administered as ferrous citrate or as any other commercially available salt.

6. A scintillation detector and counter suitable for measuring ^{59}Fe is required.

TECHNIQUE

A minimum of four mice should be used for the assay of each sample.

TRANSFUSION POLYCYTHEMIA

Day 0   The mice are injected i.p. with 0.9 ml of packed red cells.

Day 1   The mice are injected i.p. with 0.9 ml of packed red cells.

Day 6   0.5 to 1 ml of the material to be assayed is injected s.c.

Day 7   0.5 to 1 ml of the material to be assayed is injected s.c.

Day 8   0.2 ml of saline containing about 0.5 µCi of ^{59}Fe is infused i.p. The exact amount of radioactivity ad-

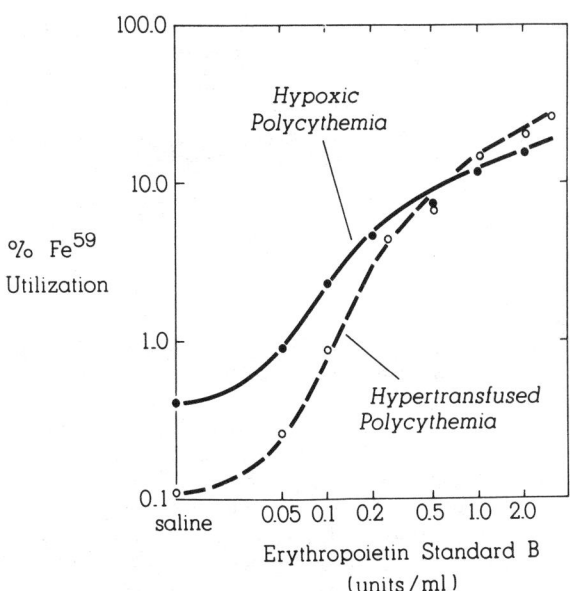

FIGURE A17-1 Dose-response curves for human urinary erythropoietin (Standard B) assayed in mice with either hypertransfused polycythemia or hypoxia-induced polycythemia. The 66-h utilization of ^{59}Fe is used as a measure of erythropoietic response.

ministered is determined by counting a suitable aliquot of the ^{59}Fe solution.

Day 11   The mice are weighed. Blood is then obtained for determination of 66-h ^{59}Fe utilization and hematocrit. For collection of blood the mice are lightly anesthetized with ether and the carotid artery severed with a scalpel. The blood is collected on a square of Parafilm, without anticoagulant. As rapidly as possible 0.2 ml of blood is transferred to 2.0 ml of saline, using a "to contain" pipette. The solution is thoroughly mixed by drawing the solution into the pipette and discharging it several times. This mixture is used to determine the ^{59}Fe concentration as counts per minute (cpm) per milliliter of blood. An aliquot of the blood on the Parafilm is also drawn into a capillary tube containing anticoagulant for subsequent determination of the microhematocrit.

HYPOXIC POLYCYTHEMIA

Day 0   The mice are placed at 0.4 atmospheric pressure for 16 h every day, including weekends.

Day 14   The mice are removed from the chambers.

Day 19   0.5 to 1 ml of the material to be assayed is injected s.c.

Day 20   0.5 to 1 ml of the material to be assayed is injected s.c.

Day 21   0.2 ml of saline with 0.5 μCi of ^{59}Fe is infused i.p. The exact amount of radioactivity administered is determined by counting a suitable aliquot of the ^{59}Fe solution.

Day 24   The mice are weighed. Blood is then obtained for determination of 66-h utilization of ^{59}Fe and hematocrit, as described above.

CALCULATION OF RESULTS

All results from mice with hematocrit readings of less than 55 percent are discarded. The blood volume of polycythemic mice is assumed to be 7 percent of body weight.

$$66\text{-h utilization of }^{59}\text{Fe} = \frac{\text{cpm of 1 ml blood} \times \text{blood volume}}{\text{cpm of injected }^{59}\text{Fe}} \times 100$$

INTERPRETATION

Using a curve relating various concentrations of a standard erythropoietin[1] to the 66-h utilization of ^{59}Fe (Fig. A17-1), it is possible to estimate the content of erythropoietin in milliunits per milliliter of sample and then to calculate its titer per milliliter of plasma or its urinary excretion in units per 24 h. A minimum of four mice should be used for each assay, and repeated assays may be needed to gain reproducible data from these crude bioassay techniques. The transfusion polycythemic mice are more sensitive to low concentrations of erythropoietin than the hypoxia-induced polycythemic mice. The hypoxia techniques are more convenient, however, and less expensive. Figures A17-2 and A17-3 give ranges for erythropoietin titers

[1] Standard B. International Reference Preparation, Medical Research Council Division of Biological Standards, National Institute for Medical Research, Mill Hill, London, N.W. 7, England.

FIGURE A17-2 The range of plasma erythropoietin concentration in patients with anemias uncomplicated by renal impairment or debilitating illnesses.

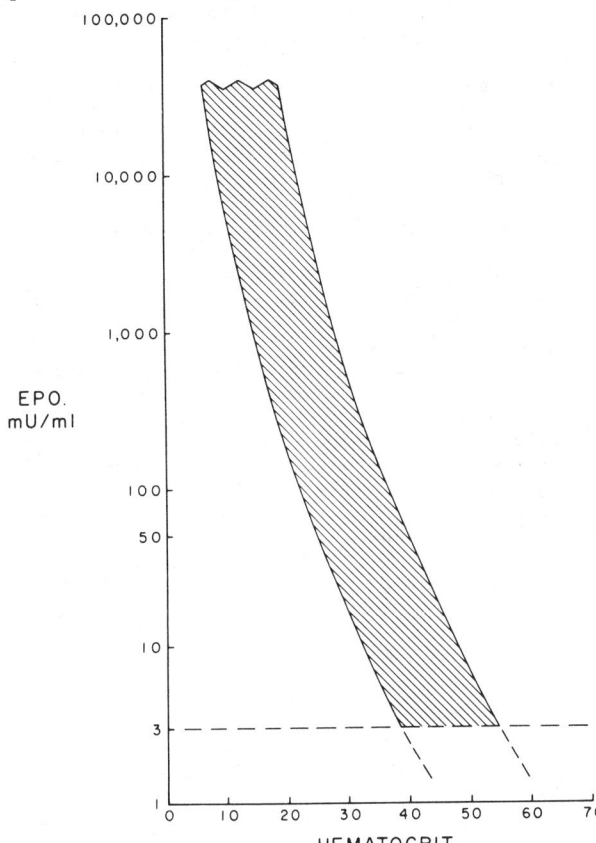

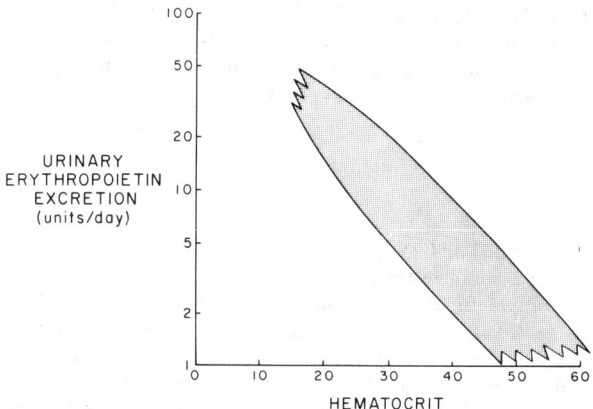

FIGURE A17-3 The range of urinary erythropoietin excretion in patients with anemias at various hemoglobin concentrations. (Adapted from Adamson et al. [10].)

in plasma and for 24-h urinary excretion of erythropoietin in individuals with anemias and polycythemias uncomplicated by renal impairment or debilitating illnesses.

SOURCE OF REAGENTS
The source of special reagents is indicated in the text.

References

1. Erslev, A. J., Caro, J., Miller, O., and Silver, R.: Plasma erythropoietin in health and disease. *Ann. Clin. Lab. Sci. 10*:250, 1980.
2. Cotes, P. M., and Bangham, D. R.: Bio-assay of erythropoietin in mice made polycythemic by exposure to air at a reduced pressure. *Nature 191*:1065, 1961.
3. Fried, W., Plzak, L., Jacobson, L. O., and Goldwasser, E.: Studies on erythropoiesis. III. Factors controlling erythropoietin production. *Proc. Soc. Exp. Biol. Med. 94*:237, 1957.
4. Erslev, A. J.: Effect of erythropoietin on the uptake and utilization of iron by bone marrow cells in vitro. *Proc. Soc. Exp. Biol. Med. 110*:615, 1962.
5. Dunn, C.D.R., Jarvis, J. H., and Greenman, J. R.: A quantitative bioassay for erythropoietin using mouse fetal liver cells. *Exp. Hematol. 3*:65, 1975.
6. Hågå, P., and Falkanger, B. B.: In vitro assay for erythropoietin: Erythroid colony formation in methylcellulose used for the measurement of erythropoietin in plasma. *Blood 53*:1172, 1979.
7. Lange, R. D., Jordan, T. A., and McDonald, T. P.: Partial characterization of an antiserum to erythropoietin. *Isr. J. Med. Sci. 7*:877, 1971.
8. Sherwood, J. B., and Goldwasser, E.: A radioimmunoassay for erythropoietin. *Blood 54*:885, 1979.
9. Erslev, A. J., Caro, J., Kansu, E., Miller, O., and Cobbs, E.: Plasma erythropoietin in polycythemia. *Am. J. Med. 66*:243, 1979.
10. Adamson, J. W., Alexanian, R., Martinez, C., and Finch, C. A.: Erythropoietin excretion in normal man. *Blood 28*:354, 1966.

Haptoglobin assay

JEAN ATWATER
ALLAN J. ERSLEV

PURPOSE OF THE TEST
Haptoglobin (Hp), discovered by Polonovski and Jayle [1] in 1938, is a heterogeneous plasma protein which migrates on electrophoresis with the α_2 fraction. In 1955 Smithies [2] described three genetically determined types of haptoglobin which he classified as Hp 1-1, Hp 2-1, and Hp 2-2 according to the bands separating on electrophoresis in starch gel. All haptoglobins have the capacity to bind with free hemoglobin in a constant ratio, forming a haptoglobin-hemoglobin complex which is readily removed by the monocyte-macrophage system. This prevents the intravascular accumulation of free hemoglobin in hemolytic anemia and renders the level of haptoglobin a sensitive indicator of intravascular hemolysis. The haptoglobin assay is of clinical importance in the differential diagnosis of jaundice and hemolytic anemia and in blood banking as an aid in determining the presence of hemolytic reactions to transfusions [3].

PRINCIPLES OF THE TEST
Several techniques have been used to measure the amounts of haptoglobin present, all showing good correlation. These include chemical [4], gel filtration on Sephadex [5], and radial immunodiffusion [6] procedures, as well as electrophoretic techniques on paper [7], starch gel [2], acrylamide gel [8], and agar gel [9]. Since free hemoglobin separates clearly from the haptoglobin-hemoglobin complex, this property has been used to measure the unbound haptoglobin in serum. Serum is added to hemoglobin solutions of known concentrations, and the mixture of Hp-Hb complex and free hemoglobin is separated. The presence of any free hemoglobin indicates that the binding capacity of haptoglobin has been exceeded at that concentration, thereby giving an indirect measurement of the haptoglobin concentration. A fast, simple, inexpensive method using agar-gel electrophoresis is described, modified from the procedure of Rowe [9].

REAGENTS AND EQUIPMENT
1. Agar gel. Add bacto agar to 0.05 *M*, pH 7.0 sodium phosphate buffer to a concentration of 0.8 percent.
2. Hemoglobin solutions. Make a stock solution from washed human red cells lysed by the addition of an approximately equal volume of distilled water. Determine the hemoglobin concentration of the lysate and adjust to a concentration of exactly 10 mg/ml (1 g/dl). Then make nine dilute stock solutions by diluting with distilled water to concentrations of 0.1, 0.2, 0.4, 0.6, 0.8, 1.0, 1.2, 1.4, and 1.6 mg/ml. These solutions are adequate for low- or normal-range concentrations of haptoglobin. If higher concentrations are anticipated or found, the serum may be diluted or higher concentration of hemoglobin solution may be used. The stock solution is stable for about 1 month under refrigeration. Discard if red color turns brownish.
3. *o*-Tolidine stain (Fisher Scientific, King of Prussia, Pa.). Make a stock solution by dissolving 6 g of *o*-tolidine in 100 ml of glacial acetic acid. Store in the dark at room temperature.

Working solution. Immediately before use, diulte 20 ml of the stock solution to 100 ml with distilled water. Then add 2 to 3 drops of 30% hydrogen peroxide and mix.

4. Electrophoretic equipment. A power supply capable of 250 V and a current of 50 mA and two buffer vessels are required. Each vessel should have a capacity of 500 ml and contain a platinum wire electrode. A 7- by 10-cm glass or plastic plate with a 3-mm lip is used as support for the agar gel. Plastic plates used for packaging agar plates have a convenient size and shape. A support for the plate can be a wooden block slightly narrower than the plate and slightly higher than the height of the buffer reservoirs. The agar gel is connected to the buffer by bridges of Whatman 3-MM filter paper. These bridges should be the same width as the glass plate.

TECHNIQUE

Melt 50 ml of the agar suspension by immersion in boiling water, cool slightly, and pour 25 ml onto each of two plates. When the agar has hardened, use a 4-mm cork borer to punch out 10 holes equally spaced along the midline of the longer dimension of the gel. A narrow-tipped spatula will facilitate lifting out the cut agar plug. To eight small test tubes (10 × 75 mm), each containing 0.02 ml of the dilute hemoglobin stock solutions (from 0.2 to 1.6 mg/ml), add an equal volume of serum, giving mixtures containing from 0.2 to 1.6 mg of hemoglobin per milliliter of serum. With a micropipette, carefully introduce 0.02 ml from each tube into one of the holes in the agar, beginning with the second hold (Fig. A18-1). To the first hole add 0.02 ml of the 0.1-mg/ml hemoglobin stock solution as a hemoglobin control. The bottom well contains 0.02 ml of the serum alone. Lay the plate across the support block placed between the two buffer reservoirs, each containing 500 ml of the phosphate buffer. Dip the filter paper bridges into the buffer and place them in position overlapping the long side of the gel by about 1.5 cm and dip them into the buffer about 1.5 cm. After connecting the electrodes, adjust the voltage to 240 V and allow electrophoresis to proceed for 50 min. Migration is toward the cathode. At the end of electrophoresis, remove the gel plate to a shallow staining dish and carefully pour the o-tolidine staining solution over the gel. After about 10 min the blue-black color is sufficiently developed and the stain is decanted or aspirated. Cover with distilled water. The gel may remain in the water for several days, or, if preferred, the gel plate may be removed after several hours and allowed to dry to a thin hard film on the plate for a permanent record.

CALCULATION OF THE RESULTS

The free hemoglobin in the first well will migrate toward the cathode about 1.5 cm. Hemoglobin bound to available haptoglobin forms a complex which will migrate only slightly toward the cathode, if at all. The last well, containing serum only, should show no migration or o-tolidine staining unless the serum contains free hemoglobin due to intravascular hemolysis, or possibly hemolysis from the process of collecting the serum sample. The hemoglobin-binding capacity of the serum, and therefore indirectly of the haptoglobin, is recorded as the highest level of hemoglobin at which no free hemoglobin is observed. For example, if free hemoglobin is migrating in the well containing 0.8 mg per millimeter of hemoglobin but none is seen in the well containing 0.6 mg per millimeter of hemoglobin, the haptoglobin is reported as 60 mg per deciliter of serum. If all wells show free hemoglobin migration, this indicates that the haptoglobin concentration is less than 10 mg per deciliter serum. When no free hemoglobin is seen in any but the first well, more than 160 mg per deciliter of haptoglobin

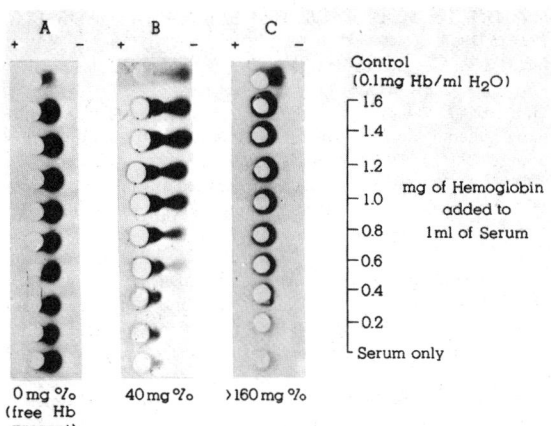

FIGURE A18-1   Agar-gel electrophoresis of various amounts of hemoglobin added to serum with (*A*) no haptoglobin, (*B*) 40 mg of haptoglobin per deciliter of serum, and (*C*) >160 mg of haptoglobin per deciliter of serum.

is present. The test can be rerun with more hemoglobin added to the serum or with the serum diluted to get a more accurate value.

INTERPRETATION

Normal haptoglobin levels range from 28 to 192 mg of Hb bound per deciliter of serum or 6 to 28 μmol of Hb bound per deciliter of serum. This wide range is due in part to the fact that haptoglobin is found in three distinct types, genetically controlled. There is a different range for each type. Nyman [10] found that type 1-1 had a mean haptoglobin level of 136 ± 37 mg/dl, type 2-2 a mean of 82 ± 34 mg/dl while the mean for type 2-1 fell between these two at 108 ± 37 mg/dl.

Low levels of haptoglobin have been reported in almost all conditions in which hemolysis occurs and also in some hemolytic anemias and hepatocellular disease.

Increased haptoglobin levels occur in a variety of diseases associated with inflammation, infection, or neoplasia. However, a wide variation of levels occurs within these groups.

Newborn infants have no haptoglobin for the first 6 weeks; thereafter the level increases with age. There is a sex difference also, with females showing a lower level than males.

For more detailed information on haptoglobin, a review by Javid [11] is recommended.

SOURCE OF REAGENTS AND EQUIPMENT

Reagents may be purchased from any supply house. Most supply houses also carry a satisfactory power supply for electrophoresis. Electrophoresis vessels (catalog No. 3-1074 B or 31074-T) may be obtained from Buchler Instruments, Fort Lee, N.J.

References

1. Polonovski, M., and Jayle, M. F.: Existence dans le plasma sanguin d'une substance activant l'action peroxydasique de l'hémoglobine. *C. R. Soc. Biol. (Paris) 129*:457, 1938.

2. Smithies, O.: Zone electrophoresis in starch gels: Group variations in the serum proteins of normal human adults. *Biochem. J. 61*:629, 1955.

3. Fink, D. J., Petz, L. D., and Black, M. B.: Serum haptoglobin. *JAMA* 199:615, 1967.
4. Jayle, M. F.: Methode de dosage de l'haptoglobine sérique. *Bull. Soc. Chim. Biol. (Paris)* 33:876, 1951.
5. Lionetti, F. J., Valerie, C. R., Bond, J. C., and Fortier, N. L.: Measurement of hemoglobin binding capacity of plasma by means of dextran gels. *J. Lab. Clin. Med.* 64:519, 1963.
6. Schultz, H. E., and Heremans, J. F.: Molecular biology of human proteins, in *Analytical Methods in Protein Chemistry*. Elsevier, New York, 1966, vol. 1, chap. 2.
7. Javid, J., and Horowitz, H. I.: An improved technic for the quantitation of serum haptoglobin. *Am. J. Clin. Pathol.* 34:35, 1960.
8. Ferris, T. G., Easterling, R. E., Nelson, K. J., and Budd, R. E.: Determination of serum-hemoglobin binding capacity and haptoglobin-type by acrylamide gel electrophoresis. *Am. J. Clin. Pathol.* 46:385, 1966.
9. Rowe, D. S.: A rapid method for the estimation of serum haptoglobin. *J. Clin. Pathol.* 14:205, 1961.
10. Nyman, M.: Serum haptoglobin: Methodological and clinical studies. *Scand. J. Clin. Lab. Invest. (Suppl. 39)* 11, 1959.
11. Javid, J.: Human serum haptoglobins: A brief review. *Semin. Hematol.* 4:35, 1967.

CHAPTER *A19*

Erythrokinetics

ALLAN J. ERSLEV

PURPOSE OF THE TEST

Diagnosis and management of patients with anemia or polycythemia depend on a knowledge of the total mass of red cells and the rate of their production and destruction. These erythrokinetic parameters can usually be assessed quite adequately from history, physical examination, and such routine laboratory tests as hemoglobin concentration, hematocrit, red cell indices, reticulocyte count, bilirubin concentration, and marrow morphology. In some patients, however, several of these parameters may be difficult to interpret or actually quite misleading. For example: (1) red cell values do not always reflect the red cell mass in severe anemia with heart failure or severe polycythemia with blood volume expansion; (2) the reticulocyte count may not reflect the rate of red cell production in patients with extramedullary hemopoiesis, ineffective red cell production, or severe hemolytic anemia; (3) the small marrow specimen obtained by aspiration may not represent overall marrow activity because of the presence of islands of overactivity in aplastic anemia and of fatty replacement in older people; (4) bilirubin concentration and spleen size are often signs of hepatic disease rather than evidence of increased red cell destruction. In all these conditions, measurements of the kinetics of iron labeled with ^{59}Fe [1,2] and red cells labeled with ^{51}Cr [3–9] will provide important information as to the production, distribution, and destruction of the red cells. These measurements can be fairly complex if they have to take into account the exchanges of isotopes which take place continuously between many different tissue compartments [10,11]. However, such tests demand multiple sampling and computer-assisted analysis and so far have not provided much more clinically

useful information than have the relatively simple tests described here.

PRINCIPLES OF THE TEST

Radioactive iron injected intravenously will uniformly label the circulating pool of iron and permit measurement of its turnover rate. Under normal conditions most of the radioactive iron cleared from the circulation will reappear in the hemoglobin of circulating red cells and the iron turnover rate will closely reflect the total mass of erythropoietic tissue. External serial scanning for radioactivity will indicate the sites of this tissue, and the speed and extent of radioactive iron incorporation into red cells will provide information about its functional capacity.

Radioactive chromium in the form of the chromate ion (^{51}CrO$_4$) readily enters and labels red cells. When red cells labeled with chromium in vitro are injected intravenously, the extent of their immediate dilution provides a direct and accurate measure of the total red cell mass. The subsequent rate of disappearance of radioactivity is a measure of red cell life-span, and external serial scanning for radioactivity may reveal the major sites of red cell destruction.

Because of the different energies of gamma rays emitted by ^{59}Fe and ^{51}Cr, it is possible to utilize these radioisotopes simultaneously.

EQUIPMENT AND REAGENTS

1. Single- or double-channel gamma scintillation scaler with discriminator.
2. Sodium iodide crystal detector.
3. Body-scanning probe.
4. Radioactive iron as ^{59}FeCl$_3$ or ^{59}Fe citrate and radioactive chromium as Na$_2$^{51}CrO$_4$. No radioisotope license is needed for the procurement of tracer amounts of these isotopes.
5. Reagents for the measurement of plasma iron and plasma iron-binding capacity.

TECHNIQUE

1. Inject approximately 40 ml of the patient's venous blood into a sterile, siliconized, capped vial containing 10 ml of ACD solution. Add approximately 50 μCi of ^{51}Cr as sodium chromate. Keep the vial at room temperature for 30 min with frequent, gentle agitation and then inject 100 mg of sterile ascorbic acid into the vial to reduce the chromate ions to chromic ions. Since chromic ions do not penetrate the red cell membrane, no further red cell labeling will occur in vitro or in vivo. Alternatively, excess chromate can be removed by washing red cells in sterile saline. This will avoid the use of ascorbic acid, which may be potentially damaging to red cells, particularly red cells which are deficient in glucose-6-phosphate dehydrogenase.

2. Withdraw exactly 2 ml of chromated whole blood from the vial with a syringe and dilute to 250 ml with 0.9% NaCl in a volumetric flask. Save a 2-ml aliquot of this suspension for counting (Cr-1).

3. Withdraw about 8 ml of chromated whole blood from the vial with a syringe, centrifuge, and obtain plasma. Dilute exactly 2 ml of plasma to 50 ml with 0.9% NaCl in a volumetric flask. Save a 2-ml aliquot of this diluted plasma for counting (Cr-2).

4. Withdraw exactly 30 ml of chromated whole blood from the vial with a syringe and inject intravenously. 10 to 15 min later obtain 10 ml of anticoagulated blood from the opposite arm. Save exactly 2 ml of this sample for counting (Cr-3).

Centrifuge the remainder of this sample and save exactly 2 ml of plasma for counting (Cr-4).

5. Determine the hematocrit on the labeled blood remaining in the vial (Hct-1) and on each subsequent blood sample obtained.

6. Add 10 μCi of ^{59}Fe to 15 ml of sterile saline, save an accurately measured 2-ml aliquot for counting, and inject exactly 10 ml of the radioactive iron solution intravenously.

7. Insert an indwelling scalp vein needle in a vein in the opposite arm and keep it open with a heparinized saline well or with a constant, slow saline drip. Collect 6 ml of anticoagulated blood 10, 20, 30, 45, and 60 min after the initial injection of ^{59}Fe. Centrifuge the blood samples and save 2-ml plasma aliquots for determination of radioactivity and for subsequent plasma iron determination.

8. Collect anticoagulated blood twice a day for 4 days and then every 2 or 3 days for the next 10 to 14 days. Save 2-ml samples for counting.

9. In vivo determination of sites of red cell production is carried out for 10 days by scanning, at suitable intervals, the sacrum, spleen, and liver for ^{59}Fe gamma emission [1]. In vivo determination of sites of red cell destruction is carried out for 5 days by daily scanning of spleen, liver, and precordium for ^{51}Cr gamma emission [8,9] (Fig. A19-1). The probe should be positioned almost directly over the center of the mass of the organ. For sacral counting, the probe is centered in the midline between the spinous process of L5 and a line between the posterior-superior iliac spines. For splenic counting, the probe is placed in the left posterior axillary line at the level of T10 pointing toward the center of the body. If the spleen is palpable, the probe is placed over the presumed center of the organ or at the level of highest radioactivity. For liver counting, the probe is placed at the center of hepatic dullness in the right anterior axillary line and vertical to the skin. For precordial counting, the probe is placed at the left sternal edge in the fourth intercostal space. These areas should be marked with India ink for serial counting.

CALCULATIONS

RED CELL MASS

$$\text{Red cell mass (ml)} = \frac{\text{total red blood cell cpm injected}}{\text{cpm per ml red blood cell withdrawn}}$$

$$= \frac{30 \times \left[\text{cpm (Cr-1)} \times 125 - \text{cpm (Cr-2)} \times 25 \ \dfrac{100 - \text{Hct}}{100} \right]}{\left[\text{cpm (Cr-3)} - \text{cpm (Cr-4)} \times \dfrac{100 - \text{Hct}}{100} \right] \times \dfrac{100}{\text{Hct}}}$$

$$\text{Blood volume (ml)} = \frac{\text{red cell mass} \times 100}{\text{Hct} \times 0.92}$$

RED CELL LIFE-SPAN

2-ml whole-blood samples, collected serially over a 10- to 14-day period are counted for ^{51}Cr gamma activity, and the count per minute is plotted against days on semilogarithmic paper. The half-life ($T_{1/2}$) is the time in days required for 50 percent of the radioactive red cells to disappear.

RADIOACTIVE IRON CLEARANCE RATE

The 2-ml plasma samples obtained serially within the first hour after the injection of ^{59}Fe are counted for ^{59}Fe radioactivity and the cpm plotted against minutes on semilogarithmic paper.

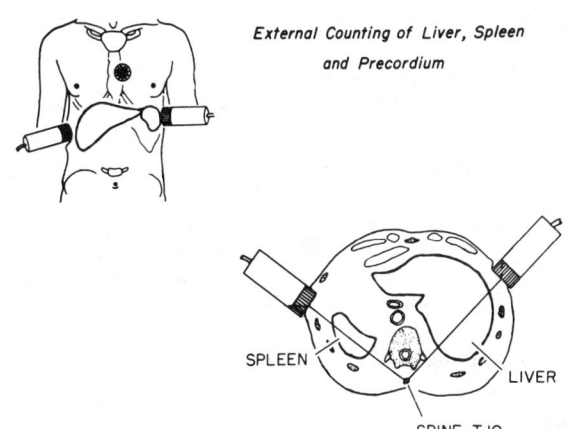

External Counting of Liver, Spleen and Precordium

SPLEEN LIVER

SPINE T 10

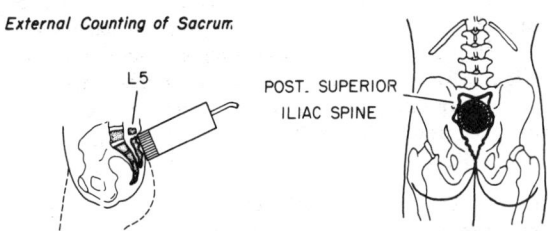

External Counting of Sacrum.

L5 POST. SUPERIOR ILIAC SPINE

FIGURE A19-1 The positioning of probes for external counting of liver, spleen, and marrow for ^{59}Fe radioactivity and of liver, spleen, and precordium for ^{51}Cr radioactivity. (Redrawn after Pollycove and Mortimer [1].)

The halftime ($T_{1/2}$) of radioactive iron is the time in minutes required for 50 percent of the extrapolated initial radioactivity to be cleared from the plasma.

PLASMA IRON TURNOVER RATE

The turnover rate of plasma iron depends on the rate of iron clearance and on the size of the circulating iron pool (plasma iron concentration in mg/ml $\times$ total plasma volume).

Plasma iron turnover rate in milligrams of iron can be expressed in a number of ways according to the point of reference (hemoglobin mass, blood volume, weight), but the most convenient and useful expression appears to be per deciliter of whole blood per day:

Plasma iron turnover rate (mg iron/dl blood/24 h)

$$= \frac{\text{plasma iron } (\mu g/dl) \times (100 - \text{Hct})}{T_{1/2} \text{ (min)} \times 100}$$

RED CELL IRON UTILIZATION RATE

2-ml whole-blood samples collected serially over a 10- to 14-day period are counted for ^{59}Fe radioactivity.

Red cell iron utilization rate (%)

$$= \frac{\text{cpm of 1 ml blood} \times \text{blood volume} \times 100}{\text{cpm of } ^{59}\text{Fe injected}}$$

RED CELL IRON TURNOVER RATE

Red cell iron turnover rate (mg iron/dl blood/24 h)
  = plasma iron turnover × maximal red cell iron utilization

ERYTHRON TURNOVER RATE

Erythron turnover rate (mg iron/dl blood/24 h)
  = plasma iron turnover − nonerythron turnover
  $= \dfrac{\text{plasma iron}}{\text{turnover}} - \dfrac{\text{plasma iron} \times (100 - \text{Hct}) \times 0.0035}{100}$

where plasma iron is measured in μg/dl.

MARROW TRANSIT TIME

The time required for intramedullary maturation of immature red cells is difficult to measure directly. An approximation may be reached by measuring the time needed for the release of 50 percent of the radioiron-labeled red cells from the marrow into circulating red cells. This time, called the *marrow transit time,* can be found by plotting daily red cell iron utilization against time and determining the point at which 50 percent of maximum red cell iron utilization has occurred.

SITES OF RED CELL PRODUCTION

All measurements of ^{59}Fe gamma emission over sacrum, liver, and spleen are related to the initial radioactivity in each tissue by dividing the observed cpm by the cpm measured immediately after the injection of radioactive iron. These values are plotted against time on standard graph paper.

SITES OF RED CELL DESTRUCTION

All measurements of ^{59}Cr gamma emission over spleen and liver are related to precordium (whole blood) by dividing the observed cpm by the cpm measured over the precordium at the same time. These values are plotted against time on standard graph paper.

INTERPRETATION

RED CELL MASS

Mixing time   A 10- to 15-min interval between the infusion of chromated red cells and sampling is usually adequate for complete mixing. In patients with splenomegaly a longer interval (30 to 45 min) should be allowed in order to secure uniform dilution of the tagged cells.

Blood volume   When red cell mass is used in the calculation of blood volume, total body hematocrit rather than venous hematocrit should be used in the equation (Chap. 41):

Total body hematocrit = venous hematocrit × 0.92

Normal values   A normal red cell mass is a value more difficult to define or establish than a normal hematocrit or hemoglobin concentration. It depends primarily on body weight and body composition, but body surface, muscular development, and age may play a role. Because of these variables, it does not appear warranted to express the red cell mass in more accurate terms than per kilogram of body weight.

Normal values:

Children	23 to 29 ml per kg body weight [12]
Adult females	23 to 29 ml per kg body weight [4]
Adult males	26 to 32 ml per kg body weight [3]

RED CELL LIFE-SPAN

Elution rate   Because of a constant loss of chromium label from red cells of about 1 percent a day, the $T_{1/2}$ of ^{51}Cr-tagged normal red cells is less than the theoretic $T_{1/2}$ of 60 days (Chap. 41). Correction charts have been published [13,14], but since the elution of chromium from abnormal red cells may vary, it is advisable to use the observed value and merely report the red cell life-span as $T_{1/2}$ of ^{51}Cr-labeled red cells. Since the curves are usually exponential, they should be charted on semilogarithmic paper in order to determine $T_{1/2}$ accurately.

The elution rate of chromium from red cells with SC hemoglobin has been reported to be considerably higher than for normal cells, but the elution rates from red cells containing AS, AC, or fetal hemoglobins are normal [15]. Immature red cells (reticulocytes) have a greater affinity for ^{51}Cr than mature red cells, providing a potential error in the measurement of red cell life-span in patients with hemolytic anemia [16]. In hemoglobin H disease life-span measurements may also be erroneous because the four β chains have a greater affinity for chromium than the two β chains in hemoglobin A [17]. The addition of ascorbic acid may damage cells with an intrinsic metabolic defect, such as glucose-6-phosphate dehydrogenase deficiency. In such conditions, excess chromium should be removed by washing rather than by ascorbate conversion.

Normal values $T_{1/2}$ of ^{51}Cr-tagged red cells is 25 to 32 days.

RADIOACTIVE IRON CLEARANCE RATE

Preincubation of ^{59}Fe with plasma   The direct intravenous injection of ^{59}Fe as a salt is usually acceptable, since unbound transferrin is normally available for almost instantaneous binding [18]. If previous studies have shown a nearly complete saturation of transferrin, ^{59}Fe should be preincubated with plasma from a normal, hepatitis-free donor prior to injection. However, the injection of plasma from another individual always carries a certain risk, so the indications for performing this study should be carefully justified. The same is true for the potential risk from radiation exposure.[1] It appears to be negligible and of no concern, but any introduction of radiochemicals to children or pregnant women should be avoided.

Interpretation   The clearance rate of radioactive iron is not a direct measure of erythropoietic tissue because it is dependent on the size of the pool of circulating iron. The clearance is fast if the serum iron is low or the plasma volume small, and slow if the serum iron is high or the plasma volume expanded. Furthermore, the clearance rate is linear only for the first few hours. After that it curves because of iron reflux from labile pools, and the clearance no longer reflects iron uptake alone. Calculations of the plasma turnover rate take the pool of circulating unlabeled iron into consideration and are based on the early linear disappearance rate. It is therefore a more accurate measure of erythroid activity than is the clearance rate.

[1] The i.v. injection of 50 μCi of ^{51}Cr and 10 μCi of ^{59}Fe will provide a total body exposure of about 0.3 rads and a splenic exposure of about 3.3 rads. This is similar to the exposure encountered in radiographic fluoroscopic examination of the abdomen.

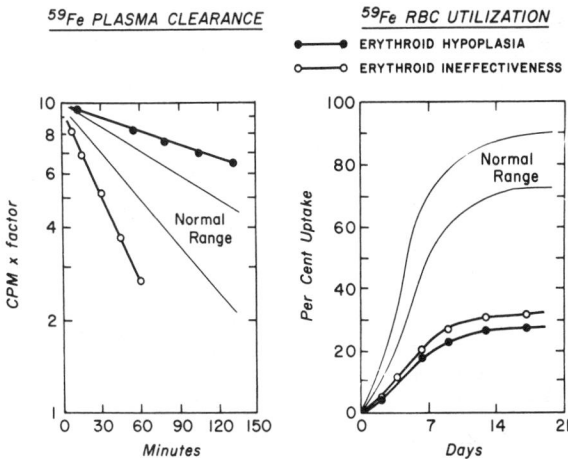

FIGURE A19-2 The plasma clearance and red cell utilization of ^{59}Fe in normal persons, in patients with erythroid hypoplasia such as aplastic anemia, and in patients with ineffective erythropoiesis, such as pernicious anemia. Although the utilization of ^{59}Fe in these two latter conditions may be equally reduced, the plasma clearance rate clearly separates them from each other.

Nevertheless, prolongation of the radioactive iron clearance is a very useful indication of decreased marrow activity. Since the normal plasma iron turnover rate is low, a decrease may be difficult to recognize, whereas a prolongation of the clearance is easily measured.

Normal values The $T_{1/2}$ of ^{59}Fe is 60 to 100 min.

PLASMA IRON TURNOVER RATE

The plasma iron turnover is used to measure the total mass of erythropoietic tissue. When it is expressed in relation to a fixed volume of blood (1 dl), one must be certain that the total blood volume bears a constant relationship to body size or body weight. Under conditions of severe dehydration or hydremia, the plasma iron turnover expressed in milligrams per deciliter of blood for 24 h may give misleading information about the size of the erythropoietic organs. As mentioned above, plasma iron turnover rates provide the most accurate information in patients with accelerated red cell production or expanded marrow. In patients with hypoplastic marrow, the radioactive iron clearance rate may be a more useful measure than the turnover rate.

The plasma iron turnover expressed as milligrams per deciliter of blood for 24 h measures the total amount of iron cleared from 1 dl of whole blood per day. If all iron cleared was used in the synthesis of hemoglobin, the normal values would be about 0.38 mg per deciliter blood per 24 h.[2] The observed normal value is higher because some iron cleared from the circulation is directed into parenchymal tissues and into labile, non-erythropoietic pools.

Normal values 0.4 to 0.8 mg per deciliter blood per 24 h.

[2] In order to maintain the red cell mass in 1 dl of blood [(Hct/100) × 100 ml = 45 ml packed red cells], the daily red cell production must equal the daily red cell destruction (1/120 × 45 ml = 0.38 ml packed red cells). Since 1 ml of packed red cells contains about 1 mg of iron, a daily plasma iron turnover rate of 0.38 mg is needed by 1 dl of blood to maintain homeostasis.

RED CELL UTILIZATION RATE

Because the normal red cell utilization of radioactive iron may be as high as 90 percent, a further increase has little significance. A decreased utilization, however, is an important finding and suggests that mature red cells are destroyed shortly after their release from the marrow (hemolysis), that immature red cells are destroyed in the marrow before their release to the

FIGURE A19-3 The distribution of ^{59}Fe radioactivity in the body within the first 10 days after injection. The radioactivity is expressed relative to the radioactivity measured in the same organ 15 min after the intravenous administration of the isotope.

In normal subjects, there is a rapid clearance of ^{59}Fe from the blood with a subsequent almost complete incorporation of the isotope into circulating red cells. The splenic radioactivity changes correspondingly, but the liver, with its relatively lower blood supply, is less affected by the changes in circulating blood. The marrow shows an initial uptake, with a subsequent decrease because of marrow release of red cells with radioactive hemoglobin.

In patients with hypersplenism, such as hereditary spherocytosis, the splenic and to a lesser degree the hepatic uptake of radioactivity reflects red cell sequestration and destruction in these organs.

In patients with ineffective erythropoiesis, such as pernicious anemia, the incorporation of ^{59}Fe into circulating red cells is diminished, although the ^{59}Fe is incorporated at a rapid rate into the marrow. Destruction of short-lived erythroblasts and erythrocytes provides labeled hemoglobin for uptake into liver and spleen.

In patients with erythroid hypoplasia, such as aplastic anemia, a slow clearance of ^{59}Fe from plasma provides iron for parenchymal uptake in the spleen and the liver. The marrow shows a decreased uptake and the blood a correspondingly decreased red cell ^{59}Fe utilization. (Redrawn after Hillman and Finch [21].)

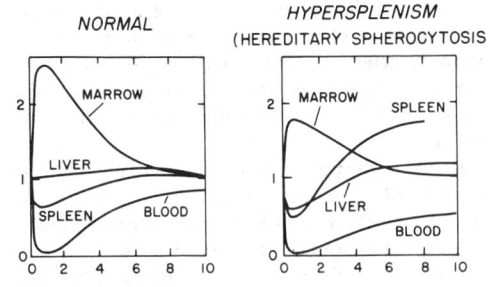

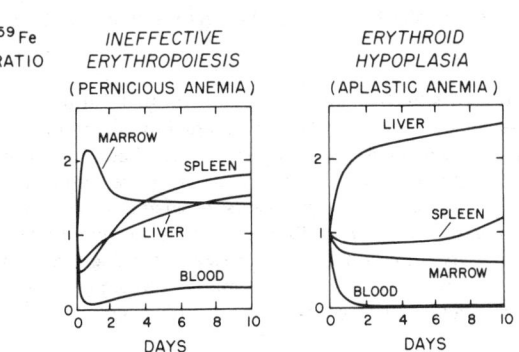

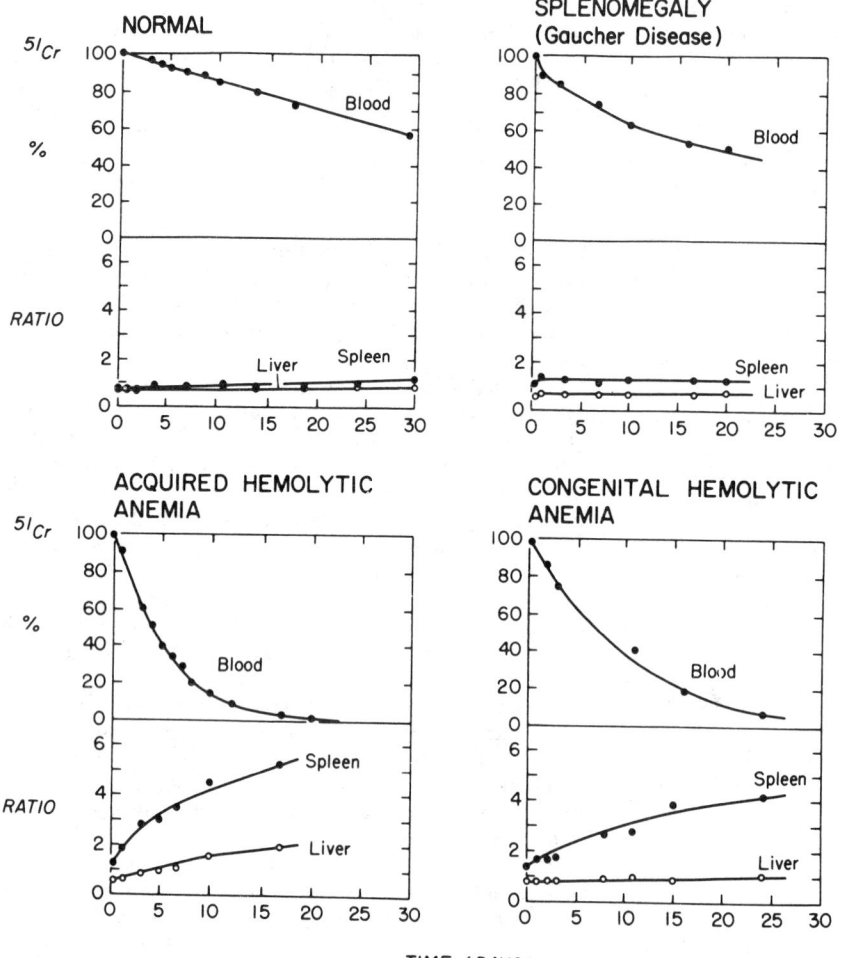

FIGURE A19-4   Distribution of ^{51}Cr in blood, spleen, and liver after the infusion of ^{51}Cr-labeled red cells. The radioactivity of blood is expressed in percent of radioactivity measured 15 min after the infusion of labeled cells. The radioactivity of the spleen and liver is expressed relative to the radioactivity determined simultaneously over the precordium.

In normal subjects, the half-life of blood radioactive chromium is about 30 days and the radioactivity over the hepatic and splenic areas is about the same as over the precordium and reflects tissue vascularity.

In patients with splenomegaly but no hypersplenism, as in some patients with Gaucher disease, the half-life of circulating blood cells may be shorter but there is no excessive uptake into the spleen or liver. The higher but stable splenic uptake presumably reflects pooling of blood rather than sequestration and destruction of red cells.

In patients with antibody destruction of red cells, such as acquired hemolytic anemia, the red cell half-life is short and the uptake in both liver and spleen enhanced.

In patients with hypersplenism, such as hereditary spherocytosis, the splenic uptake is progressive and far greater than the uptake over the liver. (Redrawn after Jandl et al. [8].)

circulation (ineffective erythropoiesis), or that serum iron, because of slow marrow uptake, is diverted to nonerythropoietic tissues (marrow hypoplasia). Severe peripheral hemolysis can be recognized from the shape of the red cell utilization curve, which displays an early rise (shortened marrow transit time), an early maximum utilization, and a subsequent falloff. Ineffective erythropoiesis is characterized by a shortened radioactive iron clearance rate and marrow hypoplasia by a prolonged radioactive iron clearance rate (Fig. A19-2).

Normal values   70 to 90 percent at 10th to 14th day.

RED CELL TURNOVER RATE
A convenient measure of effective red cell production is the red cell iron turnover. It records only that fraction of iron utilized in the synthesis of viable mature red cells.

Normal values   0.30 to 0.70 mg per deciliter blood per 24 h.

ERYTHRON TURNOVER RATE

The disappearance curve of radioactive iron shows that the initial exponential clearance of iron is not sustained but slows after 80 to 90 percent of the tracer has disappeared. Radioactive iron can be demonstrated in plasma for many days and presumably represents reflux of iron from lymphatics and tissues. Careful measurements of the magnitude of this reflux and of the iron fixed in nonerythroid parenchymal tissues have disclosed that there is a close relationship between the plasma iron level and the nonerythron turnover rate. Consequently, it is possible to assess the erythron turnover by subtracting from the plasma iron turnover an amount determined by the plasma iron level, the plasmatocrit reading, and a constant (0.0035). The erythron turnover value has been claimed to be a highly quantitative measurement of the number of nucleated red cells in the marrow and their hemoglobin synthesizing capacity [19].

Normal values 0.60 ± 0.20 mg per deciliter blood per 24 h.

MARROW TRANSIT TIME

The marrow transit time depends on the speed of erythroid maturation and/or on the early release of immature red cells from the marrow [20]. A short transit time is found in conditions with erythroid hyperactivity and may be caused by early reticulocyte release because of inadequate marrow capacity or by a direct action of erythropoitin on the rate of erythroid maturation and marrow release. A prolonged transit time suggests erythroid hypoactivity.

Normal values   3 to 4 days.

SITES OF RED CELL PRODUCTION

The in vivo scanning for sites of erythroid activity is of importance in the diagnostic workup of patients suspected of myeloid metaplasia or extramedullary erythropoiesis. It appears likely that this laborious test will be replaced by whole-marrow scanning as described in Chap. 4.

Normal values   See Fig. A19-3.

SITES OF RED CELL DESTRUCTION

The in vivo scanning for sites of red cell destruction is of importance in the diagnostic evaluation of patients with anemia and splenomegaly. A progressive increase in radioactivity over the splenic area suggests splenic destruction of red cells. An initial high level of radioactivity with little subsequent increase is more compatible with splenomegaly without red cell sequestration and destruction [8,22]

Normal values   See Fig. A19-4.

References

1. Pollycove, M., and Mortimer, R.: Quantitative determination of iron kinetics and hemoglobin synthesis in human subjects. *J. Clin. Invest.* 40:753, 1961.
2. Finch, C. A., et al.: Ferrokinetics in man. *Medicine (Baltimore)* 49:17, 1970.
3. Wennesland, R., et al.: Red cell, plasma and blood volume in healthy men measured by radiochromium (^{51}Cr) cell tagging and hematocrit: Influence of age, somatype and habits of physical activity on the variance after regression of volumes to height and weight combined. *J. Clin. Invest.* 38:1065, 1959.
4. Brown, E., Hooper, J., Jr., Hodges, J. L., Jr., Bradley, B., Wennesland, R., and Yamauchi, H.: Red cell, plasma and blood volume in healthy women measured by radiochromium cell-labeling and hematocrit. *J. Clin. Invest.* 41:2182, 1962.
5. Standard techniques for the measurement of red-cell and plasma volume: A report by the International Committee for Standardization in Haematology. *Br. J. Haematol.* 25:801, 1973.
6. Mollison, P. L.: Further observations on the normal survival curve of ^{51}Cr-labelled red cells. *Clin. Sci.* 21:21, 1961.
7. Recommended method for radioisotope red-cell survival studies: A report by the International Committee for Standardization in Haematology. *Br. J. Haematol.* 45:659, 1980.
8. Jandl, J. H., Greenberg, M. S., Yonemoto, R. H., and Castle, W. B.: Clinical determination of the sites of red cell sequestration in hemolytic anemia. *J. Clin. Invest.* 35:842, 1956.
9. Recommended methods for surface counting to determine sites of red-cell destruction: A report by the International Committee for Standardization in Haematology. *Br. J. Haematol.* 30:249, 1975.
10. Ricketts, C., Cavill, J., Napier, J. A. F., and Jacobs, A.: Ferrokinetics and erythropoiesis in man: An evaluation of ferrokinetic measurements. *Br. J. Haematol.* 35:41, 1977.
11. Cazzola, M., et al.: The use of ^{59}Fe for estimating red cell production and destruction: A comparative evaluation of two methods for the analysis of experimental data. *Hematology* 64:696, 1979.
12. Sukarochana, K., Parenzan, L., Thakurdas, N., and Klesewetter, W. B.: Red cell mass determinations in infancy and childhood, with the use of radio-active chromium. *J. Pediatr.* 59:903, 1961.
13. Bentley, S. A., Glass, H. J., Lewis, S. M., and Szur, L.: Elution correction in ^{51}Cr red cell survival studies. *Br. J. Haematol.* 26:179, 1974.
14. The International Committee for Standardization in Haematology: Recommended methods for radioisotope red cell survival. *Blood* 38:378, 1971.
15. Pearson, H. A.: The binding of Cr^{51} to hemoglobin. II. In vivo elution rates of Cr^{51} from Hb CC, Hb CS and placental red cells. *Blood* 28:563, 1966.
16. Danon, D., Marikovsky, Y., and Gasko, O.: 51-Chromium uptake as a function of red cell age. *J. Lab. Clin. Med.* 67:70, 1966.
17. Gabuzda, T. G., Nathan, D. G., and Gardner, F. H.: The metabolism of the individual C^{14}-labeled hemoglobins in patients with H-thalassemia, with observations on radio-chromate binding to the hemoglobins during red cell survival. *J. Clin. Invest.* 44:315, 1965.
18. Loeffler, R. K., Rappoport, D. A., and Collins, V. P.: Radio-iron citrate as tracer to determine disappearance rate of plasma iron in normal subjects. *Proc. Soc. Exp. Biol. Med.* 88:441, 1955.
19. Cook, J. D., Marsaglia, G., Eschbach, J. W., Funk, D. D., and Finch, C. A.: Ferrokinetics: A biologic model for plasma iron exchange in man. *J. Clin. Invest.* 49:197, 1970.
20. Labardini, J., et al.: Marrow radiation kinetics. *Haematologia (Budapest)* 7:301, 1973.
21. Hillman, R. S., and Finch, C. A.: Erythropoiesis: Normal and abnormal. *Semin. Hematol.* 4:327, 1967.
22. Najean, Y., Cacchione, R., Dresch, C., and Rain, J. D.: Methods of evaluating the sequestration site of red cells labelled with ^{51}Cr: A review of 96 cases. *Br. J. Haematol.* 29:495, 1975.

Detection of pyrimidine nucleotides

ERNEST BEUTLER

PURPOSE OF THE TEST

In pyrimidine-5'-nucleotidase deficiency (Chap. 59) high levels of pyrimidine nucleotides accumulate in erythrocytes. Examination of the ultraviolet spectrum of red cell extracts serves as a useful screening test for pyrimidine-5'-nucleotidase deficiency [1].

PRINCIPLE OF THE TEST

The nucleotides of normal red cells consist largely of purine (adenine and small amounts of guanine) derivatives. Normally the levels of pyrimidine nucleotides, cytidylic acid and uridylic acid, are extremely low. Acidic solutions of cytidine nucleotides have an absorption maximum at approximately 280 nm, while adenine, guanine, and uridine nucleotides absorb maximally at about 260 nm. The ratio of UV absorption at 260 nm to that at 280 nm reflects the relative abundance of cytidine nucleotides, with the absorbance ratio decreasing as cytidine nucleotides accumulate. Since the bulk of the nucleotides which accumulate are cytosine derivatives [2], the 260/280 absorbance ratio is a sensitive means for the diagnosis of pyrimidine-5'-nucleotidase deficiency.

REAGENTS AND EQUIPMENT

1. 1 M glycine buffer, pH 3.0. 7.51 g of glycine is dissolved in nearly 100 ml of water, the pH is adjusted to 3.0 with concentrated HCl, and the volume is adjusted to 100 ml.

2. 4% perchloric acid (PCA). 28.6 ml of a 70% perchloric acid solution is diluted to a final volume of 500 ml with distilled water.

3. Ultraviolet spectrophotometer and quartz cuvettes.

TECHNIQUE

Blood freshly collected in EDTA anticoagulant is centrifuged, the plasma removed, and the cells washed three times in 0.9% NaCl solution. Then 3 ml of a 50% suspension of the washed erythrocytes is added to 12 ml of ice-cold 4% PCA solution, and the clear supernatant obtained after centrifugation is transferred to a small test tube. A "sham" extract to be used as the blank is prepared by adding 3 ml of 0.9% NaCl solution to 12 ml of the PCA solution. 500 μl of water and 300 μl of 1 M glycine buffer, pH 3.0, are added to each of two cuvettes. In order to correct for any differences in the cuvettes, the sample cuvette is read against the blank at 260 and 280 nm, giving readings 260_B and 280_B. Then 200 μl of the sham PCA extract is added to the blank cuvette, and the PCA extract made from the red cells is added to the sample cuvette. The reading of the blank cuvette is adjusted to zero at 260 nm, and the sample cuvette is read, giving the value 260_S. The process is then repeated at 280 nm, giving the reading 280_S.

INTERPRETATION

The OD_{260}/OD_{280} absorbance ratio R is calculated by subtracting the cuvette blank readings (positive or negative) at 260 nm and 280 nm from the readings obtained on the red cell extract when blanked against the sham extract:

$$R = \frac{260_S - 260_B}{280_S - 280_B}$$

The absorbance ratio of freshly collected washed red cells from 19 normal individuals was found to be 3.11 ± 0.41 (mean ± 1 standard deviation). Absorbance ratios of less than 2.29 imply that the concentration of cytidine nucleotides is increased. Using similar techniques, a normal mean R of 3.42 has been reported with R values ranging from 0.95 to 1.12 in four enzyme-deficient patients [1].

The determination of the ultraviolet absorption ratio should be considered only a screening test, however. Definitive diagnosis of pyrimidine-5'-nucleotidase deficiency depends upon performance of a quantitative enzyme assay [3].

References

1. Valentine, W. N., Fink, K., Paglia, D. E., Harris, S. R., and Adams, W. S.: Hereditary hemolytic anemia with human erythrocyte pyrimidine 5'-nucleotidase deficiency. *J. Clin. Invest.* 54:866, 1974.
2. Torrance, J. D., and Whittaker, D.: Distribution of erythrocyte nucleotides in pyrimidine 5'-nucleotidase deficiency. *Br. J. Haematol.* 43:423, 1979.
3. Torrance, J., West, C., and Beutler, E.: A simple rapid radiometric assay for pyrimidine-5'-nucleotidase. *J. Lab. Clin. Med.* 90:563, 1977.

Erythrocyte protoporphyrin

FRANK A. OSKI

PURPOSE OF THE TEST

The measurement of erythrocyte free protoporphyrin is designated to provide a rapid and simple means of screening individuals to identify subjects with iron deficiency or lead poisoning.

PRINCIPLE OF THE TEST

In the standard methods, protoporphyrin is extracted from erythrocytes in a solvent mixture of ethyl acetate and acetic acid and reextracted in hydrochloric acid and the fluorescence of the protoporphyrin determined in a fluorometer. The technique employs a very high solvent-to-erythrocyte ratio to ensure virtually complete extraction of the protoporphyrin. In both lead poisoning and iron deficiency, the protoporphyrin in the erythrocytes is the zinc chelate, zinc protoporphyrin, and is not really unbound, or "free" [1]. In the chemical extraction procedure it is converted to the unbound form. In the direct measurements it is estimated as zinc protoporphyrin. The values obtained are equivalent.

REAGENTS

1. 5% Celite in saline. Prepare a 5-g/dl suspension Celite in saline (9 g NaCl per liter).

2. Ethyl acetate/glacial acetic acid. Mix 4 parts of ethyl acetate with 1 part glacial acetic acid.

3. 1.5 N HCl. Dilute 125 ml of concentrated hydrochloric acid to 1 liter with distilled water.

4. Coproporphyrin I standard. Preweighed vials containing 5 μg of coproporphyrin I are commercially available. Add 10 ml of 1.5 N HCl to the vial and heat 5 min in boiling water. Further dilutions are made from this stock solution in 1.5 N HCl in the range of 0.005 μg/ml to 0.05 μg/ml for a standard curve.

TECHNIQUE [2,3]

1. Pipette 20 μl of blood to the bottom of a small test tube containing 0.1 ml of a 5% Celite suspension in 0.9% NaCl.

2. Add 2 ml of a mixture of ethyl acetate and acetic acid (4:1) and agitate the tube for 10 s on a Vortex mixer.

3. Centrifuge for 30 s at approximately $500 \times g$. Transfer the supernatant into another test tube.

4. Add 2 ml of 1.5 N HCl and agitate the tube for 10 s on a Vortex mixer.

5. With a capillary pipette, transfer a sufficient amount of the lower HCl phase into a cuvette to read.

6. Read the concentration of protoporphyrin directly in micrograms in a fluorometer calibrated with a standard solution of coproporphyrin I at an excitation wavelength of 405 nm and the emission at 610 nm.

7. Calculation of results:

$$EP \ (\mu g \text{ per deciliter of whole blood}) = \frac{F_x}{F_s} \times C_s \times \frac{2.5}{0.02} \times \frac{100}{1.11}$$

where F_x = fluorescence of the unknown, F_s = fluorescence of the standard, C_s = concentration of the standard, 2.5 = final volume of HCl, 0.02 = volume of blood used, 100 = factor to convert to 1 dl of blood, and 1.11 = factor to convert fluorescence of porphyrins in the extract to fluorescence of coproporphyrin I in the 1.5 N HCl. The ratio of protoporphyrin to coproporphyrin fluorescence varies with each fluorometer; it should be determined once for each instrument. An alternative is to use protoporphyrin standards, which are, however, stable for only 1 to 2 days in the dark.

ALTERNATIVE METHOD

Red cell zinc protoporphyrin may be determined directly employing a commercially available portable filter fluorometer which utilizes "front-face" optics, internal standards, and digital computer capabilities [4]. Such fluorometers have been specifically designed for the rapid assay of erythrocyte zinc protoporphyrin in unprocessed blood. A small drop of blood, obtained by finger puncture, is placed on a disposable cover slip and inserted in the sample holder of the instrument. Zinc protoporphyrin concentration is quickly computed by the instrument, and the value is displayed digitally as micrograms of zinc protoporphyrin per deciliter of blood. These instruments should be calibrated frequently against the extraction procedure.

INTERPRETATION OF RESULTS

The normal range using the microfluorometric method is 49.6 ± 14.9 μg per deciliter of red blood cells (mean ± 1 standard deviation) [2]. Values in the range of 35 to 60 μg per deciliter of whole blood are usually observed in patients with iron defi-

ciency, and values in excess of 100 μg per deciliter of whole blood generally signify the presence of an increased body lead burden and a blood lead concentration equal to or greater than 40 μg per deciliter of whole blood. When these values are converted to micrograms per deciliter of red blood cells, they represent substantial elevation over normal. Modest elevations in erythrocyte protoporphyrin may also be observed in patients with hemolytic anemias, sideroblastic anemias, the anemia of chronic disease, and secondary polycythemia [5]. Extremely high levels of erythrocyte protoporphyrin found with the extraction procedure are indicative of either lead poisoning or erythropoietic protoporphyria. Increases in the serum bilirubin concentration will produce spuriously high values for zinc protoporphyrin as determined by the front-faced fluorometer procedure [6].

SOURCE OF REAGENTS

Acetic acid, ethyl acetate, hydrochloric acid, coproporphyrin I, and sodium chloride may be obtained from various commercial suppliers, such as Sigma Chemical Co., P.O. Box 14508, Saint Louis, MO 63178. A Vortex mixer may be purchased from American Scientific Products, McGaw Park, IL 60085. Celite is obtained from Fisher Scientific, 711 Forbes Ave., Pittsburgh, PA 15219.

Instruments for direct estimation of zinc protoporphyrin are available from Aviv Associates, Lakewood, NJ 08701, and Environmental Sciences Associates, Burlington, MA 01803.

References

1. Lamola, A. A., and Yamane, T.: Zinc protoporphyrin in the erythrocytes of patients with lead intoxication and iron deficiency anemia. *Science* 186:936, 1974.
2. Piomelli, S.: A micromethod for free erythrocyte porphyrins. The FEP test. *J. Lab. Clin. Med.* 81:932, 1973.
3. Piomelli, S.: Free erythrocyte porphyrins in the detection of undue absorption of Pb and of Fe deficiency. *Clin. Chem.* 23:264, 1977.
4. Blumberg, W. E., Eisinger, J., Lamola, A. A., and Zuckerman, D. M.: The hematofluorometer. *Clin. Chem.* 23:270, 1977.
5. Lamon, J. M.: Clinical aspects of porphyrin measurement, other than lead poisoning. *Clin. Chem.* 23:260, 1977.
6. Burhmann, E., Mentzer, W. C., and Lubin, B. H.: The influence of plasma bilirubin on zinc protoporphyrin measurement by a hematofluorometer. *J. Lab. Clin. Med.* 91:710, 1978.

Leukocyte studies

CHAPTER *A22*

Leukocyte peroxidase

DOUGLAS A. NELSON
FREDERICK R. DAVEY

PURPOSE OF THE TEST

The peroxidase reaction is positive in cells of the neutrophilic and eosinophilic series and weakly positive in monocytes, and can be used to differentiate cells of these types from lymphoid or erythroid cells, which are peroxidase-negative.

PRINCIPLE OF THE TEST

The peroxidase activity of leukocytes transfers hydrogen from various substrates to hydrogen peroxide, yielding a blue or brown derivative of the dye which is localized at the site of enzyme activity [1]. Benzidine has been widely used in this test [1]. However, U.S. governmental regulations require stringent safety precautions when using benzidine [2], and a method using 3-amino-9-ethylcarbazole is recommended [3].

REAGENTS

1. Fixative. A mixture of 25 ml of 37% formaldehyde solution, 45 ml of acetone, and 30 ml of water containing 20 mg of Na_2HPO_4 and 100 mg of KH_2PO_4. The final pH is about 6.6.
2. Staining mixture. Prepare a solution of the following reagents:

0.02 M acetic acid adjusted to pH 5.0 to 5.2 with 1 N NaOH	50 ml
Dimethylsulfoxide	6 ml
3-Amino-9-ethylcarbazole	10 mg
0.3% hydrogen peroxide	0.4 ml

The solution is filtered before use. The final pH is 5.5.
3. Mayer's hematoxylin counterstain.

TECHNIQUE

1. Fix thin blood films in the buffered formalin acetone solution at room temperature for 15 s.
2. Rinse gently in distilled water.
3. Immerse the fixed film in the staining mixture at room temperature for 2½ min.
4. Wash in running tap water.
5. Stain in Mayer's hematoxylin for 8 min.
6. Wash in tap water, air-dry, and mount in glycerine jelly.

INTERPRETATION [4,5]

All nuclei are stained blue. In the neutrophilic series the peroxidase activity is indicated by red-brown granules within the cells. Peroxidase activity is present at all stages of neutrophil development, localized in the azurophilic (nonspecific) granules, according to studies using ultrastructural cytochemistry and ultracentrifugation. Eosinophil granules show an intense peroxidase reaction. Mature basophils do not stain.

Monocytes do not stain as intensely as granulocytes and show either tiny red-brown granules or faint, diffuse cytoplasmic staining.

Lymphocytes and erythrocytes do not show peroxidase activity at any stage of maturation.

In *acute myelogenous leukemia* more than 5 percent of the primitive cells are positive, usually more than 85 percent. Auer rods, derivatives of the azurophilic granules, are peroxidase-positive. Even in blast cells which lack azurophilic granules the reaction in the cytoplasm may be positive, presumably staining peroxidase which is not yet "packaged" into granules. Less than 5 percent (and usually none) of the blasts in *acute lymphocytic leukemia* are positive for the peroxidase reaction. In *acute myelomonocytic leukemia* the monocyte precursors are sometimes weakly positive but are most often peroxidase-negative.

The peroxidase reaction may be negative or deficient in some of the mature neutrophils in *dysmyelopoietic syndromes* [6], in *acute myelogenous leukemia*, and in severe *infections* characterized by toxic granules in neutrophils.

In *hereditary myeloperoxidase deficiency*, all neutrophils and monocytes are deficient but eosinophil peroxidase is unaffected [7]. Inheritance is probably autosomal. In complete deficiency (homozygote) neutrophil peroxidase is virtually undetectable, whereas in partial deficiency (heterozygote) all neutrophils appear to be affected and have decreased but not absent activity [8]. In *chronic myelogenous leukemia*, peroxidase activity in mature neutrophils is increased [9].

SOURCE OF REAGENTS

The reagents required may be obtained from most scientific supply houses. 3-Amino-9-ethylcarbazole may be obtained from the Aldrich Chemical Co., Inc., Milwaukee, WI 53233.

References

1. Kaplow, L. S.: Simplified myeloperoxidase stain using benzidine dihydrochloride. *Blood* 26:215, 1965.
2. *Federal Register* 39(20):3756, Jan. 29, 1974.
3. Kaplow, L. S.: Substitute for benzidine in myeloperoxidase stains. *Am. J. Clin. Pathol.* 63:451, 1975.
4. Hayhoe, F. G. J., Quaglino, D., and Doll, R.: *The Cytology and Cytochemistry of Acute Leukaemias.* H. M. Stationery Office, London, 1964.
5. Hayhoe, F. G. J., and Cawley, J. C.: Acute leukaemia: Cellular morphology, cytochemistry and fine structure. *Clin. Haematol.* 1:49, 1972.
6. Breton-Gorius, J., Houssay, D., and Dreyfus, B.: Partial myeloperoxidase deficiency in a case of preleukemia. I. Studies of fine structure and peroxidase synthesis of promyelocytes. *Br. J. Haematol.* 30:273, 1975.
7. Lehrer, R. I., and Cline, M. J.: Leukocyte myeloperoxidase deficiency and disseminated candidiasis: The role of myeloperoxidase in resistance to candida infection. *J. Clin. Invest.* 48:1478, 1969.
8. Kitahara, M., Eyre, H. J., Simonian, Y., Atkin, C. L., and Hasstedt, S. J.: Hereditary myeloperoxidase deficiency. *Blood* 57:888, 1981.
9. Hayhoe, F. G. J., and Quaglino, D.: *Haematological Cytochemistry.* Churchill Livingstone, Edinburgh, 1980, chap. 10, p. 200.

CHAPTER *A23*

Leukocyte alkaline phosphatase

ERNEST BEUTLER

PURPOSE OF THE TEST

Estimation of leukocyte alkaline phosphatase activity is useful in the differentiation of chronic myelogenous leukemia from leukemoid reactions as seen in severe infections, polycythemia vera, and agnogenic myeloid metaplasia.

PRINCIPLE OF THE TEST

The substrate, naphthol AS-BI phosphate, is hydrolyzed to phosphate and an aryl naphtholamide by alkaline phosphatase. The aryl naphtholamide is coupled to the diazonium salt, such as fast red violet LB (diazotized 5-benzamide-4-chloro-2-toluidine), forming an insoluble dye.

REAGENTS

1. Naphthol AS-BI phosphate
2. Fast red violet salt LB or fast violet B salt
3. Dimethylformamide, reagent grade
4. 2-amino-2 methyl-1,3-propanediol
5. 0.03 M sodium citrate
6. 0.03 M citric acid
7. Absolute acetone
8. 0.1 M HCl
9. Hematoxylin powder
10. Sodium iodate
11. Aluminum potassium sulfate·12 H_2O

The following solutions are prepared from these reagents:

1. Fixative. Add 300 ml of absolute acetone, while stirring, to a mixture of 32 ml of 0.03 M sodium citrate and 168 ml of 0.03 M citric acid.
2. Buffer. Prepare a propanediol stock solution by dissolving 21 g of 2-amino-2-methyl-1,3-propanediol in distilled water and diluting to 1 liter. The buffer is prepared by adding 50 ml

of 0.1 M HCl to 250 ml of propanediol stock solution and diluting to 1000 ml with distilled water. The stock solution and the buffer are stored at 4°C but the buffer should be warmed to room temperature before using.

3. Staining mixture. Dissolve approximately 5 mg of naphthol AS-BI phosphate in 0.2 to 0.3 ml of dimethylformamide in a 125-ml Erlenmeyer flask. Add 60 ml of buffer, followed by approximately 40 mg of fast red violet salt LB. The mixture must be filtered and used at once.

4. Counterstain. Add 1 g of hematoxylin to 500 ml of distilled water. Heat to the boiling point and add another 500 ml of water; add 200 mg of sodium iodate and 50 g of aluminum potassium sulfate, shake the mixture well, and store at room temperature in a brown bottle. Filter just prior to use.

TECHNIQUE [1,2]

Blood films prepared from capillary blood or heparinized venous blood may be used. The films, less than 24 h old, are fixed for 30 s in the fixative solution at room temperature. They are then washed gently in running tap water for 30 to 60 s and air-dried or blotted. It is preferable to stain the smears immediately; however, fixed smears may be held at freezer temperature for 2 to 3 weeks, with loss of only approximately 10 percent of activity. The slides are stained for exactly 10 min at room temperature in the staining mixture. The slides are washed in running tap water for 30 to 60 s and counterstained for 5 to 8 min in the hematoxylin solution. After being washed in running tap water from 1 to 2 min, the slides are air-dried or blotted carefully and examined microscopically under an oil immersion lens.

CALCULATION OF RESULTS

Using the criteria summarized in Table A23-1, 100 neutrophilic leukocytes are scored from 0 to 4+ on the basis of the intensity of the precipitated dye in their cytoplasm. The scores of the 100 cells are added. It is important to score only mature polymorphonuclear leukocytes and stab forms. Lymphocytes, basophils, and eosinophils should not be included in the score.

INTERPRETATION

Healthy adults generally have a leukocyte alkaline phosphatase score of 13 to 130. However, the normal range should be determined in each laboratory and may vary with different coupling dyes and with different dye lots. Untreated chronic myelogenous leukemia patients usually have a score between 0 and 13, while the scores of patients with polycythemia vera and the

TABLE 23-1 Scoring criteria for rating neutrophils stained for alkaline phosphatase activity

| Cell rating* | Amount, %† | Precipitated azo dye in cytoplasm | | Background of cytoplasm |
		Size of granule	Intensity of staining	
1+	<50	Small	Faint to moderate	Colorless to very pale pink
2+	50–80	Small to medium	Moderate to strong	Colorless to pale pink
3+	80–100	Medium to large	Strong	Colorless to pink
4+	100	Medium and large	Brilliant	Not visible

*When there is no precipitate azo dye in the cytoplasm and the cytoplasm background is not stained, the cells are read as "zero."
†Percent of volume of cytoplasm occupied by azo dye precipitate.

leukocytosis of infection or with myeloid metaplasia are usually in the upper portion of the normal range or frankly elevated. Patients with paroxysmal nocturnal hemoglobinuria uniformly have a very low leukocyte alkaline phosphatase score.

SOURCE OF REAGENTS
Naphthol AS-BI phosphate may be obtained from Sigma Chemical Co. Fast red violet salt LB is not always commercially available and as an alternative fast violet B salt obtained from Sigma Chemical Co. may be used as the coupling dye. Formaldehyde (37%) and aluminum potassium sulfate may be obtained from J. T. Baker Chemical Co.; dimethylformamide from Eastman Chemicals; hematoxylin from Allied Chemicals; sodium iodate from Mallinckrodt; and 2-amino-2-methyl-1,3-propanediol from J. T. Baker Chemical Co.

References
1. Kaplow, L. S.: Cytochemistry of leukocyte alkaline phosphatase: Use of complex naphthol as phosphates in azo dye-coupling techniques. *Am. J. Clin. Pathol.* 39:439, 1963.
2. Kaplow, L. S., and Burstone, M. S.: Acid-buffered acetone as a fixative for enzyme cytochemistry. *Nature* 200:690, 1963.

CHAPTER *A24*

Sudan black B staining

DOUGLAS A. NELSON
FREDERICK R. DAVEY

PURPOSE
The Sudan black B reaction is useful in differentiating acute granulocytic leukemia, acute myelomonocytic leukemia, and acute lymphocytic leukemia.

PRINCIPLE OF THE TEST
Sudan black B stains a variety of lipids, including neutral fat, phospholipids, and sterols. It also stains some cellular components which are not lipid, as evidenced from failure to extract the dye completely with lipid solvents such as acetone [1]. In leukocytes, sudanophilia roughly parallels the peroxidase reaction. Lymphocytes and lymphoblasts very rarely stain with Sudan black B, while nucleolated granulocyte precursors and immature monocytes show characteristic staining patterns.

REAGENTS
1. Formalin. A 37% aqueous solution of formaldehyde is used.
2. Sudan black B stock solution. Dissolve 0.3 g of Sudan black B powder in 100 ml of absolute ethanol. This may require 1 to 2 days at room temperature.
3. Buffer solution. Mix 16 g of phenol with 30 ml of absolute alcohol and add to a solution of 0.3 g of $Na_2HPO_4 \cdot 12H_2O$ in 100 ml of distilled water. (Care should be used in preparing this solution, since phenol will cause skin burns.)

4. Staining solution. Mix 60 ml of the Sudan black B stock solution with 40 ml of the buffer. Filter by suction. The working solution is stable for several weeks at room temperature.
5. Hematoxylin. Harris's hematoxylin solution obtained commercially is satisfactory.

TECHNIQUE [2]
1. Air-dried peripheral blood or marrow films may be either freshly made or old; films several years old have been stained satisfactorily. Fix the films in formalin vapor for 10 min. This is accomplished by placing the dried slides in a closed staining dish containing a small amount of 37% formaldehyde solution. A layer of glass beads in the bottom of the staining dish will protect the slides from direct contact with the formalin solution.
2. Immerse the fixed film in the Sudan black B staining solution in a Coplin jar for 30 to 60 min.
3. Wash in 70% ethanol for 2 or 3 min to remove excess dye.
4. Wash in tap water.
5. Counterstain for 10 min in hematoxylin.
6. Wash in running tap water for 5 min.
7. Air-dry and examine microscopically.

INTERPRETATION [3]
Lymphocytes and erythroblasts are not stained with Sudan black B. Normal granulocyte precursors from blast cells onward show increasing sudanophilia corresponding roughly to the granules present. Promyelocytes contain a few sudanophilic granules, while mature polymorphonuclear neutrophils contain large numbers of sudanophilic granules. Eosinophil granules are also sudanophilic, especially at the rim of the granules. Monocytes and marrow macrophages may be unstained or may contain a few discrete sudanophilic granules.

In *acute granulocytic leukemia* more than 5 percent and often more than 85 percent of the nucleolated cells are Sudan black B–positive. Some of the nucleolated cells stain intensely in a pattern similar to normal polymorphonuclear neutrophils, while others show localized cytoplasmic positivity of variable intensity. A few may contain discrete granules such as are seen in normal monocytes. Auer bodies are intensely sudanophilic. In *acute myelomonocytic leukemia* 5 percent or more of the nucleolated cells contain fine, scattered granules resembling those seen in normal monocytes. Other primitive cells in acute myelomonocytic leukemia show staining similar to that seen in differentiated granulocytes. In *acute lymphocytic leukemia* 5 percent or less of the nucleolated (blast) cells are Sudan-positive; most commonly, all are negative. Sudanophilia of neoplastic cells from the lymphoid series is rarely reported. We have observed moderate sudanophilia in neoplastic cells from one case of T-cell lymphoma, and sudanophilia was described in 1 of 200 cases of multiple myeloma [3].

In general the Sudan black B stain is similar to the peroxidase reaction in distinguishing acute lymphocytic from acute myelogenous leukemia. Both staining reactions may be positive when the Romanowsky stain reveals no granules and therefore are more sensitive in detecting early granulocytic cells. In our experience sudanophilia appears in some cases to be more sensitive in this regard than peroxidase activity.

References
1. Lillie, R. D., and Burtner, H. J.: Stable sudanophilia of human neutrophil leukocytes, in relation to peroxidase and oxidase. *J. Histochem. Cytochem.* 1:8, 1953.

2. Sheehan, H. L., and Storey, G. W.: An improved method of staining leukocyte granules with Sudan black B. *J. Pathol. Bacteriol. 59*:336, 1947.

3. Hayhoe, F. G. J., and Quaglino, D.: *Haematological Cytochemistry.* Churchill Livingstone, Edinburgh, 1980, chap. 5.

CHAPTER *A25*

Periodic acid–Schiff (PAS) stain

FREDERICK R. DAVEY
DOUGLAS A. NELSON

PURPOSE OF THE TEST

The PAS reaction may be helpful in the diagnosis of some cases of erythroleukemia and acute lymphocytic leukemia.

PRINCIPLE OF THE TEST

Periodic acid oxidizes carbohydrates and similar compounds to aldehydes. The aldehydes can then react with the Schiff reagent (leuko-fuchsin) to release fuchsin and stain the cellular components containing the oxidizable compounds [1]. A variety of intracellular compounds react with the PAS reagents, but in blood and marrow cells glycogen appears to be the compound primarily responsible, because the staining can be blocked by digestion with amylase [2–5].

REAGENTS

1. Alcoholic formalin. Mix 10 ml of 36% formaldehyde with 90 ml of 95% ethanol.

2. Amylase. Human saliva stimulated by chewing paraffin and clarified by centrifugation is satisfactory, or a solution of 0.1 to 1.0 g of commercial malt diastase in 100 ml of 0.02 M sodium phosphate buffer at pH 6.0 may be used.

3. Periodic acid. Add 0.69 g of KIO_4 to 100 ml of distilled water, followed by 0.3 ml of concentrated HNO_3 [6]. The KIO_4 crystals are dissolved by heating. The solution may be stored at room temperature.

4. Schiff reagent [7]. Bring 1000 ml of distilled water to a boil, remove from heat, and immediately add 1 g of basic fuchsin. A small amount of the dye should be added first and stirred into the water, followed by addition of the remainder, in order to avoid violent bubbling upon addition of a large amount of fine particles to water near the boiling point. Allow the mixture to cool to 60°C and filter it. Add 2 g of $NaHSO_3$ or $Na_2S_2O_5$ and 20 ml of 1 N HCl to the filtrate. Place the solution in a stoppered bottle and hold at room temperature for 18 to 26 h. Then add 300 mg of activated charcoal (e.g., Norit A) and shake the mixture for 1 min. Filter and store the filtrate at 4° in the dark. The solution may be used until it becomes slightly pink.

5. Sodium metabisulfite. Dissolve 0.5 g of sodium metabisulfite in 100 ml of water. This rinse solution must be freshly prepared daily.

6. Hematoxylin counterstain. Harris's hematoxylin obtained commercially is satisfactory.

If cover slips are used they may be placed in a porcelain holder and the reagents placed in staining jars (Chen). If slides are used they may be placed in Coplin jars.

TECHNIQUE

1. Peripheral blood or marrow films are air-dried and then fixed in alcoholic formalin for 5 min.

2. The fixed films are washed in running tap water for 15 min.

3. If the films are to be digested, they are covered with saliva or diastase solution for 30 min at room temperature and then rinsed in running tap water for 10 min.

4. The films are treated with periodic acid at room temperature for 10 min and then washed in running tap water for 5 min. Films previously stained with Wright's or Giemsa stain can be stained with PAS, beginning with this step.

5. The films are immersed in the Schiff reagent for 10 min. They are then transferred rapidly through three successive baths of sodium metabisulfite, following which they are washed 5 min in running water.

6. The nuclei are stained by immersing the films in Harris's hematoxylin for 10 min.

7. The films are washed in running tap water for 5 min.

8. The films are air-dried and examined microscopically.

INTERPRETATION

In the peripheral blood the cytoplasm of polymorphonuclear leukocytes stains intensely pink or red, with a granular appearance in some cells. Monocyte cytoplasm stains faintly pink and may contain fine or coarse granules. A small number of lymphocytes contain a few small red or pink granules. Erythrocytes do not stain. Platelets are stained intensely. In normal marrow, the earliest granulocyte precursors do not stain. Both diffuse and granular cytoplasmic staining increases with increasing maturity of the myeloid cells. Megakaryocytes stain diffusely and intensely pink or red. Erythrocyte precursors do not stain. The nuclei of all cells stain blue. Digestion with amylase has been reported to remove the staining material from the cytoplasm of all types of blood cells [2–5].

In *erythroleukemia*, variable numbers of erythrocytic precursors may show intense PAS reaction in the cytoplasm. The staining is usually granular in the early erythroid precursors and diffuse in the more mature erythroid precursors [4,5,8]. Erythroid precursors are negative in normal marrows and in most hematologic disorders, including nutritional megaloblastic anemias [4]. PAS positivity does occur in erythroid precursors, however, in thalassemia, occasionally in iron deficiency anemia, and in some cases of sideroblastic refractory anemia [4,9]. With the exception of these conditions, PAS activity in erythroid precursors is very suggestive of erythroleukemia [8].

In *acute lymphocytic leukemia* (ALL), lymphoblasts show great variability in PAS activity. In most cases, at least some of the lymphoblasts contain coarse granules or large blocks of PAS-positive, diastase-sensitive material. It is the coarsely positive reaction and not a fine, diffuse stain that has diagnostic significance. In one study the degree of PAS reactivity found in ALL tended to be higher in younger children and had no significant prognostic value when effects of age and initial leukocyte count were considered [10]. In another study of childhood ALL, however, PAS-negative lymphoblasts were associated with males, with patients with high blast count, and with a poor prognosis [11]. In addition, there is some evidence that in adults characteristic PAS-positive ALL has a better prognosis than ALL in which the blasts are PAS-negative [12].

In *acute myeloblastic leukemia*, the blasts generally are negative; less often they contain faint diffuse or granular PAS positivity. In *acute monocytic leukemia*, the PAS reaction may be negative in some cases and strongly positive in others. When positive, however, numerous small granules are observed throughout the cytoplasm of the monoblasts.

An increased number of lymphocytes containing small granular PAS-positive reactivity are present in chronic lymphocytic leukemia, lymphosarcoma, and Hodgkin's disease, as well as in such benign disorders as infectious mononucleosis; it is therefore of no diagnostic significance in these conditions [13]. The relationship between PAS positivity and the various lymphocyte subpopulations is as yet unclear. Although some have described a correlation between PAS reactivity and B-cell lymphomas and leukemias, others have shown PAS positivity in Sézary cells, a T-cell proliferation [14–18]. In addition, increased PAS activity is observed in lymphocytes following incubation with phytohemagglutinin, suggesting that PAS may be a histochemical marker for T-blast cells [18,19].

References

1. Hotchkiss, R. D.: A microchemical reaction resulting in the staining of polysaccharide structures in fixed tissue preparations. *Arch. Biochem.* 16:131, 1948.
2. Wislocki, G. B., Rheingold, J. M., and Dempsey, E. W.: The occurrence of the periodic acid–Schiff reaction in various normal cells of blood and connective tissue. *Blood* 4:562, 1949.
3. Astaldi, G., and Verga, L. :The glycogen content of the cells of lymphatic leukaemia. *Acta Haematol.* 17:129, 1957.
4. Quaglino, D., and Hayhoe, F. G. J.: Periodic-acid–Schiff positivity in erythroblasts with special reference to di Guglielmo's disease. *Br. J. Haematol.* 6:26, 1960.
5. Hayhoe, F. G. J., and Quaglino, D.: Refractory sideroblastic anemia and erythaemic myelosis: Possible relationship and cytochemical observations. *Br. J. Haematol.* 6:381, 1960.
6. Lillie, R. D., and Fullmer, H. M.: *Histopathologic Technique and Practical Histochemistry*, 4th ed. McGraw-Hill, New York, 1954, p. 231.
7. Lillie, R. D.: Studies on the preservation and histologic demonstration of glycogen. *Bull. Int. Assoc. Med. Museum* 27:23, 1947.
8. Hayhoe, F. G. J., and Cawley, J. C.: Acute leukaemia: Cellular morphology, cytochemistry and fine structure. *Clin. Haematol.* 1:49, 1972.
9. Astaldi, G., Ronanelli, E. G., Birnardelli, E., and Strosselli, E.: An abnormal substance present in the erythroblasts of thalassemia major: Cytochemical investigations. *Acta Haematol.* 12:145, 1954.
10. Humphrey, G. B., Nesbit, M. E., and Brunning, R. D.: Prognostic value of the periodic-acid–Schiff (PAS) reaction in acute lymphoblastic leukemia. *Am. J. Clin. Pathol.* 61:393, 1974.
11. Raney, R. B., Festa, R. S., Waldman, M. T. G., Manson, D., and Hann, H. W. L.: The periodic acid–Schiff reaction and prognosis in children with acute lymphoblastic leukemia. *Am. J. Hematol.* 6:27, 1979.
12. Schmalzl, F., Huhn, D., Abbrederis, K., and Braunsteiner, H.: Acute lymphocytic leukemia: Cytochemistry and ultrastructure. *Blut* 29:87, 1974.
13. Quaglino, D., and Hayhoe, F. G. J.: Observations on the periodic acid Schiff reaction in lymphoproliferative diseases. *J. Pathol. Bacteriol.* 78:521, 1959.
14. Catovsky, D., Galetto, J., Okos, A., Miliani, E., and Galton, D. A. G.: Cytochemical profile of B and T leukemic lymphocytes with special reference to acute lymphoblastic leukemia. *J. Clin. Pathol.* 27:767, 1974.
15. Stein, H., Lennert, K., and Parwaresch, M. R.: Malignant lymphomas of B-cell type. *Lancet* 2:855, 1972.
16. Taswell, H. F., and Winkelman, R.K.: Sézary syndrome: A malignant reticulemic erythroderma. *JAMA* 177:465, 1961.
17. Flandrin, G., and Brouet, J. C.: The Sézary cell: Cytochemical and immunologic studies. *Mayo Clin. Proc.* 49:575, 1974.
18. Quaglino, D., Hayhoe, F. G. J., and Flemans, R. J.: Cytochemical observations on the effect of phytohemagglutinin in short-term tissue cultures. *Nature* 196:338, 1962.
19. Stathopoulos, G., et al.: Immunological studies in a case of T-cell leukemia. *J. Clin. Pathol.* 27:851, 1974.

CHAPTER *A26*

Leukocytic acid phosphatase

FREDERICK R. DAVEY
DOUGLAS A. NELSON

PURPOSE OF THE TEST

The demonstration of tartrate-resistant acid phosphatase in leukemic cells can be used as an enzyme marker in confirming the diagnosis of hairy cell leukemia. Acid phosphatase also may be useful in identifying the T-cell subset of acute lymphocytic leukemias, particularly when other methods of identifying T cells are not available.

PRINCIPLE OF THE TEST

Acid phosphatase in hemopoietic cells can hydrolyze a variety of hydroxynaphthoic anilides, releasing insoluble naphthols which couple efficiently at acidic pH with diazonium salts [1]. The resultant product forms a colored precipitate and gives good microscopic enzyme localization. L(+)-Tartaric acid inhibits acid phosphatase isoenzymes 1 to 4, but isoenzyme 5 is resistant [2].

REAGENTS [2]

1. Fixative. Add 10 ml of methanol to 90 ml of a mixture of 60 ml of acetone and 40 ml of 0.03 M citric acid which has been adjusted to pH 5.4 with 1 N NaOH.
2. Substrate stock solution. Dissolve 10 mg of naphthol AS-BI phosphoric acid in 0.5 ml of *N,N*-dimethyl formamide and add 0.1 M acetate buffer of pH 5.0 to a volume of 100 ml. The substrate solution is stable at 4 to 10°C for 2 months.
3. Substrate staining solution. Mix 10 ml of substrate solution with 5 mg of fast garnet GBC and filter before use.
4. Mayer's hemalum obtained commercially is satisfactory for use.
5. Tartaric acid solution. Dissolve 75 mg of L(+)-tartaric acid in 10 ml of 0.1 M acetate buffer at pH 5.0 (final concentration 0.05 M) containing 1 mg of naphthol AS-BI phosphoric acid. Shake the mixture well and adjust pH to 5.0 with concentrated sodium hydroxide. Add 5 mg of fast garnet GBC and filter before use [5].

TECHNIQUE [2]

1. Place fresh films in fixative at 4 to 10°C for 30 s.
2. Wash fixed films three times with distilled water.
3. Dry films at room temperature for 10 to 30 min.
4. Incubate films in substrate staining solution and tartaric acid solution at 37°C for 45 min.
5. Wash in tap water.
6. Counterstain with Mayer's hemalum for 1 to 3 min.
7. Mount in glycerine jelly.

INTERPRETATION

Acid phosphatase activity is indicated by a red granular precipitate and is demonstrable in most cells of the hemopoietic system [2–4]. Intense activity is present in osteoclasts and some macrophages. Moderate staining is seen in plasma cells, megakaryocytes, and monocytes. Weak reactions are noted in neutrophils, bands, metamyelocytes, myelocytes, and promyelocytes. Very little acid phosphatase activity is present in normal lymphocytes and erythroblasts. In tissue sections of normal human lymph node and spleen, acid phosphatase activity is localized in the thymus-dependent but not the bursa-dependent areas [4].

Increased acid phosphatase activity is observed in the abnormal mononuclear cells of patients with hairy cell leukemia, lymphocytes from patients with macroglobulinemia, atypical lymphocytes from infectious mononucleosis, lymphoblasts from patients with T-cell leukemias, and tissue sections infiltrated with Hodgkin's disease [5–9]. In lymphoblasts from patients with T-lymphoblastic leukemias, acid phosphatase is characteristically strong and localized to the Golgi zone [10]. Tartrate-resistant acid phosphatase isoenzyme is prominent in the neoplastic cells of hairy cell leukemia. In occasional cases, tartrate-resistant acid phosphatase is present in the atypical cells of infectious mononucleosis and in focal areas of Hodgkin's tumor [6,8].

No difference in acid phosphatase activity is seen between normal plasma cells and neoplastic plasma cells present in patients with myeloma. In addition, no consistent change in the neutrophil acid phosphatase activity is seen between normal persons and patients with chronic myeloproliferative disorders [2].

Decreased acid phosphatase is present in the neoplastic cells of chronic lymphocytic leukemia, lymphosarcoma cell leukemia, reticulum cell sarcoma, and lymphocytic lymphomas [2,6,8,11]. Following tartrate inhibition, no discernable acid phosphatase activity is present. Thus the demonstration of the tartrate-resistant isoenzyme of acid phosphatase can usually be used cytochemically to differentiate hairy cell leukemia from chronic lymphocytic leukemia and lymphomas.

SOURCES OF REAGENTS

The reagents may be obtained from many scientific supply companies. The following sources have proved satisfactory for the less widely available reagents. *Naphthol AS-BI phosphoric acid* and *fast Garnet GBC*: Sigma Chemical Co., St. Louis, Mo. *N,N-dimethyl formamide*: Eastman Kodak Co., Rochester, N.Y.

References

1. Burstone, M. S.: Histochemical demonstration of acid phosphatase with naphthol AS-phosphates. *J. Natl. Cancer Inst.* 21:523, 1958.
2. Li, C. Y., Yam, L. T., and Lam, K. W.: Acid phosphatase isoenzyme in human leukocytes in normal and pathologic conditions. *J. Histochem. Cytochem.* 18:473, 1970.
3. Kaplow, L. S., and Burstone, M. S.: Cytochemical demonstration of acid phosphatase in hematopoietic cells in health and in various hematological disorders using azo dye techniques. *J. Histochem. Cytochem.* 12:805, 1964.
4. Tamaoki, N., and Essner, E.: Distribution of acid phosphatase, β-glucuronidase and N-acetyl-β-glucosaminidase activities in lymphocytes of lymphatic tissues of man and rodents. *J. Histochem. Cytochem.* 17:238, 1969.
5. Yam, L. T., Li, C. Y., and Lam, K. W.: Tartrate-resistant acid phosphatase isoenzyme in the reticulum cells of leukemic reticuloendotheliosis. *N. Engl. J. Med.* 284:357, 1972.
6. Yam, L. T., Li, C. Y., and Finkel, H. T.: Leukemic reticuloendotheliosis: The role of tartrate-resistant acid phosphatase in diagnosis and splenectomy in treatment. *Arch. Intern. Med.* 130:248, 1972.
7. Catovsky, D., Galetto, J., Okos, A., Miliani, E., and Galton, D. A. G.: Cytochemical profile of B and T leukaemic lymphocytes with special reference to acute lymphoblastic leukaemia. *J. Clin. Pathol.* 27:767, 1974.
8. Katayama, I., Li, C. Y., and Yam, L. T.: Histochemical study of acid phosphatase isoenzyme in leukemic reticuloendotheliosis. *Cancer* 29:157, 1972.
9. Brouet, J. C., Flandrin, G., Sasportes, M., Preud'Homme, J. L., and Seligmann, M.: Chronic lymphocytic leukaemia of T-cell origin: Immunological and clinical evaluation in eleven patients. *Lancet* 2:890, 1975.
10. Catovsky, D.: T-cell origin of acid-phosphatase positive lymphoblasts. *Lancet* 2:327, 1975.
11. Douglas, S. D., Cohnen, G., Koing, E., and Brittinger, G.: Lymphocyte lysosomal enzymes in chronic lymphocytic leukemia. *Blood* 41:511, 1973.

CHAPTER *A27*

Leukocyte esterases

DOUGLAS A. NELSON
FREDERICK R. DAVEY

PURPOSE OF THE TESTS

Cytochemical reactions for esterases using different substrates allow a distinction to be made between cells of the monocyte series and cells of the neutrophil series. The reaction for nonspecific esterases using the substrates α-naphthyl acetate or α-naphthyl butyrate is strongly positive in monocytes and weak or negative in neutrophils. The reaction using naphthol AS-D chloroacetate as a substrate is positive in neutrophils and precursors and weak or negative in monocytes and precursors. These reactions can be used to distinguish both normal and leukemic cells of these two series.

PRINCIPLE OF THE TESTS

The leukocyte esterase hydrolyzes a synthetic substrate, an ester which is a derivative of naphthalene. A naphthol (or naphthyl) compound is liberated and rapidly couples with a diazonium salt present in the mixture, resulting in a brightly colored precipitate at or near the site of the enzyme activity.

REAGENTS AND TECHNIQUE [1]

Fixation is the same for all the following methods.

1. Fixative. Buffered formalin-acetone mixture, pH about 6.6. Mix 20 mg of Na_2HPO_4, 100 mg of KH_2PO_4, 30 ml of distilled water, 45 ml of acetone, and 25 ml of 37% formaldehyde solution.

2. Blood or marrow films may be freshly prepared or may be stored unfixed in the dark at room temperature for at least 2 weeks without significant loss of enzyme activity.

3. Place the films in the fixative for 30 s at 4 to 10°C.

4. Wash the films in three changes of distilled water and allow them to air-dry at room temperature for 10 to 30 min.

CHLOROACETATE ESTERASE [1]

Incubation mixture

1. Phosphate buffer ($M/15$, pH 7.6), 47.5 ml.
2. Hexazotized new fuchsin, freshly prepared, 0.25 ml:

   a. Dissolve 1 g of new fuchsin in 25 ml of 2 N HCl. This solution will keep indefinitely.

   b. Dissolve 4 g of sodium nitrite in distilled water to a total volume of 100 ml, a 4% solution. Make a fresh solution each week and store at 4°C.

   c. Allow equal volumes of the new fuchsin solution and the 4% sodium nitrite solution to react for 1 min before use. This is hexazotized new fuchsin.

3. Naphthol AS-D chloroacetate, 5 mg in 2.5 ml N,N-dimethyl formamide.

4. The solutions of hexazotized new fuchsin and naphthol AS-D chloroacetate are added to the phosphate buffer. The pH is checked and adjusted to 7.4, if necessary, and the mixture is used without filtration.

Counterstain Harris hematoxylin (alum solution), to which 4 ml of glacial acetic acid is added per 100 ml of stain solution.

Rinse solution Dilute NH$_4$OH. Mix 0.2 to 0.3 ml of concentrated NH$_4$OH (28%) with 100 ml of tap water.

Technique

1. Immerse fixed blood or marrow films in the incubation mixture for 10 min at room temperature in a Coplin jar.
2. Wash in tap water.
3. Counterstain with Harris hematoxylin for 10 min in a Coplin jar.
4. Rinse slides in dilute NH$_4$OH until the color of the film changes from red to blue.
5. Wash briefly in water, air-dry, and mount in Permount.

NONSPECIFIC ESTERASE: α-NAPHTHYL ACETATE [1]

Incubation mixture

1. Phosphate buffer ($M/15$, pH 7.6), 44.5 ml.
2. Hexazotized pararosanilin, freshly prepared, 3.0 ml:

   a. Pararosanilin solution: Dissolve 1 g of pararosanilin hydrochloride in 20 ml of distilled water and 5 ml of concentrated HCl while gently warming. After the solution cools, filter and store at room temperature [2].

   b. Mix equal volumes of the pararosanilin solution and the 4% sodium nitrite solution and allow to react for 1 min. The sodium nitrite solution should be no more than 1 week old and may be kept at 4°C.

3. α-Naphthyl acetate, 50 mg, in 2.5 ml of ethylene glycol monomethyl ether.

4. Add the solutions of hexazotized pararosanilin and α-naphthyl acetate to the phosphate buffer. Adjust the pH to 6.1 ± 0.3 with 1 N NaOH and filter the mixture before use.

Technique

1. Immerse fixed blood or marrow films in the incubation mixture for 45 min at room temperature in a Coplin jar.
2. Wash in water.
3. Counterstain with Harris hematoxylin (above) for 10 min.
4. Rinse slide in dilute NH$_4$OH until blue color appears (as above), wash with water, air-dry, and mount in Permount.

NONSPECIFIC ESTERASE: α-NAPHTHYL BUTYRATE [3]

Incubation mixture

1. Phosphate buffer ($M/15$, pH 6.3), 47.5 ml.
2. Hexazotized pararosanilin (freshly prepared, as in incubation mixture above), 0.25 ml.
3. α-Naphthyl butyrate, 50 mg in 2.5 ml of ethylene glycol monomethyl ether.
4. Add the solutions of hexazotized pararosanilin and α-naphthyl butyrate to the phosphate buffer and filter before use.

Technique

1. Immerse fixed blood or marrow films in the incubation mixture for 45 min at room temperature in a Coplin jar.
2. Wash in water.
3. Counterstain with Harris hematoxylin (above) for 10 min.
4. Rinse slides in dilute NH$_4$OH until blue color appears (as above), wash with water, air-dry, and mount in Permount.

INTERPRETATION

Cytochemical study of two groups of esterases is useful in the differential diagnosis of acute myeloblastic and acute myelomonocytic leukemias. The reaction product for chloroacetate esterase is red, and that for both nonspecific esterases is orange-brown.

Chloroacetate esterase has an optimum pH between 7.0 and 7.6 and is insensitive to fluoride inhibition [3]. It is present in the nonspecific granules of promyelocytes and of neutrophils [4]. Normal myeloblasts are negative, but myeloblasts in some cases of acute myelogenous leukemia are positive. Auer rods are usually positive [5,6]. Eosinophils, lymphocytes, plasma cells, erythroblasts, megakaryocytes, and mature monocytes are negative, but mast cells are positive. The reactions of chloroacetate esterase are parallel to those of Sudan black B and peroxidase, both in normal granulocytes and in the acute leukemias (Table A27-1). The Sudan black B and peroxidase reactions are more sensitive and reliable than chloroacetate esterase in cells of the granulocytic series; chloroacetate esterase, however, has the advantage of being more consistently negative in monocytes [7].

Nonspecific esterases react best at a pH between 6.0 and 6.3 and are inhibited by fluorides [3]. α-Naphthyl acetate esterase is strongest in monocytes, macrophages, megakaryocytes, and platelets. It is also positive in basophils and plasma cells, focally positive in the cytoplasm of resting T lymphocytes, and weakly positive in the erythroblasts of some normal individuals [5,8]. The activity in monocytes, megakaryocytes, platelets, and plasma cells is inhibited by sodium fluoride, but that in lymphocytes and granulocytes is not [3]. Fluoride inhibition studies, however, are usually not necessary to differentiate granulocytes from monocytes because granulocytes very rarely give a positive reaction with α-naphthyl acetate. α-Naphthyl butyrate esterase is also strongly reactive in monocytes and macrophages; it is somewhat less sensitive than α-naphthyl acetate esterase, but has the advantage of being more specific [3]. When the reaction is performed at pH 8, α-naphthyl butyrate esterase can be used to discriminate mononuclear cells into subpopulations of T lymphocytes, B lymphocytes, null cells, and monocytes [9].

Both nonspecific esterases find their principal utility in differentiating the positive-reacting blasts and monocytes in acute myelomonocytic leukemia from the negative-reacting blasts and promyelocytes of acute myeloblastic leukemia (Table A27-1). All monocytic leukemias appear to be derived from the

TABLE A27-1   Cytochemical reactions in normal blood cells and blasts of acute leukemias [3,5,6,10,14]

| | Peroxidase Sudan black B | Esterases | | | PAS | Acid phos-phatase |
		α-Naphthyl acetate	α-Naphthyl butyrate	Naphthol–AS-D chloroacetate		
Promyelocyte	+/++	−/±	−	+/++	±/+	+/++
Neutrophil	++	−/±	−	+/++	+++	+
Monocyte	−/±	+++	++/+++	−/±	±	++
Lymphocyte	−	−/±[a]	−/±[a]	−	−/+	−/++
Erythroblast	−	−/±[b]	−	−	−[d]	±/−
Megakaryocyte	−	+++	±	−	++	++
ALL	−	−/+[c]	−	−	+/++[e]	−/+
AML	+/++	−	−	+/++	−/±	+
APL	+++	±	−	+++	±/+	++
AMML	−/++	+/+++	+/+++	±/++	−/++	+/++
AUL	−	−	−	−	−	−

Key:
 − Negative
 ± Weak or few positive cells
 + Moderate
 ++ Moderately strong
+++ Strongly positive (most cells)

  ALL = acute lymphocytic leukemia
  AML = acute myeloblastic leukemia
  APL = acute promyelocytic leukemia
AMML = acute myelomonocytic leukemia
  AUL = acute undifferentiated leukemia
[a] Positivity is focal, not diffuse.
[b] In erythroleukemia and in some erythroid maturation defects, positivity is strong.
[c] Focal cytoplasmic positivity in a small proportion of ALLs.
[d] Positive in erythroleukemia and to a lesser degree in iron deficiency and thalassemia.
[e] Coarse blocks are typical.

same myeloid stem cells from which acute myeloblastic leukemia arises. Acute myelomonocytic leukemia is a continuum ranging from almost pure acute myeloblastic leukemia, with a small proportion of monocytes, to almost pure monocytic leukemia, in which there is usually some granulocytic involvement [10]. It is not uncommon for morphologic abnormalities to confuse the distinction between promyelocytes and promonocytes in Romanowsky-stained preparations; here the esterase reactions will frequently decide the questions of acute myeloblastic versus acute myelomonocytic leukemia [11]. In addition, the esterase reactions allow one to determine the proportion of primitive cells of the monocytic and granulocytic series in any given case of myelomonocytic leukemia.

The α-naphthyl acetate esterase reaction is focally positive in the cytoplasm of blasts in a small percentage of cases of acute lymphocytic leukemias or leukemic lymphomas [12]. In some cases the focally positive reaction product is associated with a T-lymphocyte neoplasm [13]. Erythroid precursors in diGuglielmo's syndrome, as well as in megaloblastic anemia, are often strongly reactive for α-naphthyl acetate esterase [5].

Careful attention must be paid to the details of the technique [3]. For example, increasing the time or pH of the incubation may result in hydrolysis of the nonspecific esterase substrates

by the chloroacetate esterase in the cells, resulting in apparent nonspecific esterase activity in granulocytic cells.

SOURCES OF REAGENTS
The common reagents may be obtained from many scientific supply companies. The following may be less widely available; the sources listed have been found satisfactory.

New fuchsin: Allied Chemical Co., Biological Stains and Reagents Dept., Morristown, N.J.

Naphthol AS-D chloroacetate: Sigma Chemical Co., St. Louis, Mo.; Nutritional Biochemicals Corp., Cleveland, Ohio.

Pararosanilin: Fisher Scientific Co., Chemical Manufacturing Division, Fair Lawn, N.J.

α-Naphthyl acetate: Sigma Chemical Co., St. Louis, Mo.; Nutritional Biochemicals Corp., Cleveland, Ohio.

α-Naphthyl butyrate: Sigma Chemical Co., St. Louis, Mo.

N,N-dimethyl formamide: Eastman Kodak Co., Rochester, N.Y.

References

1. Yam, L. T., Li, C. Y., and Crosby, W. H.: Cytochemical identification of monocytes and granulocytes. *Am. J. Clin. Pathol.* 55:283, 1971.

2. Barka, T., and Anderson, P. J.: Histochemical methods for acid phosphatase using hexazonium pararosanilin as coupler. *J. Histochem. Cytochem.* 10:741, 1962.

3. Li, C. Y., Lam, K. W., and Yam, L. T.: Esterases in human leukocytes. *J. Histochem. Cytochem.* 21:1, 1973.

4. Moloney, W. C., McPherson, K., and Fliegelman, L.: Esterase activity in leukocytes demonstrated by the use of naphthol AS-D chloroacetate substrate. *J. Histochem. Cytochem.* 8:200, 1960.

5. Rosenszajn, L., Leibovich, M., Shoham, D., and Epstein, J.: The esterase activity in megaloblasts, leukemic and normal hematopoietic cells. *Br. J. Haematol.* 14:605, 1962.

6. Schmalzl, F., and Braunsteiner, H.: The application of cytochemical methods to the study of acute leukemia. *Acta Haematol.* 45:209, 1971.

7. Flandrin, G., and Daniel, M. T.: Practical value of cytochemical studies for the classification of acute leukemias, in *Recent Results in Cancer Research: Acute Leukemias,* edited by G. Mathé, P. Povillart, and L. Schwarzenberg. Springer-Verlag, New York, 1973, p. 43.

8. Davey, F. R., Dock, N. L., and MacCallum, J.: Cytochemical reactions in resting and activated T-lymphocytes. *Am. J. Clin. Pathol.* 74:174, 1980.

9. Higgy, K. E., Burns, G. F., and Hayhoe, F. G. J.: Discrimination of B, T and null lymphocytes by esterase cytochemistry. *Scand. J. Haematol.* 18:437, 1977.

10. Hayhoe, F. G. J., and Cawley, J. C.: Acute leukaemia: Cellular morphology, cytochemistry and fine structure. *Clin. Haematol.* 1:49, 1972.

11. Glick, A. D., and Horn, R. G.: Identification of promonocytes and monocytoid precursors in acute leukemia of adults: Ultrastructural and cytochemical observations. *Br. J. Haematol.* 26:395, 1974.

12. Shaw, M. T., and Ishmael, D. R.: Acute lymphocytic leukemia with atypical cytochemical features. *Am. J. Clin. Pathol.* 63:415, 1975.

13. Higgy, K. E., Burns, G. F., and Hayhoe, F. G. J.: Identification of the hairy cells of leukaemic reticuloendotheliosis by an esterase method. *Br. J. Haematol.* 38:99, 1978.

14. Clein, G. P.: The classification of acute leukaemia, in *Advances in Acute Leukaemia,* edited by F. J. Cleton, D. Crowther, and J. S. Malpas. North-Holland, Amsterdam, 1974, chap. 2, p. 51.

CHAPTER *A28*

Terminal deoxynucleotidyl transferase

ERNEST BEUTLER
WANDA KUHL

PURPOSE OF THE TEST

Terminal transferase activity is present in cells of thymic origin. Activity is elevated in nearly all cases of acute lymphocytic or acute undifferentiated leukemia, whereas it is usually normal or only very slightly elevated in acute and chronic myelogenous leukemia, except in some cases of blastic crisis. It can therefore be of value in determining treatment when morphologic identification is somewhat unclear.

PRINCIPLE OF THE TEST

In the presence of terminal deoxynucleotidyl transferase, tritiated (^{3}H) deoxyadenosine triphosphate is added to the 3' end of the primer oligodeoxyadenylic acid, increasing the length of the oligonucleotide on each addition and rendering it radioactive. The radioactive product is then precipitated with acid and

the radioactivity quantitated. Histochemical determinations of the enzyme may be performed using a kit available from Bethesda Research Laboratories. Some laboratories have not found this procedure to be satisfactory, and an enzyme-linked modification has been reported [1]. Only the well-established biochemical method is presented in detail here.

REAGENTS AND EQUIPMENT

1. Ficoll-Hypaque. Mix 2.4 parts of 9% w/v Ficoll with 1 part of 34% Hypaque (sodium diatrizoate). There are commercially available preparations for mononuclear cell separation which can be used.

2. 0.25 M potassium phosphate buffer, pH 7.5, containing 1 mM β-mercaptoethanol. Dissolve 4.89 g pf $K_2HPO_4 \cdot 3H_2O$ and 0.49 g of KH_2PO_4 in distilled water and make up to 100 ml. Add 0.007 ml of β-mercaptoethanol and store refrigerated. Prepare fresh each month.

3. 0.2 M cacodylate buffer, pH 6.8, with 40 mM magnesium chloride, 2 mM zinc sulfate, and 2.5% bovine serum albumin. Dissolve 3.20 g of sodium cacodylate in approximately 80 ml of distilled water in a beaker and adjust the pH to 6.8 with hydrochloric acid. Add 0.81 g of $MgCl_2 \cdot 6H_2O$, 58 mg of $ZnSO_4 \cdot 7H_2O$, and 2.5 g of bovine serum albumin. Mix to dissolve and dilute to 100 ml with distilled water. When stored frozen in 5 to 10 ml aliquots, this buffer is stable for over 1 year.

4. Oligodeoxyadenylic acid, p(dA)$_{10}$, 10 OD units/ml in water. Add 0.5 ml of distilled water directly to the bottle containing 5 units of p(dA)$_{10}$ as purchased. Store frozen.

5. ^{3}H-dATP:dATP (50 μCi/ml:2.5 mM). Pipette 0.2 ml of ^{3}H-deoxyadenosine-5'-triphosphate (sodium salt) (500 μCi/ml, 50 nmol/ml in ethanol) into a test tube and dry under a stream of nitrogen or in a vacuum desiccator. Prepare 2 ml of nonradioactive 2.5 mM deoxyadenosine-5'-triphosphate (sodium salt) in aqueous solution, add to the tube containing the dried ^{3}H-dATP, and mix well. Store at $-20°C$.

6. Yeast RNA, 25 mg/ml in water. Store frozen.

7. 0.6% trichloroacetic acid (TCA). Prepare fresh on day of use.

8. 0.1 N sodium hydroxide.

9. 0.025 N hydrochloric acid.

10. 0.9% NaCl.

11. 2.0% NaCl.

12. Suitable scintillation fluid for counting radioactivity of aqueous samples, e.g., Handifluor (Mallinckrodt).

TECHNIQUE [2]

SAMPLE PREPARATION

Blood (7 ml) or marrow (1 to 2 ml) collected in a commercially available lavender stoppered EDTA-Na$_2$ tube is layered over 3 ml of Ficoll-Hypaque and centrifuged at 400 × g for 25 min at 4°C in a swinging bucket rotor. Between 14 and 20 ml of blood may be needed when the leukocyte count is less than 5000 per microliter. The interface layer between the plasma and the Ficoll-Hypaque contains the lymphocytes, monocytes, platelets, and blast cells, and the erythrocytes and polymorphonuclear leukocytes are deposited at the bottom of the tube. The interface layer is removed with a Pasteur pipette, and cells are collected by centrifugation and washed twice with 0.9% NaCl solution. When macroscopically contaminated with erythrocytes, the cells are shock-lysed with 2 ml of ice-cold water for 50 s, 2 ml of 2% NaCl is rapidly added, and the cells are collected by centrifugation and washed twice with 0.9% NaCl solution. Three to five volumes of 0.25 M potassium phosphate buffer, pH 7.5, containing 1 m*M* β-mercaptoethanol is added and mixed with the cells. The protein content of the suspension is determined according to the method of Lowry [3]. A commercially available micro-Lowry kit may be used according to the instruction of the manufacturer. Protein concentrations are preferably between 5 and 20 mg/ml, but suspensions with protein concentrations as low as 2 mg/ml can be assayed. After freezing three times in a dry ice–acetone bath and thawing in water at room temperature, the suspension is centrifuged at 100,000 × *g* for 60 min and the terminal transferase assay performed on the supernate. Either the leukocyte suspension or the supernate after high-speed centrifugation may be stored at −20°C for several months without significant loss of activity.

TERMINAL DEOXYNUCLEOTIDYL TRANSFERASE ASSAY

The following reagents are pipetted into 1.5-ml plastic centrifuge tubes labeled "system": 10 µl of 0.2 *M* cacodylate buffer, pH 6.8, containing 40 m*M* MgCl₂, 2 m*M* ZnSO₄, and 2.5% bovine serum albumin; 20 µl of ³H-dATP/dATP, 50 µCi/ml, 2.5 m*M*; 10 µl of p(dA)₁₀, 10 OD units/ml; and 10 µl of the supernate. A tube labeled "blank" contains the same reagents except for the substitution of 10 µl of water in place of the p(dA)₁₀. The tubes are tightly stoppered, mixed well, and incubated in a water bath at 37°C. After 15 min, two 20-µl aliquots are removed from each of the tubes into iced 12-ml centrifuge tubes containing 20 µl of yeast RNA. Five ml of ice-cold 0.6% TCA is added to the tubes, and they are allowed to stand in ice for a minimum of 10 min, but no longer than 2 h. The precipitates are sedimented by centrifugation at 1000 × *g* for 10 min at 4°C. The supernate is removed by aspiration, and the pellet is washed twice by addition of 5 ml of ice-cold 0.6% TCA, recentrifuging after each wash. It should be noted that resuspension of the pellet is very difficult and not necessary. Simply flooding the tube and pellet surface with TCA followed by centrifugation is sufficient. After the final wash the pellet is dissolved in 0.3 ml of 0.1 *N* NaOH. The solution is transferred in its entirety to a counting vial, and the tube is washed out with 1.2 ml of 0.025 *N* HCl, which is also transferred to the same counting vial. After 10 ml of scintillation fluid is added, the vial contents are mixed. The aqueous capacity of the scintillation fluid should be determined from the manufacturer's specifications, and, if necessary, the volume should be adjusted to fit that capacity. A 100% count is taken by placing into a counting vial 5 µl of the 2.5 m*M* ³H-dATP/dATP, 0.3 ml of 0.1 *N* NaOH, 1.2 ml of 0.025 *N* HCl, and 10 ml of scintillation fluid. All samples are counted for 20 min.

CALCULATION

The counts of duplicates of the blanks and systems are averaged. Activity (*A*) is presented as microunits per milligram protein (pmol dATP incorporated per minute per milligram protein).

$$A = \frac{(CPM_S - CPM_B)}{(CPM_{100\%})(4)(\frac{20}{50})} \times \frac{50,100}{(15)(P)(0.01)}$$

or

$$A = \frac{(CPM_S - CPM_B)208,750}{(CPM_{100\%})(P)}$$

where CPM_S is counts per minute of the system, CPM_B counts per minute of the blank, $CPM_{100\%}$ counts per minute of the substrate, and *P* the protein concentration in milligrams per milliliter of leukolysate. $CPM_{100\%}$ is multiplied by 4 because only 5 µl of the 20 µl used in the assay is counted, and it is multiplied

by 20/50 because the other two counts are derived from 20 µl of the 50 µl of reaction mixture. The ratio of counts then represents the fraction of ³H-dATP transferred to polymer. This is then multiplied by 50,100, the number of picomoles of dATP present in the system. The 15 is the time in minutes and 0.01 is the volume, in milliliters, of leukolysate added to the system. The protein content of 10⁸ leukocytes is approximately 7.5 mg. The results can therefore be approximated as units per 10⁸ leukocytes by multiplying by 7.5. Conversion to nanomoles per 10⁸ leukocytes per hour (the units used in some laboratories) is achieved by multiplying by 0.45.

INTERPRETATION

Normal values for terminal deoxynucleotidyl transferase in peripheral blood calculated from 15 subjects are 0.59 ± 2.09 µU per milligram protein (mean ± 1 standard deviation). The activity from nine normal marrow samples was determined to be 7.69 ± 7.34 µU per milligram protein (mean ± 1 standard deviation).

SOURCE OF REAGENTS

Histopaque (Ficoll-Hypaque), cacodylic acid (sodium salt), bovine serum albumin, yeast RNA (type VI), and the reagent kit for colorimetric microdetermination of total protein may be obtained from Sigma Chemical Co., St. Louis, Mo. Oligodeoxyadenylic acid [p(dA)₁₀] and deoxyadenosine-5'-triphosphate (sodium salt) were obtained from P-L Biochemicals, Milwaukee, Wis. ³H-deoxyadenosine-5'-triphosphate (sodium salt) may be obtained from Schwarz/Mann, Orangeburg, N.Y.

References

1. Hecht, T., et al.: Histochemical demonstration of terminal deoxynucleotidyl transferase in leukemia. *Blood 58*:856, 1981.
2. Beutler, E., and Kuhl, W.: An assay for terminal deoxynucleotidyl transferase in leukocytes and bone marrow. *Am. J. Clin. Pathol. 70*:733, 1978.
3. Lowry, O. H., Rosebrough, N. Y., Farr, A. L., and Randall, R. J.: Protein measurement with the folin phenol reagent. *J. Biol. Chem. 193*:265, 1951.

CHAPTER *A29*

Lymphocyte markers

FREDERICK R. DAVEY

PURPOSE OF THE TESTS

Lymphocyte markers can be used to identify and enumerate T lymphocytes, B lymphocytes, pre-B lymphocytes, and plasma cells. These assays are helpful in the immunologic classification of lymphoproliferative diseases and in the diagnosis of many immunologic deficiency disorders.

PRINCIPLE OF THE TESTS

T lymphocytes form spontaneous or nonimmune rosettes with sheep erythrocytes [1,2]. B lymphocytes and monocytes do not have membrane receptors for sheep erythrocytes. B lymphocytes—but not T cells, monocytes, pre-B lymphocytes, or plasma cells—synthesize surface membrane immunoglobulin (SMIg) [3–6]. SMIg can be detected by incubating a suspension of viable lymphocytes with fluorescein-conjugated antihuman immunoglobulin serum. After appropriate washing steps, the lymphocyte suspension is observed for membrane fluorescence using an epi-illuminated fluorescence microscope. Pre-B cells are characterized by small amounts of cytoplasmic IgM, whereas plasma cells contain abundant cytoplasmic immunoglobulin (CIg) not restricted to the IgM class [4]. CIg is detected by incubating cell buttons fixed on glass slides with fluorescein-conjugated antiserum. Following appropriate washing steps, the cell preparation is observed for cytoplasmic fluorescence.

Sheep erythrocyte rosette assay

REAGENTS AND EQUIPMENT

1. Lymphocyte separation medium (LSM). A solution containing 9.4 g of sodium diatrizoate and 6.2 g of Ficoll in 100 ml. The density of 1.077 to 1.080 g/ml at 20°C.
2. Fetal calf serum (FCS) is adsorbed by mixing one part packed washed sheep erythrocytes with four parts FCS and incubating at 37°C for 4 h. The suspension must be mixed thoroughly and adsorption continued at 4°C overnight. The red cells are removed by centrifugation at $600 \times g$ for 20 min and the supernatant used as noted below. This is adsorbed FCS.
3. Hanks balanced salt solution (HBSS).
4. Sheep erythrocytes stored in Alsever's solution.
5. 13×100 mm plastic tubes with screw tops.
6. Centrifuge.
7. Hemocytometer.
8. Pasteur pipettes.
9. Incubator at 37°C.
10. Refrigerator at 4°C.
11. Cytocentrifuge.

MONONUCLEAR CELL SEPARATION TECHNIQUE [7]

1. 10 to 20 ml of heparinized blood is collected from the patient in a syringe previously rinsed with a small volume of preservative-free heparin, 1000 units/ml. The blood is then transferred to a 50 ml conical plastic centrifuge tube with cap and mixed with an equal volume of HBSS.
2. The mixture is underlayered with a volume of LSM equal to one-fourth that of the diluted blood, with care taken to maintain a sharp interface between the LSM and the blood, and centrifuged at $400 \times g$ for 30 min at 18 to 20°C [7]. During centrifugation red cells and polymorphonuclear leukocytes form a layer at the bottom of the tube. Lymphocytes and monocytes collect at the interface between the plasma and the LSM, forming a narrow, cloudy band located just below the middle of the column of liquid in the tube.
3. The upper plasma layer is removed to a level about 3 to 5 mm above the layer of mononuclear cells and discarded. The mononuclear cells are collected along with about 5 ml of the tube contents, transferred to a 50-ml centrifuge tube, and mixed with sufficient HBSS to bring the total volume to 40 ml. The tube is centrifuged at $200 \times g$ for 10 min to collect the cells. The supernatant is discarded and the washing repeated twice. The washed cells are suspended in a volume of HBSS equal to one-tenth the starting volume of blood. The concentration of cells is determined by counting an aliquot in a standard count-

ing chamber. The cell suspension is adjusted to 10×10^6 per milliliter.

SHEEP ERYTHROCYTE ROSETTE TECHNIQUE (BACH) [1]

1. Combine, in a 13×100 mm tube, 5×10^6 cells in 0.5 ml of HBSS with 25% absorbed FCS and 0.05 ml of a 15% suspension of sheep erythrocytes in 0.9% saline, yielding a ratio of approximately 30 sheep erythrocytes to 1 mononuclear cell.
2. Mix this suspension by gently rocking the tube.
3. Incubate the mixture at 37°C for 1 h.
4. Centrifuge for 5 min at $200 \times g$.
5. Incubate overnight at 4°C.
6. Resuspend the cell pellet gently using a pasteur pipet.
7. Load a hemocytometer with the cell suspension and allow the suspension to settle (about 2 min).
8. Count 200 leukocytes, including both rosette-forming cells (three or more sheep erythrocytes attached to a lymphocyte) and non-rosette-forming cells. Calculate the percentage of rosette-forming cells.
9. Add an approximately equal volume of HBSS to the remaining rosette cell suspension and remix.
10. Make cytocentrifuge slides with the rest of the rosette cell suspension. (It takes about 5 to 8 drops per slide.)
11. Stain the cytocentrifuge-prepared slides with Wright-Giemsa or other appropriate cytochemical stains. Count 200 leukocytes including both rosette-forming cells and non-rosette-forming cells. Identify the cell types of the rosette-forming cells, especially in preparations from patients with leukemia or lymphoma.

Surface membrane and cytoplasmic immunoglobulin

REAGENTS AND EQUIPMENT

1. 0.016 M phosphate-buffered saline (PBS), pH 7.0 to 7.2. Dissolve 0.1 g of $CaCl_2$ in 100 ml of distilled water and dissolve 0.2 g of KCl, 0.2 g of KH_2PO_4, 0.047 g of $MgCl_2$, 8.0 g of NaCl, and 1.15 g of Na_2HPO_4 in 500 ml of distilled water. After reagents have been dissolved in both solutions, mix together and adjust to a total volume of 1 liter with distilled water.
2. $F(ab')_2$ fluorescein-conjugated antisera against human immunoglobulins (γ, μ, α, δ heavy chains; κ and λ light chains; polvalent and ϵ are optional). Before use, centrifuge aliquots of antiserum at $100,000 \times g$ (Beckman Microfuge) for 10 min to remove aggregated protein. The specificity, antibody protein, total protein, and fluorescein-protein ratio should be previously documented by the manufacturer. Because the titer of the antibody may vary among lots of antisera, it is recommended that the dilution of the antiserum be optimized before use. Make 1:1, 1:2, 1:4, 1:8, 1:16, 1:32, and 1:64 dilutions of the conjugated antiserum in PBS and incubate with mononuclear cells as described below. Determine the percentage of positive cells for each dilution of antiserum. The percentage of positive cells will be nearly constant over a range of dilutions and then decrease with further dilution. The optimal dilution of the antiserum is the second from last dilution before the percentage of positive cells is reduced.
3. Glycerin.
4. Pasteur pipettes.
5. 1-ml disposable plastic tubes for use in the microcentrifuge.

6. Microcentrifuge, Beckman Microfuge.

7. Tabletop centrifuge, Fisher Model 59.

8. Sodium azide, 0.2% in PBS containing 5% FCS.

9. Epi-illuminated fluorescence microscope.

10. Cytocentrifuge.

11. Clear nail polish; microscope slides; micro cover slips, 22 mm square.

TECHNIQUE FOR SURFACE MEMBRANE IMMUNOGLOBULIN (PAPAMICHAIL) [6,8]

1. Adjust the mononuclear cell suspension to 10×10^6 per milliliter in cold PBS and 5% FCS containing 0.2% sodium azide.

2. Label disposable 1-ml centrifuge tubes as needed (IgM, IgA, IgG, etc.).

3. Add 0.1 ml of cell suspension to each tube (1×10^6 cells per tube).

4. Centrifuge for 45 s in the tabletop centrifuge at $3500 \times g$ and then decant the supernatant.

5. Add 2 drops of antisera to the appropriate centrifuge tube, cap, and suspend the cells by vigorously agitating the tube by hand.

6. Incubate for 45 min at 4°C, centrifuge for 45 s in the microcentrifuge, and decant the supernatants.

7. Wash the cells with cold PBS containing 0.2% sodium azide and 5% FCS. Thoroughly disperse the cells by vigorously agitating the suspension by hand. Collect the cells by centrifuging for 45 s in the tabletop centrifuge at $3500 \times g$. Repeat the washing procedure twice, for a total of three washes.

8. After the third wash and centrifugation, resuspend the cells in 1 drop of 50% glycerin in PBS.

9. Draw a circle with a marking pencil on an appropriately labeled glass slide. Place 1 drop of cell mixture within the circle on the slide, carefully place a cover slip over the drop, and seal with nail polish. Slides can be stored at −20°C for at least 1 month.

10. Examine this preparation using an epi-illuminated fluorescence microscope.

11. Count at least 200 cells and determine the proportion with membrane fluorescence.

TECHNIQUE FOR CYTOPLASMIC IMMUNOGLOBULIN [9]

1. Prepare smears by centrifuging 5 to 6 drops of a suspension of mononuclear cells (2×10^6 per milliliter) in PBS or HBSS.

2. After the smear has air-dried, fix in acetone for 10 min at 4°C.

3. Allow the smear to air-dry again.

4. Add 1 drop of the appropriate fluorescein-conjugated antiserum to the specimen.

5. Incubate for 45 min at 37°C in a moist chamber.

6. Rinse the slides twice in PBS for 10 min and once in distilled water for 10 min with constant stirring.

7. Allow the slides to air-dry in the dark to avoid loss of fluorescence.

8. Mount each slide with a drop of 50% glycerin in PBS, top with a cover slip, and seal with nail polish. Slides can be stored at −20°C for at least 1 month.

9. Examine the preparation using an epi-illuminated fluorescence microscope.

10. Count at least 200 cells and determine the percentage of cells with cytoplasmic fluorescence.

INTERPRETATION

The normal range for T cells extends from 50 to 80 percent of peripheral blood mononuclear cells [10–14]. There is some disagreement with regard to the relative proportion of T lymphocytes in normal elderly people. In some studies the absolute number of T cells and the percentage of lymphocytes which are T cells were unchanged, while in others both were decreased [10–14]. The absolute number of T cells decreases significantly in the first decade of life [13].

Receptors for sheep erythrocytes are present on human thymocytes as well as on peripheral blood T lymphocytes. However, thymocytes form stable rosettes with sheep erythrocytes at 37° and 4°C, whereas peripheral blood T lymphocytes form stable rosettes only at 4°C [5].

There are numerous factors which can alter the proportion of lymphocytes which will bind to sheep erythrocytes. Antilymphocyte serum, sodium cyanide, antimycin, iodoacetamide, trypsin, phospholipase A, and ficin can inhibit the formation of rosettes [5]. The proportion of sheep erythrocyte-forming cells can be enhanced by previously treating the sheep erythrocytes with neuraminidase or 2-amino-ethylisothiouronium bromide hydrobromide (AET). "Active" rosettes are formed when lymphocytes incubated with fetal calf serum are mixed with sheep erythrocytes at a 1:20 ratio for a brief period of time at room temperature [2]. Under these conditions approximately 25 to 30 percent of peripheral blood lymphocytes bind to sheep erythrocytes.

Cytocentrifuge preparation of nonimmune rosette-forming cells is particularly useful when neoplastic lymphoid cells are being studied. In T-cell malignancies, morphologically abnormal cells will form rosettes with sheep erythrocytes.

B cells are determined by the presence of SMIg. In normal individuals approximately 10 to 15 percent of the peripheral blood lymphocytes have SMIg [13]. In population studies of normal individuals neither the percentage nor the absolute number of B cells varies significantly among various age groups. The surface of most of the B cells contain IgM, whereas IgG, IgA, and IgE are present on a minority of the B lymphocytes. IgD can be found normally on the same cell as IgM. Only one type of light chain is found on an individual cell. In normal populations the ratio of κ to λ positive cells is usually 2:1. In B cell malignancies the SMIg on the neoplastic cells is usually restricted to one heavy and one light chain [15,16]. In these disorders the κ:λ ratio is markedly abnormal. This "monoclonal" expansion of lymphoid cells helps to differentiate a malignant from a reactive lymphocytosis.

Technical factors can alter the percentage of SMIg positive cells. Dead cells have a solid green cytoplasmic stain instead of a granular membrane fluorescence. The use of cold buffer and sodium azide inhibits the capping of SMIg and eventually the loss of immunoglobulin from the membrane. It is preferred to use fluorescein conjugated $F(ab')_2$ reagents to detect SMIg. Monocytes, neutrophils, and "the third population" [16] of lymphoid cells may contain a high concentration of high-affinity Fc receptors. Thus nonspecific binding of fluorescein-conjugated antisera can be avoided by the use of $F(ab')_2$ reagents.

Pre-B lymphocytes are characterized by cytoplasmic IgM without surface-bound IgM. Pre-B lymphocytes are present in 1 percent of marrow cells and are not present in the peripheral blood of normal individuals. Approximately 20 percent of the cases of acute lymphocytic leukemia are pre-B-cell proliferations [17,18].

Plasma cells also contain CIg but usually have no SMIg.

Plasma cells may contain IgM, IgG, IgD, and IgA, in contrast to the restriction to IgM found in pre-B cells. Only one type of heavy chain is observed in any one plasma cell. Multiple myeloma is characterized by the proliferation of plasma cells containing only one type of heavy and/or light chain.

SOURCE OF REAGENTS

LSM—Litton Bionetics, Kensington, MD 20795

HBSS—Gibco, Island Biological Co., Grand Island, NY 14072

Fluorescein-conjugated antisera—Cappel Laboratories, Cochranville, PA 19330

Sodium azide—Sigma Chemical Co., St. Louis, MO 63178

PBS—Gibco, Grand Island Biological Co., Grand Island, NY 14072

References

1. Bach, J. F.: Evaluation of T-cells and thymic serum factors in man using the rosette technique. *Transplant. Rev.* 16:196, 1973.
2. Wybran, J., and Fudenberg, H. H.: Thymus-derived rosette-forming cells in various human disease states: Cancer, lymphoma, bacterial and viral infections, and other diseases. *J. Clin. Invest.* 52:1026, 1973.
3. Fu, S. M., Winchester, R. J., and Kunkel, H. G.: Occurrence of surface IgM, IgD and free light chains on human lymphocytes. *J. Exp. Med.* 139:451, 1974.
4. Gathings, W. E., Lawton, A. R., and Cooper, M. D.: Immunofluorescent studies of the development of pre-B cells, B lymphocytes and immunoglobulin isotype diversity in humans. *Eur. J. Immunol.* 7:804, 1977.
5. Gupta, S., and Good, R. A.: Markers of human lymphocyte subpopulations in primary immunodeficiency and lymphoproliferative disorders. *Semin. Hematol.* 17:1, 1980.
6. Papamichail, M., Brown, J. C., and Holborow, E. J.: Immunoglobulins on the surface of human lymphocytes. *Lancet* 2:850, 1971.
7. Böyum, A.: Isolation of mononuclear cells and granulocytes from human blood. *Scand. J. Clin. Lab. Invest.* 21 (Suppl. 97):77, 1968.
8. Lyerla, H. C., and Forrester, F. T.: *Immunofluorescence Methods in Virology.* U.S. Department of Health, Education, and Welfare, Public Health Service, Center for Disease Control, Bureau of Laboratories, Atlanta, Ga., 1979.
9. Palmer, D. F., et al.: *Quantitation and Functional Assay of T and B Cells. Part E. Quantitation of Lymphocytes with Surface Immunoglobulin.* Immunology Series No. 8. U.S. Department of Health, Education, and Welfare, Public Health Service, Center for Disease Control, Bureau of Laboratories, Atlanta, Ga., 1978.
10. Weksler, M. E., and Hütteroth, T. H.: Impaired lymphocyte function in aged humans. *J. Clin. Invest.* 53:99, 1974.
11. Augener, W., Cohnen, E., Reuter, A., and Brittinger, G.: Decrease of T lymphocytes during ageing. *Lancet* 1:1164, 1974.
12. Diáz-Jouanen, E., Strickland, R. G., and Williams, R. C., Jr.: Studies of human lymphocytes in the newborn and the aged. *Am. J. Med.* 58:620, 1975.
13. Davey, F. R., and Huntington, S.: Age-related variation in lymphocyte subpopulations. *Gerontology* 23:381, 1977.
14. Inkeles, B., Innes, J. B., Kuntz, M. M., Kadish, A. S., and Weksler, M. E.: Immunological studies of aging. III. Cytokinetic basis for the impaired response of lymphocytes from aged humans to plant lectins. *J. Exp. Med.* 145:1176, 1977.
15. Aisenberg, A. C., and Long, J. C.: Lymphocyte surface characteristics in malignant lymphoma. *Am. J. Med.* 58:300, 1975.
16. Davey, F. R., Goldberg, J., Stockman, J., and Gottlieb, A. J.: Immunologic and cytochemical cell markers in non-Hodgkin's lymphomas. *Lab. Invest.* 35:430, 1976.
17. Vogler, L. B., Crist, W. M., Bockman, D. E., Pearl, E. R., Lawton, A. R., and Cooper, M. D.: Pre-B cell leukemia: A new phenotype of childhood lymphoblastic leukemia. *N. Engl. J. Med.* 298:872, 1978.
18. Greaves, M., et al.: Antigenic and enzymatic phenotypes of the pre-B subclass of acute lymphoblastic leukemia. *Leuk. Res.* 3:353, 1979.

CHAPTER *A30*

Assay of serum and urine lysozyme (muramidase)

JEAN ATWATER
ALLAN J. ERSLEV

PURPOSE OF THE TEST

Lysozyme (muramidase) is a bacteriolytic enzyme present in low concentrations in normal serum and urine. Histochemical studies of the formed elements of blood have demonstrated lysozyme activity in all stages of the granulocytic series except for myeloblasts, eosinophils, or basophils. Monocytes contain large amounts, whereas the lymphocytes, erythrocytes, and platelets are virtually devoid of the enzyme. Serum lysozyme is derived mainly from the degradation of granulocytes [1]. Urinary lysozyme may represent filtered serum lysozyme, but since the concentration of the enzyme is high in kidney tissue, renal injury per se can also lead to significant lysozymeuria [2,3].

Some reports indicate that the levels of serum and urine lysozyme activity are useful indices of granulocyte and monocyte turnover and may be of diagnostic and prognostic significance in leukemia [4,5].

PRINCIPLE OF THE TEST

The bacterium *Micrococcus lysodeikticus* is used as substrate. When lysozyme is added to a suspension of the bacteria, it hydrolyzes the β-1,4 linkages between N-acetyl muramic acid and 2-acetamido-2-deoxy-D-glucose residues in mucopolysaccharides, thereby causing the cloudy suspension to become clear. The rate of clearing of the suspension is measured in a spectrophotometer and is directly proportional to the amount of lysozyme present.

REAGENTS AND EQUIPMENT

1. Substrate. *M. lysodeikticus* cells suspended at a concentration of 100 μg per milliliter of 0.06 M sodium phosphate buffer at pH 6.2 containing 0.15 M sodium chloride.

2. Standard. Egg white lysozyme, 40 μg per milliliter of distilled water. (A lysosome assay kit containing both the substrate and the standard lysozyme in a dried form can be obtained from Worthington Biochemical Corporation, Freehold, NJ 07728.)

3. Spectrophotometer or nephelometer with cuvettes capable of holding a 3-ml sample. A Coleman junior spectrophotometer and 12-mm cuvettes fulfill these requirements.

4. Serum or aliquot of 24-h urine specimen. Store at −20°C until time to assay.

TECHNIQUE

1. Prepare dilute standards of lysozyme in six small test tubes as follows:

ml standard	ml H₂O	Lysozyme conc., µg/ml
0.05	0.95	2
0.10	0.90	4
0.20	0.80	8
0.30	0.70	12
0.40	0.60	16
0.50	0.50	20

2. In a cuvette, pipette 3 ml of a well-mixed suspension of substrate bacteria. Allow the suspension to come to room temperature.

3. Add 0.3 ml of serum or urine and mix rapidly by inversion.

4. Read the optical density (OD) 30 s and again 180 s after adding the enzyme in a spectrophotometer set at 600 nm with a water blank. Calculate the difference in OD between the 30-s and the 180-s reading.

5. Prepare a standard curve by testing each dilution of standard enzyme listed above, using the same technique as for the urine or serum. Plot the change in OD against each standard concentration of lysozyme on regular graph paper. An exponential curve is obtained.

6. Estimate the concentration of lysozyme in the serum or urine sample from the standard curve and express in micrograms per milliliter.

The diluted enzyme standards and the substrate are stable under refrigeration at 4°C. A new standard curve should be constructed for each batch of substrate.

Serum or urine should be diluted with distilled water if the values are higher than those obtained with standard enzyme solutions.

Plasma from EDTA-anticoagulated blood may be used instead of serum. However, heparin must be avoided since it forms a complex with lysozyme.

INTERPRETATION

Normal serum levels range from 5 to 15 µg/ml. Urine levels are normally less than 2 µg/ml. The normal levels have been found to be slightly but significantly higher in males (11 ± 2.75 standard deviation) than in females (9.6 ± 1.3 standard deviation) [6].

Newborn infants have a normal adult level of serum lysozyme. The level drops temporarily to a lower level after the seventh postnatal day, returning to normal adult levels after the thirtieth day. In premature infants the lysozyme level is low at birth but then follows the pattern of term babies [7].

Serum and urine lysozyme levels are increased in most myeloproliferative disorders, including both Philadelphia chromosome negative and positive chronic myelogenous leukemia [8,9]. In polycythemia vera the levels are also elevated in contrast to the normal levels in various secondary polycythemias [10].

Decreased serum levels are seen in neutropenia when accompanied by hypoplasia of the marrow but are normal or increased when the marrow is hypercellular and the neutropenia is due to peripheral cell destruction [11,12].

The levels are low or normal in acute or chronic lymphocytic leukemia, moderately increased in acute myelomonocytic leukemia, and markedly increased in acute and chronic monocytic leukemia [8,13]. In acute granulocytic leukemia the levels may be low, normal, or moderately increased [8]. In histiocytic medullary reticulosis and in "hairy-cell" leukemia the serum and urine lysozyme levels have been reported variously to be low, normal, and even high [8,13–15]. Useful information about remissions and relapses in acute leukemias has been obtained by some investigators using serial estimation of serum lysozyme [6]. However, most reports indicate that serum levels do not correlate with the clinical course [6,16,17].

Increased serum lysozyme levels have been found in isolated cases of tuberculosis, Boeck's sarcoid, Hodgkin's disease, and multiple myeloma [11]. Crohn's disease (regional enteritis) produces increased serum lysozyme levels, and here the test may be of diagnostic significance, since ulcerative colitis does not produce an elevation in serum lysozyme levels [18]. Circulating lysozyme levels are high in patients with Chédiak-Higashi syndrome. This may be the result of intramedullary destruction of the granulocytes [19].

Renal disease has been associated with markedly increased levels of urine lysozyme even in the complete absence of marrow disorders. It has been reported that with a level of more than 5 µg per milliliter of urine there is always evidence of renal disease [2]. However, it is still unresolved whether the high level of urinary lysozyme is due to renal disease or whether renal disease can be caused by high levels of lysozyme in blood.

References

1. Briggs, R. S., Perillie, P. E., and Finch, S. C.: Lysozyme in bone marrow and peripheral blood cells. *J. Histochem. Cytochem.* 14:167, 1966.
2. Prockop, D. J., and Davidson, W. D.: A study of urinary and serum lysozyme in patients with renal disease. *N. Engl. J. Med.* 240:269, 1964.
3. Pruzanski, W., and Platts, M. E.: Serum and urinary proteins, lysozyme (muramidase), and renal dysfunction in mono- and myelomonocytic leukemia. *J. Clin. Invest.* 49:1694, 1970.
4. Osserman, E. F., and Lawlor, D. P.: Serum and urinary lysozyme (muramidase) in monocytic and monomyelogenous leukemia. *J. Exp. Med.* 124:921, 1966.
5. Hansen, N. E.: Lysozyme in haematology: Pathophysiology and clinical use. *Scand. J. Haematol.* 14:160, 1975.
6. Zucker, S., Hanes, D. J., Vogler, W. R., and Eanes, R. Z.: Plasma muramidase: A study of methods and clinical applications. *J. Lab. Clin. Med.* 75:83, 1970.
7. Xanthou, M., Agathopoulos, A., Sakellariou, A., Economou-Mavrou, C., Tsingoglou, S., and Matsaniotis, N.: Serum levels of lysozyme in term and preterm newborns. *Arch. Dis. Child.* 50:304, 1975.
8. Firkin, F. C.: Serum muramidase in haematological disorders: Diagnostic value in neoplastic states. *Aust. N.Z. J. Med.* 1:28, 1972.
9. Finch, S. C., Castro, O., Lippmann, M. E., Donadio, J. A., and Perillie, P. E.: Lysozyme in leukopathic states, in *Lysozyme*, edited by E. F. Osserman, R. E. Canfield, and S. Beychok. Academic, New York, 1974, p. 335.
10. Malmquist, J.: Serum and urinary lysozyme in leukemia and polycythemia vera. *Scand. J. Haematol.* 9:258, 1972.
11. Hansen, N. E.: Plasma lysozyme—a measure of neutrophil turnover: An analytical review. *Ser. Haematol.* 7:1, 1974.
12. Vietske, W. M., Perillie, P. E., and Finch, S. C.: Serum muramidase in patients with neutropenia. *Yale J. Biol. Med.* 45:457, 1972.
13. Bearman, R. M., et al.: Chronic monocytic leukemia in adults. *Cancer* 48:2239, 1981.
14. Klockars, M., and Selroos, O.: Elevated muramidase levels in histiocytic medullary reticulosis. *N. Engl. J. Med.* 294:901, 1976.

15. Burns, C. P.: Serum-muramidase in leukaemic reticuloendo-theliosis. *Lancet* 2:964, 1974.
16. Youman, J. D., Saarni, M. I., and Linman, J. W.: Diagnostic value of muramidase (lysozyme) in acute leukemia and preleukemia. *Mayo Clin. Proc.* 45:219, 1970.
17. Catovsky, D., Galton, D. A. G., and Griffin, C.: The significance of lysozyme estimations in acute myeloid and chronic monocytic leukaemia. *Br. J. Haematol.* 21:565, 1971.
18. Falchuk, K. R., Perrotto, J. L., and Isselbacher, K. J.: Serum lysozyme in Crohn's disease and ulcerative colitis. *N. Engl. J. Med.* 292:395, 1975.
19. Quie, P. G.: Pathology of bactericidal power of neurophils. *Semin. Hematol.* 12:143, 1975.

CHAPTER *A31*

Serum viscosity

WILLIAM J. WILLIAMS

PURPOSE OF THE TEST

Clinical manifestations of hyperglobulinemia appear to result from impaired blood flow due to increased viscosity of the blood. The viscosity of whole blood measured at low rates of shear correlates well with clinical manifestations [1]. However, whole-blood viscosity is a complex function of several variables, especially the hematocrit and plasma protein properties and concentration [1,2]. Special instruments are required to measure blood viscosity accurately [1,2] while serum viscosity can be measured easily and provides clinically useful information. Serum viscosity is frequently increased to clinically significant levels in patients with macroglobulinemia [3]. It is sometimes increased in patients with multiple myeloma, because of either aggregation of the IgG [4] or IgA [5] or an unusually high concentration of IgG [6].

PRINCIPLE OF THE TEST

The relative viscosity is determined by comparing the times required for a known amount of serum and water to flow through a capillary tube. The Ostwald viscosimeter is used for this determination. This apparatus is a glass U tube with one limb a capillary and the other of larger diameter. The larger tube is expanded near the bottom to a bulb which functions as a reservoir. The capillary side is expanded to a bulb near the open end. On either side of this bulb the capillary is scored to provide two measuring lines. The time required for the top of the fluid column to pass between these measuring lines is a function of the viscosity of the fluid.

REAGENTS AND EQUIPMENT

1. Ostwald viscosimeter
   a. Alternatively, a 0.1- or 1.0-ml volumetric pipette or a blood cell diluting pipette [7]
2. Stopwatch
3. Water bath at 37°C
4. Support stand with a clamp to hold the viscosimeter
5. Rubber tubing
6. Pipettes

PERFORMANCE OF THE TEST

1. The viscosimeter is placed in a vertical position in the water bath so that the lower half is immersed in the water.

2. Serum should be centrifuged at $3000 \times g$ for 10 min or more to remove particulate matter.

3. 5 ml of serum is added to the viscosimeter through the larger opening and allowed to equilibrate to 37°C.

4. Suction is applied to the capillary side of the viscosimeter through an attached piece of rubber tubing so that the serum fills the capillary and bulb and rises above the upper measuring line.

5. The suction is released and the serum allowed to flow through the capillary. A stopwatch is started when the meniscus crosses the upper measuring line, and the time required for the meniscus to pass the lower measuring line is determined. The measurement should be repeated three times and the average taken.

6. The serum is removed from the viscosimeter, which is then rinsed twice with 0.15 M NaCl and twice with distilled water.

7. The viscosimeter is returned to the water bath and 5 ml of distilled water is added; the viscosity of the water is determined in the same manner as for the serum.

8. If a water bath is not available, the viscosity may be determined at room temperature. If a viscosimeter is not available, the viscosity may be determined by measuring the time required for serum and water to flow from a 0.1 ml- or 1.0-ml pipette or a blood-cell diluting pipette [7] supported in a vertical position.

CALCULATION OF RESULTS

The relative viscosity is the ratio:

$$\frac{\text{Flow time of serum}}{\text{Flow time of water}}$$

INTERPRETATION

The normal range for relative viscosity is between 1.4 and 1.8. Symptoms of the hyperviscosity syndrome may appear with a relative viscosity of 4, while a relative viscosity of between 6 and 7 or more is usually accompanied by symptoms [1].

SOURCES OF EQUIPMENT

The necessary equipment is readily available from scientific supply houses.

References

1. McGrath, M. A., and Penny, R.: Paraproteinemia: Blood hyperviscosity and clinical manifestations. *J. Clin. Invest.* 58:1155, 1976.
2. Dintenfass, L.: *Rheology of Blood in Diagnostic and Preventive Medicine: An Introduction to Clinical Rheology.* Butterworths, London, 1976.
3. Fahey, I. L., Barth, W. F., and Solomon, A.: Serum hyperviscosity syndrome. *JAMA* 192:464, 1965.
4. Smith, E., Kochwa, S., and Wasserman, L. R.: Aggregation of IgG globulin in vivo. I. The hyperviscosity syndrome in multiple myeloma. *Am. J. Med.* 39:35, 1965.
5. Vaerman, J. P., Johnson, L. B., Mandy, W., and Fudenberg, H. H.: Multiple myeloma with two paraprotein peaks: An instructive case. *J. Lab. Clin. Med.* 65:18, 1965.
6. Kopp, W. L., Beirne, G. J., and Burns, R. O.:Hyperviscosity syndrome in multiple myeloma. *Am. J. Med.* 43:141, 1967.
7. Wright, D. J., and Jenkins, D. E., Jr.: Simplified method for estimation of serum and plasma viscosity in multiple myeloma and related disorders. *Blood* 36:516, 1970.

Hemostasis studies

CHAPTER *A32*

Whole-blood coagulation time test and clot observation

CECIL HOUGIE

PURPOSE OF THE TEST

The whole-blood clotting time is a very insensitive test and should never be used for screening purposes. It is often used for monitoring heparin therapy, but the results obtained are frequently unreliable, and other tests, such as the activated partial thromboplastin time test, may therefore be preferred. Nevertheless, the whole-blood clotting time is still performed because much useful information may be obtained by periodic inspection of the clot.

PRINCIPLE OF THE TEST

The time required for blood to clot in a glass tube is a measure of the overall activity of the intrinsic system in blood coagulation (Chap. 137). Periodic inspection of the clot permits evaluation of the physical properties of the clot (size, appearance, and mechanical strength), its stability, and the rate and extent of its retraction.

REAGENTS

No reagents are required for the test.

TECHNIQUE

Venous blood is used in this test. For all coagulation tests venous blood obtained by a clean venipuncture is withdrawn into a plastic syringe, using care to avoid frothing of the blood. Before transferring the blood into tubes the needle should be removed. The bore of the needle should be related to the quantity of blood required: the larger the amount of blood required, the greater the bore of the needle. Thus if 10 ml of blood is required, a size 20 needle is satisfactory, whereas a size 18 needle should be used if 30 to 50 ml of blood is needed. Blood which has been withdrawn with difficulty from a bad venipuncture should not be used. If a good sample cannot be obtained, the results must be interpreted with great caution. A two-syringe technique is preferred by many coagulation laboratories. After 1 or 2 ml of blood has been withdrawn into the first syringe, it is disconnected from the needle and the syringe and its contents discarded; only blood withdrawn into the second syringe is used.

A venipuncture is performed, and a stopwatch is started as soon as the blood enters the syringe. One-milliliter aliquots of whole blood are delivered immediately into three 12- by 75-mm glass tubes. The tubes are placed in a water bath at 37°C. The tubes are gently tilted every 30 s until a clot is seen in one of the tubes; the stopwatch is stopped at this point and the time recorded. This is considered to be the clotting time. (In the original Lee-White method, the first tube is tilted at intervals of 30 s until a solid clot has formed. The second and third tubes are then treated similarly in sequence. The clotting time is the time required for a solid clot to form in the third tube.) Each tube is then examined at the end of 1 h and again on the following morning.

INTERPRETATION

The normal value obtained by this method is between 4 and 8 min. With great care and meticulous attention to detail, this range can be reduced, but even then large, uncontrollable variations occur. Prolongation of the clotting time is due to marked coagulation factor deficiencies or to the presence of circulating anticoagulants, including heparin.

In normal blood the clot at the end of the first hour should be firm and should have retracted from the sides of the tube, occupying approximately half the original volume of blood ("clot retraction"). Retraction should be recorded as normal, equivocal, or defective, based on a normal retraction of about 50 percent. Clot retraction is impaired if there is thrombocytopenia or thrombasthenia. Erythrocytosis will also interfere with clot retraction, as will an increase in fibrinogen concentration. Anemia will facilitate clot retraction.

In intravascular coagulation (Chap. 158) or α_2-antiplasmin deficiency [1], the clot is often small and ragged and may be partially disintegrated. These changes are often more pronounced the following day. Occasionally no clot is seen after 1 h at 37°C. Dissolution of the clot is considered evidence of excessive fibrinolysis, provided a good solid clot formed initially. Marked clot retraction, with expression of the red cells from the clot, may lead to confusion because the remaining clot is not readily seen. It may be necessary to pour the blood into a Petri dish to make certain that no clot remains.

Reference

1. Aoki, N., Saito, H., Kamiya, T., Koie, K., Sakata, Y., and Kobakura, M.: Congenital deficiency of α_2-plasmin inhibitor associated with severe hemorrhage tendency. *J. Clin. Invest.* 63:877, 1979.

Recalcification time test and its modifications (partial thromboplastin time, activated partial thromboplastin time, and expanded partial thromboplastin time)

CECIL HOUGIE

Recalcification time test

PURPOSE OF THE TEST

This test measures coagulant activity generated in the intrinsic system. It is primarily used to estimate platelet thromboplastic function.

PRINCIPLE OF THE TEST

Platelet-rich plasma contains all the coagulation factors necessary for the formation of intrinsic prothrombinase or plasma thromboplastin, with the exception of calcium ions. When calcium is added to the plasma, intrinsic prothrombinase is generated; this activates prothrombin, and the thrombin thus formed converts fibrinogen to fibrin. The rate of clotting is a measure of the overall coagulant activity developed and is decreased if there is a marked deficiency of any component.

The extent of the exposure of plasma to glass surfaces and the number of platelets in the plasma have marked effects on this test; for this reason the various modifications of the test have been developed (see below and Chap. 137). The number of platelets present in the plasma is difficult to control since the platelet concentration depends not only on the patient's platelet count but, more importantly, also on the speed of centrifugation of the blood, the number of platelets decreasing with the higher centrifugal forces. The test is primarily used for platelet thromboplastic function and is performed using platelet-rich and platelet-poor plasma. If the platelets are normal, the clotting time of the platelet-rich plasma should be shorter than that of the platelet-poor plasma.

REAGENTS

1. Anticoagulants. Two parts of 0.1 M citric acid [21 g citric acid ($H_3C_6H_5O_7 \cdot H_2O$) dissolved in sufficient water to make 1 liter of solution] are mixed with three parts of 0.1 M trisodium citrate [29.4 g of trisodium citrate ($Na_3C_6H_5O_7 \cdot 2H_2O$) dissolved in sufficient water to make 1 liter of solution]. Alternatively, 3.2 or 3.8% (w/v) solutions of trisodium citrate ($Na_3C_6H_5O_7 \cdot 2H_2O$) in distilled water may be used, but the control plasma must be similarly collected.

2. Calcium chloride. A 0.025 M solution is prepared by dissolving 2.8 g of the anhydrous salt in sufficient distilled water to make 1 liter of solution.

TECHNIQUE

1. A venipuncture is performed using the technique described in Chap. A32.

2. Preparation of platelet-rich and platelet-poor plasma. Nine volumes of whole blood are placed in a disposable polystyrene tube containing one volume of citrate anticoagulant. After mixing by inversion several times, the tube is immediately centrifuged at $2000 \times g$ for 15 min or longer if platelet-poor plasma is required, or at $100 \times g$ for 10 min if platelet-rich plasma is required. The plasma is carefully pipetted from the tube, using a wide-bore, silicone-coated, glass Pasteur pipette or a disposable plastic pipette. It is also advisable, if there is sufficient platelet-poor plasma, to place 1 to 2 ml of the plasma in a small snap-closing polyethylene container and freeze it immediately; this may be kept as a reference or used later if preliminary tests are inconclusive.

3. Measurement of recalcification time. One-tenth milliliter of the plasma (platelet-poor or platelet-rich) is placed in a 12-by 75-mm glass tube, 0.1 ml of 0.85% NaCl is added, and the mixture is incubated at 37°C for 1 min. The mixture is then recalcified by the addition of 0.1 ml of 0.025 M CaCl₂ warmed to 37°C. A stopwatch is started when the calcium is added. The tube is incubated at 37°C for 60 to 80 s. The reaction mixture is then examined at intervals of 1 or 2 s for clotting by tilting the tube slowly so that the reaction mixture runs about halfway up the side of the tube. The clotting time is recorded as the interval from the addition of calcium to the appearance of the first detectable fibrin threads in the reaction mixture. The clotting time is influenced by the amount of glass surface with which the blood comes in contact; the greater the amount of contact, the shorter the time. It is therefore important to use glass tubes of the same size from one manufacturer. The test should be performed as soon as possible after collection of the blood.

INTERPRETATION

With the above technique, using 12- by 75-mm test tubes, the clotting times of normal platelet-rich plasmas have ranged from 100 to 150 s, while the clotting times of normal platelet-poor plasma have ranged from 135 to 240 s. Clotting time of the platelet-rich plasma should be at least 20 s shorter than that of the platelet-poor plasma; otherwise a defect in platelet function should be suspected.

Partial thromboplastin time test (PTT)

PURPOSE OF THE TEST

This test may be used to screen for deficiencies of plasma coagulation factors except factors VII and XIII.

PRINCIPLE OF THE TEST

This test is essentially a recalcification time in which the variable of platelet concentration is controlled by adding an optimal amount of platelet substitute (phospholipid emulsion) to platelet-poor plasma. The extent of the exposure of the plasma to glass surfaces is not controlled in this test.

REAGENTS

1. Phospholipid emulsion (platelet substitute):

a. Chloroform extract of brain. The following method was reported by Bell and Alton [1]. One gram of commercial acetone-dried rabbit brain is washed twice with acetone to free it of cholesterol and then dried. The dried powder is suspended in approximately 50 ml of chloroform at room temperature and shaken at frequent intervals. The mixture is filtered and the chloroform evaporated at 37°C. A gummy residue results, and this is homogenized in 50 ml of 0.85% NaCl. An approximately 1:100 dilution of this concentrate in 0.85% NaCl substituted for a platelet suspension in the recalcification time test gives times of 50 to 80 s. When frozen, a concentrated suspension in 0.85% NaCl remains stable for long periods and may be thawed and refrozen repeatedly without loss of activity. The exact dilution for use is determined for each batch of extract.

b. Asolectin. This is a soybean phosphatide which can be obtained commercially. It is used at a concentration of about 0.20 g per deciliter of 0.85% NaCl containing 0.01 M tris(hydroxymethyl)aminomethane[1] or imidazole[2] adjusted to pH 7.4 with 1 N HCl. The material has to be shaken vigorously for several minutes to obtain an adequate emulsion. It is usual to make a solution containing 1 g/dl and to prepare several dilutions from an aliquot of this emulsion. The optimal concentration is determined by performing partial thromboplastin times on each dilution. The bulk is then diluted to the optimal concentration and stored frozen at −20°C in small amounts in glass tubes.

c. Commercial phospholipid emulsions. These are available, are stable, and give satisfactory results. Sources of these emulsions are listed at the end of this chapter.

d. Other reagents. These are described above under "Recalcification Time Test."

TECHNIQUE

1. Platelet-poor plasma is prepared as described for the recalcification time test.

2. Performance of the test. It is essential to use at least one normal control and perform all tests in triplicate. Two-tenths milliliter of a phospholipid emulsion (platelet substitute) is added to 0.2 ml of the test plasma in a 12- by 75-mm glass test tube. The mixture is then incubated at 37°C for 30 s. Recalcification is effected by the addition of 0.2 ml 0.025 M calcium chloride warmed to 37°C. A stopwatch is started when the calcium is added, and the tube is incubated at 37°C for 40 s. The reaction mixture is examined for clot formation as described under "Recalcification Time Test" and the clotting time is recorded. The simplicity of the test is deceptive, and reliable results can be obtained only by experienced workers. Special caution is required with respect to glassware. The test must be performed as soon as possible after collection to minimize glass activation effects. It is important to perform the test at the same time on a normal control subject under the same conditions. Aliquots of fresh pooled plasma may be placed in small containers and stored at −20°C for use as additional controls and as a check on day-to-day variations.

INTERPRETATION

The normal range for the partial thromboplastin time, or PTT, test is 60 to 85 s. The test is prolonged when there is a

---

deficiency in one or more of the following: factors XII, XI, X, IX, VIII, V, prothrombin, and fibrinogen. The PTT is also prolonged by inhibitors of any one or more of these factors or by lupus-like anticoagulants. It is prolonged if the fibrinogen is below 100 mg/dl, by fibrinogen- or fibrin-split products, or by heparin. Shorter-than-normal values are often seen following a poor venipuncture, if the plasma contains platelets, when the factor VIII level is high, or in disseminated intravascular clotting.

Activated partial thromboplastin time test [2]

PURPOSE OF THE TEST

This test is used to screen for deficiencies of the plasma coagulation factors except factors VII and XIII. It is generally more sensitive than the PTT, although in some patients with mild hemophilia or acquired factor VIII antibodies the activated PTT may be within the normal range while the PTT is abnormal. The test may also be used to monitor heparin therapy.

PRINCIPLE OF THE TEST

One of the chief variables in the PTT test is the amount of surface to which the blood is exposed. Blood is usually collected in glass, and in a clinical laboratory an hour or two may elapse before the test can be performed. The plasma is thus exposed to a variable amount of glass contact. By exposing the plasma to maximal surface activation, this variable is reduced. Kaolin, Celite, and ellagic acid have been used as activating agents. The principle of the test is otherwise the same as that of the original PTT test as described above.

REAGENTS

1. Activating agents. The activating agent usually used is kaolin (2 g kaolin in 100 ml of 0.85% NaCl) or Celite (3 to 5 g in 100 ml 0.85% NaCl).

2. Phospholipid emulsions. These are described under "Partial Thromboplastin Time Test."

3. The other reagents are those described under "Recalcification Time Test."

TECHNIQUE

1. Platelet-poor plasma is prepared as described under "Recalcification Time Test."

2. Performance of the test. To 0.2 ml plasma in a 12- by 75-mm glass tube are added 0.1 ml of activating agent and 0.1 ml of phospholipid emulsion (platelet substitute). The activating agent and phospholipid emulsion may be premixed and 0.2 ml of the mixture used. As kaolin settles rapidly, this reagent must be well mixed before pipetting. The mixture of plasma, activating agent, and phospholipid emulsion is incubated at 37°C for 3 min, and then 0.2 ml of 0.025 M CaCl$_2$ warmed to 37°C is added and a stopwatch started. The tube is shaken once immediately after adding the calcium and then gently tilted 30 s later and at successive 1-s intervals. The end point is taken at the first clumping of kaolin. The tests should be performed in triplicate and a normal control included.

INTERPRETATION

This is similar to that of the original PTT test. The normal range using a semiautomated instrument is relatively narrow (for example, 26 to 33 s) provided (1) all individuals with less than 60

---

[1] 1.21 g tris base per liter of solution equals 0.01 M.
[2] 0.68 g imidazole per liter of solution equals 0.01 M.

or more than 150 percent of factor VIII, IX, XI, or XII are excluded from the pool of control subjects, (2) blood is collected into plastic tubes, and (3) the test is performed within 1 h of collection. As most routine laboratories use glass tubes and samples are left for variable periods on the bench, often several hours, before being tested (in batches), the range is therefore considerably wider (for example, 22 to 38 s). The normal range will be somewhat different depending on the reagents used, etc. The test is usually abnormal with levels of factor VIII or IX below 30 to 50 percent of normal.

The activated PTT is sometimes used to monitor heparin therapy. It has been recommended that when heparin is given continuously by intravenous drip for the treatment of venous thromboembolism the activated PTT be prolonged to 1.5 to 2.5 times the control levels [3]. However, the sensitivity of the method to heparin is dependent on the type and concentration of the activator and phospholipid used [4]. The results are not always reliable, and this is particularly true when the blood sample is withdrawn through the intravenous catheter used to infuse the heparin. The Lee and White clotting time is no better, and the best means of monitoring heparin therapy, or whether it needs to be monitored at all, remains an unsettled issue.

Expanded partial thromboplastin time test

PURPOSE OF THE TEST

This test is used to give more specific information regarding those factor deficiencies in plasma which give an abnormal activated PTT.

PRINCIPLE OF THE TEST

Addition to the deficient factor(s) to plasma giving an abnormal coagulation test will correct the abnormality. Thus, if addition of a reagent containing factors IX and X corrects an abnormal activated PTT, it may be assumed that the plasma is deficient in one or both of these factors. These substitution experiments are of great practical value, but final determination of which factor is deficient requires either specific factor assays or comparison with plasmas with known deficiencies.

REAGENTS

1. Serum. Serum may be obtained by placing approximately 1 ml of blood into each of three or four glass tubes which are roughly 10 mm in internal diameter. Each tube is gently tilted three times through an angle of 45 to 70 degrees so that the blood comes into contact with the glass sides. The tubes are placed in a bath at 37°C for 2 h and are then removed. After the tubes have been at room temperature for another hour, the clot is removed, the remaining blood centrifuged at approximately $1000 \times g$ for 10 min, and the serum separated. The blood used to perform the modified Lee and White clotting time described in Chap. A32 may be used; the tubes are left in the water bath for 2 h and the serum separated as described above. Whatever method is chosen, the important point is always to treat the control and the patient's serum in an identical manner. The unknown and control serums are diluted 1:10 and 0.85% NaCl. The diluted sera should be allowed to stand at room temperature for at least 1 h before testing because the activity increases on standing.

2. Adsorbed plasma. Adsorbed plasma is prepared by adding 0.1 ml of aluminum hydroxide gel to 2 ml of platelet-poor plasma. Aluminum hydroxide gel is available commercially. The mixture is allowed to stand at 37°C for 3 min; the gel is then removed by centrifuging at $2000 \times g$ for 20 min. The prothrombin time (Chap. A34) of the supernatant plasma is tested and should be between 45 and 300 s, with a normal control of 12 s. The actual amount of the gel required and the time of incubation will vary with different batches of the gel and is determined by trial and error. Alternatively, plasma may be adsorbed with reagent-grade barium sulfate, 0.1 g per milliliter of plasma. The plasma must be obtained from oxalated blood if $BaSO_4$ is used. The mixture of $BaSO_4$ and plasma is incubated at 37°C for 15 min; otherwise the treatment is the same as described for $Al(OH)_3$.

3. The other reagents are those described for the activated PTT test.

TECHNIQUE

1. Platelet-poor plasma is prepared from normal blood and the blood of the patient, using the technique described under "Recalcification Time Test."

2. Performance of the test. A series of tests is performed in parallel on the normal plasma and the patient's plasma. The tests should be performed in triplicate.

One-tenth milliliter of test plasma is placed in each of three 12- by 75-mm glass test tubes. To the first tube is added 0.1 ml of 0.85% NaCl, to the second tube 0.1 ml of normal serum diluted 1:10 with 0.85% NaCl, and to the third tube 0.1 ml of adsorbed plasma diluted 1:10 with 0.85% NaCl.

The activated PTT is then performed on the mixtures exactly as described above.

INTERPRETATION

The mixture of 0.85% NaCl, normal serum (diluted 1:10), or normal adsorbed plasma (diluted 1:10) with normal plasma does not markedly or consistently change the activated PTT. Addition of 0.85% NaCl to the patient's plasma may or may not further prolong the activated PTT. The activated PTT of the patient's plasma mixed with 0.85% NaCl is the reference point for the effect of serum and adsorbed plasma on this test. The extent of correction of the prolonged activated PTT by serum or adsorbed plasma will depend on the degree of the deficiency. Corrective reagents should return the activated PTT nearly to normal. If correction is equivocal, serum or adsorbed plasma diluted 1:5 or 1:2 should be tested.

If serum but not adsorbed plasma corrects the deficiency in the patient's plasma, then the deficient factor must be either IX or X. If adsorbed plasma but not serum corrects the deficiency, the deficient factor may be fibrinogen or factor V or VIII. If either corrects the deficiency, it may be due to factor XI or XII.

Additional tests are useful in deciding between a deficiency of factor IX or X when the abnormality in the patient's plasma is corrected by serum. Factor X is a reactant in the one-stage prothrombin time, while factor IX is not (Chap. A34); therefore if the prothrombin time of the patient's plasma is normal, the deficiency corrected by serum is due to factor IX. If the prothrombin time is abnormal, the abnormality in the activated PTT is due to at least a deficiency of factor X, but there may be other deficiencies as well. Similarly the prothrombin time helps differentiate between factors V and VIII as the deficient factor responsible for a prolonged activated PTT. If the prothrombin time is normal and the abnormal activated PTT is corrected by adsorbed plasma, the deficient factor is factor VIII. If the prothrombin time is abnormal, fibrinogen or factor V is implicated, although other factors may also be deficient. Fibrinogen deficiency may be detected by a direct determination (Chap. A35).

If either adsorbed plasma or serum corrects the abnormal activated PTT, a deficiency of either factor XI or XII is suggested, and further study in these cases requires comparison of the patient's plasma with plasma from patients known to have deficiencies of either factor XI or XII.

It must be emphasized that correction by serum or adsorbed plasma using both the activated PTT and prothrombin time does not provide final definition of the deficient factor or factors. In *all* instances specific determination of which factor is deficient requires specific factor assays or comparison of the patient's plasma with other plasmas with known deficiencies.

SOURCE OF REAGENTS

Most of the reagents may be purchased from any manufacturer. However, a few are special items available from a limited number of sources. These are as follows:

1. *Dried rabbit brain* may be purchased as "Tissue Thromboplastin" from the manufacturers listed in Chap. A34.

2. *Asolectin* may be purchased from Associated Concentrates, 32–30 61st St., Woodside, NY 11377, or P.O. Box 4056, Atlanta, Ga.

3. *Phospholipid emulsions (platelet substitutes).* The following reagents have been found satisfactory:

Activated Platelet Factor Reagent, Baltimore Biological Laboratories, Box 6711, Baltimore, MD 21204.

Activated Cephaloplastin, Dade Reagents, Inc., 1851 Delaware Parkway, Miami, Fla.

Hyland Partial Thromboplastin, Hyland Laboratories, 4587 Brazil St., Los Angeles, Calif.

Thrombofax, Ortho Pharmaceutical Corporation, Diagnostic Division, Route 202, Raritan, NJ 08869.

Platelin, Warner-Chilcott Laboratories, P.O. Box W, Morris Plains, NJ 07950.

4. *Aluminum hydroxide gel* prepared by Harleco, 60 St. and Woodland Ave., Philadelphia, PA 19143, may be purchased from Scientific Products, 1210 Leon Place, Evanston, IL 60201. Cutter Laboratories, Berkeley, Calif., also makes a satisfactory preparation.

5. *Barium sulfate*, powder, reagent grade, from any manufacturer is satisfactory.

References

1. Bell, W. N., and Alton, H. G.: A brain extract as a substitute for platelet suspensions in the thromboplastin generation test. *Nature* 174:880, 1954.
2. Proctor, R. R., and Rapaport, S. I.: The partial thromboplastin time with kaolin; simple screening test for first stage plasma clotting factor deficiencies. *Am. J. Clin. Pathol.* 36:212, 1961.
3. Basu, D., Gallus, A., Hirsh, J., and Cade, J.: A prospective study of the value of monitoring heparin treatment with the activated partial thromboplastin time. *N. Engl. J. Med.* 287:324, 1972.
4. Poller, L.: Quality control in blood coagulation, in *Blood Coagulation and Haemostasis*, 2d ed., edited by J. M. Thomson. Churchill Livingstone, New York, 1980, p. 331.

CHAPTER *A34*

One-stage prothrombin time

CECIL HOUGIE

PURPOSE OF THE TEST

This test measures the coagulant activity of the "extrinsic" system, including fibrinogen, prothrombin, and factors V, VII, and X. It is widely used to monitor the effects of the coumarin anticoagulants, as well as to study patients with congenital or acquired coagulation disorders.

PRINCIPLE OF THE TEST

When calcium and an extract of tissue such as brain are added to plasma, the factor VII in the plasma reacts with the tissue factor to form a reaction product which converts factor X to its activated form, factor Xa; this in turn reacts with factor V, calcium, and the phospholipid in the tissue extract to form extrinsic prothrombinase, which converts prothrombin to thrombin. Thrombin then converts fibrinogen to fibrin. The rate of fibrin formation depends on the concentration of factors V, VII, and X, prothrombin, and fibrinogen, and the test measures the overall activity of these factors.

REAGENTS

1. Tissue "thromboplastin" (tissue factor):

a. Owren's buffer is used for the final dilution of the thromboplastin. It is prepared by mixing 11.75 g sodium diethyl barbiturate, 14.67 g sodium chloride, and 400 ml 0.1 N hydrochloric acid. The pH is measured, and sufficient acid is added to bring it to 7.3 (usually a total of 430 ml of acid will be required). Distilled water is then added to bring the total volume to 2000 ml. The resultant solution should have a pH of 7.35.

b. Saline extract of human brain. A whole human brain is freed from blood vessels and meninges. The tissue is washed under tap water and then emulsified by means of a mechanical homogenizer (blender) for 60 s in 1.5 liters of 0.85% NaCl which has been heated to 45°C. The emulsion is then centrifuged for 15 min at $500 \times g$ and the sediment discarded. A small amount of supernatant is removed and diluted 1:2, 1:4, and 1:8 with 0.85% NaCl. The activity of the undiluted material and each of the dilutions is then tested by using them as the source of thromboplastin in the one-stage prothrombin time test with normal plasma. The remainder of the supernatant suspension is then diluted with 0.85% NaCl (adjusted to pH 7 by addition of 0.5 N NaOH, if necessary) so that it will be equivalent to the concentration which gave the minimum one-stage prothrombin time; this should be between 12 and 15 s. Finally a volume of Owren's buffer (prepared as described above) equal to one-tenth of the total volume of the extract is added. The extract is then distributed into containers in amounts suitable for a day's supply. These are tightly stoppered and stored frozen at −20°C.

c. Commercial tissue thromboplastins are nearly all ex-

TABLE A34-1 Relative sensitivities of commercial reagents compared with the British comparative thromboplastin* [2]

Thromboplastin	Mean ratio
British comparative thromboplastin	2.96
Thrombotest	2.47
Thromborel	1.91
Diagen (phenolized)	1.87
Simplastin A	1.83
Diagen (freeze-dried)	1.74
Ortho	1.63
Dade thromboplastin "C"	1.61
Boehringer	1.57
Hyland	1.55
Simplastin	1.52
Dade activated (liquid)	1.48
Dade (freeze-dried)	1.47

*The mean prothrombin time ratios of 12 coumarin-treated patients were determined using a variety of commercial reagents and the BCT. The ratio is obtained by dividing the patient's prothrombin time by the control prothrombin time. Fresh normal plasmas were collected from six healthy adult males on the day of testing.

tracts of acetone-dried rabbit brain or lung, or both. Sources of these preparations are listed at the end of this chapter.

2. Calcium chloride solution. This solution is described under "Recalcification Time Test," Chap. A33.

TECHNIQUE

1. Platelet-poor plasma is prepared as described under "Recalcification Time Test," Chap. A33.

2. Performance of the test. One volume of a brain suspension is mixed with an equal volume of 0.025 M calcium chloride and the mixture placed in a water bath at 37°C. One-tenth milliliter of the test plasma is pipetted into a 12- by 75-mm tube immediately prior to testing. The tube is placed in the water bath at 37°C for 1 min. Two-tenths milliliter of the brain suspension–calcium chloride mixture is added to the plasma, and a stopwatch is started immediately. The clotting time is determined by observing the appearance of the first fibrin strands in the reaction mixture while tilting the tube so that the mixture runs about halfway up the side.

Alternatively, 0.1 ml of brain extract may be added to 0.1 ml of the test plasma and, exactly 1 min later, 0.1 ml of 0.025 M calcium chloride added.

Each test should be performed in triplicate and the three results averaged. It is essential to have a normal control for each series of unknowns. While it is preferable to use fresh normal blood collected at approximately the same time as the test plasma, frozen platelet-poor citrated plasma obtained from three or more normal subjects may be used. This plasma should be separated as soon as possible after collection and frozen in small aliquots, each sufficient for four or five tests. The prothrombin time of this plasma may remain constant for as long as 28 days, but it is important to test an aliquot of it at regular intervals against a fresh normal control. Commercial plasma controls may also be used. Sources are listed at the end of this chapter.

The brain extract should give a normal control value between 12 and 16 s. This value should be consistently the same on a day-to-day basis and should not vary more than 0.5 from the mean value. This result can be readily achieved if a satisfactory standardized brain extract is used [1].

METHODS OF RECORDING RESULTS

The simplest and perhaps the best method of recording the results of this test is to give the patient's time together with that of the control. A method which is not recommended is to express the results as a percentage concentration.

The most useful parameter in monitoring anticoagulant therapy with vitamin K antagonists is the ratio of the patient's prothrombin time to that of the normal control [2]. There are important differences in the sensitivity of the various types of tissue thromboplastin, and so the ratio obtained with them on a plasma sample from a patient taking coumadin will vary. Comparative ratios with the different types of thromboplastin are shown in Table A34-1. In general, saline extracts of human brain, such as the British comparative thromboplastin (BCT), are the most sensitive and activated rabbit brain extracts are the least sensitive. The ratio with the BCT should not exceed 4:1, but with most of the other preparations the ratio should not exceed 2:1. The lower limit is more difficult to define and varies with the clinical disorder under treatment, but a ratio of 2:1 with the BCT is probably the lowest effective level. The therapeutic range of most of the rabbit brain preparations, and these are the most widely used in the United States, is very narrow compared to the BCT. This allows a margin of only a few seconds in the prothrombin time between a level of anticoagulation which is ineffective therapeutically and one which suggests the patient is overdosed and in danger of bleeding.

INTERPRETATION

The prothrombin time is prolonged when one or more of the following events occur: factor V, VII, X, or prothrombin is deficient; the fibrinogen is below 100 mg/dl; heparin or fibrin- or fibrinogen-split products are present. In polycythemia the prothrombin time may be prolonged as a result of a disproportionately high ratio of anticoagulant to plasma. Another cause is nonspecific shortening of the prothrombin time of the control plasma, which may be as much as 2 s in 3 or 4 h. Thus if the test plasma is collected several hours after the control plasma and both tested simultaneously, the test plasma, if normal, will appear to have a longer prothrombin time than that of the control.

Different values on the same plasma sample are sometimes obtained with extracts of brains from different animal species, and even with those of the same species, although the latter differences are not marked. In hemophilia B^M, the one-stage prothrombin time is normal with human brain, but with bovine brain the prothrombin time is at least twice that of the normal control (Chap. 152). The same observation has been made on some patients with cirrhosis.

SOURCES OF REAGENTS

1. Tissue thromboplastin (tissue factor) may be purchased from the following sources:

Calsoplastin, Baltimore Biological Laboratories, Box 6711, Baltimore, MD 21204

Activated Thromboplastin, Dade Reagents, Inc., 1851 Delaware Parkway, Miami, Fla.

Bacto Thromboplastin, Difco Laboratories, 920 Henry St., Detroit, MI 48201

Hyland Thromboplastin, Hyland Laboratories, 4587 Brazil St., Los Angeles, Calif.

Ortho Brain Thromboplastin (OBT), Ortho Pharmaceutical Corporation, Diagnostic Division, Route 202, Raritan, NJ 08869

Simplastin, Warner-Chilcott Laboratories, P.O. Box W, Morris Plains, NJ 07950

2. Control plasmas may be purchased from the following sources:

Ortho Plasma Coagulation Control (PCC), Ortho Pharmaceutical Corporation, Diagnostic Division, Route 202, Raritan, NJ 08869

Verify Normal Citrate, Warner-Chilcott Laboratories, Box W, Morris Plains, NJ 07950

References

1. Quick, A. J.: *Hemorrhagic Diseases and Thrombosis,* 2d ed. Lea & Febiger, Philadelphia, 1966.
2. Thomson, J. M.: Laboratory control of anticoagulant therapy, in *Blood Coagulation and Haemostasis,* edited by J. M. Thomson, Churchill Livingstone, New York, 1980, p. 249.

CHAPTER *A35*

Methods for estimating fibrinogen concentration

CECIL HOUGIE

Thrombin time test

PURPOSE OF THE TEST
The thrombin time test is used to screen for marked reductions in fibrinogen concentration and for the presence of fibrin or fibrinogen split products.

PRINCIPLE OF THE TEST
Fibrinogen can be assayed by several methods based on different principles [1]. The principle used in the thrombin time test is that thrombin attacks fibrinogen directly to convert it to fibrin. The time taken for plasma to clot on addition of thrombin is referred to as the *thrombin time.* Calcium accelerates this reaction but is not added in the thrombin time test. The rate of clotting with thrombin is a function of fibrinogen concentration or of the concentration of inhibitors that prevent the thrombin-fibrinogen reaction.

REAGENTS
1. Thrombin. The thrombin may be of either bovine or human origin. The dried powder should be reconstituted in 0.85% NaCl so that a clotting time of 9 to 11 s is obtained with pooled normal plasma when the test is carried out as outlined below. Usually the strength of the thrombin is 5 to 10 units per milliliter so a vial containing 5000 units of bovine thrombin would yield 50 to 100 ml of solution, which can be diluted 1:10 prior to use. A weaker thrombin solution giving a normal time

between 25 and 35 s should also be used. The two thrombin solutions are then placed in small tubes and stored at $-20°C$; they are remarkably stable under these conditions.

2. Normal plasma. Small aliquots of a batch of pooled normal citrated plasma which have been frozen and stored at $-20°C$ may be used as the control whenever a test is to be performed.

TECHNIQUE
1. The patient's platelet-poor citrated plasma is prepared as described in Chap. A33.
2. Performance of the test. Mixtures of 0.1 ml of the patient's citrated plasma and 0.1 ml of 0.85% NaCl are warmed to 37°C in a water bath. One-tenth milliliter of thrombin solution warmed to 37°C is added to the mixture. A stopwatch is started on the addition of the thrombin, and the clotting time is recorded. The thrombin time should be determined with both concentrations of thrombin. Tubes of the thrombin solutions should be maintained in melting ice and warmed to 37°C just prior to use. Controls are run at the same time on mixtures of 0.1 ml of normal plasma and 0.1 ml of 0.85% NaCl. If the thrombin time is prolonged, a mixture of equal parts of the patient's plasma and normal plasma should be tested in the same manner as the patient's plasma.

INTERPRETATION
With the stronger solution, a value of 3 s or more longer than that of the normal control is considered abnormal; with the weaker solution, the corresponding value is 5 s or more longer than that of the control for that strength. The test is abnormal if there is a qualitative change in fibrinogen (Chap. 153), if there is a fall in fibrinogen concentration to below 100 mg/dl, or if an antithrombic substance such as heparin or breakdown products of fibrinogen or fibrin is present.

If the test is abnormal, the thrombin time of 0.1 ml of a mixture of equal parts of normal and patient's plasma should be tested. If the thrombin time of the mixture is 4 s or more longer than that of the normal plasma alone, the presence of an antithrombic substance should be considered. The clot should be inspected at the end of 10 min and compared with that of the normal control; if a very fragile clot is seen, a low fibrinogen level is indicated.

Fibrinogen titer test

PURPOSE OF THE TEST
This test is used to estimate the concentration of fibrinogen in plasma.

PRINCIPLE OF THE TEST
The concentration of fibrinogen in plasma is such that when thrombin is added to serial dilutions of the plasma in buffered saline, a clot is normally visible at a final dilution of 1 in 64 and usually at 1 in 128.

REAGENTS
1. Thrombin. The more concentrated thrombin solution prepared for the thrombin time test (see above) should be used.
2. Buffered saline. A solution is prepared of 8.5 g of NaCl and 1.21 g of tris base dissolved in 950 ml of water. The pH is adjusted to 7.2 with 1 N HCl and the volume brought to 1 liter.

TECHNIQUE

1. Citrated platelet-poor plasma is prepared from the patient's blood as described in Chap. A33. Frozen pooled normal plasma may be used as the control.

2. Performance of the test. The following serial dilutions of patient and control plasma are prepared in buffered saline: 1 in 8, 1 in 16, 1 in 32, and 1 in 64. One milliliter of the thrombin solution is added to 1 ml of each dilution of plasma. Having been mixed, the tubes are left undisturbed in a 37°C water bath and inspected approximately 15 and 30 min after the addition of the thrombin. To evaluate systemic fibrinolysis, the clots which form may be observed after incubation at 37°C for 2 h.

INTERPRETATION

If a clot is seen in the 1 in 32 dilution of patient plasma (final dilution 1 in 64), a clinically significant quantitative abnormality in fibrinogen can be excluded (fibrinogen concentration > 100 mg/dl). Lysis of the clots after 2 h at 37°C indicates increased systemic fibrinolysis.

SOURCE OF REAGENTS

Thrombin. Bovine thrombin may be purchased as Thrombin, Topical, from Parke, Davis & Company, Detroit, MI 48232.

Human thrombin may be purchased as Fibrindex from Ortho Pharmaceutical Corporation, Diagnostic Division, Route 202, Raritan, NJ 08869.

Reference

1. Exper, T., Burridge, J., Power, P., and Rickard, K. A.: An evaluation of currently available methods for plasma fibrinogen. *Am. J. Clin. Pathol.* 71:521, 1979.

CHAPTER *A36*

Latex particle agglutination test for fibrin or fibrinogen degradation products

CECIL HOUGIE

PURPOSE OF THE TEST

The test detects the presence of fibrin or fibrinogen degradation products (FDP) in serum and is helpful in the diagnosis of disseminated intravascular clotting (DIC).

PRINCIPLE OF THE TEST

Antisera to highly purified preparations of human fibrinogen fragments D and E are adsorbed onto latex particles. These clump in the presence of fibrinogen or FDP.

REAGENTS

1. Latex suspension. This is a 0.5% suspension of polystyrene latex particles coated with rabbit antibody to FDP.

2. Positive and negative control sera. The positive control is normal human plasma diluted with normal human serum so that the fibrinogen concentration is 5 to 10 μg/ml. The negative control is normal serum containing less than 2 μg of FDP per milliliter.

3. Sample collection tubes. Each tube contains soybean trypsin inhibitor (approximately 3600 NF units) and bovine thrombin (20 NIH units), sufficient for the collection of 2 ml whole blood or urine.

4. Glycine-saline buffer. Glycine 7.5 g, NaCl 8.5 g, and sodium azide 1.0 g are dissolved in 900 ml of water. The pH is adjusted to 8.2 with 0.2 N NaOH, and the solution is diluted to 1 liter with distilled water. The buffer is stored at 4°C.

TECHNIQUE

Two milliliters of blood collected in a syringe by clean venipuncture is placed in a sample collection tube and immediately mixed by inverting several times. The blood clots within a few seconds and then is incubated at 37°C for approximately 30 min. If the patient has received heparin and the blood fails to clot, 0.2 ml of Reptilase should be added to the specimen. The serum is separated by centrifugation. It is then diluted 1:5 and 1:20 with the glycine buffer and a drop of each dilution placed on a slide. After the latex suspension is mixed by vigorous shaking, one drop is added to each of the diluted serum samples on the slides. The diluted serum/latex mixture is stirred with a mixing rod and the slides rocked gently for exactly 2 min while macroscopic agglutination is watched for. This, if present, is readily appreciated visually. A known negative and positive control should be run with each test.

INTERPRETATION

The normal serum level of FDP is less than 10 μg/ml [1], and the reagents are so adjusted that serum with less than this concentration will give no agglutination with either 1:5 or 1:20 dilutions of normal serum. In DIC the level of FDP exceeds 10 μg and in acute cases may exceed 40 μg. However, similar increases may be found in other states involving enzymatic (other than thrombin) or nonenzymatic degradation of fibrinogen [2]. Increased levels are sometimes found in deep-vein thrombosis and pulmonary embolism, but such increases are very transient.

SOURCE OF REAGENTS

A kit containing all the necessary supplies and reagents is available from Wellcome Reagents Division, Burroughs Wellcome Co., Research Triangle Park, NC 27709.

Reptilase is available from Abbott Laboratory Diagnostic Division, North Chicago, IL 60064.

References

1. Merskey, C., Johnson, A. J., Kleiner, G. J., and Wohl, H.: The defibrination syndrome: Clinical features and laboratory diagnosis. *Br. J. Haematol.* 13:528, 1967.
2. Merskey, C.: Defibrination syndrome or ? *Blood* 41:599, 1973.

CHAPTER *A37*

Immunoprecipitation assay for factor VIII–related antigen (von Willebrand's factor antigen)

CECIL HOUGIE

PURPOSE OF THE TEST

The test measures the concentration of factor VIII–related antigen (FVIIIR:Ag), also known as von Willebrand's factor antigen, and is used for the diagnosis of von Willebrand's disease.

PRINCIPLE OF THE TEST

Antibodies prepared in rabbits against crude factor VIII/von Willebrand factor (FVIII/vWF) preparations give a precipitin reaction with a factor that is present in normal plasma but decreased or absent in von Willebrand's disease [1,2]. The immunoassay is performed by the Laurell technique, which is an electroimmunodiffusion method for the quantitation of proteins [3], in which rocket-shaped anodic immunoprecipitates are formed. The area enclosed by the precipitate or, for practical purposes, the height of the "rocket," is proportional to the concentration of FVIIIR:Ag (von Willebrand's factor antigen).

REAGENTS

1. Buffer. This is 0.05 M barbital sodium containing 0.1% sodium azide. The solution is adjusted to pH 8.4 with HCl and NaOH. It is used for dissolving the agarose and as the electrophoresis buffer.

2. Antibody. This is prepared by immunizing rabbits with a cryoprecipitate prepared from normal plasma or with the void volume material from a Sepharose 4B or 6B column following application of cryoprecipitate or plasma. Suitable preparations are available commercially. Sources are listed at the end of this chapter.

3. Agarose plates. One gram of agarose is dissolved in 100 ml of the barbital buffer by heating in boiling water. When the agarose solution is clear, it is dispensed in 5-ml aliquots into stoppered tubes and stored at 4°C. The agarose is liquefied by placing the tube in a bath of boiling water. It is then allowed to cool at 56°C, when the antibody is added and mixed well by inverting the tube several times. The amount of antibody to be added depends on the titer and is determined by trial and error; it is usually 50 to 100 μl for 5 ml of agarose, and this amount of agarose is sufficient to cover a 2- by 3-in. glass slide. The agarose-antibody mixture is poured on the slide and allowed to solidify; surface tension holds the mixture on the slide, and no special device is needed. Ten 3-mm holes are then punched about 6 mm apart in a line 15 mm from the edge along the longer side of the slide, either by hand or with a commercial puncher. The gel plugs are aspirated with suction.

TECHNIQUE

The plate is placed in the electrophoresis chamber, and moistened filter-paper wicks are applied to the longer sides. These overlap the agarose by about 1 cm and extend into the electrophoresis buffer (0.05 M sodium barbital containing 0.1% sodium azide; pH 8.4). The wells are filled with 10-μl samples (see below), and a constant current of 6.5 mA per slide is applied for 15 to 16 h at room temperature. During the run the voltage may drop slightly.

Pooled normal plasma which has been divided into small aliquots and frozen is used as the standard. This is diluted 1:2, 1:4, 1:8, and 1:16 in saline, and a sample of each dilution is placed in a well. Either plasma or serum from the patient may be used, and these samples are tested after dilution 1 in 2 with saline. The specimens may be kept frozen at −20°C for several months. Each diluted patient sample is tested in duplicate.

When the electrophoresis run is completed, the plate is removed and examined over a side-lighted dark background. The rockets are often hard to see, and the visibility can be increased by immersing the plate in 1 to 2% tannic acid in distilled water for a few minutes. The heights of the rockets are measured from the center of the well to the tip of the rocket. To draw the standard curve from which the percent concentrations of the unknown values are determined, the rocket length on an arithmetic scale is plotted against concentration of plasma in percent on a log scale. The percent of von Willebrand's antigen in the patient's plasma or serum is then determined from the calibration curve.

INTERPRETATION

A value below 50 percent is consistent with von Willibrand's disease, 50 to 60 percent is borderline, and values above 60 percent are normal. A high value may be found at times in patients with known von Willebrand's disease (for example, after hepatitis or during pregnancy [4]). This test should therefore be repeated at least twice after an interval of several weeks or even months if a normal result is obtained on a patient strongly suspected of having the disease. Rare variants of the disease are reported in which the von Willebrand's factor is present but inactive [5].

SOURCE OF REAGENTS

1. Sepharose 4B or 6B, Pharmacia Fine Chemicals, Inc., 800 Centennial Ave., Piscataway, NJ 08854.

2. Lyophilized cryoprecipitate, Armour Pharmaceutical Company, 2319 N. Hathaway St., Santa Ana, CA 92701, or Abbot Scientific Products Division, 820 Mission St., South Pasadena, CA 91030.

3. Agarose, Sea-Kem Industries, distributed by Bausch and Lomb, Rochester, N.Y.

4. Factor VIII antibody, Nordic Immunological Laboratories, Langestraat 57-61, Tilburg, The Netherlands, or Behring Diagnostics, American Hoechst Corporation, Somerville, NJ 08876, or Calbiochem-Behring Corporation, P.O. Box 12087, San Diego, CA 92112.

5. Electrophoresis equipment, LKB #2117 Multiphore Electrophoresis Apparatus, LKB Instruments, Inc., 12221 Parklawn Drive, Rockville, MD 20852, and Buchler Regulated Power Supply, Scientific Products, 17111 Red Hill Ave., Irvine, CA 92714.

6. Alumina gel (C-γ, A Grade), Calbiochem, P.O. Box 12087, San Diego, CA 92112.

References

1. Zimmerman, T. S., Ratnoff, O. D., and Powell, A. E.: Immunologic differentiation of classic hemophilia (factor VIII deficiency) and von Willebrand's disease. *J. Clin. Invest. 50:*244, 1971.
2. Olson, J. D., Brockway, W. J., Fass, D. N., Magnuson, M. A., and Bowie, E. J.: Evaluation of ristocetin–Willebrand factor assay and ristocetin-induced platelet aggregation. *Am. J. Clin. Pathol. 63:*210, 1975.
3. Laurell, C. B.: Quantitative estimation of proteins by electrophoresis in agarose gel containing antibodies. *Anal. Biochem. 15:*43, 1966.
4. Bennett, B., and Ratnoff, O. D.: Antihemophilic factor (AHF, factor VIII) procoagulant activity and AHF-like antigen in normal pregnancy and following exercise and pneumonoencephalography. *J. Lab. Clin. Med. 80:*256, 1972.
5. Kernoff, P. B. A., Gruson, R., and Rizza, C. R.: A variant of factor VIII related antigen. *Br. J. Haematol. 26:*435, 1974.

forms. The tubes are maintained at 37°C and the clots observed for lysis at intervals. The end point is total lysis of the clot, and the euglobulin lysis time is the interval between clotting and complete lysis.

INTERPRETATION

The normal value for complete lysis by this procedure ranges from 90 min to 6 h. The test is not specific and is believed to reflect activator activity primarily. The results may be difficult to interpret when the fibrinogen concentration is decreased, for under these circumstances normal fibrinolytic activity may dissolve a small clot somewhat more rapidly than normal, thus giving a false impression of the level of fibrinolytic activity. The test may be of value in monitoring treatment with urokinase or streptokinase.

CHAPTER *A38*

Euglobulin lysis time

CECIL HOUGIE

PURPOSE OF THE TEST
This test is utilized to evaluate systemic fibrinolysis.

PRINCIPLE OF THE TEST
The euglobulin fraction of plasma prepared by dilution and acidification is relatively free of inhibitors of the fibrinolytic enzyme system, and therefore lysis of the clot formed from the fibrinogen in the euglobin precipitate occurs relatively rapidly. The time it takes for the clot to lyse is referred to as the *euglobulin lysis time.*

REAGENTS
1. Acetic acid. A solution is made by diluting 13.5 ml of 1% (v/v) acetic acid to 1000 ml with distilled water; the final pH of this solution should be 3.65 to 3.70.
2. Borate buffer. A borate buffer solution (pH 9.0) is prepared by placing 9 g of sodium chloride and 1 g of sodium borate in a 1-liter volumetric flask and bringing the solution to volume with distilled water.

TECHNIQUE
Four and one-half milliliters of whole blood is collected in a chilled centrifuge tube containing 0.5 ml of 0.1 M sodium citrate. The mixture is placed on ice and as soon as possible centrifuged in the cold at $2000 \times g$ for 10 min. The plasma is separated and kept on ice.

The test is performed in duplicate. One-half milliliter of plasma is added to 9.5 ml of acetic acid solution and thoroughly mixed. The tubes are refrigerated for 30 min at 4°C and then centrifuged at $2000 \times g$ for 10 min. The supernatant fluid is discarded and the precipitate reconstituted in 0.5 ml of the borate buffer, using a glass stirring rod. When the precipitate is fully dissolved, the solution is placed in a water bath at 37°C for 2 min. One-half milliliter of 0.025 M CaCl$_2$ is added, which will cause the solution to clot. A timer is started when the clot

CHAPTER *A39*

Screening test for factor XIII deficiency

CECIL HOUGIE

PURPOSE OF THE TEST
This test detects a clinically significant deficiency of factor XIII activity.

PRINCIPLE OF THE TEST
Clots formed in normal plasma are insoluble in 5 M urea because of the action of factor XIII.

REAGENTS
1. Either platelet-poor or platelet-rich plasma may be used (see Chap. A33).
2. A 5-M solution of urea (300 g of reagent-grade urea dissolved in water to make 1 liter of solution).
3. A 0.85% NaCl solution.

TECHNIQUE
The recalcification time test is performed in duplicate as outlined in Chap. A33, using platelet-poor or platelet-rich plasma. Twenty to thirty minutes after formation of a clot, 1 ml of 5 M urea is added to one tube, and to the other 1 ml of 0.85% NaCl is added. A similar test is performed on a normal control. The four tubes are left in the water bath at 37°C overnight and inspected the following morning.

INTERPRETATION
Disappearance of the clot is abnormal and is evidence of factor XIII deficiency.

Reference

1. Alami, S. Y., Hampton, J. W., Race, G. J., and Speer, R. J.: Fibrin stabilizing factor (factor XIII). *Am. J. Med. 44:*1, 1968.

Bleeding time

CECIL HOUGIE

PURPOSE OF THE TEST

The bleeding time is used as a screening test for disorders of platelet function, both congenital and acquired, and for von Willebrand's disease.

PRINCIPLE OF THE TEST

The time taken for bleeding from a standardized skin wound to cease is referred to as the *bleeding time*. It is a measure of platelet function and is independent of the coagulation mechanism, although with severe impairment of clotting the bleeding time may be prolonged.

REAGENTS

No reagents are required for these tests.

TECHNIQUE

In all these methods, the bleeding time is the interval between puncture of the skin and cessation of bleeding.

DUKE'S METHOD

A puncture is made in the lobe of an ear to a depth of about 3 mm with a disposable lancet. The ear lobe should be warm but should not be cleansed with alcohol or rubbed vigorously. As soon as the puncture is made, a stopwatch is started. The blood should flow freely, and the lobe must not be squeezed. At 15-s intervals the drops of blood which have exuded from the wound are absorbed into a piece of filter paper, which is held so that it will not touch the surface of the ear.

IVY METHOD

A blood-pressure cuff is placed around the patient's upper arm and the pressure raised to 40 mmHg. Three small punctures are made along the outer surface of the patient's forearm, taking care to avoid superficial veins. The drops of blood issuing from the three bleeding points are absorbed at intervals of 10 s into three filter paper discs, one for each puncture wound, until bleeding ceases. The average of the times required for bleeding to stop from the three puncture wounds is taken as the bleeding time. A spring lancet set at 3 mm is usually recommended, but a disposable lancet or Hagedorn needle is better. It should be noted that setting the lancet at 3 mm does not ensure that the puncture will be 3 mm deep, as the depth of the wound depends on several other variables. A spring lancet must be autoclaved after each use.

MODIFIED IVY METHOD USING A SIMPLATE [1]

This method utilizes a disposable, spring-loaded device that has either one (Simplate I) or two (Simplate II) blades that are released when the activating trigger is pressed. The single-blade model makes a single incision 6 mm long by 1 mm deep, and the two-blade device makes two such incisions. An area of forearm about 5 cm distal to the antecubital fossa and free of superficial veins is selected, cleaned with alcohol, and allowed to dry. A blood pressure cuff is placed above the antecubital fossa and the pressure maintained at 40 mmHg throughout the procedure. The Simplate device is placed firmly on the arm without pressure so that the incision(s) will be parallel to the fold of the elbow. The trigger is depressed and the stopwatch started. At 30-s intervals, the blood is absorbed as described for the Ivy technique. The patient must be warned that there may be some faint scarring.

INTERPRETATION

Aspirin and a large number of other drugs (see Chap. 147) can cause prolongation of the bleeding time, and this may be the explanation of some of the high upper limits of normal quoted in the literature. The patient must therefore be instructed to avoid all medications if possible, especially aspirin or any preparation containing aspirin, for 1 week before the test. If aspirin has been ingested, the test should be postponed for 1 week. Acetaminophen may be taken as an analgesic, if necessary.

The normal range using the Duke method is 1 to 3½ min, with a value of 4 min or more being definitely abnormal. The upper limit of the normal range with the Ivy method is 5 min, but a value up to 7 min is accepted as normal by some workers. With the modified Ivy method, the normal range is 2½ to 7½ min, with a mean of 5 min; after ingestion of aspirin the range is 4 to 21 min [1].

Reference

1. Kumar, R., Ansell, J. E., Canoso, R. T., and Deykin, D.: Clinical trial of a new bleeding device. *Am. J. Clin. Pathol. 70*:642, 1978.

Platelet adhesiveness (retention)

HARVEY J. WEISS

PURPOSE OF THE TEST

The adhesion of platelets to the surfaces of an injured blood vessel constitutes one of the earliest stages in the hemostatic process. Platelet adhesion also plays a significant role in the formation of a thrombus. A number of tests have been introduced which measure the adhesive properties of platelets. Decreased adhesiveness has been reported in some patients with bleeding disorders, and increased adhesiveness has been reported in some patients who were predisposed to thrombosis.

PRINCIPLE OF THE TEST

The adhesion of platelets to "foreign surfaces" has been measured by a variety of methods which have been reviewed [1,2]. The methods which have been used most frequently are the roller flask technique of H. P. Wright, the use of glass wool columns, and various modifications of tests in which blood is filtered through glass bead columns. The latter are frequently referred to as the Salzman method. Borchgrevink has also devised a test in which the adhesion of platelets at the site of a small skin incision is determined [3]. The principle of all these tests is the same. The decrease in platelet count which occurs when blood is allowed to contact a foreign surface for a standardized period of time is determined. This decrease is indicative, in part, of the number of platelets which have adhered to the foreign surface, and this value, expressed as a percentage of the original platelet count, has been called the platelet adhesiveness. It should be emphasized, however, that some of the loss of platelets in glass bead filters is also due to platelet aggregation, and it has been suggested that *platelet retention* be used as an alternative term [4–6]. A method for measuring the adhesion of platelets in anticoagulated blood to the subendothelium of rabbit aorta under arterial flow conditions has been developed (Baumgartner method [7]) but is used primarily for research purposes.

REAGENTS AND EQUIPMENT
The tests most commonly used at present are those in which blood is filtered through glass bead columns [4]. The principle of this test is simple, but the number of variations is wide, and the ability to obtain meaningful results depends on a number of poorly understood technical factors, such as flow rate, column length, and bead characteristics [8,9]. A method using heparinized blood has also been reported [8]. The method described below is only one of many variations which have been described.

1. Scalp vein infusion set. Abbott, 19-G Thinwall Needle (18-G bore), Abbott Laboratories, North Chicago, Ill.
2. Glass beads. "Superbrite" glass beads, Type 070-5005, average diameter 0.0185 in., Minnesota Mining and Manufacturing Co.
3. Plastic tubing. Polyvinyl tubing (I.D. 0.113 in.), Insulon Medical Tubing, Insul-Tab, Inc., Woburn, Mass.
4. Metal connectors. Becton-Dickinson adapter ML/ML.
5. Bead filter. A piece of nylon mesh is glued (Duco cement) to one end of a metal connector and is then inserted into one end of a length of plastic tubing. The tubing is packed with 0.7 g of unwashed beads, and the other end is then sealed with a second, similarly constructed connector. One end of the filter is connected by a small length of plastic tubing to a 35-ml syringe (Roehr, Monoject). When completed, the male adapter at the free end of the filter is ready for attachment to the scalp vein infusion set.
6. Infusion-withdrawal pump. Harvard Apparatus, Dover, Mass., model 1100, 8 rpm.
7. 15% tripotassium EDTA solution.

TECHNIQUE
A tourniquet is placed around the arm, the needle of the scalp vein infusion set is inserted into the antecubital vein, and a 2-ml sample of blood is obtained and placed in a tube containing 0.02 ml of 15% K_3EDTA (first "no-glass" specimen). The female adapter of the scalp vein set is quickly attached to the male adapter on the free end of a glass bead filter which is attached, by the syringe, to the infusion-withdrawal pump. Beginning with the first appearance of blood at the tip of the syringe, blood is collected for 30 s and filtered blood is then expelled into a second EDTA tube (first "glass" specimen). A second filter is then affixed to the pump and the process repeated. Fi-

nally, a second no-glass sample is obtained. The platelets in each tube are counted by any standard technique.

CALCULATION OF RESULTS
The platelet counts in the two no-glass specimens are averaged. The difference between this value, which is the platelet count of venous blood, and that in the filtered (i.e., glass) specimens, indicates the number of platelets which have been retained in the filter. This value, expressed as a percentage of the venous platelet count, is the platelet adhesiveness.

INTERPRETATION
In 58 normal subjects tested by the method described above, the mean value for platelet adhesiveness was 56.3 percent with a standard deviation of 13.1. The 95 percent confidence limits for these values were 31 and 83 percent [5].

As indicated earlier, the number of platelets which are retained in the glass bead filters depends, among other things, on the length of the filter, the quality and quantity of the beads, and the flow rate. A decrease in platelet adhesiveness in patients with von Willebrand's disease [4] has been repeatedly confirmed [5,6]. The flow rate of the blood through the filter is of critical importance, and some of the problems which have been encountered in filtering the blood into Vacutainer tubes may have been the result of inconstancy of the vacuum provided in these tubes. If the flow rates are too high, low adhesiveness values may be obtained in normal subjects; with rates that are too low, the values in von Willebrand's disease may be normal [5]. Whatever method is used, it is advisable that each laboratory establish its own range of normal values. The use of this test in diagnosing von Willebrand's disease is discussed in Chap. 155. Decreased values may be found in patients with intrinsic platelet disorders as well as in those with von Willebrand's disease (see Chaps. 146 and 147). Thus, abnormalities are not diagnostic of any one disorder. Increased values of platelet adhesiveness have been reported in some patients predisposed to venous or arterial thrombosis. In general, however, abnormalities in platelet adhesiveness have been reported with less frequency in patients predisposed to thrombosis than in those with bleeding disorders.

SOURCES OF REAGENTS AND EQUIPMENT
These are indicated under "Reagents and Equipment," above. A convenient source of nylon mesh (opening 0.002 in.) is the filter from a clinical-blood-solution administration set. Nylon mesh may also be obtained commercially.

References

1. Hartmann, R. C.: Tests of platelet adhesiveness and their clinical significance. *Semin. Hematol.* 5:60, 1968.
2. Hellem, A. J.: Platelet adhesiveness. *Ser. Haematol.* 1:2, 1968.
3. Borchgrevink, C. F.: A method for measuring platelet adhesiveness *in vivo. Acta Med. Scand.* 168:157, 1960.
4. Salzman, E. W.: Measurement of platelet adhesiveness: A simple *in vitro* technique demonstrating an abnormality in von Willebrand's disease. *J. Lab. Clin. Med.* 62:724, 1963.
5. Weiss, H. J.: Von Willebrand's disease: Diagnosis criteria. *Blood* 32:668, 1968.
6. Salzman, E. W.: Von Willebrand's disease: A platelet disorder, in *The Platelet,* edited by K. M. Brinkhous, R. W. Shermer, and F. K. Mostofi. Williams & Wilkins, Baltimore, 1971, p. 251.
7. Baumgartner, H. R.: The role of blood flow in platelet adhesion, fibrin deposition and formation of mural thrombi. *Microvasc. Res.* 5:167, 1973.

8. Bowie, E. J. W., Owen, C. A., Jr., Thompson, J. H., Jr., and Didisheim, P.: Platelet adhesiveness in von Willebrand's disease. *Am. J. Clin. Pathol.* 52:69, 1969.

9. Bowie, E. J. W., and Owen, C. A., Jr.: Some factors influencing platelet retention in glass bead columns including the influence of plastics. *Am. J. Clin. Pathol.* 56:479, 1971.

CHAPTER *A42*

Platelet factor 3 availability test

CECIL HOUGIE

PURPOSE OF THE TEST

This test measures the availability of the component of platelets required for the coagulation mechanism and is used to evaluate disorders of platelet function, both congenital and acquired.

PRINCIPLE OF THE TEST

Phospholipid (platelet factor 3) is required at two stages in the formation of intrinsic prothrombinase and is normally derived from platelets. Only after the platelets have been altered by some appropriate stimulus will phospholipid become available for participation in blood coagulation. Preincubation of platelet-rich plasma with kaolin provides this stimulus, and the kaolin clotting time of platelet-rich plasma is a measure of platelet factor 3 availability [1].

REAGENTS

1. Kaolin. A suspension of 4 g of kaolin in 100 ml of 0.85% NaCl is used in this test.

2. Calcium chloride. A 0.035 M solution of $CaCl_2$ is prepared by dissolving 3.9 g of the anhydrous salt in sufficient water to make 1 liter of solution.

TECHNIQUE

1. Platelet-rich and platelet-poor plasma are prepared from both the patient and a normal control as described in Chap. A33.

2. Platelet counts should be performed on the platelet-rich plasmas of the patient and the control; the platelet counts should be brought to approximately the same level by diluting the plasma having the higher platelet concentration with the corresponding platelet-poor plasma.

3. The test should be performed in duplicate. Mixtures of equal parts of the following plasma samples are prepared: (1) platelet-rich from the patient and platelet-poor from the normal control, (2) platelet-rich from the normal control and platelet-poor from the patient, (3) platelet-rich and platelet-poor from the patient, and (4) platelet-rich and platelet-poor from the control. Then 0.2 ml of well-mixed kaolin suspension is added to 0.2 ml of each of these mixtures. The resulting mixture is placed in a water bath at 37°C and a stopwatch started. Each of the

tubes is then incubated for exactly 20 min with occasional shaking. Then 0.2 ml of the calcium chloride solution is added, a stopwatch started, and the clotting time recorded. The end point is the first clumping of the kaolin.

INTERPRETATION

Mixtures 1 and 2 differ only in the source of platelets. If the clotting time of the mixture containing the patient's platelets (Mixture 1) exceeds that containing normal platelets (Mixture 2) by 5 s or more, there is a defect in platelet factor 3 availability. Mixtures 3 and 4 permit detection of the presence of a coagulation defect in the patient. Defects in platelet factor 3 are found in some cases of congenital qualitative platelet disorders (Chap. 146) and in some patients with uremia, myeloproliferative disorders, macroglobulinemia, etc. (Chap. 147).

Reference

1. Hardisty, R. M., and Ingram, G. C.: *Bleeding Disorders: Investigation and Management.* Blackwell Scientific, Oxford, 1965.

CHAPTER *A43*

Platelet aggregation

HARVEY J. WEISS

PURPOSE OF THE TEST

Platelets participate in primary hemostasis by forming aggregates at the site of injured blood vessels. One of the agents that is responsible for platelet aggregation is adenosine diphosphate (ADP), which may be derived from injured tissue and erythrocytes or released from the platelets themselves by, among other substances, collagen, thrombin, and epinephrine. In some patients with bleeding disorders and in normal subjects following the ingestion of some drugs, platelet aggregation by one or more of these agents may be impaired. This impairment of platelet aggregation may be the cause of the prolonged bleeding time which is often obtained in these patients.

PRINCIPLE OF THE TEST

Citrated platelet-rich plasma (PRP) is stirred in a cuvette, and the transmittance of incident light, relative to a platelet-poor plasma (PPP) blank, is recorded. When an aggregating agent is added, the formation of increasingly large platelet aggregates is accompanied by an increase in transmittance, which may be used as an index of platelet aggregation [1–3].

REAGENTS AND EQUIPMENT

1. Citrated PRP. Venous blood is mixed with one-tenth volume of 3.2 to 4% sodium citrate and centrifuged at either 250 × g for 10 min or 1600 × g for 3 min in a swinging-bucket rotor to obtain PRP. The remaining blood is centrifuged to obtain platelet-poor plasma (PPP) (see Chap. A33), which is used as a blank. Lipemic samples should be avoided. The temperature at

which the blood is centrifuged and the PRP stored may strongly affect the results obtained in aggregation studies. In general, centrifugation and storage at ambient temperature (22 to 25°C) is to be preferred. Either silicone-coated or plastic equipment may be used, but not interchangeably since the effects of these surfaces on platelets may not be identical.

2. Aggregating agents:

a. ADP. This may be conveniently dissolved in water in concentrations of 100 to 1000 μg/ml. ADP is available commercially as several different salts. The monosodium dihydrate form has a molecular weight of 485. Therefore a concentration of 970 μg/ml is 2 m*M*. This can be diluted 1:50 to give a concentration of 40 μ*M*. ADP solutions may be stored at −60°C for 3 to 6 months without significant loss of activity. The compound is less stable when stored at −20°C.

b. Collagen. Either a crude suspension of connective tissue or collagen preparations of varying degrees of purity and polymerization may be used. Suspensions of crude connective tissue are usually prepared from tendons or subcutaneous tissue [4]. The latter, which may be conveniently obtained from radical mastectomy specimens, is washed three times in an equal volume of ice-cold 0.85% NaCl. The extracts may then be prepared by homogenizing 200 g of washed tissue with 400 ml of cold saline solution at high speed for 3 min in a blender. After centrifuging the homogenate for 20 min at 2000 × *g*, the material in the upper third of the tube, which contains the bulk of the fat, and that in the lower third, containing the larger sedimented fragments, are discarded. The turbid material in the middle third of the tube is retained and may be frozen in aliquots at −50°C. The suspension may have to be diluted to obtain optimum aggregation. Collagen may also be prepared from commercial sources. This may be either homogenized to yield a suspension of collagen [5] or treated to obtain an acid-soluble preparation which, upon addition to PRP at 37°C, is transformed into insoluble collagen fibrils that are capable of aggregating platelets [6]. Commercial preparations of soluble collagen are also available (see below).

c. Epinephrine. Any commercially available solution is satisfactory. A 1:1000 concentration is 5.5 m*M* and can be diluted 1:55 to give a solution that is 100 μ*M*.

d. Thrombin. A solution of either human or bovine thrombin of known unitage may be used. See Chap. A35 for instructions regarding dilution of commercial bovine thrombin. A stock solution of 3 units per milliliter is convenient.

e. Ristocetin. This may be dissolved in 0.85% NaCl (w/v) or in buffer consisting of 1 part of 0.15 *M* tris adjusted to pH 7.3 with HCl and 2 parts of 0.85% NaCl, to give concentrations of 20 to 40 mg/ml. This solution is added to PRP to achieve concentrations of 1.2 to 2.0 mg/ml.

f. Other agents. Platelet aggregation may also be induced by serotonin, aggregated gamma globulin, bovine factor VIII, antiplatelet antibodies, polylysine, and other agents.

3. Aggregometer. Any spectrophotometer can be adapted to measure platelet aggregation. Several which have been constructed specifically for the purpose are available commercially (see below).

TECHNIQUE

The blank value is first obtained using PPP from the patient being tested. PRP is then introduced into the cuvette of the aggregometer, which has been prewarmed to the desired temperature, and stirred magnetically by means of the Teflon-coated bar which is provided with the commercially available apparatus. The rate of stirring is critical, and the optimum rate for obtaining platelet aggregation may have to be determined in preliminary experiments. With most instruments in current use, a stirring rate of 600 to 1200 is optimal. The transmittance of the PRP relative to the PPP blank may be recorded automatically, using any suitable recorder connected to the aggregometer. Upon addition of the aggregating agent (a volume of 1/10 to 1/20 the volume of PRP is convenient), the formation of platelet aggregates of increasing size results in an increase in transmittance, which may be used as an index of platelet aggregation (Figs. 126-10 and 129-5). Aggregation with most agents is usually maximal in less than 10 min and, with some agents at optimal concentration, may occur in 2 min. In studying patients suspected of having a defect in platelet aggregation, the reaction of platelets with several aggregating agents at different concentrations should be studied. Table A43-1 summarizes agents and conditions recommended for initial study

TABLE A43-1 Aggregating agents suggested for study of patients suspected of having a qualitative platelet defect

Agent	Final concentration*	Normal result
ADP	4 μ*M*	Double wave†
Collagen or connective tissue	Variable‡	Single wave
Thrombin	0.15 units/ml	Single wave followed by clot formation
Epinephrine	5 μ*M*	Small primary wave followed by large secondary wave
Ristocetin	1.2–2.0 mg/ml	Two waves sometimes, particularly at lower concentrations

*Tests may be performed by adding one-twentieth volume of test agent to citrated PRP.

†With some subjects, higher or lower concentrations may be required to produce a double wave.

‡These preparations vary in their ability to aggregate platelets, and the potency should be determined for each batch.

of such patients. Additional studies may be necessary, as discussed below under "Interpretation."

CALCULATION OF RESULTS

The degree of aggregation has been recorded in several ways, including slope of the curve, absolute magnitude of the transmittance change, and percentage change of the transmittance or optical density (OD).

INTERPRETATION

If possible, all drugs should be proscribed for 1 week before platelet aggregation studies are performed [7]. Acetaminophen may be used as an analgesic, but all aspirin-containing medications must be avoided. When the test is performed at 37°C, two waves of aggregation may be observed with some agents [8,9]. With epinephrine (5 to 50 μM), for example, the initial small wave of aggregation is followed by a second, usually larger wave, which is associated with the release of platelet ADP and the synthesis of thromboxane A_2. With ADP, either a single wave followed by disaggregation or a double wave is observed. The concentrations of ADP required to produce this double wave may vary from individual to individual, and the results may change markedly after storage of the PRP for several hours. A single wave of aggregation is usually obtained with collagen.

Abnormalities in platelet aggregation have been reported in several clinical disorders and in association with the administration of a variety of drugs (see Chap. 147). In thrombasthenia the platelets do not aggregate with any concentration of ADP, nor do they aggregate with any other agent except ristocetin.

In a variety of other primary and secondary platelet disorders, aggregation by collagen is abnormal, in most cases because of decreased release of platelet ADP (see Chap. 146). This abnormality is often not absolute and can be overcome by adding higher concentrations of collagen. A useful method is to use the minimum concentration which will give "good" aggregation (for example, 60 to 90 percent) in most normal subjects. The second wave of epinephrine-induced aggregation may be absent in patients with platelet defects; this is also associated with defective ADP release.

Abnormalities in both collagen- and epinephrine-induced aggregation may be produced by a variety of drugs, including aspirin and other anti-inflammatory drugs and many psychotropic agents (see Chap. 147), and it is essential that patients suspected of having intrinsic platelet disorders be requested to abstain from all drug ingestion for at least 1 week prior to testing.

Ristocetin-induced aggregation is decreased or absent in von Willebrand's disease and in the Bernard-Soulier syndrome. With lower concentrations of ristocetin (1.0 to 1.2 mg/ml), some decrease may sometimes be observed after ingestion of aspirin. The abnormality of ristocetin-induced platelet aggregation in von Willebrand's disease can be corrected by the addition of normal plasma or factor VIII/von Willebrand factor in vitro, and this correction is probably specific for von Willebrand's disease [10].

SOURCES OF REAGENTS AND EQUIPMENT

1. *ADP* can be purchased from several suppliers, including Sigma Chemical Company, 3500 DeKalb St., St. Louis, Mo., and Calbiochem, 3625 Medford, Los Angeles, Calif.

2. *Thrombin*. See Chap. A35, "Source of Reagents."

3. *Epinephrine*. Solutions may be purchased from any pharmacy.

4. *Collagen*. Tendon collagen may be obtained from Sigma Chemical Co., St. Louis, Mo.; soluble collagen from Worthington Biochemical Corp., Freehold, N.J., or Hormon-Chemie Munchen, Munich 45, West Germany.

5. *Ristocetin* can be obtained from Lundbeck, Copenhagen, Denmark.

6. *Aggregometer*. A satisfactory instrument may be obtained from Chrono-Log, Broomall, PA 19008; Payton Associates, Buffalo, NY 14202; or Bio-Data Corporation, Hatboro, PA 19040.

References

1. Born, G. V. R.: Aggregation of blood platelets by adenosine diphosphate and its reversal. *Nature* 194:927, 1962.
2. Mustard, J. F., Negardt, B., Rowsell, H. C., and MacMillan, R. K.: Effect of adenine nucleotides on platelet aggregation and clotting time. *J. Lab. Clin. Med.* 64:548, 1964.
3. O'Brien, J. R.: Platelet aggregation. 2. Some results from a new method of study. *J. Clin. Pathol.* 15:452, 1962.
4. Weiss, H. J., Aledort, L. M., and Kochwa, S.: The effects of salicylates on the hemostatic properties of platelets. *J. Clin. Invest.* 47:2169, 1968.
5. Packham, M. A., Warrior, E. S., Glynn, M. F., Senyi, A. S., and Mustard, J. F.: Alteration of the response of platelets to surface stimuli by pyrazole compounds. *J. Exp. Med.* 126:171, 1967.
6. Holmsen, H., and Weiss, H. J.: Further evidence for a deficient storage pool of adenine nucleotides in platelets from some patients with thrombocytopathia—"storage pool disease." *Blood* 39:197, 1972.
7. Weiss, H. J.: Platelet function tests and their interpretation. *J. Lab. Clin. Med.* 87:909, 1976.
8. MacMillan, D. C.: Secondary clumping effect in human citrated platelet-rich plasma produced by adenosine diphosphate and adrenaline. *Nature* 211:140, 1966.
9. Mills, D. C. B., and Roberts, G. C. K.: Membrane-activated drugs and the aggregation of human platelets. *Nature* 213:35, 1967.
10. Weiss, H. J.: Abnormalities of factor VIII and platelet aggregation: Use of ristocetin in diagnosising the von Willebrand syndrome. *Blood* 45:403, 1975.

CHAPTER *A44*

Detection of antiplatelet antibodies—inhibition of clot retraction

RICHARD H. ASTER

PURPOSE OF THE TEST

Detection of antibodies that react with platelets is more difficult than detection of antierythrocyte antibodies. The available techniques fall into one of three classifications: those that utilize conventional immunologic reactions, those that are based on the way in which antibody affects some specific aspect of platelet function, and those in which immunoglobulin molecules situated on the surface or interior of platelets are assayed using immunoglobulin-specific antibodies or agents

TABLE A44-1 Detection of drug-dependent antibodies by inhibition of clot retraction

Tube	Incubation mixture			Clot retraction
1	0.4 ml patient serum	0.1 ml drug solution	1 ml fresh blood (ABO-compatible)	Inhibited if antibodies are present
2	Same as above	0.1 ml distilled water	Same as above	Normal
3	0.4 ml normal serum	0.1 ml drug solution	Same as above	Normal
4	Same as above	0.1 ml distilled water	Same as above	Normal

such as staphylococcal protein A. In the first category are agglutination [1], complement fixation [2–4], and platelet cytolysis [5,6]; in the second are "release" of platelet factor 3 [7], release of radioactive serotonin [8], induction of platelet aggregation [9], and inhibition of clot retraction [10]; in the third are the enzyme-linked immunoassay (ELISA) [11] and methods dependent on immunoprecipitation [12], adherence of staphylococcal protein A [13], inhibition of the lysis of immunoglobulin-coated red cells by anti-IgG [14], immunofluorescence [15,16], and binding of radioactive anti-immunoglobulin [17–19]. Many other approaches have been tried [20–28]. None of the available techniques appears to be capable of detecting all types of platelet antibodies, although methods for directly measuring platelet-bound immunoglobulin may eventually make this possible [11–19]. Of the various techniques available for platelet antibody detection, only *inhibition of clot retraction* is sufficiently rapid and simple to be performed routinely by the physician attending a patient with thrombocytopenia. For more sophisticated investigations, the serum should be referred to a laboratory with competence in platelet serology.

PRINCIPLE OF THE TEST

Damage to 90 percent or more of the platelets in freshly collected normal blood, due to their interaction with antibody and complement, prevents retraction of the clot that forms. Sensitivity of the test can be increased by allowing an incubation period to precede clotting so that antibody and complement have additional time to affect platelets (see below under "Delayed Test").

REAGENTS AND EQUIPMENT

1. 12- by 75-mm glass tubes, clean.
2. Wooden applicator sticks.
3. Patient's serum to be tested for antibodies (3 ml).
4. Normal serum to be used as a control.
5. Normal donor blood, 5 ml, collected without anticoagulant immediately before use. The donor blood should be compatible with the ABO antibodies of the patient's serum.
6. Drugs (if appropriate). For detection of quinidine- or quinine-dependent antibodies, quinidine or quinine sulfate (or other salt of these alkaloids) should be made to a concentration of 1 mg/ml in distilled water. If a purified salt is not available, a 200-mg tablet may be crushed and dissolved with agitation in about 100 ml of warm distilled water, and the insoluble material removed by centrifugation. Excessive concentrations of quinidine or quinine may inhibit clot retraction nonspecifically and should be avoided. Inhibition of clot retraction by drug-dependent antibodies has rarely been demonstrated with drugs other than quinidine or quinine. Possible exceptions are digitoxin and diphenylhydantoin (Chap. 142). If other drugs are to be tested, the *Merck Index* or some other source book should be consulted for information on their solubility.
7. For the modification described below under "Delayed Test," 5% disodium ethylenediaminetetraacetate (EDTA), 0.1

M magnesium chloride, and 0.1 M calcium chloride are required.

TECHNIQUE

IMMEDIATE TEST

A blood sample from a patient suspected of having antibodies is allowed to clot and is then incubated for 1 h at 37°C. The serum is separated by centrifugation, and 0.4 ml is placed in each of two test tubes. Then 0.4 ml of fresh normal serum is placed in two control test tubes. If a drug antibody is suspected, 0.1 ml of a solution containing the appropriate drug is added to one tube containing the patient's serum and one tube containing control serum and 0.1 ml of distilled water is added to the other tubes (Table A44-1). Fresh normal blood is drawn from an ABO-compatible donor, and 1 ml is added to each tube and mixed with the contents. A wooden applicator stick is inserted, and the tubes are incubated at 37°C. As soon as clotting occurs, the clot should be separated from the walls of the tube so that clot retraction is not hindered by adhesion of the clot to the glass. This can be accomplished by gently flicking the tubes. After 1 h, the stick should be gently withdrawn and retraction of the clot assessed visually.

DELAYED TEST

Four tubes are set up as described under "Immediate Test," except that 0.10 ml rather than 0.4 ml of patient or normal serum is added to each, and 0.02 ml of 0.1 M magnesium chloride is then placed in each tube. For drug antibodies, 0.02 ml of the appropriate drug solution is added to two tubes as described in the preceding paragraph. Fresh normal blood is anticoagulated with 5% EDTA (0.3 ml per 10 ml of blood) and centrifuged at $100 \times g$ for 10 min and the supernatant platelet-rich plasma (PRP) removed. For maximum sensitivity, PRP should be diluted with platelet-poor plasma (PPP) to a final concentration of 200,000 platelets per cubic microliter. Next, 0.3 ml of PRP is added to each of the four tubes and incubated for 60 min at 37°C. Free magnesium ion is present in sufficient concentration to permit complement activity but not coagulation. Following incubation, 0.02 ml of 0.1 M calcium chloride is added to each tube to produce clotting. After coagulation occurs, each tube is flicked at the tip to loosen the clot and incubated for an additional hour at 37°C, after which the degree of clot retraction is observed.

CALCULATION OF RESULTS

Usually the degree of clot retraction in the tubes containing antibody can be compared visually with that of the control tubes. The technique may be made semiquantitative by measuring the amount of free fluid in each tube.

INTERPRETATION

Failure of clots exposed to the patient's serum, or the patient's serum plus drug in the case of drug antibodies, to retract as fully as clots exposed to normal serum suggests the presence of lytic antiplatelet antibodies. Only the most potent complement-fixing antibodies, notably those found in quinidine and quinine thrombocytopenia and in posttransfusion purpura (Chap. 142), inhibit clot retraction using the immediate test. Perhaps 50 percent of such antibodies may be detected in this way. The delayed test is more sensitive and gives a higher percentage of positive results. In addition to detecting antibodies associated with drug sensitivity and posttransfusion purpura, it is capable of detecting some isoantibodies reacting with histocompatibility antigens.

References

1. Dausset, J., Colin, M., and Colombani, J.: Immune platelet isoantibodies. *Vox Sang.* 5:4, 1960.
2. Shulman, N. R., Aster, R. H., Leitner, A., and Hiller, M. C.: Immunoreactions involving platelets. V. Post-transfusion purpura due to a complement-fixing antibody against a genetically-controlled platelet antigen: A proposed mechanism for thrombocytopenia and its relevance in "auto-immunity." *J. Clin. Invest.* 40:1597, 1961.
3. Aster, R. H., Cooper, H. E., and Singer, D.: Simplified complement fixation test for the detection of platelet antibodies in human serum. *J. Lab. Clin. Med.* 63:161, 1964.
4. Colombani, J., D'Amaro, J., Gabb, B., Smith, G., and Svejgaard, A.: International agreement on a microtechnique of platelet complement fixation (Pl. CFix.). *Transplant. Proc.* 3:121, 1971.
5. Aster, R. H., and Enright, S. E.: A platelet and granulocyte membrane defect in paroxysmal nocturnal hemoglobinuria: Usefulness for the detection of platelet antibodies. *J. Clin. Invest.* 48:1199, 1969.
6. Lizak, G. E., and Grume, F. C.: A new micromethod for the *in vitro* detection of antiplatelet antibodies: C-FDA thrombocytotoxicity. *Human Immunol.* 1:87, 1980.
7. Hirschman, R. J., Gralnick, H. R., and Schaff, F.: A simplified platelet factor 3 (PF-3) assay for the rapid detection of platelet isoantibodies and an antiplatelet factor in ATP and SLE. *J. Lab. Clin. Med.* 84:292, 1974.
8. Gockerman, J. P., Bowman, R. P., Conrad, M. E., and Eckley, S. L.: Detection of platelet isoantibodies by ³H-serotonin platelet release and its clinical application to the problem of platelet matching. *J. Clin. Invest.* 55:75, 1975.
9. Deykin, D., and Hellerstein, L. J.: The assessment of drug-dependent and isoimmune antiplatelet antibodies by the use of platelet aggregometry. *J. Clin. Invest.* 51:3142, 1972.
10. Zucker, M. D., Ley, A. B., Borrelli, J., Mayer, K., and Firmat, J.: Thrombocytopenia with a circulating platelet agglutinin, platelet lysin and clot retraction inhibitor. *Blood* 14:148, 1959.
11. Leporrier, M., Dighiero, G., Auzemery, M., and Binet, J. L.: Detection and quantification of platelet-bound antibodies with immunoperoxidase. *Br. J. Haematol.* 42:605, 1979.
12. Morse, B. S., Giuliani, D., and Nussbaum, M.: Quantitation of platelet-associated IgG by radial immunodiffusion. *Blood* 57:809, 1981.
13. Kekomaki, R.: Detection of platelet-bound IgG with ¹²⁵I-labelled staphylococcal protein A. *Med. Biol.* 54:112, 1977.
14. Dixon, R., Rosse, W., and Ebbert, L.: Quantitative determination of antibody in idiopathic thrombocytopenic purpura. *N. Engl. J. Med.* 292:230, 1975.
15. von dem Borne, A. E. G. K., et al.: A simple immunofluorescence test for the detection of platelet antibodies. *Br. J. Haematol.* 39:195, 1978.
16. Sugiura, K., Steiner, M., and Baldini, M.: Platelet antibody in idiopathic thrombocytopenic purpura and other thrombocytopenias. *J. Lab. Clin. Med.* 96:640, 1980.
17. Soulier, J. C., Paterrau, C., and Drouet, J.: Platelet indirect radioactive Coombs' test: Its utilization for Pl^A1 grouping. *Vox Sang.* 29:253, 1975.
18. Mueller-Eckhardt, C., Mahn, I., and Mueller-Eckhardt, G.: Detection of platelet autoantibodies by a radioactive anti-immunoglobulin test. *Vox Sang.* 35:357, 1978.
19. Cines, D. B., and Schreiber, A. D.: Immune thrombocytopenia: Uses of a Coombs' antiglobulin test to detect IgG and C3 on platelets. *N. Engl. J. Med.* 300:106, 1979.
20. Kissmeyer-Nielsen, F.: Demonstration of platelet antibodies by haemagglutination of antigen coated tanned erythrocytes. *Vox Sang.* 3:123, 1953.
21. Nachman, R. L., and Engle, R. J., Jr.: Amino acid generation following platelet-antibody interaction. *Vox Sang.* 10:416, 1965.
22. Kamoun, P. T., and Hamberger, J.: Measurement of antiplatelet activity of antilymphocyte sera based on the inhibition of 5-hydroxytryptamine uptake of blood platelets. *Transplantation* 10:53, 1970.
23. Polasek, J., and Duckert, F.: Diagnosis of quinine hypersensitivity: Use of platelet factor 3 and acid phosphatase availability tests. *Acta Haematol.* 45:35, 1971.
24. Handin, R. I., Piessens, W. F., and Moloney, W. C.: Stimulation of nonimmunized lymphocytes by platelet-antibody complexes in idiopathic thrombocytopenic purpura. *N. Engl. J. Med.* 289:714, 1973.
25. Handin, R. I., and Stossel, T. P.: Phagocytosis of antibody-coated platelets by human granulocytes. *N. Engl. J. Med.* 290:989, 1974.
26. Boxtel, C. J., Vander Weedt, C. M., and Engelfreit, C. P.: Cell electrophoresis for the detection of platelet antibodies. *Vox Sang.* 27:489, 1974.
27. Duquesnoy, R. J., Lorentz, D. F., and Aster, R. H.: Platelet migration inhibition: A new method for detection of platelet antibodies. *Blood* 45:741, 1975.
28. McMillan, R., Longmire, R. L., Yelonoski, R., Donnel, R. L., and Armstrong, S.: Quantitation of platelet-binding IgG produced in vitro by spleens from patients with idiopathic thrombocytopenic purpura. *N. Engl. J. Med.* 291:812, 1974.

SI UNIT CONVERSION TABLE

Constituent*	Traditional units	Multiplication factor†	SI units‡
δ-Aminolevulinic acid (U)	mg per day	7.63	μmol per day
Bilirubin			
Direct (S)	mg per 100 ml	17.1	μmol per l
Total (S)	mg per 100 ml	17.1	μmol per l
Calcium (S)	mg per 100 ml	0.25	mmol per l
Coproporphyrin (U)	μg per day	1.5	nmol per day
Erythrocyte count (B)	number per μl	10^6	number per l
Fibrinogen§ (Factor I) (P)	mg per 100 ml	0.01	g per l
	mg per 100 ml	0.029	μmol per l
Folic acid (S)	ng per ml	1.0	μg per l
	ng per ml	2.27	nmol per l
Haptoglobin (S)	mg per 100 ml	0.01	g per l
Hematocrit (B)	%	0.01	ratio
Hemoglobin¶ (B)	g per 100 ml	1.0	g per dl
Iron (S)	μg per 100 ml	0.179	μmol per l
Iron-binding capacity (S)	μg per 100 ml	0.179	μmol per l
Leukocyte count (B)	number per μl	10^6	number per l
Mean corpuscular hemoglobin	pg	1.0	pg
Mean corpuscular hemoglobin concentration	%	1.0	g per dl
Mean corpuscular volume	μm^3	1.0	fl
Packed cell volume (B)	%	0.01	ratio
Phosphorus (S)	mg per 100 ml	0.323	mmol per l
Platelet count (B)	number per μl	10^6	number per l
Prophobilinogen (U)	mg per day	4.42	μmol per day
Protoporphyrin (erythrocyte)	μg per 100 ml	0.018	μmol per l
Reticulocyte count (B)	%	0.01	ratio
	number per μl	10^6	number per l
Transferrin (S)	mg per 100 ml	0.01	g per l
Urea nitrogen (B)	mg per 100 ml	0.36	mmol per l
Uric acid (S)	mg per100 ml	0.0595	mmol per l
Urophorphyrin (U)	μg per day	1.2	nmol per day
Vitamin B_{12} (S)	pg per ml	1.0	ng per l
	pg per ml	0.738	pmol per l

*The following abbreviations are used: B = blood; S = serum; P = plasma; U = urine.

†Conventional units multiplied by this factor will yield SI units.

‡The following units are used:

fl = femtoliter (10^{-15} liter)	fmol = femtomole	fg = femtogram
pl = picoliter (10^{-12} liter)	pmol = picomole	pg = picogram
nl = nanoliter (10^{-9} liter)	nmol = nanomole	ng = nanogram
μl = microliter (10^{-6} liter)	μmol = micromole	μg = microgram
ml = milliliter (10^{-3} liter)	mmol = millimole	mg = milligram
dl = deciliter (10^{-1} liter)		
l = liter		

§The molar concentration is calculated assuming a molecular weight of 340,000.

¶Hemoglobin is not usually expressed in molar terms because of uncertainty regarding the polymeric state of the molecule. If the unit molecular weight is assumed to be 16,000, the multiplication factor is 0.62 to convert g per dl to mmol per L[2]. If a molecular weight of 64,500 is assumed, the conversion factor is 0.155 [3].

SOURCES:
1. Baron, D. N., Broughton, P. M. G., Cohen, M., Lansley, T. S., Lewis, S. M., and Shinton, N. K.: The use of SI units in reporting results obtained in hospital laboratories. *J. Clin. Path.* 27:590, 1974.
2. Young, D. S.: "Normal laboratory values" (case records of the Massachusetts General Hospital) in SI units. *New Engl. J. Med.* 292:795, 1975.
3. Lehmann, H. P.: Metrication of clinical laboratory data in SI units. *Amer. J. Clin. Path.* 65:2, 1976.

Index

Index